Harrison's
PRINCIPLES OF INTERNAL MEDICINE

EDITORS OF PREVIOUS EDITIONS

T. R. Harrison, Editor-in-Chief, Editions 1, 2, 3, 4, 5

W. R. Resnik, Editor, Editions 1, 2, 3, 4, 5

M. M. Wintrobe, Editor, Editions 1, 2, 3, 4, 5
Editor-in-Chief, Editions 6, 7

G. W. Thorn, Editor, Editions 1, 2, 3, 4, 5, 6, 7
Editor-in-Chief, Edition 8

R. D. Adams, Editor, Editions 2, 3, 4, 5, 6, 7, 8

P. B. Beeson, Editor, Editions 1, 2

I. L. Bennett, Jr., Editor, Editions 3, 4, 5, 6

E. Braunwald, Editor, Editions 6, 7, 8

K. J. Isselbacher, Editor, Editions 6, 7, 8

R. G. Petersdorf, Editor, Editions 6, 7, 8

Harrison's
PRINCIPLES OF INTERNAL MEDICINE
Ninth Edition

Editors

KURT J. ISSELBACHER, A.B., M.D.
Mallinckrodt Professor of Medicine, Harvard
Medical School; Physician and Chief,
Gastrointestinal Unit, Massachusetts General
Hospital, Boston

RAYMOND D. ADAMS, B.A., M.A., M.D.,
M.A. (Hon.), D.Sc. (Hon.), M.D. (Hon.)   Bullard
Professor of Neuropathology, Emeritus, Harvard
Medical School; Consultant Neurologist and
Formerly Chief of Neurology Service,
Massachusetts General Hospital; Director, Eunice
K. Shriver Research Center, Boston; Médicin
Adjoint, L'Hôpital Cantonale de Lausanne,
Lausanne

EUGENE BRAUNWALD, A.B., M.D., M.A.
(Hon.)   Hersey Professor of the Theory and
Practice of Physic (Medicine), Harvard Medical
School; Physician-in-Chief, Peter Bent Brigham
Hospital, Boston

ROBERT G. PETERSDORF, A.B., M.D.,
D.Sc. (Hon.)   Professor of Medicine, Harvard
Medical School, Boston; President, Affiliated
Hospitals Center

JEAN D. WILSON, B.A., M.D.   Professor of
Internal Medicine and Director, McDermott Center
for Growth and Development, University of Texas
Health Science Center at Dallas, Dallas

McGRAW-HILL BOOK COMPANY   *New York   St. Louis   San Francisco   Auckland   Bogotá
Hamburg   Johannesburg   London   Madrid   Mexico
Montreal   New Delhi   Panama   Paris   São Paulo   Singapore
Sydney   Tokyo   Toronto*

Harrison's
Principles of Internal Medicine

Copyright © 1980, 1977, 1974, 1970, 1966, 1962, 1958 by McGraw-Hill, Inc. All rights reserved. Copyright 1954, 1950 by McGraw-Hill, Inc. All rights reserved. Copyright renewed 1978 by Maxwell Myer Wintrobe and George W. Thorn. Printed in the United States of America. No part of this publication may be reproduced, stored in a retrieval system, or transmitted, in any form or by any means, electronic, mechanical, photocopying, recording, or otherwise, without the prior written permission of the publisher.

1234567890 DODO 7832109

Foreign Editions
FRENCH (Seventh Edition)—Flammarion, © 1975
ITALIAN (Seventh Edition)—Casa Editrice Dr. Francesco Vallardi, © 1976
POLISH (Fifth Edition)—Panstwowy Zakland Wydawnictw Lekarskich, © 1971
PORTUGUESE (Eighth Edition)—Editora Guanabara Koogan, S.A., © 1981 (est.)
SPANISH (Eighth Edition)—La Prensa Medica Mexicana, © 1979
JAPANESE (Eighth Edition)—Hirokawa, © 1978
GREEK (Eighth Edition)—G. Parissianos © 1979

This book was set in Times Roman by Rocappi, Inc.
The editors were J. Dereck Jeffers, Richard S. Laufer, and Timothy Armstrong. The indexer was Philip James; the designer was Merrill Haber; the production supervisor was Jeanne Selzam.
R. R. Donnelley & Sons Company was printer and binder.

Library of Congress Cataloging in Publication Data

Harrison, Tinsley Randolph, date   ed.
  Harrison's Principles of internal medicine.

  Includes bibliographies and index.
    1. Internal medicine. I. Isselbacher, Kurt J.
II. Title. III. Title: Principles of internal medicine.
RC46.H32 1980   616'.026   79-20855
ISBN 0-07-032068-3

        LC CIP DATA (2 vol. ed)
RC46.H32 1980b   616'.026   79-21372
ISBN 0-07-032069-1 (set)

This edition is dedicated to the Editor-in-Chief of this text during its first five editions, Tinsley R. Harrison.

From time to time a personality scintillates across the medical firmament who dazzles all beholders. Tinsley Harrison was such a person. A delightful, vivacious, passionate physician, he stimulated everyone with whom he came in contact, and he placed an indelible stamp on the medical events of his day.

As a thoughtful physician he excelled in the care of the sick, and the words which he penned for the first edition of this book reflect the importance which he attached to his role as a physician:

No greater opportunity or obligation can fall the lot of a human being than to be a physician. In the care of the suffering he needs technical skill, scientific knowledge, and human understanding. He who uses these with courage, humility, and wisdom will provide a unique service for his fellow man and will build an enduring edifice of character within himself. The physician should ask of his destiny no more than this, and he should be content with no less.

These words express the philosophy of the original editors and of all those who have followed. The patient was always in the center of the stage. To put the disease first, to refer to the patient as "a case" would arouse Tinsley's wrath.

Few people of his generation surpassed him as a bedside teacher. He had the remarkable ability to objectify an important clinical finding and to cite all relevant literature without disquieting the patient. Indeed his clinical analysis usually gained the confidence and respect of his patient in a most reassuring manner.

His originality in selecting clinical problems and investigating them by the available physiological methods, especially disorders of the heart and circulation, are familiar to all contemporary scholars. His accounts of his observations and studies were, and continue to be, models of lucid exposition.

To those of us who had the privilege of working with Tinsley on successive editions of this book, he was an unforgettable colleague and friend. It was he and his friend Morris Fischbein, then editor of the *Journal of the American Medical Association,* who saw the need of a textbook suited to the curriculum of American medical schools and resident training programs. It was Ted Philips, then an officer of the Blakiston Publishing Company, who translated Tinsley's ideas into a new type of textbook which soon was to have worldwide influence. Under his superb editorship each edition was a kind of experiment in ways to meet the changing needs of elementary and advanced students of medicine.

In the late summer of 1978, as this edition was being prepared, Tinsley succumbed to a long and distressing illness. It is to the memory of this great physician, whose life and works have so inspired us, that this, the ninth edition of *Harrison's,* is dedicated.

THE EDITORS

ABBREVIATED CONTENTS

CONTENTS

Plates 1 to 8   **254**

1-1 Dermatofibroma   1-2 Acrochordon   1-3 Angiokeratomas   1-4 Café au lait macules   1-5 Acne

2-1 Dermatophytosis   2-2 Eczematous dermatitis   2-3 Localized lichenification   2-4 Melasma (chloasma)   2-5 Milia   2-6 Psoriasis

3-1 Perleche   3-2 Rosacea   3-3 Seborrheic dermatitis   3-4 Seborrheic keratosis   3-5 Senile angioma ("cherry red spot")   3-6 Senile lentigo

4-1 Senile sebaceous adenoma   4-2 Solar keratosis   4-3 Spider nevus   4-4 Tinea versicolor   4-5 Verruca vulgaris   4-6 Xanthelasma

5-1 Necrobiosis lipoidica diabeticorum   5-2 Pretibial myxedema   5-3 Pyoderma gangrenosum   5-4 "Palpable" purpura with inflammation occurring in gonococcemia   5-5 Peutz-Jeghers syndrome   5-6 Contact eczematous dermatitis

6-1 Lentigo maligna melanoma   6-2 Superficial spreading melanoma   6-3 Nodular melanoma   6-4 Superficial spreading melanoma, superficially invasive

7-1 Normal optic nerve and retina   7-2 Glaucomatous optic disk with secondary atrophy   7-3 Drusen of the optic nerve head   7-4 Angioid streaks   7-5 Primary optic atrophy   7-6 Early papilledema   7-7 Retentive pigmentosa   7-8 Band keratopathy

8-1 Schemic optic neuritis with temporal arteritis   8-2 Cholesterol embolus in retinal arteriole   8-3 Diabetic retinopathy microaneurysm   8-4 Retinitis proliferans in diabetes mellitus   8-5 Roth spot with subacute bacterial endocarditis   8-6 Central retinal vein thrombosis   8-7 Dislocated lens in Marfan's disease   8-8 Kaiser-Fleisher ring in Wilson's disease

Plates 9 and 10   **285**

9-1 Normal marrow   9-2 Megaloblastic marrow   9-3 Erythroid hyperplasia   9-4 Sideroblastic anemia   9-5 Normal blood smear   9-6 Megaloblastic anemia   9-7 Iron-deficiency anemia   9-8 β thallasemia intermedia   9-9 Myeloid metaplasia   9-10 Uremia   9-11 Liver disease   9-12 Spur-cell anemia   9-13 Hereditary spherocytosis   9-14 Immunohemolytic anemia   9-15 Traumatic hemolysis   9-16 Sickle-cell anemia

10-1 A Normal granulocyte   B Normal monocyte and lymphocyte   10-2 A Normal eosinophil   B Normal basophil   10-3 Normal granulocyte precursors in marrow   10-4 Neutrophils with toxic granulation   10-5 Band with Döhle body   10-6 Hypersegmentation   10-7 A Chédiak-Higashi anomaly   B Pelger-Hüet anomaly   10-8 Reactive lymphocytes (infectious mononucleosis)   10-9 Chronic granulocytic leukemia   10-10 Acute myelogenous leukemia: myeloblast with Auer rod   10-11 Chronic lymphocytic leukemia   10-12 Acute lymphoblastic leukemia (marrow)   10-13 Hodgkin's disease: Reed-Sternberg cell in marrow   10-14 Non-Hodgkin's nodular lymphoma (lymph node)   10-15 Multiple myeloma (marrow)

LIST OF CONTRIBUTORS

RAYMOND D. ADAMS, B.A., M.A., M.D., M.A. (Hon.), D.Sc. (Hon.), M.D. (Hon.)
Bullard Professor of Neuropathology, Emeritus, Harvard Medical School; Consultant Neurologist and Formerly Chief of Neurology Service, Massachusetts General Hospital; Director, Eunice K. Shriver Research Center, Boston; Médicin Adjoint, L'Hôpital Cantonale de Lausanne, Lausanne

JOHN W. ADAMSON, M.D.
Professor of Medicine, University of Washington School of Medicine; Head, Division of Hematology, Veterans Administration Medical Center, Seattle

RAYMOND ALEXANIAN, M.D.
Professor of Medicine, The University of Texas M. D. Anderson Hospital and Tumor Institute, Houston

ELLIOT ALPERT, M.D.
Associate Professor of Medicine, Harvard Medical School; Assistant Physician, Gastrointestinal Unit, Massachusetts General Hospital, Boston

JOSEPH S. ALPERT, M.D.
Professor of Medicine, University of Massachusetts Medical School; Director, Division of Cardiovascular Medicine, University of Massachusetts Medical Center, Worcester

ROBERT J. ANDERSON, M.D.
Associate Professor of Medicine, Division of Renal Diseases, University of Colorado Medical Center, Denver

ARTHUR K. ASBURY, M.D.
Professor of Neurology, University of Pennsylvania School of Medicine; Chairman, Department of Neurology, Hospital of the University of Pennsylvania, Philadelphia

KARL-ERIK ÅSTRÖM, M.D.
Associate Professor of Neuropathology, Harvard Medical School; Associate Neuropathologist, Massachusetts General Hospital, Boston

K. FRANK AUSTEN, M.D.
Theodore B. Bayles Professor of Medicine, Harvard Medical School; Physician-in-Chief, Robert Breck Brigham Hospital, A Division of the Affiliated Hospitals Center, Inc., Boston

ROBERT AUSTRIAN, M.D.
Professor and Chairman, Department of Research Medicine, University of Pennsylvania School of Medicine, Philadelphia

BERNARD M. BABIOR, M.D.
Professor of Medicine, Tufts University School of Medicine; Division of Adult Hematology, New England Medical Center, Boston

JOSEPH H. BATES, M.D.
Chief, Medical Service, Veterans Administration Hospital; Professor of Medicine, University of Arkansas School of Medicine, Little Rock

HARRY N. BEATY, M.D.
Professor and Chairman, Department of Medicine, University of Vermont College of Medicine, Burlington

ARTHUR L. BEAUDET, M.D.
Associate Professor of Pediatrics and Cell Biology, Baylor College of Medicine; Investigator, Howard Hughes Medical Institute, Houston

JOHN E. BENNETT, M.D.
Head, Clinical Mycology Section, LCI, National Institute of Allergy and Infectious Disease, National Institutes of Health, Bethesda

EDWIN L. BIERMAN, M.D.
Professor of Medicine and Head, Division of Metabolism and Endocrinology, Department of Medicine, University of Washington School of Medicine, Seattle

ALAN L. BISNO, M.D.
Professor of Medicine and Chief, Division of Infectious Disease, Department of Medicine, University of Tennessee College of Medicine, Memphis

AREND BOUHUYS, M.D., D.Sc. (Med.), M.A. (Hon.) (deceased)
Professor of Physiology, Physiological Laboratory, University of Utrecht, The Netherlands; Clinical Professor of Environmental Medicine, New York University School of Medicine, New York

ROBERT M. BOYAR, M.D. (deceased)
Associate Professor of Internal Medicine, University of Texas Health Science Center at Dallas, Dallas

WALTER G. BRADLEY, M.D.
Professor of Neurology, Tufts University School of Medicine; Associate Director, Neurology Service, New England Medical Center, Boston

EUGENE BRAUNWALD, A.B., M.D., M.A. (Hon.)
Hersey Professor of the Theory and Practice of Physic (Medicine), Harvard Medical School; Physician-in-Chief, Peter Bent Brigham Hospital, Boston

BARRY M. BRENNER, M.D., M.A. (Hon.)
Samuel A. Levine Professor of Medicine, Harvard Medical School; Physician and Director, Renal Division, Peter Bent Brigham Hospital, Boston

MICHAEL S. BROWN, M.D.
Paul J. Thomas Professor of Genetics, University of Texas Health Science Center at Dallas; Senior Attending Physician, Parkland Memorial Hospital, Dallas

H. FRANKLIN BUNN, M.D.
Professor of Medicine, Harvard Medical School; Director, Hematology Division, Peter Bent Brigham Hospital, Boston

GEORGE P. CANELLOS, M.D.
Associate Professor of Medicine, Harvard Medical School; Chief, Division of Medical Oncology, Sidney Farber Cancer Center; Senior Associate in Medicine, Peter Bent Brigham Hospital, Boston

CHARLES B. CARPENTER, M.D.
Associate Professor of Medicine, Harvard Medical School; Senior Associate in Medicine, Peter Bent Brigham Hospital, Boston

CHARLES C. J. CARPENTER, M.D.
Professor and Chairman, Department of Medicine, Case Western Reserve University School of Medicine; Physician-in-Chief, University Hospitals, Cleveland

WILLIAM A. CAUSEY, M.D.
Associate Professor of Medicine, University of Mississippi School of Medicine; Chief, Medical Service, Veterans Administration Hospital, Jackson

KEITH H. CHIAPPA, M.D.
Instructor in Neurology, Harvard Medical School; Director, EEG Laboratories, Massachusetts General Hospital, Boston

BAYARD CLARKSON, M.D.
Associate Chairman and Chief, Hematology Lymphoma Service, Department of Medicine, Memorial Hospital, Memorial Sloan-Kettering Cancer Center, New York

LEIGHTON E. CLUFF, M.D.
Vice President, The Robert Wood Johnson Foundation, Princeton

FREDRIC L. COE, M.D.
Professor of Medicine and Physiology, Pritzker School of Medicine, University of Chicago; Director, Division of Renal Medicine, Michael Reese Hospital and Medical Center, Chicago

ALAN S. COHEN, M.D.
Chief of Medicine and Director, Thorndike Memorial Laboratory, Boston City University; Conrad Wesselhoeft Professor of Medicine, Boston University School of Medicine, Boston

PETER F. COHN, M.D.
Associate Professor of Medicine, Harvard Medical School; Director, Clinical Cardiology Service, Peter Bent Brigham Hospital, Boston

MAX D. COOPER, M.D.
Professor of Pediatrics and Microbiology, Department of Pediatrics, University of Alabama in Birmingham, The Medical Center, Birmingham

RICHARD A. COOPER, M.D.
Professor of Medicine, University of Pennsylvania School of Medicine; Chief, Hematology-Oncology Section, Hospital of the University of Pennsylvania; Director, University of Pennsylvania Cancer Center, Philadelphia

LAWRENCE COREY, M.D.
Assistant Professor, Laboratory Medicine and Microbiology; Adjunct Assistant Professor, Medicine and Pediatrics, University of Washington School of Medicine; Head, Virology Division, Laboratory Medicine, Childrens Orthopedic Hospital, Seattle

EUGENE P. CRONKITE, M.D.
Chairman, Medical Department, Brookhaven National Laboratory, Associate Universities, Inc., Upton

DAVID C. DALE, M.D.
Professor of Medicine and Associate Chairman, Department of Medicine, University of Washington School of Medicine, Seattle

JAMES E. DALEN, M.D.
Professor and Chairman, Department of Medicine, University of Massachusetts Medical School; Physician-in-Chief, University of Massachusetts Hospital, Worcester

CHANDLER R. DAWSON, M.D.
Professor of Ophthalmology, Francis I. Proctor Foundation for Research in Ophthalmology, University of California, San Francisco; Director, WHO Collaborating Center for Prevention of Blindness and Trachoma, San Francisco

G. ROBERT DELONG, M.D.
Assistant Professor of Neurology, Harvard Medical School; Associate Neurologist and Associate Pediatrician, Massachusetts General Hospital, Boston

VINCENT T. DeVITA, JR., M.D.
Director, Division of Cancer Treatment, National Cancer Institute, National Institutes of Health, Bethesda

JULES L. DIENSTAG, M.D.
Assistant Professor of Medicine, Harvard Medical School; Assistant in Medicine, Gastrointestinal Unit, Massachusetts General Hospital, Boston

JAMES J. DINEEN, M.D.
Assistant Professor of Medicine, Harvard Medical School; Associate Physician, Massachusetts General Hospital, Boston

ROBERT G. DLUHY, M.D.
Associate Professor of Medicine, Harvard Medical School; Senior Associate in Medicine, Peter Bent Brigham Hospital, Boston

KENDALL EMERSON, JR., M.D.
Clinical Professor of Medicine, Emeritus, Harvard Medical School; Physician, Emeritus, Peter Bent Brigham Hospital, Boston

KARL ENGELMAN, M.D., M.A. (Hon.)
Associate Professor of Medicine and Pharmacology, University of Pennsylvania School of Medicine; Chief, Hypertension and Clinical Pharmacology Section, and Director, Clinical Research Center, Hospital of the University of Pennsylvania, Philadelphia

MURRAY J. FAVUS, M.D.
Assistant Professor of Medicine, Pritzker School of Medicine, University of Chicago; Attending Physician, Division of Endocrinology and Metabolism, Michael Reese Hospital and Medical Center, Chicago

ALEXANDER FEFER, M.D.
Professor of Medicine, University of Washington School of Medicine; Head, Division of Oncology, University of Washington Hospital, Seattle

PHILIP J. FIALKOW, M.D.
Professor and Vice-Chairman, Department of Medicine, and Professor of Genetics, University of Washington; Chief, Medical Service, Veterans Administration Medical Center, Seattle

JAMES B. FIELD, M.D.
Rutherford Professor of Medicine and Head, Division of Endocrinology and Metabolism, Baylor College of Medicine; Director, Diabetes Research Laboratory, St. Luke's Episcopal Hospital, Houston

C. MILLER FISHER, M.D.
Professor of Neurology, Harvard Medical School; Neurologist and Neuropathologist, Massachusetts General Hospital, Boston

ALFRED P. FISHMAN, M.D.
William Maul Measey Professor of Medicine, University of Pennsylvania School of Medicine; Director, Cardiovascular-Pulmonary Division, Hospital of the University of Pennsylvania, Philadelphia

THOMAS B. FITZPATRICK, M.D., Ph.D.
Edward Wigglesworth Professor and Chairman, Department of Dermatology, Harvard Medical School; Chief, Dermatology Service, Massachusetts General Hospital, Boston

DANIEL W. FOSTER, M.D.
Professor of Internal Medicine, University of Texas Health Science Center at Dallas, Dallas

PAUL A. FRIEDMAN, M.D.
Assistant Professor of Clinical Pharmacology, Harvard Medical School, Boston

WILLIAM F. FRIEDMAN, M.D.
Professor and Chairman, Department of Pediatrics, Center for the Health Sciences, University of California, Los Angeles; J. H. Nicholson Professor of Pediatric Cardiology, University of California, Los Angeles School of Medicine, Los Angeles

PIERCE GARDNER, M.D.
Professor of Medicine and Pediatrics, Division of Biological Sciences, Department of Medicine, Pritzker School of Medicine, University of Chicago, Chicago

J. BERNARD L. GEE, M.D.
Associate Professor of Medicine, Yale University School of Medicine; Attending Physician, Yale-New Haven Hospital, New Haven

JAMES GERMAN, M.D.
Adjunct Professor, The Rockefeller University; Senior Investigator, The Lindsley F. Kimball Research Institute of the New York Blood Center, New York

ELOISE R. GIBLETT, M.D.
Research Professor of Medicine, University of Washington School of Medicine; Head, Immunogenetics, Puget Sound Blood Center, Seattle

WILLIAM GILL, M.D.
Associate Professor, Department of Surgery (Urology), University of Chicago Hospitals and Clinics, Chicago

BRUCE C. GILLILAND, M.D.
Professor of Medicine and Laboratory Medicine, University of Washington School of Medicine; Medical Director, Providence Hospital, Seattle

RICHARD J. GLASSOCK, M.D.
Professor of Medicine, University of California, Los Angeles School of Medicine; Chief, Division of Nephrology and Hypertension, Harbor-University of California, Los Angeles Medical Center, Los Angeles

GERALD GLICK, M.D.
Senior Consultant, Cardiovascular Institute, Michael Reese Hospital and Medical Center; Clinical Professor of Medicine, Pritzker School of Medicine, University of Chicago, Chicago

ROBERT M. GLICKMAN, M.D.
Associate Professor of Medicine, Columbia University College of Physicians and Surgeons; Chief of Gastroenterology, Presbyterian Hospital, New York

STEPHEN E. GOLDFINGER, M.D.
Associate Professor of Medicine and Associate Dean of Continuing Education, Harvard Medical School; Physician, Gastrointestinal Unit, Massachusetts General Hospital, Boston

PAUL GOLDHABER, D.D.S.
Dean and Professor of Periodontology, Harvard School of Dental Medicine, Boston

JOSEPH L. GOLDSTEIN, M.D.
Paul J. Thomas Professor and Chairman, Department of Molecular Genetics, University of Texas Health Science Center at Dallas; Senior Attending Physician, Parkland Memorial Hospital, Dallas

HARVEY M. GOLOMB, M.D.
Associate Professor of Medicine, Section of Hematology/Oncology, Department of Medicine, Pritzker School of Medicine, University of Chicago, Chicago

ROBERT W. GRAEBNER, M.D.
Assistant Clinical Professor, Department of Neurology, University of Wisconsin, Madison

J. THOMAS GRAYSTON, M.D.
Vice President for Health Affairs, Professor of Epidemiology, School of Public Health and Community Medicine, University of Washington, Seattle

NORTON J. GREENBERGER, M.D.
Professor and Chairman, Department of Medicine, University of Kansas Medical Center, College of Health Sciences, Kansas City

JAMES E. GRIFFIN III, M.D.
Assistant Professor of Internal Medicine, University of Texas Health Science Center at Dallas, Dallas

RICHARD L. GUERRANT, M.D.
Associate Professor of Medicine, Department of Medicine, University of Virginia Medical Center, Charlottesville

JAMES P. HARNISCH, M.D.
Clinical Assistant Professor, Department of Medicine, University of Washington School of Medicine, Seattle

DONALD H. HARTER, M.D.
Charles L. Mix Professor and Chairman, Department of Neurology, The Medical School, Northwestern University, Chicago

HARLEY A. HAYNES, M.D.
Associate Professor of Dermatology, Harvard Medical School; Director, Dermatology Division, Peter Bent Brigham Hospital, Boston

THOMAS R. HENDRIX, M.D.
Professor of Medicine and Chief, Gastroenterology Division, The Johns Hopkins University School of Medicine, Baltimore

JAN V. HIRSCHMANN, M.D.
Assistant Professor of Medicine, University of Washington School of Medicine; Medical Comprehensive Care Unit, Veterans Administration Hospital, Seattle

FRED HOCHBERG, M.D.
Assistant Professor of Neurology, Harvard Medical School; Assistant Neurologist, Massachusetts General Hospital, Boston

PAUL D. HOEPRICH, M.D.
Professor of Medicine and Pathology and Chief, Section of Infectious and Immunologic Diseases, Department of Internal Medicine, University of California-Davis, Sacramento

JOHN H. HOLBROOK, M.D.
Associate Professor of Medicine, Division of General Internal Medicine, Department of Internal Medicine, University of Utah Medical Center, Salt Lake City

MICHAEL F. HOLICK, M.D., Ph.D.
Assistant Professor of Medicine, Harvard Medical School; Clinical Assistant in Medicine, Massachusetts General Hospital, Boston

O. BRYAN HOLLAND, M.D.
Assistant Professor of Internal Medicine, University of Texas Health Science Center at Dallas, Dallas

NORMAN K. HOLLENBERG, M.D.
Professor and Director of Physiologic Research, Department of Radiology, Harvard Medical School; Senior Associate in Medicine, Peter Bent Brigham Hospital, Boston

KING K. HOLMES, M.D.
Professor of Medicine, University of Washington School of Medicine; Head, Infectious Diseases, U.S. Public Health Service Hospital, Seattle

EDWARD W. HOOK, M.D.
Mulholland Professor of Medicine and Chairman, Department of Medicine, University of Virginia Medical Center; Physician-in-Chief, University of Virginia Hospital, Charlottesville

THOMAS H. HOSTETTER, M.D.
Instructor in Medicine, Harvard Medical School; Junior Associate in Medicine, Peter Bent Brigham Hospital, Boston

H. DAVID HUMES, M.D.
Assistant Professor of Medicine, University of Michigan Medical School, Ann Arbor

SIDNEY H. INGBAR, M.D.
William Bosworth Castle Professor of Medicine, Harvard Medical School; Director, Thorndike Laboratory, Beth Israel Hospital, Boston

ROLAND H. INGRAM, JR., M.D.
Associate Professor of Medicine, Harvard Medical School; Physician and Chief, Respiratory Division, Peter Bent Brigham Hospital, Boston

ELI IPP, M.D.
Instructor, Department of Medicine, Pritzker School of Medicine, The University of Chicago, Chicago

KURT J. ISSELBACHER, A.B., M.D.
Mallinckrodt Professor of Medicine, Harvard Medical School; Physician and Chief, Gastrointestinal Unit, Massachusetts General Hospital, Boston

PAUL I. JAGGER, M.D.
Adjunct Professor of Medicine, University of California, San Diego School of Medicine; Codirector, Clinical Research Center, University Hospital, University of California, San Diego Medical Center, San Diego

KHURSHEED N. JEEJEEBHOY, M.B.B.S., Ph.D., F.R.C.P. (Lond.), F.R.C.P. (Edin.), F.R.C.P. (C)
Professor of Medicine, University of Toronto; Head, Gastrointestinal Division, Toronto General Hospital, Toronto

CAROL J. JOHNS, M.D.
Associate Professor of Medicine, The Johns Hopkins University School of Medicine; Physician, The Johns Hopkins Hospital, Baltimore

JOSEPH E. JOHNSON III, M.D.
Professor and Chairman, Department of Medicine, Bowman-Gray School of Medicine, Winston-Salem

BYRON A. KAKULAS, M.D., F.R.A.C.P., M.R.C., Path., F.R.C.P.A.
Professor of Neuropathology, University of Western Australia, Perth; Senior Neuropathologist, Royal Perth Hospital, Perth

SATISH KATHPALIA, M.D.
Instructor in Medicine, Pritzker School of Medicine, University of Chicago; Attending Physician, Division of Renal Medicine, Michael Reese Hospital and Medical Center, Chicago

WILLIAM N. KELLEY, M.D.
Professor and Chairman, Department of Internal Medicine, University of Michigan Medical School, Ann Arbor

WILLIAM M. M. KIRBY, M.D.
Professor of Medicine, Division of Infectious Disease, University of Washington School of Medicine, Seattle

VERNON KNIGHT, M.D.
Professor and Chairman, Department of Microbiology and Immunology, Baylor College of Medicine; Senior Attending Physician, The Methodist Hospital, Houston

RAYMOND S. KOFF, M.D.
Professor of Medicine, Boston University School of Medicine; Chief, Hepatology Section, Boston University Medical Center and Veterans Administration Medical Center, Boston

PETER O. KOHLER, M.D.
Professor and Chairman, Department of Medicine, University of Arkansas for Medical Sciences; Chief, Medical Service, University Hospital, Little Rock

STEPHEN M. KRANE, M.D.
Professor of Medicine, Harvard Medical School; Physician and Chief, Arthritis Unit, Massachusetts General Hospital, Boston

J. THOMAS LaMONT, M.D.
Assistant Professor of Medicine, Harvard Medical School; Associate in Medicine, Division of Gastroenterology, Peter Bent Brigham Hospital, Boston

ALEXANDER R. LAWTON III, M.D.
Professor of Pediatrics and Microbiology, The Medical Center, The University of Alabama in Birmingham, Birmingham

J. MICHAEL LAZARUS, M.D.
Associate Professor of Medicine, Harvard Medical School; Associate in Medicine, Peter Bent Brigham Hospital, Boston

G. RICHARD LEE, M.D.
Professor of Medicine and Dean, University of Utah College of Medicine; University of Utah Hospital, Salt Lake City

A. MARTIN LERNER, M.D.
Professor of Medicine and Head, Division of Infectious Disease, Department of Medicine, Wayne State University School of Medicine; Chief, Hutzel Hospital Medical Unit, Detroit

NORMAN G. LEVINSKY, M.D.
Wade Professor and Chairman, Division of Medicine, Boston University School of Medicine; Physician-in-Chief and Director, Evans Memorial Department of Clinical Research, University Hospital, Boston

BERNARD LOWN, M.D.
Professor of Cardiology, Harvard School of Public Health; Physician, Peter Bent Brigham Hospital, Boston

WALTER C. MacDONALD, M.D.
Professor of Medicine and Head, Division of Gastroenterology, University of British Columbia, Vancouver

JAMES D. MADDEN, M.D.
Clinical Associate Professor of Obstetrics and Gynecology, Health Science Center, University of Texas at Dallas, Dallas

LEONARD L. MADISON, M.D.
Professor, Department of Internal Medicine, University of Texas Health Science Center at Dallas, Dallas

HENRY J. MANKIN, M.D.
Edith M. Ashley Professor of Orthopedic Surgery, Harvard Medical School; Chief, Orthopedic Service, Massachusetts General Hospital, Boston

MART MANNIK, M.D.
Professor of Medicine, Adjunct Professor of Microbiology, and Head, Division of Rheumatology, Department of Medicine, University of Washington School of Medicine, Seattle

ROGER J. MAY, M.D.
Instructor in Medicine, Harvard Medical School; Assistant in Medicine, Gastrointestinal Unit, Massachusetts General Hospital, Boston

JANET W. McARTHUR, M.D.
Professor of Obstetrics and Gynecology, Harvard Medical School; Gynecologist, Massachusetts General Hospital, Boston

E. R. McFADDEN, JR., M.D.
Associate Professor of Medicine, Harvard Medical School; Associate Physician, Peter Bent Brigham Hospital, Boston

J. DENIS McGARRY, Ph.D.
Professor of Internal Medicine and Biochemistry, University of Texas Health Science Center at Dallas, Dallas

JAMES E. McGUIGAN, M.D.
Professor and Chairman, Department of Medicine, University of Florida College of Medicine, Gainesville

RIMA McLEOD, M.D.
Assistant Professor of Medicine, Division of Infectious Disease, Department of Medicine, Michael Reese Hospital and Medical Center, Chicago

JOHN P. MERRILL, M.D.
Professor of Medicine, Harvard Medical School; Director Emeritus, Cardiorenal Section, and Physician, Peter Bent Brigham Hospital, Boston

URS A. MEYER, M.D.
Professor of Clinical Pharmacology, Department of Medicine, University of Zurich Hospital, Zurich

MARTIN C. MIHM, JR., M.D.
Associate Professor of Pathology, Harvard Medical School; Associate Pathologist and Dermatologist, Massachusetts General Hospital, Boston

MYRON MILLER, M.D., F.A.C.P.
Professor of Medicine, State University of New York Upstate Medical Center; Chief, Medical Service, Veterans Administration Medical Center, Syracuse

JAY P. MOHR, M.D.
Professor of Neurology, University of South Alabama; Chief, Neurology Service, South Alabama University Hospital, Mobile

KENNETH M. MOSER, M.D.
Professor of Medicine, University of California, San Diego School of Medicine; Director, Pulmonary Division, University of California, San Diego Medical Center, San Diego

ARNOLD M. MOSES, M.D.
Director of Clinical Research Center and Professor of Medicine, State University of New York Upstate Medical Center; Chief, Endocrinology, Veterans Administration Medical Center, Syracuse

DAVID B. MOSHER, M.D.
Clinical Instructor in Dermatology, Harvard Medical School; Assistant in Dermatology, Massachusetts General Hospital, Boston

JOHN F. MURRAY, M.D.
Professor of Medicine, University of California, San Francisco; Chief, Chest Service, San Francisco General Hospital, San Francisco

ROBERT J. MYERBURG, M.D.
Professor of Medicine and Director, Division of Cardiology, Department of Medicine, University of Miami School of Medicine, Miami

JAMES C. NIEDERMAN, M.D.
Associate Clinical Professor of Epidemiology and Medicine, Department of Epidemiology and Public Health, Yale University School of Medicine, New Haven

HYMIE L. NOSSEL, M.D.
Professor of Medicine, College of Physicians and Surgeons, Columbia University; Attending Physician, Presbyterian Hospital, New York

JOHN A. OATES, M.D.
The Joe and Morris Werthan Professor of Investigative Medicine, Department of Medicine and Pharmacology, Vanderbilt University Hospital, Nashville

JERROLD M. OLEFSKY, M.D.
Professor of Medicine and Head, Division of Endocrinology and Metabolism, University of Colorado Medical Center, Denver

ROBERT A. O'ROURKE, M.D.
Professor of Medicine and Director, Division of Cardiovascular Diseases, University of Texas Health Science Center at San Antonio, San Antonio

JOHN A. PARRISH, M.D.
Associate Professor of Dermatology, Harvard Medical School; Assistant Dermatologist, Massachusetts General Hospital, Boston

MADHUKAR A. PATHAK, M.B., Ph.D.
Senior Associate in Dermatology, Harvard Medical School; Biochemist, Massachusetts General Hospital, Boston

LAWRENCE L. PELLETIER, JR., M.D.
Associate Professor of Internal Medicine, University of North Dakota School of Medicine; Chief, Infectious Diseases Section, Fargo Veterans Administration Hospital, Fargo

PETER L. PERINE, M.D.
Director, Yaws Control Assistance Programs, Research and Development Division, Bureau of Smallpox Eradication, Center for Disease Control, Atlanta

ROBERT G. PETERSDORF, A.B., M.D., D.Sc. (Hon.)
Professor of Medicine, Harvard Medical School, Boston; President, Affiliated Hospitals Center

KIRK L. PETERSON, M.D.
Associate Professor of Medicine, University of California, San Diego School of Medicine; Director, Cardiac Catheterization Laboratory, University of California, San Diego Medical Center, San Diego

JAMES J. PLORDE, M.D.
Professor of Medicine and Laboratory Medicine, University of Washington School of Medicine; Chief, Microbiology Laboratory, Veterans Administration Hospital, Seattle

JOHN W. POPP, JR., M.D.
Clinical Assistant Professor of Medicine, University of South Carolina School of Medicine, Columbia

DAVID C. POSKANZER, M.D., M.P.H.
Associate Professor of Neurology, Harvard Medical School; Associate Neurologist and Epidemiologist, Massachusetts General Hospital, Boston

JOHN T. POTTS, JR., M.D.
Professor of Medicine, Harvard Medical School; Chief, Endocrine Unit, Massachusetts General Hospital, Boston

LAWRIE W. POWELL, M.D.
Professor of Medicine, Department of Medicine, University of Queensland; Physician, Royal Brisbane Hospital, Brisbane

JOEL M. RAPPEPORT, M.D.
Assistant Professor of Medicine, Harvard Medical School; Associate in Medicine, Peter Bent Brigham Hospital, Boston

C. GEORGE RAY, M.D.
Professor of Pathology, Department of Pathology, Microbiology Section, Clinical Laboratories, University of Arizona College of Medicine, Tucson

JEAN J. REBEIZ, M.D.
Assistant Professor of Neurology and Neuropathology, American University of Beirut; Neurologist and Neuropathologist, American University Hospital, Beirut

PETER REICH, M.D.
Associate Professor of Psychiatry, Harvard Medical School; Chief, Psychiatric Services, Affiliated Hospitals Center, Boston

JACK S. REMINGTON, M.D.
Professor of Medicine, Division of Infectious Disease, Department of Medicine, Stanford University School of Medicine; Chief, Division of Allergy, Immunology, and Infectious Disease, Palo Alto Medical Research Foundation, Palo Alto

EDWARD P. RICHARDSON, JR., M.D.
Professor of Neuropathology, Harvard Medical School; Neuropathologist, Massachusetts General Hospital, Boston

ALAN R. RONALD, M.D.
Professor and Head, Department of Medical Microbiology, University of Manitoba, Winnipeg

LEON E. ROSENBERG, M.D.
Professor of Human Genetics, Medicine, and Pediatrics and Chairman, Department of Human Genetics, Yale University School of Medicine; Attending Physician, Yale-New Haven Hospital, New Haven

JOHN ROSS, JR., M.D.
Professor of Medicine, University of California, School of Medicine; Director, Cardiovascular Division, Department of Medicine, University of California, San Diego Medical Center, La Jolla

RICHARD S. ROSS, M.D.
Professor of Medicine (Cardiology) and Dean of the Medical Faculty, The Johns Hopkins University School of Medicine, Baltimore

ARTHUR H. RUBENSTEIN, M.D.
Professor of Medicine, Pritzker School of Medicine, The University of Chicago Medical Center, Chicago

CYRUS E. RUBIN, M.D.
Professor of Medicine, Division of Gastroenterology, University of Washington School of Medicine, Seattle

DANIEL RUDMAN, M.D.
Professor of Medicine and Surgery, Emory University School of Medicine; Director, Clinical Research Facility, Emory University Hospital, Atlanta

FUAD SABRA, M.D., F.A.C.P.
Professor of Neurology and Head, Division of Neurology, Medical School, American University of Beirut; Neurologist, American University Hospital, Beirut

MARIA SALAM-ADAMS, M.D.
Assistant Professor of Neurology, Harvard Medical School; Clinical and Research Fellow in Children's Neurology, Massachusetts General Hospital, Boston

MERLE A. SANDE, M.D.
Professor of Medicine and Vice Chairman, Department of Medicine, University of Virginia Medical Center, Charlottesville

JAY P. SANFORD, M.D.
Dean, Uniformed Services University of the Health Sciences, Bethesda

NICHOLAS A. SAUNDERS, M.B.B.S., F.R.A.C.P., F.R.C.P. (C)
Senior Lecturer, Department of Medicine, University of Newcastle, Newcastle

DENNIS SCHABERG, M.D.
Assistant Professor of Medicine, University of Michigan School of Medicine, Ann Arbor

I. HERBERT SCHEINBERG, M.D.
Professor of Medicine, Albert Einstein College of Medicine; Attending Physician and Head, Division of Genetic Medicine, Hospital of the Albert Einstein College of Medicine, New York

R. NEIL SCHIMKE, M.D., F.A.C.P.
Professor of Medicine and Pediatrics and Chief, Division of Metabolism, Endocrinology, and Genetics, University of Kansas Medical Center, College of Health Sciences, Kansas City

LESLIE J. SCHOENFIELD, M.D.
Professor of Medicine, University of California, Los Angeles; Director, Division of Gastroenterology, Cedars-Sinai Medical Center, Los Angeles

ROBERT W. SCHRIER, M.D.
Professor and Chairman, Department of Medicine, University of Colorado Health Sciences Center, University of Colorado Hospitals, Denver

DAVID A. SHAFRITZ, M.D.
Associate Professor of Medicine and Cell Biology, Albert Einstein College of Medicine, New York

DAVID G. SHAND, Ph.D., M.B.
Professor of Pharmacology and Medicine and Chief, Division of Clinical Pharmacology, Duke University Medical Center, Durham

CHARLES C. SHEPARD, M.D.
Chief, Leprosy and Rickettsia Branch, Center for Disease Control; Adjunct Associate Professor of Microbiology, Emory University School of Medicine, Atlanta

LOUIS M. SHERWOOD, M.D.
Professor of Medicine, Pritzker School of Medicine, University of Chicago; Physician-in-Chief and Chairman, Department of Medicine, Michael Reese Hospital and Medical Center, Chicago

ELIZABETH M. SHORT, M.D.
Assistant Professor of Medicine, Stanford University School of Medicine; Attending Physician, Stanford University Medical Center, Stanford

HARRY L. SHWACHMAN, M.D.
Professor of Pediatrics, Emeritus, Harvard Medical School; Senior Associate in Medicine, Children's Hospital Medical Center, Boston

WILLIAM SILEN, M.D.
Johnson and Johnson Professor of Surgery, Harvard Medical School; Surgeon-in-Chief, Beth Israel Hospital, Boston

FRED E. SILVERSTEIN, M.D.
Associate Professor of Medicine, Division of Gastroenterology, Department of Medicine, University of Washington School of Medicine, Seattle

DAVID W. SMITH, M.D.
Professor and Chairman, Department of Pediatrics, University of Rochester School of Medicine, Rochester

BURTON E. SOBEL, M.D.
Professor of Medicine and Director, Cardiovascular Division, Washington University; Cardiologist-in-Chief, Barnes Hospital, St. Louis

ARTHUR J. SOBER, M.D.
Assistant Professor of Dermatology, Harvard Medical School; Assistant Dermatologist, Massachusetts General Hospital, Boston

EDMUND H. SONNENBLICK, M.D.
Professor of Medicine and Chief, Division of Cardiology, Department of Medicine, Albert Einstein College of Medicine, New York

WESLEY W. SPINK, M.D., D.Sc. (Hon.)
Emeritus Regents' Professor of Medicine and Comparative Medicine, University of Minnesota Health Sciences Center, Minneapolis

WALTER STAMM, M.D.
Assistant Professor of Medicine, Division of Infectious Diseases, University of Washington School of Medicine; Physician, Harborview Medical Center, Seattle

WILLIAM W. STEAD, M.D.
Professor of Medicine, University of Arkansas School of Medicine, Little Rock; Director, Tuberculosis Program, Division of Communicable Diseases, Arkansas Department of Health

DANIEL J. STECHSCHULTE, M.D.
Professor of Medicine, Division of Allergy, Clinical Immunology, and Rheumatology, Department of Medicine, University of Kansas Medical Center, College of Health Sciences, Kansas City

GENE H. STOLLERMAN, M.D.
Professor and Chairman, Department of Medicine, University of Tennessee College of Medicine, Memphis

D. EUGENE STRANDNESS, JR., M.D.
Professor of Surgery, University of Washington School of Medicine, Seattle

DAVID H. P. STREETEN, M.B., D.Phil., F.R.C.P.
Professor of Medicine and Head, Section of Endocrinology, State University of New York Upstate Medical Center, Syracuse

E. DONNALL THOMAS, M.D.
Professor of Medicine and Head, Division of Oncology, University of Washington School of Medicine; Head, Division of Medical Oncology, Fred Hutchinson Cancer Research Center, Seattle

GEORGE W. THORN, M.D., M.A. (Hon.), LL.D (Hon.), D.Sc. (Hon.), M.D. (Hon.), F.R.C.P.
Hersey Professor of the Theory and Practice of Physic, Emeritus, and Samuel A. Levine Professor of Medicine, Emeritus, Harvard Medical School; Physician-in-Chief, Emeritus, Peter Bent Brigham Hospital, Boston

GENNARO M. TISI, M.D.
Associate Professor of Medicine, University of California, San Diego School of Medicine; Chief, Pulmonary Section, Veterans Administration Hospital, San Diego

PHILLIP P. TOSKES, M.D.
Professor of Medicine, University of Florida College of Medicine; Chief, Division of Gastroenterology, Gainesville Veterans Administration Medical Center, Gainesville

MARVIN TURCK, M.D.
Professor of Medicine, University of Washington School of Medicine; Physician-in-Chief, Harborview Medical Center, Seattle

DAVID D. ULMER, M.D.
Professor and Chairman, Department of Medicine, Charles R. Drew Postgraduate Medical School; Physician, Martin Luther King Hospital, Los Angeles

JOHN E. ULTMANN, M.D.
Professor of Medicine, Section of Hematology/Oncology, Department of Medicine; Director, University of Chicago Cancer Research Center; Associate Dean for Research Programs, Biological Sciences Division, Pritzker School of Medicine, University of Chicago, Chicago

ROGER H. UNGER, M.D.
Professor of Internal Medicine, University of Texas Health Science Center at Dallas; Senior Medical Investigator, Dallas Veterans Administration Medical Center, Dallas

HENRI VANDER EECKEN, H.M., M.D.
Professor of Neurology, Faculty of Medicine, University of Ghent; Head of the Department of Neurology, Akademisch Zeikenhuis, Ghent

MAURICE VICTOR, M.D.
Professor of Neurology, Case Western Reserve University School of Medicine; Director, Neurology Service, Cleveland Metropolitan General Hospital, Cleveland

JAMES F. WALLACE, M.D.
Professor of Medicine, University of Washington School of Medicine; Associate Physician-in-Chief, University of Washington Hospital, Seattle

PATRICK C. WALSH, M.D.
Professor and Director, Department of Urology, The Johns Hopkins University School of Medicine; Urologist-in-Chief, James Buchanan Brady Urological Institute, The Johns Hopkins Hospital, Baltimore

JACK R. WANDS, M.D.
Assistant Professor of Medicine, Harvard Medical School; Assistant Physician, Gastrointestinal Unit, Massachusetts General Hospital, Boston

HENRY deF. WEBSTER, M.D.
Head, Section Cellular Neuropathology, National Institute of Neurological Disease and Stroke, National Institutes of Health, Bethesda

LOUIS WEINSTEIN, M.D., Ph.D., Sc.D. (Hon.)
Visiting Professor of Medicine, Harvard Medical School; Physician and Director, Clinical Services, Infectious Diseases Division, Peter Bent Brigham Hospital, Boston

JOHN B. WEST, M.D., Ph.D.
Professor of Medicine, University of California, San Diego School of Medicine; Physician, University Hospital, University of California, San Diego Medical Center, San Diego

GRANT R. WILKINSON, Ph.D.
Professor of Pharmacology, Vanderbilt University School of Medicine, Nashville

GORDON H. WILLIAMS, M.D.
Associate Professor of Medicine, Harvard Medical School; Peter Bent Brigham Hospital, Boston

JEAN D. WILSON, M.D.
Professor of Internal Medicine and Director, McDermott Center for Growth and Development, University of Texas Health Science Center at Dallas, Dallas

MAXWELL M. WINTROBE, B.A., M.D., B.Sc. (Med.), Ph.D., D.Sc. (Hon. Manitoba), D.Sc. (Hon. Utah), M.A.C.P.
Distinguished Professor of Internal Medicine, University of Utah College of Medicine, Salt Lake City

KENNETH A. WOEBER, M.D.
Professor of Medicine, University of California, San Francisco School of Medicine; Chief, Department of Medicine, Mount Zion Hospital and Medical Center, San Francisco

SHELDON M. WOLFF, M.D.
Professor and Chairman, Department of Medicine, Tufts University School of Medicine, Boston

ALASTAIR J. J. WOOD, M.D., M.R.C.P.
Assistant Professor of Medicine and Pharmacology, Vanderbilt University School of Medicine; Attending Physician, Vanderbilt University Hospital, Nashville

THEODORE E. WOODWARD, M.D.
Professor of Medicine and Head, Department of Medicine, University of Maryland School of Medicine, Baltimore

RICHARD J. WURTMAN, M.D.
Professor of Endocrinology and Metabolism and Director, Laboratory of Neuroendocrine Regulation, Massachusetts Institute of Technology; Clinical Associate in Medicine, Massachusetts General Hospital, Boston

SING HEIM YAP, M.D., Ph.D.
Consultant, Division of Gastroenterology and Liver Disease, Department of Medicine, St. Radboud Hospital, University of Nijmegen, Nijmegen

ROBERT R. YOUNG, M.D.
Associate Professor of Neurology, Harvard Medical School; Associate Neurologist and Chief, Clinical Neurophysiology, Massachusetts General Hospital, Boston

PREFACE

Prefaces are always written but they are not frequently read. Hopefully, the readers of this textbook will judge its merits by the substance of its contents and not by the pretexts offered by its editors. Why then a foreword to this ninth edition?

This preface is intended to indicate the ways in which the present edition adheres to the original objectives of this book and at the same time to note some substantive changes which have been made since the last edition.

When the first group of editors met together almost thirty-four years ago, they decided to write a textbook of medicine that would conform to the *clinical method* they had found most useful both as students and as teachers. It was thought that such a book should recapitulate the steps in the process of thinking by which a physician reaches a diagnosis, these being the recording of the patient's symptoms and signs, the consideration of the various disorders that can give rise to them, and the effective utilization of measures which will support and confirm or alter the first impressions and lead ultimately to a firm diagnosis.

The logical first step consistent with this clinical approach is the consideration of the *cardinal manifestations of disease.* Patients present with symptoms, not diagnoses. Consequently, it is basic to good clinical medicine to appreciate the different causes of various manifestations of disease and to understand how they may be produced. This requires an understanding of normal physiology and of the ways in which deviations from the normal lead to disease. For this reason material of fundamental biological importance was incorporated in the first edition and has been regarded as an essential component ever since.

The revolutionary changes in the curricula of many American medical schools, particularly the abbreviation of the standard courses in the sciences basic to clinical medicine and the substitution of shorter "core" courses, has imposed, we believe, additional responsibilities on the modern teacher of clinical medicine and on the modern textbook of medicine. The students who embark on their clinical training now, although far more sophisticated in many ways than their predecessors of even one generation ago, may not possess as much understanding of the mechanisms of symptoms and disease processes as is required to deal intelligently with clinical problems. This book recognizes the challenge to education posed by such curricula. Clinical biochemistry and pathophysiology form an integral part of this book but, insofar as possible, are considered within the clinical setting.

The interpretation of symptoms usually is most effectively achieved by proceeding from the general to the particular. Symptoms often can be grouped as syndromes. Syndromes are the consequence of a variety of etiologic factors or disease mechanisms and, if these can be recognized and understood, measures to restore the normal physiological state can be designed and carried out in a logical, systematic fashion. Furthermore, the method of approaching a diagnosis which is based on an analysis of the symptoms, recognition of the syndrome, and consideration of the various disease mechanisms which may have produced it ensures consideration of the many possible interpretations of the clinical picture which the patient presents. By pursuing such an approach, it is less likely that a disorder which should be considered will be overlooked.

The plan of the book is consistent with this approach. In Part 1, "Introduction to Clinical Medicine," the Editors discuss their general philosophy regarding the approach to the patient. In Part 2, "Cardinal Manifestations of Disease," the mechanisms whereby various symptoms are produced are discussed, an approach to the recognition of the diseases of which these may be manifestations is outlined, and laboratory findings are discussed in relation to the clinical manifestations. Part 3, "Biological Considerations in the Approach to Clinical Medicine," summarizes the important considerations on the following: (1) the genetics of human disease, with discussions of cytogenetics and the prevention and treatment of genetic disorders, including genetic counseling; (2) clinical immunology, which is reviewed in depth; (3) clinical pharmacology and the principles of drug therapy, adverse reactions to drugs, and the clinical pharmacology of the autonomic nervous system; (4) nutritional disorders, with discussions of nutritional requirements, malnutrition and overnutrition (obesity), dietary therapy, and parenteral nutrition; and (5) metabolic disorders, with discussions of derangements of nucleic acid, carbohydrate, and lipid metabolism as well as fluid and electrolyte pathophysiology, including considerations of acidosis and alkalosis. In Part 4, "Disorders Caused by Biological and Environmental Agents," will be found the major discussions of the approach to the diagnosis and treatment of infectious diseases. Chemotherapy of infections and the specific diseases caused by microbial agents are discussed in detail. In addition, disorders of uncertain etiology (such as sarcoidosis and familial Mediterranean fever) and diseases due to environmental hazards such as tobacco smoking, radiation injury, drug overdosage, and alcoholism are considered.

The remainder of the book is concerned with specific disorders and disease entities. In all these sections, the syndromic approach is emphasized insofar as possible. The reader will find at the beginning of most of the sections, either in the introduction or in the first chapter, a discussion of the approach to the patient whose clinical manifestations suggest the type of disease considered in that section.

A deliberate attempt has been made to avoid long bibliographies. The references at the end of the chapters are largely to reviews and monographs. Others refer to a few of the most significant recent articles.

In this ninth edition the editors have attempted to keep pace with the dynamic and ever-changing field of medicine. Since the publication of the last edition only three years ago, new diseases have been discovered (e.g., Legionnaires' disease) and new diagnostic modalities (such as ultrasound, computerized tomography, and endoscopy) have become routine in most medical centers. Consequently, the chapters and sections of this ninth edition have been updated or completely revised as follows.

The section on the *approach to clinical problems* has been extensively updated, especially the chapters on gain and loss in weight and alterations in urinary function. The section dealing with reproductive and sexual functions is completely new, and the dermatology chapters, especially those dealing with skin pigmentation, photosensitivity, and other reactions to light, have been completely revised.

The section on *clinical pharmacology and toxicology* has been revised and updated. The chapter on the clinical pharmacology of the autonomic nervous system is new, and the chapters dealing with the principles of drug therapy and adverse reactions to drugs have been expanded.

The current section on *nutrition,* including the chapters on nutritional problems of the ill patient, anorexia, obesity, and derangements of vitamin metabolism, has been completely revised, and the newest approaches to dietary therapy and parenteral nutrition are discussed.

In the area of *infectious diseases* there are many new chapters, including those on diagnostic procedures, infectious diarrheas and bacterial food poisoning, sexually transmitted infections, immunization practices, Legionnaires' disease, fungus diseases, and urinary tract infections.

In the section on *disorders of the heart,* echocardiography, radionuclide angiography, and other noninvasive methods of cardiac examination have been discussed in greater detail. Major revisions and updating have been carried out in the chapters dealing with the cardiomyopathies, atherosclerosis, and hypertension, with emphasis placed on modern methods of treating the latter two conditions.

The section on *lung diseases* includes new chapters on hypersensitivity pneumonitis and cystic fibrosis in the adult, and the discussions of environmental lung disease and the adult respiratory distress syndrome have been substantially revised. Significant emphasis has been placed on the role of newer diagnostic procedures such as fiberoptic bronchoscopy in the examination of the respiratory system.

The entire *renal section* has been rewritten. The reader will find an up-to-date description of disturbances of renal function and major new chapters on the immunopathogenetic mechanisms of renal injury, glomerulopathies, interstitial diseases of the kidney, and hereditary tubular disorders.

The section on *gastroenterology* includes completely new and up-to-date chapters on peptic ulcer, disorders of the pancreas, and diseases of the gallbladder. The chapters on viral hepatitis (acute and chronic) have also been updated in order to provide the latest information on viral antigens and antibodies and their usefulness in clinical diagnosis of liver diseases. The chapters on intestinal absorption, malabsorption, and inflammatory bowel disease have also been extensively revised.

The sections on *disorders of the hematopoietic system* and *neoplasia* include revisions of the chapters on megaloblastic anemias, bone marrow transplantation, cancer chemotherapy, and Hodgkin's disease. Color plates of disorders of erythrocytes and leukocytes are included in this edition for the first time.

The section on *endocrine and metabolic disorders* has been completely revised. New chapters will be found on the pituitary, hypothalamus, diabetes mellitus, and hypoglycemia. In addition, there are new chapters on disorders of sexual differentiation, diseases of the testes, and disorders of the breast and milk formation.

The section on *disorders of bone and mineral metabolism* has been extensively revised with new illustrations and an updated chapter on vitamin D.

The section dealing with *disorders of the nervous system* includes new and revised chapters on epilepsy and Parkinson's disease. The chapter dealing with cerebrovascular diseases includes an in-depth discussion on the approach to diagnosis and therapy. The section dealing with *diseases of striated muscle* has also been completely revised.

The *Appendix* presents the latest complete set of important laboratory values of clinical importance. Where possible we have also included, for the convenience of the reader, values in *SI units* as well as in conventional units.

With the publication of the eighth edition of this textbook, one of the original editors and the Editor-in-Chief for that edition, Dr. George W. Thorn, retired. We, his colleagues and coeditors, are all indebted to Dr. Thorn, not only for his tremendous contributions to this textbook but also for his major contributions to the field of internal medicine. His distinguished leadership and his creative genius will be sorely missed. His influence will undoubtedly continue to be felt in future editions of this textbook. With this ninth edition we take pleasure in welcoming as a new editor Dr. Jean D. Wilson, an academic colleague who is recognized internationally as an outstanding scholar, teacher, and clinician-scientist.

We also wish to express our appreciation and gratitude to our many associates and colleagues, who as experts in their fields have helped us by providing constructive and valuable criticisms of the chapters in this ninth edition. In addition to the authors and contributors who also reviewed many manuscripts, we wish to thank the following for their many helpful suggestions: David J. Baylink, William J. Bremner, George F. Cahill, George P. Cannelos, Martin C. Carey, Earl Davie, David Donaldson, Thomas D. DuBose, John Ensinck, Z. Myron Falchuk, Donald Farrell, Daniel Federman, Bernard Fields, Clement A. Finch, Stephen Fricker, Ruben Gittes, Charles J. Goodner, Judith G. Hall, Laurence Harker, Holger W. Hoehn, Edward Kass, Juha P. Kokko, Guenter J. Krejs, Robert Labbe, S. Laksminarayan, Lewis Landsberg, Mark Leshin, Lee Levitt, Joseph Martin, James McArthur, George McDonald, Mark McPhee, Donald Miller, Donald E. Moore, Gilbert S. Omenn, C. Alvin Paulsen, James Pennington, Arnold S. Relman, R. Paul Robertson, David S. Rosenthal, David Saunders, Michael Schuffler, C. Donald Scott, Donald Sherrard, Peter Simkin, J. Donald Smiley, R. Graham Smith, George Stamatoyannopoulos, Morton A. Stenchever, Gary E. Striker, Philip D. Swanson, Ira B. Tager, Jerry S. Trier, Shirley Wray, and Joseph E. Zerwekh.

As always, we wish to express our appreciation to our dedicated secretarial coworkers who have been of immeasurable help. We are especially indebted to Mrs. Hilda Gardner, Mrs. Freda Foster, Ms. Patricia Kadlick, Mrs. Mary Jackson, Mrs. Trudy Geissler, Mrs. Cynthia Reid, Mrs. Diane Tasian, and Mrs. Raye Ann Hondroulis.

KURT J. ISSELBACHER
RAYMOND D. ADAMS
EUGENE BRAUNWALD
ROBERT G. PETERSDORF
JEAN D. WILSON

Harrison's
PRINCIPLES
OF INTERNAL
MEDICINE

VOLUME 1

1
THE PRACTICE OF MEDICINE

THE EDITORS

APPROACH TO THE PATIENT

No greater opportunity, responsibility, or obligation is given to an individual than that of serving as a physician. In treating the suffering, there is need for technical skill, scientific knowledge, and human understanding. The person who uses these with courage, with humility, and with wisdom will provide a unique service and will build an enduring edifice of character. The physician should ask of destiny no more than this and be content with no less.

Thirty years ago, the Editors of this book defined what is expected of the physician. Their eloquent words ring as true now as they did then:

Tact, sympathy and understanding are expected of the physician, for the patient is no mere collection of symptoms, signs, disordered functions, damaged organs, and disturbed emotions. He is human, fearful, and hopeful, seeking relief, help and reassurance. To the physician, as to the anthropologist, nothing human is strange or repulsive. The misanthrope may become a smart diagnostician of organic disease, but he can scarcely hope to succeed as a physician. The true physician has a Shakespearean breadth of interest in the wise and the foolish, the proud and the humble, the stoic hero and the whining rogue. He cares for people.

THE ART OF MEDICINE In the practice of medicine the physician employs a discipline which seeks to utilize scientific methods and principles in the solution of its problems, but it is one in which, in the end, both science and art are wedded. The crucial importance of understanding the scientific base of modern medicine is well known; the significance of the art of medicine is not as well appreciated. Thus, to extract from a mass of conflicting physical signs and laboratory data the ones that are of crucial significance, to know in a borderline case when to initiate and when to refrain from a line of investigation or treatment involves judgments based on "assimilated" experience. Skill in accomplishing these necessities of medical art is not usually the outcome of laboratory study alone.

Intuition and maturing wisdom are called upon in developing the more personal relations with patients and the understanding and capacity to peer beneath surface motivations into their behavior. Astute physicians will recognize when the casual mention of an apparently trivial complaint is a device for seeking reassurance regarding a feared disorder such as cancer or heart disease. They will know at once when to probe the more intimate aspects of the patient's life and when to leave them undiscussed, and they will realize when to express a bright and reassuring prognosis and when and how to utter doubt and caution.

Medicine is an art also in the sense that physicians can never be content with the sole aim of endeavoring to clarify the laws of nature; they cannot proceed in their labors with the cool detachment of the scientist whose aim is the winning of the truth, and who, in doing so, conducts a "controlled experiment." It is essential that they maintain objectivity in the study and care of their patients, for this is in the patients' interests; they must use wise judgment and must never forget that their primary and traditional objectives are utilitarian—the prevention and cure of disease and the relief of suffering, whether of body or of mind.

THE PHYSICIAN AND THE PATIENT

An aspect of illness that influences the physician-patient relationship is the real or implied significance of disease in the mind of the patient. Any departure from good health involves a potential threat of physical disintegration or crippling disability, and even the most intelligent and best-informed patients should not be considered immune to forebodings just because they refrain from mentioning them. In fact, most patients are more concerned with the possibility of being rendered dependent by illness than with the disease itself. It is especially important that these fears be borne in mind when dealing with the elderly patient, who is rarely unmindful that "the trap is laid" and death is always near.

The attitude of the patient approaching the doctor must always be tinged, for the most part unconsciously, with distaste and dread; his deepest desire will tend to be comfort and relief rather than cure, and his faith and expectation will be directed towards some magical exhibition of these boons. Do not let yourselves believe that however smoothly concealed by education, by reason, and by confidential frankness these strong elements may be, they are ever in any circumstances altogether absent.

Wilfred Trotter

Illness also constitutes a threat to the individual's status in a social group. Prolonged invalidism during childhood tends inevitably to leave behind an excessive egocentricity, which may become the basis of a lifelong neurosis. In the adult, illness often enforces a return to a posture of dependency, a change usually accompanied by feelings of apprehension and discouragement, sometimes leading to frank anxiety and depression. This explains a number of common psychologic defenses which patients exercise against illness. They may refuse medical aid; or, if they summon the courage to consult a physician, they may minimize or even fail to mention the very symptom about which they are most deeply concerned. Then, too, there are persons whose emotional stability has been tenuous and uncertain, so that the position of dependency imposed by illness comes as a welcome relief from adult responsibility. They appear to enjoy illness and to resent anything that menaces their state of invalidism. Lesser degrees of this tendency are seen among those who consult the physician at the appearance of every new symptom and who are continuously preoccupied with their past illnesses and operations.

During examination in the relatively neutral domain of the hospital ward a patient's emotional life may seem relatively unimportant. Organic lesions have a way of compelling attention to themselves, and further, it may be less exhausting to limit one's focus to the sphere of physical disease. More time, energy, and experience frequently are necessary to view the patient as an active participant in an enormous moving pageant which includes the personal eccentricities of one's forebears, one's own fears and patterns of reaction, the roles of poverty, insecurity, and perhaps poor vocational and domestic relations. Yet every experienced physician knows that to explain many of the manifestations of illness, it is necessary to view the patient comprehensively as an organism with a vast repository of past experiences, many of which are vaguely remembered, yet have become the foundation of one's current system of meeting daily problems.

THE PHYSICIAN'S RESPONSIBILITIES The physician seeks to respond to and alleviate the patient's complaints, to search out signs of ill health not yet apparent to the patient or abnormalities which may lead to ill health, and to maintain the patient in a state of well-being. To achieve these goals requires a broad orientation. Illness is never limited to one system, nor necessarily to a single disease, and whether the physician is a family practitioner, an internist who provides "primary care," or a subspecialist, the patient must be viewed not as an organ system but as a person.

EXAMINATION OF THE WELL PERSON AND PREVENTION OF DISEASE The intelligent practice of preventive medicine is often considered undramatic; yet few areas of medicine are of greater importance to a single individual or to an entire population. In this aspect of medical practice, the physician deals with individuals or groups who are not overtly ill or whose complaints may be unrelated to the disease process which is to be prevented. The use of the periodic physical examination and the ready availability of multiphasic screening tests allow the physician to detect and to intervene in disease processes early in their course, often before the first symptom becomes manifest.

Physicians who examine well individuals are not "wasting their training." More skill is required to recognize the early signs of ill health than to deal with what is obvious to patients or their families. The discovery and cure of potentially serious disease represent a far greater service to one's patient than ministrations in the course of an incurable condition.

The finding of an elevated arterial blood pressure or an elevated blood sugar, serum uric acid, or cholesterol level in an asymptomatic person or the discussion of milder degrees of nervousness or depression provides an unparalleled opportunity to prevent or retard events of serious consequence. It is not always easy to persuade asymptomatic persons to face situations they had hoped to avoid or to alter their habits or diet in order to follow a therapeutic program throughout the rest of their lives. Nevertheless the value of these efforts is so great that it fully justifies the effort and attention of every physician.

CHANGING PATIENT-PHYSICIAN RELATIONSHIPS The one-to-one patient-physician relationship which traditionally has been the goal of all physicians is changing, primarily because of the changing setting in which medicine is being practiced. In many cases the management of the individual patient requires the active participation of a variety of trained professional personnel—not only physicians, but also nurses, physicians' assistants, dietitians, biochemists, psychologists, and other health care personnel. The patient can benefit greatly from such collaboration, but it is the duty of the physician to guide the patient through an illness. In order to carry out this increasingly difficult task, the physician must have some familiarity with the techniques, skills, and objectives of colleagues in the fields allied to medicine. Their findings must be interpreted not as isolated phenomena, but rather in terms of the total clinical

picture. In giving the patient an opportunity to receive all the benefits of the important advances of science, the physician must retain responsibility for the crucial decisions concerning diagnosis and treatment.

An increasing number of patients is being cared for by groups of physicians, clinics, hospitals, and health-maintenance organizations (HMOs) rather than by a single, independent practitioner. There are many potential advantages in the use of such organized medical groups, but there also are hazards, both to the patient and the physician. The identity of the physician who is primarily and continuously responsible for each particular patient must be clearly defined. It is this physician who must have an overview of a patient's problems and who must maintain familiarity with the patient's reaction to illness, to drugs, and to the challenges of daily living. In addition, since a number of physicians may, at any one time, contribute to the care of a particular patient, and since patients as well as physicians are becoming increasingly mobile, accurate and detailed record keeping assumes progressively greater importance. It is imperative that the physician promptly commit all pertinent data obtained from the clinical and laboratory examinations to the patient's permanent medical record. Only in this way can continuity and high quality in the care of the patient be provided.

THE PHYSICIAN AS A PERSON The examining physician is first a human instrument, subject to reactions arising from events in his or her own biography. This background will strongly influence the physician's responses to and understanding of the patient. The student receives much expert coaching in the methods of physical and laboratory diagnosis, and in these areas will most easily develop the skills that permit a comfortable relationship with the patient. The young physician may feel inadequate in dealing with the patient's problems; a sense of insecurity is inevitable. Moreover, the newly acquired role of authority and responsibility may be threatening. Some reactions may be difficult to control: lack of interest in a patient who presents no fascinating problems of organic disease, irritation at the patient's verbosity or lack of clarity and consistency in reciting his or her history, or even disappointment because the patient's illness fails to respond to treatment in the expected manner.

To perceive and understand the problems of the patient, the physician requires not simply instruction but emotional maturity and an interest in and concern for other human beings. The physician must learn to be at ease and to establish rapport with persons of every walk of life, realizing that everyone is born with manifold potentialities determined by their genes and has a personality and character shaped by the emotional climate in which they grow and develop. The physician must relate as much to the person who is ill as to the illness for which he or she seeks relief.

The physician has a special function in society and should be skilled as a psychologist as well as a biologist. With the highly technical knowledge and skills needed to affect the patient's physiologic functions there should also be a feeling of humaneness, a sense of confidence and security based upon the conviction that all will be done that can be done. Such an atmosphere will allow a wholesome personal relationship to develop. The patient must be allowed to feel that his or her unique individuality is recognized and that life's problems are appreciated. This is as important to patients with well-defined organic disease as to those suffering primarily from psychiatric illness.

APPROACH TO DISEASE

HISTORY The written history of an illness should embody all the facts of medical significance in the life of the patient up to the time that the physician is consulted, but of course, the most recent diseases attract the most attention, for these, obviously, are the reason that a person seeks medical advice. Ideally the narration of symptoms should be in the patient's own words, the principal events being presented in the temporal order in which they occurred. However, few patients possess the necessary powers of observation and talent for lucid, coherent description. Hence, guiding questions from the physician may be required, though one must avoid suggesting answers.

Often a symptom which has concerned a patient has little significance, whereas a seemingly minor complaint may be of importance. Therefore the physician must be constantly alert to the possibility that any event related by the patient, any symptom however trivial or apparently remote, may be the key to the solution of the medical problem. As data are gained from the physical and laboratory examinations, the problems which are presented should be clearly identified.

An informative history is more than an orderly listing of symptoms. Something always is gained by listening to patients and noting the way in which they talk about their symptoms. Inflections of voice, facial expression, and attitude may betray important clues to the meaning of the symptoms to a patient. In listening to the history, the physician discovers not only something about the disease but also something about the patient.

With experience the pitfalls of history taking become apparent. What patients relate for the most part consists of subjective phenomena filtered through minds that vary in their background of past experience. Patients obviously differ widely in their responses to the same stimuli. Their remarks are variably colored by fear of disease, disability, and death, and by concern over the consequences of illness to their families. Additional difficulties are created by language barriers, by failing intellectual powers which deprive the patient of accurate recall, or by disorders of consciousness that make them unaware of their illness. It is not surprising, then, that even the most careful physician may at times despair of collecting factual data and be forced to proceed with evidence that represents little more than an approximation of the truth.

Viewed in another way the symptom marks, in the patient's mind, a departure from normal health; in the physician's mind, it initiates a process of inductive and deductive reasoning that culminates in diagnosis. In pondering the various possible explanations of a given symptom or clinical state, the physician begins a search for other data, elicited by further questioning of the patient and the family, by physical examination, or by laboratory tests. The symptoms alone sometimes will provide the most certain clue, as in angina pectoris or epilepsy, where physical findings and laboratory data collected between attacks may give no evidence of the existence of disease even when it is present with certitude. In most illnesses, however, the history will not be so decisive, though it may narrow the number of diagnostic possibilities and guide the subsequent investigation.

It is in taking the history that the physician's skill, knowledge, and experience are most clearly in evidence. Each symptom is evaluated according to its nature and context; there are times for questioning its credibility and turning to more reliable sources of information, but skepticism must not cause an unusual symptom or manifestation of some new condition to be overlooked. Moreover, there are times when an interrogation must be pressed more deeply in a search for further details and times when the questions must be broader, because "disease often tells its secrets in a casual parenthesis." And finally, the physician knows how to take advantage of the interview in which the history is gathered to obtain the confidence of the patient and allay apprehension and fear, the first steps in therapy.

The family history, all too often obtained in a routine, cursory fashion, is a leading tool of clinical genetics and can provide important evidence regarding the nature of the patient's complaints. Information regarding symptoms like those of the patient which have occurred in blood relatives, or "run in the family," and knowledge of the ethnic origin of the parents and of consanguinity may be exceedingly helpful. The information must be obtained with tact, however, for patients may be embarrassed by such inquiries. The best family history is one which is supported by actual examination of other members of the family. Frequently it is found that some physical deviation from the normal, too subtle to be recognized by a lay person, is quite apparent to the trained observer and that a minor deviation in laboratory data assumes significance when evaluated within a family constellation.

PHYSICAL EXAMINATION Little need be said about the importance of the physical examination, for early in their training physicians learn that physical signs are the objective and verifiable marks of disease. The physical sign represents a solid, indisputable fact. However, its significance is enhanced when it confirms a functional or structural change already evidenced by the patient's history. At other times, the physical sign may stand as the only evidence of disease, especially in those instances in which the history has been inconsistent, confused, or completely lacking.

If full advantage is to be gained from the physical examination, it must be performed methodically and thoroughly. Although attention has usually been directed by the history to the offending organ or part of the body, the examination must extend to all parts of the body. The patient must be scrutinized literally from head to toe in an objective search for abnormalities that may yield information concerning present and possible future illnesses. Unless the examination procedure is systematic, important parts of it may be forgotten, an error against which even the most skilled clinician must guard. The results of the examination, like the details of the history, should be recorded at the time they are elicited, not hours later when they are subject to the distortions of memory. Many inaccuracies stem from the careless practice of writing or dictating notes long after the examination has ended.

Skill in physical diagnosis is acquired with experience, but it is not merely technique that determines success in eliciting signs. The detection of a few scattered petechiae, a faint diastolic murmur, or a small mass in the abdomen is not a question of keener eyes and ears or more sensitive fingers, but of a mind directed to be alert to these findings. Skill in physical diagnosis reflects a way of thinking more than a way of doing.

LABORATORY EXAMINATIONS The marked increase in the number and availability of laboratory diagnostic procedures has inevitably augmented reliance on the knowledge gained from these studies in the solution of clinical problems. It is essential, however, to bear in mind the limitations of such procedures, which by virtue of their impersonal quality and complexity often gain an aura of authority regardless of the fallibility of the individuals or their instruments. More importantly, the accumulation of laboratory data cannot release the physician from the necessity of careful observation and study of the patient. The wise physician understands the merits and limitations of each source of information, whether it be history, physical examination, or laboratory investigation. The physician also must weigh carefully the hazards and the expense involved in every laboratory procedure.

Nowadays, laboratory tests rarely are ordered and reported singly. Rather they are produced as "batteries." A common combination is the M6, which consists of determinations of serum sodium, potassium, carbon dioxide combining power, chloride, blood urea nitrogen, and blood glucose. Even more common is the M12, which reports simultaneously serum calcium, phosphate, proteins, albumin, uric acid, cholesterol, and several enzymes. Some laboratories now perform batteries of 24 and even 40 tests! The various combinations of laboratory tests are often useful. For example, they may provide the clue to such nonspecific symptoms as generalized weakness and increased fatigability by revealing an elevated serum calcium which, in turn, would suggest the diagnosis of hyperparathyroidism.

The thoughtful use of screening tests is not to be confused with indiscriminate laboratory testing; it is based on the fact that a group of laboratory determinations which are known to be frequent harbingers of disease can now be carried out on a single specimen of blood at relatively low cost. Biochemical measurements, together with simple laboratory examinations such as blood count, urinalysis, and sedimentation rate, often provide the major clue to the presence of a pathologic process. This is particularly helpful in identifying organic disease in a patient with evident psychologic or emotional problems. At the same time the physician must learn to evaluate occasional abnormalities among the screening tests that may not necessarily connote significant disease. There is nothing more costly and unproductive than an in-depth work-up following the reporting of an isolated laboratory abnormality in an otherwise well patient.

Discrimination in the ordering of laboratory procedures and judgment in appraising their risk, expense, and possible benefit are important indicators of the effectiveness with which the art and science of medicine have been fused by the individual physician.

THE CLINICAL METHOD AND THE SYNDROMIC APPROACH TO DISEASE The clinical method has as its object the collection of accurate data concerning all the diseases to which human beings are subject, namely, all conditions that "limit life in its powers, enjoyment, and duration." But much more is required in making a diagnosis. Each datum must be interpreted in the light of the known facts of anatomy, physiology, and chemistry. The synthesis of these interpretations yields information concerning the affected organ or body system. Further, from the vantage point afforded by such an anatomic diagnosis the physician may then turn to other data, such as the mode of onset and clinical course of the illness, and to the results of laboratory tests, in order to ascertain the cause of the disease and degree of physiologic impairment.

The clinical method always proceeds in a series of logical steps. The perceptive student will note certain similarities between the clinical method and the scientific method. Each begins with observational data which suggest a series of hypotheses. These are then tested in the light of further observations, some of which are made in the clinic and others in the laboratory. Finally, a conclusion is reached, which in science is called a *theory* and in medicine a *working diagnosis*. The modus operandi of the clinical method, like that of the scientific method, cannot be reduced to a single principle or a type of inductive or deductive reasoning. It involves both analysis and synthesis, the essential parts of cartesian logic. The physician does not start with an open mind any more than does the scientist, but armed with the knowledge of recent cases, the patient's first statement directs one's thinking to certain channels.

It is particularly in the study of more difficult patients that the logical order of the clinical method becomes most important. Here in particular the physician must carefully list each problem indicated by the patient's complaints and physical and laboratory findings and seek answers to each. Anatomic diagnosis regularly precedes etiological diagnosis. The cause and mechanism of a disease can seldom be determined before ascertaining which organ is involved. An intermediate step is syndromic diagnosis. Most physicians attempt consciously or unconsciously to fit a given problem into one of a series of syndromes. The syndrome, in essence, is a group of symptoms and signs of disordered function, related to one another by means of some anatomic, physiologic, or biochemical peculiarity. It embodies a hypothesis concerning the deranged function of an organ, organ system, or tissue. Congestive heart failure, Cushing's disease, and dementia are examples. In congestive heart failure dyspnea, orthopnea, cyanosis, dependent edema, engorged neck veins, pleural effusion, pulmonary rales, and enlarged liver are known to be connected by a single pathophysiologic mechanism—failure of the heart, leading to salt and water retention and high venous pressure. In Cushing's disease the moon faces, hypertension, diabetes, and osteoporosis are the recognized effects of excess corticosteroids acting on many target organs. In dementia deterioration of memory, incoherent thinking, and faulty judgment are related to impairment of the function and destruction of the association areas of the cerebrum.

A syndromic diagnosis does not necessarily identify the precise cause of an illness, but it greatly narrows the number of possibilities and, thus, suggests whatever further clinical and laboratory studies are required. The derangements of each organ system in human beings are reducible to a relatively small number of syndromes. Diagnosis is greatly simplified if a given clinical problem conforms neatly to a well-defined syndrome, because a list of the various diseases that may cause it may be all that is required to make the diagnosis. The search for the cause of an illness that does not conform to a syndrome is much more difficult, for a seemingly infinite number of diseases may then have to be considered. Nevertheless, the principle remains: the clinical method is an orderly intellectual activity which proceeds almost invariably from symptom, to sign, to syndrome, to disease.

THE COMPUTER IN MEDICINE The uses of the computer in managing the economic aspects of medical practice are already well established. However, the role of the computer in clinical medicine is still in an evolutionary stage. It has been used successfully in the clinical laboratory for processing data from automated chemical and microbiological determinations. Several centers have successfully developed computerized medical records for hospital and outpatient use. Automated information systems in pharmacies are becoming sophisticated and are able to assist in prevention of drug-drug interactions and improved monitoring of therapy. Interpretation of electrocardiograms by computer is commonplace. Although these newer developments are noteworthy, computer management of medical data is still in its infancy.

The role of the computer in medical decision making remains elusive but challenging. Considerable progress has been made in using the computer to facilitate differential diagnosis and to evaluate clinical decision-making.

The advantages to the physician who can use computer technology are obvious. Much time and effort can be saved, and more accurate and reliable clinical information can be brought quickly into the hands of the physician.

ACCOUNTABILITY Traditionally, physicians, once licensed to practice medicine, have not had to account for their actions except to their peers. In the past decade, however, there have been increasing demands for physicians to account for the way in which they practice medicine by meeting certain standards prescribed by federal and state governments. Hospitalized patients whose health care is sponsored by the government (Medicare and Medicaid) have been subjected to utilization review. This means that the physician must defend the duration of a patient's hospitalization if it exceeds preset criteria. This concept has been extended in the form of Professional Standard Review Organizations (PSRO) under whose direction norms and standards for the care of patients are developed. The purpose of these regulations is ostensibly to improve the quality of patient care, and, in some instances, this will undoubtedly happen. An equally important reason for implementing these regulations, however, is to contain spiraling health care costs. There is no question but that the insertion of this type of review will be extended to all phases of medical practice and will inevitably alter not only the practice of medicine but the traditional patient-physician relationship.

Physicians also will be expected to give account of their continuing competence by mandatory continuing education, patient record audit, recertification by examination, and relicensure. The American Board of Internal Medicine has administered two voluntary recertification examinations to over 5000 physicians. The American Board of Family Practice is also administering a recertification examination to its recent diplomates.

COST-EFFECTIVENESS IN MEDICAL CARE   As society undertakes greater responsibility for health care, and as the cost of medical care continues to skyrocket, it has become necessary to establish stringent priorities in the expenditure of health dollars. Preventive measures often offer the greatest return per dollar; outstanding examples include vaccination, immunization, reduction in accidents and occupational hazards, and improved environmental control. The cost of "newborn screening" for metabolic diseases is being evaluated. For example, the detection of phenylketonuria by screening of large populations can save many thousands of dollars in hospital costs.

As experience is gained, it will become necessary to weigh the justifiability of performing prohibitively costly operations which provide only a limited life expectancy against the pressing need for more primary care centers for the large segments of population who do not have adequate access to medical services. At the level of the individual patient it has become extremely important to minimize costly hospital admissions as far as possible, if total health care is to be provided at a figure which most can afford. This, of course, implies and depends upon a close cooperative effort between patients, their physicians, third-party carriers, and government, and a constant surveillance of those types of procedures which can be conducted safely and effectively on an ambulatory basis. Equally important in reducing total health care expenditures is the need for individual physicians to monitor carefully both the cost and effectiveness of the drugs they prescribe. In the last analysis the public should depend upon the medical profession for leadership and guidance in matters of health services legislation. It is equally important, however, that consideration of these important socioeconomic aspects of the health care delivery system not be permitted to interfere with the primary humane concern of physicians for the welfare of their patients.

CARE OF THE PATIENT

THE ROLE OF THERAPEUTICS   The care of the patient begins with the development of an interpersonal relationship between the patient and the physician. In the absence of a sense of trust and confidence on the part of the patient, the effectiveness of most therapeutic measures is diminished. In many instances, when there is confidence in the physician reassurance is the best treatment and is all that is needed. Likewise, in those cases

which do not lend themselves to easy solutions or for which no effective remedy is available, a feeling on the part of the patient that the physician is doing all that is possible is one of the most important therapeutic measures that the physician can provide.

The discovery of therapeutic agents capable of exerting decisive influence on the course of disease has made it essential that the physician have some understanding not only of the disturbed functions induced by disease, but of the actions of many new drugs, their beneficial effects, and their risks.

Ideally, treatment should strive for the complete restoration of the patient's physical and mental health. When this goal is not attainable, remedies may still be available which will alleviate symptoms and make incurable diseases tolerable to the patient and the family.

IATROGENIC DISORDERS   It is the responsibility of the physician to use the new and powerful therapeutic measures wisely, with due regard for their action, cost, and potential dangers. Every medical procedure, whether diagnostic or therapeutic, has the potentiality of harm, but it would be impossible to afford the patient all the benefits of modern scientific medicine if reasonable steps in diagnosis and therapy were withheld because of possible risks. "Reasonable" implies that the physician has weighed the pros and cons of a procedure and has concluded on rational grounds that it is advisable or essential for the relief of discomfort or the cure or amelioration of disease. When the deleterious effects of the physician's action exceed the advantages that could have been anticipated, one is justified in designating these undesirable effects as iatrogenic. It is necessary only to recall the dangerous or fatal drug reactions that occasionally follow the use of antibiotics given for trivial respiratory infections, the gastric hemorrhage or perforation caused by cortisone administered for mild arthritis, the fatal hepatitis B that may follow needless transfusions of blood or plasma, or the arterial thrombosis or arrhythmia that may complicate coronary angiography.

But the harm that a physician can do to a patient is not limited to the imprudent use of medication. Equally important are ill-considered or unjustified remarks. Since the patient, no matter how apparently placid, approaches the physician with apprehension, anxiety may be enhanced by a too-serious demeanor, a flippant remark, or an unexplained conference concerning the patient's illness. Many persons have developed a cardiac neurosis because the physician expressed a grave prognosis on the basis of a misinterpreted electrocardiogram. Not only the treatment itself but the physician's words and behavior are always capable of causing injury.

The physician must never become so absorbed in the disease as to forget the patient who is its victim. As the science of medicine advances, it is all too easy to become so fascinated by the manifestations of disease that the ailing person's fears and concerns about job and family, the cost of medical care, and the specter of economic insecurity are disregarded. Treatment of a patient consists of more than the dispassionate confrontation of a disease. It embodies also the exercise of warmth, compassion, and understanding. In the now famous words of Peabody,

One of the essential qualities of the clinician is interest in humanity, for the secret of the care of the patient is in caring for the patient.

INFORMED CONSENT   In an era of rapidly advancing technology, patients progressively will require diagnostic and therapeutic procedures that are painful and that pose some risk. These include all surgical procedures, e.g., biopsies of tissues, radiographic maneuvers involving the insertion of catheters, endoscopy, and many others. In most hospitals and clinics, patients undergoing such procedures are required to sign a form consenting to them. More important, however, is the notion that the patient must understand clearly the risk entailed in these procedures; this is the definition of *informed consent.* It is incumbent upon the physician to explain to the patient, in a clearly understandable fashion, the procedures which he or she faces. By doing this conscientiously much of the dread of the unknown that is inherent in hospitalization will be mitigated.

INCURABILITY AND DEATH No problem is more distressing than that presented by the patient with incurable disease, particularly when death is imminent and inevitable. What should the patient and family be told, what measures should be taken to maintain the patient's life, and how is death to be defined?

There is no ironclad rule that the patient must be told "everything," even if he or she is an adult and the head of a family. How much the patient is told will depend upon the patient's own desires and character, the wishes of the family, the state of the patient's affairs, and perhaps religious convictions. First of all the patient must be given an opportunity to speak to the physician and to ask questions. Patients may find it easier to share their feelings about death with their physician who they realize is likely to be more objective and less emotional than their own family members.

One thing is certain: it is not for you to don the black cap and, assuming the judicial function, take hope away from any patient . . . hope that comes to us all.

William Osler

Even when the patient directly inquires, "Doctor, am I dying?" the physician must be circumspect and must attempt to determine whether this is a request for information, a demand for reassurance, or even an expression of hostility. Only further exchanges between the patient and the physician can resolve these questions and guide the physician in what to say and how to say it.

The physician should provide or arrange for emotional, physical, and spiritual support, and must be compassionate, unhurried, and open. Pain should be adequately controlled, human dignity maintained, and isolation from family avoided. The last two, in particular, tend to be overlooked in hospitals, where the intrusion of life-sustaining apparatus can so easily detract from attention to the whole person and instead concentrate on the life-threatening disorder.

The physician must also be prepared to deal with the expiatory attitude of the family when a member becomes gravely or hopelessly ill. The meager resources that may represent the savings of a lifetime may be dissipated in weeks of payment for needlessly expensive rooms, nursing services, and futile therapeutic measures. It is difficult for the physician to oppose these gestures too strenuously, for they serve more to bring consolation to the family than to assuage the distress of the patient, but they need not be encouraged.

Physicians also must be prepared to deal with the feelings of guilt that almost invariably afflict the members of a family when parent or child or spouse has died. They must be assured that everything possible has been done.

Apart from the anguish of facing the terminal phases of disease, to which patient and family react in highly individual ways according to temperament, personal philosophy, and religion, important biologic and medical problems arise as death approaches. At each stage in an illness, the physician must ascertain whether a fatal outcome is inevitable and also whether the surviving patient will suffer a degree of disability that would make life unbearable for the patient and family.

New concepts of death must also be considered. Traditionally, in every society, arrest of heart action has been taken as the only valid medical criterion of death. Lawbooks cite this as the only certain proof that human life has ended. But, as every modern physician knows, the heart may sometimes be restored to action, seemingly miraculously, minutes after it has stopped. On the other hand, other vital organs such as the brain may be destroyed, leaving the individual emotionally and psychologically dead.

When viewed at a cellular level, life is an intricate process of growth and decay in varying proportions at different ages. When decay exceeds growth in organs composed of postmitotic cells such as the musculature and nervous system, where each cell must endure for the lifetime of the individual, death proceeds gradually. This might be termed *cellular death,* and in its most advanced forms organ function may be impaired to a point incompatible with useful life. Of all the organs of humans it is the brain that imparts a meaningful quality to life. Without a functioning cerebrum humans have none of the attributes that distinguish them from other individuals of their own species or from beasts. All awareness of self is permanently effaced; no longer can one think, respond to the physical or social environment, speak, or move. Most thoughtful physicians and many lay people concede that such a state is equivalent to death even though the heart still beats.

Clinical and electrographic criteria are at hand which permit the reliable diagnosis of cerebral death. According to the report of the staff of the Massachusetts General Hospital and the Harvard Committee on Brain Death, one may assume that death has occurred when, as a consequence usually of hypoxia and hypotension, all signs of receptivity and responsivity are in abeyance, including all brainstem and spinal reflexes (pupillary reactions, ocular movement, blinking, swallowing, breathing, tendon and other spinal reflexes), and also, the electroencephalogram is isoelectric. Occasionally, intoxications and metabolic disorders may simulate this state; hence the diagnosis requires expert medical evaluation. Under the aforementioned circumstances, to continue with heroic, highly costly, supportive measures merely for the purpose of preserving cardiac function is in actuality against the best interests of patient, family, and society.

Here, physicians, on contemplating the broad implications of their actions, must either involve themselves in fruitless supportive care or may have to make the difficult decision to abandon their traditional roles of making every effort to preserve life at any cost. If the medical profession, in accord with social sanction, can be brought to redefine life as a state in which cerebral action subserves awareness of environment and the possibility of expressing intellect, emotion, personality, and character, and if it can equate the opposite of this with death, the dilemma can be avoided.

A practice which has been adopted and which has proved most acceptable is as follows:

1 The diagnosis of brain death, based on the above criteria, should be corroborated by another physician, and the clinical examination and EEG should be repeated one or more times over a period of 24 h.
2 The family and nurses should be informed of the irreversibility of brain function but should not be asked or permitted to make the decision whether medical treatment should be discontinued.
3 The physician may withdraw supportive medical measures, assuming that nothing more can be offered and that extraordinary measures to maintain heart function need not be em-

ployed (in agreement with recommendations of Pope Pius XII and others of the clergy).

4 The possibility that such patients may become sources of organs for grafting should not enter into such decisions, although prior to the cessation of heart action the family may be approached by surgeons and asked whether this would be their wish, or the family may suggest that organs be used for this purpose.

It is likely that these criteria will change with the further development of technology to "keep patients alive." In approaching these difficult problems, the physician must combine the art of medicine with its science.

2
PROBLEM-ORIENTED MEDICAL RECORD

STEPHEN E. GOLDFINGER
JAMES J. DINEEN

Whatever can be said, can be said clearly.
Whereof one cannot speak, thereof one ought remain silent.

Ludwig Wittgenstein

Medical records, as kept for years, have often failed the purposes of lucid communication, education, and rapid retrieval of stored information. Poorly supported diagnoses, incomplete progress notes, chaotically entered laboratory results, and inadequately expressed plans of management are embarrassingly common findings in records existing at some of the most sophisticated medical institutions. In response to this the problem-oriented medical record (POMR) has been devised to provide a method whereby the medical record will better reflect the health problems of patients and the professional responses to them on the part of physicians, nurses, and other major participants in care.

Central to its formulation is the view that the patient's record must be designed so that it expresses specifically what physicians deal with most frequently—the *problems* of patients. While the ultimate goal of clinical taxonomy is directed toward identification of etiology, pathology, and pathologic physiology, in view of their importance as guides to therapy, it would be both unrealistic and dangerous to require a specific diagnosis for a severely dyspneic patient in the absence of reasonably convincing information concerning the reason for the dyspnea. Until the cause can be established, all diagnostic modalities and therapeutic interventions are oriented to the real and immediate problem—*dyspnea*. The same is true of a great variety of symptoms, signs, and laboratory findings which are derived in the process of patient care. A high serum calcium reported in a smooth-muscle antibodies (SMA) screening study, a suspicious pigmented skin lesion, or a sudden unexplained deterioration of intellect are examples of worrisome findings that are most appropriately expressed initially as *problems*. In each instance, a more refined diagnosis in the absence of further data can only represent guesswork; hence, it may be wrong. As data pertaining to each problem become available, the problem may then be expressed at a higher level of understanding, i.e., hyperparathyroidism, malignant melanoma, or subdural hematoma. By offering the physician a system of record keeping compatible with the most frequent focus of attention in the practice of medicine—the problem—an opportunity is provided to reduce distortion and error.

The second and more fundamental aspect of problem orientation is the systematized display of patient care embodied in records. This is best described by considering the elements of medical care and their dynamic interrelationship, as proposed by Weed (Fig. 2-1).

THE DATA BASE All clinical care must start with a data base. A careful and complete history and a physical examination are of fundamental value to the physician. The POMR stresses the importance of this traditional approach to data collection. However, there may be instances when full information is unobtainable as, for example, in the case of an unidentified unconscious patient brought into the emergency room. Management of such a case is nevertheless contingent on data, even though incomplete—primarily the initial physical examination, lumbar puncture, and laboratory results. At the other extreme, one might safely argue that no data base can be absolutely complete on any patient, for a lifetime of psychic and biological events can never be fully recalled, much less transcribed. The POMR brings into focus a defined data base, highlights its deficiencies, and serves as the nucleus for its expansion when desirable. Elements of the data base include:

1 Identifying information (i.e., name, age, sex, race, religion, insurance information, etc.)
2 Patient profile (i.e., occupation, education, marital status, children, hobbies, worries, moods, sleep patterns, habits, etc.)
3 Medical history
   a Chief complaints
   b History of present illnesses
   c Past medical history
   d Review of systems
   e Family history
   f Medications

FIGURE 2-1

4 Physical examination

5 Laboratory data and physiologic tests (i.e., complete blood count, electrocardiogram, chest x-ray, creatinine, urinalysis, vital capacity, tonometry, etc.)

It is evident that these components do not constitute anything new to conscientious physicians. In using the POMR, they are asked to *define* the data base and to highlight the abnormalities revealed by it as *problems* with which they must deal. Admittedly, an *ideal* data base has not yet been conceived. Such a construct would depend in part on the population served, the resources at hand, and, most importantly, on the relative cost-benefit of various screening studies in regard to prevention of morbidity. Studies of the value of such tests in these terms may lead to the development of a series of risk-related data bases, each applicable to different groups of individuals. Material obtained for each part of the data base is often organized in the record by standardized formats for display. Although some rather sophisticated examples of such data sheets have been designed, it must be emphasized that the ultimate value of a data base depends on the validity of the information that is entered. An inaccurate history, careless examination of the heart, or a faulty piece of laboratory equipment will yield inaccurate data no matter how clearly the results are recorded. Moreover, it should be recognized that the data base must constantly be supplemented by later entries into the record.

THE PROBLEM LIST From the data at hand, a master problem list is formulated. It should include those features in the patient's psychobiological makeup that require continuing attention by the physician and other members of the health team. Thus, the problem list may contain entries relating to social history (e.g., marital discord), risk factors (e.g., familial polyposis of the colon), symptoms (e.g., hemoptysis), physical findings (e.g., splenomegaly), laboratory tests (e.g., anemia), etc. All problems are expressed at a level of highest understanding. For example, if the cause of gastrointestinal bleeding is known to be a duodenal ulcer, the latter becomes the appropriate entry unless severe bleeding in itself constitutes a major health hazard.

FIGURE 2-2

PROBLEM LIST

No.	Active	Date	Inactive	Date
1	Hypertension	1953		
2	Recurrent bronchitis	1958		
3	Penicillin allergy	1958		
4			S/P pyelonephritis	1960
5	Gallstones	Oct 1978	resolved → Cholecystectomy	Mar 1979
6	Arthralgias	Mar 1979	resolved → #9	June 1979
7	Pleurisy	Mar 1979	resolved → #9	June 1979
8	Proteinuria	Apr 1979	resolved → #9	June 1979
9	SLE	Jun 1979		
10	Unemployment	Nov 1979		

The problem list is a *dynamic* entity which is altered as new information and events dictate. All entries are dated, and a separate column permits the recording of resolved and inactive problems (Fig. 2-2).

When kept in this manner, a problem list featured at the beginning of a patient record provides a succinct summary of all important health matters and, moreover, serves as a table of contents for entries within the record which are properly labeled according to problem (see below). Satisfactory problem listing clearly requires periodic revision of this inventory. Also necessary is a sense of proportion, so that a variety of minor, self-limited problems (e.g., colds, sprains, minor gastrointestinal upsets) are excluded from the master problem list, which might otherwise be unduly cluttered with trivial illnesses. When a number of clearly psychosomatic complaints predominate, they may be grouped together as a single entry, e.g., functional symptoms.

PROBLEM-RELATED PLANS Problems regarded as "active" generally require planning for their proper management. The display of these plans, separately listed for each problem, is of critical importance as a reflection of the physician's response to the problems that have been identified. Plans are recorded under three categories:

1 *Diagnostic (Dx),* i.e., laboratory tests, radiological studies, consultations, continued observation, etc.
2 *Therapeutic (Rx),* i.e., medications, diet, physiotherapy, corrective surgery, etc.
3 *Patient education (Pt ed),* i.e., instruction of the patient in various aspects of self-care, education regarding the goal of therapy, the prognosis that has been given, etc.

It is not necessary that all three sections be completed for each problem, inasmuch as planning may at times be concerned with only one or two of them. For example:

1 Diarrhea
   Dx   Stool for occult blood, culture, ova, and parasites, microscopic fat, and muscle fibers
           Sigmoidoscopy
           Barium enema if persistent
   Rx   Avoid foods that exacerbate
           Propantheline 30 mg tid
   Pt ed Informed that more information is needed to make a diagnosis, will aim for symptomatic therapy for now
2 Pyuria
   Dx   BUN
           Repeat urinalysis
           Urine culture
3 Obesity
   Rx   1500 kcal diet
           Weight Watchers
   Pt ed Dangers of obesity cited. *Goal:* 170 lb

PROGRESS NOTES Progress notes are structured on the basis of those problems which have received attention during the office or hospital visit. (Thus, all problems on the list need not be entered.) In a sense, these notes update the course and management of the problem, following the same general schema already described. They are structured in the following manner:

Problem No.
   Subjective (S)   Interval history
                    Adherence to program

Problem No.
   Objective (O)   Physical findings
                      Reports of laboratory, x-ray, other tests
   Assessment (A)   Appraisal of progress, interpretation of
                      new findings, etc.

   Plan (P)
      Diagnostic
      Therapeutic
      Patient education

Example:

   3   RHD with mitral stenosis
   S   2 flight dyspnea, mild fatigue. No orthopnea, hemop-
       tysis, ankle edema. Child has strep throat.
       Medications: chlorothiazide, 500 mg qd.
   O   BP 120/70. P 78 regular.
       Neck veins normal, lungs clear.
       Grade iii diastolic rumble, wide opening snap. P_2
       slightly ↑.
       ECG: Early pulmonary mitral; otherwise normal.
   A   Stable. Catheterization still not indicated. Risk of
       strep throat present.
   P
       Dx   Cardiac fluoroscopy
       Rx   Continue chlorothiazide and penicillin V, 250
                 mg bid, 2 weeks
       Pt ed   Reinstructed about antibiotic coverage for tooth
                 extractions, scheduled for next month. (Will
                 contact oral surgeon.)

DATA FLOW SHEETS   At times, the course and management
of a particular problem may be succinctly recorded by using
data flow sheets. Many physicians are familiar with this
method of making brief-interval record entries on patients with
diabetic ketoacidosis or acute gastrointestinal hemorrhage. A
number of other conditions—both acute and chronic—lend
themselves to this manner of sequential description. Data flow
sheets for such problems as hypertension, renal failure, and
respiratory insufficiency serve as excellent adjuncts to effective
patient care within the POMR.

CLINICAL JUDGMENT   This intangible element of patient
care is so crucial that it is cited to emphasize that the style of
recording in itself is no guarantee of excellence. The *content* of
the record—the problems selected from the data base, the nature of the plans evolved, the choice of therapeutic programs—reflects the true quality of the care provided. In this
respect, the initials CJ might appropriately be placed alongside
every arrow in Fig. 2-1 to represent the absolute need for clinical judgment to effectively catalyze the process of sound medical care.

**POTENTIAL BENEFITS OF THE PROBLEM-ORIENTED MEDICAL
RECORD   Allied health personnel**   Several aspects of the
POMR facilitate the team approach to patient care. First, the
requirement that all members of the health team systematically display their thoughts and actions improves communications and potentiates supervision. Second, the existence of a
list of the patient's problems that the health team must manage
reduces errors of omission and treatment out of context. Furthermore, the establishment of a plan for each problem leads
to clearer assignment of specific tasks to each of its members.
Most importantly, the dissection of the health care process into
gathering a data base, formulating problems, and designing a
plan for the management of each problem provides a useful
road map for the intelligent expansion of the role of various
allied health personnel. This breakdown helps physicians as

team leaders to rethink their role in the health care process and
concentrate on the more difficult aspects such as identifying
problems from the data base and organizing approaches to
these problems, while assigning more routine tasks to other
members of the team. Practical experiences in clinical settings
as varied as large hospital clinics and rural offices have suggested the value of the POMR in the team approach to patient
care.

Education and audit   In addition to facilitating patient care, a
good medical record should educate its readers and also be
subject to audit in its own right. By clearly outlining the physician's logic, the POMR reveals the process of patient care in a
manner which can be evaluated. This, in itself, is an educational process. It deemphasizes rote memory and substitutes a
record of the logical steps which are being taken to recognize
the patient's problems and the physician's capacity to act as a
guide in attempting to solve them. Such an endeavor, if begun
early, can set the stage for a lifelong educational process of self
and peer evaluation through effective record audit.

Clinical research   Any record system that clarifies the details
of patient-physician interaction can be a powerful tool in clinical research. A clear data base, an organized system for record
entries, and the use of data flow sheets serve to facilitate rapid
extraction and analysis of clinical information. Efforts to com-
puterize the POMR, if successful, will amass a spectrum of
clinical and epidemiologic data that may prove extremely
valuable in our understanding of illness and the process of
health care.

THE ROLE OF THE POMR IN PATIENT CARE   The POMR is a
system of record keeping which greatly facilitates data retrieval and at the same time highlights the decision-making
role of physicians as they respond to the problems of patients.
It should be evident, nevertheless, that it can only serve the
goal of improved health care when it is used with a sound
intellectual appreciation of disease, based on a full understanding of pathophysiology and a scientific approach to therapy.
The tendency for the POMR to compartmentalize problems
must not preclude creative, synthetic thinking. At some institutions an Initial Assessment entry is placed before the Problem
List to provide an opportunity for the physician to express an
overall perspective and to distinguish the major problems from
others which are less important. Finally, as emphasized in the
preceding chapters, compassion is an element of medical care
that can never be adequately displayed by any record system.
A possible danger of the POMR is that the emotional needs of
patients may receive even less attention from a busy physician
who is intent on writing excellent notes. The patient and not
the record must remain the primary focus of physician care.

REFERENCES

BJORN JC, CROSS HD: *Problem Oriented Practice.* Chicago, Modern
   Hospital Press, McGraw-Hill, 1970
FEINSTEIN AR: The problems of the "problem-oriented medical rec-
   ord." Ann Intern Med 78:751, 1973
GOLDFINGER SE: The problem-oriented record: A critique from a be-
   liever. N Engl J Med 288:606, 1973
HURST W, WALKER HK: *The Problem Oriented System.* New York,
   Medcom Press, 1972
WEED LL: *Medical Records, Medical Education and Patient Care.*
   Cleveland, Case University Press, 1969

3
GENERAL CONSIDERATIONS

RAYMOND D. ADAMS

Pain, it has been said, is one of "Nature's earliest signs of morbidity." Few will deny that it stands preeminent among all the sensory experiences by which humans judge the existence of disease within themselves. There are relatively few maladies that do not have their painful phases, and in many of them pain is a characteristic without which diagnosis must always be in doubt. It seems appropriate, therefore, to begin a section on the cardinal manifestations of disease with a discussion of the more general aspects of pain.

The painful experiences of the sick pose manifold problems for practitioners of medicine, and students should know something of these problems in order to prepare themselves for the task ahead. They must be ready to diagnose disease in patients who have felt only the first rumblings of discomfort, before other symptoms and signs of disease have appeared. To cope effectively with problems of this type requires a sound knowledge of the sensory supply of the viscera and a familiarity with the typical symptoms of many diseases. They will be consulted by some patients who seek treatment for pains that appear to have no obvious structural basis, and further inquiry will disclose that worry, fear, and other troubled emotional states may have aggrandized relatively minor aches and pains. To understand problems of this type requires insight into the psychologic factors which influence behavior and a knowledge of psychiatric disease. Next, they must manage the "difficult pain cases," in which no amount of investigation will bring to light either medical disease or psychiatric illness, and it is here that they will sense the need of a sound and assured clinical approach to the pain problem. Finally, they must care for the patients with intractable pain, often from an established and incurable disease, who demand relief either by drug or by the "less moderate means of surgery." Assessing the possibilities of the latter requires a comprehension of the anatomic pathways of pain.

END ORGANS, AFFERENT TRACTS, AND NUCLEI OF TERMINATION OF PAIN PATHWAYS Pain is a sensation which has its own sensory apparatus. The receptors in the skin and deep structures are fine, freely branching nerve endings which form an intricate network throughout the body. A single primary pain neuron with its cell body in the posterior root ganglion subdivides into many small peripheral branches to supply an area of skin of several square millimeters. The cutaneous area of each neuron overlaps with those of other neurons, so that every spot of skin lies within the domain of two to four neurons. These freely branching nerve endings are also found in many of the other specialized sensory receptors in the skin, such as Krause's end bulbs, the ruffinian plumes, and the pacinian corpuscles, which may explain why the extremes of hot, cold, and pressure sensation become painful. Free nerve endings may also serve as receptors for other types of sensa-

tion. They are the only end organ in the cornea, where touch and temperature as well as pain are felt.

The sensory nerve fibers for pain, as they course through somatic and visceral nerves, are mixed with other sensory and motor fibers. All sensory fibers enter the spinal cord through the posterior roots and enter the brainstem through certain of the cranial nerves. The pain fibers are of two sizes, one very small (2 to 4 μm in diameter), called *C fibers* with a slow conducting velocity, the other somewhat larger (6 to 8 μm), called *A-delta fibers,* with more rapid transmission rates. As the posterior root enters the spinal cord, it separates into two divisions, medial and lateral. The medial division, heavily myelinated, synapses either with large secondary sensory neurons in the posterior horn or with anterior horn cells (serving segmental reflexes), or it passes upward in the posterior columns, with some fibers reaching the medulla. The lateral division, of thinly myelinated and nonmyelinated fibers, travels in the tract of Lissauer to reach the substantia gelatinosa, where it synapses with (1) many small neurons whose axons pass into the posterior and anterior horns of the same and adjacent segments of the spinal cord, also effecting reflex connections and (2) large secondary sensory neurons, some of which form the lateral spinothalamic tract and some of which ascend for varying distances near the gray matter as a polysynaptic pathway. The neurons on which the afferent root fibers terminate lie in the first and fifth laminae of the posterior horn, and it is postulated that their reactivity is influenced by large afferent touch fibers or by other inhibitory neurons within the spinal gray matter. Through a mechanism still rather obscure two secondary ascending pathways for pain are activated. One is the lateral spinothalamic tract, the cell bodies of which lie in the posterior horns, with axons crossing through the anterior commissure of the spinal cord within one to two segments of the level of entry. The other is a less well-defined, multineuronal chain which extends upward along the reticular part of the gray matter. The lateral spinothalamic tract, joined in the brainstem by the trigeminothalamic tract, courses through the lateral part of the medulla, pons, and midbrain, giving off many collaterals before terminating in the nucleus ventralis posterolateralis, the posterior nuclear group, and intralaminar thalamic nuclei (Fig. 3-1). The reticular chain of neurons extends cephalad and finally makes connections through the interlaminar nuclei of the thalamus and with the limbic portions of the cerebrum (Bonica).

The secondary spinothalamic and trigeminothalamic tracts synapse with the tertiary sensory neurons of the thalamus whose axons extend to the cortex of the parietal lobe. Physiologists are not agreed as to the cortical terminus for the pain fibers, for electrical stimulation of the cortex in the conscious human being seldom produces a painful sensation, and parietal lobe lesions seldom cause central pain. Presumably their cortical termination is rather diffuse and bilateral in both parietal and frontal regions. Only a few end in the primary somatosensory cortex. The secondary somatosensory cortex receives more fibers than the primary. Most of the pain fibers from the periphery cross to the opposite side of the brain; only a small contingent remains ipsilateral. (See Adams and Victor for more detailed descriptions of pain neurons and tracts.)

Segmental innervation As a means of quick orientation to the anatomy of the peripheral pain pathways it should be remembered that the facial structures and anterior cranium lie in the field of the trigeminal nerves; the back of the head, second cervical; the neck, third cervical; epaulet area, fourth cervical; deltoid area, fifth cervical, radial forearm and thumb, sixth cervical; index finger, seventh cervical; middle finger, eighth cervical; little finger and inner forearm, first thoracic; nipple segment, fifth thoracic; umbilical, tenth thoracic; groin, first lumbar; medial side of knee, third lumbar; great toe, fifth lumbar; little toe, first sacral; back of thigh, second sacral; genitosacral areas, third, fourth, and fifth sacral. The first to fourth thoracic nerve roots are the important sensory pathways for the intrathoracic viscera; the sixth to eighth thoracic, for the upper abdominal organs (Fig. 19-1).

PHYSIOLOGY AND PSYCHOLOGY OF PAIN The stimuli that arouse pain vary for each tissue. Generally the adequate stimuli for skin are those which injure tissue, i.e., pricking, cutting, crushing, burning, and freezing. Interestingly, these same forms of stimulation have little effect when applied to the stomach and intestine. Pain in the gastrointestinal tract is produced instead by local trauma of an engorged or inflamed mucosa, distention or spasm of smooth muscle, and traction on the mesenteric attachment. Pain is induced in skeletal muscles by ischemia (the basis for the condition known as intermittent claudication), as well as by tears of connective tissue sheaths, necrosis, hemorrhage, or the injection of irritating solutions. Prolonged contraction of muscles evokes an aching type of pain. Ischemia, the only proved source of pain in the heart muscle, is responsible for angina pectoris and for the pain of myocardial infarction. Joints are insensitive to pricking, cutting, and cautery, but pain is induced in the synovial membrane by hypertonic saline solution and inflammation. Arteries give rise to pain when pierced with a needle, when induced to pulsate excessively (as in migraine), and in certain diseases of their walls such as exemplified by atherosclerotic thrombosis and arteritis of cranial arteries. Traction and displacement of intracranial vessels and the meningeal structures by which they are supported may cause headache.

In these painful lesions which damage tissues, proteolytic enzymes are released which act on gamma globulins to liberate irritating substances that stimulate nerve endings. Bradykinins, serotonin, acetylcholine, 5-hydroxytryptamine, histamine, prostaglandins, and other similar polypeptides or acid metabolites released by tissue injury have been found to elicit pain when injected intraarterially or applied to the base of a blister. Such substances are viewed as the "mediators" for pain. Strong pressure may also mechanically stimulate free nerve endings.

The sensory experiences resulting from these several modes of stimulation in the skin and in deep skeletomuscular and visceral structures differ in quality. Integumentary stimuli, at the lowest levels of intensity, evoke sensations of touch, pressure, warmth, cold, or tickle. When increased to the point approaching tissue destruction, pain is added, and the resulting experience is thereafter a mixed one. The painful experience itself is one of pricking or burning. The threshold for burning pain from a thermal stimulus is approximately 2000 times the threshold for warmth. This relationship of pain to tissue destruction is the basis of a biologic principle—that pain has a protective, or self-preserving, value to the organism.

A new chapter is being written on the pharmacology of nociception. Salicylates, which are peripherally acting analgesics, exert an inhibitory effect on the synthesis of prostaglandins (potent stimulators of nociceptive endings). Salicylates fail to antagonize other of the putative neurohumors such as bradykinin and histamine. Opiates have a major central analgesic effect. High densities of specific opiate receptors (presumably on the presynaptic terminals of the C and other pain fibers) have been demonstrated in the posterior horns of spinal cord and trigeminal nuclei; others have been demonstrated in the peri-aqueductal gray matter, medial thalamus, infundibulum, amygdaloid nuclei, caudate nuclei, and frontotemporal cortex. Their distribution would appear to account for both the sensory and affective aspects of pain experience. At these receptor sites one expects to find inhibitory and excitatory transmitters. These synaptosomal receptors are blocked by opiates and their antagonists. The identification of these neurotransmitters is incomplete. One type, called the beta endorphin polypeptides, has been isolated from brain tissue; these appear to be the natural CNS transmitters or modulators of opiate action. γ-Aminobutyric acid (GABA) and glycine are potent inhibitory substances. At the cellular level opiates have been shown to inhibit function by causing a decrement in cyclic AMP.

One must ask why the brain contains alkaloid receptors which when blockaded impair the neurologic experience of pain. Guillemin suggests that these receptors were not put there to receive "the poppy" but to recognize and accept some endogenous substance serving the physiology of pain experience, and that because of the configuration of the receptor

FIGURE 3-1

Radiation and sites of reference of cardiac pain (upper) *and gallbladder pain* (lower).

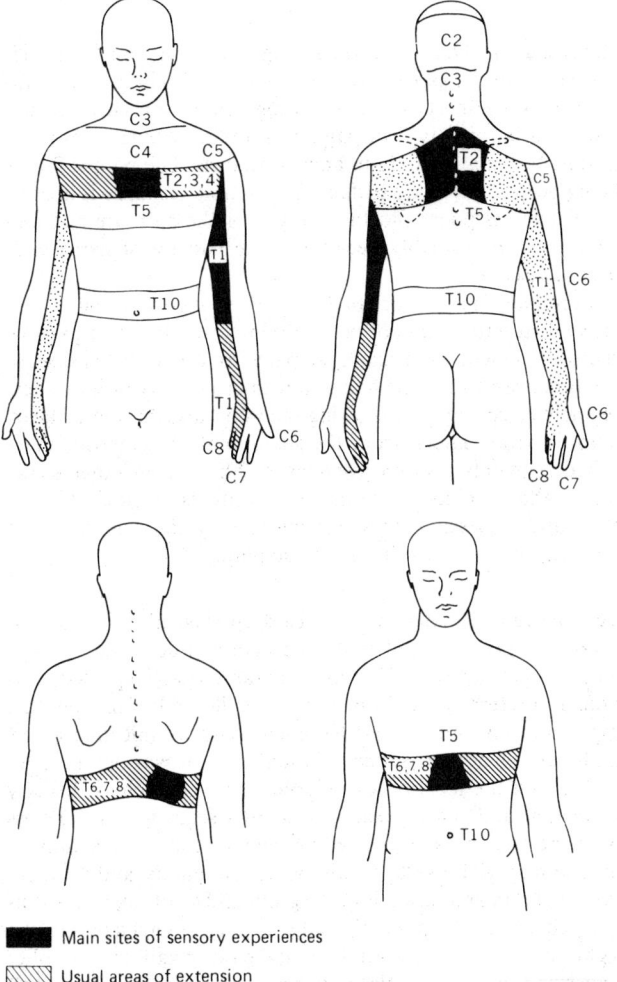

■ Main sites of sensory experiences

▨ Usual areas of extension

▒ Less common areas of extension

binding site both the endogenous substance and opiates are equally effective. Indeed, it has recently been shown that beta endorphins relieve pain and counteract withdrawal symptoms.

The threshold for the perception of pain, i.e., the lowest intensity of stimulus recognized as pain, is approximately the same in all persons. It is lowered by inflammation and raised by local anesthetics (e.g., procaine), lesions of the nervous system, and certain centrally acting analgesic drugs. Distraction and suggestion by turning attention away from the painful part reduce the awareness of and the response to pain. Strong emotion (fear or rage) suppresses pain. Neurotic patients in general have the same pain threshold as normal subjects, but their reaction may be excessive or abnormal. The pain thresholds of frontal lobotomized subjects are also unchanged, but they react briefly if at all to pain. The degree of emotional reaction and the verbalization (complaint) also vary with the personality and character of the patient.

Superficial pain Sensory impulses subserving pricking pain, being transmitted by larger pain fibers, have a more rapid rate of conductivity to the nervous system than burning pain. A hot needle applied to the toe, for example, produces a quick, pricking pain and, only 1 to 2 s later, a burning pain. Together they constitute the "double response" of Lewis. Ischemia of nerve by the application of a tourniquet to a limb abolishes pricking pain before burning pain. Both types of dermal pain are localized with precision (local sign), made possible by the overlap of sensory neurons. Analgesia means the interruption of all pain neurons to an area, and hypalgesia, the interruption of only part of them.

Visceral pain Deep pain (including that of visceral and skeletal structures) has basically the quality of aching, but if intense may be sharp and penetrating (knifelike). Occasionally there is a burning type of pain, as in the heartburn of esophageal irritation and rarely in angina pectoris. The pain is felt as being deep to the body surface. The double response is absent, localization is poor, and the margins of the pain are not well delineated, presumably because of the paucity of nerve endings in viscera.

Actually, the pain originating in deep skeletomuscular and visceral structures cannot be localized closer than two to three sensory segments. For example, pain from myocardial disease is felt to arise within the first to fourth or possibly fifth thoracic segments (see Fig. 3-1, showing theoretic distribution of heart pain). Unfortunately, from the standpoint of diagnosis, these spinal segments also receive sensory fibers from other structures—the esophagus, mediastinal contents, bones, muscles, etc.—and diseases of these structures may cause pain that is difficult to distinguish from cardiac pain.

Deep musculoskeletal pain Since deep skeletal pain and visceral pain are mediated through a common deep sensory system, it is not surprising that their characteristics (type, localization, and referral) should be similar. Kellgren has mapped the topography of muscle and tendinous pain by injecting a few milliliters of normal saline solution into the various muscles and noting the location of induced pain. The ache is usually segmental and may spread one to two segments above (less often below) the site injected. A tear or injury in a lumbar muscle may give rise to a pain which, in quality and localization, including radiation into the groin and scrotum, is indistinguishable from the pain of renal colic. A hemorrhage into the right upper rectus muscle mimics the pain of gallbladder colic; and a lesion in a muscle or ligament deep in the chest wall causes pain referred to the left arm, like that of angina. The

differentiation of these pains must be made on grounds other than location and reference.

Referred pain Deep visceral and somatic pains tend always to be referred superficially to those structures within a given spinal segment that have the most extensive nerve ramifications and therefore the widest cerebral representation (e.g., there are more sensory nerves in the integument than in the viscera, hence the pain in the latter is projected to the body surface). In the case of myocardial pain, sensory impulses entering the first to fourth thoracic nerves activate a pool of sensory neurons, the largest number of which also receive afferents from the skin of the inner side of the arm (T_1 and T_2) and the anterior precordium (T_3 and T_4). More of the sensory neurons from the heart enter the left side of the spinal cord than the right. These anatomic and physiologic data explain why cardiac pain is referred predominantly to the substernal, left precordial, and inner brachial zones.

Aberrant reference of pain occurs not infrequently and is explained in terms of the physiologic status of the spinal pool of sensory neurons. As was stated, a single sensory neuron entering one spinal root presynaptically depolarizes to a varying degree a pool of spinal neurons over four or five spinal segments. Pain then should spread to segments adjacent to the painful lesion, where it also causes cutaneous hyperesthesia and, by activating motor neurons, involuntary muscle contraction. If some preexistent disease in *adjacent* somatic segments has already partially depolarized the spinal pool of sensory neurons, a new painful disease which will further depolarize them causes the pain to spread to them. For example, if gallbladder disease which activated sensory fibers entering at the sixth to eighth thoracic nerve root, or cervical arthritis (at the second to eighth cervical nerve root) were present before a myocardial infarct, the cardiac pain might then be referred to the upper part of the abdomen or neck, respectively. Generally these aberrant referrals occur in segments that are cephalad to the normal segmental distribution of pain because their inhibitory connections are more abundant than those of caudal ones.

Hyperesthesia, hyperalgesia, hyperpathia, involuntary spasms, and other responses It has been customary to use the first two of these terms to designate a lowering of the threshold to touch and pain stimuli and the third for a state of pain with a normal or raised threshold but overreaction. Hyperpathia may even occur with anesthesia, as in *anesthesia dolorosa*. Any real distinction between these states is ephemeral. Probably only with inflammation of the skin is the pain threshold consistently lowered. What is most characteristic of all chronically painful states, and these frequently implicate nerves or central nervous structures, is that the part is unusually sensitive to all stimuli, even those which normally do not evoke pain; and the elicited pain is unnatural, radiant, outlasts the initiating stimulus, and is unusually modifiable by fatigue, emotion, etc. One sees listed here many of the characteristics of causalgia, spinal cord pain, phantom pain, zoster neuralgia, thalamic pain, etc. The explanation currently offered for these states is that at the peripheral as well as the central level the system of pain fibers is no longer in equilibrium with other sensory fibers. A kind of inhibition is exerted on the pain system at all times by the small neurons in the substantia gelatinosa, under the control of other afferent as well as descending pathways. Since the largest afferent peripheral nerve fibers suppress the secondary spinal neurons receiving pain impulses, nerve injury, which tends often to destroy some of the larger fibers, then permits their overresponse. According to Melzack and Wall, the small neurons of the substantia gelatinosa constitute a kind of "gate control system" which modulates input. The activation of large afferent fibers in a peripheral nerve is said to inhibit the gateway cells. While much of the recent physiological evidence has failed to confirm this gateway hypothesis, it has called attention to some type of mechanism that controls the pain threshold and painful states. Some such segmental mechanism must also be under the influence of descending pathways from the cerebrum and from other spinal segments. One might suppose that the activation of some of the sensory fibers controlling "gateway neurons" could be the basis of the effectiveness of *acupuncture;* the psychological mechanism of suggestion may also play a role in acupuncture therapy. There is a wide range of responses to pain to which attention is drawn. Strong, acute pain causes a startle reaction. Intense, persistent pain is usually accompanied by segmental flexion reflexes (e.g., spasm of a segment of the abdominal wall with visceral disease, flexion of knees and hips with peritoneal irritation, extension of neck with meningitis), autonomic responses, postural adjustments, avoidance movements, and vocalization. The obvious biologic function of segmental spasms is to splint the diseased part and to facilitate healing. The altered state of receptivity of the spinal gray matter accounts for stimuli of nonreceptive-type evoking pain, e.g., for subcutaneous pressure being painful.

As pain sensation may be induced by stimulation of the receptors or by irritation of peripheral nerves or roots, it may be abolished by diseases which affect the peripheral or central nervous system, or by a surgical procedure which accomplishes the same result. Pain in a circumscribed region may be terminated by section of the nerve which supplies that region (neurotomy) or by section of the spinal roots (posterior rhizotomy); pain in a limb or one side of the trunk may be abolished by section of the anterolateral spinothalamic tracts (lateral spinal tractotomy in the spinal cord or tractotomy in the lateral medulla or mesencephalon).

Perception of pain Only upon the arrival of pain impulses at the thalamocortical level of the nervous system is there conscious awareness of the pain stimulus. Clinical study has not informed us of the exact localization of the nervous apparatus for this mental process. It is not entirely abolished by a total hemispherectomy, including the thalamus on one side. It is often said that impulses reaching the thalamus create awareness of the attributes of sensation and that the parietal cortex is necessary for the appreciation of the intensity and localization of the sensation. This seems to be an oversimplification. Probably a close and harmonious relationship between thalamus and cortex must exist in order for a sensory experience to be complete. The traditional separation of sensation (in this instance awareness of pain) and perception (awareness of the nature of the painful stimulus) has been abandoned in favor of the view that sensation, perception, and the various conscious and unconscious responses to a pain stimulus comprise an indivisible process.

Although similar to other sensory or perceptive phenomena in certain respects, such as predictable response to given intensity of stimulus, pain differs in other ways. One of its most remarkable characteristics is the strong feeling tone, or affect, with which it is endowed, nearly always one of unpleasantness. Furthermore, pain does not appear to be subject to negative adaptation. Most stimuli, if applied continuously, soon cease to be effective, whereas pain may persist as long as the stimulus is operative; and, by establishing a central excitatory state, may even outlast the stimulus.

Stereotaxic surgery on the thalamus in cases of intractable pain permits dissection of the anatomy of the pain experience. Lesions in the terminus of the lateral spinothalamic tract in the posterolateral nucleus are said to abolish pain and temperature sensation in the contralateral side of the body while leaving the patient with all the misery or affect of pain. Lesions in the centrum medianum relieve the painful state without altering pain and temperature sensation. Thus, at this level there must also be a balance of inhibitory and facilitatory sensory systems, for one cannot explain intractable pain simply in terms of continuous stimulation of chains of pain neurons.

Psychologic aspects of pain A discussion of this problem could hardly be complete without some reference to the influence of emotional states or to the importance of racial, cultural, and religious factors on the pain response, especially its overt expressions. It is common knowledge that some individuals, by virtue of training, habit, or phlegmatic character, are relatively stoical, and that others are excessively responsive to pain. And there are rare individuals who are totally incapable of experiencing pain throughout their lifetime, either from a lack of sensory endings or peripheral sensory apparatus, or from some peculiarity of central reception.

Lastly, it is important to keep in mind the devastating effects of chronic pain. As Ambroise Paré remarked, "There is nothing that abateth so much the strength as paine." Continuous pain can be observed to have an adverse effect on the entire nervous system. There are increased irritability, fatigue, troubled sleep, poor appetite, and loss of emotional stability. Courageous individuals are reduced to a whimpering, pitiable state that may arouse only the scorn of a healthy person. They are irrational about illness and may make unreasonable demands on family and physician. The degree of disability exceeds the physical findings. This condition, termed *pain shock*, once established, requires delicate but firm management. Depression (reactive?) is common. Of course, demand for and dependency on narcotic drugs often complicate the picture.

CLINICAL APPROACH TO THE PATIENT WITH PAIN AS THE PREDOMINANT SYMPTOM One of the first points to keep in mind is that not all pain is the consequence of serious disease. Otherwise healthy individuals have thousands of pains which are part of their daily sensory experience. To mention but a few, there is the momentary, hard pain over an eye, in the temporal region, or in the ear or jaw, which strikes with alarming suddenness; the more persistent ache which arises in some fleshy part, such as the shoulder, neck, thigh, or calf, the darting pain in an arm or leg, the fleeting precordial discomfort that arouses momentarily the thought of heart disease, the breathtaking catch in the side from diaphragmatic cramp, the cluster of abdominal pains with their associated intestinal rumblings, and the brief discomfort upon movement of a joint. These *normal pains,* as they should be called, occur at all ages, tend to be brief, and depart as obscurely as they come. They acquire medical significance only when elicited by an inquiring physician, or when presented as a complaint by a worried patient; and, of course, they must always be distinguished from the *abnormal pains* of disease.

When pain, by its intensity, duration, and the circumstance of its occurrence, appears to be abnormal or constitutes one of the principal symptoms of disease, an attempt should be made to reach a tentative decision as to its cause and the mechanism of its production. This can usually be accomplished by thoroughly questioning and encouraging the patient to relate as accurately as possible the main characteristics of the pain and the circumstances under which it occurs. The physical examination is directed toward a search for evidences of suspected disease and the reproduction of the pain.

Location of pain When the pain is caused by a superficial lesion, the cause and effect are usually so obvious that no problem is posed. It is the deep lesion, whether involving somatic or visceral structures, that causes trouble, and here exact localization becomes especially important. We have already seen that the pain originating from such tissues is no longer sensed as coming from them, but is instead only roughly segmental, i.e., within the territory of the cord segments innervating the structure. The identification of the segments involved is of value, for it sets the limit on the diagnostic possibilities that must be considered, i.e., they are limited to those structures having a corresponding innervation. Thus an epigastric or subxiphoid pain, or one in the opposite region in the back, obliges one to search for its cause in all those structures innervated by the sixth through eighth thoracic cord segments, i.e., the esophagus, stomach, duodenum, pancreas, biliary tract, the upper retroperitoneal structures, as well as the deep somatic tissues in this region. Also, one must consider the possibility that a lesion in a viscus innervated by spinal segments above or below the sixth through eighth thoracic cord segments may at times be the source of pain that has spread outside its normal boundaries and involved the epigastrium (Fig. 3-1).

Provoking and relieving factors These factors are of greater value than quality of pain in providing important data concerning its mechanism. Pain related to breathing, swallowing, and defecation focuses attention on the respiratory apparatus, the esophagus, and the lower part of the intestinal tract, respectively. A pain coming on a few minutes after the beginning of general bodily movement and relieved almost at once by rest indicates ischemia or a neural mechanism as the probable cause (see Chaps. 9 and 10). Pain occurring several hours after meals and relieved by food or alkali suggests the irritative effect of acid on the raw lining of the stomach or duodenum. Pain that is brought on or relieved by certain movements or postures of parts of the body is usually due to diseased skeletal structures (bones, muscles, ligaments). Pain that is enhanced by cough, sneeze, and strain is usually radicular in origin or arises in ligamentous structures. Pain that is increased or altered by cutaneous stimuli is due to disease in sensory tracts in the peripheral or central nervous system.

Quality and time-intensity characteristics of pain Much reliance is put on the patient's choice of words and account of the intensity of pain. Unfortunately this will depend, in part at least, on the patient's intelligence, vocabulary, and concept of what is taking place. "Crushing" and "squeezing" are commonly employed to describe an anginal pain, and this implication of pressure has some significance since the pain may depend on an associated involuntary contraction of the pectoral muscles. Another patient with the same disease, however, may describe the pain as "exploding" or "burning." Far more important than the adjective used for pain is the information that it is steady and does not fluctuate. Similarly, the pain of peptic ulcer is frequently designated as "gnawing," but again, the deep, steady quality is more important than the word used to denote it. Gallbladder colic and renal colic are misnomers, if by colic is meant a "paroxysmal abdominal pain due to spasm, obstruction, or distention of any of the hollow viscera." *In both these disorders, the pain tends to be steady.* The aching quality of all deep pains is usually characteristic, but there are also several other informative attributes. A true colicky pain, one that is rhythmic and cramping, suggests an obstructive lesion in a hollow viscus. If the patient is a woman who has had children, it is a good idea to ask whether her "cramp" resembles the pains she had during childbirth. A pain that is steady and varies little or not at all from moment to moment means that the stimulus to pain is steady and unwavering, as in angina pectoris and peptic ulcer. Thus, a pain in the anterior midsternal region whose intensity fluctuates appreciably within the space of a minute or two is not due to angina, even

though the history may appear to suggest a relation to exertion. Similarly, a high epigastric pain appearing several hours after a meal and even apparently relieved by food is not caused by an ulcer if the pain fluctuates perceptibly within seconds or a few minutes. The stimulus to ulcer pain does not quickly vary in intensity. A throbbing pain indicates that an arterial pulsation is giving rise to painful stimuli. Sharp, recurrent stabs of pain are caused by disease of nerve roots or sensory ganglions, as exemplified by tic douloureux or tabes, or a single episode may be due to a tear of a muscle or ligament. Once started, in each instance there may be a background of dull, aching pain. Particularly noteworthy here is the abrupt intensification of the dull ache of root pain by cough, sneeze, or strain which momentarily stretches or alters the position of the root.

Mode of onset of pain This factor is also important. A pain reaching its full intensity almost immediately after its appearance suggests a rupture of tissue. The pain of a dissecting aortic aneurysm often develops in this manner. In fact, the suddenness and the severity of the pain, reaching a peak of intensity within seconds or minutes, sometimes provides the first clue in differentiating this type of chest pain from that caused by myocardial infarction. A similarly rapid accession of pain may occur with the rupture of a peptic ulcer.

Duration of pain This is another useful diagnostic attribute. Anginal pain, for example, rarely lasts less than 2 or 3 min or more than 10 to 15 min. Ulcer pain may continue for an hour or more, unless terminated by the ingestion of food or alkali or a tumbler of water.

Severity of pain In any given disease, the severity of pain is subject to wide variation, and patients differ in their tolerance to it. Therefore, one cannot judge the gravity of an illness solely by the patient's report of the intensity of pain. As a rule, pains that completely interrupt work or pleasurable activity, require opiates for relief, enforce bed rest, or awaken the patient from sound sleep are to be taken more seriously than those which have the opposite characteristics.

Time of occurrence An accurate determination must be made of the temporal aspects of the pain. The relationship of ulcer pain to the preceding meal has already been mentioned. Postural aches come after prolonged activity and disappear with rest; arthritic pains are usually most severe during the first movements after prolonged inactivity. The mechanisms for this latter phenomenon are not known, nor do we understand why painful lesions of the bone, such as those caused by metastatic cancer, are likely to be most disturbing during the night. It is possible that the occurrence or aggravation of the latter types of pain is due to enhanced awareness of painful stimuli at a time when the mind is not distracted by other stimuli, or it may be that the pains are now more easily evoked by unconscious movements made during sleep when protective reflexes are in abeyance.

It should be obvious from these remarks that the full significance of a pain is usually not revealed by any one single characteristic. It is only by combining all these data that one can determine its anatomic site and its mechanism. In general, *the most important and revealing clues are obtained from the answers to the questions: What brings on the pain? What relieves it?* Pain is a subjective manifestation, not a state to be observed or measured. The accuracy of our data depends on the skill with which we frame our questions and on the powers of observation and memory of the person answering them.

Finally, the diagnostic value of measures which *reproduce* and *relieve the pain* should be stressed. Not only are they important for diagnosis, but they convince the patient that the physician understands and can control pain and the illness behind it. Climbing several flights of stairs under the physician's supervision may settle the question of the presence or absence of angina pectoris. An injection of procaine into the tender area in the chest wall or some other skeletal structure, with complete disappearance of the pain, may establish its skeletal origin and exclude the possibility of visceral disease. Reproducing the distress sometimes caused by aerophagia merely by distending the esophagus or stomach with air, or reproducing the vague but sometimes alarming sensation of pressure in the chest caused by unconscious hyperventilation by having the patient deliberately hyperventilate are other examples of how the principle of the reproduction of pain may be usefully employed.

A systematic interrogation of the patient will not lead to accurate diagnosis in every instance, but the habit of searching for the identifying characteristics of pain will enable physicians to increase their skill in this difficult field. Furthermore, after becoming familiar with the customary responses to these questions, one becomes more alert to the anxious, the hysterical, or the depressed patient who while complaining of pain seems incapable of describing any of its details, or is unwilling to do so. Instead, there is preoccupation with theories of what is wrong or with the treatments or mistreatments already given.

Obscure and intractable pains Finally, there will always be cases that defy solution, and the physician must develop a systematic clinical approach to them. There are four discernible groups of such pains: (1) the pain of medical and surgical diseases yet undiagnosable; (2) "psychiatric" pains; (3) "neurologic" pains; (4) pains of indeterminate types.

With respect to group 1, neoplasms in retropharyngeal, posterior mediastinal, and retroperitoneal regions and the spine are among the more frequent causes of pain, lasting months before being revealed by the usual methods of diagnosis. In group 2, four psychiatric conditions are associated with pain which may dominate the clinical picture: psychotic depression, hysteria, compensation "neurosis," and constitutional psychopathy; any one of them may be complicated by drug addiction. Since psychiatric illnesses do not preclude another painful disease, the clinical analysis must of necessity rule out the latter while establishing on the basis of history and physical findings the existence and nature of the former. In group 3, neurologic diseases of painful type (causalgia, spinal cord injury, discogenic root disease, and thalamic pain syndrome) are usually diagnosable on the basis of the clinical findings (see Chaps. 19 and 365), but the difficult problems are those in which the neurologic disease is accompanied by depression, malingering, compensation "neurosis," or opiate or other drug addiction. The fourth group includes the cases that are left when the first three are excluded. They defy solution. The physician can proceed only by repeatedly reexamining the patient, explaining the need for continued observation, and enlisting the patient's aid and forbearance during this trying period. Asking the patient to tolerate a certain amount of pain without the use of powerful analgesics is usually effective, particularly when the possibility of drug addiction is explained.

In the relatively rare circumstances when all manner of investigation has failed to throw light on the cause and mechanism of the pain, demands for pain-relieving surgery may become increasingly insistent. The physician may in desperation turn to measures which are more dangerous than the disease. Here the commonest source of error is to operate unnecessarily on the hysterical patient (see Chap. 11), only to discover too late that each operative procedure is followed by a new pain, often at a higher level than the first. Or depressive psychosis may have masqueraded as a painful state and is operated upon

when antidepressant medication, electric shock therapy, or other therapy would have dramatically terminated the illness. Sometimes a half dozen or more operations are unsuccessfully performed on a single patient. The safest rule to follow in these cases is not to use opiates continuously or to recommend operation for the relief of pain unless a reasonable diagnosis has been made. For the pains of metastatic cancer, the thalamic pain of vascular disease of the brain, and other incurable diseases, the relative advantages of the controlled use of opiates versus lateral spinothalamic tractotomy or frontal lobotomy must be carefully weighed in each patient. The age of the patient, other diseases, life expectancy, and mental state are all of importance in selecting the treatment procedure. Too often an operation on the spinal cord or brain is chosen in preference to narcotics and the controlled use of drugs. Forgotten is the fact that many patients with cancer were formerly kept relatively comfortable and active by the judicious use of morphine and its analogues and were never subjected to costly operations or deprived of any of those qualities of mind and character which are so treasured by their families.

TREATMENT Superficial pain arising in integumentary structures rarely presents a problem in therapy. Acetylsalicylic acid, 0.30 to 0.60 g, or acetaminophen (Tylenol), 0.30 to 0.60 g, orally every 4 h usually suffices. Acetophenetidin may be added. These two drugs are particularly effective when one element of pain is integumentary. Commercial proprietary preparations of these drugs containing caffeine (e.g., ASA compound, Empirin compound, and aspirin) or amphetamine (e.g., Edrisal) are available in most pharmacies. The caffeine or amphetamine is particularly useful if there is central nervous system depression, and often there is advantage to adding a sedative drug. When this type of pain is not effectively controlled by nonnarcotic analgesics, codeine should be given. Usually the addition of small amounts (8 to 30 mg) of codeine phosphate to the standard dose of acetylsalicylic acid and acetophenetidin is effective. A preparation containing codeine phosphate 8 to 30 mg, acetylsalicylic acid 0.23 g, acetophenetidin 0.16 g, and caffeine 0.032 g is commercially available (Empirin compound with codeine phosphate). Codeine, 20 to 45 mg every 3 h, gives fairly effective analgesia with minimal side effects. Adequate rest and relief of muscle tensions should also be encouraged. The application of moist heat is usually beneficial. Occasionally cold applications are preferred, but with the exception of cooling packs applied to an inflamed, burning skin or to a causalgia, cold is more likely to aggravate than to soothe the painful condition.

Occasionally integumental and deep pains of skeletal structures are of such severity as to require more powerful narcotic analgesics, such as meperidine hydrochloride (Demerol) in doses of 50 to 100 mg orally or intramuscularly, methadone hydrochloride, 5 to 10 mg orally or subcutaneously, or dihydromorphine hydrochloride (Dilaudid), 1 to 2 mg orally and subcutaneously. These drugs are most useful when sedation is not required. When pain is unusually severe and some degree of euphoria is desired, one of the new drugs such as pentazocine hydrochloride (Talwin) should be given in doses of 50 mg orally or subcutaneously every 3 to 4 h. Morphine, although still a valuable drug in doses of 8 to 15 mg, is not used much because of its habit-forming tendency and the frequently associated nausea and vomiting. Since all these narcotic analgesics are, for the most part, detoxified by the liver, they either should not be used or should be given in only half the usual dosage in cases of liver disease, myxedema, adrenal insufficiency, and other states in which the metabolic rate is reduced. Morphine and related narcotic analgesics tend to cause pruritus and should therefore be used with care in patients with skin irritability. The possibility of initiating addiction in susceptible persons must be carefully evaluated in every instance (cf. Chap. 227).

If the patient exhibits mental tension, insomnia, and restlessness, a sedative drug such as phenobarbital or Amytal Sodium may be given with the analgesic agents. Sedative medications, especially the quick-acting barbiturates, should not be used alone for the control of pain, because they sometimes cause excitement and confusion under these circumstances. If endogenous depression is the underlying illness, it should be managed as outlined in Chap. 25.

Visceral pain originating in the stomach, gallbladder, intestines, or heart is usually very poorly controlled by the nonnarcotic analgesics. The narcotic analgesics are the agents of choice, but of course, they should never be given until the physician is certain that the relief of the pain will not mask the state of the patient. If sedation is not desirable and if constipation is a troublesome problem, the newer synthetic analgesics, such as meperidine in doses of 50 to 100 mg orally or intramuscularly or methadone 5 to 10 mg by mouth or subcutaneously every 4 to 6 h, are recommended. Like morphine, these drugs are habit-forming but less so because they induce milder analgesia, sedation, and euphoria. Patients with severe visceral pain who are also anxious or fearful and unable to relax or sleep should be given morphine sulfate in doses of 8 to 15 mg subcutaneously. The well-known spasmogenic effects of morphine are partially counteracted by atropine sulfate, 0.3 to 0.4 mg. Aminophylline, 0.5 g intravenously, also overcomes much of this undesirable spastic action; a rectal suppository of 0.5 g, although less effective, may be substituted. When pain is due to benign, chronic diseases, every effort should be made to avoid opiate addiction. Here the judicious use of propoxyphene (Darvon), 65 mg every 4 to 6 h; oxycodone hydrochloride (Percodan), 4.5 mg every 6 h, or pentazocine hydrochloride (Talwin), 50 mg every 3 to 4 h, may prove adequate.

Intractable pain due to incurable diseases, such as metastatic carcinoma, is one of the most difficult therapeutic problems. As a rule, one resorts to narcotic drugs because of their strong analgesic action, and habituation is accepted as the lesser of two evils. An alternative is pain-relieving surgery. Section of peripheral nerves, the lateral spinothalamic tracts in the spinal cord (cordotomy) or the lateral part of the medulla, stereotaxic thalamotomy, and lobotomy are relatively safe procedures which have advantages over the continuous use of opiates in selected cases.

REFERENCES

ADAMS RD, VICTOR M: *Principles of Neurology.* New York, McGraw-Hill, 1977, chap 6
BONICA JJ (ed): *Advances in Neurology.* New York, Raven Press, 1974, vol 4
DYKES RW: Nociception. Brain Res 99:229, 1975
GUILLEMIN R: Endorphins, brain peptides that act like opiates. N Engl J Med 296:226, 1977
HARDY JD et al: *Pain Sensations and Reactions.* Baltimore, Williams & Wilkins, 1952
LEWIS T: *Pain.* New York, Macmillan, 1942
MELZACK R, WALL PD: Interaction of fast and slow conducting fiber systems involved in pain and analgesia, in *Pharmacology of Pain,* RKS Lim et al (eds). London, Pergamon, 1968
SNYDER SH, SIMANTOV R: The opiate receptor and opioid peptides. J Neurochem 28:13, 1977
WHITE JC, SWEET WH: *Pain and the Neurosurgeon—A Forty Years Experience.* Springfield, Ill, Charles C Thomas, 1969

4
HEADACHE

RAYMOND D. ADAMS

The term *headache* should encompass all aches and pains located in the head, but in common language its application is restricted to unpleasant sensations in the region of the cranial vault. Facial, pharyngeal, and cervical pain are presented in Table 4-2 and will be described in Chaps. 8 and 376.

Headache, along with fatigue, hunger, and thirst, represents the most frequent human discomforts. Medically speaking, its significance is often abstruse, for it may stand as a symptomatic expression of disease or of some minor tension or fatigue, incident to the affairs of the day. Fortunately, in most instances it reflects the latter, and only exceptionally does it warn of serious disease seated in intracranial structures. But it is this dual significance, benign and potentially malignant, that keeps the physician on the alert. Systematic approach to the headache problem necessitates a broad knowledge of the medical and surgical diseases of which it is a symptom and a clinical methodology which leaves none of the common and treatable causes unexplored.

GENERAL CONSIDERATIONS In the introductory chapter on pain, reference was made to the necessity, when dealing with any painful state, of determining its quality, location, duration and time course, and conditions which produce, exacerbate, or relieve it. When headache is considered in these terms, a certain amount of useful information is obtained by careful history, but perhaps less than one might expect. Unfortunately, physical examination of the head itself is seldom useful.

As to quality of cephalic pain, the patient is rarely helpful in describing it. In fact persistent questioning on that point occasions surprise, for the patient usually assumes that the word *headache* should have conveyed enough information to the examiner about the nature of the discomfort. Most headaches are dull, deeply located, and of aching character, a pain recognizable as of the type that usually arises from structures deep to the skin. Seldom is there reported the superficial burning, smarting, or stinging type of pain localized to the skin. When asked to analogize the sensation to another sensory experience, the patient may make some allusion to tightness, pressure, or bursting feeling, terms which then give clue to a muscular tension or psychologic state.

Queries about the intensity of the pain are seldom of much value since they reflect more the patient's attitude toward the condition and a customary way of reporting things that happen than the true severity. As usual the bluff, hearty person tends to minimize discomfort, whereas the neurotic dramatizes it. Degree of incapacity is a better index. A severe migraine attack seldom allows performance of the day's work. The pain which awakens the patient from sleep at night, or prevents sleep, is also more likely to have a demonstrable organic basis. As a rule, the most intense cranial pains are those which accompany subarachnoid hemorrhage and meningitis, which have grave implications, or migraine and paroxysmal nocturnal orbitotemporal (cluster) headaches, which are benign.

Data regarding *location* of the headache are apt to be more informative. If the source is in deep structures (extracranial, subdermal, or intracranial), as is usually the case, the correspondence with the site of the pain is fairly precise. Inflammation of an extracranial artery causes pain well localized to the site of the vessel. Lesions of paranasal sinuses, teeth, eyes, and upper cervical vertebrae induce less sharply localized pain but one that is still referred in a regional distribution that is fairly constant. Intracranial lesions in the posterior fossa cause pain in the occipital-nuchal region, homolateral if the lesion is one-sided. Supratentorial lesions induce frontotemporal pains, again homolateral to the lesion if it is on one side. But localization can also be very uninformative or misleading. Ear pain, for example, although it may mean disease in the ear, more often is referred from other regions, and eye pain may be referred from parts as remote as the occiput or cervical spine.

Duration and *time-intensity curve* of headaches in both the attack itself and their life profile are most useful. Of course the headache of bacterial meningitis or subarachnoid hemorrhage occurs usually in single attacks over a period of days. Single, brief, momentary (1 to 2 s) pains in the cranium are presently uninterpretable and are significant only because they indicate no serious underlying disease. Migraine of the classic type has its onset in the early morning hours or daytime, reaches its peak of severity in a half hour or so, lasts, unless treated, for several hours up to 1 to 2 days, and is often terminated by sleep. In the life history a frequency of more than a single attack every few weeks is exceptional. A migraine patient having several attacks per week usually proves to have a combination of migraine and tension headaches. In contrast to this is the nightly occurrence (2 to 3 h after onset of sleep) over a period of several weeks to months of the rapidly peaking, nonthrobbing orbital or supraorbital pain of cluster headache, which tends to dissipate within an hour. The headache of intracranial tumor characteristically can occur at any time of day or night, can interrupt sleep, varies in intensity, and lasts a few minutes to hours. The life profile is one of increasing frequency and intensity over a period of months. Tension headache, once commenced, may persist continuously for weeks or months, though waxing and waning from hour to hour.

Headache that bears a more or less constant relationship to certain biologic events and also to physical environmental changes may prove to be informative. Premenstrual headaches most typically relate to premenstrual tension during the period of oliguria and edema formation; they usually vanish after the first day of vaginal bleeding. The headaches of cervical arthritis are most typically intense after a period of inactivity, and the first movements in the morning are both difficult and painful. Hypertensive headaches, like those of cerebral tumor, tend to occur on waking in the morning, but, as with all vascular headaches, excitement and tension may provoke them. Headache from infection of nasal sinuses may appear, with clocklike regularity, upon awakening and in midmorning, and is characteristically worsened by stooping and jarring of the head. Eyestrain headaches naturally follow prolonged use of the eyes, as in reading, peering for a long time against glaring headlights in traffic, or watching the cinema. Atmospheric cold may evoke pain in the so-called "fibrositic" or "nodular" headache or when the underlying condition is arthritic or neuralgic. Anger, excitement, or irritation may initiate common migraine in certain disposed persons; this is more typical of common migraine than of the classic type. Change of position, stooping, straining, cough, and sexual intercourse are each known to produce a special type of headache. Exertional headaches, another well-known type, are usually benign (only 1 in 10 will have an intracranial lesion) and disappear within weeks to months.

PAIN-SENSITIVE STRUCTURES AND MECHANISMS OF HEADACHE Understanding of headache has been greatly augmented by the observations of surgeons during operations. They inform us that the following cranial structures are sensitive to mechanical stimulation: (1) skin, subcutaneous tissue, muscles, arteries, and periosteum of skull; (2) delicate structures of eye, ear, and nasal cavity; (3) intracranial venous sinuses and their tributary veins; (4) parts of the dura at the base of the brain and the arteries within the dura mater and piarachnoid; and (5) the trigeminal, glossopharyngeal, vagus, and first three cervical nerves. The bony skull, much of the piarachnoid and dura, and the parenchyma of the brain lack sensitivity. Interestingly, pain is practically the only sensation produced by stimulation of the listed structures.

The pathways whereby sensory stimuli, whatever their source, are conveyed to the central nervous system are the trigeminal nerves for structures above the tentorium in the anterior and middle fossae of the skull, and the first three cervical nerves for those in the posterior fossa and infradural structures. The ninth and tenth cranial nerves supply part of the posterior fossa and refer the pain to the ear and throat. The tentorium is the border zone between the trigeminal and cervical innervation. The central connections through spinal cord and brainstem to thalamus have already been described in Chap. 3 and will be depicted in Chap. 19.

The pain of intracranial disease is referred, by a mechanism already discussed, to some part of the cranium lying within the areas supplied by the aforementioned nerves (the fifth, ninth, and tenth cranial nerves and the first three cervicals). There may be an associated local tenderness of the scalp at the site of reference. Dental or jaw pain may also have cranial reference. The pain of disease in other parts of the body is not referred to the head, although it may initiate headache by other means.

By analysis of several types of headache, Wolff and his colleagues have demonstrated that most "spontaneous" cranial pains can be traced to the operation of one or more of the following mechanisms:

1 Distention, traction, and dilatation of the intracranial or extracranial arteries
2 Traction or displacement of large intracranial veins or the dural envelope in which they lie
3 Compression, traction, or intrinsic disease of cranial and spinal nerves
4 Voluntary or involuntary spasm and possibly interstitial inflammation and trauma of cranial and cervical muscles
5 Meningeal irritation and raised intracranial pressure

Appenzeller would add to the list hysteria and some "psychogenic" disorders.

More specifically, intracranial mass lesions cause headache only if in a position to deform, displace, or exert traction on vessels and dural structures at the base of the brain, and this may happen long before intracranial pressure rises. In fact, the artificial induction of high intraspinal and intracranial pressure by the subarachnoid or intraventricular injection of sterile saline solution does not result in headache. Some have interpreted this to mean raised intracranial pressure does not cause headache, a conclusion which is called into question by the demonstrable relief of headache by lumbar puncture and lowering the cerebrospinal fluid (CSF) pressure in some patients. Actually, most patients with high intracranial pressure complain of recurrent bioccipital and bifrontal headache, probably due to traction on vessels or dura. As to localization, the pains follow the patterns mentioned above; those lesions deflecting the falx or pressing on superior longitudinal or straight sinuses induce pain behind or above the eye; if the lateral part of the lateral sinus is involved, the pain is felt in the ear. Displacement of tentorium elicits pain felt in the supraorbital region.

Dilatation of the extracranial, temporal, and intracranial arteries with stretching of surrounding sensitive structures is believed to be the mechanism of most of the pain of migraine. Extracranial, temporal, and occipital arteries, when involved in giant cell arteritis (cranial or "temporal" arteritis), a disease which usually afflicts individuals over 50 years of age, give rise to headache of dull aching and throbbing type, at first localized and then more diffuse. Characteristically it is severe and persistent over a period of weeks or months. The offending artery, strangely, is not always tender to pressure, yet section of it, as in biopsy, may relieve the pain (Chap. 67). Evolving atherosclerotic thrombosis of internal carotid, anterior, and middle cerebral arteries is sometimes accompanied by pain in the forehead or temple; with vertebral artery thrombosis the pain is postauricular, and basilar artery thrombosis causes pain to be projected to the occiput and sometimes the forehead.

In *infection or blockage* of *paranasal sinuses*, accompanied usually by pain over the antrum or in the forehead (from the ethmoid and sphenoid sinuses the pain localizes around the eyes on one or both sides or in the vertex or other part of the cranium, especially in disease of the sphenoid sinuses), the mechanism involves changes in pressure and irritation of pain-sensitive sinus walls. Usually it is associated with tenderness of the skin in the same distribution. The pain may have two remarkable properties: (1) When throbbing, it may be abolished by compressing the carotid artery on the same side. (2) It tends to recur and subside at the same hours, i.e., on awakening, with gradual disappearance when the person is upright, and coming again in the late morning hours. The time relations are believed to yield information concerning the mechanism; morning pain is ascribed to the sinuses filling at night, and its relief on arising to emptying after the erect posture has been assumed. Stooping intensifies the pain by pressure change, as do blowing the nose and jarring the head sometimes; and inhalant sympathomimetic drugs such as Neo-Synephrine, which reduce swelling and congestion, tend to relieve the pain. Some believe that the highly sensitive orifice of the sinus is the source, but more probably the pain arises in the sensitive mucous membrane of the sinus. However, it may persist after all purulent secretions have disappeared, probably because of mechanism of blockage of the orifice by boggy membranes and a vacuum or suction effect on the sinus wall (*vacuum sinus headaches*). The condition is relieved when aeration is restored. During air flights both earache and sinus headache tend to occur on descent, when the relative pressure in the blocked viscus falls.

Headache of ocular origin, located as a rule in the orbit, forehead, or temple, is of steady, aching type and tends to follow prolonged use of the eyes in close work. Ocular muscle imbalance is believed to be the mechanism. The main faults are hypermetropia and astigmatism (not myopia), which result in sustained contraction of extraocular as well as frontal, temporal, and even occipital muscles. Convergence insufficiency is another common disorder. Correction of the refractive error abolishes the headache. Traction on the extraocular muscles during eye surgery, particularly on the iris, will evoke pain. Another mechanism is involved in the raised intraocular pressure seen in acute glaucoma or iridocyclitis, which causes steady, aching pain in the region of the eye. When intense, it may radiate throughout the distribution of the ophthalmic division of the trigeminal nerve. As for ocular pain in general, it is important that the eyes should always be refracted, but eyestrain is probably not as frequent as one would expect from the wholesale dispensing of spectacles. The pain of diabetic third nerve palsy, intracranial aneurysm, cavernous sinus thrombosis, and Reader's paratrigeminal syndrome may also be referred to the eye.

The mechanism of *headaches accompanying disease of ligaments, muscles, and apophyseal joints* in the upper part of the spine, which are referred to occiput and nape of neck on the same side, can be in part reproduced by the injection of hypertonic saline solution into these structures. Such pains are especially frequent in late life in rheumatoid and hypertrophic arthritis and tend also to occur after whiplash injuries to the neck. If the pain is arthritic in origin, the first movements after being still for some hours are both stiff and painful. In fact,

evocation of pain by active and passive motion of the spine should indicate traumatic or other disease of movable parts. The pain of myofibrositis, evidenced by tender nodules near the cranial insertion of cervical and other muscles, is more obscure. There are no pathologic data as to the nature of these vaguely palpable lesions, and it is uncertain whether the pain actually arises in them. They may represent only the deep tenderness felt in the region of referred pain or the involuntary secondary protective spasm of muscles. Characteristically, the pain is steady (nonthrobbing) and spreads from one to both sides of the head. Exposure to cold or draft may precipitate it. Though severe at times, it seldom prevents sleep. Massage of muscles and heat have unpredictable effects but relieve the pain in some cases.

The *headache of meningeal irritation* (infection or hemorrhage), which is of acute onset, severe, generalized, deep-seated, constant, especially intense at the base of the skull, and associated with stiffness of neck on bending forward, has been ascribed by some authorities to increased intracranial pressure. Indeed the withdrawal of cerebrospinal fluid may afford some relief. But dilatation and congestion of inflamed meningeal vessels must also be a factor. It seems more probable, therefore, that the pain is due to the chemical irritation of nerve endings in the meninges.

Lumbar puncture headache, which is characterized by a steady occipital-nuchal pain and also by frontal pain coming on a few minutes after arising from a recumbent position and relieved within a few minutes by lying down, has as its cause a persistent leakage of CSF into the lumbar tissues through the needle site. The CSF pressure is low (often 0 in the lateral decubitus position), and the injection of sterile isotonic saline solution intrathecally relieves it. The headache is usually increased by compression of the jugular veins and is unaffected by digital obliteration of one carotid artery. It seems probable that in the upright position a low intraspinal and negative intracranial pressure exerts traction on dural attachments and dural sinuses by caudal displacement of the brain. Understandably, then, headache following cisternal puncture is rare. As soon as the leakage of CSF stops and CSF pressure is gradually restored (usually from a few days up to a week or so), the headache disappears. "Spontaneous" low-pressure headache may follow a sneeze or strain, presumably because of rupture of the spinal arachnoid along a nerve root.

The mechanism of the throbbing or steady headache which accompanies febrile illnesses, located in frontal or occipital regions or generalized, is probably vascular. It is much like histamine headache in being relieved on one side by carotid artery compression and on both sides by jugular vein compression or the subarachnoid injection of saline solution. It is increased by shaking the head. It seems probable that the meningeal vessels pulsate unduly and stretch pain-sensitive structures around the base of the brain. In certain cases, however, the pain may be lessened by compression of temporal arteries, and in these cases a component of the headache seems to be derived from the walls of extracranial arteries, as in migraine.

The claims of insufferable headaches by the hysteric are undecipherable. The so-called tension headaches of patients with anxiety states and depression are allegedly due to chronic spasm of cranial and cervical muscles. Combinations of the tension and vascular headaches give rise to the "mixed headaches" of many psychiatric patients.

PRINCIPAL CLINICAL VARIETIES OF HEADACHE Usually there is no difficulty in diagnosing the headache of glaucoma, purulent sinusitis, bacterial meningitis, and brain tumor, and a fuller account of these special headaches will be found where these diseases are described in later sections of the book. It is when headache is chronic, recurrent, and unattended by other important signs of disease that the physician faces one of the most difficult medical problems.

The following types of headache should then be considered.

Migraine   The term *migraine* refers to periodic, hemicranial, throbbing headaches which usually begin in childhood, adolescence, or early adult life and recur with diminishing frequency during advancing years.

Two closely related clinical syndromes have been identified. The first is called "neurologic" migraine, the second common. The classic syndrome is ushered in by a disturbance of neurologic function (hemianopsia or central blindness, hemiparesthetic disturbance, slight speech abnormality or aphasia, or hemiparesis) followed in a few minutes by hemicranial headache, nausea, and vomiting, all of which last for hours or as long as a day or two. The other syndrome is characterized by an unheralded onset of hemicranial or generalized headache with or without nausea and vomiting but following the same temporal pattern. Both headache syndromes respond to ergot preparations, if administered early in the attack. Their genetic nature is evidenced by concurrence in several members of the family of the same and successive generations in 60 to 80 percent of cases; but inheritance is somewhat less clear in the common than the classic variety, perhaps because diagnosis is less accurate.

Neurologic migraine presents such a dramatic and at times confusing sequence of events that it merits further description. On awakening in the morning, or at any time of the day, the patient may have a kind of vague premonition of an attack. Then abruptly there is a disturbance of vision consisting usually of bright spots or dazzling zigzag lines which give way within minutes to scotomatous defects; usually they are bilateral and often of homonymous and congruent pattern (corresponding parts of the field of vision of each eye). Soon thereafter, numbness and tingling of lips, face, hand (on one or both sides), slight confusion of thinking, weakness of an arm or leg, mild aphasia, dizziness and uncertainty of gait, drowsiness, or confusion (rarely coma) are added to the clinical picture. Only one or a few of these neurologic phenomena are present in any given patient, and they tend to occur in the same combination in each attack. They last 5 to 15 min or more, and if the weakness or numbness spreads from one part of the body to another or one symptom follows another, it does so slowly in a period of minutes (not in seconds as in a convulsion). Just as inexplicably as they come, they soon begin to recede, and within minutes they are followed by a unilateral throbbing headache, usually on the side of the cerebral disturbance, which slowly increases in intensity. At its peak, in an hour or so, nausea and vomiting may occur. The headache lasts hours or a day or two and is usually the most unpleasant feature of the illness.

Much variation occurs. When this "sick headache," as it is called, is most severe, the patient is forced to lie down and to shun light and noise. Milder forms, especially if partially controlled by medication, do not force withdrawal from accustomed activities. Any one of the three principal components— neurologic derangement, headache, or vomiting—may be absent or occur in different sequence than is described above. Particularly with advancing age there is a tendency for the headache and vomiting to become less severe, finally leaving only the neurologic abnormality. The neurologic symptomatology is also subject to variation. Although visual disturbances are far and away the most common manifestation, they differ in detail from patient to patient; numbness and tingling of the lips and fingers of one hand are probably next in frequency, with transient aphasia or a thickness of speech following in that order. A relatively rare syndrome of vertigo, staggering, drowsiness, and stupor has been delineated by Bickerstaff and called *basilar artery migraine.* Also, he has reported the loss of consciousness at the onset, especially in migrainous young women. Recurrent unilateral headaches associated with extraocular muscle palsies have been called *opthalmoplegic migraine.* A transient third nerve palsy with associated ptosis of one eyelid is the usual picture; rarely, the abducens nerve is affected and lateral movement is impaired. Hemifacial paralysis is another rare variant. Disturbances of the mind may appear—strange excitement, unaccountable irritability or depression, or episodes of mental confusion, which are more common. The headache, though typically hemicranial (the word *migraine* is said to be derived from *megrim,* meaning hemicrania), may be frontal, temporal, or generalized. In children abdominal pain and vomiting, sometimes cyclical, may accompany the headache (abdominal migraine). Another childhood variant is paroxysmal vertigo; this may occur as a prelude to a "sick headache" or without headache (benign paroxysmal vertigo of childhood). The attacks, instead of beginning in childhood and recurring in the usual fashion every few weeks or months with diminishing frequency in middle and late adult years, may begin in adult life or even middle age or suddenly increase in frequency during menopause or when hypertension and vascular disease develop. The neurologic symptoms, instead of being transitory, may leave a permanent deficit (e.g., a homonymous visual field defect) reminiscent of an ischemic stroke or a bleeding vascular malformation. The use of hormones to prevent pregnancy has increased the frequency and severity of migraine and in several reported instances has resulted in a permanent neurologic deficit.

Between attacks the migrainous patient is essentially normal. For a time, when psychosomatic medicine was much in vogue, there was insistence on a migrainous personality characterized by tenseness, rigidity in thinking, meticulousness, and perfectionism. The migrainous attack was said to occur often during the let-down period, after many days of hard work or stress. But further personality analyses have not borne out these ideas, and the temporal relations between headache and the day's activities have not been consistent. Moreover, the fact that the headaches may begin in early childhood, when the personality is relatively amorphous, would argue against this idea.

During an attack, the electroencephalogram reveals a nonspecific slowing of wave frequencies in one-third to one-half of all patients. The cerebral circulation is found by blood flow studies to be slowed early in the attack and speeded up once headache begins.

Migraine is frequent, found in an estimated 5 percent of the general population; women are slightly more susceptible than men, and there is a tendency for the headaches to occur during the period of premenstrual tension and fluid retention. The migrainous attacks usually cease during pregnancy. Reserpine treatment and estrogens and progesterone may increase their frequency. A few patients have linked their attacks to certain articles of diet, such as chocolate, cheese, and wine or other alcoholic beverages. Phenylethylamine, a constituent of such foods and drinks, has been shown to precipitate headaches in migraine patients; tyramine, another constituent, does not. The platelets of migraine patients are deficient in monoamine oxidase, responsible for degrading phenylethylamine. There is no clear relationship, despite many statements to the contrary, between migraine and vascular malformations of the brain and psychoneurosis. The relationship to epilepsy is less clear; convulsions are slightly increased in frequency in migrainous patients and their relatives.

Vasodilatation and excessive pulsation of branches of the external carotid artery have been observed during the headache. Further, as the pulsation decreases, either spontaneously or after the administration of ergotamine, the headache disappears. Vasoconstriction was early postulated as the basis of the neurologic symptoms; it has been confirmed in at least one chance carotid arteriogram and has been inferred from prompt abolition of the visual or neurologic disorder upon administration of nitrites. Thus the vascular theory of migraine has come to be accepted, supported further by surgical observations, that the extracranial arteries can be a source of pain. However, it is quite apparent that the theory does not explain why the intracranial and extracranial arteries should periodically undergo spasm and dilatation in the migrainous individual, nor does it account for the nausea and vomiting (infrequent in all other headaches except those due to tumor) or the tenderness and swelling of the temporal vessels and surrounding tissues.

A hypothesis of current interest postulates that the observed vasospasm and later hyperemic pulsations are induced by a release of amines such as norepinephrine, epinephrine, and serotonin in individuals whose vessels are peculiarly sensitive. These substances are known to be powerful vasoconstrictors. It was found that some migraine patients during their attack excrete increased amounts of the terminal metabolites of the catecholamines, particularly 5-hydroxyindoleacetic acid (5-HIAA) derived from serotonin, and of vanillylmandelic acid (VMA), a product of norepinephrine and epinephrine. A corresponding reduction in serotonin levels in the blood has also been detected. Other observations in line with this are that (1) reserpine, which reduces the level of serotonin in platelets, brain, and other tissues, may provoke migraine; (2) the injection of serotonin gives partial or complete relief of headache, and (3) a serotonin antagonist, methysergide, wholly prevents attacks in many instances. However, it is still difficult to reconcile these data with the finding that a heat-stable polypeptide with some of the properties of bradykinin (one of the plasma kinins) not only can be aspirated from the edematous subcutaneous tissue on the side of the headache but, if reinjected at another site, will cause increased capillary permeability, pain, and lowered skin threshold in the overlying skin. Its algogenic action is potentiated by serotonin. Whether this substance, called *neurokinin,* escapes secondarily during the phase of vasodilatation or initiates the vasodilatation is not known. While this humoral amine theory is incomplete and several of the findings need verification, it nonetheless does promise clarification of the migraine syndrome and possibly other forms of vascular headache. Couch and Hassanein have found an increase in platelet aggregability in migraine patients, especially during an attack of headache, and they suggest that it may be responsible for the stroke that rarely complicates migraine. Clover and his associates have measured a transitory decrease in platelet monoamine oxidase activity during attacks.

DIAGNOSIS Classic migraine should occasion no difficulty in diagnosis if the above facts are kept in mind and if a good history is obtained. That is possible, as a rule, for migraine patients tend to be intelligent.

The real difficulties come from three sources: (1) ignorance of the fact that a progressively unfolding neurologic syndrome may be migrainous in origin; (2) lack of appreciation that the neurologic disorder may occur without headache; (3) lack of awareness that recurrent headaches, which may be an isolated phenomenon, may take many forms, some of which may prove difficult to distinguish from the other common types of headache described in this chapter.

Some of these problems merit further elaboration because of their practical importance, as follows:

The neurologic part of the migraine syndrome may resemble focal epilepsy, the clinical picture of a vascular malformation such as an angioma or aneurysm, or some other vascular disease such as a thrombotic or embolic stroke. Here it is the pace of the neurologic symptoms of migraine more than their character that reliably distinguishes the condition from epilepsy. The clinical profile of the aura of epilepsy is measured in seconds, for it depends on spreading neural excitation, in contrast to the slow progression of migraine, which is based on spreading vascular spasm.

Ophthalmoplegic migraine will always suggest a carotid aneurysm, but in relatively few cases has carotid arteriography revealed such an abnormality. Despite many claims that the question of a vascular malformation should be raised in cases of hemicranial painful attacks occurring invariably on the same side of the head (unlike migraine), in a large series of cases this has only rarely been confirmed by arteriography. Of course, focal epilepsy, protracted headache, stiff neck and bloody cerebrospinal fluid, a persistent neurologic deficit, and cranial bruit would be indicative of a vascular type of headache associated with angioma or aneurysm. Only in the earlier stages, when periodic throbbing headache is the sole symptom, might it be confused with true migraine.

Attacks indistinguishable from epilepsy may also appear in association with the hypertensive and cerebral arteriosclerotic vascular diseases of late life. Here one is aided by late age of onset, more persistent and frequent headaches, and the evidence of vascular disease of heart, lower extremities, and brain.

A special problem relates to paroxysms of throbbing headache, not hemicranial in distribution, not preceded by a neurologic aura, and not accounted for by other known cause. Are they examples of common migraine? Unfortunately, since diagnosis depends on the interpretation of the patient's description of symptoms and since there is as yet no biologically valid confirmatory laboratory test, the controversy as to where migraine begins and ends is of the armchair type. Favoring the diagnosis of migraine are life-long history, childhood onset, positive family history, and response of the headache to ergot derivatives.

A variety of episodic attacks have been described as migraine equivalents: attacks of abdominal pain with nausea, vomiting, and diarrhea; pain localized in the thorax, pelvis, and extremities; bouts of fever; paroxysmal vertigo; transient disturbances in mood (psychic equivalents); recurrent nocturnal orbital (cluster) headache, or migrainous neuralgia. Watson and Steele attribute these associated conditions to a paroxysmal disequilibrium which they find in approximately one-third of migrainous children. The only advantage of considering such attacks as migrainous is that this view protects some patients from unnecessary diagnostic procedures and surgical intervention—but it may also prevent necessary surgery.

From all this discussion the reader should be left with the idea that the migraine syndromes are rather larger and more protean than the rigid stereotyped descriptions we have given would suggest. In these days of complicated diagnostic procedures it is tempting to take x-rays or do computerized tomography (CT scan) of the skull and perform arteriography and electroencephalography on every patient. A conservative approach would lead to temporization, reserving CT scan or EEG for the exceptional case.

Cluster headache This headache is also called *paroxysmal nocturnal cephalalgia, migrainous neuralgia, histamine headache* and Horton's syndrome. It is characterized by a fourfold higher incidence in men than in women, constant, unilateral orbital localization, and onset usually within 2 or 3 h after falling asleep, during the phase of rapid eye movement (REM) sleep (it is infrequent during the waking hours). The pain is intense and steady (nonthrobbing) with lacrimation, blocked nostril, then rhinorrhea, and sometimes flush, miosis, ptosis, and edema of cheek, all lasting approximately an hour or two.

It tends to recur nightly for several weeks or a few months (hence the term *cluster*), followed by complete freedom for years. The pain of a given attack may leave as rapidly as it began. Clusters may recur over the years, being possibly more likely in times of stress, prolonged strain, overwork, and with upsetting emotional experiences. Occasionally alcohol, nitroglycerine, or tyramine-containing foods precipitate an attack. Rarely, the condition may occur in daytime and may not cluster but continue.

The picture is so characteristic that it cannot be confused with any other disease, though to those unfamiliar with it the possibility of a carotid aneurysm, hemangioma, brain tumor, or sinusitis may be suggested. Appropriate roentgenograms and carotid arteriography will always exclude such conditions but usually are unnecessary. In the differential diagnosis orbital, nasociliary, supraorbital, Sluder's sphenopalatine, and neuralgias must also be considered (see Chap. 376).

In the life history profile the clusters of headache may last for weeks. The clusters may be single or recur two, three, or more times, with years of freedom in between, during which such precipitating factors as alcohol are no longer effective. Often the pain involves the same orbit in each cluster. Examples are seen in which the same type of headache may last a year or more or even for a period of 10 to 20 years.

The relationship of the cluster headache to migraine remains conjectural. A portion of the cases have a background of migraine, which led to the earlier postulation of migrainous neuralgia, but the majority do not. The face of the patient with cluster headache turns red (by infrared photography), whereas that of the migraine patient is pale. Some investigators have found a drop in the blood pressure of migraine patients; none occurs in cluster headaches.

Tension headache and various other cranial pains with psychiatric disease The headache is usually bilateral, often with diffuse extension over the top of the cranium. Occipital-nuchal localization is also common. Although the sensation may be described as pain, close questioning may uncover other sensations, viz., fullness, tightness, or pressure (as if the head is surrounded by a band or in a vise), on which waves of aching pain are superimposed. The onset of a given attack is more gradual than in migraine and not infrequently a throbbing "vascular" type of headache is added intermittently to a pressure ache. Tension headache may occur acutely under conditions of emotional excitement or intense worry and lasts for hours or a day or two. More often it persists unremittingly for weeks or months. In fact, this is the only type of headache that exhibits the peculiarity of being absolutely continuous day and night for long periods of time. Although sleep may be possible, whenever the patient awakens, the headache is present; the common analgesic remedies have no beneficial effect unless the pain is intense and of aching type.

As to mechanism, the ascription of it to sustained muscle activity, shown by the electromyogram, is only a partial explanation. The continuous pressing quality of milder cephalic sensations at times when the patient is relaxed hardly seems to be attributable to physiologic stimulation and suggests instead that the condition is maintained by focused attention on the head (occasioned sometimes by worry and fear of intracranial disease). Moreover, it must be remembered that all types of headache in their late stages may give rise to muscle tension, and that this is of an aching rather than a pressure type. In contrast to migraine, in which pain is periodic and lifelong, with tendency to lessen in late adult years, tension headache occurs more often in middle age and usually coincides with anxiety and depression in the trying times of life. Many premenstrual headaches are of this type, and there is an increased incidence of this type of tension headache at menopause.

Psychologic studies of groups of patients with tension headaches have revealed prominent symptoms of depression, anxiety, and to a lesser extent hypochondriasis. Kudrow records that 65 percent of depressed patients have this type of headache and that over 60 percent of his patients with tension headaches were depressed. When psychiatric syndromes are searched for in headache patients, it is evident that the majority of those with anxiety neurosis, hysteria, obsessive-compulsive neurosis, and schizophrenia, in which anxiety is a prominent symptom, exhibit this type of headache. Migraine and traumatic headaches may be complicated by tension headache.

Other odd cephalic pains, e.g., boring pains, "clavus hystericus," may occur in hysteria and raise perplexing problems in diagnosis. Their bizarre character, persistence in the face of every known therapy, absence of other signs of disease, and the presence of the stigmata of the hysterical personality provide the basis for correct diagnosis (see Chap. 11).

Headache of angioma and aneurysm The temporal profile of any given attack shows the onset to be sudden or very acute, with the pain reaching a peak within minutes. Neurologic disturbances such as scintillations, defects in vision, unilateral numbness, weakness, or aphasia may precede or occur after the onset of headache and outlast it. Should hemorrhage occur the headache is often extremely severe and localizes more toward the occiput and neck, lasting many days in association with stiff neck. A cranial or cervical bruit and, of course, blood in the cerebrospinal fluid establish the diagnosis, but it may require verification by arteriography. The claim that vascular malformations may give rise to migraine is probably untenable. Statistical data show migraine to be no more frequent in this group of patients than in the general population. There are however, a few notable exceptions to this statement. Of course, vascular lesions may exist for long periods of time without headache, or the latter may develop many years after other manifestations, such as epilepsy and hemiplegia (see Chap. 365).

Traumatic headaches Severe, chronic, continuous, or intermittent headaches appear as the cardinal symptom of three posttraumatic syndromes, separable in each instance from the headache that immediately follows head injury (i.e., that of scalp laceration and contusion with sanguineous cerebrospinal fluid and increased intracranial pressure). The latter lasts several days or a week or two (see Chap. 366).

Headache of chronic subdural hematoma Headache and dizziness of fluctuating severity, followed by drowsiness, stupor, coma, and hemiparesis, are the usual manifestations of chronic subdural hematoma. The head injury may have been minor and forgotten by patient and family. The headaches are deep-seated, steady, unilateral or generalized, and respond to the usual analgesic drugs. The typical attack profile of the headache and other symptoms is one of increasing frequency and severity over several weeks or months. Diagnosis is now established by CT scan and arteriography (see Chap. 366).

Headache of posttraumatic nervous instability See Chap. 366.

Posttraumatic dysautonomic cephalalgia This term was given by Vijayan and Dreyfus to severe, episodic, throbbing, unilateral headaches accompanied by ipsilateral mydriasis and excessive facial sweating. The condition followed injury to the neck in the region of the carotid sheath. It was postulated that the sympathetic nervous supply of the cranium had been disinhibited, and there was clinical and pharmacologic evidence of sympathetic dysfunction.

Headaches of brain tumor Headache is the outstanding symptom of cerebral tumor. Unfortunately, the quality of the pain has no specific feature. It tends to be deep-seated, nonthrobbing (or throbbing), and aching or bursting. Attacks last a few minutes to an hour or more and occur once or many times during the day. Activity and frequently change in the position of the head may provoke pain, while rest in bed diminishes its frequency. Nocturnal awakening because of pain, although typical, is by no means diagnostic. Unexpected forceful (projectile) vomiting may punctuate the illness in its later stages. As the tumor grows the pain becomes more frequent and severe; it sometimes is nearly continuous terminally. But there are exceptions: some headaches are mild and tolerable, others as agonizing as that of the headache of bacterial meningitis and subarachnoid hemorrhage. If unilateral, the headache is homolateral to the tumor in 9 out of 10 patients. Supratentorial tumors are felt anterior to the interauricular circumference of the skull; posterior fossa tumors behind this line. Bifrontal and bioccipital headache, coming on after unilateral headache, signifies the development of increased intracranial pressure.

HEADACHES RELATED TO MEDICAL DISORDERS Experienced physicians are aware of many conditions in which headache figures as a dominant symptom. These include fevers of any cause, carbon monoxide exposure, chronic lung disease with hypercapnia (headaches often nocturnal), hypothyroidism, Cushing's disease, withdrawal of corticosteroid medication, chronic nitrite exposure, occasionally Addison's disease, aldosterone-producing adrenal tumors, use of "the pill" in some instances, acute rises in blood pressure, e.g., from pheochromocytoma, and acute anemia with hemoglobin below 10 g.

With reference to chronic hypertension the relation to headache is less clear. Approximately 50 percent of patients with hypertension complain of headaches. Wolff and colleagues state that except with hypertensive encephalopathy where the intracranial pressure may be increased, the mechanism of the headache is similar to that of migraine, i.e., it is vascular, and in such individuals the headache develops not at a time when the pressure is highest, as in time of stress, but after it has fallen. Perhaps the headache is due to the release of vasodilating prostaglandins. The headaches of renal dialysis tend to increase as the blood pressure falls and sodium and osmolality decrease. Vasoconstricting drugs such as ergotamine often are as effective in hypertensive headaches as in migraine.

An erythromelalgic syndrome (flushing, red hands, numb fingers, blotchy skin) with severe headaches has been described in association with serotonin-secreting tumors, carcinoid tumors, and mastocytosis. In one type reported by Streeter and associates there were high levels of circulating bradykinin.

APPROACH TO THE PATIENT WITH HEADACHE Obviously very different possibilities are raised by a patient who presents for the first time with severe headache and a patient who has had recurrent headache over a period of years. The chances of uncovering the cause in the first instance are much greater than in the latter, and some of the potential underlying conditions (meningitis, subarachnoid hemorrhage, epidural hematoma, glaucoma, and purulent sinusitis) are more serious. The simple rules to follow are that severe, persistent headache with stiff neck and fever always means meningitis and the same combination without fever, subarachnoid hemorrhage. A lumbar puncture is mandatory. Acute persistent headache over a period of hours or days may occur in systemic infections such as influenza (febrile) or as a manifestation of an acute tension state. The first attack of migraine may present in this way.

In searching for the cause of recurrent headache one should investigate the status of cardiovascular and renal systems by blood pressure and urine examination, eyes by fundoscopic, intraocular pressure, and refraction, the sinuses by transillumination and x-rays, the cranial arteries by palpation (and biopsy?), the cervical spine by effect of passive movement of the head and x-rays, the nervous system by neurologic examination, and psychic function by mental status.

Hypertension is, of course, frequent in the general population and when present is always difficult to prove as a cause of recurrent headaches. Minor elevations of blood pressure may be a result rather than the cause of nervous tension. No doubt severe hypertension with diastolic blood pressures of over 110 mmHg is more regularly associated with headache than is moderate hypertension. If headache is severe and frequent, one should always consider the possibilities of underlying anxiety, tension state, or a common migraine syndrome exacerbated by blood vessel disease. The mechanism of the puzzling hypertensive phenomenon of occipital pain, present on awakening in the morning and wearing off during the day, is uncertain.

The adolescent with daily frontal headaches represents a special type of problem. Often their relationship to eyestrain is unclear, and refraction of the eyes and new eyeglasses do not relieve the condition. Anxiety or tension is probably a factor in such cases, but it is difficult to be certain of a causal relationship. Some of the most persistent and inexplicable headaches, which have led to a survey by a battery of diagnostic procedures for tumor, have proved in the end to be caused by depression.

Equally puzzling is the somber, tense adult whose primary complaint is headache, or the migrainous person who in late life or at menopause begins to have daily headaches. Here it becomes important to assess mental status along the lines suggested in Chaps. 11 and 25, looking for evidences of anxiety, depression, and hypochondriasis. The quality and persistence of the headache are suggestive of the possibility of psychiatric illness. Sometimes a direct question as to the patient's idea of what is the matter may elicit suspicion and fear of brain tumor. Antidepressant drugs given as an empirical test may relieve the headache, thus clarifying the diagnosis.

The most worrisome type of patient is the one who has headache of increasing frequency and severity over a period of months or a year or so. Since an intracranial mass lesion (tumor, abscess, subdural hematoma) is a leading possibility, it becomes necessary to resort to a complete neurologic survey, including careful inspection of optic disk, roentgenograms of skull, electroencephalogram, CT scan, and radioactive isotope.

Every elderly person with severe headache of some few days or weeks duration should be considered as possibly having cranial arteritis. Increased sedimentation rate, fever, and anemia may be conjoined, but only in a minority of cases, unfortunately. The finding of a thickened temporal artery is important, and arterial biopsy and response to corticosteroids establish the diagnosis; treatment with corticosteroids often relieves the pain.

TREATMENT The most important steps in the treatment of headache are those measures which uncover and remove the underlying disease or functional disturbance.

For the common everyday headache due to fatigue, stuffy atmosphere, or excessive use of alcohol and tobacco, it is simply enough to advise avoidance of the offending activity or agent, and symptomatic therapy in the form of acetylsalicylic acid, 0.6 g (some brand of aspirin such as Anacin), or acetaminophen (Tylenol), 0.6 g, will suffice. Some patients who invariably have headache when constipated and hypochondriacs who not infrequently suffer incapacitating headache, fatigue, and depression whenever bowel elimination does not meet their expectation are not easily helped. Certainly, simple explanation, an anticonstipation regimen, and drugs which counteract depression (see Chap. 11) are preferable to the continuous use of analgesics. Premenstrual headache, if troublesome, can usually be helped by the use of a diuretic compound for the week preceding the menstrual period and a mixture of mild analgesic and tranquilizing medications (acetylsalicylic acid or acetaminophen, 0.6 g, and phenobarbital, 30 mg). If the headaches are severe and incapacitating, they should be treated as common migraine.

Migraine may require no treatment at all, other than an explanation of its nature to the patient and a reassurance that it will do no harm. Some patients know, or allege to know, that certain acts induce attacks, and it is obvious enough that they should be urged to avoid these acts, if possible. In certain instances alcoholic drinks, particularly red wine, are invariably followed by a migraine. Others claim reduction of attacks of headache by an elimination diet, correction of refractive error, or by psychotherapy. However, this is so exceptional that a cause and effect relationship must be doubted in view of the variability of the disease itself.

Treatment of the neurologic aura of migraine is rarely required or possible because of its brevity. If the deficits are lasting, inhalation of an ampul of amyl nitrate should be tried as a preventive measure; it should be used at the first premonition of the attack. The time to initiate treatment of the oncoming headache is during the neurologic disorder. If many of the headaches are mild, the patient may already have learned that 0.6 g acetylsalicylic acid and possibly 5 mg dextroamphetamine sulfate (Dexedrine) will suffice to control the pain. More severe attacks also respond to simple analgesic medication and rest in a quiet, darkened room. Success has been claimed with ergot preparations, and indeed ergotamine tartrate, 0.25 mg by intravenous injection or 1 to 3 mg held under the tongue until dissolved, will interrupt a headache in 80 to 90 percent of cases if given near the onset of the headache. Sometimes the combination of caffeine, 100 mg with 1 mg ergotamine (Cafergot), is preferred. It may be taken in the form of a tablet (two at the onset of headache and a third in half an hour) or as a rectal suppository (2 mg ergotamine and 100 mg caffeine) if vomiting prevents oral administration.

Because of the danger of prolonged vascular spasm in patients who have vascular disease or are pregnant, ergot preparations must be used cautiously, if at all. Even in healthy individuals more than 10 to 15 mg ergotamine per week is risky, for it may in itself produce headache. For the frequent atypical migraine headaches, some of which respond poorly to ergot, one should prescribe a preparation containing 150 mg acetylsalicylic acid, 160 mg acetophenetidin, and dextroamphetamine sulfate, 5 mg, with phenobarbital, 30 mg. This can be repeated once or twice in a severe attack. Once the headache has become intense (after 30 min), ergot is of little help, and one must resort to codeine sulfate, 30 mg, or meperidine (Demerol), 50 mg, as the only means of terminating the pain. If sleep customarily terminates headache, 50 mg of promethazine (Phenergan) orally is helpful; it also relieves vomiting.

In individuals with frequent migrainous attacks (more than one to three times a month), efforts at prevention are worthwhile. Some success has been obtained with preparations of ergot, 0.5 mg, atropine, 0.3 mg, and phenobarbital (Bellergol), 15 mg, two or three times a day for a few weeks. Propranolol (Inderal), 40 mg. tid, has been effective in reducing the frequency and intensity of attacks in approximately one-third of cases. For the most severe forms of the disease, methysergide (Sansert) in a dose of 6 to 8 mg per day given for several weeks or months has proved to be most promising in reducing the frequency of or abolishing attacks. The main contraindication has been retroperitoneal fibrosis; this complication has been reported in several dozen cases when the patient has been treated continuously for more than 4 to 5 months. Discontinu-

ing treatment for 1 month out of every 6 has greatly reduced the incidence of this complication. Recently, claims have been proposed for cloridine hydrochloride (Dixarit), 0.025 to 0.05 mg tid, as a preventative, but it may cause depression in some patients.

All experienced physicians appreciate the importance of helping patients rearrange their schedules so as to control tensions and hard-driving ways of living, so often a feature of many migrainous patients. There is no one way of accomplishing this, but in general, long and costly psychotherapy has not been helpful, or at least one can say there are no substantial data as to its value.

Cluster headaches have proven to be most resistant to treatment. One capsule of Cafergot or 1.0 mg of ergotamine tartrate at bedtime is most widely recommended. However, if the headaches are frequent, severe, and diurnal as well as nocturnal, the intake of ergot may reach dangerous levels. Success has also been claimed for amitryptyline (Elavil), 25 to 100 mg tid, and methysergide, 6 to 8 mg per day, as means of interrupting a cluster. Histamine desensitization, originally proposed by Horton, has been little used in recent years because of inconsistent results. In rare cases of persistent cluster headaches lasting for 10 to 20 years spectacular success has been obtained by indomethacin (Indocin).

Hypertensive headaches respond to agents which lower blood pressure and relieve muscle tension. Chlorothiazide (Diuril), 250 to 500 mg twice a day, and methyldopa (Aldomet), 250 to 500 mg per day, when combined with a small amount of phenobarbital, 15 mg tid, or propranolol (Inderal) 40 mg tid, have given the best results. Meprobamate, 200 mg tid, or chlordiazepoxide hydrochloride (Librium), 5 mg tid, may be administered in place of phenobarbital. For the morning occipital ache a capsule containing sodium nitrite, 30 mg, caffeine sodium benzoate, 0.5 g, and acetophenetidin, 0.6 g, has been useful. A simplified method of treating this kind of headache is to supply the caffeine in a cup of strong black coffee and to give with it acetylsalicylic acid. Blocks under the head of the bed may be helpful.

The muscle tension headaches respond best to massage, relaxation, and a combination of drugs which relieve depression [e.g., amitryptaline (Elavil) or imiprimine (Tofranil)] and anxiety (e.g., phenobarbital, amobarbital, meprobamate, and chlordiazepoxide hydrochloride). Pain-relieving medicine of non-habit-forming type [e.g., acetylsalicylic acid and propoxyphene hydrochloride (Darvon)], should be added when throbbing headache is present. Stronger analgesic medication (codeine or meperidine hydrochloride) should be avoided. Psychotherapy may be helpful in this group of patients.

The headache of the syndrome of posttraumatic nervous instability requires supportive psychotherapy in the form of reassurance and frequent explanation of its benign and transient nature, a program of increasing physical activity, and drugs which allay anxiety and depression. However, the tricyclic antidepressants are generally less effective than in the mixed tension and throbbing headaches of anxious depressions. Tender scars from scalp laceration may be novocainized repeatedly (subcutaneous injection of 5 ml of 1% procaine) with some degree of success. Settlement of litigation as soon as possible works to the patient's advantage.

Heat, massage, salicylates, and indomethacin (Indocin) or phenylbutazone (Butazolidin) usually effect some improvement in those arthritic diseases of the cervical spine which are associated with cervicocranial pain (see Chap. 356).

Corticosteroid therapy is indicated in cranial arteritis to prevent disastrous blindness by occlusion of the ophthalmic

TABLE 4-1
Common types of headache

Type	Site	Age and sex	Clinical characteristics	Diurnal pattern	Life profile	Provoking factors	Associated features	Treatment
Common migraine	Frontotemporal Uni- or bilateral	Children, young to middle-aged adults both sexes	Throbbing and/or dull ache; worse behind one eye or ear Becomes generalized	Upon awakening or later in day Duration: hours to 1-2 days	Irregular interval, weeks to months Tends to disappear in middle age and during pregnancy	Bright light, noise, tension, alcohol Dark room and sleep relieve Scalp sensitive Pressure helps	Nausea in some cases	Ergot preparation at onset Phenergen in established phase Inderal and Bellargol Methysergide (Sansert) for prevention
"Neurologic" migraine	Same as above	Same as above	Same as above	Same as above	Same as above	Same as above	Blindness and scintillating lights Unilateral numbness Disturbed speech Vertigo Confusion	Same as above
Cluster, histamine headache, or migrainous neuralgia	Orbital Temporal Unilateral	Adolescent and adult males (80–90%)	Intense, nonthrobbing pain	Usually nocturnal; occurs one or more hours after falling asleep Rarely diurnal	Nightly for several weeks to months (cluster) Recurrence: years and later	Alcohol in some	Lacrimation, congested eye	Ergot preparation at bedtime Amytryptaline (Elavil) and lithium carbonate for prevention
Tension headaches	Generalized	Adolescents and adults, both sexes	Pressure (nonthrobbing); tightness Aching	Continuous, variable intensity, for weeks and months	One or more periods of months to years	Fatigue and nervous strain	Depression, nervousness, anxiety, insomnia	Antianxiety and antidepressant drugs
Meningeal irritation (meningitis subarachnoid hemorrhage)	Generalized	Any age, both sexes	Intense, steady deep pain, may be worse in neck	Duration: days to a week or more	Single episode	None	Neck stiff on forward bending Kernig and Brudzinski signs	For meningitis or bleeding (see text)
Brain tumor	(See text)	Any age, both sexes	Variable in intensity May awaken patient Steady pain	Lasts minutes to hours; increasing severity	Once in a lifetime: weeks to months	None Sometimes position	Papilledema Vomiting Slow mentation	Corticosteroids Mannitol Glycerol sargicine Treatment of tumor
Temporal arteritis	Unilateral, temporal, or occipital	Over 50 years, either sex	Persistent burning, aching	Continuous or intermittent	Persists for weeks to a few months	Scalp sensitive Tender arteries	Intermittent or permanent loss of sight Rheumatic myalgia Fever	Corticosteroid therapy

SOURCE: *After J Patten, Neurological Differential Diagnosis, London, Harold Starke, Springer-Verlag, 1977.*

TABLE 4-2
Types of facial pain

Types	Site	Clinical characteristics	Aggravating-relieving factors	Diseases	Treatment
Trigeminal neuralgia (tic douloureux)	Second to third division of trigeminal nerve, unilateral	Men: women = 1:3 Over 50 years Paroxysms (10–30 s) of stabbing, burning pain Trigger points, intermittent ache No sensory or motor paralysis	Touching face, chewing, smiling, talking, blowing nose	Idiopathic If in young adults and bilateral, multiple sclerosis Vascular anomaly Tumor of fifth cranial nerve	Carbamazepine (Tegretol) Phenytoin Surgical section of nerve
Atypical facial neuralgia	Unilateral or bilateral	Predominantly female 30–50 years Continuous intolerable pain Mainly maxillary areas	None	Depressive and anxiety states Hysteria Idiopathic	Antidepressant and antianxiety medication
Supraorbital ciliary, infraorbital, sphenopalatine neuralgias	Unilateral in eye, cheek, ear, neck	Persistent, aching pain	Occasional nasal obstruction	Idiopathic Paranasal sinus disease	Decongestant nasal medication ?Nerve section and injection
Postzoster neuralgia	Unilateral Any one of trigeminal divisions	History of zoster Aching, burning pain; jabs of pain Paresthesia, slight sensory loss Dermal scars	Contact, movement	Herpes zoster	Carbamazepine and phenytoin and antidepressants
Costen's syndrome	Unilateral, near temporomandibular joints	Elderly females Severe aching pain, intensified by chewing Tenderness over joints Malocclusion	Chewing, pressure over temporomandibular joint	Loss of teeth, rheumatoid arthritis	Bite correction and surgery
Tolosa-Hunt syndrome	Unilateral, mainly orbital	Intense sharp, aching pain; associated ophthalmoplegias of varying degree Intense sharp, aching pain Pupil inequality, sensory loss	None	?Arteritis and granulomatous lesions	Corticosteroids Nerve section (trigeminal)
Raeder's paratrigeminal syndrome	Unilateral, frontotemporal and maxilla	Intense sharp, aching pain Pupil inequality, sensory loss	None	Tumors, granulomatous lesions, injuries	Depends on type of lesion
Migrainous neuralgia	Orbitofrontal	See cluster headache, Table 4-1	None		Ergot

SOURCE: *After J Patten, Neurological Differential Diagnosis, London, Harold Starke, Springer-Verlag, 1977.*

arteries. The headaches of cranial tumor often respond surprisingly well to large doses of methylprednisolone acetate and like compounds.

In conclusion, it is well to mention the importance of general hygienic measures. Young physicians in particular are apt to seek a specific therapy for each headache syndrome and give little thought to the general health of the patient. We have observed that most of the recurrent and chronic headaches are likely to be more severe and disabling whenever the patient becomes nervous, sick, and tired. A well-rounded diet, adequate rest, a reasonable amount of physical exercise, and a balanced view of the sources of daily anxieties and how to cope with them should be the goal of all therapeutic programs.

REFERENCES

APPENZELLER O: *Pathogenesis and Treatment of Headache.* New York, Spectrum, 1976

CHAPMAN LF: A humoral agent implicated in vascular headache of the migraine type. Arch Neurol 3:223, 1960

CLOVER V et al: Transitory decrease in platelet monoamine oxidase activity during migraine attacks. Lancet 1:391, 1977

COUCH JR, HASSANEIM RS: Platelet aggregability in migraine. Neurology 27:843, 1977

FRIEDMAN AP: *Research and Clinical Studies in Headache.* Baltimore, Williams & Wilkins, 1967

LANCE JW: *The Mechanism and Management of Headache.* London, Butterworth, 1969

LANCE JW, HINTZENBERGER H: The control of cranial arteries by humoral mechanisms and its relation to the migraine syndrome. Headache 7:93, 1967

PARRY CH: *Collections from the Unpublished Medical Writing of the Late Caleb Hillier Parry.* London, Underwood, 1825, vol 1

SICUTERI F: Vasoneuroactive substances and their implication in vascular pain, in A Friedman (ed): *Research and Clinical Studies of Headache.* Baltimore, Williams & Wilkins, 1967, chap 2

SMITH R: *Background of Migraine.* New York, Springer, 1967

STREETER DHP et al: Hyperbradykinism, a new orthostatic syndrome. Lancet 2:1048, 1972

VIJAYAN N, DREYFUS PM: Posttraumatic dysautonomic cephalalgia: Clinical observations and treatment. Arch Neurol 32:649, 1976

VINKEN PJ, BRUYN GW: *Handbook of Clinical Neurology,* vol 5: *Headache and Cranial Neuralgias.* Amsterdam, North-Holland, 1968

WATSON P, STEELE JC: Paroxysmal dysequilibrium in the migraine syndrome of childhood. Arch Otolaryngol 99:177, 1974

5
CHEST PAIN AND PALPITATION

EUGENE BRAUNWALD

CHEST PAIN

There is little parallelism between the severity of chest pain and the gravity of its cause. Therefore, a frequent problem in patients who complain of chest pain is distinguishing trivial disorders from coronary artery disease and other serious disorders. An incorrect positive diagnosis of a hazardous condition such as angina pectoris is likely to have harmful psychologic and economic consequences, while failure to recognize a serious disorder, such as coronary artery disease or mediastinal tumor, may result in the dangerous delay of much-needed treatment.

The apparently bizarre radiation of pain arising in the thoracic viscera can usually be explained in terms of the known facts concerning nerve supply (Chap. 3). One occasionally sees a patient with extension of pain to a location which cannot be logically explained. In most instances, such a person will be found to have more than one disorder capable of causing pain in the chest. The presence of one condition may affect the radiation of the pain produced by the other disorder. For example, when the pain of angina pectoris extends to the back or abdomen, the patient may be found to have also a significant degree of spinal arthritis or an upper abdominal disorder, such as hiatus hernia, disease of the gallbladder, pancreatitis, or peptic ulcer. The common tendency to assume that the presence of an objective abnormality, such as a hiatus hernia or an electrocardiographic abnormality, necessarily means that an atypical chest pain arises in the stomach or the heart is to be strongly condemned. Such an assumption is justified only if a careful history indicates that the behavior of the pain is entirely compatible with the site of origin suggested by the objective finding.

THE LEFT-ARM MYTH There is a long tradition, widely accepted by physicians and laymen, that pain in the left arm, especially when appearing in conjunction with chest pain, has a unique and ominous significance as being almost certain evidence of the presence of ischemic heart disease. This is a myth that has neither theoretic nor clinical foundation. From a theoretic standpoint, any disorder involving the deep afferent fibers of the left upper thoracic region should be capable of causing pain in the chest, the left arm, or both areas. Hence a pain of trivial significance arising in skeletal tissues innervated by upper (first to fourth) thoracic nerves may produce left-arm-area pain; almost any condition capable of causing pain in the chest may induce radiation to the left arm. Such localization is common not only in patients with coronary disease but also in those with numerous other types of chest pain. Although pain due to myocardial ischemia most frequently is substernal, radiates down the ulnar aspect of the left arm (Chap. 244), and is pressing and constricting in nature, the location, radiation, and quality of pain are of less diagnostic significance than the behavior of the pain, in terms of the conditions which induce it and relieve it.

Most persons also believe that cardiac pain is situated in the region of the left breast, and therefore left inframammary pain is one of the common symptoms that bring the patient to seek medical advice. It differs radically from the pain due to myocardial hypoxia, i.e., angina pectoris, in that it is either momentary, sharp and lancinating, or a long-lasting, dull ache, occasionally accentuated by sharp stabs. Such pain is frequently observed in patients who are tense, easily fatigued, unusually anxious, or psychoneurotic, or who have neurocirculatory asthenia. In contrast to angina pectoris, such precordial pain has no relationship to exertion and may be accompanied by tenderness over the precordium.

PAIN DUE TO OXYGEN DEFICIENCY OF THE MYOCARDIUM
Physiologic considerations of the coronary circulation Pain due to myocardial ischemia occurs when the oxygen supply to the heart is deficient in relation to the oxygen need. The oxygen consumption of this organ is closely related to the physiologic effort made during contraction. It is dependent primarily on three factors: (1) the tension developed by the myocardium, (2) the contractile (inotropic) state of the myocardium, and (3) the heart rate. When these three factors remain constant, or almost so, an elevation of stroke volume produces an efficient type of response because it leads to an increase in the external work of the heart (i.e., in the product of cardiac output and arterial pressure) with little accompanying augmentation of myocardial oxygen requirements. Thus, a rise in flow load causes less increment in myocardial oxygen consumption than does a comparable increase in cardiac work per minute brought about by elevation either of pressure or of heart rate. However, the net effects of these hemodynamic variables depend not on oxygen need alone, but rather on the balance between the demand and the supply of oxygen. The heart is always active, and the coronary venous blood is normally much more desaturated than that draining other areas of the body. Thus the removal of more oxygen from each unit of blood, which is one of the adjustments commonly utilized by exercising skeletal muscle, is already employed in the heart in the basal state. Therefore, the heart must rely on an increase in the coronary blood flow for obtaining additional oxygen.

It follows, from hydrodynamic considerations, that the flow of blood through the coronary arteries is directly proportional to the pressure gradient between the aorta and the ventricular myocardium during systole and the ventricular cavity during diastole, but is proportional to the fourth power of the radius of the coronary arteries. Thus a relatively slight alteration in coronary diameter will produce a large change in coronary flow, provided that other factors remain constant. In the normal heart, coronary blood flow occurs primarily during diastole, when it is unopposed by myocardial constriction of the coronary vessels. Coronary flow is regulated primarily by myocardial oxygen needs, probably through the release of vasodilator metabolites, such as adenosine, and through variations in myocardial P_{O_2}. Although changes in coronary blood flow occur with activation of autonomic nerves to the coronary vessels, these alterations result primarily from the effects of these nervous stimuli on myocardial contraction and therefore on the heart's oxygen consumption. The role of direct neural regulation of the coronary vascular bed is controversial.

The coronary dilatation which normally occurs during exercise and emotion results from the increased myocardial metabolism during these conditions and is impaired in patients with fixed coronary narrowing due to coronary arteriosclerosis. Thus, any condition in which increased heart rate, arterial pressure, or myocardial contractility occurs tends, particularly in the presence of coronary obstruction, to precipitate anginal attacks by increasing myocardial oxygen needs. Bradycardia, when not severe, usually has the opposite effects, and this apparently explains the rarity of angina in patients with complete heart block, even when this disorder is associated with coronary disease.

Causes of myocardial hypoxia By far the most frequent underlying cause is organic narrowing of the coronary arteries secondary to coronary atherosclerosis. Less frequently, narrowing of the coronary orifices due to syphilitic aortitis or to distortion by a dissecting aneurysm may be responsible. There is no evidence that systemic arterial constriction or increased cardiac contractile activity (rise in heart rate or blood pressure, or increase in contractility due to liberation of catecholamines or adrenergic activity) due to emotion can precipitate angina unless there is also structural narrowing of the coronary vessels. While this is usually on an organic basis and secondary to arteriosclerosis, recently it has become clear that coronary artery spasm, with or without accompanying atherosclerosis, can also precipitate angina.

Aside from conditions which narrow the lumen of the coronary arteries, the only other frequent causes of myocardial hypoxia are disorders, such as aortic stenosis and/or regurgitation (Chap. 242), which cause a marked disproportion between the perfusion pressure and the ventricular work. Under such conditions the rise in left ventricular systolic pressure is not, as in hypertensive states, balanced by a corresponding elevation of aortic perfusion pressure. Therefore, an increase in heart rate is especially harmful in patients with aortic stenosis, because it shortens diastole more than systole and thereby decreases the total available perfusion time per minute.

Patients with marked *right ventricular hypertension* may have exertional pain which is, in most respects, identical with that of the common type of angina. It is likely that this discomfort results from relative ischemia of the right ventricle brought about by the increased oxygen needs and by the elevated intramural resistance, with sharp reduction of the normally large systolic pressure gradient which perfuses this chamber. Angina is common in patients with *syphilitic aortitis,* and the relative roles of aortic regurgitation and of coronary ostial narrowing are difficult to assess. The importance of tachycardia, decline in arterial pressure, thyrotoxicosis, or diminution in arterial oxygen content (such as occurs in anemia or arterial hypoxemia) in the production of myocardial hypoxia will be apparent from the above discussion. However, these are precipitating and aggravating factors rather than the underlying cause of angina; as already noted, the latter is, in almost all instances, coronary atherosclerosis.

Effects of myocardial hypoxia The most common of these is anginal pain, which is considered in some detail in Chap. 244. It is usually described as a heavy pressure or squeezing, a sensation of strangling or constriction in the chest, a "burning" or "heavy feeling," or difficulty in breathing, and it occurs particularly on walking, especially after meals, on cold days against a wind or uphill. It is not a stabbing pain. It occurs during exertion, following heavy meals, and with anger, excitement, and other emotional states; it is not precipitated by coughing or respiratory movements. When anginal pain is induced by walking, it forces the patient to stop or to reduce his speed; it is characteristically relieved by rest and nitroglycerin. The exact mechanism of the pain stimulus is still unknown, but it is probably related to an accumulation of metabolites within the heart muscle. Anginal pain occurs most typically in the substernal region, anteriorly across the midthorax; it may radiate to or rarely occur alone in the interscapular region, in the arms, shoulders, and teeth. The more severe the attack, the greater the radiation from the substernal areas to the left arm, especially its ulnar aspect. There is considerable variability in the amount of effort required to bring on anginal pain.

As a rule, myocardial infarction is associated with a pain similar in quality and distribution to that of angina but of greater intensity and longer duration. The pain of myocardial infarction is not relieved by rest or by coronary dilator drugs and may require large doses of narcotics. It may be accompanied by diaphoresis, nausea, and hypotension (Chap. 245).

In addition to chest pain, a second effect of myocardial ischemia consists of electrocardiographic changes (Chaps. 232, 244, and 245). Many patients with angina have normal tracings between attacks, and the record may even remain normal during the episode of pain. However, often depression of the ST segments appears in leads I, II, aVL, or in those from the left precordium during exertion. The finding of ST-segment depressions of a deep, ischemic type during an attack of pain, with a return to normal after the pain subsides, strongly suggests that the pain is anginal in origin. There is strong experimental evidence that such depressions, as well as the elevations which are usually seen in patients with infarction and are observed in a few patients during anginal attacks, are related to alterations in cellular ionic balance (Chap. 232). The value and limitation of electrocardiographic changes occurring after exercise in the diagnosis of angina pectoris are discussed in Chap. 244.

A third effect of myocardial hypoxia is an alteration in myocardial contraction. It has been shown that the left ventricular end-diastolic and pulmonary vascular pressures may rise during anginal attacks, particularly if they are prolonged. This indicates transient depression of left ventricular function, which is presumably induced by the decreased contractility of the ischemic areas. On auscultation a fourth heart sound is also frequently heard during the anginal episode; paradoxic pulsations may be evident on palpation of the precordium and can be recorded by apex cardiography.

Another characteristic effect of myocardial hypoxia is liability to sudden death (Chap. 32). This may never occur, despite thousands of anginal episodes. However, it may supervene early in the disease and even in the first attack. The usual mechanism is probably ventricular fibrillation, but occasionally in patients with impaired atrioventricular conduction sudden death may be due to ventricular standstill.

PAIN DUE TO IRRITATION OF SEROUS MEMBRANES OR JOINTS Pericarditis The visceral surface of the pericardium is ordinarily insensitive to pain, as is the parietal surface, except in its lower portion, which has a relatively small number of pain fibers carried in the phrenic nerves. The pain associated with pericarditis is believed to be due to inflammation of the adjacent parietal pleura. These observations explain why noninfectious pericarditis (that associated with uremia and with myocardial infarction) and cardiac tamponade with relatively mild inflammation are usually painless or accompanied by mild pain, whereas infectious pericarditis, being nearly always more intense and spreading to the neighboring pleura, is usually associated with pain having some pleuritic features, i.e., it is aggravated by breathing, coughing, etc. Since the central part of the diaphragm receives its sensory supply from the phrenic nerve (which arises from the third to fifth cervical segments of the spinal cord), pain arising from the lower parietal pericardium and central tendon of the diaphragm is felt characteristically at the tip of the shoulder, the adjoining trapezius ridge, and the neck. Involvement of the more lateral part of the diaphragmatic pleura, supplied by branches from the sixth to ninth intercostal nerves, causes pain not only in the anterior part of the chest but also in the upper part of the abdomen or corresponding region of the back, thus sometimes simulating the pain of acute cholecystitis or pancreatitis.

Pericarditis causes three distinct types of pain (Chap. 249):

1 By far the commonest is the pleuritic pain, related to respiratory movements and aggravated by cough or deep inspiration. It is sometimes brought on by swallowing, because the esophagus lies just beyond the posterior portion of the heart. It is often altered by a change of bodily position, becoming sharper and more left-sided. It is frequently referred to the neck or flank and lasts longer than the pain of angina pectoris. This type of pain is due to the pleuritic component of the pleuropericarditis so commonly present in the infectious forms.

2 The next commonest pericardial pain is the steady, crushing substernal pain which mimics that of acute myocardial infarction. The mechanism of this steady substernal pain is not certain, but the pain may arise from marked inflammation of the relatively insensitive inner parietal surface of the pericardium, or from irritated afferent cardiac nerve fibers lying in the periadventitial layers of the superficial coronary arteries.

3 The third type of pain, which is quite uncommon, is synchronous with the heartbeat and is felt at the left border of the heart and left shoulder.

Occasionally two and rarely all three types of pain may be present simultaneously.

The painful syndromes which may follow trauma to or operations on the heart (i.e., the postcardiotomy syndrome) or myocardial infarction are discussed in later chapters (Chaps. 245 and 249). Such pains often but not always arise in the pericardium.

Pleural pain is very common; it generally results from stretching of inflamed parietal pleura and may be identical with that of pericarditis. It occurs in fibrinous pleurisy, as well as when pneumonic processes reach the periphery of the lung. Pneumothorax and tumors involving the pleural space may also irritate the parietal pleura and cause pleural pain; the latter is sharp, knifelike, superficial in quality, and its aggravation by each breath and by coughing readily distinguishes it from the deep, dull, steady unwavering pain of myocardial ischemia.

The pain resulting from *pulmonary embolism* may resemble that of acute myocardial infarction, and in massive embolism it is located substernally. In patients with smaller emboli the pain is located more laterally, is pleuritic in nature, and may be associated with hemoptysis (Chap. 266). Massive pulmonary emboli and other causes of acute pulmonary hypertension may cause severe, persistent substernal pain, presumably due to distention of the pulmonary artery. The pain of mediastinal emphysema (Chap. 269) may be intense and sharp and may radiate from the substernal region to the shoulders; often a distinct crepitus is heard. The pain associated with mediastinitis and mediastinal tumors usually resembles that of pleuritis but is more likely to be maximal in the substernal region, and the associated feeling of constriction or oppression may cause confusion with myocardial infarction. The pain due to *acute dissection of the aorta* or to an expanding aortic aneurysm results from stimulation of the adventitia; it is usually extremely severe, is localized to the center of the chest, lasts for hours, and requires unusually large amounts of analgesics for relief. It often radiates into the back but is not aggravated by changes in position or respiration (Chap. 252).

The *costochondral and chondrosternal articulations* are the commonest sites of anterior chest pain. Objective signs in the form of swelling (Tietze's syndrome), redness, and heat are rare, but sharply localized tenderness is common. The pain may be "neuritic," i.e., darting and lasting for only a few seconds, or a dull ache enduring for hours or days. An associated feeling of tightness due to muscle spasm (see below) is frequent. When the discomfort persists for a few days only, a story of minor trauma or of some unaccustomed physical effort can often be obtained. The variety of this discomfort is common in persons with arthritis of the spine and also in patients with ischemic heart disease, but in many instances no associated disorder is found. It should be emphasized that *pressure on the chondrosternal and costochondral junctions is an essential part of the examination of every patient with chest pain.* A large

percentage of patients with costochondral pain, especially those who also have minor and innocent T-wave alterations (Chap. 232), are erroneously labeled as having coronary disease. The dire consequences of such a mistake have already been emphasized.

Pain secondary to *subacromial bursitis* and *arthritis of the shoulder and spine* may be precipitated by exercise of the local area but not by general exertion. It may be brought about by passive movement of the involved area as well as by coughing.

PAIN DUE TO TISSUE DISRUPTION Rupture or tear of a structure may give rise to pain that sets in abruptly and reaches its peak of intensity almost instantly. Such a story should arouse the suspicion of dissecting aortic aneurysm, pneumothorax, mediastinal emphysema, a cervical disk syndrome, or rupture of the esophagus. However, the patient may be too ill to recall the precise circumstances, or the pain may be atypical and increase gradually in severity. Likewise, other and more benign conditions, such as a slipped costal cartilage or an intercostal muscle cramp, may also produce pain with an abrupt onset.

Dissecting aortic aneurysm usually causes very severe persistent pain located in the anterior chest. It often radiates into the back, and is not intensified by breathing or motion.

CLINICAL ASPECTS OF THE COMMONER CAUSES OF CHEST PAIN Some of the features of pericarditis have already been described, and those of the more serious causes of chest pain such as myocardial ischemia (angina pectoris and infarction), dissecting aneurysm, and disorders of the pleura, esophagus, stomach, duodenum, and pancreas are considered in the appropriate chapters dealing with these problems. Here, we are concerned with the discussion of those causes which are not considered in more detail elsewhere.

Pain arising in the chest wall or upper extremity This may develop as a result of muscle or ligament strains brought on by unaccustomed exercise and felt in the costochondral or chondrosternal junctions or in the chest wall muscles. We mention the upper extremities and especially the left because of the deeply ingrained legend that pain in the left arm has a specific significance in indicting the heart. Other causes are *osteoarthritis* of the dorsal or thoracic spine and *ruptured cervical disks.* Pain in the left upper extremity and precordium may be due to compression of portions of the brachial plexus by a cervical rib or by spasm and shortening of the scalenus anticus muscle secondary to high fixation of the ribs and sternum. Finally, pains in the upper extremity (shoulder-hand syndrome) and in the pectoral muscles may, through unknown mechanisms, occur in patients with ischemic heart disease.

Skeletal pains in the chest wall or shoulder girdles or arms are usually recognized quite easily. Localized tenderness of the affected area is usually present, and the pain is sometimes clearly related to movements involving the painful locus. Thus deep breathing, turning or twisting of the chest, and movements of the shoulder girdle and arm will elicit and duplicate the pain of which the patient complains. The pain may be very brief, lasting only a few seconds, or full and aching and enduring for hours. The duration is, therefore, likely to be either longer or shorter than untreated anginal pain, which usually lasts for only a few minutes.

These skeletal pains often have a sharp or sticking quality. In addition, there is frequently a feeling of tightness, which is probably due to associated spasm of intercostal or pectoral muscles. This may produce the "morning stiffness" seen in so many skeletal disorders. The discomfort is unaffected by nitroglycerin but often is abolished by infiltration of the painful areas with procaine. When chest wall pain is of recent origin and follows trauma, strain, or some unusual activity involving the pectoral muscles, it presents no problem in diagnosis. However, long-standing skeletal pain is frequent in persons who also have angina pectoris. Since both disorders are very common, this association may be coincidental. In other instances, the coronary disease appears to be responsible for the chest wall pain; the exact mechanism is uncertain but probably is similar to that responsible for the well-known shoulder-hand syndrome. This coexistence of the two different types of chest pain in the same patient is a frequent cause of a confusing history, because in the patient's mind the anginal needle may be hidden in the skeletal haystack. Thus every middle-aged or elderly patient who has long-standing anterior chest wall pain merits careful study for the presence of ischemic heart disease.

Detailed questioning may reveal that what was originally thought by the patient to be a single type of discomfort actually comprises two different pains, which, though similar in quality and area, differ in duration and initiating factors. When the history is inconclusive, the exercise electrocardiogram may furnish useful information concerning the existence of myocardial ischemia. In rare instances coronary arteriography may be required. It may be necessary also to learn by direct observation whether exercise alone or postprandial exertion is capable of producing it. Repeated tests may be required, comparing the relative effects of preceding placebos and nitroglycerin on the amount of exertion required to induce the pain. *The confusion created by the presence of innocent skeletal pain impairs the reliability of the history and is probably the commonest cause of errors—both positive and negative—in the diagnosis of angina pectoris.*

Esophageal pain This usually presents as deep thoracic pain; it results from chemical (acid) irritation of the esophageal mucosa or from spasm of the esophageal muscle in the presence of an intraluminal obstruction, and characteristically follows deglutition. Accompanying dysphagia, regurgitation of undigested food, and weight loss direct attention to the esophagus (see Chaps. 34 and 289).

Emotional disorders These are also common causes of chest wall pain. Usually, the discomfort is experienced as a sense of "tightness," sometimes called "aching," and occasionally it may be sufficiently severe as to be designated a pain of considerable magnitude. Since the discomfort has almost always the additional quality of tightness or constriction, and, furthermore, since it is often localized beneath the sternum, although it may be felt in other areas of the anterior part of the chest, it is not surprising that this type of pain is frequently confused with that of myocardial ischemia. Ordinarily, it lasts for a half hour or more and may persist for a day or less with slow fluctuation of intensity. The association with fatigue or emotional strain is usually clear, although this may not be recognized by the patient until called to his attention. The pain probably develops through unconscious and prolonged increase of muscle tone (as in frowning in the face, or as can be quickly produced in the hand by rigidly clenching the fist), often enhanced by an accompanying hyperventilation (by causing a contraction of the chest wall muscles similar to the painful tetany of the extremities). When the hyperventilation and/or the associated andrenergic effect due to anxiety also causes innocent changes in the T waves and ST segments, the confusion with coronary disease is strengthened. However, the long duration of the pain, the lack of any relation to exertion but association rather with fatigue or tension, and the usually periodic occurrence on successive days without any limitation of capacity for exercise usually make the differentiation from ischemic pain quite clear.

As compared with these two causes (the chest wall muscle and ligament strains and the contraction of the pectoral muscles due to reflex influences, fatigue, or tension), the various

other conditions that may cause skeletal discomfort are uncommon and readily recognized after appropriate observation: spinal arthritis, herpes zoster, anterior scalene and hyperabduction syndromes, malignant disease of the ribs, etc.

Other causes of chest pain The several *abdominal disorders* which may at times mimic anginal pain may usually be suspected from the history, which, as in esophageal pain, ordinarily indicates some relationship to swallowing, eating, belching, etc. Pain resulting from gastric or duodenal ulcer (Chap. 290) is epigastric or substernal, commences about 1 to 1½ h after meals, and is usually promptly relieved by antacids or milk. The gastrointestinal roentgenogram is of crucial significance, and roentgenographic examination is also often helpful in differentiating biliary, gastrointestinal, aortic, pulmonary, and skeletal disease pain from angina pectoris. It should be emphasized again that the demonstration of the presence of a coexistent abdominal disorder such as a hiatus hernia does not constitute proof that the chest pain of which the patient complains is due to this. Such disorders are frequently asymptomatic and are not at all uncommon in patients who also have angina pectoris.

Substernal discomfort also frequently occurs in the presence of *tracheobronchitis;* it is described as a burning sensation accentuated by coughing. A variety of *disorders involving the breast,* including inflammatory breast disease, benign and malignant tumors, as well as mastodynia, are common causes of thoracic pain. The localization and superficial swelling and tenderness are of diagnostic importance.

APPROACH TO THE PATIENT WITH PAIN IN THE CHEST Most persons with this complaint will fall into one of two general groups. The first consists of persons with prolonged and often severe pain without obvious initiating factors. Such persons will frequently be gravely ill. The problem is that of differentiating such serious conditions as myocardial infarction, dissecting aneurysm, and pulmonary embolism from each other and from less grave causes. In some such instances, the careful history will provide significant clues, while objective evidence of crucial importance will appear within the subsequent 2 or 3 days. Thus, when the initial examinations are not decisive, a watch-and-wait policy, with repeated electrocardiograms coupled with measurements of serum enzymes, lung scans, and chest roentgenograms, will commonly provide the correct answer.

The second group of patients comprises those who have brief episodes of pain and are otherwise in apparently excellent health. Here, the resting electrocardiogram will rarely supply decisive information, but records taken during or immediately after exercise will often reveal characteristic changes (Chap. 244). However, in many instances it is the study of the subjective phenomenon, i.e., of the pain itself, that will lead to the diagnosis. Of the several methods of investigation which are available for such patients, three are of cardinal importance.

A detailed and *meticulous history* of the behavior of the pain is the most important method. The location, radiation, quality, intensity, and, especially, duration of the episodes are important. Even more so is the story of the aggravating and alleviating factors. Thus a history of sharp aggravation by breathing, coughing, or other respiratory movements will usually point toward the pericardium (because of the associated pleuropericarditis) or mediastinum as the site, although chest wall pain is likewise affected by respiratory motions. Similarly, a pain which regularly appears on rapid walking and vanishes within a few minutes upon standing still suggests the diagnosis of angina pectoris, although here, once again, a similar story will rarely be obtained from patients with skeletal disorders.

When the history is inconclusive, the *study of the patient at the time of the spontaneous episode* will often supply crucial information. Thus the electrocardiogram, which may be normal both at rest and even during or after exercise in the absence of pain, will occasionally demonstrate striking changes when recorded during an anginal episode. Similarly, radiographic study of the esophagus or of the stomach may show no evidence of cardiospasm or of hiatal hernia except when the observation is made during the pain.

The third method of study represents the *attempt to produce and alleviate the pain at will.* This procedure is necessary only when doubt exists following the history or when needed for psychotherapeutic purposes. Thus the demonstration that a localized pain, which can be reproduced by pressure on the chest, is completely relieved by local infiltration with procaine will often be of conclusive importance in convincing the patient that the heart is not the site.

When, as is not rarely the case, the history is atypical, the correct diagnosis of angina pectoris will often depend in large measure on the response to nitroglycerin. Here, a number of pitfalls should be avoided. If the patient has previously had the drug, careful questioning may be necessary to avoid errors. Thus, relief of pain after its sublingual administration does not necessarily prove that there is a cause-and-effect relationship. It is necessary to be certain that the pain vanishes more rapidly (usually within 5 min) and more completely when the drug is used than when it is not employed. A false negative impression concerning the effect of nitroglycerin may be the result of the use of a deteriorated preparation which has been exposed to light. In doubtful instances, repeated exercise tests, with and without preceding administration of nitroglycerin, are necessary. The demonstration that the time required for a given exercise to produce pain is consistently and considerably longer when it is undertaken within a few minutes after a sublingual nitroglycerin pill than after a placebo may, in some instances, represent the sole method for accurate recognition of angina pectoris. A completely negative response to such repeated tests constitutes almost conclusive evidence against angina.

In patients in whom the question of whether there is coronary disease cannot be resolved despite the aforementioned clinical and laboratory tests, including exercise electrocardiography (Chap. 244), cardiac catheterization and coronary arteriography may be required. A useful stress test that can be carried out at the time of catheterization is to elevate the heart rate in stepwise fashion by electrical pacing; the development of ST-segment depressions on the electrocardiogram and the reproduction of the pain support the diagnosis of myocardial ischemia. Coronary arteriography will show severe (more than 75 percent) reduction of the lumen in patients with obstructive coronary artery disease (Chaps. 234 and 244).

PALPITATION

Palpitation is a common, disagreeable subjective phenomenon which may be defined as an awareness of the beating of the heart, an awareness most commonly brought about by a change in the heart's rhythm or rate or by an augmentation of its contractility. Palpitation is not pathognomonic of any particular group of disorders; indeed, often it signifies not a primary physical disorder but rather a psychic disturbance. Even when it occurs as a more or less prominent complaint, the diagnosis of the underlying disease is made largely on the basis of other associated symptoms and data. Nevertheless, palpitation is frequently of considerable importance in the minds of

patients, who fear that it may indicate heart disease. Concern is all the more pronounced in patients who know or who have been told that they may have heart disease; to them palpitation may seem to be an omen of impending disaster. Since the resulting anxiety may be associated with increased activity of the autonomic nervous system, with consequent increases of the cardiac rate and rhythm and the vigor of contraction, the patient's awareness of these changes may then lead to a vicious cycle, which may ultimately be responsible for his incapacitation.

Palpitation may be described by the patient in various terms, such as "pounding," "fluttering," "flopping," and "skipping," and in most cases it will be obvious that the complaint is of a sensation of disturbed heartbeat. The wide variability in the sensitivity to alterations in cardiac activity among different individuals must be appreciated. Some patients seem to be unaware of the most serious and chaotic dysrhythmias; others are seriously troubled by an occasional extrasystole. Patients with anxiety states often exhibit a lowered threshold at which disorders of rate and rhythm result in palpitation. Indeed, it is not unusual for palpitation to be the major manifestation of the emotional disorder. The awareness of the heartbeat also tends to be more common at night and during introspective moments, but is less marked during activity. Patients with organic heart disease and chronic disorders of cardiac rate, rhythm, or stroke volume tend to accommodate to these abnormalities and are often less sensitive than normal persons to such events. Persistent tachycardia and/or atrial fibrillation may not be accompanied by continual palpitation, in contrast to a sudden, brief alteration in cardiac rate or rhythm which often causes considerable subjective discomfort. Thus, palpitation is particularly prominent when the precipitating cause for increased heart rate or contractility or arrhythmia is recent, transient, and episodic. Conversely, in emotionally well-adjusted individuals palpitation becomes progressively less disconcerting as the cause (e.g., anemia, frequent extrasystoles, complete atrioventricular block) persists.

PATHOGENESIS OF PALPITATION Under ordinary circumstances the rhythmic heartbeat is imperceptible to the healthy individual of average or placid temperament. Palpitation may be experienced by normal persons who have engaged in strenuous physical effort or have been aroused emotionally or sexually. This type of palpitation is physiologic and represents the normal awareness of an overactive heart—i.e., a heart that is beating at a rapid rate and with an increased contractility. Since palpitation due to overactivity of the heart may occur also in certain pathologic states, e.g., high fever, severe anemia, or thyrotoxicosis, it is commonly assumed that it is the overactivity per se that is responsible for the symptom.

When palpitation is heavy and regular, it is usually caused by an augmented stroke volume, and it should raise the question of aortic or mitral regurgitation, ventricular septal defect, or of a variety of hyperkinetic circulatory states (anemia, arteriovenous fistula, thyrotoxicosis, and the so-called "idiopathic hyperkinetic heart syndrome"). It may also occur immediately after the onset of cardiac slowing, as with the sudden development of heart block, or upon the conversion of sinus rhythm from atrial fibrillation. But unusual movements of the heart within the thorax are also frequently the mechanism of palpitation. Thus, the ectopic beat and/or the compensatory pause may be appreciated, since both are associated with alterations in cardiac motion.

IMPORTANT CAUSES OF PALPITATION See also Chap. 237.

Extrasystoles In most cases the diagnosis will be suggested by the patient's story. The premature contraction and postpremature beat are often described as a "flopping," or the patient may say that he feels as if "the heart turns over." The pause following the premature contraction may be felt as an actual cessation of the heartbeat, in contrast with the complete unawareness of pauses of similar duration when atrial fibrillation with a slow ventricular rate occurs. The first ventricular contraction succeeding the pause may be felt as an unusually vigorous beat and will be described as "pounding" or "thudding."

When extrasystoles are numerous, clinical differentiation from atrial fibrillation can be made by any procedure that will bring about a definite increase in the ventricular rate; at increasingly rapid heart rates, the extrasystoles usually diminish in frequency and then disappear, whereas the ventricular irregularity of atrial fibrillation increases.

Ectopic tachycardias These conditions, which are considered in some detail in Chap. 237, are common and medically important causes of palpitation. Ventricular tachycardia, one of the most serious arrhythmias, rarely is manifested as palpitation; this may be related to the abnormal sequence, and hence impaired coordination and vigor, of ventricular contraction. If the patient is seen between attacks, the diagnosis of ectopic tachycardia and its type will have to depend on the history, but of course the precise diagnosis can be made only when an electrocardiogram and observations on the effect of carotid sinus pressure are made during the episode. The mode of onset and offset gives the most important lead in distinguishing sinus from one of the various forms of ectopic tachycardias; sinus tachycardia commences and ceases over the course of minutes or seconds, but not instantaneously as is characteristic of ectopic rhythms. Monitoring of the electrocardiogram with a portable tape recording system and asking the patient to record the time of onset and cessation of the palpitations are extremely helpful in determining their cause. The technique of ambulatory electrocardiography is discussed in Chap. 237.

Thyrotoxicosis In its fully developed form, thyrotoxicosis will usually be evident and offers little difficulty in the way of diagnosis except in the elderly, in whom so-called "apathetic hyperthyroidism" may be present. Thyrotoxicosis is particularly likely to be overlooked in the presence of myocardial failure (Chap. 335).

Anemia When mild, anemia may cause palpitation during exertion; when severe, palpitation may be present at rest. Palpitation is more prominent the more rapidly the anemia develops. Appropriate studies of the blood will clarify the situation.

Fever Palpitation may be present in acute infections, particularly in the early stages, but here the symptom is merely an insignificant phenomenon in the midst of other obviously more important ones. Palpitation may be a prominent but not usually the principal presenting symptom in an individual suffering from one of the chronic and sometimes more obscure febrile illnesses, such as tuberculosis, chronic brucellosis, subacute infective endocarditis, or acute rheumatic fever with carditis and relatively few or no joint manifestations.

Hypoglycemia Palpitation is often a prominent feature of this condition and appears to be related to release of catecholamines. The diagnosis is confirmed by appropriate blood sugar estimations at the time of symptoms, by reproduction of the symptom following fasting or a 5-h glucose tolerance test, and by prompt relief of all symptoms on the administration of glucose (Chap. 340).

Tumors of the adrenal medulla (pheochromocytomas) Such tumors may give rise to recurrent attacks, including paroxysms

of hypertension and palpitation which are identical with those seen following the injection of epinephrine or norepinephrine. This type of tumor is a rather uncommon cause of palpitation and is mentioned chiefly because cure may be effected by surgical removal (Chap. 337).

Drugs The relationship between the development of palpitation and the use of tobacco, coffee, tea, alcohol, epinephrine, ephedrine, aminophylline, atropine, or thyroid extract is obvious.

Palpitation as a manifestation of the anxiety state Persons who are healthy physically and well adjusted emotionally may have palpitation under certain circumstances. Thus, during or immediately after vigorous physical exertion or during sudden emotional tension, palpitation is common and is usually associated with sinus tachycardia. In poorly conditioned persons without organic heart disease, the sinus tachycardia of exercise may be excessive and associated with palpitation.

In some patients, palpitation may be one of the outstanding manifestations of an episode of acute anxiety. In other persons the palpitation may, with other symptoms, represent prolonged anxiety neurosis or a lifelong disorder characterized by volatile autonomic function. The latter condition has been called *neurocirculatory asthenia.* Whether these illnesses are simply an expression of a chronic, deep-seated anxiety state superimposed on a normal autonomic nervous system or whether they depend on instability of the autonomic nervous system is not clear. At any rate, the clinical significance of the differentiation between the transitory and the enduring forms is that the former is often dissipated by firm reassurance from the physician, whereas the latter is usually resistant even to the most thorough and expert psychiatric care. In the latter case, the patient must be treated with most carefully planned psychologic support and tranquilizing medications. This chronic form of palpitation is known by various names such as *Da Costa's syndrome, soldier's heart, effort syndrome, irritable heart, neurocirculatory asthenia,* and *functional cardiovascular disease.* Aside from palpitation, the chief symptoms are those of an anxiety state.

Physical examination usually reveals the typical findings of the hyperkinetic syndrome. These include a left parasternal lift, a precordial or apical systolic murmur, a wide pulse pressure, rapidly rising pulse, and excessive perspiration. The electrocardiogram may display minor depressions of the ST junction and inversion of T waves and so occasionally lead to a mistaken diagnosis of coronary disease; this is particularly likely to occur when these findings are associated with complaints by the patients of an aching feeling of substernal tightness, commonly present in emotional stress. The presence of any kind of organic disease is one of the commonest causes of the underlying anxiety which frequently precipitates this functional syndrome.

Even when a patient presents undoubted objective evidence of structural cardiac disease, the possibility that a superimposed anxiety responsible for the symptoms when the clinical picture is that which has been described should be considered. Palpitation associated with organic cardiac disease is nearly always accompanied by arrhythmia or by marked tachycardia, whereas the symptom may exist with regular rhythm and with a heart rate of 80 beats per minute or less in patients with the anxiety state. It is noteworthy that an anxiety state, in contrast to heart disease, causes a sighing type of dyspnea. Also pain localized to the region of the apex, either brief and lancinating

TABLE 5-1
Items to be covered in history

Does the palpitation occur:	If so, suspect:
As isolated "jumps" or "skips"?	Extrasystoles
In attacks, known to be of abrupt beginning, with a heart rate of 120 beats per minute or over, or regular or irregular rhythm?	Paroxysmal rapid heart action
Independent of exercise or excitement adequate to account for the symptom?	Atrial fibrillation, atrial flutter, thyrotoxicosis, anemia, febrile states, hypoglycemia, anxiety state
In attacks developing rapidly though not absolutely abruptly, unrelated to exertion or excitement?	Hemorrhage, hypoglycemia, tumor of the adrenal medulla
In conjunction with the taking of drugs?	Tobacco, coffee, tea, alcohol, epinephrine, ephedrine, aminophylline, atropine, thyroid extract, monoamine oxidase inhibitors
On standing?	Postural hypotension
In middle-aged women, in conjunction with flushes and sweats?	Menopausal syndrome
When the rate is known to be normal and the rhythm regular?	Anxiety state

in character or lasting for hours or days and accompanied by hyperesthesia, is due usually to an anxiety state, not to structural cardiac disease. Giddiness due to this syndrome can usually be reproduced by hyperventilation (Chap. 13) or by change from the recumbent to the erect posture.

The *treatment* of the anxiety state with palpitation is difficult and depends on removal of the cause. In many instances a thorough examination of the heart and a statement that it is normal will suffice. Instructions to take more rather than less physical exercise will reinforce these statements. Frequently, the demonstration that the physician can reproduce not only the palpitation but many other symptoms of the anxiety state merely by the subcutaneous injection of 0.5 to 1.0 ml of 1:1000 epinephrine serves to convince the patient that the symptoms are not the result of some mysterious disorder but are rather the effect of a well-understood physiologic mechanism. This is especially true when the initial anxiety has been mainly the result of fear of heart disease. When the anxiety state is a manifestation of chronic anxiety neurosis or depressive psychosis, the symptoms are more likely to persist.

Management of patients with palpitation and the anxiety cardiac syndrome is facilitated by a clear understanding on the physician's part of the mechanisms of the symptoms. The palpitation is probably related to adrenergic stimulation of the heart and to the lower perception threshold. The pain may arise in the intercostal tissues as a result of the pounding of the heart. The hyperventilation with its ensuing train of symptoms (Chap. 13) is analogous to sighing. Explanation of these physiologic mechanisms to the patient and reassurance that they are not indicative of serious disease is one of the most important therapeutic steps.

Table 5-1 summarizes the main points of information to be ascertained in the history in elucidating the significance of palpitation. The recording of the electrocardiogram using a portable tape recorder in an ambulatory subject, and the precise temporal correlation of the cardiac rate and rhythm with the presence of palpitation are extremely useful in the identification or exclusion of a rhythmic disturbance. The effectiveness of antiarrhythmia treatment can also be assessed objectively in this manner, without the necessity of relying only on the patient's subjective symptoms. Beta-adrenergic blockade with propranolol, beginning with 40 mg per day in divided doses, and ranging as high as 240 mg per day, can be extremely effective in patients with palpitation and sinus rhythm or sinus tachycardia. The indications and contraindications for this drug are presented in Chap. 238.

One point merits special emphasis. *As a rule palpitation produces anxiety and fear out of all proportion to its seriousness.* When the cause has been accurately determined and its significance explained to patients, their concern is often ameliorated and may disappear entirely.

REFERENCES

BRAUNWALD E: Control of myocardial oxygen consumption: Physiologic and clinical considerations. Am J Cardiol 27:416, 1971

—— et al: *Mechanisms of Contraction of the Normal and Failing Heart,* 2d ed. Boston, Little, Brown, 1976

BURCH GE et al: Cardiac causalgia. Am Heart J 76:725, 1968

COHN PF: Coronary artery disease, in *Heart Disease,* E Braunwald (ed). Philadelphia, Saunders, 1980, chap 38

DRESSLER W: *Clinical Aids in Cardiac Diagnosis.* New York, Grune & Stratton, 1970

HILLIS DF, BRAUNWALD E: Myocardial ischemia. N Engl J Med 296:971, 1034, 1093, 1977

——, ——: Coronary artery spasm. N Engl J Med 299:695, 1978

HURST JW: Symptoms due to diseases of the heart and blood vessels, in *The Heart,* 4th ed, JW Hurst et al (eds). New York, McGraw-Hill, 1978, p 153

LEVENE DL: *Chest Pain.* Philadelphia, Lea & Febiger, 1977, p 203

WOOD P: The chief symptoms of heart disease, in *Diseases of the Heart and Circulation,* 3d ed. Philadelphia, Lippincott, 1968

6
ABDOMINAL PAIN

WILLIAM SILEN

The correct interpretation of acute abdominal pain is one of the most challenging demands made of any physician. Since proper therapy often requires urgent action, the luxury of the leisurely approach suitable for the study of other conditions is frequently denied. Few other clinical situations demand greater experience and judgment, because the most catastrophic of events may be forecast by the subtlest of symptoms and signs. Nowhere in medicine is a meticulously executed detailed history and physical examination of greater importance. The etiologic classification in Table 6-1, although not complete, forms a useful frame of reference for the evaluation of patients with abdominal pain.

The diagnosis of "acute or surgical abdomen" so often heard in emergency wards is not an acceptable one because of its often misleading and erroneous connotation. The most obvious of "acute abdomens" may not require operative intervention, and the mildest of abdominal pains may herald the onset of an urgently correctable lesion. Any patient with abdominal pain of recent onset requires early and thorough evaluation with specific attempts at accurate diagnosis.

SOME MECHANISMS OF PAIN ORIGINATING IN THE ABDOMEN Inflammation of the parietal peritoneum The pain of parietal peritoneal inflammation is steady and aching in character and is located directly over the inflamed area, its exact reference being possible because it is transmitted by overlapping somatic nerves supplying the parietal peritoneum. The intensity of the pain is dependent upon the type and amount of foreign substance to which the peritoneal surfaces are exposed in a given period of time. For example, the sudden release into the peritoneal cavity of a small quantity of *sterile* acid gastric juice causes much more pain than the same amount of grossly contaminated neutral fecal material. Enzymatically active pancreatic juice incites more pain and inflammation than does the same amount of sterile bile containing no potent enzymes. Blood and urine are often so bland as to go undetected if exposure of the peritoneum has not been sudden and massive. In the case of bacterial contamination, such as in pelvic inflammatory disease, the pain is frequently of low intensity early in the illness until bacterial multiplication has caused the elaboration of irritating substances.

So important is the rate at which the irritating material is applied to the peritoneum that cases of perforated peptic ulcer may be associated with entirely different clinical pictures dependent only upon the rapidity with which the gastric juice enters the peritoneal cavity.

The pain of peritoneal inflammation is invariably accentuated by pressure or changes in tension of the peritoneum, whether produced by palpation or by movement, as in coughing or sneezing. Consequently, the patient with peritonitis lies quietly in bed, preferring to avoid motion, in contrast to the patient with colic, who may writhe incessantly.

Another of the characteristic features of peritoneal irritation is tonic reflex spasm of the abdominal musculature, localized to the involved body segment. The intensity of the tonic muscle spasm accompanying peritoneal inflammation is dependent upon the location of the inflammatory process, the

rate at which it develops, and the integrity of the nervous system. Spasm over a perforated retrocecal appendix or perforated ulcer into the lesser peritoneal sac may be minimal or absent because of the protective effect of overlying viscera. As in pain of peritoneal inflammation, a slowly developing process often greatly attenuates the degree of muscle spasm. Catastrophic abdominal emergencies such as a perforated ulcer have been repeatedly associated with minimal or occasionally no detectable pain or muscle spasm in obtunded, seriously ill, debilitated elderly patients or in psychotic patients.

Obstruction of hollow viscera The pain of obstruction of hollow abdominal viscera is classically described as intermittent, or colicky. Yet the lack of a truly cramping character should not be misleading, because distention of a hollow viscus may produce steady pain with only very occasional exacerbations. Although not nearly as well localized as the pain of parietal peritoneal inflammation, some useful generalities can be made concerning its distribution.

The colicky pain of obstruction of small intestine is usually periumbilical or supraumbilical and is poorly localized. As the intestine becomes progressively dilated with loss of muscular tone, the colicky nature of the pain may become less apparent. With superimposed strangulating obstruction, pain may spread in the lower lumber region if there is traction on the root of the mesentery. The colicky pain of colonic obstruction is of lesser intensity than that of the small intestine and is often located in the infraumbilical area.

Sudden distention of the biliary tree produces a steady rather than colicky type of pain; hence the term "biliary colic" is misleading. Acute distention of the gallbladder usually causes pain in the right upper quadrant with radiation to the right posterior region of the thorax or to the tip of the right scapula, and distention of the common bile duct is often associated with pain in the epigastrium radiating to the upper part of the lumbar region. Considerable variation is common, however, so that differentiation between these may be impossible. The typical subscapular pain or lumbar radiation is frequently absent. Gradual dilatation of the biliary tree as in carcinoma of the head of the pancreas may cause no pain or only a mild aching sensation in the epigastrium or right upper quadrant. The pain of distention of the pancreatic ducts is similar to that described for distention of the common bile duct but in addition is very frequently accentuated by recumbency and relieved by the upright position.

Obstruction of the urinary bladder results in dull suprapubic pain, usually low in intensity. Restlessness without specific complaint of pain may be the only sign of a distended bladder in an obtunded patient. In contrast, acute obstruction of the intravesicular portion of the ureter is characterized by severe suprapubic and flank pain which radiates to the penis, scrotum, or inner aspect of the upper region of the thigh. Obstruction of the ureteropelvic junction is felt as pain in the costovertebral angle, whereas obstruction of the remainder of the ureter is associated with flank pain, which often extends into the corresponding side of the abdomen.

Vascular disturbances A frequent misconception, despite abundant experience to the contrary, is that pain associated with intraabdominal vascular disturbances is sudden and catastrophic in nature. The pain of embolism or thrombosis of the superior mesenteric artery or that of impending rupture of an abdominal aortic aneurysm certainly may be severe and diffuse. Yet just as frequently, the patient with occlusion of the superior mesenteric artery has only mild continuous diffuse

TABLE 6-1
Some important causes of abdominal pain

I Pain originating in the abdomen
  A Parietal peritoneal inflammation
    1 Bacterial contamination, e.g., perforated appendix, pelvic inflammatory disease
    2 Chemical irritation, e.g., perforated ulcer, pancreatitis, mittelschmerz
  B Mechanical obstruction of hollow viscera
    1 Obstruction of the small or large intestine
    2 Obstruction of the biliary tree
    3 Obstruction of the ureter
  C Vascular disturbances
    1 Embolism or thrombosis
    2 Vascular rupture
    3 Pressure or torsional occlusion
    4 Sickle-cell anemia
  D Abdominal wall
    1 Distortion or traction of mesentery
    2 Trauma or infection of muscles
    3 Distention of visceral surfaces, e.g., hepatic or renal capsules
II Pain referred from extraabdominal sources
  A Thorax—e.g., pneumonia, referred pain from coronary occlusion
  B Spine—e.g., radiculitis from arthritis
  C Genitalia—e.g., torsion of the testicle
III Metabolic causes
  A Exogenous
    1 Black widow spider bite
    2 Lead poisoning and others
  B Endogenous
    1 Uremia
    2 Diabetic coma
    3 Porphyria
    4 Allergic factors (C'1 esterase inhibitor deficiency)
IV Neurogenic causes
  A Organic
    1 Tabes dorsalis
    2 Herpes zoster
    3 Causalgia and others
  B Functional

pain for 2 or 3 days before vascular collapse or findings of peritoneal inflammation appear. The early, seemingly insignificant discomfort is caused by hyperperistalsis rather than peritoneal inflammation. Indeed, absence of tenderness and rigidity in the presence of continuous diffuse pain in a patient likely to have vascular disease is quite characteristic of occlusion of the superior mesenteric artery. Abdominal pain with radiation to the sacral region, flank, or genitalia should always signal the possible presence of a rupturing abdominal aortic aneurysm. This pain may persist over a period of several days before rupture and collapse occur.

Abdominal wall Pain arising from the abdominal wall is usually constant and aching. Movement and pressure accentuate the discomfort and muscle spasm. In the case of hematoma of the rectus sheath, now most frequently encountered in association with anticoagulant therapy, a mass may be present in the lower quadrants of the abdomen. Simultaneous involvement of muscles in other parts of the body usually serves to differentiate myositis of the abdominal wall from an intraabdominal process which might cause pain in the same region.

REFERRED PAIN IN ABDOMINAL DISEASES Pain referred to the abdomen from the thorax, spine, or genitalia may prove a vexing problem in differential diagnosis, because diseases of the upper part of the abdominal cavity such as acute cholecystitis, perforated ulcer, or subphrenic abscesses are frequently associated with intrathoracic complications. A most important, yet often forgotten, dictum is that the possibility of intrathoracic disease must be considered in every patient with abdominal pain, especially if the pain is in the upper part of the abdomen. Systematic questioning and examination directed toward detecting the presence or absence of myocardial or pulmonary infarction, pneumonia, pericarditis, or esophageal disease (the intrathoracic diseases which most often masquerade as abdominal emergencies) will often provide sufficient clues to establish the proper diagnosis. Diaphragmatic pleuritis resulting from pneumonia or pulmonary infarction may cause pain in the right upper quadrant and pain in the supraclavicular area, the latter radiation to be sharply distinguished from the referred subscapular pain caused by acute distention of the extrahepatic biliary tree. The ultimate decision as to the origin of abdominal pain may require deliberate and planned observation over a period of several hours, during which time repeated questioning and examination will provide the proper explanation.

Referred pain of thoracic origin is often accompanied by splinting of the involved hemithorax with respiratory lag and decrease in excursion more marked than that seen in the presence of intraabdominal disease. In addition, apparent abdominal muscle spasm caused by referred pain will diminish during the inspiratory phase of respiration, whereas it is persistent throughout both respiratory phases if it is of abdominal origin. Palpation over the area of referred pain in the abdomen also does not usually accentuate the pain and in many instances actually seems to relieve it. The frequent coexistence of thoracic and abdominal disease may be misleading and confusing, so that differentiation might be difficult or impossible. For example, the patient with known biliary tract disease often has epigastric pain during myocardial infarction, or biliary colic may be referred to the precordium or left shoulder in a patient who has suffered previously from angina pectoris. For the explanation of the radiation of pain to a previously diseased area, see Chap. 3.

Referred pain from the spine, which usually involves compression or irritation of nerve roots, is characteristically intensified by certain motions such as cough, sneeze, or strain and is associated with hyperesthesia over the involved dermatomes. Pain referred to the abdomen from the testicles or seminal vesicles is generally accentuated by the slightest pressure on either of these organs. The abdominal discomfort is of dull aching character and is poorly localized.

METABOLIC ABDOMINAL CRISES Pain of metabolic origin may simulate almost any other type of intraabdominal disease. Here several mechanisms may be at work. In certain instances, such as hyperparathyroidism, the metabolic disease itself may produce an intraabdominal process such as pancreatitis. Primary hyperlipemia may also be accompanied by severe pancreatitis, which can lead to unnecessary laparotomy unless recognized. C'l esterase deficiency associated with angioneurotic edema is also often associated with episodes of severe abdominal pain. Whenever the cause of abdominal pain is obscure, a metabolic origin must always be considered. Abdominal pain is also the hallmark of familial Mediterranean fever (Chap. 217).

The problem of differential diagnosis is often not readily resolved. The pain of porphyria and of lead colic usually is difficult to distinguish from that of intestinal obstruction, because severe hyperperistalsis is a prominent feature of both. The pain of uremia or diabetes is nonspecific, and the pain and tenderness frequently shift in location and intensity. Diabetic acidosis may be precipitated by acute appendicitis or intestinal obstruction, so that if prompt resolution of the abdominal pain does not result from correction of the metabolic abnormalities, an underlying organic problem should be suspected. Black widow spider bites produce intense pain and rigidity of the abdominal muscles and of the back, an area infrequently involved in disease of intraabdominal origin.

NEUROGENIC CAUSES Causalgic pain may occur in diseases which injure nerves of sensory type. It has a burning character and is usually limited to the distribution of a given peripheral nerve. Normal stimuli such as touch or change in temperature may be transformed into this type of pain, which is also frequently present in a patient at rest. A helpful finding is the demonstration that cutaneous pain spots are now irregularly spaced, and this may be the only indication of an old nerve lesion underlying causalgic pain. Even though the pain may be precipitated by gentle palpation, rigidity of the abdominal muscles is absent, and the respirations are not disturbed. Distention of the abdomen is uncommon, and the pain has no relationship to the intake of food.

Pain arising from spinal nerves or roots comes and goes suddenly and is of a lancinating type (see Chap. 7). It may be caused by herpes zoster, impingement by arthritis, tumors, herniated nucleus pulposus, diabetes, or syphilis. Again it is not associated with food intake, abdominal distention, or changes in respiration. Severe muscle spasm, as in the gastric crises of tabes dorsalis, is common but is either relieved or is not accentuated by abdominal palpation. The pain is made worse by movement of the spine and is usually confined to a few dermatome segments. Hyperesthesia is very common.

Psychogenic pain conforms to none of the aforementioned patterns of disease. Here the mechanism is hard to define. The most common problem is the hysterical adolescent or young woman who develops abdominal pain; she frequently loses an appendix and other organs because of it. Ovulation or some other natural event that causes brief mild abdominal discomfort may be maximized as an abdominal catastrophe.

Psychogenic pain varies enormously in type and location but usually has no relation to meals. It is often at its onset markedly accentuated during the night. Nausea and vomiting are rarely observed, although occasionally the patient reports these symptoms. Spasm is seldom induced in the abdominal musculature and if present does not persist, especially if the attention of the patient can be distracted. Persistent localized tenderness is rare, and if found, the muscle spasm in the area is inconsistent and often absent. Restriction of the depth of respiration is the most common respiratory abnormality, but this is in the nature of a smothering or choking sensation and is part of an anxiety state (see Chap. 11). It occurs in the absence of thoracic splinting or change in the respiratory rate.

APPROACH TO THE PATIENT WITH ABDOMINAL PAIN There are few abdominal conditions which require such urgent operative intervention that an orderly approach need be abandoned, no matter how ill the patient. Only those patients with exsanguinating hemorrhage must be rushed to the operating room immediately, but in such instances only a few minutes are required to assess the critical nature of the problem. Under these circumstances, all obstacles must be swept aside, adequate access for intravenous fluid replacement obtained, and the operation begun. Many patients of this type have died in the radiology department or the emergency room while awaiting such unnecessary examinations as electrocardiograms or films of the abdomen. *There are no contraindications to operation when massive hemorrhage is present.* Although exceedingly important, this situation fortunately is relatively rare.

Nothing will supplant an orderly painstakingly *detailed history,* which is far more valuable than any laboratory or roentgenologic examination. This kind of history is laborious and time-consuming, making it not especially popular even though a reasonably accurate diagnosis can be made on the basis of the history alone in the majority of cases. The *chronological sequence of events* in the patient's history is often more important than emphasis on the location of pain. If the examiner is sufficiently open-minded and unhurried, asks the proper questions, and listens, the patient will often provide the diagnosis. Careful attention should be paid to the extraabdominal regions which may be responsible for abdominal pain. An accurate menstrual history in a female patient is essential. Narcotics or analgesics should be withheld until a definitive diagnosis or a definitive plan has been formulated, because these agents often make it more difficult to secure and to interpret the history and physical findings.

In the examination, simple critical inspection of the patient, e.g., of facies, position in bed, and respiratory activity, may provide valuable clues. The amount of information to be gleaned is directly proportional to the *gentleness* and thoroughness of the examiner. Once a patient with peritoneal inflammation has been examined in a brusque manner, accurate assessment by the next examiner becomes almost impossible. For example, eliciting rebound tenderness by sudden release of a deeply palpating hand in a patient with suspected peritonitis is cruel and unnecessary. The same information can be obtained by gentle percussion of the abdomen (rebound tenderness on a miniature scale), a maneuver which can be far more precise and localizing. Asking the patient to cough will elicit true rebound tenderness without the need for placing a hand on the abdomen. Furthermore, the brusque demonstration of rebound tenderness will startle and induce protective spasm in a nervous or worried patient in whom true rebound tenderness is not present. A palpable gallbladder will be missed if palpation is so brusque that voluntary muscle spasm becomes superimposed upon involuntary muscular rigidity.

As in history taking, there is no substitute for sufficient time spent in the examination. It is important to remember that abdominal signs may be minimal but nevertheless, if accompanied by consistent symptoms, may be exceptionally meaningful when carefully assessed. Signs may be virtually or actually totally absent in cases of pelvic peritonitis, so that careful *pelvic and rectal examinations are mandatory in every patient with abdominal pain.* The presence of tenderness on pelvic or rectal examination in the absence of other abdominal signs must not lead the examiner to exclude such important operative indications as perforated appendicitis, diverticulitis, twisted ovarian cyst, and many others.

Much attention has been paid to the presence or absence of peristaltic sounds, their quality, and their frequency. Auscultation of the abdomen is probably one of the least rewarding aspects of the physical examination of a patient with abdominal pain. Severe catastrophes, such as strangulating small-intestinal obstruction or perforated appendicitis, may occur in the presence of normal peristalsis. Conversely, when the proximal part of the intestine above an obstruction becomes markedly distended and edematous, peristaltic sounds may lose the characteristics of borborygmi and become weak or absent even when peritonitis is not present. It is usually the severe chemical peritonitis of sudden onset which is associated with the truly silent abdomen. Assessment of the patient's state of hydration is important. The hematocrit and urinalysis permit an accurate estimate of the severity of dehydration, so that adequate replacement can be carried out.

Laboratory examinations may be of enormous value in the assessment of the patient with abdominal pain, yet with but a few exceptions they rarely establish a diagnosis. Leukocytosis should never be the single deciding factor as to whether or not operation is indicated. A white blood cell count greater than 20,000 per cubic millimeter may be observed with perforation of a viscus, but pancreatitis, acute cholecystitis, pelvic inflammatory disease, and intestinal infarction may be associated with marked leukocytosis. A normal white blood cell count is by no means rare in cases of perforation of abdominal viscera. The diagnosis of anemia may be more helpful than the white blood cell count, especially when combined with the history.

The urinalysis is also of great value in indicating to some degree the state of hydration or to rule out severe renal disease, diabetes, or porphyria. Determination of the blood urea nitrogen, blood sugar, and serum bilirubin levels may also be helpful. The serum amylase determination is overrated, since in carefully controlled series of patients with proved pancreatitis where the determination has been done within the first 72 h, amylase was less than 200 Somogyi units in one-third of the cases, between 200 and 500 in another one-third of the cases, and greater than 500 in one-third. Since many diseases other than pancreatitis, e.g., perforated ulcer, strangulating intestinal obstruction, and acute cholecystitis, may be associated with very marked increase in the serum amylase, great care must be exercised in denying an operation to a patient solely on the basis of an elevated serum amylase level. The determination of the amylase-to-creatinine clearance ratio is of much greater accuracy than either serum amylase or lipase determinations in the diagnosis of pancreatitis.

Abdominal paracentesis has proved to be a safe and effective diagnostic maneuver in patients with acute abdominal pain. It is of special value in patients with blunt trauma to the abdomen where evaluation of the abdomen may be difficult because of other multiple injuries to the spine, pelvis, or ribs and where blood in the peritoneal cavity produces only a very mild peritoneal reaction. The gallbladder is the only organ which may continue to seep fluid following accidental perforation, so that the region of this organ must be assiduously avoided. Determination of the pH of the aspirated fluid to ascertain the site of a perforation is misleading, because even highly acid gastric juice is rapidly buffered by peritoneal exudate.

Plain and upright or lateral decubitus roentgenograms of the abdomen may be of the greatest value. They are usually unnecessary in patients with acute appendicitis or strangulated external hernias. However, in cases of intestinal obstruction, perforated ulcer, and a variety of other conditions, films may be diagnostic. During a search for free air, the patient should be kept in the decubitus or upright position for at least 10 min before the appropriate film is taken lest a small pneumoperitoneum be missed. In rare instances, barium or water-soluble medium examination of the upper part of the gastrointestinal tract may demonstrate partial intestinal obstruction which may elude diagnosis by other means. If there is any question of obstruction of the colon, oral administration of barium sulfate should be avoided. On the other hand, barium enema is of inestimable value in cases of colonic obstruction and should be used with greater frequency where the possibility of perforation does not exist.

Sometimes, even under the best of circumstances with all available auxiliary aids and with the greatest of clinical skill, a definitive diagnosis cannot be established at the time of the initial examination. Nevertheless, despite lack of a clear anatomic diagnosis it may be abundantly clear to an experienced and thoughtful physician and surgeon on clinical grounds alone that operation is indicated. Should that decision be questionable, watchful waiting with repeated questioning and examination will often elucidate the true nature of the illness and indicate the proper course of action.

REFERENCES

BONICA JJ: Neurophysiologic and pathologic aspects of acute and chronic pain. Arch Surg 112:750, 1977

COPE Z: *The Early Diagnosis of the Acute Abdomen,* 14th ed. Fairlawn, NJ, Oxford University Press, 1972

LASSER RB et al: The role of intestinal gas in functional abdominal pain. N Engl J Med 293:524, 1975

LEEK BF: Abdominal and pelvic visceral receptors. Br Med Bull 33:163, 1977

STANILAND JR et al: Clinical presentation of acute abdomen: Study of 600 patients. Br Med J 2:393, 1972

7
PAIN IN THE BACK AND NECK

HENRY J. MANKIN
RAYMOND D. ADAMS

The following remarks concern mainly the lower part of the back, since it is most frequently the site of disabling pain. The lower portions of the spine and pelvis, with their many muscular and tendinous attachments, are relatively inaccessible to palpation and inspection. Although certain physical signs and radiographs are helpful, it is often necessary to depend on the patient's description of a pain (which may not be altogether accurate) and behavior during the execution of certain maneuvers to fully assess the nature of the problem. Seasoned clinicians, for these reasons, come to appreciate the need of a systematic clinical approach the description of which is one of the main purposes of this chapter.

ANATOMY AND PHYSIOLOGY OF THE LOWER PART OF THE BACK

The bony spine is a complex structure, anatomically divisible into two parts. The anterior part consists of a series of cylindrical vertebral bodies articulated by the intervertebral disks and held together by the anterior and posterior longitudinal ligaments. The posterior part consists of more delicate elements that extend from the vertebral body as pedicles and laminae, fused by ligaments to form the vertebral canal. Stout transverse and spinous bony processes project laterally and posteriorly and serve as the attachments of muscles which support and protect the vertebral column. The stability of the spine depends on two types of support: that provided by the bony articulations (principally the posterior elements) and a second type provided by the ligamentous (passive) and muscular (active) supporting structures. The ligamentous structures are quite strong, but because neither they nor the vertebral body-disk complexes have sufficient integral strength to resist the enormous forces acting on the column during even simple movements, voluntary and reflex contractions of the sacrospinalis, abdominal, gluteal, psoas, and hamstring muscles afford most of the stability.

The vertebral and paravertebral structures derive their innervation from the recurrent branches of the spinal nerves. Pain endings and fibers have been demonstrated in the ligaments, muscles, periosteum of bone, outer layers of annulus fibrosus, and synovium of the articular facets. The sensory fibers from these structures and the sacroiliac and lumbosacral joints join to form the sinovertebral nerves which pass via the recurrent branches of the spinal nerves of the first sacral and the fifth to first lumbar vertebrae into the gray matter of the corresponding segments of the spinal cord. Efferent fibers emerge from these segments and extend to the muscles through the same nerves. The sympathetic nerves contribute only to the innervation of blood vessels and appear to play no part in voluntary and reflex movement, though they do contain sensory fibers.

The parts of the back that possess the greatest freedom of movement, and hence are most frequently subject to injury, are the lumbar and cervical. In addition to the voluntary motions required for bending, twisting, and other movements, many actions of the spine are reflex in nature and are the basis of posture.

GENERAL CLINICAL CONSIDERATIONS

TYPES OF LOW BACK PAIN Of the several symptoms of disease of the spine (pain, stiffness or limitation of movement, and deformity), pain is of foremost importance by virtue of its frequency and its disabling effects. Four types of pain may be differentiated: local, referred, radicular, and that arising from secondary (protective) muscular spasm. One must identify these several types of pain by the patient's description, and here reliance is placed mainly on the character, location, and the conditions which modify them. The mechanism of the several types of pain has already been described in Chap. 3.

Local pain is caused by any pathologic process which impinges upon or irritates sensory endings. Involvement of structures which contain no sensory endings is painless. The central, medullary portion of the vertebral body may be destroyed by tumor, for example, without evocation of pain, whereas cortical fractures, or tears and distortions of the periosteum, synovial membranes, muscles, annulus fibrosus, and ligaments are often exquisitely painful. Although painful states are often accompanied by swelling of the affected tissues, this may not be apparent if a deep structure of the back is the site of disease. Local pain is often described as steady but may be intermittent, varying considerably with position or activity. The pain may be sharp or dull and although often diffuse is always felt in or near the affected part of the spine. Reflex splinting of the spine segments by paravertebral muscles is frequently noted, and certain movements or postures that alter the position of the injured tissues aggravate the pain. Firm pressure or percussion upon superficial structures in the region involved usually evokes tenderness, which is of aid in identifying the site of the abnormality.

Referred pain is of two types, that projected from the spine into regions lying within the area of the lumbar and upper sacral dermatomes and that projected from the pelvic and abdominal viscera to the spine. Pain due to diseases of the upper part of the lumbar spine is usually referred to the anterior aspects of the thighs and legs; that from the lower lumbar and sacral segments is referred to the gluteal regions, posterior thighs, and calves. Pain of this type, although of deep, aching quality and rather diffuse, tends at times to be superficially projected. In general the referred pain parallels in intensity the local pain in the back. In other words, maneuvers which alter local pain have a similar effect on referred pain, though not with such precision and immediacy as in radicular, or "root," pain. Referred pain may be confused with pain from visceral disease, but the latter is usually described as "deep" and tends to radiate from the abdomen through to the back. Also, visceral pain is usually unaffected by movement of the spine, does not improve with recumbency, and may be modified by the activity of the involved viscus.

Radicular, or "root," *pain* has some of the characteristics of referred pain but differs in its greater intensity, distal radiation, circumscription to the territory of a root, and the factors which excite it. The mechanism is distortion, stretching, irritation, or compression of a spinal root, most often central to the intervertebral foramen. Although the pain itself is often dull or aching, various maneuvers which increase the irritation of the root may greatly intensify the pain. Nearly always the radiation of pain is from a central position near the spine to some part of the lower extremity. Cough, sneeze, and strain are characteristically evocative maneuvers; but since they may also jar or move the spine, they may aggravate local pain as well. Any motion which stretches the nerve, e.g., forward bending with the knees extended or "straight-leg raising" in disease of the lower part of the lumbar spine, excites radicular pain; jugular vein compression, which raises intraspinal pressure and may cause a shift in the position of the root, may have a similar effect. The fourth and fifth lumbar and first sacral roots, which form the sciatic nerve, cause pain which extends mainly down the posterior aspects of thigh, the postero- and anterolateral aspects of the leg, and into the foot, in the distribution of this nerve—so called "sciatica." Tingling, paresthesias, and numbness or sensory impairment of the skin, soreness of the skin, and tenderness along the nerve usually accompany radicular pain. Also reflex loss, weakness, atrophy, fascicular twitching, and often stasis edema may occur if motor fibers of the anterior root are involved.

Pain resulting from muscular spasm is usually mentioned in relation to local pain. Muscle spasm may be associated with many disorders of the spine and can produce significant distortions of the normal posture. Chronic tension in muscles may give rise to a dull and sometimes cramping ache. One can in this instance feel the tautness of the sacrospinalis and gluteal muscles and demonstrate by palpation that the pain is localized to them.

Other pains often of undetermined origin are sometimes described by patients with chronic disease of the lower part of the back. In the legs, drawing, pulling, cramping sensations (without involuntary muscle spasm), tearing, throbbing, or jabbing pains, or feelings of burning or coldness are difficult to interpret and, like paresthesias and numbness, should always suggest the possibility of nerve or root disease.

Since it is often difficult to obtain physical or laboratory confirmation of painful disease of the lower region of the spine, it is extremely important to obtain an accurate history. In addition to assessing the character and location of the pain, one should determine the factors which aggravate and relieve it, its

constancy, and its relationship to recumbency and such stereotyped movements and maneuvers as forward bending, cough, sneeze, and strain. Frequently the most important lead comes from the knowledge of the mode of onset and circumstances which initiated the pain. Inasmuch as many painful afflictions of the back are the result of injury incurred during work or in an accident, the possibility of exaggeration or prolongation of pain for purposes of compensation or other personal reasons, or because of hysteria or malingering, must always be kept in mind.

EXAMINATION OF THE LOWER PART OF THE BACK

Much information may be gained by "inspection" of the back, buttocks, and lower extremities in various positions and movements. The normal spine shows a dorsal kyphosis and lumbar lordosis in the saggital plane, which in some individuals may be somewhat exaggerated (swayback). Normally the spine is relatively straight in the coronal plane, although slight curvature is frequent, particularly in females. In spinal disorders, one should observe the spine closely for excessive curvature, list, flattening of the normal lumbar arch, presence of a gibbus (a short, sharp, kyphotic angulation usually indicative of a fracture), pelvic tilt or obliquity, or asymmetry of the paravertebral or gluteal musculature. In severe sciatica, one may observe abnormalities of posture of the affected leg, presumably to reduce tension on the irritated part.

The next step in the examination is observation of the spine, hips, and legs during certain motions. During the procedure it is well to remember that no advantage accrues from trying to find out how much the patient can be hurt. Instead, it is much more important to determine when and under what conditions the pain commences. One looks for limitation of the natural motions of the patient while he or she is disrobing, standing, and reclining. When standing, the motion of forward bending normally produces flattening and reversal of the lumbar lordotic curve and exaggeration of the dorsal curve. With lesions of the lumbosacral region which involve the posterior ligaments, articular facets, or sacrospinalis muscle and with ruptured lumbar disks, protective reflexes prevent stretching of these structures. As a consequence, the sacrospinalis muscles remain taut and limit motion in the lumbar part of the spine. Forward bending then occurs at the hips and at the lumbar-thoracic junction. With disease of the lumbosacral joints and spinal roots, the patient bends in such a way as to avoid tensing the hamstring muscles and putting undue leverage upon the pelvis. In unilateral "sciatica," with its increased curvature toward the side of the lesion, lumbar and lumbosacral motions are splinted, and bending is mainly at the hips; at a certain point the knee on the affected side is flexed to relieve hamstring spasm and tilting of the pelvis and to slacken the lumbosacral roots and sciatic nerve.

It is sometimes of value to record the degree of flexion achieved either by measuring the distance between the fingertips and the floor or by estimating the degree of bending of the spine. Lateral bending is usually less instructive than forward bending. However, in unilateral ligamentous or muscular strain, bending to the opposite side aggravates the pain by stretching the damaged tissues. Moreover, in lateral disk lesions, bending of the spine toward the side from which the trunk lists is restricted. In diseases of the lower part of the spine, flexion while sitting with the hips and knees flexed can normally be performed easily, even to the point of bringing the knees in contact with the chest. The reason is that knee flexion relaxes the tightened hamstring muscles and also relieves stretch of the sciatic nerve.

The study of motions in the supine position yields the same information as study of motions in the standing and sitting positions, with the difference that there is less intradiskal pressure. With lumbosacral lesions and sciatica, passive lumbar flexion causes little pain and is not limited as long as the hamstrings are relaxed and there is no stretching of the sciatic nerve. With lumbosacral and lumbar spine disease (e.g., arthritis), passive flexion of the hips is free, whereas flexion of the lumbar spine may be impeded and painful. Passive straight-leg raising (possible in most normal individuals up to 90° except in those who have unusually tight hamstrings), like forward bending in the standing posture with the legs straight, places the sciatic nerve and its roots under tension, thereby producing pain. It may also cause an anterior rotation of the pelvis around a transverse axis, increasing stress on the lumbosacral joint, and thus causing pain if this segment is arthritic or otherwise impaired. Consequently, in diseases of the lumbosacral joints and lumbosacral roots, this movement is limited on the affected side and to a lesser extent on the opposite side. Lasègue's sign (pain and limitation of movement during elevation of the leg when the knee is extended) is a useful test of this condition. Straight-leg raising of the opposite leg may also cause contralateral pain but of lesser degree and is believed by some to be a sign of a more extensive lesion, such as an extruded disk fragment, rather than a simple prolapse or protrusion. It is important to remember, however, that the evoked

FIGURE 7-1

(1) Costovertebral angle. (2) Spinous process and interspinous ligament. (3) Region of the articular fifth lumbar to the first sacral facet. (4) Dorsum of sacrum. (5) Region of iliac crest. (6) Iliolumbar angle. (7) Spinous processes of fifth lumbar to first sacral vertebrae (tenderness = faulty posture or occasionally spina bifida occulta). (8) Region between posterior superior and posterior inferior spines. Sacroiliac ligaments (tenderness = sacroiliac sprain, often tender with fifth lumbar to first sacral disk.) (9) Sacrococcygeal junction (tenderness = sacrococcygeal injury, i.e., sprain or fracture). (10) Region of sacrosciatic notch (tenderness = fourth to fifth lumbar disk rupture and sacroiliac sprain). (11) Sciatic nerve trunk (tenderness = ruptured lumbar disk or sciatic nerve lesion).

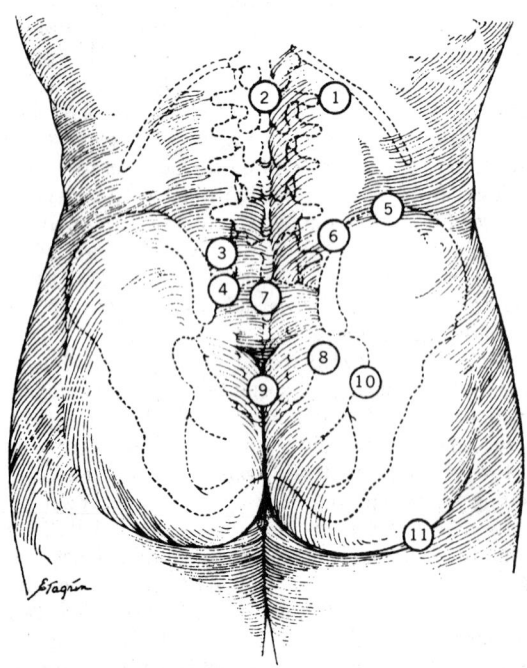

pain is always referred to the diseased side, no matter which leg is flexed.

The motion of hyperextension is best performed with the patient standing or lying prone. If the condition causing back pain is acute, it may be difficult to extend the spine in the standing position. A patient with lumbosacral strain or disk disease can usually extend or hyperextend the spine without aggravation of pain. If there is an active inflammatory process or fracture of the vertebral body or posterior elements, hyperextension may be markedly limited.

Palpation and percussion of the spine are the last steps in the examination. The approach must always be gentle since rough percussion of the designated area of pain may antagonize the patient and only serve to confuse the physician. It is preferable to palpate first those regions which are the least likely to evoke pain. At all times the examiner should know what structures are being palpated (see Fig. 7-1). Localized tenderness is seldom pronounced in disease of the spine because the involved structures are so deep that they rarely give rise to surface tenderness. Mild superficial and poorly localized tenderness signifies only a disease process within the affected segment of the body, i.e., dermatome.

Tenderness over the costovertebral angle often indicates genitourinary disease, adrenal disease (Rogoff's sign), or an injury to the transverse processes of the first or second lumbar vertebra [Fig. 7-1 (1)]. Hypersensitivity on palpation of the transverse processes of the other lumbar vertebrae as well as the overlying sacrospinalis muscles may signify fracture of the transverse process or a strain of muscle attachments. Tenderness of a spinous process or aggravation of pain by the jarring of gentle percussion may be nonspecific but frequently indicates the presence of a disk lesion at the site deep to it, inflammation (as in disk space infection), or pathologic fracture.

In palpation of the spinous processes, it is important to note any deviation in the lateral plane (this may be indicative of fracture or arthritis) or in the anteroposterior plane. A "step-off" forward displacement of the spinous process may be an important clue to a spondylolisthesis, one segment below the displaced level.

Tenderness in the region of the articular facets between the fifth lumbar and first sacral vertebrae is consistent with disease of a lumbosacral disk [Fig. 7-1 (3)]. It is also frequent in rheumatoid arthritis.

Abdominal, rectal, and pelvic examination and assessment of the status of the peripheral vascular system are important parts of the examination of the patient with complaints in the lower back and should not be omitted. They may provide evidence for vascular, visceral, neoplastic, or inflammatory disorders which may extend to the spine or cause pain to be referred to this region.

Finally, a careful neurologic examination should be performed, with special attention given to motor, reflex, and sensory changes (see "Protrusion of Lumbar Intervertebral Disks," below), particularly in the lower extremities.

SPECIAL LABORATORY PROCEDURES Useful laboratory tests, depending on the nature of the problem and the circumstances, include a complete blood count, erythrocyte sedimentation rate (especially helpful in screening for infection or myeloma), measurement of serum calcium, phosphorus, alkaline phosphatase, acid phosphatase (the last mentioned is of importance if one suspects metastatic carcinoma of the prostate), protein electrophoresis, immunoglobulin electrophoresis, tuberculin test, and tests for febrile agglutinins and rheumatoid factor. Roentgenograms of the lumbar part of the spine should be taken in every case of low back pain and sciatica (preferably with the patient standing) in the anteroposterior, lateral, and oblique planes. Special spot views or stereoscopic or laminographic films may provide further information in certain cases. Bone scans are of aid in revealing some fractures and neoplastic and inflammatory lesions. Computerized tomography (CT) scan of the spine and adjacent soft tissues may be particularly helpful in identifying a narrow canal, soft tissue mass, or destructive lesion of the body or posterior elements. Examination of the spinal canal with a contrast medium (air or other contrast myelogram) is often of great value, especially if a spinal cord tumor is suspected or if a patient is thought to have a disk herniation and fails to improve on a conservative regimen. Myelography can be combined with tests of dynamics of the cerebrospinal fluid, and a sample of the fluid should always be removed for cytologic and chemical examination prior to the instillation of the contrast medium (Pantopaque, Myodil, air, or some of the newer contrast media which are resorbed). Injection and removal of Pantopaque require special skill and should not be attempted without previous experience with the procedure. If done properly, the procedure has a very low incidence of significant complications. Injection of contrast medium directly into the intervertebral disk (diskograms) has waxed and waned in popularity over the years but remains controversial. The technique of this procedure is more complicated than that of myelographic examination, and the risk of damage to the disk or nerve roots and the possibility of introduction of infection is not inconsiderable. In the authors' opinion, such a procedure is indicated only under very special circumstances.

PRINCIPAL CONDITIONS WHICH GIVE RISE TO DISABLING PAIN IN THE LOWER PART OF THE BACK

CONGENITAL ANOMALIES OF THE LUMBAR SPINE Anatomic variations of the spine are not at all infrequent, and although rarely of themselves the source of pain and functional derangement, they may predispose an individual to excessive stress because of the altered mechanics or alignment of the spine.

There may be a lack of fusion of the laminae of the neural arch (spina bifida) of one or several of the lumbar vertebrae or of the sacrum. Hypertrichosis or hyperpigmentation in the sacral area may betray the condition, but in most patients the spine defect remains entirely occult until disclosed by x-ray. The anomaly has greater potentiality for pain if accompanied by malformation of vertebral joints. Usually the pain is induced by injury. There are many other congenital anomalies which affect the lower lumbar vertebrae such as asymmetrical facetal joints, abnormalities of the transverse processes, sacralization of the fifth lumbar vertebra (in which L_5 appears to be firmly fixed to the sacrum), or lumbarization of the first sacral vertebra (in which the first sacral resembles a sixth lumbar). Any one of these is occasionally observed in patients with symptoms referable to the low back, but they occur with equal frequency in individuals with no evidence of low back problem. Their role in the genesis of low back derangement is unclear, but in the authors' opinion, they are rarely the cause of specific symptomatology.

Spondylolysis consists of a bony defect, probably congenital, in the pars interarticularis (a segment near the junction of the pedicle with the lamina) of the lower lumbar area. The defect is best visualized on oblique projections. In some individuals the defect is bilateral. Under the circumstance of single or multiple injuries, the vertebral body, pedicle, and superior articular facet move anteriorly, leaving the posterior elements behind. This latter abnormality, known as *spondylolisthesis*, usually results in symptoms. The patient complains of pain in the low back radiating into the thighs, and there is limitation of motion. Often tenderness is elicited near the segment which has "slipped" forward (most often L_5 or occasionally L_4), and

one can feel a "step" on deep palpation of the posterior elements. The pelvis is sometimes rotated and hip flexion limited by hamstring spasm; a variety of neurologic deficits indicative of radiculopathy complete the clinical syndrome. In exceptionally severe cases, the trunk may be shortened and the abdomen protrude, both the result of the forward shift of L_5 on S_1.

TRAUMATIC AFFLICTIONS OF THE LOWER PART OF THE BACK Trauma constitutes the most frequent cause of low back pain.

In severe acute injuries, the examining physician must be careful to avoid further damage. In tests of mobility, all movements must be kept to a minimum until a diagnosis has been made and adequate measures have been instituted for the proper care of the patient. A patient complaining of back pain and inability to move the legs may have a fractured spine. The neck should not be flexed, nor should the patient be allowed to sit up. (See Chap. 375 for further discussion of spinal cord injury.)

Sprains, strains, and derangements The terms lumbosacral *sprain* and *strain* are used loosely by most physicians, and it is probably impossible to distinguish between them. The authors prefer the term *low back derangement* or *strain* for minor, self-limited injuries usually associated with lifting a heavy object, a fall, or a sudden deceleration as may occur in an automobile accident. Occasionally, these syndromes are more chronic in nature, suggesting that postural, muscular, or arthritic factors may play a role. The patients with low back derangement or strain are often acutely discomfited and may assume unusual postures related to spasm of the sacrospinalis muscles. The pain is usually confined to the lower back and is almost invariably relieved by rest. What formerly was regarded as sacroiliac strain or sprain is now known to be due to disk disease in most instances. This is caused by lifting heavy objects with the spine in a position of imperfect mechanical balance, as when lifting and turning at the same time. Sudden, unexpected motion is particularly likely to cause this injury.

The diagnosis of lumbosacral and sacroiliac strains with injury of the various structures of the lower part of the back depends upon the description of the injury, the localization of the pain by the patient, the finding of localized tenderness, and the augmentation of pain when tension is exerted on the involved structures by the appropriate maneuvers. The prompt alleviation of the pain by rest and relaxation indicates the existence of a strain. The rate of recovery depends on the degree of damage, preexisting disk disease, etc. Pain may be immediately relieved by local infiltration of an anesthetic agent, a finding which is also helpful in diagnosis.

Vertebral fractures Most fractures of the lumbar vertebral body are usually the result of flexion injuries and consist of anterior wedging or compression. With more severe trauma the patient may sustain a fracture dislocation, "bursting" fracture, or asymmetrical fracture involving not only the body but the posterior elements. The initiating trauma which causes fractures of the vertebrae is usually a fall from a height (in which case the calcanei may also be fractured) or may result from an automobile accident or other violence. When fractures occur with minimal trauma (or spontaneously), the bone is presumed to have been previously weakened by some pathologic process. Most of the time, particularly in older individuals, the cause of such an event is idiopathic osteoporosis, but there are many other underlying systemic disorders such as osteomalacia, hyperparathyroidism, hyperthyroidism, multiple myeloma, metastatic carcinoma, and a large number of local conditions that may play a role in weakening the vertebral body. Spasm of the lower lumbar muscles, limitation of motion of the lumbar section of the spine, and the roentgenographic appearance of the damaged lumbar portion (with or without neurologic abnormalities) are the basis of clinical diagnosis. The pain is usually immediate, though occasionally it may be delayed in onset for a few days. The patient may develop a mild paralytic ileus or urinary retention during the acute period.

Fractures of the transverse processes are almost always associated with tearing of the paravertebral muscles, principally the psoas. They may cause significant retroperitoneal hemorrhage resulting in a marked depression in hematocrit and, in extensive fractures, hypovolemic shock. Such injuries may be diagnosed by the finding of deep tenderness at the site of the injury, local muscle spasm on one side, and limitation of all movements which stretch the lumbar muscles. Radiologic evidence including body CT scan provides the final confirmation. Fractures of multiple transverse processes, although seemingly trivial, should be the object of considerable concern, and the patient should be carefully watched over the initial period for internal hemorrhage.

Protrusion of lumbar intervetebral disks   This condition is now recognized as the major cause of severe and chronic or recurrent low back and leg pain. It is most likely to occur between the fifth lumbar and first sacral vertebrae, and, with lessening frequency, between the fourth and fifth lumbar, the third and fourth lumbar, the second and third lumbar, and the first and second lumbar vertebrae. Rare in the thoracic portion of the spine, it is next most frequent between the sixth and seventh and fifth and sixth cervical vertebrae. The cause is usually a flexion injury, but in a considerable proportion of cases no trauma is recalled. Degeneration of the posterior longitudinal ligaments and the annulus fibrosus, which occurs in most adults of middle and advanced years, may have taken place silently or have been manifested by mild, recurrent lumbar ache. A sneeze, lurch, or other trivial movement may then cause the nucleus pulposus to prolapse, pushing the frayed and weakened annulus posteriorly. In more severe cases of disk disease, the nucleus may protrude through the annulus or become extruded to lie as a free fragment in the vertebral canal.

The fully developed syndrome of ruptured lumbar intervertebral disk consists of backache, abnormal posture, and limitation of motion of the spine (particularly flexion). Nerve root involvement is indicated by radicular pain, sensory disturbances (paresthesias, hyper- and hyposensitivity in dermatome pattern), coarse twitching and fasciculation, muscle spasms, and impairment of a tendon reflex. Motor abnormalities (weakness and muscle atrophy) may also occur but are usually less prominent than the pain and sensory disorder. Since herniation of the intervertebral lumbar disks most often occurs between the fourth and fifth lumbar vertebrae and the fifth lumbar and first sacral vertebrae with irritation and compression of the fifth lumbar and first sacral roots, respectively, it is important to recognize the clinical characteristics of lesions of these two roots. *Lesions of the fifth lumbar root* produce pain in the region of the hip, groin, posterolateral thigh, lateral calf to the external malleolus, dorsal surface of the foot, and the first or second and third toes. Paresthesias may be in the entire territory or only in the distal parts of these territories. The tenderness is in the lateral gluteal region and near the head of the fibula. Weakness, if present, involves the extensors of the great toe and of the foot. The knee and ankle reflexes are seldom altered, although occasionally, the ankle jerk is moderately depressed. Walking on the heels may be more difficult,

because of weakness of dorsiflexion of the foot, and more uncomfortable than walking on the toes. In *lesions of the first sacral root* the pain is felt in the midgluteal region, posterior part of the thigh, posterior region of the calf to the heel, and the plantar surface of the foot and fourth and fifth toes. Tenderness is most pronounced over the midgluteal region (sacroiliac joint), posterior thigh area, and calf. Rarely it may be referred to the rectum, testicles, or labia. Paresthesias and sensory loss are mainly in the lower leg and outer toes, and weakness, if present, involves the flexor muscles of the foot and toes, abductors of the toes, and hamstring muscles. The ankle reflex is diminished to absent in the majority of cases. Walking on the toes is more difficult, because of weakness of plantar flexors, and more uncomfortable than walking on the heel. With lesions of either root there may be limitation of straight-leg raising during the acute, painful stages.

Degeneration of the intervertebral disk without frank extrusion of a fragment of disk tissue may give rise to low back pain, or the disk may herniate into the adjacent vertebral body, giving rise to a Schmorl's node (seen on x-ray). Such cases often show no signs of nerve root involvement though the back pain may be referred to the thigh and leg.

The rarer *lesions of the fourth and third lumbar roots* give rise to pain in the anterior part of the thigh and knee, with corresponding sensory loss. The knee-jerk is diminished or abolished. An inverted Lasègue sign (pain with hypertension of the limb in relation to the trunk, best elicited with the patient in the prone position) is positive when the third lumbar root is affected.

The lumbar disk syndromes are usually unilateral. Only with massive derangements of the disk or the extrusion of a large, free fragment into the canal do bilateral symptoms and signs occur, and these may sometimes be associated with paralysis of the sphincters. The pain may be mild or severe. All or part of the above syndrome may be present. There may be back pain with little or no leg pain; rarely only leg pain may be experienced. The rupture of multiple lumbar or lumbar and cervical disks is not infrequent, suggesting a diffuse disorder of the connective tissue of the disks, including both the annulus fibrosus and the nucleus pulposus.

When all components of the syndrome are present, the diagnosis is easy; when only one part is present (particularly backache), it may be difficult, especially if there has been a clearly remembered initiating traumatic event. Since similar symptoms may occur without demonstrable disk rupture, other diagnostic procedures are required. Plain roentgenograms usually show no abnormality or at most a narrowing of the intervertebral space, sometimes more on the side of the rupture. Traction spurs, which are indicative of disk degeneration, may be present; in extreme cases, there may be a "vacuum" disk sign, in which a gas-density shadow is present in the intervertebral space, usually on lateral roentgenogram. Frequently however, one must resort to Pantopaque or air myelography, which in most cases will reveal an indentation of the lumbar subarachnoid space or deformity of the root sleeve. Occasionally, with large lesions there is a complete interruption of the flow of contrast material. Conversely, a small ruptured disk may not show any abnormality in the myelogram, especially at the fifth lumbar to first sacral level where there is a large space between the spinal canal and dura. Some clinics use diskograms (opaque material is injected into the disk) to reveal any evidence of extrusion, but the procedure is risky, and the results are difficult to interpret. The electromyogram is helpful in showing denervation of leg muscles (see Chap. 378). The protein level of the cerebrospinal fluid may be elevated in some instances.

Tumor of the spinal canal, epidural or intradural, may produce a syndrome similar to that of ruptured disk (see Chap. 375).

ARTHRITIS Arthritis of the spine is a major cause of back-ache, cervical pain, and occipital headache.

Osteoarthritis This more frequent type of osteoarthritic spinal disease occurs usually in later life and may involve any part of the spine. It is most prevalent in the cervical and lumbar regions, however, and the exact location determines the localization of the symptoms. Patients often complain of pain centered in the spine, which is increased by motion and is almost invariably associated with complaints of stiffness and limitation of motion. There is a notable absence of systemic symptoms such as fatigue, malaise, and fever, and the pain usually can be relieved by rest. The severity of the symptoms often bears little relation to the radiologic findings; pain may be present when there are minimal findings on an x-ray, and, conversely, marked osteophytic overgrowth with spur formation, ridging, and bridging of vertebrae can be seen in asymptomatic patients in middle and later life. Osteoarthropathic changes in the cervical spine and to a lesser extent in the lumbar spine may by their location compress roots or even the cauda equina or spinal cord, giving rise to the spondylitic form of myelopathy (see Chaps. 375 and 377).

Spondylitic caudal radiculopathy (SCR) is another variant of hypertrophic arthritis. A congenital smallness of the lumbar canal, especially at the L_4 to L_5 level, renders the individual susceptible to either a rupture of an intervertebral disk or arthrosis. The latter condition further narrows the anteroposterior diameter of the canal and leads to compression of lumbosacral roots and even to a block of the spinal canal. The roots are actually caught between the posterior surface of the vertebral body and the ligamentum flavum posterolaterally. Lumbosacral pains are followed by weakening of the lower legs, impairment of ankle and knee reflexes, and numbness and paresthesia in the feet and legs. Extension of the lumbar spine during walking and standing produces or aggravates the neurologic symptoms, and flexion relieves them. The clinical picture and its intermittency correspond to the so-called "intermittent claudication" of the spinal cord. The diagnosis may be suspected on the basis of history and radiographic findings but may be confirmed by myelography or CT scan, both of which will demonstrate the narrowed lumbar canal. Decompression of the spinal canal relieves the symptoms in a considerable proportion of the cases but should be approached with caution since it may lead to instability, necessitating an arthrodesis. SCR is the lumbar equivalent of spondylitic cervical myelopathy (SCM), described below. SCR is a cauda equina syndrome, and its differential diagnosis is discussed in Chap. 375, "Diseases of the Spinal Cord."

Rheumatoid arthritis and ankylosing spondylitis Arthritic disease of the spine takes two distinct forms, ankylosing spondylitis (the more common) and rheumatoid arthritis.

Patients with *ankylosing spondylitis* (also called Marie-Strümpell arthritis) are usually young men who complain of mild to moderate pain, which early in the course of the disease is centered in the back, and on occasion radiates to the back of the thighs. The symptoms may be vague at first (tired back, "catches" up and down the back, sore back) and the diagnosis may be overlooked for a considerable period. Although the pain is often intermittent, the finding of limitation of movement is constant and progressive and over a period of time tends to dominate the picture. Early in the course, this finding is described as "morning stiffness" or increasing stiffness after periods of inactivity, and may be present long before radiologic changes are manifest. Limitation of chest expansion, tenderness over the sternum, and decreased motion and flexion contractures of the hips may also be present early in the course. The radiologic hallmarks of the disease are destruction and subsequent obliteration of the sacroiliac joints, development of

syndesmophytes on the margins of the vertebral bodies, followed by bridging by bone to produce the characteristic "bamboo spine." The entire spine becomes immobilized, often in a flexed position, and usually the pain then subsides. Patterns of restricted movement, indistinguishable from those of ankylosing spondylitis, may accompany Reiter's syndrome, psoriatic arthritis, and inflammatory diseases of the intestine. Patients with these disorders rarely show the joint manifestations of peripheral rheumatoid arthritis, and seldom do they display involvement of the hips or knees. The rheumatoid factor is usually absent, but the sedimentation rate is often rapid, and many of the patients are found to have a HLA-B27 antigen.

Occasionally ankylosing spondylitis is complicated by progressively destructive vertebral lesions. This complication should be suspected whenever the pain returns, after a period of quiescence, or becomes localized. The etiology of these lesions is not known, but they may represent an exaggerated healing response to fracture or excessive production of fibrous inflammatory tissues. Rarely they may result in collapse of a segment of the spine and compression of the spinal cord. Another complication of severe ankylosing spondylitis is bilateral ankylosis of the ribs to the spine, which, coupled with a decrease in the height of axial thoracic structures, causes marked impairment of respiratory function.

Spinal rheumatoid arthritis tends to be localized to the cervical apophyseal joints and atlantoaxial articulation; the pain, stiffness, and limitation of motion are then in the neck and back of the head. Unlike ankylosing spondylitis, rheumatoid arthritis is rarely confined to the spine, and it does not lead to significant degrees of intervertebral bridging. Because of major affection of other joints, the diagnosis is relatively easy to make, but significant involvement of the neck may be overlooked. In the advanced stages of the disease, one or several of the vertebrae may be displaced anteriorly, or a synovitis of the atlantoaxial joint may damage the transverse ligament of the atlas, resulting in forward displacement of the atlas on the axis, i.e., atlantoaxial subluxation. In either instance serious and even life-threatening compression of the spinal cord may occur gradually or suddenly (see Chaps. 356 and 375). Lateral roentgenograms in flexion and extension, performed cautiously, are necessary to visualize dislocation or subluxation.

OTHER DESTRUCTIVE DISEASES **Neoplastic, infectious, and metabolic diseases** Metastatic carcinoma (breast, lung, prostate, thyroid, kidney, gastrointestinal tract), multiple myeloma, Hodgkin's disease, and reticulum cell sarcoma are the malignant tumors which most frequently involve the spine. Since the primary site may be overlooked or asymptomatic the presenting complaint in such patients may be pain in the back. The pain tends to be constant and dull, and is often unrelieved by rest. Indeed, it may be worse at night. Radiographic changes may be absent early in the disease, but when they appear, usually are manifest as destructive lesions in one or several vertebral bodies with little or limited involvement of the disk space, even in the face of a compression fracture. A ^{99m}Tc diphosphonate bone scan is helpful in lighting up "hot spots," indicating areas of increased blood flow and reactive bone formation associated with destructive inflammatory or arthritic lesions.

Infection of the vertebral column is usually the result of pyogenic organisms (staphylococci or coliform bacilli) or tubercle bacilli and is often difficult to distinguish on the basis of clinical findings. Patients complain of pain in the back of subacute or chronic nature that is exacerbated by motion but not materially relieved by rest. There is limitation of motion, tenderness over the spine of the involved segments, and pain with jarring of the spine, such as occurs with walking on the heels. Usually, these patients are afebrile and often do not have a leukocytosis although the erythrocyte sedimentation rate is almost invariably elevated. Radiographs may demonstrate narrowing of a disk space with erosion and destruction of the two adjacent vertebrae. A paravertebral soft tissue mass may be present, indicating an abscess, which may in the case of tuberculosis drain spontaneously, at sites quite remote from the vertebral column. In addition to a bone scan, a gallium scan is somtimes helpful in identifying a soft tissue inflammatory or infectious lesion even when overt bone destruction is not visible in x-rays.

Special mention should be made of the spinal *epidural abscess* (usually staphylococcal), which necessitates urgent surgical treatment. The symptoms are a localized pain, occurring spontaneously, aggravated by percussion and palpation. The patient is febrile and usually has severe radicular complaints, often bilateral, progressing rapidly to a flaccid paraplegia (see Chap. 368 and 375).

In so-called "metabolic bone diseases" (osteoporosis or osteomalacia) a considerable degree of loss of bone substance may occur without any symptoms whatsoever. Many patients with such conditions do, however, complain of aching in the lumbar or thoracic area. This is most likly to occur following an injury, sometimes of trivial degree, which leads to collapse or wedging of a vertebra. Certain movements greatly enhance the pain, and certain positions relieve it. One or more spinal roots may be involved. Paget's disease of the spine is nearly always painless but may lead to compression of the spinal cord or roots because of encroachment on the canal or foramina by the pagetoid bone. The recognition of these bone disorders is discussed in some detail elsewhere (Chaps. 352 and 353).

In general, patients thought to have neoplastic, infectious, or metabolic disease of the spine should be thoroughly evaluated by means of radiographs, bone scans, myelography, and appropriate laboratory studies (see above).

REFERRED PAIN FROM VISCERAL DISEASE The pain of disease of the plevic, abdominal, or thoracic viscera is often felt in the region of the spine; i.e., it is referred to the more posterior parts of the spinal segment which innervates the diseased organ. Occasionally back pain may be the first and only sign. The general rule is that pelvic diseases are referred to the sacral region, lower abdominal diseases to the lumbar region (centering around the second to fourth lumbar vertebrae), and upper abdominal diseases to the lower thoracic spine (eighth thoracic to the first and second lumbar vertebrae). Characteristically there are no local signs or stiffness of the back, and motion is of full range without augmentation of the pain. However, some positions, e.g., flexion of the lumbar area of the spine in the lateral recumbent position, may be more comfortable than others.

Low thoracic and upper lumbar pain in abdominal disease Peptic ulceration or tumor of the wall of the stomach and of the duodenum most typically induces pain in the epigastrium (see Chaps. 290 and 309); but if the posterior wall is involved, and particularly if there is retroperitoneal extension, the pain may be felt in the region of the spine. The pain may be central in location or more intense on one side, or it may be felt in both locations. If very intense, it may seem to encircle the body. It tends to retain the characteristics of pain from the affected organ; e.g., if due to peptic ulceration, it appears about 2 h after a meal and is relieved by food and antacids.

Diseases of the pancreas (peptic ulceration with extension to the pancreas, cholecystitis with pancreatitis, cyst, or tumor) are apt to cause pain in the back, being more to the right of the spine if the head of the pancreas is involved and to the left if the body and tail are implicated.

Diseases of retroperitoneal structures, e.g., lymphomas, sarcomas, and carcinomas, may evoke pain in this part of the spine with some tendency toward radiation to the lower part of the abdomen, groins, and anterior thighs. A secondary tumor of the iliopsoas region on one side often produces a unilateral lumbar ache with radiation toward the groin and labia or testicle; there may also be signs of involvement of the upper lumbar spinal roots. An aneurysm of the abdominal aorta may induce pain which is localized to this region of the spine but may be felt higher or lower, depending on the location of the lesion.

The sudden appearance of obscure lumbar pain in a patient receiving anticoagulants should arouse the suspicion of retroperitoneal bleeding.

Lumbar pain with lower abdominal diseases Inflammatory diseases of segments of the colon (colitis, diverticulitis) or tumor of the colon cause pain which may be felt in the lower part of the abdomen between the umbilicus and pubis, in the midlumbar region, or in both places. If very intense, the pain may have a beltlike distribution around the body. A lesion in the transverse colon or first part of the descending colon may be central or left-sided, and its level of reference to the back is to the second to third lumbar vertebrae. If the sigmoid colon is implicated, the pain is lower, in the upper sacral region and anteriorly in the midline suprapubic region or left lower quadrant of the abdomen.

Sacral pain in pelvic (urologic and gynecologic) diseases Although gynecologic disorders may manifest themselves by back pain, the pelvis is seldom the site of a disease which causes obscure low back pain. For the most part the diagnosis of painful pelvic lesions is not difficult, for a thorough palpation of structures by abdominal, vaginal, and rectal examination may be supplemented by methods (sigmoidoscopy, barium enema, pyelography, and culdoscopy) which permit adequate visualization of all these parts.

Menstrual pain itself may be felt in the sacral region. It is rather poorly localized, tends to radiate down the legs, and is of a crampy nature. The most important source of chronic back pain from the pelvic organs, however, is the uterosacral ligaments. Endometriosis or carcinoma of the uterus (body or cervix) may invade these structures, while malposition of the uterus may pull on them. The pain is localized centrally in the sacrum below the lumbosacral joint but may be more on one side. In endometriosis the pain begins during the premenstrual phase and often continues until it merges with menstrual pain. Malposition of the uterus (retroversion, descensus, and prolapse) is thought by some to lead to sacral pain, especially after the patient has been standing for several hours. One may observe the effect of postural influences here as when a fibroma of the uterus pulls on the uterosacral ligaments. Carcinomatous pain due to involvement of nerve plexuses is continuous and becomes progressively more severe; it tends to be more intense at night. The primary lesion may be inconspicuous, being overlooked upon pelvic examination. Papanicolaou smears, pyelogram and CT scan are the most useful diagnostic procedures. X-ray therapy of these tumors may produce sacral pain consequent to swelling and necrosis of tissue. Low back pain with radiation into one or both thighs is a common phenomenon during the last weeks of pregnancy.

Chronic prostatitis, evidenced by prostatic discharge, burning and frequency of urination, and slight reduction in sexual potency, may be attended by a nagging sacral ache; it may be mainly on one side, with radiation into one leg if the seminal vesicle is involved on that side. Carcinoma of the prostate with metastases to the lower part of the spine is another more common cause of sacral or lumbar pain. It may be present without urinary frequency or burning. Spinal nerves may be infiltrated by tumor cells, or the spinal cord itself may be compressed if the epidural space is invaded. The diagnosis is established by rectal examination, roentgenograms of the spine, and measurement of acid phosphatase (particularly the prostatic phosphatase fraction). Lesions of the bladder and testes are usually not accompanied by back pain. When the kidney is the site of disease, the pain is ipsilateral, being felt in the flank or lumbar region.

Visceral derangements of whatever type may intensify the pain of arthritis, and the presence of arthritis may alter the distribution of visceral pain. With disease of the spine in the lumbosacral region, for example, distention of the ampulla of the sigmoid by feces or a bout of colitis may aggravate the arthritic pain. In patients with arthritis of the cervical or thoracic spine the pain of myocardial ischemia may radiate to the back.

OBSCURE TYPES OF LOW BACK PAIN AND THE QUESTION OF PSYCHIATRIC DISEASE The practitioner is frequently consulted by persons who complain of low back pain of obscure origin. Usually the disorder is benign in nature and results from some minor derangement, muscular strain, or diskal prolapse. This is particularly true for those lesions which are of acute onset, aggravated by motion, and relieved by rest. Considerably more difficult are patients with chronic pain, especially those who have had prior back surgery or chronic visceral disease, or those who have severe and progressive pain in which neoplasia or infection is considered.

Even when exhaustive studies have been performed, there remains a group of patients in whom no anatomic or pathologic lesion can be found. These patients generally fall into two categories: those with postural back pain and those with psychiatric illness.

Postural back pain Many slender asthenic individuals and some obese middle-aged individuals have discomfort in the back. Their backs ache much of the time, and the pain interferes with effective work. The physical examination is negative except for slack musculature and poor posture. The pain is diffuse in the mid or low region of the back and characteristically is relieved by bed rest and induced by the maintenance of a particular posture over a period of time. Pain in the neck and between the shoulder blades is a common complaint among thin, tense, active women and seems to be related to taut trapezius muscles.

Psychiatric illness Low back pain may be encountered in compensation hysteria and malingering, in anxiety or neurocirculatory asthenia (formerly called neurasthenia), in depression and hypochondriasis, and in many nervous persons whose symptoms and complaints do not fall within any category of psychiatric illness. It is probably correct to assume that pain in the back in such patients usually signifies diseases of the spine and adjacent structures, and one should always search for a specific cause. However, even when organic factors are found, the pain may be exaggerated, prolonged, or woven into a pattern of invalidism or disability because of coexistent psychologic factors. This is especially true when there is the possibility of secondary gain (notably compensation). Patients seeking compensation for protracted low back pain without obvious structural disease, tend, after a time, to become suspicious, uncooperative, and hostile toward the medical profession or anyone who might question the authenticity of their illness. One notes in them a tendency to describe their pain poorly and to prefer, instead, to discuss the degree of their disability and their mistreatment at the hands of the medical profession. These features and a negative examination of the back should

lead one to suspect a psychologic factor. A few patients, usually frank malingerers, adopt the most bizarre attitudes, such as being unable to straighten up or walking with the trunk flexed at almost a right angle (camptocormia) (see Chap. 11).

The depressed and hypochondriac patient represents a troublesome problem, and a common error is to minimize the importance of anxiety and depression or to ascribe them to worry over the illness and its social effects. The more common and minor back ailments, e.g., those due to osteoarthritis and postural ache, are enhanced and rendered intolerable by irritable moodiness and self-concern. Such patients are often subjected to surgical procedures which prove ineffective. The disability seems excessive for the degree of spinal malfunction, and misery and despair are the prevailing features of the syndrome. One of the more reliable diagnostic measures is the favorable response to drugs that alleviate the depression (see Chaps. 11 and 25).

PAIN IN THE NECK AND SHOULDER

This topic is discussed to some extent in Chap. 5, and further references are found in Chap. 8.

It is useful to distinguish here three major categories of painful disease—of the spine, brachial plexus (thoracic outlet), and shoulder. Although pain in these three regions of the body may overlap, the patient usually can indicate the site of origin. Pain arising from the cervical spine is felt in the neck and back of the head (though it may be projected to the shoulder and arm), is evoked or enhanced by certain movements or positions of the neck, and is accompanied by tenderness and limitation of motions of the neck. Similarly, pain resulting from abnormalities of the thoracic outlet is experienced in and around the shoulder in the supraclavicular region, or between the shoulders; is induced by the performance of certain tasks and by certain positions; and is associated with tenderness of structures above the clavicle. There may be a palpable abnormality above the clavicle (aneurysms of the subclavian artery, tumor, cervical rib). The combination of circulatory symptoms and signs referable to the lower part of the brachial plexus, manifested in the hand by obliteration of pulse when the patient holds a full breath with the head tilted back or turned (Adson's test), unilateral Raynaud's phenomenon, trophic changes in the fingers, and sensory loss over the ulnar side of the hand with or without interosseous atrophy complete the clinical picture. Roentgenograms showing a cervical rib, deformed thoracic outlet, or superior sulcus tumor of the lung (Pancoast's syndrome) corroborate disease in this location. Electromyography and conduction studies along the plexus from points stimulated above and below the clavicle, and studies of arterial and venous circulation (venograms, noninvasive Doppler techniques) are especially helpful in evaluating this problem.

Pain localized to the shoulder region, often worse at night, associated with tenderness and aggravated by abduction, internal rotation, and extension points toward a lesion of the tendinous structures about the shoulder. Most often these are in the form of a calcific tendonitis or bursitis usually affecting the supraspinatus tendon and the adjacent subdeltoid bursa; occasionally the lesion is more extensive and consists of a rupture of the rotator cuff, in which case the patient may have weakness on abduction and forward flexion. In some such patients there is an adhesive capsulitis, leading to profound limitation of motion, designated as a "frozen shoulder." Shoulder pain may radiate into the arm or hand, but the sensory, motor, and reflex changes which indicate disease of nerve roots, plexus, or peripheral nerves are absent.

Osteoarthritis of the cervical part of the spine may cause pains which radiate into the back of the head, shoulders, and arms on one or both sides of the thorax. Coincident involvement of nerve roots is manifested by paresthesias, sensory loss, weakness, or deep tendon reflex change. Should bony ridges form in the spinal canal (spondylosis) the spinal cord may be compressed (see Chap. 375). A myelogram or CT scan may reveal the degree of encroachment on the spinal canal (narrowing of the canal to less than 11 mm in the anteroposterior diameter) at the level at which the spinal cord is affected. The authors have experienced difficulty in distinguishing spondylosis with or without disk rupture and spinal cord compression from primary neurologic diseases (syringomyelia, amyotrophic lateral sclerosis, or tumor) with an unrelated osteoarthritis of the cervical portion of the spine, particularly at the fifth to sixth and sixth to seventh cervical vertebrae, where the disk spaces are often narrowed in the adult. A combination of nervous tension with osteoarthritis of the cervical part of the spine or a painful injury to ligaments and muscles after an accident in which the neck is forcibly extended and flexed (e.g., whiplash injury to spine) raises extremely vexatious clinical syndromes. If the pain is persistent and limited to the neck, the problem will sometimes prove to have been due to disruption of a disk, but it is often complicated by psychologic factors.

RUPTURED CERVICAL DISKS One of the commonest causes of neck, shoulder, and arm pain is disk herniation in the lower cervical region. As with rupture of the lumbar disks, the complete syndrome includes the disorder of spinal function and evidence of neural involvement. It may develop after trauma either major or minor (sudden hyperextension of the neck, diving, forceful manipulations, etc.). Virtually every patient exhibits an abnormality in range of motion of the neck (limitation and pain). Hyperextension is the movement that most consistently aggravates the pain, although one occasionally sees patients whose principal limitation is in flexion. With laterally situated disk lesions between the fifth and sixth cervical vertebrae, the symptoms and signs are referred to the sixth cervical roots. The full syndrome is characterized by pain felt at the trapezius ridge, tip of the shoulder, anterior upper part of the arm, radial forearm, and often in the thumb; paresthesias and sensory impairment or hypersensitivity in the same regions; tenderness in the area above the spine of the scapula and in the supraclavicular and biceps regions; weakness in flexion of the forearm; diminished to absent biceps and supinator reflexes (triceps retained or exaggerated). When the protruded disk lies between the sixth and seventh cervical vertebrae, the seventh cervical root is involved. Under these circumstances, in the patient with the complete syndrome, the pain is in the region of the shoulder blade, pectoral region and medial axilla, posterolateral upper arm, elbow and dorsal forearm, index and middle fingers, or all the fingers; tenderness is most pronounced over the medial aspect of the shoulder blade opposite the third to fourth thoracic spinous processes, in the supraclavicular area and triceps region; paresthesias and sensory loss are most pronounced in the second and third fingers or tips of all the fingers; weakness is seen in extension of the forearm, in the extension of the wrist, and in the hand grip; the triceps reflex is diminished to absent, and the biceps and supinator reflexes are preserved. Either of these syndromes may be incomplete in that only one of several of the typical findings (e.g., pain) is present. Usually the patient states that cough, sneeze, and downward pressure on the head in the hyperextension position exacerbate pain and traction (even manual) tends to relieve it.

Unlike lumbar disks, the cervical ones, if large and centrally situated, may result in compression of the spinal cord (central disk, all the cord; paracentral disk, part of the cord). The central disk is often nearly painless, and the cord syndrome may simulate a degenerative disease (amyotrophic lateral sclerosis, combined system disease). A common error is to fail to think of a ruptured disk in the cervical region in patients with obscure symptoms in the legs. The diagnosis of ruptured cervical disk should be confirmed by the same laboratory procedures that were mentioned under "Spondylosis," above.

OTHER CONDITIONS Metastases to the cervical spine are fortunately less common than to other parts of the vertebral column. They are frequently painful and the cause of disordered root function. Compression fractures or extension of the tumor posteriorly may lead to rapid development of quadriplegia.

Shoulder injuries (rotator cuff), subacromial or subdeltoid bursitis, the frozen shoulder (periarthritis or capsulitis), tendonitis, and arthritis may develop in patients who are otherwise well, but these conditions are also frequent in hemiplegics or in individuals suffering from coronary heart disease. The pain is often severe and extends toward the neck and down the arm into the hand. The dorsum of the latter may tingle without other signs of nerve involvement. Vasomotor changes also may occur in the hand (shoulder-hand syndrome), and after a time, osteoporosis and atrophy of cutaneous and subcutaneous structures occur (Sudeck's atrophy or Sudeck-Leriche syndrome). These conditions fall more within the province of orthopedics than of medicine and are not discussed here in detail. The physician, however, must know that they can often be prevented by proper exercises (Chap. 253).

The *carpal tunnel syndrome*, with paresthesias and numbness in palmar distribution of the median nerve and aching pain which extends up into the forearm, may be mistaken for disease of the shoulder or neck. Similarly, other less common forms of nerve entrapment may involve the ulnar, radial, or median nerves and lead to a mistaken diagnosis of brachial plexus lesion or cervical syndrome. Electromyography and conduction studies are especially helpful in such conditions (Chap. 377).

MANAGEMENT OF BACK PAIN

Without doubt the preventive aspects of back pain are important. There would be many fewer back problems if adults kept their trunk muscles in optimal condition by regular exercise such as swimming, bicycle riding, walking briskly, running, or calisthenic programs. Morning is the ideal time since the back of the older adult tends to stiffen during the night because of inactivity. This happens regardless of whether a bed board or a stiff mattress is used. Sleeping with back hyperextended and sitting for long times in an overstuffed chair or a badly designed auto seat are particularly risky. It is estimated that pressures between disks are increased 200 percent by changing from a recumbent to a standing position and by 400 percent by sitting slumped in an easy chair. Correct sitting posture lessens this. Long trips in a car or plane without change in position put maximal strain on disk and ligamentous structures in the spine. Lifting from a position of flexed trunk, as in removing a suitcase from the trunk of a car, is dangerous (always lift with the object close to the body). Sudden strenuous activity without conditioning and warm-up also is likely to cause trouble to disks and their ligamentous envelopes (the commonest sources of back pain); certain families seem disposed.

The following diagrams are useful guides in strengthening trunk muscles (Figs. 7-2 to 7-6).

Muscular and ligamentous strains and minor disk prolapses are usually self-limited, responding to simple measures in a relatively short period of time. The basic principle of therapy is rest in a recumbent position for several days to weeks. When weight bearing is resumed, a light lumbosacral support is usu-

FIGURE 7-2

A. With knees bent, feet flat on floor, and hands clasped behind head, pinch buttocks together, pull in abdomen, and flatten back against floor. At first, hold position for a count of 5, relax for 5, then gradually increase to counts of 20. B. Next do this same exercise with legs extended and arms raised straight overhead. (From U.S. News & World Report. Copyright 1975 U.S. News & World Report).

ally helpful in continuing the immobilization until the patient is restored to full health. Physical measures such as heat, cold, diathermy, or massage are of limited value; of considerably greater importance are active exercises to both reduce the spasm and improve muscle tone. Analgesic medication should be given liberally during the first few days: codeine, 30 mg, and aspirin, 0.6 g, or pentazocine (Talwin), 50 mg, propoxyphene (Darvon), 65 mg, or meperidine (Demerol), 50 mg. Muscle relaxants are often a valuable adjunct, particularly in that such drugs as Valium, 8 to 40 mg in divided doses, and carisoprodol (Soma), 350 mg, twice daily, make bed rest more tolerable. If an inflammatory component is suspected, indomethacin, 75 mg per day (in divided doses), or ibuprofen (Motrin), 400 mg 3 or 4 times daily, may be helpful.

In the treatment of an acute or chronic rupture of a lumbar or cervical disk, complete bed rest is essential, and strong analgesic medication may be required. Traction is of little value in lumbar disk disease, and it is best to permit the patient to find the most comfortable position. Cervical traction with a halter may be of considerable benefit to patients with cervical disk syndrome. It can be administered with the patient in recumbency, or after sufficient improvement to allow ambulation, can be performed intermittently in the erect position using special equipment. During the recumbent phase of treatment of lumbar disk disease, exercises to reduce spasm, muscle relaxants, and anti-inflammatory agents as described above may be

FIGURE 7-3

A. Keeping shoulders flat on floor, draw knees toward chest, clasp hands around knees, and pull knees tightly against chest. B. Next bring forehead up to knees (From U.S. News & World Report. Copyright 1975 U.S. News & World Report.)

FIGURE 7-4

A. With knees bent, keep feet flat on floor and held or hooked under a heavy piece of furniture to provide leverage. B. Cross arms on chest, raise head and shoulders, and curl up to a sitting position. Keep back round and pull with abdominal muscles. Lower self slowly. (From U.S. News & World Report. Copyright 1975 U.S. News & World Report.)

of considerable value. After 2 to 3 weeks in bed, the patient can be allowed to slowly resume activities, usually with the protection of a brace or light spinal support. Exercise programs designed to increase the strength of the abdominal and gluteal muscles are helpful at this point. The patient may suffer some minor recurrence of the pain but be able to carry on his or her usual activities, and eventually most individuals will recover. If the pain and neurologic findings do not disappear on prolonged, conservative management, or if the patient suffers frequently recurring acute episodes, surgical management may be indicated. This should always be preceded by a myelogram to localize the lesion (and rule out the presence of intra- or extradural tumors). The surgical procedure most often indicated is a hemilaminectomy with excision of the disk involved. Arthrodesis of the involved segments is indicated only in cases in which there is extraordinary instability usually related to an anatomic abnormality (such as spondylolysis) or in the cervical region when an extensive laminectomy has rendered the spine unstable.

Spondylosis of the cervical part of the spine, if painful, is helped by bed rest and traction; if signs of spinal cord involvement are present, a collar to limit movement may halt the progression and even lead to improvement. Decompressive

FIGURE 7-5

A. Bend knees, keeping feet flat on floor and arms straight forward. Raise up and touch head to knees. B. Lower self, then pull knees up tightly against chest and bring forehead up to knees. (From U.S. News & World Report. Copyright 1975 U.S. News & World Report.)

FIGURE 7-6

A. Place hands at edge of chair. B. Bend forward to bring head to knees, pulling in abdomen as you curl forward. Keep weight well back on hips. Release abdominal muscles slowly as you come up. (From U.S. News & World Report. Copyright 1975 U.S. News & World Report.)

laminectomy or anterior fusion is reserved for severe instances of the disease with advancing neurologic symptoms. The shoulder-hand syndrome may benefit from stellate ganglion blocks or ganglionectomy, but the basic treatment is physiotherapy, with or without prednisone, and surgical procedures are used only as measures of last resort.

REFERENCES

ARMSTRONG JR: *Lumbar Disc Lesions,* 3d ed. Baltimore, Williams & Wilkins, 1965

BRADY LP et al: An evaluation of the electromyogram in the diagnosis of lumbar disk lesion. J. Bone Joint Surg 51A:539, 1969

CONVENTRY MB: Anatomy of the intervertebral disk. Clin Orthop 67:9, 1969

EDEIKEN J, PITT MJ: The radiologic diagnoses of disk disease. Orthop Clin N Amer 2:405, 1971

FRIEDENBERG AB, MILLER WT: Degenerative disk disease of the cervical spine. J Bone Joint Surg 45A:1171, 1963

GOLUB B et al: Cervical and lumbar disk disease: A review. Bull Rheum Dis 21:635, 1971

NAYLOR A: The changes in the human intervertebral disk in degeneration and nuclear prolapse. Orthop Clin N Am 2:343, 1971

WATTS C et al: Chymopapain treatment of intervertebral disk disease. J Neurosurg 42:374, 1975

8
PAIN IN THE EXTREMITIES

D. EUGENE STRANDNESS, JR.

APPROACH TO THE PATIENT Pain in the extremities occurs from a wide variety of diseases of the skin, musculoskeletal, vascular, and nervous systems. In approaching a patient with an extremity problem, it is first necessary to establish which of the above systems is most likely the basis for the complaint. Once this has been accomplished, a more detailed clinical and laboratory evaluation will usually provide a specific diagnosis. In this chapter, the cardinal manifestations without specific emphasis on etiology are presented in Table 8-1. It is important to recognize some of the major distinguishing features of the various problems causing the pain since these will at least lead the observer in most instances to the system involved.

In the diagnosis of pain of the limbs it is important to classify the pain and localize the site of involvement. Pain may be classified as superficial, deep, and referred. *Superficial pain* either arising from the skin or spreading from adjacent structures such as joints is well localized and is associated with tenderness and hyperalgesia. *Deep pain* arising from fascia, vessels, periosteum, joints, and supporting structures is often poorly localized and dull, and may be associated with muscular rigidity and deep tenderness. *Referred pain* is usually well localized and similar to pain arising from deep structures (Chap. 3). In persons with acute ischemia of the limbs, with threatened loss of viability, both superficial and deep pain are present.

A thorough examination of the limbs must include inspection for evidence of cutaneous manifestations, palpation for masses and tenderness, and auscultation for arterial bruits. Examination of the peripheral pulses at their accessible sites must always be done. A careful neurologic examination looking for changes in reflexes and sensation is also essential.

In most instances an accurate diagnosis can be made or strongly suspected from the history and physical examination. Special tests such as arteriography, myelography, and nerve conduction studies are often helpful but are primarily reserved for accurate localization of the disease and determination of the extent of involvement.

Acute arterial insufficiency regardless of the cause produces the greatest changes in the *distal* limb. This simple fact, often overlooked, has been a source of confusion to many physicians. It is also important to recognize that the degree of ischemia is a reflection of the available collateral circulation. The dramatic presentation with pain, pallor, and paralysis is rarely missed but lesser symptoms such as transient numbness and a reduction in skin temperature are often overlooked. If there are any questions about the diagnosis, the measurement of the systolic pressure at the ankle and wrist will establish the diagnosis with certainty.

Chronic arterial occlusion produces pain in three circumstances:

1 With exercise (intermittent claudication). The location of the muscle pain depends on the level of occlusion.
2 Pain at rest. As with acute arterial occlusion, the distal limb is most affected, and the condition is recognized by the coexisting dependent rubor, loss of pulses, and improvement in the pain with dependency.
3 Ulceration combined with infection. These patients are often treated for cellulitis without proper attention to the underlying ischemia.

While it is common to lump all cases of acute venous occlusion under the title of *thrombophlebitis,* this is not a wise practice. Involvement of the superficial veins does have a prominent inflammatory component, with marked tenderness, erythema, and local edema. The vein is *always* thrombosed and recognized as a palpable, tender cord. While this condition may be secondary to bacterial infection, this is usually not the case, but the clinical picture is easily confused with cellulitis. The key diagnostic feature is the presence of the thrombosed vein, a condition which does not occur with cellulitis or lymphangitis.

Thrombosis of the deep veins does not have a prominent

inflammatory component and thus is often missed on clinical examination. Tenderness, edema, fever, and prominent superficial veins are so variable that they cannot be relied upon for certainty in establishing the diagnosis. The major point to remember when deep venous thrombosis is suspected is that the diagnosis *must* be established by some independent means, such as noninvasive testing or venography.

Chronic venous disorders of the lower limb are commonly considered in two categories, *varicose veins* and the *postphlebitic syndrome.* Varicose veins, of course, are easily recognized by inspection alone with the patient upright. The most serious sequelae occur secondary to deep vein thrombosis with destruction of the venous valves, which leads to edema, pain in the distal limb, and the stasis skin changes in the vicinity of the medial malleolus. Repeated injury with infection can produce similar skin changes.

PAINFUL SKIN DISEASE The common bacterial and fungous infections may occasionally produce pain, and it can occur in or remote to the involved areas. This is especially true when bacteria have entered the dermis and subcutaneous tissues via the base of the nails or interdigital areas. Depending upon the infecting agent, cellulitis with or without lymphangitis may rapidly ensue and produce local swelling, pain, erythema, and systemic signs of toxicity. If the infection develops in areas such as the pulp of the digits or in plantar or palmar spaces, the pain is severe, throbbing, and may secondarily extend to tendons and joints.

Fungous infections, particularly those of the interdigital areas of the feet, may also become secondarily infected by bacteria, resulting in a spreading cellulitis and lymphangitis. There are also nonbacterial forms of cellulitis. The lymphangitis is diagnosed by the presence of the "red lines" in the involved areas. Pain may also occur in the region of the lymph nodes which drain the infected area and may be the first sign of secondary infection.

Cellulitis, particularly of the lower extremities, may be confused with thrombophlebitis. Differentiating features supporting the diagnosis of cellulitis include: (1) rapidity of onset, (2) prominent cutaneous hyperemia and tenderness, (3) presence of a portal of entry for the infective agent, and (4) the nature of the systemic response (fever, leukocytosis), which is usually much more severe than with thrombophlebitis.

Erythema nodosum (Chap. 49) should be suspected when tender erythematous nodules appear in or under the skin and are associated with fever and joint pains. The articular manifestations often precede the appearance of the nodules. These lesions can be associated with a wide variety of diseases, some of which include tuberculosis, sarcoidosis, coccidioidomycosis, streptococcal infections, and ulcerative colitis. However, in the majority of cases, no underlying disease is found.

MUSCULOSKELETAL PAIN Bursitis and tendonitis *Inflammation* of one or more of the bursae may occur as a result of trauma, rheumatoid arthritis, gout, connective tissue disorders, and bacterial infection. The commonly involved bursae are the subdeltoid, olecranon, trochanteric, calcaneal, and prepatellar. When the process is acute, it is characterized by severe local pain and tenderness with marked limitation of activity and mobility. In long-standing cases the symptoms and physical findings are less pronounced. Calcific deposits within the involved bursa develop in some patients and may be seen in an x-ray.

Tenosynovitis of the tendon sheaths of hands or wrists produces pain in restricted regions. Tenosynovitis may arise in association with infection, rheumatoid arthritis, osteoarthritis, or trauma, or occur without explanation. When the sheath of the thumb's abductor longus and extensor brevis tendons at the radial styloid are affected, the condition is called *de Quer-*

vain's disease. The flexor tendons in the palm and finger and the extensor sheaths on the dorsum of the wrist may also be the site of the inflammation. Typically, the pain and tenderness occur in the region of the tendon, and the pain is aggravated by stretching the involved tendons as their muscles contract.

An important variant of tenosynovitis is the *carpal tunnel syndrome,* the symptoms of which may be confused with the thoracic outlet syndrome, cervical disk disease, and local vascular insufficiency. Thickening or swelling of the tendons as they pass through the flexor compartment at the wrist, amyloid deposit with multiple myeloma, or bone enlargement (acromegaly) can exert pressure on the median nerve, causing nocturnal paresthesias and pain in the fingers, wrist, and forearm. As the condition worsens, atrophy of the thenar eminence develops, as well as weakness and sensory loss in the territory of the median nerve. There may be tenderness on pressure over the carpal ligament and electrical tingling in the fingers when the wrist is tapped (Tinel's sign). Nerve conduction may be delayed at the wrist, confirming the diagnosis.

Calcific and *noncalcific tendonitis* is common in the bicipital and supraspinatus tendons, and in the common tendon of origin for the forearm extensors and flexors at the lateral and medial epicondyle of the humerus, respectively (tennis elbow). The diagnosis is suspected by the location of the pain and the painful limitation of motion involved by movement of these tendons.

Painful synovial cysts Cysts of the popliteal space (Baker's cysts) can be an obscure source of pain in the leg. The lesion consists of a cyst in the popliteal fossa, which frequently communicates with the knee joint. While the cause is unknown, such cysts are frequently associated with rheumatoid or osteoarthritis. Trauma may be an inciting factor. Unruptured cysts produce only mild aching in the popliteal space with associated stiffness of the joint. If the cyst ruptures, there is an acute, extensive inflammation of the lower leg with swelling and pain which may be severe. The clinical picture is commonly confused with thrombophlebitis. The diagnosis can easily be made by instilling radiopaque material into the knee joint.

Painful arthritis of extremities Most causes of arthritis can be classified into one of five major groups: (1) infectious, (2) degenerative, (3) posttraumatic, (4) metabolic, and (5) unknown etiology. The synovial membranes and periarticular structures are primarily involved in rheumatoid disease, infectious arthritis, and gout, whereas the cartilage and bone are mainly affected in osteoarthritis and rarer varieties. With acute pyogenic arthritis, gout, and rheumatic fever, the pain is severe even at rest and greatly intensified by even the slightest motion. The local findings of swelling, redness, and heat may be pronounced.

The principal symptom of *osteoarthritis* is pain which is brought on by use and is relieved by rest. Stiffness after sitting and immediately upon rising in the morning is common but seldom persists for more than a few minutes. Some of the more common locations are the terminal phalanges, knees, hips, and spine.

Rheumatoid arthritis most commonly involves the proximal interphalangeal and metacarpophalangeal joints, toes, wrists, ankle, knee, elbow, hip, and shoulder. The onset is often insidious with general fatigue, paresthesias in the extremities, joint pain, and stiffness. The most common symptoms include joint pain at rest which is aggravated by motion. Thickening of the periarticular structures may be marked and accompanied by atrophy of adjacent muscles. Subcutaneous nodules are often

TABLE 8-1
Pain in the extremities

	Chap.	Pain			Physical findings			Lab findings
		Location	Nature	Duration	Inspection	Palpation	Auscultation	
SUDDEN ONSET								
Arterial occlusion (large–medium-sized vessels)	253	Distal limb	Severe	Variable	Pale distal limb	Cool, absent pulses; look for aneurysm	Cardiac arrythmia, murmur, bruits	Positive cardiac findings, ECG abnormal; enzymes normal; decreased ankle, wrist systolic pressure
Arteriovenous fistula acquired	253	At site of fistula	Mild	Acute phase	Look for site of injury	False aneurysm, palpable thrill	Bruit over fistula	Decrease in systolic pressure distal to fistula
Ruptured synovial cysts		Adjacent to ruptured cyst	Severe	Acute phase	Swelling may be marked	Exquisite tenderness in involved area		Positive arthogram; look for associated rheumatoid arthritis
Nocturnal muscle cramps	383	Muscle group	Severe cramp	Several minutes	Normal	Local tenderness during attack		Not associated with any known disorder
SUDDEN OR GRADUAL ONSET (SEVERAL HOURS)								
Thrombophlebitis (superficial)	253	Involved veins	Severe	Acute phase	Erythema prominent	Severe local tenderness		Elevated WBC count; positive blood culture if septic
Acute venous thrombosis (deep veins)	253	Within involved segments	Mild to moderate	Transient	Usually normal	Edema, degree variable; mild tenderness		Positive noninvasive tests with major venous occlusion; phlebogram diagnostic
Cellulitis		Involved area	Moderate	With inflammation	Marked hyperremia	Local edema, tenderness		Those associated with bacterial infection
Lymphangitis	253	Involved segment	Moderate to severe	Acute phase	"Red streak"	Local edema, tenderness		Those associated with bacterial infection
Arthritis (articular)	355 361	Affected joints	Severe at rest	Acute phase	Joint may be reddened, swollen	Pain increases with motion		Depends on cause
Herniated nucleus pulposus	7	Poorly localized; may radiate	Moderate to severe	Worse with motion	Usually normal	Paravertebral muscle spasm; positive neurologic findings		Narrowing disk space, positive myelogram
Osteomyelitis	360	Affected bone	Severe with motion	Inflammatory phase	Normal to swelling over involved area	Severe pain with motion, palpation		Neutrophilic leukocytosis; elevated sedimentation rate; positive blood cultures; positive x-ray usually evident after second week

TABLE 8-1 *(continued)*
Pain in the extremities

		Pain			Physical findings			
	Chap.	Location	Nature	Duration	Inspection	Palpation	Auscultation	Lab findings
GRADUAL ONSET (DAYS TO MONTHS)								
Chronic arterial occlusion, moderate	253	Muscle group(s)	Cramp	With exercise	Normal or dependent rubor	Absent pulses	Bruits often present	Decreased ankle systolic pressure; further drop with exercise
Chronic arterial occlusion, severe	253	Distal foot	Severe	Constant	Tissue necrosis; loss of hair; nail changes	Distal limb cool; absent pulses	Bruits often present	Ankle systolic pressure index <0.5
Erythromelalgia	253	Foot; distal leg	Severe burning	During attack only	Foot, distal leg bright red	Increased temperature affected area		Rare cases secondary to myeloproliferative disorders
Sympathetic dystrophy (major)	3	In distribution of injury to nerve	Hyperalgesia; hyperesthesia	Persistent	Normal, late trophic changes	Increased sweating; hyperesthesia		Sympathetic block gives immediate relief
Causalgia (minor reflex dystrophy)	363	As above			Same as above			May accompany many illnesses, myocardial infarction, neurologic (central and peripheral) infections, severe ischemia
Carpal tunnel syndrome	363	Fingers, wrist, and forearm	Paresthesia burning	Persistent	Possible thenar atrophy			Nerve conduction delayed
Interdigital neuroma		Plantar aspect of foot	Moderate	With pressure or walking	Normal	Pain produced by lateral foot compression		Nothing diagnostic
Bursitis; tendonitis; fibrositis	363	Affected area only	Moderate	Until treated	Normal muscle atrophy, longstanding cases	Local tenderness		Calcium may be seen on x-ray, particularly in cases of bursitis
Rheumatoid arthritis	356	Proximal interphalangeal joints	Moderate	Variable	Periarticular thickening, muscle atrophy	Local tenderness; subcutaneous nodules		Positive rheumatoid factor; antinuclear antibodies; x-ray abnormality
Osteoarthritis	361	Involved joints	Moderate	With exercise	Terminal phalanges may be deformed, enlarged	Minimal tenderness over joints		No specific chemical abnormality; joint space narrow; osteophytes
Erythema nodosum	49	Nodules	Mild	Variable	Reddened subcutaneous nodule	Moderate tenderness with surrounding edema		Usually secondary; extensive workup may be required
Neuritis	377	Along affected nerves	Burning, tearing	Persistent	Usually normal	Areflexia		Nerve conduction delayed

TABLE 8-1 (continued)
Pain in the extremities

	Chap.	Pain			Physical findings			Lab findings
		Nature	Location	Duration	Inspection	Palpation	Auscultation	
GRADUAL ONSET (MONTHS TO YEARS)								
Primary varicose veins	253	Mild	Distal leg	Only with dependency	Dilated superficial veins	Edema if present mild, distal limb		Valvular incompetence confined to superficial veins
Postphlebitic syndrome (secondary to varicose veins)	253	Moderate	Distal leg	Only with dependency	Stasis dermatitis: varicose veins; ulcers often present	Edema, induration in ulcer-bearing zone		Valvular incompetence, superficial and deep veins
Arteriovenous fistula, congenital	253	Mild	Affected limb	With dependency	Prominent venous pattern; increased limb length and girth	Edema variable	Bruits rarely present	Arteriography may show feeding vessels with early venous filling
EPISODIC OR WITH CHANGE OF POSITION								
Thoracic outlet syndromes	253	Moderate	Along distribution of compressed nerve root	Relieved with arm in neutral position	Normal	Decrease in radial pulse in position that produces symptoms, bruit in supraclavicular area		X-ray: cervical rib; osseous abnormality of clavicle, first rib
Vasospastic disorders	253	Mild	Fingers, toes	Transient	Color changes with attack	Pulses usually present	Usually normal	Raynaud's disease, digital circulation normal; secondary form, digital artery occlusions common

found over pressure points. Many of the patients are also subject to cold sensitivity of Raynaud's type. (See Chap. 356.)

Gout, a disease usually of men over 30 years of age, manifests itself often in acute episodes. Most frequently the metatarsophalangeal joint is involved; the affected joint is extremely painful and swells markedly within a few hours, becoming hot and dusky red. The process, particularly in the acute form, may be difficult to distinguish from acute rheumatic fever, gonococcal arthritis, atypical rheumatoid arthritis, traumatic arthritis, cellulitis, suppurative arthritis, and Reiter's syndrome. The presence of tophi and an elevated uric acid clarify the diagnosis. Finding the rodlike crystals of sodium urate in a tophus or synovial fluid establishes the diagnosis with certainty. (See Chap. 92.)

Pyogenic arthritis localizes usually in large joints (hip, knee, and shoulder). Such infections are usually metastatic in origin and remain monoarticular. The cardinal signs of infection, pain, and swelling, and a local increase in temperature with cutaneous hyperemia and fever, usually leave little doubt about the nature of the condition. In suspected cases the joint must be aspirated to identify the organism by Gram's stain and culture. (See Chap. 360.)

Hypertrophic osteoarthropathy, with its characteristic clubbing, periostitis at the ends of long bones, arthritis, and autonomic disorder, causes pain which varies from mild to severe. The pain is deep and aching and along with tenderness is localized to the involved joints and adjacent long bones. This syndrome usually appears in relation to malignancies or suppurative conditions of the lungs, mediastinum, or pleura.

Osteomyelitis Osteomyelitis may occur following open fractures, open surgical reduction of fractures, or from a distant infective focus. Usually the symptoms commence abruptly with severe pain (aggravated by motion), local swelling, exqui-

site tenderness, chills, and fever. There is nearly always a neutrophilic leukocytosis and elevated sedimentation rate, and blood cultures may be positive. X-ray changes may not be evident until the second week or later. The differential diagnosis includes acute pyogenic arthritis, hemarthrosis (particularly in children), cellulitis, and erysipelas. (See Chap. 360.)

Painful disorders of muscle Disorders of muscles are common causes of severe pain in the limbs. Localized tenderness and pain with motion is most commonly seen after trauma or severe exercise. An acute suppurative myositis is nearly always associated with injury and direct inoculation with bacteria. Clostridial myositis (Chap. 141) must be considered in every case of a deep infection occurring secondary to a puncture wound.

A condition frequently confused with ischemic rest pain is the *nocturnal muscle cramp.* This process of unknown cause occurs in both sexes at all ages but is most often a source of complaints in pregnant women, the middle-aged, and the elderly. Unusually strenuous activity in the daytime increases the liability to cramp at night, especially when the feet are cold. The onset is sudden, usually in one of the muscles of the foot or leg, and it may awaken the patient. The pain subsides with vigorous massage and stretching (Chap. 383) of the part. If frequent and troublesome, 50 mg benadryl taken at bedtime will usually prevent the cramps.

When there is generalized muscle tenderness, weakness, increasing fatigability, and other systemic symptoms, the possibility of polymyositis and dermatomyositis must be considered.

section 2 | Alterations in body temperature

9
DISTURBANCES OF HEAT REGULATION

ROBERT G. PETERSDORF

CONTROL OF BODY TEMPERATURE

INTRODUCTION In health, the body temperature of human beings is maintained within a narrow range despite extremes in environmental conditions and physical activity. This is also true for most birds and mammals, and such animals are termed *homeothermic,* or warm-blooded. An almost invariable accompaniment of systemic illness is a disturbance in temperature regulation, usually an abnormal elevation, or *fever.* In fact, fever is such a sensitive and reliable indicator of the presence of disease that thermometry is probably the commonest clinical procedure in use. Even in the absence of a frank febrile response, interference with heat regulation by disease is evident. This may take the form of flushing, pallor, sweating, shivering, and abnormal sensations of cold or warmth, or it

may consist of erratic fluctuations of body temperature within normal limits when a patient is at bed rest.

HEAT PRODUCTION The major source of basal heat production is through thyroid thermogenesis and the action of adenosine triphosphatase (ATPase) on the sodium pump of all membranes. The muscles are most important in promoting increased heat production with exercise through increased shivering. Heat production by muscle is of particular importance because the quantity can be varied according to the need. In most circumstances this variation consists of small increases and decreases in the number of nerve impulses to the muscles, causing inapparent tensing or relaxing. When, however, there is a strong stimulus for heat production, muscle activity may increase to the point of shivering, or even to a generalized rigor.

HEAT LOSS Heat is lost from the body in several ways. Small amounts are used in warming food or drink and in the evaporation of moisture from the respiratory tract. Most heat is lost from the surface of the body, by *convection,* i.e., the transfer of heat to a fluid medium. Heat loss by convection depends on the existence of a temperature gradient between the body surface and the ambient air. A second mechanism for heat loss is *radiation,* which may be defined as an exchange of electromagnetic energy between the body and the radiant environment. *Evaporation* is the third major mechanism for dissipating heat and is particularly important when the ambient temperature exceeds that of the body.

The principal method of regulating heat loss is by varying the volume of blood flowing to the surface of the body. A rich circulation in the skin and subcutaneous tissues carries heat to the surface, where it can escape. In addition, sweating increases heat loss by providing water to be vaporized. The sweat, or eccrine, glands are under the control of the sympathetic nerves which, in this instance, mediate cholinergic stimuli. Heat loss by sweating may be tremendous, and as much as 1 liter per h of sweat may be evaporated. The amount of heat loss through sweating is also dependent upon the humidity in the air. The greater the humidity, the less the ability to lose heat through sweat.

When there is need for conservation of heat, adrenergic autonomic stimuli cause a sharp reduction in the blood flow to the surface. This causes vasoconstriction and transforms the skin and subcutaneous tissue into layers of insulation.

HEAT TRANSFER WITHIN THE BODY This depends upon *conduction,* i.e., the transfer of heat between adjacent organs, and upon *circulatory convection,* which is governed by bulk movement of body fluids and which is responsible for the transfer of heat between the cells and the bloodstream. It is useful, although oversimplified, to visualize the body as a central core at uniform temperatures surrounded by an insulating shell. The role of the shell as a mediator for heat conservation and heat loss is determined in part by its blood supply and by vasoconstriction or vasodilatation. Although insulation is relatively uniform throughout the body, some parts, such as the digits, are particularly susceptible to cold because of the increased surface-to-volume ratio. Moreover, blood that reaches the digits has already been cooled on the way. Insulation may be enhanced by the addition of clothing.

NEURAL CONTROL OF TEMPERATURE The control of body temperature, integrating the various physical and chemical processes for heat production or loss, is a function of cerebral centers located in the hypothalamus. A high-decerebrate animal displays a normal temperature if the hypothalamus is left intact. On the other hand, an animal whose brainstem has been sectioned loses ability to control body temperature, which consequently tends to vary with the environment, a condition referred to as *poikilothermia.* Animal experiments suggest that the preoptic anterior hypothalamus and some centers in the spinal cord have neurons which respond directly to local temperature and act as a sensor for internal temperature. This function is distinct from the integrative function which responds to temperature-sensitive structures all over the body.

Factors affecting neural control of temperature The temperature-regulating system is a negative feedback control system, and possesses three elements essential to such a system: (1) receptors which sense the existing central temperatures; (2) effector mechanisms, consisting of the vasomotor, sudomotor, and metabolic effectors, and (3) integrative structures which determine whether the existing temperature is too high or too low and which activate the appropriate motor response. It is a negative feedback system because a rise in central temperature initiates mechanisms for losing heat while a fall in central temperature activates mechanisms for heat production and heat

conservation. The activation of these effector responses is governed by a central integrative mechanism which may be compared with a thermostat and which responds to a variety of stimuli, such as the sensory impulses engendered in flushing or sweating, behavioral impulses, exercise, endocrine influences, and probably the temperature of the blood circulating through the hypothalamic centers. In a sense all these stimuli reset the thermostat.

A classic example of the endocrine influence on temperature is the effect of menstruation. The mean body temperature of women is higher during the second half of the menstrual cycle than it is between the onset of menstruation and the time of ovulation. The sensations of intense heat followed by diaphoresis that characterize the vasomotor instability experienced by some women at the menopause are undoubtedly the result of endocrine imbalance. The activation of the adrenal medulla in response to cold is another example of the relationship between the endocrine system and the thermoregulatory apparatus.

NORMAL BODY TEMPERATURE It is not practical to designate an exact upper level of normal body temperature because there are small differences among normal persons. There are rare individuals whose temperatures are always elevated slightly above accepted "normal" levels, and there is considerable variation in temperature in a given individual. In general, however, it is safe to regard an oral temperature above 99°F (37.2°C) in a person at bed rest as probable indication of disease. The temperature may be as low as 96.5°F (35.8°C) in healthy persons. Rectal temperature is usually 0.5 to 1.0°F higher than oral temperature. In very hot weather the body temperature may be elevated by 0.5 or even 1.0°F.

There is a distinct diurnal variation in body temperature in healthy human beings. Oral readings of 97°F (36.1°C) are relatively common on arising in the morning. Body temperature rises steadily through the day, reaches a peak of 99°F (37.2°C) or greater between 6 P.M. and 10 P.M., and then drops slowly to reach a minimum at 2 A.M. to 4 A.M. Although it has been postulated that this diurnal variation is dependent upon increasing activity during the day and rest at night, the pattern is not reversed in individuals who work at night and sleep during the day for long periods of time. The febrile patterns of most human diseases also tend to follow this normal diurnal pattern. Fevers tend to be higher, to "spike," in the evening, and many patients with febrile disease have relatively normal temperatures in the early morning hours.

Body temperature is more labile in young children, and transient elevations after relatively slight exertion in warm weather are frequently observed in them.

Severe or prolonged exercise can produce considerable elevation in body temperature. For example, marathon runners often have temperatures between 103.2 and 105.8°F (39 and 41°C). Although this marked increase in temperature with exercise tends to be balanced by compensatory cutaneous vasodilatation, resulting in loss of heat, and hyperventilation, these compensatory mechanisms may fail, leading to hyperpyrexia and, if uncontrolled, to heat stroke. Many of the adverse effects of long-distance running can be prevented by holding races only if the ambient temperature is below 82°F (27.8°C), preferably in the early morning or early evening, and by assuring ample fluid intake both before and during a race.

DISORDERED THERMOREGULATION In exercise, there is a temporary imbalance between heat production and heat loss with prompt reestablishment of normal temperatures at rest due to continuing activation of heat loss mechanisms. In fact, in prolonged exercise, cutaneous vasodilatation in response to an increase in central body temperature stops in order to preserve central temperature. Less adaptation occurs in fever because once a stable body temperature is reached, heat production equals heat loss, but both are greater than in the basal state. Cutaneous blood flow plays a greater role in controlling heat production and heat loss in fever than does sweating. At the beginning of fever, the body temperature as sensed by the thermoreceptors is low and the individual responds physiologically as if he were cold. *Heat production* is increased by shivering, and *heat loss* is decreased by vasoconstriction. These events explain the sensation of cold or chills that characterize the beginning of fever. Conversely, when the cause of fever is removed, the temperature returns to normal, and the individual responds as if he were warm. Cutaneous vasodilatation, sweating, and inhibition of shivering are the compensatory responses.

Deviations of 5°F (approximately 3.5°C) from the normal body temperature do not interfere appreciably with most bodily functions. Convulsions are common at temperatures higher than 106°F (41.1°C) in children, and irreversible brain damage, presumably due to protein denaturation (impairment of normal enzymic functions), is common when temperatures of 108°F (42.2°C) are reached. Fortunately, when hyperthermia reaches dangerous levels, the mechanisms for heat loss are suddenly activated; consequently, oral temperatures above 106°F (41.1°C) are relatively rare in humans. Conversely, when temperatures are lowered to 91°F (32.8°C), loss of consciousness occurs; at 86°F (30°C) poikilothermia sets in, and between 83 and 84°F (28.5°C) slow atrial fibrillation supervenes. Ventricular fibrillation occurs at extremely hypothermic temperatures.

The systemic symptoms accompanying deviations in temperature are poorly understood. For example at temperatures of 102°F (39°C) many patients have malaise, drowsiness, weakness, and generalized aches and pains. Many others, however, feel entirely well. Why some individuals are able to tolerate fever so well while others become markedly ill remains an enigma. Perhaps the inciting stimulus rather than fever per se is the major determinant of systemic complaints.

Diseases of the nervous system   Disease of the regulatory centers in the hypothalamus may affect body temperature. Cases have been observed in which there was destruction of the centers controlling heat-conserving mechanisms, with resulting hypothermia. More commonly, cerebral lesions are manifested by hyperthermia; this may occur with tumors, degenerative diseases, vascular accidents, particularly cerebral hemorrhage, or infections involving the hypothalamus, such as encephalitis. All these may result in loss of neurons and gliosis. Central fever is accompanied by lack of a diurnal variation, absence of sweating, resistance to antipyretic drugs, excessive response to external cooling, and loss of consciousness.

There are several diseases, of which heat stroke is the cardinal example, in which the central mechanisms for cooling suddenly fail and the patient ceases to sweat, despite the fact that his temperature is rising. Some of the highest temperatures ever observed in human beings [112 to 113°F (44.4°C)] have been in cases of heat stroke. A temperature higher than 114°F (45.6°C) is probably not compatible with life.

Increased heat production   Patients with thyrotoxicosis show exaggerated heat production, and their temperature is often 1 to 2°F above the normal range. Dinitrophenol, a drug once used for weight reduction, causes elevation of temperature; this, too, seems to be caused by increased metabolic activity.

Impairment of heat loss   Patients with *congestive heart failure* often have an elevation of body temperature between 0.5 and 1.5°F. Perhaps this elevation is caused by impairment of heat dissipation as a result of diminished cardiac output, decline in cutaneous blood flow (with increasing insulation of the central

temperature core), the insulating effect of edema, and the increased heat production incident to the muscular activity of dyspnea. On the other hand, patients with congestive heart failure are likely to have other causes of fever, such as venous thrombosis, pulmonary embolism and infarction, myocardial infarction, pneumonia, and urinary tract infection. However, since slight fever is so regularly present even in the absence of such complications, the circulatory disturbance may be responsible.

Patients with skin disorders such as *ichthyosis* and *congenital absence of sweat glands* may have fever in a warm environment because of inability to lose heat from the surface of the body. Similarly, individuals taking *drugs which impair sweating,* such as atropine, scopolamine, phenothiazines, monoamine oxidase inhibitors, glutethimide, lysergic acid diethylamide (LSD), amphetamines, and inhalation anesthetics, to mention just some, may have fever in warm weather.

Patients with severe burns tend to be hyperthermic, probably because occlusive dressings interfere with heat loss despite large areas of denuded skin.

PATHOGENESIS OF FEVER

Fever is a consequence of many stimuli, including bacteria and their endotoxins, viruses, yeasts, antigen-antibody reactions, hormonal substances, exemplified by etiocholanolone, drugs, and synthetic polynucleotides like poly I:poly C. These substances, which have been termed collectively *exogenous pyrogens,* are both diverse and complex. It has been postulated that they act through an intermediary substance termed *endogenous pyrogen* (EP). Most of the knowledge concerning EP has come from work in experimental animals.

Endogenous pyrogen is a basic protein of low molecular weight that is derived from leukocytes and macrophages, including Kupffer cells, splenic sinusoidal cells, alveolar macrophages and peritoneal-lining cells. Endogenous pyrogen has not been isolated from lymphocytes, but these cells may react with antigens and, through the action of lymphokines, may stimulate neutrophils and macrophages to release EP.

When stored in cells, such as polymorphonuclear leukocytes, EP is not present in active form. Rather, its release requires synthesis of new messenger ribonucleic acid (RNA) and protein. Because it is present in such small amounts, EP has been difficult to detect in human serum or exudates. However, a radioimmunoassay to detect EP is being developed.

Once released, EP probably acts on the thermosensitive neurons in the preoptic region of the hypothalamus. These neurons control the constancy of body temperature and are the point where fever is initiated.

The action of EP on the hypothalamus is by no means simple. It appears as if there must be a release of 5-hydroxytryptamine (serotonin), a thermogenic amine, to mediate the febrile response. In addition, EP induces synthesis of prostaglandins E_1 and E_2 in the hypothalamus, where they function as central transmitters in the initiation of fever. The action of antipyretics, such as aspirin, has been shown to be the result of their ability to block prostaglandin synthesis. The prostaglandins, in turn, lead to an increase in cyclic AMP, which may be important in the metabolic processes—heat conservation and increased oxygen consumption—that are operative in fever.

All these observations make for a cohesive explanation of the pathogenesis of fever, at least at the level of peripheral tissues, but more studies are needed to elucidate the mechanism of the action of EP in the central nervous system.

DISORDERS ASSOCIATED WITH HIGH TEMPERATURES

CAUSES OF HYPERPYREXIA The incidence of hyperpyrexia, defined as a temperature above 106°F (41.1°C), in adults is not known. In a series of 28 such patients studied at the Massachusetts General Hospital, 11 had infections, 9 had infections plus failure to dissipate heat adequately, such as autonomic dysfunction or occlusive burn dressings, 5 had thermoregulatory failure due to cerebral hemorrhage and heat stroke, and in 3 the cause was not determined. The majority of the hyperpyrexic episodes occurred in summer when the ambient temperature and humidity were high. The mortality was 29 percent and was related primarily to underlying disease; only two deaths were attributed to hyperpyrexia per se. In most patients, the high temperature responded to antipyretic drugs and cooling devices. The good outcome in this series of hospitalized patients was due in part to the early recognition of the high temperature and its intensive treatment.

HEAT SYNDROMES Three clinical syndromes are associated with high environmental temperature: *heat cramps, heat exhaustion,* and *heat pyrexia.* Although each entity may be identified clinically, there is considerable overlap in the changes produced by a high environmental temperature. These alterations are especially prevalent during the first days of a heat wave before effective acclimatization can occur. Prophylaxis by augmenting sodium chloride and fluid intake prior to exposure; by ensuring that susceptible individuals, particularly the elderly or the very young, wear light clothing, take frequent cool baths, and remain in a cool environment; or by restoring a physiologic balance prior to the onset of overt morbidity can help prevent the full-blown syndrome, especially heat pyrexia.

Strenuous physical activity or the presence of an acute or chronic disease may hasten the development of one of the heat syndromes.

Acclimatization The basic mechanism by which humans accommodate to excessive temperatures is unknown. Acclimatization does not increase the threshold for sweating. However, sweating is the most effective natural means of combating heat stress and can occur with little or no change in the core temperature of the body. As long as sweating continues, humans can withstand remarkably high temperatures, provided water and sodium chloride, the most important physiologic constituents of sweat, are replaced. The concentration of sodium chloride varies between that of interstitial fluid and very low concentrations, and the ability to secrete sweat with low sodium chloride content, as well as to increase the quantity of sweat, is a major mechanism for the conservation of salt in hot weather. Dilatation of the peripheral blood vessels in an attempt to dissipate heat is another major way for the body to acclimatize to hot temperatures. Other alterations include a decrease in total circulating blood volume, a decrease in renal blood flow, an increase of antidiuretic hormones (ADH) as well as aldosterone, a decrease in urine sodium, and an increase in respiratory and pulse rates. Ordinarily, acclimatization takes from 4 to 7 days. The hyperaldosteronism may result in severe potassium loss, which may be aggravated by replacement of sodium without concomitant repletion of potassium. Initially there is an increase in cardiac output but as heat stress persists, venous return diminishes and heart failure may occur. If environmental temperatures in excess of the body's temperature persist, heat is retained and hyperpyrexia develops.

Heat cramps Heat cramps, called "miner's cramps" and "stoker's cramps," are the most benign heat syndrome. Cramps are characterized by painful spasms of the voluntary muscles and usually follow strenuous exercise. In general, only individuals in good physical condition develop this syndrome. External temperatures need not exceed the body temperature, and direct exposure to the sun is not necessary. The body temperature is usually not elevated. Muscle cramps usually occur after excessive sweating and may even be precipitated by strenuous exercise in cold environments in untrained persons heavily clothed. Muscles of the extremities bear the brunt of physical activity and hence show the highest incidence of cramps. Physical examination of the patient is normal between the paroxysms. Examination of the blood reveals a concentration of the formed elements and a decreased sodium and chloride concentration. Excretion of these ions in the urine is characteristically low. Treatment consists of sodium chloride; cessation of cramps with replacement of sodium chloride and water is striking and supports the hypothesis that the cause of heat cramps is depletion of these essential electrolytes. Occasionally cramps involve the abdominal musculature, mimicking an intraabdominal emergency. Such patients have had mistaken exploratory surgery performed, often with disastrous results. Replacement of saline prior to surgery would have obviated such operations.

Heat exhaustion Heat prostration, or heat collapse, is probably the most common heat syndrome. It represents a failure of the cardiovascular responses to high external temperatures and is particularly common in elderly individuals who are receiving diuretics. Weakness, vertigo, headache, anorexia, nausea, vomiting, the urge to defecate, and faintness may precede collapse. Heat collapse occurs in both physically active and sedentary individuals. The onset is usually sudden and the duration of collapse brief. During the acute stage, the patient looks ashen-gray. The skin is cold and clammy. The pupils are dilated. The blood pressure may be low and the pulse pressure elevated. Since prostration develops before exposure to heat is prolonged, body temperature is subnormal or normal. The duration of exposure and the extent to which sweat is lost determine the degree of hemoconcentration. Treatment consists of removal of the patient to a cool area and placing him in the recumbent position. Spontaneous recovery then usually takes place. Intravenous administration of saline solution or whole blood is necessary only rarely. Although the pathogenetic mechanism of heat prostration is not primarily a depletion of water and salt, it is likely that maintenance of these electrolytes will prevent heat prostration in individuals exposed to high temperatures.

Heat pyrexia ETIOLOGY Heat hyperpyrexia, heat stroke, or sunstroke is most common in elderly individuals with preexisting chronic disease. Among these are arteriosclerosis and congestive heart failure, particularly when patients receive diuretics. Other predisposing factors include diabetes mellitus, alcoholism, the use of atropinelike drugs, and skin disorders in which it may be difficult to lose heat such as ectodermal dysplasia, congenital absence of the sweat glands, or severe scleroderma. Direct exposure to the sun is not a necessary prerequisite. Heat pyrexia may develop during any period of hot weather, but the incidence in temperate climates increases during prolonged heat waves and at temperatures of 90°F (32.2°C) or higher. High humidity in the range of 60 to 75 percent is a prerequisite to heat stroke. The major pathogenic mechanism of heat stroke is "sweat fatigue," and patients usually stop sweating before the onset of acute symptoms. The cessation of sweating is due to an intrinsic breakdown of the heat regulatory mechanism for reasons not known.

MANIFESTATIONS There may be few premonitory symptoms of heat stroke, and loss of consciousness may be the first sign. Other patients may complain of headache, vertigo, faintness, abdominal distress, confusion, or hyperpnea. Delirium may develop in more severe cases.

Pyrexia and prostration are the significant findings on physical examination. A rectal temperature greater than 106°F (41.1°C) is common and is a grave prognostic sign. Internal body temperatures as high as 112 to 113°F (44.4°C) have been recorded. The skin is hot and dry, and sweating is absent. The pulse rate is increased, and respirations are rapid and weak. The systolic blood pressure may be elevated. The muscles are flaccid, and tendon reflexes may be diminished. Lethargy, stupor, or coma, depending on the severity, is present. Shock is common in fatal cases.

Examination of the blood and urine may show few abnormalities. Leukocytosis is characteristic as are proteinuria, cylinduria, and an elevation in BUN. There is usually a respiratory alkalosis, hypokalemia, and severe hypophosphatemia. The electrocardiogram may show, in addition to tachycardia and sinus arrhythmia, flattening and subsequent inversion of the T wave and depression of the ST segment. Diffuse myocardial necrosis with ECG evidence of myocardial infarction has been reported. Other major laboratory abnormalities include thrombocytopenia; prolonged bleeding, clotting, and prothrombin times; afibrinogenemia and fibrinolysis; and consumptive coagulopathy. All these may be responsible for diffuse bleeding. Liver damage is common; it appears 24 to 36 h after admission and is characterized by clinically apparent jaundice and, often, by abnormalities in hepatocellular enzymes. Renal failure is a common complication of heat stroke.

Patients with heat stroke may die within a few hours after being discovered, or may die of complications such as acute renal failure. However, a number of patients will die several weeks after the acute episode, usually of myocardial infarction, heart failure, renal failure, bronchopneumonia, or complicating bacteremia. In them autopsy may show extensive parenchymal damage to various organs, either from hyperpyrexia per se or from petechial hemorrhages in the brain, heart, kidneys, or liver.

TREATMENT Heat stroke requires heroic emergency measures. Time is most important. The patient should be placed in a cool place with adequate circulation of fresh air and with most of the clothing removed. Because the pathogenesis of heat stroke involves failure of the heat-regulating mechanism with cessation of sweating, external means of heat dissipation must be employed. The most effective measure is to immerse the patient in an ice-water bath, and there is no effective substitute for this seemingly drastic treatment. An ice-water bath does not induce shock or stimulate significant cutaneous vasoconstriction. The bath should be given with a minimum of delay. The patient should be watched constantly by a nurse or physician and the rectal temperature monitored. The bath may be discontinued when the rectal temperature falls below 101°F (38.3°C), but treatment should be resumed if there is a febrile rebound. Compared with immersion in ice water, other forms of therapy are less effective, but covering the patient with cold wet towels under a fan may be satisfactory if a bath is not available. After the bath the patient should be placed in a cool, well-ventilated room. Massage of the skin aids the acceleration of heat loss and stimulates return of the cool peripheral blood to the overheated brain and viscera. Phenothiazine may be given to reduce shivering. Stimulants such as epinephrine and narcotics are contraindicated. Intravenous fluids should be given with monitoring of the central venous pressure and urinary output. Both dehydration and heart failure must be avoided. Fresh blood should be given in case of bleeding, and clear-cut evidence of disseminated intravascular coagulation calls for heparin (7500 units per hour). Persistent oliguria is an indication for early dialysis.

Malignant hyperthermia ETIOLOGY Malignant hyperthermia is an inherited disorder that is characterized by a rapid increase in temperature to 102.2 to 107.6°F (39 to 42°C) in response to inhalational anesthetics such as halothane, methoxyflurane, cyclopropane, and ethyl ether or muscle relaxants, notably succinyl choline. Two forms of the disease exist; in one, where the mechanism of inheritance is autosomal dominant, the individuals are normal between attacks. A second form, which is recessive, occurs in young boys with a number of congenital abnormalities including short stature, undescended testes, lumbar lordosis, thoracic kyphosis, pectus carinatum, webbed neck, winged scapulae, small chin, low-set ears, and an antimongoloid obliquity of the palpebral fissures. The incidence of the autosomal dominant form is 1:50,000 to 1:100,000.

PATHOGENESIS The triggering anesthetic releases calcium from the membrane of the muscle cell's sarcoplasmic reticulum, which is defective in storing this ion. The result is a sudden increase in myoplasmic calcium. The calcium activates myosin ATPase which converts adenosine triphosphate (ATP) to adenosine diphosphate, phosphate, and heat. There are also inhibition of tropanin, uncoupling of oxidative phosphorylation, activation of phosphorylase kinase, and increased glycolysis. Muscular contraction occurs, and it, as well as the chemical events, leads to production of heat.

MANIFESTATIONS Existence of malignant hyperthermia can be suspected if less relaxation is noted during induction of anesthesia and muscle fasciculations when succinyl choline is given. If the temperature is not monitored, the first signs may be a hot skin and tachycardia or a cardiac arrhythmia. In addition to the high fever, there is muscle rigidity, hypotension, and mottled cyanosis.

Early laboratory abnormalities include respiratory and metabolic acidosis, hyperkalemia and hypermagnesemia, and elevation in blood lactate and pyruvate. Late complications include massive skeletal muscle swelling, pulmonary edema, disseminated intravascular coagulation, and acute renal failure.

TREATMENT Malignant hyperthermia is a medical emergency. Surgery must be interrupted and the patient cooled with ice. One hundred percent oxygen should be given, along with sodium bicarbonate, to combat the severe metabolic acidosis. A diuresis should be induced with fluids and diuretics to reduce myoglobinemia and hyperkalemia. Specific treatment consists of procainamide 10 mg/kg [0.5 to 1.0 (mg/kg)/min]. An experimental drug, dantroline sodium, is also effective.

PREVENTION While the best way to detect this syndrome is to monitor the temperature of all patients under anesthesia, the best way to avert it altogether is to take a thorough family history. Examining patients preoperatively is often not helpful because, between attacks, persons susceptible to malignant hyperthermia may be entirely normal. Some have increased muscle bulk, some have localized areas of muscle weakness, some spontaneous muscle cramps, and a few have generalized muscle weakness. In some of these patients, the creatine phosphokinase (CPK) is elevated, but in many this test is entirely normal. Microscopy of muscle shows marked variation in fiber diameter. In susceptible patients, surgery should be performed under spinal, epidural, or regional anesthesia. If this is not possible, a combination of pentothal and diazepam is probably safest.

DISORDERS ASSOCIATED WITH LOW TEMPERATURES

COLD ACCLIMATIZATION This state of increased resistance to cold injury is the result of exposure to a cold but tolerable environment. Adaptive responses consist of circulatory adjustments protecting the temperatures of exposed portions of the body, metabolic adaptation providing greater heat production to compensate for increased heat loss, and behavioral and neural adaptations minimizing either the actual cold stress or the discomfort resulting from physiologically tolerable hypothermia. In contrast with heat acclimatization, it is not possible to delineate adaptive physiologic changes to cold. Nevertheless, primitive people live at zero temperatures wearing little or no clothing; pain perception is less in persons, such as fishermen, who work periodically with their hands in ice water; and military personnel shiver less during cold exposure after training in the Arctic. Adaptation may take place either by shivering, with production of excess heat, or, as is the case with Australian aborigines, by a drop of internal temperature with only minimal shivering.

HYPOTHERMIA Although far less common than is elevation in temperature, hypothermia is of considerable importance because it represents a medical emergency which lends itself to treatment.

Accidental hypothermia This is a well-known complication of exposure and has been reported frequently during the winter months. It usually occurs in elderly individuals after prolonged exposure, not necessarily to excessively low external temperatures. It is attributed not only to exogenous factors such as a cold external environment but also to unknown endogenous factors. The diagnosis of hypothermia has proved elusive largely because *clinical thermometers do not record temperatures below 95°F (35°C). Whenever a patient presents with a temperature below this level, the true temperature should be determined with an incubator thermometer or a thermocouple.* Accidental hypothermia has been found in association with myxedema, pituitary insufficiency, Addison's disease, hypoglycemia, cerebrovascular disease, myocardial infarction, cirrhosis, pancreatitis, and ingestion of drugs or alcohol. For example, it is not uncommon to find a derelict in a railroad yard or under a bridge following an alcoholic debauch with a temperature between 85 and 90°F (28.5 and 32.3°C) or lower. These patients usually appear cold and pale and, when their temperatures are very low, give the appearance of having rigor mortis, so stiff is their musculature. Patients with temperatures less than 80°F (26.7°C) are usually unconscious. The pupils are usually miotic, respirations tend to be shallow and slow, there is bradycardia, and most patients are hypotensive. Generalized edema is often present. Laboratory data tend to show hemoconcentration, mild azotemia, and metabolic acidosis. The acidosis is due in part to hypoxemia in peripheral tissues. At cold temperatures, the hemoglobin dissociation curve is shifted to the left, and there is decreased unloading of oxygen in the peripheral tissues. Some patients have hypoglycemia while others show evidence of diabetes mellitus. Thyroid function tests may give results typical of myxedema. Some patients have elevations in serum amylase, and a few show pancreatitis at autopsy. The electrocardiogram is distorted by muscular tremors and may show bradycardia or slow atrial fibrillation and a characteristic J wave (occurring at the junction of the QRS complex and ST segment). Other arrythmias are common; ventricular fibrillation is usually a terminal event.

TREATMENT Hypothermia is a medical emergency, and therapy should be instituted at once. The following steps are indicated:

1 An airway must be established and maintained, and the patient should be well oxygenated.
2 Blood gases should be monitored; they should be corrected for temperature.
3 Blood volume should be expanded with glucose and saline, low-molecular-weight dextran, or albumin. Maintenance of blood volume is necessary to prevent the infarctions which have been a hallmark in fatal cases and to avert "rewarming shock."
4 Because of the tendency to arrythmias, serum potassium should be monitored carefully; a transvenous pacemaker may be indicated.
5 Sodium bicarbonate should be given if pH ≤ 7.25.
6 Although external rewarming with blankets or warm baths may be appropriate in patients with mild hypothermia, patients who are severely hypothermic require reestablishment of core temperature. External rewarming does this poorly because, while it tends to dilate the constricted peripheral blood vessels, it diverts blood from the visceral organs. On the other hand, restoration of the core temperature by hemodialysis, during which the blood is warmed externally, or by peritoneal dialysis, during which the dialysate is warmed to 98.6°F (37°C), is the method of choice. It is particularly important to rewarm the myocardium because, in cases of ventricular fibrillation, defibrillation will not be successful until myocardial temperature is raised to near normal levels.
7 There is a tendency for these patients to develop pneumonia which should be treated promptly with antibiotics.
8 Finally, resuscitative efforts should be vigorous and prolonged despite the poor prognosis which is related primarily to the advanced age and associated debilitating disease of these patients. In younger individuals, some remarkable rescues have been recorded; one young woman was resuscitated even after her temperature had dropped to 69°F (20.6°C).

Hypothermia secondary to acute illness There is a group of patients who develop moderate hypothermia in association with acute diseases including congestive heart failure, uremia, diabetes mellitus, drug overdose, acute respiratory failure, and hypoglycemia. These patients are generally elderly and upon admission to the hospital are found to have temperatures of 92 to 93.9°F (33.3 to 34.4°C). They also have a severe metabolic acidosis, due to increased production of lactic acid, and cardiac arrhythmias. Most of these patients are comatose. This entity differs from accidental hypothermia only in the absence of exposure; these cases have all occurred at normal ambient temperatures. The mechanism appears to be an acute failure of thermoregulation; shivering did not occur in any of these patients. Usually these patients have been rewarmed within a few hours by means of an alcohol-circulating blanket. Upon return to normal temperature, cardiac arrythmias, which were present in most of these patients, responded to treatment, and the sensorium returned to normal. With the exception that core rewarming could be established by external means, other facets of therapy should follow the steps outlined above. In addition, treatment of the underlying disease such as diabetes with insulin, uremia with dialysis, or congestive heart failure with appropriate cardiac drugs and diuretics is essential. The prognosis is good provided the syndrome is recognized early and treatment is instituted at once.

Immersion hypothermia Responses to cold-water immersion may be classified as (1) stimulatory, with deep body temperature normal to 95°F (35°C); (2) depressant, with deep body temperature 95 to 86°F (35 to 30°C); and (3) critical, with deep body temperature 86 to 77°F (30 to 25°C).

The long-distance swimmer is able to maintain a normal body temperature for periods of 15 to 25 h or more in water that may plunge skin temperature to 59°F (15°C) or lower, which is some 28°F below deep body temperature, lending support to the concept of a body core insulated by a body shell. The vasoconstriction operative in cold water greatly reduces heat loss. However, there is great individual variability in heat loss in cold water. The relatively obese swimmer may maintain a normal rectal temperature for 2 h without shivering in 61°F (16°C) water. A lean person under the same conditions, despite violent shivering, may experience a fall in rectal temperature of several degrees and become incapacitated from the rigor. In hypersensitive persons, immersion in cold water may be followed by vascular spasm, vomiting, and syncope.

Other compensatory responses include bradycardia, a slight rise in blood pressure, and an early rise in rectal temperature followed by a fall. At 86°F (30°C), atrial fibrillation is common.

TREATMENT   Although rewarming in hot water has been recommended in the treatment of immersion hypothermia, the same objections to sudden diversion of cardiac output to peripheral tissues described above apply. Individuals with this problem should be covered with a light blanket and placed in a room with a moderate ambient temperature. The other measures described for the treatment of accidental hypothermia, including hemodialysis or peritoneal dialysis, should be instituted depending on the clinical picture.

LOCAL COLD INJURIES Mechanisms of freezing injury
These can be divided into phenomena which affect cells and extracellular fluids (direct effects) and those which disrupt the function of organized tissues and the integrity of the circulation (indirect effects).

DIRECT EFFECTS   When tissue freezes, ice crystals form and, concomitantly, solutes in the residual liquid become concentrated. The physical dislocation during slow freezing is extreme. Ice crystals many times the size of individual cells form but only in the extracellular spaces. Large ice crystals can develop between cells in soft tissue without producing irreversible injury as long as the percentage of water frozen does not exceed a critical amount. A major source of damage to living cells during freezing and thawing appears to be the strong salt solutions which develop during formation and dissolution of ice; changes in the proportions of lipids and phospholipids in the cell membrane are also of great importance. The discovery of the protective value of such substances as glycerol and dimethylsulfoxide, which enter cells and prevent freezing injury during comparatively slow cooling to low temperatures and rewarming from them, represents a significant advance. This method has been used extensively in banking spermatozoa for subsequent artificial insemination. It has not been possible, however, to protect organs in this manner since the protective substance must be delivered to all cells.

INDIRECT EFFECTS   The fulminating vascular reaction and stasis which supervene are associated with production of histamine-like substances which increase the permeability of the capillary bed. Within blood vessels, cellular elements aggregate. Irreversible occlusion of small blood vessels by cell masses has been demonstrated in thawed tissue following freezing injury. The damaged frozen tissue simulates tissue damage produced by burns.

Manifestations   The mildest form of cold injury is called *frostnip* and tends to occur in organs farthest removed from the core of the body such as the earlobes, nose, cheeks, fingers and toes, and hands and feet. It can be prevented by warm clothing and treated with simple rewarming. More consequential, local cold injuries may be divided into freezing (frostbite) and nonfreezing (immersion-foot) injuries. The two types may be observed in the same extremity or in different extremities in the same individual, e.g., trench foot and freezing of the hands but not the feet of shipwreck survivors. The diagnosis of freezing versus nonfreezing injury generally can be made on the basis of history and clinical manifestations.

IMMERSION FOOT   This entity is observed in shipwreck survivors or in soldiers (trench foot) whose feet have been wet but not freezing cold for prolonged periods. There is primarily injury to nerve and muscle tissue, but no gross or irreparable pathologic changes occur in blood vessels and skin. The clinical picture reflects primary hypoxic trauma giving rise to three clearly recognizable conditions: (1) *ischemia,* denoted by a pale, pulseless extremity; (2) *hyperemia,* characterized by a bounding pulsatile circulation in red, swollen, painful feet; and (3) the *posthyperemic* or recovery period. The initial cold-induced vasoconstriction, increased blood viscosity, and impaired oxygen transport in the ischemic state are aggravated by such factors as malnutrition, general hypothermia, dehydration, and trauma from relatively fixed, pendant extremities. The problem of rewarming is critical in these patients during the stage of ischemia, when overheating of tissue may lead to gangrene. In the state of hyperemia, the red, swollen feet require judicious cooling. Severe cases may show muscular weakness, atrophy, ulceration, and gangrene of superficial areas. Sensitivity to cold and pain on weight bearing, which may cause discomfort for many years, are sequelae even of milder injuries.

FROSTBITE   In contrast with immersion foot, in frostbite the blood vessels may be severely and irreparably injured, the circulation of blood ceases, and the vascular bed of the frozen tissue is occluded by agglutinated cell aggregates and thrombi. The cutaneous injury consists in part of separation of the epidermal-dermal interface. Early, the intravascular clumping is reversible. However, with the passage of time, clumped red blood cells within vessels in injured tissue lose their morphologic identity and take on the appearance of a homogenous, hyalinaceous plug. It has been shown in some, but not all, experimental studies that much of the intravascular aggregation following freezing injury can be reversed and microcirculatory perfusion improved if low-molecular-weight dextran is given intravenously shortly after injury. Frostbitten tissues unfortunately are often neglected and with thawing become macerated; if this is the situation, the method of rewarming is not important. The method of rewarming has been a matter of controversy. It seems most rational to warm the core of the body before treating the local area of frostbite. Following restoration of the core temperature to normal, warming of a frostbitten limb should begin in water at 50 to 59°F (10 to 15°C), which is then increased 9°F (5°C) every 5 min to a maximum of 104°F (40°C).

Most cold injuries do not require warming, and treatment should be conservative and consists of bed rest, elevation of the injured part, tetanus antitoxin, and antibiotics, when indicated; early drainage of blebs and bullae; daily washes with pHisoHex; and early institution of physiotherapy. Alcohol and cigarettes are strongly contraindicated. Surgical amputation and reconstruction is usually not necessary. Regional sympathectomy performed 24 to 48 h after thawing is followed by rapid resolution of edema, earlier demarcation of destroyed tissue, and faster healing. The effect of regional sympathectomy is probably due to ablation of persistent vasospasm and to restoration of cold perception. Intraarterial reserpine has effects similar to sympathectomy, with marked decrease in local vasospasm and decrease in pain and edema.

Some patients with frostbite have residua consisting of excessive sweating, pain, cold feet, numbness, abnormal color, and pain in the joints. The symptoms are generally worse in the winter and following exposure to cold. These patients also often show abnormal nails, discoloration and pigmentation, hyperhydrosis, and, by x-ray, osteoporosis and cystic defects near the joints. These abnormalities tend to be milder in patients who have had sympathetic blockade. Most cold injuries are preventable by graded exposure to cold, as well as appropriate clothing in freezing temperatures.

REFERENCES

Brengelman G: Temperature regulation, in *Physiology and Biophysics,* TC Ruch and HD Patton (eds). Philadelphia, Saunders, 1973

Clowes GHA Jr, O'Donnel TF Jr: Current concepts: Heat stroke. N Engl J Med 291:564, 1974

Dinarello CA, Wolff SM: Pathogenesis of fever in man. N Engl J Med 298:607, 1978

Edelman IS: Thyroid thermogenesis. N Engl J Med 290:1303, 1974

Goulding MR et al: The role of sympathectomy in frostbite, with a review of 68 cases. Surgery 57:774, 1965

Knochel JP et al: The renal, cardiovascular, hematologic and serum electrolyte abnormalities of heat stroke. Am J Med 30:299, 1961

Lask RF et al: Accidental profound hypothermia and barbiturate intoxication: A report of rapid "core" rewarming by peritoneal dialysis. JAMA 201:123, 1966

MacLean D et al: Metabolic aspects of spontaneous recovery in accidental hypothermia and hypothermic myxedema. Q J Med (n.s.) 43(171):371, 1974

O'Donnel TF Jr, Clowes GHA Jr: The circulatory abnormalities of heat stroke. N Engl J Med 287:734, 1972

Penn I, Schwartz SI: Evaluation of low molecular weight dextran in the treatment of frostbite. J Trauma 4:784, 1964

Shibolet S et al: Heat stroke: A review. Aviat Space Environ Med 47:280, 1976

Simon HB: Extreme pyrexia. JAMA 236:2419, 1976

Stephen RC: Malignant hyperthermia. Annu Rev Med 28:153, 1977

Whittle JL, Bates JH: Thermoregulatory failure secondary to acute illness: Complications and treatment. Arch Intern Med 139:418, 1979

Wickstrom P et al: Accidental hypothermia. Am J Surg 131:622, 1976

Wyndham CH: Heat stroke and hyperthermia in marathon runners. Ann NY Acad Sci 301:128, 1977

10
CHILLS AND FEVER

ROBERT G. PETERSDORF

In view of the extensive knowledge of physiologic mechanisms controlling body temperature mentioned in Chap. 9, it is surprising that so little is known about the ways in which disease upsets thermoregulation.

Some bacteria, particularly gram-negative species, produce endotoxins which are pyrogenic, and a few viruses also cause fever when injected into humans or animals. Many microorganisms, however, possess no demonstrable pyrogenic toxin and, of course, fever accompanies diseases which do not involve invasion of the body by any known parasite. Omitting disorders which may involve cerebral thermoregulatory centers directly, such as brain tumors, intracranial hemorrhage or thrombosis, or heat stroke, the following disease states may be accompanied by fever:

1 All *infections,* whether caused by bacteria, rickettsias, viruses, or more complex parasites, cause fever.
2 *Mechanical trauma,* e.g., a crushing injury, frequently gives rise to fever lasting 1 or 2 days. Not infrequently, however, complicating infection sets in.
3 Many *neoplastic diseases* are associated with fever. In most patients, fever in patients with cancer is related to obstruction or infection produced by the tumor. In some solid tumors, however, fever may be due to the tumor per se, particularly following metastasis to the liver. Tumors which are associated with fever include hypernephroma, carcinoma of the pancreas, lung, or bone, and hepatoma. In tumors of the reticuloendothelial system, including Hodgkin's disease, lymphosarcoma, reticulum cell sarcoma, and acute leukemias, fever may be one of the prominent early manifestations.
4 *Hematopoietic disorders,* e.g., acute hemolytic episodes, may be characterized by pyrexia.
5 *Vascular accidents* of any magnitude, e.g., myocardial, pulmonary, and cerebral infarctions, nearly always cause fever.
6 *Diseases due to immune mechanisms* are almost always febrile. These include the collagen diseases, drug fevers, and serum sickness.
7 Certain *acute metabolic disorders,* such as gout, porphyria, hypertriglyceridemia, Fabry's disease, and Addisonian or thyroid crises, sometimes are associated with fever.

ACCOMPANIMENTS OF FEVER Systemic symptoms The perception of fever by patients varies enormously. Some persons can tell with considerable accuracy whether their body temperatures are elevated; others, notably patients with tuberculosis, may be wholly unaware of body temperature as high as 103°F (39.4°C). Often, also, patients may pay no attention to fever because of other unpleasant symptoms such as headache and pleuritic pain. Pain in the back, generalized myalgias, and arthralgia without arthritis are common in fever. Whether these symptoms reflect the presence of an infectious agent or are merely a nonspecific accompaniment of pyrexia is not clear.

Chills Abrupt onset of fever with a *chill* or *rigor* is characteristic of some diseases and, in the absence of antipyretic drugs, rare in others. Although repeated rigors are typical of pyogenic infection with bacteremia, a similar pattern of fever may occur in noninfectious diseases such as lymphoma. It is important to differentiate a true chill, which is accompanied by teeth chattering and bed shaking, from the chilly sensation which occurs in almost all fevers, particularly those in viral infections. In some instances, however, a true rigor occurs in viremia. Chills may be evoked or perpetuated by the intermittent administration of aspirin or other antipyretics. These agents may cause a sharp depression in temperature, which is followed by compensatory involuntary muscular contractions, i.e., a chill. This unpleasant side effect of antipyretic drugs can be averted by administering these agents frequently, around the clock, in low doses, rather than by prescribing them only for elevations in temperature above a certain level.

Herpes labialis So-called "fever blisters" result from activation of the herpes simplex virus by elevation in temperature. For reasons which are obscure, fever blisters are common in pneumococcal infections, streptococcosis, malaria, meningococcemia, and rickettsioses but are rare in mycoplasma pneumonia, tuberculosis, brucellosis, smallpox, and typhoid.

Delirium This may result from elevation of body temperature and is particularly common in patients with alcoholism, cerebral arteriosclerosis, or senility.

Convulsions These are not infrequent in febrile children, especially those with a family history of epilepsy, although febrile convulsions do not, in general, reflect serious cerebral disease.

CLINICAL IMPORTANCE OF FEVER The temperature is a simple, objective, and accurate indicator of a physiologic state and is much less subject to external and psychogenic stimuli than the other vital signs, i.e., the pulse, respiratory rate, and blood pressure. For these reasons, determination of the body temperature assists in estimating the severity of an illness, its course and duration, and the effect of therapy, or even in deciding whether a person has an organic illness.

Benefit of fever There are a few infections of humans in which pyrexia appears definitely to be beneficial to the host, such as neurosyphilis and perhaps chronic brucellosis. Certain other diseases, such as uveitis and rheumatoid arthritis, sometimes improve after fever therapy. In experimental animals some pneumococcal and cryptococcal infections have been influenced in favor of the host animal by raising the body temperature. Aged and debilitated patients with infection may have little or no fever, and this is generally interpreted as a bad prognostic sign. In the great majority of infectious diseases, however, there is no reason to believe that pyrexia accelerates phagocytosis, antibody formation, or other defense mechanisms.

Detrimental aspects of fever Fever accelerates all metabolic processes and accentuates weight loss and nitrogen wastage. The work and the rate of the heart are increased. Sweating aggravates loss of salt and water. There may be discomfort due to headache, photophobia, general malaise, or unpleasant sensation of warmth. Fever may precipitate seizures in epileptic patients. The rigors and profuse sweats of hectic fevers are particularly unpleasant for the patient. In elderly individuals with overt or potential cardiac or cerebral vascular disease, fever may be particularly deleterious.

MANAGEMENT OF FEVER Since fever ordinarily does little harm and imposes no great discomfort, antipyretic drugs are rarely necessary and may obfuscate the effect of a specific therapeutic agent or of the natural course of the disease. There are situations, however, in which lowering of the body temperature is of vital importance; e.g., heat stroke, postoperative hyperthermia, delirium due to hyperpyrexia, epileptic seizures, or shock associated with fever and heart failure. Under these circumstances lowering the temperature is indicated. Cooling blankets which can be set at hypothermic temperatures are a highly effective means for external cooling. Alternatively, sponging the body surface with cool saline solution or the application of cool compresses to the skin and forehead may be employed. There is no advantage in sponging with alcohol, which, because of its pungent odor, makes some patients ill. When high internal temperature is combined with cutaneous vasoconstriction, as in heat stroke or postoperative hyperthermia, the cooling measures should be combined with massage of the skin in order to bring blood to the surface, where it may be cooled. Immediate immersion in a tub of ice water should be considered a lifesaving emergency procedure in patients with heat stroke if the internal body temperature is in excess of 108°F (42.2°C). If cooling blankets are available, they are preferable to immersion in ice in most instances.

If antipyretic drugs, such as aspirin (0.3 to 0.6 g), are employed to bring about a fall in temperature, ill effects such as unpleasant diaphoresis, sometimes associated with an alarming fall in blood pressure and the subsequent return of fever and occasionally accompanied by a chill, may occur. These can be mitigated by enforcing a liberal fluid intake and by administering the drug regularly and frequently at 2- to 3-h intervals. Although adrenal steroids are also potent antipyretics, they must be used with caution because of their tendency to precipitate abrupt falls in temperature accompanied by hypotension. The capacity of these drugs to mask other manifestations of infection also constitutes a relative contraindication to their use.

The discomfort of a rigor can be alleviated in many patients by the intravenous injection of calcium gluconate. This procedure will stop the shivering and chilliness but has no influence on the ultimate height of the fever. Severe disruptive rigors sometimes need to be abolished with morphine sulfate (10 to 15 mg subcutaneously) or with parenteral chlorpromazine.

DIAGNOSTIC CONSIDERATIONS IN FEVER

In many illnesses fever is the most prominent and often the only manifestation of disease. It is not an indication of any particular type of disease; rather it should be considered a reaction to injury comparable with an elevated leukocyte count or a rapid erythrocyte sedimentation rate.

TYPES OF FEVER Fever is classically described as intermittent, remittent, sustained, and relapsing.

Intermittent fever With *intermittent fever* the temperature falls to normal each day. When the variation between the peak and the nadir is very large, the fever is called *hectic* or *septic*. Intermittent fevers are characteristic in pyogenic infections, particularly abscesses, lymphomas, and miliary tuberculosis.

Remittent fever With *remittent fever* the temperature falls each day but does not return to normal. Most fevers are remittent, and this type of febrile response is in no way characteristic.

Sustained fever A *sustained fever* is characterized by persistent elevation without significant diurnal variation. It is exemplified by the fever of untreated typhoid or typhus.

Relapsing fever With *relapsing fever* short febrile periods occur between one or several days of normal temperature. Examples of relapsing fever are seen in the following conditions:

Malaria (Chap. 200) had vanished from the United States almost completely, but for several years Vietnam war veterans constituted an important and sizable reservoir of this infection, as do other persons recently arrived from foreign countries. It is most unusual, however, for malaria to recur after a symptom-free interval of 1 year or more. Febrile bouts recur at 2- or 3-day intervals, or more irregularly in falciparum infections, depending on the maturation cycle of the parasite. The diagnosis depends on demonstration of the parasites in the blood.

Relapsing fever (Chap. 149) occurs in the southwest part of the United States, as far east as Texas, and in many other parts of the world. The recurrences are related to the cyclic development of parasites. Diagnosis is by demonstration of the spirochetal organisms in stained films of the blood.

Rat-bite fever (Chap. 130) is brought about by two agents—*Spirillum minus* and *Streptobacillus moniliformis,* both transmitted by the bite of a rat. Both may cause an illness characterized by periodic exacerbations of fever. The clue to the diagnosis depends on obtaining a history of rat bite 1 to 10 weeks prior to the onset of symptoms. The cause can be established by appropriate laboratory procedures.

Localized *pyogenic infections* in rare instances give rise to periodic bouts of fever separated by afebrile and relatively symptom-free intervals. The so-called "Charcot's intermittent biliary fever," i.e., cholangitis with biliary obstruction due to stones, is an example. *Urinary tract infection,* with episodes of ureteral obstruction due to small stones or inspissated pus, can also cause recurrent fever.

Approximately 5 percent of patients with Hodgkin's disease at some time have so-called "Pel-Ebstein fever"—bouts of fever lasting 3 to 10 days, separated by afebrile and asymptomatic periods of 3 to 10 days. These cycles may be repeated regularly over a period of several months. In rare instances this periodicity of the fever has been sufficiently striking to suggest the correct diagnosis before lymphadenopathy or splenomegaly became evident. However, relapsing fevers indistinguishable from Pel-Ebstein fever usually have causes other than Hodgkin's disease.

EPIDEMIOLOGY OF FEVER   The diagnosis of febrile illnesses must take into consideration the context of the epidemiologic setting. For example, an acute 6-day febrile illness in Southeast Asia is probably due to dengue or Chikungunya fever (Chap. 190), malaria (Chap. 200), scrub typhus (Chap. 169), or leptospirosis (Chap. 148); in a college student in the United States it may result from infectious mononucleosis or some other viral infection; and in an octogenarian following prostatectomy it is probably an indication of urinary tract infection, wound infection, pulmonary infarction, or aspiration pneumonia. In children, infections are more likely to be responsible for prolonged fevers than in adults. Likewise, travelers returning from short trips to foreign countries are much more likely to have febrile illnesses indigenous to their home than to the foreign country they have visited.

RARE VERSUS COMMON DISEASES   Most of the time fever is a manifestation of a common disease, and fever associated with a pulmonary infiltrate is much more likely to be due to pneumococcal than to pneumocystis pneumonia. Failure to appreciate this cardinal principle has led to many prolonged and futile diagnostic work-ups.

FEBRILE ILLNESSES OF SHORT DURATION   Acute febrile illnesses of less than 2 weeks' duration are a common occurrence in medical practice. In many instances they run their course, progressing to complete recovery, and a precise diagnosis is not made. In most instances, however, it is safe to assume that the illness is of infectious origin. Although short febrile illnesses may be noninfectious (e.g., allergic fevers due to drugs, thromboembolic disease, hemolytic crises, or gout), they are decidedly in the minority.

Most undiagnosed acute febrile infectious diseases are probably viral and remain undiagnosed because diagnostic methods are unavailable or cumbersome. It is not practical to carry out tests needed to identify all the known viruses, and, furthermore, there must be a considerable number of still unidentified viruses pathogenic for humans. In bacterial infections, on the other hand, laboratory diagnosis is simpler, and

these infections are often rapidly controlled with chemotherapy.

The following characteristics, though not restricted solely to acute infections, are highly suggestive that infection is present:

1 Abrupt onset
2 High fever, i.e., 102 to 105°F (38.9 to 40.6°C), with or without chills
3 Respiratory symptoms—sore throat, coryza, cough
4 Severe malaise, with muscle or joint pain, photophobia, pain on movement of the eyes, headache
5 Nausea, vomiting, or diarrhea
6 Acute enlargement of lymph nodes or spleen
7 Meningeal signs, with or without spinal fluid pleocytosis
8 Leukocyte count above 12,000 or below 5000 per cubic millimeter
9 Dysuria, frequency, and flank pain

None of the symptoms or signs listed is encountered only in infection. Many of these features could be seen in acute leukemia or disseminated lupus erythematosus. Nevertheless, in a given instance of acute febrile illness with some of or all the manifestations listed, the probabilities strongly favor infection, and the patient may be given reasonable reassurance that he will probably recover in a week or two, regardless of a precise diagnosis.

It is desirable, of course, to establish an accurate diagnosis, and whatever steps are practicable in the circumstances to establish the cause should be taken. Cultures of the throat, blood, urine, or feces should be obtained before institution of antibacterial chemotherapy. Skin and/or serologic tests should be carried out when indicated.

There is a tendency to rely immediately and excessively on the laboratory in ascertaining the cause of fever. In many instances, a thorough history and a complete and, if necessary, repeated physical examination, along with a complete blood count (CBC), urinalysis, and sedimentation rate will provide the answer. Often a little patience, in the form of watchful waiting, before plunging into an expensive and extensive laboratory work-up, will lead to the diagnosis.

PROLONGED FEBRILE ILLNESSES   Some of the knottiest problems in the field of internal medicine are found in cases of prolonged fever in which the diagnosis remains obscure for weeks or even months. Eventually, however, the true nature of the illness usually reveals itself, since a disease which causes injury sufficient to evoke temperature elevations to 101°F (38.3°C) or higher for several weeks does not often subside without leaving some clue as to its nature. The elucidation of problems of this sort calls for skillful application of all diagnostic methods—careful history, thorough physical examination, and the carefully considered use of laboratory examinations and roentgenograms.

Fever of unknown origin (FUO)   In some patients fever becomes the dominant sign or symptom in a patient's illness, and when its cause escapes detection it is defined as fever of unknown origin (FUO). It is appropriate to use this term only in patients who have elevations in temperature [>101°F (38.3°C)] for a prolonged period (at least 2 to 3 weeks) and in whom the diagnosis cannot be made during at least 1 week of intensive studies. These rigid criteria eliminate from this diagnostic category patients with common bacterial or viral infections, those in whom the diagnosis is obvious, and those whose fever is due to a sequential occurrence of etiologically unrelated diseases. An example is a patient who is febrile following a myocardial infarction, who then develops thrombophlebitis that is associated with fever, and in whom this is followed by multiple pulmonary emboli, also a febrile disease. Much of the confusion in the literature concerning causes of FUO is due to failure to define the criteria employed in classifying patients who have had fever of unknown origin.

DISEASES CAUSING PROLONGED FEVERS

Table 10-1 lists some of the diseases which are responsible for prolonged fever. Some of these disorders must initially be considered to be FUO; in others the diagnosis comes to mind readily.

INFECTION Infections occupy a less prominent position among causes of prolonged fever now than formerly because of the common practice of administering antibiotics to any patient in whom fever persists for more than a few days. Consequently, many infections are at present being eradicated by more or less "blind" therapy without accurate determination of their nature or location. Nevertheless, patients with infections compose approximately 40 percent of any group with FUO. Many times these infections take the form of localized abscesses, osteomyelitis, or bacterial endocarditis; or the organisms are located intracellularly and present as bacteremias.

Tuberculosis (Chap. 143) Tuberculosis remains the most prominent cause of FUO. The diagnosis should be considered strongly in dark-skinned persons. Most of these patients do not have pulmonary tuberculosis but extrapulmonary or miliary disease involving the bones, lymph nodes, genital or urinary organs, peritoneum, or liver. Extrapulmonary or miliary tuberculosis may not be detectable by x-ray until late in the course of the disease. Because many of these patients are debilitated and have overwhelming disease, the skin test may be negative. A positive skin reaction, on the other hand, does not prove that tuberculosis is causing the illness but requires that the diagnosis be kept in mind until another cause for the fever is found. Occasionally, fungous infections present as FUO, but most often specific organ involvement leads to the diagnosis.

Pyogenic infections UPPER ABDOMINAL INFECTIONS These commonly occur in the right upper quadrant and are related to the gallbladder or liver. Patients with such conditions tend to have mild jaundice, abnormality of liver function, high spiking fevers, and leukocytosis. Bacteremia, often due to enteric pathogens or *Salmonella,* is common. Liver scan is a most useful diagnostic tool, although exploratory laparotomy is often necessary for diagnosis and may achieve cure as well.

LOWER ABDOMINAL INFECTIONS Appendicitis with perforation and abscess formation is a remarkably common cause of prolonged fever, particularly in elderly patients. Persistent right lower quadrant physical signs along with x-ray abnormalities require surgical exploration. Diverticulitis is also common in elderly patients. In younger women, pelvic inflammatory disease may present as FUO.

RENAL INFECTIONS Ordinary pyelonephritis is rarely accompanied by prolonged fever; if pyrexia occurs in these patients, intrarenal or perinephric abscess should be considered. Ureter-

TABLE 10-1
Common disease entities in the United States causing prolonged fever

I Infections
  A Granulomatous infections
    1 Tuberculosis
    2 Deep-seated fungous infections
  B Pyogenic infections
    1 Upper abdominal infections
      a Cholecystitis (stone), empyema of gallbladder
      b Cholangitis
      c Liver abscess
      d Subhepatic abscess
      e Lesser sac abscess
    2 Lower abdominal infections
      a Diverticulitis
      b Appendicitis
    3 Pelvic inflammatory disease
    4 Urinary tract infections
      a Pyelonephritis (rare)
      b Intrarenal abscess
      c Perinephric abscess
      d Ureteral obstruction
      e Prostatic abscess
    5 Sinusitis
  C Bacterial endocarditis (acute and subacute)
  D Bacteremias without overt primary focus
    1 Meningococcemia
    2 Gonococcemia
    3 Vibriosis
    4 Listeriosis
    5 Brucellosis
    6 Coliform bacteremia in patients with cirrhosis
  E Viral, rickettsial, and chlamydial infections
    1 Infectious mononucleosis
    2 Cytomegalovirus
    3 Group B coxsackievirus diseases
    4 Q fever (including endocarditis)
    5 Psittacosis
  F Parasitic diseases
    1 Amebiasis
    2 Malaria
    3 Trichinosis
  G Spirochetal infections
    1 Leptospirosis
    2 Relapsing fever
II Neoplasms
  A Solid (localized)
    1 Kidney

    2 Lung
    3 Pancreas
    4 Liver
    5 Large bowel
    6 Atrial myxoma
  B Metastatic
    1 From gastrointestinal tract
    2 From lung, kidneys, bone
    3 Melanoma
  C Tumors of the reticuloendothelial system
    1 Lymphoma, Hodgkin's disease
    2 Leukemias
    3 Reticulum-cell sarcoma, multiple myeloma (rare)
  D Unclassified
    1 Unclassified lymphatic diseases [immunoblastic lymphadenopathy; lymphamatoid granulomatosis; mucocutaneous lymph node syndrome (children)]
    2 Diffuse sarcoma of bone
III Connective tissue disease
  A Rheumatic fever
  B Systemic lupus erythematosus
  C Rheumatoid arthritis (including Still's disease)
  D Temporal arteritis (polymyalgia rheumatica)
  E Hypersensitivity vasculitis
  F Periarteritis nodosa
  G Wegener's granulomatosis
IV Miscellaneous
  A Drug fever
  B Multiple pulmonary emboli
  C Sarcoidosis
  D Thyroiditis
  E Hemolytic states
  F Cryptic trauma with bleeding into enclosed space
  G Regional enteritis and Whipple's disease
  H Granulomatous hepatitis
  I Dissecting aneurysm (with or without infection)
V Metabolic and inherited diseases
  A Familial Mediterranean fever
  B Hypertriglyceridemia and hypercholesterolemia
  C Fabry's disease
VI Pseudogenic fevers
  A Habitual hyperthermia
  B Factitious fever
VII Periodic fevers (e.g., cyclic neutropenia)
VIII Thermoregulatory disorders
  IX Undiagnosed

al obstruction by either a mass of leukocytes or renal epithelium, as in papillary necrosis, may be accompanied by prolonged fever. Prostatic abscess should be considered in males. These patients may not have dysuria or rectal pain.

RETROPERITONEAL INFECTION Aneurysms that have become filled with organizing clot and debris may become infected. Enteric pathogens (including *Escherichia coli,* bacteroides, and *Salmonella*), have been isolated frequently from patients with such infections. Surgery is mandatory for both diagnosis and therapy. In addition, some patients with dissecting aneurysms have fever without superimposed infections.

Bacterial endocarditis In the classic subacute form of the disease, a heart murmur is nearly always present; therefore, absence of murmur largely eliminates this disease from consideration. The correct diagnosis is likely to be missed in middle-aged or elderly patients, in whom a heart murmur may not be given much weight. For example, an elderly patient with subacute bacterial endocarditis may first come to the physician's attention following the occurrence of a cerebral embolus and may be regarded as having had a hemorrhage or thrombosis because of arteriosclerosis. The best clinical practice is to culture the blood of *every* patient who has fever and a heart murmur. Bacterial endocarditis without cardiac murmurs is seen most frequently in intravenous drug users who develop infection on the tricuspid valve; every such person with fever should be assumed to have endocarditis until proved otherwise. In addition, antibiotics mask subacute bacterial endocarditis (SBE) because they often render the blood culture negative until they have been excreted or metabolized. For this reason, patients suspected of having SBE who have received antimicrobials should have blood cultures taken for several days after administration of the drugs is discontinued.

Bacteremia NEISSERIA Although rare, chronic meningococcemia (Chap. 118) is a well-known cause of prolonged fever. The arthralgia and rash of this disease are sufficiently evanescent to be missed. When this syndrome appears in a young woman, gonococcemia is much more likely (Chap. 119).

SALMONELLA (Chap. 123) Typhoid fever is not often a cause of prolonged fever of obscure origin because cultures of feces and blood will be positive and specific antibodies will be found in the serum. Other *Salmonella* organisms may, however, cause prolonged febrile illness and may present greater diagnostic difficulties. Repeated culture of the blood or bone marrow may yield the cause of this organism. Eventually, the infection may localize in a joint, pleural cavity, or another metastatic focus. Sometimes, salmonella bacteremia occurs spontaneously in patients with cirrhosis, although most often spontaneous bacteremia is due to *E. coli*. Serologic confirmation of a salmonella infection is sometimes helpful.

Brucellosis (Chap. 127) This infection should be considered primarily in farmers, veterinarians, or slaughterhouse workers. Arthralgia and myalgia are common, but arthritis is rare. These patients tend to have normal or depressed leukocyte counts, and their sedimentation rate is often normal. In active febrile disease the blood and bone marrow cultures are frequently positive and specific agglutinins are nearly always present in the serum.

Viral, rickettsial, and chlamydial infections These are rarely the cause of prolonged fevers, but occasionally patients with Epstein-Barr or cytomegalovirus infections may have febrile illnesses, which are often characterized by spontaneous remissions and exacerbations. Cytomegalovirus (with or without *Pneumocystis*) is becoming a progressively more common cause of prolonged fever in immunocompromised hosts. Psittacosis may look much like typhoid fever, and Q-fever endocarditis has been a particularly puzzling and lethal illness that must be treated both with antibiotics and valve replacement.

Parasitic diseases Amebiasis presents as an FUO, primarily in the form of liver abscess. The diagnosis of malaria demands a history of recent exposure.

NEOPLASMS Carcinomas and sarcomas Certain malignant processes are especially likely to cause fever. Notable are sarcomas involving bone or lymphoid tissue, hypernephroma, carcinoma of the pancreas, stomach, or colon, and primary or metastatic cancer of the liver. Occasionally, the clinical picture is strongly suggestive of pyogenic infection, with hectic fever, chills, sweats, and marked leukocytosis; and patients have been subjected to laparotomy with preoperative diagnoses such as empyema of the gallbladder, localized peritonitis, or liver abscess. An elevated alkaline phosphatase level and abnormal retention of Bromsulphalein accompanied by filling defects on a liver scan are important clues to intrahepatic malignancy or other infiltrative hepatic disease.

Hodgkin's disease and lymphomas Fever may be the principal symptom and only objective finding early in the course of Hodgkin's disease, especially when the principal involvement is in the abdominal viscera or retroperitoneal regions. Pel-Ebstein fever is seen in a minority of cases of Hodgkin's disease. The diagnosis of this disorder is usually made by biopsy or occasionally by lymphangiography or staging laparotomy.

Lymphoma-like syndromes Several disease entities have been described which are similar clinically and histologically to lymphoma but which may have a better prognosis, or respond differently to steroids and antitumor agents. Among these entities, all of which may present as FUOs, are immunoblastic lymphadenopathy, lymphadenoid granulomatosis, and, in children, the mucocutaneous lymph node syndrome (Kawasaki's disease). These diseases are discussed more fully in Chap. 55.

Leukemias It is not uncommon for acute leukemia to be mistaken for acute infection at the onset. The acute leukemias are nearly always accompanied by fever, sometimes as high as 105°F (40.6°C). The correct diagnosis is suggested by rapid development of anemia and characteristic changes in peripheral blood and bone marrow. Chronic lymphatic or granulocytic leukemia may be characterized by fever, but such fever is usually due to concomitant infection. Because of the typical changes in circulating leukocytes, fever does not often cause a diagnostic problem. Before it is assumed that fever in a patient with leukemia is due to the blood dyscrasia, infection must be ruled out by appropriate tests and cultures, and often attempts to treat the "most likely" pathogen must be made.

Atrial myxoma Patients with changing heart murmurs, peripheral embolic phenomena, and joint pains are usually suspected of having bacterial endocarditis, rheumatic fever, or occasionally some other connective tissue disease such as lupus erythematosus. In the face of persistence of these symptoms and signs without a positive diagnosis, echocardiography and, if the echocardiogram is positive, angiography should be performed with the possibility that an atrial myxoma may be responsible.

CONNECTIVE TISSUE DISEASE Rheumatic fever Though rheumatic fever is generally easy to detect in children, the diagnosis in adults may be difficult. Attention to unexplained heart murmurs, arrhythmias, pleural and pericardial rubs, arthralgias, and skin rashes should call the diagnosis to mind. These findings, along with an elevated antistreptolysin titer, C-reactive protein, and other acute phase reactants, contribute to the diagnosis. A prompt response to large doses of aspirin is characteristic of rheumatic fever and provides another diagnostic clue.

Systemic lupus erythematosus Fever is a common accompaniment of this disease. Of course, in the presence of arthritis, pleuritis, pericarditis, the classic malar rash, and renal failure, the diagnosis is easy. However, often these findings are absent and fever is the major manifestation. Biopsy of many organs, including the kidney, is generally not helpful; the diagnosis must be made by detecting a high titer of antinuclear or anti-deoxyribonucleic (anti-DNA) antibody (Chap. 68).

Rheumatoid arthritis In its classic form, this disease is not difficult to recognize, but in certain patients who initially have FUO arthritis is absent early in the course of the illness; these patients have primarily fever, hepatosplenomegaly, lymphadenopathy, evanescent rashes, anemia, and leukocytosis. Joint changes do not appear until late in the disease. This disease often occurs in young adults, and may be considered the adult counterpart of juvenile rheumatoid disease. The diagnosis is made usually only after prolonged observation, in part because serologic tests for rheumatoid disease are characteristically negative. The prognosis is generally good, and patients respond well to anti-inflammatory drugs.

Temporal arteritis (polymyalgia rheumatica) This is a disease of elderly women who complain of fever, headache, and pain in the muscles and joints. Overt arthritis is unusual. At times, fever is the only symptom, and there are no abnormal physical findings. The sedimentation rate tends to be very rapid, and there may be anemia, leukocytosis, or eosinophilia. Occasionally, the temporal or occipital arteries are inflamed and tender, but usually they are normal. In either instance, the diagnosis must be made by temporal artery biopsy. There may be accompanying visual defects or blindness because of involvement of the retinal artery. This disease responds extremely well to steroids, which may be used as a therapeutic trial.

MISCELLANEOUS CAUSES OF FEVER **Sarcoidosis** Ordinarily fever is not characteristic of sarcoidosis, but it is prominent in a minority of cases, especially those characterized by arthralgia, hilar lymphadenopathy, and cutaneous lesions resembling erythema nodosum, or in those with extensive hepatic lesions. The diagnosis is suggested by lymphoid enlargement, ocular lesions, and hyperglobulinemia and is clinched by biopsy of skin, lymph nodes, muscle, and liver.

Regional enteritis Inflammatory lesions of the large and small intestine rarely present as FUO, but an occasional patient who has only fever, abdominal pain, and subtle changes in bowel habits will be found to have regional enteritis. Likewise, Whipple's disease may make itself known by fever, without arthritis or malabsorption.

Drug fever This is an important cause of cryptic fever; a careful history of drug intake should be taken in every patient with unexplained fever. Fever due to allergy to one of the antibiotics may become superimposed on the fever of the infection for which the drug was given, resulting in a very confused picture. Often fever is due to common drugs, including sulfonamides, arsenicals, iodides, thiouracils, barbiturates, and laxatives, especially those containing phenolphthalein. Any questions of drug fever can be resolved rapidly by discontinuing all medications. The diagnosis can be further substantiated by giving a test dose of the drug after fever has subsided, but this may result in a very unpleasant or even dangerous reaction.

Multiple pulmonary emboli Symptomless thrombosis of deep calf or pelvic veins may cause prolonged febrile illness either because of the thrombophlebitis or as a result of repeated small pulmonary emboli. These emboli may not be manifested by pleuritic pain or hemoptysis, but cough, dyspnea, and vague thoracic discomfort are likely to be present. Careful examination of the legs and repeated examination of the lungs should reveal the diagnosis. Sometimes these patients come to the physician's attention with a nephrotic syndrome due to renal vein thrombosis. Pelvic thrombophlebitis with or without pulmonary emboli is an important cause of FUO in postpartum patients.

Hemolytic episodes Most hemolytic diseases are characterized by bouts of fever, and acute hemolytic crises may give rise to shaking chills and marked elevations of temperature. The difficulty sometimes encountered in differentiating sickle-cell disease from acute rheumatic fever is well known. The presence of these hemolytic disorders is suggested by the more rapid development of anemia than occurs in other febrile illnesses and by the usual accompaniment of reticulocytosis and jaundice. Fever is not characteristic of severe anemia due to external blood loss or of the anemia of uremia.

Cryptic trauma Perisplenic and perivesical hematomas, with or without superimposed infection, are among the sites in which accumulated old blood and pus have resulted in prolonged fever. A history of remote trauma is a helpful clue.

Granulomatous hepatitis This disease of unknown etiology is not an uncommon cause of FUO. It is probably a manifestation of hypersensitivity. Liver biopsy shows only nonspecific granulomas. The fever generally subsides spontaneously over a period of weeks or months. Sometimes defervescence can be achieved with steroids, but because the diagnosis of tuberculosis cannot be ruled out completely, patients in whom steroid therapy is given should also be given antituberculous medication.

Habitual hyperthermia Not infrequently, a patient while not appearing acutely ill has been subject to elevation of body temperature above the "normal" range level, i.e., his temperature has been in the range of 99.0 to 100.5°F (37.2 to 38°C). Prolonged low-grade fever may be a manifestation of serious illness, or it may be a matter of no real consequence. Possibly there are some persons whose "normal" temperatures are in this range. However, there is no certain way of identifying such individuals. The possibilities to be considered in such cases vary considerably according to the age groups concerned. A special problem termed *habitual hyperthermia* is encountered in young females. The patient may have temperatures ranging from 99.0 to 100.5°F (37.2 to 38.0°C) regularly or intermittently for years and also usually has a variety of complaints characteristic of psychoneurosis, such as fatigability, insomnia, bowel distress, vague aches, and headache. Prolonged careful study and observation fail to reveal evidence of organic disease. Unfortunately, many of these people go from physician to physician and are subjected to a variety of unpleasant, expensive, and even harmful tests, treatments, and operations. The diagnosis of this syndrome can be made with reasonable certainty after a suitable period of observation and study, and if the patient can be convinced of its validity, a real service will have been rendered.

In a patient past middle age, even low-grade fever should always be regarded as a probable indication of organic disease. The possibilities to be considered in this age group are the same as those discussed earlier under "Prolonged Febrile Illness."

Factitious fever Occasionally, patients will produce purposeful false elevations in temperature. Usually these patients are young women, many of whom are allied health professionals. They fall into two groups—one infects itself with bacteria or other contaminated materials and a second finds a way to cause the thermometer to register higher than the true temperature. If malingering is suspected, all that is necessary to prove it is to repeat the temperature determination immediately after a high reading has been obtained, with someone remaining at the bedside while the thermometer is in place. Other clues to false elevations in the temperature are a dissociation between pulse and temperature, absence of the normal diurnal variation in temperature, and excessively high fevers [greater than 106°F (41.1°C) in adults] and the absence of chills, sweats, or tachycardia. These patients fall into the psychiatric diagnostic category of "borderline syndrome," a state between neurosis and psychosis, in which the prognosis is guarded. Others, mostly young girls, falsify their temperatures to ask for psychiatric help and do well with psychotherapy.

Metabolic causes of fever These include familial Mediterranean fever, hypertriglyceridemia and hypercholesterolemia, Fabry's disease, and, rarely, gout, thyrotoxicosis, and Addison's disease.

Thermoregulatory disorders Rare patients have fever due to an abnormality in their temperature-regulating mechanism. They may be febrile without any other cause or may have exaggerated responses in temperature during the course of other fever-producing diseases. The diagnosis is made by exclusion. Some patients have responded to chlorpromazine.

Cyclic neutropenia See Chap. 56.

DIAGNOSTIC PROCEDURES IN FEVER

With so large a number of possibilities, it is obvious that no single plan can be outlined for the systematic study of every problem in unexplained fever. In any given patient, the history, physical examination, and, most importantly, epidemiologic setting must determine the diagnostic approach. If the features suggest infectious disease, the main dependence will be upon bacteriologic and immunologic methods, whereas when a person in the "cancer age group" has an obscure febrile disorder, the best chance of early diagnosis may lie in x-ray studies, scans, and biopsy.

HISTORY Careful attention to the patient's past history and the chronologic development of symptoms may provide important leads. Places of recent residence, contact with domestic or wild animals and birds, preceding acute infectious diseases such as diarrheal illness or boils, and contact with persons with tuberculosis may provide clues to infection. Localizing symptoms may provide a lead to the affected organ system.

PHYSICAL EXAMINATION Careful search is made for skin lesions and for petechial hemorrhages in the ocular fundi, conjunctivas, nail beds, and skin. The lymph nodes are carefully palpated, with special attention to the supraclavicular, axillary,

and epitrochlear areas. The finding of a heart murmur may be important. Detection of an abdominal mass may be the first lead to the diagnosis of neoplastic disease. Palpable enlargement of the spleen suggests infection, leukemia, or lymphoma and points away from a diagnosis of solid tumors. Enlargement of the liver and spleen suggests lymphoma, leukemia, chronic infection, or cirrhosis. A large liver without a palpable spleen points to liver abscess or metastatic cancer. The rectum and the female pelvic organs may reveal masses or abscesses; the testicles may reveal teratoma or tuberculosis.

LABORATORY TESTS Useful examinations include:

1 Cultures of blood, bone marrow (*Brucella* or *Salmonella*), or other body fluids.
2 Serum enzymes, particularly *alkaline phosphatase* and corroborating enzymes such as 5'-nucleotidase and enzymes that measure hepatocellular function, and serum and urinary amylase.
3 Blood smears for abnormal morphology of red or white blood cells or platelets, or for demonstration of parasites.
4 Bone marrow examination for tumor cells, granulomas, lupus erythematosus cells, and abnormal red or white blood cells. Bone marrow biopsy is superior to aspiration for detection of granulomas and tumor cells.
5 Immunologic tests, i.e., antistreptolysin O titers, and other acute-phase reactants, antinuclear and related antibodies, latex fixation tests, and a variety of febrile agglutinins.

ROENTGENOGRAMS The following should be considered:

1 Chest films, which need to be repeated at intervals.
2 Bone x-rays are useful for detecting foci of osteomyelitis or primary or metastatic bone tumors.
3 Intravenous urograms are helpful in finding tumors of the kidney or perinephric or intrarenal abscesses. However, if a renal tumor is suspect on clinical grounds, a negative intravenous pyelogram does not rule out the diagnosis, and renal scan and aortogram should be performed.
4 Abdominal aortography is useful for diagnosing tumors of the kidney, retroperitoneal mass lesions, and, if selective arterial catheterization is performed, tumors of the liver, pancreas, and gut.
5 Intravenous or transhepatic cholangiograms may be helpful in delineating right upper quadrant pathologic changes if the patient is not jaundiced.
6 Visualization of the gallbladder, common bile duct, hepatic ducts, and pancreas may be best accomplished by instilling contrast medium through a flexible endoscope following cannulation of the ampulla of Vater (endoscopic retrograde choledochopancreatography).
7 Echocardiograms should be performed to screen for atrial myxoma; if positive or suggestive, they should be confirmed with angiography.
8 Lymphangiograms are helpful in the diagnosis of abdominal or retroperitoneal lymphomas and may be the only abnormality in these disorders.
9 Upper gastrointestinal x-rays are rarely useful; films of the small intestine may provide clues to Whipple's disease or regional enteritis, and a barium enema may show diverticulitis or tumor.

ULTRASONOGRAPHY This technique has come into vogue to detect abdominal, renal, retroperitoneal, or pelvic mass lesions. Both false-positive and false-negative results are common. Radioactive scanning techniques are usually superior in providing anatomic clues.

RADIOACTIVE SCANS *The liver/spleen scan is the single most useful test in the diagnosis of disease in the right upper quadrant.*

Lung scans may reveal pulmonary emboli, and simultaneous liver and lung scans are useful in delineating subphrenic abscess. Bone scans may detect osseous metastases more readily than x-rays. Renal scans are helpful in the diagnosis of hypernephroma. Gallium scan may be useful in identifying a cryptic focus of infection or infiltration but is rarely the only means for doing so.

There has not been sufficient experience to evaluate the role of total body computerized tomography (CT scan) in the diagnosis of FUO. It is probably most useful in delineating retroperitoneal lesions.

BIOPSIES Often the best means of definitive diagnosis is a biopsy.

1 Bone marrow biopsy may be helpful not only in clarifying the histologic nature of the marrow but also for occasional demonstration of other disease processes such as metastatic carcinoma or granulomas, and for culture.
2 Needle biopsy of the liver is a very helpful procedure and can be done with reasonable safety. It may lead to the diagnosis not only in primary or metastatic disease of the liver, but also may reveal existence of other diseases such as histoplasmosis, schistosomiasis, brucellosis, tuberculosis, sarcoidosis or lymphoma, or granulomatous hepatitis. There has been some controversy about the value of liver biopsy, but it remains very useful when the enzymes indicating infiltrative liver disease are elevated.
3 Lymph node biopsy is helpful in the diagnosis of many diseases, including the lymphomas, metastatic cancer, tuberculosis, and mycotic infections. However, inguinal nodes are notoriously unsatisfactory for biopsy and are too frequently chosen because of their easy accessibility. Axillary, cervical, and supraclavicular nodes are much more likely to yield helpful information, and the node excised need not necessarily be large.
4 Skin and muscle biopsy may be of assistance in the recognition of dermatomyositis, periarteritis nodosa, sarcoidosis, and trichinosis.
5 Lung biopsy may be performed with a needle under direct fluoroscopy or through the bronchoscope. It is of value primarily in solitary mass lesions; diffuse pulmonary disease is rarely diagnosed by needle biopsy; instead, open lung biopsy should be performed.
6 Renal biopsy is rarely helpful, even in connective tissue disease.
7 Pleural and pericardial biopsy with the hook needle technique should be attempted in the presence of effusion.
8 Biopsy of the temporal artery should be considered in elderly women with fever, anemia, hypoalbuminemia, and a rapid sedimentation rate, even though the temporal arteries are not palpable.
9 Biopsy of other accessible masses should not be neglected.

EXPLORATORY LAPAROTOMY Exploratory laparotomy has been advocated as the most definitive diagnostic maneuver in connection with FUO but is valuable only when other investigations including history, physical examination, x-rays, and laboratory data point to the abdomen as a possible source of disease. The clues to intraabdominal disease are often subtle, but they are present nonetheless. Blind exploration of the abdomen simply because the diagnosis is obscure is poor practice. Moreover, often the tissue that is obtained at laparotomy could just as easily have been sampled by external biopsy techniques.

THERAPEUTIC TRIALS It is common practice to give a trial of antibiotic therapy to patients with unidentified febrile disorders. Occasionally, this kind of marksmanship is effective, but in general, "blind" therapy does more harm than good. Undesirable features include drug toxicity, superinfection due to resistant pathogenic bacteria, and interference with accurate diagnosis by cultural methods. Furthermore, a coincidental fall in temperature not due to therapy is likely to be interpreted as response to treatment, with the conclusion that an infectious disease is present. If therapeutic trials are instituted, they should be as specific as possible. Examples are *isoniazid* or *ethambutol* for tuberculosis; *aspirin* for rheumatic fever; *metronidazole* for hepatic amebiasis; *penicillin* and *gentamicin* for enterococcal endocarditis; and *chloramphenicol* for *Salmonella* bacteremia. Shotgun broad-spectrum therapy is contraindicated, because it is unlikely to yield useful information and is more likely to be toxic. Similarly, steroid therapy is often nonspecific. These drugs do have an antipyretic effect and produce euphoria in many persons, but the apparent improvement induced by them tells little about the nature of the underlying disease. Temporal arteritis is an exception to this statement.

PROGNOSIS IN FUO The intelligent application of appropriate diagnostic maneuvers should provide the answer in approximately 90 to 95 percent of patients with prolonged obscure febrile illness. Fortunately, most of the remainder recover spontaneously. Because many of the procedures involved in the diagnosis of FUO are painful, time-consuming, and expensive, it is essential that they be chosen with thoughtfulness and care.

REFERENCES

ADUAN RP et al: Factitious fever and self-induced infection. Ann Intern Med 90:230, 1979

BAKER RR et al: The value of exploratory laparotomy in fever of undetermined etiology. Johns Hopkins Med J 125:159, 1969

BUJAK JS et al: Juvenile rheumatoid arthritis presenting in the adult as fever of unknown origin. Medicine 52:431, 1973

DINARELLO CA, WOLFF SM: Pathogenesis of fever in man. N Engl J Med 298:607, 1978

GHOSE MK et al: Arteritis of the aged (giant cell arteritis) and fever of unexplained origin. Am J Med 60:429, 1976

JACOBY GA, SWARTZ MN: Fever of undetermined origin. N Engl J Med 289:1407, 1973

MITCHELL DP et al: Fever of unknown origin: Assessment of the value of percutaneous liver biopsy. Arch Intern Med 137:1001, 1977

MURRAY HW et al: Fever with dissecting aneurysm of the aorta. Am J Med 61:140, 1976

PETERSDORF RG, BEESON PB: Fever of unexplained origin: Report of 100 cases. Medicine 40:1, 1961

———, WALLACE JF: Fever of unknown origin, in *Diagnostic Approaches to Presenting Syndromes,* JA Barondess (ed). Baltimore, Williams & Wilkins, 1971, p 301

SIMON HB, WOLFF SM: Granulomatous hepatitis and prolonged fever of unknown origin: A study of 13 patients. Medicine 52:1, 1973

VICKERY DM, QUINNELL RK: Fever of unknown origin: An algorithmic approach. JAMA 238:2183, 1977

WOLFF SM et al: Unusual etiologies of fever and their evaluation. Annu Rev Med 26:277, 1975

section 3 | Alterations in nervous function

INTRODUCTION

RAYMOND D. ADAMS

The symptoms and signs of nervous disease are probably the most frequent and complex in all of medicine. To present a lucid exposition of all the many diverse neurologic manifestations is difficult in part because the more complex phenomena may be viewed from either a neurologic or psychologic standpoint. The neurologic physician is inclined to assume that all are manifestations of diseases of the nervous system. The psychiatrically minded physician thinks of many of them in terms of abnormal psychologic reactions. Naturally, our bias is more toward the neurologic for it draws on all the accepted principles of medicine and biologic science. But each extreme can be criticized. The aim, therefore, throughout this section is to avoid entanglement in such theoretical problems, to describe as accurately as possible all the more common expressions of disordered nervous function, and to offer the most generally accepted explanations in terms of anatomy, physiology, biochemistry, and psychology. However, in discussing some of the more abstruse, complex cerebral derangements, a particular effort will be made to present both the neurologic and psychologic conceptions, for the latter have received much attention in recent years.

To provide an initial orientation toward the broad field of neuropsychiatry, it is helpful to think of the subject matter as divisible into two main categories: diseases of the nervous system and disorders based on abnormal psychologic reactions. By *disease* we mean any condition which produces a visible lesion in the nervous system or in which there is actual or presumptive evidence of such. By *abnormal psychologic reaction* we mean a disorder in psychic life and behavior occasioned by abnormal life experiences and maladjustments in social relations. A brain tumor, delirium tremens, and a confusional psychosis would be considered examples of disease; unusually protracted grief, unexplained anxiety, and a character disorder would fall in the category of a reactive psychologic abnormality or one due to the formation of unusual personality traits after repeated psychic traumas and environmental stresses. All diseases of the neuromuscular apparatus, spinal cord, brainstem, and cerebellum and many of those of the cerebrum, fall within the province of neurology, whereas other of the cerebral diseases (especially if they disturb intellect, emotions, and behavior) are of concern to both neurology and psychiatry, and all abnormal psychologic reactions are within the province of psychiatry.

Many nervous disorders are not so easily classified. A psychopathic personality, an anxiety neurosis, or a depression could be considered either as a manifestation of a disease of the brain or an abnormal psychologic reaction. Schizophrenia and manic-depressive psychosis would presently be classified as genetically determined diseases by neurologists and many psychiatrists even though a lesion has never been demonstrated by the conventional techniques of pathology. Other psychiatrists believe psychogenic factors to be important and therefore we have listed these two psychoses as reactive states.

Our objective in the early part of this book is to single out all the common symptoms and signs of diseases of the nervous system as well as the manifestations of certain abnormal psychologic states. In the section on diseases of organ systems, we shall present in one section all the common diseases of the nervous system. The major psychiatric disorders will be subdivided. The neuroses will be presented in Chap. 11 and the two major psychoses, manic-depressive disease and schizophrenia, in Chap. 25.

There are two areas of neuropsychiatry which in a way are even more controversial—the psychosomatic diseases and the sociopathic states. Included under psychosomatic disorders are such conditions as Raynaud's disease, peptic ulcer, ulcerative colitis, bronchial asthma, dysmenorrhea, hypertension, hyperthyroidism, neurodermatitis, rheumatoid arthritis, migraine, and paroxysmal tachycardia. These diseases have been set apart on the basis of three lines of evidence: (1) a large series of observations which have revealed that the malfunctioning organ is excited and possibly deranged by strong emotion and restored to relative normality by tranquility and feelings of security; (2) the discovery in the biographies of such patients of an inordinately high incidence of resentment, hostility, suppressed emotionality, etc.; (3) a demonstrable relationship between onset and exacerbation of the disease and disturbing and frustrating incidents in the patient's life. These psychosomatic diseases differ from the psychoneuroses in that they exhibit different symptoms, are of longer duration, have a known pathologic basis and often a known cause (e.g., allergy in asthma, atopic dermatitis, and hay fever). Finally, the incidence of frank neuroses in this group of diseases is no greater than in the population at large, and neurotics are not more liable to them than normal individuals. For many reasons, not the least of which is that a psychogenic basis has never been proved in any of these diseases, we have chosen to present the relevant facts in the organ systems involved. They are not discussed further in the sections on neurology and psychiatry.

The sociopathies which include those individuals who from childhood exhibit impulsivity, aggressiveness, and various antisocial behaviors (running away, truancy, repeated thefts, alcohol and drug abuse, etc.) involve so many sociologic, educational, economic, and political factors that they fall almost beyond the orbit of medicine. While a medical position is often of value, particularly if there are questions of nervous disease or major psychiatric disorder, there is no clear evidence that medical opinion contributes significantly to the understanding and management of these problems. For these and other reasons such sociopathic states are also eliminated from this section of the book.

11

NERVOUSNESS, ANXIETY, DEPRESSION, PERSONALITY DISORDERS, AND NEUROSES

RAYMOND D. ADAMS

The majority of patients who enter a physician's office or hospital will admit to being or having been nervous, anxious, or depressed. The stress of contemporary life or the prospect of real or imaginary illness is thought to induce these reactions. If they stand in clear relationship to a stressful event or situation, such as worry over economic reverses or grief over the death of a loved one, such states can be accepted as normal. Only when excessively intense and uncontrollable or when accompanied by obscure derangements of visceral function do they become the basis for medical consultation.

Such problems become more abstruse when similar symptoms occur in persons who are not being subjected to immediately stressful or unhappy experiences, and awareness of such threatening situations, if it exists at all, lies buried in the subconscious mind of the patient. One may assume that it either has been suppressed from consciousness or is part of an elaborate subjective interpretation of which the patient is unaware. The relationship between social stimulus and prevailing anxiety or nervousness, if there is any such association, can then be discovered only by gentle probings by the psychologically sophisticated physician. But once the connection is established and the problem dealt with realistically, the symptoms allegedly become understandable and disappear. One recognizes here all the elements of a *psychoneurotic reaction.* The line of separation between the latter and normal emotional reactions is admittedly ambiguous.

There is still another category of nervousness, anxiety, and depression wherein the emotional states are intense and prolonged, and may occur in cycles, but again without obvious explanation. Such states may overwhelm the individual and cause derangement of all that individual's activities. Delving into the unconscious mind or studying lifelong reaction patterns fails to reveal a plausible psychogenesis. One recognizes here all the elements of a more complete, pervasive *psychotic reaction.* In many such instances a genetic factor appears to operate, and the features of the illness are so stereotyped as to indicate a disease of the parts of the nervous system which control the affective, emotional life. Yet a consistent biochemical change in the blood or brain tissue has not been found, and no lesion has been discerned. Treatment must proceed empirically, along nonpsychologic lines.

The problem confronting every physician is to recognize all these nuances of reaction, personality disorder, and disease, which obviously shade into one another, and to determine to what extent they figure in the medical condition of the patient. Some type of therapeutic maneuver must then be initiated, varying from simple reassurance and realistic management of existing personal difficulties, to suppression of symptoms by drugs. Often, referral to a psychiatrist is necessary for more expert management, including electrotherapy.

In this chapter we shall first consider the cardinal features of these common reactive states and then the personality and character disorders from which they are believed to arise, together with currently accepted views of their origins. The major neuroses of which they may be a part are discussed further on, and the psychoses are discussed in Chap. 25.

NERVOUSNESS By this vague term the lay person usually refers to a state of restlessness, tension, uneasy apprehension, irritability, or hyperexcitability. But it may connote other states, such as thoughts of suicide, fear of killing one's child or spouse, a distressing hallucination, a paranoid idea, or a frankly hysterical outburst. Careful inquiry as to what the patient means when complaining of nervousness is always a necessary first step.

In its most common signification, a period of nervousness may represent no more than a psychic and behavioral state in which an organism is maximally challenged by difficult personal problems, and there are periods in normal life when this is more likely to happen. For example, adolescence rarely passes without its period of turmoil as the person attempts emancipation from parental dominance or adjustment to demands of a scholastic or social nature. The menses are regularly accompanied by increased tension and moodiness, and, of course, the menarche and menopause are other critical periods. Some persons, because of early patterning or character formation, claim to have been nervous in all their social relationships throughout life; one should then suspect a psychoneurosis or unstable character formation or an oncoming psychosis, even though performance within the family unit, at school, and at work were adequate. When nervousness is a recent development, one must consider such conditions as an upheaval in personal affairs, the first attack or exacerbation of a psychoneurosis, an endogenous depression, an endocrine disease (hyperthyroidism, adrenal corticism, or corticosteroid therapy), or withdrawal from a sedative drug (alcohol, barbiturate). Some patients complain of a nervousness that attends or follows the onset of a medical or neurologic disease; and it would then appear to be secondary, occasioned by fear of disability, dependency, or death.

Nervousness, even in its simplest form, is reflected in many important activities of the human organism. There are often a mild somberness of mood and an increased tendency to tears and anger (irritability). Fatigue that bears no proper relationship to activity and rest is frequent, and sleep is often disturbed, as are eating and drinking habits. Headaches may increase in number and intensity. There is a tendency to sweat, tremble, be aware of heart action, feel a bit "queer in the head" or giddy, have an upset stomach, and urinate more often, though these recognized autonomic accompaniments of anxiety are seldom as conspicuous as in anxiety neurosis. Thus, it would appear that nervousness and anxiety constitute a graded series of reactions, the latter in many instances being only a more intense and protracted form of nervousness.

ANXIETY Anxiety is "the fundamental phenomenon and central problem of the neurosis . . . a nodal point, linking up all kinds of most important questions, a riddle of which the solution must cast a flood of light upon our whole mental life" (Freud). From the viewpoint of the social historian, anxiety is said to be "the most prominent mental characteristic of Occidental civilization" (Willoughby). These comments should inform the reader of the broad implications of this reaction.

The more strictly medical meaning of the term *anxiety,* and the one used in this chapter, is a state characterized by a subjective feeling of fear and uneasy anticipation (apprehension), usually with a definite topical content and associated with the physiologic accompaniments of strong emotion, i.e., breathlessness, choking sensation, palpitation, restlessness, increased muscular tension, tightness in the chest, giddiness, trembling, sweating, and flushing. By *topical content* is meant the idea, person, or object about which the person is anxious. The several vasomotor and visceral alterations that underlie the symptoms are mediated through the autonomic nervous system, particularly the sympathetic part of it, and involve also the thyroid and adrenal glands.

Forms of anxiety Anxiety is manifested in acute episodes, each lasting a few minutes and clearly related to a disturbing event in the patient's life; or it may represent an inexplicable protracted state that may last for weeks, months, or years. There may be a succession of acute *attacks,* or *panics* as they are called; the patient is plunged into an inexplicable mental state and fears death, loss of reason or self-control, and insanity, or feels that he or she may commit some horrible crime. The patient is breathless, has a racing heart, chokes, sweats, trembles, and feels gastric distress and anorexia. In a persistent, protracted state the patient experiences lesser and fluctuating degrees of nervousness, restlessness, irritability, fatigue, insomnia, intolerance of physical exertion, and pressure or tension headaches. Discrete anxiety attacks and chronic states of anxiety merge into one another.

Episodic anxiety without disorder of mood (i.e., depression) is usually classified as *anxiety neurosis.* The chronic form with prominent exercise intolerance is called *neurocirculatory asthenia.* Anxiety may, however, be combined with other somatic symptoms in hysteria and may be the restraining factor in *phobic neurosis.* Persistent anxiety with insomnia, lassitude, and fatigue, regardless of mood, should always raise suspicion of a *depressive psychosis,* especially if it begins late in life. Panic attacks are said to occur at the beginning of a schizophrenic illness, but this is rare in our experience. Both anxiety and depression are prominent features of the syndrome of posttraumatic nervous instability (see Chap. 366).

Thus, the differential diagnosis of an anxiety state requires that the physician consider all the major syndromes in psychiatry. Often it is but one component of a far more serious condition, one which may result in suicide or some other antisocial act. Also, without the psychic counterparts of fear and apprehension, the visceral symptoms alone should arouse suspicion of thyrotoxicosis, epilepsy, corticosteroid overdosage, pheochromocytoma, hypoglycemia, or menopause.

DEPRESSION (UNHAPPINESS, GLOOM, AND GRIEF) There are few persons who do not experience periods of discouragement and despair, and these periods become manifestly more frequent in modern society where individual freedom is constrained and one's impulses must be inhibited. As with nervousness and anxiety, depression of mood that is appropriate to a given situation in life is a natural, healthy reaction and seldom is the basis of medical complaint. The patient tends to seek help only when grief or unhappiness becomes uncontrollable. But there are numerous instances in which the patient is miserable, unhappy, and hopeless for reasons which are not apparent. Many of the symptoms are interpreted as ill health, being so similar to those of many disease states as to bring the patient first to the internist. Sometimes another disease is found (such as chronic hepatitis, brucellosis, or postinfluenzal asthenia) or infections in which chronic fatigue is confused with depression, but often an endogenous depression is itself the essential problem. Since the risk of suicide is not inconsiderable, if the illness is mistaken for another or overlooked as a complication, an error in diagnosis may be life-threatening.

Information about depression, like that about all psychiatric syndromes, is gained from three sources: the history obtained from the patient, the history obtained from the family or close friend, and the findings on examination.

From the patient and family it is learned that the patient has been "feeling unwell," "low in spirits," "blue," "glum," "unhappy," or "morbid." There has been a change in emotional reactions of which the patient may not be fully aware.

Activities that were formerly pleasurable are no longer so. Often, however, change in mood is less conspicuous than reduction in psychic and physical energy. Fatigue is almost invariable; not uncommonly, it is worse in the morning after a night of restless sleep. The words "loss of pep," "weak," "tired," "no energy to work," "my job seems more trying and difficult" appear in the language of the patient. The outlook is pessimistic. The patient is preoccupied with uncontrollable worry over trivialities. With excessive worry the ability to think with accustomed efficiency is reduced; there is complaint that the mind does not function properly, of being forgetful and unable to concentrate. If the patient is naturally of suspicious nature, paranoid tendencies may assert themselves.

Particularly troublesome in medical diagnosis is the patient's tendency to become hypochondriacal about associated diseases. Indeed, most cases formerly diagnosed as hypochondriasis are now regarded as depression. Pain from whatever cause—a stiff joint, a toothache, fleeting abdominal pains, or other troubles such as constipation, frequency of urination, insomnia, pruritus, burning tongue, weight loss—may become an obsessive focus of complaint. The patient passes from doctor to doctor seeking relief from symptoms that would not trouble the average person, and no amount of reassurance relieves this state of mind. The nervousness and anxiety felt by many of these persons may be obscured by their preoccupation with visceral functions.

When examined, the patient's facial expression is often plaintive, troubled, pained, or anguished. The attitude and manner betray a prevailing mood of depression, discouragement, and despondency. In other words, the affective response, which is the outward expression of feeling, is consistent with the depressed mood. During the interview the patient's eyes may be tearful, or he or she may cry openly. In some there is a kind of immobility of the face that mimics parkinsonism, though others are restless and agitated (pacing the floor, wringing their hands, etc.). Occasionally the patient will smile, but the smile impresses one as more of a social gesture than an expression of feeling.

The stream of speech, from which the ideational content is determined, is slow. At times the patient is mute and speaks neither spontaneously nor in response to questions. Again there may be a long pause between questions and answers. The latter are brief and may be monosyllabic. There is a paucity of ideas. The retardation extends to all topics of conversation and affects movement of limbs as well. The most extreme forms of decreased motor activity, rarely seen in the medical clinic, border on stupor.

Content of speech is found to be abnormal if examined carefully. Conversation is replete with pessimistic thoughts, fears, expressions of unworthiness, inadequacy, inferiority, and sometimes guilt. In severe depressions bizarre ideas, delusions about the body ("blood drying up," "bowels are blocked with cement," "I am half dead") may be expressed.

Etiology and mechanism (see Chap. 25) Like anxiety, depression is a state which may stand as a simple reaction to an environmental circumstance, a form of neurosis or a major psychosis. It is the writer's belief that depression is one of the most commonly overlooked diagnoses in clinical medicine. Part of the trouble is with the word itself, which implies being unhappy about something. The persistent or recurrent endogenous depression or involutional depression should be suspected in all chronic states of ill health, hypochondriasis, multiple complaints involving many organ systems, disability that exceeds manifest signs of a medical disease, neurasthenia, and suicide attempts. Inasmuch as recovery is the rule, the suicide is a tragedy for which the medical profession must often share responsibility.

Personality disorders

Type of disorder	Characteristics
1 Paranoid	Chronic wariness, suspiciousness, litigiousness; lack of insight or humor; tendency to blame others; sense of self-importance and entitlement
2 Cyclothymic	Recurring periods of depression and elation not readily explained by circumstances; severe moodiness
3 Schizoid	Isolation, seclusiveness, secretiveness; discomfort in relationships; often eccentric and lacking in energy; few friends
4 Explosive	Outbursts of rage and aggression not in keeping with usual personality, often in response to minor provocation; sense of loss of control followed by regret
5 Obsessive-compulsive	Chronic worries about standards; excessive concern about self-image; tension in relationships, leading to isolation; inability to relax and excessive inhibitions; predisposition to depression
6 Hysterical	Immaturity, histrionic behavior, sexualization of relationships, low frustration tolerance, and shallow interpersonal ties; dependency
7 Asthenic	Chronic weakness, easy fatigability, sense of vulnerability, poor response to stress, little ambition or aggression
8 Passive-aggressive	Obstructive behavior, stubbornness, intentional errors or omissions; intolerance of authority with struggles over control, often creating difficulties in medical settings; externalization of conflicts and blaming others for untoward events
9 Inadequate	Chronic inability to meet ordinary life demands in the absence of mental retardation; severe dependency on others; tendency to become institutionalized or to become dependent on institutions
10 Antisocial	Unsocialized or antisocial behavior in conflict with society; selfishness, callousness, impulsiveness, lack of loyalty, and little guilt; frustration tolerance is low; tendency to blame others and have a long history of interpersonal and social difficulties and arrests

PERSONALITY DISORDERS When the above nervous states occur repeatedly and without explanation, there is likelihood that they derive from chronic lifelong patterns of maladaptation and peculiarities of character. Psychiatrists speak of such states as *borderline character disorders,* implying that they account for the ways different individuals cope with life.

The origins of these peculiarities of character are obscure. To avoid the dispute as to whether they are conditioned by early life experiences or are the product of genetic factors, the adjective "constitutional" is sometimes used in reference to them. The formal types of neuroses are believed to originate in these personality disorders.

If one examines Table 11-1, the specific personality types clearly shade into particular neuroses, and one wonders if they are not merely milder forms of neurosis, differing from the latter in that they less frequently present as medical problems. Personality disturbances are important to recognize, however, for the perceptive physician must take account of them as well as of the related neuroses in the diagnosis of disease and the management of patients with medical illnesses. Such patients may sabotage a needed diagnostic test or therapy. Actually, it is the physician's knowledge of human nature and skill in the care of these difficult and often exasperating patients that enable him or her to be the leader of a therapeutic team.

NEUROSES When nervousness, anxiety, and depression are persistently or episodically joined with various combinations of irrational fears, obsessive thoughts, compulsions, lassitude and fatigue, insomnia, preoccupation with trivial symptoms, and a number of different somatic disturbances for which no

cause can be found, the condition is properly called *neurosis* or *psychoneurosis.*

The neuroses represent a specific group of mental disorders appearing in adolescence and early to middle adulthood in individuals who have already achieved relatively adequate mental function. Since these disorders have no demonstrable organic basis, they are often called "functional," a term that is incorrect, for all functional disorders must have a physical basis. In all instances the neurotic patients are normally alert and correctly oriented, have considerable insight into their troubles, and manifest *"unimpaired reality testing,"* meaning that they do not confuse their subjective experiences and fantasies with external reality, more explicitly that they are not deluded and do not suffer hallucinations. The personality remains organized, and conduct is within socially acceptable limits. Neurotic patients can usually study, work, and function in the family and social circle even though assailed by doubts, loss of self-confidence, and despondency. They know that the troublesome symptoms originate within the mind, but are incapable of overcoming them by force of will, and hence they feel ashamed and inadequate. In these several ways neuroses are to be distinguished from the more pervasive and disorganizing psychoses.

Within this multitude of symptoms certain natural clusterings occur, and these are the basis of the classification in Table 11-2, which has been sanctioned by an international committee of psychiatrists.

In general medicine we have frequently encountered types 1 to 4, whereas type 6 (neurasthenia) and type 8 (hypochondriasis) will usually prove to be manifestations of a depressive state. Type 5 (depressive neurosis) will be difficult to distinguish from the nonpsychotic depression. Type 7 (depersonal-

TABLE 11-2
The neuroses

Type of neurosis	Characteristics
1 Anxiety neurosis	Episodic diffuse anxiety in attacks or waves; somatic complaints such as palpitations, paresthesias, weakness, dizziness; pessimism and irritability
2 Hysterical neurosis:	
a Conversion type	Physical symptoms involving voluntary musculature and sensory system, such as paradoxic paralyses, seizures, sensory deficits, and pain; attitude of indifference
b Dissociative type	Alterations in consciousness and sense of identity, such as fugue states, amnesias, somnambulism; anxiety not evident
3 Phobic neurosis	Intense irrational fears of objects or situations; anxiety attacks may occur with corresponding physical symptoms
4 Obsessive-compulsive neurosis	Persistent or intrusive thoughts, often distressing in content, and uncontrollable minor acts, often to expiate, cleanse, or counteract evil; depression and guilt are prominent; preoccupations with disease may occur
5 Depressive neurosis	Episodic excessive self-criticism, low self-esteem, and lowered vitality, often accompanied by physical complaints
6 Neurasthenic neurosis	Weakness, fatigability, exhaustion, with low self-esteem but little self-criticism
7 Depersonalization neurosis	Feelings of unreality and estrangement from self, body, and surroundings; panic may occur
8 Hypochondriacal neurosis	Morbid preoccupations with bodily processes and diseases, accompanied by multiple physical complaints; anxiety and agitation may occur; depression is common

ization neurosis), a relatively rare condition in the author's experience, probably is a form of depression or pseudoneurotic schizophrenia.

For clarity of concept the term neurosis should be reserved for these particular groupings of symptoms and signs, and not loosely applied to individuals who are transiently upset by some circumstance or are emotional or eccentric. Each type may occur in relatively pure form, but often there are overlappings of symptoms. Anxiety, for example, may occur in pure form with a depressive reaction, in hysteria, and with phobic states. These combinations of neuroses are called "mixed neuroses."

The diagnosis of a neurosis depends largely on a thorough history that covers much of the medical biography of the patient. The physical examination seldom yields abnormal findings. Moreover, there is no laboratory test to which one can turn for final confirmation of diagnosis, which is true also of manic-depressive psychosis and schizophrenia. Subjective impressions supersede objective data, reducing accuracy of diagnosis.

Most psychiatrists hold the opinion that the neuroses have their genesis in the early life experiences that mold character and personality; that is, the neurosis stems from a neurotic character (hysterical, hypochondriacal, etc.). Reich and Kelly, who wrote the chapter on neuroses in the eighth edition of this textbook, regard them as psychologic decompensations of a neurotic personality that are basically maladaptive and inappropriate to the level of stress. The form of the neurotic episode is believed to be determined by the personality structure of the patient. But such explanations do not seem relevant to the most frequent of all the neuroses, the anxiety neurosis, which may strike a well-balanced person at any time during life. Furthermore, the stress of urban living conditions seems not to be a factor in the development of neurosis, for surveys of urban and rural populations show approximately the same incidence of neurotic behavior. The lifetime prevalence, regardless of social environment, is approximately 15 percent.

Neuroses vary in severity from mild periods of uneasiness that may not come to medical attention to episodes of severe, incapacitating illnesses that may require hospitalization. Since neuroses are frequent and may masquerade as medical illnesses with which the internist must contend, or complicate certain disease states, the following descriptive data should be fixed in mind.

Anxiety neurosis When anxiety occurs in pure form and is persistent and without explanation as a reaction, whether in an acute self-limiting form or as a chronic state with wavelike intensification of symptoms, it is called anxiety neurosis. The physical manifestations of rapid heart action, smothering, and hyperventilation have already been described. Such patients are seen more frequently by cardiologists than other specialists. Phobias, obsessions, compulsions, and hypochondriacal concerns may appear but are usually transitory and unimportant. Depression of mood is not part of the illness, but herein lies a difficult theoretical problem. Many psychiatrists hold that all persistent anxiety states that do not respond to simple explanation and reassurance are basically *anxious depressions*. The suicide rate in that group is distressingly high, and in not a few instances patients have ended their lives while receiving psychotherapy. The author has known of families afflicted with hereditary endogenous depressions or manic-depressive disease in which one member has developed a typical anxiety neurosis.

Of more general medical importance is the fact that both anxiety and depression can surface in patients hospitalized for a medical illness. The fears that naturally attend a myocardial

infarction, a mild stroke, or a tumor may be exaggerated, and the patient may become so agitated as to become unable to listen to explanations or accept reassurance. Unreasonable anger may force the patient to attempt to leave the hospital. Convalescence may be prolonged by "weakness," persistent fatigue, and unwillingness to return to customary activities.

Physiologic and psychologic basis The cause, mechanism, and biologic meaning of anxiety have been the subjects of much speculation, and completely satisfactory explanations are not possible. The psychologist regards anxiety as anticipatory behavior, i.e., a state of uneasiness about something which may happen in the future. William McDougall spoke of it as "an emotional state arising when a continuing strong desire seems likely to miss its goal." The primary emotion, somewhat muted perhaps, is that of fear, and its arousal under conditions not overtly threatening may be explained by conditioning to some recondite component of a formerly threatening stimulus.

The only well-systematized theory is that put forth by the school of psychoanalysis, which looks upon anxiety as a response to a situation that in some manner undermines the security of the individual. The topical content or cause of potential danger lies in the unconscious mind. The postulated danger is internal rather than external; a primitive drive has been aroused that is not compatible with current social practices, and it can be relieved only at risk of harm to the person. In other words, the anxiety protects the individual by preventing the execution of the unacceptable action.

Physicians have searched for evidence of impairments of visceral function without success. The neurocirculatory asthenic is in poor physical condition, has an elevated blood lactate level after exercise, and will not tolerate the work or exercise needed to build up stamina. And even in the resting state lactic acid levels in the blood may be elevated, and infusions containing lactic acid are said to make the symptoms worse. The urinary excretion of epinephrine has been found elevated in some patients; in others, there is an increased urinary excretion of norepinephrine. Aldosterone excretion is raised to two or three times the normal level during intense anxiety. Medical students experiencing fear and anxiety while preparing for an examination also excrete increased amounts of aldosterone. The interpretation of these data (whether as primary or secondary effects) is not certain, but it is becoming increasingly evident that prolonged and diffuse anxiety is a pattern of behavior related to certain biochemical abnormalities of blood, and probably of the brain. A genetic factor seems operative in many cases. Anxiety neurosis and endogenous depressions, which are closely related, tend to run in families.

Easton and Sherman have reviewed the subject of anxiety in relation to adrenergic hyperresponsivity. It has been claimed that in susceptible individuals isoproterenol, when administered by intravenous infusion, induced an anxiety attack. Propranolol (Inderal) gives symptomatic relief. Other investigators have not been able to corroborate these observations and caution against the indiscriminate prescription of propranolol, for it is potentially hazardous in patients with congestive heart failure, atrioventricular block, and asthma (we have found it harmless to most individuals). These observations do, however, emphasize the role of the sympathetic nervous system in anxiety neurosis.

Treatment In the management of acute anxiety states, it is important to explain to patients that they suffer from a real medical illness and not just "nerves," or an imaginary condition. They should be allowed to express their feelings, doubts, and fears. Superficial psychotherapy, involving support, insight, and reeducation proves to be the most practical. Often, as the patient is mobilized and returned to usual activities, the symptoms subside. If the anxiety is persistent and severe, one should be alert to the risk of suicide and be prepared to send the patient to a psychiatric hospital for treatment of depression. If mild, antianxiety drugs such as meprobamate 400 mg tid, chlordiazepoxide 10 to 20 mg tid, diazepam 5 to 10 mg tid, propranolol 40 mg tid, or sodium amytal 100 to 200 mg tid, prescribed in the lowest possible dose, may suffice to bring the symptoms under control.

Hysterical neurosis   Unlike anxiety neurosis, where males and females are equally affected, chronic hysterical neurosis is almost exclusively a female illness. Beginning in late childhood (earliest age around 9 to 10 years), adolescence, or early adulthood, the patient begins to present a variety of inexplicable episodes of illness. Abdominal pains leading to appendectomy or ovariectomy (for cysts), severe and disabling dysmenorrhea, urinary retention requiring catheterization (sometimes followed by permanent injury to bladder), fainting spells and bizarre seizures, recurrent vomiting without weight loss, inexplicable fevers, paraplegias, hemiplegias, ataxias, blindness, deafness, intractable headaches and dizziness, and trancelike states and amnesias (the woman who appears in the emergency ward with lost identity) are some of the principal problems that bring these patients to internists and neurologists. Since these episodes of illness recur over years, one must distinguish between them and all the diseases that are common to this age period. More of these patients are seen on the neurology services of a general hospital than on any other service. By adult years it is not unusual for the patient to have had several unnecessary abdominal operations and many hospitalizations.

Psychiatrists, on the basis of psychoanalytic theory, subdivide the hysterical neurosis into two types, the conversion and the dissociative. All the forms of illness in which there are gross neuromuscular and other somatic derangements are called conversions, with the implication that suppressed anxiety has been converted into the physical symptom. Dissociative states include an alteration of self-awareness resulting in amnesia, fugue states, somnambulism, and split personality. But there are no basic differences between these two forms, and most patients will at some time exhibit both. Strangely, the attitude of the patient is often one of unconcern and apparent indifference to a major physical disability, but typical anxiety symptoms are not infrequent. Most of our patients have been of rather average or low average intelligence. Women working in health care organizations (practical nurses, ward attendants) show a particular susceptibility.

At times, the patient appears to be gaining something by being ill, but this is hard to prove. Nevertheless, it leads to a suspicion of malingering. However, most students of mental illness believe that hysterical symptoms are not under conscious control. And, despite the fact that nurses, ward attendants, and physicians perceive the disability as obviously spurious, the patient seems totally unaware of the unconvincing nature of the symptoms. True malingering usually occurs in immature, sociopathic males who have been in trouble from childhood.

The line between conversion symptoms and malingering is especially vague in a closely related condition called "compensation neurosis" where, following a civilian accident or a frightening experience (an army assignment, a threat of disability) the patient becomes paralyzed or has some other symptom of obscure origin. Such patients differ from the chronic hysterical neurotic in that the potential gain is easily discovered, there is not the history of neurotic illness prior to injury, the patient's lack of insight is less convincing, and males and females are equally susceptible. The author prefers to regard this as a separate illness.

As a rule, a careful physical examination will usually distinguish the hysterical disorders from physical ones, though physicians inexperienced with some of the subtleties of rare medical and neurologic diseases may be misled.

In the management of such patients, prolonged psychotherapy has seldom produced successful results. Often, any suggestion that the illness is psychiatric arouses a hostile reaction, and the patient may refuse to see a psychiatrist. The author has obtained the best results by explaining to the patient and the family that the illness is really a chronic constitutional nervous weakness which is now abating. After all tests for other physical ailments are concluded, the patient is urged to begin walking and resuming normal activities. Sometimes this positive approach can overcome a paralysis within a few minutes, but if it has been present a long time, a vigorous physical program will be needed to restore lost function. Subjective complaints are disregarded, and if the patient continues to emphasize them, reassurance is offered that they will soon recede. Hypnosis, electric stimulation, and dramatic curative methods (Lourdes, acupuncture, etc.) have no advantage. Once rid of the pressing complaint, the patient is best managed by a kindly, understanding physician, sensitive to the nuances of this psychologic disorder, who will analyze each new illness to make sure it is hysterical and not some new intervening disease. Hysterical symptoms should be treated symptomatically, with simple non-habit-forming drugs.

The treatment of compensation neurosis requires a thorough medical survey, reassurance, symptomatic therapy, and early settlement of the compensation claims. The results in the older worker are far from satisfactory.

Phobic and obsessive-compulsive neuroses   These two neuroses, together called psychesthenia by Janet, are relatively rare and need not be described in detail. Individuals with neuroses of this type are rigid and perfectionist; otherwise capable of functioning effectively, they have their lives dominated by a single irrational fear (e.g., of being away from their own home or neighborhood) or by a series of obsessive thoughts or compulsive rituals. Any departure from their restricted mode of life occasions intense anxiety. Overwhelmed by physical symptoms, ashamed and despondent, the patient limps through life with this handicap.

Opinion is divided among psychiatrists as to the efficacy of psychotherapy, including psychoanalysis. Cures have been reported. Several of the author's patients whose phobic state had recently increased to the point where they were disabled, were brought again under partial control by the use of amitryptaline or imipramine. Presumably a depressive state had supervened.

Neurasthenic neurosis   Persistent weakness, fatigability, and exhaustion are common to many mental illnesses, particularly anxiety neurosis and depression. In some instances it seems to be a character type and is lifelong—the asthenic psychopathy of Kahn. This problem will be discussed in Chap. 12.

Hypochondriacal neurosis   Morbid preoccupation with bodily functions and physical symptoms is a frequent condition. Such patients make up a sizeable segment of every medical outpatient clinic. They seem possessed with worries about their bowel functions, tinnitus, arthritic and postzoster pains, old-age vertigo, and many of the other symptoms to which middleaged and elderly adults are prey. Every minute detail is studied and described, recounted again and again. It is difficult to turn them to any other topic of conversation. Unlike hysteria and anxiety neurosis, one can find no physiologic or somatic derangements.

Most of these patients have a depression, and a few express

frankly delusional ideas about their viscera. Severe hypochondriasis in a young person should always suggest schizophrenia. But there are many individuals who have no other mental illness. They go through life being concerned and worried about disease in themselves and their families. Often, one finds that they have been raised in a family atmosphere of overconcern about health. It has become part of their character.

In hypochondriacal patients, after the proper physical examination procedure and laboratory tests have eliminated serious disease, the physician should tell them that they have a neurosis and need help. Symptomatic therapy, a regulated program of daily activities, frequent visits with an understanding physician for explanation and reeducation, and group psychotherapy are all beneficial. But whenever there is suspicion of despondency and depression, a psychiatric opinion should be sought and antidepressive measures as outlined in Chap. 25 should be initiated.

Depressive neurosis Many patients with any one of the above neuroses may feel trapped, hopeless, and gloomy—a natural reaction to the symptomatology over which they have no control. Unlike the endogenous and involutional depressions, the mood change may be transitory and variable from day to day, and vegetative symptoms such as loss of appetite, weight loss, constipation, loss of libido and impotence do not occur. Many psychiatrists distinguish this neurotic type of depression and the reactive depression from the endogenous or organic types, and they caution that the drugs and electroconvulsive therapy used in the endogenous and organic types are usually unsuccessful in neurotic depressions. The line between the two types is thin, however, and the physician is well advised to let a psychiatric consultant stand responsible for separating them and making sure the patient is not suicidal.

COMMON PROBLEMS IN DIAGNOSIS OF PSYCHIATRIC ILLNESSES THAT PRODUCE PHYSICAL SYMPTOMS The physician's greatest concern is misdiagnosis, and physicians rightly appreciate the difficulty of deciding when mental symptoms appear to accompany, mask, or mimic physical disease. There is often the impression that diagnosis is reduced to inspired guesswork. Shulman, in a discussion of psychogenic illness with physical manifestations, states that the common problems are relatively few and not difficult to recognize. He believes the most frequent source of error to be the too strict application of the law of parsimony, which tries to subsume all symptoms under one diagnosis. At least one-fourth to one-half of all adult medical problems represent a cluster or complex of functional-organic or physical-psychosocial illnesses. Most astute physicians can separate the effects of diseases from the associated psychologic reactions.

Probably the largest and most serious diagnostic error may be committed when there are recurrent symptoms in many organ systems for which no obvious cause can be found. Here one must suspect the *masked depression,* i.e., the form of endogenous illness in which the leading complaint is pain (headache, precordial pain, backache, etc.) or exhaustion, and it is a mistake to consider the despondency a secondary reaction. A safe rule to follow is that whenever an unexplained syndrome is accompanied by complaints in two or three other organ systems, a serious psychiatric illness with anxiety and depression should be suspected. Complications of pharmacologic therapy and chronic liver or pancreatic disease may rarely give rise to a similar picture.

Another perplexing problem is the anxiety state that is misdiagnosed as menopause, thyrotoxicosis, hypoglycemia, pheochromocytoma, carcinoid tumor, left-sided heart failure, or temporal lobe epilepsy. Each of these diseases causes visceral derangements not unlike those of anxiety. But the latter differs descriptively in that there is always a prominent psychic component of fear and apprehension. It is the combination of mental and autonomic symptoms that should always lead to the suspicion of an anxiety state or anxious depression.

And finally there is the problem of misdiagnosing a neurologic disease (e.g., multiple sclerosis) in a patient who has the conversion form of hysteria or a compensation problem. The lifelong history, the context of the illness, and discrepancy between symptoms and signs should direct thinking along the right path.

In all these problems, a good history is the cornerstone of diagnosis, especially if it includes a kind of life chart of key personal events, medical illnesses, and psychologic derangements. The history is more important than the physical examination and laboratory tests. Incongruities between complaints and between symptoms and physical findings and disabilities are the most important leads. It is "the old crock" with a long history of ill health that is most subject to misdiagnosis.

REFERENCES

NICHOLI AM (ed): *The Harvard Guide to Modern Psychiatry.* Cambridge, Mass, Harvard University Press, 1978

SHULMAN R: Psychogenic illness with physical manifestations: A practical approach. Lancet 1:524, 1977

EASTON D, SHERMAN DG: Somatic anxiety attacks and propranolol. Arch Neurol 33:689, 1976

12
LASSITUDE AND ASTHENIA

RAYMOND D. ADAMS

The terms *weakness* and *fatigue* are used by patients to describe a variety of subjective complaints which vary in their import and prognostic significance. The different meanings can usually be fitted into the following classification:

1 Lassitude, fatigue, lack of energy, listlessness, and languor. These terms, though not synonymous, shade into one another. All refer to a weariness and a loss of that sense of well-being typically found in persons healthy of body and mind.
2 Weakness, loss of strength, paresis, paralysis. These may be persistent or episodic.
   a Persistent weakness: This may be (1) restricted to certain muscles or groups of muscles (see Chap. 15) or (2) more or less generalized, i.e., involving the entire musculature (see Chaps. 381 and 382).
   b Episodic, often recurrent: Attacks of weakness may occur in the periodic paralyses. [Many patients confuse "attacks of weakness" with a diminished sense of alertness, lightheadedness, feeling of faintness. These usually turn out to be episodes of partial or threatening syncope, attacks of anxiety or vertigo, or seizures (see Chaps. 11, 14, and 23).]

LASSITUDE AND FATIGUE Of all the symptoms in this group these are among the most frequent and abstruse. More than half of all patients entering a general hospital register direct complaint of fatigability or admit to it when questioned. During the Second World War fatigue was so prominent as to be given a separate place in medical nosology, viz., "combat fatigue," which came to refer to all acute psychiatric illnesses that happened on the battlefield. The common clinical antecedents and accompaniments of fatigue, its significance, and its physiologic and psychologic bases should, therefore, be matters of common medical knowledge.

Patients who complain of weariness and tiredness have a more or less characteristic way of describing their condition. They say that they "are all in," "have lost pep," "have no ambition" or "no interest," are "turned off" or "fed up." They manifest their condition by showing an indifference to the tasks at hand, by talking much about how hard they are working; they are inclined to sit around or lie down, occupying themselves with trivial tasks. On closer analysis one observes that they have a difficulty in initiating activity and also in sustaining it.

This condition is the familiar aftermath of prolonged labor or great physical exertion, and under such circumstances it is accepted as a normal, physiologic reaction. When, however, the same symptoms or similar ones appear in no relation to such antecedents, they are suspected to be the manifestations of disease.

The physician's task begins, then, with an attempt to determine whether the patient is merely suffering from the physical and mental effects of overwork without realizing it. Overworked, overwrought people are everywhere observable in our society. Their actions are both instructive and pathetic. They seem to be impelled by notions of duty and refuse to think of themselves. Or, as is often the case, some personal inadequacy seems to prevent them from deriving pleasure from any activity except their work, in which they indulge themselves as a kind of defense mechanism. Such persons show their fatigue by other symptoms, such as irritability, restlessness, and sleeplessness. Their symptoms and behavior are best understood by referring to psychologic studies of the effect of fatigue on the normal individual.

Effects of fatigue on the normal person   According to several authoritative sources, fatigue has both explicit and implicit effects, logically grouped under (1) a series of biochemical and physiologic changes in many organs of the body, (2) an overt disorder in behavior, a reduced output of work, known as *work decrement*, and (3) an expressed dissatisfaction and a subjective feeling of tiredness.

As to the biochemical and physiologic changes, continuous muscular work leads to depletion of muscle glycogen and an accumulation of lactic acid and other metabolites, which in themselves reduce the power of contraction and delay recovery. Extreme degrees of muscle work, in which activity exceeds provision of substrate, results in necrosis of fibers and rise in serum levels of creatine phosphokinase and aldolase even in normal persons. The muscles are slightly swollen and sore for several days. It is said that the injection of blood from a fatigued animal into a rested one will produce overt manifestations of fatigue in the latter. During repeated contractions of muscle, its action is observed to become tremulous, movements are less adept, and the coordination of agonist, antagonist, and synergic muscles is less perfect. The rate of breathing increases, the pulse quickens, the blood pressure rises and pulse pressure widens, and the white blood cell count and metabolic rate are increased. These alterations bear out the hypothesis that fatigue is in part a manifestation of altered metabolism.

The decreased capacity for work or productivity which is a direct consequence of fatigue has been investigated by industrial psychologists. Their findings show clearly the importance of the motivational factor on work output, whether it be in manual or clerical tasks. Individual differences in energy potential appear also to be important, as are differences in physique, intelligence, and temperament.

The subjective feelings of fatigue have been carefully recorded. Aside from feeling weary tired persons are unable to deal effectively with complex problems and tend to be unreasonable, often about trivialities. The number and quality of

their associations in psychologic tests are reduced. The ability to deliberate and to reach judgments is impaired; decisions made late at night may appear unsound the next day. The worker after a long, hard day is unable to perform adequately his or her duties as head of a household; the example of the tired businessperson who becomes the proverbial tyrant of the family circle is well known. A disinclination to try and the appearance of ideas of inferiority are other characteristics of the fatigued mind.

Instances of fatigue and lassitude resulting from overwork are not difficult to recognize. Descriptions of patients' daily routines and talks with associates and family will usually suffice. Moreover if they can be persuaded to live at a more reasonable pace and allow time for outside pleasurable activities, their symptoms will promptly subside. A common error in diagnosis, however, is the ascription of fatigue to overwork when actually it is a manifestation of a psychoneurosis or depression.

Fatigue as a manifestation of psychiatric disorder   The great majority of patients who enter a hospital because of unexplained chronic fatigue and lassitude have been found to have some type of psychiatric illness. Formerly this state was called *neurasthenia;* but since fatigue rarely exists as an isolated phenomenon, the current practice is to label such cases according to the total clinical picture. The usual associated symptoms are nervousness, irritability, anxiety, depression, insomnia, headaches, difficulty in concentrating, sexual disorders, and loss of bodily appetites. In one series in a general hospital 75 percent of persons admitted because of chronic fatigue and nervousness were diagnosed, finally, as having *anxiety neurosis* and *tension states.* Depression accounted for another 10 percent, and the remainder of the patients had a miscellany of medical and psychiatric illnesses.

Several features are common to the psychiatric group. The fatigue may be worse in the morning. There is an inclination to lie down and rest, but sleep does not come. The fatigue relates more to some activities than to others. Inquiry as to what was happening when the fatigue was first experienced may reveal an unpleasant event, a grief reaction, a surgical operation, or a medical illness. The feeling of fatigue interferes with mental as well as physical activities. The psychic aspects are manifested as difficulty in concentrating on the solution of a problem or in carrying on an involved conversation.

Depressing emotion, as was remarked in the previous chapter, has its characteristic effect on impulse life and energy. Also, it impairs sleep, with a tendency to early-morning waking. Such persons are at their worst in the morning, both in spirit and in energy output. Their tendency is to improve as the day wears on, and they may even feel fairly normal by evening. It is often difficult in them to decide whether the fatigue is a primary manifestation of the depression or is secondary to a lack of interest.

Many physicians question whether all chronically fatigued individuals deviate enough from normal to justify the diagnosis of psychoneurosis or depression. Many people in society, because of circumstances beyond their control, have no purpose in life and much idle time. They are bored with the monotony of their routine. Such circumstances are conducive to fatigue, just as the opposite is also true—that a new enterprise that excites optimism and enthusiasm will dispel fatigue. Other individuals seem normal until some adversity is encountered, arousing worry or fear, and then it becomes apparent that their adjustment is unstable. Such reactions are understandable to anyone who has ever had stage fright or "buck fever" and who remembers the sense of physical weakness, the utter incapacity to act, the intellectual chaos that overwhelms the previously well-ordered mind, and the exhaustion which follows.

Psychologic theories The enervating effect of a strong emotion such as anxiety is well known, and it might be supposed that the simple prolongation of the emotional experience would provide a rational explanation for a chronic fatigue of anxiety. But even if true, however, this explanation does not account for the occurrence of emotion at a time when there is no reason for it.

The dynamic schools of psychiatry, particularly the psychoanalytic, have postulated that chronic fatigue, in the broadest sense, is like the anxiety from which it derives; it is a danger signal that something is wrong—that some attitude or activity has been too intense or too persistent. The fatigue is self-preservative, serving not merely as a protection against physical injury but also as a protection of the individual's self-esteem and confidence in self. As to mechanism, it is claimed that the fatigue is the result of exhaustion of the store of psychic energy required to maintain repression of unacceptable ideas. Others, however, claim to have evidence that fatigue is not a negative symptom, a lack or depletion of energy, but an unconscious desire for inactivity. A reciprocal relationship is said to exist between fatigue and anxiety. Both are protective, but anxiety is the more imperative. It calls for the individual to take some positive action to extricate him- or herself from a predicament, whereas fatigue calls for inactivity. Both operate blindly, however, for the person cannot perceive what it is that must be done or not done. All this happens at the unconscious level.

It is also observed that some persons are low in impulse and energy throughout life, being more so at times of stress. Some psychiatrists believe that they have a constitutional inadequacy. Kahn classifies such individuals as "psychopaths weak in impulse," and points out in his description their inability throughout life to play games vigorously, to compete successfully, to work hard without exhaustion, to withstand or recover quickly from illness, or to assume a dominant role in a social group. The physician caring for them expects greater disability and more prolonged convalescence from every illness.

It is obvious that these several psychologic hypotheses could not all be correct, nor could they be applicable to all situations in which chronic fatigue is the complaint. Undoubtedly there are persons who are underactive and weak because of genetic factors or early life experiences. It is equally clear that psychic and physical energy are closely linked to mood. The more chronic varieties of acquired fatigue, without a basis in medical disease, have in nearly all instances a psychologic basis.

Lassitude and fatigue in chronic infection and in endocrine and other medical diseases Infection is another cause of chronic fatigue, though a much less frequent one. Everyone has at some time or other sensed the abrupt onset of extreme exhaustion, the tired ache in the muscles, an inexplicable listlessness, only to discover later that one is "coming down with the flu." In chronic infections such as hepatitis, tuberculosis, brucellosis, infectious mononucleosis, the infection may not be at once evident. But it should always be suspected when the fatigue is out of proportion to other symptoms such as mood change, nervousness, and anxiety. Often this syndrome will begin with an obvious infection but will persist for several weeks after it should have terminated, and it may then be difficult to decide whether there is still a lingering infection or the infection has been complicated by psychiatric illness during convalescence. In many diseases such as infectious hepatitis, brucellosis, infectious mononucleosis, and a host of other systemic viral infections, long-standing neurotic symptoms appear to have been uncovered. Nevertheless it is difficult to dismiss an obscure secondary metabolic disorder consequent to the infection.

Metabolic and endocrine diseases (see Chaps. 332 and 334) of various types may cause inordinate degrees of lassitude and fatigue. Sometimes there is in addition a true muscular weakness (see Chaps. 13 and 357). In Addison's disease and Simmonds' disease fatigue may dominate the clinical picture. Aldosterone deficiency is another established cause of fatigue (see Chap. 335). In persons with hypothyroidism, with or without frank myxedema, lassitude and sluggishness are frequent complaints. These same symptoms may also be present in patients with hyperthyroidism but are usually less troublesome than nervousness. Uncontrolled diabetes mellitus may be accompanied by excessive fatigability, as are hyperparathyroidism, hypogonadism, and Cushing's disease.

Anemia, when moderate or severe (hematocrit less than 25) should be considered as a possible cause of unexplained lassitude. Mild grades of anemia are usually asymptomatic; lassitude is far too often ascribed to it.

Any type of nutritional deficiency may, when severe, cause lassitude, and in its earlier stages this may be the chief complaint. Weight loss and the history of dietary inadequacy may provide the only other clues to the nature of the illness. Many patients feel weak and tired after a myocardial infarct, but usually there is an accompanying depression.

Among neurologic diseases in which fatigability is a prominent symptom should be mentioned the posstraumatic nervous instability syndrome, Parkinson's disease, and multiple sclerosis. The fatigue of Parkinson's disease may precede the recognition of neurologic signs by months or even years. It is probably a reaction to the increasing disability occasioned by subjective awareness of the akinesia. The majority of patients who recover from a stroke complain of being weak and tired. Hot temperatures worsen the fatigue and other symptoms of the multiple sclerotic patient.

Differential diagnosis If one looks critically at the patients who enter a hospital because of lassitude and fatigability (sometimes incorrectly called weakness), it is clear that the most commonly overlooked diagnoses are psychoneurosis and depression. The correct conclusion can usually be reached by keeping these illnesses in mind as one elicits the principal symptoms of these psychiatric illnesses from patient and family. Difficulty arises when such symptoms are so inconspicuous as not to be appreciated; one comes then to suspect the psychiatric diagnosis only by having eliminated the common medical causes. Observations in the hospital may bear out the existence of a tension state or gloomy mood, as the patient resists attempts to be mobilized. Strong reassurance in combination with a therapeutic trial of 2.5 to 5.0 mg dextroamphetamine morning and noon and 100 to 200 mg sodium amobarbital three times a day may suppress symptoms of which the patient was barely aware and may clarify diagnosis. The danger of mistaking a depression for a neurosis has already been mentioned. Of course, asthenic psychopaths are recognized by their actions as revealed in biographies.

Obscure infections such as pulmonary tuberculosis, brucellosis, subclinical hepatitis, subacute bacterial endocarditis, malaria, hookworm, and parasitic infections should be recognizable, by the characteristic symptoms and signs described elsewhere in the book. An endocrine survey particularly for adrenal insufficiency and thyroid disease, is in order in all obscure cases. There should also be a search for occult tumors. If one has no access to hormone assays, the use of a simple "water excretion test" may prove very helpful in identifying an organic component in a patient's fatigue syndrome, since a wide variety of systemic disorders is associated with a delayed diuresis following the ingestion of water. It is thought that the "sick cell" with impaired permeability of cell membrane "traps" water and then releases it slowly. The test consists in the administration of 500 ml water at 8:00, 8:15, and 8:30 A.M. for a total intake of 1500 ml with the patient fasting and lying in a horizontal position. Smoking is not permitted. The water should be room temperature, *not cold*. Urine volume is measured hourly for 3 to 4 h. A normal response will usually include a diuresis of 400 to 600 ml in the first, second, and third hours, with a total volume of at least 80 percent in 3 to 4 h (1200 ml). An impaired response in the horizontal position suggests *organic disease*. It should be remembered that chronic intoxications with barbiturates, alcohol, or bromides, some of which are given to suppress nervousness, may contribute to fatigability.

Finally, when onset of fatigue is rapid and recent, the cause is likely to be an infection, a disturbance in fluid balance, or rapidly developing circulatory failure of either peripheral or cardiac origin.

GENERALIZED WEAKNESS AND ASTHENIA   As can be judged from the foregoing remarks, weakness must be distinguished from lassitude and fatigue. The demonstration of reduced muscular power sets the case analysis along rather different lines, for it raises consideration more particularly of diseases of the nervous system or of the musculature.

True neural or myopathic weakness is probably never due to psychologic factors, though the hysteric or malingering patient may claim weakness. Usually this can be detected by the criteria outlined in Chap. 11. In anemia, chronic infection, malignancy, and nutritional depletion (except when polyneuropathy is present), the thin muscles are always stronger during tests of peak contraction than one would expect, though of course strength falls short of that of a healthy individual (see Chap. 378 for description of tests of peak power and endurance of muscles).

The proper ascertainment of muscular weakness depends on two lines of inquiry: (1) a history of reduced efficiency; and (2) demonstrable failure in ability to contract the muscles forcefully one or more times. If one proceeds to test each of the major groups of muscles from head to foot, comparing the patient's performance with one's idea of normalcy for man or woman, one may ascertain whether all or certain groups fall below standard. Quantitative and qualitative changes (myasthenia, inverse myasthenia, myotonia, paramyotonia, pathologic cramping) may also be detected by the methods outlined in Chap. 378. The topography of weakness and associated neurologic findings permit distinction between the various types of spinal, peripheral nerve, and myopathic pareses. Rare diseases, difficult to diagnose, that cause inexplicable muscle weakness are masked hyperthyroidism, hyperparathyroidism, ossifying hemangiomas with hypophosphatemia, some of the kalemic periodic paralyses, and hyperinsulinism.

REFERENCES

ADAMS RD: *Pathology of Muscle Diseases,* 3d ed. New York, Harper & Row, 1976

MAYER-GROSS W et al: *Clinical Psychiatry,* 3d ed. Baltimore, Williams & Wilkins, 1969

WALTON JN (ed): *Disease of Voluntary Muscle,* 3d ed. London, Churchill, 1975

13
FAINTNESS, SYNCOPE, AND EPISODIC WEAKNESS

RAYMOND D. ADAMS
EUGENE BRAUNWALD

Episodic faintness, lightheadedness or giddiness, and reduced alertness are frequently difficult to distinguish, tending to shade into one another. And the difference between faintness and frank syncope is only quantitative. Types of episodic weakness, such as myasthenia gravis, cataplexy, and familial periodic paralysis, which cause striking reduction of muscular strength but no impairment of consciousness, should be set apart (see Chaps. 381 and 382); epilepsy, which is also associated with episodic unconsciousness, differs from syncope in most other respects and is discussed in Chap. 23.

CARDINAL FEATURES

Syncope comprises a generalized weakness of muscles, with inability to stand upright, and a loss of consciousness. The term *faintness*, in contrast, refers to lack of strength, with sensation of impending loss of consciousness. At the beginning of a syncopal attack the patient is nearly always in the upright position, either sitting or standing [the Stokes-Adams attack (see Chap. 237) is exceptional in this respect]. Usually an individual is warned of the impending faint by a sense of "feeling bad." The patient is assailed by giddiness, the floor seems to move, and surrounding objects begin to sway. The senses become confused; the patient yawns or gapes, there are spots before the eyes, vision may dim, and the ears may ring. Nausea and sometimes vomiting accompany these symptoms. There is a striking pallor or ashen grey color of the face, and very often the face and body are bathed in cold perspiration. The deliberate onset may often allow the patient time for protection against injury; a hurtful fall is exceptional. If the patient can lie down promptly, the attack may be averted without complete loss of consciousness.

The depth and duration of unconsciousness vary. Sometimes the patient is not completely oblivious of the surroundings, or there may be profound coma with complete lack of awareness and of capacity to respond. The patient may remain in this state for seconds to minutes or even as long as half an hour. Usually the patient lies motionless with skeletal muscles relaxed, but a few clonic jerks of the limbs and face may occur shortly after the beginning of the unconsciousness. Generalized tonic-clonic convulsions are never a part of syncope. Sphincter control is usually maintained. The pulse is feeble or cannot be felt; the blood pressure may be low and breathing almost imperceptible. Once the patient is in a horizontal position, perhaps from having fallen, gravitation no longer hinders the flow of blood to the brain. The strength of the pulse then improves, color begins to return to the face, breathing becomes quicker and deeper, and consciousness is regained. There is from this moment onward a correct perception of the environment. The patient is, nevertheless, keenly aware of physical weakness, and rising too soon may precipitate another faint. Headache and drowsiness, which, with mental confusion, are the usual sequelae of a convulsion, do not follow a syncopal attack.

ETIOLOGY

The list of causes in Table 13-1 is based on established or assumed physiologic mechanisms. The commoner types of faint are reducible to a few simple mechanisms. Syncope results essentially from a sudden impairment of brain metabolism usually brought about by a hypotensive reduction of cerebral blood flow.

Nature has provided humans with several mechanisms by which circulation adjusts to the upright posture. Approximately three-fourths of the systemic blood volume is contained in the venous bed, and any interference with venous return may lead to a reduction in cardiac output. Cerebral blood flow may still be maintained, as long as systemic arterial vasoconstriction occurs; but when this adjustment fails, serious hypotension with resultant cerebral underperfusion to less than half of normal results in syncope. Normally, the pooling of blood in the lower parts of the body is prevented by (1) pressor reflexes which induce constriction of peripheral arterioles and venules; (2) reflex acceleration of the heart by means of aortic and carotid reflexes; and (3) improvement of venous return to the heart by activity of the muscles of the limbs and by increased rate of respiration. Placing a normal person on a tilt table to relax the muscles and tilting upright slightly diminishes cardiac output, and allows the blood to accumulate in the legs to a

TABLE 13-1
Causes of recurrent weakness, faintness, and disturbances of consciousness

I Circulatory (deficient quantity of blood to the brain)
  A Inadequate vasoconstrictor mechanisms
    1 Vasovagal (vasodepressor)
    2 Postural hypotension
    3 Primary autonomic insufficiency
    4 Sympathectomy (pharmacologic or surgical)
    5 Diseases of central and peripheral nervous systems, including autonomic nerves (Chap. 377)
    6 Carotid sinus syncope (see also Bradyarrhythmias, below)
  B Hypovolemia
  C Mechanical reduction of venous return
    1 Valsalva maneuver
    2 Cough
    3 Micturition
    4 Atrial myxoma, ball valve thrombus
  D Reduced cardiac output
    1 Obstruction to left ventricular outflow: aortic stenosis, hypertrophic subaortic stenosis
    2 Obstruction to pulmonary flow: pulmonic stenosis, primary pulmonary hypertension, pulmonary embolism
    3 Myocardial: massive myocardial infarction with pump failure
    4 Pericardial: cardiac tamponade
  E Arrhythmias (Chap. 237)
    1 Bradyarrhythmias
      a Atrioventricular (AV) block (11° and 111°), with Stokes-Adams attacks
      b Ventricular asystole
      c Sinus bradycardia, sinoatrial block, sinus arrest
      d Carotid sinus syncope (see also Inadequate Vasoconstrictor Mechanisms, above)
      e Glossopharyngeal neuralgia (and other painful states)
    2 Tachyarrhythmias
      a Episodic ventricular fibrillation with or without associated bradyarrhythmias
      b Ventricular tachycardia
      c Supraventricular tachycardia without AV block
II Other causes of weakness and episodic disturbances of consciousness
  A Altered state of blood to the brain
    1 Hypoxia
    2 Anemia
    3 Diminished carbon dioxide due to hyperventilation (faintness common, syncope seldom occurs)
    4 Hypoglycemia (episodic weakness common, faintness occasional, syncope rare)
  B Cerebral
    1 Cerebrovascular disturbances (cerebral ischemic attacks, see Chap. 365)
      a Extracranial vascular insufficiency (basilar-vertebral, carotid)
      b Diffuse spasm of cerebral arterioles (hypertensive encephalopathy)
    2 Emotional disturbances, anxiety attacks, and hysterical seizures (see Chaps. 11 and 25)

slight degree. This may then be followed by a slight transitory fall in systolic arterial pressure and, in patients with defective vasomotor reflexes, may be a means of reproducing faints.

TYPES OF SYNCOPE

VASOVAGAL (VASODEPRESSOR) SYNCOPE This is the common faint that may be experienced by normal persons; it is frequently recurrent and tends to take place during emotional stress (especially in a warm, crowded room), after an injurious, shocking accident, and during pain. Mild blood loss, poor physical condition, prolonged bed rest, anemia, fever, organic heart disease, and fasting are other factors which increase the possibility of fainting in susceptible individuals. A short premonitory phase is characterized by nausea, perspiration, yawning, epigastric distress, hyperpnea, tachypnea, weakness, confusion, tachycardia, and pupillary dilatation. Physiologically, there is first a marked fall in arterial pressure and systemic vascular resistance which is most notable in the skeletal muscular beds. Cardiac output may be within normal limits, but it fails to exhibit the expected increase which normally occurs with hypotension. It declines when vagal activity leads to marked bradycardia, replacing tachycardia, resulting in further lowering of arterial pressure and reduction of cerebral perfusion. Assumption of the supine posture with elevation of the legs and removal of the offending stimulus will rapidly restore consciousness.

POSTURAL HYPOTENSION WITH SYNCOPE This type of syncope affects persons who have a chronic defect in or variable instability of vasomotor reflexes. Though the character of the syncopal attack differs little from that of the vasovagal or vasodepressor type, the effect of posture is its cardinal feature; sudden arising from a recumbent position or standing still are the circumstances under which it is most likely to happen.

Postural syncope tends to occur under the following conditions: (1) in otherwise normal persons who for some unknown reason have defective postural reflexes (this may be familial); (2) rarely, as part of a syndrome named *primary autonomic insufficiency,* which includes chronic orthostatic hypotension either in pure form or in association with symptoms of peripheral preganglionic autonomic and cerebellar or extrapyramidal disorder; (3) after physical deconditioning, e.g., after prolonged illness with recumbency, especially in elderly individuals with flabby muscles; (4) after a sympathectomy that has abolished vasopressor reflexes; (5) in diabetic, alcoholic, and other neuropathies, tabes dorsalis, syringomyelia, subacute combined sclerosis, and diseases of the nervous system which cause muscular atrophy and paralysis of vasopressor reflexes; (6) in patients receiving antihypertensive and vasodilator drugs as well as those who may be hypovolemic because of diuretics, excessive sweating or adrenal insufficiency.

In the otherwise normal individuals who faint if tilted on a table, it has been found that at first the blood pressure diminishes slightly and then stabilizes at a lower level. Shortly thereafter the compensatory reflexes suddenly fail, and the arterial pressure falls precipitously. This reaction also may be observed in some of the conditions listed above. In others, e.g., after pharmacologic sympathectomy, in diseases of the sympathetic nervous system, and in the unusual condition known as chronic orthostatic hypotension, the arterial pressure never stabilizes after tilting but falls steadily to a level at which cerebral circulation cannot be maintained.

ORTHOSTATIC HYPOTENSION Here a critical fall in blood pressure on assumption of upright posture is due to a loss of vasoconstrictor reflexes in resistance and capacitance vessels of the lower extremities. Peripheral (postganglionic) or central (preganglionic) neurons may be defective.

The most common form of neurogenic orthostatic hypotension is that which accompanies diseases of the peripheral nervous system. Diabetic polyneuropathy, beriberi, amyloid polyneuropathy, and the Adie syndrome are examples. Usually the orthostatic hypotension is associated with disturbances in sweating, impotence, and sphincter difficulties. Presumably the lesion involves postganglionic, nonmedullated fibers in peripheral nerves (see Chap. 377).

There are other forms of severe orthostatic hypotension which occur in the absence of all signs of sensory-motor nerve involvement. These are called *primary autonomic insufficiencies* or *dysautonomias*. At least three syndromes have been delineated.

1 *Acute or subacute dysautonomia.* In this disease an otherwise healthy adult or child is afflicted over a period of a few days or weeks with a partial or complete paralysis of the parasympathetic and sympathetic nervous systems. Pupillary reflexes are lost, as are lacrimation, salivation, and sweating; and there is impotence, paresis of bladder and bowel musculature, and orthostatic hypotension. The CSF protein is increased. Sensory and motor nerve fibers are demonstrably intact, but nonmedullated autonomic ones have degenerated. Recovery occurs within a few months, possibly hastened by prednisone therapy. The disease is believed to represent a variant of acute idiopathic polyneuritis, akin to Landry-Guillain-Barré syndrome (Young et al.).

2 *Chronic postganglionic autonomic insufficiency.* This is a disease of middle-aged and elderly individuals who gradually become troubled by chronic orthostatic hypotension, sometimes in conjunction with anyhydrosis, impotence, and sphincter disturbances. Upon standing for 5 to 10 min the blood pressure decreases at least 35 torr and the pulse pressure narrows, both without increase in pulse rate, pallor, or nausea. Men are more often affected than women. The condition is relatively benign and seemingly irreversible.

3 *Chronic preganglionic autonomic insufficiency.* In this condition orthostatic hypotension with variable anyhydrosis, impotence, and sphincter disturbances is combined with any one of three or more disorders of the central nervous system. These include (*a*) tremor, extrapyramidal rigidity, and akinesia (Shy-Drager syndrome); (*b*) progressive cerebellar degeneration, some instances of which are familial; and (*c*) a more variable extrapyramidal and cerebellar disorder (strionigral degeneration). These syndromes lead to disability and often death within a few years.

The differentiation of the chronic peripheral postganglionic and central preganglionic insufficiency is based on pathologic and pharmacologic evidence. In the postganglionic type, neurons of the sympathetic ganglia degenerate, whereas in the central type, the lateral horn cells of the spinal cord degenerate. In the postganglionic peripheral type, the resting levels of norepinephrine are subnormal because of failure of release from postganglionic endings, and there is hypersensitivity to injected norepinephrine. In the central type, the resting levels of norepinephrine are normal. On standing, unlike the normal individual, there is little if any rise in norepinephrine levels in either type. And in both types, the levels of plasma dopamine β-hydroxylase (the enzyme that converts dopamine to norepinephrine) are subnormal (Ziegler et al.).

This distinction of types has therapeutic significance. In the peripheral postganglionic type, the most effective treatment of the orthostatic hypotension is a 9α-fluorohydrocortisone (oral dose 0.5 to 2.0 mg per day) and salt loading to increase blood volume, supplemented by mechanical devices to prevent pooling of blood in the legs and lower trunk (g suit). For the central preganglionic type, there has been greater success with use of a sympathomimetic amine such as tyramine (which releases norepinephrine from intact postganglionic endings) supplemented by a monoamine oxidase inhibitor (to prevent destruction of the amine), and possibly propranolol (Inderal).

Micturition syncope, a condition usually seen in the elderly during or after urination, particularly after arising from the recumbent position, is probably a special type of postural syncope. It has been suggested that release of intravesicular pressure causes sudden vasodilatation, augmented by standing and that vagally medicated bradycardia is a contributory factor (Johnson and Spaulding).

SYNCOPE OF CARDIAC ORIGIN (CARDIAC SYNCOPE) Cardiac syncope results from a sudden reduction in cardiac output, caused most commonly by a cardiac arrhythmia. In normal individuals slow ventricular rates, but above 35 to 40 beats per minute, and fast ones not exceeding 180 beats per minute do not reduce cerebral blood flow, especially if the person is in the supine position, but changes in pulse rate outside these limits may impair cerebral circulation and functions. The upright posture, cerebrovascular disease, anemia, and coronary, myocardial, or valvular disease all reduce the tolerance to alterations in rate.

Complete atrioventricular block is the commonest arrhythmia that leads to fainting, and syncopal episodes associated with this arrhythmia are known as the Stocks-Adams-Morgagni syndrome. The etiology of disturbances in atrioventricular conduction is considered elsewhere (Chap. 237), but in patients with these attacks the block may be persistent or intermittent; it is often preceded or followed by disturbed conduction in one or two of the three fascicles through which the ventricles are normally activated, by second degree atrioventricular block (Mobitz type II), or bifascicular or trifascicular block. When the block is complete and the pacemaker below the block fails to function, syncope occurs. A brief bout of ventricular tachycardia or fibrillation may also be responsible for the syncopal episode. Recurrent syncope due to ventricular fibrillation, characterized by a prolonged QT interval (sometimes associated with congenital deafness), has been reported; this condition may be familial or sporadic.

Stokes-Adams attacks occur usually without more than a momentary sense of weakness, the patient suddenly losing consciousness. After cardiac standstill of more than several seconds, the patient turns pale, falls unconscious, and, as in other types of fainting, may exhibit a few clonic jerks. With longer periods of asystole, the ashen gray pallor gives way to cyanosis, stertorous breathing, fixed pupils, incontinence, and bilateral Babinski signs. Prolonged confusion and neurologic signs due to cerebral ischemia may occur in some patients, and permanent impairment of mental function may also occur, although focal neurologic signs are rare. Cardiac faints of this type may recur several times a day. Occasionally the heart block is transitory, and the electrocardiogram taken later may not show any arrhythmia.

Less commonly, a decreased rate of discharge of the sinoatrial node leads to syncope. Recurrent attacks of tachyarrhythmias—including atrial flutter and paroxysmal atrial and ventricular tachycardia with normal AV conduction—may also suddenly reduce cardiac output to a degree sufficient to cause syncope.

In another form of cardiac syncope the heart block is reflexive and is due to irritation of the vagus nerves. Examples of this phenomenon have been observed in patients with esophageal diverticula, mediastinal tumors, gallbladder disease, carotid sinus disease, glossopharyngeal neuralgia, and pleural and pulmonary irritation. However, in these conditions reflex bradycardia is more commonly of the sinoatrial than the atrioventricular type.

Cardiac syncope may also result from *acute massive myocardial infarction,* particularly when associated with cardiogenic shock. *Aortic stenosis* often sets the stage for exertional syncope, most commonly by limiting cardiac output in the face of peripheral vasodilatation, but sometimes during exertion, with resultant myocardial and cerebral ischemia and occasionally arrhythmias. *Idiopathic hypertrophic subaortic stenosis* may also lead to exertional syncope, because of intensified obstruction and/or ventricular arrhythmias (Chap. 237). In *primary pulmonary hypertension* a relatively fixed cardiac output and bouts of acute right ventricular failure may be associated with syncope (Chap. 265). However, vagal reflexes may be involved in this condition as well as in the syncope that occurs with *pulmonary embolism.* Ball valve thrombus in the left atrium, left atrial myxoma, or thrombosis or malfunction of a prosthetic valve may produce sudden mechanical obstruction of the circulation and syncope. *Tetralogy of Fallot* is the congenital cardiac malformation most commonly responsible for syncope. In this condition systemic vasodilatation, perhaps associated with infundibular spasm, greatly increases the right-to-left shunt and produces arterial hypoxia, which leads to syncope (Chap. 240).

CAROTID SINUS SYNCOPE The carotid sinus is normally sensitive to stretch and gives rise to sensory impulses carried via the nerve of Hering, a branch of the glossopharyngeal nerve, to the medulla oblongata. Massage of one or both of the carotid sinuses, particularly in elderly persons, causes (1) a reflex cardiac slowing (sinus bradycardia, sinus arrest, or even atrioventricular block), the so-called vagal type of response, (2) a fall of arterial pressure without cardiac slowing, the so-called "depressor" type of response, and (3) an interference with the circulation of the ipsilateral cerebral hemisphere, the so-called "central" type. Two or three types of carotid sinus response may coexist.

Syncope due to carotid sinus sensitivity may be initiated by turning of the head to one side, by a tight collar, or, as in a few reported cases, by shaving over the region of the sinus. But the absence of such stimuli is of no aid in diagnosis, since spontaneous attacks may occur. The attack nearly always begins when the patient is in an upright position, usually when standing. The period of unconsciousness seldom lasts longer than a few minutes. The sensorium is immediately clear when consciousness is regained. The majority of the reported cases have been in men. In a patient displaying faintness on compression of one carotid sinus, it is important to distinguish between the benign disorder (hypersensitivity of one carotid sinus) and a much more serious condition—atheromatous narrowing of the opposite carotid or of the basilar artery (see Chap. 365).

Other forms of vasovagal syncope have been described. Exceptionally intense pain of visceral origin may inhibit cardiac action through vagal stimulation, e.g., cardiac standstill during an attack of gallbladder colic, a lesion of the esophagus or mediastinum, bronchoscopy, pleural or peritoneal taps, intense vertigo from labyrinthine or vestibular disease, and needling of body cavities.

VAGAL AND GLOSSOPHARYNGEAL NEURALGIA Occasionally this induces a reflex type of fainting. Again the sequence is always pain, then syncope; in this instance the pain is localized to the base of the tongue, pharynx or larynx, tonsillar area, and ear. It may be triggered by pressure at these sites. Section of the appropriate branches of the ninth or tenth cranial nerve relieves the condition. The cardiovascular effects are attributable to excitation of the dorsal motor nucleus of the vagus via collateral fibers from the nucleus of the tractus solitarius.

TUSSIVE SYNCOPE (LARYNGEAL VERTIGO) This is a rare condition that results from a paroxysm of coughing, usually in men with chronic bronchitis. After hard coughing the patient suddenly becomes weak and loses consciousness momentarily. The intrathoracic pressure becomes elevated and interferes with the venous return to the heart, as does the Valsalva maneuver (exhaling against a closed glottis). Episodes of faintness and lightheadedness are not infrequent in pertussis and chronic laryngitis.

SYNCOPE ASSOCIATED WITH CEREBROVASCULAR DISEASE This is usually caused by partial or complete occlusion of the large arteries in the neck. Physical activity may then critically reduce blood flow to the upper part of the brainstem, causing abrupt loss of consciousness (see Chap. 365).

PATHOPHYSIOLOGY OF SYNCOPE

In the final analysis the loss of consciousness in these different types of syncope is caused by a change in the nervous elements in those parts of the brain which subserve consciousness. Syncope resembles epilepsy in this respect; yet there is an important difference. In epilepsy, whether major or minor, the arrest in mental function is almost instantaneous, and, as revealed by the electroencephalogram, it is accompanied by a paroxysm of activity in certain groups of cerebral neurons. Syncope, on the other hand, is not so sudden. The difference relates to the essential pathophysiology—a sudden spread of an electric discharge in epilepsy, and the more gradual failure of the cerebral circulation in syncope.

During syncopal attacks, there are demonstrable reductions in cerebral blood flow, cerebral oxygen utilization, and cerebral vascular resistance. The electroencephalogram reveals high-voltage slow waves, two to five per second, coincident with the loss of consciousness. If the ischemia lasts only a few minutes, there are no lasting effects on the brain. If it persists for a longer time, it may result in necrosis of the border zones between the major cerebral and cerebellar arteries.

DIFFERENTIAL DIAGNOSIS OF CONDITIONS INVOLVING EPISODIC WEAKNESS AND FAINTNESS BUT NOT SYNCOPE

ANXIETY ATTACKS AND THE HYPERVENTILATION SYNDROME These are discussed in detail in Chaps. 11 and 25. The giddiness of anxiety is frequently interpreted as a feeling of faintness without actual loss of consciousness. Such symptoms are not accompanied by facial pallor and are not relieved by recumbency. The diagnosis is made on the basis of the associated symptoms, and part of the attack can be reproduced by hyperventilation. Two of the mechanisms known to be involved in the attacks are reduction in carbon dioxide as the result of hyperventilation and the release of epinephrine. Hyperventilation results in hypocapnia, alkalosis, increased cerebrovascular resistance, and decreased cerebral blood flow.

HYPOGLYCEMIA When severe, hypoglycemia is usually traceable to a serious disease, such as a tumor of the islets of Langerhans or advanced adrenal, pituitary, or hepatic disease, or to excessive administration of insulin. The clinical picture is one of confusion or even a loss of consciousness. When mild, as is usually the case, hypoglycemia is the reactive type (Chap. 339), occurring 2 to 5 h after eating, and is not usually associated with a disturbance of consciousness. The diagnosis depends on the history, the documentation of reduced blood sugar during an attack, and the reproduction by an injection of insulin of a symptom complex exactly similar to that occurring in the spontaneous attacks.

ACUTE HEMORRHAGE Acute blood loss, usually within the gastrointestinal tract, is an occasional cause of syncope. In the absence of pain and hematemesis the cause of the weakness, faintness, or even unconsciousness may remain obscure until the passage of a black stool.

CEREBRAL ISCHEMIC ATTACKS These occur in some patients with arteriosclerotic narrowings or occlusion of the major arteries of the brain. The main symptoms vary from patient to patient and include dim vision, hemiparesis, numbness of one side of the body, dizziness, and thick speech, and to these may be added an impairment of consciousness. In any one patient all attacks are of identical type and indicate a temporary deficit of the function in a certain region of the brain due to inadequate circulation.

HYSTERICAL FAINTING Hysterical fainting is rather frequent and usually occurs under dramatic circumstances (Chap. 11). The attack is unattended by any outward display of anxiety. The evident lack of change in pulse and blood pressure or color of the skin and mucous membranes distinguishes it from the vasodepressor faint. The diagnosis is based on the bizarre nature of the attack in a person who exhibits the general personality and behavioral characteristics of hysteria.

DIFFERENTIAL DIAGNOSIS OF SEIZURE AND SYNCOPE

Most typical varieties of syncope must be distinguished from other disturbances of cerebral function, the most frequent of which is akinetic or some other form of epilepsy (see Chap. 23). The epileptic attack may occur day or night, regardless of the position of the patient; syncope rarely appears when the patient is recumbent, the only common exception being the Stokes-Adams attack. The patient's color does not usually change in epilepsy; pallor is an early and invariable finding in all types of syncope, except chronic orthostatic hypotension and hysteria, and it precedes unconsciousness. Epilepsy is more sudden in onset, and if an aura is present, it rarely lasts longer than a few seconds before consciousness is abolished. The onset of syncope is usually more deliberate and without aura. Injury from falling is frequent in epilepsy and rare in syncope, for the reason that only in epilepsy are protective reflexes instantaneously abolished. Tonic-convulsive movements with upturning eyes are a feature of epilepsy and not syncope. The period of unconsciousness tends to be longer in epilepsy than in syncope. Urinary incontinence is frequent in epilepsy and rare in syncope, but since it may be observed occasionally in syncope, it cannot be used as a means of excluding epilepsy. The return of consciousness is prompt in syncope, slow in epilepsy. Mental confusion, headache, and drowsiness are common sequelae in epilepsy; physical weakness with clear sensorium characterizes the postsyncopal state. Repeated spells of unconsciousness in a young person at a rate of several per day or month are more suggestive of epilepsy than of syncope. No one of these points will absolutely differentiate epilepsy from syncope, but taken as a group and supplemented by electroencephalograms, they provide a means of distinguishing the two conditions.

DIFFERENT TYPES OF SYNCOPE Differentiation of the several conditions that diminish cerebral blood flow is discussed in greater detail in Chap. 30.

When faintness is related to reduced cerebral blood flow

resulting directly from a disorder of cardiac function, there is likely to be a combination of pallor and cyanosis. When, on the other hand, the peripheral circulation is at fault, pallor is usually striking but is not accompanied by cyanosis or respiratory disturbances. When the primary disturbance lies in the cerebral circulation, the face is likely to be florid and the breathing slow and stertorous. During the attack a heart rate faster than 150 beats per minute indicates an ectopic cardiac rhythm, while a striking bradycardia (rate of less than 40 beats per minute) suggests complete heart block. In a patient with faintness or syncope attended by bradycardia, one has to distinguish between the neurogenic reflex and the cardiogenic (Stokes-Adams) types. The electrocardiogram is decisive, but even without it, the Stokes-Adams seizures can be recognized clinically by their longer duration, by the greater constancy of the slow heart rate, by the presence of audible sounds synchronous with atrial contraction, by atrial contraction (A) waves in the jugular venous pulse, and by marked variation in intensity of the first sound, despite the regular rhythm (Chap. 237).

It is of primary importance to know the circumstances and the precipitating and alleviating factors in a given episode of weakness or fainting.

TYPE OF ONSET When the attack begins over the period of a few seconds, carotid sinus syncope, postural hypotension, sudden atrioventricular block, ventricular standstill, or fibrillation is likely. When the symptoms develop gradually during a period of several minutes, hyperventilation or hypoglycemia should be considered. Onset of syncope during or immediately after exertion suggests aortic stenosis or idiopathic hypertrophic subaortic stenosis and, in elderly subjects, postural hypotension. Exertional syncope is seen occasionally in persons with aortic insufficiency and with severe occlusive disease of cerebral arteries. In patients with ventricular standstill or ventricular fibrillation, loss of consciousness occurs several seconds later, followed rapidly by cessation of electroencephalographic activity and then often by brief clonic contractions.

POSITION AT ONSET OF ATTACK Epilepsy and syncopal attacks due to hypoglycemia, hyperventilation, or heart block are likely to be independent of posture. Faintness associated with a decline in blood pressure (including carotid sinus attacks) and with ectopic tachycardia usually occurs only in the sitting or standing position, whereas faintness resulting from orthostatic hypotension is apt to set in shortly after change from the recumbent to the standing position.

ASSOCIATED SYMPTOMS Palpitation is likely to be present when the attack is due to anxiety or hyperventilation, to ectopic tachycardia, or to hypoglycemia. Numbness and tingling in the hands and face are frequent accompaniments of hyperventilation. Genuine convulsions during the attack, although characteristic of epilepsy, may occasionally occur with heart block, ventricular standstill, or fibrillation.

DURATION OF ATTACK When the duration is very brief, i.e., a few seconds to a few minutes, carotid sinus syncope or one of the several forms of postural hypotension is most likely. A duration of more than a few minutes but less than an hour suggests hypoglycemia or hyperventilation.

SPECIAL METHODS OF EXAMINATION

In many patients who complain of recurrent weakness or syncope but do not have a spontaneous attack while under observation of the physician, an attempt to reproduce attacks is of great assistance in diagnosis.

When hyperventilation is accompanied by faintness, the pattern of symptoms can be reproduced readily by having the subject breathe rapidly and deeply for 2 to 3 min. This test is often of therapeutic value also, because the underlying anxiety tends to be lessened when the patient learns that the symptoms can be produced and alleviated at will simply by controlling breathing.

Among other conditions in which the diagnosis is commonly clarified by reproducing the attacks are carotid sinus hypersensitivity (massage of one or the other carotid sinus), orthostatic hypotension and orthostatic tachycardia (observations of pulse rate, blood pressure, and symptoms in the recumbent and standing positions), and tussive syncope (by inducing the Valsalva maneuver). In all these instances the crucial point is not whether symptoms are produced (the procedures mentioned frequently induce symptoms in healthy persons) but whether the exact pattern of symptoms that occurs in the spontaneous attacks is reproduced in all the artificial ones. Careful, continuous monitoring of the electrocardiogram in the hospital or the recording of the electrocardiogram over 1 or 2 days using a portable lightweight tape recorder in an ambulatory patient may be extremely useful in identifying an arrhythmia responsible for the syncopal episode. Monitoring is most helpful if it shows that the syncopal episode is characterized by a bout of cardiac standstill, extreme bradycardia, or tachyarrhythmia.

The electroencephalogram may be helpful in differentiating syncope from epilepsy. In the interval between epileptic seizures it may show some degree of abnormality in 40 to 80 percent of cases. In the interval between syncopal attacks it should be normal.

TREATMENT

Fainting in most instances is relatively benign. In dealing with patients who have fainted, the physician should think first of those causes of fainting that consitute a therapeutic emergency. Among them are massive internal hemorrhage and myocardial infarction, which may be painless, and cardiac arrhythmias. In elderly persons a sudden faint, without obvious cause, should arouse the suspicion of complete heart block, even though all findings are negative when they are seen by a physician.

Patients seen during the preliminary stages of fainting or after they have lost consciousness should be placed in a position which permits maximal cerebral blood flow, i.e., with head lowered between the knees, if sitting, or in the supine position. All tight clothing and other constrictions should be loosened and the head turned so that the tongue does not fall back into the throat, blocking the airway. Peripheral irritation, such as sprinkling or dashing cold water on the face and neck or the application of cold moist towels, is helpful. If the temperature is subnormal, the body should be covered with a warm blanket. If available, aromatic spirit of ammonia may be given cautiously by inhalation. Since emesis is frequent, one should be prepared for a possible aspiration. Nothing should be given by mouth until the patient has regained consciousness. Then one-half a teaspoon of aromatic spirit of ammonia in one-half a glass of cold water, or a sip of brandy or whiskey, may be given. Patients should not be permitted to rise until the sense of physical weakness has passed, and they should be watched carefully for a few minutes after rising.

The *prevention* of fainting depends on the mechanisms involved. In the usual vasovagal faint of adolescents, which tends to occur in periods of emotional excitement, fatigue, hunger, etc., it is enough to advise the patient to avoid such circumstances. In postural hypotension, patients should be cautioned against arising suddenly from bed. Instead, they should first exercise their legs for a few seconds, then sit on the edge of the bed and make sure they are not lightheaded or dizzy before starting to walk. Sleeping with the headposts of the bed elevated on wooden blocks 8 to 12 in high and wearing snug elastic abdominal binder and elastic stockings are often helpful. Drugs of the ephedrine group may be useful if they do not cause insomnia. If there are no contraindications, a high intake of sodium chloride, which expands the extracellular fluid volume, may be beneficial.

In the syndrome of chronic orthostatic hypotension, special corticosteroid preparations (Florinef acetate tables, 1 to 2 mg per day in divided doses) have given relief in some cases. Binding of the legs (g suit) and sleeping with head and shoulders elevated are helpful.

The treatment of carotid sinus syncope involves first of all instructing the patient in measures that minimize the hazards of a fall (see below). Loose collars should be worn, and the patient should learn to turn the whole body, rather than the head alone, when looking to one side. Atropine or the ephedrine group of drugs should be used, respectively, in patients with pronounced bradycardia or hypotension during attacks. If atropine is not successful, a demand pacemaker should be inserted into the right ventricle. Radiation or surgical denervation of the carotid sinus has apparently yielded favorable results in some patients, but it is rarely necessary. Once it has been concluded that the attacks are due to a narrowing of major cerebral arteries, some of the surgical measures discussed in Chap. 365 must be considered.

The treatment of the various cardiac arrhythmias which may induce syncope is discussed in Chap. 237. The treatment of hypoglycemia will be found in Chap. 339 and of the hyperventilation syndrome and hysterical fainting in Chaps. 11 and 12, respectively.

The chief hazard of a faint in most elderly persons is not the underlying disease but rather fracture or other trauma due to the fall. Therefore, patients subject to recurrent syncope should cover the bathroom floor and bathtub with rubber mats and should have as much of their home carpeted as is feasible. Especially important is the floor space between the bed and the bathroom, because faints are common in elderly persons when walking from bed to toilet. Outdoor walking should be on soft ground rather than hard surfaces, and the patient should avoid standing still, which is more likely than walking to induce an attack.

REFERENCES

HICKLER R: Fainting, in *Signs and Symptoms,* 6th ed, RS Blacklow (ed). Philadelphia, Lippincott, 1977, chap 33

JOHNSON RH, SPAULDING JMK: *Disorders of the Autonomic Nervous System.* Philadelphia, Davis, 1974

LEE JE et al: Episodic unconsciousness, in *Diagnostic Approaches to Presenting Syndromes,* JA Barondess (ed). Baltimore, Williams & Wilkins, 1971, pp 133–167

WEISSLER AM, WARREN JV: Syncope and shock, in *The Heart,* 4th ed, JW Hurst (ed). New York, McGraw-Hill, 1978, p 705

WRIGHT KE JR., MCINTOSH MD: Syncope: Review of pathophysiological mechanisms. Prog Cardiovasc Dis 13:580, 1971

YOUNG RR et al: Pure pandysautonomia with recovery. Trans Am Neurol Assoc 94:355, 1969

ZIEGLER MG et al: The sympathetic nervous system defect in primary orthostatic hypotension. New Engl J Med 296:293, 1977

DIZZINESS AND VERTIGO

MAURICE VICTOR
RAYMOND D. ADAMS

Dizziness and other sensations of unbalance occur in a wide variety of diseases. In many instances the clue to an important medical disorder is afforded by the correct analysis of the complaint.

The term *dizziness* covers a number of different sensory experiences—true vertigo, which refers to a feeling of whirling or rotation, as well as nonrotatory swaying, weakness, faintness, and lightheadedness. Blurring of vision, feelings of unreality, syncope, and even petit mal may be incorrectly called dizzy spells; hence a close questioning as to how the patient is using the term becomes a necessary first step in clinical study. A distinction is sometimes drawn between subjective vertigo, meaning a sense of turning one's body, and objective vertigo, an illusion of movement of objects in the environment, but its validity is doubtful.

In this chapter the term *vertigo* is used to refer to all subjective and objective illusions of rotation. *Giddiness* refers to a swaying type of dizziness. *Equilibrium,* the state of equipoise whereby the posture of the body is maintained against the forces of gravity, is deranged in vertigo but is also affected by other disorders as well, e.g., loss of joint or muscle sense (sensory ataxia), cerebellar disease (cerebellar ataxia), and motor abnormalities (spasticity and rigidity, myotonia, and the pseudomyotonia of hypothyroidism).

ANATOMIC, PHYSIOLOGIC, AND PSYCHOLOGIC CONSIDERATIONS Several mechanisms maintain balanced posture and awareness of the body's positions in relation to its surroundings. The most important of these are:

1 Impulses from the retinas of the eyes which are coordinated by ocular motor mechanisms to supply information about the position and movement of the body and its surroundings.
2 Impulses from the labyrinths of the inner ears—specialized spatial proprioceptors whose primary function is to register changes in the direction of motion (either acceleration or deceleration) and position of the body. [*Note:* The semicircular canals respond to movement and angular momentum, whereas the otoliths (sense organs of the utricle and saccule) are mainly concerned with orienting the organism with reference to gravitational force.]
3 Impulses from the proprioceptors of joints and muscles—essential to all reflex, postural, and volitional movements. Those of the neck are of special importance in relating the position of the head to that of the rest of the body.

The cerebellum and certain ganglionic centers in the brainstem (particularly the vestibular nuclei, oculomotor nuclei, and red nuclei) and in the basal ganglia are the important coordinators of these sensory data and provide for postural adjustment, upright stance, and locomotion.

Important psychophysiologic mechanisms are also involved in the maintenance of equilibrium and the proper relationship of our bodies to the external world. Early in life we come to coordinate the parts of our body in relation to one another and to perceive that portion of space occupied by our bodies. The construct of these integrated sensory data has been designated by Russell Brain as the *body schema.* The space around our body is said to be represented by another set of data, the *environmental schema.* These two schemata are dynamic and interdependent, since both are simultaneously changed in every activity. For example, we learn to see objects as being stationary when we are moving. Thus, the motion of ourselves and of objects in space is always relative. At times, when sensory information is incomplete, we mistake movement of our surroundings for those of our own body, as in the illusion caused by motion of a neighboring train. A disturbance in the awareness of one's own body schema is postulated by some psychiatrists as the basis of neurotic disorientation and psychotic feelings of unreality.

CLINICAL CHARACTERISTICS OF VERTIGO AND GIDDINESS
The clinical recognition of *vertigo* proves to be relatively easy when the patient states that objects in the environment turned or moved in one direction or that the head and body whirled. Often, however, the patient is not so explicit. The feeling may be described as oscillation, or of veering, of being pulled to one side or to the ground, as though drawn by a magnet (impulsion). Again, the floor or walls may seem to tilt, sink, or rise up. The feeling of impulsion is particularly characteristic of vertigo.

All but the mildest forms of vertigo are accompanied by perspiration, pallor, nausea, and vomiting. The nystagmus which is invariably present causes objects in the field of vision to move rhythmically in one direction. As a rule the patient can walk only with difficulty or not at all, should the vertigo be intense. A sudden attack may even catapult the patient to the ground, and only when down is vertigo experienced. Forced to lie down the patient realizes that one position, usually on one side with eyes closed, reduces the vertigo and nausea, and that the slightest motion of the head aggravates them. One form of vertigo, the benign positional vertigo of Bárány, occurs only for a few seconds after lying down and sitting up. If the vertigo is less severe, the patient can walk unsteadily but may veer to one side. The ataxia of gait with vertigo (vertiginous ataxia) is recognized always as being a "dizziness in the head," not a trouble in the control of the legs and trunk. It is noteworthy that in these circumstances the coordination of the individual movements of the limbs is not impaired—a point of difference from cerebellar disease. There may be headache, especially in the region of the offending ear. Loss of consciousness as part of a vertiginous attack nearly always signifies another type of disorder (seizure or faint).

Giddiness and other types of pseudovertigo are usually described as feelings of swaying, lightheadedness, a swimming sensation, and, more rarely, as though walking on air, "queer in the head," uncertain, about to fall or "pass out." These sensory experiences are particularly common in psychiatric illnesses featured by anxiety attacks. They may be reproduced by hyperventilation, and then it is appreciated that panic and apprehensiveness, palpitation, breathlessness, trembling, and sweating are concurrent.

Other pseudovertiginous symptoms are less definite. In severe anemic states weakness and languor may be attended by a lightheadedness related to postural change and exertion. In the emphysematous patient physical effort may be associated with weakness and peculiar cephalic sensations, and coughing may lead to giddiness and even fainting (tussive syncope) because of impaired return of venous blood to the heart. The dizziness that so often accompanies hypertension is more difficult to evaluate. Sometimes it is an expression of anxiety, or it may be due to an unstable adjustment of cerebral blood flow. *Postural dizziness* is another example of unstable vasomotor reflexes preventing a constancy of cerebral circulation and is notably frequent in persons recently bedfast, in the weak and ill, and the elderly. Abrupt arising from a recumbent or sitting position is followed immediately by a swaying type of dizziness, dimming of vision, and spots before the eyes which last a few seconds. The patient is forced to stand still and hold onto a nearby object until steady. A syncopal attack may occur at this time (see Chap. 13).

In practice it is not difficult to separate these types of pseudovertigo from true vertigo, for there is none of the feeling of rotation or impulsion so characteristic of the latter. Lacking also are the other ancillary symptoms of true vertigo, namely, nausea, vomiting, tinnitus and deafness, nystagmus, and staggering.

NEUROLOGIC AND OTOLOGIC CAUSES OF VERTIGO Vertigo may constitute the aura of an epileptic seizure, but this event is rare. The lesion is then on the posterolateral aspects of the temporal lobe near the sylvian fissure. A sensation of movement, either of the body away from the side of the lesion or of the environment in the opposite direction, lasts for a few seconds before being submerged in other seizure activity. Vertiginous sensations may rarely serve as a stimulus for *reflex epilepsy* (see Chap. 23), and the test for this form of vertigo provokes the seizure.

Oculomotor disorders are a source of a spatial disorientation simulating dizziness. This is maximal when the patient looks in the direction of action of the paralyzed muscle; it is attributable to the receipt of two conflicting visual images. In fact some normal individuals even experience dizziness for a time when adjusting to bifocal glasses or when looking down from a height.

Whether lesions of the cerebellum can produce vertigo seems to depend on the part of it involved. Large destructive processes in the cerebellar hemispheres and vermis may cause no vertigo whatsoever, unless they extend to central vestibulocerebellar connections. However, Duncan, Parker, and Fisher report definite vertigo in verified lesions of the posterior-inferior part of the hemisphere due to occlusion limited to the cerebellar branch of the inferior cerebellar artery.

Labyrinthine (aural) lesions are the usual causes of paroxysmal vertigo. In the classic variety, that of Ménière's disease, the onset is abrupt, the vertigo is clearly of the rotary type, and it lasts a few minutes to hours. Concomitant tinnitus, fullness in the ear, high-tone deafness with auditory recruitment (see Chaps. 18 and 376), nystagmus, nausea, vomiting, and staggering constitute the full syndrome. The patient preferentially lies with the faulty ear uppermost and is disinclined to look toward the normal side because of exaggeration of the nystagmus and dizziness. The nystagmus is fine, rotatory, and most pronounced when the eyes are turned away from the offending ear. Vertiginous attacks of this type may recur and give rise to mild, chronic states of disequilibrium which may persist for days. Seldom does the vertigo last, however, for central mechanisms compensate for permanent deficits of one labyrinth. Chronic vertigo may be complicated by the giddiness of a secondary anxiety state. *Vestibular neuronitis* is a term that refers to severe vertigo, often of several days' duration, without tinnitus or deafness. Its pathologic basis is uncertain. Episodic vertigo occurs in the syndrome known as *Bárány's benign positional vertigo* and the more malignant positional vertigo of posterior fossa tumors and other lesions, and lasts only a few seconds (Chap. 376).

Vertigo of acoustic nerve origin, the commonest cause of which is an acoustic neuroma, tends usually to be mild and intermittent (lasting weeks or months). Seldom does it come in discrete attacks separated by free intervals. Vertigo has rarely been observed as the initial symptom with eighth nerve tumors, but the usual sequence is deafness of high-frequency

type (without recruitment), followed some time later by a sense of imbalance and impaired caloric responses, then cranial nerve palsies (involving the eighth, fifth, and tenth nerves), ipsilateral ataxia of limbs, and headache, the other common signs of a cerebellopontine angle tumor (see Chap. 367).

A number of ototoxic drugs may result in labyrinthine and auditory symptoms, sometimes permanent (see Chap. 376).

Vertigo of brainstem origin implicates vestibular nuclei and their connections. In these cases auditory function is nearly always spared, since the vestibular and cochlear fibers separate upon entering the medulla and pons. The nystagmus which accompanies such central lesions tends to be coarse, protracted, and variable; it is more marked on lateral gaze to one side than the other. There may also be a nonrotary vertical component. The central localization is evidenced further by the attendant signs of involvement of other structures within the brainstem (cranial nerves, sensory and motor tracts, etc.) Mode of onset, duration, and other features of the clinical picture depend upon the nature of the causative disease, usually vascular (basilar artery, vertebral artery, or labyrinthine artery occlusion), traumatic, neoplastic, or demyelinative.

Electronystagmography is often helpful in the diagnosis of central vertigo. It will reveal vertical nystagmus with eyes closed, types I and II positional nystagmus, perverted nystagmus on caloric stimulation, and ocular deviations with eyes closed.

APPROACH TO THE PATIENT WITH DIZZINESS As already stated, a careful history and physical examination of the dizzy patient usually afford a basis for separating true vertigo from the swaying dizziness of the hyperventilating, anxious patient and from the other types of pseudovertigo (such as partial syncope and feelings of unreality). If the patient is unobservant or imprecise in descriptions, a helpful tactic is to provoke a number of dissimilar sensations by rotating the patient, irrigating the ears with warm or cold water, by asking the patient to stoop for a minute and straighten up, by hyperventilating for 3 min, and by measuring the blood pressure as the patient changes from a recumbent to a standing position and remains upright for 3 to 4 min. Should the patient be unable to distinguish among these several types of induced sensation or to ascertain the similarity of one of the types to his or her own condition, the history is probably too inaccurate for purposes of diagnosis.

When vertigo is mild or difficult for the patient to describe, small items of the history, such as disinclination to walk during an attack, tendency to list to one side, aggravation by riding in a vehicle, preference for one position, are helpful. They distinguish vertigo from giddiness.

In some patients an attack of vertigo is so abrupt and violent that they are virtually flung to the ground, sometimes with a serious injury. These attacks have been called by the quaint term "otolithic crises of Tumarken," but without proof of involvement of the utricle or saccule. The diagnosis is usually substantiated by the presence of vertigo, nausea, and vomiting while on the ground, distinguishing it from a seizure, faint, or cataplexy. Probably it differs from other forms of labyrinthine vertigo only in its severity.

In the differentiation of types of labyrinthine and vestibular nerve disease, inspection of eardrums, x-rays of mastoids, middle ears, and inner ears, and auditory and caloric tests are useful, especially in excluding labyrinthitis. In caloric testing, the patient's head is tilted forward 30° from the horizontal (bringing the horizontal semicircular canal into a vertical plane), which is the position of maximal sensitivity to thermal stimuli. The external auditory meati are irrigated in turn for 40 s with water at 30 and 44°C (7°C below and above body temperature). Cold water induces nystagmus to the opposite side (direction of the fast phase), and warm water to the same side.

The nystagmus begins in 20 s and should persist 90 to 120 s. Comparison of the two ears reveals which one is paretic or hypersensitive. Special rotational chairs and electronystagmography are other more refined means of assessing disordered labyrinthine function. The diagnosis of benign positional vertigo is settled at the bedside by reproducing a brief vertigo and nystagmus (lasting up to a minute) by moving the patient from the sitting position to recumbency with head to one side in one trial and to the other in the second. Going from a recumbent to a sitting position reverses the direction of vertigo and nystagmus. This specific pattern and its reversibility are not observed in the more malignant positional vertigo of posterior fossa tumors and other lesions. The application of some of the maneuvers designed to elicit weakness and syncope (see Chap. 13) will distinguish these forms of pseudovertigo.

The association of vertigo with auditory signs and symptoms always signifies a disease process of end organ or eighth nerve. Labyrinthine and auditory tests and the presence or absence of neurologic signs of structures adjacent to the eighth cranial nerve nuclei are useful in their differentiation.

Pure vertigo as a manifestation of disease of the brainstem is rare, and the rule we have found trustworthy is that unless other symptoms and signs appear within 1 to 2 weeks, one can nearly always postulate an aural origin and exclude vascular disease of the brainstem. This is also true of multiple sclerosis, which may be the explanation of a persistent vertigo in some adolescents or young adults.

REFERENCES

ADAMS RD, VICTOR M: *Principles of Neurology.* New York, McGraw-Hill, 1977

ALTMANN F: Diagnostic significance of vertigo, in *The Vestibular System and Its Diseases,* RJ Wolfson (ed). Philadelphia, University of Pennsylvania Press, 1966, p 353

DIX MR: Modern tests of vestibular function, with special reference to their value in clinical practice. Br Med J 3:317, 1969

DUNCAN GW et al: Acute cerebellar infarction in the PICA territory. Arch Neurol 32:364, 1975

FISHER CM: Vertigo in cerebrovascular disease. Arch Otolaryngol 85:529, 1967

SPECTOR M: *Dizziness and Vertigo.* New York, Grune & Stratton, 1967

15
MOTOR PARALYSIS

RAYMOND D. ADAMS

Impairments of motor function may be subdivided into (1) paralysis due to affection of lower motor neurons, (2) paralysis due to disorder of upper motor (corticospinal and corticobrainstem) neurons, (3) abnormalities of coordination (ataxia) due to lesions in the cerebellum, (4) abnormalities of movement and posture due to disease of the extrapyramidal motor system, and (5) apraxic or nonparalytic disturbances of purposive movement due to involvement of the cerebrum. The first two types of motor disorder and the cerebral disorders of movement are discussed briefly in the following pages; purely muscular weakness and paralysis will be discussed in Chap. 378; cerebellar ataxia and extrapyramidal motor abnormalities are considered in Chap. 16.

DEFINITIONS When applied to voluntary muscles, *paralysis* means loss of contraction due to interruption of one of the motor pathways from the cerebrum to the muscle fiber. Lesser degrees of paralysis are sometimes spoken of as *paresis,* but in everyday medical parlance motor paralysis usually stands for either partial or complete loss of function. The word *plegia* comes from the Greek word meaning stroke; and the word *palsy,* from an old French word, has the same meaning as paralysis. It is preferable to use paresis for slight and paralysis or plegia for severe loss of motor function.

PARALYSIS DUE TO DISEASE OF THE LOWER MOTOR NEURONS Each motor nerve cell, through the extensive arborization of the terminal part of its fiber, comes into contact with 100 to 200 or more muscle fibers; altogether they constitute "the motor unit." All the variations in force, range, and type of movement are determined by differences in the number and size of motor units called into activity and the frequency of their action. Feeble movements recruit few units, stronger ones many more units of increasing size. Histochemical methods show that motor units involved in slow, tonic contractions (type I) have muscle fibers rich in oxidative enzymes and mitochondria, and those involved in fast, phasic contractions (type II), more phosphorylase. When a motor neuron becomes diseased, as in progressive muscular atrophy, it may manifest increased irritability, and all the muscle fibers that it controls may discharge sporadically, in isolation from other units. The result of the contraction of one or several such units is a visible twitch, or *fasciculation,* which can be seen and recorded in the electromyogram as a large diphasic or multiphasic action potential. If the motor neuron is destroyed, all the muscle fibers to which it is attached undergo a profound atrophy, namely, denervation atrophy. For some unknown reason the individual denervated muscle fibers now begin to be hypersensitive and to contract spontaneously, though they can no longer do so in response to a nerve impulse as a part of the motor unit. This isolated activity of individual muscle fibers is called *fibrillation* and is so fine that it cannot be seen through the intact skin and can be recorded only as a repetitive short-duration spike potential in the electromyogram. The motor nerve fibers of each anterior root intermingle with adjacent roots as they join to form plexuses, and although the innervation of the muscles is roughly according to segments of the spinal cord, each large muscle comes to be supplied by two or more roots. In contrast, a single peripheral nerve usually provides the complete motor innervation of a muscle or group of muscles. For this reason the distribution of paralysis due to disease of the anterior horn cells or anterior roots differs from that which follows a lesion of a peripheral nerve.

All motor activity, even the most elementary reflex type, requires the cooperation of several muscles. The analysis of a relatively simple movement, such as clenching the fist, affords some idea of the complexity of the underlying neural arrangements. In this act the primary movement is a contraction of the flexor muscles of the fingers, the flexor digitorum sublimis and profundus, the flexor pollicis longus and brevis, and the abductor pollicis brevis. These muscles act as *agonists,* or *prime movers,* in this act. In order for flexion to be smooth and forceful, the extensor muscles (antagonists) must relax at the same rate at which the flexors contract. The muscles which flex the fingers also flex the wrist; and since it is desired that only the fingers flex, the muscles which extend the wrist must be brought into play to prevent its flexion. The action of the wrist extensors is *synergic,* and these muscles are called synergists in this particular act. Lastly the wrist, elbow, and shoulder must be stabilized by appropriate flexor and extensor muscles, which serve as *fixators.* The coordination of agonists, antagonists, synergists, and fixators involves reciprocal innervation and is managed entirely by segmental spinal reflexes under the guidance of proprioceptive sensory stimuli. Only the agonist movement in a voluntary act is believed to be initiated at a cortical level.

In addition, there are many basic motor activities, such as the maintenance of certain postures and stepping movements, which do not involve reciprocal innervation. For these activities agonists and antagonists contract simultaneously. The alternating movements of spinal stepping represent an even more elaborate type of coordination. Also in the support of the body in an upright posture, when the limb must be as rigid as a pillar, and in shivering the agonists and antagonists must act together. In general, the more delicate the movement, the more precise the coordination between agonist and antagonist muscles.

If all or practically all peripheral motor nerves supplying a muscle are destroyed, all voluntary, postural, and reflex movements are abolished. The muscle becomes soft and yields excessively to passive stretching, a condition known as flaccidity. Muscle tone—the slight resistance that normal relaxed muscle offers to passive movement—is reduced (hypotonia or atonia). The denervated muscles undergo extreme atrophy, usually being reduced to 20 to 30 percent of their original bulk within 3 months. The reaction of the muscle to sudden stretch, as by tapping its tendon, is lost. And, finally, it may be demonstrated that the muscle will no longer respond to electric stimuli of short duration, i.e., faradic stimuli, but still responds to currents of long duration, i.e., to galvanic stimuli. This alteration of electric response is known as *Erb's reaction of degeneration*. If only a part of the motor units in the muscles is affected, partial paralysis will ensue. Quantitative testing by determination of strength-duration curves is a means of showing partial denervation, and electromyographic evidence of fibrillations may also be obtained.

The tonus of muscle and the tendon reflexes are known to depend on the muscle spindles and the afferent fibers to which they give origin and on the small anterior horn cells whose axons terminate on the small muscle fibers within the spindles. These small spinal motor neurons are called *gamma neurons*, in contrast to the large *alpha neurons*. Two different gamma neurons are now recognized, one, connected with nuclear bag spindle muscle fibers for phasic actions; the other, with nuclear chain spindle muscle fibers for tonic actions. A tap on a tendon, by stretching the spindle muscle fibers, activates afferent neurons which transmit impulses to alpha motor neurons. The result is the familiar brief muscle contraction or tendon reflex. The spindle muscle fibers are then relaxed (unloaded), which terminates the reflex. Thus the setting of the spindle fibers and the state of excitability of the gamma neurons (normally inhibited by the corticospinal fibers and other supranuclear neurons) determine the level of activity of the tendon reflexes and the responsiveness of muscle to stretch. Other mechanisms of an inhibitory nature, involving Golgi tendon organs, are brought into play in more powerful stretching of muscle.

Lower motor neuron paralysis is the direct result of physiologic arrest or destruction of anterior horn cells or their axons in anterior roots and nerves. The signs and symptoms vary according to the location of the lesion. Probably the most important question for clinical purposes is whether sensory changes coexist. The combination of flaccid, areflexic paralysis and sensory changes usually indicates involvement of mixed motor and sensory nerves or affection of both anterior and posterior roots. If sensory changes are absent, the lesion must be situated in the gray matter of the spinal cord, in the anterior roots, in a purely motor branch of a peripheral nerve, or in motor axons alone. The distinction between nuclear (spinal) and anterior root (radicular) lesions may at times be impossible to make. Retention of reflexes and spasticity in muscles

weakened by a spinal lesion point to a lesion of the corticospinal tracts and integrity of the segments below the level of the lesion.

PARALYSIS DUE TO DISEASE OF THE CORTICOSPINAL AND CORTICO-BRAINSTEM NEURONS It was formerly believed that the corticospinal tract originated from the large motor cell of Betz in the fifth layer of the precentral convolution. However, there are only about 25,000 to 30,000 Betz cells, whereas the corticospinal tract at the level of the medulla contains approximately 1 million axons. This tract must, therefore, contain many fibers that arise not from the giant Betz cells of the motor cortex (area 4 of Brodmann) but rather from the smaller Betz cells of area 4, the cells of the adjacent precentral cortex (area 6), as well as those of the secondary motor cortex in the superior frontal convolution and postcentral cortex (areas 1, 2, 3, 5, 7). The most critical degeneration studies of van Crevel have shown that when areas 4, 6, 1, 2, 3, 5, and 7 are removed in the cat, if one waits several months, all of the pyramidal fibers will be found to have degenerated. The corticospinal tract is the only long-fiber connection between the cerebrum and the spinal cord. At the level of the internal capsule these corticospinal fibers are intermingled with many others destined to end in the globus pallidus, substantia nigra, red nucleus, and reticular substance and with others ascending from the thalamus. The fibers to the cranial nerve nuclei become separated at about the level of the midbrain and cross the midline to the contralateral cranial nerve nuclei (Fig. 15-1). These fibers form the corticomesencephalic, corticopontine, and corticobulbar tracts, and since they have functions similar to those of the corticospinal tract, they may be included in the pyramidal system of motor neurons. The decussation of the corticospinal tract at the lower end of the medulla is variable in different persons. Most of the crossing fibers come to occupy a position in the posterolateral part of the lateral funiculus; a few cross to form an anterior fasciculus. A small number of fibers, 10 to 20 percent, do not cross but descend ipsilaterally as the uncrossed

FIGURE 15-1
Diagram of the corticospinal and corticobulbar tracts. Lesion at A produces ipsilateral oculomotor palsy and contralateral paralysis involving face, arm, and leg. Lesion at B causes ipsilateral facial paralysis of peripheral type and contralateral paralysis of arm and leg. Lesion at b results in ipsilateral facial weakness of upper motor neuron of central type and contralateral paralysis of arm and leg. (Courtesy of Bergmann and Staehln, Krankheiten des Nervensystems, Berlin, Springer-Verlag, 1939.)

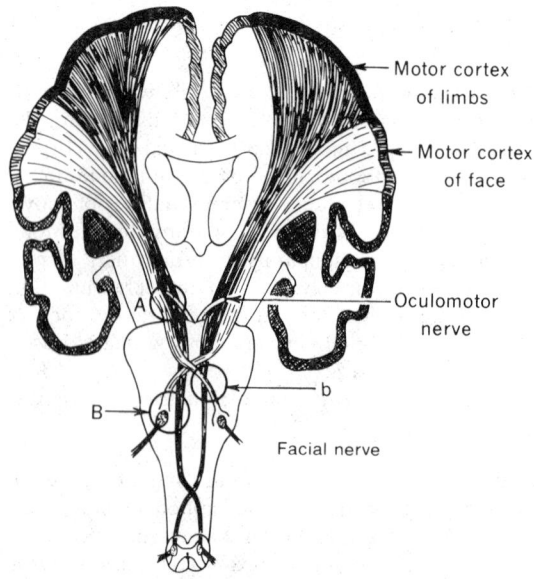

corticospinal tract. Exceptionally, all of them cross; rarely, none. The termination of the corticospinal tract is in relation to nerve cells in the intermediate zone of gray matter, and not more than 10 to 15 percent establish direct synaptic connection with anterior horn cells. These facts, derived from degeneration studies, must of necessity modify current views of the anatomy of the corticospinal tract and suggest new interpretations.

The motor area of the cerebral cortex is difficult to define. It includes that part of the precentral convolution which contains Betz cells (area 4), but, as already mentioned, it probably extends anteriorly into area 6 and the secondary motor area of the superior frontal convolution and posteriorly into the anterior parietal lobe, where it overlaps the sensory areas. Physiologically it is defined as the region of electrically excitable cortex from which isolated movements can be evoked by stimuli of minimal intensity. The muscle groups of the contralateral face, arm, trunk, and leg are represented in the motor cortex, those of the face being at the lower end of the precentral convolution and those of the leg in the paracentral lobule on the medial surface of the cerebral hemisphere. The parts of the body capable of the most delicate movements have, in general, the largest cortical representation. Very strong stimuli elicit movements from a wide area of premotor frontal and parietal cortex, and the same movements may be obtained from several points. From this it may be assumed that one of the functions of the motor cortex is to synthesize simple movements into an infinite variety of finely graded, highly differentiated patterns.

Corticospinal motor neuron paralysis may be due to lesions in the cerebral cortex, subcortical white matter, internal capsule, brainstem, or spinal cord. Usually much more is involved than the corticospinal, or pyramidal, tract. There has been a dispute as to the effects of a pure lesion of the corticospinal system. A lesion which severs the corticospinal system at midbrain level is said to cause only hemiparesis. However, in the 11 proven cases of destruction of the pyramid in the medulla, a flaccid then spastic hemiplegia was observed. In part, difference in the degree of dysfunction is a function of completeness of the corticospinal lesions (Trelles et al.). The distribution of the paralysis varies with the locale of the lesion, but there are certain common features. Paralysis due to a lesion of these supranuclear motor neurons always involves a group of muscles, never individual muscles. If any volitional movement is possible, the maximum effort is attained more slowly than in the normal limb, and there is a lesser degree of multiple motor unit recruitment and frequency of single-unit discharge. The paralysis never involves all the muscles on one side of the body, even in the hemiplegia resulting from a complete lesion of the internal capsule. Movements that are invariably bilateral, such as those of the eyes, jaw, pharynx, larynx, neck, thorax, and abdomen, are little if at all affected. The hand and arm muscles suffer most severely, the leg muscles next, and of the cranial musculature only the muscles of the lower part of the face and tongue are involved to any significant degree. Clinical observation informs us that the cortical control of all movements is to some extent bilateral. Examples that prove this are hemiplegias that worsen when the other corticospinal tract is interrupted by disease. Corticospinal motor paralysis is rarely complete for any long period of time; in this respect it differs from the total and absolute paralysis due to a complete destruction or interruption of anterior horn cells and their axons. The paralyzed arm may suddenly move during yawning and stretching, and various spinal reflexes can be elicited at all times.

Acute disorders of the corticospinal motor system, at lower levels such as the cervical cord, may not only cause a paralysis of voluntary movement but may also abolish temporarily the spinal reflexes subserved by segments below the lesion. This condition is known as *spinal shock*. After a few days to weeks

the shock disappears and gives way to a phenomenon known as *spasticity*. The latter is a feature of all acute and chronic lesions of the pyramidal system at cerebral, capsular, midbrain, and pontine levels. In cerebral and brainstem lesions it does not usually appear immediately, and in exceptional cases the paralyzed limbs remain flaccid but with reflexes. Spasticity is related to the excessive activity of the released or disinhibited spinal motor neurons. The tendon reflexes are hyperactive, and clonus may appear. The posture of the arm and leg inform us that certain spinal neurons are more active than others. The arm, for example, is maintained in a pronated, flexed position and the leg in an adducted, extended position. Any attempts to extend the arm or flex the leg passively will encounter, after a brief free interval, a resistance which quickly yields (clasp-knife phenomenon). When the limb is left in the new position, the resistance reappears (lengthening and shortening reactions). Actually the clasp-knife type of spasticity is infrequent. It is more usual for corticospinal lesions to produce a sustained resistance to movement, as pointed out by Colne. But the tendon reflexes are hyperactive and the muscles weakened. The nocifensive spinal flexion reflexes, of which Babinski's sign is a part, are also released, and the cutaneomuscular abdominal and cremasteric reflexes abolished. The flexion reflexes are not actually a component of spasticity. In the hemiplegic patient they are less prominent than in the spinal paraplegic or quadriplegic patient. With cerebral lesions exaggerated stretch and cutaneous cranial reflexes can also be elicited in cranial as well as limb and trunk muscles, and when the corticospinal disorder is bilateral, there is pseudobulbar paralysis (dysarthria, dysphonia, and dysphagia with bifacial paralysis). Prolonged flexor and extensor spasms may occur with lesions of the spinal cord; they are due to a release of tonic myotatic reflexes.

Spasticity may be present when the limbs are not paralyzed but only paretic, and it then produces interesting effects on voluntary movements. As the patient flexes and then extends the forearm, for example, the contraction of the biceps and brachioradiales persists during extension. It would appear that there is not only a diminution of anterior horn cell activation (the negative effect), but also a deficit in the "dynamic range and degree of reciprocal motor neuron control" (Sohrman and Norton). Moreover attempts by the patient to move the hemiplegic limbs voluntarily may result in a variety of associated movements. When asked to rotate one arm, the quadriparetic patient makes the same movement in the other (mirror movement). Flexion of the arms results in involuntary pronation; flexion of the leg causes the foot to dorsiflex and invert automatically (Strumpell's tibialis sign) and the thigh to flex on the trunk. Flexion of one leg is associated with involuntary extension of the other.

Table 15-1 shows the main differences between corticospinal and lower motor neuron syndrome.

Not all hemiplegias of cerebral origin are spastic.

APRAXIC OR NONPARALYTIC DISORDERS OF MOTOR FUNCTION Aside from upper and lower motor neuron paralysis with cerebral lesions, there may be loss of purposive movement without paralysis. This is called *apraxia* and may be explained as follows. Many simple actions are acquired by learning or practice. These depend on the formation of movement patterns, particularly those which involve the use of tools and instruments as well as gestures. Once established, they are remembered and may be reproduced under the proper circumstances. Any purposive act may be conceived as occurring in several stages. First, the idea of an act must be aroused in the mind of the subject by an appropriate stimulus situation, perhaps by a spoken command to do something. This idea is then translated into action by excitation of patterns of premotor or motor cortical neurons in proper sequence, which are transmitted to lower centers by the corticospinal tracts. These initiate particular movements of individual muscle groups but also modify or suppress the subcortical mechanisms that control the basic attitudes and postures of the body. In right-handed and most left-handed persons the neural mechanisms for the formulation of an idea of an act (motor schema or image) in response to a spoken command or a verbal stimulus and its reproduction are believed to be centered in the posterior and inferior parts of the left parietal lobe; these areas, near the language mechanism, are connected with the left premotor regions for the control of the right hand and thence with the motor areas of the right cerebral hemisphere through the corpus callosum for the control of the left side.

A failure to execute certain acts in the correct context while retaining the ability to carry out the individual movements upon which such acts depend is the main feature of *apraxia*. The most adequate clinical test of motor deficits of this type is to observe a series of self-initiated actions such as using a comb, a razor, a toothbrush, or a common tool, or gesturing, e.g., waving goodbye, saluting, shaking the fist as though angry, or blowing a kiss. These actions may be called forth by a command or a request to imitate the examiner. Of course, failure to follow a spoken or written request may be due to an aphasia that prevents understanding of what is asked, or an agnosia may prevent recognition of the tool or object to be used. But when these difficulties are excluded, there remains a peculiar motor deficit in which the patient appears to understand but has lost the memory of how to perform a given act, especially if it is called for in an unnatural setting. The patient may have the idea of what to do, but cannot translate the idea of the sequence of movements into a precise, well-executed act. This is sometimes called *ideomotor apraxia*. The failure may be evident both after a spoken command and in requests to imitate the gestures of the examiner. Sometimes these two conditions may be dissociated; the patient, while not aphasic, cannot execute a spoken command but can still imitate the act if it is called forth by gesture. Also if merely given the tool the patient may use it properly in an automatic fashion.

Apraxia may be limited to one group of muscles, such as tongue or lips, as in Broca's aphasia (Chap. 24), or the loss of commanded actions of the left arm and leg in right-sided hemiplegics (sympathetic apraxia). (See Chap. 25.)

If this motor disorder can be singled out, it reflects a specific loss of certain learned patterns of movement (a "specific amnesia," so to speak, analogous to the amnesia of words in aphasia). The added element of mental confusion tends often to obscure the disorder.

DIFFERENTIAL DIAGNOSIS OF PARALYSIS The diagnostic consideration of paralysis may be simplified by the following subdivisions, which relate to the location and distribution of weakness.

Monoplegia The examination of patients who complain of weakness of one extremity often discloses an unnoticed weakness in another limb, and the condition is actually hemiplegia or paraplegia. Or instead of weakness of all the muscles in a limb, only isolated groups are found to be affected. Ataxia, sensory disturbances, or pain in an extremity will often be interpreted by the patient as weakness, as will the mechanical limitation resulting from arthritis or the rigidity of parkinsonism.

In general, the presence or absence of atrophy of muscles in a monoplegic limb can be of diagnostic help.

PARALYSIS WITH LITTLE OR NO ATROPHY Long-continued disuse of a limb may lead to atrophy, but this is usually not so marked as in diseases that denervate muscles; the tendon reflexes are normal, and the response of the muscles to electric stimulation and the electromyogram are unaltered.

The most frequent cause of monoplegia without muscular wasting is a lesion of the cerebral cortex. Only occasionally does it occur in diseases which interrupt the corticospinal tract at the level of the internal capsule, brainstem, or spinal cord. A vascular lesion (thrombosis or embolus) is the commonest cause, and, of course, a tumor or abscess may have the same effect. Multiple sclerosis and spinal cord tumor, early in their course, may cause weakness of one extremity, usually the leg. Weakness due to damage to the corticospinal system is usually accompanied by spasticity, increased reflexes, and an extensor plantar reflex (Babinski's sign), and the electric reactions and electromyogram are normal. However, acute diseases that destroy the motor tracts in the spinal cord may at first (for several days) reduce the tendon reflexes and cause hypotonia (*spinal shock*). This does not occur in partial or slowly evolving lesions and occurs only to minimal degree, if at all, in lesions of brainstem and cerebrum. In acute diseases affecting the lower motor neurons the tendon reflexes are always reduced or abolished, but atrophy may not appear for several weeks. Hence one must take into account the mode of onset and the duration of the disease in evaluating the tendon reflexes, muscle tone, and degree of atrophy before reaching an anatomic diagnosis.

PARALYSIS WITH MUSCULAR ATROPHY This is more frequent than paralysis without muscular atrophy. In addition to the paralysis and reduced or abolished tendon reflexes, there may be visible fasciculations. If completely paralyzed, the muscles exhibit an electric reaction of degeneration, and the electromyogram shows reduced numbers of motor units (often of large size), fasciculations at rest, and fibrillations. The lesion may be in the spinal cord, spinal roots, or peripheral nerves. Its location can usually be decided by the distribution of the palsied muscles (whether the pattern is one of nerve, spinal root, or spinal cord involvement), by the associated neurologic symptoms and signs, and by special tests (cerebrospinal fluid examination, roentgenogram of spine, and myelogram).

Brachial atrophic monoplegia is relatively rare, and when present, it should suggest in an infant a brachial plexus trauma, in a child poliomyelitis, in an adult poliomyelitis, sy-

TABLE 15-1
Differences between paralysis of corticospinal and lower motor neurons

Upper, corticospinal motor paralysis	Lower, spinomuscular, or nuclear-infranuclear paralysis
Muscle groups affected diffusely, never individual muscles	Individual muscles may be affected
Atrophy slight and due to disuse	Atrophy pronounced, 70 to 80 percent of total bulk
Spasticity with hyperactivity of the tendon reflexes	Flaccidity and hypotonia of affected muscles with loss of tendon reflexes
Extensor plantar reflex, Babinski's sign	Plantar reflex, if present, is of normal flexor type
Fascicular twitches not produced	Fascicular twitches may be present
Normal reactions to galvanic and faradic current	Loss of faradic reaction, retention of galvanic action (reaction of degeneration)

ringomyelia, amyotrophic lateral sclerosis, or other brachial plexus lesions. Crural monoplegia is more frequent and may be caused by any lesion of thoracic or lumbar cord, i.e., trauma, tumor, myelitis, multiple sclerosis, etc. Multiple sclerosis almost never causes atrophy, and ruptured intervertebral disk and the many varieties of neuritis rarely paralyze all or most of the muscles of a limb. Muscle dystrophy may begin in one limb, but by the time the patient is seen the typical more or less symmetric pattern of proximal limb and trunk involvement is evident. A unilateral retroperitoneal tumor may paralyze the leg by implicating the lumbosacral plexus.

Hemiplegia   Loss of strength in arm, leg, and sometimes face on one side of the body is the most frequent distribution of paralysis in humans. With rare exceptions (a few unusual cases of poliomyelitis or motor system disease) this pattern of paralysis is due to involvement of the corticospinal tract.

LOCATION OF LESION-PRODUCING HEMIPLEGIA   The site or level of the lesion can usually be deduced from the associated neurologic findings. Diseases localized in the cerebral cortex, cerebral white matter (corona radiata), and internal capsule usually evoke weakness or paralysis of the face, arm, and leg on the opposite side. The occurrence of convulsive seizures or the presence of a defect in speech (aphasia), a cortical type of sensory loss (astereognosis, loss of two-point discrimination, etc.), anosognosia, or defects in the visual fields suggest a cortical or subcortical location. A pure, isolated hemiplegia affecting simultaneously the face, arm, and leg indicates a lesion in the posterior limb of the internal capsule, often a vascular lacuna.

Damage to the corticospinal and cortico-brainstem tracts in the upper portion of the brainstem (see Fig. 15-1) may cause paralysis of the face, arm, and leg on the opposite side. The lesion in such cases is localized by the presence of a paralysis of the muscles supplied by the oculomotor nerve on the same side as the lesion (Weber's syndrome) or other neurologic findings. With low pontine lesions a unilateral abducens or facial palsy is combined with a contralateral weakness or paralysis of the arm and leg (Millard-Gubler syndrome). Lesions of the lowermost part of the brainstem, i.e., in the medulla, affect the tongue and sometimes the pharynx and larynx on one side and arm and leg on the other side. These "crossed paralyses," so common in brainstem diseases, are described in Chap. 376. Ataxic hemiplegia with or without dysarthria also indicates lesion in the contralateral basis pons. Here Fisher has traced the involvement to the uncrossed corticospinal, corticobulbar, and corticopontocerebellar tracts.

Rarely, a homolateral hemiplegia (sparing cranial muscles) may be caused by a lesion in the lateral column of the cervical spinal cord. At this level, however, the pathologic process often induces bilateral signs, with resulting quadriparesis or quadriplegia. Homolateral paralysis, if combined with a loss of vibratory and position sense on the same side and a contralateral loss of pain and temperature (Brown-Séquard syndrome), signifies disease of the spinal cord on one side (Chaps. 19 and 375).

Muscle atrophy of minor degree often follows lesions of the corticospinal system but never reaches the proportions seen in diseases of the lower motor neurons. The atrophy is due to disuse. When the motor cortex and adjacent parts of the parietal lobe are damaged in infancy or childhood, the normal development of the muscles and the skeletal system in the affected limbs is retarded. The palsied limbs and even the trunk on one side are small. This does not occur if the paralysis begins after the greater part of skeletal growth is attained (after puberty). In the hemiplegia due to spinal cord injury, muscles at the level of the lesion may undergo atrophy if there is associated damage to anterior horn cells or ventral roots.

CAUSES OF HEMIPLEGIA   In this condition vascular diseases of the cerebrum and brainstem exceed all others in frequency. Trauma (brain contusion, epidural and subdural hemorrhage) ranks second, and other diseases such as brain tumor, brain abscess and encephalitis, demyelinative diseases, complications of meningitis, tuberculosis, and syphilis are of decreasing order of importance.

Paraplegia   Paralysis of both lower extremities may occur in diseases of the spinal cord and the spinal roots or of the peripheral nerves. If the onset is acute, it may be difficult to distinguish spinal from neural paralysis, for in any acute myelopathy spinal shock may result in abolition of reflexes and flaccidity. As a rule in acute spinal cord diseases with involvement of corticospinal tracts, the paralysis affects all muscles below a given level; and often, if the white matter is extensively damaged, sensory loss below a particular level (loss of pain and temperature sense with lateral spinothalamic tracts and loss of vibratory and position sense with posterior columns) is conjoined. Also, in bilateral disease of the spinal cord, the bladder and bowel sphincters are paralyzed. Alterations of cerebrospinal fluid (dynamic block, increase in protein or cells) are frequent. In peripheral nerve diseases both sensory loss and motor loss tend to involve the distal muscles of the legs more than the proximal ones (an exception is acute idiopathic polyneuritis), and the sphincters are spared or only briefly deranged in function. Sensory loss, if present, is more likely to consist of distal impairment of touch, vibration, and position sense, with pain and temperature sense spared in many instances. The cerebrospinal fluid protein level may be normal or elevated.

Acute paraplegia beginning at any age is relatively infrequent. Fracture dislocation of the spine with traumatic necrosis of the spinal cord, spontaneous hematomyelia with bleeding from a vascular malformation (angioma, telangiectasis), thrombosis of a spinal artery with infarction (myelomalacia), and dissecting aortic aneurysm or atherosclerotic occlusion of nutrient spinal arteries arising from the aorta with resulting infarction (myelomalacia) are the commonest varieties of sudden paraplegia (or quadriplegia, if the cervical cord is involved). Postinfectious or postvaccinal myelitis, acute demyelinative myelitis (Devic's disease if the optic nerves are affected), necrotizing myelitis, and epidural abscess or hemorrhage with spinal cord compression tend to develop somewhat more slowly, over a period of hours or days, or they may have an acute onset. Poliomyelitis, a purely motor disorder with meningitis, must be distinguished from the other acute myelopathies.

In adult life multiple sclerosis, subacute combined degeneration, spinal cord tumor, ruptured cervical disk and cervical spondylosis, syphilitic meningomyelitis, chronic epidural infections (fungous and other granulomatous diseases), Erb's spastic paraplegia and motor system disease, familial spastic paraplegia, and syringomyelia represent the most frequently encountered forms of spinal paraplegia. (See Chap. 375 for discussion of these spinal cord diseases). The several varieties of polyneuritis and polymyositis must be considered in their differential diagnosis, for they, too, may cause paraparesis. Friedreich's ataxia and familial paraplegia, progressive muscular dystrophy, and the chronic varieties of polyneuritis tend to appear during late childhood and adolescence and are slowly progressive.

Quadriplegia   All that has been written about the common causes of paraplegia applies to quadriplegia. The lesion is usually in the cervical rather than the thoracic or lumbar segments of the spinal cord. If it is situated in the low cervical segments and involves the anterior half of the spinal cord, as in occlusion of the anterior spinal artery, the arm paralysis may be flaccid and areflexic and the leg paralysis spastic (anterior spinal syndrome). There are only a few points of difference between the common paraplegic and quadriplegic syndromes. Repeated cerebral vascular accidents may lead to bilateral hemiplegia, usually accompanied by pseudobulbar palsy.

Isolated paralysis Paralysis of isolated muscle groups usually indicates a lesion of one or more peripheral nerves. The diagnosis of a lesion of an individual peripheral nerve is made on the presence of weakness or paralysis of the muscle or group of muscles and impairment or loss of sensation in the distribution of the nerve in question (Chap. 337). Complete transection or severe injury to a peripheral nerve is usually followed by atrophy of the muscles it innervates and by loss of their tendon reflexes. Trophic changes in the skin, nails, and subcutaneous tissue may also occur. It is of considerable importance to decide whether the lesion is a temporary one of conduction only (neuropraxia) or whether there has been a pathologic dissolution of continuity, requiring nerve regeneration for recovery. Electromyography may be of value here.

EXAMINATION SCHEME FOR MOTOR PARALYSIS AND APRAXIA The first step is to inspect the paralyzed limb, taking note first of its posture and of the presence or absence of muscle atrophy, hypertrophy, and fascicular twitchings. The patient is then called upon to move each muscle group, and the power and facility of movement are graded and recorded. The range of passive movement is then determined by moving all the joints. This provides information concerning alterations of muscle tone, i.e., hypotonia, spasticity, and rigidity. Dislocations, diseased joints, and ankyloses may also be revealed by these same maneuvers. Muscle bulk is then inspected. Slight atrophy may be due to disuse from any cause, i.e., pain, fixation as the result of a cast, or any type of paralysis. Pronounced atrophy usually occurs only with denervation of several weeks' or months' standing.

The tendon reflexes are then tested. The usual routine is to try to elicit the jaw jerk (increased in pseudobulbar palsy) and the supinator, biceps, triceps, quadriceps, and Achilles tendon reflexes. Two cutaneous reflexes are then tested, the abdominal and plantar reflexes.

If there is no evidence of upper or lower motor neuron disease, but certain acts are nonetheless imperfectly performed, one should look for a disorder of postural sensibility or of cerebellar coordination or rigidity with abnormality of posture and movement due to disease of the basal ganglions (Chap. 16). In the absence of these disorders, the possibility of an apraxic disorder may be investigated by watching the patient's own movements and those called forth by specific command and gesture.

Hysterical paralysis may pose problems. Usually it is easily distinguished from chronic lower motor neuron disease by absence of areflexia and severe atrophy. Diagnostic difficulty arises only in certain acute cases of upper motor neuron disease that lack all the usual changes in reflexes and muscle tone. In hysterical paralysis one arm or one leg or all one side of the body may be affected. The hysterical gait is sometimes diagnostic (Chap. 17). Often there is loss of all forms of sensation (touch, pain, smell, vision, and hearing) in the paralyzed side, a group of sensory changes that is never seen in organic brain disease. The patient should be asked to move the affected limbs; the movement is seen to be slow and jerky, often with contraction of both agonist and antagonist muscles simultaneously or intermittently. Hoover's sign and Babinski's com-

bined leg flexion test are helpful in distinguishing hysterical from organic hemiplegia. To elicit Hoover's sign, the patient, lying on the back, is asked to raise one leg from the bed against resistance; in a normal individual the back of the heel of the contralateral leg is pressed firmly down, and the same is true when the patient with organic hemiplegia attempts to lift the paralyzed leg. The hysteric will contract the good leg more strongly under these circumstances than as a primary willed action. To carry out Babinski's combined leg flexion test, a patient with an organic hemiplegia is asked to sit up without using the arms; in doing this, the paralyzed or weak leg flexes at the hip, and the heel is lifted from the bed while the heel of the sound leg is pressed into the bed. This sign is absent in hysterical hemiplegia.

MUSCULAR PARALYSIS AND SPASM UNATTENDED BY VISIBLE CHANGE IN NERVE OR MUSCLE A group of diseases appears to have no basis in visible structural change in motor nerve cells, nerve fibers, motor end plates, and muscular fibers. This group is composed of myasthenia gravis, myotonia congenita (Thomsen's disease), familial periodic paralysis, disorders of potassium, sodium, calcium, and magnesium metabolism, tetany, tetanus, botulinus poisoning, black widow spider bite, and the thyroid myopathies. In these diseases, each of which possesses a fairly distinctive clinical picture, the abnormality is purely biochemical, and even if the patient survives for a long time, no visible microscopic changes develop. An understanding of these diseases requires knowledge of the processes involved in nerve and muscle excitation and the contraction of muscle. They are discussed in Chaps. 378 and 383.

REFERENCES

BRODAL A: *Neurological Anatomy in Relation to Clinical Medicine.* New York, Oxford, 1969

CALNE DB: Drug treatment of spasticity and rigidity, in *Modern Trends in Neurology,* 6th ed, D Williams (ed). London, Butterworths, 1975

FISHER CM: Ataxic hemiparesis—a pathological study. Arch Neurol 35:126, 1978

SOHRMAN SA, NORTON BJ: The relationship of voluntary movement to spasticity in the upper motor neuron syndrome. Ann Neurol 2:460, 1977

TRELLES JO et al: Spasticity in hemiplegia due to lesion of anterior pyramid. Rev Neurol 129:105, 1973

16

TREMOR, CHOREA, ATHETOSIS, ATAXIA, AND OTHER ABNORMALITIES OF MOVEMENT AND POSTURE

RAYMOND D. ADAMS

In this chapter are discussed the automatic, static, and less modifiable postural activities of the human nervous system. These are believed, on good evidence, to be an expression of the function of the *older motor system,* meaning the motor structures in the basal ganglia and brainstem.

In health, the activities of the motor systems of basal ganglia and cerebellum are blended and modulate the corticospinal and cortico-brainstem-spinal systems. The static postural activities of the former are indispensable to the voluntary or willed movements of the latter.

This close association of the corticospinal (formerly pyramidal) and extrapyramidal systems is shown by human disease. Lesions of the corticospinal tracts result not only in paralysis of volitional movements of the contralateral half of the body but in the appearance of a fixed posture or attitude in which the arm is maintained in flexion and the leg in extension (predilection type of Wernicke-Mann or hemiplegic dystonia of Denny-Brown). Similarly, decerebration from a lesion in the upper pons or midbrain releases another posture in which all four extremities are extended and the cervical and thoracolumbar spine is dorsiflexed. In these released action patterns one has evidence of extrapyramidal postural and righting reflexes which are mediated through bulbospinal and other brainstem-spinal systems.

The student may be dismayed to read in current articles trenchant criticism of the validity of the concept of the corticospinal tract and the division of the motor system into corticospinal and extrapyramidal. Extremists claim the corticospinal tract may be severed in animals and even in humans without lasting motor deficits. But it must be remembered that this tract is so puny in most mammals, even in small monkeys, that it can hardly be compared with that of humans, and there has yet to be a pathologically proved example in humans of complete interruption of this tract with preserved voluntary motor function.

If an oversimplification may be permitted for clarity of exposition, the extrapyramidal motor system may be subdivided into two parts: (1) the striatopallidonigral and (2) the cerebellar. Disease in either of these parts will result in disturbances of movement and posture without significant paralysis. These two major systems and the symptoms that result when they are diseased are reviewed on the following pages.

BASAL GANGLIA: PATHOLOGIC ANATOMY

As an anatomic entity the basal ganglia have no precise definition. The list of basal structures originally thought to have some part in motor function, such as the caudate and lenticular nuclei, has been greatly expanded by physiologists to include the field of Forel and zona incerta, subthalamic nucleus of Luys, substantia nigra, red nucleus, dentate nucleus of cerebellum, and the reticular formation of the brainstem.

For the convenience of the reader, a diagram (Fig. 16-1) is included to show the principal structures and their connections. Attention is drawn to the wide range of corticostriate connections; the caudate nucleus and putamen (striatal) connections with the outer and inner segments of the globus pallidus; the direct striatonigral and nigrostriatal circuit; the globus

pallidus–ventrolateral thalamus (ansa and striatal lemnisci) pathway; the striatothalamic and thalamostriatal circuit; and the connection between outer pallidum and subthalamic nucleus. The details of these relationships are well presented in Carpenter's neuroanatomy monograph, but unfortunately a fine map of the connections of the individual cell types, their chemical transmitters, and their philosophy in the workings of the motor system have yet to be established.

The principal new anatomic datum to emerge in recent years is the central physiologic role of the ventrolateral (and anterior) nucleus of the thalamus. It is a vital link in an ascending fiber system from the lenticular nucleus and cerebellum to the motor cortex. Indeed, it would seem that most of the basal ganglionic and cerebellar influence on the motor system is funneled through the ventral plane of thalamic nuclei, thus effecting a number of corticocortical circuits. Descending pathways to the spinal cord are disputed; probably there are polysynaptic descending fibers through the reticular formation of the pons and medulla to the motor neurons of the spinal cord. It is noteworthy that these ascending thalamocortical fibers pass through the internal capsule and cerebral white matter; hence lesions in these parts may simultaneously affect both corticospinal and extrapyramidal systems.

NEUROPHARMACOLOGY

In recent years it has been discovered that the neurons of these several striatopallidothalamic, striatonigral, striatothalamic, and pallidosubthalamic circuits are activated by chemical transmitters. Acetylcholine (ACh), norepinephrine (NE), 5-hydroxytryptamine (5-HT), dopamine (DA), and the inhibitory transmitter γ-aminobutyric acid (GABA) have been localized to certain neurons of the basal nuclei and hypothalamus.

Particular neurotransmitters appear to figure prominently in extrapyramidal diseases. In Parkinson's disease, which is manifested by a combination of akinesia, tremor, rigidity, and flexed posture, the DA content of the striatum is depleted, presumably due to a loss of neurons in the substantia nigra and degeneration of the nigrostriatal tract to which they give rise. This loss of DA is believed to upset the normal balance between DA and ACh. Restoration of this equilibrium, by giving L-dopa and anticholinergic medication (belladonna alkaloids) has been shown to suppress this neurologic disorder (see Fig.

FIGURE 16-1

Basal ganglia in the coronal plane, illustrating major connections between the nuclear groups. (From RD Adams and M Victor, Principles of Neurology, New York, McGraw-Hill, 1977.)

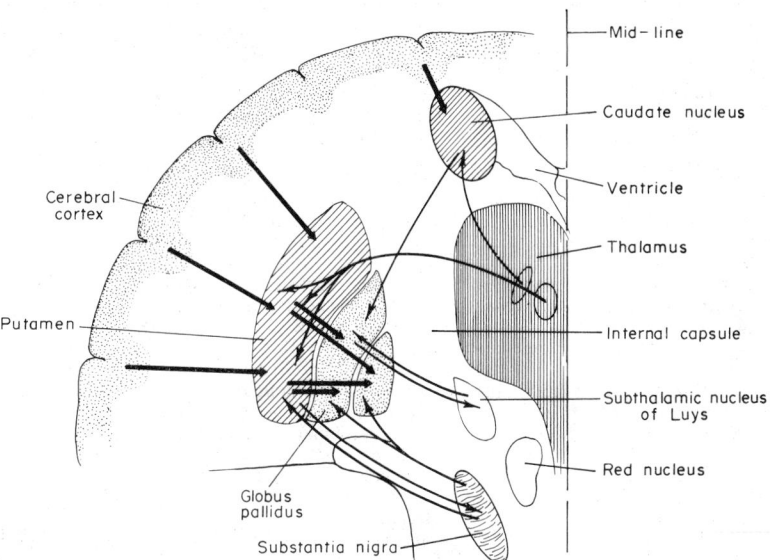

Mid-line

Caudate nucleus

Ventricle

Thalamus

Internal capsule

Subthalamic nucleus of Luys

Red nucleus

Cerebral cortex

Putamen

Globus pallidus

Substantia nigra

337-1 for diagram of metabolic pathways of DA). Reserpine and tetrabenzine, which cause a more or less typical parkinsonian syndrome, also reduce the content of DA in this part of the brain (and also its NA and 5-HT).

Another point of interest is the observation that an excess of L-dopa in the patient with Parkinson's disease, probably by the stimulation of receptors in the striatum, induces a wide variety of abnormal movements. This seems to be dose-related. The most frequent of these is craniofacial athetosis, but a more generalized choreoathetosis, facial and cervical spasms, tremors and myoclonic jerks (see below) may also occur. Presumably certain striatal neurons, not the ones causing the Parkinson's syndrome, have been rendered hypersensitive, for L-dopa appears not to have this effect on normal individuals. Moreover, drugs of the phenathiazine and butyrophenone groups (Chap. 229), for reasons that are unclear, are capable of evoking acute dystonic reactions, akathesia (motor restlessness, repetitive tapping and fiddling with hands and feet, and facial mannerisms) and tardive dyskinesias. In Huntington's chorea, L-dopa worsens the chorea. Physostigmine enhances the activity of the cholinergic transmitters by blocking cholinesterase and is said to lessen it. This may be explained by the reduction in acetylcholine transferase, the enzyme necessary for acetylcholine formation, in the caudate nuclei in this disease. GABA is also reduced.

While these findings cannot be integrated into a coherent theory of central neurotransmitters, they nonetheless offer prospects of a new pathophysiology of extrapyramidal chemical phenomena and of basal ganglionic diseases. (Further information concerning the biochemistry of norepinephrine and serotonin may be found in Chaps. 91 and 373.)

Some of the most significant facts about clinicopathologic relationships in humans are indicated in Table 16-1, which presents clinicopathologic correlations accepted by many neurologists; however, there is still much uncertainty as to finer details.

The symptoms that lend themselves best to clinical analysis are akinesia, rigidity, chorea, athetosis, dystonia, myoclonus, and tremor.

TABLE 16-1
Clinicopathologic correlations

Symptoms	Principal location of morbid anatomy
Unilateral plastic rigidity with static tremor and regular slowness of movement (Parkinson's syndrome)	Contralateral substantia nigra plus (?) other structures
Unilateral hemiballismus and hemichorea	Contralateral subthalamic nucleus of Luys, prerubral area, and Forel's fields
Chronic chorea of Huntington's type	Caudate nucleus, putamen
Athetosis and dystonia	Contralateral putamen or thalamus
Cerebellar ataxia, i.e., intention tremor; irregular slowness in starting and stopping alternating voluntary movements; hypotonia; rebound phenomenon	Homolateral cerebellar hemisphere or middle and inferior cerebellar peduncles, superior brachium conjunctivum (ipsilateral if below the decussation, contralateral if above)
Decerebrate rigidity, i.e., opisthotonos, extension of arms and legs	Lesion usually bilateral in tegmentum, involving upper brainstem, particularly red nucleus or structures between red nucleus and vestibular nuclei
Palatal and facial myoclonus (rhythmic)	Lesion in the central tegmental tract, inferior olivary nucleus, and olivodentate connections
Diffuse myoclonus	Cerebellar cortex (?), thalami (?)

AKINESIA

When extrapyramidal disease is analyzed along classic neurologic lines into primary functional deficits and secondary release effects, akinesia stands as the principal negative or deficit symptom. By the term *akinesia* one refers to the disinclination of the patient to use an affected part of the body, to engage it freely in all the natural actions of the body. In contrast to paralysis, the negative symptom of corticospinal lesions, strength is relatively undiminished in the part, and it can be used effectively in the desired movement under conditions of maximal motivation. In this respect, too, it is unlike apraxia, where movements are lost because of a lesion which erases the memory of the motor schema that forms a sequence of movements for intended action. Parkinsonian patients exhibit the phenomenon of akinesia most clearly in their extreme underactivity. They sit motionless for long times. In looking to the side they move the eyes, not the head. In arising from a chair they fail to make all the little adjustments needed (putting feet back, putting hands on arms of chair, etc.). They neglect the affected arm. Yet they are not weak (paretic) or apraxic. Formerly, akinesia was attributed to rigidity, which could reasonably hamper all movements, but now that stereotaxic surgery has been shown to abolish both tremor and rigidity, it becomes clear that the motor deficit, or akinesia, is still there. Strictly interpreted, it would appear that apart from their contribution to the maintenance of postures, the basal ganglia must provide something essential to the performance of the large variety of semiautomatic actions that make up the full repertoire of natural human motility.

ALTERATIONS OF MUSCLE TONE (SPASTICITY, RIGIDITY, HYPOTONIA)

It has been pointed out that muscle tone (the small resistance to muscle stretch offered by healthy muscle) is enhanced in the many conditions that cause a paralysis of voluntary movement by interrupting the corticospinal tract. The special distribution of the increased tone (i.e., greater in antigravity muscles—leg extensors and arm flexors in humans), the sudden augmentation of tone with gradual yielding upon quick movement (the lengthening reaction or clasp-knife phenomenon), the absence of resistance upon slow movement and its disappearance in relaxed muscle with "electromyographic silence when relaxed," and exaggerated tendon (phasic myotatic) reflexes are the identifying characteristics of spasticity. This type of hypertonus is believed to be due in some instances to hyperactivity of the small gamma motor neurons, resulting in increase in the sensitivity of the spindle muscle fibers to stretch. In other instances especially when a voluntary movement evokes a persistent, diffuse resistance to active and passive movement (tonic myotatic reflex activity), it seems clearly related to excessive activity (or disinhibition) of the larger alpha motor neurons. The "gamma spasticity" is abolished by procaine injection of the motor nerve, which paralyzes the small gamma motor and sensory fibers, leaving the larger ones intact, without weakening the willed contractions of the muscle; the "alpha spasticity" is not affected by procaine.

In the state known as *rigidity* the muscles are continuously or intermittently firm, tense, and prominent; and the resistance to passive movement is intense and even, like that noted in bending a lead pipe or in stretching a strand of toffee. Although rigidity is present in all muscle groups, both flexor and extensor, on the whole it tends to be more prominent in those which maintain a flexed posture, i.e., the flexor muscles of trunk and limbs. It appears to be somewhat greater in the large muscle groups, but this may be merely a question of muscle mass. Certainly the smaller muscles of the face and tongue and even those of the larynx are often affected. Nevertheless, like "gamma spasticity," this rigidity is said to be abolished by procaine, and Foerster earlier demonstrated that it is eradicated by posterior root section. In the electromyographic tracing, motor unit activity tends to be more continuous than in spasticity, persisting even after relaxation (Table 16-2).

A special type of rigidity is the *cogwheel phenomenon*. When the hypertonic muscle is passively stretched, the resistance may be rhythmically jerky, as though the resistance of the limb were controlled by a ratchet. A number of different explanations of this phenomenon have been suggested. Wilson postulated that it might be due to a minor form of the lengthening-shortening reaction, but a more likely explanation is an associated static tremor that is masked by rigidity during an attitude of repose but emerges faintly during manipulation.

Rigidity is prominent in extrapyramidal diseases such as paralysis agitans, postencephalitic Parkinson's syndrome, and dystonia musculorum deformans.

The *tension hypertonus of athetosis* differs from both spasticity and rigidity. Strictly speaking, it takes two forms, one which occurs during the involuntary athetotic movement, and another which appears in the absence of any involuntary motion. Clinically these forms of hypertonus are variable from one moment to the next and are paradoxic in that they some-

times disappear during a rapid passive movement or when the limb is passively shaken. The tendon reflexes may be normal or brisk. The lengthening and shortening reactions are absent. This form of variable hypertonus is found in double athetosis and choreoathetosis and in some cases of dystonia musculorum deformans. Usually in Sydenham's and Huntington's chorea a state of hypotonia prevails, sometimes as strikingly as in sensory polyneuropathies and lower motor neuron paralyses.

INVOLUNTARY MOVEMENTS

CHOREA Derived from the Greek word meaning "dance," *chorea* refers to widespread arrhythmic movements of a forcible, rapid, jerky type. These movements are involuntary and are noted for their irregularity, variability, relative speed, and relatively brief duration. They may be simple or quite elaborate and of variable distribution. In some respects they resemble a voluntary movement in their complexity, yet they are never combined into a coordinated act. The patient may, how-

TABLE 16-2
Nontremorous extrapyramidal movement disorders

Type	Physiologic characteristics	Pathologic anatomy	Common diseases	Treatment
Plastic rigidity, static tremor, slowness of movement (Parkinson's syndrome)	Present during rest and activity Worsened by excitement No change in tendon or cutaneous reflexes unilateral or bilateral See Table 16-3	Substantia nigra- and nigrostriatal pathway Contralateral if one-sided	Paralysis agitans (Parkinson's disease) Postencephalitic parkinsonism Wilson's disease Hallevorden-Spatz disease Phenothiazine effect	Anticholinesterase drugs L-Dopa Amantadine Stereotaxic thalamic surgery
Chorea and choreoathetosis: Generalized	Moderately fast, arrhythmic, usually with hypotonia but without change in reflexes or ataxia	Striatum, caudate nucleus, and putamen	Rheumatic (Sydenham's chorea) Huntington's chorea Senile chorea Tardive dyskinesia Rarely thyrotoxicosis, "the pill," lupus erythematosus, polycythemia vera, hypernatremia Sydenham's chorea	Prednisone Haloperidine Diazepam
Unilateral or localized	Same	Contralateral striatum	Infarct or hemorrhage in thalamus or striatum (contralateral)	Rest, quiet, sedatives Stereotaxic thalamic surgery
Athetosis and dystonia: Generalized	Present at rest, worse on willed movement Aggravated by excitement Reflexes normal or abnormal	Anterior thalamus or venticular nuclei with intact pyramidal tracts	Cerebral palsy Wilson's disease Rigid form of Huntington's chorea Overdose of L-dopa Postanoxic sequela Other degenerative diseases Dystonia musculorum deformans	Stereotaxic thalamic surgery
Unilateral (restricted dystonias, see text)	Same	Same	Posthemiplegic states	As above Surgical denervation of affected muscles
Hemiballismus	Arrhythmic; large excursion; usually unilateral; no weakness or pyramidal signs	Contralateral subthalamic nucleus	Vascular lesions (hemorrhage or infarct) Posttraumatic (rare)	Surgical section of cerebral peduncles Stereotaxic thalamic surgery Diazepam and other sedatives
Myoclonus: Arrhythmic	Movements quicker than chorea Associated ataxia (often) or dementia and seizures	Cerebellum, ?cortex, ?dentate nuclei, ?thalamus	Postanoxic Lipidoses Jakob-Creutzfeld disease Subacute sclerosing encephalitis Familial myoclonic epilepsy and other degenerative diseases	5-Hydroxytryptophane Anticonvulsant and sedative medications
Rhythmic (restricted, palatal myoclonus)	Continuous, awake and asleep; other brainstem signs	Central segmental tracts of pons, medulla, and inferior olivary nuclei	Vascular lesions, gliomas	None known

ever, incorporate them into a deliberate movement, as if to make them less noticeable. When superimposed on voluntary movements, these may take on a grotesque and exaggerated character. Grimacing and peculiar respiratory sounds may be other expressions of the movement disorder. Usually the movements are discrete, but if very numerous, they may flow into one another; the resultant picture then resembles athetosis. They may be limited to a limb or one side of the body (hemichorea), or they may involve all parts of the body. Normal volitional movements are, of course, possible, for there is no paralysis, but they too may be excessively quick and poorly sustained. The limbs are often unusually slack, or hypotonic. A choreic movement may be superimposed on a tendon reflex, giving rise to the "hung-up reflex." The tendon reflexes tend to be pendular because of the associated hypotonia; when the knee jerk is elicited with the patient sitting, the leg swings back and forth four or five times, like a pendulum, rather than one or two times as in a normal person. (See Table 16-2 for list of common pathologies.)

A special variety of chorea (sometimes choreoathetosis or dystonia) is clearly paroxysmal and sometimes familial (dominant inheritance). Paroxysms lasting minutes to hours appear during childhood or adolescence and continue throughout life. In one special subtype the chorea is kinesogenic, meaning that it is initiated by a sudden voluntary movement. Alcohol, hypernatremia, and diphenylhydantoin (especially in patients who have had Sydenham's chorea in childhood) are other factors in paroxysmal chorea. Lance has discussed this in terms of a dopaminergic "sensitivity." In some cases anticonvulsive drugs (clonazepam, phenobarbital) have prevented attacks and in others L-dopa has been effective.

ATHETOSIS This term is from a Greek word meaning "unfixed" or "changeable." The condition is characterized by an inability to sustain the fingers and toes, tongue, or any other group of muscles in one position. The maintained posture is interrupted by continuous, slow, sinuous, purposeless movements. These are most pronounced in the digits and the hands but often involve the tongue, throat, and face. One can detect as basic patterns of movement an extension and pronation and flexion and supination of the arm, and alternating flexion and extension of the fingers. They may be unilateral, especially in children who have suffered a hemiplegia at some previous date (posthemiplegic athetosis). The movements are slower than those of chorea, but in many cases gradations between the two (choreoathetosis) are seen. Most athetotic patients exhibit variable degrees of motor deficit due in some instances to associated corticospinal tract disease. Discrete individual movements of the tongue, lips, and hand are often impossible, and attempts to perform such voluntary movements result in a contraction of all the muscles in the limb and other parts of the body (*intention spasm*). Variable degrees of rigidity are generally associated, and these may account for the slower quality of athetosis, in contrast to chorea. It must be admitted, however, that in some cases it is almost impossible to distinguish between chorea and athetosis.

TORSION SPASM OR DYSTONIA Torsion spasm is closely allied to athetosis, differing only in that the larger axial muscles (those of the trunk and limb girdles) rather than appendicular muscles are involved. It results in bizarre, grotesque movements and positions of the body. The word *dystonia* has been given to these movements but, unfortunately, is also applied to any fixed posture which may be the end result of a disease of the motor system. Thus Denny-Brown speaks of hemiplegic dystonia, the flexion dystonia of parkinsonism, and extensor dystonia with retraction of the head and arching or twisting of

the back. If the latter meaning is given, it would be better to speak of athetosis of the trunk as torsion spasms or phasic dystonia, in contrast to fixed dystonia. The former, like athetosis, may show remarkable fluctuations; sometimes the whole musculature of the body may be thrown into spasm by an effort to move an arm or to speak. If mild, the torsion spasm may be limited to the lumbar or cervical muscles or those of one limb and may cease when the body is at rest (see below).

Torsion spasm may be seen in the condition of double athetosis after hypoxic damage to the brain, in kernicterus, in chronic manganese intoxication, and, rarely, in Wilson's hepatolenticular degeneration. It is most characteristic of the syndrome designated *dystonia musculorum deformans* but also occurs in other conditions such as the postphenothiazine dyskinesias and Hallevorden-Spatz disease (Chap. 373).

Chorea, athetosis, and torsion spasm are all closely related. The movements are elaborate and depend for their expression on cortical mechanisms. Paralytic lesions involving the corticospinal tract abolish these involuntary movements. The hypotonia in chorea and some cases of athetosis, the pendular reflexes, and some degree of interference with natural movements are also reminiscent of the syndrome that follows disease of the cerebellum. Lacking, however, are intention tremor and true incoordination or ataxia.

MYOCLONUS This term refers to several different motor disorders, some localized, others diffuse. As in chorea, the myoclonic movement is involuntary and arrhythmic, but it is much faster than chorea, being concluded in a few hundred milliseconds or less. Variations in degree are noteworthy; it may consist of no more than a flick of a single muscle or part of a muscle, but the larger movements always betray its nature, involving as they do a group of muscles. Thus myoclonus may be distinguished from fasciculation. Sensory relationships are another prominent attribute. Flickering light, a series of loud sounds, or abrupt contact with some part of the body in some instances may regularly initiate a jerk, sometimes as a direct sensorimotor effect, again through the mechanism of startle. One special variety is evoked by willed movement, presumably through a proprioceptive mechanism. Hence, one may speak of action or intention myoclonus, auditory or visual myoclonus. A series of intense stimuli may recruit a series of myoclonic jerks that progress to a full-blown seizure, as happens often in the familial myoclinic epilepsy syndrome of Unverricht-Lundborg. The pathologic disturbance in the latter is usually a lipid storage disease or an amyloid Lafora body inclusion disease (Chap. 373). See Table 16-2 for list of common causes.

The term *myoclonus* unfortunately has also been assigned to a rather different motor phenomenon—that of repetitious, rhythmic clonus of some part of the "branchial cleft" or craniocervical musculature. Examples are "nystagmus of the palate" (rhythmic contractions at the rate of 10 to 50 or more per minute of the soft palate) and rhythmic contractions of the pharyngeal muscles, vocal cords, facial muscles, and diaphragm. The lesions producing this state, which we would prefer to designate as a form of continuous *bulbar, facial,* or *diaphragmatic clonus,* have been situated in all instances in the central tegmental tract, inferior olivary nucleus, or olivocerebellar tract. The causative lesions have been infarcts, tumors, and encephalitic processes.

The main fault with our concept of myoclonus is that it covers too many motor disorders. When movements are grouped according to their brevity or involuntary nature, one must include the normal dormescent start or jerk of a limb as one falls asleep, and the motor components of a natural startle reaction. The obligatory Moro response also falls within the group, as well as the form of epilepsy known as infantile or salaam spasms and the falling spells of the petit mal triad. Metrazol injections cause myoclonus of the limbs, which has been shown to depend on a lower brainstem (medullary reticular) mechanism. Another problem arises on the clinical side in distinguishing diffuse myoclonus from other abrupt involuntary movements such as tremors, chorea, and restricted forms of epilepsy (epilepsia partialis continua). Speed of movement, lack of rhythmicity, and relationships to sensory stimulation prove to be the most reliable identifying features of the larger group of myoclonic disorders. There is an advantage in separating the arrhythmic diffuse form from the rhythmic restricted form in that each stands as a diagnostic attribute of a separate category of nervous diseases.

TREMOR This consists of a more or less regular rhythmic oscillation of a part of the body around a fixed point. The rate varies from three to eight oscillations per second; in a particular person the rate is fairly constant in all affected parts, regardless of the size of the muscle or of the part of the body. Tremors usually involve the distal part of the limbs, the head, tongue, or jaw, and rarely the trunk.

There are many different types of tremor, and only a few are recognized as bearing any meaningful relationship to disease of the extrapyramidal motor system; but since tremors have not been discussed elsewhere, all the different types will be considered here.

Tremors may be subdivided according to their distribution, amplitude, regularity, and relationship to volitional movement. The tremors described in the following paragraphs should be familiar to every physician (Table 16-3).

Static (parkinsonian) tremor This is a coarse, rhythmic tremor, with an average rate of four to five beats per second,

most often localized in one or both hands, and, occasionally, in the jaw or tongue. Its most characteristic feature is that it occurs when the limb is in an attitude of repose, and willed movement at least temporarily suppresses it. If the tremulous limb is completely relaxed, the tremor usually disappears, but the average patient rarely achieves this state. In some cases the tremor is constant; in others it varies from time to time and with the progress of the disease extends from one group of muscles to another. In paralysis agitans the tremor tends to be rather gentle and more or less limited to the distal muscles, whereas in postencephalitic parkinsonism and hepatolenticular degeneration it often has a wider range and involves proximal muscles. In many cases there is a variable degree of rigidity of a plastic type in the tremulous limb or elsewhere. The tremor interferes with voluntary movements surprisingly little; it is not uncommon to see a patient who has been trembling violently raise a full glass of water to the lips and drain the contents without spilling a drop. The handwriting of these patients is often small and cramped (micrographia). The gait may be of festinating type (see Chap. 17). It is the combination of static tremor, slowness of movement, rigidity, and flexed postures without true paralysis that constitutes Parkinson's syndrome (also called *amyostatic* syndrome).

The exact pathologic anatomy of static tremor is unknown. In paralysis agitans and postencephalitic Parkinson's syndrome, the visible lesions are predominantly in the substantia nigra. In hepatocerebral degeneration, where this syndrome is

TABLE 16-3
Tremors

Types	Physiologic characteristics	Anatomic pathology	Common diseases	Treatment
Fast frequency (7–10 per second), slightly arrhythmic action tremor	Generalized (usually) Present during activity; increased in precise movement and excitement; ceases during full relaxation Increased by epinephrine	Unknown ?Peripheral or spinal	One of hereditary types Hyperthyroidism Intense fright Corticosteroid and lithium therapy Pheochromocytoma and carcinoid Alcoholic withdrawal	Reduced by propranolol (Inderal) and beta-blocking agents Reduced by alcohol Sometimes helped by diazepam
Medium frequency (5–7 per second), rhythmic action tremor	Same as above except for rhythmic alternations of agonists and antagonists	Unknown ?Central (spinal or higher centers)	One of hereditary types General paresis (syphilis) Rare in other diseases Some cases of corticosteroid therapy	Variably reduced by Inderal and alcohol Reduced by diazepam
Ataxic intention tremor (4–6 per second)	Present in terminal phase of projected (willed) movement; absent during relaxation May be unilateral Associated with cerebellar ataxia	Cerebellum—especially dentatothalamic tracts (superior cerebellar peduncle and brachium conjunctivum)	Multiple sclerosis Cerebellar and brainstem tumors Vascular lesions	None Drugs ineffective
Combined rest and intention tremor (4–6 per second, erroneously called "rubral tremor")	Wide range and rhythmic; worse during willed movement, but present at rest Associated with cerebellar ataxia and/or parkinsonism May be unilateral	Tegmentum of midbrain and subthalamus ?Brachium conjunctivum	Multiple sclerosis Wilson's disease Vascular lesions and traumatism	Stereotaxic surgery of ventromedial nucleus may help Drugs ineffective
Tremor at rest (4–5 per second, static tremor or "parkinsonian tremor")	Rhythmic alternation of agonist-antagonist muscles Present in attitude of repose; temporarily abolished by willed movement May be combined with fast-frequency tremor Usually associated with rigidity and slowness of movement	Lesions in substantia nigra and nigrolenticular pathway	Paralysis agitans (Parkinson's disease) Postencephalitic parkinsonism Wilson's disease Senile syndromes Postphenothiazine (tardive) dyskinesia	Reduced by anticholinergic drugs and L-dopa Reduced by stereotaxic surgery (ventral thalamus and pallidum)

mixed with cerebellar ataxia, the lesions are more diffuse. A similar tremor, without rigidity, slowness of movement, flexed postures, or masked facies, is seen in senile persons. Unlike Parkinson's disease, it does not progress to motor disability and does not respond to antiparkinson drugs.

Action tremor This term refers to a tremor present when the limbs are actively maintained in a certain position, as when outstretched, and throughout voluntary movement. It may increase slightly as the action of the limbs becomes more precise, but it never approaches the degree of augmentation in fine movement seen in intention tremor. It is easily made to disappear when the limbs are relaxed. Probably some of the *action tremors* are but an exaggeration of normal or physiologic tremor, which ranges from six to eight per second, being slower in childhood and old age. In adults the tremor is of small excursion, has a frequency of seven to eight per second, and is somewhat irregular. The tremor involves the outstretched hand, head, and, less often, the lips and tongue, and it interferes little with voluntary movements such as handwriting and speech. This type of tremor is seen in numerous medical, neurologic, and psychiatric diseases and is therefore more difficult to interpret than static tremor. There are somewhat slower frequencies of action tremor, and instead of rather irregular potentials in both agonist and antagonist muscles (as in the aforementioned type), their activity alternates. Either form, when occurring as the only neurologic abnormality in several members of a family, is known as *familial* or *hereditary tremor*. Familial tremor may begin in childhood, but usually comes on later and persists throughout adult life. Being worse when the patient is under observation, it becomes a source of embarrassment because it suggests to the onlooker that the patient is nervous. A curious fact about familial tremors is that one or two drinks of an alcoholic beverage may abolish them, and they may become worse after the effects of the alcohol have worn off. Similar fast-frequency action tremors are seen in delirious states, such as delirium tremens, in chronic alcoholism as an isolated symptom (the morning shakes), and in general paresis. An action tremor, usually more rapid than the above, is also characteristic of hyperthyroidism and other toxic states, and a similar tremor is frequently observed in patients suffering intense anxiety. In fact it can be reproduced by injections of epinephrine. Severe action tremor may also accompany certain diseases of the basal ganglia, including parkinsonism. Some of the fast-frequency action tremors are suppressed by beta-adrenergic blocking agents such as propranolol (Inderal, 40 mg tid).

Intention tremor The word *intention* is ambiguous in this context because the tremor itself is not intentional. The term means, instead, that the tremor requires for its full expression the performance of an exacting, precise, willed movement. The term *ataxic tremor* has been suggested because it is always combined with and adds to cerebellar ataxia. The tremor is absent when the limbs are inactive and during the first part of a voluntary movement, but as the action continues and greater precision is demanded (e.g., in touching a target such as the patient's nose or the examiner's finger), a jerky, more or less rhythmic interruption of forward progression, with side-to-side oscillation, appears. It continues for a fraction of a second or so after the act is completed. The tremor may seriously interfere with the patient's performance of skilled acts. Sometimes the head is involved (titubation). This type of tremor invariably indicates disease of the cerebellum and of its connections. When the disease is very severe, every movement, even the lifting of a limb, results in a wide-ranging tremor of such violence as to throw the patient off balance. This latter state is

occasionally seen in multiple sclerosis, Wilson's disease, and vascular, traumatic, and other lesions of the tegmentum of the midbrain and subthalamus but not of the cerebellum.

OTHER INVOLUNTARY MOVEMENTS There are other abnormalities of movement, about which only a few words can be said. They vary from simple irritative phenomena to complex psychologically related disorders, such as compulsions, mannerisms, etc.

The first group are the isolated or restricted dystonias (dyskinesias) of adult life. These include idiopathic spasmodic torticollis, oromandibular dystonia, blepharospasm, spastic dysphonia, and dystonic writer's cramp.

Spasmodic torticollis This is an intermittent or continuous spasm of sternomastoid, trapezius, and other neck muscles, usually more pronounced on one side, with turning or tipping of the head. It is involuntary and cannot be inhibited and thereby differs from habit spasm or tic. This condition should be considered a form of dystonia. It is worse when the patient sits, stands, or walks, and usually contactual stimulation of the chin or of the back of the head partially alleviates the muscle imbalance.

Women are affected twice as often as men and the average age of onset is 40 years. Rarely is it seen in early adult life or adolescence. Extranuchal dystonia, tremor, and facial masking are seen in some cases.

Various modes of therapy have been tried with inconsistent results. L-Dopa (1 g per day) or carbidopa, carbamazepine (Tegretol, 200 to 1200 mg per day), haloperidal (2 to 12 mg per day) and biofeedback therapy have each been beneficial in certain cases. Psychiatric treatment is ineffectual. In severe cases muscle sectioning, neurectomy, or section of the anterior cervical roots has given favorable results.

Other craniocervical spasms Blepharoclonus (inability to keep the eyes open), lingual spasms, "spastic" dysphonia, facial spasms, cervicothoracic spasms, and writer's cramp are all special varieties of involuntary movement, appearing usually in late middle life and the senium. Such facial, cervical, and thoracic spasms have occurred with striking frequency during phenothiazine medication, but they also appear de novo. Marsden refers to them as restricted dystonias. Nonprogressivity, unresponsiveness to psychotherapy, and uncertain amelioration by all pharmacologic agents characterize most of them. Exceptionally, when these disorders are induced by drugs of the phenothiazine class, they persist after discontinuance of the drug (tardive or postphenothiazine dyskinesias). Once started they tend to persist indefinitely, and the only therapy of value has been surgical denervation of the affected muscles (C_1 to C_3 and unilateral C_4 roots) in spasmodic torticollis.

Tics and habit spasms Many persons throughout life are given to habitual movements, such as sniffing, clearing the throat, protruding the chin, or blinking, whenever they become tense. The patient admits that the movements are voluntary and that he or she feels compelled to make them in order to relieve tension; they can be inhibited for a time by an effort of will but reappear when attention is diverted. Children between five and ten years of age are especially likely to have habit spasms. The movements are often purposive coordinated acts which normally serve the organism; it is only their incessant repetition when uncalled for that constitutes a habit. In certain cases they become so ingrained that the person is unaware of them and unable to control them. Stereotypy purposelessness, and repetitiveness at irregular intervals are their main identifying features. Multiple convulsive tics with coprolalia (compulsive utterance of vile words; *Gilles de la Tourette's disease*) constitute a more severe and often unremitting form of the same condition. In children with transitory habit spasms it is best to ignore the habit spasm and at the same time to arrange for more rest and calmer environment. In adults, relief of nervous tension by tranquilizing drugs (chlorpromazine, 25 to 75 mg tid) and psychotherapy is helpful, but the disposition to tic formation persists. In the chronic tic or Tourette's syndrome large doses of haloperidol (10 to 20 mg per day orally) have been beneficial in some cases.

Mentally backward children and adults often display, when idle, a wide variety of rhythmic body-rocking, head-bobbing, arm-and-finger movements. These are of the nature of mannerisms and have no known basal ganglion pathology.

It would be a mistake to assume that each of the above disorders of movement occurs separately in specific relationships to certain diseases. This may happen, as in paralysis agitans; but there is sometimes much overlap in the degenerative diseases and birth injuries.

EXTRAPYRAMIDAL MOTOR DISTURBANCES DUE PRIMARILY TO DISEASES OF THE CEREBELLUM

Isolated lesions in the midline flocculonodular lobe result in grave disturbances of equilibrium. Often the symptoms are exhibited only when the patient attempts to stand and walk. Then sways, staggers, titubates, and reels occur (see "Disturbance of Movement and Posture," below). There may be no disturbance in coordination and no intention tremor of the limbs. A midline tumor of the cerebellum such as medulloblastoma, hemorrhage, or other lesion usually produces this syndrome.

Extensive lesions of one cerebellar hemisphere, especially the anterior lobe, cause disturbances in coordination of volitional movements of the ipsilateral arm and leg. This is known as *ataxia*. The movements are characterized by an inappropriate range, rate, and strength of each of the various components of a motor act and by an improper combination of those components. Electromyographic analysis has shown that ataxia is manifested as a decomposition of movement consisting of abnormal duration and timing of bursts of contraction and relaxation of agonists and antagonists of a joint, usually a large one. This incoordination is also called *asynergia*. The defects are particularly noticeable in acts that require rapid alternation of movements. Irregular slowness in acceleration and deceleration, which is almost invariably present, impedes the performance (dysdiadochokinesis). The direction of projected (purposive) movement is frequently inaccurate. Owing to delay in arresting a movement, the patient may overshoot the mark. The antagonist muscles do not come into play at the proper time, possibly because of the hypotonia that is almost always present. This may be demonstrated by having the patient flex the arm against a resistance that is suddenly released. The patient with cerebellar disease will sometimes strike the face because of failure to check the flexion movement. In movements requiring accurate direction, as the limb approaches its destination it may stop short and then advance by a more or less rhythmic series of jerks and oscillations (intention tremor). In addition to hypotonia, there may be, in acute cerebellar lesions, some slight weakness.

A similar ataxia, asynergia, and dysmetria, usually with hypotonia and only a little intention tremor, may accompany lesions of the lateral and inferior parts of the cerebellar hemisphere. Bilateral lesions of the cerebellar hemispheres and midline flocculonodular lobe lead to such a severe disturbance in all movements that the patient may be unable to stand or walk or use the limbs effectively. In addition, there are ocular and speech disturbances, namely, nystagmus, dysmetria and skew deviation of the eyes, and dysarthria. Lesions of the cerebellar peduncles have the same effect as extensive hemispheral lesions. This syndrome, due to involvement of one cerebellar hemisphere, may be observed in a tumor or abscess or in vascular lesions of the brainstem and cerebellar peduncles. The ataxia tends to be bilateral and symmetric in primary atrophy or degeneration of the cerebellum.

There have been numerous attempts to explain in physiologic terms the hypotonia, mild degrees of weakness and fatigability, and abnormalities in the rate and regularity of projected movement that accompany cerebellar lesions in humans. It has been found that depression of fusimotor (spindle) efferent activity in the spinal cord leads to decreased spindle afferent discharge and lessened tonic facilitation of alpha motor neuron activity. The cerebellar facilitation that is lost with acute lesions is normally mediated through two systems of fibers—the fastigioreticulospinal and the dentatorubrothalamocortical. The latter, acting specifically on cortical areas 4 and 6, is the more important in humans. Although the corticospinal tract is probably essential for expression of cerebellar deficits in humans, in the primate any pathway subserving specifically projected movements into environment may support tremor and other parts of the syndrome. Tremor, ataxia, and hypotonia seem to be separable, independent entities, but all are believed related to the disturbed fusimotor activity.

A kind of pseudoataxia, especially of gait, may be caused by the improper timing of the components of complex actions, e.g., with defects in postural sense (sensory ataxia) and with slow relaxation of muscles in hypothyroidism (myxedema with ataxia).

SOME GENERAL FEATURES OF ALL EXTRAPYRAMIDAL MOTOR DISTURBANCES

From the above discussion of many special types of motor disorder the reader must not think that they always appear in pure form. Various combinations occur in diseases. For example, Wilson's disease usually presents with a Parkinson-like picture of tremor, rigidity, slowness of movement, and flexion dystonia of trunk, but exceptionally there is athetosis, tonic innervation (inability to relax a voluntary movement), phasic dystonia, and intention tremor. Hallevorden-Spatz disease may take the form of universal rigidity and flexion dystonia or choreoathetosis. Occasionally the degeneration of Huntington's chorea leads to rigidity rather than choreoathetosis. Corticospinal and various of these extrapyramidal disorders may be associated in patients with cerebral diplegia. Nonetheless certain combinations tend to occur with greater or lesser frequency in certain diseases, as discussed in Chaps. 373 and 374.

In broad terms all the extrapyramidal disorders should be viewed in terms of the primary deficit (negative symptom) and of the new phenomena (movements, abnormal postures, tremors, etc.) which have appeared. These latter positive symptoms are presently ascribed to release from or disequilibrium of undamaged motor parts of the nervous system. The clearest negative effect is usually evidenced as an akinesia, or disinclination to use the affected muscles. The difficulty in rapid alternating sequences of movement stands as another negative effect in diseases of both the basal ganglia and the cerebellum. In fact this latter symptom, presenting as a clumsiness, may be the only fault manifest in certain congenitally maladroit children. Stress and nervous tension characteristically worsen both the motor deficiency and the abnormal movements in all these extrapyramidal syndromes, just as relaxation helps the motor performance. All the movement disorders are abolished in sleep.

One of the most remarkable discoveries of recent years, to

be credited largely to the pioneering efforts of neurosurgeons (Cooper), has been the abolition of tremors, rigidity, and involuntary movements of the limbs by a surgical lesion in the medial segment of the globus pallidus or the ventrolateral nucleus of the thalamus. The effects are contralateral. Usually the lesion has been made first by the injection of procaine (Novocain) and then by use of alcohol, cooling and freezing (Cooper), or electrocoagulation. The operation has been successful in temporarily alleviating tremor or rigidity (or both) on one side. The procedure is successful in approximately 80 percent of cases of paralysis agitans, and the postural abnormality in dystonia musculorum deformans and double athetosis has responded somewhat less consistently. The operations have been perfected to the point at which the mortality rate is less than 1 percent, and the risk of hemiplegia or some other sequel is less than 10 percent. Of course, as the disease progresses, the beneficial effects are lost. The therapeutic procedure indicates that the pallidum and ventrolateral nucleus, probably through their connections with the cerebral cortex (motor cortex and its corticospinal pathway), are essential for the expression of these extrapyramidal syndromes. The indications for these surgical procedures are discussed in Chap. 373.

DISTURBANCE OF MOVEMENT AND POSTURE: EXAMINATION AND DIFFERENTIAL DIAGNOSIS

In Chap. 15 the methods of examining the motor system are described at some length, so only a few additional remarks concerning extrapyramidal disorders need be made here. These abnormalities are best demonstrated by seeing the patient in action. Patients who complain of a limp after walking a distance or of difficulty in climbing stairs should be observed under these conditions. Tests of rate, regularity, and coordination of voluntary movement must be sufficiently varied and demanding of the patient's motor coordination to bring out the defect. The physician must cultivate the habit of accurately observing and describing abnormalities of movement and must not be content merely to give the condition a name or to force it into some category such as chorea, tic, or myoclonus. The main postures of the body in all common acts should be noted. Aside from the assessment of muscle power and of gait, the usual test applied to the upper limb is to ask the patient to touch the examiner's fingertip and then the tip of his or her own nose repeatedly (*finger-to-nose test*). To test the leg, the patient is asked to place a heel on one knee and then to run it down the shin and back to the knee (*heel-to-knee-to-shin test*). Finer movements of the hand may be tested by having the patient successively touch each finger to the thumb, pat a thigh rapidly, or use tools or handle objects. Rapidly alternating movements such as repeatedly touching the index finger with the thumb, pronation and supination of wrist, or opening and closing the hands are valuable tests.

The fully developed extrapyramidal motor syndromes can be recognized without difficulty once the physician has become familiar with the typical pictures. The mental picture of Parkinson's syndrome, with its slowness of movement, poverty of facial expression, and static tremor and rigidity should be fixed in mind. Similarly, the gross distortions and postural abnormalities of dystonia, whether widespread in trunk muscles or involving only neck muscles, as in spasmodic torticollis, once seen should thereafter be familiar. Athetosis, with its instability of postures and ceaseless movements of fingers and hands; intention spasm, chorea, with its more rapid and complicated movements; and the abrupt movements of myoclonus that flit over the body are other standard syndromes. Characteristic of all is a mild defect in the voluntary use of the affected parts.

The clinical differences between corticospinal and extrapyramidal disorders are summarized in Table 16-2.

Early or mild forms of these conditions, like all medical diseases, may offer special difficulties in diagnosis. Cases of paralysis agitans, seen before the appearance of tremor, are often overlooked. The patient may complain of being nervous and restless or may have experienced an indescribable stiffness and aching in certain parts of the body. Because of the absence of weakness or of reflex changes, the case may be considered psychogenic or rheumatic. It is well to remember that Parkinson's syndrome often begins in a hemiplegic distribution, and for this reason the illness may be misdiagnosed as cerebral thrombosis. A slight masking of the face, a suggestion of a limp, blepharoclonus (uninhibited blinking of eyes when the bridge of the nose is tapped), a mild rigidity, failure of an arm to swing naturally in walking, or loss of certain movements of cooperation will help in diagnosis at this time. Every case presenting the syndrome of Parkinson or other abnormality of movement and posture in adolescence or early adult life should be surveyed for hepatolenticular degeneration by tests of liver function and slit-lamp examination for corneal pigmentation (Kayser-Fleischer ring); if facilities are available, urinary amino-nitrogen excretion and copper excretion should be determined.

Mild or early chorea is often mistaken for simple nervousness. If one sits for a time and watches the patient, the diagnosis will often become evident. There are cases, nonetheless, in which it is impossible to distinguish simple nervousness from early Sydenham's chorea, especially in children, and there is no laboratory test upon which one can depend. The first postural manifestation of dystonia may suggest hysteria, and it is only later, when the fixity of the postural abnormality, the lack of the usual psychologic picture of hysteria, and the relentlessly progressive character of the illness become evident, that accurate diagnosis is reached. Another common error is to assume that a bedfast patient who has complained of dizziness, staggering, and headaches and exhibits no other neurologic abnormality is suffering from hysteria. The flocculonodular cerebellar syndrome is demonstrable only when the patient attempts to stand and walk.

The uncertainty of balance and short-stepped gait (*marche à petit pas*) in the elderly is often incorrectly attributed to loss of confidence and fear of falling.

REFERENCES

CARPENTER M: Anatomy of the basal ganglia and related nuclei: A review, in *Advances in Neurology*, vol 14: *Dystonia*, D Williams (ed). London, Butterworths, 1975

COOPER IS: *Involuntary Movement Disorders*. New York, Hoeber, 1969

CUMINGS JN: Biochemistry of the basal ganglia, in *Handbook of Clinical Neurology*, vol 6, PJ Vinken, GW Bruyn (eds). Amsterdam, North-Holland, 1968, p 116

DENNY-BROWN D: Clinical symptomatology of disease of the basal ganglia, in *Handbook of Clinical Neurology*, vol 6, PJ Vinken, GW Bruyn (eds). Amsterdam, North-Holland, 1968, p 133

LANCE JW: Familial paroxysmal dystonic choreoathetosis and its differentiation from related syndromes. Ann Neurol 2:285, 1977

MARSDEN CD: The neuropharmacology of abnormal involuntary movement disorders (the dyskinesias), in *Modern Trends in Neurology*, D Williams (ed). London, Butterworths, 1975

DISTURBANCES OF EQUILIBRIUM AND OF GAIT

MAURICE VICTOR
RAYMOND D. ADAMS

All that has been said previously in Chap. 14, "Dizziness and Vertigo," refers in large measure to the patient's awareness of a disorientation in space; however, there are forms of neurologic abnormality with a prominent disequilibrium of the body but no dizziness whatsoever. Since these are manifested most clearly as an impairment of upright stance and locomotion, their evaluation depends on a knowledge of the nervous mechanisms underlying these peculiarly human functions.

Since normal body posture and locomotion require visual information, labyrinthine function, and proprioception, it is of interest to note the effect of deficits in these senses on normal function. Blind persons or persons with sight who are blindfolded may walk very well. They move cautiously, to avoid collision with objects, and on smooth pavement shorten their step slightly; with the shortening there is less rocking of the body, and they seem unnaturally stiff. A person deprived of labyrinthine function shows a slight unsteadiness in walking and an inability to descend stairs without holding onto a banister. Running is also difficult. Characteristically, there is great difficulty in focusing on a stationary object when the individual is moving, so that he or she cannot drive a car. Proof of dependence on visual cues comes from blindfolded performance, when unsteadiness and staggering increase to some extent, but usually not to the point of falling. A loss of proprioception, as in a complete lesion in the posterior columns of the spinal cord in the high cervical region, abolishes for a long time the capacity for independent locomotion. After years of training, the patients will still have difficulty in starting to walk and in propelling themselves forward. As Purdon Martin has illustrated, they hold the hands in front of the body, bend body and head forward, walk with a wide base with irregular uneven steps but do rock the body. If they lose balance, they show no reaction to the altered posture. If they fall, they cannot arise without help, and they cannot get up from a chair. They are unable to crawl or to get into an all-fours posture. When standing, if blindfolded, they immediately fall. Thus the postural reactions are demonstrably more dependent on proprioceptive than on visual or labyrinthine information.

CLINICAL APPROACH TO GAIT DISORDERS When confronted with a disorder of gait, the examiner must observe the patient's natural stance and the attitude and dominant positions of the legs, trunk, and arms. Questions about coexistent vertigo and giddiness should be asked. If present, one proceeds as outlined above. It is good practice to watch while patients walk into the examining room, because they are apt to walk more naturally then than during special tests. They should be asked to stand with the feet together, head erect, with eyes first open and then closed. Swaying due to nervousness may be overcome by diverting the patient's attention as in asking the patient to touch the tip of the nose with the finger of first one hand and then the other. Next the patient should be asked to walk forward and backward, with the eyes first open and then closed. Any tendency to reel to one side, as in cerebellar disease, can be checked by having the patient walk around a chair. When the affected side is toward the chair, the patient tends to walk into it; when it is away from the chair, the patient veers outward in ever-widening circles. More delicate tests of gait are walking a straight line heel to toe or having the patient arise quickly from a chair, walk briskly, and then stop

or turn suddenly. If all these tests are successfully executed, it may be assumed that any difficulty in locomotion is not due to disease of the proprioceptive mechanisms or cerebellum. Detailed neurologic examination is then necessary in order to determine which of the many other possible diseases is responsible for the patient's disorder of gait.

The following abnormal gaits are so distinctive that with a little practice they can be recognized at a glance.

Cerebellar gait The main features of this gait are *wide base* (separation of legs), *unsteadiness, irregularity,* and *lateral reeling.* Steps are uncertain, some are shorter and others longer than intended, and the patient may lurch to one side or the other. The unsteadiness is more prominent on quickly arising from a chair and walking, on stopping suddenly while walking, or on turning abruptly. If the ataxia is severe, the patient cannot stand without assistance. If it is lesser in degree, standing with feet together and head erect, with eyes either open or closed, may be difficult. In its mildest form the ataxia is best demonstrated by having the patient walk a line heel to toe. After two or three steps there is loss of balance and the patient must place one foot to the side to avoid falling. Romberg's sign, i.e., marked swaying or falling with the eyes closed but not with the eyes open, is not a feature of cerebellar disease. Compensation may be effected by shortening the step and shuffling, i.e., keeping both feet simultaneously on the ground. The defect in the cerebellar gait is not in antigravity support, steppage, or propulsion but in the coordination of proprioceptive, labyrinthine, and visual information in reflex coordination of movements. The abnormality of gait may or may not be accompanied by other signs of cerebellar incoordination and intention tremor of the arms and legs. The presence of the latter signs depends on involvement of the superior midline structures as distinct from cerebellar hemispheres; if the lesion is unilateral, the signs are always on the same side.

Cerebellar gait is in some instances the major symptom in multiple sclerosis, cerebellar tumors, particularly medulloblastoma of the cerebellar vermis, paraneoplastic diseases, and the cerebellar degenerations. In certain forms of cerebellar degeneration (e.g., the type associated with chronic alcoholism) the disease process reaches a plateau and then remains stable for many years, and the gait disorder, in these circumstances, becomes altered to some extent. The base is wide and the steps are still short, but more regular; the trunk is inclined slightly forward, the arms are held away from the sides, and the gait assumes a somewhat rhythmic quality. In this way the patient can walk for long distances but lacks the capacity to make the necessary postural adjustments in response to sudden changes in position.

A slowness in muscle relaxation as in myxedema may also lead to a kind of gait disorder that simulates a cerebellar defect.

Gait of sensory ataxia This gait is due to an impairment of proprioception resulting from interruption of afferent nerve fibers in the peripheral nerves, posterior roots, posterior columns of the spinal cords, or medial lemnisci; it may also be produced occasionally by a lesion of both parietal lobes. Whatever the location of the lesion, the patient is deprived of knowledge of the position of the limbs. The principal features of the resulting gait disorder are *uncertainty, irregularity,* and the *stamp* of the feet. Hunt characterized this type of gait very well when he said that the ataxic patient is recognized by "his stamp and stick." More explicitly, there are varying degrees of difficulty in standing and walking, and in advanced cases a complete failure of locomotion, even though muscular power is retained. The legs are kept far apart to correct the instability, and the patient carefully watches the ground and the feet. As the patient steps out, the legs are flung abruptly forward and outward, often lifted higher than necessary. The steps are of variable length, and many are attended by an audible stamp as the foot is banged down on the floor. The body is held in a slightly flexed posture, and the weight may be supported on the cane that the severely ataxic patient usually carries. The incoordination is greatly exaggerated when the patient is deprived of visual cues, as in walking in the dark. Most patients, when asked to stand with feet together and eyes closed, show greatly increased swaying or actual falling (Romberg's sign). It has been said that a lame person whose shoes are not worn in any one place is probably suffering from sensory ataxia. There is invariably a loss of vibratory and position sense in the feet and legs. A disordered gait of this type is observed in tabes dorsalis, Friedreich's ataxia, subacute combined degeneration, syphilitic meningomyelitis, chronic polyneuritis, and those cases of multiple sclerosis in which posterior column disease predominates.

Hemiplegic and paraplegic (spastic) gait   In hemiplegia the leg is held stiffly and does not flex freely and gracefully at the knee and hip. It tends to rotate outward and describes a semicircle, first away from and then toward the trunk (circumduction). The foot scrapes along the floor, and the toe and outer side of the sole of the shoe are worn. One can diagnose the hemiplegic gait by hearing the slow rhythmic scuff of the foot along the floor. The other muscles of the body on the affected side are weak and stiff to a variable degree, particularly the arm, which is carried in a flexed position and does not swing naturally. This type of gait disorder is most frequently associated with vascular disease of the brain.

The spastic paraplegic gait is entirely different from the gait of sensory ataxia, though the two may be combined. Each leg is advanced slowly and stiffly with restricted motion at the knee and hip. The patient looks as though wading in water. The legs are extended or slightly bent at the knees and may be strongly adducted at the hips, tending almost to cross ("scissors" gait). The steps are regular and short. Movements of the legs are slow, and the patient may be able to advance only with great effort. An easy way to remember the main features of the hemiplegic and paraplegic gait is by the letter S, which begins each of its descriptive adjectives—spastic, slow, scuffing. The defect is in the stepping mechanism and in propulsion, not in support or equilibrium. Cerebral spastic diplegia, multiple sclerosis, syringomyelia, spinal syphilis, combined system disease, spinal cord compression, and familial spinal spastic ataxia are the common causes of spastic paraparesis.

Festinating gait   The term *festinating* comes from the Latin *festinare,* to hasten, and appropriately describes the involuntary increase or hastening of the gait that characterizes both paralysis agitans and postencephalitic Parkinson's syndrome (see Chap. 373). *Rigidity* and *shuffling,* in addition to *festination,* are the cardinal features of this gait. When they are joined to the typical tremors, rigidity, and slowness of movement, there can be little doubt as to the diagnosis.

The general attitude of the patient is one of flexion; rigidity and immobility of the body are other conspicuous features. There is a paucity of the automatic movements made in sitting, standing, and walking; the head does not turn in looking to one side, the arms are seldom folded, and the legs are rarely crossed. The arms are held stiffly as though in preparation for writing, and the facial expression is unblinking and masklike.

This slight, generalized stiffening is common in psychiatric patients treated with phenothiazine drugs.

In walking, the trunk is bent forward and the arms are carried ahead of the body and do not swing. The legs are stiff and bent at the knees and hips. The steps are short, and the feet barely clear the ground as the patient shuffles along. Once forward or backward locomotion is started, the upper part of the body advances ahead of the lower part, as though the patient were chasing the center of gravity. Steps become more and more rapid, and the patient may fall if not assisted. This is the festination, and it may occur when the patient is walking forward or backward, taking the form of either propulsion or retropulsion. The defect is in rocking the body from side to side so as to clear the floor and in moving the legs quickly enough to catch the center of gravity in forward propulsion. Other unusual gaits are sometimes observed in postencephalitic patients. For example, they may be unable to take the first step forward because they cannot lift one foot, or they may be unable to step forward until they hop or take one step backward; walking may be initiated by a series of short steps that give way to a more normal gait; occasionally such a patient may run better than walk or walk backwards better than forward. Choreoathetotic movements may be added to the festinating gait in the L-dopa-treated patient with Parkinson's disease.

Athetotic, dystonic, and choreic gaits   Diseases that are characterized by involuntary movements and abnormal postures seriously affect gait. In fact, a disturbance of gait may be the initial and dominant manifestation of these diseases, and the testing of gait often serves to provoke abnormalities of movement and posture that are otherwise not conspicuous. The *athetotic* patient often assumes the most grotesque postures. One arm may be held aloft and the other one behind the body with wrist and fingers alternately undergoing slow flexion, extension, and rotation. The head may be inclined in one direction, the lips alternately retract and then purse as part of a grimace, and the tongue intermittently protrudes from the mouth. The legs advance slowly and awkwardly, the result of superimposed involuntary movements and postures. Sometimes the foot is plantar-flexed at the ankle, and the weight is carried on the toes; or it may be dorsiflexed or inverted or flung to one side. This type of gait is typical of congenital athetosis and Huntington's chorea.

In *dystonia musculorum deformans* the first symptom may be a limp due to inversion or plantar flexion of the foot or a distortion of the pelvis. The patient stands with one leg rigidly extended or one shoulder elevated. The trunk may be in a position of exaggerated lordosis, and the hips are partly flexed, with a tilting forward of the pelvis. Because of the muscle spasms that deform the body in this manner, the patient may have to walk with knees flexed. The gait may seem normal as the first steps are taken, but as the patient walks, one or both legs become flexed, giving rise to the "dromedary gait." In the more advanced stages walking becomes impossible, owing to torsion of the trunk or the continuous flexion of one leg.

In *Sydenham's chorea* the gait is often bizarre (see Chap. 373). As the patient stands or walks, there is a continuous play of irregular "choreic" movements affecting the face, neck, hands, and, in the advanced stages, the large proximal joints and trunk. The positions of the trunk and upper parts of the body vary with each step. There are jerks of the head, grimacing, squirming, twisting movements of the trunk and limbs, and peculiar respiratory noises.

Drop-foot, steppage, or equine gait   This is caused by paralysis of the pretibial and peroneal muscles. The legs must be lifted abnormally high in order for the feet to clear the ground. There is a slapping noise as the foot strikes the floor. The anterior and lateral borders of the sole of the shoe become worn. The steps are regular and even; otherwise, walking is not remarkable. Foot drop may be unilateral or bilateral and occurs in diseases that affect the peripheral nerves of the legs or motor neurons in the spinal cord, such as poliomyelitis, progressive muscular atrophy, and Charcot-Marie-Tooth disease (peroneal muscular atrophy). It may also be observed in patients with peripheral types of muscular dystrophy. The most common cause of unilateral foot drop is compression of the anterior tibial nerve, where it crosses the head of the fibula (see Chap. 377).

Waddling gait This gait is characteristic of progressive muscular dystrophy. The attitude of the body may be straight, but more often the lumbar lordosis is accentuated. The steps are regular but a little uncertain. With each step there is an exaggerated elevation of one hip and depression of the other; once the weight is on the hip it yields to an abnormal degree, so that the upper trunk then inclines to that side. This alternation of lateral trunk movements results in the rolling gait, or *waddle*, a term suggested by Oppenheim. The gluteal musculature is weak and inefficient, although leg muscles may appear well developed. Muscular contractures leading to an equinovarus position of the foot may complicate childhood cases, so that the waddle is combined with circumduction of the legs and "walking on the toes."

Staggering or drunken gait This is characteristic of alcoholic and barbiturate intoxication. The drunken patient totters, reels, tips forward and then backward, threatening each moment to lose balance and fall. Control over trunk and legs is greatly impaired. The steps are irregular and uncertain. The patient appears stupefied and indifferent to the quality of performance, but under certain circumstances can momentarily correct the defect.

The frequently used adjectives *drunken* and *reeling* do not describe aptly the gait of cerebellar disease, except, perhaps, the most acute and severe cases. The intoxicated patient reels in many different directions, unlike the patient with cerebellar disease, and no effort is made to correct the staggering by watching the legs or the ground, as in cerebellar or sensory ataxia. In the drunken patient, despite a wide diversity of excursions of all parts of the body, balance may be exquisitely maintained. In contrast, patients with cerebellar disease have great difficulty in maintaining balance if they sway or lurch too far to one side.

Hysterical gait This may take one of several forms—monoplegic, paraplegic, or hemiplegic. The monoplegic or hemiplegic patient does not lift the foot from the floor while walking; instead, it is dragged as a useless member or pushed ahead as though it were a skate. The characteristic circumduction is absent in hysterical hemiplegia, and the typical hemiplegic posture, hyperactive tendon reflexes, and Babinski sign are missing. The hysterical paraplegic cannot very well drag both legs, and usually depends on a crutch or remains helpless in bed; the muscles may be rigid with pseudocontractures or flaccid. The gait may be quite dramatic. Some patients look as though they were walking on stilts, and others lurch wildly in all directions, actually demonstrating by their gyrations a remarkable ability to make rapid postural adjustments.

Astasia-abasia, in which the patient, though unable to either stand or walk, retains normal use of the legs while in bed, is nearly always hysterical. When such patients are placed on their feet, they take a few normal steps and then become unable to advance the feet; they lurch widly to and crumple to the floor if not assisted.

Frontal lobe ataxia Equilibrium and the capacity to stand and walk may be severely disturbed by diseases that affect the frontal lobes, particularly their medial parts. Although this disorder of gait is sometimes spoken of as an ataxia or as an *apraxia,* since the difficulty in walking cannot be accounted for by weakness or loss of sensation, it is probably neither. It most likely represents a loss of integration at the cortical and basal ganglionic level of the essential elements of stance and locomotion which were acquired in infancy and are often lost in senility.

These patients assume a posture of slight flexion, with the feet placed farther apart than normal. They advance slowly, with small, shuffling, hesitant steps. At times they halt, unable to advance without great effort, although they do much better with a little assistance. Turning is accomplished by a series of tiny, uncertain steps which are made with one foot, the other being planted on the floor as a pivot. The initiation of walking becomes progressively more difficult, and in advanced cases patients may be unable to take a step, as though the feet were glued to the floor. Finally they become unable to stand or even to sit, and without support fall backward or to one side.

Some patients are able to make complex movements with their legs, such as drawing imaginary figures, at a time when their gait is seriously impaired. Eventually, however, all movements of the legs become slow and awkward, and the limbs, when passively moved, offer variable resistance (gegenhalten). An inability to turn and sit in a chair or to lie down on a bed is highly characteristic, and may eventually become complete. These motor disabilities are usually associated with dementia, but there need be no parallelism in their evolution. Grasping, groping, hyperactive tendon reflexes, and Babinski signs may or may not be present. The end result in many cases is a "cerebral paraplegia in flexion" (Yakovlev), in which the patient lies curled up in bed, immobile and mute, the limbs fixed by contractures in an attitude of flexion.

Senile gait Elderly persons often complain of difficulty in walking, and examination may disclose no abnormality other than the slightly flexed posture of the senile and short uncertain steps, *marche à petit pas.* Speed, balance, and all the graceful, adaptive movements are lost. The exact nature of this gait disorder is not understood. Probably it is a combination frontal lobe and basal ganglionic defect. It should be noted, however, that a short-stepped, cautious gait lacks specificity, being a general defensive reaction to all forms of defective locomotion.

REFERENCES

ADAMS RD, VICTOR M: *Principles of Neurology.* New York, McGraw-Hill, 1977

DIX MR: Modern tests of vestibular function, with special reference to their value in clinical practice. Br Med J 3:317, 1969

18
COMMON DISTURBANCES OF VISION, OCULAR MOVEMENT, AND HEARING

MAURICE VICTOR
RAYMOND D. ADAMS

Diseases of the eyes and ears, by virtue of their frequency, unusual nature, and serious consequences, make up separate medical specialties and, therefore, fall outside the field of internal medicine. Yet disturbances of visual and auditory function may be the initial or leading manifestations of many systemic diseases. Of more general interest is the fact that these two senses represent the most finely developed parts of the entire afferent apparatus of the nervous system; hence the study of their disorders may yield important information about neurologic diseases.

THE EYE AND DISORDERS OF VISION

The eye, with its diverse epithelial, vascular, collagenous, neural, and pigmentary components, is a medical microcosm, susceptible to manifold diseases. Moreover, its transparency makes it accessible to direct inspection by the ophthalmoscope, an instrument found in the consulting room of every physician, and affords an opportunity to observe many of the specific lesions of medical diseases.

Since the eye is the organ of vision, it is obvious that impairment of visual acuity of varying degree should stand as the most frequent symptom of eye disease. Strabismus and diplopia, ocular pain, irritation, redness and photophobia, inability to read or recognize objects and people, and drooping or closure of the eyelids are also important. The impairment of eyesight may be unilateral or bilateral, sudden or gradual, episodic or enduring. The common causes vary with age. In late childhood and adolescence increasing difficulty in focusing the eyes and in seeing clearly usually can be traced to *myopia,* though an optic nerve disorder or suprasellar tumor must be excluded. In middle age *presbyopia* is almost invariable and requires refraction and eyeglasses. Still later in life *cataracts, glaucoma,* and *retinal hemorrhages* and *detachments* are the most frequent causes of visual disturbance. Episodic blindness in early life is usually due to migraine; later, amaurosis fugax is caused by stenosis of the carotid artery or cranial arteritis. Cerebrovascular disease deranges vision with increasing frequency in late life.

Thus failing eyesight may be due to an abnormality of the refractive media of the eye or to a lesion of the retina or optic nerve or the parts of the brain with which they are connected. In approaching this problem one begins always by inquiring as to precisely what patients mean when they say they cannot see properly, for they may be referring to symptoms as varied as excessive tearing, diplopia, partial syncope, or even giddiness or dizziness. Fortunately these statements can be checked by the measurement of visual acuity, a technique which is the single most important part of the ocular examination. If visual acuity is less than 20/20 and cannot be improved by refraction and if the media of the eye are transparent, there is some sensory defect, the nature of which must be ascertained.

In the measurement of visual acuity the *Snellen chart,* which contains rows of letters of diminishing size (those of each row subtending 5 min of an arc when held at various distances from the eye), is utilized. The letters at the top of the chart subtend 5 min of an arc at a distance of 200 ft; those at the bottom subtend an arc of 5 min at 20 ft. Thus if the patient can see only the top letters at 20 ft, rather than 200 ft, vision is 20/200; if those letters at the bottom are seen at this distance, the acuity is 20/20. The patient with a corrected refractive error should wear eyeglasses for the test; if the visual acuity is then less than 20/20, either the refractive error has not been properly corrected or there is some other reason for it. The former possibility can be ruled out if the patient sees clearly while looking through a pinhole of 2 to 3 mm in a cardboard with the glasses still on. The pinhole permits a narrow shaft of light to fall on the fovea without being refracted.

Light entering the eye is focused on the outer layer of the retina (the rods and cones). Consequently the media (tissues and fluids) through which the light passes must be transparent. These media are the cornea, the aqueous humor of the anterior chamber, the lens, the vitreous humor of the vitreous cavity, and the retina itself. The clarity of these media can be determined ophthalmoscopically, but this examination requires that the pupil be dilated to at least 6 mm in diameter. This is best accomplished by instilling a few drops of 10% phenylephrine (Neo-Synephrine) in each eye after the visual acuity is measured, the pupillary response recorded, and the intraocular pressure estimated. *An attack of angle-closure glaucoma may be precipitated by pupillary dilatation, but this happens rarely;* this complication should be treated by the intravenous administration of mannitol (50 g of a 20% solution) and oral administration of the carbonic anhydrase inhibitor, acetazolamide (Diamox, 250 mg qid), followed by the topical instillation of 4% pilocarpine. The cycloplegic action of phenylephrine lasts only an hour or two. Looking through a +6 ophthalmoscopic lens from a distance of 15 to 20 cm permits the visualization of any opacity in refractive media against the diffuse bright red of reflected light from the retina. By adjusting the lens of the ophthalmoscope from high + to 0 or −, one can "depth-focus" from the cornea to the retina. Clarity of all media means that reduced vision uncorrected by glasses must be due to a lesion in the macula, optic nerve, or structures further back in the visual system.

More specifically, the alterations in the refractile media that affect vision have certain medical implications, as follows.

CORNEAS In hypercalcemia secondary to sarcoid (Chap. 216), hyperparathyroidism (Chap. 350), and vitamin D intoxication (Chap. 351), calcium phosphates and carbonates precipitate, primarily beneath the corneal epithelium in a plane corresponding to the interpalpebral tissue—so-called *band keratopathy* (see Plate 7-8); cystine crystals are deposited in cystinosis (Chap. 90), cholesterol esters in hypercholesterolemia (*arcus senilis*) (Chap. 100), chloroquine crystals in treatment of discoid lupus by this drug, and copper in hepatolenticular degeneration [Kayser-Fleischer ring (Plate 8-8 and Chap. 95)]. Opacification of the cornea (keratitis) may also occur after herpes simplex and herpes zoster infections (Chaps. 193 and 185); or it may be combined with uveitis and iritis in Behçet's disease, Reiter's disease (Chap. 358), Stevens-Johnson disease (Chap. 67), and idiopathic infections, Keratitis may be a manifestation also of congenital syphilis (Chap. 146) and of more innocent states such as drying and injury of eyes during coma.

AQUEOUS HUMOR The common problem is one of high pressure due to impediment of the outflow of the aqueous fluid. This is termed *glaucoma.* In 90 percent of cases (of the wide-angle type) the cause is unknown; in 5 percent the angle between pupil and lateral cornea is narrow and blocked when the pupil is dilated; and in the remaining 5 percent the condition is secondary to some disease process that blocks outflow channels (inflammatory debris of uveitis, or red blood cells from hemorrhage in the anterior chamber, i.e., hyphema). Glaucoma occurs in 2 percent of all patients over the age of 40; it may be asymptomatic and go unrecognized for years before it progresses to rapid loss of vision. Therefore, the intraocular pressure should be measured routinely, using a Schiotz tonometer. This is a simple procedure which should be practiced by every physician. With the patient supine, a drop of local anesthetic is put into each eye and the tonometer is then placed on the cornea so that the instrument is perfectly vertical. When the tonometer is pressed against the eye, the scale is read and the units are converted into millimeters of mercury from the chart in the tonometer case. The normal pressure is about 15 mmHg. Pressures of 20 to 30 mmHg may damage the optic nerve, leading first to a nasal quadrant defect and finally to blindness. With the ophthalmoscope one can see also that the optic disk is excavated and, in some instances, atrophic (Plate 7-2).

THE LENS Opacities form in diabetes mellitus (Chap. 337) and galactosemia ("sugar cataracts") from sustained high levels of blood glucose and galactose, which are changed to sorbitol or dulcitol (the accumulation of which leads to a high osmotic gradient within the lens fibers); in hypoparathyroidism (Chap. 350), which by lowering the concentration of calcium in the aqueous humor opacifies newly forming lens fibers; after prolonged high doses of chlorpromazine and corticosteroid therapy, which are believed to result in lenticular opacities; and in myotonic dystrophy (Chap. 380), which is associated with a special type of cataract. Weakening of the zonular ligaments of the lens allows a dislocation (iridodenesis) in both Marfan's syndrome and homocystinuria (Plate 8-7 and Chap. 58).

VITREOUS HUMOR Hemorrhage may occur from rupture of a retinal vessel, causing a shower of black or red dots. It is also seen in diabetes mellitus, where it may occur following rupture of newly formed retinal vessels, i.e., *retinitis proliferans,* or after a retinal tear which may progress to retinal detachment. The vitreous humor may also be affected by deposition of calcium soaps (seen as small white opacities with the ophthalmoscope)—so-called "asteroid hyalosis" of diabetes mellitus.

RETINA AND OPTIC NERVE The search for neurologic explanations of reduced vision begins with an ophthalmoscopic examination of the retina. This thin (0.4 mm) sheet of transparent tissue and the optic nerve head into which the visual information is channeled are the only parts of the central nervous system that can be inspected during life.

Light entering the eye passes through the full thickness of the retina to reach the receptor layer of rods and cones. Impulses arising in these photoreceptors are transmitted via secondary neurons, the bipolar cells, to the innermost ganglion cell layer, the axons of which in turn travel through the optic nerve head, optic nerve, chiasm, and optic tracts to the lateral geniculate bodies. These retinal neurons normally acquire a myelin sheath only after piercing the lamina cribrosa. The macular region, which lies two disk diameters or 3 mm lateral to the optic disk, is the most sensitive part of the retina. The vascular supply comes from the ophthalmic branch of the internal carotid artery, which in turn gives origin to the central retinal artery. The latter, upon issuing from the optic disk, divides into four arterioles, which supply the four quadrants of the retina (Plate 7-1). The ganglion cells and bipolar cells receive their blood supply from these arterioles and their capillaries, whereas photoreceptor elements receive nourishment from the underlying choroidal vascular bed.

These small vessels react in disease states like vessels of corresponding size in the brain. Since the walls of the retinal arterioles are transparent to the ophthalmoscope, what is seen is a column of blood. In arteriosclerosis (usually coexistent with hypertension), the lumens of the vessels are narrowed because of fibrous tissue replacement of the media and thickening of the basement membrane. The light reflection from the vessel then has a different refractive index than the adjacent retinal tissue. Tortuosity of vessels, arteriole-venous compressions, and narrowed segments are other signs of hypertension and arteriolosclerosis. In malignant hypertension there are, in addition, cotton-wool exudates, splinter hemorrhages, and papilledema, changes that may also be present in the intracranial arterioles. Atheromatous deposits, which form in larger arteries, are observed in the retina only with extreme degrees of hyperlipemia because of the small size of the vessels. Occasionally atheromatous and other emboli from the carotid and aorta

may lodge in them. Capillary-venular aneurysms may develop, most often in diabetes mellitus (Plate 8-3). Since the central retinal vein and artery share a common adventitial sheath, atheromatous plaques in the artery may result in thrombosis of the vein. Round or oval hemorrhages always lie in the outer plexiform layer and linear or flame-shaped ones in the superficial layer of the retina, as occurs in conditions with extremely high intracranial pressure, such as ruptured intracranial saccular aneurysm and hemangioma; occasionally brain hemorrhage or cranial trauma permits blood to cover the retina and extend beneath the vitreous humor (subhyaloid hemorrhage).

The systemic coagulopathies of thrombotic thrombocytopenia and disseminated intravascular coagulopathy may cause clotting, preferentially in the submacular choriocapillaries. Sometimes this is associated with choroidal hemorrhage and detachment of the retina. The patient will complain of blurred vision because of a scotoma.

Aside from visible vascular lesions, other more specific alterations of the retina may impair vision. The most important of these are tears and separations and detachments and degenerations.

1 *Degeneration of the outer receptor layer and subjacent pigment epithelium* occurs as a hereditary trait in *retinitis pigmentosa* (Plate 7-7), and also in Laurence-Moon-Biedl syndrome, progressive ophthalmoplegia, Bassen-Kornzweig disease (Chap. 100), Refsum's disease (Chap. 377), Batten-Mayou juvenile lipid storage disease, and idiopathic senile macular degeneration (Chaps. 100 and 373).
2 *Degeneration in Bruch's membrane* (which supports the layer of pigment epithelium next to the rods and cones) and its repair by fibrosis give rise to angioid streaks (Plate 7-4) typical of pseudoxanthoma elasticum (Chap. 363), Paget's disease (Chap. 353), hyperphosphatemia, and acromegaly.
3 *Deposits of phenothiazine conjugate with the melanin* of the pigment layer result in degeneration of the outer retinal layers. When these drugs are used, the doses should be kept low and the central visual fields tested with small colored test objects.

Sarcoidosis, toxoplasmosis, and *histoplasmois* involve both the retina and the choroid. The latter is the site of noninfective inflammatory reactions, often in association with iridocyclitis.

The optic nerves, chiasm, and tracts which constitute the third visual neuron can be inspected only in part, from the foveal or macular region to the optic disk. The latter reflects raised intracranial pressure (papilledema or choked disk), papillitis (disease of the optic nerve close to the disk), optic nerve atrophy, and glaucoma (Plates 7-2, 7-5, and 7-6).

Central visual disturbances (caused by defects in the retina, optic nerves and tracts, lateral geniculate bodies, geniculocalcarine path, and striate cortex of occipital lobes) are evidenced by changes in the visual fields. In good light, if one of the patient's eyes is covered and the other aligned with the corresponding eye of the examiner and a cottom pledget or white disk on a stick is brought from the outside toward the center, the periphery of the patient's visual field can be compared with that of the examiner. The types of visual field defect resulting from lesions in different parts of the visual pathways are shown in Fig. 18-1. A prechiasmal lesion causes either a scotoma (an island of impaired vision within the visual field) or a cut in the peripheral part of the visual field. A small scotoma in the macular part of the visual field may seriously impair visual acuity in the early stages of macular disease, giving rise to a central scotoma; patients may complain of distortion of vision, particularly for straight lines (metamorphopsia). One may test for this at the bedside by asking the patient to look at the center of a checkerboard or a jigsaw puzzle. The straight lines in the center appear curved or kinked. Metamorphopsia is diagnostic of retinal disease and aids in the distinction between a macular lesion and one in the optic nerve or occipital lobe. Demyelinative, toxic (methyl alcohol, quinine, and certain of the phenothiazine tranquilizing drugs), nutritional (so-called "tobacco-alcohol" amblyopia), and vascular diseases are the usual causes of scotomas. The toxic states are characterized by symmetric bilateral scotomas, and the nutritional disorders by more or less symmetric central scotomas (involving the fixation point) or centrocecal scotomas (involving both the fixation point and the blind spot). These latter scotomas are predominantly in the distribution of the papillomacular bundle, but their presence does not establish whether the primary effect is on the nerve fibers or the ganglion cells. Demyelinative diseases are characterized by unilateral or asymmetric bilateral scotomas. If the lesion is near the optic disk, there may be swelling of the optic nerve head, i.e., *papillitis,* which can usually be distinguished from papilledema by the marked impairment of vision it produces. Vascular lesions as a rule give rise to unilateral scotomas. The lesions take the form of retinal hemorrhages, hard exudates, or occluded vessels which cause infarction of the retina. The common cotton-wool patches are in reality small retinal infarcts. Large zones of retinal infarction may follow occlusion of a branch of the central retinal artery (Plates 8-1, 8-2, 8-4, and 8-5).

FIGURE 18-1

Diagram showing the effects on the fields of vision produced by lesions at various points along the optic pathway. A. Complete blindness in left eye. B. Bitemporal hemianopsia. C. Nasal hemianopsia of left eye. D. Right homonymous hemianopsia. E and F. Right upper and lower quadrant hemianopsia. G. Right homonymous hemianopsia with preservation of central vision. (From Homans, A Textbook of Surgery, Springfield, Ill, Charles C Thomas, 1945.)

Ischemic optic neuropathy is another well-recognized entity. The onset is abrupt, usually in an elderly person. It may be painful. Vision may be abolished completely, or there may be an altitudinal or segmental defect in one eye. Examination of the fundus may show no abnormality, but later the optic disk may become pale; rarely there is congestion, hemorrhage, and swelling of the disk. The pathologic basis of this disturbance is thrombosis or embolism of the posterior ciliary artery. If preceded by headache, pain on chewing, and arthralgia, the diagnosis is usually temporal arteritis. Both eyes may be affected simultaneously or in succession. Prognosis for recovery of vision is poor. Fluorescein retinography (see below) is a valuable method for revealing retinal vascular abnormalities.

Another common defect encountered on visual field examination is concentric constriction. This may be due to papilledema, in which case it is usually accompanied by an enlargement of the blind spot. A concentric constriction of the visual field, at first unilateral and later bilateral, and pallor of the optic disks (optic atrophy) should suggest chronic syphilitic meningo-optic neuritis. Glaucoma is another cause of this type of field defect. Tubular vision, i.e., constriction of the visual field to the same degree regardless of the distance of the visual test stimulus from the eye, is a sign of hysteria. In organic disease, for example, chorioretinitis, the area of the constricted visual field naturally enlarges as the distance between the patient and the stimulus increases.

With most diseases of the optic nerve, the nerve will eventually become pale (optic atrophy). This may require several weeks or months to occur, as illustrated by the delay between the sudden blindness of a traumatic severance of one optic nerve and the pallor. If the optic nerve degenerates [e.g., in multiple sclerosis, Leber's hereditary optic atrophy (Chap. 373), or syphilitic optic atrophy], the disk becomes chalk-white, with sharp, clean margins. If the atrophy is secondary to papillitis or papilledema, the margins are obscure and irregular, with pigment deposits in the adjacent retina.

Hemianopsia means blindness in one-half of the visual field. *Bitemporal hemianopsia* indicates a lesion of the decussating nasal retinal fibers of the optic chiasm and is due usually to tumor of the pituitary gland or of the infundibulum or third ventricle, to meningioma of the diaphragm of the sella, or occasionally to a large suprasellar aneurysm of the circle of Willis. *Homonymous hemianopsia* (a loss of vision in corresponding halves of the visual fields) signifies a lesion of the visual pathway behind the chiasm and, if *complete,* gives no more information than that. *Incomplete homonymous hemianopsia* has more localizing value: if the field defects in the two eyes are identical (*congruous*), the lesion is likely to be in the calcarine cortex; if *incongruous,* the visual fibers in the parietal or temporal lobe are more likely to be implicated. Since the fibers from the peripheral lower quadrants of the retina extend for a variable distance into the temporal lobe, lesions of this lobe may be accompanied by a homonymous upper quadrantic field defect. Parietal lobe lesions may affect the lower quadrants more than the upper.

If the entire optic tract or calcarine cortex on one side is destroyed, there is complete homonymous hemianopsia, including that part of the field supplied by the macula. Incomplete lesions of the optic tract and radiation usually spare central (macular) vision. Apparent macular sparing is frequently due to imperfect fixation of gaze. A lesion of the tip of one occipital lobe produces central homonymous hemianopsia because half the macular fibers of both eyes terminate there. Lesions of both occipital poles (as in embolization of the posterior cerebral arteries) result in bilateral central scotomas; if all the calcarine cortex on both sides is completely destroyed, there is "cortical" blindness. Altitudinal or horizontal hemianopsias are more often due to lesions of the occipital lobes below or above the calcarine sulcus than to lesions of the optic chiasm.

In addition to blindness, i.e., "visual anesthesia," there is another category of visual impairment, which consists of a defect of visual perception, i.e., *visual agnosia*. These patients can see but cannot recognize objects unless they hear, smell, taste, or palpate them. The failure of visual recognition of words alone is called *alexia*. The ability to recognize visually presented objects and words depends upon the integrity not only of the visual pathways and primary areas of the cerebral cortex but also of those secondary and tertiary visual cortical areas which lie just anterior to them and the angular gyrus of the dominant hemisphere. Visual-object agnosia and alexia result from lesions of these latter areas or from a lesion of the left calcarine cortex combined with one which interrupts the fibers crossing from the right occipital lobe. These subjects are discussed further in Chaps. 19 and 25.

Other disturbances of vision include various types of distortion in which the perceived objects appear too small (micropsia), too large (macropsia), or askew. If this disturbance is in only one eye, a local retinal lesion should be suspected. When bilateral, such phenomena suggest disease of the temporal lobes, in which case the visual disturbances tend to occur in attacks and are accompanied by complex visual hallucinations and other manifestations of temporal lobe seizures (Chap. 23).

The optic nerves also contain the afferent fibers for the pupillary reflexes. These fibers leave the optic tract and terminate in the pretectal region of the midbrain. A lesion of the optic nerve or tracts may abolish the pupillary light reflex; the pupil is dilated and unreactive. Cerebral lesions, on the other hand, leave the pupillary light reflex unaltered. The lack of direct reflex in the blind eye and of consensual reflex in the sound one means that the afferent limb of the reflex arc (optic nerve) is the site of the lesion. A lack of direct light reflex with retention of the consensual reflex places the lesion in the efferent limb of the reflex (the homolateral oculomotor nucleus or nerve). Loss of light reflex without visual impairment or ocular palsy (Argyll Robertson pupillary phenomenon) is thought to be due to a lesion in the superior colliculi or periaqueductal region (see "Alterations of Pupils," below).

Amaurosis refers to blindness from any cause. *Amblyopia* refers to an impairment or loss of vision which is not due to an error of refraction or to other disease of the eye. *Nyctalopia* means poor twilight or night vision and is associated with either vitamin A deficiency or pigmentary degenerations of the retina.

Papilledema (choked disk) refers to venous congestion and edema and elevation of disk margins. The depression of the optic disk is obliterated. The elevation ranges from 1 to 4 mm and when extreme may be surrounded by hemorrhages. Visual acuity is little affected until late, except for constriction of visual fields and enlargement of blind spots, which is in contrast to papillitis where visual loss occurs early. The cause is raised intracranial pressure (tumors, abscesses, hemorrhages) which is transmitted to the subarachnoid space around optic nerves. This leads, after some days, to obstruction of venous outflow from the retinas, usually more so on the side of the lesion (see Plates 7-3 and 8-6).

Minor degrees of disk swelling are difficult to distinguish from the disk of the normal hyperopic eye. Lack of vein pulsation suggests increased pressure. Fluorescein retinography reveals early papilledema by the leakage of the dye into the disk and surrounding retina. Myelination of optic nerve fibers and drusen must not be confused with papilledema.

In the analysis of retinal, optic nerve and tract, and geniculocalcarine lesions, two other techniques are especially valuable—the electroretinogram (ERG) and the patterned stimulus visual-evoked responses (VER) to light flash. The human ERG is a mass response that is reduced only in diseases of the retina.

The VER provides evidence of the speed of visual impulse conduction between the retina and occipital lobe. With diseases of the optic nerve, even with normal visual acuity and a normal appearance of the retina, it may be abnormal.

DIPLOPIA, STRABISMUS, AND DISORDERS OF THE THIRD, FOURTH, AND SIXTH NERVES *Strabismus* (squint) refers to a muscle imbalance that results in improper alignment of the two eyes. It may be due to paralysis of an eye muscle or the ocular deviation resulting from the unrestrained activity of the opposing muscle; or it may be due to inequality of tone in the muscles that yoke the two eyes together in a central position. The former is called *paralytic strabismus* and is primarily a neurologic problem; the latter is *nonparalytic strabismus* (referred to as comitant strabismus if the angle between the visual axes is the same in all fields of gaze) and is an ophthalmologic problem. Once binocular fusion is established, any type of ocular muscle imbalance causes diplopia, for the reason that images then fall on disparate or noncorresponding parts of the two retinas. After a time, however, the patient learns to suppress the image of one eye. This almost invariably happens early in comitant strabismus of congenital nature, and the person may then have a diminished visual acuity in that eye (*amblyopia ex anopsia*). The vision may remain normal in both eyes when the eyes are used alternately for fixation; this is *alternating strabismus*.

The oculomotor, trochlear, and abducens nerves innervate the extrinsic musculature of the eye. A knowledge of their origin and anatomic relationships is essential to an understanding of the various paralytic ocular syndromes. The oculomotor nucleus consists of several groups of nerve cells ventral to the aqueduct of Sylvius, at the level of the superior colliculi. All nuclear neurons send fibers to the ipsilateral eye except those innervating the superior rectus muscle, which are contralateral like those of the trochlear nucleus. The nerve cells that innervate the iris and ciliary body are situated dorsally in the so-called "Edinger-Westphal nucleus." Ventral to this nucleus are the cells for the levator of the lid, superior and inferior recti, inferior oblique, and medial rectus muscles, in this dorso-ventral order. Convergence is under the control of an unpaired medial group of cells. The cells of origin of the trochlear nerves are just inferior to those of the oculomotor nerves. The sixth nerve arises at a considerably lower level, from a paired group of cells in the floor of the fourth ventricle at the level of the lower pons. The intrapontine portion of the facial nerve loops around the sixth nerve nucleus before it turns anterolaterally to make its exit; a lesion in this locality usually causes a homolateral paralysis of both the lateral rectus and facial muscles.

All three nerves, after leaving the brainstem, course anteriorly and pass through the cavernous sinus, where they come into close proximity with the ophthalmic division of the fifth nerve, and together they enter the orbit through the superior orbital fissure. The oculomotor nerve supplies all the extrinsic ocular muscles except two—the superior oblique and the external rectus—which are innervated by the trochlear and the abducens nerves, respectively. The levator palpebrae muscle is also supplied by the oculomotor nerve, the involuntary part being under the control of autonomic fibers. Parasympathetic fibers of the oculomotor nerve supply the sphincter pupillae and the ciliary muscles (muscles of accommodation).

Although all the extraocular muscles probably participate in every movement of the eyes, particular muscles move the eyes in certain fields. The lateral rectus deviates the eye outward; the medial rectus, inward. The function of the vertical recti and the oblique muscles varies according to the position of the eye. When the eye is turned outward, the elevators and depressors of the eye are the superior and inferior recti; when the eye is turned inward, they are the inferior and superior oblique muscles, respectively. In contrast, torsion of the eyeball is effected by the oblique muscles when the eye is turned outward.

Accurate binocular vision is achieved by the associated action of the ocular muscles, which allows a visual stimulus to fall on exactly corresponding parts of the two retinas. Conjugate movement of the eyes is controlled by centers in the cerebral cortex and brainstem. Area 8 in the frontal lobe is the center for voluntary conjugate movements of the eyes to the opposite side. In addition, there is a center in the occipital lobe concerned with contralateral following movements. Fibers from these centers pass to the opposite sides of the brainstem, where they connect with lower centers for conjugate movements: those for right lateral gaze are thought to be in the proximity of the right abducens nucleus; those for left lateral gaze are near the left abducens. Simultaneous innervation of one internal rectus and the other external rectus during lateral gaze is mediated through the medial longitudinal fasciculus which connects one abducens nucleus with the opposite oculomotor nucleus. The arrangements of nerve cells and fibers for vertical gaze and convergence are situated in the pretectal areas and paramedian zones of the midbrain tegmentum.

The coordination of eye movement by those cerebral and brainstem structures involves the interaction of five physiologic systems: those for voluntary, saccadic, pursuit, vergence, and vestibular and fixation. The clinical importance of this subdivision relates to the fact that each system may be affected independently by disease (Bach-y-Rita and Collins).

OCULAR MUSCLE AND GAZE PALSIES   There are three types of paralysis of extraocular muscles: (1) paralysis of isolated ocular muscles, (2) paralysis of conjugate movements (gaze), and (3) syndromes of mixed gaze and ocular muscle paralysis.

Characteristic clinical disturbances result from single lesions of the third, fourth, or sixth cranial nerves. A complete third nerve lesion causes ptosis (since the levator palpebrae is supplied mainly by the third nerve), an inability to turn the eye upward, downward, or inward; a divergent strabismus due to unopposed action of the lateral rectus muscle; a dilated nonreactive pupil (iridoplegia); and paralysis of accommodation (cycloplegia). When only the muscles of the iris and ciliary body are paralyzed, the condition is termed *internal ophthalmoplegia.* Fourth nerve lesions result in an extorsion of the eye and a weakness of downward gaze most marked when the eye is

TABLE 18-1
Comparison of lesions within and outside the brainstem

Effect	Lesions within the brainstem	Lesions external to the brainstem
Involvement of multiple contiguous nerves	±	+
Involvement of sensorimotor tracts	+, often "alternating" or crossed sensory motor palsies	±
Disturbance of consciousness	+	0 (+ late)
Evidence of other segmental disturbances of the brainstem such as decerebrate rigidity, tonic neck reflexes, pseudobulbar palsy	+	0 (+ late)
X-ray evidence of erosion of cranial bones or enlargement of foramens	0	+

turned inward, so that patients commonly complain of special difficulty in going downstairs. Head tilting, to the opposite shoulder, is especially characteristic of a fourth nerve lesion. Such patients may also have difficulty in reading with their bifocal glasses. When the difficulty is bilateral, there is often a V-pattern isotropia that is most marked on looking down and minimal on looking up. The patient compensates for this by keeping the chin down to minimize the diplopia. This maneuver puts the eye in a position where the superior oblique is relaxed, thereby facilitating binocular vision. Lesions of the sixth nerve result in paralysis of abduction and a convergent strabismus, owing to the unopposed action of the internal rectus muscles. With incomplete sixth nerve palsies, turning the head toward the side of the paretic muscle may overcome diplopia by relaxing the affected lateral rectus muscle. (The foregoing signs may occur with various degrees of completeness, depending on the severity and site of the lesion or lesions.)

Ocular palsies may be central, i.e., due to a lesion of the nucleus or the intramedullary portion of the cranial nerve, or peripheral. Opthalmoplegia due to a lesion in the brainstem is usually accompanied by involvement of other cranial nerves or long tracts. Peripheral lesions, which may or may not be solitary, have a great variety of causes; the most common are *aneurysm of the circle of Willis,* tumors of the base of the brain, carcinomatosis of the meninges, herpes zoster, *syphilitic* and other chronic forms of *meningitis.* A practical rule is that any nontraumatic oculomotor palsy with a dilated, unreactive pupil will usually be traced to a tumor or aneurysm. The third nerve palsy that occurs with diabetes is most often due to infarction of the third nerve, and the prognosis for recovery in such cases, as with other nonprogressive diseases of the peripheral nerve, is usually excellent. The points of difference between lesions within and outside the brainstem are tabulated in Table 18-1, and the various intramedullary and extramedullary cranial nerve syndromes are described in Tables 376-1 and 376-2. See also the diagrams in Chap. 365.

Paralysis of conjugate movement (gaze)   The term *conjugate gaze,* or *conjugate movement,* refers to the simultaneous movement of the two eyes in the same direction. An acute lesion, such as an infarct, in one frontal lobe may cause paralysis of contralateral gaze, and the eyes will turn toward the side of the lesion. The ocular disorder in this circumstance is temporary (several days' duration). In bilateral frontal lesions the patient may be unable to turn the eyes voluntarily in any direction—up, down, or to the side—but retains fixation and following movements, which are believed to be occipital lobe functions. Gaze paralysis of cerebral origin is not attended by strabismus or diplopia. The usual causes are vascular occlusion with infarction, hemorrhage, and abscess or tumor of the frontal lobe. With certain extrapyramidal disorders, e.g., postencephalitic parkinsonism, Huntington's chorea, and progressive supranuclear palsy, ocular movements may be limited in all directions, especially upward. Lesions of the superior colliculi and tegmentum, near the posterior commissure, interfere with voluntary upward gaze, and often movements of convergence as well as the pupillary light reflex are abolished (Parinaud's syndrome). There also exists a pontine center for conjugate lateral gaze, probably in the vicinity of the abducens nucleus. A lesion here causes ipsilateral gaze palsy, with the eyes turning to the opposite side. Vertical and lateral gaze palsies are combined in Steele-Richardson disease. The palsy is persistent, unlike that of cerebral lesions, and is frequently accompanied by other signs of midbrain disease. Fully developed forms of gaze paralysis are readily discerned, but lesser degrees may be overlooked unless one pays special attention to the predominant position of the eyes at rest and the ability to sustain conjugate movement.

Ocular apraxia is another special gaze disorder. Normally, on looking to the side, the eyes and head turn together, but in this condition the head turns and the eyes actually go in the opposite direction. The head is flung too far, in order not to lose sight of the target, and then the eyes "catch up." This may be a solitary congenital abnormality (Cogan), the anatomy of which is unknown, or it may be acquired as in ataxia telangiectasia (see Chap. 374).

In skew deviation, a poorly understood disorder of gaze, the eyes diverge, one looking down, the other up. The deviation is constant in all fields of gaze. It may occur with any lesion of the posterior fossa but particularly with one in the brainstem. The lesion is on the side of the lower eye.

Mixed gaze and ocular paralyses These are always a sign of intrapontine or mesencephalic disease. A lesion of the lower pons in or near the sixth nerve nucleus causes a homolateral paralysis of the lateral rectus muscle and a failure of adduction of the opposite eye, i.e., a combined paralysis of the sixth nerve and of conjugate lateral gaze. Lesions of the medial longitudinal fasciculi interfere with lateral conjugate gaze in another way. When the patient looks to the right, the left eye fails to adduct; when looking to the left, the right eye fails to adduct. The abducting eye may show nystagmus. This condition is referred to as *internuclear ophthalmoplegia* and should always be suspected when only adduction of the eyes is affected. It may be unilateral or bilateral. If unilateral, the lesion is always on the side of the weak adducting eye. If the lesion is in higher (midbrain) part of the medial longitudinal fasciculus, convergence may be lost, occurring with paralysis of the medial recti on attempted lateral gaze (anterior internuclear ophthalmoplegia); if the lesion is in the lower (pontine) part, convergence is normal, but there may be some degree of associated limitation of conjugate lateral gaze or sixth nerve palsy (posterior internuclear opthalmoplegia).

NYSTAGMUS AND OTHER INVOLUNTARY EYE MOVEMENTS
Nystagmus refers to involuntary rhythmic movements of the eyes. It is usually subdivided into two types, oscillating (pendular) and rhythmic (jerk). Although practical, this classification is an oversimplification. In jerk nystagmus, the movements are distinctly faster in one direction than the other; in pendular nystagmus, the oscillations are roughly equal in rate for the two directions, although on conjugate lateral gaze the pendular type may resemble the jerk type, with the fast component to the side of the gaze.

In testing for nystagmus, the eyes should first be examined in the central position and then during upward, downward, and lateral movements. If nystagmus is monocular, each eye should be tested separately, with the other one covered. Labyrinthine nystagmus is most obvious when visual fixation is prevented by shielding the eyes; and brainstem nystagmus and cerebellar nystagmus are brought out best by having the patient fixate on a finger. Labyrinthine nystagmus may vary with the position of the head; hence, these various tests should be performed with the head in several different positions. In particular, the postural nystagmus of Bárány is evoked by hyperextension of the neck, with the patient supine. A series of moving visual stimuli also evoke nystagmus. This optokinetic nystagmus should be tested by asking the patient to look at a rotating cylinder on which several stripes have been painted or at a striped cloth moved across the field of vision.

A few irregular jerks are observed in many normal individuals when the eyes are turned far to the side. These so-called "nystagmoid movements" are probably similar to the tremulousness of a muscle that is contracted maximally. Occasionally a fine rhythmic nystagmus may be found in extreme lateral gaze, but if it is bilateral and disappears as the eyes move a few degrees toward the midline, it usually has no clinical significance.

Pendular nystagmus is found in a variety of conditions in which central vision is lost early in life, such as albinism and in various other diseases of the retina and refractive media. Occasionally it is observed in patients with multiple sclerosis and as a congenital abnormality, even without poor vision. The syndrome of miners' nystagmus, formerly a common cause of industrial disability, occurs after many years of work in comparative darkness. The oscillations of the eyes are very rapid, increase on upward gaze, and are often associated with vertigo, head tremor, and intolerance of light.

Jerk nystagmus is the commoner type. It may be lateral or vertical, particularly on ocular movement in these planes, or it may be rotary. By custom, the direction of the nystagmus is named according to the direction of the fast component. There are several varieties of jerk nystagmus. When one is watching a moving object—e.g., the passing landscape from a train window or a rotating drum with vertical stripes— rhythmic jerk nystagmus, *optokinetic nystagmus,* normally appears. The slow phase is a result of visual fixation; the quick phase is compensatory. With unilateral cerebral lesions, particularly in the parietooccipital region, optokinetic nystagmus is lost when the moving stimulus, e.g., the drum, moves toward the side of the lesion.

Aside from optokinetic nystagmus, lateral and vertical nystagmus are most frequently due to barbiturate intoxication. Jerk nystagmus may signify disease of the labyrinthine-vestibular apparatus. Labyrinthine stimulation or irritation by cold water in the external auditory meatus produces a nystagmus with the fast phase to the opposite side. The slow component reflects the effect of impulses derived from the semicircular canals, and the fast component is a corrective movement. Vestibular-labyrinthine nystagmus may be horizontal, vertical, or, most characteristically, rotary. Vertigo, nausea, vomiting, and staggering are the usual accompaniments (Chap. 14). Brainstem lesions often cause a coarse unidirectional nystagmus, which may be horizontal or vertical; the latter is brought out usually on upward gaze and rarely on downward gaze. The presence of vertical nystagmus is pathognomic of disease in the tegmentum of the brainstem and possibly of cerebellar connections. Vertigo is inconstant, and signs of disease of other nuclear structures and tracts in the brainstem are frequent. Upward jerk nystagmus of this type is frequent in demyelinative or vascular disease, in tumors, and in Wernicke's disease and syringobulbia. Vertical downward nystagmus is most often associated with lesions at the cervicomedullary junction, such as meningeal cysts, meningiomas, and the Arnold-Chiari malformation. Cerebellopontine angle tumors cause a coarse bilateral horizontal nystagmus, coarser to the side of the lesion. We have also observed nystagmus with a single lesion of the inferior cerebellar hemisphere. Periodic alternating nystagmus (horizontal nystagmus on straight-ahead gaze in one direction for 1 or 2 min and then reversing direction) has been observed with lesions of the fastigial nuclei and flocculonodular lobe of the cerebellum. The nystagmus that occurs only in the abducting eye and is said to be a pathognomonic sign of multiple sclerosis probably represents an incompletely developed form of internuclear opthalmoplegia.

Convergence nystagmus is a rhythmic oscillation in which a quick movement of adduction is followed by a slow abduction of the eyes in respect to each other. It is usually accompanied by other types of nystagmus and by one or more features of Parinaud's syndrome. Occasionally there is also a rhythmic retraction movement of the eyes (*nystagmus retractorius*) or eyelids, or a maintained spasm of convergence, best brought out on attempted elevation of the eyes to command. These unusual phenomena all point to a lesion of the upper midbrain tegmentum and are usually manifestations of vascular disease or of pinealoma. *Seesaw nystagmus*—one eye moving up, the other down—is occasionally observed in conjunction with bitemporal hemianopia. Its mechanism is unknown. In children it occurs with gliomas of the optic chiasm; in adolescents and adults it is most frequent with craniopharyngiomas and pituitary adenomas.

Oscillopsia refers to illusory movement of the environment, in which objects seem to move back and forth, to jerk, or to wiggle. It may or may not occur with turning of the eyes and consequent displacement of the image on the retina. Such movement of all objects in the environment appears with coarse central nystagmus or opsoclonus. Movement or distortion of position of single visualized objects may be part of a metamorphopsia from cerebral lesions.

Opsoclonus is the term applied to either sustained, irregular, conjugate "dancing" movements of the eyes in a horizontal, rotary, and vertical direction or a fast-frequency flutter. The neurologic basis for these movements is not clear, but in most cases they are associated with signs of cerebellar disease, a viral infection, or occult neuroblastoma. In some viral infections causing stupor or coma, the eye movements are constant and chaotic. Slow downward movement of both eyes with a fast upward movement (called "ocular bobbing" by Fisher) is characteristic of pontine lesions such as hypertensive hemorrhage.

Ocular dysmetria consists of an overshoot of the eyes on attempted fixation, followed by several cycles of oscillations of diminishing amplitude until precise fixation is attained. The overshoot may occur on eccentric fixation or on refixation in the primary position of gaze. This sign occurs in disease of the cerebellum or its pathways and is analogous to cerebellar dysmetria of the limbs.

ALTERATIONS OF PUPILS   Pupil size is determined by the balance of innervation between the dilator and constrictor fibers. The pupillodilator fibers arise in the posterior part of the hypothalamus and descend in the lateral tegmentum of the midbrain, pons, medulla, and cervical spinal cord to the eighth cervical and first thoracic segments, where they synapse with the lateral horn cells. These give rise to preganglionic fibers that synapse in the superior cervical ganglion; the postganglionic fibers course along the internal carotid artery and traverse the cavernous sinus to join the first division of the trigeminal nerve, finally reaching the eyes as the long ciliary nerves. The pupilloconstrictor fibers arise in the nucleus of Edinger-Westphal, join the oculomotor nerve, and synapse in the ciliary ganglion with the postganglionic neurons that innervate the iris and ciliary body.

The pupils are usually equal in size, though if the eyes are turned to one side, the pupil of the abducting eye dilates slightly. Pupil size varies with light intensity; as one pupil constricts under a bright light (direct reflex), the other unexposed pupil does likewise (consensual reflex). Pupillary constriction is also part of the act of convergence and accommodation for near objects.

Interruption of the sympathetic fibers either centrally, between the hypothalamus and their point of exit from the spinal cord (first thoracic segment), or peripherally (superior or cervical ganglion in the neck or along the carotid artery) results in miosis and ptosis (because of paralysis of Müller's muscle), with loss of sweating of the face, and occasionally enophthalmos (Bernard-Horner syndrome). Stimulation or irritation of the pupillodilator fibers has the opposite effect, i.e., lid retraction, slight proptosis, and dilatation of the pupil. The ciliospinal pupillary reflex, evoked by pinching the neck, is effected

through these efferent sympathetic fibers. Abnormal dilatation of the pupils (mydriasis), often with loss of pupillary light reflexes, may result from midbrain lesions and is a frequent finding in cases of deep coma. Extreme constriction of the pupils (miosis) is commonly observed with pontine lesions, presumably because of bilateral interruption of the pupillodilator fibers.

The functional integrity of the sympathetic and parasympathetic nerve endings in the iris may be determined by the use of certain drugs. Atropine and homatropine dilate the pupils by paralyzing the parasympathetic nerve endings; physostigmine and pilocarpine constrict them, the former by inhibiting cholinesterase activity at the neuromuscular junction, and the latter by direct stimulation of the sphincter muscle of the iris. Cocaine dilates the pupils by preventing the reuptake of norepinephrine into the nerve endings. Morphine acts centrally to constrict the pupils.

In chronic syphilitic meningitis and other forms of late syphilis, particularly tabes dorsalis, the pupils are usually small, irregular, and unequal; they do not dilate properly in response to mydriatic drugs and fail to react to light, although they do constrict on accommodation. In some cases there is an associated atrophy of the iris. This is known as the *Argyll Robertson pupil*. The exact locality of the lesion is not certain; it is generally believed to be in the tectum of the midbrain proximal to the oculomotor nuclei, where the descending pupillodilator fibers are in close proximity to the light-reflex fibers. A dissociation of the light reflex from the accommodation-convergence reaction is sometimes observed with other midbrain lesions, e.g., pinealoma, multiple sclerosis, and diabetes mellitus; in these diseases miosis, irregularity of pupils, and failure to respond to a mydriatic are not constantly present. However, in the usual Argyll Robertson pupillary abnormality of tabes and of diabetic and amyloid polyneuropathy the lesion is probably peripheral, in the oculomotor nerve or ciliary ganglion. Another interesting pupillary abnormality is the myotonic reaction, sometimes referred to as *Adie's pupil*. The patient may complain of blurring of vision or may have suddenly noticed that one pupil is larger than the other. The reaction to light and convergence are absent if tested in the customary manner, although the size of the pupil will change slowly on prolonged stimulation. Once contracted or dilated, the pupils remain in that state for some minutes. The affected pupil reacts promptly to the usual mydriatic and miotic drugs but is usually sensitive to a $\frac{1}{16}\%$ solution of pilocarpine or a 2.5% solution of methacholine (Mecholyl), a strength that will not affect a normal pupil. The myotonic pupil usually appears during the third or fourth decade of life; it may be associated with absence of knee or ankle jerks and hence be mistaken for tabes dorsalis.

Ocular movement, pupillary contraction, and visual acuity may be affected by diseases which alter the contents of the orbit. Usually this is accompanied by bilateral exophthalmos, as in thyroid or pituitary disease (Chap. 334). Unilateral exophthalmos may occur with orbital tumors (dermoids, adenoma of lacrimal gland, optic nerve glioma, neurofibroma, metastatic carcinoma, meningioma) or granuloma, or cavernous sinus thrombosis (Chap. 368). Sometimes thyroid disease will have an asymmetric effect with more exophthalmos and/ or limitation of motion on one side than the other. Progressive paralysis of the eyelids, which may obstruct vision, occurs separately or as part of an external paralysis, as in ocular dystrophy or in oculopharyngeal dystrophy.

DISTURBANCES OF HEARING

Tinnitus and *deafness* are frequent symptoms and always indicate disease of the ear or of the auditory nerve and its central connections.

Tinnitus, or ringing in the ears, is a purely subjective phenomenon and may also be reported as a buzzing, whistling, hissing, or roaring sound. It is a very common symptom in adults. Low-frequency vibratory clicks, pops, roarings, etc., are invariably due to diseases of the middle ear and eustachian tube. High-pitched tonal, nonvibratory tinnitus means disease of the cochlea and eighth nerve. Severe and prolonged tinnitus in the presence of normal hearing is very rare. If tinnitus is localized to one ear and is described as having a low-pitched tonal character, such as ringing or a bell-like tone, and particularly if there is reduced hearing with the recruitment phenomenon (see below), it is probably cochlear in origin. Clicking sounds are caused by intermittent contraction of the tensor tympani. A pulsating tinnitus synchronous with the pulse may be related to an intracranial vascular malformation; however, this symptom must be carefully judged, since introspective persons often report hearing their pulse when lying with one ear on a pillow. Certain drugs such as salicylates and quinine produce tinnitus and transient deafness. Nervous persons are less tolerant of tinnitus than more stable ones; depressed or anxious patients may demand relief from tinnitus that has existed for years.

Examination of hearing should always begin with inspection of the external auditory canal and the tympanic membrane. A ticking watch or whispered words are suitable means of testing hearing at the bedside, the opposite ear being closed by the finger. If there is any suspicion of deafness or a complaint of tinnitus or vertigo, or if the patient is a child with a speech defect, then hearing must be tested further. This can be done with the use of tuning forks of different frequencies, but the most accurate results are obtained by the use of an electric audiometer and the construction of an audiogram which reveals the entire range of hearing at a glance.

Deafness is frequent. In the United States it is estimated that there are more than 6 million persons with hearing loss; in one-third to one-half of these persons the loss is hereditary. Deafness is of two types: (1) nerve deafness (also called perceptive or sensorineural), due to disease of the cochlea or of the cochlear division of the eighth cranial nerve, and (2) conductive deafness, due to disease of the middle ear, such as otosclerosis or chronic otitis, or to occlusion of the external auditory canal or eustachian tube. In differentiating these two types, the tuning fork tests are of value. When a tuning fork vibrating at 256 Hz is held about one inch from the ear (the test for air conduction), sound waves can be appreciated only as they are transmitted through the middle ear and are reduced with disease in this location. When the fork is applied to the skull (test for bone conduction), the sound waves are conveyed directly to the cochlea, without the intervention of the middle ear apparatus, and are therefore not reduced or lost. Normally air conduction is better than bone conduction. These principles form the basis for several tests of auditory function.

In *Weber's test,* the vibrating fork is applied to the forehead in the midline. In middle ear deafness the sound is localized in the affected ear; in nerve deafness, in the normal ear. In *Rinné's test,* the vibrating fork is applied to the mastoid process, the other ear being closed by the observer's finger. At the moment the sound ceases, the fork is held at the auditory meatus. In middle ear deafness the sound cannot be heard by air conduction after bone conduction has ceased (abnormal or negative Rinné's test). In nerve deafness the reverse is true (normal or positive Rinné's test), although both air and bone conduction may be quantitatively decreased. In *Schwabach's test,* the patient's bone conduction is compared with that of a normal observer. In general, high-pitched tones are lost in nerve deafness and low-pitched ones in middle ear deafness, but there are frequent exceptions to this rule.

The following audiologic tests, taken together, help distinguish between cochlear and retrocochlear (nerve) lesions:

1 *Auditory recruitment:* the difference in hearing between the two ears is estimated, and the loudness of the stimulus delivered to each ear is then increased by regular increments. In nonrecruiting deafness (characteristic of nerve trunk lesion) the original difference in hearing persists in all comparisons of loudness above threshold. In recruiting deafness (as occurs in Ménière's disease) the more defective ear gains in loudness and finally is equal to the better one.
2 *Speech discrimination:* retrocochlear lesions are indicated by a failure to recognize more than 30 percent of phonetically balanced monosyllabic words (e.g., *thin and sin*) at suprathreshold levels.
3 *Short-increment sensitivity index* (SISI), in which the patient responds to a series of twenty 1-decibel (dB) increments in amplitude superimposed on a steady tone of the same frequency presented at a sensation level of 20 dB. The patient's score is the percentage of these 20-dB increments which he or she is able to detect at a given frequency. Low SISI scores, below 60 percent, point to an end-organ lesion.
4 *Threshold sensitivity* recorded via *Békésy audiometry* for both continuous and interrupted tonal stimuli. Four types of tracing may be obtained; the type II tracing is obtained in patients with end-organ lesions, and type III or IV, usually the former, characterizes retrocochlear lesions.
5 *Threshold tone decay:* this test quantifies auditory adaptation and requires only a conventional pure tone audiometer. Retrocochlear lesions yield greater amounts of decay than cochlear ones.

The common causes of middle ear deafness are otitis media, otosclerosis, and rupture of the eardrum. Nerve deafness has many causes. The internal ear may be aplastic from birth (hereditary deaf-mutism), or it may be damaged by rubella in the pregnant mother. Acute purulent meningitis or chronic infection spreading from the middle ear may cause nerve deafness in childhood. The auditory nerve may be involved by tumors of the cerebellopontine angle or by syphilis. Deafness may also result from a demyelinative plaque in the brainstem. A large series of genetically determined syndromes which feature a neural type of deafness, some congenital, others progressive, has come to light (see article by Konigsmark). The most interesting of these are dominant progressive nerve deafness, dominant unilateral deafness, dominant low-frequency hearing loss, recessive congenital deafness, sex-linked congenital neural deafness, several types of deafness (neural and conductive) with malformations of external ears, face, and neck (Treacher-Collins disease and Engelmann's diaphyseal dysplasia); hereditary deafness with goiter (Pendred's disease); hereditary heart disease with deafness; hereditary deafness with various combinations of mental retardation, retinitis pigmentosa, and polyneuropathy (as in Hallgren's disease, Alstrom's disease, Refsum's disease); hereditary deafness with skin abnormalities such as albinism, lentigines, piebaldness, white forelock (Waardenburg's disease), onchydystrophy and pegged teeth, atopic dermatitis, and anhydrosis.

Of the types of progressive conduction deafness, hereditary otosclerosis is the most frequent (cause of 50 percent of deafness in adulthood). Hysterical deafness may be difficult to distinguish from organic disease. In the case of bilateral deafness, the distinction can be made by observing a blink (cochleoorbicular reflex) or an alteration in skin sweating (psychogalvanic skin reflex) in response to a loud sound. Unilateral hysterical deafness may be detected by an audiometer, with both ears connected, or by whispering into the bell of a stethoscope attached to the patient's ears, closing first one tube and then the other without the patient's knowledge.

In otosclerosis and hereditary sensorineural deafness, vestibular function is usually retained (caloric responses are normal).

REFERENCES

ASHWORTH B: Neuro-ophthalmology, in *Recent Advances in Clinical Neurology*, WB Mathews (ed). Edinburgh, Churchill-Livingstone, 1975

BACH-Y-RITA P, COLLINS CC: *The Control of Eye Movements.* New York, Academic, 1971

BENDER MB: Neurophthalmology, in *Clinical Neurology*, AB Baker (ed). New York, Hoeber-Harper, 1962, vol 1, chap 4

COGAN DG: *Neurology of the Ocular Muscles,* 2d ed. Springfield, Ill, Charles C Thomas, 1956

GLASER JM: *Neuro-ophthalmology.* New York, Harper & Row, 1978

KONIGSMARK BW: Medical progress. Hereditary deafness in man. N Engl J Med 281:713, 774, 827, 1969

TILLMAN TW: Special hearing tests in otoneurologic diagnosis. Arch Otolaryngol 89:25 1969

19
DISORDERS OF SENSATION

MAURICE VICTOR
RAYMOND D. ADAMS

Loss or perversion of somatic sensation not infrequently is the principal manifestation of disease of the nervous system. The reason for this is clear enough, since the major anatomic pathways of the sensory system are distinct from those of the motor system and may be selectively disturbed by disease. An understanding of these sensory disorders may provide important leads to neurologic diagnosis.

GENERAL CONSIDERATIONS Unfortunately, space does not permit here a more detailed review of the anatomy of the sensory system or of its physiology. The interested reader may turn to the references at the end of the chapter. The cutaneous distribution of sensory spinal roots may be observed in Fig. 19-1 (see also Chap. 3).

Disorders of the somatic sensory apparatus pose special problems for these patients. They are confronted with derangements of sensation which may be unlike anything they have previously experienced, and they have few words in their vocabulary to describe what they feel. They may say that a limb feels "numb" and "dead" when in fact they mean it is weak. Observant individuals may occasionally discover a loss of sensation, for example, inability to feel discomfort on touching an object hot enough to blister the skin or unawareness of articles of clothing and other objects in contact with the skin. But more often disease has induced a new and unnatural series of sensory experiences. If nerves, spinal roots, or spinal tracts are only partially interrupted, a touch may arouse tingling or pricking, meaning presumably that at least some of the remaining touch and pain fibers are functional but are acting abnormally. Tightness and drawing and pulling sensations, a feeling of a band or girdle around the limb or trunk, are common with partial involvement of pressure fibers. Similarly, burning and pain (causalgia) may represent overactivity of surviving thermal and pain fibers. The responsible lesion may be in the peripheral nerve, the lateral spinothalamic tract in the spinal cord or brainstem, or the thalamus. Also, hyperesthesia and hyperpathia are frequent. These abnormal sensations are called *paresthesias,* or *dysesthesias,* if they are unpleasant; and their character and distribution inform us of the anatomy of the lesion involving the sensory system.

EXAMINATION OF SENSATION The examination of sensation is the most difficult part of the neurologic examination. For one thing, test procedures are relatively crude and inadequate. And, embarrassingly often, no objective sensory loss can be demonstrated despite symptoms that clearly indicate the presence of such a deficit. Also, a response to a sensory stimulus is difficult to evaluate objectively, since the examiner's conclusions depend on the patient's interpretations of sensory experiences. This presupposes a general responsiveness, alertness, and a desire to cooperate, as well as intelligence and a certain level of education. Hypersuggestibility and fatigue may interfere with the obtaining of accurate test data.

The detail in which sensation is tested will be determined by the clinical situation. If the patient has no sensory complaints, it is sufficient to examine vibration and position sense in the fingers and toes, to test the appreciation of pain over the face, trunk, and extremities, and to determine whether the sensory findings are the same in symmetric parts of the body. A rough survey of this sort may detect sensory defects of which the patient is unaware. On the other hand, more thorough testing is in order if the patient has complaints referable to the sensory system or if there is localized atrophy or weakness, ataxia, trophic changes of joints, or painless ulcers.

A few other general principles should be mentioned. One should not press the sensory examination in the presence of fatigue, for an inattentive patient is a poor witness. The exam-

FIGURE 19-1

Distribution of the sensory spinal roots on the surface of the body. (From G Holmes, Introduction to Clinical Neurology, 2d ed, Baltimore, Williams & Wilkins, 1952.)

iner must also avoid suggesting symptoms to the patient. After having explained in the simplest terms what is required, as few questions and remarks should be interposed as possible. Consequently, patients must not be asked, "Do you feel that?" each time they are touched; they should simply be told to say "yes" or "sharp" every time they have been touched or feel pain. The patient should not be permitted to see the part under examination. For short tests it is sufficient to close the eyes; during more detailed testing it is preferable to screen the eyes from the part being examined. Quantitative methods are available, utilizing graded sensory stimuli (Dyck et al.). Finally, the findings of the sensory examination should be accurately recorded on a chart.

Sensation is frequently classified as *superficial* (cutaneous, exteroceptive) and *deep* (proprioceptive); the former comprises the modalities of light touch, pain, and temperature; the latter includes the sense of position, passive motion, vibration, and deep pain.

Sense of touch   This is usually tested with a wisp of cotton. The patient is first made acquainted with the nature of the stimulus by applying it to a normal part of the body and is then asked to say "yes" each time various other parts are touched. A patient simulating sensory loss may say "no" in response to a tactile stimulus. Cornified areas of skin, such as the soles and palms, will require a heavier stimulus than normal, and the hair-clad parts a lighter one because of the numerous nerve endings around the hair follicles. The patient is more sensitive to a moving contactual stimulus of any kind than a stationary one. The gentle movement of the examiner's or preferably the patient's finger tip over the skin is a useful method of mapping out an area of tactile loss.

Sense of pain   This is most efficiently estimated by pinprick, although it may be evoked by a great diversity of noxious stimuli. The patient must understand that he or she is to report the degree of sharpness of the pin, not simply the feeling of contact or pressure of the point or even a special sensation due to penetration of the skin. If the pinpricks are applied rapidly, their effects may be summated and excessive pain may result; therefore, they should be delivered not too rapidly, about one per second, and not over the same spot.

If an area of diminished or absent touch or pain sensation is encountered, its boundaries should be demarcated to determine whether it has a segmental or peripheral nerve distribution or whether sensation is lost below a certain level. Such areas are best delineated by proceeding from the region of impaired sensation toward the normal, and the changes may be confirmed by dragging a pin lightly over the skin.

Deep pressure sense   One can estimate this sense simply by pinching gently or pressing deeply on the tendons and muscles. Pain can often be elicited by heavy pressure even when superficial sensation is diminished; conversely, in some diseases, such as tabetic neurosyphilis, the loss of deep pressure sense may be more prominent.

Thermal sense   The following procedure for testing thermal sensation is suggested. The areas of skin to be tested should be exposed for some time before the examination. The test objects should be large, preferably Erlenmeyer flasks containing hot and cold water. Thermometers which extend into the water through the flask stoppers indicate the temperature of the water at the moment of testing. At first, extreme degrees of heat and cold (e.g., 10 and 45°C) may be employed to delineate roughly an area of thermal sensory disturbance; the patient will report that the flask feels "less hot" or "less cold" over such an area than over a normal part. If areas of impaired sensation are found, the borders may be accurately determined

by moving the flask along the skin from the insensitive to the normal region. The qualitative change should then be quantitated as far as possible by estimating the *differences in temperature* which the patient is able to recognize. The patient is asked to report whether one stimulus is *warmer or colder* than another not whether a given stimulus is warm or cold, since the cooler of the two may be interpreted as warm. The range of temperature difference between the two flasks is gradually narrowed by mixing their contents. A normal person is capable of detecting a difference of 1°C when the temperature of the flasks is in the range of 28 to 32°C. In the warm range one should readily recognize differences between 35 and 40°C, and in the cold range, between 10 and 20°C. In many normal older persons and in others with poor peripheral circulation (especially in cold weather), the responses may be modified.

The sensation of heat or cold depends not only on the temperature of the stimulus but also on the duration of the stimulus and the area over which it is applied. This principle may be employed to detect slight degrees of sensory impairment; the patient may be able to distinguish small differences in temperature when the bottom of the flask is applied for 3 s but unable to do so if only the side of the flask is applied for 1 s. Throughout the test procedure, especially when small temperature differences are involved, the area of sensory disturbance should be continually checked against perception in normal parts.

Postural sense and the appreciation of passive movement   These modalities are usually lost together, although in any particular case one may be disproportionately affected.

Abnormalities of postural sensation may be revealed in several ways. When the patient extends the arms forward and closes the eyes, the affected arm will wander from its original position; if the fingers are spread apart, they may undergo a series of slow-changing postures ("piano-playing" movements, or *pseudoathetosis*). In attempting to touch the tip of the nose with the index finger, the patient may miss the target repeatedly.

The lack of position sense in the legs may be demonstrated by displacing the limb from its original position and asking the patient to point to the large toe. If postural sensation is defective in both legs, the patient will be unable to maintain balance with feet together and eyes closed (Romberg's sign). This sign should be interpreted with caution. Even a normal person in the Romberg position will sway slightly more with the eyes closed than open. A patient with lack of balance due to motor disorders or cerebellar disease will also sway more if visual cues are removed. Only if there is a marked discrepancy between the state of balance with eyes open and closed can one confidently state that the patient shows Romberg's sign, i.e., loss of joint-position sense. Mild degrees of unsteadiness in nervous or suggestible patients may be overcome by diverting their attention, e.g., by having them alternately touch the index finger of each hand to their nose while standing with their eyes closed.

The appreciation of passive movement is first tested in the fingers and toes, and the defect, when present, is reflected maximally in these parts. It is important to grasp the digit firmly at the sides opposite the plane of movement; otherwise the pressure applied by the examiner in displacing the digit may allow the patient to identify the direction of movement. This applies to the testing of the more proximal segments of the limb as well. The patient should be instructed to report each movement as "up" or "down" in relation to the previous stationary position. It is useful to demonstrate the test with a large and easily identified movement, but once the idea is clear to the patient, the smallest detectable changes in position should be tested. The range of movement normally appreciated in the digits is said to be as little as 1°. Clinically, however, defective appreciation of passive movement is judged by comparison with a normal limb or, if bilaterally defective, on the basis of what the examiner has through experience learned to regard as normal. Slight impairment may be disclosed by a slow response or, if the digit is displaced very slowly, by a relative unawareness that movements have occurred; or after the digit has been displaced in the same direction several times, the patient may misjudge the first movement in the opposite direction; or after the examiner has moved the toe, the patient may make a number of small voluntary movements of the toe, in an apparent attempt to determine its position or the direction of the movement.

The sense of vibration   This is a composite sensation comprising touch and rapid alterations of deep pressure sense, the end organ of which is the pacinian corpuscle. Its conduction depends on both cutaneous and deep afferent fibers which ascend in the dorsal columns of the cord. It is therefore rarely affected by lesions of single nerves but will be disturbed in cases of polyneuritis and disease of the dorsal columns, medial lemniscus, and thalamus. For this reason, vibration and position sense are usually lost together, although one of them (usually vibration sense) may be affected disproportionately. With advancing age, vibration sense may be diminished at the toes and ankles.

Vibration sense is tested by placing a tuning fork with a low rate (and long duration) of vibration (128 Hz) over the bony prominences. The examiner must make sure that the patient responds to the vibration, not simply to the pressure of the fork. Although there are mechanical devices to quantitate vibration sense, it is sufficient for clinical purposes to compare the point tested with a normal part of the patient or the examiner. Thus, if the fork is allowed to run down until vibration is no longer appreciated but is still felt at an analogous point on the opposite limb, and if this finding is consistent, one can be certain of a significant impairment of vibration sense. In a similar way, the appreciation of vibration at the tibial tuberosity after it has disappeared in the ankle, or at the iliac portion of the spine after it has disappeared at the tibial tuberosity, is an indication of a peripheral nerve lesion. The level of vibration-sense loss due to spinal cord lesions may be estimated by placing the fork over successive vertebral spines.

DISCRIMINATIVE SENSORY FUNCTIONS   Damage to the sensory cortex or to the sensory projections from thalamus to cortex results in a special type of disturbance that affects mainly the patient's ability to make sensory discriminations. Lesions in these structures may disturb postural sense but leave the so-called "primary modalities" (touch, pain, temperature, and vibration sense) relatively little affected. In such a situation, or if a cerebral lesion is suspected on other grounds, discriminative function should be tested further in the following ways:

Two-point discrimination   The ability to distinguish two points from one is tested by using a compass, the points of which should be blunt and applied simultaneously and painlessly. The distance at which such a stimulus can be recognized as double varies greatly; 1 mm at the tip of the tongue, 2 to 3 mm on the lips, 3 to 5 mm on the dorsa of the hands and feet, and 4 to 7 cm on the body surface. It is characteristic of the patient with a lesion of the sensory cortex to mistake two points for one, although occasionally the opposite occurs.

Cutaneous localization and number writing   The ability to localize cutaneous stimuli is tested by touching various parts of

the patient's body and asking the patient to point to the part touched or the corresponding part on the examiner's limb. Recognition of numbers or letters (these should be larger than 4 cm) or of the direction of lines drawn on the skin also depends on localization of tactile stimuli.

Appreciation of texture, size, and shape   Appreciation of texture depends mainly on cutaneous impressions, but the recognition of shape and size of objects is based on impressions from deeper receptors as well. The lack of recognition of shape and form, therefore, though frequently found with cortical lesions, may also be present with lesions of the spinal cord and brainstem because of interruption of tracts transmitting postural and tactile sensation. The latter type of sensory defect, called stereoanesthesia, should be distinguished from astereognosis, which connotes an inability to identify an object by palpation, the primary sense data (touch, pain, temperature, and vibration) being intact. In practice, a pure astereognosis is rarely encountered, and the term is employed where the impairment of superficial and vibratory sensation in the hands is of insufficient severity to account for the defect. Defined in this way, astereognosis may be the product of a lesion in *either* hemisphere, in the postcentral gyrus or the thalamoparietal projections. Astereognosis may be confused with *tactile agnosia*. The latter disorder is due to a lesion lying posterior to the postcentral gyrus of the *dominant* parietal lobe, and causes an inability to recognize an object by touch or handling in one or both hands. In contrast, the patient with astereognosis may not appreciate the size, form, consistency, and weight of an object placed in the hand, and therefore cannot identify it.

Extinction of sensory stimuli and sensory inattention   In response to bilateral simultaneous testing of symmetric parts, the patient may acknowledge only the stimulus on the sound side or may improperly localize the stimulus on the affected side, whereas stimuli applied to each side separately are properly appreciated. This phenomenon of extinction, or cortical inattention, is characteristic of parietal lobe lesions, the symptoms of which are considered in Chap. 25.

A few other terms require definition, since they may be encountered in descriptions of sensation. *Anesthesia* refers to a loss of all forms of sensation, and *hypesthesia* to a diminution of all sensation. Loss or impairment of specific cutaneous sensations is indicated by an appropriate prefix or suffix, e.g., thermoanesthesia or thermohypesthesia, analgesia (loss of pain) or hypalgesia, tactile anesthesia (loss of sense of touch), and pallanesthesia (loss of vibratory sense). The term *hyperesthesia* requires special mention; although it implies a heightened receptiveness of the nervous system, careful testing will usually demonstrate an underlying sensory defect, i.e., an elevated threshold to tactile, painful, or thermal stimuli; once the stimulus is perceived, however, it may have a severely painful or unpleasant quality (hyperpathia).

SYNDROMES OF SENSORY ABNORMALITY   **Sensory changes due to single nerve involvement**   Sensory changes may be due to interruption of a single peripheral nerve. These changes will vary with the composition of the nerve involved, depending on whether it is predominantly muscular, cutaneous, or mixed. In lesions of cutaneous nerves, the area of tactile anesthesia is more extensive than the one for pain, because of greater overlapping of pain fibers. Also, because of overlap from adjacent nerves, the area of sensory loss following division of a cutaneous nerve is always less than its anatomic distribution. If a large area of skin is involved, the sensory defect characteristically consists of a central portion, in which all forms of cutaneous sensation are lost, surrounded by a zone of partial loss, which becomes less marked as one proceeds from the center to the periphery. The senses of deep pressure and passive movement are intact because they are carried by special nerve fibers from subcutaneous structures and joints. Along the margin of the hypesthetic zone the skin becomes excessively sensitive. According to Weddell, this is because of collateral regeneration from surrounding healthy nerves into the denervated region (see Chap. 3).

Particular types of lesions differentially affect the fibers in a sensory nerve. Compression paralyzes large touch and pressure fibers more than the small pain, thermal, and autonomic motor fibers; procaine and cocaine have opposite effects.

In lesions involving the brachial and lumbosacral plexuses, the sensory disturbance is no longer confined to the territory of a single nerve and is almost invariably accompanied by muscle weakness and reflex change.

Sensory changes due to multiple nerve involvement (polyneuropathy) In most instances of polyneuropathy the sensory changes are accompanied by varying degrees of motor and reflex loss. Usually the sensory impairment is symmetric, with notable exceptions in some instances of diabetic and periarteritic neuropathy. Since the longest and largest fibers tend to be the most affected, the sensory loss is most severe over the feet and legs and less severe over the hands. The abdomen, thorax, and face are spared except in the most severe cases. The sensory loss usually involves all the modalities, and although it is manifestly difficult to equate the impairment of pain, touch, temperature, vibration, and position sense, one of these may seemingly be impaired out of proportion to the others. One cannot accurately predict from the patient's symptoms which mode of sensation will be disproportionately affected. The term *glove-and-stocking anesthesia* is frequently employed to describe the sensory loss of polyneuropathy and draws attention to the predominantly distal pattern of involvement. It is an inaccurate term insofar as the border between normal and impaired sensation is not so sharp; the sensory loss shades off gradually. In hysteria, by contrast, the border between normal and absent sensation is usually sharp. (See Chap. 377 for description of special varieties of sensory changes in polyneuropathies.)

Sensory changes due to involvement of single or multiple spinal nerve roots Because of considerable overlap from adjacent roots, division of a single sensory root does not produce complete loss of sensation in any area of skin. Compression of a single sensory cervical or lumbar root (e.g., in herniated intervertebral disks) causes varying degrees of impairment of cutaneous sensation in a segmental pattern, however. When two or more roots have been completely divided, a zone of sensory loss can be found in which reduction of pain perception is greater in extent than touch. Surrounding the area of complete loss is a narrow zone of partial loss, in which a raised threshold accompanied by overreaction (*hyperpathia*) may or may not be demonstrated. The presence of muscle paralysis, atrophy, and reflex loss indicates involvement of ventral roots as well.

Tabetic syndrome This, too, is a radicular syndrome, resulting from damage to the large proprioceptive and other fibers of the posterior lumbosacral roots. It is usually caused by neurosyphilis, less often by diabetes mellitus, meningeal tumors, etc. Numbness or paresthesias and lightning pains are frequent complaints, and areflexia, atonicity of the bladder, abnormalities of gait (Chap. 17), and hypotonia without muscle weakness are found on examination. The sensory loss may consist only of loss of vibration and position sense in the lower extremities, but in severe cases, loss or impairment of superficial or deep pain sense or of touch may be added. The feet and legs are most affected, much less often the arms and trunk.

Complete spinal sensory syndromes In a complete transverse lesion of the spinal cord, all forms of sensation are abolished below a level that corresponds to the lesion. There may be a narrow zone of "hyperesthesia" at the upper margin of the anesthetic zone. During the evolution of such a lesion there may be a discrepancy between the level of the lesion and that of the sensory loss, the latter ascending as the lesion progresses. This can be understood if one conceives of a lesion evolving from the periphery to the center of the cord, affecting first the outermost fibers carrying pain and temperature sensation from the legs. Conversely, a lesion advancing from the center of the cord may affect these modalities in the reverse order. (See Chap. 375 for more complete discussion.)

Partial spinal sensory syndromes (hemisection of the spinal cord, Brown-Séquard syndrome) In rare instances disease is confined to one side of the spinal cord; pain and heat sensation are affected on the opposite side, and proprioceptive sensation is affected on the same side as the lesion. The loss of pain and temperature sensation begins two or three segments below the lesion. An associated motor paralysis on the side of the lesion completes the syndrome. Tactile sensation is not involved, since the fibers from one side of the body are distributed in tracts on both sides of the cord.

Lesions of the central gray matter (syringomyelic syndrome) Since fibers conducting pain and temperature cross the cord in the anterior commissure, a lesion in this location will characteristically abolish these modalities on one or both sides but will spare tactile sensation. The commonest cause of such a lesion is syringomyelia, less often tumor and hemorrhage. This type of dissociated sensory loss usually occurs in a segmental distribution (the sensation is normal above and below the affected segment), and since the lesion frequently involves other parts of the gray matter, varying degrees of segmental amyotrophy and reflex loss may be added. If the lesion has spread to the white matter, signs of involvement of corticospinal and spinothalamic tracts and posterior columns will be present as well.

Posterior column syndrome There is loss of vibratory and position sense below the lesion, but the senses of pain, temperature, and touch are affected relatively little or not at all. This condition may be difficult to distinguish from an affection of large fibers in sensory roots (tabetic syndrome). In some diseases vibratory sensation may be involved predominantly, whereas in others position sense is more affected. An interruption of proprioceptive fibers may interfere with discriminative sensory function, such as two-point discrimination and recognition of size, shape, and weight; and impairment of these functions may occur with posterior column disease alone. Paresthesias in the form of tingling and "pins-and-needles" sensations or girdle sensations are a common complaint with diseases of posterior columns, and pain stimuli may also produce unpleasant sensations.

The "anterior spinal artery syndrome" With occlusion of the anterior spinal artery or other destructive lesions that predominantly affect the ventral portion of the cord, there is a relative or absolute sparing of the posterior column functions and only a loss of pain and temperature sensation below the level of the lesion. Since the corticospinal tracts and the ventral gray matter also fall within the area of distribution of the anterior spinal artery, paralysis of motor function forms a prominent part of this syndrome.

Disturbances of sensation due to lesions of the brainstem A characteristic feature of lesions of the medulla and lower pons is crossed sensory disturbance, i.e., loss of pain and temperature sensation of one side of the face and of the opposite side of the body. This is accounted for by involvement of the trigeminal tract or nucleus and the lateral spinothalamic tract on one side of the brainstem. This is nearly always due to a lateral medullary infarction (Wallenburg's syndrome). In the upper pons and midbrain, where the spinothalamic tracts and the medial lemniscus become confluent, an appropriately placed lesion may cause a loss of all superficial and deep sensation over the contralateral side of the body. Cranial nerve palsies, cerebellar ataxia, or motor paralysis are often associated (see Chap. 376).

Sensory loss due to a lesion of the thalamus (syndrome of Dejerine-Roussy) Involvement of the nucleus ventralis posterolateralis of the thalamus, usually due to a vascular lesion or tumor, causes loss or diminution of all forms of sensation on the opposite side of the body. Position sense is affected more frequently than any other sensory function, and deep sensory loss is usually, but not always, more profound than cutaneous loss. Sooner or later, often as sensation improves, spontaneous pain or discomfort ("thalamic pain"), sometimes of the most torturing and disabling type, appears on the affected side of the body; and any form of stimulus may acquire a diffuse, unpleasant, lingering quality. Emotional disturbance also aggravates the painful state. The thalamic pain syndrome may occasionally accompany lesions of the white matter of the parietal lobe (Chap. 25).

Sensory loss due to lesions in the parietal lobe There is a unique disturbance mainly of discriminative sensory functions on the opposite side of the body, particularly the face, arm, and leg. Loss of position sense, impaired ability to localize touch and pain stimuli, elevation of two-point threshold, a general inattentiveness to sensory stimuli on one side of the body, and astereognosis (if the lesion is in the dominant hemisphere) are the most prominent findings. With cortical lesions, the patient's reports are variable; one examination may disclose no sensory abnormalities, whereas another does. This type of response is often attributed to hysteria. As to the anatomic localization of lesions that impair tactile discrimination, they have been found consistently in the postcentral gyrus of the contralateral parietal lobe (Roland). Other features of parietal lobe symptomatology and the differences between dominant and nondominant parietal lobe syndromes are considered in Chap. 25. More frequent with lesions of the parietal lobe is a global reduction of all forms of somatic sensation on the opposite side of the body.

Sensory loss due to suggestion and hysteria Hysterical patients almost never complain spontaneously of cutaneous sensory loss, although they may use the term *numbness* to indicate a paralysis of a limb. Complete hemianesthesia, often with reduced hearing, sight, smell, and taste, as well as impaired vibration sense over only half the skull, is a common finding in hysteria. Anesthesia of one entire limb or a sharply defined sensory loss over part of a limb, not conforming to the distribution of root or cutaneous nerve, is also frequently observed. Postural sensation is rarely affected. The diagnosis of hysterical hemianesthesia is best made by eliciting the other relevant symptoms of hysteria or, if this is not possible, by noting the discrepancies between this type of sensory loss and that which occurs as part of the usual sensory syndromes.

REFERENCES

BRODAL A: The somatic afferent pathways, in *Neurological Anatomy*. New York, Oxford, 1969, chap 2

DYCK PJ et al: Clinical vs. quantitative evaluation of cutaneous sensation. Arch Neurol 33:651, 1976

MAYO CLINIC: *Clinical Examinations in Neurology*, 3d ed. Philadelphia, Saunders, 1972

MOUNTCASTLE VB: Central nervous mechanisms in sensation, in *Medical Physiology*, 12th ed, VB Mountcastle (ed). St. Louis, Mosby, 1968, vol 2, chaps 61–63

ROLAND PE: Astereognosis: Tactile discrimination after localized hemispheric lesions in man. Arch Neurol 33:543, 1976

20
COMA AND RELATED DISTURBANCES OF CONSCIOUSNESS

RAYMOND D. ADAMS

The practitioner of medicine is frequently called upon to treat patients whose principal abnormality is an impairment of consciousness, which varies from inattentiveness and simple confusion to coma. In large municipal hospitals it is estimated that as many as 3 percent of total admissions to the emergency ward are due to diseases that have caused coma; although this figure seems high, it serves to emphasize the importance of this class of neurologic diseases and the necessity for every student of medicine to acquire a theoretic as well as practical knowledge of them.

The terms *consciousness, confusion, stupor, unconsciousness,* and *coma* have been endowed with so many meanings that it is almost impossible to avoid ambiguity in their usage. They are not strictly medical terms, but literary, philosophic, and psychologic ones as well. The word *consciousness* is the most difficult of all. William James once remarked that everyone knew what consciousness was until attempting to define it. To the psychologist consciousness denotes a state of awareness of one's self and one's environment. Knowledge of one's self, of course, includes all "feelings, attitudes and emotions, impulses, volitions, and the active or striving aspects of conduct"—in short, an awareness of all one's own mental functioning, particularly of the cognitive processes. These can be judged only by the patient's verbal account of introspections and, indirectly, by actions. Physicians, being practical persons for the most part, have learned to place greater confidence in their observations of the patient's general behavior and reactions to overt stimuli than in what the patient says. For this reason when they employ the term *consciousness*, they usually do so in its commonest and simplest signification, namely, a state of awareness of the environment. This narrow definition has another advantage in that the word *unconsciousness* is its exact opposite—a state of unawareness of environment or a suspension of those mental activities by which humans are made aware of their environment. To add to the ambiguity, psychoanalysts have given the word *unconscious* a still different meaning; for them it stands for the repository of impulses and memories of previous experiences that cannot immediately be recalled to the conscious mind.

Description of states of normal and impaired consciousness
The following definitions, though admittedly unacceptable to most psychologists, are of service to medicine, and they will provide the students with a convenient terminology for describing the mental states of their patients.

Normal consciousness This is the condition of the normal person when fully awake, who is responsive to psychologic stimuli and "indicates by his behavior and speech that he has the same awareness of himself and his environment as ourselves." This normal state may fluctuate during the course of the day from keen alertness or deep concentration with a marked constriction of the field of attention to general inattentiveness and drowsiness.

Sleep Sleep is a state of physical and mental inactivity from which the patient may be aroused to normal consciousness. A person in sleep gives little evidence of being aware of self or environment and in this respect is unconscious. Yet such a person differs from a comatose patient in that the former may still respond to unaccustomed stimuli and at times is capable of some mental activity in the form of dreams, which leave their traces in memory. Also, he or she is arousable.

Inattention, confusional, and cloudy states of consciousness In these conditions the patient does not take into account all elements of the immediate environment. As in delirium, there is always an element of sensorial clouding or imperceptiveness and distractibility of attention. The term *confusion* lacks precision, for often it is meant to denote an inability to think with customary speed and coherence. Here the difficulty is in defining *thinking,* a term which invariably refers to problem solving and coherence of ideas about a subject.

An inattentive, severely confused person is usually unable to do more than carry out a few simple commands. Few if any thought processes are in operation. The capacity for speech may be limited to a few words or phrases, or the patient may be voluble. These patients are unaware of much that goes on around them and do not grasp the immediate situation. Moderately confused persons can carry on simple conversations for short periods of time, but their thinking is slow and incoherent, and they are unable to stay on one topic. They are distractible and at the mercy of every stimulus. Usually they are disoriented in time and place. In mild degrees of confusion, the disorder may be so slight that it is overlooked unless the examiner is scrutinizing the patient's behavior and conversation. The patient may even be roughly oriented as to time and place and able to speak freely on almost any subject. Only occasional irrelevant remarks betray an incoherence of thinking. Patients with mild or moderately severe confusion may be subjected to psychologic testing. The degree of confusion often varies from one time of day to another and tends to be least pronounced in the early morning. Severe confusion or stupor may resemble semicoma during periods when the patient is drowsy or asleep. Many events that happen to the confused patient leave no apparent trace in the memory; in fact, capacity to recall later the events that transpired in any given period is one of the most delicate tests of mental clarity. However, careful analysis will show the defect to be one of inadequate registration and fixation of items rather than a fault in retentive memory.

Some neurologists regard *delirium* as a state of confusion with excitement and hyperactivity, and in some medical writings the terms *delirium* and *confused-cloudy states* are used interchangeably. It is undoubtedly true that the delirious patient is nearly always confused. However, the inability to sleep, vivid hallucinations, the relative inaccessibility of the patient to other events than those to which he or she is reacting at any one moment, extreme agitation and tremulousness, and the tendency to convulse, all of which characterize delirious states, suggest a cerebral disorder of a somewhat different type. The clearest evidence of the relationship of inattention, confusion, stupor, and coma is that the patient may pass through all these states while becoming comatose or emerging from coma. The

author has not observed any such relationship between coma and delirium. These distinctions are drawn with greater clarity in Chap. 25.

At times a patient with certain types of aphasia, especially jargon aphasia, may create the impression of confusion, but close observation will reveal that the disorder is confined to the sphere of language and that behavior is otherwise natural.

Stupor In stupor mental and physical activity are reduced to a minimum. Although inaccessible to many stimuli, the patient opens the eyes, looks at the examiner, and does not appear to be unconscious. Response to spoken commands is either absent or slow and monosyllabic. As a rule tendon or plantar reflexes are not altered. On the other hand, tremulousness of movement, coarse twitching of muscles, restless or stereotyped motor activity, and grasping and sucking reflexes are not infrequent, depending on the way in which disease affects the nervous system. In psychiatry the term *stupor* means a state in which impressions of the external world are normally received but activity is suspended or marked by negativism, e.g., catatonic stupor of schizophrenia and mania.

Coma The patient who appears to be asleep and is at the same time incapable of sensing (unreceptive) and responding adequately to either external stimuli or inner needs (unresponsive) is in a state of coma. Coma may vary in degree, and in its deepest stages no reaction of any kind is obtainable. Corneal, pupillary, pharyngeal, tendon, and plantar reflexes are all absent, and there may or may not be extensor rigidity of the limbs and opisthotonos, signs which, as Sherrington showed, indicate decerebration. Respirations are often slow or rapid and may be periodic, i.e., Cheyne-Stokes breathing. With lesser degrees of coma, pupillary reflexes and ocular movements and other brainstem reflexes are preserved; in still lighter stages, referred to as *semicoma,* most of the above reflexes can be elicited, and the plantar reflexes may be either flexor or extensor (Babinski's sign). Moreover, pricking or pinching the skin, shaking and shouting at the patient, or an uncomfortable distention of the bladder may cause the patient to stir or moan and respirations to quicken. Coma differs from akinetic mutism (a state in which a patient is awake but lacking in impulse to speech and action) and the "locked-in" syndromes (a global paralysis of limbs and cranial musculature) in which the patient is still receptive but unresponsive.

ELECTROENCEPHALOGRAM AND DISTURBANCES OF CONSCIOUSNESS One of the most delicate confirmations of the fact that these states of altered consciousness are expressions of neurophysiologic changes is the electroencephalogram. In the normal waking state the electric potentials of the cortical neurons are integrated into regular waves of two frequency ranges, from 8 to 15 per second (alpha rhythm) and from 16 to 25 per second (beta rhythm). These waveforms are established by the time one reaches adolescence, but certain individual differences in general pattern and dominance of alpha waves are maintained throughout adult life. With sleep these cortical potentials slow down, and amplitude (voltage) of the individual waves increases. At one stage in light sleep characteristic bursts of 14 to 16 waves per second appear, the so-called "sleep spindles," and in deep [nonrapid eye movement (NREM)] sleep all the waves of normal frequency and amplitude are replaced by slow ones of high voltage ($1\frac{1}{4}$ to 3 per second). In rapid eye movement (REM) sleep the brain waves return to normal (see Chap. 22). Similarly, some alteration in brain waves occur in all disturbances of consciousness except the milder degrees of confusion. This alteration usually consists of a disorganization of the electroencephalographic pattern, which shows random, slow waves of high voltage in stages of confusion; more regular, slow, 2- to 3-per-second waves of high voltage in stupor and semicoma; and slow waves or even suppression of all organized electric activity (isoelectric state) in the deep coma of hypoxia and ischemia, the so-called "brain-death syndrome." The electroencephalograms of deep sleep and of light coma resemble each other. However, not all diseases that cause confusion and coma have the same effect on the electroencephalogram. Some, such as barbiturate intoxication, may cause an increase in frequency and amplitude of the brain waves. In epilepsy the disturbance of consciousness is usually attended by paroxysms of "spikes" (fast waves of high amplitude) or by the characteristic alternating slow waves and spikes of petit mal. Other diseases, such as hepatic coma, characteristicially cause a slowing in frequency and an increasing amplitude of "brain waves" and special triphasic waves. Whether all metabolic diseases of the brain induce similar changes in the electroencephalogram has not been determined. Probably there are differences among them, some of which may be significant (see Chap. 371).

MORBID ANATOMY AND PHYSIOLOGY OF COMA In recent times there has been some clarification and amplification of earlier neuropathologic observations that the smallest lesions associated with protracted coma are always to be found in the midbrain and thalamus. The essence of more recent neurophysiologic studies, to be found in the writings of Bremer, of Morison and Dempsey, and of Moruzzi and Magoun, is that a systematic series of destructive lesions of spinal cord, medulla, pons, and cerebellum has no effect on the state of consciousness until the level of midbrain and diencephalon (thalamus) is reached. High brainstem transections invariably induce states of prolonged unresponsiveness, whereas stimulation of the upper brainstem reticular formation causes a drowsy or sleeping animal to become suddenly alert and its EEG to change correspondingly. As anesthetic agents abolish consciousness, they are found to suppress the activity of the upper reticular activating system, without interfering, at least at certain levels, with the transmission of specific sensory impulses en route to parietal lobe cortex.

Anatomic studies show the reticular activating system of the upper brainstem to receive collaterals from the specific sensory pathways and to project, not just to the sensory cortex of the parietal lobe, as do the thalamic relay nuclei for somatic sensation, but to the whole of the cerebral cortex. The latter has corticofugal connections which feed back nerve impulses to the reticular formation. Sensory stimulation, it would seem, then, has the double effect of conveying to the brain information about the outside world and also of providing some of the energy for activating those parts of the nervous system on which consciousness depends.

These new data are in line with the older ideas of Herbert Spencer and Hughlings Jackson—that the diencephalon and cerebral cortex always function together as a unit and represent the highest levels of integrative nervous activity, called by Penfield *centrencephalic*. Though anatomic details have yet to be worked out and the precise physiology of the reticular activating system leaves much to be desired, being more complicated than this simple formulation woud suggest, nevertheless, as a working idea it will make some of the following neuropathologic observations more comprehensible.

The study of a large series of human cases in which coma has preceded death by several days will bring to light two major types of lesion. In the first group a macroscopically visible lesion such as a tumor, abscess, intracerebral, subarachnoid, subdural, or epidural hemorrhage, massive infarct, or meningitis is demonstrable; usually the lesion involves a portion only of the cortex and white matter, leaving much of the cerebrum intact. Rarely, it is located in the thalamus or midbrain, which would make the coma understandable. In the mass-type lesions the coma will always be related to a *temporal lobe–tentorial herniation* with compression, ischemia, and secondary hemorrhage in the midbrain and lower thalamus or with downward displacement of the brainstem (see Chap. 367). A detailed clinical record will show the coma to have coincided with these secondary displacements and herniations. Exceptionally, widespread bilateral damage to the cortex and subcortical white matter will be found—the result of bilateral infarcts or hemorrhages, viral encephalitis, hypoxia, or ischemia—without thalamic or midbrain lesions. In the second group (and this is larger than the first) no visible lesion is seen by the naked eye, and often no abnormality is divulged by any technique of pathology. The lesion here is caused by a metabolic or toxic state which may be impossible to detect morphologically. In some instances the grossly normal brain will reveal a demonstrable cellular change under the light microscope which may be characteristic, e.g., hepatic coma. Usually, in these latter instances the microscopic lesions are too diffuse for clinicoanatomic correlation. Thus, pathologic changes are compatible with physiologic deductions—that the state of prolonged coma correlates with lesions of all parts of the cortical-diencephalic systems of neurons, but it is only in the upper brainstem that they may be small and discrete.

MECHANISMS WHEREBY CONSCIOUSNESS IS DISTURBED IN DISEASE Knowledge of diseases of the nervous system is so limited that is is not possible to identify all the different mechanisms by means of which consciousness is disturbed. Already several different ways in which the mesencephalic-diencephalic-cortical systems are deranged have been identified; there are probably many others.

In a number of disease processes there is evidence of direct interference with the metabolic activities of the nerve cells in the cerebral cortex and central thalamic nuclei of the brain and depletion of putative transmitters (serotonin, dopamine, acetylcholine, norepinephrine, γ-aminobutyric acid, choline, and glutamic acid). Hypoxia, hypoglycemia, hyper- and hypo-osmolar states, acidosis, alkalosis, hyper- and hypokalemia, hyperammonemia, and deficiencies of thiamine, nicotinic acid, vitamin B_{12}, pantothenic acid, and pyridoxine are well-known examples (see Chap. 371). Relevant points for our discussion are that cerebral metabolism or blood flow is reduced in all the metabolic disorders leading to coma. Oxygen values below 2 ml per 100 g brain tissue per minute are incompatible with an alert state. In hypoglycemia the cerebral blood flow is normal or above normal, whereas the cerebral metabolic rate is diminished, owing to deficiency of substrate. In thiamine and vitamin B_{12} deficiency the cerebral blood flow is normal or slightly diminished, and the cerebral metabolic rate is diminished, presumably because of insufficiency of coenzymes. Extremes of body temperature, either hyperthermia (temperature over 41°C) or hypothermia (temperature below 35°C), probably induce coma by exerting a nospecific effect on the metabolic activity of neurons.

Diabetic acidosis, uremia, hepatic coma, and the coma of systemic infections are examples of endogenous intoxications. The identity of the toxic agents is not entirely known. In diabetes acetone bodies (acetoacetic acid, β-hydroxybutyric acid, and acetone) are present in high concentration or in the nonketotic form a lactic acidosis, and in uremia there is probably accumulation of dialyzable toxins, perhaps phenolic derivatives of the aromatic amino acids. In both conditions "dehydration" and serum acidosis (pH < 7.3, $P_{CO_2} < 35$ mmHg, [HCO_3^-] < 10 meq per liter) may also be significant. In many cases of hepatic coma, elevation of blood NH_3 to levels five to six times normal has been found. Lactic acidemia and other organic acids may affect the brain by lowering its pH. The mode of action of bacterial toxins is unknown. In all these conditions the cerebral metabolic rate tends to be reduced, whereas cerebral blood flow remains normal. Extreme hypoglycemia (blood glucose concentration <10 to 15 mg per 100 ml) critically reduces substrate for cerebral function, and hyperglycemia (500 mg per 100 ml) affects cerebral function by causing hyperosmolality. In water intoxication hypoosmolality the membrane excitability of nerve cells is altered by hyponatremia and changes in intracellular K levels. In respiratory acidosis (serum $[HCO_3^-] > 20$ meq per liter, $P_{CO_2} > 45$ mmHg, $pH < 7.30$) from depressant drug poisoning or chronic pulmonary disease, coma is caused by a combination of hypercapnia and hypoxia. In respiratory alkalosis and metabolic alkalosis ($pH > 7.45$) from cardiopulmonary disease, central neurogenic hyperventilation, alkali ingestion, etc., cerebral function is disturbed because of altered neuronal membrane activity.

Drugs such as barbiturates, bromides, diphenylhydantoin (Dilantin), alcohol, glutethimide, and phenothiazines induce coma by their direct suppressive effect on the neurons of the cerebrum and diencephalon. Others such as methyl alcohol, paraldehyde, and ethylene glycol result in metabolic acidosis. Many additional pharmacologic agents have no direct action on the nervous system but may lead to coma through the mechanism of circulatory collapse and inadequate cerebral blood flow. In toxic and metabolic diseases, although the patient usually approaches coma through stages of drowsiness, confusion, and stupor, and the reverse sequence occurs while emerging from it, each disease has its special effects, manifesting itself by a characteristic clinical picture. This means that the mechanism and topography of the lesion will be different.

A critical fall in blood pressure, usually to a systolic level below 70 mmHg, affects neural structures by causing a critical decrease in oxygenation, which reduces cerebral blood flow by half, and secondarily, a diminution in cerebral metabolic rate. If decline in blood pressure is episodic, the corresponding clinical picture is one of physical weakness usually preceding and following the loss of consciousness, i.e., syncope, the whole process being acute and promptly reversible. Cardiac arrest completely interrupts cerebral circulation and abolishes consciousness in 5 to 10 s.

The sudden, violent, and excessive discharge of *epilepsy* is another mechanism. Usually a Jacksonian convulsion has little effect on consciousness until it spreads from one side of the body to the other. Coma immediately ensues, presumably because the spreading of the seizure discharge to central neuronal structures paralyzes their function. Other types of seizure in which consciousness is interrupted from the very beginning are believed to orginate in the diencephalon.

Concussion exemplifies still another special pathophysiologic mechanism. In "blunt" head injury it has been shown that there is an enormous increase in intracranial pressure of the order of 200 to 700 lb/in², lasting a few thousandths of a second. Either the vibration set up in the skull and transmitted to the brain or this sudden high intracranial pressure is believed to be the basis of the abrupt paralysis of the nervous system that follows head injury. A separate rotatory motion of the brain within the skull is another more likely possibility. Raising the intraventricular pressure to a level approaching diastolic blood pressure has abolished all vital functions in the experimental animal.

As was pointed out above, large, destructive, supratentorial, space-consuming lesions of the brain, such as hemorrhage, tumor, or abscess, interfere with consciousness in two ways. One is by direct destruction of the midbrain and diencephalon; the other, far more frequent, is by producing herniation of the

medial part of the temporal lobe through the opening of the tentorium and crushing the upper brain against the opposite free edge of the tentorium or lateral and downward displacement of brainstem. Here the mechanism is again mechanical, and probably circulatory as well.

CLINICAL APPROACH TO THE COMATOSE PATIENT Coma is not an independent disease entity but is always a symptomatic expression of disease. Sometimes the underlying disease is perfectly obvious, as when a healthy individual is struck on the head and rendered unconscious. All too often, however, the patient is brought to the hopsital in a state of coma, and little or no information is immediately available. The physician must then subject the clinical problem to careful scrutiny from many directions. To do this efficiently requires a broad knowledge of disease and a systematic approach that leaves none of the common and treatable causes of coma unexplored.

It should be pointed out that when the comatose patient is seen for the first time, simple therapeutic measures take precedence over diagnostic procedures. In a quick survey one makes sure that the comatose patient has a clear airway and is not in shock (circulatory collapse) or, if trauma has occurred, that the patient is not bleeding from a wound. In patients who have suffered a head injury there may be a fracture of the cervical vertebrae, and therefore one must be cautious about moving the head and neck lest the spinal cord be inadvertently crushed. There must be an immediate inquiry as to the previous health of the patient: whether he or she had suffered a head injury or had been seen in a convulsion, and the circumstances in which the patient was found. The persons who accompany the comatose patient to the hospital should not be permitted to leave until they have been questioned.

Diagnosis The temperature, pulse, respiratory rate and pattern, and blood pressure are of aid in diagnosis. Fever suggests a severe systemic infection such as pneumonia, bacterial meningitis, or a brain lesion that has disturbed the temperature-regulating centers. An excessively high body temperature, 41 to 44°C, associated with dry skin should arouse the suspicion of heat stroke. Hypothermia is frequently observed in alcoholic or barbiturate intoxication, extracellular fluid deficit, peripheral circulatory failure, or myxedema. Slow breathing points to morphine, barbiturate intoxication, central alveolar hypoventilation, metabolic alkalosis, or hypothyroidism, whereas deep, rapid breathing suggests pneumonia but may occur in diabetic or uremic acidosis or exogenous organic acid intoxication (Kussmaul's respiration) or with intracranial diseases, as in central neurogenic hyperpnea. The rapid breathing of pneumonia is often accompanied by an expiratory grunt, cyanosis, and fever. Diseases that elevate the intracranial pressure or damage the brain, especially the brainstem or cerebrum, often cause slow, irregular, or periodic (Cheyne-Stokes) breathing. The pulse rate is less helpful, but if exceptionally slow, it should suggest heart block, or if combined with periodic breathing and hypertension, an increase in intracranial pressure. A tachycardia of 140 heartbeats per minute or above calls attention to the possibility of an ectopic cardiac rhythm with insufficiency of cerebral circulation. Marked hypertension occurs in patients with cerebral hemorrhage and hypertensive encephalopathy and, at times, in those with increased intracranial pressure, whereas hypotension is the usual finding in the coma of alcohol or barbiturate intoxication, or internal hemorrhage, myocardial infarction, gram-negative bacillary septicemia, and Addison's disease.

Inspection of the skin may also yield valuable information.

Cyanosis of the lips and nail beds means inadequate oxygenation. Cherry-red coloration indicates carbon monoxide poisoning. Multiple bruises, and in particular a bruise or boggy area in the scalp, favor cranial trauma. Bleeding from an ear or the nose or orbital hemorrhage also raises the possibility of trauma. Puffiness and hyperemia of face and conjunctivas and telangiectasia are the usual stigmas of alcoholism; marked pallor suggests internal hemorrhage. The presence of a maculo-hemmorrhagic rash indicates the possibility of meningococcal infection, staphylococcus endocarditis, typhus, or Rocky Mountain spotted fever. Pellagra may be diagnosed from the typical skin lesions on face and hands. The myxedematous appearance of the face is indicative of hypothyroid stupor or coma. In pituitary hypoadrenalism the skin is sallow. Excessive sweating suggests hypoglycemia or shock, and dry skin diabetic acidosis and uremia. Skin turgor is reduced in dehydration. Hemorrhagic blisters will have formed over pressure points if the patient has been motionless for a time.

The odor of the breath may provide clues to the nature of a disease causing coma. The odor of alcohol is easily recognized (except for vodka, which is odorless). The spoiled-fruit odor of diabetic coma, the uriniferous odor of uremia, and the musty fetor of hepatic coma are distinctive enough to be identified by physicians who possess a keen sense of smell.

The next step in the physical examination should give special attention to the status of the nervous system. Although the examination is limited in many ways, careful observation of the stuporous or comatose patient may yield considerable information concerning the function of different parts of the nervous system. One of the most helpful procedures is to sit at the bedside for 5 to 10 min and observe what the patient does. The predominant postures of the body, the position of the head and eyes, the rate, depth, and rhythm of respiration, and the pulse should be noted. The state of responsiveness should then be estimated by noting both the reaction when the patient's name is called and the capacity to execute a simple command or to respond to painful stimuli. The most effective painful stimuli are supraorbital pressure, sternal pressure, or pinching the side of the neck or inner parts of the upper arms or thighs. By grading these stimuli, one may titrate the response, so to speak, and evaluate both the degree of coma and changes from hour to hour in the course of the disease. Vocalization may persist in stupor and light coma and is the first response to be lost. Deft avoidance movements of parts stimulated, and grimacing are preserved in light coma and substantiate the integrity of corticomedullary and corticospinal tracts.

Usually it is possible to determine whether the coma is accompanied by meningeal irritation or focal disease in the cerebrum or brainstem. With meningeal irritation from either bacterial meningitis or subarachnoid hemorrhage, there is resistance to active and passive flexion of the neck but not to extension, turning, or tipping the head. Resistance to movement of the neck in all directions indicates disease of the cervical spine or is part of generalized rigidity. In infants, bulging of the anterior fontanel is at times a more reliable sign of meningeal irritation than stiff neck. A temporal lobe or cerebellar pressure cone or decerebrate rigidity may also limit passive flexion of the neck and may be confused with meningeal irritation.

Evidence of disease of a cerebral hemisphere, diencephalon, midbrain, pons, or medulla can be obtained even though the patient is comatose by noting the residual movement, prevailing postures of the body, respiratory rhythm and frequency, and status of cranial nerves. This is of more than passing importance, because severe and persistent derangements of these functions are frequent with mass lesions of the brain and rare in metabolic disorders (except in terminal stages). A hemiple-

gia, in most instances, reflects a contralateral hemispheral lesion and is revealed by lack of restless movements, grasp reflex, and avoidance movements. The paralyzed limbs are slack and remain in uncomfortable positions. If lifted from the bed, they "fall flail." The cheek puffs out in expiration on the paralyzed side, and the eyes are often turned away from the paralysis (toward the lesion). Painful stimuli may provoke a moan or grimace on one side and not the other, reflecting a hemianesthesia. A homonymous hemianopia in a stuporous patient is revealed by attraction of eyes to visual stimuli presented on one side and not the other or lack of blink in reaction to threat on one side.

Of the various tests of brainstem function those which have been most useful are pattern of breathing, pupillary size and reactivity, and ocular movement and oculovestibular reflexes. As to patterns of abnormal breathing in progressive lessions which reduce the state of consciousness from confusion and inattention to stupor and coma, the earliest abnormality with cerebral lesions is the appearance of posthyperventilation apnea (period of apnea after 5 to 10 deep breaths). Its presence indicates bifrontal disease, wherein lies the mechanism, according to Plum, for activating rhythmic breathing when CO_2 is reduced. In coma due to massive cerebral lesions the rate of respiration increases slightly, and as it progresses an irregularity appears which gives way to the waxing-waning Cheyne-Stokes respiration (CSR). This means that the centers in the brainstem, now isolated from the cerebrum, are rendered more sensitive than usual to CO_2 (hyperventilation drive); and by intermittently reducing plasma CO_2 to low levels, a temporary apnea follows. With midbrain–upper pontine lesions a state of central neurogenic hyperpnea (CNH), rather like Kussmaul breathing, supervenes. Here respirations are increased in rate (up to 100 per minute) and in depth, to the extent that respiratory alkalosis may result. The reflex mechanisms for respiratory control in the lower brainstem have in this instance been released, and the threshold of respiratory activation is low. This respiratory drive continues despite low arterial CO_2 tensions and elevated pH. Oxygen therapy (unlike the hyperventilation of pneumonia, pulmonary congestion, etc.) does not modify the pattern. Low pontine-level lesions sometimes cause apneustic breathing (where there is a pause of 2 to 3 s after full inspiration) or other abnormal patterns, such as short cycle clusters [three to four respirations without a waxing or waning followed by a pause (Biot respirations)]; or respiration alternans, in which a few breaths are omitted from time to time. With lesions of the medulla the rhythm of breathing is chaotic, being irregularly interrupted, the breath varying in rate and depth. This has been called "ataxic breathing," not a very appropriate term. The latter progresses to apnea, as may also CSR or CNH; in fact, respiratory arrest is the mode of death of most patients with serious central nervous system disease. As Plum and Fisher both point out, when certain supratentorial brain lesions progress to the point where the temporal lobe and cerebellum herniate, one may observe a succession of respiratory patterns (CSR–CNH–Biot breathing to ataxic breathing), indicating extension of the functional disorder from upper to lower brainstem.

With midbrain lesions the pupils dilate to 4 or 5 mm and become unreactive to light; with severe destruction of the tissue at this level (anoxic pannecrosis), they will finally dilate widely to 8 to 9 mm and not respond. Pontine and midbrain tegmental lesions cause miotic pupils with only slight reaction to strong light. Thus, normal-sized pupils and the preservation of pupillary light reflexes indicate integrity of the pupillary dilatation and constrictive mechanisms in the midbrain. Ciliospinal pupillary dilatation is also lost in brainstem lesions (see Chap. 18). Unilateral Horner's syndrome (miosis, ptosis, exophthalmos, and reduced sweating) may be observed homolateral to a predominantly one-sided lower brainstem lesion, usually medullary. The pupillary reactions are of great importance, because drug intoxications and metabolic disorders which cause coma leave the pupils unaffected. Exceptions are glutethimide (Doriden) and deep ether anesthesia, which cause the pupils to be of medium size or slightly enlarged and unreactive for several hours; opiates (heroin and morphine), which cause pinpoint pupils with light reflex so small that it can be seen only with a magnifying glass, and atropine poisoning, in which the pupils are widely dilated and fixed.

Ocular movements are altered in a variety of ways. In light coma from metabolic abnormalities the eyes rove from side to side in random fashion like the slow eye movements of light sleep. They disappear as brainstem function becomes depressed. Oculocephalic reflexes (doll's eye movements), elicited by briskly turning or tilting the head, with eyes moving conjugately in the opposite direction, are easily elicited. They are not present in the normal person, and if they are elicitable, evidence is obtained of release from cerebral control and integrity of the tegmental structures of the midbrain and pons, which integrate ocular movements, and of the third, fourth, and sixth cranial nerves. Irrigation of each ear with 30 to 100 ml ice water (or just cold water if the patient is not completely comatose) will normally cause nystagmus away from the stimulated side (see Chap. 18). In comatose patients in whom the fast corrective "cortical" phase of nystagmus is lost, the eyes are deflected to the side irrigated with cold water or away from the side irrigated with hot water. The position is held for 2 to 3 min. These vestibuloocular reflexes are also lost in brainstem lesions. If only one eye abducts and the other fails to adduct in the lateral conjugate movement, there is indication of interruption of the medial longitudinal fasciculus (on the side of adductor paralysis). Irrigating both ears with ice water with the head extended to 60° will sometimes induce vertical conjugate movements. An abducens palsy (sixth nerve) is reflected by a turning in of the eye because of unopposed action of the abducens muscle. The eyes may be held conjugately to one side at all times in a coma—away from the side of the paralysis with large cerebral lesions (looking at the lesion) and toward the side of the paralysis with unilateral pontine lesions (looking away from the lesion). And during a one-sided seizure, the eyes jerk toward the convulsing side of the face, arm, and leg (opposite the irritative focus). The eyes may be turned down and inward (looking at the nose) in thalamic and upper midbrain lesion (Parinaud's syndrome, see Chap. 18). Retraction and convergence nystagmus and ocular bobbing [brisk downward movements of both eyes with slow elevation to the original position (2 or 3 times a minute)] occur with lesions in the midrain tegmentum and lower pons, respectively. The major brainstem structural lesions, including temporal lobe herniation, abolish most, if not all, conjugate ocular movements when producing coma, whereas metabolic disorders do not. Barbiturates and diphenylhydantoin (Dilantin) are the only common intoxicating drugs which affect ocular movements, but they leave pupillary reactions intact.

As to the meaning of the forced postures and movements in the comatose patient, it may be said that restless, grasping, picking movements of one arm or arm and leg or all four extremities signify that the corticospinal tract(s) is intact; variable resistance to passive movement (paratonic rigidity) and strong grasping or complex avoidance movements have the same signification, and if they are bilateral, the coma usually is not deep. Focal seizures require an intact corticospinal motor system and are seldom seen in the paralyzed side with massive destruction of a cerebral hemisphere. Often these elaborate forms of semivoluntary movement are present on the "good side" in patients with extensive disease in one hemisphere and probably represent some type of disequilibrium of cortical and subcortical movement patterns. Definite choreic, athetotic, or even hemiballismic movements indicate disorder of the subtha-

lamic and basal ganglionic structures, just as they do in the alert patient. *Decerebrate rigidity,* with jaw clenched, neck retracted, arms and legs stiffly extended and internally rotated, appears in the condition of diencephalic-midbrain compression by temporal lobe pressure cone, with hemorrhages and infarction of the upper pons and midbrain and with certain metabolic disorders such as hypoglycemia and hypoxia. Occasionally the mechanism of the decerebrate posture is unclear, as with certain bilateral subacute encephalitic, demyelinative, and infarctive cerebral lesions. In some instances the lesions are clearly in the cerebral white matter or basal ganglia. *Decorticate rigidity,* with arm or arms in flexion and adduction and leg(s) extended, signifies higher lesions in cerebral white matter, internal capsules, and thalamus. *Diagonal postures,* opposite arms and legs flexed and extended, probably mean supratentorial lesions; extended arms and flexed legs are probably fragments of decerebrate postures and point to midpontine lesions. *Abolition of all postures and movements* indicates acute bilateral corticospinal interruption and low pontine-medullary lesions involving reticular facilitatory (extrapyamidal) mechanisms. The coma is usually profound.

Lower brainstem reflexes are seldom helpful in the analysis of coma. Only in the most profound metabolic comas and intoxications and in the hypoxemic pannecrosis of the entire brain (brain-death syndromes) are blinking, coughing, swallowing, and spontaneous respirations all abolished. Further, the tendon and plantar reflexes give little indication of what is happening. Tendon reflexes may be preserved until late and may be normal or slightly reduced on the hemiplegic side. The plantar reflexes may be absent or extensor. Only in deep coma or in states of decerebrate rigidity will a cerebral hemiplegia not be detected by flaccidity and motionless arm and leg.

A history of headache before or at the onset of coma, recurrent vomiting, and papilledema afford the best clues to increased intracranial pressure. The lesion is most safely evidenced by computerized tomography (CT scan); however, if there is a question of subarachnoid hemorrhage or meningitis, a lumbar puncture will help. It is usually safe unless there is a herniation of the temporal lobe through the tentorium or of the cerebellum through the foramen magnum. In the latter instance the cerebrospinal fluid pressure may not reflect intracranial pressure. Papilledema may develop within 12 to 24 h in brain trauma and brain hemorrhage but, if pronounced, usually signifies a lesion of longer duration such as a brain tumor or abscess. Multiple retinal or large subhyaloid hemorrhages are usually associated with ruptured saccular aneurysm or hemorrhage from an angioma. Papilledema, with widespread retinal exudates, hemorrhages, and arteriolar changes, is an almost invariable accompaniment of hypertensive encephalopathy. See Chap. 18 for further discussion of retinal changes.

Laboratory procedures Unless the diagnosis is established at once by history and physical examination, it is necessary to carry out a number of laboratory procedures. If poisoning is suspected, the gastric contents must be aspirated and saved for later chemical analysis. A catheter is passed into the urinary bladder, and a specimen of urine is obtained for determination of specific gravity, sugar, acetone, and albumin content. Urine of low specific gravity and high protein content is nearly always found in uremia, but proteinuria may also occur for 2 or 3 days after a subarachnoid hemorrhage or with fever. Urine of high specific gravity, glycosuria, and acetonuria are almost invariable in diabetic coma; but glycosuria and hyperglycemia may result from a massive cerebral lesion. If diphenylhydantoin, bromide, or barbiturate or other intoxication is suspected, it can be verified by special tests for these substances in the blood. A blood count is made, and in malarial districts a blood smear is examined for malarial parasites. Neutrophilic leukocytosis occurs in bacterial infections and also with brain hemorrhage and softening. A blood sample should be examined for glucose, BUN, P_{CO_2}, P_{O_2}, pH, NH_3, Na, K, Cl, and Ca. The cerebrospinal fluid must be drawn if there are no lateralizing signs (CT scan if there are), and the pressure, presence of blood, white cell count, and results of Pandy's test should be recorded. Bloody cerebrospinal fluid (CSF) occurs in cerebral contusion, subarachnoid hemorrhage, brain hemorrhage, and occasionally with hemorrhagic infarcts due to arterial embolism and thrombophlebitis. If there is pleocytosis, a stained smear of the sediment should be searched for bacteria, and a rough quantitative sugar determination should be done. The standard cerebrospinal fluid formula in bacterial meningitis is elevated pressure, high white cell count (5000 to 20,000 per cubic millimeter), elevated protein level, and subnormal sugar values, but exceptionally bacteria may be seen with relatively low white cell counts. The fluid should be saved for quantitative tests for sugar and protein, and a bacterial culture and Wassermann reaction should be performed. If it is suspected that the pressure is elevated, a No. 22 needle should be used. A very high pressure must be slowly reduced by removal of 10 to 15 ml over a period of 15 to 20 min, and urea, mannitol, or other hypertonic solutions should be given to reduce brain swelling over a longer period of time. Jugular compression tests are obviously contraindicated. X-rays of the skull and CT scan should be obtained immediately if there is clinical evidence of mass lesion (one-sided neurological signs with or without papilledema), preferably between the emergency ward and the hospital room. Tests to be done later are: liver function tests, blood and CSF culture, full electrolyte evaluation, and EEG.

CLASSIFICATION OF COMA AND DIFFERENTIAL DIAGNOSIS

The demonstration of focal brain disease or meningeal irritation with cerebrospinal fluid abnormality helps in differential diagnosis. The disease that frequently cause coma may be conveniently divided into three classes, as follows:

I Diseases that cause no focal or lateralizing neurologic signs or alteration of the cellular content of the cerebrospinal fluid
  A Intoxications (alcohol, barbiturates, opiates, etc.) (Chaps. 226 to 227)
  B Metabolic disturbances (diabetic acidosis, uremia, Addisonian crises, hepatic coma, hypoglycemia, hypoxia) (Chap. 371)
  C Severe systemic infections (pneumonia, typhoid fever, malaria, Waterhouse-Friderichsen syndrome) (Chaps. 115 and 118)
  D Circulatory collapse (shock) from any cause, and cardiac decompensation in the aged (Chaps. 30 and 109)
  E Epilepsy (Chap. 23)
  F Hypertensive encephalopathy and eclampsia (Chap. 365)
  G Hyperthermia or hypothermia (Chap. 9)
  H Concussion (Chap. 366)
II Diseases that cause meningeal irritation, with either blood or an excess of white cells in the cerebrospinal fluid, usually without focal or lateralizing signs
  A Subarachnoid hemorrhage from ruptured aneurysm, occasionally trauma (Chap. 365)
  B Acute bacterial meningitis (Chap. 368)
  C Some forms of virus encephalitis (Chap. 369)
  D Acute hemorrhagic leukoencephalitis (Chap. 370)

III Diseases causing focal or lateralizing neurologic signs, with or without changes in cerebrospinal fluid
  A Brain hemorrhage (Chap. 365)
  B Brain softening due to thrombosis or embolism (Chap. 365)
  C Brain abscess (Chap. 368)
  D Epidural and subdural hemorrhage and brain contusion (Chap. 366)
  E Brain tumor (Chap. 367)
  F Miscellaneous, i.e., thrombophlebitis, some forms of virus encephalomyelitis (Chap. 369)

With the clinical laboratory tests outlined above clearly in mind, one can usually ascertain whether a patient with coma falls in one of these three classes. Concerning the group of comas without focal, lateralizing, or meningeal signs, which includes most of the secondary metabolic diseases of the brain, intoxications (both exogenous and endogenous), concussion, and postseizure states, it should be point out that a previous neurologic disease may have left residues which confuse the clinical picture. An earlier hemiparesis from vascular disease or trauma may reveal itself in an alcoholic or hepatic coma, uremia, or hyperglycemic encephalopathy. Also, in hypertensive encephalopathy transitory focal signs may sometimes be present. And occasionally, for no understandable reason, one leg may seem to move less or one plantar reflex be extensor in a metabolic coma. In actuality, the diagnosis of postepileptic coma or concussion depends on observation of the precipitating event or indirect evidence thereof; usually the diagnosis is not too long obscure, for another fit may occur and recovery of consciousness, once the seizures cease, is usually prompt. The final determination of the exact toxic or metabolic disorder requires a variety of clinical and laboratory tests, which are described in other parts of the book.

With respect to the comas of group II, the signs of meningeal irritation (head retraction, stiffness of neck on forward bending, Kernig and Brudzinski leg flexion signs) can usually be elicited in both bacterial meningitis and subarachnoid hemorrhage. However, if the coma becomes deep, stiff neck may disappear or be absent from the beginning. In such cases diagnosis is established by CSF examination. In the coma of bacterial meningitis, unless it is associated with brain swelling and cerebellar herniation, the CSF pressure is not exceptionally high (usually less than 400 mmHg); if the pressure is high, as death approaches there are signs of compression of the medulla, with fixed, dilated pupils, arrest of respiration, and fall in arterial blood pressure. Patients in coma from ruptured aneurysms also have high CSF pressure and often a massive hemispheral and ventricular extension of the hemorrhage.

In patients with group III type of coma it is the inequality of sensorimotor disturbances in the two arms and legs and the aforementioned changes in respiratory pattern, pupillary and ocular reflexes, and the remaining postural states that provide clues to serious structural lesions in the cerebrum and segmental brainstem apparatus. As the latter become prominent, they may obscure earlier signs of cerebral disease. It is noteworthy that bilateral cerebral infarction or hemorrhage or traumatic necrosis and hemorrhage may resemble the comatose state of metabolic and toxic disease, since brainstem mechanisms may be preserved; contrariwise, hepatic, hypoglycemic, and hypoxic coma will sometimes look like the coma of brainstem lesion by causing decerebrate postures. Usually, however, the CSF pressure is elevated and the fluid sanguineous in massive cerebral hemorrhage. Unilateral infarction due to anterior, middle, or posterior cerebral artery occlusion seldom produces more than a stupor or light coma; if infarction is bilateral, however, coma may be profound. Evidence of brainstem displacement and temporal lobe herniation is manifested by increased or altered ventilation (CSR, CNH), bilateral Babinski signs, dilated pupil and drooped eyelid on the side of the lesion, decerebrate postures, later dilated pupils, and loss of full ocular movements. The coma itself gives no clue to the nature of the original mass lesion. The terminal pattern of a descending gradient of diencephalic, mesencephalic, pontomedullary paralysis of nervous system is identical in all. Differential diagnosis must depend on the other data.

An error which must be cautioned against is the diagnosis of irreversible coma (brain-death syndrome) on the basis of complete abolition of all brainstem and cerebral activity and isolectric (flat) EEG if there is hypothermia or evidence of intoxication. Only with hypoxia and cerebral ischemia can this diagnosis be made securely.

Diagnosis has as its prime purpose the direction of therapy, and it matters little to the patient if we diagnose a disease for which we have no treatment. The treatable forms of coma are drug intoxications, toxemia from systemic infections, epidural and subdural hematoma, brain abscess, bacterial and tuberculous meningitis, diabetic acidosis, and hypoglycemia.

RELATIVE INCIDENCE OF DISEASES THAT CAUSE COMA
There have been only a few attempts to determine the relative incidence of diseases that lead to coma. A report from the Boston City Hospital (Solomon and Aring) included the largest series of clinical cases but was heavily skewed by the large local problem of chronic alcoholics, which made up 60 percent of all admissions in coma. Trauma (13 percent), cerebral vascular disease (10 percent), poisonings (3 percent), epilepsy (2.4 percent), diabetes, bacterial meningitis, pneumonia, uremia, and eclampsia followed in that order. In a series of 386 cases of coma of uncertain cause Plum and Posner observed that approximately 40 percent turned out to be metabolic; 25 percent, drug intoxications; and the remainder, neurologic disease of supra- or infratentorial structures.

Of course, figures like these do not provide information concerning coma caused by multiple factors. For example, a patient with a cerebral vascular lesion, old or recent, and diabetes mellitus may lapse into coma during an insulin reaction at a time when there is still sugar in the urine. Only by appreciating the interplay of these several common factors is one likely to reach the correct diagnosis.

The differential diagnosis of diseases that cause focal or lateralizing signs and meningitis is taken up under the dicussions of traumatic, neoplastic, vascular, and infective diseases of the brain.

CARE OF THE COMATOSE PATIENT Impaired states of consciousness, regardless of their cause, are often fatal because they not only represent an advanced stage of many diseases but also add their own characteristic burden to the primary disease. The main objective of therapy is, of course, to find the cause of the coma, by utilization of procedures already outlined, and to remove it. Often, however, the disease process is one for which there is no specific therapy; or, as in hypoxia or hypoglycemia, the disease process may already have expended itself before the patient comes to the attention of the physician. Again, the problem may be infinitely complex, for the disturbance may be attributable not to a single cause but to several possible factors acting in unison, no one of which could account for the total clinical picture. In lieu of direct therapy, supportive measures must be used, and, indeed, it may be said that the patient's chances of surviving the original disease often depend in large measure on their effectiveness.

The physician must give attention to every vital function in the insensate patient. A brief outline of the more important procedures follows. In order for them to be carried out successfully, a well-coordinated team of nurses under constant guidance of a physician is needed.

1 If the patient is in shock, this takes precedence over all other abnormalities. The treatment of shock is discussed in Chap. 30.

2 Shallow and irregular respirations and cyanosis require the establishment of a clear airway and oxygen. The patient should be placed in a lateral position so that secretions and vomitus do not enter the tracheobronchial tree. Pharyngeal reflexes are usually suppressed, and therefore an endotracheal tube can be inserted without difficulty. Stagnant secretions should be removed with a suction apparatus as soon as they accumulate, since they will lead to atelectasis and bronchopneumonia. Oxygen can be administered by mask in a 100% concentration for 6 to 12 h, alternating with 50% concentration for 4 h. The depth of respiration can be increased by the use of 5 to 10% carbon dioxide for periods of 3 to 5 min every hour. Atropine should not be given; edema of the lungs and fluid in the tracheobronchial passages are not glandular secretions. Furthermore, atropine thickens the fluid and also may disturb temperature regulation of the body. Aminophylline is helpful in controlling Cheyne-Stokes breathing. Respiratory paralysis dictates the use of endotracheal intubation and a positive pressure respirator, but in the author's experience neither has been effective in comatose states in which there is disorganization of respiratory centers.

3 The temperature-regulating mechanisms may be disturbed, and extreme hypothermia, hyperthermia, or an unrecognized poikilothermia may occur. In hyperthermia, removal of blankets and use of alcohol sponges and cooling solutions are indicated. An optimal temperature is 1 to 2°C below the normal level.

4 The bladder should not be permitted to become distended. If the patient does not void, a retention catheter should be inserted. If more than 500 ml urine is found in the bladder, decompression must be carried out slowly over a period of hours. Urine excretion should be kept between 500 and 1000 ml per day. The patient should not be permitted to lie in a wet or soiled bed.

5 Diseases of the central nervous system may upset the control of water, glucose, and salt. The unconscious patient can no longer adjust the intake of food and fluids by hunger and thirst. Salt-losing and salt-retaining syndromes have both been described with brain disease. Water intoxication and severe hyponatremia may of themselves prove fatal. The maintenance of water and electrolytes is discussed in Chap. 84. If coma is prolonged, the insertion of a stomach tube will ease the problem of feeding the patient and maintaining fluid and electrolyte balance.

6 Aspiration pneumonitis should be avoided by prevention of vomiting (stomach tube), position, and restriction of oral fluids. Should it occur, corticosteroid therapy is beneficial. The legs should be examined each day for signs of thrombophlebitis.

7 If the patient is capable of moving, suitable restraints should be used to prevent a possible fall out of bed.

8 Convulsions should be controlled by measures outlined in Chap. 23. However, anticonvulsant medication should be used cautiously. An occasional seizure is less harmful than is deep coma from excessive medication.

REFERENCES

FISHER CM: Neurological examination of the comatose patient. Acta Neurol Scand 45(suppl 36):5, 1969

PLUM F, POSNER J: *Diagnosis of Stupor and Coma*, 2d ed. Philadelphia, Davis, 1975

21

DELIRIUM AND OTHER ACUTE CONFUSIONAL STATES

RAYMOND D. ADAMS
MAURICE VICTOR

All physicians sooner or later discover through clinical experience the need for special competence in assessing the mental faculties of their patients. They must be able to observe with detachment and complete objectivity their character, intelligence, mood, memory, judgment, and other attributes of personality, in much the same fashion as they observe the nutritional state and the color of the mucous membranes. The systematic examination of these affective and cognitive functions permits the physician to reach certain conclusions regarding patients' mental status, and these are also of value in understanding the patient and the illness. Without data obtained from the study of mental status, errors will be made in evaluating the reliability of the patients' histories, in diagnosing the neurologic or psychiatric diseases from which they suffer, and in conducting any proposed therapeutic program.

DEFINITION OF TERMS

The definition of normal and abnormal states of mind is difficult because the terms used to describe these states have been given so many different meanings in both medical and non-medical writings. Compounding the difficulty is the fact that the pathophysiology of the confusional states, delirium and dementia, is not fully understood, and the definitions depend on their clinical relationships, with all the lack of precision which this entails. The following nomenclature, though tentative, is useful, and is employed throughout this textbook.

Confusion is a general term denoting an incapacity of the patient to think with customary speed and clarity. This abnormality may depend on any one of several factors. In delirium, for example, inattention and the intrusion of illusory and hallucinatory experiences are mainly responsible. At certain stages in the evolution or devolution of stupor and coma, as indicated in Chap. 20, confusion is aligned with a disorder of conscious awareness and perception. In patients with dementia, confusion is related to a derangement of intellectual function, i.e., an inability to learn, remember, calculate, make appropriate deductions from given premises, reason abstractly, etc.

The term *delirium* is used here to denote a special type of confusional state, acute in onset and transient in nature, and characterized by gross disorientation in the presence of alertness and vigilance, disorder of perception in which illusions and vivid hallucinations are prominent, and overactivity of psychomotor and autonomic nervous functions. Implicit in the definition are certain nonmedical connotations of the term—intense agitation, frenzied excitement, and creations of the imagination. Most stuporous and some demented patients, in contrast to those with delirium, show a *reduced* state of alertness and attentiveness, *decreased* psychomotor activity, and a *relatively slight* tendency to hallucinate. For these reasons, and also because of the particular clinical settings in which they occur, it seems worthwhile to set the delirious states apart from those of depressed consciousness on the one hand and of dementia and amnesia on the other. Such a concept is far from new. To a greater or lesser extent, the terms exogenous reaction type, symptomatic psychosis, toxic psychosis, infective-exhaustive psychosis, and drug, traumatic, or fever delirium all have reference to the syndrome of delirium. All these terms convey the idea of an acute and transient (reversible) confusional state, occurring in a particular clinical setting and carrying a serious prognosis, by virtue of adding its burden to an already serious medical illness.

It should be pointed out that not all neuropsychiatrists agree with our distinction between *confusion* and delirium. There are some, such as Engel and Romano, and Lipowski, who use the term delirium in reference to both conditions. Our insistence on their separation is based on their different clinical manifestations and the clinical settings in which they occur.

The term *amnesia* refers to a loss of past memories coupled with an inability to form new memories, i.e., to learn. It presupposes an alert state of mind, an ability to grasp the problem, to use language normally, and to maintain adequate motivation. The failure is mainly one of retention, recall, and reproduction, and it should be distinguished from the loss of memory that accompanies states of drowsiness and acute confusion, in which information seems never to have been adequately registered in the first place or assimilated.

Dementia means loss of reason or, more particularly, a deterioration of all intellectual or cognitive functions, without clouding of consciousness or disturbance of perception. Implied in the word is the idea of a gradual enfeeblement of mental powers in a person who formerly possessed a normal mind and in most instances irreversibility. *Amentia*, by contrast, indicates a congenital feeblemindedness.

OBSERVABLE BEHAVIOR AND ITS RELATION TO CONFUSION, DELIRIUM, AMNESIA, AND DEMENTIA

The components of mentation and behavior that lend themselves to bedside examination are (1) the processes of sensation and perception; (2) the capacity for memorizing; (3) the ability to think, reason, and form logical conclusions; (4) temperament, mood, and emotion; (5) initiative, impulse, and drive; (6) insight. Of these (1) is sensorial, (2) and (3) may be considered cognitive, (4) affective, and (5) conative or volitional. Insight includes all introspective observations made by patients concerning their own normal or disordered functioning. Each component of behavior and intellection has its objective side, expressed in the manifest effects of certain stimulus conditions on patients and their behavioral responses, and its subjective side, expressed in what patients say they think and feel in relation to the stimuli.

DISTURBANCES OF PERCEPTION Perception, i.e., the processes utilized in acquiring through the senses a knowledge of the "world about" or of one's own body, involves many things aside from the simple sensory phenomenon of being aware of the attributes of a stimulus. It includes the selective focusing and maintaining of attention, elimination of all extraneous stimuli, and recognition of the stimulus by knowing its relationship to personal remembered experience. The perception of an object undergoes predictable types of derangement in disease. Most often one finds a reduction in the number of perceptions in a given unit of time and failure to synthesize them properly and relate them to the ongoing activities of the mind. There may be inattention or fluctuations of attention, distraction (pertinent and irrelevant stimuli now having equal value), and inability to persist in an assigned task. Qualitative changes also appear, mainly in the form of sensory distortions and misinterpretation and misidentification of objects and persons (illusions). These changes, at least in part, form the basis of hallucinatory experience in which the patient reports and reacts to stimuli not present in the environment. There is also an inability to perceive simultaneously all elements of a large complex of stimuli, which is referred to by some as a "failure of subjective reorganization." These major disturbances in the perceptual sphere, sometimes called "clouding of the sensorium," occur most often in acute confusional states and deliria, but quantitative deficiency may also become evident in the advanced stages of amentia and dementia.

DISTURBANCES OF MEMORY Memory, i.e., the retention of learned experiences, is involved in all mental activities. It may be arbitrarily subdivided into several parts, namely, (1) registration, which includes all that was mentioned under perception; (2) mnemonic integration and retention; (3) recall; and (4) reproduction. In disturbances of perception and attention there may be a complete failure of learning and consequently of memory for the reason that the material to be learned was never registered and assimilated. In Korsakoff's amnesic syndrome, newly presented material appears to be temporarily registered but cannot be retained for more than a few minutes, and there is always an associated defect in the recall and reproduction of memories formed some days, weeks, or months before the onset of the illness (retrograde amnesia). Dislocation of events in time and the fabrication of stories, *confabulation,* constitutes a third, but not invariable feature of the syndrome. Sound retention with failure of recall is at times a normal state; when it is severe and extends to all events of past life, it is usually due to hysteria or malingering. Proof that the processes of registration and retention are intact under these circumstances comes from hypnosis and suggestion, and questioning under amytal or pentothal narcosis, whereby the lost items are fully recalled and reproduced. In Korsakoff's amnesic state the patient fails on all tests of learning and recent memory, and behavior accords with the deficiencies of information. Since some aspect of memory is involved to some extent in all mental processes, it becomes the most testable component of mentation and behavior.

DISTURBANCES OF THINKING Thinking, which is central to so many important intellectual activities, remains one of the most elusive of all mental operations. If by thinking we mean selective ordering of symbols for problem solving and capacity to reason and form sound judgments (the usual definition), obviously the working units of most complex experiences of this type are words and numbers. The activity of substituting word and number symbols for the objects for which they stand (symbolization) is a fundamental part of the process. These symbols are formed into ideas or concepts, and the arrangement of new and remembered ideas into certain orders or relationships, according to the rules of logic, constitutes another intricate part of thought. One test is problem solving—the capacity to formulate a problem into several hypotheses, to analyze critically the evidence for and against each hypothesis, and to make a correct choice. In a general way one may examine thinking for speed and efficiency, ideational content, coherence and logical relationships of ideas, quantity and quality of associations to a given idea, and the propriety of the feeling and behavior engendered by an idea.

Information concerning the thought processes and associative functions is best obtained by analyzing the patient's spontaneous verbal productions and by engaging him or her in conversation. If the patient is taciturn or mute, one may then have to depend on the responses to direct questions or upon written material, i.e., letters, etc. One notes the prevailing trends of the patient's thoughts; whether the ideas are reasonable, precise, and coherent or vague, circumstantial, tangential, and irrelevant; and whether the thought processes are shallow and fragmented. Disorders of thought are frequent in confusional states and in degenerative and other types of cerebral disease. The organization of thought may be disrupted with fragmentation, repetition, and perseveration. This is spoken of as *incoherence* and characterizes many acute confusional and delirious states. The patient may be excessively critical, rationalizing, and hairsplitting; this is a type of thinking often manifest in depressive psychoses. Derangements of thinking may also take the form of a flight of ideas. The patient moves nimbly from one idea to another, and associations are numerous and loosely linked. This is a common feature of hypomanic or manic states. The opposite condition, poverty of ideas, is characteristic both of depression, where it is combined with gloomy thoughts, and of dementing diseases, where it is part of a general reduction in intellectual activity. Thinking may be distorted in such a way that the patient fails to check his or her ideas against reality. When a false belief is maintained in spite of normally convincing contradictory evidence, the patient is said to have a *delusion.* Delusions are common to many illnesses, particularly manic-depressive and schizophrenic states. Ideas may seem to the patient to have been implanted in the mind by some outside agency such as radio, television, or atomic energy. These reflect the passivity feelings characteristic of schizophrenic psychoses. Other distortions of thinking, such as gaps or condensations of logical associations are also typical of schizophrenia, of which they constitute a diagnostic feature.

DISTURBANCES OF EMOTION, MOOD, AND AFFECT The emotional life of the patient is expressed in a variety of ways. In the first place, rather marked individual differences in basic temperament are to be observed in the normal population; some persons are throughout their life cheerful, gregarious, optimistic, and free from worry, whereas others are just the opposite. The unusually volatile, cyclothymic person is believed to be liable to manic-depressive psychosis, and the suspicious, withdrawn, introverted person to schizophrenia and paranoia. Strong, persistent emotional states such as fear and anxiety may occur as reactions to life situations and may be accompanied by derangements of visceral function. If excessive and disproportionate to the stimulus and persistent, they are usually manifestations of an anxiety neurosis, depression, or autism and schizophrenia. Variations in the degree of responsiveness to emotional stimuli are also frequent and, when excessive and persistent, assume importance. In depression all stimuli tend to enhance the somber mood of unhappiness. Emotional response that is excessively labile, variable from moment to moment, and poorly controlled or uninhibited is a condition common to many diseases of the cerebrum, particularly those involving the corticopontine and corticobulbar pathways. It constitutes a part of the syndrome of pseudobulbar palsy. All emotional expression may be lacking, as in apathetic states or severe depressions, or the patient may be a victim of every trivial problem in daily life; i.e., cannot control worries. Finally, the emotional response may be inappropriate to the stimulus, e.g., a depressing or morbid thought may seem amusing and be attended by a smile or arouse no emotional reaction, as in schizophrenia.

Since there are relatively few overt manifestations of temperament, mood, and other emotional experiences described above, the physician must evaluate these states by the appearance of the patient and by verbalized accounts of feelings. For these purposes it is convenient to divide emotionality into mood and feeling or affect. By *mood* is meant the prevailing emotional state of the individual without reference to the stimuli immediately impinging upon him or her. It may be pleasant and cheerful or melancholic. The language, e.g., the adjectives used, and the facial expressions, attitudes, postures, and speed of movement most reliably betray the patient's mood. By contrast, *feelings* (or *affect*) are said to be emotional experiences evoked by particular stimuli.

DISTURBANCES IN IMPULSE Impulse, that basic biologic urge, driving force, or purpose, by which every organism is directed to reach its full potentialities, appears to be another extremely important and observable, though somewhat neglected, dimension of behavior. Again, one notes wide normal variations from one person to another in strength of impulse to action and thought, and these individual differences are present throughout life. One of the most conspicuous pathologic deviations is an apparent constitutional weakness in impulse in certain neurotic persons. Moreover, with many types of cerebral disease (particularly those which involve the posterior orbital parts of the frontal lobes, medial forebrain tracts, and lateral hypothalamus), a reduction in impulse is coupled with an indifference or lack of concern about the consequences of actions. In such cases all other measurable aspects of psychic function may be normal. Extreme degrees of lack of impulse, or *abulia,* may take the form of mutism and immobility, a state sometimes called *akinetic mutism.* Psychomotor retardation is a lesser degree of the same state and is a feature of both cerebral disease and depression. In the latter instance mood alteration and extreme fatigability are conjoined.

LOSS OF INSIGHT Insight, the state of being fully aware of the nature and degree of one's deficits, becomes manifestly impaired or abolished in relation to all types of cerebral disease that cause complex disorders of behavior. Rarely does the patient with any of these disorders seek advice or help for the illness. Instead, the family usually brings the individual to the physician. Thus, it appears that the diseases which produce many of the high-order or complex mental abnormalities not only evoke observable changes in mentation and behavior but also alter or reduce the patient's capacity for self-observation.

DELIRIUM

CLINICAL FEATURES These are most perfectly depicted in the alcoholic patient. The symptoms usually develop over a period of 2 or 3 days. The first indications of the approaching attack are difficulty in concentrating, restless irritability, tremulousness, insomnia, and poor appetite. One or several generalized convulsions are the initial major symptom in almost 30 percent of the cases. The patient's rest becomes troubled by unpleasant and terrifying dreams. There may be momentary disorientation or an occasional inappropriate remark.

These initial symptoms rapidly give way to a clinical picture that, in severe cases, is one of the most colorful and dramatic in medicine. The state of consciousness becomes altered ("clouded"); it is clouded in that the patient is inattentive and unable to perceive all elements of the situation. There may be incessant talking, and the patient may be incoherent and look distressed and perplexed; his or her expression is in keeping with vague notions of being annoyed or pursued by some threatening person. From the patient's manner and from the content of his or her speech it is evident that the patient misinterprets the meaning of ordinary objects and ambient sounds and has vivid visual, auditory, and tactile hallucinations, often of a most unpleasant type. At first the patient can be brought momentarily into touch with reality and may in fact answer questions correctly; but almost at once there is a relapse into the preoccupied, confused state; the patient gives wrong answers, is unable to think coherently, and is incapable of proper self-orientation. Before long the patient is unable to shake off the hallucinations even for a second and does not recognize family or physician. Tremor and restless movements are usually present and may be violent. Sleep is impossible or occurs only in brief naps. The countenance is flushed, the pupils are dilated, and the conjunctivas are injected; the pulse is rapid,

and the temperature may be raised. There is much sweating, and the urine is scanty and of high specific gravity. The signs of overactivity of the autonomic nervous system, more than any other, distinguish delirium from all other confusional states.

The symptoms abate, either suddenly or gradually, after 2 or 3 days, although in exceptional cases they may persist for several weeks. The most certain indication of the end of the attack is the occurrence of sound sleep and of lucid intervals of increasing length. Recovery is usually complete.

Delirium is subject to all degrees of variability, not only from patient to patient but in the same patient from day to day and hour to hour. The entire syndrome may be observed in one patient and only one or two components in another. In its mildest form, as so often occurs in febrile diseases, it consists of an occasional wandering of the mind and incoherence of verbal expression, interrupted by periods of lucidity. This form, lacking motor and autonomic overactivity, is sometimes referred to as a *quiet delirium* (or *hypokinetic delirium*) and is difficult to distinguish from other confusional states. The most severe form, best exemplified by delirium tremens, may progress to a "muttering stupor" and in about 10 percent of patients ends fatally.

MORBID ANATOMY AND PATHOPHYSIOLOGY The brains of patients who have died in delirium tremens usually show no pathologic changes of significance. A number of diseases, however, may cause delirium and also give rise to focal lesions in the brain, such as focal embolic encephalitis, viral encephalitis, Wernicke's disease, or trauma. The topography of these lesions is of particular interest. They tend to be localized in the midbrain and subthalamus and in the temporal lobes, where they involve the reticular activating and limbic systems.

Penfield's studies of the human cortex during surgical exploration clearly indicate the importance of the temporal lobe in producing visual, auditory, and olfactory hallucinations. With subthalamic and midbrain lesions there may be visual hallucinations that are not unpleasant, animated, and accompanied by good insight (the peduncular hallucinosis of Lhermitte).

The electroencephalogram in delirium may show nonfocal slow activity in the 5- to 7-per-second range, a state that rapidly returns to normal as the delirium clears. In other cases only low voltage, fast activity in the fast beta frequency range is seen, and in milder degrees of delirium there is usually no abnormality at all.

An analysis of the several conditions conducive to delirium suggests at least three different physiologic mechanisms. The withdrawal of alcohol, barbiturates, or other sedative hypnotic drugs, following a period of chronic intoxication is the most common cause of delirium (Chaps. 226 and 228). These drugs are known to have a strong depressant effect on certain areas of the central nervous system; presumably the release and overactivity of these parts, after withdrawal of the drug, are the basis of delirium. In the case of bacterial infections and poisoning by certain drugs, such as atropine and scopolamine, the delirious state probably results from the direct action of the toxin or chemical agent on these same parts of the brain. Thirdly, destructive lesions, such as acute inclusion body encephalitis of the temporal lobes, may cause delirium by disturbing the function of certain areas, particularly the inferotemporal portions of the temporal lobes.

ACUTE CONFUSIONAL STATES ASSOCIATED WITH REDUCED MENTAL ALERTNESS AND RESPONSIVENESS

In the most typical examples, all mental functions are reduced to some degree, but alertness, attentiveness, and the ability to grasp all elements of the immediate situation suffer most. In the mildest form the patient may pass for normal, and only failure to recollect and reproduce happenings of the past few hours or days reveals the inadequacy of mental function. The more obviously confused patient spends much time in idleness, and what is done may be inappropriate and annoying to others. Only the more automatic acts and verbal responses are properly performed, but these may permit the examiner to obtain from the patient a number of relevant and accurate replies to questions about age, occupation, and residence. Reactions are slow and indecisive, and it is difficult for the patient to sustain a conversation. There may be dozing during the interview and the patient may sleep more hours each day than is natural or the same number at more irregular intervals. Responses tend to be rather abrupt, brief, and mechanical. Disturbances of perception are frequent, and voices, common objects, and the actions of other persons are frequently misinterpreted. Often one cannot discern whether the patient hears voices and sees things that do not exist, i.e., whether the person is hallucinating, or merely misinterpreting stimuli in the environment. Inadequate perception and forgetfulness result in a constant state of bewilderment. Failing to recognize the surroundings and having lost all sense of time, the patient repeats the same question and makes the same remarks over and over again. Irritability may or may not be present. Some patients are extremely suspicious, demanding, and aggressive; in fact, a paranoid trend may be the most pronounced and troublesome feature of the illness.

As the confusion deepens, conversation becomes more difficult, and at a certain stage the patient no longer notices or responds to much of what is occurring. Replies to questions may be with a single word or a short phrase spoken in a soft tremulous voice or whisper. The patient may be mute. In its most advanced stages confusion gives way to stupor and finally to coma. As the patient improves, there may again be a stage of stupor and confusion, occurring in the reverse order. All this informs us that at least one category of confusion is but a manifestation of the same disease processes that in their severest form cause coma.

In the most typical cases, this type of confusional state is readily distinguished from delirium; in others with more than the usual degree of irritability and restlessness, one cannot fail to notice the resemblance to delirium. Similarly, certain cases of delirium, in which tremor, vivid hallucinations, vigilant excited attitude, and insomnia, are relatively inconspicuous, are difficult to distinguish from other acute confusional states. The same diagnostic difficulty arises when a delirium is complicated by an illness that superimposes stupor (e.g., delirium tremens with pneumonia or meningitis).

When clouding of consciousness is minimal and the confusion is of insidious onset and several weeks duration, it may mimic dementia. Lipowski has called it "reversible dementia," claiming it to be an intermediate state between delirium and dementia and still potentially reversible. We would classify it as a protracted confusional state.

SENILE DEMENTIA AND OTHER CEREBRAL DISEASES COMPLICATED BY MEDICAL OR SURGICAL ILLNESS (BECLOUDED DEMENTIA)

Many elderly patients who enter the hospital with medical or surgical illness are mentally confused. Presumably the liability to this state is determined by preexisting brain disease, in this instance senile dementia, which may or may not have been obvious to the family before the onset of the complicating illness. Other cerebral diseases (vascular, neoplastic, demyelinative) may have the same effect of increasing the patient's liability to confusion.

All the clinical features of hypokinetic delirium or of acute confusion may be present. The severity may vary greatly. The confusion may be reflected only in the patient's inability to relate sequentially the history of the illness, or it may be so severe that the patient is virtually *non compos mentis.*

Although almost any complicating illness may bring out the confusion, it is particularly frequent with infectious disease; with posttraumatic and postoperative states, notably after concussive brain injuries; with the removal of cataracts (in which case the confusion is probably related to being temporarily deprived of vision); and with congestive heart failure, chronic respiratory disease, and severe anemia, especially pernicious anemia. Often it is difficult to determine which of several possible factors is responsible for the confusion in this heterogeneous group of illnesses, and there may be more than one. A cardiac patient with a confusional psychosis may be febrile, have marginally reduced cerebral blood flow, be intoxicated by one or more drugs, and be in electrolyte imbalance.

When these patients recover from a medical or surgical illness, they usually return to their premorbid state, though their shortcomings, now drawn to the attention of the family and physician, may be more obvious than before.

CLASSIFICATION AND DIAGNOSIS (See Table 21-1)

The first step in *diagnosis* is to recognize that the patient is confused. This is obvious in most cases, but, as pointed out above, the mildest form of confusion, particularly when some other acute alteration of personality is prominent, may be overlooked. In these mild forms a careful analysis of the thought patterns as the patient gives the history of the illness and the details of personal life will usually reveal an incoherence. Digit span and serial subtraction of 3s and 7s from 100 are useful bedside tests of the patient's capacity for sustained mental activity. Memory of recent events is one of the most delicate tests of adequate mental function and may be accomplished by having the patient relate all the details of entry into the hospital, laboratory tests, etc.

A certain proportion of psychoses of the schizophrenic or manic-depressive type first become manifest during an acute medical illness or following an operation or parturition. A causal relationship between the two is usually sought but cannot be established. Usually the psychosis began long before but was not recognized. The diagnostic studies of the psychiatric illness must proceed along the lines suggested below. Close observation will usually reveal a clear sensorium and relatively intact memory, which permits differentiation from the acute confusional states.

Once it is established that the patient is confused, the differential diagnosis must be made among delirium, acute confusional states associated with psychomotor underactivity, and a beclouded dementia. This can be done usually by careful attention to the patient's degree of alertness and wakefulness, capacity to solve new problems, memory, accuracy of perception, and hallucinations. The distinction between confusional states and dementia may be difficult at times.

CARE OF THE DELIRIOUS AND CONFUSED PATIENT

The physician must be secure in the ability to manage the delirious and confused patient because such illnesses are observed almost daily on the medical and surgical wards of a general hospital. Occurring as they do during an infective fever, in the course of another illness such as cardiac failure, or following an injury, operation, or withdrawal from alcohol, they never fail to create grave problems. The physician's program of treatment may constantly be threatened by the patient's agitation, sleeplessness, and uncooperative attitude. The nursing personnel are often sorely taxed by the necessity of providing a satisfactory environment for the convalescence of the patient and, at the same time, maintaining a tranquil atmosphere for the other patients. And the family is appalled by the sudden specter of insanity and all that it entails.

The primary therapeutic effort is directed to the control of the underlying medical disease. Other important objectives are to quiet the patient and protect him or her against injury. A private nurse, an attendant, or a member of the family should be with the patient at all times, if this can be arranged. Depending on how active and vigorous the patient is, a locked room, screened windows that cannot be opened by the patient, and a low bed or mattress on the floor should be arranged. It is often better for the patient to be allowed to walk about the room rather than be tied into bed, which may excite or frighten him or her into struggling to the point of complete exhaustion and collapse. If less active, the patient can usually be kept in bed by leather wrist restraints, a restraining sheet, or a net thrown over the bed. Unless it is contraindicated by the primary disease, the patient should be permitted to sit up or walk about the room part of the day.

TABLE 21-1
Classification of delirium and acute confusional states

I Delirium
  A In a medical or surgical illness (no focal or lateralizing neurologic signs; cerebrospinal fluid usually clear)
    1 Typhoid fever
    2 Pneumonia
    3 Septicemia, particularly erysipelas and other streptococcal infections
    4 Rheumatic fever
    5 Thyrotoxicosis and ACTH intoxication (rare)
    6 Postoperative and posttraumatic states
  B In neurologic disease that causes focal or lateralizing signs or changes in the cerebrospinal fluid
    1 Vascular, neoplastic, or other diseases, particularly those involving the temporal lobes and upper part of the brainstem
    2 Cerebral contusion and laceration (traumatic delirium)
    3 Acute bacterial and tuberculous meningitis
    4 Subarachnoid hemorrhage
    5 Viral encephalitis
  C The abstinence states, exogenous intoxications, and postconvulsive states; signs of other medical, surgical, and neurologic illnesses absent or coincidental
    1 Withdrawal of alcohol (delirium tremens), barbiturates, and nonbarbiturate sedative drugs, following chronic intoxication (Chaps. 226 and 228)
    2 Drug intoxications: camphor, caffeine, ergot, bromides, scopolamine, atropine, amphetamine
    3 Postconvulsive delirium
II Acute confusional states associated with psychomotor underactivity
  A Associated with a medical or surgical disease (no focal lateralizing neurologic signs; cerebrospinal fluid clear)
    1 Metabolic disorders: hepatic stupor, uremia, hypoxia, hypercapnea, hypoglycemia, porphyria
    2 Infective fevers
    3 Congestive heart failure
    4 Postoperative and posttraumatic psychoses
  B Associated with drug intoxication (no focal or lateralizing signs; cerebrospinal fluid clear): opiates, barbiturates, bromides, Artane, etc.
  C Associated with diseases of the nervous system (the focal or lateralizing neurologic signs and cerebrospinal fluid changes of these conditions are commoner than in delirium)
    1 Cerebral vascular disease, tumor, abscess
    2 Subdural hematoma
    3 Meningitis
    4 Encephalitis
  D Beclouded dementia, i.e., senile or other brain disease in combination with infective fevers, drug reactions, heart failure, or other medical or surgical disease

All drugs that could possibly be responsible for delirium—particularly opiates, barbiturates, bromides, atropine, hyoscine, cortisone, adrenocorticotropic hormone (ACTH), and salicylates in large doses—should be discontinued (unless withdrawal effects are believed to underlie the illness). Paraldehyde and choral hydrate are trustworthy sedatives under these circumstances. Paraldehyde, which is preferred, may be given orally or rectally in doses of 10 to 12 ml. For oral administration, mixing it with fruit juices makes it more palatable. Chlorpromazine, chlordiazepoxide, and diazepam are often extremely effective if given in full doses, and should be continued until natural sleep is restored. One must be cautious in attempting to suppress agitation completely. To accomplish this may require very large doses of drugs, and vital functions may then be dangerously impaired. The purpose of sedation is to ensure rest and sleep so that the patient does not become exhausted.

Confusional states related to antidepressant drugs, e.g., amitriptyline, are said to be reversed by a 2-mg dose of physostigmine.

A fluid intake and output chart should be kept, and any fluid and electrolyte deficit should be corrected. The pulse and blood pressure should be recorded at intervals of 2 h in anticipation of circulatory collapse. Transfusions of whole blood and vasopressor drugs may be lifesaving.

Finally, the physician should be aware of many small therapeutic measures that may allay fear and suspicion and reduce the tendency to hallucinations. The room should be kept dimly lighted at night, and if possible the patient should not be moved from one room to another. Every procedure should be explained in detail, even such simple ones as the taking of blood pressure or temperature. The presence of a member of the family may enable the patient to maintain contact with reality.

Most delirious patients tend to recover if they are placed in good hygienic surroundings and competently nursed. The family should be reassured on this point and must also understand that the abnormal behavior and irrational actions of the patient are not willful but rather are symptomatic of a brain disease. Once recovered, the patient will be at least partly amnesic for the period of the delirium or confusion, a gap which must be filled by information provided by physician and family.

REFERENCES

Adams RD, Victor M: *Principles of Neurology.* New York, McGraw-Hill, 1977

Benson FD, Blumer D: *Psychiatric Aspects of Neurologic Disease.* New York, Grune & Stratton, 1975, chap 2

Lipowski ZJ: Delirium, clouding of consciousness and confusion. J Nerv Ment Dis 145:227, 1967

22

SLEEP AND ITS ABNORMALITIES

RAYMOND D. ADAMS

NORMAL SLEEP The pattern of sleeping varies in the different epochs of life. A nocturnal predominance begins to appear after the first few weeks of postnatal life, resulting in the biphasic pattern of sleeping and waking which persists throughout adolescence and adult years, unless altered by disease. Not until old age does it break down progressively. Night awakenings then increase in frequency, and the daytime waking period becomes interrupted frequently by paroxysmal bursts of sleep lasting 1 to 10 s (microsleep) and by longer naps. Throughout most of life females are said to need about an hour more sleep than males.

Physiologic mechanisms By means of electroencephalographic analysis five stages of sleep, associated with two alternating physiologic mechanisms, have been defined. Relaxed wakefulness is found to be accompanied by sinusoidal alpha waves of 8 to 12 cycles per second (cps) and low-voltage fast activity of mixed frequency in the EEG; there are the usual associated blinks, eye and limb movements, and moderate tone in all the skeletal muscles. As a person falls asleep and the muscles relax, the eyelids droop, the eyes begin to roll from side to side, and the EEG pattern changes to one of progressively lower voltage and mixed frequency. This is called stage I sleep. As sleep deepens into stage II, bursts of 12- to 14-cps waves (sleep spindles) and high-amplitude, sharp, slow-wave (*k*) complexes appear. By now eye movements have ceased, but muscle tone is maintained. The deep sleep of stages III and IV is featured by an increasing proportion of high-voltage, slow-wave activity in the EEG. In stage V, rapid eye movements return and muscle tension increases in the jaw, whereas the neck, trunk, and limb muscles, after a few quivering, tremulous, or myoclonic movements, become completely slack. The first four stages are called *nonrapid eye movement sleep* (NREMS); the last stage is variously designated as *rapid eye movement sleep* (REMS), *paradoxic sleep* (PS), or *activated sleep* (AS).

In a typical night the normal drowsy adult passes successively through stages I, II, III, and IV of NREMS. After about 70 min, mostly spent in stages III and IV, the first REMS period occurs, usually heralded by an increase in body movements and a shift in the EEG pattern from stage IV to II. This NREMS-REMS cycle (activity-rest cycle of Kleitman) is repeated at about the same interval four to six times during the night, depending on the length of sleep. The first REMS cycle may be brief, and the later cycles include less stage IV NREMS.

There is some evidence that the two alternating physiologic sleep mechanisms for NREMS and REMS lie in the brainstem and are influenced by biogenic amines, particularly 5-hydroxytryptamine (serotonin) and norepinephrine. The serotoninergic neurons are known to be located in the medial tegmentum of the medulla, pons, and lower midbrain and to project upward to the hypothalamus and thalamus and to the orbital frontal and medial temporal (limbic) cortex. Activation of serotoninergic neurons, presumably by factor S (see below), suppresses the higher reticular formation subserving consciousness and causes hypersomnia with increase in NREMS and REMS; their destruction or pharmacologic suppression by serotonin antagonists results in insomnia, with disappearance of both NREMS and REMS. Another group of neurons, presumably responsive to dopamine and norepinephrine, lies in the lateral tegmentum of the pons, the locus ceruleus, substantia nigra, and hypothalamus and are necessary for REMS. Their activation increases REMS and their destruction or suppression by norepinephrine antagonists reduces or abolishes it. However, REMS is primed by NREMS serotoninergic neurons, and the two types of sleep are always closely related. Only under conditions of narcolepsy, cataplexy, and sleep paralysis (see below) is REMS separated from NREMS. Monoamine oxidase inhibitors selectively diminish or abolish REMS. Thus, normal sleep involves both a serotoninergic mechanism and a catecholaminergic or adrenergic mechanism.

The details of the neuropharmacology of sleep have not yet been fully ascertained. In some mysterious way, a product(s) of fatigue or some obscure hypnotoxin activates the serotoninergic neurons subserving NREMS and at the same time suppresses the effects of afferent stimulation of the upper reticular

formation. It is not known how neuronal systems of REMS are suppressed for a time during NREMS and periodically become active and interrupt it. The plasma of drowsy or sleeping animals has been shown by Monnier to contain factor delta, a substance with properties that induce somnolence and increase NREMS in alert animals. More recently Pappenheimer and his associates have isolated a factor S from the cerebrospinal fluid and brain of animals deprived of sleep. When injected into rats and rabbits, it induces slow-wave sleep lasting 4 to 6 h. Its molecular weight is about 350, and it is destroyed by pronase, indicating the presence of peptides. Probably it is similar if not identical to the sleep-promoting factor isolated by Nagasaki.

EFFECTS OF SLEEP LOSS Of all the conditions that make for human efficiency and sense of well-being, sleep is one of the most important. Deprived of sleep, experimental animals will die within a few days, no matter how well they are fed, watered, and housed; under similar circumstances human beings suffer a variety of unpleasant symptoms that must be separated from the diseases that cause insomnia.

Human beings deprived of sleep (NREM and REM) for periods of 60 to 200 h experience increasing fatigue and irritability and find it difficult to concentrate, to perceive accurately, and to maintain their orientation. Illusions and hallucinations intrude into consciousness, primarily in the visual and tactile sensory fields, becoming more intense as the period of sleeplessness is prolonged. Performance of motor tasks deteriorates. If the tests are of short duration and of slow pace, the subject can keep up, but cannot if speed and perseverance are demanded. Incentive to work weakens, and sustained action is interrupted by lapses of attention. Neurologic signs include mild and fleeting nystagmus, a slight tremor of the hands, ptosis of eyelids, expressionless face, and thickness of speech, with mispronunciation and incorrect choice of words. A decrement of alpha waves appears in the EEG, and closing of the eyes no longer generates alpha activity. The concentration of 17-hydroxycorticosteroids increases in the blood, and catecholamine output rises.

Recovery after prolonged sleep deprivation shows that the amount of sleep required to recuperate is never equal to the amount lost. At first, the subject rapidly falls into stage IV of NREMS, often with "supernormal" slow waves in the EEG and remains there, at the expense of stage II sleep; stage IV is interrupted from time to time by REMS which remains in the usual proportion. But by the second night, REMS rebounds and exceeds that of the predeprivation period. Stage IV NREMS seems, then, to be the most valuable stage in restoring the flagging functions of the nervous system.

The effects of partial and differential deprivation are somewhat different. If prevented night after night from having REMS, subjects show a greater tendency to become hyperactive and emotionally labile, and less able to control their impulses, a state which corresponds to the heightened activity, excessive appetite, and oversexuality of REMS-deprived animals. Differential deprivation of NREMS (stages III and IV) leads, instead, to hyporesponsiveness.

Of course, since the need for sleep is known to vary from person to person in everyday life, it is difficult to decide what is partial sleep deprivation. Some individuals function perfectly on as little as 3 to 4 h per night, and others, who sleep long hours, claim not to obtain the maximum benefit from it.

DERANGEMENTS OF SLEEP Insomnia This word signifies want of sleep, and is used popularly to indicate any impairment in its duration, depth, or restorative properties. Quantitative precision as to what constitutes insomnia is impossible because of the uncertainty as to the natural requirement of sleep and also its role in the economy of the human body.

Two classes of insomniacs may be defined: one in which there appears to be a primary disturbance of the normal sleep mechanism, the other in which sleep impairment is secondary to another disease or condition. The latter is encountered frequently in medical practice and may usually be ascribed to pain or some other annoying sensation, or to nervousness, anxiety, and worry.

The term *primary insomnia* should be reserved for those persons who throughout their lives have never enjoyed restful slumber, and in whom none of the usual symptoms of neurosis, depression, or other psychiatric or medical diseases can be elicited. Unlike the rare individuals who seem to thrive on 3 to 4 h sleep a night, they suffer the effects of partial sleep deprivation and resort to drugs and various techniques to induce or maintain sleep. Their life comes so obviously to revolve around sleep that they have been called "sleep pedants" or "sleep hypochondriacs." They sleep for shorter periods than normal persons, awaken more often, spend less time in REMS and more in stage II NREMS, move more often, have more rapid pulse, peripheral vasoconstriction, and higher body temperature, and show a heightened physiologic arousal. Thus their sleep is both quantitatively and qualitatively different from that of "good sleepers."

While there is no doubt that the victims of insomnia, regardless of the cause of their wakefulness, are likely to exaggerate the amount of sleep lost, *primary insomnia* should be recognized as an entity and not passed off as a neurotic quirk.

Of the sensory disorders conducive to abnormal wakefulness, pain in the spine with or without nerve root involvement stands out, as does abdominal discomfort from peptic ulcer and carcinoma. Tired, aching, restless legs, an obscure benign state known as the "restless leg syndrome" (anxietas tibialis), may regularly delay the onset of sleep. Excessive fatigue may give rise to many abnormal muscular sensations of similar nature. Acroparesthesias, peculiar nocturnal tingling and numbness of palms and fingers due to tight carpal ligaments (carpal tunnel syndrome), may awaken the patient at night, as does cluster or histamine headache, which nearly always occurs 2 to 3 h after falling asleep.

Severe insomnia is a frequent complaint of patients suffering from psychiatric disease (more than 85 percent of a group of insomniacs in one series). Its simplest form occurs in a reactive nervous state in which domestic and business worries keep the patient's mind in a turmoil. Also, vigorous mental activity late at night or excitement which leaves the muscles tense counteracts drowsiness and sleep. Under these circumstances there is difficulty in falling asleep and a tendency to sleep late in the morning.

Sleeplessness is also commonly recorded in the histories of patients suffering from psychoneuroses and psychoses. Illnesses in which anxiety and fear are prominent symptoms usually result in difficulty in falling asleep and light, fitful, or intermittent sleep. Also, disturbing dreams are frequent and may awaken the patient; exceptionally, the patient may even try to stay awake in order to avoid them. The diurnal-nocturnal timing of sleep is altered, but quality and quantity are little if at all changed. In contrast, the depressive illnesses, particularly the manic-depressive or involutional type, cause either light sleep in the early part of the night or early morning waking and inability to return to sleep. Quantity of sleep is reduced, and nocturnal mobility is increased. The REMS, although not reduced, comes earlier in the night; this is termed the *increased pressure of REMS*. If anxiety is combined with depression,

both the above patterns are observed. In states of mania, sleep diminishes and REMS may be abolished. The sleep rhythm may be totally deranged in acute confusional states and delirium, and REMS increases. In the latter the patient may only doze for short periods, both day and night. The total amount and depth of sleep in a 24-h period are reduced. Frightening hallucinations may prevent sleep. The senile and arteriosclerotic patient tends to catnap during the day and then refuses to go to bed at night. The nocturnal sleep is intermittent; its total amount may be either increased or decreased.

Disturbances in the transitional period of sleep As sleep comes on, certain nervous centers may be excited to a burst of insubordinate activity. The result is a sudden start that arouses the incipient sleeper. It may involve one or both legs or the trunk, less often the arms. If the start occurs repeatedly during the process of falling asleep and is a nightly event, it may become a matter of great concern to the patient.

Sensory centers may be disturbed in a similar way, either as an isolated phenomenon or in association with phenomena that induce motion. The patient may drop off to sleep but be aroused by a sensation that darts through the body. Or a sudden clang or crashing sound disturbs commencing sleep. Sometimes there is a sudden flash of light or a sensation of being lifted and dashed to earth or of being turned. These symptoms are probably similar sensory paroxysms involving the labyrinthine mechanism.

Sleep palsies and acroparesthesias Curious and at times distressing paresthetic disturbances develop during sleep. Everyone is familiar with the phenomenon of an arm or leg "falling asleep." The immobility of the limbs and the maintenance of uncomfortable postures without being aware of them permit pressure to be applied to exposed nerves. The ulnar, radial, and peroneal nerves are quite superficial in places; pressure of the nerve against an underlying bone may interfere with intraneural circulation of the compressed segment. If such pressure is continued for half an hour or longer, a sensory and motor paralysis sometimes referred to as *sleep palsy* may develop. This condition usually lasts only a few minutes or hours, but if the compression is prolonged, the nerve may be severely damaged so that functional recovery awaits remyelination or regeneration. Unusually deep sleep, as in alcoholic intoxication, renders the patient especially liable to sleep palsies merely because the patient does not heed the discomfort of an unnatural posture.

Acroparesthesias are frequent in adult women and are not unknown to men. The patient complains of being awakened by an intense numbness, tingling, prickling, a feeling of "pins and needles" in the fingers and hands after being asleep for a few hours. There are also aching, burning pains or tightness and other unpleasant sensations. At first there is a suspicion of having slept on the arm, but the usual bilaterality and the occurrence regardless of the position of the arms dispel this notion. Usually the paresthesias are in the distribution of the median nerves. Vigorous rubbing of the hands restores normal sensation, and the paresthesias subside within a few minutes, only to return later upon first awakening in the morning. The condition seldom occurs during the daytime unless the patient is lying down or sitting with the arms and hands in one position. When acroparesthesias are frequent, the hands may at all times feel swollen, stiff, clumsy, slightly numb, and sometimes distressingly painful. More severe degrees of this condition merge with the compression syndrome of the median nerve (carpal tunnel syndrome) described in Chaps. 19 and 377.

Nightmares and night terrors (pavor nocturnus) Awakening in a state of terror has happened to nearly everyone. Children are especially susceptible. Fever disposes to it, as may many other conditions, such as indigestion. Bad dreams, stimulated directly by the reading of blood-curdling stories or seeing exciting television programs before bedtime, may be followed by a nightmare. Nightmares differ from night terrors only in the greater intensity of the anxiety and extreme degree of autonomic discharges in the latter. In addition there is more vocalization and motor activity, even to the point of running as if pursued. Then night terror and somnambulism are combined. Gastaut and his associates, who have compared nightmares and night terrors, found the latter to occur in stage IV NREMS often within a half hour of falling asleep. The patient suddenly develops an arousal response (imperfect) with return of alpha rhythm in the EEG and a pattern of extreme motility. Vocalizations, walking, screams, tachycardia (130 to 170 beats per min) and increase in respiratory rate, all lasting a few minutes, may occur.

Such phenomena are of little significance as isolated events in childhood. Indeed, few children have escaped the more frequent experience of nightmare. Only if persistent and frequent do they become matters of pressing medical complaint. Of greater importance is the differentiation of both the nightmare and night terror from nocturnal epilepsy, which also may have a tendency to occur only during a specific stage of sleep. Pharmacologic agents which interfere with the metabolism of either serotonin or norepinephrine offer a possible therapeutic approach to both nightmares and night terrors.

Somnambulism and sleep automatism Examples of sleepwalking occasionally come to the attention of the practicing physician. This condition likewise occurs more often in children than in adults. After being asleep for a time, the patient arises from bed, walks about the house, and may turn on a light or perform some other familiar act. There is no outward sign of emotion; the eyes are open, and the sleeper is guided by vision, thus avoiding familiar objects. The sight of an unfamiliar object may awaken the sleeper. If spoken to, there is no response; if told to return to bed, the sleeper may do so but more often must be led back to it. Sometimes strange phrases or sentences are muttered over and over. The following morning there is usually no memory of the episode. Talking in one's sleep is probably a minor variant.

Nocturnal epilepsy Paroxysmal abnormalities of the brain waves of the type seen in epilepsy tend to occur in epileptic patients during or shortly after the onset of sleep. Not infrequently an individual subject to grand mal attacks will have them only at night during sleep.

Nocturnal jerks of the legs, also called *nocturnal myoclonus*, are another troublesome symptom because they interfere with sleep night after night. This condition differs from the restless leg syndrome in that involuntary movements occur. Only recently has it been classified as a myoclonic form of epilepsy. It is unaccompanied by all other epileptic manifestations. Anticonvulsant drugs are said to control it, though in two cases the author has had better success with an occasional dose of purified opium alkaloids (Pantopon). Obviously an opiate cannot be prescribed for its control.

THE HYPERSOMNIAS *Prolonged states of sleep* are characteristic of patients suffering from encephalitis lethargica (Chap. 369), trypanosomiasis, and a variety of other diseases localized to the floor and walls of the third ventricle. Small tumors in the posterior hypothalamus and midbrain have been associated with arterial hypotension, diabetes insipidus, and somnolence lasting many weeks. Such patients can be aroused, but if left alone, immediately fall asleep. Tumors of the brain, in general, show a tendency to cause drowsiness and increase in time spent in sleep, but those of the diencephalon more so than any others (e.g., more so than those of the posterior fossa). Trau-

matic brain lesions and other diseases have been found to produce similar clinical pictures. Myxedema, if severe, may cause hypersomnia.

There are two special varieties of hypersomnia, the Kleine-Levin and Pickwickian syndromes. The Kleine-Levin syndrome consists of periodic hypersomnolence lasting for periods of 2 to 3 weeks and hyperphagia (bulimia). The attacks occur two or three times a year. Onset is usually during adolescence with a striking male predominance. The pathogenesis is obscure. The Pickwickian syndrome of obesity, dyspnea, hypercapnea, and drowsiness are discussed in Chap. 371. This condition may be accompanied by a distressing *sleep apnea.*

NARCOLEPSY AND CATAPLEXY The essential characteristic of narcolepsy is uncontrollable sleepiness. Many times a day the individual is assailed by an uncontrollable desire to sleep. The eyes close, muscles relax, breathing slows, and the person appears to be dozing. A noise or a touch is enough to awaken these individuals, and they may feel refreshed momentarily. As a rule the condition begins in adolescence or early adult life. The periods of sleep may occur at any time of day, especially when the patient is physically inactive. The impulse to sleep is so insistent that the victim may be unable to sit through a single class in school or a meeting without at once falling asleep. A given period of sleep usually lasts up to 15 min, seldom as long as an hour unless lying down. At the onset there may be blurring of vision, diplopia, and ptosis which may raise the question of an ophthalmologic disorder. The condition is often associated with cataplexy (70 percent of cases), sleep paralysis (50 percent), and hypnagogic hallucination (25 percent).

Cataplexy consists of the sudden loss of muscle tone provoked by exaggerated emotion such as excessive laughter or anger. Approximately 70 percent of patients with narcolepsy, if questioned carefully, will admit to having cataplexy. Reference here is made to the curious circumstance that hearty laughter, sadness, or anger will cause the patient's head to fall forward, the jaw to drop open, the knees to buckle, even with falling to the ground, and all with preservation of consciousness. The attack lasts only a minute or two.

The other components of the narcoleptic tetrad are sleep paralysis and hypnagogic hallucinations. In sleep paralysis individuals, while falling asleep or awakening, become conscious of an inability to move or speak. They have the helpless feeling that a word from someone or a touch would break the spell. Recovery occurs in a minute or two. Vivid hallucinations may also occur in this period or separately in a brief nap.

Narcolepsy and cataplexy usually begin in adolescence or early adult life and, once started, continue throughout the adult period, possibly being less frequent in old age. Males are affected more than females, and there is suggestion of a genetic factor. The attack of narcolepsy resembles REMS, as is also true of cataplexy, sleep paralysis, and the hallucinations. The night sleep pattern may also begin with REMS. The EEG is usually normal. No complete pathologic studies are available. There are no other neurologic abnormalities. The condition must be distinguished from the somnolence of obesity, hypothyroidism, heart failure, and excessive use of drugs and alcohol. In these latter cataplexy is always absent.

OTHER CAUSES OF EXCESSIVE DAYTIME DROWSINESS Diurnal hypersomnia of nonnarcoleptic type is another common complaint. Idleness and imposed inactivity due to medical disease increase the amount of daytime sleep, especially in certain parts of the day—after breakfast, after lunch, around dinner time. In part it may be occasioned by poor nocturnal sleep or drugs. Certain medical conditions such as cardiac decompensation, pulmonary disease with hypercapnea, hypothyroidism, and brain tumor cause diurnal drowsiness.

In an analysis of more than 200 cases of diurnal hypersomnia, Guilleminault and Dement found more than half had narcolepsy and the rest heavy snoring with "upper airway sleep apnea," narcolepsy with sleep apnea, drug dependency, or other disorders.

SLEEP IN RELATION TO MEDICAL DISEASES Patients with a variety of nocturnal medical complaints have been found to undergo other important physiologic changes in relation to certain phases of sleep. Anginal attacks at night appear usually with REMS and peptic ulcer pain increases during REMS when production of hydrochloric acid increases. On the other hand, attacks of bronchial asthma during the night may appear in any phase of sleep.

TREATMENT OF SLEEP DISORDERS Insomnia In general, there are three varieties of wakefulness. For best management, treatment should be based on the type exhibited by the patient. One type, infrequently observed in younger patients, is the inability to fall asleep. Individuals affected by this type have become more and more tense during the day and are unable to relax. This type of insomnia usually lasts from 1 to 3 h, and then the individual sinks into an exhausted, deep sleep which continues through the night. For these patients any fairly quick-acting, rapidly destroyed hypnotic such as secobarbital (Seconal), 0.1 g, flurazepam (Dalmane), 30 to 60 mg, chloral hydrate (Noctec), 500 to 1000 mg, glutethimide (Doriden), 500 mg, or methaqualone (Sopor), 150 to 300 mg, given 15 to 30 min before going to bed is useful in inducing and maintaining sleep. After a week or two, however, their effect wanes. Kales and Kales found only flurazepam to retain its power of reducing sleep latency and awake time after sleep onset.

The second type of insomnia is exhibited by patients who are able to go to sleep but who awaken in 2 or 3 h and lose sleep in the middle of the night. They awaken during the period when sleep normally lightens, and some are alternately awake and asleep all the rest of the night. Often these are sick persons with a debilitating or painful illness which generates more pain and restlessness as muscles relax and leave painful areas unsplinted. In others, fever, sweats, dyspnea, or other distressful symptoms develop and demand attention. Frequently, these patients secure relief from pentobarbital (Nembutal), 0.1 g, or flurazepam (Dalmane), 30 to 60 mg, given at bedtime. For cardiac patients who have Cheyne-Stokes respiration or moderate orthopnea, a rectal suppository of aminophylline, 0.5 g given at bedtime, will frequently relieve the respiratory distress and promote sleep. When pain is a factor in insomnia, acetylsalicylic acid, 0.3 to 0.6 g, should be given with the sedative. Occasionally, codeine phosphate, 30 mg, meperidine (Demerol), 50 mg, or morphine sulfate, 10 to 15 mg, may be required when pain is severe.

The third type of insomnia is seen in patients who go to sleep promptly and sleep well most of the night, only to awaken too early in the morning. Most of these individuals are older persons who turn night into day. They go to bed and get up earlier and earlier so that soon they are sleeping during the day and are alert during the night. Into this category also fall those individuals who are under great tension, worry, or anxiety or are overworked and exhausted. These people sink into bed and sleep through sheer exhaustion, but around 4 or 5 A.M. they awaken with their worries and are unable to get back to sleep. Most of these patients are benefited by barbital, 0.3 g,

given with fruit juice or milk at bedtime. For debilitated patients the compressed tablets of insoluble material should be crushed to ensure proper absorption, or sodium barbital should be substituted. Chloral hydrate, 500 mg given with fruit juice at bedtime, is also effective and may be substituted for barbital.

Patients with serious mental agitation, delirium, or excitement who require prompt, easily controlled, relatively safe sedation should receive whiskey, 30 to 60 ml by mouth, or paraldehyde, 15 to 30 ml by mouth in iced fruit juice, or the same dose of the latter by rectum but diluted with 200 ml physiologic saline or 120 ml olive oil. For frankly delirious patients 25 to 50 mg chlorpromazine tid or a similar psychotropic drug has been a most helpful medication. Generally, it is wise to avoid barbiturates with highly agitated patients, since occasionally they may precipitate serious mental confusion, excitement, or even manic tendencies. Chloral hydrate, 1 to 2 g by mouth, is also useful in the management of these individuals and frequently proves more satisfactory than the barbiturates.

A word of caution about oversedation is wise in any discussion of sedative drugs. All too frequently they are abused in that they are given when not needed, the dosage is too great, or the wrong preparation is chosen. These drugs are a common source of constipation, lead to fatigue and lack of energy and strength, and interfere with the patient's recovery from illness.

When large dosages of quicker-acting barbiturates, 0.4 to 0.6 g daily, or other of the soporific drugs are given for more than a few weeks, there is real danger of habituation, which, once developed, is pernicious in character. Withdrawal, unless accomplished skillfully and in graded steps, may cause serious mental disturbance or precipitate convulsions. The chronic insomniac who has no other symptoms should not be permitted to use sedative drugs as a crutch on which to limp through life. The solution to the problem is rarely to be found in medication. One should search out and correct the underlying difficulty, using medication only as a temporary helpful tool. A good book, pleasure in staying awake, and belief that the human organism will always get as much sleep as needed are helpful.

Since psychologic factors have not been demonstrated in such cases, a conservative program of medical management and pharmacologic treatment is indicated. Diazepam (Valium), which suppresses stage IV NREMS, is helpful in controlling night terrors, and if their differentiation from nocturnal epilepsy is impossible, a trial on diphenylhydantoin (Dilantin) and phenobarbital is indicated. (See Chap. 23 for further information concerning anticonvulsant medication.)

Narcolepsy and cataplexy For narcolepsy and cataplexy there is no therapy which will control all the symptoms. The narcoleptic responds best to (1) strategically placed naps (during lunch hour, before or after dinner, etc.) and (2) the use of analeptic drugs, such as amphetamine sulfate (Benzedrine), methylphenidate (Ritalin), or pipradrol (Meratran). The time of medication should be adjusted to the study or work habits of the patient. The usual dose of amphetamine varies from 5 to 10 mg given three to five times a day. This is ordinarily well tolerated and does not cause wakefulness at night. The dose of Ritalin is 10 to 20 mg thrice daily, and of Metratran, 2.5 to 5.0 mg 2 or 3 times daily. These have rather little effect on cataplexy but are partially effective in the Kleine-Levin syndrome. Fortunately the latter is less frequent, and some psychiatrists have claimed that it can be controlled by avoidance of emotionally charged situations. The newest addition to the pharmacology of cataplexy is imipramine (Tofranil), which, in doses of 25 mg three to four times a day, markedly reduces attacks, presumably by abolishing REMS.

REFERENCES

ADAMS RD, VICTOR M: *Principles of Neurology.* New York, McGraw-Hill, 1977

GUILLEMINAULT C, DEMENT W: Two hundred thirty-five cases of excessive daytime sleepiness: Diagnosis and tentative classification. J Chronic Dis 29:733, 1976

KALES A, KALES JD: Recent findings in the diagnosis and treatment of disturbed sleep. N Engl J Med 290:487, 1974

PAPPENHEIMER JR, SETCHELL BP: The measurement of cerebral blood flow in the rabbit and sheep. J Physiol (Lond) 226:48P, 1972

23
THE CONVULSIVE STATE AND IDIOPATHIC EPILEPSY

MARIA SALAM-ADAMS
RAYMOND D. ADAMS

The magnitude of the problem of convulsion as a leading manifestation of a medical or neurologic disease can hardly be overstated. The statistics of Hauser and Kurland show that at least 1 million persons in the United States are subject to recurrent seizures and that at least ten times that number consult a physician or go to a hospital at some time in their lives because of a seizure.

A solitary or brief outburst of convulsions may occur during the course of many medical illnesses; its significance derives from the fact that it indicates involvement of the nervous system and by its very nature, if repeated every few minutes, as in status epilepticus, may threaten life. Recurrent convulsions over long periods of life, most of the episodes being more or less identical in type, represent a different sort of problem. On the one hand they may be a manifestation of an ongoing primary neurologic disease that demands diagnosis and therapy, as in brain tumor. On the other hand, they may call attention to a long-standing, occult, episodic, corticothalamic derangement that began some time in the distant past and remains in some instances as a fibroglial scar. Not infrequently the original disease was unnoticed; perhaps it occurred in utero, at birth, or during childhood in parts of the brain that were too immature to test; or it may have affected a silent area of the mature brain. Patients with such old lesions, who make up the majority of those with recurrent seizures, are necessarily classified as having "idiopathic epilepsy," because it is impossible to obtain data regarding the original disease. The seizure may be the only sign of the brain abnormality.

The convulsive disorder is the expression of a sudden, excessive, disorderly discharge of neurons in either a structurally normal or diseased cortex. The discharge results in an almost instantaneous disturbance of sensation, loss of consciousness, convulsive movement, or some combination thereof. A terminologic embarrassment arises from the diversity of the clinical manifestations. It seems improper to call a condition a "convulsion" when only an alteration of sensation or of consciousness takes place. The word "seizure" is preferable, as a generic term, and also lends itself to qualification. Motor or convulsive seizure is not, therefore, tautologic, and one may also speak of sensory seizure.

COMMON TYPES OF CONVULSIVE DISORDER The generalized convulsion ranks as the most frequent type, being both a common expression of a number of ongoing diseases and the lasting mark of some obscure disease in the past. As in petit mal, another special type of spell noted for its brevity, the cause of the lesion and its location are unknown. Presumably the generalized seizure involves the entire cerebral cortex and diencephalon. Various other patterns of seizure, such as the psychomotor, which is associated with disease of the temporal lobe, usually have a demonstrable cortical focus, either actively progressing or stationary.

When the idiopathic recurrent types of convulsive disorder are analyzed as a group, as in the survey of nearly 2000 patients by Lennox, it was found that 51 percent had generalized convulsions; 8 percent, petit mal; and the remaining 41 percent, focal and mixed types, of which psychomotor was the most frequent.

Generalized convulsion (other than grand mal) Certain intercurrent medical diseases manifest themselves at one stage by a seizure or a series of seizures beginning as immediate loss of consciousness, with stiffening, then clonic rhythmic jerking of the limbs or only with the latter. The focality of the initiating lesion may be indicated by tonic or clonic spasm of the muscles of only one part of the body or a turning of eyes and head to one side. Consciousness tends to be reinstated soon after the cessation of the generalized motor activity. A single myoclonic jerk or multiple ones may be a prelude to the major seizure or may follow it or be interspersed between seizures. In some instances, especially in metabolic disorders of the brain, the focal motor seizures may appear first on one side of the body, then on the other, progressing to a generalized seizure.

Generalized convulsion (grand mal) The recurrent generalized seizure of grand mal type is more elaborate and demonstrates more clearly the effect of the epileptic discharge on the physiology of the nervous system. It begins with a sudden loss of consciousness, a cry, a fall to the ground, tonic then clonic movements of muscles of cranium and limbs, sometimes sphincteric incontinence, and other autonomic disorders. The motor activity soon terminates, leaving the patient in a state of coma, which lasts for many minutes or even as long as a half-hour. As the coma recedes, mental confusion, drowsiness, and headache become evident.

Petit mal (minor epilepsy, l'absence) This type of seizure, occurring most frequently between the fourth year of life and adolescence, comes without warning and is notable for its brevity and minimal motor accompaniment. It consists essentially of a brief loss of consciousness, lasting a few seconds. A few 3-per-second blinks or jerks of eyelids and sometimes arms may be conjoined. Petit mal may be more variable (atypical) with 2-per-second motor and EEG pattern and then is more likely to be combined with sudden falling episodes or single, brief, generalized myoclonic contractions of limbs or other types of seizures (laughing or "gelastic" spells, unilateral tonic or clonic spasms). These mixed types are especially difficult to control.

COMMON FOCAL SEIZURE PATTERNS **Psychomotor epilepsy** Certainly this is the most frequent and interesting type of focal seizure pattern. The aura, if it occurs, often takes the form of a complex hallucination or perceptual illusion. There may be an unpleasant smell or taste, or the revival of a complicated visual scene involving people, dwellings, etc., usually taken from past experiences and resembling a dream. There may be recurrence of a certain thought. Furthermore, the patient's perception of what is seen and heard and relationship to the outside world are altered. Objects appear to be far away or unreal (*jamais vu*); or strange objects or persons may seem familiar (*déjà vu phenomenon*). Hughlings Jackson applied the term *dreamy state* to these psychic disturbances. In the seizure patients behave as though partially conscious. They may get up and walk about, unbutton or remove clothes, attempt to speak, or even continue such habitual acts as driving a car. If asked a specific question or given a command, it is evident that they are out of contact with the examiner and do not understand. When restrained, they may resist with great energy and at times may be violent. This type of behavior is said to be *automatic*, presumably because the patient behaves like an automaton. Convulsive movements, when present, are likely to consist of chewing, smacking and licking of the lips, and, less often, tonic spasms of the limbs or turning of the head and eyes to one side.

In any given case one or several of these phenomena may be observed. In the series studied by Lennox and Lennox, which numbered 414 cases, 43 percent of patients displayed some of these motor or psychomotor phenomena; 32 percent, the automatic state; and 25 percent, the psychic changes. Some psychomotor seizures are very brief, lasting only for seconds, and others continue for hours. This calls to mind that the duration of the seizure is an unsatisfactory criterion for classification.

LOCALIZED MOTOR SEIZURES A lesion in one or the other frontal lobe may give rise to a generalized or major convulsive seizure of the type described above, without an introductory aura. In some cases there is a turning movement of the head and eyes to one side, simultaneously with loss of consciousness. It has been postulated that in both types of seizure, the one with and the one without contraversive movements, the discharge from the frontal lobe spreads rapidly into an integrating center such as the thalamus, with immediate loss of consciousness.

The *Jacksonian motor seizure* begins usually with a tonic contraction or a clonic rhythmic twitching of the fingers of one hand, the face on one side, or one foot. The twitching may occur in bursts, or paroxysms. The disorder then spreads, or marches, from the part first affected to other muscles on the same side of the body—from the face to the neck, hand, forearm, arm, trunk, and leg; if the first movement is in the foot, the order is reversed. A high incidence of onset in the lips, fingers, and toes probably is related to the greater cortical representation of these parts of the body. The disease process or focus of excitation is usually the rolandic cortex, area 4 (Fig. 25-1) on the opposite side; in a few cases it has been found in the postrolandic convolution. Lesions confined to the premotor cortex (area 6) are said to induce tonic contractions of an arm, face, neck, or all of one side of the body. Perspiration and piloerection, sometimes only of the parts of the body involved in a focal motor seizure, suggest that these autonomic functions have cortical representation in the rolandic area.

Another type of focal motor epilepsy consists of rhythmic clonic movements of one group of muscles, usually in the face, arm, or leg. These may continue for a variable period of time, from minutes to weeks or months (epilepsia, partialis continua). The seizure does not occur in bursts or paroxysms and usually does not "march" to other parts of the body. Its localizing value has not been settled. Some patients have a lesion in the opposite sensorimotor areas of the cerebral cortex.

SOMATIC, VISUAL, AND OTHER SENSORY SEIZURES Somatic sensory seizures, either focal or marching to other parts of the body on one side, nearly always indicate a parietal lobe lesion. The usual *sensory disorder* is described as a numbness, a tingling, or a "pins-and-needles" feeling. Other variations are sensations of crawling (formication), buzzing, electricity, or vibration. Pain and thermal sensations are infrequent. The onset is in the lips, fingers, and toes in the majority of cases, and the spread to adjacent parts of the body follows a pattern determined by sensory arrangements in the postcentral (postro-

landic) convolution of the parietal lobe. In the series of Kristiansen and Penfield the seizure focus was found in the postcentral convolution in 24 of 55 cases; it was central (both pre- and postrolandic) in 18, and precentral in 7 cases. If localized in the cranial muscles, the focus is in the lowest part of the convolution, near the sylvian fissure; if in the foot or leg, the upper part near the superior sagittal sinus is involved.

Lesions in or near the striate cortex of the occipital lobe usually produce a sensation of lights, of darkness, or of color. The patient may tell of seeing stars or moving lights in the visual field on the side opposite the lesion. Sometimes they appear to be straight ahead of the patient. Often, if they occur on only one side of the visual field, the patient believes only one eye to be affected, the one opposite the lesion, probably because the average person is unaware that there are two corresponding visual fields. It is curious that a seizure arising in one occipital lobe may cause momentary blindness in both eyes. It has been noted that seizures arising in the lateral surface of the occipital lobes (Brodmann's areas 18 and 19) are more likely to cause twinkling or pulsating lights. Complex visual hallucinations are usually due to a focus more anterior in the visual association areas at the junction of occipital, parietal, and the posterior part of the temporal lobe, and they may be associated with auditory hallucinations. Often the visual images, either those of the hallucination or of objects seen, are distorted or seem too small (*micropsia*) or unnaturally arranged.

Auditory hallucinations are rather infrequent as an initial manifestation of a seizure. Occasionally a patient with a focus in the superior temporal convolution on one side will report a buzzing or a roaring in the ears. A human voice sometimes repeating recognizable words has been reported a few times by patients with lesions in the more posterior part of the dominant temporal lobe.

Vertiginous sensations of a type suggesting vestibular stimulation may be the first symptom of a seizure. The lesion is usually localized in the superior posterior temporal region or at the junction between the parietal and temporal lobes. Occasionally, with a temporal focus, vertigo is followed by an auditory sensation.

Olfactory hallucinations are often associated with disease of the inferior and medial parts of the temporal lobe, usually in the region of the hippocampal convolution or the uncus (hence the term *uncinate seizures*, after Jackson). Usually the smell is exteriorized, i.e., projected to someplace in the environment, and is of a disagreeable nature. Gustatory hallucinations have also been recorded in proved cases of temporal lobe disease. Sensations of thirst and salivation may be associated. Seizures arising in and stimulation of the upper surface of the temporal lobe in the depths of the sylvian fissure during neurosurgical operations have produced peculiar sensations of taste.

Visceral sensations arising in the thorax, epigastrium, and abdomen are among the most frequent of the auras. They are described as a vague, indefinable feeling, a sinking sensation in the pit of the stomach, and a weakness in the epigastrium or substernal area that rises to the throat and head. The seizure discharge may be localized to the upper bank of the sylvian fissure or in the upper intermediate or medial frontal areas near the cingulate gyrus. Palpitation and acceleration of pulse at the beginning of the attack have also been related to a temporal lobe focus.

PSYCHIC PHENOMENA A close relationship between psychic changes and temporal lobe foci has been established. Disease of either temporal lobe may be accompanied by seizures that have many of the characteristics of psychomotor epilepsy. In addition, complex visual and auditory hallucinations with feelings of unreality, and partial or complete interruption of consciousness, may be observed more often in the dominant than the nondominant temporal lobe. Compulsive thought or action may recur in a fixed pattern during each seizure. Automatic behavior or even frank psychoses resembling confusional states or schizophrenia, and lasting for hours or days, may be induced by seizure discharges or electrical stimulation of the temporal lobe.

The various motor, sensory, or psychic phenomena may be combined in many different sequences. These presumably indicate the spread of a seizure discharge from one cortical area to another. A flash of light followed by tingling of one side of the body suggests that the epileptic discharge began in the occipital lobe and extended to the somatic sensory areas in the parietal lobe. A smell of something burning, followed by chewing and smacking movements, and then loss of speech would be interpreted as a spread of the seizure discharge from the region of the uncus to the upper parts of the temporal and the inferior frontal lobes. A focal motor seizure followed by a tonic contraction of one side of the body and then by turning of the head and eyes contralaterally would indicate a successive involvement of the motor, premotor, and contraversive cortical field for head and eyes. Little is known about the factors that facilitate or inhibit the spread of seizure discharges from one part of the brain to another.

EVOCATION OF SEIZURES (REFLEX EPILEPSY) Seizures can sometimes be evoked in susceptible persons by a physiologic or psychologic stimulus. Approximately 1 in every 15 patients will have remarked that their seizures occur under special circumstances, such as being exposed to flickering light, passing from darkness to light or the reverse, being startled by a loud noise, hearing a series of monotonous sounds or music, touching, rubbing, or hurting a particular part of the body, making certain movements (e.g., eating, reading, carrying out some complex mental task), or being subjected to fright or other strong emotion. The evoked seizure may be focal (beginning often in the part of the body that has been stimulated) or generalized. In a few instances this reflex epilepsy, as it is called, has been due to a focal cerebral disease, such as a tumor, but more often its cause cannot be ascertained. A special type of reflex myoclonic epilepsy with a strong tendency to familial incidence can be elicited by photic stimulation (photic epilepsy). Another point of interest in these cases of evoked seizure has been the phenomenon of willfully averting the seizure by undertaking some mental task, e.g., thinking about some distracting subject or counting, or by initiating some physical activity.

PATHOPHYSIOLOGY OF THE CONVULSION Reflex epilepsy suggests that epilepsy is a natural state, a physiologic event resulting from excitation and subsequent inhibition of a damaged part of the cerebrum. Eventually the physiologic event that initiates the seizure is a high-voltage discharge of an assemblage of cortical neurons. There need not be a visible lesion for, under the proper circumstances, it can be initiated in entirely normal cerebral cortex, as when the cortex is functionally altered by low-intensity electric stimulation that does not in itself produce seizures but leaves an epileptic focus (kindling effect of Goddard), or is activated by a drug or injured by hypoxia. But it is the visible focal lesion that has been the most thoroughly investigated. Some of the electric properties of the cortical focus suggest that its neurons have been deafferented. Deafferented neurons are known to be hypersensitive; they remain chronically in a state of partial depolarization, and the cytoplasmic membranes have an increased permeability which renders them susceptible to activation by hyperthermia, hypoxia, hypoglycemia, and hyponatremia, as well as by repeated sensory (e.g., photic) stimulation and during certain phases of sleep (when hypersynchrony of neurons is known to occur). Another hypothesis is that the lesion of the cortex has

resulted in the removal of a normal diencephalic inhibitory effect. An excellent review of these and other pathophysiologic mechanisms is to be found in the monograph of Jasper et al.

The biochemical studies of the involved clone of neurons of a seizure focus have suggested some interesting possibilities. Epileptic foci are known to be sensitive to the facilitatory transmitter substance acetylcholine and to be slower in binding and removing it than normal cerebral cortex; a deficiency of γ-aminobutyric acid (GABA), the inhibitory transmitter, a disturbance of cytochrome oxidase with decrease in ATP production, a reduction in the Krebs cycle function with a shift to GABA-succinate shunt, and disturbance in local regulation of extracellular K, Na, Ca, Mg are other hypotheses. An interesting proposal is that astrocytes adjacent to neurons and presynaptic terminals have altered relationships in cortical scars and are no longer able to modulate fluxes of extracellular potassium.

Once the intensity of the seizure discharge exceeds a certain point, it spreads to adjacent cortical and to thalamic and brainstem nuclei. It is then that the first clinical manifestation of the convulsion begins. Presumably the excitatory activity is fed back from the thalamus to the original focus and to other parts of the forebrain, giving rise to the characteristic high-frequency discharge in the EEG, and there is propagation downward to spinal neurons via corticospinal and reticulospinal pathways. Shortly thereafter a diencephalocortical inhibition begins and intermittently interrupts the focal and generalized seizure discharge, changing it from the persistent discharge of the tonic phase to the intermittent bursts of the clonic phase. These become less and less frequent and finally cease altogether, leaving in their wake strong inhibition or paralysis of the neurons of the epileptic focus. This latter is the presumed basis of *Todd's postepileptic paralysis* which is accompanied by diffuse slow waves in the EEG in all parts of the cerebrum. In petit mal it is thought that the high-voltage spike-slow-wave discharge originates in the thalamus, and this may also be true of some cases of grand mal, in both of which consciousness is at once abolished. On the other hand, atypical petit mal and possibly the typical type as well can be induced by a mesial frontal lesion. Temporal lobe seizures are known to arise in foci in the medial temporal lobe, amygdaloid nuclei, and hippocampus. Electric stimulation in these areas reproduces a partial loss of conscious contact with environment, feelings of depersonalization, and automatic behavior.

A discovery of no little importance is that a seizure focus, if active for a time, may establish via commissural and corticocortical connections, a secondary focus in the corresponding area of cortex in the opposite hemisphere (mirror focus) or in adjacent regions. The nature of this development is not fully understood, but probably it is similar to the kindling effect. This becomes a source of confusion in trying to identify electrographically the side of the primary lesion.

Severe seizures may disturb the chemistry of the brain by causing hypoxia, acidosis with rise in P_{CO_2}, and an accumulation of lactic acid. Some of these effects are secondary to respiratory spasm, blockage of airway, and excessive muscular activity at a time when the metabolic activity of the involved cerebral tissue is maximal. These biochemical changes give rise to secondary cerebral lesions. The latter are especially frequent in the temporal lobes and cerebellum and may themselves later become epileptic foci. Ohmsted and others explain the rising frequency of temporal lobe foci in the epileptic individual in this way. A violent epileptic discharge of the brain may cause respiratory arrest or cardiac standstill, with death ensuing immediately or if there is survival, a severe hypoxic (postepileptic) encephalopathy.

The electroencephalogram provides a delicate proof of Hughlings Jackson's theory of epilepsy—that it is an excessive, disorderly discharge of cortical neurons. At the onset of the focal seizure this is registered in or near the focus as a series of spikes or sharp waves interrupting the normal alpha and beta waves. The clinical spread of the seizure has its electroencephalographic equivalent in the extension of the abnormal electrical waves; with generalization of the seizure (grand mal), the entire electroencephalographic recording surface of the brain exhibits spikes of high voltage. Petit mal is accompanied by a characteristic 3-per-second wave-spike complex occurring simultaneously in all cortical leads and presumably taking origin from a diencephalic focus. At first there was thought to be a characteristic electroencephalographic picture for psychomotor epilepsy, but further studies have not confirmed this. The postseizure state, sometimes called *postconvulsive paralysis of cerebral function*, also has its electroencephalographic correlate in random generalized slow waves. With recovery of normal mentation the electroencephalogram returns to normal. If the electroencephalographic tracing is obtained during the interval between seizures, it is abnormal to some degree in approximately 40 percent of fully conscious and 75 percent of sleeping patients.

The epileptic lesion   Of the innumerable diseases that are epileptogenic it has not been possible to distinguish the component of the lesion that is responsible for the seizures from one that is not. In other words one cannot say from microscopic examination whether any given lesion was epileptic. Gliosis, fibrosis, vascularization, meningocerebral cicatrix have all been incriminated, but they occur as well in nonepileptic foci. Partial disconnection of groups of cortical neurons from those of neighboring cortex, of the other cerebral hemisphere, and of the thalamus seems likely to have occurred. Or certain systems of inhibiting neurons may have been destroyed. Once a gliotic focus of whatever cause, bordered by groups of discharging neurons, becomes epileptogenic, it may remain so throughout the lifetime of the patient. Of course, none of these remarks apply to the "kindled focus" in which the structurally normal cortical neurons are capable of giving rise to seizures for a year or more.

DISEASES CAUSING SYMPTOMATIC SEIZURES   Among the medical diseases which may be complicated by a burst of seizures, the following are the most frequent.

Generalized convulsions mixed in some instances with unilateral muscular contractions of clonic type appear prominently during an abstinence or withdrawal period in patients addicted to *alcohol* or *barbiturates*. Suspicion of this mechanism is raised by the telltale marks of alcoholic excesses or the history of a prolonged nervousness requiring sedation. Also disturbances of sleep, disorientation, illusions, and visual hallucinations often precede and follow the convulsive phase of the illness. The convulsive period lasts several days and is accompanied and followed for several more by a confusional state.

Bacterial meningitis is another type of illness with a strong convulsive tendency, more pronounced in children than in adults. Fever and stiff neck usually provide the clue, and lumbar puncture yields the salient laboratory data.

Uremia is another condition with a prominent convulsive aspect. Of interest is the sequence of events in complete anuria. This condition is tolerated for 2 to 3 days without neurologic signs, and then there is a rapid onset of twitching, trembling, myoclonic jerks, and generalized motor seizures. Tetany may

be added (see Chap. 275). The motor display, one of the most dramatic in medicine, lasts several days until the patient sinks into terminal coma or recovers. When this syndrome accompanies lupus erythematosus, delirium tremens, idiopathic epilepsy, or generalized neoplasia, one can nearly always be sure that it has a basis in renal failure.

Cardiac arrest, suffocation or respiratory failure, NO_2 anesthesia, CO poisoning—the common causes of hypoxic encephalopathy—usually induce a diffuse myoclonic jerking of all the musculature and generalized seizures as soon as cardiac function is resumed. The convulsive phase of this condition may last only a few days, in association with coma, stupor, or confusion; or it may persist indefinitely as an intensive myoclonic-convulsive state.

Other acute illnesses complicated by generalized and multifocal motor seizures are hyponatremia and water intoxication, thyrotoxic storm, hypertensive encephalopathy, porphyria, hypoglycemia, pyridoxine deficiency, argininosuccinic aciduria, and phenylketonuria. Picrotoxin and pentylenetetrazol (Metrazol) are two of the most highly convulsant drugs in use, and lead and arsenic the most frequent convulsive metallic intoxicants.

Generalized seizures with or without twitching may occur in the terminal phases of many other illnesses, such as gram-negative septicemias with shock, liver coma, and intractable congestive heart failure.

There are several primary diseases of the brain which are announced by an acute convulsive state. Myoclonic jerking and seizures appear early in acute inclusion-body encephalitis and other forms of viral, treponemal, and parasitic encephalitis, subacute sclerosing encephalitis, as well as in lipid storage diseases, Jakob-Creutzfeldt disease, and diffuse gliomatosis of the brain.

It seems strange that difficult problems of a convulsive nature seldom occur in patients suffering from cerebrovascular disease. Seizures hardly ever occur in limbs paralyzed by cerebral infarction and hemorrhages, and limbs that are involved in seizures in a comatose patient will later prove to have retained their normal power. However, old cortical infarcts, usually of embolic origin or due to an old subcortical hemorrhage, become epileptogenic in approximately 20 percent of cases. The rupture of an aneurysm is occasionally marked by one or two generalized convulsions. Thrombotic occlusions of cerebral arteries are almost never convulsive in the opening phases of the stroke. The rare thrombophlebitis with cortical ischemia and infarction is probably the most highly convulsive vascular lesion. Tumor, on the other hand, is a frequent cause of focal or generalized seizures, the latter present in more than 30 percent of cases if located in the central parts of the cerebrum. Nearly 40 percent of cerebral abscesses have in their wake recurrent convulsions. Cerebral traumatism is the other common convulsive disease. Thirty to forty percent of all penetrating and contusing cerebral injuries will be followed by focal epilepsy. (See Chaps. 366 to 368.)

IDIOPATHIC EPILEPSY   Idiopathic epilepsy tends to express itself with maximal frequency at two periods in life, between the ages of 2 and 5 years and around puberty. More often than not the first seizure is generalized, though a series of petit mal, "staring spells," may precede its appearance. Up to this moment development may have been normal, and a neurologic examination is likely to disclose no other abnormality. In a smaller proportion other types of seizures (neonatal, infantile spasms, severe febrile seizures, etc.) have occurred earlier in life. Although the seizures may be either of generalized motor type (51 percent of cases) or petit mal (8 percent) in the beginning, as the years pass and the seizures continue, approximately 40 percent of patients will have both these types or psychomotor seizures.

The severity of the convulsive state varies from a single attack every several years to many per day. If the generalized seizures are at all frequent, they pose a constant threat of injury and social embarrassment, often preventing the further education of the child or the gainful occupation of the adult, and they may interfere with the development of a stable, mature personality. Of the milder form of disorder, however, sufficient medical control may be achieved so that there is no interference with normal life activities. In enlightened communities no longer is an intelligent epileptic ostracized by teachers or employers, and virtually all patients without other neurologic abnormalities can find their place in society. If there is evidence of mental retardation, character changes, hemiparesis, etc., as not infrequently happens, the other problems may be as important as the idiopathic epilepsy.

The common diagnostic procedures performed in the interval between seizures are usually uninformative, i.e., the cerebrospinal fluid is normal, x-rays of skull are normal, pneumoencephalogram and arteriograms, where they have been done, are negative. Only the electroencephalogram will demonstrate an abnormality in 40 to 75 percent of cases, either a generalized paroxysmal 3-per-second spike-slow-wave complex (dart-dome), sharp waves, or some other less specific alterations.

Without doubt the appearance of a convulsion poses a serious problem for the patient, family, and physician. There is first of all the possibility of its being the initial manifestation of a neurologic disease which will take the life of the patient (e.g., infiltrating glioma). But even if the convulsion is due to a stationary, healed lesion, life expectancy is slightly reduced owing to the danger of injury or, rarely, unexplained death. If seizures are frequent or difficult to control, mentation may be altered: the patient is dull, vague, querulous, often hyperreligious, and illogically argumentative. If seizures are infrequent and the EEG relatively normal between attacks, prognoses for successful schooling, occupational adjustment, and marriage are excellent. Mental deterioration, fortunately, occurs rarely, contrary to lay opinion, and when it becomes evident over a few weeks, months, or years one must suspect (1) wrong initial diagnosis (not idiopathic epilepsy but seizures due to some definable cerebral disease), (2) drug intoxication from anticonvulsant medication, (3) recurrent subclinical seizures, (4) hypoxic-hypotensive crisis during a bout of prolonged seizures, (5) subdural hematoma resulting from head injury.

APPROACH TO THE CLINICAL PROBLEM OF RECURRENT SEIZURES A history of recurrent attacks of loss of consciousness or awareness associated with abnormal movements or confusion is usually sufficient to establish a diagnosis of epilepsy. With such patients a thorough history, a complete physical and neurologic examination, testing of the visual fields, and laboratory studies, including computerized tomography (CT scan) of the skull and an electroencephalogram, should be done. The results of these essential procedures will determine to which of the categories in the above classification the case belongs or whether one is justified in making the diagnosis of idiopathic epilepsy.

If a patient not known to have been epileptic has an acute illness with frequent generalized or one-sided seizures, a search must be conducted for clinical and laboratory signs of infection, metabolic and endocrine diseases, and intoxications.

If convulsions have occurred in the past, an inquiry as to epilepsy in the family history and occurrence of head trauma or cerebral infections in the past must be made; careful description of the seizure itself, including prodromata, aura, manifestations during the seizure and the postictal period, must be obtained. Seizures in other members of the family favor slightly the diagnosis of *idiopathic epilepsy*. Signs of pulmonary or ear infection or of congenital heart disease with a right-to-left shunt should suggest, in a patient with recently acquired seizures, the possibility of a *brain abscess*. The presence of a heart murmur and fever or of atrial fibrillation favors embolism. Head trauma of a serious nature, followed by seizures after an interval of several weeks to 2 years, indicates that an injury may have given rise to convulsions. A regularly recurring aura, especially of a focal nature, may indicate a localized lesion in the brain. Similarly, a focal convulsive movement at the onset of the seizure probably indicates a localized cerebral lesion. A transient monoplegia or hemiplegia or aphasia or hemisensory loss (Todd's paralysis) in the postictal period also has considerable significance in localizing a lesion. In fact, its presence may provide the best clue to a focal brain lesion. A history of other neurologic symptoms such as headache, localized paralysis, or mental changes often indicates the need for special diagnostic studies.

A general physical examination may provide clues to the legion of conditions associated with epilepsy. Protuberances over the skull may suggest an underlying pathologic condition. Vascular nevi over the body, especially over the face and in the retina, may be associated with vascular abnormalities within the skull. Small tumors, often pedunculated, distributed over the body surface bring to mind the diagnosis of von Recklinghausen's disease and, when associated with seizures, may indicate an intracranial glioma or neurofibroma. White spots over the trunk and limbs and sebaceous adenomas of the face point to the diagnosis of tuberous sclerosis. Smallness of an arm or leg indicates a lesion acquired at an early age. Cranial nerve disturbances are also helpful in diagnosis; thus, a sixth-nerve paralysis is often associated with increased intracranial pressure. Localized weakness, differences in reflexes, or the presence of abnormal reflexes, such as Babinski's response, all have localizing value.

The question of what laboratory procedures should be done in cases of epilepsy can be answered only on the basis of the clinical findings. With recent onset of generalized convulsions simple blood chemistry tests are among the first measures to be carried out. The determination of blood glucose helps orient the examiner in instances of hypoglycemia and hyperglycemia; the calcium level provides the main clue to hypocalcemia, the blood urea nitrogen (BUN) to kidney disease, and sodium and potassium levels to multiple metabolic disturbances, including dilutional hyponatremia. X-rays of the skull, and more particularly a CT scan, if available, should be taken in all cases. Significant findings related to increased intracranial pressure include erosion of the clinoid processes and, in infants and children, separation of the sutures. Hyperostoses, erosions of the skull, abnormal vascular markings, and intracranial calcifications are other findings of importance that may appear in skull x-rays. In the CT scan one looks for defects in cerebral tissue, ventricular distortion, and areas of enhancement (with contrast techniques). Because of the frequency of cerebral metastases from primary carcinoma of the lung, chest x-rays should be made in all patients suspected of having intracranial neoplasm.

Lumbar puncture can be of considerable value in elucidating the causes of epilepsy. If the history, neurologic examination, or skull x-rays show any abnormality, especially if a focal lesion in the brain is suggested, then a lumbar puncture is mandatory (unless there are signs of high intracranial pressure). Of special importance are determination of the pressure, cell count, total protein, and serologic tests. An abnormal cell count usually indicates an infectious process. An elevation only of total protein (greater than 100 mg per 100 ml) favors the diagnosis of a tumor. If the pressure is normal but other symptoms or signs point to a recently acquired, localized brain lesion, an arteriogram, radionuclide scans, or pneumoencephalogram may be needed to supplement the findings on CT scan. The visualization of the cerebral hemisphere by these procedures may be of particular help to the neurosurgeon in localizing the lesion and in planning a surgical approach to it.

The electroencephalogram, although now routinely employed in the definitive diagnosis of cases with epilepsy, is not absolutely conclusive, since it may be normal in some patients, particularly if the seizures are relatively infrequent, or abnormal in diseases that do not cause epilepsy. The test is of particular value in diagnosing petit mal, for here clinical or subclinical attacks are apt to be frequent enough to register during the electroencephalographic test. Abnormal electric waves may manifest themselves in other types of epilepsy as well, and the electroencephalogram may be abnormal during the interseizure period, demonstrating either focal or generalized abnormalities of cortical activity. Activation of the electroencephalogram by photic stimulation and drug-induced sleep is now standard procedure in many laboratories (see Chap. 364).

The type of clinical study in any given case is dictated to some extent by the age of the patient and the length of time the patient has been having seizures. Up until early adulthood most patients turn out to have idiopathic epilepsy. With increasing age, the incidence of idiopathic epilepsy becomes less and that of symptomatic epilepsy increases. Thus the appearance of convulsions for the first time in early or middle adult life should be presumptive evidence of brain tumor until every effort has been made to rule it out (see Table 23-1). If seizures have been occurring for 15 to 20 years or more, the likelihood of tumor or other progressive neurologic disease is so remote that most diagnostic tests are not worthwhile.

DIFFERENTIAL DIAGNOSIS The clinical differences between a seizure and a syncopal attack are presented in Chap. 13 and need not be repeated here. It must be emphasized once again that there is no single criterion for distinguishing between them. The author has erred in calling akinetic seizures simple faints and in mistaking cardiac or carotid sinus faints for seizures. Petit mal may be difficult to identify because of the brevity of attacks. One helpful maneuver is to have the patient count for 5 to 10 min. If having petit mal, the patient will blink or stare, pause in counting, or skip one or two numbers. Hyperventilation is a useful way of evoking this type of seizure. Psychomotor seizures are the most difficult of all to diagnose. These attacks are so variable in character and so likely to induce minor disturbances in conduct rather than obvious interruptions of consciousness that they may be misdiagnosed as temper tantrums, hysteria, psychopathic behavior, or acute psychosis.

A special problem in diagnosis is offered by states of mental dullness and confusion. Epileptic patients as seen in hospital and office practice usually show no mental deterioration, regardless of the type of seizure. Therefore, the appearance of dementia, confusion, or some other derangement of mental function should suggest the possibility of recurrent subclinical seizures not controlled by medication, drug intoxication, postseizure psychosis, or a brain disease that has caused both dementia and seizures. To distinguish these clinical states may require careful observation, along the lines suggested in Chap. 21, and electroencephalography (Chap. 364).

TREATMENT AND MANAGEMENT OF THE CONVULSING AND EPILEPTIC PATIENT Status epilepticus Rarely does a single seizure terminate life, although instances do occur presumably from a cardiac arrhythmia, suffocation, or aspiration. Recovery from a single seizure is usually prompt and requires no special treatment.

It is necessary to protect the convulsing patient from injury and to make sure that there is a clear airway. A soft object that cannot be swallowed may be placed between the teeth to protect the tongue, but once the jaws are set in a tonic spasm, one should not try to force them open because of the risk of breaking teeth.

Once the seizures are under control, further anticonvulsant therapy depends on the nature of the disease. If a causative lesion is eliminated by medication, e.g., meningitis, no further therapy is needed. When seizures are associated with a surgically removable lesion of the brain, such as a tumor or abscess, its excision may eradicate the discharging focus. This is unpredictable, however, for convulsive seizures are relieved in only about 50 percent of cases of meningioma and an even smaller percentage of cases of glioma or abscess of the cerebrum.

A series of seizures without restoration of consciousness between (status epilepticus) is more dangerous and demands admission to a hospital and prompt pharmacotherapy. Often the patient is already receiving a maintenance dose of anticonvulsant medication, but if not, intravenous therapy should be initiated at once. Diphenylhydantoin (Dilantin) in a loading dose of 1000 mg (in single or divided doses) should be given, supplemented by diazepam (5 mg) or sodium phenobarbitol (100 mg). Intravenous injection of diazepam (Valium) should be made slowly over the period of a minute into a large vein and repeated every 2 to 4 h if necessary. Rapid injection may cause apnea or cardiac arrest. The alternative, sodium phenobarbital, may also be given intravenously, in a dose of 200 mg, to be repeated if necessary every 4 h. For *focal* status epilepticus paraldehyde, 1 to 3 ml given slowly by intravenous route or 5 to 10 ml intramuscularly (avoiding nerves), is sometimes useful. Once the cycle of status epilepticus is broken, one may rely on the standard oral anticonvulsant medications. If the seizures are not responsive to the above doses of Valium or sodium phenobarbital, it is better for the patient to have a few seizures than to be rendered comatose by increasing doses of medication.

The type of disease causing the seizures and its treatment is another important consideration. Antibiotic medication usually arrests the seizure tendency in bacterial meningitis. NaCl in a 3% solution usually terminates the seizures in hyponatremia, and 5% glucose solution has a similar effect in hypoglycemic seizures. $MgSO_4$ and calcium gluconate often help in uremic seizures. Abstinence seizures cease usually within a few days and are rarely severe and frequent. In all these conditions or in idiopathic epilepsy if status epilepticus occurs, occasional seizures are of less serious consequence than a deepening drug-induced coma from excessive doses of anticonvulsant medication.

Recurrent seizures including idiopathic epilepsy Of course success in the management of patients with epilepsy depends in large measure on the deployment of drugs for the prevention

TABLE 23-1
Causes of recurrent convulsion in different age groups

Age of onset, years	Probable cause
Infancy, 0–2	Congenital maldevelopment, birth injury, metabolic disorder (hypocalcemia, hypoglycemia), vitamin B_6 deficiency, phenylketonuria
Childhood, 2–10	Birth injury, trauma, infections, thrombosis of cerebral arteries or veins, beginning of idiopathic epilepsy
Adolescence, 10–18	Idiopathic epilepsy, trauma, congenital defects
Early adulthood, 18–35	Trauma, neoplasm, idiopathic epilepsy, alcoholism, drug addiction
Middle age, 35–60	Neoplasm, trauma, vascular disease, alcoholism, drug addiction
Late life, over 60	Vascular disease, degeneration, tumor

of seizures. If managed well with anticonvulsants, fully 75 percent of patients may have their seizures controlled or reduced in frequency.

The drugs in common use for this purpose are the barbiturates, hydantoins, and oxazoladinediones, and to a lesser extent acetylureas and benzodiazepams. The available products which have received a thorough clinical trial and their daily dosages are listed in Table 23-2.

Certain drugs are more effective in one type of seizure than in another, and it is necessary to use the proper drugs in the optimum dosages for the different types of seizures. If satisfactory results are not obtained with one of the drugs, the others should be tried, but frequent shifting of drugs is not advisable, and each should be given in adequate trial before another is substituted. In some patients a combination of two or more drugs will produce better results than one alone.

Intelligent administration of drugs depends on having the patients chart daily their medication and the number, time, and circumstances of their seizures. Ideally such a baseline should be established before medication is begun, since each patient tends to have an individual pattern of seizures, but often this is impractical. Changes in medication should be made only when a given program is shown to be inadequate. Frequent measurements of blood levels of diphenylhydantoin, barbiturate and other drugs are useful. For Dilantin, the therapeutic level is 10 to 15 μg/ml, and one-half of patients have side effects at 30 or more μg/ml. These consist of ataxia, slurred speech, staggering, nystagmus, diplopia, mental dullness, forgetfulness, and confusion. Stupor or coma may occur when the level exceeds 50 μg/ml. Clinical and electroencephalographic improvement are not usually obtained if the level is below 10 μg/ml. The therapeutic level for phenobarbital is probably about 10 to 15 μg/ml, though the range varies with the type of barbiturate used. Side effects appear in patients on long-term treatment with phenobarbital levels above 30 μg/ml.

When changing medication, the dosage of the new drug should be gradually increased to an optimum level at the same time as the dosage of the old drug is gradually decreased. The sudden withdrawal of a drug may lead to status epilepticus, even though a new drug is substituted. Once an anticonvulsant or a combination of anticonvulsants is found to be effective, its use should be maintained for a period of years.

The therapeutic dose for any patient must be determined to some extent by trial and error. Not uncommonly a drug is discarded as being ineffective, when a slightly increased dosage would have led to a complete disappearance of the seizures. It is, however, inadvisable to administer a drug to the point where the patient is so dull and stupid as to be more incapacitated by the toxic effects than by the seizures. There is no evidence to prove that the prolonged administration of anticonvulsant medication is a factor in the development of the mental deterioration that occurs in a small percentage of the patients with convulsive seizures. It is not uncommon to note an improvement in the mental faculties of some patients following control of the seizures by the use of anticonvulsant drugs.

An antifolate effect on blood serum and a reduction of protein-bound iodine (without lowering of the BMR) have been reported. Some of the anticonvulsant drugs [primidone (Mysoline) or Dilantin] cause hirsutism, gum hypertrophy (Dilantin), and coarsening of the features of a growing child. Mild polyneuropathy (abolition of reflexes in legs and numb feet) has also been reported. Some adult males complain of reduced sexual potency and both Dilantin and carbamazepine (Tegretol) have been shown to decrease 17-corticosteroids (Luhdorf et al.). When this happens, the drug should be changed.

TABLE 23-2
Anticonvulsant medications*,†

Generic name	Trade name	Total daily dose per kg body wt and usual adult dose	Principal therapeutic purposes	Serum half-life, h	Effective blood level, μg per 100 ml	Toxic level, μg per 100 ml
Phenobarbital	Luminal	1–5 mg; 60–200 mg	Major seizures; partial seizures; psychomotor seizures; and petit mal	96 ± 12	15	40
Diphenylhydantoin	Dilantin	4–7 mg; 200–500 mg	Major seizures; psychomotor seizures; partial epilepsy	24 ± 12	10	20
Primidone	Mysoline	10–25 mg; 750–1500 mg	Major seizures; psychomotor seizures; partial epilepsy	12 ± 6	5	12
Ethosuximide	Zarontin	20–30 mg; 1000–1500 mg	Petit mal	30 ± 6	40	100
Trimethadione	Tridione	10–25 mg; 500–1250 mg	Petit mal			
Paramethadione	Paradione	10–25 mg; 500–1250 mg	Petit mal			
Mephenytoin	Mesantoin	7–12 mg; 300–600 mg	Major seizures; psychomotor seizures; focal epilepsy			
Mephobarbital	Mebaral	2.5–10 mg; 200–500 mg	Same as phenobarbital; myoclonic epilepsy			
Methsuximide	Celontin	10–20 mg; 500–1000 mg	Petit mal			
Phensuximide	Milontin	10–20 mg; 500–1250 mg	Petit mal			
Acetazolamide	Diamox	5–15 mg; 250–750 mg	Petit mal; infantile spasms; major seizures			
Diazepam	Valium	0.15–2 mg; 15–30 mg	Petit mal; major seizures; status epilepticus			
Nitrazepam	Mogadon	0.15–2 mg; 10–100 mg	Infantile spasms; myoclonic epilepsy			
Ethotoin	Peganone	10–20 mg; 500–1000 mg	Major seizures; focal seizures			
ACTH		40–60 units per day	Infantile spasms			
Carbamazepine	Tegretol	10–20 mg; 1000–1200 mg	Tonic-clonic seizures; complex partial seizures	12 ± 3	4	8
Clonazepam	Rivotril	1–12 mg per day	Atypical petit mal			
Sodium valproate		400 mg qid	Intractable epilepsy of all types, especially atypical petit mal			

* *Children usually need larger doses than adults, if dose is calculated according to body weight. Excessive drowsiness can often be diminished by dextroamphetamine (Dexedrine), methamphetamine (Desoxyn), or methylphenidate (Ritalin).*
† *This table lists only drugs in common use; for a complete list and discussion consult JK Penry (ed), Epilepsy: Eighth International Symposium, New York, Raven Press, 1977.*

Indications for use of specific drugs GRAND MAL SEIZURES
For those patients with infrequent grand mal seizures (from one to four per year), phenobarbital can be tried first because of its high therapeutic index and its relatively low toxicity. When the seizures are more frequent, Dilantin is the drug of choice. A combination of Dilantin (0.3 to 0.4 g) and phenobarbital (0.1 to 0.2 g) is more often effective than either of the drugs used alone. When these drugs are used in combination, a full therapeutic dose of each drug must be given. Occasionally, mephenytoin (Mesantoin) or a combination of this drug with the Dilantin or Mysoline will succeed where Dilantin alone has failed. In the more difficult cases carbamazepine, 400 mg tid, clonazepam, 2 mg tid, and sodium valproate, 400 mg qid, have controlled the seizures, though the carbamazepine is more effective in minor seizures.

The toxic effects of phenobarbital, which are drowsiness and mental dullness, nystagmus, and staggering, should be used as indications of excess dosage. Only skin eruption is a contraindication to its further use; otherwise these symptoms can be controlled by reducing the dose. Dilantin almost always leads to hypertrophy of gums, and, as was stated above, ataxia, stupor, or coma if given in excess dosages. If skin rashes and other hypersensitivity phenomena (polyarteritis) occur, discontinuation of the medication is necessary. Reduction of dose controls the other symptoms. The most important side effects of clonazepam and sodium valproate are drowsiness and lassitude. Nausea, vomiting, and diarrhea occur in approximately 10 percent of patients receiving clonazepam.

PSYCHOMOTOR ATTACKS Drugs effective in the treatment of grand mal seizures are effective in the treatment of patients with psychomotor attacks. Dilantin, 300 to 400 mg per day, and Mysoline, 750 to 1000 mg per day, have given the best results. The results on the whole are not as good as in grand mal epilepsy. Carbamazepine has had a notable success in many patients with this type of seizure. One should begin with a low dosage (100 mg bid or tid) and increase to 1200 mg per day.

PETIT MAL ATTACKS As a rule, drugs effective in the treatment of grand mal and psychomotor seizures are relatively ineffective in the treatment of patients with petit mal attacks. Ethosuximide (Zarontin), 750 to 1500 mg per day, has been most successful and has the advantage over trimethadione (Tridione), paramethadione (Paradione), and phensuximide (Milontin) in producing fewer side effects. It is wise to begin with a single dose of 250 mg per day and increase it every week until therapeutic effect is achieved. Toxic symptoms to Tridione and Paradione are skin eruptions and photophobia. Aplastic anemia has been reported; hence monthly blood counts during the first year are indicated. Methsuximide (Celontin; adult dose 0.3 g three or four times a day) and acetazolamide (Diamox; adult dose 0.25 to 0.75 g per day) have been useful in controlling difficult cases of petit mal and massive myoclonus in children. Atypical varieties of petit mal (2-per-second wave and spike EEG paroxysms) in association with myoclonus and akinetic falling spells or brief focal tonic or clonic seizures may be exceedingly resistant to medication. Methsuximide (Celontin) and acetazolamide (Diamox) or carbamazepine (Tegretol; adult dose 1.0 to 1.2 g per day) have had some success. Clonazepam, recently introduced (1.0 to 4.0 mg tid) and particularly sodium valproate (400 mg qid), are reported to have controlled atypical petit mal better than Zarontin.

MINOR SEIZURES AND FOCAL ATTACKS The same drugs effective in the treatment of grand mal and psychomotor seizures are effective against minor seizures and focal attacks. Minor seizures, which appear in patients whose grand mal attacks have been controlled, can occasionally be checked by simply increasing the dose of the drug or drugs that the patient is already taking. If the minor attacks are very infrequent and nonincapacitating, no great effort need be made to treat them.

PETIT MAL PLUS OTHER TYPES When patients are subject to petit mal seizures as well as grand mal or psychomotor seizures, they should receive Zarontin plus diphenylhydantoin sodium, phenobarbital, or sodium valproate.

MYOCLONIC EPILEPSY Mephobarbital (Mebaral), 0.2 to 0.5 g, and phenobarbital, 0.1 to 0.2 g, have been the most effective agents in this type of seizure, but in intractable cases clonazepam and sodium valproate should be tried. In the treatment of massive myoclonus in infants, ACTH or a combination of nitrazepam (Mogadon) and Diamox have been most effective.

Other treatments and management Surgery has been advocated for the removal of cortical scars secondary to cerebral trauma, of vascular lesions, and birth injuries on the assumption that such scars are surrounded by irritable foci which act as a trigger mechanism for the seizures. Reduction in the frequency of seizures has been reported as a sequel to these operations by a number of neurosurgeons. This treatment should be limited to the group of patients with focal attacks which do not respond to medical therapy. In addition, such lesions should be excised only by neurosurgeons who have facilities for the adequate localization of the lesion. Further medical treatment will still be required for most of these patients after operation.

The anterior tip of the temporal lobe and the amygdaloid nuclei have been removed or destroyed by stereotaxis in patients with psychomotor seizures who have failed to respond to medical therapy and in whom it was possible to demonstrate a temporal lobe focus by electroencephalography. Favorable results have been reported with this procedure by some neurosurgeons, but experience is too limited to evaluate its efficacy. The same may be said of implantation of cerebellar stimulators and section of the corpus callosum to prevent spread of seizure.

Biofeedback in which the patient is warned of the abnormal brainwaves and is trained to control them has attracted attention in the lay press, but the studies are so poorly controlled and so limited that no conclusions can be drawn.

Since epilepsy is a long-term medical problem, general hygienic measures are important, for they tend to stabilize the neurophysiologic state of the cerebrum. They should include regular hours of sleep, balanced diet, daily exercise, avoidance of constipation, and abstinence from alcohol. With proper safeguards even the more dangerous sports such as swimming and football may be permitted. The uncontrolled epileptic obviously should not be allowed to drive a car, operate unguarded machines, climb to heights, and so forth. Patients whose seizures are under medical control are no more dangerous on the highways than the average nonepileptic citizen.

Psychotherapy will help prevent or overcome feelings of inferiority and self-consciousness or shame. Both the patient and family will benefit from such therapy, and proper attitudes may be established. Oversolicitude and overprotection are to be discouraged. It is important for the patient live as normal a life as possible.

Every effort should be made to keep children in school, and adults should stay at work. Many communities have a branch of the American Committee against Epilepsy or a vocational rehabilitation center, and advantage should be taken of such facilities. Patients should participate in available recreational activities such as movies, dancing, and parties.

Not infrequently the convulsive disorder is but one manifestation of a widespread static cerebral disease that in itself interferes with education and work. Then realistic planning for activities that lie within the patient's scope is desirable.

As with all medications there are side effects. Toxic levels may cause confusion, stupor, or coma. Diphenylhydantoin may induce cerebellar ataxia, nystagmus, ocular palsies, asterixes, chorea, or choreoathetosis; chronic overdose may leave in its wake a permanent cerebellar ataxia due presumably to degeneration of Purkinje cells. Chronic usage of barbiturates leads to addiction and withdrawal effects (see Chap. 228).

REFERENCES

ADAMS RD, VICTOR M: *Principles of Neurology.* New York, McGraw-Hill, 1977

GLAZER GH: Epilepsy, in *Recent Advances in Clinical Neurology*, WB Mathews (ed). Edinburgh, Churchill Livingstone, 1975, pp 23–68

HAUSER WA, KURLAND LT: The epidemiology of epilepsy in Rochester, Minnesota. Epilepsia 16:1, 1975

JASPER HH et al (eds): *Basic Mechanisms of the Epilepsies.* Boston, Little, Brown, 1969

LENNOX W, LENNOX M: *Epilepsy and Related Disorders.* Boston, Little, Brown, 1960

LÜHDORF K et al: Epilepsy, in *Eighth International Symposium*, JF Penry (ed). New York, Raven Press, 1977, pp 209–214

SCHMIDT RP, WILDER BJ: *Contemporary Neurology Series*, vol 5: *Epilepsy*, F Plum, FH McDowell (eds). Philadelphia, Davis, 1968

24
AFFECTIONS OF SPEECH

JAY P. MOHR
RAYMOND D. ADAMS

Language and speech are of fundamental significance to humanity both in social intercourse and private intellectual life. When disordered as a consequence of disease of the brain, the loss exceeds in gravity even blindness, deafness, and paralysis.

GENERAL CONSIDERATIONS

The terms *speech* and *language* refer to some of the most complex and poorly understood integrating activities of the cerebrum. The terms are not synonymous.

Speech involves the execution of acquired skills by which vocal, manual, auditory, and visual systems are utilized to permit the conveyance of communicative efforts. These skills include: pronunciation of words, variations in stress, intonation, and melody; the production of graphic marks in the accepted spatial orientation; the discrimination of spoken speech and its classification as to speaker; the discrimination of handwritten or printed speech, the visual search patterns involved in scanning a text; and the use of other, less specifiable behaviors. Deficiencies in these skills impede interpersonal communication apart from any separate impairment in language usage; when intact, these skills do not suffice for any but elemental communication, such as that between two individuals who speak languages unfamiliar to each other.

Language has a wider connotation and refers to the selection and serial ordering of individual words according to accepted rules that permit a person using the speech modalities to modify the behavior of another and to externalize that poorly understood cerebral activity referred to as *thinking*. A disturbance of language usage, usually accompanied by a disturbance in speech from cerebral dysfunction, is referred to as *aphasia*, or more properly as *dysphasia* (see below).

CEREBRAL DOMINANCE AND ITS RELATIONSHIP TO SPEECH AND HANDEDNESS

The functional supremacy of one cerebral hemisphere is crucial to language function. There are three ways of determining that the left side of the brain is dominant: (1) the loss of speech when disease occurs in certain parts of the left hemisphere and its preservation in diseases involving corresponding parts of the right hemisphere; (2) the greater facility in the use of the right hand, foot, and eye; (3) the arrest of speech immediately after the injection of amobarbital (Amytal sodium) or some other drug in the left internal carotid artery. Only (2) and (3) are of use in deciding the cerebral dominance of a living, healthy patient. Unfortunately the Amytal sodium, or Wada, test does not reproduce the syndrome of major hemisphere inactivation. There is only mutism, followed by a brief period of groping for names. Presumably it gives information about the localization of motor output areas rather than of sensory ones.

Of the general population approximately 90 to 95 percent are right-handed; the remainder prefer the left hand. A person who chooses the right hand for intricate, complex acts and is more skillful with it is said to be right-handed. The preference is more complete in some persons than in others. Most individuals are neither right-handed nor completely left-handed but favor one hand for more complicated tasks.

The reason for hand preference is still controversial. There is strong evidence of a hereditary factor, but the mode of inheritance is uncertain. Learning is also a factor; many children are shifted at an early age from left to right (shifted sinistrals) because it is a handicap to be left-handed in a right-handed world. Many right-handed persons sight with the right eye, and it has been said that eye preference determines hand preference.

Anatomic differences between the dominant and the minor cerebral hemispheres have recently attracted attention. The left planum temporale, part of Wernicke's language zone, in the left hemisphere, is larger, and other evidence of asymmetries elsewhere are being uncovered; it is suggested that they are related to functional hemispheral differences.

Left-handedness may result from disease of the left cerebral hemisphere in early life; this fact probably accounts for its higher incidence among the feebleminded and brain-injured. Presumably the neural mechanisms for language then become centered in the right cerebral hemisphere. Handedness and cerebral dominance may fail to develop in some individuals; this is particularly true in certain families.

In studies of groups of left-handed individuals who suffer cerebral derangements of speech, it has been noted that approximately 75 percent have had lesions in the left cerebral hemisphere. Further, in those extremely rare cases of aphasia due to right cerebral lesions, the patient is nearly always left-handed, and the speech disorder tends to be less severe and enduring. The latter may take the form of an expressive disturbance, with prominent faults in calculation, implicit unawareness of the neurologic deficits (anosognosia), and visuoconstructive troubles.

The functional capacities of the minor hemisphere in speech are not fully understood despite careful anatomic studies. An additional problem in assessment is the uncertainty as to whether any residual function after lesions of the major hemisphere is due to recovery of parts of its language zones or to the activity solely of the minor hemisphere. The following functions are not disturbed in lesions of the left hemisphere: motor responses of mimicry, social anticipation (smiling, hand-shaking, modesty reactions) and self-care (washing and feeding), avoidance behavior to noxious stimuli, and capability of training in performances of cross-matching visually presented simple words with pictures.

TYPES OF LANGUAGE DISORDERS ENCOUNTERED IN MEDICAL PRACTICE

These may be divided into four categories:

1 *Cerebral disturbances* in which there is a loss more or less exclusively of the production and/or comprehension of spoken and/or written speech and language. Such a condition is called *aphasia,* or, in milder degrees, *dysphasia.*
2 *Defects in articulation* with intact mental functions and normal comprehension and memory of words. These are pure motor disorders of the muscles of articulation and may be due to flaccid or spastic paralysis, rigidity, repetitive spasms (stuttering), or ataxia. The terms *anarthria* and *dysarthria* have been applied to some of these conditions.
3 *Loss of voice* due to a disease of the larynx or its innervation, with resultant *aphonia* or *dysphonia.*
4 *Disturbances of speech* that occur with diseases affecting the higher nervous integrations, namely delirium and dementia (see Chaps. 21 and 25). Speech is seldom lost in these conditions but is instead merely deranged as part of a general impairment of all elements of language.

APHASIA OR DYSPHASIA In the scientific study of aphasia one faces formidable problems since there are no experimental models; this prevents the easy testing of hypotheses of speech and language function. The only reliable source materials are humans with cerebral disease, and the study of such cases is hampered by a number of uncontrollable variables such as the difficulty in delineating the basic functional deficit and the changes in symptomatology at different periods in the time-course of the disease. The anatomic site of the lesion is often imprecisely characterized which makes for difficulty in clinicoanatomic and clinicopathologic correlation. And, finally, of theoretical importance is the problem of ascribing normal function to a part of the cerebrum by a study of the abnormal diseased brain.

As a general orientation, most of the lesions that lead to aphasia are known to be located in the perisylvian or *opercular* regions (frontal, temporal, and parietal) that cover the insula of the dominant cerebral hemisphere, i.e., the left in right-handed individuals.

The clinical deficit is most easily demonstrated in the acute phase. The changes that occur with time make estimation of lesion site and size more difficult later on, especially with the smaller lesions. Lesions one or more centimeters in diameter are often found at autopsy in cases whose clinical deficit was evanescent and had faded to functional insignificance within weeks or months. Diseases affecting the cerebral surface gray matter produce a more significant deficit than those more confined to the white matter; tumors, for example, confined as they are largely to the white matter, may reach discouragingly large size before speech or language deficit is evident. The site is more significant than the size of the lesion, for the former determines the qualitative features of the deficit, but the size determines the quantitative features and, in the larger lesions, appears to produce additional qualitative features not present in the smaller lesions. In particular, deficits in speech function are more evident in smaller lesions, while deficits in language as well as speech functions occur in the larger lesions.

The importance of site of lesion is well illustrated by a study of the types of aphasia observed in diseases affecting the

sylvian territory. Those that lie anteriorly produce deficits in the acts of speaking. These disorders include mutism, impaired articulation, disordered transitions from syllable to syllable, and defective stress, intonation, and melody. Those located more posteriorly produce malpositioning of the oral cavity and some anticipatory errors out of sequence that result in gross mispronunciations of the intended syllables and words, more evident when the expected utterance is lengthy. Lesions grouped around the posterior sylvian fissure including the superior temporal lobe and its auditory gyri are manifested by disordered discrimination of spoken words, resulting in poor repetition of speech sounds and faulty understanding of spoken language.

Language deficits are well understood and less well correlated with anatomic pathology. Many formulations of aphasia envision only one "true" language deficit, the detection of which by any method of testing suffices to label the patient as aphasic. But those formulations based more on pathoanatomic correlations are leaning more toward separation of two large categories of disorder. That disorder reflecting large lesions involving the bulk of the frontal operculum and insula shows *agrammatism,* which features sharply contracted sentence structure, lacking most small grammatic words, often with faulty use of grammar in the words remaining, the surviving words serving mainly a predicative or substantive function. Large posterior sylvian lesions show almost the opposite, with substantive elements missing or substituted by errors in which the desired response is only approximated (paraphasias). These latter may consist of faulty pronunciations (literal paraphasias) or faulty word selections (verbal paraphasias). Disturbances in understanding language through auditory and visual speech forms reflect both types of major paraphasias.

Lesions in other parts of the cerebrum either cause no disturbance of human communicative skills or alter them only secondarily. An example of the latter is the lesion of the frontal lobes, especially the medial and orbital parts which impairs all motor activities, and often results in abulia, verging on akinetic mutism. The speech is laconic with long pauses between utterances, and there is an inability to sustain monologue and narrative. Extensive occipital lesions impair reading and reduce the utilization of all visual, lexic stimuli. Thalamic and deep cerebral lesions impair alertness and cause fluctuant states of inattention and disorientation, thereby inducing fragmentation of words (neologisms) and phrases, and protracted uncontrollable talking (logorrhea). Strong stimulation which momentarily stabilizes behavior and speech informs us of the essential integrity of language mechanisms.

In the initial formulations of cerebral function in the last century, it was easily concluded that lesions of the frontal (motor) regions produced syndromes independent from those of the posterior (sensory) regions, that the dysphasias could be classified as motor (Broca's) or sensory (Wernicke's), and could be further specified as subcortical, cortical, or transcortical in type. Subcortical lesions were envisioned to cut off the main efferent or afferent projections of the cortical "center." Cortical lesions involved the "centers" themselves. Transcortical lesions isolated the "centers" from one another, i.e., a kind of "conduction" aphasia, or from other regions of the brain. In modern times, the difficulties in attempting to understand the disorders of language that usually accompany the disorders of speech in focal brain disease, the improvements in techniques to document the extent of the lesion, and data available in longitudinal studies have led to a greater awareness of the complexity of these relationships.

TYPES OF APHASIA The examination of patients with disturbances of speech and language discloses a number of different abnormalities. Attempts have been made to classify them in terms of their predominant form, their presumed physiologic or psychologic bases, or the anatomy of the underlying diseases. No one of the many schemes has been accepted, and the leading students of language have railed against the premature acceptance of incomplete simplistic theories of language.

The most readily recognized type of aphasia is one that is complete or global, in which all modes of expression (spoken word, written word, and gesture) as well as the capacity for reading and understanding of spoken words are abolished. If more or less permanent, large perisylvian lesions of the left cerebral hemisphere are demonstrable, they usually reflect involvement of both divisions of the left middle cerebral artery. A second major type involves the motor, verbal, and executive side of the language and is named *Broca's aphasia.* The lesion is large, involving the bulk of the anterosuperior sylvian operculum and insula, in the territory of supply of the upper division of the left middle cerebral artery. A third major type involves the receptive, sensory, and central aspects of language and is named *Wernicke's aphasia.* The syndrome is ascribed to a large lesion involving the left posterior temporal and parietal regions, in the territory of supply of the lower, posterior division of the left middle cerebral artery. There are in addition a number of so-called "dissociative" aphasias such as "conduction" aphasia, "pure" word deafness, "pure" word blindness, "amnestic" aphasia, and "pure" agraphia, each attributed to smaller lesions within the speech areas or in their afferent and efferent connections. Scrutiny of these syndromes has shown that their anatomy is poorly established, and ideas about them are more in tune with theory of language than observed fact.

The practical student might question the purpose of these classifications. There are several. Many of these syndromes have fairly specific anatomic localizing value and are of clinical assistance to the physician in cases having surgical implications. In addition, the different prognoses attached to several syndromes are helpful in management and in the use of different corrective measures in therapy. And, finally, such data might become the basis of a unified theory of language.

Complete (global) aphasia This syndrome is due to a lesion that destroys a large part of the speech areas of the major cerebral hemisphere. As such, it represents the maximal aphasic deficit possible and shows the least improvement of all aphasic syndromes. Since the middle cerebral artery nourishes all the speech areas, nearly all aphasic syndromes due to vascular occlusion are caused by involvement of this artery or its branches. In complete aphasia, occlusion of the left internal carotid or the middle cerebral artery at its origin is usually responsible. Less often, the syndrome may be caused by a large hemorrhage, tumor, other lesions, or even temporarily as a postictal effect of grand mal epilepsy.

Most patients with total aphasia can say at most a few words; they cannot read or write, and they understand only a few words and phrases of the speech of others. Related signs include right hemiplegia, hemianesthesia, and homonymous hemianopia. The state of consciousness may vary from full alertness to semicoma. The alert patient may participate in common gestures of greeting, may show modesty and avoidance reactions, and is able to engage in self-help activities. With the passage of time some degree of understanding of spoken speech may be evident, and a few spoken words may emerge. Early appearance of clearly vocalized stereotyped words, such as "hi," are often falsely encouraging signs and may reflect the uninhibited function of the right hemisphere. Rapid improvement frequently occurs when the main cause is edema, postconvulsive paralysis, or transient metabolic derangements such as infection, or hyponatremia, which worsen old aphasic lesions. Although speech loss from a disintegrating embolus of the left middle artery may be transient, some part of the deficit may persist, being easily demonstrated by presenting the patient with complex words or double negatives in sentences.

Broca's aphasia (major motor aphasia) This term is used to designate a complex syndrome, predominantly a failure of motor aspects of speaking and writing, with an accompanying *agrammatism* and a variable impairment in language comprehension. Although commonly thought due to a circumscribed lesion in the inferior frontal convolution (Broca's area), this major syndrome is usually the result of a larger lesion, involving cortical and subcortical structures along the frontal and superior sylvian fissure including the insula, in the territory of supply of the upper division of the left middle cerebral artery.

The large extent of the lesion, and involvement of the sensorimotor rolandic region, account for the more or less dense right hemiparetic and hemisensory syndrome that almost invariably accompanies the aphasia and usually persists. Initially, a transient right hemianopia and an ipsilateral deviation of the eyes are observed.

In the acute phase of the syndrome, the entire language mechanism appears inactivated, and the helplessly mute, noncommunicative, and uncomprehending patient presents the syndrome of *total aphasia,* indistinguishable by present methods from the previously described form of total aphasia coming from infarction of the whole left middle cerebral artery territory. Within weeks to years, the disorder of comprehension abates somewhat but remains forever easily detected by formal testing. This improvement in comprehension exceeds that in speaking and writing, where deficits are sufficient to stamp the syndrome traditionally as *motor aphasia.*

In the chronic stage of the syndrome, the patient will have severe difficulties in speaking aloud. The lower part of the face on the right side is weak and sags, and the tongue also deviates to the weak side, usually accompanied by weakness of the right arm and leg. For a time, despite satisfactory comprehension of spoken words and ability to read simple commands, an apraxia of the linguooropharyngeal apparatus is manifested in faulty efforts to smack the lips and to make other purposeful or commanded movements. In these circumstances imitation of the examiner's actions are better performed than execution of acts on command. Self-initiated actions, by contrast, are often normal. The patient who speaks at all may repeat a few remaining words over and over, as if compelled to do so. Certain stereotyped phrases such as "hi," "good morning," "how are you" seem to be more easily emitted, as are the words of popular songs when sung. When angered or excited, the patient may curse. Thus, it is evident that although "speechless" the person is not "wordless." The patient's efforts and facial expressions suggest an awareness of his or her own ineptitudes and mistakes. Repeated failures cause exasperation and despair.

As improvement occurs and in the milder forms of motor aphasia, the patient is able to speak aloud to some degree. Words are enunciated slowly and laboriously. Articulation and the melody of speech (prosody) are impaired. This dysfluency takes the form of improper accent or stress on certain syllables, incorrect phrasing of words in a series, pacing of the speed of word sequences, and even a stammering stuttering quality to the uttered phrases. Speech is sparse and consists mainly of nouns, transitive verbs, and important adjectives; many of the small words (articles, prepositions, conjunctions) are omitted, giving the speech an agrammatic and telegraphic character. The substantive content allows the patient to communicate to some extent despite the gross mechanical and language difficulties. Once fully established, these speech impediments persist and improve only slightly despite years of speech therapy.

Most patients with Broca's aphasia have a correspondingly severe impairment in writing. Should their right hand be paralyzed, they cannot print with their left one; if manual mobility is spared, they fail as completely in writing out their commands or replies to questions as in speaking them. Writing from dictation is severely impaired, though letters and words can still be copied. On careful testing, communication by writing can be shown superior to that of speaking, suggesting a certain independence between these two acts as vehicles of language.

The lesion of Broca's aphasia is most often an infarction of frontal, anterior parietal, and anterior insular parts of the cerebrum due to embolic occlusion of the upper division of the left middle cerebral artery. Major putaminal hypertensive hemorrhage is also a common cause. A huge frontal lobe tumor or abscess is occasionally responsible; metastatic lesions, subdural hematoma, and encephalitis only rarely cause the syndrome.

Minor motor aphasia Sharp focal lesions along the anterior and superior sylvian operculum and insula produce remarkably circumscribed effects on the mechanical elaboration of speech which can be observed alone or in combinations, depending on the site and extent of the lesion. However, *none of these focal lesions produces significant or lasting deficits in language usage;* the experienced listener can easily detect the error patterns in speech and, through them, discern the communicative efforts of the sufferer, who is acutely aware of and discouraged by the deficit. The effects on speech of focal opercular lesions take several forms. *Broca's area infarction* involves the lower premotor cortex adjacent to the motor cortex for the oropharynx, larynx, and respiratory apparatus; the infarct interrupts skilled movements of these muscle groups, and the resultant dyspraxia in speech takes the form of impaired transitions between syllables and words, and disruption of the melodic intonation of phrases (dysprosody). Involvement of this region appears insufficient to produce the major syndrome referred to as Broca's aphasia. *Rolandic infarction* involves the sensorimotor cortex itself; poor articulation, lowered volume and pitch of speech, and a nasal quality to the voice reveal the pareses of the involved musculature. *Postcentral, anterior parietal infarction* appears to be associated with errors in the positioning of the oral cavity for individual sounds, syllables, and whole words; the acoustic features of the utterance are often distorted by these malpositions of the oral cavity and strike the listener's ear as literal paraphasias. Since they are easily produced in tests of repeating and reading aloud and occur in conversation, the patient could be labeled as having "conduction" aphasia. The important point with all these minor motor aphasias is that at first they may resemble major motor aphasia except for the satisfactory understanding of spoken and written words. The prognosis for nearly full recovery is excellent.

Most lesions sufficiently focal as to produce such circumscribed deficits are embolic in nature. The sequential branching of the upper division of the middle cerebral artery provides a series of separate sites for emboli to lodge. Deeper, larger lesions, or larger emboli involving the stem of the upper division, encompass several deficit types in a single patient, making these individual distinctions less clear, and blend with the major syndromes of Broca's aphasia. Facial, lingual, and sometimes brachial paresis and ideomotor dyspraxia of the face and *left,* nondominant limbs commonly accompany the speech disorder. Most of these syndromes fade in clinical significance within weeks or months.

Wernicke's aphasia (major central or sensory aphasia) This term encompasses a wide range of syndromes reflecting lesions from the posterior perisylvian structures to the posterior parietooccipital regions supplied by the lower division of the middle cerebral artery. There is disruption of the whole array of language behavior. When more restricted to the temporal lobe, the main disturbance is most evident in language tasks involving words heard; when more parietooccipital, in words seen.

In brief, spoken and written efforts at communication as well as in auditory and visual comprehension are affected, a combination which justifies the term *central aphasia.* The older term, *sensory aphasia,* was formerly used to accentuate the contrast from motor (Broca's) aphasia; instead of the difficult articulation, faulty transitions, dysmelodic speaking, and disproportionate condensation of grammatical forms that characterize Broca's aphasia, the speech of Wernicke's aphasia is fluent. Hence the name "fluent aphasia." We prefer the eponym, *Wernicke's aphasia,* for it serves to encompass all the syndromes while avoiding the many sharp controversies that still surround unsuccessful attempts to characterize these aphasias by a single functional term.

In severe cases, the patient utters a series of incomprehensible syllables, makes illegible marks on a page in attempts at writing, cannot be made to repeat aloud or copy at sight correctly, and treats the examiner's attempts at written and verbal communication as if they were in a wholly unfamiliar foreign language. In less severe cases, the patient can be made to repeat aloud and copy, but in so doing frequently echoes the words heard with faulty pronunciation, or copies the words seen in a slavish manner, imitating even the examiner's handwriting style. It is as though the test words were unfamiliar. Clearly the disturbance in language does not simply reflect a disturbance in hearing or in vision. In the mildest cases, the deficits are reflected in errors in word comprehension and usage that show some approximation to the desired response, the words often belonging to the same functional class (i.e., "cow" for "pig," but not "cow" for "yellow"); errors in word structure, with improper tenses, prefixes, suffixes (i.e., "beautifuling"); and other errors that resemble performances by normal people unfamiliar with the language in question. Some such patients pass for normal in casual conversation. Their speech resembles the performance of people tired or distracted, and their abnormality is detected only on tests of complex language function. This state is often the residual of a more severe initial deficit.

As a rule, the syndrome is due to an embolic occlusion of the lower division of the left middle cerebral artery. A "slit hemorrhage" in the subcortex of the temporoparietal region or involvement of the temporal isthmus and adjacent white matter by tumor, abscess, or extension of a small putaminal or thalamic hemorrhage may have similar effects. The posterior sylvian region, comprising posterosuperior temporal, opercular supramarginal, and posterior insular gyri, appears to encompass a variety of language functions, since seemingly minor changes in size and locale of the lesion are associated with important variations in the elements of Wernicke's aphasia detailed below.

Minor central aphasia syndromes In time the patient with Wernicke's aphasia improves, and in so doing a number of lesser syndromes appear. These latter, however, may be present in comparatively pure form from the beginning, when only small restricted lesions involve some part of the territory of the lower division of the middle cerebral artery. Depending on the exact locale of lesion, language behavior dependent on auditory function (hearing spoken words, echoing sounds and speech, relating the spoken to the written word, and finally repeating and writing it) may be deranged partially or in its entirety. The same is true of language behavior dependent upon visual function, when the left posterior parietal lobe is involved.

These partial syndromes have been traditionally labeled as conduction aphasia, pure word deafness, and pure word blindness.

Attempts to correlate complete and partial posterior sylvian syndromes with arteriographic findings during life frequently fail. Since most partial vascular aphasias are due to cerebral embolism, the latter may have lodged in the artery long enough to cause infarction and then disintegrate. The arteriogram done after this happens is normal. Or a fragment of the disintegrating embolus may drift distally and permanently block only a more distal branch, sometimes permitting part of the ischemic tissue to recover. Computerized tomography (CT scan) has proved a helpful addition to attempts to delineate the areas involved.

Dissociative speech syndromes These disorders are characterized by an interruption of afferent nervous impulses to the language mechanism or efferent ones from these centers to other motor structures. This concept is an interesting one and has had the heuristic value of indicating certain lines of anatomicophysiologic separation of language functions. However, the anatomy of several of the following conditions is far from proved, and the theories that derive from such data as are available lead one to a naïve conception of the language mechanisms in terms of a kind of telephonic circuitry. With these reservations we present the following syndromes.

CONDUCTION APHASIA: SEPARATION OF WERNICKE'S AND BROCA'S LANGUAGE AREAS   Here the principal abnormality resembles Wernicke's aphasia in certain respects. There is the same paraphasia in self-initiated speech, in repeating what is heard, and in reading aloud. In contrast, no difficulty is shown in comprehending words that are heard or seen. Nor is any element of dysarthria or dysprosody detected. The patient is alert and aware of the deficit. One of the best ways of eliciting the defect is to have the patient repeat nonsense syllables. The mistakes are then manifestly of a type observed in literal paraphasia, i.e., close similarity but detectably different sounds occasioned by improper positioning of the oropharyngeal apparatus. The disorder in repeating from dictation becomes more apparent when the rate of presentation of auditory material is increased and as the uttered words become more polysyllabic. Since nouns are the longest words in the sentence, one may gain an impression that they are specifically affected.

The lesion in autopsied cases is located in the cortex and subcortical white matter in the upper bank of the sylvian fissure, involving the supramarginal gyrus of the inferior parietal lobule and occasionally the posterior part of the superior temporal region. Presumably fiber systems in the insula are interrupted. The usual cause is an embolus in the ascending parietal or posterior temporal branch of the middle cerebral artery. Deeper, larger lesions in position to interrupt the arcuate fasciculus connecting the temporal and frontal lobes usually involve other pathways as well, giving rise to a more extensive speech deficit (central, Wernicke's aphasia, or amnestic aphasia). However, these latter types of aphasia, as they regress, may resolve into conduction aphasia. More anterior insular lesions usually include some degree of Broca's aphasia.

"PURE" WORD DEAFNESS   This syndrome could be considered the auditory form of Wernicke's aphasia, in which the most obvious findings are an impaired auditory comprehension and inability to repeat what is said or to write to dictation. Spoken language is far better performed but is rarely normal, and occasionally the patient is initially diagnosed as having Wer-

nicke's aphasia. By audiometric testing no hearing defect is found, or minor abnormalities appear which may well reveal the underlying deficit in individual cases. Ordinary sounds can be distinguished. The patient is forced to depend heavily on visual cues in understanding the remarks of others and frequently uses these cues well enough to obviate much of the difficulty. But tests which prevent the use of visual cues readily uncover the deficit. Comprehension of visually presented material, for example, printed matter such as newspapers, is far better than auditory comprehension; it occasionally approaches normal, and justifies use of the traditional term, *pure word deafness.*

In most recorded autopsy studies the lesion has been embolic, bilateral in the superior temporal gyrus, and in position to damage the primary auditory cortex in the transverse gyrus of Heschl and its relations to the association areas of the superior, posterior part of the temporal lobe. The few unilateral lesions are localized in this part of the major (dominant) temporal lobe and encroach on those regions whose involvement precipitates the larger syndrome of Wernicke's aphasia.

DYSLEXIA WITH DYSGRAPHIA   This syndrome features a language disturbance most evident in reading and writing. The errors take a form typical of those encountered in the larger syndrome of Wernicke's aphasia. Yet auditory comprehension is so much superior to visual comprehension that the syndrome could be considered the visual form of Wernicke's aphasia. Since conversational testing frequently is the extent of many casual clinical evaluations of such patients, satisfactory auditory comprehension, ability to repeat aloud, and mild paraphasic errors in spontaneous speech frequently lead to a diagnosis of very mild Wernicke's aphasia. Detailed testing of reading aloud and for comprehension, and tests of spontaneous writing and writing in response to dictated and visually presented material, will reveal a far greater disturbance on these tasks and expose the syndrome. This type of aphasia is often the late sequel of the larger syndrome of Wernicke's aphasia.

The parietooccipital region is the anatomic site of this deficit. A lesion here is unusual in embolism, which more often affects structures more proximal in the territory of the lower division of the middle cerebral artery. Tumors, abscess, and the like disrupt other structures as well, and this syndrome is often a less conspicuous part of a larger clinical picture. Systemic hypotension and hypoxia may leave as a residual abnormality dyslexia with dysgraphia; but more often they have produced a more severe defect described below under "Isolation of speech areas."

"PURE" WORD BLINDNESS   In this state literate persons lose their ability to read and often to name colors. They can no longer name or point on dictated command to visual letter stimuli or the words of which they are composed. However, understanding spoken language, repetition of what is heard, writing to dictation, and conversation are all intact. Often the patient is unaware of the difficulty and registers no complaint; it is discovered almost by accident. In lesser degrees of the affection, reading aloud is possible, but the patient manages only a single letter at a time (this may be seen in otherwise normal patients who have bilateral hemianopia with only central vision remaining); commonly letter or name responses that seem to have little connection with the presented ones are expressed. The response may be corrected and the defect obscured if other visual cues are available, such as the bottle on which the words Coca-Cola appear. The naming of common colors presented singly and of objects is also impaired. When the dominant hemisphere is involved, as it usually is in such cases, there may be a right homonymous hemianopia, an amnestic defect (see Chap. 25), and a hemisensory defect on the right due to involvement of the left occipital lobe, the left fornix and its decussation, and the left thalamus, respectively, a combination which nearly always signifies thrombosis or embolism of the left posterior cerebral artery.

The autopsy of such lesions has usually demonstrated a lesion that destroys the left visual striate cortex (area 17) and visual association areas (18 and 19), as well as the connections of the right visual cortex and association areas with the temporoparietal region. This latter "disconnection" usually is due to interruption of the fibers passing through the posterior part (splenium) of the corpus callosum, which connect the visual association areas of the two hemispheres. A lesion deep in the left parietooccipital region may also prevent visual information from both occipital lobes reaching the left angular gyrus. In this case the right homonymous hemianopia may be absent. With purely left cerebral lesions, aside from vascular lesions there may be a primary or secondary tumor, or, rarely, multifocal leukoencephalopathy may be the underlying disease.

ISOLATION OF SPEECH AREAS Following prolonged hypotension or carbon monoxide poisoning, widespread cerebral ischemia affects the vascular anatomic border zones linking the major cerebral arteries and their distal branches on the cerebral surfaces, and spreads centripetally into their adjacent territories. The central fields of supply of these arteries are spared. In the middle cerebral artery territory, this sparing leaves largely intact the sylvian region and its speech areas. With much of the rest of the brain out of action in patients who have survived such hypoxic-hypotensive accidents, the speech mechanism is preserved and can be activated by spoken words. There is parrot-like repetition of words and sounds (echolalia) and similar findings which indicate that the auditory-vocal loop remains functional. Scant evidence of comprehension or self-initiated conversation has been observed, findings that are thought to reflect the widespread injury outside the speech regions. The syndrome is of great theoretic interest, and may prove common in cases surviving cardiac arrest.

Amnestic-dysnomic aphasia This may be a relatively early or an isolated manifestation of disease of the nervous system. The patient loses only the ability to produce names on demand, including nouns, adjectives, and other descriptive parts of speech. There are typical pauses in speech, groping for words, and substitution of another word or phrase that conveys the meaning (circumlocution). When shown a series of common objects, the patient may tell of their use instead of giving their names. The difficulty applies not only to objects seen but to the names of things heard or felt. By contrast, other verbal tasks, including recall of the names for letters, digits, reading, writing, spelling, etc., are almost invariably preserved. That the deficit is principally one of naming is shown by the patient's correct use of the object and, usually, by an ability to point to the correct object on hearing or seeing the name. There is a tendency among patients to attribute their failure to forgetfulness, or to give some other lame excuse for the disability, suggesting that they are not completely aware of the nature of their difficulty.

The causative lesion is usually deep in the temporal lobe, in position, probably, to interrupt connections of sensory speech areas with the hippocampal-parahippocampal regions concerned with learning and memory. Mass lesions, such as a tu-

mor or an otogenic abscess, are the most frequent, and as they enlarge, an upper contralateral quadrantic visual field defect or Wernicke's aphasia is added. Occasionally, dysnomia appears with diseases which occlude the temporal branches of the posterior cerebral artery. Alzheimer's disease and senile dementia may begin with a dysnomic or amnestic type of aphasia. By the time the patient's difficulty is fully recognized, other disorders of speech and indifference, apathy, and abulia are conjoined. This deficit may also be discovered in testing patients with a confusional state caused by metabolic, infectious, intoxicative, or other acute medical illnesses, but then it has no certain localizing value.

DISORDERS OF ARTICULATION AND PHONATION In simple dysarthria there is no abnormality of the cortical centers. Dysarthric patients are able to understand perfectly what they hear, and if literate, read and have no difficulty in writing, even though they are unable to utter a single intelligible word. This is the strict meaning of being inarticulate.

The act of speaking is a highly coordinated sequence of contractions of the larynx, pharynx, palate, tongue, lips, and respiratory musculature. These are innervated by the hypoglossal, vagal, facial, and phrenic nerves. The nuclei of these nerves are controlled through the corticobulbar tracts by both motor cortices. As with all movements, there are also extrapyramidal influences from the cerebellum and basal ganglia. A current of air is produced by expiration, and the force of it is finely regulated by the activity of the various muscles engaged in speech. *Phonation,* or the production of vocal sounds, is a function of the larynx. Changes in the size and shape of the glottis and in the length and tension of the vocal cords are controlled by the action of the laryngeal muscles. Vibrations are set up and transmitted to the column of air passing over the vocal cords. Sounds thus formed are modified as they pass through the nasopharynx and mouth, which act as resonators. Articulation consists of contractions of the tongue, lips, pharynx, and palate, which interrupt or alter the vocal sounds. Vowels are of laryngeal origin, as are some consonants, but the latter are formed for the most part during articulation. For instance, the consonants *m, b,* and *p* are labial, *l* and *t* are lingual, and *nk* and *ng* are nasoguttural.

Defective articulation and phonation are recognized at once by listening to patients during ordinary conversation or while they are reading aloud from a newspaper or book. Test phrases or attempts at rapid repetition of lingual, labial, and guttural consonants (e.g., la-la-la-la or me-me-me-me) bring out the particular abnormality. Disorders of phonation call for a precise analysis of the voice and its apparatus. The movements of the vocal cords should be inspected with the aid of a hand mirror, or, even better, a laryngoscope, and those of the tongue, palate, and pharynx by direct observation.

Defects in articulation may be subdivided into several types; paretic dysarthria, spastic and rigid dysarthria, choreic, myoclonic, and ataxic dysarthria.

Paretic dysarthria This is due to a neural or bulbar (medullary) weakness or paralysis of the articulatory muscles (lower motor neuron paralysis). In the latter condition the shriveled tongue lies inert on the floor of the mouth, and the lips are relaxed and tremulous. Saliva constantly collects in the mouth because of dysphagia, and spills over the lips causing drooling. Speech becomes less and less distinct. There is a special difficulty in the correct utterance of vibratives, such as *r;* as the paralysis becomes more complete, lingual and labial consonants are finally not pronounced at all. Degrees of this abnormality are observed in myasthenia gravis. Bilateral paralysis of the palate may occur with diphtheria, poliomyelitis, and progressive bulbar palsy. Bilateral paralysis of the lips, as in the facial diplegia of idiopathic polyneuritis, interferes with enunciation of labial consonants; *p* and *b* are slurred and sound more like *f* and *v*.

Spastic and rigid dysarthria These are more frequent than the paralytic variety. Diseases that involve the corticobulbar tracts, usually vascular disease or motor system disease, result in the syndrome of pseudobulbar palsy. The patient may have had a minor stroke some time in the past affecting the corticobulbar fibers on one side; but since the bulbar muscles are probably represented in both motor cortices, there is no impairment in speech or swallowing from a unilateral lesion. Should another stroke then occur, involving the other corticobulbar tract and possibly the corticospinal tract at the pontine, midbrain, or capsular level, the patient immediately becomes anarthric or dysarthric and dysphagic. Often the muscles of facial expression on both sides are weakened as well. Unlike bulbar paralysis due to lower motor neuron involvement, this condition entails no atrophy or fasciculation of the paralyzed muscles; the jaw jerk and other facial reflexes soon become exaggerated; the palatal reflexes are retained; emotional control is poor (pathologic laughter and crying); and sometimes breathing becomes periodic (Cheyne-Stokes). When the frontal operculum alone is involved, the speech deficit may be a pure dysarthria but usually without the impairment in emotional control. In the beginning, the patient may be totally anarthric and aphonic, but as improvement occurs or in mild degrees of the same condition, speech is notably slow, thick, and indistinct, much like that of partial bulbar paralysis.

In paralysis agitans, or postencephalitic Parkinson's syndrome, one observes an extrapyramidal disturbance of articulation. The patient speaks hastily and articulates poorly, slurring over many syllables and trailing off the end of sentences. The words are pronounced hastily. The voice is low-pitched, monotonous, and lacks inflection; voice volume diminishes. In advanced cases speech is almost unintelligible; only whispering is possible. It may happen that the patient finds it impossible to talk while walking but can speak if sitting or lying down.

Pyramidal and extrapyramidal disturbances of speech may be combined in generalized cerebral diseases such as general paresis, in which slurred speech is one of the cardinal signs.

In many cases of capsular hemiplegia or partially recovered Broca's aphasia the patient is left with a dysarthria that may be difficult to distinguish from a pure articulatory defect. Careful testing of other language functions, especially writing, will reveal the aphasic quality.

Choreic and myoclonic dysarthria In chorea and myoclonus, speech may also be affected in a highly characteristic way. Unlike the defect of pseudobulbar palsy or paralysis agitans, chorea and myoclonus abruptly interrupt the pronunciation of words by the abnormal movements. The idea is best conveyed by the phrase "hiccup speech," in that the breaks are as unexpected as in singultus. Grimacing and other characteristic motor signs must be depended upon for diagnosis.

Ataxic dysarthria This is characteristic of acute and chronic cerebellar lesions. It may be observed in multiple sclerosis, Friedreich's ataxia, cerebellar atrophy, and heat stroke. The principal speech abnormality is slowness; imprecise enunciation, monotony, and unnatural, irregular separation of the syllables of words (scanning) are other features. Coordination of speech and respiration are poor. There may not be enough breath to utter certain words, and others may be ejaculated explosively. *Scanning dysarthria* is distinctive, but in some cases, especially if there is a possibility of spastic weakness of the tongue from corticobulbar tract involvement, it is impossible to predict the anatomy of disease from analysis of speech alone. Myoclonic jerks involving the speech musculature may be superimposed on cerebellar ataxia in a number of diseases.

APHONIA AND DYSPHONIA Finally, a few points should be made concerning the group of speech disorders involving disturbances of voice.

Paresis of the respiratory movements, as in poliomyelitis and acute infectious polyneuritis, may affect voice because insufficient air is provided for phonation and speech. Also, disturbances in the rhythm of respiration may interfere with the fluency of speech. This is particularly noticeable in so-called "extrapyramidal diseases," where one may observe that the patient does not allow sufficient air during expiration to complete a phrase. In the latter conditions reduced volume of speech due to limited excursion of the breathing muscles is another common feature; the patient is unable to speak above a whisper or to shout. Whispering speech is also a feature of stupor, but strong stimulation may make the voice audible.

Paresis of both vocal cords causes complete aphonia. There is no voice, and the patient can speak only in whispers. Since the vocal cords normally separate during inspiration, their failure to do so when paralyzed may result in an inspiratory stridor. If one vocal cord is paralyzed, the voice becomes hoarse, low-pitched, and rasping. Involvement of one of the tenth cranial nerves by tumor, for example, may also cause a certain nasality of voice because the posterior nares do not close during phonation. Certain consonants such as *b*, *p*, *n*, and *k* are followed by escape of air into the nasal passages. The abnormality is sometimes less pronounced in recumbency and increases when the head is thrown forward. Hoarseness may also be due to structural changes in the vocal cords caused by cigarette smoking, chronic inflammation, polyps, etc.

Another curious condition about which little is known is *spastic dysphonia*. The authors have seen many patients, middle-aged or elderly men and women, otherwise healthy, who gradually lose the ability to speak quietly and fluently. Any effort to speak results in contraction of all the speech musculature so the patient's voice is strained and phonation is labored. This is apparently a neurologic disorder similar to writer's cramp, i.e., a kind of restricted dystonia. The patients are not neurotic, and psychotherapy and speech therapy have been ineffective. This condition differs from the stridor caused by spasm of the laryngeal muscles in tetany. It is nonprogressive but in some instances is combined with other of the restricted extrapyramidal disorders such as blepharospasm and spasmodic torticollis.

CLINICAL APPROACH TO LANGUAGE DISORDERS Aphasia
In investigating a case of aphasia, it is first necessary to inquire into the patient's native language, handedness, and previous education. Many naturally left-handed children are trained to use their right hand for writing; therefore, in determining this point we must ask which hand is used for throwing a ball, threading a needle, or using a spoon and common tools such as a hammer, saw, or bread knife. It is important before the beginning of the examination to determine whether the patient is alert and can be made to participate reliably in testing, as accurate assessment of language depends on these factors. One should quickly ascertain whether the patient has other signs of a gross cerebral lesion such as hemiplegia, facial weakness, homonymous hemianopia, or cortical sensory loss. When hemiplegia, hemianesthesia, and homonymous hemianopia coexist, the aphasic disorder is usually complete or global. Such a constellation of major neurologic signs is seldom associated with the less complete forms of language disorder, the posterior sylvian syndromes, or one of the dissociative syndromes. Dyspraxia of limbs and speech musculature, in response to spoken commands or to visual mimicry, is generally associated

with Broca's aphasia and sometimes with Wernicke's aphasia. Bilateral or unilateral homonymous hemianopia without motor weakness tends often to be linked to "pure" word blindness (alexia or dyslexia) or to amnestic-dysnomic aphasia. Bilateral hemiplegias due to extensive frontal lesions are accompanied not infrequently by "pure" word muteness. The special types of aphasia—alexia, "pure" word deafness, etc.—are often associated with evidence of embolism to other parts of the brain or other organs.

Conversational testing permits quick assessment of the motor aspects of speech (praxis and prosody) and apparent language formulation and auditory comprehension.

Disabilities in the purely motor aspects of speech suggest a motor aphasia, and this possibility can be pursued further by tests of repeating from dictation and by special tests of praxis of the oropharyngeal and respiratory apparatus. Disabilities in language formulation in the form of literal paraphasias with impaired comprehension are indicative of Wernicke's aphasia. Impaired comprehension but perfectly normal formulated speech suggest the rare syndrome of pure word deafness. Disorders confined to naming, generally without paraphasias, when other language functions (reading, writing, spelling, etc.) are found adequate, are diagnostic of amnestic dysnomia.

When conversation shows virtually no disabilities, other tests may still be revealing. Reading aloud single letters, words, and text may reveal the dissociative syndrome of pure word blindness, while tests of writing in this syndrome will show little abnormality. Literal and verbal paraphasic errors may appear in milder cases of Wernicke's aphasia as the patient reads aloud from text or from words in the examiner's handwriting. Similar errors appear even more frequently when the patient is asked to explain the text, read aloud, or give explanations in writing. Should such tests still be unrevealing of deficits, the examiner may find it useful to increase the complexity of the tests. If the patient then succeeds, one may be sure that there is no disorder of adequacy of reception. Adequacy of response channels is next determined by presenting the patient with tasks that permit a response physically identical with the test stimulus. Copying visual stimuli and repeating aloud from auditory stimuli are examples of this kind of testing. Inadequacy of receptive or response channels will then preclude further analysis of the deficit involving that channel in more complex types of tests, except in the unlikely instance that the more complex test is better performed. If reception and response channels are found adequate in these initial tests, they may then be used in tests requiring all types of language function, such as writing from dictation, vocal naming of visual stimuli, matching physically dissimilar stimuli having a name in common (i.e., the word "cow" and a picture of a cow). By utilizing the same test material used in the earlier tests, direct comparison of performances in spoken naming, written naming, and matching can be compared from visual, auditory, and palpated stimuli. A performance profile can be constructed separately for each type of stimulus material tested (i.e., objects, pictures, words, letters, numbers, colors, etc.). The resultant profile can then be used to determine whether the main deficits fall across one or more input or response channels. These data then provide a baseline against which later changes may be compared.

Articulatory-phonation disorders Disturbances of articulation point to involvement of a different set of neural structures, such as the motor cortices, the corticobulbar pathways, the seventh, ninth, and tenth nuclei, the brainstem, and extrapyramidal nuclei and tracts. Often it is necessary to use other neurologic findings to decide which of these are implicated in any given case. The important distinction between the

pseudobulbar or supranuclear palsies and the bulbar palsies is grasped only with difficulty by the average student. The information obtained by localizing these two major types of dysarthria is extremely helpful in differential diagnosis.

Dysphonia should lead to an investigation of laryngeal disease, either primary or secondary to an abnormality of innervation. Inspection of vocal cords is a necessary step in the clinical study.

TREATMENT The sudden loss of speech would be expected to cause great apprehension, but except for almost pure motor defects, most patients show remarkably little concern. It appears that the very lesion that deprives them of speech also causes a partial loss of insight into their own disability. This reaches almost a ludicrous extreme in some cases of Wernicke's aphasia, in which patients become indignant when others cannot understand their jargon. Nonetheless, as improvement occurs, many patients do become discouraged. Reassurance and a positive program of speech rehabilitation are the best ways of helping the patient at this stage.

Most aphasic difficulties are due to vascular disease of the brain, and nearly always this is accompanied by some degree of spontaneous improvement in the days, weeks, and months that follow the stroke. Sometimes recovery is complete within hours or days; at times not more than a few words are regained after a year or two of assiduous speech training. Nevertheless, it is the opinion of many experts in the field that speech training is worthwhile.

One must decide for each patient whether speech training is needed and when it should be started. As a rule, therapy is not advisable in the first few days of an aphasic illness, because one does not know how lasting it will be. Also, if the patient suffers a severe global aphasia and can neither speak nor understand spoken and written words, the speech therapist is helpless. Under such circumstances, one does well to wait a few weeks until some one of the language functions has begun to return. Then the physician may begin to encourage and help the patient to use the function to a maximal degree. In milder aphasic disorders the patient may be sent to the speech therapist as soon as the illness has stabilized.

The methods of speech training are specialized, and it is advisable to call in a person who has been trained in this field.

There is no special treatment for the dysarthric disturbance of speech.

PROGNOSIS The outcome of aphasia depends on the nature of the underlying disease and the magnitude of the lesion within the speech areas. Global aphasias lasting more than a week or two usually have a bad outcome. Seldom is there enough recovery of communicative speech to permit resumption of occupation or profession. Partial aphasias frequently improve, sometimes to a gratifying degree, if of vascular or encephalitic origin. Aphasias due to embolism, whether global or restricted, may disappear in hours to days, like all cerebral embolic deficits, or persist.

REFERENCES

BRAIN R: Aphasia, apraxia, agnosia, in *Neurology*, 2d ed, SAK Wilson, N Bruce (eds). Baltimore, William & Wilkins, 1955, vol 3, chap 83

GESCHWIND N: Disconnection syndromes in animals and man. Brain 88:237, 585, 1965

MOHR JP: Broca's area and Broca's aphasia, in *Studies in Neurolinguistics*, H Whitaker (ed). New York, Academic, 1975, chap 6

———, SIDMAN M: Aphasia: Behavioral aspects, in *American Handbook of Psychiatry*, vol 4, M Reiser (ed). New York, Basic Books, 1975, pp 279–298

NIELSEN JM: *Agnosia, Apraxia, Aphasia: Their Value in Cerebral Localization*, 2d ed. New York, Hafner, 1962

DERANGEMENTS OF INTELLECT, MOOD, AND BEHAVIOR, INCLUDING SCHIZOPHRENIA AND MANIC-DEPRESSIVE STATES

RAYMOND D. ADAMS
MAURICE VICTOR

Increasingly, as mental, emotional, and behavioral disorders are recognized as manifestations of diseases of the brain, the internist is consulted because an otherwise healthy person begins to lose the capacity to function effectively as a student, a worker, or head of a family. This may have several meanings—the beginning of a brain tumor, the formation of chronic subdural hematoma, the development of chronic drug intoxication, chronic meningoencephalitis (syphilis), degenerative cerebral disease, or a schizophrenic psychosis. In former times, when there was little that could be done about any of these clinical states, no great premium was attached to diagnosis, but modern medicine now offers the means of treating several of these conditions and in some instances of restoring the patient to normal health and effectiveness. Early recognition of the underlying pathologic process improves the chances of recovery.

In this chapter we consider first the global deterioration of mental functions subsumed under the term dementia and then certain special impairments such as Korsakoff's amnesic state, schizophrenia, and manic-depressive psychosis. The last part of the chapter will be devoted to the clinical manifestations of focal cerebral diseases, exclusive of aphasia and convulsions.

THE CLINICAL SYNDROME OF DEMENTIA

The term *dementia* usually denotes a clinical state composed of failing memory and loss of other intellectual functions due to chronic progressive degenerative disease of the brain. It may or may not be associated with signs of disease in one or more of the motor, sensory, or language areas of the cerebrum. The chronicity of the process is ordinarily emphasized, but the illogic of setting apart any one constellation of cerebral symptoms on the basis of their speed of onset, rate of evolution, or duration is obvious. We would insist that the state of dementia is a generic syndrome of multiple causation and mechanism, and that a diffuse degeneration of neurons is only one of the types.

Clinical findings The earliest signs of dementia may be so subtle as to escape the notice of even the most discerning physician. Often an observant relative of the patient or an employer is the first to become aware of certain lack of initiative, irritability, loss of interest, and inability to perform up to the usual standard. Later there is distractibility of attention, inability to think with accustomed clarity, reduced general comprehension, perseveration in speech, action, and thought, and defective memory, especially for recent events. Frequently a change in mood becomes apparent, deviating more often toward depression than elation. The direction of this deviation is said to depend on the previous personality of the patient rather than upon the character of the disease. Excessive lability of mood may be observed, i.e., easy fluctuation from laughter to tears on slight provocation. Lapses in social graces and conduct occur, and judgment becomes impaired, early in some cases and late in others. Paranoid ideas and delusions may develop. As a rule, the patient has little or no realization of these changes in behavior and lacks insight into their meaning.

As the condition progresses, there is loss of almost all intellectual faculties. Dysarthria, aphasia, and sphincteric incontinence, reduced responsivity, and finally mutism may be added to the clinical picture. In a late stage a secondary physical deterioration also takes place. Food intake, which may be increased in the beginning of the illness, is in the end usually limited, with resulting emaciation. Any febrile illness or metabolic upset induces a marked increase in confusion and even stupor or coma, indicating the precarious state of cerebral compensation. Finally, the patient remains in bed most of the time and dies of pneumonia or some other intercurrent infection. This whole process may evolve over a period of months or years, usually the latter.

Many of the alterations of behavior are the direct result of disease of the nervous system; expressed in another way, the symptoms are the primary manifestations of neurologic disease. Others are secondary; i.e., they are reactions to the catastrophe of losing one's mind. For example, the dement is said to seek solitude to hide the affliction and may thus appear asocial or apathetic. Again, excessive orderliness may be an attempt to compensate for failing memory; apprehension, gloom, or irritability may reflect general dissatisfaction with a necessarily restricted life. It would appear that even in a state of fairly advanced deterioration the patient is still capable of reacting to the illness and to the persons who care for him or her.

Degenerative diseases may terminate in virtually complete decortication. The patient is unaware of what is happening but lies with eyes open. He or she no longer responds to spoken commands or speaks. There is no interest in food or drink, though they are swallowed if placed in the mouth. The facial and limb muscles are stiff with increased tendon reflexes and Babinski signs. Grasping and sucking are prominent. The sphincters are incontinent.

Morbid anatomy and pathologic physiology of dementia Dementia is related usually to obvious structural disease of the cerebrum and the diencephalon. In some, such as the Alzheimer-senile dementia complex and Pick's disease, the main process appears to be a degeneration and loss of nerve cells in the association areas, with secondary changes in the cerebral white matter. A degeneration of neurons confined to the thalamus may also cause dementia. In others, such as Huntington's chorea and certain of the cerebral-basal ganglionic degenerations, loss of neurons in the cerebral cortex is accompanied by a similar degeneration of neurons in the putamen and caudate nuclei and cerebellum. Arteriosclerotic vascular disease may result in multiple foci of infarction throughout the thalami, basal ganglia, brainstem, and cerebrum. Cerebral involvement may include the motor, sensory, or visual projection areas as well as the association areas. Severe trauma may cause contusions of cerebral convolutions and white matter as well as necroses and hemorrhages in the midbrain, lesions which are responsible for protracted stupor, coma, or dementia. Most diseases that produce dementia are quite extensive, and the frontal lobes are affected more often than other parts of the cerebrum.

Mechanisms other than the destruction of brain tissue may be operative in some cases. Chronic increased intracranial pressure or chronic hydrocephalus (with large ventricles the pressure may not exceed 180 mmHg), regardless of cause, is often associated with a general impairment of mental function. Compression of cerebral white matter is the main factor. The compression of one or both of the cerebral hemispheres by chronic subdural hematomas may cause a widespread disturbance of cortical function. A diffuse inflammatory process is at least in part the basis for dementia in syphilis and in certain virus infections such as "inclusion body encephalitis"; presumably there is loss of some neurons as well as inflammatory derangement of the function of other neurons. Lastly, several of the toxic and metabolic diseases discussed in Chap. 371 may interfere with nervous function over a period of time and create a clinical picture similar to, if not identical with, that of dementia. One must suppose that the altered biochemical environment has affected the excitability of the neurons.

Bedside classification of dementia

I Diseases in which dementia is usually the only evidence of neurologic or medical disease
  A Alzheimer's disease and senile dementia
  B Pick's disease
II Diseases in which dementia is associated with other neurologic signs but not with other obvious medical disease
  A Invariably associated with other neurologic signs
    1 Huntington's chorea (choreoathetosis)
    2 Schilder's disease, metachromatic leukodystrophy, and related demyelinative diseases (spastic weakness, pseudobulbar palsy, blindness, deafness)
    3 Lipofuscinosis and other lipid-storage diseases (myoclonic seizures, blindness, spasticity, cerebellar ataxia)
    4 Myoclonic epilepsy (diffuse myoclonus, generalized seizures, cerebellar ataxia)
    5 Jakob-Creutzfeldt disease (diffuse myoclonus and cerebellar ataxia)
    6 Cerebrocerebellar degeneration (cerebellar ataxia of olivopontocerebellar type and others)
    7 Cerebral-basal ganglionic degenerations (apraxia-rigidity)
    8 Dementia with spastic paraplegia
    9 Basal ganglia calcification (idiopathic and hypoparathyroidism)
    10 Hallervorden-Spatz disease
    11 Dementia with Parkinson's disease
  B Often associated with other neurologic signs
    1 Cerebral arteriosclerosis
    2 Brain tumor
    3 Brain trauma, such as cerebral contusion, midbrain hemorrhage, chronic subdural hematoma
    4 Marchiafava-Bignami disease (often with apraxia and other frontal lobe signs)
    5 Low-pressure hydrocephalus (always with ataxia of gait and often with sphincteric incontinence)
III Diseases in which dementia is usually associated with clinical and laboratory signs of other medical disease
  A Hypothyroidism
  B Cushing's disease
  C Nutritional deficiency states such as pellagra, the Wernicke-Korsakoff syndrome, and subacute combined degeneration of spinal cord and brain (vitamin B_{12} deficiency)
  D Neurosyphilis: general paresis and meningovascular syphilis
  E Hepatolenticular degeneration, familial and acquired
  F Bromidism, chronic barbiturate intoxication

The degenerative diseases that cause dementia are discussed in Chap. 373. The special features of the dementia that accompanies arteriosclerotic, senile, syphilitic, traumatic, nutritional, and degenerative diseases are discussed in the appropriate chapters.

Differential diagnosis The first task in dealing with this class of patients is to make sure that the central problem is one of general deterioration of intellect and personality change. It may be necessary to examine the patient several times before one is confident of the clinical findings.

An easy mistake is to assume that mental function is normal if there is complaint only of nervousness, fatigue, insomnia, or vague somatic symptoms, and to label such patients as psychoneurotic. *This will be avoided if one keeps in mind that psychoneuroses rarely begin in middle or late adult life.* A practical rule is to assume that all mental illnesses beginning during this period are due either to structural disease of the brain or to a depressive psychosis.

A mild dysphasia must not be mistaken for dementia. Aphasic patients appear uncertain of themselves, and their speech may be incoherent. Furthermore, they may be anxious and depressed over this ineptitude. Careful attention to the language performance of these patients will lead to the correct diagnosis in most instances. Further observation will disclose that their behavior, except that which is related to the language disorder, is within normal limits.

Depressed patients present another type of problem. They may remark that their mental function is poor or that they are forgetful and cannot concentrate. Scrutiny of these remarks will show, however, that they actually remember the details of their illness and that no qualitative change in mental ability has taken place. The difficulty is either a lack of energy and interest or an anxiety that prevents the focusing of attention on anything except their own problems. Even during mental tests their performance may be impaired by their emotions in much the same way as the performance of worried students is impaired during examinations. This condition of emotional blocking is called *experiential confusion.* When patients are calmed by reassurance and given more time in the performance of tests, mental function improves, indicating that intellectual deterioration has not occurred. Hypomanic patients fail in tests of intellectual function because of restlessness and distractibility. It is helpful to remember that demented patients, except in the early phases of their illness, rarely have sufficient insight to complain of mental deterioration and those who admit to poor memory seldom realize the degree of their disability. The physician must never rely on patients' statements of the efficiency of mental function and must always evaluate a poor performance on tests in the light of the emotional state and motivation at the time the test is given.

The neurologic syndromes associated with metabolic or endocrine disorders, i.e., ACTH therapy, hyperthyroidism, Cushing's disease, Addison's disease, or the postpartum state may be difficult to separate from that of dementia because of the wide variety of clinical pictures by which they manifest themselves. Some such patients appear to be suffering from a dementia, others from an acute confusional psychosis; or if mood change or negativism predominates, a manic-depressive psychosis or schizophrenia is suggested. In these conditions some degree of clouding of sensorium and impairment of intellectual function can usually be recognized, and these findings alone should be enough to exclude schizophrenia and manic-depressive psychosis. It is well to remember that acute onset of mental symptoms always suggests confusional psychosis or delirium. Inasmuch as many of these conditions are completely reversible, they must be distinguished from the dementia of degenerative diseases (see Chap. 21).

Once it is decided that the patient suffers from a dementing disease, the next step is to determine by careful physical examination whether there are other neurologic signs or indications of a particular medical disease. This enables the physician to place the case in one of the three categories in the bedside classification. X-rays of the skull, electroencephalogram, lumbar puncture, and computerized tomography (CT) scans should be carried out in most cases. Usually these procedures necessitate admission to a hospital. The final step is to determine by the total clinical picture which disease within any one category the patient has.

SPECIAL TYPES OF INTELLECTUAL IMPAIRMENT

KORSAKOFF'S PSYCHOSIS (AMNESIC CONFABULATORY PSYCHOSIS) Clinical findings These terms are used interchangeably to designate a unique but common disorder of cognitive function, in which memory is deranged out of all proportion to other components of mentation and behavior. It possesses two salient features which may vary in severity but are always conjoined: (1) an impaired ability to recall events and other information that has been recorded in the mind before the onset of the illness (retrograde amnesia); and (2) an impaired ability to acquire new information, i.e., to learn or to form new memories (anterograde amnesia). Other cognitive functions (particularly the capacity for concentration, spatial organization, visual and verbal abstraction), which depend little or not at all on memory, may also be impaired but to a relatively minor degree. The patient tends to be lacking in initiative and spontaneity. *Confabulation,* meaning false or fabricated accounts of recent events, is present in most cases, especially in the acute phase of the illness.

The definition of Korsakoff's psychosis demands also that certain aspects of behavior and mental function be intact. The patient should be alert, attentive, responsive, and capable of understanding the written and spoken word, of making appropriate deductions from given premises, and of solving such problems as can be concluded within the his or her forward memory span. These "negative" features are of particular importance because they help to distinguish Korsakoff's psychosis from a number of other disorders in which the basic defect is not necessarily in retentive memory but in some other psychologic mechanism, e.g., in attention and perception (as in the delirious, confused, or stuporous patient), in recall (as in the hysterical patient), or in volition (as in the patient with frontal lobe disease).

Pathologic anatomy The anatomic structures of particular importance in memory function are the diencephalon (specifically the medial portions of the medial dorsal nuclei of the thalamus) and the inferomedial portions of the temporal lobes, particularly the hippocampal formations and underlying white matter. Bilaterally placed lesions in either of these regions derange memory and learning out of all proportion to other cognitive functions, and even unilateral lesions in the dominant hemispheres produce a lesser degree of the same effect. It would appear that the aforementioned anatomic structures are involved in all forms of learning and integration of newly formed memories and that they form a tenuous but vital link between the high brainstem reticular formation (the integrity of which is necessary to maintain an alert state of mind, a prerequisite for any learning) and the cerebral cortex, which is the locus for special memories such as words, geometric figures, and numbers.

Classification of diseases characterized by an amnesic syndrome

I Amnesic syndrome of sudden onset—usually with gradual but incomplete recovery
   A Bilateral hippocampal infarction due to atherosclerotic-thrombotic or embolic occlusion of the posterior cerebral arteries or their inferior temporal branches
   B Trauma to the diencephalic or inferomedial temporal regions

   C Spontaneous subarachnoid hemorrhage
   D Carbon monoxide poisoning and other hypoxic states (rare)
II Amnesia of sudden onset and brief duration with full recovery
   A Temporal lobe seizures
   B Postconcussive states
   C "Transient global amnesia"
III Amnesic syndrome of subacute onset with varying degrees of recovery, usually leaving permanent residue
   A Wernicke-Korsakoff disease
   B Inclusion body (herpes simplex) encephalitis
   C Tuberculous and other forms of meningitis characterized by a granulomatous exudate at the base of the brain
IV Slowly progressive amnesic states
   A Tumors involving the walls of the third ventricle and temporal lobes
   B Alzheimer's disease and other degenerative disorders (early stage only)

The differentiation of the diseases that give rise to the amnesic syndrome proceeds along the lines indicated in Chaps. 265, 366, 369, 372, and 373.

THE DELUSIONAL-HALLUCINATORY (SCHIZOPHRENIFORM) SYNDROME AND RELATED MENTAL STATES (PSYCHOSES) From the neurologist's standpoint this syndrome is basically a subtle disorder in attention and thinking associated with hallucinatory experiences, delusions, and an inability to distinguish subjective experience from reality. Conjoined often are disturbances in affect, verbal expression, motor activity, and social behavior.

Originally Kraepelin, one of the pioneers in German psychiatry, referred to this syndrome as *dementia praecox,* but it soon became evident that it bore little resemblance to the general intellectual deterioration described above under dementia. Indeed, memory function, lost early in the latter syndrome, is usually preserved except in the most advanced stages. Even then the sensorium tends to remain clear, and language functions, arithmetic ability, and all gnosic and praxic activities of the brain are preserved. Bleuler decided that the term schizophrenia, meaning a splitting of the mind (or dissociation of content of thought and affect) was more appropriate. He emphasized disturbances in the association of ideas, an inclination to withdraw from reality, and a preference for rumination and fantasy (autism) as the fundamental derangements.

Discerning analyses of abnormal mentation, mood, and behavior inform us that this more or less unique syndrome, readily recognizable in its most typical form, has multiple causes. While characteristic of a genetic disease known to the medical world as *schizophrenia,* the syndrome may also be the clinical expression of manic-depressive psychosis, alcoholic auditory hallucinosis, *amphetamine psychosis, temporal lobe epilepsy,* some of the *puerperal* and *endocrine psychoses,* and rarely a focal cerebral disease of other type.

Clinical aspects of the syndrome This clinical state is the most abstruse of any in the realm of neuropsychiatry. Thinking and behavioral abnormalities are both present. In some instances they may be so obvious that diagnosis offers no difficulty whatsoever, but in many others the symptoms may be subtle, vague, and difficult to elicit. The clinician must always depend for diagnosis on the verbal expressions and actions of the patient. If the patient is mute, taciturn, incapable of freely expressing his or her thoughts, or reluctant to talk because of hostility and suspicion toward the examiner, the primary disorder of thought may not be discovered or may be only inferred from his or her actions. A detailed account of the patient's speech and behavior by an observant member of the family then is particularly helpful.

The most striking feature of the syndrome is a curious alteration of awareness of what is going on. Such patients are seemingly preoccupied with their own thoughts so that their responses to questions are neither constant nor prompt. In their replies to questions and spontaneous remarks, one finds that orientation to time, place, and person is intact, and usually the names of doctors, nurses, medications, etc., can be given accurately. In other words, the general aspects of formal intelligence are preserved. However, during the most intense phases of the syndrome, in which mental disorganization is profound, there may be inattentiveness to ambient surroundings.

The thoughts of these patients are often interrupted by hallucinations (usually auditory) and unreal dreamlike experiences. Sometimes the hallucinations consist of voices coming from outside the body, but often no clear distinction is drawn between a hallucination and an idea that has been planted in the mind. In the struggle to retain sanity, patients try vainly to separate their own thoughts and perceptual experiences from those of others who are ostensibly trying to control them. Communication of this melange of confusing experiences is difficult. Even when obviously preoccupied with voices, the patients may be reluctant or unable to admit that they are hallucinating.

The patients may feel that their thoughts are being read by others or that they are under outside control. When extraneous ideas are forced upon them they may feel powerless, as though they are passive recipients of the ideas of others (passivity feelings). They may believe these ideas have been transmitted to them by wireless electronic devices, laser beams, or whatever is culturally in vogue. Sometimes they may believe that their own thoughts are made known to others by similar devices. Trying to cope with this confusion of strange and disturbing ideas, patients become so self-absorbed that simple questions may evoke no reply or only one that seems tangential, inappropriate, and incomplete.

Psychologists have attempted for decades to categorize this thought disorder and to educe its essential character. They have remarked on the apparent "disregard for the logical limits of time and space," the "confusion of parts for wholes," "the lumping and condensation of separate items," the acceptance of "the identity of opposites," and the inability to think abstractly. None of these attributes appear to be inclusively descriptive.

Associated with this thought disorder are delusions. These are expressed at some time in the majority of cases. Patients may come to believe they have a disease, that their lives are in danger, that they have been singled out or are threatened for some obscure reason, or that they have suddenly gained remarkable insight into world events. The delusions, based as they are on accusatory or controlling hallucinatory and imagined experiences, cannot be eradicated by logical argument. Such thoughts may be acted upon and occasionally lead to suicide or homicide.

This disorder of thought may vary in intensity from time to time. If it is severe and persistent, patients appear overwhelmed; they may lie mute and frozen in a state of suspended activity (catatonia), or they may be found wandering aimlessly, perplexed, and fearful or excited. The mental state then may resemble a confusion or delirium but without the characteristic clouding of consciousness. If the thought disorder is mild, there are periods when patients appear relatively normal and only withdrawal, disregard of social customs, and preoccupations prevent adequate school or work performance. However, at any time the thought disorder may break through, and seemingly well persons may for no obvious reason once again become vague, preoccupied, and deluded.

The typical and allegedly characteristic affect of the delusional-hallucinatory syndrome is difficult to interpret. Often it seems to be a reflection of the patients' mental state and content of thought. When they are preoccupied, they appear to be detached and indifferent to surroundings. Irritability and undue sensitivity are prominent in some patients and are expressed as resentment toward the therapist and sometimes as unreasonable hostility. If voices and ideas threaten, they first excite patients, but later, if the threats continue, patients become more or less inured to them. While some of the emotional reactions seem inappropriate to the immediate situation, it is usually discovered that they are not inappropriate to the patients' thoughts and mental preoccupations. If one can probe the content of thought, one may then find that the emotions are not at all incongruous, but in some instances the incongruity of thought and feeling is obvious and impossible to understand.

In summary, it is the combination of a subtle *alteration of clear awareness and the intrusion of hallucinatory and dreamlike experiences,* occurring all during the waking hours and making separation of fantasy and reality impossible, and *the delusional systems of ideas* that identifies this psychotic syndrome. Semiologically it falls between delirium on one side and a vague personality and character disorder on the other.

Schizophrenia   This is a hereditary lifelong disease of the nervous system which begins in early life, pursues a recurrent course without full remissions, and is characterized by the above syndrome or some variant thereof.

The disease is frequent and worldwide. Prevalence rates are in the order of 0.2 to 0.5 percent, and life expectancy rates (chance of manifesting schizophrenic symptoms sometime during life) are at least 1.0 percent. New cases each year number about 0.05 to 0.1 percent of the total population. World prevalence is 10 to 20 million cases. Males and females are equally affected. Family studies show that the closer a person is related to a schizophrenic, the greater the risk of the disease for that person. If both parents have schizophrenia, the risk to a child is approximately 50 percent; this holds whether the child is raised with the biologic parents or in a foster home. A monozygotic twin has three to four times the risk of a dizygotic twin or sibling. However, the hereditary pattern does not conform to any known mendelian type, and the importance of environmental stress, which is emphasized by many psychiatrists, is difficult to evaluate.

CLINICAL FINDINGS   The onset of the clinical manifestations occurs usually during adolescence or early adult life, but in approximately half the cases the psychotic episode occurs in an individual who throughout childhood is known to have been eccentric, timid, aloof, or socially maladjusted in some way. In some instances the onset is acute and at a time of stress, and the disease is so disturbing to the patient and family as to require hospitalization. The symptoms subside within a few weeks or months, especially under the influence of medication. Equally as frequent is a gradual onset with drift into an inactive, withdrawn, delusional state where the beginning of the illness is impossible to date. Even after recovery from an acute episode, patients tend not to be normal and are unable to function up to their previous intellectual level. These patients tend to be vague, poorly motivated, worried, and concerned about matters of little importance to a healthy mind. Relapse is frequent throughout the remainder of their lives.

The psychosis may vary in its outward manifestations.

Some patients are strikingly paranoid, others catatonic or remarkably disorganized and silly in their delusional behavior (hebephrenia); or the illness may resemble a severe and persistent neurosis (pseudoneurotic) or a pervasive character disorder. One may question whether these are variations of a single disease or several diseases, closely related in their clinical expression (cf., *Harvard Guide in Modern Psychiatry*).

In this disease complete recovery after an acute episode of the schizophrenic syndrome is said to occur in approximately 30 percent of cases, but this is disputed. Probably many of the complete recoveries are in patients who have the delusional-hallucinatory syndrome but not schizophrenic disease. For example, an acute hypomania or mixed manic-depressive state in an adolescent, as will be pointed out below, may be virtually indistinguishable from the psychosis of schizophrenia.

According to Robins and Guze the diagnosis of schizophrenia becomes reliable only when, over a period of at least 6 months, a patient exhibits the delusional-hallucinatory syndrome (with clear consciousness and orientation), along with a type of "verbal production that makes communication difficult because of lack of logical or understandable organization." Usually the individual is unmarried and has had poor premorbid social adjustment and work history, and a family history of schizophrenia. The onset of illness before the age of 40 years and the absence of drug or alcohol abuse and of manic and depressive symptoms increase the probability of accuracy of this diagnosis to over 90 percent.

ETIOLOGY AND PATHOGENESIS Theories are legion, but a textbook of medicine is hardly the place to discuss them. Many psychiatrists are committed to a psychogenic etiology, but this remains entirely unproved. In recent years attention has been focused largely on biological factors, particularly chemical derangement of certain structures in the limbic portions of the brain (nucleus accumbens, bed nucleus of stria terminalis, ventral septum, and mammillary bodies). In several cases of chronic paranoid schizophrenia the norepinephrine levels in these regions have been significantly increased (McCullough et al.). This finding, if verified, would incriminate a disorder in neurotransmitter dynamics as the chemical pathology of this hereditary disease.

The morphologic substratum of this disease has eluded all neuropathologic techniques. The possible ways in which a genetic factor can be translated into disordered function of certain parts of the brain without visibly altering neuronal structure has been reviewed by Kety. He finds all current biochemical hypotheses to be unsubstantiated.

TREATMENT The treatment of schizophrenia is relatively unsatisfactory and is usually left to the psychiatrist. Chlorpromazine (Thorazine) in a dose usually of 200 to 300 mg per day (range 200 to 2000 mg per day) is the most widely used medication for acute psychotic episodes. However, it carries the risk of extrapyramidal side effects, some of which are permanent (tardive dyskinesia), even when treatment is combined with antiparkinson drugs. There are now many new drugs, some of which are modifications of the original phenothiazines, including the piperazine derivatives, which are higher in their per milligram potency [e.g., fluphenazine (Prolixin), trifluoperazine (Stelazine), and perphenazine (Trilafon)]. Other drugs in common use are chlorprothixene (Taractan), butyrophenone (Haldol), and loxapine (Loxitene). These medications do not merely tranquilize, but suppress hallucinations and delusions and improve the organization of thought. Electroconvulsive therapy (ECT) is sometimes used for stuporous or agitated patients, but its general efficacy is questionable. The value of psychotherapy is unproved, and most psychiatrists agree with Baldessarini, who stated that it has little to offer "as a primary mode of treatment." A few psychoanalysts claim to have suc-

cessfully treated schizophrenia. Active supportive medical and psychotherapy directed to helping the patient maintain a grasp on reality and to readjust to home and work situations are clearly indicated. In combination with drug therapy, a large proportion of schizophrenic patients are now able to leave psychiatric hospitals and return to a sheltered existence in the community.

Psychotic form of manic-depressive disease Descriptions of manic-depressive disease and dementia praecox, from the earliest ones by Kraepelin, cannot fail to impress the readers with the similarities between these disease states. Contemporary psychiatrists attest to the difficulty in distinguishing some cases of these two diseases by positing a category of *schizoaffective* or *schizothymic* states in which are combined attributes of both. Pope and Lipinski, after a review of the literature and a 4-year personal experience with admissions to the McLean Hospital, and Robins and Guze and their associates, observe that the full delusional-hallucinatory psychotic syndrome of schizophrenia occurs frequently in manic-depressive disease. They insist that this syndrome when viewed in "cross section" is not diagnostic of either schizophrenia or manic-depressive disease; i.e., it is nonspecific. If it occurs acutely in association with a prominent affective or mood disorder in a previously well-adjusted individual, especially if it is preceded by euphoria, hyperactivity, flight of ideas, pressure of speech, grandiosity, hostility and sleeplessness (the usual symptoms and signs of mania), the diagnosis will usually turn out to be manic-depressive disease. The hypomanic patient often will have a family history of manic-depressive disease, and over 70 percent will respond to lithium therapy and make a full recovery within a few months. Schizophrenia differs in the lack of manic-depressive disease in the family, lack of affective symptoms and an emotional state incongruent with thought content, a more gradual onset, incomplete recovery, and little or no response to lithium. Depressive states of nonpsychotic type are more fully discussed below.

Alcoholic auditory hallucinosis This disease begins as a withdrawal or abstinence syndrome in the chronic alcoholic. Usually it subsides in 1 to 2 weeks, but in some the hallucinosis persists indefinitely. The illness comes in time to resemble schizophrenia (see Chap. 226). Affected individuals do not have a premorbid schizoid personality and have no family history of schizophrenia. Such cases reinforce the authors' argument that a slightly altered consciousness, delusions, and hallucinatory experiences stand as the primary abnormalities in the schizophrenic syndrome and are not of themselves diagnostic of the disease schizophrenia.

Schizophrenic psychosis in patients with temporal lobe epilepsy Quite apart from the psychomotor seizures, which in themselves induce curious behavioral abnormalities, such patients may develop an acute psychosis with prominent thought disorder, hallucinations and delusions, ideas of reference, remoteness, and a disorganization of activity and social relations that simulates schizophrenia. The psychosis appears not to be due to continuous subclinical firing of a seizure focus, for the EEG contains no paroxysmal discharge. The patients respond to antipsychotic drugs and recover within a few weeks.

Amphetamine psychosis High dosage and prolonged usage of amphetamines can induce a typical paranoid psychosis with characteristic autistic thought disorder, delusions, and hallucinations. Once started it may continue for several weeks and is said to respond to antipsychotic drugs. A similar syndrome is occasionally observed in a metabolic disease, and after marijuana and lysergic acid overdosage. The authors have had little experience with these states and cannot document the similarity of such syndromes to the one under consideration.

Puerperal psychosis Brief psychologic disturbances are not infrequent in the puerperium. The most typical reaction is a depression which may last for days, weeks, or months, and may recur after the next pregnancy. There is another type of psychosis featured by variable degrees of confusion and autistic thought disorder. The deluded mother may claim the baby not to be her own, and there are tragic instances where she has killed the infant. Recovery occurs over many weeks or months, and opinion is divided as to whether this is a confusional psychosis or delirium or is a delusional-hallucinatory psychosis of either schizophrenic or manic type.

Endocrine psychosis In patients receiving high-dose corticosteroid or ACTH therapy and occasionally in a person suffering from hyperthyroidism, there may occur poor sleep, hallucinations, delusions, disordered thought, and frenzied excitement in varying combinations. Discontinuation of the steroid or treatment of the thyrotoxicosis usually restores the patient to normalcy within a few weeks. Here once again is an example of an illness that overlaps the acute confusional and delirious state where there is clouding of consciousness on the one hand and the more protracted delusional-hallucinatory syndrome with relatively clear consciousness on the other.

Differential diagnosis At times a schizophrenic illness that never explodes into an overt psychosis but leads to persistent inability to function in school, at work, or as a member of a family unit may be difficult to distinguish from one in which there is adolescent turmoil, maladjustment, preoccupation with philosophical ideas and Eastern religions, and involvement in the activist affairs of the counterculture. Abuse of drugs adds to the problem. Suspiciousness, dramatic behavior, unreasonable attitudes, and indifference to conventional practices are common to both conditions. Only by identification of the basic cognitive disorders of the schizophrenic syndrome with the added stipulation that it persist for many months will the diagnosis of schizophrenia be established, and this may require a period of observation in the neutral environment of a hospital. It is said that some social derelicts, vagrants, chronic drug abusers, and sociopathic individuals are actually suffering from simple schizophrenia.

The elderly patient who becomes paranoid while still mentally intact and who is not depressed presents another difficult clinical problem. Such cases need to be studied over a period of time before one can eliminate the possibility of a dementing illness or a depressive psychosis. Only if the latter are excluded is one justified in the conclusion that they have the rare and special psychiatric illness known as pure *paranoia*.

SYNDROMES OF EMOTIONAL (AFFECT AND MOOD) DISTURBANCE The term *emotion* is used in medical practice in so many ways that it virtually loses all meaning. It refers indiscriminately to the nervous, the neurotic, the unhappy and maladjusted, and to the patient with obscure medical disease. The neurologist assigns to it a more precise definition—a complex state of the organism comprised of a mental component of fear, anger, love, or hate in association with certain visceral changes that are mainly under the control of the autonomic nervous system and lead to a certain pattern of motor expression. Intense emotion may disturb rational thought, and the

resulting behavior, while apparently degraded and stereotyped, is nonetheless protective of the organism. Mild emotion may take the form of anxiety, depression, or elation with only the most subtle visceral accompaniments and somatic manifestations.

Human emotion upon strict analysis consists of a stimulus, the accurate perception of which requires the memory of specific associations drawn from previous experience. The psychic state aroused by the perception includes a *feeling* or *affect* known only to the experiencing individual and manifested through verbal expressions and behavior. Thus, on the one side, an emotion includes the same perceptive-cognitive processes as does any induced sensory experience, but it differs with respect to its affective component with the associated visceral reactions and with respect to certain specific patterns of behavior.

Cannon and Bard and their associates studied the ways in which the two parts of the autonomic nervous system participate in the emotional state—the parasympathetic mediating trophotropic, restorative, and reproductive functions, viz., the general homeostatic functions; and the sympathetic (including the adrenal glands) mediating self-protective or ergotropic functions. Hess and Bard localized the central control mechanisms in the hypothalamus which are ideally situated to send impulses via descending tracts to the parasympathetic and sympathetic segmental apparatus and via releasing factors to the pituitary-adrenal-thyroid system. This entire complex of emotional activities, including visceral, glandular, and motor reactions, could be elicited from decerebrate animals as long as the hypothalamus remained intact. Papez postulated that the limbic parts of medial temporal and orbital-frontal lobes, which have rich connections with the hypothalamus, could sustain and modulate the long-acting emotional states.

Clinical observations The affective and emotional apparatus is known to be disordered in a number of ways by diseases of the brain. There may be an unnatural *apathy* and *placidity*, wherein the usual stimuli of fear, anger, love, and anxious concern have little or no effect on the patient. Bilateral temporal lesions may result in this condition, along with a remarkable failure of visual recognition, a tendency to examine every object by touch or oral exploration, and either hyper- or hyposexuality. This entire complex is known as the *Kluver-Bucy syndrome*. The right parietal (nondominant) lobe seemed very important in emotional experience, and large lesions here result in an unusual blunting of all emotional reactions. In contrast, a focal lesion in the dominant temporoparietal region rarely may plunge the patient into a state of frenzied excitement, rage, and fear; every stimulus, even innocuous ones, excite the individual, who may lash out blindly at everyone who approaches. One may imagine that the dominant cerebral lesion has disinhibited the intact right parietal lobe. Inferior bifrontal lesions may cause either apathy along with abulia or, rarely, excitement and aggressive behavior, depending on their anatomy. Complete disinhibition of the facial-respiratory apparatus for laughter and crying (syndrome of forced or pathologic laughter and crying) is a frequent accompaniment of pseudobulbar palsy. Here it is the apparatus for emotional expression and not the mental state that is out of control. Lesser degrees of this, in the forms of emotional lability, occur in many cerebral diseases.

The emotional disorders that are the most subtle and difficult to comprehend are *acute* and *chronic anxiety, depression,* and *mania*. They stand as separate syndromes that may appear as the dominant features of certain mental disturbances. They bear no clear relationship to the circumstances which may have occurred in the patient's life. In some instances the prevailing emotional state, on close examination, has been induced by a hallucination or delusion. In a delirium or the schizophreniform syndrome, for example, voices which threaten the patient's life naturally excite fear. In other mental illnesses, the patient experiences an overwhelming anxiety or depression. Unlike the normal person, in whom anxiety, depression, and elation are the natural reactions to life situations such as loss of livelihood or grief over the death of a loved one, or the winning of a coveted treasure, these patients have no conscious awareness of any provocative stimulus. In this sense their emotional state is endogenous. Manic-depressive psychosis, involutional melancholia, and anxiety neurosis (actually a form of depression in most instances) are the most familiar examples, and in the opinion of most neurologists and many psychiatrists they represent diseases of the brain.

Manic-depressive disease Manic-depressive psychosis is a disease characterized by a cyclic disorder of mood. There may be episodes of depression or of mania, appearing once or many times during the lifetime of the patient. Depression is more frequent than mania, and some patients have only depressions. Thus, the mood disorder may be subdivided into monopolar or bipolar type; but in some individuals, there may be both features within a given episode, i.e., mixed manic-depressive.

The disease was given its name by Kraepelin in 1896, and he fully delineated its most distinctive features. Unlike schizophrenia, which usually leaves the patient permanently disabled, between attacks of manic-depressive disease the patient is usually entirely normal.

The incidence of this disease is difficult to determine because of inaccuracy of diagnosis. As pointed out above, many young adults who are said to have recovered from schizophrenia actually have had a manic psychosis. In the author's clinical experience manic-depressive disease is several times more frequent than schizophrenia, at least on the wards of a general hospital. The worldwide incidence is 3 to 4 per 1000 population. In certain countries as many as 5 percent of males and 8 to 9 percent of females will have symptoms of this disease sometime in their lifetime.

The onset is most frequent in middle adult life, but typical episodes may be seen in children, adolescents, and young adults. In fact, it is the most frequent cause of admission of adolescents and young adults to a psychiatric hospital. Any one episode may last months or years, being shortened by therapy.

CLINICAL PICTURE The fully developed depression may evolve within a few days or develop more slowly. The symptoms and signs have already been described in Chap. 11. It need only be restated that the patient, without obvious cause, begins to feel helpless, discouraged, and despondent. Life seems worthless and without purpose, and there is self-blame for the condition. Energy for both mental and physical activity is reduced; the powers of concentration and capacity to maintain interest in the ordinary tasks of the day are lowered, and the least effort is exhausting. It becomes impossible to cope with everyday worries and concerns. Indecisiveness, pain, and many of the bodily effects of frank anxiety are other prominent symptoms. Thoughts of suicide assert themselves. As the depression worsens the patient talks less and finally becomes motionless and mute. Delusions of a somatic or paranoid type often appear and are a source of distress. Finally there is indifference even to nutritional needs; anorexia, weight loss, constipation, insomnia, and loss of libido are the most prominent vegetative effects and will last until the patient begins to emerge from the depression.

In the manic phase the symptoms are the opposite to those of depression. The patient becomes more energetic and is full of enthusiasm and the joy and zest for life. New schemes are embarked upon with great drive and confidence but are seldom carried to completion. New ideas flood the mind, and

there is a great pressure of speech. Judgment is poor, and irritability may become apparent even to the point of hostility if the patient is thwarted or criticized. The euphoria and expansiveness may increase and give way to delusions of grandeur, supernatural power, and self-importance. As in depressive psychosis, paranoid and somatic delusions may appear along with hallucinations. In a more advanced phase of the disease, the patient may have ideas of reference, look disheveled, and neglect personal hygiene. In a *delirious mania*, as was pointed out above, behavior is totally disorganized; the patient is disoriented, hallucinates, and may lapse into catatonia. This extreme form is rare. *Hypomania* refers to the milder degrees of mania.

First attacks of either mania or depression usually last an average of 6 months, but treatment may reduce this by half. Over 90 percent of patients recover from their first attack. Episodes tend to be longer in old age.

ETIOLOGY AND PATHOGENESIS The hereditary factor is the most important biologic attribute of the disease. If one parent has the disease, there is at least one chance in five that one of the children will have it. Not infrequently it can be traced through three or four generations, involving as many as a dozen individuals. If one of identical twins has the disease, the chances are over three out of four that the other will have it, whereas the coincidence in dizygotic twins is about 20 percent.

The discoveries that reserpine may cause depression, that iproniazid may cause elation, and that certain tricyclic drugs and monoamine oxidase inhibitors may relieve depression has aroused great interest in the role of biogenic amines (norepinephrine, serotonin, dopamine) in the causation of hereditary manic-depressive disease. This subject has been reviewed by Maas, who points out that one group of depressive patients (bipolar type) have a consistently low urinary excretion of 3-methoxy-4-hydroxyphenethyleneglycol, one of the major metabolites of brain norepinephrine. This group, interestingly, responds well to imiprimine (Tofranil), desipramine, and dextroamphetamine. A central adrenergic disorder is postulated. In another group excretion of this metabolite is normal or increased, and there is little or no response to these drugs. Instead, amitriptyline (Elavil), which acts on serotonin metabolism, is more effective. These studies of biogenic amine metabolism suggest a biochemical heterogeneity of depressive illness, a concept which is also in line with clinical data.

Psychoanalytic theory postulates a personality type that is prone to depressive illness and attempts to discover a psychogenesis, but there is no convincing proof of this hypothesis. Further, psychotherapy has been of no apparent value in terminating an episode of either depression or mania or in preventing another episode.

Involutional melancholia This form of depression, probably a variant of manic-depressive disease, differs from that disease in several ways: later age of onset (more or less), more prominent anxiety and agitation, higher incidence in women, absence of manic phase, possibly greater frequency of obscure pains, and hypochondriasis.

DIFFERENTIAL DIAGNOSIS Endogenous depression and involutional melancholia, conditions that are closely related if not identical, are among the most frequently misdiagnosed of all diseases. Chronic pains of obscure type (headache, atypical facial pain, backache, uncomfortable and fatigable muscles, pseudoangina pectoris at rest (without ECG change) in the middle-aged and elderly usually turn out to be "masked depressions." Hypochondriasis of persistent type is so frequently a manifestation of depression that it no longer stands as a separate nosologic entity in psychiatry. Chronic anxiety symptoms (giddiness and dizziness, rapid heart action, smothering, trembling, and uneasy apprehension) of longer than a month's duration and unresponsive to reassurance are virtually always due to depression, especially in the middle-aged and elderly. Paranoid and somatic delusions should be regarded as having a depressive origin until proved otherwise. At any age an acute episode of hallucinations and disorganization of thought and delusions in a person whose consciousness is unclouded and who has been previously well-adjusted and is not abusing alcohol or drugs is more likely to be manic-depressive disease than schizophrenia. Persistent weakness and fatigability in association with multiple complaints in various organ systems, often mistakenly attributed to chronic infection (brucella, viral hepatitis, postinfluenzal asthenia), mild anemia, hypothyroidism, and adrenal insufficiency, frequently prove to be due to a depressive illness. Thoughts of or frank attempts at suicide are always to be judged as expressions of a depression, though schizophrenics may also commit suicide and hysterics may make dramatic but not serious attempts. Persistent depression should not be passed off as a natural reaction to some circumstance in life unless the relationship is convincing.

Treatment For the depressed phase of manic-depressive psychosis and for involutional melancholia the plan of therapy embraces five points.

1 *Enlisting the help of a psychiatrist.* The untrained physician would be rash to attempt the management of these patients without psychiatric assistance.
2 *The prevention of suicide.* This involves the question of hospitalization. If there is any doubt about the patient's intention of suicide, it is better to hospitalize the individual than to take a chance. In manic-depressive illness, attacks of depression or elation are remarkably similar in the same individual. Thus one can predict the course and content of the present spell on the basis of the last. If suicide attempts were made then, the chance is they will be made again.
3 *Antidepressant medication.* There are two categories of antidepressants, the tricyclic compounds and the monoamine oxidase (MAO) inhibitors. Representing the former are imipramine (Tofranil) and amitriptyline (Elavil), and the latter, phenelzine (Nardil) and tranylcypromine (Parnate). In the treatment of depression, most psychiatrists start with the tricyclic antidepressants because they are far safer. With imipramine and amitriptyline, doses range from 100 to 200 mg each day. The starting dose is usually 100 mg per day, which is then raised in stepwise fashion as needed. The therapeutic effect of tricyclic medication is often not evident for 2 or 3 weeks after treatment has been initiated, so that it would be premature to stop the drug before that time. Common side effects are orthostatic hypotension, dry mouth, constipation, tachycardia, and urinary retention. Because of their effect on the cardiovascular system, the tricyclic compounds should not be given to patients who have coronary heart disease. If these are not effective, they are discontinued for 2 weeks and administration of an MAO inhibitor is started. Phenelzine is regarded as the least likely of the MAO inhibitors to produce serious side effects. The usual starting dose is 15 mg tid, which is gradually increased as needed to a maximum of 45 mg tid. The most serious side effect of this class of antidepressants is hypertensive crisis. As a consequence, all MAO inhibitors should be dispensed with extreme caution in patients with a history of cardio- or cerebrovascular disease. Patients taking MAO inhibitors should avoid foods with high tyramine content. The latter is

a pressor amine that is normally inactivated by MAO, and ingestion under such circumstances may result in a hypertensive crisis. Proscribed foods (aged cheese, pickled herring, chicken liver, etc.) are always listed on the manufacturer's information insert.

Since patients are usually responsive to one or the other but not to both, it is important to find out whether tricyclics or MAO inhibitors have been more helpful in the past. This will guide one in current management. Interestingly enough, it has been found that members of the same family are apt to have a similar response to the same antidepressant. Thus, if a patient's mother was helped by an MAO inhibitor, then her children would probably react well to drugs in this category.

4 *Lithium carbonate.* Lithium carbonate has been used since 1949. It is the drug of choice in treating the manic phase of manic-depressive illness. Because it takes a few days to weeks to act effectively against mania, the patient should be hospitalized and sedated with chlorpromazine or haloperidol until the lithium has taken effect. Lithium carbonate has been found to be an effective prophylactic against further attacks of mania and possibly depression. Since it is not a specific antidepressant, the depression must be controlled by either an antidepressant or electroconvulsive therapy before lithium can be started. The blood level of lithium must be followed closely, both to ensure that a therapeutic dose is being given and to guard against toxicity.
5 *Electroconvulsive therapy (ECT).* Electroconvulsive therapy is an effective treatment for the depressed phase of manic-depressive psychosis and involutional melancholia and can also be used to interrupt manic excitements. The last disorder often requires only two or three treatments. The technique is quite simple. The patient is premedicated with a muscle relaxant (Anectine) and then anesthetized by an intravenous injection of a short-acting barbiturate (Brevital). An electrode is then placed over each temple, and an alternating current of about 400 mA and 70 to 120 V is passed between them for $\frac{1}{10}$ to $\frac{1}{2}$ s. The Anectine prevents strong and sometimes injurious muscle spasm. The patient is awake within 5 to 10 min and is up and about in $\frac{1}{2}$ h. Convulsions can also be induced chemically by injecting Metrazol or by inhaling the gas Indoklon. The mechanism by which convulsive therapy works is not known. In treating depression, ECT is usually given every other day for 14 to 20 treatments. The only absolute contraindication is the presence of an intracranial mass such as a neoplasm or hematoma. Its one major drawback is a transient impairment of recent memory for the period of treatment and the days which follow, the degree of impairment being related to the number of treatments given. Placing both electrodes on the nondominant side (unilateral ECT) produces less memory disturbance but is thought to be less effective against the depression.

In manic-depressive illness the best program of management relies on a physician who is willing to follow the patient's course over a long period of time and who is known to the family. Although the prognosis for any individual attack is relatively good, it is wise to arrange for a plan of action which is set in operation as soon as the first symptoms of a recurrence become manifest. A physician who works in conjunction with the family and who has ready access to a psychiatrist would be helpful in arranging for the early treatment of each recurrence.

The manic phase of manic-depressive psychosis also usually requires hospitalization to prevent patients from impulsive and often aggressive behavior which might jeopardize their career or standing in the community. Judgment is so poor in mania that patients may gamble away fortunes or make reckless investments. Chlorpromazine (Thorazine) or haloperidol (Haldol) can be used to control the mania while lithium carbonate is started. If tranquilizers are ineffective in slowing hyperactivity, ECT can be used.

SYNDROMES CAUSED BY DISEASES OF SPECIAL PARTS OF THE CEREBRUM

FRONTAL LOBES   In Fig. 25-1, it is seen that the frontal lobes lie anterior to the central, or rolandic, sulcus and superior to the sylvian fissure. They consist of several functionally different parts, which are conventionally designated in the neurologic literature by numbers (according to a scheme devised by Brodmann) and by letters (according to a scheme of von Economo and Koskinas).

The posterior parts, areas 4 and 6 of Brodmann, are specifically related to motor function. Voluntary movement in humans depends on the integrity of these areas, and lesions in them produce spastic paralysis of the contralateral face, arm, and leg. This is discussed in Chap. 15. Lesions limited more or less to the premotor areas (area 6) are accompanied by prominent grasp and sucking reflexes. Lesions in area 8 of Brodmann interfere with the mechanism concerned with turning the head and eyes contralaterally. Lesions in area 44 (Broca's area) of the dominant cerebral hemisphere, usually the left one, have often resulted in at least a temporary loss of verbal expression. Lesions in the medial limbic or piriform cortex (areas 23 and 24), wherein are bilaterally organized the mechanisms controlling respiration, circulation, and micturition, have relatively unclear clinical effects.

The remaining parts of the frontal lobes (areas 9 to 13 of Brodmann), sometimes called the *prefrontal areas,* have less specific and measurable functions. In contrast to the motor areas of the frontal lobes and other areas of the brain, stimulation of the prefrontal areas in humans has yielded a paucity of findings. Many patients with gunshot wounds of these areas have shown only mild and inconsistent abnormalities of behavior. Nevertheless, the following groups of symptoms have been observed in patients with large lesions of one or both of the frontal lobes or of the central white matter and the anterior part of the corpus callosum by which they are joined:

1 Lack of initiative and spontaneity in conjunction with diminished speech and motor inactivity (apathetic-akinetic-abulic state). Necessary daily activities are neglected. Interpersonal social reactions are reduced and shallow.
2 Change of personality, usually expressed as lack of concern over the consequences of any action, which may take the form of a childish excitement, an inappropriate joking and punning, or an instability and superficiality of emotion, or irritability. This puerility and euphoria may at times assume a pseudopsychopathic form.
3 Slight impairment of intelligence, usually described as lack of concentration, vacillation of attention, inability to carry out planned activity, difficulty in changing from one activity to another, or slight loss of recent memory. According to Luria, who views the frontal lobe as a regulating mechanism of the organism's activities, planned action is deficient with respect to steady control and goal-orientation.
4 Motor abnormalities such as decomposition of gait and upright stance, wide base, flexed posture, and small shuffling steps, culminating in an inability to stand (truncal ataxia of Bruns), abnormal postures, reflex grasping or sucking, and incontinence of sphincters.

Some differences have been noted between the dominant (left) and right frontal lobes. In psychologic tests left frontal lesions impair verbal fluency and right frontal the learning of visual spatial patterns (see Hecaen and Albert for further details).

TEMPORAL LOBES   The boundaries of the temporal lobes may be seen in Fig. 25-1. The sylvian fissure separates the superior surface of each temporal lobe from the frontal and anterior parts of the parietal lobes. There is no definite anatomic boundary between the temporal and occipital lobes or between posterior temporal and parietal lobes. The temporal lobe includes the superior, middle, and inferior temporal, fusiform, and hippocampal convolutions and the transverse convolutions of Heschl, which are the auditory receptive area present on the superior surface within the sylvian fissure. The hippocampal convolution was once believed to be related indirectly to the olfactory bulb, but now it is known that lesions here do not cause anosmia. The lower fibers of the geniculocalcarine pathway (from the inferior retina) swing in a wide arc over the temporal horn of the ventricle into the white matter of the temporal lobe en route to the occipital lobes, and lesions that interrupt them characteristically produce a contralateral homonymous upper quadrant defect of visual fields. Hearing, also localized in the temporal lobes, is bilaterally represented, which accounts for the fact that unless both temporal lobes are affected, there is little or no demonstrable loss of hearing. Loss of equilibrium has not been observed with temporal lobe lesions. Extensive disease in the superior and middle convolutions of the left temporal lobe in right-handed individuals results in Wernicke's aphasia. This syndrome, discussed in Chap. 24, consists of jargon aphasia and inability to read, to write, or to understand the meaning of spoken words.

FIGURE 25-1

Diagram to show cortical areas, numbered according to the scheme of Brodmann. The speech areas are in black, the three main ones of which are 39, 41, and 45. The zone marked by vertical stripes in the superior frontal convolution is the secondary motor area which, like Broca's area 45, if stimulated, causes vocal arrest. (After Handbuch der Inneren Medizin, Berlin, Springer-Verlag, 1939.)

Between the auditory and olfactory projection areas there is a large expanse of temporal lobe which has no assignable function. This is the temporal association area. Dysnomia has been the most frequent symptom in lesions of the dominant hemisphere. The most careful psychologic studies have shown a difference between cases involving loss of the dominant and nondominant temporal lobe. With lesions of the dominant side there is impairment in learning auditorially presented material; with nondominant lesions there is a similar failure in tests with visually presented material. In addition, about 20 percent of both right and left lobectomy patients have shown a syndrome similar to that described for the prefrontal parts of the brain; but more significant is the fact that the other cases exhibited little or no alteration of personality. The study of cases of uncinate epilepsy, with the characteristic dreamy state, olfactory or gustatory hallucinations, and masticatory movements, suggests that all these functions are organized through the temporal lobes. Similarly, stimulation of the posterior parts of the temporal lobes of fully conscious epileptic patients during surgical procedures has brought to light the interesting fact that complex memories and visual and auditory images, some with strong emotional content, can be aroused. Studies of the effect of stimulation of the amygdaloid nucleus, which is in the anterior and medial part of the temporal lobe, have shed additional light on this subject. Symptoms not unlike some of those of schizophrenic and manic patients may be evoked. Complex emotional experiences that have occurred previously may be revived. There are remarkable autonomic effects: blood pressure rises, pulse increases, respirations increase in frequency and depth, and the patient looks frightened. In temporal lobe epilepsy, recently reviewed by Geschwind, there may be an intensification of the patient's emotional reactions, an intense concern about moral and religious issues, a tendency to write excessively, and sometimes aggressiveness. Ablation of the amygdaloid nuclei has eliminated uncontrollable rage reactions in psychotic patients. Hippocampal and adjacent convolutions have been excised bilaterally, with a disastrous loss of ability to learn or to establish new memories (Korsakoff's psychosis). Bilateral destruction of the temporal lobes in both humans and monkeys results in placidity, loss of visual recognition, tendency to examine objects by touch and mouthing, and hypersexuality (Kluver-Bucy syndrome). All this indicates an important role of the temporal lobes in auditory and visual perception and imagery, in learning and memory, and in the emotional life of the individual.

I Effects of unilateral disease of the dominant temporal lobe
  A Homonymous quadrantanopia
  B Wernicke's aphasia
  C Impairment in verbal tests of material presented through the auditory sense
  D Dysnomia or amnesic aphasia
II Effects of unilateral disease of nondominant temporal lobe
  A Homonymous quadrantanopia
  B Impairment of mental function with inability to judge spatial relationships in some cases
  C Impairment in nonverbal tests of visually presented material
III Effects of bilateral disease
  A Korsakoff's amnesic defect
  B Apathy and placidity
  C Loss of sexual capacity
  D Loss of other of the unilateral functions
  E Kluver-Bucy syndrome

PARIETAL LOBES The postcentral convolution is the terminus of somatic sensory pathways from the opposite half of the body. However, destructive lesions here do not abolish cutaneous sensation but instead cause mainly a defect in sensory discrimination with variable impairment of primary sensation. In other words, the perception of painful, tactile, thermal, and vibratory stimuli is more or less normal, whereas stereognosis, sense of position, distinction between single and double contacts (two-point threshold), and the localization of sensory stimuli are impaired or lost. There is also the phenomenon of extinction; i.e., if both sides of the body are touched simultaneously, only the stimulus on the normal side is perceived. This type of sensory disturbance, sometimes called *cortical sensory defect*, is discussed in Chap. 19. Extensive lesions deep in the white matter of the parietal lobes produce an impairment of all forms of sensation contralaterally as well as a contralateral homonymous hemianopia, often incongruous and greater in the inferior quadrants. Lesions in the angular gyrus of the dominant hemisphere result in an inability to read.

More recent investigations have centered on the function of the parietal lobes in the perception of one's position in space and of the relationship of the various parts of the body to one another. Since the time of Babinski it has been known that patients with a large lesion of the minor parietal lobe are often unaware of their hemiplegia and hemianesthesia. Babinski called this condition *anosognosia*. Related psychologic disorders are lack of recognition of the left arm and leg, neglect of the left side of the body (as in dressing) and of external space on the left side, and constructional apraxia (an inability to perform the movements of constructing simple figures). All these disorders of parietal lobe function may occur with left-sided lesions as well but are observed only infrequently, since aphasic difficulties with lesions of the left hemisphere make it difficult to adequately test these functions.

Another frequent constellation of symptoms, usually referred to as *Gerstmann's syndrome*, occurs only with lesions of the dominant parietal lobe. This consists of inability to write (agraphia), inability to calculate (acalculia), failure to distinguish right from left, and loss of recognition of various fingers and toes. This is a true *agnosia*, since it represents a defect in the formulation and use of symbolic concepts, including the significance of numbers and letters and the names of parts of the body. An ideomotor apraxia may or may not be associated. *Apraxia and agnosia* are discussed in Chaps. 15 and 19.

The effects of disease of the parietal lobes may be organized into three major categories:

I Effects of unilateral disease of the parietal lobe, right or left
  A Cortical sensory syndrome and sensory extinction (or total hemianesthesia with large acute lesions of white matter)
  B Mild hemiparesis, unilateral muscular atrophy in children
  C Homonymous hemianopia or visual inattention, and sometimes anosognosia, neglect of one-half of the body and of extrapersonal space
  D Abolition of opticokinetic nystagmus to one side
II Effects of unilateral disease of the dominant parietal lobe (left hemisphere in right-handed patients), additional phenomena
  A Disorders of language (especially alexia)
  B Gerstmann's syndrome
  C Bimanual astereognosis (tactile agnosia)
  D Bilateral apraxia of the ideomotor type
III Effects of nondominant parietal lobe (additional phenomena)
  A Dressing apraxia
  B Constructional apraxia
  C Misidentification of left arm and leg
  D Bland mood, indifference to illness, or neurologic defects

In all these lesions, if the disease is sufficiently extensive, there may be a reduction in the capacity to think clearly, inattentiveness, and impaired memory.

OCCIPITAL LOBES The occipital lobes are the terminus of the geniculocalcarine pathways and are essential for visual sensation and perception. Lesions in one occipital lobe result in homonymous defects in the contralateral visual fields. Most often the defect takes the form of loss of vision in part or all of the homonymous fields. Occasionally patients complain of changes in the form and contour of visually perceived objects (metamorphopsia), as well as illusory displacement of images from one side of the visual field to another (visual allesthesia), or of abnormal persistence of the visual image after the object has been removed (palinopsia). Bilateral lesions cause "cortical" blindness, a state of blindness without change in optic fundi or pupillary reflexes. Visual illusions, hallucinations, and metamorphopsias (distortion of form, size, movement, and color) may also occur.

Lesions in Brodmann's areas 18 and 19 of the dominant hemisphere (Fig. 25-1) cause a loss of visual recognition with retention of some degree of visual acuity, a state termed *visual agnosia.* In the classic form of this blindness individuals with intact mental powers are unable to recognize objects, even though by tests of visual acuity and perimetry they appear to see sufficiently well to do so; they are able to recognize objects by tactile or other extravisual sense. In these terms, *alexia,* or inability to read, represents a visual verbal agnosia or "word blindness." Patients can see letters and words but cannot recognize their meaning, although they can still recognize them through tactile or auditory senses. Other types of agnosia for recognition of faces (prosopagnosia), for a complex of objects the elements of which are perceived but not the whole (simultanagnosia), color agnosia, and Balint's syndrome (inability to look at and grasp an object and inattention) are observed with unilateral and bilateral occipital lesions (see Adams and Victor).

CORPUS CALLOSUM AND THE DISCONNECTION SYNDROMES Considerable attention has been devoted to the study of each of the two cerebral hemispheres in isolation. This is possible only when the corpus callosum which forms a bridge between the two hemispheres is congenitally defective, surgically sectioned (for epilepsy), or destroyed by infarction or tumors. From these studies emerges the well-known fact that the left hemisphere is dominant in all language functions and auditory perception and the right hemisphere is superior in spatial and visual perception. Partial lesions of the corpus callosum or of the long tracts in the cerebral white matter are found to be associated with a number of interesting syndromes (commissural and intrahemispheric) which will be described below. (See reference to disconnection syndromes by Dimond.)

When the entire corpus callosum is missing because of a congenital defect or destroyed by a surgical procedure or anterior cerebral artery occlusion (anterior four-fifths), the speech and perceptual areas of the left hemisphere are isolated from those of the right hemisphere. These patients, if blindfolded, are unable to match an object held in one hand with that in the other hand. Further, they cannot match an object seen in the right half of the visual field with one in the left half. If given verbal commands to execute, they perform correctly with the right hand but not with the left. Without vision, objects placed in the right hand are named correctly, but not those in the left. In lesions confined to the posterior fifth of the corpus callosum (splenium), only the visual part of the disconnection syndrome occurs. Occlusion of the left posterior cerebral artery provides the best examples of the latter. Since infarction of the left occipital lobe causes a right homonymous hemianopia, thereafter all visual information needed for activating the speech areas of the left hemisphere must come from the right occipital lobe and cross the splenium of the corpus callosum. If there is a lesion in the corpus callosum the patient cannot read or name colors because the visual information cannot reach the left angular gyrus. There is no difficulty in copying words (though the patient cannot read what has been written); apparently the visual information for activating the left motor area crosses the corpus callosum more anteriorly. Matching of colors without naming them is done without error.

A disconnection in the anterior third of the corpus callosum, where fiber systems between right and left motor areas pass, results only in failure of the left hand to obey commands, the right one performing perfectly (left-sided apraxia). The left one can still imitate the examiner's movements.

Of intrahemispheric disconnections, those listed below are the most important:

1 Conduction (also called "central") aphasia. The patient has fluent but paraphasic speech and writing with nearly perfect comprehension of spoken or written language. Repetition is severely affected. The lesion is presumably in the arcuate fasciculus, which connects Wernicke's area with Broca's area.
2 Sympathetic apraxia in Broca's aphasia. A lesion in the subcortical white matter, underlying Broca's area, by destroying the origin of the fibers that connect the left and right motor association cortices causes an apraxia of command movements of the left hand.
3 Pure word deafness. Although the patient is able to hear and to identify nonverbal sounds, there is loss of ability to comprehend spoken language. The patient's speech remains normal. This defect has been attributed to a subcortical lesion sparing Wernicke's area.
4 Alexia and inability to name colors without agraphia. This is due to a lesion in the left occipital lobe and splenium of corpus callosum.

OTHER BEHAVIORAL DISORDERS ASSOCIATED WITH CEREBRAL DISEASE

When one attempts to categorize all the patients with relatively acute or subacute disorders of mentation and behavior under the section headings above, there are still a considerable number that remain difficult to classify. They present themselves as an almost infinite variety of syndromes in which the following abnormalities of function may occur: reduced or increased levels of speech, thought, and action; disorientation as to time and place; idleness and lack of interest; loss of spontaneity and sense of humor; muteness and hypokinesia, resistiveness and negativism; hostility, lack of observance of social customs, use of abusive and vulgar language; inexplicable fright, euphoria, and lack of proper concern; complaint of visual distortion, of excess sensitivity to sounds; distortions of smell and taste; inability to find the names of objects, to follow a conversation, to think coherently; sexual indiscretion, lack of modesty, and other signs of disinhibition; seizures; disturbances of sleep. Obviously these many symptoms do not all have the same basic significance, and the majority possess only relative localizing value. They may be associated with definite hemiparesis, hemihypesthesia, frank aphasia, or homonymous hemianopia, but even without these lateralizing signs they point to the existence of cerebral disease.

Syndromes comprising these elements may be observed in subacute sclerosing panencephalitis, listeriosis with meningoencephalitis, Behçet's meningoencephalitis, adult toxoplasmosis, infectious mononucleosis, acute or subacute demyelinative diseases (acute or subacute recurrent multiple sclerosis), granulomatous and other forms of angiitis, gliomatosis cerebri, carcinomatosis with encephalopathy of multifocal type, multiple tumor metastases, acute and subacute bacterial endocarditis, and thrombopenia with multiple-platelet thromboses in small vessels (Moschkowitz's disease). A fuller account of some of the cerebral symptoms enumerated above is found in chapters dealing with these diseases.

APPROACH TO THE PATIENT

The physician presented with a patient suffering from delirium, confusional states, dementia and psychoses of manic-depressive or schizophrenic type must adopt an examination technique designed to expose fully the intellectual defect. Abnormalities of posture, movement, sensation, and reflexes cannot be relied upon for the full demonstration of the neurologic deficit, for it must be remembered that the association and limbic areas of the brain may be severely damaged without demonstrable neurologic signs of this type.

Three sources of data are required for the recognition and differential diagnosis of these mental disorders:

1 A reliable history of the illness
2 Findings on mental examination, i.e., so-called "mental status," as well as on the rest of the neurologic examination
3 Special laboratory procedures, lumbar puncture, x-rays of the skull, electroencephalogram, CT and radionuclide scanning of the brain, and sometimes pneumoencephalogram

The history should always be supplemented by information obtained from a person other than the patient. Through lack of insight, patients are often unaware of their illness; indeed, they may be ignorant even of their chief complaint. Special inquiry should be made about the patient's general behavior, social adjustment, capacity for work, personal habits, etc., and family history.

This examination of the mental status must be systematic. At a minimum it should provide answers to the questions listed below.

I Insight (patients' replies to questions about their chief symptoms): What is your difficulty? Are you ill? When did your illness begin?
II Orientation (knowledge of personal identity and present situation): What is your name? What is your occupation? Where do you live? Are you married? Where are you now?
  A Place: What is the name of the place where you are now? How did you get here? What floor is it on? Where is the bathroom? What are you doing now?
  B Time: What is the date today? What time of day is it? What meals have you had? When was the last holiday?
III Memory:
  A Remote: Tell me the names of your children and their birth dates. When were you married? What was your mother's maiden name? What was the name of your first school teacher? What jobs have you held?
  B Recent past: Tell me about your recent illness (compare with previous statements). What did you have for breakfast today? What is my name or the nurse's name? When did you see me for the first time? What tests were done yesterday? What were the headlines in the newspaper today? Give patients a simple story, oral or written, and ask him to recall it after 3 to 5 min.
  C Immediate recall (short-term memory): Repeat these numbers after me (give a series of 3, 4, 5, 6, 7, and then

8 digits at the speed of one per second). Now when I give a series of numbers, repeat them in reverse order.
  D Visual span: Show patients a picture of several objects, ask them to name what they have seen and note any inaccuracies.
IV General information: Ask about names of presidents, well-known historic dates, the names of large rivers or cities, etc.
V Capacity for sustained mental activity:
  A Calculation: Test ability to add, substract, multiply, and divide. Serial subtraction of 7s or 3s from 100 is a good test of calculation as well as of concentration.
  B Abstract thinking: See if patients can detect similarities and differences between classes of objects, or explain a proverb or a fable.
VI General behavior: Attitudes, general bearing, attentiveness, manner of dress, etc.
  A Content of thought: What ideas occupy the thoughts of patients? Do they believe that their thoughts and actions are controlled or are being broadcast to others? Are there hallucinations and/or delusions? Is there a press of speech or lack of speech?
  B Mood: Do patients appear gay or sad? How do they feel? Are they nervous and worried or apprehensive? What feeling is revealed through speech, attitude, facial expression?
VII Special tests of localized cerebral functions: grasping, sucking, aphasia battery, praxis with both hands, cortical sensory function, drawing of clock face, map of United States or Europe, floor plan of patient's house, etc.

In order to enlist the full cooperation of patients, physicians must prepare them for questions of this type. Otherwise, their first reaction will be one of embarrassment or anger because of the implication that their mind is not sound. It should be pointed out to patients that some individuals are rather forgetful and that it is necessary to ask specific questions in order to form some impression about their degree of nervousness when being examined. Reassurance that these are not tests of intelligence or of sanity is helpful. A more formal and reliable method of examining the mental capacity of adults is the Wechsler-Bellevue test.

Correct diagnosis of treatable forms of mental disease (e.g., general paresis, subdural hematoma, brain tumor, bromide or other chronic drug intoxication, normal-pressure hydrocephalus, pellagra and other deficiency states, and hypothyroidism) is of greater practical importance than the diagnosis of the untreatable ones.

The separation of the Korsakoff amnesic syndrome and dementia depends on the relative integrity of all cognitive functions except retentive memory. The two major so-called "functional psychoses," schizophrenia and manic-depressive disease, are distinguished from the amnesic state and dementia on the basis of the retention of an alert state of mind, retention of all cognitive functions including retentive memory, and the identification of disordered thinking with prominent hallucinations, delusions, and/or alteration of mood. The separation of these two latter types of mental illness, both of which are chronic, is based on the presence or absence of premorbid psychic peculiarity, age of patient, mode of onset, duration of illness, recovery, recurrence, etc. If of recent onset while using drugs and alcohol, or associated with temporal lobe seizures or an endocrine disease, a period of observation may be required before the diagnosis can be settled.

MANAGEMENT OF THE PATIENT

These major mental derangements and psychoses are clinical states of the most serious nature, and usually it is worthwhile to admit the patient to the hospital for a period of observation. The physician then has an opportunity to see the patient several times in a neutral and fairly constant hospital environment, and certain special procedures such as x-rays of the skull, lumbar puncture, analysis of blood for drugs, basal metabolic rate, an electroencephalogram, CT scan, and sometimes a pneumoencephalogram can be carried out at this time. The management of the demented patient in the hospital may be relatively simple if the person is quiet and cooperative. If the disorder of mental function is severe, i.e., the patient is psychotic, a nurse, attendant, or member of the family must stay with the patient at all times. Provision must be made for adequate food and fluid intake and control of infection, using the same measures outlined for the delirious patient (see Chap. 21).

Once it is established that the patient has an untreatable dementing, amnesic, schizophrenic, or manic-depressive brain disease, a responsible member of the family should be apprised of the medical facts. The patient should be told that he or she has a nervous condition for which rest and treatment has been prescribed. Nothing is accomplished by telling the individual more. The family should be given diagnosis and prognosis if the diagnosis is sufficiently certain for this to be done. If the psychic or mood abnormalities are slight and circumstances are suitable, the patient should remain at home, continue appropriate activities, and receive appropriate medication. If he or she is depressed and suicidal, the patient should remain in a psychiatric hospital. The individual should be spared responsibility and guarded against injury that might result from imprudent action. If the patient becomes demented while still at work, plans for occupational retirement should be carried out. In more advanced stages of disease, mental and physical enfeeblement become pronounced and institutional care should be advised. Seizures should be treated symptomatically. Nerve tonics, vitamins, and hormones are of no value in checking the course of dementia or in regenerating decayed tissue. They may, however, offer some support to the patient and family.

Sometimes, stimulants in the form of dextroamphetamine, caffeine, and nicotinic acid cause transitory improvement in mental function. Undesirable restlessness, nocturnal wandering, belligerency, or anxiety may be reduced by some of the "minor" tranquilizing drugs (see Chap. 227).

REFERENCES

ADAMS RD, VICTOR M: *Principles of Neurology.* New York, McGraw-Hill, 1977

ARMAND MN (ed): *Harvard Guide to Modern Psychiatry.* Cambridge, Mass, Harvard University Press, 1978

BENSON L, BLUMER D: *Psychiatric Aspects of Neurologic Disease.* New York, Grune & Stratton, 1975

DIMOND SJ: The disconnection syndrome, in *Modern Trends in Neurology,* E Williams (ed). London, Butterworths, 1975

GESCHWIND N: Temporal lobe epilepsy. Arch Neurol 34:454, 1977

HECAEN H, ALBERT ML: Disorders of mental functioning related to frontal lobe, in *Modern Trends of Neurology,* E Williams (ed). London, Butterworths, 1975

HOREL JA: The neuroanatomy of amnesia. A critique of the hippocampal memory hypothesis. Brain 101:403, 1978.

LURIA AR: *Higher Cortical Functions* in *Man.* New York, Basic Books, 1966

MAAS JW: The clinical and biochemical heterogeneity of the depressive disorders. Ann Intern Med 88:556, 1978

MCCULLOUGH E et al: Norepinephrine in chronic paranoid schizophrenia: Above-normal levels in limbic forebrain. Science 200:456, 1978

POPE HG, LIPINSKI JF: Diagnosis in schizophrenia and depressive illness. Arch Gen Psychiatry (in press)

ROBINS E et al: Diagnostic criteria for use in psychiatric research. Arch Gen Psychiatry 26:57, 1972

section 4 | Alterations in circulatory and respiratory function

26
COUGH AND HEMOPTYSIS

GENNARO M. TISI
EUGENE BRAUNWALD

COUGH

Cough, one of the most frequent cardiorespiratory symptoms, is an explosive expiration which provides a means of clearing the tracheobronchial tree of secretions and foreign bodies.

MECHANISM Coughing may be initiated either voluntarily or reflexly. As a defensive reflex it has both afferent and efferent pathways. The *afferent limb* includes cough receptors within the sensory distribution of the trigeminal, glossopharyngeal, superior laryngeal, and vagus nerves. The *efferent limb* includes the recurrent laryngeal nerve (which causes glottic closure) and the spinal nerves (which cause contraction of the thoracic and abdominal musculature). The *sequence of a cough* includes an appropriate stimulus which initiates a deep inspiration. This is followed by glottic closure, relaxation of the diaphragm, and muscle contraction against a closed glottis so as to produce maximally positive intrathoracic and intraairway pressures. These positive intrathoracic pressures result in a narrowing of the trachea, produced by an infolding of its more compliant posterior membrane. Once the glottis opens, the combination of a large pressure differential between the airways and the atmosphere coupled with this tracheal narrowing produces flow rates through the trachea close to the speed of sound. The shearing forces which are developed aid in the elimination of mucus and foreign materials. A tracheostomy short-circuits glottic closure and therefore decreases the effectiveness of the cough mechanism.

ETIOLOGY Cough is produced by inflammatory, mechanical, chemical, and thermal stimulation of the cough receptors. *Inflammatory* stimuli are initiated by edema and hyperemia of the respiratory mucous membranes, and by irritation from exudative processes. Such stimuli may arise either in the airways (as in laryngitis, tracheitis, bronchitis, and bronchiolitis) or in the alveoli (as in pneumonitis and lung abscess). *Mechanical* stimuli are produced by inhalation of particulate matter, such as dust particles, and by compression of the air passages and pressure or tension upon these structures. Lesions associated with airway compression may be either extramural or intramural in type. The former include aortic aneurysms, granulomas, pulmonary neoplasms, and mediastinal tumors; intramural lesions include bronchogenic carcinoma, bronchial adenoma, foreign bodies, granulomatous endobronchial involvement, and contraction of airway smooth muscle (bronchial asthma). Pressure or tension upon the air passages is usually produced by lesions associated with a decrease in pulmonary compliance. Examples of specific causes include acute and chronic interstitial fibrosis (Chap. 264), pulmonary edema, and atelectasis. *Chemical* stimuli may result from inhalation of irritant gases, including cigarette smoke and chemical fumes. Finally, *thermal* stimuli may be produced by inhalation of either very hot or cold air.

DIAGNOSTIC EVALUATION When one is considering the above list of causes, answers to the following general questions will significantly narrow the diagnostic possibilities: Is the cough acute or chronic? Is it productive of sputum or nonproductive? A chronic productive cough may be caused by diseases such as chronic bronchitis, pulmonary tuberculosis, and pulmonary neoplasms. Are the findings on physical examination of the chest normal or abnormal? Is the chest roentgenogram normal or abnormal?

Features of the history, physical examination, chest roentgenogram, screening pulmonary function studies (static lung volumes and dynamic flow rates), and sputum examination may indicate a specific cause. The *history* may indicate specific diagnoses. Acute episodes of cough may be associated with such viral infections as acute tracheobronchitis or pneumonitis or with bacterial bronchopneumonia. Cough associated with an acute febrile episode and associated with hoarseness is usually produced by viral laryngotracheobronchitis. The character of the cough may suggest the anatomic site of involvement: the patient with a "barking" type of cough may have epiglottal involvement, while the cough associated with tracheal or major airway involvement is often loud and "brassy." Cough associated with generalized wheezing may be produced by acute bronchospasm. The time of occurrence of a cough may indicate a specific cause: a cough which occurs selectively at night suggests congestive heart failure; one related to meals suggests a tracheoesophageal fistula, a hiatal hernia, or an esophageal diverticulum; a cough precipitated by a change in position suggests a lung abscess or a localized area of bronchiectasis. The description of sputum or secretions produced in conjunction with the cough may also be helpful: putrid sputum suggests a lung abscess; bloody sputum, bleeding (see "Hemoptysis," below); frothy and pink-tinged sputum, pulmonary edema; mucoid and massive sputum, alveolar cell carcinoma; purulent and/or large amounts of sputum, lung abscess and bronchiectasis.

On *physical examination* the character of the auscultatory findings may suggest the site of disease: inspiratory stridor and wheezing may be present in laryngeal disease; inspiratory and expiratory rhonchi favor tracheal and major airway involvement; coarse subcrepitant inspiratory rales may indicate interstitial fibrosis and/or edema; fine crepitant rales may indicate

a process such as pneumonitis or pulmonary edema, which fills the alveoli with fluid. The *chest roentgenogram* may reveal the cause of the cough; it may show an intrapulmonary mass lesion which may be either central or peripheral (Chap. 268), an alveolar filling process which may be pneumonic or nonpneumonic, an area of honeycombing and cyst formation which may indicate an area of localized bronchiectasis, or bilateral hilar adenopathy which may indicate sarcoidosis or a lymphoma.

Screening pulmonary function studies may also indicate specific diagnoses. Significant expiratory obstruction to airflow (as determined from a forced expiratory flow maneuver), coupled with a history of cough and significant sputum production, suggests that irrespective of other lesions the patient has significant bronchitis. Decreased lung volume (as determined from the static lung volumes) indicates that a restrictive type of lung disease is present—reduction of lung volumes produced by thoracic, pleural, alveolar, or interstitial disease. Finally, a careful *sputum examination* may be more enlightening than a patient's description of the character of the sputum. Examination shows whether the sputum is thin or viscid, purulent or not, foul-smelling or not, blood tinged or not, scant or copious. Gram stain and culture of the deep-cough specimen may reveal a specific bacterial, fungal, or mycoplasmal causation, while sputum cytology may result in a positive diagnosis of a pulmonary neoplasm.

Two features of cough should be highlighted: (1) A cough is often so common in the cigarette smoker as to be ignored or minimized. *Any changes in the nature and character of a chronic cigarette cough should initiate immediate diagnostic evaluation, with particular attention directed to detection of bronchogenic carcinoma.* (2) Female patients are inclined to swallow sputum and not to expectorate as male patients do. This tendency may lead to the incorrect conclusion that a cough in a female patient is irritative and nonproductive.

COMPLICATIONS Three complications may be produced by the coughing mechanism: paroxysms of coughing may precipitate syncope (cough syncope, Chap. 13), and strenuous coughing may produce rupture of an emphysematous bleb and rib fractures. A potential mechanism for cough syncope includes the development of markedly positive intrathoracic and alveolar pressures which decrease venous return, producing a decrease in cardiac output and resultant syncope. Although cough fractures of the ribs may occur in otherwise normal patients, their occurrence should at least raise the possibility of pathologic fractures, which are seen in multiple myeloma, osteoporosis, and osteolytic metastases.

THERAPY Specific treatment of cough depends upon the underlying cause. An irritative, nonproductive cough may be suppressed by an antitussive agent, such as codeine or dextromethorphan, 15 mg qid. These drugs are particularly useful in interrupting prolonged, self-perpetuating paroxysms. However, a cough productive of significant quantities of sputum should not be suppressed, since retention of sputum in the tracheobronchial tree may interfere with alveolar aeration and impair the ability of the lung to resist infection. When secretions are tenacious and thick, adequate hydration, expectorants (such as potassium iodide), and humidification of the air with an ultrasonic nebulizer may be helpful.

HEMOPTYSIS

For purposes of definition hemoptysis includes both blood-streaked sputum and gross hemoptysis. It is apparent that any patient with gross hemoptysis should be given appropriate diagnostic tests so that a specific cause may be found. The patient with blood-streaked sputum should also be studied unless one can be certain that this type of hemoptysis is due to a benign condition. A major pitfall in dealing with hemoptysis is to ascribe recurrent episodes of hemoptysis to a previously established diagnosis, such as chronic bronchiectasis or bronchitis. Such an approach may result in missing a serious but potentially treatable lesion. The safest approach to a recurrent episode of hemoptysis is to treat it as if it were the initial episode and proceed with a complete diagnostic evaluation.

ETIOLOGY AND INCIDENCE Prior to embarking upon an extensive diagnostic workup of hemoptysis, it is essential to determine that the blood is in fact coming from the respiratory tract, not from the nasopharynx or gastrointestinal tract. Once this point is established, the diagnostic tests for hemoptysis may proceed. Although there are numerous single case reports of diseases which have been associated with hemoptysis, Table 26-1 presents the more common disorders.

The incidence of the diagnoses listed in Table 26-1 depends upon the nature of the series reported and whether one includes both gross bleeding and blood streaking of the sputum. If both types of bleeding are included, then the major causes (approximately 60 to 70 percent) are chronic bronchitis and bronchiectasis. If the definition is restricted to gross bleeding (greater than several tablespoons) then the incidence depends upon the type of series reported. Surgical series favor the incidence of mass lesions and operable lesions (carcinoma, 20 percent; localized, segmental, or lobar bronchiectasis, 30 percent). Those from centers with a large tuberculosis population favor this condition (incidence varying between 2 and 40 percent). Combined medical-surgical series include a wider representation of those lesions which present with hemoptysis (carcinoma, 20 percent; bronchiectasis, 30 percent; bronchitis, 15 percent; other inflammatory lesions including tuberculosis, 10 to 20 percent; other lesions including the vascular, traumatic, and hemorrhagic etiologies listed in Table 26-1, 10 percent). Despite the most extensive of evaluations, 5 to 15 percent of cases entailing gross hemoptysis remain undiagnosed.

Two points should be highlighted with reference to diseases associated with hemoptysis: (1) *hemoptysis is rare in metastatic carcinoma to the lung;* (2) *although hemoptysis may occur at some time during the course of a viral or pneumococcal pneumonia, it is usually scanty and its occurrence should always raise the question of a more serious underlying process.*

DIAGNOSIS The *history* may suggest specific diagnoses: recurrent, chronic hemoptysis in a young, otherwise asymptomatic female favors the diagnosis of a bronchial adenoma; recurrent hemoptysis with chronic, marked sputum production associated with ring shadows, tram lines (abnormal air bronchograms), and cyst formation on the roentgenogram suggests a diagnosis of bronchiectasis; putrid sputum production suggests a lung abscess; weight loss and anorexia in a male smoker over the age of 40 raises the possibility of a bronchogenic carcinoma; a recent history of blunt trauma to the chest suggests a lung contusion; and acute pleuritic chest pain raises the possibility of pulmonary embolism with infarction or some other pleurally based lesion (lung abscess, coccidiomycosis cavity, and vasculitis). Several findings on the *physical examination* may also suggest a specific diagnosis: a pleural friction rub suggests those diagnoses just mentioned in connection with pleuritic pain; the findings of pulmonary hypertension raise the diagnostic possibilities of primary pulmonary hypertension, mitral stenosis, recurrent or chronic thromboembolism, and Eisenmenger's syndrome; a localized wheeze over a major lobar airway suggests an intramural lesion such as a bronchogenic carcinoma or a foreign body; systemic arteriovenous communications or the presence of a murmur over the lung fields suggest the diagnosis of Osler-Weber-Rendu disease with pulmonary atrioventricular malformation; evidence of signifi-

cant expiratory obstruction to airflow coupled with sputum production suggests that whatever other lesion may be present, the patient has significant bronchitis. Finally, the *chest roentgenogram* is critical to diagnosis. The presence of ring shadows favors a diagnosis of bronchiectasis; an air-fluid level, the diagnosis of a lung abscess; and a mass lesion, the diagnosis of a central or peripheral pulmonary neoplasm. A mass lesion which may cause hemoptysis should be distinguished from an area of blood pneumonitis caused by aspiration of blood into contiguous areas.

One of the most demanding diagnostic problems is the identification of the side of bleeding in a patient with normal findings on physical examination and a normal roentgenogram of the chest. A patient with hemoptysis tends to keep the bleeding side dependent. Otherwise, gravitational drainage would cause aspiration into the noninvolved dependent lung. The patient may also be able to give a history of a burning or deep pain which may localize the side of bleeding; bronchoscopy may then be useful. This procedure generally is most helpful when the bleeding is scant, and of least help when the bleeding is massive, since blood may be aspirated into contiguous airways.

Following the history and physical examination, the diagnostic approach to a patient with hemoptysis includes whatever specialized studies and procedures are required to make a specific diagnosis. The first step is to obtain a roentgenogram. Usually bronchoscopy is the procedure employed next. The recent introduction of fiberoptic bronchoscopy (Chap. 256) has improved visualization of the upper lobes and included within the range of visualization airways as small as several millimeters in diameter. This endoscopic technique may provide definitive visual, biopsy, or cytologic information. Since direct visualization of more peripheral portions of the airway system is now possible, the indications for bronchography in the evaluation of hemoptysis are being modified. The principal indications for bronchography in such patients are (1) to establish the presence of localized bronchiectasis (including a sequestered lobe) and (2) to rule out the presence of more generalized bronchiectasis in a patient with localized disease who is regarded as a surgical candidate because of either repetitive hemoptysis or recurrent infections. The majority of patients with bronchiectasis have a normal chest roentgenogram. If bronchoscopy in such patients is also negative, bronchography is the only means of establishing an anatomic diagnosis of bronchiectasis. If the chest roentgenogram is abnormal, revealing

TABLE 26-1
Causes of hemoptysis

   I Inflammatory
     A Bronchitis
     B Bronchiectasis
     C Tuberculosis
     D Lung abscess
     E Pneumonia, particularly *Klebsiella*
  II Neoplastic
     A Lung cancer: squamous cell, adenocarcinoma, oat cell
     B Bronchial adenoma
 III Other
     A Pulmonary thromboembolism
     B Left ventricular failure
     C Mitral stenosis
     D Traumatic, including foreign body and lung contusion
     E Primary pulmonary hypertension; arteriovenous malformation; Eisenmenger's syndrome; pulmonary vasculitis including Wegener's granulomatosis and Goodpasture's syndrome; idiopathic pulmonary hemosiderosis; and amyloid
     F Hemorrhagic diathesis including anticoagulant therapy

either ring shadows or tram lines, a diagnosis of bronchiectasis may be made without the need for bronchography.

THERAPY Since hemoptysis is such an alarming symptom, there is a tendency to overtreat the patient. Usually hemoptysis is scant and will stop spontaneously without specific therapy. If the hemoptysis is substantial, the mainstays of therapy include keeping the patient calm, instituting complete bed rest, excluding unnecessary diagnostic procedures until the hemoptysis has begun to subside, and suppressing cough if it is present and an aggravating feature of the hemoptysis. The emergency care of such a patient demands that intubation and suctioning equipment be at the bedside. In patients in danger of asphyxiation by flooding of the lung contralateral to the site of hemorrhage, intubation by a technique which isolates the hemorrhaging lung and prevents contralateral aspiration of blood should be carried out. This can be accomplished by strategic location of a balloon catheter whose introduction into the bronchus in question is facilitated by direct visualization through a fiberoptic bronchoscope.

The management of potentially lethal massive hemoptysis remains controversial. The choice between a medical approach and surgical intervention hinges on the words *potentially lethal.* Massive hemoptysis, usually defined as greater than 1000 ml in 24 h, is an alarming clinical situation in which asphyxiation due to aspiration of blood represents the principal threat to life. The choice between surgical and medical management relates most often to the anatomic basis for the massive hemoptysis. In patients with cavitary tuberculosis, anaerobic lung abscess, and lung cancer, the risk of mortality is far greater than when the cause for the hemoptysis is bronchitis or bronchiectasis. Operation may occasionally be necessary in the former, but virtually never in the latter group. In either case the initial management should include the conservative measures suggested above. With such management, spontaneous cessation of bleeding usually occurs. Surgical intervention should be considered in that small group of patients with a definable lesion or chest roentgenogram (i.e., cavitary disease, lung abscess, lung cancer) who have evidence of uncontrollable respiratory or hemodynamic compromise. If a patient is a surgical candidate, bronchoscopy should be performed to identify the specific site of bleeding. Otherwise bronchoscopy should be deferred for several days because of the tendency of this procedure to aggravate cough and thereby perpetuate the hemoptysis. Bronchial arterial catheterization and embolization are new modalities of treatment currently under evaluation for the nonsurgical control of massive hemoptysis, especially in patients with nonresectable lung cancer.

REFERENCES

BATES DV et al: *Respiratory Function in Disease.* Philadelphia, Saunders, 1971, p 584ff

COMMITTEE ON ETIOLOGY OF CHRONIC BRONCHITIS, MEDICAL RESEARCH COUNCIL: Definition and classification of chronic bronchitis. Lancet 1:775, 1965

COMMITTEE ON THERAPY, AMERICAN THORACIC SOCIETY: The management of hemoptysis. Am Rev Resp Dis 93:471, 1966

KARY RC, SMITH JR: Medical history and physical examination in the assessment of pulmonary disease, in *Textbook of Pulmonary Diseases*, 2d ed, GL Baum (ed). Boston, Little, Brown, 1974, p 3

LOUDON RG, SHAW GB: Mechanics of cough in normal subjects and in patients with obstructive respiratory disease. Am Rev Resp Dis 96:666, 1967

PIERCE J: Cough and hemoptysis, in *Signs and Symptoms*, 6th ed, RS Blacklow (ed). Philadelphia, Lippincott, 1979, chaps 17, 18

WOLFE JD, SIMMONS DH: Hemoptysis: Diagnosis and management (medical progress). West J Med 127:383, 1977.

27
DYSPNEA AND PULMONARY EDEMA

ROLAND H. INGRAM, JR.
EUGENE BRAUNWALD

DYSPNEA

INTRODUCTION For an average 70-kg adult at rest the normal breathing pattern consists of an average frequency of 14 breaths per minute and has a mean tidal volume of 600 ml. It is not surprising that a normal, resting person is unaware of the act of breathing since it originates in the more vegetative portions of the central nervous system and is modulated by both lower central and peripheral vagal pathways. The breathing pattern is changed by a series of higher central and peripheral control mechanisms which can increase ventilation in excess of metabolic demands in conditions such as anxiety and fear, and can increase ventilation appropriate to increased metabolic demands during physical activity. Although a person may become conscious of breathing during mild to moderate exertion, no discomfort is experienced. However, during and following exhausting exertion an individual may become unpleasantly aware of breathing, yet feel reasonably assured that the sensation will be transitory and is appropriate to the level of exercise. Therefore, as a cardinal symptom of diseases affecting the cardiorespiratory system, dyspnea is defined as an *abnormally uncomfortable awareness of breathing.*

Although dyspnea is not painful in the usual sense of the word, it is, like pain, involved with both the perception of a sensation and the reaction to that perception. Thus, since it is a symptom, dyspnea is present whenever a patient experiences it. Patients experience a number of uncomfortable sensations related to breathing and use an even larger number of verbal expressions to describe these sensations, such as "cannot get enough air," "air does not go all the way down," "smothering feeling in the chest," "tightness in the chest," "fatigue in the chest," and a "choking sensation." It may be necessary, therefore, to review meticulously the patient's history in order to ascertain whether the more abstruse descriptions do, in fact, represent dyspnea. Once it is established that a patient does have dyspnea, it is of paramount importance to define the circumstances in which it occurs and to assess associated symptoms. There are situations in which breathing appears labored but in which dyspnea does not occur. For example, the hyperventilation in association with metabolic acidemia is rarely accompanied by dyspnea. On the other hand, patients with apparently normal breathing patterns may complain of shortness of breath.

QUANTITATION OF DYSPNEA The gradation of dyspnea may usefully be based upon the amount of physical exertion required to produce the sensation. In actual practice the major functional classifications of patients with heart or lung disease are based largely on dyspnea in relation to degree of exertion. However, in assessing the severity of dyspnea, it is important to obtain a clear understanding of the patient's general physical condition, work history, and recreational habits. For example, the development of dyspnea in a trained runner upon running 2 mi may signify a more serious disturbance than a similar degree of breathlessness on running a fraction of this distance in a sedentary person. It is also important to note that some patients with lung or heart disease may have such reduced capabilities due to other disease that exertional dyspnea is precluded despite serious impairment of pulmonary or cardiac function; in contrast, others who decrease their physical activities gradually may avoid dyspnea because they do not stress themselves.

Some patterns of dyspnea are not directly related to physical exertion. Sudden and unexpected dyspneic episodes at rest can be associated with pulmonary emboli, spontaneous pneumothorax, or anxiety. Nocturnal episodes of severe paroxysmal dyspnea and diaphoresis are characteristic of congestive heart failure in association with hypertensive cardiovascular disease. Dyspnea upon assuming the supine posture, *orthopnea* (see below), thought to be mainly characteristic of congestive heart failure, may also occur in some patients with asthma and chronic obstruction of the airways and is a regular finding in the rare occurrence of bilateral diaphragmatic paralysis. The term *trepopnea* is used to describe the unusual circumstance in which dyspnea occurs only in the left or right lateral decubitus position, most often in patients with heart disease, while *platypnea* is dyspnea which occurs only in the upright position. Both of these patterns remain to be fully explained but may be related to positional alterations in ventilation-perfusion relations.

MECHANISMS OF DYSPNEA Physicians usually relate the symptom of dyspnea to a process such as obstruction of the airways or congestive heart failure and generally proceed with further diagnostic and/or therapeutic attempts, having satisfied themselves that they understand the mechanism of the dyspnea. In fact, elucidation of the *actual* mechanism(s) of dyspnea has eluded clinical investigators.

It is well known that dyspnea occurs whenever the work of breathing is excessive. Increased force generation is required of the respiratory muscles to produce a given volume change if the chest wall or lungs are less compliant or if resistance to airflow is increased. Although it is true that an individual is more apt to become dyspneic when the work of breathing is increased, the work theory does not account for the perceptual difference between a deep breath with a normal mechanical load and a normal-sized breath with an increased mechanical load. The work might be the same with both breaths, but the normal one with the increased load will be associated with discomfort. In fact, with respiratory loading, such as adding a resistance at the mouth, there is an increase in respiratory center output, as gauged by newer indices, that is disproportionate to the increase in work of breathing. Hence, a more appealing theory is one that links inappropriate length to tension in the respiratory muscles. Campbell has proposed that a sense of discomfort arises when there is misalignment of the nerve spindles, which are sensing tension, in relation to muscle length. This misalignment would lead to the sensation that a person is getting an insufficient breath for the tension generated by the respiratory muscles. Such a theory is difficult to test and, if tested and proved in some circumstances, would still not explain why patients who are completely paralyzed, either by cord transections or neuromuscular blockade, experience dyspnea although aided by a mechanical ventilator. It is probable, in these circumstances, that signals from the lungs and/or airways travel via the vagus nerve to the central nervous system to account for the sensation.

In all likelihood a number of different mechanisms operate to different degrees in the various clinical situations in which dyspnea occurs. Perhaps, in some circumstances, dyspnea is evoked by stimulation of receptors in the upper respiratory tract; in others it may originate from receptors in the lungs, airways, respiratory muscles, or some combination of those structures. In general, there is a reasonably good correlation between the severity of dyspnea and the disturbances of pulmonary or cardiac function which are responsible.

DIFFERENTIAL DIAGNOSIS **Obstructive disease of airways** (see also Chaps. 257 and 263) Obstruction to airflow can be present anywhere from the extrathoracic airways out to the small airways in the periphery of the lung. Large extrathoracic airway obstruction can occur acutely, as with aspiration of food or a foreign body or with angioneurotic edema of the glottis. Circumstantial evidence or testimony from witnesses should cause the physician to suspect aspiration, and an allergic history together with a few scattered hives should raise the possibility of glottic edema. The acute form of upper airway obstruction is a medical emergency. More chronic forms can occur with tumors or with fibrotic stenosis following tracheostomy or prolonged endotracheal intubation. Whether acute or chronic, the cardinal symptom is dyspnea, and the characteristic signs are stridor and retraction of the supraclavicular fossae with inspiration.

Obstruction of intrathoracic airways can occur acutely and intermittently or can be present chronically with worsening during respiratory infections. Acute intermittent obstruction with wheezing is typical of *asthma*. Chronic cough with expectoration is typical of *chronic bronchitis* and *bronchiectasis*. Most often there is a prolongation of expiration and coarse rhonchi which are generalized in chronic bronchitis and may be localized in the case of bronchiectasis. Intercurrent infection results in worsening of the cough, increased expectoration of purulent sputum, and more severe dyspnea. During such episodes the patient may complain of nocturnal paroxysms of dyspnea with wheezing relieved by cough and expectoration of sputum.

Many years of exertional dyspnea progressing to dyspnea at rest characterize the patient with predominant *emphysema*, a condition which is defined as dilatation of the terminal air sacs with disruption of alveolar septa. Although a parenchymal disease by definition, emphysema is invariably accompanied by obstruction of airways. The signs are prominent usage of accessory muscles which lift the anterior thorax, retraction of the lower intercostal spaces with inspiration, distant breath sounds with a hyperresonant percussion note, and end-expiratory wheezes.

With severe chronic bronchitis and/or emphysema, the signs of cor pulmonale may either appear or increase during a respiratory infection. Spirometry and measurements of lung volumes and arterial blood gases (Chap. 255) not only are helpful in establishing a diagnosis but also serve to assess the severity of the process in guiding therapy.

Diffuse parenchymal lung diseases (see also Chap. 264) This category includes a large number of diseases ranging from acute pneumonia to chronic disorders such as sarcoidosis and the various forms of *pneumoconiosis*. History, physical findings, and radiographic abnormalities often provide clues to the diagnosis. The patients are often tachypneic with arterial P_{CO_2} and P_{O_2} values below normal. Exertion often further reduces the arterial P_{O_2}. Lung volumes are decreased and the lungs are stiffer, i.e., less compliant.

Pulmonary vascular occlusive diseases (see also Chap. 266) Whether due to repeated emboli or intrinsic vascular disease, right ventricular hypertrophy or signs of right ventricular failure in the absence of obvious parenchymal lung disease should suggest the possibility of pulmonary vascular occlusive disease. Repeated episodes of dyspnea at rest often occur with repeated emboli. A source for emboli, such as phlebitis of a lower extremity or the pelvis, is quite helpful in leading the physician to suspect the diagnosis. Arterial blood gases are almost invariably abnormal, but lung volumes are frequently normal or only minimally abnormal.

Diseases of the chest wall or respiratory muscles (see also Chap. 270) The physical examination establishes the presence of a chest wall disease such as severe kyphoscoliosis, pectus excavatum, or spondylitis. Although all three of these deformities may be associated with dyspnea, only severe kyphoscoliosis regularly interferes with ventilation sufficiently to produce chronic cor pulmonale and respiratory failure.

Both weakness and paralysis of respiratory muscles can lead to respiratory failure, but most often the signs and symptoms of the neurologic or muscular disorder are more prominently manifested in other systems. A reduction in total lung capacity and vital capacity along with an increased residual volume in the absence of apparent heart or lung disease suggests the diagnosis. Such a pattern can be explained by muscle weakness, which can be confirmed by measuring maximal voluntary static pressures.

Anxiety neurosis Dyspnea experienced by someone with an anxiety neurosis is a difficult symptom to evaluate. The signs and symptoms of acute and chronic hyperventilation do not serve to distinguish between anxiety neurosis and other processes, such as recurrent pulmonary emboli. A rather extensive series of pulmonary and cardiac function tests, carried out both at rest and during exercise, may be needed to be certain that anxiety is, in fact, the cause of the dyspnea. Certain clues are helpful in leading one to suspect a psychogenic origin. Frequent sighing respirations and a bizarre, irregular breathing pattern are helpful. Often the breathing pattern returns to normal during sleep.

Heart disease In patients with cardiac disease exertional dyspnea occurs most commonly as a consequence of an elevated pulmonary capillary pressure; aside from uncommon causes such as obstructive disease of the pulmonary veins (Chap. 240), pulmonary capillary hypertension is a consequence of left atrial hypertension, which in turn may be due to left ventricular dysfunction (Chaps. 235 and 236), reduced left ventricular compliance, and mitral stenosis. The elevation of hydrostatic pressure in the pulmonary vascular bed tends to upset the Starling equilibrium (see "Pulmonary Edema" below) with resulting transudation of fluid into the interstitial space, reducing the compliance of the lungs. A diminution in compliance increases the work of breathing which, to some degree, is minimized by both an increase in frequency of respirations and a reduction in tidal volume. In severe heart disease, usually involving elevation of both pulmonary and systemic venous pressures, hydrothorax develops, further interfering with pulmonary function and intensifying dyspnea. Less commonly, in patients with heart disease, dyspnea is due to a severely diminished cardiac output, resulting in inadequate perfusion of the respiratory muscles and hence their fatigue; dyspnea may also be associated with severe systemic and cerebral anoxia, as occurs during exertion in patients with congenital heart disease and right-to-left shunts.

Cardiac dyspnea usually begins as breathlessness on strenuous exertion and, over the course of months or years, progresses until the patient is dyspneic at rest. Occasionally, as in patients with massive acute myocardial infarction, the course may be associated with a nonproductive cough developing in the recumbent position, particularly at night.

ORTHOPNEA Orthopnea, i.e., dyspnea in the recumbent position, is characteristic of those forms of heart failure associated with elevations of pulmonary venous and capillary pressures. While orthopnea is usually a symptom of more advanced heart failure than exertional dyspnea, in patients who are physically inactive its onset may actually precede that of exertional dyspnea. Orthopnea is associated with the redistribution of blood from the lower extremities and splanchnic bed to the lungs as

the result of the alteration of gravitational forces when the recumbent position is assumed. This augmentation of intrathoracic blood volume elevates pulmonary venous and capillary pressures which increases the pulmonary closing volume and reduces the vital capacity. An additional factor associated with recumbency is the elevation of the diaphragm, which results in a lower end-expiratory lung volume. This combination of lower end-expiratory lung volume and increase in closing volume results in a significant alteration of alveolar-capillary gas exchange.

PAROXYSMAL (NOCTURNAL) DYSPNEA Also known as *cardiac asthma,* this condition is characterized by attacks of severe shortness of breath which generally occur at night and usually awaken the patient from sleep. The attack is precipitated by stimuli which aggravate the previously existing pulmonary congestion; frequently the total blood volume is augmented at night because of the reabsorption of edema from dependent portions of the body during recumbency; the redistribution of blood volume which takes place results in an increase in intrathoracic blood volume and therefore produces pulmonary congestion. A sleeping patient can tolerate relatively severe pulmonary engorgement and may awaken only when actual pulmonary edema and bronchospasm have developed, with the feeling of suffocation and with wheezing respirations.

CHEYNE-STOKES RESPIRATION See Chap. 236.

DIAGNOSIS The diagnosis of cardiac dyspnea depends on the recognition of heart disease on the basis of the history and physical examination. There may be a history of antecedent myocardial infarction, third and fourth sound gallops may be audible, and/or there may be evidence of left ventricular enlargement, jugular neck vein distention, and/or peripheral edema. Often there are radiographic signs of heart failure, with evidence of interstitial edema, pulmonary vascular redistribution, and accumulation of fluid in the septal planes and pleural cavity (Chap. 233). Cardiomegaly is often present, but the overall heart size may be normal, particularly in patients with dyspnea due to acute myocardial infarction or mitral stenosis; an enlarged left atrium is usually evident in the latter condition. The electrocardiogram (Chap. 232) is rarely specific for heart disease and cannot specifically indicate whether a patient's dyspnea is caused by heart disease; however, it is rarely normal in patients with cardiac dyspnea.

Differentiation between cardiac and pulmonary dyspnea In most patients with dyspnea there is obvious clinical evidence of disease of either heart or lungs. The dyspnea of chronic obstructive lung disease tends to develop more gradually than that of heart diseases; exceptions, of course, occur in patients with obstructive lung disease who develop an episode of infectious bronchitis, pneumonia, or pneumothorax, or an exacerbation of asthma. Like patients with cardiac dyspnea, patients with chronic obstructive lung disease may also waken at night with dyspnea, but this is usually associated with sputum production; the dyspnea is relieved after these patients rid themselves of secretions.

The difficulty in the distinction between cardiac and pulmonary dyspnea may be compounded by the coexistence of diseases involving both organ systems. Patients with a history of chronic bronchitis or asthma who develop left ventricular failure tend to develop recurrences of bronchoconstriction and wheezing in association with bouts of paroxysmal nocturnal dyspnea and pulmonary edema. This condition, i.e., cardiac asthma, usually occurs in patients with overt clinical evidence of heart disease. Acute cardiac asthma is further differentiated from acute attacks of bronchial asthma by the presence of diaphoresis, more bubbly airway sounds, and the more common occurrence of cyanosis.

It is desirable to carry out pulmonary function testing in patients in whom the etiology of dyspnea is not clear, for these tests should be helpful in determining whether dyspnea is produced by heart disease, lung disease, abnormalities of the chest wall, or anxiety. In addition to the usual means of assessing patients for heart disease (Chap. 230), the arm-to-tongue circulation time may be useful, since in patients with dyspnea on a cardiac basis it usually exceeds the upper normal limit of 16 s by 4 s or more. Careful observation during the performance of an exercise treadmill test will often help in the identification of the patient who is malingering or whose dyspnea is secondary to anxiety. Under these circumstances the patient usually complains of severe shortness of breath but appears to be breathing either effortlessly or totally irregularly.

PULMONARY EDEMA

An increase in pulmonary venous pressure, which results initially in the engorgement of the pulmonary vasculature, is common in most instances of dyspnea in association with congestive heart failure. The lungs become less compliant, the resistance of small airways increases, and there is an increase in lymphatic flow which apparently serves to maintain a constant pulmonary extravascular fluid volume. At this early stage there is usually mild tachypnea, and if arterial blood gases are measured, the arterial P_{O_2} and P_{CO_2} are both lowered with an increase in the alveolar-to-arterial oxygen difference. Tachypnea itself, which might result from stimulation of receptors in the pulmonary interstitium, apparently increases lymphatic flow by augmenting ventilatory pumping of lymphatic vessels. The changes described are seen well in advance of auscultatory findings or radiographic signs pointing to congestive heart failure. If sufficient both in magnitude and duration, the increase in intravascular pressure results in a net gain of fluid in the extravascular space despite further increases in lymphatic flow. It is at this point that symptoms worsen, tachypnea increases, gas exchange deteriorates further, and radiographic changes, such as Kerley B lines and loss of distinct vascular margins, are seen. Even at this intermediate stage, the capillary endothelial intercellular junctions have been shown to widen and allow passage of macromolecules into the interstices. Up to and including this stage, the edema is purely *interstitial.* Sufficient further elevations in intravascular pressure result in disruption of the tighter junctions between alveolar lining cells, and alveolar edema ensues with outpouring of fluid, which contains both red blood cells and macromolecules. At this point *alveolar edema* is present. Although originally considered an early and subtle radiographic sign of interstitial edema, recent evidence suggests that an antigravity redistribution of pulmonary blood flow occurs only after the onset of alveolar edema. With yet more severe disruption of the alveolar-capillary membrane, edematous fluid floods the alveoli and airways. At this point, full-blown clinical pulmonary edema with bilateral wet rales and rhonchi will occur, and the chest radiograph may show diffuse haziness of the lung fields. Typically, the patient is anxious and perspires freely, and the sputum is frothy and blood-tinged. Gas exchange is more severely compromised with worsening hypoxemia and possibly hypercapnia. Without effective treatment (Chap. 236) progressive acidemia, hypoxemia, and respiratory arrest ensue.

The earlier sequence of fluid accumulation described above follows the Starling law of capillary–interstitial fluid exchange:

$$\text{Fluid accumulation} = K[(P_c + \pi_{IF}) - (P_{IF} + \pi_{pl})] - Q_{lymph}$$

where K = permeability coefficient
P_c = mean intracapillary pressure
π_{IF} = oncotic pressure of interstitial fluid
P_{IF} = mean interstitial fluid pressure
π_{pl} = oncotic pressure of the plasma
Q_{lymph} = lymphatic flow

The pressures tending to move fluid out of the vessel are P_c and π_{IF}, which are normally more than offset by pressures tending to move fluid back into the vasculature, i.e., the algebraic sum of P_{IF} and π_{pl}. Implicit in the above equation is that lymphatic flow can increase in the case of imbalance of forces and result in no net accumulation of interstitial fluid. However, in later sequences, with opening of first the endothelial and then the alveolar intercellular junctions, the permeability coefficient changes strikingly. Thus, the initial process of hemodynamic pulmonary edema is one of fluid filtration and clearance. With further increasing pressures, disruption of both the structure and the function of the alveolar-capillary membrane occurs.

There are several clinical conditions which are associated with pulmonary edema based upon an imbalance of Starling forces other than through primary elevations of pulmonary capillary pressure. Although diminished plasma oncotic pressure in hypoalbuminemic states (e.g., severe liver disease, nephrotic syndrome, protein-losing enteropathy) might be expected to lead to pulmonary edema, the balance of forces normally so strongly favors resorption that even under these conditions some elevation of capillary pressure is necessary before interstitial edema develops. Increased negativity of interstitial pressure has been implicated in the genesis of unilateral pulmonary edema following rapid evacuation of a large pneumothorax. In this situation the findings are apparent only by radiography. It has been recently proposed that large negative intrapleural pressures during acute severe asthma may be associated with the development of interstitial edema. If this proposal can be supported by sufficient clinical data, then asthma would represent an additional example of edema due to increased negativity of interstitial pressure. Lymphatic blockade secondary to fibrotic and inflammatory diseases or lymphangitic carcinomatosis may lead to interstitial edema. In such instances both clinical and radiographic manifestations are dominated by the underlying disease process.

There are other conditions characterized by increases in the interstitial fluid content of the lungs which begin neither with an imbalance between intravascular and interstitial forces nor with alterations in lymphatics, but rather appear to be associated primarily with disruption of the alveolar-capillary membranes. Experimentally the prototype for such conditions is the pulmonary edema following alloxan administration. Any number of spontaneously occurring or environmental toxic insults are associated with diffuse pulmonary edema which clearly does not have a hemodynamic origin. These conditions are discussed in Chap. 271.

There are three forms of pulmonary edema which have not been clearly related to increased permeability, inadequate lymphatic flow, or an imbalance of Starling forces; hence their precise mechanism remains unexplained. *Narcotic overdose* is a well-recognized antecedent to pulmonary edema. Although illicit use of parenteral heroin has been the most frequent cause, parenteral and oral overdoses of legitimate preparations of morphine, methadone, and dextropropoxyphene have also been associated with pulmonary edema. Thus the earlier idea that injected impurities lead to the disorder is untenable. Available evidence suggests that there are alterations in the permeability of alveolar and capillary membranes rather than elevation of pulmonary capillary pressure. *Exposure to high altitude* in association with severe physical exertion is a well-recognized setting for pulmonary edema in unacclimatized, yet otherwise healthy, persons. Recent data show that acclimatized high-altitude natives also develop this syndrome upon return to high altitude after a relatively brief sojourn at low altitudes. The mechanism for high-altitude pulmonary edema remains obscure, and studies have been conflicting, some suggesting pulmonary venous constriction and others indicating pulmonary arteriolar constriction as the prime mechanisms. *Neurogenic* pulmonary edema has been suspected in patients with central nervous system disorders and without apparent preexisting left ventricular dysfunction. Although most experimental equivalents have implicated sympathetic nervous system activity, the mechanism whereby sympathetic efferent activity leads to pulmonary edema is a matter of speculation. It is known that a massive adrenergic discharge leads to peripheral vasoconstriction with elevation of blood pressure and shifts of blood to the central circulation. In addition, it is probable that a decrease in left ventricular compliance also occurs, and both factors serve to increase left atrial pressures sufficiently to induce pulmonary edema on a hemodynamic basis.

Treatment of pulmonary edema   See Chap. 236.

REFERENCES

Campbell EJM et al: *Breathlessness.* Oxford, Blackwell, 1966
——— et al: *The Respiratory Muscles: Mechanisms and Neural Control.* Philadelphia, Saunders, 1970
Fishman AP, Renkin EM (eds): *Pulmonary Edema.* Washington, DC, American Physiological Society, 1979
Gold W: Dyspnea, in *Signs and Symptoms,* 6th ed, RS Blacklow (ed). Philadelphia, Lippincott, 1979, chap 19
McFadden ER, Ingram RH Jr: Relationship between diseases of the heart and lungs, in *Heart Disease,* E Braunwald (ed). Philadelphia, Saunders, 1980, chap 53
Scoggin CH et al: High altitude pulmonary edema in the children and young adults of Leadville, Colorado. N Engl J Med 297:1269, 1977
Staub NC: State of the art review: Pathogenesis of pulmonary edema. Am Rev Respir Dis 109:358, 1974
Szidon JP et al: The alveolar-capillary membrane and pulmonary edema. N Engl J Med 286:1200, 1972

28
CYANOSIS, HYPOXIA, AND POLYCYTHEMIA

EUGENE BRAUNWALD

CYANOSIS

Cyanosis refers to a bluish color of the skin and mucous membranes resulting from an increased amount of reduced hemoglobin, or of hemoglobin derivatives, in the small blood vessels of those areas. It is usually most marked in the lips, nail beds, ears, and malar eminences. The "red cyanosis" of polycythemia vera (Chap. 320) must be distinguished from the true cyanosis discussed here. A cherry-colored flush, rather than cyanosis, is caused by carboxyhemoglobin (Chap. 224). In *argyria,* the skin is bluish because of the deposition of silver salts, and the discoloration persists despite pressure, unlike cyanotic skin which blanches. The degree of cyanosis is modified by the quality of cutaneous pigment, the color of the blood plasma, and the thickness of the skin, as well as by the state of the cutaneous capillaries. The accurate clinical detection of the presence and degree of cyanosis is difficult, as proved by oxi-

metric studies. Some observers can reliably detect central cyanosis when the arterial saturation has fallen to 85 percent; others may not detect it until the saturation has reached 75 percent.

The increase in the amount of reduced hemoglobin in the cutaneous vessels, which produces cyanosis, may be brought about either by an increase in the quantity of venous blood in the skin as the result of dilatation of the venules and venous ends of the capillaries, or by a decrease in the oxygen saturation in the capillary blood. In general, cyanosis becomes apparent when the mean capillary concentration of reduced hemoglobin exceeds 5 g per 100 ml. It is the *absolute* rather than the *relative* amount of reduced hemoglobin which is important in producing cyanosis. Thus, in a patient with severe anemia the relative amount of reduced hemoglobin in the venous blood may be very large when considered in relation to the total amount of hemoglobin. However, since the latter is markedly lowered, the absolute amount of reduced hemoglobin may still be small, and therefore patients with severe anemia and marked arterial desaturation do not display cyanosis. Conversely, the higher the total hemoglobin content, the greater the tendency toward cyanosis; thus, patients with marked polycythemia tend to be cyanotic at higher levels of arterial oxygen saturation than patients with normal hematocrit values. Likewise, local passive congestion, which causes an increase in the total amount of reduced hemoglobin in the vessels in a given area, may cause cyanosis. Cyanosis also is observed when nonfunctional hemoglobin is present in the blood; as little as 1.5 g per 100 ml methemoglobin or 0.5 g sulfhemoglobin is sufficient to produce cyanosis (Chap. 315).

True cyanosis may be subdivided into *central* and *peripheral* categories. In the *central* type, there is arterial blood unsaturation or an abnormal hemoglobin derivative, and the mucous membranes and skin are both affected. *Peripheral* cyanosis is due to a slowing of blood flow to an area and abnormally great extraction of oxygen from normally saturated arterial blood. It results from vasoconstriction and diminished peripheral blood flow, such as occurs in cold exposure, shock, congestive failure, and peripheral vascular disease. Often, in these conditions, the mucous membranes of the oral cavity or those beneath the tongue may be spared. Clinical differentiation between central and peripheral cyanosis may not always be simple, and in conditions such as cardiogenic shock with pulmonary edema there may be a mixture of both types.

DIFFERENTIAL DIAGNOSIS (See Table 28-1)   **Central cyanosis** Decreased arterial oxygen saturation results from a marked reduction in the oxygen tension in the arterial blood. This may be brought about by a decline in the tension of oxygen in the inspired air without sufficient compensatory alveolar hyperventilation to maintain alveolar oxygen tension. Cyanosis does not occur in a significant degree in an ascent to an altitude of 8000 ft but is marked in a further ascent to 16,000 ft. The reason for this becomes clear on studying the S shape of the oxygen dissociation curve (Fig. 53-4). At 8000 ft the tension of oxygen in the inspired air is about 120 mmHg, the alveolar tension is approximately 80 mmHg, and the hemoglobin is nearly completely saturated. However, at 16,000 ft the oxygen tensions in atmospheric air and alveolar air are about 85 and 50 mmHg, respectively, and the oxygen dissociation curve shows that the arterial blood is only about 75 percent saturated. This leaves 25 percent of the hemoglobin in the reduced form, an amount likely to be associated with cyanosis in the absence of anemia. Similarly, a mutant hemoglobin with a low affinity for oxygen (Hb Kansas) causes lowered arterial oxygen saturation and resultant central cyanosis (Chap. 315).

Seriously *impaired pulmonary function,* through alveolar hypoventilation or perfusion of unventilated or poorly ventilated areas of the lung, is a common cause of central cyanosis

(Chap. 255). This may occur acutely, as in extensive pneumonia or in pulmonary edema, or with chronic pulmonary diseases (e.g., emphysema). In the last situation clubbing of the fingers and polycythemia are generally present. However, in many types of chronic pulmonary disease with fibrosis and obliteration of the capillary vascular bed, cyanosis does not occur because there is relatively little perfusion of underventilated areas.

Another cause of decreased arterial oxygen saturation is shunting of systemic venous blood into the arterial circuit. Certain types of congenital heart disease are associated with cyanosis (Chap. 240). Since blood normally flows from a high-pressure to a low-pressure region, in order for a cardiac defect to result in a right-to-left shunt, it must ordinarily be combined with an obstructive lesion distal to the defect or with elevated pulmonary vascular resistance. The commonest congenital cardiac lesion associated with cyanosis is the combination of ventricular septal defect and pulmonary outflow tract obstruction (tetralogy of Fallot). The more severe the obstruction, the greater the degree of right-to-left shunting and resultant cyanosis. The mechanisms for the elevated pulmonary vascular resistance which may produce cyanosis in the presence of intra- and extracardiac communications without pulmonic stenosis are discussed elsewhere (Chap. 240). In patients with patent ductus arteriosus, pulmonary hypertension, and right-to-left shunt, differential cyanosis results; i.e., cyanosis occurs in the lower extremities but not in the upper extremities.

Pulmonary arteriovenous fistulas may be congenital or acquired, solitary or multiple, microscopic or massive. The degree of cyanosis produced by these fistulas depends upon their size and number. They occur with some frequency in hereditary hemorrhagic telangiectasia (Chap. 317). Arterial oxygen unsaturation also occurs in some patients with cirrhosis, presumably as a consequence of pulmonary arteriovenous fistulas or portal vein-pulmonary vein anastomoses.

In patients with cardiac or pulmonary right-to-left shunts, the presence and severity of cyanosis depend on the size of the shunt relative to the systemic flow as well as on the oxyhemoglobin saturation of the venous blood. In patients with central cyanosis due to arterial oxygen unsaturation, the severity of cyanosis increases with exercise. With increased extraction of oxygen from the blood by the exercising muscles, the venous blood returning to the right side of the heart is more unsaturated than at rest, and shunting of this blood or its passage through lungs incapable of normal oxygenation intensifies the cyanosis. Also, since the systemic vascular resistance normally decreases with exercise, the right-to-left shunt is augmented by

exercise in patients with congenital heart disease and communications between the two sides of the heart. Secondary polycythemia occurs frequently in patients with arterial unsaturation and contributes to the cyanosis.

Cyanosis can be caused by small amounts of circulating methemoglobin and by even smaller amounts of sulfhemoglobin (Chap. 315). Although they are uncommon causes of cyanosis, these abnormal hemoglobin pigments should be sought by spectroscopy when cyanosis is not readily explained by malfunction of the circulatory or respiratory systems. Generally, clubbing does not occur with them. The diagnosis of methemoglobinemia can be suspected, if, on mixing the patient's blood in a test tube, it remains brown.

Peripheral cyanosis Probably the most common cause of peripheral cyanosis is generalized vasoconstriction resulting from exposure to cold air or water. This is clearly a normal response to the stimulus and is transient. When cardiac output is low, as in severe congestive heart failure or shock, cutaneous vasoconstriction occurs as a compensatory mechanism, so that blood is diverted to more vital areas [central nervous system, heart (Chap. 236)], and intense cyanosis associated with cool extremities may result. Even though the arterial blood is normally saturated, the reduced volume flow through the skin and the reduced oxygen tension at the venous end of the capillary result in cyanosis.

Arterial obstruction to an extremity generally results in pallor and coldness, but there may be associated slight cyanosis. If there is venous obstruction, the extremity is usually congested and markedly cyanotic, and there is true stagnation of blood flow. Venous hypertension, which may be local (as in thrombophlebitis) or generalized (as in tricuspid valve disease or constrictive pericarditis), dilates the subpapillary venous plexuses and intensifies cyanosis.

APPROACH TO THE PATIENT WITH CYANOSIS Certain features are important in arriving at the proper cause of cyanosis:

1 The history, particularly the duration (cyanosis present since birth is usually due to congenital heart disease); possible exposure to drugs or chemicals which may produce abnormal types of hemoglobin.

2 Clinical differentiation of central as opposed to peripheral cyanosis. Objective evidence by physical or radiographic examination of disorders of the respiratory or cardiovascular systems. Massage or gentle warming of a cyanotic extremity will increase peripheral blood flow and abolish peripheral but not central cyanosis.

3 The presence or absence of clubbing of the fingers. Clubbing without cyanosis is frequent in patients with subacute bacterial endocarditis and in association with ulcerative colitis, it may occasionally occur in healthy persons, and in some instances it may be occupational, e.g., in jackhammer operators. Slight cyanosis of the lips and cheeks, without clubbing of the fingers, is common in patients with well-compensated mitral stenosis and is probably due to minimal arterial hypoxia resulting from fibrotic changes in the lungs secondary to long-standing congestion combined with reduction of cardiac output. The combination of cyanosis and clubbing is frequent in many patients with certain types of congenital cardiac disease and is seen occasionally in persons with pulmonary disease such as lung abscess or pulmonary arteriovenous shunts. On the other hand, peripheral cyanosis or acutely developing central cyanosis is not associated with clubbed fingers.

TABLE 28-1
Causes of cyanosis

I Central cyanosis
  A Decreased arterial oxygen saturation
    1 Decreased atmospheric pressure—high altitude
    2 Impaired pulmonary function
      a Alveolar hypoventilation
      b Uneven relationships between pulmonary ventilation and perfusion
      c Impaired oxygen diffusion
    3 Anatomic shunts
      a Certain types of congenital heart disease
      b Pulmonary arteriovenous fistulas
      c Multiple small intrapulmonary shunts
    4 Hemoglobin with low affinity for oxygen
  B Hemoglobin abnormalities
    1 Methemoglobinemia—hereditary, acquired
    2 Sulfhemoglobinemia—acquired
    3 Carboxyhemoglobinemia (not true cyanosis)
II Peripheral cyanosis
  A Reduced cardiac output
  B Cold exposure
  C Redistribution of blood flow from extremities
  D Arterial obstruction
  E Venous obstruction

4 Determination of arterial blood oxygen tension or oxygen saturation. Spectroscopic and other examinations of the blood for abnormal types of hemoglobin.

HYPOXIA

The fundamental purpose of the cardiorespiratory system is to deliver oxygen (and substrates) to the cells and to remove carbon dioxide (and other metabolic products) from them. Proper maintenance of this function depends on intact cardiovascular and respiratory systems and a supply of inspired gas containing adequate oxygen. Changes in oxygen and in carbon dioxide tension as well as changes in the intraerythrocytic concentration of certain *organic phosphate compounds*, especially 2,3-diphosphoglyceric acid (2,3-DPG), cause shifts in the oxygen dissociation curve. These are discussed in detail in Chap. 53 and are illustrated in Fig. 53-4. When hypoxia results as a consequence of respiratory failure, arterial P_{CO_2} usually rises (Chaps. 263 and 271), and the oxygen dissociation curve tends to be displaced to the right. Under these conditions the percentage saturation of the hemoglobin in the arterial blood at a given level of alveolar oxygen tension declines. Thus arterial hypoxia and cyanosis are likely to be more marked in proportion to the degree of depression of alveolar oxygen tension when such depression results from pulmonary disease than when the depression occurs as the result of a decline in the partial pressure of oxygen in the inspired air, in which case arterial P_{CO_2} falls and the oxygen dissociation curve is displaced to the left.

DIFFERENTIAL DIAGNOSIS   Anemic hypoxia   Any decrease in hemoglobin concentration is attended by a corresponding decline in the oxygen-carrying power. The P_{O_2} in the arterial blood remains normal, but the absolute amount of oxygen transported per unit volume of blood is diminished. As the anemic blood passes through the capillaries, and the usual amount of oxygen is removed from it, the P_{O_2} in the venous blood declines to a greater degree than would normally be the case.

Carbon monoxide intoxication (Chap. 224)   This condition is accompanied by the equivalent of anemic hypoxia in that the hemoglobin which is combined with the carbon monoxide (carboxyhemoglobin) is unavailable for oxygen transport. In addition, the presence of carboxyhemoglobin increases the affinity of normal hemoglobin for oxygen at low levels of P_{O_2} (i.e., shifts the lower portion of the dissociation curve of hemoglobin to the left), so that the oxygen can be unloaded only at lower tensions. By such formation of carboxyhemoglobin a given degree of reduction in oxygen-carrying power produces a far greater degree of tissue hypoxia than the equivalent reduction in hemoglobin due to simple anemia.

Circulatory hypoxia   As in anemic hypoxia, arterial P_{O_2} is normal but venous and tissue P_{O_2} are reduced as a consequence of reduced tissue perfusion in the face of normal tissue oxygen consumption. For this reason the term *stagnant hypoxia* may be used for this condition. Generalized circulatory hypoxia occurs in heart failure, as discussed in Chap. 236.

Specific organ hypoxia   Decreased circulation to a specific organ resulting in localized stagnant hypoxia may be due to organic arterial or venous obstruction or may occur as a reflex phenomenon. The latter may occur when vasoconstriction of, for instance, the limbs results from an attempt to maintain adequate perfusion to more vital organs, as in severe congestive heart failure. When organic arterial obliterative disease develops, ischemic hypoxia results, with accompanying pallor. Localized hypoxia may also result from venous obstruction which results in congestion. Edema, which increases the distance through which oxygen diffuses before it reaches the cells, can also cause localized hypoxia.

Increased oxygen requirements   Even if oxygen diffusion into blood perfusing the pulmonary capillary bed is unhampered and the hemoglobin is qualitatively and quantitatively normal, the P_{O_2} in venous blood (hence, capillary and tissue P_{O_2}) may be reduced if the oxygen consumption of the tissues is elevated without a corresponding increase in volume flow per unit of time. Such a situation may be encountered in febrile states and in thyrotoxicosis. Under such conditions the circulation may be considered deficient relative to the metabolic requirements. Thus, this type of metabolic hypoxia is comparable to circulatory hypoxia, in that in both conditions the volume flow of blood is decreased relative to the needs of the tissues; the difference is that in one case the primary defect is the volume flow of blood and in the other the primary defect is an increased oxygen need by the tissues.

Ordinarily, the clinical picture of patients with hypoxia due to an elevated basal metabolic rate is quite different from that in other types of hypoxia; the skin is warm and flushed, owing to increased cutaneous blood flow which dissipates the excessive heat produced, and cyanosis is absent in these patients.

Exercise is a classic example of increased tissue oxygen requirements. The increased demands are normally met by several mechanisms: (1) increasing the cardiac output and thus oxygen delivery to the tissues; (2) preferentially directing the blood to the exercising muscles and away from resting muscles (by changing vascular resistances in various circulatory beds, in some areas by direct effects, in others reflexly); (3) increasing oxygen extraction from the delivered blood and widening the arteriovenous oxygen differences. If the capacity of these mechanisms is exceeded, then hypoxia, especially of the exercising muscles, will result.

Improper oxygen utilization   The administration of cyanide (Chap. 224) and several other similarly acting poisons leads to a paradoxic state in which the tissues are unable to utilize oxygen and as a consequence the venous blood tends to have a high oxygen tension. This condition has been termed *histotoxic hypoxia*. Cyanide produces cellular hypoxia by paralyzing the electron-transfer function of cytochrome oxidase so that it cannot pass electrons to oxygen, whereas diphtheria toxin is believed to inhibit the synthesis of one of the cytochromes and thus interfere with oxygen consumption and energy production by the cells involved.

EFFECTS OF HYPOXIA   When hypoxia is general, all parts of the body may suffer some impairment of function, but those parts which are most sensitive to the effects of hypoxia give rise to symptoms which dominate the clinical picture. The *changes in the central nervous system*, particularly the higher centers, are especially important. Acute hypoxia produces impaired judgment, motor incoordination, and a clinical picture closely resembling that of acute alcoholism. When hypoxia is long-standing, the symptoms consist of fatigue, drowsiness, apathy, inattentiveness, delayed reaction time, severe fatigue, and reduced work capacity. As hypoxia becomes more severe, the centers of the brainstem are affected, and death usually results from respiratory failure. With reduction of arterial oxygen tension, cerebrovascular resistance decreases and cerebral blood flow increases, which tends to minimize the cerebral hypoxia. On the other hand when the reduction of arterial P_{O_2} is accompanied by hyperventilation and diminution of P_{CO_2}, cerebrovascular resistance rises, blood flow falls, and hypoxia is enhanced. Compared with the brain, the phylogenetically older spinal cord and peripheral nerves are relatively insensitive to hypoxia. Hypoxia also causes pulmonary arterial constriction, which serves the useful function of shunting blood away from poorly ventilated areas toward better-ventilated portions of the lung. However, it has the disadvantage of causing increased pulmonary vascular resistance and an increased burden on the right ventricle.

A complex disturbance of cellular functions results from the metabolic effects of severe acute hypoxia. In liver and muscles the breakdown of the primary foodstuff, carbohydrate, normally proceeds anaerobically (i.e., without oxidation) to the stage of formation of pyruvic acid. The breakdown of pyruvate requires oxygen, and when this is deficient, increasing proportions of pyruvate are reduced to lactic acid, which cannot be further broken down (Chap. 86). Hence, there is an increase in the blood lactate, with decrease in bicarbonate and a corresponding acidosis. Under these circumstances the total energy obtained from foodstuff breakdown is greatly reduced, and the amount of energy available for continuing resynthesis of energy-rich phosphate compounds becomes inadequate. Impairment of the myriad anabolic reactions which take place in tissues follows. The deficiency of energy-rich phosphate compounds produces a complex disturbance of cellular function.

Most of the useful respiratory response to hypoxia originates in special chemosensitive cells in the carotid and aortic bodies, although the respiratory center is also stimulated directly by oxygen lack. The peripheral chemoreceptors are extremely rugged and continue to function after other tissues have been damaged by hypoxemia. The chemoreceptors are stimulated by a reduction in their oxygen supply below their needs, either by lowered arterial P_{O_2} or by lowered blood flow to them. If respiration is stimulated by hypoxia, the resulting increase in ventilation, with loss of carbon dioxide, tends to make the blood more alkaline. On the other hand, the diffusion of additional quantities of lactic acid from the tissues into the blood tends to make the blood more acid. In either case the total amount of bicarbonate, and hence the carbon dioxide–combining power, tends to be diminished. With mild hypoxia there is likely to be respiratory alkalosis; severe hypoxia is attended by metabolic acidosis.

The heart, although relatively sensitive to hypoxia as compared with most of the structures of the body, is less sensitive than the nervous system. Consequently, in the absence of severe coronary artery disease, serious manifestations arising in the nervous system dominate the picture. Diminished oxygen tension in any tissue results in local vasodilatation, and the diffuse vasodilatation which occurs in generalized hypoxia results in an elevation of total cardiac output (Fig. 53-5). In patients with preexisting heart disease, particularly coronary artery disease, the combination of hypoxia and the requirements of the peripheral tissues for an increase of cardiac output may precipitate congestive heart failure. Prolonged or severe hypoxia may also impair hepatic and renal function.

One of the important mechanisms of compensation for prolonged hypoxia is an increase in the amount of hemoglobin in the blood (Fig. 53-5). This is due not to direct stimulation of the bone marrow but to the effect of an erythropoiesis-stimulating factor (erythropoietin) which originates primarily in the kidneys. Assayable levels of erythropoietin are increased by hypoxia, and its production has been found to be regulated by the balance between tissue oxygen supply and demand.

POLYCYTHEMIA

The term *polycythemia* signifies an increase above the normal in the number of red corpuscles in the circulating blood. This increase is usually, though not always, accompanied by a corresponding increase in the quantity of hemoglobin and in the volume of packed red corpuscles. The increase may or may not be associated with an increase in the total quantity of red blood cells in the body. It is important to distinguish between *absolute* polycythemia (an increase in the total red corpuscle mass) and *relative* polycythemia, which occurs when, through loss of blood plasma, the concentration of the red corpuscles becomes greater than normal in the circulating blood. This may be the consequence of abnormally lowered fluid intake, of the loss of plasma into the interstitial fluid, and of the marked loss of body fluids, such as occurs in persistent vomiting, severe diarrhea, copious sweating, or acidosis (Chap. 85).

Because the term polycythemia is used loosely to refer to all varieties of increase in the number of red corpuscles, the terms *erythrocytosis* and *erythremia* are preferred in referring to two forms of absolute polycythemia. Erythrocytosis denotes absolute polycythemia which occurs in response to some known stimulus (secondary polycythemia); erythremia (polycythemia rubra vera) refers to the disease of unknown etiology, which is discussed elsewhere (Chap. 320). An approach to the differential diagnosis of erythrocytosis should begin with a consideration of its mechanisms (Table 28-2). Erythrocytosis develops as a consequence of a variety of factors and represents a physiologic response to conditions of hypoxia. Sojourn at high altitudes leads to defective saturation of arterial blood with oxygen and stimulates the production of more red corpuscles. The oxygen saturation, rather than oxygen tension, appears to be the more important determinant of the erythropoietic response to chronic hypoxia (Fig. 28-1). A disorder may set in insidiously after several years of continued residence at high altitudes, leading to the development of a condition known as *chronic mountain sickness* or *seroche* (Monge's disease). Prominent manifestations are a florid color which turns to cyanosis on mild exertion, mental torpor, fatigue, and headache. Those affected are usually in the fourth to sixth decades. Return to sea level promptly relieves the symptoms. *Brisket disease of cattle*, a disorder of calves grazing at high altitudes in Utah and Colorado, which is characterized by pulmonary hypertension and subsequent failure of the right side of the heart, is not a true counterpart of Monge's disease, since it is not associated

FIGURE 28-1

Relationship between mean arterial oxygen saturation (percent) and the mean hemoglobin content (grams per 100 ml) in healthy male residents at various altitudes. (From Hurtado, by permission of Annals of Internal Medicine.)

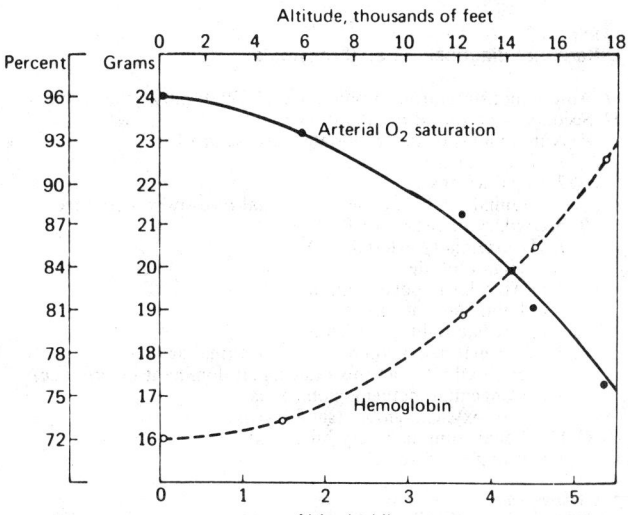

with sustained oxygen unsaturation or polycythemia. Living at high altitudes also evokes a number of compensatory reactions which act to increase oxygen delivery to the tissues. These include hyperventilation, which reduces the oxygen gradient between ambient and alveolar air, an augmentation of pulmonary capillary blood volume, a reduction of diffusing capacity, and an increase in cardiac output.

Any chronic pulmonary disease which alters ventilation-perfusion relationships or seriously impairs gas diffusion may produce chronic hypoxemia and lead to erythrocytosis. *Pulmonary arteriovenous fistulas* or *cavernous hemangioma of the lung* may lead to impaired saturation of arterial blood with oxygen, with the consequent development of erythrocytosis and of a clinical picture resembling closely that of certain types of congenital heart disease. The increased blood viscosity secondary to the polycythemia elevates pulmonary arterial pressure and, combined with the elevation of pulmonary vascular resistance resulting from hypoxia, further elevates right ventricular pressure, contributing to the development or intensification of cor pulmonale (Chap. 246).

The *abnormal ventilatory conditions* present in very obese individuals may cause alveolar hypoventilation and result in arterial unsaturation, erythrocytosis, hypercapnia, and somnolence (the Pickwickian syndrome, Chap. 270). This syndrome is observed less commonly in nonobese persons, in whom decreased sensitivity of the respiratory center to CO_2 may play a role.

The partial shunting of blood from the pulmonary circuit, such as occurs in *congenital heart disease,* causes the most striking erythrocytosis resulting from abnormalities in the heart or lungs. Erythrocyte counts as high as 13 million per mm^3, which are possible only when the red corpuscles are smaller than normal, have been observed in such cases, with volumes of packed red blood cells even as high as 86 ml per 100 ml of blood. As the polycythemia develops, there is a progressive rise in blood viscosity, the sharpest increase beginning when the volume of packed red blood cells reaches 65 to 70 percent. The commonest defect producing such polycythemia is pulmonary stenosis associated with a right-to-left shunt that allows venous blood to enter the systemic arterial tree without traversing the lungs. Other conditions include transposition of the great arteries, tricuspid atresia, persistent truncus arteriosus, and other less common anomalies, discussed in Chap. 240.

Reduction in red blood cell volume (phlebotomy with reinfusion of the plasma) is sometimes performed in severely symptomatic patients with extremely high hematocrit levels, but it must be carried out slowly and with great caution. It

TABLE 28-2
Differential diagnosis of erythrocytosis

I Autonomous erythroid proliferation ($\downarrow$ EP*); polycythemia vera
II Secondary erythroid proliferation
  A Autonomous or inappropriate increase in EP
    1 Neoplasm
    2 Renal lesions
    3 Familial erythrocytosis (autosomal recessive inheritance)
  B Secondary increase in EP
    1 Hypoxemia ($\downarrow$ arterial P_{O_2})
      a High altitude
      b Alveolar hypoventilation
      c Pulmonary disease
      d Cardiac right-to-left shunt
    2 Abnormal hemoglobin function (normal arterial P_{O_2})
      a High-affinity variants (autosomal dominant inheritance)
      b Congenital methemoglobinemia
      c Carboxyhemoglobin (smokers)
  C Hormonal stimulus to erythropoeisis
    1 Cushing's syndrome

* *Erythropoietin.*
SOURCE: *HF Bunn et al, Human Hemoglobins, Philadelphia, Saunders, 1977.*

results in a reduction of the elevated blood viscosity which decreases the impedance to flow. When pulmonary blood flow is derived largely from the systemic circuit, as in patients with tetralogy of Fallot and severe pulmonary outflow obstruction, this maneuver reduces systemic O_2 saturation. On the other hand, if pulmonary blood flow is independent of the systemic circuit, as in D-transposition of the great arteries, an increase in pulmonary blood flow occurs.

The polycythemia of cyanotic congenital heart disease may lead to spontaneous thrombosis at any site, including the central nervous system. It may also be accompanied by a variety of blood coagulation defects, including reduced fibrinogen and prothrombin concentrations, as well as thrombocytopenia.

The excessive use of coal-tar derivatives and other forms of chronic poisoning, by producing abnormal hemoglobin pigments such as methemoglobin and sulfhemoglobin (Chap. 315), also may cause erythrocytosis. Carriers of certain abnormal hemoglobins which displace the oxygen dissociation curve to the left and interfere with oxygen unloading in the tissues stimulate the production of erythropoietin and a secondary erythrocytosis unassociated with leukocytosis or thrombocytosis (Chap. 315).

Erythrocytosis is found in *Cushing's syndrome* (Chap. 336) and can be produced by the administration of large amounts of adrenocortical steroids. Especially intriguing are the instances of polycythemia observed in association with various *tumors.* These have been chiefly of two varieties, *infratentorial* and *renal.* The tumors in the posterior fossa of the skull have usually been vascular (hemangioblastomas). The renal tumors have included hypernephroma, adenoma, and sarcoma. Other tumors that have been associated with polycythemia include uterine myoma and hepatic carcinoma. Polycythemia also has been reported in association with polycystic disease of the kidneys and hydronephrosis. However, only a small proportion (0.3 to 2.6 percent) of the various renal disorders mentioned above have been associated with polycythemia. Plasma erythropoietin levels have been found to be elevated in a number of these patients. Erythropoiesis-stimulating activity has been demonstrated in tumor extracts and in renal cyst fluid, and polycythemia has disappeared after the associated tumor was removed.

The term *stress erythrocytosis* has been applied to the polycythemia seen occasionally in very active, hard-working persons in a state of anxiety, who appear florid but who have none of the characteristic signs of erythremia—no splenomegaly or leukocytosis with immature cells in the blood. In such persons the total red blood cell mass is normal, and the plasma volume is below normal.

The differential diagnosis of polycythemia is discussed in Chap. 320. However, it should be pointed out that in secondary polycythemia with hypoxia, arterial P_{O_2} is reduced, erythropoietin levels are elevated, while levels of leukocyte alkaline phosphatase and serum vitamin B_{12} are normal. In polycythemia vera, erythropoietin levels are normal or decreased and leukocyte alkaline phosphatase and vitamin B_{12} levels are elevated.

REFERENCES

DENNIS RC et al: Improved myocardial performance following high 2,3-DPG red cell transfusions. Surgery 77:741, 1975
GOLD W: Cyanosis, in *Signs and Symptoms,* 6th ed, RS Blacklow (ed). Philadelphia, Lippincott, 1979
HARKNESS DR: The regulation of hemoglobin oxygenation, in *Advances in Internal Medicine,* GH Stollerman (ed). Chicago, Year Book, 1971, p 189
HURTADO A: Some clinical aspects of life at high altitudes. Ann Intern Med 53:247, 1960
JEPSON JH, FRANKL W: *Haematological Complications in Cardiac Practice.* Philadelphia, Saunders, 1975

Rosenthal A, Tyler DC: Effect of red cell volume reduction or pulmonary blood flow in polycythemia of cyanotic congenital heart disease. Am J Cardiol 33:410, 1974

Smith JR, Landaw SA: Smokers' polycythemia. N Engl J Med 298:6, 1978

Williams EJ (ed): Erythrocyte disorders—polycythemia, in *Hematology*, 2d ed. New York, McGraw-Hill, 1977, p 624

29
EDEMA

EUGENE BRAUNWALD

Edema is defined as an increase in the extravascular (interstitial) component of the extracellular fluid volume, which may increase by several liters before the abnormality is recognized. Therefore, a weight gain of several kilograms usually precedes overt manifestations of edema, and a similar weight loss resulting from diuresis can be induced in a slightly edematous patient before "dry weight" is achieved. *Ascites* (Chap. 40) and *hydrothorax* refer to accumulation of excess fluid in the peritoneal and pleural cavities, respectively, and are considered to be special forms of edema. *Anasarca,* or "dropsy," refers to gross, generalized edema. Depending on its etiology and mechanism, edema may be localized or have a generalized distribution; it is recognized in its generalized form by puffiness of the face, which is most readily apparent in the periorbital areas, and by the persistence of an indentation of the skin following pressure; this is known as "pitting" edema. In its more subtle form, it may be detected by the fact that the rim of the bell of the stethoscope leaves an indentation on the skin of the chest that lasts a few minutes. One of the early symptoms a patient may note is the ring on a finger fitting more snugly than in the past, or difficulty in putting on shoes, particularly in the evening.

PATHOGENESIS (A more detailed discussion of the volume and distribution of body fluids is presented in Chap. 84.) About one-third of the total body water is confined to the extracellular space. This compartment, in turn, is composed of the plasma volume and the interstitial space. Under ordinary circumstances the plasma volume represents about 25 percent of the extracellular space, and the remainder is interstitial fluid. The forces that regulate the disposition of fluid between these two components of the extracellular compartment are frequently referred to as the Starling forces (see "Pulmonary Edema" in Chap. 27). In general terms, two forces, the hydrostatic pressure within the vascular system and the colloid oncotic pressure in the interstitial fluid, tend to promote a movement of fluid from the vascular to the extravascular space. In contrast, the colloid oncotic pressure contributed by the plasma proteins, and the hydrostatic pressure within the interstitial fluid, referred to as the *tissue tension,* promote a movement of fluid into the vascular compartment. As a consequence of these forces there is a large movement of water and diffusible solutes from the vascular space at the arteriolar end of the microcirculation and back into the vascular compartment at the venous end. In addition, fluid is returned from the interstitial space into the vascular system by way of the lymphatics, and unless these channels are obstructed, lymph flow tends to increase if there is a tendency toward a net movement of fluid from the vascular compartment to the interstitium. All these forces are usually balanced so that a steady state exists in the size of the intravascular and interstitial compartments, and yet a large exchange between them is permitted. However, should any one of these factors be altered significantly, a net move-

ment of fluid from one component of the extracellular space to the other will occur.

An increase in capillary pressure may readily result from an increase in venous pressure due to local obstruction in venous drainage, to congestive heart failure, or rarely to the simple expansion of the vascular volume by the administration of large volumes of fluid at a rate in excess of the ability of the kidneys to excrete these excesses. The colloid oncotic pressure of the plasma may be reduced, owing to any of the factors that may induce hypoalbuminemia, such as malnutrition, liver disease, and loss of protein into the urine or into the gastrointestinal tract, or to a severe catabolic state.

Edema may also result from damage to the capillary endothelium, which increases the permeability of these vessels, permitting the transfer to the interstitial compartment of a fluid containing more protein than usual. Injury to the capillary walls may be the result of chemical, bacterial, thermal, or mechanical agents. Increased capillary permeability may also be a consequence of a hypersensitivity reaction and is characteristic of immune injury. Damage to the capillary endothelium is presumably responsible for inflammatory edema, which is nonpitting, usually localized, and readily recognized by the presence of other signs of inflammation—redness, heat, and tenderness.

In an attempt to formulate a hypothesis about the pathophysiology involved in edematous states, it is important to discriminate between the *primary* events, such as venous or lymphatic obstruction, reduction of cardiac output, hypoalbuminemia, or trapping of fluid in spaces such as the peritoneal cavity, and the predictable *secondary* consequences, which include the renal retention of salt and water. There are instances in which an abnormal positive balance of salt and water may, in fact, be the primary disturbance. In these circumstances the edema is a secondary manifestation of the generalized increase in extracellular fluid volume. These special instances are usually related to conditions characterized by an acute reduction in renal function, such as acute tubular necrosis or acute glomerulonephritis (Fig. 29-1).

These circumstances aside, a hypothesis can be advanced, which, although admittedly incomplete, leads to improved understanding of the events in a variety of edematous states and enhances the perception of their pathophysiology. The basic premise is that the primary disorder concerns one or more alterations in the Starling forces so that there is a net movement of fluid from the vascular system into the interstitium or into a "third space," or from the arterial compartment of the vascular space into the chambers of the heart or into the venous circulation itself. The *effective arterial blood volume,* an as yet poorly defined parameter of the filling of the arterial tree, is reduced, and a series of physiologic responses which are designed to restore it to normal are set into motion. A key element of these responses is the retention of an increment of salt and water, and in many instances this repairs the deficit of the effective arterial blood volume; often this occurs without the development of overt edema. If, however, the retention of salt and water is insufficient to restore and maintain the effective arterial blood volume, the stimuli are not dissipated, the retention of salt and water continues, and edema develops. The sequence of events described above is operative in a variety of circumstances, including dehydration and hemorrhage. Although there is a reduction of effective arterial blood volume and activation of the entire sequence shown on the right side of Fig. 29-1, including the retention of salt and water, edema does not occur because the total extravascular fluid volume is reduced.

Certain data suggest that the increase in volume of some component(s) of the extracellular space normally promotes the secretion of a natriuretic hormone, also referred to as "third factor." The unambiguous demonstration of such a hormone, its site(s) of secretion, and its characterization is yet to be presented. The retention of sodium is accompanied by an increased reabsorption of water. This is attested to by (1) the usual failure to accumulate edema if sodium is not available in the diet, and (2) the successful use of pharmacologic agents and other measures that promote the excretion of sodium chloride in the urine. In most circumstances the mechanisms responsible for maintaining a normal effective osmolality in the body fluids continue to operate efficiently so that sodium retention promotes thirst and secretion of the antidiuretic hormone, which, in turn, lead to the ingestion and retention of approximately 1 liter of water for each 140 mmol sodium retained. Similarly, measures which promote the loss of sodium into the urine are accompanied by the net loss of an equivalent volume of water from the body.

Obstruction of venous and lymphatic drainage of a limb In this condition the hydrostatic pressure in the capillary bed increases so that more fluid is transferred from the vascular to the interstitial space than can be reabsorbed at the venous end of the capillaries; since the alternate route (i.e., the lymphatic channels) is obstructed as well, this event must of necessity cause an increased volume of interstitial fluid in the limb, i.e.,

FIGURE 29-1
Sequence of events leading to the formation and retention of salt and water and the development of edema.

a trapping of fluid in the extremity, at the expense of the blood volume in the remainder of the body, thereby reducing effective arterial blood volume and leading to the consequences shown in Fig. 29-1.

As fluid accumulates in the interstitium of the limb, in which venous and lymphatic drainage are obstructed, tissue tension rises until it is great enough to counterbalance the primary alterations in the Starling forces, at which time no further fluid will accumulate in that limb. At this point the additional accumulation of fluid will repair the deficit in plasma volume, and the stimuli to retain more salt and water are dissipated. The net effect is an increase in the volume of interstitial fluid in a local area, and the secondary responses repair the plasma volume deficit incurred by the primary event. This same sequence may be translated to many other edematous states.

Congestive heart failure (see also Chap. 236) In this disorder it is postulated that the defective systolic emptying of the chambers of the heart promotes an accumulation of blood in the heart and venous circulation at the expense of the arterial volume, and the aforementioned sequence of events (Fig. 29-1) is initiated. In many instances of mild heart failure a small increment of volume may be achieved, which repairs the volume deficit and establishes a new steady state because through the operation of Starling's law of the heart, up to a point an increase in the volume of blood within the chambers of the heart promotes a more forceful contraction and may thereby increase the volume ejected in systole (Fig. 235-4). However, if the cardiac disorder is more severe, retention of fluid cannot repair the deficit in effective arterial blood volume. The increment accumulates in the venous circulation, and the increase in hydrostatic pressure therein promotes the formation of ede-

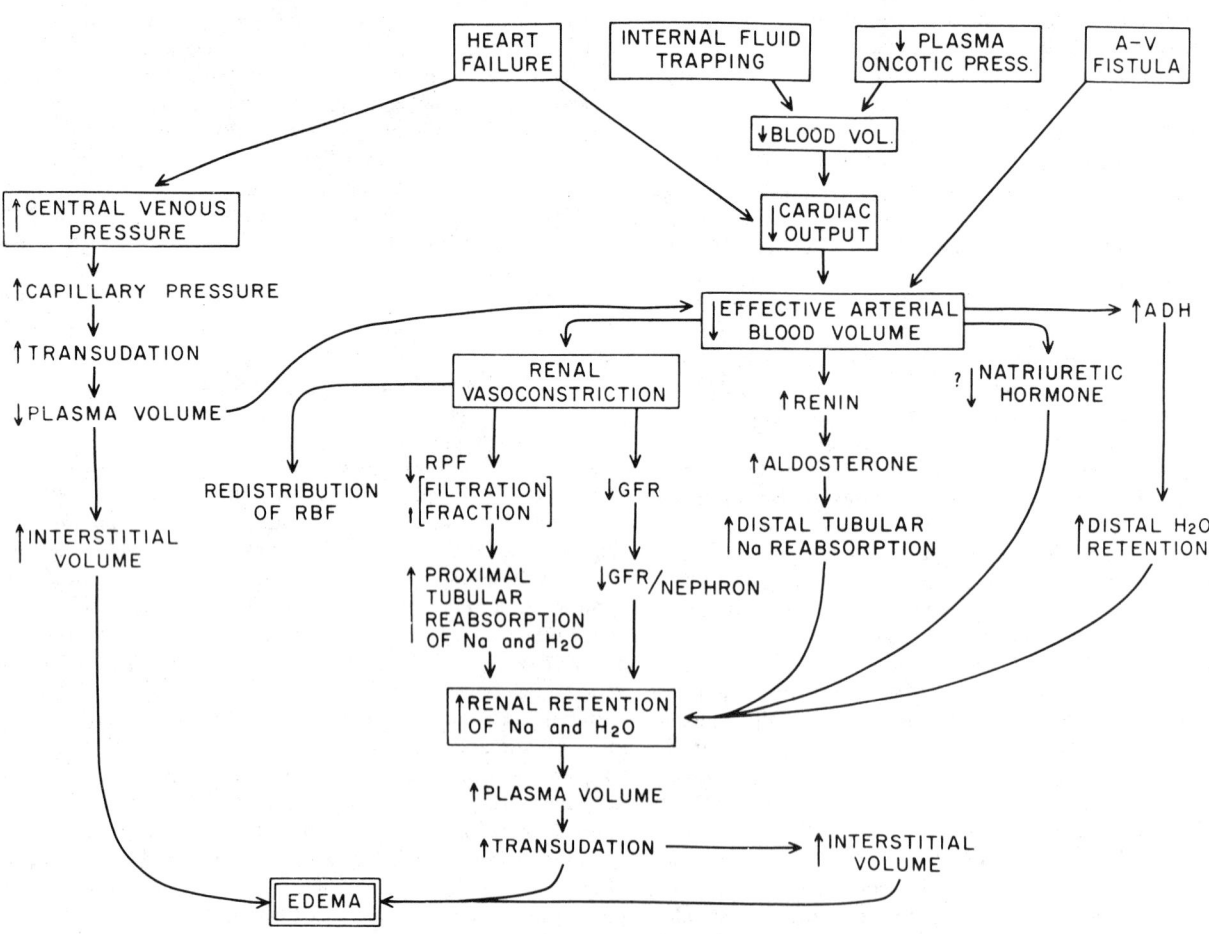

ma. The formation of edema in the lungs (Chap. 27) impairs gas exchange and may induce hypoxia, which embarrasses cardiac function still further.

In addition to the sequence shown on the right-hand side of Fig. 29-1, incomplete ventricular emptying leads to an elevation of ventricular end-diastolic pressure. If the impairment of cardiac function involves the right ventricle primarily, then incomplete ventricular emptying leads to an elevation of right ventricular end-diastolic volume and pressure; as a consequence pressures in the systemic veins and capillaries also rise, thereby augmenting transudation of fluid into the interstitial space and enhancing the likelihood of peripheral edema. If the impairment of cardiac function involves the left ventricle, then pulmonary venous and capillary pressures rise [leading in some instances to pulmonary edema (Chap. 27)], as does pulmonary artery pressure; this in turn interferes with the systolic emptying of the right ventricle, leading to an elevation of right ventricular end-diastolic and central and systemic venous pressures, enhancing the likelihood of edema formation.

A reduction of cardiac output is associated with a reduction of the effective arterial blood volume as well as of renal blood flow and an elevation of the filtration fraction, i.e., the ratio of glomerular filtration rate to renal plasma flow. In severe heart failure the blood flow to the outer renal cortex, in particular, is significantly reduced with less depression in the more central regions of the kidney, and there is a reduction in the glomerular filtration rate. This constriction of renal cortical vessels appears to play an important role in the retention of salt and water and the formation of edema in heart failure. Indirect evidence suggests that at different stages of heart failure, activation of the sympathetic nervous system and of the renin-angiotensin systems is responsible for renal vasoconstriction. Activation of the former can be counteracted by the administration of alpha-adrenergic blocking agents, a finding which indicates that the elevated renal vascular resistance in heart failure is mediated, at least in part, by sympathetic stimuli.

It is generally agreed that an increase in the tubular reabsorption of glomerular filtrate plays a principal role in the salt and water retention of heart failure. However, the precise site(s) in the system composed of the renal tubules, loops of Henle, and collective ducts which is involved is not clear, nor have the responsible mechanism(s) been identified. Alterations in intrarenal hemodynamics appear to play a significant role. Heart failure, by augmenting renal arteriolar constriction, reduces the hydrostatic pressure and raises the colloid osmotic pressure in the peritubular capillaries, thus enhancing salt and water reabsorption in the proximal tubule. The aforementioned distribution of intrarenal blood flow characteristic of heart failure may be responsible for augmentation of sodium reabsorption in the ascending limb of the loop of Henle.

In addition, the diminished renal blood flow characteristic of all states in which the effective arterial blood volume is reduced is translated by the renal juxtaglomerular cells into a signal for increased renin release (Chap. 336). The specific nature of the signal is complex. One factor involves a baroreceptor mechanism, in which reduced renal perfusion results in incomplete filling of the renal arterioles and diminished stretch of the juxtaglomerular cells, a signal that provides for the elaboration or release, or both, of renin. A second mechanism involves the macula densa; as a result of reduced glomerular filtration the sodium load reaching the distal renal tubules is reduced. This is sensed by the macula densa, which in an as yet undefined manner signals the neighboring juxtaglomerular cells to secrete renin. A third mechanism involves the sympathetic nervous system and circulating catecholamines. Activation of the beta-adrenergic receptors in the juxtaglomerular

cells stimulates them to release renin. These three mechanisms generally act in concert.

Renin, an enzyme that has a molecular weight of about 40,000, acts on its substrate, angiotensinogen, an α_2 globulin synthesized by the liver, resulting in the elaboration of angiotensin II, an octapeptide with vasoconstrictor properties. The intrarenal production of angiotensin II may also contribute to renal vasoconstriction in heart failure and to the salt and water retention in this state. Angiotensin II also passes through the circulation and stimulates the production of aldosterone by the zona glomerulosa region of the adrenal cortex. In patients with heart failure, not only is aldosterone secretion elevated, but the biologic half-life of aldosterone is prolonged, indicating a reduced catabolic rate and further increasing the plasma level of the hormone. A depression of hepatic blood flow, particularly during exercise, secondary to a reduction in cardiac output, is responsible for the reduced hepatic catabolism of aldosterone.

Although increased quantities of aldosterone have been demonstrated to be secreted during heart failure and other edematous states, augmented levels of aldosterone (or other mineralocorticoids) do not always promote the accumulation of edema, as witnessed by the lack of striking fluid retention in most instances of primary aldosteronism. Furthermore, although normal subjects will retain some salt and water under the influence of a potent mineralocorticoid, such as deoxycorticosterone acetate or 9α-fluorohydrocortisone, the accumulation appears to be self-limiting, despite continued exposure to the steroid and to salt and water. It is probable that the failure of normal subjects to accumulate large quantities of fluid is a consequence of an increase in glomerular filtration rate, other hemodynamic influences, and most importantly the increase in volume which promotes an increased excretion of salt independent of the filtered load of sodium, i.e., through the action of natriuretic substance(s). The role of aldosterone in the accumulation of fluid in edematous states may be more important because these patients are unable to repair the crucial deficit in volume.

Nephrotic syndrome and other hypoalbuminic states (see also Chap. 278) The primary alteration in this disorder is a diminished colloid oncotic pressure due to massive losses of protein into the urine. This should promote a net movement of fluid into the interstitium and hypovolemia, and initiate the sequence of events described above. As long as the hypoalbuminemia is severe, the salt and water retained cannot be restrained within the vascular compartment, and hence the stimuli to retain salt and water are not abated. A similar sequence of events occurs in other conditions which lead to severe hypoalbuminemia, including severe nutritional deficiency states, protein-losing enteropathy, congenital hypoalbuminemia, and severe, chronic liver disease.

Cirrhosis (see also Chaps. 40 and 304) The total blood volume in cirrhosis of the liver is commonly increased when the disorder is accompanied by a system of dilated venous radicles and multiple small arteriovenous fistulas. Effective systemic perfusion and the effective arterial blood volume appear to be diminished, probably as a consequence of the passage of blood through these fistulas. The enlarged abdominal venous system resulting from obstruction of the lymphatic drainage of the liver, as well as from portal vein obstruction, also promotes a deficit in the arterial component. These alterations are frequently complicated by the reduced serum albumin characteristic of cirrhosis, which tends to reduce the effective arterial blood volume even further. Initially, the excess interstitial fluid is localized preferentially behind the congested portal venous system and obstructed hepatic lymphatics, i.e., in the peritoneal cavity. In late stages of the disease, particularly when there is hypoalbuminemia, peripheral edema may also be noted.

Idiopathic cyclic edema This syndrome, which occurs predominantly in women, particularly those with psychosocial difficulties, is characterized by periodic episodes of edema, frequently accompanied by abdominal distention. Fairly large, diurnal alterations in weight occur, so that the patient may well weigh several pounds more in the evening than in the morning after having been in the upright posture most of the day. Such large diurnal weight changes suggest an increase in capillary permeability which appears to fluctuate in severity. The fact that it occurs most commonly in women and appears to have some temporal relation to the menstrual cycle suggests that there may be some hormonal influence in the permeability of the vessels which permits the loss of plasma volume into the interstitial space and the sequence of events secondary to a contraction in plasma volume.

The treatment of idiopathic cyclic edema includes a reduction in salt intake, education in the use of rest in the supine position for several hours each day, the wearing of elastic stockings which are put on before arising in the morning, and an attempt to understand the underlying emotional problems. Diuretics are initially effective but may lose their effectiveness with continuous administration; accordingly, they should be employed sparingly. It has been reported that the plasma concentration of cyclic adenosine monophosphate (AMP) is high in patients with idiopathic edema in both the recumbent and upright positions, and its renal clearance, unlike that of creatinine, is low. If a relationship between extracellular cyclic AMP and the action of hormones on beta-adrenergic receptors could be established, the favorable therapeutic effect of propranolol in cases where diuretics alone did not satisfactorily control the disease could be explained.

DIFFERENTIAL DIAGNOSIS As a rule, localized edema can be readily differentiated from generalized edema. The great majority of patients with noninflammatory generalized edema of significant degree suffer from advanced cardiac, renal, hepatic, or nutritional disorders. Consequently, the differential diagnosis of generalized edema should be directed toward implicating or excluding these several conditions.

Localized edema Edema originating from inflammation or hypersensitivity is usually readily identified. Localized edema due to venous or lymphatic obstruction may be caused by thrombophlebitis, chronic lymphangitis, resection of regional lymph nodes, filariasis, etc. Lymph edema is particularly intractable because restriction of lymphatic flow results in increased protein concentration in the interstitial fluid, a circumstance which severely impedes removal of retained fluid.

Edema of heart failure Evidence of heart disease, as manifested by cardiac enlargement and gallop rhythm together with evidence of cardiac failure, such as dyspnea, basilar rales, diminished vital capacity, prolonged circulation time, venous distention, increased venous pressure, and hepatomegaly, usually provides an indication of the pathogenesis of edema resulting from heart failure (see also Chap. 236).

Edema of the nephrotic syndrome Massive proteinuria, severe hypoproteinemia, and in some instances hypercholesterolemia are present. This syndrome may occur during the course of a variety of kidney diseases, which include glomerulonephritis,

diabetic glomerulosclerosis, and hypersensitivity reactions. A history of previous renal disease may or may not be elicited (see also Chap. 278).

Edema of acute glomerulonephritis The edema occurring during the acute phases of glomerulonephritis is characteristically associated with hematuria, proteinuria, and hypertension. Although some evidence supports the view that the fluid retention is due to increased capillary permeability, in most instances the edema in this disease results from primary retention of sodium and water by the kidneys owing to renal insufficiency. This state differs from congestive heart failure in that it is characterized by a normal or increased cardiac output, normal or diminished circulation time, a reduction in the packed cell volume, a normal arteriovenous oxygen difference, and failure to respond to a digitalis preparation. Patients commonly have evidence of pulmonary congestion on chest roentgenograms before cardiac enlargement is significant and do not develop orthopnea. If one cannot discriminate between the congested state and congestive heart failure, use of a cardiac glycoside is appropriate, but special care should be taken to avoid digitalis intoxication in a patient with impaired renal function (see also Chap. 278).

Edema of cirrhosis Ascites and evidence of hepatic disease (collateral venous channels, jaundice, and spider angiomas) characterize edema of hepatic origin. The ascites is frequently refractory to treatment because it collects as a result of a combination of obstruction of hepatic lymphatic drainage, portal hypertension and hypoalbuminemia. Edema may also occur in other parts of the body in these patients as a result of hypoalbuminemia. Furthermore, the sizable accumulation of ascitic fluid may be expected to increase intraabdominal pressure and impede venous return from the lower extremities; hence, it tends to promote accumulation of edema in this region as well (see also Chap. 304).

Edema of nutritional origin An inadequate diet over a prolonged period may produce hypoproteinemia and edema, which may be intensified by beriberi heart disease, in which multiple peripheral arteriovenous fistulas result in reduced effective systemic perfusion and effective arterial blood volume, thereby enhancing edema formation. More striking edema is commonly observed when these famished subjects are provided with an adequate diet. The mechanism responsible for this latter phenomenon is not clear, but the ingestion of more food may increase the quantity of salt ingested, which is then retained along with water. Edema of nutritional origin may be more apparent than under other circumstances, because the subcutaneous tissue is so depleted of fat that modest collections of edema may be more obvious than they would be in a well-nourished subject.

Distribution The distribution of edema is an important guide to the cause. Thus, edema of one leg or of one or both arms is usually the result of venous and/or lymphatic obstruction. Edema resulting from hypoproteinemia characteristically is generalized, but it is especially evident in the eyelids and face and tends to be most pronounced in the morning because of the recumbent posture assumed during the night. Edema associated with heart failure, on the other hand, tends to be more extensive in the legs and to be accentuated in the evening, a feature also determined largely by posture. In the rare types of cardiac disease, such as tricuspid stenosis and constrictive pericarditis, in which orthopnea may be absent and the patient actually prefers the recumbent posture, the factor of gravity may be equalized and facial edema observed. Less common causes of facial edema include trichinosis, allergic reactions, and myxedema. Unilateral edema occasionally results from lesions in the central nervous system affecting the vasomotor fibers on one side of the body; paralysis also reduces lymphatic and venous drainage on the affected side.

Additional factors in diagnosis The color, thickness, and sensitivity of the skin are significant. Local tenderness and increase in temperature suggest inflammation. Local cyanosis may signify a venous obstruction. In individuals who have had repeated episodes of prolonged edema, the skin over the involved areas may be thickened, hard, and often red.

Measurement of the venous pressure is also of great importance in evaluating edema. Elevation in an isolated part of the body usually reflects localized venous obstruction. Generalized elevation of systemic venous pressure suggests the presence of congestive heart failure, although it may be present in the congested state that accompanies acute renal insufficiency. Ordinarily, significant increase in venous pressure can be recognized by the level at which cervical veins collapse; in doubtful cases and for accurate recording, the central venous pressure should be measured. In patients with obstruction of the superior vena cava, edema is confined to the face, neck, and upper extremities, where the venous pressure is elevated compared with that in the lower extremities. Measurement of venous pressure in the upper extremities is also useful in patients with massive edema of the lower extremities and ascites; it is elevated when the edema is on a cardiac basis (e.g., constrictive pericarditis or tricuspid stenosis), but is normal when it is secondary to cirrhosis.

Determination of the concentration of serum proteins, and especially of serum albumin, clearly differentiates those patients in whom edema is due entirely or in part to diminished intravascular colloid osmotic pressure. The presence of proteinuria affords useful clues. The complete absence of protein in the urine is evidence against, but does not exclude, either cardiac or renal disease as a cause of edema. Slight to moderate proteinuria is the rule in patients with heart failure, whereas persistent massive proteinuria usually reflects the presence of the nephrotic syndrome. Valuable information can also be obtained from other features of the examination. Some of these are the presence or absence of heart disease, the character of the urinary sediment, the dietary history, and a history of alcoholism.

APPROACH TO THE PATIENT WITH EDEMA A significant question to ask is whether the edema is localized or generalized. If it is localized, those phenomena alluded to above that may be responsible should be concentrated upon. In this context, localized edema may include hydrothorax, ascites, or both, in the absence of congestive heart failure or hypoalbuminemia. Either of these collections may be a consequence of local venous or lymphatic obstruction, as in inflammatory disease or carcinoma. It is a frequent accompaniment of an inflammatory process which involves the pleura or peritoneum, and the cause of the inflammatory process may vary from bacterial invasion to infarction or underlying parenchyma to a diffuse connective tissue disease with vasculitis, etc. In instances of either hydrothorax or ascites, an examination of the characteristics of the fluid is extremely important. This should include bacterial culture, smear with stains for ordinary and less common infectious agents, determination of protein concentration, cell count, and the presence or absence of blood; the cells should be concentrated by centrifugation and preparation for histologic examination for evidences of malignancy and other characteristics.

If the edema is generalized, it should be determined, first, if there is hypoalbuminemia of significant degree, e.g., serum albumin concentration less than 2.5 g per 100 ml. If there is, a history, physical examination, and other laboratory data will help evaluate the question of cirrhosis, severe malnutrition, protein-losing gastroenteropathy, or the nephrotic syndrome as the underlying disorder. It should then be determined if there is evidence of congestive heart failure of a severity to promote generalized edema even in the absence of hypoalbuminemia, or if there is evidence of both congestive heart failure and some degree of hypoalbuminemia. Finally, it should be ascertained whether the patient has an adequate urine output, or is there significant oliguria or even anuria? These abnormalities are discussed in Chaps. 43, 275, and 276. The major differential diagnosis in these instances is frequently the discrimination between overload with fluid and a congested state as opposed to congestive heart failure.

REFERENCES

BRAUNWALD E et al: *Mechanisms of Contraction of the Normal and Failing Heart*, 2d ed. Boston, Little, Brown, 1976

BRENNER BM, STEIN JH (eds): *Sodium and Water Homeostasis.* New York, Churchill Livingstone, 1978

COGGINS CP: Edema, in *Signs and Symptoms,* 6th ed, RS Blacklow (ed). Philadelphia, Lippincott, 1977, chap. 36

DE WARDENER HE: The control of sodium excretion, in *Handbook of Physiology,* vol 8: *Renal Physiology,* J Orloff et al (eds). Washington, The American Physiological Society, 1973, chap 21, p 677

EARLEY LE, SCHRIER RW: Intrarenal control of sodium excretion by hemodynamic and physical factors, in *Handbook of Physiology,* vol 8: *Renal Physiology,* J Orloff et al (eds). Washington, The American Physiological Society, 1973, chap 22, p 721

GUYTON AC: Edema, in *Textbook of Medical Physiology,* 5th ed. Philadelphia, Saunders, 1976, p 403

LARAGH JH, SEALEY JE: The renin-angiotensin-aldosterone hormonal system and regulation of sodium, potassium and blood pressure homeostasis, in *Handbook of Physiology,* vol 8: *Renal Physiology,* J Orloff et al (eds). Washington, The American Physiological Society, 1973, chap 26, p 831

LEVY M, SEELY J: Pathophysiology of edema formation, in *The Kidney,* 2d ed, BM Brenner, FC Rector Jr (eds). Philadelphia, Saunders, 1980, chap 15

30
HYPOTENSION AND THE SHOCK SYNDROME

KARL ENGELMAN
EUGENE BRAUNWALD

The differential diagnosis of hypotensive states and the development of a rational plan of therapy require understanding of the normal regulation of arterial pressure.

CONTROL OF ARTERIAL PRESSURE Arterial pressure must be maintained at levels sufficient to permit adequate perfusion of the extensive capillary networks in the systemic vascular bed. The level of pressure in the central arterial bed is in a large measure dependent on two factors—the volume of blood ejected by the left ventricle per unit of time, i.e., the cardiac output, and the resistance to blood flow offered by the vessels in the peripheral vascular bed. The resistance of a blood vessel, in turn, varies inversely as the fourth power of its radius, and at any given level of cardiac output arterial pressure is therefore largely dependent upon the degree of constriction of the smooth muscle in the walls of the arterioles. Though resistance to flow also varies with the viscosity of the fluid and the length of the vessels, alterations in these factors are ordinarily of only secondary importance.

Cardiac output is controlled largely by factors which regulate ventricular end-diastolic volume, the level of myocardial contractility, and heart rate (Chap. 235). The autonomic nervous system plays a major role in the maintenance of arterial pressure by its influences on the cardiac output and on the degree of constriction of the resistance (arterioles) and capacitance (venules and veins) vessels. The afferent limbs of the autonomic reflex arcs regulating arterial pressure acutely arise in stretch receptors in the carotid sinuses, the aortic arch, the chambers of the heart, and the lungs. Impulses are transmitted along afferent fibers in the glossopharyngeal and vagus nerves to extensive central autonomic connections in the medulla. Synapses connect not only the sympathetic and parasympathetic nuclei and efferent arcs, but also the cerebral cortex and hypothalamic nuclei which control hormonal secretion via the pituitary gland.

A rapid reduction of arterial pressure diminishes the stimulation of pressoreceptors, which in turn activates sympathetic outflow and inhibits parasympathetic activity. As a result, the vascular smooth muscle in arterioles and veins constricts, while heart rate and myocardial contractility are augmented. In addition, as arterial pressure falls, adrenal medullary secretion increases, along with the output of antidiuretic hormone (ADH), adrenocorticotropic hormone (ACTH), renin, and aldosterone; all these effects act to restore the arterial pressure to control levels. Opposite changes occur if arterial pressure is raised acutely. Thus, the operation of the pressoreceptor and a number of humoral systems normally serve to buffer the body from a variety of influences which would otherwise produce marked alterations in arterial pressure.

MEASUREMENT OF ARTERIAL PRESSURE Arterial pressure is determined clinically with a pneumatic cuff; ordinarily, this indirect method provides slight underestimation of the true arterial pressure. Considerable error may be introduced if proper precautions are not taken in determining blood pressure by this method. The arterial pressure may be significantly underestimated if the air in the cuff is released too rapidly, especially in the presence of bradycardia or an irregular rhythm, or if inadequate inflation of the cuff does not result in complete vascular occlusion. This indirect method is most accurate when, in normal-sized adults, cuffs 12 to 14 cm in width are employed. However, when a cuff of this size is used on children or adults with unusually thin arms, blood pressure may be seriously underestimated, or conversely, it may be overestimated when employed on an arm or thigh greater than 20 cm in girth. Marked vasoconstriction resulting in severely attenuated limb blood flow and/or marked reductions in pulse pressure may also result in serious underestimation of arterial pressure by the auscultatory method. Direct intraarterial recordings may reveal a normal or even an elevated pressure, while the absence of Korotkov sounds makes the pressure unobtainable by the indirect methods.

THE "NORMAL" BLOOD PRESSURE The "normal" blood pressure is difficult to define. Traditional statistical approaches define normality on the basis of values included within two standard deviations of the mean of pressures obtained in a large population of presumably healthy individuals. On this basis 95 percent of the population are defined as being normotensive, the remaining 5 percent evenly divided between the hypertensive and hypotensive groups. A better definition of abnormality would be based on demonstrated deleterious effects of blood pressure levels exceeding certain limits. If such

criteria are used, chronic hypotension would seem to occur very rarely. However, the incidence of hypertension based on casual blood pressure levels exceeding 160/95 (widely accepted as hazardous) is estimated to be approximately 15 percent in the adult population of the United States, the incidence in the black population exceeding that in the nonblacks by 50 to 100 percent. Even these statistics may understate the prevalence of hypertension if one accepts the validity of actuarial data indicating that longevity is shortened progressively in adults whose blood pressures exceed 100/60. The hazard of hypertension and its major complication, widespread vascular disease, appears to be a function of the level of blood pressure; the hazard rises more steeply with higher levels, especially as they exceed diastolic values of 90 to 95 mmHg (Chap. 251).

ACUTE HYPOTENSION AND SHOCK

Not uncommonly, physicians are called upon to treat patients who acutely develop severe hypotension or shock. These two terms are not synonymous; although shock is usually associated with hypotension, a previously hypertensive patient may be in shock despite an arterial pressure within normal limits, and hypotension may occur in the absence of shock. *Shock* may be defined as a state in which there is widespread, serious reduction of tissue perfusion, which, if prolonged, leads to generalized impairment of cellular function.

CAUSES The most common clinical causes of shock are listed in Table 30-1. Since arterial pressure is dependent on

TABLE 30-1
Etiologic factors in shock

I Hypovolemia
  A External fluid losses
    1 Hemorrhage
    2 Gastrointestinal
      a Vomiting (pyloric stenosis, intestinal obstruction)
      b Diarrhea
    3 Renal
      a Diabetes mellitus
      b Diabetes insipidus
      c Excessive use of diuretics
    4 Cutaneous
      a Burns
      b Exudative lesions
      c Perspiration and insensible water loss without replacement
  B Internal sequestration
    1 Fractures
    2 Ascites (peritonitis, pancreatitis, cirrhosis)
    3 Intestinal obstruction
    4 Hemothorax
    5 Hemoperitoneum
II Cardiogenic
  A Myocardial infarction
  B Arrhythmia (paroxysmal tachycardia or fibrillation, severe bradycardia)
  C Severe congestive heart failure with low cardiac output
III Obstruction to blood flow
  A Pulmonary embolus
  B Tension pneumothorax
  C Cardiac tamponade
  D Dissecting aortic aneurysm
  E Intracardiac (ball valve thrombus, atrial myxoma)
IV Neuropathic
  A Drug induced
    1 Anesthesia
    2 Ganglion-blocking or other antihypertensive drugs
    3 "Ingestion" (barbiturates, glutethimide, phenothiazines)
  B Spinal cord injury
  C Orthostatic hypotension (primary autonomic insufficiency, peripheral neuropathies)
V Other
  A Infection
    1 Gram-negative septicemia (endotoxin)
    2 Other septicemias
  B Anaphylaxis
  C Endocrine failure (Addison's disease, myxedema)
  D Anoxia

cardiac output and peripheral vasomotor tone, marked reductions in either of these variables without a compensatory elevation of the other results in systemic hypotension. Reduction of cardiac output due to hypovolemia or acute myocardial infarction is among the most frequently encountered and easily categorized causes of shock. Failure of neurogenic mechanisms resulting in decreased vasoconstrictor impulses is another well-defined category; in many patients, particularly in the late stages of shock, multiple factors figure in the development of circulatory failure.

Hypovolemia has been studied much more extensively than any other cause of shock; the mechanism of development is usually readily evident and well understood, and therapy, i.e., restoration of blood volume, is both simple and effective if applied before irreversible tissue damage occurs. Whether the primary insult is the external loss of blood, plasma, or water and salt or the internal sequestration of these fluids in a hollow viscus or body cavity, the general effect is similar, i.e., reduced venous return and decreased cardiac output. For purposes of a general discussion of shock, hemorrhagic hypovolemia will be used as the model, but the consequences of general reduced tissue perfusion are similar in other forms of shock.

Stages of hypovolemic shock Depending upon the severity and rate of development of hypovolemia, the shock syndrome may develop abruptly or evolve gradually. If the precipitating factors progress unabated, the endogenous defense mechanisms, while initially competent to maintain adequate circulation, eventually are extended beyond their capacity for compensation. The development of the shock syndrome may be thought to evolve through several stages which merge with one another:

1 The period in which the blood volume deficit is relatively minor and in which the patient may be asymptomatic. In a previously healthy individual compensation for an acute blood loss of as much as 10 percent of the normal blood volume (as with venesection of 500 ml blood from a donor) is achieved acutely by constriction of the arteriolar bed and an augmentation of heart rate, effects mediated by reflex increases in sympathetic neural discharge of norepinephrine from sympathetic nerve endings and of both norepinephrine and epinephrine from the adrenal medulla. Other responses with more gradual effects include the increased secretion of antidiuretic hormone and the activation of the renin-angiotensin-aldosterone axis (Chap. 336). Arterial pressure is maintained and cardiac output is normal, or only slightly reduced, primarily as a consequence of selective reductions of blood flow to the skin and muscle beds.

2 With a reduction of blood volume of 15 to 25 percent, cardiac output falls markedly, and despite intense arteriolar constriction in most vascular beds, arterial pressure declines, although proportionately less than cardiac output. Generalized venoconstriction occurs, increasing the fraction of the total blood volume in the central circulation and tending to sustain venous return. Accompanying this massive reflex adrenergic discharge are tachycardia, tachypnea, intense cutaneous vasoconstriction, pallor, diaphoresis, piloerection, oliguria, apprehension, and restlessness. The latter mental signs relate to primary reduction in cerebral circulation due to decreased perfusion pressure rather than to local vasoconstriction. Angina may occur in patients who have intrinsic coronary vascular disease.

3 Once the patient has achieved this state of maximal mobilization of compensatory mechanisms, small additional losses of blood result in rapid deterioration of the circulation, with life-threatening reductions of cardiac output, blood pressure, and tissue perfusion. The duration of this shock state, the severity of tissue anoxia, and the age and underlying phys-

ical state of the patient are of primary importance in determining the ultimate outcome. If tissue perfusion is restored rapidly, recovery may be expected. However, if shock persists, the severe vasoconstriction may itself become a complicating factor, and by reducing tissue perfusion even further may initiate a vicious cycle leading to an irreversible state due to widespread cellular injury. Blood flow to the brain, heart, and kidneys is further reduced, and severe ischemia of these vital organs leads to irreversible tissue damage which may result in impaired function of the organ and, eventually, death. Impaired coronary perfusion depresses cardiac function, particularly in patients with some coronary vascular obstruction, and this may lead to further lowering of cardiac output, thus perpetuating a vicious cycle. Cardiac function is also depressed by the release of myocardial *depressant factor(s)* from other hypoperfused organs. Reduced flow to the medullary vasomotor center late in the stage of shock depresses the activity of compensatory reflexes. Anoxia, hypercapnia, and lactic acidosis result from hypoperfusion of tissues and anaerobic metabolism. These metabolic derangements ultimately result in failure of the energy-requiring active transport systems of cell membranes. The cellular high-energy phosphate reserves are depleted. The integrity of the cells is compromised, and potassium ions, intracellular lysosomal enzymes, peptides, and other vasoactive compounds are released into the circulation. The integrity of capillary membranes is disrupted, and fluid, proteins, and cellular constituents of the blood seep into the extravascular space of tissues.

In profound shock from any cause an additional important factor which may exacerbate the status of microcirculation is widespread disseminated intravascular coagulation (DIC) in the bowel, kidney, and other organs. The resultant ischemia produced in the bowel may further complicate the circulatory compensation as a result of breakdown of the mucosal barrier, leading to entry of bacteria and toxic bacterial products into the circulation. Similar changes in the capillary network of the lungs result in interstitial and alveolar edema and impaired respiratory gas transfer. Because many bacterial substances are potent vasodilators, vasoconstrictor mechanisms may be inhibited, with a further decrease in blood pressure despite intense sympathetic activity.

Just as tissue perfusion may fall to dangerous or even fatal levels because of actual fluid losses or sequestration with diminished venous return, cardiac failure or intrathoracic obstruction to blood flow may have a similar effect. Furthermore, even in the presence of a normal blood volume and cardiac function, "vasomotor collapse" due to drug-induced or neuropathic failure of sympathetic vasomotor activity can result in shock because of reduction of peripheral resistance and the pooling of blood in the venous bed.

Other forms of shock A complex form of shock may result from infection, especially gram-negative bacteremia with endotoxin release. This form of shock is associated with vascular pooling, diminished venous return, and reduced cardiac output. Sometimes there is inadequate vasoconstriction with a decline in perfusion pressures. At other stages there is intense vasoconstriction with tissue damage secondary to reduced perfusion. In anaphylactic shock, release of histamine or a histaminelike substance causes venous dilatation and an attendant increase in vascular capacity and reduction in cardiac output. Also, it results in arteriolar dilatation and a reduction of perfusion pressure, as well as increased capillary permeability with loss of intravascular volume.

TREATMENT This should be directed toward the rapid restoration of cardiac output and tissue perfusion. General supportive measures must be undertaken immediately, sometimes even before the cause of the shock state has been identified. Whether shock results from decreased cardiac output due to a primary reduction in intravascular volume or from a reduction of "effective blood volume" with pooling of blood in certain vascular beds, the most effective means of restoring adequate circulation is by the rapid infusion of volume-expanding fluids (whole blood, plasma, plasma substitutes, or isotonic electrolyte solutions). However, when shock is secondary to, or is accompanied by, cardiac failure with increased pulmonary vascular and central venous pressures, the infusion of volume-expanding fluids may result in pulmonary edema. Here attention must be directed toward restoring cardiac function with cardiotonic drugs such as digitalis glycosides and isoproterenol, and an attempt should be made to support arterial pressure at levels sufficient to maintain the coronary perfusion pressure (Chap. 245). Arrhythmias, which may also contribute to the low cardiac output, should be corrected (Chap. 237).

The appearance of the external jugular veins may be helpful in differentiating between shock with high or low central venous pressure. However, catheters inserted into the superior vena cava and, if possible, into the pulmonary artery (a Swan-Ganz balloon-tipped catheter) are the best means for continuously monitoring venous pressure and of considerable value in guiding therapy; such catheters should be inserted in patients with shock whenever possible. Serial measurements of central venous pressure, urine flow rate, heart rate, and the clinical and mental state of the patient often provide more important indexes of the efficacy of therapy than arterial pressure changes do. In patients with shock and impaired left ventricular function, e.g., cardiogenic shock due to massive acute myocardial infarction, the balloon-tipped catheter "floated" into the pulmonary artery at the bedside without the aid of fluoroscopy is essential in guiding treatment (Chap. 245).

There is considerable debate concerning the efficacy of vasoconstrictor drugs in shock. In patients with severe peripheral constriction these agents are often ineffective and may actually reduce the already lowered tissue perfusion. However, these drugs are usually helpful in patients with inadequate vasoconstrictor responses. The use of alpha-adrenergic blocking agents or massive doses of adrenal glucocorticoids in shock secondary to gram-negative septicemia with endotoxin release is also a matter of considerable controversy and cannot yet be considered a routine procedure. Following immediate attention to improvement of perfusion, attention should be directed to treating the underlying etiologic factor, such as diabetic acidosis, pneumothorax, or septicemia (Table 30-1).

CHRONIC HYPOTENSION

Although many patients have been treated for chronic "low blood pressure," most of them, with systolic pressures in the range of 90 to 110 mmHg, are normal and may actually have a greater life expectancy than those with higher pressures. Patients with true chronic hypotension may complain of lethargy, weakness, easy fatigability, and dizziness or faintness, especially if arterial pressure is lowered further when the erect position is assumed. These symptoms are presumably due to a decrease in perfusion of the brain, heart, skeletal muscle, and other organs.

Chronic hypotension occasionally results from severe re-

ductions of the cardiac output. The major endocrine causes of chronic hypotension are associated with deficient gluco- and mineralocorticoid secretion and resultant reductions of the intravascular and interstitial fluid volume. Hypotension is usually more pronounced in patients with primary adrenocortical insufficiency than in those with hypopituitarism because secretion of the salt-retaining adrenocortical hormone, aldosterone, is partially preserved in pituitary insufficiency (Chap. 336).

Malnutrition, cachexia, chronic bed rest, and a variety of neurologic disorders may result in chronic hypotension, especially in the standing position. Interference with the neural pathways anywhere between the vasomotor center and the efferent sympathetic nerve endings on the blood vessels or heart may prevent the vasoconstriction and increase in cardiac output which occur as a normal response to a reduction in arterial pressure. Multiple sclerosis, amyotrophic lateral sclerosis, syringomyelia, syphilitic or diabetic tabes dorsalis, peripheral neuropathies, spinal cord section, diabetic neuropathy, extensive lumbodorsal sympathectomy, and the administration of drugs interfering with nerve transmission in the sympathetic nervous system are all associated with orthostatic hypotension. In addition, *idiopathic orthostatic hypotension* (primary autonomic insufficiency), a rare condition in which there is degeneration of central and/or peripheral autonomic nervous structures, may result in such severe orthostatic hypotension that syncope or seizures occur when the patient arises from recumbency. This condition is progressive and characterized by ascending anhidrosis and loss of hair, decreased basal metabolic rate (BMR), reduced norepinephrine production, deficient secretion of lacrimal and salivary glands, ileus, bladder atony, and absence of tachycardia on standing despite the marked reduction of blood pressure.

Those patients with central nervous system disease have normal resting plasma norepinephrine levels, while those with only peripheral autonomic disease have depressed levels at rest. Both groups fail to increase their circulating concentrations of the neurotransmitter during standing and exercise. Thus, it appears that patients with orthostatic hypotension and central nervous system disease have an intact peripheral sympathetic nervous system, but are unable to activate it, while those without central disease have true insufficiency of the peripheral autonomic nervous system.

Specific therapy is not available for most of the neurologic causes of orthostatic hypotension, and treatment with sympathomimetic drugs has not proved effective over prolonged periods. However, the expansion of extracellular volume, which may be achieved with a high-salt diet (10 to 20 g per day), and/or the potent synthetic salt-retaining steroid, 9α-fluorohydrocortisone (0.1 to 0.5 mg per day) may be helpful. Tight, full-length elastic supportive hose to reduce orthostatic pooling of blood in the legs may also be helpful in sustaining arterial pressure, and in the most severe cases pressurized aviator suits may be necessary to permit ambulation.

REFERENCES

ANDERSON RW: Shock and circulatory collapse, in *Gibbon's Surgery of the Chest*, 3d ed, DC Sabiston, FC Spencer (eds). Philadelphia, Saunders, 1976, chap 5, p 107

CHRISTY JH: Pathophysiology of gram-negative shock. Am Heart J 81:694, 1971

GUYTON AC: Circulatory shock and physiology of its treatment, in *Textbook of Medical Physiology*, 5th ed. Philadelphia, Saunders, 1976, chap 28, p 357

NICKERSON M: Vascular adjustments during the development of shock. Can Med Assoc J 103:853, 1971

SOBEL BE: Shock, in *Heart Disease*, E Braunwald (ed). Philadelphia, Saunders, 1980, chap 18

WEIL MH et al: Treatment of circulatory shock. JAMA 231:1280, 1975

ZIEGLER MG et al: The sympathetic nervous system defect in primary orthostatic hypotension. N Engl J Med 296:293, 1977

31
ELEVATION OF ARTERIAL PRESSURE

GORDON H. WILLIAMS
KARL ENGELMAN
EUGENE BRAUNWALD

DIAGNOSIS OF HYPERTENSION Patients with elevations of arterial pressure are usually asymptomatic, and the blood pressure abnormality often arouses attention only incidentally during military, life insurance, or other periodic physical examinations. Because hypertension results in secondary organ damage and a reduced life span, it should be evaluated fully and, when appropriate, treated.

Often, however, the first question is whether patients with a moderately elevated routine blood pressure recording are truly hypertensive. It is well established that anxiety, discomfort, physical activity, or other stress can acutely and transiently raise arterial pressure. Most persons have a higher pressure when initially examined than after several measurements made in the course of a single visit; in order to establish the diagnosis of hypertension, it is necessary to document in the course of several examinations that arterial pressure remains elevated (Chap. 251). This precaution need not be taken in patients with markedly elevated blood pressure and/or in those in whom significant target organ damage is already manifest. Patients with transient or "labile" hypertension may not require immediate treatment but should be reexamined periodically, since over the course of time they often develop sustained hypertension.

Systolic hypertension is most commonly seen in elderly patients with decreased compliance of the aortic wall and, like diastolic hypertension, is a risk factor for the development of atherosclerosis (Chap. 251). When systolic hypertension is due to an elevated stroke volume, as in patients with severe bradycardia, thyrotoxicosis, severe anemia, aortic valvular regurgitation, arteriovenous shunts or fistulae, patent ductus arteriosus, or the hyperkinetic heart syndrome, it is usually accompanied by a reduced diastolic pressure and a normal mean pressure, and under these circumstances it does not appear to be a risk factor for atherosclerosis.

Regardless of the primary cause, the hemodynamic abnormality in most patients with increased systolic, mean, and diastolic arterial pressures is increased vascular resistance, especially at the level of the smaller muscular arteries and arterioles, though a small number of patients may have an increased cardiac output, particularly in the early stages of the illness. In some patients, hypertension is associated with hypervolemia.

MECHANISM OF HYPERTENSION Arterial pressure is the product of cardiac output and peripheral resistance. Cardiac output in turn is dependent on four interrelated factors (Chap. 235): (1) myocardial contractile state (contractility, inotropic state, or the position of the heart's force-velocity curve); (2) preload—i.e., the length of cardiac muscle at the onset of contraction; (3) afterload—the tension which the muscle is called upon to develop during contraction; and (4) heart rate.

Peripheral resistance is determined by the intrinsic physical characteristics of the resistance vessels, i.e., the ratio of lumen to wall thickness, as well as the neurohumoral influences that act on vascular smooth muscle; the latter include the neurotransmitters norepinephrine, a vasoconstrictor, and in some vessels, acetylcholine, a vasodilator. Humoral and locally acting substances include angiotensin II (a vasoconstrictor) and prostaglandins and kinins (vasodilators). Hypoxia and products of metabolism, such as H^+, lactic acid, and perhaps most important, adenosine, also exert potent *local* vasodilating influences.

For arterial pressure to rise, there must be an increase either in cardiac output or peripheral resistance, or both. Theories of the pathogenesis of essential hypertension have suggested increases in either cardiac output or peripheral resistance as the initiating events.

In 1963, Borst and Borst de Geus proposed that "hypertension is part of a homeostatic reaction to deficient renal sodium output." The proposed abnormality in renal function, i.e., reduced sodium excretion at normal arterial pressure, might be secondary to (1) a primary (perhaps genetic) tubular defect, (2) mild increases in mineralocorticoid activity, (3) decreased renal kallikrein-kinin or prostaglandin activity, or (4) *local* increases in vasoconstrictor activity (angiotensin II or sympathetic nervous system), reducing renal blood flow and secondarily sodium excretion. Regardless of the mechanism of salt retention, according to this concept, blood volume rises because of the decreased sodium excretion, raising central venous pressure and preload, and thereby, cardiac output, i.e., systemic blood flow. However, tissues have the intrinsic capacity to regulate this overperfusion down to appropriate levels by increasing local vascular resistance. When resistance is increased in many vascular beds, arterial pressure rises and serves as negative feedback by increasing cardiac afterload, thereby depressing stroke volume and cardiac output (Fig. 235-6). As has been shown by Guyton, and others, the elevated arterial (renal perfusion) pressure also increases the urinary excretion of sodium, thereby serving as a source of negative feedback and reducing blood volume, central venous pressure, preload, and ultimately cardiac output. Thus, the end result of this process would be increased peripheral resistance and arterial pressure, with all other parameters, including blood volume, cardiac output, and renal sodium excretion, remaining normal. Indeed, this sequence has been documented in experimental human (desoxycorticosterone) and animal (renal artery stenosis) hypertension. However, in patients with essential hypertension, most investigations have reported only a normal cardiac output and elevated peripheral resistance, suggesting either that the studies have not been performed early enough in the course of the disease or that this theory is incorrect in that a change in peripheral resistance is actually a *primary* rather than secondary event.

Such a primary elevation in peripheral resistance can occur either because of an increase in factors tending to produce vasoconstriction, a reduction in factors producing vasodilation, or a change in the arterial smooth muscle—i.e., an increase in muscle mass or an increase in its responsiveness and/or sensitivity to vasoconstrictor stimuli. Each theory has it advocates. Thus, the hypertension associated with emotional stress, some neurologic disorders, and perhaps early essential hypertension is accompanied by increased plasma or urine levels of norepinephrine. Presumably, this reflects augmented neural releases of the vasoconstrictive adrenergic neurotransmitter which is responsible for the increased arterial pressure. Secondly, there is an increased vascular response to vasoconstrictor agents (e.g., angiotensin II, norepinephrine) in many patients with essential hypertension. Finally, since the early 1930s, hypertensive patients have been noted to exhibit a decrease in the urinary excretion of kinins, and thus it is possible that reduced vasodilator activity could also result in increased peripheral resistance and arterial pressure.

The "primary increase in peripheral resistance" hypothesis and the "deficient renal sodium output" theory are not necessarily mutually exclusive. For example, an increased retention of sodium enhances vascular reactivity, at least to angiotensin II, even in normotensive subjects. Thus, a primary defect of sodium excretion could simultaneously increase both cardiac output and peripheral resistance. It appears that all the factors mentioned above play some role in the development of essential hypertension; individual patients may differ in the relative importance of each. Thus, essential hypertension might be best regarded as a multifactorial disease related to abnormalities of the regulatory mechanisms normally concerned with the control of systemic vascular resistance, sodium excretion, blood volume, cardiac output, and ultimately arterial pressure. The specific parameter which is improperly regulated may differ from patient to patient.

ETIOLOGY OF HYPERTENSION A specific cause for the elevated arterial pressure cannot be defined for most patients with hypertension. The percentage of patients with so-called "idiopathic," essential, or primary hypertension is high, varying from 80 to 95 percent depending on both the patient population and how extensive the "routine" evaluation is.

TABLE 31-1
Classification of arterial hypertension

I Systolic hypertension with wide pulse pressure
  A Decreased compliance of aorta (arteriosclerosis)
  B Increased stroke volume
    1 Arteriovenous fistula
    2 Thyrotoxicosis
    3 Hyperkinetic heart disease
    4 Fever
    5 Psychogenic factors
    6 Aortic valvular insufficiency
    7 Patent ductus arteriosus
II Systolic and diastolic hypertension (increased peripheral vascular resistance)
  A Renal
    1 Chronic pyelonephritis
    2 Acute and chronic glomerulonephritis
    3 Polycystic renal disease
    4 Renovascular stenosis or renal infarction
    5 Most other severe renal disease (arteriolar nephrosclerosis, diabetic nephropathy, etc.)
    6 Renin-producing tumors
  B Endocrine
    1 Oral contraceptives
    2 Adrenocortical hyperfunction
      a Cushing's disease and syndrome
      b Primary hyperaldosteronism
      c Congenital or hereditary adrenogenital syndromes (17α-hydroxylase and 11β-hydroxylase defects)
    3 Pheochromocytoma
    4 Myxedema
    5 Acromegaly
  C Neurogenic
    1 Psychogenic
    2 "Diencephalic syndrome"
    3 Familial dysautonomia (Riley-Day)
    4 Poliomyelitis (bulbar)
    5 Polyneuritis (acute porphyria, lead poisoning)
    6 Increased intracranial pressure (acute)
    7 Spinal cord section
  D Miscellaneous
    1 Coarctation of aorta
    2 Increased intravascular volume (excessive transfusion)
    3 Polyarteritis nodosa
    4 Hypercalcemia
  E Unknown etiology
    1 Essential hypertension (>90% of all cases of hypertension)
    2 Toxemia of pregnancy
    3 Acute intermittent porphyria

More specific etiologic relationships have been established for a smaller group of patients with systemic hypertension (Table 31-1). Primary renal diseases associated with the development of serious hypertension (as distinguished from renal damage secondary to hypertension) have been recognized for years, although in many cases the exact mechanism of blood pressure elevation is unknown. In some instances it is due to activation of the renin-angiotensin-aldosterone axis; in others, perhaps it is related to a reduced ability to excrete sodium and the sequence already described. Hypertension may develop suddenly during the course of acute glomerulonephritis, and it is usually a prominent feature in the late stages of renal damage due to chronic glomerulonephritis or pyelonephritis. Polycystic renal disease, renal infarction, and partial occlusion of the renal artery due to congenital or acquired vascular defects are also implicated as etiologic factors, the last of these being clearly related to activation of the renin-angiotensin-aldosterone system.

The most clearly defined etiologic relationships in the development of hypertension are found among the endocrine disorders. Adrenocortical hormones have also been implicated in the hypertensive syndromes associated with tumors or hyperplasia of the anterior pituitary (Cushing's syndrome, primary hyperaldosteronism, Chap. 336), as well as with various congenital or hereditary enzyme defects (hypertensive adrenogenital syndromes). Secretion of excessive quantities of the pressor catecholamines, norepinephrine and epinephrine, associated with pheochromocytomas, i.e., chromaffin cell tumors arising from the adrenal medulla or sympathetic ganglia, is also commonly associated with hypertension (Chap. 337). Up to 50 percent of patients with acromegaly (Chap. 333) may have hypertension, but the mechanism of their blood pressure elevation is less clear. The presence of these endocrinopathies is usually readily recognizable and distinguishable from essential hypertension by their distinctive clinical and biochemical features. The clinical differences between the primary form and the various forms of secondary hypertension are detailed in Chap. 251.

EFFECTS OF HYPERTENSION For nearly 70 years it has been known that patients with hypertension die prematurely. The most common cause of death is heart disease, with strokes and renal failure also frequently occurring, particularly in those patients with significant retinopathy.

Effects on heart (see also Chap. 251) Cardiac compensation for the excessive workload imposed by increased arterial pressure is at first sustained by the development of left ventricular hypertrophy. Ultimately, the function of this chamber deteriorates; it dilates, and the symptoms and signs of heart failure appear (Chap. 236). Angina pectoris may also occur because of accelerated coronary arterial disease and/or increased myocardial oxygen requirements as a consequence of the increased myocardial mass, which exceeds the capacity of the coronary circulation. On physical examination the heart is enlarged and has a prominent left ventricular impulse. The sound of aortic closure is accentuated, and there may be a faint murmur of aortic insufficiency. Presystolic (S_3) gallop sounds appear frequently in hypertensive heart disease, and a protodiastolic (S_4, summation) gallop rhythm may be present. Electrocardiographic changes of left ventricular hypertrophy are common; evidence of ischemia or infarction may be observed late in the disease. The majority of deaths due to hypertension result from myocardial infarction or congestive heart failure.

NEUROLOGIC EFFECTS (See also Chap. 365) The neurologic effects of long-standing hypertension may be divided into retinal and central nervous system changes. Because the *retina* is the only tissue in which the arteries and arterioles can be examined directly, repeated ophthalmoscopic examination provides the opportunity to observe the progress of the vascular effects of hypertension. The Keith-Wagener-Barker classification of the retinal changes in hypertension has provided a simple and excellent means for serial evaluation of the hypertensive patient. Increasing severity of hypertension is associated with focal spasm and progressive general narrowing of the arterioles, as well as the appearance of hemorrhages, exudates, and papilledema. These retinal lesions often produce scotomata, blurred vision, and even blindness, especially in the presence of papilledema or hemorrhages of the macular area. Hypertensive lesions may develop acutely, and if therapy results in significant reduction of blood pressure, may show rapid resolution. Rarely, these lesions resolve without therapy. In contrast, retinal arteriolosclerosis results from endothelial and muscular proliferation, and it accurately reflects similar changes in other organs. Sclerotic changes do not develop as rapidly as hypertensive lesions, nor do they regress appreciably with therapy. As a consequence of increased wall thickness and rigidity, sclerotic arterioles distort and compress the veins as they cross within their common fibrous sheath, and the reflected light streak from the arterioles is changed by the increased opacity of the vessel wall.

Central nervous system dysfunction also occurs frequently in patients with hypertension. Occipital headaches, most often in the morning, are among the most prominent early symptoms of hypertension. Dizziness, lightheadedness, vertigo, tinnitus, and dimmed vision or syncope may also be observed, but the more serious manifestations are due to vascular occlusion or hemorrhage.

The pathogenesis of each of these disorders is quite different. Cerebral infarction is secondary to the increased atherosclerosis observed in hypertensive patients, while cerebral hemorrhage is the result of both the elevated arterial pressure and the development of cerebral vascular microaneurysms (Charcot-Bouchard aneurysms). Only age and increased arterial pressure are known to influence the development of the microaneurysms. Thus, it is not surprising that the correlation of arterial pressure with cerebral hemorrhage is so much better than with either cerebral or myocardial infarction. The former is two-factorial while the latter are multifactorial.

Renal effects (see also Chap. 282)   Arteriolosclerotic lesions of the afferent and efferent arterioles and the glomerular capillary tufts are the most common renal vascular lesions in hypertension and result in decreased glomerular filtration rate and tubular dysfunction. Proteinuria and microscopic hematuria occur because of glomerular lesions, and approximately 10 percent of the deaths secondary to hypertension result from renal failure. Blood loss in hypertension occurs not only from renal lesions; epistaxis, hemoptysis, and metrorrhagia also occur more frequently in these patients.

APPROACH TO THE PATIENT WITH HYPERTENSION   The physician's first task is to determine whether or not a patient with a given level of arterial pressure has hypertension. Then, determinations of the extent of pretreatment evaluation, whether or not to treat, how to treat, and how frequently to reevaluate are necessary. In general, it is preferable to measure arterial pressure on several occasions prior to starting therapy using a mercury sphygmomanometer with the patient seated.

Initial history, physical examination, and laboratory evaluation should be directed at (1) uncovering correctable secondary forms of hypertension (Table 31-1), (2) establishing the base-line status of the patient, and (3) assessing factors which may influence the type of therapy or which therapy may adversely modify.

An assessment of the following areas in the medical history is particularly important: family or personal history of hyper-

tension; drugs or dietary factors which may aggravate the hypertension, e.g., high salt intake, oral contraceptives, and hormones; cardiovascular risk factors including diabetes mellitus, smoking, lipid abnormalities, or strokes; cardiac or renal disease; and symptoms suggestive of secondary forms of hypertension, e.g., muscle cramps and weakness associated with primary aldosteronism (Chap. 336) or episodic headaches, palpitations, and sweating associated with pheochromocytoma (Chap. 337).

The *physical examination* should include: a standing blood pressure, height, weight, funduscopic examination, assessment of thyroid size, bruits in neck or abdomen, peripheral pulses including determination of synchrony between upper and lower extremities, examination of the heart for size, rate, murmurs, gallops, auscultation of the lungs, examination of the abdomen for masses, and particularly kidney size, and a neurologic examination to assess the presence of deficits associated with a stroke.

The basic *laboratory evaluation* should consist of hematocrit, urinalysis, blood urea nitrogen or creatinine, serum potassium, ECG, and chest x-ray. Often blood glucose, uric acid, and cholesterol determinations and a blood count are also useful, particularly since they may be part of a battery of automated blood tests that as a group are about the same price as the individual tests listed above. Other studies to identify secondary forms of hypertension may be indicated on the basis of the initial therapy or physical examination.

If the average diastolic pressure is greater than 105 mmHg, therapy is almost always indicated. In an adult, if the diastolic pressure is less than 90 mmHg, no other therapy than a change in diet or exercise is usually needed. Individualization is necessary for patients with intermediate elevations of arterial pressures (diastolic pressure between 90 and 105 mmHg), since documentation that therapy is beneficial is lacking. Thus, ancillary factors such as age, sex, and family history need to be considered before starting therapy. In most instances, therapy is indicated in patients with pressures in this range.

Therapy should be directed at reducing the arterial pressure to or near normal levels, since studies have documented that morbidity and mortality are reduced particularly if the initial diastolic pressure is greater than 105 mmHg. In order to minimize drug side effects in achieving this goal, a "step-care approach" has been advocated. The principle involves initiating therapy with a small dose of a single drug, usually a thiazide diuretic, increasing the dose of that drug, and then adding other drugs as needed, one at a time (Chap. 251). The therapeutic regimen should be revised as dictated by the arterial pressure measured at periodic intervals. The frequency of reevaluation should be as often as weekly while blood pressure is being lowered in patients with initial diastolic pressures greater than 115, and approximately every 4 months in symptom-free patients on stable treatment programs.

The specific drugs are discussed elsewhere (Chap. 251). However, it is important to emphasize here that control of arterial pressure is a lifelong endeavor the success of which is often dependent on the physician's ability to motivate the patient to adhere to the therapeutic program and to recognize the pharmacologic interactions and adverse reactions of antihypertensive agents.

REFERENCES

Borst JGG, Borst de Geus A: Hypertension explained by Starling's theory of circulatory homeostasis. Lancet 1:677, 1963

GENEST J et al: Role of the adrenal cortex and sodium in the pathogenesis of human hypertension. Can Med J 118:538, 1978

GUYTON AC: Regulation of arterial pressure, in *Textbook of Medical Physiology*, 5th ed. Philadelphia, Saunders, 1976, pp 265–294

HUNT JC: Management and treatment of essential hypertension in *Hypertension: Physiopathology and Treatment*, J Genest et al (eds). New York, McGraw-Hill, 1977, pp 1068–1085

KAPLAN NM: *Clinical Hypertension*, 2d ed. Baltimore, Williams & Wilkins, 1978

MOSER M et al: Report of the joint national committee on detection, evaluation, and treatment of high blood pressure. JAMA 237:255, 1977

PICKERING G: *Hypertension*, 2d ed. New York, Churchill Livingstone, 1974

32
SUDDEN CARDIOVASCULAR COLLAPSE AND DEATH

BURTON E. SOBEL
EUGENE BRAUNWALD

Sudden death claims more than 400,000 lives annually in the United States alone. It is a major health problem in the Western world. Despite the liberality of the definition of sudden death according to the Joint American Heart Association-International Society of Cardiology Committee (death occurring instantaneously or within an estimated 24 h of the onset of acute symptoms or signs), about half of all sudden deaths are virtually instantaneous. A brief period of time, usually only several minutes, elapses between sudden cardiovascular collapse (without effective cardiac output) and irreversible ischemic changes in the central nervous system. Prolonged survival without functional impairment may be the reward for prompt treatment of certain forms of cardiovascular collapse.

MECHANISMS Sudden cardiovascular collapse may be due to (1) dysrhythmia (Chap. 237); (*a*) most commonly, ventricular tachycardia or fibrillation, sometimes occurring following a bradyarrhythmia, or (*b*) less frequently, ventricular asystole or severe bradycardia; (2) a marked, abrupt reduction in cardiac output, such as occurs with mechanical blockade of the circulation; massive pulmonary thromboembolism (Chap. 266) and cardiac tamponade are two examples of this form; (3) sudden ventricular (pump) failure, which may occur in the presence of critical aortic stenosis (Chap. 242) or acute myocardial infarction ("nonarrhythmic cardiac death") with or without ventricular rupture (Chap. 245); (4) activation of vasodepressor reflexes, which may contribute to sudden reductions in arterial pressure and heart rate, and which are activated in diverse conditions, including primary pulmonary hypertension (Chap. 265), pulmonary thromboembolism, and the hypersensitive carotid sinus syndrome (Chap. 13).

Sudden death and coronary atherosclerosis Sudden death is primarily a complication of coronary atherosclerosis. More than two-thirds of the cases result from this disorder. In the vast majority of such patients sudden death results from precipitous ventricular fibrillation. However, evidence of coronary occlusion and, indeed, of acute myocardial infarction may not be found at autopsy; nonetheless, acute myocardial ischemia appears to be the precipitating event. Only approximately 40 percent of patients dying from coronary artery disease survive long enough to be hospitalized. The remainder (approximately

300,000 patients per year in the United States) die suddenly before they reach the hospital. In fact, in 25 percent of patients with coronary artery disease, death is the first indication of the presence of the disorder (Chap. 245). By extrapolation from experience in coronary care units, in which control of electrical activity of the heart has affected the mortality rate favorably, it would appear that the incidence of sudden death in the community might be reduced substantially by prophylactic therapy in populations at particularly high risk, if such therapy could be demonstrated to be effective, of low toxicity, and convenient to the patient. However, sudden death may be but one mode of expression of coronary artery disease, and effective prevention of sudden death will almost certainly require reduction in the incidence and severity of this disease.

Factors associated with increased risk of sudden death in nonhospitalized persons When electrocardiograms are recorded for 24 h during the course of normal activities, supraventricular premature contractions are found to occur in most American men over 50 years of age, ventricular premature contractions and complex ventricular dysrhythmias in almost two-thirds, and persistent or transient conduction defects in less than 10 percent. Supraventricular dysrhythmias do not appear to be associated with increased risk of sudden death except when they are a manifestation of ventricular dysfunction or atrial infarction accompanying extensive myocardial infarction. Conduction abnormalities and certain types of ventricular premature beats, such as those originating from the left ventricle (recognizable by their terminal anterior and rightward vectors), those occurring during the vulnerable period, and those occurring in pairs or salvos have been thought to be associated with an increased risk. However, among patients with myocardial infarction, late ventricular ectopic beats are particularly prone to be associated with complex malignant ventricular dysrhythmia.

Ventricular premature beats may precipitate ventricular fibrillation, particularly with concomitant myocardial ischemia. On the other hand, they may be manifestations of common fundamental electrophysiologic disturbances predisposing to both ventricular premature beats and ventricular fibrillation or totally independent phenomena associated with electrophysiologic mechanisms different from those responsible for fibrillation. Thus, it is not surprising that, in more than 75 percent of patients with recurrent ventricular fibrillation, after resuscitation from primary ventricular fibrillation warning ventricular dysrhythmias are absent.

In general, ventricular dysrhythmias are of greater significance and more ominous in the presence of acute ischemia than in its absence. In the asymptomatic patient, ventricular premature contractions, particularly when they are relatively frequent (more than 20 per hour), should alert the physician to look for more definitive evidence of heart disease, such as other electrocardiographic abnormalities, mitral valve prolapse, hypertension, or a history of angina.

Overt coronary artery disease, hypertension, or diabetes mellitus is present in more than 75 percent of persons dying suddenly, and perhaps more significantly, the incidence of sudden death in persons with at least one of the three abnormalities is substantially increased. Severe coronary artery disease, not necessarily accompanied by morphologic evidence of an acute event, is consistently present in victims of sudden, unexpected death. More than 75 percent of men without known prior coronary artery disease who die suddenly exhibit at least two of the following four risk factors: hypercholesterolemia, hypertension, hyperglycemia, and cigarette smoking. Obesity and electrocardiographic criteria of left ventricular hypertrophy are also associated with an increased incidence. The incidence of sudden death is higher in cigarette smokers than in nonsmokers, perhaps because of the elevation of circulating catecholamines and fatty acids and the production of increased circulating carboxyhemoglobin with consequently diminished oxygen-carrying capacity by the blood. The proclivity of cigarette smoking to cause sudden death is not cumulative and appears to be reversible when smoking is discontinued.

Ventricular premature contractions may be increased or made overt by exercise, and sudden death appears sometimes to follow unusual exertion. On the other hand, their incidence appears to be diminished in subjects engaged in regular, intermittent, strenuous physical activity in comparison with controls in the same socioeconomic group with a more sedentary existence. Cardiovascular collapse on exertion occurs only rarely in patients with ischemic heart disease undergoing exercise testing, and with appropriate personnel and facilities these episodes respond promptly to electrical defibrillation. Acute emotional stress may precipitate acute myocardial infarction and sudden death, findings which are in keeping with recent experimental observations of increased susceptibility to ventricular tachycardia and ventricular fibrillation after coronary occlusion in emotionally stressed animals or those with augmented sympathetic activity.

Two major clinical syndromes may be recognized in patients who die suddenly and unexpectedly; both are generally associated with ischemic heart disease. In the larger group, the dysrhythmia, which may be termed *primary ventricular fibrillation,* occurs totally unexpectedly and without preceding symptoms or prodromata. This form is *not* associated with acute myocardial infarction; following resuscitation, there is a propensity for early recurrence, probably reflecting the myocardial electrical instability responsible for the intitial episode, and a relatively high 2-year mortality rate (approximately 50 percent). Clearly, these patients can be salvaged only by a rapidly responsive system, and pharmacologic prophylaxis is required to enhance survival. The second, smaller group consists of patients who, following resuscitation, exhibit evidence of acute myocardial infarction. These patients often exhibit prodromal symptoms—chest pain, dyspnea, and syncope—and show a much lower recurrence and 2-year mortality rate (15 percent). Survival in this subgroup is similar to that following resuscitation from ventricular fibrillation complicating acute myocardial infarction in the coronary care unit. Thus, the propensity for developing ventricular fibrillation at the time of acute infarction is of short duration, while ventricular fibrillation in the absence of acute infarction may be related to a chronic process and is likely to recur.

Other causes of sudden death Sudden cardiovascular collapse may result from a number of disorders other than coronary atherosclerosis (Table 32-1). Severe aortic stenosis (congenital or acquired) with sudden dysrhythmias or pump failure, idiopathic hypertrophic subaortic stenosis, and myocarditis or cardiomyopathy associated with dysrhythmia may be responsible. Massive pulmonary embolism leads to circulatory collapse and death within minutes in approximately 10 percent of patients; some of the remainder succumb gradually with progressive right ventricular failure. Acute circulatory collapse may be presaged by smaller emboli occurring at variable intervals before the lethal attack. Accordingly, implementation of therapy during the premonitory sublethal phase, including anticoagulant administration, may be lifesaving (Chap. 266). Sublethal emboli are common in hospitalized patients and can be recognized in at least 40 percent of postmortem examinations when specialized pulmonary arterial injection techniques are utilized. Their clinical manifestations include unexplained or disproportionate dyspnea or tachypnea, hypoxemia, respiratory alkalosis, and hypocapnia. Sinus tachycardia is common. Atrial flutter, chaotic atrial rhythms, and multiple premature atrial beats are compatible with the diagnosis; thrombophlebi-

tis or conditions predisposing to this are also helpful, suggestive signs.

Sudden death with cardiovascular collapse is a rare but always potential complication of infective endocarditis (Chap. 243). In this condition it is usually due to relentless progression of congestive heart failure, but it may also result from ventricular fibrillation, complete atrioventricular block, rupture of a sinus of Valsalva, or a septic embolus to the cerebral or coronary vessels. Sudden, unexpected death in infants, so-called "crib death," is responsible for approximately 10,000 deaths per year in the United States. A defect in the regulation of ventilation may be responsible.

A number of less common causes of sudden death have been recognized increasingly in recent years. Primary degeneration of the atrioventricular conduction system, with or without deposition of calcium or cartilage, may lead to sudden death in the absence of severe coronary atherosclerosis. Trifascicular atrioventricular (AV) block is often seen in these conditions, which account for more than two-thirds of the cases of chronic AV block in adults (Chap. 237). Patients in whom the degree of block is unstable are particularly susceptible to more serious brady- or tachyarrhythmias. Electrocardiographic QT-interval prolongation, nerve deafness, and autosomal recessive inheritance seem to be associated with a high proportion of cases of ventricular fibrillation. The same electrocardiographic abnormality and electrophysiologic instability without nerve deafness appear to be inherited in an autosomal dominant mode. Electrocardiographic changes in these disorders may be manifest only after exercise, and so they may be more important causes of sudden death than has been generally recognized. Other conditions with QT prolongation and increased temporal dispersion of repolarization, such as hypothermia and phenothiazine, emetine, or quinidine toxicity, are rarely associated with sudden death. Sinoatrial arrest or block with depression of lower pacemakers or the sick sinus syndrome, usually accompanied by conduction system dysfunction as well, may also lead to asystole. Sudden rupture of a papillary muscle, the ventricular septum, or free wall, usually occurring within the first few days following acute myocardial infarction, occasionally causes sudden death (Chap. 245). Sudden cardiovascular collapse is also a major, and frequently the terminal,

TABLE 32-1
Conditions associated with cardiovascular collapse and sudden death in adults

Ischemic heart disease secondary to coronary atherosclerosis (including acute myocardial infarction)
Prinzmetal's variant angina; coronary artery spasm
Congenital coronary artery disease
Coronary embolism
Wolff-Parkinson-White syndrome
Hereditary QT-interval prolongation (with or without congenital deafness)
Sinoatrial node disease
Atrioventricular block (Stokes-Adams syndrome)
Secondary disease of the conduction system (e.g., amyloid, sarcoid, hemochromatosis, thrombotic thrombocytopenic purpura, myotonia dystrophica)
Drug toxicity or idiosyncrasy (e.g., digitalis, quinidine)
Valvular heart disease, especially aortic stenosis
Infective endocarditis
Myocarditis
Cardiomyopathies, particularly idiopathic hypertrophic subaortic stenosis
Pericardial tamponade
Cardiac tumor
Ruptured or dissecting aortic aneurysm
Pulmonary thromboembolism
Cerebrovascular accident, particularly hemorrhage

event in patients with major cerebrovascular accidents, sudden alterations of intracranial pressure, or lesions affecting the brainstem. It may also occur with asphyxia, and the toxicity of cardioactive drugs such as digitalis and quinidine may result in life-threatening arrhythmias, leading to sudden cardiovascular collapse and, if treatment is not immediate, to death (Chap. 238).

Electrophysiologic mechanisms underlying ventricular fibrillation Potentially lethal ventricular dysrhythmias in patients with acute myocardial infarction may result from reentry, enhanced automaticity, or both. It would appear that reentry plays a dominant role in early dysrhythmia, for example, within the first hour, and that increased automaticity is an important contributing factor later. Analysis of electrophysiologic changes after experimental coronary occlusion in dogs supports this differentiation, since slowed conduction, asynchronous depolarization, and alterations in recovery time compatible with reentry occur early in ischemic zones.

Several factors appear to set the stage for ventricular fibrillation and other rhythms dependent upon reentry early after the onset of ischemia. Local accumulation of hydrogen ions, an increased ratio of extra- to intracellular potassium, and regional adrenergic stimulation tend to shift diastolic transmembrane potentials toward zero and facilitate slow-current depolarizations. Such depolarizations, sometimes mediated by calcium currents, are characterized by a slow rate of rise of the action potential, low amplitude, diminished duration of the plateau phase of the action potential, and repetitive reponses triggered by a single depolarization. It appears likely that the prominence of depolarizations of this type within ischemic zones of myocardium, in contrast to the fast, sodium-mediated depolarizations evident under physiologic conditions, contribute to slowed conduction required for the development of reentry early after the onset of ischemia.

Another mechanism implicated in reentry early after ischemia is focal reexcitation. Anoxia results in marked abbreviation of the duration of the action potential. Accordingly, during electrical systole, cells within an ischemic zone may be repolarized before cells in adjacent nonischemic tissue. The consequent disparity between prevailing transmembrane potentials may give rise to an uneven depolarization of adjacent cells and hence contribute to dysrhythmia dependent upon reentry.

Among some patients with ischemic heart disease, concomitant pharmacologic or metabolic factors may predispose toward reentry. For example, quinidine may depress conduction velocity, thereby facilitating dysrhythmias dependent upon reentry early after the onset of ischemia.

The so-called "vulnerable period," corresponding to the ascending limb of the T wave (Chap. 239), represents that portion of the cardiac cycle when temporal dispersion of ventricular refractoriness is maximum under physiologic conditions and, accordingly, when reentrant rhythms leading to sustained, repetitive activity can be initiated most readily. In patients with severe myocardial ischemia, the vulnerable period is prolonged and the intensity of stimulus required to evoke repetitive tachycardia or ventricular fibrillation is reduced, so that a single ventricular premature contraction may initiate the rhythm. Electrical shocks of low energy or even a blow struck over the precordium ("thump version") may terminate ventricular tachycardia, presumably by interrupting a reentrant pathway. Since paroxysms of ventricular ectopic beats progressively increase asynchrony of recovery, such paroxysms frequently augur ventricular fibrillation.

Temporal dispersion of refractoriness may be increased in nonischemic tissue in the presence of a slow heart rate. Ac-

cordingly, profound bradycardia due to decreased automaticity of the sinus node or AV block may also be particularly dangerous in patients with acute myocardial infarction since it may potentiate reentry.

Malignant ventricular dysrhythmia occurring later after the onset of ischemia appears to be dependent in part on enhanced automaticity of Purkinje fibers and possibly of myocardial cells as well. Reduction of diastolic transmembrane potential in response to regional biochemical alterations induced by ischemia may contribute to the enhanced automaticity by facilitating repetitive depolarizations of Purkinje fibers triggered by a single depolarization. Since catecholamines facilitate propagation of such slow-current responses, enhanced regional adrenergic stimulation may be an important contributing factor. The apparent efficacy of beta-adrenergic blockade in suppressing some ventricular dysrhythmias and the relative inefficacy of conventional antiarrhythmic agents such as lidocaine in patients with sympathetic hyperactivity may be reflections of the importance of regional adrenergic stimulation to enhanced automaticity.

Electrophysiologic derangements tend to occur with greatest frequency early following the onset of myocardial ischemia or infarction. They may be accentuated by widely distributed ischemia, concomitant metabolic derangements, and deleterious effects of cardioactive drugs. These derangements cause the majority of instantaneous deaths, but they may also occur suddenly and unexpectedly later in the course of an otherwise uncomplicated hospitalization. Since slow-current depolarizations, mediated by calcium under some conditions, have been implicated as factors contributing to malignant ventricular dysrhythmias early after the onset of ischemia depend in part on reentry and to dysrhythmias occurring later, apparently reflecting enhanced automatcity as well, electrical stability of the ischemic heart might be enhanced by administration of antiarrhythmic agents, such as verapamil (currently under investigation in the United States), which selectively block slow-current, calcium-mediated responses.

Asystole is a less common electrophysiologic mechanism underlying sudden death due to coronary atherosclerosis. It may occur when impulse formation in the sinus node is impaired or AV block impedes transmission and subsidiary pacemakers fail to function effectively.

PREVENTION OF SUDDEN DEATH The difficulties entailed in ambulatory electrocardiographic monitoring or other procedures for mass screening to detect candidates at risk for sudden death are formidable, since the population at risk comprises more than one-third of all men 35 to 74 years of age. At greatest risk are patients who have previously experienced primary ventricular fibrillation without associated acute myocardial infarction. Also, patients with ischemic heart disease who exhibit bouts of rapid ventricular tachycardia as well as those within 6 months after recovery from acute myocardial infarction with frequent, early, and/or multifocal ventricular premature contractions at rest, during physical activity, or during psychologic stress are particularly susceptible to sudden death. Patients with prolonged QT intervals and frequent premature contractions, particularly those who present with a history of syncope, represent another vulnerable group. Although identification of patients at high risk is particularly important, selection of an effective prophylactic regimen remains difficult, and none has clearly demonstrated effectiveness in reducing the risk. For example, although procainamide is effective in suppressing ventricular dysrhythmias in patients in the coronary care unit, drug toxicity militates against its routine prolonged use in a general ambulatory population.

It is reasonable to propose a trial of prophylactic treatment, on an individual basis, for patients with known or suspected coronary artery disease with recurrent or complex dysrhythmias. Quinidine gluconate, 330 mg by mouth every 6 h, may be effective in suppressing these dysrhythmias. The dosage may be increased up to 3 g per day if found necessary, unless gastrointestinal disturbances or electrocardiographic evidence of toxicity occurs. The long-acting preparation has the obvious advantage of requiring relatively infrequent dose schedules (bid or tid). Patients who tolerate quinidine poorly may do well with procainamide, 500 mg by mouth every 4 h. Ambulatory electrocardiographic monitoring may be particularly helpful in documenting the efficacy of treatment, since the incomplete knowledge regarding the pathogenesis of sudden death makes rational prophylactic drug selection and dosage difficult and a stereotyped regimen for all patients impractical. However, since the fundamental electrophysiologic derangements underlying ventricular fibrillation and premature ventricular beats may not be the same, documented suppression of premature beats provides no real assurance of prevention of sudden death.

Decreased incidence of sudden death in a random selection of patients surviving acute myocardial infarction has been documented in prospective double-blind studies utilizing beta-adrenergic blocking agents, although the effect of treatment on dysrhythmia was not quantified and the mechanism of apparent protection has not yet been identified. Similarly, it has been suggested that sulfinpyrazone, a uricosuric agent that inhibits platelet aggregation, reduces the incidence of sudden death in patients who had experienced myocardial infarction.

Delays by the patient, physician, and transportation system and in the emergency room after the occurrence of acute myocardial infarction are significant impediments to prevention of sudden death. The median elapsed time between onset of symptoms and hospitalization averages 5 to 8 h in most areas of the United States. Denial by the patient of the seriousness of the condition and indecision by both the patient and physician contribute most to total delay.

Experience gained in Seattle, Washington, has shown that in order to deal effectively on a community-wide basis with the problem of sudden cardiovascular collapse and death, it is necessary to develop a system that provides rapid and effective response for these emergencies. Important elements of the system include a city-wide emergency call number through which the system can be activated, a well-trained group of paramedical personnel such as fire fighters to respond, a short average time of response (under 4 min), and a large number of lay people trained in techniques of resuscitation. Clearly, the success in immediate resuscitation and for long-term survival is directly related to how soon following collapse resuscitation efforts are initiated. The availability of special ambulances (mobile coronary care units) equipped and staffed to handle acute cardiac emergencies appears to reduce delay by increasing community and physician awareness of the urgency of prompt medical attention. Such a system can be effective in resuscitating more than 40 percent of patients who have undergone cardiovascular collapse, and more than 25 percent of such patients are discharged from the hospital.

Therefore, providing instructions to susceptible persons on how to seek medical care on an emergency basis upon the development of symptoms of myocardial infarction is of great importance in the prevention of sudden cardiac death. This strategy includes instructing the patient that prompt entry into an effective emergency care system is not only correct but also what the physician expects of the patient, regardless of whether symptoms suggestive of myocardial infarction occur during the day or night (Chap. 245); this concept also means instructing the patient to bypass the physician and to contact the emergency care system directly. Unsupervised physical stress, such as jogging, should be discouraged in patients with known ischemic heart disease and prohibited in those at high risk of sudden death, as defined above.

APPROACH TO THE PATIENT WITH SUDDEN CARDIOVASCULAR COLLAPSE Sudden death can often be averted even when cardiovascular collapse has occurred. In patients experiencing sudden onset of ventricular fibrillation without prior ventricular failure (primary ventricular fibrillation) while they are under observation in the operating room, the cardiac catheterization laboratory, or the coronary care unit, correction of the dysrhythmia is the rule, and the outcome is usually favorable. However, prompt application of definitive therapy for sudden cardiovascular collapse in the community entails formidable practical obstacles, as outlined above.

The development of transvenous and transthoracic cardiac pacemakers (Chap. 237) and the improvement of cardiopulmonary resuscitative maneuvers, including external cardiac massage coupled with artificial respiration, have contributed to effective therapy.

When a patient under close medical observation develops sudden collapse from a dysrhythmia, the immediate goal must be restoration of effective cardiac rhythm. Circulatory collapse must be recognized and confirmed immediately. Its cardinal features are (1) loss of consciousness, syncope, and seizures, (2) absent peripheral arterial pulses, and (3) absent heart sounds. Since external cardiac massage can provide only limited cardiac output, no more than 30 percent of the lower limit of normal, definitive restoration of effective rhythm should be the immediate goal, and in the absence of evidence to the contrary, abrupt circulatory collapse should be assumed to be due to ventricular fibrillation. If the physician sees the patient within 1 min of the collapse, time should not be wasted by attempting to achieve oxygenation. An immediate blow to the precordium ("thump version") may be attempted, since this is occasionally effective and takes only seconds. Electrical defibrillation (Chap. 239) should be attempted immediately thereafter, without necessarily even pausing first to record an electrocardiogram on separate equipment, although use of portable defibrillators capable of electrocardiographic recording directly from the defibrillating electrodes may be helpful. Maximum electrical output, usually 400 W·s, should be used. If these immediate attempts are unsuccessful, external cardiac massage and complete cardiopulmonary resuscitation should be implemented.

If collapse is due to unequivocal asystole, transthoracic or transvenous electrical pacing should be implemented immediately. Intracardiac epinephrine, 1 ml of 1:1000 solution diluted 1:10 with intracavitary blood, may facilitate the heart's response to artificial pacing or be helpful when a slow ventricular focus is present but ineffective. If these initial definitive measures fail despite adequate technical performance, prompt restitution of a favorable metabolic milieu and monitoring are necessary. This is best accomplished by these three procedures: (1) External cardiac massage. (2) Correction of acid-base balance, often requiring intravenous sodium bicarbonate administration in an initial dose of 1 mg/kg repeated once within 5 to 10 min. Administration of subsequent doses of bicarbonate should be guided by frequent determinations of arterial pH, particularly since intracellular pH may paradoxically decrease, despite a rise in extracellular pH, because permeability to carbon dioxide is so much greater than to bicarbonate. (3) Assessment and correction of electrolyte imbalance. Definitive efforts to restore an effective cardiac rhythm should be attempted again as soon as possible, certainly within minutes. When effective cardiac rhythm is restored but rapidly degenerates again into ventricular tachycardia or fibrillation, lidocaine should be administered as a bolus, 1 mg/kg intravenously, then continued by intravenous infusion at a rate up to 1 to 5 (mg/kg)/h, and countershock repeated.

A   B   C

FIGURE 32-1
External cardiac massage. A. Position of hands during application of external cardiac massage. B. When pressure is applied, the lower portion *of the sternum is displaced posteriorly with the palm of the hand. C. In order to apply maximal downward pressure, the resuscitator leans forward so that both arms are at right angles to the patient's sternum.*

Cardiac massage External cardiac massage is designed to lead to the ejection of blood from the heart by manual compression of the ventricles between the sternum and the spine, and cyclic passive ventricular filling. Adherence to several aspects of technique is essential (Fig. 32-1). (1) The patient should be placed supine on a firm surface (a wooden board serves well). (2) Compression of the chest should be performed with the heel of one hand on the lower third of the sternum cephalad to the xiphoid process (to avoid lacerations of the liver) and the other hand applied on top of the first. (3) The frequency of external massage should approximate one per second to permit adequate time for ventricular filling. (4) The resuscitator's waist must be higher than the patient's chest in order to permit the resuscitator to administer the approximately 100-lb force required to depress the anterior chest wall of an adult male the necessary 5 cm per beat. (5) Depression and release of the chest wall should be smooth, with each occupying 50 percent of the cycle, since sudden compression may elicit a pressure wave palpable at the femoral or carotid artery but able to eject little blood. (6) Massage should not be interrupted, even momentarily, since cardiac output increases cumulatively during the first 8 to 10 compressions and even brief interruptions are detrimental. (7) Effective ventilation must be carried out. To accomplish this, the chin must be retracted and the neck fully extended. Mouth-to-mouth or mouth-to-nose technique must be continued throughout the resuscitative effort at a frequency of about 12 per minute and monitored by arterial blood gas analyses. If the latter are clearly abnormal, endotracheal intubation should be carried out expeditiously.

Each external cardiac compression limits venous return, and the optimal anticipated cardiac index during external massage approximates only 40 percent of the lower limit of normal, well below that seen in most patients after spontaneous ventricular contractions have returned or have been induced by ventricular pacing. Therefore, prompt restoration of effective cardiac rhythm is essential. Rarely, organized electrocardiographic activity unaccompanied by effective cardiac contraction (electromechanical dissociation) may occur and respond to intracardiac epinephrine (1 ml of 1:1000 solution diluted 1:10 with blood) or calcium gluconate (1 g). Cardiac massage should be terminated as soon as effective cardiac contractions, initiated spontaneously or by ventricular pacing, serve to produce a detectable pulse and systemic arterial blood pressure. Subsequent treatment of dysrhythmias and hypotension and adjustment of intravascular volume should be guided by the same general principles underlying their management in circulatory collapse due to cardiogenic shock (Chap. 245).

The therapeutic approach outlined above is based on several considerations: (1) irreversible brain damage often occurs after a few (approximately 4) minutes of circulatory collapse; (2) the likelihood of restoring effective cardiac rhythm and successfully resuscitating the patient diminishes rapidly with time;

(3) 80 to 90 percent survival can be anticipated in patients developing primary ventricular fibrillation, as when undergoing cardiac catheterization or exercise testing, in whom definitive treatment is prompt; (4) survival rates in the general hospital setting are much lower, approximately 20 percent, depending in part on the coexisting or underlying disease process; (5) survival rates in the community approach zero, unless special emergency care systems have been perfected, probably because of unavoidable delays in initiating definitive therapy and limitations of equipment and available personnel; and (6) external cardiac massage can provide only a limited cardiac output. When ventricular fibrillation occurs, the earliest application of electrical countershock is the one most likely to succeed. Thus, when circulatory collapse is a primary event, therapy must be directed toward prompt restoration of effective cardiac rhythm.

Complications External cardiac massage is not free from significant complications, including rib fracture, hemopericardium and tamponade, hemothorax, pneumothorax, liver laceration, fat embolus, and ruptured spleen with late, occult blood loss. However, these complications can be minimized by proper technique and, if appropriately considered, can be readily recognized and often managed effectively. The decision to terminate unsuccessful cardiopulmonary resuscitation is always difficult. In general, if effective cardiac rhythm has not been restored and if the patient's pupils are fixed and dilated despite 30 min or more of cardiac massage, a successful resuscitation cannot be expected.

An important challenge to the medical system is to provide trained medical or paramedical personnel immediately for patients who develop sudden cardiovascular collapse. The development of appropriately staffed "rescue stations" in large factories, office buildings, and sports arenas is one approach that has been proposed since aggressive precoronary care can reduce the mortality rate. However, it is likely that the identification of individuals at high risk and the application of effective preventive measures to this segment of the population will be more satisfactory.

REFERENCES

THE AUTURANE REINFARCTION TRIAL RESEARCH GROUP: Sulfinpyrazone in the prevention of cardiac death after myocardial infarction. N Engl J Med 298:289, 1978

CORDAY E, DODGE HT (eds): Symposium on Identification and Management of the Candidate for Sudden Cardiac Death. Am J Cardiol 39:813, 1977

HAYNES RE et al: Repolarization abnormalities in survivors of out-of-hospital ventricular fibrillation. Circulation 57:654, 1978

KANNEL WB et al: Precursors of sudden coronary death: Factors related to the incidence of sudden death. Circulation 51:606, 1975

LOWN B: Cardiovascular collapse and sudden death, in *Heart Disease*, E Braunwald (ed). Philadelphia, Saunders, 1980, chap 22

MULTICENTRE INTERNATIONAL STUDY: Improvement in prognosis of myocardial infarction by long-term beta-adrenoreceptor blockade using practolol. Br Med J 217:35, 1975

OLDHAM HN JR: Cardiopulmonary arrest and resuscitation, in *Gibbon's Surgery of the Chest,* 3d ed, DC Sabiston, FC Spencer (eds). Philadelphia, Saunders, 1976, chap 10, pp 239-255

PANTRIDGE JF et al: *The Acute Coronary Attack.* New York, Grune & Stratton, 1975

PRINEAS RJ, BLACKBURN H (eds): Sudden coronary death outside hospital. Circulation 52(suppl 3):287, 1975

RAIZES G et al: Instantaneous nonarrhythmic cardiac death in acute myocardial infarction. Am J Cardiol 39:1, 1977

SCHULZE RA et al: Sudden death in the year following myocardial infarction. Relation to ventricular premature contractions in the late hospital phase and left ventricular ejection fraction. Am J Med 62:192, 1977

section 5 | Alterations in gastrointestinal function

33
ORAL MANIFESTATIONS OF DISEASE

PAUL GOLDHABER

DISTURBANCES OF THE TEETH AND DENTAL TISSUES

DENTAL CARIES, PULPAL AND PERIAPICAL INFECTION, AND SEQUELAE Dental caries, the principal cause of tooth loss up to the fourth decade of life, is characterized by a bacteria-induced progressive destruction of the mineral and organic components of the outer enamel and underlying dentin. Numerous long-term studies have clearly shown that the artificial fluoridation of drinking water supplies to a level of 1 part per million leads to a 50 to 75 percent reduction in the occurrence of dental caries in permanent teeth of children, presumably because of an alteration of the developing enamel crystals during tooth formation which makes them more resistant to acid dissolution.

If the carious lesion progresses unchecked, there is eventual infection of the dental pulp, giving rise to an *acute pulpitis.* During the early stages of pulpitis moderately severe pain may result from thermal changes, particularly with cold drinks. As more of the pulp becomes involved because of advanced caries, heat or reclining may stimulate the onset of even more severe and continuous pain. At this stage, damage to the pulp is irreversible, and treatment consists of either extraction or thorough removal of the remaining contents of the pulp chamber and root canals followed by sterilization and filling with an inert material (root canal therapy).

If the pulpitis is not treated, infection may spread beyond the apex of the tooth into the periodontal ligament, giving rise to pain on chewing or percussion. The most common manifestation of periapical disease is the *periapical granuloma,* a localized mass of chronic granulation tissue which slowly expands at the expense of the surrounding alveolar bone. The *chronic periapical granuloma* may present the above symptoms or may be asymptomatic. If allowed to persist untreated, the periapical granuloma may give rise to a *periapical cyst* or a *periapical abscess*—all three lesions appearing as radiolucent areas on roentgenograms. The acute periapical abscess may extend into the surrounding bone marrow, resulting in an *osteomyelitis.* More frequently, the abscess perforates the cortical plate and, following the path of least resistance, spreads through various tissue spaces, giving rise to cellulitis and bacteremia, or discharges into the oral cavity, into the maxillary sinus, or through the skin.

The symptoms produced by cellulitis depend on which tissue space is affected. For example, *Ludwig's angina* originates from an infected mandibular molar, involves the submaxillary space, and subsequently extends into the sublingual and submental spaces. Clinically, this is manifested by swelling of the floor of the mouth, elevation of the tongue, and difficulty in swallowing and breathing. With continued swelling, there may be edema of the glottis, necessitating an emergency tracheotomy. Spread of the infection to the parapharyngeal spaces may lead to cavernous sinus thrombosis.

PERIODONTAL DISEASE

After the third decade chronic destructive periodontal disease *(periodontitis)* is responsible for the loss of more teeth than dental caries. It begins as a marginal inflammation of the gingivae (gingivitis), which slowly spreads to involve the underlying alveolar bone and periodontal ligament. As the disease progresses, the alveolar bone is resorbed, resulting in loss of periodontal ligament fiber attachment from the tooth to the bone. The separation of the soft tissue from the tooth surface results in "pocket" formation, the inner aspect of which bleeds readily on probing or spontaneously during chewing. Frank pus sometimes exudes from under the gingival margin, accounting for the use of the now outmoded term "pyorrhea." With continued loss of alveolar bone the involved teeth become mobile. As the periodontal pockets deepen, the pocket orifice may become occluded, leading to the formation of a *periodontal abscess.* The prognosis for teeth with advanced bone loss, extreme mobility, and recurrent abscess formation is usually poor or hopeless, and the usual treatment is extraction.

The most important local etiologic factors associated with this disease are thought to be *poor oral hygiene,* resulting in the accumulation of grossly visible adherent masses of bacteria *(bacterial plaque),* calculus (mineralized bacterial plaque), and food impaction. The margins of overextended fillings also play a role as local irritating factors. Occlusal trauma, particularly trauma due to grinding and clenching habits, may be involved. Therapy is aimed at elimination of these factors and the development of a local environment which can be maintained in health by good oral hygiene.

Systemic factors are thought to modify the response of the host to the local factors, but their nature is more obscure. Reduced neutrophil functions, such as chemotaxis and phagocytosis, appear to predispose to *juvenile periodontitis*, a form of periodontitis characterized by early and severe alveolar bone loss. Similar periodontal destruction is found in youngsters with the *Papillon-Lefèvre syndrome*, which includes keratotic lesions of the palms and soles. Individuals with *Down's syndrome* seem to be particularly susceptible to periodontal disease and may demonstrate advanced alveolar bone loss around the permanent mandibular incisors and maxillary first molars. Severe chronic periodontal disease may be present in uncontrolled *diabetes mellitus*. In some instances, however, there are characteristic alterations in the gingiva in response to a number of specific systemic conditions. For example, during *pregnancy* the gingiva may become edematous and friable, with a raspberry-like appearance of the interdental papillae. Occasionally, a tumorlike mass may develop in an interdental area; this usually regresses following parturition. Oral contraceptives may lead to an increase in gingival inflammation. The use of the anticonvulsant drug *phenytoin* (Dilantin) frequently results in fibrous hyperplasia of the gingiva, which may actually cover the teeth, interfere with mastication, and cause a serious aesthetic problem. A similar clinical picture, although usually more generalized and extensive, occurs in *idiopathic familial fibromatosis*. The latter condition appears to be hereditary.

A relatively common gingival disease, found predominantly in young adults, is *acute necrotizing ulcerative gingivitis* (Vincent's infection, trench mouth). This disease is characterized by tender or painful gingivae, bleeding on pressure, and the pathognomonic sign of papillary or marginal gingival necrosis and ulceration. Clinical evidence suggests that the cause of this disease has a psychosomatic component. Vincent's infection differs from *acute herpetic gingivostomatitis*, with which it is most frequently confused, in that fever or malaise rarely develops, and patients respond rapidly to penicillin or broad-spectrum antibiotics.

It should be noted that both infected periapical lesions and periodontal disease provide potential sources of infection which may spread to other sites. Transient bacteremias have been demonstrated after simple massage of inflamed gingivae or use of an oral irrigative device, as well as during tooth extraction. The frequent association of tooth extraction with the subsequent occurrence of subacute bacterial endocarditis has led to the prophylactic use of antibiotics in dental patients with a history of rheumatic fever or other evidence of valvular disease. Similar precautions should be taken with dental patients having heart valve or joint prostheses. Prophylactic extraction of healthy teeth in leukemic patients is not justified.

DISEASES OF THE ORAL MUCOSA AND TONGUE

HEMATOLOGIC DISTURBANCES Oral manifestations are common in both the acute and chronic forms of all types of leukemia, particularly *monocytic leukemia*. They consist of local gingival bleeding, enlargement, and necrosis. Petechiae and ulceration of the oral mucosa may also be evident. Extensive ulcerations of the gingivae, buccal mucosa, lips, soft palate, pharynx, and tonsils may also occur in *agranulocytosis*. In thrombocytopenic states multiple petechiae, ecchymoses, and bleeding gingivae may be observed. The mucous membranes of the oral cavity, including the papillae of the tongue, are atrophic in the *Plummer-Vinson syndrome* (see Chaps. 34 and 289). As a result, the tongue is red, smooth, and sore, and there is difficulty in swallowing. Of interest is the finding that the atrophic mucous membranes have a predisposition toward the development of oral carcinoma. The oral symptoms in *pernicious anemia* are similar (see Chap. 311). Ulceration, mucositis, xerostomia, and infection (bacterial or fungal) are relatively common oral complications among patients receiving chemotherapy and/or radiotherapy for malignancies not involving the head or neck.

VITAMIN DEFICIENCIES *The oral effects of deficiency of the B group of vitamins* involve the soft tissues primarily, giving rise to reddening and ulceration of the oral mucosa and tongue, swelling and burning of the tongue, and fissuring at the corners of the lips (*angular cheilosis*). Severe vitamin C deficiency (*scurvy*) is manifested by petechiae in the oral mucosa; swollen, ulcerated, bleeding gingivae; and loosening of teeth.

PIGMENTATIONS (See Table 33-1) The spread of irregular spots or blotches or brown pigment throughout the oral mucosa, primarily the buccal mucosa, may be the first sign of *Addison's disease*. The pigmentation associated with the *Peutz-Jeghers syndrome* is readily differentiated because of its characteristic distribution around the lips, eyes, and nostrils, as well

TABLE 33-1
Pigmented lesions of the oral mucosa

Condition	Usual location	Clinical features	Course
Black, hairy tongue	Dorsum of tongue	Elongation of filiform papillae of tongue, which take on a brown to black coloration	Long-lasting but may disappear spontaneously
Heavy metal pigmentation (bismuth, mercury, lead)	Gingival margin	Thin blue-black pigmented line along gingival margin due to prior treatment for syphilis with bismuth or mercury or from accidental absorption of lead	Long-lasting
Drug ingestion (tranquilizers, oral contraceptives, antimalarials)	Any area in mouth	Brown, black, or gray areas of pigmentation	Disappears following cessation of drug
Amalgam tattoo	Gingiva and mucobuccal fold	Small blue-black pigmented areas associated with embedded amalgam particles in soft tissues; these will show up on radiographs as radiopaque particles	Remains indefinitely
Fordyce's disease	Buccal and labial mucosa	Aggregation of numerous, small yellowish spots just beneath mucosal surface; no subjective symptoms	Remains without apparent change indefinitely
Addison's disease	Any area in mouth but mostly on buccal mucosa	Blotches or spots of bluish black to dark brown pigmentation occurring early in the disease accompanied by diffuse pigmentation of skin; other symptoms of adrenal insufficiency	Condition controlled by steroid therapy
Peutz-Jeghers syndrome	Any area in mouth	Dark brown spots on lips, buccal mucosa, and palate with characteristic distribution of pigment around lips, nose, eyes, and on hands; concomitant intestinal polyposis	Lesions remaining indefinitely
Malignant melanoma	Any area in mouth	May appear as a raised, painless, brown-black lesion or may be amelanotic; may be ulcerated and infected	Early metastasis leading to death

TABLE 33-2
Vesicular, bullous, or ulcerative lesions of the oral mucosa

Condition	Usual location	Clinical features	Course
VIRAL DISEASES			
Acute herpetic gingivostomatitis (herpes simplex, type I)	Lip and oral mucosa	Labial vesicles which rupture and crust, and intraoral vesicles which quickly ulcerate; extremely painful to pressure; acute gingivitis, fever, malaise, foul odor, and cervical lymphadenopathy; occurs primarily in infants and children	Heals spontaneously in 10-14 days unless secondarily infected
Recurrent herpes labialis	Mucocutaneous junction of lip	Eruption of groups of vesicles which may coalesce, then rupture and crust; painful to pressure or spicy foods	Lasts about 1 week, but condition may be prolonged if secondary infection occurs
Primary herpes, type II	Mouth, oral pharynx, and genitalia	Large, painful, discrete vesicles on zone of erythema; anterior cervical glands enlarged	Lasts several weeks; may recur
Herpangina (coxsackievirus A; also possibly coxsackievirus B and echovirus)	Oral mucosa, pharynx, tongue	Sudden onset of fever, sore throat, and oropharyngeal vesicles usually in children under 4 years, during summer months; diffuse pharyngeal injection and vesicles (1-2 mm), grayish white surrounded by red areola; vesicles enlarge and ulcerate	Incubation period 2-9 days; fever for 1-4 days; recovery uneventful
Hand, foot, and mouth disease (type A coxsackieviruses)	Oral mucosa, pharynx, palms, and soles	Fever, malaise, headache with oropharyngeal vesicles which become painful, shallow ulcers	Incubation period 2-18 days; lesions heal spontaneously in 2-4 weeks
Chickenpox	Gingiva and oral mucosa	Skin lesions may be accompanied by small vesicles on oral mucosa that rupture to form shallow ulcers; may coalesce to form large bullous lesions that ulcerate; mucosa may have generalized erythema	Lesions heal spontaneously within 2 weeks
Herpes zoster	Cheek, tongue, gingiva, or palate	Unilateral vesicular eruption and ulceration in linear pattern following sensory distribution of trigeminal nerve	Gradual healing without scarring
Infectious mononucleosis	Oral mucosa	Fatigue, sore throat, malaise, low-grade fever, and enlarged cervical lymph nodes; numerous small ulcers usually appear several days before lymphadenopathy; gingival bleeding and multiple petechiae at junction of hard and soft palates	Oral lesions disappear during convalescence
Warts	Any place on skin and oral mucosa, primarily lips and vestibule	Single or multiple papillary lesions, with thick, white, keratinized surfaces containing many pointed projections	Lesions grow rapidly and spread
BACTERIAL OR FUNGAL DISEASES			
Acute necrotizing ulcerative gingivitis ("trench mouth," Vincent's infection)	Gingiva	Painful, bleeding gingiva characterized by necrosis and ulceration of gingival papillae and margins plus lymphadenopathy and foul odor	Continued destruction of tissue followed by remission, but may recur
Prenatal (congenital) syphilis	Palate, jaws, tongue, and teeth	Gummatous involvement of palate, jaws, and facial bones; Hutchinson's incisors, mulberry molars, glossitis, mucous patches, and fissures of corners of mouth	Tooth deformities in permanent dentition irreversible
Primary syphilis (chancre)	Lesion appears where organism enters body; may occur on lips, tongue, or tonsillar area	Small papule developing rapidly into a large, painless ulcer with indurated border; unilateral lymphadenopathy; chancre and lymph nodes containing spirochetes; serologic tests positive by third to fourth weeks	Healing of chancre in 1-2 months, followed by secondary syphilis in 6-8 weeks
Secondary syphilis	Oral mucosa frequently involved with mucous patches, primarily on palate but also at commissures of mouth	Maculopapular lesions of oral mucosa, about 5-10 mm in diameter with central ulceration covered by grayish membrane; eruptions occurring on various mucosal surfaces and skin accompanied by fever, malaise, and sore throat	Lesions may persist from several weeks to a year
Tertiary syphilis	Palate and tongue	Gummatous infiltration of palate or tongue followed by ulceration and fibrosis; atrophy of tongue papillae may produce characteristic bald tongue and glossitis	Gumma may destroy palate, causing complete perforation
Gonorrhea	Lesions may occur in mouth at site of inoculation or secondarily by hematogenous spread from a primary focus elsewhere	Earliest symptoms are burning or itching sensation, dryness, or heat in mouth followed by acute pain on eating or speaking; tonsils and oropharynx most frequently involved; oral tissues may be diffusely inflamed or ulcerated; saliva develops increased viscosity and fetid odor; submaxillary lymphadenopathy with fever in severe cases	Lesions resolve with appropriate antibiotic therapy
Tuberculosis	Tongue, tonsillar area, soft palate	A solitary, irregular ulcer covered by a persistent exudate; ulcer has an undermined, indurated border	Lesion may persist
Cervicofacial actinomycosis	Swellings in region of face, neck, and floor of mouth	Infection may be associated with an extraction, jaw fracture, or eruption of molar tooth; in acute form resembles an acute pyogenic abscess, but contains yellow "sulfur granules" (gram-positive mycelia and their hyphae)	Acute form may last a few weeks; chronic form lasts months or years; prognosis excellent; actinomycetes respond to antibiotics (tetracyclines or penicillin) but not to antifungal drugs

TABLE 33-2 *(continued)*
Vesicular, bullous, or ulcerative lesions of the oral mucosa

Condition	Usual location	Clinical features	Course
BACTERIAL OR FUNGAL DISEASES *(continued)*			
Histoplasmosis	Any area in mouth, particularly tongue, gingiva, or palate	Numerous small nodules which may ulcerate; hoarseness and dysphagia may occur because of lesions in larynx, usually associated with fever and malaise	May be fatal
DERMATOLOGIC DISEASES			
Mucous membrane pemphigoid	Primarily mucous membranes of the oral cavity, but may also involve the eyes, urethra, vagina, and rectum	Painful, grayish white collapsed vesicles or bullae with peripheral erythematous zone; gingival lesions desquamate, leaving ulcerated area	Protracted course with remissions and exacerbations; involvement of different sites occurs slowly; corticosteroids may control severe cases
Erythema multiforme (Stevens-Johnson syndrome)	Primarily the oral mucosa and skin of hands and feet	Intraoral ruptured bullae surrounded by an inflammatory area; lips may show hemorrhagic crusts; the "iris" or "target" lesion on the skin is pathognomonic; patient may have severe signs of toxicity	Onset very rapid; condition may last 1–2 weeks; may be fatal
Pemphigus vulgaris	Oral mucosa and skin	Ruptured bullae and ulcerated oral areas; mostly in older adults	With repeated recurrence of bullae, toxicity may lead to cachexia, infection, and death within 2 years
NEOPLASTIC DISEASES			
Squamous cell carcinoma	Any area in mouth, most commonly on lower lip, tongue, and floor of mouth	Ulcer with elevated, indurated border; failure to heal, pain not prominent; lesions tend to arise in areas of leukoplakia or in smooth or atrophic tongue	Invades and destroys underlying tissues or may metastasize to regional lymph nodes
Acute leukemia	Gingiva	Gingival swelling and superficial ulcerations followed by hyperplasia of gingiva with extensive necrosis and hemorrhage; deep ulcers may occur elsewhere on the mucosa complicated by secondary infection	Fatal
Lymphosarcoma	Gingiva, palate, tongue, and tonsillar area	Elevated, ulcerated area which may proliferate rapidly, giving the appearance of a traumatic inflammatory lesion; swelling of regional lymph nodes	Fatal
OTHER CONDITIONS			
Recurrent aphthous stomatitis	Any place on oral mucosa	Single or clusters of painful ulcers with surrounding erythematous border, found anywhere on mucosa; lesions may be 1–15 mm in diameter	Lesions heal in 1–2 weeks but may recur monthly or several times a year
Behçet's syndrome	Oral mucosa, eyes, and genitalia	Multiple aphthouslike ulcers in mouth; inflammatory ocular changes and ulcerative lesions on genitalia	Ulcers may persist for several weeks and heal without scarring
Traumatic ulcers	Any place on oral mucosa; dentures frequently responsible for ulcers in vestibule	Localized, discrete ulcerated lesion with red border; produced by accidental biting of mucosa, penetration by a foreign object, or chronic irritation by a denture	Lesion usually heals in 7–10 days when irritant is removed, unless secondarily infected

TABLE 33-3
White lesions of oral mucosa

Condition	Usual location	Clinical features	Course
Pachyderma oris	Any area in mouth	Elevated white lesion due to hyperkeratosis and thickening of the oral epithelium secondary to chronic irritation	Removal of irritant leads to healing in 2–3 weeks
Leukoplakia	Any area in mouth	White patch or raised plaque with sharply defined borders; in more severe cases the lesion is indurated and rough, and may be fissured and eroded; pain not present in early lesions	Carcinoma frequently arises in the more severe type of lesion
Lichen planus	Any area in mouth but most often on buccal mucosa	Varied appearance of lesion due to arrangement of grayish white papules which coalesce to make up the pattern; a reticular network is most common; oral lesions may precede skin lesions	May disappear spontaneously
Moniliasis (thrush)	Any area in mouth	Creamy white curdlike patches which reveal a raw, bleeding surface when scraped; found in sick infants, debilitated elderly patients, or patients receiving high doses of corticosteroids or broad-spectrum antibiotics	Responds favorably to antifungal therapy after correction of predisposing causes
Chemical burns	Any area in mouth	White slough due to necrosis of epithelium and underlying connective tissue caused by contact with agents (e.g., aspirin) applied locally or the use of undiluted sodium perborate or hydrogen peroxide as a mouthwash; removal of slough leaves a raw, painful surface	Lesion heals in several weeks if not secondarily infected

as its intraoral distribution. Both *lead poisoning* and *bismuth poisoning* may be manifested by a dark line along the gingival margin, particularly in individuals who have poor oral hygiene. Bismuth poisoning may also demonstrate pigmented patches elsewhere in the oral mucosa.

INFECTIONS   See Tables 33-2 and 33-3.

DERMATOLOGIC DISEASES   See Tables 33-2 and 33-3 and Chaps. 48 to 52.

TONGUE ALTERATIONS   See Table 33-4.

MALODOROUS BREATH   A distinctly unpleasant odor of the breath (halitosis) may emanate from any patient with *infections of the upper part of the respiratory tract,* especially in bronchiectasis and lung abscess. Halitosis may occur with oral sepsis as in *stomatitis, gingivitis,* or extensive *caries.* Some persons who smoke excessively may have halitosis. Occasionally otherwise normal persons will have halitosis without obvious cause. A *fishy odor* of the breath is found in patients with hepatic failure, an *ammoniacal or urinary odor* is found in azotemia, and a *sweet, fruity odor* is typical of diabetic acidosis.

DISEASES OF THE SALIVARY GLANDS

Conditions affecting the salivary glands include mumps parotitis (Chap. 188), Mikulicz's disease, Sjögren's syndrome (Chap. 356), and sarcoidosis. Inflammation of the salivary glands (*sialadenitis*) is usually associated with the presence of a salivary stone (*sialolithiasis*) in the duct of one of the major salivary glands. The classic history of pain and swelling of the gland at mealtimes is due to the partial blockage of salivary flow by the

stone. Localization of the stone may be accomplished by palpation or by roentgenograms with or without the use of an intraductal injection of radiopaque material (*sialography*). Acute or recurrent parotitis, with or without a defined microorganism, may occur in children and is marked by sudden onset of swelling of the whole gland or side of the face, accompanied by suppuration from Stensen's duct.

Xerostomia, or dryness of the mouth, is due to salivary gland dysfunction and may be temporary or permanent. Among the factors which cause temporary dryness are emotional factors (such as fear), infection of the glands, and administration of drugs, such as atropine, antihistamines, or tricyclic antidepressants and phenothiazines. Radiation of the area may produce a more permanent xerostomia because of atrophy of the glands. A similar dryness may occur in Sjögren's syndrome. The dry mouth may give rise to rampant caries, particularly if sugar-containing candies are sucked in an attempt to stimulate salivary flow. Extensive dental caries, especially around the gum margins of the teeth, may be seen in drug addicts and alcoholics, presumably due to xerostomia and lack of oral hygiene and dental care. Xerostomia-induced caries may be prevented or arrested by the daily topical application of a 1% sodium fluoride gel.

Benign or malignant tumors may arise in the major or minor salivary glands. The benign *mixed tumor* accounts for the vast majority of all salivary gland tumors and has a relatively high recurrence rate. Malignant tumors of the parotid gland may affect the facial nerve.

ORAL CANCER

Oral cancer constitutes more than 5 percent of all human cancers. *Squamous cell carcinoma* is the most common malignant oral tumor, accounting for approximately 90 to 95 percent of all oral malignant tumors. Most of these tumors occur on the lips, primarily the lower lip, rather than intraorally. About half the intraoral tumors involve the tongue, primarily the posterior two-thirds and the lateral borders. The major etiologic factor in lip cancer appears to be exposure to intense sunlight. Predisposing factors for intraoral carcinoma include tobacco (usually in the form of cigar or pipe smoking, or snuff placed in the mucobuccal fold), excessive consumption of alcohol, syphilitic glossitis, and the atrophic mucosa of the Plummer-Vinson syndrome. Although numerous instances of carcinoma of the tongue adjacent to a sharp tooth or dental appliance have been reported, animal studies with chronic irritation per se, as well as epidemiologic studies, cast doubt on this apparent relationship. The most common *precancerous lesion* in the oral cavity is *leukoplakia,* a whitish patch on the mucosa that histologically shows hyperkeratosis, acanthosis, and dyskeratosis. Recent evidence suggests that the asymptomatic, red velvety (erythroplastic) lesion of the floor of the mouth, ventrolateral aspect of the tongue, or soft palate–anterior pillar complex is more likely to be carcinoma in situ or invasive carcinoma than is the white lesion. *All chronic ulcerative lesions which fail to heal within 1 to 2 weeks should be considered potentially malignant* and must be biopsied in order to make the definitive diagnosis. It is noteworthy that in their early stages intraoral epidermoid carcinomas are rarely painful, in contrast to similar-appearing inflammatory lesions.

The prognosis for patients with carcinoma of the lip is usually good, since these malignant tumors are noted sooner and apparently metastasize later. Patients with carcinoma of the tongue have a poorer prognosis, particularly as the tumor occurs more posteriorly on the tongue. Intraoral carcinomas may

TABLE 33-4
Alterations of the tongue

Type of change	Clinical features
SIZE OR MORPHOLOGY CHANGES	
Macroglossia	Enlarged tongue which may be part of a syndrome found in developmental conditions such as Down's syndrome; may be due to tumor (hemangioma or lymphangioma), metabolic disease (such as primary amyloidosis), or endocrine disturbance (such as acromegaly or cretinism)
Fissured ("scrotal") tongue	Dorsal surface and sides of tongue covered by painless shallow or deep fissures which may collect debris and become irritated
Median rhomboid glossitis	Congenital abnormality of tongue with ovoid, denuded area in the median posterior portion of the tongue
COLOR CHANGES	
"Geographic" tongue ("wandering rash")	Asymptomatic inflammatory condition of the tongue, with rapid loss and regrowth of filiform papillae, leading to appearance of denuded red patches "wandering" across the surface of the tongue
Hairy tongue	Elongation of filiform papillae of the medial dorsal surface area due to failure of keratin layer of the papillae to desquamate normally; brownish black coloration may be due to staining by tobacco, food, or chromogenic organisms
"Strawberry" and "raspberry" tongue	Appearance of tongue during scarlet fever due to the hypertrophy of fungiform papillae plus changes in the filiform papillae
"Bald" tongue	Complete atrophy of papillae which may occur in pernicious anemia, severe iron-deficiency anemia, pellagra, or syphilis; may be accompanied by painful, burning sensations

spread by direct invasion to the underlying bone. Depending on the site of origin of the intraoral carcinoma, metastases usually spread to the submaxillary or cervical lymph nodes. Death may result from recurrent or uncontrollable disease above the clavicles; metastatic disease beyond the neck; treatment complications; or a second primary cancer, usually in the oral cavity or the upper parts of the gastrointestinal or respiratory tract.

NEUROLOGIC DISTURBANCES

A number of neurologic disturbances have a direct effect on oral and paraoral structures. *Trigeminal neuralgia* (tic douloureux) is an example of a syndrome involving the trigeminal nerve. It is characterized by extremely severe, unilateral, lancinating pain of the face occurring spontaneously or set off by pressure on a "trigger zone" on the face (see Chap. 376). Facial palsy is a unilateral disturbance of the motor branch of the facial nerve due to either trauma, surgical sectioning, or tumor involvement. When it is of acute onset and unknown cause, possibly a localized infection in the nerve, it is called *Bell's palsy*. It may be due to cranial herpes zoster in some instances. The condition is manifested by drooping of the corner of the mouth, inability to close the eye on the same side, and difficulty in speech and eating. In mild cases the symptoms may disappear spontaneously within a month. Alteration in taste sensation in the anterior two-thirds of the tongue due to disturbance of the sensory component of the facial nerve occurs in some cases and indicates a more central location of the lesion in the nerve (see Chap. 376).

The pain associated with the *glossopharyngeal neuralgia syndrome* is similar in type and intensity to that found in trigeminal neuralgia, being set off by a trigger zone in the pharynx and affecting the posterior region of the tongue, pharynx, soft palate, and ear. Disturbance of the hypoglossal nerve leads to dysfunction of the tongue musculature and atrophy. Bilateral nerve involvement prevents protrusion of the tongue; unilateral involvement leads to deviation of the protruded tongue toward the affected side.

DISTURBANCES OF THE TEMPOROMANDIBULAR JOINT

Pain in the area of the temporomandibular joint frequently causes the patient to seek therapy. It may be due to posterior displacement of the condyle in the fossa leading to displacement of the meniscus and chronic trauma. *Dislocation of the condyle anteriorly* beyond the articular eminence due to sudden stretching or tearing of the capsular ligament may result in a locking of the mandible in an open position. In *osteoarthritis* the clinical signs and symptoms may be minimal despite extensive changes in the condyle. Temporomandibular joint involvement occurs less frequently in *rheumatoid arthritis*. When affected, the joints are swollen and painful, leading to limitation of movement, particularly on arising in the morning. In children the disease may lead to malocclusion. *Ankylosis* on the joint may occur eventually, necessitating a condylectomy (see Chap. 356).

The myofascial pain syndrome, the most common disorder of the temporomandibular joint, is characterized by facial pain and mandibular dysfunction. The pain is often localized in the ear or jaw and may extend to the neck and shoulder. The mandibular dysfunction is manifested by limitation of movement, particularly an inability to open the jaw to the fullest extent. It is thought that such patients have increased musculature tension and hyperexcitable reflexes related to emotional tension. The precipitating factor appears to be the stretching of

an abnormal focus of pain which initiates a self-sustaining pain-spasm-pain cycle. Treatment of the pain-dysfunction syndrome involves the use of drugs to relieve the pain, lessen cortical excitability, and relax the muscles. Local anesthetics are used intramuscularly in the region of the trigger zone or as superficial sprays in an attempt to break the pain-spasm-pain cycle.

REFERENCES

BHASKAR SN: *Synopsis of Oral Pathology,* 5th ed. St Louis, Mosby, 1977

CIANCIOLA LJ et al: Defective polymorphonuclear leukocyte function in a human periodontal disease. Nature 265:445, 1977

GOLDMAN HM, COHEN DW (eds): *Periodontal Therapy,* 6th ed. St Louis, Mosby, 1978

MASHBERG A: Erythroplasia: The earliest sign of asymptomatic oral cancer. J Am Dent Assoc 96:615, 1978

SHAFER WG et al: *A Textbook of Oral Pathology,* 3d ed. Philadelphia, Saunders, 1974

SHAW JH et al: *Textbook of Oral Biology.* Philadelphia, Saunders, 1978

SHKLAR G, MCCARTHY PL: *The Oral Manifestations of Systemic Disease.* Woburn, Mass, Butterworths, 1976

34
DYSPHAGIA

THOMAS R. HENDRIX

Dysphagia, or difficulty in swallowing, is a most reliable symptom and indicates the presence of disease or dysfunction. Dysphagia should never be dismissed as an emotional disturbance or be confused with globus hystericus, a term used to indicate the sensation of a lump or tightness in the throat independent of swallowing.

The most characteristic manifestation of dysphagia is the sensation of food "sticking" somewhere in its passage to the stomach, usually at the level of the obstruction but sometimes referred to the suprasternal notch, even though the obstruction may be at the lower end of the esophagus. Pain may accompany dysphagia, especially if esophageal spasm is induced by the peristaltic waves attempting to force the bolus through the obstruction. If the pain is mild, it tends to be localized to the site of obstruction; if more severe, it radiates more widely, into the base of the neck, angles of the jaw, arms, epigastrium, or back. Sometimes pain, in a sense, may even cause dysphagia, as when the throat is so sore that swallowing is difficult. For further details regarding these symptoms, see Chap. 289.

Normal swallowing is a complex function dependent upon coordination of voluntary muscular structures of the oropharynx, striated muscles protecting the larynx and respiratory passages, as well as relaxation of the esophageal sphincters and the peristaltic wave itself; hence dysphagia may occur as a consequence of derangement or incoordination of any of the elements of the swallowing act as well as narrowing of the lumen by inflammatory stricture or tumor.

For clinical purposes it is useful to consider dysphagia as having either an oropharyngeal or an esophageal origin, because symptoms, etiology, and treatment are usually different for the two types.

OROPHARYNGEAL DYSPHAGIA Symptoms associated with dysphagia caused by disorders of oropharyngeal structures include aspiration with swallowing, regurgitation of fluid into the nose, pharyngeal pain with swallowing, and inability of the tongue to move the bolus into the pharynx. Dilatation and atony of piriform sinuses and pharynx and retention of contrast media in the valleculae are characteristic radiographic findings in patients with pharyngeal dysfunction. In addition, aspiration of contrast medium into the trachea or regurgitation into the nasopharynx and apparent obstruction at the upper esophageal sphincter (cricopharyngeus) may be found.

Neuromuscular disorders are the most common causes of oropharyngeal dysphagia, which, however, is usually only part of the symptom complex. Examples of these disorders are cerebrovascular accidents which cause pseudobulbar palsy (see Chap. 15) or bulbar palsy, poliomyelitis, motor system disease, diphtheritic polyneuritis, myasthenia gravis, myotonic dystrophies and restricted muscular dystrophies (oculopharyngeal and laryngoesophageal), and dermatomyositis. Ulcerative lesions such as pharyngitis, Vincent's angina, monilia stomatitis, viral infections with herpetic lesions, and retropharyngeal abscess interfere by causing pain and thereby inhibiting the initiation of deglutition. Plummer-Vinson syndrome (Paterson-Kelly syndrome, or sideropenic dysphagia) may also be listed here, since the difficulty in swallowing in this disorder resembles that due to a neuromuscular disorder, although pain may be an additional disturbing feature. Limited pathologic studies have shown both epithelial and muscle atrophy. It is clear that the dysphagia is not due to the characteristic web, or mucosal fold, of the anterior aspect of the cricopharyngeal area, because the web often persists long after the symptoms have been relieved by iron replacement.

Oropharyngeal dysphagia may be caused by narrowing of the lumen of the pharynx or upper esophagus by tumor, granulomatous disease, Zenker's diverticulum, or an enlarged thyroid.

ESOPHAGEAL DYSPHAGIA Symptoms indicating that the cause of dysphagia is to be found in the esophagus range from retrosternal fullness with swallowing to failure of the bolus to pass through the esophagus associated with pain relieved only by regurgitation of the offending bolus. Barium swallows in patients with dysphagia of esophageal origin show segmental narrowing of the esophageal lumen, failure of peristalsis, or both. Abnormalities of peristalsis may be characterized more precisely by intraluminal manometric studies.

Mechanical narrowing of the esophageal lumen is most frequently caused either by carcinoma of the squamous type, arising from the esophagus itself, or by adenocarcinoma of the cardia extending up into the esophagus. Rarely, benign tumors may reach sufficient size to cause dysphagia. Inflammatory strictures most commonly result from reflux esophagitis but are also caused by ingestion of corrosive substances, such as lye, or by trauma from foreign bodies or instrumentation. In addition, a lower esophageal ring may produce dysphagia by obstructing the esophageal lumen. Extrinsic pressure from aneurysms, vascular anomalies, mediastinal tumors, or paraesophageal diaphragmatic hernias may compress the esophageal lumen sufficiently to cause dysphagia. Finally, the motility disturbances associated with diffuse esophageal spasm, achalasia, and esophageal reflux may be the basis of dysphagia. Although esophageal peristalsis is absent in the majority of patients with scleroderma, dysphagia does not become a prominent symptom until reflux esophagitis has led to an inflammatory stricture.

DIFFERENTIAL DIAGNOSIS Determination of the basic mechanism responsible for dysphagia is usually a simple matter, but identification of the exact disorder responsible for it may be quite difficult. For example, cancer of the esophagus sometimes presents suddenly rather than gradually, and the roentgenogram may have a smooth, symmetric appearance such as is more commonly seen with benign stricture or achalasia; even esophagoscopy may be inconclusive, and biopsy

may yield deceptive results if the tissue shows only inflammatory reaction and does not include neoplastic cells. Similarly, neuromuscular disorders and disturbances of esophageal motility interfering with swallowing may be difficult to classify.

Certain symptoms associated with dysphagia, however, have diagnostic value. Hiccups, together with difficulty in swallowing, suggest a lesion at the terminal portion of the esophagus, such as carcinoma, achalasia, or hiatal hernia. Dysphagia followed, after an interval of some duration, by hoarseness usually means extension of a malignant growth beyond the walls of the esophagus and the involvement of a recurrent laryngeal nerve. When the hoarseness comes first and the dysphagia later, the primary lesion is almost always in the larynx. This combination of laryngeal and pharyngeal symptoms may also occur in polymyositis or dermatomyositis or with any disease causing bilateral involvement of vagus nerves or nuclei (poliomyelitis and polyneuritis). In motor system disease, the most common cause of a mixture of bulbar and pseudobulbar palsy, dysphagia is usually combined with dysphonia and dysarthria; the jaw jerk is hyperactive and the tongue atrophic. Dysphagia and unilateral wheezing virtually always indicate a mediastinal mass involving the esophagus and a main or large bronchus. Coughing with each swallow of food or drink means a fistulous communication between the esophagus and the trachea or a motor disorder in which the larynx is not effectively closed. Coughing occurring some time after swallowing may be due to regurgitation of food, most common in achalasia and Zenker's diverticulum.

DIAGNOSTIC PROCEDURES Examination of the mouth and pharynx should disclose those lesions which impede the transfer of food from the mouth to the esophagus, because of pain or mechanical interference. When lesions of the hypopharynx (e.g., *chronic abscess secondary to tuberculosis of the spine*) or of the larynx (e.g., *tuberculosis* or *carcinoma*) are suspected, examination with a mirror is necessary.

The most important diagnostic technique in the evaluation of dysphagia is a *barium swallow,* which makes it possible to determine whether dysphagia is caused by mechanical obstruction or by esophageal motor abnormality. Absence of esophageal peristalsis can best be demonstrated by barium swallows with the patient in Trendelenburg's position. If there is no peristalsis, barium will remain in the esophagus until the patient is tilted upright. Since the muscular action of the pharynx is so rapid, swallows must be recorded by *cineradiography.* Projection of the film at slow speed permits detection and analysis of abnormalities of pharyngeal function.

If barium swallow shows a lesion within the esophagus or a narrowing of the lumen, *esophagoscopy* is the most direct method for establishing the nature of the lesion. In addition to inspecting the lesion, one should perform biopsies and brushings of the lesion for cytologic examination to differentiate inflammatory from neoplastic lesions. A malignant stricture is not ruled out with certainty, however, if the biopsy shows only normal tissue or chronic inflammation, because tumors of the esophagus often spread beneath the mucosa and may be missed by a superficial biopsy. In such circumstances repeated biopsies or exfoliative cytologic examination is necessary. Cytologic studies by experienced personnel are very accurate in the diagnosis of esophageal cancer.

Since dysphagia usually is first experienced with solid food and only later with liquids, a normal swallow with liquid barium must not be taken as evidence that significant esophageal disease has been excluded. To simulate the situation in

NORMAL   ACHALASIA   DIFFUSE SPASM

5 sec

FIGURE 34-1

Esophageal manometric records from patients with normal esophageal function, achalasia, and diffuse esophageal spasm. Intraluminal pressure is recorded in the lower esophageal sphincter (lowest tracings) and 5 and 10 cm above the sphincter. Normally, a swallow of water (ws) is followed by relaxation of the lower esophageal sphincter, then the esophagus is cleared by a peristaltic wave proceeding abroad, and finally the sphincter closes. In achalasia, the resting pressure in the sphincter is elevated, and the sphincter does not relax completely in response to a swallow. The simultaneous elevation of pressure in the esophagus is caused by the pharynx propelling the bolus into an esophagus that is closed because of incomplete relaxation of the sphincter. In diffuse spasm, a swallow triggers a simultaneous series of repetitive high-amplitude esophageal contractions. In this record sphincter pressure and relaxation are normal. Relaxation is prolonged in association with continuing motor activity in the body of the esophagus. Some patients with diffuse spasm have sphincter dysfunction with elevated pressure and intermittent incomplete relaxation.

which the patient experiences dysphagia, the passage of a solid bolus, such as a radiopaque marshmallow, is observed. A solid bolus swallow most often demonstrates peristaltic disorders missed by liquid swallow but occasionally provides the first indication of early cancer of the esophagus.

Motor abnormalities of the pharynx and esophagus may be suspected by viewing the movement of a swallowed radiopaque bolus by fluoroscopy, but to characterize these abnormalities definitely, the motor response of pharynx and esophagus to swallowing must be studied by recording intraluminal pressure from several points simultaneously. Records are best obtained by use of a train of water-filled, perfused catheters connected to external pressure transducers or strain gauges. Examination of manometric records of swallows will demonstrate whether the wave is normally propagated over the length of the esophagus, whether the pressure generated by the peristaltic wave is normal and sufficient to propel the bolus, and finally, whether sphincter relaxation is complete, of adequate duration, and properly coordinated with the peristaltic wave (Fig. 34-1). Combining manometric with cineradiographic techniques has added greatly to understanding pharyngoesophageal function.

REFERENCES

CASTELL DO et al: Dysphagia. Gastroenterology 76:1015, 1979

COHEN BR, WOLF BS: Cineradiographic and intraluminal pressure correlations in the pharynx and esophagus, in *Handbook of Physiology*, sec 6, vol IV, CF Code (ed). Washington, American Physiological Society, 1968, p 1841

KILMAN WJ, GOYAL RK: Disorders of pharyngeal and upper esophageal sphincter motor function. Arch Intern Med 136:592, 1976

MUKHOPADHYAY AK, GRAHAM DY: Esophageal motor dysfunction in systemic disease. Arch Intern Med 136:583, 1976

PHILLIPS MM, HENDRIX TR: Dysphagia. Postgrad Med 50:81, 1971

POPE CE: Esophageal motility—Who needs it? Gastroenterology 74:1337, 1978

35
INDIGESTION

KURT J. ISSELBACHER

Indigestion is a term frequently used by patients to describe a multitude of symptoms generally appreciated as distress associated with the intake of food. The term is thus nonspecific and may not have the same meaning for the patient and the physician. In approaching the patient with indigestion, it is important for the physician first to elicit a good description of this complaint. To some patients indigestion refers to a feeling that digestion has not proceeded naturally. They may describe a sense of abdominal fullness, pressure, or actual pain. Others may use the term to describe heartburn, belching, distention, or flatulence. These complaints are considered in this chapter. Discussed elsewhere are the closely related symptoms of dysphagia, nausea and vomiting, and anorexia (Chaps. 34 and 36).

Indigestion may occur as a result of disease of the gastrointestinal tract or in association with pathologic states in other organ systems. As a result of systematic clinical and laboratory tests, a definable pathophysiologic process often can be shown to be responsible for the symptoms in a given case of indigestion. Frequently, however, clear etiologic explanation for the patient's complaints of indigestion are not established. Such cases are often designated as "functional indigestion," with a strong implication that psychosomatic factors underlie the complaints. Although it is clear that psychic factors may lead to symptoms of indigestion, the designation of "functional indigestion" is rarely, if ever, a satisfactory explanation, serving only to rephrase the patient's description of the symptoms. A psychogenic cause should not be assumed until organic causes of indigestion have been thoroughly excluded.

After having ascertained the patient's definition of indigestion, it is also important to determine (1) the location and duration of the discomfort, (2) the temporal relation of the symptoms to the ingestion of food, and (3) the possible relation of the symptoms to the ingestion of specific types of food (e.g., fatty foods, milk, and drugs).

PAIN PATTERNS True visceral abdominal pain as seen in indigestion is mediated over visceral afferent nerves which accompany the abdominal sympathetic pathways (see Chap. 6). Visceral pain is generally described as dull and aching in nature (with a diffuse midline localization) or as fullness or pressure. The location of the discomfort corresponds generally to the segmental level of the affected organ. Abdominal visceral pain can be produced experimentally by artificially increasing pressure in a hollow viscus. Usually this pain is the result of distention or exaggerated muscular contraction of a viscus. Inflammation generally lowers the threshold to such stimuli.

The visceral pain of indigestion should be distinguished from the sharp, lateralized, and localized pain patterns seen in many acute abdominal processes involving the peritoneum. In contrast to true visceral pain, this pain is mediated over cerebrospinal afferent nerves. Again it is of a dull, aching type, whether from inflammation of the viscera or of peritoneal surfaces.

In view of the diffuse nature of true visceral abdominal pain, the main clue comes from the segmental level of the viscus; in any given segmental region there is no way of determining which of several viscera are the source of it (Table 35-1). The following rules, already given in Chap. 6, are useful: *Substernal pain* of gastrointestinal origin usually arises from disorders in the esophagus or cardia of the stomach. Because pain in this area is frequently of cardiac origin, heart disease must be considered carefully and excluded. *Epigastric pain* is generally of gastric, duodenal, biliary, or pancreatic origin. As the pathologic process in the biliary tract and pancreas becomes more intense, it tends to lateralize and localize, e.g., biliary pain to the right upper quadrant and tip of the right scapula and pancreatic pain to the epigastrium, left upper quadrant, and back. *Periumbilical pain* is generally associated with small-intestinal disease. *Pain below the umbilicus* is often of appendiceal, large-intestinal, or pelvic origin.

TEMPORAL RELATIONSHIPS OF PAIN AND INDIGESTION
The unraveling of the temporal relationships of the patient's symptoms often provides the most significant diagnostic information. It is important to ascertain whether the symptoms are *constant* (continually present over extended periods of time), as may occur, for example, with an infiltrating gastric carcinoma, or *intermittent,* as in acute gastritis following an alcoholic binge or in association with the use of certain drugs. The symptoms may have a *diurnal* pattern; e.g., pain occurring *nocturnally* and with *recumbency* is seen in esophagitis and hiatus hernia. Symptoms are occasionally *seasonal;* this may occur in peptic ulcer disease, in which some patients experience more discomfort in the spring and autumn.

Another important and often diagnostic feature is the relation of pain or indigestion to ingestion of food. This relationship is especially significant or helpful if symptoms occur either during or minutes after the meal or if they occur several hours (4 or more) after eating. *Early postprandial symptoms* may reflect esophageal disease, because they may be associated with disordered swallowing function. In such instances, the distress or other symptoms of indigestion often are experienced substernally. Early postprandial complaints occur also in gastric disorders such as acute gastritis or carcinoma. *Late postprandial indigestion,* i.e., that occurring several hours after eating, may reflect failure of the stomach to empty adequately, as in pyloric stenosis or gastric atony. It may also be a symptom of duodenal ulcer, in which case it classically occurs several hours after the meal, when the ulcerated mucosa is exposed to acid secretions of the stomach unbuffered by food. Conversely,

the relief of pain following food ingestion is also seen in patients with peptic ulcer and is presumably due to the neutralization of the acid by the ingested food. Such pain also is typically alleviated quickly by oral antacids. Late postprandial indigestion also may result from impaired digestive and absorptive processes, as in pancreatic insufficiency.

FOOD INTOLERANCE In a number of situations specific foods or types of foods appear to be related to indigestion. Careful documentation of this relationship is sometimes of great help in arriving at an etiologic diagnosis.

Some foods may be poorly tolerated because of their consistency. Patients with esophageal stricture or carcinoma may tolerate liquids well, but the ingestion of solids may be associated with discomfort, especially substernal distress (see Chap. 289). Certain foods may be tolerated poorly because the intestinal tract cannot assimilate them adequately. This may occur following the ingestion of fatty foods in patients with pancreatic or biliary tract disease. Citrus fruits, with their relatively low pH, often provoke symptoms in patients with peptic ulcer disease.

Individuals may lack a specific enzyme required for assimilation of a certain nutrient. Patients may have a deficiency of the mucosal enzyme lactase, which catalyzes the hydrolysis of lactose. When lactase deficiency exists on a hereditary or acquired basis (e.g., in sprue, ulcerative colitis) (Chap. 292), the ingestion of milk (which contains lactose) results in abdominal cramps, distention, flatulence, and diarrhea.

There are a number of other conditions or disorders in which specific foods are poorly tolerated. Foods may be poorly tolerated because they initiate *allergic reactions* or exert a deleterious or *toxic effect* on the intestinal tract of susceptible persons (e.g., gluten in patients with nontropical sprue). Finally, certain substances may lead to systemic effects because of biochemical defects in the patient which render the substances particularly hazardous. An example of the latter is galactose intolerance in galactosemia (Chap. 98).

The above mechanisms do not explain the majority of clinical situations in which indigestion is associated with the eating of specific foods. For example, a history of fatty-food intolerance or an inability to eat cabbage, cucumbers, or spicy foods

TABLE 35-1
Distribution of visceral pain and examples of disorders frequently involving the specific organ

Organ	Location of referred pain	Frequent disorders
Esophagus	Substernum, epigastrium	Peptic esophagitis, hiatus hernia, stricture, carcinoma
Stomach	Epigastrium	Gastritis, peptic ulcer, carcinoma
Duodenum (first and second portions)	Epigastrium	Peptic ulcer
Duodenum (third portion, jejunum, and ileum)	Periumbilical	Regional enteritis, lymphoma, gastroenteritis (infectious), intestinal obstruction
Gallbladder	Epigastrium, right upper quadrant, right side of back	Cholelithiasis, cholecystitis
Pancreas	Epigastrium, left side of back	Pancreatitis, pancreatic carcinoma
Liver	Right upper quadrant	Passive congestion of liver, hepatitis, cirrhosis
Colon	Below umbilicus	Ulcerative colitis, carcinoma, partial obstruction

is commonly obtained from patients with indigestion. However, the mechanisms underlying the production of symptoms in these circumstances are still unclear.

ADDITIONAL SYNDROMES COMMONLY DESCRIBED AS INDIGESTION **Gaseousness, flatulence, aerophagia** A number of common clinical syndromes which may be described by the patient as "indigestion" appear to be related to increased quantities of gas in the intestinal tract. About 20 to 60 percent of intraluminal gas represents swallowed air. A degree of air swallowing, or *aerophagia*, occurs in normal persons, and the swallowed air can be observed at fluoroscopy. Under certain circumstances, such as chronic anxiety, poor eating habits, or actual intestinal disease itself, aerophagia may increase in magnitude and lead to symptoms in its own right.

The combination of early postprandial fullness and pressure, relieved by eructation and accompanied by a large amount of air seen in the gastric fundus on roentgenogram, is often referred to as the *magenblase* (i.e., gastric bubble) *syndrome*. Acute gastric distention by swallowed air can occasionally produce sharp pains which may mimic angina pectoris. This sequence of events may be especially perplexing in older patients with coronary artery disease, because it is well recognized that true angina pectoris may itself be precipitated by the ingestion of a large meal. Fatty meals delay gastric emptying and hence the passage of swallowed air in the intestine. This relationship may explain, in part, the prolonged sense of fullness and eructations experienced by many individuals after a fatty meal.

Swallowed air that is not eructated passes on in the intestinal tract and may either produce diffuse abdominal distention or become trapped in the splenic flexure of the colon. Distention of this segment of the colon produces a sensation of left upper quadrant fullness and pressure with radiation to the left side of the chest. This is known as the *splenic flexure syndrome*. Patients will often describe relief of pain with defecation or with the expulsion of flatus. Diagnosis may be made by demonstrating, on physical examination, a note of increased tympany in the extreme left lateral portion of the upper part of the abdomen or by the visualization of large amounts of air in the splenic flexure of the colon by radiography.

A second major source of intestinal gas is the fermentative action of bacteria on carbohydrates and proteins within the lumen. Increased amounts of intraluminal gas production due to this mechanism have been demonstrated in conditions associated with abnormal bacterial colonization of the small intestine and in patients with carbohydrate malabsorption.

Increased gas production may occur following the ingestion of certain foods (e.g., the legumes) which contain significant quantities of nonabsorbable sugars. As in the case of swallowed air, increased amounts of intraluminally produced gas can produce symptoms by causing distention, pain, increased motility (with diarrhea), or flatulence.

Heartburn Heartburn, or pyrosis, is a sensation of warmth or burning located substernally or high in the epigastrium. Experimental studies in human beings have shown that esophageal distention or increased motor activity is associated in most subjects with a feeling of fullness and burning in this area.

Heartburn may occur with organic disease of the intestinal tract and is usually associated with gastroesophageal reflux. This is frequently the case in hiatus hernia. In this setting, heartburn occurs after a large meal or with stooping or bending. Esophageal reflux of acid contents at these times leads to symptoms by either the production of abnormal motor activity or direct mucosal irritation (i.e., esophagitis). Heartburn may arise following the ingestion of certain foods or drugs (e.g.,

alcohol and aspirin). It may also be seen in the absence of a demonstrable anatomic or motor pathologic condition, in which case it is frequently accompanied by aerophagia and for lack of other explanation is often attributed to psychological factors.

INDIGESTION DUE TO DISEASE OUTSIDE THE INTESTINAL TRACT A multitude of extraintestinal disease processes may result in indigestion by mechanisms which are poorly understood. Indigestion may be the presenting complaint, for example, in congestive heart failure, uremia, pulmonary tuberculosis, and neoplastic disease. Under these circumstances the symptoms of indigestion may present with no unique features to suggest that they are in fact due to some other systemic disease process. Drugs such as aspirin, corticosteroids, indomethacin, and phenylbutazone affect gastric secretion and are ulcerogenic; thus they may lead to symptoms of indigestion.

DIAGNOSTIC APPROACH TO THE PATIENT WITH INDIGESTION Indigestion represents a challenging and difficult diagnostic problem because of the nonspecific nature of its manifestations. The evaluation of indigestion must include initially a thorough medical workup, with ultimate confirmation or exclusion of pathophysiologic derangements by the appropriate diagnostic procedures.

A careful history should include an assessment of the patient's general medical health, including the possibility of diseases in extraintestinal organ systems which may produce indigestion. Careful evaluation of psychological factors is crucial, because they often play an etiologic or contributory role in the patient's problem. Of particular importance are anxiety, depressive reactions, and hysteria (Chap. 11). Evaluation of the patient's intestinal problem must include an assessment of nutritional status, changes in weight, and appetite.

A clear and detailed description of the specific symptoms should be obtained, particularly the patient's definition of the term "indigestion." The nature of the pain, its frequency and time of occurrence, its relationship to meals, and the special circumstances which lead to its exacerbation or relief should be elicited. Associated intestinal symptoms such as nausea and vomiting, abnormal bowel habits, steatorrhea, diarrhea, and melena should also be sought. Physical examination rarely establishes the specific diagnosis, but it may be useful in detecting disease in other organ systems (e.g., congestive heart failure) which can affect intestinal physiology.

X-ray examination of the alimentary tract is crucial to the evaluation of indigestion. This may involve examination of the esophagus, stomach, small intestine, colon, and biliary tract. Esophagoscopy, gastroscopy, colonoscopy, or sigmoidoscopy also may be helpful or necessary. Stools should be examined for appearance, occult blood, fat, and muscle fibers. As stated above, careful attempts must be made to exclude nonintestinal disease, especially cardiac disease.

Unfortunately, even after completion of careful diagnostic studies, many cases of indigestion will turn out to have no clear explanation. Some of these are psychogenic and may respond to appropriate psychiatric measures. Others represent physiologic derangements which are undetectable by currently available diagnostic methods. Still others represent actual disease processes in early stages which may be diagnosable by conventional methods at a later date. The ultimate evaluation of indigestion requires, therefore, the utmost in sensitivity, diligence, and patience on the part of the examining physician.

REFERENCES

BOND JH, LEVITT MD: A rational approach to intestinal gas problems. Viewpoints Digestive Dis vol 9, no 2, 1977

COGHILL NF: Dyspepsia. Br Med J 4:97, 1967

Lasser RB et al: The role of intestinal gas in functional abdominal pain. N Engl J Med 293:524, 1975

Levitt MD: Methane production in the gut. N Engl J Med 291:528, 1974

36
ANOREXIA, NAUSEA, AND VOMITING

KURT J. ISSELBACHER

ANOREXIA   Anorexia, or loss of the desire to eat, is a prominent symptom in a wide variety of intestinal and extraintestinal disorders. It must be clearly differentiated from satiety and from specific food intolerance. Anorexia occurs in many disorders and as a result *by itself is of little specific diagnostic value.* The mechanisms whereby hunger and appetite are modified in various disease states are poorly understood. Normally food intake is regulated by two hypothalamic centers—a lateral "feeding center" and a ventromedial "satiety center." The latter inhibits the feeding center following a meal leading to the sensation of satiety.

Anorexia is commonly seen in diseases of the gastrointestinal tract and liver. For example, it may precede the appearance of jaundice in hepatitis, or it may be a prominent symptom in gastric carcinoma. In the setting of intestinal disease, anorexia should be clearly differentiated from *sitophobia,* or fear of eating because of subsequent or associated discomfort. In such circumstances, appetite may persist, but the ingestion of food is curtailed nonetheless. Sitophobia may be seen, for example, in regional enteritis (especially with partial obstruction) or in patients with gastric ulcer following partial or total gastrectomy.

Anorexia may also be a prominent feature of severe extraintestinal diseases. For example, anorexia may be profound in severe congestive heart failure and is often associated with cardiac glycoside intoxication. It may be a major symptom in patients with uremia, pulmonary failure, and various endocrinopathies (e.g., hyperparathyroidism, Addison's disease, and panhypopituitarism). Anorexia also often accompanies psychogenic disturbances, such as anxiety or depression. For a discussion of anorexia nervosa, see Chap. 77.

NAUSEA AND VOMITING   Nausea and vomiting may occur independently of each other, but generally they are so closely allied that they may conveniently be considered together. *Nausea* denotes the feeling of the imminent desire to vomit, usually referred to the throat or epigastrium. *Vomiting* refers to the forceful oral expulsion of gastric contents; *retching* denotes the labored rhythmic respiratory activity that frequently precedes emesis. Extremely forceful *projectile vomiting* is a special form of vomiting which has significance because it connotes the presence of increased intracranial pressure.

Nausea often precedes or accompanies vomiting. It is usually associated with diminished functional activity of the stomach and alterations of the motility of the duodenum and small intestine. Accompanying severe nausea there is often evidence of altered autonomic (especially parasympathetic) activity: pallor of the skin, increased perspiration, salivation, and the occasional association of hypotension and bradycardia (vasovagal syndrome). Anorexia is also often present.

Following a period of nausea and a brief interval of retching, a sequence of involuntary visceral and somatic motor events occurs, resulting in emesis. The stomach plays a relatively passive role in the vomiting process, the major ejection force being provided by the abdominal musculature. With relaxation of the gastric fundus and gastroesophageal sphincter, a sharp increase in intraabdominal pressure is brought about by forceful contraction of the diaphragm and abdominal wall. This, together with concomitant annular contraction of the gastric pylorus, results in the expulsion of gastric contents into the esophagus. Increased intrathoracic pressure results in the further movement of esophageal contents into the mouth. Reversal of the normal direction of esophageal peristalsis may play a role in this process. Reflex elevation of the soft palate during the vomiting act prevents the entry of the material into the nasopharynx, whereas reflex closure of the glottis and inhibition of respiration help to prevent pulmonary aspiration.

Repeated emesis may have deleterious effects in a number of different ways. The process of vomiting itself may lead to traumatic rupture or tearing in the region of the cardioesophageal junction, resulting in massive hematemesis, the Mallory-Weiss syndrome. Prolonged vomiting may lead to dehydration and the loss of gastric secretions (especially hydrochloric acid), resulting in metabolic alkalosis with hypokalemia. Finally, in states of central nervous system depression (coma, etc.), gastric contents may be aspirated into the lungs, with a resulting aspiration pneumonitis.

Vomiting mechanism   The act of vomiting is under the control of two functionally distinct medullary centers: the *vomiting center* and the *chemoreceptor trigger zone.* They lie close to each other near other brainstem centers regulating vasomotor and autonomic functions. The vomiting center controls and integrates the actual act of emesis. It receives afferent stimuli from the intestinal tract and other parts of the body, from higher cortical centers, especially the labyrinthine apparatus, and from the chemoreceptor trigger zone. The important efferent pathways in vomiting are the phrenic nerves (to the diaphragm), the spinal nerves (to the abdominal musculature), and visceral efferent nerves (to the stomach and esophagus).

The chemoreceptor trigger zone is also located in the medulla but by itself is incapable of mediating the act of vomiting. Activation of this zone results in efferent impulses to the medullary vomiting center, which in turn initiates the act of emesis. The chemoreceptor trigger zone can be activated by many stimuli, including drugs such as apomorphine, cardiac glycosides, and ergot alkaloids. Certain of the phenothiazine derivatives appear to antagonize the effects of the above-mentioned drugs on the chemoreceptor trigger zone.

Clinical classification   Nausea and vomiting are common manifestations of organic and functional disorders. The precise mechanisms triggering vomiting in the various clinical states are poorly understood, making classification of mechanisms difficult. The categories mentioned below serve to illustrate some of the many disorders which may be accompanied by nausea and vomiting.

Many *acute abdominal emergencies* which lead to the "surgical abdomen" are associated with nausea and vomiting. Notably, vomiting may be seen with inflammation of a viscus as in acute appendicitis or acute cholecystitis, obstruction of the intestine, or acute peritonitis (see Chap. 6).

In many of the disorders involving *chronic indigestion* (see Chap. 35) nausea and vomiting may be prominent. Emesis may be either spontaneous or self-induced and may lead to relief of symptoms, as, for example, in uncomplicated peptic ulcer. Nausea and vomiting may accompany the distention and pain seen in the aerophagic syndromes. Often in patients with chronic indigestion, nausea and vomiting may be provoked by specific foods (e.g., fatty foods), for reasons that are poorly understood.

Acute systemic infections with fever, especially in young children, are frequently accompanied by vomiting and often by severe diarrhea. The mechanism whereby infections remote from the gastrointestinal tract produce these manifestations is unclear. Viral, bacterial, and parasitic infections of the intestinal tract may be associated with severe nausea and vomiting, often with diarrhea. Severe nausea and vomiting may be prominent in viral hepatitis, even before the appearance of jaundice.

Central nervous system disorders which lead to increased intracranial pressure may be accompanied by vomiting, often projectile. Brain swelling due to inflammation, anoxemia, acute hydrocephalus, neoplasms, etc., may thus be complicated by vomiting. Disorders of the labyrinthine apparatus and its central connections which underlie vertigo may be accompanied by vomiting with nausea and retching. Acute labyrinthitis and Ménière's disease are examples of such disturbances. Migraine headaches, tabetic crises, and acute meningitis are additional examples of disorders of the nervous system which may lead to vomiting. In the reactive phase of hypotension with syncope, there may also be nausea and vomiting.

Severe nausea and vomiting may be present in *acute myocardial infarction*, especially of the posterior wall of the heart. Nausea and vomiting may also be seen in *congestive heart failure*, perhaps in relation to congestion of the liver. The possibility that these symptoms may be due to drugs (e.g., opiates or digitalis) should always be borne in mind in patients with cardiac disease.

Nausea and vomiting commonly accompany several *endocrinologic disorders*, including diabetic acidosis and adrenal insufficiency, especially adrenal crises. The morning sickness of early pregnancy is another instance of nausea and vomiting possibly related to hormonal changes.

The *side effects of many drugs and chemicals* include nausea and vomiting. In some instances this is because of gastric irritation which stimulates the medullary vomiting center.

Psychogenic vomiting means vomiting which may occur as part of any emotional upset on a transitory basis or more persistently as part of a psychic disturbance. Close observation will usually disclose the condition to be one of regurgitation rather than of vomiting, and weight loss may not correspond at all to the patient's description of the frequency and severity of vomiting. As discussed in Chap. 77, anorexia nervosa is an emotional disturbance which may be associated not only with anorexia but also with vomiting. Often patients with emotional disorders and vomiting maintain a relatively normal state of nutrition because a relatively small amount of the ingested food is vomited.

Differential diagnosis Vomiting should be distinguished from *regurgitation*, which refers to the expulsion of food in the absence of nausea and without abdominal diaphragmatic muscular contraction which is part of vomiting. Regurgitation of esophageal contents may occur with esophageal stricture or diverticula. Regurgitation of gastric contents is generally seen with gastroesophageal sphincter incompetence, especially with hiatus hernia or in association with peptic ulcer, usually when pylorospasm supervenes.

The temporal relationships of vomiting to eating may be of help diagnostically. Vomiting which occurs predominantly in the morning is often seen early in pregnancy and uremia. Alcoholic gastritis is commonly accompanied by early-morning emesis, the so-called "dry heaves." Vomiting which occurs shortly after eating may suggest pylorospasm or gastritis. On the other hand, vomiting which occurs 4 to 6 h or longer after eating and involves the elimination of large quantities of undigested food often indicates gastric retention (e.g., diabetic gastric atony or pyloric obstruction).

The character of the vomitus offers clues to the diagnosis. If the vomitus contains free hydrochloric acid, the obstruction may be due to an ulcer; absence of free hydrochloric acid is more compatible with gastric malignancy. A feculent or putrid odor reflects the results of bacterial action on the intestinal contents. Such vomiting may be seen with low-intestinal obstruction, peritonitis, or gastrocolic fistula. Bile is commonly present in gastric contents whenever vomiting is prolonged. It has no significance unless constantly present in large quantities, when it may signify an obstructive lesion below the ampulla of Vater. The presence of blood in the gastric contents usually denotes bleeding from the esophagus, stomach, or duodenum.

REFERENCES

HALL RJC: Normal and abnormal food intake. Gut 16:744, 1975

LUMSDEN K, HOLDEN SW: The act of vomiting in man. Gut 10:173, 1969

SWANSON DW et al: Persistent nausea without organic cause. Mayo Clin Proc 51:257, 1976

37
CONSTIPATION, DIARRHEA, AND DISTURBANCES OF ANORECTAL FUNCTION

STEPHEN E. GOLDFINGER

NORMAL COLONIC FUNCTION Each day one to two liters of semiliquid material composed of undigested dietary residue, intestinal secretions, and cellular debris passes across the ileocecal valve to the colon. Little of nutritional value remains following the extensive digestive processing and absorption that occurs in the small intestine. This liquid ileal effluent is converted to solid feces in the colon before it is advanced to the rectum and evacuated. To accomplish this, many important physiologic processes underly normal colonic function; among these are *absorption* of fluid and electrolytes; *peristaltic contractions* that facilitate mixing, dessication, and passage of feces to the rectum; and finally, *defecation*.

Absorption of fluid and electrolytes (see also Chap. 292) In Western societies the average daily stool weight is less than 200 g, of which 60 to 80 percent is water. Thus, the colon normally absorbs more than 90 percent of the fluid it receives, and this occurs well within its absorptive *capacity* of 6 liters water and 800 meq sodium per day. The primary absorptive sites are the ascending and transverse colon. Water absorption occurs passively, osmotically following the active transport of sodium and chloride ions. In addition, bicarbonate is secreted in exchange for chloride, and there is a small net efflux of potassium across the colonic mucosa into the lumen. The secreted bicarbonate is converted, in part, to carbon dioxide by reacting with acids produced by colonic bacteria. Analysis of fecal electrolyte concentrations in normal subjects reveals considerable variation, but average values for sodium, potassium, chloride, and bicarbonate are 32, 75, 16, and 40 meq per liter, respectively. The hyperosmolality of normal stool, which averages 375 mosmol, is largely due to osmotically active organic compounds produced by bacteria.

Factors which tend to cause diarrhea include:

1 Excessive outpouring of fluid from the small intestine into the colon. This may occur in association with viral and bacterial enteritis, various malabsorptive diseases of the small intestine, pancreatic tumors secreting gastrin or vasoactive intestinal peptide, and resection of the terminal ileum.

2 Reduced amount or deficient function of colonic mucosa (e.g., subtotal colectomy, diffuse ulcerative colitis).

3 Neural and hormonal stimuli which decrease to-and-fro peristalsis or promote massive propulsive activity (see below) and thus reduce mucosal surface contact time (e.g., exaggerated postprandial motility).

4 Impaired colonic reabsorption of water and electrolytes due to the presence of excessive bile salts and fatty acids. When ileal reabsorption of bile salts is defective (e.g., ileal resection, regional ileitis), increased amounts of dihydroxy bile salts reach the colon where they inhibit sodium absorption and promote secretion. Increased intraluminal hydroxylated fatty acids, which are present in sprue and pancreatic malabsorption, produce diarrhea by a similar effect upon mucosal cells.

5 Excessive colonic secretion distal to reabsorptive sites (e.g., villous adenoma of the rectum).

6 Increased luminal concentrations of nonabsorbed molecules exerting significant osmotic effect (e.g., magnesium-containing cathartics, lactose when individuals with lactase deficiency eat milk products).

Excessively hard stools are usually due to increased absorption of fluid as a result of prolonged contact of the luminal contents with the colonic mucosa consequent to delayed transit. In some instances ingested material such as calcium carbonate can explain "rock-like" feces.

Motility (contraction) patterns of the colon The colon and rectum are innervated by sympathetic and parasympathetic fibers, as well as by nonadrenergic, noncholinergic nerves that may release bioactive amines, peptides, or nucleotides. Impulses transmitted via these nerve fibers, local neural reflex arcs, and intrinsic contractile responses of smooth muscle all play a part in the coordination of colonic motility. Parasympathetic nerves, which stimulate peristaltic contraction, dominate the regulation of colonic motor activity; adrenergic tone inhibits cholinergic stimulation. The precise integration of all neural and nonneural mediators of colonic motility remains poorly understood.

Basal colonic motor activity consists mainly of nonpropulsive contractions of circular smooth muscle which move luminal contents back and forth across relatively short segments of bowel. Since no net aboral advance is achieved, it is presumed that the main purpose of these movements is to maximize mucosal surface contact for absorption. With increased parasympathetic tone, such as occurs postprandially, more propulsive activity occurs. This may take the form of aboral contractions across short segments of colon or involve massive peristalsis, which begins in the right or transverse colon and rapidly moves luminal contents to the sigmoid colon and rectum. Massive peristalsis may occur only several times a day. Resultant distention of the rectum initiates the defecatory urge.

Since colonic motility plays an important role in both absorption and movement of contents to the rectum, alterations of bowel tone occurring as a result of disease, stress, or various drugs tend to have an important influence on bowel movements. In view of the number of pharmacologic agents that may influence smooth muscle contractility, it is essential to take a careful drug history when evaluating patients with constipation or diarrhea of recent onset.

Defecation The defecatory reflex is initiated by acute distention of the rectum. When it is allowed to progress by supraspinal centers, sigmoidal and rectal contractions heighten the pressure within the rectum and also obliterate the rectosigmoidal angle. Concomitant relaxation of the internal and external anal sphincters then permits the evacuation of feces. This can be augmented by an increase in intraabdominal pressure created by the Valsalva maneuver (i.e., voluntary closure of the glottis, diaphragmatic fixation, and abdominal-wall contraction). Conversely, defecation may be consciously prevented by the forceful contraction of the striated muscles of the pelvic diaphragm and external anal sphincter. The functional value of voluntary control of defecation requires little elaboration, but the opportunity for individuals to resist the defecatory urge, when abused, may lead to chronic rectal distention, reduced afferent signals, lax motor tone, and chronic constipation.

DIARRHEA AND CONSTIPATION The bowel habits of apparently healthy persons vary widely. For this reason, the terms *diarrhea* and *constipation* have most meaning when viewed as a change from an individual's customary pattern. Reasonably detailed information is important in evaluating either abnormality. When patients complain of diarrhea, it is important to obtain an estimate of the volume as well as frequency of fecal output and, in addition, to directly examine a stool sample for consistency, blood, oiliness, and malodor. For example, the repeated elimination of small quantities of solid material admixed with gas has a far different connotation than the same number of movements of voluminous blood-tinged feces. The term *constipation* may be used by the patient to refer to a variety of changes including reduction in frequency of defecation, a constant sensation of rectal fullness with incomplete evacuation of feces, and sometimes painful defecation due to hard stools or perianal pathology. In an assessment of complaints of diarrhea or constipation, it is important to consider the patient's emotional state since in many instances the recent onset of psychological stress is the major reason for altered bowel habits. However, it can be hazardous to assume this to be the case, even when the relationship seems convincing. For this reason, the judicious use of laboratory, proctoscopic, and radiologic procedures is recommended to make certain that organic disease will not be overlooked.

Acute diarrhea Diarrhea of abrupt onset occurring in otherwise healthy persons is most often related to an infectious process. A variety of accompanying symptoms are often observed, including fever, headache, anorexia, vomiting, malaise, and myalgia, but they cannot be used to distinguish with certainty among viral, bacterial, and protozoal causes. In most instances, identifiable pathogens are not recovered from the feces. For this reason so-called "nonspecific" diarrhea is usually considered to be of viral etiology. However, the demonstration of enterotoxins produced by strains of *Escherichia coli* and other bacteria, which are not distinguishable from "normal flora" on routine culture, suggests that this assumption may sometimes be incorrect and that these bacteria may account for a number of cases that are usually ascribed to viral infection.

Acute diarrhea presumed to be of viral etiology typically persists for a period of 1 to 3 days; death is extremely rare except in previously debilitated individuals who become severely dehydrated. Abnormal small-intestinal morphology including villous shortening, increase in the number of crypt cells, and increased cellularity of the lamina propria has been described in experimentally infected human volunteers who have also demonstrated transient malabsorption of fat and xylose. Unfortunately, immune electron microscopy, the technique frequently used for viral identification in stool, is generally not available clinically. The diagnosis of viral diarrhea is supported (but not confirmed) by the absence of polymorphonuclear leukocytes and erythrocytes in stool samples after preparation with Loeffler's methylene blue. Bacterial diarrhea may be suspected if there is a history of a similar and simultaneous illness in individuals who shared contaminated food with the patient. Diarrhea developing within 12 h of the meal is most likely due to ingestion of a preformed toxin (e.g., staphylococcal exotoxin). A lag period of up to 3 days after consumption of contaminated food can occur with salmonellosis.

The pathogenesis of bacterial diarrhea is due to two principal mechanisms, *mucosal invasion* and *enterotoxin-induced hypersecretion.* Bacterial invasion of the colonic wall leads to mucosal hyperemia, edema, leukocytic infiltration, and frank ulceration. Lower abdominal cramps and tenderness are prominent, as are tenesmus and rectal urgency. In severe cases the stool is grossly bloody. At other times, microscopic examination of the stool will reveal erythrocytes along with pus cells. In *shigellosis* diarrhea is mainly due to mucosal destruction by the invading microorganisms, but small-intestinal hypersecretion may also occur with some enterotoxin-producing strains of *Shigella.* The prototype of hypersecretory bacterial diarrhea is *cholera,* in which the organism *Vibrio cholerae* adheres to, but does not invade, the surface epithelial cells and releases an enterotoxin which stimulates massive secretion of fluid and electrolytes by the small intestine. This may be produced experimentally in animals by placing the enterotoxin, free of the organism itself, into isolated intestinal loops. Hypersecretion reaches a peak at 4 to 6 h and is mediated by the stimulation of mucosal adenylate cyclase by the toxin. It should be emphasized that in cholera, mucosal morphology is essentially normal, and intestinal absorptive capacity is preserved. This provides the basis for oral rehydration therapy with solutions containing glucose and sodium chloride, the former stimulating absorption of the latter. Because other species of bacteria, such as *E. coli, Clostridium,* and *Salmonella,* have been shown to produce enterotoxins, the finding of an exudate-free stool does not preclude bacterial infection as the cause of diarrhea.

Protozoal infections may also be responsible for acute diarrhea. *Entamoeba histolytica,* prevalent in some areas of the United States, produces an inflammatory colitis which can closely mimic idiopathic ulcerative colitis. Giardiasis is a cause of prolonged, watery diarrhea that often afflicts travelers returning from endemic areas where the water supply has been contaminated. In some patients giardiasis is associated with an underlying immunoglobulin deficiency of the IgA type. Careful examination of fresh stools by experienced technicians is required for the diagnosis of protozoal infection. Duodenal samples in the form of aspirate and biopsy touch preparations may be necessary to make the diagnosis of giardiasis.

Travelers' diarrhea may result from any one or several of the pathogens described above. However, often no known agent is identified, and the etiology is assumed to be viral or due to enterotoxin-producing coliform organisms. Not infrequently prolonged bowel irregularity will occur following the acute illness.

Ulcerative colitis and *regional enteritis* (Crohn's disease) may begin as acute diarrhea (Chaps. 293 and 294). Bloody stools and generalized abdominal cramping and tenderness are more apt to occur in the patients with ulcerative colitis; in regional enteritis, the diarrhea tends to be milder, is usually nonbloody, and is associated with right lower quadrant pain and tenderness. Diarrhea may be caused by a variety of *drugs,* including cholinergic agents, magnesium-containing antacids, antimetabolites used in cancer chemotherapy, and broad-spectrum antibiotics. Diarrhea due to *diverticulitis* is usually ac-

companied by fever, tenesmus, and rectal urgency, together with cramps and tenderness in the left lower quadrant (Chap. 294). When there is no evidence of acute inflammation, diarrhea in the presence of colonic diverticula is probably due to a spastic (irritable) colon which may set the stage for the development of diverticula. In elderly and debilitated individuals with *fecal impaction,* the presenting symptom may be the frequent expulsion of small amounts of liquid stool overflowing from colonic distention behind the impaction. Acute *psychological stress* can cause diarrhea at any age.

DIAGNOSTIC APPROACH   The appropriate tempo and approach in the evaluation of acute diarrhea depend so heavily on the clinical setting in which it occurs that only very general guidelines can be offered. It is entirely reasonable to withhold studies in mild, self-limited cases such as are seen as part of an epidemic viral illness. When dealing with sporadic severe diarrhea or when a suggestive epidemiologic history is obtained, bacterial cultures and microscopic examination of the stool for parasites and inflammatory cells are appropriate. Proctoscopy is generally reserved for patients with bloody diarrhea, or those who do not show improvement within 5 days. Likewise, radiologic studies should usually be deferred until the initial course of the illness has been observed. In cases of massive fluid loss, measurement of serum electrolytes is useful to aid in determining replacement therapy.

TREATMENT   General and nonspecific treatment of acute diarrhea includes rest, encouragement of fluid intake, and prescription of opiate-containing agents by mouth. Intravenous fluid and electrolyte replacement may be desirable and necessary in infants and the elderly. As a result of success achieved with cholera patients, the use of oral glucose-electrolyte solutions is being extended to the treatment of patients with acute diarrhea considered to be due to other enterotoxin-producing bacteria.

Chronic diarrhea   Diarrhea persisting for weeks or months, whether constant or intermittent, may be a functional symptom or a manifestation of serious illness. For this reason, it is incumbent upon the physician to search carefully for evidence of organic disease, such as fever, weight loss, malnutrition, anemia, or an increased erythrocyte sedimentation rate. Abdominal tenderness and fever suggest the presence of inflammation. When there is involvement of the large bowel, the major diseases to be considered include ulcerative colitis, Crohn's disease of the colon, amebiasis, and diverticulitis. Crohn's disease of the small intestine may involve one or more of its segments. The ileum is most frequently affected. Other diarrheal conditions which may resemble Crohn's disease radiographically include tuberculous and fungal enteritis, lymphosarcoma, amyloidosis, and argentaffin (carcinoid) tumors of the small bowel.

Prolonged diarrhea without evidence of inflammation may reflect impairments of absorption, secretion, or digestion. Selective derangements, such as those due to *bile salt enteropathy* and *lactase deficiency,* are usually not accompanied by weight loss or malnutrition. *Mucosal disorders,* best exemplified by sprue, are frequently associated with weight loss, malodorous stools, abdominal distention, and anemia, and, when more severe, with osteomalacia, hypoprothrombinemia, avitaminotic neuropathies, and tetany. *Pancreatic insufficiency* resulting from chronic pancreatitis, carcinoma, or resection produces steatorrhea and weight loss of varying severity. A number of mechanisms may be responsible for *postgastrectomy diarrhea* (see Chap. 290). These include the dumping syndrome, postvagotomy motility derangements, inadequate stimulation of pancreatic digestive enzymes, and incomplete mixing of these enzymes with food. On rare occasions severe postgastrectomy diarrhea and malnutrition are due to the inadvertent creation by the surgeon of a gastroileostomy instead of a gastrojejunostomy. *Bacterial overgrowth* in the small intestine, as may occur with extensive diverticulosis and prolonged bowel stasis secondary to disorders of peristalsis (e.g., scleroderma, diabetic visceral neuropathy), can also lead to chronic diarrhea and weight loss. This has been attributed to bacterial deconjugation of bile salts and hydroxylation of long-chain fatty acids, to consumption of nutrients by the organisms, and to mucosal abnormalities believed to be caused by bacteria or their metabolites (see Chap. 292). At times, diarrhea may accompany stasis in the absence of bacterial overgrowth.

Endocrine disorders that may be accompanied by chronic diarrhea include thyrotoxicosis, diabetes mellitus, adrenal insufficiency, and hypoparathyroidism. The release of potent secretagogues from neoplastic tissue in the Zollinger-Ellison syndrome (gastrin), medullary carcinoma of the thyroid (calcitonin, prostaglandins), and pancreatic cholera syndrome (vasoactive intestinal peptide) makes diarrhea a prominent feature of these disorders. The passage of excessive amounts of clear liquid, at times sufficient to cause dehydration, occurs in some patients with large villous adenomas of the rectum.

Habitual *cathartic abuse* must be suspected when the cause of prolonged diarrhea remains perplexing. Even if this is denied by the patient, a stool sample should be alkalinized with sodium hydroxide; this will produce a burgundy color if phenolphthalein-containing laxatives have been surreptitiously ingested. The observation of melanosis coli by sigmoidoscopy indicates chronic usage of anthraquinone laxatives.

Constipation Constipation is a common complaint often resulting from the inordinate expectation of "regularity" in bowel-conscious individuals. Stools are described as infrequent, incomplete, or unduly hard; unusual straining may be required to achieve defecation. A review of the patient's habits often reveals contributory and correctable causes, such as insufficient dietary roughage, lack of exercise, suppression of defecatory urges arising at inconvenient moments, inadequate allotment of time for full defecation, and prolonged travel. Appropriate adjustments of these patterns and reassurance are preferable to the prescription of laxatives and may be all that is required for improvement. When the patient also has symptoms such as fatigue, malaise, headaches, or anorexia, the possibility should be considered that such symptoms reflect an underlying depression of which constipation is but one component. Decreased colonic motility is responsible for the constipation associated with the use of parasympatholytic drugs, spinal cord injury, scleroderma, and Hirschsprung's disease.

Hemorrhoids, anal fissures, perineal abscesses, and rectal strictures often prevent easy and adequate stool evacuation. When constipation and tenesmus of recent onset are reported, the possibility of carcinoma of the rectum or descending colon must be seriously considered. In such instances sigmoidoscopic and barium enema examinations should be obtained early and are virtually obligatory if fecal blood has been observed or if occult blood is detected on any of three successive stool specimens. Stools of abnormally thin caliber occur in patients with rectal or sigmoid colon carcinoma but are even more commonly due to an irritable colon. Other mechanical causes of constipation include volvulus of the sigmoid colon, diverticulitis, intussusception, and hernias. A variety of metabolic abnormalities, such as hypothyroidism, hypercalcemia, hypokalemia, porphyria, lead poisoning, and dehydration are often associated with constipation. Tremendous fecal retention and impaction may occur in certain neurologic disorders (e.g., spinal cord injury, multiple sclerosis, cerebral palsy, senility), and in these instances, when autonomous regulation of evacuation is unachievable, vigorous and sustained enema programs are often necessary.

IRRITABLE BOWEL The irritable bowel syndrome (also referred to as *spastic colon* and *mucous colitis*) is one of the most frequent gastrointestinal disorders (see Chap. 294). This condition is characterized by periodic or chronic symptoms of diarrhea, constipation, and abdominal pain. These symptoms are generally associated with psychologic stresses, but the anxiety produced by the bowel disturbance is sometimes regarded by the patient as the fundamental cause of the emotional upset. Stools tend to be thin, fragmented, or pelletlike, and accompanied by excessive mucus and gas. Efforts to ameliorate symptoms with mild cathartics or antispasmodic drugs may yield adverse and exaggerated responses. An increased sigmoidal motility has been demonstrated in association with the clinical pattern of pain and constipation, whereas hypomotility is characteristic of painless diarrhea. A variety of therapeutic approaches, including the avoidance of foods which tend to upset the patient, addition of bulk-forming agents, judicious use of antispasmodics and tranquilizers, and gentle psychotherapy may provide some relief. If the patient's life goals can be shifted away from the quixotic search for the perfect stool, much can be accomplished. At the same time, it must be remembered that such individuals are not exempt from developing bowel cancer, and any worrisome deviation from their general pattern of derangement must be seriously evaluated.

FLATULENCE A significant amount of flatus is passed each day by normal persons, and the complaint of flatulence often reflects a heightened and embarrassing awareness of this natural occurrence. Many who complain of gas are, in reality, experiencing symptoms ascribable to disordered motility. Excessive passage of intestinal gas may be the result of aerophagia or the formation of increased amounts of gas by intestinal bacteria. The latter process can be associated with malabsorption syndromes or significant constipation but is more frequently a consequence of eating foods such as beans, broccoli, and cabbage which have a high content of nondigestible polysaccharides. The oligosaccharides stachyose and raffinose, isolated from beans, are particularly effective substrates for fermentation to carbon dioxide, hydrogen, and methane by colonic flora. The treatment of flatulence is generally undertaken to reduce embarrassment and consists of measures to decrease aerophagia along with avoidance of foods that cause excessive gas.

REFERENCES

DAVENPORT HW: *Physiology of the Digestive Tract*, 4th ed. Chicago, Year Book, 1977

DEBONGNIE JC, PHILLIPS SF: Capacity of the human colon to absorb fluid. Gastroenterology 74:698, 1978

DROSSMAN DA et al: The irritable bowel syndrome. Gastroenterology 73:811, 1977

GORBACH SL et al: Travellers' diarrhea and toxigenic *Escherichia coli*. N Engl J Med 292:933, 1975

LASSER RB et al: The role of intestinal gas in functional abdominal pain. N Engl J Med 293:524, 1975

PHILLIPS SF: Diarrhea: A current view of the pathophysiology. Gastroenterology 63:495, 1972

PLOTKIN GR et al: Gastroenteritis: Etiology, pathophysiology and clinical manifestations. Medicine 58:95, 1979

SCHREIBER DS et al: Recent advances in viral gastroenteritis. Gastroenterology 73:174, 1977

38

HEMATEMESIS AND MELENA

KURT J. ISSELBACHER
JOHN W. POPP, JR.

Hematemesis is defined as the vomiting of blood, and *melena* as the passage of stools rendered black and tarry by the presence of altered blood. These symptoms of gastrointestinal hemorrhage should bring the patient to medical attention and, within certain limits, suggest the anatomic site of bleeding. Exsanguinating gastrointestinal hemorrhage will rarely occur without the appearance of altered or gross blood passed by mouth or rectum. The color of vomited blood will vary depending on the concentration of hydrochloric acid in the stomach and its admixture with the blood. Thus, if vomiting occurs shortly after the onset of bleeding, the vomitus appears red; if there is a delay in vomiting, the appearance will be dark red, brown, or black. Precipitated blood clots in the vomitus will produce a characteristic "coffee grounds" appearance. Hematemesis usually indicates bleeding proximal to the ligament of Treitz, since blood entering the gastrointestinal tract below the duodenum rarely reenters the stomach.

While bleeding sufficient to produce hematemesis usually results in melena, less than half of patients with melena have hematemesis. *Melena* usually denotes bleeding from the esophagus, stomach, or duodenum, but lesions in the jejunum, ileum, and even ascending colon may cause melena provided the gastrointestinal transit time is sufficiently prolonged. Approximately 60 ml of blood is required to produce a single black stool; acute blood loss greater than this may produce melena for up to 3 days. After the stool color returns to normal, tests for occult blood may remain positive for up to a week or longer.

The black color of stools secondary to intestinal bleeding results from contact of the blood with hydrochloric acid to produce hematin. Characteristically, such stools are tarry ("sticky"). This tarry consistency is in contrast to black or dark stools occurring after the ingestion of iron, bismuth, or licorice. Similarly, red stools may result from the ingestion of beets or intravenous administration of sulfobromophthalein. Gastrointestinal bleeding, even if detected only by positive tests for occult blood, indicates potentially serious disease and must be further investigated.

Hematochezia, the passage of bright red blood per rectum, generally signifies bleeding from a source distal to the ligament of Treitz. However, since blood must remain in the gut for approximately 8 h to produce melena, rapid hemorrhage into the esophagus, stomach, or duodenum may also result in hematochezia.

The clinical manifestations of gastrointestinal bleeding depend upon the extent and rate of hemorrhage, and the presence of coincidental diseases. Blood loss of less than 500 ml is rarely associated with systemic signs; exceptions include bleeding in the elderly or in the anemic patient in whom smaller amounts of blood loss may produce hemodynamic alterations. Rapid hemorrhage of greater volume results in decreased venous return to the heart, decreased cardiac output, and increased peripheral resistance due to reflex vasoconstriction. Orthostatic hypotension greater than 10 mmHg usually indicates a 20 percent or greater reduction in blood volume. Concomitant symptoms include syncope, lightheadedness, nausea, sweating, and thirst. When blood loss approaches 40 percent of blood volume, shock frequently ensues with pronounced tachycardia and hypotension. Pallor is prominent, and the skin is cool.

It is important to recognize that the hematocrit, when determined immediately after the onset of bleeding, may not accurately reflect blood loss, since equilibration with extravascular fluid and hemodilution require several hours. Common laboratory findings include mild leukocytosis and thrombocytosis which develop within 6 h after the onset of bleeding. The blood urea nitrogen may be mildly elevated, particularly in upper gastrointestinal bleeding, due to breakdown of blood proteins to urea by intestinal bacteria as well as from a mild reduction in the glomerular filtration rate. Blood in the gut may also produce a low-grade fever.

ETIOLOGY OF UPPER GASTROINTESTINAL BLEEDING A careful history and physical examination of the oropharynx should serve to exclude swallowed blood as a source of hematemesis or melena.

The three most common causes of upper gastrointestinal hemorrhage are (1) peptic ulceration, (2) erosive gastritis, and (3) variceal bleeding. These entities account for up to 90 percent of all cases of upper gastrointestinal hemorrhage in which a definite lesion can be found.

Peptic ulcer Peptic ulcer is probably the most common cause of upper gastrointestinal bleeding; the majority of such ulcers are found in the duodenum. Approximately 20 to 30 percent of patients with documented ulcers will have significant bleeding sometime during the course of their disease. Since hemorrhage may be the initial manifestation of a peptic ulcer, this lesion should be seriously considered even when a history characteristic of ulcer disease is not obtained.

Gastritis Gastritis may be associated with recent alcohol ingestion or with the use of anti-inflammatory drugs, such as aspirin or indomethacin. Another frequent setting is the development of gastric erosions in stressful situations such as following major trauma or surgery, or in association with severe systemic disease. The occurrence of gastritis in burn victims and patients with increased intracranial pressure is also common. Since there are no characteristic physical findings, the diagnosis of gastritis must be suspected when the appropriate clinical setting is encountered. Gastroscopy is usually needed to confirm the diagnosis since radiologic examination generally lacks the sensitivity required to detect gastritis.

Variceal bleeding Variceal bleeding is characteristically abrupt and massive; chronic gastrointestinal blood loss is unusual. Bleeding from esophageal or gastric varices is usually the result of portal hypertension, secondary to hepatic cirrhosis. Although alcoholic cirrhosis is the most prevalent cause of esophageal varices in the United States, any condition producing portal hypertension, even in the absence of hepatic disease (i.e., portal vein thrombosis or idiopathic portal hypertension), may result in variceal bleeding. Further, while the presence of varices usually connotes long-standing portal hypertension, acute hepatitis or severe fatty infiltration of the liver may occasionally produce varices which disappear once the hepatic abnormality resolves. It should be emphasized that although upper gastrointestinal bleeding in a patient with cirrhosis suggests a variceal source, approximately half those patients will be bleeding from other lesions (e.g., gastritis, ulcers). Consequently, it is essential to exclude nonvariceal causes of bleeding so that the appropriate treatment can be instituted. Finally, since varices may occur at any site in the gastrointestinal tract, angiography may be required to identify hemorrhage from varices distal to the duodenum.

Other lesions With the advent of esophagogastroduodenoscopy, the Mallory-Weiss syndrome has been demonstrated with increasing frequency as a cause of acute upper gastrointestinal hemorrhage. This syndrome refers to laceration in the region of the esophagogastric junction characterized by retching or nonbloody vomiting followed by hematemesis. Less common bleeding esophageal lesions include esophagitis (with or without hiatus hernia) and carcinoma; these generally cause chronic blood loss and rarely produce massive bleeding.

Gastric carcinoma may result in chronic gastrointestinal bleeding. Lymphoma, polyps, and other tumors of the stomach and small bowel are uncommon and, consequently, are infrequent causes of hemorrhage. Leiomyoma and leiomyosarcoma are likewise rare, but they can lead to massive hemorrhage. Bleeding from duodenal and jejunal diverticula is relatively unusual. Vascular insufficiency of the mesenteric vessels, including occlusive and nonocclusive disease, may lead to bloody diarrhea.

Arteriosclerotic aortic aneurysms may rupture into the small intestine; such an event is almost always fatal. Rupture may also occur following arterial reconstructive surgery with fistula formation between synthetic graft and bowel lumen. Sudden bleeding may also occur after trauma resulting in hepatic laceration; this may result in blood loss into the bile ducts (i.e., hemobilia).

Primary blood dyscrasias, including leukemia, thrombocytopenic states, the hemophilias, and disseminated intravascular coagulation may result in significant gastrointestinal bleeding. Polycythemia vera, although associated with an increased incidence of peptic ulceration, may also result in gastrointestinal bleeding due to mesenteric or portal vein thrombosis. Periarteritis nodosa, Henoch-Schönlein purpura, and other forms of vasculitis may lead to gastrointestinal blood loss.

Mild gastrointestinal bleeding may be seen with amyloidosis, Osler-Weber-Rendu disease, pseudoxanthoma elasticum, Turner's syndrome, intestinal hemangiomas, neurofibromatosis, Kaposi's sarcoma, and Peutz-Jeghers syndrome. Uremia may produce gastrointestinal blood loss; the most common presentation is chronic, occult bleeding from diffuse involvement of the mucosa of the stomach and small bowel.

ETIOLOGY OF LOWER GASTROINTESTINAL LESIONS Anal and rectal lesions Small amounts of bright red blood on the surface of the stool and toilet tissue are often caused by hemorrhoids; such bleeding is generally precipitated by the strained passage of a hard stool. Anal fissures and fistulas may present in a similar fashion. Proctitis is another source of rectal bleeding; it is frequently seen in young adults, especially in male homosexuals. In the latter situation, proctitis may be nonspecific or due to gonorrheal infection. Rectal trauma is a cause of hematochezia, and the placement of foreign objects in the rectal vault may precipitate perforation as well as acute rectal hemorrhage. It must be emphasized that anal pathology does not preclude other sources of blood loss, and these must be sought and excluded.

Colonic lesions Carcinoma of the colon, as well as colonic polyps, may produce chronic blood loss. Frankly bloody diarrhea is common and may be the presenting symptom in patients with ulcerative colitis; it is less frequent in granulomatous colitis, but occult blood may be present in the stool. Bleeding may also accompany diarrhea due to infections such as shigellosis, amebiasis, and rarely, salmonellosis. In the elderly patient, ischemic colitis may be a cause of bloody diarrhea; this lesion may also be seen in the younger age group associated with the use of oral contraceptive agents. Angiodysplastic lesions, usually involving the ascending colon, can be a major source of bleeding in elderly patients, especially those with aortic stenosis; such vascular lesions can be identified by angiography or colonoscopy.

Diverticula Colonic diverticula are most often located in the sigmoid colon; however, most episodes of diverticular bleeding originate in the ascending colon. Bleeding from colonic diverticula is one of the most common causes of massive lower gastrointestinal hemorrhage. The usual presentation of a diverticular hemorrhage is that of painless passage of a maroon-colored stool. Mild blood loss is more often associated with diverticulitis. Meckel's diverticulum, a congenital anomaly of the distal ileum, is present in about 2 percent of the population and may cause bleeding. Although only about 15 percent of these diverticula contain gastric mucosa, the lesions which cause acute bleeding contain gastric mucosa half the time. This anomaly is an important cause of acute hemorrhage in children and young adults.

APPROACH TO THE PATIENT WITH GASTROINTESTINAL BLEEDING The approach to the bleeding patient depends upon the site, extent, and rate of bleeding. Patients with hematemesis have usually bled greater amounts (often greater than 1000 ml) than those who have melena alone (usually 500 ml or less), and mortality with the former is about twice that of the latter. When first seen, the patient may be in shock. Prior to taking a history and performing a thorough physical examination, vital signs should be noted, blood sent for typing and cross-matching, and a large-bore intravenous line placed for infusion of saline or other plasma expanders. The physician initiating the evaluation of the bleeding patient must be aware that the primary consideration is the necessity of maintaining adequate intravascular volume and hemodynamic stability during the diagnostic workup.

History A history of prior ulcer disease or symptoms suggestive thereof may provide a useful clue. Similarly, recent abuse of alcohol or ingestion of anti-inflammatory drugs should make erosive gastritis more suspect. If alcohol abuse has been long-standing, esophageal varices may be a more likely source of hemorrhage. Aspirin use may also cause bleeding by aggravating a preexisting lesion (e.g., peptic ulceration). Prior history of gastrointestinal bleeding may be helpful, as may a family history of intestinal disease or hemorrhagic diathesis. Recent retching followed by hematemesis should suggest the possibility of the Mallory-Weiss syndrome. The acute onset of bloody diarrhea may indicate the presence of inflammatory bowel disease or infectious involvement of the colon. It is also important to exclude associated systemic illnesses or recent trauma, since bleeding from erosive gastritis is frequently seen under such conditions.

Physical examination Following evaluation for orthostatic changes in pulse and blood pressure and institution of volume repletion, the patient should be examined for clues to the underlying illness. A nonintestinal bleeding source should be excluded by careful examination of the nasopharynx. Dermatologic examination may disclose the characteristic telangiectasia of Osler-Weber-Rendu disease (although these will not be visible if severe anemia is present), the perioral pigmentation of Peutz-Jeghers syndrome, the dermal fibromas of neurofibromatosis, the sebaceous cysts and bony tumors of Gardner's syndrome, the palpable purpura frequently seen with vasculitis, or the diffuse pigmentation seen in hemochromatosis. Stigmata of chronic liver disease such as spider angiomata, gynecomastia, testicular atrophy, jaundice, ascites, and hepatosplenomegaly should suggest portal hypertension resulting in bleeding from esophageal or gastric varices. Significant lymph node enlargement or abdominal masses may reflect underlying intraabdominal malignancy. Careful rectal examination is important to exclude local pathology as well as to observe the color of the stool.

Laboratory studies Initial studies should include the hematocrit, hemoglobin, careful assessment of red blood cell morphologic features (hypochromic, microcytic red blood cells suggest that blood loss is chronic), white blood cell count, differential, and platelet count. Prothrombin time, partial thromboplastin time, and other coagulation studies may be in order to exclude primary or secondary clotting defects. A radiograph of the abdomen is rarely helpful in establishing a diagnosis unless a perforated viscus is suspected. Though the initial studies are valuable and essential, repeated evaluation of the laboratory data is important as one follows the clinical course of the bleeding.

Diagnostic approach The diagnostic approach to the patient with gastrointestinal hemorrhage must be individualized. The initial management of gastrointestinal bleeding may be under the direction of the internist, but it is prudent to consult a surgeon in the event that the bleeding cannot be controlled by medical means. It must be emphasized that demonstration of a lesion in a patient with gastrointestinal bleeding should also be accompanied by evidence that this lesion is the site of bleeding. In recent years the availability of experienced endoscopists as well as radiologists with facilities for selective arteriography has increased to the extent that in many medical centers it is possible to have emergency endoscopic, angiographic, and barium studies performed within hours of the patient's admission to the hospital. It is to be hoped that this "vigorous diagnostic approach" will serve to decrease the morbidity and mortality rates associated with upper gastrointestinal bleeding.

When there is a history of melena or hematemesis or the suspicion of bleeding from the upper part of the gastrointestinal tract, the patient should have a nasogastric tube passed to empty the stomach and to determine whether the bleeding is in the upper part of the gastrointestinal tract. If the initial nasogastric aspirate is clear, the tube should be left in place until bile-stained material appears, since active duodenal bleeding may occur with a clear nasogastric aspirate. The latter situation is due to failure of duodenal contents to reflux into the stomach secondary to pyloric irritability and spasm. If the aspirate is bile-stained and negative for occult blood, one can assume that active bleeding is not occurring in the gastroduodenal region, and the nasogastric tube can be removed.

If red blood or "coffee grounds" material is aspirated from the nasogastric tube, iced saline irrigation of the stomach should be initiated. Irrigation serves two purposes: it provides the clinician with an assessment of the rapidity of the bleeding, and its vasoconstricting effect often diminishes bleeding due to erosive gastritis. Subsequent diagnostic maneuvers will depend on whether bleeding continues; this can be assessed by vital signs, transfusion requirements, and the number and consistency of stools.

If the nasogastric aspirate suggests that bleeding has stopped, one may proceed with either esophagogastroduodenoscopy or upper gastrointestinal barium studies. Although *endoscopy* provides a higher diagnostic yield, it has not been proved conclusively that survival is increased by early endoscopy. *Barium examination* often identifies a potential source of hemorrhage, but there are important limitations to such x-rays. First, lesions such as erosive gastritis and Mallory-Weiss lacerations are not visualized by x-ray. Second, if the patient rebleeds following a barium exam, the retained contrast material will make endoscopy difficult and angiography impossible. Clearly the approach in this setting must be individualized. The decision to employ esophagogastroduodenoscopy or barium studies will depend on several variables, including the availability of an experienced endoscopist and the condition of the patient. The two procedures should be viewed as complementary in the diagnostic evaluation of upper gastrointestinal hemorrhage.

Persistent upper gastrointestinal hemorrhage must be viewed differently, and most clinicians would proceed immediately to esophagogastroduodenoscopy. Determination of the site and cause of bleeding is essential for appropriate therapy, particularly if varices are responsible. Such information is beneficial both to the surgeon, who may be asked to intervene, and to the angiographer, should injection of vasoconstricting agents into the artery supplying the lesion be deemed appropriate. Thus, anticipation of surgery, angiography, or the suspicion of bleeding varices are strong indications for esophagogastroduodenoscopy in the evaluation of the patient with persistent upper gastrointestinal bleeding.

In contrast, esophagogastroduodenoscopy is less vital in the evaluation of *massive* hemorrhage, since large amounts of blood obscure visualization of mucosal pathology. In such a setting, selective arteriography or surgery is more appropriate.

Should bleeding continue and gastric aspiration fail to reveal fresh blood, the site of hemorrhage may be beyond the ligament of Treitz. In this situation angiography is frequently valuable in establishing a diagnosis. Angiographic demonstration of the bleeding site requires blood loss at a rate of at least 0.5 ml/min. Clinical correlates reflecting this degree of blood loss include postural hypotension and the necessity for blood transfusion to maintain stable vital signs. Emergency angiography may localize the site of bleeding; however, the cause of the bleeding may not be determined unless varices, vascular malformations, or aneurysms are present. Therapeutic angiography is a promising approach to the control of persistent hemorrhage. Continuous intraarterial infusion of vasoconstrictor agents, such as vasopressin, is often successful in controlling hemorrhage (Fig. 38-1). Additionally, embolic material may be injected directly into the artery perfusing the bleeding site. This technique has been performed successfully with autologous clot as well as with commercially available hemostatic material such as gelatin powder (Gelfoam). At present embolization therapy is regarded as a temporizing measure for bleeding varices and peptic lesions, and eventual surgery is to be expected.

If bleeding esophageal varices are identified on upper endoscopy, peripheral infusions of vasopressin (Pitressin) may control the bleeding. The ability to respond to such therapy depends upon the general condition of the patient as assessed by certain clinical and laboratory parameters (Child's criteria). It has been shown that intraarterial vasopressin is no more effective than intravenous administration in the control of variceal bleeding. This is not the case, however, for arterial bleeding where selective angiographic catheter placement is mandatory to achieve hemostasis. Varices may also be controlled by balloon tamponade with a Sengstaken-Blakemore tube. Unlike vasopressin, this technique is generally used as a stabilizing preoperative measure which should be followed by surgical decompression of the portal system within 48 h whenever possible.

In the evaluation of *rectal* bleeding the most important procedures are the digital examination, anoscopy, and sigmoidoscopy. The last of these may identify a bleeding site or document bleeding coming from above the range of the instrument. If brisk bleeding continues, arteriography may serve to localize the bleeding site and allow local infusion of vasoconstrictor agents to control bleeding. Several investigations are currently being conducted to assess the efficacy of colonoscopy in identifying bleeding lesions proximal to the sigmoid colon. This procedure has therapeutic promise as well, since direct visualization may allow the colonoscopist to excise the bleeding lesion or cauterize it with an electrosurgical device. As with esophagogastroduodenoscopy, massive hemorrhage precludes effective use of colonoscopy, and in such instances it should not be

A

B

FIGURE 38-1

Angiographic findings on a patient with massive upper gastrointestinal bleeding. Angiographic studies revealed the bleeding to be secondary to hemorrhagic gastritis; it was controlled by the selective left gastric arterial infusion of vasopressin. A. Selective left gastric arteriography demonstrates massive extravasation of contrast material (arrow) from a branch of the left gastric artery. B. Selective left gastric arteriography during the infusion of 0.1 unit of vasopressin per minute demonstrates a marked decrease in the caliber of the left gastric artery and cessation of hemorrhage.

attempted. Finally, a barium enema has a limited role in the evaluation of acute rectal bleeding. A barium-filled colon may localize potential bleeding sources, but will not necessarily define the bleeding site. Furthermore, if brisk bleeding recurs, subsequent colonoscopy or angiography will be difficult to interpret due to retained contrast material. Therefore, it is advisable to withhold barium studies of both the upper and lower bowel for at least 24 h after the cessation of active bleeding.

REFERENCES

ATHANASOULIS CA: Angiography. Its contribution to the emergency management of gastrointestinal hemorrhage. Radiol Clin North Am 14:265, 1976

———: Angiodysplasia of the intestinal tract as a cause of recurrent bleeding. Prog Gastroenterol 3:857, 1977

CONN HO et al: Intraarterial vasopressin in the treatment of upper gastrointestinal hemorrhage: A prospective, controlled clinical trial. Gastroenterology 68:211, 1975

DRONFIELD MW et al: A prospective, randomised study of endoscopy and radiology in acute upper-gastrointestinal-tract bleeding. Lancet 1:1167, 1977

HASTINGS PR et al: Antacid prophylaxis of bleeding in the critically ill. N Engl J Med 298:1041, 1978

HEDBERG SE: Endoscopy in gastrointestinal bleeding. A systematic approach to diagnosis. Surg Clin North Am 54:549, 1974

TERES J et al: Upper gastrointestinal bleeding in cirrhosis: Clinical and endoscopic correlations. Gut 17:37, 1976

39
JAUNDICE AND HEPATOMEGALY

KURT J. ISSELBACHER

JAUNDICE

Jaundice, or *icterus,* refers to the yellow pigmentation of the skin or scleras by bilirubin. This in turn is a result of elevated levels of bilirubin in the bloodstream. Jaundice may be brought to clinical attention by a darkening of the urine or a yellow discoloration of the skin or sclera; the latter often is the site where clinical icterus may first be detected. Scleral pigmentation is attributed to richness of this tissue in elastin, which has a special affinity for bilirubin. Jaundice must be distinguished from other causes of yellow pigmentation such as carotenemia (see Chaps. 51, 80, and 335), which is due to carotenoid pigments in the bloodstream and is associated with a yellowish discoloration of the skin but not of the sclera. Atabrine treatment (see Chap. 200) may produce a yellow color of the skin and urine, but the scleras are usually only minimally discolored, and when pigment is present, it is seen only in the regions of the scleras exposed to light.

Normal serum bilirubin concentrations range from 0.5 to 1.0 mg per 100 ml, and normally most of this is unconjugated (see Fig. 39-1). The precise level at which jaundice becomes clinically evident varies, but usually it can be recognized when the total serum bilirubin exceeds 2 to 2.5 mg per 100 ml. Not infrequently in deep jaundice the skin may take on a greenish hue because of the conversion of bilirubin to biliverdin, an oxidation product of bilirubin. Oxidation occurs more readily with conjugated bilirubin, and hence a greenish hue is seen more frequently in conditions with pronounced conjugated hyperbilirubinemia. When bilirubin is exposed to visible light (from 430 to 470 nm) the pigment undergoes photooxidation leading to water-soluble and colorless breakdown products. Ultraviolet light can also produce isomers of bilirubin (IXα) that may not require conjugation for hepatic excretion (see below).

PRODUCTION AND METABOLISM OF BILIRUBIN Normal sources of bilirubin (Fig. 39-2)   The greater part of the bilirubin is derived from the catabolism of hemoglobin present in senescent red blood cells. This normally accounts for about 80 to 85 percent of the daily bilirubin production. When a circulating red blood cell reaches the end of its normal life span of approximately 120 days, it is destroyed in the reticuloendothelial system. In the catabolism of hemoglobin, globin is first dissociated from heme, after which the heme moiety (ferroprotoporphyrin IX) is oxidatively cleaved and converted to bili-

$$O_6H_9C_6-OOC \qquad COO-O_6H_9C_6^*$$

A

B

FIGURE 39-1

The chemical structures of conjugated (A) and unconjugated (B) bilirubin. Abbreviations: M = methyl, V = vinyl, P = propionic acid. The asterisk (*) refers to glucuronic acid.

verdin by a microsomal heme oxygenase. This enzyme system requires oxygen and a cofactor, reduced nicotinamide adenine dinucleotide phosphate (NADPH). Bilirubin (in the chemical form of bilirubin IXα) is then formed from biliverdin by biliverdin reductase.

About 15 to 20 percent of the bilirubin is derived from sources other than senescent erythrocytes. One source is the *destruction of maturing erythroid cells in the bone marrow,* or so-called "ineffective erythropoiesis" (see Chap. 312). The other is *nonerythroid components,* especially in the liver, and involves

FIGURE 39-2

The sources and precursors of bilirubin and steps in its subsequent metabolism and excretion.

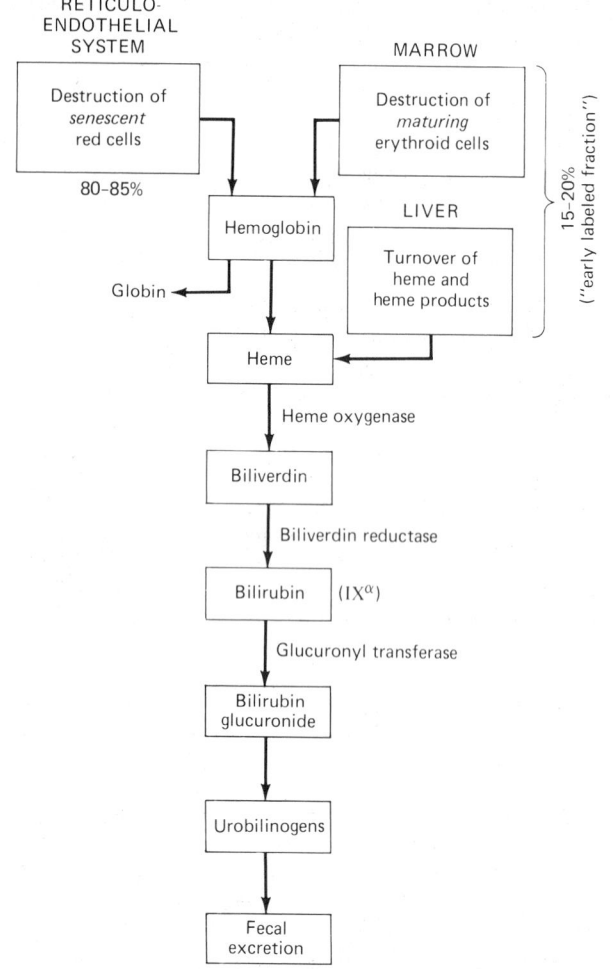

the turnover of heme and heme proteins (such as cytochrome, myoglobin, and heme-containing enzymes). These two sources of bilirubin are collectively referred to as the *early labeled fraction,* a term derived from experiments with labeled glycine and Δ-aminolevulinic acid (ALA). Thus when labeled glycine is administered to a normal subject, approximately 15 percent of the label appears in stool urobilinogens in the first 3 to 5 days; 85 percent of the label appears at about 120 days and reflects the bilirubin produced from the normal destruction of senescent red blood cells.

Transport of bilirubin Following liberation of bilirubin into the plasma, virtually all the pigment is tightly *bound to albumin.* The maximum binding capacity is 2 mol bilirubin per mole of albumin. Because in a normal adult this corresponds to plasma unconjugated bilirubin concentrations of 60 to 80 mg/ml, saturation of the binding capacity of the plasma almost never occurs. It is clinically relevant that certain organic anions, such as sulfonamides and salicylates, compete with bilirubin for common binding sites on albumin and may displace bilirubin from albumin, permitting it to enter tissues such as the central nervous system. Most of the evidence for albumin binding has been obtained from studies using unconjugated bilirubin. The conjugated pigment also appears to be bound primarily to albumin, although the binding to albumin is much weaker than with unconjugated bilirubin. This may account for the fact that conjugated, but not unconjugated, bilirubin may be filtered by the renal glomeruli.

Bilirubin is found in body fluids (cerebrospinal fluid, joint effusions, cysts, etc.) in proportion to the albumin content of the fluids and is absent from true secretions such as tears, saliva, and pancreatic juice. Scar tissue is rarely bilirubin-stained. The appearance of jaundice is also influenced by blood flow and edema. Paralyzed extremities and edematous areas tend to remain uncolored, and "unilateral" jaundice in patients with hemiplegia and edema may be seen if jaundice develops.

Hepatic metabolism of bilirubin (Fig. 39-3) The liver occupies a central role in the metabolism of the bile pigments. Three distinct phases are recognized: (1) *hepatic uptake,* (2) *conjugation,* and (3) *excretion* into bile. Of these three steps, excretion appears to be the rate-limiting step and the one most susceptible to impairment when the liver cell is damaged.

UPTAKE Unconjugated bilirubin bound to albumin is presented to the liver cell, and upon entry the pigment and albumin become dissociated. The uptake phase is believed to involve the binding of bilirubin to certain cytoplasmic anionic binding proteins (ligandins). Hepatic uptake appears to be reversible.

CONJUGATION Unconjugated bilirubin is water-insoluble and must be converted to a *water-soluble derivative* in order to be excreted by the liver cell into bile. This is accomplished by conjugation whereby bilirubin is predominantly converted to bilirubin glucuronide. The reaction occurs in the endoplasmic reticulum of the hepatocytes by action of bilirubin glucuronyl transferase. As shown in Fig. 39-3, this appears to be a two-step reaction, resulting first in the formation of the monoglucuronide followed by the production of the diglucuronide. It has recently been suggested that the conversion of the monoglucuronide to the diglucuronide may be mediated by a separate enzyme, a plasma membrane transesterase (or transglucuronidase), rather than glucuronyl transferase. However, other studies suggest glucuronyl transferase may also mediate the conversion of monoglucuronide to diglucuronide. Normally, bile contains 85 percent of bilirubin diconjugates and 15 percent monoconjugates. Unconjugated bilirubin usually is *not* ex-

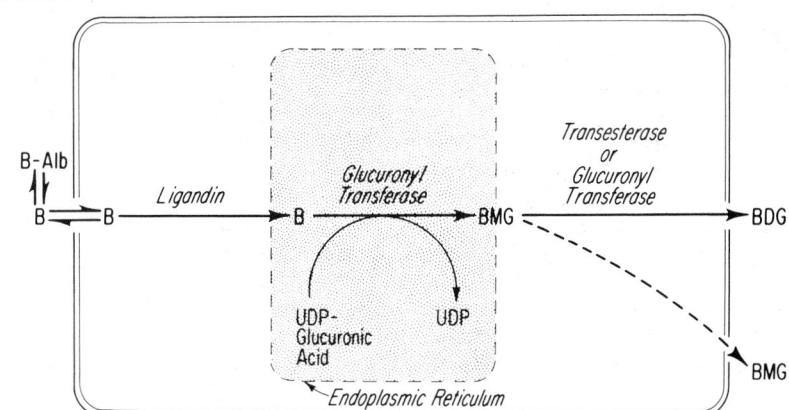

PLASMA HEPATOCYTE BILE

FIGURE 39-3
Scheme of bilirubin uptake, conjugation, and excretion by the liver cell. Abbreviations: B = bilirubin, BMG = bilirubin monoglucuronide, BDG = bilirubin diglucuronide, UDP = uridine diphosphate.

creted by the liver into the bile (except following photooxidation, see below). Bile also contains small amounts of bilirubin conjugated with other sugars (e.g., with xylose and aldobiuronic acid). The physiologic significance of these nonglucuronide conjugates is not known.

EXCRETION OR SECRETION INTO BILE   Normally, for bilirubin to be excreted into bile, *the pigment must be in the conjugated form.* Although the overall process is not well understood, the excretion of conjugated bilirubin into bile appears to be an energy-dependent process and the *rate-limiting* step in the hepatic metabolism of bilirubin. When this step is compromised, two consequences occur: (1) decreased excretion of bilirubin into the bile, and (2) "regurgitation," or reentry of conjugated bilirubin from the liver cells into the bloodstream.

It should be noted that bilirubin (i.e., IXα, Z isomer) is readily photooxidized to an isomer (IXα, E isomer), which does not need to be conjugated in order to be excreted by the liver cell. Hence after phototherapy unconjugated bilirubin (as the E isomer) can be excreted into bile.

Intestinal phase of bilirubin metabolism   After its appearance in the intestinal lumen, bilirubin glucuronide may be excreted in the stool or metabolized to urobilinogen and related products. Because of its polarity, *conjugated bilirubin is not reabsorbed* by the intestinal mucosa, a mechanism which may serve to rid the body of this pigment. The formation of urobilinogen from conjugated bilirubin requires the action of bacteria and occurs in the lower part of the small intestine and colon.

In contrast to conjugated bilirubin, *urobilinogen is reabsorbed* from the small intestine into the portal blood and is thus subject to enterohepatic circulation. Some urobilinogen is reexcreted by the liver into the bile; the rest is excreted in the urine in an amount usually not exceeding 4 mg daily. When the hepatic excretory mechanism is impaired (e.g., in hepatocellular disease) or the production of bilirubin is greatly increased (e.g., in hemolytic anemia), the urinary urobilinogen may increase significantly.

The normal output of fecal urobilinogen ranges from 50 to 280 mg per day. Under conditions of decreased excretion of conjugated bilirubin into the intestine (e.g., liver disease, bile duct obstruction) or suppression of intestinal flora by antibiotics, fecal output will be diminished. In hemolytic anemia, urinary and fecal urobilinogen excretion is greatly increased.

In a normal person with a blood volume of 5 liters and a hemoglobin concentration of 15 g per 100 ml, the total circulating hemoglobin is 750 g. Because approximately 0.8 percent of the red blood cells are destroyed daily, 6.3 g hemoglobin is released for catabolism. Assuming a quantitative degradation of heme to bilirubin and to urobilinogen, the expected daily output of urobilinogen would be approximately 250 mg plus

the additional 15 to 30 mg which would be derived from the other sources described above (i.e., ineffective erythropoiesis, nonhemoglobin heme precursors). Often, however, the amount excreted is considerably less, and it appears likely that there are alternative pathways for hemoglobin degradation not involving bilirubin formation.

Renal excretion of bilirubin   Normally the urine contains no bilirubin that can be detected by the methods usually employed, although traces may be detectable by sensitive spectrophotometric procedures. Unconjugated bilirubin, being tightly bound to albumin, is not filtered by the renal glomeruli, and because there is no tubular secretory process for bilirubin, *unconjugated bilirubin is not excreted in urine.* On the other hand, conjugated bilirubin is less tightly bound to albumin, and a small fraction (about 5 percent) is unbound. The unbound fraction is dialyzable and is filtered by the renal glomeruli. Thus, in contrast to the unconjugated pigment, a fraction of plasma *conjugated bilirubin appears in the urine.* Bile salts enhance the dialyzability of conjugated bilirubin, and in obstructive jaundice, the elevated level of plasma bile acids may account for an increased renal excretion of conjugated bilirubin. This may also explain why in biliary tract obstruction, serum conjugated bilirubin levels tend to plateau and not to exceed 30 to 40 mg per 100 ml, while with severe hepatocellular injury bilirubin levels higher than this may occur.

CHEMICAL TESTS FOR BILE PIGMENTS   The most widely employed chemical test for the bile pigments in serum is the van den Bergh reaction. In this reaction the bilirubin pigments are diazotized with sulfanilic acid, and the chromogenic products are measured colorimetrically. The van den Bergh reaction can be used to distinguish between unconjugated and conjugated bilirubin because of the different solubility properties of the pigments. When the reaction is carried out in an *aqueous* medium, the water-soluble conjugated bilirubin reacts to give the so-called "direct" van den Bergh reaction. When the reaction is carried out in *methanol,* both conjugated and unconjugated pigments react, giving a measure of the *total* bilirubin level. The total minus the direct-reacting bilirubin give the *indirect* value, which is a measure of the unconjugated bilirubin level.

In the direct van den Bergh reaction, the most accurate measurements are those carried out at 1 min. If the reaction is allowed to proceed longer, a small amount of the unconjugated pigment may begin to react in the aqueous medium. As a result, if the reaction is carried out at 30 min in a patient with unconjugated hyperbilirubinemia, falsely low values for the indirect-reacting bilirubin may be obtained. This serves to emphasize that the direct and indirect van den Bergh reactions represent *approximations* (not absolute measurements) of the conjugated and unconjugated pigments. A summary of the key differences in the properties and reactions of the bilirubin pigments is presented in Table 39-1.

The measurement of bilirubin in the urine may be carried out by the Harrison spot test or with Ictotest tablets. The foam test is also a simple and qualitatively valid procedure. When normal urine is vigorously shaken in a test tube, the foam is absolutely white. In a urine containing bilirubin, the foam will be yellow. This difference may be subtle and may become evident only by comparing a normal urine specimen and one containing bilirubin side by side. Urine urobilinogen may be estimated by the semiquantitative Watson-Schwartz test or the qualitative Diamond test. Fecal measurement must be quantitative to be of value.

Except for concentrated urine, the most common cause of a deep yellow-brown or dark urine is bilirubinuria. However, other mechanisms and diseases associated with a dark urine need to be considered. These include yellow urine due to drugs (e.g., sulfasalazine); red urine due to porphyria, hemoglobinuria, myoglobinuria, or drugs (e.g., pyridium); and dark brown or black urine due to homogentisic acid (in ochronosis) or melanin (with melanoma).

APPROACH TO THE PATIENT WITH JAUNDICE Once jaundice is recognized clinically or chemically, it is important to determine whether it is predominantly due to unconjugated or conjugated hyperbilirubinemia. *A simple clue in this regard is to determine whether bilirubin is present in the urine.* Its absence in the urine suggests unconjugated hyperbilirubinemia (since this pigment is not filtered by the glomerulus); its presence indicates conjugated hyperbilirubinemia. One can then proceed to the direct chemical measurement of the bilirubin pigments in the serum. In predominantly unconjugated hyperbilirubinemia, 80 to 85 percent of the total serum bilirubin is unconjugated (i.e., less than 15 to 20 percent is conjugated). The patient is considered to have predominantly conjugated hyperbilirubinemia when more than 50 percent of the serum bilirubin is of the conjugated type.

An approach to the classification of jaundice based on this important distinction is presented in Table 39-2. Derangements of bilirubin metabolism may occur through any of four mechanisms: (1) overproduction, (2) decreased hepatic uptake, (3) decreased hepatic conjugation, and (4) decreased excretion of bilirubin into bile (due to both intrahepatic and extrahepatic factors). Jaundice may also be described on the basis of the pathogenetic mechanisms or disease processes leading to increased bilirubin levels. Thus, the terms *hemolytic jaundice, hepatocellular jaundice,* and *obstructive* (or cholestatic) *jaundice* are often used.

Though these classifications and terms are helpful, in any one patient more than a single derangement or more than one "type" of jaundice may be present. For example, a patient with cirrhosis may have not only impaired liver cell function (and hence hepatocellular jaundice) but also hemolysis. Furthermore, obstructive jaundice may be due to either *mechani-*

TABLE 39-1
Comparison of the major differences between conjugated and unconjugated bilirubin

Properties and reactions	Unconjugated	Conjugated
Water solubility	0	+
Affinity for lipids	+	0
Bound to serum albumin	+ + +	+
Renal excretion	0	+
Van den Bergh reaction	Indirect (total minus direct)	Direct
Lipid membrane permeability	+	0

TABLE 39-2
Classification of jaundice based on underlying derangement of bilirubin metabolism

I Predominantly *unconjugated* hyperbilirubinemia
  A Overproduction
    1 Hemolysis (intra- and extravascular)
    2 Ineffective erythropoiesis
  B Decreased hepatic uptake
    1 Drugs (e.g., flavaspidic acid)
    2 Prolonged fasting (< 300 cal per day)
    3 Sepsis
  C Decreased bilirubin conjugation (decreased glucuronyl transferase activity)
    1 Gilbert's syndrome (*mild* decrease in transferase)
    2 Crigler-Najjar type II (*moderate* decrease in transferase)
    3 Crigler-Najjar type I (absent transferase)
    4 Neonatal jaundice
    5 Acquired transferase deficiency
      a Drug inhibition (e.g., pregnanediol, chloramphenicol)
      b Hepatocellular disease (hepatitis, cirrhosis)*
    6 Sepsis
II Predominantly *conjugated* hyperbilirubinemia
  A Impaired hepatic excretion (intrahepatic defects)
    1 Familial or hereditary disorders
      a Dubin-Johnson syndrome; Rotor syndrome
      b Recurrent (benign) intrahepatic cholestasis
      c Cholestatic jaundice of pregnancy
    2 Acquired disorders
      a Hepatocellular disease* (e.g., viral or drug-induced hepatitis)
      b Drug-induced cholestasis (e.g., oral contraceptives, methyltestosterone)
      c Sepsis
  B Extrahepatic biliary obstruction (mechanical obstruction, e.g., stones, stricture, tumor of bile duct)

* *In hepatocellular disease (hepatitis and cirrhosis) there is usually interference in the three major steps of bilirubin metabolism—uptake, conjugation, and excretion. However, excretion is the rate-limiting step and is usually impaired to the greatest extent. As a result, conjugated hyperbilirubinemia predominates.*

cal obstruction of the biliary radicles or *functional* factors causing impaired hepatic excretion of bilirubin into bile.

In the present chapter a brief description of the major types of jaundice is given. A more detailed discussion of the individual disease entities is found in Chap. 301.

Jaundice with predominantly unconjugated bilirubin in the serum OVERPRODUCTION OF BILIRUBIN When an increased amount of hemoglobin is released from red blood cells into either the bloodstream or tissues, increased bilirubin production occurs. Hyperbilirubinemia develops when the capacity of the liver to remove the pigment from the circulation is exceeded. In most cases of hemolysis, the total serum bilirubin concentration ranges from 3 to 5 mg per 100 ml. A slight increase in direct-reacting pigment may also be found, but this usually constitutes less than 15 percent of the total serum bilirubin. This finding is probably analogous to the slight elevations of direct-reacting bilirubin which occur when normal subjects are infused with unconjugated bilirubin. Both instances appear to be a reflection of the fact that the rate-limiting step in hepatic bilirubin metabolism is excretion and that when the excretory capacity of the liver is exceeded, some reentry of conjugated bilirubin into the bloodstream occurs. For a detailed description of the causes of increased bilirubin production, see Chap. 301.

IMPAIRED HEPATIC UPTAKE OF BILIRUBIN As indicated previously, the uptake of bilirubin by the liver cell involves dissociation of the pigment from albumin, and presumably binding to certain cytoplasmic proteins (i.e., ligandins). In some cases of drug-induced jaundice (e.g., due to flavaspidic acid) and possibly in some patients with Gilbert's syndrome, there may be a derangement in this phase of bilirubin metabolism (see Chap. 301).

IMPAIRED GLUCURONIDE CONJUGATION Both acquired and genetic derangements in hepatic glucuronyl transferase occur.

In the fetus and at birth, glucuronyl transferase activity is low and appears to account in part for the *neonatal jaundice* normally found between the second and the fifth days of life. *Mild* decreases in glucuronyl transferases occur in Gilbert's syndrome, *moderate* decreases are found in Crigler-Najjar syndrome type II, and the enzyme is totally absent in the rare Crigler-Najjar syndrome type I (see Chap. 301).

Acquired defects in bilirubin glucuronyl transferase activity may be produced by drugs (i.e., enzyme inhibition) or intrinsic liver disease. However, with liver cell damage, the excretory capacity of the liver is impaired to a greater extent than is the conjugating capacity. Therefore in most hepatocellular diseases, the hyperbilirubinemia is predominantly of the conjugated type (see Chap. 301).

Jaundice with predominantly conjugated bilirubin in the serum
IMPAIRED EXCRETION OF BILIRUBIN BY THE LIVER   The impaired excretion of bilirubin into the biliary canaliculi, whether due to functional or mechanical factors, results in predominantly conjugated hyperbilirubinemia and bilirubinuria. The presence of *bilirubin in the urine is evidence of conjugated hyperbilirubinemia* and is a most important point in the differential diagnosis of jaundice. Such findings are identical to those occurring in complete obstruction of the bile duct, emphasizing that *jaundice due to hepatocellular disease can seldom be differentiated from that due to extrahepatic obstruction solely on the basis of changes in bile pigment metabolism.* Indeed there are often instances when the two conditions are not distinguishable by any biochemical criteria, and liver biopsy or other diagnostic procedures are needed for the definitive diagnosis.

When there is interference in the excretion of conjugated bilirubin into bile, by what mechanism does this pigment enter the systemic circulation? Several postulates have been proposed for this "reentry": (1) rupture of the bile canaliculi secondary to the necrosis of the hepatic cells that constitute their walls; (2) occlusion of the canaliculi by inspissated bile or their compression by swollen hepatic cells; (3) obstruction of the terminal intrahepatic bile ducts (cholangioles) by inflammatory cells; (4) altered hepatic cell permeability; and (5) as a result of impaired excretion, accumulation of conjugated bilirubin in the hepatocytes and secondary diffusion into the plasma. Although some of these postulates are speculative, it is likely that several of these mechanisms occur. For example, occasionally in histologic sections, escape of bile through rents in the walls of canaliculi in areas of necrosis is apparent. Also, microscopic studies of the liver of rats injected with fluorescent dyes have shown reflux of bile from canaliculi into sinusoids. However, no anatomic damage needs to be invoked, because when unconjugated bilirubin is infused into normal subjects at high rates, conjugated hyperbilirubinemia occurs; this is explained most logically by passive diffusion.

EXTRAHEPATIC BILIARY OBSTRUCTION   Complete obstruction of the extrahepatic bile ducts leads to jaundice with predominantly conjugated hyperbilirubinemia, bilirubinuria, and clay-colored stools. Failure of bile to reach the intestine results in virtual disappearance of urobilinogen from the stool and urine. The concentration of bilirubin rises progressively but then usually plateaus at a level of 30 to 40 mg per 100 ml. To some extent this plateau may be explained by a balance between renal excretion and diversion of bilirubin to other metabolites. In hepatocellular jaundice, such a plateau tends not to occur, and bilirubin levels in excess of 50 mg per 100 ml may be found.

Partial obstruction of the extrahepatic bile ducts can also give rise to jaundice but only if the intrabiliary pressure is increased, because the excretion of bilirubin does not diminish until the intraductile pressure approaches the maximal secretory pressure of approximately 250 mmHg bile. Jaundice may occur at much lower pressures if the obstruction is complicated by infection of the ducts or hepatocellular injury. Therefore, jaundice, bilirubinuria, and clay-colored stools are inconstant findings in partial biliary obstruction, and the amount of urobilinogen in urine and stool varies with the degree of occlusion.

The functional reserve of the liver is so great that *occlusion of the intrahepatic bile ducts* does not give rise to jaundice unless the drainage of bile from a large segment of the parenchyma is interrupted. Either of the two major hepatic ducts or a large number of secondary radicles may be occluded without production of jaundice. In experimental animals the ducts draining at least 75 percent of the parenchyma must be occluded before jaundice appears.

Additional points of terminology   In clinical practice, a patient may be described as having *obstructive,* or *cholestatic,* jaundice. By this is meant that clinically, and especially biochemically, there is little to suggest hepatocellular damage and that the main features point to interference with, or obstruction in, the flow of bile. Typically one would expect such a patient to show (1) predominantly conjugated hyperbilirubinemia, (2) minimal biochemical changes of parenchymal liver damage, and (3) a moderate to a marked increase in the serum alkaline phosphatase level [usually three or four times normal (greater than 15 Bodansky units or greater than 250 IU per liter)]. As emphasized in Chaps. 299 and 300, an *elevated alkaline phosphatase level* in a patient with jaundice or liver disease, in the absence of other disorders such as bone disease, is most suggestive of interference with bile secretion or an infiltrative process in the liver. However, *laboratory tests alone may not permit differentiation of intrahepatic from extrahepatic cholestasis.*

Some clinicians reserve the term obstructive jaundice for those situations in which anatomic obstruction can be demonstrated and use the term cholestatic jaundice for cases of parenchymal liver disease in which the obstructive phase is on a junctional basis. Nevertheless, because these two entities frequently are indistinguishable by clinical and biochemical criteria, the terms obstructive jaundice and cholestatic jaundice are often used interchangeably.

Hepatocellular disorders in which jaundice associated with an obstructive, or cholestatic, phase occurs include (1) occasional cases of viral hepatitis, (2) drug reactions, especially those due to chlorpromazine and methyltestosterone, (3) some cases of alcoholic hepatitis or alcohol-induced fatty liver, (4) jaundice in the last trimester of pregnancy, (5) most cases of Dubin-Johnson or Rotor syndrome, (6) benign recurrent intrahepatic cholestasis, and (7) certain types of postoperative jaundice. These and other conditions are discussed in Chaps. 301 and 302.

In summary, all forms of conjugated hyperbilirubinemia have by definition an impairment in the excretion of bilirubin into bile. In most cases of parenchymal liver disease, a broad derangement is shown by the biochemical tests of liver function. However, when the major detectable alterations of liver function tests include (1) conjugated hyperbilirubinemia and (2) moderate to marked elevation of the serum alkaline phosphatase level, the terms obstructive or cholestatic jaundice may be appropriate. Additional procedures, including operation, are often needed to determine the cause of the cholestasis (see Chaps. 298 and 300).

HEPATOMEGALY

In the supine position, the major part of the liver lies beneath the right rib cage. In some normal persons the liver edge may be palpable 1 to 2 cm below the right costal margin, and a palpable liver edge by itself does not necessarily indicate hepatomegaly. In evaluating liver size by physical examination, two factors other than ability to palpate the liver edge need to be considered, namely, (1) the location of the upper border of liver dullness by percussion, and (2) the body habitus.

Normally, the upper edge of liver dullness on the right side in the midclavicular line is at the level of the fifth rib, but in asthenic habitus it may be lower. The liver edge normally descends 1 to 3 cm with deep inspiration. In hypersthenic subjects, the liver may extend over to the left side of the abdominal wall, with the lower edge high and not palpable; in hyposthenic subjects with a very acute costal angle, the liver may lie in the right half of the abdomen, the edge being palpable by as much as 6 to 8 cm below the right costal margin lateral to the right rectus abdominis muscle. Thus, palpability does not necessarily imply hepatomegaly.

In determining liver enlargement by palpation, one should be certain that the liver is being palpated rather than other right upper quadrant masses such as gallbladder, colonic neoplasm, or fecal material in the colon. Liver enlargement is often confirmed by radiologic studies, including hepatic scintiscans, celiac axis angiography, and echography.

In many cases of generalized liver enlargement, the left lobe will be felt in the epigastrium between the xiphoid and umbilicus. The liver should be carefully palpated during deep inspiration to determine whether the edge is tender, regular or irregular, firm or soft, rounded and thickened, or sharp. The edge is tender and often rounded with hepatic inflammation, as in hepatitis, or when the liver is acutely congested, as in cardiac decompensation. Pulsation of the liver may be found with tricuspid valvular incompetence. A carcinomatous liver may be rocklike in hardness; the cirrhotic liver is very firm in consistency. The largest livers are often found with carcinoma (primary or metastatic), marked fatty infiltration, congestive cardiac decompensation, Hodgkin's disease, and amyloidosis. Rapid decrease in liver size may occur with improvement of congestive failure, mobilization of fat from the liver, or massive hepatic necrosis.

TABLE 39-3
Causes of a palpable liver and hepatomegaly

I Palpable liver without hepatomegaly
  A Right diaphragm displaced downward (e.g., emphysema, asthma)
  B Subdiaphragmatic lesion (e.g., abscess)
  C Aberrant lobe of liver (Riedel's lobe)
  D Extremely thin or relaxed abdominal muscles
  E Occasionally present in normal persons
II Hepatomegaly
  A Vascular congestion (e.g., congestive heart failure, hepatic vein thrombosis)
  B Bile duct obstruction (e.g., lesion in common duct leading to hepatomegaly and subsequently biliary cirrhosis)
  C Infiltrative disorders
    1 Bone marrow and reticuloendothelial cells
      a Extramedullary hematopoiesis
      b Leukemia
      c Lymphoma
    2 Fat
      a Fatty liver (e.g., secondary to alcohol, diabetes, or toxins)
      b Gaucher's disease and some other lipidoses
    3 Glycogen (e.g., diabetes, especially after insulin excess)
    4 Amyloid
    5 Iron (hemochromatosis and hemosiderosis)
    6 Granuloma (tuberculosis, sarcoid)
  D Inflammatory disorders
    1 Hepatitis—due to drugs or infectious agents
    2 Cirrhosis—except in late stages when prolonged scarring may lead to a *small,* shrunken liver
  E Tumors—primary or metastatic
  F Cysts—polycystic disease, congenital hepatic fibrosis

In a patient with hepatomegaly, auscultation is sometimes helpful. A friction rub may be audible (and palpable) in the right upper quadrant; it is usually due to a recent biopsy, tumor, or perihepatitis. In portal hypertension a venous hum may be audible between the umbilicus and the xiphoid. An arterial murmur or bruit over the liver may indicate tumor, usually hepatoma.

Some of the causes of a palpable liver and hepatomegaly are given in Table 39-3.

REFERENCES

BERK PD et al: Inborn errors of bilirubin metabolism. Med Clin North Am 59:803, 1975

BISSELL DM: Formation and elimination of bilirubin. Gastroenterology 69:519, 1975

FEVERY J et al: Unconjugated bilirubin and an increased proportion of bilirubin monoconjugates in the bile of patients with Gilbert's syndrome and Crigler-Najjar disease. J Clin Invest 60:970, 1977

GORESKY CA, FISHER MM: *Jaundice.* New York, Plenum, 1975

SCHMID R: Bilirubin metabolism: State of the art. Gastroenterology 74:1307, 1978

SCHMID R, McDONAGH AF: Hyperbilirubinemia, in *The Metabolic Basis of Inherited Disease,* 4th ed, JB Stanbury et al (eds). New York, McGraw-Hill, 1978

40
ABDOMINAL SWELLING AND ASCITES

ROBERT M. GLICKMAN
KURT J. ISSELBACHER

ABDOMINAL SWELLING Abdominal swelling or distention is a common problem in clinical medicine and may be the initial manifestation of a systemic disease or of otherwise unsuspected abdominal disease. *Subjective* abdominal enlargement, often described as a sensation of fullness or bloating, is usually transient and is often related to a functional gastrointestinal disorder when it is not accompanied by objective physical findings of increased abdominal girth or local swelling. *Obesity* and lumbar lordosis, which may be associated with prominence of the abdomen, may usually be distinguished from true increases in the volume of the peritoneal cavity by history and careful physical examination.

Clinical history Abdominal swelling may first be noticed by the patient because of a progressive increase in belt or clothing size, the appearance of abdominal or inguinal hernias, or the development of a localized swelling. Often, considerable abdominal enlargement has gone unnoticed for weeks or months, either because of coexistent obesity or because the ascites formation has been insidious, without pain or localizing symptoms. Progressive abdominal distention may be associated with a sensation of "pulling" or "stretching" of the flanks or groins and vague low back pain. Localized *pain* usually results from involvement of an abdominal organ (e.g., a passively congested liver, large spleen, or colonic tumor). Pain is uncommon in cirrhosis with ascites and when it is present pancreatitis, hepatoma, or peritonitis should be considered. Tense ascites or abdominal tumors may produce increased intraabdominal pressure, resulting in *indigestion* and *heartburn* due to gastroesophageal reflux or *dyspnea, orthopnea,* and *tachypnea* from elevation of the diaphragm. A coexistent pleural effusion, more commonly on the right, presumably due to leakage of ascitic fluid through lymphatic channels in the diaphragm, may also contribute to respiratory embarrassment. The patient with diffuse abdominal swelling should be questioned about increased alcoholic intake, a prior episode of jaundice or hematuria, a change in bowel habits, or a past history of rheumatic heart disease. Such historic information may provide the clues that will lead one to suspect an occult cirrhosis, a colonic tumor with peritoneal seeding, congestive heart failure, or nephrosis.

Physical examination A carefully executed *general physical examination* can yield valuable clues concerning the etiology of abdominal swelling. Thus palmar erythema and spider angiomas suggest an underlying cirrhosis, while supraclavicular adenopathy (Virchow's node) should raise the question of an underlying gastrointestinal malignancy. *Inspection* of the abdomen is an important but often cursorily performed aspect of the abdominal examination. By noting the abdominal contour, one may be able to distinguish localized from generalized swelling. The tensely distended abdomen with tightly stretched skin, bulging flanks, and everted umbilicus is characteristic of ascites. A prominent abdominal venous pattern with the direction of flow away from the umbilicus often is a reflection of portal hypertension; venous collaterals with flow from the lower part of the abdomen toward the umbilicus suggests obstruction of the inferior vena cava; flow downward toward the umbilicus suggests superior vena cava obstruction. "Doming" of the abdomen with visible ridges from underlying intestinal loops is usually due to intestinal obstruction or distention. An epigastric mass, with evident peristalsis proceeding from left to right, usually indicates underlying pyloric obstruction. A liver with metastatic deposits may be visible as a nodular right upper quadrant mass moving with respiration.

Auscultation may reveal the high-pitched, rushing sounds of early intestinal obstruction or a succussion sound due to increased fluid and gas in a dilated hollow viscus. Careful auscultation over an enlarged liver occasionally reveals the harsh bruit of a vascular tumor, especially a hepatoma, or the leathery friction rub of a surface nodule. A venous hum at the umbilicus may signify portal hypertension and an increased collateral blood flow around the liver. A fluid wave and flank dullness which shifts with change in position of the patient are important signs that indicate the presence of peritoneal fluid. In obese patients, small amounts of fluid may be difficult to demonstrate; on occasion the fluid may be detected by abdominal percussion with patients on their hands and knees. Doubt about the presence of peritoneal fluid may be resolved by careful paracentesis with a small-gauge (No. 19 or 20) needle. Careful percussion should serve to distinguish generalized abdominal enlargement from localized swelling due to an enlarged uterus, ovarian cyst, or distended bladder. Percussion can also outline an abnormally small or large liver. Loss of normal liver dullness may result from massive hepatic necrosis; it may also be a clue to free gas in the peritoneal cavity, as from perforation of a hollow viscus.

Palpation is often difficult with massive ascites, and ballottement of overlying fluid may be the only method of palpating the liver or spleen. A slightly enlarged spleen in association with ascites may be the only evidence of an occult cirrhosis. When there is evidence of portal hypertension, a soft liver suggests that obstruction to portal flow is extrahepatic; a firm liver suggests cirrhosis as the likely cause of the portal hypertension. A very hard or nodular liver is a clue that the liver is infiltrated with tumor, and when accompanied by ascites, it suggests that the latter is due to peritoneal seeding. A pulsatile liver and ascites may be found in tricuspid insufficiency.

An attempt should be made to determine whether a mass is solid or cystic, smooth or irregular, and whether it moves with respiration. The liver, spleen, and gallbladder should descend with respiration unless they are fixed by adhesions or extension of tumor beyond the organ. A fixed mass not descending with respiration may indicate that it is retroperitoneal. Tenderness, especially if localized, may indicate an inflammatory process

such as an abscess; it may also be due to stretching of the visceral peritoneum or tumor necrosis. Rectal and pelvic examinations are mandatory; they may reveal otherwise undetected masses due to tumor or infection.

Radiographic and laboratory examinations are essential for confirming or extending the impressions gained on physical examination. Upright and recumbent films of the abdomen may demonstrate the dilated loops of intestine with fluid levels characteristic of intestinal obstruction or the diffuse abdominal haziness and loss of psoas margins suggestive of ascites. A plain film of the abdomen may reveal the distended colon of otherwise unsuspected ulcerative colitis and give valuable information as to the size of the liver and spleen. An irregular and elevated right side of the diaphragm may be a clue to a liver abscess or hepatoma. Studies of the gastrointestinal tract with barium or other contrast media are usually necessary in the search for a primary tumor.

ASCITES In most cases the clinical and laboratory evaluation of the patient with ascites is sufficient to reveal the cause of the fluid accumulation. Often the ascites is a component or complication of cirrhosis, congestive heart failure, nephrosis, or disseminated carcinomatosis. However, even when the cause of ascites seems obvious, it is often important to determine whether another separate or related disease process has supervened. For example, when the patient with compensated cirrhosis and minimal ascites develops progressive ascites that is increasingly difficult to control with sodium restriction or diuretics, the obvious temptation is to attribute the worsening of the clinical picture to progressive liver disease. However, an occult hepatoma, portal vein thrombosis, spontaneous bacterial peritonitis, or even tuberculosis may be responsible for the decompensation. The disappointingly low success of diagnosing tuberculous peritonitis or hepatoma in the patient with cirrhosis and ascites reflects the too-low index of suspicion for the development of such superimposed conditions. Similarly, the patient with congestive heart failure may develop ascites from a disseminated carcinoma with peritoneal seeding. The thorough evaluation of each patient with ascites, even in the presence of an "obvious" cause, will help avoid these errors.

Diagnostic paracentesis (50 to 100 ml) should be part of the routine evaluation of the patient with ascites. The fluid should be examined for its gross appearance, protein content, cell count, and differential cell count, as well as Gram's and acid-fast stains and culture. Cytologic and cell-block examination may disclose an otherwise unsuspected carcinoma. Table 40-1 presents some of the features of ascitic fluid typically found in various disease states. In some disorders, such as cirrhosis, the fluid has the characteristics of a transudate (less than 2.5 g protein per 100 ml and a specific gravity less than 1.016); in others, such as peritonitis, the features are those of an exudate. Although there is variability of the ascitic fluid in any given disease state, some features are sufficiently characteristic to suggest certain diagnostic possibilities. For example, blood-stained fluid with more than 2.5 g protein per 100 ml is unusual in uncomplicated cirrhosis but is consistent with tuberculous peritonitis or neoplasm. Cloudy fluid with a predominance of polymorphonuclear cells and a positive Gram stain are characteristic of bacterial peritonitis; if most cells are lymphocytes, tuberculosis should be suspected. The complete examination of each fluid is most important, for occasionally only *one* finding may be abnormal. For example, if the fluid is a typical transudate but contains more than 250 white blood cells per cubic millimeter, the finding should be recognized as

TABLE 40-1
Ascitic fluid characteristics in various disease states

Condition	Gross appearance	Specific gravity	Protein, g/100 ml	Cell count Red blood cells, >10,000/mm³	White blood cells, per mm³	Other tests
Cirrhosis	Straw-colored or bile-stained	<1.016 (95%)*	<2.5 (95%)	1%	<250 (90%);* predominantly endothelial	
Neoplasm	Straw-colored, hemorrhagic, mucinous, or chylous	Variable, >1.016 (45%)	>2.5 (75%)	20%	>1000 (50%); variable cell types	Cytology, cell block, peritoneal biopsy
Tuberculous peritonitis	Clear, turbid, hemorrhagic, chylous	Variable, >1.016 (50%)	>2.5 (50%)	7%	>1000 (70%); usually >70% lymphocytes	Peritoneal biopsy, stain and culture for acid-fast bacilli
Pyogenic peritonitis	Turbid or purulent	If purulent, >1.016	If purulent, >2.5	Unusual	Predominantly polymorphonuclear leukocytes	+Gram's stain, culture
Congestive heart failure	Straw-colored	Variable, <1.016 (60%)	Variable, 1.5–5.3	10%	<1000 (90%); usually mesothelial, mononuclear	
Nephrosis	Straw-colored or chylous	<1.016	<2.5 (100%)	Unusual	<250; mesothelial, mononuclear	If chylous, ether extraction, Sudan staining
Pancreatic ascites (pancreatitis, pseudocyst)	Turbid, hemorrhagic, or chylous	Variable, often >1.016	Variable, often >2.5	Variable, may be blood-stained	Variable	Increased amylase in ascitic fluid and serum

* *Since the conditions of examining fluid and selecting patients were not identical in each series, the percentage figures (in the parentheses) should be taken as an indication of the order of magnitude rather than as the precise incidence of any abnormal finding.*
SOURCES: *Berner et al; Borhanmanesh et al; Coder and Olander; Malagelada et al.*

atypical for cirrhosis, nephrosis, or congestive heart failure and should warrant a search for tumor or infection. This is especially true in the evaluation of cirrhotic ascites where occult peritoneal infection may be present with only minor elevations in the white blood cell count of the peritoneal fluid (300 to 500 cells per cubic millimeter). Since Gram's stain of the fluid may be negative in a high proportion of such cases, careful culture of the peritoneal fluid is mandatory.

Chylous ascites refers to a turbid, milky, or creamy peritoneal fluid due to the presence of thoracic or intestinal lymph. Such a fluid shows Sudan-staining fat globules microscopically and an increased triglyceride content by chemical examination. A turbid fluid due to leukocytes or tumor cells may be confused with chylous fluid, and it is often helpful to carry out alkalinization and ether extraction of the specimen. Alkali will tend to dissolve cellular proteins and thereby reduce turbidity; ether extraction will lead to clearing if the turbidity of the fluid is due to lipid. Chylous ascites is most often the result of lymphatic obstruction from trauma, tumor, tuberculosis, filariasis (see Chap. 209), or congenital abnormalities. It may also be seen in the nephrotic syndrome.

Rarely, ascitic fluid may be *mucinous* in character, suggesting either pseudomyxoma peritonei (Chap. 297) or rarely a colloid carcinoma of the stomach or colon with peritoneal implants.

On rare occasions a syndrome may be seen of fever and ascites, without infection, occurring several weeks after abdominal surgery. This seems to result from starch (from surgical gloves) introduced into the peritoneum at the time of surgery, with a subsequent foreign-body reaction and ascites formation. Given the proper index of suspicion, diagnosis can be made by paracentesis and finding double refractile particles (i.e., starch) when polarized light is used (Fig. 40-1).

The etiology of ascites may remain uncertain even after the all these conditions pronounced weight loss, wasting, anorexia, and fever may be found, and hepatomegaly, splenomegaly, and deranged liver function tests may be present. Procedures such as peritoneal biopsy, peritoneoscopy, liver biopsy, splenoportography, or laparotomy may be necessary to provide the diagnosis. Other less common causes of ascites include constrictive pericarditis, hepatic vein obstruction, myxedema and benign tumors of the ovary, particularly fibroma (Meigs's syndrome, with ascites and hydrothorax). The physiologic and metabolic factors involved in the production of ascites are described in Chap. 304.

REFERENCES

BAR-MEIR S: Analysis of ascitic fluid in cirrhosis. Dig Dis Sc 24:136, 1979

BERNER C et al: Diagnostic probabilities in patients with conspicuous ascites. Arch Intern Med 113:687, 1964

FIGURE 40-1

Starch peritonitis. Examination of ascitic fluid under polarized light reveals doubly refractile starch granules.

BORHANMANESH F et al: Tuberculous peritonitis: Prospective study of 32 cases in Iran. Ann Intern Med 76:567, 1972

CODER DM, OLANDER GA: Granulomatous peritonitis caused by starch glove powder. Arch Surg 105:83, 1972

CONN HO: Spontaneous bacterial peritonitis: Multiple revisitations. Gastroenterology 70:455, 1976

———, FESSEL JH: Spontaneous bacterial peritonitis in cirrhosis: Variations on a theme. Medicine 50:161, 1971

MALAGELADA JR et al: Origin of fat in chylous ascites of patients with liver cirrhosis. Gastroenterology 67:878, 1974

WARSHAW AL: Diagnosis of starch peritonitis by paracentesis. Lancet 2:1054, 1972

section 6 | Alterations in body weight

41
GAIN AND LOSS IN WEIGHT

DANIEL W. FOSTER

GENERAL PRINCIPLES

In normal persons weight is maintained stable because caloric intake is matched to caloric expenditure by the coordinated activities of the feeding and satiety centers located in the brainstem. Energy costs fall into three categories: (1) calories needed for maintenance of basal metabolism, (2) calories necessary for food absorption (specific dynamic action), and (3) calories required for physical activity. *Basal metabolism* is defined as the total caloric requirement when the body is in the supine position, motionless except for quiet respiration. It can be translated as the energy required to maintain structural and functional integrity of the organism in the absence of physical activity. Under normal circumstances about half the total daily caloric intake is consumed by basal processes. In nonobese, nonsedentary subjects another 10 percent of the total intake is used for food absorption. The remainder is spent in physical activity. In active persons this represents about 40 percent of daily intake, though athletes may use greater than 50 percent of calories for physical activity.

Gain or loss in tissue mass is determined by the net balance between caloric intake and caloric expenditure. Change in body weight as a consequence of voluntary alteration in diet or exercise is never worrisome; change in weight that is not deliberately sought, on the other hand, is a frequent reason for consultation with the physician and often indicates the presence of disease. It is important to recognize that changes in weight may reflect alteration in either tissue mass or body fluid content. Rapid swings almost always indicate the latter. Even when tissue mass is changing, fluid loss or gain plays a major role in the measured change in weight, particularly over the short run. This point is well illustrated by the data of Table 41-1 where the composition of weight loss was estimated during a 24-day period of semistarvation in 13 normal soldiers (daily intake 1010 cal). During the first 3 days 70 percent of the weight loss was due to water, while in subsequent stages protein and fat accounted for essentially all the decreased mass. This varying contribution of fluid accounts for the fact that one cannot use a fixed formula for predicting weight loss or gain. It is frequently stated that a net change of 7700 cal will be accompanied by a 1-kg change in body mass (3500 cal/lb). While this figure is reasonable as an estimate for long-term

changes in caloric intake, obviously the apparent caloric cost per kilogram of weight lost or gained will vary with the accompanying fluid shifts. In the experiment summarized in Table 41-1, for example, a negative balance of only 2596 cal resulted in the loss of a kilogram of weight between days 1 and 3, while between days 22 and 24, loss of a kilogram required a deficit of 8700 cal. In general if weight loss or gain has occurred over a period of weeks or months, it is safe to assume that change in tissue mass has occurred; weight loss or gain limited to a several-day period may be due to fluid shifts alone. Occasionally true loss of tissue mass is obscured by fluid retention as in the case of the cirrhotic patient who develops ascites or the patient with anorexia nervosa and edema.

WEIGHT GAIN

While obesity is a major public health concern (see Chap. 76), its diagnosis is usually uncomplicated. Obese subjects often deny overeating, but the true situation can usually be assessed either by tabulating actual food intake and determining its caloric content from standard tables or by interviewing the patient's family and friends. Regardless of history, excess caloric intake is the cause of obesity in the overwhelming majority of cases. Pathological causes of obesity are rare. In the adult, Cushing's syndrome can result in acquired obesity in a previously nonobese patient, but usually the diagnosis suggests itself by the pattern of fat distribution and the clinical picture. Other endocrine diseases such as hypothyroidism, hypogonadism, and insulin-secreting tumors are frequently listed in the differential diagnosis of acquired obesity but in fact do not represent significant diagnostic problems. Congenital diseases such as the Prader-Willi and Laurence-Moon-Biedl syndromes are usually readily recognizable and appear early in life. Rarely neoplastic disease involving the hypothalamus, particularly

TABLE 41-1
Percentage composition of mean daily weight loss in 13 young men during caloric restriction for 24 days

Days	Mean weight loss, kg/day	Water, %	Fat, %	Protein, %	Calorie equivalents of weight loss, cal/kg
1–3	0.80	70	25	5	2596
11–13	0.23	19	69	12	7043
22–24	0.17	0	85	15	8700

SOURCE: *After Brožek et al.*

craniopharyngioma, may be a cause of acquired obesity. Extensive workup of the central nervous system in obesity is not indicated, however, in the absence of suspicious symptoms (headache, visual difficulties, vomiting, or endocrine changes).

WEIGHT LOSS

Weight loss in the absence of deliberate dieting is a more serious problem than weight gain simply because there is a high chance that organic disease is present. Mechanisms include decreased appetite, accelerated tissue metabolism, and loss of calories in urine or stool, acting singly or in combination. No attempt will be made to list all the diseases capable of causing weight loss. The majority of cases will fall into one of the seven following categories.

DIABETES MELLITUS   Initial weight loss with the onset of diabetes is largely fluid and is due to the osmotic diuresis induced by hyperglycemia. Subsequently loss of tissue mass occurs in the insulin-dependent form of the disease due to both caloric wastage (the consequence of glycosuria) and the hormonal abnormalities that characterize the illness. Insulin deficiency and glucagon excess result in impaired synthesis of protein and fat and simultaneously cause accelerated proteolysis and lipolysis such that the net energy state is catabolic. Weight loss in diabetes is frequently associated with increased food intake.

ENDOCRINE DISEASE   The most important endocrine disease causing weight loss is thyrotoxicosis. While weight loss is not inevitable (indeed, thyrotoxicosis may rarely be found in a patient who has gained weight), it is extremely common. Increased appetite and food intake are the rule, and patients often spontaneously choose a very high carbohydrate diet. Caloric expenditure is enormous, primarily because of an increased metabolic rate, but increased motor activity also plays a role. The molecular mechanism whereby thyrotoxicosis causes weight loss is not settled, but thyroid hormone is thought to increase sodium-potassium adenosine triphosphatase (ATPase) activity in many tissues, suggesting that the diminished efficiency of ingested calories is due to a futile cycle of adenosine triphosphate (ATP) synthesis and breakdown with energy lost as heat. Panhypopituitarism and adrenal insufficiency may also be associated with weight loss, probably primarily as a consequence of diminished appetite secondary to cortisol deficiency.

GASTROINTESTINAL DISEASE   A variety of gastrointestinal diseases may cause weight loss. Overt or occult steatorrhea due to sprue, chronic pancreatitis, or cystic fibrosis may produce wasting despite major increases in food intake. Chronic diarrhea due to inflammatory bowel disease (with or without fistulas) or parasites, esophageal disease with reflux or vomiting, even ordinary peptic ulcer have to be considered in the differential diagnosis. The mechanism of weight loss in alimentary tract disease is generally either decreased food intake or mal-absorption, though inflammation per se probably plays a major role in ulcerative colitis and regional enteritis.

INFECTION   Hidden infection must always be sought in patients with unexplained weight loss. Tuberculosis, fungal diseases, amebic abscess, and subacute bacterial endocarditis should be high on the list of suspects. The mechanism probably involves both anorexia and inflammation-induced acceleration of cellular metabolic demands. It has been suggested that glucagon plays a major role in the induction of negative nitrogen balance and tissue wastage in inflammation, but it is likely that the catabolic state also requires changes in a number of other hormones.

MALIGNANCY   Occult malignancy is probably the number one cause of weight loss occurring in the absence of major signs and symptoms. In the search for malignancy particular emphasis must be placed on the gastrointestinal tract, pancreas, and liver. Lymphoma and leukemia should also be considered. While silent (except for weight loss) malignancy can occur in any organ, statistically the gastrointestinal tract is the most common site.

PSYCHIATRIC DISEASE   The classic psychiatric illness associated with profound weight loss is anorexia nervosa (Chap. 77). However, anorexia may also occur in depressive states and schizophrenia. The presence of anorexia is usually clear from the history. While organic disease causing both anorexia and depression has to be ruled out, ordinarily the psychiatric nature of the problem will be clear.

RENAL DISEASE   One of the earliest manifestations of uremia is anorexia. As a consequence all patients with unexplained weight loss should be given screening renal function tests.

SUMMARY

Weight loss is more often a diagnostic problem than weight gain and much more often a sign of serious organic illness. If the weight loss is associated with increased food intake, the diagnosis will likely be diabetes, thyrotoxicosis, or a malabsorption syndrome. If food intake is normal or decreased, malignancy, infection, renal disease, psychiatric syndromes, or endocrine deficiency will more commonly be found.

REFERENCES

Brožek J et al: Changes in body weight and body dimensions in men performing work on a low calorie carbohydrate diet. J Appl Physiol 10:412, 1957

Konishi F: Food energy equivalents of various activities. J Am Diet Assoc 46:186, 1965

Runcie J, Hilditch TE: Energy provision, tissue utilization and weight loss in prolonged starvation. Br Med J 2:352, 1974

Yang M-U, Van Itallie TB: Composition of weight loss during short-term weight reduction. Metabolic responses of obese subjects to starvation and low calorie ketogenic and non-ketogenic diets. J Clin Invest 58:722, 1976

42

PROTEINURIA, HEMATURIA, AZOTEMIA, AND OLIGURIA

FREDRIC L. COE

PROTEINURIA

Normal adults may excrete up to 150 mg protein daily. Of this, only 10 to 15 mg is albumin; the rest is composed of over 30 different plasma proteins and of glycoproteins that derive from the renal cells. Tamm-Horsfall mucoprotein, the most prevalent of the urine proteins that do not arise from plasma, is produced by the cells of the ascending limb of the loop of Henle and is excreted at the rate of 25 mg per day. Daily excretion of more than 150 mg protein is properly termed *pathological proteinuria,* but in common usage the word *proteinuria* suffices. Protein excretion above 3.5 g per 24 h is termed *massive* proteinuria and usually occurs when glomeruli have been damaged enough to allow plasma proteins, especially albumin, to enter the urine. Urinary albumin loss lowers serum albumin concentration, and the consequent fall in intracapillary oncotic pressure fosters the accumulation of tissue edema (Chap. 29); serum lipids rise. The combination of *massive proteinuria, hypoalbuminemia, edema,* and *hyperlipidemia* is often called the *nephrotic syndrome,* but this term is becoming synonymous with massive urinary protein loss alone. Hypoalbuminemia, elevated blood lipids, and edema are pathophysiologic consequences of massive proteinuria and occur only when hepatic albumin synthesis, though normal or even increased, fails to compensate for urine albumin losses; they are not a direct result of renal disease.

DETECTION OF PROTEINURIA Detection of proteinuria is usually by urine "dipsticks" that register a trace result in response to as little as 50 mg protein per liter, and a distinct color change of the 1+ level at about 300 mg per liter. Since proteinuria can be missed if the urine is very dilute, fasting morning samples that tend to be concentrated are usually studied. Dipsticks respond best to albumin, so that a negative result can occur when large amounts of other protein, or protein fragments such as light chains, are being excreted. Dipstick proteinuria requires additional evaluation by the measurement of 24-h excretion rate. If total protein excretion is abnormal, it is helpful to characterize the proportions of albumin and globulins in the urine by cellulose acetate electrophoresis or other methods. Immunoelectrophoresis is required to identify immunoglobulin fragments, kappa or lambda light chains, when their presence is suggested by a monoclonal peak on routine urine electrophoresis.

MECHANISMS OF PROTEINURIA Tubular proteinuria Normal low-molecular-weight serum proteins below 40,000 daltons, such as β_2 microglobulin (11,600 mol wt), lysozyme (14,000 mol wt), or light chains (22,000 mol wt) are readily filtered by the glomeruli but are normally present in urine in only trace amounts because tubular reabsorption of them is very efficient. Diseases that selectively damage the tubules more than glomeruli (Chap. 281) cause excessive excretion of these small proteins with little or no increase in albumin excretion. The resulting proteinuria is usually between 1 and 3 g per 24 h, and edema and lipid disorders do not occur because albumin losses are small. Bence-Jones protein, which is probably a dimer of two light chains, light chains themselves, and myoglobin are examples of proteins whose plasma concentrations may increase as a consequence of disease. If their filtered load rises enough to exceed tubular reabsorptive capacity, "overflow" proteinuria may occur.

Glomerular proteinuria When glomerular damage is present, albumin and even larger globulin molecules may be filtered excessively because normal selective filtration is lost. The glomerular capillary endothelial cells form a barrier penetrated by pores of about 1000 Å diameter that holds back cells and other particles but offers no impediment to most proteins. The glomerular basement membrane traps molecules above 50 Å in effective radius. These usually have a molecular weight above 100,000 daltons. The *foot processes (podocytes)* of the visceral epithelial cells (Fig. 42–1) cover the urinary aspect of the glomerular basement membrane and produce a series of narrow channels through which molecules that traverse the basement membrane must pass. Anionic molecules, like albumin, are filtered less freely than are neutral or positively charged molecules of the same size, so little albumin enters the filtrate. This charge selectivity appears to be due to anionic glycoproteins that cover the surfaces of the foot processes and contribute to the matrix structure of the basement membrane (Chap. 274). The glycoproteins are anionic because they contain the dicarboxylic amino acids, glutamic and aspartic acid, and sialic acid. At the pH of blood (7.4) or urine (4.5 to 7.5) carboxylic and sialic acid residues are dissociated and, therefore, have a negative charge. Albumin also carries an overall negative charge. The negatively charged portions of the glycoproteins repel those of albumin and retard filtration.

Glomerular disease can disrupt any of these filtration barriers. Injury limited to the polyanion glycoproteins would tend to produce selective losses of anionic proteins, such as albumin, that would be filtered more completely by the normal glomerulus but for their charge. Extensive injury that involves the entire basement membrane, not only its polyanion components, may increase losses of very large proteins, as well as albumin.

The selectivity of proteinuria varies with the extent of glomerular injury. However, the clinical value of measuring selectivity has not been fully defined. The basis of such measurements is to express the excretion rate of a protein as a fraction of its theoretical maximum filtered load, which is the product of its serum concentration and the glomerular filtration rate (GFR). This fraction must reflect the relative filtration efficiency of the protein to that of a completely filtered GFR marker, usually inulin or creatinine, provided that tubular reabsorption and renal production or catabolism are negligible. The slope of a plot of such a clearance ratio against molecular weight for a variety of serum proteins is one index of filtration selectivity. A more practical version of this test is based upon the ratio of the clearance fractions of two proteins of different molecular weight. For example, the IgG transferrin clearance fraction ratio is below 0.1 in most children with lipoid nephrosis, a proteinuric disorder in which fusion of foot processes is the only detectable glomerular abnormality (Chap. 278). In chronic membranous glomerulopathy (Chap. 278) the basement membrane is filled with immune complex deposits, and progressive renal failure occurs. Here, the clearance ratio usually is between 0.1 and 0.2. The ratio usually is above 0.2 in membranoproliferative glomerulonephritis, a severe renal disease that can progress rapidly to renal failure and in which glomerular architecture is severely disturbed (Chap. 278). These and other aspects of the relationship between glomerular pathology and proteinuria are considered in greater detail in Chaps. 277 to 279.

APPROACH TO THE PATIENT WITH PROTEINURIA Given dipstick proteinuria of the 1+ level or more, 24-h urine protein excretion must be measured. If it is above 150 mg, electrophoresis should be carried out to determine the proportions of albumin and other proteins. Excretion mainly of albumin signifies a glomerular lesion. When the total daily protein excretion exceeds 3.5 g, by definition the nephrotic syndrome is considered to be present; milder albuminuria is called an *asymptomatic urinary abnormality*. Tubular proteinuria usually reflects a hereditary or acquired tubular disorder or tubulointerstitial nephropathy (Chap. 281). The presence of large amounts of Bence-Jones protein suggests that multiple myeloma may be present (Chap. 63).

ISOLATED HEMATURIA Urinary tract bleeding from the urethra to the renal pelvis produces isolated hematuria, without significant proteinuria, cells, or urinary casts. Total hematuria, which occurs evenly throughout voiding, means that blood has had the opportunity to mix fully with the bladder urine. When bleeding occurs mainly at the beginning or end of micturition, a prostatic or urethral origin is more likely.

Common causes of *isolated* hematuria are urinary tract stones, benign and malignant neoplasms of the urinary tract, tuberculosis, trauma, and prostatitis; few primary renal diseases cause it. As discussed in Chaps. 273 and 278, *focal glomerulitis,* in the syndrome of benign recurrent hematuria or in Berger's disease, i.e., IgA nephropathy, is usually associated with red blood cell casts. Analgesic nephropathy and sickling states cause isolated hematuria, but modest proteinuria, papillary necrosis, or azotemia often is present and suggests a renal origin. Hemoglobin electrophoresis is appropriate whenever a sickling disorder is suspected.

Prostatic and external urethral examination is the basic first step in the evaluation of isolated hematuria. Intravenous pyelography is the next. If no lesion is found, cystoscopy and retrograde pyelography may become necessary. At cystoscopy, blood may be found to issue from only one ureter, a helpful clue which indicates a localized lesion rather than a primary renal disease. Disorders of coagulation, and thrombocytopenia, as well as urinary infection, must be excluded. Because

FIGURE 42-1

Top. Diagram showing normal structures separating the capillary lumen and urinary space in the glomerulus. In the process of glomerular filtration, an ultrafiltrate of plasma traverses the glomerular capillary wall through endothelial fenestrae, basement membrane, and slit diaphragms. Macromolecules in the plasma are believed to be restricted from entry into glomerular urine by each of these wall structures. In addition, circulating polyanions (e.g., albumin) are thought to be retarded by negatively charged glycosialoproteins, which, as shown by the shaded area in the upper panel, are distributed throughout the glomerular wall. Bottom. A corresponding electron micrograph of the same structures. (Drawing by NL Gahan from BM Brenner, R Beeuwkes, Hosp Prac, vol 13, no 7, 1978. Reproduced with permission.)

infection with tuberculosis and fungi may be difficult to detect, multiple urine samples must be cultured and examined by microscopy. Renal arteriography may be needed to disclose anatomic lesions such as cysts or tumors.

HEMATURIA ASSOCIATED WITH URINARY TRACT INFECTION
Bacterial infection of the lower urinary tract or of the kidneys occasionally causes hematuria. The presence of associated pyuria suggests the diagnosis of infection and the demonstration of pathogenic bacteria in concentrations above 10^5 colonies per milliliter of urine establishes it. Acute cystitis or urethritis in women is an especially common cause of gross hematuria. Urinary tuberculosis can produce isolated hematuria, but pyuria often is present as well.

HEMATURIA WITH EVIDENCE OF RENAL DISEASE **Nephronal hematuria** Blood may enter the tubular fluid anywhere along the nephron, from the glomerulus to the end of the collecting duct. Tamm-Horsfall protein tends to gel when concentrated at a low pH, as occurs during dehydration, or when exposed to myoglobin, hemoglobin, albumin, Bence-Jones protein, and pyelographic contrast media. Red blood cells in the tubule lumens can be trapped in a cylindrical mold of the gelled protein to produce red blood cell casts, which provide conclusive evidence of bleeding into the nephron. Degenerated red blood cells and clumps of hemoglobin can produce deeply pigmented casts that have the same significance as red blood cell casts.

Bleeding from the nephron itself, like glomerular proteinuria, always connotes significant renal disease such as glomerulonephritis, tubulointerstitial injury, or a vasculitis that has damaged the circulation of the nephron. Glomerular or tubular proteinuria often accompanies renal bleeding, as a consequence of nephron injury. As a rule, renal bleeding or proteinuria alone arises from diseases that have a better prognosis than those in which proteinuria and hematuria occur in combination.

Hematuria with proteinuria or casts Frequently, hematuria is accompanied by proteinuria, but red blood cell and deeply pigmented granular casts are absent. The presumption then is that bleeding is of nephronal origin, but a coincident independent lesion of the urinary tract must always be considered, because common renal diseases, such as diabetic glomerulosclerosis and arteriolar nephrosclerosis associated with hypertension, produce mainly proteinuria.

Heavy albuminuria or dehydration can cause showers of transparent, refractile "hyaline" casts. During heavy proteinuria tubule cells fill with cholesterol-rich lipid droplets that display a Maltese-cross appearance in polarized light. Casts that incorporate these cells are called *fatty casts* because the lipid droplets are prominent. The same lipid-rich cells free in urine are called *oval fat bodies*.

White blood cell and *epithelial cell casts* can occur in any inflammatory state that involves the nephrons. White blood cell casts are particularly common in pyelonephritis, nephritis associated with systemic lupus erythematosus, and during transplant rejection. When white blood or epithelial cells degenerate, they form granular nonpigmented casts that contain cellular debris and aggregated proteins. So-called *waxy* casts, with few granules and very distinct margins, arise when cell debris has broken down to a fine dispersion so that granules are no longer visible.

Broad casts, of unusual width, are thought to arise in the dilated tubules of enlarged nephrons that have undergone compensatory hypertrophy in response to a reduction of functioning renal mass. A urine sample that contains a combination of broad and waxy casts as well as cellular or granular casts or red blood cells indicates a chronic smoldering process and has been termed a *telescoped* urine. This abnormality, first

described in polyarteritis nodosa and systemic lupus erythematosus, can also be found in many chronic forms of glomerulonephritis with active glomerulitis.

APPROACH TO THE PATIENT WITH HEMATURIA The most important step is to determine whether the hematuria is isolated or associated with other features of primary renal disease, i.e., cells, casts, or proteinuria. Many urinalyses may be needed to define the casts, cells, and proteins which accompany the hematuria, and the magnitude and type of associated proteinuria should be determined. As a general rule intravenous pyelography should be performed, if it can be done safely, even when the hematuria is of definite nephronal origin. Not only lesions of the urinary tract, but renal tumors or cysts, discrete areas of papillary necrosis, or signs of renal venous obstruction may be present. The source of isolated hematuria must always be ascertained, and this means a progressively detailed examination of the urinary tract by cystoscopy, retrograde pyelography, and arteriography to disclose tumor, stone, cysts, or other cause. If all the studies disclose normal structures, a nephronal origin of hematuria is likely even if no red blood cell casts are present. Hematuria with infection or overt renal disease usually requires no steps beyond intravenous pyelography.

AZOTEMIA, OLIGURIA, AND ANURIA

AZOTEMIA Measurements of urea and creatinine concentrations in serum are often obtained to assess the GFR. Both substances are produced at a reasonably constant rate, by the liver and muscles, respectively. As discussed in Chap. 274, they undergo complete glomerular filtration and are not reabsorbed extensively by the renal tubules; hence their clearances tend to reflect the GFR. An increase in their serum concentrations, termed *azotemia* (*azo*, "containing nitrogen"), occurs as the GFR falls. Renal failure is reflected by a high blood nitrogen level. Of the two substances, creatinine is a more reliable index of GFR because of its lower back diffusion from tubule lumen to peritubular blood. Although azotemia is a laboratory finding, rather than a symptom, it is an almost universal clue to the presence of abnormal renal function and often of renal disease, now that multiple-test biochemical screening of blood has become a common practice.

Glomerular filtration rate may be reduced by a fall in the filtration rates of individual functioning nephrons, or by a reduction in the total number of functioning nephrons. (See Table 42-1.)

Reduced single-nephron glomerular filtration rate TUBULAR FUNCTION NORMAL The physiological response of the normal kidney to a sodium-conserving stimulus is reduction of the single-nephron glomerular filtration rate (SNGFR) and subsequent reabsorption of an increased fraction of the reduced amounts of NaCl and water that enter the tubules. Depletion of extracellular fluid volume is a most instructive example of such a stimulus. Azotemia occurs and urine Na concentration falls below 20 (often below 1 meq per liter). Secretion of vasopressin is stimulated by depletion of extracellular fluid volume, and as a consequence, the distal tubules and collecting ducts become fully permeable to water. The concentrating mechanisms in the inner medulla (Chap. 274) are very efficient when flow rates through the loops of Henle and the collecting ducts are low. As a result, the filtrate that escapes reabsorption in the proximal tubule undergoes maximal osmotic concentration, the urine volume becomes small, and it has a high osmolality, above 500 mosmol per kilogram of water. Most of the filtered creatinine escapes tubular reabsorption, and so the ratio of the urine-to-plasma (U/P) creatinine concentrations is very high, 40 or more. Because urea can back-diffuse more completely than creatinine, the urea U/P ratio is less elevated, above 8, and the blood urea nitrogen (BUN) level rises more than the serum creatinine concentration. Normally, the ratio of BUN to serum creatinine concentration is 10:1; with depletion of the extracellular fluid volume the ratio rises.

The pattern of renal response to extracellular fluid volume depletion appears in any edema-forming condition during the phase of NaCl and water accumulation. Typical examples include the nephrotic syndrome and hepatic cirrhosis with ascites (Chaps. 29 and 278). When a diuretic is being administered to inhibit the tubular reabsorption of NaCl, urine volume and sodium concentration may be normal or elevated, even though SNGFR falls in response to the combination of the underlying edema-forming stimulus and further extracellular fluid volume depletion from the drug. Severe oliguria may appear upon withdrawal of the drug as the renal tubules resume intense reabsorption of NaCl and water. The pattern of low SNGFR with well-preserved tubule function may also be seen when renal blood flow is reduced, by systemic hypotension, incomplete renal arterial or venous occlusion, or other cause (Chap. 282). Acute incomplete obstruction of the ureter and acute glomerular injury may also reduce SNGFR and leave tubule function relatively intact, but whenever chronic obstruction or glomerulonephritis damages nephrons extensively, the high urinary osmolality, U/P ratios for creatinine or urea, and low urinary sodium concentrations disappear.

TUBULAR FUNCTION IMPAIRED Certain acute renal diseases which produce azotemia lower SNGFR and at the same time damage the tubules sufficiently to reduce or even abolish their reabsorptive functions. Acute tubular necrosis, exposure to nephrotoxic agents, and all forms of acute tubulointerstitial disease are excellent examples. Azotemia and oliguria appear, but the urine sodium concentration is above 20 meq per liter and usually above 40 meq per liter, the U/P ratios for urea and creatinine are below 2 and 20, respectively, and urine osmolality is below 350 mosmol per kilogram of water. The ratio of BUN to serum creatinine is not elevated.

Reduced nephron number INCREASED SNGFR If one kidney is removed, the other grows larger, its nephrons enlarge, and the SNGFR increases until the total GFR becomes nearly normal for two kidneys. The tubules are overperfused with filtrate, but they appear to cope well with their increased reabsorptive burdens, perhaps in part because they are longer and wider and possess more cells. If more kidney tissue is removed, the remnant nephrons enlarge further, and their SNGFR rises. Extreme overperfusion of the tubules interferes with sodium conservation. At the same time, total GFR comes to depend more and more upon expansion of the extracellular fluid volume largely because the increase in SNGFR is due not only to anatomic growth of the glomeruli but also to a relatively high rate of blood flow per glomerulus.

Azotemia occurs because the total GFR, the product of the elevated SNGFR and the markedly reduced nephron number, is low. The ratio of BUN to serum creatinine concentration is approximately 10. Urine-to-plasma ratios for creatinine and urea are usually between 3 and 10, urine sodium concentration is above 40 meq per liter, and urine osmolality approaches that of plasma. Tubule conservation of filtered water and sodium conservation are poor, so fluid and salt intake must be liberal. Clinical states that produce this picture include surgical loss of renal substance because of trauma, neoplasm, stone, and destruction of kidneys by bacterial infection or tuberculosis, polycystic and medullary cystic renal diseases, and all the

TABLE 42-1
Pathophysiologic mechanisms of azotemia

Mechanism of reduced GFR	Clinical examples	Laboratory findings					
		Oliguria	Urine osm, mosmol/kg	Urine [Na+], meq/L	$\left(\dfrac{U}{P}\right)_{creat}$	$\left(\dfrac{U}{P}\right)_{urea}$	$\dfrac{BUN}{Serum\ creat}$
REDUCED SNGFR							
Tubules normal	Severe dehydration, edema-forming states, diuretic agents, systemic hypotension, acute glomerular disease, acute urinary obstruction, incomplete renal vascular obstruction	Often present	>500	<20	>40	>8	>10
Tubules damaged	Acute tubular necrosis, nephrotoxic agents, glomerulonephritis with tubule injury	Usually present	<350	>40	<20	<2	10
REDUCED NEPHRON NUMBER							
Elevated SNGFR	Chronic tubulointerstitial/renal disease Surgical loss of renal tissue	Rare*	290	>40	3–10	3–10	10
Normal SNGFR	Diffuse chronic glomerulonephritis Diabetic nephropathy	Rare†	100–350‡	10–100‡	>3	>20	>10
Reduced SNGFR	Any of the factors that can reduce SNGFR (listed above) may lower SNGFR in a patient who has a reduced number of functioning nephrons	Usually present	290	>20	<10	<3	>20

* Occurs only when total GFR is below 5% normal.
† Rare as long as GFR is above 5% normal.
‡ Varies with diet and with the level of GFR. When GFR is below 20% normal, osmotic concentration of the urine is usually impossible.
NOTE: osm = osmolality; creat = creatinine concentration; U = urine; P = plasma.

chronic tubulointerstitial nephropathies (Chaps. 281 and 283). In each of these disorders, the nephrons that remain viable are either fully intact or behave as though the SNGFR is better preserved than tubule function.

SNGFR NORMAL The SNGFR does not appear to increase despite a reduction of nephron number in diseases such as glomerulonephritis and diabetic glomerulosclerosis, where the glomerulus is the primary site of damage. In these diseases total GFR falls directly with nephron number and is not supported by elevated SNGFR. Since the tubules are not confronted with an excessive reabsorptive burden, sodium conservation is adequate. In these disorders, superimposed conditions that lower SNGFR, such as depletion of extracellular fluid volume, can cause oliguria with low urine sodium concentration and U/P ratios for creatinine and urea above 3 and 20, respectively. The serum urea to creatinine ratio will rise distinctly.

SNGFR REDUCED In patients with chronic renal disease in whom total GFR has been sufficient to support life only because of a very high SNGFR, inadvertent dehydration or any other factor that lowers the SNGFR can provoke oliguria and severe azotemia. Under these circumstances, urine sodium concentration will fall, but not below 20 meq per liter, as in the normal person, because SNGFR, though reduced, may still be above normal. The U/P ratios for creatinine and urea will be low, usually below 3 and 10, respectively, despite oliguria, and urine osmolality will not rise above the plasma level. The serum urea to creatinine ratio may rise, but not above 20. In less extreme situations, reduction of SNGFR will worsen azotemia and alter urine chemistry in the same directions but to a lesser extent.

OLIGURIA In this condition urine volume is insufficient to sustain life in a steady state; it is usually less than 400 ml per 24 h (16.6 ml/h) in an adult of average size. Daily urine volume is difficult to measure when flow rate is low, because small absolute errors of volume measurement, in the range of 50 to 100 ml of urine each day, or of timing of collection, may represent large percentage errors.

APPROACH TO THE PATIENT WITH AZOTEMIA OR OLIGURIA
Clinical history, physical examination, and urinalysis often disclose an obvious reason for azotemia or oliguria. The most discriminating additional measurements include serum urea and creatinine concentrations, and the sodium, urea, and creatinine concentrations and osmolality of a concurrent urine sample. Reduction of SNGFR with well-preserved tubular function is usually present when urine osmolality exceeds 500 mosmol per kilogram of water, sodium is below 20 meq per liter, the U/P ratios for urea and creatinine exceed 8 and 40, respectively, and the BUN is more than 10 times the serum creatinine concentration. The prognosis for recovery of adequate GFR is good, if the cause of reduced SNGFR can be reversed. When urine osmolality is below 350 mosmol per kilogram of water, sodium is above 40 meq, the U/P values for urea and creatinine are below 2 and 20, respectively, and the BUN exceeds the serum creatinine by only tenfold, tubule function has been lost, and some form of acute or chronic renal failure usually is present.

ANURIA This extreme condition is uncommon. Urinary obstruction is the main cause and must be excluded as a first step (Chap. 285). Complete renal arterial and venous occlusion are other important causes. Few severe renal diseases produce anuria in the adult, and anuria should never be ascribed to a primary renal disease until patency of the urinary tract and major renal blood vessels has been established.

REFERENCES

BRENNER BM et al: Molecular basis of proteinuria of glomerular origin. N Eng J Med 298:826, 1978

DE WARDENER HE: Tests of glomerular functional integrity, in *The Kidney*, HE de Wardener (ed). London, Churchill Livingstone, 1973

GLASSOCK RJ, BENNETT CM: The glomerulopathies, in *The Kidney*, BM Brenner, FC Rector Jr (eds). Philadelphia, Saunders, 1980

MORRISON RBI: Urinalysis and assessment of renal function, in *Renal Disease*, D Black (ed). Oxford, Blackwell, 1972

POLLAK VE, PESCE AJ: Proteinuria: A review of glomerular permeability in the normal and in various disease states, in *Seminars in Nephrology*, E Becker (ed). New York, Wiley, 1977

43
POLYURIA AND NOCTURIA

FREDRIC L. COE

Though considered together in this chapter because they are superficially similar, polyuria and nocturia have little in common pathophysiologically. True polyuria that is not due to a deliberate, habitual high fluid intake always points to an important defect of renal water handling or of the secretion of vasopressin. Nocturia is less specific. It can arise from defective renal water conservation, excretion of an abnormal fraction of the daily salt load at night, low bladder capacity, irritable bladder, or partial bladder obstruction.

Patients cannot always distinguish urinary frequency from polyuria. Voiding of small volumes is typical of frequency, whereas large volumes characterize the polyuric states. Since voiding volumes may not be clear from the history, polyuria must be substantiated by 24-h urine collection before beginning an investigation of causes. The presence of nocturia is best established by the history alone.

POLYURIA

PHYSIOLOGY OF URINE FORMATION Adaptation to life on dry land requires efficient renal water conservation, and even though modern life no longer requires it, the normal person enjoys the convenience of a modest urine volume. When an individual is in water balance, urine volume is the difference between water intake and insensible water losses. Polyuria implies the production of more urine than normal; if it is chronic, there is also high water intake. A reasonable definition of polyuria is a urine volume above 3 liters per day, but should be qualified to exclude normal individuals who desire a large fluid intake and therefore form large volumes of urine.

NORMAL RENAL WATER CONSERVATION (See also Chap. 274) Between 20 and 30 percent of NaCl and water filtered at the glomerulus reach the thick ascending limb of Henle's loop in the outer medulla where NaCl is reabsorbed but most of the water and urea are not. As a result of this process, the outer medullary interstitial fluid becomes hypertonic to plasma, about 400 mosmol/kg compared with 290 mosmol/kg, as NaCl is transported from the tubular lumen of the thick ascending limb of Henle's loop without a corresponding transport of water. Therefore, the fluid that leaves the thick ascending limb of Henle's loop to enter the distal convoluted tubule is hypotonic to plasma.

The dilute tubular fluid equilibrates to isotonicity with plasma by losing water into the cortical interstitium as it traverses the terminal portion of the distal convoluted tubule and cortical collecting tubule, provided that vasopressin is present. Without vasopressin the water permeability of the entire distal convoluted tubule is low. Though it becomes isotonic to plasma, late distal convoluted tubule fluid has a composition different from that in the thick ascending limb of Henle's loop. Much of its osmolality is due to urea, not to NaCl, because urea is lost from the fluid to only a small extent whereas NaCl is reabsorbed in the thick ascending limb of Henle's loop and beginning of the distal convoluted tubule. By the time it reaches the end of the distal convoluted tubule the fluid is appreciably reduced in volume. Like the end of the distal convoluted tubule, the cortical collecting tubule in the presence of vasopressin is permeable to water but not to urea (Fig. 274-2).

The urea-rich fluid then enters the inner medulla in the papillary portion of the collecting duct. The inner medullary interstitium is very hypertonic to plasma because of high urea and NaCl concentrations. Water is extracted from the papillary collecting duct segments to create the final urine. Unlike the thick ascending limb of Henle's loop, distal convoluted tubule, and cortical collecting tubules, the permeability to urea of the papillary portion of the collecting duct epithelium is high, but urea losses from the tubule are low because of a high prevailing interstitial urea concentration.

How the inner medulla comes to have an interstitium so hypertonic is still a matter of controversy, but a *passive counterflow model* seems reasonable and is widely accepted as a working hypothesis at present. If the medullary interstitium were empty, without an accumulation of surplus urea or NaCl urea would diffuse out of the papillary collecting duct and enter the interstitium, because the luminal fluid has been rendered hypertonic in the outer medulla. The urea would be removed by the ascending vasa recta, but counterflow exchange between ascending and descending vasa recta lowers the efficiency of solute removal and allows a high interstitial urea concentration to develop. The urea concentration will be distributed as a gradient, with a peak level at the papillary tips. This is true because the trapping efficiency of the counterflowing vasa recta loop increases with its length. In other words, the concentration of solute in vasa recta can exceed that in the blood that enters the vasa recta more and more as the solute approaches the tip of the loop.

Given a urea gradient, NaCl accumulation could be passive. The descending limb of the loop of Henle appears very permeable to water, less so to urea, and even less to NaCl. Water can leave the descending limb because of the urea gradient in the medullary interstitium, so that intratubular NaCl concentration rises progressively down to the bend of the loop. The thin ascending limb appears to very permeable to NaCl, less so to urea, and least to water, so that in the presence of a favorable electrochemical gradient, the accumulated NaCl can diffuse into the interstitium until its interstitial concentration rises to the equilibrium dictated by its entry and washout rates. In other words, transport of NaCl in the thick ascending limb of Henle's loop can lead to urea and NaCl accumulation in the inner medulla.

When the process is fully established, the inner medulla is in a complex steady state. Urea and NaCl deliveries from papillary collecting ducts and descending limbs balance total washout in the thin ascending limb of Henle's loop and the vasa recta. Water that is lost from papillary collecting ducts in the process of creating an osmotically concentrated urine must be carried away in the ascending vasa recta, so that total flow in the ascending vasa recta must exceed that in the descending vasa recta. The process can be disrupted by changes in tubular or vascular flow rates, or by structural abnormalities that prevent normal equilibration between capillary loops, tubules, and interstitium. In particular, increased rates of blood flow diminish the efficiency of solute trapping by the vasa recta and promote medullary washout. Excessive delivery of water into the papillary collecting ducts or into the descending limb of Henle's loop has the same effect.

CAUSES Polyuria can arise from inadequate secretion of vasopressin, failure of the renal tubules to respond to vasopressin, solute diuresis, or natriuresis (Table 43-1). It may also occur as a physiological adaptation to deliberate excessive water drinking.

Diabetes insipidus (see also Chap. 334) The term *diabetes insipidus* is applied to situations in which renal water conservation is so inadequate that polyuria occurs. Either vasopressin insufficiency (central diabetes insipidus) or renal unresponsiveness to vasopressin (nephrogenic diabetes insipidus) produces severe polyuria and secondary thirst. In both, water reabsorption is reduced all along the distal nephron, because passive water movement from tubules into the hypertonic outer and inner medullary interstitium is slow. But even though the rate of water movement out of the collecting ducts is low for a given osmotic difference between the tubule lumen and interstitial fluid, the fluid that enters the collecting ducts is so abnormally dilute and copious in volume that more water enters the inner medulla than under normal circumstances and medullary solutes are washed out into the vasa recta. Washout is incomplete and vasopressin administration can lead to formation of an osmotically concentrated urine, but the maximum urine osmality that can be attained is below normal.

Vasopressin-sensitive (central) diabetes insipidus may be idiopathic or secondary to hypophysectomy or trauma or to neoplastic, inflammatory, vascular, or infectious causes (Table 43-1). Idiopathic diabetes insipidus can be familial, and then it is usually inherited as an autosomal dominant trait; but more commonly it is sporadic and appears in childhood. In both forms there is selective destruction of the neurons that produce vasopressin in the supraoptic nucleus.

Failure of the kidney to respond to vasopressin, i.e., nephrogenic diabetes insipidus, may be acquired or congenital. Nephrogenic diabetes insipidus acquired from renal disease (Table 43-1) probably is the most common form; the familial form is rare. Hypercalcemia and hypokalemic nephropathy are important reversible causes of nephrogenic diabetes insipidus.

TABLE 43-1
Causes of polyuria

I Inadequate renal water conservation
   A Diabetes insipidus
      1 Vasopressin-sensitive (posthypophysectomy; posttrauma; postpituitary ablation; idiopathic, supra- or intrasellar tumors or cysts; histiocystosis or granuloma; encroachment by aneurysm; Sheehan's syndrome, meningoencephalitis; Guillain-Barré's syndrome; fat embolus; empty sella)
      2 Nephrogenic
         a Acquired tubulointerstitial renal disease (pyelonephritis, analgesic nephropathy, multiple myeloma, amyloidosis, obstructive uropathy, sarcoidosis, hypercalcemic or hypokalemic nephropathy, Sjögren's syndrome, sickle cell anemia, renal transplantation)
         b Drugs or toxins (lithium, demeclocycline, methyoxyflurane, ethanol, diphenylhydantoin, propoxyphene, amphotericin)
         c Congenital (hereditary nephrogenic diabetes insipidus, polycystic or medullary cystic disease)
   B Solute diuresis (glucosuria, high-protein tube feedings, urea or mannitol infusion, radiographic contrast media, chronic renal failure)
   C Natriuretic syndromes (salt-losing nephritis, diuretic phase of acute tubular necrosis, diuretic agents)
II Primary polydipsia

Lithium carbonate, methoxyflurane (1,1-difluoro-2,2-dichlor-ethyl methyl ether) anesthetic, and demeclocycline, a tetracycline derivative, can also produce nephrogenic diabetes insipidus.

Solute diuresis Excessive filtration of a poorly resorbed solute such as glucose, mannitol, or urea can depress reabsorption of NaCl and water in the proximal tubule and cause their loss in the urine, producing polyuria. Urine sodium concentration is below that of blood, so that more water than salt is lost from the body and serum hypertonicity can be produced. Glucosuria in diabetes mellitus is a common cause of solute diuresis. Iatrogenic solute diuresis may arise from mannitol infusion, angiographic contrast media, and high-protein gavage feedings, which produce excessive excretion of urea.

Natriuretic syndromes Excessive chronic sodium loss may occur during the course of tubulointerstitial or cystic renal diseases. Polyuria and polydipsia are accompanied by an unusually large daily sodium requirement. Examples of this phenomenon include medullary cystic disease, Bartter's syndrome, and the diuretic phase of acute tubular necrosis, in which sodium and water losses are very large.

Primary polydipsia Whether because of habit, predilection, psychiatric disorder, or a specific lesion in the brain, some people drink enough water every day to produce polyuria. The body and the kidneys rarely if ever are injured by chronic polydipsia, but the condition can be confused with diabetes insipidus, which it resembles closely. During deliberate polydipsia, extracellular fluid volume is normal or high, and vasopressin secretion is reduced to a basal level because serum osmolality tends to be near the lower limits of normal. Reabsorption of water from the end distal convoluted tubule and collecting ducts is reduced so that all the surplus water can be excreted into the urine. The inner medulla loses its urea and NaCl gradients because of washout, as in diabetes insipidus. Washout may be more severe than in diabetes insipidus because primary polydipsia tends to cause expansion of the extracellular fluid volume, whereas primary renal water loss does the opposite. Volume expansion raises total delivery of NaCl and water to the thick ascending limb of Henle's loop and therefore to the inner medulla, all things being equal. It also raises renal blood flow, and increased flow through the vasa rectae reduces their ability to trap solutes in the medulla.

APPROACH TO THE PATIENT Solute diuresis and natriuretic syndromes usually are apparent from the history, physical examination, urinalysis, clinical setting, blood count, and serum creatinine or the BUN. Diagnostic problems occur mainly when stable, chronic polyuria and polydipsia of uncertain origin are present. Here, one must try to distinguish between vasopressin-sensitive diabetes insipidus, nephrogenic diabetes insipidus, and primary polydipsia; and the best way to do this is by measuring the response of urine osmolality to water deprivation and the administration of vasopressin.

The patient should have free access to water and receive a normal diet that provides approximately 100 mmol NaCl per day for 3 days; then a total fast is instituted. During the fast, pulse and blood pressure should be measured every 30 min and body weight every hour, using an accurate balance. When 3 percent of the initial body weight has been lost or 14 h has elapsed, urine and serum osmolality are measured. A normal subject will lower urine volume below 0.5 ml/min and raise urine osmolality to above 700 mosmol per kilogram of water. In complete diabetes insipidus, nephrogenic or vasopressin-sensitive, the urine osmolality will remain below 200 mosmol/kg and urine flow will remain above 0.5 ml/min, but some rise in osmolality and fall in flow will occur given incomplete dia-

betes insipidus. If urine osmolality is below 700 mosmol/kg, by the end of the fasting period, 5 milliunits per minute of aqueous vasopressin is administered by intravenous drip. Patients with complete or partial vasopressin-sensitive diabetes insipidus will raise their urine osmolality above the level achieved by fasting alone. No increase will occur given complete nephrogenic diabetes insipidus, although incomplete forms of nephrogenic diabetes insipidus will permit some response to vasopressin.

The response of patients with primary polydipsia is quite different. During fluid restriction the secretion of vasopressin increases, and at the completion of the test the flow rate and osmolality of the urine will reflect a physiological level of vasopressin acting upon normal tubules that traverse a medullary interstitium whose urea and NaCl concentrations have been reduced by chronic washout. In other words, the washout will set the upper limit on urine osmolality, and patients with primary polydipsia thus demonstrate a submaximal concentrating ability in spite of intact vasopressin secretion. Exogenous vasopressin can increase urine osmolality very little, if at all, because medullary washout, not vasopressin insensitivity, is the main limiting factor. Usually the urine osmolality will be above 400 mosmol/kg by the end of the fluid deprivation test, in contrast to the lower values of approximately 200 mosmol/kg encountered in patients with nephrogenic diabetes insipidus; but it may be impossible to distinguish incomplete nephrogenic diabetes insipidus from primary polydipsia, in some cases, by using the fluid deprivation test alone.

NOCTURIA

Whether an individual sleeps through the night without urinating depends upon a diurnal rhythm in which the volume of urine formed during sleep does not exceed bladder capacity. Nocturia results when nocturnal urine volume exceeds bladder capacity, or it results from reduced renal osmotic concentration, high sodium excretion, solute diuresis, or low bladder capacity.

All the polyuric states may cause nocturia. Urinary concentrating ability falls in most renal diseases (Chap. 274), often at an early stage. Even though overt polyuria may be absent, overnight urine volume frequently exceeds bladder capacity. Nocturia also occurs in edema-forming states. In congestive heart failure, nephrotic syndrome, and hepatic cirrhosis with ascites, fluid accumulates preferentially in dependent portions of the body during the day. At night, with recumbency, tissue capillary forces change and some edema fluid is mobilized, producing the effect of an intravenous saline infusion. Venous insufficiency may produce dependent edema of the legs that is often also mobilized at night, causing nocturia.

Reduced bladder capacity is present when infection, tumor, or stone, causes inflammation or increased irritability. Chronic partial bladder-outflow obstruction, from prostatic hypertrophy, urethral stricture, or benign or malignant neoplasm or stone, causes a frequent stimulus to void and also a thickening of the muscular wall that reduces its compliance. Frequent small voidings may be a clue to this lower urinary tract cause of nocturia, but in its earlier phases chronic obstruction may lead to only one nocturnal voiding of reasonable volume.

REFERENCES

ANDREOLI TE et al (eds): *Disturbances in Body Fluid Osmolality.* Baltimore, Williams & Wilkins, 1977

KLEEMAN CR: Water metabolism, in *Clinical Disorders of Fluid and Electrolyte Metabolism*, MH Maxwell, CR Kleeman (eds). New York, McGraw-Hill, 1972

HAYS RM, LEVINE SD: Pathophysiology of water metabolism, in *The Kidney*, 2d ed, BM Brenner, FC Rector Jr (eds). Philadelphia, Saunders, 1980

BERL T et al: Clinical disorders of water metabolism. Kidney Int 10:117, 1976

44

DYSURIA, INCONTINENCE, AND ENURESIS

WILLIAM GILL
FREDRIC L. COE

NORMAL BLADDER FUNCTION

The detrusor muscle, which provides the propulsive force for emptying the bladder, consists of interlacing fibers of smooth muscle that are under parasympathetic autonomic control through the pelvic nerves from sacral spinal cord segments S2, S3, and S4. The smooth muscle of the trigonal portion of the bladder, between the ureteral orifices and the posterior area of the bladder outlet, is innervated by motor fibers from thoracolumbar segments (T11 to L2) of the sympathetic nervous system, in which alpha receptor sites predominate. This layer of muscle extends into the posterior urethra and acts as an involuntary internal sphincter that helps maintain urinary continence even in the absence of voluntary control. The external urethral sphincter and perineal muscles are under voluntary control via the pudendal nerves.

Sensory tracts for pain, temperature, and distention pass from the bladder via the pelvic nerves to sacral spinal levels S2, S3, and S4, creating a simple spinal voiding reflex between the bladder and the sacral spinal cord. The sensory tracts from the bladder further ascend through sacrobulbar pathways to the medulla of the brain and ultimately to cortical centers (superomedial portion of the frontal lobes), from which impulses arise, pass back down the lateral and ventral reticulospinal tracts, and normally suppress the sacral spinal reflex arc controlling bladder emptying.

The normal adult bladder can accommodate as much as approximately 400 ml fluid without a significant increase in intravesical pressure (< 20 cmH$_2$O). Above this point, sensations of fullness are transmitted to the sacral cord. If not suppressed by cortical control, the sacral cord reflexly discharges motor impulses that cause powerful sustained detrusor contraction. Urination can be prevented by cortical suppression of the reflex arc or by voluntary contraction of the external sphincter and perineal muscles. Infants, and adults with spinal cord damage above S2, urinate spontaneously when the bladder fills sufficiently.

Normal micturition is initiated by voluntary suppression of cortical inhibition of the reflex arc and by relaxation of the muscles of the pelvic floor and the external sphincter. The base of the bladder falls; then the trigone contracts, an action that occludes the ureters as they pass through the bladder wall and helps to prevent vesicoureteral reflux of urine during voiding. Finally, the detrusor contracts and voiding occurs.

DYSURIA

Dysuria refers to anything abnormal having to do with urination, such as urinary frequency, nocturia, hesitancy in starting urination, straining to urinate, burning upon urination, urgency, decreased size of urinary stream, dribbling at the end of urination, and combinations of these symptoms. Some clinicians restrict the use of the term dysuria to burning or pain upon urination, but the broader definition is preferable.

MECHANISMS OF DYSURIA Reduced bladder compliance When the bladder has a decreased ability to expand, frequency, nocturia, and urgency usually result. When decreased expansion is due to inflammation of the mucosa (cystitis) from infection, radiation, chemicals, or foreign bodies (catheters, stones), burning usually is more prominent than when it is due to infiltration of the muscle by tumors of the bladder or from adjacent organs (prostate, rectum, uterus). Any upper motor neuron lesion that interferes with cortical inhibition of the voiding reflex produces a spastic hypertonic bladder, and incontinence is then a frequent manifestation.

Impaired bladder emptying Increased outflow resistance because of obstruction of the bladder neck or urethra causes hesitancy, reduced caliber of the stream, and dribbling. Damage to the sacral nerves involved in vesical emptying can produce a completely autonomous bladder, or a sensory paralytic or motor paralytic neurogenic bladder. Thus, the individual whose bladder has lost all sensory and motor innervation must rely for emptying upon distention of the organ leading to muscle stretching and automatic contraction, because the sacral voiding reflex is absent. Hesitancy, incomplete emptying, and even gross retention of urine can result. Symptoms of bladder fullness will depend upon whether the sensory tracts are intact. Since the bladder cannot empty itself properly in the worst cases of deficient innervation, gross overflow incontinence occurs.

CAUSES OF DYSURIA Infection *Acute bacterial cystitis*, which occurs more frequently in women, usually causes great frequency day and night, burning on urination, and, not infrequently, gross hematuria. *Prostatitis* or *prostatocystitis* in men can cause a picture similar to acute cystitis in women. When only the prostate is involved, milder symptoms such as vague pain or discomfort in the lower abdomen, groin, perineum, rectum, testes, or penis occur. The symptoms may be associated with urination, but more frequently are noticed at times other than during micturition or ejaculation.

Benign prostatic hypertrophy This condition afflicts upwards of 75 percent of older men. It is manifested by nocturia, reduced size and force of the urinary stream, straining to urinate, and terminal dribbling, all due to outflow obstruction.

Psychosomatic cystitis The functional bladder syndrome and chronic glandular urethrotrigonitis are synonyms for a very common but poorly understood affliction of middle-aged and older women, in which pain is usually vague, aching in nature, and in the lower abdomen or vagina. There is daytime frequency without nocturia; pyuria is absent. A complete urological evaluation usually becomes necessary because symptoms are chronic and hard to eradicate. The functional bladder syndrome must be distinguished from the effects of a cystocele, which can be repaired surgically. (See also Chap. 280.)

APPROACH TO THE PATIENT The medical history should focus on past as well as present urinary problems. A pelvic examination in women and prostatic examination in men are necessary components of the physical examination. Microscopic examination of a two-glass urinary sediment in all patients and of the prostatic fluid in men is also necessary. The first 20 ml of a voiding, if collected separately, may contain a higher concentration of leukocytes and bacteria than the remainder of the voided urine, when the urethra is the principal site of inflammation or infection. Normal prostatic fluid, not subjected to centrifugation, contains less than 10 leukocytes per high-power field; excessive leukocytes in the prostatic fluid are an important clue to prostatitis and may, when prostatitis is chonic, be the only detectable abnormality. Further diagnostic studies will depend upon such positive findings as a history of chronic or recurrent episodes or associated fever, which are rare in lower urinary tract infections except in acute prostatitis, or an abnormality on physical examination such as a pelvic or rectal mass or tenderness, hematuria or pyuria, or excessive leukocytes and macrophages in the prostatic fluid. Serum acid phosphatase may be elevated when carcinoma of the prostate has extended beyond the boundary of the prostatic capsule.

Additional evaluation of dysuria, when the cause is not evident from clinical examination, may include cultures of urine and prostatic fluid for aerobic and anerobic bacteria, tubercle bacilli, and mycoplasma, excretory urography and voiding cystourethrography. If these examinations do not reveal the diagnosis, but the symptoms are sufficiently troublesome, urologic consultation should be sought. The urologist may carry out cystoscopy and urethroscopy with endoscopic biopsies where abnormalities are found. Functional urodynamic studies, gas cystometry, sphincter electromyography, urethral pressure profile, uroflometry, and urine spectrometry may be needed in special cases.

INCONTINENCE

Incontinence refers to the inability to retain urine in the bladder. The diagnostic approach to the evaluation of the patient should be the same as that used for dysuria.

Stress incontinence is common in postmenopausal parous women. The structures of the female urethra atrophy when deprived of estrogen and many become unable to resist the passage of urine under the stress of increased intraabdominal pressure during coughing, sneezing, climbing stairs, and other physical activity. Parturition may damage the pelvic support of the bladder so that the bladder and urethra can slip downward from their normal position above the pelvic diaphragm. As they do, the urethra shortens, and the normal urethrovesical angle, important in closing the urethral sphincter, is lost. In men, stress incontinence usually is secondary to prostatic surgery for benign prostatic hypertrophy or prostatic carcinoma. If the external sphincter has also been damaged during operation, total, complete incontinence may result.

Inflammatory lesions of the bladder mucosa, especially in the trigone area, can cause uncontrollable detrusor contractions and unwanted passage of urine, often called *urgency incontinence.* Common inflammatory lesions include infection, stones in the intravesical ureter, bladder tumors, and catheters in the bladder. Upper motor neuron lesions of the spinal cord or brain may produce a hypertonic, spastic, neurogenic bladder with frequent, uncontrollable, urgency incontinence.

Overflow or paradoxical incontinence arises from large residual volumes of urine secondary to obstruction at the bladder neck or along the urethra (urethral stricture) or from neurological damage. Hypotonic neurogenic bladders may occur in diseases which produce autonomic peripheral neuropathy, such as diabetes mellitus, uremia, hypothyroidism, chronic alcoholism, Guillain-Barré syndrome, collagen vascular diseases, and toxic neuropathies associated with some carcinomas (espe-

cially lung and kidney). It may also occur because of prolonged overdistention of the bladder. Hydronephrosis and impaired renal function can occur in patients with chronic overflow incontinence.

Some congenital anomalies, extrophy of the bladder, patent urachus, and ectopic ureteral openings distal to the vesical neck cause *mechanical incontinence.* Acquired mechanical incontinence can follow transurethral resection of the prostate in which damage has occurred to both the internal and external sphincter mechanisms. Pelvic surgery or irradiation of the uterus or rectum may cause incontinence because of vesicovaginal, ureterovaginal, vesicoperineal, or ureteroperineal fistulae.

Children, and even some young adults, draw attention to themselves by feigning incontinence and thereby derive some secondary emotional satisfaction. A complete diagnostic evaluation usually is necessary to rule out organic disease even when *psychogenic incontinence* is strongly suspected.

ENURESIS

Enuresis refers to the involuntary passage of urine at night or during sleep—hence, the synonym *bed-wetting.* Some clinicians reserve the term enuresis for those bed-wetters who have no gross urological abnormalities, but it should be used for bed-wetting in general.

The sacral spinal reflex arc alone controls urination in the infant; therefore, enuretic incontinence is normal under the age of 2 years. As the nervous system matures, cortical control over the spinal reflex arc results in the voluntary control over urination and defecation by the age of 2½ years. Even so, enuresis beyond the age of 3 years occurs to some degree in approximately 10 percent of all otherwise normal children and probably is due to a delay in maturation of bladder control, which may be familial.

Although the majority of bed-wetters will be dry by the age of puberty, organic diseases, especially infections of the urinary tract, obstructive lesions with overflow incontinence, neurovesical dysfunction, and polyuric conditions that overload the bladder must be suspected in any child who is enuretic beyond the age of 3 years. Patients with organic disease usually, but not always, are incontinent during the day as well as at night. The approach to the patient with enuresis is the same as that used for dysuria or incontinence.

REFERENCES

BRADLEY WE: Autonomic neuropathy and the genitourinary system. J Urol 119:299, 1978

―――, SCOTT FB: Physiology of the urinary bladder, in *Urology,* 4th ed, JH Harrison et al (eds). Philadelphia, Saunders, 1978, vol 1, chap 4, p 87

HARRISON JH et al (eds): Infections and inflammations of the genitourinary tract, in *Urology,* 4th ed. Philadelphia, Saunders, 1978, vol 1, sec IV, p 451

LAPIDES J (ed): *Symposium on Neurogenic Bladder: The Urologic Clinics of North America.* Philadelphia, Saunders, 1974

WHITESIDE CG, ARNOLD EP: Persistent primary enuresis: A urodynamic assessment. Br Med J 1:364, 1975

45
DISTURBANCES IN MENSTRUATION, SEXUAL FUNCTION, AND REPRODUCTION IN WOMEN

JAMES D. MADDEN
JEAN D. WILSON

Since normal reproductive physiology depends upon the integrated action of the central nervous system, the endocrine glands, and the reproductive organs, it is to be expected that abnormalities in the menstrual cycle, sexual function, and reproductive capacity occur in association with a variety of systemic and psychological disorders as well as with primary disease in the endocrine system and reproductive organs.

MENSTRUATION

MENARCHE During the prepubertal years, the anterior pituitary can respond to hypothalamic luteinizing hormone-releasing hormone (LHRH) by secreting gonadotropins [follicle-stimulating hormone (FSH), luteotropic hormone (LH)]. The prepubertal ovaries are capable of responding to exogenous gonadotropin stimulation as evidenced by maturation of follicles and production of estrogen. Puberty in the female probably commences as a result of increased synthesis and release of LHRH and the subsequent increase in the secretion of ovarian hormones. Sexual maturation occurs as an orderly sequence beginning with breast development, early growth of genital and axillary hair, and increase in the rate of growth. There is ordinarily a 2-year interval between the commencement of sexual maturation and menarche.

During early puberty gonadotropins are released principally during sleep (see Chap. 342). There appears to be a relationship between the onset of the pubertal process and a "critical body weight." For American girls of European ancestry, the average weight at which menarche occurs is 48 kg. However, weight increase alone is not sufficient, and a critical combination of weight and percent body fat is required. In some unknown manner the amount of body fat determines the minimum weight for height necessary for the onset and maintenance of menstrual cycles. Earlier acquisition of the critical body composition, the result of improved nutrition, is believed to have led to earlier sexual maturation in recent generations. In the United States menarche now occurs on the average approximately two years earlier than at the beginning of this century. It is uncertain whether the critical changes in body composition are the cause or only a correlate of the neuroendocrine events initiating puberty.

THE NORMAL CYCLE At the time of menarche, the increase in gonadotropin release is no longer limited to the time of sleep. FSH and LH are secreted episodically by the anterior pituitary throughout the day. A young woman enters reproductive life with approximately 300,000 follicles in the ovaries. The normal menstrual cycle is discussed in Chap. 342. In brief, owing to the precise biochemical messages conveyed to the gonad by FSH and LH, a cohort of follicles within one ovary begins to mature in each cycle. It is uncertain what determines which follicles will mature, nor is it known why a single member of the cohort gains ascendancy (becoming the "dominant follicle") while the remainder of the follicles in the cohort undergo atresia. A burst of estradiol secreted from the mature "dominant follicle" operating through a positive feedback mechanism causes a surge in the secretion of LH from the anterior pituitary. The latter begins approximately 24 h prior to ovulation and is responsible for the release of the ovum and its surrounding cumulus mass from the ovary. LH also causes luteinization of the ovarian granulosa and theca cells remaining behind in the follicle after ovulation. This collection of luteinized cells, known as the *corpus luteum,* secretes progesterone at an increasing rate for approximately one week. Progesterone, in addition to causing qualitative changes in the endometrium favorable for implantation of a fertilized ovum, causes elevation of basal body temperature and an increase in breast volume. The life span of the corpus luteum appears to be fixed (14 ± 3 days) unless it is "rescued" by the luteotropin human chorionic gonadotropin (HCG) arising from the implanting trophoblast. Thus, pregnancy is the only normal cause of a persistent corpus luteum. The corpus luteum continues to produce progesterone for the first 8 weeks of pregnancy and thus maintains a secretory endometrium as well as ensures myometrial quiescence. The placenta then takes over the task of progesterone production and retains this function for the remainder of the pregnancy.

Corpus luteum death and progesterone/estrogen withdrawal lead to spasm of the spiral arterioles of the endometrium. It is likely that prostaglandins and related metabolites formed in the endometrium cause myometrial contractions during menstruation. Such contractions cause discomfort but are likely useful in expelling the menstrual content. Menstrual blood does not normally clot, and the amount of blood lost per spontaneous cycle varies from 10 to 80 ml in normal women. The duration of menses varies from 2 to 8 days.

As judged by relative infertility and the relative infrequency of biphasic basal body temperature patterns in early postmenarchal girls, many of the cycles in early reproductive life are anovulatory. A similar pattern is characteristic of the perimenopausal woman.

DISORDERS OF MENSTRUATION **Primary amenorrhea** The average age of menarche in the United States is 12½ years with a range of 9 to 16 years. Constitutional delay of menarche often correlates with delay in acquisition of critical body composition. The age at which the diagnosis of primary amenorrhea should be made is arbitrary. Evaluation should be performed by age 14 when primary amenorrhea is associated with a failure of breast development or at any age when the lack of menstruation becomes of concern to a patient or her parents, recognizing that many such patients will prove to have only a delayed onset of puberty. The two most common causes of true primary amenorrhea at age 18 (gonadal dysgenesis and congenital absence of the uterus and vagina) can both be diagnosed by physical examination and laboratory tests several years before that age. Other causes of primary amenorrhea in declining order of frequency are polycystic ovarian disease, CNS disorders that interfere with gonadotropin secretion (such as craniopharyngioma or pituitary tumor), male or female pseudohermaphroditism, and pregnancy.

Secondary amenorrhea Cessation of menses in a woman who has previously experienced spontaneous vaginal bleeding is termed *secondary amenorrhea*. Any disruption in the hypothalamic-pituitary-ovarian-uterine interrelationships described above may lead to secondary amenorrhea, but the disorder must be considered to be due to pregnancy until proved otherwise. In the past it was common to attempt to induce withdrawal bleeding with progestational agents to rule out pregnancy. This procedure is to be discouraged because of the increase in congenital malformations (limb reduction defects, congenital heart disease, hypospadias, and neural tube defects) that appear to be associated with the use of progestational agents during pregnancy.

The common causes of secondary amenorrhea are conveniently categorized as chronic acyclic endogenous estrogen production and a profound deficiency of estrogen production. In the former category are patients with partial (often temporary) disruption in the hormonal relationships between the brain and ovary leading to ovarian estrogen production but not ovulation. Also in this category are patients with the rare granulosa–theca cell tumors of the ovary which secrete estradiol. The remaining patients in this category are victims of excessive extraglandular estrogen production and include those with polycystic ovarian disease (Stein-Leventhal syndrome), liver disease, and obesity (see dysfunctional uterine bleeding below).

Those patients with absence of estrogen production have either primary or secondary ovarian failure. The former situation is termed *premature menopause* and is diagnosed by detecting castrate levels of FSH and LH in serum. The cause of primary ovarian failure is seldom apparent, and there is little hope for fertility in these patients. Secondary ovarian failure is the result of decreased gonadotropin production and is caused by psychogenic (stress) and organic/endocrinologic disorders influencing hypothalamic pituitary function (craniopharyngioma, prolactin-secreting pituitary microadenoma, severe systemic illness, malnutrition, "post-pill oversuppression").

Rarely secondary amenorrhea may be the consequence of loss of functioning endometrium, due to endometrial tuberculosis or endometrial scarring following pregnancy-related uterine curettage (Asherman's syndrome). Occasional cases of secondary amenorrhea are accompanied by acquired virilization, and the cause of ovarian or adrenal androgen excess must be sought (Chap. 46).

Abnormal uterine bleeding Any woman in the reproductive age group with abnormal uterine bleeding has a pregnancy-associated disorder (abortion, ectopic pregnancy) until proved otherwise. Continuing improvements in the specificity and sensitivity of pregnancy tests make it easier for the clinician to exclude complications of pregnancy as a cause of abnormal bleeding. The second major cause is iatrogenic due to exogenous hormone administration.

Organic lesions of the uterus (submucous leiomyoma, adenomyosis, endometritis, endometrial polyp) usually produce menorrhagia (heavier bleeding than usual at the expected time of menses). Carcinoma of the endometrium is primarily a disease of postmenopausal women but should also be considered in cases of abnormal bleeding during the "perimenopause" or in individuals with predisposing conditions such as morbid obesity, liver disease, chronic oligoanovulation from the time of puberty, or a strong family history of cancer. In the woman who has never had a previous episode of abnormal menstruation, the possibility of a bleeding diathesis (e.g., idiopathic

thrombocytopenic purpura, acute leukemia) must be considered.

The term *dysfunctional uterine bleeding* is intended to describe bleeding from an endometrium which has not progressed through full maturation under the influence of a dominant ovarian follicle that passes through full follicular and luteal phases. This is "anovulatory bleeding" and is seen in two broad classes of patients: (1) Individuals who usually ovulate but who have suffered a transient disruption in the synchronous hypothalamic-pituitary-ovarian relationships that are necessary for monthly ovulation; this occurs most commonly at the extremes of reproductive life but may occur at any time. (2) Patients with *chronic estrus*. The most common entity in this group is patients with polycystic ovarian disease (Stein-Leventhal syndrome). Characteristically, these patients give a history of relative infertility and oligoanovulation dating from puberty and often exhibit cutaneous manifestations of androgen excess (hirsutism, acne). A predominant feature of the pathophysiology of this disorder is increased ovarian production of androstenedione which is converted to estrone in extragonadal sites, resulting in chronic excess endogenous estrogen production. Since androstenedione is also a precursor of testosterone, overproduction of androstenedione is also ultimately responsible for the androgenic manifestations. Two other causes of a chronic estrous state due to excessive estrogen (estrone) production at extragonadal sites are liver disease and obesity. In these two disorders the production of androstenedione is normal, but the extent of conversion to estrone is increased. It should be noted that certain previously designated "nonendocrine" epithelial, germ cell, or metastatic ovarian neoplasms (e.g., mucinous cystadenoma, mature teratoma, or Krukenberg tumor) can also secrete excessive androstenedione which may lead to overproduction of testosterone. Infrequently (since it is an uncommon tumor, occurring most often in postmenopausal women), unilateral granulosa–theca cell tumors of the ovary secrete estradiol and cause premenopausal women to present with chronic estrus and abnormal bleeding. These tumors are usually sizable and, therefore, palpable on bimanual examination.

Ordinarily a careful history and physical examination will disclose the likely etiology of the anovulatory bleeding. Endometrial biopsy is not part of the standard management of patients with dysfunctional uterine bleeding. The only exceptions are individuals who are at high risk for endometrial carcinoma.

PAIN Mittelschmerz The term applied to ovulatory pain is *mittelschmerz*. This is typically a dull aching pain at midcycle in one lower quadrant lasting from a few minutes to 8 h. The etiology of the pain is unknown but may be inflammation of the ovulation site itself or peritoneal irritation from follicular fluid released at ovulation. The principal clinical importance of mittelschmerz is that it must be distinguished from more serious organic diseases such as appendicitis, pelvic inflammatory disease, and ectopic pregnancy.

Premenstrual syndrome The premenstrual syndrome consists of a variety of somatic symptoms occurring in the postovulatory phase of the cycle and ordinarily terminating with the onset of menses. These symptoms include edema, breast engorgement, abdominal bloating, headache, and exacerbation of acne. There is, in addition, a psychological component known colloquially as "premenstrual tension" consisting of cyclic irritability, depression, and lethargy. The severity varies. The biochemical events responsible for the somatic symptoms and for the psychological component are not known.

Painful menstruation Virtually all menses subsequent to ovulation are associated with some pelvic discomfort if only for the first few hours of bleeding. This is so because myometrial contraction is an essential part of the process. *Dysmenorrhea* refers to excessive and incapacitating pain at the time of menstruation. In patients with such complaint, careful search for congenital uterovaginal malformation, pelvic infection, tumor, endometriosis, or other pelvic nongenital pathology should be made. The majority of cases of dysmenorrhea are deemed "primary" in that no discernible organic cause for the pain can be discovered. It is likely that primary dysmenorrhea is caused by an exaggeration of the biochemical events leading to the synthesis of prostaglandin and related uterotonic metabolites and their action on the myometrium or by an alteration in the individual's response to the genuine discomfort of myometrial contraction—or a combination of the two. Careful inquiry will often disclose precipitating or aggravating psychological factors.

Explanation of the physiology of primary dysmenorrhea, reassurance, and general measures such as rest and local heat will suffice in many instances. More potent analgesics and sedatives are sometimes required. Prostaglandin inhibitors such as aspirin may be useful if begun during the week prior to menses. In cases where the episodes are recurrent and the degree of incapacitation is significant, low-dose, combination oral contraceptive therapy (estrogen plus progestin) is ordinarily effective. Such therapy probably reduces the amount of prostaglandin precursors present in the endometrium at the end of the cycle and decreases the volume of blood lost during menses with the consequence that myometrial contractions are reduced.

MENOPAUSE Cessation of menstruation is a significant event in the life of most women. The loss of this physiologic function is a dramatic reminder that aging is relentless, and the psychological impact is maximal in a culture that prizes youth. The term *climacteric* refers to the time of life during which menopause occurs. Many other significant events relating to a woman's career or her role as spouse and parent may occur during the climacteric.

The average age of menopause is 47 years. The postmenopausal ovary is on an average two-fifths of its previous weight, is virtually devoid of follicles, and no longer secretes estrogen. An auxiliary mechanism of estrogen production becomes manifest during the postmenopausal years. Androgens of adrenal origin are converted in peripheral tissues to estrone. While estrone is a less potent estrogen than estradiol, it is nonetheless biologically active. Thus, the postmenopausal woman is only *relatively* deficient in estrogen. The efficiency of this mechanism of estrogen production increases with aging and with excess weight. Estrogen therapy is indicated only in the postmenopausal woman with complaints of vasomotor instability or urogenital atrophy. The role of estrogens in the prevention of osteoporosis in postmenopausal women remains controversial. Ordinarily estrogens should be given orally and in the smallest effective dose for the shortest possible time. Personality change, easy fatigability, insomnia, and depression are symptoms more likely related to events in the climacteric other than ovarian failure.

SEXUAL FUNCTION

Patients consult physicians more and more frequently because of disturbances in sexual function. In general, women request help more frequently than men, and they usually complain of lack of arousal during intercourse or failure to achieve orgasm. (See also Chap. 345, "Sexual Counseling.") The term *frigidity* has been used for centuries in connection with female sexual problems. Recent classifications of female sexual problems have moved away from the term because of its imprecision.

LIBIDO Libido or sexuality is not governed exclusively by sex hormones. While the normal action of certain hormones appears to be important for human libido, cultural, emotional, and other influences on behavior affect sexuality to variable degrees. A reduction in libido is rarely caused solely by ovarian or adrenal insufficiency. Augmented or diminished libido is most often the consequence of psychological events rather than an endocrinopathy.

SEXUAL RESPONSE The female sexual response consists of two distinct components: (1) a local genital vasocongestive response analogous to erection in the male and (2) orgasm. Vasocongestion of the vagina, under autonomic nervous control, leads to vaginal lubrication in preparation for intromission. The lubrication is due principally to a transudate from the glandless vaginal mucosa. There is also a general increase in pelvic and vulvar vascularity. Healthy vaginal tissue is a prerequisite to normal lubrication, but the neurogenic reflex leading to genital congestion and vaginal lubrication is initiated by psychic sexual stimuli. Fatigue, interpersonal conflicts between the couple, depression, anxiety, or stress may lead to failure of the vasocongestive response.

Orgasm is a cortical sensory phenomenon in which involuntary rhythmic contractions of skeletal muscles and engorged tissues surrounding the vaginal outlet as well as some deeper pelvic muscles are perceived as pleasurable. Direct or indirect stimulation of the clitoris is as critical in producing female orgasm as stimulation of the penis for male orgasm. The female can physically participate in sexual intercourse without experiencing either component of sexual response and may enjoy nonorgasmic sexual encounters particularly with a loving partner, presumably because of the pleasure derived from physical closeness in a cherished relationship. Exploitation of a woman's capacity to participate in sexual intercourse without sexual response can, however, be destructive to a couple's general relationship and may be a source of frustration manifested on occasion by psychosomatic complaints. Failure of orgasm in spite of normal vaginal lubrication is most often the consequence of insufficient clitoral stimulation. Organic diseases that preclude normal vascularity and sensation in the genitalia may also cause failure of sexual response. (See Chap. 345.)

DYSPAREUNIA Painful intercourse is termed *dyspareunia;* it can ordinarily be localized by the patient to the vagina or deeper within the pelvis. Dyspareunia is most commonly due to the failure of vaginal lubrication but may be due to organic pathology of the vagina or pelvis. Failure of the appearance of the vaginal transudate may be the result of estrogen deficiency or failure of the autonomic nervous mechanisms which lead to vasocongestion. The latter is analogous to male impotence and like impotence most often indicates a psychological conflict. Pelvic dyspareunia may be due to pathology such as infection, endometriosis, or tumor. In instances where relief cannot be anticipated as a result of restoration of more normal pelvic anatomy, changes in coital technique which limit the extent of vaginal penetration may prevent the discomfort.

VAGINISMUS Vaginismus is the painful, involuntary contraction of the musculature surrounding the entrance to the vagina. This rare but disabling disorder prohibits intromission and usually is a conditioned response related to some previous real or imagined adverse sexual experience. Treatment consists of eliminating the conditioned response by progressive dilation of the vaginal entrance by the patient. In only the most recalcitrant cases is it profitable to subject a patient to psychotherapy in search of the etiologic sexual conflict.

REPRODUCTION

The scarcity of infants for adoption has aggravated the plight of couples in whom the reproductive process has failed. While not an illness, infertility can be devastating in that it is the unexpected denial of the personal and often powerful drive to reproduce. A systematic approach to the problem in an atmosphere of empathy and honesty will be most rewarding to infertile couples.

Infertility is always a problem involving two people. The physician's initial encounter with an infertile couple should be used to gather historical data relative to the reproductive process. Frequency of intercourse, relationship of time of intercourse to time of ovulation, use of potentially spermicidal lubricants, general health of the individuals, and use of medications that might be detrimental to the reproductive process should be reviewed.

Because it is the simplest, safest, and least expensive part of an infertility evaluation, a semen analysis is the first laboratory test performed (see Chap. 341). Unfortunately, there is no opportunity to scrutinize directly the female germ cells.

The preovulatory postcoital test is a second useful procedure for the evaluation of infertility; during the immediate preovulatory time of the cycle an aspirate of cervical mucus is taken within 2 h after intercourse. A normal test should disclose several motile spermatozoa per high-power microscopic field and implies successful male erection, intromission, and ejaculation, as well as presumably normal cervical function. Infections or alterations in cervical mucus production subsequent to surgery or cryotherapy of the cervix are the most common causes of abnormal postcoital tests when the male is normal.

Basal body temperature graphs, endometrial biopsy, and plasma progesterone 1 week prior to expected menses are indirect methods useful for determining ovulation and the adequacy of corpus luteum function. An occasional short luteal phase is likely a normal event in many women; it remains conjectural whether repeated corpus luteum insufficiency can be responsible for infertility or repeated spontaneous abortion. The list of therapeutic alternatives useful in inducing ovulation in some ovulatory disorders is slowly expanding and includes clomiphene citrate, human menopausal gonadotropins, bromocriptine mesylate, and wedge resection of the ovary.

Hysterosalpingography is the accepted method of determining tubal patency. The oviduct plays several roles in the reproductive process including pickup of the ovum from the site of ovulation, spermatozoan and ovum transport to the site of fertilization in the ampullary portion of the oviduct, and nourishment and transportation of the early zygote. A radiographic study showing patency of the oviduct does not assess these aforementioned aspects of tubal function. Infection, endometriosis, and adhesions due to previous pelvic surgery are the most frequent causes of distortions of tubal anatomy and function. Though recent advances in microsurgical techniques have improved the likelihood of reversing surgical sterilization, surgical restoration of normal tubal function in the aforementioned disorders is less than satisfactory. Pharmacological superovulation of a female who had no oviducts, harvesting of the ovum through laparoscopy, in vitro fertilization, and transfer of the embryo to the mother's uterus resulted in the delivery of an apparently normal infant in England in 1978. It remains to be seen whether this technique in the coming decade will continue to be a medical curiosity or will have widespread application in the management of the infertile couple.

We understand only a small part of the story of reproduction, and our diagnostic tests are inadequate to perceive many impediments to conception (for example, to assess tubal function). These limitations likely account for the fact that at least 10 percent of barren couples have no discernible cause for

infertility. In some of these the impediment is relative, for after a variable and sometimes lengthy period of time, conception may occur.

REFERENCES

AIMAN J et al: The origin of androgen and estrogen in a virilized postmenopausal woman with bilateral benign cystic teratomas. Obstet Gynecol 49:695, 1977

FORDNEY DS: Dyspareunia and vaginismus. Clin Obstet Gynecol 21:205, 1978

FRISCH RE, McARTHUR JW: Menstrual cycles: Fatness as a determinant of minimum weight for height necessary for their maintenance or onset. Science 185:949, 1974

KAPLAN HS: *The New Sex Therapy: Active Treatment of Sexual Dysfunctions.* New York, Brunner/Mazel, 1974

LEVINE SB, ROSENTHAL M: Marital sexual dysfunction: Female dysfunctions. Ann Intern Med 86:588, 1977

SHOEMAKER E et al: Estrogen treatment of postmenopausal women, benefits and risks. JAMA 238:1524, 1977

SIITERI PK, MACDONALD PC: Role of extraglandular estrogen in human endocrinology, in *Handbook of Physiology: Endocrinology II,* part I, RO Greep, EB Astwood (eds). Washington, DC, The American Physiological Society, 1973, chap 28, p 615

46
HIRSUTISM AND VIRILIZATION

JEAN D. WILSON

Hirsutism in women, the growth of hair in a pattern characteristic of men, is a common and perplexing problem in medicine. Numerous factors—genetic, endocrine, and undefined—influence the growth and distribution of hair so that there is considerable overlap between normal men and women. As a consequence abnormal hair growth is difficult to define; an unbearable burden to one woman may be an unnoticed amount of hair in another. However, if the patient thinks that hair growth is excessive, no amount of reassurance, persuasion, or argument will convince her otherwise. The central issue in dealing with such patients is the separation of those infrequent instances in which hirsutism is one manifestation of an underlying virilizing or defeminizing syndrome from the vast majority of individuals in which it is fundamentally a cosmetic problem.

CONTROL OF NORMAL HAIR GROWTH AND DISTRIBUTION
Endocrinology There are three principal circulating androgens in women—dehydroepiandrosterone derived from the adrenal, androstenedione derived equally from adrenal and ovary, and testosterone which is both secreted from the ovary and formed by peripheral conversion from circulating dehydroepiandrosterone and androstenedione. The production of adrenal androgen is regulated primarily by adrenocorticotropic hormone (ACTH), while ovarian androgen secretion is regulated by the gonadotropins. Dehydroepiandrosterone and androstenedione are weak androgens, but they can be converted into physiologically potent hormones in nonendocrine (peripheral) tissues; by this process dehydroepiandrosterone is converted to androstenediol, and androstenedione is transformed into testosterone and dihydrotestosterone. Androgens are the major determinants of hair distribution in both sexes.

In simple terms four types of androgen response can be defined:

1 No androgen dependence: lanugo, eyebrows, eyelashes
2 Dependence upon adrenal androgen and hence equal growth in men and women: axillary and lower pubic hair
3 Dependence upon testicular androgen: upper pubic, facial, ear, extremity, and truncal hair
4 Inhibition by testicular androgen: scalp hair

Why different body regions respond differently to the same or similar androgen is uncertain. Theoretically, the metabolism of androgens might differ in the various sites, or hormone receptors might vary. Evidence against the former possibility comes from studies of patients with single gene mutations influencing androgen action (Chap. 344). The hair follicle, like other androgen-responsive cells, requires conversion of testosterone to dihydrotestosterone for expression of testicular androgen action, and hair follicles from all regions of the body perform this conversion equally well. Moreover, the same cytoplasmic receptor that is essential for androgen action in other cells (Chap. 341) is necessary for the action of adrenal and testicular androgens in the hair follicle. Genetic disorders with normal testosterone production but absent receptor have deficient or absent axillary, pubic, facial, truncal, and limb hair. Regional differences in androgen responsiveness of hair are probably the consequence of regional differences in the level of androgen receptor in hair follicles.

Genetic factors Despite similar hormone levels, there is considerable diversity in the distribution of hair among individuals and among racial groups in regard to facial, truncal, and pubic hair. It is generally agreed that dark-haired, darkly pigmented whites of either sex tend to be more hirsute than blonde or fair-skinned persons. Orientals, American Indians, and blacks are less hirsute than whites. Orientals rarely have facial or body hair except in the pubic and axillary regions, and American Indians, in addition, rarely develop baldness in either sex. There is also considerable heterogeneity of hair patterns within family groups. The inheritance of hair patterns is obviously complex and is probably polygenic in nature.

Other factors Aging is a prerequisite for the expression of some types of hair development, whether mediated by androgens or otherwise. For example, in men hair on the trunk and extremities frequently increases for several years after maximal levels of plasma androgens have been reached. Conversely, loss of androgens rarely results in diminution of normal hair or reverses hirsutism. The appearance of pubic hair is frequently the heralding event of puberty in females. Women in the first trimester of pregnancy commonly observe increased hairiness of the face, extremities, and breasts. Menopause is often associated with the loss of hair in the pubic area, axillae, and extremities, whereas growth of hair on the face increases in postmenopausal women. The physiological basis for these changes is unclear and cannot be explained entirely by changes in androgen levels.

PATHOLOGICAL HAIR GROWTH OR DISTRIBUTION Drugs

Drug-induced hirsutism is a frequent complication of modern therapy. It may be an isolated symptom or part of a virilizing syndrome. If the onset is subtle, it may go unrecognized by the physician. Drugs that produce hirsutism without actual virilization include phenytoin, Minoxidil, diazoxide, hexachlorobenzene, and ACTH. Steroidal drugs that are capable of inducing virilization as well as hirsutism include progestins (which may also cause virilization of infants born to mothers given them) and androgens.

Virilizing syndromes In an evaluation of patients for hirsutism, the most important feature is whether virilization or defeminization is also present (Table 46-1). In patients with androgen overproduction defeminizing signs are more consistent than are the signs of virilization, although the latter, if present, are valuable, since they indicate either ovarian or adrenal pathology. Two reservations should be kept in mind in interpreting the presence or absence of virilization. First, virilization is indicative of androgen excess at some time in the patient's life but does not mean that active disease is present at the time of evaluation. This can be ascertained by measurement of plasma androgen levels and/or production rates. Second, severe over-androgenization may exist in the absence of a true virilization syndrome; i.e., at the same level of androgen production clitoromegaly may be present in one patient and not another.

Two types of virilizing syndromes can occur—ovarian and adrenal—but it should be emphasized that these disorders account for only a small fraction of patients who complain of hirsutism.

OVARIAN ANDROGENIZATION Polycystic ovary disease is the commonest cause of ovarian hyperandrogenism (see Chap. 342). The disorder has a wide clinical spectrum that varies from apparently normal menses and mild hirsutism to complete amenorrhea and virilization; hyperthecosis of the ovary characterized by the presence of luteinized theca-like cells in the ovarian stroma is a varient of the disorder. Luteinizing hormone (LH) is almost invariably elevated, and there is considerable overproduction of androgens by the ovary. Other causes of ovarian virilization include stromal hyperplasia, luteomas, hilar-cell hyperplasia, and a variety of androgen-secreting tumors including arrhenoblastoma and Krukenberg tumor; in these disorders plasma testosterone levels are elevated, frequently to the male range; the tumors may be so small as to be undetectable by pelvic examination or laparoscopy.

ADRENAL ANDROGENIZATION Adrenal androgen-secreting tumors (adenoma or carcinoma) are generally accompanied by elevated urinary 17-ketosteroid excretion. Plasma testosterone levels may be elevated but not as high as in ovarian disease. Hirsutism can also be a manifestation of congenital adrenal hyperplasia and Cushing's disease.

Idiopathic or simple hirsutism This term applies to those hirsute women in whom a specific etiologic diagnosis cannot be made. The diagnosis should be restricted to patients in whom the urinary 17-ketosteroid level is not elevated, the ovaries are not enlarged, adrenal function is normal, there is no evidence of an adrenal or ovarian tumor, and menstruation is normal. Slight elevations of plasma androstenedione and/or testosterone are usual, and testosterone secretion rates may be increased above the mean; whether these abnormalities represent the extreme end of a normal continuum or a distinct pathological group is unclear. However, substantial evidence indicates that in the majority of such women the increased plasma androgens are derived from the ovaries. In some the underlying diagnosis may be mild or early polycystic ovarian

TABLE 46-1
Clinical signs of defeminization and virilization

Signs of defeminization	Signs of virilization
Amenorrhea	Frontal balding
Decrease in breast size	Increase in size of shoulder girdle muscles
Loss of female body contours	Clitoromegaly
	Coarsening of the voice
	Acne

SOURCE: *After Karp and Herrmann.*

disease, but in most the hormone abnormalities are not accompanied or followed by signs of ovarian dysfunction. Thus, it is possible that these patients are variants of normal. Since androgens are a major determinant of hair distribution and growth, it is to be expected that within the normal range higher androgen levels would be associated on average with greater androgen-mediated hair growth. Therefore, the belief of many endocrinologists that the majority of hirsute women have no associated endocrinopathy may still be valid.

TREATMENT In the case of drugs and tumors of the ovaries or adrenal glands, treatment is straightforward—stop the drugs or remove the tumors. In polycystic ovarian disease and idiopathic hirsutism, effective therapy is ovarian suppression using a combination-type oral contraceptive; improvement in hirsutism can frequently be documented in 6 months to a year. Whether the risks of contraceptive therapy are justified in simple hirsutism is an individual judgment. If fertility is desired, other forms of therapy are indicated (Chap. 342). Since coarsened hairs usually do not return completely to normal, local therapy for hirsutism including depilatory agents, shaving, tweezing, and electrolysis is often required. Other evidences of virilization such as balding, clitoromegaly, and coarsening of the voice rarely improve following cure of the overandrogenization.

REFERENCES

GIVENS JR: Hirsutism and hyperandrogenism. Adv Intern Med 21:221, 1976

KARP L, HERRMANN WL: Diagnosis and treatment of hirsutism in women. Obstet Gynecol 41:283, 1973

KIRSCHNER MA, BARDIN CW: Androgen production and metabolism in normal and virilized women. Metabolism 21:667, 1972

MULLER SA: Hirsutism. Am J Med 46:803, 1969

ROSENFIELD RL: Relationship of androgens to female hirsutism and infertility. J Reprod Med 11:87, 1973

47
DISTURBANCES OF SEXUAL FUNCTION AND REPRODUCTION IN MEN

PATRICK C. WALSH
JEAN D. WILSON

A coordinated sequence of physiological events (psychic, endocrine, vascular, and neurological) controls normal sexual and reproductive function in men. In this chapter, the discussion is focused on the clinical presentation of sexual disorders in men. (Also see Chaps. 341, "Diseases of the Testis," and 345, "Sexual Counseling.")

SEXUAL FUNCTION

NORMAL SEXUAL FUNCTION Simply stated, normal male sexual function can be divided into five phases, each of which is under diverse regulation: libido, erection, ejaculation, orgasm, and detumescence.

The first, sexual desire or libido, is regulated by poorly understood psychic factors and by testicular androgens. Castration produces a decline in libido that can be restored by treatment with testosterone.

The second phase, erection, is primarily a neurological event that results in modification of the vascular supply to the penis, causing it to become engorged with blood. The neurological aspect of erection is controlled by both reflex and psychic stimuli. The sensory portion begins with fibers that originate in pacinian corpuscles of the penis and pass via the pudendal nerve to the S_2 to S_4 dorsal root ganglia. The efferent limb begins with parasympathetic preganglionic fibers from the S_2 to S_4 dorsal root ganglia, which synapse in the perivesicular, prostatic, and cavernous plexuses. From there, postganglionic fibers pass to blood vessels of the corpora cavernosa. Efferent fibers from S_3 and S_4 ganglia also travel in the pudendal nerve to the ischiocavernosus and bulbocavernosus muscles. There is also sympathetic innervation of the male genitalia. These fibers originate from the lateral columns of the spinal cord at the levels of T_{12} and L_1, the so-called "thoracolumbar erection center," and synapse in the pelvic and perivesicular plexuses. Postganglionic fibers innervate the smooth muscle of the vas deferens, seminal vesicle, and internal sphincter of the bladder. Sympathetic innervation can act synergistically with the sacral parasympathetics to mediate erection initiated by psychic stimuli. For example, some patients with sacral cord transection who cannot have erection with tactile "reflex" stimulation can become erect in response to psychic stimuli. On the other hand, sympathetic innervation is not mandatory for erection. This is demonstrated by continued potency in most patients after bilateral complete sympathectomy. The central nervous system modulates erectile response via pathways thought to descend in the lateral columns of the spinal cord. The effect of the central nervous system on erection can be either stimulatory or inhibitory; thus the importance of psychic stimulation for erection.

While erection is primarily controlled by the parasympathetic system, the transformation of the penis from a flaccid to an erect state is a vascular phenomenon. Blood reaches the penis via terminal branches of the right and left internal pudendal arteries. The erectile tissue of the penis consists of two corpora cavernosa lying side by side on the dorsal aspect of the penis and the corpus spongiosum that surrounds the urethra. This tissue consists of an irregular sponge-like system of valvular spaces interspersed between arteries and veins. These valve-like structures (called *polsters*) are located in the arterioles, and in the flaccid state are constricted, causing blood to be shunted away from the corpora directly into the veins. Under the influence of the autonomic erection centers, the polsters relax and allow blood to fill the vascular spaces of the corpora and expand the penis to the erect state. It is not clear whether venous valves impede flow and thus further promote erection. Passive venous obstruction undoubtedly occurs.

The third phase, ejaculation, is under control of the sympathetic nervous system and consists of two processes, seminal emission and true ejaculation. Emission results from the contraction of the vas deferens, prostate, and seminal vesicles which causes seminal fluid to enter the urethra. True ejaculation results from contraction of the muscles of the pelvic floor including the bulbocavernosus and ischiocavernosus muscles. Retrograde ejaculation is prevented by partial bladder neck closure mediated by the sympathetic nerves.

The fourth phase, orgasm, is a cortical sensory phenomenon in which the rhythmic contraction of the bulbocavernosus and ischiocavernosus muscles is perceived as pleasurable. It is purely psychic. The fact that orgasm can occur without either ejaculation or bladder neck closure explains why some drugs that prevent ejaculation do not interfere with erection or orgasm.

The mechanism for detumescence after orgasm and ejaculation is poorly understood but may be related to vasoconstriction of the arterioles supplying blood to the erectile tissue, thus allowing venous drainage to empty the sinuses and the penis to become flaccid. Following orgasm, there is a refractory period that varies with age, physical condition, and psychic factors during which erection and ejaculation are inhibited.

IMPOTENCE Male sexual dysfunction, often termed *impotence,* may be manifested in various ways: loss of desire, inability to obtain or maintain an erection, premature ejaculation, absence of emission, inability to achieve orgasm. Many subjects complain of more than one abnormality simultaneously. These complaints can be secondary to other chronic or debilitating diseases, the consequence of specific disorders of the urogenital or endocrine systems, or the result of psychiatric disturbance. It is mandatory in all instances to exclude organic (and in some instances potentially correctable or treatable) causes.

Loss of desire Because androgens have a major influence on sexual desire in men, a decrease in libido may indicate androgen deficiency arising from either pituitary or testicular disease. This possibility can be tested by the measurement of plasma testosterone and gonadotropins. However, since the testosterone required to maintain libido is usually less than the amount necessary for full stimulation of the prostate and seminal vesicles, the patient should also complain of absence of emission when the loss of libido is on an endocrine basis. Conversely, if patients have normal semen volume, it is unlikely that endocrine factors are responsible for their sexual dysfunction.

Loss of erection Some of the organic causes of erectile impotence are listed in Table 47-1. Several types of neurological disorders can cause impotence including lesions in the anterior temporal lobe, spinal cord disorders, insufficiency of sensory input as can occur in diabetic neuropathy and tabes dorsalis, or damage to parasympathetic nerves, for example following surgical procedures such as total prostatectomy. Transurethral prostatectomy, in contrast, probably does not cause organic impotence. If spinal cord injury is above the thoracolumbar region, reflex erections may occur. Injury at the level of the

TABLE 47-1
Some organic causes of erectile impotence in men

I Neurological diseases
  A Anterior temporal lobe lesions
  B Diseases of the spinal cord
  C Loss of sensory input
    1 Diabetes mellitus and various polyneuropathies
    2 Tabes dorsalis
    3 Disease of dorsal root ganglia
  D Disease of nervi erigentes
    1 Complete prostatectomy
    2 Rectosigmoid operations
    3 Aortic bypass surgery
II Endocrine causes
  A Testicular failure (primary or secondary)
  B Hyperprolactinemia
III Drugs
  A Phenothiazines
  B Thioridazine
  C Imipramine
  D α-Methyldopa
  E Guanethidine
  F Reserpine
  G Spironolactone
  H Alcohol
  I Heroin, methadone
  J Estrogen
IV Vascular diseases: Leriche syndrome
V Failure of detumescence, priapism
VI Penile diseases
  A Previous priapism
  B Penile trauma
  C Peyronie's disease

sacral cord or cauda equina does not interfere with psychogenic erections but prevents reflex or tactile erections. Diffuse injury of the spinal cord results in total impotence. Diabetes mellitus deserves special comment. As many as half of diabetic men develop impotence within 6 years of the onset of diabetes, and impotence may be the first clinical manifestation of diabetic neuropathy. However, when careful neurological examination is performed including the cystometrogram, other evidences of neurological disturbance are usually uncovered. Many of the other polyneuropathies described in Chap. 377, and the paralytic states of the autonomic nervous system described in Chap. 13, have similar effects.

Endocrine causes of testicular failure that result in impotence usually bring about such profound changes that the disorders are not difficult to recognize (Chap. 341). Recent studies suggest that hyperprolactinemia may be a cause for impotence in some patients with pituitary tumors (see Chap. 333). As many as 90 percent of men with increased prolactin levels are impotent; gonadotropins and testosterone values are in the low normal range, and there is a normal pituitary response to luteinizing hormone–releasing hormone (LHRH). Bromocriptine mesylate, a dopamine agonist, lowers prolactin levels and reverses impotence in most such patients.

Drugs are a common cause of impotence. The usual explanation is neurological blockade, and this may well be the case for those drugs with peripheral parasympatholytic actions such as the tricyclic antidepressants. Others may act by enhancing prolactin secretion. In addition, the drugs of addiction such as alcohol, methadone, and heroin frequently lead to impotence. Whether the impotence in the latter instances is caused by reduced testosterone levels or the general condition of the patient is unclear.

One can readily understand vascular causes of impotence since continued high flow into the vascular network of the penis is necessary to maintain the erect state. The prototype of impaired penile blood supply is the Leriche syndrome. Here impedance to the blood flow into the penis occurs as the result of obstruction of the distal aorta at the bifurcation of the common iliacs. This usually presents as claudication and impotence; either can occur separately. Likewise, occlusion in smaller vessels supplying the penis can also lead to impotence. Recently several noninvasive methods have been devised to detect decreased blood flow to the penis using the Doppler technique. Differences between brachial pressure and systolic pressure in the penis should not be greater than 30 to 40 mmHg. There is a good correlation between vascular obstruction as the cause for impotence and failure to meet these criteria.

Premature ejaculation This disorder seldom has an organic cause. It is usually related to anxiety in the sexual situation, unreasonable expectations about performance, or an emotional disorder. A variety of successful therapeutic modalities have been described by Levine.

Absence of emission Three disorders may produce this symptom: (1) retrograde ejaculation, (2) sympathetic denervation, or (3) androgen deficiency. Retrograde ejaculation may occur following surgery on the bladder neck or may develop spontaneously in diabetic men. Examination of a postcoital urine specimen will establish the diagnosis. Following sympathectomy or occasionally after extensive retroperitoneal surgery, the autonomic innervation of the prostate and seminal vesicles is lost, resulting in absence of smooth-muscle contraction at the time of ejaculation. Finally, androgen deficiency may lead to absence of secretions from the prostate and seminal vesicles.

Absence of orgasm If libido and erectile function are normal, the absence of orgasm is almost always due to a psychiatric disorder.

Failure of detumescence *Priapism* is a persistent painful erection, often totally unrelated to sexual activity. The etiology of priapism is usually idiopathic, but the disorder can be associated with sickle-cell anemia, chronic granulocytic leukemia, or spinal cord injury. The disorder is thought to be secondary to clotting within the penile vascular network. The persistent erection disrupts this network and can lead to fibrosis and subsequent erectile impotence.

Penile diseases Finally, in addition to priapism, penile trauma and Peyronie's disease of the penis can also cause impotence (Table 47-1).

Evaluation of impotence Although the failure of erectile function is frequently the result of psychological disturbances, every effort must be made to exclude a remedial, organic cause (Table 47-1). Usually, the history is informative. Normally, from early childhood through the eighth decade, erections occur during sleep. This phenomenon, termed *nocturnal penile tumescence* (NPT), occurs during rapid eye movement sleep, and the total time of NPT usually averages 100 min per night. Consequently, if the patient gives a history of turgid erections under any circumstances (often when awakening in the early morning), the psychic, efferent neurological, and circulatory systems that mediate erection are intact, and dysfunction is probably due to a psychiatric disorder. In these patients the physical and laboratory examinations should be limited. (Occasional patients with sensory neuropathy may have nocturnal erections.) If the history of nocturnal erections is questionable, measurements of NPT can be made with the use of a strain gauge attached to a recorder.

Factors in favor of organic impotence include a similar degree of erectile dysfunction under all circumstances, onset not associated with any particular psychiatric symptomatology, a previous uninterrupted period of normal erectile function, and persistent sexual desire. Questions should be directed toward specific etiologies. These should include symptoms of diabetes, symptoms of peripheral neuropathy or bladder dysfunction, and symptoms referable to the vascular system such as intermittent claudication or history of priapism. A thorough drug history should be obtained, and inquiry concerning past operations that may have produced neurological damage should be made.

Physical examination should include a thorough genital examination to rule out any abnormalities of the penis itself. The testes should be palpated for size or abnormal masses; if the length is less than 4 cm, hypogonadism should be considered. Evidence of feminization should be looked for such as gynecomastia and abnormal body hair distribution. All pulses should be palpated, including the penile pulse, which can be felt by pressing both corpora between the thumb and forefinger and palpating to either side of the midline. If possible, penile blood pressure should be measured. If there is an indication from either history or physical examination of a vascular etiology, an aortogram may be indicated.

A neurological examination to evaluate the erectile reflex is advisable including anal sphincter tone, perineal sensation, and the bulbocavernosus reflex. This reflex is obtained by squeezing the glans penis and noting the degree of anal sphincter constriction. An examination for peripheral neuropathy, including distal muscle weakness, loss of tendon reflexes in the legs, and tests for impairment of vibratory, position, tactile, and pain sensation, should also be performed (see Chap. 377).

A frequent cause of prolonged impotence is an anxiety or depression state. These closely related conditions can be diagnosed by the criteria enumerated in Chaps. 11 and 25. Other psychological factors such as disinterest in the sexual partner, fear of sexual incompetence, marital discord, deviant sexual

attitudes, worry, fatigue, and ill health often operate in various combinations to reduce sexual impulse.

Laboratory evaluation is probably of minimal value. Measurement of serum testosterone in the absence of evidence of feminization or hypogonadism is seldom helpful.

Treatment of impotence Medical therapy with androgens offers little more than placebo benefit except in hypogonadal men. If a pituitary tumor producing high prolactin levels is present, however, either surgical removal or treatment with bromocriptine mesylate will usually result in return of potency. Surgical therapy may be useful in the treatment of decreased potency related to aortic obstruction; however, potency can be lost rather than improved after aortic operation if the autonomic nerve supply to the penis is damaged. This complication is minimized if an endarterectomy is done or, if a graft is required, the reconstruction of the distal end is performed above the origin of the external iliac arteries. Early surgical relief of priapism by shunting procedures, such as corpora spongiosum shunting, might prevent subsequent impotence.

A useful surgical technique for improvement of potency in refractory patients such as individuals with diabetic neuropathy is the implantation of a penile prosthesis, that is, the insertion within the corpora of a small, blunt silastic rod. The patient must be made aware that full erection is not produced and that the device only prevents buckling during intercourse. More recently, an inflatable prosthetic device has been devised for implantation on either side of the corpora. A connecting reservoir of material is placed in the perivesicular space, and pumps are located in the scrotum. By means of these pumps the penis can be made to become nearly fully erect at the appropriate time and then be made to relax after intercourse.

In the larger group of anxiety states and depressive illnesses measures directed at their alleviation will usually restore sexual potency, and sexual counseling, education, and psychotherapy are beneficial in alleviating psychogenic factors.

REPRODUCTION

Approximately a tenth of marriages in the United States are barren, and another tenth result in fewer children than desired. The husband is the cause of the infertility in about a third of these marriages.

Infertility in the male can be due to disorders of the hypothalamic-pituitary system, disorders of the testes, or abnormalities of the ejaculatory system (Table 341-1). When a history is obtained, information should be sought about the duration of infertility, fertility in other marriages of either the husband or wife, acquired or congenital disease that may lead to infertility, technique and frequency of intercourse, and family history of infertility. To exclude the presence of gross abnormalities of the endocrine system, the physical examination should evaluate the distribution of body hair, the presence of gynecomastia, the development of the scrotum and penis, the location of the urethral meatus, and the presence of normal vasa deferentia and epididymides. The size of each testis should be estimated with care. Because the seminiferous tubules account for more than 75 percent of the testicular mass, a reduction in testicular size (less than 4 cm in length) indicates a severe deficiency in the spermatogenic function of the testis. Finally, with the patient standing in the upright position, the Valsalva maneuver should be utilized to test for the presence of a varicocele.

The next step in the evaluation of the male partner is the semen analysis. This provides a semiquantitative estimation of the severity of the dysfunction. The findings are usually considered normal if: the semen coagulates and then liquefies, the volume is 2 to 5 ml, the spermatozoa count is greater than 20 million per milliliter, more than 60 percent of the spermatozoa are actively motile, and more than 60 percent have normal morphology. If no spermatozoa are present, the term *azoospermia* is used; if spermatozoa are present but the count is less than 20 million per milliliter, the patient is considered to have oligospermia. In the azoospermic male with normal-sized testes, the differential diagnosis includes hyalinization of the seminiferous tubules, Sertoli cell–only syndrome, gonadotropin deficiency, ductal obstruction, or maturation arrest. Plasma testosterone and serum LH and follicle-stimulating hormone (FSH) measurements are helpful in distinguishing among these conditions. In patients with hyalinization of the seminiferous tubules LH and FSH are elevated, and plasma testosterone is low or borderline normal. Patients with Sertoli cell–only syndrome usually have normal LH and testosterone levels, but FSH levels are characteristically elevated. In gonadotropin deficiency LH, FSH, and testosterone are low, and in ductal obstruction or maturation arrest all studies are normal. To differentiate between the last two disorders, a testicular biopsy is necessary. In oligospermic patients, if the history

and physical examination are normal, it is unlikely that any further laboratory investigation will be useful in defining the etiology. These patients are usually classified in the large group having *idiopathic oligospermia*.

REFERENCES

AMELAR RD et al: *Male Infertility.* Philadelphia, Saunders, 1977, p 153

FITZPATRICK T: A cavernosogram study on the valvular competence of the deep human dorsal vein. J Urol 113:497, 1975

FURLOW WL: Surgical management of impotence using the inflatable penile prosthesis: Experience with 103 patients. Br J Urol 50:114, 1977

KARACAN I et al: Sleep-related penile tumescence as a function of age. Am J Psychiatry 132:9, 1975

KOLODNY RC et al: Sexual dysfunction in diabetic men. Diabetes 23:306, 1974

LAROCQUE M et al: Priapism: A review of 46 cases. J Urol 112:770, 1974

LEVINE SB: Marital sexual dysfunction: Ejaculation disturbances. Ann Intern Med 84:575, 1976

WEISS H: The physiology of human penile erection. Ann Intern Med 76:793, 1972

section 9 | Alterations in the skin

48
INTERPRETATION OF ALTERATIONS IN THE SKIN

THOMAS B. FITZPATRICK
HARLEY A. HAYNES

CLINICAL EXAMINATION OF THE SKIN

The identification of skin lesions, or alterations, is a problem similar to the recognition of cells in a blood smear: the minute details are of the greatest importance. The individual type of skin lesion (e.g., papule, nodule) can be considered as a letter in the alphabet, forming the basic element for the identification of the pathologic change and often leading to the clinical diagnosis. Lesions may be the presenting complaint of the patient or may be incidental findings during the routine physical examination; or they may be incidental to some major presenting complaint such as fever, cough, arthralgia, and the like. The recognition of the important and nonimportant skin lesions commonly encountered during the routine physical examination of the skin is a requisite part of the physician's task (Plates 1 to 6).

Inasmuch as the identification of skin lesions is the *sine qua non* of dermatologic diagnosis, the examiner's eye is undoubtedly the most valuable instrument at his or her disposal. Adequate illumination, preferably with natural light, is necessary. The observation of the skin should begin with an overall, "low-power" general assessment of the completely disrobed patient. The systematic approach to the examination of skin should be as follows: first the fingernails and then the anterior and posterior aspects of the arm; then, in sequence, the scalp, the face, the trunk, the lower extremities and the skin between the toes;

and then the mucous membranes, including the mouth and anogenital areas. The examiner of dermatologic lesions should consider: (1) the specific *type* of lesion, (2) the *configuration*, or *shape* of the lesion, and (3) the *arrangement* of the groups of lesions, such as linear, arciform, annular, polycyclic, herpetiform, zosteriform, and serpiginous.

Types of skin lesions can be classified by determining the topographic level of the lesions in relation to the normal skin (Table 48-1). For example, it is possible to distinguish lesions that are in or that protrude or are superimposed above or below the level of the normal skin. The lesions that are encom-

TABLE 48-1
Types of skin lesion

Flat lesions (in plane of skin)	Elevated lesions (above plane of skin)	Depressed lesions (below plane of skin)
Macule	Vesicle and bulla	Atrophy§
Infarct*	Pustule	Sclerosis§†
Sclerosis*†	Abscess‡	Erosion
Telangiectasia†	Cyst†	Excoriation
	Papule	Scar†
	Wheal	Ulcer
	Plaque	Sinus‡
	Nodule‡	Gangrene§
	Vegetation	
	Keratosis	
	Desquamation (scales)	
	Exudate* (crusts)	
	Lichenification	

* May also be below the plane of the skin.
† May also be above the plane of the skin.
‡ May also be in or below the plane of the skin.
§ May also be in the plane of the skin.
SOURCE: *TB Fitzpatrick, in Dermatology in General Medicine, 2d ed, TB Fitzpatrick et al (eds), New York, McGraw-Hill, 1979.*

passed within the scope of dermatology are listed in Fig. 48-1 and Table 48-1, and the histologic aspects are illustrated in Figs. 48-2 through 48-13.

The *shape* of the individual lesion and the *arrangement* of two or more lesions in relation to each other sometimes constitute important diagnostic clues. A linear arrangement of lesions often is indicative of an exogenous cause; also, linear lesions may occur because the pathologic process involves a vein, a lymphatic component, or an arteriole. Linearity can often be seen in various types of cutaneous hamartoma involving epidermal cells or melanocytes or even dermal connective tissue. In contrast, annular and arciform lesions and annular and arciform arrangements are relatively common and therefore only rarely lead to a specific diagnosis. The *iris* lesion, however, a special and important type of annular lesion, is an erythematous annular macule or papule with either a purplish papule or vesicle in the center. Iris lesions are characteristic of the erythema-multiforme syndrome. Annular macules may be observed in drug eruptions, secondary syphilis, and lupus erythematosus. Annular lesions with scale often suggest dermatophytosis or pityriasis rosea or psoriasis. The wheals that occur in creeping eruptions as well as the nodules in the late syphilis are arranged in a *serpiginous* (snake-like) pattern.

Lesions that are contiguous are described as *grouped*, and are of relatively little diagnostic value except in the special pattern, *herpetiform*, which is pathognomonic for herpes simplex or herpes zoster. Similarly, the special arrangement, *zosteriform*, follows a dermatome in a bandlike pattern and is characteristically seen in herpes zoster; a zosteriform arrangement of skin nodules is occasionally seen in metastatic carcinoma of the breast. A *reticular* arrangement often results from vascular dilatation and is observed in cutis marmorata and livedo reticularis.

The *distribution* of sites of localization of skin eruptions has been greatly overemphasized in dermatologic diagnosis; of far more importance are the type, shape, and arrangement of the lesions. The distribution of eruptions can be classified as *isolated*, *regional*, or *generalized*; the term *total* (universal) denotes an involvement of all the skin, including the hair and the nails.

When the eruption occurs in a bilateral and symmetric distribution, the pathologic stimulus is usually endogenous or is hematogenously disseminated. Bilateral symmetry is characteristic of hypersensitivity and is a common response to a drug. In photosensitivity eruptions, lesions are localized to the parts of the body that are exposed to sunlight. The exposed areas of the face that are usually spared include the fold of skin in the upper eyelids, the skin of the hair-covered scalp, and the region below the chin.

LABORATORY AND OTHER AIDS IN EXAMINATION OF THE SKIN

There are certain technical, clinical, and laboratory aids and procedures that are indispensable in the clinical examination and interpretation of skin conditions.

VISUAL AIDS Magnification Certain diagnostic signs can be revealed only by magnification of the skin lesions, e.g., the follicular plugging indicative of lupus erythematosus, the fine telangiectasia and raised border indicative of basal cell carcinoma, and, if present, the bluish color indicative of early primary malignant melanoma. A pocket magnifier (2 to 7×) is necessary for proper identification.

Transillumination Transillumination, or sidelighting, of skin lesions, which is done in a darkened room, is often required to detect slight degrees of elevation or depression, and is also sometimes useful in estimating the extent of the eruption.

Diascopy Diascopy is an essential technique for the examination of skin because it permits the differentiation of purpura from erythematous macules. Diascopy consists of firmly press-

FIGURE 48-1

Common lesions, shown on anterior and posterior views of the patient, encountered during the physical examination of the skin. See also Plates 1 to 6. [From TB Fitzpatrick, DP Johnson, in Dermatology in General Medicine, TB Fitzpatrick et al (eds), New York, McGraw-Hill, 1971.]

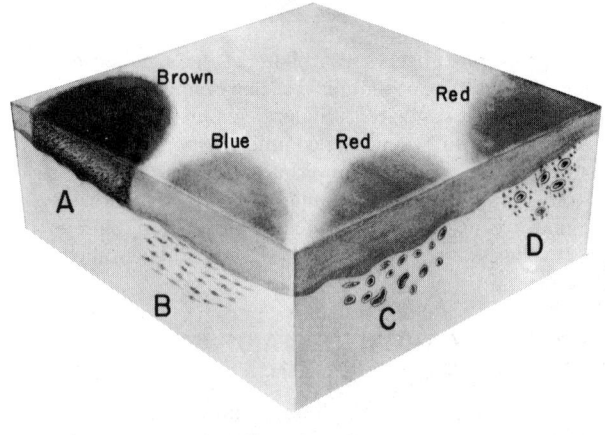

MACULE

FIGURE 48-2

A macule *is a circumscribed area of change in normal skin color without elevation or depression of the surface relative to the surrounding skin. The macules may be of any size and are the result of hypopigmentation (e.g., vitiligo) or hyperpigmentation—melanin (A) or hemosiderin (D)—such as café au lait spots and Mongolian spots (B), or permanent vascular abnormalities of the skin, as in a capillary hemangioma or transient capillary dilation (erythema) (C). Pressure of a glass slide (diascopy) on the border of a red lesion is a simple and reliable method for detecting the extravasation of red blood cells. If the redness remains under the pressure of the slide, the lesion may be purpuric (D); if the redness disappears, the lesion is erythematous and is due to vascular dilation (C).*

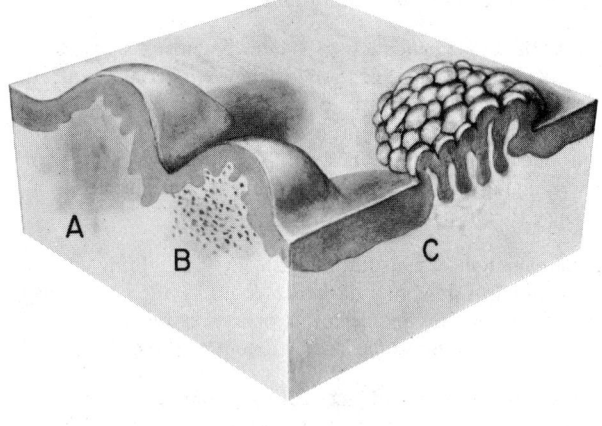

PAPULE

FIGURE 48-3

A papule *is a solid lesion, generally considered as less than 1 cm in diameter. Most of it is elevated above, rather than deep within, the plane of the surrounding skin. The elevation is caused by metabolic deposits (A) in the dermis or by localized infiltrates (B) in the dermis or by localized hyperplasia of cellular elements (C) in the dermis or epidermis. Superficial papules with distinct borders are seen when the lesion is the result of an increase in the number of epidermal cells (C) or melanocytes. Deeper dermal papules resulting from cellular infiltrates have indistinct borders. The topography of a papule or plaque may consist of multiple, small, closely packed, projected elevations that are known as a vegetation (C).*

ULCERS

FIGURE 48-4

An ulcer *is a lesion in which there has been destruction of the epidermis and the upper papillary layer of the dermis. Certain features that are helpful in determining the cause of ulcers include location, borders, base, discharge, and any associated topographic features of the lesions, such as nodules, excoriations, varicosities, hair distribution, presence or absence of sweating, and adjacent pulses.*

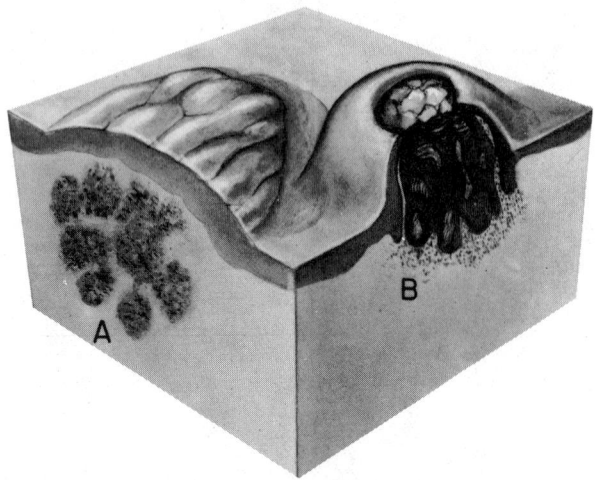

NODULE

FIGURE 48-5

A nodule *is a palpable solid, round, or ellipsoidal lesion deeper than a papule and is in the dermis or subcutaneous tissue (A) or in the epidermis (B). The depth of involvement rather than the diameter primarily differentiates a nodule from a papule. Nodules result from infiltrates (A), neoplasms (B), or metabolic deposits in the dermis or subcutaneous tissue and often indicate systemic disease. Late syphilis, tuberculosis, the deep mycoses, lymphoma, and metastatic neoplasms, e.g., can present as cutaneous nodules. Therefore, biopsy should be performed on unidentified persistent nodules, and a portion of excised tissue should be ground in a sterile mortar and cultured for fungi. Nodules can develop as a result of a benign or malignant proliferation of keratinocytes, as in keratoacanthoma (B), verruca vulgaris, and squamous-cell and basal-cell carcinoma.*

WHEAL

FIGURE 48-6

A wheal *is a rounded or flat-topped, pale-red elevation in the skin that is characteristically evanescent, disappearing within hours. Observation of the borders of wheals that have been traced with a skin-marking pencil reveals that the wheals shift relatively rapidly from the involved to the uninvolved adjacent areas. Wheals are the result of edema in the upper layer of the dermis.*

VESICLE

FIGURE 48-7

A vesicle *(less than 0.5 cm) or a* bulla *(more than 0.5 cm) is a circumscribed elevated lesion containing fluid. Often the walls are so thin that they are translucent, and the serum, lymph fluid, blood, or extracellular fluid can be seen. Vesicles and bullae arise from a cleavage at various levels of the skin; the cleavage may be within the epidermis (i.e., intraepidermal vesication), or at the epidermal-dermal interface (i.e., subepidermal).*

BULLA (A, subcorneal; B, spongiotic)

FIGURE 48-8

When the cleavage is just beneath the stratum corneum, a subcorneal vesicle *or* bulla *results (A), as seen in impetigo and subcorneal pustular dermatosis. Intraepidermal vesication may result from intercellular edema, or* spongiosis *(B), as characteristically seen in delayed hypersensitivity reactions of the epidermis (e.g., in contact eczematous dermatitis), and in dyshidrotic eczema (B).* Spongiotic vesicles *may or may not be seen clinically as vesicles.*

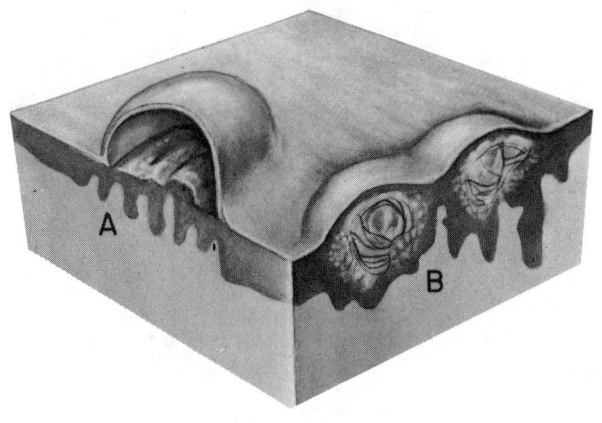

VESICLE (A, acantholytic; B, viral)

FIGURE 48-9

Loss of intercellular bridges, or desmosomes, is known as acantholysis *(A), and this type of intraepidermal vesication is seen in the vesicles or bullae of pemphigus vulgaris; the cleavage is usually just above the basal layer, as in pemphigus vulgaris, but may occur just below the subcorneal layer, as in pemphigus foliaceus. Viruses cause a curious "ballooning degeneration" of epidermal cells (B), as in herpes zoster, herpes simplex, variola, and varicella. Vital bullae often have a depressed ("umbilicated") center.*

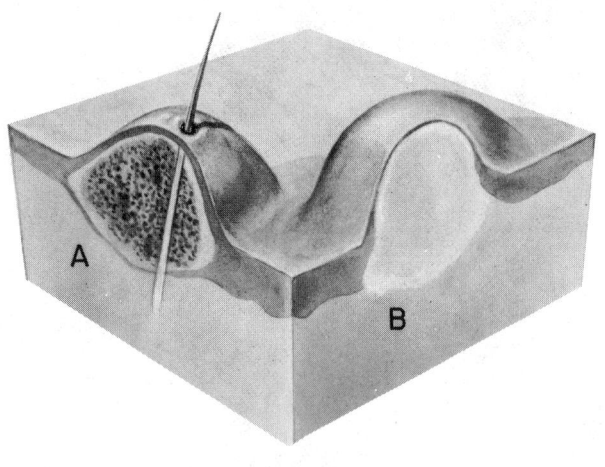

PUSTULE

FIGURE 48-10

A pustule *is a circumscribed elevation of the skin that contains a purulent exudate that may be white, yellow, or greenish yellow. This process may arise in a hair follicle (A) or independently (B). Pustules may vary in size and shape; follicular pustules, however, are always conical and usually contain a hair in the center. The vesicular lesions of the viral diseases (varicella, variola, vaccinia, herpes simplex, and herpes zoster) may secondarily become pustular. A Gram's stain and culture should be done on all pustules.*

PLAQUE

FIGURE 48-11

A plaque *is an elevation above the skin surface that occupies a relatively large surface area in comparison with its height above the skin. Frequently, it is formed by a confluence of papules, as in psoriasis and mycosis fungoides. Lichenification is a proliferation of keratinocytes and stratum corneum forming a plaquelike structure. The skin appears thickened, and the skin markings are accentuated. The process results from repeated rubbing, and frequently develops in persons with atopy. Lichenification occurs in eczematous dermatitis.*

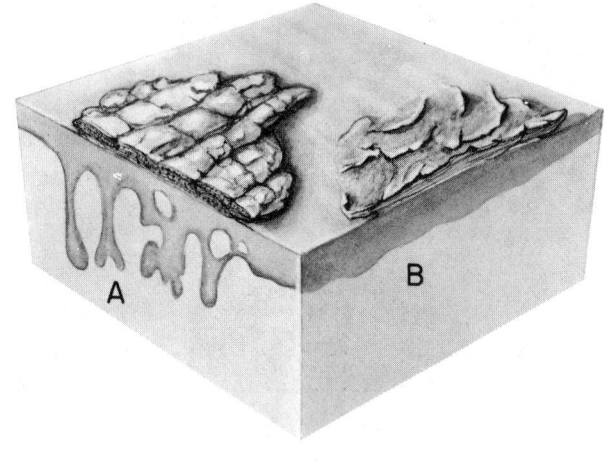

SCALES

FIGURE 48-12

Epidermal cells are completely replaced every 27 days. The end product of this holocrine process is the stratum corneum. This outermost layer of skin, the stratum corneum, normally does not contain nuclei and is imperceptibly lost. With an increased rate of proliferation of epidermal cells, as in psoriasis, the stratum corneum is not formed normally, and the outermost layers of the skin retain the nuclei. These desquamating layers of skin are seen clinically as scales. *Densely adherent scales that have a gritty feel (like sandpaper) result from a localized increase in the stratum corneum and are typically seen in solar keratosis (B).*

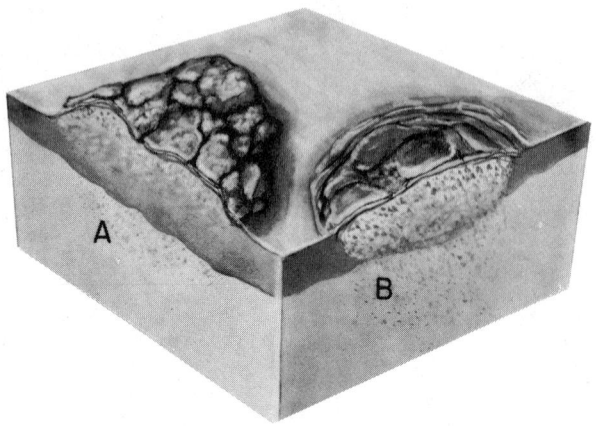

CRUSTS

FIGURE 48-13

Crusts, *resulting when serum, blood, or purulent exudate dries on the skin surface, are the hallmark of pyogenic infection. Crusts may be thin, delicate, and friable (A) or thick and adherent (B). Crusts are yellow when formed from dried serum, green or yellow-green when formed from purulent exudate, or brown or dark red when formed from blood. Superficial crusts occur as honey-colored, delicate, glistening particulates on the surface (A) and are typically seen in impetigo. When the exudate involves the entire epidermis, the crusts may be thick and adherent, and this condition is known as* ecthyma (B).

ing a microscope slide or a piece of clear plastic over the skin lesion; if the lesion is erythematous, the pressure will reveal capillary dilatation rather than an extravasation of blood. Sarcoidosis, lymphoma, and tuberculosis of the skin are suggested if diascopy of the nodules shows either a characteristic hyaline, yellowish brown, or an "apple-jelly" appearance.

Long-wave ultraviolet light, or Wood's lamp Long-wave ultraviolet light (360 nm), or Wood's lamp, is a necessary source of illumination for examination of the skin. Wood's lamp consists of a high-pressure mercury arc lamp with a specially compounded glass filter made of nickel oxide and silica (Wood's filter). This filter permits the passage of a band of radiation of 360 nm, which will reveal fluorescence when light passed through the filter impinges upon certain structures.

Wood's lamp is important for the detection of the pinkish red fluorescence of the urine of patients with porphyria cutanea tarda; the addition of 5% hydrochloric acid greatly intensifies the fluorescence, owing to the oxidation of porphyrin precursors to porphyrins.

Wood's lamp is also a great help in estimating variation in the pigmentation of the skin; it reveals both increased and decreased pigmentation. Inasmuch as melanin is a universal absorber of ultraviolet light, areas of increased melanin will show an increased intensity under Wood's lamp; conversely, areas of decreased melanin will show a decrease in intensity (or an increased reflection) because the ultraviolet light is not absorbed. In this respect, Wood's lamp may be the only means of recognizing the sometimes indistinguishable hypomelanotic macules in tuberous sclerosis, a dominantly inherited trait associated with mental retardation and seizures. The white spots are present at birth and remain throughout life, and therefore represent important markers of this serious genetic disorder. The Wood's lamp can be used in mass screening for detection of the fluorescence of dermatophytosis *in the hair shaft* in ringworm of the scalp.

CLINICAL TESTS Patch testing Patch testing is primarily used by dermatologists to detect contact sensitivity. The contactants are listed in Fisher's 1973 monograph on the subject.

Darier's sign One very useful clinical response of the skin, Darier's sign, is used as a test for urticaria pigmentosa, and is evoked by the vigorous rubbing of a pigmented macule with the blunt end of a pen. In urticaria pigmentosa (mastocytosis), a palpable red wheal occurs within a few minutes after the physical trauma, owing to the release of histamine by the mast cells in the skin.

LABORATORY PROCEDURES Examination for bacteria in crusts and biopsy specimens Gram's stains and bacterial cultures of exudates should be performed on all lesions consisting of crusts and purulent exudates. Ulcers and nodules should be biopsied by removal of a wedge of tissue that extends from the surface down to the subcutaneous fat. The biopsy specimen should be minced in a sterile mortar and cultured for bacteria (including typical and atypical mycobacteria) and fungi.

Examination for mycelia The presence of mycelia may be ascertained by the application of 10% potassium hydroxide to a single tiny portion of scale, which is then gently heated. For fungi and yeasts, scales and hair should be cultured on Sabouraud's medium.

Tzanck test The Tzanck test, or the microscopic examination of cells from the base of vesicles, determines the presence of giant epithelial cells and multinucleated giant cells that occur in herpes simplex, herpes zoster, and varicella. Material taken from the base of a vesicle by gentle curettage with a scalpel is

spread gently on a glass slide and prepared with Giemsa's or Wright's stain for the examination.

Dark-field examination of serum for *Treponema pallidum* Dark-field examination of serum from ulcers and erosions on the male and female genitalia is essential for the detection of *Treponema pallidum*. Dark-field examination of material obtained from the oral cavity is not diagnostic because of the presence of nonpathogenic treponemas that are indistinguishable from *T. pallidum*.

BIOPSY Microscopic examination of tissue is particularly applicable in dermatology because biopsies of the lesions can be easily obtained. Although the classic method is an elliptical incision followed by suturing, a satisfactory method for diagnostic purposes is "punch" biopsy. Biopsy of the skin enables correlation of gross and microscopic pathology. For punch biopsy, a small, 3.0- to 4.0-nm, disposable tubular blade is rotated between the thumb and index finger to cut through the entire thickness of the abnormal skin; the resulting cylinder of

TABLE 48-2
Approach to dermatologic diagnosis

I Initial clinical impression.
II Physical examination.
  A Detailed examination of skin, hair, nails, and mucous membranes, including transillumination and disascopy.

> Seven cardinal signs:
> *1* Type of lesion: macule, papule, nodule, vesicle, etc.?
> *2* Color:
>   *a* If diffuse: red, brown, gray-blue, white, purple, orange-yellow?
>   *b* If circumscribed: red, orange, yellow, brown, blue or white? (Use Wood's lamp.)
>   *c* Does color blanch with diascopy?
> *3* Palpation of lesion: soft, doughy, firm, hard, "infiltrated," dry, moist, change in temperature?
> *4* Shape of individual lesion: round, oval, ash-leaf, annular, iris, arciform, linear, umbilicated?
> *5* Arrangement of multiple lesions: isolated, grouped, herpetiform, zosteriform, annular, arciform, linear, reticular?
> *6* Distribution (examine scalp and mouth):
>   *a* Extent of involvement: circumscribed, regional, generalized, universal?
>   *b* Pattern and location: symmetry, exposed areas, sites of pressure, intertriginous areas?
>   *c* Characteristic patterns: scabies, secondary syphilis, erythema multiforme, psoriasis, seborrheic dermatitis, atopic dermatitis, lichen planus, pityriasis rosea, dermatitis herpetiformis?
> *7* Morphologic component of skin primarily affected (see Table 48-3).

  B Does the patient appear ill?
  C Examination for lymphadenopathy and hepatosplenomegaly.
III History of skin lesions and system review as indicated by differential diagnosis. Two key questions:
  A How long?
  B Does it itch?
IV Laboratory procedures.
  A Special.
    1 Material (crusts, scales, or exudate) for Gram's stain for bacteria and KOH preparation for yeast or fungi.
    2 If vesicle, direct smear of base for giant cells (herpes simplex or varicella zoster).
    3 Biopsy: for an inflammatory nodule, obtain tissue for mycologic and bacterial culture.
    4 Wood's lamp examination of urine for porphyrins, and of hair for fluorescence.
    5 Hematologic, chemical, urine, serologic, and roentgenologic studies.
    6 Reexamination over *time* and a biopsy of the skin may be required for definitive diagnosis.
  B General.
V Final diagnosis.

SOURCE: *TB Fitzpatrick, in Dermatology in General Medicine, 2d ed, TB Fitzpatrick et al (eds), New York, McGraw-Hill, 1979.*

TABLE 48-3
Clinical classification of skin lesions and syndromes according to the component of the skin primarily involved

I Epidermis (keratinocytes and melanocytes)
  A Keratinocytes
    1 Scaling macules, papules, or plaques
    2 Vesicles and bullae
    3 Pustules
    4 Exudative (impetiginized) lesions
    5 Eczematous dermatitis
    6 Erythroderma syndrome (exfoliative dermatitis)*
    7 Atrophy, diffuse* or circumscribed
  B Melanocytes
    1 Hypomelanotic macules
    2 Diffuse hypomelanosis*
    3 Hypermelanotic (brown) macules
    4 Diffuse brown hypermelanosis*
II Dermis (connective tissue and blood vessels)
  A Connective tissue component
    1 Papules and nodules (with and without inflammation)
    2 Ulcers
    3 Sclerosis, diffuse* or circumscribed
    4 Edema*
    5 Atrophy, diffuse* or circumscribed
  B Blood vessels
    1 Morbilliform and scarlatiniform eruptions
    2 Urticarial syndromes
    3 Erythema multiforme syndrome
    4 Purpura (with and without inflammation)
    5 Infarcts
    6 Telangiectasia
III Panniculus adiposus (connective tissue and blood vessels)
  A Connective tissue component
    1 Nodules, noninflammatory, usually nontender
    2 Atrophy
  B Blood vessels
    1 Nodules, inflammatory, usually tender and red
     a Erythema nodosum syndrome

* *Pathologic changes affect large areas of skin, and there are no discrete, circumscribed lesions.*
SOURCE: *TB Fitzpatrick, in Dermatology in General Medicine, 2d ed, TB Fitzpatrick et al (eds), New York, McGraw-Hill, 1979.*

skin is then lifted out with forceps, and the skin is cut off at its base with a pointed scissors. This simple operation is done under local anesthesia, and the bleeding can be stopped by the use of pressure or absorbable foam; suturing is not usually necessary. This technique is as harmless and simple as a venipuncture, and supplies enough tissue to permit a definitive histologic diagnosis in most cases.

APPROACH TO DIAGNOSIS In Tables 48-2 and 48-3 an orderly sequence is suggested as a method of establishing a diagnosis in a patient presenting with skin lesions.

REFERENCES

FISHER AA: *Contact Dermatitis.* Philadelphia, Lea & Febiger, 1973
FITZPATRICK TB et al (eds): *Dermatology in General Medicine,* 2d ed. New York, McGraw-Hill, 1979
ROOK A, WILKINSON DS: The principles of diagnosis, in *Textbook of Dermatology,* A Rook et al (eds). Oxford, Blackwell Scientific Publications, 1972, p 37

49
SKIN LESIONS OF GENERAL MEDICAL SIGNIFICANCE

THOMAS B. FITZPATRICK
HARLEY A. HAYNES

The skin is one of the best indicators of serious disease; even an untrained eye can recognize the ashen pallor of shock, or cyanosis, or jaundice. The competent physician must be able to detect the subtle skin signs of life-threatening diseases and the skin clues to diseases in other organs. Skin lesions are frequently critical in the final resolution of puzzling diagnostic medical problems.

The skin (Fig. 49-1) is composed of three layers: (1) the *epidermis,* the outermost part, which consists of two main cell types, keratinocytes and melanocytes; (2) the *dermis,* upon which the epidermis rests, which is composed of a mélange of connective tissue elements, nerves, blood and lymph vessels, glands, appendages, and a few cells (mast cells, histiocytes); and (3) the *panniculus adiposus* (subcutaneous tissue), which acts as a cushion between the epidermis and dermis and the underlying bone. The specialized cells of the epidermis, the keratinocytes, produce and retain in their cytoplasm the scleroprotein keratin. They are constantly turning over, about 27 days being required to complete differentiation and maturation. Maturation of keratinocytes consists of loss of the nucleus, leaving only the cytoplasm. The latter is made up of a highly ordered, two-phase system of keratin filaments embedded in an amorphous matrix, much like the cellulose-lignin system of wood fiber, which is known to be well adapted to withstand shearing and compression forces. The anucleate outermost portion of the epidermis is the *stratum corneum,* which acts as a tough, keratinous membrane. The stratum corneum functions structurally as a "waterproof" wall between the internal fluid milieu and the environment, and is the major barrier of the skin, protecting the body against loss of fluids and entrance of toxic agents. It also serves as a passive membrane—substances move across the skin by passive diffusion in the direction of the concentration gradient.

The skin has a relatively limited number of pathologic responses. If the letters of the alphabet are taken to represent individual skin lesions (see Table 48-1), then words or phrases can be said to represent groups of lesions. The lesions in the majority of patients seen by the general physician can be classified in one of the groups of clinical reactions (see Table 48-3) or types of skin lesions listed in Table 48-1. These skin lesions

FIGURE 49-1

Anatomy of the skin. (Copyright 1967 CIBA Pharmaceutical Company, division of CIBA-Geigy Corporation. Reproduced, with permission from the Clinical Symposia, illustrated by Frank H. Netter, M.D. All rights reserved.)

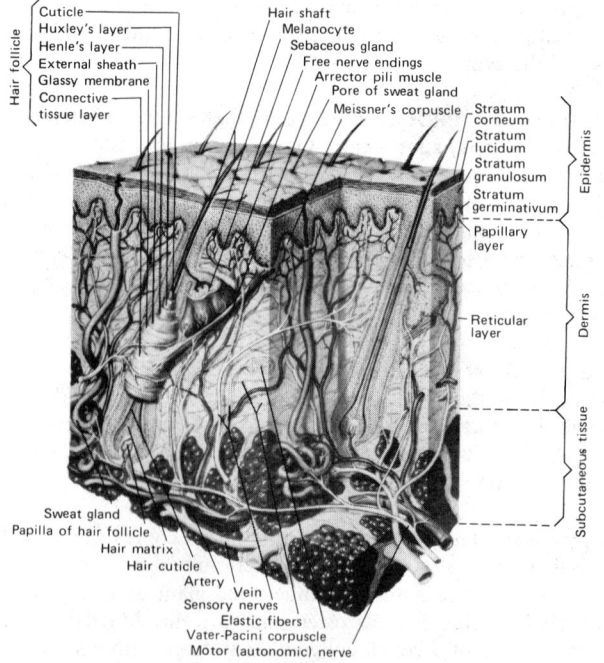

or clinical reactions may consist of one type of lesion, such as a vesicle or a nodule, or aggregates of various types of lesions, such as papules or vesicles, as in erythema multiforme. Just one lesion or several solitary lesions or one or more groups of lesions may be distributed any place on the body. A pathologic process may involve the skin in the form of isolated lesions, as just mentioned, or the pathologic process may involve all the skin so that the borders of the lesions may not be defined; this latter type of diffuse involvement occurs in systemic sclerosis and in pigmentation disorders.

In the physician's attempts to identify the specific types of lesions, it is therefore essential to try to estimate the component of the skin that is *primarily* affected, as the epidermis, the dermis, the blood vessels, or the panniculus adiposus. Inasmuch as there are a finite number of disorders that produce pathologic changes in the various individual components, this method of approach will improve the physician's diagnostic acumen. For example, even though erythema multiforme involves the dermis and the epidermis, the *primary component* affected is the blood vessel, and it is this involvement that explains the erythematous macules; the inflammatory process leads subsequently to the development of the cellular infiltrates seen clinically as papules and to destruction of the basement membrane and the development of bullae.

CLASSIFICATION OF LESIONS ACCORDING TO THE COMPONENT OF THE SKIN PRIMARILY AFFECTED

EPIDERMIS **Scaling macules, papules, or plaques** Generalized scaling macules, papules, or plaques are frequent and important diagnostic problems and are usually a presenting complaint of the patient (see Figs. 48-2, 48-3, and 48-11).

Sudden onset of symmetrical, scaling, erythematous macules or papules should suggest that drugs are the etiologic agents. Scaling erythematous papules on the scalp and extensor aspects of the arms and legs are suggestive of *psoriasis;* psoriatic lesions often are accentuated on the sites of repeated trauma, such as the elbows and knees. The papules or plaques of psoriasis often contain a silvery white micaceous scale that is relatively easily removed in layers (see Plate 2-6). In psoriasis, there is a severalfold increase in the normal number of the basal cells of the epidermis. This increase in the basal cell population reduces the turnover time of the epidermis from the normal 27 days to 3 to 4 days. With this shortened interval of epidermal cell migration from the basal layer to the skin surface, the normal events of cell maturation and keratinization do not occur (see A in Fig. 48-12); this failure of maturation is reflected by an array of abnormal morphologic and biochemical changes. In association with the basal cell hyperplasia, there is enhanced metabolism and accelerated synthesis and degradation of nucleoproteins, resulting in an elevated urinary excretion of nucleic acid metabolites such as uric acid. In addition, there is a proliferation of the subepidermal vasculature that is necessary to support the increased rate of cell division. These numerous cytologic, histologic, histochemical, and biochemical alterations are now known to be the result, rather than the cause, of the disease process. The only main fact known at this time about the fundamental cause of psoriasis is that the predisposition to its development is genetically transmitted. An erosive joint disease, *psoriatic arthritis,* is discussed in Chap. 358.

The treatment of psoriasis still remains the province of the dermatologist. The most effective treatment in the control of localized psoriasis, for most patients, is the use of topical corticosteroids with plastic wrap, topical coal-tar preparations, and ultraviolet light or sunlight exposures. Corticosteroids can also be injected directly into small, resistant plaques. Systemic corticosteroids not only are ineffective in psoriasis but may cause

generalization of the process and are absolutely contraindicated. With certain patients who are resistant to topical therapy, it has been necessary to use a variety of systemic chemotherapeutic agents, especially methotrexate; the latter has the capacity to inhibit cell replication without a proportionate inhibition of cell function, i.e., keratinization. In 1974, a new form of photochemotherapy was introduced which uses oral methoxsalen and a high-intensity, long-wave ultraviolet light source. This approach may replace many of the other forms of therapy.

In this so-called "PUVA" treatment, psoralen (P) is administered by mouth 2 h before total-body irradiation with a special light system that emits predominantly long-wave (320- to 400-nm) ultraviolet light (UV-A). The light alone is ineffective in producing erythema or remission of psoriatic lesions; however, in the presence of one of the psoralens (methoxsalen) the UV-A becomes a potent photoactive agent and produces an erythematous response and a remission of psoriatic lesions after several exposures. The mechanism of action is probably related in part to the binding of psoralen to DNA by the action of UV-A. Large, multicenter, clinical trials involving over 3000 patients have shown that oral methoxsalen photochemotherapy is highly effective in the control of severe psoriasis; in over 80 percent of such patients the psoriasis completely cleared in 3 to 4 weeks of treatment using two or three exposures per week. After clearing, the patients were given maintenance exposures once per week or less frequently. While methoxsalen photochemotherapy is effective, it requires specialized knowledge and lighting systems, delivering precise measured amounts of UV-A. Therefore, the treatment is available at present in only a few hundred centers in the United States and Europe, and PUVA treatment is recommended only for patients with disabling psoriasis because long-term sequelae will not be known for a decade; such adverse effects could include skin cancers, skin aging, and cataracts.

The general physician does not always appreciate the impact of psoriasis as a major cause of disability and of disfigurement. Psoriasis affects between 2 and 8 million persons in the United States.

Psoriasiform lesions occurring on the face, lower abdomen, buttocks, groin, perineum, and legs occur in *glucagonoma syndrome.* The lesions may be almost indistinguishable from subacute psoriasis, but often they have necrosis in the center of the plaques; also stomatitis, anemia, and marked weight loss are present. Hyperglycemia may or may not be present. The eruption disappears rapidly on removal of the glucagon-secreting tumor of the pancreas.

Symmetrical scaling macules or papules localized on the palms and soles often are presenting signs of *secondary syphilis;* very frequently there is generalized lymphadenopathy and there may be mouth lesions occurring as erosions.

A relatively common and often baffling generalized scaling eruption is seen in *pityriasis rosea.* In this condition, the scale at the periphery of the lesion is very thin and forms a collarette; the center of the lesion may or may not be scaly. Pityriasis rosea typically has a "fir-tree" type of distribution, especially evident on the back. Very often, but not always, a preceding, single, isolated scaling lesion is present for several days before generalization of the lesions.

Scaling macules and papules are seen in *dermatophytosis* (Plate 2-1) and *candidiasis,* and it is therefore necessary that some of the scales be examined for the presence of mycelia (see "Laboratory Procedures" in Chap. 48).

From the clinician's point of view, *mycotic infections of the skin* may be separated into two major categories, each of which has a different etiology, associated systemic disease, and response to treatment, with only one category responding to the oral antifungal, griseofulvin.

The various types of *dermatophytosis* (so-called "ringworm" infections) constitute one category, and all (except tinea versicolor) respond to oral griseofulvin and are confined to the epidermis, hair, toenails, and fingernails. Dermatophytosis is due to three types of fungus: *Microsporum, Epidermophyton,* and *Trichophyton. Microsporum audouini,* a parasite of humans, is the principal pathogen causing epidemic urban fungous infection of the scalp. *Microsporum canis,* which affects the scalp and also the face, where it causes boggy nodules, is a parasite of animals and originates largely from young (usually) farm animals and pets (kittens, puppies, and calves). *Trichophyton rubrum, T. mentagrophytes,* and *E. floccosum,* which also are parasites of humans, are the agents usually causing dermatophytosis of the feet, the most common site of mycotic infection. The type of fungus infecting upper extremities, face, and trunk can be *Trichophyton* or *Microsporum* or *Epidermophyton.*

Inasmuch as *Trichophyton, Microsporum,* and *Epidermophyton* are parasites in humans, factors other than mere contact might be implicated. Variation in the host response, for instance, based on hereditary factors and mediated, possibly, through increased susceptibility or related to immune factors, has yet to be clearly defined.

The response of these three types of fungus to oral griseofulvin varies. Griseofulvin is effective, even in short courses, in fungous infection of the scalp, trunk, and groin, but even prolonged therapy rarely controls infection of the hands, fingernails, or toenails. Topical treatment with any of the antifungals is quite effective in infection of the feet, trunk, and groin, but is ineffective for infections of the fingernails or toenails.

The other major category of mycotic infections is represented by candidiasis (monilial infections). These infections do not respond at all to oral griseofulvin and are caused chiefly by *Candida albicans,* although occasionally by *C. tropicalis, C. krusei,* and *C. stellatoidea. C. albicans* can exist as a harmless saprophyte in the gastrointestinal tract and in the vagina. It is more common in females, and is most often present in those who are pregnant or who are taking oral contraceptives or broad-spectrum antibiotics. The association with diabetes mellitus, however, is so common that all patients (regardless of sex) with candidiasis should be screened for this disease.

Despite the fact that *C. albicans* is a normal saprophytic fungus in the vagina and gastrointestinal tract, it is rarely isolated from the exposed surface of the normal skin. *C. albicans* can invade the epidermis when the skin is exposed to high humidity and when the skin becomes macerated; therefore, candidiasis commonly occurs in the intertriginous areas (under the breasts and in the umbilicus, groin, and axillae) and in the oral, as well as the vaginal, mucous membranes. Chronic paronychia is usually caused by *C. albicans.* Candidiasis also may involve the lungs, urinary tract, and heart (see Chap. 158).

The treatment of candidiasis of the skin and mucous membranes depends on the site of the infection and the type of lesion. Maceration of the skin should be treated by air-drying of the area. Lotions and dusting powders containing nystatin are also very useful for intertriginous areas. Oral administration of nystatin is not of value in cutaneous moniliasis. Unless the sexual partner is treated when candidiasis is present, there will be constant retransfer of the infection. For monilial paronychia, 2% alcohol solutions of gentian violet are still the best treatment.

Differentiation between dermatophytosis caused by any of the three types of fungus already mentioned and candidiasis may be difficult, if not impossible, without cultures of the fungus. Direct examination of the scales from a scaling eruption in the intertriginous area is not diagnostic because it may reveal mycelia in both dermatophytosis and candidiasis; spores, however, are seen only in candidiasis. Too often, the general physician starts treatment with topical antifungal agents or with griseofulvin without establishing whether the eruption is a type of dermatophytosis or candidiasis. Inasmuch as candidiasis does not respond to systemic griseofulvin or to most of the topical antifungal agents, prescribing these agents for an eruption that is actually candidiasis results in prolonged disability for the patient. Newer agents such as haloprogin and miconazole are effective against both dermatophytosis and candidiasis.

In the past few years, fungous diseases have assumed a new significance in medicine because of the increased number of patients under treatment with chemotherapeutic agents for leukemia and other neoplasms. Almost all of the saprophytic fungi are now known to invade the tissues of patients who are being treated with chemotherapeutic agents or who have had kidney transplants.

Vesicles and bullae Some diseases may occasionally be associated with vesicles or bullae, such as erythema multiforme or porphyria cutanea tarda, but blisters (vesicles and bullae) are the major feature of a number of disorders: certain bacterial and viral infections; allergic contact dermatitis (such as poison ivy); trauma from mechanical, thermal, or chemical agents; and most important, the bullous diseases of unknown cause (such as pemphigus and pemphigoid).

Grouped vesicles occur in herpes zoster and herpes simplex, whereas scattered, discrete vesicles occur in varicella. A helpful sign in determining the nautre of the vesicles is the Tzanck test (see "Laboratory Procedures" in Chap. 48). In herpes simplex, herpes zoster, and varicella, there will be clusters of epithelial giant cells, which are absent in vaccinia and variola. Skin biopsy will also establish the nature of the vesicle or bulla; that is, whether it is an intraepidermal (as seen in virus infections and pemphigus) or a subepidermal bulla (as seen in bullous pemphigoid) (see Figs. 48-7 to 48-9).

Vesicles arranged in linear streaks are characteristic of poison ivy dermatitis. The most reliable clue to the diagnosis of both allergic and primary-irritant contact dermatitis is the localization of vesicles to the skin areas likely to have been exposed to the agent in question. Isolated vesicles and bullae on the pressure areas of the dorsa of the hands and the face may be the only sign of porphyria cutanea tarda; the diagnosis is immediately confirmed by examination of the urine, using the Wood's lamp. These patients do not present with photosensitivity.

Scattered, isolated bullae in adults represent a special and serious problem in diagnosis and treatment. *Bullous pemphigoid* and *pemphigus* are chronic and occur primarily in adults; one of them, pemphigus, has serious consequences for the patient. These two disorders need to be distinguished by biopsy of the skin and by the newly available immunofluorescence techniques. It is impossible on the basis of clinical diagnosis alone to distinguish between bullous pemphigoid, which is a chronic and relatively benign disorder and often of limited duration, and *pemphigus vulgaris,* which is a serious disease leading in a relentless course to death, unless treatment with immunosuppressive agents or steroids is instituted. Pemphigus has been divided into four separate entities, but pemphigus vulgaris is the most important for the general physician to recognize. Pemphigus vulgaris may begin in the nasal or oral mucous membrane, and the patient may consult the dentist or otolaryngologist first for persistent erosions of the larynx (hoarseness), the mouth, or a bloody nasal discharge. The lesions tend to involve in an unpredictable fashion other parts of the body, but localize chiefly on the umbilicus, scalp, and trunk, although there is no specific distribution pattern. Pemphigus vulgaris affects primarily the middle-aged, particularly between the ages of 40 and 60. It rarely occurs before the age of 17 or after the age of 75. The clinical lesions appear as flaccid bullae from the beginning; they break easily and rarely become very large. The denuded areas that form at the site of the ruptured bullae increase in size as the epidermis detaches itself. Occasionally, almost the entire surface may be involved by large, denuded areas; this involvement represents a serious problem in the management of secondary infection and in maintenance of fluid balance—more or less the same problems that occur in a severely burned patient. Oral or nasal mucosal lesions occur in nearly all the patients, and more than half have lesions in the mucous membrane of the mouth as the first manifestation of the disease. The disease often starts with only a few lesions in the mouth and may remain limited in extent for several weeks; it then gradually spreads to other parts of the body.

The diagnosis of pemphigus is made on the basis of the light-microscopic examination of the biopsy of an early vesicle. The earliest change in pemphigus vulgaris consists of intercellular edema followed by disappearance of intercellular bridges in the lower epidermis (see A in Fig. 48-9). This results in loss of cohesion between the epidermal cells (acantholysis) and leads to the formation of clefts and then bullae that are predominantly in the suprabasal locations; in other words, the basal cells, although separated from one another, remain attached to the dermis much like a "row of tombstones."

Immunofluorescence allows detection of IgG antibodies specific for an intercellular substance of the skin and mucosa in the serum of patients with pemphigus, and makes possible a differentiation of pemphigus and pemphigoid by the localization of the antibody. The antibodies, which are in the IgG fraction of serum, react with a specific intercellular antigen. The fluorescence is localized precisely to the site of acantholysis in pemphigus; IgG is confined to the glycocalyx of epidermal cells. In bullous pemphigoid, however, the antibodies react with the basement membrane, and the fluorescence is localized there.

Treatment of pemphigus with systemic corticosteroids, sometimes in combination with azathioprine, is quite successful. Azathioprine alone can control the disease in some patients.

Pustules This skin reaction (see Fig. 48-10) may result from infections or from sterile inflammation. Pustules may arise from preexisting vesicles of any etiology. Infection by pyogenic bacteria, especially staphylococci, as well as by certain fungi and mycobacteria, can produce pustules without a preceding vesicular stage. Noninfectious causes of pustules include acne, pustular psoriasis, and hypersensitivity to drugs, particularly sulfonamides, iodides, or bromides.

Exudative (impetiginized) lesions Acute infection with grampositive cocci can occur as a primary process or may be superimposed on eczematous dermatitis or occasionally on any of the vesicular bullous diseases, and is characterized by the presence of crusts (see Fig. 48-13). Such infection on the skin has the same implications as a streptococcal pharyngitis, inasmuch as acute glomerular nephritis develops in a significant percentage of patients with impetiginized dermatitis. Patients with impetiginized dermatitis must be treated with full courses of systemic antibiotics.

Eczematous dermatitis Eczematous dermatitis (Plates 2-2 and 5-6) is not a specific disease entity but a characteristic inflammatory response of the skin due to both endogenous and exogenous agents that cause a delayed hypersensitivity reaction. Eczematous dermatitis therefore requires a qualifying etiologic term, e.g., *atopic eczematous dermatitis*. Eczematous dermatitis is sufficiently serious to account for the highest incidence of

skin disease, being responsible for incalculable losses of time and productivity in industry; approximately one-third of all patients in the United States seen by dermatologists have eczema. In Tables 49-1 and 49-2 some of the types of eczematous dermatitis are summarized (see also B in Fig. 48-8 and Fig. 48-11). For the general physician, atopic eczematous dermatitis is the most important disease of this group of disorders. Over 30 percent of patients develop respiratory allergic manifestations. Furthermore, the disease may persist for 15 to 20 years. Cataracts develop in 15 percent of young patients. Finally, patients with atopic eczematous dermatitis are susceptible to infections with herpes simplex and vaccinia. The majority of patients with severe atopic eczematous dermatitis have elevated serum levels of IgE. The control of the intractable pruritus in this disease is difficult, and best results are obtained by judicious use of topical corticosteroids, tar gels, oil baths, lubrication with emollients, and limitation of emotional stress.

Erythroderma syndrome (exfoliative dermatitis) The erythroderma syndrome is an important dermatologic complication that may occur as the result of an extension of a drug reaction, as a generalized spreading of a preexisting dermatitis, such as psoriasis or atopic dermatitis, or in association with lymphoma and leukemia. This syndrome consists of a generalized, erythematous, scaling eruption involving all of the skin surface, and has important implications in general medicine because of the systemic effects occasioned by the massive and continuous exfoliation of the skin. The severity of the metabolic response to exfoliation depends on the duration and severity of the process itself. Patients with extensive exfoliative dermatitis may have negative nitrogen balance, edema, hypoalbuminemia, and loss of muscle mass. Another salient feature in these patients is the large extrarenal water loss, due to the defective cutaneous barrier that leads to markedly increased transepidermal water loss. Serious metabolic effects of chronic exfoliative dermatitis occur when the rate of scaling reaches 17 g/m^2 per 24 h. The etiology of exfoliative dermatitis determines its course: the disease eventually clears in patients with psoriasis or atopic dermatitis, whereas the prognosis is relatively poor in patients with lymphoma and leukemia. Approximately 60 percent of patients with exfoliative dermatitis recover within 8 to 10 months, 30 percent die, and 10 percent have a persistent problem unresponsive to therapy.

Atrophy, diffuse or circumscribed Epidermal atrophy is manifested by an almost transparent epidermis and is associated with a decrease in the number of epidermal cells. An atrophic epidermis may or may not retain the normal skin markings. Circumscribed epidermal atrophy occurs in discoid lupus erythematosus, in necrobiosis lipoidica diabeticorum, and in striae cutis distensae; diffuse epidermal atrophy occurs with aging and in scleroderma.

The most important atrophic-type disorder is *necrobiosis lipoidica diabeticorum* (NLD) (Plate 5-1). These lesions, which are usually asymptomatic, occur more frequently in women and *on the areas subject to trauma* such as the anterior and lateral surfaces of the lower legs. Lesions may also occur on the arms and even on the face. The lesion begins as a small, reddish, elevated nodule with a sharply circumscribed border, gradually enlarges, and becomes flattened and depressed as the skin becomes atrophic. The brownish yellow color is prominent, and blood vessels are readily seen because of the atrophic epidermis that is smooth and loses its skin markings entirely. The lesions of NLD are extremely indolent, and shallow ulcerations that are very slow to heal may develop. NLD may apparently occur when diabetes mellitus cannot be detected, but in these patients full tests of glucose tolerance, such as the cortisone-glucose tolerance test, have not been done. It is characterized by focal changes in the dermis that present as acellular and intense eosinophilic areas of necrosis bordered by inflammation. The inflammatory cells are granulomatous and include epithelioid cells, histiocytes, and multinucleated giant cells. The blood vessels are always involved, with endothelial proliferation and sometimes even occlusion of the arterioles and arteries deep within the dermis; the capillary walls are thickened with focal deposits of PAS-positive material. NLD can be controlled with intralesional injections of suspensions of triamcinolone acetonide in some patients.

Hypomelanotic macules   See Chap. 51.

Diffuse hypomelanosis   See Chap. 51.

Hypermelanotic macules   See Chap. 51.

Diffuse brown hypermelanosis syndrome   See Chap. 51.

DERMIS   Papules and nodules (with and without inflammation)
Papules and nodules without epidermal change (i.e., scaling) may be either skin color, erythematous, or even slightly pigmented (yellow or brown). Dermal papules and all nodules require a biopsy for definitive diagnosis because they often represent either processes that have general medical significance, such as sarcoidosis or histiocytosis X, or tuberculosis or lymphoma. Inasmuch as dermal nodules may be present in deep mycotic infections such as coccidioidomycosis, it is necessary to obtain a biopsy, not only to rule out malignancy but to culture a portion of the excised tissue for fungi. Cultures of nodules must be made from minced tissue. The histologic specimen should be carefully studied for the presence of acid-fast bacilli, since nodules are the presenting feature of leprosy

or tuberculosis; nodules removed from the common areas of localization for leishmaniasis (face and arms) should be carefully examined for the presence of parasites.

Papules and nodules with and without inflammation can occur in disorders of the sebaceous glands. Sebaceous glands are distributed largely on the face and scalp, although they can also occur in the labia minora and on the scrotal skin, trunk, nipples, and eyelids. The sebaceous gland is a holocrine gland in which the entire cell is cast off into the excretory stream. Sebum is a complex lipid mixture of squalene (a major product of the steroid pathway), triglycerides, and wax ester. Sebaceous glands are controlled by direct hormonal stimulation with androgens, derived largely from the gonads in both sexes; in the female, but not in the male, adrenal androgens may be important factors in maintaining sebum production. The major disease of the sebaceous gland in humans is *acne vulgaris* (Plate 1-5), which occurs predominantly on the face and, to a lesser degree, on the back, chest, and shoulders. It is characterized by a variety of clinical lesions. These lesions may be either noninflammatory or inflammatory papules and nodules. The noninflammatory papules are called comedones, and these may be either open (blackheads) or closed (whiteheads). The closed comedones are the precursors of large inflammatory nodules and of papules and pustules. In addition, cysts and scars of various sizes may occur, the typical acne scar being a sharply punched-out pit. In the pustular and cystic lesions, despite a large amount of purulent exudate that may be recovered following incision, the lesions are usually sterile but may contain *Propionibacterium acnes*. It is believed that acne develops as a result of a primary inflammation in the follicle wall, and that the follicle partly ruptures, leading to a spilling out of its components and the development of a perifollicular inflammatory process. The inflammatory infiltrate is lymphocytic, but later, as a result of the presence of keratinous material, gram-positive diphtheroids, and sebum, the infiltrate consists essentially of a foreign-body giant-cell reaction.

The initial stimulus to the formation of comedones (both

TABLE 49-1
Various types of eczematous dermatitis* of uncertain etiology

Clinical type	Suspected pathogenesis	Diagnostic considerations
Atopic eczematous dermatitis	Hereditary predisposition plus precipitating factors	Eczematous dermatitis, especially localized to the antecubital and popliteal fossae and to the face
Lichen simplex chronicus	Hereditary predisposition plus repeated local trauma	One or more lichenified plaques (see Fig. 48-11), especially on neck
Prurigo nodularis	Repeated local trauma	One or more nodules, especially on extremities
"Neurodermatitis"	Hereditary predisposition plus repeated scratching	Generalized or localized eczematous eruption at sites of repeated trauma
Stasis dermatitis	Chronic venous insufficiency	Signs of venous insufficiency
Nummular eczematous dermatitis	Various precipitating factors (contact irritants, xerosis, emotional stress, etc.)	Discrete coin-shaped patches, usually on extremities and trunk
"Dyshidrotic" eczematous dermatitis	Emotional stress plus other factors‡	Vesicles and bullae on palms and soles
Seborrheic dermatitis	Constitutional diathesis	Greasy scaling patches on scalp, eyebrows, and nasolabial area
Various patterns of eczematous dermatitis	Association with gastrointestinal malabsorption	Eczematous eruption in patient with steatorrhea and abnormal biopsy specimens of the jejunal mucosa
"Eczematous-like eruptions"† with systemic disease: Wiskott-Aldrich syndrome X-linked agammaglobulinemia Phenylketonuria Ahistidinemia Hurler's syndrome Hartnup disease Acrodermatitis enteropathica	Metabolic and immunologic disorders	Related features of clinical syndrome plus immunologic deficiency or biochemical abnormality

* This term is used by many clinicians for at least four types of eczematous dermatitis that may be exclusively localized to the hands (atopic eczematous dermatitis, allergic contact eczematous dermatitis, nummular eczematous dermatitis, and "dyshidrotic" eczematous dermatitis). Possibly, contact irritants to which the hands are frequently exposed may precipitate or aggravate one of the above-mentioned basic types of eczematous dermatitis.
† These eruptions are reported in the literature as eczematous dermatitis, but clear, careful clinical descriptions with cutaneous biopsy specimens are frequently lacking.
‡ Such as constitutional diathesis and contact dermatitis.

the closed and open types) is not precisely known at this time, but the initial histologic event in comedone formation is excessive keratinization within the follicular canal. It is currently believed that *Propionibacterium acnes* is responsible for lipolysis with a release of fatty acids; it is thought that these fatty acids are capable of producing an inflammatory process in the follicle wall. Acne vulgaris is a serious problem, especially common during adolescence, and its therapy is complex and prolonged. Moderate to severe acne vulgaris is best treated by a dermatologist who has a number of modalities: topical agents, incision and drainage of the cystic lesions, ultraviolet light therapy, and judicious use of systemic antibiotics; x-ray therapy has no place in the treatment of acne vulgaris.

The mechanism of action of antibiotics such as tetracycline is not completely understood, but these drugs are known to suppress the number of propionibacteria and to cause a reduction of free fatty acids recoverable from the skin. Because the organisms have been shown to have lipolytic activity in vitro, it is presumed that the antibiotic causes this reduction of free fatty acids. Benzoyl peroxide lotions and gels probably act as antibacterial agents and decrease the bacterial population; these agents are very effective and are widely used by dermatologists.

Estrogens combined with progestins (oral contraceptives) were initially considered to be effective in controlling acne; however, they have been of only limited value in the treatment of acne in females and cannot be given to males. There is no evidence suggesting that diet has any effect on the course or severity of acne vulgaris. Acne vulgaris may begin as early as the eighth year or may not appear until the twentieth. It lasts for several years and then subsides spontaneously, usually when the patients are in their early twenties. In some patients, however, acne vulgaris may continue into the third and fourth decades. Topical antibiotic solutions such as clindamycin or erythromycin are effective new agents for treatment of acne vulgaris.

Pretibial myxedema (PM) also may cause nodules on the legs and dorsa of the feet (Plate 5-2). The lesions are usually bilateral and consist of elevated, firm, dermal nodules and plaques that are not easily movable. They may be skin color, pink, or, rarely, brown, and, when diascoped, appear yellow and waxy. The epidermis over the nodules may appear normal or may have a marked verrucous (warty) surface. The pathogenesis of pretibial myxedema is not clear. Pretibial myxedema may occur with or without hyperthyroidism (Graves' disease) or before or after treatment of hyperthyroidism, and its development does not parallel the ocular changes (if present). The nodules in pretibial myxedema are accumulations of mucopolysaccharides, which can be demonstrated by special staining of the histopathologic material. LATS (long-acting thyroid stimulator), which is associated in the plasma with immunoglobulin G (7S gamma globulin), has been implicated in the pathogenesis of pretibial myxedema, exophthalmos, and acropachy; the role of LATS in the pathogenesis of pretibial myxedema has not been established.

Ulcers   Ulcers occur as a result of destruction of the epidermis and, at least, the papillary layer of the dermis (see Fig. 48-4). All ulcers of the skin that do not heal within a period of a month must be assumed to be carcinoma until proved otherwise, and it is essential that a biopsy be obtained to rule out malignancy. Ulcers can be divided into two categories: lesions that occur on the legs and feet, and lesions that occur elsewhere on the body. Ulcers not occurring on the legs are rather rare except in primary cancer of the skin or in malignant metastases to the skin. Ulcers arising in nodules with inflammation should be approached in the manner suggested previously for nodules—that is, a biopsy should be obtained, and the tissue examined for bacterial, mycotic, and parasitic diseases. Chancre-like ulcerations and noduloulcerative lesions with regional lymphadenopathy may occur in primary syphilis and primary tuberculosis and in tularemia, anthrax, glanders, and bubonic plague. Isolated noduloulcerative lesions may be seen in sporotrichosis, coccidioidomycosis, leishmaniasis, cryptococcosis, and tertiary syphilis. Serologic studies are necessary in the diagnosis of syphilis.

The most prominent etiologic factors in ulceration on the legs and feet are disturbances of circulation. Chronic venous insufficiency leads to ulceration, especially on the medial aspect of the ankle or lower leg, and the ulcers develop in areas of skin with brownish hemosiderin pigmentation and occasionally where there is edema or sclerosis of the area. Hypertensive or ischemic ulcerations tend to start on the lateral aspect of the ankle. Ulceration can also occur as a result of tissue infarction in areas supplied by either large or small blood vessels (arteries, arterioles); this infarction may occur as the result of occlusion or constriction due to a variety of etiologic factors, in addition to those already mentioned: emboli, thrombosis, cryoagglutinins, macroglobulinemia, cryoglobulinemia, thrombotic thrombocytopenic purpura, polycythemia, systemic lupus erythematosus, Raynaud's phenomenon, arteriosclerosis obliterans, and thromboangiitis obliterans. Ulceration of the lower extremities also occurs in hemolytic anemia, including sickle-cell anemia, thalassemia, and hereditary spherocytosis.

Some ulcers show extensive necrosis of the edges, such as those in *pyoderma gangrenosum* (Plate 5-3), an indolent ulcer usually on the lower extremities and often associated with ulcerative colitis or regional ileitis. The ulcers in pyoderma gan-

TABLE 49-2
Various types of eczematous dermatitis* of known etiology

Clinical type	Pathogenesis	Diagnostic considerations
Allergic contact eczematous dermatitis	Chemical allergens (plants, medicaments, cosmetics, metals, fabrics, etc.)	Site and configuration are clues to causal agent; patch tests may confirm diagnosis; avoidance of cause cures eruption
Photoallergic contact eczematous dermatitis	Ultraviolet radiation plus topical chemicals (in soaps, perfumes, citrus fruits, etc.), which then become allergens	Occurs on exposed skin; photopatch tests confirm diagnosis
Polymorphous light-induced eruption—eczematous type	Ultraviolet radiation; sometimes visible light	Occurs on exposed skin; diagnosis implies that all known causes of light-induced eruptions have been eliminated
"Infectious eczematoid dermatitis"	Bacterial products from draining focus (e.g., ear infection)	Occurs near site of infection; responds to treatment of primary infection
Eczematous dermatophytosis	Fungus	Fungi demonstrated in scales or exudate

* *This term is used by many clinicians for at least four types of eczematous dermatitis that may be exclusively localized to the hands (atopic eczematous dermatitis, allergic contact eczematous dermatitis, nummular eczematous dermatitis, and "dyshidrotic" eczematous dermatitis). Possibly, contact irritants to which the hands are frequently exposed may precipitate or aggravate one of the above-mentioned basic types of eczematous dermatitis.*

grenosum have ragged bluish red overhanging edges and a necrotic base. These lesions often start as pustules or tender red nodules at the site of trauma, and then gradually increase in size until liquefaction necrosis occurs and an irregular ulcer develops. The ulcers are often multiple and may cover large areas of the leg. The histopathologic findings are not specific. The healing of the ulcers usually parallels the activity of the ulcerative colitis, and, inasmuch as the ulceration extends into and involves the reticular layer of the dermis and the subcutis, scarring occurs.

The term *"tropical" ulcer,* in addition to cutaneous leishmaniasis, now also includes ulceration due to cutaneous diphtheria, treponemal disorders (syphilis, yaws, and bejel), and phagedenic ulcer, a chronic ulcer of the feet and legs caused by mixed bacteria that occurs in persons suffering from starvation and neglect.

Ulcers can be associated with peripheral neuropathy ("neuropathic" ulcer, or malum perforans) seen in diabetes mellitus, tabes dorsalis, polyneuritis, leprosy, congenital anesthesia, or hereditary sensory radicular neuropathy.

Anal and perianal ulcers are seen in histiocytosis X and in amebiasis. A hanging-drop preparation is necessary to detect *Entamoeba histolytica.*

Ulcers with artificial and bizarre shapes must be suspected of being self-induced by means of destructive agents such as acid and lighted cigarettes. Factitial ulcers are overstudied and, unfortunately, underdiagnosed by most physicians.

Stony-hard, noduloulcerative lesions, particularly around joints (elbows, knees, and fingers) are suggestive of calcinosis cutis or gout; roentgenographic examination enables the detection of calcinosis cutis but shows no opaque bodies in gout.

Sclerosis, diffuse or circumscribed Diffuse sclerosis of the skin is most often seen on the upper extremities, chest, and face in systemic scleroderma (sometimes called progressive systemic sclerosis). Initially, the skin appears yellowish and shows slight nonpitting edema; later, however, it becomes indurated, bound down, and may be markedly hyperpigmented. Calcinosis cutis and Raynaud's phenomenon commonly occur.

Circumscribed sclerosis occurs in *morphea,* which consists of one or more round or oval, firm, reddish plaques up to several centimeters in diameter that become white or yellow centrally, often with a lilac-colored, telangiectatic border. This disorder is not associated with any other organ involvement and is a localized cutaneous form of scleroderma. Another type of localized scleroderma is *linear scleroderma,* in which the morphologic change is the same as that seen in morphea except that the process occurs in bands extending parallel to the long axis of the extremity or along the paramedian line of the forehead and scalp. This form of scleroderma has no relationship to progressive systemic sclerosis.

Edema In addition to the various causes of localized edema and generalized edema, there is a type of edema of the lower extremities that is not often recognized by the physician. This is a bilateral pedal edema which is common in patients with subacute or chronic dermatitis of the lower extremities. This type of edema is most often seen with chronic eczematous dermatitis but is unrelated to cardiac failure or lymphatic obstruction. It is most probably due to an increased permeability as a result of local capillary damage, which is part of the inflammatory process in the skin. The increased capillary permeability leads to an increased transfer of fluid from the intravascular to the extravascular component of the extracellular fluid space. This type of pitting edema disappears completely when the dermatitis has resolved.

Atrophy, diffuse or circumscribed Dermal atrophy results from a decrease of the papillary or reticular connective tissue and is manifested in the skin as a depression. Circumscribed dermal atrophy may follow trauma, or may occur in association with epidermal atrophy, as in the striae of pregnancy or in Cushing's disease.

PANNICULUS ADIPOSUS (SUBCUTIS) Nodules (inflammatory, usually tender, red) Nodules in the subcutis may be recognized by the fact that the skin is usually movable over the nodule; occasionally, however, in inflammatory processes, the nodule may involve both the dermis and panniculus adiposus, and the skin will then not be movable over the nodule. Acute, tender, red nodules on the leg are characteristically found in two disorders: *erythema nodosum syndrome* and *nodular subcutaneous fat necrosis* associated with pancreatitis.

The erythema nodosum syndrome refers to the occurrence of multiple bilateral tender nodules appearing principally on the anterior aspect of the lower extremities and occasionally on the upper extremities and face. The erythema nodosum syndrome is associated with a number of disorders that are unrelated to each other.

The nodules in erythema nodosum are only slightly elevated, edematous, and sometimes exquisitely tender. Bruising is a characteristic feature of the disease and is due to hemorrhage, leading to the formation of contusions. The lesions never ulcerate or become indurated and very seldom leave any scarring or atrophy. Erythema nodosum is associated with primary tuberculosis and primary coccidioidomycosis, histoplasmosis, *Yersinia* infection, beta-hemolytic streptococcal infections, lymphogranuloma venereum, leprosy, sarcoidosis, ulcerative colitis, Crohn's disease, regional enteritis, drugs (penicillin, sulfonamides, bromides, iodides), and oral contraceptives containing ethynylestradiol and norethynodrel.

Tender, red subcutaneous nodules may also appear on the legs in association with acute pancreatitis and with pancreatic neoplasms and are often erroneously called erythema nodosum. This disorder has been termed *nodular liquefying panniculitis* (NLP). These lesions are distinctive. Their morphologic features are different from those of classic erythema nodosum. The lesions in NLP vary in size from a few millimeters to several centimeters, and, in contrast to the lesions of erythema nodosum, are movable. The lesions of NLP involute in 2 to 3 weeks and may leave a hyperpigmented scar that is slightly depressed. The nodules are often associated with abdominal pain and may also be accompanied by fever and arthralgia. Rarely, lesions may be present on other parts of the body besides the legs. Some of the larger nodules may undergo an abscess-like change, becoming fluctuant, and may rupture, exuding a whitish, creamy, or oily viscous material; abscess formation with drainage rarely, if ever, occurs in erythema nodosum. The most common pancreatic neoplasm associated with NLP is an acinous adenocarcinoma of the pancreas. In *Weber-Christian panniculitis,* the subcutaneous nodules, which at first are slightly mobile, become adherent to the overlying skin; then, as the edema subsides in the area of induration, a central depression occurs.

In addition to the above-mentioned entities, various types of vasculitis may also produce tender subcutaneous nodules. Therefore, diagnosis of these lesions often requires an excisional or incisional biopsy.

Nodules (noninflammatory, usually nontender, nonerythematous) Movable, painless, noninflammatory-appearing nodules occur around joints in rheumatic fever, rheumatoid arthritis, and in certain metabolic diseases such as xanthoma, gout, and calcinosis. Metastatic carcinoma or metastatic malignant melanoma may appear as movable, nontender subcutaneous nodules. Sarcoidosis may be manifested in the skin solely as subcutaneous nodules on the lower extremities. Subcutaneous nodules also occur in onchocerciasis and loiasis. *Lipomas,* relatively common causes of subcutaneous nodules, are benign tumors composed of adipose tissue and may be single or multiple and are frequently lobulated; they are often rubbery or compressible and occur most often on the trunk and back of the neck and forearms. Occasionally, subcutaneous lipoma may be painful and associated with marked obesity; this condition, known as *Dercum's disease,* is most common in middle-aged females.

Atrophy, diffuse or circumscribed Atrophy of the panniculus adiposus produces depressions in the skin; these depressions are seen in progressive lipodystrophy, in liquefying panniculitis, and in the localized fat atrophy that occurs at the site of injections of insulin. About 25 percent of diabetics who receive insulin (most often females under the age of 20) have this type of atrophy. The depressed areas of localized fat atrophy show a complete absence of the panniculus, and there is no inflammation. In lipodystrophy, diffuse atrophy of the skin may involve large portions of the body.

BLOOD VESSELS Morbilliform and scarlatiniform eruptions Morbilliform (measlelike) and scarlatiniform eruptions are macular and papular exanthems and can be due to drug hypersensitivities, measles, German measles, erythema infectiosum, viral exanthems, rickettsial diseases including endemic murine typhus and Rocky Mountain spotted fever, scarlet fever, and secondary syphilis. Many of the diseases manifested by macules or papules and occurring in acutely ill patients with a fever are listed in Table 49-3.

TABLE 49-3
Rash and fever in the acutely ill patient: Diagnosis according to type of lesion

DISEASES MANIFESTED BY MACULES OR PAPULES

Drug hypersensitivities	Rocky Mountain spotted fever
Scarlet fever	(early lesions)*
Erythema infectiosum (fifth disease)	Pityriasis rosea
	Erythema multiforme
Measles (rubeola)	Erythema marginatum
German measles (rubella)*	Systemic lupus erythematosus*
Enterovirus (echo- and coxsackievirus) infections	Dermatomyositis
	"Serum sickness"* (manifested only as wheals)
Adenovirus infections	
Typhoid fever	Urticaria, acute (viral hepatitis)
Secondary syphilis	
Typhus, murine (endemic)	

DISEASES MANIFESTED BY VESICLES, BULLAE, OR PUSTULES

Drug hypersensitivities	Eczema vaccinatum†
Dermatitis from plants	Variola†
Rickettsialpox	Enterovirus (echo- and coxsackievirus) infections, including hand-foot-mouth disease
Varicella (chickenpox)†	
Generalized herpes zoster†	
Disseminated herpes simplex†	Toxic epidermal necrolysis
Eczema herpeticum†	Staphylococcal scaled-skin syndrome
Disseminated vaccinia†	Erythema multiforme bullosum

DISEASES MANIFESTED BY PURPURIC MACULES, PURPURIC PAPULES, OR PURPURIC VESICLES

Drug hypersensitivities	Enterovirus (echo- and coxsackievirus) infections
Bacteremia:‡	Rickettsial diseases:
Meningococcemia (acute or chronic)*	Rocky Mountain spotted fever*
Gonococcemia*	Typhus, louse-borne (epidemic)
Staphylococcemia	"Allergic" vasculitis*,‡
Pseudomonas bacteremia	Purpura fulminans‡
Subacute bacterial endocarditis	

* *May have arthralgia or musculoskeletal pain.*
† *One characteristic lesion of these exanthems is an umbilicated papule or vesicle.*
‡ *Often present as infarcts.*
SOURCE: *TB Fitzpatrick, RA Johnson, in Dermatology in General Medicine, 2d ed, TB Fitzpatrick et al (eds), New York, McGraw-Hill, 1979.*

Urticaria Urticaria is characterized by wheals, of which the outstanding feature is their persistence for only a few hours (see Fig. 48-6). This short duration differentiates urticarial wheals from the otherwise almost identical papules of erythema multiforme, which persist for more than 1 or 2 days rather than for a few hours. An acute onset of urticaria is usually related to ingestion of drugs or certain types of foods (shellfish, fresh berries).

Chronic recurrent urticaria is a special problem, and its causes are not easily established. Most patients with this disorder require a careful examination for cryptic diseases such as lymphoma, systemic lupus erythematosus, primary or metastatic carcinoma, intestinal parasites, acute hepatitis, systemic vasculitis, or dermatomyositis. It is especially important, even in chronic urticarias, to carry out a painstaking interrogation of the patient in search of a history of drugs. Aspirin is one of the most common causes of chronic urticaria and can often be missed even in a careful drug history because many patients do not consider aspirin a drug. It is probably true that some patients with chronic urticaria can relate their problem to emotional stress, but this should be considered only after excluding all possible organic causes.

Erythema multiforme syndrome Erythema multiforme syndrome is a characteristic response of the skin and mucous membranes that is related to a number of possible etiologies, including infectious agents (herpesvirus hominis, *Mycoplasma pneumoniae*) and drugs (especially penicillin, antipyretics, barbiturates, hydantoins, and sulfonamides). In 50 percent of patients no etiology is ascertained. The major pathologic change is an acute lymphohistiocytic inflammatory infiltrate around blood vessels and may include degenerative changes in the endothelial cells of the capillaries and marked papillary dermal edema. There is some evidence for an immune-complex etiology with hypocomplementemic vasculitis.

The lesions occur in a characteristic symmetrical distribution and favor the extensor areas of the distal parts of the limbs, the backs of the hands, and the dorsa of the feet; the palms and soles are often involved, even to the exclusion of the dorsal surfaces. Oral lesions, first as blisters and then erosions, occur on the buccal mucous membrane, gums, and tongue, and there is often swelling and crusting of the lips. The syndrome may also include severe toxemia and prostration, high fever, cough, and "patchy" inflammation of the lungs. The skin lesions are often characterized by a vivid redness that gradually becomes duller, and they become more indurated, with the development of centers that are pale or may have bullae; these "target" or "iris" lesions, which are characteristic of erythema multiforme but do not invariably occur, are identified by the clear red area at the periphery that surrounds a pale pink zone and a central livid area, which may contain a bulla. The efficacy of systemic corticosteroids has not been proved, but this therapy is commonly used.

Purpura (with and without inflammation) A purpuric eruption demands immediate exploration for its etiology. Purpura arises in the skin of the vascularized dermis and is almost always confined to the dermis. The purpuric macules gradually disappear after days or weeks, depending on their size. Punctate or tiny purpuric spots are termed *petchiae,* larger (>2.0 cm) macules are spoken of as *suggillations,* and extensive purpuric macules are called *ecchymoses* (see D in Fig. 48-2).

Purpura with inflammation is usually "palpable," i.e., papular, and is seen in systemic vasculitis and in bacteremias such as staphylococcemia, gonococcemia (Plate 5-4), and meningococcemia. In these bacteremias and in vasculitis, the examination of biopsied skin may establish a diagnosis within 8 h (the time required for processing the tissue). Gentle scraping of the purpuric lesions will produce enough material for a Gram's stain; intracellular gram-negative diplococci are occasionally found in the lesions in acute, but not in chronic, meningococcemia, and are rarely found in acute gonococcemia. The differential diagnosis of papable purpuric lesions and infarcts occurring in *systemic vasculitis* (necrotizing vasculitis) as compared with those in chronic meningococcemia is not easy. The skin lesions in systemic vasculitis are usually bilateral, and almost symmetrical, in their distribution. They tend to be concentrated on the lower extremities, especially on the lower portion and around the ankles and the dorsa of the feet. The lesions in chronic meningococcemia are more randomly distributed, with occurrence on the trunk, lower and upper extremities, and face. Nevertheless, in meningococcemia, lesions can occur in a bilateral distribution, which makes the distinction between chronic meningococcemia and systemic vasculitis difficult, if not impossible, at times. The individual lesions in both chronic meningococcemia and systemic vasculitis may be identical, consisting of a mixture of palpable purpura and urticarial-type papules without purpura. Unfortunately, the histologic findings in biopsy specimens of the lesions in both diseases do not permit a distinction. Therefore, a patient with bilaterally distributed palpable purpuric lesions and fever is best treated with antibiotics before the results of blood cultures are available.

Purpura without inflammation is completely macular, and examination of a blood smear can quickly establish the presence of platelets; if platelets are seen in the smear, thrombocytopenic purpura can be safely ruled out as a possibility.

On the lower legs of older people, a great variety of inflammatory skin diseases, including various types of contact dermatitis, may be associated with purpura; under these circumstances, the purpura does not have the same importance as it does when present on the trunk or upper extremities. Perifollicular purpura, however, on the lower extremities (usually accompanied by a follicular hyperkeratosis) is almost pathognomonic of scurvy.

Purpura frequently develops in amyloidosis when the lesions (waxy macules and papules) are pinched. This "pinch" purpura, however, may also occur in the normal skin of patients with thrombocytopenic purpura or in the skin of apparently normal elderly persons. (For a full discussion of the classification and differential diagnosis of purpura, see Chaps. 54 and 316.)

Infarcts Infarcts in the skin are usually not pale like those that occur in the kidney but have a variegated dusky red, grayish hue. They are irregularly shaped macules, sometimes slightly depressed below the plane of the skin, and often surrounded by a pink zone of hyperemia. Infarcts are usually slightly tender.

Cutaneous infarctions are important and often diagnostic signs of serious multisystem disease, including both acute and chronic meningococcemia, streptococcal and staphylococcal septicemia, gonococcemia, pseudomonas septicemia, systemic vasculitis, purpura fulminans, systemic lupus erythematosus, and, rarely, dermatomyositis.

Telangiectasia Redness of the skin is most freqently caused by transient dilatation of blood vessels (erythema). In contrast to the color produced by fixed blood pigments, as in purpura, the erythema will disappear under the pressure of a glass or plastic slide (see "Diascopy" in Chap. 48). Telangiectasia is the condition in which the redness of the skin is the result of a permanent enlargement in the caliber of the blood vessels (which will be revealed by examination with a hand lens) and an increase in the number of the vessels. Telangiectasia may be composed of fine linear branches of blood vessels appearing distinctly red (i.e., not blue), which are often seen on the nose and face, or of confluent macular areas that appear as a permanent erythema. Telangiectasia is the cause of the erythema in discoid and systemic lupus erythematosus, dermatomyositis, and psoriasis.

Telangiectasia may also occur in a scattered, discrete fashion on the upper trunk or on the extremities and is seen characteristicaly in progressive systemic sclerosis (systemic scleroderma). Telangiectasia occurring around the nail beds, i.e., periungual telangiectasia, is an important diagnostic sign in lupus erythematosus (both discoid and systemic) and in dermatomyositis; these lesions are seen rarely, if at all, in systemic scleroderma or rheumatoid arthritis.

Sharply outlined, red macules or papules 1 to 2 mm in diameter, with an area of radiating telangiectasia, are seen in *hereditary hemorrhagic telangiectasia* (Chap. 318). These occur on the lips, tongue, nasal mucosa, face, and hands.

Generalized telangiectasia occurring in the form of red macules over most of the body surface may be the presenting sign of mastocytosis or urticaria pigmentosa.

Telangiectasia is a prominent and diagnostic feature of *ataxia telangiectasia,* or Louis-Bar syndrome. Telangiectasia may be present as early as the second year of life but usually develops by the fifth year; it appears first on the bulbar conjunctiva and subsequently involves the ears, the eyelids, the butterfly area of the face, the upper aspect of the chest, and the extremities.

Telangiectasia may occur in a characteristic form known as the *arterial spider,* or spider nevus, spider angioma, or naevus araneus. The main vessel of the spider is an arteriole, and it is usually faintly pulsating, which will show under the diascope. A less common skin lesion usually found with vascular spiders in liver disorders is the telangiectatic *mat* or net, a small red patch composed of intermeshed fine vessels that blanch on pressure. Spider angiomas, usually three or fewer, occur not infrequently in normal children and adults. Numerous spider angiomas often develop during pregnancy or after the ingestion of progestational agents or in rheumatoid arthritis or thyrotoxicosis. Most patients with numerous and prominent vascular spiders, however, have some form of underlying diffuse liver disease, e.g., alcoholic cirrhosis. The progression of subacute hepatitis is often paralleled by the appearance of crops of spiders, and in alcoholic and postnecrotic cirrhosis, almost half the patients have multiple vascular spiders. The mechanism responsible for the development of spider angiomas in liver disease is not known, nor has it been firmly established that the lesions result from disordered metabolism of estrogens by the liver.

REFERENCES

FARBER EM, COX AJ (eds): *Psoriasis: Proceedings of the Second International Symposium.* New York, Yorke Medical Books, 1977

FITZPATRICK TB: Fundamentals of dematologic diagnosis, in *Dermatology in General Medicine,* 2d ed, TB Fitzpatrick et al (eds). New York, McGraw-Hill, 1979

———, JOHNSON RA: Atlas of differential diagnosis of rashes in the acutely ill febrile patient and in life-threatening diseases, in *Dermatology in General Medicine,* 2d ed, TB Fitzpatrick et al (eds). New York, McGraw-Hill, 1979

PARRISH JA et al: Photochemotherapy of psoriasis with oral methoxsalen and longwave ultraviolet light. N Engl J Med 291:1207, 1974

WOLFF K et al: Photochemotherapy for psoriasis with orally administered methoxsalen. Arch Dermatol 67:669, 1976

50
GENERALIZED PRURITUS

THOMAS B. FITZPATRICK
HARLEY A. HAYNES

Generalized pruritus is a frequent and important problem in differential diagnosis for the general physician. In many patients, intense generalized pruritus is the only symptom. Unfortunately, there are no good studies that have described in detail the special qualities of pruritus that permit a specific diagnosis; in other words, it is not really known what type of pruritus is seen, for example, in obstructive biliary disease as opposed to lymphoma. In the absence of these data, the clinician must rely on the history, physical examination, and laboratory studies to establish the nature of the pruritus.

An important cause of pruritus is psychogenic, that is, a reaction to stress and strain. This type of pruritus often affects the skin of the scalp, and may be associated with other sensory complaints such as a bitter taste in the mouth or burning of the tongue. Some patients with psychogenic pruritus are convinced that the itching is caused by some sort of parasite in their skin that cannot be seen by themselves or the physician. Such patients may scratch their skin until the lesions become excoriated, and then assert that the itching has disappeared, owing, they believe, to removal of the parasite or "germ" by the appearance of bleeding.

Older persons in whom dry skin is a common occurrence may have generalized pruritus unrelated to multisystem disease. Some other older persons, however, usually more than 60 years of age, who do not have obvious dry skin may also have generalized ("senile") pruritus that is intense and does not seem to be caused by emotional stress. This pruritus is usually most severe when the patients disrobe to go to bed, and usually begins in one area, particularly the back, and spreads to involve the entire body. Neither psychogenic nor senile pruritus leads to a loss of sleep.

A subtle and important cause of pruritus without a visible rash may be a reaction to drugs, such as aspirin and, especially, opiates and their derivatives, and quinidine.

The itching that is associated with pediculosis corporis may be so intense that it will interfere with the patient's sleep. This type of eruption is usually relatively easy to diagnose by the linear excoriations that occur along the back and often the insect can be found in the clothing, particularly along the seams.

For a list of conditions in which generalized pruritus occurs without any evidence of primary skin disease, see Table 50-1.

The pruritus in hepatic disease has no special qualities. Generalized pruritus may frequently be the first sign of biliary cirrhosis and may occur many months before the onset of jaundice. It may be the first sign also of lymphoma, and, rarely, of carcinoma. The pruritus may be of sudden onset and may be very severe from the beginning.

Patients with pruritus associated with obvious skin lesions, such as vesicles and papules, should be referred to a dermatologist. Some of the dermatologic disorders in which pruritus is a common symptom include scabies, dermatitis herpetiformis, lichen planus, urticaria, mycosis fungoides, insect bites, psoriasis, and eczematous dermatitis including atopic dermatitis. Many of these disorders require specialized dermatologic approaches, particularly biopsy of the skin, in order to establish the diagnosis.

The itching patient without an apparent skin eruption, with or without the sequelae of chronic scratching (linear excoriations) and rubbing (lichenification, polished nails), poses a diagnostic challenge. Initially, a search should be undertaken for subtle evidence of a cutaneous disorder.

Thorough evaluation of the patient with generalized pruritus in an attempt to discover an underlying systemic disease should include, in addition to history and physical examination, the following basic laboratory screening tests: complete blood count; sedimentation rate; urinalysis; blood glucose; liver, thyroid, and renal function tests; chest x-ray; Papanicolaou smear; and stool test for ova, parasites, and occult blood. Additional tests such as serum protein electrophoresis, serum calcium, and radiologic surveys should be performed when indicated. A psychological assessment is helpful. Attributing generalized pruritus of uncertain etiology to a psychological disturbance is hazardous.

The treatment of generalized pruritus is unsatisfactory. Not one of the systemic medications has been shown to be effective in generalized pruritus. A topical preparation containing 0.5% menthol and 1% phenol in Nivea oil is somewhat helpful in relieving pruritus temporarily. The topical anesthetics containing benzocaine should be avoided because of the high risk of allergic sensitization. When the patient with pruritus also has insomnia, a hypnotic or a sedative should be prescribed. Antihistamines are of little value except in pruritus due to urticaria. It is a general clinical impression that aspirin is helpful in pruritus of any origin, but this has not been proved. The development of drugs that control pruritus remains one of the great challenges of medical research, and it is paradoxical that, at this juncture, severe pain can be immediately controlled with a variety of agents but there is not one single agent that is so effective for generalized pruritus. The receptors for the itch stimuli reside in the papillary layer of the dermis, but there are

TABLE 50-1

Conditions with generalized pruritus without diagnostic skin lesions

Psychogenic states:
    Transitory: periods of emotional stress
    Persistent: delusions of parasitosis
Metabolic and endocrine conditions:
    Hyperthyroidism
    Diabetes mellitus*
    Carcinoid syndrome
Malignant neoplasms:
    Lymphoma and leukemia
    Abdominal cancer*
    CNS tumors*
    Multiple myeloma*
Drug ingestion:
    Opium derivatives
    Subclinical drug sensitivities
Infestations:
    Pediculosis corporis
    Scabies†
    Hookworm (ancylostomiasis)
    Onchocerciasis
Renal disease:
    Chronic renal failure
Hematologic disease:
    Polycythemia vera‡
Hepatic disease:
    Obstructive biliary disease
    Pregnancy (intrahepatic cholestasis)
Miscellaneous conditions:
    Dry skin§
    "Senile" pruritus§

* *Not definitely proved.*
† *Diagnostic lesions may be present.*
‡ *Especially after a bath.*
§ *Unexplained intense pruritus in patients over 65 years old without obvious "dry skin" and with no apparent emotional stress.*
SOURCE: *TB Fitzpatrick, in Dermatology in General Medicine, 2d ed, TB Fitzpatrick et al (eds), New York, McGraw-Hill, 1979.*

no specific end organs for itching. Itching is a sensation carried principally by unmyelinated slowly conducting fibers of the C group to central neuronal pools in the spinal cord. The stimuli are then carried by the posterior roots of the spinal nerves, and, from the anterolateral spinothalamic tracts, enter the thalamus and then proceed to the sensory area of the gyrus postcentralis of the cortex.

REFERENCE

CAIRNS RJ: The skin and the nervous system, in *Textbook of Dermatology*, A Rook et al (eds). Oxford, Blackwell Scientific Publications, 1972, p 1791

51
PIGMENTATION OF THE SKIN AND DISORDERS OF MELANIN METABOLISM

THOMAS B. FITZPATRICK
DAVID B. MOSHER

THE MELANOCYTE SYSTEM

DEFINITION OF MELANIN The presence of melanin, oxyhemoglobin, reduced hemoglobin, and carotene accounts for the kaleidoscope of normal human skin colors, but melanin is the principal pigment responsible for the color of human skin, hair, and eyes. Melanin is also a filter that decreases the harmful effects of ultraviolet light on the dermis and thereby provides protection against acute sunburn reaction and chronic actinic damage, including skin cancer.

Derived from the Greek word *melas*, "black," melanin is a protein-bound polymer formed by the oxidation of tyrosine by tyrosinase to dihydroxyphenylalanine (dopa) within melanocytes, which are specialized epidermal dendritic cells of neural crest origin. The precise chemical nature of melanin is unknown because it is so insoluble that all attempts to degrade it into identifiable fragments have failed. However, all animal melanins are known to contain indoles and are composed basically of indole 5,6-quinone units, in contrast to plant melanins which contain catechols. Radioactive dopa studies have shown that melanin is a copolymer of dopa quinone, indole 5,6-quinone, and indole 5,6-quinone 2-carboxylic acid in a ratio of 3:2:1.

Skin color is derived from the presence of melanin within the keratinocytes, which are receptor cells for melanocyte-formed melanin-containing organelles called *melanosomes*. Normal skin color is "constitutive"—that of habitually unexposed skin, as the buttocks—and "facultative"—that resulting from the sun-induced tanning reaction or from increased pigmentation by pituitary melanocyte-stimulating hormones (MSH).

BIOSYNTHESIS OF MELANIN The melanocyte system is composed of melanocytes found at the dermoepidermal interface, in the hair bulb, uveal tract, retinal pigment epithelium, inner ear, and leptomeninges (Fig. 51-1). The melanocyte system is analogous to, but not known to be related to, the chromaffin system, the cells of which are also derived from the neural crest and which possess biochemical mechanisms for the hydroxylation of tyrosine to dopa. However, in the latter system the enzyme is not tyrosinase but tyrosine hydroxylase, and dopa is converted to adrenochrome and not to tyrosine melanin.

The melanocytes present in the epidermis at the dermoepidermal interface are dendritic cells that are functionally linked to a number of keratinocytes; they constitute the epidermal melanin unit (Fig. 51-2). This functional unit permits organized transfer of specialized tyrosinase-containing organelles, or melanosomes, to associated keratinocytes. Melanosomes are spherical vesicles which are thought to arise in the area of the endoplasmic reticulum and Golgi apparatus; they are formed as unmelanized spherical structures that darken and become more dense and oval in shape with increasing melanization.

Tyrosinase is one of a large group of copper-containing aerobic oxidases that catalyze the oxidation of both monohydroxy and *o*-dihydroxy phenols to orthoquinones. In humans and other mammals, this oxidase catalyzes the hydroxylation of the melanin precursor, tyrosine, to dopa and dopa quinone (Fig. 51-3). Tyrosinase is required only for the first step in the biosynthesis of tyrosine melanin, i.e., the orthohydroxylation of tyrosine. It is noteworthy that zinc ions catalyze the conversion of dopachrome to 5,6-dihydroxyindole and that melanosomes have been shown to contain high concentrations of zinc.

BIOLOGY OF MELANIN PIGMENTATION Melanin pigmentation (Fig. 51-4), from the clinical point of view, results from the melanin present in the keratinocytes and also in the melanocytes. Inasmuch as the ratio of keratinocytes to melanocytes in the epidermis is 36:1, it is apparent that the amount of melanin present in the keratinocytes must be the predominant factor in the determination of skin color. The relationship of skin color

FIGURE 51-1

Diagram showing the embryonic origin, dispersal, and developmental fate of melanocytes in humans. (By permission from JB Stanbury et al (eds), The Metabolic Basis of Inherited Disease, 2d ed, New York, McGraw-Hill, 1966.)

Neural crest

Embryo

Miscellaneous sites

Mucous membrane
Internal ear
Orbital cavity
Mesentery

to the location of melanin in the epidermis was studied with the light microscope in Negro Americans of various hues of brown coloration. In lightly pigmented skin, there was a great variation in both the number and location of melanin particles within the epidermis; only scanty melanin deposits were in the malpighian layer, and no deposits were in the stratum corneum. In fact, in the most lightly pigmented skin, the only melanin particles were in the keratinocytes of the basal layer.

In the most heavily pigmented skin, there were melanin particles in the keratinocytes of the basal layer, throughout the malpighian cells, and in the stratum corneum.

It is apparent, therefore, from studies of normal skin and of pigmentary disorders, that the intensity of pigmentation, as viewed clinically, depends not only on the rate of melanosome production but also on the number of melanosomes that are transferred to the keratinocytes (Fig. 51-2). Another factor that determines normal and abnormal melanin pigmentation is the degree of melanization of the individual melanosomes. Until recently, three factors—melanosome formation, melanosome melanization, and melanosome secretion—were considered to be the major variables in normal and abnormal melanin pigmentation. In the past few years, however, a fourth variable has been implicated in melanin pigmentation, i.e., the phenomenon of aggregation and degradation of melanosomes that occurs during their transport in the keratinocytes.

Melanosomes are present in melanocytes mainly as nonaggregated (single), membrane-delimited, discrete organelles. In keratinocytes, however, melanosomes occur either as single, or nonaggregated, particles or as aggregates of three or more within a membrane-delimited organelle. These melanosome-containing organelles resemble the melanosome-containing organelles within macrophages that have been identified as lysosomes. In the epidermal keratinocyte, melanosomes appear to undergo a gradual degradation. In heavily pigmented skin, however, intact melanosomes remain in the stratum corneum, indicating that some melanosomes are apparently not degraded with the lysosomes in the epidermis. Numerous studies in recent years have shown that there appears to be a considerable variation in the arrangement of melanosomes in the

FIGURE 51-2

Epidermal melanin unit. Four biologic processes in melanin pigmentation underscore the differences in melanosome formation and packaging between Negroes and Caucasians: (1) Formation of melanosomes in melanocytes; (2) melanization of melanosomes in melanocytes; (3) secretion of melanocytes by keratinocytes; and (4) transport of melanocytes by keratinocytes, either with degradation of melanosomes within lysosome-like organelles (in Caucasoids) or without apparent degradation of melanosomes (in Negroids). Note the difference in size between the melanosomes in the Negroid and Caucasoid epidermal keratinocytes. In the Negroid keratinocytes, the melanosomes are nonaggregated. In the Caucasoid keratinocytes, groups of several melanosomes are aggregated within membrane-limited lysosome-like organelles, and the melanosomes often appear fragmented (G, Golgi apparatus; N, nucleus; I to IV, the four stages in the development of the melanosome). The epidermal melanin unit is shown at the top. The melanocyte supplies melanosomes to a group of keratinocytes.

FIGURE 51-3

Biosynthesis of tyrosine melanin.

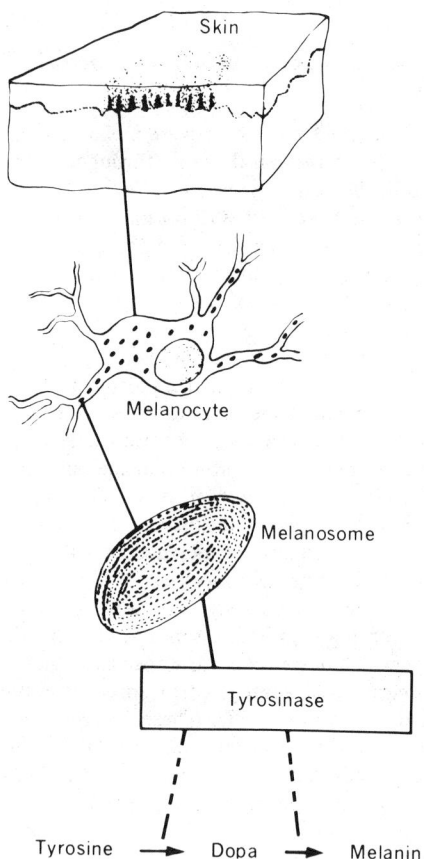

FIGURE 51-4

Melanogenesis in human skin, as seen in the light and the electron microscopes and at the molecular level.

nonfollicular keratinocytes in different racial groups. In the keratinocytes of the hair follicle in all racial groups, there are, in the growing phase of the hair growth cycle, single, or nonaggregated, melanosomes. In Negroids and Australian aborigines, however, melanosomes are found, in the epidermal keratinocytes, to be nonaggregated (single), whereas in Caucasoids, Mongoloids, and American Indians, melanosomes are found, in the keratinocytes, to be mostly aggregated, and there is often a suggestion of fragmentation of the melanosomes within these lysosome-like organelles. Some recent observations have shown that the size of the melanosome determines whether a melanosome becomes aggregated in the keratinocytes. Melanosomes that are smaller than 1 μm can aggregate in the form of a phagosome and undergo degradation—a process that could gradually decrease the intensity of the coloration.

Melanin pigmentation of the skin is related to 11 biologic processes as shown in Fig. 51-5. Aggregation[1] and dispersion of melanosomes probably play little part in the pigmentary anomalies of humans. Such movement has thus far been observed only in specialized effector cells, *melanophores,* present only in vertebrates below mammals in the phylogenic scale; this movement of melanosomes is under neural and hormonal control in these animals.

DISORDERS OF THE MELANOCYTE SYSTEM; HYPOMELANOSES AND HYPERMELANOSES

Disorders of melanin pigmentation have been increasingly found to be markers for diseases of other organ systems (Table

---

[1] *Aggregation in this sense refers to the clustering of melanosomes around the nucleus of the melanocyte, e.g., the phenomenon that occurs when a frog is placed on a white background; when the frog is placed on a dark background, however, there is movement, or dispersion, of the melanosomes into the dendrites.*

51-1). Such disorders (Table 51-2) may be classified as hypomelanoses (decreased or absent epidermal melanin) or hypermelanoses (increased epidermal or dermal melanin). Hypomelanoses, in general, result from the absence of melanocytes, failure of formation of normal melanosomes, or failure of transfer of melanosomes to keratinocytes. The hypermelanoses are further classified as epidermal disorders which present as brown, or as dermal disorders which are blue, blue-gray, or gray. Brown hypermelanoses arise from increased melanin in the epidermis, resulting from increased melanocyte activity, increased numbers of secretory melanocytes, increased numbers of melanosomes, or increased size of melanosomes. The blue-gray hypermelanoses represent a virtual "melanin tattoo"—the presence of melanin in the dermis in ectopic dermal melanocytes or in dermal macrophages which, because of the Tyndall effect, imparts a characteristic slate, blue, or gray color to the skin. Blue or slate-gray coloration of the skin may also arise from nonmelanin sources—ochronosis, tattoos, and deposition of other foreign materials in the dermis.

Clinical recognition of hypomelanosis and of gray or slate or blue hypermelanosis is usually not difficult. When the degree of hypomelanosis is very slight, when the patient's normal skin color is very light, or when the patient's skin is untanned, the lesions may be inapparent, and the diagnosis may be facilitated by the use of black light (Wood's lamp; see Chap. 48). This maneuver will heighten the contrast between abnormal epidermal pigmentation and normal skin but will not increase the contrast between increased dermal pigmentation and normal skin. Differentiation between abnormal diffuse brown hyperpigmentation and normal pigmentation frequently poses a

TABLE 51-1
Pigmentary disturbances as diagnostic signs in general medicine

Complaint or presenting problem	Pigmentary change	Diseases
Darkening skin	Generalized diffuse brown melanosis	Addison's disease; hemochromatosis; ACTH-producing tumors; systemic scleroderma
Abdominal pain; brown spots on lips, fingers	Circumscribed small dark brown macules	Peutz-Jeghers syndrome
Brown spots; hypertension	Circumscribed uniformly brown macules	Neurofibromatosis; Albright's syndrome
Mole	Circumscribed polychromic macules and papules (red, white, and blue admixed with brown)	Early primary malignant melanoma
White spots	Circumscribed white macules	Leukoderma associated with vitiligo, Addison's disease, pernicious anemia, thyrotoxicosis
Seizures; mental retardation	Circumscribed leaf-shaped white macules present at birth; poliosis	Tuberous sclerosis
Uveitis; deafness	Circumscribed white macules; poliosis	Vogt-Koyanagi-Harada disease
Deafness	White forelock; circumscribed white macules	Waardenburg's syndrome
Sun sensitivity; decreased vision	Generalized diffuse hypomelanosis of skin, hair, and uveal tract	Oculocutaneous albinism

FIGURE 51-5

Morphological and metabolic pathway of epidermal melanin pigmentation.

Within the figure:

1 Migration of Melanoblasts

2 Differentiation of Melanoblasts into Melanocytes

3 Mitotic Division of Melanocytes

MELANOCYTE

KERATINOCYTE

MELANOSOME

Melanin Removal with Loss of Stratum Corneum

10 Melanosome Degradation

9 Melanosome Transfer

8 Melanosome Melanization

7 Melanosome Formation

6 Tyrosinase Transport

5 Melanosome Matrix Synthesis

4 Tyrosinase Synthesis

problem because there is such a wide range of skin coloration in normal individuals. Diffuse color changes may be insidious; often patients themselves have been unaware of an unusual or unexplained progressive or gradual deepening of their skin color, such as a summer tan which is fading. The degree of hypermelanosis that develops pathologically appears to be related to the basic skin color of the patient involved. With the onset of primary Addison's disease, a patient of Mediterranean extraction (such as Italian, French, or Spanish) may become intensely pigmented, whereas a light-skinned individual may have only a minimal degree of hypermelanosis that may or may not be apparent. Localized pigmentation that develops in mucous membranes and in specific areas, such as axillae and palmar creases, is usually easier to identify as an abnormality than is generalized brown hyperpigmentation.

GENETIC FACTORS *Oculocutaneous albinism* is an autosomal recessive trait characterized by congenital, decreased, uniform hypomelanosis of skin and hair; albinism involving the skin alone has not been reported, but ocular albinism with minimal or no cutaneous involvement has been observed. The classic constellation of findings in oculocutaneous albinism includes marked hypomelanosis or amelanosis of skin, white or faintly blondish hair, photophobia, nystagmus, hypopigmented fundus oculi, and translucent irides. Oculocutaneous albinism may be classified according to the presence or absence of tyrosinase in plucked hair follicles of the scalp (the hair bulb incubation test). In normal individuals hair bulbs darken when incubated with tyrosine; in some persons with oculocutaneous albinism the hair follicles darken when incubated in tyrosine, i.e., *tyrosinase-positive,* while in others no such darkening occurs, i.e., *tyrosinase-negative.* These two types of albinism are known to have separate gene loci. In oculocutaneous albinism melanocytes are present, but formation of melanosomes is interrupted in the early stages so that few mature melanosomes

are present in albino skin or hair. Whatever tyrosinase is present must be functionally defective and unable to convert enzymatically tyrosine to dopa. Other variants of oculocutaneous albinism include yellow mutant, Cross-McKusick-Breen syndrome (oculocerebral-hypopigmentation syndrome), Hermansky-Pudlak syndrome (hemorrhagic diathesis secondary to storage pool platelet defect), and Chédiak-Higashi syndrome (recurrent infections, hematologic and neurologic abnormalities, and early death from lymphoma). The deficiency of melanin in oculocutaneous albinism has two disturbing consequences for humans: decreased visual acuity and an abnormal degree of intolerance to sunlight. The sensitivity of human albinos to ultraviolet light often leads to the development of carcinoma in exposed areas of the skin. Nearly all albinos in the tropics are said to have actinic keratoses or skin cancers by the third decade. Daily use of effective topical sunscreens and avoidance of unnecessary sun exposure are indicated for all albinos.

Phenylketonuria is an autosomal recessive disorder of phenylalanine metabolism in which there is a single metabolic block in the conversion of phenylalanine to tyrosine. There is pigmentary dilution of the skin, hair, and irides. The lightening of hair, which is characteristically light blond to dark brown, may be appraised only by comparison with uninvolved siblings. The melanocytes are normal but lack a full complement of melanosomes. Decreased melanin formation results from the fact that excess phenylalanine and its metabolites, present in serum and extracellular fluid, act as competitive inhibitors of tyrosinase and block melanin synthesis. Institution of universal screening programs of neonates has resulted in early detection of cases of phenylketonuria. Early treatment with a low phenylalanine diet prevents development of mental retardation which, once established, is not reversible.

Vitiligo is an idiopathic, acquired, circumscribed hypomelanosis which is familial in about 30 percent of cases and is

TABLE 51-2
Disturbances of human melanin pigmentation

Hypomelanosis[a]	Hypermelanosis[a]	Hypomelanosis[a]	Hypermelanosis[a]
White	Brown, gray, slate, or blue[b]	White	Brown, gray, slate, or blue[b]
GENETIC FACTORS		**CHEMICAL AND PHARMACOLOGIC AGENTS**	
Piebaldism[c]	Café au lait and freckle-like macules in neurofibromatosis[c]	Hydroquinone, monobenzyl-ether[c]	Arsenical intoxication[f]
Waardenburg's syndrome[c]	Melanotic macules in polyostotic fibrous dysplasia (Albright's syndrome)[c]	Hydroquinone[c,e]	Busulfan administration[f]
Vitiligo[c,d]		Miscellaneous catechol and phenol compounds[f]	Photochemical agents (topical or systemic drugs)[f]
Hypomelanotic macules in tuberous sclerosis[c,e]	Ephelides (freckles)[c]	Chloroquine and hydroxychloroquine[h]	5-Fluorouracil, systemic[f]
Nevus depigmentosus[c,e]	Lentigines[c]	Arsenical ingestion[c]	Cyclophosphamide[f]
Ziprkowski-Margolis syndrome[c]	Lentigines with cardiac arrhythmias[c]	Mercaptoethyl amines[c]	Nitrogen mustard, topical[c]
Albinism, oculocutaneous:[f,g]	Melanocytic nevus[c]	Corticosteroids, topical and intradermal[c,e]	Bleomycin[c]
Tyrosinase-negative	Neurocutaneous melanosis[c]	Retinoic acid, topical[c,e]	Fixed (drug) eruption[b,c]
Tyrosinase-positive	Xeroderma pigmentosum[c]		
Yellow mutant	Acanthosis nigricans	**PHYSICAL AGENTS**	
Hermansky-Pudlak syndrome	Dyskeratosis congenita[c]	Burns: Thermal, ultraviolet, ionizing radiation[c,m]	Ultraviolet light (suntanning)[c]
Chédiak-Higashi syndrome	Fanconi's syndrome[c]	Trauma[c,m]	Thermal radiation[c]
Cross-McKusick-Breen syndrome	Oculodermal melanocytosis		Alpha, beta, and gamma ionizing radiation[c]
Albinism, ocular[c,g,h]	Nevus of Ota[b,c]		Trauma (e.g., chronic pruritus)[c]
Albinoidism, oculocutaneous[f,g,h]	Dermal melanocytosis (Mongolian spot)[b,c]		
Phenylketonuria[f,g,h]	Blue melanocytic nevus[b,c]	**INFLAMMATION AND INFECTION**	
Fanconi's syndrome[h]	Incontinentia pigmenti[b,c]	Sarcoidosis[c,e]	Postinflammation melanoses (exanthems, drug eruptions)[c]
Homocystinuria[f,h]	Franceschetti-Jadassohn syndrome[b,c]	Pinta[c]	Lichen planus[c]
Histidinemia[f]		Yaws[c]	Lupus erythematosus, discoid[c]
Menkes' kinky hair syndrome[h]		Syphilis, secondary[c]	Lichen simplex chronicus[c]
Canities, premature[h]		Syphilis, endemic, nonvenereal[c]	Atopic dermatitis[i]
		Onchocerciasis[c]	Psoriasis[c]
METABOLIC FACTORS		Leoprosy[c,e]	Tinea versicolor[c]
	Hemochromatosis[f]	Tinea versicolor[c,e]	Pinta in exposed areas[b,c]
	Hepatolenticular disease (Wilson's disease)[f]	Post-kala azar[c]	Erythema dyschromicum perstans[c,n]
	Porphyria (congenital erythropoietic, variegata and cutanea tarda)[f]	Eczematous dermatitis[c,e]	
	Gaucher's disease[i]	Psoriasis[c]	
	Niemann-Pick disease[i]	Discoid lupus erythematosus[c]	
	Hemochromatosis[f]	Vagabond's leukoderma[c]	
	Amyloidosis, cutaneous macular[b,c]	Miscellaneous postinflammatory hypomelanoses[c,e]	
ENDOCRINE FACTORS		**NEOPLASMS**	
Hypopituitarism[f]	ACTH-producing and MSH-producing pituitary and other tumors[f]	Leukoderma acquisitum centrifugum (including halo nevus)[c]	Malignant melanoma[c,h]
Addison's disease[c]	ACTH therapy[f]	Malignant melanoma	Mastocytosis (urticaria pigmentosa)[c]
Hyperthyroidism[c]	Pregnancy[i]	Around primary neoplasms[c]	Acanthosis nigricans, with adenocarcinoma and lymphoma[c]
	Addison's disease[f]	Vitiligo-like hypomelanosis[c,e]	Slate-gray dermal pigmentation with metastatic melanoma and melanogenuria[f]
	Estrogen therapy[j]	Around nevi and metastatic melanoma[c]	
	Melasma[c,k]		
NUTRITIONAL FACTORS		**MISCELLANEOUS FACTORS**	
Chronic protein deficiency or loss:[h,l]	Kwashiorkor[c]	Vogt-Koyanagi-Harada syndrome[c]	Scleroderma, systemic[f]
Kwashiorkor	Pellagra[i]	Scleroderma, circumscribed or systemic[c]	Chronic hepatic insufficiency[f]
Nephrosis	Sprue[i]	Canities[h]	Whipple's syndrome[f]
Ulcerative colitis	Vitamin B_{12} deficiency[i]	Alopecia areata[o]	Encephalitis, chronic[c]
Malabsorption	Chronic nutritional insufficiency[c]	Horner's syndrome, congenital and acquired[g]	Lentigo, senile ("liver spots")[c]
Vitamin B_{12} deficiency[h]		Idiopathic, guttate hypomelanosis[c]	Cronkhite-Canada syndrome[c]
			Catatonic schizophrenia[c]

[a] Listing includes the pigmentation disorder itself or the condition with which it is associated.
[b] Gray, slate, or blue color results from the presence of dermal melanocytes or phagocytized melanin in the dermis.
[c] Pigment change is circumscribed.
[d] Total loss of pigment in the skin and hair may occur.
[e] Loss of pigmentation is usually partial (hypomelanosis); viewed with Wood's lamp, the lesions are not completely devoid of pigment (amelanosis), as in vitiligo.
[f] Pigment change is diffuse, not circumscribed, and there are no identifiable borders.
[g] Pigment is decreased in the iris.
[h] Pigment is decreased in the hair.
[i] Pigment change may be diffuse or circumscribed.
[j] Nipples are affected.
[k] Idiopathic or due to progestational agents.
[l] Hair is gray or reddish.
[m] There is a loss of melanocytes.
[n] Areas of brown may be admixed with the slate-gray and blue discoloration.
[o] Regrown hair is white.

SOURCE: *DB Mosher et al, in Dermatology in General Medicine, 2d ed, TB Fitzpatrick et al (eds), New York, McGraw-Hill, 1979.*

characterized by progressively enlarging amelanotic macules (Table 51-3). Vitiligo may be localized, segmental (one or more dermatomes), or generalized. On occasion, vitiligo may become so extensive that all or nearly all the skin becomes white. Characteristic distribution patterns of vitiligo involve extensor surfaces and bony prominences (elbows, knees), the small joints in the hands, and the area around the eyes and mouth. The low back, axillae, and flexor wrists may also be involved. Genitalia, palms and soles, and mucous membranes are often affected. Typically, the vitiligo macules gradually enlarge centrifugally, and new macules appear. In up to 30 percent of cases some minimal spontaneous repigmentation occurs, particularly in sun-exposed areas of skin. White hairs are common in macules of vitiligo, but may also be seen on normally pigmented skin and scalp. Most vitiligo patients are generally healthy, although thyroid disease, diabetes mellitus, Addison's disease, and pernicious anemia occur with increased frequency. Thyroid disease—hyperthyroidism, thyroiditis, hypothyroidism, and nontoxic goiter—may, in fact, be a common coexisting disorder with vitiligo in patients over the age of fifty. Syndromes with multiple endocrinopathies and with hyperthyroidism, hypoparathyroidism, Addison's disease, chronic mucocutaneous candidiasis, and alopecia areata have been described. Circulating complement-binding antimelanocyte antibodies have been found in two such patients.

Electron microscope studies show a total absence of melanocytes in the white vitiligo macules and decreased numbers of melanocytes in trichrome areas (macules or margins of vitiligo patches in which a color intermediate between the normal skin color and the vitiligo white is present).

In over half the patients treated with psoralens and ultraviolet A [UV-A (sunlight or an artificial UV-A light system; see Chap. 52)] significant repigmentation occurs, particularly on the face and neck, and usually on the trunk, upper arms, and legs. Up to 200 or more treatments may be required, however. In some older patients with extensive areas of depigmentation, irreversible depigmention with topical monobenzylether of hydroquinone cream is a more practical and feasible approach. These persons look essentially normal but need to use sun-protective lotions.

Piebaldism is a congenital, autosomal dominant, stable, circumscribed hypomelanosis which resembles vitiligo except that it has a characteristic distribution pattern different from vitiligo and does not usually progress or resolve over time. The hypomelanosis in piebaldism occurs in circumscribed areas on

TABLE 51-3
Circumscribed vitiligo-type hypomelanosis of skin

Presentation	*Delayed onset*
ASSOCIATED WITH GENETIC DISORDERS	
Piebaldism	Vitiligo
Waardenburg's syndrome	
Nevus depigmentosus	
Tuberous sclerosis	
Neurofibromatosis	
Ataxia telangiectasia	
ASSOCIATED WITH CHEMICALS (OCCUPATIONAL OR THERAPEUTIC)	
Phenolic germicides (O-Syl, Phebocide, etc.)	
Hydroquinone	
Hydroquinone, monobenzylether of	
Hydroquinone, monomethylether of	
ASSOCIATED WITH METABOLIC OR ENDOCRINE DISORDERS	
Addison's disease	
Hyperthyroidism	
Pernicious anemia	
Hypoparathyroidism-Addison's disease-candidiasis syndrome	
ASSOCIATED WITH NEOPLASMS	
Malignant melanoma (in sites of regression)	
Melanocytic nevi (halo nevi)	
ASSOCIATED WITH INFECTIONS	
Leprosy	
Pinta	
Tinea versicolor	
ASSOCIATED WITH IDIOPATHIC CONDITIONS	
Vogt-Koyanagi-Harada syndrome	
Postinflammation: atopic dermatitis, pityriasis alba, psoriasis	
Sarcoidosis	

the extremities and anterior surface of the thorax. A white forelock is typical. The eyes are normal, and the patients are otherwise healthy.

Waardenburg's syndrome, an autosomal dominant trait, has a characteristic appearance similar to that of piebaldism, but also present are congenital deafness, wide-spaced inner canthi, heterochromia irides, and hypertelorism. Electron microscope studies of the white macules in piebaldism and in Waardenburg's syndrome show an absence of identifiable melanocytes.

Tuberous sclerosis is an autosomal dominant disease which manifests itself by the presence of congenital, circumscribed, white macules in up to 98 percent of cases, and classically by the development by the fourth year of seizures, mental retardation, and adenoma sebaceum. The white macules are characteristically on the trunk or buttocks, hypomelanotic, number from 3 to 100, and of typical shape—oval, lance-ovate, or polygonal, like a "thumbprint." The most characteristic, though not the most frequent, is the lance-ovate or American mountain "ash-leaf" macule, which is usually less than 3 cm in its longest dimension and off-white, not pure white, in color. The macules are usually oriented transversely on the trunk and axially on the extremities. The size and color of these lesions do not change over time. The presence of three or more circumscribed macules in a patient is strongly suggestive of tuberous sclerosis. Examination with Wood's lamp is often necessary to visualize the lesions. Histologically, these macules contain melanocytes which have decreased numbers of small melanosomes. All persons with unexplained seizures or mental retardation should be screened with a Wood's lamp examination for the presence of white spots to exclude tuberous sclerosis. In addition, examination of parents and siblings is necessary for genetic counseling.

Neurofibromatosis (von Recklinghausen's disease) is an autosomal dominant trait characterized by the appearance, usually by the age of three and primarily on the trunk and the extremities, of numerous pale yellow-brown macules (Plate 1-4), or café au lait spots, that vary in diameter from less than 1 cm to more than 15 cm. Spotty generalized pigmentation and axillary freckling may also be present. Often, a few or many soft, rounded, cone-shaped, or pendulous cutaneous tumors covered by normal skin appear by the second or third decade.

The presence of six or more café au lait spots—which are uniformly hypermelanotic, circumscribed, oval macules with a diameter greater than 1.5 cm—is characteristic of neurofibromatosis even in the absence of a positive family history. In *Albright's disease* (polyostotic fibrous dysplasia), however, there are rarely more than three or four such macules, which are usually unilaterally distributed on the buttocks or cervical areas. A single, large, isolated café au lait spot of neurofibromatosis resembles the macule of Albright's disease. It is possible, however, using light microscopy, to detect large pigmented globules in whole amounts of epidermis prepared from café au lait macules of neurofibromatosis; these pigmented globules, or macromelanosomes, are usually not found in the macular pigmented areas present in Albright's disease or in the café au lait macules observed in 10 percent of the normal population. Café au lait spots have also been associated with pulmonic stenosis (Watson's syndrome).

Generalized *lentigines* may be a feature of Moynahan's syndrome, or the "leopard" syndrome, which is an autosomal dominant trait in which the diffuse presence of multiple, small, circumscribed hypermelanotic macules has been associated with ECG abnormalities and, in its fully expressed form, with other findings (*l*entigines, *E*CG abnormalities, *o*cular hypertelorism, *p*ulmonary stenosis, *a*bnormal genitalia, *r*etardation of growth, and *d*eafness).

Peutz-Jeghers syndrome is an autosomal dominant disorder in which hyperpigmented, brown to blue macules on the lips and buccal mucosa are associated with similar cutaneous lesions and gastrointestinal polyps. The cutaneous macules may fade by adulthood. Chronic gastrointestinal blood loss may occur.

METABOLIC FACTORS Generalized brown hypermelanosis of the skin is a characteristic manifestation of hemochromatosis and of porphyria cutanea tarda. The hyperpigmentation observed in hemochromatosis may be grayish brown or brown and indistinguishable from that of Addison's disease. The diagnosis of hemochromatosis may be established from a skin biopsy which shows hemosiderin deposition in the sweat glands of the skin. Porphyria cutanea tarda may be diagnosed by the clinical presence of vesicles, bullae, atrophic macules, sclerodermoid changes, and milia on the skin of the dorsal hands and face, and in the laboratory by red fluorescence of acidified urine, or the presence of increased urinary uroporphyrins (uroporphyrin to coproporphyrin ratio usually is greater than 3:1). Similar changes may be seen in patients with variegate porphyria which has a distinctive porphyrin profile including a urinary uroporphyrin to coproporphyrin ratio around 1:1.

NUTRITIONAL FACTORS In chronic nutritional deficiency, in general, splotches of dirty-brown hyperpigmentation appear, especially on the trunk. In selective deficiencies, such as protein deficiency in kwashiorkor, or when there is protein loss as in chronic nephrosis, ulcerative colitis, and malabsorption syndrome, there is sometimes dilution of hair color so that the hair becomes a reddish brown and eventually gray. In other selective deficiencies, such as sprue, there may be a brown hypermelanosis over any area of the body. In pellagra, however, the abnormality is limited to areas of skin exposed to light or to irritation. In vitamin B_{12} deficiency, there is premature graying of hair and a hypermelanosis most apparent overlying the small joints of the hands.

ENDOCRINE FACTORS Diffuse brown hypermelanosis is a striking feature of primary adrenocortical insufficiency (Addison's disease). There is a marked accentuation of pigmentation over certain areas, namely, the pressure points (vertebrae, knuckles, elbows, and knees), and in body folds, palmar creases, and gingival mucous membrane. An identifiable type of diffuse hyperpigmentation has also been reported to follow adrenalectomy in patients with Cushing's disease. In these patients, there usually are signs and symptoms of pituitary tumors; all tumors recorded have been chromophobe adenomas. A third example of the Addisonian type of melanosis has also been observed in patients with pancreatic and lung tumors. The generalized brown hypermelanosis found in all these conditions results from overproduction of melanocyte-stimulating hormone (MSH) and adrenocorticotropic hormone (ACTH), which share common amino acid sequences. It appears that an excess of α-MSH plays a dominant role in the abnormal pigmentation that occurs in Addison's disease. Both MSH and ACTH are increased in adrenal insufficiency as a result of decreased output of cortisol by the adrenals. Hypermelanosis of the Addisonian type can be produced in adrenalectomized human subjects by the administration of large amounts of homogeneous ACTH and α-MSH.

Melasma, or the "mask of pregnancy," is found in pregnant women, women on oral contraceptives, and in some otherwise normal women and men. This is a circumscribed hypermelanosis, usually of the forehead, cheeks, upper lip, and chin, probably secondary to progestational effects. MSH levels are normal in these patients. Melasma-like hyperpigmentation has also been observed in patients taking phenytoin or mesantoin.

CHEMICAL FACTORS Use of various chemicals, particularly phenol derivatives and sulfhydryl compounds, may cause depigmentation. Topical use of hydroquinone induces a temporary lightening which may be useful in some patients with melasma; monobenzylether of hydroquinone, however, causes a permanent vitiligo-like leukoderma, even remote from the site of application, and is used only to depigment completely the normal skin in patients with extensive vitiligo. Addisonian-like hypermelanosis of the skin follows busulfan therapy, and hypermelanosis may also be seen after use of cyclophosphamide and nitrogen mustard. Inorganic trivalent arsenicals may also produce generalized Addisonian-like hypermelanosis as well as scattered macular hypomelanosis and punctate keratosis of the palms and soles.

PHYSICAL FACTORS Mechanical trauma, as well as burns caused by heat, ultraviolet light, or alpha, beta, and gamma radiation, can lead to hypomelanosis or hypermelanosis. The effects of these physical agents on pigmentation are determined by the intensity and duration of exposure and are limited to the site of injury. Hypomelanosis results from destruction of melanocytes.

INFLAMMATORY AND INFECTIOUS FACTORS Many epidermal proliferative processes resolve and leave aberrations of pigmentation at the sites of involvement; both postinflammatory hypermelanosis (blue-gray, brown, or both) and hypomelanosis may occur following resolution of eczema, psoriasis, lichen planus, drug reactions, pemphigus, viral exanthems, etc. Usually these hypermelanoses disappear spontaneously within several months. White halos surrounding psoriatic plaques (Wornoff rings) are a result of abnormal prostaglandin synthesis and are not an abnormality of melanin biology.

Tinea versicolor, a hypomelanotic, not amelanotic, scaling, circumscribed eruption of the upper anterior and posterior chest in young people, results from the presence in the skin of *Pityrosporum orbiculare* which contains an enzyme that forms azelaic acid, a tyrosinase inhibitor, and results in decreased melanin pigmentation. Repigmentation with sun exposure follows appropriate topical therapy.

Tuberculoid and lepromatous leprosy have hypomelanotic macules that are anesthetic. The color, unlike vitiligo, is not pure white, rather, off-white, and the margins of these macules are characteristically indiscrete.

NEOPLASTIC FACTORS Disorders of melanin pigmentation are uncommon features of neoplasms. Hypomelanosis has been found around benign nevi (halo nevi) in healthy patients but may also be found in or around malignant melanoma, primaries, or metastases; vitiligo-like hypomelanotic macules remote from the melanoma may also occur. A Vogt-Koyanagi-Harada syndrome has been reported following bacillus Calmette-Guérin (BCG) therapy of melanoma. During terminal stages of malignant melanoma, striking development of blue hypermelanosis may be observed, associated with large amounts of a conjugated derivative of 5,6-dihydroxyindole excreted in the urine (melanogenuria). This intermediate in the metabolic pathway from tyrosine to melanin can be oxidized to melanin in the absence of tyrosinase; therefore, melanin can be synthesized at almost any site in which oxidation can take place. Consequently, diffuse black pigmentation may develop

4-1 Senile sebaceous adenoma occurs on the face in patients over 40 and is often diagnosed as basal-cell carcinoma. The lesions are soft, small, flat-topped papules, varying in size from 1 to 8 mm, and are characterized by a minute central depression from which sebaceous material can be exuded by lateral compression.

4-2 Solar keratosis (1) occurs usually in persons with light skin prone to sunburn or with darker skin after chronic excessive exposure; (2) is strictly limited to exposed skin, especially on the face and dorsal surfaces of the hands; (3) is more easily felt than seen (gritty and sandpaperish); (4) in fair-skinned persons, consists of skin-colored or light brown macules or slightly raised papules with superficial adherent scales not easily removed; and (5) is associated with marked wrinkling, telangiectasia, and often diffuse, tiny, pale yellow papules indicating solar degeneration of connective tissue ("turkey skin").

4-3 Spider nevus consists of a central, punctate, bright red macule or papule (the body) from which fine red lines radiate like spider legs. There is often a red flare between the radiating vessels. On diascopy, the central body pulsates.

4-4 Tinea versicolor is a relatively common disorder occurring primarily on the trunk and appearing in two forms: as scattered, 3- to 5-mm, very slightly scaling brown macules or as whitish macules that may be confused with vitiligo. The fungal spores and hyphae can be easily demonstrated on direct examination of the scales using Swartz stain.

4-5 Verruca vulgaris may occur at any age, but it is most common in children. The lesions, which vary in size from 0.5 to 2.0 cm, are round or oval, firm, skin-colored papules with multiple tiny keratotic, rounded or filiform projections covering the surface (vegetation). They occur most frequently on the hands and soles.

4-6 Xanthelasma consists of one or more bright yellow, sharply marginated plaques with no epidermal change, usually occurring on the eyelids. All patients with xanthelasma should be investigated for evidence of plasma lipid abnormalities.

3-1 **Perlèche** consists of painful small fissures at the angles of the mouth, often covered with yellow crusts. Perlèche most often occurs with poorly fitting dentures and in moniliasis and secondary syphilis.

3-2 **Rosacea,** usually limited to the face, consists of tiny, erythematous papules and pustules 1 to 5 mm in size. The pustules, often tiny and sometimes hardly visible, sit on the dome of the papules. The diffuse redness of the face is due to vasodilatation, as well as to myriad telangiectases. In men, rhinophyma, a disfiguring enlargement of the nose, may occur.

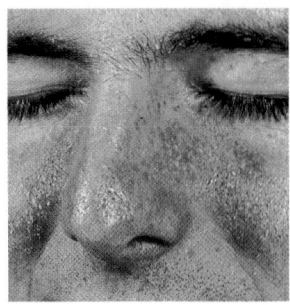

3-3 **Seborrheic dermatitis,** a common disorder found in all age groups, occurs most frequently on the scalp, eyebrows, and nasolabial folds and behind the ears. Scaling is the prominent feature and is loose and branny; it may be yellow and oily or dry and white. The lesion may become exudative and crusted or eczematous.

3-4 **Seborrheic keratosis** appears in middle life and may occur on exposed or unexposed areas but is especially common on the trunk. The lesions are irregularly round or oval flat-topped papules or plaques that seem "stuck" on the skin. The margins are distinct, and the surface is often warty or consists of multiple tiny projections (vegetation). In fair-skinned persons, the lesions are light brown at first but, enlarging, become more heavily pigmented and may be confused with malignant melanoma.

3-5 **Senile angioma ("cherry red spot")** appears in the third decade. On the lip, the lesion is usually singular and consists of a bluish red round nodule. On the trunk, the lesions are small (2 to 3 mm), bright red, globular papules.

3-6 **Senile lentigo** occurs as a single macule or as a group of isolated, sharply circumscribed macules on the exposed areas, especially on the dorsal surfaces of the hands and arms and on the forehead and cheeks. The macules are usually light yellowish brown, but may be dark brown; the color is somewhat variegated, rather than uniform as it is in a café au lait macule. Rarely, dark brown *papules* develop in these lesions, and then the condition is called *lentigo maligna,* which may slowly develop, over a period of years, into a melanoma *(lentigo maligna melanoma).*

2-1 **Dermatophytosis** is identified by the striking polycyclic, annular shape of the scaling, especially on the feet and hands, where there is often a scalloped pattern. A positive diagnosis of dermatophytosis is quickly established by direct examination of scales from the advancing border; the mycelia are revealed when the scales are immersed in 10% potassium hydroxide or Swartz stain.

2-2 **Eczematous dermatitis** is a very common cutaneous reaction that is localized to the hands of housewives, to the legs in patients with chronic venous insufficiency, and behind the ears in patients with seborrheic dermatitis. In subacute eczematous dermatitis, there are mild erythema, dry scales, and often small red papules, many of which are excoriated. In chronic eczematous dermatitis, lichenification is the most prominent feature.

2-3 **Localized lichenification** results from repeated rubbing of the skin and consists of isolated, circumscribed plaques. These single lesions vary in size from 2 to 10 cm and occur most often on the extensor aspect of the forearm and in the scrotal, nuchal, inguinal, and anogenital areas. The perianal and vulvar areas may become diffusely lichenified. Lichenification is thought to be more frequent in persons with an atopic background.

2-4 **Melasma (chloasma)** is the so-called "mask" of pregnancy, but it also occurs in men and in women taking progestational agents. The pigmentation is uniform and is limited to the exposed areas of the face. There is no scaling or epidermal change. In fair-skinned persons, the pigment may be any shade from light tan to a very dark brown. It is most often seen on the cheeks and upper lip, as here, and on the forehead.

2-5 **Milia** are a collection of lesions, occurring most commonly on the face, and consist of tiny (1 to 2 mm), white, hard, rounded, superficial papules. There is no orifice, and the keratinous contents are easily expressed by lateral compression after the making of a tiny incision in the dome of the lesion.

2-6 **Psoriasis,** affecting more than 2 percent of the population, consists of isolated scaling papules or plaques and is quite commonly observed in the routine physical examination. The lesions occur most frequently on the scalp, elbows, and knees. The color and type of scales are the identifying features of the lesions. The scales are either dense and lamellated with peripherally detached edges or loose and branny. The plaques are pink to deep red, and the borders are distinct.

Atlas of common lesions encountered during the physical examination of the skin

The skin and mucous membrane may frequently contain a variety of lesions that are rarely a major complaint (see Fig. 48-1). They are, therefore, incidental findings in the general physical examination. The recognition of "bumps and blemishes" is a necessary first step for physicians inasmuch as they will be required to distinguish the trivial from the serious and important skin changes. For example, such a serious lesion as a malignant melanoma may be incidentally discovered during a routine physical examination (see Plates 6-1 to 6-4 and the discussion in Chap. 330).

The common disorders of the skin that every physician should be able to recognize are presented in this series of color photographs (Plates 1 to 4).

A   B

1-1 **Dermatofibroma** is especially common in middle life and in women. The lesions, when pigmented, are occasionally confused with malignant melanoma. They appear as isolated, slightly elevated, hard, button-like nodules *(A)*. In fair-skinned persons, the lesions are not usually skin color, but are pink or dark red, yellowish brown, or gray-black. They are usually less than 1 cm in diameter. A diagnostic sign is that a dermatofibroma dimples or becomes depressed *(B)* when it is laterally compressed; melanocytic nevus and melanoma, however, with which dermatofibroma may be easily confused, become elevated with lateral compression.

1-2 **Acrochordon** (skin tag) is very common after middle life and appears on the neck, especially in women, in the axillae, and on the upper part of the trunk. The lesions are small (1 to 5 mm), soft, pedunculated papules, usually of normal skin color.

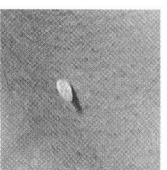

1-3 **Angiokeratomas** are bizarre vascular dilatations that occur under the tongue and on the scrotum and consist of myriads of 2- to 3-mm purplish red papules. They are of no known significance. When they occur on the trunk and extremities, a biopsy is indicated to rule out glycolipid lipidosis or Fabry's disease.

1-4 **Café au lait macules** are found in about 10 percent of the normal population and, in fair-skinned persons, are light yellowish brown macules, which may also be markers of neurofibromatosis and polyostotic fibrous dysplasia (Albright's syndrome). The presence of six or more café au lait macules with a diameter of 1.5 cm or greater is diagnostic of neurofibromatosis.

1-5 **Acne** is a condition in which the most characteristic lesion is the comedo, or "blackhead," that later becomes a conical erythematous papule or pustule. A third type of lesion is the "blind boil," which is a dermal cyst without an orifice. This lesion is often associated with atrophic or hypertrophic scarring. Cystic acne may appear with only a very few comedones; also, comedo-like acne may occur with few cysts or erythematous papules.

5-1 **Necrobiosis lipoidica diabeticorum.** Note the vivid colors (brown and yellow) and fine, arborizing blood vessels traversing the atrophic skin.

5-2 **Pretibial myxedema.**

5-3 **Pyoderma gangrenosum** in a patient with ulcerative colitis.

5-4 **"Palpable" purpura with inflammation occurring in gonococcemia.** An identical lesion may be seen in meningococcemia, staphylococcemia, and systemic vasculitis.

A   **B**

5-5 **Peutz-Jeghers syndrome.** *A.* Macules on the buccal mucosae that are blue or blue-black and are pathogonomonic. *B.* Punctate dark brown macules that typically occur on the lips, around the mouth, and on the fingers. The pigmented macules may disappear on the lips but not on the buccal mucosa.

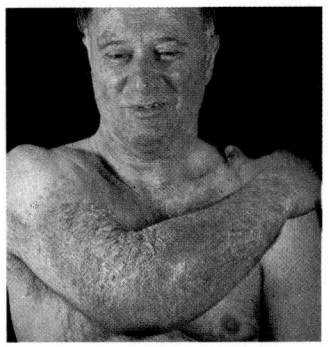

5-6 **Contact eczematous dermatitis.** The diagnosis is made by detailed history in the manner of a detective and also by the periodicity of the attacks. The artificial configuration (sharp borders, etc.) indicates an "outside job."

6-1 In **lentigo maligna melanoma,** the lesion is predominantly flat, but there may be a few nodules or papules. The color consists mainly of shades of brown and black, admixed with whitish gray and, occasionally, with reddish brown, bluish gray, and bluish black.

6-3 In **nodular melanoma,** the lesion is always raised and may be dome-shaped or polypoid. The color is usually uniform bluish black, but there may rarely be shades of reddish blue (purple) or an admixture of bluish black with brown or black.

6-2 In **superficial spreading melanoma,** the lesion is usually slightly raised in its entirety and is punctuated with papules and, sometimes, nodules. The color consists mainly of brown and black, admixed with bluish red (violaceous), bluish gray, bluish black, reddish brown, and often whitish pink. The presence of a notched border is distinctive.

6-4 **Superficial spreading melanoma, superficially invasive.** At this very early stage in the evolution of this tumor, the variegation of color is the clue to the diagnosis.

7-1 **Normal optic nerve and retina.**

7-2 **Glaucomatous optic disk with secondary atrophy.**

7-3 **Drusen of the optic nerve head.**

7-4 **Angioid streaks.**

7-5 **Primary optic atrophy.**

7-6 **Early papilledema.**

7-7 **Retentive pigmentosa.**

7-8 **Band keratopathy.**

8-1 **Schemic optic neuritis with temporal arteritis.**

8-2 **Cholesterol embolus in retinal arteriole.**

8-3 **Diabetic retinopathy microaneurysm.**

8-4 **Retinitis proliferans in diabetes mellitus.**

8-5 **Roth spot with subacute bacterial endocarditis.**

8-6 **Central retinal vein thrombosis.**

8-7 **Dislocated lens in Marfan's disease.**

8-8 **Kayser-Fleischer ring in Wilson's disease.** (*Note:* The ring is the golden brown pigment at the periphery of the cornea and is characteristically broader superiorly and inferiorly than it is medially and laterally.)

in peritoneum, liver, heart, muscle, and dermis of patients during the late stages of malignant melanoma. The brown melanin in the dermal phagocytes appears clinically as blue in the skin because of the Tyndall light-scattering phenomenon. Velvety textured hypermelanotic (brown) macules, representing acanthosis nigricans, may be found in the axillae and other areas in patients with various carcinomas, particularly adenocarcinomas of the gastrointestinal tract. Acanthosis nigricans may also be congenital or benign and associated with diabetes mellitus, Cushing's disease, Addison's disease, pituitary adenoma, and other disorders.

The multiple, irregular, round or oval, yellowish brown to reddish brown macules and papules characteristic of urticaria pigmentosa are related to the presence of melanin in the epidermis overlying clusters of mast cells. Vigorous stroking of such lesions results in the development of urticarial wheals. Systemic mastocytosis, in which mast cells infiltrate diffusely into the liver, spleen, gastrointestinal system, and bones, is a rare condition. Mast-cell leukemia occasionally develops. In children, the skin lesions usually appear in infancy and often spontaneously disappear in several years. The usual course is quite benign, but symptoms of flushing, itching, and urticaria occur in about 30 percent of patients; less than 15 percent experience vomiting, syncope, or shock. The symptoms are presumed to be due to histamine release from mast cells and often coincide with increased urinary excretion of free histamines and metabolites. Urinary levels of 5-hydroxyindoleacetic acid are normal. Antihistamines are of little value.

UNKNOWN CAUSES Generalized brown hypermelanosis of the type seen in Addison's disease may be associated with systemic scleroderma, even early in the course of the disorder. Generalized hyperpigmentation occasionally develops in patients with chronic hepatic insufficiency, especially that due to portal cirrhosis. The pathogenesis of the pigmentation in both conditions is unknown; MSH levels are not elevated. Hypomelanotic macules may also be found in a small percentage of patients with sarcoidosis. These macules are characteristically not pure white and are circumscribed with indiscrete margins. They may overlie dermal nodules, particularly on the extremities but also at times on the trunk.

REFERENCES

DEMIS DJ: Mast cell disease (urticaria pigmentosa), in *Clinical Dermatology,* DJ Demis et al (eds). New York, Harper & Row, 1974, vol 1, units 4–11, p 1

FITZPATRICK TB et al: Biology of the melanin pigmentary system, in *Dermatology in General Medicine,* 2d ed, TB Fitzpatrick et al (eds). New York, McGraw-Hill, 1979

JIMBOW K et al: Congenital circumscribed hypomelanosis: A characterization based on electron microscopic study of tuberous sclerosis, nevus depigmentosis, and piebaldism. J Invest Dermatol 64:50, 1975

MOSHER DB et al: Abnormalities of pigmentation, in *Dermatology in General Medicine,* 2d ed, TB Fitzpatrick et al (eds). New York, McGraw-Hill, 1979

TODA K et al: Alteration of racial differences in melanosome distribution in human epidermis after exposure to ultraviolet light. Nature [New Biol] 236:143, 1972

WITKOP CV et al: Albinism, in *The Metabolic Basis of Inherited Diseases,* 4th ed, JB Stanbury et al (eds). New York, McGraw-Hill, 1978, p 283

52
PHOTOSENSITIVITY AND OTHER REACTIONS TO LIGHT

MADHUKAR A. PATHAK
THOMAS B. FITZPATRICK
JOHN A. PARRISH

Humans have evolved in sunlight and depend upon it for much more than an indirect source of food and maintenance of the earth's temperature. The natural light has always been recognized for, and endowed with, health-giving powers. Our skin, eyes, blood vessels, and certain endocrine gland functions respond to radiation from the electromagnetic spectrum of the sun. The formation of vitamin D from sterol precursors in the skin by solar ultraviolet (UV) exposure has long been recognized in the management of rickets. Certain of our daily biorhythms are dependent upon the cycles of sunlight. Yet, sunlight can be harmful and damage or kill living cells. Sunlight causes sunburn, damage to deoxyribonucleic acid (DNA), skin cancer, wrinkling and aging of the skin, eye inflammation, and possibly cataracts. During the last decade, interest in the reaction of human skin to light has been renewed as a result of (1) the public's obsession with sunbathing, resulting in premature "aging" of the skin (solar elastosis); (2) demographic data indicating that exposure to sunlight is an important cause of basalcell and squamous-cell carcinoma and even melanoma of the sun-exposed parts of the body; (3) the widespread use of certain drugs such as phenothiazines, thiazides and related sulfonamide diuretics, and antibiotics (demethylchlortetracycline), which alter the cutaneous responses to sunlight and cause undesirable photosensitivity reactions; (4) the increased recognition of, and better diagnostic and therapeutic approaches to, various skin eruptions (papules, plaques, and eczematous and urticarial reactions) of unknown cause and differing morphologic features (i.e., polymorphic photodermatitis) that follow exposure to UV and visible light; and (5) increased awareness that sunlight is a major cause of discomfort and photosensitivity reactions in patients with certain types of porphyria, especially for those with erythropoietic protoporphyria.

In spite of these negative factors, UV radiation and visible light can be advantageously used in phototherapy and control of certain skin diseases and to prevent brain damage (kernicterus) due to neonatal hyperbilirubinemia. Considerable interest has been generated in recent years in a new type of treatment called *photochemotherapy;* this involves the oral or systemic administration of a drug (methoxsalen) and subsequent exposure of skin to UV radiation (320 to 400 nm). This regimen has been found to be highly effective in clearing psoriasis in over 90 percent of persons treated.

There are more than 25 human disorders that are either caused by or aggravated by exposure of the skin to sunlight. These range from degenerative and neoplastic changes to disability and discomfort associated with chemically induced photosensitivity reactions. These abnormal reactions to light in humans are briefly presented in Table 52-1.

This chapter will be concerned with (1) common conditions such as sunburn, the degenerative and neoplastic conditions associated with solar radiation [basal-cell carcinoma, squamous-cell carcinoma, malignant melanoma, solar keratoses (Plate 4-2)] and chronic sun-induced degeneration; (2) photosensitivity related to drugs and to increased blood or plasma levels of photosensitizing porphyrins in patients with all types of porphyria (except acute intermittent porphyria); (3) photochemotherapy; and (4) photoprotection.

The unit of wavelength most commonly used to measure

and express nonionizing UV radiation or visible light is the nanometer (1 nm = 10^{-9} m = 10 Å). Electromagnetic emanations from the sun comprise a wide range of radiation and include electric waves, radio waves, infrared rays, visible light, UV radiation, roentgen rays (x-rays), gamma rays, and cosmic rays. The shortest wavelengths that reach the surface of the earth through the atmosphere are about 286 to 290 nm. Wavelengths shorter than 286 nm are principally absorbed by ozone in the stratosphere. The solar radiation that reaches the earth's surface ranges from around 286 nm in the UV region, through the visible (400 to 760 nm) and infrared region and well beyond to include electric and radio waves. The solar spectrum that can affect human skin includes wavelengths of 290 to 720 nm; however, infrared radiation (1.5 to 1000 μm) can produce thermal effects (including burn) and potentiate the photochemical and biologic reactions initiated by UV or visible radiation.

For practical reasons, UV radiation is often arbitrarily subdivided into three bands designated as (1) UV-A (320 to 400 nm or long-wave ultraviolet), (2) UV-B (290 to 320 nm or sunburn spectrum), and (3) UV-C (below 290 nm or germicidal radiation).

The amount and type of solar radiation that may reach a given part of the earth at any given time are determined by a great variety of factors, including latitude, time of day, season, altitude, local atmospheric conditions (smog, cloudiness, haze, smoke, dust, fog, humidity, aerosol particles), variations in the thickness of the ozone layer, and height of the sun above the horizon.

Approximately 50 percent of the sun's radiant energy is in the visible portion of the spectrum (400 to 760 nm), about 40 percent in the infrared region, and about 10 percent in the UV region. The damage to skin (sunburn, skin cancer) is evoked by 3 percent of the ultraviolet radiation wavelengths, namely, from 290 to 320 nm.

The transmission of radiant energy varies with wavelength and different areas of the human skin; it may range from 0 to 70 percent. Shorter wavelengths (< 285 nm) are mostly absorbed by the dead-cell layer of the stratum corneum; wavelengths that produce sunburn (290 to 315 nm) are also mostly absorbed in the epidermis. Longer wavelengths (320 to 760 nm) penetrate more deeply into the dermis. Transmission of different wavelengths depends upon (1) the regional thickness of the epidermis, (2) the degree of hydration, (3) the concentration of UV and visible light-absorbing components such as melanin, proteins (keratin, elastin, collagen), nucleic acid, urocanic acid, carotenoids, and hemoglobin, and (4) the number and spatial arrangement of melanosomes and of blood vessels. In fair-skinned individuals, about 85 to 90 percent of 290- to 315-nm radiation is absorbed by the epidermis and only about 10 to 15 percent can penetrate through the epidermis to reach the dermis. In dark-skinned individuals, nearly 90 to 95 percent of 290- to 315-nm radiation is absorbed by the epidermis. The transmission through the epidermis of long-wave UV radiation (320 to 400 nm) and visible radiation (400 to 760 nm) may range from 20 to 70 percent.

The most detrimental effect of UV radiation is cell death. Other effects include mutagenesis, carcinogenesis, interference or inhibition in the synthesis of DNA, ribonucleic acid (RNA), and protein. The mutagenic and carcinogenic effects appear to be mediated largely though the action of UV-B radiation on DNA. The most common reactions, such as sunburn, tanning or melanin pigmentation, keratosis, and skin aging are also caused by UV-B radiation. Although the longer wavelengths (UV-A or 320 to 400 nm and visible or 400 to 760 nm) penetrate more deeply into the skin, they are much less effective at causing these types of photobiologic phenomena. However, in the presence of certain chemical agents (e.g., drugs that are given orally or endogenous porphyrins in certain porphyrias), these wavelengths become highly damaging and cause severe skin photosensitization reactions.

Protection against this damage to the "normal" skin has been the subject of much investigation, and many commercially available sunscreens can be recommended in the prevention of sunburn, skin cancer, aging of skin, and in various types of photosensitivity disorders.

SUNBURN AND TANNING

CLINICAL CHANGES Erythema, or sunburn reaction Erythema is caused principally by 290- to 320-nm radiation, maximum solar effectiveness being from 300 to 307 nm. Ultraviolet radiation, emitted by artificial light sources, produces erythema maximally at 297 and 254 nm. Light of wavelengths greater than 320 nm (320 to 760 nm) is generally considered to be nonerythemogenic, although prolonged exposure to radiation of 320 to 400 nm (2 h of midday summer sun in northern latitudes) can produce mild sunburn in normal subjects. Wavelengths of 290 to 320 nm are thought to accelerate aging (wrinkling) of the skin and to lead to the development of solar keratoses, carcinoma, and, possibly, some types of malignant melanoma.

The sunburn reaction is a complex inflammatory process. The observed histologic changes include the appearance of dyskeratotic cells (containing pyknotic nuclei), spongiosis, vacuolation of keratinocytes, and edema. The dermal changes include an inflammatory infiltrate (mostly neutrophils), endothelial swelling, and capillary leakage manifested by extravasation of red blood cells. The severity of these changes and the rate at which they evolve depend on the exposure dose, the incident wavelength, and the type of skin. Hypopigmented, fair-skinned individuals (e.g., red-haired, freckled individuals such as the Irish or Scottish) are more susceptible than pigmented individuals who tan well. The nature of the chromophore that absorbs the light energy which initiates the primary photochemical responses is not well established, although the bulk of evidence suggests that nucleic acids (DNA) are primary targets for the absorption of the 290- to 320-nm radiation. Vasodilatation which accompanies the sunburn reaction

TABLE 52-1
Diseases induced or exacerbated by light

I By light alone
  A Genetic: ephelides (freckles)
  B Idiopathic
    1 Acute solar skin damage (sunburn)
    2 Connective tissue degeneration (wrinkling)
    3 Telangiectasia
    4 Solar keratoses and solar lentigo
    5 Basal-cell carcinoma
    6 Squamous-cell carcinoma
    7 Malignant melanoma
    8 Polymorphous photodermatosis
    9 Solar urticaria
II By light plus exogenous agents
  A Chemical or drug
    1 Phototoxic reactions
    2 Phytophotodermatitis
    3 Lupus erythematosus (with hydralazine, procainamide)
  B Chemical and immunologic: photoallergic reactions
III By light plus metabolite(s)
  A Porphyrias
  B Porphyria cutanea tarda associated with hexachlorobenzene, estrogens, alcohol
IV By light plus preexisting disease
  A Genetic
    1 Xeroderma pigmentosum
    2 Oculocutaneous albinism
    3 Vitiligo
    4 Hartnup syndrome
  B Nutritional or metabolic
    1 Pellagra
    2 Malignant carcinoid
  C Viral: herpes simplex
  D Unknown: lupus erythematosus (cutaneous, systemic)

appears to result from the activation and release of one or more chemical mediators (e.g., kinins, serotonin, histamine).

There has been considerable focus on the role of prostaglandins and related derivatives of arachidonic acid. These are low-molecular-weight, oxygenated, fatty acid structures synthesized by microsomal enzymes present in all mammalian cells, including epidermal cells. Increased levels of prostaglandins (PGE series) have been observed in widely different types of inflammation, including the UV-induced sunburn reaction. Indomethacin, a nonsteroidal anti-inflammatory agent, when applied topically or given intradermally, can decrease a delayed sunburn response of human skin produced by UV-B radiation. Since indomethacin is known to inhibit prostaglandin synthesis, these findings support the possible role of prostaglandins as mediators of the delayed erythemal response to UV-B radiation. Ultraviolet radiation may also have a direct effect on the blood vessels of the upper layer of the dermis (capillaries, venules, and arterioles). The formation of peroxides or free radicals may play an important role in the damage to lysosomal membranes associated with lipid peroxidation. In fair skin 290- to 320-nm spectrum is known to produce damaging free radicals (molecules with unpaired electrons).

Melanin pigmentation, or tanning   Tanning (increase in melanin pigment) that follows exposure of the skin to solar radiation involves two distinct photobiologic processes. The first, *immediate pigment darkening* (IPD), or darkening of preformed pigment in the epidermis, is elicited by wavelengths of 320 to 720 nm. The second, *melanogenesis,* is an intricate process that consists of the *erythema response (sunburn)* followed usually in 3 to 4 days by formation of new pigment. Immediate pigment darkening results from oxidation of melanin through the production of semiquinone-like free radicals in the melanin polymer; transfer of melanosomes from melanocytes and redistribution of already existing melanosomes within the keratinocytes also may occur.

Melanogenesis involves (1) an increase in the number of functional melanocytes, resulting from increased proliferation of melanocytes, and activation of dormant melanocytes; (2) increased arborization of melanocytic dendrites; (3) an increase in the number of melanosomes in proliferating melanocytes; (4) an increase in tyrosinase activity; and (5) an increase in the transfer of melanosomes from melanocytes to keratinocytes. The degree of melanin pigmentation, however, that can be achieved in an individual by exposure to solar radiation is genetically predetermined. People with fair skin who burn easily but do not tan or tan poorly (skin types I and II) cannot with repeated sun exposures achieve that degree of tanning which can be easily achieved by someone genetically able to tan profusely with minimal exposure.

CELLULAR AND MOLECULAR CHANGES Hyperplasia Within 72 h after exposure, there is an increase in the number of epidermal cells with a high rate of mitotic activity. The rate of cell proliferation decreases after 7 to 10 days, and the thickness of the epidermis gradually returns to normal within the next 30 to 60 days.

DNA and RNA changes   Damage to DNA by sunburn-producing UV light (290 to 320 nm) may result in cell death. The principal epidermal DNA photoproducts are pyrimidine dimers (e.g., thymine dimers); these are of the cyclobutane type and are formed between adjacent pyrimidine bases. DNA and RNA synthesis in the epidermis is inhibited within 1 h after irradiation. New synthesis is evident by 24 h and is maximal by 60 to 70 h.

Mitosis   Inhibition of epidermal mitosis and retardation of basal-cell turnover occur within 1 h after irradiation. The epidermal cell cycle is interrupted at the S phase of DNA synthesis. Inhibition of mitosis can persist for 7 to 24 h; it is followed by an acceleration of mitotic rate and basal-cell turnover that reaches a peak by 48 to 72 h and is associated with epidermal hyperplasia. The mitotic cycle appears to be interrupted in the G_2 stage, in the prophase stage, or in both. The increased mitotic activity and the associated hyperplasia may last for 30 to 60 days. This hyperplasia appears to be due to a combination of the removal of the epidermal mitotic inhibitors (chalones) and stimulation of growth by the action of cyclic adenosine monophosphate (AMP) and guanosine 5′-monophosphate (GMP).

SUN-INDUCED CARCINOMA

Epidemiologic evidence clearly implicates solar radiation as a factor in the induction of human skin cancer. Some studies have established that carcinoma of the skin occurs more frequently on the parts of the body habitually exposed to sunlight; thus, the lesions of the head and hands are concentrated on the nose, central portions of the cheeks, eyelids, and dorsum of the hands. In fair-skinned Caucasoids who sunburn easily, these cancers are limited almost exclusively to the exposed portions of the face, head, neck, arms, and hands. Negroid skin, on the other hand, is remarkably resistant to the development of skin cancer on the exposed surfaces, and a similar resistance is seen among the pigmented Caucasoids (e.g., East Indians), American Indians, and Asiatics.

Carcinoma of the exposed skin is more prevalent among persons who are outdoors a great deal and is the common cause of cancer in Caucasoids in Australia, South Africa, and the southern parts of the United States. The action spectrum for photocarcinogenesis is similar to that of sunburn reaction.

Several studies based on the distribution of local populations in the United States, Australia, and Ireland have emphasized that skin cancer develops earlier and more frequently in people who have light skin and freckles, who burn easily and do not tan on exposure to the sun, and who are of mostly Celtic ancestry (people with skin types I and II). *Australia, with the highest reported incidence of skin cancer* in the world, has a population largely descended from British stock, with about 25 percent claiming Celtic (i.e., Irish, Scottish, and Welsh) extraction. In all three countries surveyed, persons of Celtic ancestry were found to have a disproportionately high incidence of skin cancer. Dark-pigmented races and people who tan well (skin types IV to VI) are least susceptible to skin cancer.

All varieties of skin cancer develop in patients with *xeroderma pigmentosum*, an autosomal recessive disorder. This rare defect represents, in the extreme, the basic problem of solar radiation and skin cancer. Patients with this disease have a greatly increased susceptibility to malignant tumors of the skin in the light-exposed areas. The characteristic skin manifestations are atrophy, telangiectasia, hyperpigmented macules, keratoses, and ulcerations, all occurring in sun-exposed areas. Within the first few years of life, basal-cell or squamous-cell carcinomas or sarcomas or malignant melanomas develop. An inherited enzyme defect may be responsible, at least in part, for the cancer-forming potential in patients with xeroderma pigmentosum. Cultured fibroblasts from patients with xeroderma pigmentosum are incapable of releasing thymine dimers from DNA and, in consequence, are deficient in their ability to repair their UV-damaged DNA. Xeroderma pigmentosum is the most notable human disease in which there is a defect in the excision repair process involving the removal of UV-induced dimers followed by the synthesis and re-forming of new segments of DNA. This enzymatic deficiency may result in a high somatic mutation rate of skin cells after sun exposure and, eventually, in cancer formation.

DEGENERATIVE CHANGES OF THE SKIN

Degenerative skin changes (wrinkling, telangiectasia, keratoses) are more frequent in white-skinned people living in areas where the intensity of UV radiation is great (e.g., southwestern United States, Australia, South Africa). The term *solar degeneration* implies a group of changes in the exposed areas of the skin, including wrinkling, atrophy, hypermelanotic and hypomelanotic macules, telangiectasia, yellow papules and plaques, and keratoses. The furrowed and leathery condition of the skin is seen particularly in persons who have fair skin and poor tanning ability and are constantly exposed to the sun. The most conspicuous and characteristic change may result from biochemical and structural alterations of connective tissue (elastin as well as collagen). The generative changes are caused by sunburn-producing (290 to 320 nm) and UV-A (320 to 400 nm) radiation that can penetrate deeply into the dermis.

Chronically light-damaged human epidermis shows shortening or flattening of the rete ridges, thinning of the epidermis (decrease in malpighian cells), and many abnormal cells in disorderly arrangement. There is a progressive degeneration in the papillary and subpapillary zones of the dermis. Other changes include (1) the development of vascular ectasia, (2) accumulation of acid mucopolysaccharides, (3) appearance of abnormal fibrocytes, (4) loss of collagen, (5) degeneration of elastic tissue ("actinic elastosis") and disorganization of the connective tissue into amorphous masses. These changes are irreversible and can be minimized by daily topical application of effective sunscreens.

PHOTOTOXICITY AND PHOTOALLERGY

Sensitivity to sunlight is a common clinical problem. Continuous daily exposure to sun alone may be the major factor responsible for irreversible skin changes (e.g., freckles, telangiectasia, wrinkling, keratoses, atrophy, hypermelanotic and hypomelanotic macules, and carcinomas in the sun-exposed regions). Apart from these chronic changes, human skin can also become hypersensitive to UV and visible light. The interface between humans and their environment is the skin, and the physical (light) and chemical agents acting directly on it are important etiologic or precipitating factors in photosensitivity disorders.

EFFECT OF DRUGS AND OTHER CHEMICALS IN ASSOCIATION WITH LIGHT EXPOSURE Some chemicals and drugs by themselves may not act as contact irritants and are generally innocuous to skin in the absence of light exposure. However, when the skin is challenged with proper concentrations of the agent and the appropriate light wavelengths, these agents can induce undesirable skin reactions.

Cutaneous photosensitivity is a general term used to refer to the abnormal reaction of the human skin to the stimulus of light. Drug photosensitivity reactions may be defined clinically as adverse skin responses resulting from the combination of exposure to certain therapeutic or chemical agents and UV radiation of 320 to 400 nm. Adverse cutaneous reactions can occur in some individuals who either have ingested certain drugs or have been in contact with certain chemicals (Tables 52-2 and 52-3). These reactions may include an acute, abnormal sunburn response, namely, edema, papules, macules, vesicles, bullae, or acute eczematous or urticarial reactions. There may be desquamation and hyperpigmentation or hypopigmentation. These adverse photosensitivity reactions are classified into two broad categories: (1) phototoxic reactions and (2) photoallergic reactions.

TABLE 52-2
Contact photosensitizers: Chemicals that induce photosensitivity reactions in humans

Name	Use	Reported clinical observations
Halogenated salicylanilides; 3,3',4',5-tetrachlorosalicylanilide; 3,4',5- and 3,3',5-trichlorosalicylanilide; 3,4',5- and 3,3',5-tribromosalicylanilide; 3,5- and 4,5'-dibromosalicylanilide	Deodorant, bacteriostatic agents in soaps	Phototoxic and eczematous photoallergic reactions, burning, itching, cross-photosensitivity reactions
Hexachlorophene	Antimicrobial, antiseptic	Phototoxic reactions
Bithionol or bis(2-hydroxy-3,5-dichlorophenyl) sulfide	Antimicrobial, antiseptic	Photoallergic reactions
Fentichlor (2,2'-dihydroxy-5,5'-dichlorodiphenyl sulfide); multifungin (bromochlorosalicylanilide); Jadit (4-chloro-2-hydroxybenzoic acid *N-n*-butylamide)	Antifungal	Phototoxic and photoallergic reactions
5-Flurouracil	Antineoplastic	Acceleration of inflammatory process
p-Aminobenzoic acid (PABA) and esters of PABA	Sunscreen	Photoallergic reactions
4,4'-Bis(3-phenylureido)-2,2'-stilbenedisulfonic acid or blankophor	Fluorescent brightening agent for cellulose, nylon, or wool fibers	Phototoxic and photoallergic reactions
Cadmium sulfide	In tattoos	Erythema
Furocoumarins: psoralen, 8-methoxypsoralen, 5-methoxypsoralen, 4,5',8-trimethylpsoralen	In vitiligo for increased pigment formation and sun tolerance	Marked erythema, vesicles, bullae, hyperpigmentation
Essential oils: oil of bergamot, oil of lime, oil of cedar, oil of lavender, oil of citron, oil of sandalwood	Cosmetics and beauty aids	Phototoxic reactions and postinflammatory hyperpigmentation
Plants: Umbelliferae, Rutaceae	Used in perfumes or flavorings or as spices	Phytophotodermatitis, hyperpigmentation, vesicles, bullae
Dyes: fluorescein, rose bengal, eosin, erythrocine, trypaflavin, orange red, paraphenylenediamine, methylene blue, toluidine blue, trypan blue	Cosmetics and dye industry	Erythema, edema, vesicles, pigmentation, phototoxic reaction
Coal tar and coal tar derivatives containing anthracene, phenanthrene, naphthalene, thiophene, and many phenolic agents; pitch	In therapy for psoriasis and chronic eczema; in hair shampoos	Smarting, exaggerated sunburn, urticarial wheals, tar melanosis

SOURCE: *TB Fitzpatrick et al, in Sunlight and Man: Normal and Abnormal Photobiologic Responses, MA Pathak et al (eds), Tokyo, University of Tokyo Press, 1974.*

Phototoxic reactions are those that can be elicited in almost everyone with enough light energy of the appropriate wavelengths and when appropriate concentrations of the agent are either applied topically or given orally. Light plus the offending agent leads to an exaggerated sunburn reaction, with or without painful edema. The reaction can occur within 5 to 18 h after exposure to the sun and is usually maximum at 36 to 72 h. Hyperpigmentation and desquamation can also occur. The reaction is usually confined to the site of exposure. If the applied concentration of the implicated agent is high, bullae or small vesicles may develop.

Certain *phototoxic reactions* require the presence of molecular oxygen (e.g., hematoporphyrin, several dyes). The oxygen-dependent reactions are referred to as *photodynamic reactions.* On the other hand, many phototoxic reactions can occur in the absence of oxygen (e.g., psoralen photosensitization). Most reactions have been reported to require UV-A (320 to 400 nm) radiation; however, certain phototoxic reactions can be initiated by the UV-B (290 to 320 nm) as well as by the visible (400 to 700 nm) spectra. The phototoxic reactions in general should be regarded as the undesirable sequelae of augmentation of the primary photochemical reactions that underlie the inflammatory response of skin evoked by UV radiation. It is believed that a deleterious amount of radiant energy is absorbed by the skin and the photosensitizing agents. This absorbed energy can directly cause cell damage by creating a covalent linking of the sensitizing molecule to the pyrimidines (e.g., thymine) in the cellular DNA. This linkage (the formation of cyclobutane photoadducts of the sensitizer and the pyrimidines) can be lethal to the cell. Photosensitizers like the psoralens selectively intercalate between two base pairs and produce interstrand crosslinks with epidermal DNA. In addition, the photosensitizing molecule can transfer the absorbed energy and promote formation of free radicals (molecules with unpaired electrons that are highly reactive) and cause damage to the cell membranes and lysosomes. In the presence of certain porphyrins (e.g., hematoporphyrin, protoporphyrin), a reactive singlet form of oxygen can be generated by these photosensitizing molecules. Drug-induced phototoxic reactions may thus involve damage to the DNA, RNA, lysosomes, cell membranes, and other organelles.

Photoallergy to drugs is an acquired and altered capacity of the skin to respond to light in the presence of a photosensitizer, and involves the immune system. The absorbed light energy seems to promote a photochemical reaction between the drug and the skin proteins. The drug acts to form a haptenic group and either combines directly with the protein to form a photoantigen or is altered by the absorbed energy; this altered haptenic group then reacts with the proteins to form an antigen.

The clinical manifestations in drug-induced photoallergic reactions may range from acute urticarial lesions, developing

TABLE 52-3
Systemic photosensitizers: Chemicals that induce photosensitivity reactions in humans

Name	Uses	Clinical observations	Action spectrum, nm
SULFONAMIDES			
Sulfanilamide, sulfathiazole, sulfapyridine, sulfamethazine, sulfaguanidine, sulfisoxazole, monochlorphenamide	Chemotherapy, antibacterial agents	Phototoxic and photoallergic reactions	290–320
SULFONYLUREA			
Carbutamide, tolbutamide (Orinase), chlorpropamide (Diabinese)	Hypoglycemic or antidiabetic drugs	Phototoxic reactions	290–360
CHLORTHIAZIDES			
6-Chloro-7-sulfamyl-3,4-dihydro-1,2,4-thiodiazine 1,1-dioxide (HydroDiuril)	Diuretics, antihypertensive	Papular and edematous eruption, plaques	290–320
Quinethazone (Diuril)	Antihypertensive	Phototoxic and photoallergic reactions	320–400
PHENOTHIAZINES			
Chlorpromazine (Thorazine), promethazine (Phenergan), mepazine, Stelazine, trimeprazine, Compazine, promazine (Sparine)	Tranquilizer, nematode infestation agent, urinary antiseptic, antihistamine	Exaggerated sunburn, maculopapular and urticarial eruptions, gray-blue hyperpigmentation	290–400
ANTIBIOTICS			
Demethylchlortetracycline (Declomycin), chlortetracycline, oxytetracycline, doxycycline	Broad-spectrum antibiotic	Exaggerated sunburn, phototoxic reaction	320–400
Griseofulvin	Antimycotic	Exaggerated sunburn, phototoxic and photoallergic reactions	320–400
Nalidixic acid (NegGram)	Antibacterial	Erythema, bullae	320–400
FUROCOUMARINS			
4,5′,8-Trimethylpsoralen (trioxsalen), 8-methoxypsoralen (methoxsalen), psoralen	In photochemotherapy of psoriasis and vitiligo; for sun tolerance and increased pigment formation	Erythema, bullae, hyperpigmentation	320–400
ESTROGENS AND PROGESTERONES			
Mestranol and norethynodrel, diethylstilbesterol	Oral contraceptives	Melasma, phototoxic reactions	?290–320
Chlordiazepoxide (Librium)	Tranquilizer, psychotropic	Eczematous eruption	290–360
Triacetyldiphenolisatin	Laxative	Eczematous photoallergic reaction	290–320
Cyclamates, calcium cyclamate, sodium cyclohexylsulfamate	Artificial sweeteners	Phototoxic and photoallergic reactions	290–360

SOURCE: *TB Fitzpatrick et al, Sunlight and Man: Normal and Abnormal Photobiologic Responses, MA Pathak et al (eds), Tokyo, University of Tokyo Press, 1974.*

within a few minutes after exposure, to eczematous or papular lesions appearing within 24 h or later. The eruption may extend beyond the exposed areas. In recurrent cases, flare-ups of distant, previously uninvolved sites may also occur. Some edema and vasodilatation are common in most of these eruptions. The action spectrum is generally in the long-wave range (320 to 400 nm), and less energy is required than is necessary for the production of phototoxic reactions.

The various systemic therapeutic agents and their effects on the skin in the presence of light (whether phototoxic or photoallergic reactions) are listed in Table 52-3. The biologic action spectra that induce either the phototoxic or photoallergic reactions are also given.

EFFECT OF PLANTS PLUS LIGHT *Phytophotodermatitis* (phototoxic reactions) can develop as the result of contact with many plants (belonging principally to the families Rutaceae and Umbelliferae, e.g., certain limes, parsley, celery, bishop's weed, figs) and subsequent exposure of the skin to sunlight. The photodermatitis involves a mild-to-severe erythematous reaction with or without vesicles or bullae. Dense postinflammatory hyperpigmentation is visible within 3 to 5 days. Perfumes and colognes containing oil of bergamot are also known to induce hyperpigmentation with or without erythema. The pigmentation in berloque dermatitis occurs in configurations that seem bizarre but actually represent the areas to which the scent was applied; sometimes the hyperpigmentation may be droplike or pendant-like, and has therefore been named accordingly (*berloque* or *berlock*, meaning trinket or pendant). This phytophotodermatitis, as well as that which follows contact with various other plants, is thought to be caused by furocoumarins (e.g., 5-methoxypsoralen, 8-methoxypsoralen, and other psoralens) characteristically present in these plants. The combination of exposure to long-wave UV radiation (320 to 400 nm) and furocoumarins greatly enhances the erythema and the pigmentation response.

Treatment Therapy of acute phototoxic reactions induced by topical or systemic agents is best achieved by removal of the offending agent and avoidance of exposure to the sun, or both. If necessary, the usual dermatologic procedures for minimizing the discomforts of the inflammatory response should be undertaken. However, in instances in which continued systemic use of the drug is vital, cutaneous photoreactions can be prevented by instructing the patient to remain indoors or by avoiding exposure to sunlight between 10 A.M. and 4 P.M. Generally the problem subsides within a week after discontinuation of the stress (sun and the drug). Sunscreens listed in Table 52-4 also should be prescribed.

EFFECT OF LIGHT PLUS ENDOGENOUS PHOTOSENSITIZERS
This category includes several photosensitivity reactions in patients with various types of porphyria (see Chap. 96). The photosensitivity reactions are related to the overproduction in vivo of either photo-, uro-, or coproporphyrins and their precursors.

TABLE 52-4
Topical sunscreens

Formulation ingredient	Concentration	Commercial name	PF*	Recommended for skin type nos.
PABA SUNSCREENS				
Aminobenzoic acid in 50–70% ethyl alcohol	5%, clear lotion	PreSun	>10–15	I and II
		Pabanol	>10–15	I and II
		Coppertone SuperShade	6	III and IV
ESTERS AND DERIVATIVES OF PABA				
Isoamyl-*p*-*N*,*N*-dimethyl aminobenzoate (Escalol 506, Padimate A)	2.5% or 3.3%, clear lotion	Block Out	6	III and IV
		PABA Film	6	III and IV
		Spectraban	6	III and IV
Glyceryl PABA + octyldimethyl PABA or 2-ethylhexyl ester of dimethylaminobenzoate (Escalol 507)	2.5% + 2.5%, milky lotion	Eclipse	>8–10	I and II
Escalol 507 + dioxybenzone	2.5% + 3%, clear lotion	Sungard	6	III and IV
Escalol 507 (octyldimethyl PABA) in ammonium acrylate-acrylate polymer	3.3%, milky lotion	Sundown	4–5	IV
Homomenthyl salicylate + *p*-dimethylaminobenzoate	5%, clear lotion	Aztec	6	III and IV
NON-PABA CHEMICAL SUNSCREENS				
2-Hydroxy-4-methoxybenzophenone 5-sulfonic acid	10%, milky lotion	UVAL	7	III and IV
Ethylhexyl-*p*-methoxycinnamate + 2-hydroxy-4-methoxybenzophenone + 2-phenylbenzamidazole sulfonic acid (G6)	5% + 3% + 4%, cream	Piz Buin Exclusiv Piz Buin Extrem Cream	11	I and II
Ethylhexyl-*p*-methoxycinnamate	4%–4.5% cream or lotion	Piz Buin	>6	I and II
Ethylhexyl-*p*-methoxycinnamate + 2-hydroxy-4-methoxybenzophenone	5% + 3% milky lotion	Piz Buin	>8	I and II
PHYSICAL SUNSCREENS				
Titanium dioxide, zinc oxide, kaolin, talc, iron oxide, etc.	Heavy cream or paste	A-fil RVPaque Shadow Reflecta Covermark	>4–8	All skin types—protection against UV-A, UV-B, and visible light.

* *PF = Protection factor established under field conditions with natural sunlight.*
NOTE: *Eyes should be always protected with ultraviolet-opaque goggles or sunglasses while sunbathing or skiing.*

In the prophyrias, endogenously synthesized porphyrin molecules, when exposed to light, cause burning, itching, urticaria, edema, crusting and scarring, vesiculation, atrophy, and many other disabling cutaneous changes. The light-absorbing molecules involved in evoking the cutaneous reactions are the irreversibly oxidized porphyrins present in abnormal amounts in red blood cells, plasma, skin, liver, stool, and urine. The photodermatitis is produced by a narrow band of light in the region of 400 to 410 nm, which corresponds to one of the absorption peaks of porphyrins. Patients, however, are sensitive to wavelengths from 380 to 600 nm. The most disabling type of photosensitivity reactions are encountered in erythropoietic (congenital) porphyria and in erythropoietic protoporphyria (Chap. 96). Symptoms and signs of sensitivity to sunlight occur in early childhood.

The adverse cutaneous responses to sunlight in patients with erythropoietic protoporphyria (EPP) have been found to be ameliorated by oral ingestion of β-carotene (Chap. 96). Patients who take β-carotene are able to withstand prolonged exposures to sunlight and experience relief from their usual photosensitivity reactions. A recommended treatment is the daily oral ingestion of β-carotene (Solatene) sufficient to maintain blood levels of 600 to 800 μg per 100 ml (usually adults receive a dose of 120 to 180 mg per day; children under 12 years receive 30 to 90 mg per day). Photoprotective effect of β-carotene is observed after 4 to 6 weeks, and the therapy is generally continued throughout the year. In vitro, β-carotene has been found to be an effective quencher for the "singlet" oxygen generated in certain photosensitivity reactions. During porphyrin-mediated photosensitivity reactions, peroxides are generated which damage the lipid membranes. It is presumed that β-carotene is preferentially oxidized and that by quenching the "singlet" oxygen, it inhibits lipid peroxide formation.

POLYMORPHOUS LIGHT ERUPTIONS

Polymorphous light eruption (PMLE) is an idiopathic, acquired syndrome characterized by a delayed abnormal response to light and varied morphology. The clinical patterns are pleomorphic or polymorphic in nature. The most common pattern consists of multiple small papules, or papules and vesicles that may become confluent and present at times an eczematous clinical picture. Lichenification due to scratching of the pruritic lesions commonly supervenes. Less frequently, the primary lesion is a large papule that may present an erythema multiforme–like pattern or become confluent to form plaques. This variety is usually, but not exclusively, confined to the face and neck. The only consistent histologic feature in all cases is a dense perivascular infiltrate in the upper and middle dermis. Typically the lesions appear in early spring and after each exposure. The latent period between exposure and the appearance of rash may range from a few hours to 2 days, with the most common interval being 24 to 36 h. Itching is frequent and may occur during sun exposure and even preceding the eruption.

The sunburn-producing spectrum (UV-B, or 290 to 320 nm) is the most effective waveband for eliciting abnormal PMLE responses. However, in many instances, the action spectrum may extend into the UV-A (320 to 400 nm) region; in some instances it may extend into the visible region. Even alpha particles, x-rays, and germicidal radiation (290 nm) may produce PMLE. Although the mechanisms underlying these reactions are not known, the evidence suggests a delayed hypersensitivity reaction to an antigen induced by radiation.

TREATMENT Photoprotection, either through avoidance or with the use of highly effective sunscreens (Table 52-4), may be adequate to control symptoms and appearance of new lesions. The synthetic antimalarials are effective in PMLE, but they must be used with great caution to prevent retinopathy and optic nerve atrophy. The lesions of PMLE are often responsive to topical corticosteroids; systemic steroids are rarely indicated. Desensitization by repeated graduated exposure to sunlight or to artificial radiation (UV-A) in combination with psoralens (methoxsalen) has been successful in a limited number of cases. Oral administration of β-carotene (Solatene) has been found to be of limited value.

PHOTOTHERAPY AND PHOTOCHEMOTHERAPY

Phototherapy refers to the therapeutic effectiveness of UV (usually 290 to 320 nm) or visible radiation without the systemic use of a drug. Photochemotherapy, on the other hand, involves the combination of nonionizing electromagnetic radiation and a systemically administered, photochemically reactive agent. Generally in the doses used, neither the drug alone nor the radiation alone has any therapeutic response; only the combination of the photoactive drug and the radiation, administered at the appropriate time, is therapeutic. Indications for phototherapy include various dermatoses, uremic pruritus, and neonatal hyperbilirubinemia. Phototherapy with blue visible light (430 to 500 nm) enhances the photodegradation and excretion of bilirubin in neonatal jaundice. Psoriasis, eczema, and pityriasis rosea may improve with controlled sun exposures. UV-B radiation (290 to 320 nm) is, therefore, a part of the therapeutic regimen for these dermatoses.

The treatment of psoriasis and other proliferative diseases of the skin has involved attempts to inhibit cellular proliferation and DNA synthesis.

The topical application of crude coal tar products followed by subsequent UV exposure has been a standard treatment for severe generalized psoriasis. Although tar-induced phototoxicity affecting DNA synthesis is believed to be responsible for therapeutic effects, it is not yet clear whether the beneficial effects are due to the chemical ingredients of tar alone or the photosensitizing action of UV-A (320 to 400 nm) or UV-B.

ORAL PSORALEN PHOTOCHEMOTHERAPY Psoralens are naturally occurring furocoumarins that are tricyclic compounds, many of which are photochemically reactive [e.g., 8-methoxypsoralen (methoxsalen) and 4,5′,8-trimethylpsoralen (trioxsalen)]. It has been shown that in the presence of psoralens irradiation with UV-A (320 to 400 nm) can result in covalent binding of psoralens to pyrimidine bases in DNA. This photoconjugation may lead to interstrand cross-linking of psoralen between base paired strands of DNA, inhibition of DNA synthesis, and cell death. Methoxsalen is now widely used in treating psoriasis, vitiligo, eczema, and mycosis fungoides. Two hours after ingestion of methoxsalen (0.6 to 0.9 mg/kg), patients are exposed to a measured dose of UV-A radiation. The initial dose depends on the patient's skin reactivity to ultraviolet radiation (sunburn history) and degree of melanin pigmentation of skin. Repeated psoralen plus UV-A treatments cause disappearance of psoriatic lesions; a total of 10 to 20 treatments given two or three times weekly will usually result in clearance of psoriasis. Maintenance treatments are recommended, and it appears that gradually tapering the frequency of treatments is most effective. The scalp and areas to which UV-A does not penetrate do not respond to therapy.

In vitiligo, a disease characterized by amelanotic macules of varying sizes and absence of melanocytes, methoxsalen plus UV-A treatment can be used in restoring the normal skin color to pigmentless areas of vitiligo macules. Over 100 to 200 treatments are needed, and this long duration of treatment can often be frustrating, especially when the pigment response is slow, unpredictable, and subject to the presence of functional melanocytes.

The long-term concerns of photochemotherapy include premature aging (irreversible changes in connective tissue, blood vessels, and keratinocytes), cataract, and skin cancer. Oral methoxsalen photochemotherapy using long-wave UV radiation sources is a new approach. Although over 2000 patients with psoriasis and thousands of patients with vitiligo have been treated, well-documented examples of actinic keratoses or early squamous-cell carcinoma have been observed. However, there is no evidence of cataractogenesis in humans treated with psoralens and sunlight or high-intensity ultraviolet radiation over the past 25 years. Photochemotherapy is an effective treatment which, when compared with other available treatments for generalized psoriasis or vitiligo, appears to have the most acceptable risk/benefit ratio.

TOPICAL SUNSCREENS IN HEALTH AND DISEASES

Sunscreens protect viable cells of the skin by absorbing and reflecting the radiation impinging on the skin. The majority of sunscreens are designed to protect the user against UV-B (290 to 320 nm). In counseling people in the prevention of sunburn, skin cancer, aging of the skin, actinic elastosis, and various forms of sun sensitivity, the choice and recommendations of sunscreen depend upon several factors. The most important consideration should be the individual's reactivity to sunlight. People with fair skin, blue eyes, with or without freckles, who burn easily and tan poorly (skin types I and II) should be given those sunscreens that have a high protection index (Table 52-4) i.e., a protection factor of 6 or more. Individuals with skin types III and IV, who burn moderately or minimally but tan well, may be recommended sunscreens with a protection factor of 4.

For the greatest protection patients should apply 5.0 percent *p*-aminobenzoic acid (PABA) lotions in 50 to 70 percent ethyl alcohol 1 h before exposure. PABA esters in 2.5 percent concentration in ethanol are less effective than PABA. Most sunscreens should be reapplied after swimming or during prolonged sunbathing. In many instances patients may be exquisitely sensitive, irrespective of skin type, and they may require combination therapy with two or more sunscreens (preferably an opaque sunscreen). The drug-induced photosensitization reactions can be minimized or prevented by prescribing topical sunscreens containing benzophenones (Table 52-4). Sunscreens containing PABA or its derivatives should *not* be prescribed for individuals who are photosensitive to certain drugs and manifest phototoxic or cell-mediated delayed hypersensitivity reactions. In patients receiving antihypertensive thiazide diuretics or sulfonamides there may be a cross-reaction with PABA leading to eczematous dermatitis. These patients should be prescribed sunscreens containing benzophenones or opaque sunscreens containing zinc oxide, titanium oxide, and other light-scattering agents such as kaolin.

Individuals with acute sunburn reaction manifesting severe erythema, edema, and painful blistering reaction may be treated with systemic corticosteroids. Oral prednisone, beginning with 40 to 60 mg and tapering over 4 to 8 days, will help to control the severe sunburn reaction.

REFERENCES

MAGNUS IA: *Dermatological Photobiology.* Oxford, Blackwell, 1976

PARRISH JA et al: Photomedicine, in *Dermatology in General Medicine,* 2d ed, TB Fitzpatrick et al (eds). New York, McGraw-Hill, 1979

PATHAK MA et al (eds): *Sunlight and Man: Normal and Abnormal Photobiologic Responses.* Tokyo, University of Tokyo Press, 1974

———, EPSTEIN JH: Normal and abnormal reactions of man to light, in *Dermatology in General Medicine,* TB Fitzpatrick et al (eds). New York, McGraw-Hill, 1971

——— et al: Evaluation of topical agents that prevent sunburn. N Engl J Med 280:1459, 1969

section 10 | Hematologic alterations

53
PALLOR AND ANEMIA

H. FRANKLIN BUNN

PALLOR

Pallor is the physical finding most commonly associated with anemia. However, the usefulness of this sign is limited by other factors that affect the color of the skin. The thickness and texture of the skin vary widely among individuals. Furthermore, the blood flow to the skin can undergo wide fluctuations. Normal individuals will appear sallow when blood is shunted away from the skin, whereas anemic patients may appear flushed when overheated or during periods of excitement. The concentration of melanin in the epidermis is another important

determinant of skin color. Individuals with a fair complexion may look pale even though they are not anemic. Conversely, pallor is difficult to detect in deeply pigmented individuals. Furthermore, acquired disorders of melanin pigmentation (e.g., Addison's disease, hemochromatosis) or jaundice may interfere with detection of pallor. Nevertheless, even in blacks, the presence of anemia may be suspected by the color of the palms or of noncutaneous tissues such as oral mucous membranes, nail beds, and palpebral conjunctivas. The color of the creases of the palm is a useful sign. When they are as pale as the surrounding skin, the patient usually has a hemoglobin of less than 7 g per 100 ml.

Two factors contribute to the development of pallor in patients with anemia. There is, of course, a decrease in the hemoglobin concentration of blood perfusing the skin and mucous membranes. Also, blood is shunted away from the skin and other peripheral tissues, permitting enhanced blood flow to vital organs. Redistribution of blood flow is an important mode of compensation in anemia (see Fig. 53-5).

ANEMIA

By definition patients with anemia have a significant reduction in red cell mass and a corresponding decrease in the oxygen-carrying capacity of the blood. Normally, blood volume is maintained at a nearly constant level. Therefore, anemia entails a decrease in the concentration of red cells or hemoglobin in peripheral blood. Measuring the packed cell volume (PCV) or hematocrit is the simplest and one of the most precise ways to ascertain the concentration of red cells in the blood; the result is termed the *hematocrit*. Generally, a small sample of anticoagulated blood is drawn into a capillary tube which is sealed at one end and centrifuged. The PCV is the ratio of the volume of packed red cells to the total volume. Alternatively, the concentration of hemoglobin can be determined spectrophotometrically from the absorbance of the cyanmethemoglobin form at a specific wavelength. With the advent of automated red blood cell counting technology, very precise measurements became readily available in nearly all hospitals and well-equipped clinical laboratories. The electronic counter makes a direct measurement of the red cell count (RBC/μl) and the mean red cell volume (MCV):

$$MCV \text{ (fl)} = \frac{PCV \text{ (liters/liters)}}{(RBC/\mu l) \times 10^{-9}}$$

This instrument calculates the PCV from the direct measurement of MCV and RBC/μl. In addition, hemoglobin concentration is measured directly on a separate channel. The mean corpuscular hemoglobin concentration (MCHC) is then computed as follows:

$$MCHC \text{ (g per 100 ml)} = \frac{Hb \text{ (g per 100 ml)}}{PCV \text{ (liters/liters)}}$$

A third red blood cell index, the mean corpuscular hemoglobin (MCH), is determined as follows:

$$MCH \text{ (pg)} = \frac{Hb \text{ (g per 100 ml)}}{(RBC/\mu l) \times 10^{-7}}$$

Generally, an automated system provides a printout which includes hemoglobin concentration, red cell count, packed cell volume, and the three red cell indexes (MCV, MCHC, and MCH). Normal values for individuals of various ages are shown in the Appendix. In women in the childbearing age group the normal blood values are 10 percent lower than in men. At high altitudes, higher values are found, roughly in proportion to the elevation above sea level. Anemia may be defined as a reduction of more than 10 percent below the mean values for the sex. However, since the variations in normal hemoglobin values approach this limit, the documentation of mild anemia may be uncertain.

RED BLOOD CELL PRODUCTION Red cells are derived from an undifferentiated progenitor cell in the bone marrow called the *pluripotent stem cell* (Fig. 53-1). A stem cell is one which is capable of both self-renewal and differentiation. *Pluripotent* implies that granulocytes, monocytes, and platelets also evolve from this ancestor cell. The pluripotent stem cell probably has the morphological characteristics of a mature lymphocyte. The control of proliferation into differentiated cell lines is poorly understood. Experiments have been hampered by difficulty in isolating early red cell precursors from the bone marrow. However, in the past 5 years, considerable advances have been made in culturing erythroid progenitor cells in vitro. As Fig. 53-1 shows, the most primitive erythroid progenitor which has been cultured from both bone marrow and peripheral blood is called the *erythroid burst-forming unit* (BFU$_e$). After 10 to 15 days in tissue culture it produces a large colony of recognizable red cell precursors. The BFU$_e$ is responsive only to high doses of the erythroid-promoting hormone, erythropoietin. A more developed cell, the *erythroid colony-forming unit* (CFU$_e$), develops a smaller clone of erythroid cells after 4 to 7 days in culture and is very sensitive to erythropoietin. A number of other factors have been proposed to influence erythroid cell differentiation including catecholamines, steroids, thyroid hormone, growth hormone, and cyclic nucleotides. In addition, helper T lymphocytes may also play a role. Well-designed experiments involving erythroid cells in culture should provide considerably more information about the mechanism underlying the differentiation and maturation of erythroid cells, as well as insights into certain disorders involving erythroid precursor cells.

Erythropoietin, a glycoprotein having a molecular weight of about 32,000 has been purified nearly to homogeneity. Original experiments indicated that this hormone is produced primarily by the kidneys. Alternatively, the kidneys may produce a substance, renal erythropoietic factor, which converts a biologically inactive plasma protein into erythropoietin, analogous to the formation of angiotensin. Erythropoietin production is stimulated by hypoxia. Currently, erythropoietin is

FIGURE 53-1
Differentiation and morphological maturation of erythroid cells. Erythroid cells are derived from pluripotent stem cells shown on left. Under the influence of erythropoietin, erythroid stem cells (BFU$_e$ → CFU$_e$) differentiate into proerythroblasts, the earliest recognizable red blood cell precursor in the bone marrow. During further maturation, globin mRNA accumulates, directing the cell to synthesize hemoglobin. (After Nienhuis and Benz.)

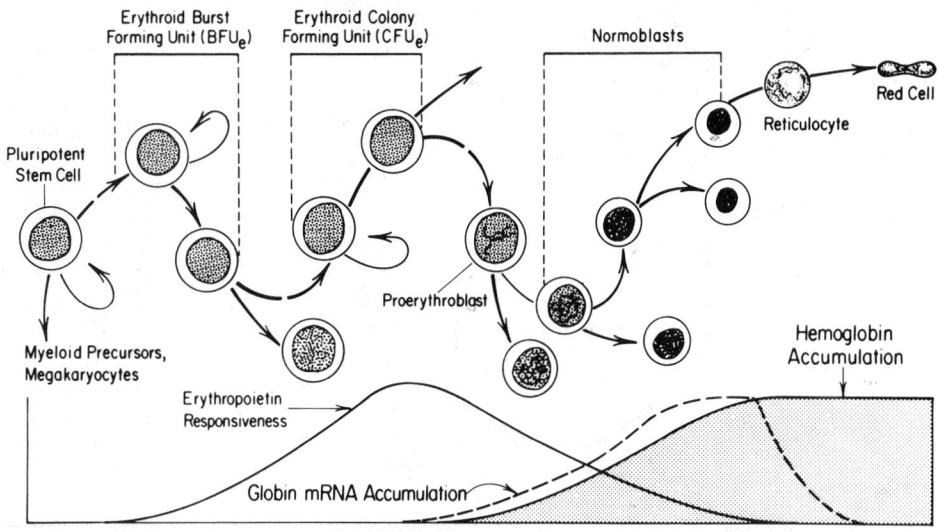

measured by rather crude bioassays. Its recent purification should permit the development of a more accurate and sensitive radioimmune assay. Reliable measurements of erythropoietin would have a number of diagnostic applications and also provide new information about the pathogenesis of several types of anemias.

Erythropoietin probably interacts with specific receptors on the surfaces of committed erythroid stem cells, inducing them to differentiate into pronormoblasts, the earliest red cell precursor that can be recognized on examination of the bone marrow. In addition, erythropoietin acts on later red cell precursors, stimulating cell division as well as hemoglobin synthesis. Normally the transition from the proerythroblast to the most mature normoblast involves three or four cell divisions over a 4-day period (Fig. 53-1). During this time, the nucleus becomes smaller, and an increasing amount of hemoglobin is produced in the cytoplasm. Following the last division, the pyknotic nucleus is removed from the normoblast, forming the reticulocyte which stays in the bone marrow for about two days. The reticulocyte is then released into the general circulation, where it remains for another 24 h before it loses its mitochondria and ribosomes and assumes the morphologic appearance of a mature red cell.

Erythroid precursor cells ranging from the pronormoblast to the reticulocyte possess a specific surface receptor for the iron-transferrin complex, enabling them to incorporate sufficient iron for hemoglobin production (Fig. 53-2). Normally, about 80 percent of circulating iron bound to plasma transferrin goes to erythroid cells in the marrow. After 4 to 6 days the iron reappears in circulating erythrocytes. The use of a radioactive iron label such as ^{59}Fe permits a quantitative assessment of erythropoiesis. From the rate at which injected ^{59}Fe-labeled transferrin disappears from the plasma, plasma iron turnover can be calculated. This parameter is generally proportional to the total developing erythroid cell mass. The extent to which circulating red cells acquire the label provides an index of the efficiency or effectiveness of erythropoiesis.

Under maximal stimulation, the normal marrow is capable of increasing its red cell production about six- to eightfold. As the erythroid marrow expands, fat is replaced by erythroid cells, and formerly inactive or "yellow" marrow becomes active or "red."

HEMOGLOBIN BIOSYNTHESIS Erythroid cell development is directed toward the production of hemoglobin-containing cells. About 98 percent of the protein in the cytoplasm of circulating red cells is hemoglobin. This protein is a tetramer composed of two pairs of polypeptide chains designated α, β, γ, and δ, each of which is covalently linked to a heme group. The synthesis of a particular globin subunit is directed by a corresponding gene inherited from each parent. As shown in Fig. 53-1, there is a marked amplification in the transcription of globin chain mRNA during the development of proerythroblasts.

In the red cells of normal adults, hemoglobin A ($\alpha_2\beta_2$) composes about 97 percent of the total hemoglobin. The remaining 3 percent is primarily hemoglobin A_2 ($\alpha_2\delta_2$). As discussed in Chap. 315, this minor component is increased in patients with β thalassemia. Hemoglobin F or fetal hemoglobin ($\alpha_2\gamma_2$) is found in trace amounts in adult red cells localized to about 1 to 7 percent of red cells. It is the main hemoglobin component of fetal red cells. During the last 3 months of gestation, γ-chain synthesis switches to β-chain synthesis. However, in certain types of congenital hemolytic anemias such as the β thalassemias and sickle-cell anemia, the production of γ chains (and therefore of hemoglobin F) persists. In addition, increased levels of hemoglobin F may also be encountered in certain acquired anemias in which there is disordered red cell proliferation.

Normally α- and β-chain synthesis in erythroid precursors is evenly balanced. The thalassemias (Chap. 315) are characterized by imbalance in globin chain synthesis.

The synthesis of *heme* in red cell precursors is closely matched to globin chain production. As shown in Fig. 53-3 the initial and rate-limiting step is the condensation of succinyl CoA and glycine to form δ-aminolevulinic acid. This reaction which takes place in mitochondria requires that glycine be activated by pyridoxal phosphate. Accordingly, patients with sideroblastic anemia in whom heme synthesis is usually defective may sometimes respond to pyridoxine therapy (Chap. 310). The next steps of heme synthesis take place in the cytosol. Two molecules of δ-aminolevulinic acid condense to form a ring structure, porphobilinogen. The concentration of this colorless pyrrole is elevated in acute intermittent porphyria and can be detected in urine by the Watson-Schwartz test. The subsequent steps in porphyrin synthesis are also shown in Fig. 53-3. The

FIGURE 53-2

Erythrocyte production, circulation, and destruction. Circulating iron-bound transferrin (TF) is bound to specific receptors on the surface of red blood cell precursors in the marrow. Most of this iron is incorporated into hemoglobin; the remainder is stored as ferritin. Following maturation of the erythroid precursor, the nucleus is shed and the red blood cell emerges from the marrow into the plasma where it circulates for approximately 120 days. The senescent red blood cell is taken up by the mononuclear-macrophage system and is destroyed. The heme-iron is initially incorporated into ferritin. This storage iron is available for transport to the marrow via transferrin.

last three reactions take place in mitochondria. Iron is inserted into protoporphyrin IX to form heme. In iron deficiency, as well as in lead poisoning, increased levels of protoporphyrin can be detected in red cells. Disorders of porphyrin synthesis and metabolism are discussed in Chap. 96.

HEMOGLOBIN STRUCTURE AND FUNCTION The primary role of red cells is to transport oxygen from lungs to tissues and to transport carbon dioxide in the reverse direction. Both of these functions are assumed by hemoglobin. The three-dimensional structure of human hemoglobin has been determined from x-ray crystallographic analysis. The important functional properties of hemoglobin such as heme-heme interaction, the pH dependency of oxygen affinity (the Bohr effect), and the interaction with 2,3-diphosphoglycerate can now be understood on a stereochemical basis. This structural information has also been useful in explaining the abnormal functional properties of a number of human hemoglobin variants which are associated with clinical and hematologic manifestations (see Chap. 315).

During the circulation through the lungs, hemoglobin becomes almost fully saturated with oxygen (1.34 ml O_2 per gram of hemoglobin). As red cells perfuse the capillary beds, oxygen is extracted. Efficient unloading of oxygen at relatively high oxygen tensions is possible because of the sigmoid shape of the oxygen dissociation curve (heme-heme interaction) (see Fig. 53-4). The affinity of hemoglobin for oxygen is modified by three intracellular cofactors: hydrogen ion, carbon dioxide, and 2,3-diphosphoglycerate (2,3-DPG). Increasing concentrations of each of these three effectors results in a "shift to the right" in the oxygen dissociation curve. In human red cells, 2,3-DPG appears to be an important regulator of hemoglobin

function. One molecule of 2,3-DPG binds to the β chains of deoxyhemoglobin, thereby decreasing oxygen affinity. Elevated levels of 2,3-DPG have been noted in various states of hypoxia. The resulting decrease in oxygen affinity permits enhanced oxygen release. The oxygenation of a particular organ or tissue depends on three main factors (depicted in Fig. 53-5): blood flow, oxygen-carrying capacity of the blood (hemoglobin concentration), and the difference between arterial and venous oxygen saturation. The last factor is dependent on the shape and position of the oxygen dissociation curve. Patients with a primary abnormality of one of these three factors depend on adjustments in one or both of the other two in order to maintain optimal tissue oxygenation. For example, patients with anemia have two available modes of compensation: enhanced blood flow and decreased oxygen affinity, mediated by increased levels of 2,3-DPG. Conversely, individuals with a hemoglobin variant having increased oxygen affinity have a primary defect in oxygen unloading. As discussed in Chap. 315, such patients compensate by developing secondary erythrocytosis.

RED BLOOD CELL METABOLISM As the red cell emerges from the bone marrow, it loses its nucleus, ribosomes, and mitochondria and therefore all capability for cell division, protein synthesis, and oxidative phosphorylation. Compared with other cells, the erythrocyte has a rather simple scheme of intermediary metabolism. Glucose is virtually the only fuel utilized

FIGURE 53-3

The biosynthesis of heme. The following abbreviations are used: CoA, coenzyme A; GTP, guanosine triphosphate; GDP, guanosine diphosphate; Pi, inorganic phosphorus; GSH, glutathione; Δ-ALA-DH, Δ-aminolevulinate dehydrase; UIS, uroporphyrinogen I synthetase; UIII CoS, uroporphyrinogen III cosynthetase; UD, uroporphyrinogen decarboxylase; CO, coproporphyrinogen oxidase; HS, heme synthetase. Enzymatic steps that occur in mitochondria are shown.

FIGURE 53-4

The oxyhemoglobin dissociation curve of normal blood. The major factors influencing the position of the curve are pH, temperature, and the intracellular concentration of 2,3-DPG. An increase in plasma pH or a decrease in temperature and 2,3-DPG causes an increase in oxygen affinity (shift to the left) and a relative decrease in oxygen unloading when going from an arterial P_{O_2} of 95 mmHg to a venous P_{O_2} of 40 mmHg. Conversely, a decrease in pH or an increase in temperature and 2,3-DPG causes a decrease in oxygen affinity (shift to the right) and a relative increase in oxygen unloading.

by the red cell. It readily enters the red cell by facilitated diffusion and is then phosphorylated to glucose 6-phosphate. There are two major pathways available for glucose 6-phosphate (Fig. 314-2). About 80 to 90 percent of this intermediate is converted to lactate by means of the glycolytic (or Embden-Meyerhof) pathway. Two moles of adenosine triphosphate (ATP) are generated for every mole of glucose that is metabolized. The intracellular mediator of hemoglobin function, 2,3-diphosphoglycerate, is synthesized in a side reaction shown in Fig. 314-2. About 10 percent of intracellular glucose 6-phosphate may undergo oxidation by means of the hexose-monophosphate shunt. This pathway maintains glutathione in the reduced form, thereby protecting sulfhydryl groups in hemoglobin and the red cell membrane from oxidation by peroxides and superoxide as well as by certain drugs and toxins. Such oxidant stress can compromise red cell function and viability in patients with a deficiency in glucose 6-phosphate dehydro-

FIGURE 53-5

Oxygen delivered to an organ or tissue is directly proportional to (1) blood flow, (2) hemoglobin concentration, and (3) the difference in oxygen saturation of the arterial and venous blood. Patients with various types of hypoxia may compensate in the following ways: (1) The distribution of blood flow is altered to maintain oxygenation of vital organs; total cardiac output increases when hypoxia is severe. (2) Increased erythropoietin production stimulates erythropoiesis. (3) Oxygen unloading is enhanced by a shift to the right in the oxygen dissociation curve, mediated by red blood cell pH and 2,3-DPG.

genase, the first enzymatic step in the hexose monophosphate shunt (see Chap. 314). Less commonly, individuals may have a deficiency in one of the enzymes of the glycolytic pathway or in one of the other enzymes of the hexose monophosphate shunt.

The red cell has rather modest metabolic obligations in keeping with its simplified structure. A significant portion of the ATP generated by glycolysis is spent in operating the sodium-potassium pump, necessary to preserve the ionic milieu in the cytoplasm and prevent colloid osmotic lysis. In addition, some metabolic energy is expended on maintenance and repair of the red cell membrane. Certain proteins in the membrane become phosphorylated by means of ATP and protein kinases, but the physiologic significance of this process is not yet understood. Finally, a small amount of metabolic currency is spent on maintaining hemoglobin iron atoms in the reduced form (Fe^{2+}).

The 120-day survival of the circulating red cell is dependent on preservation of the pliability of its membrane. The red cell membrane is composed of 50 percent protein, 40 percent lipid, and 10 percent carbohydrate. According to the most widely accepted model, it is a bilayer consisting of molecules of phospholipid and cholesterol in a 1.2:1 molar ratio oriented in a stacked array so that the hydrophobic portions of the molecules are oriented toward the interior while the polar side groups are either on the external surface of the cell (the plasma membrane) or on the inner cytoplasmic surface (see Fig. 53-6). The distribution of phospholipids differs significantly in the two portions of the bilayer. The outer surface is relatively rich in lecithin and sphingomyelin while the inner surface has relatively more phosphatidyl serine and phosphatidyl ethanolamine. The lipids on the outer surface exchange freely with plasma lipids.

The red cell membrane contains about eight major proteins (depicted in Fig. 53-6) and a large number of minor components. These proteins can be divided into two groups. A few span the lipid bilayer so that one end of the polypeptide is on the external cell surface and the other is on the inner surface. Examples include glycophorin which contains a number of polysaccharide blood group antigens and band 3, which serves as a channel for the passage of anions in and out of the red cell. Other proteins bind only to the inner surface of the red cell membrane. These include several enzymes as well as two structural proteins, spectrin and actin, which interact to form a meshwork that laminates the cytoplasmic surface of the membrane.

It is likely that the physiologic demise of 120-day-old red cells is due to a loss of membrane flexibility preventing them from negotiating the narrow-bore channels of the microcirculation including the sinusoids of the spleen. The factors responsible for red cell senescence are poorly understood. Experimental evidence indicates that deterioration of the red cell's metabolic machinery, sufficient to deplete it of ATP, can cause the cell to become spiculated (ecchinocytic) and lose its normal pliability. Depletion of ATP disrupts the spectrin and actin meshwork lining the inner membrane surface, resulting in aggregation of these proteins. Other factors such as enhanced rigidity due to accumulation of calcium and, perhaps, alterations in charge on the external surface of the membrane may also contribute to the recognition of the senescent red cell by the mononuclear-phagocyte system. In contrast to normal red cells, there is a large and well-documented body of information on the mechanisms responsible for red cell destruction in various hemolytic anemias. These will be discussed in Chap. 314.

Once the senescent red cell is sequestered (Fig. 53-2), hemoglobin is readily catabolized. Amino acids are released by proteolytic digestion and subsequently neutralized or metabolized. The heme group is catabolized by a microsomal oxidizing system. The porphyrin ring is converted to bile pigments which are excreted almost quantitatively by the liver. One mole of carbon monoxide is formed per mole of heme that is broken down. Measurement of endogenous carbon monoxide production is a rather precise indication of erythroid cell destruction. As Fig. 53-2 shows, the iron that is released during heme catabolism may be initially incorporated into the storage protein, ferritin, but it is eventually transported to marrow erythroid precursors by transferrin, the plasma-iron-binding protein.

If red cell production is disordered, there may be significant destruction of erythroid cells within the bone marrow. A number of anemias are characterized by *ineffective erythropoiesis,* particularly those in which erythroid maturation is morphologically abnormal and the circulating red cells are abnormal in size. Examples discussed in detail elsewhere include megaloblastic anemias, sideroblastic anemias, and β-thalassemia major. Such disorders are characterized by erythroid hyperplasia in the bone marrow and rapid uptake of labeled iron into the marrow but a low recovery of the labeled iron in circulating red cells. Endogenous carbon monoxide production and plasma levels of unconjugated bilirubin are generally elevated in ineffective erythropoiesis.

SIGNS AND SYMPTOMS OF ANEMIA The clinical presentation of the anemic patient depends on the underlying disease as well as on the severity and chronicity of the anemia. The manifestations of anemia per se can be explained by the pathophysiologic principles outlined in this chapter. Most of these signs and symptoms represent cardiovascular and ventilatory adjustments which compensate for the decrease in red cell mass.

The degree to which symptoms occur in an anemic patient depends on several contributing factors. If the anemia has developed rapidly, there may not be adequate time for compensatory adjustments to take place, and the patient may have more marked symptoms than if an anemia of equivalent severity had developed insidiously. Furthermore, the patient's complaints may depend on the presence of local vascular disease. For example, angina pectoris, intermittent claudication, or transient cerebral ischemia may be unmasked by the development of anemia.

Individuals with mild anemia are often asymptomatic.

They may complain of fatigue as well as dyspnea and palpitation, particularly following exercise. Severely anemic patients will often be symptomatic at rest and unable to tolerate significant exertion. When the hemoglobin concentration falls below 7.5 g per 100 ml, resting cardiac output rises significantly with an increase in both heart rate and stroke volume. The patient may be aware of this hyperdynamic state and complain of palpitation or a pounding pulse. Symptoms of cardiac failure may develop if the patient's myocardial reserve is reduced.

The clinical manifestations of severe anemia extend to other organ systems. Patients often complain of dizziness and headache and may experience syncope, tinnitus, or vertigo. Many patients are irritable and have difficulty sleeping or concentrating. Because of decreased blood flow to the skin, patients may become hypersensitive to cold. Gastrointestinal symptoms such as anorexia, indigestion, and even nausea or bowel irregularity are attributable to shunting of blood away from the splanchnic bed. Females commonly develop abnormal menstruation, both amenorrhea and increased bleeding. Males may complain of impotence or loss of libido.

The *physical findings* associated with anemia include pallor, discussed at the beginning of the chapter, tachycardia, wide pulse pressure, and a hyperdynamic precordium. A systolic ejection murmur is often heard over the precordium, particularly at the pulmonic area. In addition, a venous hum may be detected over the neck vessels. These cardiac findings disappear when the anemia is corrected. Patients with hemolytic anemia often have icterus and splenomegaly and occasionally develop superficial skin ulceration over the ankle bones.

APPROACH TO THE PATIENT WITH ANEMIA

In evaluating the anemic patient, the physician should proceed in an orderly fashion so that the correct diagnosis can be established with a minimum of laboratory tests and procedures. As in other clinical disciplines, a comprehensive history and meticulous physical examination are of paramount importance in

FIGURE 53-6
Diagram of a cross section of the red blood cell membrane. Spectrin and actin form a meshwork which laminates the inner surface of the membrane. Several other proteins of varying sizes including the enzyme glyceraldehyde 3-phosphate dehydrogenase (G3PD) also bind to the inner surface. In contrast, other proteins such as the glycophorins A and B (GP–A and GP–B) and the anion transport protein traverse the lipid bilayer.

Long polysaccharide chains are covalently attached to these proteins on the outer surface of the cell and also to glycolipid. Phospholipids include phosphatidyl choline (PC) and sphingomyelin (SM), which are located primarily on the outer surface of the membrane, and phosphatidyl serine (PS) and phosphatidyl ethanolamine (PE), which are located primarily on the inner surface of the membrane. (This figure was prepared by Dr. Samuel Lux IV.)

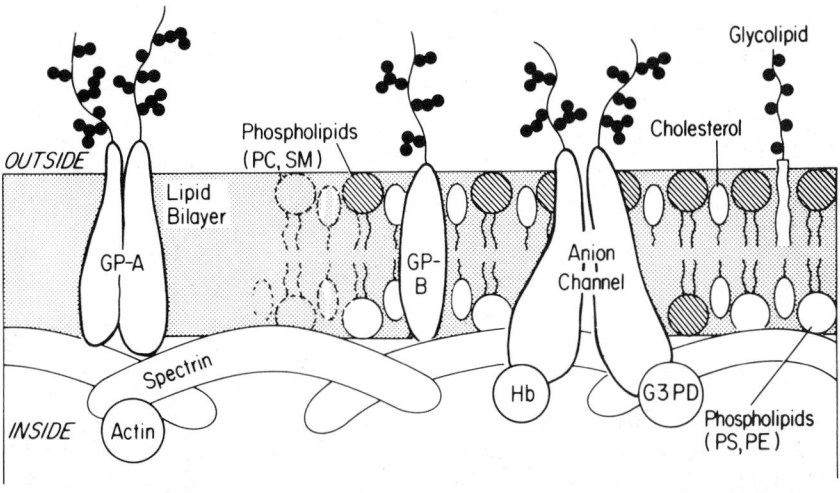

the initial work-up of the anemic patient. For example, a family history which reveals a dominant inheritance pattern provides strong support for the diagnosis of hereditary spherocytosis. The discovery of a heart murmur and splenomegaly raises the possibility that the anemic patient may have subacute bacterial endocarditis.

The work-up of the anemic patient should be based on a firm understanding of the pathophysiologic principles outlined earlier in this chapter. Table 53-1 shows an overview of the laboratory tests that are useful in the diagnosis of anemias. The clinician must first ask whether the anemia is due to a decreased production of red cells or enhanced destruction. In addition, the possibility of blood loss either as the sole etiology or as a contributing factor must always be considered. At this crossroad, laboratory information can be gathered which will establish whether the patient is failing to produce an adequate number of red cells or is undergoing accelerated cell breakdown.

The *reticulocyte count* is the most useful laboratory test in answering this question. When an appropriate supravital stain is applied to a sample of peripheral blood, the 1- to 2-day-old red cells exhibit a network of purple strands, which are aggregates of ribosomes. On a routinely prepared peripheral smear, these young red cells appear larger than average and have a purplish hue, so-called polychromatophilia. Reticulocytosis is a reflection of the release of an increased number of young cells from the bone marrow. The degree of increased erythropoiesis can be assessed more quantitatively by determining the reticulocyte index, which uses the hematocrit or PCV and is calculated as follows:

$$\text{Reticulocyte index} = \text{reticulocyte \%} \times \frac{\text{patient's PCV}}{\text{normal PCV}}$$

This measure fails to consider the distribution of reticulocytes between the bone marrow and the peripheral blood. When the marrow is greatly stimulated, marrow reticulocytes enter the circulation prematurely. Since the circulation of these "shift reticulocytes" in the peripheral blood is prolonged, the reticulocyte index should be divided by 2. This correction should always be made if normoblasts are encountered in the peripheral blood since this finding indicates the premature release of red cell precursors into the circulation.

A failure to produce red cells is reflected in an inappropriately low reticulocyte count. In contrast, a significant elevation of reticulocytes is suggestive of hemolysis. Exceptions include (1) the brisk reticulocyte response that is seen in a patient with hemorrhage, (2) reticulocytosis encountered in patients recovering from a suppression of erythropoiesis (e.g., an individual with pernicious anemia who received an injection of vitamin B_{12} 1 week earlier), and (3) mild to moderate elevations in reticulocytes (3 to 7 percent) encountered in myelophthisic anemia in which cells may be prematurely released because of irritative foci within the bone marrow such as tumor or granulomata. These exceptions are often readily appreciated in the initial evaluation of the patient. Furthermore, a number of ancillary laboratory tests described below are useful in determining to what extent hemolysis is occurring. The measurement of unconjugated bilirubin in the serum is a particularly

TABLE 53-1
Laboratory evaluation of anemias

	Reticulocytes	Peripheral smear	Marrow	Additional lab tests	Diagnosis
↓ Hematocrit	Normal, decreased	Hypochromic: Microcytic	0 Iron	↓ Fe, ↑ TIBC	Iron deficiency
			+ Iron Ring sideroblasts	↑ Hb A₂, ↑ Hb F ↓ Hb A₂	β thalassemia Sideroblastic anemia
		Macrocytic	Megaloblastic	↓ Serum B_{12} achlorhydria ↓ Serum folate	Vitamin B_{12} deficiency, pernicious anemia Folic acid deficiency
		Normochromic: Normocytic	Normal	↓ Fe, ↓ TIBC	Anemia of chronic inflammation
				↑ Creatinine Abnormal LFT ↓ T₄	Anemia of uremia Anemia of liver disease Anemia of myxedema
		Normoblasts, teardrops	Aplastic Infiltrated: Tumor, lymphoma, etc. Fibrosis	↑ LAP	Aplastic anemia Myelophthisic Myeloid metaplasia
	Increased	Polychromatophilia + Schistocytes, helmet cells	Erythroid hyperplasia	+ Sucrose lysis	Paroxysmal nocturnal hemoglobinuria Traumatic hemolytic anemia
		Spherocytes		+ Coombs' test ↑ Osmotic fragility	Immunohemolytic anemia Hereditary spherocytosis
		Spur cells Sickle cells		Abnormal LFT Positive sickle prep	Spur-cell anemia Sickle-cell syndromes
		Target cells		Abnormal Hb electrophoresis	Hb C, D, etc.
		Heinz bodies		Abnormal Hb electrophoresis ↓ G6PD	Congenital Heinz body hemolytic anemia G6PD deficiency
				Blood in stomach, stool	Blood loss anemia

NOTE: *Fe, iron; TIBC, total iron-binding capacity; Hb, hemoglobin; LAP, leukocyte alkaline phosphatase; G6PD, glucose 6-phosphate dehydrogenase, LFT, liver function tests.*

useful guide to the presence of accelerated red blood cell breakdown. Once this information is obtained, the work-up can be directed toward the establishment of a specific etiology.

Four additional base-line studies are of critical importance in the initial work-up of the patient with anemia: *measurement of red cell indexes, examination of the peripheral blood smear, testing the stool for occult blood,* and, in many patients, *bone marrow examination.*

RED CELL INDEXES As Table 53-2 shows, two indexes, the MCV and MCHC, are particularly useful in classifying the anemias due to decreased red cell production. Microcytic, hypochromic anemias have low values for MCV. On microscopic examination, the red cells appear small and pale. In contrast, in the macrocytic anemias the MCV is elevated and large oval cells (macroovalocytes) are seen on microscopic examination. Unlike the anemias of underproduction, nearly all the hemolytic anemias are normochromic and normocytic. Exceptions include the severe forms of thalassemias in which hypochromic microcytic red cells are accompanied by brisk hemolysis. In addition, hereditary spherocytosis is the one commonly encountered hemolytic anemia in which red cells are hyperchromic with a significantly increased MCHC.

EXAMINATION OF THE BLOOD SMEAR In the evaluation of patients with anemia, the physician should take the time to examine a well-stained peripheral blood film. Plate 9 shows examples of abnormalities in red cell morphology encountered in various types of anemia. Many subtleties escape the attention of the technologist whose primary purpose in examining the slide is to obtain a white cell differential count. Furthermore, the clinician can approach the specimen with a prepared mind and can scrutinize it for specific abnormalities. As suggested above, the examination can confirm the size and color of red cells as estimated by RBC indexes. Furthermore, while these indexes provide mean statistical values, the microscopic examination can reveal variation in red cell size (anisocytosis) or shape (poikilocytosis), changes which are helpful in the diagnosis of specific anemias. Examination of the blood smear is particularly important in evaluating a patient with hemolysis. Most hemolytic anemias have characteristic morphologic abnormalities. Finally, this practice may yield unexpected dividends. The finding of rouleaux may indicate the presence of dysproteinemia as occurs in multiple myeloma. The examination may provide the initial clue that the patient has significant thrombocytopenia.

TABLE 53-2
Anemias due to decreased red cell production

  I Microcytic-hypochromic anemias
    A Iron deficiency (Chap. 310)
    B Sideroblastic anemias (Chap. 310)
    C Thalassemias (Chap. 314)
  II Macrocytic (megaloblastic) anemias (Chap. 311)
    A Vitamin B_{12} deficiency, including pernicious anemia
    B Folic acid deficiency
    C Others: Drug-induced, orotic aciduria, some refractory anemias, erythroleukemia
  III Normocytic-normochromic anemias
    A Primary bone marrow failure (Chap. 312)
      1 Aplastic anemia
        (rare: pure red cell anemia)
      2 Myelophthisic anemias: leukemia and lymphoma, other neoplasms, myelofibrosis, granulomas
    B Secondary anemias (Chap. 313)
      1 Anemias of chronic inflammation
        (infections, connective tissue disorders, etc.)
      2 Anemia of uremia
      3 Anemias associated with endocrinopathies
      4 Anemia of chronic liver disease

BONE MARROW EXAMINATION A microscopic examination of the bone marrow is generally indicated in the work-up of any *unexplained* anemia. The more severe the anemia, the more likely that the procedure will be informative. An assessment of the quantity and quality of red cell precursors may determine whether there is a primary defect in cell production. A marrow biopsy is particularly useful in estimating overall cellularity. The normal differential of nucleated cells in the marrow is shown in the Appendix. The ratio of myeloid (M) to erythroid (E) precursors is normally 3:1. The ratio is increased in patients with infection, a leukemoid reaction, or neoplastic proliferation of myeloid cells. Rarely, a high M:E ratio is due to selective aplasia of the red cell precursors. A decreased M:E ratio indicates erythroid hyperplasia (seen in hemolysis or hemorrhage) or ineffective erythropoiesis (megaloblastic and sideroblastic anemias). The morphology of the precursors may reveal a maturation deficit such as megaloblastic anemia. The bone marrow examination is also important in demonstrating the presence of cellular infiltrates such as those found in leukemia, lymphoma, or multiple myeloma. The demonstration of tumor, fibrosis, or granulomata usually requires a biopsy. A portion of the marrow specimen should routinely be stained with Prussian blue. In addition to providing an assessment of iron stores, the iron stain is required for the identification of sideroblasts.

ANEMIA DUE TO BLOOD LOSS This form of anemia varies considerably in its clinical presentation depending upon the site, severity, and rapidity of the hemorrhage. At opposite extremes are acute fulminant bleeding producing hypovolemic shock and chronic occult blood loss leading to iron-deficiency anemia.

Patients who have sustained an acute hemorrhage generally present with signs and symptoms secondary to hypoxia and hypovolemia. Depending on the severity of the process, the patient will have weakness, fatigue, light-headedness, stupor, or coma. He will often appear pale, diaphoretic, and irritable. Vital signs are a reflection of cardiovascular compensation to the acute blood loss. The patient will have hypotension and tachycardia in proportion to the degree of hemorrhage. Elicitation of postural signs is useful in the initial evaluation of patients with acute blood loss. If the pulse rises 25 percent or more, or the systolic blood pressure falls 20 torr or more upon going from a supine to sitting position, the patient is likely to have significant hypovolemia (blood loss > 1000 ml) and requires prompt replacement. Acute blood loss in excess of 1500 ml usually leads to cardiovascular collapse.

If the blood loss has been acute and recent, the peripheral blood may not reveal a significant decrease in packed cell volume or hemoglobin, since the red cell mass and plasma volume are contracted in parallel. There often is a moderate leukocytosis and a "shift to the left" in the white cell differential count. Thrombocytosis may be encountered in both acute and chronic blood loss. During the first few days following an acute hemorrhage there is usually an increase in reticulocytes. Occasionally nucleated red cells may appear in the peripheral blood. Since young red cells are larger than old ones, the patient may develop slightly macrocytic red cell indexes (MCV = 100 to 105 fl). As mentioned above, sustained reticulocytosis will be seen if significant blood loss continues, until iron stores have been exhausted. Internal bleeding may be accompanied by an increase in unconjugated bilirubin and even in methemalbumin (see below). These abnormalities are a reflection of an increase in catabolism of heme from extravasated red cells.

Patients with large amounts of blood in the gut will often have an elevation of blood urea nitrogen.

It is of critical importance to assess these patients promptly and institute treatment without delay. A large-bore intravenous line should be placed. While blood is being typed and cross matched, saline, Ringer's lactate, or, preferably, a colloid such as 5% albumin should be infused to correct hypovolemia. Whole blood is then administered as soon as it is available. Monitoring of vital signs and central venous pressure is useful in determining the appropriate amount of volume replacement. During and following these emergency measures, diagnostic studies may reveal the site or sites of bleeding. If there appears to be generalized hemorrhage from skin, mucous membranes, urine, etc., an emergency coagulation profile should be obtained. Demonstration of bleeding from the gastrointestinal tract may require the insertion of a nasogastric tube. Appropriate radiologic studies may be indicated to determine sites of internal bleeding such as retroperitoneal hemorrhage.

Chronic blood loss is usually due to lesions in the gastrointestinal tract or the uterus. The testing of stool specimens for occult blood is an essential, though frequently overlooked, part of the evaluation of anemia. It may be necessary to examine serial specimens over a prolonged period of time since gastrointestinal bleeding is often intermittent. The hematologic manifestations of chronic blood loss are those of iron-deficiency anemia, discussed in detail in Chap. 310.

ANEMIAS DUE TO DECREASED RBC PRODUCTION As shown in Table 53-2, red cell indexes are useful in classifying the anemias due to underproduction of red cells. They can be conveniently grouped into three major categories: microcytic-hypochromic, macrocytic (normochromic), and normocytic-normochromic.

The *microcytic-hypochromic* anemias include iron-deficiency anemia (Chap. 310), some sideroblastic anemias (Chap. 310), and the thalassemias (Chap. 314). Collectively, they represent a decrease in the availability or synthesis of one of the three major constituents of the hemoglobin molecule: iron, porphyrin, and globin. Since hemoglobin composes over 90 percent of the protein within the erythrocyte, it is not surprising that these defects in hemoglobin synthesis result in the formation of small, pale red cells. As mentioned above, these disorders involve a variable degree of ineffective erythropoiesis. In addition, the anemias of chronic inflammation and malignancy may be slightly microcytic and hypochromic (Chap. 313). This phenomenon may be due to a poorly understood defect in the availability of iron. However, these disorders are more often normocytic-normochromic and have been so classified in Table 53-2. As shown in Table 53-1, measurement of serum iron and iron-binding capacity and evaluation of marrow iron stores are particularly useful in distinguishing between these anemias.

The *macrocytic* anemias generally are associated with megaloblastic morphology in the bone marrow. In most cases, a deficiency of either vitamin B_{12} or folic acid results in an impairment of the replication of DNA, particularly in cells having a high turnover rate. Because nuclear maturation lags behind cytoplasmic development, large red cells tend to be produced in the bone marrow. Megaloblastic anemias are discussed in detail in Chap. 311. Like the microcytic-hypochromic anemias, these disorders are maturation defects associated with ineffective erythropoiesis. Macrocytosis, generally of a lesser degree, may also be encountered in patients with liver disease and hypothyroidism. However, in these two conditions, the red cell precursors in the bone marrow do not appear megaloblastic. The macrocytes in liver disease and hypothy-

roidism may be related to an increased deposition of lipid in the red cell membrane.

The *normocytic-normochromic* anemias of underproduction[1] comprise a diverse group of disorders. As shown in Table 53-2, this group can be conveniently subdivided into two categories: those due to intrinsic pathology within the bone marrow and those secondary to some other underlying disease.

The primary disorders of the bone marrow are best approached by microscopic examination of a marrow aspirate. In addition, biopsy of the bone marrow is particularly useful in the evaluation of these patients. For example, a biopsy may reveal the presence of fibrosis, granulomata, or tumor deposits which may not be detected in a marrow aspirate. This group of anemias is often accompanied by leukopenia and thrombocytopenia. Pancytopenia, usually to a lesser degree, can also be seen in hypersplenism and in the megaloblastic anemias. Aplastic anemia and the myelophthisic anemias are discussed in Chap. 312.

The diagnosis of anemia secondary to some underlying disease is usually quite straightforward. Conversely, the presence of an unexplained normocytic-normochromic anemia should prompt the search for an underlying disorder such as chronic renal failure, infection, or myxedema. If the presence of such an illness is established, the physician is obliged to investigate whether other factors such as blood loss or a nutritional deficiency contribute to the patient's anemia. Generally, the anemias due to liver disease, chronic inflammation, or an endocrinopathy are of only moderate severity. Unlike the other "secondary" anemias, that due to chronic renal failure can be severe. All these anemias are discussed in more detail in Chap. 313.

HEMOLYTIC ANEMIAS Hemolytic anemias are encountered much less frequently than the anemias due to decreased red cell production. Although they are a diverse group, the hemolytic anemias have a number of clinical features in common. Signs and symptoms of patients with hemolysis are discussed above.

A number of laboratory tests are available to establish the presence of accelerated breakdown of red cells. This group of tests, shown in Table 53-3, is useful in determining the extent of hemolysis but provides no information on specific etiology.

---

[1] As mentioned above, the hemolytic anemias are also normocytic-normochromic.

TABLE 53-3
Laboratory evaluation of hemolysis

	Moderate hemolysis (RBC life span 20–60 days)	Severe hemolysis (RBC life span 5–20 days)
HEMATOLOGIC		
Routine blood film	Polychromatophilia	Polychromatophilia
Reticulocyte index	↑	↑↑
Bone marrow examination	Erythroid hyperplasia	Erythroid hyperplasia
PLASMA OR SERUM		
Bilirubin	↑ Unconjugated	↑ Unconjugated
Haptoglobin	↓, absent	Absent
Hemopexin	Normal, ↓	↓, absent
Plasma hemoglobin	↑	↑↑
Lactate dehydrogenase	↑ (variable)	↑↑ (variable)
Methemalbumin	0	+ (intravascular)
URINE		
Bilirubin	0	0
Urobilinogen	Variable	Variable
Hemosiderin	0	+
Hemoglobin	0	+ (intravascular)

As mentioned previously, the reticulocyte count is the single most useful test in the initial work-up. Patients with hemolytic anemia generally have a brisk reticulocytosis. The bone marrow predictably reveals erythroid hyperplasia. Since it seldom provides useful additional information, a bone marrow examination is generally not indicated in the evaluation of a patient with hemolytic anemia, unless an associated disorder such as lymphoma is suspected.

A variety of serum tests are useful in establishing the presence of hemolysis (see Table 53-3), among them the test for bilirubin, a tetrapyrrole formed from the oxidative catabolism of heme. *Unconjugated* or *"indirect" bilirubin* circulates in the plasma in transit from the mononuclear-phagocyte system to the liver where it is conjugated. When measured accurately, unconjugated bilirubin is a very reliable guide to the presence of increased heme catabolism and is predictably elevated in patients with hemolysis. The serum level of conjugated or "direct" bilirubin is normal unless the patient has associated hepatic or biliary dysfunction. Unconjugated bilirubin is also increased in patients with ineffective erythropoiesis where there is enhanced destruction of red cell precursors within the bone marrow. Since circulating unconjugated bilirubin is tightly bound to albumin, it does not pass through renal glomeruli. Thus, patients with hemolytic anemia have acholuric jaundice, whereas the hyperbilirubinemia of liver disease is associated with bilirubin in the urine.

Other serum tests are also useful in the assessment of hemolysis. *Haptoglobin* is an α globulin which is present in high concentration (~100 mg per 100 ml) in the plasma (and serum). It binds specifically and tightly to the protein (globin) in hemoglobin. The hemoglobin-haptoglobin complex is cleared within minutes by the mononuclear-phagocyte system, while free haptoglobin has a prolonged circulation time ($T_{1/2} = 4$ days). Thus, patients with significant hemolysis, either intravascular or extravascular, have low or absent levels of serum haptoglobin. Haptoglobin synthesis is decreased in patients with hepatocellular disease. Conversely, synthesis is enhanced in inflammatory states. Haptoglobin, like α_1-antitrypsin, orosomucoid, and the third component of complement are acute phase reactants. These facts must be considered in the interpretation of serum haptoglobin. *Hemopexin* is a plasma β globulin which binds specifically to heme. It becomes depleted in patients with moderate and severe hemolysis. The usefulness of the test is limited by the fact that in vitro hemolysis during the collection of the specimen will give a falsely elevated result. In addition to that bound by hemopexin, some of the heme from circulating free hemoglobin is transferred to albumin, resulting in the formation of *methemalbumin*. This complex is encountered only in severe intravascular hemolysis.

The urine should be tested in patients suspected of having intravascular hemolysis. Once the haptoglobin binding capacity of the plasma is exceeded, free hemoglobin will permeate renal glomeruli, primarily as $\alpha\beta$ dimers with a molecular weight of 32,000. This filtered hemoglobin is reabsorbed by the proximal tubule. The molecule is catabolized in situ, and the heme iron is incorporated into storage proteins, ferritin and hemosiderin. The presence of hemosiderin in the urine, detected by staining the sediment with Prussian blue, indicates that a significant amount of circulating free hemoglobin has been filtered by the kidneys. When the absorptive capacity of the tubular cells is exceeded, hemoglobinuria will ensue. The presence of hemoglobinuria indicates severe intravascular hemolysis. Sometimes the clinician is faced with the dilemma of whether benzidine-positive heme pigment in the urine is hemoglobin or myoglobin. The easiest way to distinguish between these alternatives is to examine an anticoagulated blood specimen after centrifugation. Patients with myoglobinuria have normal-appearing plasma. Conversely, the plasma of patients with hemoglobinuria always has a reddish brown color. Because of its higher molecular weight, hemoglobin has a lower glomerular permeability than myoglobin and is less rapidly cleared by the kidneys.

Tagging red cells with an appropriate isotopic label provides the most direct and precise measure of cell survival. The most commonly used labels are sodium [^{51}Cr]chromate and diisopropylfluoro[^{32}P]phosphate. Such studies are not necessary or indicated in the diagnostic work-up of the majority of patients with hemolytic anemia. However, scanning with a collumnated detector can be employed to monitor the sequestration of ^{51}Cr-tagged red cells in the liver and spleen. This approach has proved useful in evaluating patients for possible splenectomy.

Classification of hemolytic anemias A large battery of laboratory tests is available for establishing the specific diagnosis in a patient with hemolytic anemia. No other area of internal medicine is better suited to detailed and fruitful diagnostic probing. In the interest of time and money, the clinician should use the available tests in an orderly fashion. This complex group of disorders is easier to approach diagnostically if a concise and workable classification is used. The hemolytic anemias can be grouped in several ways: congenital versus acquired, intracorpuscular versus extracorpuscular, or by anatomic site of the erythrocyte defect. In Table 53-4, all three ways of classifying these anemias are shown. As stressed earlier in this chapter, the laboratory work-up should begin with careful scrutiny of a well-stained peripheral blood smear. All the hemolytic anemias are normocytic-normochromic except for the thalassemias. However, many of the hemolytic anemias have characteristic red cell morphology. Often the information gleaned from a careful history and physical examination coupled with an inspection of the blood film is sufficient to suggest a working diagnosis which can then be confirmed by appropriate laboratory tests. In this way, a large number of unnecessary diagnostic studies can be circumvented. The various kinds of hemolytic anemia are discussed in Chap. 314.

THERAPEUTIC CONSIDERATIONS The effective treatment of anemia, like other disorders, is predicated upon a thorough diagnostic evaluation. There is no reason to administer hematinics such as iron, vitamin B_{12}, or folic acid unless a specific deficiency of these substances has been demonstrated or is anticipated. Although the indiscriminate administration of vitamin B_{12} is not deleterious per se, it lulls both the patient and the physician into false security. In contrast, the inappropriate use of iron preparations over a prolonged period of time can be

TABLE 53-4
Hemolytic anemias

Extracorpuscular	*I* Environmental factors *A* Antibody: Immunohemolytic anemias *B* Mechanical trauma: Microangiopathic hemolytic anemia *C* Direct toxic effect: Malaria, clostridial infection, etc. *II* Membrane abnormalities *A* Spur-cell anemia	Acquired
Intracorpuscular	*B* Paroxysmal nocturnal hemoglobinuria *C* Hereditary spherocytosis (rare: elliptocytosis, stomatocytosis) *III* Abnormalities of red blood cell interior *A* Enzyme defects *B* Hemoglobinopathies	Hereditary

directly harmful, leading to a state of iron overload. Pyridoxine is indicated only in the treatment of sideroblastic anemias.

Many kinds of anemias can be corrected if a precipitating cause can be uncovered and reversed. If a drug or toxin can be incriminated, its withdrawal may allow full recovery. The outcome of the "secondary" anemias is dependent on whether the underlying condition can be corrected. Anemias due to an endocrinopathy or infection should respond favorably to appropriate treatment. Occasionally, the anemia of malignancy is corrected by the removal of the primary tumor. One of the most dramatic sequelae of a successful renal transplant is the prompt correction of the "anemia of uremia." In chronic disorders such as hepatic cirrhosis or rheumatoid arthritis, the anemia is likely to persist, along with the underlying disease.

Primary disorders of the bone marrow such as aplastic anemia or myelophthisic anemia are often irreversible and are treated with supportive measures. *Androgens* are sometimes employed in this group of anemias, but their efficacy is marginal. Many of these patients require transfusions of red cells and platelets. Because prognosis is so bleak in these disorders, a radical approach to treatment seems justified. As described in Chap. 312, bone marrow transplantation is now a reasonable therapeutic alternative in selected cases of severe aplastic anemia and possibly in refractory leukemia.

Several factors should be weighed in determining whether an anemic patient should be transfused. The risks and complications of the administration of blood products are discussed in Chap. 319. Patients with chronic or long-standing anemias are able to compensate in several ways, discussed earlier in this chapter. A considerable reduction in red cell mass can be surprisingly well tolerated, especially if the patient is young or sedentary. Transfusion is seldom indicated in a patient with a chronic anemia whose hemoglobin is 9 g per 100 ml or greater. Those who are expected to respond to the administration of a specific agent such as iron, folic acid, or vitamin B_{12} can usually be spared transfusions. If the anemia has precipitated an episode of congestive heart failure or myocardial ischemia, prompt but cautious administration of packed red cells is indicated. In general, whole blood should be given only if the patient is hypovolemic.

Corticosteroids have only a limited role in the treatment of anemia. These agents are not effective in stimulating erythropoiesis. High doses of a glucocorticoid are indicated in the treatment of immunohemolytic anemia, thrombotic thrombocytopenic purpura, and pure red cell anemia. Otherwise, steroids should be prescribed sparingly unless some coexisting condition dictates their use.

Splenectomy is indicated in the treatment of certain hemolytic anemias. The efficacy of splenectomy correlates with the degree to which the abnormal or defective red cells are sequestered. Splenectomy is virtually curative in hereditary spherocytosis. The operation may be beneficial in selected patients with immunohemolytic anemia, congestive splenomegaly, spur-cell anemia, and certain hemoglobinopathies and enzymopathies. Splenectomy has also been recommended early in the treatment of thrombotic thrombocytopenic purpura. The operative morbidity and mortality from elective splenectomy is very low. Occasional patients develop a left subphrenic abscess. Following splenectomy, young children are at risk of developing overwhelming septicemia. This complication is much rarer in adults. Thrombocytosis generally develops promptly following splenectomy. However, in most cases, it is transient. In patients with continued hemolysis, the thrombocytosis usually persists and may occasionally be associated with thromboembolic phenomena.

REFERENCES

Bunn HF et al: *Human Hemoglobins.* Philadelphia, Saunders, 1977

Erslev AJ, Gabuzda TG: *Pathophysiology of Blood.* Philadelphia, Saunders, 1975

Harris JW, Kellermeyer RW: *The Red Cell.* Cambridge, Harvard University Press, 1970

Hillman RS, Finch CA: *Red Cell Manual.* Philadelphia, Davis, 1974

Nienhuis AW, Benz EJ: Regulation of hemoglobin synthesis during the development of the red cell. N Engl J Med 297:1318, 1371, 1430, 1977

Rapaport SI: *Introduction to Hematology.* New York, Harper & Row, 1971

Schmid R (ed): Physiology and disorders of hemoglobin degradation. Semin Hematol 9:1, 1972

Weed RI: *Hematology for Internists.* Boston, Little, Brown, 1971

Wintrobe MM: *Clinical Hematology,* 7th ed. Philadelphia, Lea & Febiger, 1974

54
BLEEDING

HYMIE L. NOSSEL

Bleeding is one of the most serious and significant of the cardinal manifestations of disease. It may occur from a local site or may be generalized. Bleeding associated with a local lesion may be superimposed on either a normal or a defective hemostatic mechanism; in contrast, general bleeding is usually associated with a hemorrhagic diathesis. Spontaneous bleeding also suggests defective hemostasis.

LOCAL BLEEDING

In the evaluation of local bleeding, the site, appearance of the blood, signs of blood loss, and evidence for disordered hemostasis should be considered. The sites and common causes of bleeding are listed in Table 54-1. The appearance of the blood may provide a clue as to the cause of the bleeding. Bleeding from the lungs and bronchi is influenced by the degree of aeration and the presence of mucus and pus. In pneumococcal pneumonia the sputum is characteristically rusty. In tuberculosis it is usually bright red. Pus is usually mixed with the blood when infection is present. Massive hemorrhage occasionally occurs in mitral stenosis when a bronchial varicosity ruptures or in tuberculosis when a vessel is eroded. In pulmonary infarction the blood is usually dark red. Blood derived from the gastrointestinal tract may be darkened because of conversion of hemoglobin to brown hematin by gastric acid. Blood vomited from the stomach may be dark ("coffee ground") or bright red if the vomiting is sufficiently rapid. When it appears in the stool, it may be pitch black (melena). Blood derived from the colon is red or brown, and, if inflammation is the cause, mucus or pus is mixed with it (see Chap. 38). If bleeding from the urinary tract is profuse, clots or bright blood may be present in the urine. Small amounts of blood impart a smoky appearance to urine, whereas lesser degrees of hematuria may be detected only by microscopy.

The signs and symptoms of blood loss depend on the amount and rate of bleeding. If very acute, syncope occurs rapidly; with a slower rate of loss, signs and symptoms of peripheral circulatory collapse occur. Shock may occur without external blood loss if a large amount of blood is lost into a serous cavity. Slow and prolonged blood loss will gradually result in symptoms of iron-deficiency anemia.

TABLE 54-1
Causes of localized bleeding

273

CHAPTER 54
BLEEDING

Locations	Commonest causes
Skin (petechiae, purpura, ecchymoses)	Thrombocytopenia
Limbs:	
Joints	Hemophilia
Intramuscular and subcutaneous hematomas	Hemophilia
Central nervous system	Trauma, hypertension, congenital vascular malformations
Head and neck:	
Nose and sinuses	Trauma, inflammation, hypertension, polyps and tumors, hereditary telangiectasia
Ears	Trauma
Optic fundi	Hypertension, nephritis, diabetes, thrombocytopenia, trauma
Chest:	
Respiratory tract	Tumors, infections, bronchiectasis, pulmonary embolism, mitral stenosis
Serous cavity	Tumors, tuberculosis, pulmonary infarction
Nipples	Fissure, tumor
Gastrointestinal tract	Esophageal varices, hiatal hernia, peptic ulcer, gastritis, tumors, colitis, hemorrhoids, hereditary telangiectasia
Abdominal cavity	Trauma, splenic rupture, ectopic gestation
Urinary tract	Calculi, infections, glomerulonephritis, tumors, cystitis, prostatic hypertrophy
Vagina	Obstetric and endocrine disorders, tumors

Local bleeding which is out of proportion to the injury suggests a hemostatic defect. For example, when a patient suffers bleeding following dental extraction sufficient to require blood transfusion, a defect of the coagulation or platelet systems can almost always be defined.

HEMOSTASIS AND ITS DISORDERS

The successful management of patients with a disorder of the hemostatic mechanism depends on accurate diagnosis. Correct diagnosis and rational therapy depend on an understanding of the normal mechanisms for preserving hemostasis.

Normal hemostasis comprises mechanisms operative immediately following an injury and those acting over a longer period to maintain hemostasis. The immediate mechanism consists principally of two components: *vasoconstriction* due to active contraction of the smooth muscle of the vessel wall, and *plug formation* by masses of aggregated platelets. The maintenance mechanism consists of the *fibrin* (and fibrin clot) produced by the coagulation system.

Platelet plug formation is especially important in capillary hemostasis, while vasoconstriction and fibrin formation seem to be more important in larger vessel hemostasis. These several mechanisms involved in achieving normal hemostasis are interconnected at several points, but for the sake of clarity they will be described as separate entities.

PLATELETS The normal platelet count is 150,000 to 400,000 per cubic millimeter. The most accurate method of counting platelets is by electronic particle counting or by phase-contrast microscopy. An estimate of platelet number may be made by examination of the stained peripheral blood smear. With a normal platelet count, several (3 to 10) platelets (individually or in small clumps) should be visible in each oil-immersion field.

Structure Normal platelets are anucleate bodies 2 to 3 μm in diameter which appear light blue and contain small purple-red granules when stained with Giemsa's solution. With the electron microscope, three distinct structural zones may be identified in the platelet, each related to specific platelet functions. The unique quality of the platelet is its ability to adhere to foreign surfaces and form aggregates in response to a variety of stimuli including thrombin, adenosine diphosphate (ADP), and catecholamines. The *peripheral* zone is involved in adhesion, the *cytoplasm* (sol-gel zone) in contraction, and the *organelle* zone in secretion.

The peripheral zone comprises a surface coat of acid mucopolysaccharides (the glycocalyx) and glycoproteins, the trilaminar plasma unit membrane, and a submembranous area. The surface coat is involved in adhesion, and the membrane provides a trigger mechanism whereby stimuli are transmitted from the exterior into the interior. Specific binding sites for thrombin and ADP are present.

The submembranous area and cytoplasmic zone contain the contractile protein *actomyosin* (also termed *thrombosthenin*) in the form of a number of fibrous elements. In the submembranous area, bundles of microtubules encircle the platelet forming a cytoskeleton that stabilizes the cell, permitting it to circulate as a flattened disk. The microtubules are composed of subfilaments which are indistinguishable from microfilaments present in the cytoplasm. The microfilaments are responsible for the centripetal movement and coalescence of granules occurring during platelet aggregation, the contraction of pseudopods, and clot retraction.

Distinct components in the organelle zone include granules, mitochondria, glycogen-containing particles, and, in an occasional platelet, stacks of flattened saccules resembling a Golgi apparatus. Three types of membrane-enclosed granules can be distinguished: (1) alpha granules which contain a number of proteins including platelet factor 4 which has heparin-neutralizing activity, beta thromboglobulin, fibrinogen, and a factor(s) which stimulates the mitosis of smooth muscle cells and fibroblasts; (2) dense granules in which calcium, ADP, serotonin, and catecholamines are localized; and (3) lysosomal granules with enzymes such as phosphatase, β-glucuronidase, and cathepsin. The three granule populations constitute the secretory organelles of the platelet and release their contents in response to stimuli such as thrombin, collagen, ADP, and epinephrine. The threshold for release for each type of granule is different; the sequence in order of increasing threshold is alpha granules, dense granules, and lysosomal granules. Active intermediary metabolism occurs in the mitochondria. ATP is generated from both glycolysis and the tricarboxylic acid cycle. Glycogen and lipid are also synthesized.

Distribution and fate Platelets are formed in the marrow and released into the circulation. At any moment, about 80 percent of the platelets are in the circulation and 20 percent are in the spleen; free movement occurs between these two pools. If the spleen enlarges markedly, the distribution shifts and up to 80 percent of the platelets may be pooled in the spleen. Survival curves of ^{51}Cr-labeled platelets are linear and suggest that most platelets become senescent and die after a life span of about 10 days.

Some platelets appear to be consumed in repairing the minor vascular injuries of daily life. There is evidence that younger platelets are physiologically more active and have higher enzyme concentrations than old platelets. This distinction is most apparent when thrombopoiesis is accelerated in response to increased platelet destruction. Senescent platelets are probably removed by the reticuloendothelial system. In thrombocytopenia due to increased platelet destruction, the destruction is random. Damaged platelets may be removed primarily in the spleen or in both the spleen and the liver. The bone marrow does not contain a reserve of platelets, and if circulating platelets are rapidly destroyed or lost, thrombocytopenia persists for several days until enough new platelets are formed. Governing normal platelet production are one or more humoral factors that appear to regulate platelet production.

Function in hemostasis   The platelet contributes to hemostasis by forming platelet plugs and by promoting thrombin production. Platelet plug formation may be divided into a number of stages (Fig. 54-1).

ADHESION   Platelets adhere to subendothelial structures exposed by trauma. Such structures include collagen fibers and basement membranes. Regularly spaced free amino groups on the collagen molecule are required for platelet adhesion. In addition, a number of plasma proteins, including fibrinogen and von Willebrand factor, are required for normal platelet adherence.

RELEASE REACTION   Following adherence to collagen, platelets extrude the contents of their granules—a process termed the *release reaction*. This reaction is also induced by thrombin, and in physiologic hemostasis very likely both collagen and throm-

bin initiate release. Epinephrine and ADP also promote platelet aggregation and release.

Detailed understanding of the mechanism of release is incomplete, but certain facts are clear. The reaction has an absolute requirement for energy derived from glycolysis and the Krebs cycle. A major control mechanism for both aggregation and release is the platelet concentration of cyclic adenosine 3′, 5′-monophosphate (AMP) which is produced from ATP by adenylate cyclase and degraded by phosphodiesterase. Release is inhibited by substances which increase the platelet concentration of cyclic AMP. These agents include prostacyclin (PGI$_2$, a potent prostaglandin produced only in endothelial cells and not in platelets), which stimulates adenylate cyclase, and theophylline, which inhibits phosphodiesterase. Epinephrine, on the other hand, lowers platelet cyclic AMP levels and promotes release.

It has been shown that an intermediate of platelet prostaglandin synthesis plays a major role in mediating the release reaction (Fig. 54-2). When platelets are stimulated by a release-inducer, such as thrombin or ADP, phospholipase A$_2$ cleaves free arachidonic acid from platelet phospholipids. Arachidonic acid, under the influence of a cyclooxygenase, is sequentially converted to the cyclic endoperoxides PGG$_2$ and PGH$_2$, the latter of which is transformed to thromboxane A$_2$ by thromboxane synthetase. Thromboxane A$_2$ directly induces the release reaction but is unstable and is rapidly transformed to thromboxane B$_2$, which is inactive. Aspirin leads to acetylation of cyclooxygenase, rendering it inactive; thus aspirin inhibits formation of endoperoxide and thromboxane A$_2$. Inhibition of cyclooxygenase prevents platelet release resulting from

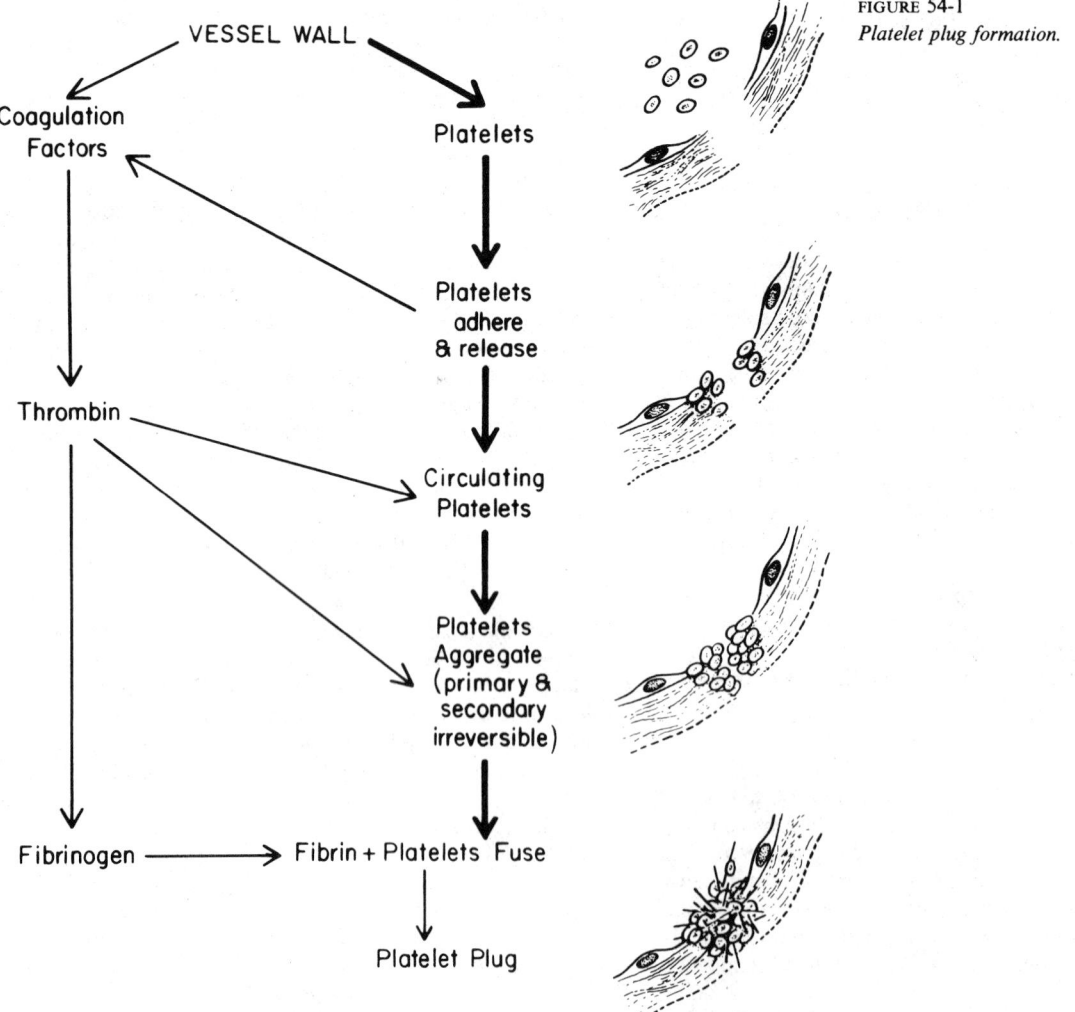

FIGURE 54-1
Platelet plug formation.

weak or moderate stimulation. High concentrations of collagen or thrombin will overcome the inhibitory effect of aspirin and produce full release, indicating the presence of an alternative release mechanism. Calcium ionophores, which allow movements of calcium ions between subcellular compartments, may induce release by still another mechanism.

AGGREGATION The released ADP causes additional platelets to aggregate and is thus a key component for amplifying the extent of platelet aggregation. How ADP produces aggregation is as yet unclear. Low concentrations of ADP ($\sim 10^{-6}$ M) cause only primary platelet aggregation, which is reversible, whereas two- to threefold higher concentrations of ADP produce irreversible aggregation. Low concentrations of thrombin or collagen, in addition to causing primary aggregation, stimulate the release of ADP, which promotes secondary irreversible aggregation.

Platelets participate in coagulation factor reactions leading to thrombin formation by providing a lipoprotein surface (so-called "platelet factor 3") on which coagulation enzymes and substrates interact. Factor X_a is bound via factor V to the platelet lipoprotein membrane and there activates prothrombin. "Activation" of the platelet is necessary for factor X_a binding and consequent promotion of coagulation (Fig. 54-5). Hence, a defect in platelet activation will be detected as a defect in the activity of platelet factor III coagulant activity.

FUSION The action of thrombin produced by the coagulation mechanism leads to coalescence. Fibrin (also a product of thrombin action) and fused platelets form a stable hemostatic plug.

CLOT RETRACTION Following in vitro coagulation of blood or platelet-rich plasma, platelets retract the fibrin threads of the clot into a contracted volume and express the fluid trapped in the clot. It is uncertain to what extent clot retraction is a necessary component of hemostasis, but the test is simple to do and provides useful information. Clot retraction is readily tested in whole blood or by adding thrombin to platelet-rich plasma and noting the extent of clot retraction 1 h later. Clot retraction is defective in a severe congenital defect of platelet function termed *thrombasthenia,* or when either the platelet count or the fibrinogen concentration is very low.

Tests of platelet function Platelet plugs rapidly stop bleeding from ruptured capillaries and small vessels. The integrity of the platelet plug-forming mechanism is tested by measuring the *bleeding time.* This is most commonly determined by the Ivy bleeding time technique, in which the time is measured for bleeding to cease from three incisions 1 cm long and 1 mm deep in an avascular area of the forearm. Venous return is obstructed by a blood pressure cuff set at 40 mmHg pressure over the upper forearm. The bleeding time is normal in disorders of the coagulation system but is abnormal in the presence of severe thrombocytopenia, defects of platelet function, deficiency of the von Willebrand plasma protein, or total absence of blood fibrinogen. Generally, clinically significant defects in platelet function are found only if the bleeding time is prolonged. Platelet aggregation, a measure of platelet function, may be studied by recording the increase in light transmitted through a cuvette containing continuously stirred platelet-rich plasma when aggregating agents are added to the plasma. The aggregating agents usually tested are collagen, epinephrine, adenosine diphosphate, thrombin, and ristocetin.

FIGURE 54-2

Generation of thromboxane A_2 in platelets and prostacyclin PGI_2 in endothelial cells and effects on platelet activation and release.

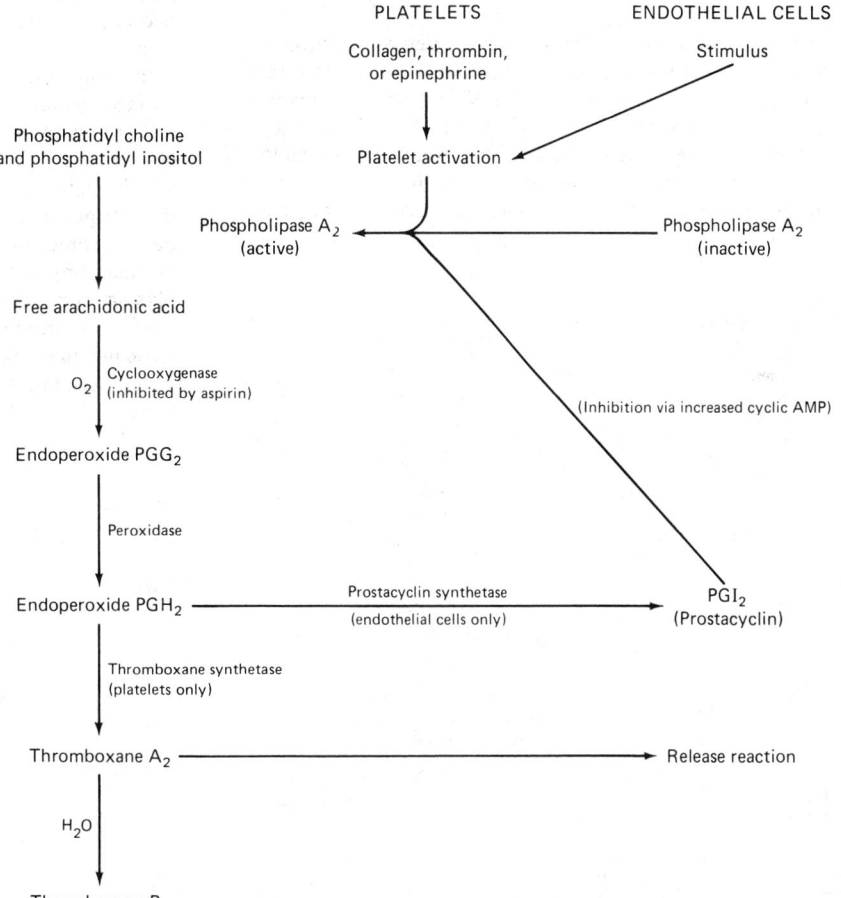

BLOOD COAGULATION: MECHANISM AND FUNCTION The two main functions of the blood coagulation mechanism are as follows:

1 Production of thrombin which stabilizes the platelet plug
2 Formation of fibrin which, by rendering the platelet plug permanent, mechanically blocks the flow of blood through ruptured vessels

A number of discrete proenzymes and proteins (termed *coagulation factors*), platelets, and calcium participate in the coagulation process. The process consists of several stages and ends with fibrin formation.

Fibrin formation Fibrinogen is a 340,000-dalton dimeric protein, each half of which contains three polypeptide chains termed Aα, Bβ, and γ. The first step in fibrin formation is cleavage by thrombin of fibrinopeptides A and B from the fibrinogen molecule to produce fibrin monomer (Fig. 54-3). Fibrinopeptide A is cleaved first, and following its release, the fibrin molecules polymerize to form visible coagulum. When the concentration of fibrin relative to fibrinogen is low, the fibrin forms a complex with fibrinogen and remains in solution. When the ratio of fibrin to fibrinogen molecules becomes greater, the fibrin precipitates to form the clot. The approximate ratio above which clot formation occurs is one fibrin molecule per five fibrinogen molecules.

Polymerized fibrin is soluble in acid and concentrated urea solutions and is hemostatically ineffective. Fibrin polymer is cross-linked by the action of activated factor XIII, which, in the presence of calcium, forms covalent peptide bonds between glutamyl and lysyl amino acid residues of adjacent molecules. The resulting product is highly insoluble and is hemostatically very effective.

Prothrombin activation Thrombin is formed by the proteolytic cleavage of a proenzyme, prothrombin. The process results from the action of activated factor X (X_a) which binds to the surface of activated platelets via factor V and cleaves prothrombin in the presence of calcium. Activation of factor X may occur by either of two separate pathways, the extrinsic and the intrinsic. Clinical experience suggests that effective he-

FIGURE 54-3
Steps in cross-linked fibrin formation.

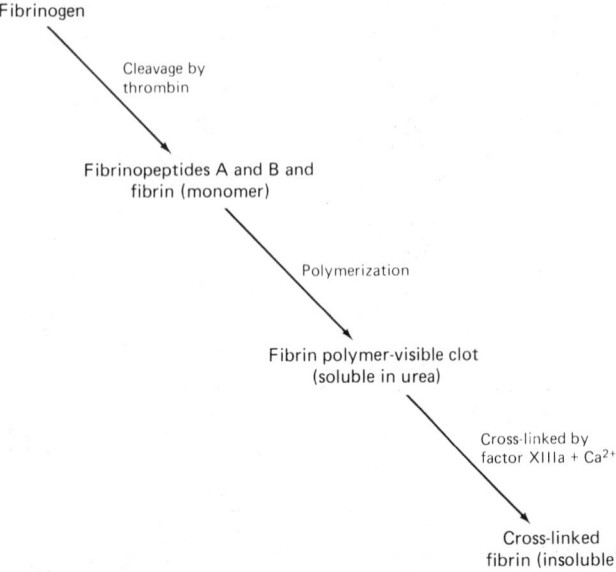

mostasis requires the participation of both. In the *extrinsic pathway*, a tissue factor (tissue thromboplastin), released from damaged cells, activates factor X in the presence of factor VII and calcium (Fig. 54-4). In the *intrinsic* or *cascade pathway* (Fig. 54-5), the contact of blood with a "foreign" surface, such as collagen or skin, activates factor XII. Activated factor XII, in the presence of prekallikrein and high-molecular-weight kininogen, activates factor XI which, in the presence of calcium, cleaves a peptide from factor IX producing activated factor IX. Activated factor IX proteolytically converts factor X into the activated form (X_a) in the presence of platelet membrane lipoprotein, factor VIII, and calcium.

Tests of the coagulation mechanism The intrinsic pathway of blood coagulation including fibrin polymerization is tested by measuring the *whole-blood clotting time* and *partial thromboplastin time* (Fig. 54-6). The whole-blood clotting time is the time taken for 1 ml of whole blood to clot at 37°C with controlled temperature and exposure of the blood to the glass surface of the test tube. The test is influenced by gross defects in the intrinsic clotting system. The partial thromboplastin time (celite or kaolin cephalin time) is the time required for recalcified citrated plasma to clot. A standardized platelet substitute (cephalin or "partial thromboplastin") and standard surface activation (provided by celite or kaolin) are used to eliminate variability due to the platelet count and surface factors. The test is influenced by moderate defects in the intrinsic clotting system.

The activity of any of the coagulation factors involved in the intrinsic pathway (i.e., factors XII, XI, IX, and VIII) may be measured by comparing the ability of control and test plasma samples to shorten the partial thromboplastin time of a plasma sample known to be deficient in the specific factor.

The extrinsic clotting system is tested by the *one-stage prothrombin time*. In this test, the time taken for recalcified citrated plasma to clot in the presence of tissue thromboplastin is measured. The test is sensitive to defects in the extrinsic clot-

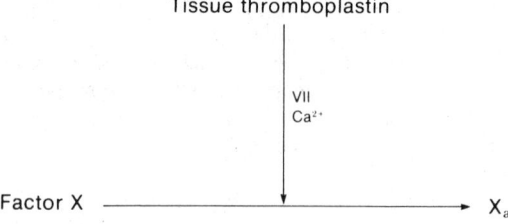

FIGURE 54-4
Activation of factor X by steps in the extrinsic coagulation pathway.

FIGURE 54-5
Activation of factor X by the steps in the extrinsic coagulation pathway.

FIGURE 54-6
Coagulation tests.

FIGURE 54-7
Plasminogen activation in plasma and in a thrombus and digestion of fibrinogen and fibrin.

ting system (Figs. 54-4 and 54-6). The activity of factor VII and the common pathway coagulation factors (factors II, V, and X) may be measured by comparing the ability of control and test plasma samples to shorten the prothrombin time of plasma deficient in the specific factor.

The polymerization of fibrinogen is tested by measuring the *thrombin clotting time.* This test measures the time for citrated plasma to clot in the presence of added thrombin. The test is abnormal in the presence of heparin or of congenital or acquired abnormalities of the fibrinogen molecule such as disseminated intravascular coagulation.

Blood fluidity system (regulator mechanisms) In addition to the coagulation factors, several mechanisms exist in the circulation for maintaining the blood in a fluid state. In the absence of this system, sufficient thrombin would be generated by the clotting of only 1 ml blood to coagulate all the fibrinogen in 3 liters blood. The fluidity-maintaining system consists of both cellular and humoral components.

The cellular component comprises the reticuloendothelial system and the liver, both of which specifically remove activated clotting factors and fibrin without affecting precursor (unactivated) coagulation factors. The humoral component consists of several proteins which specifically inactivate the activated coagulation factors. These proteins include antithrombin III and α_2 macroglobulin. Antithrombin inactivates thrombin and each of the activated intermediates of the clotting mechanism.

The humoral system also includes the fibrinolytic mechanism for dissolving fibrin. Fibrinolysis is produced by the action of an enzyme, plasmin, which is formed from a precursor, plasminogen. Plasminogen is proteolytically converted to plasmin by an extrinsic system in which the activator is supplied by damaged cells present in the blood vessel wall or by an intrinsic system in which the components are all present in the blood. The intrinsic plasmin system is initiated by the contact of factor XII with a foreign surface; by way of a number of intermediates, including prekallikrein and high-molecular-weight kininogen, an activator is formed which converts plasminogen to plasmin (Fig. 54-7).

Initially polypeptides from the C-terminal part of the Aα chain and from the N-terminal part of the Bβ chain are cleaved. The remaining part of the molecule is often termed *fragment X* and is still clottable by thrombin. Subsequent stages of digestion are not clottable. An intermediate stage is often termed *fragment Y,* and final stages are termed *D* and *E.* These products of plasmin digestion are termed *fibrinogen-fi-*

brin degradation products. The degradation products have significant physiologic effects. They inhibit the clotting of normal blood by acting as anticoagulants. They delay the polymerization of fibrin and thus prolong the thrombin clotting time. The fibrinogen-fibrin degradation products may also interpose between fibrin polymers as they are forming. This results in a weak, disordered fibrin clot. Platelet aggregation by ADP is also inhibited. Plasmin also digests factors V and VIII. A number of powerful inhibitors are present in normal blood, and these control plasmin action and prevent proteolysis of fibrinogen. The most important of these inhibitors is a 63,000-dalton α_2 globulin which rapidly and irreversibly inactivates plasmin.

As fibrin is deposited, plasminogen becomes incorporated in the growing thrombus, and is thereby separated from the circulating inhibitors of plasminogen activation so that the plasmin formed is localized at the site of fibrin formation. Thus freed from the inhibitors, it is able to digest fibrin. In this way, discrete local lysis of fibrin can occur without proteolysis of circulating fibrinogen. Clot lysis following fibrin deposition results in release of *fibrin degradation products* into the blood. In those pathologic conditions with extensive intravascular clotting, fibrin degradation products may accumulate in the blood without detectable plasmin levels in the blood sampled from a distant site such as an arm vein.

Production, distribution, and life span of coagulation factors Because the concentrations of all plasma clotting factors, except factor VIII, are depressed in patients with massive liver necrosis, it is thought that hepatic parenchymal cells synthesize all factors except factor VIII. There is evidence that von Willebrand protein, which is closely related to factor VIII, is synthe-

TABLE 54-2
Properties of coagulation factors

Factor	Plasma concentration, $\mu g/ml$	Hemostatic level, % of normal	In vivo recovery, % of infused material	$T_{1/2}$, h
Fibrinogen	3000	100 mg per 100 ml	50	100
Prothrombin	150	?40	50	72
V	10	25	?50–100	16
VII	0.5	10	?100	6
VIII (antihemophilic)	?	30	80	12
IX	3	25	50	24
X	15	20	50–100	48
XI	6	?25	100	60
XII	29	—	—	60
XIII	20	3	50–100	120

TABLE 54-3
Clinical distinction between blood coagulation defects and capillary and platelet defects

	Coagulation defects	Capillary and platelet defects
Family history	Usually positive	Usually negative
Sex predominance	Males	Females
Type of bleeding	Visceral and intra-muscular deep he-matomas; usually after trauma	Skin and mucosal surfaces; petechiae and ecchymoses; spontaneous
Duration	Delayed after trauma and persis-tent	Immediate after trauma; short-lived
Local pressure	Not effective	May stop bleeding

sized by endothelial cells. It is not known where factor VIII coagulant activity is synthesized. It does not appear to be made in endothelial cells. Levels of factor VIII rise sharply after a burst of muscular exercise or an infusion of epineph-rine. The rise apparently reflects the release of stores of factor VIII into the circulation. Stress, fever, and infection elevate fibrinogen and factor VIII levels by an unknown mechanism. Gram-negative bacterial endotoxin also stimulates fibrinogen production. Levels of factors VII, VIII, and X and fibrinogen are elevated in pregnancy and in patients using oral contraceptives.

The plasma clotting factors have short intravascular half-lives compared with other plasma proteins. These can be grouped (in order of decreasing intravascular half-life) as follows (see also Table 54-2):

1 Fibrinogen, factor XIII: 4 to 5 days
2 Prothrombin, factors V, IX, X, XI, and XII: 1 to 3 days
3 Factor VIII: 12 h
4 Factor VII: 5 h

Because of these relatively short half-lives, postoperative prophylaxis or control of bleeding following trauma in a pa-tient with a severe clotting-factor deficiency usually requires repeated replacement therapy during the period of healing.

DIAGNOSTIC APPROACH TO DISORDERS OF HEMOSTASIS

The diagnosis of coagulation disorders is based on both clinical and laboratory evidence. A careful and knowledgeably col-lected history is essential if the results obtained from labora-tory studies are to be properly interpreted.

CLINICAL HISTORY (Table 54-3) A history taken to evaluate hemostasis should answer these questions: (1) Has *abnormal bleeding* or *bruising* occurred either spontaneously or after in-jury, dental extraction, or surgery? Was there *delayed* or *pro-longed* bleeding, suggesting a coagulation disorder, or immedi-ate and transient bleeding, suggesting a platelet disorder? (2) Was there bleeding from the umbilical stump or after circum-cision? (3) Is there a history of *prolonged nose bleeds?* Brief epistaxis, stopping within minutes, even if frequent, is usually associated with normal tests of hemostasis.

One should try to determine the degree and frequency of the following:

1 *Bruising.* Spontaneous bruises larger than the palm of the hand are generally significant; a history of hematomas and bruises at the sites of injections or immunizations may like-wise be suggestive of a hemostatic disorder.
2 *Excessive bleeding from small cuts.* Specific details as to the size of laceration and duration of bleeding should be elic-ited.

One should question the patient for (1) evidence of an un-derlying *systemic disorder* that may be accompanied by defec-tive hemostasis, such as liver disease, systemic lupus erythema-tosus, uremia, or a hematologic malignancy; (2) a *family history* of bleeding and, if present, the hereditary pattern of transmission; and (3) *drug ingestion.* Drugs that interfere with hemostasis fall into two categories: (1) drugs that impair for-mation of the hemostatic plug by inhibiting platelet function or causing thrombocytopenia and (2) drugs that interfere with blood coagulation.

Drugs that impair plug formation include aspirin in ordi-nary doses, but such prolongation in bleeding time usually re-mains within the normal range unless platelet function is al-ready abnormal; aspirin should be discontinued several days before surgery. Other drugs which interfere with platelet func-tion are dipyridamole, clofibrate, phenylbutazone, antihista-mines, and tranquilizers. The clinical significance of these drugs with respect to hemostasis has yet to be clearly docu-mented.

Drugs that interfere with blood coagulation include heparin and the oral coumarin drugs. Although preoperative patients are rarely receiving parenteral heparin, patients on long-term oral anticoagulant therapy are frequently encountered.

TABLE 54-4
Diagnosis of bleeding disorders involving coagulation

Disorders	Tests					
	Prothrombin time	Partial thromboplastin time	Thrombin time	Fibrinogen concentration	Fibrinogen proteolysis	Factor assays
Congenital deficiency of factor VII	Abnormal	Normal	Normal	Normal	Normal	Specific factor abnormal
Congenital deficiency of factors VIII, IX, XI, XII, high-molecu-lar-weight kininogen or prekalli-krein	Normal	Abnormal	Normal	Normal	Normal	Specific factors abnormal
Deficiency of prothrombin, factor V, factor X, or vitamin K; or coumarin or warfarin effect	Abnormal	Abnormal	Normal	Normal	Normal	Specific factor abnormal
Dysfibrinogenemia, heparin effect	Abnormal	Abnormal	Abnormal	Normal	Normal	Normal
Disseminated intravascular coagu-lation, liver failure, congenital hypofibrinogenemia	Abnormal	Abnormal	Abnormal	Decreased	Abnormal	Abnormal

TABLE 54-5
Diagnosis of bleeding disorders involving platelets

| | Tests | | | | |
| | Bleeding time | Platelet count | Platelet function | | |
Disorders			Clot retraction	PF III*	Platelet aggregation
Thrombocytopenia	Prolonged	Decreased	Abnormal		
Thromboasthenia	Prolonged	Normal	Abnormal	Abnormal	Abnormal with ADP and other aggregating agents
Release defects	Prolonged	Normal	Normal	Abnormal	Primary normal, secondary abnormal
von Willebrand's disease (also has low factor VIII coagulant activity and antigenic activity)	Prolonged	Normal	Normal	Normal	Abnormal only with ristocetin, normal with ADP, epinephrine, thrombin, collagen

* *Activity of platelet factor III.*

PHYSICAL FINDINGS The patient should be examined for the following.

1 *Abnormal bleeding in the skin.* Ecchymoses suggest abnormal bleeding from relatively large vessels due to a defect in blood clotting. Petechiae, which may be small, require a careful search, particularly around the ankles. Petechiae suggest increased vascular fragility secondary to thrombocytopenia.
2 *Mucosal bleeding.* Look for purpura of the buccal mucosa and the conjunctival surfaces of the eyelids. Hemorrhagic bullae in the mouth are found only in the presence of thrombocytopenia. Hemorrhages in the optic fundi, however, may reflect local eye disease, hypertension, diabetes, severe anemia, or thrombocytopenia. The presence of telangiectasia on or under the tongue should be noted.
3 *Hemarthrosis and ankylosis.* These suggest a deficiency of factor VIII or IX.
4 *Hereditary connective tissue disorder.* Abnormal elasticity of the skin and hyperextensibility of the joints (Ehlers-Danlos syndrome) may be associated with vascular bleeding.
5 *Chronic liver disease,* including spider angiomas, palmar erythema, dilated abdominal veins, hepatomegaly, or splenomegaly.

LABORATORY STUDIES Screening tests A careful history is the best screening test. Nevertheless, laboratory tests for the integrity of the coagulation and platelet components of the hemostatic mechanism are indicated under a number of circumstances, including (1) historical or physical evidence of abnormal hemostasis; (2) family history of abnormal hemostasis; (3) presence of a disorder which may be associated with abnormal hemostasis, e.g., liver disease, systemic lupus erythematosus; and (4) prior surgical procedures known to be associated with a high incidence of hemorrhage.

Coagulation system tests (Table 54-4) A commonly used set of screening tests for coagulation defects include (1) *prothrombin time,* (2) *partial thromboplastin time,* (3) *thrombin clotting time,* and (4) *fibrinogen concentration* (most tests of fibrinogen depend on measuring the concentration of thrombin-clottable protein in the plasma). If one or more of these tests are abnormal, an assessment is made, based on the history as well as the test results, as to the most likely defect. The factor(s) most likely to be abnormal should be specifically assayed, including factor XIII. If all the coagulation system screening tests are normal, no further tests are necessary unless the history strongly suggests abnormal hemostasis.

Platelet system tests (Table 54-5) Basic screening tests include (1) the *bleeding time* and (2) the *platelet count.*

Tests which screen for defects of platelet function include (1) clot retraction; (2) activity of platelet factor III; and (3) platelet aggregation.

If the bleeding time is prolonged and thrombocytopenia is detected, the etiology of the thrombocytopenia should be pursued by a careful history of drug or toxin exposure, physical examination for splenomegaly and systemic disease, a complete blood count, examination of the bone marrow, and tests for systemic lupus erythematosus and platelet antibodies. If the bleeding time is prolonged and the platelet count is normal, tests for von Willebrand's disease and for platelet function should be undertaken (see Chaps. 316 and 318).

REFERENCES

BIGGS R (ed): *Human Blood Coagulation, Haemostasis and Thrombosis,* 2d ed. Oxford, Blackwell, 1976

Haemostasis. Br Med Bull, vol 33, no 3, 1977

MONCADA S, VANE JR: Arachidonic acid metabolites and the interactions between platelets and blood vessel walls. N Engl J Med 300:1142, 1979

WILLIAMS WJ et al (eds): *Hematology,* 2d ed. New York, McGraw-Hill, 1977, chaps 128–162

55
ENLARGEMENT OF LYMPH NODES AND SPLEEN

ALEXANDER FEFER

LYMPH NODES

STRUCTURE AND FUNCTION The principal cells in lymph nodes are the lymphocytes in the lymphoid follicles and the reticuloendothelial cells which line nodal sinuses. Each follicle, located in the cortex of the node, has a germinal center which contains rapidly dividing large lymphocytes (B cells) and macrophages. Surrounding the germinal center is a cuff of densely packed small lymphocytes (T cells) which proliferate at a slower rate and which ultimately leave the node. The chief function of lymphocytes is to respond to antigens presented to the node from the structures being drained. The cells either differentiate into plasma cells and produce antibody (B cells) or enlarge, proliferate, and generate a T-cell-mediated response. The reticuloendothelial cells (histiocytes or macrophages), which can also proliferate, participate in immunity but function chiefly in the phagocytosis of cellular debris and foreign material such as microorganisms which may have gained access to the node from the area being drained by it.

MECHANISMS OF LYMPH NODE ENLARGEMENT Lymphadenopathy may be due to an increase in the number and size of lymphoid follicles with proliferation of lymphocytes or reticuloendothelial cells or to infiltration of the node by cells normally not present in it. Nodal cells proliferate in response to antigens, to other stimuli which evoke greater phagocytic activity, and to unknown stimuli which cause nodal cells to become transformed to lymphoma cells and to proliferate autonomously. Nodes can be infiltrated by leukemia or metastatic carcinoma cells, by polymorphonuclear cells in lymphadenitis, or by metabolite-laden macrophages in the lipid storage diseases.

SIGNIFICANCE OF LYMPHADENOPATHY In normal persons nodes are not palpable or barely palpable. Whether a palpable node is clinically significant depends partly on its location and on the age and occupation of the patient. The number and size of nodes are greater at puberty. Children are far more likely than adults to respond with lymphoid hyperplasia and generalized adenopathy even to relatively minor stimuli, such as mild infections of the upper respiratory tract or skin, and develop appendicitis, mesenteric adenitis, and tonsillitis far more often than do adults.

Lymphadenopathy reflects significant disease more often in adults than in children. However, palpable nodes do not always connote serious disease. They may reflect merely minor trauma to and infections of the structures being drained, such as the hands of a manual laborer (epitrochlear nodes), the upper extremities (axillary), upper respiratory tract and teeth (cervical), and, most frequently, the lower extremities (inguinal). Although usually benign, enlargement of the inguinal nodes may at times reflect significant disease, and enlarged posterior auricular, supraclavicular, epitrochlear (not in a manual laborer), popliteal, mediastinal, and abdominal nodes must always be considered pathological.

DISEASES ASSOCIATED WITH LYMPHADENOPATHY Enlarged nodes may reflect no significant disease, a self-limited benign disease, or a severe or even fatal one. Table 55-1 presents a partial list of the conditions associated with enlarged nodes. The likelihood of each diagnosis varies with age, sex,

TABLE 55-1
Conditions associated with lymph node enlargement

I Neoplastic
  A Hematologic: Lymphomas, acute leukemia, chronic lymphocytic leukemia, myeloproliferative syndromes, histiocytoses
  B Nonhematologic: Carcinomas of head and neck, lung, breast, kidney
II Immunologic or inflammatory
  A Infections: Pyogenic streptococcal, staphylococcal, and salmonella infections, brucellosis, tuberculosis, syphilis, infectious mononucleosis, cytomegalovirus, infectious hepatitis, rubella, lymphogranuloma venereum, toxoplasmosis, histoplasmosis, coccidioidomycosis, malaria
  B Connective tissue diseases: Rheumatoid arthritis, systemic lupus erythematosus, dermatomyositis
  C Serum sickness
  D Reaction to hydantoins
  E Sarcoidosis
  F Miscellaneous: Giant (angiofollicular) lymph node hyperplasia, sinus histiocytosis, dermatopathic lymphadenitis, immunoblastic lymphadenopathy
III Endocrine: Hyperthyroidism, Addison's disease
IV Lipid storage diseases: Gaucher's and Niemann-Pick's diseases

and geography. Although most patients with significant adenopathy will have either a malignancy, an infection, or a connective tissue disease, the likelihood of each of those conditions is greatest, respectively, in the old, the young, and the female.

PHYSICAL CHARACTERISTICS OF ENLARGED NODES Some nodal characteristics provide clues to the diagnosis. Nodes involved by lymphomas or by chronic lymphatic leukemia tend to be large, symmetric, rubbery, firm, movable, discrete, and nontender, whereas nodes in acute leukemia are often tender because of rapid enlargement and concurrent infection. Nodes containing metastatic carcinoma are stony-hard, nontender, well-localized, and bound to surrounding tissues and, therefore, nonmovable. In acute infections, nodes are firm, tender, asymmetric and matted, and the overlying skin may be red and edematous, whereas in chronic infections the nodes are nontender and there is no edema. However, these nodal characteristics are only modestly helpful clues, not pathognomonic signs.

LOCATION OF ENLARGED NODES The extent and location of enlarged nodes also provide diagnostic clues. Generalized adenopathy, i.e., involving more than two separate node groups, is common in non-Hodgkin's lymphomas, chronic lymphocytic leukemia, the histiocytoses, and immunoblastic lymphadenopathy but not with nonhematologic malignancies. Generalized adenopathy is uncommon in adults with infections except in infectious mononucleosis, brucellosis, cytomegalovirus, tuberculosis, infectious hepatitis, secondary syphilis, toxoplasmosis, and histoplasmosis.

In the absence of generalized adenopathy, enlargement of specific lymph node groups can be helpful diagnostically. Posterior auricular adenopathy suggests rubella. Unilateral anterior auricular adenopathy is associated with lesions of the conjunctiva and eyelids with a resultant oculoglandular syndrome as is seen with trachoma, tularemia, cat-scratch fever, tuberculosis, syphilis, epidemic keratoconjunctivitis, and swimming pool outbreaks of adenovirus type III pharyngoconjunctival fever. Oropharyngeal or dental infections can occasionally cause cervical adenopathy. Bilateral cervical adenopathy is prominent in tuberculosis, coccidioidomycosis, infectious mononucleosis, toxoplasmosis, sarcoid, lymphomas, and leukemias. However, a unilateral cervical mass often represents a metastasis from an undetected asymptomatic nasopharyngeal tumor. In one study of 1600 patients admitted to surgery with a nonthyroid neck mass, 88 percent of the patients had a malignancy, most often a metastatic tumor or a lymphoma. Therefore, a nonthyroid neck mass in adults, but not children, should be considered neoplastic until proved otherwise and is a strong indication for examination of the mouth, pharynx, nasopharynx, and larynx in search of a malignancy.

Palpable supraclavicular nodes are always abnormal and, in the absence of generalized adenopathy, reflect neoplastic disease in the abdomen or chest. The right node drains parts of the lungs and mediastinum and is involved by intrathoracic lesions especially of the lung and esophagus, whereas the left (Virchow's) node is close to the thoracic duct and is involved by intraabdominal tumor, especially from the stomach, ovary, testis, and kidney. Axillary nodes drain part of the breast and are favorite sites for metastatic breast carcinoma. Epitrochlear nodes often are chronically enlarged bilaterally in secondary lues. Inguinal adenopathy is especially common in lymphogranuloma venereum, chancroid, and syphilis.

Enlarged nodes in certain areas cannot be palpated but are suspected in the presence of characteristic clinical problems. For example, enlarged mediastinal or hilar nodes detectable on routine chest x-ray may be asymptomatic or may cause tracheobronchial compression with cough and wheezing, recurrent laryngeal nerve compression with hoarseness and stridor, paralysis of the left leaf of the diaphragm, esophageal compression with dysphagia, superior vena caval compression with swelling of the neck and face, and subclavian vein compression with swelling of the arm. Hilar nodes are often asymmetrically involved by metastatic carcinoma from the lungs and, rarely, from the testis and kidney. Bilateral asymmetric mediastinal adenopathy is common with non-Hodgkin's lymphomas and is characteristic of nodular sclerosing Hodgkin's lymphoma. Hilar adenopathy is rarely associated with bacterial or viral pneumonias. It is seen, however, in tuberculosis (usually unilateral) and in coccidioidomycosis (usually bilateral). Bilateral hilar adenopathy is characteristic of sarcoidosis, although tuberculous involvement must be excluded. One study of 100 patients with bilateral hilar adenopathy documented its very frequent association with sarcoidosis and revealed that such adenopathy in patients without symptoms or only with erythema nodosum or uveitis was nearly diagnostic for sarcoidosis. Unlike lymphomatous nodes, hilar nodes in sarcoidosis, coccidioidomycosis, and tuberculosis often show roentgenographically detectable calcification.

Abdominal nodes can enlarge in any disorder which causes generalized adenopathy. However, the cause of intraabdominal or retroperitoneal adenopathy in adults is most often neoplastic, especially lymphomatous. The nodes may cause abdominal pain, nausea, constipation, intestinal obstruction, urinary complaints, backache, fever, ascites, or peripheral edema. If sufficiently large, they can be detected by abdominal, pelvic, or rectal examination, but they are most often detected only by lymphangiography; ultrasonography and, more particularly, computerized tomography (CT) scan are often helpful in detecting abdominal and retroperitoneal lymph nodes.

APPROACH TO THE PATIENT WITH ENLARGED LYMPH NODES
In most patients, a diagnosis can be made by a careful history and physical examination, hematologic and other laboratory tests, skin tests, and routine x-rays. The association of some diagnoses with age and sex is helpful, e.g., systemic lupus erythematosus in the young female, breast carcinoma in the older female, infectious mononucleosis in the young adult, and chronic lymphocytic leukemia in the old. A history of exposure to potential sources of infection, and of constitutional complaints such as fever, malaise, fatigue, and weight loss, which accompany hematologic malignancies and systemic infections, is important. The duration of symptoms and signs is suggestive. Patients whose nodes are neoplastic tend to present with a longer history—often months—of adenopathy, whereas patients with painful infectious or inflammatory adenopathy often present within days after the nodes appear.

Physical examination should include a search for associated findings of special significance, e.g., splenomegaly for its myriad implications (see below), hepatomegaly for hepatitis and malignancies, skin rashes for viral infections, heart murmurs as in subacute bacterial endocarditis, and evidence of local infection such as chancre. An oral and nasopharyngeal examination for tumor is essential in any patient with a neck mass.

Routine hematologic studies may be diagnostic. The immature cells of leukemia or the atypical lymphocytes of infectious mononucleosis and other viral infections may be detected. A chest x-ray might reveal mediastinal nodes with or without pulmonary nodules or infiltrates. A liver and spleen scan using radioactive material might reveal increased size and defects associated with neoplasia. Cultures of blood, throat, sputum, urine, bone marrow, and other possible infectious sites should be obtained when appropriate, as should special serologic tests such as a test for syphilis, antibody titers for toxoplasmosis and cytomegalovirus, and a heterophil test for infectious mononucleosis. A marrow aspiration is indicated for anemia, thrombocytopenia, or leukopenia and may reveal leukemia or metastatic carcinoma or, when cultured, tuberculosis or other

infections. A marrow biopsy is more likely than an aspirate to reveal a lymphoma.

If the above work-up is not diagnostic and a neoplasm or infection for which treatment should not be delayed is suspected, than a lymph node should be biopsied, examined, and cultured. It is best to biopsy cervical or supraclavicular nodes and to avoid axillary or inguinal nodes which are subject to local trauma and infections. Excision biopsy of an entire node provides a look at the nodal architecture. A node biopsy can be diagnostic in lymphoma, carcinoma, immunoblastic lymphadenopathy, infections such as tuberculosis or histoplasmosis, or a granuloma without caseation suggestive of sarcoidosis.

However, in 40 to 60 percent of patients the node biopsy will reveal only reactive hyperplasia and will not yield a specific diagnosis. This failure has been attributed to inability to differentiate histologically conditions such as hydantoin-induced hyperplasia from a true lymphoma, to noninvolvement of the node obtained, or to distortion of the involved node by other processes. If another node is palpable or detectable on chest x-ray, an open biopsy or biopsy via mediastinoscopy should be obtained. If no nodes are evident and lung carcinoma, sarcoidosis, or tuberculosis is considered likely, a biopsy of the scalene node and fat pad in the supraclavicular area should be obtained. However, if despite a nondiagnostic biopsy lymphoma remains a strong possibility, no other nodes are accessible, and progressive disease is apparent, a lymphangiogram is indicated. If abnormal abdominal or retroperitoneal nodes are detected, abdominal laparotomy may be necessary for diagnostic biopsies. However, if the patient with the nondiagnostic biopsy is otherwise well or improving and has no other accessible nodes, watchful waiting is acceptable. Adenopathy secondary to infections will almost always regress within 2 to 3 weeks. However, in several long-term follow-up studies, 25 to 60 percent of patients with nondiagnostic lymph node biopsies were found within a very few months to have lymphomas or carcinomas and, less often, connective tissue disease or infection. The need for careful and frequent follow-up evaluations of such patients and for a node biopsy as nodes become available is obvious.

Lymph node syndromes In addition to the diagnostic entities cited, several new diseases of lymph nodes, with or without involvement of other organs, have been discovered. These include the combination of fever, rash, and lymphadenopathy, also termed the *mucocutaneous lymph node syndrome* (*Kawasaki's disease*), in children (Chap. 180) and a lymphoproliferative and granulomatous disease involving predominantly the lungs called *lymphomatoid granulomatosis*. This process usually spares the lymph nodes, spleen, and bone marrow, although sometimes generalized atypical lymphoid hyperplasia may antedate for pulmonary lesions.

IMMUNOBLASTIC LYMPHADENOPATHY This is a disease characterized by the morphological triad of (1) predominant infiltration of immunoblasts, (2) proliferation of arborizing small blood vessels, and (3) deposition of acidophilic material in the lymph nodes, liver, spleen, and other organs. Clinically, the disease is characterized by weakness, fever, sweats, weight loss, generalized lymphadenopathy, and often hepatosplenomegaly. Rashes, which vary from maculopapular to urticarial, are common. An autoimmune hemolytic anemia is a commonly associated finding as is polyclonal hypergammaglobulinemia, involving at one time or another gamma-G, gamma-M, and gamma-A immunoglobulins. One report describes a subset of these patients who also have interstitial pulmonary infiltrates, vasculitis, and hypocomplementemia. Most of these patients are elderly; the majority have had progressive disease and have died within 18 months but, in a few, the course has been much more benign, and they have done well with modest doses of steroids. According to some authors, aggressive chemotherapy is contraindicated in these patients.

The pathophysiology of this process remains a matter of speculation. Because many cases have followed in the wake of drug ingestion, it has been suggested that this disease is a hyperimmune response of the B-cell system, which escapes from T-cell suppressor control resulting in an exaggerated transformation to immunoblasts and plasma cells. This hypothesis remains to be confirmed.

ENLARGEMENT OF THE SPLEEN

STRUCTURE OF THE SPLEEN Splenic function reflects the specialized cells and unique circulation of this organ. The spleen has a capsule and trabeculae which enclose the white and red pulp. The white pulp consists of periarterial sheaths of lymphocytes with follicles containing germinal centers in which there are plasma cells and macrophages. The red pulp consists of cords of reticulum containing phagocytic macrophages separated from sinuses by a basement membrane. The narrow, tortuous splenic circulation sequesters blood within the pulp and exposes the traversing blood cells to phagocytic cells and to metabolic and immunologic hazards, as well as to barriers which make it necessary for the cells to change their size and shape in order to squeeze through the cords and sinuses and return into the circulation.

FUNCTION OF THE SPLEEN The spleen functions as the largest lymph node. It responds to antigens with proliferation of T lymphocytes in the lymphatic sheath and of the antibody-forming B cells in the germinal centers, as well as with proliferation of phagocytic cells. The phagocytic function of the spleen includes "culling" and "pitting" which occur mostly in the tortuous red pulp. Culling refers to phagocytosis of abnormal whole red blood cells which have been damaged physically or immunologically and of cells containing nuclei or Howell-Jolly bodies, reticulocytes, siderocytes, target cells, and spherocytes. Pitting refers to the removal of inclusions, e.g., red blood cell nuclei, Heinz bodies, and malarial parasites from red blood cells without destroying the cells. The spleen serves as a reservoir of platelets but not of red blood cells or leukocytes. It normally sequesters 30 to 40 percent of the blood platelets. The spleen is normally the site of blood formation through the fifth fetal month, but not after birth—except in some abnormal conditions.

MECHANISMS OF SPLENIC ENLARGEMENT Like other lymph nodes, the spleen enlarges with reactive hyperplasia in infection and inflammation and with proliferation of lymphoma cells or with infiltration by other neoplastic cells, mostly in chronic leukemias, or by lipid-laden macrophages. The spleen also enlarges with extramedullary hemopoiesis, with proliferation of phagocytic cells in response to increased destruction of blood cells, and, uniquely, by vascular congestion in the presence of portal hypertension.

DISEASES ASSOCIATED WITH SPLENOMEGALY Table 55-2 lists the principal conditions associated with splenomegaly, some of which require a brief comment. Any condition which causes generalized lymphadenopathy can cause splenomegaly.

TABLE 55-2
Conditions associated with splenomegaly

I Immunologic-inflammatory
  A Infections: Subacute bacterial endocarditis, brucellosis, tuberculosis, infectious mononucleosis, cytomegalovirus, syphilis, histoplasmosis, malaria, kala azar, schistosomiasis
  B Connective tissue diseases: Rheumatoid arthritis, Felty's syndrome, systemic lupus erythematosus
  C Sarcoidosis
II Hematologic disorders
  A Neoplastic: Lymphomas, histiocytoses, myeloproliferative syndromes (chronic myelocytic leukemia, polycythemia vera, myelofibrosis, and myeloid metaplasia), chronic lymphocytic leukemia, acute leukemia
  B Nonneoplastic: Hemolytic anemias, e.g., hereditary spherocytosis, autoimmune hemolytic anemia, hemoglobinopathies, immunoblastic lymphadenopathy
III Congestive splenomegaly due to portal hypertension: Hepatic cirrhosis, portal or splenic vein thrombosis or stenosis, myeloid metaplasia, vinyl chloride
IV Metabolic-infiltrative: Gaucher's and Niemann-Pick's disease, amyloidosis
V Miscellaneous: Cyst, splenic abscess, aneurysm of splenic artery, cavernous hemangioma

Splenomegaly is frequent in infectious mononucleosis, subacute bacterial endocarditis, brucellosis, histoplasmosis, malaria, kala azar, and other parasitic infections. It occurs in 10 to 20 percent of patients with systemic lupus erythematosus and in rheumatoid arthritis which, when associated with splenomegaly and anemia, thrombocytopenia, or, most often, leukopenia, is designated *Felty's syndrome*. The cytopenia often responds to splenectomy. Splenomegaly also occurs in most patients with immunoblastic lymphadenopathy.

Lymphomas often involve the spleen even when it is not palpable, and laparotomy to determine the extent of a lymphoma—especially in Hodgkin's disease—always includes splenectomy. The spleen is massively enlarged in myeloproliferative syndromes, especially chronic myelogenous leukemia and myelofibrosis. Splenomegaly may also be prominent in chronic lymphocytic leukemia and may be associated with autoimmune hemolytic anemia. Splenomegaly associated with increased destruction of red blood cells occurs with many hemolytic anemias some of which like hereditary spherocytosis and, sometimes, autoimmune hemolytic anemia, respond dramatically to splenectomy.

Chronic congestive splenomegaly due to portal hypertension (Banti's syndrome; see Chap. 322) is associated with gastrointestinal bleeding and pancytopenia. It is usually secondary to cirrhosis of the liver or, less commonly, to portal vein thrombosis. Splenomegaly is often accompanied by the syndrome of hypersplenism (Chap. 322), consisting of a large spleen, anemia, leukopenia or thrombocytopenia, and hyperactivity of the bone marrow. It is often reversed by splenectomy. Hypersplenism may occur in most splenomegalic states (Table 55-2). Its severity does not correlate with the degree of splenic enlargement. However, splenomegaly does not always cause hypersplenism.

APPROACH TO THE PATIENT WITH AN ENLARGED SPLEEN
Splenomegaly is common, yet a palpable spleen in an adult is almost always clinically significant. In one study, the spleen was palpable in only 3 percent of students entering an American college and persisted in only a third of them. The spleen is even less likely to be palpable in normal persons beyond college age. Therefore, patients with a palpable spleen but without other signs or symptoms should have at least a spleen scan and complete blood count. Colloid tagged with technetium 99 injected intravenously is taken up by reticuloendothelial cells and visualizes splenic size, shape, and defects suggestive of tumor or abscess. The scan is the best method for detecting an

enlarged spleen and for ruling out a nonsplenic mass, e.g., cyst or metastatic tumor, which might cause splenic displacement rather than enlargement. A complete blood count and smear are often helpful or even diagnostic in asymptomatic splenomegalic patients with chronic myelogenous or lymphocytic leukemia.

Since most conditions which cause splenomegaly also cause lymphadenopathy, the approach to diagnosis is that presented in the section on adenopathy (above). The cause of splenomegaly should be determined not by tests on the spleen itself but by tests—possibly including a lymph node biopsy—for diseases known to cause splenomegaly and lymphadenopathy. Splenomegaly in acute leukemia is usually a minor clinical feature—the diagnosis is made by blood count and marrow examinations. Splenomegaly in lymphomas is almost always associated with adenopathy, and the diagnosis made by node biopsy or at laparotomy.

Most conditions which cause splenomegaly without adenopathy can also be suspected and diagnosed by history and physical and laboratory examination. For example, a hemolytic anemia is detectable by routine laboratory tests for anemia and for hemolysis, including reticulocyte counts and serum bilirubin. Specific causes for hemolysis can then be determined by other procedures such as Coombs' test, osmotic fragility, and hemoglobin electrophoresis. Similarly, splenomegaly and hypersplenism secondary to portal hypertension caused by cirrhosis of the liver are readily diagnosed by a history of alcoholism or previous liver disease, physical signs of liver dysfunction and portal hypertension, laboratory abnormalities consistent with liver dysfunction and hypersplenism, and radiological evidence of esophageal varices. The diagnosis of the rare vascular causes of portal hypertension requires angiography.

Some patients with splenomegaly may have systemic symptoms but no nodes available for biopsy. If an underlying lymphoma or serious infection is considered likely but is not detected by the usual examinations, including lymphangiograms, a laparotomy with biopsy of the liver and abdominal nodes, and splenectomy, may be necessary. Appropriate cultures and pathological examinations are essential. Such laparotomies on patients with splenomegaly of unknown cause have revealed lymphoma in one-third, congestive splenomegaly in one-fourth, and inflammatory disease in one-fifth of patients.

REFERENCES

CHRISTENSEN BE: Pathophysiology of "hypersplenism syndrome." Scand J Haematol 11:5, 1973

FRIZERRA G et al: Angio-immunoblastic lymphadenopathy. Am J Med 59:803, 1975

LIEBOW AA et al: Lymphomatoid granulomatosis. Hum Pathol 3:457, 1972

LUKES RJ, TINDLE BH: Immunoblastic lymphadenopathy. N Engl J Med 292:1, 1975

MCINTYRE OR, EBAUGH FG JR: Palpable spleens in college freshmen. Ann Intern Med 66:310, 1967

SINCLAIR S et al: Biopsy of enlarged, superficial lymph nodes. JAMA 228:602, 1974

SKANDALAKIS JE et al: Tumors of the neck. Surgery 48:375, 1960

WEINSTEIN IM: Lymph node enlargement and splenomegaly, in *Hematology,* WJ Williams et al (eds). New York, McGraw-Hill, 1977, chap 106, p 950

WEISENBURGER D et al: Immunoblastic lymphadenopathy with pulmonary infiltrates, hypocomplementemia and vasculitis. Am J Med 63:849, 1977

WINTERBAUER RH et al: A clinical interpretation of bilateral hilar adenopathy. Ann Intern Med 78:65, 1973

WINTROBE MM et al: *Clinical Hematology,* 7th ed. Philadelphia, Lea & Febiger, 1974

ZUELZER WW, KAPLAN J: The child with lymphadenopathy. Semin Hematol 12:323, 1975

section 11 | Alterations in laboratory findings

56
ABNORMALITIES OF LEUKOCYTES

DAVID C. DALE

Alterations of leukocyte counts and functions occur in a wide variety of hematologic, infectious, inflammatory, metabolic, and neoplastic diseases. Because leukocytes are affected by so many diseases, the routine laboratory evaluation of many patients begins with determination of the leukocyte count and the examination of a stained blood smear. From the clinical examination and these blood studies, certain diagnoses can be made or strongly suspected, e.g., leukemia, agranulocytosis, infectious mononucleosis, systemic mastocytosis, and the Chédiak-Higashi syndrome. In patients with infectious and inflammatory diseases, the leukocyte count usually serves as a useful guide to the severity of the disease process. The leukocyte count and blood smear examination plus special studies of leukocyte function also will identify certain patients with heightened susceptibility to infections.

Five types of circulating leukocytes can be identified by their morphology on blood smears: neutrophils, lymphocytes, monocytes, eosinophils, and basophils. It is generally accepted that all these leukocyte types, along with erythrocytes and platelets, derive from a common pluripotent stem cell. However, beyond this common origin, independent regulatory mechanisms govern the production, distribution, and function of each type of leukocyte. For simplicity, inferences are often made about the presence or severity of illness from the total leukocyte count and the differential leukocyte count expressed as a percentage. It is more precise to express the counts of each type of leukocyte in terms of the concentration or absolute count per cubic millimeter of blood. This is usually determined simply by multiplying the total leukocyte count by the percent value. Normal values for blood leukocyte counts are shown in Table 56-1.

NEUTROPHILS

NORMAL PHYSIOLOGY The primary function of neutrophils is phagocytosis, killing, and digestion of microorganisms. The cells develop the capacity to perform these special functions in the bone marrow. Early neutrophil precursors, myeloblasts and promyelocytes, differentiate from hematopoietic stem cells by developing an active Golgi apparatus and endoplasmic reticulum and beginning the formation of cytoplasmic granules. The initial or *primary granules* stain reddish-purple with azure dyes; hence they are also called *azurophilic granules*. They contain myeloperoxidase, acid hydrolases, lysozyme, and cationic antibacterial proteins. With further development the cells become myelocytes. At this stage the cytoplasm becomes packed with characteristic secondary or *specific granules* which stain faintly pink with the usual blood stains. These granules contain alkaline phosphatase, collagenase, lactoferrin, lysozyme, and aminopeptidase. Beyond the myelocyte stage, neutrophilic cells do not divide; instead their nuclear chromatin becomes condensed, the cell diminishes modestly in size, and cytoplasmic glycogen accumulates. Normally neutrophils are not released to the blood until the nucleus is segmented, that is, the cells have matured beyond the metamyelocyte and "band" stages.

Approximately 8 to 14 days are required for a cell to move through the sequence of four to six cell divisions and complete maturation, that is, from the myeloblast stage to a mature blood neutrophil. Measurement of the time required for the early developmental stages is difficult, but it is clear that there are normally 3 to 4 days of neutrophil maturation after cell division is finished. During this time the maturing cells can be released from the bone marrow to the blood under sufficient stress, and therefore they are described as being in the marrow neutrophil reserves. Morphologic and radioisotopic studies on bone marrow indicate that there are normally about 10 times as many nearly mature neutrophils in the marrow as in the blood. The size of the marrow neutrophil reserves can be estimated by administration of endotoxin, etiocholanolone, or glucocorticosteroids and measuring the increase in the neutrophil counts. In normal individuals, these agents roughly double the count or increase blood neutrophils by a minimum of 2000 cells per cubic millimeter.

The regulation of neutrophil production and release remains poorly understood. Normal individuals maintain their own characteristic neutrophil count, but this is subject to substantial day-to-day variation and is greatly affected by activity and many other factors. A humoral substance has been identified which will stimulate neutrophil release from the bone marrow (neutrophilia-inducing factor). Colony-stimulating factor, a substance present in serum and urine which will stimulate neutrophilic bone marrow cells to grow in tissue culture systems, is another possible neutrophil regulator. The precise physiologic role of these substances is not clear.

The blood serves to transport neutrophils to areas of acute inflammation as well as to the mucosal surfaces of the body where these cells serve to maintain the normal defensive barrier to microbial invasion. Normally only about half of the neutrophils in the vascular system are circulating freely and are described as being in the circulating neutrophil pool. Only these cells are counted in routine blood samples. The other half of the blood neutrophils are loosely adherent to the walls of blood vessels throughout the body in the marginal neutrophil pool. In response to inflammation, neutrophils are shifted to the marginal pool. Certain drugs, i.e., epinephrine, glucocorticosteroids, and other anti-inflammatory agents, may reduce margination.

The neutrophil blood half-disappearance time (blood half-life) is only about 6 to 7 h. Neutrophils leave the vascular compartment by passing between endothelial cells presumably because they are attracted to sites of inflammation by chemotactic factors. Bacteria can release low molecular weight chemotactic substances. A well-characterized chemotactic factor, C5a, is generated from the complement system when plasma reacts with endotoxin, antigen-antibody complexes, and other foreign substances. Kallikrein, plasminogen activator, transfer factor, and other substances will also attract neutrophils.

At the inflammatory site, phagocytosis is facilitated by humoral substances, opsonins, which have coated the surface of the foreign material to be ingested. Immunoglobulins (IgG) and complement (C3) are the best-characterized opsonins. Phagocytosis stimulates numerous intracellular events including increased oxygen consumption, glycogenolysis, glucose oxidation via the hexosemonophosphate shunt, and hydrogen peroxide production. Within the cell, the phagocytized particle is held in a vacuole, and the contents of the secondary and then the primary granules are sequentially emptied into this vacuole. The vacuolar pH is dramatically lowered, and the granule enzymes are activated. The neutrophil possesses a variety of bactericidal mechanisms giving it an "overkill" capacity. The best characterized bactericidal mechanism involves myeloperoxidase, hydrogen peroxide, and a halide such as iodide or chloride. The highly reactive oxygen derivatives, superoxide ($O_2\bar{v}$), singlet oxygen ($^1O_2$), and hydroxyl radical (OH·) may also participate in the microbicidal system of the cell. An interesting result of the cell's respiratory burst and the generation of these oxygen derivatives is the emission of light, or chemiluminescence. The neutrophil usually degenerates after it digests the phagocytized material. Neutrophils, cellular debris, and digested foreign matter become the pus which characterizes acute inflammation, and to which the residual myeloperoxidase imparts the slightly greenish color.

NEUTROPHIL DISORDERS

A branching diagram for evaluating patients with neutrophil disorders is shown in Fig. 56-1. Neutrophil abnormalities are readily separated into those in which the number or morphology of the cells is abnormal and those in which the cell number and morphology are usually normal. The data base for evaluating disorders of neutrophils includes a complete history, with particular emphasis on drug usage and the frequency and severity of infections, and physical examination, especially noting the presence or absence of lymphadenopathy, splenomegaly, bone tenderness, and signs of inflammation. Basic laboratory data should include complete blood counts with

TABLE 56-1
Normal values for concentration of blood leukocytes*

Cell type	Mean, cells/mm³	95% confidence limits, cells/mm³
Neutrophil	3650	1830–7250
Lymphocyte	2500	1500–4000
Monocyte	430	200–950
Eosinophil	150	0–700
Basophil	30	0–150

* *Total leukocyte counts from venous blood samples were done in a Coulter counter, and 200 leukocytes were differentiated on Wright-stained blood smears made on cover glass.*

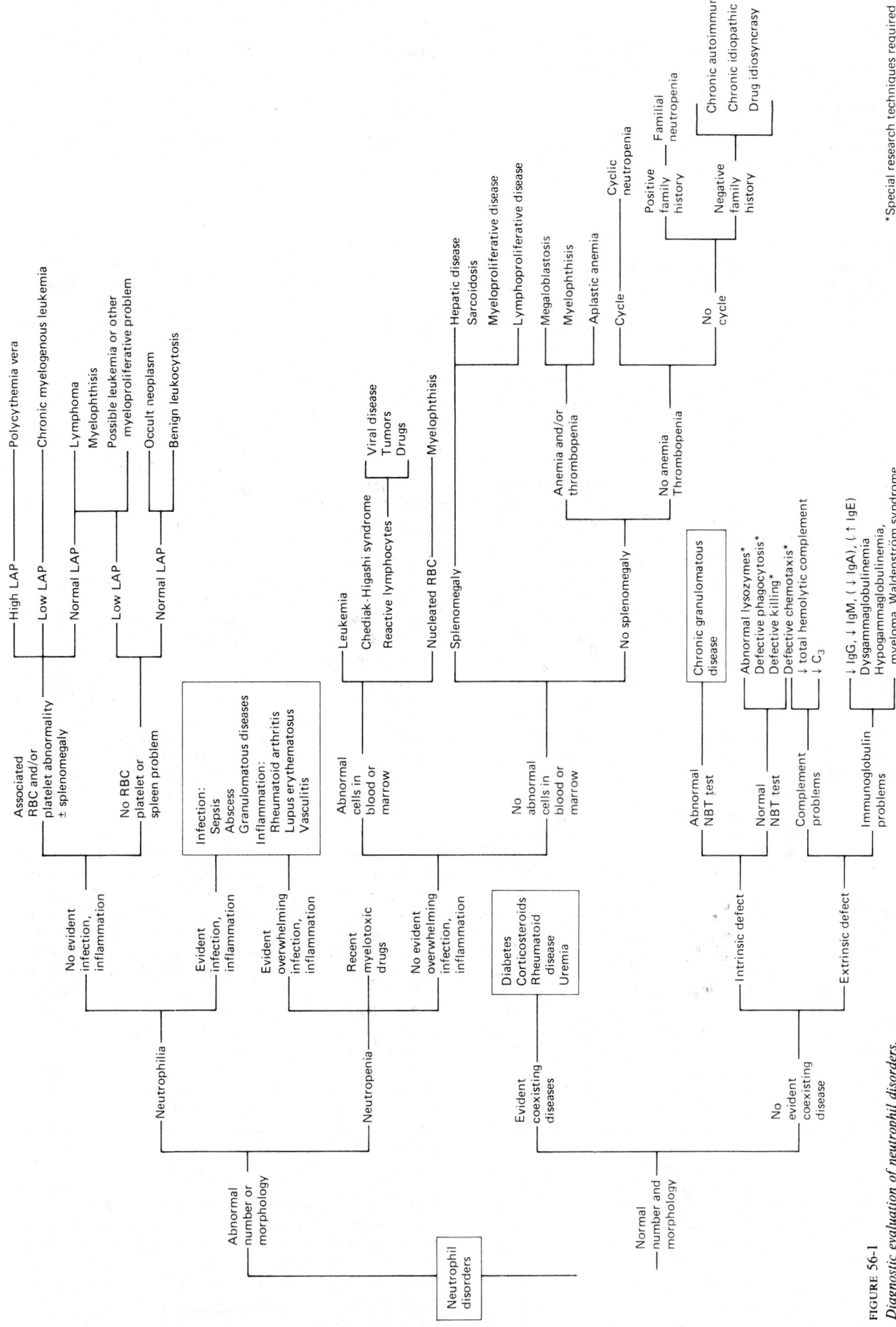

FIGURE 56-1

Diagnostic evaluation of neutrophil disorders.

*Special research techniques required

careful observation of leukocyte morphology and bone marrow aspirate and biopsy. In patients with neutrophilia, measurement of the leukocyte (neutrophil) alkaline phosphatase activity is very helpful for distinguishing between leukemoid reactions, chronic myelogenous leukemia, and other myeloproliferative states. In patients with frequent infections, immunoglobulins and complement are measured and nitroblue tetrazolium reduction (NBT) tests are done as base-line investigations before other studies of neutrophil function are made.

NEUTROPHILIA An absolute neutrophil count of greater than 10,000 per cubic millimeter should be regarded as elevated in most patients, although for a few individuals neutrophil counts of 10,000 to 15,000 per cubic millimeter are normal. The causes of neutrophilia are listed in Table 56-2. Exercise, excitement, epinephrine administration, or stress of any sort will increase the count up to twice the resting level within a few minutes. The duration of this neutrophilia is brief. It is largely due to a shift of cells from the marginal to circulating pool and is not accompanied by an increase in the number of nonsegmented blood neutrophils. Most acute bacterial infections are associated with neutrophilia, especially those that are accompanied by bacteremia, involve substantial amounts of tissue, and are localized in a closed space. This neutrophilia initially occurs because of accelerated release of cells from the bone marrow reserves and is often accompanied by an increase in the number of nonsegmented neutrophils in the blood, i.e., a "shift to the left." With prolonged inflammation from any cause, neutrophil production is stimulated and the bone marrow shows granulocytic hyperplasia. Toxic granulation, due to increased staining of the primary granules, and cytoplasmic vacuolization also occur under these circumstances. In all the usual conditions causing neutrophilia, the counts are generally between 10,000 and 25,000 per cubic millimeter. Persisting neutrophilia with counts greater than 30,000 to 50,000 per cubic millimeter is called a *leukemoid reaction*. This term is sometimes used to describe any persisting high leukocyte count because this degree of leukocytosis suggests leukemia. Characteristically in a leukemoid reaction the raised count is due predominantly to an increase in mature neutrophils with some increase of band neutrophils and metamyelocytes. Blood myelocytes are rare. The leukocyte alkaline phosphatase is generally high, and the cells do not contain Auer rods. The erythrocyte and platelet counts also are usually not strikingly abnormal. The differentiation between leukemoid reactions, leukemia, and myeloproliferative diseases is discussed further in Chaps. 321 and 326.

NEUTROPENIA Neutrophil counts of less than 2000 per cubic millimeter are relatively uncommon in normal individuals although some healthy resting adults, particularly black persons and Yemenite Jews, may have counts as low as 1000 per cubic

TABLE 56-2
Causes of neutrophilia

Physiologic: Exercise, excitement, stress, epinephrine
Infections: Chiefly bacterial, also fungal, parasitic, and some viral diseases
Inflammation: Burns, tissue necrosis as in myocardial and pulmonary infarction, collagen vascular diseases, hypersensitivity states, other inflammatory diseases
Metabolic disorders: Ketoacidosis, acute renal failure, eclampsia, acute poisoning
Myeloproliferative diseases: Myelocytic leukemia, myeloid metaplasia, polycythemia vera
Other: Metastatic carcinoma, acute hemorrhage or hemolysis, glucocorticosteroids, lithium therapy, idiopathic

TABLE 56-3
Clinical conditions characterized by neutropenia

Hematologic diseases: Chronic idiopathic neutropenias; cyclic neutropenia, lazy-leukocyte syndrome; Chédiak-Higashi syndrome; leukemia; aplastic anemia
Drug-induced conditions: Agranulocytosis; myelotoxic drugs
Nutritional deficiencies: Vitamin B_{12}; folate, especially in alcoholics; copper
Secondary to other diseases: Infections including typhoid, infectious mononucleosis, malaria, overwhelming sepsis; diseases with splenomegaly, Felty's syndrome, congestive splenomegaly, Gaucher's disease, sarcoidosis; malignancies with marrow infiltration

millimeter with no apparent disease. Neutropenia occurs in a wide variety of clinical circumstances (Table 56-3). In general, as the count declines below about 1000 per cubic millimeter, the risk of infection increases. However, the risk of infection is related to both the nature of the primary disease process and the cell count. For instance, many patients with chronic idiopathic neutropenia have counts of less than 500 per cubic millimeter for years without infections, whereas few patients with leukemia or aplastic anemia will survive for even a few weeks at these levels without developing an infection.

It is not possible to describe the neutropenias on the basis of kinetic mechanisms analogous to the mechanisms of anemia and thrombocytopenia. Most patients encountered will fit into the following general clinical categories.

Chronic neutropenia without splenomegaly (Chronic idiopathic neutropenia or granulocytopenia, familial benign neutropenia, chronic hypoplastic neutropenia, and chronic benign neutropenia of childhood) Isolated individuals and families are occasionally observed with neutropenia as their sole hematologic abnormality. Characteristically, the spleen is not enlarged. Onset may occur at any age; frequently, the syndrome is recognized on an incidental blood count. In adults, there is a striking female predominance, whereas in children both males and females are affected. Neutrophil counts may be as low as 50 to 200 per cubic millimeter with only infrequent infections, usually involving the upper respiratory tract. Bacteremia is rare. The blood usually contains normal-appearing mature neutrophils in reduced numbers; blood monocytes are often increased, and hypergammaglobulinemia may be present. The marrow is normocellular and shows few or no mature neutrophils. In a few cases, not readily distinguished from the rest of these patients on clinical grounds, leukoagglutinating antibodies to normal neutrophils have been detected and may be of etiologic significance (chronic idiopathic immunoneutropenia). The disease mechanisms otherwise remain largely unknown. In periods of observation up to 25 years, evolution to leukemia has been reported only extremely rarely. A few children with this disorder have had spontaneous remissions. In a few patients with frequent infections and extremely low counts, alternate-day glucocorticosteroids have elevated the neutrophil counts and reduced infections.

Several other groups of patients with chronic neutropenia without splenomegaly can be recognized which have distinctly different clinical characteristics. *Infantile genetic agranulocytosis* is usually a rapidly fatal disorder associated with anemia and atypical, vacuolated marrow precursor cells. *Neutropenia associated with hypogammaglobulinemia* leads to fatal infections at an early age. In *cyclic neutropenia, lazy-leukocyte syndrome,* and *Chédiak-Higashi syndrome,* chronic neutropenia is present but additional neutrophil abnormalities have been observed. Other patients are occasionally encountered with episodic severe neutropenia associated with febrile illnesses. Many other unusual neutropenic disorders have been observed; undoubtedly these neutropenias will be categorized further as their etiologies are better understood.

9-1 **Normal marrow.**

9-2 **Megaloblastic marrow.**

9-3 **Erythroid hyperplasia.**

9-4 **Sideroblastic anemia.**

9-5 **Normal blood smear.**

9-6 **Megalobastic anemia.**

9-7 **Iron-deficiency anemia.**

9-8 **β thallasemia intermedia.**

9-9 **Myeloid metaplasia.**

9-10 **Uremia.**

9-11 **Liver disease.**

9-12 **Spur-cell anemia.**

9-13 **Hereditary spherocytosis.**

9-14 **Immunohemolytic anemia.**

9-15 **Traumatic hemolysis.**

9-16 **Sickle-cell anemia.**

PLATE 9
Normal and abnormal bone marrow smears (top row) and peripheral blood smears (bottom three rows). The size of normal red blood cells is about the same as that of the nucleus of a mature lymphocyte. Cell specimens were prepared with Wright's stain except the sideroblastic anemia marrow (9-4) which was stained with Prussian blue. 760×. (Courtesy of C von Kapff.)

10-1 A. **Normal granulocyte.** *B.* **Normal monocyte and lymphocyte.**

10-2 A. **Normal eosinophil.** *B.* **Normal basophil.**

10-3 **Normal granulocyte precursors in marrow.**

10-4 **Neutrophils with toxic granulation.**

10-5 **Band with Döhle body** (center).

10-6 **Hypersegmentation.**

10-7 A. **Chédiak-Higashi anomaly.** *B.* **Pelger-Hüet anomaly.**

10-8 **Reactive lymphocytes** (infectious mononucleosis).

10-9 **Chronic granulocytic leukemia.**

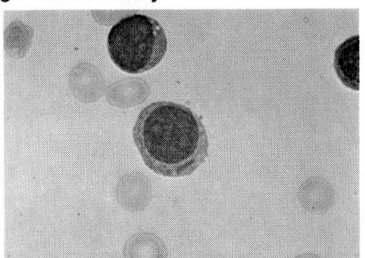

10-10 **Acute myelogenous leukemia:** myeloblast with Auer rod (center).

10-11 **Chronic lymphocytic leukemia.**

10-12 **Acute lymphoblastic leukemia** (marrow).

10-13 **Hodgkin's disease:** Reed-Sternberg cell in marrow (center).

10-14 **Non-Hodgkin's nodular lymphoma** (lymph node).

10-15 **Multiple myeloma** (marrow).

Cyclic neutropenia This disorder is characterized by the periodic absence of neutrophils from the blood and bone marrow associated with fever, malaise, mouth ulcers, and cervical adenopathy. These findings recur regularly at approximately 21-day intervals. Between episodes the patients are usually well. Symptoms characteristically begin in early childhood, although adult onset has been described. Cyclic fluctuations of other blood leukocytes, platelets, and reticulocytes occur, and bone marrow investigations indicate that the disease is due to a defect in the regulation of hematopoietic cell proliferation. Treatment with glucocorticosteroids, androgens, or splenectomy is not of predictable benefit, although cases improving with each of these treatments have been reported. Early recognition and prompt treatment of infectious complications are very important.

Neutropenia in the leukemias and aplastic anemia In leukemia, particularly the acute leukemias, neutropenia is frequently present at the time the disease is recognized. The predisposition to infection is severe, in part because the neutrophils which are present may not be functionally normal. The number of neutrophils and other host defenses are further suppressed by chemotherapy. When the neutrophil count is less than 500 per cubic millimeter, especially in patients in relapse, fever and infection should be expected (Chap. 107).

In aplastic anemia, the infection risk is probably roughly proportional to the neutrophil count with the chance of a severe and possibly fatal infection being substantially increased with neutrophil counts below 500 per cubic millimeter. The monocytopenia observed in these patients coupled with their neutropenia contributes substantially to the predisposition to infection.

Agranulocytosis (Schultz syndrome) Severe neutropenia occurs as an occasional or rare reaction to a great variety of drugs (Table 56-4). In most instances the patient is seen by the physician several weeks or months after beginning the offending agent and presents acutely ill with fever, sore throat, and oral or perianal ulceration. The total leukocyte count is often 1000 to 2000 per cubic millimeter, and neutrophils are absent from the blood and bone marrow. Marrow examination generally will exclude leukemia as the cause. Marrow recovery is the rule if the patient can be sustained long enough after the drug is discontinued. The pathophysiologic mechanisms for these reactions remain poorly understood. Both toxic effects of drugs on neutrophil formation and immunologic mechanisms causing accelerated cell destruction have been proposed and demonstrated in a few instances.

With some drugs, e.g., chloramphenicol, phenothiazines, carbamazepine (Tegretol), and propylthiouracil, patients may have a gradually declining neutrophil count, probably due to suppressed neutrophil production. It is not absolutely certain that these patients will develop agranulocytosis if the drug is not discontinued. However, as a rule, the presumed offending agent should be discontinued if the neutrophil count falls below 3000 per cubic millimeter.

Neutropenia and hematotoxic drugs In sufficient doses, a great number of therapeutic agents predictably cause leukopenia and neutropenia. This is particularly true for the agents used in cancer chemotherapy and for immunosuppressive therapy of nonmalignant, inflammatory diseases (Chap. 324). These drugs reduce neutrophil production. If the neutrophil count is not allowed to drop below 1000 to 2000 cells per cubic millimeter or if the period of neutropenia is brief, infectious complications are infrequent.

Neutropenia and nutritional deficiencies Vitamin B_{12} and folic acid deficiencies are sometimes accompanied by neutropenia as well as neutrophil hypersegmentation, particularly when folate deficiency is coupled with alcoholism. Copper deficiency, which may occur with chronic hyperalimentation, also reduces blood neutrophils.

Neutropenia with infections Certain infections may be accompanied by neutropenia. These include typhoid and paratyphoid fevers (Chap. 123), brucellosis (Chap. 127), tularemia (Chap. 128), infectious mononucleosis (Chap. 195), infectious hepatitis (Chap. 302), yellow fever (Chap. 190), measles (Chap. 181) and many other viral infections, malaria (Chap. 200), kala azar (Chap. 201), and rickettsial diseases (Chaps. 163 to 171). For the most part, these neutropenias are mild and their precise mechanisms are not known. It is postulated that they are largely due to redistribution of cells out of the circulating pool into an enlarged marginal pool. In certain overwhelming infections, for example, gram-negative bacteremia, pneumococcal pneumonia, and miliary tuberculosis, the occurrence of neutropenia portends a poor prognosis. This is particularly true in alcoholics, malnourished individuals, and patients with preexisting hematopoietic diseases.

Neutropenia with splenomegaly Neutropenia occurs in Felty's syndrome (Chap. 55), congestive splenomegaly (Chap. 55), Banti's syndrome (Chap. 55), Gaucher's disease (Chap. 102), and sarcoidosis (Chap. 216) as well as in infectious diseases with splenomegaly. There are often an associated mild thrombocytopenia and anemia. Splenic sequestration, as well as increased peripheral utilization, are proposed mechanisms. The predisposition to infection with these disorders is quite variable. Splenectomy to attempt to alter the neutropenia should be reserved for patients with repeated severe infections.

NEUTROPHIL DYSFUNCTION The normal functions of mature neutrophils are chemotaxis, phagocytosis, microbicidal action, and digestion of foreign material. There are a few specific diseases and syndromes in which these functions are abnormal. More commonly, defects in neutrophil function are observed which are secondary to other diseases such as alcoholism, diabetes mellitus, uremia, rheumatoid arthritis, and lupus erythematosus. Other defects occur secondary to abnormalities of complement and immunoglobulin metabolism.

Chemotaxis Accumulation of neutrophils in response to inflammation is most often deficient because of neutropenia. The tissue neutrophil response is also reduced by drugs, such as alcohol and glucocorticosteroids, which impair neutrophil adherence to the vascular endothelium. Chemotactic defects due

TABLE 56-4
Drugs producing neutropenia

INFREQUENTLY CAUSE NEUTROPENIA

Analgesics: Aminopyrine, dipyrone, salicylates
Anticonvulsants: Dilantin, carbamazepine
Anti-inflammatory drugs: Phenylbutazone
Antimicrobial agents: Chloramphenicol, penicillins, sulfonamides, organic arsenicals
Antithyroid agents: Propylthiouracil, methimazole
Phenothiazine: Chlorpromazine, promazine
Tranquilizers: Meprobamate

REGULARLY CAUSE NEUTROPENIA

Alkylating agents: Nitrogen mustard, busulfan, chlorambucil, cyclophosphamide
Antibiotics: Daunomycin
Antimetabolites: Methotrexate, 6-mercaptopurine, 5-fluorocytosine

to complement abnormalities have been observed chiefly in patients with either C3 or C5 deficiency. In general, defects permitting complement activation and C3 generation by the alternate complement pathway, for example, C1r, C2, and C4 deficiency, are associated with only a temporary delay in generation of chemotactic factor, and these patients have comparatively few infections. Defects in chemotaxis also may occur because of complement depletion in essential C3 hypercatabolism and possibly in acute glomerulonephritis and systemic lupus erythematosus. Chemotactic factor inactivators and inhibitors have been described in Hodgkin's disease, cirrhosis, uremia, and a few other circumstances. In patients with these complement-related disorders, the cells are usually normal when tested with normal serum. Cellular defects in chemotaxis have been described in the Chédiak-Higashi syndrome, lazy-leukocyte syndrome, newborn infants, and some patients with congenital ichthyosis, diabetes mellitus, rheumatoid arthritis, burns, hypogammaglobulinemia, and acute infections. In the *lazy-leukocyte syndrome,* the patients have gingivitis, stomatitis, and otitis with relatively few severe infections. They also have severe neutropenia, but the bone marrow shows ample mature neutrophils. The marrow neutrophils are not mobilized with endotoxin administration, and the cells show defective chemotaxis and random migration in vitro. In *Job's syndrome,* characterized by recurrent staphylococcal abscesses, eczema, and high IgE levels, a cellular defect in chemotaxis is also observed. Abnormal chemotaxis and defective phagocytosis have been recognized with hypophosphatemia and consequently diminished intracellular ATP. A specific chemotactic defect has been described resulting from the lack of the normal cellular contractile proteins necessary for cell movement.

Phagocytosis Reduced serum opsonic activity is the best-known cause for abnormal phagocytosis. This occurs in hypo- and agammaglobulinemia and certain complement disorders, including most of those with reduced chemotaxis, especially if activated C3 is not generated normally. Defective opsonic activity has been documented in premature infants, sickle-cell anemia, lupus erythematosus, and cirrhosis.

Microbicidal defects A few patients have reduced killing mechanisms because of isolated lysozomal enzyme deficiencies. In hereditary and acquired myeloperoxidase deficiency the leukocytes are morphologically normal except that specific staining shows decreased or absent myeloperoxidase. Eosinophil peroxidase is normal. The bactericidal and fungicidal defect is not as severe as in chronic granulomatous disease, and severe infections have been infrequent. Neutrophil lysozyme deficiency and total absence of secondary granules have been described with accompanying subnormal bactericidal activity.

CHRONIC GRANULOMATOUS DISEASE (CGD) This inherited disorder is characterized by severe recurrent infections of the skin, lymph nodes, lungs, liver, and bones. The infections are caused chiefly by staphylococci and certain gram-negative bacteria (particularly *Escherichia coli, Serratia marcescens,* and *Salmonella*). Histologically the tissues usually show a granulomatous reaction, lipid-filled macrophages, and multiple small abscesses. The neutrophils are morphologically normal. Neutrophil production, blood counts, and chemotaxis are also normal. Other measures of host defenses, including delayed hypersensitivity and lymphocyte functions, are normal, but immunoglobulins may be increased. The neutrophils, as well as the monocytes, have a greatly impaired ability to kill the types of microorganisms with which these patients usually become infected. Phagocytosis of bacteria is normal, but the metabolic burst which follows ingestion is markedly blunted. Superoxide

and H_2O_2 are not generated normally, and chemiluminescence is not observed. When CGD neutrophils phagocytize streptococci or pneumococci, these bacteria are killed normally because the bacteria contribute reactive oxygen derivatives from their own metabolism to the intracellular environment. This observation emphasizes the key role of oxygen and its derivatives in the intracellular bactericidal mechanism. Chronic granulomatous disease is most easily diagnosed by determining the amount of nitroblue tetrazolium (NBT) reduction which occurs when the patient's cells are incubated with this dye. Normally NBT is reduced intracellularly to a blue-black substance, blue formazan, which precipitates in the cell and can be seen as black intracellular particles. In CGD cells this reaction does not occur. The diagnosis is confirmed by observing that postphagocytic O_2 consumption, glucose C-1 oxidation, or the iodination reaction is reduced.

NADPH oxidase is probably the critically deficient enzyme in CGD. However, deficiencies of NADH oxidase and glutathione peroxidase, have been described in patients having typical CGD. The genetic heterogeneity indicated by family studies and the variable clinical presentations of CGD suggest that several different molecular lesions may result in this clinical picture. In *familial lipochrome histiocytosis* the neutrophils have a similar defect, but this disorder is described only in women, has a late onset, and presents very striking lipid-laden histiocytes in many tissues. Severe *deficiency of leukocyte glucose 6-phosphate dehydrogenase* with G6PD levels less than 5 percent of normal is also accompanied by neutrophil dysfunction similar to CGD. The management of CGD and its variants depends upon careful observation and detection of infections as early as possible. Cultures of affected tissues are critical for the correct diagnosis and selection of the appropriate antibiotic. Prophylactic antibiotics have probably been useful for some cases but may be accompanied by the usual problems of superinfections and emergence of resistant organisms (Chap. 114).

CHÉDIAK-HIGASHI SYNDROME This rare autosomal recessive disease is characterized by partial albinism, giant lysosomal granules in most granule-containing cells (neutrophils, monocytes, hepatocytes, renal tubular cells), and increased susceptibility to infections. The abnormal blood cells are readily seen on routine blood smears. The disease is usually recognized in children. There are several neutrophil abnormalities including moderately severe neutropenia, reduced marrow neutrophil reserves, and reduced neutrophil chemotaxis. In addition, in microbicidal studies, the giant primary granules are observed to degranulate slowly and thereby delay the killing of phagocytized bacteria. The disease is also accompanied by an accelerated phase with lymphohistiocytic infiltration in the liver, spleen, nerves, and other tissues with accompanying dysfunctions. Treatment is limited to prompt antimicrobial therapy of infections which usually resolve slowly. In the accelerated phase, vincristine and prednisone have been used to retard organ infiltration.

Other neutrophil abnormalities Unusual morphologic abnormalities of neutrophils include hereditary hyposegmentation (Pelger-Huet anomaly); hereditary hypersegmentation; retained remnants of endoplasmic reticulum, chiefly composed of RNA (May-Hegglin anomaly and Doehle bodies); and abnormally large azurophilic granules (Alder-Reilly anomaly). These abnormalities apparently do not interfere with neutrophil function.

OTHER LEUKOCYTIC CELLS

LYMPHOCYTES The chief functions of lymphocytes are production of immunoglobulins and expression of cellular immunity. Immunoglobulins react directly with foreign substances,

TABLE 56-5
Characteristics of T and B cells

	T cells	B cells
Origin	Bone marrow (with thymic influence)	Bone marrow
Life span	Long (months to years)	Short (probably days to weeks)
Circulating pattern	Chiefly recirculating	Chiefly nonrecirculating
Major location		
Lymph nodes	Deep cortical Perifollicular	Germinal centers Subcapsular
Spleen	Periarteriolar	Red pulp
Receptors	Sheep erythrocyte (rosettes) Mitogens (phyto-hemagglutinin)	Immunoglobulin (Fc) Complement (C3)
Functions		
Cellular immunity	4+	±
Antibody synthesis	0	4+

hastening their removal from the body by many mechanisms (Chap. 61). Cellular immunity is involved in delayed hypersensitivity and homograft rejection. Lymphocytes also can directly damage some foreign cells (cellular cytotoxicity).

On the blood smear, lymphocytes are a reasonably homogeneous collection of mononuclear cells with a small amount of blue cytoplasm containing a few granules. Through the analysis of surface receptors and responses to antigenic and mitogenic stimuli, it has been learned that there are two main types of lymphocytes, T and B cells, with strikingly different biological properties (Table 56-5). Approximately 80 percent of blood lymphocytes are T cells and 12 to 15 percent are B cells in normal individuals; these percentages are altered in many disease states. Different proportions of T and B cells are found also in the various lymphoid organs, i.e., lymph nodes, spleen, and bone marrow. Human lymphocytes are formed chiefly in the bone marrow. Normal T cells develop only in the presence of a normally functioning thymus (Chap. 62). Labeling studies indicate that there is a huge overproduction or ineffective production of lymphocytes by the lymphoid organs but that a substantial portion of the cells which reach the blood may live for years. These long-lived cells are principally T cells. They recirculate through the spleen and lymph nodes, thoracic duct, and bone marrow, leaving and reentering the circulation repeatedly. There are subpopulations of T cells which serve to enhance (helper T) or reduce (suppressor T) B-cell responses. It is not yet known precisely how the various surface receptors on T and B cells influence cell function, but they are probably involved in antigen recognition and cell-to-cell interactions with macrophages and other lymphocytes.

Lymphocytosis An increase in the absolute lymphocyte count occurs in certain infections: infectious mononucleosis, infectious hepatitis, infectious lymphocytosis, pertussis, tuberculosis, brucellosis, syphilis, thyrotoxicosis, and adrenal insufficiency. A lymphocyte count of greater than 10,000 per cubic millimeter usually indicates chronic lymphocytic leukemia especially in older patients (Chap. 326). The term "relative lymphocytosis" is sometimes used to describe situations where neutrophils are decreased with an increase in the percentage, but not absolute number, of lymphocytes. This term is misleading and should not be used.

Lymphocytopenia An absolute lymphocyte count of less than 1000 per cubic millimeter is observed in less than 5 percent of normal individuals but commonly occurs with acute, stressful illnesses such as myocardial infarction, pneumonia, or sepsis.

A transient lymphocytopenia regularly occurs even with very small doses of glucocorticosteroids. Chronic lymphocytopenia occurs in a variety of malignancies, uremia, congestive heart failure, lymphomas (especially Hodgkin's disease), aplastic anemia, lupus erythematosus, intestinal lymphangiectasia, and other immunologic deficiency syndromes (Wiskott-Aldrich syndrome, ataxia telangiectasia, Di George's syndrome, Swiss-type agammaglobulinemia, and thymic alymphoplasia) (Chap. 62). It also occurs following treatment with antilymphocyte globulin and certain chemotherapeutic agents.

MONOCYTES Monocytes are phagocytic cells with bactericidal capacities similar to neutrophils but with distinctive physiologic characteristics. They form in the bone marrow from promonocytes and have lysosomal granules containing myeloperoxidase, lysozyme, and acid phosphatases. They spend less time in the marrow than neutrophils and enter the blood with mitochondria and protein synthetic capacity intact, able to complete their differentiation as the circumstances demand. Monocytes leave the blood more slowly than neutrophils with a half-disappearance time estimated to be 12 to 24 h. They accumulate after neutrophils in acute inflammations in response to monocyte chemotactic factors.

In response to pinocytosis of serum proteins or ingestion of foreign material, monocytes enlarge and synthesize increased amounts of lysosomal enzymes and thereby are transformed to more active phagocytes called *macrophages*. Blood monocytes are the precursors of the pulmonary alveolar macrophages, spleen macrophages, and fixed macrophages of the monocyte-macrophage system (sometimes less precisely called the *reticuloendothelial system*). This system serves chiefly to remove foreign matter from the blood, e.g., bacteria, fungi, injected colloidal substances, and damaged or effete blood cells. During differentiation in each tissue site, monocytes acquire unique characteristics for that particular site. For instance, alveolar macrophages utilize chiefly oxidative phosphorylation to meet energy requirements, whereas peritoneal macrophages may chiefly utilize glycolysis. Generally, in all tissue sites these cells maintain the capacity to divide.

Monocytes have surface receptors for IgG, IgM, and complement, form rosettes with antibody-coated (IgG) erythrocytes, and are capable of synthesizing components of the complement system, transferrin, interferon, endogenous pyrogen, and colony-stimulating factor. In chronic inflammation they are probably responsible for the high serum and urine lysozyme concentrations. Monocytes serve a critical role in processing of antigen essential for both cellular and humoral immunity. They respond to lymphocyte-derived chemotactic and immobilizing factors (migration inhibitory factor, MIF). The incompletely catabolized endogenous materials generated in Gaucher's, Niemann-Pick's, and Fabry's diseases also accumulate in monocytes.

Monocytosis Increases in blood monocytes are observed in certain infections: tuberculosis, subacute bacterial endocarditis, brucellosis, Rocky Mountain spotted fever, malaria, and kala azar; in granulomatous diseases: sarcoidosis, regional enteritis; in some collagen vascular diseases; and in malignancies. Monocytosis may occur in leukemia and preleukemia, lymphomas, myeloproliferative syndromes, hemolytic anemias, and chronic idiopathic neutropenia.

Monocytopenia Reduced blood monocyte counts are seen acutely with stress and following glucocorticosteroid administration. Monocytopenia is observed in many acute infections, with aplastic anemia and acute leukemia, and as a direct effect of myelotoxic and immunosuppressive drugs.

EOSINOPHILS Many diseases are encountered where blood or tissue eosinophils are increased (Table 56-6). Eosinophils develop in the bone marrow similar to neutrophils. Their characteristic red-staining granules contain a unique peroxidase. Eosinophils have microbicidal capacities, and although these cells are chiefly involved in allergic and immune responses, their precise function in these responses is not known. Eosinophils are selectively attracted by an eosinophilic chemotactic factor elaborated by lymphocytes in response to certain stimuli. Eosinophils also accumulate in the skin in response to the topical application of allergens in allergic individuals. Animal studies indicate that the blood pool of eosinophils is relatively small compared with the number of these cells in various tissues. Significant tissue eosinophilia may occur in many inflammatory states, not necessarily accompanied by marked blood eosinophilia.

Eosinophilia More than 500 eosinophils per cubic millimeter of blood is infrequent in normal individuals. The most common cause for mild eosinophilia in hospitalized patients is probably some form of drug allergy. Parasitic infections, principally helminthic infections, cause eosinophilia, especially during the invasive phase. Some parasites may be difficult to recognize, e.g., strongyloides (Chap. 207), trichinella (Chap. 208), toxocara (Chap. 207), and filariae (Chap. 209). In these diseases the eosinophil count is rarely greater than 25,000 per cubic millimeter with the highest counts probably occurring in trichinosis. Protozoan infections generally do not cause eosinophilia. Eosinophilia is usually mild and irregularly present in allergic and collagen vascular diseases and malignancies and is not necessarily a clear guide to disease activity. The hypereosinophilic syndromes cause the highest eosinophil counts, occasionally in the 50,000 to 100,000 per cubic millimeter range or higher. Many tissues become infiltrated by eosinophils, a condition leading to organ dysfunction, particularly congestive heart failure.

Eosinopenia A reduction in eosinophils occurs with any stress or following corticosteroid administration. No known adverse effects result.

BASOPHILS These are the least common blood leukocytes; usually none are seen in the routine examination of a blood smear. The distinctive deep-blue granules, characteristically obscuring the cell nucleus, are rich in histamine. These cells are thought to be involved in certain acute allergic responses. Basophils are increased in chronic myelogenous leukemia, myelofibrosis, and polycythemia vera. This finding helps to distinguish these diseases from leukemoid reactions. Basophilia

may also be observed occasionally in some chronic inflammatory conditions.

REFERENCES

BABIOR BM: Oxygen dependent microbial killing by phagocytes. N Engl J Med 298:659, 721, 1978

CHUSID MJ et al: The hypereosinophilic syndrome. Medicine 54:1, 1975

CRADDOCK CG et al: Lymphocytes and the immune response. N Engl J Med 285:324, 1971

DALE DC et al: Chronic neutropenia. Medicine 58:128, 1979

GOLDE DW, CLINE MJ: Regulation of granulopoiesis, N Engl J Med 291:1388, 1974

KLEBANOFF SJ: Antimicrobial mechanisms in neutrophilic polymorphonuclear leukocytes. Semin Hematol 12:117, 1975

MORETTA L et al: Functional analysis of two human T cell subpopulations: Help and suppression of B-cell responses by T cells bearing receptors for IgM or IgG. J Exp Med 146:184, 1977

PRICE TP, DALE DC: The selective neutropenias. Clin Hematol 7:501, 1978

QUIE PG: Pathology of bactericidal power of neutrophils. Semin Hematol 12:143, 1975

ROWLANDS DT, DANIELE RP: Surface receptors in the immune response. N Engl J Med 293:26, 1975

STOSSEL TP: Phagocytosis. N Engl J Med 290:717, 774, 833, 1974

VAN FURTH R (ed): *Mononuclear Phagocytes in Immunity, Infection and Pathology.* Oxford, Blackwell, 1975

WILLIAMS WJ et al: *Hematology.* New York, McGraw-Hill, 1977

WINTROBE MM et al: *Clinical Hematology,* 7th ed. Philadelphia, Lea & Febiger, 1974

57
BIOCHEMICAL ABNORMALITIES AS A PRESENTING COMPLAINT

JEAN D. WILSON

INTRODUCTION Until a few years ago the majority of laboratory tests were performed at the discretion of clinicians. In the recent past the use of routine laboratory screening procedures has become more widespread, and the measurement of a biochemical profile, which includes some assays made formerly on a discretionary basis, is now a standard part of the clinical evaluation of patients.

Problems inherent in the interpretation of such screening tests constitute only a magnification of issues inherent in the understanding of all laboratory tests. Indeed, the unsuspected, unexplained abnormal laboratory result is a common, recurring problem in practice. It is also true that performing tests for which there is no obvious clinical indication is not solely a concern of laboratory medicine; the routine taking of blood pressure, examination of the heart, and roentgenography of the chest also fall into the category of screening procedures. However, the implications of admission biochemical profiles for the identification of asymptomatic disease constitute a particular challenge. [The problems inherent in population screening and of screening groups at high risk for certain diseases are beyond the scope of this discussion (see Chaps. 87 to 90).]

The vast majority of unanticipated abnormal results in medicine can be explained as due to laboratory error, a lack of recognition of the so-called "normal" range of values, or the presence (or presumed presence) of previously unrecognized disease.

LABORATORY ERROR One reason for unexpected, unexplained abnormal results is laboratory error, either random or

---

TABLE 56-6
Causes of blood eosinophilia

Drug reactions: Iodides, aspirin, sulfonamides, nitrofurantoin (see Chap. 71)

Parasitic infections: Hookworm disease, strongyloidiasis, toxocariasis, trichuriasis, trichinosis, filariasis, schistosomiasis, echinococcosis, cysticercosis

Allergic diseases: Hay fever, asthma, angioedema, serum sickness, allergic vasculitis, eczema, pemphigus

Collagen vascular diseases: Rheumatoid arthritis, dermatomyositis, periarteritis nodosa

Malignancy: Hodgkin's disease, carcinomatosis, mycosis fungoides, chronic myelogenous leukemia

Hypereosinophilic syndromes: Loeffler's syndrome, Loeffler's endocarditis, eosinophilic leukemia systematic. The random error may be caused by incorrect labeling, switching of specimens, or error at any stage in the process of reception, analysis, or reporting; the frequency of random error is difficult to assess, but it may occur in 1 percent or more of analyses. Systematic error is more common; it may represent a generalized decrease in or general lack of precision within the laboratory. Lack of precision may be due to poorly trained personnel, but even in well run laboratories systematic errors occur from time to time and may carry whole groups of measurements from the normal to the abnormal range. Constant vigilance is required to detect the appearance of such errors.

LACK OF UNDERSTANDING OF NORMAL VALUES There is no absolute method for defining either normal values or normal ranges for laboratory tests. For example, if a normal population is surveyed for 16 independent factors, each of which is normally distributed (gaussian), and if the limit of normal is accepted as ± 2 standard deviations (SD) of the mean, then 40 percent of the population will have at least one abnormally high result. In practice many factors are not normally distributed, and a range of normal greater than ± 2 SD is used. Furthermore, so-called "normal" values are usually not corrected for age or sex (glucose, albumin, uric acid, calcium, creatinine, alkaline phosphatase, bilirubin, cholesterol, potassium). Changes with age are a particular problem, since mean values may either increase (glucose, alkaline phosphatase) or decrease (calcium) in the elderly. If the whole distribution of values shifts to a different mean with age while the standard deviation remains unchanged, it can be assumed that the increase in the number of elevated or lowered values is due to a physiological change rather than to more frequent disease in the older population. Abnormal results due to failure to correct for age and sex usually fall just outside the normal range.

Another factor that influences interpretation of normal values is lack of appreciation of the magnitude of variation with time in the same individual. These variations are often due to the operation of a series of biological rhythms that influence the levels of plasma constituents, particularly hormones. Such rhythms operate over a period of minutes (plasma luteinizing hormone, testosterone), as diurnal or sleep-related variations during a 24-h cycle (cortisol, growth hormone, luteinizing hormone), or as monthly cycles (estradiol, progesterone, gonadotropins in women). Furthermore, biological rhythms may be more significant at certain times of life (secretion of growth hormone and luteinizing hormone at night in adolescents and preadolescents).

Other plasma constituents are subject to major day-to-day variations of unknown cause and without evident rhythmicity (urea, uric acid, phosphate, bilirubin, creatine kinase, and calcium). Although the magnitude of such changes is usually less than differences between individuals, in specific instances it may be the source of confusion. The degree of intraindividual variation in disease can be either less than normal (serum cortisol in Cushing's disease) or greater than normal (serum calcium in hyperparathyroidism).

DETECTION OF DISEASE In instances in which an unanticipated laboratory result is truly abnormal, such a finding may have any of several diagnostic implications.

Expansion of understanding in a recognized disease Analyses of biochemical profiles have provided insights into certain diseases that are not afforded by discretionary measurements. For example, in the past, serum uric acid was measured only in those patients with suspected gout, whereas determination of uric acid in all patients entering the hospital has led to elucidation of the pathophysiology of uric acid changes in many disorders other than gout (see Chap. 92). Likewise, as the result of

routine measurements, it is now clear that serum alkaline phosphatase is frequently elevated in hyperthyroidism.

Suspected but undocumented disease Abnormal tests may be found in patients who have no evidence of disease; this may pose little problem. In one 5-year follow-up of 241 patients with asymptomatic monoclonal elevations of serum globulins, development of associated disease was documented in only 18 percent. The presence of such an abnormality in the asymptomatic individual requires long-term follow-up, but no therapeutic intervention is indicated when disease is suspected but not proved.

Presymptomatic disease or disease with early manifestations In some patients biochemical abnormalities are initially unaccompanied by symptoms or signs but later prove to be early evidence of a specific disease. Examples include high serum transaminase in patients with unsuspected hepatitis, elevated blood urea in patients with unrecognized renal failure, and elevated serum alkaline phosphatase values in patients who have unsuspected liver or bone disease. Diagnosis by serendipity has always been a part of medicine.

The therapeutic implications of such a diagnosis depend on the disease in question, the extent of the manifestations, and the treatment modalities available. For example, in a 4-year follow-up of 20 patients with elevated serum alkaline phosphatase values who proved to have asymptomatic biliary cirrhosis, only half developed symptoms of the disease. Thus, in this case long-term follow-up is warranted, but since no effective treatment is available, the recognition of asymptomatic disease is probably of no benefit to the patient.

In other instances the issues are more complicated, as is perhaps best illustrated by the problem of hyperparathyroidism (see Chap. 350). Whereas previously only about 1 percent of cases were considered to be asymptomatic, with the widespread use of the biochemical profile large numbers of patients with unanticipated, persistent hypercalcemia are now being detected. In one large series only about 15 percent of such hypercalcemic patients developed symptomatic hyperparathyroidism over a 3-year period, and consequently many patients with hypercalcemia must be classified as having suspected but undocumented hyperparathyroidism.

Nevertheless, the fortuitous finding of hypercalcemia is so common that the 15 percent who do have hyperparathyroidism now constitute a significant fraction of patients in whom the diagnosis is made. Some of these patients are clinically asymptomatic but have biochemical or roentgenographic evidence of the disease (change in bone density or hypercalciuria) on careful examination. When a potentially serious disorder such as hyperparathyroidism is metabolically manifest—even mildly—it is generally assumed that surgical intervention is indicated. Such patients with purely laboratory manifestations now account for one-fifth or more of patients coming to surgery in many hospitals. Whether routine intervention in such cases is appropriate will not be clear until more is known about the natural history of the process.

In *summary,* the finding of unanticipated abnormal laboratory results is increasingly common because of the availability of routine laboratory screening procedures. In some instances, the presence of disease is established after a complete evaluation, and therapeutic intervention is warranted; in other cases, patients have either suspected disease or asymptomatic disease and should simply be followed closely long term. In still other instances, particularly in that group of borderline patients who are clinically asymptomatic but have some laboratory or metabolic evidence of disease, therapy is commonly undertaken. Whether this is actually justified is unknown.

REFERENCES

BARZEL US: The changing face of hyperparathyroidism. Hosp Prac 12:89, November 1977

KYLE RA: Monoclonal gammopathy of undetermined significance. Natural history in 241 cases. Am J Med 64:814, 1978

LONG RG et al: Presentation and course of asymptomatic primary biliary cirrhosis. Gastroenterology 72:1204, 1977

MARTIN HF et al: *Normal Values in Clinical Chemistry*. New York, Marcel Dekker, 1975

MURPHY EA, ABBEY H: The normal range—a common misuse. J Chron Dis 20:79, 1967

SUNDERMAN FW JR: Current concepts of "normal values," "reference values," and "discrimination values" in clinical chemistry. Clin Chem 21:1873, 1975

WHITEHEAD TP: Multiple analyses and their use in the investigation of patients. *Advan Clin Chem* 14:389, 1971

WILSON JMG: Current trends and problems in health screening. J Clin Pathol 26:555, 1973

WINKEL P, STATLAND BE: Using the subject as his own referrent in assessing day-to-day changes of laboratory test results, in *Contemporary Topics in Analytical and Chemical Chemistry*, DM Hercules et al (eds). New York, Plenum, 1977, p 287

section 1 | Genetics and
human disease

58

GENETIC ASPECTS OF HUMAN DISEASE

JOSEPH L. GOLDSTEIN
MICHAEL S. BROWN

GENETIC PRINCIPLES

More than one-fifth of the proteins (and hence genes) in each human being exist in a form that differs from the one present in the majority of the population. This remarkable degree of genetic variability, or polymorphism, among "normal" people accounts for much of the naturally occurring variation in body traits such as height, intelligence, and blood pressure. Moreover, these genetic differences produce marked variations in the ability of individuals to handle every environmental challenge, including those that produce disease. Thus, every human disease can be considered to occur as a result of an interaction between a given individual's genetic makeup and the environment. In certain diseases, however, the genetic component is so overwhelming that it expresses itself in a predictable manner without a requirement for extraordinary environmental challenges. Such diseases are termed *genetic disorders.*

MOLECULAR BASIS OF GENE EXPRESSION All hereditary information is transmitted from parent to offspring through the inheritance of specific molecules of deoxyribonucleic acid (DNA). DNA is a linear polymer composed of purine and pyrimidine bases whose sequence ultimately determines the sequence of amino acids in every protein molecule made by the body. The four types of bases in DNA are arranged in groups of three, each group forming a code word, or codon, that signifies a particular amino acid. A *gene* represents the total sequence of bases in DNA that specifies the amino acid sequence of a single polypeptide chain of a protein molecule.

In order to be translated into a polypeptide, each DNA region corresponding to a gene must first be transcribed within the cell nucleus into a molecule called *messenger ribonucleic acid* (mRNA). The mRNA represents a sequence of purine and pyrimidine bases that is "complementary" to that of the DNA. Hence, each adenine of DNA becomes a uridine of RNA, each cytosine of DNA becomes a guanine of RNA, each thymine of DNA becomes an adenine of RNA, and each guanine of DNA becomes a cytosine of RNA. Figure 58-1

shows the DNA and mRNA code words for each of the 20 amino acids that are utilized to form proteins.

The mRNA leaves the cell nucleus and enters the cytoplasm where it becomes associated with *ribosomes* and thereby serves as a template for the ribosomal synthesis of proteins. Each of the 20 precursor amino acids for protein synthesis is attached in the cell cytoplasm to specific molecules called *transfer RNA* (tRNA). Each tRNA contains a sequence of purine and pyrimidine bases that is "complementary" to a specific codon in the mRNA. These tRNA molecules with their attached amino acids line up along the mRNA molecule in the precise order dictated by the mRNA code. Under the action of a variety of cytoplasmic enzymes (initiation factors, elongation factors, and termination factors), peptide bonds are formed between the various amino acids, and the completed protein is released from the ribosome. A schematic diagram of the genetic control of protein synthesis is shown in Fig. 58-2.

MAINTENANCE OF GENETIC DIVERSITY THROUGH TRANSMISSION AND SEGREGATION OF GENES It is estimated that the amount of DNA in the nucleus of each human cell is sufficient to code for more than 100,000 genes and hence to specify more than 100,000 polypeptide chains. The genes are arranged in a linear sequence of DNA that together with certain histone proteins form rod-shaped bodies called *chromosomes*. Each somatic cell contains 46 chromosomes, arranged in 23 pairs, one of each pair derived from each of the individual's parents. Thus, each individual inherits two copies of each chromosome and hence two copies of each gene. The chromosomal location of the two copies of each gene is termed the *genetic locus*. When a gene occupying a genetic locus exists in two or more different forms, these alternate forms of the gene are referred to as *alleles*.

In humans, a given gene resides at a specified genetic locus on one particular chromosome. For example, the genetic locus for the Rh blood group is on chromosome 1; at this chromosomal site there are two Rh genes, one on chromosome 1 derived from the mother and the other on chromosome 1 derived from the father. When two genes at the same genetic locus are identical, the individual is a *homozygote*. When the two genes differ (i.e., two alleles are present at the locus), the individual is a *heterozygote*. Each normal human is heterozygous at approximately 20 percent of genetic loci and homozygous at 80 percent. Figure 58-3 shows a map of human chromosome 1, illus-

Second nucleotide

First nucleotide	A or U			G or C			T or A			C or G			Third nucleotide
A or *U*	**AAA** *UUU*	Phe		**AGA** *UCU*	Ser		**ATA** *UAU*	Tyr		**ACA** *UGU*	Cys		A or *U*
	AAG *UUC*			**AGG** *UCC*			**ATG** *UAC*			**ACG** *UGC*			G or *C*
	AAT *UUA*	Leu		**AGT** *UCA*			**ATT** *UAA*	Stop		**ACT** *UGA*	Stop		T or *A*
	AAC *UUG*			**AGC** *UCG*			**ATC** *UAG*			**ACC** *UGG*	Trp		C or *G*
G or *C*	**GAA** *CUU*	Leu		**GGA** *CCU*	Pro		**GTA** *CAU*	His		**GCA** *CGU*	Arg		A or *U*
	GAG *CUC*			**GGG** *CCC*			**GTG** *CAC*			**GCG** *CGC*			G or *C*
	GAT *CUA*			**GGT** *CCA*			**GTT** *CAA*	Gln		**GCT** *CGA*			T or *A*
	GAC *CUG*			**GGC** *CCG*			**GTC** *CAG*			**GCC** *CGG*			C or *G*
T or *A*	**TAA** *AUU*	Ile		**TGA** *ACU*	Thr		**TTA** *AAU*	Asn		**TCA** *AGU*	Ser		A or *U*
	TAG *AUC*			**TGG** *ACC*			**TTG** *AAC*			**TCG** *AGC*			G or *C*
	TAT *AUA*			**TGT** *ACA*			**TTT** *AAA*	Lys		**TCT** *AGA*	Arg		T or *A*
	TAC *AUG*	Met		**TGC** *ACG*			**TTC** *AAG*			**TCC** *AGG*			C or *G*
C or *G*	**CAA** *GUU*	Val		**CGA** *GCU*	Ala		**CTA** *GUA*	Asp		**CCA** *GGU*	Gly		A or *U*
	CAG *GUC*			**CGG** *GCC*			**CTG** *GAC*			**CCG** *GGC*			G or *C*
	CAT *GUA*			**CGT** *GCA*			**CTT** *GAA*	Glu		**CCT** *GGA*			T or *A*
	CAC *GUG*			**CGC** *GCG*			**CTC** *GAG*			**CCC** *GGG*			C or *G*

Note: The DNA codons appear in boldface type; the complementary RNA codons are in italics. A = adenine, C = cytosine, G = guanine, T = thymine, U = uridine (replaces thymine in RNA). In RNA, adenine is complementary to thymine of DNA; uridine is complementary to adenine of DNA; cytosine is complementary to guanine, and vice versa. "Stop" = termination. The amino acids are abbreviated as follows:

Ala = alanine	*Cys = cysteine*	*His = histidine*	*Met = methionine*	*Thr = threonine*
Arg = arginine	*Gln = glutamine*	*Ile = isoleucine*	*Phe = phenylalanine*	*Trp = tryptophan*
Asn = asparagine	*Glu = glutamic acid*	*Leu = leucine*	*Pro = proline*	*Tyr = tyrosine*
Asp = aspartic acid	*Gly = glycine*	*Lys = lysine*	*Ser = serine*	*Val = valine*

FIGURE 58-1

The genetic code.

trating the location of those genes that have been assigned loci on this chromosome.

The genetic information carried on chromosomes is transmitted to daughter cells under two different sets of circumstances. One of these occurs whenever a somatic cell (i.e., a nongerm cell) divides. This process, called *mitosis,* functions to transmit identical copies of each gene to each daughter cell, thus maintaining a uniform genetic makeup in all cells of a single organism. The other set of circumstances prevails when genetic information is to be transmitted from one individual to an offspring. This process, called *meiosis,* functions to produce germ cells (i.e., ova or spermatozoa) that possess only one copy of each parental chromosome, thus allowing for new combinations of chromosomes to occur when ovum and sperm cell fuse during fertilization.

During the process of meiosis, the 46 chromosomes of an immature germ cell arrange themselves in 23 pairs at the center of the nucleus, each pair being composed of one chromosome derived from the mother and its homologous chromosome derived from the father. At a specified point in the meiotic process, the two partner chromosomes separate, only one of each pair going into each daughter cell, or gamete. Thus, meiosis produces gametes with a reduction in the number of chromosomes from 46 to 23, each gamete having received one chromosome from each of the 23 pairs. The assortment of the chromosomes within each pair is random so that each germ cell receives a different combination of maternal and paternal chromosomes. During the process of fertilization,

FIGURE 58-3

Gene map of human chromosome 1. The black bands represent those genetic regions of the chromosome that stain brightly by a fluorescent dye such as quinacrine; the white bands are the negatively staining regions; the hatched area is a variable region that stains differently (i.e., either brightly or negatively) in the chromosomes of different individuals. Each gene that has been localized to this chromosome is listed opposite its genetic locus on the right. (Data provided by FH Ruddle and VA McKusick.)

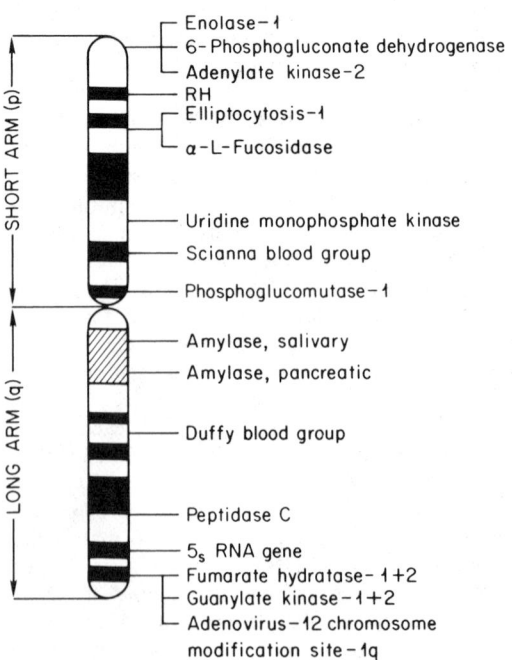

FIGURE 58-2

A schematic diagram of the genetic control of protein synthesis, illustrating the flow of genetic information from DNA to messenger RNA (mRNA) to the polypeptide chain of a protein molecule. Although DNA exists in a double-stranded form, only one of the two strands is used as a template for transcribing mRNA.

the fusion of ovum and sperm cell, each of which has 23 chromosomes, results ultimately in an individual with 46 chromosomes.

The independent assortment of chromosomes into gametes during meiosis produces an enormous diversity among the possible genotypes of the progeny. For each 23 pairs of chromosomes, there are 2^{23} different combinations of chromosomes that could occur in a gamete, and the likelihood that one set of parents will produce two offspring with the identical complement of chromosomes is one in 2^{23} or one in 8.4 million (assuming no monozygotic or identical twins).

RECOMBINATION Adding even further to the enormous genetic diversity in humans is the phenomenon of *genetic recombination.* During meiosis, when homologous chromosomes are paired, bridges frequently form between corresponding regions of the chromosome pair. These bridges, or *chiasmata,* are regions in which the two chromosomes break at identical points along their length and subsequently rejoin, the distal segments having been switched from one homologous chromosome to another. This process is designated *crossing over.* Although no net change in the amount of genetic material occurs during crossing over, a recombination of genes does occur. For example, consider a chromosome with two loci, A and B, located at opposite ends of the same chromosome. On this particular chromosome, the A locus has a rare allele *x* and the B locus also has a rare allele *y*. Without the phenomenon of recombination every offspring that inherited the *x* allele at the A locus would also inherit the *y* allele at the B locus. However, if recombination occurs, the A locus with the *x* allele would then be on the opposite chromosome from the B locus with the *y* allele. In this case any offspring that inherited the *x* allele at the A locus could not inherit the *y* allele at the B locus.

Crossing over in humans occurs with great frequency in every meiosis, and the resultant recombination of genes may occur at any point on a chromosome. The farther apart two genes are on the same chromosome, the greater is the likelihood that a crossing over will occur in the space between them. When two genes are on the opposite ends of a long chromosome, the probability of recombination is so great that their respective alleles are transmitted to offspring almost independently of one another, just as if the two gene loci were on different chromosomes. On the other hand, gene loci that are close together on the same chromosome are said to be *linked* so that there is a great likelihood that offspring will inherit the same combination of alleles that are present on the parental chromosome.

Several examples of *gene linkage* can be seen from the map of human chromosome 1 (Fig. 58-3). For example, the locus for the gene specifying the Rh blood group factor and the locus for the gene producing one form of the dominant trait, hereditary elliptocytosis, occur in close proximity on this chromosome. Thus, if a subject with hereditary elliptocytosis transmits the disease to an offspring, the offspring will usually inherit the allele that is present at the Rh locus on this chromosome. If the Rh allele happens to be a rare one in the population (such as *r'*), one can assume that whichever offspring inherits the *r'* allele at the Rh locus will also inherit the abnormal allele at the elliptocytosis locus. On the other hand, if an offspring does not exhibit the *r'* allele, he or she will not usually have elliptocytosis. The concept of linkage does not imply an association between any particular set of Rh alleles and the disease state elliptocytosis, rather between the two genetic loci. Thus, in different families the abnormal elliptocytosis allele may be linked to the R^1, R^0, r_2, or any other allele at the Rh locus, depending on the allele that happened to be at that locus when the elliptocytosis mutation occurred. Stated another way, the elliptocytosis locus is linked to the Rh locus in every family, but the particular Rh allele with which it is associated will differ from family to family.

MUTATION Broadly defined, a *mutation* is a stable, heritable alteration in DNA. Although the causes of mutation in humans are largely unknown, a variety of environmental agents, such as radiation, viruses, and chemicals, are among the factors that are implicated.

Mutations can involve a visible alteration in the structure of a chromosome, such as a deletion or translocation of a portion of a chromosome, or they can involve a minute change in one of the purine or pyrimidine bases of a single gene. Most commonly, such "point" mutations consist of the substitution of one base for another, changing the meaning of the codon containing that base, hence their designation as *missense mutations.* For example, in the gene coding for the β chain of hemoglobin, the sixth position normally contains either the nucleotide triplet CTT or CTC, both of which code for the amino acid glutamic acid (Fig. 58-1). The mutation that gives rise to hemoglobin C produces a change of the first base of this triplet from cytosine to thymine, changing the triplet to TTT or TTC, either of which codes for lysine. On the other hand, the mutation that gives rise to hemoglobin S produces a change in the second base of the same triplet (from thymine to adenine), producing either CAT or CAC, which codes for valine. Thus, in the sixth position of the β chain of hemoglobin, the normally occurring glutamic acid may be replaced with either lysine (producing hemoglobin C) or valine (producing hemoglobin S). More than 84 such single-base mutations in the hemoglobin β chain have been identified in different population groups, and many of these mutations produce distinct clinical syndromes. Of all the mutations so far elucidated in humans, the vast majority involve such single-base changes.

Besides producing an amino acid substitution, a single-base substitution can also cause another abnormality in protein synthesis—premature chain termination. Three mRNA code words (UAA, UAG, and UGA) normally do not specify an amino acid but constitute the signal that the message has ended and that the protein chain should be released from the ribosome (Fig. 58-1). If a change occurs in DNA that produces one of these mRNA code words [for example, a switch in an mRNA triplet from UAU (tyrosine) to UAA (termination)], the polypeptide chain would be terminated prematurely when translation had reached that point. Such mutations, called *nonsense mutations,* produce short fragments of proteins that have reduced function.

CELLULAR MECHANISM BY WHICH MUTANT GENES PRODUCE DISEASES Critical to the modern understanding of heredity is the concept that the only information transmitted from generation to generation is the sequence of bases in DNA and that these sequences in turn specify only the primary structure of RNA and protein molecules. All other chemical reactions within a cell—such as the synthesis of complex lipids and carbohydrates, the formation of membranes and other cellular organelles, and the accumulation and partitioning of inorganic ions—occur as a secondary consequence of the action of specific proteins. Many of these proteins are enzymes that catalyze the biochemical conversion of one molecule into another. Others are structural proteins such as collagen and elastin, and still others are regulatory proteins that dictate how much of each enzyme and each structural protein is to be made.

Since proteins are the cellular molecules whose structures are encoded by genes, mutations in genes exert their deleterious effects by altering the structure of enzymes, structural proteins, or regulatory proteins. For example, in a disease such as glycogen storage disease, type I (von Gierke's disease), massive accumulation of glycogen in the liver is due not to a primary structural abnormality in the polysaccharide glycogen but to a structural abnormality in a protein, glucose 6-phosphatase, an enzyme that is required to liberate glucose from glycogen. Other examples of the biochemical mechanisms by which mutant genes alter cellular metabolism are discussed below in "Simply Inherited Disorders."

GENETIC HETEROGENEITY When two or more mutations can produce a similar clinical syndrome, genetic heterogeneity is said to exist. Hemophilia is one example of such a genetically heterogeneous syndrome. A clinically similar bleeding disorder can be caused by mutations at either of two different loci on the X chromosome, one leading to a deficiency of factor VIII (classic hemophilia) and the other causing a deficiency of factor IX (Christmas disease). It is now generally believed that most, if not all, hereditary diseases, when carefully analyzed, will be shown to be genetically heterogeneous.

Genetic heterogeneity may result from the existence of a series of different mutations at a single genetic locus (allelic mutations) or from mutations at different genetic loci (nonallelic mutations). For example, drug-induced hemolysis of red blood cells can occur in patients with several different types of allelic mutations at the glucose 6-phosphate dehydrogenase locus. On the other hand, hemophilia is an example of a syndrome in which nonallelic mutations can produce a similar clinical picture (see above).

In some cases of heterogeneity, both the genetic locus and the mode of inheritance will differ, depending on the mutation. Diseases such as spastic paraplegia, Charcot-Marie-Tooth peroneal muscular atrophy, and retinitis pigmentosa are inherited as autosomal dominant traits in some families, as autosomal recessives in others, and as X-linked recessives in still others. The identification of such genetic heterogeneity in these disorders is of obvious importance for correct genetic counseling.

TAKING THE FAMILY HISTORY

The investigation of a patient with a possible genetic disorder begins with the *family history*. The first step in obtaining an accurate family history involves obtaining certain information on the *proband* or *index case* (i.e., the clinically affected person who has brought the family to attention) and on each of the *first-degree relatives* (i.e., the parents, siblings, and offspring of the proband). This information includes the given name, surname, maiden name, birth date or current age, age at death, cause of death, and name or description of any disease or defect.

The second step includes asking six questions designed to survey the family for the presence of disease or defect. (1) Has any relative an identical or similar trait? (2) Has any relative a trait that is absent in the proband but is known to occur in some patients with the same disease? This question requires that the physician have some knowledge about the manifestations of the disease in question. For example, when obtaining the family history from a proband with dissecting aneurysm caused possibly by Marfan's syndrome, one should ask about the occurrence of eye abnormalities, cardiac abnormalities, and skeletal abnormalities in the proband's relatives. (3) Has any relative a trait that is recognized to be genetically determined? The purpose of this question is to ascertain the occurrence of hereditary disease in the family even though the particular patient may not be involved. (4) Has any relative an

unusual disease, or has any relative died of a rare condition? The purpose of this question is to identify a condition that might be genetically determined though not recognized as such by the informant. In addition, this question may help to identify conditions in relatives that might be etiologically related to the patient's problem. For example, a patient with pheochromocytoma should be suspected of having von Recklinghausen's disease who has a brother with scoliosis and mental retardation, both of which can be manifestations of the neurofibromatosis (von Recklinghausen's) gene. (5) Is there any consanguinity in the family? This inquiry should be made directly, but in addition one should ask whether common last names appear in the families of husband-wife pairs. Consanguineous marriage may be the source of a rare autosomal recessive syndrome, and sometimes its presence in the family may not be known by the proband. (6) What is the ethnic origin of the family? Persons of various ethnic origins, such as blacks, Jews, and Greeks, have increased chance of specific genetic diseases. Table 58-1 lists examples of simply inherited disorders that are found with increased frequency in various ethnic groups.

CATEGORIES OF GENETIC DISORDERS

Genetic diseases generally fall into one of three categories: (1) *Chromosomal disorders* involve the lack, excess, or abnormal

TABLE 58-1
Examples of simply inherited disorders that occur with increased frequency in specific ethnic groups

Ethnic group	Simply inherited disorder
African blacks	Hemoglobinopathies, especially Hb S, Hb C, persistent Hb F, α and β thalassemias Glucose 6-phosphate dehydrogenase deficiency
Armenians	Familial Mediterranean fever
Ashkenazi Jews	Abetalipoproteinemia Bloom's syndrome Dystonia musculorum deformans (recessive form) Factor XI (PTA) deficiency Familial dysautonomia (Riley-Day syndrome) Gaucher's disease (adult form) Neimann-Pick disease Pentosuria Tay-Sachs disease
Chinese	α thalassemia Glucose 6-phosphate dehydrogenase deficiency Adult lactase deficiency
Eskimos	Pseudocholinesterase deficiency Adrenogenital syndrome
Finns	Congenital nephrosis Mulibrey nanism
French Canadians	Tyrosinemia
Japanese	Acatalasemia
Lebanese	Homozygous familial hypercholesterolemia
Mediterranean peoples (Italians, Greeks, Sephardic Jews)	β thalassemia Glucose 6-phosphate dehydrogenase deficiency Familial Mediterranean fever Glycogen storage disease, type III
Northern Europeans	Cystic fibrosis
Scandinavians	α_1-Antitrypsin deficiency LCAT (lecithin: cholesterol acyltransferase) deficiency
South African whites	Porphyria variegata

SOURCE: *After McKusick.*

arrangement of one or more chromosomes, producing excessive or deficient genetic material. (2) *Mendelian or simply inherited disorders* are determined primarily by a single mutant gene. This is indicated by the fact that these disorders display simple (mendelian) inheritance patterns which can be classified into autosomal dominant, autosomal recessive, or X-linked types. (3) *Mulifactorial disorders* are caused by an interaction of multiple genes and multiple exogenous or environmental factors. Although many of these multifactorial disorders, such as essential hypertension and cleft lip and palate, are said to run in families, the inheritance pattern is complex and the risk to relatives is much less than that seen in the single-gene (mendelian) disorders. Each of these three categories of genetic disease presents different problems with respect to causation, prevention, diagnosis, genetic counseling, and treatment.

CHROMOSOMAL DISORDERS The karyotype of an individual (i.e., the number and structure of the chromosomes) can be ascertained from readily accessible body tissues, such as peripheral blood lymphocytes or skin, by growing them in tissue culture until active cell proliferation occurs and then preparing single cells for examination of chromosomes by microscopy. Recent developments have made it possible to identify accurately each individual chromosome by special staining of DNA sequences, by the affinity of fluorescent dyes (such as quinacrine hydrochloride) for certain chromosomal segments that can be visualized by fluorescence microscopy, and by treatment with special dyes (Giemsa) and proteolytic enzymes (trypsin). These techniques produce characteristic *banding patterns* for each chromosome (Fig. 58-4).

The number of chromosomes in normal individuals is 46, of which 44 are the 22 pairs of *autosomes* and the other two are the *sex chromosomes*. Females have two X chromosomes (XX), and males have one X chromosome and one Y chromosome (XY). Each of the 22 pairs of autosomes and the two sex chromosomes can be distinguished on the basis of size, location of the centromere (which divides the chromosome into arms of equal or unequal length), and the unique banding pattern (Fig. 58-4). The relative length of the arms and the position of the centromere are used as further criteria to divide the human

FIGURE 58-4

The karyotype of a normal male showing the chromosomes of a single somatic cell in the metaphase stage of cell division. The photographic images of the chromosomes have been cut out and arranged according to descending length and varying arm ratio. The chromosomes have been stained by the Giemsa technique, which allows each chromosome pair to be identified by its unique banding pattern. Chromosomes 1 to 22 are the autosomes. The sex chromosomes in this normal male are an X and a Y. The normal female has an identical karyotype except for the absence of the Y chromosome and the presence instead of a second X chromosome. (Courtesy of K Hirschhorn.)

chromosomes into seven groups (designated A to G) (Fig. 58-4).

For a complete discussion of the etiology and clinical features of chromosomal abnormalities affecting humans, the reader is referred to Chap. 60.

SIMPLY INHERITED DISORDERS Disorders caused by the transmission of a single mutant gene show one of three simple (or mendelian) patterns of inheritance: (1) autosomal dominant, (2) autosomal recessive, or (3) X-linked. The distinction between "dominant" and "recessive" is one of convenience in pedigree analysis and does not imply a fundamental difference in genetic mechanism. The term *dominant* implies that a mutation will be clinically manifest when an individual has a single dose of this mutation (or is *heterozygous* for it), while *recessive* implies that a double dose (or *homozygosity*) is required for clinical detection. Genes are never dominant or recessive; their effects, however, produce clinical patterns that are classified as dominant or recessive. Despite their overall clinical "normality," individuals who are heterozygous for "recessive" genes often have biochemical abnormalities that are demonstrable in the laboratory; on the other hand, those who are homozygous for "dominant" genes are usually more severely affected than are the heterozygotes.

With few exceptions, each of the approximately 1200 or so mendelian diseases is rare. However, as a group these disorders constitute an important cause of morbidity and death, accounting directly for more than 5 percent of all hospital admissions.

The demonstration that a particular disease or syndrome shows one of the three mendelian patterns of inheritance implies that its pathogenesis, no matter how complex, is due to an abnormality in a single protein molecule. For example, in sickle-cell anemia, the entire clinical syndrome, including such seemingly unrelated disturbances as anemia, pain crises, nephropathy, and predisposition to pneumococcal infections, are all the physiologic consequences of having thymine instead of adenine at a specific site in the gene that codes for the β chain of hemoglobin, producing a substitution of a valine for a glutamic acid in the sixth amino acid position in the protein sequence.

In many mendelian disorders, especially in those with dominant inheritance, it is not possible to demonstrate directly the protein that is primarily altered by the mutation. In such cases (e.g., adult polycystic kidney disease and tuberous sclerosis) only the distal physiologic effects of the mutation are recognizable. Nevertheless, it is safe to assume that a single primary defect exists whenever a disease is transmitted by a single gene mechanism and that the various manifestations of the disease all can be related to the mutational event by a more or less complicated "pedigree of causes." Table 58-2 lists the most commonly encountered mendelian disorders affecting adults.

Autosomal dominant disorders Dominant diseases are those manifest in the heterozygous state, that is, when only one abnormal gene (*mutant allele*) is present and the corresponding partner allele on the homologous chromosome is normal. The gene responsible for an autosomal dominant disorder is located on one of the 22 autosomes, and both males and females can be affected. Since alleles segregate independently at meiosis, there is a 1 in 2 chance that the offspring of an affected heterozygote will inherit the mutant allele and, similarly, a 1 in 2 chance of the offspring inheriting the normal allele.

Figure 58-5 shows a typical pedigree involving an autosomal dominant trait. The following features are characteristic:

TABLE 58-2
Some relatively frequent mendelian disorders affecting adults

AUTOSOMAL DOMINANT DISORDERS

Familial hypercholesterolemia
Hereditary hemorrhagic telangiectasia
Marfan's syndrome
Hereditary spherocytosis
Adult polycystic kidney disease
Huntington's chorea
Acute intermittent porphyria
Osteogenesis imperfecta tarda
von Willebrand's disease
Myotonic dystrophy
Hemochromatosis
Idiopathic hypertrophic subaortic stenosis (IHSS)
Noonan's syndrome
Neurofibromatosis
Tuberous sclerosis

AUTOSOMAL RECESSIVE DISORDERS

Deafness
Albinism
Wilson's disease
Sickle-cell anemia
β thalassemia
Cystic fibrosis
Hereditary emphysema (α_1-antitrypsin deficiency)
Homocystinuria
Familial Mediterranean fever
Friedreich's ataxia
Phenylketonuria

X-LINKED DISORDERS

Hemophilia A
Glucose 6-phosphate dehydrogenase deficiency
Fabry's disease
Ocular albinism
Testicular feminization
Chronic granulomatous disease
Hypophosphatemic rickets
Color blindness

(1) Each affected individual has an affected parent (unless the condition arose by a new mutation in the given individual or is mildly expressed in the affected parent); (2) an affected individual will bear, on the average, both normal and affected offspring in equal proportions; (3) normal children of an affected individual will have only normal offspring; (4) males and females are affected in equal proportions; (5) each sex is equally likely to transmit the condition to male and female offspring, with male-to-male transmission occurring; and (6) vertical transmission of the condition through successive generations occurs, especially when the trait does not impair reproductive capacity.

While half of the offspring of an individual with an autosomal dominant condition will inherit the disease, it is not necessarily true that each affected person must have an affected

FIGURE 58-5
Pedigree pattern of an autosomal dominant trait. Note the vertical *pattern of inheritance.*

■ ● Affected male, female

□ ○ Unaffected male, female

parent. In every autosomal dominant disease a certain proportion of affected persons owe their disorder to a new mutation rather than to an inherited mutation. Since the estimated frequency of mutation is 5×10^{-6} mutations per gene per generation and since a dominant trait, by definition, requires a mutation in only one of a pair of alleles, one would expect that about 1 in 100,000 newborn persons would possess a new mutation at any given genetic locus. Many of these mutations either will not impair the function of the gene product or will involve a recessive function so that the mutation will be clinically silent. Others, however, will cause a defective gene product that gives rise to a dominant trait. The parent in whose germ cells the mutation arose will be clinically normal. Likewise, the siblings of the affected individual will be normal since the mutation will affect only a single germ cell. However, the affected individual will be able to transmit the disease, and half of his or her children will be affected.

The proportion of patients with dominant disorders who represent new mutations is inversely proportional to the effect of the disease in question on biologic fitness. The term *biologic fitness* refers to the ability of an affected individual to produce children who survive to adult life and reproduce. In the extreme case, if a dominant mutation produced absolute infertility, then all observed cases would of necessity represent new mutations, and it would be impossible to prove the genetic transmission of the trait. In less severe disorders, as in tuberous sclerosis, the severe mental retardation reduces biologic fitness to about 20 percent of normal, and the proportion of cases due to new mutations is about 80 percent. Other examples of the relation between biologic fitness and the proportion of new mutations in dominant disorders are shown in Table 58-3.

Many new mutations appear to occur in the germ cells of fathers who are of relatively advanced age. Such a "paternal age effect" is seen, for example, in Marfan's syndrome in which the average age of fathers of sporadic or "new mutation" cases (37 years) is in excess of the mean age of fathers generally (30 years) and also in excess of the age of fathers who transmit Marfan's disease due to an inherited mutation (30 years).

Before one concludes that a dominant disorder in a given patient with unaffected parents is the result of a new mutation, it is important to consider two other possibilities: (1) that the gene may be carried by one parent in whom the disease is of low expressivity (discussed below), and (2) that extramarital paternity may have occurred, since such is found in about 3 to 5 percent of randomly studied children in the United States.

Most autosomal dominant disorders show two characteristic features that are not usually seen in recessive syndromes: (1) *delayed age of onset* and (2) *variability in clinical expression.* Delayed age of onset is seen in disorders such as Huntington's chorea and adult polycystic kidney disease. These disorders do not manifest clinically until adult life, even though the mutant gene is present from the time of conception. Variability in clinical expression is illustrated dramatically by the multiple endocrine adenoma–peptic ulcer syndrome. Patients in the

TABLE 58-3
Approximate proportion of patients affected by new mutations in some autosomal dominant disorders

Disorder	Percentage
Achondroplasia	80
Tuberous sclerosis	80
Neurofibromatosis	40
Marfan's syndrome	30
Myotonic dystrophy	25
Huntington's chorea	4
Adult polycystic kidney disease	1
Familial hypercholesterolemia	Very low

FIGURE 58-6

Pedigree of a family affected with the multiple endocrine adenoma–peptic ulcer syndrome, a disorder inherited as an autosomal dominant trait. Circles denote females; squares, males. Open circles and squares denote unaffected relatives; closed circles and squares denote affected relatives. Deceased relatives are indicated by the oblique line. The age of each relative is indicated above his or her symbol. Note the marked variation in clinical expression among living affected heterozygotes.

1 Islet cell adenomas
Parathyroid adenomas
Lipomas
2 Lipomas, kidney stones

3 Islet cell adenomas
Parathyroid adenomas
Pituitary adenoma
Lipomas

4 Peptic ulcer disease
5 Pituitary adenoma

same family inheriting the same abnormal gene may have hyperplasia or neoplasia of one or all of a wide variety of endocrine tissues such as the pancreas, parathyroid glands, pituitary gland, or adipose tissue. The resulting clinical manifestations are extremely diverse; different members of the same family may develop peptic ulcers, hypoglycemia, kidney stones, multiple lipomas of the skin, or bitemporal hemianopsia. The recognition that each family member suffers from the same genetic abnormality can be very difficult, as illustrated by the family pedigree in Fig. 58-6.

Since dominant mutations involve a type of gene product that in a 50 percent deficiency is capable of producing clinical symptoms in heterozygotes, the responsible mutations are likely to involve abnormalities in two classes of proteins: (1) those that regulate complex metabolic pathways, such as membrane receptors and rate-limiting enzymes in pathways under feedback control, and (2) key structural proteins, such as hemoglobin or collagen.

The basic biochemical defects have been identified in only a handful of the approximately 600 autosomal dominant disorders. These include familial hypercholesterolemia (abnormal cell surface receptor that binds plasma low-density lipoprotein and thereby regulates cholesterol metabolism); hereditary methemoglobinemia and several hemolytic anemias due to unstable forms of hemoglobin (abnormal hemoglobin molecule); hereditary angioneurotic edema (abnormal protein inhibitor of an enzyme involved in the serum complement system); and acute intermittent porphyria (abnormal enzyme that catalyzes a rate-limiting step in the heme biosynthetic pathway).

Autosomal recessive disorders Autosomal recessive conditions are those that are clinically apparent only in the homozygous state, that is, when both alleles at a particular genetic locus are mutant alleles. By definition, the gene responsible for an autosomal recessive disorder must be located on one of the 22 autosomes; thus, both males and females can be affected.

Figure 58-7 shows a pedigree in which an autosomal recessive trait is present in the family. The following features are characteristic: (1) the parents are clinically normal; (2) only siblings are affected, and vertical transmission does not occur; and (3) males and females are affected in equal proportions.

The relative infrequency of recessive genes in the population and the requirement for two abnormal genes for clinical expression combine to create special conditions for autosomal recessive inheritance: (1) the more infrequent the mutant gene in the population, the stronger the likelihood that affected individuals are the product of consanguineous matings (see below); (2) if a husband and a wife are both carriers for the same autosomal recessive gene, 25 percent of the children will be normal, 50 percent will be heterozygous carriers, and 25 percent will be homozygous and affected with the disease; (3) if an affected individual marries a heterozygote (as may occur with consanguineous marriage), half the children will be affected, and a pedigree simulating dominant inheritance will result; and (4) if two individuals with the same recessive disease marry, all their children will be affected.

The clinical picture in autosomal recessive disorders tends to be more uniform than that of dominant diseases, and the age of onset is often early in life. As a general rule, recessive disorders are more commonly diagnosed in children, while dominant diseases are more frequently encountered in adults.

Since with recessive inheritance only one of four children in a sibship is expected to be affected, multiple cases in a family may not occur. This is especially true in a society in which small families are common. Consider, for example, 16 families in which both parents are heterozygous for the same recessive disorder. If each family has two children, 9 of the families will have no affected children, 6 will have one affected and one normal child, and only 1 of the 16 families will have two affected children. In the United States physicians usually see

FIGURE 58-7

Pedigree pattern of an autosomal recessive trait. Note the horizontal pattern of inheritance.

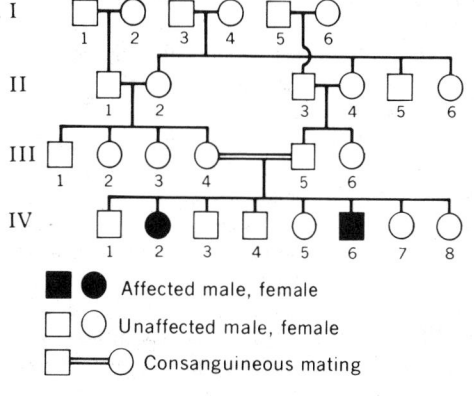

■ ● Affected male, female
□ ○ Unaffected male, female
□═○ Consanguineous mating

sporadic or isolated cases of a recessive disorder without an affected sibling to alert them to the possibility of a genetic disorder. Fortunately, because of the relatively uniform clinical picture of recessive disorders and because most can be diagnosed directly by biochemical tests, the correct diagnosis can usually be made even when no other members of a family are clinically affected.

The basic biochemical lesions underlying many autosomal recessive disorders have been identified. Of the three types of proteins in which mutations could occur (i.e., enzymes, structural proteins, and regulatory proteins), the one most easy to study has been the enzymes. A mutation that destroys the catalytic activity of an enzyme generally does not impair the health of a heterozygote (i.e., an individual who has one mutant allele specifying a functionless enzyme and one normal allele on the partner chromosome specifying a normal enzyme). In this situation each cell in the body usually produces about 50 percent of the normal number of active enzyme molecules. However, normal regulatory mechanisms function to avert any clinical consequences of this 50 percent deficiency, and so heterozygotes usually are clinically normal. On the other hand, when an individual inherits functionless alleles at both loci specifying an enzyme, the reduction in enzyme activity is too great for a compensatory mechanism to overcome the deficiency, and a disease results. For example, heterozygotes for phenylketonuria who have half the normal activity of phenylalanine hydroxylase are clinically asymptomatic because the body compensates for the half-normal level of the enzyme by raising the substrate concentration approximately twofold. Under these conditions a normal amount of phenylalanine can be metabolized with no symptoms. On the other hand, the homozygote for phenylketonuria has such a severe reduction in phenylalanine hydroxylase activity that enormous levels of phenylalanine and its derivatives accumulate, causing detrimental brain development. As in the case of phenylketonuria, the majority of enzyme deficiency states produce *simultaneously* both a simple accumulation of one or more metabolites preceding the enzymatic block and a deficient production of other metabolites distal to the block in the metabolic pathway.

Most of the genetic enzyme deficiencies that have been elucidated are not only inherited as recessive traits, but also tend to involve enzymes that participate in catabolic pathways. Frequently these enzymes degrade organic molecules that are ingested in the diet, such as galactose (galactosemia), phenylalanine (phenylketonuria), and phytanic acid (Refsum's syndrome). A special class of such catabolic diseases is that in which the deficiency affects an acid hydrolase that occurs within lysosomes. In these *lysosomal storage disorders* the substrate, usually a complex lipid or polysaccharide, accumulates within swollen lysosomes in specific organs, giving the cells a foamy appearance. Examples of such lysosomal diseases include the mucopolysaccharidoses such as Hurler's syndrome (α-iduronidase deficiency) and the lipid storage diseases such as Gaucher's disease (glucocerebrosidase deficiency).

In general, recessive diseases are rare because the reduced biologic fitness of homozygotes acts to remove the mutant gene from the population. However, a few recessive disorders, such as cystic fibrosis and sickle-cell anemia, are very common. To explain this paradox, it has been postulated that the biologic fitness of heterozygotes is greater than that of noncarriers for these genes. In such a case the frequency of the gene in the population depends on the balance between the increased fitness of the relatively numerous heterozygotes and the reduced fitness of the less common homozygotes. A small selective advantage of the heterozygote over the normal results in a high gene frequency and hence a high birth frequency of homozygotes even when the disease is lethal. Thus, about 1 in 22 Caucasians is a heterozygous carrier for the genetically lethal disease cystic fibrosis, and the disease occurs in about 1 in 2000 Caucasian births. In order to maintain such a high gene frequency, heterozygotes for cystic fibrosis must have a definite reproductive advantage over noncarriers, but the nature of this advantage is unknown. However, in sickle-cell anemia, another recessive disorder with high frequency among certain populations, heterozygotes appear to have increased resistance to malaria.

Inasmuch as recessive diseases require the inheritance of a mutation at the same genetic locus from each parent, when the genes are rare, the likelihood of any two parents being carriers for the same defect becomes very small. However, if the parents have a common ancestor and if that ancestor was a carrier for the same recessive gene, then the likelihood that two of the descendants would each have inherited the gene becomes relatively great. The rarer the recessive gene, the stronger becomes the likelihood that an affected individual will have resulted from such a consanguineous mating. On the other hand, certain recessive genes are so common in the population that the likelihood of two random parents being carriers is great enough to eliminate the need for consanguinity. For common traits such as sickle-cell anemia, phenylketonuria, cystic fibrosis, and Tay-Sachs disease, all of which have a high carrier frequency in certain populations, consanguinity is usually not present in the parents.

In general, consanguinity is an infrequent finding clinically in families with recessive diseases in the United States. This is because the background rate of consanguinity in the general population is very low. In most of the United States (as opposed to areas with relative geographic isolation such as northern Norway and Switzerland), a disorder must indeed be rare before it is associated with an important frequency of consanguinity. For example, consanguinity is expected in a large proportion of families having children with very rare disorders such as the Laurence-Moon-Biedl syndrome and abetalipoproteinemia.

Genetic compounds represent a special type of recessively inherited disorder in which the affected individual's two mutant genes, although derived from the same genetic locus, are not identical. The mutations in the paternal and maternal alleles presumably involve different alterations in the DNA of the same gene. Sickle-cell-C hemoglobinopathy is an example of such a *heteroallelic* compound state in which individuals have a gene for sickle-cell hemoglobin on one chromosome and a gene for hemoglobin C on the homologous chromosome.

X-linked disorders The genes responsible for X-linked disorders are located on the X chromosome; therefore, the clinical risk and severity of the disease are different for the two sexes. Since a female has two X chromosomes, she may be either heterozygous or homozygous for a mutant gene, and the trait may therefore demonstrate either recessive or dominant expression. Males, on the other hand, have only one X chromosome, so they can be expected to display the full syndrome whenever they inherit the gene regardless of whether the gene behaves as a recessive or as a dominant trait in the female. Thus, the terms *X-linked dominant* or *X-linked recessive* refer only to the expression of the gene in women.

An important feature of all X-linked inheritance is the absence of male-to-male (i.e., father-to-son) transmission of the trait. This follows because a male must always contribute his Y chromosome to his sons; hence, he can never contribute his X chromosome. On the other hand, a male contributes his one X chromosome to all his daughters.

The pedigree in Fig. 58-8 illustrates the characteristic features of X-linked recessive inheritance. (1) In contrast to the vertical transmission in dominant traits (parents and children affected) and the horizontal transmission in autosomal reces-

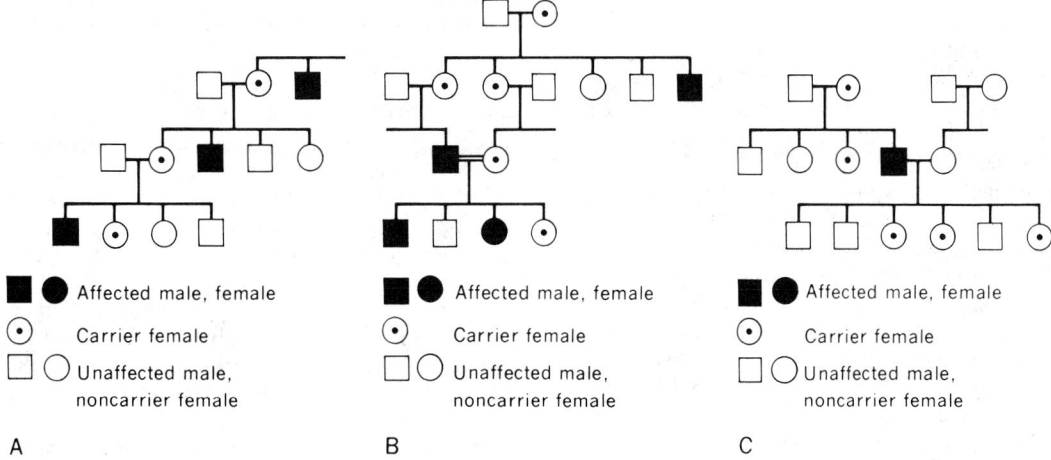

FIGURE 58-8

Pedigree patterns of an X-linked recessive trait. A. Note the oblique pattern of inheritance. B. An affected female can result from the mating of an affected male and a carrier female, as in the consanguineous marriage

shown here. C. An affected male mating with a normal noncarrier female has all normal sons and all carrier daughters. (Courtesy of V A McKusick.)

sive traits (siblings affected), the pedigree pattern in X-linked recessive traits tends to be oblique because of the occurrence of the trait in the sons of normal carrier sisters of affected males (uncles and nephews affected) (Fig. 58-8A); (2) male offspring of carrier women have a 50 percent chance of being affected; (3) all female offspring of affected males are carriers, and affected males do not transmit the disease to their sons (Fig. 58-8C); (4) unaffected males do not transmit the trait to any offspring; and (5) affected homozygous females occur only when an affected male fathers the child of a carrier female (Fig. 58-8B).

Examples of X-linked recessive disorders in humans include hemophilia A, nephrogenic diabetes insipidus, the Lesch-Nyhan syndrome, Duchenne form of muscular dystrophy, glucose 6-phosphate dehydrogenase deficiency, testicular feminization, and Fabry's disease. Color blindness is also inherited as an X-linked recessive trait, but it is sufficiently frequent (occurring in about 8 percent of Caucasian males) that the occurrence of homozygous color-blind females is no rarity.

X-linked dominant inheritance is illustrated by the pedigree in Fig. 58-9. Its characteristic features are as follows: (1) Females are affected about twice as often as males; (2) an affected female transmits the disorder to half of her sons and half of her daughters; (3) an affected male transmits the disorder to all his daughters and to none of his sons; and (4) the syndrome

is more variable and less severe in heterozygous affected females than in hemizygous affected males. One common trait, the Xg(a+) blood group, is inherited as an X-linked dominant trait, as are diseases such as vitamin D-resistant rickets (hypophosphatemic rickets) and pseudohypoparathyroidism.

Some rare conditions may be inherited as X-linked dominant traits in which there is lethality in the hemizygous male. The characteristics of this form of inheritance are illustrated by the pedigree in Fig. 58-10: (1) The disorder occurs only in females who are heterozygous for the mutant gene; (2) an affected mother transmits the trait to half of her daughters; (3) an increased frequency of abortions occurs in affected women, the abortions representing affected male fetuses. Conditions that appear to be transmitted by this mode of inheritance include incontinentia pigmenti, focal dermal hypoplasia, orofaciodigital syndrome, and hyperammonemia due to ornithine transcarbamylase deficiency.

Understanding of the mechanisms of gene expression of X-linked traits in females has been greatly advanced by the so-called "Lyon hypothesis" or "X-inactivation hypothesis." (The term *hypothesis* is used for historical reasons only; Lyon's hypothesis can now be regarded as proved fact.) This hypothesis states that early in embryonic development one of the two X chromosomes in each somatic cell of a female is inactivated. The inactivation process is random, so that for each cell there

FIGURE 58-9

Pedigree pattern of an X-linked dominant trait.

FIGURE 58-10

Pedigree pattern of an X-linked dominant trait lethal in the hemizygous male.

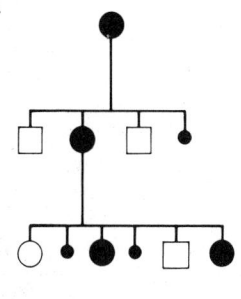

is an equal probability that the paternally or maternally derived X chromosome will be inactivated. The inactivated X chromosome is rendered permanently nonfunctional, so that all progeny of the initial cell inherit the same active and inactive X chromosomes. Thus, each female is a mosaic; on the average, half of her cells express the X chromosome of the father, and half express the X chromosome of the mother. If a mutation in a gene is carried on one of her X chromosomes, about one-half of the cells in each tissue will be normal and the other half will manifest the mutant phenotype. However, chance or selection of one or the other set of clones of cells may disturb these proportions in any given individual. Depending on the proportions of mutant and normal X chromosomes in each tissue, a genetically heterozygous female may either be clinically normal or have mild or severe manifestations of the disease. To illustrate, mothers of boys with the X-linked recessive Duchenne form of muscular dystrophy may occasionally show mild manifestations of the disease, such as limb girdle weakness or hypertrophied calves.

In each female cell the nonfunctional X chromosome can be visualized by several techniques. By ordinary staining, the inactivated X chromosome in metaphase appears heteropyknotic (very condensed in appearance), and it replicates late in the mitotic cycle ("late-labeling" with tritiated thymidine). In nondividing cells the inactivated X chromosome can be observed as a clump of chromatin at the periphery of the nucleus—the so-called "X chromatin" or "Barr body." In abnormal states with more than two X chromosomes such as 47 XXX, all but one of the X chromosomes are inactivated, so female cells may have multiple X chromatin bodies (see Chap. 60).

Since a single mutant allele is sufficient for the expression of X-linked recessive disorders, consanguinity does not increase the likelihood of expression in males, unlike the case in the rare autosomal recessive disorders. On the other hand, just as in the dominantly inherited disorders, new mutations can be a factor. In general, if an X-linked recessive condition reduces biologic fitness to zero, one-third of affected males will be born as a result of new mutations and an additional one-third will be born to mothers who themselves are carriers as a result of a new mutation. Thus, only one-third will come from a classic pedigree manifesting oblique transmission. An example of such a disease is the Duchenne form of muscular dystrophy in which affected hemizygous males are so severely disabled that they never reproduce. In hemophilia A, in which the biologic fitness is greater than zero, about 20 percent of affected males represent new mutations.

In families in which only one male is affected with an X-linked recessive disease and there is no other family history of the trait, it is essential for proper genetic counseling that the mother undergo biochemical tests or other relevant studies to determine whether she is a carrier. If she is a carrier, half of her daughters will be carriers and half of her sons will be affected. On the other hand, if her affected son represents a new mutation, only his daughters will inherit the gene. At present, biochemical tests can identify female carriers for several X-linked diseases including the Lesch-Nyhan syndrome, Fabry's disease, Hunter's syndrome, hemophilia, and the Duchenne form of muscular dystrophy.

The distinction between X-linked inheritance and *sex-influenced autosomal dominant inheritance* is important. Both baldness and hemochromatosis are probably inherited as autosomal dominant traits, yet both disorders occur mainly in men and rarely in women. Heterozygous females rarely manifest the hemochromatosis gene because of menstruation and pregnancy, which mitigate against the overaccumulation of iron, and they express the baldness gene only when a source of testosterone becomes available as occurs with a masculinizing tumor of the ovary.

MULTIFACTORIAL GENETIC DISEASES The common chronic diseases of adults (such as essential hypertension, coronary heart disease, diabetes mellitus, peptic ulcer disease, and schizophrenia) as well as the common birth defects (such as cleft lip and palate, spina bifida, and congenital heart disease) have been long known to "run in families." They fit best into the category of *multifactorial genetic diseases.* The genetic element in these disorders rarely manifests itself in an all-or-none fashion as it does in the simply inherited (mendelian) disorders and in chromosomal aberrations. Instead, it is the interaction of multiple genes with multiple environmental factors that produces the familial aggregation.

In the multifactorial genetic diseases, there is a *polygenic component* consisting of a series of genes that interact in a cumulative fashion. An individual who inherits just the right combination of these genes passes beyond a "threshold of risk," at which point an *environmental component* determines whether and to what extent that person is clinically affected. In order for another individual in the same family to express the same syndrome, the same or a very similar combination of genes must be inherited. Since the first-degree relatives of an affected individual (i.e., parents, siblings, and offspring) each share half of that person's genes, they are all at increased risk of exhibiting the same polygenic syndrome. Second-degree relatives (uncles, aunts, and grandparents) share on the average one-fourth of an individual's genes $(\frac{1}{2})^2$, and third-degree relatives (cousins) share one-eighth $(\frac{1}{2})^3$. Thus, as the degree of relation becomes more distant, the likelihood of a relative inheriting the same combination of genes becomes less. Moreover, the chances of any relative inheriting the right combination of risk genes decrease as the number of genes required for the expression of a given trait increases.

Since the precise number of genes responsible for polygenic traits is unknown, the risk of inheritance for a relative of an affected individual is difficult to calculate, and the standard is based on empiric risk figures (i.e., a direct tally of the proportion of affected relatives in previously reported families). In contrast to the simply inherited disorders in which 25 or 50 percent of the first-degree relatives of an affected proband are at genetic risk, multifactorial genetic disorders are generally observed empirically to affect no more than 5 to 10 percent of first-degree relatives. Moreover, in contrast to mendelian traits, the recurrence risk of multifactorial conditions varies from family to family, and its estimation is significantly influenced by two factors: (1) the number of affected persons already present in the family, and (2) the severity of the disorder in the index case. The greater the number of affected relatives and the more severe their disease, the higher the risk to other relatives. For example, the risk of cleft lip in the siblings of a child with unilateral cleft lip is about 2.5 percent, but if the lesion in the index case is bilateral, the risk in the siblings rises to 6 percent. Table 58-4 lists the empirical risk figures for the familial recurrence of a number of multifactorial genetic diseases.

The hypothesis of a polygenic component in the inheritance of multifactorial diseases has been given a sound basis in recent years by the demonstration that at least one-third of all gene loci harbor polymorphic alleles that vary among individuals. Such a large degree of variation in normal genes undoubtedly provides the substrate for variations in genetic predisposition with which environmental factors can interact. So far, the genetic loci most strikingly associated with predisposition to specific diseases are those that constitute the HLA system. The HLA gene complex is located on the short arm of chromosome 6. It consists of four closely linked but distinct

TABLE 58-4
Empiric risks for some common multifactorial genetic diseases affecting adults

Disorder in index case	Estimated absolute risk for first-degree relatives, %
Cleft lip and/or palate	3
Congenital heart disease	4
Coronary heart disease	8 for male relatives
	3 for female relatives
Diabetes mellitus	5–10
Epilepsy	5–10
Hypertension	10
Manic-depressive psychosis	10–15
Psoriasis	10–15
Schizophrenia	15
Thyroid disease (autoimmune disorders including hyperthyroidism, thyroiditis, primary myxedema, simple goiter)	10

TABLE 58-5
Alleles at the HLA loci associated with multifactorial genetic diseases

Disease	HLA locus	Specific allele	Relative risk*
Ankylosing spondylitis	B	B27	121
Reiter's syndrome	B	B27	40
Psoriasis with arthritis	B	B27	5
Celiac disease	B	B8	10
Chronic active hepatitis	B	B8	4
Myasthenia gravis	B	B8	4
Diabetes mellitus (insulin-dependent)	B	B8, B15	3
	D	D3	3
Hyperthyroidism	D	D3	4
Addison's disease	B	B8	7
	D	D4	10
Multiple sclerosis	D	D2	7

* Relative risk *is the probability of the disease developing in an individual with the specific allele, divided by the probability of its development in an individual who does not possess this specific allele.*

loci (A, B, C, and D). The products of these genes are proteins that are found on the surface of body cells and that enable an individual's immune system to distinguish its own cells from those of someone else. Each HLA locus in the population consists of multiple alleles, each of which produces an immunologically distinct protein. For example, an individual may inherit any 2 of 20 alleles at the HLA-B locus.

An important observation of recent years has been the finding that certain alleles at the HLA loci predispose individuals to certain specific diseases. For example, if the B27 allele at the HLA-B locus is inherited by an individual, that person has a 121-fold greater chance of developing ankylosing spondylitis than an individual who lacks this allele (Table 58-5). Ankylosing spondylitis remains a multifactorial disease, however, because its development clearly requires one or more other factors in addition to the B27 allele. Thus, less than 15 percent of people who inherit this allele develop this disease. Table 58-5 lists some of the diseases associated with alleles at the HLA loci. Several of them in the past have been suspected to be of viral etiology, suggesting that the HLA loci may dictate the mode of expression of certain viral diseases.

Multifactorial disorders are heterogeneous in the sense that

TABLE 58-6
Examples of inherited disorders involving an abnormal response to drugs

Disorder	Molecular abnormality	Mode of inheritance	Frequency	Clinical effect	Drugs producing abnormal response
Slow inactivation of isoniazid	Isoniazid acetylase in liver	Autosomal recessive	~50% of U.S. population	Polyneuritis	Isoniazid, sulfamethazine, sulfamaprine, phenelzine, dapsone, hydralazine
Suxamethonium sensitivity	Pseudocholinesterase in plasma	Autosomal recessive	Several mutant alleles; most common affects 1 in 2500	Apnea	Suxamethonium, succinylcholine
Coumadin	? Altered receptor or enzyme in liver with increased affinity for vitamin K	Autosomal dominant	Rare	Inability to achieve anticoagulation with usual doses of drug	Coumadin
Glaucoma	Unknown	? Autosomal dominant	Common	Increased intraocular pressure	Corticosteroids
Malignant hyperthermia	Unknown	Autosomal dominant	~1 in 20,000 anesthesized patients	Severe hyperpyrexia, muscle rigidity, death	Such anesthetics as halothane, succinylcholine, methoxyflurorane, ether, cyclopropane
Unstable hemoglobins: Hemoglobin Zurich	Arginine substitution for histidine at sixty-third position of β chain of hemoglobin	Autosomal dominant	Rare	Hemolysis	Sulfonamides
Hemoglobin H	Hemoglobin composed of four β chains	Autosomal dominant	Rare	Hemolysis	Sulfisoxazole
Glucose 6-phosphate dehydrogenase deficiency	Glucose 6-phosphate dehydrogenase in erythrocytes	X-linked recessive	$\sim 1 \times 10^8$ affected persons in world; common in persons of African, Mediterranean, Asiatic origin; multiple mutant alleles	Hemolysis	Analgesics, sulfonamides, antimalarials, nitrofurantoin, other drugs

SOURCE: *ES Vesell, N Engl J Med 287:904, 1972.*

the relative contribution of the polygenic factors ("risk genes") and environmental factors to the etiology will vary greatly from patient to patient. However, it is important to remember that among common phenotypes which are largely multifactorial, often a small proportion will be created by major mutant genes. For example, although coronary heart disease is usually of multifactorial etiology, about 5 percent of subjects with premature myocardial infarctions are heterozygotes for familial hypercholesterolemia, a single-gene disorder that produces atherosclerosis in the absence of any other predisposing factor. Similarly, in a small proportion of patients with other common diseases such as peptic ulcer disease or "essential" hypertension, the condition is not multifactorial but determined by a single gene, as in the multiple endocrine adenoma–peptic ulcer syndrome or the medullary thyroid carcinoma–pheochromocytoma syndrome, respectively.

INTERACTION BETWEEN SINGLE GENETIC AND ENVIRONMENTAL FACTORS

Many diseases are now recognized to result from an interaction between a specific genotype and a specific environmental factor. In particular, inherited single-gene mutations have been shown to produce clinically significant and often life-threatening idiosyncratic responses to certain drugs.

Table 58-6 lists the most important of these *pharmacogenetic disorders,* which encompass all the mendelian modes of inheritance. Perhaps the most common is glucose 6-phosphate dehydrogenase deficiency, an X-linked recessive trait in which a variety of drugs may precipitate a hemolytic anemia. Plasma pseudocholinesterase deficiency and hepatic transacetylase deficiency are examples of autosomal recessive traits which alter drug catabolism so that when the muscle relaxant suxamethonium or the antituberculous drug isoniazid is administered, apnea or peripheral neuropathy, respectively, may ensue. Malignant hyperthermia is an autosomal dominant trait in which acute hyperpyrexia, muscle rigidity, and hyperkalemic cardiac arrest may be induced by administration of any one of several anesthetic agents. Acute intermittent porphyria is another example of a genetic disorder that is exacerbated by drugs, such as barbiturates.

Misinterpretation of adverse drug reactions may result in serious harm to patients. In general, all unusual idiosyncratic reactions should be considered to be genetically determined until proved otherwise. Fortunately, the pharmacogenetic disorders are a group of diseases for which therapy is straightforward: avoidance of the noxious drug by patient and relatives.

In addition to drugs, other factors in the environment may aggravate specific genetic traits. Cigarette smoke may have deleterious effects on persons homozygous and possibly heterozygous for α_1-antitrypsin deficiency, who are predisposed to the development of emphysema. Patients with xeroderma pigmentosa and anhydrotic ectodermal dysplasia are unusually sensitive to sunlight and high temperatures, respectively. Avoidance of milk at an early age prevents many of the complications ordinarily seen in persons with galactosemia.

Genetic-environmental interactions are particularly important in pregnancy. Women who are affected with phenylketonuria may develop high plasma phenylalanine levels during pregnancy, and thus their offspring may suffer from a variety of phenylalanine-induced birth defects even though the offspring may not themselves have phenylketonuria. Other examples of diseases resulting from an adverse genetic relation between the mother and fetus include erythroblastosis caused by Rh incompatibility and diabetic embryopathy, a term that re-

fers to a series of major birth defects occurring in about 5 percent of the offspring of women who are clinically diabetic during pregnancy.

REFERENCES

Brown MS, Goldstein JL: New directions in human biochemical genetics: Understanding the manifestations of receptor deficiency disorders. Prog Med Genet 1:103, 1976

Carter CO: Genetics of common disorders. Br Med Bull 25:52, 1972

Cavalli-Sforza LL, Bodmer WF: *The Genetics of Human Populations.* San Francisco, Freeman, 1971

Childs B, Der Kaloustian VM: Genetic heterogeneity. N Engl J Med 279:1205, 1267, 1968

Harris H: *The Principles of Human Biochemical Genetics,* 2d ed. New York, American Elsevier, 1975

McKusick VA: *Mendelian Inheritance in Man: Catalogs of Autosomal Dominant, Autosomal Recessive and X-linked Phenotypes,* 5th ed. Baltimore, Johns Hopkins, 1978

———, Claiborne R: *Medical Genetics.* New York, HP Publishing, 1973

Nora JJ, Fraser FC: *Medical Genetics: Principles and Practice.* Philadelphia, Lea & Febiger, 1974

Schaller JG, Omenn GS: The histocompatibility system and human disease. J Pediat 88:913, 1976

Stanbury JB et al: *The Metabolic Basis of Inherited Disease,* 4th ed. New York, McGraw-Hill, 1978

Watson JD: *Molecular Biology of the Gene,* 3d ed. New York, Benjamin, 1976

59
PREVENTION AND TREATMENT OF GENETIC DISORDERS

JOSEPH L. GOLDSTEIN
MICHAEL S. BROWN

APPROACHES TO PREVENTION

In view of the present trend for couples to have smaller families, there is increasing concern that children should be healthy and free of genetic diseases, and primary-care physicians are called upon to play a more active role in the prevention and treatment of hereditary diseases. In most clinical situations, genetic advice can be given by the primary physician once the relatively simple principles of medical genetics (Chap. 58) and genetic counseling (discussed below) have been mastered.

RETROSPECTIVE GENETIC COUNSELING   The prevention of genetic diseases requires the identification of matings that are capable of producing defective genotypes. These may involve matings in which one of the two individuals is carrying a dominant or X-linked gene mutation or a balanced translocation, or matings in which both individuals are carriers of a deleterious recessive gene. Such individuals are usually identified through an affected child or near relative, in which case retrospective genetic counseling can be provided.

When advising family members about the risk of transmitting a disorder that has already affected someone in the family, the counselor's first step is to be certain of the *correct diagnosis*—in particular, to make certain that the problem in question is really of genetic origin. This is especially important in disorders that may have either a genetic or a nongenetic etiology, such as deafness or mental retardation. Second, if the disease has a hereditary element, the possibility of *genetic heterogeneity,* i.e., a situation in which clinically similar genetic disorders show varying patterns of inheritance, must be considered. For example, there are two types of hereditary methemoglobinemia that resemble each other quite closely, but one shows autosomal recessive and the other autosomal dominant inheritance.

To estimate the *recurrence risk,* one must initially determine what is known of the genetic mechanisms controlling the relevant disorder. When more than one genetic mechanism exists, or when environmental factors can cause clinically indistinguishable traits, the *relative probabilities* of the different mechanisms operating in the particular family are computed. For conditions determined by simple mendelian inheritance, there is no difficulty in predicting the probability of an offspring being affected, provided that the genotypes of the parents can be recognized. Identification of the parental genotype is easiest for autosomal recessive and X-linked disorders since the basic lesions in these two forms of mendelian inheritance usually involve simple enzyme deficiencies for which biochemical tests are now available.

For autosomal dominant disorders, identification of the parental genotype is considerably more difficult since the basic defect is known for only a few of these disorders, and the diagnosis of the heterozygote for a dominant disorder depends almost exclusively on the clinical evaluation and a careful pedigree analysis. In counseling a family in which one relative is affected with a dominant disorder, it is important that appropriate clinical examination of all first-degree relatives and appropriately selected distant relatives be carried out. If relatives appear unaffected, there is the possibility that the clinical symptoms may be masked by *delayed age of onset* and *variability in expression.* When no relatives are affected, the possibility of a new dominant mutation must be entertained. Table 59-1

TABLE 59-1
Methods for detection of asymptomatic heterozygotes in frequently encountered dominantly inherited disorders

| Disorder | *Method of heterozygote detection* | | Therapeutic advantage of early diagnosis |
	Physical findings	*Laboratory tests*	
GASTROINTESTINAL, LIVER, AND PANCREAS			
Hemochromatosis		Serum iron	Prevent cirrhosis, heart failure, and diabetes
Gilbert's disease		Serum bilirubin	Avoid confusion with more serious forms of liver disease
Peutz-Jeghers syndrome	Melanin spots on lips, buccal mucosa, and digits	X-ray of small intestine	Clarify cause of gastrointestinal bleeding
Familial polyposis		X-ray of colon; colonoscopy	Prevent colon carcinoma
Gardner's syndrome	Multiple sebaceous cysts; lipomas; fibromas; osteomas; dental abnormalities; desmoid tumors	X-ray of colon and small intestine; colonoscopy	Prevent colon carcinoma
METABOLIC AND ENDOCRINE			
Medullary thyroid carcinoma-pheochromocytoma syndrome		Serum calcitonin; measurement of blood pressure	Prevent thyroid carcinoma and complications of hypertension
Multiple endocrine adenomatosis	Multiple lipomas	Serum calcium, gastrin, blood sugar; x-rays of sella turcica, stomach, and small intestine	Prevent complication of hyperparathyroidism, hypoglycemia, peptic ulcer, metastatic cancer
Familial hyperparathyroidism		Serum calcium, parathyroid hormone	Prevent renal damage and other complications of hypercalcemia
Familial hypercholesterolemia	Tendon xanthomas, xanthelasma, arcus corneae	Serum cholesterol; low-density lipoprotein receptor activity of cultured fibroblasts	Prevent premature coronary heart disease
HEART AND VASCULAR			
Holt-Oram syndrome	Abnormality of thumb and carpals; murmur of atrial septal defect	X-ray of hands; cardiac evaluation	Prevent complications of atrial septal defect
Noonan's syndrome	Hypertelorism; small chin; low-set ears; ptosis; pectus deformity; cryptorchidism; murmur of pulmonic stenosis	Cardiac evaluation; x-ray of skeleton; intravenous pyelogram (renal anomalies)	Prevent heart failure
Idiopathic hypertropic subaortic stenosis (asymmetric septal hypertrophy)	Presystolic gallop; characteristic carotid arterial pulse	ECG; echocardiogram	Prevent sudden death, syncope, angina, heart failure
Dominantly inherited form of atrial septal defect	Heart murmur	ECG showing first degree heart block, right bundle branch block, right axis deviation	Prevent complications of atrial septal defect
HEMATOLOGIC			
Hereditary spherocytosis	Splenomegaly; jaundice	Blood smear; reticulocyte count; hemoglobin; osmotic fragility test	Prevent anemia, cholethiasis
Hereditary hemorrhagic telangiectasia	Telangiectasia of tongue, lips, conjunctiva, ears, fingers; pulmonary AV fistula	X-ray of lungs	Clarify cause of nosebleeds and gastrointestinal bleeding

TABLE 59-1 (continued)
Methods for detection of asymptomatic heterozygotes in frequently encountered dominantly inherited disorders

Disorder	Method of heterozygote detection		Therapeutic advantage of early diagnosis
	Physical findings	Laboratory tests	
HEMATOLOGIC (continued)			
Von Willebrand's disease		Immunologic and functional assays of plasma antihemophilic globulin levels; bleeding time	Prevent gastrointestinal and urinary bleeding
CONNECTIVE TISSUE AND BONE			
Ehler-Danlos syndromes (types I, II, III)	Loose-jointedness; fragile, stretchable, bruisable skin; subcutaneous calcified spherules		
Marfan's syndrome	Ectopic lens; mitral and aortic murmurs; excessive length of extremities	Slit-lamp examination; metacarpal index by x-ray	Reduce risk of aortic dissection; prevent blindness
Osteogenesis imperfecta	Multiple fractures; loose-jointedness; blue scleras; deafness; aortic regurgitation	X-ray of bones	
RENAL			
Alport's syndrome	Nerve deafness; cataracts, lenticonus, spherophakia	Urinalysis, slit-lamp examination	Prevent uremia
Nail-patella syndrome	Dysplastic nails; absent patellas	X-ray of pelvis (iliac horns); urinalysis	Clarify cause of hematuria and azotemia
Polycystic kidney disease		Urinalysis; intravenous pyelogram; renal arteriogram; measurement of blood pressure	Prevent uremia and complications of hypertension
Renal tubular acidosis		X-ray of kidneys (nephrocalcinosis); urine pH, calcium; serum electrolytes, calcium	Prevent acidosis, osteoporosis, kidney stones
RESPIRATORY			
Hereditary angioneurotic edema		Serum level of Cl esterase inhibitor of complement	Reduce risk of sudden death caused by laryngeal edema and clarify cause of acute abdominal pain
DERMATOLOGIC			
Neurofibromatosis	Café au lait spots; neurofibromas; scoliosis		Prevent malignant degeneration of neurofibromas
Waardenburg syndrome	Wide bridge of nose; frontal white blaze of hair; heterochromia iridis; white eyelashes; deafness		Clarify cause of deafness
Basal-cell nevus syndrome	Multiple basal-cell carcinomas; jaw cysts; pits on palms and soles; skeletal defects (ribs, spina bifida, scoliosis)	X-rays of skull (calcification of falx cerebri) and skeleton	Removal of cutaneous cancers; provide cosmetic surgery
NEUROLOGIC			
Charcot-Marie-Tooth disease	Pes cavus; atrophy of anterior tibial and calf muscles ("stork legs"); absence of deep tendon reflexes	Biopsy of muscle and of sural cutaneous nerve	Improve walking by corrective shoes and orthopedic measures
Myotonic dystrophy	Myotonia; muscle wasting of temporal and sternocleidomastoid muscles; cataracts; frontal baldness; signs of hypogonadism	Slit-lamp examination; electromyography; measurement of serum immunoglobulins; electrocardiogram	Anticipate complete heart block
Acute intermittent porphyria		Measurement of uroporphyrinogen synthetase activity in red blood cells	Reduce risk of neuropathic attacks by avoidance of aggravating drugs such as barbiturates
Tuberous sclerosis	Adenoma sebaceum; cutaneous white macules; shagreen patch; periungual fibromas		Prevent seizures
Huntington's chorea	Paranoia, other personality changes; choreic movements; dementia		
Periodic paralysis syndromes (hypo-, hyper-, and normokalemic types)	Cold-induced myotonia	Electromyogram; serum potassium	Reduce frequency of attacks by avoidance of aggravating agents such as high-carbohydrate diet and exposure to cold
PHARMACOGENETIC			
Malignant hyperthermia		Serum creatine phosphokinase	Prevent fatal episode of hyperthermia induced by general anesthesia

lists the most commonly encountered dominant disorders affecting adults and the best clinical methods currently available for detection of the heterozygote.

When advising families about multifactorial genetic diseases, such as diabetes mellitus, in which the inheritance pattern is not clear-cut, the physician must resort to empiric risk estimates that have been derived from retrospectively assembled data (Table 58-4).

Once the parental genotypes are determined, the genetic prognosis is usually presented in terms of probability that a given couple will produce an affected offspring. The physician providing genetic counseling must make certain that the couple understands not only the meaning of such absolute risk figures, but also the severity of the disease and the variability in clinical expression. In other words, in dealing with a disorder such as neurofibromatosis, it is important for the parents to realize not only that they have a 50 percent risk of producing a child with this disorder but also that a certain proportion of patients with the disorder have severe disease, a certain proportion have mild disease, etc. They should also have an understanding of the potential impact of the disease on their family; a disease that is lethal at birth might be classified by some as more "severe" than one that is lethal at age 16, but the latter is likely to have a much more profound impact on the family.

Although different families initially react in different ways to the same risk, most couples who seek genetic advice can be expected to take a responsible course of action that is based on the information quoted. Generally, the physician should avoid giving direct advice to the couple as to whether they "should" or "should not" have children. For serious genetic disease, with a recurrence risk equal to or greater than 1 in 10, most parents are usually deterred from planning further children. When the risk is less than 1 in 10, most parents usually continue with additional pregnancies.

PROSPECTIVE GENETIC COUNSELING In contrast to retrospective genetic counseling in which advice is given after the birth of at least one affected family member, in prospective genetic counseling advice is provided to possible carriers of recessive genes before an affected individual is born. As a first step, this requires the identification of heterozygous individuals by a population-screening procedure. Second, unmarried heterozygotes are instructed about the risk of their having affected children if they marry another heterozygote for the same gene. Finally, if two heterozygotes are already married, there is the possibility of interrupting the birth of affected infants if the disease can be diagnosed in utero by amniocentesis.

Population screening for heterozygote detection is possible for several autosomal recessive disorders (such as sickle-cell anemia, thalassemia major, and Tay-Sachs disease) that occur in certain populations with high frequency. For example, 8 percent of the American black population are carriers of the sickling gene, and 4 percent of the American Jewish population of Eastern and Central European extraction are carriers of the Tay-Sachs gene.

Screening programs raise many ethical and social problems. Informing a healthy person that he or she is carrying a specific mutant gene that may cause disease in the children if a certain type of mate is chosen differs from counseling parents who have already had an affected child. Very little is known about the social and psychologic effects as well as occupational discrimination that may result from discovering that a person carries a "bad" gene.

PRENATAL DIAGNOSIS The use of transabdominal amniocentesis permits diagnosis of certain genetic diseases at a stage early enough to terminate a pregnancy and to prevent the birth of a defective child. This procedure gives high-risk couples the opportunity to have unaffected children provided they are willing for the pregnancy to be terminated in the event that an abnormal fetus is detected. Amniocentesis consists of the transabdominal aspiration of amniotic fluid from the uterus. The procedure is preferably performed between the fourteenth and sixteenth weeks of pregnancy. When performed by a trained gynecologist, the technique is relatively safe for both mother and fetus.

Direct examination of the amniotic fluid itself may be diagnostic. For example, an elevated level of α-fetoprotein is a relatively good indicator of the presence of spina bifida or some other related neural tube abnormality. More frequently, prenatal diagnosis requires culture of the fetal cells in vitro, a process which usually takes 3 weeks. By this means the karyotype of the fetus can be determined, to ascertain fetal sex and to detect various chromosomal aberrations. Moreover, many inborn errors of metabolism can be detected by suitable assays of specific enzyme activities in the cultured fetal cells. Table 59-2 lists those enzyme deficiency states for which prenatal diagnosis is currently feasible. More disorders are constantly being added to this list.

TABLE 59-2
Inborn errors of metabolism for which prenatal diagnosis is feasible

LIPIDOSES

Cholesteryl ester storage disease
Fabry's disease
Gaucher's disease
Krabbe's disease (globoid cell leukodystrophy)
Metachromatic leukodystrophy
Neimann-Pick disease
Refsum's syndrome
Tay-Sachs disease and other gangliosidoses
Wolman's syndrome

MUCOPOLYSACCHARIDOSES

β-Glucuronidase deficiency
Hunter's syndrome
Hurler's syndrome
Sanfilippo's syndrome
Scheie's syndrome

AMINO ACID AND RELATED DISORDERS

Argininosuccinicaciduria
Citrullinemia
Cystathionine synthetase deficiency (homocystinuria)
Cystinosis
Histidinemia
Maple syrup urine disease
Methylmalonic aciduria

DISORDERS OF CARBOHYDRATE METABOLISM

Fucosidosis
Galactosemia
Glucose 6-phosphate dehydrogenase deficiency
Glycogen storage diseases, types II, III, and IV
Mannosidosis

MISCELLANEOUS DISORDERS

Adenosine deaminase deficiency
Familial hypercholesterolemia, homozygous form
Hypophosphatasia
I-cell disease
Lesch-Nyhan syndrome
Lysosomal acid phosphatase deficiency
Orotic aciduria
Sickle-cell anemia
Testicular feminization
Thalassemia
Xeroderma pigmentosa

SOURCE: *Milunsky.*

TABLE 59-3
Major indications for prenatal diagnosis

TABLE 59-3
Major indications for prenatal diagnosis

Clinical situation	Estimated risk to fetus, %	Method of detection of abnormal fetus
Couples having a previous child with spina bifida or anencephaly	5	Measurement of α-fetoprotein in amniotic fluid
Couples having a previous child with a chromosomal disorder such as the trisomy 21 form of Down's syndrome	2	Chromosomal analysis of cultured amniotic fluid cells
Couples in whom either the husband or wife carries a balanced translocation for Down's syndrome	5–20	Chromosomal analysis of cultured amniotic cells
Pregnant women 38 years of age and older whose risk of having a child with Down's syndrome is increased	1–2	Chromosomal analysis of cultured amniotic fluid cells
Couples at risk for having a child with a detectable inborn error of metabolism (see Table 59-2)	25 or 50	Biochemical analysis of cultured amniotic fluid cells

Prenatal diagnosis by amniocentesis is currently indicated in the following high-risk situations: (1) couples having a previous child with spina bifida or anencephaly, (2) couples having a previous child with a chromosomal aberration such as the trisomy 21 form of Down's syndrome, (3) couples in whom either the husband or wife carries a balanced translocation

chromosome for Down's syndrome, (4) couples at high risk for having a child with a detectable inborn error of metabolism, and (5) pregnant women 38 years of age and older. Table 59-3 lists the major indications for prenatal diagnosis, the risks involved, and methods by which the abnormal fetus can be detected.

APPROACHES TO TREATMENT

The goal of treatment for genetic diseases is to modify the natural history of the genetic trait so that an affected person may live a comfortable and healthy life despite a mutant genotype. Such treatment can be achieved for a number of inherited diseases using a variety of approaches, including (1) the exclusion or restriction of toxic foods, (2) metabolic supplementation, (3) removal of toxic products, (4) surgery, and (5) organ transplantation. Table 59-4 lists examples of hereditary diseases affecting adults that can be successfully treated at the present time.

REFERENCES

Epstein CJ: Prenatal diagnosis of genetic disorders. Adv Intern Med 20:325, 1975

Milunsky A: *The Prevention of Genetic Disease and Mental Retardation.* Philadelphia, Saunders, 1975

Stanbury JB et al: *The Metabolic Basis of Inherited Disease,* 4th ed. New York, McGraw-Hill, 1978

World Health Organization: *Genetic Disorders: Prevention, Treatment, and Rehabilitation.* WHO Tech Rep 497, 1972

TABLE 59-4
Some treatable hereditary disorders affecting adults

Method of treatment	Disorder
REDUCTION OF TOXIC FOOD	
Lactose	Lactase deficiency
Galactose	Galactosemia
Fructose	Fructose intolerance
Neutral fats	Familial lipoprotein lipase deficiency
Cholesterol and saturated fats	Familial hypercholesterolemia
Phytanic acid	Refsum's syndrome
Phenylalanine	Phenylketonuria
METABOLIC SUPPLEMENTATION	
Vitamin D and phosphate	Hypophosphatemic rickets
Gamma globulin	Agammaglobulinemia
Factor VIII (AHG)	Hemophilia
Cortisol	Adrenogenital syndromes
Thyroxine	Familial goiters
Growth hormone	Pituitary dwarfism
REMOVAL OF TOXIC PRODUCT	
Cystine removal by D-penicillamine	Cystinuria
Copper removal by D-penicillamine	Wilson's disease
Iron removal by phlebotomy	Hemochromatosis
SURGERY	
Splenectomy	Hereditary spherocytosis
Portacaval shunt	Glycogen storage disease, type I
Colectomy	Familial polyposis of the colon
Thyroidectomy	Medullary thyroid carcinoma syndrome
ORGAN TRANSPLANTATION	
Kidney	Fabry's disease
Kidney	Adult polycystic kidney disease

60
CYTOGENETIC ASPECTS OF HUMAN DISEASE

JAMES GERMAN

The chromosome complement of humans, like that of other species, is guarded carefully against change; most chromosome mutations, either structural or numerical, are deleterious. Only rarely is a balanced structural rearrangement (one that results in neither deficiency nor duplication of significant chromosome segments) introduced into the population and transmitted from generation to generation. (Figure 60-1 shows the normal human chromosome complement. In the legend of the figure several terms used in human cytogenetics are defined.) As a rule an abnormal number of autosomes results in early death, except for trisomy of the shortest chromosome. In contrast, an abnormal number of sex chromosomes is often tolerated reasonably well, although infertility or subfertility usually is present. Nevertheless, among human embryos abnormalities in chromosome structure and number are common and are, in fact, the major known cause of embryonic and early fetal wastage. However, not every fetus with an abnormal chromosome complement is aborted, and those that survive constitute the material of medical cytogenetics.

Clinical disorders resulting from chromosome imbalance present varying features including abnormal anatomic development, mental retardation, behavioral disorders, and disturbances in growth and sexual development. Sometimes infertility, repeated abortion, or the birth of malformed children is the presenting complaint of persons with abnormal chromosome complements whose own general development is normal.

The disorders just referred to are due to chromosome imbalance that affects tissues throughout the body. In addition, change can occur in the chromosome complement in a single cell of some somatic tissue. Such a mutant cell may have a proliferative advantage over normal cells, in which case a clone bearing the abnormal chromosome complement can develop amid otherwise normal cells. Although such mutant clones are in many cases clinically insignificant, much evidence suggests that they are also important in the etiology of cancer.

This chapter is addressed to those aspects of normal chromosome structure and function that constitute the basis for an understanding of the chromosome alterations in human disease. In addition, the classes of alterations important in adult medicine and their consequences are summarized.

CHROMOSOME STRUCTURE AND FUNCTION The human autosomes are numbered 1 through 22, and the sex chromosomes are denoted X and Y (Fig. 60-1). Each is recognizable microscopically by morphological features such as relative length and position of the centromere and by staining characteristics (banding pattern). Each mammalian chromosome is believed to be composed of one double-stranded chain of deoxyribonucleic acid (DNA) that extends from one end through the centromere to the other end.

FIGURE 60-1
Normal human lymphocyte chromosomes arrested in metaphase and stained for G bands (G standing for Giemsa). The inset shows the arrangement of chromosomes in an intact cell, and the remainder of the figure shows their ordered arrangement into a karyotype. By the time mitosis begins, each chromosome consists of two identical parts called sister chromatids and is identified by the relative length, the location of the centromere, and a distinctive sequence of bands of varying lengths and depth of staining. Normally, the G-band patterns of the two chromosomes of a pair are alike, with the exception of certain polymorphic regions, examples of which are shown in Fig. 60-3.

The centromere of a chromosome divides it into a short arm (p) and a long arm (q). Numbers 13 to 15, 21, 22, and Y are called acrocentric because of the nearly terminal positions of their centromeres; the minute p of each acrocentric autosome bears a nucleolus-organizing region which

often causes a secondary constriction in the metaphase chromosome (the constriction at the centromere is the primary constriction). Telomeres are the nonvisible, somewhat theoretical, "structures" at the ends of each chromosome.

By standard nomenclature, this karyotype is described as 46,XY, indicating that its chromosome number is 46, its sex chromosomes are an X and a Y, and the autosomes (those besides the X and Y) number 44. The following examples show the general use of this nomenclature: A normal female karyotype is described as 46,XX. A female cell with an extra chromosome 18 (trisomic for 18) would be described as 47,XX,+18. A cell with only one sex chromosome, an X, and with deletion in the short arm of chromosome 5 would be described as 45,X,5p−. A male cell with a translocation between the long arm of chromosome 2 and the short arm of chromosome 3 would be described as 46,XY,t(2q;3p); exact breakpoints could be indicated by additional characters and symbols.

FIGURE 60-2

Schematic representation of the mitotic and meiotic cell division cycles, as described in the text. G_1 and G_2 = time gaps before and after S, the period in which DNA replicates. Each of these intervals is several hours in duration; together they constitute interphase. M = mitosis; I and II = the two divisions of meiosis. The DNA content of the cycling cells is indicated on the vertical axis: $1c$ = the content in a gamete; $2c$ = that in either an egg immediately postfertilization or a somatic cell emerging from mitosis; $4c$ = the amount in a cell which has completed chromosome duplication and is ready to enter mitosis or meiosis.

Cell division cycle Chromosomes must duplicate before cell division can occur. This duplication occurs over a period of several hours prior to the onset of mitosis or meiosis in a phase of the cell cycle termed S, for synthesis of DNA (Fig. 60-2). Thus, from the completion of S to the completion of metaphase, each chromosome contains two identical double-stranded chains of DNA, and the nucleus contains four times as much DNA as a spermatozoan or ovum. During mitosis chromosomes are condensed, and the two sister chromatids can be visualized by late prophase or early metaphase (Fig. 60-1). (Metaphase is the stage in the cell division cycle ordinarily employed for cytogenetic analysis.)

At the onset of anaphase the centromeric regions of each chromosome separate, and the two chromatids move quickly to opposite poles of the mitotic spindle. As soon as each pole receives one full complement of chromatids (chromosomes), a nuclear membrane (disassembled late in prophase) is reassembled about each cluster to complete formation of the nuclei of the two sister cells that emerge at telophase. The sister cells emerge in what is usually called the G_1 phase of the cell cycle, in which they remain unreplicated unless another division is to be prepared for, whereupon they enter the S phase. Cells engaged in some differentiated function ordinarily remain unreplicated.

Most normal cells in the human body are diploid; i.e., they have twice the haploid number (the number in a gamete) of chromosomes (haploid = 23, diploid = 46). In the germ cell line, which is devoted to gamete formation, cells destined eventually to differentiate into spermatozoa or ova undergo mitotic cell cycles until they enter the two specialized divisions termed *meiosis*. In meiosis, pairing of homologous chromosomes occurs (the paternally derived chromosome 1 with the maternally derived chromosome 1, and so on), and genetic recombination takes place (see Chap. 58). At the first meiotic division homologous chromosomes are segregated, and the diploid chromosome number is reduced to the haploid; i.e., each cell then contains one each of the 22 (duplicated) autosomes plus one

(duplicated) sex chromosome. No S phase takes place between the first and second meiotic divisions (depicted in Fig. 60-2, right) so that at the second division, in which sister chromatids separate, emerging cells maintain the haploid number of chromosomes but are reduced in their content of DNA to half the amount of diploid G_1 cells of somatic tissues. With fertilization of an ovum by a spermatozoan, both the chromosome constitution and the DNA content of the zygote are restored to that of a G_1 somatic cell. An S period in the zygote then permits reinstitution of regular cell-division cycles characteristic of the somatic cells.

Chromosome differentiation A chromosome is differentiated along its length, and some aspects of this differentiation are resolvable in the light microscope. The DNA is complexed with a number of proteins in a highly specific way. The DNA-protein complex together with some associated ribonucleic acid (RNA) is referred to as *chromatin*. The fine structure and the manner in which the DNA is compacted and interacted with proteins are thought to pertain to the control of RNA production and DNA replication, perhaps to cellular differentiation itself.

The sequences of nucleotide bases in DNA that constitute the genes and that can be transcribed into messenger RNA are distributed throughout the length of the various chromosomes. (These sequences are too short to be resolved microscopically.) Over a hundred genes have been mapped to specific chromosomes, in many cases to specific regions of a chromosome; for example, the Rh blood group locus is on the short arm of chromosome 1, and the ABO blood group locus has been assigned to a band near the end of the long arm of chromosome 9.

Certain segments of at least 12 chromosomes vary in length among individuals. These segments can be delineated by their staining characteristics (Fig. 60-3). The variable segments consist of nontranscribed, highly repetitive nucleotide sequences of DNA and are transmitted from parent to child in a straightforward mendelian fashion. Variations in these segments are unassociated with detectable phenotypic effect. (They can serve as useful cell markers in determination of zygosity of twins, paternity, and survival of transplants.)

FIGURE 60-3

Metaphase chromosomes stained for C bands (C standing for centromeric or constitutive heterochromatin), showing inherited variation in lengths of C bands in chromosome 1 (arrows).

Other microscopically recognizable segments in the short arms of the acrocentric autosomes are devoted to the production of ribosomal RNA and nucleoli. As mitosis progresses, these nucleolus-organizer regions tend to remain relatively uncondensed later than other regions. Consequently, at metaphase they appear understained and thereby demarcate condensed segments of chromatin distal to them on the chromosome arms—*satellites*. (Satellites are examples of the polymorphic segments just mentioned.) Other examples of segmental specialization along the chromosome include regions known as *telomeres* and *centromeres*. Telomeres, the distal termini of each arm, have some relationship to the nuclear membrane and probably are important in the maintenance of the order of the interphase nucleus; centromeric regions are sites of microtubule attachment at metaphase.

A further example of chromosome differentiation is the established sequence by which various segments replicate during S; certain segments replicate early, others late. In general, late replication of a chromosome segment correlates with genetic inertness. This correlation is exemplified by one of the two X chromosomes in female cells; the chromosome inactivated by the Lyon effect is almost entirely late-replicating (see Chap. 58 for an explanation of the Lyon hypothesis).

A little-understood type of chromatin is that which has long been referred to as *heterochromatin*. It is tightly condensed, not just at metaphase but throughout interphase. Such condensation of chromatin correlates positively with genetic inactivity and also with late replication. Some regions are condensed and inactive in all cells (constitutive heterochromatin), while others, for example, the X chromosome, may be either condensed and inactive or unwound and active (facultative heterochromatin). Many chromosome imbalances that permit viability beyond intrauterine life involve chromosome segments that are rich in this apparently inactive, or inactivatable, type of chromatin, e.g., chromosomes that can be trisomic in live-born individuals or, in the case of X, monosomic. The activity of genes can sometimes be affected, even inactivated, if they are positioned near regions of heterochromatin.

Therefore, in chromosomal imbalance both the specific genetic loci and the particular types of chromatin deleted or duplicated are important. Also, the significance of a structural rearrangement probably depends on the new and abnormal positioning of structural and regulatory genes in relation to each other and to heterochromatin.

Fortunately for the cytologist, several differentiated features of the chromosome correlate with cytological artifacts that can be produced and visualized in the laboratory. A number of techniques are now in use to display a pattern of bands of various lengths and staining characteristics (Figs. 60-1 and 60-3). These patterns are identical in each chromosome 1, each chromosome 2, etc., varying only in the inert polymorphic regions mentioned above, so that they can be used in clinical cytogenetics to identify chromosomes and to detect and define structural rearrangements.

Sources of error Every aspect of the cell division cycle is complicated. Doubtless a large number of genetic loci must be active to produce the numerous enzymes and structural proteins required to initiate and complete a cycle. Remarkable precision and accuracy are demanded over and over in matters such as the passage of a cell from G_1 into S, orderly progression of replication, assembly of the mitotic spindle, and spindle function in segregating chromatids during mitosis. An additional battery of loci is activated to permit a cell of the germ line to pass successfully through the complicated stages of meiotic prophase, including pairing of homologous chromosomes, genetic recombination, and then disjoining of chromosomes. Probably all these mechanisms and processes are subject to

FIGURE 60-4

Breaks and rearrangements (arrows) in metaphase chromosomes of a blood lymphocyte that received γ-ray irradiation before being stimulated by phytohemagglutinin to enter S and divide.

errors, some spontaneous, others promoted by some unfavorable environmental influence (Fig. 60-4) or by the presence of deleterious mutations involving one of the many steps just mentioned. Furthermore, the genetic material itself is subject to damage, and an unrepaired or erroneously repaired lesion in DNA theoretically may predispose to chromosome rearrangement. Errors at many of these steps lie behind chromosome imbalance. Errors that occur in germ cells, during fertilization, and in early postfertilization divisions are important in relation to embryonic maldevelopment and infertility; errors in somatic cells may be important in relation to neoplasia.

CHROMOSOME ABNORMALITIES Mutations of a single base in a gene and small chromosome deletions and duplications are not visible to the cytogeneticist. In fact, for the normal chromosome banding pattern to be detectably disturbed, a lengthy segment of DNA must be deleted, duplicated, or transposed. This means that a microscopically detectable chromosome mutation must involve relatively huge amounts of DNA. It is noteworthy, however, that the same environmental agents known to produce point mutations (mutagens in the usual sense) are in general also chromosome-breaking agents and vice versa. Thus, it seems safe to assume the existence of a spectrum extending from mutations visible to the cytogeneticist to those that must be defined by nucleotide sequencing. Mutations visible to the cytogeneticist ordinarily exert a more widespread effect on development than do point mutations; ordinary genes—often many of them—as well as other specialized types of chromatin, whose function is unknown, are involved in cytologically visible mutations.

If an entire chromosome is affected in an imbalance, the genome is said to be either trisomic or monosomic for the chromosome (thus, trisomy 13, monosomy X). Genes and chromatin carried on the affected chromosome then are present in triple or single dose, respectively, rather than the normal double dose. Abnormal dosage affecting less than an entire chromosome, the result of chromosome breakage and rearrangement, is often termed *partial trisomy* or *partial monosomy*, to indicate that segments rather than entire chromosomes are involved (thus, partial trisomy 13q, partial monosomy 4p).

Incidence The frequency with which chromosomal imbalance is detectable depends on the population investigated. It is estimated that a minimum of 1 in 10 recognized conceptions has a chromosome abnormality. In human embryos and fetuses aborted spontaneously, the incidence of chromosome imbalance is higher the earlier in pregnancy the sampling is made. The contribution of imbalance to late abortion and stillbirth, though not well studied yet, probably also is significant. In the more than 50,000 consecutive or random live-born babies that have now been examined in different laboratories, approximately 1 in 200 has a significant chromosome abnormality, either numerical or structural. In such studies, at least 1 in 700 newborns is trisomic for one of the autosomes 21, 18, or 13; about 1 in 350 newborn males has the complement 47,XXY or 47,XYY. One in every several thousand newborns has monosomy X. One in five hundred has some structural rearrangement, most of which are genetically balanced. Samplings of the general adult population reveal an occasional inherited balanced structural rearrangement as well as the expected number of XXY, XYY, and XXX complements; the inherited, apparently innocuous segmental polymorphisms (e.g., Fig. 60-3) and minor structural rearrangements demonstrable by banding techniques are found in abundance.

In populations of individuals with mental retardation, 10 to 15 percent have a chromosome abnormality, the proportion being greater if there also are anatomic malformations. In some groups of male criminals and in all infertile men, an increased incidence of individuals with an extra sex chromosome, an X or a Y, is found. Infertile women also include many individuals with extra or missing sex chromosomes and an appreciable number with structural chromosome rearrangement; approximately one-fourth of women with primary amenorrhea have some abnormality of the X chromosome. Among infertile men and women, individuals with genes that interfere with meiosis, so-called "meiotic mutants," are also found occasionally.

Numerical abnormalities Trisomy (47 chromosomes) is the most common chromosome imbalance in early spontaneous abortuses, followed by monosomy (45 chromosomes) and triploidy (69 chromosomes). The extra or missing chromosomes can be either paternal or maternal in origin, and the error in segregation of chromosomes can occur in the germ line, fertilized egg (zygote), or early embryo. Trisomy of every chromosome has been observed in spontaneous abortions, trisomy 16 most frequently.

Sex chromosomal trisomy (XXY, XYY, and XXX) is compatible with intrauterine survival; in contrast, autosomal trisomy rarely permits survival to term. However, a small proportion of autosomal trisomics is live-born. For practical purposes these are only trisomy 21, 18, and 13, in decreasing frequency. Trisomies 18 and 13 cause death during infancy. Trisomies of significance in adults are trisomy 21, XXY, XXX, and XYY. A few other autosomal trisomies, such as trisomy 8, have occasionally been reported, usually in mosaicism with a normal cellular component. (Mosaicism is the coexistence of multiple, genetically different populations of cells, derived originally from a single zygote.)

Autosomal monosomy is rare even among abortion material. In contrast, monosomy X (45,X) occurs in approximately 1.5 percent of recognized conceptions. It is common (approximately 10 percent) among spontaneously aborted human embryos and is present in one in every several thousand live-born babies. The reason for the death of 45,X embryos and fetuses is unknown, although developmental abnormalities doubtless contribute to it; cardiovascular and renal anomalies are common in the few that survive. In monosomy X, the missing sex chromosome can be either a Y or an X and is either paternal or maternal in origin. Often the second sex chromosome is not completely absent but is replaced by a structurally rearranged Y or X. Mosaicism is common in live-borns with monosomy X; here, tissues are populated not only by cells with a 45,X complement but by other cells, perhaps with a normal complement, either 46,XY or 46,XX, or with a complement in which the second sex chromosome is rearranged in some way.

Triploidy is rare in live-born babies and usually leads to early death, even when in a mosaicism with normal cells: 46,XY/69,XXY. The phenotypic effects of the autosomal trisomies, of 47,XXY, and of monosomy X (45,X) are characteristic and well defined so that their diagnosis usually is not difficult. The effects of the 47,XYY and 47,XXX constitutions are less striking, and therefore these complements are underdiagnosed. Mosaicism with coexistence of abnormal and normal populations of cells can cause an abnormal phenotype to approach the normal.

The mechanisms responsible for the numerical abnormalities are undefined and may be multiple. A striking but unexplained maternal age effect exists in trisomies 21, 18, 13, XXY, and XXX. Over one-third of babies with trisomy 21 are born to women over 35, whereas only one-tenth of all births occur in this group. The frequency of trisomy 21 rises from 0.5 to 0.7 per 1000 live births between ages 21 and 23 to 3.1 per 1000 at age 35, 10.5 per 1000 at age 40, and 33.6 per 1000 at age 45. (A paternal age effect may also exist in trisomy 21.) Maternal x-ray irradiation in low dosage is also associated with an increased incidence of trisomy 21. After a child with trisomy 21 is born, the risk to the parents of recurrence in future pregnancies is increased to approximately 1 percent. As to the etiology of monosomy X, the frequent association of the 45,X complement in mosaicism with normal complements and with structural rearrangements of the X and Y suggests that the zygote or early embryo may often be the target of a chromosome-breaking event.

Structural abnormalities Some structural chromosome rearrangements are inherited, and others represent new mutations. The etiology of the new rearrangements is unknown, although they are assumed to be partly spontaneous and partly the effect of environmental agents such as mutagenic chemicals or ionizing radiation acting on the germ line, zygote, or early embryo (Fig. 60-4).

Many of the known chromosome rearrangements have been detected only once or a few times. Others are detected repeatedly, the same one occurring in unrelated individuals and families. For example, the commonest translocation, one that can occur either as a result of de novo mutation or by inheritance, affects one chromosome 13 and one 14 at or near their centromeres. In this translocation, only inert chromatin is lost from the tiny short arms. A similar translocation affecting chromosomes 14 and 21 is also common.

Chromosome complements bearing rearrangements can be genetically balanced or effectively so, thus imparting no unfavorable phenotypic effect to their bearers; about two-thirds of rearrangements detected during surveys of consecutive live-born babies are balanced. Or the complement can be unbalanced and affect development unfavorably, the usual case when rearrangements are detected during surveys of spontaneous abortuses or of individuals with multiple anomalies and mental retardation.

Some balanced rearrangements are transmitted from generation to generation without producing clinical effects. In other cases, however, they are profoundly important to members of the kindred transmitting them, by being responsible for the conception of embryos with unbalanced genomes. For example, bearers of some 13;14 translocations are at risk of having children with the trisomy 13 syndrome, and inherited translocations involving chromosome 21 predispose to the trisomy 21 syndrome. Approximately 5 percent of live-borns with the trisomy 21 syndrome have a translocation, and in about a fifth of those it is detectable in one of the parents. Because most babies with the trisomy 21 syndrome due to translocation are born to women under 30, a search for a translocation is important when a child with this clinical syndrome is born to young parents.

Different translocations bestow on their carriers different risks of having offspring with unbalanced rearrangements. These risks cannot be predicted on the theoretical basis of the way the translocation might be expected to behave during meiosis. Useful empiric risk figures have been accumulated for common translocations; e.g., the 14;21 translocation bestows a 2 percent risk on a balanced male carrier and more than a 10 percent risk on a female carrier of having a child with the trisomy 21 syndrome. In constrast, the balanced carrier of a 21;21 translocation can expect only unbalanced offspring. Information of this type is indispensable to those undertaking genetic counseling in relation to chromosome disorders.

Although the phenotypic effects of many of the different segmental chromosome imbalances which can occur are varied and nonspecific, the resulting anomalies sometimes compose a recognizable clinical syndrome. Two examples are the following: (1) If a rearrangement causes partial trisomy of the distal band of the long arm of 21, the clinical features composing the full syndrome associated with an extra chromosome 21 develop. (A triple dose of other segments of the long arm of chromosome 21 also produces adverse effects but not the trisomy 21 syndrome.) (2) Partial monosomy of a short segment within the short arm of chromosome 5 causes mental retardation, a characteristic facies, and a characteristic cry during infancy. This group of signs is known as the *5p−* or *cri-du-chat syndrome*.

Because of the large number of karyotype-phenotype correlations made in recent years, additional specific syndromes produced by imbalance of many different segments now are known, e.g., the 4p−, 9p partial trisomy, 13q−, and 18q− syndromes, to name a few. Rearrangements not previously described and their corresponding clinical syndromes are still being recognized. Any of these syndromes may appear as result either of de novo chromosome rearrangement or through formation of a genetically unbalanced gamete in a person carrying in balanced state a rearrangement affecting the segment involved. Families transmitting an unusual rearrangement in balanced form are said, because of the recurrence of individuals with the same specific imbalance, to have *private syndromes*.

In most individuals with chromosome imbalance, regardless of which segments are affected, a degree of phenotypic similarity is present. These recurring and nonspecific features include mental retardation, growth retardation, dysmorphic ears, nose, and mouth, cardiac malformations of standard types, abnormalities of dermal ridges and creases, and dysmorphic digits. (As a rule, autosomal imbalance need not be considered in the etiology of anatomic defects unaccompanied by mental retardation.) Why similar abnormalities occur with so many different segmental imbalances is unknown, but when several such features are observed in a single individual, they can be a valuable clinical indication for cytogenetic analysis. Imbalance affecting certain segments also causes specific phenotypic changes; an example is the anomalous cry in the 5p− syndrome mentioned above. Another example of specificity is retinoblastoma, which may develop when one particular band of chromosome 13 is present in single dose. Whereas the nonspecific changes serve to call the clinician's attention to the possibility of some chromosome imbalance, the specific features can suggest the exact segment of the genome affected.

DISEASE ASSOCIATIONS Various combinations of abnormalities in malformed and defective individuals have been correlated with variations in the chromosome complement. In this way, clinical syndromes due to specific chromosome imbalances have been defined. (Many of the pediatric conditions are of little significance in adult medicine because of their lethality in infancy or early childhood.)

Autosome imbalance Of the three autosomal trisomies found in live-born babies, only trisomy 21 is compatible with survival past infancy. The phenotype produced by the presence of an extra chromosome 21, formerly known as *mongolism* but now termed the *Down syndrome* or *trisomy 21 syndrome,* is characteristic and easily diagnosed from birth: mental retardation, short stature, muscular hypotonia, brachycephaly, short neck, typical facies (oblique orbital fissures, flat nasal bridge, small simple or folded ears, nystagmus, mouth hanging open), narrow palate, short broad hands with incurving fifth fingers, gaps between the first and second toes, and characteristic dermatoglyphics. Additional findings may include congenital heart disease, blepharitis and conjunctivitis, Brushfield's spots of the iris, straight pubic hair, abnormal teeth, protruding furrowed tongue, high-arched palate, loose skin of the neck, transverse palmar creases, and hyperflexibility of the joints. Cardiac malformations lead to death in infancy in a third of individuals with trisomy 21, and other malformations and infections may also cause early death. However, subjects who survive infancy often reach adulthood, and some even old age. The proneness to develop leukemia in affected infants is not maintained in later life. Females occasionally become pregnant, and, as expected, approximately half their children have trisomy 21.

Mosaicism of trisomy 21 with normal cells $(46/47, +21)$ may occur in individuals with modified features of the trisomy 21 syndrome, and it is probable that many individuals with this mosaicism go unrecognized. The risk of such persons having trisomic children is increased, but unfortunately their mosaicism is usually detected only after they have had an affected child. Partial trisomy, partial monosomy, or a combination of the two explains many of the instances in both children and adults of multiple developmental defects combined with mental retardation. Sometimes a balanced autosomal translocation is detected in normally developed adults who have repeated spontaneous abortion or subnormal fertility, with or without abnormal live-born children.

Sex chromosome imbalance (see also Chap. 344) In contrast to autosome imbalance, sex chromosome imbalance has relatively mild phenotypic effects. This is because X chromosomes beyond one in the complement of somatic cells are usually inactivated and because the Y chromosome bears few if any genes other than the testis determinants. X-linked loci (in contrast to autosomal loci) function normally in single dose: the male is hemizygous for X-linked genes, having only one X chromosome (with the possible exception of a few loci on the Y that may be homologous to a segment on the X); the female is functionally hemizygous through the Lyon effect. The addition of an extra sex chromosome to the normal male or female complement has a phenotypic effect but insufficient to interfere with intrauterine survival. Since major anatomic defects are usually absent, individuals with the complements 47,XXY and 47,XYY, both of whom are males, and 47,XXX, who are females, ordinarily go unrecognized till adolescence or later, often never to be diagnosed at all.

The *Klinefelter syndrome* (Chap. 344), which in classic form consists of small testes, infertility, gynecomastia, and variable degrees of underandrogenization, sometimes with mild mental retardation, antisocial behavior, or both, is the consequence of the addition of an extra X to the male complement: 47,XXY. The extra X interferes in some way with the survival of germ cells, and atrophy of the spermatogenic tubules and azoospermia are the consequence. Sometimes the phenotypic effects are surprisingly mild, the testicular atrophy being the only noteworthy feature in otherwise healthy and socially well-adjusted men. The mosaicism 46,XY/47,XXY sometimes occurs and may ameliorate the phenotypic effect of the extra X. More extreme phenotypic effects and mental retardation result when more than one extra sex chromosome is added to the normal male complement: 48,XXXX or 49,XXXXX.

The phenotypic effect of 47,XYY is less well defined; although increased height, behavioral difficulties, and infertility are common, the extra Y is sometimes found in otherwise normal men. The rare complement 48,XXYY results in infertility, probably because of the extra X, as in the 47,XXY Klinefelter's syndrome. The phenotype associated with 47,XXX is also poorly defined, but women with mild mental retardation, psychosis, and menstrual abnormalities are increased in frequency; this complement is sometimes detected in normal, healthy women. Further clarification is needed concerning the effects on personality and behavior of all three complements: 47,XXY, 47,XYY, and 47,XXX.

Loss of the Y or of the second X has drastic effects on development. If it does not cause abortion, it may or may not be recognizable at birth. Loose nuchal folds and edema of the hands and feet in a newborn girl, with or without renal or cardiovascular anomalies, may point to the diagnosis of the 45,X complement. The *Turner syndrome* is the manifestation in subsequent life (Chap. 344): short stature resistant to all treatment, infantilism of otherwise normal female external and internal genitalia, germ-cell-free gonads referred to as *gonadal streaks,* and variable renal, cardiovascular, skeletal, and ectodermal anomalies. Without estrogen administration breast development remains infantile, and menstruation does not occur. Although mental retardation is not a feature, a poorly defined emotional immaturity and difficulty with spatial perception are common.

The Turner syndrome may be the developmental consequence of several chromosome constitutions besides 45,X. Mosaicism as well as structural abnormalities of a second sex chromosome, either a Y or an X, cause a spectrum of disorders at both the clinical and cytogenetic levels. A normal male or normal female cellular component may be present along with the 45,X cellular component, or one component may bear a structurally abnormal chromosome. Common abnormalities of the Y and X are isochromosome formation (one arm deleted and the other duplicated) or deletion of part of or all one arm. In some affected individuals, all cells have 46 chromosomes, with one normal X plus an abnormal Y or X, for example, 46,XXp− deletion from the short arm of one of the X chromosomes. In others, a second or third cellular component may be present as well, for example, 45,X/46,XX/46,XXp−. Clinically pure Turner syndrome may be found in association with various combinations of these karyotypes if one of them is either monosomic or partially monosomic for X. However, when Y-bearing cells coexist with the 45,X cells, for example, 45,X/46,XY, genital ambiguity often develops, and gonads may vary from streaks to functional testes (the syndrome of *mixed gonadal dysgenesis*); here the risk of malignant gonadal tumors is significant. When 46,XX cells coexist with 45,X, varying degrees of ovarian function may be maintained, including ovulation. Although the phenotype may approach a normal male or female pattern when normal and abnormal

cells coexist, the effects of mosaicism are unpredictable. Thus, the clinical syndrome associated with monosomy X and structurally abnormal Ys or Xs ranges from a predominantly male phenotype through Turner syndrome to an almost normal female phenotype.

Two other rare conditions deserve mention—*true hermaphroditism* and the *46,XX male* (see also Chap. 344). *True hermaphroditism* is present when both testicular and ova- and follicle-containing ovarian tissue exist in the same individual. In most cases, 46,XX is the chromosome complement, and it appears normal by banding; here the most plausible explanation is that an occult translocation of the testis-determining segment of the Y to an X or autosome has occurred. Sometimes true hermaphrodites have the complement 46,XY; rarely the chimerism 46,XY/46,XX is found, the two cellular components having been derived from two zygotes.

Males occasionally have the complement 46,XX. As in 47,XXY men, the second X interferes with meiosis, and azoospermia results. In both the 46,XX true hermaphrodite and the *46,XX male* the rule that a Y is required for testicular differentiation appears to break down. However, the two conditions may have the same etiologic basis, undetected translocation of Y material onto another chromosome.

Chromosome change in cancer The theory that an alteration in the chromosomal complement may be the cause of cancer was advanced almost seven decades ago, but the matter is still unsettled. Chromosome changes are plentiful in cancer, but this very fact—too many changes—has been a major reason many have rejected them as of etiologic significance. However, support for the idea that chromosome alteration is significant in the etiology of human cancer has come from two observations: (1) the known environmental "causes" of human cancer (carcinogenic chemicals and ionizing radiation) are also chromosome-breaking agents (Fig. 60-4); and (2) three recessively inherited disorders result in increased chromosome breakage and rearrangement in cells in culture, and in each the risk of cancer is increased—Bloom's syndrome, Fanconi's anemia, and ataxia-telangiectasia (the Louis-Bar syndrome). Thus, the known environmental and the known genetic causes of increased chromosome mutation all predispose to cancer.

Many human cancers have altered chromosome complements. In the leukemias, lymphomas, and certain myeloproliferative disorders, the alterations are less extensive than in solid tumors and, therefore, easier to define. In certain lymphomas, chromosome 14 is often found to have undergone structural rearrangement. In over 80 percent of chronic granulocytic leukemias, a translocation affecting chromosome 22 (usually chromosome 9 is the other chromosome affected) is detected, the so-called "Ph[1] chromosome"; if the disease progresses into a "blastic" phase, the karyotype often evolves, certain additional chromosome changes being added stepwise in a nonrandom sequence. In this leukemia and in a few others, the various chromosome changes appear to have some value in prognosis and choice of therapy. In most other leukemias, detectable karyotypic specificity is less impressive so far.

Solid tumors, which generally are studied later in their course than conditions affecting the bone marrow, show extensive karyotypic changes, both structural and numerical. Different cells from a single tumor have similar numerical changes and structural rearrangements, but in the same type tumor from another person the changes are usually different. This apparent lack of specificity is partly due to the complexity of the changes, however, and a few examples of chromosome alterations specific for a solid tumor are known; for example, meningiomas are associated with a deletion of chromosome 22 in almost every case. The findings in both solid tumors and leukemias demonstrate the clonal nature of human cancer.

TECHNICAL CONSIDERATIONS Human metaphase chromosomes can be examined in any tissue in which sufficient cells are cycling. Preparations can therefore be made directly from almost any embryonic tissue and from adult bone marrow, lymphoid tissue, and malignant tissues. In searches for mosaicism, the study of multiple tissues is often required. Some tissues unlikely to yield cells in metaphase can be placed in culture, and chromosome preparations can be made after many cells have been brought into mitosis. Blood lymphocytes stimulated to enter cell division cycles by phytohemagglutinin are the standard material for diagnosing constitutional chromosome imbalance. In some myeloproliferative disorders and leukemias, unstimulated circulating blood cells divide spontaneously after a few hours in culture. Long-term cultures of fibroblasts can be derived from minute skin biopsies or from most any tissue, although more elaborate laboratory facilities and a longer period of time are required before cytogenetic preparations can be made. Amniotic fluid is among the sources of cells suitable for culture, and these embryonic cells are widely used in the diagnosis of fetal chromosome imbalance.

Nucleated cells in interphase can be used for the study of sex chromatin. Cells from buccal mucosa and hair follicles are perhaps the most readily obtained, but surgical and autopsy specimens or cells in culture are at times useful also. X chromatin (formerly called the Barr body), a condensed body of chromatin characteristically apposed to the nuclear membrane, is present in normal female cells. The X responsible for X chromatin in any particular cell is the one genetically inactivated and late-replicating. The number of X-chromatin masses is an indication of the number of X chromosomes in excess of 1. Y chromatin, a condensed segment of the Y demonstrated by quinacrine staining and fluorescence microscopy, is present in interphase nuclei of Y-bearing cells (for example, 48,XXYY cells contain one X-chromatin plus two Y-chromatin masses).

Meiotic chromosome preparations from testicular biopsies are sometimes useful in obscure cases of infertility. Here translocations and genetically determined disturbances in meiotic pairing may be identified.

section 2 | Clinical immunology

61
INTRODUCTION TO CLINICAL IMMUNOLOGY

BRUCE C. GILLILAND

Clinical immunology is a rapidly expanding field with increasing practical application to medicine. The scope of immunology covers defense against infections, prevention of diseases by immunization, organ transplantation, blood banking, deficiencies of the immune system, and a variety of disorders that are mediated by immunologic mechanisms. Besides the clinical relevance of immunology, immunologic techniques are frequently used in the clinical laboratory, as in the measurement of hormones and drugs.

The intent of this chapter is to provide the reader with a review of the essential fundamentals of immunology. The cellular components of the immune system, lymphocytes, plasma cells, and macrophages, along with their role in antibody-mediated or humoral immunity and in cell-mediated or cellular immunity, will be discussed first. This will be followed by a review of the immunoglobulins, cellular immunity, the interrelationship of the B and T lymphocytes and macrophages in the immune response, tolerance, and autoimmunity. The last sections cover the complement system and types of immunologically mediated inflammation and tissue damage.

CELLS OF THE IMMUNE SYSTEM

The principal cells of the immune system are lymphocytes, plasma cells, and macrophages which are collectively organized into lymphoid tissue. The thymus, lymph nodes, and spleen are examples of highly developed lymphoid tissues. Other lymphoid tissue is found along the gastrointestinal tract (tonsils, Peyer's patches, appendix) and also may accumulate at sites of inflammation.

The large body of experimental evidence has affirmed the existence of two populations of lymphocytes. These two populations were first demonstrated in chickens by removal of the thymus or by removal of the bursa of Fabricius (a lymphoid organ near the cloaca) during the neonatal period. Excision of the bursa resulted in low immunoglobulin levels and impaired antibody synthesis. Lymphoid nodules did not develop in lymph nodes and spleen, and only a few plasma cells were present. Cell-mediated immunity, however, remained intact as demonstrated by delayed hypersensitivity and allograft rejection. Evidence for two populations of immunocompetent cells in humans has largely come from study of congenital and acquired defects of immunity (Chap. 62) and from development of techniques for identification of populations of lymphocytes. These observations clearly indicate the existence of two separate systems for the differentiation of lymphoid cells involved in humoral and cellular immunity (Fig. 61-1). The two populations of immunocompetent lymphocytes are referred to as B cells and T cells (Table 61-1). The designation *B cell* was used originally because these cells depend for their development on the presence of the bursa in birds or its equivalent in humans. The equivalent of the bursa in humans remains unknown but might be the fetal liver, spleen, or bone marrow. The designation *T cell* connotes the role of the thymus in the development of these cells.

B CELLS B cells represent approximately 15 to 20 percent of the normal peripheral blood lymphocytes, 50 percent of the splenic lymphocytes, and 75 percent of the lymphocytes in the bone marrow. They are the principal cells in the cortical germinal centers and medullary cords of lymph nodes. Their chief role is the production of antibodies.

The B cells carry membrane-bound immunoglobulins as demonstrated by immunofluorescence staining with anti-immunoglobulin antiserum. The main immunoglobulin classes on

TABLE 61-1
Characteristics of T and B lymphocytes

	T cells	B cells
Function	Delayed hypersensitivity	Humoral immunity
Product	Lymphokines	Immunoglobulins
Identification	Sheep RBC rosettes	Surface Ig Fc and activated complement receptors
Assessment	Proliferative response to PHA, Con A Delayed skin test	Immunoglobulin levels Antibody response to immunization Blastogenic response to PWM

NOTE: *Ig, immunoglobulin; PHA, phytohemagglutinin; Con A, concanavalin A; PWM, pokeweed mitogen.*

the surface of peripheral blood B cells are IgM, present in the low-molecular-weight (7S subunit) monomeric form, and IgD. Approximately three-quarters of the peripheral blood B cells carry these two immunoglobulins; the remaining cells stain mostly for IgG, while about 1 percent stain for IgA. The membrane-bound immunoglobulin molecule is attached by its crystallizable fragment (Fc) portion to the plasma membrane, leaving the antigen-binding sites freely available. Upon contact with specific antigen and with modulatory signals from other cells, B cells bearing the complementary antigen binding site will evolve through a series of events leading to clonal expansion and differentiation into antibody-synthesizing plasma cells.

The most widely accepted theory of antibody formation is clonal selection, which suggests that there are large numbers of precommitted lymphocytes, each with its specific membrane receptor capable of reacting with specific immunogen. The selective binding of immunogens is followed by clonal expansion and antibody production.

Most of the B cells have a membrane receptor for the Fc portion of IgG in the form of either antigen-antibody complexes or aggregated IgG. Approximately one-half of the B cells also carry membrane receptors for the activated third component of complement (C3b). Receptors for other complement components (C3d, C4, and Clq) have also been identified on B cells. These various membrane receptors and membrane-bound immunoglobulins have membrane mobility and can undergo redistribution and capping. For example, when membrane-bound immunoglobulin binds with specific antigen, the immunoglobulin molecules reorganize into patches on the membrane and then these molecules localize at one pole of the membrane (capping). The polar cap of molecules is interiorized by endocytosis. As this process is occurring, the B cell is synthesizing new immunoglobulins for insertion into its membrane. These events may be important in the initiation of cell proliferation and antibody production. It has also been suggested that the capping process may serve only to remove excess antigen from the cell surface.

T CELLS Approximately 70 to 80 percent of normal peripheral blood lymphocytes and 90 percent of lymphocytes in thoracic duct fluid are T cells. They circulate primarily as long-lived small lymphocytes. These cells are the principal lymphocytes in the deep cortical areas of lymph nodes and in the periarteriolar areas of the splenic white pulp. The T cells are the main effectors of cell-mediated immunity and also are involved as helper or suppressor cells in modulating the immune response.

The T cells possess antigens that are identified with specific anti-T-cell antiserum by use of immunofluorescence or cytotoxic assays. The similarity of a T-cell antigen to the theta antigen identified on the lymphocyte in the thymus of mice has led to the following concept of T-cell differentiation in humans. Stem cells proliferate in the bone marrow and migrate to the thymus, where, under the influence of the epithelial cells of thymus, they acquire the characteristics of T cells, including the theta antigen or its equivalent in humans. Once the T cell has left the thymus, this gland may continue to exert an effect on T cells by secretion of thymic hormones.

The T cells in humans are usually identified by the presence of membrane receptors for sheep red blood cells which form rosettes around T cells when they are incubated together. Several subpopulations of T cells are recognized on the basis of differences in function, surface antigens, and membrane receptors for immunoglobulins. The various subsets of T cells function as helper cells, suppressor cells, or cytotoxic effector cells (see "Immune Response" below). The nature of the antigen-binding receptor on T cells is uncertain. One candidate for antigen receptor is a monomeric IgM-like molecule which has been identified on the T-cell membrane by some investigators. Other candidates include the cell membrane product of histocompatibility genes and the membrane product of immune response genes (Ir genes).

A small number of lymphocytes in blood (2 to 10 percent) do not have the usual surface membrane markers for B or T cells and are referred to as *null cells.* Some of these cells may represent incompletely differentiated B or T cells. Others have an Fc receptor for IgG and are referred to as *K* or *killer cells,*

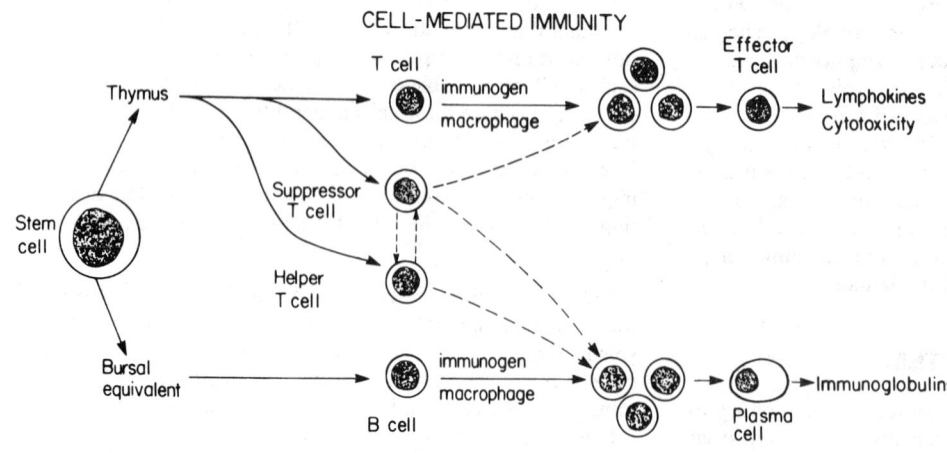

CELL-MEDIATED IMMUNITY

HUMORAL IMMUNITY

FIGURE 61-1
Schematic representation of the development of the immune system and the immune response. Upon exposure to immunogen, T cells proliferate and become sensitized lymphocytes that form the basis of cell-mediated immunity. The B cells proliferate and evolve to antibody-synthesizing plasma cells that constitute the basis of humoral immunity. Macrophages process and present immunogen to T and B cells. Subsets of T cells function as helper T cells which stimulate B-cell activity, or as suppressor T cells which suppress humoral and cell-mediated immune responses.

since they are the effector cell in antibody-dependent cell-mediated cytotoxicity (see "Immune Mechanisms of Tissue Injury" below).

MACROPHAGES Macrophages originate from promonocytes in the bone marrow and are released into the circulation as monocytes. Monocytes comprise 3 to 8 percent of the circulating leukocyte population. An even greater number of monocytes, estimated to be approximately three times the circulating population, exists in a marginal pool consisting of monocytes adhering to endothelial surfaces. Upon entering tissue, monocytes develop into macrophages. Tissue sites where macrophages are commonly found include the liver (where they are called *Kupffer cells*), peritoneum, lung, spleen, and lymph nodes. Macrophages have surface receptors for IgG1 and IgG3, and also a receptor for C3b. Through these receptors, macrophages can effectively bind and interiorize antigen-antibody complexes consisting of IgG antibodies or immune complexes which contain activated C3. Macrophages kill bacteria, fungi, and tumor cells. They also function in the induction of the immune response by processing and presenting immunogenic material to lymphocytes (see "Immune Response" below).

IMMUNOGLOBULINS

Immunoglobulins are synthesized by the B-cell series and have common structural features and structural units. Immunoglobulin molecules are composed of two kinds of polypeptide chains (Fig. 61-2); each molecule consists of larger identical polypeptide chains referred to as *heavy chains* (H chains) and two identical smaller ones referred to as *light chains* (L chains). These polypeptide chains are held together by disulfide bonds and by noncovalent bonds, which are primarily hydrophobic. The heavy and light polypeptide chains are synthesized on separate ribosomes, assembled in the cell, and secreted as an intact molecule. A slight to moderate excess of light chains is synthesized and secreted as free light chains.

The understanding of the structure and function of immu-

noglobulins was facilitated by studies of fragments produced by enzymatic cleavage of the antibody molecule (Fig. 61-3). For example, treatment of antibody molecules with papain results in two Fab fragments, which are the antigen binding fragments of the molecule, and one Fc fragment, which is responsible for the biologic activities discussed below. The amino-terminal half of the light chains and the amino-terminal quarter of the heavy chains of the immunoglobulin molecules vary in their amino acid sequence and are termed the *variable region* (V region) of the polypeptide chains. Portions of the V region of one heavy and one light polypeptide chain contribute the site for antigen binding. Considerable variation of the amino acid sequence must exist in this portion of the immunoglobulin molecule in order to explain the estimated 1 million antibody specificities. The constant region of H chains allows their differentiation into a class or subclass and confers to the immunoglobulins certain biological properties such as the ability to activate complement, to cross the placenta, and to bind to polymorphonuclear leukocytes or macrophages.

Five immunoglobulin classes (IgG, IgA, IgM, IgD, and IgE) are recognized on the basis of structural differences of their heavy chains including the amino acid sequence and length of the polypeptide chain. The antigenic determinants on the heavy chains also permit the identification and quantitation of the immunoglobulin classes by immunochemical techniques. On protein electrophoresis at a pH of 8.6, the immunoglobulins migrate mainly in the gamma region. Significant amounts of immunoglobulins also may be found in the beta region. The bulk of the gamma globulin consists of IgG immunoglobulin. The wide range in which immunoglobulins can migrate on protein electrophoresis is due to amino acid differences in the variable region of the molecules. A narrow band of protein staining in the gamma to beta region usually indicates the presence of a monoclonal population of immunoglobulins, the product of a single clone of cells as in multiple myeloma or macroglobulinemia (Chap. 63). Antibodies to a given antigen may be detected in all or several classes of immunoglobulins or may be restricted to a single class or subclass of immunoglobulin. Autoantibodies likewise may belong to one or several classes of immunoglobulins. For example, rheumatoid factors (antibodies to IgG) are most often recognized as an IgM immunoglobulin, but can also consist of IgG or

FIGURE 61-2

Schematic model of the variable and constant regions of an antibody molecule. The blackened areas represent the variable regions in the amino terminal half of each L chain and the amino terminal quarter of each H chain. The remainder of the molecules constitutes the constant regions. Amino acid sequences in the variable regions provide the basis for antibody specificity.

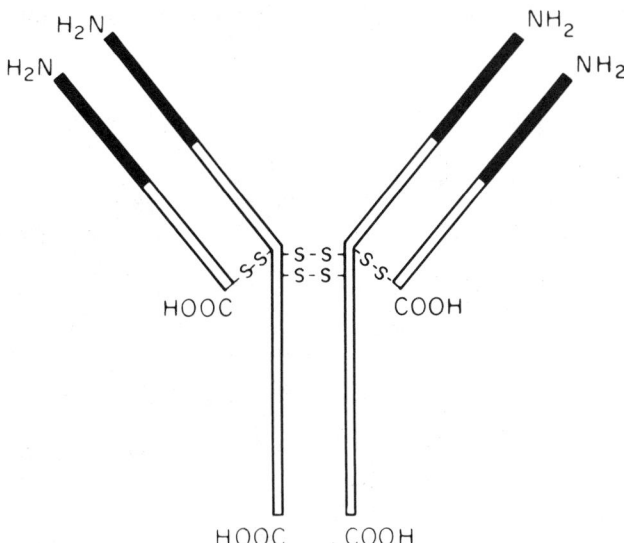

FIGURE 61-3

Schematic representation of enzyme cleavage of immunoglobulin molecules. Papain cleaves the molecule into three parts, two Fab fragments with antigen-binding sites and one Fc fragment. Pepsin produces a bivalent F(ab')₂ fragment, and the Fc portion is cleaved into small peptides.

IgA. The physical and biologic properties of immunoglobulins are listed in Table 61-2.

IgG The most abundant immunoglobulin is IgG; approximately 50 percent of its distribution is in the intravascular compartment. It has a molecular weight of 150,000 daltons. IgG is the only immunoglobulin that crosses the placenta and thereby provides maternal antibodies to the neonate. The structural features that mediate the transport across the placenta reside in the Fc fragment of IgG molecules. Four subclasses of IgG have been defined. While each has a common antigenic determinant for IgG, some differences in their amino acid sequences provide antigens that permit separation into subclasses. IgG1 and IgG3 are able to activate the complement system upon formation of immune complexes and to react with IgG receptors on monocytes and polymorphonuclear leukocytes. Both of these properties of IgG reside in the Fc portion of the molecule. Approximately 70 percent of the total IgG is IgG1, 18 percent is IgG2, 8 percent is IgG3, and 4 percent is IgG4.

IgA The predominant immunoglobulin in external secretions of the respiratory tree, gastrointestinal tract, and genitourinary system, and in tears, saliva, and colostrum is IgA. The IgA-producing plasma cells are the predominant plasma cells in the submucosa. For example, in the lamina propria of the intestine, approximately 20 IgA-producing plasma cells exist for each IgG-producing cell, compared with a 1:3 ratio in the peripheral lymph nodes and spleen. Secretory IgA is composed of two IgA molecules bound to a secretory piece by disulfide bonds. The secretory piece is a polypeptide chain with a molecular weight of 70,000 daltons that is synthesized by epithelial cells. The dimeric IgA is held together by a single J chain which is also synthesized by submucosal plasma cells and has a molecular weight of 15,000 daltons. Once the dimeric IgA leaves the plasma cell, it enters the epithelial cell and becomes covalently bound to a secretory piece. It is then secreted into the lumen. Secretory IgA has a molecular weight of approximately 400,000 daltons. Low concentrations of secretory IgA sometimes are found in the normal serum. Secretory IgA is more resistant to digestion by most proteolytic enzymes than monomeric IgA. An IgA protease that specifically cleaves human IgA in secretions has been discovered. This protease occurs in certain microorganisms such as *Neisseria gonorrhoeae* and *Streptococcus sanguis,* both of which are known to invade mucosal membranes in spite of prior immunity. Secretory IgA

can have antibody activity to bacterial and viral antigens, toxins, and dietary macromolecules. Secretory antibodies bind microorganisms and prevent their attachment to epithelial cells, and administration of antigens by either the gastrointestinal or respiratory route results in enhanced production of secretory IgA in these organ systems.

In the serum, IgA exists as a monomer with a molecular weight of 160,000 daltons, and to a lesser extent in polymeric forms. Two subclasses of IgA have been identified; approximately 75 percent of the total IgA is IgA1, and 25 percent IgA2. No biological differences are known to exist between IgA1 and IgA2 except that IgA2 appears to be resistant to cleavage by the specific IgA proteases.

IgM Approximately 10 percent of the serum immunoglobulins are IgM, which is a pentamer of the usual four polypeptide chain structure of immunoglobulins, having a molecular weight of 900,000 daltons. The five IgM subunits are linked by disulfide bonds in association with a single J chain to constitute the IgM molecule. While the J chain apparently assists in the polymerization of IgM, polymers form in the absence of the J chain. Even though the pentameric IgM has 10 antigen binding sites, these antibodies have a functional valence of 5 with large antigenic molecules. The distribution of IgM is predominantly intravascular. Activation of the complement system requires only one molecule of IgM antibody to react with antigen. IgM antibody is prominent in the early immune response and is the major class of antibodies to blood group substances A and B. Autoantibodies, such as rheumatoid factor (anti-IgG) and cold agglutinins, are also predominantly IgM immunoglobulins. A natural subunit of IgM is called *low-molecular-weight IgM* and has a molecular weight of 180,000 daltons. It is found on the surface of B cells, in fetal blood, and in certain diseases such as rheumatoid vasculitis, systemic lupus erythematosus, ataxia telangiectasia, progressive muscular atrophy and idiopathic chronic neuropathy, Waldenström's macroglobulinemia, and lymphoma. The biological significance of this molecule in the circulation is not known.

IgD IgD has a molecular weight of 180,000 daltons and is found mainly in the intravascular space and on resting B cells as a cell surface immunoglobulin. IgD is easily degraded by proteolytic enzymes and by heat. The function of free IgD in blood is not known, but the IgD on B cells may, in association with monomeric IgM, play an important role in the binding of antigen to B cells.

IgE The distinctive biological feature of IgE is its role in the immediate allergic or hypersensitivity reaction (reagenic prop-

TABLE 61-2
Properties of immunoglobulins

	IgG	IgA	IgM	IgD	IgE
Molecular weight, daltons	150,000	160,000	900,000	180,000	190,000
Average serum concentration, mg per 100 ml	1200	280	100	3	0.025*
Percent of total body pool in intravascular compartment	50	40	75	75	
Half-life days	23	5.5	5.1	2.8	2.3
Complement fixation by classic pathway	Yes†	No‡	Yes	No	No
Reagenic properties	No	No	No	No	Yes
Selective secretion by mucous membranes	No	Yes	No	No	No
Placental transfer	Yes	No	No	No	No
Macrophage binding	Yes¶	No	No	No	No

* Serum concentration in normal nonatopic individuals is less than 0.025 mg per 100 ml.
† IgG4 does not activate complement and IgG2 only weakly.
‡ IgA activates complement system only by the alternative pathway.
¶ Only IgG1 and IgG3.

erty) (Chap. 65). IgE has a molecular weight of 190,000 daltons and binds to basophils and mast cells through its Fc region. When a specific antigen combines with the antigen-binding sites on IgE, histamine and serotonin are released from these cells. The allergen must bind to two or more adjacent molecules of IgE to evoke the release of histamine. These pharmacological mediators lead to the characteristic wheal and flare reaction in the skin. In the lung, the same sequence of events leads to the release of slow reactive substance of anaphylaxis. The bulk of the body's pool of IgE is bound to basophils and mast cells, and the serum concentration of this immunoglobulin is extremely low, in the order of 0.1 to 0.2 μg/ml.

CELL-MEDIATED IMMUNITY (DELAYED TYPE OF HYPERSENSITIVITY)

The principal effectors of cell-mediated immunity are T cells that have become sensitized to foreign substances. These specifically sensitized T cells, along with macrophages, play a very important role in the defense of the host against a variety of infectious microorganisms including *Mycobacterium tuberculosis*, fungi, viruses, and protozoa. Cell-mediated immunity is most prominent in infections due to intracellular organisms. The killing of tumor cells and rejection of allografts such as kidney transplants are also expressions of cell-mediated immunity (Chap. 69).

Cell-mediated immunity is exemplified by the delayed type of hypersensitivity reaction in skin. The intradermal or subcutaneous injection of antigen into an individual previously sensitized to that antigen results in a reaction that consists of erythema followed by induration and reaches a peak in approximately 2 days. Lymphocytes and macrophages are the predominant cells in the lesion. If the inflammation is intense, necrosis of the skin may occur. Cell-mediated immunity can be transferred to a previously unimmunized individual with T cells but not with serum. In addition, cell-mediated immunity can also be transferred to a normal recipient with *transfer factor*, a low-molecular-weight material derived from disrupted sensitized lymphocytes or from the supernatant of a stimulated lymphocyte culture.

The events of cell-mediated immunity are initiated as the result of interaction of antigen with a few specifically sensitized T cells. The sensitized T cells, activated by antigen, elaborate soluble products referred to as *lymphokines,* which have several biological activities. Lymphokines mediate and amplify cell-mediated immune reactions by affecting the activities of macrophages, polymorphonuclear leukocytes, B cells, and other T cells. Several of the products of activated lymphocytes are listed in Table 61-3. While the T cell is considered the principal cell in cell-mediated immunity, the concept of cell-mediated immunity has taken on a broader connotation with the observation that B cells also release lymphokines, including macrophage chemotactic factor, macrophage activating factor, and macrophage inhibitory factor.

The development of the cell-mediated immune reaction in vivo may occur as follows: Antigen activates specifically sensitized T cells resulting in the elaboration of lymphokines. One of these factors, macrophage chemotactic factor, attracts macrophages to the site of immunologically induced inflammation where they are activated by macrophage-activating factor which is either identical or similar to macrophage migration inhibitory factor (MIF). Properties of the activated macrophages include an increase in their size and number of lysosomes, greater phagocytic ability, and enhanced killing of bacteria or tumor cells. The biological property of MIF is most likely to reduce the random migration of macrophages, thereby keeping them at the site of inflammation. Mitogenic factors amplify the response by increasing the number of acti-

vated lymphocytes. The sensitized T cells kill antigen-specific target cells, such as tumor cells, either by direct cell-to-cell contact or by the elaboration of lymphotoxin. Bacteria or tumor cells are also killed by macrophages, and polymorphonuclear leukocytes are then attracted to the site of inflammation.

For the clinical assessment of cell-mediated immunity, skin tests continue to be useful. The diagnosis of several infectious diseases is aided by the finding of a positive skin test which indicates prior exposure and T-cell sensitization to the particular organisms but not necessarily active disease. Since at least 80 percent of the population have been sensitized to *Candida, Trichophyton,* or streptokinase-streptodornase, these antigens are suitable for determining the general status of cell-mediated immunity. The absence of a response to a battery of antigens that previously elicited a cell-mediated immune response is termed *anergy* and may signify an underlying disorder such as lymphoma or sarcoidosis. Several drugs, diseases, and other conditions may suppress skin tests of the delayed type. These include glucocorticosteroids, malignant diseases such as Hodgkin's disease or lymphoma, sarcoidosis, infections (measles, infectious mononucleosis, miliary tuberculosis), old age, malnutrition, acquired and congenital immunodeficiency disorders, and, in some instances, fever.

The ability of an individual to develop cell-mediated immunity de novo can be determined by applying directly to the skin a chemical such as dinitrochlorobenzene (DNCB) to which the individual has not been previously exposed. The chemical combines with skin proteins to form an immunogenic substance that stimulates the sensitization of T cells to DNCB. Ten to fourteen days following this initial exposure to DNCB, the reapplication of DNCB on the skin will result in a positive skin test if cell-mediated immunity is intact. In suspected anergic patients, a negative test with DNCB confirms a cutaneous anergic state.

Cell-mediated immunity can be assessed in vitro by stimulating lymphocytes with specific antigens, unrelated lymphocytes, or nonspecific substances such as the plant lectins, phytohemagglutinin or concanavalin A. The functional capacity of T cells is determined by culturing lymphocytes with phytohemagglutinin or concanavalin A. These lectins bind to the carbohydrate moieties of cell membrane receptors and stimulate transformation or blastogenesis of lymphocytes which is measured by the incorporation of radioactive precursors (tritiated thymidine) into DNA. These two lectins are primarily T-cell mitogens; however, they stimulate different subsets of T cells.

T cells previously sensitized to an antigen will also undergo blastogenesis when cultured with the specific antigen. The blastogenic response of T cells on exposure to antigen in vitro

TABLE 61-3
Products of activated lymphocytes

I Affecting macrophages
  A Migration inhibitory factor (MIF)
  B Macrophage-activating factor (identical to MIF?)
  C Chemotactic factor for macrophages
II Affecting lymphocytes
  A Mitogenic factor
  B Transfer factor
III Affecting polymorphonuclear leukocytes
  A Chemotactic factors for neutrophils, eosinophils, and basophils
  B Migration-inhibiting factor
IV Affecting other cell types
  A Cytotoxic factors (lymphotoxin)
  B Interferon
  C Growth inhibitory factors (inhibits proliferation of target cells)
  D Osteoclast activation factor

corresponds fairly well with the in vivo skin tests of delayed hypersensitivity. The response of T cells to specific antigens can also be determined by measuring the biologic activity of the various soluble mediators or lymphokines released from the activated T cells (e.g., quantitating the amount of inhibition of macrophage migration resulting from the release of MIF). The release of soluble mediators from T cells may occur without the cells undergoing blastogenesis.

The mixed lymphocyte culture (MLC) is an assay widely used in the field of transplantation for the typing of histocompatibility antigens (Chap. 69). The test is usually performed in unidirectional method by treating the stimulating lymphocyte population with either radiation or mitomycin C which prevents these cells from responding without affecting their stimulatory properties. When the lymphocytes from a normal individual are cultured with these treated lymphocytes, the individual's T cells will undergo blastic transformation if the antigens on the stimulatory cells are sufficiently different. The cell antigens recognized in the MLC reaction are the products of genes at the HLA-D locus. The absence of a response indicates the presence of identical antigens in the two cell populations. The MLC reaction can also be used to assess the functional capacity of T cells.

IMMUNE RESPONSE

Upon exposure to a foreign substance, an individual can respond by producing specific antibodies, by developing cell-mediated immunity (delayed hypersensitivity), or by becoming immunologically unresponsive. The substances that elicit an immune response are termed *immunogens,* and their ability to evoke this response is called *immunogenicity.* Antigens are substances that will react specifically with available antibodies or sensitized lymphocytes. Certain small molecules with molecular weights of less than 1000 daltons usually are not capable of inducing an immune response but can interact as antigens with available antibodies and are called *haptens.* However, an immune response can be elicited with haptens if they are coupled to a larger carrier molecule which is immunogenic in the host.

The route of administration, the dose of the immunogen, and the response of the host are all factors determining the immune response. For example, the oral administration of poliomyelitis virus leads to effective immunization by stimulating the production of IgA antibodies in the gastrointestinal tract. Skin contact with chemicals (e.g., resins of poison ivy) evokes primarily a cell-mediated or delayed hypersensitivity reaction involving the skin. The dose of immunogen also affects the immune response. Both very high doses and low doses of immunogen may produce tolerance. The failure to detect an immune response, therefore, is not conclusive, since a substance may be immunogenic at a different dose or by a different route of administration.

One of the most exciting areas in immunology is the role of genetic factors in the immune response. Evidence for a genetic influence on the immune response to a given immunogen is based on studies in inbred strains of mice and other laboratory animals. Genetic differences within a species are associated with an immune response to a given immunogen in one strain and with no response in another. These differences may also lead to a high level of antibody production in one strain and to low levels in another strain. In several species including humans, the ability of an individual to respond to a specific immunogen is under the control of immune response genes that are located in the chromosomal region referred to as *major histocompatibility gene complex.* Genes within this region code for molecules that are involved in the initiation, stimulation, and suppression of the immune response.

CELL COOPERATION Many immunogens require an interaction of B and T cells to generate a humoral immune response. These immunogens are referred to as being *thymus dependent.* Examples of some thymus-dependent antigens are glycoproteins, natural proteins, heterologous serum proteins, and erythrocytes. The interaction of T cells with B cells is termed *cooperation,* and the T cells that function in this context are called *helper T cells.* Other immunogens, referred to as being *thymus independent,* are able to initiate B-cell proliferation and antibody production without the help of T cells. The biochemical characteristics that differentiate thymus-independent from thymus-dependent immunogens have not been fully identified, but some differentiating features are the repeating linear polymeric structure of the thymus-independent immunogens and the slow degradation of these molecules in the host. Examples of thymus-independent immunogens include pneumococcal polysaccharides, polymerized *Salmonella* flagellin, dextran, and lipopolysaccharides.

T cells play a central role in the induction and regulation of the immune response. Various subsets of T cells function as helper cells, suppressor cells, or cytotoxic cells. In mice, these functions of T cells have been shown to be genetically programmed. The subsets of T cells are identified by surface antigens belonging to the Ly system of T-cell alloantigens. T cells expressing the surface phenotype $Ly1^+$ are helper cells and cooperate with B cells to induce antibody production. They also stimulate proliferation of T cells expressing the surface phenotype $Ly2, 3^+$ which function as cytotoxic effector cells in cell-mediated immunity. Other $Ly2, 3^+$ cells have suppressor activity. The third subset of T cells, $Ly1, 2, 3^+$, represents resting cells that have receptors for antigen but are not yet committed to either helper or suppressor activity. A set of these resting $Ly1, 2, 3^+$ cells can be activated by antigen-stimulated $Ly1^+$ helper cells to produce suppressor activity. These observations suggest that $Ly1^+$ helper cells, when activated by specific antigen, induce B cells to produce antibody and also stimulate $Ly1, 2, 3^+$ to exert suppression of helper T cell activity. The suppression of helper T cell activity, in turn, would lead to a reduction in antibody formation as well as suppressor cell activity. The interaction of these subsets of T cell provides a mechanism for self-regulation and homeostasis of the immune response. Similar systems of immunoregulation are undoubtedly present in humans. In them, a subpopulation of T cells that carry receptors for the Fc portion of IgM and that may represent helper T cells has been recognized. Another group has membrane receptors for the Fc portion of IgG and may represent suppressor T cells. The distinguishing features of helper and suppressor T cells are being investigated intensively, and the field is very much in flux. In a clinical context, hyperactivity of the suppressor T-cell system in patients with common variable hypogammaglobulinemia may induce low levels of immunoglobulins by suppressing B-cell proliferation and antibody production (Chap. 62). Hypergammaglobulinemia, on the other hand, may represent too much helper T cell activity owing to loss of suppressor T cell function.

Macrophages are also critical cells in the immune response and especially involve thymus-dependent antigens. An important function of the macrophage is the presentation of immunogenic material to B and T cells. In this setting, immunogens may interact directly with the surface of macrophages. Macromolecules or particulate substances, however, require digestion by macrophages to become immunogenic. A few immunogenic molecules of the digested material are retained on the surface of the macrophages. Macrophages also elaborate soluble biologic substances that stimulate both T and B cells.

MODELS OF ANTIBODY PRODUCTION Several models of antibody production involving T and B cell cooperation have emerged from studies in animals. In one such model, immunogenic material may be initially processed by macrophages or may directly bind with a specific antigen receptor on T cells. As mentioned above, the nature of the antigen receptor on T cells may be an IgM-like molecule. This T cell antigen receptor and the antigen dissociate as a complex from the T cell and bind to the macrophage, perhaps through the Fc receptor on the macrophage. As a result of this binding, the necessary density and frequency of antigenic determinants are created for the interaction with antigen receptors on B cells and subsequent stimulation of antibody production. The antigen-activated T cells may also elaborate nonspecific factors that stimulate antibody production.

Other models for antibody production take into greater consideration the genetic control of the immune response. The antigen receptor on T cells in one such model is referred to as the *T-cell recognition factor* and is coded for by an immune response gene. The T cell, through its recognition factor, can directly bind immunogen or can interact with immunogen presented on the surface of a macrophage. The recognition factor is associated with an interaction factor which is coded for by an I-region gene. I-region genes are located within the major histocompatibility complex and control immune responsiveness. The complex of antigen, recognition factor, and interaction factor dissociates from the T cell and binds to B cells carrying the specific immunoglobulin receptor for antigen and the complementary receptor site for interaction factor. The receptor site for interaction factor on these B cells is also coded for by the same I-region gene. Antigen-stimulated T cells may also react directly with the B cells carrying the complementary antigen receptor and site for interaction factor. The interactions between T cells, B cells, and macrophages may depend on the sharing of common histocompatibility antigens.

PRIMARY AND SECONDARY IMMUNE RESPONSES On a first exposure to a new immunogen, several days are required before humoral and cell-mediated immunity are detected. This initial response to a new immunogen is termed the *primary* immune response. When the immunogen is thymus dependent, IgM and IgG classes of antibody are initially secreted by the B cells, and IgM appears first. As the titer of IgG rises during the second week following immunogenic stimulation, the IgM titer falls. The antibody titer reaches a peak in approximately two weeks and then falls gradually. However, low levels of antibody can be demonstrated for months and even years. The switch from IgM synthesis to predominantly IgG synthesis in B cells requires T-cell cooperation. The synthesis of IgA and IgE also is dependent on T-cell cooperation. In the absence of T-cell cooperation, the B cells stimulated by thymus-dependent antigens produce low levels of antibody belonging to the IgM classes. The thymus-independent immunogens such as pneumococcal polysaccharides and *Salmonella* O stimulate the production of antibodies belonging to the IgM class even after repeated injections.

Following a second exposure to the same immunogen, heightened cell-mediated or humoral responses are observed. This is termed a *secondary* or *anamnestic* response. These responses occur sooner than the primary response, usually in 4 to 5 days in humans, and depend on a marked proliferation of antibody-producing cells or effector T cells of cell-mediated immunity. The antibody produced is of the IgG class and has a greater affinity for antigen than the antibody synthesized initially during the primary immune response. The secondary response depends on immunologic memory that must be demonstrated by both T and B cells.

TOLERANCE A state of specific immunologic unresponsiveness to substances that would normally evoke an immune response is termed *tolerance*. It is an active physiologic process

and not merely the lack of an immune response. Humoral immunity, cell-mediated immunity, or both may be suppressed. Tolerance provides the essential mechanism for the prevention of immunologically induced self-injury. The impairment of self-tolerance is presently considered the basic pathogenic mechanism in autoimmune diseases.

Tolerance can be induced in several ways. The physical form and dose of an antigen are important factors determining whether tolerance or an immune response develops. In experimental models, the administration of soluble antigen in monomeric form produces tolerance, while the same antigen in aggregated or polymeric form leads to an immune response. High doses of antigen lead to tolerance of both B and T cells. In comparison with B cells, tolerance in T cells is induced with lower doses of antigen and persists longer. Tolerance is more readily achieved in the neonate than in the adult. The maintenance of tolerance requires repeated or chronic exposure to the tolerogenic antigen. Tolerance may also be induced and maintained by the stimulation of suppressor T-cell activity which can suppress both humoral and cell-mediated immunity.

Immunologic unresponsiveness also can be caused by antibody. Antibody binding to antigen may produce conformational changes in the antigen, preventing its interaction with lymphocytes. Antibody in the form of an immune complex can also suppress the immune response by interacting with suppressor T cells enhancing suppressor activity.

AUTOIMMUNITY The development of immunologic responsiveness to self is called *autoimmunity* and reflects the impairment of self-tolerance. Immunologic, environmental, and genetic factors are closely interrelated in the pathogenesis of autoimmunity. Clinical disorders in which autoimmune responses play a role in the pathogenesis of the illness are referred to as *autoimmune diseases*. Autoantibodies, however, are found in some normal persons without evidence of autoimmune disease. The frequency of autoantibodies in the general population increases with age, suggesting a breakdown of self-tolerance with aging. Autoantibodies also may develop as an aftermath of tissue damage. The spectrum of autoimmune disorders ranges from thyroiditis, which is organ specific, to systemic lupus erythematosus, which is characterized by an array of autoantibodies to cell and tissue antigens.

The development of autoimmunity usually involves the breakdown or circumvention of self-tolerance. The potential for the development of autoantibodies probably exists in most individuals. For example, normal human B cells are capable of reacting with several self-antigens (e.g., thyroglobulin) but are suppressed from producing autoantibodies by one or more mechanisms of tolerance. Precommitted B cells in tolerant individuals can be stimulated in several ways. Tolerance involving only T cells, induced by persistent low levels of circulating self-antigens, may be circumvented by substances such as endotoxin. Such substances would stimulate the B cells directly to produce autoantibodies, thus obviating the need for helper T cells. A decrease in suppressor T cell activity could also lead to production of autoantibodies (see below).

Autoimmunity may develop to antigens that were sequestered or anatomically separated from the immune system during embryonic development. For example, in the absence of low levels of circulating antigen, both B and T cells are immunocompetent. In later life, exposure to such antigens through trauma or infection results in autoimmune responses (e.g., release of myelin in experimental allergic encephalomyelitis).

Viruses also play an important role in the pathogenesis of autoimmunity. Several animal models of autoimmunity such as F_1 hybrids of the New Zealand black (NZB) and white (NZW) mice have persistent viral infections from birth (Chap. 68). It is difficult to determine whether the viral infection interferes with the immune system or if preexisting abnormal immunity permits chronic viral infection. In any event, these animals develop circulating immune complexes, composed of antibodies to nuclear antigens and to viral antigens, which deposit in the glomerular basement membrane and other tissue sites, leading to the manifestations of immune complex disease. The expression of viral antigens on the surfaces of the host's cells may elicit autoantibodies to cell membrane antigens. Furthermore, autoantibodies may develop from exposure to exogenous viral antigens that cross-react with autoantigens. Bacteria or other foreign substances may also act as cross-reacting antigens.

It has been proposed that autoimmunity is a disorder of abnormal immunologic regulation resulting in excessive B-cell activity and diminished T-cell activity. A decrease in suppressor T-cell activity or an increase in helper T-cell activity would result in uncontrolled excessive production of autoantibodies. The strongest support for this concept of autoimmunity comes from studies in animal models and human autoimmune disorders in which the loss of suppressor T-cell function and excessive B-cell antibody production can be demonstrated.

A role for genetic factors in the pathogenesis of autoimmunity has been clearly demonstrated in animal models and clinical autoimmune disorders. New Zealand black mice manifest autoimmune hemolytic anemia, whereas the NZB/NZW F_1 hybrids develop a disease analogous to systemic lupus erythematosus (SLE). The relatives of patients with SLE may have clinical and serologic abnormalities of SLE: a high concordance of SLE is also found in monozygotic twins. Associations with histocompatibility antigens are noted in several clinical autoimmune disorders. Chronic active hepatitis, Graves' disease, and Addison's disease occur more often in individuals who are HLA-B8 positive. An association with genes located at the HLA-D locus has been noted in adult rheumatoid arthritis, Sjögren's syndrome, and multiple sclerosis. These associations may be significant because of the close relationship between genes determining histocompatibility antigens and genes controlling the type and magnitude of the immune response.

COMPLEMENT SYSTEM The complement system consists of a group of at least 15 plasma proteins which interact sequentially, producing substances that mediate several functions of inflammation (see Table 61-4). The activated complement components and the enzymatically cleaved fragments of components exert many of their biologic activities by interaction with cell membranes. The actions of complement system include cell lysis, release of histamine from mast cells and platelets, vascular permeability, contraction of smooth muscle, chemotaxis of leukocytes, and neutralization of certain viruses. The complement system also is interrelated with the coagulation, fibrinolytic, and kinin systems. Complement is involved in the pathogenesis of tissue injury observed in many immuno-

logically mediated diseases which include SLE, rheumatoid arthritis, glomerulonephritis, and immunohemolytic anemia.

The activation of complement is initiated either by the classic pathway or by the alternative (properdin) pathway (Fig. 61-4). Both pathways lead to activation of a common terminal sequence of complement components. The complement components of the classic pathway are C1, C4, and C2. C1 is composed of three subunits, C1q, C1r, and C1s, which are held together by calcium. The classic pathway is activated by immune complexes containing IgG or IgM, and by aggregates of IgG (IgG1, IgG3, and IgG2), which bind to C1q by their Fc fragments. The binding of C1q activates C1r, which in turn activates C1s, resulting in formation of an esterase. The esterase cleaves C4 into a small fragment, C4a, and a large fragment, C4b, which binds to the immune complex or cell membrane. Activated C1s and C4b act together to split C2 into a small fragment, C2a, which has kinin-like properties and a larger fragment. The larger fragment of C2 combines with C4b to form C3 convertase, a magnesium-dependent enzyme that acts on C3.

The alternative (properdin) complement pathway produces activation of C3 by a series of reactions that bypass C1, C4, and C2. The components of the alternative complement system include factor D, which is an esterase similar to C1s, factor B, properdin, and C3. This pathway is activated by endotoxin, other polysaccharides, aggregated IgA, immune complexes, or nephritic factors. The latter are most likely IgG immunoglobulins which function by binding to the alternative pathway C3 convertase and may be autoantibodies to this enzyme complex. Nephritic factors are present in the serum of some patients with membranoproliferative glomerulonephritis or with partial lipodystrophy. The C3 convertase of the alternative pathway is formed by the interaction of factor D or nephritic factors, factor B and C3, and requires divalent Mg^{2+} ions. The C3 convertase is stabilized by properdin. Cleavage of C3 by either pathway results in a small peptide, C3a, and a large molecule, C3b. The latter interacts with components of the alternative complement pathway, resulting in C3 activation with formation of C3b which leads to more activation of C3, and amplification of complement activity. Regulators of this pathway are C3b inactivator and its cofactor, $\beta 1H$.

The two complement pathways converge at C3. Activation of the terminal complement components (C5 to C9) is initiated by C5 convertase, which consists of C3b in association with C3 convertase from either pathway. The C5 convertase cleaves a small fragment C5a from C5, and the remaining larger fragment C5b along with C6 to C9 self-assemble on the cell membrane. The insertion of these components into the membrane results in hydrophobic characteristics and reorientation of the lipid bilayer leading to membrane injury and disruption of the cell.

The regulation of the complement system is through the rapid decay of C2 to C5 once they have been activated. There is also decay of C3 convertase of both the classic and alternative pathways. C1 inhibitor (C1 INH) inhibits activated C1r and C1s by combining with these enzymes. The inactivation of C3b by C3b inactivator and its cofactor $\beta 1H$ is important in preventing the continued formation of C3b which interacts with components of the alternative pathway to produce a functional C3 convertase and thus more cleavage of C3 to C3b.

The peptides C3a and C5a are referred to as *anaphylatoxins*. C5a and the trimolecular complex of C5 to C7 are chemotactic for neutrophils, eosinophils, and monocytes. The presence of C3b on the cell membranes enhances phagocytosis by interaction with phagocytic cells possessing receptors for C3b. The interaction of C5b with neutrophils causes these cells to become adherent and to release lysosomal enzymes. Neutralization of certain viruses, such as herpes simplex, occurs by coating the virus with C1, C4, and C2. A peptide generated from

TABLE 61-4
Biological functions of complement

Biological function	Complement components
Chemotaxis	C3a, C5a, $\overline{C5}$, $\overline{C6}$, $\overline{C7}$
Histamine release (anaphylatoxin)	C3a, C5a
Opsonization	C3b
Cytolytic	C5 to C9
Kinin-like activity	C2 fragment
Viral neutralization	C1, C4

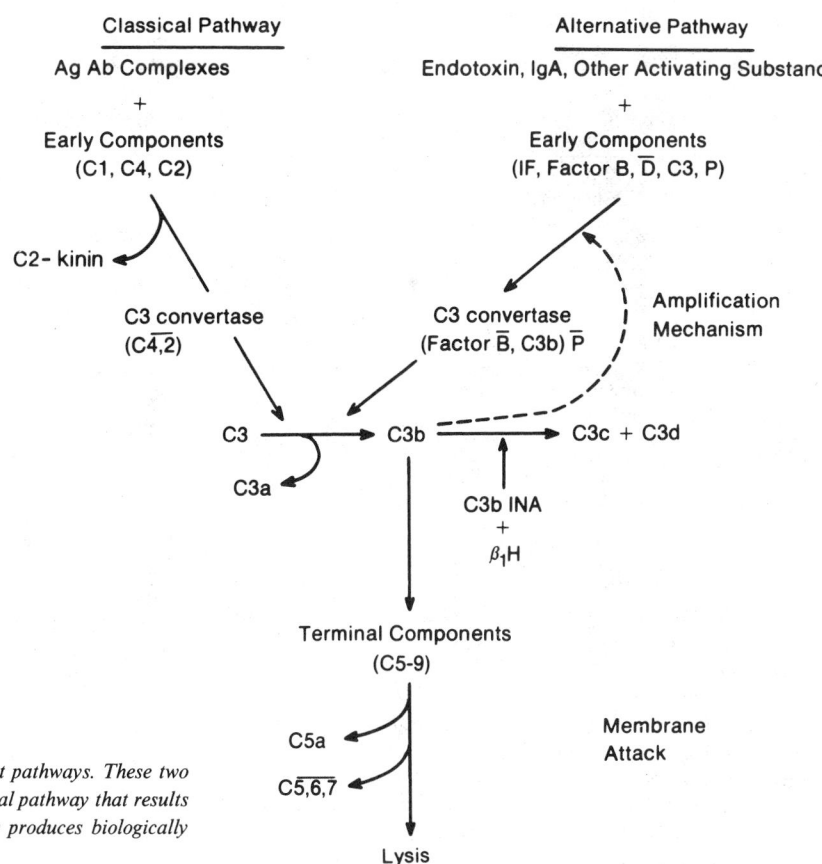

Classical Pathway
Ag Ab Complexes
+
Early Components
(C1, C4, C2)

Alternative Pathway
Endotoxin, IgA, Other Activating Substances
+
Early Components
(IF, Factor B, $\overline{D}$, C3, P)

C2- kinin

C3 convertase
(C$\overline{4,2}$)

C3 convertase
(Factor $\overline{B}$, C3b) $\overline{P}$

Amplification
Mechanism

C3 → C3b → C3c + C3d
C3a
C3b INA
+
β_1H

Terminal Components
(C5-9)

Membrane
Attack

C5a
C$\overline{5,6,7}$

Lysis

FIGURE 61-4

Diagram of the classic and alternative complement pathways. These two pathways converge at C3 to form a common terminal pathway that results in cell lysis. Cleavage of complement components produces biologically active fragments. (See text for details.)

activated C2 has been shown to have kinin-like properties and is probably responsible for the swelling observed in hereditary angioedema.

The complement system interacts with the coagulation, fibrinolytic, and kinin-generating systems. The activation of Hageman factor (factor XII) not only leads to clotting but also to the formation of plasmin, a fibrinolysin. Plasmin also activates C1 and cleaves C3 to produce C3a (anaphylatoxin). Plasmin also cleaves Hageman factor to produce Hageman factor fragments which convert prekallikrein to kallikrein. Kallikrein cleaves kininogen to bradykinin. Lysosomal enzymes can activate C1 and cleave C5 to form C5a.

Measurement of complement may be useful in diagnosis, assessment of disease activity, and evaluation of treatment. The serum level of complement depends on the balance of synthesis, catabolism, and consumption of the various complement components. Evidence for complement activation may be reflected in a low hemolytic complement level, decreased levels of individual components, or the finding of cleavage fragments of complement components. Low complement levels, however, may be the result of decreased synthesis or an inherited deficiency of a complement component. Normal or elevated complement levels do not exclude the participation of complement since synthesis of complement may equal or exceed consumption. Serum complement levels do not necessarily reflect intense local consumption of complement as might occur in synovial and pleural fluid. Further evidence of complement activation in disease can be adduced by the demonstration of complement components in lesions by immunofluorescence microscopy.

Complement is measured by its hemolytic activity expressed in CH_{50} units. Normal hemolytic activity depends on optimum concentrations of all the major components, C1 through C9. If any one component is markedly reduced or absent, little or no hemolytic activity is measured. The C3 and

C4 components are readily measured immunochemically. In most instances, the measurements of C3 and C4 and hemolytic complement activity provide sufficient clinical information. Measurements of C1q and factor B may also be useful. For example, low levels of C1q, C4, C3, and CH_{50} indicate activation of complement primarily through the classic pathway. Immune complex disease such as systemic lupus erythematosus may show this complement profile. Reduced C3, CH_{50}, and factor B with a normal C4 reflect activation of complement by the alternative complement pathway, and may be seen in patients with membranoproliferative glomerulonephritis and in patients with bacterial endotoxin shock. The absence of CH_{50} may signify a hereditary deficiency of a complement component.

HEREDITARY DEFICIENCIES OF COMPLEMENT The most common hereditary deficiency of complement is C2 deficiency which is inherited as an autosomal recessive trait (Table 61-5). Homozygous C2 deficiency has been recognized in normal individuals and in patients with SLE and other syndromes with a comparable clinical picture. Heterozygous C2 deficiency may also be associated with rheumatic disorders. Inherited as well as acquired deficiencies of the early components (C1, C4, C2) appear to be more common in diseases resembling SLE. Lupus-like illness has also been noted in persons with hereditary angioedema who lack C1 inhibitor. Serum levels of C4 and C2 are often low in these individuals. Systemic lupus erythematosus has been observed in patients with the homozygous deficiency of C5 or C8. Severe recurrent bacterial infections occur in patients with homozygous C3 deficiency and in those patients with low levels of C3 secondary to the absence of C3b inactivator. In addition, acquired or hereditary deficiencies of early complement components may predispose individuals to infection because of inefficient activation of C3. The homozygous deficiency of a terminal complement component (C5 to C8) has been noted in patients with disseminated *Neisseria*

TABLE 61-5
Clinical disorders associated with hereditary complement deficiencies

Complement component	Clinical disorders
Clr, Cls	SLE-like syndrome
C2	SLE-like syndrome, dermatomyositis, vasculitis, glomerulonephritis, normal persons
C3	Recurrent infections
C4	SLE-like syndrome
C5	SLE-like syndrome
C5 dysfunction	Recurrent infections with gram-negative bacteria and eczema (Leiner's syndrome)
C6	Gonococcal, meningococcal infections
C7	Raynaud's phenomenon, normal persons
C8	Gonococcal, meningococcal infections, SLE-like syndrome
C1 inhibitor	Hereditary angioedema, SLE-like syndrome
C3b inactivator	Recurrent infections

NOTE: *SLE, systemic lupus erythematosus.*

infections. These persons may be more susceptible to infection with bacteria which are normally killed by complement-mediated cell lysis, a function which depends on the terminal complement components.

Hereditary deficiencies of C2 and C4 are linked to histocompatibility antigens (HLA). The genes determining immune responses are located near the genes for the HLA system. This has raised the possibility that relationships exist between inherited deficiencies of the complement system, HLA, the immune response, and the development of SLE or lupus-like illnesses. In view of the current hypothesis of a viral etiology for SLE, it has been suggested that the inherited deficiencies of early complement components predispose these individuals to viral infections. The development of lupus-related illnesses in patients with acquired deficiencies of early complement components also supports this notion and makes the possibility less likely that a direct causative relationship exists between HLA and SLE. Another explanation is that inherited deficiency of C2 or C4 is more closely associated with a particular type of immune response that predisposes these individuals to autoimmune disease. Further work is needed to elucidate the meaning of the associations between complement synthesis and SLE or lupus-like illnesses.

Hereditary angioedema is characterized by acute episodes of circumscribed edema involving skin, gastrointestinal tract, and upper respiratory tract and an imminent danger of life-threatening laryngeal edema. The basic abnormality is the absence of C1 inhibitor. The disorder has an autosomal dominant pattern of inheritance, and the affected heterozygote has low levels of C1 inhibitor. In approximately 10 to 15 percent of these individuals, normal amounts of C1 inhibitor can be measured immunochemically, but the protein does not possess C1 inhibitor activity (Chap. 65).

IMMUNE MECHANISMS OF TISSUE INJURY

The immune system protects the individual from the attacks of microorganisms by preventing their entry or facilitating their removal. The same immunologic mechanisms that protect the individual, however, may cause damage to normal tissue, especially if the immune response is excessive or prolonged. Moreover, damage to normal cells and tissue occurs in autoimmune disorders because immune responses are directed against autoantigens. The mechanisms of immune injury have been divided into four types: anaphylactic (type I), cytotoxic (type II), immune-complex-mediated (type III), and cell-mediated reactions (type IV). An additional mechanism interferes with the function of biologically active substances and is referred to as type V. Clinical manifestations of disease may be the conse-

quence of one or any combination of these five mechanisms of tissue injury.

ANAPHYLACTIC REACTION (TYPE I) This reaction is characterized by the release of pharmacologically active substances from mast cells or basophils as a result of the binding of antigen to IgE antibody attached to the surface of these cells. Histamine, slow-reacting substances of anaphylaxis, and eosinophil chemotactic factor of anaphylaxis are the major substances released from the mast cells in this reaction. The anaphylactic reaction is also referred to as *immediate hypersensitivity*. Clinical features of the anaphylactic reaction include generalized anaphylaxis, urticaria, angioedema, and atopic disorders (allergic rhinitis or hay fever, bronchial asthma, atopic dermatitis) (Chap. 65).

CYTOTOXIC REACTIONS (TYPE II) In the cytotoxic mechanism of injury, antibodies belonging to either IgG or IgM class react with antigenic determinants on cell membranes or tissue. The antigens may be intrinsic or result from the firm binding of free antigens to cell membranes or tissues. The ensuing tissue damage from antigen-antibody reactions occurs through the activation of the complement system when the antibody belongs to the IgM class. Receptors for IgM are not present on phagocytic cells, and complement activation is necessary for generation of inflammation. Antigen-antibody reactions involving IgG antibodies, however, can lead to tissue damage with or without the activation of complement. Since macrophages and neutrophils have receptors for IgG, these phagocytic cells will bind to the IgG antibodies that are attached to cell membranes or tissue. Examples of type II reactions include immune hemolytic anemia, transfusion reactions, erythroblastosis fetalis, immune thrombocytopenia, and Goodpasture's syndrome. In immune hemolytic anemia of the warm antibody type, IgG antibody coated red blood cells become bound to macrophages mainly in the spleen and in other reticuloendothelial tissues. A portion of the red blood cell membrane is removed by the macrophage. The red blood cell with its decreased membrane returns to the circulation as a spherocyte which has both increased mechanical and osmotic fragility. Penicillin-induced hemolytic anemia is an example of a cytotoxic reaction in which free antigen (penicillin) becomes firmly bound to the red blood cell membrane. If patients on high doses of penicillin form anti-penicillin antibodies of the IgG class, these antibodies will react with the penicillin antigens bound to the red blood cell membrane and lead to increased red blood cell destruction by the process of erythrophagocytosis. In Goodpasture's syndrome, antibodies develop that are specific for antigens intrinsic to the glomerular basement membrane and for antigens in the walls of pulmonary blood vessels. The inflammation generated by these antigen-antibody reactions leads to glomerulonephritis and pulmonary vasculitis, and these patients often present with hemoptysis as their initial complaint.

ANTIGEN-ANTIBODY COMPLEX-MEDIATED REACTIONS (TYPE III) The deposition of circulating antigen-antibody complexes in tissue leads to inflammation (Chap. 66). An understanding of immune complex disease has come largely from studies of experimental serum sickness. Many human diseases in which immune complexes play a pathogenetic role are now recognized. Circulating immune complexes have been identified in SLE, subacute bacterial endocarditis, and malignancies, to name only a few. Immune complex disease may develop locally at a tissue site such as in the rheumatoid joint or in the lung in patients with hypersensitivity pneumonitis. The systemic form of immune complex disorders such as SLE is characterized by deposition of circulating immune complexes in various sites such as the glomerular basement membrane, pleura, pericardium, synovium, and in cutaneous blood vessels. The process by which immune complexes generate inflammation involves the following steps: (1) antigen-antibody complexes deposit at tissue sites, (2) complement activation provides chemotactic factors and vasoactive peptides which dilate blood vessels and attract neutrophils, and (3) interaction of phagocytic cells with immune complexes leads to release of lysosomal enzymes which damage surrounding tissue.

CELL-MEDIATED REACTIONS (TYPE IV) This form of immune injury, also referred to as *delayed type of hypersensitivity*, centers on the role of the cytotoxic effector T cell (see "Cell-mediated Immunity" above). Sensitized T cells activated by antigen become cytotoxic cells capable of killing bacteria, tumor cells, or other target cells. They also release lymphokines, which stimulate macrophages, neutrophils, and other lymphocytes. The T cell is also capable of inducing cytotoxicity. Macrophages attracted to the site of immunologically mediated inflammation by T cells also cause tissue damage. Cell-mediated reactions play a significant role in the development of immunity and/or formation of lesions in tuberculosis, mycotic infections, and certain viral infections such as mumps, hepatitis, vaccinia, and herpes. Cell-mediated reactions are also involved in the pathogenesis of rheumatoid synovitis, Hashimoto's thyroiditis, and contact dermatitis resulting from exposure to oily resins of plants (e.g., poison oak) or to a variety of simple chemicals in the home or work environment. Renal allograft rejection and the graft versus host reaction observed in bone marrow transplantation are also in part a consequence of cell-mediated reactions (Chap. 69).

Another form of cell-mediated tissue injury is antibody-dependent cell-mediated cytotoxicity (ADCC). First, antibodies of the IgG class react with antigens on target cells such as tumor cells. Effector lymphocytes or macrophages through their receptors for the Fc portion of IgG then bind to IgG antibodies on the target cells without involving immunologic specificity. This interaction of lymphocytes or macrophages with target cells results in the killing of target cells. Only small amounts of antibody are required to initiate this form of immune injury. The type of lymphocyte participating in ADCC is not clear. While these cells have receptors for the Fc fragment of IgG, other markers that would distinguish them as B or T cells are absent. As noted in the description of T cells (above), these lymphocytes are referred to as *K* or *killer cells* and may be the same as the null cell which lacks T- and B-cell markers.

INTERFERENCE WITH FUNCTION OF BIOLOGICALLY ACTIVE SUBSTANCES (TYPE V) The interaction of antibodies with biologically active substances can interfere with their function. Antibodies to clotting factors, in particular factor VIII, may lead to serious bleeding abnormalities. Antibodies to intrinsic factors in patients with pernicious anemia may interfere with the absorption of vitamin B_{12}. In patients with myasthenia gravis, antibodies to acetylcholine neural receptors may be responsible for the block of neural transmission. In most diabetic patients receiving foreign insulin, antibodies to insulin develop. Anti-insulin antibodies are responsible for the insulin resistance observed in some patients. In other patients, antibodies to cell membrane receptors for insulin produce severe insulin resistance. These examples illustrate the potential clinical importance of recognizing this form of immune reaction.

REFERENCES

BELLANTI JA (ed): *Immunology II*. Philadelphia, Saunders, 1978

FUDENBERG HH et al (eds): *Basic & Clinical Immunology*. Los Altos, Lange, 1978

ROITT IM: *Essential Immunology*. Philadelphia, Lippincott, 1977

SAMTER M (ed): *Immunological Diseases*. Boston, Little, Brown, 1979

TALAL N (ed): *Autoimmunity. Genetic, Immunologic, Virologic and Clinical Aspects*. New York, Academic, 1977

Diseases of under- and overproduction of immune globulins

62
IMMUNE DEFICIENCY DISEASES

ALEXANDER R. LAWTON III
MAX D. COOPER

INTRODUCTION Immunologic functions are mediated by two developmentally divergent, but functionally interacting, families of lymphocytes. The activities of B and T lymphocytes, and their products, in host defense are closely integrated with the functions of other cells of the reticuloendothelial system. Fixed and wandering macrophages play an important role in the trapping and processing of antigens and become effector cells, especially when activated by products of T lymphocytes. The scavenger activity of polymorphonuclear leukocytes is directed and made specific by antibodies in concert with prod-ucts of the complement system (Chap. 61). The interaction of basophils and tissue mast cells with IgE antibodies in causation of immediate hypersensitivity is discussed in Chap. 65. Consideration of these interrelationships is an important part of the analysis of patients with suspected immune deficiency.

CLINICAL DISEASE FEATURES COMMON TO IMMUNE DEFICIENCY Immunodeficiency syndromes, whether congenital, spontaneously acquired, or iatrogenic, are characterized by unusual susceptibility to infection and, sometimes, to autoimmune disease and lymphoreticular malignancies. The types of infection often provide the first clue to the nature of the immunologic defect.

Patients with defects in humoral immunity have recurrent or chronic sinopulmonary infection, meningitis, and bacteremia, most commonly caused by pyogenic bacteria such as *He-*

mophilus influenzae, Streptococcus pneumoniae, and staphylococci. This spectrum of infections is similar to that occurring in patients with normal immune responses, but with either neutropenia or a deficiency of the pivotal third component of complement (C3), suggesting that a tripartite collaboration involving antibody, complement, and phagocytes exists as the chief mechanism of host defense against pyogenic organisms. Binding of antibody to the bacterial surface causes activation of the complement system. One cleavage product of activated C3 serves as a chemotactic factor for polymorphonuclear leukocytes. Activated C3b fixed to bacterial surfaces facilitates phagocytosis by interaction with C3b receptors on neutrophils.

Agammaglobulinemic patients in whom cell-mediated immunity is intact have an interesting response to viral infections. The clinical course of primary infection with viruses such as varicella zoster or rubeola, unless complicated by bacterial infection, does not differ significantly from that of the normal host. However, long-lasting immunity may not develop, and as a result multiple bouts of chickenpox and measles may occur. Such observations suggest that intact T cells may be sufficient for control of established viral infections, while antibodies are primarily important in limiting the initial dissemination of virus. Exceptions to this generalization are becoming more widely recognized. Agammaglobulinemic patients fail to clear hepatitis B virus from their circulation and have a progressive, and often fatal, course. Chronic encephalitis, which may progress over a period of months to years, is being observed with apparently increasing frequency. Echoviruses and adenoviruses have been isolated from brain biopsies or spinal fluid from some patients; in others no agent has been detected. Immunologic injury resulting from a partial and ineffective immune response may contribute as much to the pathogenesis of these diseases as the direct effects of the viruses.

The occurrence of unusual serious infection, for example, *H. influenzae* meningitis in an older child or adult, warrants consideration of humoral immune deficiency. Bacterial infections in certain sites may also suggest this possibility. Chronic otitis media occurs frequently in patients with hypogammaglobulinemia, and is significant because of its relative rarity in normal adults. Pansinusitis, although almost invariably present in immunoglobulin deficiency, is a less helpful finding because it is not rare in apparently normal people. Bacterial infections of the skin or urinary tract are less frequent problems in hypogammaglobulinemic patients.

Abnormalities of cell-mediated immunity predispose to *disseminated virus infections,* particularly with latent viruses such as herpes simplex (Chap. 193), varicella zoster (Chap. 185), and cytomegalovirus (Chap. 195). Patients so affected also almost invariably develop mucocutaneous candidiasis and frequently acquire widely disseminated fungal infections.

Pneumonia caused by the protozoan *Pneumocystis carinii* is also common (Chap. 204).

Infestation with the intestinal parasite *Giardia lamblia* is a frequent enough cause of diarrhea in antibody-deficient patients to warrant diagnostic duodenal aspiration and intestinal biopsy when the organism cannot be demonstrated in the stool.

T-cell deficiency is probably always accompanied by some abnormality of antibody responses, although this may not be reflected by hypogammaglobulinemia. This may explain in part why patients with primary T-cell defects are also subject to overwhelming bacterial infection.

The most severe form of immune deficiency occurs in individuals, usually infants, who lack both cell-mediated and humoral immune functions. They are susceptible to the whole range of infectious agents including organisms not ordinarily considered pathogenic. Multiple infections with viruses, bacte-

ria, and fungi occur, often simultaneously. Because donor lymphocytes cannot be rejected by the recipients, blood transfusions can produce fatal graft-versus-host disease.

DIFFERENTIATION OF T AND B CELLS The functional deficits which occur in both congenital and acquired immunodeficiencies are most usefully viewed as defects at various points along the differentiation pathways of immunocompetent cells. For this reason certain features of the development and differentiation of T and B cells that are especially relevant to the analysis of immunodeficiency are briefly presented here; Chap. 61 provides a general account of their roles in cellular and humoral immunity.

A subpopulation of hematopoietic stem cells may become restricted to lymphoid differentiation prior to migration to the thymus, where T cells are generated, or to the fetal liver and adult bone marrow, where B-cell development occurs (Fig. 62-1). A major function of central lymphoid tissues is to generate the clonal diversity characteristic of the immune system. Each T or B lymphocyte is induced to express surface receptor molecules of a unique specificity for antigen. The receptors of B lymphocytes are immunoglobulins. The nature of T-cell receptors is not yet precisely defined, but they may be similar or identical to the variable regions of immunoglobulins. Generation of clonal diversity depends upon cellular proliferation, such that each of the different receptor specificities encoded in the genome comes to be expressed in individual cells. Thus a clone contains all cells that express the identical antigen-binding receptors. Estimates for the total number of B-cell clones usually vary between 1 and 100 million. This process of clonal development is independent of antigen and reflects a genetically programmed sequence of differentiation analogous to that of primary erythropoiesis or myelopoiesis. This phase, termed *primary differentiation,* begins early in human fetal development but probably continues into adult life.

The first recognizable step in development of B cells is the emergence of lymphoid cells which contain small amounts of intracytoplasmic IgM but lack the surface immunoglobulin receptors characteristic of mature B lymphocytes. These pre-B cells are found almost exclusively in the bone marrow of adults but are first generated in fetal liver. Pre-B cells proliferate rapidly and spawn immature B lymphocytes which express surface IgM receptors and divide rarely. Young B lymphocytes differ from their more mature counterparts in an important physiologic characteristic; they are highly susceptible to inactivation when their receptors bind antigen. This phenomenon almost certainly is an important mechanism in the development of tolerance to self-antigens.

The developmental sequence for expression of diverse immunoglobulin classes by human B lymphocytes begins with expression of IgM. The expression of IgD on IgM-bearing cells occurs later. Lymphocytes committed to synthesis of IgG, IgA, and IgE are all derived from IgM-bearing precursors through a genetic switch mechanism.

There is increasing evidence suggesting that the diversity of T-lymphocyte function is associated with developmentally divergent subpopulations of T cells. T lymphocytes which, as helpers or suppressors, regulate B-lymphocyte differentiation are distinguishable by the presence of cell surface receptors which bind IgM or IgG antibodies, respectively, and also on the basis of histochemical markers and fine-structural features. Membrane antigenic differences, recognized by antiserums prepared in animals or by antibodies occurring in certain autoimmune states, are also being used to identify subpopulations of T cells having different functions. This developmental heterogeneity may explain some immunodeficiencies in which T-cell functions are impaired selectively.

In addition to generating T cells, the thymus apparently secretes hormonal products which regulate cellular maturation

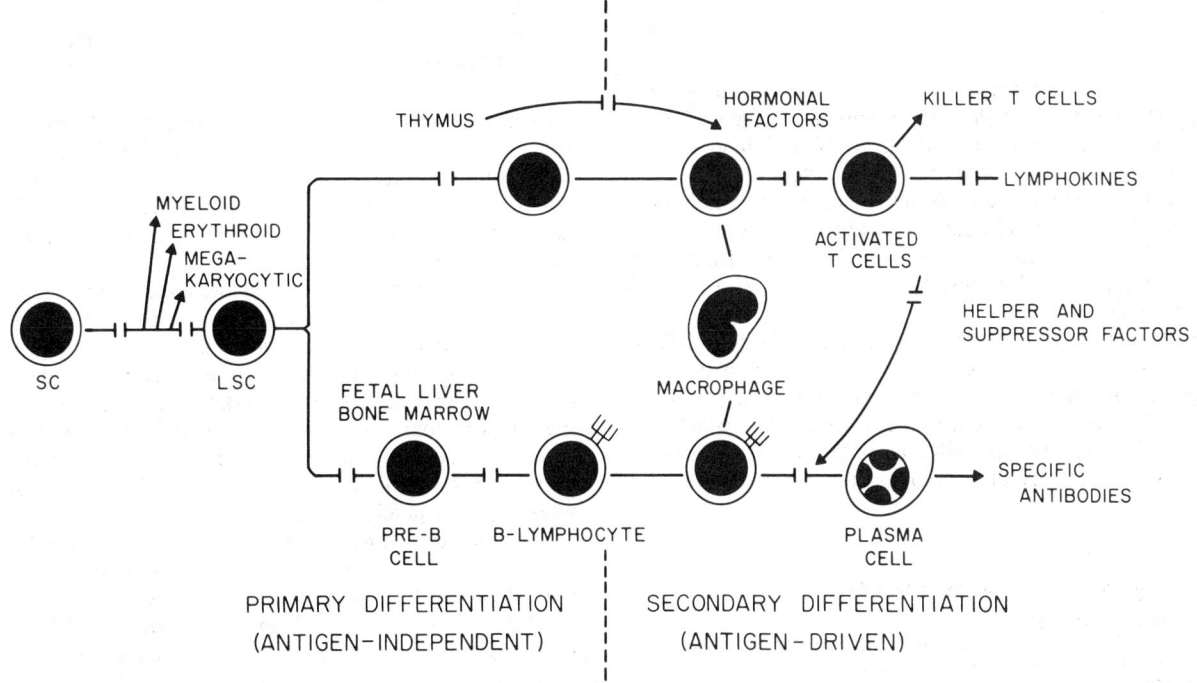

THYMUS — HORMONAL FACTORS — KILLER T CELLS — LYMPHOKINES

ACTIVATED T CELLS

HELPER AND SUPPRESSOR FACTORS

MYELOID ERYTHROID MEGA-KARYOCYTIC

SC   LSC

MACROPHAGE

FETAL LIVER BONE MARROW

PRE-B CELL   B-LYMPHOCYTE

PLASMA CELL

SPECIFIC ANTIBODIES

PRIMARY DIFFERENTIATION (ANTIGEN-INDEPENDENT)

SECONDARY DIFFERENTIATION (ANTIGEN-DRIVEN)

FIGURE 62-1
Failure to develop T and B cells may result from defective stem cells or from inborn metabolic errors affecting both cell types. Rarely, other hematopoietic cell lines are also absent. Absence of either T or B cells suggests malfunction of central lymphoid tissues, including the thymus and the fetal liver–bone marrow complex. B-cell deficiency may result from failure to generate pre-B cells from their stem-cell precursors or from failure of pre-B cells to give rise to their B-lymphocyte progeny. Agammaglobulinemia and deficiencies of some T-cell functions may occur despite the presence of normal numbers of B or T cells in the circulation. Failure of B lymphocytes to differentiate to plasma cells can be due to intrinsic cellular abnormalities or to faulty T-cell regulation.

in peripheral lymphoid tissues. These hormones have been called *thymosin* or *thymopoetin;* deficiencies of these factors have been implicated in some immunodeficiencies.

The events designated *secondary differentiation* (Fig. 62-1) follow stimulation of specific clones of lymphocytes by antigen. These processes are synonymous with the immune response (Chap. 61). Particularly important in consideration of immunodeficiencies are the collaborative interactions among macrophages, T cells, and B cells. B lymphocytes can proliferate in response to thymus-dependent antigens without the help of T cells, and may differentiate to IgM-secreting plasma cells when stimulated by thymus-independent antigens such as polysaccharides. However, production of normal quantities of antibodies, particularly those of the IgA and IgG classes, requires the collaboration of T cells.

Differentiation of T or B cells may be arrested at either the primary or secondary stage (Fig. 62-1). Reflecting the complex cellular interactions involved in immune responses and the pivotal role played by T lymphocytes, immune deficiencies primarily involving T cells are usually also associated with abnormal B-cell function. Conversely, immunodeficiencies manifested primarily by inability to produce antibodies may be caused by T-cell defects not associated with abnormal cell-mediated immunity.

EVALUATION OF IMMUNODEFICIENT PATIENTS Many of the laboratory assays used for precise evaluation of immunologic functions in humans are available only in specialized centers; nevertheless, most immunodeficiencies may be diagnosed by thoughtful use of tests available in most clinical laboratories. Table 62-1 presents a résumé of laboratory investigations roughly in order of increasing complexity.

A careful history will usually indicate whether the major problem involves the antibody-complement-phagocyte system or cell-mediated immunity. A history of a normal response to smallpox vaccination or of contact dermatitis due to poison ivy suggests intact cellular immunity. Lymphopenia and the absence of palpable lymph nodes may be important findings. However, patients with profound immunodeficiency may have diffuse lymphoid hyperplasia.

Humoral immunity With rare exceptions, deficiency of humoral immunity is accompanied by diminished serum concentration of one or more classes of immunoglobulin. Normal values vary with age, and adult concentrations of IgM (100 mg per 100 ml) are reached at about 1 year, of IgG (1000 mg per 100 ml) at 5 to 6 years, and of IgA (200 mg per 100 ml) at puberty (Chap. 61). Also, the wide range of values among normal adults creates difficulty in defining the lower limits of normal. Reasonable estimates for low normal values are 40 mg per 100 ml for IgM, 500 mg per 100 ml for IgG, and 50 mg per 100 ml for IgA. In the presence of borderline hypogammaglobulinemia, assessing the patient's capacity to produce specific antibodies becomes particularly important. Most hospital laboratories can measure isohemagglutinins, antistreptolysin O, and "febrile agglutinins." Typhoid H and O agglutinins can be measured before and after immunization with standard typhoid vaccine. Many state public health laboratories can perform titrations for antibodies to common viral agents.

Since antibody deficiency may be mimicked clinically by deficiency of complement components, measurement of total hemolytic complement (CH_{50}) should be a part of the evaluation of host defense. Measurement of C3 (β1C) alone is inadequate for screening, since deficiencies of both early and late complement components may predispose to bacterial infection (Chap. 61). Estimation of numbers of circulating B lymphocytes has been of great value in determining the pathogenesis of certain types of immune deficiency. B lymphocytes are identified by the presence of membrane-bound immunoglobulins;

additional markers include receptors for aggregated IgG (Fc receptor), receptors for the third component of complement (C3 receptor), and receptors which specifically bind the Epstein-Barr virus. Fc receptors and C3 receptors are also found on circulating monocytes. Morover, not all B lymphocytes bear the C3 receptor. The Epstein-Barr virus receptor appears to be highly specific for B lymphocytes. They can also be identified and enumerated by specific heterologous antiserums, although these are difficult to prepare.

Pokeweed mitogen (PWM), an extract of the plant *Phytolacca americana,* has the capacity to induce B lymphocytes in culture to proliferate and differentiate to plasma cells. This activity requires the presence of T lymphocytes, which also proliferate in response to PWM. Thus, this assay can measure not only the capacity of B lymphocytes to differentiate, but

TABLE 62-1
Laboratory evaluation of host defense defects

I Preliminary screen*
  A Complete blood count with differential smear
  B Quantitative immunoglobulin levels
II Readily available studies†
  A B-cell function
    1 Natural or commonly acquired antibodies: isohemagglutinins, "febrile" agglutinins, antibodies to common viruses (rubella, rubeola, influenza), and toxins (diphtheria, tetanus)
    2 Response to immunization (typhoid, polio, diphtheria-tetanus vaccines)
  B T-cell function
    1 Skin tests (PPD, mumps, *Candida, Trichophyton,* histoplasmin), streptokinase-streptodornase (Varidase, 1:200), tetanus toxoid
    2 Contact sensitization with dinitrochlorobenzene
    3 Chest x-ray (thymus shadow in infants, thymoma in adults)
  C Complement
    1 C3 (β1C globulin)
    2 CH_{50} (total hemolytic complement)
  D Phagocyte function
    1 Reduction of nitroblue tetrazolium
    2 Inflammatory skin window (Rebuck)
III In-depth investigation
  A B cell
    1 Pre-B cell examination in bone marrow samples
    2 B-lymphocyte membrane markers: IgM, IgD, IgG, IgA; receptors for aggregated IgG (Fc receptor), C3, Epstein-Barr virus; antigens detected by anti-B antiserum
    3 Induction of B-lymphocyte differentiation in vitro stimulated by pokeweed mitogen
    4 Kinetics and immunoglobulin class of antibody produced in response to specific primary and secondary immunization
    5 Measurement of IgG subclasses and κ/λ ratio
    6 Histologic and immunofluorescent examination of biopsy specimens (intestinal mucosa, lymph node, bone marrow)
  B T cell
    1 Surface markers: binding of sheep erythrocytes (E rosettes), anti-T antiserum, T cells bearing receptors for IgM (T_M) and IgG (T_G)
    2 In vitro correlates of delayed hypersensitivity
      a Proliferative response to mitogens: phytohemagglutinin, concanavalin A specific antigens (PPD, *Candida*); allogeneic cells (one-way mixed lymphocyte response)
      b Quantification of lymphokines (migration inhibitory factor, etc.)
      c Induction of killer cells by stimulation with allogeneic lymphocytes
    3 Measurement of thymus hormones
    4 Assays for T-cell "helper" function using supernatants of antigen-activated T cells or T cells plus PWM or antigens to trigger B-lymphocyte differentiation
    5 Skin graft rejection
  C Phagocytes and complement
    1 Chemotactic response in vitro
    2 Bactericidal function
    3 Classic and alternative complement components
  D Miscellaneous: lymphocytotoxic antibodies to T or B cells

* *Together with a history and physical examination, these tests will identify more than 95 percent of patients with primary immunodeficiencies.*
† *These assays are generally available in either hospitals or state public health laboratories. With rare exceptions, information gained from tests in categories I and II is sufficient to diagnose and treat those immunodeficiencies amenable to conventional treatment with gamma globulin or plasma.*

can also assess the "helper" or "suppressor" function of patients' T lymphocytes.

Cellular immunity Human T lymphocytes can be most easily enumerated by their capacity to bind sheep erythrocytes in the cold, forming what are called *E rosettes.* The nature and function of these receptors are unknown, but they are not related to the antigen-specificity of T cells. T cells can also be enumerated by use of specific antiserums.

T-lymphocyte function can be measured in vivo by delayed hypersensitivity skin testing, using a variety of antigens to which the majority of older children and adults have been sensitized. Among the most useful are purified protein derivative (PPD), histoplasmin, *Candida* extract, *Trichophyton* extract, mumps, streptokinase-streptodornase, and tetanus toxoid. The capacity to become sensitized to a new antigen may be tested by application of dinitrochlorobenzene to the skin, followed 2 weeks later by patch testing at a different site.

T-lymphocyte function may be estimated in vitro by the capacity of cells to proliferate in response to antigens to which the patient has been sensitized, to lymphocytes from an unrelated donor, or to the T-cell mitogens, which include phytohemagglutinin, concanavalin A, and pokeweed mitogen. The response is usually quantified by measurement of incorporation of radioactive thymidine into newly synthesized DNA. It is also possible to measure the production of lymphokines, particularly migration inhibition factor, by activated T cells. Finally, the ability of T cells activated in mixed lymphocyte culture to lyse target cells sensitized by phytohemagglutinin can be measured.

The capacity of T lymphocytes from immunologically normal persons to be activated in vitro with antigens or mitogens may be abolished or markedly diminished by acute febrile illness, treatment with corticosteroids, or stress. Except for these situations, there are relatively few instances in which normal numbers of T lymphocytes, as measured by the E rosette test, are not associated with relatively normal function in the aforementioned in vitro assays.

CLASSIFICATION Primary immunodeficiencies may be either congenital or acquired, and are currently classified according to mode of inheritance and whether the defect involves T cells, B cells, or both. Unfortunately, the best current classification, established by an expert committee of the World Health Organization, still places the majority of immunodeficiency diseases in an undefined category called *common variable immunodeficiency.* In general, this classification will be followed in the following discussion, which emphasizes three related concepts; first, that immunodeficiencies are most logically viewed as defects of cellular differentiation; second, that these defects may involve either primary development of T or B cells or the antigen-dependent phase of their differentiation; and third, that defects of secondary B-cell differentiation may in some instances reflect T-cell abnormalities resulting from faulty T-B collaboration.

Secondary immunodeficiencies are those not caused by intrinsic abnormalities in development or function of T and B cells. Examples are immune deficiency associated with malnutrition, protein-losing enteropathy, and intestinal lymphangiectasia. Also considered secondary are immunodeficiencies resulting from hypercatabolic states such as occur in myotonic dystrophy, immunodeficiency associated with lymphoreticular malignancy, and immunodeficiency resulting from treatment with x-rays, antilymphocyte serum, or cytotoxic drugs.

Incidence As a group, the immunodeficiency syndromes discussed in this chapter are relatively common. Isolated IgA deficiency occurs in approximately 1 in 600 individuals; no other specific category approaches this frequency, but the cumulative total is not insignificant. The incidence of diagnosed immunodeficiency diseases is clearly a function of the awareness of physicians in a community. An epidemic of immunodeficiency diseases commonly follows the addition of a clinical immunologist to a medical center staff.

The more severe forms of primary immunodeficiency have their onset early in life and all too frequently result in death during childhood. Immunodeficiencies may be acquired at any age, however, and a substantial number of patients with congenital hypogammaglobulinemia survive to middle age or beyond. In a referral center for patients with immunodeficiency diseases, approximately two-thirds of the immunodeficient patients under care are adults. Improved methods of diagnosis and treatment can be expected to increase this ratio in the future.

Severe combined immunodeficiency (SCID) This syndrome is characterized by gross functional impairment of both humoral and cell-mediated immunity. It is usually congenital, may be inherited either as an X-linked or autosomal recessive defect, or may occur sporadically. Affected infants rarely survive beyond one year. This syndrome has been associated with a diversity of defects in development of immunocompetent cells, some of which may be related to specific enzymatic abnormalities.

The classic example of SCID, *Swiss-type agammaglobulinemia,* is characterized by severe lymphopenia involving both T and B cells, and is inherited with an autosomal recessive pattern. Rarely, other hematopoietic cell lines fail to develop. The cellular defect in these forms of SCID logically rests with the precursor common to both T and B cells. The immunologic defects in a few of these patients have been repaired following transplantation of fetal liver as a source of stem cells, confirming the hypothesis that they have a thymus and bursa equivalent capable of supporting differentiation of normal stem cells. About half of patients with autosomal recessive SCID are deficient in an enzyme involved in purine metabolism, adenosine deaminase (ADA). These patients have varying degrees of lymphopenia, T cells usually being more deficient than B cells. The pathophysiologic relationship of ADA deficiency to lymphoid differentiation is slowly being unraveled. The best current evidence suggests that intracellular accumulation of deoxy-ATP, by inhibiting ribonucleotide reductase enzymes, interferes with synthesis of DNA precursors, particularly deoxycytidine. Improvement of both clinical status and immunologic function has occurred in some but not all patients treated with a source of exogenous ADA; therapy with deoxynucleosides is currently being investigated.

SCID may also occur with an X-linked inheritance pattern. Affected boys may not have severe lymphopenia; some have had normal numbers of B lymphocytes with few or no circulating T lymphocytes. This developmental pattern (which may also occur with autosomal recessive inheritance) suggests the possibility of a faulty thymus epithelium. Mononuclear cells from such patients have been induced to express T-cell characteristics by coculture on normal thymus epithelium or by treatment with thymus hormones.

A number of individuals with SCID have been successfully treated by transplantation of histocompatible bone marrow from sibling donors. The same treatment has been used in children and adults with leukemia or aplastic anemia (Chaps. 69 and 312) following purposeful destruction of the immune system by irradiation and cytotoxic drugs. Other modes of treatment, including fetal liver and thymus transplants, have been successful in restoring immunocompetence, but as yet there are only short-term survivors. Treatment of these patients should probably be attempted only in centers with a strong research interest in this problem. It is crucial that these patients be

recognized early and not be given blood transfusions which may cause fatal graft-versus-host disease.

T-cell immunodeficiency Primary T-cell defects are extremely difficult to define. Reflecting the diversity of T-cell functions, abnormalities of T-cell development may be responsible for a wide spectrum of immune deficiencies including severe combined immunodeficiency, apparently isolated defects in cell-mediated immunity, and syndromes presenting as antibody deficiency with apparently normal cell-mediated immunity. These defects may be acquired as well as congenital. Until very recently, laboratory assays of T-lymphocyte function were limited to correlates of cell-mediated immunity; no means were available for studying T-cell regulation of B-cell differentiation. With the development of appropriate methodology it will undoubtedly be found that clinically significant abnormalities of T cells are much more common and heterogeneous than is now appreciated.

DI GEORGE SYNDROME This is the classic example of isolated T-cell deficiency and results from maldevelopment of organs derived embryologically from the third and fourth pharyngeal pouches. Affected infants usually present with congenital cardiac defects, particularly those involving the great vessels, hypocalcemic tetany due to failure of parathyroid development, and absence of the thymus. Other associated abnormalities may include abnormal ears, shortened philtrum, and hypertelorism. Serum immunoglobulin concentrations are usually normal. Lymphocyte counts may be normal, but virtually all the lymphocytes are B cells. Carefully performed autopsies have often revealed a tiny, histologically normal thymus, usually in an ectopic location. With time, a few patients developed functional T cells. Patients with Di George's syndrome have had transplants of fetal thymus and subsequently have developed normal cell-mediated immunity, associated with T cells of host origin.

Children lacking the congenital anomalies associated with Di George's syndrome may present with severe impairment of cell-mediated immunity. Some have normal or even increased immunoglobulin levels, while others have selective deficiencies of one or more immunoglobulin classes. Specific antibody responses are usually impaired even in patients with normal concentrations of immunoglobulins. This ill-defined entity has been called the *Nezelof syndrome.*

Inherited deficiency of the enzyme purine nucleoside phosphorylase (PNP) is associated with an often severe and selective deficiency of T-lymphocyte function. This enzyme functions in the same purine salvage pathway as ADA; toxic effects of its deficiency are attributed to reduction in synthesis of deoxycytidine by mechanisms similar to those involved in ADA deficiency.

A few patients with isolated T-cell deficiency have been treated with fetal thymus grafts. Some have shown improvement in numbers of circulating T cells, in vitro reactivity to mitogens, and clinical condition, while others have had no change in status. A patient treated with thymosin developed increased numbers of circulating T cells and delayed hypersensitivity skin reactions associated with clinical improvement. Transfer factor has been reported to benefit a few patients.

ATAXIA-TELANGIECTASIA This is an autosomal recessive genetic disorder characterized by cerebellar ataxia, oculocutaneous telangiectasia, and immunodeficiency. Onset of truncal ataxia usually occurs in infancy and is progressive. Immunodeficiency is clinically manifest by recurrent and chronic sinopulmonary infection leading to bronchiectasis. The two most frequent causes of death are chronic pulmonary disease and malignancy. Lymphomas are most common, although carcinomas have also occurred.

The immunologic abnormalities seem to be related to maldevelopment of the thymus. If found at all, the thymus in autopsied patients has been markedly hypoplastic and similar in appearance to an embryonic thymus. Patients' lymphocytes frequently respond poorly to T-cell mitogens in vitro. Cutaneous anergy and delayed rejection of skin grafts are common. Although the number and class distribution of B lymphocytes are usually normal, most patients are deficient in serum IgE and IgA, and a smaller number have reduced serum levels of IgG. IgM and IgD are usually normal. This suggests a maturational arrest of B lymphocytes secondary to T-cell dysfunction. Indeed, in one IgA-deficient patient, peripheral lymphocytes were triggered by pokeweed mitogen to develop into IgA-synthesizing plasma cells.

There is circumstantial evidence that ataxia-telangiectasia may involve a generalized defect in cellular differentiation. Ovarian agenesis occurs frequently. Persistence of very high levels of oncofetal proteins, including α-fetoprotein and carcinoembryonic antigen, has been found in patients' serum. At the other end of the age spectrum are signs of progeria, including premature graying and early development of senile keratoses and vitiligo. These patients may have a defect in DNA repair mechanisms. Such a defect might underly their unusual susceptibility to irradiation injury, a high frequency of chromosomal breaks in some patients, and the increased incidence of malignancy.

Only symptomatic treatment is available. Unless severe deficiency of IgG is present, therapy with gamma globulin is not indicated. Transplantation with histocompatible bone marrow was followed in one patient by increased synthesis of IgA and transient improvement of cellular immune responsiveness, but chimerism could not be demonstrated. Unusual sensitivity to x-irradiation should be kept in mind in planning therapy for patients who develop cancer.

Immunoglobulin deficiency syndromes X-LINKED AGAMMA-GLOBULINEMIA

This syndrome was long thought to represent a central failure of development of all elements of the B-cell lineage. Recent evidence has modified this concept. Affected males have very few immunoglobulin-bearing B lymphocytes in their circulation and lack primary and secondary lymphoid follicles. However, pre-B cells are found in normal frequency in their bone marrow. This developmental block contrasts with earlier and later arrests in B-cell differentiation characterizing other immunodeficiencies (see below and Fig. 62-1). Patients usually have a substantial number of small mononuclear cells bearing receptors for aggregated immunoglobulin and C'3. Although resembling B lymphocytes, these cells have been shown to have markers characteristic of the monocyte line and to lack the B-lymphocyte specific surface antigen(s) and receptors for Epstein-Barr virus. A few patients with well-documented X-linked agammaglobulinemia have had a normal number of B lymphocytes, suggesting that there may be two distinct forms of this disease.

Agammaglobulinemia is a misnomer, as most patients with this and other forms of severe panhypogammaglobulinemia synthesize some immunoglobulins, primarily of the IgG class. Within the same family some affected males have had substantial levels of IgM, IgG, and IgA, while others have been nearly agammaglobulinemic. All these patients were markedly deficient in circulating B lymphocytes. This observation suggests that the few B lymphocytes which are generated are fully capable of differentiating to plasma cells and secreting immuno-

globulins. A form of arthritis with some of the features of rheumatoid disease occurs in some of these patients and may remit following treatment with gamma globulin.

TRANSIENT HYPOGAMMAGLOBULINEMIA OF INFANCY This is a reversible syndrome in which normal physiologic hypogammaglobulinemia of infancy is unusually prolonged and severe. IgG levels of normal-term infants commonly drop to levels of 300 to 400 mg per 100 ml between 3 and 6 months of age as maternally derived IgG is catabolized; levels subsequently rise reflecting the infants' increased synthetic capacity. In transient hypogammaglobulinemia, the rate of synthesis of IgM, IgG, and IgA remains low for long periods. Some of these infants have a reduced number of B lymphocytes while others have a normal number.

ISOLATED DEFICIENCY OF IgA This is by far the most commonly encountered immunodeficiency, occurring with a frequency of approximately 1 in 600 individuals. With rare exceptions, both serum and secretory IgA are involved. Many adults with isolated IgA deficiency do not seem to have unusual problems with infection. Nevertheless, this condition is not benign. A substantial proportion of IgA-deficient individuals develop precipitating antibodies to IgA. These patients may have severe anaphylactic reactions when transfused with normal blood from a blood bank.

As a group, individuals with IgA deficiency have an increased number of respiratory infections of varying severity, and a few have had severe pulmonary disease such as bronchiectasis. Chronic diarrheal disease also occurs. The incidence of asthma and other atopic diseases among IgA-deficient patients is high, and, conversely, the incidence of IgA deficiency among atopic children has been found to be twenty to forty times that in the normal population. In one study it was found that combined deficiency of IgE and IgA (or IgE deficiency alone) did not predispose to recurrent respiratory infections, while IgA-deficient patients with normal or elevated IgE had recurrent sinopulmonary disease. IgA deficiency is also significantly associated with autoimmune diseases such as rheumatoid arthritis and systemic lupus erythematosus.

IgA deficiency may be familial, but no single pattern of inheritance has been encountered consistently. It has occurred in association with congenital intrauterine infections, such as toxoplasmosis, rubella, and cytomegalovirus infection. Several patients with abnormalities of chromosome 18 have had isolated IgA deficiency. Most commonly, the syndrome appears as a sporadic defect. It may be transient or acquired late in life.

The pathogenesis of IgA deficiency, whether genetic or caused by environmental insult, apparently involves a block in terminal differentiation of B lymphocytes. The great majority of patients studied have had normal numbers of circulating B lymphocytes bearing surface IgA determinants. In vitro stimulation with pokeweed mitogen cells from some patients has resulted in differentiation of IgA-secreting plasma cells, while in others selective T-cell suppression of IgA plasma cell differentiation may exist. Although peripheral lymphocytes from IgA-deficient patients generally respond normally to T-cell mitogens, diminished numbers of circulating T cells as detected by the E rosette test and abnormal production of lymphokines by stimulated T cells have been described. Thus, it seems likely that the failure of IgA-bearing B lymphocytes to mature to secretory plasma cells in many patients may reflect abnormalities in T-cell function, the nature of which could reflect either deficiencies in helper T cells or excessive activity of suppressor T cells. A primary T-cell defect, rather than IgA deficiency per se, may help to explain the striking association of IgA deficiency with other immunologically related diseases.

Treatment of IgA deficiency is symptomatic. IgA cannot be effectively replaced by exogenous gamma globulin or plasma, and use of either would greatly increase the risk of development of antibodies to IgA. IgA-deficient patients in need of transfusion should be screened for the presence of antibodies to IgA, and ideally should be given blood only from IgA-deficient donors. All patients known to be IgA-deficient should be warned of the risk of severe transfusion reactions which may occur following infusion of only a few milliliters of blood.

X-LINKED IMMUNODEFICIENCY WITH INCREASED LEVELS OF IgM This is a specific syndrome only because of its inheritance pattern. IgG levels are usually very low, and IgA low or undetectable, while IgD levels may be high. The clinical patterns of infection are similar to those occurring with other hypogammaglobulinemic states. The number and distribution of B lymphocytes bearing IgM, IgG, and IgA have been normal, suggesting that this type of immunodeficiency may also involve a block in terminal differentiation of B lymphocytes. Neutropenia often occurs in affected males and can increase their vulnerability to infections.

ISOLATED DEFICIENCY OF IgM This syndrome has been reported rarely in this country but was detected frequently in a British population. Approximately 20 percent of these patients were asymptomatic while 60 percent had severe recurrent infections, often with bacteremia. Pneumococcal pneumonia and meningitis have often been noted in IgM-deficient patients. Other associated conditions included gastrointestinal disease, atopy, splenomegaly, and development of malignancy. The condition was frequently familial, and was four times more common in males than females. The number of circulating B lymphocytes has varied from very low to normal.

Common variable immunodeficiency This represents a heterogeneous group of syndromes which may be congenital or acquired, sporadic or familial, and which occur in both males and females. These patients have in common the clinical manifestations of antibody deficiency associated with panhypogammaglobulinemia, with deficiency of IgG and IgA, or rarely, with selective IgG deficiency.

Approximately one-third of these patients have few or no circulating B lymphocytes, suggesting a central failure of development of this cell line. The remainder have B lymphocytes, and more than half have a normal number and class distribution. In the few patients studied, B lymphocytes capable of binding specific antigens were present and increased in frequency following immunization. Consistent with the evidence that B lymphocytes in these patients are able to recognize antigens and proliferate, but fail to differentiate to plasma cells, is the fairly common finding of lymphoid hyperplasia, including splenomegaly and nodular lymphoid hyperplasia of the gut.

In agammaglobulinemic patients having B lymphocytes, the pathogenesis of immune deficiency must involve the failure of these cells to differentiate to plasma cells. By use of assays capable of measuring B-lymphocyte differentiation to plasma cells in vitro, three major types of defect have been tentatively identified. First, and most common, is an intrinsic abnormality of B lymphocytes. B lymphocytes from these patients cannot differentiate into immunoglobulin-secreting plasma cells even when provided with help from normal T cells. In other instances, plasma cells containing intracytoplasmic immunoglobulin develop but fail to secrete this product. Second, there is evidence that in some patients the T cells, or their products, may actively suppress terminal differentiation of autologous or normal B lymphocytes. The increase in suppressor activity could be either a primary or secondary abnormality; the latter could explain the increase in T-cell suppressor activity in patients with abnormal B lymphocytes and others in whom B lymphocytes are congenitally absent. Third, quantitative deficiency of helper T-cell function has been observed in some

patients, usually also in association with defective B-cell function.

Cells from some agammaglobulinemic patients having normal B-lymphocyte numbers respond normally to pokeweed mitogen in vitro. Studies of their separated T and B lymphocytes have shown no distinctive abnormalities of the types described above.

Patients with common variable immunodeficiency may present with signs and symptoms highly suggestive of lymphoid malignancy, including fever, weight loss, splenomegaly, generalized lymphadenopathy, and lymphocytosis. Routine histologic examination of lymphoid tissues usually reveals germinal center hyperplasia which may be extremely difficult to distinguish from nodular lymphoma (Chapter 327). Demonstration of a normal distribution of immunoglobulin isotypes and light chain classes on circulating and tissue B lymphocytes can serve to distinguish these patients from those having a monoclonal B-cell malignancy with secondary hypogammaglobulinemia. Treatment of several patients with gamma globulin has resulted in relief of symptoms and reversal of lymphoid hyperplasia.

IMMUNODEFICIENCY WITH THYMOMA Recognition of this condition provided one of the early clues as to the role of the thymus in immunobiology. Although T-cell numbers and cell-mediated immunity are frequently intact, several T-cell abnormalities have been identified. Patients' T cells suppress differentiation of normal B lymphocytes in the pokeweed mitogen assay and may also suppress development of erythroid precursors. Suppressor T-cell activity is mediated by the subset of T cells bearing receptors for IgG, which are found in increased numbers. These patients are very deficient in circulating B lymphocytes, frequently have eosinopenia, and may develop erythroid aplasia. Failure to produce B lymphocytes has been traced to the stem-cell level, since pre-B cells could not be found in their bone marrow. The relationship between the thymoma, T-cell dysfunction, and apparent abnormalities of hematopoietic stem cells remains conjectural.

WISKOTT-ALDRICH SYNDROME This is an X-linked genetic disease characterized by eczema, thrombocytopenia, and repeated infections. Affected boys often present with bleeding in infancy. Most do not survive childhood, dying of complications of bleeding, infection, or lymphoreticular malignancy. The immunologic defects in this disease are well characterized but poorly understood. Serum concentrations of IgM are usually decreased, while IgA and IgG are normal. However, synthetic rates for all three classes may be elevated, indicating a significant element of hypercatabolism. The number and class distribution of B lymphocytes usually have been normal. Some patients acquire a diminished number of T cells as evaluated by the E rosette test and appraisal of lymph node biopsies. Functionally, these boys are unable to make antibodies to polysaccharide antigens normally; responses to protein antigens are often not impaired. They are frequently anergic, and their T cells do not respond normally to challenge with ubiquitous antigens. However, responses to T-cell mitogens, such as phytohemagglutinin, are generally normal. Serial appraisal of affected males suggests that the defects in T-cell function are secondary. It is possible that the Wiskott-Aldrich syndrome reflects a primary defect in the B lymphocyte.

A number of patients with this syndrome have been treated with transfer factor obtained from leukocytes of normal donors. About half appear clinically improved, as judged by a decreased number of infections, clearing of eczema, and, in a few, increased platelet counts. Clinical improvement has been correlated with transfer of delayed hypersensitivity skin reactions to antigens to which the donor was sensitive. It has been difficult to assess the value of transfer factor in the treatment of patients with this syndrome because controlled studies are only now being done. However, fatal infections, severe eczema, hemolytic anemia, nephrotic syndrome, and development of lymphoreticular malignancy have all occurred in patients with and without transfer factor treatment. Greater success has been obtained with transplantation of histocompatible sibling bone marrow in a few patients. The first, treated nearly 10 years ago, has sustained marked improvement in immunologic function but remains thrombocytopenic. Two other boys have apparently had both hematologic and immunologic abnormalities corrected by elimination of their own lymphopoietic system before matched marrow transplantation.

Miscellaneous immunodeficiency syndromes Infection with *Candida albicans* is the almost universal accompaniment of severe deficiencies in cell-mediated immunity. The syndrome of *chronic mucocutaneous candidiasis* is different because superficial candidiasis is usually the only major manifestation of immunodeficiency. These patients rarely develop systemic infection with *Candida* or other fungal agents and are not unusually susceptible to virus or bacterial disease. The syndrome is often congenital and may be associated with single or multiple endocrinopathies as well as iron deficiency. Treatment of associated conditions may lead to improvement or even cure of *Candida* infection.

No uniformity of immunologic defects has been identified in these patients, although defects of antibody formation have been detected occasionally. Humoral immunity, including ability to make specific anti-*Candida* antibodies, is usually normal. Many patients are anergic, some to a variety of antigens and some only to *Candida;* anergy in some patients has been related to inability of their lymphocytes to produce migration inhibition factor.

Results of treatment with antifungal agents, such as amphotericin B, have been variable but generally not encouraging. In some patients, clearing of the *Candida* lesions by treatment with antifungal agents has been maintained sometimes with surgical removal of affected nails and sometimes without periodic administration of transfer factor.

IMMUNODEFICIENCY ASSOCIATED WITH SERUM LYMPHOCYTO-TOXINS This syndrome has been reported in a few patients with recurrent bacterial and fungal infections. Most have had fluctuating lymphopenia. Both cellular immunity and specific antibody responses were impaired, although immunoglobulin levels were usually normal. Antibodies specific for B-cell antigens have also been reported as a cause of selective elimination of B cells and resultant hypogammaglobulinemia.

IMBALANCES OF IgG SUBCLASSES Some patients with repeated infections and only moderately decreased serum IgG levels may have an imbalance of IgG subclasses. A few such patients appeared to benefit from administration of gamma globulin. *Kappa light-chain deficiency* has also been reported in association with recurrent infections, and doubtless many more subtle gaps in antibody diversity, which may be clinically significant, will be elucidated.

Metabolic abnormalities associated with immunodeficiency The relation of deficiencies of the purine salvage enzymes, adenosine deaminase and purine nucleoside phosphorylase, to immunodeficiency was discussed earlier. Other inherited metabolic defects should be briefly mentioned because of their po-

tential importance in understanding the molecular basis of immunologic function. Inherited *deficiency of transcobalamin II,* the serum carrier molecule responsible for transport of vitamin B_{12} to tissues, was associated with failure of immunoglobulin production as well as megaloblastic anemia, leukopenia, thrombocytopenia, and severe malabsorption. All abnormalities were reversed by administration of pharmacologic doses of vitamin B_{12}. The syndrome of *acrodermatitis enteropathica* includes severe desquamating skin lesions, intractable diarrhea, bizarre neurologic symptoms, variable combined immunodeficiency, and an often fatal outcome. This disease is apparently caused by an inborn error of metabolism resulting in malabsorption of dietary zinc, and can be effectively treated by parenteral or large oral doses of zinc. Similar disease manifestations have occurred in mice and cattle with different inherited defects leading to zinc malabsorption. Zinc deficiency might in part account for the immunodeficiency which accompanies severe malnutrition.

TREATMENT OF IMMUNODEFICIENCIES Treatment of immunodeficiency diseases involving severe abnormalities of T-cell function, with or without hypogammaglobulinemia, is currently limited in effectiveness and extremely complicated. Experimental approaches, including transplantation of bone marrow, fetal liver, and thymus, were mentioned in preceding sections. Also under investigation is the use of thymic hormones and of pharmacologic agents which may correct defects in lymphoid function caused by inherited metabolic disorders.

Replacement therapy with human gamma globulin should be used in patients who have recurrent bacterial infections and are deficient in IgG. Maintenance of serum IgG levels between 100 and 300 mg per 100 ml is sufficient to prevent most overwhelming infections, although chronic sinusitis, otitis media, and bronchitis often persist. These serum levels usually can be achieved by intramuscular injection of IgG, 100 mg/kg, at monthly intervals, following a loading dose of twice this amount given over a period of several days. Forty milliliters of 16% gamma globulin, given in two or more sites at one time, is about the maximum tolerable in adults. If more is needed, it is preferable to increase the frequency of injections. Many hypogammaglobulinemic patients and their physicians normally prefer division of the monthly doses into bimonthly injections. In patients with mild to moderate IgG deficiency (300 to 400 mg per 100 ml), the decision to treat must be based on clinical symptoms and on failure to respond to antigenic challenge, because injection of gamma globulin at the recommended doses will not significantly elevate serum IgG levels. Gamma globulin treatment is of no value in patients with deficiencies of immunoglobulins other than IgG. This form of treatment is not benign. Many patients become intolerant, having symptoms of diaphoresis, tachycardia, and hypotension immediately following injections. This reaction is thought to be mediated by aggregates of IgG in the gamma globulin preparation, but why it develops after years of treatment in some patients, and never in others has not been adequately explained. Most patients intolerant of gamma globulin injections can be treated successfully with plasma.

Infusion of fresh plasma, 10 to 20 ml/kg at intervals of 3 to 4 weeks, has the advantages of being less painful and of replacing IgM and IgA as well as IgG; however, both IgM and IgA have a half-life of only a few days. The major disadvantage of plasma is the risk of transmitting hepatitis, which is particularly devastating in immunodeficient patients. This risk can be minimized by use of selected donors, usually family members, carefully screened for the absence of Australia antigen or antibody.

Therapy with exogenous IgG usually does not prevent chronic sinopulmonary infection and its all too frequent progression to pulmonary fibrosis and bronchiectasis. Therefore, maintenance of good pulmonary toilet with regular postural drainage is an especially important part of patient management. The principles of antibiotic therapy are not different in these than other patients, except that the index of suspicion of bacterial infection should remain very high.

REFERENCES

AIUTI F et al: Identification, enumeration, and isolation of B and T lymphocytes from human peripheral blood. Scand J Immunol 3:521, 1974

BERGSMA D et al (eds): *Immunodeficiency in Man and Animals, Birth Defects,* Original Article Series, vol XI, no 1. The National Foundation–March of Dimes, Sunderland, Mass, Sinauer Associates, 1975

COOPER MD et al: Meeting Report 2nd International Workshop on Primary Immunodeficiency Diseases in Man. Clin Immunol Immunopathol 2:416, 1974

JAPAN MEDICAL RESEARCH FOUNDATION (eds): *Immunodeficiency: Its Nature and Etiological Significance in Human Disease.* Tokyo, University of Tokyo Press, 1978

MEISCHER PA, MÜLLER-EBERHARD HJ (eds): *Seminars in Immunopathology,* vol 1: *Immunodeficiency Diseases.* Berlin, Springer-Verlag, 1978

STIEHM ER, FULGINITI VA (eds): *Immunologic Disorders in Infants and Children,* 2d ed. Philadelphia, Saunders, 1979

63
PLASMA CELL NEOPLASMS AND RELATED DISORDERS

RAYMOND ALEXANIAN

Plasma cell diseases constitute a group of related disorders in which a single clone of cells produces large quantities of an immunoglobulin molecule that is usually recognized as a peak on serum or urine electrophoresis. The most important entity is multiple myeloma; other related conditions include Waldenström's macroglobulinemia, idiopathic monoclonal gammopathy, primary amyloidosis, and the heavy-chain diseases. A combination of clinical and electrophoretic studies is necessary to distinguish these entities, to stage the extent of disease, and to evaluate change in tumor mass with or without therapy.

The distinction between these disorders requires an understanding of normal and abnormal immunoglobulin synthesis. Normal immunoglobulins are produced by differentiated plasma cells and consist of two heavy chains linked to two light chains by disulfide bonds. In normal humans, a very large number of different plasma cells produce a wide range of different immunoglobulins that have been grouped into five major classes depending on their heavy chain type: IgG, IgA, IgM, IgD, and IgE. Light chains are of either kappa or lambda type; because of a slightly excessive rate of light chain synthesis, normal humans excrete in urine up to 10 mg per day of a mixture of kappa and lambda light chains. Fig. 63-1 depicts the electrophoretic pattern of normal serum and urine.

Among the different plasma cell disorders, the frequency of a specific abnormality in a globulin is proportional to the number of cells producing that particular type of protein and is reflected by the concentration of the different immunoglobulins in serum. Monoclonal gammopathies of IgG type are more common than those of IgA or IgM classes. A monoclonal gammopathy is usually recognized on electrophoresis when about 10^{11} cells of a single clone are present, as in idiopathic gammopathy or primary amyloidosis. Tumor growth usually occurs when about 10^{12} malignant cells are produced, as in multiple myeloma, macroglobulinemia, or the heavy chain

diseases. In addition to the markedly increased production of a monoclonal protein, the quality of immunoglobulin synthesis may also be defective. For example, there may be a markedly excessive rate of monoclonal light chain production, and some patients excrete up to 40 g protein (Bence-Jones protein) a day in the urine. In fact, about 20 percent of the patients with multiple myeloma show only light chain production, although immunofluorescent studies of the involved cells indicate that a low level of heavy chain synthesis also may occur. Some patients produce only the Fc fragments of heavy chains, and have heavy chain disease. Others with myeloma or macroglobulinemia have smaller deletions of segments of their heavy or light chains. The autonomously proliferating cells in these malignant disorders are capable of producing immunoglobulins that are structurally normal in some patients, and a few even demonstrate immunological reactivity. In contrast, still other patients produce a distorted proportion of heavy and light chains, or an excessive quantity of defective globulins.

MULTIPLE MYELOMA Multiple myeloma is a disseminated malignancy of plasma cells that may be associated with bone destruction, bone marrow failure, hypercalcemia, renal failure, and recurrent infections. The disease is most common in the middle-aged and elderly; the median age of occurrence is 60 years. Males are affected slightly more frequently than females. The annual incidence of the disease is about 3 per 100,000 population.

Clinical and laboratory findings The clinical manifestations of multiple myeloma result primarily from the damage produced by plasma cell tumors in the bone marrow and from the effects of abnormal proteins. There is a wide spectrum of pathologic features, and the complications of the disease as well as the modes of therapy required vary markedly among patients.

FIGURE 63-1

Electrophoretic patterns of normal serum and urine. Normal humans produce a mixture of gamma globulins with different heavy and light chain types. In hypergammaglobulinemia, an increased number of plasma cells produce larger quantities of different globulins so that a broad elevation is apparent.

Bone pain from pathologic fractures constitutes the most common symptom and usually is due to compression fractures of the thoracic or lumbar spine. Typically, the pain is well localized, sometimes radicular, and is usually aggravated by movement, as on arising. In about 5 percent of patients, extradural plasmacytomas arising from a vertebra may produce spinal cord compression, paraplegia, and bladder dysfunction. Pathologic fractures of the ribs and proximal bones of the extremities are common. In about two-thirds of the patients, skeletal radiographs demonstrate punched-out lesions that are best seen on lateral skull films, but demineralization without focal destruction or even a normal skeletal structure may be present. Isotopic bone scans are sometimes useful when radiographic bone surveys fail to demonstrate bony lesions and vice versa. Osteolysis appears to result from the increased production by the malignant plasma cells of a factor that stimulates osteoclast proliferation. Rarely, a diffuse osteoblastic bone reaction may occur. In about 15 percent of patients, firm plasmacytomas grow from areas of underlying bone destruction; these lesions usually develop over the skull, sternum, and clavicles where the skin is contiguous to the involved bones. Multiple vertebral compression fractures frequently result in a painless kyphosis of the dorsal spine and a diminution in height of as much as 6 in.

In about 90 percent of patients, the bone marrow infiltration by plasma cells produces a normochromic, normocytic anemia at the time of diagnosis, and the anemia becomes more severe as the number of malignant cells increases. Other factors that contribute to anemia include the hypoferremia of chronic disease, renal failure, chemotherapy, and radiotherapy. The globulins of myeloma may coat the red blood cells, causing rouleaux formation, a markedly increased erythrocyte sedimentation rate, and increased hemolysis. When there is marked hyperglobulinemia the plasma volume may be increased to an extent to reduce the hematocrit by as much as 6 volume percent lower than the value expected for the red blood cell volume. Occasionally, plasma cells may be present in the peripheral blood, but plasma cell leukemia with more than 1000 cells per cubic millimeter is unusual. Granulocytopenia or thrombocytopenia occurs in less than 10 percent of untreated patients. Some myeloma globulins may produce an increased bleeding tendency by interfering with platelet function or by interactions with specific coagulation factors. When

present in high concentrations, IgG or IgA myeloma globulins may result in a symptomatic hyperviscosity syndrome or in cold hypersensitivity from cryoglobulinemia.

Bone marrow aspirates usually contain prominent focal collections of immature plasma cells. The cells are usually large, ovoid, and basophilic, and contain an eccentric nucleus with finely clumped chromatin. Multinucleated cells, prominent nucleoli, and intracytoplasmic deposits of protein may be present. Electron microscopy always reveals a highly developed endoplasmic reticulum characteristic of cells elaborating extracellular protein, even in those few patients without apparent evidence of a monoclonal globulin on electrophoretic studies. Yet, there are no pathognomonic cytologic features that will always distinguish malignant from normal plasma cells.

A variety of chemical abnormalities may result from bone or kidney damage. Hypercalcemia with levels in excess of 11.5 mg per 100 ml is found in about one-fourth of the patients at the time of diagnosis and is due to increased bone resorption. Symptoms due to hypercalcemia, such as nausea, mental confusion, and constipation, may constitute the patient's major complaint. Mild or severe renal failure with elevations of blood urea nitrogen to more than 40 mg per 100 ml is a serious complication that occurs in about 20 percent of the patients. Although tubular damage from large quantities of filtered light chains is considered the major factor, other important causes include hypercalcemia, uric acid nephropathy, and amyloidosis. Renal failure may be precipitated by dehydration, as is induced by some radiographic procedures. In rare patients, an adult Fanconi syndrome may result from derangement of specific tubular functions. An elevated serum uric acid level may occur as a consequence of an increased plasma cell turnover, increased cell destruction from chemotherapy, and/or decreased uric acid clearance from renal impairment. A symmetrical peripheral neuropathy that most frequently involves the lower extremities has been described in some patients. An increased susceptibility to bacterial infection results primarily because the levels of normal immunoglobulins are decreased in about 85 percent of the patients. Cell-mediated immunity is also impaired. Pneumonia, urinary tract infection, and bacteremia may develop, particularly when the myeloma has not been controlled by chemotherapy. Herpes zoster occurs in about 10 percent of the patients.

One of the major features of the disease that is seen in about 98 percent of patients is a homogeneous globulin peak on electrophoresis of the serum, urine, or both (Fig. 63-2). This

FIGURE 63-2

Serum and urine electrophoresis in upper and lower panels from two patients with multiple myeloma. On the left, increased production of a complete monoclonal globulin is reflected in a serum peak; excessive light chains are excreted and produce a urine peak of different mobility. A second patient on the right has a normal serum electrophoresis with evidence only of light chain excretion in the urine.

is present in the serum of about 80 percent of patients and is usually a complete gamma globulin, with immunoelectrophoresis usually revealing monoclonal IgG or IgA heavy chains combined with either kappa or lambda light chains (for example, IgGK, IgAL). Abnormal globulins of IgG type are about three times more frequent than those of IgA type. Monoclonal globulins of IgD or IgE heavy chain type are rare, and Bence-Jones proteinemia has been detected primarily when renal failure inhibits the normal catabolism and excretion of monoclonal light chains. In about 20 percent of patients, only the light chain portion of a gamma-globulin molecule is evident —Bence-Jones protein. Because of its lower molecular weight of about 20,000, light chains of either kappa or lambda type are excreted in the urine and detected as a monoclonal peak on urine electrophoresis (Fig. 63-2). All patients suspected of having multiple myeloma or one of its variants should have electrophoretic studies of both serum and urine. In about 2 percent of patients, a monoclonal globulin cannot be detected in either serum or urine, but immunofluorescent studies almost always confirm the production of a monoclonal globulin by plasma cells.

Diagnosis The diagnosis should be suspected when one or more of the following abnormalities is present: bone pain from pathologic fractures of the spine or ribs, anemia, proteinuria, azotemia, hypercalcemia, recurrent infection, or spinal cord compression. In patients with severe bone pain and anemia who demonstrate bone marrow plasmacytosis, the presence of lytic bone lesions and a peak on serum or urine electrophoresis is diagnostic. Both serum and urine electrophoresis must be evaluated in patients suspected of having myeloma, and electrophoresis of concentrated urine may be necessary for the detection of small amounts of light chains. Examination of the marrow alone may not distinguish the plasma cell infiltration of multiple myeloma from the reactive plasmacytosis found in chronic infection, chronic liver disease, or collagen diseases. In these disorders, the generalized plasma cell reaction will usually produce a diffuse hypergammaglobulinemia on electrophoresis (Fig. 63-1). The occurrence of hypercalcemia or azotemia is also not specific, but the finding of markedly depressed normal immunoglobulins may help to distinguish myeloma from other nonmalignant plasma cell dyscrasias. In patients with equivocal findings, the presence of large IgG or IgA peaks in the serum (>3.0 g per 100 ml), depressed values of normal serum immunoglobulins, or a detectable quantity of Bence-Jones protein in the urine supports the diagnosis of myeloma. The excretion of monoclonal light chains of either kappa or lambda type usually signifies myeloma, macroglobulinemia, or primary amyloidosis, but the patient may not be clinically symptomatic for a prolonged period when this is the only abnormality. Diseases that must be distinguished from myeloma include idiopathic monoclonal gammopathy, primary amyloidosis, Waldenström's macroglobulinemia, the heavy chain diseases, and metastatic bone tumors. In addition, patients with localized plasmacytoma or indolent multiple myeloma need to be identified because in them chemotherapy is not indicated.

Treatment and prognosis The best treatment for multiple myeloma requires the prevention and control of the complications of this disease, as well as simultaneous efforts to reduce the number of malignant plasma cells. In disabled patients, increased physical activity should be encouraged by the rational use of analgesics, corsets, and walkers. Radiation therapy is useful for disabling bone pain from pathologic fractures, particularly when there is little improvement after the first course of chemotherapy. Immediate radiotherapy to areas of spinal cord compression may prevent the need for decompressive laminectomy after tumor masses are identified by prompt my-

elography. Adequate hydration is essential in order to prevent and control renal complications from the precipitation of Bence-Jones protein in the renal tubules; dehydration must be avoided in preparing patients for radiologic procedures. For patients with severe renal failure, hemodialysis may maintain life for the period required to reduce Bence-Jones protein production with chemotherapy. Hypercalcemia in previously untreated patients is almost always reversible with fluids, increased activity, and chemotherapy with drug combinations that include prednisone. If a bacterial infection develops, prompt and rational use of antibiotics is essential. Prophylactic gamma globulin has no value, and vaccinations with live organisms must be avoided in these immunosuppressed patients.

For symptomatic patients with multiple myeloma and asymptomatic patients with rising myeloma proteins or progressive lytic bone lesions, chemotherapy is required in order to reduce the number of plasma cells. Serial assessments of myeloma protein levels in serum and/or urine are essential for evaluating changes in tumor mass. Before each course of drug therapy, blood counts must be monitored to ensure adequate recovery of granulocytes to a level of 2000 per cubic millimeter and platelets to a level of 100,000 per cubic millimeter. Intermittent courses of an alkylating agent–corticosteroid combination, repeated at 4- to 6-week intervals, will produce tumor reductions of greater than 75 percent in about one-half of previously untreated patients. Melphalan (8 mg/m^2 per day for 4 days) and prednisone (60 mg/m^2 per day for 4 days) are the drugs most commonly used for patients with multiple myeloma. The addition of intravenous vincristine (1.0 mg) with a 3-week treatment interval may produce a 15 percent higher response rate and a median survival time about 5 months longer than previously achieved. Recalcification of lytic bone lesions and an elevation of low immunoglobulin levels occur in 15 percent of patients who respond. Intermittent treatment should be continued for at least 18 months because many patients respond slowly. After 18 months, patients who have responded and whose abnormal globulins have disappeared from the serum can be followed without chemotherapy. Serial electrophoretic measurements must continue to be made because tumor recurrence, recognized by the reappearance of myeloma proteins, can usually be controlled with chemotherapy. When relapses fail to respond despite continued treatment with alkylating agents and steroids, repeated courses of doxorubicin (Adriamycin) combinations can produce significant tumor reductions in about 25 percent of patients resistant to alkylating agents. A representative program consists of intravenous vincristine (1.0 mg) and intravenous doxorubicin (25 mg/m^2 on day 1) combined with cyclophosphamide (100 mg/m^2 per day) and prednisone (60 mg/m^2 per day for 4 days). Patients who have not responded previously to an alkylating agent–corticosteroid combination rarely respond to doxorubicin.

The median survival time for patients who receive combinations of alkylating agents, corticosteroids, and vincristine is about 30 months. But there is a wide variation in prognosis that depends on the extent of tumor mass at the time of diagnosis and the maximum degree of tumor reduction with chemotherapy. The pretreatment tumor mass can be estimated from such laboratory data as the degree of anemia, hypercalcemia, and bone lesions; the degree of tumor mass reduction can be assessed by the rate of reduction in myeloma proteins. The median survival is less than 1 year for patients with a high cell mass and no response, about 4 years for those with a low tumor mass and a marked response, and various intermediate responses depending on the number of plasma cells. When severe irreversible renal failure is present, the median survival is short regardless of the tumor mass and the degree of remission. About 2 percent of all patients and about 6 percent of responding patients who live longer than 2 years will develop acute myelogenous and monocytic leukemia; the long-term treatment with alkylating agents is probably the major cause.

INDOLENT MYELOMA   An increasing number of asymptomatic patients with multiple myeloma in an indolent phase have been recognized. In many patients, the diagnosis was first suspected after routine biochemical studies revealed an elevated total protein level which on serum electrophoresis is found to be due to a monoclonal gammopathy. Further studies usually confirm bone marrow plasmacytosis and depressed normal immunoglobulins; mild anemia and lytic bone lesions may also be present. Chemotherapy should be withheld in patients unlikely to experience major morbidity, but changes in the level of myeloma protein, hemoglobin, and bone lesions must be monitored to detect tumor mass progression. Patients with Bence-Jones proteinuria, compression fractures of the vertebrae, recurrent infection, or rising myeloma proteins should receive chemotherapy without delay.

LOCALIZED MYELOMA   In occasional patients considered to have a localized plasmacytoma, only one or two plasma cell tumors can be identified without other areas of bone destruction or bone marrow plasmacytosis. All the major disease complications usually associated with myeloma, such as severe anemia and hypercalcemia, are absent. About one-half of the patients do not show a monoclonal globulin peak in the serum or urine; even when present, the level is always low. Normal serum immunoglobulins are usually not depressed. Local radiotherapy in a dose of about 4000 rads is recommended for treatment, but prophylactic chemotherapy is not indicated. Periodic evaluation of serum and urine globulins and of skeletal radiographs in those without abnormal globulins is necessary to detect the presence of multiple myeloma.

WALDENSTRÖM'S MACROGLOBULINEMIA   Waldenström's macroglobulinemia is a chronic lymphoproliferative disorder with a wide range of manifestations. This disease affects the middle-aged and elderly and has a slightly higher frequency in men than women. The presence of a monoclonal peak on electrophoresis which is found to be of IgM type by immunoelectrophoresis is a prerequisite for the diagnosis (Fig. 63-3). Aside from uncommon patients with idiopathic IgM peaks, most patients have evidence of an underlying lymphoma which is characterized by bone marrow infiltration, enlargement of lymph nodes and/or spleen, chronic lymphocytic leukemia, or a combination of these features. Conversely, in about 80 percent of patients with chronic lymphocytic leukemia or lymphocytic lymphoma, the affected cells show evidence of monoclonal IgM production by immunofluorescent studies; about 5 percent of patients with these diseases also have an IgM peak on serum electrophoresis.

Clinical and laboratory features   The most common clinical presentations include anemia, lymphadenopathy, chronic lymphocytic leukemia, and the hyperviscosity syndrome. The anemia usually results from a marked bone marrow infiltration by lymphocytes, plasma cells, and lymphocytes that resemble plasma cells. Histologically, the nodes are infiltrated diffusely in a pattern that resembles a lymphocytic lymphoma, although the picture may be closer to that of a histiocytic lymphoma. Because of the large molecular weight of the pentametric IgM molecule (Fig. 63-3), increased serum concentrations of mono-

clonal IgM may produce marked hyperviscosity of the blood. The symptoms of the hyperviscosity syndrome are most commonly lassitude and confusion, segmental dilatation of retinal veins with retinal hemorrhages, and an increased bleeding tendency due to an interaction of the monoclonal IgM with coagulation factors and interference with platelet function. Sometimes the macroglobulin may show the characteristics of a cold agglutinin and produce a chronic hemolytic anemia. Renal failure is rare in macroglobulinemia, probably because Bence-Jones proteinuria is absent or the protein is excreted at low levels. About 2 percent of patients show lytic bone destruction, as seen in myeloma. Normal IgG and IgA are usually not reduced to the degree found in multiple myeloma. Cryoglobulins have been described in patients who have both macroglobulinemia and multiple myeloma. These consist of monoclonal globulins that precipitate at temperatures below 37°C (98.6°F). Raynaud's phenomenon, ulcers of the fingers and toes, and other manifestations of cold sensitivity may develop. In the work-up of patients with cryoglobulinemia, serum should be collected and separated at warm temperatures before precipitation is studied in the cold.

Treatment   For most patients, the best management includes the reduction of the tumor mass with chemotherapy and the simultaneous control of complications. Red blood cell transfusions should be given only after considering that a markedly increased plasma volume due to the IgM globulin may produce severe hemodilution and reduce the hematocrit up to 6 volume percent and that raising the hematocrit with transfusions may increase blood viscosity to symptomatic levels. For patients with symptoms due to cryoglobulinemia, protection of the extremities from the cold is necessary. When fatigue or neurologic changes occur, and serum viscosity measurements

FIGURE 63-3

In macroglobulinemia, the excessive production of a single pentameric globulin is demonstrated as a peak and requires immunoelectrophoretic studies for identification. With heavy chain disease, IgG heavy chains are present in serum and urine without monoclonal kappa or lambda light chains.

Macroglobulinemia

Heavy Chain Disease

that exceed five times normal are present, plasmapheresis is indicated. This procedure is carried out most expeditiously with an automatic blood cell separator. Because about 80 percent of the macroglobulin is located within the circulation, efficient removal of IgM molecules is possible.

Intermittent courses of a chlorambucil (8 mg/m² per day for 10 days) and prednisone (30 mg/m² per day for 10 days) combination, repeated at 6-week intervals, are effective in reducing the tumor mass by at least 50 percent in approximately three-fourths of the patients. As in myeloma, periodic monitoring by serum electrophoresis is necessary because changes in the monoclonal IgM concentration are helpful in assessing the change in tumor mass. Irradiation may be necessary for aggregates of large lymph nodes. After 18 months, chemotherapy can be withheld from selected patients who achieve a marked reduction in tumor and can be resumed should relapse occur. When there is progressive tumor growth despite repeated courses of alkylating agents and prednisone or when the histologic features of a histiocytic lymphoma are present, other drug combinations that include doxorubicin (Adriamycin) and bleomycin may be helpful. The prognosis is considered slightly better than for multiple myeloma; the median survival is about 3 years.

IDIOPATHIC MONOCLONAL GAMMOPATHY About 0.5 percent of normal individuals over the age of 40 years show a small monoclonal peak on serum electrophoresis. The incidence increases with advancing age so that about 3 percent of individuals over the age of 70 show this abnormality. Usually, monoclonal gammopathy is not suspected when the electrophoresis is ordered, and none of the laboratory or radiographic abnormalities associated with myeloma are present. The concentration of the monoclonal protein is almost always less than 3.0 g per 100 ml, and Bence-Jones proteinuria is rarely present. The protein consists of IgG in about 85 percent of patients, and IgA and IgM globulins account for the remainder. In contrast to myeloma, immunoglobulin levels are usually normal.

When a peak is detected, appropriate studies should rule out the presence of myeloma, macroglobulinemia, or amyloidosis. Most authorities agree that any relationship between monoclonal peaks and other specific underlying diseases, such as an occult solid tumor, is probably coincidental. Periodic long-term follow-up usually shows no changes in the level of the abnormal globulin for the remainder of the patient's life. Less than 20 percent of these individuals have developed multiple myeloma, lymphoma, or amyloidosis after many years of evaluation. Prophylactic chemotherapy, as is used in myeloma, is unjustified. Some benign peaks are transient, particularly those associated with acute hepatitis and other viral infections.

PRIMARY AMYLOIDOSIS (Chap. 64) Amyloidosis is a disease in which major organs become damaged by a homogeneous material that probably results from the interaction of light-chain fragments with tissue polysaccharides. The organs most commonly affected are the kidneys (nephrotic syndrome), heart (congestive failure), joints (carpal tunnel syndrome), tongue (macroglossia), nerves (peripheral neuropathy), and gastrointestinal tract (malabsorption syndrome). "Secondary" amyloidosis occurs in association with prolonged chronic infection or inflammation, such as familial Mediterranean fever or rheumatoid arthritis. "Primary" amyloidosis with the organ involvement described above has no apparent inflammatory basis and occurs in about 15 percent of patients with overt myeloma or macroglobulinemia; usually it is recognized in these patients only on postmortem examination. In addition, about 90 percent of patients with primary amyloidosis and without evidence of myeloma have a small monoclonal peak on serum or urine electrophoresis. Fragments of light chains are present in amyloid fibrils both in myeloma-associated and

in primary amyloidosis without myeloma. Therefore, primary amyloidosis must be considered a monoclonal gammopathy. The disease apparently results from a single clone of plasma cells that has expanded to a stable size of about 10^{11} cells, as in idiopathic monoclonal gammopathy, but with an excess secretion of free light chains that produces tissue damage in the form of amyloidosis. Biopsies of skin lesions, gums, and rectum provide the best histologic evidence for the disease. All histologic material should be stained with Congo red, and the presence of green birefringence should be sought by polarized microscopy. Because of the risks of hemorrhage, liver and renal biopsies should be employed only when biopsies of other sites are negative. In patients with a monoclonal gammopathy, the excretion of more than 1.0 g albumin in the urine should suggest the diagnosis of amyloidosis. Chemotherapy with melphalan and prednisone is ineffective in resolving amyloid infiltration but may slow the rate of amyloid production by reducing the size of the plasma cell clone.

HEAVY CHAIN DISEASES These rare malignant disorders are characterized by an excessive production of heavy chain fragment, related mainly to the Fc portion of the gamma-globulin molecule. Each of the three described types (gamma, alpha, and mu) have different clinical features and requires immunoelectrophoretic and other special studies for diagnosis.

Patients with *gamma heavy chain disease* are elderly and have easy fatigability, recurrent infections, lymphadenopathy, and splenomegaly. The clinical picture resembles a diffuse lymphoma. Palatal edema may be present because the nodes of Waldeyer's ring are frequently enlarged. Anemia, thrombocytopenia, and eosinophilia are often present, and the bone marrow and lymph nodes are replaced by plasma cells or lymphocytes that resemble plasma cells. The diagnosis requires the demonstration of a monoclonal globulin in both serum and urine of identical electrophoretic mobility and a positive immunoelectrophoretic reaction to IgG antibody (Fig. 63-3). An IgG globulin is present simultaneously in both serum and urine because the Fc fragment of the heavy chain molecule has a molecular weight of about 60,000. No light chains are present. In the presence of a monoclonal peak in serum the diagnosis should be considered when a monoclonal urine globulin does not react with antibody to kappa or lambda light chains. Chemotherapy has usually been ineffective and the prognosis is poor; most patients die of infection within a year of the diagnosis.

Alpha chain disease is the most common of the heavy chain diseases, and afflicted patients have an extensive plasmacytic infiltrate throughout the small intestinal mucosa. The result is a severe malabsorption syndrome with all its attendant complications. Chronic diarrhea, abdominal pain, nausea, and weight loss are common. Young adults between 20 and 30 years of age who live in the Mediterranean region are affected most commonly. There is no sexual preponderance. The diagnosis requires the demonstration of a monoclonal gammopathy in serum or urine that consists only of alpha heavy chains and that is devoid of light chains. Because serum electrophoresis may appear normal, sensitive immunoelectrophoretic procedures and other special studies are often necessary to establish the diagnosis. The disease is progressive in most patients, although spontaneous remissions in some patients have suggested that the disease may represent an unusual reaction to infection.

Very few patients with *mu chain disease* have been described. Most have had a chronic lymphocytic leukemia with a small monoclonal component that is usually difficult to detect on serum electrophoresis. The diagnosis requires the demonstration by serum immunoelectrophoresis of an IgM monoclonal globulin that is devoid of light chains, although free light chains may be present in the urine. Insufficient data are available to determine whether the natural history of this disease differs from that of chronic lymphocytic leukemia.

REFERENCES

ALEXANIAN R et al: Prognostic factors in multiple myeloma. Cancer 36:1192, 1975

————: Combination therapy for multiple myeloma. Cancer 40:2765, 1977

AXELSSON U et al: Frequency of pathologic proteins (M-components) in 6995 sera from an adult population. Acta Med Scan 179:235, 1966

FRANGIONE B, FRANKLIN EC: Heavy chain diseases: Clinical features and molecular significance of the disordered immunoglobulin structure. Semin Hematol 10:53, 1973

ISOBE T, OSSERMAN EF: Patterns of amyloidosis and their associations with plasma cell dyscrasia, monoclonal immunoglobulins and Bence-Jones proteins. N Engl J Med 290:473, 1974

KYLE RA, BAYRD ED: Amyloidosis: Review of 236 cases. Medicine 54:271, 1975

————, ————: The Monoclonal Gammopathies. Springfield, Ill, Charles C Thomas, 1977

MACKENZIE MR, FUDENBERG HH: Macroglobulinemia: An analysis of 40 patients. Blood 39:874, 1972

64
AMYLOIDOSIS

ALAN S. COHEN

DEFINITION AND CLASSIFICATION Amyloidosis may be defined as the extracellular deposition of the fibrous protein amyloid in one or more sites of the body. This protein has unique ultrastructural, x-ray diffraction, and biochemical characteristics. It can be deposited locally where it has no clinical consequences or may involve virtually any organ system of the body leading to severe pathophysiologic changes, or the disease may fall between these two extremes. The natural history of amyloidosis is poorly understood, and the clinical diagnosis is often not made until the disease is far advanced. The following classification is clinically the most useful: (1) primary amyloidosis (no evidence for preexisting or coexisting disease); (2) amyloid associated with multiple myeloma; (3) secondary amyloidosis associated with chronic infectious diseases (e.g., osteomyelitis, tuberculosis, leprosy) or chronic inflammatory diseases (e.g., rheumatoid arthritis and ankylosing spondylitis); (4) heredofamilial amyloidosis, the amyloidosis associated with familial Mediterranean fever and a variety of neuropathic, renal, cardiovascular, and other syndromes; (5) local amyloidosis (local, often tumor-like, deposits occur in isolated organs without evidence of systemic involvement); and (6) amyloidosis associated with aging.

PATHOLOGY AND STRUCTURE Amyloid is amorphous, eosinophilic, hyalin, extracellular, and ubiquitous in distribution. The involved organs may have a rubbery firm consistency and a waxy, pink or grey appearance. Organ enlargement, especially of the liver, kidney, spleen, and heart, may be prominent.

Microscopically, amyloid stains pink with the hematoxylineosin stain and shows metachromasia with crystal violet or methyl violet. The Congo red stain imparts a unique green birefringence when sections are viewed in the polarizing microscope. This is the single most useful procedure for establishing the presence of amyloid. Amyloid deposits may be focal in almost any area of the body but are most often perivascular.

The heart may show focal or diffuse interstitial deposits in the myocardium, endocardium, or pericardium.

In the kidney, the glomerulus is primarily affected although interstitial, peritubular, and vascular amyloid occur. In early lesions, small nodular or diffuse deposits appear near the basement membrane and, as the disease progresses, the glomerulus may be massively laden with amyloid, and its capillary bed will be occluded.

In the gastrointestinal tract, there may be perivascular deposits only, or irregular or diffuse deposits may be found in the submucosa, in the muscularis mucosa, or subserosa. The amyloid may appear at any level or portion of the gastrointestinal tract including the gallbladder and pancreas.

In the nervous system, amyloid has been described along peripheral nerves, in autonomic ganglia, and in senile plaques as well as blood vessels of the central nervous system. It may be found in any portion of the orbit including the vitreous humor and cornea.

In summary, there is virtually no area of the body that is spared. This ubiquitous distribution elicits a wide variety of clinical symptoms and signs.

All types of human amyloid consist of fine, nonbranching rigid fibrils that in tissue sections measure approximately 100 Å in diameter. The amyloid fibrils are usually seen earliest in the mesangial cell in the kidney and Kupffer cell in the liver. Isolated amyloid fibrils have a delicate, thin, nonbranching fibrous character. The individual fibril (or filament) has a diameter of about 70 Å and tends to aggregate laterally. Each fibril (filament) has subunit protofibrils of 30 to 35 Å diameter.

A second component, the plasma component or pentagonal unit (P component) with a different ultrastructure, x-ray diffraction pattern, and chemical characteristics, has also been isolated from amyloid and is identical with a circulating α globulin present in very minute amounts. It is not responsible for the characteristic tinctorial properties or ultrastructure of amyloid.

BIOCHEMISTRY OF AMYLOID FIBRILS The bulk of amyloid deposits consists of fibrils. The homology of the fibril of primary and myeloma amyloid to the N-terminal region of the variable fragment of an immunoglobulin light chain and subsequently, in a limited number of cases, to a homogeneous light polypeptide chain, has been demonstrated. These light chain–related proteins range in size from about 5000 to 25,000 daltons and are now termed amyloid light chain (AL) or A_κ or A_λ (Table 64-1). Amino acid sequence analysis indicates that most primary amyloid proteins contain the N-terminal amino acid residue identical to the variable regions of the light chain (Asp-Ile-Gln-Ser-Pro-Ser-Ser-Leu-...).

Another protein that is unrelated to any known immunoglobulin has been described in the secondary amyloid deposits. This protein, amyloid A (AA) protein, can be isolated from the amyloid of patients with secondary amyloidosis and from that associated with familial Mediterranean fever. It is a unique protein with a molecular weight of about 8500 daltons made up of 76 amino acid residues arranged in a single chain, and an amino acid sequence beginning with Arg-Ser-Phe....

Antiserums to alkali-degraded amyloid fibrils of the AA protein have detected an antigenically related serum component, SAA. Amino acid analysis, peptide maps, and sequence studies suggest that AA protein is an amino terminal fragment of SAA and is derived from it by proteolysis. SAA appears to behave as an acute phase reactant and is elevated in infection, inflammation, and with aging. In addition, SAA is elevated in amyloid-resistant animals suggesting that the appearance of

TABLE 64-1
Helsinki nomenclature of amyloid

Current usage	New nomenclature
TISSUE ISOLATES	
Amyloid fibril protein related to immunoglobulin light chains	AL (or A_κ or A_λ) subtype when known, for example, A_{Kl}
Amyloid of unknown origin, nonimmunoglobulin amyloid, amyloid A, A protein	AA
Pentagonal unit of amyloid, plasma component of amyloid, P component	AP
SERUM ISOLATES	

To designate the serum-related component, simply add S as a prefix; i.e., the serum-related AA would now be SAA (instead of amyloid serum component, ASC, etc.). It is recognized that the serum-related component of AL may simply be designated as kappa or lambda light chains or Bence-Jones proteins.

SOURCE: *Cohen AS, Rheumatology-Immunology: The Scientific Basis of Clinical Medicine, New York, Grune & Stratton, 1979, with permission.*

amyloid is not solely determined by the level of SAA. SAA appears to suppress antibody response, suggesting that it might act as an immune regulator.

P component of amyloid In addition to the characteristic fibrils described above, a minor second component, the P component, has been noted in most amyloid deposits. P component (AP) has been recognized by electron microscopy as a pentagonal-shaped structured unit having an outside diameter of about 90 Å and an inside diameter of about 40 Å. On immunoelectrophoresis it migrates as an alpha globulin, and it possesses antigenic identity with a constituent of normal human plasma. The amino acid sequence is distinct from that of the amyloid fibrils. Its pentagonal ultrastructure is similar to C-reactive protein (CRP), but the latter is one-half the molecular weight of AP and has other well-defined differences despite a similar amino acid sequence.

IMMUNOBIOLOGY OF AMYLOID The etiology and pathogenesis of amyloidosis are unknown. Electron microscopic autoradiographic studies have revealed high concentrations of fibrils adjacent to reticuloendothelial cells, suggesting that these cells may synthesize as well as degrade the fibrils.

An excess antigenic stimulus has been shown to induce amyloid in animals. However, the basic conditions for the experimental induction of amyloidosis have not been clearly defined. Marked depression of T cells with maintenance of normal or hyperactive B-cell function has been described. These findings suggest that disturbances in immunoregulatory mechanisms may be an important step in the pathogenesis of amyloid disease.

CLINICAL MANIFESTATIONS The clinical manifestations of amyloidosis are varied and depend entirely on the area of the body which is involved.

Kidney Renal involvement may consist of mild proteinuria or frank nephrosis. In some cases, the urinary sediment may show only a few red blood cells. The renal lesion is usually not reversible and in time leads to progressive azotemia and death. The prognosis does not appear to be related to the degree of the proteinuria; when azotemia finally develops, the prognosis is grave. In one series the mean survival of patients with renal amyloid from the time of biopsy was 29 months, but in a few cases there was presumptive evidence of regression of the renal amyloid. Hypertension is rare except in long-standing amyloi-

dosis. Renal tubular acidosis or renal vein thrombosis may occur. Localized accumulation of amyloid may be noted in the ureter, bladder, or other parts of the genitourinary tract.

Liver While hepatic involvement is common, liver function abnormalities are minimal and occur late in the disease. The two tests most useful in indicating hepatic amyloid are the Bromsulphalein (BSP) extraction and serum alkaline phosphatase activity. Liver scans produce variable and nonspecific results. Portal hypertension occurs but is uncommon. In a series of 54 patients in which liver tissue was available for examination, all 54 had some amyloid present either in the parenchyma or blood vessels, irrespective of the type of amyloidosis (primary or secondary). Amyloidosis of the spleen characteristically is not associated with leukopenia and anemia.

Heart Cardiac manifestations consist primarily of congestive failure and cardiomegaly (with or without murmurs) and a variety of arrhythmias. Although the cardiac manifestations reflect predominantly diffuse myocardial amyloid, the endocardium, the valves, and the pericardium may be involved as well. Pericarditis with effusion is very rare, although the differential diagnosis of constrictive pericarditis versus restrictive cardiomyopathy frequently arises. Echocardiography has demonstrated symmetrical thickening of left ventricular wall, hypokinesia and decreased systolic thickening of the interventricular septum and left ventricular posterior wall, and left ventricular cavities of small to normal size. Hearts which are heavily infiltrated with amyloid may or may not show an enlarged silhouette. Fluoroscopy usually shows decreased mobility of the ventricular wall; angiographic studies usually demonstrate thickened ventricular wall, decreased ventricular mobility, and absence of rapid ventricular filling in early diastole. Cardiac amyloidosis can present as intractable heart failure. Electrocardiographic abnormalities include a low-voltage QRS complex and abnormalities in atrioventricular and intraventricular conduction, often resulting in varying degrees of heart block. Owing to their propensity to develop conduction defects and arrhythmias, patients with cardiac amyloidosis appear to be especially sensitive to digitalis, and this drug should be used with caution.

Skin Involvement of the skin is one of the most characteristic manifestations of so-called "primary" amyloidosis. The lesions may consist of slightly raised, waxy papules or plaques which usually are clustered in the folds of the axillae, anal, or inguinal regions, the face and neck, or mucosal areas such as ear or tongue. The lesions are seldom pruritic. Involvement of the skin or mucosa may not be apparent clinically but may be disclosed by biopsy. Gentle rubbing of the skin may induce bleeding into the skin, leading to purpura. Cutaneous involvement also can occur in secondary amyloidosis; in one series it was found in 42 percent of such patients, in 55 percent of a group of patients with primary disease, and in all eight patients with hereditary amyloid neuropathy.

Gastrointestinal tract Gastrointestinal symptoms are common in amyloidosis. They may result from direct involvement of the gastrointestinal tract at any level or from infiltration of the autonomic nervous system with amyloid. The symptoms include those of obstruction, ulceration, malabsorption, hemorrhage, protein loss, and diarrhea. Infiltration of the tongue occasionally leads to macroglossia. When not enlarged, the tongue may become stiffened and firm to palpation. While infiltration of the tongue is characteristic of primary amyloidosis or amyloidosis accompanying multiple myeloma, it is occasionally seen in the secondary form of the disease.

Gastrointestinal bleeding may occur from any of a number of sites, notably the esophagus, stomach, or large intestine, and may be severe. Amyloid infiltration of the esophagus may lead to abnormal motility patterns. Small-bowel lesions may lead to clinical and x-ray changes of obstruction. A malabsorption syndrome is seen at times. Amyloidosis may develop in association with other entities involving the gastrointestinal tract, especially tuberculosis, granulomatous enteritis, lymphoma, and Whipple's disease; differentiation of these conditions, which give rise to secondary amyloidosis, from diffuse primary amyloidosis of the small bowel may be difficult. Similarly, amyloidosis of the stomach may closely mimic gastric carcinoma, with obstruction, achlorhydria, and the radiologic appearance of tumor masses.

Nervous system Neurologic manifestations may include peripheral neuropathy, postural hypotension, inability to sweat, Adie pupil, hoarseness, and sphincter incompetence. These manifestations are especially prominent in the heredofamilial amyloidoses. The cranial nerves are generally spared except for those involving the pupillary reflexes. The protein concentration in the cerebral spinal fluid may be increased. Infiltrates of the cornea or vitreous body may be present in hereditary amyloid syndromes. Certain of these syndromes are characterized by a bilateral scalloping appearance of the pupil. Amyloid may infiltrate the thyroid or other endocrine glands but rarely causes endocrine dysfunction. Local amyloid deposits almost invariably accompany medullary carcinoma of the thyroid. Amyloid infiltration of muscle may lead to a pseudomyopathy.

Joints Amyloid can directly involve articular structures by its presence in the synovial membrane and synovial fluid or in the articular cartilage. Amyloid arthritis can mimic a number of rheumatic diseases because it can present as a symmetrical arthritis of small joints, including nodules, morning stiffness, and fatigue. Most patients with amyloid arthropathy eventually are found to have multiple myeloma. The synovial fluid usually has a low white blood cell count, a good to fair mucin clot, a predominance of mononuclear cells, and no crystals.

Respiratory system The nasal sinuses, larynx, and trachea may be involved by accumulations of amyloid which block the ducts, in the case of the sinuses, or the air passages. Amyloidosis of the lung involves the bronchi and alveolar septa diffusely. The lower respiratory tract is affected most frequently in primary amyloidosis and in the disease associated with dysproteinemia. Pulmonary symptoms attributable to amyloid are present in about 30 percent of these patients and in some are the most serious manifestations of the disease. In secondary amyloidosis, pulmonary disease is a frequent histopathologic accompaniment but seldom gives rise to clinically significant symptoms. Amyloid may also be localized in the bronchi or pulmonary parenchyma and may resemble a neoplasm. In these cases, local excision should be attempted and, when successful, may be followed by prolonged remissions.

Hematopoietic system Hematologic changes may include fibrinogenopenia, increased fibrinolysis, and selective deficiency of clotting factors.

HEREDOFAMILIAL AMYLOIDOSIS There is no generally accepted nosology for the heredofamilial amyloid syndromes. Some reports emphasize the site of predominant organ involvement as neuropathic, nephropathic, or cardiopathic amyloidosis, while others stress the genetic aspects. To date, virtually all analyses of pedigrees have shown that, with one major exception, the mode of inheritance is autosomal dominant. The exception is amyloidosis of familial Mediterranean fever which is inherited as an autosomal recessive disorder (Chap. 217). Since there are no specific biochemical, hematologic, or immunologic tests that enable the differentiation of one type of amyloid from another, the specific and recognizable clinical patterns form the basis for classification. Table 64-2 proposes a tentative classification and is based largely on the major site of organ involvement, in addition to genetic data and ethnic background.

The heredofamilial amyloidoses include a group primarily involving the nervous system. Among these are lower limb neuropathy, first described in Portugal, which has a poor prognosis and is characterized by progressively severe neuropathy including marked autonomic nervous system involvement. This variety also has been described in Japan and in a family of Greek origin in the United States and probably exists in several other kinships. In some of these individuals, bilateral "scalloped" pupils are pathognomonic of the disease. The second type of neuropathy has been found in families of Swiss origin in Indiana and of German origin in Maryland. It is a milder disease and is often associated with a carpal tunnel syndrome and vitreous opacities. A more severe variety of generalized neuropathy associated with renal amyloidosis has been described in Iowa in a family of English-Irish-Scottish ancestry.

Several types of severe familial renal disease in association with amyloid have been described. Possibly the most remarkable is familial Mediterranean fever (FMF), a disorder subdivided into phenotype I, with irregularly occurring fever and abdominal, chest, or joint pain, preceding or accompanying renal amyloid, and phenotype II, in which amyloidosis is the first or only manifestation of the disease (Chap. 217). Sporadically, other hereditary forms of renal amyloidosis have been described, including the curious association of urticaria, deafness, and renal amyloid.

Severe familial amyloid heart disease has been described in a Danish family, and familial persistent atrial standstill with amyloid in a family of Mexican-American origin. Miscellaneous hereditary amyloid syndromes include hereditary multiple endocrine neoplasms type II (including medullary carcinoma of the thyroid with amyloid) as well as others listed in Table 64-2.

DIAGNOSIS The specific diagnosis of amyloidosis depends upon obtaining a tissue specimen by biopsy and the demonstration of amyloid with appropriate stains. First, of course, the disease must be suspected. When a patient with a chronic disorder predisposing to amyloid such as rheumatoid arthritis,

TABLE 64-2
Heredofamilial amyloidoses

I Neuropathy
  A Lower limb (Portuguese, Japanese, Swedish, other)
  B Upper limb (Swiss-Indiana, German-Maryland)
II Nephropathy
  A Familial Mediterranean fever
  B Fever and abdominal pain (Swedish, Sicilian)
  C Urticaria, deafness, and renal disease
  D Renal disease and hypertension
III Cardiopathy
  A Progressive heart failure (Danish)
  B Persistent atrial standstill (Mexican-American)
IV Miscellaneous
  A Medullary carcinoma of the thyroid
  B Lattice corneal dystrophy and cranial neuropathy (Finland)
  C Cerebral hemorrhage (Iceland)

SOURCE: *Cohen AS, Rheumatology-Immunology: The Scientific Basis of Clinical Medicine, New York, Grune & Stratton, 1979, with permission.*

tuberculosis, paraplegia, multiple myeloma, bronchiectasis, or leprosy develops hepatomegaly, splenomegaly, malabsorption, cardiac disease, or, most importantly, proteinuria, amyloid should come to mind. In addition, in any heredofamilial syndromes, especially those which have a dominant autosomal mode of inheritance and are characterized by peripheral neuropathy, nephropathy, or cardiopathy, the diagnosis of amyloid should be considered. Finally, primary systemic amyloid should be considered in any individual with a diffuse noninflammatory infiltrative disease involving either mesenchymal tissues—blood vessels, heart, gastrointestinal tract—or parenchymal tissues—kidney, liver, spleen, adrenal.

When the diagnosis is suspected, it is good practice to perform a rectal biopsy. If there is a specific reason for not carrying out this procedure, other sites including skin, gums, or the suspected organ—kidney, liver—may be biopsied. All tissues obtained must be stained with Congo red and examined in the polarizing microscope for green birefringence.

In order to establish the relationship of immunoglobulin-related amyloid to multiple myeloma, electrophoretic and immunoelectrophoretic studies on serum or urine should be performed, when the biopsy reveals amyloid deposition. Most of these patients will have only relatively small paraprotein components and only a few will have frank multiple myeloma. The therapeutic implications of these findings are discussed in greater detail in Chap. 63.

PROGNOSIS AND TREATMENT The course of amyloidosis is difficult to document since dating the time of origin of the disease is rarely possible. When amyloidosis develops in patients with rheumatoid arthritis, it seldom becomes evident when the arthritis is less than 2 years in duration. The mean duration of arthritis before amyloidosis was detected was 16 years in one series. When amyloidosis develops in patients with multiple myeloma, manifestations leading to initial hospitalization are more apt to be related to amyloid disease than to myeloma. In these cases prognosis is very poor, and life expectancy is usually less than 6 months.

Instances have been reported of amyloidosis accompanying treatable infections, such as osteomyelitis, in which at least partial remission has occurred following treatment of the primary disease. There have been similar experiences following successful treatment of tuberculosis or drainage of chronic empyema. However, many such reports are not substantiated by biopsy proof of resorption.

Generalized amyloidosis is usually a slowly progressive disease and leads to death in several years, but it may have a better prognosis than was suspected in the past. The average survival in most large series is 1 to 4 years, but a number of individuals with amyloid have been followed 5 to 10 years and longer.

The major cause of death is renal failure. Sudden death, presumably due to arrhythmias, is also quite common. Occasionally, gastrointestinal hemorrhage, respiratory failure, in-tractable heart failure, and superimposed infections are the terminal events.

There is no specific therapy for any variety of amyloidosis. Rational therapy should be directed at (1) decreasing chronic antigenic stimuli that produce amyloid, (2) inhibition of the synthesis and extracellular deposition of amyloid fibrils, and (3) promoting lysis or mobilization of existing amyloid deposits.

A variety of agents have been used to treat amyloidosis. Proof of their efficacy is not available. The finding that a portion of the immunoglobulin light chain is incorporated in the amyloid of patients with primary amyloidosis and its presumed synthesis by plasma cells has led to the use of alkylating agents. However, these agents cause bone marrow depression, and there are reports of acute leukemia developing in patients receiving melphalan. Moreover, there is experimental evidence that immunosuppressive agents may enhance the deposition of preexisting amyloid. Hence, conservative and supportive measures provide the mainstay of management. It is important to provide these patients with a more optimistic outlook.

Two patients with severe renal amyloidosis and azotemia were subjected to bilateral nephrectomy and renal transplantation followed by immune therapy. One patient died of infection 5 months after surgery. The donor kidney showed no evidence of amyloidosis. The second patient is in clinical remission 7 years after receiving a transplanted kidney. Notwithstanding the hazards of operating upon patients with systemic amyloidosis who may have cardiac involvement, carefully selected azotemic patients could benefit from transplantation.

Colchicine has been shown to be effective in preventing acute attacks in patients with familial Mediterranean fever, and two groups of investigators independently have reported the inhibition of amyloid deposition in the mouse model by colchicine. It is conceivable, therefore, that colchicine is effective in blocking amyloid deposition. However, the exact mechanism of its action is unknown, and no controlled human clinical study has been reported.

REFERENCES

COHEN AS: Amyloidosis. N Engl J Med 277:522, 1967

———: Diagnosis of amyloidosis, in *Laboratory Diagnostic Procedures in the Rheumatic Diseases,* 2d ed, AS Cohen (ed). Boston, Little, Brown, 1975, p 395

——— et al: Amyloidosis: Current trends in its investigation. Arthritis Rheum 21:153, 1978

FRANKLIN EC, ZUCKER-FRANKLIN D: Current concepts of amyloid. Adv Immunol 15:249, 1972

GLENNER GG et al: Amyloid fibril proteins: Proof of homology with immunoglobulin light chains. Science 172:1150, 1971

Diseases of immune-mediated injury

65
DISEASES OF IMMEDIATE TYPE HYPERSENSITIVITY

K. FRANK AUSTEN

INTRODUCTION The capacity of a toxic substance, when injected repeatedly, to elicit an adverse reaction rather than a protected state was recognized and designated *anaphylaxis* by Portier and Richet in 1902. Von Pirquet, perceiving that immunity and hypersensitivity were intimately linked, coined the term *allergy* in 1906 to imply a state of changed reactivity. The inadvertent passive transfer of the capacity to develop an acute allergic response to horses by blood transfusion from an allergic to a nonallergic subject was recognized in 1919 by Ramirez. Passive transfer of serum from a patient allergic to fish to the skin of a normal recipient followed by the antigen-induced appearance of wheal and flare at that site was accomplished by Prausnitz and Küstner in 1921, and this technique became the reference for defining a specific allergy. The association of allergic rhinitis and asthma in the same patient, often with a familial background, and the presence in serum of passive transfer activity to the clinical allergen led Coca and Cooke in 1923 to introduce the concept of *atopy* to imply a propensity to develop the altered state without an unusual exposure to the relevant allergens. As presently used, the term *atopic allergy* implies a familial tendency to manifest alone or in combination such conditions as asthma, rhinitis, urticaria, and eczematous dermatitis (atopic dermatitis). However, individuals with an atopic background may also develop hypersensitivity reactions, particularly urticaria and anaphylaxis, associated with the same class of antibody found in atopic individuals. Thus, the designation *diseases of immediate type hypersensitivity* presents a more suitable framework than the broad term *allergy* or the restrictive definition of atopy.

The passively transferred activity in human serum belongs to a unique immunoglobulin class, IgE; a myeloma protein with skin-fixing capacity was independently recognized and shown to be of the same class. The fixation of IgE to human basophils has been demonstrated by radioautography and electron microscopy and to intraepithelial and perivenular mast cells in tonsils, adenoids, and nasal polyps of humans by immunofluorescence. The biochemical characteristics of mast-cell activation, mediator generation, and secretion of both preformed and newly derived mediators are considered elsewhere (Chap. 61) utilizing information gained from studies with human lung slices or peripheral blood leukocytes rich in basophils. IgE-dependent mediator generation and release also occur in the mast cells of human nasal polyps or skin and thus have been observed in those tissues most involved in diseases of immediate type hypersensitivity.

The physicochemically and functionally diverse mast-cell–derived mediators, presented in Chap. 257 include: histamine, which increases venular permeability and elicits both direct and reflex alterations in pulmonary mechanics; eosinophil chemotactic factor of anaphylaxis (ECF-A) which contains acidic tetrapeptides with preferential chemotactic activity for eosinophils; slow-reacting substance of anaphylaxis (SRS-A) with permeability-enhancing and smooth-muscle–contracting activity; platelet activating factors (PAFs), lipids capable of initiating platelet secretion and aggregation; a heparin proteoglycan; and diverse enzymes with degradative capacity, including a chymotrypsin-like protease termed chymase. Thus the mast cell, bearing a specific recognition unit in the form of IgE, and positioned in tissues, has the capacity to respond to a foreign substance by eliciting a local increase in venular permeability and by initiating the influx of certain cell types from the marginated cell pool; this response allows plasma proteins such as antibody and complement and various phagocytic cells to be recruited to the reaction site without the necessity for extensive local tissue injury. On the other hand, an uncontrolled response could proceed from a physiologic local reaction to a self-perpetuating inflammatory state.

Consideration of the mechanism of immediate type hypersensitivity diseases in the human has focused largely on the IgE-dependent recognition of otherwise nontoxic substances. Support for this thesis has come from the finding that clinical atopic allergy is associated with elevated total levels of IgE and in some instances with a specific immune response that is linked to the histocompatibility locus. Populations of allergic Caucasians have a significantly higher total serum level of IgE than nonallergic individuals, and highly atopic persons with asthma have significantly higher serum levels of IgE than those with fewer allergic manifestations. Further, IgE distribution in families is consistent with the dominant inheritance of the low IgE phenotype. Thus, as a result of the action of a single IgE regulator gene the majority of family members would have elevated IgE levels as a possible basis for their atopic state. The association between HLA histocompatibility type and the immediate hypersensitivity response has been noted in persons of the low IgE phenotype who were studied with highly purified allergens, generally of small size. Such presumptive evidence of immune response (Ir) genes by linkage disequilibrium, that is, the association of the hypersensitivity response with a particular histocompatibility haplotype, represents an additional element in the polygenic atopic allergic state. Nonetheless, all the studies taken together, both of families and of populations, seem to indicate that the genetically determined elevated IgE levels found in about three-fourths of atopic allergic subjects exert the predominant influence on most specific IgE responses. It is also likely that diseases of immediate type hypersensitivity may occur because of deficient intracellular controls of mediator generation or release, or both, or that the extracellular controls directed against mediator inactivation may be impaired.

ANAPHYLAXIS **Definition** The life-threatening anaphylactic response of a sensitized human appears within minutes after administration of specific antigen and is manifested by respiratory distress often followed by vascular collapse, or shock without antecedent respiratory difficulty. Cutaneous manifestations exemplified by pruritus and urticaria with or without angioedema are characteristic of such systemic anaphylactic reactions.

Predisposing factors and etiology There is no convincing evidence that age, sex, race, occupation, or geographic location predisposes a human being to anaphylaxis except through exposure to some immunogen. According to some studies, but not others, atopy predisposes individuals to penicillin anaphylaxis.

The materials capable of eliciting the systemic anaphylactic reaction in the human include the following: heterologous proteins in the form of antiserum, hormones, enzymes, *Hymenoptera* venom, pollen extracts, and foods; polysaccharides such as iron dextran; and most commonly diagnostic agents and drugs such as antibiotics and even vitamins. The diagnostic and therapeutic agents are generally of low molecular weight and are considered to function as haptens which form immunogenic conjugates with host proteins. The conjugating hapten may be the parent compound, a nonenzymatically derived storage product, or a metabolite formed in the host.

Pathophysiology and manifestations Individuals differ in the time of appearance of perception of symptoms and signs, but the hallmark of the anaphylactic reaction is the onset of some manifestation within seconds to minutes after introduction of the antigen, generally by injection or less commonly by ingestion. There may be upper or lower airway obstruction or both. Laryngeal edema may be experienced as a "lump" in the throat, hoarseness, or stridor, while bronchial obstruction is associated with a feeling of tightness in the chest or audible wheezing. A particularly characteristic feature is the eruption of well-circumscribed, discrete cutaneous wheals with erythematous, raised, serpiginous borders and blanched centers. These urticarial eruptions are intensely pruritic and may be localized or distributed. They may coalesce to form giant hives, and seldom persist beyond 48 h. A localized, nonpitting, deeper edematous cutaneous process, angioedema, may also be present. It may be asymptomatic or cause a burning or stinging sensation.

In fatal cases with clinical bronchial obstruction, the lungs show marked hyperinflation on gross and microscopic examination. The microscopic findings in the bronchi, however, are limited to luminal secretions, peribronchial congestion, submucosal edema, and eosinophilic infiltration, and the acute emphysema is attributed to intractable bronchospasm which subsides with death. The angioedema resulting in death by mechanical obstruction occurs in the epiglottis and larynx, but the process is also evident in the hypopharynx and to some extent the trachea; on microscopic examination there is wide separation of the collagen fibers and the glandular elements; vascular congestion and eosinophilic infiltration are also present. Patients dying of vascular collapse without antecedent hypoxia from respiratory insufficiency have visceral congestion but no major shift in the distribution of blood volume. Whether the associated electrocardiographic abnormalities, with or without infarction, noted in such patients reflect a primary cardiac event or are secondary to a critical reduction in plasma volume has not been established.

The manifestations of the anaphylactic syndrome have been attributed to release of endogenous histamine. The role of SRS-A in altering pulmonary mechanics by causing marked bronchiolar constriction awaits further definition. Vascular collapse without respiratory distress in response to experimental challenge with the sting of a hymenopteran was associated not only with marked and prolonged elevations in blood histamine but also with evidence of intravascular coagulation.

Diagnosis The diagnosis of an anaphylactic reaction depends largely upon an accurate history revealing the onset of the appropriate symptoms and signs within minutes after the responsible material is encountered. When only a portion of the full syndrome is present, such as isolated urticaria, sudden bronchospasm in an asthmatic patient, or vascular collapse after intravenous administration of an agent it is difficult to exclude a nonimmunologic, toxicologic, or idiosyncratic response. For example, intravenous administration of a chemical mast-cell–degranulating agent elicits generalized urticaria, angioedema, and a sensation of retrosternal oppression without clinically detectable bronchoconstriction or hypotension. Furthermore, nonsteroidal anti-inflammatory agents such as indomethacin, aminopyrine, mefenamic acid, and acetylsalicylic acid may precipitate a life-threatening episode of obstruction of upper or lower airways in asthmatic subjects which is clinically reminiscent of anaphylaxis but is not associated with a detectable IgE response.

The presence of a labile reagin (IgE) in the heart blood of a patient dying of systemic anaphylaxis has been demonstrated at postmortem by passive transfer of the serum intradermally into a normal recipient, followed in 24 h by antigen challenge into the same site, with subsequent development of a wheal and flare, the Prausnitz-Küstner reaction. Indeed, such a reagin can be transiently identified in the serum of most patients who develop systemic anaphylaxis to a variety of different agents. In order to avoid the hazards of transferring hepatitis to the recipient in the Prausnitz-Küstner reaction, it is preferable to employ the less sensitive monkey recipient or a human leukocyte suspension enriched with basophils for subsequent antigen challenge. It is presumed that the activity responsible for most cases of systemic anaphylaxis resides with the IgE class, since the Prausnitz-Küstner activity in the serums of patients with systemic reactions to Hymenoptera venom or human seminal plasma protein can be removed by IgE immunosorbent columns. Furthermore, radioimmunoassays have demonstrated specific IgE antibodies in patients with anaphylactic reactions to insulin and to parathromone, but such approaches require purified antigens. In the transfusion anaphylactic reaction which occurs in patients with IgA deficiency, the responsible specificity resides in IgG anti-IgA rather than in IgE; the mechanism of the reaction is presumed to be complement activation with secondary mast cell participation.

Treatment and prevention Early recognition of an anaphylactic reaction is mandatory, since death occurs within minutes to hours after the first symptoms. Mild symptoms such as pruritus and urticaria can be controlled by administration of 0.2 to 0.5 ml of 1:1000 epinephrine subcutaneously, with repeated doses as required at 3-min intervals for a severe reaction. If the antigenic material was injected into an extremity, the rate of absorption may be reduced by prompt application of a tourniquet proximal to the reaction site, administration of 0.2 ml of 1:1000 epinephrine into the site, and removal without compression of an insect stinger, if present. An intravenous infusion should be initiated to provide a route for administration of epinephrine, diluted 1:50,000, volume expanders, and vasopressive agents if intractable hypotension occurs. Whether epinephrine acts to prevent mediator release, to reverse the action of mediators on target tissues, or both is not established; but its early administration appears critical. When epinephrine fails to control the situation, hypoxia due to airway obstruction or related to a cardiac arrhythmia, or both must be considered. Oxygen via a nasal catheter or intermittent positive pressure breathing of oxygen with 0.5 ml isoproterenol diluted 1:200 in saline may be helpful, but either endotracheal intubation or a tracheostomy is mandatory if progressive hypoxia exists. Ancillary agents such as the antihistamine diphenhydramine, 50 to 80 mg intramuscularly or intravenously, and aminophylline, 0.25 to 0.5 g intravenously, are appropriate for urticaria-angioedema and bronchospasm, respectively. Intravenous corticosteroids are not effective for the acute event but may be considered for persistent bronchospasm and hypotension.

Prevention of anaphylaxis must take into account the sensitivity of the recipient, the dose and character of the diagnostic or therapeutic agent, and the effect of the route of administration on the rate of absorption. If there is a definite history of a past anaphylactic reaction, even though mild, it is advisable to select another agent or procedure. A skin test should be performed before the administration of certain materials producing a high incidence of anaphylactic reactions, such as horse serum or allergenic extracts, or when the nature of the past adverse reaction is unknown. Since even a skin or conjunctival test can produce a serious reaction, a scratch test should precede these tests in a high-risk situation. With regard to penicillin, two-thirds of patients with a positive reaction history and positive intradermal skin tests to benzylpenicilloyl-polylysine (BPL) and/or the minor determinant mixture (MDM) of benzylpenicillin products experience allergic reactions with treatment, and these are almost uniformly of the anaphylactic type in those patients with minor determinant reactivity. Even patients without a history of previous clinical reactions have a 6 percent incidence of positive skin tests to the two test materials, and about 3 per 1000 with a negative history experience anaphylaxis with therapy with a mortality of about 1 per 100,000. The value of skin testing is both to permit therapy with the agent in question when the risk does not exist and to emphasize the hazards where the sensitivity is confirmed. In the event that an agent must be used despite a positive history, a positive skin test, or both, the following precautionary measures should be taken. An intravenous infusion should be started, with intubation equipment and a tracheostomy set at hand; the material should be given intradermally, then subcutaneously, and then intramuscularly in increasing doses at 20- to 30-min intervals so that the initial dose by the next route does not exceed the final dose by the previous route. It is difficult to be certain that the mediator-containing cells have been exhausted, and therapeutic use of the agent may be accompanied by untoward consequences. It may be critical to give the therapeutic agent at regular intervals to prevent the reestablishment of a sensitized cell pool of large size. A different form of protection involves the development of blocking antibody of the IgG class which is protective against Hymenoptera venom–induced anaphylaxis by interacting with antigen so that less reaches the sensitized tissue mast cells; to be effective this immunotherapy requires the use of specific or cross reacting Hymenoptera venom rather than whole insect body extracts.

URTICARIA AND ANGIOEDEMA **Definition** Urticaria and angioedema may appear separately or together as cutaneous manifestations of localized nonpitting edema; a similar process may occur at mucosal surfaces of the upper respiratory or gastrointestinal tract. *Urticaria* involves only the superficial portion of the dermis presenting as well-circumscribed wheals with erythematous raised serpiginous borders with blanched centers which may coalesce to become giant wheals. *Angioedema* is a well-demarcated localized edema involving the deeper layers of the skin including the subcutaneous tissue. Recurrent episodes of urticaria and/or angioedema of less than 6 weeks duration are considered acute, while attacks persisting beyond this period are designated chronic.

Predisposing factors and etiology The occurrence of urticaria and angioedema is probably more frequent than usually described because of the evanescent, self-limited nature of such eruptions, which seldom require medical attention when limited to the skin. Although persons in any age group may expe-

rience acute or chronic urticaria and/or angioedema, these lesions increase in frequency after adolescence, with the highest incidence occurring in persons in the third decade of life; indeed, one survey of college students indicated that some 15 to 20 percent had experienced a pruritic wheal reaction.

The classification of urticaria/angioedema presented in Table 65-1 focuses on the different mechanisms for eliciting clinical disease. Only the IgE-dependent and the IgG-mediated reactions in IgA-deficient persons should be considered immediate hypersensitivity. However, the other mechanisms are important for differential diagnosis, and most cases of chronic urticaria are idiopathic. The appearance of urticaria and angioedema in atopic persons in the absence of a specific exposure is attributed to the atopic diathesis and implies an IgE mechanism. Urticaria and/or angioedema occurring during the appropriate season in patients with seasonal respiratory allergy or as a result of exposure to animals or molds is attributed to inhalation of pollens, animal dander, and mold spores, respectively. However, urticaria and angioedema secondary to inhalation are relatively uncommon compared with ingestion of fresh fruits, shellfish, chocolate, nuts, tomatoes, and various drugs, including penicillin-contaminated milk products, which may elicit not only the anaphylactic syndrome with prominent gastrointestinal complaints but also chronic urticaria. Additional etiologies include physical stimuli such as cold, solar rays, exercise, and mechanical irritation (dermographism). Angioedema without urticaria occurs with C1 inhibitor (C1 INH) deficiency that can be inborn as an autosomal dominant characteristic or can be acquired in association with lymphoproliferative disorders. The urticaria and angioedema associated with classical serum sickness or with idiopathic cutaneous necrotizing angiitis is believed to be an immune complex disease when hypocomplementemia is a concomitant. The idiosyncratic drug reactions to mast cell granule-releasing agents and to nonsteroidal anti-inflammatory drugs can be systemic, resembling anaphylaxis, or limited to cutaneous sites.

Pathophysiology and manifestations Urticarial eruptions are distinctly pruritic, involve any area of the body from the scalp to the soles of the feet, and appear in crops of 24- to 72-h duration with old lesions fading as new ones appear. The most common sites are the extremities, external genitalia, and face, particularly the region of the eyes and lips. Although self-limited in duration, angioedema of the upper respiratory tract may be life-threatening due to laryngeal obstruction, while gastrointestinal involvement may present with abdominal colic, with or without nausea and vomiting, and may precipitate unnecessary surgical intervention. No residual discoloration occurs with either urticaria or angioedema unless there is an underlying process leading to superimposed extravasation of erythrocytes.

TABLE 65-1
Classification of urticaria with angioedema

I IgE-dependent
  A Atopic diathesis
  B Specific antigen sensitivity (pollens, foods, drugs, therapeutic agents, Hymenoptera venom, helminths)
  C Physical: dermographism; cold; light; cholinergic; vibratory
II Complement-mediated urticaria
  A Hereditary angioedema
  B Acquired angioedema with lymphoproliferative disorders
  C Necrotizing vasculitis
  D Serum sickness
  E Reactions to blood products
III Nonimmunologic urticaria
  A Direct mast cell–releasing agents: opiates; antibiotics; curare, D-tubocurarine; radiocontrast media
  B Agents which presumably alter arachidonic acid metabolism: aspirin and nonsteroidal anti-inflammatory agents; azo dyes and benzoates
IV Idiopathic urticaria

The pathology of urticaria and angioedema is usually characterized by massive edema of the dermis in urticaria, and the subcutaneous tissue as well as dermis in angioedema. Collagen bundles in affected areas are widely separated, and the venules are sometimes dilated. The perivenular infiltrate may consist of lymphocytes, eosinophils, and neutrophils that are present in varying combination and number throughout the dermis. Allergen-induced wheal and flare reactions are characterized by mast-cell degranulation and an accumulation of eosinophils over hours to days. The elicitation of a wheal and flare response upon injection of the relevant allergen into a patient with urticaria and/or angioedema, or into a site in a normal recipient prepared with serum from the patient, the Prausnitz-Küstner reaction, indicates an IgE-dependent, mast-cell–mediated reaction.

Perhaps the best-studied example of mast-cell–mediated urticaria and angioedema is *cold urticaria*. Acquired cold urticaria is a disorder in which patients exposed to cold experience an urticarial eruption that may evolve into angioedema and be associated with syncope. Cryoglobulins, cryofibrinogens, cold agglutinins, or hemolysins may be recognized, but not in the majority of patients. The finding in a number of patients of a serum factor, characterized as being of the IgE class, that is capable of transferring the cold urticaria reaction to a skin site of a normal recipient has focused attention upon the mast cell in this condition. Immersion of an extremity in an ice bath precipitates angioedema of the distal portion with urticaria at the air interface within minutes of the challenge. Histologic studies reveal marked mast cell degranulation with associated edema of the dermis and subcutaneous tissues. The venous effluent of the cold-challenged and angioedematous extremity reveals a marked rise in plasma content of histamine, low-molecular-weight eosinophilotactic activity, and high-molecular-weight neutrophil chemotactic activity which are presumably of mast cell origin, whereas the venous effluent of the contralateral normal extremity contains none of these mediators.

Diagnosis The rapid onset and self-limited nature of urticarial and angioedematous eruptions are distinguishing features. Additional characteristics are the occurrence of the urticarial crops in various stages of evolution and the asymmetric distribution of the angioedema. Urticarial and/or angioedema involving IgE-dependent mechanisms are often appreciated by historical considerations implicating specific allergens, by seasonal incidence, by exposure to certain environments, or by physical stimuli such as cold, exercise, sunlight (solar urticaria), or trauma (dermographism). Direct reproduction of the lesion with physical stimuli is particularly valuable because it so often establishes the cause of the lesion. The diagnosis can be confirmed by careful testing with the putative foreign substance to determine if a local wheal and flare results, and by passive transfer of such a reaction with serum of the patient to a skin site in a normal recipient, the Prausnitz-Küstner phenomenon. Passive transfer to the skin of a nonhuman primate or in vitro to human basophils may also be attempted. IgE-mediated urticaria and/or angioedema may or may not be associated with an elevation of total IgE or with peripheral eosinophilia. Fever, leukocytosis, or an elevated sedimentation rate are characteristically absent.

The classification of urticarial and angioedematous states noted in Table 65-1 in terms of possible mechanisms necessarily includes some differential diagnostic points. Hypocomplementemia is not observed in IgE-mediated mast cell disease and can reflect either an acquired abnormality generally attributed to the formation of immune complexes or a genetic deficiency of C1 INH. Chronic recurrent urticaria and angioedema, generally in females, associated with arthralgias, an elevated sedimentation rate, and hypocomplementemia suggest an underlying cutaneous necrotizing angiitis. Confirmation depends upon a biopsy which reveals cellular infiltration, nuclear debris, and fibrinoid necrosis of the venules.

Hereditary angioedema is an autosomal dominant state associated with the absence of functional C1 INH. The diagnosis is suggested not only by family history but also by the lack of urticarial lesions, the prominence of recurrent gastrointestinal attacks of colic, and episodes of laryngeal edema. Laboratory diagnosis depends upon demonstrating the antigenic lack of C1 INH in most kindreds, but some kindreds have an antigenically intact nonfunctional protein and require a functional assay to establish the diagnosis. The natural substrates of uninhibited C$\bar{1}$, C4, and C2 are chronically depleted but fall further during attacks due to the activation of additional C1 to C$\bar{1}$. The pathogenetic peptide is cleaved from the C2 substrate and then fully activated by the additional proteolysis of plasmin. An acquired form of C1 INH deficiency, associated with lymphoproliferative disorders, has the same clinical manifestations and differs only in the lack of a familial element and in the reduction of C$\bar{1}$/C$\bar{1}$ as well as C1 INH, C4, and C2.

Urticaria and angioedema must be differentiated from contact sensitivity, an acute vesicular eruption that progresses to chronic thickening of the skin with continued allergenic exposure. They must also be differentiated from atopic dermatitis, a condition that may present as erythema, edema, papules, vesiculation, and oozing proceeding to a subacute and chronic stage in which vesiculation is less marked or absent, and in which scaling, fissuring, and lichenification predominate in a distribution that characteristically involves the flexor surfaces.

Prevention and treatment Identification of the etiologic factor(s) and their elimination provide the most satisfactory therapeutic program; this approach is feasible to varying degrees with IgE-mediated allergens or physical stimuli. Topically applied steroids are of no benefit in the management of urticaria and/or angioedema, and while systemic steroids have no proved value, they are helpful in an occasional patient with necrotizing cutaneous angiitis or even ordinary urticaria and angioedema. Antihistamines and sympathomimetic agents often provide symptomatic relief; cyproheptadine, hydroxyzine, and similar drugs are held to be even more beneficial. The therapy of C1 INH deficiency has been simplified by the finding that attenuated androgens correct the biochemical defect and afford prophylactic protection. Since the use of such agents for children and pregnant women is not yet accepted, the antifibrinolytic agent ε-aminocaproic acid may be used to control spontaneous attacks or for preoperative prophylaxis in some patients.

ALLERGIC RHINITIS **Definition** Allergic rhinitis is characterized by sneezing, rhinorrhea, obstruction of the nasal passages, conjunctival and pharyngeal itching, and lacrimation. Although commonly seasonal owing to its relation to airborne pollens, other patterns and etiologies occur. The use of the term "hay fever" to describe seasonal allergic rhinitis is a common convention but is literally inappropriate because the symptom complex is neither produced by hay nor associated with fever.

Predisposing factors and etiology Allergic rhinitis generally presents in atopic individuals, that is, in persons with a family history of a similar or related symptom complex and a personal history of collateral allergy expressed as eczematous dermatitis, urticaria, and/or asthma (Chap. 257). Symptoms generally appear before the fourth decade of life and tend to diminish gradually with aging, although complete spontaneous remissions are uncommon. A relatively small number of weeds which depend upon wind rather than insects for cross-pollination, as well as certain grasses and trees, produce sufficient quantities of pollen suitable for wide distribution by air currents to elicit seasonal allergic rhinitis. The dates of pollination of these species generally vary little from year to year in a particular locale but may be quite different in another climate. Molds, which are widespread in nature because they occur in soil or decaying organic matter, may propagate spores in a pattern dependent upon climatic conditions. Perennial allergic rhinitis occurs in response to allergens that are present throughout the year such as in desquamating epithelium in animal dander, the plant materials processed or chemicals utilized in an industrial setting, or the dust accumulating at work or at home. Dust has a diverse content including mites, and many patients with allergic rhinitis are sensitive only to house dust. Moreover, in many patients with this disease, no clear-cut allergen can be demonstrated. When present, the ability of allergens to cause rhinitis rather than lower respiratory symptoms may be attributed to their size, 10 to 100 μm. When inhaled, they are retained within the nose without progressing to the lower respiratory tract.

Pathophysiology and manifestations Episodic rhinorrhea, sneezing, and obstruction of the nasal passages with lacrimation and pruritus of the conjunctiva, nasal mucosa, and oropharynx are the hallmarks of allergic rhinitis. The nasal mucosa is pale and boggy, but the nares are not reddened or excoriated. The conjunctiva may be congested and edematous; the pharynx is generally unremarkable but may appear injected. Swelling of the turbinates and mucous membranes with obstruction of the sinus ostia and eustachian tubes precipitates secondary infections of the sinuses and middle ear, respectively, commonly in perennial but rarely in seasonal disease. Nasal polyps often arise concurrently with edema and/or infection within the sinuses and increase obstructive symptoms.

The nose presents a large mucosal surface area through the folds of the turbinates and thus serves to adjust the temperature and moisture content of inhaled air and to filter out particulate materials. The convoluted nasal passages readily filter out particles above 10 μm in size by impingement in a mucous blanket at bends in their course; ciliary action then moves the entrapped particles toward the pharynx. Entrapment of pollen and digestion of the outer coat by mucosal enzymes such as lysozymes release protein allergens generally of 10,000 to 40,000 molecular weight. Although the initial interaction occurs between the allergen and intraepithelial mast cells sensitized with specific IgE, the bulk of the mast cells are located beneath the mucosal surface and are recruited secondarily. During the symptomatic season when the mucosa are already swollen and hyperemic, there is enhanced adverse reactivity to the seasonal pollen as well as to antigenically unrelated pollens for which there is underlying hypersensitivity. This priming effect is attributed to improved penetration of the allergens to the deeper perivenular mast cells. Biopsy specimens of nasal mucosa during an episodic allergic reaction show profound submucosal edema with infiltration predominantly by eosinophils, although some neutrophil polymorphonuclear leukocytes are present. Polyps, a feature in perennial rhinitis, are mucosal protrusions containing chiefly edema fluid with variable degrees of eosinophilic infiltration.

The muscosal surface fluid contains not only IgA that is present preferentially because of its secretory piece, but also IgE, which apparently arrives by diffusion from plasma cells distributed in proximity to mucosal surfaces. IgE fixes to mucosal and submucosal mast cells, and the intensity of the clini-

cal response to inhaled allergens is quantitatively related to the naturally occurring or experimentally defined pollen dose. Specific IgE is distributed not only to tissue mast cells but also to circulating basophilic leukocytes; patients with more severe clinical disease have basophils which release histamine in response to lesser concentrations of allergen in vitro than do cells from patients with milder disease. Human nasal polyps from ragweed-sensitive patients release histamine, ECF-A, and SRS-A upon challenge with ragweed allergen in vitro. Polyps from nonallergic patients with cystic fibrosis or chronic sinusitis, passively sensitized by interaction with serum of a ragweed-sensitive patient, release the same mediators upon challenge with the allergen. Thus, the mast cells of nasal polyp tissue, and presumably of the nasal mucosa and submucosa, generate and release mediators through IgE-dependent reactions which are capable of producing tissue edema and eosinophilic infiltration.

Diagnosis The diagnosis of seasonal allergic rhinitis depends largely upon an accurate history of occurrence coincident with the pollination of the offending weeds, grasses, or trees. The continuous character of perennial allergic rhinitis due to contamination of the home or place of work makes historical analysis difficult, but there may be a variability in symptoms that can be related to animal exposure or work habits. Patients with perennial rhinitis commonly develop the problem in adult life, are more often women than men, and manifest nasal polyps and thickening of the sinus membranes by x-ray. The term *vasomotor rhinitis* designates a symptom complex resembling perennial allergic rhinitis without an established allergic basis. Other entities to be excluded are exposure to irritants, upper respiratory infection, pregnancy with prominent nasal mucosal edema, prolonged topical use of alpha-adrenergic agents in the form of nose drops, and the use of certain therapeutic agents such as rauwolfia. Nasal polyps are a characteristic of perennial allergic rhinitis and are often associated with sinus infection.

The nasal secretions of allergic patients are rich in eosinophils, and peripheral eosinophilia with elevations in relation to clinical exacerbations is a common feature. Local or systemic neutrophilia implies infection. Total serum IgE is frequently elevated, but the demonstration of immunologic specificity for IgE is critical to an etiologic diagnosis. Some normal individuals will exhibit a wheal and flare skin response to intracutaneous inoculation of high concentrations of common airborne allergens. The diagnosis rests not only on the skin test alone, but also on the correlation of the clinical history with skin reactivity to concentrations of allergen selected by controlled testing. This provides the best balance of selectivity with specificity. Scratch tests with food allergens are unreliable but are not dangerous, while intracutaneous testing may be, and elimination diets are the best approach to the diagnosis. Regardless of method of testing, food allergy is uncommon as a significant cause of allergic rhinitis.

Although standard radioimmunodiffusion techniques can be used to screen for patients with markedly elevated levels of IgE, their sensitivity of less than 1000 ng/ml is insufficient to detect the elevations in most atopic allergic patients. A commonly employed technique, sensitive to about 50 ng/ml, is known as the competitive radioimmunosorbent test (RIST). In this procedure, the IgE of the serum competes with radiolabeled IgE for solid-phase-bound anti-IgE; the displacement of radiolabeled IgE is compared to a standard curve to yield the IgE concentration of the serum. Other assays, such as the noncompetitive RIST and double antibody radioimmunoprecipitin test (RIP), have greater sensitivity and reproducibility, respectively, and, like the competitive RIST, establish a normal geometric mean serum IgE for nonallergic Caucasians of less than 120 ng/ml. Even more useful is the measurement of specific anti-IgE in serum by its binding to a solid-phase allergen and quantitation by the subsequent uptake of radiolabeled anti-IgE. This radioallergosorbent technique (RAST) correlates satisfactorily with the bioassay of specific IgE by skin test or histamine release from peripheral blood leukocytes and is convenient for the patients; however, it requires defined allergens and full standardization.

Prevention and treatment Avoidance of exposure to the offending allergen is the most effective means of controlling allergic diseases; removal of pets from the home to avoid animal danders, utilization of air filtration devices to minimize the concentrations of airborne pollens, travel to nonpollinating areas during the critical periods, and even a change of domicile to eliminate a mold spore problem may be necessary. *Immunotherapy,* often termed *hyposensitization* consists of repeated subcutaneous injections of gradually increasing concentrations of the allergen(s) considered to be specifically responsible for the symptom complex. Controlled studies in ragweed and grass allergic rhinitis have established that patients are partially relieved of their symptoms by such treatments applied over a period of years. Improvement appears to be dose-related, and the end point is based either on severe adverse local or systemic reactions to the allergen injection or on satisfactory relief of symptoms. The immunologic characteristics of a response include a rise in antibodies of the IgG class, a small increase in specific IgE early in the treatment course followed by a plateau or decline, and a decline in the percentage of histamine released from peripheral blood basophilic leukocytes challenged with a fixed concentration of the allergen. The antibodies of the IgG class might well reduce or neutralize the quantity of allergen available for interaction with the tissue mast cells but, more importantly, could modify the seasonal booster response in specific IgE synthesis. None of the individual parameters of the response to immunotherapy correlates well with the assessments of clinical efficacy, suggesting that benefit is derived from a complex of effects. Immunotherapy should be reserved for clearly documented seasonal diseases that cannot be managed with drugs because of their side effects.

Management with pharmacologic agents offers a diverse approach. Antihistamines are the only specific end-organ antagonists available for control of a mast-cell–derived reaction and are limited to competition with but one mediator. Nonetheless, antihistamines are very effective for some patients, and the side effects such as drowsiness and gastrointestinal distress, which limit the dosage of a particular preparation, can sometimes be circumvented by use of an agent of different structure. An orally active agent with alpha-adrenergic activity is often employed for its decongestant effects and to partially counteract the drowsiness produced by antihistamines. Topical administration of alpha-adrenergic agents may be helpful but has the immediate disadvantage of rebound vasodilatation and prolonged usage may produce a chronic rhinitis. The topically active steroids of the beclamethasone class ameliorate symptoms of both seasonal and perennial rhinitis without detectable adrenal suppression and may represent a major advance in therapy in view of the earlier favorable results with certain other steroids which were more readily absorbed. Cromolyn sodium inhaled nasally has also given encouraging prophylactic results and is of particular merit because it acts to prevent mast-cell activation.

REFERENCES

AUSTEN KF: Systemic anaphylaxis in the human being. N Engl J Med 291:277, 1973

BIAS WB, MARSH DG: The genetic basis of asthma: current studies of the genetics of the IgE-mediated immune response in man, in *Asthma: Physiology, Immunopharmacology and Treatment. Second International Symposium,* LM Lichtenstein, KF Austen (eds). New York, Academic, 1977, p 21

GREEN GR et al: Evaluation of penicillin hypersensitivity: value of clinical history and skin testing with penicilloyl-polylysine and penicillin G. J Allerg Clin Immunol 60:339, 1977

KALINER M et al: Immunologic release of chemical mediators from human nasal polyps. N Engl J Med 289:277, 1973

KAPLAN AP et al: In vivo studies of mediator release in cold urticaria and cholinergic urticaria. J Allergy Clin Immunol 55:394, 1975

LICHTENSTEIN LM, NORMAN PS: Pathogenesis of allergic rhinitis, in *Immunological Diseases,* 2d ed, M Samter (ed). Boston, Little, Brown, 1971, p 825

NORMAN PS, LICHTENSTEIN LM: Allergic rhinitis: Clinical course and treatment, in *Immunological Diseases,* 2d ed, M Samter (ed). Boston, Little, Brown, 1971, p 840

SOTER NA et al: Urticaria and arthralgias as manifestations of necrotizing angiitis (vasculitis). J Invest Dermatol 63:485, 1974

66
IMMUNE-COMPLEX DISEASES

BRUCE C. GILLILAND
MART MANNIK

DEFINITION Immune-complex diseases are characterized by the deposition of antigen-antibody complexes in vascular and glomerular basement membranes and by the presence of these complexes in the circulation and in other body fluid compartments. The localization of immune complexes in tissues initiates immunologically mediated inflammation with resultant tissue damage. Immune-complex diseases have a common pathogenic mechanism, but the etiology is variable since the sources of antigens differ from disease to disease. The immune-complex diseases constitute a clinical syndrome which includes glomerulonephritis, arthritis, skin eruptions, pericarditis, pleuritis, and vasculitis at diverse sites.

PATHOGENESIS Upon the first exposure to a foreign substance, the host develops an antibody response after a week or 10 days. The synthesized antibodies result in formation of antigen-antibody complexes, which facilitate removal of the antigen. Normally, the majority of immune complexes are removed by cells in the reticuloendothelial system (also called the mononuclear phagocyte system). However, when complexes are deposited at other sites, such as along vascular and glomerular basement membranes, inflammation may develop at these sites, leading to the signs and symptoms of immune-complex disease.

The concepts of immune-complex disease in humans have evolved largely through study of animal models, including both spontaneous and experimentally induced disease. Acute serum sickness can be induced in experimental animals by injection of a foreign protein such as bovine serum albumin. Antigen disappears from the circulation in three phases: the first represents equilibration of the antigen between the intra- and extravascular compartments; the second is produced by catabolism of the antigen; the third involves the immune clearance of the antigen due to newly made specific antibodies. During the initial part of the immune-clearance phase, small circulating immune complexes are formed. As more antibody is synthesized, the lattice structure of the immune complexes increases until the complexes reach a critical lattice structure. Then the complexes are rapidly removed from the circulation by the reticuloendothelial system in the liver and elsewhere. Once the circulating immune complexes reach a critical size, the complement system is activated. This is manifested by a decrease in total hemolytic complement or individual complement components. This event does not ensue if the complexes are formed by antibodies incapable of complement activation. The overwhelming bulk of the antigen in the form of immune complexes is removed from the circulation by the reticuloendothelial system. For example, in experimental animals less than 1 percent of the circulating immune complexes becomes entrapped in the kidneys as determined in chronic serum sickness models or by intravenous injection of preformed immune complexes. Yet these small quantities of immune complexes suffice to cause glomerulonephritis. In human diseases no data are available on the total burden of circulating immune complexes or on the amount deposited in kidneys. The exact nature of the complexes that become deposited in the vascular or glomerular basement membranes is not certain, but persistence of complexes in the circulation is a requirement for development of renal disease. In rabbits, the release of vasoactive amines facilitates the deposition of immune complexes in the glomeruli, but in humans this mechanism has not been demonstrated. Coincident with circulating immune complexes and complement utilization, clinical abnormalities develop in experimental animals (Fig. 66-1). These abnormalities include glomerulonephritis, vasculitis, arthritis, skin eruptions, pleuritis, and pericarditis. Once the antigen is completely cleared, the complement levels return to normal, and gradually the lesions in target organs subside. Thus, acute serum sickness is a limited disease and progresses only as long as antigen persists in the recipient.

In experimental animals the acute serum sickness model can be converted to a chronic serum sickness or immune-complex disease model by repeated administration of antigen. The development of clinical abnormalities in such models can be achieved by frequent (daily or several times a week) administration of an appropriate dose of antigen. For development of maximal lesions the total dose of antigen should result in slight antigen excess in relation to the specific antibody pool. In such

FIGURE 66-1

Schematic presentation of events in experimental acute serum sickness. In this experimental animal, antibody production began on the eighth day with the appearance of circulating immune complexes and subsequent decrease in serum complement (C). Vasculitis, glomerulonephritis, and arthritis develop after deposition of immune complexes. With the clearance of immune complexes by the reticuloendothelial system, the pathogenic process ceases, free antibody can be detected, and the inflammatory events run their course and gradually abate.

a model, renal failure due to chronic proliferative glomerulonephritis can be achieved. These animals also develop vasculitis in other locations, and extensive antigen, antibody, and C3 deposits are identifiable.

A chronic immune-complex disease can develop spontaneously in animals with viral or other microbial infection that provides a continued source of antigen for immune-complex formation. Glomerulonephritis develops in mice with persistent lymphocytic choriomeningitis virus, Maloney sarcoma virus, or lactic dehydrogenase virus infection and in Aleutian disease of mink. Immune complexes consisting of antivirus antibody, virus antigen, and complement components (mainly C3) can be identified in the kidney and serum of these animals. Immune-complex nephritis resembling closely that of systemic lupus erythematosus occurs in the F_1 hybrid of New Zealand black and New Zealand white mice. Deoxyribonucleic acid (DNA), antibodies to DNA, and C3 deposits are found in the glomerular basement membrane. The role of viruses in the etiology and pathogenesis of this disease model remain under investigation.

A localized experimental immune-complex disease can be generated by repeated injection of a foreign substance into the same location of an immunized animal. For example, rabbits immunized with a foreign protein, such as bovine serum albumin, develop arthritis when the same protein is injected into the joint cavity. Intense inflammation can be induced in a similar manner in the pericardial and pleural cavities. Again, the local immunologically induced inflammation progresses as long as antigen is present. The synovitis of rheumatoid arthritis appears to be a local immune-complex disease of joints.

Immune complexes activate complement components, leading to formation of vasoactive peptides and chemotactic factors. Neutrophils accumulate in the involved area and phagocytize the immune complexes, resulting in release of lysosomal enzymes and subsequent damage to structural components of tissue. Later in the course of the lesions monocytes, T cells, and B cells accumulate because of specific chemotactic factors. Newly arrived B cells evolve to plasma cells that synthesize antibodies to the antigen present at the site. For example, if bovine serum albumin is used to induce arthritis in the rabbit, the bulk of plasma cells in the synovium of this animal will synthesize antibodies to bovine serum albumin.

PATHOLOGY Light microscopy of the renal lesion of acute serum sickness or immune-complex disease reveals swelling of endothelial cells and the presence of a few leukocytes. In the chronic form, thickening of the basement membrane is accompanied by accumulation of neutrophils and proliferation and swelling of endothelial cells. Epithelial cells proliferate to form crescents with eventual obliteration of Bowman's space. The renal lesions may be classified as showing mesangioproliferative, focal proliferative, diffuse proliferative, or membranous glomerular involvement, depending on the extent of the disease and the characteristics of the inflammatory response. Immunofluorescent studies of the kidney in both the acute and chronic forms of disease reveal granular deposits of immunoglobulin and complement (C3) in the mesangial matrix or along the glomerular basement membrane. Transmission electron microscopy shows electron-dense deposits in the mesangial matrix, the subendothelial space, the subepithelial space, and the glomerular basement membrane.

This history of the vascular lesion initially shows accumulation of neutrophils and proliferation of endothelial cells. This is followed by disruption of the internal elastic lamina and fibrinoid necrosis of the vessel wall. Mononuclear cells appear later. The vasculitis may vary from an intense inflammatory lesion consisting mainly of polymorphonuclear cells to one in which only perivascular cuffing with mononuclear cells is seen at the time of biopsy. If the examination is made early in the course, granular deposits of immunoglobulin and complement may be identified by immunofluorescence. However, within hours, these immune deposits are removed by the inflammatory response.

ETIOLOGY For any given immune-complex disease the etiology depends on the nature and source of the antigens that form immune complexes as well as the immunogens that incite the immune response. In most immune-complex diseases the antigen and immunogen are the same substance, but in certain autoimmune diseases they may differ. Thus, in immune complex diseases the etiologic factors may be drugs, microorganisms, tumors, or the host's own tissues. If strict criteria are employed, the etiology of an immune-complex disease is defined when the specific antigens and antibodies causing the tissue inflammation are identified. This has been achieved largely by elution of antigens and antibodies from the target tissues or by immunofluorescent microscopy using specific antigens and antibodies. The list of established immune-complex diseases has grown steadily (Table 66-1). A number of diseases, particularly glomerulonephritis and vasculitis, have all the hallmarks of immune-complex diseases in terms of the clinical pattern of the disorder and the deposition of immunoglobulins at sites of inflammation, but the involved antigens are not defined—therefore, these disorders are often listed as "probable" immune-complex diseases.

Drugs produce immune-complex disease either by acting as immunogens or by inducing synthesis of autoantibodies by an unknown mechanism. Numerous drugs and foreign proteins (e.g., penicillins, sulfonamides, horse antitoxin to tetanus, and horse antihuman lymphocyte serum) are potentially immunogenic and cause immune-complex disease. Binding of a drug or its metabolite to a serum protein may be necessary for its immunogenicity.

A form of immune-complex disease restricted to the destruction of platelets or red blood cells is occasionally observed after administration of stibophen, phenacetin, quinine, or quinidine. Antibodies made in response to one of these drugs combine with the drug to form immune complexes. These complexes are absorbed to the blood cell surface and activate complement, leading to either hemolytic anemia or thrombocytopenia. Some drug-induced neutropenias may also develop by this mechanism.

Other drugs do not act as immunogens but instead stimulate the synthesis of autoantibodies, especially those with specificity to nuclear antigens. Patients receiving drugs such as procainamide, hydralazine, or hydantoins may form antibodies to nuclear antigens and manifest features of systemic lupus erythematosus. Several months of drug administration may be required before the onset of symptoms. The autoantibodies persist for months after administration of the drug has been discontinued.

Several types of infections are accompanied by immune-complex disease, and many have glomerulonephritis as a common feature. Antigens derived from the responsible microorganisms are presumed to be released at the site of bacterial growth and then are deposited as immune complexes in glomeruli. Examples include poststreptococcal glomerulonephritis, the glomerulonephritis of bacterial endocarditis, infected ventriculoatrial shunt, osteomyelitis, quartan malaria, and hepatitis B infection.

Manifestations of immune-complex disease may accompany viral infections. For example, the preicteric phase of hepatitis B infection can be recognized by the appearance of fever, arthritis, and skin eruptions along with low serum complement and circulating hepatitis-associated antigen. As the arthritis and rash subside and complement levels return to normal, the hepatitis-associated antigen disappears from the circulation, and antibodies to the antigen can then be demonstrated

with the onset of clinical manifestations of hepatitis. In this disorder the immune complexes consist of viral surface antigens (HBsAg) and the specific antibody.

Fungal diseases such as coccidioidomycosis may be accompanied by erythema nodosum and arthritis, most likely due to immune complex deposition.

Patients with malignancies may develop arthritis, arthralgia, and skin eruptions. Renal biopsies in some patients with nephrotic syndrome associated with adenocarcinoma of the colon have shown IgG, complement components, and carcinoembryonic antigen in the glomerular basement membrane. As methods are developed for identifying other tumor antigens, examples of immune complex disease will increase.

The autoimmune group of disorders is characterized by immune complexes composed of autologous antigens and their specific antibodies. The prototype of this group is systemic lupus erythematosus characterized by formation of antibodies to nuclear antigens (Chap. 68). In particular, deposition of immune complexes consisting of native DNA, and antibodies to native DNA, in the glomerular basement membrane and other tissue leads to inflammation at these sites. Another example is mixed cryoglobulinemia in which immune complexes composed of IgG–anti-IgG can be identified in the cryoprecipitate. The antibody in these immune complexes consists of IgG, IgA, or IgM, and the antibody specificity is directed to IgG. These complexes are soluble at body temperatures and show progressive insolubility as the temperature is lowered. Upon deposition, they produce glomerulonephritis, arthritis, and vasculitis. Cutaneous lesions may also develop owing to precipitation of complexes at reduced temperatures in the extremities. Immune complexes of IgG–anti-IgG are also found in rheumatoid arthritis and in hypergammaglobulinemic purpura of Waldenström, in which joint inflammation, pleuritis, pericarditis, and vasculitis are not uncommon.

Autologous antigens may be released by prior tissue damage to serve first as immunogens and later as antigens in the generation of immune-complex disease. For example, in sickle-cell disease, renal tubular cell antigens are released from damaged tubular cells, antibodies to these antigens are synthesized, and the resultant immune complexes are deposited in the glomerular basement membrane.

Many forms of vasculitis, especially small-vessel vasculitis, are caused by deposition of immune complexes (Chap. 67). Biopsy of an involved site may reveal immunoglobulins along

TABLE 66-1
Immune-complex diseases in humans

I Administered (exogenous) antigens
   A Serum sickness (animal antitoxins, antiserums, hormones, drugs)
   B Drug-induced hemolytic anemia and thrombocytopenia (stibophen, quinine, quinidine, phenacetin)
   C Hypersensitivity pneumonitis (e.g., farmer's lung)
II Microbial antigens
   A Poststreptococcal glomerulonephritis
   B Glomerulonephritis of bacterial endocarditis, infected ventriculoatrial shunts, syphilis, typhoid fever, toxoplasmosis, quartan malaria, schistosomiasis, infectious mononucleosis
   C Arthritis, polyarteritis, glomerulonephritis of hepatitis B infection
III Autologous antigens
   A Systemic lupus erythematosus
   B Rheumatoid arthritis
   C Mixed cryoglobulinemia
   D Thyroiditis
   E Glomerulonephritis due to renal tubular antigen
IV Tumor antigens
   A Glomerulonephritis with colonic carcinoma, bronchogenic carcinoma, clear-cell renal carcinoma

with complement components. The absence of these substances, however, does not exclude an immune-complex pathogenesis because immune complexes may be destroyed by the inflammatory process within hours of their deposition. The nature and source of antigens that lead to immune-complex–induced vasculitis are largely unknown. In some patients with periarteritis nodosa, hepatitis-associated antigen is found in the serum. Furthermore, the antigen, antibodies, and complement components are present in the involved vessel wall, suggesting a pathogenic role for these specific immune complexes.

A localized form of immune-complex disease occurs when antibodies come in contact with their antigens at or near the site where antigen is being released or where it is being absorbed. The gingivitis of periodontal disease is thought to be generated by complexes composed of bacterial antigens from the plaque and the specific antibodies. Studies of experimental thyroiditis indicate that antibodies specific to thyroglobulin react with this antigen as it is released from the follicular cells. Immune complexes are formed between the follicular basement membrane and the follicular cells, leading to interstitial inflammation. Thyroiditis in humans may be produced by a similar mechanism. The synovitis of rheumatoid arthritis also represents a localized immune-complex disease, in part attributed to antibodies to IgG (rheumatoid factors) that are produced in the synovium. Hypersensitivity pneumonitis, such as pigeon breeder's lung and farmer's lung, results from antibodies uniting with the respective inhaled antigen in the alveolar wall (Chap. 258).

CLINICAL MANIFESTATIONS Since immune-complex diseases have a common pathogenic mechanism, many of the clinical manifestations are similar even though the responsible antigens may be quite different. Glomerulonephritis, arthritis, and skin lesions are frequently observed, either individually or in various combinations. The characteristics of skin lesions can be indicative of the size of involved blood vessels. The involvement of small vessels causes palpable purpura, urticaria, morbilliform eruptions, and maculopapular eruptions. The inflammation of arterioles and small arteries leads to small infarcts, ulcerations, and bullous lesions. The involvement of even larger vessels leads to digital gangrene. Renal involvement may not be apparent clinically or by urinalysis; however, biopsy may show immune deposits in the mesangium or in the glomerular capillary loop. Pleuritis, pericarditis, and small-vessel vasculitis also occur. The number and severity of clinical manifestations vary among patients, even when the disorder is produced by a single etiologic agent. The reasons for this variability are not apparent.

The clinical manifestations and course of the acute, self-limited form of immune-complex disease are best exemplified by serum sickness following injection of a foreign protein such as horse antitoxin to diphtheria or tetanus. In the person who has not been previously exposed to the antitoxin, the first manifestation is reddening and swelling at the site of injection, occurring 1 to 2 weeks after antitoxin administration. This is followed within a few days by fever, myalgia, skin lesions, arthralgias or arthritis, gastrointestinal symptoms, and lymphadenopathy including nausea, vomiting, and abdominal pain. The skin lesions are most commonly urticarial; but petechial, erythematous, macular, or morbilliform lesions may be seen. Arthritis usually begins in one or two joints and rapidly progresses to include many joints. The wrists, ankles, knees, and small joints of the hand are most commonly involved. Acute glomerulonephritis with red blood cell casts, proteinuria, and decreasing renal function may develop. Vasculitis of the vasa nervorum produces peripheral neuropathy. Rarely meningoencephalitis may develop. In a person with previous exposure to the antitoxin, the above manifestations may appear 3 to 4 days following exposure. The same syndrome may occur after administration of a drug or in association with infection.

An anaphylactoid reaction may follow administration of a drug or foreign protein in a previously immunized patient who has preformed circulating antibodies to the specific antigen (Chap. 65). This reaction begins minutes after exposure and is characterized by urticaria, bronchospasm, dyspnea, diarrhea, hypotension, and shock. This reaction may be fatal. It is caused by the release of large amounts of vasoactive peptides.

Chronic forms of immune-complex disease occur in patients who have prolonged or repeated availability of the antigen. Such conditions are seen when the antigen is released from a persistent microorganism or a persistent tumor, or when the antigen is a normal constituent of the host. Examples include bacterial endocarditis, adenocarcinoma of the colon, and systemic lupus erythematosus.

DIAGNOSIS Immune-complex disease should be suspected in a patient presenting with arthritis, skin eruptions, and glomerulonephritis. It should also be considered in patients with pericarditis, pleuritis, vasculitis, and/or neuropathy. When the presence of an immune-complex disease is suspected, the offending antigen must be identified by historical or laboratory inquiry. A detailed history of drug exposure is extremely important. The presence of chronic bacterial or viral infections must be sought by history and by physical and laboratory examinations.

Several diseases with diffuse vascular involvement in many organ systems may mimic immune-complex disease. Patients with a left atrial myxoma may have showers of skin lesions due to small emboli of myxomatous tissue. Similarly, patients with nonbacterial thrombotic endocarditis have peripheral embolization to small blood vessels. These patients may also have arthralgias. Patients with thrombotic thrombocytopenic purpura develop skin lesions, arthralgias, or arthritis, central nervous system abnormalities, and renal failure. The severity of the thrombocytopenia and absence of an inflammatory component in the purpuric skin lesions help to distinguish this entity from immune-complex disease.

LABORATORY FINDINGS The laboratory abnormalities in patients with immune-complex disease include an elevated erythrocyte sedimentation rate, anemia, mild leukocytosis, and occasionally eosinophilia. The cerebrospinal fluid often shows pleocytosis. The urine may contain protein, red blood cells, and red blood cell casts. Serum complement may be low. Conduction abnormalities may be present on the electrocardiogram.

In the patient suspected of having immune-complex disease, the search for antigen should include blood cultures for detection of bacteria that may release the antigens and serologic tests for viral antigens, such as the hepatitis B antigen. Serologic tests for detection of antibody to microbial antigens may be useful in detecting the underlying etiology. These include heterophil, antistreptolysin O, and fluorescent treponemal antibody absorption tests, to mention just some. Tumor antigens, such as the carcinoembryonic antigen, should be sought. In the autoimmune diseases, antibodies to nuclear antigens and antibodies to IgG (rheumatoid factors) point to the underlying disorder. Tests for cryoglobulins should be performed; if they are found, specific antigens and antibodies can be characterized. Measurements of serum complement can be helpful in supporting the diagnosis initially and in following the course of immune-complex diseases. Since immune complexes primarily activate the classic complement pathway, both the early and late components of complement will be consumed. A normal complement level does not exclude the presence of immune-complex disease because the rate of synthesis may compensate for the degree of complement consumption.

The biopsy and routine histological examination of suspected vasculitic skin lesions is relatively innocuous and useful in the diagnosis of immune-complex diseases with vasculitis (Chap. 67). Examination of tissue by immunofluorescence or by electron microscopy may be helpful in establishing the diagnosis of immune-complex disease. Demonstration of IgG and complement components in the glomerular basement membrane by immunofluorescence indicates deposition of immune complexes. They stain in a granular or "lumpy" pattern. In contrast, a linear pattern of staining is seen when antibody is directed to antigens of the glomerular basement membrane (e.g., in Goodpasture's syndrome). Also, the detection of immunoglobulin and complement in the wall of involved blood vessels suggests an immune-complex etiology. Phagocytosis of these deposited complexes results in the finding of immunoglobulins and complement in the phagolysosomes of neutrophils and macrophages.

The finding of decreased total hemolytic complement, decreased complement components, immunoglobulin and complement tissue deposits, or elevated titers of specific antibodies provides only inferential evidence for the presence of circulating immune complexes.

The detection and quantification of circulating immune complexes is possible with specialized techniques. Immune complexes can be identified by analytical ultracentrifugation, but this technique is insensitive. Certain monoclonal rheumatoid factors (anti-IgG antibodies) are effective in combining and precipitating with immune complexes containing IgG. Also, the first component of complement (C1q) can be used to detect complexes containing IgG since this molecule combines firmly with IgG in large-latticed immune complexes. It is also possible to detect circulating immune complexes by the use of a human lymphoblastoid cell line (called the Raji cell line). Complement-fixing immune complexes bind to these cells through complement (C3b, C3d, and C1q) receptors. These techniques are limited by the requirement to form an immune complex lattice of a critical size, in order to facilitate binding of complement or interaction with cell receptors, and by the subclass of antibody. The presence of antibodies to lymphocytes may cause false-positive tests for immune complexes in the Raji cell assay. The presence of circulating DNA or endotoxin may cause false-positive tests for immune complexes in the assay with C1q.

TREATMENT The principles of therapy for immune-complex diseases are to remove the offending antigen and to reduce the inflammation when it threatens to compromise organ function. When a drug is suspected of causing immune-complex disease, its administration should be stopped immediately. In patients with immune-complex disease associated with an infection, such as bacterial endocarditis, adequate doses of the appropriate antibiotic should be given.

The treatment of anaphylactic reactions is considered in Chap. 65.

In acute or subacute immune-complex disease, anti-inflammatory drugs such as salicylates will usually reduce joint pain. Antihistamines or small doses of epinephrine will relieve urticaria. In some patients the severity of disease warrants the use of corticosteroids which help to minimize clinical manifestations. Prednisone, 40 mg per day, can be given over a 2-week period with gradual tapering. Tissue damage may be slowed in chronic immune-complex disease by the use of corticosteroids alone or in combination with immunosuppressive drugs. Treatment of the chronic forms of immune-complex disease is discussed in detail in the chapters dealing with the specific disorders.

REFERENCES

BEAUFILS M et al: Glomerulonephritis in severe bacterial infections with and without endocarditis. Adv Nephrol 7:217, 1978

COCHRANE CB, KOFFLER D: Immune complex disease in experimental animals and man. Adv Immunol 16:185, 1963

HAAKENSTAD AO, MANNIK M: The biology of immune complexes, in *Autoimmunity,* N Talal (ed). New York, Academic, 1977

KENNETH SR et al: Application of the solid phase C1q and Raji cell radioimmune assay for the detection of circulating immune complexes in glomerulonephritis. J Clin Invest 62:61, 1978

LAMBERT PH et al: A WHO collaborative study for the evaluation of eighteen methods for detecting immune complexes in serum. J Clin Lab Immunol 1:1, 1978

ROY LP et al: Etiologic agents of immune-deposit disease, in *Progress in Clinical Immunology,* RS Schwartz (ed). New York, Grune & Stratton, 1972

THEOFILOPOULOS AN et al: The Raji cell radioimmune assay for detecting immune complexes in human sera. J Clin Invest 57:169, 1976

ZUBLER RH, LAMBERT PH: Detection of immune complexes in human diseases. Prog Allergy 24:1, 1978

67
VASCULITIS

*MART MANNIK
BRUCE C. GILLILAND*

Many clinical syndromes of necrotizing inflammation of blood vessels exist. In most of these conditions the etiology is not known, but several descriptive classifications have been offered, depending on the size of the involved blood vessels, the anatomic sites, the stage of the inflammation, and the histologic characteristics of the lesions. In these conditions cellular infiltration, necrosis, and fibrinoid deposits are present in the walls of blood vessels and perivascular areas. The cellular infiltrates are composed of polymorphonuclear leukocytes in acute stages; with progression of the lesion, monocytes, lymphocytes, and plasma cells appear. Giant cells are encountered in some types of vasculitis. Endothelial edema and proliferation, together with hemorrhage, contribute to diminution or occlusion of the vascular lumen and subsequent ischemic symptoms and signs.

Most forms of vasculitis are thought to be caused by immunologic phenomena. Multiple reasons exist for this belief. Necrotizing inflammation of blood vessels is a common finding in experimentally induced immune-complex diseases (Chap. 66). Vasculitis is a known manifestation of human serum sickness and occurs frequently in several known immune-complex diseases. For example, in systemic lupus erythematosus DNA, antibodies to DNA and complement components have been identified in vascular lesions. In mixed cryoglobulinemia IgG, antibodies to IgG and complement components have been seen in involved vessels. Furthermore, in some patients with polyarteritis the hepatitis-associated antigen has been implicated as the causative agent with the finding of antigen, immunoglobulins, and complement in the lesions. In other types of necrotizing inflammation, immunoglobulins and complement components have been visualized with immunofluorescence microscopy, but antigens have not been identified. Future work should identify the etiologic factors in many forms of vasculitis. Until then, however, the histologic and clinical features of the vasculitides serve to classify them.

Periarteritis nodosa was delineated by Kussmaul and Maier in the last century. In the early 1950s Zeek's careful descriptive work laid the foundation for most of the classifications of vasculitides. The descriptive classifications of vasculitides have been helpful in predicting the prognosis and response to therapy of individual patients. Upon careful microscopic examination of the lesions, the vasculitides can usually be placed in one of the five categories indicated in Table 67-1. However, at times the clinical problem defies categorization, and even within each of these categories variability from patient to patient is common. The nature of the antigen, the type of antibodies produced, the size of immune complexes formed, and cellular immunity are factors that may play a role in the pleomorphism of the clinical picture in the various vasculitides.

PERIARTERITIS NODOSA Pathology In periarteritis nodosa (polyarteritis nodosa) the necrotizing inflammation involves medium and small arteries, adjacent veins, occasionally arterioles and venules, but not capillaries. The lesions involve segments of vessels, at times affecting only part of the circumference, and there is a predilection for the bifurcation of arteries. These areas may form small aneurysms, which may rupture. During the active disease each patient has acute lesions that show predominantly polymorphonuclear leukocytic infiltration of the vessel walls and perivascular areas, as well as chronic lesions with mononuclear cell infiltration and partial healing. These observations suggest that the disease process is continuous, with repeated insults, and if it is caused by immune mechanisms, there must be repeated or continuous availability of antigen(s).

The lesions of periarteritis nodosa are widespread throughout the body; they are commonly found in such places as the coronary arteries, mesenteric arteries, kidneys, muscles, and vasa nervorum. The extent and location of lesions dictate the severity of clinical symptoms. Central nervous system involvement is unusual. The lungs are usually not involved, but this question has caused controversy and confusion among those contributing to literature in the field. Necrotizing inflammation and granuloma formation in blood vessels accompanied by lung involvement and eosinophilia should be classified as allergic granulomatosis.

Clinical manifestations Periarteritis nodosa is usually a disease of adulthood, but it occurs in childhood and senescence. It affects two to three men for every woman. The onset of the disease is extremely variable. Often an antecedent history of upper respiratory tract infection or reaction to drugs is recorded.

The early complaints of patients with polyarteritis nodosa include fever, weakness, anorexia, weight loss, myalgias, and arthralgias. With the progression of the disease several organs may show involvement. Small, 5- to 10-mm nodules occur along the course of the arteries as a result of aneurysm formation. Involvement of vessel walls leads to occlusion, ecchymoses, ulceration (often secondarily infected), and gangrene of fingers or toes. Muscle weakness may evolve. Arthralgias are common, but severe and persistent arthritis is uncommon. Mononeuritis multiplex develops because of involvement of the vasa nervorum. Asymmetric and multiple nerve trunks may be involved. Retinal exudates and hemorrhages may occur.

Pericarditis and pleuritis, with or without effusions, are common. Involvement of coronary arteries may lead to myocardial ischemia or infarction, but electrocardiographic abnormalities may be recorded in the absence of symptoms.

Abdominal complaints are frequent (in 60 to 70 percent of patients) and include abdominal pain, nausea, vomiting, diarrhea, and bleeding. All these symptoms are related to the involvement of the mesenteric arteries. The mesenteric vasculitis may lead to mucosal ulceration, with hemorrhage, perforation, and infarction. The acute abdominal symptoms early in the disease lead to erroneous diagnoses of intraabdominal catastrophies of other causes, often resulting in unavoidable but unnecessary laparotomy. The liver may be involved, and massive hepatic infarction has been reported. Periarteritis of the gallbladder may cause cholecystitis and perforation.

Renal involvement occurs in over half the patients, and affects predominantly arteries and arterioles. Glomerulosclerosis occurs with severe involvement. Hypertension may evolve along with renal failure. However, hypertension may occur early in the disease when renal function is normal. Rupture of intrarenal aneurysms may cause renal infarcts or perinephric hematomas.

The causes of death in polyarteritis nodosa include renal failure, myocardial infarction, infections, congestive heart failure, and gastrointestinal bleeding.

Laboratory findings and diagnosis No specific chemical or serologic tests exist for periarteritis nodosa. The leukocyte count is elevated in about 80 percent of patients, principally because

TABLE 67-1
Classification of vasculitis

Periarteritis nodosa	Allergic granulomatosis	Wegener's granulomatosis	Hypersensitivity vasculitis	Giant-cell arteritis
SIZE OF INVOLVED BLOOD VESSELS				
Medium and small arteries, adjacent veins	Small arteries, adjacent veins, occasional arterioles	Small arteries, arterioles, venules, some capillaries	Arterioles, venules, capillaries	Large and medium arteries
HISTOLOGY AND STAGE OF LESIONS				
Necrotizing inflammation, coexistence of acute and healing lesions, no giant cells	Necrotizing inflammation with extravascular granulomas, coexistence of acute and healing lesions, giant cells in granulomas, abundant eosinophils	Necrotizing inflammation with granulomas, coexistence of acute and healing lesions, giant cells in granulomas	Necrotizing inflammation, all lesions in same stage, no giant cells	Inflammation without necrosis, no neutrophils, giant cells present
ANATOMIC PREDILECTIONS				
Widespread, common to branching points of arteries; lungs rarely involved	Widespread, but lungs frequently involved	Upper and lower respiratory tract involved; necrotizing glomerulitis	Widespread but common to skin, serosal surfaces, glomeruli	All large arteries, including aorta, coronary, vertebral, carotid, temporal, mesenteric

of neutrophilia. Anemia may be present because of blood loss and the inflammatory process. The erythrocyte sedimentation rate is often elevated. Other abnormalities depend on the organ involvement, e.g., hematuria, proteinuria, and decreased renal function due to kidney involvement or abnormal electrocardiogram (ECG) due to coronary artery vasculitis.

Angiography has become useful in documenting the diagnosis of periarteritis nodosa. The characteristic aneurysms at branching points of arteries occur in the kidneys, mesentery, liver, pancreas, and elsewhere during the acute phase of the disease. In late stages of the disease narrowing and thrombosis of arteries predominate in the same areas. In a number of reports the finding of arterial aneurysms on angiography has been employed to support the diagnosis of periarteritis nodosa. A large-scale study of the prevalence of these aneurysms during the course of the disease has not been reported.

The diagnosis of periarteritis nodosa often causes difficulties. This disease should be suspected in patients with involvement in several of the systems mentioned above, particularly in adult males. Infections, systemic lupus erythematosus, trichinosis, heart failure, Hodgkin's disease, and most other syndromes can be ruled out. Histologic examination of tissue is essential for proper diagnosis and for distinction from other vasculitides. Clinically involved tissue is best for histologic examinations, and tender subcutaneous nodules, tender muscles, and skin infarcts are suitable. Each tissue should be examined thoroughly because of the segmental nature of the lesions. Blind muscle biopsy has yielded positive information only in one-third of patients shown to have periarteritis later. Since vasculitis may involve the testes, testicular biopsy may be of diagnostic value.

Hepatitis-associated antigen has been found in the circulatory systems of 30 to 40 percent of patients with periarteritis nodosa. The same substance has been identified in vascular lesions along with immunoglobulins and complement, suggesting that in these patients the vasculitis is caused by immune complexes containing the hepatitis antigen. The liver involvement in these patients may be mild and overlooked unless liver function studies are performed. Some patients with this form of vasculitis have chronic liver disease, which may progress to hepatic failure. The evaluation of a patient with polyarteritis should include a search for the hepatitis B antigen.

In some patients the necrotizing vasculitis appears to follow a bout of serous otitis media. The basis of this association has not been established.

Treatment The prognosis of periarteritis nodosa with involvement of many organ systems is grim. Hypertension and renal involvement are thought to predict rapid progression of the disease. In untreated patients one-half to two-thirds have died within a year, but these statistics are heavily biased by postmortem studies and selective inclusion of severely ill patients. Treatment with corticosteroids frequently leads to rapid symptomatic improvement (initial dose 40 to 60 mg prednisone or prednisolone per day, tapered subsequently). In one study 5-year survival in untreated patients was estimated at 13 percent. Controlled studies on the use of cytotoxic (immunosuppressive) drugs have not been recorded, but some experiences suggest that these agents may help when other drugs have failed.

ALLERGIC GRANULOMATOSIS Allergic granulomatosis is separated from periarteritis nodosa because of prominent eosinophilia in the lesions, the presence of perivascular granulomas, and the clinical association with bronchial asthma.

Pathology In allergic granulomatosis small arteries and veins are most commonly involved in segmental fashion. Prominent eosinophilia is seen, epithelioid cells are numerous, giant cells

are present, and a marked accumulation of inflammatory cells occurs, thus leading to the granulomatous appearance. At times extravascular granulomas are present. The organ involvement is comparable to that of periarteritis nodosa, except that pulmonary involvement is seen with granuloma formation in the vessel walls and perivascular areas.

Manifestations Patients with allergic granulomatosis frequently give a history of an antecedent respiratory infection. Many have asthma that precedes evidence of vasculitis. In contrast to polyarteritis nodosa, fever is common. Fifty-four percent of these patients have peripheral eosinophilia, with eosinophils in excess of 1500 per cubic millimeter. The radiologic examination is not diagnostic, but parenchymal lung lesions include consolidation in small and large areas. Pleural effusions are not common.

The clinical findings due to involvement of other organs is quite similar to that in periarteritis nodosa, and includes the heart, kidneys, intestine, and peripheral nerves.

Treatment This has not been evaluated systematically. Sporadic reports and analogy to other forms of necrotizing vasculitis indicate that corticosteroids, in the same doses used for periarteritis, are the drugs of choice. Cytotoxic (immunosuppressive) drugs might be tried in patients unresponsive to corticosteroids.

WEGENER'S GRANULOMATOSIS See Chap. 218.

HYPERSENSITIVITY VASCULITIS (SMALL-VESSEL VASCULITIS) Hypersensitivity vasculitis has been given many names because of its varied clinical picture. The role of immunity in its pathogenesis is inferred by similarity to experimental models, and in some patients with this disorder the involvement of antigen-antibody complexes is documented. Basically, the arterioles, venules, and capillaries of many organs are involved by necrotizing inflammation. All lesions tend to be of the same age. The clinical picture depends on the extent of the disease and on the primary target organ. Systemic lupus erythematosus, rheumatoid arthritis, and mixed cryoglobulinemia are excellent examples of this type of vasculitis in which immune mechanisms have been implicated in the pathogenesis of the blood vessel inflammation. The finding that the cryoprecipitates from many patients with mixed cryoglobulinemia contain the hepatitis B surface antigen or its antibody suggests that this syndrome may be related to hepatitis B virus. Drugs and microbial infections have also been implicated as the causative agents. Small-vessel vasculitis is also seen in some patients with hyperglobulinemic purpura of Waldenström. These patients have characteristic purpura of the lower extremities, marked elevation of gamma globulin on serum protein electrophoresis, and intermediate complexes on ultracentrifugation of serum.

Pathology Hypersensitivity vasculitis (small-vessel vasculitis) is the most frequently encountered vasculitis. The inflammation and necrosis involve arterioles and capillaries, and not medium and large arteries. In some studies the lesions have been confined to venules. As a result, the clinical symptoms do not evolve from large vessel ischemia and infarction but result from hemorrhagic and exudative lesions and microinfarcts. Many organs may be involved, including skin, mucous membranes, brain, lungs, heart, gastrointestinal tract, kidneys, and muscle. Neutrophils have accumulated in small-vessel walls and in perivascular areas. Necrosis, edema, and extravasation of blood are present. Many neutrophils are fragmented; hence some prefer to call this form of vasculitis "leukocytoclastic angiitis." These patients may have detectable hypocomplementemia. In contrast, when the inflammatory lesions consist entirely of lymphocytes during the active phase of the disease, the serum complement levels are normal. Healing and hyalinization occur late. Focal or diffuse glomerulonephritis occurs in some patients. Characteristically all vascular lesions are in the same stage of evolution, in contrast to what occurs in periarteritis nodosa. This observation suggests episodic, rather than continuous, exposure to immune complexes, if indeed this is the mechanism of injury. Immunopathologic studies have shown deposits of immunoglobulins and complement components in active vasculitic skin lesions, if examined within 24 h of their development.

Clinical manifestations The clinical manifestations and onset of hypersensitivity vasculitis are variable, and the reasons for this variability are not known. In some patients the skin manifestations are extensive; systemic manifestations and involvement of other organs predominate throughout the course of the illness in others. In some the disease follows a quick course that leads to death, but most patients survive for years and may recover without recurrences.

In youngsters and in some adults hypersensitivity vasculitis may present as the Henoch-Schönlein syndrome, with prodromal headache, anorexia, fever, abdominal pain and bleeding, arthralgias, purpuric eruptions, and evidence of renal involvement. In adults the criteria for the Henoch-Schönlein syndrome are not usually fulfilled; however, in a group of adults with refractory urticaria and arthralgias, small-vessel vasculitis was present in the skin lesions.

The history of an antecedent respiratory infection may be obtained; drugs may have been ingested. (The list is long and includes penicillin, sulfonamides, other antibiotics, salicylates, phenylbutazone, phenacetin, propylthiouracil, busulfan, iodides, vaccines, and phenothiazines.) Fever is a common systemic symptom. The skin lesions include urticaria, purpura, ecchymoses, papules, nodules, vesicles, and necrotic ulcerations. Lesions may occur anywhere, but they tend to have some symmetry, and the lesions predominate in lower extremities—the legs, ankles, and feet. Patients frequently complain of itching, burning, stinging, and pain in the skin lesions. They may have myalgia, arthralgia, and arthritis. The joints may be warm, red, and painful with acute effusions. However, synovitis of long duration with synovial hypertrophy is unusual, and bony erosions do not develop, unless rheumatoid arthritis is present. Pulmonary infiltrates and pleural effusions may be found on chest roentgenograms. Pericarditis and myocarditis may develop, accompanied by electrocardiographic abnormalities. These patients may have peripheral neuropathy and encephalopathy, manifested by confusion, delirium, and coma. Diffuse electroencephalographic abnormalities may be present. Renal involvement becomes apparent, with microscopic hematuria, proteinuria, and decreasing renal function. Abdominal and gastrointestinal bleeding pain occur.

Similar clinical manifestations accompany the vasculitis associated with systemic lupus erythematosus, rheumatoid arthritis, and mixed cryoglobulinemias. Patients with subacute bacterial endocarditis may have small-vessel vasculitis, as manifested by the Osler's nodes, Roth's spots, arthralgias, and glomerulonephritis, although some of these lesions may be embolic in origin.

Laboratory findings Elevation of the erythrocyte sedimentation rate is the most common abnormality. Mild anemia and moderate leukocytosis occur. Complement levels may be reduced, particularly when neutrophilic infiltrates predominate

in the lesions. The finding of a positive test for antibodies to nuclear antigens suggests that the vasculitis is a feature of systemic lupus erythematosus. Similarly, the finding of a positive test for rheumatoid factor might indicate underlying rheumatoid arthritis, mixed cryoglobulinemia, or subacute bacterial endocarditis with vasculitis. Examination of the urinary sediment and evaluation of proteinuria and renal function are indicated for initial evaluation and follow-up of these patients. Biopsy of lesions is important.

Treatment The mortality figures for this disorder are variable because many series are based on autopsy findings. Spontaneous improvement occurs in some patients; in others the disease lingers. If drugs, toxins, or other environmental factors are suspected, all these exposures should be eliminated. If this disorder is immunologically mediated, then removal of the antigen would be the best treatment. Uncontrolled observations suggest that corticosteroids favorably influence the course of this disorder. The optimal dosages have not been determined; 40 to 60 mg prednisone or prednisolone seems reasonable at the onset, but the dose should be reduced when symptoms, signs, and laboratory tests show improvement. The dose should be increased when flare-ups occur. By analogy to systemic lupus erythematosus and Wegener's granulomatosis, cytostatic (immunosuppressive) drugs might be used in desperate situations. However, the results of controlled clinical trials with this therapy are not yet available.

GIANT-CELL ARTERITIS Giant-cell arteritis (also called *temporal or cranial arteritis*) is an inflammation of arteries in elderly persons. The cause of the disorder is unknown, and the pathogenesis of arterial inflammation has not been elucidated. However, some evidence for both humoral and cellular immunity to elastic arterial tissue has been presented. Any large or medium-sized artery may be involved, including the superficial temporal artery. Giant-cell arteritis responds dramatically to treatment with corticosteroids.

Pathology The inflammatory changes of giant-cell arteritis affect the large and medium-sized arteries without involving the arterioles and capillaries. Histiocytes, epithelioid cells, multinucleated giant cells, lymphocytes, and plasma cells accumulate in the intima and media adjacent to the internal elastic lamina of medium-sized arteries. The elastic lamina is highly fragmented and absent in some areas. In large arteries and the aorta, the media tends to be prominently involved with inflammation and fragmentation of the elastic fibers. The intima is thickened more than expected from age alone. The lesions are spotty and do not involve long stretches of the arteries. Thrombosis may occur at sites of inflammation.

The segmental lesions of giant-cell arteritis may involve any arteries, including the superficial temporal artery. The aorta is frequently involved, and aneurysms and dissection have been recorded. The external and internal carotid arteries and the vertebral artery systems are involved. Inflammation and occlusion of the ophthalmic or central retinal artery lead to blindness. Involvement of iliac, femoral, mesenteric, and coronary arteries may cause ischemia and infarction in the respective sites. The distribution and histopathology of the lesions in giant-cell arteritis resemble the pathology of pulseless disease or Takayasu's syndrome (see Chap. 252), but in the latter the lesions tend to be confined to the aorta and the disease starts in early life, particularly in women during the second and third decade.

Clinical manifestations Giant-cell arteritis is a disease of the elderly that affects both sexes nearly equally. This illness has rarely been diagnosed before the age of 50 or 60, and it is rare among blacks. The symptomatic involvement of arteries is frequently preceded by systemic symptoms, including fever, sweats, malaise, fatigue, anorexia, and weight loss. The fever tends to be low grade but may be striking. A fever of unknown origin in an elderly person, accompanied by a very high erythrocyte sedimentation rate, should always raise the diagnostic possibility of giant-cell arteritis.

Patients with giant-cell arteritis often have the *polymyalgia rheumatica* syndrome. This is characterized by an aching pain and stiffness in the neck and shoulders, which may extend to the upper arms and less frequently to the forearms. The hips and thighs may be similarly involved. Aching is increased with motion. Marked morning stiffness may be present. The muscles may be tender, and disuse atrophy may ensue. Joint pain in the shoulders, hips, and, less commonly, peripheral joints is reported, but objectively the joints are usually not inflamed and do not show synovial hypertrophy, even though small effusions may be present. Biopsy of asymptomatic temporal arteries will establish a histologic diagnosis of giant-cell arteritis in some patients with polymyalgia rheumatica. The segmental occurrence of the lesions must be considered in interpreting the results of the biopsies. The frequency of positive temporal artery biopsies varies from series to series, but the true prevalence of giant-cell arteritis in polymyalgia rheumatica remains unknown.

Headache is a frequent symptom, particularly in patients who have clinical temporal arteritis, with tender and thickened temporal arteries. The headache has no typical pattern, but marked scalp tenderness is often prominent. Furthermore, these patients may complain of intermittent claudication of the jaws and tongue upon mastication or talking.

Loss of vision is a serious complication of giant-cell arteritis. Blindness usually develops suddenly without significant warning, but mild visual disturbances may herald total visual loss. Usually for months or weeks these patients will have had other complaints suggestive of giant-cell arteritis or polymyalgia rheumatica. Aortic aneurysms, aortic dissection, mesenteric arteritis, myocardial ischemia, and infarction and claudication of the lower extremities have been attributed to giant-cell arteritis.

Laboratory findings The significant abnormalities in laboratory tests include a very high erythrocyte sedimentation rate (ESR), mild to moderate hypoproliferative anemia, and elevation of the α globulins and fibrinogen. The ESR exceeds 50 mm/h (by Westergren's method) and often reaches values above 100 mm/h. Important negative findings include normal serum levels of muscle enzymes and normal electromyograms, even in the presence of severe polymyalgia. Muscle biopsies disclose no characteristic changes.

In the absence of specific diagnostic tests, the diagnosis of giant-cell arteritis or polymyalgia rheumatica has to rest on clinical findings and a positive biopsy. Any one of the symptoms discussed above, in the presence of a high ESR in an elderly person, should raise the question of giant-cell arteritis or polymyalgia rheumatica. A temporal artery biopsy should be considered early in the evaluation of such patients. Other causes of high ESR must, of course, be considered, including occult neoplasms and chronic infections.

Treatment Though patients with the polymyalgia rheumatica syndrome and giant-cell arteritis may obtain some relief from their symptoms with salicylates, indomethacin, or phenylbutazone, the basic process of arteritis does not seem to improve. Patients with this disorder, however, have a remarkable response to corticosteroid treatment. The clinical symptoms abate in a few days, the ESR and the hypoproliferative anemia return toward normal within 2 weeks, and the reversal of arterial lesions has been documented by arteriography. Several dosage schedules have been recommended. For patients with proved giant-cell arteritis a daily starting dose of 60 mg prednisone is recommended. A dramatic improvement in symptoms can be expected in a few days. The dose should be reduced gradually when symptoms have abated and the ESR has decreased. The maintenance dose is usually 10 mg prednisone per day or less. In patients with polymyalgia rheumatica a starting dose of prednisone from 10 to 20 mg per day can give striking relief of symptoms. Higher doses can be considered if fever, anemia, or profound symptoms are debilitating to the patient. Alternate-day corticosteroids are not useful for patients with these disorders. Ultimately, corticosteroids can be discontinued in the majority of patients. The hazards of corticosteroids should be considered, and the prolonged use of high doses of corticosteroids should be discouraged.

REFERENCES

CHUMBLEY LC et al: Allergic granulomatosis and angiitis (Churg-Strauss syndrome): Report and analysis of 30 cases. Mayo Clin Proc 52:477, 1977

CHURG J, STRAUSS L: Allergic granulomatosis, allergic angiitis and periarteritis nodosa. Am J Pathol 27:277, 1951

FISHER RG et al: Polyarteritis nodosa and hepatitis-B surface antigen: Role of angiography in diagnosis. Am J Roentgenol 129:77, 1977

HAMILTON CR JR et al: Giant cell arteritis: Including temporal arteritis and polymyalgia rheumatica. Medicine 50:1, 1971

HAMRIN B: Polymyalgia arteritica. Acta Med Scand (suppl): 533, 1973

KLEIN RG et al: Large artery involvement in giant cell (temporal) arteritis. Ann Intern Med 83:806, 1975

LEVO Y et al: Association between hepatitis B virus and essential mixed cryoglobulinemia. N Engl J Med 296:1501, 1977

MICHALAK T: Immune complexes of hepatitis B surface antigens in the pathogenesis of periarteritis nodosa. Am J Pathol 90:619, 1978

PARK JR, HAZLEMAN BL: Immunological and histological study of temporal arteries. Ann Rheum Dis 37:238, 1978

SERGENT JS, CHRISTIAN CL: Necrotizing vasculitis after acute serous otitis media. Ann Intern Med 81:195, 1974

SOTER NA et al: Two distinct cellular patterns in cutaneous necrotizing angiitis. J Invest Dermatol 66:344, 1976

ZEEK PM: Periarteritis nodosa and other forms of necrotizing angiitis. N Engl J Med 148:764, 1953

68
SYSTEMIC LUPUS ERYTHEMATOSUS

MART MANNIK
BRUCE C. GILLILAND

INTRODUCTION Systemic lupus erythematosus (SLE) is a disease of unknown cause. However, abundant evidence shows that immunologic mechanisms of tissue injury are important in its pathogenesis. The clinical presentation and the course of SLE are variable. A hallmark of this disease is the presence of a number of antibodies to nuclear components, but other immunologic abnormalities exist as well. Some patients with SLE have spontaneous remissions, others respond favorably to treatment with corticosteroids, and in some patients the course is unresponsive to available medications. On the basis of detailed studies of animal models that resemble SLE, viral infections and genetic predisposition appear etiologically important.

PATHOGENESIS The serum of patients with SLE contains many antibodies; among them are the antibodies to deoxyribonucleic acid (DNA), nucleoprotein, histones, nuclear ribonucleoprotein, and other nuclear constituents. These antibodies are collectively termed antibodies to nuclear antigens (ANA). The antibodies to nuclear antigens alone are harmless; their presence in vivo or in tissue cultures does not harm living cells, since antibodies do not penetrate the membrane of living cells. However, the ANA participate in the pathogenesis of SLE by forming antigen-antibody complexes with their specific antigens. DNA and antibodies to DNA, nucleoprotein and antibodies to nucleoprotein, as well as complement components, have been demonstrated in the renal glomerular basement membrane and in the vascular basement membrane of patients with SLE. These observations resemble the findings in experimental serum sickness (Chap. 66). During the active phase of SLE, serum complement is decreased and circulating immune complexes can be detected with sensitive techniques. For these reasons SLE has been classified as an immune-complex disease. Even though DNA and nucleoprotein have been identified in tissue lesions, the source of these antigens has not been clarified. Other antigen-antibody systems may also be involved.

In experimental immune-complex diseases of animals and in human serum sickness, inflammation of joints, pleura, and pericardium occurs because of the presence of antigen and subsequent immune-complex formation. Similar mechanisms may well explain the multitude of clinical manifestations in patients with SLE.

ETIOLOGY The reasons for development of the antinuclear and other antibodies in SLE are not clear. Furthermore, the origin of the antigens in tissue lesions has not been elucidated—they may be autologous nuclear components, or they may originate from invading microorganisms. The hypothesis that SLE results from a viral infection in genetically predisposed persons is supported by several observations. The strongest support for this hypothesis comes from studies on the F_1 hybrids of New Zealand black (NZB) and white (NZW) mice that develop a syndrome analogous to SLE. These mice develop among other manifestations renal lesions, antinuclear antibodies, antibodies to DNA, and decreased serum complement. DNA and antibodies to DNA exist in the renal deposits of immune complexes. Furthermore, in certain colonies of dogs SLE-like disease can be transmitted with cell-free extracts, and C-type viruses have been identified in these animals in association with the disease. In a very high percentage of patients with SLE, cytoplasmic virus-like tubuloreticular structures are found by electron microscopy in endothelial cells of glomerular and other capillaries. These structures initially were thought to represent viruses, but now are thought to represent an unidentified response to cell injury. Similar inclusions are seen in other disorders, but with lesser frequency.

In humans and mice with SLE, abnormalities exist in the regulatory mechanisms of the immune response. A suppression of cell-mediated immunity is apparent with an enhanced activity of humoral immunity. These observations suggest a diminution of the T-cell suppressor mechanism on B-cell functions. These abnormalities may account for the multitude of antibodies to intracellular components as mentioned above, but the reasons for the existence of these abnormalities remain obscure.

A genetic predisposition for SLE has been suggested by the subclinical abnormalities in relatives of patients with SLE and by the high concordance of clinical SLE in monozygotic twins. On the other hand, the finding of a high prevalence of lymphocytotoxic antibodies among household contacts, including but not limited to blood relatives, raises the possibility of nongenetic transmission of SLE. The occurrence of SLE and lupus-

like syndromes in patients with several inborn errors of complement (predominantly deficiencies of C1, C4, and C2) has been noted but not explained.

PATHOLOGY The pathologic changes in SLE are variable and depend on the stage of the disease. Fibrinoid deposits are commonly seen in blood vessels, among collagen fibers, and on serosal surfaces. Hematoxylin bodies are specific for SLE and are defined as hematoxylin-stained round or oblong masses in areas of inflammation. Hematoxylin bodies are thought to represent degenerated nuclei that have interacted with antibodies to nuclear antigens.

The renal lesions in patients with SLE have been classified into *focal glomerulonephritis, diffuse glomerulonephritis,* and *membranous lupus nephritis.* In focal glomerulonephritis some glomeruli show focal hypercellularity, accumulation of inflammatory cells, and thickening of the basement membrane. Immunofluorescence microscopy shows the presence of immunoglobulins and the third component of complement (C3) in involved areas as well as in the mesangium of uninvolved areas. In diffuse glomerulonephritis the same changes are present in all glomeruli, but frequently in an uneven manner. The basement membrane may be considerably thickened. On immunofluorescence microscopy, extensive "lumpy-bumpy" deposits of immunoglobulin and C3 are seen along the basement membrane. On electron microscopy, the electron-dense deposits are found on the endothelial side of the basement membrane and in the mesangium.

In membranous lupus nephritis hypercellularity is not present, but the basement membrane is diffusely thickened. Immunofluorescence microscopy discloses granular deposits of immunoglobulins and C3. By electron microscopy these deposits are localized on the epithelial side of the basement membrane and within the basement membrane. The mechanisms for these differences in renal involvement have not been elucidated.

Over the years a number of lupus patients with normal renal function and normal urine have had renal biopsies. Histologically these specimens may be normal, show increased mesangial cellularity, or have minimal glomerulonephritis. On immunofluorescence microscopy mesangial deposits of immunoglobulins and complement components are commonly seen. By electron-microscopic examination, electron-dense deposits are in the mesangial matrix and to a small extent in the subendothelial area of the glomerular basement membrane. These observations indicate that glomerular abnormalities are ubiquitous in patients with SLE, even when renal function and urine sediment are entirely normal by the usual clinical criteria. With follow-up only some of these patients progress to overt renal involvement and renal failure.

In addition to glomerular damage, immune complexes also lead to interstitial nephritis in SLE. Over half of biopsied patients show focal or diffuse interstitial cellular infiltrates, tubular damage, or interstitial fibrosis. The finding of immunoglobulins, complement components, and electron-dense deposits along the tubular basement membrane and in the interstitium indicate that immune complexes initiate these lesions. The immune-complex interstitial nephritis is most common in patients with diffuse proliferative glomerulonephritis and less frequent in the other glomerulonephritides associated with SLE.

The pathological findings in skin lesions vary according to the clinical stage of the lesions. The histology of the erythematous, maculopapular eruptions, as seen in the butterfly distribution on the face, are not diagnostic. Edema, extravasation of red cells, and some perivascular inflammation are early alterations. More chronic lesions show hyperkeratosis, epidermal atrophy, and small vessel inflammation in the dermis. The lesions in discoid lupus erythematosus will show atrophy, epidermal hyperkeratosis, and keratotic plugging. The dermis is edematous and infiltrated variably with lymphocytes, plasma cells, and histiocytes. On immunofluorescent staining, the epidermal-dermal junction of patients with SLE has IgG and C3 deposits. Similar changes are frequently present in clinically uninvolved skin. The mechanism for development of these deposits has not been clarified, but antibodies to nuclear antigens, including antibodies to DNA, have been identified in these deposits.

Widespread small-vessel vasculitis may be present in many organs. Such lesions exist in the synovium and show both mononuclear and polymorphonuclear infiltration. Autopsy studies on SLE patients with central nervous system abnormalities may show necrotizing vasculitis of arterioles and capillaries in many parts of the brain. Microinfarcts of brain tissues may be apparent. In some patients abundant deposits of immunoglobulins and complement components occur at the basement membrane of vessels in the choroid plexus analogous to glomerular deposits of immune complexes. The spleen shows marked intimal proliferation of penicillar and central arteries, which gives an "onion skin" appearance to these vessels. The heart valves and chordae tendineae have at times nonbacterial verrucous vegetations (Libman-Sacks endocarditis).

CLINICAL MANIFESTATIONS   SLE is predominantly a disease of women (9 women to 1 man) in the second to fifth decades of life, but it spares neither children nor persons of advanced age. The prevalence of SLE is 2 to 3 per 100,000. Most recent estimates indicate that 77 percent of patients with SLE survive 5 years. The presence of renal disease and central nervous system involvement decrease survival. The most frequent causes of death are uremia, heart failure, hemorrhage, central nervous system disease, and intercurrent bacterial infections.

Patients with SLE may present with a variety of abnormalities, including arthritis and arthralgias, cutaneous manifestations, nephritis, fever, central nervous system manifestations, Raynaud's phenomenon, pleurisy, pericarditis, hemolytic anemia, leukopenia, or thrombocytopenia (Table 68-1).

The course of SLE is highly variable from patient to patient. The observations on outcome and prognosis are largely based on patient populations studied at medical centers and therefore would exclude patients with mild and uncomplicated disease. SLE is not always a fatal disease as was thought years ago.

Arthritis and *arthralgias* are the most frequent presenting as well as the most common complaints during the course of the illness. The arthralgias are fleeting; they involve the hands or feet and also large joints. Redness, warmth, tenderness, and synovial effusions are frequently present. However, deformities are rare, and the erosions so characteristic of rheumatoid arthritis are unusual. The synovial fluid white blood cell counts are relatively low (less than 3000 per mm^3), and mononuclear cells predominate. Aseptic necrosis may occur, in part because of therapy with corticosteroids. Profound muscle weakness and tenderness reflect myositis in some patients.

Fever is frequent during the course of SLE. Fatigue, malaise, anorexia, and weight loss also occur. However, systemic complaints may be totally absent in some patients.

Cutaneous manifestations of SLE include a variety of lesions. A facial eruption, with butterfly distribution over the malar areas and bridge of the nose, consists of erythema and edema during the acute phase; atrophy and telangiectasia appear in chronic lesions. This characteristic rash occurs in about 40 percent of patients. Similar eruptions may occur in other parts of the body, particularly in the exposed areas. At times skin eruptions are precipitated or worsened by exposure to ultraviolet rays. Patchy alopecia occurs with similar frequency and is found only if sought under coiffures or wigs. Patients with SLE may have short broken hairs above the forehead, the

so-called "lupus hairs." Dermal vasculitis can be found in about 20 percent of patients, usually as small infarcts of the digital skin. In some patients only erythema due to excessively large or numerous capillaries around the digits and fingernails is seen. Ulcers may be encountered on nasal or oral mucous membranes. Other cutaneous manifestations include purpura, bullae, hives, and angioneurotic edema. Raynaud's phenomenon is seen in about one-fifth of patients with SLE.

Discoid lupus is a chronic skin ailment with lesions usually confined to face, neck, arms, and scalp. Scaling is prominent, with atrophy, telangiectasia, and keratotic plugging. Deep scars remain when the lesions subside. Only a few of these patients go on to develop systemic lupus erythematosus. On the other hand, some patients with SLE also have discoid lesions.

Renal involvement is one of the most serious manifestations in SLE. Clinically detectable evidence of renal involvement is seen in about one-half of all patients with SLE. These abnormalities extend from minimal proteinuria and few red blood cell casts to massive hematuria, proteinuria, and frank nephrotic syndrome. In some patients renal involvement goes on to total renal failure; in others there is a course of exacerbations and remissions, with eventual renal failure. Some patients respond well to treatment or improve spontaneously, but minimal proteinuria and decreased creatinine clearance may persist as evidence of irreversible damage.

The development of superimposed urinary tract infection should always be kept in mind, since these patients seem liable to such infections.

Cardiopulmonary abnormalities are moderately frequent in patients with SLE. Symptoms and signs of pericarditis or other cardiac abnormalities are encountered in almost 50 percent of them. Pericarditis may be the presenting complaint, with the usual physical and electrocardiographic findings. Tamponade due to SLE pericarditis is unusual. Myocarditis may occur. The nonbacterial verrucous endocarditis is rarely diagnosed clinically but should be suspected when new murmurs develop in the absence of bacterial endocarditis. Symptomatic or asymptomatic pleural involvement occurs in nearly half the patients. Patchy and transient parenchymal infiltrates have been noted, and occasionally severe lupus pneumonitis may occur. The cause of these abnormalities is not known, and they are difficult to distinguish from infiltrates caused by infections.

Neurologic manifestations represent another serious aspect of SLE. A variety of central nervous system manifestations has been noted in 20 to 50 percent of patients. Among these are convulsive disorders, followed in frequency by abnormalities in mental functions and cranial nerves and by transverse myelitis. Peripheral neuropathies are infrequent. Occasionally pa-

TABLE 68-1
Clinical manifestations during the course of systemic lupus erythematosus

Manifestation	Cumulative percentage of patients
Arthritis and arthralgias	92
Fever	84
Skin eruptions	72
Lymphadenopathy	59
Renal involvement	53
Anorexia, nausea, vomiting	53
Myalgia	48
Pleuritis	45
Central nervous system abnormalities	26

SOURCE: *After Dubois.*

tients present with primarily mental dysfunction, e.g., emotional lability, psychosis, or organic brain syndrome, without other significant symptoms. Cerebrospinal fluid of patients with central nervous system involvement may show slight to moderate increase in protein concentration and mild increase in lymphocytes; usually these occur late in the disease. The electroencephalogram is abnormal, with diffuse nonspecific changes. The brain scan may show focal increased uptake of isotope during active central nervous system involvement. Computerized tomography may reveal infarcts due to cerebral vasculitis.

Lymph node enlargement occurs in many patients with SLE. Such abnormalities may be diffuse or local. Characteristically the nodes are not tender. The enlargement of nodes is thought to occur because of increased activity of the immune system. Splenomegaly occurs in about 10 percent of patients and may be associated with hemolytic anemia. *Hepatomegaly* is found in about 25 percent of patients. Lupoid hepatitis is a syndrome of chronic active hepatitis associated with positive tests for LE cells or antibodies to nuclear antigens (Chap. 303).

LABORATORY FINDINGS A variety of abnormalities in *hematologic* and *immunologic* tests may be encountered in SLE (Table 68-2).

A mild, normochromic, normocytic *anemia* is seen frequently. Most likely this is the hypoproliferative anemia that accompanies many inflammatory processes. Less frequently patients have severe immune-hemolytic anemia that requires steroid therapy or splenectomy. *Leukopenia* is seen in over half the patients. The mechanisms for leukopenia and thrombocytopenia are not fully delineated, but intravascular immune complexes as well as antibodies directed to leukocytes and platelets may contribute to these abnormalities. A potentially serious but infrequent problem is the occurrence of *clotting defects* due to antibodies to factors VII, IX, or X or to the presence of an inhibitor to prothrombin activation. Prior to a renal biopsy, the integrity of the clotting mechanism must be evaluated.

Urinalysis and renal function studies indicate that over half the patients with SLE have mild to severe damage to the kidneys. With early or focal glomerulonephritis the creatinine clearance may be normal, and only mild proteinuria and microscopic hematuria may exist. With more extensive renal involvement proteinuria may become significant (>0.5 per day), and the urine sediment may contain abundant red and white blood cells and red blood cell casts as indicators of glomerular damage.

The serum albumin/globulin ratio becomes reversed because of an increase in immunoglobulins, particularly IgG. Serum electrophoresis reveals that the major elevation is in globulin. Small amounts of cryoglobulins, composed of immunoglobulins and complement components, may be present. The erythrocyte sedimentation rate (ESR) tends to be high in patients with active disease.

The most characteristic laboratory abnormalities in SLE are the autoantibodies. The presence of antibodies to nuclear antigens (ANA) in a patient with active SLE is almost a sine qua non for the diagnosis. These tests are now widely available as a diagnostic aid. The ANA are usually detected by rat or mouse liver sections (other tissues with nucleated cells may also be used); the test serum is applied to the tissue section, antibodies to nuclear antigens interact with the nuclei, other proteins are washed away, and the ANA are detected with an antiserum to human immunoglobulins (these antibodies are coupled with fluorescein isothiocyanate that permits their detection with appropriate microscopy). The patterns of nuclear staining were attributed to the presence of specific antibodies to certain nuclear antigens. These interpretations, however, were fraught with difficulties and tests are now available for specific antibodies. The ANA include antibodies to single-stranded DNA, double-stranded (native) DNA, deoxyribonucleoprotein, histones, nuclear ribonucleoprotein (abbreviated RNP), and an acidic nuclear protein (also called the Sm antigen). Patients with SLE also have antibodies to RNA, ribosomes, lysosomes, and other cytoplasmic constituents. The reasons for such a large number of antibodies are not clear. Many of these antibodies persist even when the disease is quiescent, except that the titers of antibodies to native DNA tend to be higher during exacerbations of the disease. Antibodies to native DNA in high titers are most specific for SLE with a low prevalence in other disorders. The lupus erythematosus cell test (LE cell test) is positive less frequently than the test for ANA because more antibodies are required for positivity. The listed antibodies to nuclear antigens are not specific for SLE, but when three or more of these antibodies are present, the likelihood of SLE in a given patient is very high. In end-stage renal disease due to SLE, the tests for ANA may become negative.

During flare-ups of SLE the total serum hemolytic complement (expressed in 50 percent hemolytic units—CH_{50}) or individual components of complement are decreased owing to activation by immune complexes. The most frequently used measurements of complement components are the immunochemically determined C3 and C4 levels. These measurements are useful in following the response to therapy or for detecting exacerbations. Occasionally the complement levels remain low in spite of apparent full clinical remission; the reasons for this are not known. In addition, during clinically active disease, circulating immune complexes can be detected.

About 20 percent of patients with SLE develop positive tests for rheumatoid factors, but the titers tend to be lower than in rheumatoid arthritis. False positive tests for syphilis are encountered, at times prior to clinical onset of SLE. Antibodies to nuclear antigens occur in many other diseases (rheumatoid arthritis, 20 percent; Sjögren's syndrome, 60 percent; scleroderma, 40 percent) and are induced by several drugs (see below).

DIAGNOSIS The possibility of SLE should be considered in any young or middle-aged female in the presence of three or four of the symptoms or signs listed in Table 68-1 or in the presence of glomerulonephritis, hemolytic anemia, leukopenia, or thrombocytopenia. A positive test for ANA is essential for diagnosis. Other diseases that cause positive tests for ANA must be considered, and they must often be excluded on the basis of clinical observations alone. Major consideration must be given to rheumatoid arthritis, scleroderma, Sjögren's syndrome, and the history of ingestion of drugs that might have

TABLE 68-2
Laboratory abnormalities in systemic lupus erythematosus

Abnormality	Percent of patients
HEMATOLOGIC	
Anemia (Hb < 11 g/100 ml)	72
Leukopenia (WBC $< 4500/\text{mm}^3$)	61
Thrombocytopenia (platelets $< 100,000/\text{mm}^3$)	15
Positive direct Coombs test	14
Circulating anticoagulants	Rare
IMMUNOLOGIC	
Positive tests for ANA	99
Positive LE cell tests	60–80
Hypocomplementemia	75
Increased γ globulin (> 1.5 g/100 ml)	60–77
Positive tests for rheumatoid factors	20
Biologic false positive tests for syphilis	15

induced a positive test for ANA. The mixed connective tissue disease (Chap. 362) is distinguished from SLE by sclerodermatous skin changes, active myositis, lack of significant glomerulonephritis, and cerebritis. The finding of very high titers of antibodies to nuclear ribonucleoprotein is the most helpful distinguishing characteristic.

Drug-induced SLE Hydralazine and procainamide clearly induce a syndrome similar to SLE in some patients. This syndrome includes arthralgias, arthritis, myalgias, pleurisy, pericarditis, fever, skin eruptions, lymphadenopathy, and positive tests for ANA. Renal disease and central nervous system involvement are very unusual in drug-induced SLE. Prospective studies have shown that about 70 percent of patients receiving procainamide develop positive tests for ANA within weeks or months. A much smaller proportion become symptomatic. Once the drug is discontinued, the symptoms abate in a few weeks but occasionally may smolder on for months; recovery may be hastened by treatment with corticosteroids. The ANA tests revert to negative in a few months. Isoniazid alone or with *p*-aminosalicylic acid (PAS), several anticonvulsants (Dilantin, Mesantoin), phenothiazine derivatives, γ-methyldopa, and levodopa have also been associated with positive tests for ANA. In some patients the administration of sulfonamides, penicillin, and oral contraceptives has been associated with exacerbations of SLE.

TREATMENT A cure for SLE is not available. However, abundant experience indicates that appropriate therapy may suppress flare-ups and prolong life. The optimal treatment programs for various manifestations of SLE have not been defined. Adequately designed studies have been difficult to perform because of the variability in the manifestations and course of the disease and the lack of adequate prognostic parameters. Corticosteroids remain the cornerstone of therapy, even though the "immunosuppressive" drugs seem to be helpful in some patients.

Arthralgias, arthritis, myalgias, and fever may respond adequately to rest and salicylates. Antimalarials have been used successfully for the same symptoms, as well as for control of skin eruptions. Chloroquine was used widely in mild SLE, but potential retinal toxicity has decreased its usage. Hydroxychloroquine in small dosages (200 mg per day) seems safe, but the patient should be cautioned about potential toxicity, and careful examination by the ophthalmologist should be conducted at least twice a year. Exposure to ultraviolet light should be avoided, particularly with active and recurrent skin lesions. If skin involvement becomes debilitating and does not respond to conservative therapy, corticosteroids in small to moderate dosages should provide relief.

Central nervous system involvement, pericarditis, myocarditis, pleurisy, severe myositis, severe hemolytic anemia, clotting problems, significant leukopenia, and thrombocytopenia are indications for use of corticosteroids. In desperate situations, particularly in central nervous system involvement with seizures or psychosis, relatively high doses should be used (even up to 2 mg prednisone or prednisolone per kg body weight). With central nervous system involvement a high (60 mg or more per day) dose of prednisone should be used up to about 2 weeks. Once improvement has occurred, the dose should be tapered and adjusted to maintain control of symptoms. Many of the above manifestations can be controlled with 10 mg prednisone or less per day as a maintenance dose. If a flare-up occurs and is recognized by the patient and the physician, only a moderate (5 to 10 mg) increase of the prednisone dose may provide control of symptoms. Careful follow-up of patients, with judicious use of laboratory tests, is essential in treatment of the above manifestations of SLE. Psychosis or other mental disturbances may be difficult to evaluate in a patient who is receiving steroids for SLE, since such symptoms may be caused by the steroids or by the SLE. No single laboratory test, including cerebrospinal fluid complement levels, can distinguish between these two possibilities. With further increase of the steroid dosage the symptoms should decrease if they are due to central nervous system involvement by SLE. In the use of corticosteroids the side effects, such as increased risk of infections and osteopenia, must always be considered in relation to the anticipated benefits.

Several approaches to the treatment of SLE nephritis have been advocated, but no currently available program is useful in all patients. Renal biopsy is recommended for establishing the nature of glomerular lesions, since those with focal lupus glomerulonephritis respond to treatment well or improve spontaneously. Perhaps the most useful program is to start with 40 to 60 mg prednisone or prednisolone per day until all clinical symptoms have abated. This may take a few weeks; the urinary sediment should improve, and complement should return toward normal. Thereafter the steroid dose should be reduced gradually to the minimal dose to keep the patient free of symptoms. With severe focal involvement and with diffuse lupus glomerulonephritis or membranous glomerulonephritis, higher doses (up to 150 to 200 mg prednisone or prednisolone) have been tried and found helpful for some patients, with subsequent improvement of renal function. However, the diffuse and membranous lesions do not respond well. For these reasons azathioprine (1 to 2 mg per kilogram of body weight) or cyclophosphamide (100 to 150 mg per day) has been added to prednisone. Cyclophosphamide and prednisone appear to be the most effective combination, but many serious side effects are encountered, including marrow toxicity, hemorrhage cystitis, alopecia, and sterility; their long-term risks are not fully known. The search for better combinations of drugs and new medications for treatment of severe SLE continues.

Plasmapheresis has been suggested as an adjunct to treatment with corticosteroids. The rationale for plasmapheresis is to remove sufficient immune complexes from the circulation to allow endogenous clearance mechanisms to cope with the load of immune complexes until other forms of therapy control the disease manifestations.

Any intercurrent infections must be recognized and treated with appropriate therapy. Patients with SLE, either because of their disease or as a consequence of treatment, are liable to bacterial infections, which are a leading cause of death among them.

Exacerbations of SLE tend to occur during the third trimester of pregnancy or in the immediate postpartum period. Nevertheless, many patients with SLE can be carried to term and successful delivery with appropriate therapy. Therefore, SLE is not an absolute indication for therapeutic abortion, but the procedure is recommended during life-threatening active disease.

REFERENCES

BRENTJENS JR et al: Interstitial immune complex nephritis in patients with systemic lupus erythematosus. Kidney Int 7:342, 1975

CAVALLO T et al: Immunopathology of early and clinically silent lupus nephropathy. Am J Pathol 87:1, 1977

DECKER JL et al: Cyclophosphamide or azathioprine in lupus glomerulonephritis. A controlled trial: Results at 28 months. Ann Intern Med 83:606, 1975

DUBOIS EL (ed): *Lupus Erythematosus,* 2d ed. Los Angeles, University of Southern California Press, 1974

FRIES JF, HOLMAN HR: *Systemic Lupus Erythematosus: A Clinical*

Analysis, vol 6: *Major Problems in Internal Medicine,* LH Smith (ed). Philadelphia, Saunders, 1975

GRIGOR R et al: Systemic lupus erythematosus: A prospective analysis. Ann Rheum Dis 37:121, 1978

NOTMAN DD et al: Profiles of antinuclear antibodies in systemic rheumatic diseases. Ann Intern Med 83:464, 1975

PHILLIPS PE: The virus hypothesis in systemic lupus erythematosus. Ann Intern Med 83:709, 1975

POLLACK VE et al: The clinical course of lupus nephritis: Relationship to the renal histological findings, in *Perspectives in Nephrology and Hypertension,* P Kincaid-Smith et al (eds). New York, Wiley, 1973, vol 1, p 1167

STEINMAN CR et al: Binding of synthetic double-stranded DNA by serum from patients with systemic lupus erythematosus: Correlation with renal histology. Am J Med 62:319, 1977

VERRIER-JONES J et al: Plasmapheresis in the management of acute systemic lupus erythematosus? Lancet 1:709, 1976

69
HISTOCOMPATIBILITY AND TRANSPLANTATION

CHARLES B. CARPENTER
JOHN P. MERRILL

INTRODUCTION Transplantation of the human kidney is now a justified procedure for the treatment of advanced chronic renal failure. Tens of thousands of such procedures have been performed, and occur at the rate of 50 or more per year in some medical centers. The results with properly matched familial donors are superior to those obtained with organs from cadaveric donors, with 75 to 80 percent compared to 45 to 50 percent graft survival rates at 1 year, respectively. Grafts functioning at 1 year are rejected at a much slower rate over the subsequent years, although occasionally a graft may suffer an acute irreversible rejection episode after many months of good function. The most striking improvement in clinical renal transplant results in recent years is in patient morbidity and mortality, the latter declining to less than 5 percent in a number of units. These findings represent an increasing tendency on the part of transplant teams to decrease immunosuppressive therapy so that in the case of severe rejection the kidney rather than the patient may be lost. The figures for graft survival, however, show no improvement since 1970, suggesting that methods of immunosuppressive therapy which have been uniformly utilized from 1970 to the present time remain inadequate. There are increasing numbers of second and even third transplants being performed, and the overall results are comparable to those with first transplants; in other words, rejection of a graft does not necessarily prejudice the results of another transplant attempt. Human liver, pancreas, bone marrow, heart, and endocrine glands have been transplanted, but with less success. The results of cardiac transplantation in one of the largest and best-studied series in the United States show a better than 50 percent 1-year survival.

IMMUNOLOGIC CONSIDERATIONS Necessary to the understanding of transplantation immunity are the following terms: *autograft*—the transplantation of tissue from one part of an individual to another part of the same individual; *isograft*—the transplantation of tissues between two individuals of the same inbred strain. Because in these cases the antigens of the donor and recipient are identical, no histocompatibility difference exists and no immune response to the graft occurs. A case in

point in humans is transplantation between identical twins. In an *allograft,* i.e., a graft of tissues between two individuals of the same species, histocompatibility differences may be strong or weak, depending on the individual and the species. A *xenograft* is a graft between individuals of two different species. The term "heterograft" is still used synonymously with xenograft.

NATURE AND ROLE OF THE MAJOR HISTOCOMPATIBILITY GENE COMPLEX (HLA) The fate of transplanted tissues and organs depends upon a number of factors, but the recipient's immune response to graft antigens is the central event. Definition of antigenic systems which serve as strong barriers to transplantation has therefore become a major investigative interest, having both practical application in clinical transplantation and theoretical value in understanding the natural role of the histocompatibility antigens in immunobiology.

A single chromosomal gene complex codes for the major histocompatibility antigens in all vertebrate species investigated so far. The mouse is the most completely studied species because of the availability of numbers of inbred and recombinant strains which can be employed in studies to determine the precise role of each of the gene products of the histocompatibility (H-2) chromosomal segment. Except for some details of the ordering of the genes on the chromosomal segment, the human HLA system is thus far quite analogous to the H-2. In a general sense, incompatibility for major locus antigens constitutes a strong barrier to transplantation of tissues and organs, and in clinical experience matching for major locus antigens affords excellent transplantation results, since the minor mismatches are easily suppressed by immunosuppressive drug therapy. The HLA gene complex is a portion of the short arm of the C6 human chromosome and consists of several series of paired alleles which are inherited from generation to generation in a dominant fashion, segregating randomly from other important antigens such as the ABH red blood cell type groups.

Antigens of the HLA system CLASS I The development of antileukocyte antibodies after multiple blood transfusions and as a result of pregnancy was first recognized as involving a series of antigens distinct from red cell blood group antigens. HLA antigens are defined serologically by serums from human sources, principally multiparous females, and are present in varying densities in most body tissues, including B cells, T cells (see "Immunology of Rejection," below), and platelets but not in mature red blood cells. The number of serologically defined specificities is very large, and the HLA system is at present the most polymorphic genetic system known in humans. There are known to be three clearly defined loci within the HLA complex for class I serologically defined (SD), HLA antigens. Each class I antigen consists of an 11,600-dalton β_2 microglobulin subunit and a 44,000-dalton heavy chain which carries the antigenic specificity (Fig. 69-1). The A and B loci were recognized as such in 1970, and the C locus shortly thereafter. There are over 50 clearly defined A and B specificities, while over five C-locus specificities are known. Antigens of the major complex are all prefixed by HLA, but this may be omitted when the context is clear. Antigens tentatively accepted as a result of World Health Organization workshops have a w after the locus designation. The HLA antigens of African, Asian, and Oceanic peoples are not as well defined at present, although they include some of the antigens commonly found in Caucasians. The distribution of HLA antigens is distinctive for certain racial groups and can serve as anthropologic markers in the study of migration patterns.

Since chromosomes are paired, each individual has six serologically defined HLA-A, HLA-B, and HLA-C antigens, three from each parent. Each of these chromosomal sets is termed a

FIGURE 69-1

Short arm of the human sixth chromosome. The HLA region contains genes for three class I loci (A, B, C) and the D locus region defined by the mixed lymphocyte reaction (MLR). Class II serologically defined antigens on B lymphocytes and monocytes exist which are D-related (DR). Some of the enzyme and complement polymorphisms are also shown. C2 and C4 deficiency and allotypic variants of C2 and Bf are HLA-linked. C6 linkage is suggested by some data, but not established. (cM = centimorgan map unit.) (From CB Carpenter, in Kidney International, New York, Springer-Verlag, 1978.)

haplotype, and by simple mendelian inheritance 25 percent of siblings will have identical haplotypes, 50 percent will share a haplotype, and the remaining 25 percent will be completely incompatible (Fig. 69-2). Evidence that this gene complex plays the major role in the transplantation response comes from the fact that haplotype-matched sibling donor-recipient combinations show excellent results in kidney transplantation, in the vicinity of 85 to 90 percent long-term survival.

CLASS II   Linked to the serologically defined antigens, but distinct from them, is another locus which determines the in vitro proliferative response of lymphocytes to mismatched haplotypes. Because haplotype-matched identical siblings have negative mixed lymphocyte culture responses, it was initially assumed that the antigens were responsible for the proliferative response of lymphocytes mixed in tissue culture. However, a number of recombinants in families have shown clearly that a distinct locus, called D, exists for the mixed lymphocyte response (MLR), and is responsible for a vigorous mixed lymphocyte culture (MLC) proliferative response, even in the presence of HLA-A, HLA-B, and HLA-C antigen identity (Fig. 69-2). The recombinant rate in human families is around 1

percent between B and D loci, and it is also approximately 1 percent between the A and B loci. HLA-D antigens are defined by reference stimulating lymphocytes which are homozygous for HLA-D, and inactivated by x-irradiation or mitomycin C to make the reaction unidirectional. Although D-locus antigens, sometimes called MLF-S (stimulating), are not as yet clearly identifiable by serotyping techniques, serologically defined specificities closely related to the D locus have been defined. They have the special property of not being expressed on platelets or T lymphocytes. These specificities are termed class II, having two glycoprotein chains of 29,000 and 34,000 daltons, and lacking β_2 microglobulin. They are termed HLA-DR (D-related), and are markers for closely linked D-locus determinants and putative immune response (Ir) genes. The precise relationship between HLA-D and class II serologically defined antigens (HLA-DR) has yet to be established. They could be part of the same molecule, or the products of closely linked genes. In addition, preliminary evidence exists for class II antigens unrelated to HLA-D type; hence, a complex series of loci encompassing the HLA-D region may be ultimately discerned. Two additional methods are under investigation for defining histocompatibility antigens. In the primed lymphocyte test (PLT), responder cells which have completed a proliferative response in MLC are restimulated with the same or different stimulating cells. The secondary response of primed lymphocytes is rapid (24 to 36 h, instead of 5 to 6 days), and the specificity of restimulation is a test for antigenic similarity between priming and restimulating cells. Data thus far indicate that PLT antigens are more closely related to class II HLA-DR than to HLA-D. In the cell-mediated lympholysis (CML) test the specificity of killer T cells, which arise as a result of proliferation in MLC, is determined upon target cells from donors other than those providing the MLC-stimulating cells. Antigen systems defined by this method show a close, but imperfect, correlation with class I antigens. Since killer T cells may play a crucial role in some types of allograft rejection, the definition of CML antigens may prove to be of some practical importance in clinical transplantation (Fig. 69-3).

Other sixth chromosome genes   There are at least two additional major classes of genes within the HLA region; one is for complement, with structural genes for C2 and C4 and factor B (GBG), and the other involves immune responsiveness to ragweed antigen and possibly to measles virus and *Mycobacterium leprae*. The latter findings are of enormous importance in relation to the analogy to mouse H-2 systems where the MLR region is closely linked to a number of genes responsible for certain immune responses (Ir region). There are, therefore, a number of genes in this complex which are related to the immune response, ranging from the immunogenicity of certain antigens to the proliferative response (MLR) of the immune

FIGURE 69-2

Inheritance of HLA haplotypes. Each chromosomal segment of linked genes is termed a haplotype, and each individual inherits one haplotype from each parent. The A, B, C, and D antigens of haplotypes a and b are shown for this hypothetical individual in chromosomal order on the diagram, and also below as they would be written in text. If individual ab were to marry cd, their offspring would be of four types only, as far as HLA is concerned. Occasionally (dotted cross) recombination occurs in the germ line (meiosis) of a parent, resulting in an altered haplotype. The frequency of recombinant children is a measure of the map distance (1 percent recombination frequency = 1 cM; see Fig. 69-1). (From CB Carpenter, in Kidney International, New York, Springer-Verlag, 1978.)

HLA REGION, CHROMOSOME 6

HAPLOTYPES:

a = Al, Cw3, B8, Dw3
b = A29, Cw4, Bw35, Dw1
a_r = Al, Cw3, B8, Dw1
b_r = A29, Cw4, Bw35, Dw3

INHERITANCE:

ab   x   cd

ac   ad   bc   bd

system. Furthermore, the serologically defined antigens serve as targets for alloimmune effector mechanisms, while components of the complement mediator system can play a role in the effector phase. It is apparent therefore that the major histocompatibility gene complex has evolved to play a major role in body defense and has a significance far in excess of its relationship to current efforts in clinical transplantation. Recombinant rates among all these loci are low enough in most cases to ensure that within a family the HLA antigens will serve as markers for the entire haplotype, including the D locus. A recombinant frequency of approximately 1 percent indicates that there is considerable room for a large number of genes within the complex, and a number of undefined antigens may exist. However, they are all inherited en bloc within a family, and HLA serotyping is therefore a valuable system for marking family haplotypes. In the outbred human population, however, HLA antigens are much less likely to predict compatibility for other genes in the complex.

Disease associations If the major histocompatibility complex serves a critical natural biological function, what might that be? Hypotheses have been put forth relating to immune surveillance against neoplastic cells which develop in the course of an individual's lifetime. It is apparent also that the system could play an important role in pregnancy because of the histoincompatibility that always exists between the mother and the fetus. Work in inbred mouse models indicates the importance of some of the gene products of this locus during the phase of antigen recognition of cell-to-cell cooperation in initiation of an immune response. It is possible also that the high degree of polymorphism present ensures the survival of the species in relation to the large numbers of microbiological agents present in the environment. Self-tolerance which happens to cross react with microbiological agents would produce a high degree of susceptibility, resulting in lethal infection, whereas the high degree of polymorphism present in the HLA system provides assurance that segments of the population will recognize the offending agent as foreign and initiate the appropriate response. All these hypotheses relate to the survival value of the system under selective evolutionary pressures, and there is some evidence for each of them.

The most striking circumstantial evidence of the role of the major histocompatibility complex in human immunobiology comes from the finding that a number of disease processes are positively associated with certain HLA antigens within the population. The search for such associations has been stimulated by the discovery of immune response genes linked to the H-2 complex in the mouse, and also by the H-2 complex-linked susceptibility to murine oncogenic viruses. Although surveys of human malignancies, including leukemias and lymphoproliferative disorders, have not shown consistent associations with serologically defined HLA phenotypes, some very striking correlations exist between HLA antigens of the second locus and a number of diseases in which the pathogenesis is unclear (Table 69-1). Most striking is the increased frequency of HLA-B27 in certain rheumatic diseases, particularly ankylosing spondylitis, a condition already known to have a strong familial tendency. B27 is present in about 7 percent of the Caucasian population, while it appears in 87 percent of 286 patients combined from five studies. Expressed as a relative risk, the antigen B27 confers a susceptibility to the development of ankylosing spondylitis which is 127 times that in the general population. Similarly, Reiter's syndrome and reactive arthritis to at least three bacterial infections (yersinia, salmonella, and gonococcus) show a high degree of association with B27. Furthermore, acute anterior uveitis has a similar high association with the same antigen. Since it is well known that significant overlap exists among these three conditions (spondylitis, Reiter's syndrome, and uveitis), it seems likely that B27 is a marker for a clustering of connective tissue responses to a number of infectious agents, or unknown environmental factors. It was suggested initially that juvenile rheumatoid arthritis (JRA) might also show a similar B27 association, but this is due in part to inclusion of coexistent spondylitis in these studies. Nevertheless, true JRA does show some B27 association. The increased incidence of B27 in cases of psoriatic arthritis is also highly significant and contrasts with the increased incidence of HLA-B13 and HLA-Bw17 in psoriasis per se. Patients with degenerative arthritis or gout show no alteration in antigen frequencies. Rheumatoid arthritis patients show an association with Dw4.

Gluten-sensitive enteropathy (celiac disease, nontropical sprue) in both children and adults shows a clear-cut association with HLA-B8. The actual percentage of such patients having this antigen ranges from 66 to 88 percent in five studies in which B8 was present in 16 to 29 percent of controls. The same antigen is also present in increased frequency in patients

ALLOGRAFT RESPONSE

HLA ANTIGEN | HOST LYMPHOCYTE | RESPONSE

Anti-A,B,C cytotoxic T lymphocytes Ⓐ

MIXED LYMPHOCYTE RESPONSE

primarily proliferative

T-CELL DEPENDENT ALLOANTIBODY RESPONSE

IgM and IgG Anti-A,B,C,D antibodies Ⓑ

FIGURE 69-3
Schema of the relative roles of HLA-A, HLA-B, HLA-C, and HLA-D antigens in initiation of the alloimmune response and in the development of effector cells and antibodies. Two main classes of T lymphocytes recognize antigens: T_c, the precursors to the cytotoxic "killer" cells, and T_H, the helper cells for amplification of the cytotoxic response. T_H also provide help to B lymphocytes for production of a fully mature IgG response. Note that T_c generally recognize class I antigens, while the T_H signal is provided principally by HLA-D, which has class II antigens closely associated. (From CB Carpenter, in Kidney International, New York, Springer-Verlag, 1978.)

TABLE 69-1
Associations between HLA antigens and disease

Disease	Antigen	Relative risk*
RHEUMATIC		
Ankylosing spondylitis	B27	127
Reiter's syndrome	B27	71
Acute anterior uveitis	B27	31
Psoriatic arthritis	B27	4.7
Reactive arthritis (yersinia, salmonella, gonococcus)	B27	150 (estimated)
Rheumatoid arthritis	Dw4	6.1
	DRw4	6.0
GASTROINTESTINAL		
Gluten-sensitive enteropathy	B8	9.5
Chronic active hepatitis	B8	3.6
Hemachromatosis	A3	8.2
	B14	26.7
	A3, B14	90
SKIN		
Dermatitis herpetiformis	B8	4.3
Psoriasis vulgaris	B13, Bw17	4.3
Pemphigus	A10	3.1
ENDOCRINE		
Juvenile diabetes mellitus	B8	3.3
	Bw15	3.0
	Dw3	4.5
	Dw4	3.7
	DRw3	2.8
	DRw4	5.3
Graves's disease	B8	3.6
Addison's disease	B8	6.4
	Dw3	10.5
NEUROLOGIC		
Myasthenia gravis	B8	4.4
Multiple sclerosis	Dw2	5.0
	DRw2	3.9

$$* \ \frac{Relative}{risk} = \frac{(\% \ antigen\text{-}positive \ patients) \ (\% \ antigen\text{-}negative \ controls)}{(\% \ antigen\text{-}negative \ patients) \ (\% \ antigen\text{-}positive \ controls)}$$

with chronic active hepatitis or dermatitis herpetiformis. Pemphigus is a disease in which a first-series antigen, HLA-A10, has shown an increased incidence.

Three endocrinopathies have been under intensive investigation following initial reports of increases in HLA-B8 frequency. Juvenile (insulin-dependent) diabetes mellitus has also shown an HLA-Bw15 association. With techniques for typing of D-locus antigens by performance of mixed lymphocyte cultures with homozygous stimulating cells and by serologic DR typing, a greater degree of association with the HLA-Dw3, DRw3, Dw4, and DRw4 has been reported. These antigens are often linked to HLA-B8 and HLA-Bw15, respectively, but these results would indicate that the loci related to juvenile diabetes are closer to the D locus than to B. Similar results have been obtained with Addison's disease. MLR typing has revealed an association with HLA-Dw2 and multiple sclerosis, while the frequently linked HLA-B7 antigen is less frequently associated.

Hence, disease associations with the HLA complex describe a spectrum, ranging from an extremely high degree of correlation with a serologically defined B locus HLA antigen, through diseases in which both B- and D-locus markers correlate, to a disease in which only the D-locus determinant is disease-associated. It is clear that definition of this spectrum is still in its early stages. It is likely that the development of more precise typing systems for identification of products of genes of the "left" of the B locus series, encompassing the D and related regions, may mark susceptibility in a number of diseases, such as leukemia, lymphoma, other malignancies and lupus erythematosus, in which HLA typing has been inconclusive.

LINKAGE DISEQUILIBRIUM Before reviewing the possible mechanisms of HLA gene complex influences in disease susceptibility, it is necessary to point to the most salient feature of the population genetics of HLA antigens, namely, the presence of linkage disequilibria among certain antigens of the A and B, B and C, and B and D loci. A linkage disequilibrium means that antigens of closely linked loci appear together more frequently than predicted by random association. The classic example is the linkage disequilibrium present between the A-locus antigen, HLA-A1, and B-locus antigen, HLA-B8, in Caucasian populations of Western Europe and America. One expects the coincidence of A1 and B8 to be the product of their individual gene frequencies, or 0.17 times 0.11 equals approximately 0.02. The observed frequency of A1 and B8 in Caucasians is 0.06, three times that expected, and an increase of 0.04. The latter value is termed Δ (delta), and is a measure of the disequilibrium. Other A and B locus haplotype disequilibria have been recognized, and include (A3, B7), (A2, B12), (A29, B12), and (A11, Bw35). Furthermore, some D-locus determinants are now known to be in linkage disequilibrium with second-series antigens (for example, Dw3 and B8), and C-locus antigens often have a Δ with B-locus antigens. Just as the serologically defined HLA antigens can serve as markers for the genes of an entire haplotype within a family, they may also serve as markers within a whole population for specific genes, but only where a linkage disequilibrium exists.

The development of linkage disequilibria is a matter of some importance because such gene associations may have some bearing on their function. For example, it has been proposed that selective pressures during the course of evolution have been the major factor in the survival of certain gene combinations in a haplotype. Such a theory would suggest, for example, that A1 and B8, along with certain D-locus and other determinants, conferred a selective advantage in the face of epidemics such as the plague or smallpox. It would go on to conclude that the descendants of the survivors now display susceptibility to certain diseases because of their unique gene complex which happens to confer an abnormal response to nonlethal environmental agents. The major difficulty with this hypothesis is the assumption that selection would have to work on several genes simultaneously in order to account for the observed deltas; however, the need for complex interactions among the products of the several loci of the major histocompatibility complex is only beginning to be appreciated, and it is possible that selection could force multiple linkage disequilibria.

On the other hand, one does not require the selection hypothesis to establish deltas in a population. With fusion of a population lacking certain antigens with one having a high frequency of antigens in equilibrium, a Δ can develop within a very small number of generations. For example, the increasing Δ value for A1, B8, found as one samples populations from East to West, from India to Western Europe, can be explained on the basis of migration and fusion. In smaller groups, consanguinity, a founder effect, and gene drift may account for disequilibria. Finally, certain linkage disequilibria could occur as a result of a nonrandomness in crossing over during gametic meiosis, because of chromosomal segments which are either more or less likely to break. In any event, the facts strongly suggest that a large number of nonrandom associations exist throughout the HLA gene complex, and the reasons for their existence, when they are better understood, may relate closely to the mechanism underlying certain disease susceptibilities.

MECHANISMS   There are three main hypotheses regarding the mechanisms by which histocompatibility complex genes influence disease susceptibility. The first is termed *molecular mimicry* and would propose that immunochemical similarities between HLA glycoproteins and microbiologic agents result in an impaired immune response because of cross-reacting tolerance of self-antigens. In order to be consistent with the observed facts of the dominance of disease susceptibility in the heterozygous state (e.g., ankylosing spondylitis occurs with B27 on one haplotype only), such a hypothesis would lead to the conclusion that the diseases in question are the result of chronic infection with a depressed immune response. However, there are no clearly demonstrated HLA and microbial cross-reactions. Most telling with regard to B27 and ankylosing spondylitis is the finding that B27 usually associates with this disease only when it is on a haplotype with the first series antigens, A2 or A9, providing evidence that B27 per se is most likely a marker for a linkage disequilibrium with other HLA region genes.

The second hypothesis suggests that HLA antigens may serve as *receptors for specific viruses,* resulting in an increased susceptibility to infection. This hypothesis has problems similar to the first, and direct attempts to show predilections for cell invasion by a variety of known viruses and cells of various HLA types have been unrewarding to date.

The third hypothesis, one which is gaining increased acceptance, is that important *immune response (Ir) genes* are present in the HLA gene complex, and that HLA antigens are markers for genes in linkage disequilibrium with them. The degree of association would then depend upon the distance between the marker and disease genes on the chromosome, and the degree to which crossing over between them may be restricted. An example is the finding that dermal responsiveness to ragweed antigen segregates with HLA haplotypes in atopic families, although the HLA antigens themselves may not be the same. A suggestive association with a D-locus gene and ragweed antigen E reactivity now exists, indicating that the gene(s) for a heightened immediate hypersensitivity response is placed far enough into the putative Ir region so that B-locus series HLA antigens are not good markers. When one considers the association of HLA-B8 and HLA-Dw3 markers with so many diseases (juvenile diabetes, Addison's disease, Graves' disease, gluten sensitivity, myasthenia gravis), it is tempting to conclude that a control mechanism for immune responsiveness, particularly with regard to autoimmunity, is involved. Since the etiologic agent is known in one of these diseases (gluten), and suspected in another (viral infection in juvenile diabetes mellitus), carefully designed studies should provide evidence regarding immune responsiveness to the agent versus an exaggerated secondary response to damaged tissue antigens. The distinction between association and linkage of a disease to HLA needs emphasis. The population studies summarized in Table 69-1 show associations to varying degrees, but linkage is not proved until family studies show segregation of the disease with HLA haplotypes. There is increasing evidence that at least some forms of juvenile-onset diabetes mellitus are not only linked to HLA, but that a recessive mode of inheritance may be involved, since there is a preponderance of HLA haplotype identical siblings among diabetic children, indicating that an HLA-linked gene(s) is required from both parents. A similar situation exists with idiopathic hemochromatosis and also 21-hydroxylase deficiency (Chap. 336 and Table 69-1) in which a preponderance of HLA identity among affected siblings also exists. The latter diseases illustrate the fact that an HLA-linked gene need not be an antigen of the HLA system itself, nor even related to any currently understood parameter of the immune response. The

numbers of genes involved and the variety of ways in which the final patterns of various diseases present may well be highly variable. Nevertheless, the way is now open to a better understanding of the genetic control of immune responsiveness in disease states.

Tissue typing for transplantation   Study of the HLA gene complex has, at present, limited direct clinical application, but its relationship to transplantation efforts is central. Siblings matched for the major antigens are easily treated with conventional drug therapy, and renal transplant results are in the range of 85 to 90 percent long-term success. A small number of A- and B-locus identical, but D-locus incompatible, transplants have been performed, and although not statistically significant, the majority of these have been rejected. The general experience in bone marrow transplantation also emphasizes the importance of matching for the D-locus region even when, due to recombination, the serologically defined A- and B-locus antigens are mismatched. Since the degree of linkage disequilibrium between HLA serologically defined antigens and other genes, including the D locus, is variable, and in many cases absent, matching of HLA-A and -B antigens for cadaveric renal transplantation is poorly predictive of graft success. Some series in Europe have provided evidence for improved survival with increasing numbers of A- and B-locus antigen matches, but these results have not been completely confirmed in North America, possibly because the greater degree of racial inhomogeneity in the New World reduces the amount of linkage disequilibrium between A, B, D, and other loci of the major histocompatibility gene complex. In contrast, some evidence exists for the importance of D-locus matching as assessed by retrospective results in MLC responses between cadaver and recipient lymphocytes. Since the MLC takes 5 to 7 days for the development of measurable degrees of proliferation ([^{3}H]thymidine incorporation), more rapid means (<24 h) of typing for these antigens are needed. Typing for DR antigens allows for rapid assessment of the D region and may prove to be useful in cadaveric organ matching.

HLA serologically defined A- and B-locus differences are clearly of major importance once an alloimmune response has been initiated, as these determinants are the major, though not the sole, targets for both humoral and cellular effector mechanisms. Forty to fifty percent of patients exposed to blood products while on chronic hemodialysis develop complement-dependent cytotoxic antibodies to allogenic lymphocytes. The "high responder" sensitized patients may make a selective response against certain HLA antigens, or may develop such a polyspecific response that they react with 90 to 100 percent of a randomly selected population. Transplants are not performed when the specific cross matches of recipient serums with donor lymphocytes are positive, because of a very high likelihood of an immediate "hyperacute" rejection. Furthermore, sensitized patients receiving cadaveric renal grafts may have a high failure rate, even though the specific donor cross match is negative, indicating either a lack of sensitivity in the test or the absence of the relevant antibodies at that particular time. Evidence for the latter comes from the reported improvement in kidney survival rates when additional serums, obtained at monthly intervals while on dialysis, are used at the time of cross match, or if analyses of anti-HLA specificities in the serums are made. Either way, mismatches can be avoided by assessment of past, as well as present, reactivities. In other words, a profile of the patient's immunologic memory is developed in order to avoid anamnestic responses. Further improvement in practical matching techniques, employing more sensitive cross matches and techniques for assessment of direct and antibody-dependent, cell-mediated cytotoxicity may offer further refinement in solving this major problem in cadaveric renal transplantation. Avoidance of sensitization would appear to offer a logical approach; however, a number of female patients have been sensitized by prior pregnancies, and occasionally the development of such cytotoxins is not explained by either pregnancy or blood transfusion. More important is the absence of data to confirm the notion that patients who never receive blood will have improved graft results; in fact, several studies show an increased failure rate in nontransfused patients. Taken together, these results suggest that genetic control of the alloimmune response also exists in humans, although no correlation can be made with HLA phenotypes. Prior exposure to alloantigens provides a definition of who is a "low responder" and who is a "high responder," and in the latter case it is now possible to avoid, in many instances, the specific mismatches to which a response has already been made, selecting a "new" incompatibility which, as a primary response, is more amenable to conventional drug therapy. The clinical significance of preexisting antidonor B-cell antibodies, generally though not exclusively anti-DR, is unclear. Several units report no deleterious effect when this cross-match barrier is crossed, while others find that true anti-DR responses may be harmful, although other specificities are not. The latter antibodies are usually reactive only in the cold (4 to 20°C), are of the IgM class, and frequently behave as autoantibodies.

Although minor transplantation antigen incompatibilities may on occasion be of importance in renal transplantation, the only other major antigenic system of proved importance is the ABH red blood cell system, a genetic system which segregates randomly from HLA. For example, HLA identical siblings can be mismatched for ABH. The rules of blood transfusion apply with regard to group O being a universal donor and group AB being a universal recipient. The clinical importance of non-HLA, non-ABH systems in bone marrow transplantation is greater than with organ grafts because of the graft-versus-host reactivity which commonly occurs in HLA-matched marrow recipients, and, in fact, has become the major limiting factor in clinical marrow grafting.

Another important application of HLA typing is in matching for platelet transfusions in individuals sensitized by prior blood component exposure. Platelets express most of the HLA serologic specificities (A and B loci), but not the D- and DR-locus antigens. Matching donor and recipient lymphocyte HLA-A and -B loci is of proved value in improving survival of transfused platelets in sensitized recipients.

IMMUNOLOGY OF REJECTION Knowledge of the immunology of tissue transplantation stems largely from animal experimentation. However, enough evidence has accumulated in humans, particularly in kidney transplantation, to indicate that the evidence is similar though not identical for the different species. The following observations describe reasonably accurately the events that transpire during the rejection of most human tissue transplants. Spleen and bone marrow grafts differ because in these instance cells capable of reacting against the recipient (graft-versus-host reaction) are transplanted.

From data derived both from animal and human experience, it appears that the rejection of transplanted tissue results from the antigenic stimulus of a two-component lymphoid system (Fig. 69-4). The lymphocytes involved are the offspring of marrow-derived stem cells. As these stem cells mature under the direct or humoral influence of (1) the thymus or (2) a human equivalent to the cells of the avian bursa, they develop antigen receptors so that they can respond in a cooperative manner to make an immune response when stimulated by antigen. The mature lymphocytes comprising the two distinct populations are for convenience abbreviated as (1) thymus-dependent (T) and (2) bone marrow (bursa)-dependent (B). Cooperative interaction between T and B cells, through the mediation of a factor furnished by the T cells after antigenic stimulation, is necessary for initiation of the immune response.

This cell interaction may take place upon the dendrites of tissue macrophages. In the case of the renal allograft, donor antigen may stimulate either T or B cells by way of antigen liberated from the kidney and reaching the lymphocytes by the bloodstream or lymphatics; or by contact between the recipient's lymphocytes and donor antigen as the former circulate through the kidney.

Some T cells are long-lived, circulating in the peripheral blood but "homing" in on lymphoid organs. They are responsible for cell-mediated immunity (CMI) such as graft rejection, delayed hypersensitivity (tuberculin skin test), the immune response to intracellular organisms, and possible "surveillance" which protects against growth of spontaneously occurring neoplasia. B cells are shortlived, noncirculating cells, largely responsible for the production of immune globulins, often referred to as "circulating antibody" or "humoral antibody" (Fig. 69-3). Both cell types are involved in immunity to transplants. A third effector system, involving the cooperative effort of graft-specific IgG antibodies and a nonimmune non-T cell, tentatively called a K cell, is now recognized. These effector cells are distinct from the specifically sensitized "killer" T cells. K cells interact with the Fc portion of the target-cell-bound IgG to mediate antibody-dependent cell-mediated cytotoxicity. Both lymphocytes and monocyte subpopulations may have K-cell activity. Even the polymorphonuclear leukocyte can damage IgG-coated target cells. Allografts to recipients previously unexposed to donor antigen are rejected as a "first-set" graft, largely through the T-cell system. Recipients who have previously been immunized to donor allografts by exposure to donor antigens by blood transfusions or by a previous transplant, or who have been the recipients of xenografts, have circulating preformed humoral antibody, and such grafts undergo "humoral rejection" in which the B-cell mechanism predominates. Because unrelated individuals may share one or more specific HLA determinants, a recipient may become immunized to the tissues of a donor by previous exposure to transfused white blood cells or platelets from another individual whose tissues contain the same antigens as the allograft donor. Once a kidney has been in place for several days in a previously unsensitized recipient, humoral immunity may become superimposed upon the cellular rejection; therefore, both types of immune processes may mediate the rejection of an allograft, with one or the other predominating; furthermore, the K-cell mechanism provides a potential link between humoral and cell-mediated immunity.

The rejection of an allograft by an individual who has not previously been exposed to donor antigens occurs first by way of the CMI pathways in which the sensitized T lymphocytes predominate. In the case of the kidney, the sensitized lymphocyte first combines with an antigen on vascular endothelium. Very early in the rejection process cells can be seen in contact with the small venules. The precise mechanism of the damage induced by the sensitized "killer" T lymphocytes awaits elucidation, but immunoglobulins and complement are not required. Rather, a cyclic nucleotide (cAMP and cGMP)-dependent process which follows direct cell-to-cell contact has been implicated. Similarly, the interaction of sensitized lymphocytes and antigens at the graft site is likely to release migration inhibitory factor (MIF) which may account for the accumulation of mononuclear (histiocytic) cells at the graft site. Some of these cells migrate through the vessel wall and are seen as perivascular accumulations. Intravascular accumulations result in slowing of flow, stasis, and graft ischemia. B lymphocytes, specifically sensitized, or K cells nonspecifically recruited by the prior formation of immune complexes of antibody and histocompatibility antigens, may also appear in the graft along the endothelial lining of vessels. Recovery of infiltrating cells from rejecting organs for study has shown that B cells, T cells, K cells, and monocytes may all be present. Of importance is the fact that donor-specific "killer" cells have been recovered from both animals and human allografts. When significant amounts of circulating antibodies, principally IgG and IgM, appear, the complement sequence is initiated. If intense, such activation may release significant amounts of polymorphonuclear (PMN) chemotactic factors, and PMNs are attracted to the graft, where the release of lysosomal enzymes from the leukocytes may result in damage to the vascular wall. In addition, the deposition of platelets is facilitated, with the release of vasoactive kinins and the deposition of fibrinogen and fibrin. This sequence of events is corroborated by histologic observations of rejection demonstrating interstitial infiltration of cells and damage to vascular endothelium with the deposition of fibrin, complement, and immune globulins. It can be shown also that the earliest evidence of renal allograft rejection is redistribution of blood flow from the cortex to the corticomedullary area, reflecting the primary role of the influence of vascular damage in the rejection process.

When a kidney is transplanted into a heterologous species or an individual previously sensitized to donor antigen, it is immediately perfused by "preformed" humoral antibody directed specifically against graft antigen. Again, the sequence of events which takes place reflects primarily the vascular site of injury. In such an instance little cellular infiltrate may be seen, but destruction to the vessel wall is violent and immediate, occurring in a matter of minutes in some instances. Platelet thrombi, the deposition of fibrin, and necrosis of vascular endothelium are prominent, and flow through the graft may cease within minutes or hours. Presumably, the same humoral mechanisms discussed above participate, but the sequence of events is accelerated; thus, the term "hyperacute rejection" has been applied.

The failure of transplanted kidneys after 2 or even 3 years of adequate function is due to a form of "chronic rejection." In such kidneys the development of nephrosclerosis, with proliferation of the vascular intima of renal vessels, and intimal fibrosis with marked decrease in the lumen of the vessels take place (Fig. 69-5). The result is renal ischemia, hypertension, widespread tubular atrophy, interstitial fibrosis, and glomerular atrophy with eventual renal failure. Occasionally, lobular or proliferative glomerulonephritis may be the initiating factor and may progress to renal failure. Most long-term vascular lesions and glomerular lesions are probably the result of subclinical episodes of rejection with damage to capillary and vascular epithelium and resultant healing fibrosis and sclerosis.

Finally, there is evidence that humoral antibody, in all probability some fraction of IgG, may actually play a role in promoting the *survival* of the allograft. This enhancing anti-

FIGURE 69-4

Overall scheme of the development of effector mechanisms in graft rejection. Bone marrow stem cells differentiate under the influence of the thymus gland into mature thymus-derived (T) lymphocytes, or under the influence of an equivalent to the avian bursa of Fabricius into mature bone-marrow-derived (B) lymphocytes. Exposure to antigen (Δ) results in an interaction between T cells and B cells, and often involves macrophages. The sensitized B cells, after mitoses, develop into immunoglobulin-secreting cells (e.g., plasma cells), illustrated here by IgG and IgM. Such immunoglobulins may form immune complexes with antigen in the circulation which activate the complement sequence, or they may react directly with antigens on the blood vessel surface. Elaboration of secondary mediators, including the products of complement activation, results in vascular damage as illustrated. Sensitized T lymphocytes are the primary effector cells in cell-mediated immunity (CMI) and may react directly with antigens in the graft to exert a cytotoxic effect. In addition, T cells release factors, such as macrophage migration inhibition factor (MIF) which may accelerate the rate of mononuclear cell infiltration. It has also been shown that unsensitized non-T cells (K cells) can be activated to exert cytotoxic effects by the fixation of IgG to target cells, followed by interaction of the IgG (Fc portion) with a receptor on the K cell. Nonimmune B cells may have K-cell activity, but since other mononuclear cells can react with IgG on target cells, the K cell is shown as having a separate lineage. Finally, platelet aggregation and thrombosis can occur following the endothelial damage induced by any of these mechanisms.

FIGURE 69-5

Biopsy of the renal cadaveric allograft illustrating obliterative endarteritis. Loss of the media is associated with intimal thickening. The elastic tissue shows dissolution of the elastica. The evidence for arteritis with subsequent thrombosis is typically the gaps in the elastica and media. The intimal thickening probably represents organization of a thrombus formed in response to the arteritis. [From GJ Dammin, JP Merrill, in Structural Basis for Renal Disease, EL Becker (ed), New York, Hoeber-Harper, 1968.]

body may block the action of cytotoxic "killer" lymphocytes, thus preventing the disastrous effects of the immune onslaught against the graft or may alter the presentation of antigen to responding B and T cells (Fig. 69-3).

IMMUNOSUPPRESSIVE TREATMENT When histocompatibility differences exist between donor and recipient, it is necessary to modify or suppress the immune response in order to enable the recipient to accept a graft. Immunosuppressive therapy in general suppresses all immune responses, including those to bacteria, fungi, and even malignant tumors. Agents used in humans to suppress the immune response are the following:

Drugs *Azathioprine (Imuran)*, an analogue of 6-mercaptopurine, is the keystone to immunosuppressive therapy in humans. This agent can inhibit synthesis of deoxyribonucleic acid (DNA), ribonucleic acid (RNA), or both. Because cell division and proliferation result as part of the immune response to antigenic stimulation, suppression may be mediated by the inhibition of mitosis of immunologically competent lymphoid cells interfering with synthesis of DNA. Alternatively, inhibition may be brought about by blocking the synthesis of ribonucleic acid (possibly messenger RNA), which is thought to play an

immunologic role in the processing of antigens prior to lymphocyte stimulation. Therapy with azathioprine is generally instituted 2 to 5 days prior to transplantation in the recipient of a living donor kidney and on the day of transplantation in the case of a cadaver donor kidney recipient. The drug is continued at levels of 2 to 3 mg/kg per day, as long as the allograft functions. Because the drug is rapidly metabolized by the liver, its dose need not be varied directly in relation to renal function, even though renal failure results in retention of the metabolites of azathioprine. Some patients are unusually sensitive to this drug, particularly when renal function is compromised, and reduction in dosage is required because of leukopenia and occasionally thrombocytopenia. Excessive amounts of azathioprine may also cause jaundice, anemia, and alopecia.

The *corticosteroids,* usually in the form of prednisone, are important adjuncts to immunosuppressive therapy. Of all the agents employed, prednisone has effects that are easiest to assess, and in large doses it is unquestionably the most effective agent for the reversal of rejection. In general, 150 to 200 mg prednisone is given immediately prior to or at the time of transplantation, and the dosage is reduced to maintenance levels over a period of 2 weeks. The well-known side effects of the corticosteroids, particularly impairment of wound healing and predisposition to infection, make it desirable to taper the dose as rapidly as possible in the immediate postoperative period. Customarily methylprednisolone, 1 to 2 g, intravenously, is administered immediately upon diagnosis of beginning rejection. When the drug is effective, the results are usually apparent within 48 to 96 h, and the dose may be subsequently tapered over a 5-day period and oral prednisone resumed. Such "pulse" doses are less effective in the slow rejection process which may not become apparent until 2 to 3 years after transplantation. Although most patients whose renal function is stable after 6 months or a year do not require large doses of prednisone, maintenance doses of 20 mg per day are the rule. Many patients tolerate an alternate-day course of steroids better without an increased risk of rejection.

When jaundice or nephritis appears in patients maintained on azathioprine, *cyclophosphamide* may be substituted. It appears to be as effective in the maintenance of renal allografts as Imuran and somewhat more effective in hepatic allografts. Leukopenia, alopecia, cystitis, ovarian fibrosis, and aspermia may result if the dosage is not carefully regulated. In one series of cadaver allografts the prospective donor was treated with massive doses of cyclophosphamide and methylprednisolone in an attempt to decrease the antigenicity of the graft by eliminating "passenger leukocytes." The preliminary results of this technique are encouraging.

Antilymphocyte globulin (ALG) When serums from animals made immune to host lymphocytes are injected into the recipient, a marked suppression of cellular immunity to the tissue graft results. The action upon CMI is considerably more effective than upon humoral immunity. A globulin fraction of the serum is the agent generally employed. For use in humans, peripheral human lymphocytes, thymocytes, lymphocytes from cadaver spleens, or those harvested from thoracic duct fistulas have been utilized. More recently, cultured human lymphoblasts, which can be produced in large quantities, offer the advantage of availability. These cells are injected into horses, rabbits, or goats to produce antilymphocyte serum, from which the globulin fraction is then separated. The globulin is injected intramuscularly, or preferably intravenously, 5 days to 1 week prior to transplantation and continued for 2 to 3 weeks thereafter. Although ALG, or ATG (antithymocyte globulin) is unquestionably effective in prolonging grafts in experimental animals, its efficacy in the transplantation of human tissue is somewhat less clear, even though an effective preparation of ALG may result in the disappearance of a previously positive delayed type of skin reaction. ALG should be used with caution in human beings; it cannot now be considered part of routine immunosuppressive therapy. Further exploration of this preparation, particularly employing larger doses, may result in the development of an effective agent which can be used with relatively little hazard of serum sickness or nephrotoxic nephritis.

Other techniques Of the alternate techniques of immunosuppression, thymectomy and splenectomy have not favorably influenced the course of human kidney transplants. Local irradiation to the transplanted kidney in two or three doses of 350 rads each has also been utilized. This technique may result in fewer early rejection episodes in cadaveric transplants than in nonirradiated controls.

COMPLICATIONS OF RENAL TRANSPLANTATION The complications of human renal transplantation often result from the use of *immunosuppressive therapy.* Wound infection with gram-negative organisms is common, as is breakdown of wounds, particularly the ureteral anastomosis. Pulmonary infections with a variety of unusual organisms, including *Candida* (Chap. 158), *Aspergillus* (Chap. 159), *Nocardia* (Chap. 152), *Pneumocystis* (Chap. 204), and cytomegalovirus (Chap. 194) also occur. Their relationship to a general defect in immunologic integrity is clear. The complications of *corticosteroid* therapy are well known and include gastrointestinal bleeding, hemorrhagic pancreatitis, impairment of wound-healing, osteoporosis, diabetes, and cataract formation. Leukopenia, anemia, and jaundice may occur as a result of azathioprine administration.

Even identical twins who do not require immunosuppressive therapy develop complications. In 18 sets of identical twins whose original disease was glomerulonephritis, 11 developed a similar histologic lesion in the transplanted kidney. The glomerular lesion is not, however, limited to the isograft, nor is it necessarily a question of "catching" the disease in the transplant because of continuing antiglomerular activity. A number of patients with true allografts treated with immunosuppressive therapy have developed typical glomerular lesions over a period of years. One patient who received a successful allograft from his mother developed a classic nephrotic syndrome with glomerulonephritis 2½ years after transplantation. Because the reason for transplantation initially was the accidental removal of a single normal ectopic kidney, the development of glomerulonephritis in the transplant cannot be attributed to "continuing activity."

Glomerular lesions occur in some 10 to 15 percent of allografts. In many of these the lesions so resemble those of the patient's own original disease that they must be considered recurrences of the original disease. The recurrence of the nephrotic syndrome with "nil disease" in transplanted kidneys whose recipient's original nil disease has progressed to renal failure with focal sclerosis, the recurrence in renal allografts of the classic lesions of IgA nephropathy, and those of membranoproliferative glomerulonephritis with electron-dense deposit disease are classic examples. In the last of these, the incidence of recurrence has been reported as high as 30 to 40 percent. In many instances, however, the recurrence of the original renal lesions may represent no threat to the patient's immediate prognosis, and an established diagnosis of glomerulonephritis is rarely taken as a contraindication to transplantation. Finally, in at least one case, glomerulonephritis has developed apparently de novo in a patient who has survived 5 years with a normally functioning allograft.

Sensitization of the human recipient to the antigens of the renal allograft may occur because of exposure to these antigens via blood transfusions or pregnancy. When the cytotoxic antibodies are directed against the antigens of the donor, rapid rejection of the graft occurs, and even when the cytotoxic antibodies in the recipient's serum are not specific for those of the donor, the prognosis for graft survival is poorer than in unsensitized individuals. This is discussed elsewhere in this chapter.

The incidence of *tumors* arising in patients on immunosuppressive therapy in one well-studied group was 5.6 percent, or approximately 100 times greater than that observed in the general population in the same age range. These figures correspond with those in the world experience in well over 27,000 cases. The most common lesions were cancer of the skin and lips and carcinoma in situ of the cervix. These lesions were easily treated. There was a high incidence of lymphomas, particularly reticulum cell sarcoma of the nervous system. The prognosis was poor when these lesions occurred. Two possibilities are suggested for the high incidence of cancer in transplant recipients: (1) immunosuppressive therapy impairs the "immunologic surveillance" of the lymphoreticular system, in consequence of which potentially malignant cellular mutations are not detected and destroyed; (2) immunosuppressed individuals frequently harbor viruses, some of which may be oncogenic. The chronic immunostimulation produced by the resident allograft may be more important than the drug-induced immunosuppression, particularly since such stimulation may activate some viruses.

Tumor cells have been transplanted inadvertently with kidneys taken from cadaver donors and occasionally from living donors. The immunosuppressive therapy which allows the kidney to be tolerated in the recipients also apparently permits survival and propagation of the malignant tumor. In two instances cessation of immunosuppressive therapy resulted in rejection of both the graft and the tumor with its metastases.

Urinary fistula requiring nephrostomy may be the result of rejection of the ureter, disruption of the ureteral blood supply, infection, or a combination of all three. Wound infection and failure of the wound to heal are not uncommon, particularly when the higher doses of steroids are required.

Hypercalcemia may develop within days or weeks after transplantation and persist for as long as 7 years. In many instances this appears to be due to markedly enlarged parathyroid glands which have developed during the uremic phase and do not spontaneously regress with the resumption of normal renal function. In other instances no elevation of blood levels of parathyroid hormone can be found. Although several instances of renal and vascular calcification have been reported, renal function in general does not appear to suffer. However, when bone disease occurs or persists in the presence of hyperparathyroidism, subtotal parathyroidectomy is indicated. Glucocorticoid administration may contribute to the hypercalcemia.

Aseptic necrosis of the head of the femur has been reported in 10 to 20 percent of the posttransplant patients. This complication is probably due to preexisting uremic bone disease or hyperparathyroidism, plus the large doses of corticosteroid. With improved management of calcium and phosphorus metabolism during periods of dialysis, however, the incidence of aseptic necrosis following transplantation has fallen dramatically.

There has been considerable improvement in patient morbidity and mortality rates during the mid-1970s, attributable to more judicious use of immunosuppressive agents and antibiotics. It is customary now to use steroid pulses only twice, or rarely three times, and to allow the patient to return to dialysis. Although graft survival is not improved by this protocol, it has not worsened, while patient mortality has dropped from around 20 percent to less than 5 percent per year, a rate which is comparable to that for hemodialysis. Urinary fistulae are also much less common, partly because aberrant polar arteries which nourish the renal pelvis and upper ureter are no longer ligated, but are anastomosed by microsurgical techniques. Concomitant with improved mortality, the incidence of bacterial infection has declined to less than 15 percent, and units which formerly had major problems with fungal and viral diseases now must deal with these in only a small minority of transplant recipients.

The incidence of death from *myocardial infarction* and *cerebrovascular accidents* is considerably higher in transplant recipients than in the population at large. The contributing factors are preexisting hypertension, vascular disease, and hypertriglyceridemia, which occurs in uremic patients and persists in the posttransplant period. There is possibly a contribution by hypercalcemia. *Gastrointestinal hemorrhage* is also a complication.

SELECTION OF RECIPIENTS FOR KIDNEY TRANSPLANTATION

Table 69-2 lists practical considerations in the selection of a recipient for a human renal allograft. Such a procedure should be undertaken only when conservative treatment has failed, when there are no reversible elements in the patient's renal failure, and when the patient is too sick to be maintained comfortably with the usual methods of treatment. However, the considerable success with kidneys transplanted from blood relatives, reports of success with second or third kidney transplants, and the ability to maintain patients who have had transplant failures on hemodialysis justify consideration of kidney transplantation before the patient is critically ill and possibly even before it is obvious that hemodialysis is the only other course. Transplantation should not be utilized in an attempt to salvage patients from failure to thrive on dialysis. On the other hand, when no well-matched related donor is available, the patient and physician should carefully consider the relative risks against those of continued dialysis. Approximately 10 percent of dialysis patients receiving cadaver transplants cannot be successfully returned to dialysis if the graft fails. The attrition rate in most well-run dialysis programs is about 4 to 7 percent per year. Each case, of course, must be individualized before the statistics have pertinence. The recipient should be free of life-threatening extrarenal complications such as cancer, severe coronary artery disease, and cerebrovascular disease. Provided that diffuse vascular involvement is not present, diabetes itself is not a contraindication. Although age may be a limiting factor, the "physiologic" age rather than the chronologic age contraindicates transplantation. A cadaver transplant into an 82-year-old patient is on record, and adult renal allografts have been transplanted into recipients as young as 3. Although abnormalities of the bladder and urethra present additional hazards, successful renal allografts have been placed in individuals with these abnormalities by prior construction of an artificial bladder (i.e., ileal conduit) into which the donor ureter is placed. The demonstration of "preformed antibodies" in the potential recipient prior to transplantation is a contraindication when in the standard lymphocytotoxicity test these antibodies react specifically to donor cells.

DONOR SELECTION Donor sources are cadavers or volunteer blood-related living donors. Living volunteer donors should be found completely normal on physical examination and should be of the same major ABO blood group, because there is good evidence that crossing major blood group barriers prejudices survival of the allograft. It is, however, possible to transplant a kidney of a type O donor into an A or B recipient. Selective renal arteriography should be performed on volunteer donors to rule out the presence of multiple or abnormal renal arteries, because the surgical procedure is inordinately difficult and the ischemic time of the normal kidney prohibitively long when vascular abnormalities exist. Cadaver donors should be free of malignant neoplastic disease because of possible transmission of cancer to the recipient.

Although tissue typing for A- and B-locus HLA antigens is of limited value for cadaver donors, direct cross matching for the presence of preformed antibodies against specific donor tissue is mandatory. The chances of finding a perfect A- and B-locus 4-antigen match between unrelated donor and recipient are calculated to be between 1 in 300 and 1 in 1000, varying with the incidence of HLA antigens in the population. If, in addition, antigens of the D locus are found to be of practical importance, matching will require a large recipient pool, maintained on hemodialysis. A coordinated regional or national system of computerized information sharing and logistical support for the transportation of cadaver kidneys to the suitable recipient is under development. It is now possible to remove cadaver kidneys and to maintain them up to 48 h on cold pulsatile perfusion or simple flushing and cooling. This should permit adequate time for various typing, cross matching, transportation, and selection problems to be solved.

CLINICAL COURSE AND MANAGEMENT OF THE RECIPIENT Bilateral nephrectomy at some point prior to transplantation is performed for specific cause but not as a routine. Hypertension which is difficult to control or infection involving the end-stage kidneys are the two most common indications. Nephrectomized patients maintain a much lower hematocrit level, but this is no longer considered a disadvantage per se, because blood transfusions are not to be avoided in preparation for transplantation. When comparing the overall results with nephrectomized vs. nonnephrectomized recipients, no significant difference has emerged, except for the fact that nontransfused recipients of cadaveric grafts are more likely to reject their grafts. It should be ascertained also that the recipient has a normally functioning bladder and lower outflow tract.

Adequate hemodialysis should be performed within 48 h prior to surgery, and care should be taken that the serum potassium level is not markedly elevated so that intraoperative cardiac arrhythmias can be averted. In patients who have been presensitized to donor tissue, hyperacute rejection may take place on the operating table. Within minutes the kidney will become swollen, tense, and a mottled purple in color, and blood flow may cease soon thereafter. Thrombotic obliterative lesions may be seen by frozen section, and if they are extensive the kidney should be removed. Postoperatively the diuresis that occurs must be carefully monitored; in many instances it

TABLE 69-2
Contraindications to human kidney transplantation

I Absolute contraindications:
  A Reversible renal involvement
  B Ability of conservative measures to maintain useful life
  C Major extrarenal complications (cerebrovascular or coronary disease; neoplasia)
  D Active infection
  E Active glomerulonephritis
  F Previous sensitization to donor tissue
II Relative contraindications (see text):
  A Age
  B Presence of vesical or urethral abnormalities
  C Iliofemoral occlusive disease
  D Diabetes mellitus
  E Inactive lupus erythematosus
  F Psychiatric problems

may be massive, reflecting the inability of ischemic tubules to regulate sodium and water excretion. Massive potassium losses may occur and occasionally result in cardiac arrhythmias. The chronically uremic patient undoubtedly has some excess of extracellular fluid, and some degree of negative balance should be accomplished provided circulatory hemodynamics remain stable.

Although immunosuppressive regimens vary, a typical program would be the following:

Azathioprine in a dose of 4 mg/kg is given for 2 days preoperatively to recipients of a living donor transplant; on the day of operation it is administered by the intravenous route, and it is continued for about 1 week, depending upon renal function. It is then reduced to 3 mg/kg, and the maintenance dose is 1½ mg/kg by mouth. In recipients of kidneys from living donors the equivalent of 300 to 500 mg cortisone is given on the day of operation; this dose is maintained for 2 days and is decreased gradually to a maintenance dose of 50 to 100 mg cortisone, usually administered as the prednisone equivalent. For rejection episodes, 1 to 2 g soluble corticosteroid in the form of methylprednisolone is administered intravenously daily for a 3-day period. This is decreased to 800, 600, and 400 mg over the next 10-day period while oral prednisone dosage is maintained at 25 to 50 mg.

The rejection episode Early diagnosis of rejection is imperative, because prompt institution of vigorous therapy may reverse renal function and prevent irreversible damage due to fibrosis. Clinical evidence of rejection is characterized by fever, swelling, and tenderness over the allograft, and by significant reduction in urine volume. In patients whose renal function is good initially, oliguria may be accompanied by decreased urinary sodium concentration and increased osmolarity. These changes may not be present in the more chronic stages of rejection or when renal function is impaired at the onset of rejection. A transplanted cadaver kidney frequently undergoes a period of anuria which may last as long as 3 weeks without prejudicing the eventual function of the graft. In this instance, the reversible lesion is presumably due to ischemia, and the diagnosis of rejection becomes more difficult. Renal arteriography and radioactive Hippuran renograms may be useful in ascertaining changes in the renal vasculature and in renal blood flow, even in the absence of urinary flow. Diagnostic ultrasound has become the procedure of choice to rule out urinary obstruction or to confirm the presence of perirenal collections of urine, blood, or lymph. When renal function has been good initially, a rise in the serum creatinine level and a decrease in the creatinine clearance may herald the onset of rejection. The serum creatinine or its clearance is more reliable than the blood urea nitrogen because fever and the administration of prednisone may influence the concentration of blood urea nitrogen without necessarily reflecting a decrease in urea clearance. Increase in the 24-h excretion of urinary lysozyme has been helpful. Increase in proteinuria may reflect rejection, but when it occurs later in the course of the postoperative period, predominant glomerular disease may be present. Hypertension is also a concomitant of rejection. When hypertension responds to prednisone, it is likely that rejection has been responsible for the elevation of blood pressure, because other forms of hypertension usually do not improve with corticosteroid therapy. A number of tests have been posed for the diagnosis of rejection which depend upon the measurements of variation in expressions of cellular or humoral immunity; persistent antidonor antibody activity, as detected by complement-dependent cytotoxicity or by antibody-dependent cell-mediated cytotoxicity (K cells), often correlates with irreversible rejection with vasculitis in the graft. Appearance of circulating cytotoxic T cells ("killer" cells) is more likely to relate to a cell-mediated rejection process. Other tests, such as the measurement of lysozyme excretion and that of fibrin-split products reflect nonspecific renal damage, although the latter test may have somewhat more pertinence to the rejection mechanism.

Modification of the usual clinical manifestations of infection by immunosuppressive therapy is a major problem in the posttransplant period. The signs and symptoms of infection may be masked and distorted, and fever without obvious cause is common. Only after days or weeks will it become apparent that it has a viral or fungal origin. The importance of blood cultures in such patients cannot be overemphasized, because systemic infection without obvious external foci is frequent. Particularly important are rapidly occurring pulmonary lesions, which may result in death within 5 days of onset. When these become apparent, immunosuppressive agents should be discontinued except for maintenance doses of prednisone. In the case of *Pneumocystis carinii*, trimethoprim-sulfa or pentamidine is the treatment of choice; amphotericin B has been used effectively in systemic fungal infections. Involvement of the oropharynx with *Candida* may be treated with local nystatin. Small doses (a total of 300 mg) of amphotericin given over a period of 2 weeks may be effective in refractory oral candidiasis. The treatment of jaundice in transplant patients should include cessation of azathioprine therapy. It is surprising that total cessation of azathioprine therapy often does not result in rejection of a graft. In some instances of jaundice, cyclophosphamide may be substituted for azathioprine. Antiplatelet agents and anticoagulants, although effective in theory, have not been strikingly successful in the prevention of the chronic vascular lesion.

The condition of patients who have been discharged from the hospital should be closely observed in a specialized outpatient clinic whose physicians are familiar with the problems and complications of the posttransplant patient. When, in spite of repeated efforts to reverse the rejection, renal function progressively fails, the philosophy should be to save the patient, not the graft. Excessive immunosuppressive therapy may lead to fatal infection or bleeding. A biopsy of the graft may establish the irreversibility of the lesion. When such irreversibility is established, the graft should be removed and the patient started again on hemodialysis. Infection and hemorrhage at the operative sites days and even months following removal of the graft occasionally occur and must be carefully watched. Psychological complications following transplantation are common. Depression and anxiety may reflect both the difficult, stressful postoperative course and the anxiety and uncertainty of the physician.

In spite of the potential teratogenic effects of immunosuppressive agents, both women and men have become parents after transplantation. The incidence of congenital abnormalities in the offspring is not unusual. The major problems with pregnancy are related to the concomitant development of rejection activity in the graft causing uremia and hypertension. In one series of over 400 pregnancies in transplant recipients 25 percent required therapeutic abortion. Although one-half of the live births had no complications, the others were either premature or underweight, and there was an increased incidence of the respiratory distress syndrome. There is an impression that pregnancy may provoke rejection activity in some previously stable patients, a point of interest because the fetus itself is an allograft. Although obstruction of the transplant ureter by extrinsic compression is a potential problem, its actual incidence is rare; furthermore, urinary infections do not seem to be more frequent in pregnant transplant recipients.

It is evident that immunosuppressive therapy as currently used in renal transplantation is inadequate. What is badly needed is a solution to the problem of producing specific immunologic unresponsiveness to the antigens of the donor without affecting the recipient's immune potential for infective agents. Such techniques have been successfully developed for the experimental animal, and their safe application to humans is eagerly awaited.

TRANSPLANTATION OF OTHER TISSUES Organs other than the kidney which have a potential for clinical transplantation are the liver and heart. Two possible indications for *liver transplantation* are chronic hepatic failure and malignancy which is localized to the liver. Two techniques for liver transplantation have been utilized in humans: (1) *orthotopic*—the recipient's own liver is removed and the transplant is substituted for it in the anatomic positon; (2) *auxiliary*—the recipient's liver is left in place and the allograft is placed in the right paravertebral gutter. The donor's vena cava then is interposed in the recipient terminal inferior vena cava, and the hepatic artery is anastomosed to the right common iliac artery. Finally, the end of the allograft portal vein is anastomosed to the recipient's superior mesenteric vein.

Immunosuppressive regimens are similar to those in kidney transplantation. There is some suggestion that the use of antilymphocyte globulin is more effective in liver allografting. Obviously, the donor source must be a cadaver. Complications of liver transplantation have been strikingly different from those encountered with renal allografts. In many instances an initial hemorrhagic diathesis with fibrinolysis occurs. This is followed by a phase of hypercoagulability in the successfully transplanted recipient, which in one instance resulted in fatal pulmonary emboli. Infections also seem to present a greater problem than with renal allografts. These complications are not insurmountable, however, and there are now a number of liver-transplant recipients who have survived for 2 years or more. Although at this time liver transplantation is not as clinically feasible a procedure as kidney grafting, in a few centers with expertise and experience in this technique liver transplants continue to be performed, it is hoped with steady improvement in the results.

Transplantation of the heart has been accomplished successfully in humans in a number of instances. Current results suggest that it is comparable to transplantation of the cadaver kidney and that results probably will improve. Indications for cardiac transplantation are myocardial insufficiency, usually due to severe coronary artery disease and myocardial fibrosis, and failure to respond to the most rigorous medical measures. The donor must be a cadaver and is usually an individual whose death has resulted from trauma or suicide. The question of the ethics and morals raised by the removal of a heart capable of sustaining life in another individual has been discussed by many medical and lay authors. It seems eminently reasonable that if "death" of the brain has occurred, as evidenced by lack of electrical activity in the electroencephalogram over a period of 24 to 36 h, dilated pupils, failure of spontaneous respiration, and lack of peripheral reflexes, the ability to maintain respiration or cardiac output by artificial methods is academic. Nevertheless, the decision as to when to discontinue these efforts should be made independently by the physician caring for the prospective donor in consultation with one or two colleagues. The question whether the heart is to be used for transplantation should not affect this decision. Once the decision has been made, the donor can be maintained until the recipient is prepared for operation. Recently a human "auxiliary heart" has been transplanted with initial success. The anastomosis of the donor heart to that of the recipient is made in such a way that the normal left ventricle of the donor assists the failing left ventricle of the recipient while the hypertrophied right ventricle of the recipient is allowed to continue to function in the pulmonary circuit, thus eliminating the sudden load imposed upon the normal right ventricle by the preexist-

ing pulmonary hypertension. At present, cardiac transplantation is and should be done only in specialized centers with highly skilled and experienced teams. Its future as an important therapeutic procedure is still unclear.

Human *spleen* and *pancreas* have been transplanted with limited success. If it could be shown that normal spleen can produce a useful amount of antihemophilic globulin (AHG), transplantation of that organ to some patients with hemophilia would provide a distinct advantage over standard substitution therapy. Transplantation of lymphoid tissue (including spleen) for total agammaglobulinemia has resulted in temporary improvement, but eventually the transplanted lymphoid tissue rejects the host (graft-versus-host reaction). Temporary success in transplanting pancreas in diabetics also has been reported, but substitution therapy seems more feasible.

Various other *endocrines,* including parathyroid, adrenal, and thyroid, have all been transplanted with only temporary success. A large percentage of *corneal grafts* survive as allografts in humans primarily because the cornea is not vascularized and excludes immunologically competent cells. Grafts of bone and blood vessels do not survive as living allografts but act as a "scaffolding" over which host tissue may grow.

Transplantation of allogenic bone marrow in humans (Chap. 312) is of particular interest to patients with leukemia and aplastic anemia and has resulted in a number of attempts to modify these diseases by this means. Similarly, the reconstitution of the defect in congenital or acquired agammaglobulinemia or alymphocytosis has been attempted by grafting into such recipients cells competent to produce cell-mediated immunity or humoral immunity. When the recipient and donor are identical twins, no immunosuppressive therapy is necessary, and 50 percent of the recipients transplanted have done well. Aplastic anemia has also been treated by marrow-grafting between siblings who are 4-antigen HLA matches and MLC-negative. In this case the recipient is prepared with cyclophosphamide and total body irradiation, while methotrexate is given after grafting. Some 50 percent of these patients have also done well. In the treatment of acute leukemia the object is to destroy as many of the malignant cells as possible; therefore, 1000 rads total body irradiation plus cyclophosphamide is given, and, in one protocol, in order to enhance the immune reaction of donor cells against malignant antigens, the recipient is immunized by radiation-killed malignant cells. In the instances where this was accomplished between identical twins, 10 remissions longer than 3 months and 1 greater than 49 months have occurred. The recipients of matched allogenic marrow, similarly prepared, have done increasingly well, and the probability of being in remission at 2 years is about 30 percent. Immune-competent donor cells reacting against the antigens of the host result in a "graft-versus-host reaction" in some 70 percent of the cases. This may be acute or indolent and is characterized by involvement of the skin, liver, and gastronintestinal tract. Infection, similar to that seen in kidney transplant recipients, is common. Methotrexate, cyclophosphamide, and antithymocyte globulin have been used in the treatment of this syndrome with some success. A striking and unexpected phenomenon has been malignant transformation of donor cells in two instances.

Transplantation of a normal allogenic liver to repair the metabolic defect in Wilson's disease has been reported in two instances with some preliminary success, and the transplantation of the kidney not as a functioning excretory organ but as a source of the congenitally absent enzyme has been attempted in Fabry's disease and oxalosis. The long-term results are disappointing.

ORGAN PRESERVATION If it were possible to remove ca-daver organs and to store them for a period of weeks or longer under conditions permitting their successful replantation, one of the difficult problems in organ procurement would be solved. Bone marrow is the only organ that can be stored easily for prolonged periods.

XENOGRAFTS Kidneys, lungs, and hearts have been transplanted to human beings from various primates, including chimpanzees and baboons. Although one chimpanzee kidney graft functioned well for more than 7 months, clinical efforts in this area have been abandoned.

REFERENCES

CARPENTER CB (ed): *Clinical Histocompatibility Testing*, vol 2. New York. Grune & Stratton, 1978
——— et al: The role of antibodies in the rejection and enhancement of organ allografts. Adv Immunol 22:1, 1976

DEGOS L, DAUSSET J: Human migrations and linkage disequilibrium of HLA system. Immunogenetics 3:195, 1974
GALE RP, OPELZ G (eds): *Immunobiology of Bone Marrow Transplantation.* New York, Grune & Stratton, 1978
GOTTLIEB MN et al: Bone disease following renal transplantation, in *Calcium and Bone Metabolism in Renal Disease*, DS David (ed). New York, Wiley, 1977, p 279
JERSILD C et al: The HLA system and inherited deficiencies of the complement system. Transplant Rev 32:43, 1976
MERRILL JP: Dialysis versus transplantation in the treatment of end-stage renal disease. Annu Rev Med 29:343, 1978
STRAFFON RA (ed): Renal transplantation. Urol Clin North Am 3:3, 1976
SVEJGAARD A et al: HLA and disease associations—a survey. Transplant Rev 22:3, 1978
TERASAKI PI et al: Summary of kidney transplant data, 1977—factors affecting graft outcome. Transplant Proc 10:417, 1978
——— et al: Microdroplet testing for HLA-A, B, C and D antigens. Am J Clin Pathol 69:103, 1978
VAN ROOD JJ et al: B-cell antibodies, Ia-like determinants in man. Transplant Rev 30:122, 1976

section 3 | Clinical pharmacology

70
PRINCIPLES OF DRUG THERAPY

JOHN A. OATES
GRANT R. WILKINSON

QUANTITATIVE DETERMINANTS OF DRUG ACTION

Safe and effective therapy with drugs requires their delivery to target tissues in concentrations within the narrow range that yields efficacy without toxicity. Optimal precision in achieving concentrations of drug within this therapeutic "window" can be achieved with regimens that are based on the kinetics of the drug's availability to target sites. This chapter deals with the principles of drug elimination and distribution that form the basis for loading and maintenance regimens for the average patient and considers instances in which elimination of the drug is impaired (e.g., renal failure). The kinetic basis for optimal utilization of plasma level data is also discussed.

PLASMA LEVELS AFTER A SINGLE DOSE The levels of lidocaine (Chap. 238) in plasma following intravenous administration decline in two phases as illustrated in Fig. 70-1; such a biphasic decline is typical for many drugs. Immediately following rapid injection, all the drug is in the plasma compartment, and the high initial plasma level reflects its confinement to this small volume. Subsequently, the drug is rapidly distributed from plasma into the extravascular compartment, and the period of time during which this is occurring is referred to as the *distribution phase.* For lidocaine this distribution phase is virtually complete within 30 min; then there is a slower rate of fall, referred to as the *equilibrium phase* or the *elimination phase.* During this latter phase, the drug levels in plasma and those in the tissues of the body are in pseudoequilibrium.

Distribution phase Pharmacological events during the distribution phase depend on whether the level of drug at the receptor site closely reflects that in the plasma. If this is the case, the pharmacological effects, whether favorable or adverse, may be inordinately great during this period. For example, following a small bolus dose (25 mg) of lidocaine, antiarrhythmic effects may be evident during the early distribution phase but disappear as levels rapidly fall below those that are minimally effective and even before equilibrium between plasma and tissue is reached. Thus, larger single doses or multiple small doses must be administered in order to achieve an effect that is sustained into the equilibrium phase. The toxicity of high levels of some drugs during the distribution phase precludes administration of a single intravenous loading dose that will achieve therapeutic levels during the equilibrium phase. For example, the administration of a loading dose of the anticonvulsant, phenytoin (diphenylhydantoin) as a single intravenous bolus can cause cardiovascular collapse due to the high levels during the distribution phase. For this reason, if a loading dose of phenytoin is administered intravenously, it must be given in fractions (10 to 15 percent of the total loading amount) at intervals sufficient to permit substantial distribution of the prior dose before the next is given. For similar reasons, the loading dose of many potent drugs that rapidly equilibrate with their receptors is divided into fractional doses for intravenous administration.

After an oral dose that delivers an equivalent amount of drug into the systemic circulation, plasma levels during the distribution phase do not rise nearly as steeply as they do after an intravenous bolus dose. Because the drug is not absorbed instantly after oral administration, it is delivered into the systemic circulation more slowly, and much of the drug is already distributed by the time absorption is complete. Thus, procainamide, which is almost totally absorbed after oral administration, can be given as a single 750-mg loading dose with little risk of hypotension; in contrast, loading of the drug by the

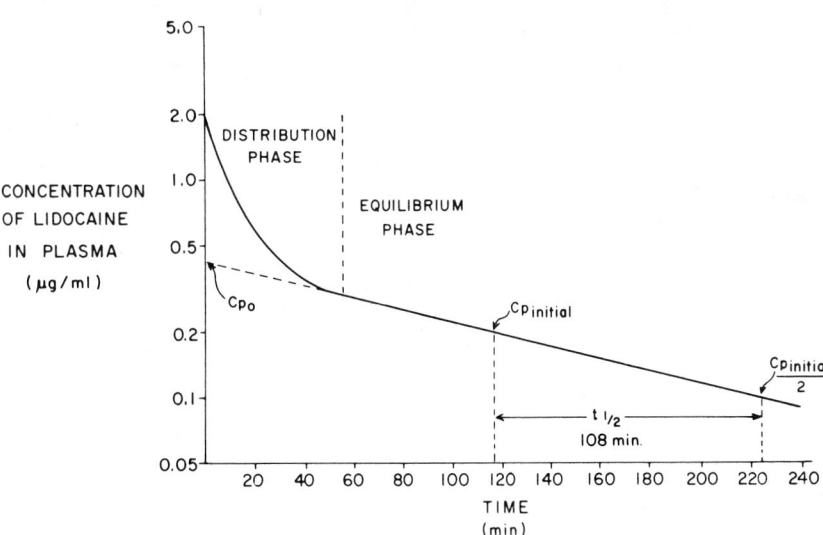

FIGURE 70-1

Concentrations of lidocaine in plasma following the administration of 50 mg intravenously. The half-life of 108 min is computed as the time required for levels to fall from any given value during the equilibrium phase ($C_{P_{initial}}$) to one-half that level. C_{P_0} is the hypothetical concentration of lidocaine in plasma at time zero if equilibrium had been achieved instantly.

intravenous route is more safely accomplished by giving the loading dose in fractions of about 100 mg at 5-min intervals in order to avoid the hypotension that would ensue during the distribution phase in some patients if the entire loading dose were given as a single bolus.

In contrast, other drugs are distributed to their sites of action only slowly during the distribution phase. For example, levels of digoxin at the receptor site (and its pharmacological effect) do not reflect plasma levels during the distribution phase (Chap. 238). Digoxin is transported (or bound) to its cardiac receptors more slowly by a process that proceeds throughout distribution. Thus, plasma levels during a distribution phase of several hours are falling while levels at the site of action and pharmacological effect are increasing. Only at the end of the distribution phase when the drug has reached equilibrium with the receptor does the concentration of digoxin in plasma reflect pharmacological effect. For this reason, there should be a 6- to 8-h wait after the distribution phase before samples for plasma levels of digoxin that are to be used as a guide to therapy are obtained.

Equilibrium phase After distribution has proceeded to the point where the concentration of drug in plasma is in equilibrium with that in the tissues outside the vascular compartment, the levels in plasma and tissues fall in parallel as the drug is eliminated from the body. Thus, the equilibrium phase is sometimes also referred to as the *elimination phase.*

Most drugs are eliminated as a first-order process. During the equilibrium phase, a characteristic of the first-order process is that the time required for the level of drug in plasma to fall to one-half the original value (the half-life) will be the same regardless of which point on the plasma level curve is chosen as a starting point for the measurement. Another characteristic of the first-order process is that a plot of the concentrations in plasma versus time during the equilibrium phase is linear on a semilogarithmic graph. From such a plot (Fig. 70-1) it can be seen that the half-life of lidocaine is 108 min.

One can readily calculate what amount of the administered dose remains in the body at any multiple of the half-life interval following administration:

Number of half-lives	Amount of dose remaining in the body, %
1	50
2	25
3	12.5
4	6.25
5	3.13

In theory, the elimination process never reaches comple-

tion. From a clinical standpoint, however, elimination can be considered as being essentially complete when it has reached 90 percent. Therefore, for practical purposes, *a first-order elimination process can be said to reach completion after 3 to 4 half-lives.*

DRUG ACCUMULATION—LOADING AND MAINTENANCE DOSES With repeated administration of a drug, the amount in the body will accumulate if the elimination of the first dose is incomplete when the second dose is given, and both the amount of drug in the body and its pharmacological effect will increase with continuing administration until they reach a plateau. The accumulation of digoxin administered in repeated maintenance doses (without a loading dose) is illustrated in Fig. 70-2. As digoxin's half-life is about 1.6 days in a patient with normal renal function, 65 percent of digoxin remains in the body at the end of 1 day. Thus, the second dose will raise the amount of digoxin in the body (and average plasma level) to 165 percent of that following the first dose. Each subsequent dose will result in greater amounts in the body until a plateau is attained. At the plateau, or *steady state,* drug intake per unit of time is the same as the rate of drug elimination. For *all* drugs with first-order kinetics, the time required to accumulate to steady-state levels can be predicted from the half-life because accumulation also is a first-order process with a half-life identical to that for elimination. Hence, accumulation will reach 90 percent of steady-state levels at the end of 3 to 4 half-lives. For digoxin, with a half-life of 1.6 days (with normal renal function), accumulation thus will be practically complete in 5 days (Chap. 238). Continuing infusion of the drug at a constant rate also will result in progressive accumulation to a steady state over a time course predictable from the elimination curve for that drug (Fig. 70-3).

When the time required to reach steady-state levels is longer than one wishes to wait, plasma levels may be achieved more rapidly by the administration of a *loading dose.* Loading entails the administration of an amount that will bring the concentration in plasma (at equilibrium) to the level present during steady state. This may be accomplished by the administration of the loading amount as a single dose, or in the case of drugs with low therapeutic indexes (the therapeutic index is the ratio of the toxic dose to the therapeutic dose) the loading amount is given in a series of fractions of the total loading amount. As the accumulation of procainamide to 90 percent of steady state by infusion would require approximately 10 h (3.3 × the half-life of 3 h), a loading regimen is almost always desirable. The load required to suppress an arrhythmia, how-

FIGURE 70-2

The time course of digoxin accumulation when a single daily maintenance dose is given without a loading dose. Note that accumulation is more than 90 percent complete by the end of 4 half-lives.

ever, varies among individuals from 300 to 1000 mg, and rapid intravenous administration of the *average loading dose* would cause hypotension during the high plasma levels in the distribution phase in some patients. Therefore, the intravenous loading dose of procainamide is given in fractions (e.g., 100 mg every 5 min) until the arrhythmia is controlled or adverse effects such as hypotension signal that no further drug should be given. Dividing the loading dose into fractions is appropriate for most drugs that, like procainamide, have a low therapeutic index. This permits better individualization of the loading amount and avoids needless adverse effects that might occur during the distribution phase of a single large dose.

The size of loading dose required to achieve the plasma levels present at steady state can be determined from the fraction of drug eliminated during the dosage interval and the maintenance dose (in the case of intermittent drug administration). For example, if the fraction of digoxin eliminated daily is 35 percent and the planned maintenance dose is to be 0.25 mg daily, then the loading dose to achieve steady-state levels should be 100/35 times the maintenance dose, or approximately 0.75 mg. Thus,

$$\frac{\text{Loading}}{\text{dose}} = \frac{100}{\frac{\% \text{ of drug eliminated}}{\text{per dosage interval}}} \times \text{maintenance dose}$$

The fraction of drug eliminated during any dosage interval can be determined from a semilogarithmic graph, in which the total body dose at time zero is set at 100 percent and the fraction remaining at the end of 1 half-life is 50 percent.[1] Conversely, if the loading dose is known, the maintenance dose can be similarly calculated.

Regardless of the size of the loading dose, *after maintenance*

FIGURE 70-3

The time course of plasma levels of a drug following a single intravenous dose (——) compared with those during a constant intravenous infusion (----). This relationship applies to all drugs that rapidly achieve equilibrium between plasma and tissues.

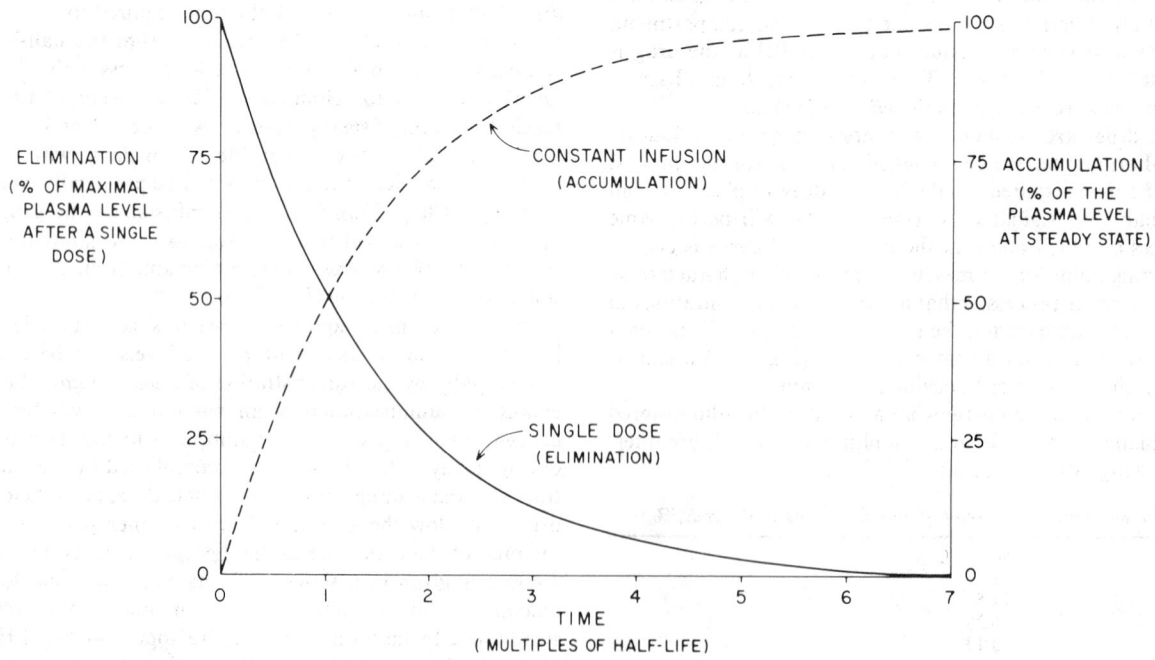

therapy has been given for 3 to 4 half-lives, the amount of drug in the body is determined only by the maintenance dose. The independence of the plasma levels at steady state from the load is illustrated in Fig. 70-3, which indicates that the elimination of any drug given at time 0 (elimination curve) would be practically complete after 3 to 4 half-lives.

DETERMINANTS OF PLASMA LEVELS DURING THE EQUILIBRIUM PHASE An important determinant of the level of drug in plasma during the equilibrium phase after a single dose is the extent to which the drug has distributed outside the plasma compartment. For example, if the distribution of a 3-mg dose of a large macromolecule is confined to a plasma volume of 3 liters, then the concentration in plasma will be 1 mg per liter. However, if a different drug is distributed so that 90 percent of it leaves the plasma compartment, then only 0.3 mg will remain in the 3-liter plasma volume, and the concentration in plasma will be only 0.1 mg per liter. The extent of extravascular distribution at equilibrium can be expressed by the term *apparent volume of distribution,* or V_d. More precisely, V_d expresses the constant relationship between the amount of drug in the body and the plasma concentration at equilibrium:

$$V_d = \frac{\text{amount of drug in body}}{\text{plasma concentration}}$$

The amount of drug in the body is expressed as mass (e.g., milligrams), and the plasma concentration is expressed as mass per volume (e.g., milligrams per liter). Thus V_d is a hypothetical volume into which a quantity of drug would distribute if its concentration in the entire volume were the same as that in plasma. Although it does not represent a real volume, it is an important quantity because it determines the fraction of total drug which is in the plasma and therefore the fraction available to the organs of elimination. An approximation of V_d in the equilibrium phase can be obtained by estimating the concentration of drug in plasma at time zero (C_{p0}) by a back-extrapolation of the equilibrium phase plot to zero time as illustrated in Fig. 70-1. Then, after intravenous administration when the amount in the body at time zero is the dose, we have

$$V_d = \frac{\text{dose}}{C_{p0}}$$

For the administration of the large macromolecule mentioned above, the measured C_{p0} of 1 mg per liter after a 3-mg dose indicates a V_d that is a real volume, the plasma volume. This example is the exception, however, for the V_d of most drugs does not relate to any real volume; many drugs are so extensively taken up by cells that cellular levels greatly exceed those in plasma water. For such drugs, the hypothetical V_d will be large, even greater than the volume of body water. For example, Fig. 70-1 indicates that the C_{p0} obtained by extrapolation following 50 mg lidocaine is 0.42 mg per liter, yielding a V_d by the above equation of 119 liters.

As elimination is carried out largely by individual organs such as the kidney and liver, it is useful to consider the elimination of drugs by these organs according to the *clearance*

concept. For example, in the kidney, regardless of the extent to which removal of drug is determined by filtration, secretion, or reabsorption, the net result is that drug removal results in a reduction of the concentration of drug in plasma as it passes through the organ. The extent to which the concentration is reduced is expressed as the *extraction ratio,* or E.

$$E = \frac{C_a - C_v}{C_a}$$

where C_a = arterial plasma concentration
C_v = venous plasma concentration

If the extraction is complete, $E = 1$. If the total plasma flow to the kidneys is Q (ml/min), the total volume of plasma from which drug is completely removed in a unit time (clearance) is determined as

$$Cl_{renal} = QE$$

If the extraction ratio of penicillin is 0.5 and renal plasma flow is 680 ml/min, then penicillin's renal clearance will be 340 ml/min. If the extraction ratio of a compound is high, as is the case for renal extraction of *p*-aminohippuric acid (PAH) or hepatic extraction of propranolol, then clearance becomes primarily a function of organ blood flow.[2]

Clearance from the total body (Cl) is the sum of clearance from all organs of elimination and is the best measure of the efficiency of the elimination processes. If a drug is removed by both renal excretion and hepatic metabolism, then

$$Cl = Cl_{renal} + Cl_{hepatic}$$

Thus, if penicillin is eliminated by both renal clearance (340 ml/min) and hepatic clearance (36 ml/min) in a normal individual, total clearance will be 376 ml/min. If renal clearance is reduced to half, total clearance = 170 + 36 = 206 ml/min. In anuria, total clearance will equal hepatic clearance.

Only the drug in the vascular compartment can be cleared during each passage through an organ. To ascertain the effect of a given plasma clearance by one or more organs on the rate of removal of drug from the body, the clearance must be related to the volume of "plasma equivalents" to be cleared, that is, the volume of distribution. If the volume of distribution is 10,000 ml and clearance is 1000 ml/min, then one-tenth of the drug in the body is eliminated per minute. This fraction, Cl/V_d, is known as a *fractional elimination constant* and is designated as k:

$$k = \frac{Cl}{V_d}$$

If the fraction k is multiplied by the total amount of drug in the body, the actual rate of elimination at any given time can be determined:

$$\text{Rate of elimination} = k \times \text{amount in body} = ClC_p$$

This is the general equation for all first-order processes and expresses the fact that rate is proportional to the declining quantity in a first-order process.

---

[1] *Alternatively, the fraction of drug lost from the body during a dosage interval can be determined nongraphically from this equation*

$$\text{Fraction of drug lost from body} = 1 - e^{-kT}$$

Values for e^{-kT} can be obtained from a table of natural exponential functions or by a calculator, where k ($= 0.693/T_{1/2}$) is the fractional elimination constant (described in the next section) and T is the time interval after drug administration.

[2] *When drug is present in the formed elements of blood, then calculation of extraction and clearance from blood is more physiologically meaningful than from the plasma.*

As half-life is a temporal expression of the exponential first-order process, half-life ($T_{1/2}$) can be related to k as follows:

$$T_{1/2} = \frac{0.693}{k}$$

Because

$$k = \frac{Cl}{V_d}$$

then

$$T_{1/2} = \frac{0.693 V_d}{Cl}$$

As will be seen in the following discussion on drug dosage in renal failure, the linear relationship of k to creatinine clearance makes k a more useful parameter upon which to base calculations of the changes in drug elimination that occur with a known reduction in creatinine clearance in renal insufficiency. Half-life is not linearly related to clearance.

The important relationship

$$T_{1/2} = 0.693 V_d/Cl$$

expresses clearly that half-life is determined by both clearance and volume of distribution. Thus, for example, half-life is shortened when phenobarbital induces the enzymes responsible for hepatic clearance of a drug, and half-life is lengthened when a drug's renal clearance is attenuated in renal failure. Also, the half-life of some drugs is shortened when their volume of distribution is reduced. If, as in the case of cardiac failure, the volume of distribution is reduced at the same time that clearance is reduced, there may be little change in drug half-life to reflect the impaired clearance, but plasma levels will be increased. In treating patients after an overdose, expectations of how hemodialysis will affect the drug's elimination are dependent on its volume of distribution. When the volume of distribution is very large, as is the case with tricyclic antidepressants (V_d of nortriptyline equals more than 2000 liters), the removal of drug, even with a high-clearance dialyzer, will proceed slowly.

The extent to which a drug is bound to plasma protein also determines the fraction of drug extracted by the organ(s) of elimination. Altered binding will change the extraction ratio significantly, however, only when elimination is limited to the free drug in plasma. The extent to which binding influences elimination depends on the relative affinity of the plasma binding versus the affinity of the drug for the extraction process. The high affinity of the renal tubular anion transport system for many drugs will lead to extraction of both bound and free drug, and the efficient process by which the liver removes propranolol will result in extraction of most of this highly bound drug from blood.

STEADY STATE With a constant infusion of drug, the infusion rate equals elimination rate at steady state. Therefore,

$$\underset{\text{(amt/unit time)}}{\text{Infusion rate}} = \underset{\text{(amt/vol)}}{C_p} \times \underset{\text{(vol/unit time)}}{Cl}$$

when the units for amount, volume, and time are consistent.

Thus, if clearance (Cl) is known, the infusion rate required to achieve a given plasma level can be calculated. An approach to estimating the clearance of a number of drugs is discussed below in the section on renal disease.

When the dose is given intermittently instead of by infusion, the above relationship between plasma concentration and the dose administered at each dosage interval can be expressed as

$$\text{Dose} = C_{p\text{av}} \times Cl \times \text{dosage interval}$$

The average plasma concentration ($C_{p\text{av}}$) implies that, as seen in Fig. 70-2, levels can be considerably higher and lower than the average during the dosage interval.

When a drug is given orally and is not completely absorbed, the calculated dose must be corrected by the fraction (F) of drug that reaches the systemic circulation following oral administration:

$$\frac{\text{Oral}}{\text{dose}} = \frac{C_{p\text{av}} \times Cl \times \text{dosage interval}}{F}$$

DRUG ELIMINATION THAT IS NOT FIRST ORDER The elimination of some important drugs such as phenytoin and salicylate does not follow first-order kinetics when amounts of drug in the body are in the therapeutic range. For these drugs, the clearance is not a constant value but changes as levels in the body fall during elimination or after changes in dose. This pattern of elimination is said to be *dose-dependent*. Accordingly, the time for the concentration to fall to one-half becomes less as plasma levels fall; this halving-time is not truly a half-life, however, because the term *half-life* applies to first-order kinetics and is a constant. The elimination of phenytoin is dose-dependent, and when very high levels are present (in the toxic range), the halving time may be longer than 72 h, whereas after the concentration in plasma has declined to lower levels, the clearance increases and the concentration in plasma will halve in 20 to 30 h.

When drug is eliminated by first-order kinetics, the plasma level at steady state is directly related to the amount of the maintenance dose, and a doubling of the dose should lead to doubling of the steady-state plasma level. However, for phenytoin and other drugs with dose-dependent kinetics, increases in the dose may be accompanied by disproportionately large increases in plasma level. Thus, if the daily dose of phenytoin is increased from 300 to 400 mg, plasma levels rise by considerably more than 33 percent. Unfortunately, the extent of increase is not predictable because of the wide interpatient variability in the extent to which clearance deviates from first order. Salicylates are eliminated by dose-dependent kinetics at high plasma levels, and in children particular caution must be taken with the administration of high doses. Ethanol metabolism also is dose-dependent, with obvious implications. The mechanisms involved in dose-dependent kinetics may include the saturation of the rate-limiting step in metabolism or a feedback inhibition of the rate-limiting enzyme by a product of the reaction.

INDIVIDUALIZATION OF DRUG THERAPY

Recognition of factors modifying drug action is essential for therapy that provides optimal benefit with minimal risk to each individual patient. Certain disease states can modify the delivery of a drug to its site of action.

RENAL DISEASE Where urinary excretion is an important route of elimination, renal failure results in decreased drug clearance and therefore slower removal of the drug from the body, so that administration according to the usual dosage regimen leads to greater accumulation and an increased likelihood of toxicity. A reasonable therapeutic goal in such cases is to modify the dosage schedule so that the average drug concentration in the plasma of the patient with renal insufficiency is the same, and steady state is reached after a similar time interval, as in the patient with normal renal function.

One approach to dosage alteration in renal insufficiency is to calculate the *fraction of the normal dose* that is to be given at the usual dosage interval. This fraction can be determined from data on either drug clearance (Cl) or the fractional rate

TABLE 70-1
Clearance of drugs

Drug	Renal clearance,* ml/min	Nonrenal clearance, ml/min
Ampicillin†	340	12
Carbenicillin	68	10
Digoxin†	110	36
Gentamicin	78	3
Kanamycin	60	0
Penicillin G‡	340	36

* The "normal" renal clearances are those associated with a clearance of creatinine of 100 ml/min.
† The fraction of digoxin absorbed after an oral dose (F) is approximately 0.6 and F for ampicillin is 0.5.
‡ One microgram of penicillin G = 1.6 units.

constant (k), based on the fact that both renal clearance and renal k are directly proportional to creatinine clearance (Cl_{cr}). Thus, the dose in renal insufficiency ($dose_{ri}$) is

$$Dose_{ri} = dose \times \frac{Cl_{ri}}{Cl}$$

where ri = renal insufficiency
 Cl = clearance from the whole body with normal renal function
 Cl_{ri} = clearance from the whole body with renal insufficiency
 Dose = maintenance dose with normal renal function ($Cl_{cr} \approx 100$ ml/min)

The normal clearance and that in renal impairment can be obtained by employing the data in Table 70-1 in the following equations:

$$Cl = Cl_{renal} + Cl_{nonrenal}$$

$$Cl_{ri} = Cl_{renal} \times \frac{measured\ Cl_{cr}}{100\ ml/min} + Cl_{nonrenal}$$

As the Cl_{renal} values in Table 70-1 are those found with

FIGURE 70-4

Nomogram for estimation of the dose fraction (k_{ri}/k) in patients with renal insufficiency. The application of the nomogram is described in the text.

TABLE 70-2
Estimated fraction of usual dose of drug required for a patient with a creatinine clearance of zero (dose fraction$_0$) and average overall fractional elimination rate constant for a patient with normal renal function (k)

Drug	Dose fraction$_0$	k, per hour
ANTIBIOTICS		
Amikacin	0.01	0.4
Amoxicillin	0.15	0.7
Ampicillin	0.1	0.6
Carbenicillin	0.1	0.6
Cephalexin	0.04	0.7
Cephaloridine	0.08	0.4
Cephalothin	0.02	1.4
Cephazolin	0.06	0.35
Chloramphenicol	0.8	0.3
Clindamycin	0.8	0.2
Cloxacillin	0.25	1.2
Colistimethate	0.3	0.2
Dicloxacillin	0.5	1.2
Doxycycline	0.8	0.03
Erythromycin	0.7	0.5
Gentamicin	0.02	0.3
Isoniazid:		
Fast inactivators	0.8	0.5
Slow inactivators	0.5	0.25
Kanamycin	0.03	0.35
Lincomycin	0.4	0.15
Methicillin	0.12	1.4
Minocycline	0.9	0.06
Nafcillin	0.4	1.2
Oxacillin	0.25	1.4
Oxytetracycline	0.2	0.08
Penicillin G	0.1	1.4
Polymyxin B	0.12	0.15
Rifampin	1.0	0.25
Streptomycin	0.04	0.25
Sulfadiazine	0.45	0.7
Sulfamethoxazole	0.85	0.07
Tetracycline	0.12	0.08
Tobramycin	0.02	0.35
Tricarcillin	0.1	0.6
Trimethoprim	0.45	0.06
Vancomycin	0.03	0.12
MISCELLANEOUS DRUGS		
Chlorpropamide	0.4	0.02
Lidocaine	0.9	0.4
Sulfinpyrazone	0.55	0.3
CARDIAC GLYCOSIDES		k, per day
Digitoxin	0.7	0.1
Digoxin	0.3	0.45

$Cl_{cr} = 100$ ml/min, then the renal clearance of drug in renal insufficiency is obtained by multiplying Cl_{renal} by the ratio of measured Cl_{cr} (in milliliters per minute) to 100 ml/min.

For gentamicin, with a normal Cl_{renal} of 78 ml/min and $Cl_{nonrenal}$ of 3 ml/min, Cl = 81 ml/min. Therefore, with a Cl_{cr} of 12 ml/min, $Cl_{ri} = 78 \times (12/100) + 3 = 12.4$ ml/min. If the dose of gentamicin for a given infection should be 1.5 mg/kg per 8 h in the presence of normal renal function, then

$$Dose_{ri} = \frac{1.5\ mg/kg}{8\ h} \times \frac{12.4\ ml/min}{81\ ml/min} = \frac{0.23\ mg/kg}{8\ h}$$

In the patient with renal insufficiency, this computation will yield an average plasma level during a dosage interval that is the same as the average plasma level during the dosage interval with normal renal function; the fluctuations between peaks and troughs, however, will be less pronounced.

All calculation of dosage is most accurately based on the clearance of a drug, because this is a direct measure of the efficiency of drug removal. However, clearance data are not available for some drugs, in which case [if it is assumed that renal disease does not affect the distribution of the drug (V_d)], the dosage fraction can be approximated from the ratio of the fractional rate constant for elimination from the total body in renal failure (k_{ri}) to that with normal renal function (k). The approach is the same as that employed with clearance data:

$$\text{Dose}_{ri} = \text{dose} \times \frac{k_{ri}}{k}$$

As the ratio k_{ri}/k is the fraction of the usual dose employed in a given degree of renal insufficiency, it is termed the *dose fraction* and may be readily estimated from the information in Table 70-2 and the nomogram (Fig. 70-4). Table 70-2 gives the fraction of the usual dose of a drug required at a creatinine clearance of zero (dose fraction$_0$). The nomogram presents the dose fraction as a linear function of creatinine clearance.

To calculate the dose fraction$_{ri}$, the dose fraction$_0$ is obtained from Table 70-2, plotted on the left ordinate of the nomogram, and connected by a straight line to the upper right hand corner of the nomogram. This line describes the dose fraction over a range of creatinine clearances from 0 to 100 ml/min. The point of intersection between the patient's measured creatinine clearance (on the lower abscissa) with this dose fraction line is a coordinate with the dose fraction (on the left ordinate) corresponding with that particular creatinine clearance. For example, if a patient with a creatinine clearance of 20 ml/min requires penicillin G for an infection that would be treated with 10 million units daily in patients with normal renal function, then an appropriate dose would be 2.8 million units daily. This estimated dose is obtained by plotting the dose fraction$_0$ for penicillin G (0.1) on the left-hand ordinate and connecting it to the top right-hand corner of the nomogram (Fig. 70-4). On this dose fraction line for penicillin G, the coordinate for a creatinine clearance of 20 ml/min corresponds on the left ordinate with a dose fraction of 0.28. Hence, the dose is 0.28×10 million units daily.

In some instances it may be desirable to calculate a dose that will yield a certain plasma level at steady state. This approach is most appropriate for constant intravenous infusions where 100 percent of the dose is delivered to the systemic circulation. When clearance of a drug in a patient with renal insufficiency is calculated as above, then

$$\begin{array}{ccc} \text{Dose}_{ri} & = & \text{Cl}_{ri} & \times & C_p \\ \text{(amt/unit time)} & & \text{(vol/unit time)} & & \text{(amt/vol)} \end{array}$$

where the time, amount, and volume terms are uniform.

If a plasma concentration of carbenicillin of 100 μg/ml is the therapeutic objective in a patient with a creatinine clearance of 25 ml/min, the infusion rate is calculated as follows. Carbenicillin clearance is

$$\text{Cl}_{ri} = 68 \times \frac{25}{100} + 10 = 27 \text{ ml/min}$$

Therefore, carbenicillin should be infused at a rate of 2700 μg/min.

Should the method of calculating dose based on the desired plasma level be applied to intermittent-dose therapy, particular attention should be given to the fact that the calculation is based on an *average* plasma level and that peak plasma levels will obviously be higher. In addition, if a drug is given orally and is not completely absorbed, the computed dose must be divided by the fraction of drug which reaches the systemic circulation following oral administration (F) (see "Steady State" above).

In all the above calculations, it is assumed that the nonrenal clearance and nonrenal k are constant in renal failure. In fact,

when cardiac failure accompanies renal failure, metabolic clearance for many drugs is reduced. Accordingly, when a drug with a narrow therapeutic index, such as digoxin, is used in cardiac failure, an appropriate precaution would be to reduce the value for nonrenal clearance (or k) to about one-half.

In addition to adjusting the maintenance dose in patients with renal failure, consideration must also be given to the necessity of a loading dose. Since this dose is designed to bring the plasma concentration, or more particularly the amount of drug in the body, rapidly to the level that is reached at steady state, there is no need to modify the usual loading dose, if one is normally used. For many drugs, however, their elimination is sufficiently rapid that the time required to reach steady state is not clinically significant and no loading dose is usually used. On the other hand, in renal failure where the half-life may be significantly prolonged, this accumulation period may become unacceptably long. In such a case, for a drug given intermittently, a loading dose may be calculated as described in "Drug Accumulation" above. For an infusion, the loading dose may be approximated (when all units are consistent)

$$\text{Loading dose}_{ri} = \frac{\text{infusion rate}_{ri}}{k_{ri}}$$

Because of the considerable individual differences in volumes of distribution and rates of metabolism, the above calculations of drug dose for patients in renal failure must be viewed as valuable approximations which prevent the use of doses that are grossly excessive or inadequate for most patients. However, *maintenance dosages are most accurate when plasma level data are employed as a feedback to enable adjustment of the dose where necessary.*

Active or toxic metabolites of drugs also may accumulate in renal failure. Meperidine, for example, is cleared largely by metabolism, and its concentration in plasma is little altered by renal insufficiency. However, the plasma concentration of one of its metabolites, normeperidine, is substantially increased when its renal elimination is impaired. As normeperidine has more convulsant activity than meperidine, its accumulation in patients with renal failure probably accounts for the signs of central nervous system excitation such as irritability, twitching, and seizures that result from the administration of multiple doses of meperidine to patients in renal insufficiency.

The metabolite of procainamide, N-acetylprocainamide, has cardiac effects that are similar to those of the parent drug. As N-acetylprocainamide is eliminated almost entirely by the kidney, its concentration in plasma is increased by renal failure. Thus, the potential of procainamide to produce toxicity in patients with renal insufficiency cannot be assessed by measuring the plasma concentration of procainamide alone.

LIVER DISEASE In contrast to the predictable decline in renal clearance of drugs when glomerular filtration is reduced, it is not possible to make a general prediction of the effect of liver disease on hepatic biotransformation of drugs (Chap. 298). Rather, in hepatitis and cirrhosis there is a spectrum of changes ranging from impaired to increased drug clearance. Even when there is advanced hepatocellular disease, the magnitude of impairment in drug clearance usually is only about two- to fivefold. The extent of such changes, however, cannot be predicted by any of the commonly available tests of liver function. Consequently, even though it may be suspected that drug elimination is altered in a patient with liver disease, there is no quantitative base upon which to adjust the dosage regimen.

Portacaval shunting creates a special situation because the effective hepatic blood flow is substantially reduced. This situation has its greatest effect on drugs that normally have a high hepatic extraction ratio so that their clearance is largely a function of blood flow; thus the clearance of such drugs (e.g., propranolol and lidocaine) will be remarkably reduced by portacaval shunting. In addition, the fraction of an administered oral dose reaching the systemic circulation will be significantly increased, because drug that is shunted around the liver during the absorption process will escape the efficient first-pass metabolism by this organ.

CIRCULATORY INSUFFICIENCY—CARDIAC FAILURE AND SHOCK Under conditions leading to decreased tissue perfusion, redistribution of the cardiac output occurs to preserve blood flow to the heart and brain at the expense of other tissues (Chap. 30). As a result, the drug is distributed into a smaller volume of distribution, higher drug concentrations are present in the plasma, and the vital organs are exposed to these higher concentrations. If either the brain or heart is sensitive to the pharmacological effect of the drug, an alteration in response will occur.

Furthermore, the decreased perfusion of the kidney and liver may impair drug clearance by these organs either directly or indirectly. Thus, in severe congestive heart failure, in hemorrhagic shock, and particularly in cardiogenic shock, the response to the usual dose of the drug may be excessive, and dosage modification may be necessary. For example, the clearance of lidocaine is reduced by about 50 percent in cardiac failure, and consequently therapeutic plasma levels are achieved at infusion rates of only about half of those usually required. In cardiac failure there also is a significant reduction in lidocaine's volume of distribution which results in the requirement of a smaller loading dose. Similar situations are thought to exist for procainamide, theophylline, and possibly quinidine. Unfortunately, predictors of these types of pharmacokinetic alterations are unavailable. Therefore, loading doses should be conservative, and continued therapy should be monitored closely, following clinical indicators of toxicity and plasma levels.

DISEASE-INDUCED CHANGES IN PLASMA BINDING Many drugs circulate in the plasma partly bound to the plasma proteins and other constituents. Since only the unbound or free drug can distribute to the site of pharmacological action, the therapeutic response should be related to the free rather than the total circulating plasma drug concentration. In most cases the degree of binding is fairly constant across the therapeutic concentration range so that significant error is not caused by individualizing therapy on the basis of measuring levels of total drug in plasma. However, several clinical states such as hypoalbuminemia, liver disease, and renal disease can decrease the extent of drug binding so that at any total plasma level there is a greater concentration of free drug and a risk of increased response and toxicity. The drugs for which such changes are important are those which are normally highly bound in the plasma ($>$ 90 percent) because a small alteration in the extent of binding produces a large relative increase in the fraction of drug in the unbound form.

The binding of phenytoin is altered in patients with chronic renal failure by several mechanisms; the percentage of unbound drug increases about fourfold from a normal of approximately 7 percent to as high as 25 to 30 percent. Similar, but less pronounced, changes are also seen in patients with viral hepatitis, jaundice, and the nephrotic syndrome, and with other drugs such as diazoxide, digitoxin, clofibrate, and certain sulfonamides.

The pharmacokinetic consequences of these binding changes, particularly with respect to total drug levels, depend on whether the clearance and distribution are dependent on the unbound or total drug. For many drugs, including those cited above, elimination and distribution are largely restricted to the free fraction, and therefore a decrease in binding leads

to an increase in the clearance and distribution of the total drug. The relative magnitudes of these changes are such that the net effect is to shorten the half-life. For example, in uremia the half-life of phenytoin may be as low as 6 to 8 h compared with a normal value of about 20 to 30 h. However, the clearance of *free* drug is unaffected, and the average steady-state plasma concentration of unbound drug is unaltered. Accordingly, the appropriate modification of the dosage regimen in clinical conditions with reduced drug binding is simply to administer the usual daily dose of the drug, but in divided doses at more frequent intervals. Individualization of therapy can then be based on either the clinical response or the plasma concentration of unbound drug. It is critical that the patient not be titrated into the usual therapeutic range for concentration of *total* drug in plasma since this will inevitably lead to supraeffective response and toxicity.

INTERACTIONS BETWEEN DRUGS

The effect of some drugs can be altered markedly by the administration of other agents. Such interactions can sabotage therapeutic intent by producing excessive drug action (with adverse effects) or decreasing the action of a drug, rendering it ineffective. Drug interactions must be considered in the differential diagnosis of unexpected responses to drugs, taking into account that ambulatory patients often come to the physician with a legacy of drugs acquired during their previous medical experiences. A meticulous drug history will minimize the unknown elements in the patient's therapeutic milieu; it should include examination of the patient's medications and calls to the pharmacist to identify prescriptions, if necessary.

There are two principal types of interactions between drugs. *Pharmacokinetic interactions* result from alteration in the delivery of drugs to their sites of action. *Pharmacodynamic interactions* are those in which the responsiveness of the target organ or system has been modified by other agents.

An index of the drug interactions discussed in this chapter is provided in Table 70-3. Included are a selected group of interactions which have verified significance in patients and a few which are of such potential danger to the patient that cognizance should be taken of experimental data or case reports suggesting their likely occurrence.

I PHARMACOKINETIC INTERACTIONS CAUSING DIMINISHED DRUG DELIVERY

A Impaired gastrointestinal absorption Aluminum ions, present in antacids, form insoluble chelates with the tetracyclines, thereby preventing absorption of these drugs. Ferrous ions similarly block tetracycline absorption. Cholestyramine, an ionic exchange resin, binds thyroxine, triiodothyronine, and the cardiac glycosides with sufficiently high affinity to impair their absorption from the gastrointestinal tract. This resin probably also interferes with the absorption of other drugs, and it is safest not to give it within 2 h of their administration. Oral administration of *p*-aminosalicylate interferes with the absorption of rifampin by a mechanism not yet determined.

All the above instances of impaired absorption result in a reduction in the total amount of drug absorption, with reduced area under the plasma level curve and reduced peak plasma levels, as well as lower steady-state concentrations of the drug involved.

B Induction of hepatic drug-metabolizing enzymes When the elimination of the drug proceeds largely via biotransformation, an increase in the rate at which it is metabolized reduces its availability to sites of action. The biotransformation of most drugs occurs largely in the liver, because of its mass, high blood flow, and concentration of enzymes that metabolize drugs. The initial step in metabolism of many drugs is executed by the mixed-function oxidase enzymes located in the hepatic endoplasmic reticulum. These enzyme systems containing cytochrome P_{450} oxidize the molecule by a variety of reactions including aromatic hydroxylations, N-demethylations, O-demethylations, and sulfoxidations. The products of these reactions are usually more polar (and more readily excreted by the kidney).

The number of mixed-function oxidase enzyme units in the liver can be increased by treatment with enzyme inducers, of which phenobarbital is the prototype. Almost all the barbiturates in clinical use increase the mixed-function oxidase enzymes. Induction with phenobarbital can occur with doses of as little as 60 mg daily. Mixed-function oxidases are also induced by glutethimide, phenytoin, and rifampin, and by occupational exposure to chlorinated insecticides such as DDT, as well as by alcohol.

The actions of a number of drugs are inhibited by treatment with inducing agents. Phenobarbital and other inducers lower plasma levels of warfarin, bishydroxycoumarin, digitoxin, quinidine, dexamethasone, and metyrapone. These interactions all

have obvious clinical significance. With the coumarin anticoagulants, the major risk occurs when an appropriate level of anticoagulation is achieved while the coumarin drug is coadministered with an inducing agent. When the inducer is discontinued, e.g., following discharge from the hospital, plasma levels of the coumarin anticoagulant will rise as the induction effect wears off, leading to excessive anticoagulation. Barbiturates have been shown to lower the plasma levels of phenytoin in some patients, but the clinical effect of reduced phenytoin levels is probably counter-balanced by the anticonvulsant effects of phenobarbital.

There is considerable variation among individuals in the extent to which drug metabolism can be induced. In some patients phenobarbital leads to marked acceleration in the rate of drug metabolism, whereas little induction is seen in others. This variability in the extent of induction of mixed-function oxidases is largely genetically determined.

In addition to inducing the mixed-function oxidase enzymes, phenobarbital has a number of other effects on hepatic function. It increases liver blood flow, bile flow, and the hepatocellular transport of organic anions. The conjugation of drugs and bilirubin is also enhanced by inducing agents.

C Inhibition of cellular uptake or binding The guanidinium antihypertensives, guanethidine and bethanidine, are transported to their site of action in adrenergic neurons by an energy-requiring membrane transport system for biogenic monoamines. Although the physiological function of the transport system is re-uptake of the adrenergic neurotransmitter, it also transports a variety of ring-substituted bases, including guanethidine and bethanidine, into the adrenergic neuron against a concentration gradient. Inhibitors of norepinephrine uptake will prevent the uptake of the guanidinium antihypertensives into adrenergic neurons and will thereby block their pharmacological effects. The tricyclic antidepressants are potent inhibitors of norepinephrine uptake. Consequently, concomitant administration of clinical doses of tricyclic antidepressants including desipramine, protriptyline, nortriptyline, and amitriptyline will almost totally abolish the antihypertensive effects of guanethidine and bethanidine. Although they are less potent inhibitors of norepinephrine uptake, doxepin and chlorpromazine, when given in doses of greater than 100 mg daily, produce dose-related antagonism of the action of the guanidinium antihypertensives. In patients with severe hypertension, the loss of control of blood pressure resulting from these drug interactions can lead to serious clinical complications such as stroke and malignant hypertension.

Amphetamine also antagonizes the antihypertensive effect of guanethidine by displacing it from its site of action within the adrenergic neuron (Chap. 251). Ephedrine, a component of many drug combinations used in asthma, also antagonizes the effect of guanethidine, probably by both inhibition of uptake and displacement from the neuron.

The antihypertensive effect of clonidine in humans is partially antagonized by the tricyclic antidepressants. Clonidine lowers arterial pressure by reducing sympathetic outflow from the blood-pressure-regulating centers in the hindbrain (Chap. 251). This central hypotensive action is antagonized by the tricyclic antidepressants.

II PHARMACOKINETIC INTERACTIONS CAUSING INCREASED DRUG DELIVERY

A Inhibition of drug metabolism If the active form of a drug is cleared largely by biotransformation, inhibition of its metabolism will lead to a prolonged half-life and to accumulation of the drug during maintenance therapy. Excessive accumulation due to inhibited metabolism leads to significant adverse effects in the case of several drugs.

TABLE 70-3
Drug interaction index

Drug	Section of chapter describing interaction
Acetohexamide	IIB
Allopurinol	IIA
p-Aminosalicylate	IA
Amphetamine	IC, III
Antidepressants, tricyclic (desipramine, nortriptyline, imipramine, doxepin, protriptyline, amitriptyline)	IC
Aspirin	IIB, III
Azathioprine	IIA
Barbiturates (class)	IB
Bethanidine	IC
Bishydroxycoumarin	IB, IIA, IIB
Chloral hydrate	IIC
Chloramphenicol	IIA, III
Chlorpromazine	IC
Cholestyramine	IA
Clofibrate	IIA
Clonidine	IC
Cyclophosphamide	IIA
Dexamethasone	IB
Digitoxin	IB
Diphenylhydantoin (see phenytoin below)	
Disulfiram	IIA
Ephedrine	IC, III
Ethanol	IIA
Furazolidone	III
Guanethidine	IC
Isoniazid	IIA
6-Mercaptopurine	IIA
Methotrexate	IIB
Metyrapone	IB
Monoamine oxidase inhibitors	III
Pargyline	III
Phenobarbital	IB
Phenylbutazone	IIA, IIB
Phenylpropanolamine	III
Phenytoin (diphenylhydantoin)	IB, IIA
Potassium	III
Quinidine	IB
Rifampin	IA, IB
Spironolactone	III
Tetracycline	IA, III
Tolbutamide	IIA
Triamterene	III
Warfarin	IB, IIA, IIC, III

The metabolism of phenytoin is inhibited by a number of drugs. Clofibrate, phenylbutazone, chloramphenicol, disulfiram, bishydroxycoumarin, and isoniazid can raise the steady-state plasma levels of phenytoin by more than two-fold. In the case of isoniazid, the extent of inhibition of phenytoin metabolism is a function of the genetically determined rate of isoniazid acetylation; substantial inhibition of phenytoin metabolism and resultant clinical toxicity are seen only in those individuals who are slow acetylators. Inhibited metabolism may lead to abrupt development of symptoms such as somnolence, mental confusion, and disturbance of gait in patients who have not changed their phenytoin dosage.

Impaired metabolism of tolbutamide with severe hypoglycemia has resulted from coadministration of clofibrate, phenylbutazone, chloramphenicol, and bishydroxycoumarin. Excessive anticoagulation by warfarin may result from inhibition of its metabolism by disulfiram or phenylbutazone, or by concurrent and copious ingestion of ethanol. Warfarin is administered as a racemic mixture, and its $S(-)$ isomer has five times the anticoagulant potency of the $R(+)$ isomer. Phenylbutazone selectively inhibits the metabolism of the $S(-)$ isomer, and only when this isomer is examined specifically can the substantial reduction in its metabolism produced by phenylbutazone be unmasked.

Azathioprine is readily converted in the body to an active metabolite, 6-mercaptopurine, which in turn is inactivated in part by xanthine oxidase which sequentially oxidizes it to 6-thiouric acid. When allopurinol, a potent inhibitor of xanthine oxidase, is administered concurrently with standard doses of azathioprine or 6-mercaptopurine, life-threatening toxicity (bone marrow suppression) can result. Therefore, it has been recommended that the doses of azathioprine and 6-mercaptopurine be reduced to one-third or one-fourth the usual amounts when allopurinol is given at the same time. These are rough approximations of the dose modifications, and the quantitative aspects of this interaction have not been determined.

B Inhibition of renal secretion

A number of drugs are secreted by the renal tubular transport systems for organic ions. Inhibition of this tubular transport system can cause excessive accumulation of a drug when this is the major pathway of its elimination. Several drugs, including phenylbutazone, probenecid, salicylates, and bishydroxycoumarin, will competitively inhibit this transport system. Patients receiving the oral antidiabetic acetohexamide have developed profound hypoglycemia when phenylbutazone was added to their drug regimen. This exaggerated hypoglycemia resulted from the inhibition by phenylbutazone of the tubular secretion of hydroxyacetohexamide, an active metabolite which is responsible for most of the hypoglycemic effect that ensues from acetohexamide administration. Renal tubular secretion contributes substantially to the elimination of penicillin, which can be inhibited by probenecid.

C Inhibition of plasma protein binding

When the binding of a drug to plasma protein is reduced by another agent, more unbound drug will be made available to receptor sites for any given level of total drug. Reduction in the binding of a drug does not have significance in vivo unless the drug is very highly bound (more than 90 percent) and the volume of distribution is small. A drug may alter the binding of another by competitive displacement or by an interaction with protein (usually albumin) to decrease binding affinity. Reduction in the extent of binding also will make more drug available to the organs of clearance, and if the drug normally has a low extraction ratio because binding sequesters the drug in plasma, then reduction of binding will increase its clearance. As a result, following a binding displacement interaction, total and free-drug levels at steady state will fall until free-drug concentration returns to the previous levels; at steady state, the average unbound warfarin levels should be independent of the degree of binding. Therefore, in most instances, any enhancement of the pharmacological effect will be transient.

Although reduction of the binding of many drugs by others has been demonstrated in vitro, the only instance where clinical significance has clearly been linked to reduced binding is the potentiation of the anticoagulant effect of warfarin by chloral hydrate in high dosage. Chloral hydrate is converted in the body to trichloroacetic acid, which displaces warfarin from albumin-binding sites. As a result there is a transient increase in the anticoagulant effect of warfarin, persisting for only a few days until the concentration of free warfarin returns to previous levels.

III PHARMACODYNAMIC AND OTHER INTERACTIONS BETWEEN DRUGS

Therapeutically useful interactions in which the combined effect of two drugs is greater than that of either drug alone are numerous. These favorable drug combinations are covered extensively in specific therapeutic sections in this text, and the following is directed toward those pharmacodynamic interactions that create unwanted effects. Two drugs may act on separate components of a common process and yield effects greater than either drug alone. For example, small doses of aspirin (less than 1 g daily) will not alter the prothrombin time appreciably in patients who are stabilized on warfarin therapy. However, the addition of aspirin to patients therapeutically anticoagulated with warfarin increases the risk of bleeding because aspirin inhibits platelet aggregation. Thus the combination of impaired functions of both the platelets and the fluid-phase clotting system increases the potential for hemorrhagic complications in patients receiving warfarin therapy.

The administration of supplemental potassium leads to more frequent and more severe hyperkalemia when potassium elimination is reduced by concurrent treatment with spironolactone or triamterene.

Occasionally, the addition of bacteriostatic antibiotics such as the tetracyclines and chloramphenicol to bactericidal agents (e.g., penicillin) may impair the cure of infections. In vitro, the combination of bacteriostatic and bactericidal agents yields a combined effect resembling that of the bacteriostatic agent alone. This may have clinical significance in meningitis, and, on the basis of studies in experimental animals, it is suggested that when bactericidal drugs need to be used, the administration of the static drug be delayed 1 h after initiating the bactericidal agent.

VARIABLE ACTIONS OF DRUGS CAUSED BY GENETIC DIFFERENCES IN THEIR METABOLISM

ACETYLATION Isoniazid, hydralazine, procainamide, and a number of other drugs are metabolized by acetylation of a hydrazino or amino group. This reaction is catalyzed by *N*-acetyl transferase, a nonmicrosomal (soluble) enzyme in the liver that transfers an acetyl group from acetyl coenzyme A to the drug. Individuals differ markedly in the rate at which drugs are acetylated, and there is a bimodal distribution of the population into "rapid acetylators" and "slow acetylators." The rate of acetylation is under genetic control; rapid acetylation is an autosomal dominant trait.

The toxic, sometimes fatal, hepatitis that occurs in about 1 percent of patients on isoniazid occurs predominantly in rapid acetylators. The greater hepatotoxicity in rapid acetylators appears to result from the synthesis of more acetylisoniazid which is further metabolized to acetylhydrazine, a potent hepatotoxin. Acetylhydrazine exerts its toxic effect through an active metabolite that binds covalently to macromolecules in the hepatic cells that produce it. Conversely, the lupus erythematosus-like syndrome produced by hydralazine (Chap. 251) occurs only in individuals who are slow acetylators.

Because these important toxic drug effects are largely predictable from the acetylation phenotype, it may in certain instances be of value to determine the rate of acetylation in patients who are to receive isoniazid, or those who would benefit from doses of hydralazine above the 200 mg per day dose that can be safely employed in the population at large. Acetylation phenotype can be determined by measuring the ratio of acetylated to nonacetylated dapsone or sulfamethazine in plasma or urine following administration of a test dose of these acetylation substrates. The ratio of monoacetyldapsone to dapsone in plasma at 6 h after dapsone administration is less than 0.35 for slow acetylators and greater than 0.35 for rapid acetylators. At 6 h following the administration of sulfamethazine, less than 25 percent of the drug in the plasma is in the acetylated form in slow acetylators (rapid acetylators, more than 25 percent); in the urine collected in the 5- to 6-h interval after administration, less than 70 percent of the drug is in the acetylated form in slow acetylators (rapid acetylators, more than 70 percent).

METABOLISM BY MIXED-FUNCTION OXIDASES In healthy individuals taking no other medications, the major determinant of the rate of metabolism of drugs by the hepatic mixed-function oxidases is genetic. In contrast to the bimodal distribution of individuals with respect to acetylation rates, there is a unimodal distribution for most drugs metabolized by enzymes of the hepatic endoplasmic reticulum, indicating control by multiple genes. The genetically controlled variation in hepatic clearance is marked for some of these drugs. Steady-state plasma levels of nortriptyline, propranolol, and chlorpromazine vary by more than tenfold among individuals. This has obvious consequences in attempting to predict effect from a given dose in those individuals who differ markedly from the average.

CONCENTRATION OF DRUGS IN PLASMA AS A GUIDE TO THERAPY

Optimal individualization of therapy is assisted by measuring the concentration of certain drugs in plasma. Genetic variation in elimination rates, interactions with other drugs, disease-induced alterations in elimination and distribution, and other factors combine to yield a wide range of plasma levels in patients given the same dose. Furthermore, the problem of noncompliance with prescribed regimens during continuing therapy is an endemic and elusive cause of therapeutic failure. There are clinical indicators that assist the titration of some drugs into the desired range, and no chemical determination is a substitute for careful observations of the patient's response to treatment. However, the therapeutic and adverse effects are not precisely quantifiable for all drugs, and in complex clinical situations estimates of the action of a drug may be misleading. For example, previously existing neurological disease may obscure the neurological consequences of intoxication with phenytoin. Because clearance, half-life, accumulation, and steady-state plasma levels are difficult to predict, the measurement of plasma levels is often useful as a guide to the optimal dose. This is particularly so when there is a narrow range between the plasma levels yielding therapeutic and adverse effects. The concept of the average dose will not benefit the patient whose levels are inadequate for therapeutic effect or in the toxic range. Adjustment of dosage based on creatinine clearance in

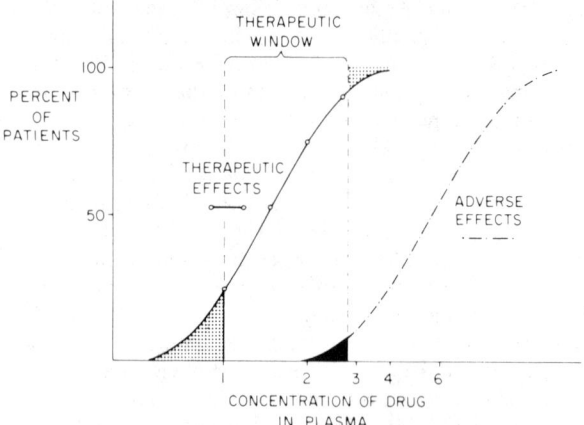

FIGURE 70-5

The cumulative percentage of patients responding to increasing levels of drug in plasma with both therapeutic and adverse effects. The therapeutic "window" defines the range of concentrations of drug that will achieve therapeutic effects in most patients with adverse effects in only a small percentage.

renal insufficiency will minimize gross over- and undertreatment, but still it is a calculation based on an average and will not yield ideal treatment for all patients.

Data on concentrations of drugs in plasma are utilized most effectively in the framework of the known kinetics of the drug, including consideration of whether the levels are likely to reflect the steady state, whether they represent the equilibrium phase (cf., the distribution phase discussed above), and the extent to which disease-induced changes in the drug binding can influence the concentration of total (bound plus unbound) drug. In addition, the variability among individual responses to given plasma levels must be recognized. This is illustrated by a hypothetical population dose-response curve (Fig. 70-5) and its relationship to the therapeutic range or therapeutic "window" of desired plasma levels. The defined therapeutic window should include the levels at which the majority of patients will achieve the intended pharmacological effect. However, there are a few people who are quite sensitive to the therapeutic effects of most drugs, responding to lower levels, whereas others are sufficiently refractory as to require levels that impose an increased likelihood of adverse effects as a potential price for therapeutic benefit. For example, a few pa-

TABLE 70-4
Concentrations of drugs in plasma: relation to efficacy and adverse effects

Drug	Efficacy*	Adverse effects†
Carbenicillin	100 µg/ml‡	300 µg/ml
Digitoxin	12 ng/ml	25–30 ng/ml
Digoxin	0.8 ng/ml	2.0 ng/ml
Gentamicin	4 µg/ml§	12 µg/ml
Lithium	0.5 meq/liter	1.3 meq/liter
Penicillin G	1–25 µg/ml¶	
Phenytoin (diphenylhydantoin)	10 µg/ml	20 µg/ml
Procainamide	4 µg/ml	8 µg/ml
Quinidine	3 µg/ml	7 µg/ml
Theophylline	8 µg/ml	20 µg/ml

* *The therapeutic effect is infrequent or slight at levels below these.*
† *The frequency of adverse effects increases sharply when these levels are exceeded.*
‡ *Minimal inhibitory concentration (MIC) for most strains of Pseudomonas aeruginosa. MIC for other, more sensitive, organisms is less.*
§ *Dependent on the MIC. Higher levels (up to 8 µg/ml) may be desired when host defenses are impaired.*
¶ *There is a wide range of MIC of penicillin for various organisms, and the MIC of all those for which penicillin is used is < 20. "Massive" penicillin therapy with 20 million units daily achieves levels of 20 to 25 µg/ml in patients with clearance of creatinine of 100 ml/min.*

tients with strong seizure foci will require plasma levels of phenytoin exceeding 20 μg/ml in order to control their seizure disorders. Increments in dosage to achieve this effect may be appropriate. However, with an elevation in dose that yields levels at which adverse effects become more frequent, one must exercise heightened sensitivity for subtle changes in higher integrative function. In addition, because phenytoin has dose-dependent kinetics, it is essential to monitor carefully the possibly large variations of plasma levels that can accompany small increases in the dosage as levels exceed 20 μg/ml.

As also illustrated in Fig. 70-5, some patients may be prone to adverse effects at levels which are well tolerated by most of the population, and therefore elevation of levels to those achieving a high probability of therapeutic effect may bring on unwanted actions in the exceptional patient.

Table 70-4 presents for a number of drugs the concentrations in plasma that are associated with probable adverse and therapeutic effects in most patients. Its use within the guidelines discussed should permit more effective and safer therapy for those patients who are not "average."

REFERENCES

DETTLI L: Elimination kinetics and dosage adjustment of drugs in patients with kidney disease. Prog Pharmacol, vol 1, no 4, 1977

SHAND DG et al: Pharmacokinetic drug interactions, in *Handbook of Experimental Pharmacology,* vol 28: *Concepts in Biochemical Pharmacology,* JR Gillette, JR Mitchell (eds). New York, Springer-Verlag, 1975, p 272

SHEINER LB, TOZER TN: Clinical pharmacokinetics: The use of plasma concentrations of drugs, in *Clinical Pharmacology: Basic Principles in Therapeutics,* 2d ed. New York, Macmillan, 1978, p 71

WILKINSON GR, SHAND DG: A physiological approach to hepatic drug clearance. Clin Pharmacol Ther 18:377, 1975

71
ADVERSE REACTIONS TO DRUGS

ALASTAIR J. J. WOOD
JOHN A. OATES

The beneficial effects of drugs are coupled with the inescapable risk that they may also cause untoward effects. The morbidity and mortality that result from these untoward effects often present diagnostic problems, for these drugs can involve every organ and system of the body.

Major advances in the investigation, development, and regulation of drugs ensure in most instances their uniformity, claims of effectiveness, and relative safety, as well as identify their recognized hazards. However, the extremely large number and variety of drugs and drug products available over the counter (OTC) or by prescription from a physician make it impossible for patient or physician to obtain or retain the knowledge necessary to use all these drugs well. It is understandable, therefore, that many OTC drugs are used unwisely by the public and that restricted drugs may be prescribed incorrectly by physicians.

Most physicians use no more than 50 drug products in their practice, gaining familiarity with their effectiveness and safety. Most patients probably use only a limited number of OTC drugs. Nevertheless, many patients receive care and drug prescriptions from more than one physician, and surveys have shown that in any 30-day period patients may consume more than three different OTC drug products containing nine or more different chemical agents.

Twenty-five to fifty percent of patients may make errors in self-administration of prescribed medicines, and this can be responsible for adverse drug effects. Elderly patients are most likely to commit such errors. One-third or more of patients also may not take their prescribed medications. It also seems likely that many patients commit similar errors in taking OTC drugs by not reading or following the directions for use of the medicines provided on the containers. Physicians must recognize that providing directions with prescriptions does not always guarantee their patients' compliance.

Every drug can produce untoward consequences, even when used according to standard or recommended methods of administration. When used incorrectly, the drug's effectiveness may be reduced, or adverse reactions can be expected to occur more frequently. The administration of several drugs during the same period of time also may result in adverse interactions between drugs (see Chap. 70).

In the hospital all the drugs a patient is given should be under the control of a physician, and patient compliance is, in general, ensured. Errors may occur nevertheless, in that the wrong drug or dose may be given, or the drug may be given to the wrong patient, although systems improving drug distribution and administration in hospitals have reduced this problem. On the other hand, there are no means for controlling how ambulatory patients take prescription or OTC drugs.

EPIDEMIOLOGY Epidemiologic studies of adverse drug reactions have been helpful in evaluating the magnitude of the overall problem, in calculating the rate of reactions to individual drugs, and in characterizing some of the determinants of adverse drug effects.

Patients receive on the average 10 different drugs while hospitalized. The sicker the patient, the more drugs are given, and as expected, there is a corresponding increase in the likelihood of adverse drug reactions. When fewer than six different drugs are given to hospitalized patients, the probability of an adverse reaction is about 5 percent, but if more than 15 drugs are given, the probability is over 40 percent. Retrospective analysis of ambulatory patients has revealed a history of some adverse drug effects in 20 percent of them.

Thus, the magnitude of the problem posed by drug-induced disease has become exceedingly large. Two to five percent of patients are admitted to the medical and pediatric services of general hospitals because of illnesses attributed to drugs. Five to thirty percent of patients experience adverse reactions to drugs during hospitalization. The case/fatality ratio from drug-induced disease in hospitalized patients varies from 2 to 12 percent. An unknown proportion of fetal or neonatal abnormalities may be due to medicines taken by the mother during pregnancy or parturition. An undetermined number of illnesses caused by drugs are responsible for visits of patients to physicians' offices.

Epidemiologic studies revealing the rates of adverse drug reactions are limited by the availability of suitable controls. Hence, both major and minor manifestations of presumed drug-induced illness are difficult to establish. Gastrointestinal signs and symptoms, particularly vomiting and diarrhea, account for approximately one-third; neurologic manifestations account for about one-fifth; cardiovascular, metabolic, and cutaneous manifestations each account for about one-tenth; and hematologic and other manifestations each account for about one-twentieth of adverse drug reactions. Women experience twice as many gastrointestinal manifestations of adverse drug effects as do men.

A small group of widely used drugs account for a disproportionate number of reactions. A number of studies have shown that aspirin, digoxin, anticoagulants, diuretics, antimicrobials, steroids, and hypoglycemic agents account for as many as 90 percent of all reactions.

ETIOLOGY Most adverse reactions to drugs may be classified into two groups. The most frequent are those that result from the exaggerated but predicted pharmacologic action of the drug. Other adverse reactions ensue from toxic effects on cells that result from mechanisms unrelated to the intended pharmacologic actions. These therefore are often unpredictable, are frequently severe, and result from a number of recognized as well as undiscovered mechanisms. Some of the mechanisms of extrapharmacologic toxicity include direct cytotoxicity, the initiation of abnormal immune responses, and the perturbation of metabolic processes in individuals rendered susceptible by genetic enzymatic defects.

EXAGGERATION OF THE INTENDED PHARMACOLOGIC EFFECT By prior consideration of the known factors that modify drug action, these adverse reactions often are preventable.

Abnormally high drug concentration at the receptor site (site of action) due to the pharmacokinetic variability discussed in Chap. 70 is the usual cause. For example, reduction in the volume of distribution, in the rate of metabolism, or in the rate of excretion all will result in higher than expected concentration of the drug at the receptor site with consequent increase in pharmacologic effect.

Alteration in the dose-response curve due to increased receptor sensitivity will result in an increase in drug effect at the same concentration. An example of this is seen in the excessive response to the anticoagulant warfarin at normal and lower than normal blood levels in the elderly.

The shape of the dose-response curve itself also determines the likelihood of the development of adverse drug reactions. These drugs with a steep dose-response curve are more likely to be associated with dose-related toxicity because of the small increase in dose required to produce a large change in pharmacologic effect. An increase in the dose of drugs which exhibit nonlinear kinetics, such as phenytoin (see previous chapter) may produce a proportionately greater increase in the blood level, resulting in toxicity.

Concomitant drug therapy may affect the pharmacokinetics or pharmacodynamics of other drugs. Pharmacokinetics may be affected by alterations in bioavailability, protein binding, or the rate of metabolism or excretion. Pharmacodynamics may be altered by competition for receptor sites, by prevention of the drug's reaching its site of action, or by antagonism or enhancement of the drug's pharmacological effect. These subjects are discussed in detail in the previous chapter.

TOXICITY UNRELATED TO A DRUG'S PRIMARY PHARMACOLOGIC ACTIVITY **Cytotoxic reactions** Our understanding of these so-called "idiosyncratic" reactions has greatly improved recently as it has become clear that many of these reactions are due to irreversible binding of drug or metabolites to tissue macromolecules by shared electron (covalent) bonds. Some chemical carcinogens such as the alkylating agents combine directly with DNA. However, it is more commonly only after metabolic activation to chemically reactive metabolites that covalent binding occurs. This metabolic activation usually occurs in the microsomal mixed-function oxidase system, the hepatic enzyme system which is responsible for the metabolism of many drugs (Chap. 70). During the course of drug metabolism by these pathways, reactive metabolites of some drugs may be produced which covalently bind to tissue macromolecules, causing tissue damage. Because of the highly reactive nature of these metabolites covalent binding often occurs close to the site of production, such as the liver, but the mixed-function oxidase system is found in other tissues as well.

An example of this type of adverse drug reaction is the hepatotoxicity associated with isoniazid, which is metabolized principally by acetylation (Fig. 71-1) to acetylisoniazid, which is then hydrolyzed to acetylhydralazine. The further metabolism of acetylhydralazine by the mixed-function oxidase system liberates reactive metabolites which covalently bind to liver macromolecules, causing hepatic necrosis. The rate of acetylation shows a bimodal distribution, the population dividing into slow and fast acetylators. Fast acetylators predominate in Orientals, who have been shown to be particularly susceptible to isoniazid hepatoxicity. The administration of drugs known to increase the activity of the mixed-function oxidase system, such as phenobarbital or rifampin, together with isoniazid, is associated with the production of increased amounts of reactive metabolites, increased covalent binding, and hepatic damage.

The liver necrosis produced by overdosage of acetominophen is caused by the covalent binding of reactive electrophilic metabolites to liver macromolecules. Normally these reactive metabolites are detoxified by combining with hepatic glutathione. When glutathione becomes exhausted, the metabolites bind instead to liver macromolecules with resultant hepatocyte damage. The hepatic necrosis produced by the ingestion of large quantities of acetaminophen can be prevented, or at least attenuated, by the administration of substances such as cysteamine, which bind the electrophilic metabolites and prevent them from reacting with hepatic proteins with resultant hepatic necrosis. The risks of hepatic necrosis are increased in patients also receiving drugs such as phenobarbital which increase the rate of drug metabolism and rate of production of toxic metabolites.

It is likely, though as yet unproved, that other "idiosyncratic" reactions are caused by the covalent binding of reactive metabolites to tissue macromolecules, with either direct cytotoxicity or via the initiation of an immunologic response.

FIGURE 71-1
Biotransformation of isoniazid to a hepatotoxic metabolite.

Immunologic mechanisms Most pharmacologic agents are poor immunogens since they consist of small molecules with molecular weights less than 2000. Stimulation of antibody synthesis or sensitization of lymphocytes by a drug or one of its metabolites usually requires in vivo activation and covalent linkage to protein, carbohydrate, or nucleic acid.

Drug stimulation of antibody production may mediate tissue injury by one of several mechanisms. The antibody may attack the drug affixed to a cell by covalent linkage and thereby destroy the cell, as occurs in penicillin-induced hemolytic anemia. Complexes of antibody-drug-antigen may be passively adsorbed by a bystander cell which is destroyed by activation of complement; this occurs in Sedormid-induced thrombocytopenia. Drugs or their reactive metabolites may alter host tissue, rendering it antigenic, and stimulate autoantibodies; for example, hydralazine and procainamide can chemically alter nuclear material, stimulate formation of antinuclear antibodies, and occasionally cause lupus erythematosus. Autoantibodies may be stimulated by drugs which neither interact with the host antigen nor have any chemical similarity to the host tissue; for example, alpha methyldopa frequently stimulates formation of antibodies to host erythrocytes, yet the drug does not itself attach to the erythrocyte nor share any chemical similarities with the antigenic determinants on the erythrocyte.

Serum sickness (Chap. 65) results from deposition of circulating drug-antibody complexes on endothelial surfaces. Complement activation occurs, chemotactic factors are generated locally, and an inflammatory response appears at the site of complex entrapment. Arthralgias, lymphadenopathy, glomerulonephritis, or cerebritis may result. Penicillin is the most common cause of serum sickness today. Many drugs, particularly the antimicrobial agents, induce production of IgE, which affixes to mast cell membranes. Contact with a drug antigen initiates a series of biochemical events within the mast cell and results in the release of mediators which may produce urticaria, wheezing, rhinorrhea, and occasionally hypotension characteristic of anaphylaxis.

Drugs may also excite cell-mediated immune responses. Topically administered substances may interact with sulfhydryl or amino groups in the skin and react with sensitized lymphocytes to produce the rash characteristic of contact dermatitis. Other types of rashes may also appear from the interaction of serum factors, drugs, and sensitized lymphocytes. The role of drug-activated lymphoctyes in the immune mechanisms governing destruction of visceral tissue is unknown.

Toxicity associated with genetically determined enzymatic defects In the porphyrias, any drugs that accelerate the activity of enzymes proximal to the deficient enzyme in the biosynthetic pathway of porphyrins can increase the quantity of porphyrin precursors that accumulate proximal to the deficient enzyme (Chap. 96). These drugs are listed in Table 71-1.

Patients with a deficiency of glucose 6-phosphate dehydrogenase (G6PD) will develop hemolytic anemia on primaquine and a number of other drugs (Table 71-1) which do not cause hemolysis in patients who have adequate quantities of this enzyme (Chap. 314).

Diagnosis The manifestations of drug-induced diseases frequently resemble those associated with other diseases, and may be produced by different and dissimilar drugs. Recognition of the role of a drug or drugs responsible for illness is dependent upon appreciation of the possible implication of adverse reactions to drugs in any disease, identification of a temporal relationship between drug administration and development of illness, and familiarity with the manifestations most often caused by particular drugs. Although specific reactions have been described as resulting from the use of particular drugs, there is always a "first," and any drug should be suspected of causing an adverse effect if the clinical setting is appropriate.

Illness related to a drug's pharmacologic action may be more easily recognized than illness attributable to immunologic or other mechanisms. For example, side effects such as cardiac arrhythmias in patients receiving digitalis, hypoglycemia in patients given insulin, and bleeding in patients receiving anticoagulants are more easily related to the prescribed drug than are symptoms like fever or rash, which may be caused by many drugs or by other factors.

Once an adverse reaction is suspected, discontinuance of the suspected drug followed by disappearance of the reaction is presumptive evidence of a drug-induced illness. Reappearance of the reaction upon cautious readministration of the drug may provide confirmatory evidence of the relationship if such confirmation adds useful information to the future management of the patient without entailing undue risk. With concentration-dependent adverse reactions, lowering the dosage may also be followed by disappearance of the reaction, and increasing the dose may cause it to reappear. When the reaction is thought to be allergic, however, readministration of the drug may be hazardous, since anaphylactic shock may develop. Readministration is unwise under these conditions unless alternate drugs are not available and treatment is mandatory.

If the patient is receiving many different drugs when an adverse reaction is suspected, the drugs most likely to be incriminated can usually be identified. All drugs may be discontinued at once, or if this is not practical, then drugs should be discontinued one at a time, starting with the drug under greatest suspicion, and the patient observed for signs of improvement. It must be remembered that the time taken for the disappearance of a concentration-dependent adverse effect will depend on the time taken for the concentration to fall below the range associated with the adverse effect, and this is turn will depend on the initial blood level and on the rate of elimination or metabolism of the drug. Adverse effects of drugs such as phenobarbital which have long half-lives will take a considerable time to disappear.

To assist in the identification of adverse reactions, a table of the drugs recognized as producing a number of reactions appears in this chapter (Table 71-1). This table is not intended to be exhaustive but rather includes well-documented reactions and some less well-documented reactions whose effects are sufficiently devastating as to require their consideration. It should be used to suggest the likely causative drug, but the absence of a drug from the table should not be interpreted to mean that it is not responsible for the reaction.

Serum antibody has been demonstrated in some persons with drug allergy involving cellular blood elements, as in agranulocytosis, hemolytic anemia, and thrombocytopenia. In other types of drug allergy, precipitation, hemoagglutination, or complement-fixation tests with drugs or drug degradation products have only rarely been clearly related to adverse reactions. Skin tests with the drug or its degradation products are often of little value in identifying the allergic individual. These poor results testify to the inadequacy of present methods of testing and are not an argument against an immunologic basis for allergic drug reactions.

Eliciting a drug history from patients is important for diagnosis. Attention must be directed to nonprescription, or OTC, as well as to prescription drugs. Each type can be responsible for adverse drug effects, and frequently adverse interactions occur between drugs purchased by patients over the counter and those prescribed by physicians. In addition, it is common for patients to be cared for by several physicians; and duplicative, additive, counteractive, or synergistic drugs may therefore

TABLE 71-1
Clinical manifestations of adverse reactions to drugs

I Multisystem
  A Fever
    1 Penicillins
    2 Novobiocin
    3 p-Aminosalicylic acid
    4 Amphotericin B
    5 Antihistamines
    6 Cephalosporins
    7 Barbiturates
    8 Phenytoin
    9 Quinidine
    10 Sulfonamides
    11 Iodides
    12 Thiouracil
    13 Phenolphthalein
    14 Methyldopa
    15 Procainamide
  B Drug-induced lupus erythematosus
    1 Hydralazine
    2 Procainamide
    3 Isoniazid
  C Serum sickness
    1 Aspirin
    2 Penicillins
    3 Streptomycin
    4 Sulfonamides
    5 Propylthiouracil
  D Anaphylaxis
    1 Bromsulphothalein
    2 Penicillins
    3 Cephalosporins
    4 Streptomycin
    5 Dextran
    6 Iron Dextran
    7 Procaine
    8 Insulin
    9 Demeclocycline
    10 Iodinated drugs or contrast media
    11 Lidocaine
II Endocrine
  A Disorders of thyroid function tests
    1 Oral contraceptives
    2 Bromsulphalein
    3 Phenindione
    4 Iodides
    5 Tolbutamide
    6 Chlorpropamide
    7 Lithium
    8 Acetazolamide
    9 Gold salts
    10 Dimercaprol
    11 Clofibrate
    12 Phenothiazines (long term)
    13 Phenylbutazone
    14 Sulfonamides
    15 Phenytoin
  B Addisonian-like syndrome
    1 Busulfan
  C Gynecomastia
    1 Estrogens
    2 Testosterone
    3 Spironolactone
    4 Digitalis
    5 Reserpine
    6 Methyldopa
    7 Isoniazid
    8 Ethionamide
    9 Griseofulvin
  D Galactorrhea (may also cause amenorrhea)
    1 Methyldopa
    2 Phenothiazines
    3 Reserpine
    4 Tricyclic antidepressants
    5 Dexamphetamine
  E Sexual dysfunction
    1 Impaired ejaculation
      a Guanethidine
      b Debrisoquin
      c Bethanidine
      d Thioridazine
    2 Decreased libido and impotence
      a Oral contraceptives
      b Sedatives
      c Major tranquilizers
      d Lithium

      e Methyldopa
      f Clonidine
III Metabolic
  A Hyponatremia
    1 Dilutional
      a Vincristine
      b Cyclophosphamide
      c Chlorpropamide
      d Diuretics
    2 Salt wasting
      a Diuretics
      b Corticosteroid (withdrawal)
      c Enemas
      d Mannitol
  B Hyperkalemia
    1 Spironolactone
    2 Triamterene
    3 Amiloride
    4 Cytotoxics
    5 Corticosteroid (withdrawal)
    6 Succinylcholine
    7 Digitalis overdose
    8 Potassium salts of drugs
    9 Potassium preparations including salt substitute
    10 Lithium
  C Hypokalemia
    1 Diuretics
    2 Laxative abuse
    3 Corticosteroids
    4 Amphotericin B
    5 Alkali-induced alkalosis
    6 Insulin
    7 Osmotic diuretics
    8 Carbenoxolone
    9 Gentamicin
    10 Degraded tetracycline
    11 Vitamin B_{12}
  D Metabolic acidosis
    1 Paraldehyde (degraded)
    2 Phenformin
    3 Acetazolamide
    4 Spironolactone
    5 Salicylates
  E Hypercalcemia
    1 Antacids with absorbable alkali
    2 Vitamin D
    3 Thiazides
  F Hyperuricemia
    1 Thiazides
    2 Chlorthalidone
    3 Ethacrynic acid
    4 Furosemide
    5 Aspirin
    6 Cytotoxics
    7 Hyperalimentation
    8 Fructose (IV)
  G Hyperglycemia
    1 Corticosteroids
    2 Oral contraceptives
    3 Chlorthalidone
    4 Ethacrynic acid
    5 Thiazides
    6 Furosemide
    7 Diazoxide
    8 Growth hormone
  H Porphyria exacerbation
    1 Barbiturates
    2 Chlordiazepoxide
    3 Meprobamate
    4 Sulfonamides
    5 Estrogens
    6 Oral contraceptives
    7 Chlorpropamide
    8 Phenytoin
    9 Glutethimide
    10 Griseofulvin
    11 Rifampin
  I Hyperbilirubinemia
    1 Rifampin
    2 Novobiocin
IV Dermatologic
  A Exfoliative dermatitis
    1 Penicillins
    2 Sulfonamides
    3 Barbiturates
    4 Phenytoin

    5 Phenylbutazone
    6 Gold salts
    7 Quinidine
  B Toxic epidermal necrolysis (bullous)
    1 Barbiturates
    2 Phenylbutazone
    3 Phenytoin
    4 Sulfonamides
    5 Phenolphthalein
    6 Penicillins
    7 Allopurinol
    8 Iodides
    9 Bromides
    10 Nalidixic acid
  C Erythema multiforme or Steven-Johnson syndrome
    1 Sulfonamides
    2 Barbiturates
    3 Phenylbutazone
    4 Chlorpropamide
    5 Thiazides
    6 Sulfones
    7 Phenytoin
    8 Ethosuximide
    9 Salicylates
    10 Tetracyclines
    11 Codeine
    12 Penicillins
  D Erythema nodosum
    1 Penicillins
    2 Sulfonamides
    3 Oral contraceptives
  E Fixed drug eruptions
    1 Phenolphthalein
    2 Barbiturates
    3 Sulfonamides
    4 Salicylates
    5 Phenylbutazone
    6 Quinine
  F Photodermatitis
    1 Tetracyclines, particularly demeclocycline
    2 Griseofulvin
    3 Sulfonamides
    4 Sulfonylureas
    5 Thiazides
    6 Furosemide
    7 Phenothiazines
    8 Nalidixic acid
    9 Oral contraceptives
    10 Chlordiazepoxide
  G Urticaria
    1 Aspirin
    2 Penicillins
    3 Sulfonamides
    4 Barbiturates
  H Nonspecific rashes
    1 Ampicillin
    2 Barbiturates
    3 Allopurinol
    4 Phenytoin
    5 Methyldopa
  I Pigment changes (hyperpigmentation)
    1 ACTH
    2 Busulfan
    3 Phenothiazines
    4 Hypervitaminosis A
    5 Oral contraceptives
    6 Gold salts
    7 Chloroquine and other antimalarials
    8 Cyclophosphamide
    9 Bleomycin
  J Alopecia
    1 Cytotoxics
    2 Ethionamide
    3 Heparin
    4 Oral contraceptives (withdrawal)
  K Purpura (see also thrombocytopenia)
    1 Corticosteroids
    2 Aspirin
  L Lichenoid eruptions
    1 Chlorpropamide
    2 Gold salts
    3 Antimalarials
    4 PAS

TABLE 71-1 *(continued)*
Clinical manifestations of adverse reactions to drugs

5 Methyldopa
6 Phenothiazines
M Eczema (contact dermatitis)
  1 Topical antimicrobials
  2 Topical local anesthetics
  3 Topical antihistamines
  4 Cream and lotion preservatives
  5 Lanolin
N Acne
  1 Anabolic and androgenic steroids
  2 Corticosteroids
  3 Bromides
  4 Iodides
  5 Oral contraceptives
  6 Isoniazid
  7 Troxidone
V Hematologic
 A Pancytopenia (aplastic anemia)
  1 Chloramphenicol
  2 Phenytoin
  3 Mephenytoin
  4 Trimethadione
  5 Phenylbutazone
  6 Oxyphenbutazone
  7 Gold salts
  8 Mepacrine
  9 Quinacrine
  10 Potassium perchlorate
  11 Cytotoxics
 B Agranulocytosis (see also pancytopenia)
  1 Chloramphenicol
  2 Sulphonamides
  3 Phenylbutazone
  4 Oxyphenbutazone
  5 Gold salts
  6 Indomethacin
  7 Propylthiouracil
  8 Methimazole
  9 Carbimazole
  10 Phenothiazines
  11 Cytotoxics
  12 Tolbutamide
  13 Cotrimoxazole
  14 Tricyclic antidepressants
 C Thrombocytopenia (see also pancytopenia)
  1 Quinidine
  2 Quinine
  3 Furosemide
  4 Chlorthalidone
  5 Thiazides
  6 Gold salts
  7 Cotrimoxazole
  8 Aspirin
  9 Indomethacin
  10 Phenylbutazone
  11 Oxyphenbutazone
  12 Chlorpropamide
  13 Acetazolamine
  14 Phenytoin and other hydantoins
  15 Methyldopa
  16 Carbamazepine
  17 Digitoxin
  18 Novobiocin
 D Megaloblastic anemia
  1 Folate antagonists
  2 Cotrimoxazole
  3 Phenytoin
  4 Primidone
  5 Phenobarbital
  6 Triamterene
  7 Trimethoprim
  8 Oral contraceptives
 E Hemolytic anemia
  1 Methyldopa
  2 Levodopa
  3 Mefenamic acid
  4 Melphalan
  5 Isoniazid
  6 Rifampin
  7 Sulfonamides
  8 Penicillins
  9 Cephalosporins
  10 Insulin
  11 Quinidine
  12 Chlorpromazine
  13 Phenacetin

14 p-Aminosalicylic acid
15 Dapsone
F Hemolytic anemia (in G6PD deficiency)
  1 Antimalarials, e.g., primaquine
  2 Chloramphenicol
  3 Dapsone
  4 Nalidixic acid
  5 Nitrofurantoin
  6 Sulfonamides
  7 Aspirin
  8 Phenacetin
  9 p-Aminosalicylic acid
  10 Quinidine
  11 Vitamin C
  12 Vitamin K
  13 Cotrimoxazole
  14 Probenecid
  15 Procainamide
G Lymphadenopathy
  1 Phenytoin
  2 Primidone
H Leukocytosis
  1 Lithium
  2 Corticosteroids
I Eosinophilia
  1 Erythromycin estolate
  2 Sulfonamides
  3 Chlorpropamide
  4 p-Aminosalicylic acid
  5 Imipramine
  6 Nitrofurantoin
  7 Procarbazine
  8 Methotrexate
VI Cardiovascular
 A Exacerbation of angina
  1 Vasopressin
  2 Oxytocin
  3 Ergotamine
  4 Methysergide
  5 Propranolol withdrawal
  6 Excessive thyroxin
  7 Alpha blockers
  8 Hydralazine
 B Cardiomyopathy
  1 Emetine
  2 Sympathomimetics
  3 Phenothiazines
  4 Lithium
  5 Sulfonamides
  6 Daunorubicin
  7 Adriamycin
 C Pericarditis
  1 Procainamide
  2 Hydralazine
  3 Methysergide
  4 Emetine
 D Fluid retention or congestive heart failure
  1 Estrogens
  2 Steroids
  3 Carbenoxolone
  4 Phenylbutazone
  5 Indomethacin
  6 Propranolol
  7 Mannitol
  8 Diazoxide
 E Arrhythmias
  1 Sympathomimetics
  2 Thyroid hormone
  3 Digitalis
  4 Quinidine
  5 Procainamide
  6 Verapamil
  7 Atropine
  8 Propranolol
  9 Guanethidine
  10 Emetine
  11 Propellants in aerosols
  12 Tricyclic antidepressants
  13 Phenothiazines, particularly thioridazine
  14 Lithium
  15 Anticholinesterases
  16 Papaverine
  17 Daunomycin
  18 Adriamycin
  19 Lincomycin (intravenous)

F Hypotension (see also arrythmias)
  1 Nitroglycerin
  2 Phenothiazines
  3 Morphine
  4 Diuretics
  5 Citrated blood
  6 Levodopa
G Hypertension
  1 Oral contraceptives
  2 Sympathomimetics
  3 Clonidine withdrawal
  4 Monoamine oxidase inhibitors with sympathomimetics
  5 Tricyclic antidepressants with sympathomimetics
  6 Corticosteroids
  7 ACTH
  8 Phenylbutazone
H Thromboembolism
  1 Oral contraceptives
VII Respiratory
 A Nasal congestion
  1 Reserpine
  2 Guanethidine
  3 Isoproterenol
  4 Oral contraceptives
  5 Decongestant abuse
 B Respiratory depression
  1 Aminoglycosides
  2 Polymixins
  3 Trimethaphan
  4 Opiates
  5 Sedatives
  6 Hypnotics
 C Airway obstruction (bronchospasm, asthma; see also anaphylaxis)
  1 Beta blockers
  2 Nonsteroidal anti-inflammatory drugs, e.g., aspirin, indomethacin
  3 Cholinergic drugs
  4 Tartrazine (drugs with yellow dye)
  5 Penicillins
  6 Cephalosporins
  7 Streptomycin
  8 Pentazocine
 D Pulmonary infiltrates
  1 Nitrofurantoin
  2 Methysergide
  3 Chlorambucil
  4 Procarbazine
  5 Busulfan
  6 Melphalan
  7 Cyclophosphamide
  8 Azothioprine
  9 Bleomycin
  10 Methotrexate
  11 Sulfonamides
 E Pulmonary edema
  1 Heroin
  2 Methadone
  3 Hydrochlorthiazide
  4 Propoxyphene
  5 Contrast media
VIII Gastrointestinal
 A Dental discoloration
  1 Tetracycline
 B Gingival hyperplasia
  1 Phenytoin
 C Oral ulceration
  1 Aspirin
  2 Isoproterenol (sublingual)
  3 Cytotoxics
  4 Pancreatin
  5 Gentian violet
 D Taste disturbances
  1 Penicillamine
  2 Biguanides
  3 Griseofulvin
  4 Metronidazole
  5 Lithium
  6 Rifampin
 E Dry mouth
  1 Anticholinergics
  2 Levodopa
  3 Tricyclic antidepressants
  4 Clonidine
  5 Methyldopa

TABLE 71-1 (continued)
Clinical manifestations of adverse reactions to drugs

    F Swelling of salivary gland
      1 Phenylbutazone
      2 Guanethidine
      3 Bethanidine
      4 Bretylium
      5 Clonidine
      6 Iodides
    G Peptic ulceration or hemorrhage
      1 Aspirin
      2 Phenylbutazone
      3 Indomethacin
      4 Ethacrynic acid
      5 Reserpine (large doses)
    H Intestinal ulceration
      1 Enteric-coated potassium chloride
    I Nausea or vomiting
      1 Digitalis
      2 Opiates
      3 Estrogens
      4 Levodopa
      5 Potassium chloride
      6 Ferrous sulfate
      7 Aminophylline
      8 Tetracyclines
    J Diarrhea or colitis
      1 Lincomycin
      2 Clindamycin
      3 Broad-spectrum antibiotics
      4 Magnesium in antacids
      5 Guanethidine
      6 Debrisoquin
      7 Methyldopa
      8 Reserpine
      9 Digitalis
      10 Colchicine
      11 Purgatives
      12 Lactose excipients
    K Constipation or ileus
      1 Ganglionic blockers
      2 Tricyclic antidepressants
      3 Phenothiazines
      4 Opiates
      5 Aluminum hydroxide
      6 Calcium carbonate
      7 Barium sulfate
      8 Ion exchange resins
      9 Ferrous sulfate
    L Malabsorption
      1 Broad-spectrum antibiotics
      2 Neomycin
      3 Cholestyramine
      4 Colchicine
      5 p-Aminosalicylic acid
      6 Biguanides
      7 Phenytoin
      8 Primidone
      9 Phenobarbital
      10 Cytotoxics
    M Pancreatitis
      1 Corticosteroids
      2 Thiazides
      3 Azathioprine
      4 Oral contraceptives
      5 Sulfonamides
      6 Opiates
      7 Furosemide
      8 Ethacrynic acid
    N Diffuse hepatocellular damage
      1 Halothane
      2 Methoxyflurane
      3 Methyldopa
      4 Isoniazid
      5 Rifampin
      6 Aminosalicylic acid
      7 Ethionamide
      8 Phenytoin and other hydantoins
      9 Acetaminophen (paracetamol)
      10 Salicylates
      11 Allopurinol
      12 Sulfonamides
      13 Tetracyclines
      14 Erythromycin estolate
      15 Propylthiouracil
      16 Methimazole
      17 Oxyphenisatin
      18 Methotrexate
      19 Pyridium

      20 Propoxyphene
      21 Monoamine oxidase inhibitors
    O Cholestatic jaundice
      1 Phenothiazines
      2 Androgens
      3 Anabolic steroids
      4 Oral contraceptives
      5 Erythromycin estolate
      6 Chlorpropamide
      7 Gold salts
      8 Methimazole
      9 Acetohexamide

IX Urinary tract
    A Nephrotic syndrome
      1 Penicillamine
      2 Gold salts
      3 Phenindione
      4 Probenecid
    B Tubular necrosis
      1 Amphotericin B
      2 Aminoglycosides
      3 Polymixins
      4 Cephaloridine
      5 Tetracyclines
      6 Colistin
      7 Sulfonamides
      8 Radioiodinated contrast medium
      9 Methoxyflurane
    C Interstitial nephritis
      1 Penicillins, particularly methicillin
      2 Sulfonamides
      3 Phenindione
      4 Furosemide
      5 Thiazides
    D Nephropathies due to analgesics (e.g., phenacetin)
    E Concentrating defect with polyuria (or nephrogenic diabetes insipidus)
      1 Vitamin D
      2 Lithium
      3 Demeclocycline
      4 Methoxyflurane
    F Renal tubular acidosis
      1 Degraded tetracycline
      2 Amphotericin B
      3 Acetazolamide
    G Calculi
      1 Acetazolamide
      2 Vitamin D
    H Obstructive uropathy
      1 Intrarenal: cytotoxics
      2 Extrarenal: methysergide
    I Hemorrhagic cystitis
      1 Cyclophosphamide
    J Bladder dysfunction
      1 Anticholinergics
      2 Monoamine oxidase inhibitors
      3 Tricyclic antidepressants
      4 Disopyramide

X Genital (see also endocrine)
    A Vaginal carcinoma
      1 Diethylstilbestrol (administered to mother)
    B Impairment of spermatogenesis or oogenesis
      1 Cytotoxics

XI Neurologic
    A Peripheral neuropathy
      1 Isoniazid
      2 Hydralazine
      3 Nitrofurantoin
      4 Vincristine
      5 Mustine
      6 Streptomycin
      7 Polymixin, colistan
      8 Clioquinol
      9 Phenelzine
      10 Tricyclic antidepressants
      11 Chloramphenicol
      12 Procarbazine
      13 Ethambutol
      14 Ethionamide
      15 Glutethimide
      16 Demeclocycline
      17 Nalidixic acid
      18 Tolbutamide
      19 Chlorpropamide

      20 Methysergide
      21 Phenytoin
    B Exacerbation of myasthenia
      1 Aminoglycosides
      2 Polymixins
    C Extrapyramidal effects
      1 Butyrophenones, e.g., haloperidol
      2 Phenothiazines
      3 Tricyclic antidepressants
      4 Methyldopa
      5 Levodopa
      6 Reserpine
      7 Metoclopramide
    D Seizures
      1 Amphetamines
      2 Analeptics
      3 Phenothiazines
      4 Isoniazid
      5 Lidocaine
      6 Theophylline
      7 Penicillins
      8 Nalidixic acid
      9 Physostigmine
      10 Tricyclic antidepressants
      11 Vincristine
      12 Lithium
    E Stroke
      1 Oral contraceptives
    F Pseudotumor cerebri (or intracranial hypertension)
      1 Corticosteroids
      2 Oral contraceptives
      3 Tetracyclines
      4 Hypervitaminosis A
    G Headache
      1 Hydralazine
      2 Bromides
      3 Glyceryl trinitrate
      4 Ergotamine (withdrawal)
      5 Indomethacin

XII Ocular
    A Corneal opacities
      1 Vitamin D
      2 Mepacrine
      3 Chloroquine
      4 Indomethacin
    B Corneal edema
      1 Oral contraceptives
    C Cataracts
      1 Phenothiazines
      2 Corticosteroids
      3 Busulfan
      4 Chlorambucil
    D Glaucoma
      1 Mydriatics
      2 Sympathomimetics
    E Retinopathy
      1 Chloroquine
      2 Phenothiazines
    F Optic neuritis
      1 Clioquinol
      2 Chloramphenicol
      3 Streptomycin
      4 Isoniazid
      5 Ethambutol
      6 Quinine
      7 Phenothiazines
      8 Penicillamine
      9 PAS
      10 Phenylbutazone
    G Alteration in color vision
      1 Troxidone
      2 Sulfonamides
      3 Streptomycin
      4 Methaqualone
      5 Barbiturates
      6 Digitalis
      7 Thiazides

XIII Ear
    A Vestibular disorders
      1 Aminoglycosides
      2 Quinine
      3 Mustine
    B Deafness
      1 Aminoglycosides
      2 Ethacrynic acid
      3 Furosemide

    4 Quinine
    5 Bleomycin
    6 Chloroquine
    7 Mustine
    8 Aspirin
    9 Nortriptyline
XIV Musculoskeletal
  A Myopathy or myalgia
    1 Corticosteroids
    2 Chloroquine
    3 Clofibrate
    4 Oral contraceptives
    5 Amphotericin B
    6 Carbenoxolone
  B Bone disorders
    1 Osteoporosis
      a Corticosteroids
      b Heparin
    2 Osteomalacia
      a Anticonvulsants
      b Glutethemide
      c Aluminum hydroxide
XV Psychiatric disorders
  A Schizophrenic-like or paranoid reactions
    1 Amphetamines
    2 Lysergic acid

    3 Levodopa
    4 Tricyclic antidepressants
    5 Monoamine oxidase inhibitors
    6 Bromides
    7 Corticosteroids
  B Depression
    1 Centrally acting antihypertensives (reserpine, methyldopa, clonidine)
    2 Propranolol
    3 Corticosteroids
    4 Amphetamine withdrawal
    5 Levodopa
  C Hypomania, mania or excited reactions
    1 Levodopa
    2 Sympathomimetics
    3 Corticosteroids
    4 MAO inhibitors
    5 Tricyclic antidepressants
  D Hallucinatory states
    1 Amantadine
    2 Narcotics
    3 Pentazocine
    4 Propranolol
    5 Levodopa
    6 Tricyclic antidepressants

    7 Meperidine
  E Delirious or confusional states
    1 Digitalis
    2 Anticholinergics
    3 Bromides
    4 Sedatives and hypnotics
    5 Phenothiazines
    6 Antidepressants
    7 Corticosteroids
    8 Isoniazid
    9 Levodopa
    10 Amantadine
    11 Penicillins
    12 Aminophylline
    13 Methyldopa
  F Sleep disturbances
    1 Anorexiants
    2 Levodopa
    3 Monoamine oxidase inhibitors
    4 Sympathomimetics
  G Drowsiness
    1 Anxiolytic drugs
    2 Major tranquilizers
    3 Tricyclic antidepressants
    4 Antihistamines
    5 Methyldopa
    6 Clonidine
    7 Reserpine

be taken if the physicians are not aware of the patients' drug histories. Every physician should determine what drugs a patient has been taking, at least during the preceding 30 days, before prescribing any medications. A history of previous adverse drug effects in patients is common. Since these patients have a predisposition to other drug-induced illnesses, familiarity with such a history should dictate added caution in prescribing drugs.

Patients with biochemical abnormalities such as erythrocyte G6PD deficiency can be identified; patients with the defect are usually blacks or of Mediterranean extraction. Drug-induced hemolytic crisis can be avoided by testing for the enzyme defect before administering these drugs. Similarly, persons with an abnormal serum pseudocholinesterase may have abnormally prolonged apnea when given succinylcholine.

General comments No drug is completely without side effects, and it is important to remember that a side effect in one patient may be the desired pharmacologic effect in another. Recent improvements in drug regulation allow physicians to prescribe drugs with considerable confidence in their purity, bioavailability, and effectiveness. However, while regulatory bodies try to ensure that drugs with serious toxic potential are not marketed, they have to constantly weigh the potential toxicity against the possible benefits. Thus toxicity which would be acceptable for an effective antineoplastic agent would not be permitted in, for example, an oral contraceptive. In addition, because of the necessarily small number of patients treated in premarketing studies, rare adverse reactions cannot be identified, so that the first responsibility for identifying and reporting these effects must rest with the practicing clinician through the use of the various national adverse reaction reporting systems, such as those operated by the Food and Drug Administration in the United States and the Committee on Safety of Medicines in Great Britain. The publication of a newly recognized adverse reaction can in a short time stimulate a very large number of similar such reports which previously had gone unrecognized.

The prevention of adverse drug reactions must first involve a high index of suspicion that the development of a new symptom or sign may be drug-related. Reduction of the dose or discontinuation of the suspected agent will usually clarify the position in concentration-dependent toxic reactions. Physi-

cians should be familiar with the common adverse effects of the drugs they use, and if they are in doubt, should consult the literature.

REFERENCES

CLUFF LE et al: *Clinical Problems with Drugs.* Philadelphia, Saunders, 1975
———, JOHNSON JE: Drug fever. Prog Allergy 8:149, 1964
DAVIES DM: *Textbook of Adverse Drug Reactions.* New York, Oxford University Press, 1977
DOWLING HF: *Medicines for Man.* New York, Knopf, 1970
GARDNER P, CLUFF LE: The epidemiology of adverse drug reactions: A review and perspective. Johns Hopkins Med J 126:77, 1970
HURWITZ N: Predisposing factors in adverse reactions to drugs. Br Med J 1:536, 1969
MITCHELL JR et al: Toxic drug reactions, in *Handbook of Experimental Pharmacology,* vol 28, no 3: *Concepts in Biochemical Pharmacology,* JR Gillette, JR Mitchell (eds). New York, Springer Verlag, 1975

72

CLINICAL PHARMACOLOGY OF THE AUTONOMIC NERVOUS SYSTEM

DAVID G. SHAND
JOHN A. OATES

FUNCTION OF THE AUTONOMIC NERVOUS SYSTEM

The autonomic nervous system comprises a series of reflex arcs which control or modulate involuntary functions, such as blood pressure, heart rate, glandular secretions, the release of renin, intestinal motility, and bladder function. The efferent nerves comprise two systems, the sympathetic and parasympathetic, that receive impulses arising in the central nervous system. Both systems form synapses at autonomic ganglia in the periphery before innervating their target tissues. The preganglionic fibers of both parasympathetic and sympathetic systems which arise in the central nervous system stimulate the ganglionic cells by releasing acetylcholine (ACh); that is, they are cholinergic. The sympathetic ganglia form a chain along the spinal column extending from the cervical to the lumbar regions. The postganglionic sympathetic fibers are adrenergic and mediate their effects by releasing norepinephrine. While most sympathetic responses are adrenergic, two exceptions exist in that the nerves stimulating the sweat glands and those causing vasodilation in skeletal muscle are both cholinergic. The final component of the sympathetic nervous system is the adrenal medulla which is derived from the same embryonic tissue as autonomic ganglia (the neural crest) and releases epinephrine into the general circulation following stimulation. This, together with the neural links in the sympathetic chain, accounts for the generalized nature of some responses to sympathetic activation. In contrast, the parasympathetic ganglia usually are situated near or in the organs they innervate, so that responses tend to be more discrete, subserving local functions, for example, in the pupil and urinary bladder. Parasympathetic postganglionic fibers are cholinergic.

The brain regulates the degree of sympathetic and parasympathetic traffic by integrating a number of input signals including those from the baroreceptors, from the perception of pain and emotional stress, and from mental and physical effort. Although a rather generalized response of the sympathetic nervous system may occur with severe stress, more often the brain controls specific autonomic functions discretely, for example, the parasympathetic control of pupillary constriction or the sympathetic reflex that evokes sexual ejaculation.

The brain plays a key role in the control of arterial pressure by regulating cardiac output, renin release, and sympathetically mediated vasoconstriction. The sympathetic impulses that lead to vasoconstriction arise from the vasomotor center in the medulla, which is the major site for integrating the excitatory and inhibitory inputs that determine the final level of traffic in peripheral sympathetic neurons. The vasomotor center is under constant stimulation by fibers arising from higher centers of the brain including the hypothalamus. This tonic level of *excitatory* impulses is heightened by wakefulness, pain, mental and muscular effort, or emotional stress. Angiotensin II also elicits stimulation of the vasomotor center by its action on neurons arising from areas in the vicinity of the third ventricle. A major *inhibitory* regulator of sympathetic activity is the baroreceptor system. With a rise in arterial pressure and accompanying stretch of the baroreceptors in the carotid sinus and aortic arch, the afferent baroreceptor fibers fire more rapidly. These baroreceptor impulses travel to the medulla where the afferent fibers form synapses with interneurons that inhibit sympathetic outflow from the vasomotor center. The synapse of these afferent baroreceptor fibers with inhibitory neurons takes place in the nucleus tractus solitarius, an area of the medulla which is a major source of the inhibitory impulses that regulate vasoconstrictor sympathetic outflow. Afferent impulses from the baroreceptors to the nucleus tractus solitarius also result in inhibition of sympathetic output to the heart and to an increase in cardiac vagal tone. Any rise in arterial pressure, therefore, results in stimulation of the nucleus tractus solitarius, which in turn inhibits the resting level of sympathetic output to resistance vessels and to the heart. In addition to the afferents from the baroreceptors, the nucleus tractus solitarius also receives fibers from other neurons, many of which are adrenergic in type. Like the baroreceptors, these adrenergic fibers also stimulate the interneurons that *inhibit* sympathetic outflow. The neurotransmitter from these neurons, either norepinephrine or epinephrine, acts through an alpha receptor to elicit inhibition of the vasomotor center. Thus, stimulation of this alpha receptor in the nucleus tractus solitarius lowers blood pressure, quite in contrast to the pressor effect of stimulating alpha receptors on arterial smooth muscle.

THE ADRENERGIC NEURON

The normal transmitter, norepinephrine, is synthesized from tyrosine by a series of steps (Fig. 72-1). The first, hydroxylation to form dihydroxyphenylalanine (dopa), is catalyzed by tyrosine hydroxylase and is rate-limiting. Dopa is then decarboxylated by aromatic L-amino acid decarboxylase to form dopamine which is taken up into the specialized neurosecretory vesicles and hydroxylated to form norepinephrine. Following stimulation, the secretory vesicles discharge their soluble contents, including norepinephrine and dopamine β-hydroxylase. The exact mechanism of this excitation-secretion coupling is unclear but involves Ca^{2+}. The nerve terminals have receptors modulating transmitter release, with stimulation of alpha receptors (alpha$_2$) decreasing and stimulation of beta receptors increasing transmitter release. It has also been postulated that prostaglandins exert a negative feedback inhibition of adrenergic transmission.

The effects of norepinephrine are terminated by three mechanisms. The first and most important involves re-uptake

FIGURE 72-1

Synthesis, storage, secretion, and disposition of the adrenergic neurotransmitter, norepinephrine (NE). A varicosity of the adrenergic neuron is depicted diagramatically. The terminal segments of peripheral adrenergic neurons have multiple varicosities along their course which are in juxtaposition with effector sites within target organs. Tyrosine is transported into the adrenergic neuron to provide substrate for the synthesis of NE. The rate-limiting enzyme is tyrosine hydroxylase, and the final enzyme, dopamine β-oxidase, is located within the neurosecretory vesicles.

1 *Depolarization of the neuron leads to release of NE by a calcium-dependent process of "excitation-secretion coupling" in which the neurosecretory vesicle fuses with the neuronal membrane and by exocytosis discharges its soluble contents that include NE and dopamine β-oxidase.*
2 *Much of the NE released into the synaptic cleft between the neuron and effector cell is removed from this area by a specialized membrane transport system known as the NE pump, which transports NE back into the neuron against a concentration gradient. This transport system is relatively unspecific and is responsible for the uptake of a number of ring-substituted amines such as tyramine, ephedrine, and guanethidine. It is competitively inhibited by the tricyclic antidepressants.*
3 *The major pathway for intraneuronal bioinactivation of NE (and dopamine) is via monoamine oxidase (MAO).*
4 *Extraneuronally, a major pathway of NE metabolism is via catechol-o-methyl transferase (COMT) to which NE is exposed at some effector cells and in remote organs such as the liver.*

into the adrenergic neuron by means of an energy-dependent norepinephrine pump. Once inside the neuron, much of the transmitter is again taken up into the neurosecretory granules and is reused. Norepinephrine which escapes into the circulation is metabolized by catechol-*o*-methyl transferase (COMT) to normetanephrine, some of which is converted to vanillylmandelic acid (VMA) via the action of monoamine oxidase (MAO) and aldehyde dehydrogenase (Fig. 72-2). Finally, some norepinephrine is converted intraneuronally to 3,4-dihydroxymandelic acid and then to VMA by COMT. In the adrenal medulla, norepinephrine is metabolized to epinephrine; adrenal cells do not have a re-uptake system for epinephrine which, after release, is metabolized similarly by MAO and COMT to form VMA and metanephrine. Measurement of the urinary catecholamines and their metabolites forms the basis for detecting enhanced catecholamine production in patients with pheochromocytoma (Chap. 337).

EFFECTS OF DRUGS Many drugs are available which affect the synthesis, release, metabolism, and re-uptake of norepinephrine. Inhibition of tyrosine hydroxylase by α-methyl-*p*-tyrosine can profoundly depress catecholamine synthesis, a property that may be useful in patients with pheochromocytoma. Competitive inhibitors of aromatic L-amino acid decarboxylase have little effect on the endogenous synthesis of norepinephrine because this enzymatic step is not rate-limiting, and almost complete inhibition of the enzyme would be required to block norepinephrine synthesis. One decarboxylase inhibitor, carbidopa, has been used clinically to prevent the breakdown of L-dopa by peripheral tissues and thereby to reduce the dosage of the latter required in the treatment of parkinsonism. As carbidopa does not gain access to the brain, it does not prevent the beneficial central effects of L-dopa in parkinsonism.

Release of the adrenergic neurotransmitter from peripheral adrenergic neurons is blocked by *guanethidine* and *bethanidine* (Chap. 251). These adrenergic neuron blockers act in part by replacing norepinephrine in the neurosecretory vesicles. Blockade of the peripheral adrenergic neuron produces a reduction in blood pressure that is much greater in the standing position and also may be associated with exercise-induced hypotension.

FIGURE 72-2
The metabolism of norepinephrine.

NOREPINEPHRINE

Monoamine Oxidase, Aldehyde Dehydrogenase

Catechol-O-Methyl Transferase

3,4-DIHYDROXYMANDELIC ACID

NORMETANEPHRINE

Catechol-O-Methyl Transferase

Monoamine Oxidase, Aldehyde Dehydrogenase

3-METHOXY-4-HYDROXYMANDELIC ACID
or VANILLYLMANDELIC ACID (VMA)

These highly polar drugs do not enter the central nervous system to any appreciable degree, and their use is generally devoid of side effects attributable to the central nervous system.

A state of pseudotolerance to guanethidine may develop as a result of fluid retention, and the drug is most effective when given with a diuretic together with restriction of dietary sodium. The drug has a long persistence within the adrenergic neuron and accordingly has a long half-life (about 5 days). Thus, guanethidine may be given only once daily in doses ranging upward from 10 mg. Guanethidine's action is selectively targeted to the peripheral adrenergic neuron because it is transported into the adrenergic neuron against a concentration gradient by the relatively nonspecific norepinephrine pump. The dependence of the pharmacological effects of guanethidine upon its concentration within the adrenergic neuron by the norepinephrine pump has two important clinical consequences: (1) Virtually all the actions of the drug in the body are targeted to the peripheral adrenergic neuron; thus, most of the side effects of guanethidine, including failure of ejaculation, result from the blockade of peripheral adrenergic neurons, and the drug is devoid of any toxic effects exclusive of this action. (2) Drugs that competitively inhibit the norepinephrine pump such as the tricyclic antidepressants, ephedrine, and the phenothiazines will compete with guanethidine's uptake and, therefore, counteract its antihypertensive action.

Reserpine is another antihypertensive which blocks adrenergic transmission, in this case by preventing norepinephrine incorporation into the neurosecretory vesicles. A similar effect in the central nervous system probably accounts for its most serious side effect, that of producing psychic depression. This effect is insidious in onset and is dose-dependent, so that only relatively mild degrees of hypertension can be treated with less than the greatest recommended dose (0.5 mg daily).

Inhibitors of MAO, such as *pargyline,* are occasionally used as antihypertensive agents chiefly in patients who also have psychic depression. As a result of MAO inhibition several amines as well as norepinephrine accumulate. One of these, octopamine, accumulates in and is released from the granules. As it has only 1 percent of the potency of norepinephrine, it serves as an inactive false transmitter. In addition to the accumulation of this false neurotransmitter in peripheral adrenergic neurons, actions of the MAO inhibitors in the central nervous system also may contribute to the inhibition of sympathetic reflexes.

ADRENERGIC RECEPTORS

The peripheral effects of the sympathetic nervous system are diverse. The integrated cardiovascular response of arteriolar constriction, tachycardia, enhanced cardiac contractility, and renin release maintains or raises arterial pressure. Metabolic functions including lipolysis, glycogenolysis, and release of antidiuretic hormone are stimulated by the sympathetic nervous system, as is mydriasis, ejaculation, and bronchodilatation. The sympathetic nervous system also participates in the regulation of body temperature and salivary secretion.

The peripheral effects mediated by catecholamine release have been classified as alpha or beta (Table 72-1). An important effect of norepinephrine is to cause vasoconstriction, an action on postsynaptic alpha receptors on vascular smooth muscle. Following the release of norepinephrine from the adrenergic neuron, it acts not only on postsynaptic alpha receptors, but also on receptors located on the neuron terminal itself. These presynaptic alpha receptors act to reduce the release of neurotransmitter. Thus, presynaptic alpha receptors

TABLE 72-1
Effects of peripheral postsynaptic adrenergic receptors

Alpha receptor	Beta$_1$ receptor	Beta$_2$ receptor
Vasoconstriction	Cardioacceleration	Vasodilatation
Pupil dilatation	Positive inotropy	Bronchial relaxation
Relaxation of gut		Uterine relaxation

serve as feedback inhibitors of the release of norepinephrine from the neuron terminal. Because of the differing potency of agonists and antagonists for these alpha receptors, it has been suggested that the postsynaptic receptor on vascular smooth muscle be designated an alpha$_1$ receptor and that the presynaptic receptor on the neuron terminal be designated an alpha$_2$ receptor.

Beta adrenoceptors are also divided into two types: beta$_1$ (mediating increased heart rate and contractility and probably renin release) and beta$_2$ (mediating relaxation of bronchial, uterine, and vascular smooth muscle). The metabolic responses to catecholamines, including hyperglycemia, are not well categorized according to receptor type. It is generally felt that stimulation of the beta receptor activates adenylate cyclase with a subsequent increase in intracellular concentrations of cyclic adenosine monophosphate (AMP). Cyclic AMP is thought to mediate the cellular response by activating protein kinases which phosphorylate intracellular proteins that control the cellular response. The enzyme phosphodiesterase catalyzes the breakdown of cyclic AMP to 5'-AMP.

The effect of norepinephrine and other beta-adrenergic agonists on cardiac rate is mediated by an increased rate of diastolic depolarization in the sinoatrial node as well as in other pacemaker cells, including those in the His-Purkinje system which pace the heart during atrioventricular block.

There is some evidence that both alpha and beta receptors can be regulated at the membrane level. For example, exposure to a stimulant such as isoproterenol may decrease the number of receptors (down regulation) by a process not involving protein synthesis. Conversely, reduced transmitter release or exposure to antagonists may increase receptor number. The relationship between these findings and denervation supersensitivity or withdrawal rebound phenomena is unclear.

SYMPATHOMIMETIC AGENTS

In addition to the catecholamines many drugs are available which mimic the effects of the sympathetic nervous system and act either directly to stimulate adrenergic receptors or indirectly by releasing stored norepinephrine. The directly acting drugs vary with respect to the preponderance of alpha or beta actions. *Phenylephrine* and *methoxamine* are almost pure alpha stimulators, and their major action is to produce arteriolar vasoconstriction. They may be used in the unusual hypotensive state (as occurs during spinal anesthesia) when increasing peripheral resistance without cardiac stimulation is required. These agents used alone are generally not considered beneficial in situations when depressed cardiac contractility contributes to hypotension, for example, in shock due to myocardial infarction. Alpha agonists also may be employed in the treatment of paroxysmal atrial tachycardia (see "Parasympathetic Regulation of Normal and Abnormal Cardiac Rhythm" below). Sympathomimetic vasoconstrictors are frequently employed as local nasal decongestants.

Norepinephrine, being the natural transmitter for sympathetic neurons, has both alpha and beta properties. When given systemically, the alpha vasoconstrictor effect seems to predominate, and the elevation in blood pressure causes reflex bradycardia. Stroke volume is increased and cardiac output is unchanged. Coronary blood flow is generally increased, but

flow to kidney, brain, gut, and skeletal muscle falls as a result of vasoconstriction. Prolonged infusions can lead to hypovolemia and tachyphylaxis which, together with the tendency to produce oliguria, require close attention to fluid balance, especially during weaning from the drug when the dose may have to be tapered and volume expanded to prevent hypotension. When extravasation from an intravenous infusion occurs, tissue necrosis and sloughing may occur. Infiltration with an alpha-blocking drug (see below) may counteract the vasoconstriction and prevent tissue necrosis. *Epinephrine* also has combined alpha and beta actions, but its beta effects are more striking than those of norepinephrine, especially in low doses. Vasoconstriction is produced in the skin and kidneys, while skeletal muscle vessels dilate and tachycardia is usual. Epinephrine may be injected directly into the cardiac ventricles during the treatment of cardiac arrest. It is also given subcutaneously to reverse anaphylaxis, urticaria, and angioneurotic edema, probably by increasing cyclic AMP levels in mast cells, thus inhibiting the release of allergic mediators. *Dopamine* is the third naturally occurring catecholamine which is thought to subserve a transmitter function in the CNS. Although it has not been established as a transmitter in the periphery, it produces some of its effects by stimulating what appear to be specific dopamine receptors, in addition to having both alpha and beta effects. Its effects are dose-dependent. At low doses [1 to 5 (μg/kg)/min, administered intravenously], it dilates mesenteric and renal vessels, producing increased renal blood flow and sodium excretion by its action on dopamine receptors. At intermediate doses [5 to 10 (μg/kg)/min)] beta stimulation increases cardiac output with relatively little tachycardia. Finally at higher doses alpha stimulation occurs, leading to obvious vasoconstriction which can compromise the circulation of the limbs and reverse renal vasodilation and naturesis. The combination of cardiac stimulation and renal vasodilation makes dopamine particularly useful in the treatment of a variety of hypotensive states and in the treatment of congestive heart failure.

Isoproterenol is a synthetic compound with pure beta-agonist activity causing a reduction in peripheral vascular resistance with an increase in heart rate and contractility and, thus, an increase in cardiac output. Isoproterenol is indicated in the treatment of a number of arrhythmias characterized by reduced automaticity and conductivity. It may be administered as a continuous intravenous infusion (1 to 6 μg/min) or sublingually (10 to 20 mg every 2 to 4 h) in patients with sinus arrest, sinoatrial block, sinus bradycardia, various forms of atrioventricular conduction defects, and Stokes-Adams attacks (Chap. 237). This amine is also useful in a variety of low cardiac output states, including those following cardiac operations and those associated with septic and hemorrhagic shock, unless the peripheral vascular bed is already dilated; during isoproterenol infusion expansion of circulating volume it is often necessary in order to maintain central venous pressure and ventricular preload. Adverse effects include the development of arrhythmias and increase in myocardial oxygen consumption due to enhanced myocardial contractility and heart rate; this may intensify myocardial ischemia. While the bronchodilator properties may be useful in asthmatics, cardiac stimulation may be troublesome even after inhalation. As a result, drugs such as *terbutaline* and *salbutamol* which are relatively more specific for bronchial beta$_2$ receptors have been developed.

Theophylline is another drug used both intravenously and orally in the treatment of bronchospasm (Chap. 257). Its major action is to inhibit phosphodiesterase and, therefore, the breakdown of cyclic AMP. It also causes cardiac stimulation and, in excessive doses, convulsions. The drug is eliminated by hepatic metabolism with little presystemic extraction, so that oral availability is good. When used intravenously, it may be given as a loading dose (5.6 mg/kg slowly) followed by an infusion.

In young adults an average rate of infusion of 0.7 to 0.9 (mg/kg)/h usually gives levels in the therapeutic range of 8 to 20 μg/ml. The infusion rate should be reduced to 70 percent of this rate in neonates and the elderly, and reduced to an even greater extent in patients with cardiac failure or liver disease. Somewhat higher doses may be needed in young children and in patients exposed to enzyme-inducing agents, including cigarettes. Because of considerable variation among individuals in the clearance of theophylline, the concentration of drug in plasma should be measured when infusions extend for more than 12 h, recognizing that a concentration obtained after 12 to 18 h of infusion may not reflect the steady-state concentration, but may provide a warning of excessive accumulation.

Certain sympathomimetic drugs act indirectly by releasing norepinephrine from storage sites as well as having some direct actions. Examples include *metaraminol* and *mephentermine.* Because they eventually cause depletion of the active chemical, norepinephrine, their prolonged use is not recommended and may explain in part the difficulties of weaning patients from these drugs. *Tyramine* acts only indirectly.

SYMPATHOLYTIC AGENTS

ALPHA-ADRENOCEPTOR BLOCKING DRUGS The use of the alpha blockers phentolamine and phenoxybenzamine is largely confined to the diagnosis and treatment of pheochromocytoma (Chap. 337), though phentolamine also has been used to reduce afterload, i.e., the impedance to left ventricular emptying in the treatment of heart failure (Chap. 236). Phentolamine has a relatively rapid onset and evanescent action, and has been used as a test for pheochromocytoma in which hypertension is caused by catecholamine excess. Chronic treatment with alpha blockers is used to control hypertension prior to the operative treatment of pheochromocytoma or in the rare patient with metastatic pheochromocytomas.

Whereas phentolamine and phenoxybenzamine block both pre- and post synaptic alpha receptors, prazosin blocks primarily the postsynaptic (alpha$_1$) receptors on arteriolar and venous smooth muscle. Thus, the feedback inhibition of neurotransmitter release at the presynaptic (alpha$_2$) receptor is less impaired. This may account for the lesser degree of cardiac sympathetic stimulation evoked by prazosin. By reducing both arteriolar and venous tone, prazosin lowers both the venous return and filling of the heart, i.e., the preload, as well as the impedance to left ventricular emptying, i.e., the afterload (Chap. 235) in patients who receive it for the treatment of cardiac failure or hypertension (Chap. 251).

BETA-ADRENOCEPTOR BLOCKING DRUGS The beta-blocking drugs have enjoyed widespread use in the treatment of hypertension, angina pectoris, and certain arrhythmias. Blockade is of the competitive type and antagonizes the effects of catecholamines and sympathetic-nerve stimulation on heart rate, cardiac output, and contractility. Therefore, it tends to reduce resting heart rate and cardiac index in normal subjects, but impairment of cardiac performance is even more pronounced during muscular exercise because of the blockade of the augmented sympathetic activity which occurs during exercise.

Propranolol, the initial beta-adrenoceptor blocker to be widely used clinically, is the prototype for this class. Subsequently, many other beta-adrenoceptor antagonists have been introduced. A number of differences between these beta blockers have been demonstrated, including relative selectivity for the beta$_1$ receptors, the presence or absence of a "membrane-stabilizing" effect, partial beta-agonist activity, and penetration of the blood-brain barrier. The difference which clearly has been shown to have clinical significance is that the rela-

tively selective beta$_1$ antagonists produce less bronchospasm in asthmatic patients at the lower end of the effective dose range, even though higher doses will block bronchial beta receptors as well. Beta agonists such as isoproterenol or salbutamol can more readily surmount the blockade of bronchial beta$_2$ receptors during treatment with the relatively selective beta$_1$ antagonists. Metoprolol, atenolol, tolamolol, and acebutolol are relatively selective beta$_1$ blockers, whereas propranolol, timolol, oxprenolol, alprenolol, sotalol, and pindolol produce essentially equivalent blockade of beta$_1$ and beta$_2$ adrenoceptors. As the brain is the target for some of the adverse effects of the beta-receptor antagonists, the lack of distribution of atenolol into the central nervous system may also be of clinical significance.

In patients with impaired myocardial function and cardiac failure, there is a compensatory reflex sympathetic stimulation of myocardial contractility (Chap. 236). In some patients with severe underlying myocardial dysfunction or excessive volume or pressure overloads, the contribution of the beta-adrenergic system to maintaining cardiac performance is critical, and beta blockade may cause serious deterioration of cardiac output and even profound hypotension. The *intravenous* administration of beta blockers is particularly dangerous in patients with compromised cardiac function. On the other hand, if the major cause of the patient's cardiac failure can be corrected, as is usually the case in hypertension, the use of beta blockers may be considered. Where there is any doubt regarding the underlying myocardial function, beta-blocking drugs should be initiated with small, orally administered doses and under careful observation, as any major problem with reduced cardiac output will be evident immediately upon absorption of the first dose.

Indications Beta-adrenoceptor antagonists, alone or in combination with nitroglycerin or long-acting nitrates, are often effective in patients with angina pectoris in whom nitrates alone have failed to provide relief (Chap. 244). Propranolol with isosorbide dinitrate is one such combination which is felt to be effective. The beneficial effects of beta blockers in angina pectoris probably are achieved by preventing the increased myocardial oxygen requirements induced by sympathetic nervous discharge during physical activity, cold, or emotion. The reduced demand for oxygen allows more prolonged exercise before pain occurs.

A second major use of beta-blocking drugs is the treatment of cardiac arrhythmias, particularly in the abolition and prevention of paroxysmal supraventricular and ventricular tachycardias. They are also useful in reducing excessive ventricular rate in patients with atrial fibrillation (Chap. 237). Their beneficial effects result from prolongation of the refractory period of the atrioventricular junction by blocking adrenergic influences on this system, and this effect of propranolol is additive to that of digitalis. Beta blockade is also efficacious in sinus tachycardia and in the ventricular arrhythmias in pheochromocytoma (Chap. 337). In patients with pheochromocytoma it is important that alpha blockade be present before propranolol administration, otherwise blocking the beta vasodilation due to epinephrine may lead to unopposed alpha vasoconstriction by the catecholamines and subsequent paradoxical hypertension. The mechanism in ventricular arrhythmias is not clearly defined, but in low doses, beta blockade is probably responsible. In some patients who require higher plasma levels, electrophysiologic effects independent of beta blockade may contribute.

Propranolol has been shown to be effective in relieving

many of the symptoms of idiopathic hypertrophic subaortic stenosis (Chap. 247). Its effects are related to a depression of myocardial contractility leading to lessening of the severity of outflow obstruction.

Finally beta blockers are useful in the treatment of hypertension, their particular advantage being to lower pressure equally well in both supine and upright positions (Chap. 251). Their mechanism of action is poorly understood, but several effects may be involved including a reduction in cardiac output and inhibition of renin release leading to a fall in the vasoconstrictor hormone, angiotensin II. The drugs appear particularly useful in young patients with high cardiac output and labile or early hypertension. High-renin essential hypertensives respond well to low doses, while low-renin patients appear to need larger doses (up to 960 mg daily) when propranolol is used as the sole drug. In clinical practice, however, such large doses are seldom required as propranolol in doses up to 240 or 320 mg daily is very effective in combination with diuretics or diuretics plus a vasodilator (Chap. 251).

Pharmacokinetics Propranolol is very efficiently cleared by the liver, so that after intravenous administration its elimination depends on liver blood flow. During chronic oral therapy hepatic extraction is somewhat less, but remains relatively high (65 percent or so), and the half-life is from 3 to 6 h. Hepatic extraction is reduced in patients with liver disease. Much larger doses are required after oral than intravenous administration, because, despite complete alimentary absorption, the drug is extracted presystemically by the liver (Chap. 70). There is considerable variation in clinical response because of differing plasma levels (up to tenfold) due to genetic variation in hepatic extraction as well as the effects of other drugs, age, and smoking habits. Variable plasma binding and the generation of active metabolites may also contribute to the differences in response. All these factors necessitate an exploration of the dose-response curve in clinical practice beginning with 40 to 80 mg daily. Although the half-life is relatively short, propranolol can be given as infrequently as twice daily in the treatment of hypertension, provided the same total daily dose is administered. Metoprolol also is eliminated primarily by hepatic metabolism, having a high degree of presystemic elimination after oral administration and variable concentration in plasma. The half-life is 3 to 4 h.

Adverse effects These occur infrequently (2 to 5 percent) and in addition to precipitation of heart failure (see above) include bizarre vivid dreams, weakness, lethargy, easy fatigability, and occasional exacerbation of psychic depression. Clinically important hypoglycemia may occur in insulin-dependent diabetics in whom the sympathetic defense of hypoglycemia has been blunted and the early warning sign of palpitation is obscured. Beta blockers are specifically contraindicated in patients with impaired cardiac impulse generation or conduction. In patients with second- or third-degree atrioventricular block, they may produce serious bradycardia or even asystole, and in the presence of slowed impulse generation within or conduction from the sinoatrial node (the "sick-sinus syndrome") removal of the influence of norepinephrine can lead to sinoatrial arrest or severe bradycardia. Nonselective beta-blocking drugs are contraindicated in patients with asthma or bronchial constriction, where relatively selective beta$_1$ antagonists are preferred, though these drugs may cause some bronchospasm. Since these drugs are competitive antagonists, their effects can be counteracted by increasing sympathetic activity with isoproterenol, employing larger than usual doses to overcome the competitive beta blockade.

Another adverse reaction is the withdrawal syndrome in which severe angina, arrhythmias, and infarction may occur in patients with angina within 1 to 2 weeks of suddenly stopping the administration of propranolol. This is more common outside the hospital in patients who have gained maximum benefits. Treatment is by bed rest and reinstitution of the drug. If the discontinuation of propranolol in such patients is required, it should be tapered over 1 to 2 weeks.

REDUCTION OF ARTERIAL PRESSURE BY DRUGS ACTING ON THE CENTRAL NERVOUS SYSTEM Two antihypertensives, *methyldopa* and *clonidine,* exert their effect on the central nervous system (Chap. 251). Methyldopa itself has no direct effect on blood pressure regulation. However, it readily crosses the blood-brain barrier and enters adrenergic neurons. Intraneuronally, methyldopa is decarboxylated to form methyldopamine, which in turn is converted by dopamine β-oxidase to α-methylnorepinephrine. α-Methylnorepinephrine, like norepinephrine itself, is stored in the neurosecretory vesicles in adrenergic neurons, and when the nerve is stimulated, this metabolite of methyldopa is released in place of the normal transmitter. In the nucleus tractus solitarius, α-methylnorepinephrine acts as a potent transmitter, stimulating the alpha receptors that evoke an inhibitory effect on sympathetic outflow. Studies with inhibitors suggest that these receptors most closely resemble alpha$_2$ receptors. Because the drug must be metabolized and transported into the granules, it takes some 4 to 6 h to have a maximal effect. Doses of the order of 500 to 2000 mg daily may be required, and a continuing control of blood pressure may be achieved by administration as infrequently as twice daily. Methyldopa does produce some orthostatic hypotension, but this is less marked than with the adrenergic neuron blockers. During treatment renal blood flow is better preserved with this than other antihypertensives. Side effects referable to the central nervous system, including drowsiness, fatigue, impotency, and depression, are usual only with larger doses and are less severe than with reserpine. The most serious toxicities are drug fever and hepatotoxicity which may on rare occasions progress to necrosis. Although 25 percent of patients receiving more than 1 g daily for greater than 6 months will develop a reversible positive direct Coombs' test, fewer than 1 percent will develop frank hemolysis. Although its potential for toxicity requires vigilance, methyldopa is a useful agent.

Clonidine acts to stimulate central alpha receptors directly, and its spectrum of activity is very similar to methyldopa, including a modest orthostatic component and preservation of renal blood flow. Common side effects include sedation, dry mouth, and impotence. The most serious adverse effect is rebound hypertension on cessation of therapy occurring 8 to 36 h later. Characteristic anxiety, headache, sweating, tachycardia, and nausea occur which mimic the sympathetic overactivity seen with pheochromocytoma. Treatment is with alpha blockade.

PARASYMPATHETIC NERVOUS SYSTEM

Drugs that act directly on the efferent limb of the parasympathetic nervous system generally have the disadvantage of acting on the diverse organs which this system innervates. Acetylcholine released from parasympathetic nerves acts on receptors that slow sinoatrial rate and atrioventricular conduction, stimulate salivary, bronchial, and gastric secretion, contract the iris and the ciliary muscle, stimulate bronchial smooth muscle contraction and intestinal motility, sustain penile erection, and promote sweating with attendant heat loss. Thus, atropine, which blocks the action of acetylcholine on parasympathetic receptors (muscarinic receptors), impairs all the above functions to varying degrees, accounting for the side effects that result from its administration.

Acetylcholine also is the neuromuscular transmitter for skeletal muscle as well as the transmitter for preganglionic autonomic neurons, acting on the nicotinic type of receptors in these locations. Thus, the therapeutic use of acetylcholine esterase inhibitors (neostigmine, pyridostigmine) to enhance neuromuscular transmission in myasthenia gravis carries with it attendant side effects on the muscarinic or parasympathetic receptors (Chap. 381). These adverse effects such as gastrointestinal cramping and bronchoconstriction can be attenuated by a careful titration of atropine or other muscarinic receptor blockers. Tolerance is developed to the muscarinic side effects so that parasympathetic receptor blockers may usually be progressively withdrawn.

In contrast to the rather general enhancement of parasympathetic activity achieved with acetylcholine esterase inhibitors, some direct muscarinic-cholinergic agonists possess a relative degree of selectivity within the parasympathetic nervous system. Thus, *bethanechol* in the usually employed doses of 5 mg subcutaneously or 10 mg orally has a relative selectivity for muscarinic receptors in the bladder and the gastrointestinal tract, providing the basis for its use in selective disorders of bladder and gastrointestinal dysfunction.

PARASYMPATHETIC REGULATION OF NORMAL AND ABNORMAL CARDIAC RHYTHM Release of acetylcholine from vagal parasympathetic fibers slows the heart rate by reducing the rate of diastolic depolarization in sinoatrial pacemaker cells, an effect which counters the action of norepinephrine on sinoatrial rate. Similarly, acetylocholine prolongs atrioventricular conduction and the atrioventricular functional refractory period in opposition to the effects of norepinephrine.

Parasympathetic impulses are delivered to the heart via the vagus nerve which arises in the nucleus of the vagus in the medulla. Here, the baroreceptor reflex regulates vagal impulses to the heart in a reciprocal direction from the sympathetic outflow. The afferent baroreceptor fibers entering the nucleus tractus solitarius synapse with interneurons that *stimulate* the vagal nucleus with a resultant increase in efferent vagal traffic and cardiac slowing.

Activation of parasympathetic stimulation of the heart by the baroreceptor reflex can be employed in the treatment of some patients with paroxysmal atrial tachycardia (Chap. 237). There is evidence that a large subset of patients with atrial tachycardia has a sustained reentry pathway that involves vagal-sensitive fibers in the atrioventricular node. In such patients, reversion of the arrhythmia may be accomplished by stimulating the afferent limb of the baroreceptor reflex to evoke parasympathetic stimulation of the heart and reciprocal sympathetic withdrawal with resultant reversion of the arrhythmia. This sometimes may be achieved by a brief Valsalva maneuver or by unilateral massage of the carotid sinus area (only in young patients). If these simple measures are ineffective, elevation of arterial pressure by intravenous administration of alpha-adrenergic agents can be employed to produce a more predictable parasympathetic stimulation of the heart. For example, methoxamine may be given slowly intravenously in doses from 2 to 10 mg with the objective of cautiously elevating systolic pressure by 20 to 40 mmHg. Such maneuvers to evoke an increase in vagal tone by baroreceptor stimulation should be reserved for patients whose left ventricular function is judged adequate to sustain the increased afterload. Cholinergic slowing of conduction in the reentrant pathways associated with paroxysmal atrial tachycardia also can be achieved by blocking the metabolism of acetylcholine released from the vagal parasympathetics. The acetylcholine esterase inhibitor most suited for this purpose is *edrophonium* which has a very brief duration of action. A total of 10 mg edrophonium is given intravenously; an initial test dose of 1 mg may be followed in 2 min by the remaining 9 mg.

Parasympathetic receptor blockers are used to counteract severe bradycardias and atrioventricular block. *Methylscopolamine* appears to have advantages over atropine for this purpose as it does not cause bradycardia at low doses (as has been reported after small intravenous doses of atropine), and it does not cause effects related to blockade of central muscarinic receptors (e.g., delirium). *Methylscopolamine bromide* may be titrated giving 0.75 µg/kg intravenously as the initial dose and repeating 0.75 or 1 µg/kg every 5 min until it is effective or to a total dose of 6 µg/kg.

GANGLION BLOCKING DRUGS

Drugs which block transmission through autonomic ganglia produce the predicted effects of both sympathetic and parasympathetic blockade. The principal drug of this class currently used in therapy is *trimethaphan* which, in addition to lowering blood pressure, also diminishes myocardial contractility and consequently reduces the rate of rise of the arterial pulse, properties that are useful in the medical treatment of aortic dissection (Chap. 252). Side effects include paralytic ileus and urinary retention. High infusion rates (more than 5 mg/min) should be avoided, because such large doses may lead to respiratory depression. Tachyphylaxis may occur if large volumes of fluid are infused concomitantly.

ASSESSMENT OF SYMPATHETIC FUNCTION IN HUMANS

The pathogenesis of sympathetic insufficiency is varied (see Chap. 30). Impairment of the sympathetic nervous system may be suspected on the basis of a substantial drop in blood pressure after 2 to 5 min of standing. Patients with a marked deficiency in blood volume also have orthostatic hypotension, but usually will have a compensatory rise in the heart rate on standing. However, as the heart rate also increases following the withdrawal of parasympathetic stimulation, some disturbances of sympathetic reflex function may be accompanied by a modest increase in cardiac rate upon standing.

The diagnosis of impaired sympathetic function may be approached with some precision, allowing an assessment not only of the intactness of baroreceptor reflex function, but also of whether the lesion resides in the peripheral adrenergic neuron or in the central nervous system. Intactness of baroreceptor reflexes may be assessed by measuring both target organ response and neurotransmitter release. The vasoconstrictor response to hypotension may be assessed by the Valsalva maneuver, in which transient hypotension is produced by increased intrathoracic pressure which diminishes filling of the right side of the heart. In the supine position, the patient exhales into a manometer, maintaining a forced expiratory pressure of 40 mmHg for 10 s. The hypotension developing at the end of the maneuver normally generates a pronounced sympathetic discharge that causes a rebound pressor overshoot in which the diastolic pressure (measured via arterial needle) rises to levels higher than in the pretest period after the hypotensive stimulus is removed. The diastolic pressor overshoot should be proportional to the reduction in pulse pressure at the end of the maneuver, and its attenuation reflects an impaired sympathetic reflex arc. As a result of the pressor overshoot, a vagally mediated reflex bradycardia also occurs normally.

Interruption of the baroreceptor reflex either at the peripheral adrenergic neuron or within the central nervous system also impairs the release of neurotransmitter and is reflected by failure of the concentration of norepinephrine in plasma to rise appropriately with upright posture or exercise. When the deficit is located in the peripheral adrenergic neuron, there also is a reduced level of circulating norepinephrine in the supine position. When the baroreceptor reflex is interrupted by processes that damage the peripheral adrenergic neuron, indirectly acting sympathomimetic amines such as tyramine are ineffective pressor agents, because they act by releasing neuronal norepinephrine. Tyramine will evoke a pressor response when the only abnormality in the sympathetic reflex arc is located proximally to the peripheral adrenergic neuron in the central nervous system as is the case in the Shy-Drager syndrome, or within the afferent limb of the baroreceptor reflex.

The afferent limb of the baroreceptor reflex may be bypassed in assessing the efferent system by employing other stimuli to pressure elevation, as in the cold pressor test. When one hand is immersed in ice-cold water for 1 min, there normally is an increase in blood pressure which averages 16/12 mmHg. An abnormal Valsalva maneuver in the presence of normal cold pressor response suggests an abnormality in the afferent limb of the baroreceptor reflex. The integrity of the efferent pathway also can be tested by measuring the pressor and cardioaccelerator effects of mental arithmetic which does not require either baroreceptor or pain afferents.

REFERENCES

GOLDBERG LI: Dopamine—clinical uses of an endogenous catecholamine. N Engl J Med 291:707, 1974

GROSS, F (ed): *Antihypertensive Agents*. Berlin, Springer-Verlag, 1977

SHAND DG: Propranolol. N Engl J Med 299:280, 1975

TARAZI RC: Sympathomimetic agents in the treatment of shock. Ann Intern Med 81:364, 1974

section 4 | Nutritional disorders

73
NUTRITIONAL REQUIREMENTS

DANIEL RUDMAN

ESSENTIAL AND NONESSENTIAL NUTRIENTS AND THEIR THRESHOLDS (REQUIREMENTS, ALLOWANCES, AND TOLERANCES)

Over the past few decades diverse factors, including increased personal income, expanded public assistance programs, and vitamin and mineral enrichment of food, have reduced the prevalence of the classic nutritional deficiency diseases in the United States. Nevertheless, malnutrition, both overt and subclinical, remains a major problem, especially among the poor, the elderly, alcoholics, the chronically ill, and hospital populations. All too often the patient's nutritional status is ignored during the initial clinical evaluation, and complete nutritional needs are not met during hospitalization. To approach nutritional care rationally, the physician must assess the preexisting nutritional status, calculate the needs for maintenance and repletion, and understand how diseases influence these needs.

The body contains many thousands of species of organic molecules but requires for health the intake of only 21 organic compounds in addition to a source of calories: eight essential amino acids, one fatty acid, eleven vitamins, and water. The vast majority of organic molecules in food, although metabolized or assimilated by the body, are "nonessential" in the sense that their deletion from the diet does not cause illness. The simplicity of the *nutritional requirements* of the healthy subject, compared with the complexity of his *chemical composition,* is the result of the remarkable capacity for endogenous biosynthesis.

Of the limited number of *inorganic* compounds in food, the majority of their constituent elements, that is, 15, are believed to be nutritionally essential: calcium, phosphorus, iodine, iron, magnesium, zinc, copper, potassium, sodium, chloride, cobalt, chromium, manganese, molybdenum, and selenium.

The *minimal daily requirement* of an essential nutrient is the smallest quantity that maintains normal mass, chemical composition, morphology, and physiological functions of the various tissues and organs of the body and prevents any clinical or biochemical sign of the corresponding deficiency state. In children, an additional criterion is a normal rate of growth. Tables 73-1 to 73-3 list the minimal requirements of the 36 essential nutrients (21 organic, 15 inorganic) needed by adults, and Table 73-4 describes the main features of the illness which ensues when each essential nutrient is deficient. In children, two additional amino acids, arginine and histidine, are required. "Macro-" and "micronutrients" are defined on the basis of a daily requirement greater or less than 100 mg, respectively.

Minimal daily requirements are determined as follows:

1 In healthy adults the minimal daily requirement of protein (or its constituent amino acids) and macrominerals can be assessed by the elemental balance technique. Daily balance of each element equals intake minus output (urinary plus fecal). The requirement of each amino acid or macromineral is the smallest intake that maintains zero balance for nitrogen or for the mineral under study. Negative balance of any essential element, if it persists long enough, leads to illness and death.
2 In the infant or growing child the requirement of calories and essential nutrients is the smallest amount of each that maintains an optimal rate of growth while all others are fed in adequate amounts.
3 For micronutrients the requirement is the smallest daily intake that prevents eventual appearance of the nutrient-specific deficiency state.

The *recommended daily allowances* (RDA) of each nutrient range from 1.5 to 10 times the minimal daily requirements. Because the requirements vary among individuals due to numerous genetic and environmental circumstances, the minimal daily requirement may provide a *suboptimal* amount of a nutrient for a substantial minority of the healthy population. Accordingly, RDAs provide a margin of safety sufficient to meet

TABLE 73-1

Adult minimal daily requirements* for "reference man"† and "reference woman"‡

Nutrient	Requirements
Water	1–5 liters
Energy	2000–2700 kcal
Protein	28–33 g
Linoleic acid	3 g
Retinol equivalents	390
Vitamin D	Sunlight
Vitamin E activity	3–6 IU
Ascorbic acid	10 mg
Folacin§	50 μg
Niacin¶	9–12 mg
Riboflavin	1–1.4 mg
Thiamine	0.7–0.9 mg
Vitamin B_6	0.6–1.3 mg
Vitamin B_{12}	1 μg
Pantothenic acid	5 mg
Calcium	200–400 mg
Phosphorus	400 mg
Iodine	58–70 μg
Iron	6.5–9 mg
Magnesium	200 mg
Zinc	8–10 mg
Copper	2 mg
Potassium	2500 mg
Sodium	400 mg
Chloride	500 mg
Cobalt	0–1 μg
Chromium	200–290 μg
Manganese	2.5–2.7 mg
Molybdenum	45–500 μg
Selenium	0.1 μg

* *No minimum presently recognized for cholesterol, biotin, vitamin K, choline, cadmium, fluoride, nickel, tin, vanadium, silicon, and boron.*
† *"Reference man": 35 years old, 70 kg in weight, 172 cm tall, moderately active, temperate climate.*
‡ *"Reference woman": 35 years old, 58 kg in weight, 162 cm tall, moderatively active, temperate climate.*
§ *The folacin allowance refers to dietary sources as determined by* Lactobacillus casei *assay. Pure forms of folacin may be effective in doses one-fourth of the requirement listed here.*
¶ *One milligram of niacin may be derived from every 60 mg dietary tryptophan.*
SOURCE: *RS Goodhart, E Shils, Modern Nutrition in Health and Diseases, 5th ed, Philadelphia, Lea & Febiger, 1973.*

difficult (e.g., protein intake of a cachectic, encephalopathic, cirrhotic patient).

PHYSIOLOGICAL FACTORS Growth, exercise, pregnancy, and lactation (Table 73-2) increase the daily requirements per kilogram of body weight for calories and most essential nutrients. Caloric requirement declines with age.

COMPOSITION OF THE DIET Given diets with identical contents of nitrogen, digestible carbohydrates, fat, vitamins, and minerals, the metabolic availability of the nutrients may vary widely. Thus all proteins are not equally effective in meeting the daily requirement because of differences in digestibility or in content of essential amino acids. Gastrointestinal absorption of some minerals is influenced by the presence in the diet of other reactive components; the utilization of vitamins may be influenced by level of intake of organic macronutrients. Examples are given in Table 73-6.

ROUTE, RATE, AND TIMING (See Chap. 78) The requirements and allowances listed in Tables 73-1 to 3 apply to *enteral* nutrition. For some nutrients, different values will be required for *parenteral* nutrition. Net gastrointestinal absorption of ingested amino acids, carbohydrates, fats, sodium, chloride, and potassium normally is greater than 90 percent (Table 73-7), and these nutrients from this point of view have the same RDAs for the intravenous as for the enteral route. For the remaining essential minerals, however, net absorption is only 50 percent or less (Table 73-7); consequently the intravenous requirement is only a fraction of the oral one. It is also likely that the requirements of amino acids are not identical by enteral and parenteral routes. After ingestion and absorption into the portal venous system, a portion of the absorbed amino acids is catabolized during the "first pass" through the liver, where many of the enzymes of amino acid degradation are located. Intravenously infused amino acids, in contrast, can bypass these catabolic pathways and directly perfuse sites of protein synthesis in muscle and other extrahepatic tissues.

Timing can be important. For example, all essential amino acids must be supplied simultaneously to support protein synthesis. If even one of the essential amino acids is administered at a different time than the other essential and nonessential acids, assimilation of all into protein is curtailed. Similarly, when amino acids, glucose, lipids, and minerals are infused at separate times during the day or week, as often happens in parenteral feeding, assimilation may be impaired. Thus omission of phosphorus or potassium from central hyperalimentation solutions impairs retention of the nitrogen furnished by the same fluid. For these reasons the requirements of several essential nutrients by the *parenteral route* remain uncertain even though parenteral nutrition is a major component of clinical therapeutics.

DISEASE Nutritional requirements and tolerances may be altered by disease through at least seven mechanisms (see also Table 73-8):

1 Increased utilization of nutrients. Fever, infection, and trauma increase resting metabolic rate and, as a consequence, daily caloric requirement. Folate is utilized more rapidly in patients with hemolysis and increased cell turnover (hemolytic anemia, psoriasis, cancer). Many nutritional

the needs of virtually the entire healthy population (Table 73-2).

Another nutritional threshold is the maximal daily tolerance of a nutrient. Just as intake of any essential nutrient *below* a specific level causes disease, likewise intake *above* a certain level for many nutrients (either essential or nonessential) disturbs body structure or function (Table 73-5). A physiologic diet provides intakes of each nutrient between the two thresholds of minimal requirement and maximal tolerance. The recognition that tolerance for a nutrient can be exceeded is particularly important during parenteral nutrition, when the gastrointestinal mechanisms (emesis, incomplete absorption, diarrhea) that ordinarily protect the patient at least partially from the ill effects of excessive nutrient intake are bypassed. Unfortunately, although requirements and allowances have been established for each of the 31 essential nutrients, the maximal tolerance for most nutrients is uncertain.

FACTORS ALTERING NUTRITIONAL THRESHOLDS

Both the minimal requirement and maximal tolerance of each essential nutrient are influenced by a host of factors: rate of growth, age, exercise, pregnancy and lactation, chemical composition of the diet, diseases, drugs. In addition, the route, rate, and timing of alimentation influence requirements and tolerances. As the "distance" between requirement and tolerance narrows, nutritional management of the patient becomes more

TABLE 73-2
Recommended daily dietary allowances[a]

Age, years	Weight, kg	Height, cm	Energy, kcal	Protein, g	Fat-soluble vitamins		Vitamin D, IU	Vitamin E activity,[c] IU
					Vitamin A activity			
					RE[b]	IU		
INFANTS								
0.0–05	6	60	kg × 117	kg × 2.2	420	1400	400	4
0.5–1.0	9	71	kg × 108	kg × 2.0	400	2000	400	5
CHILDREN								
1–3	13	86	1300	23	400	2000	400	7
4–6	20	110	1800	30	500	2500	400	9
7–10	30	135	2400	36	700	3300	400	10
MALES								
11–14	44	158	2800	44	1000	5000	400	12
15–18	61	172	3000	54	1000	5000	400	15
19–22	67	172	3000	54	1000	5000	400	15
23–50	70	172	2700	56	1000	5000		15
51+	70	172	2400	56	1000	5000		15
FEMALES								
11–14	44	155	2400	44	800	4000	400	12
15–18	54	162	2100	48	800	4000	400	12
19–22	58	162	2100	46	800	4000	400	12
23–50	58	162	2000	46	800	4000		12
51+	58	162	1800	46	800	4000		12
PREGNANCY								
			+300	+30	1000	5000	400	15
LACTATION								
			+500	+20	1200	6000	400	15

[a] *The allowances are intended to provide for individual variations among most normal persons as they live in the United States under usual environmental stresses. Diets should be based on a variety of common foods in order to provide other nutrients for which human requirements have been less well-defined. Adult RDA for water, 1 ml/cal; for linoleic acid, 1 to 2 percent of total caloric intake.*

[b] *Retinol equivalents (RE): Assumed to be all as retinol in milk during the first 6 months of life. All subsequent intakes are assumed to be half as retinol and half as β-carotene when calculated from international units. As retinol equivalents, three-fourths are as retinol and one-fourth as β-carotene.*

[c] *Total vitamin E activity, estimated to be 80 percent as α-tocopherol and 20 percent as other tocopherols.*

requirements are greater during repletion from cachexia than during maintenance of normal nutriture. In this respect, the repletion process in adults resembles growth in children.

2 *Malabsorption.* For each nutrient absorbed less efficiently than normal in malabsorption states, the daily requirement is increased correspondingly.

3 *Impaired ability to activate a nutrient.* The requirement for vitamin D is increased by renal disease which impairs hydroxylation of the vitamin; requirements for folate, thiamine, and pyridoxine in cirrhotics may be greater than normal because of impaired hepatic capacity to transform these vitamins into their active forms.

4 *Abnormally large losses of nutrients.* Impaired conservation of sodium, phosphorus, or amino acids because of renal disease, burns, blood loss, nasogastric suction, diarrhea, or hemodialysis leads to loss of nutrients. One criterion of normal nutriture for nitrogen and minerals in the adult is zero elemental balance, i.e., enteral or parenteral intake equal to urinary plus fecal output. If output of nitrogen or mineral is increased by abnormal renal or extrarenal loss, then intake must be correspondingly higher to maintain zero balance.

5 *Impaired catabolic or excretory pathways.* Metabolic defects can reduce both requirement and tolerance, because the rate of degradation or excretion of a nutrient is slowed. In children with phenylketonuria or maple syrup urine disease, the requirements for phenylalanine or branched-chain amino acids, respectively, are less than in normals. Patients with uremia have a reduced dietary requirement for nonessential amino acids.

6 *Hyperabsorption.* Increased absorption can result in a decrease in both requirement and tolerance. Examples are calcium in hyperabsorptive hypercalciuria, iron in hemochromatosis, and copper in Wilson's disease.

7 *Drugs.* Pharmacological agents can alter nutritional requirements by causing malabsorption or renal loss of a nutrient, by preventing its metabolic utilization, or by accelerating its degradation (Table 73-9).

INDIVIDUAL ESSENTIAL NUTRIENTS

WATER A reasonable allowance is 1 ml/cal for adults and 150 ml/kg for infants. The minimal daily requirement, considerably less than the customary allowance, depends on the preformed and potential solutes ingested (largely protein, sodium, chloride, and potassium), the concentrating ability of the kidney, and extrarenal losses. Normally 50 to 100 ml per day is excreted in the feces, 400 to 600 ml is lost by exhalation and

Ascorbic Acid, mg	Folacin,[d] μg	Niacin,[e] mg	Riboflavin, mg	Thiamine, mg	Vitamin B6, mg	Vitamin B12, μg	Calcium, mg	Phosphorus, mg	Iodine, μg	Iron, mg	Magnesium, mg	Zinc, mg
35	50	5	0.4	0.3	0.3	0.3	360	240	35	10	60	3
35	50	8	0.6	0.5	0.4	0.3	540	400	45	15	70	5
40	100	9	0.8	0.7	0.6	1.0	800	800	60	15	150	10
40	200	12	1.1	0.9	0.9	1.5	800	800	80	10	200	10
40	300	16	1.2	1.2	1.2	2.0	800	800	110	10	250	10
45	400	18	1.5	1.4	1.6	3.0	1200	1200	130	18	350	15
45	400	20	1.8	1.5	2.0	3.0	1200	1200	150	18	400	15
45	400	20	1.8	1.5	2.0	3.0	800	800	140	10	350	15
45	400	18	1.6	1.4	2.0	3.0	800	800	130	10	350	15
45	400	16	1.5	1.2	2.0	3.0	800	800	110	10	350	15
45	400	16	1.3	1.2	1.6	3.0	1200	1200	115	10	350	15
45	400	14	1.4	1.1	2.0	3.0	1200	1200	115	18	300	15
45	400	14	1.4	1.1	2.0	3.0	800	800	100	18	300	15
45	400	13	1.2	1.0	2.0	3.0	800	800	100	18	300	15
45	400	12	1.1	1.0	2.0	3.0	800	800	80	18	300	15
60	800	+ 2	+ 0.3	+ 0.3	2.5	4.0	1200	1200	125	10	300	20
80	800	+ 4	+ 0.5	+ 0.3	2.5	4.0	1200	1200	250	18 +[g]	450	25

[d] *The folacin allowances refer to dietary sources as determined by* Lactobacillus casei *assay. Pure forms of folacin may be effective in doses less than one-fourth of the recommended dietary allowance.*

[e] *Although allowances are expressed as niacin, it is recognized that on the average 1 mg niacin is derived from each 60 mg dietary tryptophan.*

[f] *Reasonable guides for intake of the other essential minerals, expressed as milligrams per day, are: potassium, 2500; chloride, 2000; sodium, 2500; copper, 2.*

[g] *This increased requirement cannot be met by ordinary diets; therefore, the use of supplemental iron is recommended.*

SOURCE: *Food and Nutrition Board.*

evaporation (insensible loss), and the remainder is excreted in the urine. Water intake must equal these losses for the subject to maintain water balance and avoid under- or overhydration.

Maximal tolerance normally is more than 5 liters daily because of the kidney's large capacity for free water clearance. Water requirement and tolerance are increased by factors that cause increased losses in urine, feces, or sweat. The obligatory urinary loss is proportional to the excretion of solutes (largely urea, Na^+, K^+, and Cl^-) and the kidney's concentrating capacity; it is increased in proportion to intake of protein, Na^+, K^+, and Cl^-. Water requirements are increased by deficiency of antidiuretic hormone and decreased when the hormone is secreted inappropriately. Fecal loss of water may increase to over 5 liters per day in severe diarrhea. Nasogastric suction, ileostomy, gastrointestinal fistulas, and burns similarly increase daily water requirements. Water loss is excessive during fever, heavy exercise, or exposure to high environmental temperature. Each degree Celsius of fever causes an obligatory loss of about 200 ml water per day.

CALORIES To maintain stable weight, caloric intake must equal caloric output. The output can be divided into *basal* and *activity* components. Basal metabolic rate (BMR) is usually measured in the fasting, resting subject immediately after awaking. Standard values are given in Table 73-10; values during sleep are about 10 percent less. After each meal, metabolic rate increases up to 30 percent; during each day, this "specific dynamic action" amounts to about 6 percent of the basal caloric expenditure. BMR declines with age by about 3 to 10 percent per decade. It is rarely measured except for experimental purposes.

Activity increases caloric demands. Mild, moderate, or severe exercise raises caloric expenditure by roughly 30, 50, or 100 (or more) percent, respectively. Caloric expenditures in specific types of activity are described in Chap. 76.

TABLE 73-3
Minimal daily requirements for young adult male subjects of the essential amino acids

Amino acid	Requirement, mg
L-Threonine	500
L-Valine	800
L-Methionine	1100
L-Isoleucine	700
L-Leucine	1100
L-Phenylalanine	1100
L-Lysine	800
L-Tryptophan	250

TABLE 73-4
Syndromes of undernutrition

Nutrient	Signs and symptoms of deficiency	Laboratory tests
Water	Thirst, poor tissue turgor, dry mucous membranes, vascular collapse, altered mental status	Serum electrolytes ↑, serum osmolarity ↑, total body water ↓
Calories (energy)	Weakness and physical inactivity, loss of subcutaneous fat, muscle wasting, bradycardia	Weight loss, TSF ↓, MAMC ↓, creatinine/ht ↓, BMR ↓
Protein	Psychomotor change, dyspigmented, sparse, and easily plucked hair, "flaky-paint" dermatitis, edema, muscle wasting, hepatomegaly	MAMC ↓, serum albumin and transferrin ↓, anemia, creatinine/ht ↓, serum nonessential/essential amino acids ↑, urine urea/creatinine ↓
Linoleic acid	Xerosis	Serum ratio of triene to tetraene fatty acids ↑
Sodium	Muscle weakness and cramps, confusion, apathy, anorexia, hypotension, oliguria	Serum Na^+ ↓, BUN/creatinine ↑
Chloride	Muscle cramps, apathy, anorexia	Serum Cl^- ↓
Potassium	Lassitude, polyuria, ileus, muscular weakness	Serum and urine K^+ ↓, body ^{40}K ↓, abnormal ECG
Calcium	Stunted growth, rickets, osteomalacia, convulsions	Osteopenia by x-ray, serum $Ca^\dagger$ ↓
Phosphorus	Weakness, osteomalacia	Osteopenia by x-ray, serum P ↓
Magnesium	Growth failure, behavioral disturbances, weakness, tremor, tetany, seizures, cardiac arrhythmias	Serum, urine, and RBC Mg ↓
Iron	Pallor, weakness, reduced resistance to infection, angular stomatitis, atrophic lingual papillae, koilonychia	Plasma and marrow iron ↓, microcytic hypochromic anemia
Fluorine	Higher frequency of tooth decay	
Zinc	Growth restriction, hypogonadism, delayed puberty, slow wound healing, hypogeusia	Plasma, hair, and 24-h urine zinc ↓
Copper	Pallor	Hypochromic microcytic anemia, osteopenia, plasma and urine copper ↓
Iodine	Goiter, symptoms of hypothyroidism	TSH ↑, T_4 and T_3 ↓, 24-h urine iodine ↓, RAI uptake ↑
Thiamine (vitamin B_1)	Beriberi, muscle tenderness and weakness, hyporeflexia, hypesthesia, tachycardia, cardiomegaly, congestive heart failure	Erythrocyte thiamine pyrophosphate and transketolase activity ↓ and in vitro effect thereon of thiamine pyrophosphate ↑; urinary thiamine ↓, blood pyruvate, α-ketoglutarate levels ↑
Riboflavin (vitamin B_2)	Angular stomatitis (or angular scars), cheilosis, magenta tongue, atrophic lingual papillae, corneal vascularization, angular blepharitis, dyssebacia, scrotal (vulvar) dermatosis	EGR activity ↓ and in vitro effect on EGR activity of flavin adenine dinucleotide ↑
Niacin (vitamin B_3)	Pellagra, scarlet and raw tongue, atrophic lingual papillae, tongue fissuring, mental disorders, pellagrous dermatosis, diarrhea	Urinary N^1-methylnicotinamide ↓
Pyridoxine (vitamin B_6)	Nasolabial seborrhea, glossitis, kidney stones, peripheral neuropathy, muscular twitching, convulsions, microcytic anemia	EGOT activity ↓ and in vitro effect of pyridoxal phosphate on EGOT activity ↑; tryptophan load test ↓ (urinary excretion of xanthurenic and quinolinic acids); urinary vitamin B_6 excretion ↓
Pantothenic acid	Fatigue, sleep disturbances, impaired coordination, nausea	
Folic acid	Pallor, glossitis, stomatitis, diarrhea, anemia	Erythrocyte and serum folate concentration ↓; urine formiminoglutamic acid excretion ↑ after histidine load; macrocytic anemia, polymorphonuclear leukocytes hypersegmented, megaloblastic bone marrow
Vitamin B_{12}	Pallor, mild icterus, anorexia, diarrhea, paresthesia, ataxia, optic neuritis, mental changes	Serum vitamin B_{12} ↓; peripheral blood and bone marrow morphology
Biotin	Fatigue, depression, nausea, dermatitis, muscular pains	
Vitamin C	Scurvy, petechiae, ecchymoses, perifollicular hemorrhage, spongy and bleeding gums (if not edentulous)	Ascorbic acid concentration in plasma, platelets, whole blood, and white blood cells ↓; urinary ascorbic acid ↓
Vitamin A	Xerosis of eye and skin, xerophthalmia, Bitot's spot, follicular hyperkeratosis	Plasma vitamin A ↓ Dark adaptation time ↑
Vitamin D	Rickets and growth failure in children, osteomalacia in adults	Serum alkaline phosphatase concentration ↑; plasma 25-hydroxycholecalciferol ↓; serum Ca and P ↓
Vitamin E	Anemia	
Vitamin K	Bleeding diathesis	Prothrombin time ↑

NOTE: *BMR* = basal metabolism rate; *BUN* = blood-urea nitrogen; *creatinine/ht* = 24-h urine creatinine/height ratio; *ECG* = electrocardiogram; *EGOT* = erythrocyte glutamic-oxaloacetic transaminase; *EGR* = erythrocyte glutathione reductase; *MAMC* = midarm muscle circumference; *RAI* = radioactive iodine; *RBC* = red blood cell; T_3 = triiodothyronine; T_4 = thyroxine; *TSF* = triceps skin fold; *TSH* = thyroid-stimulating hormone.

TABLE 73-5
Syndromes which can result from excessive intake or absorption of nutrients by oral route, or excessive infusion by parenteral route

Nutrient	Manifestation of overnutrition
Water	Edema, headache, nausea, hypertension
Calories	Obesity
Protein	Exacerbation of inborn errors in amino acid catabolism or "nitrogen accumulation diseases"; hepatic encephalopathy
Calcium	Hypercalcemia, mental and renal dysfunction
Potassium	Muscular weakness, arrhythmia, death
Sodium chloride	Hypertension, edema, heart failure
Magnesium	Diarrhea
Iron	Siderosis, hemochromatosis
Fluorine	Mottling of teeth, increased bone density, neurological disturbances
Zinc	Fever, nausea, vomiting, diarrhea
Copper	Wilson's disease
Manganese	Generalized disease of nervous system
Iodine	Depression of thyroid activity, goiter, occasional hyperthyroidism
Ascorbic acid (vitamin C)	Hyperoxaluria, destruction of vitamin B_{12}
Retinol (vitamin A)	Headache, vomiting, peeling of skin, anorexia, swelling of long bones, cirrhosis
Phylloquinone (vitamin K)	At high doses may cause jaundice
Vitamin D	Hypercalcemia, nephrolithiasis, impaired renal function

The daily energy requirement equals the sum of expenditures incurred by basal metabolism, specific dynamic action, and physical activity. The requirement can be estimated by assessing basal caloric expenditure per day from the subject's surface area (Table 73-10), using ideal body weight in this calculation. Subtract 10 percent from basal during the sleeping hours. Add 6 percent to the 24-h basal estimate to cover the specific dynamic action of meals. From an activity-calorie chart, such as is given in Chap. 76, calculate the caloric expenditure of the subject's physical activities during a typical day. The daily caloric output can be estimated as the sum of basal requirements (minus correction for sleep) plus specific dynamic action plus caloric requirement for physical activity. Since on average 93 percent of caloric intake is utilized and 7 percent is

TABLE 73-6
Some essential nutrients for which the daily dietary requirement is influenced by other dietary components

Nutrient	Influence by other dietary component
Calcium, magnesium, iron	Absorption decreased by phytates
Calcium	Urinary excretion increased by high protein intake
Essential amino acids	Utilization curtailed if any essential amino acid is deficient
Nonheme iron	Absorption improved by vitamin C or meat
Folic acid	Protected from destruction during cooking by ascorbic acid
Vitamin B_6	Requirement increased by protein
Vitamin E	Requirement proportional to intake of essential fatty acids
Thiamine	Requirement proportional to calories
Protein	Requirement inversely related to calories when the latter are deficient
Niacin	Requirement inversely related to tryptophan intake
Phenylalanine	Requirement inversely related to tyrosine intake
Methionine	Requirement inversely related to cystine intake
Valine, leucine, isoleucine	Requirement of each is increased by excess of the other branched chain amino acid(s)

TABLE 73-7
Net absorption of nutrients by normal adults

Element	Percent	Element	Percent
Protein	>90	Cu	~30
Carbohydrate	>90	Co	20–95
Fat	>95	Mn	<5
Na	>95	Se	40–70
K	80–90	F	80–90
Cl	>95	Cr	1–3
Ca	5–40	Mo	40–50
Mg	25–50	Zn	33
P	50–60	I	>90
Fe	5–15		
Cu	~30		

lost in feces and urine, the estimated caloric requirement for zero balance equals 107 percent of the calculated output.

In actual practice, a simpler formula can be used. Twenty-two calories per kilogram of ideal body weight are allowed for basal metabolism. For sedentary, moderate, or heavy activity, add 30, 50, or 100 percent, respectively. Weight is monitored weekly, and if weight increases or decreases, calories are adjusted accordingly.

Caloric expenditure is increased by fever (about 13 percent over basal per degree Celsius), burns (10 to 100 percent), trauma (40 to 100 percent), and hyperthyroidism (10 to 100 percent). Hypometabolism, whether of thyroidal or other cause, lowers the energy expenditure and, therefore, the energy requirement.

Patients with severe malabsorption may absorb as little as 25 percent of their ingested calories (fat, carbohydrate, protein) compared with the normal value of over 95 percent. In these patients, oral caloric requirement is higher than normal and may prove impossible to achieve if diarrhea is aggravated by increased nutrient intake. In such patients only parenteral nutrition can prevent progressive starvation.

PROTEIN Dietary protein provides the body a mixture of amino acids for endogenous protein synthesis and is also a metabolic fuel for energy (see Chap. 85). Healthy adults require eight essential amino acids in amounts varying from 250 to 1100 mg per day. About 30 g of nonessential amino acids is

TABLE 73-8
Diseases which alter nutrient requirements by the oral route

Nutrient	Increases dietary requirement	Reduces dietary requirement
Calories	Fever, hyperthyroidism, trauma, malabsorption	Coma, hypothyroidism
Protein	Fever, hyperthyroidism, trauma, azotorrhea	Nitrogen accumulation diseases, inborn errors of urea synthesis
Phenylalanine		Phenylketonuria
Branched-chain amino acids		Maple syrup urine diseases
Linoleic acid and fat-soluble vitamins	Malabsorption syndromes	
Calcium	Malabsorption syndromes	Hyperabsorptive hypercalciuria
Magnesium	Malabsorption syndromes	
Iron	Malabsorption syndromes	Hemochromatosis
Copper		Wilson's disease
Phosphorus	Malabsorption syndromes	Renal insufficiency
Folic acid	Increased cell turnover	
Carnitine*	Advanced cirrhosis	

* No requirement normally.

TABLE 73-9
Drugs capable of causing undernutrition

Drug	Nutrient	Mechanism
Diuretics	Water, Na, Cl, Ca, Mg, K	↑ renal excretion
Neomycin	Protein, Ca, Mg, linoleic acid	Malabsorption
Colchicine, cholestyramine	Fat-soluble vitamins, Fe, vitamin B_{12}	Malabsorption
Aluminum hydroxide, calcium carbonate (antacids), calomel (laxative)	P	Decreased intestinal absorption
Anticonvulsants (phenobarbital, phenytoin primidone, glutethimide, diphosphonates)	Vitamin D, Ca, folic acid	Altered metabolism
Alcohol	Folic acid, Mg, protein, thiamine	Malabsorption, anorexia, magnesuria
Chelating agents (D-penicillamine, EDTA)	Zn, Cu, Fe, Ca, Mg	↑ renal excretion
Isoniazid	Pyridoxine	Hydrazide formation
Potassium chloride	Vitamin B_{12}	Malabsorption
Mineral oil	Fat-soluble vitamins	Malabsorption

TABLE 73-11
Biologic value of food proteins*

Protein source	Biologic value
Milk	93
Egg	93
Beef	76
Peanut meal	74
Corn	72
Potato	69
Oat	65
Rice	65
Corn	50
Soy flour	41
Wheat gluten	40

* *As determined from nitrogen balance studies conducted in the rat, generally at a dietary protein concentration of 5 percent. Tests in the rat at other concentrations, or in other species, give generally similar but not identical biologic values.*

also required for protein synthesis. The requirement and allowance of dietary protein depend on the biologic value of the proteins ingested. *Biologic value* is defined as the proportion of absorbed protein retained by the body under standard test conditions. It is primarily dependent on the content of essential amino acids. Nearly optimal ratios of the eight essential and twelve nonessential amino acids are present in egg and milk proteins, which consequently have the highest biologic values for the diet, viz., 90 to 95 (Table 73-11). The biologic value of proteins in the world's major food products follows the general order: animal products > cereals (rice, wheat, corn) > legumes > roots. The adult RDA for protein given in Table 73-2, about 50 g per day, assumes a biologic value of about 80, a characteristic value when animal products are the major protein source. The lower the biologic value, the higher the daily protein requirement.

Plant proteins have low biologic value because one or more essential amino acids are deficient. Thus for corn (maize), lysine, threonine, and tryptophan are limiting; for soy beans and green peas, methionine; for rice, lysine and threonine; for wheat, lysine. Therefore, mixtures of two "complementary" vegetable proteins deficient in different essential amino acids have a higher biologic value than either protein separately.

While the usual reason for low biologic value of a particular protein or mixture of proteins is limiting content of one or

TABLE 73-10
Basal caloric requirements of normal subjects

Age, years	Males, $(cal/m^2)/h$	Females, $(cal/m^2)/h$
14–16	46.0	43.0
16–18	43.0	40.0
18–20	41.0	38.0
20–30	39.5	37.0
30–40	39.5	36.5
40–50	38.5	36.0
50–60	37.5	35.0
60–70	36.5	34.0
70–80	35.5	33.0

SOURCE: *EF DuBois, Basal Metabolism in Health and Disease, 3d ed, Philadelphia, Lea & Febiger, 1936, p 151.*

more essential amino acids, excess of an amino acid can also impair the value. For example, excessive intake of leucine increases the requirement for isoleucine; this type of influence is termed *amino acid imbalance* and is an important consideration in planning the composition of mixtures of synthetic amino acids for parenteral or enteral feeding. In addition, certain amino acids may be "spared" by chemically related amino acids. For example, tyrosine and cystine are in part converted to phenylalanine and methionine, respectively, and therefore spare the latter substances.

The daily requirement of a protein, or its constituent amino acids, is also influenced by caloric intake; the values for protein requirement and allowance given in Tables 72-1 to 72-3 assume adequate caloric intake. When the caloric requirement is met by nonprotein calories, a substantial portion of ingested amino acids is utilized for protein synthesis. If calories are deficient, amino acids are diverted from protein synthesis into pathways of oxidative metabolism and gluconeogenesis. Under these circumstances, the daily protein requirement is inversely proportional to the caloric intake. Thus, caloric undernutrition makes a person more vulnerable to protein starvation, an interaction which accounts for the high prevalence of the combined deficiency state *protein-energy undernutrition* (see Chap. 75).

The daily protein requirement per unit body weight is increased by growth, pregnancy, lactation, repletion after cachexia, fever, infection, trauma, and malabsorption.

To understand how the "nitrogen accumulation diseases," hepatic and renal insufficiency, alter the requirements and tolerances of dietary protein, consider the scheme of amino acid metabolism shown in Fig. 73-1. The daily adult requirement of about 50 g protein serves to maintain reaction 2, that is, protein synthesis, at a rate equal to protein breakdown (reaction 3). Tolerance for protein is greater than 250 g per day because of the high capacity of the degradative pathway (reactions 4, 6, 7, and 9). Note that 20 to 40 percent of urea formed in the liver is hydrolyzed by microbes within the colon and recycles at least once as ammonia (reaction 8). When step 10 is blocked (uremia), the requirement for nonessential nitrogen is reduced. Urea, instead of being excreted, recycles as ammonia and remains available for synthesis of nonessential amino acids; the carbon skeletons of these acids are readily produced by the intermediary metabolism of glucose. This pathway for endogenous synthesis of nonessential amino acids is the basis for the Giovanetti diet in uremia. If the uremic patient is fed the carbon skeletons (α-keto derivatives) of the *essential* amino acids, the requirement of the latter nutrients (except for threonine and lysine) is also reduced because of the reversibility of transamination, i.e., reaction 5 in Fig. 73-1. Similar considerations apply in advanced cirrhosis and in hereditary disorders of urea synthesis.

FIGURE 73-1
Overview of amino acid metabolism.

Not only is the daily requirement for protein in some ure- mics and cirrhotics lower than normal, but the maximal toler- ance is curtailed as well. As little as 20 g protein a day can precipitate or aggravate symptoms of hepatocerebral disease in the susceptible hepatic patient. Intakes of protein customary for healthy subjects in the United States (80 to 100 g per day) can also intensify the uremic syndrome.

FAT While the average adult in the United States eats 70 to 120 g fat per day, the only actual requirement is for about 3 g linoleic acid per day. Within the range 3 to 120 g fat, it is unclear what intake to recommend, except as dictated by body weight considerations. Palatability requires a minimum of 40 g. In patients predisposed to hyperlipoproteinemia by heredity or obesity, the distribution of calories between fat and carbo- hydrates influences the severity of the lipemia.

MINERALS AND VITAMINS The daily requirements/allow- ances and the influence of physiological and pathological cir- cumstances on these thresholds are listed in Tables 73-1, 73-2, 73-6, and 73-8. The deficiency syndromes corresponding to each nutrient are listed in Table 73-4, and some clinical effects of exceeding the daily tolerance are given in Table 73-5 (see also Chaps. 79 to 82).

REFERENCES

FOOD AND NUTRITION BOARD: *Recommended Dietary Allowances.* Washington, DC, National Academy of Sciences, 1974

HERBERT V: The five possible causes of all nutrient deficiency: Illus- trated by deficiencies of vitamin B_{12} and folic acid. Am J Clin Nutr 26:77, 1973

ROE D: Drug-induced nutritional deficiencies. Westport, Conn, Avi Publishing Company, 1976

SCRIMSHAW NW, YOUNG UR: The requirements of human nutrition. Sci Am 235:50, September 1976

SHILS E: Nutrition and neoplasia, in *Modern Nutrition in Health and Disease,* 5th ed, RS Goodhart, ME Shils (eds). Philadelphia, Lea & Febiger, 1973, pp 981–996

74

ASSESSMENT OF NUTRITIONAL STATUS

DANIEL RUDMAN

Undernutrition is a common contribution to morbidity and mortality in most hospitals. As a peculiar discrepancy, how- ever, undernutrition rarely appears on charts in the list of diag- noses or in the progress notes. Consequently, quantitative tests of nutritional status are rare in the initial clinical workup, and the progress of the nutritional state is not monitored regularly during the course of illness. As a result, undernutrition tends to be recognized late, when it is severe and difficult to treat. This chapter defines feasible methods for identifying and quantify- ing the deficiency syndromes, for investigating their cause, and for monitoring their course.

MASS AND COMPOSITION OF THE BODY COMPARTMENTS Consideration must first be given to the normal mass and chemical composition of the major body compartments, since these compartmental properties are altered by nutritional defi- ciencies in characteristic ways. The body can be viewed as consisting of four compartments: extracellular fluid, proto- plasm (intracellular compartment), bone, and adipose tissue. The first three make up the *lean body mass.*

The mass and elemental composition of the body compart- ments of a healthy "reference man," 70 kg in weight, 172 cm tall, 35 years old, are shown in Table 74-1. Typical masses of extracellular fluid, protoplasm, bone, and adipose tissue are 17, 35, 5, and 13 kg, respectively. Chloride is localized almost ex- clusively in the extracellular fluid, where its average concentra- tion is 96 meq per liter; nitrogen and potassium are largely located in protoplasm, with normal concentrations of 27 and 150 meq per kilogram of wet weight, respectively; calcium is found primarily in bone, where its concentration averages 260 g per kilogram of wet weight. The adipose tissue contains in- significant levels of these elements.

DIRECT AND INDIRECT METHODS FOR MEASURING MASS OF BODY COMPARTMENTS If one assumes that the concentra- tions of chloride, nitrogen, potassium, phosphorus, and cal- cium remain normal in extracellular fluid, protoplasm, and bone during a period of observation involving expansion or contraction of these compartments, and if one knows the bal- ance (i.e., intake and output) of each element (termed Δ nitro- gen, Δ phosphorus, etc.) during this period, then from the equations in Table 74-2 one can calculate the change (Δ) in the mass of each of these three compartments during the period under consideration. The change in adipose mass can then be estimated as

$$\Delta \text{ body weight} - (\Delta \text{ protoplasm} + \Delta \text{ extracellular fluid} + \Delta \text{ bone})$$

TABLE 74-1
Approximate mass and major elemental composition of body compartments in a 70-kg healthy "reference man"

	Protoplasm	Extracellular fluid	Bone	Adipose tissue
Mass	35 kg	17 kg	5 kg	13 kg
Body weight	50%	24%	7%	19%
Elemental composition, per kg wet wt	27 g N 97 mmol P 150 meq K	140 meq Na 96 meq Cl	260 g Ca 115 g P	

TABLE 74-2
Reifenstein equations for determining change in mass of body compartments

Δ Protoplasm (g)	$= 27 \times \Delta \text{N (g)}$
Δ ECF* (g)	$= 9.6 \times \Delta \text{Cl (meq)}$
Δ Bone (g)	$= 0.1 \times \Delta \text{Ca (meq)}$
Δ Adipose tissue (g)	$= \Delta \text{BW}^\dagger \text{ (g)} - [\Delta \text{ protoplasm (g)}$ $+ \Delta \text{ ECF (g)} + \Delta \text{ bone (g)}]$

* *Extracellular fluid.*
† *Body weight.*

The equation is based on the fact that each kilogram of extracellular fluid, protoplasm, or bone gained or lost by the body contains a characteristic amount of chloride, nitrogen, or calcium, respectively.

Metabolic balance techniques of this type provide estimates of the change in mass of each compartment during the period of observation but provide no information about the absolute mass of the compartment at the beginning and end. Several methods capable of such absolute measurements are available: whole-body counting of potassium (total body protoplasm); measurement of extracellular fluid by isotope dilution; measurement of total body water by isotope dilution; calculation of intracellular water (closely related to protoplasmic mass) as total body water minus extracellular water; measurement of adipose mass by determining whole-body density. These various methods are largely restricted to research units. Fortunately, several indirect methods for estimating the mass of body compartments are available to the clinician:

1 In the nonedematous patient, body weight as percent of ideal is a useful indicator of adipose tissue plus lean body mass. Reduction of the ratio, body weight/ideal body weight, to 80 percent in nonedematous patients usually means mild protein-energy undernutrition, a reduction to 70 to 80 percent indicates moderate protein-energy undernutrition and to 70 percent or less indicates severe protein-energy undernutrition.

2 Anthropometric analysis of the midarm requires only 1 min with a tape measure and caliper. The principle is illustrated in Fig. 74-1; the arm consists of a cylinder of muscle within a sheath of adipose tissue. From the external circumference of the midarm and the width of the adipose layer (equal to one-half the triceps skin fold), midarm muscle circumference can be calculated. Triceps skin fold and midarm muscle circumference are indicators of the body's masses of adipose tissue and skeletal muscle, respectively. Normal average values for adult men and women, respectively, are triceps skin fold, 12.5 and 16.5 mm, and midarm muscle circumference, 25.3 and 23.2 cm.

3 The ratio of 24-h creatinine excretion (in grams) to height (in centimeters), is a more accurate measure of muscle mass. Urine creatinine is related to lean body mass by the equation

$$\text{Lean body mass (kg)} = 21.0 + 21.5 \times \text{(g creatinine/24 h)}$$

The creatinine/height ratio is the best clinical laboratory test for protein starvation. In normal men and women, the ratio averages 10.5 and 5.8 mg/cm, respectively. In men, ratios in the ranges 8.4 to 9.5, 7.4 to 8.4, and less than 7.4 mg/cm signify mild, moderate, and severe degrees of protein starvation, respectively.

4 Sagittal or horizontal radiograms of an extremity also provide quantitative information about the mass of representative skeletal muscles but are more expensive.

FIGURE 74-1

Anthropometric measurement of muscle and adipose compartments of the mid-upper arm. Midarm circumference is measured with a tape measure and triceps skin fold with a caliper. (After Butterworth and Blackburn.)

Calculation of mid upper arm muscle circumference

C_1 = mid upper arm circumference in centimeters
S = triceps skinfold in centimeters
d_1 = arm diameter
d_2 = muscle diameter
Skinfold (S) = 2 × subcutaneous fat
$\qquad = d_1 - d_2$
Circumference $(C_1) = \pi d_1$
Muscle circumference $(C_2) = \pi d_2$
$\qquad\qquad = \pi[d_1 - (d_1 - d_2)]$
$\qquad\qquad = \pi d_1 - \pi(d_1 - d_2)$
$\qquad\qquad = C_1 - \pi S$

Midarm circumference (adults), cm

Sex	Normal	>90% normal	90-60% normal	<60% normal
Male	29.3	>26.3	26.3-17.6	<17.6
Female	28.5	>25.7	25.7-17.1	<17.1

Midarm muscle circumference (adults), cm

Sex	Normal	>90% normal	90-60% normal	<60% normal
Male	25.3	>22.8	22.8-15.2	<15.2
Female	23.2	>20.9	20.9-13.9	<13.9

Triceps skinfold (adults), mm

Sex	Normal	>90% normal	90-60% normal	<60% normal
Male	12.5	>11.3	11.3-7.5	<7.5
Female	16.5	>14.9	14.9-9.9	<9.9

Skeletal muscle makes up about 30 percent of the lean body mass. This organ atrophies progressively in protein-energy starvation, the most common deficiency state in American hospitals (see Chap. 75). By monitoring the creatinine/height ratio and midarm muscle circumference, the clinician can identify protein-energy starvation easily and inexpensively and monitor its course.

SYNDROMES OF UNDERNUTRITION When any of the 36 essential nutrient requirements (Chap. 73) are not met, undernutrition syndromes result. Undernutrition of such macronutrients as nitrogen, sodium, chloride, potassium, calcium, and phosphorus reduces the mass of one or more body compartments, often with associated abnormalities in compartmental chemistry, structure, and function. For example, deficiencies of nitrogen (protein), sodium, and calcium erode protoplasm, extracellular fluid, and bone, respectively. Undernutrition of a micronutrient tends to cause a specific morphological or functional abnormality in certain tissues without alteration in compartmental mass or elemental composition. While in theory there are 36 different types of human malnutrition, undernutrition syndromes usually occur in groups rather than in "pure" form.

Deficiency of each essential nutrient can be characterized in terms of symptoms, signs, and chemical and radiographic abnormalities, but deficiency syndromes have several principles in common:

1 Undernutrition can be either primary or secondary in origin. The primary form is due to inadequate supply of food containing the essential nutrients. In secondary undernutrition adequate diet is available but, because of illness or medical treatment, nutrients cannot be ingested, absorbed, or metabolized adequately, or the rate of utilization or external losses is excessive. Primary and secondary mechanisms frequently reinforce each other; for example, the hypermetabolism and anorexia of infection precipitate nutritional deficiencies more rapidly in patients who previously subsisted on marginal diets than in well-nourished individuals. To determine whether undernutrition in a particular patient is primary or secondary, the physician must obtain a dietary history, assess personal income and living conditions, and examine the patient for organic disease.

2 Nutritional deficiency syndromes tend to evolve through three stages. Many essential nutrients are stored in the tissues of the well-nourished subject: for example, iron, folate, thiamine, pyridoxine, and vitamins B_{12}, A, and D in liver; essential fatty acids in adipose tissue; nitrogen in a labile reserve in muscle and liver. When intake falls below the daily requirement, these reserves temporarily forestall deficiency manifestations and maintain normal blood levels (stage 1). In stage 2, blood levels of the nutrient or nutrient-dependent metabolic products decline, but the patient continues to be asymptomatic. In stage 3, clinical signs and symptoms develop. Methods for assessing the nutritional status should ideally be capable of detecting all three stages of each deficiency syndrome. Available techniques, however, usually reveal only stages 2 and 3.

3 Because anorexia is a major mechanism in the current endemic of protein-energy undernutrition in hospitals in the United States, the intake of nutrients must be measured in one of three ways: by recall, by diary (outpatient), or by observation (inpatient).

4 Change in weight is ambiguous. In the absence of edema various proportions of weight loss are adipose tissue and lean body mass. In the presence of edema body weight changes are even more difficult to interpret. Gain in weight can reflect accumulation of edema, masking erosion of protoplasm; loss of weight can reflect diuresis with simultaneous expansion of the protoplasmic compartment. An initially obese patient can lose 30 lb because of chronic wasting illness and present for the first medical examination with a normal body weight, the still substantial adipose organ masking a shrinkage in the lean body mass. For these reasons, direct or indirect estimation of the size of the protoplasmic compartment is essential as described above.

5 The undernourished patient is usually deficient in several nutrients. Common patterns are deficiency of both protein and energy, deficiency of two or more water-soluble vitamins (usually including folate, vitamin C, and/or thiamine), and deficiency of both Ca^{2+} and Mg^{2+} in patients with malabsorption.

The various physical, chemical, and radiographic characteristics of each type of undernutrition are summarized in Table 73-4. The most commonly used chemical indexes of nutrient deficiency are listed in Table 74-3, which gives three average concentration ranges for each test: normal, subnormal without clinical manifestations, and subnormal with clinical signs or symptoms of deficiency. Although these tests are of value in population surveys and in following the response of patients to therapy, the variation is such that they have limited diagnostic value (Chaps. 79 to 82).

The clinician must select a reasonable number of historical, physical, and laboratory items to use as a "nutritional data base" to screen patients for undernutrition. Table 74-4 presents a selection of historical and physical items that would reveal most deficiency states in hospital patients.

INVESTIGATING THE CAUSE OF MALNUTRITION The first issue is to distinguish between primary and secondary malnutrition. Socioeconomically determined primary malnutrition is the major variety worldwide. With improving socioeconomic conditions, primary malnutrition sufficient to cause symptoms is now uncommon in the United States. Subclinical deficiencies of protein, iron, folate, and ascorbate are still detectable in up to 40 percent of the population in some regions (see Chap. 75).

The prevalence of primary malnutrition is closely related to the nutrient density of the population's diet. A child or adult generally cannot ingest more than about 3000 g (or ml) of food, or 3500 cal, per day. To forestall a deficiency syndrome, recommended daily allowance (RDA) quantities of the 36 essential nutrients must be available in the food ingested. Foods meeting this requirement are said to have satisfactory nutrient density. The alarming prevalence of protein starvation (kwashiorkor) in certain African nations has been attributed to the critically low protein "density" in the bulky, root-based diet which is often available in large quantity but which can be consumed up to a limit of only about 3000 g per day. The quantity and quality of protein in this volume of root-based food are insufficient to prevent negative nitrogen balance and eventual protein starvation. Similarly, the substantial prevalence of subclinical primary nutritional deficiency in the United States may be related to the growing consumption of "snack foods" with low nutrient density ("empty calories"). Alcohol represents another type of "low nutrient density" food. For these reasons, evaluation of the undernourished patient's habitual dietary intake at home is of central importance

TABLE 74-3

Interpretation of laboratory tests for the evaluation of nutritional status (adults)

Test	Deficient (often with clinical manifestations)	Low (usually without clinical manifestations)	Acceptable	Nutrient evaluation
Serum iron, μg per 100 ml	<30	30–60	>60	Iron
Serum albumin, g per 100 ml	<3.0	3.0–3.5	>3.5	Protein
Plasma retinol, μg per 100 ml	<10	10–20	>20	Vitamin A
Serum folate, ng/ml	<3	3.0–6.0	>6.0	Folate
Erythrocyte folate, ng/ml	<140	140–160	>160	Folate
Serum vitamin B_{12}, pg/ml	<150	150–200	>200	Vitamin B_{12}
Serum ascorbic acid, mg per 100 ml	<0.20	0.20–0.30	>0.30	Vitamin C
Erythrocyte transketolase (% thiamine diphosphate stimulation)	>20	15–20	<15	Thiamine
Erythrocyte glutathione reductase activity coefficient	>1.40	1.20–1.40	<1.20	Riboflavin
Erythrocyte aminotransferase activity coefficients:				
EGPT	>1.25		<1.25	Vitamin B_6
EGOT	>2.0		<2.0	Vitamin B_6
Tryptophan load test (xanthurenic acid), mg per day	>50	25–50	<25	Vitamin B_6
N^1-Methylnicotinamide excretion, mg/g creatinine	<0.5	0.5–1.59	>1.6	Niacin
Serum Ca × P product, mg per 100 ml	<40		>40	Vitamin D
Alkaline phosphatase, King-Armstrong units per 100 ml	>40	15–40	8–14	Vitamin D
Hemoglobin, g per 100 ml	<12	12–14	>14	Protein, Fe, folate, vitamin B_{12}, pyridoxine, Cu
24-h urine K^+, meq	<20	20–40	>40	K
24-h urine Mg^{2+}, meq	<4	4–8	>8	Mg
24-h urine Ca^{2+}, mg	<50	50–100	>100	Ca
24-h urine Na^+, meq	<20	20–40	>40	Na
24-h urine P, mg	<100	100–300	>300	P
24-h urine urea N, g	<6	6–10	>10	Protein
Creatinine/height ratio	<90% of standard	90–95%	>95%	Protein

in searching for a possible primary etiology of the deficiency state.

In secondary undernutrition, a diet furnishing all the RDAs is available, but the patient becomes undernourished because of one or more problems: (1) inadequate intake (anorexia, dysphagia, coma, intestinal obstruction); (2) malabsorption; (3) inadequate utilization of nutrients (e.g., failure to activate vitamin D in renal or hepatic disease); (4) increased requirement (e.g., increased requirement for calories in fever or for folate in psoriasis or hemolytic anemia); (5) increased loss (iron in bleeding, electrolytes and calories in diarrhea); or (6) drug-nutrient interactions (see Chap. 73).

MONITORING THE COURSE OF MALNUTRITION Besides defining the type, severity, and mechanism for the development of undernutrition, it is important to ascertain its rate of pro-

FIGURE 74-2

Monitoring the course of a patient with protein-calorie depletion during repletion by nasogastric hyperalimentation.

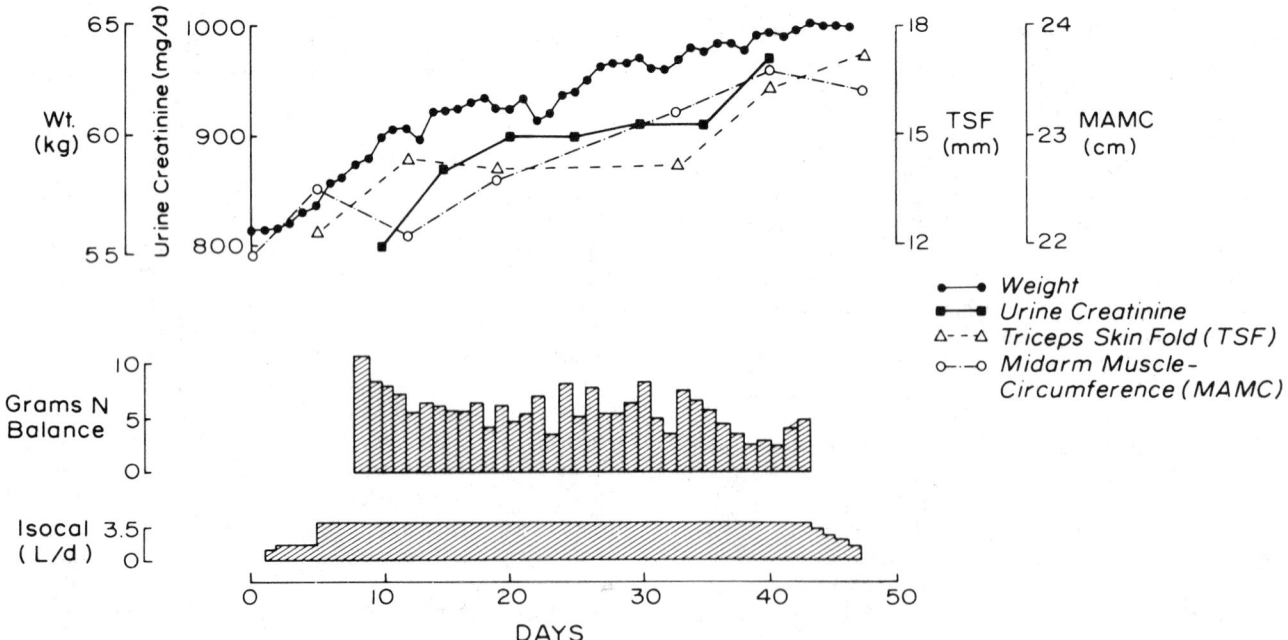

TABLE 74-4
Nutritional data base

HISTORY

Previous weight curve
Dietary intake by retrospective recall and prospective diary
Alcohol
Socioeconomic and family status, including income
Anorexia, vomiting, diarrhea
Blood loss
Pregnancy, lactation, menses
Vitamin and mineral supplements
Use of drugs which might affect nutrition

PHYSICAL EXAMINATION

General: Weight as percent of ideal body weight; triceps skin fold; midarm muscle circumference
Skin: Xerosis, follicular hyperkeratosis, pellagrous dermatitis, petechiae, ecchymoses, perifollicular hemorrhages, flaky paint dermatitis, pallor
Hair: Dyspigmentation, easy pluckability, thinning, straightening
Head: Temporal wasting, parotid enlargement
Eyes: Bitot's spots, conjunctival and scleral xerosis, keratomalacia, corneal vascularization, angular palpebritis
Mouth: Cheilosis, angular stomatitis, magenta tongue, atrophic lingual papillae, tongue fissuring, glossitis, spongy gums
Heart: Cardiomegaly, findings of congestive heart failure
Abdomen: Hepatomegaly
Extremities: Edema, koilonychia
Neurological: Irritability, weakness, calf tenderness, loss of deep tendon reflexes

gression. This is accomplished by periodic monitoring of body weight, albumin, hematocrit, creatinine excretion, midarm muscle circumference, triceps skin fold, and appropriate blood or urine concentrations of nutrition-dependent variables. An example of monitoring the course of progressive protein-energy malnutrition is shown in Fig. 74-2. A bedside estimate of daily nitrogen balance in grams can be made as follows:

$$\tfrac{1}{6} \text{ [Daily protein intake in grams (estimated by hospital dietician)]} - \text{(24-h urine urea nitrogen in grams)} + 4 \text{ g}^1$$

The more negative the nitrogen balance, the more rapidly protein depletion progresses.

REFERENCES

ARROYAVE G et al: Assessment of protein nutritional status. Am J Clin Nutr 23:807, 1970

BUTTERWORTH CE, BLACKBURN GL: Hospital malnutrition and how to assess the nutritional status of a patient. Nutr Today 10:8, March/April 1974

JELLIFFE DB: *The Assessment of the Nutritional Status of the Community.* Geneva, World Health Organization, 1966

REIFENSTEIN EC JR et al: The accumulation, interpretation and presentation of data pertaining to metabolic balances, notably those of calcium, phosphorus and nitrogen. J Clin Endocrinol Metab 5:367, 1945

SAUBERLICH HE et al: *Laboratory Tests for the Assessment of Nutritional Status: Critical Reviews in Clinical Laboratory Sciences,* JW King, R Faulkner (eds). Cleveland, CRC Press, 1973, vol 4, no 3, pp 215–340

VITERI FE, ALVARADO J: The creatinine height index: Its use in the estimation of the degree of protein depletion and repletion in protein calorie malnourished children. Pediatrics 46:696, 1970

---

[1] Four grams is the approximate sum of urinary nonurea nitrogen plus fecal and integumentary losses of nitrogen.

75
PROTEIN-ENERGY UNDERNUTRITION

DANIEL RUDMAN

RELEVANCE TO CONTEMPORARY MEDICINE

Attention was focused on this deficiency state in the 1930s by physicians in developing nations. The syndrome affects structure and function of every organ in the body. The causes, manifestations, and treatment have been intensively studied in African and Asian children, in whom the prevalence of the primary form of the disease averages 25 percent. It is recognized that the secondary varieties of protein-energy deficiency are common within hospital populations in developed nations. Subacutely or chronically ill patients living longer under the protection of modern therapeutics but handicapped by anorexia, hypermetabolism, or malabsorption may rapidly develop protein-calorie deficiency.

DEFINITION AND ETIOLOGY

The syndrome consists of progressive loss of both lean body mass and adipose tissue. It results from insufficient consumption of protein and calories, although one or the other may play the dominant role in a given individual. The inadequate intake may be primary or secondary, as discussed in Chap. 74. Synergism between the two mechanisms is common. Patients with scanty reserves of protein and energy develop clinical protein-energy starvation more rapidly than well-nourished subjects when challenged by the hypermetabolism, catabolism, and anorexia of infection or other illnesses.

On a global basis, the primary mechanism predominates. Socioeconomic factors that limit the quantity and quality of the diet are paramount. Particularly important is the poor biologic value of many vegetable proteins. The problem is accentuated if calories are deficient, because a large proportion of the dietary amino acids must then be oxidized as fuel instead of used to synthesize tissue and plasma protein. In developed countries poverty is the most important cause of the syndrome, but the low nutrient densities of alcohol and snack foods play an important role in subclinical protein deficiency regardless of economic status.

EPIDEMIOLOGY

The prevalence of protein-energy undernutrition can be assessed by measuring percent reduction from normal in triceps skin fold, midarm muscle circumference, 24-h urinary creatinine/height ratio, and serum albumin (see Chap. 74).

Estimates of prevalence of protein-energy depletion in various population groups are given in Table 75-1. It is much more prevalent in Africa than in the United States. In the United States, subclinical protein deficiency is more common in the South than in the North and in blacks and Latin Americans than in whites. In contrast to developing nations, protein-energy depletion in the general population of the United States tends to be mild and subclinical. In hospitals, on the other hand, severe as well as mild deficiencies are frequently encountered. Protein-energy starvation is frequently associated with other types of malnutrition.

PATHOPHYSIOLOGY

Calorie and protein undernutrition have been studied most extensively in children of developing nations in whom inadequate or marginal diets, the augmented nutritional require-

TABLE 75-1
Prevalence of protein-energy malnutrition in selected groups

Group	Criterion of deficiency	Prevalence of deficiency, %
Pregnant or lactating women, United States*	<3.5 g albumin per 100 ml serum	50
Children <5 years, 28 developing countries†	Body weight <80% (kwashiorkor) or <60% of standard (marasmus)	25
General surgical patients 1 week postoperative, Leeds, England‡	Midarm muscle circumference, triceps skin fold, serum albumin more than two standard deviations below normal mean	50
Heart valve recipients, postoperative, London§	Total body ^{40}K less than 87% of standard	40
General surgical patients, Boston City Hospital¶	Midarm muscle circumference, triceps skin fold, serum albumin more than two standard deviations below normal mean	48

* *J Carter, US Department of Health, Education, and Welfare Publication no (HSM) 72-8132, 1971.*
† *JM Bengou, J Trop Pediatr 13:169, 1967.*
‡ *GL Hill et al, Lancet 1:689, 1977.*
§ *RK Walesby, Lancet 1:76, 1978.*
¶ *BR Bistrain et al, JAMA 230:858, 1974.*

ments of infancy, and frequent episodes of infectious disease combine to cause florid deficiency manifestations. Two syndromes have been distinguished: (1) *marasmus,* caused primarily by deficiency of calories and manifested by stunted growth, loss of adipose tissue, and generalized wasting of lean body mass without edema; and (2) *kwashiorkor,* in which calories are adequate but protein is deficient. This syndrome is manifested by growth failure (in children), hypoalbuminemia, edema, fatty liver, and preservation of adipose tissue. Mixed forms (kwashiorkor-marasmus) are common. It is likely that similar principles apply to protein-energy malnutrition in adults.

METABOLIC AND ENDOCRINE ASPECTS Calorie deficiency
When the intake of calories falls below the daily requirement, the body responds with an orderly physiologic adaptation (see Chap. 86), engineered in large part by a reduced secretion of insulin, augmented plasma levels of glucagon and cortisol, and curtailed hepatic production of triiodothyronine (T_3) from thyroxine (T_4). The fall in plasma insulin permits free fatty acids and amino acids to be mobilized from adipose tissue and muscle to provide carbon for the continuing oxidative metabolism of the body. When energy balance is negative, oxidative metabolism claims first priority in the utilization of dietary protein. During starvation, the carbon chains of amino acids also provide substrate for gluconeogenesis, since a continuing supply of glucose is required by the central nervous system. As amino acids are diverted from protein synthesis into oxidative metabolism and gluconeogenesis, protein synthesis in the body is curtailed, particularly in muscle. The metabolic rate gradually declines, because of diminished extrathyroidal conversion of T_4 to T_3, decreased synthesis of the T_3 receptor, curtailed production and turnover of catecholamines, and loss of the specific dynamic action of the dietary components. During partial or total deprivation of calories, both lean body mass and adipose tissue contract, but the latter does so more rap-

idly. The progress of the consumption of adipose tissue and muscle can be followed at the bedside by such clinical indicators as measurement of the triceps skin fold, midarm muscle circumference, and creatinine/height ratio.

During the first week of total starvation, the average patient loses 4 to 5 kg of body weight which consists of about 25 percent adipose tissue, 35 percent extracellular fluid, and 40 percent protoplasm. Losses of nitrogen, potassium, sodium, and chloride represent 3 to 8 percent of the body content of each element. Negative balances of magnesium, phosphorus, and calcium are also considerable. During ensuing weeks, as further adaptive endocrine and enzymatic adjustments occur, losses of nitrogen and other elements continue but at a slower rate. The intracellular compartment does not contract at the same rate in all tissues. The central nervous system does not lose weight. Skeletal muscle atrophies more rapidly than cardiac muscle, while gastrointestinal tract and liver lose mass more rapidly than kidneys. Mobilization of amino acids from muscle to liver permits the latter organ to continue to synthesize some albumin and lipoproteins; as a consequence hypoalbuminemia and fatty liver are not conspicuous.

Protein deficiency Frequently the intake of protein is more limited than that of calories. This occurs because dietary protein is more expensive than carbohydrate or fat; because protein of high biologic value (chiefly animal) is more expensive than protein of low biologic value (chiefly vegetable); because high-calorie, low-protein foods (many snack foods, ethanol, starchy root-based vegetables) are in frequent use in the United States and abroad; and because physicians often use glucose as the sole organic nutrient in the intravenous feeding of the patient who cannot eat. The deficiency state under these conditions is analogous to kwashiorkor in children. The reduction of insulin secretion, which is a central mechanism in the adaptation to energy starvation, is circumvented. Insulin secreted in response to the dietary or intravenous carbohydrate promotes lipogenesis and retards lipolysis; adipose tissue is well-preserved, and free fatty acids are not available for oxidation in place of amino acids. The high-plasma insulin also impairs mobilization and redistribution of muscle amino acids from skeletal muscle to liver. Plasma amino acids fall, and the total body rate of protein synthesis declines. Fatty infiltration of the liver is common. Two biochemical mechanisms are probably involved: (1) lack of methionine limits phospholipid synthesis, secondarily impairing lipoprotein formation, and (2) hepatic synthesis of triglycerides from glucose continues. In the blood decreased concentrations of albumin, transferrin, and hemoglobin reflect severe protein starvation. Edema is characteristic of this stage.

Variable degrees of calorie and protein starvation occur together.

Mineral metabolism Protein-energy undernutrition is generally associated with depletion of body minerals. In part this reflects the contraction of protoplasmic and extracellular fluid compartments with their constituent elements (nitrogen, phosphorus, potassium, and magnesium within cells; sodium and chloride in extracellular fluid) being excreted into the urine in the same proportions as in the lean body mass. However, mineral losses are often out of proportion to the contraction of lean body mass. One reason is a shift of potassium and magnesium from muscle to plasma in exchange for sodium. In addition, potassium, magnesium, phosphorus, and calcium intakes may be even less adequate than those of protein and calories (e.g., during prolonged intravenous nutrition with magnesium- or phosphorus-free solutions). Finally, renal and extrarenal losses of these elements may be significant (diuresis, diarrhea, fistulas, etc.).

CARDIOVASCULAR-RESPIRATORY AND RENAL RESPONSES

The heart and kidneys lose mass progressively during the course of protein-energy starvation. These losses are generally proportional to the erosion of lean body mass, so that ratios of heart mass/lean body mass and kidney mass/lean body mass remain normal. Consequently functional insufficiency of these two shrunken organs is not a usual feature of protein-energy depletion. Cardiac output declines in parallel with the falling metabolic rate. Blood pressure is reduced by the fall in cardiac output. The ventilatory response to hypoxia is blunted. Glomerular filtration rate and renal blood flow are lowered. The ability of the kidney to excrete an acid load or to respond to antidiuretic hormone may be impaired. Although these changes in cardiac and renal structure and function are appropriate to the reduced lean body mass and hypometabolic state, they may become important handicaps during vigorous nutritional repletion, acute infection, or other circumstances that require rapid increases in cardiac output, metabolic rate, and urinary excretion of solutes.

BLOOD Reduced blood volume, hematocrit, albumin, and transferrin are characteristic in the wasted patient. The anemia of "pure" protein-energy depletion is normocytic and normochromic and usually results from decreased production of red blood cells, perhaps reflecting the protein requirement for globin synthesis. Frequently deficiencies of iron, folate, or pyridoxine contribute to the anemia.

STRUCTURE AND FUNCTION OF GASTROINTESTINAL TRACT AND PANCREAS The gastrointestinal tract and pancreas atrophy. In the small intestine, villous height, mitotic index, and content of disaccharidases and dipeptidases all decline. Exocrine elements of the pancreas atrophy as well, and the production of digestive enzymes is reduced. Bacterial overgrowth may occur in the small intestine. These factors combine to produce malabsorption and lactose intolerance. The structural and functional regression of the small intestine results, at least in part, from decreased oral feeding rather than systemic malnutrition, since patients fully nourished by the parenteral route exhibit the same lesion.

IMMUNE SYSTEM Lymphatic tissues atrophy. Impaired cell-mediated immunity is evident by all standard tests (blastogenic response of lymphocytes to mitogens, total lymphocyte count, and skin testing with recall antigens). Bactericidal activity of polymorphonuclear leukocytes is decreased. Plasma immunoglobulin concentrations and humoral responses to antigens are preserved. Protein-energy starved patients experience increased morbidity and mortality during common infections compared with well-nourished groups and are subject to infection by opportunistic organisms (gram-negative bacteria, *Candida,* herpes simplex). Cachectic patients do not manifest the usual reactions to infection; hypothermia, delayed healing of wounds, paucity of polymorphonuclear cells, and increased degree of tissue necrosis at sites of infection are all characteristic.

WOUND HEALING The fibroblastic response to surgical wounds is impaired by protein-energy depletion. Consequently, incisions and enteric anastomoses heal more slowly in undernourished patients; wound dehiscence is common.

TEMPERATURE REGULATION In severe protein-energy starvation in the absence of fever, basal metabolic rate is reduced. Hypothermia is frequent. The underlying mechanisms are reduced heat production due to exhaustion of carbohydrate and fat reserves, low plasma T_3, possible decreased adrenergic function, and loss of thermal insulation when subcutaneous adipose tissue is gone. Hypoglycemia is occasionally seen (see Chap. 340).

REPRODUCTION Nearly every phase of the reproductive process is impaired by protein deficiency in the mother's diet. Fertility is reduced. If implantation occurs, there is a high risk of early fetal resorption. If gestation is completed, the progeny are substandard in weight and length. Lactation is impaired by protein starvation, so that undernutrition is common postnatally. Even if postnatal nutrition is adequate, stunted growth in the infant is in part irreversible, and life-long impairment in learning capacity may result.

PATHOLOGICAL CHANGES In the child growth is stunted, weight more than height. At all ages the body is wasted and may be edematous. Ascites is common. Subcutaneous fat may be totally absent (advanced calorie depletion) or variably preserved (protein starvation). Involution is most pronounced in adipose tissue, thymolymphatic system, spleen, exocrine glands, skeletal muscle, gastrointestinal tract, and pancreas. The gastrointestinal tract is thin and distended; rectal prolapse is common. The size and fat content of the liver are variable. Heart and kidney size are decreased in proportion to the loss of nonedematous body weight. Pituitary, thyroid, and adrenal glands are atrophic. Muscle atrophy is invariable. Terminal infection is common, often with opportunistic organisms; there is less inflammatory reaction and more tissue necrosis, including gangrenous ulcers, than in well-nourished cadavers bearing evidence of terminal infection.

Skin is atrophic, dyspigmented, scaly, and frequently ulcerated. The cornea is dry, atrophic, and often ulcerated.

No microscopic lesions are specific in protein-energy starvation. Adipose tissue is atrophic. Mitotic figures in proliferating tissues are decreased compared with those of patients who die with normal nutriture. Enzyme granules and ribosomes are less prominent in exocrine glands. The liver is often fatty. Muscle and kidney show nonspecific hyalinization and cloudy swelling. Germinal centers are absent in lymph nodes. Columnar epithelium tends to become cuboidal, villi are flat, and the brush border atrophies in many cells.

CLINICAL MANIFESTATIONS

HISTORY A primary component in the etiology can be uncovered only by reviewing the intakes of protein and calories and the biological quality of the dietary protein during the months before the clinical examination. Suggestive of a primary component are poverty, alcoholism, habitual consumption of "low nutrient density" foods, solitary life-style, and old age. Suggestive of a secondary etiology are the presence of a known chronic medical problem, anorexia or other gastrointestinal symptoms (including lack of teeth), or prolonged fever.

In children, failure to gain height and weight is an early sign. In adults, weight loss usually occurs. However, in the adult a body weight equal to or greater than ideal does not rule out the presence of deficiency of calories, protein, or both. Thus progressive loss of protoplasm and adipose tissue may be masked by accumulating edema; or the patient may have been previously obese, and a substantial loss of lean body mass during the current illness may be masked by a residue of obesity. Listlessness, easy fatigability, sensation of coldness, swollen ankles, and dry, cracked skin are frequent symptoms in patients eating insufficient protein or calories.

PHYSICAL SIGNS The facies is drawn, temporal regions are concave and fleshless, intercostal spaces are excavated, and the skin hangs in folds on the wasted extremities. "Flaky paint" dermatitis and dyspigmentation of skin and hair are common. The patient is pale and may be edematous. Signs of deficiency of water-soluble or fat-soluble vitamins may be present. Decubiti and skin ulcers are typical in advanced stages.

VITAL SIGNS Blood pressure is decreased. Pulse is slow, and extremities are cool; central temperature may be decreased.

ANTHROPOMETRICS Triceps skin fold and midarm muscle circumference are reduced in varying ratios dependent on preillness nutritional state and relative severity of the energy and protein deficiencies.

LABORATORY AND X-RAY FINDINGS Twenty-four-hour urinary creatinine/height ratio is decreased. This is the most sensitive and practical clinical indicator of protein starvation and should be monitored at weekly intervals in the chronically ill hospital patient. The excretion of 3-methylhistidine has similar significance but is more difficult to measure. These analyses should be done only in afebrile patients, since urinary excretion of both creatinine and 3-methylhistidine is increased by fever. Other signs include decrease in serum albumin, serum transferrin, and hematocrit, but these changes are less specific. Nevertheless, protein depletion may be the most common cause of hypoalbuminemia in hospitalized patients, even in patients with hepatic disease. Serum essential and nonessential amino acid concentration and urine urea and creatinine levels are reduced. T-lymphocyte cell function is decreased, as revealed by cutaneous anergy and peripheral lymphopenia (absolute lymphocyte count < 1200 cells per cubic millimeter). Glucose tolerance is impaired. Plasma cortisol is often increased (in part because of retarded metabolic clearance). T_3 is decreased, reverse T_3 may be increased, and basal metabolic rate is low. Heart size is small on chest film. Echocardiography shows a small heart with decreased cardiac output. Sagittal or cross-sectional x-rays of arm show diminished muscle mass.

COURSE A typical case is illustrated in Fig. 75-1. In children, an early manifestation is slowing of growth. As the protein-energy depletion becomes more severe, pallor, fatigue, and

FIGURE 75-1

Course of a typical case of progressive protein-energy starvation.

TABLE 75-2
Undesirable practices affecting the nutritional health of hospital patients

1 Failure to record height and weight on admission.
2 Lack of a weight curve in the hospital chart.
3 Prolonged use of glucose and saline intravenous feedings.
4 Failure to measure patient's food intake.
5 Withholding meals because of diagnostic tests.
6 Use of tube feedings of inadequate amount and uncertain composition.
7 Ignorance of the composition of nutritional products.
8 Failure to recognize increased nutritional needs due to injury or illness.
9 Delay of nutrition support until the patient is in an advanced state of depletion.
10 Limited availability of laboratory tests to assess nutritional status; failure to use those that are available.
11 Failure to correct inadequate dentition or the edentulous state.

SOURCE: *After Butterworth.*

amenorrhea appear. Loss of cell-mediated immunity predisposes to infections. The hypermetabolism and anorexia of intercurrent infection accelerate the progress of the cachexia. In advanced undernutrition (triceps skin fold < 3 mm, creatinine/height ratio < 60 percent of standard), decubiti, hypothermia, and terminal infection are the rule.

RELATION TO OTHER DEFICIENCY STATES Usually other nutrients are also depleted. Folic acid, thiamine, riboflavin, nicotinic acid, pyridoxine, ascorbic acid and vitamin A deficiencies are relatively common in hospital populations in the United States (see Table 75-2). Body content of most minerals is also reduced, but a distinction must be made between absolute and relative decreases. As protoplasmic protein is consumed to supply metabolic fuel and substrate for gluconeogenesis in the underfed patient, the intracellular minerals potassium, phosphorus, magnesium and perhaps some of the microminerals are excreted in parallel with the nitrogen. Such loss is absolute but not relative, since the intracellular and extracellular concentrations of potassium, phosphorus, and magnesium usually remain normal. If the diet is specifically deficient in potassium, phosphorus, or magnesium, a further relative deficiency occurs, with the intracellular and perhaps the extracellular and urinary concentrations becoming subnormal. Similar considerations apply to the body content of essential fatty acids. Whether the depletion of potassium, phosphorus, magnesium, or essential fatty acids is absolute or relative, repletion with a feeding solution that contains little or none of that nutrient may lead to chemical and clinical manifestations of the corresponding deficiency state within a few days. Life-threatening hypokalemia, hypophosphatemia, or hypomagnesemia can occur. By similar mechanisms, plasma levels of trace minerals regularly decline during hyperalimentation if adequate rations of these nutrients are not provided.

REFERENCES

ALLEYNE GAO et al: *Protein-Energy Malnutrition.* London, Butler & Tanner, 1977

BISTRIAN BR et al: Protein status of general surgical patients. JAMA 230:858, 1974

——— et al: Prevalence of malnutrition in general medical patients. JAMA 235:1567, 1976

BOLLET AJ, OWENS S: Evaluation of nutritional status of selected hospitalized patients. Am J Clin Nutr 26:931, 1973

BUTTERWORTH CE: The skeleton in the hospital closet. Nutr Today 9:4, March/April 1974

———, BLACKBURN GL: Hospital malnutrition and how to assess the nutritional status of a patient. Nutr Today 10:8, March/April 1975

Cahill GF: Starvation in man. N Engl J Med 282:668, 1970

Geefhuysen J et al: Impaired cellular immunity in kwashiorkor with improvement after therapy. Br Med J 27:527, 1971

Hansen RG: An index of food quality. Nutr Rev 31:1, 1973

Law DK et al: Immunocompetence of patients with protein-calorie malnutrition. Ann Intern Med 79:545, 1973

Leevy CM et al: Incidence and significance of hypovitaminemia in a randomly selected municipal hospital population. Am J Clin Nutr 17:259, 1965

Nicol BM: Protein and calorie concentration. Nutr Rev 29:83, 1971

Ten-State Nutrition Survey, 1968-1970, US Department of Health, Education, and Welfare Publication no (HSM) 72-8131, 1972

Whitehead RG Alleyne GAO: Pathophysiological factors of importance in protein-calorie malnutrition. Br Med J 28:72, 1972

76
OBESITY

JERROLD M. OLEFSKY

The ability to store food energy as fat has provided significant survival value to organisms living in environments in which food supply is scarce or sporadic. Unlike glycogen or protein, triglyceride does not require water or electrolytes for storage purposes and can be retained essentially as pure fat; 1 g adipose tissue yields close to the full theoretical equivalent of 9 kcal. Because of the efficient storage of energy in adipose tissue, an individual of normal weight can survive up to 2 months of total starvation. However, Western society is generally not characterized by periodic or insufficient food supply but rather by constant and abundant food. As a consequence, the ability to store fat all too frequently becomes of negative survival value because of overconsumption and the resulting obesity.

DEFINITION AND INCIDENCE   Obesity can most easily be assessed using a subject's height and weight. One way to do this is to relate the patient's weight to an average range for his height and age. This measure of relative weight leads to an underestimation of the problem, however, since in the United States the "average" individual is somewhat obese. Tables of ideal or desirable weight provide more meaningful information and are based on actuarial estimates of what is consistent with normal life expectancy. Such tables are more useful if adjusted for differences in body build. Although relative weight correlates fairly well with the degree of adiposity, excess poundage can be either lean or fat tissue. Obviously, with this measurement, heavily muscled individuals would be considered obese. More precise measurements of obesity are based on body density or isotopic dilution methods, but these are too complicated for routine clinical use. Anthropometry is a simpler but accurate method for measuring the degree of adiposity. Skin fold thickness can be measured over various areas of the body and along with height, weight, and age can be used to assess the degree of adiposity. Triceps and subscapular skin folds are most commonly employed (see Chap. 74).

Obesity is often defined as an excess of adipose tissue, but the meaning of *excess* is hard to define. Aesthetic considerations aside, the clinical diagnosis of obesity can best be viewed as the degree of excess adiposity that imparts a health risk. This cutoff can only be approximated. The Framingham study demonstrated that a 20 percent excess over ideal weight imparted a health risk; by use of that criterion 20 to 30 percent of men and 30 to 40 percent of women are obese.

ETIOLOGY   When caloric intake exceeds expenditure, the excess calories are stored as fat tissue; the net balance between

these two variables regulates the amount of adipose tissue in the body. Many obese patients firmly believe they suffer from a "metabolic problem," but this is rarely the case. Abnormal eating behavior is the essential cause of the problem.

The regulation of eating behavior is incompletely understood. To some extent, appetite is controlled by discrete areas in the hypothalamus. A feeding center is located in the ventrolateral nucleus of the hypothalamus (VLH), and a satiety center is present in the ventromedial hypothalamus (VMH). The cerebral cortex receives positive signals from the feeding center that stimulate eating (Fig. 76-1), and the satiety center modulates this process by sending inhibitory impulses to the feeding center. Destruction of the feeding center in animals results in decreased food intake, while destruction of the satiety center leads to overeating and gross obesity. Several regulatory processes have been proposed as modulators of these hypothalamic centers. The satiety center may be activated by the surges in plasma glucose and/or insulin that follow a meal. It is of interest that the VMH contains insulin receptors and is insulin-sensitive. Meal-induced gastric distention is another possible inhibitory factor. The total adipose tissue mass may also influence the activity of the hypothalamic centers; i.e., there is a relatively fixed "set point" for the body's degree of adiposity. An elevated set point may account for the frequent recidivism in obese patients who have lost weight. How the "set point" is established and the mechanism by which the hypothalamus senses total fat stores are unknown. Glycerol release from fat cells and ascending neural impulses have been

FIGURE 76-1

The regulation of eating. The ventromedial satiety center is considered to be inhibitory, and the ventrolateral feeding center stimulatory. See text for discussion.

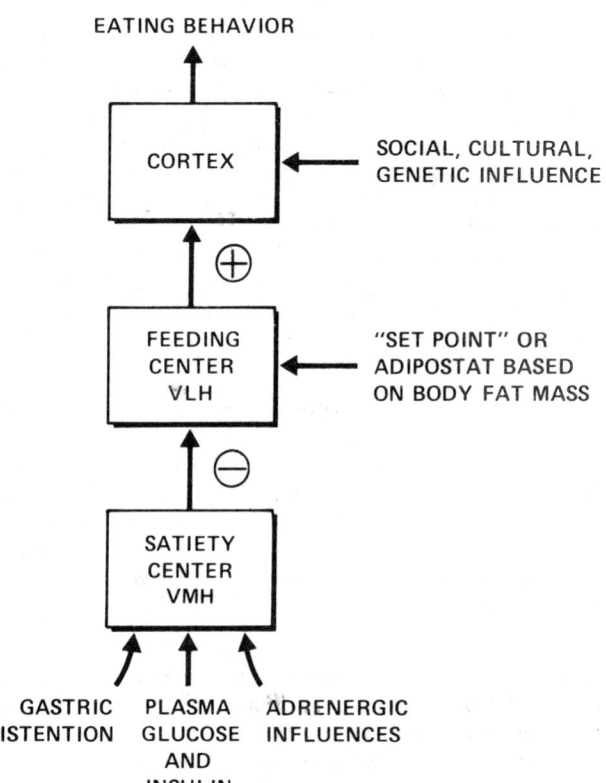

suggested as signals of adipose tissue size. Additionally, the hypothalamic centers are sensitive to catecholamines, and beta-adrenergic stimulation inhibits eating behavior. This provides at least one rationale for the anorexant effects of amphetamines.

Ultimately, the cerebral cortex controls eating behavior, and impulses from the feeding center to the cerebral cortex are only one input. Psychological, social, and genetic factors also influence food intake. In many obese subjects these influences are overriding; indeed, obese patients usually respond to external signals such as time of day, social setting, and smell or taste of food to a greater extent than do normal persons.

Although overeating is the cause of obesity in the majority of patients, other factors may participate—at least in certain individuals. Daily caloric needs range between 31 and 35 kcal per kilogram of body weight; this figure is somewhat higher in active and somewhat lower in sedentary individuals. With rare exceptions overly efficient utilization of food energy or decreased metabolic rate have not been documented in obesity. However, a distinction must be made between *static obesity* and the actual *process of gaining weight*. When normal subjects consume hypercaloric diets, less weight is gained than would be predicted on the basis of the excess calories ingested. This effect is most marked when carbohydrate is consumed and disappears when the excess calories consist of fat. Thus, humans can apparently adapt to chronic excessive carbohydrate and protein intake, and this protective effect attenuates the weight gain. Part of this adaptive response is related to an increase in thermogenesis. The mechanism of the increase in thermogenesis is unknown, but overeating of carbohydrate or mixed nutrients leads to increased plasma levels of triiodothyronine (T_3) and decreased levels of reverse T_3 (rT_3). A converse effect is seen in starvation with decreased T_3 and increased rT_3 levels. The conversion of thyroxine to T_3 occurs largely in the liver; excess food may induce adaptive thermogenesis by increasing the concentration of T_3 relative to that of T_4 and rT_3. An interesting postulate is that in certain individuals obesity results from a failure of this adaptive response.

Physical activity clearly modulates overall caloric balance, and obese individuals tend to be less active than normal subjects. This can be a contributory factor in the maintenance of excess weight, but decreased physical activity is unlikely to be important as a *cause* of major weight gain. Rather, obesity itself leads to inactivity. The modest increase in weight that often accompanies the middle years may be related more directly to diminished physical activity.

Certain animal models of obesity have clear-cut genetic causes, but the role of genetic influences in human obesity is difficult to evaluate because of confounding social and cultural factors.

SECONDARY OBESITY Hypothyroidism Obesity can result from hypothyroidism because of decreased caloric needs. However, only a minority of hypothyroid patients are truly obese, and an even smaller proportion of obese patients are hypothyroid. Indiscriminate use of thyroid hormone replacement in the treatment of obesity is to be deplored and should never be instituted without careful documentation of decreased thyroid function.

Cushing's disease Cushing's disease is a rare cause of obesity. Hyperadrenocorticism elicits a typical pattern of obesity with predominantly centripetal fat stores, characteristic rounded or moon facies, and cervical or supraclavicular fat deposits.

Insulinoma Hyperinsulinemia, secondary to an insulinoma, can occasionally cause obesity, presumably because of increased caloric intake secondary to recurrent hypoglycemia. Most patients with islet-cell tumors and hypoglycemia are not obese.

Hypothalamic disorders Froehlich's syndrome is characterized by obesity and hypogonadotrophic hypogonadism in boys with other variable features such as diabetes insipidus, visual impairment, and mental retardation. The anterior pituitary is usually normal, and the syndrome is thought to be the result of hypothalamic dysfunction. Occasionally pituitary tumors are present (as in Froehlich's original case) which may physically impair the hypothalamus. Most likely this syndrome includes a number of overlapping disorders having in common a hypothalamic lesion that leads to overeating and to hypogonadotrophism.

Other rare diseases include the Laurence-Moon-Biedl syndrome characterized by retinitis pigmentosa, mental retardation, skull deformities, polydactyly and syndactyly, and the Prader-Willi syndrome which is associated with hypotonia, mental retardation, and a predilection for diabetes mellitus. Both of these disorders also feature obesity and hypogonadism that are thought to be hypothalamic in origin.

PATHOLOGICAL SEQUELAE Increased adipose tissue stores are deposited subcutaneously around all internal organs, throughout the omentum, and in the intramuscular spaces. Obese individuals also have an expansion of lean body mass as evidenced by increased size of the kidneys, heart, liver, and skeletal muscle mass. Fatty livers are common in extreme obesity.

Adipocyte size and number Obese individuals can be classified on the basis of the relative degree of *adipocyte hypertrophy* versus *hyperplasia*. In several rodent species and in humans the capacity to increase adipocyte number exists for only a limited period in early life. Sometime prior to reaching adulthood the organism's ability to increase the number of adipocytes ceases, and after this time expansion of adipose tissue mass is accomplished solely by an increase in fat-cell size. Thus, overnutrition during the time of preadipocyte proliferation leads to a permanent change in cell number and an increase in cell size; later nutritional alterations influence only cell size. Cross-sectional studies in humans have demonstrated that *individuals with severe obesity have both increased adipocyte size and number* with a tendency toward onset of obesity early in life. Patients having mild to moderate obesity show *only fat-cell hypertrophy,* and the onset of obesity is during adult life. Impressive supporting evidence for this formulation has been provided by studies showing that when adult men are made experimentally obese by purposeful overfeeding, fat-cell size, but not number, increases. Weight reduction is accompanied only by a decrease in adipocyte size. It is possible that preadipocyte proliferation from adipoblasts, usually a phenomenon of early life, can also occur at additional critical points such as puberty and early adolescence.

METABOLIC SEQUELAE Obesity has a profound impact on diabetes mellitus and various hyperlipoproteinemias primarily through its influences on insulin secretion and insulin sensitivity (see Chaps. 100 and 338).

Hyperinsulinemia: insulin resistance Increased insulin secretion is a well-characterized feature of obesity. It occurs in the basal state and in response to a wide variety of insulinogenic agents. A correlation exists between the degree of obesity and the magnitude of the hyperinsulinemia—particularly the basal insulin levels. Some obese patients exhibit hyperglycemia or frank diabetes in the face of hyperinsulinemia. The combination of hyper- or euglycemia and hyperinsulinemia indicates an insulin-resistant state, and decreased hypoglycemic responses to insulin are common in obese humans and animals. Insulin resistance could be due to an abnormal beta-cell product, circulating insulin antagonists, or tissue insulin insensitivity. Since abnormal islet secretory products or circulating antagonists have not been identified, it is thought that the insulin resistance of obesity is primarily due to tissue insensitivity. The initial step in the cellular action of insulin involves binding to specific cell surface receptors located in target tissues. After the formation of the plasma membrane–insulin receptor complex, insulin's biological effects are initiated. Cells from obese animals and humans contain decreased numbers of insulin receptors, and this decrease in insulin receptors doubtless plays an important role in the insulin resistance of obesity. However, other factors may participate. The enlarged adipocytes of obese rats have a decrease in insulin receptors but an even greater defect in the capacity to metabolize glucose, suggesting a major biochemical abnormality distal to the receptor mechanism. Since adipose tissue accounts for only a small (< 5 percent) portion of total body glucose metabolism, a similar intracellular defect presumably exists in other major insulin target tissues such as muscle and liver. Both decreased insulin receptors and intracellular defects in glucose metabolism probably contribute to the overall tissue insulin resistance in obesity.

Diabetes mellitus Although only a minority of obese patients are diabetic, the converse is not the case. Nonketotic, insulin-independent patients compose about 90 percent of the diabetic population in the United States, and 80 to 90 percent of nonketotic diabetics are obese. Obesity is an important contributory factor in these patients, predominantly through its influences on insulin sensitivity. Obesity exacerbates the diabetic state, and in many cases diabetes can be ameliorated by weight reduction.

Hyperlipoproteinemia (see also Chap. 100) Most plasma cholesterol circulates in the low-density lipoprotein (LDL) fraction, and, in the fasting state, very low density lipoproteins (VLDL) contain most of the circulating triglyceride. The association between obesity and elevated LDL levels is modest at best, and this is especially true when the relationship is corrected for other factors such as age. Total body cholesterol is increased in obesity, but this is mainly accounted for by adipose tissue cholesterol stores. Cholesterol turnover may be increased in obesity, leading to increased biliary excretion of cholesterol. This may contribute to the increased incidence of gallstone formation in obese individuals. Obesity has a more clear-cut and pronounced effect on VLDL metabolism. Hypertriglyceridemia is frequent, and the degree of obesity correlates with the level of hypertriglyceridemia. The increased triglyceride levels are due to increased hepatic VLDL production with no defect in the removal of VLDL from plasma. As discussed above, plasma insulin levels are greatly elevated in obesity, particularly in the portal blood. Hyperinsulinemia can promote increased hepatic VLDL synthesis and secretion. In addition, increased plasma free fatty acid (FFA) turnover exists in obesity, and FFA extracted by the liver provides an important precursor for hepatic triglyceride synthesis. Thus, the hypertriglyceridemia in obesity may be secondary to increased hepatic VLDL secretion due to hyperinsulinemia and augmented FFA availability.

MANIFESTATIONS AND COMPLICATIONS Gross obesity produces mechanical and physical stresses that aggravate or directly cause a number of disorders including osteoarthritis (especially the hips) and sciatica. Additionally, varicose veins, thromboembolism, ventral and hiatal hernias, and cholelithiasis are more common than in individuals of normal weight.

Hypertension In significantly obese persons, use of the standard size blood pressure cuff leads to readings which are erroneously high; an oversize cuff should always be used. A strong association between hypertension and obesity is observed even when accurate measurements are obtained. The mechanisms whereby obesity causes hypertension are uncertain, but peripheral vascular resistance is usually normal, while blood volume is increased. Weight loss leads to significant reductions in systemic blood pressure independent of changes in sodium balance.

Hypoventilation syndrome (Pickwickian syndrome) The obesity-hypoventilation syndrome is a heterogeneous group of disorders with differing clinical manifestations. The hypersomnolence that can occur in obesity is a manifestation of nighttime sleep apnea. In these individuals, once sleep begins, upper airway obstruction leads to hypoxemia and hypercapnia, causing arousal with return of normal respiration. Many such episodes occur each night, leading to chronic sleep deprivation and daytime somnolence. The combination of the obese habitus plus sleep-induced relaxation of the pharyngeal musculature is believed to be the cause of the intermittent upper airway obstruction. Occasionally such episodes are life-threatening (causing serious cardiac arrhythmias) and require long-term tracheostomy therapy. Chronic daytime hypoventilation is common but usually is not as severe as that occurring during sleep. Abnormalities of the respiratory control centers may also be important. Patients with hypoventilation display blunted ventilatory responses to hypercapnia and hypoxia and often develop hypercapnia and hypoxemia due to decreased basal ventilation; in addition, ventilation/perfusion mismatch due to mechanical factors may be present. In severe cases polycythemia, pulmonary hypertension, and cor pulmonale can result. Weight reduction will reverse these abnormalities if instituted before permanent cardiac damage develops. Some obese patients with sleep apnea and hypersomnolence do not have daytime hypoventilation and have normal ventilatory responses to hypoxia and hypercapnia. Progestational agents have been used therapeutically in the obesity-hypoventilation syndrome since they stimulate the ventilatory response to hypercarbia and hypoxia in normal subjects. Medroxyprogesterone increases ventilation and improves heart failure and erythrocytosis in these patients, although obstructive sleep apnea continues.

Adrenal function Although Cushing's disease can usually be distinguished from simple obesity on purely clinical grounds, laboratory testing is occasionally necessary. This can lead to confusion since 24-h urinary 17-hydroxycorticoid excretion is often elevated in obesity. Less commonly, plasma cortisol levels are also increased. Corticosteroid levels are usually suppressible with dexamethasone in obesity, but occasionally suppression is incomplete, rendering the diagnosis difficult.

Growth hormone Secretory responses of growth hormone to a variety of stimuli such as hypoglycemia, exercise, and arginine infusion are reduced. Furthermore, the starvation-induced rise in plasma growth hormone levels is attenuated.

Obesity as a risk factor Obesity is a serious risk factor for the development of coronary artery disease and stroke. Most of the risk imparted by obesity is mediated through the associated hypertension, hyperlipoproteinemia, and diabetes. Nevertheless, even when these abnormalities are factored out, a residual, albeit much smaller, risk can be ascribed to obesity per se.

TREATMENT Amelioration of hyperinsulinemia, insulin resistance, diabetes, hypertension, and hyperlipidemia can occur following weight loss. These changes are significant and enduring provided the weight loss is maintained. During weight loss all adipose tissue depots diminish proportionately. This generalized loss produces unattractive cosmetic effects. Many techniques, exercises, and other maneuvers have been proposed to effect selective adipose tissue reduction over particular regions of the body, but none is effective.

Methods of weight reduction In cases where obesity is secondary, the appropriate therapy is to treat the underlying disease. Most of the time the difficult problem of primary weight reduction must be undertaken.

Diet Caloric restriction is the cornerstone of any weight reduction program. From both the patient's and the physician's standpoint this is a frustrating and demanding undertaking. The basic principles of caloric restriction are simple. If caloric intake is less than caloric expenditure, stored calories, predominantly in the form of fat, will be consumed. In general, a deficit of 7700 kcal leads to loss of about 1 kg fat. By estimating the patient's daily caloric needs (approximately 33 kcal/kg), one can calculate the daily deficit necessary to achieve a given rate of weight loss.

Dietary restriction can range from total starvation to mild caloric deprivation, and these approaches will be discussed separately. Dietary recommendations are most effective when they are specific and geared to the patient's life-style. A dietitian or a similarly trained health professional should interview each patient and estimate his average daily caloric intake, food preferences, and eating patterns. The amount of calories the patient is to consume on the restricted diet should then be carefully explained in terms of quantities of specific foodstuffs. Frequently, the therapist must balance the degree of restriction against potential patient noncompliance. The more restrictive the diet, the more rapid the weight loss, but also the more likely the noncompliance. It is preferable to design a diet with which the patient is happy and comfortable and that produces a modest but steady weight loss.

The process of weight reduction has become a multimillion dollar business in the United States, and there are almost as many diets as there are therapists. Each proponent claims that the presence or absence of certain foodstuffs is desirable for more effective weight loss. However, little evidence exists to support the claim that calorie for calorie one hypocaloric diet will lead to a greater weight loss than another. The relationship between the patient and the therapist, plus patient education and encouragement, are more important to success than are the specific dietary constituents. The major virtue of "fad" diets is that patients are usually motivated to try them, at least initially, and patient cooperation is often better. Provided a particular diet is not harmful, probably the best course for the therapist is to maintain flexibility in the treatment program. Nevertheless, diets markedly deficient in any major class of foodstuff are to be avoided. For example, whole-food diets that are exceedingly low in carbohydrate are by nature high in fat and, depending on the type and quantity of fat ingested, may lead to hypercholesterolemia. The major virtue of a low-carbohydrate diet is the attendant increase in ketosis. (Ketone bodies have a central anorexant effect.) This provides part of the rationale for the widely touted liquid or powdered protein diets. These diets have been dubbed "protein-sparing modified fasts," and claims have been made that they allow drastic long-term caloric restriction without inducing negative nitrogen balance. These claims have not been substantiated, nor has it been shown that the diets lead to a greater degree of tissue weight loss than mixed hypocaloric diets of equal caloric value. Furthermore, a number of deaths have been reported in otherwise healthy individuals participating in such long-term dietary programs, even under medical supervision. Consequently, caution is required when treating obese patients with these approaches. Basically a calorie is a calorie whether it comes from protein, carbohydrate, or fat.

Prior to therapy it is wise to forewarn patients that when caloric restriction is started there is usually a marked initial weight loss, in large part due to fluid loss. The patient should be told that such rapid rates of loss will not persist. Likewise, positive shifts in fluid balance can sometimes mask real loss of adipose mass, a fact that can sometimes be demonstrated to the patient's satisfaction by keeping a record of skin fold thickness at monthly intervals.

Total starvation diets have been advocated for the treatment of obesity; provided underlying diseases such as gout, renal insufficiency, and ketosis-prone diabetes are not present, short-term fasts are usually well tolerated. Ketonemia and hyperuricemia regularly develop during starvation but rarely lead to acidosis or gout. Because of these potential complications, total fasting should be carried out only under medical supervision. Probably the major usefulness of total fasting is as a motivational aid at the beginning of a dietary program or when weight loss has stopped. Even though much of the weight loss during short-term fasting represents fluid, this weight loss can be encouraging to frustrated patients and motivate them to increase their compliance with the long-term weight reduction program.

The major problem in the treatment of obesity is not weight reduction but maintenance of the reduced weight. Provided the therapist works hard and long enough, most motivated patients can eventually lose weight. Unfortunately, only the rare patient maintains the weight loss permanently. Obesity is an eating disorder, and the underlying mechanisms are not reversed by limiting food intake.

Behavior modification In recognition of the problems involved, the techniques of behavior modification are being used increasingly to treat abnormal patterns of eating behavior. Many studies demonstrate that obese individuals respond less well than normal individuals to internal cues which regulate eating behavior such as gastric contractions, fear, and previous food ingestion. Conversely, obese subjects overrespond to external cues such as taste, smell, food attractiveness, abundance, and the amount of work involved in obtaining food. Given the fact that the obese individual is unusually susceptible to external stimuli, food intake may be altered by changing the pattern and nature of these external cues, and this is the major premise underlying the behavior modification approach to weight reduction.

Behavior modification begins with a detailed individual history of the patient's eating episodes with respect to time of day, length of eating period, place of ingestion (restaurant, dining table, standing in front of refrigerator), simultaneous activities (watching television, reading, idleness), emotional state, companions (relatives, friends, or alone), and finally the kinds and quantities of foods ingested. Once this detailed record is obtained, the therapist and patient can design specific behavioral changes aimed at disrupting or aborting recurring behavior patterns which initiate or prolong abnormal eating activity. As examples: if a patient eats in response to certain emotional states, then other activities can be consciously substituted when the patient perceives such a state; if the patient snacks frequently from readily available food storage areas (refrigerators, cookie jars, etc.), then he is encouraged to eat only while sitting down at a table with a fixed place setting; if eating frequently occurs while watching television alone, then efforts to avoid this activity can be initiated. Obviously, many other examples of specific and general interventions could be given. Results with behavior modification techniques have been encouraging and indicate that patients can maintain long-term weight reduction providing the new behavior patterns are truly "learned."

Exercise In any weight reduction program exercise has its place. However, the importance of exercise in terms of caloric balance must be clearly understood. Table 76-1 shows that even moderate daily exercise would not lead to a large enough increase in caloric expenditure to alter significantly the initial rate of weight reduction. This does not mean exercise is unimportant in weight reduction, since even modest increases in caloric expenditure can lead to large long-term differences in caloric balance, provided exercise is performed on a regular basis. For example, a daily increase in caloric expenditure of 300 cal over a period of 4 months could lead to a 4.5-kg weight loss. More importantly, there is evidence that incorporation of regular exercise into the overall weight reduction program improves the chances that the patient will maintain his weight loss.

Drugs Two classes of drugs are frequently used in the treatment of obesity: anorexants and thyroid hormone supplements. The addition of L-thyroxine or triiodothyronine to a weight reduction program is of no benefit. These drugs are ineffective in promoting adipose tissue loss and, if anything, accentuate lean tissue loss causing negative nitrogen balance. In susceptible individuals, cardiotoxicity may occur. Thus, unless clear-cut hypothyroidism is present, thyroid supplementation has no role in the treatment of obesity.

The major anorexants are amphetamine-like agents, and these drugs presumably exert their effect at the level of the hypothalamus. It is probable that they have a modest effect in promoting short-term weight loss in certain individuals. However, they are effective for a period of only a few weeks, and problems of habituation, addiction, and generalized drug abuse limit their usefulness. Two newer anorexants, diethylpropion and fenfluramine, may be less addictive and, therefore, somewhat more useful. However, none of these agents treats the underlying eating disorder, and they are, therefore, of little use in maintenance of weight reduction.

Injections of human chorionic gonadotropin (HCG) have been popularized as an adjunct to weight reduction, but no evidence exists to indicate a beneficial effect. The primary effectiveness of the HCG-diet program is due to the calorically restricted diet, frequent physician contact, and placebo effects. Comparable weight loss is achieved if saline injections are substituted for HCG.

Jejunoileal shunt Small-bowel bypass is an effective means of achieving weight reduction in morbidly obese patients. However, it is an experimental procedure and should be attempted only in institutions where a trained team is committed to regular, systematic, and long-term follow-up.

The most common operative procedures involve end-to-end or end-to-side anastomosis of about 38 cm of proximal jejunum to 10 cm of terminal ileum. Weight loss is initially rapid, reaching a plateau at 18 to 24 months. While all patients lose weight, few return to ideal weight. In several series the mean weight loss was 30 to 50 percent of initial excess weight, leaving patients still about 50 percent overweight once a steady state was reached. Although some degree of malabsorption occurs, the major portion of the weight loss is due to decreased food intake.

TABLE 76-1
Energy equivalents of food calories expressed in minutes of activity

Food	Calories	Activity				
		Walking*	Riding bicycle†	Swimming‡	Running§	Reclining¶
Apple, large	101	19	12	9	5	78
Bacon, 2 strips	96	18	12	9	5	74
Beer, 1 glass	114	22	14	10	6	88
Bread and butter	78	15	10	7	4	60
Carbonated beverage, 1 glass	106	20	13	9	5	82
Carrot, raw	42	8	5	4	2	32
Cheese, cottage, 1 tbsp	27	5	3	2	1	21
Chicken, fried, ½ breast	232	45	28	21	12	178
Cookie, chocolate chip	51	10	6	5	3	39
Egg, fried	110	21	13	10	6	85
Ham, 2 slices	167	32	20	15	9	128
Ice cream, ⅙ qt	193	37	24	17	10	148
Mayonnaise, 1 tbsp	92	18	11	8	5	71
Milk, skim, 1 glass	81	16	10	7	4	62
Milk shake	421	81	51	38	22	324
Orange, medium	68	13	8	6	4	52
Pancake with syrup	124	24	15	11	6	95
Peas, green, ½ cup	56	11	7	5	3	43
Pizza, cheese, ⅛	180	35	22	16	9	138
Potato chips, 1 serving	108	21	13	10	6	83
Sandwiches:						
Hamburger	350	67	43	31	18	269
Tuna fish salad	278	53	34	25	14	214
Sherbet, ⅙ qt	177	34	22	16	9	136

* *Energy cost of walking for 70-kg individual = 5.2 cal/min at 3.5 mi/h.*
† *Energy cost of riding bicycle = 8.2 cal/min.*
‡ *Energy cost of swimming = 11.2 cal/min.*
§ *Energy cost of running = 19.4 cal./min.*
¶ *Energy cost of reclining = 1.3 cal/min.*

Most teams performing this surgery select patients who are at least 100 lb overweight and in whom adequate attempts at medical management have failed repeatedly. Because of postoperative morbidity, older patients ($>$ 50 years) and psychologically unstable individuals are usually excluded.

Complications of jejunoileal surgery are common. The overall surgical mortality ranges from 0.5 to 7.8 percent with an average of 3.9 percent. Mortality is inversely related to the experience of the surgical team. The major postoperative morbidity is related to wound infection and thromboembolism. The common serious medical complications are cirrhosis and hepatic failure, nephrolithiasis, electrolyte imbalances, cholelithiasis, and arthritis (Table 76-2). Severe liver disease probably occurs in only 5 percent of patients, but milder degrees of hepatic dysfunction are more common. The long-range implications of mild hepatic abnormalities are unknown. Possible causes of liver damage following small-bowel bypass include (1) protein and particularly essential amino acid deficiency, (2) accumulation of hepatotoxic, secondary bile salts, and (3) release of unknown toxic substances from the excluded bowel. Hypokalemia is most likely secondary to diarrhea. Persistent calcium and magnesium deficiency can result from malabsorption and must be treated with appropriate replacement. Transient depression of plasma 25-hydroxyvitamin D levels may also contribute to abnormal mineral metabolism. Nephrolithiasis can occur in up to 30 percent of patients and is due to hyperoxaluria secondary to calcium malabsorption (see Chap. 292). It can be treated by calcium supplements and a low oxalate intake. Migratory polyarthritis has been found in up to 6 percent of patients and may be due to circulating immune complexes.

Gastric surgery Gastroplasty establishes a small upper gastric remnant connected to a larger lower gastric pouch by a narrow 1- to 1.5-cm channel. Gastric bypass excludes the lower 90 percent of the stomach pouch and maintains intestinal continuity of the upper 10 percent via a retrocolic gastrojejunostomy. Both of these procedures cause patients to limit food intake by delaying gastric emptying and providing a small gastric reservoir so that fullness is experienced after a small meal. Weight loss with these procedures has been comparable with that achieved with small-bowel bypass operations but without the complications related to malabsorption, diarrhea, and hepatic dysfunction.

SUMMARY For most patients obesity is an eating disorder, and a major hope for effective long-term treatment of this disease lies in understanding the causes of overeating. Clearly no single etiology explains all cases, and different causes exist for different individuals. At present a variety of techniques, gimmicks, and maneuvers are available to effect initial weight loss. Unfortunately, initial weight loss is not the real therapeutic problem. Rather, the problem is that almost all obese patients eventually regain their weight. An effective means to sustain weight loss is the major challenge in the treatment of obesity today. The technique of behavioral modification, when professionally and rigorously applied, is the best tool for this task. As information develops concerning the hypothalamic "set point," or *adipostat*, and the factors that regulate it, pharmacological and perhaps physiological methods may emerge that will effect long-term correction of abnormal eating patterns.

REFERENCES

Assimacopoulos-Jeannet F, Jeanrenaud B: The hormonal and metabolic basis of experimental obesity. Clin Endocrinol Metab 5:337, 1976

Bray GA: Current status of intestinal bypass surgery in the treatment of obesity. Diabetes 26:1072, 1977

Hashim SA, Porikos K: Food intake behavior in man: Implications for treatment of obesity. Clin Endocrinol Metab 5:503, 1976

Hirsch J, Batchelor B: Adipose tissue cellularity in human obesity. Clin Endocrinol Metab 5:299, 1976

Mann GV: The influence of obesity on health. N Engl J Med 291:178, 226, 1974

Olefsky JM: The insulin receptor: Its role in insulin resistance in obesity and diabetes. Diabetes 25:1154, 1976

Printen KJ, Mason EE: Gastric surgery for relief of morbid obesity. Arch Surg 106:428, 1973

Sims EAH: Experimental obesity, dietary induced thermogenesis, and their clinical implications. Clin Endocrinol Metab 5:377, 1976

TABLE 76-2
Complications of bypass surgery

Complication	Percentage
EARLY	
Perioperative mortality	2–6
Thromboembolic disease	1–5
Wound infection	2–5
Renal failure	3
Severe nausea vomiting	3
Wound dehiscence	1–3
LATE	
Urinary calculi	3–10
Severe electrolyte imbalance	5–8
Acute cholecystitis	0–5
Progressive liver disease	2–4
Intestinal obstruction	2
Peptic ulcer	1–2
Osteoporosis	?
Tuberculosis	1
MINOR	
Diarrhea	100
Weakness	80
Hypokalemia	80
Hypoproteinemia	50
Vomiting	50
Thirst	50
Hypocalcemia	30
Arthralgias	15
Incisional hernias	3
Hyperuricemia	$<$10
Anemias (Fe, vitamin B_{12}, folate)	$<$10

77
ANOREXIA NERVOSA

ROBERT M. BOYAR

Anorexia nervosa is a disorder of previously healthy adolescent girls who become emaciated as a result of voluntary starvation. The population at risk consists largely of white girls from middle- to upper-class backgrounds. The disorder rarely occurs in black or oriental women and is almost never seen in men. Primary anorexia nervosa should be distinguished from eating disorders associated with psychiatric diseases such as schizophrenia, depression, obsessive-compulsive states, and hysteria.

CLINICAL PICTURE The anorexia syndrome usually begins before or shortly after puberty but may appear earlier or later (rarely above the middle twenties). Patients frequently communicate a history of having been overweight in childhood. Sometimes a precipitating stressful event can be identified, such as

TABLE 77-1
Criteria for the diagnosis of anorexia nervosa

I Onset prior to age 25
II Anorexia with weight loss of at least 25 percent of original body weight
III Distorted attitude toward eating, food, or weight that overrides hunger, admonitions, reassurances, and threats
IV No known medical illness that could account for the weight loss
V No other known psychiatric disorder
VI At least two of the following manifestations:
   A Amenorrhea
   B Lanugo hair
   C Bradycardia (persistent resting pulse of 60 beats per minute or less)
   D Periods of overactivity
   E Episodes of bulimia
   F Vomiting (may be self-induced)

leaving home for the first time. The characteristic clinical finding is emaciation equivalent to that seen in the concentration camps of World War II. Despite this emaciation the patients deny hunger, thinness, and fatigue. They are often physically active, and ritualized exercise programs are common. If social circumstances require them to eat, they frequently induce vomiting as soon as they can reach a bathroom. Amenorrhea is present almost invariably.

In advanced cases physical examination shows absent body fat. Body hair is often increased. Usually this is of fine, lanugo quality, but frank hirsutism may occur. Interestingly, breast tissue is often preserved. Parotid glands may be enlarged as in other forms of starvation. Edema is common. Because of edema in the legs and parotid gland enlargement, which gives a fullness to the face, the patient's true state of emaciation may be masked when she is fully dressed. The skin tends to be dry. Body temperature is often in the hypothermic range. Blood pressure is low, and the pulse is slow.

Laboratory abnormalities that may be present include anemia and leukopenia with hypocellularity of the bone marrow, hypokalemia, and hypoalbuminemia. Serum β-carotene levels tend to be elevated with a concomitant decrease in vitamin A concentration. The serum cholesterol concentration is sometimes increased. Glucose tolerance is abnormal, as would be expected in any starving subject. Other laboratory tests are usually normal. The endocrine changes of anorexia nervosa will be considered separately below.

A summary of the diagnostic criteria for anorexia nervosa is given in Table 77-1.

PSYCHOLOGICAL ASPECTS While all investigators agree that anorexia nervosa is associated with profound psychological dysfunction, there is disagreement about its nature. One interpretation is that the primary drive is the need to break away from a restrictive family environment. Often there is a history of a strong mother who has imposed eating demands on the child from an early age. The timing of the illness around puberty suggests that developing sexuality and the necessity of accommodating to a widening social circle play significant roles. Poor self-esteem and a sense of ineffectiveness have been commonly noted. Analytically oriented psychiatrists assume that the denial of hunger, the refusal to eat, the self-induced vomiting, and the ritualized exercise are symbolic expressions of the patient's need to take control over her own body. A fear of fatness also seems to play a role, particularly when one or both parents are overweight. A second school believes that the primary problem in anorexia nervosa is depression. Those holding to this view point out that loss of appetite, lack of self-esteem, disinterest in personal appearance, and self-destructive thoughts are common manifestations of depression. Some studies have shown that up to 80 percent of anorexia patients exhibit symptoms of depression. In support of this hypothesis,

a high percentage of first-degree relatives of such subjects have been reported to have a history of manic-depressive or depressive illness. A third theory, held by some biologically oriented psychiatrists, is that an abnormality exists in the satiety center of the hypothalamus in patients with anorexia nervosa. The evidence for this interpretation is not persuasive.

To summarize, while the psychiatric manifestations of anorexia nervosa are well understood at the descriptive level, the mechanisms by which they are produced remain uncertain.

ENDOCRINOLOGIC ASPECTS A number of endocrinologic abnormalities accompany anorexia nervosa. Most are probably the consequence of starvation and malnutrition.

Amenorrhea The onset of amenorrhea is usually associated with significant weight loss, but menses may cease prior to any decrease in body mass. Studies of the 24-h circadian pattern of luteinizing hormone (LH) in patients with anorexia show regression of the maturational stage of LH secretion to a pattern characteristic of prepubertal or early pubertal girls; i.e., episodic LH release is missing or occurs only during sleep (see Fig. 77-1). Administration of clomiphene citrate fails to result in a rise in plasma LH and follicle-stimulating hormone (FSH) concentrations. Normal LH secretory patterns return, and response to clomiphene reverts to normal following weight gain. It is now accepted that menarche usually does not appear (despite spontaneous gonadotropin release activity) until the percentage of body fat reaches 17 percent. Interestingly, return of menses in patients with secondary amenorrhea due to starvation does not occur until body fat reaches 27 percent, a figure some 10 percent higher than the value required for menarche.

FIGURE 77-1

Plasma LH concentration every 20 min for 24 h during acute exacerbation of anorexia nervosa (upper panel) and after clinical remission with return of body weight to normal (lower panel). (From Boyar et al, 1974. Used by permission.)

The mechanism for secondary amenorrhea occurring prior to weight loss in patients who subsequently develop anorexia nervosa is unknown. It is possible that amenorrhea with or without weight loss is due to abnormalities in the hypothalamus since injections of gonadotropin-releasing hormone in these subjects results in LH and FSH release. While the initial LH response is blunted, repeated injections are followed by normalization of the LH response. Ovulation has been induced by such treatment.

If anorexia begins before the expected onset of puberty, primary amenorrhea may be the complaint bringing the patient to the physician.

Adrenal function   Patients with anorexia nervosa have reduced urinary excretion of 17-hydroxysteroids but normal or elevated plasma cortisol concentrations. Cortisol production rates are normal or slightly elevated, while metabolic clearance is decreased. Plasma half-life of cortisol is prolonged. Some patients, particularly those with agitation or depression, show hyperresponsiveness to adrenocorticotropic hormone (ACTH) and a failure to suppress normally after dexamethasone. Urinary 17-ketosteroids are low, reflecting a decreased production of dehydroepiandrosterone sulfate, dehydroepiandrosterone, and androstenedione.

Thyroid function   Thyroid hormone levels of plasma are altered by anorexia nervosa. Both thyroxine (T_4) and 3,3′,5-triiodothyronine (T_3) concentrations are decreased, while levels of the physiologically inactive 3,3′,5′-triiodothyronine (reverse T_3, rT_3) are increased. The latter change is thought to be the consequence of decreased conversion of rT_3 to diiodothyronine. Plasma thyrotropin (TSH) concentrations are normal, and response to thyrotropin-releasing hormone (TRH) is intact. These changes are characteristic of starvation and wasting diseases; they cannot be considered specific for anorexia nervosa.

Pituitary function   Patients with anorexia nervosa have normal growth-hormone concentrations but show increased growth-hormone release after TRH, an anomalous response that is also seen in protein-energy malnutrition. Other pituitary hormones, including prolactin, seem to function normally.

TEMPERATURE REGULATION   Subjects with moderately severe anorexia nervosa appear to have a defect in temperature regulation. They fail to shiver or to increase core temperature following cold exposure and do not diminish core temperature in response to external heat. In view of the previously described abnormalities in gonadotropin regulation, it is attractive to suppose that the defect in temperature control resides in the hypothalamus. Consistent with this view is the observation that concentration of the urine following dehydration is submaximal in these subjects, a finding suggestive of a defect in release of antidiuretic hormone.

TREATMENT   Since the etiology of anorexia nervosa is unknown, there is no specific therapy. However, it is important to identify the disorder early so that supportive treatment can be initiated prior to the development of significant weight loss. The most effective treatment is the removal of the patient from the environment in which the disorder occurred. This usually requires hospitalization where active intervention can be undertaken. The supportive care of an understanding physician is usually of great benefit. If the psychiatric disturbance is significant, the coordinated effort of a psychiatrist with a special interest in the adolescent is often helpful. Antidepressant drugs

are occasionally useful. The long-term prognosis is generally good when treatment is initiated early; however, mortality in most series ranges between 2 and 5 percent. Until more is learned about etiology and pathogenesis of the disorder, treatment will be largely supportive in nature. In those instances in which starvation is extreme, parenteral nutrition may be indicated as described in Chap. 78.

REFERENCES

BOYAR RM et al: Anorexia nervosa: Immaturity of the 24 hour luteinizing hormone secretory pattern. N Engl J Med 291:861, 1974
———: Cortisol secretion and metabolism in anorexia nervosa. N Engl J Med 296:190, 1977
BRUCH H: Eating disorders: Obesity, anorexia nervosa, and the person within. New York, Basic Books, 1973
FEIGHNER JP et al: Diagnostic criteria for use in psychiatric research. Arch Gen Psychiatry 26:57, 1972
FRISCH FE, MCARTHUR JW: Menstrual cycles: Fatness as a determinant of minimum weight for height necessary for their maintenance or onset. Science 185:949, 1974
HALMI KA: Anorexia nervosa: Recent investigations. Annu Rev Med 29:137, 1978
MECKLENBURG RS et al: Hypothalamic dysfunction in patients with anorexia nervosa. Medicine 53:147, 1974
MOSHANG T JR et al: Low serum triiodothyronine in patients with anorexia nervosa. J Clin Endocrinol Metab 40:470, 1975
VIGERSKY R (ed): *Anorexia Nervosa.* New York, Raven Press, 1977
——— et al: Hypothalamic dysfunction in secondary amenorrhea associated with simple weight loss. N Engl J Med 297:1141, 1977

78
DIETARY THERAPY AND PARENTERAL NUTRITION

KHURSHEED N. JEEJEEBHOY

Regular intake of a variety of foods, necessary for survival and growth in normal humans, may be affected by a number of diseases which alter the ability to eat, absorb, or metabolize food. These diseases require dietary therapy. Diabetes mellitus, obesity, malabsorptive states, hyperlipoproteinemia, uremia, and congestive heart failure are obvious examples of illnesses where dietary manipulation plays a major role in treatment and where noncompliance with a dietary prescription may impair or even block the effectiveness of other therapeutic measures. Diets required in these and other conditions are described under the chapters devoted to each illness elsewhere in this book. Details of individual diets, including the foods required and proscribed, are readily available from dietary manuals and will not be described here. If available, a professional dietician should be utilized in initiating dietary therapy. In this chapter, after a brief review of dietary principles, emphasis will be placed on tube feeding and parenteral nutrition. Significant advances have been made in this area, and total parenteral nutrition is now recommended for growing numbers of patients in a wide variety of clinical situations. It is imperative, therefore, that the general internist be familiar with these techniques.

DIETARY THERAPY

In normal humans orally ingested nutrients provide the substrates necessary to meet energy requirements for physical and metabolic activity. Ordinarily intake matches utilization such that body composition remains relatively constant. This homeostasis may be altered by disease in several ways: (1) Intake and absorption of energy may be insufficient to meet body demands. (2) Food intake may be normal or increased but inadequate to meet increased requirements produced by the disease state. In both these situations weight loss and/or malnutrition will result if the illness is prolonged. (3) The intake of nutrients may exceed needs, causing weight gain and obesity. (4) Caloric intake may be appropriate, but specific nutrients may be deficient or present in excess.

In the planning of dietary therapy, the first step is the assessment of the operative pathophysiology, then a decision regarding the alteration of diet that will be required. For example, once the diagnosis of congestive heart failure is made, the need to restrict salt in the diet becomes obvious. Similarly, sprue requires gluten restriction; obesity, caloric limitation; diabetes, elimination of refined sugars; hepatic and renal failure, low protein intake; hypercholesterolemia, increased unsaturated fat; and phenylketonuria, a phenylalanine-free diet. Many other examples could be given. After the proper diet has been selected, other decisions become necessary. A common problem involves the degree of restriction to be prescribed. If limitation of salt is needed, should daily intake be 200 mg or 2 g? Such decisions demand more than a simple assessment of the state of the patient's disease. Also entering the equation is the likelihood of compliance by the patient and his ability to obtain the proper foods. The physician might prefer, for medical reasons, a 200-mg sodium diet but actually prescribe a 2-g sodium intake coupled with diuretic therapy because the patient does not have the economic resources to buy salt-free foods or distilled water to drink. An identical decision might be reached for a person of unlimited economic means who for psychological reasons will not eat a diet with maximum sodium restriction. Similarly the physician caring for a teen-ager with diabetes mellitus might modify the diabetic diet to allow the ingestion of a small amount of dessert on special occasions, despite its ordinary proscription, in order to keep the young person from feeling "different" from his or her peers. The patient with hypercholesterolemia might be allowed to eat eggs or steak once or twice a month in an attempt to enhance compliance with the diet on a day-to-day basis. Both of these are examples of the "treat" technique of dietary therapy. The point to be made is that diets must be prescribed realistically and not simply in accord with an abstract or theoretical ideal.

In most cases diets can be administered orally. In a number of situations, however, this is not possible. Two general problems exist. In the *first*, food cannot be swallowed normally. Examples are the comatose patient and subjects with an impairment of the swallowing mechanism. Cerebral vascular accidents are the most common cause clinically, but other neuromuscular diseases such as myasthenia gravis might act similarly. Obstruction to passage of food by esophageal cancer or scleroderma can preclude normal oral feeding. In these and similar illnesses tube feeding of defined formula diets or administration of such diets via a feeding jejunostomy may be the therapeutic avenue of choice. The *second* general category includes diseases where absorption of food in the intestinal tract is blocked or therapy demands bowel rest to allow healing of the primary pathological process. Regional ileitis and ulcerative colitis are classic examples of the latter. In these situations total parenteral nutrition by intravenous administration is required.

DEFINED FORMULA DIETS AND TUBE FEEDING

Patients unable to eat a normal diet can be nourished without resort to the parenteral route provided the diet can be modified to allow tube feeding without detrimental side effects. Such diets have now become commercially available and are composed of mixtures of precisely defined nutrients capable of being given through a fine silicone rubber feeding tube. They are called *defined formula diets* (DFD). While blenderized foods can also be used in some situations, they require a large-bore nasogastric tube for administration with attendant discomfort, risk of esophagitis, and aspiration.

COMPOSITION OF DEFINED FORMULA DIETS A selection from a vast number of available diets is given in Table 78-1. These diets can be grouped into (1) moderate-residue, lactose-containing diets, (2) low-residue, lactose-free diets with intact protein, and (3) amino acid-based lactose-free diets.

Defined formula diets differ in osmolality, palatability, absorbability, and lactose content. Diets listed in columns A and B (intact protein diets) in Table 78-1 are low in osmolality and are palatable. Amino acid-glucose-fatty acid based diets (Table 78-1, columns C) do not require digestion and hence may be absorbed in the presence of severe malabsorption. Diets in columns A can be given only to patients who do not have

TABLE 78-1
Complete nutritional preparations per 1000 kcal*

Name (Manufacturer):	A			B			C	
	Formula 2 (Cutter)	Compleat B (Doyle)	Sustacal Liquid (Mead Johnson)	Ensure (Ross)	Isocal (Mead Johnson)	Precision Isotonic (Doyle)	Flexical (Mead Johnson)	Vivonex (Eaton)
Protein, g	37.5	40.0	60.3	35.5	32.5	30.0	22.4	20.4
Protein source	Nonfat milk, beef	Nonfat milk, beef	Milk, soy protein	Milk, soy protein	Milk, soy protein	Egg white	Hydrolysed casein	Crystalline amino acids
Fat, g	40.0	40.0	23.0	35.0	42.0	31.3	34.0	1.4
Carbohydrate, g	122.5	120.0	137.8	136.7	125.0	150	154.0	226.3
Lactose, g	37.5	24.4	16.7	0	0	0	0	0
mosmol/kg	435–510	490	625	450	350	300	723	500
Volume needed to meet usual daily requirements, ml	2000	1600	1080	1920	1910	1560	2000	1800

* Composition is given only in terms of protein and energy, but these diets contain vitamins, minerals, and trace elements to meet requirements. For details see source.
SOURCE: *After Shils et al.*

lactose intolerance. All diets in columns A and B can be taken orally as well as by tube and are useful in some ambulatory patients with chronic obstructive or inflammatory bowel disease. They are more palatable than those of columns C. The latter are amino acid-glucose based and in theory should be easily absorbed. However, they cause diarrhea in patients with short-bowel syndromes, a side effect which limits their usefulness. They may also cause bloating, nausea, gastric dilatation, and hyperglycemia. Diets in columns A and B have fewer side effects. Even though they utilize intact protein instead of free amino acids, their slower intestinal transit time usually offsets any disadvantage resulting from the requirement for digestion of protein prior to absorption.

MODE OF ADMINISTRATION   Diets grouped under columns A and B in Table 78-1 can be fed orally in small quantities at frequent intervals. They are preferably served ice cold. Diets under columns C must be given as a slow intragastric or intraintestinal drip. Intragastric drip should be used in all patients with marked "intestinal hurry," malabsorption, and diarrhea in order to provide a uniform slow input of the formula. The preferred method of administration is an infusion given at the rate of 20 to 30 ml/h via a 2- to 3-mm silicone rubber nasogastric tube. The stomach is aspirated after 4 h, and if the residual volume exceeds 50 ml, the infusion is stopped temporarily. If the volume is less than 50 ml, the rate of infusion is gradually increased to 125 ml/h over a 3- to 4-day period. Blood glucose, blood urea nitrogen (BUN), electrolytes, phosphate, calcium, and magnesium should be monitored three times a week until stabilized. If diarrhea occurs, loperamide or diphenoxylate with atropine may be given. Caution is required with these drugs because of the danger of developing gastric dilatation and vomiting.

INDICATIONS   Defined formula diets given orally or by tube feeding are indicated in three general situations. The first consists of conditions where an oral diet cannot be eaten. Examples include unconsciousness, oropharyngeal abnormalities, partial esophageal obstruction, and severe anorexia. A second indication is disease characterized by discomfort after ingestion of normal food, e.g., partial bowel obstruction due to Crohn's disease or adhesions, infiltrative disease of the intestine, and chronic pancreatitis. The third category includes malabsorptive diseases, gastrointestinal fistulas, and short-bowel syndromes. Diets listed in columns C of Table 78-1 are helpful in this group of diseases.

PARENTERAL NUTRITION

This section is mainly concerned with techniques for providing nutrients in circumstances where, owing to disorders of the gastrointestinal tract, patients cannot eat a normal diet, do not absorb an oral diet efficiently, or deteriorate clinically on oral feeding. Such patients need partial or complete nourishment via the parenteral route for varying lengths of time ranging from days to years. The particular combination of nutrients and the route of infusion vary with the needs of the patient and the duration of infusion. Discussed below are the indications for parenteral nutrition and the principles and techniques necessary for rational parenteral therapy.

INDICATIONS FOR TOTAL PARENTERAL NUTRITION   The indications for total parenteral nutrition (TPN), are fairly easily recognized. They include the following situations:

1 Malnourished patients who are unable to eat or to absorb an oral diet. In such patients the diagnosis of malnutrition should be based on a number of factors including previous dietary history, evidence of muscle wasting, hypoalbuminemia, edema, reduced skin fold thickness, and body weight. Weight alone is not sufficient to make the diagnosis of malnutrition because edema or previous obesity may mask the degree of nitrogen depletion actually present.

2 For bowel rest in patients with Crohn's disease, intestinal fistulas, and pancreatitis. In these patients food ingestion often results in exacerbation of symptoms with increased inflammation and high output through fistulas, preventing healing. When they are given nothing by mouth and receive TPN, they appear to improve rapidly, heal fistulas without surgery, and maintain nutritional status.

3 For well-nourished patients entering the hospital who will be unable to eat temporarily. In these cases a judgment has to be made about the probable length of time that oral diet will not be available. If the period is likely to exceed 10 to 14 days, then total parenteral nutrition should be administered to avoid undue wasting and malnutrition during the period of starvation. This is especially important if sepsis and trauma complicate the clinical picture since both accelerate catabolism and tissue wasting.

4 Prolonged coma when tube feeding is not possible.

5 Nutritional support in patients with marked hypercatabolism, such as those with severe trauma and burns, even if some oral intake is possible.

6 Nutritional support during therapy for malignant disease. In many patients with malignant tumors weight loss is a prominent feature and is accentuated by surgery, radiation, or chemotherapy. Chemotherapy is particularly prone to cause anorexia and mucosal inflammation that may severely limit oral intake. TPN given prior to and with chemotherapy results in an improved nutritional status in these patients.

NUTRIENT REQUIREMENTS DURING TPN   Energy and fluid requirements   Afebrile patients without septicemia require about 32 kcal per kilogram of ideal body weight daily for weight maintenance and 40 to 45 kcal/kg for weight gain when malnourished. The energy requirement increases to 60 kcal/kg per day with a body temperature of 40°C. While elective surgery does not increase these requirements significantly, septicemia does increase them by 50 percent; in burns exceeding 40 percent of the surface area, the requirements may increase by about 100 percent.

Basal fluid intake should be about 1 to 1.2 ml/kcal infused. To this amount should be added a volume equivalent to losses from diarrhea, stomal output, nasogastric suction, and fistula drainage. In oliguric renal failure a basal intake of 750 to 1000 ml should be given plus a volume equal to that of urine and other losses. In patients with cardiac failure about 40 ml/kg can be infused provided that the sodium intake is restricted to between 20 and 50 meq per day.

Amino acid requirements   The efficient functioning of the body requires maintenance of the integrity of the musculoskeletal system and viscera together with normal levels of enzymes, hormones, and plasma proteins. All are dependent on new protein synthesis to meet the demands of normal turnover, and this protein synthesis in turn requires that amino acids be available. A major objective of parenteral nutrition is to provide an adequate supply of amino acids for protein synthesis. The amount required is influenced by several factors. Severe injury, sepsis, and burns dramatically increase nitrogen losses as already mentioned, requiring that larger amounts of amino acids be infused in their presence. The pattern of amino acids infused is important since unbalanced mixtures will not support protein synthesis. Finally, requirements are much larger if amino acids are given as the sole energy source than they are if caloric demands are met by fat or carbohydrate.

In pure dietary starvation the infusion of 100 g glucose per day reduces urinary nitrogen loss but will not produce positive nitrogen balance. Infusion of amino acids also reduces net nitrogen deficits and in large amounts can induce a slight positive nitrogen balance. During starvation a fall in plasma insulin coupled with a rise in glucacon, cortisol, and catecholamines shifts body metabolism toward a fat economy by elevating plasma free fatty acid concentrations and increasing ketone body production. Certain experimental evidence suggests that this elevation of plasma ketones may have a role in minimizing breakdown of muscle protein (and hence the negative nitrogen balance of prolonged starvation). On the basis of these experiments it was postulated by some investigators that the infusion of glucose together with amino acids would be detrimental since a glucose-induced rise in insulin secretion would lower plasma free fatty acids and diminish plasma ketone concentrations, with the result that protein breakdown in muscle would be accelerated. While this area remains controversial, the author believes the evidence to be persuasive that when amino acids are infused with glucose sufficient to meet caloric requirements, they are more efficiently used than when given alone. Significantly positive nitrogen balance is achieved in most malnourished patients (not suffering abnormal losses) by infusing only 0.5 to 1.0 g amino acids per kilogram of ideal body weight per day if nonprotein calories are optimal. Abnormal losses, such as protein-rich exudates in burns, or upper gastrointestinal tract contents rich in pancreatic secretions increase requirements to between 1.5 and 2.0 g/kg per day. As the input of nonprotein energy is increased, there is a concurrent augmentation of nitrogen retention at all levels of amino acid intake until the input of nonprotein energy reaches 55 to 60 kcal per kilogram of ideal body weight. Beyond this point additional calories do not seem to improve nitrogen retention significantly in adults.

Relation of nitrogen retention to the source of nonprotein energy
Both carbohydrates and lipids can be infused with amino acids to provide sufficient nonprotein energy to meet metabolic requirements of the patient. The question then arises whether glucose and lipid are comparable in improving the utilization of amino acids above the level seen in hypocaloric states. The answer, obtained from carefully controlled crossover studies, is that the two types of substrate are equal in efficacy after an initial 3- to 4-day period for adaptation to the source of the energy. Hence the source of nonprotein energy chosen for use in a patient depends on factors other than its effect on nitrogen retention.

The first factor of importance is osmotic pressure. Concentrated glucose solutions are hyperosmolar and cause thrombosis when administered by peripheral vein. TPN regimens using glucose as the primary energy source thus require placement of a catheter in the superior vena cava where rapid blood flow quickly dilutes the hypertonic infusion. A second major consideration is the metabolic state of the patient. Glucose requires insulin for utilization, and hypertonic glucose solutions are probably not ideal in diabetic subjects. Conversely triglyceride emulsions might be contraindicated in hyperlipoproteinemic states.

Glucose infusion mixtures are quite simple and consist of 25 percent dextrose containing 2 percent amino acids together with necessary vitamins and minerals. Lipid emulsions are mixtures of triglyceride, phospholipid (as an emulsifying agent), and glycerol or sorbitol which is added to maintain isotonicity. Lipid can be infused with amino acid-dextrose mixtures using a Y connector to provide 50 to 80 percent of nonprotein calories. These concentrations can be given by peripheral vein without fear of thrombosis. Insulin is not required for metabolism of the fat; indeed, insulin concentrations are low, and free fatty acids and ketones are high during

the administration of lipid when this is providing the major part of nonprotein calories. A valuable additional benefit is that lipid solutions can be discontinued abruptly without danger of hypoglycemia because insulin levels are not elevated. This aspect is particularly important in critically ill patients who may require repeated and unpredictable alterations in their infusions, especially when surgery has to be carried out upon short notice. Finally, lipid infusions meet essential fatty acid requirements since linoleic acid is present in sufficient quantities if as little as 500 ml Intralipid (the commercially available triglyceride emulsion) is given daily. While essential fatty acid deficiency is rare in adults, biochemical signs of deficiency may appear in as little as 1 week with TPN in the absence of lipid, and abnormalities of liver function and skin rash may follow.

It is also possible to carry out TPN with a 1:1 mixture of glucose and lipid calories. Substrate and hormone profiles in the blood following infusion of such a mixture are similar to those seen in the postprandial state.

Recommendations regarding source (type) of nonprotein energy
In North America, in contrast to Europe and the United Kingdom, lipid-free systems were used almost exclusively in the past because triglyceride emulsions had not been approved for nonexperimental use. At the present time lipid-free systems are required only in patients with hyperchylomicronemia. The author believes that most patients should receive lipid as a part of the regimen for total parenteral nutrition. The 80 percent lipid system can be given by peripheral vein, minimizing the threat of catheter sepsis and other catheter-related complications. The 1:1 lipid-glucose solution, given through a central venous line, simulates closely the normal diet and causes neither hyperinsulinemia nor hyperglycemia, thus almost eliminating the need for exogenous insulin.

Other requirements VITAMINS Vitamin requirements are given in Table 78-2. Amounts of vitamins sufficient to meet these needs must be added to the basic parenteral feeding solutions. It is important to avoid infusing excessive amounts of fat-soluble vitamins, in particular vitamins A and D, because of the danger of hypercalcemia and other toxic effects. A combination of 5 ml MVI with 10 ml Soluzyme plus vitamin C on alternate days will meet the requirements for vitamins A and D and will meet or exceed the need for most water-soluble vitamins. These solutions should be supplemented with vitamin K (5 mg) and vitamin B_{12} (200 μg) initially and at intervals of 3 weeks. Folate (5 mg) is given weekly.

ELECTROLYTES Electrolytes are an essential component of the fluids infused during total parenteral nutrition. Potassium, magnesium, and phosphorus are necessary for optimal nitrogen retention and tissue formation. In addition sodium and chloride should be infused to maintain osmolality and acid-base balance. Calcium is required to maintain calcium balance and prevent demineralization of bone. Recommended ranges of intake are given in Table 78-3.

TRACE ELEMENTS The need for trace elements, in particular zinc, copper, and chromium, is becoming increasingly recognized in courses of parenteral nutrition that exceed 1 to 2 weeks.

Zinc is essential for wound healing, for defense against infection, and for the activity of a number of enzymes. In its absence ageusia, loss of hair, night blindness, and a skin rash

TABLE 78-2
Vitamin input and blood or plasma vitamin levels in six patients on long-term TPN

Vitamin	Input* provided by: MVI, per 5 ml	Soluzyme + vitamin C, per 10 ml	Consequent average daily input	Daily (oral) recommended requirement	Plasma/blood vitamin level Average level observed in six patients	Normal range
A	5000 IU		2500 IU	5000 IU	41.6	25–70 µg/100 ml
D	500 IU		250 IU	400 IU	34.4	28–42 ng/ml
E	5 mg		27.5 mg†	30 mg	0.65	0.8–1.2 ng/100 ml
B_1	22 mg	10 mg	16.0 mg	1.5 mg	226	10–64 ng/ml
B_2	5 mg	10 mg	7.5 mg	2.0 mg		
Niacinamide	50 mg	250 mg	150 mg	20.0 mg	16	3–6 µg/ml
Pantothenate	12 mg	45 mg	28 mg	10.0 mg	689	150–400 ng/ml
Pyridoxine	6 mg	5 mg	5.5 mg	2.5 mg	40	30–80 ng/ml
Ascorbic acid	500 mg	500 mg	500 mg	75 mg	2.0	0.4–1 mg/100 ml
Folic acid		5 mg	2.5 mg	0.15 mg	48	4–20 ng/100 ml
B_{12}		25 µg	12.5 µg	1.0 µg	872	100–900 pg/ml
Biotin				300 µg	63	200–500 pg/ml

* Given on alternate days.
† Twenty-five milligrams of the average of 27.5 mg vitamin E per day is provided by infusing 500 ml Intralipid per day.
SOURCE: After KN Jeejeebhoy, Ann Coll Physicians Surg Can 9:287, 1976.

occur. The skin rash is often associated with superficial infection due to staphylococci and yeasts and responds only to zinc supplementation. Zinc deficiency has also been shown to interfere with delayed hypersensitivity. In the absence of excessive gastrointestinal losses, 3 mg zinc per day is sufficient to meet needs. For each liter of intestinal fluids lost through fistulas, stomal output, suction, or diarrhea in patients with extensive resection of the small bowel, an additional 12 mg should be added. If the small bowel is intact, zinc losses are greater and about 17 mg zinc is required per liter of intestinal fluids lost per day.

Deficiency of *copper* causes anemia and neutropenia. The daily requirement is estimated to be between 0.8 and 1.6 mg with the larger intake to be given patients with major losses of gastrointestinal fluid. Copper should not be given to patients with obstructive jaundice.

The estimated requirement for *manganese* is about 0.8 mg per day. This element also should not be given if obstructive jaundice is present.

Deficiency of *chromium* is associated with glucose intolerance and neuropathy. The daily requirement of chromium is about 20 µg.

ROUTES OF ADMINISTRATION   Central venous catheterization
This route allows infusion of fluids irrespective of osmolality and is comfortable for patients since repeated venipuncture is avoided. On the other hand, there is a significant risk of septicemia and thrombosis, especially if the catheter is not properly inserted and cared for during administration of the parenteral nutrition.

TABLE 78-3
Recommended electrolyte intake per day (milliosmoles)

	Na	K	Ca	Mg	P
Basal*	100–120	80–100	10–15	10–12	12–16
Cardiac failure	20–50	80–100	10–15	10–12	12–16
Renal failure	20	†	†	†	†

* To this basal intake, amounts of Na, K, Cl, and HCO_3 are added to meet losses from fistulas, nasogastric tube drainage, diarrhea, and stomal output.
† These ions are added as needed, on the basis of initial and continuing measurements of their circulating level and the clinical state of the patient.

Basic principles of catheter insertion and care are as follows:

1 Catheters should always be placed, and subsequently handled, using completely aseptic technique. Face mask and sterile gloves are required.
2 The catheter should be demonstrated radiologically to be positioned in the superior vena cava prior to commencing total parenteral nutrition with hypertonic fluids. If the tip has entered another central vein (e.g., the internal jugular), thrombosis may occur.
3 Catheters should always be introduced via puncture of a large central vein and not a peripheral vein.
4 The catheter used for TPN should not be used to withdraw blood or measure central venous pressure.
5 The skin puncture site should be cleansed weekly with a detergent, painted with a povidone iodine solution, and occluded with a dressing. A transparent plastic dressing is recommended since it is occlusive and easy to apply and allows for easy inspection of the insertion site for infection, drainage, bleeding, etc.
6 Barium-impregnated silicone rubber catheters (e.g., Silastic, made by Extracorporeal Medical Specialties, Inc., King of Prussia, Pennsylvania) should be used since they do not traumatize the central veins and are less likely to be surrounded with a fibrin clot.

Peripheral venous infusion   This route is safe and not as likely to be a source of septic or thrombotic complications. However the infused fluids must be isotonic or only mildly hypertonic. In order to achieve these conditions, nonprotein energy must be given mainly as lipid. A representative protocol is discussed below.

REPRESENTATIVE PROTOCOLS FOR ADMINISTRATION OF TOTAL PARENTERAL NUTRITION   The three sample protocols given in Table 78-4 are designed for a 60-kg individual. They are intended to be administered throughout 24 h and provide 1 g amino acids and 40 nonprotein calories per kilogram of body weight. Proportionate modifications can be made for larger or smaller persons. Nonprotein energy is provided as (1) glucose, (2) 50 percent glucose and 50 percent lipid, or (3) 85 percent lipid and 15 percent glucose. The latter is suitable for peripheral venous administration. Preparation of the infusion materi-

TABLE 78-4
Representative protocols for the administration of total paren-teral nutrition (see text)

100% GLUCOSE

8 A.M. to 8 P.M.:	
2% amino acids with 25% dextrose	1500 ml
Electrolyte additives, as needed[a]	30 ml (approx)
MVI[b] or	5 ml
Soluzyme plus vitamin C[c]	10 ml
8 P.M. to 8 A.M.:	
2% amino acids with 25% dextrose	1500 ml
Electrolyte additives, as needed[a]	30 ml (approx)
Trace element mix (1) to (4)[d]	1 ml (each)
Nutrient composition of above regimen:	
Amino acids (60 g)	240 kcal
Glucose monohydrate (750 g)	2550 kcal
Lipid	
Total nonprotein energy	2550 kcal
Total volume	3000 ml (approx)
Electrolytes:[a]	
Na	130 meq
K	80 meq
Ca	10 meq
Mg	11 meq
P	14 meq

50% GLUCOSE AND 50% LIPID

8 A.M. to 8 P.M.:	
4% amino acids with 25% dextrose[e]	750 ml
Electrolyte additives, as needed[a]	30 ml (approx)
MVI[b] or	5 ml
Soluzyme plus vitamin C[c]	10 ml
Intralipid 10%[e, f]	500 ml
8 P.M. to 8 A.M.:	
4% amino acids with 25% dextrose[e]	750 ml
Electrolyte additives, as needed[a]	30 ml (approx)
Trace element mix (1) to (4)[d]	1 ml (each)
Intralipid 10%[e, f]	500 ml
Nutrient composition of above regimen:	
Amino acids (60 g)	240 kcal
Glucose monohydrate (375 g)	1275 kcal
Lipid (100 g)	1100 kcal
Total nonprotein energy	2375 kcal
Total volume	2600 ml (approx)
Electrolyte composition: same as for	
100% glucose protocol	

85% LIPID AND 15% GLUCOSE

8 A.M. to 8 P.M.:	
6% amino acids with 12% dextrose[g]	500 ml
Electrolyte additives, as needed[a]	30 ml (approx)
MVI[b] or	5 ml
Soluzyme plus vitamin C[c]	10 ml
Intralipid 10%[f, g]	1000 ml
8 P.M. to 8 A.M.:	
6% amino acids with 12% dextrose[g]	500 ml
Electrolyte additives, as needed[a]	30 ml (approx)
Trace element mix (1) to (4)[d]	1 ml (each)
Intralipid 10%[f, g]	1000 ml
Nutrient composition of above mixture:	
Amino acids (60 g)	240 kcal
Glucose monohydrate (120 g)	408 kcal
Lipid (200 g)	2200 kcal
Total nonprotein energy	2608 kcal
Total volume	3100 ml (approx)
Electrolyte composition: same as for	
100% glucose protocol	

[a] *Total electrolytes have been calculated on the assumption that the amino acid mixture used is electrolyte-free. If another amino acid source is used, the values will be different. The total input of electrolytes given in this table has been found to be capable of maintaining balance in patients without abnormal losses of gastrointestinal secretions. However in patients with such losses appropriate replacement has to be made.*
[b] *MVI injection (USV Pharmaceutical Corp).*
[c] *Soluzyme plus vitamin C (Upjohn).*
[d] *Trace element mix: 1 ml each of (1) 1.6 mg/ml elemental Cu as cupric chloride ($CuCl_2 \cdot 2H_2O$), 20 µg/ml elemental Cr as chromic nitrate [$Cr(NO_3)_3$], and 120 µg/ml elemental Se as selenious acid, (H_2SeO_3); (2), 120 µg/ml elemental I as potassium iodide (KI); (3) 3 mg/ml elemental Zn as zinc sulfate ($ZnSO_4 \cdot 7H_2O$); and (4) 0.7 mg/ml elemental Mn as manganous chloride ($MnCl_3 \cdot 4H_2O$).*
[e] *The triglyceride emulsion and dextrose-amino acid mixture are infused concurrently through a central venous line using a Y connector for continuous mixing.*
[f] *Intralipid 10% (Cutter Laboratories).*
[g] *It is very important in this system that the amino acid-dextrose solution and Intralipid be infused in correct proportions through the Y connector so that the concentration of the former is diluted adequately by constant mixing with the Intralipid to make the dextrose noninjurious to the peripheral vein. An infusion pump is advisable.*

als must be carried out with great care. In most medical centers such preparation is done exclusively by one or more specially trained pharmacists.

HOME PARENTERAL NUTRITION (HPN) It is now possible to administer parenteral nutrition at home in patients requiring prolonged nutritional support. A permanent silicone rubber catheter is placed in the superior vena cava via a subclavian or jugular vein and led to the outside through a subcutaneous tunnel. These catheters may be left in place for years without need for replacement. The patient receives monthly supplies of prepackaged nutrients ready for infusion. The nutrients are infused during the night while the patient is sleeping. A simple pneumatic cuff placed around the plastic bags containing the prepackaged infusion fluids is safe, cheap, and less cumbersome than mechanical-electrical delivery systems. The system is disconnected in the morning after a 10-h overnight infusion, and the catheter is capped and filled with a heparin solution. The patient is then free to carry out normal social activities or work during the day. This method has revolutionized the life of persons who otherwise would be nutritional cripples because of prolonged hospitalization for TPN.

PARTIAL PARENTERAL NUTRITION Whether amino acids should replace glucose and electrolyte solutions in the management of patients unable to eat for short periods (up to 1 week) following surgery, strokes, or other acute illnesses is debatable. In 7 days a patient has (on average) a net negative nitrogen balance of 100 to 110 g when receiving only glucose replacement. If amino acids are given at a level of 1 g/kg per day, the nitrogen loss is cut to 35 to 45 g. This difference is equal to only about 3 percent of the total nitrogen content in a 60-kg man. Since there is no evidence that such a small deficit makes any difference in clinical outcome (the nitrogen loss is quickly repleted when food intake is restored) and since amino acid solutions are expensive, amino acid infusion is not recommended for fasts of up to 1 week. Beyond 1 week, full TPN should probably be given.

In some patients oral intake is possible but the amounts ingested are inadequate for full nutrition. In such cases an estimate is made of the amount taken orally, and the deficiency is made up by parenteral means. When there is a question about how much of the ingested diet is absorbed (e.g., after bowel resection or with intestinal fistulas), the amount of nutrition given parenterally will have to be determined by trial and error, with evaluation of weight gain and other signs of clinical improvement.

REFERENCES

ANDERSON GH et al: Design and evaluation by nitrogen balance and blood aminograms of an amino acid mixture for total parenteral nutrition of adults with gastrointestinal disease. J Clin Invest 53:904, 1974

———— et al: Dose-response relationships between amino acid intake and blood levels in newborn infants. Am J Clin Nutr 30:1110, 1977

BATSTONE GF et al: Metabolic studies in subjects following thermal injury. Intermediary metabolites, hormones and tissue oxygenation. Burns 2:207, 1976

BLACKBURN GL et al: Protein sparing therapy during periods of starvation with sepsis or trauma. Ann Surg 177:588, 1973

CAHILL GF JR et al: Starvation in man. N Engl J Med 282:668, 1970

CRAIG RP et al: Intravenous glucose, amino acids and fat in the postoperative period. Lancet 2:8, 1977

GREENBERG GR et al: Protein-sparing therapy in postoperative patients. Effects of added hypocaloric glucose or lipid. N Engl J Med 294:1411, 1976

JEEJEEBHOY KN: Protein sparing effect of amino acids, in *Clinical Nutrition Update: Amino Acids,* HL Greene et al (eds). Chicago, American Medical Association, 1977

———: Role of measuring albumin synthesis as a way of measuring protein body repletion, ibid.

——— et al: Metabolic studies in total parenteral nutrition with lipid in man: Comparison with glucose. J Clin Invest 57:125, 1976

——— et al: Total parenteral nutrition at home: Studies in patients surviving 4 months to 5 years. Gastroenterology 71:943, 1976

MENG HC, WILMORE DW (eds): *Fat Emulsions in Parenteral Nutrition.* Chicago, American Medical Association, 1976

MUNRO HN: General aspects of the regulation of protein metabolism by diet and by hormones, in *Mammalian Protein Metabolism,* HN Munro, JB Allison (eds). New York, Academic, 1964, vol I

RUDMAN D et al: Elemental balances during intravenous hyperalimentation of underweight adult subjects. J Clin Invest 55:94, 1975

SHILS ME et al: Liquid formulas for oral and tube feeding. Clin Bull 6:151, 1976

79
DEFICIENCY OF NIACIN (PELLAGRA)

JEAN D. WILSON
LEONARD L. MADISON

NORMAL PHYSIOLOGY OF NIACIN Biochemistry Niacin is the accepted generic description for nicotinic acid (pyridine-3-carboxylic acid) and derivatives exhibiting the nutritional activity of nicotinic acid. In one sense niacin is not a vitamin since it can be formed from the essential amino acid tryptophan. Studies in humans indicate that an average of about 1 mg niacin is formed from 60 mg dietary tryptophan. Accordingly, estimates of the adequacy of dietary intake must take into account the tryptophan content of the diet as well as the content of niacin. It should also be recognized that many foodstuffs, especially cereals, contain bound forms of niacin from which the vitamin is not nutritionally available.

The absorption, tissue distribution, and metabolism of the vitamin are poorly understood. In most species approximately a fifth of the vitamin is decarboxylated, and the remainder is excreted in the urine as methylated products, largely *n*-methylnicotinamide and its derivatives.

Mechanism of action Niacin is an essential component of nicotinamide adenine dinucleotide (NAD) and nicotinamide adenine dinucleotide phosphate (NADP), coenzymes for a multitude of important oxidation-reduction reactions in metabolism. Nicotinic acid is transaminated to nicotinamide which subsequently reacts with phosphoribosyl pyrophosphate to form nicotinamide mononucleotide; the latter then reacts with adenosine triphosphate (ATP) to form NAD, and the reaction with a second molecule of ATP results in the formation of NADP.

Requirements The requirements and recommended daily allowances for niacin and tryptophan are listed in Tables 73-1 and 73-2. In contrast to most vitamins there is no clear evidence that requirement is increased during pregnancy. As discussed below, the principal factor that influences requirements may be the amino acid composition of the diet.

EXPERIMENTAL DEPLETION Following the administration of a diet deficient in niacin and tryptophan, the urinary excretion of the metabolites of niacin decreases rapidly, reaching minimal values (< 1.5 mg per day) after 30 to 60 days and remaining constant thereafter. In most instances the first clinical evidence of deficiency is noted within a short period of time after excretion becomes stable at a low level. The symptoms and signs of niacin deficiency include dermatitis, glossitis, stomatitis, diarrhea, proctitis, mental depression, heartburn, abdominal pain, vaginitis, dysphagia, and amenorrhea, findings similar to those in pellagra.

CLINICAL DEFICIENCY Frequency and clinical context Pellagra was previously an endemic disease in the American South and in many other parts of the world. Endemic pellagra is usually associated with a high intake of maize (or sorghum) and can be cured by the administration of niacin. However, our understanding of the pathogenesis of pellagra has changed over the years from that of a pure vitamin deficiency to that of a mixed deficiency of tryptophan and available niacin in the diet to that of a vitamin and amino acid deficiency associated with an imbalance in dietary amino acids. This conclusion is based on the following facts: (1) the niacin content of maize is low, and a significant portion appears to be "bound" and unavailable for absorption; (2) however, the niacin equivalent of maize (available niacin and tryptophan) is no lower than in some cereals that are unassociated with endemic pellagra; and (3) the leucine content of common varieties of maize is high. A hybrid strain of maize, opaque 2, has recently been described which differs from the ordinary grain in having lower leucine but similar tryptophan and niacin content. Dogs fed a diet rich in conventional maize or a diet rich in opaque 2 maize supplemented with leucine develop experimental pellagra (black tongue), whereas dogs fed the opaque 2 maize alone do not. This finding presumably explains why pellagra occurs in Indians who ingest a diet rich in sorghum (jowar), which has a leucine content similar to that of maize but a niacin and tryptophan content (and availability) equivalent to that of rice. Leucine is believed to inhibit the synthesis of nicotinic acid mononucleotide and consequently the synthesis of NAD and NADP. Thus, in pathogenic terms, the development of symptoms of niacin "deficiency" depends on the amino acid content of the diet as well as upon the intake of the vitamin and its precursors.

Whatever the exact cause, endemic pellagra disappeared in the United States coincident with the improvement in nutritional education and with the institution of widespread supplementation of grain cereal products with niacin. However, pellagra is an occasional secondary manifestation of two disorders that profoundly affect tryptophan metabolism, the carcinoid syndrome in which up to 60 percent of tryptophan is catabolized by what is ordinarily a minor pathway of metabolism (see Chap. 91) and Hartnup disease, an autosomal recessive disorder in which several amino acids including tryptophan are absorbed poorly from the diet. In both disorders the symptoms of pellagra appear to be the consequence of diminished availability of effective niacin equivalents, and in both the symptoms and signs of pellagra can be cured by the administration of large amounts of the vitamin.

Manifestations The typical presentation of pellagra is that of a chronic wasting disease associated with dermatitis, dementia, and diarrhea. The dermatitis is characteristic; it is bilateral, symmetrical, seen on those parts exposed to sunlight, and due to photosensitivity. The mental changes are less discrete; fatigue, insomnia, and apathy may precede the development of an encephalopathy characterized by confusion, disorientation, hallucination, and loss of memory. Eventually, frank organic psychoses may develop. Paresthesias and polyneuritis seen in pellagra may actually be the result of other coexisting vitamin deficiencies. The diarrhea, when it occurs, is a portion of a widespread inflammation of the mucous surfaces; other manifestations include achlorhydria, glossitis, stomatitis, and vaginitis. After the development of symptoms the course is slowly progressive over a period of several years before death supervenes, usually due to secondary complications.

The exact relation between the known coenzyme functions of NAD and NADP and these various symptoms has never been defined. Levels of NAD and NADP in erythrocytes are lower in patients with pellagra than in normal persons, but the coenzymes are essential to so many reactions in intermediary metabolism that profound deficiency is incompatible with life. Some evidence suggests that the mental changes in pellagra may be associated with diminished conversion of tryptophan to serotonin.

Diagnosis Suspicion and response to replacement therapy must be the basis of diagnosis. No biochemical test is of diagnostic value. As would be predicted, the urinary excretion of the metabolites of nicotinic acid and tryptophan is lower than average but not lower than in patients with generalized malnutrition (Table 74-4). Plasma tryptophan and erythrocyte NAD and NADP levels may be low. Histopathology of the skin is characterized by hyperkeratosis, hyperpigmentation, and desquamation.

Management The administration of small amounts of niacin (10 mg per day) in the face of limiting amounts of dietary tryptophan may be sufficient to cure endemic pellagra. Large doses (40 to 200 mg per day) may be required in Hartnup disease.

REFERENCES

DARBY WJ et al: Niacin. Nutr Rev 33:289, 1977

DE LANGE DJ, JOUBERT CP: Assessment of nicotinic acid status of population groups. Am J Clin Nutr 15:169, 1964

GOLDSMITH GA: Experimental niacin deficiency. J Am Diet Assoc 32:312, 1956

GOPALAN C, RAO KSJ: Pellagra and amino acid imbalance, in *Vitamins and Hormones,* PL Munson et al (eds). New York, Academic, 1975, pp 505–528

JEPSON JB: Hartnup disease, in *The Metabolic Basis of Inherited Disease,* 4th ed, JB Stanbury et al (eds). New York, McGraw-Hill, 1978, pp 1563–1577

80
DEFICIENCY OF THIAMINE (BERIBERI), PYRIDOXINE, AND RIBOFLAVIN

JEAN D. WILSON
LEONARD L. MADISON

THIAMINE

NORMAL PHYSIOLOGY OF THIAMINE Biochemistry Thiamine consists of a pyrimidine ring and a thiazole moiety linked by a methylene bridge (Fig. 80-1). The vitamin is synthesized by a variety of plants and microorganisms but not ordinarily by animal tissues. However, rats and pigeons fed a thiamine-free diet can be protected from developing symptoms of deficiency by being given large quantities of the pyrimidine and thiazole moieties, suggesting that animal tissues have a small capacity to couple the two subunits. Limited amounts may also be synthesized by microorganisms in the gastrointestinal tract. Thiamine is absorbed from the diet by both an active transport process and passive diffusion. The capacity to absorb

the vitamin in the human intestine is limited to about 5 mg per day. In the normal individual approximately 25 to 30 mg is stored in the body, 80 percent as thiamine diphosphate (pyrophosphate), 10 percent as thiamine triphosphate, and the remainder as free thiamine and thiamine monophosphate. Large amounts are found in skeletal muscles (about half of body stores), heart, liver, kidneys, and brain. Three distinct enzymes are known to participate in the formation of thiamine phosphate esters—a pyrophosphate kinase that catalyzes the formation of thiamine diphosphate from adenosine triphosphate (ATP) and thiamine, a phosphoryl transferase that catalyzes the formation of thiamine triphosphate from ATP and the diphosphate, and a pyrophosphatase that hydrolyzes thiamine triphosphate to thiamine monophosphate. Several metabolites of thiamine are excreted in the urine, principally thiamine itself (which is secreted by the renal tubules), an acetylated derivative, and two major end products of thiamine catabolism, thiazole-acetate and pyrimidine carboxylic acid. Indeed, a number of enzymes called *thiaminases* inactivate thiamine by splitting the vitamin into its two component parts.

Mechanism of action The role of thiamine diphosphate as a coenzyme is well established. In mammals thiamine diphosphate is required for a variety of reactions that have in common the cleavage of carbon-carbon bonds—the oxidative decarboxylation of α-keto acids (pyruvate and α-ketoglutarate) and keto analogues of leucine, isoleucine, and valine and the transketolase reaction in the pentose phosphate pathway. (In bacteria thiamine diphosphate also acts as a coenzyme for certain phosphoketolase enzymes.) Thiamine triphosphate, which has no carboxylase function itself, is important in the binding of thiamine diphosphate to its various apoenzymes. Pioneering work by Sir Rudolph Peters and his associates suggested that the entire spectrum of changes in thiamine deficiency could be explained by the inhibition of these key enzymatic reactions and, in some instances, the accumulation of the proximal metabolites. However, in recent years circumstantial evidence has accrued to suggest that thiamine may have a specific role in the process of neural conduction independent of its coenzymatic function in general metabolism. It is of particular interest in this regard that thiamine and its esters are located in axonal membranes of nerves and that electrical stimulation of nerves results in the hydrolysis and release of both thiamine diphosphate and triphosphate.

Requirements The requirements and recommended daily allowances for thiamine are listed in Tables 73-1 and 73-2. The vitamin has a widespread distribution in food and is entirely absent only from oils, fats, cassava, and refined sugar. A large portion of the vitamin in vegetable products is in the form of thiamine itself. In cereal grains the vitamin is especially rich in the outer layers of the grain; hence machine-milled rice is a poor source. In animal tissues it is present largely in the form of phosphate esters. The ester is dephosphorylated by phos-

FIGURE 80-1

Thiamine pyrophosphate.

phatases present in the intestine, and only the free vitamin is absorbed. A substantial loss of the vitamin takes place during cooking above 100°C.

Several factors influence the absorption and metabolism of the vitamin (and hence alter daily requirements). One is the presence of thiaminases in foods including fresh fish, clams, shrimp, mussels, and some raw animal tissues. Some microorganisms in the colon may also contain thiaminases. Another factor that influences the requirement is the carbohydrate and caloric intake. Daily needs are reduced when fat forms a large part of the diet and are increased as carbohydrate intake increases. As is true for many vitamins, requirements are increased in pregnancy, during lactation, in thyrotoxicosis, and by fever. Accelerated loss of thiamine from the body may occur as the result of diuretic therapy, hemodialysis, peritoneal dialysis, and diarrhea. Defective intestinal absorption can occur in malabsorption states, alcoholism, chronic malnutrition, and folate deficiency.

EXPERIMENTAL DEPLETION OF THIAMINE Following the institution of a thiamine-free diet in control subjects, thiamine excretion in the urine decreases to 5 percent of the control value by the sixth day and becomes undetectable by day 18. However, the excretion of the pyrimidine and thiazole catabolites of thiamine does not change significantly for as long as 33 days on a deficient diet (about 0.8 mg per day), indicating that the body pool is slowly utilized during a period of deficient intake.

Within 9 days after the institution of a deficient diet, subjects develop a resting tachycardia, followed by the onset of muscle weakness, a decrease in the deep tendon reflexes, and (in some) the appearance of a sensory neuropathy. Subjective symptoms include generalized malaise, headache, nausea, and generalized aching of the muscles. The development of these symptoms is paralleled by a fall in the level of red blood cell transketolase activity. Within a week of thiamine repletion (2 mg per day) all abnormal physical findings disappear; the subjective symptoms clear after 2 weeks. (Experimental depletion in humans has never been carried to the point of development of severe cerebral or cardiovascular symptoms.)

CLINICAL DEFICIENCY **Frequency and clinical context** In most developed nations thiamine deficiency develops in alcoholics or in the context of special clinical situations, including refeeding after starvation, peritoneal dialysis or hemodialysis, or the administration of glucose to asymptomatic but thiamine-depleted patients. In underdeveloped countries where beriberi may be a common nutritional disease, the causes derive mainly from the consumption of milled rice and foods containing thiaminases and (possibly) other antithiamine factors.

Several factors are involved in the etiology of thiamine deficiency in chronic alcoholics including a low thiamine intake, impaired thiamine absorption, varying rates of destruction of the cofactor, and varying degrees of energy expenditure. However, clinical manifestations of thiamine deficiency develop in only a small fraction of alcoholics and other chronically malnourished persons. Studies by Blass and Gibson suggest that genetic factors are involved in the pathogenesis of clinical manifestations; they demonstrated that a thiamine-requiring enzyme (transketolase) in fibroblasts cultured from four patients with the Wernicke-Korsakoff syndrome bound thiamine diphosphate only a tenth as avidly as controls. This finding implies a genetic abnormality that would be clinically silent if the diet were adequate in thiamine but made overt if thiamine intake were low or marginal. Thus, it is possible that the development of beriberi commonly depends on the presence of an inborn error of metabolism.

Manifestations The two major syndromes of thiamine deficiency involve the cardiovascular (wet beriberi) and nervous systems (dry beriberi and the Wernicke-Korsakoff syndromes). The typical patient has mixed symptoms involving both the cardiovascular and nervous systems, but pure cardiovascular, pure polyneuritic, and pure cerebral forms also occur. The factors that determine the relative preponderance of these manifestations are poorly understood but are related at least in part to the duration and severity of the deficiency, the degree of physical exertion, and the caloric intake. Thus, severe physical exertion, high carbohydrate intake, and a moderate degree of chronic deficiency favor wet beriberi with little or no peripheral neuritis, whereas an equal deficiency with caloric restriction and relative inactivity favors the development of dry (polyneuritic) beriberi.

CARDIOVASCULAR SYSTEM Beriberi heart disease comprises three major physiologic derangements: (1) a state of peripheral vasodilatation leading to a high-output state, (2) a state of biventricular myocardial failure, and (3) retention of sodium and water leading to edema.

In the chronic form, the peripheral vasodilatation leads to increased arteriovenous shunting of blood, rapid circulation time, tachycardia, increased cardiac output, and a venous congestive state characterized by elevated peripheral venous pressure, elevated right ventricular end-diastolic pressure, decreased arteriovenous extraction of oxygen, sodium retention, and edema. Disordered flow of blood to the organs (decreased cerebral and renal blood flow and greatly increased flow to the muscles) is common. It is striking that cardiac output increases to such an extent that, notwithstanding the lowered peripheral vascular resistance, ventricular work, arterial blood pressure, and pulmonary wedge pressure tend to be elevated. Also of interest is the fact that temporary worsening of hypertension occurs during thiamine repletion, presumably due to closing of arteriovenous shunts.

In acute fulminant cardiovascular beriberi, the myocardial lesion appears to be the central feature in a course in which acute cardiovascular collapse develops with death in hours to days. The patient complains of severe dyspnea, intense thirst, restlessness, and anxiety. Physical findings include "stocking-glove" cyanosis, extreme tachycardia, marked cardiomegaly, hepatomegaly, arterial bruits, and neck vein distention. The venous pressure is high, and the circulation time is rapid. Because of the fulminant course little or no edema may be present.

Administration of thiamine rapidly restores peripheral vascular resistance, but improvement in the myocardial abnormality may be delayed so that a low-output failure may supervene during treatment.

NERVOUS SYSTEM Three types of nervous system involvement occur: peripheral neuropathy, Wernicke's encephalopathy (cerebral beriberi), and the Korsakoff syndrome. The neuropathy is characterized by a symmetrical impairment or loss of sensory, motor, and reflex function affecting the distal segments of limbs more severely than the proximal ones. It may or may not be painful. The essential lesion is a noninflammatory, degenerative change affecting the myelin sheaths primarily. No meaningful distinction can be made between this disorder and so-called "alcoholic neuropathy" on the basis of either clinical course or neurologic grounds.

The symptoms of cerebral beriberi ordinarily develop in an orderly progression and consist of vomiting, nystagmus (horizontal more commonly than vertical), palsies of the external recti leading to unilateral or bilateral ophthalmoplegia (and decrease in the nystagmus), fever, ataxia of gait, and progressive mental deterioration that eventuates in a global confusional state and may progress to coma and death. Improvement occurs after the institution of therapy, although symptoms of Korsakoff's syndrome may supervene. Thus, when thiamine therapy is instituted, the eye palsies are corrected, the nystagmus improves in half the patients, the ataxia improves or disappears in two-thirds, and the global confusion state disappears to be replaced by Korsakoff's syndrome. The latter consists of retrograde amnesia, impaired ability to learn, and confabulation (not always present). The patient is usually alert and responsive and exhibits no serious defect in social behavior. Once the Korsakoff disorder supervenes, recovery (complete or partial) can be expected in only half the patients.

In summary, the Wernicke's encephalopathy and the amnesic psychosis of the Korsakoff syndrome are not separate clinical events; instead, the changing ocular and ataxic signs, the transformation of the global confusional state into the amnesic-confabulatory syndrome, and the subsequent development of a nonconfabulatory amnesic state are successive stages in the recovery from a single disease process. The clinical spectrum, differential diagnosis, course, and pathology of cerebral beriberi are discussed in greater detail in Chap. 372.

Diagnosis Various biochemical tests based on thiamine metabolism or the biochemical functions of thiamine diphosphate have been developed to detect thiamine deficiency in humans. These include the measurement of blood thiamine, pyruvate, α-ketoglutarate, lactate, and glyoxylate; the urinary excretion of thiamine and thiamine metabolites; a thiamine-loading test; and measurement of urinary methylglyoxal content. At present the most reliable method is the measurement of whole blood or erythrocyte transketolase activity. Any enhancement in enzymatic activity resulting from added thiamine diphosphate (TPP) is referred to as the *TPP effect* (expressed in percent). If the activity of the enzyme is increased more than 15 percent by the added thiamine diphosphate, then a deficiency state is probably present (Table 74-4). Owing to wide variations in transketolase activity, absolute levels are not very useful, but an increase in activity after treatment coupled with a significant stimulation in vitro by added thiamine diphosphate suggests the presence of thiamine deficiency. Recent work in experimental animals indicates that leukocyte transketolase activity may be a more sensitive index of thiamine nutriture than the red blood cell test.

Another criterion for the diagnosis of thiamine deficiency is the assessment of clinical response to thiamine administration. Clinical improvement may be dramatic in cardiovascular beriberi; an increase in blood pressure and decrease in heart rate may be seen within 12 h after start of therapy. Diuresis and reduction in heart size may be apparent by 24 to 48 h.

Management Prompt administration of thiamine is indicated when beriberi is diagnosed or suspected. Fifty milligrams per day should be given intramuscularly for several days, after which 2.5 to 5 mg per day can be administered by mouth. Larger amounts are usually not absorbed. All patients should also receive other water-soluble vitamins in therapeutic quantities.

THIAMINE-RESPONSIVE INBORN ERRORS OF METABOLISM
A number of thiamine-responsive inborn errors of metabolism have been described in which patients respond to pharmacological doses of thiamine. These include thiamine-responsive megaloblastic anemia, for which the mechanism is unknown; thiamine-responsive lactic acidosis, which is due to low activity of pyruvate carboxylase in liver; thiamine-responsive branched-chain ketoaciduria, which is due to low activity of a ketoacid dehydrogenase; and intermittent cerebellar ataxia

which may result from an abnormal pyruvate dehydrogenase. In addition, it is possible that the autosomal recessive disorder known as *subacute necrotizing encephalomyelopathy* (Leigh's disease) may be related to a diminished amount of thiamine triphosphate in neural tissue; a factor has been isolated from urine of such patients which inhibits the enzyme that synthesizes thiamine triphosphate. The clinical response of patients with Leigh's disease to pharmacological doses of the vitamin appears to be minor, however.

PYRIDOXINE (VITAMIN B$_6$)

NORMAL PHYSIOLOGY OF PYRIDOXINE Biochemistry The biological activity of the vitamin B$_6$ group is displayed by pyridoxine, pyridoxal, and pyridoxamine and their 5-phosphate esters. The coenzyme form is pyridoxal 5-phosphate, and the other compounds owe their enzymatic activity to conversion by tissues to pyridoxal 5-phosphate. Animal tissues contain an oxidase that converts pyridoxine to pyridoxal and a potent pyridoxal kinase that synthesizes pyridoxal phosphate from pyridoxal and ATP. The vitamin is widely and uniformly distributed in all foods; muscle meats, liver, vegetables, and whole-grain cereals are among the best sources.

Mechanism of action Pyridoxal phosphate acts as a cofactor for an exceptionally large number of enzymes involved in amino acid metabolism, including transaminases, synthetases, and hydroxylases. It is of particular importance in humans in the metabolism of tryptophan, glycine, serine, glutamate, and the sulfur-containing amino acids. Pyridoxal phosphate is also required for the synthesis of the heme precursor δ-aminolevulinic acid. A large share of body pyridoxine is found in muscle phosphorylase, where it may function not catalytically but to stabilize the enzyme. It also plays a vital (but poorly understood role) in neuronal excitability, possibly as a result of its function in transsulfuration reactions or γ-aminobutyric acid metabolism.

Requirements The requirements and recommended daily allowances for the vitamin are described in Tables 73-1 and 73-2. Even more than for most vitamins, the requirement is increased in pregnancy and by the ingestion of estrogenic drugs. In both conditions abnormal tryptophan metabolites are excreted in urine, and this can be prevented by supplementation with pyridoxine. Estrogenic steroids appear to inhibit selectively the pyridoxal phosphate function in tryptophan metabolism. In addition, pyridoxine requirement may be increased by high protein intake. The ingestion of ethanol interferes with the metabolism of pyridoxal phosphate, the ethanol metabolite acetaldehyde displacing the coenzyme from proteins and thus enhancing its degradation.

EXPERIMENTAL DEPLETION OF PYRIDOXINE The feeding to experimental subjects of diets deficient in pyridoxine leads to chemical evidence of deficiency (increased xanthurenic acid and decreased pyridoxine in urine) within a week. Electroencephalographic abnormalities appear within 3 weeks in subjects with previously normal EEGs, and some subjects subsequently have grand mal seizures. Deficiency induced with the pyridoxine antagonist desoxypyridoxine causes, in addition, seborrheic dermatitis, cheilosis, glossitis, and severe systemic symptoms such as nausea, vomiting, weakness, and dizziness.

CLINICAL DEFICIENCY Frequency and clinical context The widespread occurrence of the vitamin in food is probably the reason that a naturally occurring pure pyridoxine deficiency has never been recognized except when the pyridoxine content of food is destroyed during processing, as has occurred in some processed infant formulas. Thus, it is a paradox that at present pyridoxine deficiency is frequent in the United States. This happens because many commonly used drugs act as pyridoxine antagonists. Hydrazines such as isoniazid induce peripheral neuritis that can be prevented by vitamin B_6 supplementation; these drugs appear to combine with pyridoxal or pyridoxal phosphate to form hydrazones. The hydrazones may be excreted in the urine (causing pyridoxal deficiency) but may also inhibit enzymes directly (for example, pyridoxal kinase). The hydrazones may in addition act directly as convulsants. Cycloserine, an antituberculous drug, causes an increase in the excretion of the vitamin in the urine and produces profound neurological effects; it is thought that the drug forms a complex with pyridoxal phosphate which competes with the cofactor for apoenzymes. Penicillamine acts as an antagonist by forming a thiazolidine derivative with pyridoxal phosphate; abnormal tryptophan metabolism and convulsions can be prevented by supplementation with the vitamin.

Diagnosis Estimates of vitamin deficiency have been based upon the cure of clinical signs of deficiency, the excretion of tryptophan metabolites after tryptophan-loading tests, measurement of various amino acid transferase activities in blood, and excretion of pyridoxine or its metabolites or of oxalate in the urine (Table 74-3). Because of the relative ease with which it can be done, the most common index is the measurement of tryptophan metabolites, particularly xanthurenic acid, following tryptophan loading. Alternatively cystathionine can be assayed after a methionine load. It is possible that measurement of red blood cell glutamic pyruvic transaminase in vitro in the presence and absence of pyridoxal phosphate is superior to both loading tests.

Management The appropriate management is prevention of deficiency. Supplementation of the diet with 30 mg pyridoxine normalizes tryptophan metabolism in pregnancy, in contraceptive users, and in patients taking isoniazid. Doses as high as 100 mg per day may be required in subjects taking penicillamine.

PYRIDOXINE-RESPONSIVE DISEASES There are a large number of genetic conditions in which abnormalities in vitamin B_6 metabolism occur. One group, if not provided with large daily supplements of pyridoxine during infancy, develops convulsions and brain damage and dies; these children have an apoenzyme for glutamic acid decarboxylase that has a decreased binding affinity for pyridoxal phosphate. Consequently they do not form γ-aminobutyric acid, a putative physiological inhibitor of neurological activity in the brain, at a normal rate. Another group has pyridoxine-responsive chronic anemia; although pyridoxine supplementation results in prompt hematologic remission, it does not correct the morphological abnormality in the erythrocytes.

The synthesis of cystathionine from homocystine and serine and its cleavage to cysteine and homoserine are catalyzed by two pyridoxal phosphate enzymes. The biochemical changes which occur in deficiency of these two enzymes and in xanthurenic aciduria due to kynureninase deficiency have been reviewed by Mudd. Some patients with vitamin B_6–responsive xanthurenic aciduria or cystathioninuria have a mutant apoenzyme that interacts abnormally with pyridoxal phosphate in a manner which can be largely overcome by elevated concentrations of the cofactor. In contrast, the vitamin B_6 response in patients with homocystinuria due to cystathionine synthetase

deficiency is not due to restoration of the affected enzyme to normal levels but to an enhancement of the activity of the small amount of normal enzyme present.

RIBOFLAVIN

Riboflavin is essential for all oxidation-reduction reactions involving the coenzymes flavin mononucleotide (FMN) and flavin adenine dinucleotide (FAD). In addition, covalently attached flavins are essential to the structure of such enzymes as succinate dehydrogenase and monoamine oxidase. The vitamin is absorbed from the gastrointestinal tract either as free riboflavin or the 5′-phosphate by a specific transport process. The requirements and recommended daily allowances are listed in Tables 73-1 and 73-2. Covalently linked vitamin accounts for less than a tenth of the tissue pool. The vitamin is excreted in urine predominantly in the free form, although a small fraction of the daily turnover is catabolized by microorganisms in the gastrointestinal tract.

Clinical riboflavin deficiency can be induced in human subjects either by feeding a riboflavin-deficient diet and/or by administering riboflavin antagonists such as galactoflavin. The deficiency syndrome is characterized by sore throat, hyperemia and edema of the pharyngeal and oral mucous membranes, cheilosis, angular stomatitis, glossitis, seborrheic dermatitis, and normochromic, normocytic anemia associated with pure red blood cell hypoplasia of the bone marrow. All these features can be rapidly and completely reversed after riboflavin administration.

Riboflavin deficiency almost invariably occurs in combination with other vitamin deficiencies. Certain features of the syndrome such as glossitis and dermatitis may be seen with other vitamin deficiencies as well.

REFERENCES

Pyridoxine

FRIMPTER GW et al: Vitamin B_6-dependency syndromes: New horizons in nutrition. Am J Clin Nutr 22:794, 1969

GERSHOFF SN: Vitamin B_6, in *Nutrition Reviews' Present Knowledge in Nutrition,* 4th ed, DM Hegsted et al (eds). Washington, DC, The Nutrition Foundation, 1976, p 149

HARRIS JW, HORRIGAN DL: Pyridoxine-responsive anemia-prototype and variations on a theme, in *Vitamins and Hormones: Advances in Research and Applications,* RS Harris et al (eds). New York, Academic, 1964, vol 22, pp 721–753

JAFFE IA: The antivitamin B_6 effect of pencillamine: Clinical and immunological implications, in *Advances in Biochemical Psychopharmacology,* vol 4, MS Ebodi, E Costa (eds). New York, Raven Press, 1972

LUHBY AL et al: Vitamin B_6 metabolism in users of oral contraceptive agents. I: Abnormal urinary xanthurenic acid excretion and its correction by pyridoxine. Am J Clin Nutr 24:684, 1971

LUMENG L: The role of acetaldehyde in mediating the deleterious effects of ethanol on pyridoxal 5′-phosphate metabolism. J Clin Invest 62:286, 1978

MUDD SH: Pyridoxine-responsive genetic disease. Fed Proc 30:970, 1971

SAUBERLICH HE et al: Biochemical assessment of the nutritional status of vitamin B_6 in the human. Am J Clin Nutr 25:629, 1972

Riboflavin

LANE M et al: The rapid induction of human riboflavin deficiency with galactoflavin. J Clin Invest 43:357, 1964

RIVLIN RS: Riboflavin metabolism. N Engl J Metab 283:463, 1970

Thiamine

AKBARIAN M et al: Hemodynamic studies in beriberi heart disease. Am J Med 41:197, 1966

BLASS JP, GIBSON GE: Abnormality of a thiamine-requiring enzyme in patients with Wernicke-Korsakoff syndrome. N Engl J Med 297:1367, 1977

BROWN GM: Biogenesis and metabolism of thiamine, in *Metabolic Pathways*, 3d ed, DM Greenberg (ed). Academic, New York, 1970, pp 369–381

KOZAM RL et al: Cardiovascular beriberi. Am J Cardiol 30:418, 1972

PINCUS JH et al: Thiamine derivatives in subacute necrotizing encephalomyelopathy. Pediatrics 51:716, 1973

SCRIVER CR: Vitamin-responsive inborn errors of metabolism. Metabolism 22:1319, 1973

TANPHAICHITR V et al: Clinical and biochemical studies of adult beriberi. Am J Clin Nutr 23:1017, 1970

VICTOR M et al: *The Wernicke-Korsakoff Syndrome.* Philadelphia, Davis, 1971

ZIPORIN ZZ et al: Excretion of thiamine and its metabolites in the urine of young adult males receiving restricted intakes of the vitamin. J Nutr 85:287, 1965

81
DEFICIENCY OF VITAMIN C (SCURVY)

JEAN D. WILSON

NORMAL PHYSIOLOGY OF VITAMIN C Biochemistry In most animals vitamin C can be readily synthesized from glucose. Indeed, humans, other primates, and the guinea pig are the only mammals known to be unable to synthesize L-ascorbic acid and consequently to require vitamin C in the diet to prevent scurvy. These three species can perform all the various reactions required for the biosynthesis of the vitamin from *d*-glucose except for one step, the conversion of L-glucono-γ-lactone to L-ascorbic acid. The enzyme that catalyzes this reaction (L-gluconolactone oxidase) is missing because of a mutation that has occurred in these species; thus the need for vitamin C in the diet is the result of a defect in carbohydrate metabolism.

Mechanism of action L-Ascorbic acid readily undergoes reversible oxidation and reduction as follows:

$$\text{L-Ascorbic acid} \rightleftharpoons \text{dehydro-L-ascorbic acid} + 2H^+ + 2e$$

This property of the vitamin is of paramount importance in understanding its physiological role. Indeed, several systems have been characterized in animal tissues in which L-ascorbic acid is coupled with other redox agents. However, there is no direct evidence that the vitamin acts as a conventional cofactor since its requirement can usually be replaced by other compounds with similar redox properties. The most clearly established functional role of the vitamin is in the synthesis of collagen; absence of the vitamin in vitro leads to impairment of peptidyl hydroxylation of procollagen and a reduction in collagen formation and excretion by the connective tissue cell. Nonhydroxylated collagen is unstable and cannot form the triple helix required for normal structures. Many of the clinical findings in scurvy result from this impaired collagen synthesis, including the capillary fragility that underlies the hemorrhagic features, the poor healing of wounds, and (in part) the bony abnormalities of children. Collagens which ordinarily have the highest content of hydroxyproline are most affected, accounting for the disruption of blood vessel adventitia, media, and basal laminae that is characteristic of the disease. Ascorbic acid also acts to prevent oxidation of tetrahydrofolate and thus protect the active folic acid pool. In addition it functions in some manner to regulate iron distribution and storage, probably by influencing the valence of stored iron and thus maintaining a normal ratio of ferritin to hemosiderin. Scorbutic patients also excrete incompletely oxidized products of tyrosine metabolism, but the clinical significance of these metabolites is not clear.

Requirements The requirements and recommended daily allowances for vitamin C are given in Tables 73-1 and 73-2. The vitamin is absent in many common foods but is present in milk and some meats (kidney, liver, fish) and is widely distributed in a variety of fruits and vegetables. A portion of the vitamin is lost after prolonged storage of unprocessed fruits and vegetables (for example, potatoes), but it is partially preserved (half or greater) by most means of food processing (boiling, steaming, pressure cooking, preserving jams and jellies, freezing, dehydration, and canning). As a consequence, fulfilling the recommended daily allowances is easy with even a modest intake of fruits or vegetables. Many factors increase vitamin C requirements including pregnancy, lactation, and thyrotoxicosis which increase utilization, and diarrheal states and achlorhydria which decrease absorption.

EXPERIMENTAL DEPLETION OF VITAMIN C Metabolism of vitamin C has been studied extensively in adults fed diets deficient only in vitamin C and then during repletion in the same subjects. The total body pool varies from 1.5 to 3 g, and when a deficient diet is instituted, the pool is depleted at a constant rate of decay (first order), which varies among individuals (rates as high as 4 percent per day occurring in some). Recent studies in monkeys indicate that the major catabolic pathway involves oxidation of the alcohol at carbon 6 to an aldehyde and then to an acid. Because of differences in initial pool size and rates of turnover, variability in the completeness of deficiency in experimental diets, and variability at the cellular or enzymatic level as well, the time required for the appearance of symptoms ranges from 1 to 3 months in different studies. Symptoms of deficiency correlate better with the total pool size than with plasma or blood levels. In most patients the first symptoms (petechial hemorrhages and ecchymoses) usually do not begin to appear until the pool size is less than 0.5 g; with further depletion (pool size 0.1 to 0.5 g) additional changes appear including gum abnormalities, hyperkeratosis, congested hair follicles, arthralgias, the sicca syndrome, coiled hairs, and joint effusions. When depletion becomes extreme (pool size <0.1 g), dyspnea, edema, oliguria, and neuropathy supervene. After the onset of symptoms, clinical progress of the disease may be rapid.

Symptoms do not improve until the pool size is repleted, and the larger the therapeutic dose, the more rapid the repletion. However, with doses as small as 6.5 mg per day repletion of the body pool and amelioration of symptoms eventually occur in some individuals.

CLINICAL DEFICIENCY Frequency and clinical background Clinical scurvy is an unusual disease in the United States and in most of the world today. It occurs for the most part in areas of urban poverty, and from time to time patients are admitted with it to the wards of most municipal hospitals. A peak of incidence occurs at 6 to 12 months of age in infants whose processed milk formulas are unsupplemented with citrus fruit or vegetables as the result of maternal error or neglect. Another peak occurs in middle and old age; edentulous *men* who live alone and cook for themselves are particularly prone to develop the disease. Clinical scurvy is more severe than the experimental disease, doubtlessly because affected individuals usually have deficiencies of other dietary constituents as well and because the groups at risk (infants and the elderly) are especially vulnerable. The disorder has different clinical features in adults and children.

Manifestations In adults the characteristic features include perifollicular hyperkeratotic papules in which hairs become fragmented and buried, perifollicular hemorrhages, purpura beginning on the backs of the lower extremities coalescing to become ecchymoses (Fig. 81-1), hemorrhage into the muscles of the arms and legs with secondary phlebothromboses, hemorrhages into joints, splinter hemorrhages into the nail beds, gum involvement (only in people with teeth) that includes swelling, friability, bleeding, secondary infection, and loosening of the teeth, poor healing of wounds and breakdown of recently healed wounds, petechial hemorrhages in the viscera, and emotional changes. The development of symptoms resembling those of the sicca syndrome has been noted. Terminally, icterus, edema, and fever are common, and convulsions, shock, and death may occur suddenly.

In infancy and childhood, hemorrhage into the periosteum of long bones causes painful swellings and may result in epiphyseal separation (x-ray changes may in fact be diagnostic). The sternum may sink inwardly, leaving a sharp elevation at the rib margins (scorbutic rosary). Skin purpura and ecchymoses may also occur, and gum lesions occur only if the teeth have erupted. Retrobulbar, subarachnoid, and intracerebral hemorrhages may lead to rapidly progressive illness culminating in death if treatment is delayed.

FIGURE 81-1
Hemorrhages and ecchymoses in a patient with scurvy. (Courtesy of LL Madison.)

Severe to moderate anemia is a common feature in children and adults and is usually normochromic and normocytic, the result of the bleeding into tissues. On occasion, it may be macrocytic and/or megaloblastic. Many foods which contain vitamin C also contain folate, and a diet that causes scurvy may also cause folate deficiency. However, folate metabolism is also altered in scurvy; ascorbic acid deficiency permits an increased irreversible oxidation of formyl tetrahydrofolic acid to inactive folate metabolites and may thus cause a decrease in the active metabolic pool of the vitamin. Whether changes in iron distribution and storage are involved in the pathogenesis of the anemia is unclear. Whatever the mechanism the anemia is corrected with refeeding and replenishment of vitamin C and the institution of a balanced diet.

Diagnosis In some hospitals platelet ascorbic acid levels are useful in diagnosing scurvy and are usually less than a fourth of the normal value (52 ± 22 μg per 10^{10} platelets). Plasma levels of the vitamin correlate less well with the clinical state (Table 74-3). In infants x-ray changes of the bones may be diagnostic. Indirect bilirubin is frequently elevated. Anemia is usually normochromic, normocytic but may (4 out of 21 patients in one series) be megaloblastic. Capillary fragility is abnormal. The remainder of the laboratory tests are nondiagnostic.

Management If scurvy is suspected, samples of blood should be obtained, and ascorbic acid should be administered promptly. Scurvy is potentially fatal, and treatment should never be delayed. The usual dose of the vitamin in adult patients is 100 mg three to five times a day by mouth until 4 g has been administered, then 100 mg per day. In infants and children 10 to 25 mg three times a day is adequate. A diet rich in vitamin C should be initiated in all patients. Generally, spontaneous bleeding ceases within 24 h, muscle and bone pain subsides quickly, and within 2 to 3 days the gums begin to heal. Even large ecchymoses and hematomas are resolved in 10 to 12 days, although pigmentary changes in areas of extensive hemorrhage may persist for months. Serum bilirubin becomes normal within 3 to 5 days, and the anemia ordinarily is completely corrected within 2 to 4 weeks.

THE MEGAVITAMIN QUESTION Considerable controversy has risen over the claim that large doses of vitamin C (1 g or more per day) are effective in preventing or minimizing the symptoms of the common cold. However, in adequately controlled studies, no significant differences in occurrence, severity, or duration have been demonstrated in subjects treated with a placebo as compared with the vitamin. The long-term toxicity of ascorbic acid in these doses is not known, but large doses can interfere with the absorption of vitamin B_{12}, and by enhancing the development of metabolizing enzymes in the fetus may cause development of scurvy in the offspring of mothers who have ingested large amounts of the vitamin during pregnancy. It must be concluded that common use of the vitamin in this way is both unwarranted and unwise. However, ordinary pharmacological doses (200 mg daily) may correct leucocyte abnormalities in patients with the Chediak-Higashi syndrome (Chap. 56).

REFERENCES

BAKER EM et al: Ascorbic acid metabolism in man. Am J Clin Nutr 19:371, 1966

BARNES MJ, KODICEK E: Biological hydroxylations and ascorbic acid with special regard to collagen metabolism. Vitam Horm 30:1, 1972

BARNESS LA: Nutritional aspects of vegetarianism, health foods and fad diets. Nutr 59:153, 1977

BOXEN LA et al: Correction of leucocyte function in Chediak-Higashi syndrome by ascorbate. N Engl J Med 295:1041, 1976

Burns JJ: Biosynthesis of L-ascorbic acid; basic defect in scurvy. Am J Med 26:740, 1959

Chalmers TC: Effects of ascorbic acid on the common cold. Am J Med 58:532, 1975

Hodges RE et al: Clinical manifestations of ascorbic acid deficiency in man. Am J Clin Nutr 24:432, 1971

Tolbert, BM et al: New information on synthesis and metabolism of ascorbic acid. Nutr Rev 35:22, 1977

Vilter RW: Effects of ascorbic acid deficiency in man, in *The Vitamins*, WH Sebrell Jr, RS Harris (eds). New York, Academic, 1967, vol 1, p 457

Wallerstein RO, Wallerstein RO Jr: Scurvy. Semin Hematol 13:211, 1976

82
DEFICIENCY OF VITAMINS A AND K AND HYPERVITAMINOSIS A

JEAN D. WILSON

VITAMIN A

NORMAL PHYSIOLOGY Chemistry and metabolism Vitamin A can be either ingested or synthesized within the body from dietary carotenoids. Preformed vitamin A is found almost exclusively in animals, and the best sources are liver, milk, and kidney, where it is found largely in the form of esters of fatty acids. It is hydrolyzed during the process of digestion, absorbed in the free form, resterified with fatty acids within the intestinal mucosa, and transported in association with lymph chylomicrons. The major substrates for the synthesis of vitamin A are plant carotenoids, mainly β-carotenes, that are widely distributed. β-Carotene can be either absorbed intact or cleaved at the central double bond by a dioxygenase enzyme in the intestinal mucosa (or lumen) to form two molecules of retinaldehyde. Subsequently retinaldehyde is reduced by an aldehyde reductase to retinol. Retinol from whatever source is stored as retinyl esters in the parenchymal cells of the liver. The body pool size in normal subjects varies from 300 to 900 mg.

Prior to release from the liver, the retinyl esters are hydrolyzed, and the free alcohol is mobilized bound to a specific transport protein, retinol-binding protein (RBP). This is the form in which vitamin A is transported to peripheral tissues. In vitamin A deficiency the release of RBP from the liver is inhibited, and the protein accumulates in liver; with repletion rapid release of the protein from preformed stores occurs. The mechanism(s) by which retinol is catabolized and/or excreted has not been defined; approximately equal amounts are excreted in the bile and urine.

Mechanism of action The only physiological function of vitamin A that has been clearly defined in biochemical terms is its role in vision; in the retina vitamin A forms a series of carotenoid proteins that provide the molecular basis for visual excitation. Beyond its role in the visual cycles, vitamin A is known to be required for growth, reproduction, and the maintenance of life. The recent discovery of retinol-phosphate-mannose glycolipid suggests that the vitamin may play a primary role in the synthesis of certain glycoproteins. This process may be one of several functions of the vitamin, but the importance of glycoprotein to every epithelial function implies that this may be a major function of the vitamin.

Requirements The recommended daily allowances for vitamin A are listed in Tables 73-1 and 73-2. The assumed utiliza-

tion efficiency for the conversion of β-carotene to vitamin A in the human is one-sixth (0.167). Other carotenoids with provitamin activity have, on the average, half the activity of β-carotene. Pregnancy and disease states in which there is impaired absorption or storage, excessive utilization, or increased excretion of vitamin A may lead to increased requirements.

EXPERIMENTAL DEPLETION OF VITAMIN A When experimental subjects are fed a diet deficient in both retinol and carotene, plasma levels fall progressively to less than 10 μg per 100 ml in three-fourths of subjects. The body pool simultaneously shrinks to less than half the control value. A true or manifest deficiency develops in all subjects. Follicular hyperkeratosis, impaired dark adaptation, and abnormalities of the electroretinogram are consistent findings. All these changes are corrected after supplementation with 150 μg retinol or 300 μg β-carotene per day.

VITAMIN A DEFICIENCY Clinical occurrence and context Endemic deficiency results from inadequate amounts of the vitamin and the carotene provitamins in the diet and probably never occurs except in conjunction with deficiency of other nutrients or complicating infectious diseases. In many underdeveloped countries vitamin A deficiency is a major cause of blindness in the young; failure to incorporate green leafy vegetables and other rich sources of the provitamin or vitamin into the child's diet is the root of the problem. Vitamin A deficiency may also accompany protein calorie malnutrition, and here the deficiency is due to the defective release mechanism from the liver secondary to inadequate retinol binding protein. In most developed nations, including the United States, vitamin A deficiency is almost always due to either intestinal malabsorption (sprue), abnormal storage (liver disease), or enhanced destruction or excretion of the vitamin (renal disease).

Clinical findings Night blindness is the earliest symptom of deficiency, followed by degenerative changes in the retina. The bulbar conjunctiva becomes dry (xerosis), and small, grey plaques with foamy surfaces develop (Bitot's spots). These lesions are reversible with vitamin A. The more serious effect of vitamin A deficiency is keratomalacia and involves the cornea with ulceration and necrosis, leading to perforation, prolapse, and endophthalmitis. The end result is impairment of vision. Patients may have associated dryness and hyperkeratosis of the skin.

Diagnosis Measurements of dark adaptation, rod scotometry, and electroretinography all suffer the disadvantages of requiring trained personnel and expensive equipment. Vitamin A levels in plasma are not reliable for the assessment of stores in individual cases. The diagnosis ultimately must rest upon a high index of suspicion in every malnourished child.

Treatment Night blindness and the milder conjunctival changes respond well to 30,000 IU vitamin A for a few days. Corneal damage constitutes a therapeutic emergency, and the usual treatment is 20,000 IU per kilogram of body weight per day for 5 days.

OVERDOSAGE Carotenemia Hypercarotenemia results from excessive intake of carotene-containing foods, principally carrots. Excess carotene does not appear to be injurious apart from the cosmetic effect; the fact that it never leads to hypervitaminosis A indicates that some step(s) in the conversion of carotene to vitamin A must be regulated. Carotenemia is characterized by yellowing of the skin with greatest intensity on the palms and soles and with a corresponding yellowness of serum. The yellowing of the skin can be distinguished from jaundice in that the scleras remain white. The omission of carrots from the diet always leads to the rapid disappearance of the pigmentation. Yellowness of the skin can also result on occasion from the consumption of excessive amounts of other colored fruits and vegetables. Hypothyroid patients appear to be particularly susceptible.

Vitamin A toxicity Hypervitaminosis A can result from accidental overingestion by hunters or explorers (polar bear liver), as the result of food faddism (usually caused by oversolicitous parents), or as a side effect of inappropriate therapy. It may be either acute or chronic. Acute toxicity from a single massive dose consists of abdominal pain, nausea, vomiting, severe headaches, dizziness, sluggishness, and irritability followed within a few days by generalized desquamation of the skin and recovery. Chronic toxicity occurs in people who take 40,000 units or more daily for protracted periods and is characterized by bone and joint pain, hair loss, dryness and fissures of the lips, anorexia, benign intracranial hypertension, weight loss, and hepatomegaly. The only diagnostic laboratory finding is elevation of the vitamin in serum, chiefly in the form of retinyl esters. The concentration of retinol-binding protein is normal, and the excess vitamin A circulates in association with lipoprotein. Relief is prompt on withdrawal of the vitamin from the diet.

VITAMIN K

Vitamin K occurs in nature in two major forms: vitamin K_1 (phylloquinone) which is present in most edible vegetables, particularly in green leaves, and vitamin K_2 which is produced by intestinal bacteria. All the many compounds with vitamin K activity are structurally related to the simpler compound, 2-methyl-1,4-naphthoquinone (menadione). Menadione may be formed in the gut by the action of intestinal bacteria on vitamins K_1 and K_2. After absorption, menadione is converted in the body to the active menaquinone. Vitamin K is required by humans and other animals to maintain prothrombin and clotting factors VII, IX, X, and possibly V. The vitamin is a component of a specialized microsomal electron transport system coupled to a carbon dioxide fixalin that effects the γ-carboxylation of glutamic acid in several proteins of the plasma, bone, kidney, and urine, including the precursor proteins for the above clotting factors. It is presumed that in deficiency states death from hemorrhage ensues before other abnormalities become manifest.

Under ordinary circumstances about 80 percent of vitamin K is absorbed in the small bowel into the intestinal lymph. Because the naturally occurring forms of vitamin K are fat-soluble and are poorly stored in the body, a conditioned deficiency can occur in association with diseases that interfere with fat absorption. In addition, long-term treatment with certain antimicrobial drugs may temporarily eliminate intestinal bacteria as a vitamin K source. The coumarin anticoagulant drugs appear to induce hypoprothrombinemia by inhibiting the γ carboxylation of the precursor protein.

Newborn infants tend to be deficient in vitamin K, exhibiting low plasma levels of several coagulation factors in the prothrombin complex. Such deficiencies result from minimal stores of vitamin K at birth, lack of an established intestinal flora, and a very limited dietary intake of the vitamin.

Routine determination of prothrombin should be performed before all surgical procedures and deliveries. Patients with values below 70 percent of normal should receive therapy with vitamin K; administration of 75 mg menadione is satisfactory by any route and may be repeated until body stores of vitamin K are repleted. Hypoprothrombinemia secondary to hepatic dysfunction and excessive use of anticoagulants requires multiple dosage of vitamin K_1 for optimal results.

REFERENCES

DOISY EA JR, MATSCHINER JT: Biochemistry of vitamin K, in *Fat-Soluble Vitamins,* RA Morton (ed). New York, Pergamon, 1970, vol 9, p 293

LOMBAERT A, CARTON H: Benign intracranial hypertension due to A-hypervitaminosis in adults and adolescents. Eur Neurol 14:340, 1976

OLSON RE, SUTTIE JW: Vitamin K and γ-carboxyglutamate biosynthesis, in *Vitamins and Hormones,* PL Munson et al (eds). New York, Academic, 1977, vol 35, p 59

SAUBERLICH HE et al: Vitamin A metabolism and requirements in the human studied with the use of labeled retinol, in *Vitamins and Hormones: Advances in Research and Applications,* RS Harris et al (eds). New York, Academic, 1974, vol 32

SHEARER MJ et al: Studies on the absorption and metabolism of phylloquinone (vitamin K) in man, in *Vitamins and Hormones: Advances in Research and Applications,* RS Harris et al (eds). Academic, 1974, vol 32, p 513

SMITH FR, GOODMAN DS: Vitamin A transport in human vitamin A toxicity. N Engl J Med 294:805, 1976

SMITH JE, GOODMAN DS: Vitamin A metabolism and transport, in *Present Knowledge in Nutrition,* 4th ed, DM Hegsted et al (eds), Washington, DC, The Nutrition Foundation, 1976

SRIKANTIA SG: Human vitamin A deficiency, in *World Review of Nutrition and Dietetics,* GH Bourne (ed). Basel, Karger, 1975, vol 20, p 185

WALD G: Molecular basis of visual excitation. Science 162:230, 1968

83

DISTURBANCES IN TRACE ELEMENT METABOLISM

DAVID D. ULMER

Inorganic ions are crucial to virtually all biochemical and physiologic processes. Some, present in tissues only in minute quantity, micrograms to picograms per gram of wet organ, are arbitrarily designated *trace elements.* Of these, iron, iodine, cobalt, copper, manganese, molybdenum, selenium, chromium, fluorine, silicon, nickel, zinc, tin, and vanadium are now thought to be essential for animal life.

The functions of trace elements have been defined at levels of biologic complexity ranging from isolated enzymes to intact animals. Thus, many metals participate in enzymic catalysis through substrate binding, activation of the enzyme-substrate complex, or by formation of a tight coordination complex with the enzyme such that the two are isolated together as a unit, i.e., *metalloenzyme.* Metals appear to play a role in the synthesis of both proteins and nucleic acids. Trace elements are also involved in the function of organized subcellular systems, such as mitochondria, in regulation of intracellular heme concentrations, and in membrane transport, nerve conduction, and muscle contraction. Critical biologic functions in animals are disrupted by deprivation of essential metals resulting in discrete deficiency states. Toxic manifestations owing to grossly excessive exposure to metals are also well recognized. The biologic effects of metals, both essential and toxic, are often conditioned by *metal-ion antagonism;* i.e., one metal induces a biologic effect by altering the requirement for another, usually through competition for the same biochemical sites. As a consequence, such metal-ion *imbalances* are likely among the most common and certainly the most elusive sources of either metal-deficiency or intoxication states. This phenomenon complicates investigative efforts and helps to account for the fact that proved manifestations of trace-element deficiency in human beings, except for those due to iron and iodine, are rare despite extensive documentation of deficiency syndromes in many animal species.

ZINC The average adult human body contains 1.4 to 2.3 g zinc; highest concentrations are found in liver, voluntary muscle, bone, prostate, and eye. The minimum daily requirement (about 15 mg) is easily attained in most diets since the element is widely distributed in food, particularly meat, shellfish, liver, gelatin, bread, cereals, lentils, peas, beans, and rice. However, *phytic acid* in the diet binds zinc tightly, limits its absorption, and operates as a conditioning factor to induce zinc deficiency. Zinc is crucial to growth, development, and normal function of all living forms. It is an essential component of many enzymes in the liver, pancreas, and other organs, and its importance for protein synthesis may be surmised from recent evidence that both DNA and RNA polymerases are zinc metalloenzymes. While marked changes in the zinc content of tissues, blood, and urine accompany many different human diseases, the relationship of such alterations to the underlying conditions are, for the most part, poorly understood.

Spontaneous or experimental zinc deficiency in animals results in anorexia, retarded growth, gonadal atrophy, hyperkeratotic dermatitis, loss of hair, parakeratosis of tongue and esophagus, and diarrhea. Two human syndromes exhibit features observed in zinc-deficient animals. Hypogonadal dwarfism, sometimes accompanied by hepatosplenomegaly, anemia, and geophagia, has been described in rural Iranian and Egyptian boys subsisting on diets consisting largely of bread and beans and nearly devoid of animal protein. The youths have decreased zinc concentrations in plasma, red cells, and hair and decreased activity of serum alkaline phosphatase, a zinc-dependent enzyme. Oral zinc supplements enhance growth and sexual maturation beyond that observed with administration of an adequate diet alone. However, the anemia is improved only by correction of concomitant iron deficiency. Delayed growth and sexual maturation accompanied by moderate decreases in serum zinc concentration have also been observed in this country in youths afflicted with chronic illnesses such as intestinal malabsorption and sickle-cell anemia. It is postulated that such patients may have an incomplete form of the hypogonadal dwarf syndrome.

In recent years, *acrodermatitis enteropathica* has been characterized as the first inherited human zinc-deficiency disease. This autosomal recessive disorder is manifested by severe chronic diarrhea, wasting, alopecia, and roughened, thickened, and ulcerated skin about body orifices and on the extremities. Patients exhibit a profound decrease in zinc concentrations in serum and hair, and defective leukocyte chemotaxis. They improve quickly upon administration of zinc. Whether the zinc deficiency results from an intestinal absorptive defect, excessive losses, or other factors is not yet clear. Acrodermatitis enteropathica owing to acquired zinc deficiency has also been observed in adults maintained on long-term parenteral nutrition. The response to zinc administration is equally dramatic.

Demonstration of the value of zinc replacement in patients with acrodermatitis enteropathica has prompted renewed interest in the role of this element in promoting healing of surgical wounds and chronic skin ulcers. Several investigations suggest that wound healing is delayed in patients with zinc deficiency and is restored to normal by oral administration of zinc. However, controlled studies indicate that zinc has no effect in wound-healing in normal persons.

Zinc has been postulated to play a role in the maintenance of normal taste and patients with decreased taste acuity (hypogeusia) may improve with oral administration of zinc sulfate.

Zinc toxicity may result from excessive ingestion of the element in food or drink, although the margin of safety is large. Nausea, vomiting, colic, and diarrhea are predominant manifestations. Toxicity also results from inhalation of high concentrations of zinc oxide fumes, leading to *metal-fume fever* or *brass chills*. Once a fairly common industrial hazard, this self-limited, acute illness is accompanied by fever, shaking chills, excessive salivation, headache, cough, malaise, and pronounced leukocytosis.

COPPER Copper is an essential nutrient for animals and is critical to such diverse activities as heme synthesis, connective tissue metabolism, bone development, and nerve function. Experimental copper deficiency is manifested by severe anemia, abnormalities of hair and skin pigmentation, defective elastic tissue in great vessels resulting in arterial rupture, faulty development of bone and nervous tissue, and decreased concentrations of plasma copper and the serum copper protein, *ceruloplasmin (ferroxidase)*. Ceruloplasmin catalyzes oxidation of ferrous to ferric ions and is postulated to control the rate of iron uptake by transferrin—hence, availabilitiy to reticulocytes of iron for heme synthesis. Copper is also a component of a number of other critical metalloenzymes, e.g., cytochrome oxidase, lysine oxidase, polyphenol oxidases, amine oxidases, and the cupreins—cuprozinc proteins in liver, red cells, and brain which appear to function as superoxide dismutases and may also serve in quenching highly reactive singlet oxygen in cells. Copper is important to mitochondrial function and is found frequently as a component of ribonucleic acid.

The copper concentration in adult human beings averages 1.5 to 2.4 μg per gram of fat-free tissue; the metal concentrates in liver, heart, brain, kidneys, and hair; for example, to 18 to 45 μg per gram of dry weight in liver. Balance is maintained on an average intake of 2 to 5 mg copper daily, obtained readily from meats, particularly liver and kidney, shellfish, raisins, whole-grain cereals, dried legumes, and nuts. Bile constitutes a major route of excretion.

Elevated concentrations of copper in serum are observed in a large number of acute and chronic diseases and appear to be a manifestation of response to stress. Hypocupremia is a more specific finding and is associated primarily with hepatolenticular degeneration (Wilson's disease), certain dysproteinemias of infancy, the nephrotic syndrome (secondary to renal loss of copper proteins), intestinal malabsorption, and kwashiorkor. Acute poisoning owing to ingestion of metallic copper manifests as nausea, vomiting, hematemesis, and melena, and may be accompanied by centrilobular liver necrosis. Rapid absorption of copper sulfate through the skin, as employed for therapy of burns, or through use of copper-containing dialysis equipment, has resulted in acute hemolytic anemia. Increased copper accumulation is observed in Wilson's disease (Chap. 95), primary biliary cirrhosis (Chap. 304), and prolonged extrahepatic biliary tract obstruction (Chap. 307).

Frank copper deficiency is rare in human beings, but has been reported in severely malnourished infants, premature infants, and in children and adults receiving prolonged intravenous hyperalimentation (Chap. 78). Anemia, leukopenia, and neutropenia are observed, and the bone marrow is megaloblastoid, contains increased sideroblasts, and shows a predominance of early granulocytes and cytoplasmic vacuolization of erythroid and myeloid elements (maturation arrest). The hematologic abnormalities are reversed by oral copper therapy.

An abnormality in copper transport by intestinal cells has been described in *Menkes's kinky hair disease,* a rare X-chromosome-linked inherited syndrome manifested by rapid central nervous system and arterial degeneration, bony abnormalities, and hypothermia in male infants. As is also observed in copper-deficient animals, the hair of affected patients has less crimp and has a steely texture (pili torti), presumably owing to impaired disulfide bond formation. Concentrations of serum copper and ceruloplasmin are markedly decreased and can be restored to normal by intravenous but not oral administration of copper. Thus far, however, therapeutic efforts to replace copper and prevent early death have failed.

COBALT Although colbalt deficiency occurs in ruminants, the physiologic significance of cobalt to most other animals and humans is limited to its participation in reactions of vitamin B_{12}, of which it is a component (Chap. 311). Acute cobalt poisoning in humans is manifested by nausea, vomiting, diarrhea, tinnitus, and loss of hearing, while chronic administration of cobalt induces polycythemia and, by blocking iodine uptake, may produce goiter, especially in children. During the last decade, cobalt added to beer as an antifoaming agent produced several localized epidemics of an extraordinary cardiomyopathy, often accompanied by pericardial effusion, frequently with fatal outcome.

SELENIUM Selenium deficiency has not yet been verified in humans; however, in animals deficiency results in liver necrosis, striking pallor, and degeneration of skeletal muscle, *white-muscle disease,* occasionally involving the heart. It has been recognized for many years that these alterations resemble certain of the manifestations of vitamin E deficiency in animals and can be ameliorated by dietary supplementation with sulfur-containing amino acids. The nature of these interrelationships has been partially clarified recently by findings that selenium is a component of glutathione peroxidase in red blood cells and likely other tissues. Hence, selenium, like vitamin E, appears to help protect against damage from complex intracellular peroxides.

MANGANESE Manganese activates a host of critical intracellular enzymes; among these, mitochondrial pyruvate carboxylase and superoxide dismutase from chicken liver have recently been identified as manganese metalloenzymes. The metal appears to play a role in such important metabolic functions as oxidative phosphorylation, fatty acid metabolism, and the synthesis of proteins, mucopolysaccharides, and cholesterol. Experimental manganese deficiency has been described in animals, but not as yet in humans.

NICKEL Nickel has been found to be firmly bound to RNA from several tissues and may act to stabilize nucleic acid structure. The metal is also postulated to play a general role in the maintenance of membrane structure and function. A nickel-containing α_2-macroglobulin, nickeloplasmin, has been isolated from both human and rabbit serum, but its significance is uncertain at present. Nickel carbonyl, formed from nickel and carbon monoxide, is exceedingly dangerous and produces severe lung inflammation and liver necrosis. Chronic excess industrial exposure to nickel is associated with an increased incidence of lung and nasal carcinoma.

SILICON (AND SILICA) Silicon is a component of many mucopolysaccharides and may contribute to connective tissue structure by bridging polysaccharide chains or linking polysaccharides to proteins. Inhalation of fine particles of free crystalline silica (SiO_2) produces a pulmonary inflammatory response, granuloma formation, and chronic fibrosis (silicosis).

FLUORINE In pharmacologic doses, fluorine exerts anticariogenic effects, promotes stabilization of newly synthesized bone matrix, and inhibits bone resorption, providing a rationale for its use in treatment of osteoporosis. Chronic ingestion of fluorides in moderate amounts produces mottling of dental enamel (fluorosis); in larger amounts, e.g., from ingestion of insect poisons, fluorides cause nausea, vomiting, abdominal pain, diarrhea, and tetany often resulting in death from cardiovascular collapse.

CHROMIUM Chromium, in the form of a low-molecular-weight organic complex, *glucose tolerance factor,* present in brewer's yeast, animal meats, and grains, is required for normal glucose metabolism in several animal species. The ability of mammals to synthesize glucose tolerance factor appears to be limited, and, in humans, marginal chromium deficiency may possibly accompany protein-caloric malnutrition, pregnancy, and old age. While diabetics often exhibit altered chromium metabolism, the precise relation of this metal to diabetes remains uncertain.

REFERENCES

BURCH RE, SULLIVAN JF (eds): Symposium on trace elements. Med Clin North Am 60:653, 1976

DANKS DM et al: Menkes's kinky hair syndrome: An inherited defect in copper absorption with widespread effects. Pediatrics 50:188, 1972

HALSTED JA et al: Zinc deficiency in man: The Shiraz experiment. Am J Med 53:277, 1972

HOESTRA WG et al (eds): *Trace Element Metabolism in Animals.* Baltimore, University Park Press, 1974

NELDER KH, HAMBRIDGE KM: Zinc therapy of acrodermatitis enteropathica. N Engl J Med 292:879, 1975

SCHWARTZ K: Recent dietary trace element research, exemplified by tin, fluorine, and silicon. Fed Proc 33:1748, 1974

TUCKER SB et al: Acquired zinc deficiency: Cutaneous manifestations typical of acrodermatitis enteropathica. JAMA 235:2399, 1976

ULMER DD: Trace elements. N Engl J Med 297:318, 1977

VILTER RW et al: Manifestations of copper deficiency in a patient with systemic sclerosis on intravenous hyperalimentation. N Engl J Med 291:188, 1974

84
FLUIDS AND ELECTROLYTES

NORMAN G. LEVINSKY

SODIUM AND WATER

PHYSIOLOGIC CONSIDERATIONS Both physiologically and clinically, sodium and water metabolism are closely interrelated. The sodium content of the body depends on the balance between dietary intake and renal excretion of sodium. In health, extrarenal losses of sodium are negligible. Renal sodium excretion is closely regulated to match dietary content. Within 2 to 4 days after sodium intake stops, urinary excretion decreases to 5 meq per day or less. If dietary sodium is abruptly increased, sodium excretion promptly rises. About one-half of the surfeit is excreted within the first 24 h and the remainder over the next few days. Thus, the sodium content of the body remains quite constant despite wide variations in sodium intake; over the range of 0 to 400 meq per day, total body sodium varies only by about 10 percent.

Although detailed knowledge of the mechanism of this renal response is limited, certain general points deserve emphasis because of their clinical relevance. Sodium loads tend to increase glomerular filtration and to depress proximal tubular reabsorption of sodium, while sodium deficits have the opposite effects. Thus, delivery of sodium to the distal segments of the nephron tends to vary in parallel with extracellular sodium. Reabsorption in the loop of Henle and distal convolutions appears to change proportionately with the rate of sodium delivery. This modulates variations in the amount of sodium entering the collecting ducts, where final adjustments are made. Multiple regulatory factors control these tubular adjustments. Of these, only the role of aldosterone is well established; its principal action is to stimulate sodium transport in the distal nephron. There is some evidence for a "natriuretic hormone" which inhibits sodium reabsorption, perhaps at a distal tubular site such as the collecting duct. Changes in proximal tubular reabsorption in response to altered sodium balance appear to be mediated, at least in part, by changes in hemodynamic factors in the peritubular microcirculation. Undoubtedly, other regulatory mechanisms remain to be defined. The multiplicity of control mechanisms prevents abnormalities of any single mechanism from grossly distorting the regulation of sodium excretion. For example, increased aldosterone secretion leads only to limited and transient sodium retention, because the initial accumulation of sodium stimulates opposing natriuretic factors such as increased glomerular filtration and decreased proximal tubular reabsorption.

All but 2 to 5 percent of the sodium in the body is located in the extracellular fluids. (Approximately 40 percent of total body sodium is located in bone, but this fraction does not participate significantly in most physiologic processes and will not be considered further.) Except for minor differences in concentration due to the Gibbs-Donnan effect of plasma proteins, the electrolyte compositions of plasma and interstitial fluid are essentially equal. For practical purposes, plasma composition can be considered representative of the entire extracellular compartment. Total extracellular volume approximates 20 per-

cent of body weight. Of this, 5 percent represents plasma volume and 15 percent the volume of interstitial fluids. Thus, in a 70-kg individual with plasma sodium concentration of 140 meq per liter, extracellular sodium content will approximate 2000 meq. The volume of intracellular fluid is approximately twice as great as that of extracellular fluid, i.e., about 40 percent of body weight. However, since intracellular sodium concentration is less than 5 meq per liter, total intracellular sodium content is only about 100 to 150 meq. The asymmetric distribution of sodium across cell membranes is maintained by expenditure of a large fraction of the energy derived from cell metabolism, which is required constantly to pump sodium out of cells against its electrochemical grandient. All the principal electrolytes are asymmetrically distributed across cell membranes. The principal electrolytes of the extracellular fluids are sodium, chloride, and bicarbonate. The major electrolytes of the intracellular fluids are potassium, magnesium, calcium, and organic anions, including proteins.

Since sodium salts account for more than 90 percent of the total osmolality of the extracellular fluid, variations in plasma sodium concentration are almost always reflected in equivalent changes in plasma osmolality. Exceptions due to accumulation of other solutes in plasma are discussed later. Although the electrolyte compositions of intracellular and extracellular fluids differ markedly, they are always in osmotic equilibrium, since water moves rapidly across cellular membranes to dissipate osmotic gradients. Therefore, although sodium is largely confined to extracellular fluids, plasma sodium concentration is an index of not only the relative proportions of sodium and water in those fluids but also the relation between total body solute and total body water. An example is the effect of shift of sodium from extracellular to intracellular fluid without a change in total body solute. Movement of sodium into cells would not cause hyponatremia, since water would shift into cells with the sodium. On the other hand, a primary decrease in the concentration of osmotically active solute within cells would decrease total body solute; although there would be no change in total body sodium or water, hyponatremia would result from the shift of intracellular water into the extracellular compartment.

A very effective mechanism involving the hypothalamus, the neurohypophysis, and the kidney regulates plasma osmolality. Changes of 2 percent or less in plasma osmolality can be detected by osmoreceptors in the hypothalamus. Small increases in osmolality stimulate the secretion of antidiuretic hormone (ADH) from the neurohypophysis, while small decreases suppress secretion of the hormone. Normal plasma osmolality is approximately 280 to 300 mosmol per kilogram of water; the exact level is determined by the "set" of the hypothalamic osmoreceptors in a given individual. When ADH secretion is maximal, urine volume will be about 500 ml per day, and urine osmolality will be 800 to 1400 mosmol/kg. In the absence of ADH, minimal urine osmolality is 40 to 80 mosmol/kg, and maximum water diuresis can reach 15 to 20 liters per day or more. The capacity of this receptor-effector system is sufficient to maintain plasma osmolality within narrow limits despite large variations in the volume and concentration of dietary fluids.

The total sodium *content* of the body is determined by the

renal sodium regulatory mechanisms described earlier. However, the principal determinant of plasma sodium *concentration* is water metabolism rather than total body sodium content. If excess sodium were to be ingested and retained, hypernatremia would be only transient. Water intake would increase because of thirst, and the fluid ingested would be retained because hypernatremia (hyperosmolality) would stimulate ADH secretion. Expanded extracellular volume, not hypernatremia, would be the end result. Conversely, if the osmoregulatory system is functioning normally, loss of sodium without water would not result in permanent reduction of plasma sodium concentration. The initial reduction would shut off secretion of ADH, and a water diuresis would ensue. The final outcome would be contraction of extracellular volume, while plasma sodium concentration would be restored to normal. It should be apparent that changes in total sodium content tend to cause changes in extracellular volume. In this sense, the sodium content of the extracellular fluid determines extracellular volume. On the other hand, changes in plasma sodium concentration reflect altered regulation of water excretion, not changes in total body sodium content alone. Clinically, plasma sodium concentration per se gives no information about the amount of sodium present in the body. Total body sodium content is determined by the volume of extracellular fluids as well as by the concentration of sodium in these fluids. Extracellular volume is usually the dominant factor since changes in volume tend to be greater than changes in sodium concentration. Plasma sodium concentration reflects merely the relative proportions of sodium and water (or, more exactly, of total body solute and water), not the absolute amount of sodium in the body. Either hyponatremia or hypernatremia may occur when total body sodium content is decreased, normal, or increased.

CLINICAL DISORDERS   Deficits and excesses of sodium and water occur in a great variety of clinical circumstances. The manifestations of the underlying illness may overshadow the

clinical features of the fluid and electrolyte disorder. Theoretically, disturbances of sodium and water metabolism can be classified into four categories, reflecting a primary excess or deficit of water or sodium. Practically, such isolated disturbances are uncommon. A primary excess of sodium leads to edema; it is not ordinarily considered as an electrolyte disorder but as a feature of underlying disease, such as congestive heart failure, hepatic cirrhosis, or nephrotic syndrome. Primary sodium deficits are nearly always accompanied by water depletion, leading to the clinical syndrome of extracellular volume depletion. Pure or disproportionate water excess leads to hyponatremia, relative or absolute water depletion to hypernatremia. A practical clinical classification of disorders of sodium and water metabolism is given in Table 84-1.

VOLUME DEPLETION   Combined sodium and water deficits are far more frequent than isolated deficits of either constituent. Although the term *dehydration* is often used for combined deficits, this usage is confusing. Dehydration should be used to describe relatively pure water depletion leading to hypernatremia; *volume depletion* or some similar term should be used for combined deficits.

Pathogenesis   As noted earlier, elimination of sodium from the diet will not by itself lead to sodium depletion, since urinary sodium excretion will quickly fall to very low levels. Therefore, sodium depletion is always due either to extrarenal losses or to abnormal renal losses.

GASTROINTESTINAL   The most common cause of volume depletion is loss of a significant fraction of the 8 to 10 liters of gastrointestinal fluids normally secreted daily. Since the principal secretions contain potassium and hydrogen ion or bicarbonate in large amounts, volume depletion due to gastrointestinal losses is often combined with potassium depletion and acidosis or alkalosis.

Significant volume depletion may be caused by sequestration of secretions within an obstructed gastrointestinal tract or within the peritoneal cavity in peritonitis. Rapid reaccumulation of ascites after paracentesis may cause contraction of the effective circulating blood volume.

SKIN   The sodium concentration of sweat varies from 5 to 50 meq per liter; sodium concentration increases with higher rates of sweating and in adrenal insufficiency. Because sweat is always a hypotonic solution, sweating leads to water deficits out of proportion to sodium losses. In burns, capillary damage may lead to sequestration of large amounts of sodium and water in the injured skin.

RENAL   Abnormal losses of sodium in the urine may occur in both acute and chronic renal diseases. Early in the recovery (diuretic) phase of *acute renal failure*, urinary sodium concentration tends to be high (50 to 100 meq per liter), and substantial deficits may ensue. With rare exceptions, severe sodium wasting does not persist beyond the first few days. It is important to discriminate between increased sodium excretion which represents elimination of excess salt retained during the oliguric period and true tubular sodium wasting which depletes normal extracellular sodium. Only the latter requires replacement. Acute salt wasting due to tubular damage may also occur immediately after relief of prolonged *obstruction* of the urinary tract. Although such a postobstructive diuresis may be severe, it rarely persists for more than several days as a clinically important phenomenon.

Patients with *chronic renal failure* have limited ability to decrease sodium excretion in response to decreased intake. They will become progressively volume-depleted if their intake is restricted by the anorexia, nausea, and vomiting characteris-

TABLE 84-1
Disorders of sodium and water metabolism

I Combined sodium and water depletion (volume depletion)
  A Extrarenal losses
    1 Gastrointestinal (vomiting, diarrhea, gastrointestinal suction, fistulas)
    2 Abdominal sequestration (peritonitis, rapid reaccumulation of ascites)
    3 Skin (sweating, burns)
  B Renal losses
    1 Renal disease (chronic renal failure, salt-wasting tubular disease, diuretic phase of acute renal failure)
    2 Osmotic diuresis (diabetic glycosuria)
    3 Adrenal insufficiency (Addison's disease)
II Hyponatremia
  A Associated with sodium and water depletion (volume depletion)
  B Associated with sodium retention and edema
  C Primary dilutional
  D Adrenal insufficiency
  E Syndrome of inappropriate secretion of antidiuretic hormone
    1 Spontaneous
    2 Drug-induced
  F Essential ("sick-cell syndrome")
  G Osmotic (hyperglycemia, mannitol)
  H Artifactual (hyperlipemia, hyperproteinemia, laboratory error)
III Hypernatremia
  A Extrarenal water loss
    1 Skin (insensible losses, burns, sweat)
    2 Lungs (insensible)
  B Renal water loss
    1 Diabetes insipidus (pituitary, nephrogenic)
    2 Osmotic diuresis (glycosuria, urea diuresis)
  C Primary excess of sodium (excessive salt administration without access to water)
  D Adrenal hyperfunction (Cushing's disease, primary hyperaldosteronism)

tic of uremia or because of their physician's instructions. Large deficits may develop insidiously over many days or weeks. A "vicious circle" may result, in that volume depletion will tend further to compromise renal function. Sodium-wasting renal disease, i.e., negative sodium balance when dietary sodium is normal, is very rare. It occurs in occasional patients with tubulointerstitial diseases of the kidney, especially medullary cystic disease.

Renal sodium wasting in the presence of normal intrinsic renal function occurs in three clinical circumstances. Perhaps the most common is sodium depletion due to continued administration of potent *diuretics* after edema has been relieved or to patients whose edema is sequestered and cannot be mobilized. For example, attempted treatment of cirrhotics with ascites may result in depletion of overall extracellular volume rather than mobilization of ascitic fluid. An obligatory *osmotic diuresis* may also cause renal sodium wasting despite normal renal function. Marked glycosuria in uncontrolled diabetes mellitus is the most frequent clinical example. Administration of osmotic diuretics such as mannitol and urea is a common iatrogenic cause. Volume depletion in patients receiving high-protein tube feedings may be due to an osmotic diuresis of urea formed by protein metabolism. Finally, renal sodium wasting despite normal intrinsic function occurs in *adrenal insufficiency* due to a deficiency of mineralocorticoids.

Clinical features and diagnosis The cause of volume depletion can usually be suspected from a history of inadequate salt and water intake together with vomiting, diarrhea, or excessive sweating; the symptoms of poorly controlled diabetes mellitus or of renal or adrenal disease may be elicited. The key findings on physical examination are those of plasma and extracellular volume depletion. Decreased skin turgor is usually present in patients with significant volume contraction. It can be estimated clinically by noting the slow rate of return of skin to its original position when it is raised between the examiner's fingers. An area of skin normally free of wrinkles and not subject to wide variations in the thickness of subcutaneous tissue, such as that over the sternum, should be selected for this maneuver. With moderate volume depletion, blood pressure is usually normal when the patient is recumbent, although resting tachycardia may be present. Postural hypotension, i.e., a drop of 5 to 10 mmHg in the sitting or standing position, is often present. With greater degrees of volume depletion, even recumbent blood pressure is reduced, and frank shock may occur. The patient with moderate or severe degrees of volume contraction is often lethargic, weak, confused, or obtunded. Such patients are usually oliguric, even when recumbent blood pressure is normal.

LABORATORY FINDINGS The hematocrit and plasma protein concentration are increased, but values within the normal range are interpretable only if prior values are known. Plasma sodium concentration may be decreased, normal, or increased, depending upon the proportion between deficits of sodium and of water. Plasma creatinine and urea nitrogen are usually increased, since the glomerular filtration rate is decreased ("prerenal azotemia"). Urinary sodium concentration may be of value in differentiating extrarenal and renal sources of sodium loss if the probable cause is not clear from the history. With extrarenal losses, urinary sodium concentration will be less than 10 meq per liter; the concentration will usually exceed 20 meq per liter if renal or adrenal disorders are at fault. However urinary sodium may ultimately fall below this level even in patients with renal salt wasting if sodium depletion becomes very severe.

Treatment The principal clinical manifestations of extracellular volume depletion are due to reduction of plasma and inter-

stitial fluid volume. Since there is no convenient clinical method for assessing these volumes, the effect of treatment must be determined by following the clinical response through evaluation of changes in parameters such as blood pressure, urine output, and skin turgor. Modest deficits of sodium and water can often be corrected by increased oral intake in patients not suffering from gastrointestinal disorders. Severe depletion requires therapy with intravenous solutions. Isotonic saline (0.85%) is the infusion of choice in patients whose serum sodium concentration is approximately normal. The amount to be infused can be estimated from the history of prior losses and from the severity of the physical findings of extracellular volume contraction. Patients with clinically moderate volume contraction usually require replacement with 2 to 3 liters of saline, while patients with severe depletion may require much larger volumes. The need for correction of other concurrent electrolyte abnormalities may alter the composition of the required infusion; e.g., some of the sodium may be given as bicarbonate to patients with volume contraction and metabolic acidosis, or potassium may be added in patients with concurrent potassium depletion. In estimating the total amount to be infused, allowance for ongoing losses must be included. Since the amount to be infused cannot be calculated precisely, patients should be monitored carefully to avoid fluid overload and congestive failure.

HYPONATREMIA Pathophysiology Hyponatremia indicates that the body fluids are diluted by an excess of water relative to total solute. Hyponatremia is not equivalent to sodium depletion, which is only one of a number of clinical states in which it may occur (see Table 84-1). Most types of hyponatremia can be considered to result from defective urinary dilution. The normal response to dilution of body fluids is a water diuresis, which corrects the hypoosmotic state. Normal water diuresis requires three factors: (1) Secretion of ADH must be suppressed. (2) Sufficient sodium and water must reach the diluting sites of the nephron, in the ascending limb of Henle's loop and the distal convoluted tubule. (3) These nephron segments must function normally, reabsorbing sodium while remaining impermeable to water.

Three general types of mechanisms may cause defective water diuresis in patients with hyponatremia. (1) Secretion of ADH may continue "inappropriately" despite hypotonicity of extracellular fluid, which normally shuts off secretion of the hormone. (2) Insufficient sodium may reach the diluting segments to permit the formation of an adequate amount of dilute urine. Inadequate delivery of tubular fluid to distal sites may be due to reduced glomerular filtration and/or enhanced proximal tubular reabsorption. Even in the absence of ADH, distal tubular segments are not absolutely impermeable to water; small amounts of water continue to leak from the hypotonic tubular fluid into the isotonic cortical and slightly hypertonic medullary interstitial fluid. The amount of water leaking back in this manner becomes an increasingly large fraction of the volume of dilute urine formed, as the diluting process is progressively limited by decreasing delivery. Hence, urine osmolality rises progressively. In some instances, this mechanism may even result in excretion of a urine hypertonic to plasma, despite the absence of ADH. (3) Sodium transport in the diluting segments may be defective or water permeability may be excessive at these sites even in the absence of ADH. One of these three factors can account for most types of hyponatremia. However, it must be recognized that information about actual disease states is incomplete.

Paradoxically, hyponatremia in *volume depletion* and in

edematous states appears to result from similar mechanisms. Delivery of sodium and water to the diluting segments of the nephron is reduced because of decreased gomerular filtration, increased proximal tubular reabsorption, or both. Volume-mediated secretion of ADH may also be a factor in these conditions. Contraction of plasma or extracellular volume is the stimulus to these changes in renal function and hormone secretion during salt depletion. These volumes appear to be normal or increased in most edematous patients. However, it is believed that the "effective" volume is reduced by decreased cardiac output or sequestration of fluid beyond the central circulation. Essential hyponatremia may be an additional mechanism in some edematous patients (see below).

The normal kidney can excrete 15 to 20 liters of dilute urine per day. Normal water intake, regulated by thirst and habit, is a small fraction of this maximum excretory capacity. Hence, *dilutional hyponatremia* usually occurs only when defective water diuresis or water intake unregulated by thirst is present. Oliguric patients may develop dilutional hyponatremia if the volume of oral and intravenous fluids is not limited appropriately. The ability to excrete a normal volume of dilute urine is progressively limited in advancing chronic renal failure. Hyponatremia may be precipitated in patients with advanced renal failure by instructions to force fluids. In the postoperative state, water diuresis is limited by a number of factors, such as secretion of ADH induced by pain or narcotics and extracellular volume contraction. The administration of excessive volumes of hypotonic solutions to such patients is a common cause of hyponatremia. Very rarely, psychogenic polydipsia may be so severe that the rapid ingestion of huge quantities of fluids may overwhelm normal excretory capacity and produce symptomatic dilutional hyponatremia despite normal renal diluting mechanisms.

Multiple factors appear to play a role in limiting water diuresis in patients with *adrenal insufficiency*. Deficient secretion of mineralocorticoid hormones may lead to sodium depletion, with consequent reduction of glomerular filtration and enhancement of proximal tubular sodium reabsorption. Moreover, glucocorticoid deficiency directly reduces filtration. Therefore, adrenal insufficiency will tend to decrease delivery of sodium to diluting sites. In addition, glucocorticoid deficiency directly or indirectly prevents the maintenance of normal water impermeability in distal diluting segments of the nephron. Some evidence suggests a direct effect of glucocorticoid deficiency on water permeability of distal tubular epithelium, but conflicting data indicate that inappropriate secretion of ADH may occur when glucocorticoids are deficient.

Hyponatremia in patients with chronic *inappropriate secretion* of *antidiuretic hormone* is principally due to water retention, but continued urinary losses of sodium also contribute to producing a mild negative sodium balance. Renal sodium wasting is related to volume expansion, since it can be eliminated by restricting fluid intake. The mechanisms by which extracellular expansion may increase sodium excretion have been discussed above.

A limited number of observations suggest that some patients may be hyponatremic in the absence of a defect in water diuresis. The terms "essential hyponatremia" and "sick-cell syndrome" have been applied to this category. Osmoreceptor cells in the hypothalamus are thought to be "reset" to maintain a decreased level of body fluid osmolality as though it were normal. The genesis of such a syndrome is speculative; it has been suggested that changes in cellular metabolism might lead to a primary reduction in cellular osmolality. Such a reduction in intracellular solute would result in a shift of water out of cells, thereby diluting extracellular fluids and initiating hyponatremia. Once the osmoreceptor was "reset," water and sodium metabolism would behave normally. Urine would become dilute or concentrated if plasma sodium fell or increased slightly from the new "normal" level for that patient.

Hyponatremia due to *accumulation* of *osmotically active solutes* in the plasma is the sole exception to the rule that hyponatremia means decreased plasma osmolality. In this type of hyponatremia, plasma osmolality is increased. Plasma sodium is diluted by movement of water out of cells along the osmotic gradient created by addition to the plasma of the abnormal solute, such as glucose or mannitol. It should be noted that solutes which equilibrate across cell membranes do not induce movement of water from cells. Thus, high plasma urea levels in patients with renal failure do not cause hyponatremia.

Clinical features and diagnosis In *sodium* (volume) *depletion*, hyponatremia per se is usually of little clinical significance. The major features are those of extracellular volume contraction, described above. Reduction of plasma sodium concentration by more than 10 to 15 meq per liter is rare in the absence of obvious decreases in skin turgor, postural or recumbent hypotension, and some degree of azotemia.

In *edematous states* such as congestive heart failure, cirrhosis, and the nephrotic syndrome, the severity and frequency of hyponatremia correlates to some extent with the magnitude of the edema and the seriousness of the underlying condition. Hyponatremia is usually present in patients with advanced disease unless water intake is restricted. The hyponatremia itself is often of little clinical significance. The principal features are those of the underlying disease. However, symptomatic hyponatremia may occur, most often in connection with vigorous diuretic therapy or excessive oral or parenteral intake of dilute fluids.

The diagnosis of *primary dilutional hyponatremia* is usually evident from the history. This diagnosis should be considered in postoperative patients and in patients with acute or chronic renal failure. Since extracellular fluid volume is expanded by water retention, blood pressure and skin turgor are normal. Plasma creatinine and urea are normal unless preexisting renal disease is present.

The *syndrome* of *chronic inappropriate secretion of antidiuretic hormone* (SIADH) is defined by a unique group of clinical features. (1) Urine osmolality is not maximally dilute even when marked hyponatremia is induced by water loading. In most cases, urine osmolality exceeds plasma osmolality. (The elaboration of hypertonic urine is presumptive evidence of ADH secretion if the glomerular filtration rate is normal.) (2) Plasma creatinine and urea are normal or low, indicating that the glomerular filtration rate is normal or increased. (3) During fluid loading, hyponatremia increases due to water retention and urinary sodium wasting. During restriction of fluid intake, hyponatremia and urinary sodium wasting are corrected. It should be noted that sodium wasting during volume expansion may be minimal or even absent in patients with extreme degrees of hyponatremia. In clinical testing to demonstrate these features, patients with symptomatic hyponatremia or plasma sodium concentrations below 125 meq per liter should first have their fluid intake restricted to 800 to 1000 ml per day or less. Infusion of small volumes of hypertonic saline may be appropriate in symptomatic patients. During restriction of fluid intake, hyponatremia should disappear promptly, and urinary sodium excretion should not exceed intake. Thereafter, plasma and urinary parameters should be evaluated during daily administration of 2 to 3 liters of fluids by mouth or intravenously. Urine osmolality will always exceed 100 mosmol per liter (urine specific gravity greater than 1.003); in the great majority of instances, it will exceed plasma osmolality, despite progressive dilution of body fluids. Urinary sodium excretion will usually exceed sodium intake during this phase of fluid loading. Two to three days of this regimen are ordinarily sufficient to demonstrate the requisite clinical pattern for SIADH without inducing symptomatic hyponatremia.

SIADH has been found frequently in patients with oat-cell carcinoma of the lung but has also been described in patients with a variety of other neoplasms. In some of these patients there is evidence that the tumor is secreting ADH or a substance with analogous biological activity (see also Chap. 334). The syndrome has also been reported in patients with disorders of the central nervous system, including meningitis and encephalitis. It is assumed that ADH in these patients is secreted in response to direct stimulation of the hypothalamic osmoreceptors. SIADH has also been noted in a number of apparently unrelated disorders such as acute porphyria and hypothyroidism. The stimulus to ADH in these patients is unknown.

An ever-increasing list of pharmacological agents has been reported to induce SIADH. The list includes: (1) the oral hypoglycemic agents, chlorpropamide and tolbutamide; (2) antineoplastic and immunosuppressive agents, vincristine and cyclophosphamide; (3) psychoactive drugs, carbamazepine (Tegretol) and amitriptyline (Elavil); and (4) clofibrate. These agents exert their antidiuretic effects either by potentiating the tubular action of small amounts of ADH or by stimulating inappropriate secretion of ADH. In addition, diuretics such as thiazides may induce a syndrome indistinguishable from SIADH, probably by a direct renal action to limit water excretion in patients ingesting moderate to large amounts of dilute fluids.

Since patients with *adrenal insufficiency* may have the combination of defective dilution of the urine and sodium wasting, hyponatremia due to Addison's disease can occasionally be confused with SIADH. Usually, other clinical features of adrenal insufficiency such as hyperkalemia, pigmentation, and hypoglycemia will suggest the correct diagnosis. However, specific tests of adrenal cortical function are indicated whenever the diagnosis is in doubt.

Essential hyponatremia (sick-cell syndrome) may occur in a variety of chronic illnesses, such as pulmonary tuberculosis, congestive heart failure, and hepatic cirrhosis. This type of hyponatremia is asymptomatic; skin turgor, blood pressure, and renal function are normal, unless altered by the primary disease. Definitive diagnosis of essential hyponatremia requires the demonstration of normal urinary dilution in response to water loading, normal urinary concentration during dehydration, and normal renal sodium excretory responses to sodium loading and restriction.

The diagnosis of hyponatremia due to *increased plasma concentrations of osmotically active solute* is usually apparent from the history and clinical features of uncontrolled diabetes. Plasma sodium concentration will decrease by about 1.6 meq per liter with every elevation of 100 mg per 100 ml in plasma glucose above normal. This type of hyponatremia should also be considered whenever there is a history of recent administration of mannitol, especially to oliguric patients unable to excrete it promptly. Since plasma osmolality is increased, clinical manifestations of hypotonicity are absent in this type of hyponatremia.

In patients with severe hyperlipemia or, very rarely, with extreme hyperproteinemia, hyponatremia which is clinically *artifactual* may be reported by the laboratory. In severe hyperlipemia part of any unit voume of plasma taken for analysis will be lipid, which is sodium-free. This type of hyponatremia is rarely reported unless the plasma is grossly milky. In patients with extreme hyperproteinemia, proteins occupy more than the normal 7 percent of plasma volume, thereby reducing the proportion of aqueous sodium-containing fluid per unit of plasma taken for analysis. In both cases, hyponatremia will be reported by the laboratory because the sodium concentration will be low in milliequivalents per liter of plasma. However,

sodium concentration per liter of plasma water and plasma osmolality are normal; hence, this type of hyponatremia has no clinical significance.

DIFFERENTIAL DIAGNOSIS   Although the type of hyponatremia can be defined without difficulty in many patients, differentiation among categories may be very difficult. More than one type of hyponatremia may occur in a specific disease entity. For example, hyponatremia in patients with hepatic cirrhosis is usually associated with edema or is due to excessive administration of diuretics, but essential hyponatremia may also occur in this condition. Moreover, current categories may prove artificial or inaccurate when the pathophysiology of hyponatremia is more completely understood and specific diagnostic tests such as a sensitive assay for ADH are readily available. Despite these limitations, the classification outlined above is a useful framework for diagnosis and treatment.

The history is often the most important factor in differential diagnosis. For example, prolonged vomiting, diarrhea, or nasogastric suction will suggest volume depletion. Primary dilutional hyponatremia or hypernatremia associated with sodium losses should be suspected in the postoperative period. Critical information to be derived from the physical examination includes the presence or absence of edema, signs of volume depletion, and evidence of disordered cerebral function. Initial laboratory studies of value include the plasma creatinine and urinary osmolality (specific gravity) and sodium concentration. The combination of high urine specific gravity (above 1.005), increased urinary sodium concentration, and normal or low plasma urea or creatinine in a hyponatremic patient without clinical evidence of volume depletion suggests the diagnosis of SIADH. A maximally dilute urine in a hyponatremic patient suggests psychogenic polydipsia or essential hyponatremia.

CLINICAL MANIFESTATIONS   Neurologic dysfunction is the principal clinical feature of hyponatremia. The severity of symptoms is related to the degree of hyponatremia and the rapidity with which it develops. Patients may be lethargic, confused, stuporous, or comatose. If hyponatremia develops rapidly, signs of hyperexcitability such as muscular twitches, irritability, and convulsions may occur. These are believed due to intracellular movement of water, leading to swelling of brain cells. Hyponatremia rarely causes clinical symptoms when plasma sodium is above 125 meq per liter, although symptoms may occur occasionally at higher levels if the decrease in concentration has been rapid.

Treatment   Hyponatremia itself is often of little clinical significance and requires no specific treatment. When hyponatremia is associated with volume depletion, treatment is directed to correction of the volume deficits. In the occasional patient with sodium depletion whose plasma sodium concentration is less than 125 meq per liter, some of the intravenous sodium replacement fluids should be administered as hypertonic saline. Hyponatremia associated with edema responds to effective treatment of the underlying disease. Moderate, nonprogressive hyponatremia in edematous patients usually does not cause symptoms. Attempts to correct such hyponatremia by restriction of fluid intake induce thirst and discomfort without improving the clinical picture or longevity. Patients with severe or progressive hyponatremia may require some restriction of water intake, especially during vigorous treatment with diuretics. However, moderate limitations to the range of 1000 to 1500 ml per day will often suffice to avoid symptoms or progressive hyponatremia. More severe restriction should be instituted only if specific clinical or laboratory observations warrant. Since edematous subjects have excess total extracellular sodium, hypertonic saline solution should not be administered, except in rare instances in which clinical manifestations of extreme hyponatremia, such as coma or convulsions, justify emergency measures. Dilutional hyponatremia is treated by water restriction. Only if severe symptoms occur is hypertonic saline infusion required. Hyponatremia due to SIADH responds to limitation of fluid intake; restriction to the range of 1000 to 1200 ml per day is ordinarily adequate. Occasional patients with marked hyponatremia due to this syndrome may be symptomatic and require initial therapy with hypertonic saline infusions.

When severe hyponatremia of any type is to be treated intravenously, 5% sodium chloride is the infusion of choice. The amount of sodium to be given should be calculated by multiplying the deficit in plasma sodium concentration (milliequivalents per liter) by total body water (approximately 50 to 60 percent of body weight). Although the administered sodium will remain in the extracellular compartment, the osmotic effect of the hypertonic saline will cause water to shift out of cells. The amount needed to raise plasma sodium concentration to the range of 125 to 130 meq per liter should be calculated and infused over several hours. The patient's symptoms and clinical status, especially with respect to circulatory congestion, should be carefully assessed throughout the infusion. Complete correction of hyponatremia, if clinically indicated, is usually best carried out more slowly, by water restriction or oral sodium supplementation if possible.

HYPERNATREMIA

Pathophysiology Hypernatremia is due to a deficit of body water relative to total body solute or sodium content. Without exception, hypernatremia indicates that the body fluids are hypertonic. Since hypertonicity normally stimulates thirst, severe persistent hypernatremia occurs only in patients who cannot respond to thirst by voluntary ingestion of fluid, e.g., infants or mentally obtunded patients. In such individuals, loss of dilute body fluids will progressively elevate body fluid osmolality. Initial losses of water are from the extracellular compartment, but water deficits are rapidly equilibrated throughout total body water. The rise in extracellular fluid tonicity causes intracellular water to shift into the extracellular compartment. In effect, approximately two-thirds of pure water deficits are derived from intracellular fluid. Hence, the clinical findings of extracellular volume depletion occur in patients with relatively pure deficits of water only when such deficits are large. The principal clinical features are attributable to decreased intracellular volume, especially dehydration of cells in the central nervous system. Brain cells appear to adapt to chronic hyperosmolality by accumulating increased intracellular solute. When hyperosmolality is rapidly corrected, the increase in total intracellular solute may promote brain swelling even at normal or slightly elevated plasma osmolality. These mechanisms may account for the clinical observation that rapid correction of hypertonicity sometimes causes deterioration of central nervous function. The identity of the excess brain solute is uncertain; experimental data suggest that electrolyte accumulation accounts only for part of the excess in chronic hypernatremia.

Minimal persistent hypernatremia may be seen in some patients with Cushing's disease and hyperaldosteronism. Presumably stimulation of renal tubular reabsorption by adrenal steroids initiates the hypernatremia. It is not known why the thirst mechanism fails to maintain normal body fluid osmolality.

Pathogenesis The principal causes of hypernatremia are listed in Table 84-1. The most frequent is unreplaced loss of hypotonic fluid from the skin and lungs. Insensible losses of water from these sources may reach several liters per day, especially in patients with fever or increased respirations. Since sweat is hypotonic fluid, hypernatremia will develop if sweating patients are unable to drink. Major losses of insensible water may occur in patients with extensive burns. Renal losses may lead to hypernatremia in two clinical circumstances, diabetes insipidus and solute diuresis. Alert patients with diabetes insipidus ordinarily maintain normal or only slightly hypertonic body fluids despite massive renal water wasting by increasing fluid intake appropriately. However, diabetes insipidus may develop acutely in patients who suffer cerebral trauma or undergo neurosurgical procedures. In such patients, careful attention to replacement of urinary losses is mandatory to avoid severe hypernatremia. In an osmotic diuresis, urinary sodium concentration is less than plasma concentration; therefore, hypernatremia tends to occur. Hypernatremia due to a urea diuresis may develop when patients unable to complain of thirst are placed on a high-protein tube feeding. Examples include patients with severe cerebrovascular accidents who are unable to swallow and postoperative neurosurgical patients. In the syndrome of hyperosmolar nonketotic diabetic coma, severe hyperosmolality of the body fluids is due to a combination of hyperglycemia and relative or absolute hypernatremia. The hypernatremia is a consequence of an intense glucose osmotic diuresis in patients who are unable to ingest fluids. Since hyperglycemia itself causes hyponatremia by inducing a shift of water from cells, the presence of hypernatremia in the face of extreme hyperglycemia indicates that total body water is severely depleted. Hypernatremia due to an osmotic diuresis is usually accompanied by significant extracellular volume depletion, since both sodium and water are lost.

In rare instances, hypernatremia may result from an absolute excess of sodium rather than from water depletion. Examples are hypernatremia caused by accidental substitution of salt for sugar in infant feeding formulas and administration of excessive amounts of hypertonic saline to comatose adults.

Clinical features and diagnosis The principal clinical manifestations of hypernatremia are observed in the central nervous system. Confusion, obtundation, stupor, or coma may develop, depending on the severity of the hyperosmolality. These symptoms appear to be due to dehydration of brain cells; the clinical features are similar whether hyperosmolality is due to hypernatremia or extreme hyperglycemia. In patients with pure water deficits, manifestations of extracellular volume depletion are minimal because only one-third of the deficit is derived from extracellular fluid. As already noted, combined deficits are common, especially in patients who are undergoing an osmotic diuresis; in such individuals, the signs and symptoms of volume depletion may overshadow those due to hypernatremia.

Treatment Water by mouth or intravenous administration of a dilute solution (5% dextrose or 0.45% saline) is the treatment of hypernatremia. Calculation of water requirements must be based on total body water, since water deficits are drawn from both intracellular and extracellular fluid and both must be repleted. Hypernatremia should be corrected slowly; no more than half the water deficit should be replaced in the first few hours. Excessively rapid correction of hypernatremia may cause clinical deterioration of central nervous function.

POTASSIUM

PHYSIOLOGIC CONSIDERATIONS Potassium is the principal intracellular cation. Active transport maintains a cellular concentration of approximately 160 meq per liter, 40 times that in extracellular fluid. All but 2 percent of the 2500 to 3000 meq potassium in the body is within cells. Since potassium is a large fraction of total cellular solute, it is a major determinant of the volume of the cell and the osmolality of the body fluids. Moreover, potassium is an important cofactor in a number of metabolic processes. Extracellular potassium, while a small fraction of the total, greatly influences neuromuscular function. The ratio of intracellular to extracellular potassium concentration is the principal determinant of membrane potential in excitable tissues. Since extracellular potassium concentration is low, small deviations in absolute concentration will produce large variations in this ratio; conversely, only large changes in intracellular potassium will influence the ratio significantly. These relationships have practical consequences. For example, toxic effects of hyperkalemia can be mitigated by inducing movement of potassium from extracellular fluid to cells.

The relation between plasma and cellular potassium is complex and influenced by a number of factors, prominent among them being acid-base balance. Acidosis tends to shift potassium out of cells, and alkalosis favors movement of potassium from extracellular fluid into cells. Thus, a patient with normal total body potassium will tend to be hyperkalemic if acidotic and hypokalemic if alkalotic. During potassium depletion, plasma potassium initially decreases about 1 meq per liter for each 100 to 200 meq lost. However, plasma potassium falls much more slowly after it reaches 2 meq per liter. Thus, a plasma potassium in the range of 2 to 3.5 meq per liter is a reasonably accurate guide to the magnitude of depletion, but plasma potassium concentrations less than 2 meq per liter may reflect a wide range of deficits, from moderate to very severe. Plasma concentration increases about 1 meq per liter after acute administration of 100 to 200 meq potassium. Assuming an extracellular volume of 15 liters, 150 meq would be expected to raise plasma potassium by about 10 meq per liter. Thus, it is evident that the largest fraction of administered potassium rapidly enters cells. Renal excretion also increases promptly. Chronic exposure to high potassium diets enhances both tissue uptake and renal excretion of the ion; the mechanism of these adaptations is uncertain. Sustained hyperkalemia rarely is caused by excess intake, because these mechanisms normally function so efficiently. Impaired renal excretion or cellular transfer are the usual causes of hyperkalemia.

Of the usual potassium intake of 50 to 150 meq per day, all but a few milliequivalents are excreted in the urine. Normally, stool and sweat contain only about 5 meq per day. As already noted, the kidneys respond to acute and chronic changes in potassium intake by corresponding changes in excretion. Excess potassium is excreted promptly; about half of an acute load appears in the urine within 12 h. The renal response to potassium depletion is more sluggish. Excretion does not fall to minimal levels for 7 to 14 days. During this period, a deficit of 200 meq or more may develop in an individual on a potassium-deficient diet. Renal excretory mechanisms for potassium are complex. Potassium in the urine is secreted in the distal convoluted tubule and collecting duct; filtered potassium is nearly quantitatively reabsorbed in more proximal segments. Potassium secretion appears to be determined by the potassium concentration of tubular cells and by an electrochemical gradient favoring diffusion of the ion into tubular fluid. Net excretion is the resultant of secretion and concurrent reabsorption in the distal segments. Among the key influences on this complex system are aldosterone, sodium reabsorption, and acid-base balance. Aldosterone stimulates potassium secretion. Thus, hyperkalemia increases potassium excretion by two mechanisms: it stimulates adrenal secretion of aldosterone, and it directly enhances renal secretion, presumably via increased tubular cell potassium. Sodium reabsorption in the distal tubule creates the electrical gradient which favors potassium secre-

tion. Hence, increased distal sodium reabsorption will favor potassium excretion. For example, administration of diuretics which bring more sodium distally will increase potassium excretion, especially in patients with edema and secondary aldosteronism. Conversely, a low sodium diet decreases potassium excretion even in patients with primary aldosteronism; distal secretion is limited and reabsorption of potassium in collecting ducts is stimulated. Alkalosis enhances and acidosis depresses renal potassium secretion, probably by inducing corresponding changes in cell potassium.

POTASSIUM DEPLETION AND HYPOKALEMIA **Pathogenesis**
The principal causes of potassium depletion are listed in Table 84-2. As noted earlier, renal excretion of potassium falls slowly in persons on potassium-deficient diets. During the 10 to 14 days before balance is achieved, significant deficits may occur. Thus, in contrast to sodium, moderate potassium depletion may result from *poor intake* alone. The most frequent cause of potassium deficiency is *gastrointestinal loss.* The potassium concentration of gastric fluid is approximately 5 to 10 meq per liter; significant deficits may result from direct losses of potassium in *vomitus.* The concomitant alkalosis maintains urinary potassium excretion at levels inappropriately high for the degree of potassium depletion. *Diarrhea* may also lead to large potassium deficits, since the potassium concentration of liquid stool is 40 to 60 meq per liter.

The most frequent *renal* cause of potassium depletion is probably administration of *diuretics* without adequate dietary potassium supplementation. All diuretics in common use except spironolactone, triamterene, and amiloride promote potassium excretion, especially in edematous patients with secondary aldosteronism. Potassium excretion is increased during an *osmotic diuresis.* In patients with diabetic ketoacidosis, potassium depletion due to glycosuria may be masked by the shift of potassium out of tissues caused by acidosis. Failure to recognize potassium depletion may lead to serious cardiotoxicity from sudden hypokalemia when the acidosis is corrected with insulin or alkali. A normal plasma potassium concentration in an acidotic patient strongly suggests potassium depletion.

Urinary potassium loss is often due to *excessive mineralocorticoid activity.* Hypokalemia is characteristic of *primary aldosteronism,* but may be minimal in patients with restricted sodium intake. *Secondary aldosteronism* causes renal potassium

TABLE 84-2
Causes of potassium depletion and hypokalemia

I Gastrointestinal
  A Deficient dietary intake
  B Gastrointestinal losses (vomiting, diarrhea, villous adenoma, fistulas, ureterosigmoidostomy)
II Renal
  A Diuretics
  B Osmotic diuresis (glycosuria)
  C Excessive mineralocorticoid effects
    1 Primary aldosteronism
    2 Secondary aldosteronism (including malignant hypertension, Bartter's syndrome, juxtaglomerular cell tumor)
    3 Licorice ingestion
    4 Glucocorticoid excess (Cushing's syndrome, exogenous steroids, ectopic ACTH production)
  D Renal tubular diseases
    1 Renal tubular acidosis
    2 Leukemia with lysozymuria
    3 Liddle's syndrome
III Hypokalemia due to shift into cells (no depletion)
  A Hypokalemic periodic paralysis
  B Insulin effect

wasting and hypokalemia in patients with malignant hypertension, Bartter's syndrome, and renin-secreting renal tumors. Bartter's syndrome is most frequent in children and adolescents. *Licorice* contains a compound with mineralocorticoid activity; patients who consume hugh amounts may become hypokalemic. Excessive levels of *glucocorticoids* stimulate secretion of renal potassium (and hydrogen), leading to hypokalemia and alkalosis in patients with *Cushing's syndrome* and those receiving *therapeutic steroids*.

Renal tubular potassium wasting is a feature of *renal tubular acidosis*. Some patients with monocytic or myelomonocytic *leukemia* have developed hypokalemia. Renal potassium wasting in these patients appears to correlate with lysozymuria, and it has been suggested that the enzyme may interfere with tubular function. In *Liddle's syndrome*, a rare familial disorder, renal potassium wasting is an intrinsic tubular abnormality.

Clinical features and diagnosis

The most prominent features of hypokalemia and potassium depletion are neuromuscular. Moderate degrees of depletion may be asymptomatic, especially if they develop slowly. Some patients, however, may complain of muscle weakness. With more severe or acute degrees of hypokalemia and potassium deficiency, marked and generalized weakness of skeletal muscles is prominent. Very severe or abrupt development of hypokalemia may lead to virtually total paralysis, including the respiratory muscles. Rhabdomyolysis may occur in patients with potassium depletion. On physical examination, in addition to decreased motor power, the patient may demonstrate decreased or absent tendon reflexes.

Abnormalities in the electrocardiogram are common in patients with hypokalemia and potassium depletion. The characteristic changes include flattening and inversion of the T wave, increased prominence of the U wave, and sagging of the ST segment. These alterations are not well correlated with the severity of the disturbance in potassium metabolism and cannot be relied on as indexes of the clinical significance of a potassium deficit. Although moderate potassium depletion rarely affects cardiac action, severe or rapid reduction in serum potassium may cause cardiac arrest. Potassium deficiency enhances the cardiac toxicity of digitalis preparations.

Renal tubular function is markedly impaired by potassium depletion. The most prominent abnormality is decreased concentrating ability, which may cause polyuria and polydipsia. Glomerular filtration rate is normal or only slightly reduced; moderate reductions may occur in occasional patients with chronic potassium depletion nephropathy. Renal regulation of potassium excretion remains normal. The urinalysis is benign: protein excretion is normal or minimally increased, and the urinary sediment is normal or demonstrates only a slight increase in hyaline or granular casts.

DIAGNOSIS The cause of hypokalemia and potassium depletion is usually evident from the history. However, patients whose potassium deficiency is caused by chronic abuse of laxatives or psychogenic, self-induced vomiting will rarely volunteer an accurate history. Patients with villous adenomas of the rectum sometimes report that their feces are formed; careful questioning will reveal the elimination of the characteristic mucous secretion of the tumor.

When the history is obscure, evaluation of urinary potassium excretion may be helpful in determining the origin of the potassium deficit. If gastrointestinal losses have occurred, urinary excretion will usually be less than 20 to 25 meq per liter. Although renal conservation of potassium is slow, excretion will have fallen to these levels by the time that clinically significant deficits of potassium have accumulated. On the other hand, when renal potassium wasting is the cause, urinary concentration will usually exceed 20 meq per liter. However, lower concentrations may be found in severely depleted patients, in those with excessive mineralocorticoid activity while on low sodium intake, and in patients where diuretics have been stopped at the time of examination.

Treatment When possible, potassium depletion should be corrected by increased dietary intake or supplementation with potassium salts. Potassium chloride is the salt of choice, especially in alkalotic patients. Enteric-coated potassium chloride tablets have been responsible for ulceration of the small bowel, due to release of high concentrations of potassium salts. Organic salts such as gluconate or citrate are adequate in patients who are not severely alkalotic.

Intravenous treatment is required for patients with gastrointestinal disorders or when the potassium deficiency is severe. It must be emphasized that the potassium *concentration* in commonly available intravenous solutions of potassium chloride is 2000 meq per liter. Concentrations in intravenous infusions should not exceed 40 or at the most 60 meq per liter. The rate of infusion should not exceed 20 meq/h or approximately 200 to 250 meq per day, unless the need for more rapid infusion has been demonstrated in the individual patient by evidence of continuing losses large enough to justify more intensive therapy. The results of treatment are best monitored by repeated determinations of plasma potassium and evaluation of clinical symptoms such as muscular weakness or paralysis. Disappearance of electrocardiographic abnormalities correlates only roughly with improvement in total body potassium content. However, during rapid intravenous administration of potassium, the electrocardiogram should be monitored to avoid cardiac toxicity from inadvertent hyperkalemia.

Hypokalemia and hypocalcemia may occur together, for example, in patients with malabsorption syndrome. The neuromuscular effect of each electrolyte abnormality is masked by the other. Treatment of either disorder alone may precipitate symptoms. Thus, treatment of hypokalemia alone may precipitate tetany, and conversely, treatment of hypocalcemia without correcting the hypokalemia may exacerbate the manifestations of potassium deficiency.

HYPERKALEMIA Pathogenesis The causes of hyperkalemia are shown in Table 84-3. *Inadequate renal excretion* is the most frequent cause. When oliguria or anuria is present, as in acute renal failure, progressive hyperkalemia is the rule. Plasma potassium will rise by about 0.5 meq per liter per day if there are no abnormal loads. Chronic renal failure does not cause severe

TABLE 84-3
Causes of hyperkalemia

I Inadequate excretion
  A Renal failure
    1 Acute renal failure
    2 Severe chronic renal failure (especially with marked acidosis or oliguria)
  B Adrenal insufficiency
    1 Hypoaldosteronism
    2 Addison's disease
  C Diuretics which inhibit potassium secretion (spironolactone, triamterene, amiloride)
II Shift of potassium from tissues
  A Tissue damage (muscle crush, hemolysis, internal bleeding)
  B Drugs: succinylcholine, digitalis poisoning
  C Acidosis
  D Hyperkalemic periodic paralysis
III Excessive intake
IV Pseudohyperkalemia
  A Thrombocytosis
  B Leukocytosis
  C Poor venipuncture technique
  D In vitro hemolysis

or progressive hyperkalemia unless oliguria supervenes. Adaptive changes of unknown etiology increase potassium excretion per residual nephron as chronic renal failure progresses. However, patients with chronic renal failure are functioning at the limits of their excretory capacity. Hence, hyperkalemia may develop rapidly if the potassium load is increased or excretory capacity is limited, e.g., by administration of spironolactone.

Hyperkalemia is a cardinal feature of *adrenal insufficiency* (Addison's disease) and of selective *hypoaldosteronism.* In the latter condition, cardiac toxicity (heart block) due to hyperkalemia is the principal clinical manifestation.

A kilogram of tissue such as muscle or erythrocytes contains about 80 meq potassium, and damaged cells release potassium into the plasma. Hence hyperkalemia may be seen when there is *muscle-crushing injury, hemolysis,* or *internal hemorrhage. Acidosis* drives potassium out of cells and leads to hyperkalemia. Severe progressive hyperkalemia is not ordinarily a consequence of increased release of potassium from damaged or acidotic tissues alone. However, acidosis and tissue damage often occur together with acute renal insufficiency; under these circumstances, severe hyperkalemia may develop quickly. In contrast to the increase of 0.5 meq per liter per day typical of uncomplicated anuria, plasma potassium in anuric patients with tissue damage may increase 2 to 4 meq per liter per day. Such rapidly progressive hyperkalemia may be an important cause of death in military casualties. In patients with trauma, burns, or neuromuscular diseases such as paraplegia and multiple sclerosis, the muscle relaxant *succinylcholine* may cause dangerous hyperkalemia. This agent apparently releases potassium from muscle by depolarizing cell membranes. In *hyperkalemic periodic paralysis,* the hyperkalemia is associated with repeated attacks of muscular paralysis. The mechanism of this syndrome is not understood. Ingestion of increased amounts of potassium may precipitate attacks.

Patients with extreme thrombocytosis or, more rarely, extreme leukocytosis in leukemia may demonstrate the phenomenon of pseudohyperkalemia. Platelets or white blood cells release potassium during blood clotting in vitro. While serum potassium may be grossly abnormal, plasma potassium is not increased. Artifactual elevation of plasma potassium may occur if blood is drawn after repeated fist clenching to make veins more prominent during application of a tourniquet. Artifactual hyperkalemia may be suspected when electrocardiographic abnormalities are absent despite apparently marked elevation of serum potassium.

Clinical features and diagnosis The most important toxic effects of hyperkalemia are cardiac arrhythmias. The characteristic sequence of electrocardiographic changes is shown in Fig. 84-1. The earliest manifestation is the development of high peaked T waves, especially prominent in precordial leads. Hyperkalemia does not prolong the QT interval, unlike other disorders which induce peaking of the T waves. Later changes include prolongation of the PR interval, complete heart block, and atrial asystole. As plasma potassium rises further, ventricular complexes may deteriorate. The QRS becomes progressively prolonged and finally tends to merge with the T wave in a sine wave configuration. Terminally, ventricular fibrillation and standstill may occur.

Occasionally moderate or severe hyperkalemia may have striking effects on peripheral muscles. Ascending muscular weakness can occur, progressing to flaccid quadriplegia and respiratory paralysis. Cerebral and cranial nerve function are normal, as is sensation.

Treatment In considering appropriate therapy, it is helpful to classify hyperkalemia according to degree of severity. The seriousness of hyperkalemia is best estimated by considering both the plasma potassium and the electrocardiogram. When the plasma potassium is less than 6.5 meq per liter and electrocardiographic changes are limited to peaking of T waves, hyper-

FIGURE 84-1

Electrocardiographic changes in hyperkalemia. A. Early toxicity in a patient with plasma potassium of 6.8 meq per liter. Note symmetrical peaking of T waves. B. Advanced toxicity in a patient with plasma potassium of 8.6 meq per liter. QRS complexes are abnormally widened, P waves have disappeared, and ventricular rhythm is irregular. (From NG Levinsky, Clinician, 1973.)

A

B

kalemia can be considered minimal. When the plasma potassium is 6.5 to 8 meq per liter and T-wave peaking is the only electrocardiographic abnormality, hyperkalemia may be considered moderate. Severe hyperkalemia is present if the plasma potassium exceeds 8 meq per liter or if electrocardiographic abnormalities include absent P waves, widened QRS complexes, or ventricular arrhythmias. Minimal hyperkalemia can usually be treated by elimination of a cause, such as potassium-sparing diuretics, or by treatment of accompanying acidosis. More severe or progressive hyperkalemia requires vigorous therapy. Severe cardiac toxicity responds most rapidly to infusion of calcium; 10 to 30 ml of 10% calcium gluconate may be infused intravenously within a period of 1 to 5 min under constant electrocardiographic monitoring. While calcium infusions do not alter plasma potassium, they counteract the adverse effects of potassium on neuromuscular membranes. The effect of calcium infusions, while almost immediate, is relatively transient if the hyperkalemia is not treated directly.

In moderately severe hyperkalemia, infusion of hypertonic glucose solutions will decrease toxicity by shifting potassium into cells. In the first 30 min, 200 to 500 ml of 10% glucose may be given. An additional 500 to 1000 ml may be infused over the next several hours. Ten units of regular insulin may be given subcutaneously, although this is probably necessary only in insulin-deficient diabetic patients. This treatment may reduce serum potassium by 1 to 2 meq per liter, and effects persist for a number of hours. The infusion of sodium bicarbonate will also help lower serum potassium rapidly by causing potassium to shift into cells; 44 to 132 meq alkali (two to three ampuls) may be added to a liter of glucose. Although this agent is most valuable in acidotic patients, it also is effective in individuals with normal acid-base status. The effect occurs within 1 h and persists for a number of hours thereafter. The infusion of hypertonic sodium solutions may also be effective in reversing cardiac toxicity, especially in hyponatremic or volume-depleted patients. In part the effect depends simply on dilution of plasma potassium, but there may be a direct effect of elevated plasma sodium to antagonize hyperkalemic neuromuscular toxicity as well. Glucose, bicarbonate, and sodium may be combined in a "therapeutic cocktail," formulated by adding an ampul or two of sodium bicarbonate to a liter of 5% dextrose in 0.9% saline.

None of the measures just described removes potassium from the body. Cation exchange resins such as sodium polystyrene sulfonate may be given by retention enema in the treatment of moderate or severe hyperkalemia. Enough potassium may be removed by a single enema to reduce potassium by 0.5 to 2 meq per liter within an hour, and repeated enemas can be given. These resins can also be given repeatedly by mouth to maintain low plasma potassium concentration. Twenty grams are given three or four times a day together with 20 ml of a 70% sorbitol solution, as required to ensure the passage of several loose stools daily. In patients with renal failure, hemodialysis and peritoneal dialysis will effectively control hyperkalemia. However, they are relatively slow techniques, and patients with severe hyperkalemia should be treated first with one of the methods previously discussed.

REFERENCES

Sodium and water

BARTTER FE, SCHWARTZ WB: The syndrome of inappropriate secretion of antidiuretic hormone. Am J Med 42:790, 1967

BERL T et al: Clinical disorders of water metabolism. Kidney Int 10:117, 1976

MILLER M, MOSES AM: Drug-induced states of impaired water excretion. Kidney Int 10:96, 1976

WEINER M, EPSTEIN FH: Signs and symptoms of electrolyte disorders. Yale J Biol Med 43:76, 1970

Potassium

LEVINSKY NG: Management of emergencies: VI. Hyperkalemia. N Engl J Med 274:1076, 1966

MICHELIS MF, MURDAUGH HV: Selective hypoaldosteronism. Am J Med 59:1, 1975

SCHWARTZ WB, RELMAN AS: Effects of electrolyte disorders on renal structure and function. N Engl J Med 276:283, 1967

SURAWICZ B: Relationship between the ECG and electrolytes. Am Heart J 73:814, 1967

WRIGHT FS: Sites and mechanisms of potassium transport along the renal tubule. Kidney Int 11:415, 1977

85
ACIDOSIS AND ALKALOSIS

NORMAN G. LEVINSKY

PHYSIOLOGIC CONSIDERATIONS Normal metabolism continuously produces acids. Despite the addition of some 20,000 mmol carbonic acid and 80 mmol of nonvolatile acids to body fluids daily, the free hydrogen ion concentration of these fluids is fixed within a narrow range. The pH of extracellular fluid is normally between 7.35 and 7.45 (hydrogen ion, 45 to 35 nmol per liter). The pH of intracellular fluids cannot be determined with precision, but most methods suggest a mean intracellular pH in the range of 6.9. It seems likely that hydrogen ion concentration varies among intracellular organelles and cytoplasm even within individual cells. Although the free hydrogen ion concentration of body fluids is exceedingly low, protons are so reactive that even minute changes in concentration significantly influence enzymatic reactions and physiologic processes. Immediate defense against untoward changes in pH is provided by body buffers which can take up or release protons instantaneously in response to changes in acidity of body fluids. Regulation of pH ultimately depends on the lungs and the kidneys.

The principal acid product of metabolism is carbon dioxide, equivalent to potential carbonic acid. The normal concentration of carbon dioxide in body fluids is fixed at 1.2 mmol per liter ($P_{CO_2} = 40$ mmHg) by the lungs; at this concentration, pulmonary excretion equals metabolic production. Although carbon dioxide reacts with water and body buffers during transport from cells to pulmonary alveoli, no net change in body fluid composition results, since the CO_2 excreted by the lungs is directly equivalent to the CO_2 produced by cells. When a nonvolatile acid is produced by metabolism, the protons are removed instantaneously from body fluids by reaction with buffers. In extracellular fluid, bicarbonate is converted to water and carbon dioxide, which is excreted by the lungs. Although this mechanism effectively minimizes changes in acidity, it destroys bicarbonate and uses up cell buffer capacity. The total buffer capacity of the body fluids is about 15 meq per kilogram of body weight. Thus, the normal rate of production of nonvolatile acids would be sufficient to deplete the body buffers completely in 10 to 20 days, were it not for the unique ability of the kidney to eliminate protons from the body by secretion into the urine, thereby regenerating bicarbonate and cell buffer capacity.

The principal source of nonvolatile acid appears to be metabolism of methionine and cystine in dietary proteins, which produces sulfuric acid. Additional sources include the incomplete combustion of carbohydrates and fats, which produces organic acids; the metabolism of nucleoproteins, which produces uric acid; and the metabolism of organic phosphorus compounds, which releases protons and inorganic phosphates. The diet does not normally contain significant amounts of pre-formed acids or alkalis, but significant amounts of potential acid (e.g., an excess of cationic acids, such as lysine) or alkali (e.g., citrate) may be present.

The principal functions of the kidney in acid-base metabolism can be viewed as retention of existing bicarbonate and generation of new bicarbonate to replace that used to buffer nonvolatile acids. Bicarbonate is reabsorbed in both proximal and distal segments by secretion of protons into tubular fluid. The bicarbonate concentration of extracellular fluid is, in effect, set by this process. If plasma bicarbonate rises so that filtered load exceeds renal reabsorptive capacity, bicarbonate will be excreted rapidly and normal plasma bicarbonate will be restored promptly. New bicarbonate is generated by secretion of protons onto urinary buffers. Normally, one-third is titrated onto phosphate, converting HPO_4^{2-} to $H_2PO_4^-$, the remainder onto ammonia. The amount of free acid which can be excreted in the urine is negligible, even at the minimum urine pH of 4.8. However, acidification of the urine is essential for titration of acid onto phosphate and ammonia. Changes in the pH of body fluids lead to regulatory responses by the kidney. Acidosis stimulates renal hydrogen ion secretion. Ammonia production increases, and more protons can be excreted as ammonium. In extreme acidosis, ammonia production may increase tenfold or more above the normal rate of 40 to 50 meq per day. The rate of bicarbonate reabsorption and hence plasma bicarbonate is determined, in part, by carbon dioxide concentration. Thus, hypercapnia stimulates renal bicarbonate reabsorption and elevates plasma bicarbonate, presumably because the increased concentration of carbonic acid in tubular cells enhances renal hydrogen ion secretion. Hypocapnia has the opposite effects.

The respiratory response to changes in blood pH is almost instantaneous. Acidosis stimulates and alkalosis depresses ventilation. The respiratory center in the medulla appears to respond to a pH intermediate between those of blood and cerebrospinal fluid.

EVALUATION OF ACID-BASE BALANCE In practice, classification of acid-base disorders is based on measurements of changes in the bicarbonate–carbonic acid system, the principal buffer of extracellular fluid. Because intracellular and extracellular buffers are functionally linked, measurement of the plasma bicarbonate system provides useful information about total body buffers. The relationship among the elements of the bicarbonate system is usually described in terms of the Henderson-Hasselbalch equation:

$$pH = pK + \log \frac{[HCO_3^-]}{[H_2CO_3]}$$

(The pK of carbonic acid is 6.1. $[H_2CO_3]$ is calculated as αP_{CO_2}; α, the solubility factor for carbon dioxide in body fluids, is 0.031 mmol per liter per mmHg P_{CO_2}. For a normal P_{CO_2} of 40 mmHg, $[H_2CO_3]$ is calculated to be $40 \times 0.031 = 1.2$ mmol per liter.)

Acidosis is defined as a physiologic disturbance which tends to add acid or remove alkali from body fluids, while *alkalosis* is any physiologic disturbance which tends to remove acid or add base. Since compensatory processes may minimize or prevent a change in the hydrogen ion concentration of the plasma, some authors prefer to use the terms *acidemia* and *alkalemia* to indicate those situations in which the pH of the plasma is measurably altered. *Respiratory* disorders are those in which the primary change is in the concentration of carbon dioxide (carbonic acid). As can be seen from the Henderson-Hasselbalch equation, a fall in carbon dioxide concentration will tend to cause alkalemia, while an increase in carbon dioxide con-

centration will cause acidemia. *Metabolic* disorders are those in which the primary disturbance is in the concentration of bicarbonate. Since bicarbonate appears in the numerator of the buffer salt/acid ratio in the Henderson-Hasselbalch equation, increased bicarbonate concentration causes alkalemia while a decrease in bicarbonate causes acidemia.

A major problem in the clinical assessment of acid-base disorders results from the compensatory responses of the lungs and the kidney. A primary change in carbon dioxide concentration induces a compensatory renal response which alters plasma bicarbonate in the same direction. Conversely, a primary alteration of plasma bicarbonate will induce compensatory changes in plasma carbon dioxide. Consider a patient with chronic respiratory insufficiency who has the following set of acid-base parameters: $P_{CO_2} = 70$ mmHg, $[HCO_3^-] = 33$ mmol per liter, pH = 7.30. The clinician needs to know whether the elevation of plasma bicarbonate is merely the appropriate renal response to the primary hypercapnia or a metabolic acid-base disorder is superimposed. No calculations or a priori reasoning will provide the answer to this key question. Such information can be derived only from in vivo observations in which the usual compensatory response to a given degree of chronic hypercapnia is determined.

Appropriate clinical and experimental observations in humans (and animals) have been made in all common primary acid-base disturbances. They are most readily visualized and used for analysis of clinical acid-base disorders by the "confidence band" technique, as shown in Fig. 85-1. Each band represents the mean ± 2 SD, that is, 95 percent of observations, for the compensatory response to each primary disturbance. In the example under discussion, inspection of the confidence band marked *chronic respiratory acidosis* indicates that 95 percent of individuals with chronic elevation of P_{CO_2} to 70 mmHg would have $[HCO_3^-]$ between 37 and 44 meq per liter, due to renal compensation. Thus, the $[HCO_3^-]$ of 33 meq per liter in

FIGURE 85-1

In vivo nomogram, showing bands for uncomplicated respiratory or metabolic acid-base disturbances. Each "confidence" band represents the mean ± 2 SD for the compensatory response of normal subjects or patients to a given primary disorder. (From Arbus.)

the example cannot be interpreted as solely the result of an appropriate compensatory response to chronic hypercapnia. A second acid-base disorder, presumably metabolic acidosis, must be superimposed. Obviously, the use of this figure is no panacea nor does it obviate the need for commonsense clinical evaluation of alternative possibilities. For example, if the patient under discussion had only recently developed hypercapnia, the $[HCO_3^-]$ of 33 meq per liter would be too high for a purely compensatory response to acute respiratory acidosis and would be interpreted as superimposed metabolic alkalosis. The difference between these two interpretations depends entirely on the clinical recognition of the chronicity of the primary respiratory disorder. The use of Fig. 85-1 in each type of acid-base disturbance is described in the appropriate section of this chapter.[1]

METABOLIC ACIDOSIS

PATHOPHYSIOLOGY Metabolic acidosis is caused by one of three mechanisms: (1) Increased production of nonvolatile acids; (2) decreased acid excretion by the kidney; (3) loss of alkali. In intracellular fluid excess protons replace potassium, which shifts out of cells, tending to elevate plasma levels. Extracellular bicarbonate is reduced by reaction with hydrogen ions or, in patients wasting alkali, by loss of bicarbonate in urine or stool. The decrease in pH stimulates respiration, and P_{CO_2} is lowered. Inspection of the confidence band for metabolic acidosis (Fig. 85-1) indicates that a decrease in P_{CO_2} of roughly 1 mmHg can be expected for each decrement of 1 mmol per liter in plasma bicarbonate. Complete respiratory compensation for primary metabolic acidosis does not occur. Respiratory compensation for acute acidosis tends to be somewhat greater than for chronic metabolic acidosis. The minimum level of P_{CO_2} which can be attained is approximately 10 mmHg; levels below 15 to 20 mmHg are rarely maintained in chronic metabolic acidosis. When kidney function is normal, net acid excretion increases promptly in response to metabolic acidosis. Most of the initial rise is due to increased titration of urinary phosphate as urine pH falls below 5.2. Over several days, ammonia production by the kidney increases and becomes quantitatively by far the most important mechanism for excreting excess protons. Net acid excretion may increase 5 to 10 times above normal, reaching a maximum of several hundred milliequivalents per day.

PATHOGENESIS The major causes of metabolic acidosis are shown in Table 85-1. Renal disease is the most common cause of *chronic* metabolic acidosis. In *chronic renal failure,* the principal defect is decreased ability to excrete ammonium, but some patients also waste bicarbonate, especially at plasma levels of 18 mmol per liter or above. Acidification of the urine and formation of titratable acidity are usually normal. Plasma bicarbonate tends to fall progressively as renal insufficiency becomes increasingly severe, but plasma bicarbonate usually stabilizes at levels of 12 to 18 mmol per liter; it rarely falls below 10 mmol per liter, even in advanced uremia. The mechanisms of stabilization are thought to be (1) stimulation of acid excretion by advancing acidosis, which occurs to some extent even in the diseased kidney, and (2) buffering of the daily metabolic acid load by carbonate and phosphate in bone. Chronic metabolic acidosis is the hallmark of tubular dysfunction in *renal tubular acidosis,* which may be a primary renal disease, part of

---

[1] *Although the confidence band method does not permit automatic identification of simple or complicated acid-base disorders, it is much preferable to other techniques such as "buffer base" or "base excess-deficit" for reasons discussed in detail by Schwartz and Relman. These terms are not used in this chapter.*

TABLE 85-1
Causes of metabolic acidosis

I Renal disease
  A Chronic renal failure
  B Renal tubular acidosis
  C Acute renal failure
II Increased acid production
  A Ketoacidosis
    1 Diabetic acidosis
    2 Associated with alcoholism
    3 Starvation ketosis
  B Lactic acidosis
    1 Secondary to circulatory or respiratory failure
    2 Associated with various disorders
    3 Drugs and toxins
    4 Hereditary forms
  C Poisoning and drug toxicity
    1 High anion gap: salicylates, methanol, ethylene glycol
    2 Normal anion gap: ammonium chloride, lysine and arginine hydrochloride
III Loss of alkali
  A Diarrhea
  B Ureterostomy
  C Carbonic anhydrase inhibitors

---

the Fanconi syndrome, or associated with a number of nonrenal primary disorders (see Chap. 89). In *acute renal failure,* plasma bicarbonate usually decreases by no more than 1 to 2 mmol per liter per day; greater rates of fall suggest the presence of some cause of increased acid production, such as damaged tissue or sepsis.

The most common cause of *acute* metabolic acidosis is increased production of nonvolatile acids. In *diabetic ketoacidosis,* acetoacetic and β-hydroxybutyric acids are produced more rapidly than they can be metabolized. Severe ketoacidosis may occur in *association* with *acute* and *chronic alcoholism.* Typically patients have given a history of prolonged abstention from food, protracted vomiting, and appreciable alcohol intake just before development of the ketoacidosis. β-Hydroxybutyrate, acetoacetate, and lactate accumulate in the plasma. The ketosis may be overlooked because the ratio of β-hydroxybutyrate to acetoacetate tends to be unusually high; the nitroprusside test used for clinical detection of plasma ketones responds only to the latter. Blood sugar is usually normal or mildly elevated in these patients. The mechanism of the syndrome is uncertain. *Starvation* may cause mild ketoacidosis because of increased fat metabolism.

Several types of *lactic acidosis* have been recognized. The most common is *secondary* to severe acute circulatory or respiratory failure, with poor tissue perfusion or arterial oxygen desaturation. The clinical features of shock are usually present. In these patients, lactic acidosis probably is due both to increased production of lactate by hypoxic tissues and to decreased utilization by the liver. Lactic acidosis may also be *associated* with *various disorders* such as acute hepatic necrosis, leukemia, and infections. The biguanide oral hypoglycemic agents, such as phenformin, have been the drugs most often responsible for *drug-induced* lactic acidosis; they recently were removed from general use. Certain sugars used for parenteral alimentation, such as fructose, may cause lactic acidosis. Increased lactic acid production contributes to acidosis in *poisoning* by methanol and salicylates. In infants and children, a variety of congenital defects in enzymes of carbohydrate metabolism have been identified as causes of lactic acidosis. Primary lactic acidosis in patients without an underlying disease has been reported but the existence of such a spontaneous disorder is uncertain. This disorder is discussed in greater detail in Chap. 339.

Poisoning and drug toxicity are causes of acute metabolic acidosis. Among the more common agents are salicylates, ethylene glycol, and methyl alcohol. Each of these intoxicants appears to create a metabolic block, which leads to production of a mixture of endogenous organic acids. The quantities of acid formed far exceed the amount which can be attributed to acidic properties of the drugs or their metabolites. Salicylates have the additional effect of stimulating the respiratory center directly. Respiratory alkalosis is the earliest derangement in salicylate intoxication and may be the only acid-base disorder in some patients. Several medications may induce hyperchloremic acidosis; these include ammonium chloride, lysine and arginine hydrochloride, and carbonic anhydrase inhibitors (see below).

Loss of *alkali* may be the cause of acute or chronic metabolic acidosis. Severe *diarrhea* or intestinal malabsorption usually causes mild to moderate acidosis due to the loss of bicarbonate in liquid stool, in which concentrations of 40 to 60 mmol per liter may be present. Ureterosigmoidostomy, i.e., transplantation of the ureters into the sigmoid colon, leads to metabolic acidosis both because of exchange of chloride for bicarbonate by intestinal epithelium and because renal disease (obstructive uropathy and pyelonephritis) often develops. Acidosis has virtually been eliminated as a problem by the more modern technique for urinary diversion, in which a bladder is formed from a small isolated loop of ileum. Carbonic anhydrase inhibitors, such as acetazolamide, cause mild to moderate acidosis by increasing bicarbonate loss in the urine.

CLINICAL FEATURES AND DIAGNOSIS There are few specific symptoms or signs of metabolic acidosis; diagnosis depends on recognition of the clinical setting and appropriate laboratory studies. In acute metabolic acidosis, hyperventilation is usually evident and may be extremely intense (Kussmaul respiration). However, it is ordinarily impossible to detect increased respiration by physical examination in patients with chronic metabolic acidosis, despite substantial reduction of P_{CO_2}. Acute, severe acidosis produces a variety of nonspecific symptoms ranging from fatigue through confusion, stupor, and coma; vascular collapse and shock may occur. Chronic metabolic acidosis may produce no symptoms or may be associated with fatigue and anorexia, although it is usually difficult to determine whether these symptoms reflect the acidosis per se or are related to the underlying disease.

The characteristic laboratory features are reduction of plasma bicarbonate and blood pH, together with a compensatory reduction in P_{CO_2} (see Fig. 85-1). Hyperkalemia is often present. In those instances in which the cause of metabolic acidosis is not evident from the history or clinical setting, calculation of unmeasured anions (anion gap) may help in differential diagnosis. Unmeasured anions are calculated by subtracting the sum of plasma bicarbonate and chloride from plasma sodium concentration; the normal value is 4 to 12 mmol per liter. In those instances in which acidosis is due to loss of bicarbonate or to administration of acid with chloride, the anion gap will be normal (hyperchloremic acidosis). This category includes diarrhea, loss of upper intestinal fluid, ureterosigmoidostomy, renal tubular acidosis, and administration of ammonium chloride, lysine, or arginine chloride and acetazolamide. When production of nonvolatile acids is increased or renal failure is present, the anions associated with metabolic acids will accumulate in plasma. An increase in unmeasured anions is typical of renal failure, diabetic and alcoholic ketoacidosis, lactic acidosis, and poisoning by salicylates, ethylene glycol, and methyl alcohol.

TREATMENT The treatment of metabolic acidosis depends on its cause and severity. In *chronic renal failure,* mild or moderate metabolic acidosis does not require treatment. When plasma bicarbonate falls below 15 mmol per liter, it is reasonable to treat patients with oral alkali, such as sodium bicarbonate or sodium citrate. The dose is gradually increased until plasma bicarbonate concentration rises to about 18 to 20 mmol per liter. Some patients appear to benefit symptomatically

from elevation of bicarbonate to this level, and fatigue, anorexia, and malaise tend to be alleviated. Caution must be exerted to avoid excessively rapid alkalination of the plasma, which may precipitate tetany; excess sodium given with alkali may aggravate hypertension or edema. Acidosis should be corrected as completely as possible in patients with *renal tubular acidosis;* this will avoid hypercalciuria, osteomalacia, nephrocalcinosis, and lithiasis. Patients with *acute renal failure* do not ordinarily require specific therapy for acidosis. Dialysis instituted for management of the renal failure should maintain an adequate plasma bicarbonate.

Diabetic *ketoacidosis* responds to insulin, and most patients do not require treatment with alkali. However, when acidosis is extreme (pH less than 7.1 or [HCO_3^-] less than 6 to 8 meq per liter), intravenous bicarbonate therapy is justified. The ketoacidosis associated with alcoholism responds rapidly to infusions of glucose and saline. Insulin is not required, nor should alkali be given unless acidosis is extreme. The ketoacidosis of starvation is mild and requires no specific treatment.

Lactic acidosis secondary to acute circulatory or respiratory failure is corrected if treatment of the underlying disorder is successful. Since this type of lactic acidosis is usually associated with severe acute circulatory or respiratory failure, the mortality rate is high. Lactic acidosis occurring in other disorders is usually resistant to treatment. Rapid administration of several hundred milliequivalents of alkali may raise plasma bicarbonate in some patients, but in others net production of lactic acid may be so rapid that correction of acidosis is difficult. Since vigorous administration of alkali may lead to circulatory overloading, dialysis may be a useful therapeutic measure. Despite rapid administration of alkali, the mortality rate in these patients is high.

The acidosis associated with *diarrhea* or loss of alkaline upper intestinal secretions is usually associated with other electrolyte abnormalities, including volume depletion and potassium deficiency. Treatment with intravenous infusions appropriate for all these abnormalities may be required.

Some general points about therapy with alkali are worth emphasis. Oral treatment with sodium bicarbonate should usually begin with 1 g three times daily and be increased to maintain the desired plasma bicarbonate level. Some patients find that sodium bicarbonate leads to upper gastrointestinal discomfort; a 10% sodium citrate solution may be more palatable. In treatment of acute metabolic acidosis by intravenous administration of alkali, sodium bicarbonate is the agent of choice. The concentration of bicarbonate to be given depends upon the severity of the acidosis and any associated disorders of serum sodium concentration. Typically, concentrations of bicarbonate between 44 and 132 meq per liter are achieved by adding one to three ampuls of sodium bicarbonate to a liter of dextrose in water. The concentration of bicarbonate in these ampuls is 880 meq per liter (44 meq in 50 ml); they should never be given undiluted in the treatment of acidosis, since rapid infusion may induce serious or even fatal cardiac arrhythmias, especially if given as a bolus through a central venous catheter. The total amount of alkali needed to raise plasma bicarbonate can be estimated from the effects of administration of acid loads. In experiments, approximately equal amounts of acid appear to be buffered by extracellular bicarbonate and by intracellular buffers. (In extremely severe acidosis, a greater fraction of the acid load may be buffered within cells.) Therefore, it is appropriate to calculate the amount of alkali needed by assuming that approximately half will accept protons from intracellular buffers and be destroyed; the other half will elevate plasma bicarbonate concentration. Thus, the calculation would be: millimoles of bicarbonate required equals desired increment in plasma concentration (millimoles per liter) times 40 percent of body weight. The 40 percent figure represents twice the extracellular volume. It is rarely desirable to infuse enough alkali to elevate plasma bicarbonate to normal. Possible untoward effects include hypokalemic cardiac toxicity in patients who are substantially potassium-depleted; tetany in patients with renal failure or hypocalcemia; and congestive failure due to excess sodium. Moreover, alkalosis may supervene. Cerebrospinal fluid bicarbonate does not equilibrate rapidly with plasma. Hence the respiratory center, which responds to acidity both of blood and cerebrospinal fluid, maintains some degree of hyperventilation as plasma bicarbonate is increasing. This type of respiratory alkalosis may sometimes persist for several days after correction of metabolic acidosis. In acute acidosis due to overproduction of metabolic acids, successful treatment of the primary disorder will cause rapid metabolic conversion of lactate and ketone bodies to bicarbonate. Thus, excessive administration of bicarbonate early in therapy also may lead to metabolic alkalosis at a later stage of treatment, when endogenous bicarbonate has been reconstituted by improvement in metabolism.

METABOLIC ALKALOSIS

PATHOPHYSIOLOGY Metabolic alkalosis is usually initiated by increased loss of acid from the stomach or the kidney. However, excretion of bicarbonate at high plasma concentrations is normally so rapid that alkalosis will not be sustained unless bicarbonate reabsorption is enhanced or alkali is continuously generated at a great rate. Clinically, maintenance of metabolic alkalosis is most often due to stimulation of bicarbonate reabsorption by a volume (chloride) deficit. During volume depletion, renal conservation of sodium chloride takes precedence over other homeostatic mechanisms, such as correction of alkalosis. Since in alkalosis a large fraction of plasma sodium is paired with bicarbonate, complete reabsorption of filtered sodium requires reabsorption of bicarbonate as well. Alkalosis is sustained until volume depletion is corrected by administration of sodium chloride. This diminishes tubular avidity for sodium and provides chloride as an alternative anion for reabsorption with sodium; excess bicarbonate can then be excreted with sodium.

The mechanism of metabolic alkalosis in patients with excess mineralocorticoid activity is not fully clarified. Mineralocorticoids stimulate renal hydrogen ion secretion; presumably, elevation of plasma bicarbonate is initiated by increased urinary loss of protons as ammonium and titratable acidity. Stimulation of tubular acid secretion also enhances bicarbonate reabsorption, thereby sustaining the metabolic alkalosis. Patients with excess mineralocorticoid activity are not volume- or chloride-deficient. Hence, this type of metabolic alkalosis does not respond to sodium chloride administration.

The mechanism of alkalosis associated with severe potassium depletion is incompletely understood. To some extent extracellular alkalosis may be initiated by a shift of hydrogen ions into cells as potassium is lost. Renal proton secretion is stimulated by potassium depletion. The older concept that hydrogen and potassium compete for secretion on a transport carrier in the distal nephron has been discarded. Nevertheless, part of the sodium reabsorbed distally does exchange for hydrogen or potassium, although the linkage is now understood to be indirect, in that sodium reabsorption creates a favorable electrical gradient for countermovement of cellular cation into the urine. In potassium depletion cellular potassium concentration falls, and hydrogen ion concentration appears to increase. It seems likely that this change in the intracellular ratio of the two ions in renal epithelial cells promotes hydrogen ion secretion and maintains a high renal threshold for bicarbonate.

Respiratory compensation for metabolic alkalosis is limited. Alveolar ventilation decreases, and P_{CO_2} is elevated. However, since this response is limited by hypoxia, P_{CO_2} rarely rises above 50 to 55 mmHg.

PATHOGENESIS The causes of metabolic alkalosis are outlined in Table 85-2. *Vomiting* and *gastric drainage* usually induce only minimal or moderate alkalosis, but occasional patients, especially those with increased gastric acid secretion, e.g., with acid-peptic disease or the Zollinger-Ellison syndrome, may develop very severe alkalosis.

Alkalosis may be present in patients treated with any *diuretic* except those which specifically inhibit bicarbonate reabsorption, such as acetazolamide, or those which inhibit distal cation secretion, such as spironolactone and triamterene. Alkalosis due to oral treatment with diuretics is usually mild. Acute administration of very potent intravenous diuretics such as ethacrynic acid to patients on low-sodium diets may induce more severe alkalosis due to rapid loss of sodium chloride in the urine. Sudden contraction of extracellular volume elevates plasma bicarbonate; renal excretion of excess bicarbonate is prevented by the mechanism discussed above.

Patients with chronic hypercapnia due to respiratory insufficiency maintain high plasma bicarbonate concentrations (see "Respiratory Acidosis" below). If respiration improves, P_{CO_2} will fall promptly. However, urinary excretion of excess bicarbonate previously generated by renal compensatory mechanisms will take a number of days. In patients on low-salt diets or diuretics who have a volume (chloride) deficiency, *posthypercapnic* alkalosis of this type may persist indefinitely unless sodium or potassium chloride is added to the diet. The mechanism in this condition is the same as that which causes persistent alkalosis in vomiting, described earlier.

Alkalosis is variable in patients with excess mineralocorticoid activity. Minimal or moderate alkalosis is usually present in patients with *Cushing's syndrome* or *primary aldosteronism*. More marked alkalosis may be seen in patients with extreme adrenal hyperfunction associated with ACTH-secreting tumors, such as bronchogenic carcinoma. Moderate alkalosis is typical of patients with *Bartter's syndrome*.

Although alkalosis and *potassium depletion* are often associated, mild or moderate potassium depletion is rarely the sole cause of sustained metabolic alkalosis. However, extreme degrees of potassium depletion (serum potassium usually 2 meq per liter or less) may cause metabolic alkalosis. This type of alkalosis is not corrected by administration of sodium chloride but does respond to administration of potassium.

For reasons noted earlier, alkalosis due to administration of alkali cannot be sustained unless large amounts are given. When renal function is compromised, alkalosis may be sustained by small exogenous loads. This is apparently the mechanism of alkalosis in the milk-alkali syndrome, in which hyper-

TABLE 85-2
Causes of metabolic alkalosis

I Associated with volume (chloride) depletion
  A Vomiting or gastric drainage
  B Diuretic therapy
  C Posthypercapneic alkalosis
II Associated with hyperadrenocorticism
  A Cushing's syndrome
  B Primary aldosteronism
  C Bartter's syndrome
III Severe potassium depletion
IV Excessive alkali intake
  A Acute
  B Milk-alkali syndrome

calcemic nephropathy and alkalosis develop in response to excessive intake of absorbable alkali. The nephropathy limits bicarbonate excretion, thus maintaining the alkalosis.

CLINICAL FEATURES AND DIAGNOSIS There are no specific clinical signs or symptoms. Severe alkalosis may cause apathy, confusion, and stupor. If serum calcium is borderline or low, rapid development of alkalosis may lead to tetany. The diagnosis of metabolic alkalosis depends on recognition of the clinical setting and appropriate laboratory studies. Plasma bicarbonate is increased, and elevation of P_{CO_2} is insufficient to prevent alkalemia (see Fig. 85-1). Plasma potassium concentration is often reduced, and the electrocardiogram may reveal changes in T and U waves typical of hypokalemia; it is uncertain whether these changes are due to alkalosis itself or to associated alterations in potassium metabolism. Despite elevation of plasma bicarbonate, the urine pH is usually less than 7 in patients with sustained metabolic alkalosis. This "paradoxical aciduria" reflects the fact that bicarbonate reabsorption must be increased if metabolic alkalosis is to be sustained.

TREATMENT Mild or moderate metabolic alkalosis rarely requires specific treatment. In patients with gastric alkalosis, infusion of saline solutions is usually sufficient to enhance renal bicarbonate excretion and to correct alkalosis by mechanisms discussed above. Administration of potassium chloride is also helpful in treating or preventing alkalosis in these patients and in treating those with diuretic-induced alkalosis. In patients with adrenal hyperfunction, alkalosis is corrected by specific treatment of the underlying disease. In Bartter's syndrome hypokalemia and potassium wasting may be partly corrected by treatment with prostaglandin synthetase inhibitors such as indomethacin. Whenever alkalosis and potassium depletion occur together, potassium depletion should be treated with potassium chloride, not with an organic salt of potassium.

Rarely, prolonged gastric losses in patients with metabolic alkalosis may be severe enough to require intravenous therapy with acidifying agents. Ammonium chloride or arginine hydrochloride may be given slowly under such circumstances. In most patients the use of potentially toxic acidifying agents can be avoided by appropriate treatment with saline and potassium chloride.

RESPIRATORY ACIDOSIS

PATHOPHYSIOLOGY Failure of ventilation promptly increases P_{CO_2} (carbonic acid) because metabolic production of carbon dioxide is so rapid. Acute respiratory acidosis is modulated to a limited degree by tissue buffers. As can be seen from the curve labeled *acute respiratory acidosis* in Fig. 85-1, immediate tissue buffering is insufficient to elevate plasma bicarbonate more than a few milliequivalents per liter. If hypercapnia is sustained, renal acid excretion is enhanced, and bicarbonate reabsorption stimulated. Over a period of several days, plasma bicarbonate rises approximately 3 meq per liter for each increase of 10 mmHg in P_{CO_2}, thereby minimizing the degree of acidemia. The increment in plasma bicarbonate attributable to renal activity is represented by the difference between the curves marked *chronic respiratory acidosis* and *acute respiratory acidosis*.

PATHOGENESIS *Acute* respiratory acidosis occurs whenever there is a sudden failure of ventilation. Common causes include depression of the respiratory center by cerebral disease or drugs, neuromuscular disorders, and cardiopulmonary arrest. *Chronic* respiratory acidosis occurs in pulmonary diseases such as chronic emphysema and bronchitis, in which ventilation and perfusion are mismatched and effective alveolar ventilation is decreased. Chronic hypercapnia may also result

from primary alveolar hypoventilation or from alveolar hypoventilation related to extreme obesity (Pickwickian syndrome). Acute and chronic diseases characterized principally by interference with alveolar gas exchange, such as chronic pulmonary fibrosis, pneumonia, and pulmonary edema, usually cause hypocapnia rather than hypercapnia. In these conditions, hypoxia stimulates increased ventilation; since carbon dioxide is much more diffusible than oxygen, excretion of carbon dioxide is enhanced despite the barrier to gas exchange. Hypercapnia occurs only with respiratory fatigue or extremely severe disease.

CLINICAL FEATURES AND DIAGNOSIS It is often difficult to separate the manifestations of respiratory acidosis from those of associated hypoxia. Moderate hypercapnia, especially if it develops slowly, probably has no specific clinical features. When P_{CO_2} exceeds 70 mmHg, patients progressively become confused and obtunded. Asterixis may be noted. Papilledema may occur, apparently because intracranial pressure is increased by the cerebral vasodilation characteristic of hypercapnia. Dilatation of conjunctival and superficial facial blood vessels may be noted.

The diagnosis of acute respiratory acidosis is usually evident from the clinical situation, especially if respiration is obviously depressed. Proof requires laboratory confirmation that P_{CO_2} is elevated. Acidemia is always present in patients with acute hypercapnia. Acidosis in acute cardiopulmonary arrest is usually a combination of a metabolic lactic acidosis and acute respiratory acidosis. Patients with chronic hypercapnia are usually acidemic. However, some individuals with minimal or moderate chronic hypercapnia may have normal or even slightly elevated plasma pH, as may be seen from Fig. 85-1. The mechanism of full compensation or of "overcompensation" in such individuals is unknown. However, significant elevation of pH in patients with chronic hypercapnia is almost always due to complicating metabolic alkalosis. Diuretics, low-sodium diets, and posthypercapneic alkalosis are frequent causes of this type of superimposed acid-base disorder.

Because of the differences between plasma bicarbonate in acute hypercapnia and in chronic hypercapnia, proper interpretation of acid-base parameters in respiratory acidosis depends on clinical information. This is discussed in an earlier section of this chapter.

TREATMENT The only worthwhile approach to treatment of respiratory acidosis is correction of the underlying disorder. Rapid infusion of alkali is justified in cardiopulmonary arrest. In other circumstances, attempted treatment of respiratory acidosis with infusions of alkali or with buffers such as THAM is of transient benefit and has no role in practical management.

RESPIRATORY ALKALOSIS

PATHOPHYSIOLOGY Acute reduction in carbon dioxide concentration releases hydrogen ion from tissue buffers, which minimize alkalemia by reducing plasma bicarbonate. Acute alkalosis also enhances glycolysis; increased production of lactic and pyruvic acids lowers serum bicarbonate and raises plasma concentrations of the corresponding anions by a millimole or two. Reduction in P_{CO_2} through its effect on plasma bicarbonate concentration decreases renal bicarbonate reabsorption. In chronic hypocapnia, serum bicarbonate is maintained at a reduced level because of decreased renal reabsorption.

TABLE 85-3
Causes of respiratory alkalosis

I Acute
  A Hyperventilation due to anxiety
  B Fever
  C Exercise
  D Acute hypoxia (e.g., pneumonia, acute pulmonary edema, asthma)
  E Salicylate intoxication
  F Excessive mechanical ventilation
  G Bacteremia, especially gram-negative
II Chronic
  A Cerebral disease (tumor, encephalitis, etc.)
  B Chronic hepatic insufficiency
  C Pregnancy
  D Chronic hypoxia (lung disease, cyanotic heart disease, adaptation to high altitudes)

PATHOGENESIS The causes of respiratory alkalosis are shown in Table 85-3.

CLINICAL FEATURES AND DIAGNOSIS Depending on its severity and acuteness, hyperventilation may or may not be clinically apparent. In acute respiratory alkalosis, the clinical picture is rather characteristic: patients complain of paresthesias, numbness, and tingling; of light-headedness; and, if alkalosis is sufficiently severe, of manifestations of tetany. Alkalosis directly enhances neuromuscular excitability; this effect, rather than the modest decrease in ionized plasma calcium induced by alkalosis, is probably the major cause of tetany. Severe respiratory alkalosis may cause confusion or loss of consciousness, perhaps due to cerebral vasospasm induced by hypocapnia.

The diagnosis may be suspected from the clinical setting but must be confirmed by analysis of the plasma bicarbonate system. Hypocapnia together with a variable degree of alkalemia is found; plasma bicarbonate is decreased but is rarely below 15 mmol per liter.

TREATMENT The only successful treatment for respiratory alkalosis is elimination of the underlying disorder. In the acute hyperventilation syndrome, sedation, reassurance, and if symptoms are sufficiently severe, rebreathing into a bag will usually terminate the attack.

REFERENCES

ARBUS GS: An in vivo acid-base nomogram for clinical use. Can Med Assoc J 109:291, 1973

BRACKETT NC JR et al: Acid-base response to chronic hypercapnia in man. N Engl J Med 280:124, 1969

COHEN RD, WOODS HF: *Clinical and Biochemical Aspects of Lactic Acidosis.* Oxford, Blackwell Scientific Publications, 1976

EMMETT M, NARINS RG: Clinical use of the anion gap. Medicine 56:38, 1977

LEVY LH et al: Ketoacidosis associated with alcoholism in non-diabetic subjects. Ann Intern Med 78:213, 1973

RELMAN AS: Renal acidosis and renal excretion of acid in health and disease. Adv Intern Med 12:295, 1964

SCHWARTZ WB, RELMAN AS: A critique of the parameters used in the evaluation of acid-base disorders. N Engl J Med 268:1382, 1963

SELDIN DW, RECTOR FC: The generation and maintenance of metabolic alkalosis. Kidney Int 1:306, 1972

86
INTERMEDIARY METABOLISM OF CARBOHYDRATES, LIPIDS, AND PROTEINS

DANIEL W. FOSTER
J. DENIS McGARRY

Fuel metabolism in the human is a complicated and finely regulated process. In this chapter the general principles of the intermediary metabolism of carbohydrates, lipids, and proteins will be briefly reviewed. Emphasis will be placed on the physiology of substrate flow under the influence of the endocrine system rather than on the molecular biochemistry of the various pathways.

It is helpful to consider intermediary metabolism in two phases—*anabolic* and *catabolic*. While each phase will be discussed in some detail, a preliminary overview may be useful. Under ordinary circumstances energy needs of the body are met by exogenous substrate derived from ingested food. In simple terms, oxidation of the constituent molecules of absorbed foodstuffs to carbon dioxide and water is accompanied by the generation of adenosine triphosphate (ATP), the principal high-energy compound of the body (Fig. 86-1). In one sense biological life can be defined as the continued ability to generate ATP (and related high-energy nucleotides) for the preservation of cellular integrity in all its manifestations.

When caloric intake is greater than immediate oxidative needs, as would be the case after the usual meal, excess substrate is stored as fat, structural protein, and glycogen. This stored substrate is readily mobilized for use by the various tissues of the body during fasting or caloric restriction (Fig. 86-2). From conception to adult life net substrate flux is in the anabolic direction (caloric balance is positive) to allow body growth. At maturity anabolic and catabolic cycles ideally balance such that weight is maintained constant. Deviation in a positive direction results in obesity, while prolonged fasting or semistarvation leads to unidirectional flow over the catabolic pathway and weight loss.

Anabolic and catabolic phases of metabolism are hormonally determined, and transition from one to the other is smoothly integrated. Insulin is the primary hormone mediating the anabolic phase, while a rise in plasma glucagon, coupled with a fall in insulin, initiates catabolism. Epinephrine, cortisol, and growth hormone likewise rise during the catabolic phase and doubtless contribute to the metabolic pattern. A summary of the feeding-fasting cycle is given in Table 86-1.

ANABOLIC PHASE

When food is ingested the absorptive process begins through the action of intraluminal and brush border enzymes in the intestine which break down complex carbohydrates, lipids, and proteins to constituent sugars, fatty acids, and amino acids. The normal diet is a mixture of all three components, and absorption and metabolism of carbohydrate, fat, and protein occur simultaneously. For descriptive purposes, however, each will be discussed separately.

CARBOHYDRATE Following a carbohydrate meal, absorbed sugars pass into the portal vein for transport to the liver. In the liver a significant portion of glucose (>60 percent) is retained and utilized primarily for glycogen synthesis. The remainder enters the general circulation as free glucose or, to a much lesser extent, as lactate and pyruvate, products of the hepatic

FIGURE 86-1

Anabolic pathways. Simplified scheme showing a hepatic cell with a mitochondrion. Transport systems and enzymatic details are omitted. Following a meal, a portion of ingested food is used directly to generate energy in the form of ATP while the remainder is available for storage. In the example shown glucose is oxidized via the glycolytic pathway and Krebs cycle, serves as substrate for glycogen synthesis, and is transformed to fat following conversion to citrate in the mitochondrion. Citrate is transported to the cytosol and hydrolyzed to acetyl CoA, the substrate from which malonyl CoA is formed, and oxaloacetate, which then is transported back into the mitochondrion (not shown). Exogenous amino acids and fatty acids are stored as protein and triglyceride in muscle cells and adipocytes, respectively. G-6-P, glucose 6-phosphate, F-6-P, fructose 6-phosphate, F-1,6-P, fructose-1,6-diphosphate; NAOH, nicotinamide adenine dinucleotide; ATP, adenosine triphosphate; CoQ, coenzyme Q; Cyto A$_3$, cytochrome A$_3$; CoA, coenzyme A.

oxidation of glucose. As plasma glucose concentrations rise subsequent to the meal, insulin release from the pancreas is stimulated and glucagon concentrations fall. The magnitude of the insulin response to glucose is increased through the action of other gastrointestinal hormones secreted following food intake. The latter account for the fact that glucose taken by mouth results in much greater insulin release than equivalent amounts given intravenously. Gastric inhibitory polypeptide appears to play a key role in this regard. The newly released insulin, coupled with the fall in glucagon, enhances the capacity of the liver to retain glucose as glycogen and accelerates the disposal of glucose in muscle and adipose tissue. In muscle a portion of the glucose taken up is oxidized while the remainder is stored as glycogen. In adipose tissue glucose is utilized for de novo synthesis of long-chain fatty acids which, in turn, are esterified with glucose-derived glycerol to form triglycerides. A significant amount of triglyceride is also synthesized in liver. It is transported to adipose tissue by very low density lipoprotein molecules.

PROTEIN After a protein-containing meal, absorbed amino acids also pass first to the liver via the portal vein. It is of great interest that the amino acids entering the systemic circulation

from the liver do not reflect the makeup of the ingested protein; about 60 percent of the total is accounted for by the branched-chain components valine, isoleucine, and leucine. The precise mechanism whereby selective release of these amino acids is accomplished is unknown. The branched-chain amino acids appear to play a pivotal role in overall protein metabolism in the body. They are markedly responsive to the anabolic effect of insulin in muscle, and one of them—leucine—seems to have a specific stimulatory effect on protein synthesis. It thus is likely that replenishment of protein stores in muscle following a meal is a function of branched-chain amino acid uptake. Muscle also has the capacity (not shared by liver) to oxidize the branched-chain acids for energy purposes. This capacity is important in fasting as will be mentioned below. Amino acids stimulate insulin release from the pancreas but, in contrast to glucose, also cause glucagon secretion. It has been suggested that the role of glucagon is to prevent hypoglycemia when insulin secretion is stimulated by a protein meal under circumstances where dietary carbohydrate is absent or limited.

FAT Fat absorption is much slower than that of carbohydrate or protein and follows a different course. The rate-limiting step

TABLE 86-1
The feeding-fasting cycle

Phase	Primary hormone	Plasma substrates	Substrate flux	Active process
Anabolic*	Insulin	↑ Glucose ↑ Triglycerides ↑ Branched-chain amino acids ↓ Free fatty acids ↓ Ketones	Splanchnic bed → storage and utilization sites	Glycogen storage Protein synthesis Triglyceride formation
Catabolic†	Glucagon	↓ Glucose ↓ Triglycerides ↑ Alanine and glutamine‡ ↑ Free fatty acids ↑ Ketones	Storage sites → liver and utilization sites	Glycogenolysis Gluconeogenesis Proteolysis Lipolysis Ketogenesis

Expected findings during the first several hours after ingestion of a mixed meal of fat, carbohydrate, and protein.
†*The major catabolic phase occurs during the overnight fast, although partial catabolic cycles occur between meals.*
‡*Arrows indicate plasma concentrations except for alanine and glutamine. While arterial concentrations of these amino acids are relatively constant, uptake by the liver and intestine is increased in the catabolic phase.*

FIGURE 86-2

Catabolic pathways. Simplified scheme showing a hepatic cell with a mitochondrion. Transport systems and enzymatic details are omitted. In the postabsorptive state hepatic glucose production is derived from glycogen breakdown and gluconeogenesis. The latter is largely dependent on amino acids and lactate moving to the liver from the periphery. The energy for gluconeogenesis (ATP) comes primarily from oxidation of long-chain fatty acids released from adipose tissue and from hepatic triglycerides. Fatty acids are also the substrate for ketone body synthesis (see text). PEP, phosphoenolpyruvate; other abbreviations as defined for Fig. 86-1.

is intestinal transport, which may take hours to complete. Following absorption of long-chain fatty acids, triglyceride is reformed inside the intestinal cell and packaged in the form of chylomicrons that then pass into the lymph channels and reach the systemic circulation via the thoracic duct. During transit in both lymph and plasma the apolipoprotein content of the chylomicron is altered by exchange with high-density lipoprotein (HDL). Particularly important is an increase in apoprotein CII, an activator of lipoprotein lipase. In the capillaries of a number of tissues, especially adipose and skeletal tissue and cardiac muscle, the triglycerides of chylomicrons are broken down to free fatty acids and 2-monoglycerides by lipoprotein lipase. Subsequently the monoglyceride is hydrolyzed by a monoglyceridase. The free fatty acids liberated by the two reactions pass into the cell where they may be oxidized for energy purposes or reesterified for storage as triglyceride. The latter pathway predominates in the adipocyte. Most of the triglyceride in the chylomicron is removed in a single passage through the peripheral capillary bed. The cholesterol ester—rich remnant particle then passes to the liver where it serves to regulate hepatic cholesterol synthesis.

The hormonal control of lipid metabolism is slightly more complicated than that of protein and carbohydrate. Pure fat does not stimulate insulin release in humans. However, if carbohydrate is present, triglycerides enhance the insulin response, probably via stimulation of gastric inhibitory polypeptide. Insulin plays an important, if indirect, role in the transport of triglyceride across the plasma membrane of peripheral cells since it is required for synthesis of lipoprotein lipase. Insulin also acts to stimulate fatty acid synthesis and triglyceride formation in the adipocyte and inhibits lipolysis catalyzed by the intracellular hormone-sensitive lipase. In experimental animals triglyceride stimulates secretion of glucagon and enteric glucagon-like material, but this does not appear to be a major response in humans.

SUMMARY The first few hours after a meal are characterized by an anabolic state in which ingested foods pass from the gastrointestinal tract to the liver and peripheral tissues. Under the influence of insulin some substrate is utilized immediately for energy purposes, but significant quantities are stored as glycogen, structural protein, and fat to be used as needed in the postabsorptive state or during more prolonged fasting.

CATABOLIC PHASE

Postabsorptively[1] a series of metabolic adaptations takes place which ensures adequate fuels for body tissues in the absence of exogenous substrate. Since the brain and other parts of the central nervous system can utilize only glucose or ketone bodies for energy purposes, it is obvious that during a fast plasma glucose concentrations must be sustained in a safe range until acetoacetate and β-hydroxybutyrate concentrations rise to protective levels. Three major processes are involved: (1) The liver is transformed from an organ of glucose uptake to one of net glucose production. Initially the bulk of glucose released comes from glycogen breakdown, while in later stages new glucose production is derived from peripheral precursors via gluconeogenesis. (2) Free fatty acids are mobilized from adipose tissue stores to be utilized directly for oxidative purposes in many tissues of the body and to serve as substrate for ketone body synthesis in the liver. Importantly, free fatty acids also provide the energy required for gluconeogenesis in the liver although they are not themselves substrates for glucose formation. (3) Hepatic ketogenic machinery is activated. As a result of the latter two processes, after only a few days of fasting most tissues of the body utilize free fatty acids and ketones for energy, sparing glucose for the central nervous system. Under these circumstances the enhanced endogenous production of glucose by the liver is adequate to avoid hypoglycemia. In addition the ketone bodies themselves become a major substrate for the brain, sufficient to maintain central nervous system function if for any reason glucose production is impaired. An outline of glucose homeostasis during fasting is given in Table 86-2.

All three of the adaptive processes described above are hormonally induced. In the postabsorptive state there is a fall in insulin release, probably primarily as the consequence of a decline in plasma glucose concentration. Concomitantly there

---

[1] *The term* postabsorptive *is used technically in the literature to indicate an overnight (10- to 12-h) fast. In this discussion it is used to indicate the end of the anabolic phase, which may occur much earlier.*

TABLE 86-2
Maintenance of plasma glucose during fasting

Length of fast	Source of plasma glucose	Mechanism	Tissues using glucose	Primary fuel of brain
3–4 h	Diet	Intestinal absorption	All	Glucose
4–16 h	Liver	Glycogenolysis	All except liver (↓ rates in muscle and adipose tissue)	Glucose
16–48 h	Liver	Gluconeogenesis (± glycogenolysis)	All except liver (further ↓ rates in muscle and adipose tissue)	Glucose
2–24 days	Liver, kidney	Gluconeogenesis	Brain, RBC, renal medulla	Glucose Ketones
>4 weeks	Liver, kidney	Gluconeogenesis	Brain, RBC, renal medulla (↓ rates)	Ketones Glucose

SOURCE: *After Ruderman et al.*

is a rise in four key counterregulatory hormones: epinephrine, glucagon, cortisol, and growth hormone. If hypoglycemia is rapidly induced, as by insulin injection, epinephrine appears to play the most important role since its release precedes that of glucagon, cortisol, and growth hormone. Moreover, in patients with high spinal cord transection, 2-deoxyglucose administration (which mimics hypoglycemia) is not followed by the appearance of compensatory hyperglycemia as occurs in normal subjects. The quadriplegic patients have a normal rise in glucagon, growth hormone, and cortisol but are unable to release epinephrine, again suggesting a critical role for the catecholamine in activating hepatic glyceogenolysis. When the fall in glucose is more gradual, as in the postabsorptive state, glucagon is thought to be the most important hormone controlling hepatic glucose production. Lipolysis is generally considered to be primarily the consequence of insulin deficiency, while the ketogenic capacity of liver appears to be induced by the rise in plasma glucagon.

GLYCOGENOLYSIS AND GLUCONEOGENESIS Hepatic glucose production in the immediate postabsorptive state is due almost exclusively to breakdown of preformed glycogen. Ordinarily the liver contains sufficient glycogen to maintain the plasma glucose for only 12 to 24 h (depending on activity and caloric demands). Beyond this period gluconeogenesis is required if hypoglycemia is to be avoided. The gluconeogenic substrates are lactate, glycerol, and amino acids. Lactate derived from glucose not completely oxidized in peripheral tissues normally returns to the liver and after an overnight fast accounts for up to 20 percent of hepatic glucose production (Cori cycle). This does not result in net glucose synthesis, however, since the lactate was originally derived from glucose passing to muscle and other tissues. Net glucose synthesis from lactate (as opposed to the recycling sequence) requires its production from stored muscle glycogen. Glycerol utilized for gluconeogenesis comes from triglycerides hydrolyzed in adipose tissue. Its contribution to overall glucose production is relatively minor. Amino acids represent the major substrate for gluconeogenesis, but amino acid metabolism during fasting is complicated. While there is net release of all amino acids, the output of alanine and glutamine is out of proportion to their relative concentrations in muscle protein. Glutamine is preferentially utilized by extrahepatic splanchnic tissues, while alanine uptake by the liver is greater than that of any other amino acid, suggesting a prime role for the latter in the gluconeogenic process. Moreover, alanine extraction by the liver increases during fasting. Glutamine is also taken up by the kidney, serv-

ing as substrate for NH_3 generation and renal gluconeogenesis. While liver is the primary gluconeogenic organ, measurable glucose production occurs in the kidney during prolonged fasting.

It is now thought that the bulk of the alanine released from muscle is derived from transamination of pyruvate which, in turn, is produced from muscle glycogen, glucose from plasma, and possibly directly from amino acids themselves. The source of nitrogen for the transamination of pyruvate is likely the branched-chain amino acids that are released from the breakdown of muscle protein. Following transamination, the α-keto analogues of these acids are oxidized to provide energy for the muscle. The end result is that muscle protein becomes the major source of new glucose formation by the liver, transported to that organ in the form of alanine. Presumably the advantage of alanine resides in its ready ability to enter the hepatocyte and the gluconeogenic pathways.

It is believed that the amino acids utilized in gluconeogensis come from structural protein of muscle rather than from nonfunctional storage pools. As a consequence they represent enzymes, transport molecules, and membrane proteins, all of which are vital to cellular integrity (in contrast to loss of glycogen and triglyceride which are not essential to the cell). For this reason when starvation is extended beyond a few days, limitation of protein loss becomes critical. After several weeks of total starvation (in obese subjects) a definite decrease of nitrogen excretion in the urine has, in fact, been observed. At this stage essentially all tissues of the body are sustained by the oxidation of fat—either as free fatty acids or the ketone bodies. As a result the demand for glucose (and thus the demand for protein as gluconeogenic substrate) markedly diminishes, and the negative nitrogen balance of starvation is blunted. There is suggestive evidence that the ketone bodies somehow signal the muscle to damp amino acid release. Infusion of β-hydroxybutyrate to fasting subjects decreases plasma alanine concentration and acutely lowers urinary nitrogen excretion. Presumably other factors are also involved since massive negative nitrogen balance occurs in diabetic ketoacidosis despite ketone concentrations far higher than maximal levels attained in prolonged starvation. In view of its known anabolic (anticatabolic) effects, insulin may be the required additional factor.

LIPOLYSIS The hydrolysis of adipose tissue triglycerides to free fatty acids and glycerol is mediated by an intracellular, hormone-sensitive lipase which is distinct from the extracellular lipoprotein lipase previously mentioned. This lipase appears susceptible to both positive and negative regulation. Insulin in low concentrations can effectively block lipolysis, while catecholamines activate the process. A number of hormones that increase triglyceride breakdown in rat adipose tissue [e.g., glucagon, growth hormone, adrenocorticotropin (ACTH)] appear to be much less effective in human adipocytes. Activation is thought to involve cyclic adenosine monophosphate (AMP) acting via a protein kinase that phosphorylates the hormone-sensitive lipase. On the negative side both the ketone bodies and adenosine, in addition to insulin, have been suggested to deactivate lipolysis. Free fatty acids rise early in the postabsorptive state and usually reach a maximum of about 1 mM in prolonged fasting.

The importance of lipolysis resides in the fact that body fat represents the organism's primary defense against starvation. This is true because its energy value per gram (about 9 cal) is twice that of protein and carbohydrate (about 4 cal/g) and because its mass is large. Estimates are that the average size person has approximately 140,000 cal stored as fat compared with 24,000 cal as protein and 300 cal as glycogen. If adipose tissue has been depleted (because of disease or famine) or if fatty acids cannot be normally oxidized (see Chap. 340), fatal hypoglycemia or death from protein deficiency may occur.

KETOGENESIS As noted, the ketone bodies play a critical role in the catabolic response to food deprivation. They represent an energy source that can be used by almost every tissue in the body, and they are the only effective alternative substrate for brain metabolism. Interestingly, when total ketones reach concentrations of 4 to 6 mM, hypoglycemia sufficient to cause adrenergic response and mental confusion in a nonketotic individual produces no symptoms. Presumably under these circumstances acetoacetate and β-hydroxybutyrate can meet the metabolic demands of the central nervous system despite inadequate glucose.

Significant ketosis requires changes in both liver and adipose tissue. In the fed state the capacity for fatty acid oxidation in the liver is low. Most of the fatty acid taken up by the hepatocyte is reesterified to triglyceride and either stored or released as a very low density lipoprotein particle. It is now believed that the rate of hepatic fatty acid oxidation is governed by the activity of the carnitine acyltransferase system of enzymes that transports fatty acids into the mitochondria. Present evidence suggests that in the fed state malonyl CoA, a potent inhibitor of carnitine acyltransferase I, keeps the system inactive. This inhibition is removed during fasting through the action of glucagon which lowers the malonyl CoA concentration and simultaneously increases the carnitine content of liver. With these changes the capacity for fatty acid oxidation and ketogenesis in the hepatocyte is maximally activated. (For a more detailed explanation, see Chap. 338.) Once the liver is activated, the rate of ketone body production is determined solely by the rate of delivery of free fatty acids from the periphery; i.e., the higher the free fatty acid concentration in plasma, the greater the hepatic production of acetoacetate and β-hydroxybutyrate until maximal rates are obtained.

Quantitative estimates of substrate flux after a 24-h fast are shown in Table 86-3.

SUMMARY The catabolic changes occurring in the absence of food vary with the duration of the fast. In the first few hours glycogenolysis predominates, while the adaptive response after the first day emphasizes gluconeogenesis and protein breakdown together with acceleration of fat catabolism. If the fast is prolonged, a fat economy is established with diminution of gluconeogenesis and nitrogen wastage. Provided that adipose tissue stores are adequate, prolonged survival can occur in the complete absence of food.

STARVATION AND DIABETIC KETOACIDOSIS

It has long been recognized that diabetic ketoacidosis is a catabolic illness that resembles an accelerated state of starvation. In this situation hepatic gluconeogenesis is markedly increased, plasma-free fatty acids are extremely high (2 to 4

TABLE 86-3
Substrate flux during fasting (per 24 h)*

Amino acids released	75 g
Free fatty acids released:	160 g
Used directly	120 g
Converted to ketones	40 g
Glucose produced	180 g
Ketones produced	60 g

* *Fluxes calculated after 24 h of fasting in a subject with basal energy requirements of 1800 cal.*
SOURCE: *After Cahill.*

TABLE 86-4
Typical laboratory values in fasting and diabetic ketoacidosis

	48-h fast	*Ketoacidosis*
Glucose, mg per 100 ml	65	475
Free fatty acids, mM	0.9	2.1
Acetoacetate, mM	0.8	4.8
β-Hydroxybutyrate, mM	2.2	13.7
Lactate, mM	0.7	4.6
Blood urea nitrogen, mg per 100 ml	16	25
Urinary nitrogen, g per 24 h	12	20
HCO$_3^-$, mM	22	5
pH	7.35	7.05
Insulin, μU/ml	10	<5
Glucagon, pg/ml	200	400

mM), acetoacetate and β-hydroxybutyrate concentrations are sufficient (18 to 20 mM) to cause frank acidosis, and protein wastage is massive. It seems clear that the quantitative differences between starvation and diabetic coma can be accounted for primarily by the almost complete absence of insulin in ketoacidosis-prone diabetes. As outlined above, normal persons subjected to fasting show a modest fall in plasma glucose which results in diminished insulin release from the pancreatic islets. The fall in insulin concentration, coupled with release of glucagon and other counterregulatory hormones, activates glycogen breakdown, gluconeogenesis, lipolysis, and ketogenesis. Since both ketone bodies and free fatty acids can stimulate insulin release from the beta cell, a protective feedback loop is available during fasting in the normal subject that prevents the occurrence of ketoacidosis; i.e., when total ketones and free fatty acids approach levels sufficient to produce a significant acidosis, insulin release is stimulated (or further fall in insulin is prevented), resulting in modulation of adipose tissue lipolysis and limitation of ketone formation by restriction of fatty acid flow to the liver. In the absence of an adequate insulin feedback loop, as in the juvenile diabetic, lipolysis is unrestrained and ketogenesis becomes maximal, resulting in life-threatening ketoacidosis. Ketoacidosis and the major catabolic responses so characteristic of the uncontrolled insulin-dependent patient do not occur in maturity-onset diabetes. Presumably the difference resides in the fact that insulin deficiency is not as complete in the latter state. A comparison of laboratory values in fasting and diabetic ketoacidosis is shown in Table 86-4.

REFERENCES

BRODOWS RG et al: Neural control of counter-regulatory events during glucopenia in man. J Clin Invest 52:1841, 1973

BUSE MG, REID SS: Leucine. A possible regulator of protein turnover in muscle. J Clin Invest 56:1250, 1975

CAHILL GF JR: Starvation in man. N Engl J Med 282:668, 1970

CROCKETT SE et al: The insulinotropic effect of endogenous gastric inhibitory polypeptide in normal subjects. J Clin Endocrinol Metab 42:1098, 1976

FELIG P: Amino acid and protein metabolism in diabetes mellitus. Arch Intern Med 137:507, 1977

GARBER AJ et al: The role of adrenergic mechanisms in the substrate and hormonal response to insulin-induced hypoglycemia in man. J Clin Invest 58:7, 1976

KHOO JC et al: The mechanism of activation of hormone-sensitive lipase in human adipose tissue. J Clin Invest 53:1124, 1974

MCGARRY JD, FOSTER DW: Hormonal control of ketogenesis. Biochemical considerations. Arch Intern Med 137:495, 1977

RUDERMAN NB et al: Gluconeogenesis and its disorders in man, in *Gluconeogenesis: Its Regulation in Mammalian Species*, RW Hanson, MA Mehlman (eds). New York, Wiley, 1976, pp 515–532

SAUDEK CD, FELIG P: The metabolic events of starvation. Am J Med 60:117, 1976

UNGER RH: Diabetes and the alpha cell. Diabetes 25:136, 1976

87
OVERVIEW OF INHERITED METABOLIC DISEASES

LEON E. ROSENBERG

GENE-ENVIRONMENT INTERACTION Metabolism, by definition, comprises all the processes by which living matter is built up (anabolism) or broken down (catabolism). These processes begin with the earliest chemical reactions leading to the formation of the sperm and egg; continue throughout growth, maturation, and senescence; and end inexorably with the death of cell, tissue, organ, and finally the individual. Metabolic processes are controlled by two integrated inputs: the *genes*, which delimit the capacity of any given cell (and pari passu of any organism), and the *environment*, which determines how those genes will be expressed. It follows that all metabolic disorders result from some disturbance in the interaction between genetic and environmental factors, and, in the strictest sense, that no metabolic disorder can be classified as either purely *inherited* or *acquired*. When we have little or no information about the genetic determinants of a disease, as in susceptibility to tuberculosis or to traumatic fractures of bones, we think of the condition as acquired. Conversely, when a metabolic disorder is due to a primary abnormality of a specific protein (and hence to a mutation of a specific gene) and when this abnormality is inherited as a simple mendelian dominant or recessive trait (as in acute intermittent porphyria or phenylketonuria), we consider the metabolic derangement inherited. In fact neither condition might be serious were it not for precipitating and modifying factors in the environment (drugs and hormones in porphyria; dietary phenylalanine in phenylketonuria). Appreciation of this gene-environment continuum is of more than nosologic interest. Thus, identification of genes controlling susceptibility to tuberculosis will, one day, enable us to identify individuals and groups at risk; and additional information about age-related dietary phenylalanine requirements will permit more effective nutritional treatment of phenylketonuria.

CHARACTER OF INBORN ERRORS In the chapters of the section to follow, those metabolic disorders with an "inherited" etiology are emphasized. Literally hundreds of such inherited metabolic diseases or, as they were originally designated by Garrod, "inborn errors of metabolism," are now recognized, and new ones continue to be described at a logarithmic rate. As a group, these conditions affect all phases of metabolism and have contributed enormously to the understanding of normal metabolic pathways (confirming the wisdom of the dictum "treasure your exceptions"). They share only the two common features mentioned earlier: each is inherited as a simple mendelian trait and each has been traced (or is attributed) to a functional abnormality of a specific protein. In other ways the features are diverse. Most are inherited as autosomal recessive traits, implying that a double dose of the mutant gene is required for the disorder to be phenotypically manifest (see Chap. 58); others are inherited as X-linked or autosomal dominant traits. Some have an incidence as high as 1:500 (familial

hypercholesterolemia); others have an incidence as low as 1:1,000,000 (alcaptonuria). Some demonstrate prominent racial or ethnic clustering, and others appear to be uniformly distributed in races and groups. Some produce clinical manifestations at birth (or even before), others only in adult life (or not at all). Some are uniformly lethal regardless of treatment; others are compatible with a normal life span and health.

LEVELS OF UNDERSTANDING Since it is generally assumed that the clinical and chemical abnormalities observed in patients with a given inherited metabolic disease reflect the mutational disturbance of a specific gene, it is theoretically possible to understand each inborn error at four levels: the gene, the protein coded for by the gene, the metabolic step at which the protein works, and the clinical or chemical phenotype produced by abnormalities at that step. Of all the genetic disorders, it is only in certain of the hemoglobinopathies that we can approach this level of understanding (see Chap. 315). In hemoglobin S disease (sickle-cell anemia) the specific mutant codon and the precise amino acid substitution in the β globin chain have been identified. Furthermore, physicochemical studies with hemoglobin S have shown why this mutant protein has a tendency to gel in the deoxygenated state and form the tactoids that distort the erythrocyte and lead to the hyperviscosity, sludging, tissue infarction, and hemolysis characteristic of this disorder. Such complete information is possible because hemoglobin is the only human protein that has been studied to date at the level of the gene and messenger RNA. For other loci, understanding stops at the level of the gene product and, even there, in an incomplete way. For example, in one form of galactosemia the activity of galactose 1-phosphate uridyltransferase is deficient; this deficiency leads to accumulation of galactose and galactose 1-phosphate, which results in serious hepatic and central nervous system dysfunction. However, we know little about either the molecular nature of the transferase deficiency or the means by which metabolite accumulation leads to cirrhosis and mental retardation. In other instances, such as Wilson's disease or cystinosis, the particular protein whose function is deranged is unknown, although it is recognized that copper and cystine respectively accumulate in tissues of affected patients. Even more primitive is our understanding of Huntington's disease, which can only be described clinically as an autosomal dominant disease without a known biochemical "handle" with which to grapple with the diagnostic and prognostic dilemmas. Much has been learned about inherited metabolic disorders in the past 25 years, but that quantum of knowledge is trivial compared with the enormity of our ignorance.

PROTEINS AS GENE PRODUCTS

SPECTRUM OF MUTANT PROTEINS Genes and messenger RNAs are polymers of nucleic acids often referred to as "informational macromolecules." Along similar lines proteins and polypeptides can be called "functional macromolecules." These linear polymers of amino acids convert the informational potential of genes and messengers into chemical and physiologic work. Proteins are ubiquitous. They are a vital constituent of the membranes that separate tissues, cells, and organelles from one another. In the blood, lymph, and cerebrospinal fluid they maintain osmotic pressure and selectively bind and transport a large number of small molecules. As enzymes and hormones, whether extracellular or intracellular, they catalyze or regulate reactions that allow anabolic and catabolic pathways to proceed. Proteins display almost limitless variation in size, shape, and function. Molecular weights vary from a few hundred, for the pituitary hormone releasing factors, to more than a million, for gamma macroglobulin. Some are monomeric; others are oligomers of two, three, four, or more like or unlike polypeptide chains. Some are globular while others are helical; still others have both globular and helical regions. Some have metal ions as prosthetic groups or cofactors, while others require organic constituents for activity. Each, however, owes its unique structural features and functional specificity to a single feature—the primary amino acid sequence. Since this primary sequence is dependent on the nucleotide sequence of the gene and messenger RNA that codes for the polypeptide, inherited variations in protein structure or function are the visible expression of gene mutation. Mutations occur in all genes, and hence variation must occur in all proteins. Some variants are detected easily because they lead to obvious chemical or clinical disturbance. Others are detected with great difficulty, either because they produce early lethality or because they are clinically or chemically silent.

In general, mutations responsible for inherited metabolic disorders affect the structural genes that code for the *primary structure* of the protein (see Chap. 58). Single codon changes usually lead to single amino acid substitutions and are referred to as *missense* mutations. Other point mutations (those leading to inappropriately placed terminator codons) as well as deletions and insertions (of codons, segments, or entire genes) produce *nonsense* mutations that result in complete absence of the gene product or one so incomplete or distorted as to be essentially functionless. Alternatively, mutations can modify the *rate* at which a protein is made. Such rate control may be exerted either by modifying control genes or by changing codons in structural genes in a way that leads to accelerated or retarded transcription or translation. Because the messenger RNAs and the genes controlling synthesis of the α and β globin chains of hemoglobin have been purified and characterized, impressive knowledge has been acquired regarding the chemical nature of genetic modifications in this system. Since molecular biological information is lacking for other human loci, inferences about disturbances in gene structure must be drawn from the observed effects of gene-controlled protein functions.

Inborn errors have been described for all types of proteins. In their seminal contributions, Garrod, Beadle, Tatum, and associates stressed enzymatic defects that produce a block in an anabolic or catabolic pathway. More than 100 examples of this type of defect are known (see subsequent chapters), and new enzymatic deficiencies are currently being described at a rate of about ten per year. Although dysfunction of these intracellular catalysts provides the largest body of data concerning the impact of inherited variation on homeostasis, they do not reflect the full scope of functional changes produced by genetic alterations. For example, numerous inherited disorders of cell membrane function have been described. Inborn errors of transport affecting gut and kidney may selectively impair transmembrane movement of sugars, amino acids, phosphate, vitamins, or water (see Chap. 90). Disorders like cystinuria or glycosuria are thought to reflect deficiency of specific membrane carrier proteins required for transepithelial movement of dibasic amino acids or glucose, respectively. Other transport defects lead to abnormal binding of hormones to membrane receptors as in vasopressin-resistant diabetes insipidus or of protein-ligand complexes as in the cell surface receptor defect for low-density lipoprotein in familial hypercholesterolemia (see Chap. 100). Still other mutations alter circulating proteins rather than membrane constituents or intracellular enzymes. Analbuminemia, transcobalamin II deficiency, and abetalipoproteinemia are examples of such deficiencies.

FUNCTIONAL DERANGEMENTS **Increased activity** Simply put, metabolic disorders can be thought of as resulting from too much or too little of a specific protein (or of that protein's activity). Variant forms of G6PD, pseudocholinesterase, and phosphoribosylpyrophosphate synthetase have been described in which enzyme activity is *increased*. In these instances, mutations result in an increase in intracellular enzyme content either because the mutant protein is synthesized more rapidly than normal or is degraded more slowly. In acute intermittent porphyria and familial hypercholesterolemia, rate-controlling enzymes are increased as well (see Chaps. 96 and 100). In the latter disorders, however, enzyme overactivity is a secondary event, reflecting impaired feedback regulation produced by other primary genetic disturbances.

Decreased activity All other inborn errors that have been analyzed in detail are associated with decreased activity (or content) of a protein. The deficiency may be *virtually complete* (as in the classical forms of phenylketonuria and galactosemia) or *partial* (as in the benign variants of those disorders). It should be emphasized that complete loss of enzyme activity cannot be equated with complete absence of a protein. For example, in classic galactosemia, no galactose 1-phosphate uridyltransferase activity can be detected in tissues of affected patients, but immunochemical analyses have shown that such tissues contain a protein that cross-reacts with antibody to the native transferase molecule. Numerous examples of cross-reacting material positive (CRM$^+$) abnormalities are now recognized. They indicate that the mutation has resulted in the synthesis of a protein that has lost catalytic activity but retains antigenic specificity. Other metabolic disorders characterized by complete enzyme deficiency such as muscle phosphorylase deficiency or Von Willebrand disease are CRM$^-$, implying either that no protein is made or that the gene product is so altered that both catalytic and antigenic functions have been lost.

As increasingly sensitive methods of enzyme assay have been developed, it has become apparent that most inborn errors are characterized by partial, rather than complete, loss of activity. Such partial deficiency may result from several different mechanisms. First, it may reflect reduced rate of synthesis of normal or abnormal enzyme molecules. Second, it may result from accelerated destruction of a structurally altered enzyme. Third, reduced activity may reflect reduced affinity of the active enzyme for substrate or cofactor. Fourth, for oligomeric enzymes, reduced activity could result from impaired interaction of identical or nonidentical subunits. Fifth, for those enzymes in which more than a single isoenzyme exists in a tissue, reduced activity could reflect isolated loss of one form of the enzyme. Examples of each of these mechanisms exist among inherited metabolic disorders in humans. Moreover, the same phenotypic manifestations can result from different mechanisms. For example, some G6PD variants exhibit increased lability, others abnormal affinity for substrate, and still others impaired oligomer formation. All these abnormalities result from different structural alterations in a single polypeptide chain.

CONSEQUENCES OF TRANSPORT OR ENZYMATIC DEFECTS

The effect of any given genetic alteration on cellular metabolism and clinical status depends on the role that the mutant protein plays and the severity of the defect. As mentioned earlier, most inborn errors are the result of intracellular enzymatic defects or of membrane transport abnormalities. Since these kinds of mutations are discussed repeatedly in the following chapters, it is appropriate to summarize the possible consequences of inherited transport or enzyme defects. The model reaction sequence shown in Fig. 87-1 is used for illustrative purposes. A, B, C, D, F, and G are substrates or products of a series of enzymatic reactions; T_A, E_{AB}, E_{BC}, and E_{CD} refer to specific transport systems or enzymes catalyzing specific reactions in this sequence. The major pathway involves the conversion of A to D via intermediates B and C. F and G are products of an alternate metabolic pathway. The arrow from D to E_{AB} represents negative feedback control of the first enzyme in the pathway by the final product of the sequence. Wherever possible, examples of specific inborn errors that illustrate specific consequences of transport or enzyme defects will be cited.

PRECURSOR DEFICIENCY   If T_A, the receptor or carrier system that transports A into the cell, is defective, the intracellular concentration of A may be so low that E_{AB} will not be saturated with its substrate. This could slow the entire reaction sequence and result in inadequate formation of B, C, and D. In Hartnup disease (see Chap. 90), intestinal transport of tryptophan is defective. This transport defect has important chemical and clinical consequences, since tryptophan is converted to nicotinamide intracellularly. Patients with this disorder may exhibit cerebellar ataxia and temporary or permanent dementia due to nicotinamide deficiency if they do not receive supplements of niacin in the diet. Similarly, patients with inherited defects in intestinal absorption of vitamin B_{12} develop megaloblastic anemia unless the vitamin is supplied parenterally. Precursor or substrate deficiency may also occur if the defect involves a circulating protein that transports substance A in the blood and carries it to the cell surface.

PRECURSOR ACCUMULATION   Let us next consider the effect of reduced activity of one of the intracellular enzymes, (E_{AB}, E_{BC}, or E_{CD}). Such a defect might lead to intracellular and extracellular accumulation of the immediate or remote precursors of the reaction. If E_{AB} is defective, only A will accumulate. Such a result is illustrated by the marked increase in lysosomal glucocerebroside content in Gaucher's disease (see Chap. 101) and of blood galactose concentration in galactokinase deficiency (see Chap. 98). Defects of E_{BC} may result in accumulation of A as well as B, and a defect of E_{CD} could lead to the pileup of A, B, and C. In homocystinuria due to cystathionine synthase deficiency, methionine, a remote precursor, accumulates, as does homocystine, the immediate precursor of the blocked reaction (see Chap. 88).

ALTERNATE PATHWAY UTILIZATION   If the conversion of A to B is impaired by deficiency of E_{AB}, not only will A accumulate, but the usually minor, alternate pathway to F and G may become prominent. Phenylketonuria represents an excellent example of this phenomenon. The absence of phenylalanine hydroxylase activity leads to gross overproduction and excretion of phenylpyruvic, phenylacetic, and phenyllactic acids, compounds not usually detectable in blood or urine (see Chap. 88). Such alternate pathway augmentation may have important physiologic significance if the products of the alternate pathway interfere with cell processes when present in more than minute concentrations.

PRODUCT DEFICIT   If D is the physiologically active product of the hypothetical reaction sequence, a block at any of the steps from A to D results in inadequate synthesis of D. The formation of thyroxine in the thyroid gland proceeds through just such a series of reactions, involving first the transport of iodide into the gland and then its subsequent oxidation and organification. Several enzymatic defects lead to goitrous cretinism due to impaired synthesis of thyroxine. Similarly, in some patients with congenital adrenal hyperplasia due to a defect in hydroxylation at the C_{21} position of the steroid nucleus, aldosterone production is impaired, leading to renal salt wasting and hyponatremic crises. Deficient synthesis of product may cause overproduction of precursors, as in acute intermittent porphyria, because of loss of feedback control (D → E_{AB}).

PRODUCT EXCESS   As shown in Fig. 87-1, the end product of the reaction sequence D is presumed to regulate the activity of E_{AB}, the first enzyme in this biosynthetic pathway. The phenomenon of end product inhibition (commonly called feedback inhibition) was first described in microbial systems but is now known to exist for pathways in mammalian cells as well. Several inborn errors demonstrate abnormalities in feedback regulation, but the biochemical events involved are not well understood. In some patients with primary gout urate is overproduced, presumably because the first enzyme in the purine pathway is defective and does not respond to its normal feedback inhibitors, hypoxanthine and adenine. Abnormal feedback control occurs in the congenital adrenal hyperplasias and congenital goitrous cretinism as well, presumably by different chemical mechanisms. In these disorders the formation or release of ACTH and TSH, respectively, is not impeded by their usual "servo" regulators, cortisol and thyroxine, resulting in hyperplasia and functional disturbances in the two target glands.

Faulty feedback control is not the only mechanism capable of producing product excess. In those disorders characterized

FIGURE 87-1
Schematic representation of metabolic pathway including transport system, enzymes, alternate route, and feedback regulation. (From Rosenberg.)

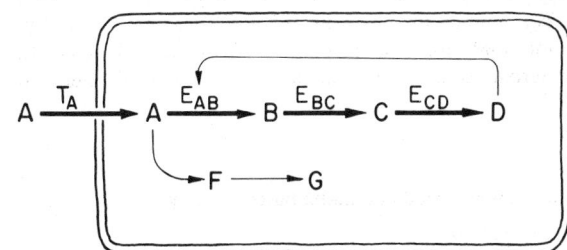

A, B, C, D - Substrate and Products of Major Pathway
F, G - Products of Minor Pathway
T_A - Transport System for A
E_{AB}, E_{BC}, E_{CD} - Enzymes Catalyzing Conversion of A to B, B to C, and C to D
- Cell Membrane

by enzyme excess, such as hyperuricemia resulting from increased PRPP synthetase activity (see Chap. 92), product excess can be explained simply by accelerated conversion of precursor to product.

GENETIC HETEROGENEITY

It is well recognized that a given abnormal phenotype may be produced by more than one genotype. This situation, referred to as genetic heterogeneity, is ubiquitous and important. Clinically, an appreciation of genetic heterogeneity has important diagnostic implications, and since diagnosis defines our approach to treatment and counseling, it is important in these matters as well. Scientifically, elucidation of the mechanisms of heterogeneity is imperative for understanding the ways in which the human genome can be modified and how such genetic manifestations can be expressed phenotypically. As noted in Table 87-1, heterogeneity has been discerned using three general methodologic approaches: clinical, biochemical, and genetic.

CLINICAL EVIDENCE In the absence of independent biochemical or genetic information, it is often impossible to determine whether subtle variations in clinical expression of a given metabolic disorder in any two affected individuals reflect the presence of different mutations or result from modification of an identical mutation by other genetic and environmental influences. However, on the basis of information gleaned from biochemical techniques, such clinical evidence suggesting heterogeneity becomes interpretable. For example, it is likely that patients with juvenile Gaucher's disease have an earlier age of onset and a more rapidly progressive downhill course than do those with adult Gaucher's disease because the mutant glucocerebrosidase in cells from the former group is distinct from and retains less catalytic activity than that in cells from the latter (see Chap. 101). It follows that tissue glucocerebroside content will increase more rapidly if glucocerebrosidase activity is 3 percent of normal than if it is 15 percent of normal. Similarly, the reason that patients with Hunter's disease do not have corneal clouding, whereas patients with the phenotypically similar Hurler's disease do, almost certainly depends on the different enzymatic dysfunctions in the two disorders: iduronate sulfatase deficiency in Hunter's, α-L-iduronidase deficiency in Hurler's.

BIOCHEMICAL TECHNIQUES More often, heterogeneity is first defined through chemical or biochemical assays. Such assays vary greatly in design and complexity—from identification of compounds in blood, urine, or CSF to molecular hybridization analyses. Illustrative examples of disorders shown to be heterogeneous by each of the four kinds of biochemical

assays noted in Table 87-1 are as follows. First, the "ketotic hyperglycinemia" syndrome, characterized by episodic ketoacidosis, protein intolerance, and hyperglycinemia, was shown by chemical analyses of blood and urine to be a feature of several different disturbances of organic acid metabolism—α-methylacetoacetic acidemia, propionic acidemia, and methylmalonic acidemia. Second, patients with an entity originally called "congenital, nonspherocytic hemolytic anemia" were found to have different deficiencies in glycolytic enzymes when assays were carried out with erythrocyte hemolysates. Third, the nature of the heterogeneity in patients with GM_2 gangliosidosis did not become apparent until the lysosomal hexoseaminidases were subdivided into A and B isozymes whose activities could be measured individually in patients with Tay-Sachs or Sandhoff's disease. The fourth approach is directed at the gene rather than the gene product. Molecular hybridization experiments employing DNA and RNA provided the evidence for two general categories of β thalassemia: $β^0$, characterized by the apparent absence of β globin mRNA, and $β^+$, characterized by reduced but clearly detectable amounts of β-globin message. Such hybridization studies were also useful in defining heterogeneity in α thalassemia and in those conditions characterized by hereditary persistence of fetal hemoglobin.

GENETIC METHODS Genetic methods have also been important in demonstrating heterogeneity (Table 87-1). One of the earliest and most convincing evidences of such heterogeneity came from the chance mating of two individuals each affected with autosomal recessively inherited nerve deafness. None of their progeny was deaf, demonstrating conclusively that the mutations that produced deafness in the parents were different and likely nonallelic. In several instances heterogeneity was suggested by different modes of inheritance of phenotypically similar (or identical) disorders. For example, Hunter's and Hurler's diseases were differentiated early because the former is inherited as an X-linked trait, the latter as an autosomal recessive. Similarly, at least three forms of spastic diplegia are now recognized: one inherited as an autosomal dominant, a second as an autosomal recessive, and a third as an X-linked trait. In a few instances heterogeneity was first appreciated by studying obligate heterozygotes for a recessive phenotype. Thus, cystinuria was shown to be heterogeneous by the observation that all obligate heterozygotes in some families excreted increased amounts of cystine and lysine, whereas in other pedigrees urinary findings in obligate heterozygotes could not be distinguished from controls. A fourth genetic tool that has revealed heterogeneity is classical linkage analysis. Through this investigation hereditary elliptocytosis was divided into two forms—one closely linked to the Rh blood group locus, the other not. Finally, heterogeneity has been demonstrated in a number of instances by application of complementation analyses as first worked out in bacteria and neurospora. The general strategy of such studies is simple. Cultured fibroblasts from two affected individuals are cocultivated in the same dish or are fused into heterokaryons with Sendai virus or polyethylene glycol. If the abnormal phenotype expressed in both parental strains remains in the mixed culture, the defect in the two patients is assumed to be identical; if correction occurs in the mixed culture, the defects in the original strains must be different. This approach has been used to define heterogeneity in a wide variety of disorders, including the mucopolysaccharidoses, the GM_2 gangliosidoses, the methylmalonic acidemias, the propionic acidemias, xeroderma pigmentosum, and branched-chain ketoaciduria. Theoretically, positive complementation tests could reflect either of two general mechanisms: intergenic complementation, in which two different loci are involved, or interallelic complementation, in which two different mutations at the same locus are mutually corrective. It

TABLE 87-1
Methods of demonstrating genetic heterogeneity

I Clinical analysis
   A Age of onset
   B Severity
   C Specific features
II Biochemical analysis
   A Constituents of blood, urine, and cerebrospinal fluid
   B Enzymatic activity
   C Protein characterization
   D DNA-RNA or DNA-DNA hybridization
III Genetic analysis
   A Chance matings
   B Mode of inheritance
   C Manifestations in heterozygotes
   D Linkage relationships
   E Complementation in mixed cells or heterokaryons

seems likely that the vast majority of positive complementation tests reflect the intergenic mechanism.

GENETIC COMPOUNDS One of the important conclusions drawn from these biochemical and genetic demonstrations of heterogeneity is that in some instances individuals with a given metabolic disorder are "genetic compounds" rather than true homozygotes. By genetic compounds we mean individuals who have received a different mutant allele at a given locus from each parent rather than identical mutant alleles. Patients with hemoglobin SC disease were the first compounds identified, having inherited the gene for hemoglobin S from one parent and that for hemoglobin C from the other. These individuals have a double dose of a mutation for β globin chain synthesis and thus make no normal β chains. They are clinically and chemically distinct from true SS or CC homozygotes. More recently, genetic compounds have been identified in patients with cystinuria, iminoglycinuria, galactose 1-phosphate uridyltransferase deficiency, and L-iduronidase deficiency. Some, but not all, genetic compounds are as severely affected as true homozygotes, depending on the nature of the mutant alleles inherited. Little direct information is available in this area, with the exception of those loci coding for globin chains.

DIAGNOSTIC TECHNIQUES AND TARGETS

PHYSIOLOGIC FLUIDS Most of the early information concerning the mechanisms of the inborn errors and their mode of detection came from chemical studies of blood or urine. Such chemical determinations did more than point out specific biochemical abnormalities; they provided the clues in many instances for the more elegant enzymatic studies that clarified the specific defect involved. They also allowed large populations to be screened for specific disorders, thereby facilitating the detection of affected subjects prior to the onset of overt clinical problems. The use of screening tests in blood and urine has allowed the detection of heterozygous carriers for many conditions. They are also often useful in monitoring the effects of specific dietary, drug, or replacement therapy.

TISSUE ANALYSES During the past 15 to 20 years, enzymatic assays and biochemical studies using human tissue obtained by biopsy made a great impact on the definition and detection of the inborn errors. Analyses of liver, muscle, brain, gut mucosa, kidney, erythrocytes, leukocytes, stratum corneum, and spleen have revealed specific enzymatic defects in more than a hundred metabolic diseases. Membrane transport defects have also been demonstrated in vitro in such disorders as hereditary spherocytosis, cystinuria, and the glucose-galactose malabsorption syndrome by the use of erythrocytes, kidney cortex, and gut mucosa, respectively. These assays have often identified the biochemical and genetic heterogeneity characteristic of the inborn errors, in addition to documenting specific gene product abnormalities. Tissue studies do not lend themselves to population surveys and have the greatest impact when combined with investigations of detectable abnormalities in blood and urine.

CELL CULTURE Within the past decade human fibroblasts grown in tissue culture have yielded important insights into the biochemistry and genetics of numerous inborn metabolic disorders. In some instances (acatalasia, galactosemia, glucose 6-phosphate dehydrogenase deficiency, glycogen storage disease type II, branched-chain ketoaciduria, and orotic aciduria) enzymatic defects initially described in other tissues were confirmed in cultured fibroblasts. In citrullinemia and Refsum's disease, specific enzymatic defects were first demonstrated in fibroblasts, while in the Lesch-Nyhan syndrome defective hy-

poxanthine-guanine phosphoribosyl transferase activity was demonstrated coincidently in erythrocytes, leukocytes, and cultured fibroblasts. Cultured cells are not only of value in defining biochemical abnormalities in affected patients; abnormalities found in cells from heterozygous carriers have also been of significance. For example, the study in obligate heterozygotes of several X-linked traits provided evidence confirming the validity of the Lyon hypothesis.

HETEROZYGOTE DETECTION The detection of heterozygous carriers contributes to the study of inborn errors in two important ways. First, such detection provides the most convincing evidence for a recessive mode of inheritance of a disorder, whether the mutation is autosomal or X-linked. Second, the identification of heterozygous carriers in a single pedigree provides valuable information for counseling family members. Counseling relates to such problems as family planning or the choice of a marriage partner. In those diseases in which clinical manifestations may be observed in the carriers (i.e., in dominantly inherited conditions such as acute intermittent porphyria or familial hypercholesterolemia) heterozygote detection has direct clinical relevance.

Identification of heterozygotes requires many of the same methods employed for the recognition of chemical or enzymatic defects in affected subjects. In a few instances, simple blood or urine screening techniques may be sufficient to detect carriers. Enzymatic assays using blood cells or serum have been helpful in several other conditions. In some disorders blood or urine analyses fail to discriminate between normal subjects and heterozygous carriers, but carriers can be detected after administration of oral or parenteral loads of the metabolic precursor involved in the chemical defect. Thus, heterozygotes for galactosemia and phenylketonuria respond to oral loads of galactose and phenylalanine, respectively, with higher plasma concentrations of these substances than observed in normal subjects.

Finally, carriers for an increasing number of diseases have been detected only by enzymatic assays or phenotypic appearance of cells in biopsy material. These techniques for carrier detection have usually been worked out and utilized in one laboratory or, in some instances, a few centers. Because of their complexity, they have not been employed for carrier detection in large populations.

PRENATAL DETECTION There is now considerable interest in the detection of genetic diseases in utero (see Chap. 58). More than 20 inherited metabolic disorders have been identified by chemical examination of amniotic fluid or enzymatic assays on amniotic fluid cells. The largest group of disorders so detected are those mucopolysaccharide or lipid storage diseases due to deficiency of particular lysosomal hydrolases, but a growing list of disorders of amino acid, organic acid, carbohydrate, and purine metabolism have been identified as well. A few inborn errors have been diagnosed by examination of fetal blood obtained by placental puncture or under fetoscopic control. Sickle-cell anemia, β thalassemia, Duchenne's muscular dystrophy, and hemophilia have been detected in this way.

GENETIC SCREENING

Genetic screening is the search in a population for persons possessing certain genotypes that are known to be associated with or to predispose to disease in the individuals or their descendants. As a research tool, screening can define the incidence of a particular genotype in the population and can be used to search for polymorphism. In the context of this discussion of inherited metabolic diseases, however, screening has two important applications: early identification of at-risk patients with treatable disease prior to onset of clinical symptoms and identification of at-risk couples who may benefit from appropriate genetic counseling. The prototypic example of the former application is neonatal screening for phenylketonuria. The features of this screening application include a relatively common disease (about 1:10,000 in Caucasians) with serious clinical consequences (severe mental retardation); clear evidence that institution of dietary phenylalanine restriction by age 30 days can return blood phenylalanine concentrations to values commensurate with normal or near normal development; and a simple, sensitive, and specific assay that can be performed in the neonatal period. More than 90 percent of neonates in North America and Western Europe are currently being screened for phenylketonuria using the bacterial inhibition assay. The human and monetary savings of this screening program have been enormous and have prompted extension to neonatal detection of other treatable diseases such as galactosemia, hypothyroidism, and homocystinuria. Such "secondary" prevention emphasizes the interaction between environment and heredity, and raises no serious ethical problems.

That statement, however, cannot be made with regard to the other screening application—identification of couples at risk for having offspring with untreatable (or nearly untreatable) disorders. The prototype is Tay-Sachs disease in Ashkenazi Jews. When two Ashkenazim marry, there is a 1:900 chance that both individuals are carriers for the Tay-Sachs gene. Theoretically, if all Ashkenazim were screened before marriage, if all pregnancies in at-risk couples were monitored by prenatal diagnosis and if all affected fetuses were aborted, the incidence of Tay-Sachs disease could be decreased to zero. However, mandatory screening is not a possibility, and compliance for voluntary testing is poor. Education, motivation, and effective follow-up are crucial to the success of such a venture. Similar programs have been mounted in the black community, where 1:100 couples are at risk for having children with sickle-cell anemia. Early results were not only ineffective but indeed counterproductive, owing to inadequate pretesting educational programs, misunderstanding about the difference between sickle trait and sickle-cell disease, and penalties for diagnosis levied by employers and insurance companies. This debacle points out the importance of ethical and social issues in such screening programs.

TREATMENT

A pessimistic approach to the treatment of inherited metabolic disorders is no longer warranted. Effective therapy is available for many of these disorders, particularly those in which the biochemical abnormalities have been defined. As more is learned about the mutational events responsible for specific disorders and about the chemical consequences of the mutations, other inborn errors will surely be controlled or modified by specific therapeutic programs. Two potential levels of treatment exist: the first is directed to means by which the basic genotype of the affected subject can be altered; the second aims to manipulate the environment so as to lessen or eradicate the harmful effect of the mutant phenotype. Successful therapy of the inborn errors has, thus far, been achieved only at the latter level. Although there is great interest in the possibility of genotypic alteration in humans, clinical application remains only a distant hope.

Several prerequisites are necessary for successful therapy. The correct diagnosis must be established. Some inborn errors such as phenylketonuria have harmless phenocopies that produce transient but similar biochemical abnormalities in the newborn. Whereas a low-phenylalanine diet mitigates the central nervous system complications of true phenylketonuria, such a diet may have catastrophic effects on the growth and development of a newborn with transient hyperphenylalaninemia due to delayed maturation of phenylalanine hydroxylase. Next, the physician must be convinced that the disorder is harmful and requires therapy. As stated earlier, some well-defined inborn errors such as pentosuria or iminoglycinuria do not appear to cause any significant clinical pathology and require no treatment. Finally, any therapeutic program must be continually scrutinized for evidence of harmful effects as well as for documentation of beneficial effects of therapy. These may be difficult parameters to dissociate. Penicillamine is an effective drug in Wilson's disease because of its ability to chelate copper; it is also efficacious in solubilizing and preventing the formation of cystine stones in cystinuria. Unfortunately, penicillamine also causes several untoward effects that limit its usefulness and demand careful medical follow-up.

MODALITIES EMPLOYED Phenotypic modification has been approached in many ways, depending on the nature of the defect and the timing of its deleterious effects. Both medical and surgical modalities have been employed, the range and experience with the former far exceeding the latter. Five medical modalities have been used and will be described briefly.

Avoidance For several disorders, clinical consequences can be mitigated or forestalled entirely by avoiding exposure to particular environmental influences. For example, the hemolytic episodes in patients with G6PD deficiency can be modified significantly by avoiding exposure to such drugs as primaquine or sulfa and to such foods as fava beans. Similarly, the prolonged apnea that occurs after succinylcholine administration in individuals deficient in pseudocholinesterase activity will not occur if this anesthetic is not used. Avoiding barbiturates and many other drugs in acute intermittent porphyria and cigarettes and other noxious fumes in α_1-antitrypsin deficiency is another example of this approach.

Restriction There are numerous disorders in which the phenotypic abnormalities result from the accumulation of a specific substrate or its metabolic by-products. Such disorders may respond to restriction of intake of the injurious substrate or its precursors, providing that the substrate is essential in the dietary sense and thus cannot be manufactured by the organism. Phenylketonuria, branched-chain ketoaciduria, homocystinuria, galactosemia, essential fructosuria, and Refsum's disease are examples of inborn errors that have been effectively treated in this way. Similarly, patients with the glucose-galactose malabsorption syndrome who develop profound diarrhea when fed lactose-containing foods do well if their source of dietary carbohydrate is changed. In contrast, dietary restriction is of no value in hyperprolinemia, hydroxyprolinemia, or citrullinemia, because these amino acids are synthesized extensively de novo. Even in those conditions in which dietary restriction is of value, doubt exists about the needed duration of such restriction. The injurious effects of excess phenylalanine, galactose, or branched-chain amino acids or keto acids may be limited to the early years of life when brain development and organization are proceeding at a maximal rate. If this is so, it should be possible to modify or even discontinue dietary restrictions after a given age. There is still considerable uncertainty regarding this matter, however, and more experience is needed before meaningful recommendations can be made.

Replacement Many disorders caused by the failure to make a specific protein or small-molecular-weight product have responded dramatically to replacement therapy. Hemophilia and agammaglobulinemia are examples of inborn errors that respond to parenteral protein replacement. These disorders are amenable to such replacement because the proteins involved normally circulate in abundance. In most instances, however, the missing protein or enzyme is confined to some intracellular organelle and is present in very small amounts. Replacement therapy in these instances may be difficult or impossible for three reasons: first, because large amounts of the protein are difficult to purify or synthesize; second, because parenteral administration of the protein will not increase its entry into the cell where it is required; and third, because the protein may initiate unfavorable immunologic reactions. Despite these drawbacks, attempts along these lines are being made. Pure human glucocerebrosidase has been administered intravenously to a few patients with Gaucher's disease. Tissue glucocerebroside content fell modestly in these patients, suggesting that some enzyme was being taken up by cells and was active intracellularly. More striking success has been reported in combined immunodeficiency due to adenosine deaminase deficit. Administration of frozen, irradiated, normal erythrocytes led to prolonged and dramatic improvement in immune status.

The clinical stigmata of a disorder may be related not to the protein whose synthesis is defective, but rather to the product of the blocked pathway. Cortisol synthesis is blocked in several variants of congenital adrenal hyperplasia, and replacement therapy with this steroid produces dramatic improvement. Similarly, administration of thyroid hormone and uridine reverses the serious clinical disturbances in familial goitrous cretinism and oroticaciduria, respectively.

Supplementation A growing list of metabolic disorders respond clinically and/or chemically to supplementary amounts of specific vitamins. Infants with seizures controlled only by supraphysiologic amounts of pyridoxine provided the first evidence for this phenomenon. Now more than 20 different disorders are known to respond to supplements of a single vitamin. Most of these disorders are caused by primary enzymatic disturbances that result in impaired affinity for cofactor. A growing list, however, are caused by primary abnormalities in the pathway of coenzyme or metabolite synthesis from vitamin precursors. Several disorders responsive to cobalamin (vitamin B_{12}), folate, or vitamin D can now be included in this category. Long-term experience with such vitamin supplements is limited but promising.

Drug administration Clinical disturbances in several inherited metabolic disorders result from deposition of a specific substance in one or more tissues. Successful treatment of these conditions may be achieved by enhancing the excretion of the stored chemical or by preventing its formation. Copper deposition in Wilson's disease can be controlled by drugs such as D-penicillamine, which chelates copper and markedly enhances its urinary excretion. The excretion of iron in hemochromatosis is augmented by phlebotomy and by the administration of desferrioxamine B. D-Penicillamine is also effective in solubilizing cystine calculi in cystinuria by reacting with cystine to form the more soluble cysteine-penicillamine disulfide. In this instance, the amount of cystine excreted is not changed, but its chemical form is altered in a therapeutically advantageous fashion. Uric acid deposition in gout responds both to drugs that enhance its excretion, such as sulfinpyrazone and probenecid, and to metabolic inhibitors like allopurinol that inhibit uric acid biosynthesis.

Surgical intervention At present, surgery is of limited value in the treatment of the inborn errors. Its use is restricted to a few conditions, such as gout, cystinuria, and oxalosis, in which nephrolithotomy or ureterolithotomy may provide important symptomatic relief while other programs of therapy are initiated. Several reports indicate that tissue transplants may be beneficial in some diseases. Thus, kidney transplants have been undertaken in cystinosis, hyperoxaluria, and Fabry's disease. Here the aim is restoration of renal function in conditions which produce progressive, and ultimately lethal, renal injury. Results have been variable. In hyperoxaluria, the transplanted kidney has been destroyed by oxalate deposition. In cystinosis, this has not occurred. A second, and quite different, goal of transplantation involves restitution of normal function. Thus, in combined immune deficiency, administration of fetal liver cells has produced clinical improvement. Similar beneficial results of bone marrow transplantation have been reported in other immune deficiency diseases. In the future, spleen transplantation may provide lasting benefit to patients with hemophilia or agammaglobulinemia by providing a constant source of antihemophilic globulin or gamma globulin, respectively. It is likewise possible that hepatic homografts may supply specific enzymes in phenylketonuria, branched-chain ketoaciduria, or the glycogen storage diseases and thus prevent the accumulation of toxic substances that lead to clinical abnormalities.

REFERENCES

HARRIS H: *The Principles of Human Biochemical Genetics,* 2d ed. Amsterdam, North-Holland, 1975

ROSENBERG LE: Inborn errors of metabolism, in *Metabolic Control and Disease,* 8th ed, PK Bondy, LE Rosenberg (eds). Philadelphia, Saunders, 1979

STANBURY JB et al: Inherited variation and metabolic abnormality, in *The Metabolic Basis of Inherited Disease,* 4th ed, JB Stanbury et al (eds). New York, McGraw-Hill, 1978

Disorders of amino acid metabolism

88

INHERITED DISORDERS OF AMINO ACID METABOLISM

LEON E. ROSENBERG

All polypeptides and proteins are polymers of 20 different amino acids. Eight of these, referred to as *essential,* cannot be synthesized by humans and must be obtained from dietary sources. The others are formed endogenously by a variety of chemical rearrangements. Although the vast bulk of the body's amino acids are "tied up" in proteins, small but critical pools of *free* amino acids are found intracellularly, and these pools are in equilibrium with extracellular reservoirs in plasma, cerebrospinal fluid, and the lumina of the gut and kidney. Physiologically, amino acids are more than mere "building blocks." Some (glycine, γ-aminobutyric acid) are neurotransmitters. Others (phenylalanine, tyrosine, tryptophan, glycine) are precursors of hormones, coenzymes, pigments, purines, or pyrimidines. Each has a unique and complicated degradative pathway by which its nitrogen and carbon components are used for the synthesis of other amino acids, carbohydrates, and lipids.

Current concepts of inherited metabolic diseases depend to a considerable degree on investigations of amino acid disorders. Three of the conditions analyzed by Garrod in his seminal descriptions of "inborn errors of metabolism" in the first decade of this century involved amino acids (alkaptonuria, albinism, and cystinuria). Although not appreciated at the time, these three conditions contain examples of the two general classes of "aminoacidopathies" now recognized: Enzymatic defects in amino acid catabolism and disorders of transmembrane transport. More than 70 inherited aminoacidopathies are now known, the catabolic defects (approximately 60) discussed in this and the following chapter far outnumbering the transport abnormalities (approximately 10) considered in Chap. 90. Each of these disorders is rare—their incidences range from 1 in 10,000 for phenylketonuria to 1 in 200,000 for alkaptonuria. Collectively, however, they occur in perhaps 1 in 500 to 1 in 1000 live births.

The salient features of inherited disorders of amino acid catabolism, arranged according to structural classes of the respective amino acids, are presented in Table 88-1. In general, these disorders are named for the compound which accumulates to highest concentration in blood (*-emias*) or urine (*-urias*). For many conditions the parent amino acid is found in excess; for others, products in the catabolic pathway accumulate. Which process takes place depends, of course, on the site of the enzymatic block, the reversibility of the reactions proximal to the lesion, and the existence of alternate pathways of metabolic "run-off." For some amino acids, such as the sulfur-containing or branched-chain molecules, defects at nearly each step in the catabolic pathway have been described. For others numerous gaps in our knowledge remain but are being filled rapidly as biochemical screening programs expand and interest in the field grows. Biochemical and genetic heterogeneity

abounds among the aminoacidopathies. At least four distinct forms of hyperphenylalaninemia, three variants of homocystinuria, and five types of methylmalonic acidemia are recognized—variants of both chemical and clinical interest.

The manifestations of these conditions differ widely as noted in Table 88-1. Some, such as sarcosinemia or hyperprolinemia, appear to produce no clinical consequences. At the other extreme, uniform neonatal lethality occurs in the untreated patient with complete deficiency of ornithine transcarbamylase or of branched-chain keto acid dehydrogenase. Central nervous system dysfunction, in the form of developmental retardation, seizures, alterations in sensorium, or behavioral disturbances, occurs in more than half of the disorders. Protein-induced vomiting, neurological dysfunction, and hyperammonemia occur in many disorders of urea cycle intermediates. Metabolic ketoacidosis often accompanied by hyperammonemia is a frequent presenting finding in the disorders of branched-chain amino acid metabolism. Occasional disorders produce focal tissue or organ involvement such as liver disease, renal failure, cutaneous abnormalities, or ocular lesions.

The clinical manifestations in many of these conditions can be prevented or mitigated significantly if diagnosis is achieved early and appropriate treatment (i.e., dietary protein or amino acid restriction or vitamin supplementation) is instituted promptly. For this reason, aminoacidopathies are screened for in mass newborn surveys which analyze blood or urine with an array of chemical and microbiological techniques. Once a presumptive diagnosis is made, confirmation can be provided by direct enzyme assay on extracts of leukocytes, erythrocytes, cultured fibroblasts, or liver. Several (cystinosis, branched-chain ketoaciduria, propionic acidemia, and methylmalonic acidemia) have been diagnosed in utero by chemical analysis on cultured amniotic fluid cells. The remainder of this and the subsequent chapter are focused on selected disorders that illustrate the problems posed by aminoacidopathies.

THE HYPERPHENYLALANINEMIAS

DEFINITION The hyperphenylalaninemias are a group of disorders (Table 88-1), each resulting from impaired conversion of phenylalanine to tyrosine. The most important is phenylketonuria, which in the untreated state is characterized by an increased concentration of phenylalanine in blood, increased concentrations of phenylalanine and its by-products (notably phenylpyruvate, phenylacetate, phenyllactate, and phenylacetylglutamine) in urine, and severe mental retardation.

ETIOLOGY AND PATHOGENESIS Each of the hyperphenylalaninemias results from reduced activity of the enzyme complex called *phenylalanine hydroxylase*. This system is found in appreciable amounts only in liver and kidney. Phenylalanine and molecular oxygen are substrates for the apoenzyme which requires a reduced pteridine, tetrahydrobiopterin, as a cofactor. Tyrosine and dihydrobiopterin are the products of this catalytic system, the latter being reconverted to tetrahydrobiopterin by a second enzyme, dihydropteridine reductase. In classic phenylketonuria activity of the hydroxylase apoenzyme is almost totally deficient. Benign hyperphenylalaninemia results from a less complete deficiency, whereas transient hyperphenylalaninemia (sometimes called transient phenylketonuria) is caused by a delayed maturation of the hydroxylase apoenzyme. In a variant of phenylketonuria, however, persistently impaired hydroxylating activity results not from abnormality in the apohydroxylase but from a lack of tetrahydrobiopterin due to virtually complete deficiency of the dihydropteridine reductase that regenerates it.

As a group the hyperphenylalaninemias occur in about 1 in 10,000 births. Classic phenylketonuria, which accounts for nearly half of these, is inherited as an autosomal recessive trait and is widely distributed among Caucasian ethnic groups and Orientals. It is rare in blacks. Phenylalanine hydroxylase activity in obligate heterozygotes is distinctly less than normal but higher than in homozygotes. Heterozygous carriers are clinically well but usually have slightly increased phenylalanine concentrations in postprandial blood plasma. Each of the other hyperphenylalaninemias also appears to be inherited as an autosomal recessive.

Phenylalanine accumulation in blood and urine and reduced tyrosine formation are direct consequences of the impaired hydroxylation. In untreated phenylketonuria and in dihydropteridine reductase deficiency, plasma concentrations of phenylalanine become sufficiently high (greater than 20 mg per 100 ml) to activate alternate pathways of metabolism and lead to formation of phenylpyruvate, phenylacetate, phenyllactate, and other derivatives that are rapidly cleared by the kidney and excreted in urine. Plasma concentrations of several other amino acids are moderately reduced, probably secondary to inhibition of gastrointestinal absorption or impairment of renal tubular reabsorption by the excess phenylalanine in body fluids. The severe brain damage observed in untreated phenylketonuria appears to be related to several consequences of phenylalanine accumulation: deprivation of other amino acids required for protein synthesis, impaired polyribosome formation or stabilization, reduced myelin synthesis, and inadequate formation of norepinephrine and serotonin. Phenylalanine is a competitive inhibitor of tyrosinase, a key enzyme in the pathway of melanin synthesis. This block plus reduced availability of the melanin precursor, tyrosine, accounts for the hypopigmentation of hair and skin.

CLINICAL MANIFESTATIONS No abnormalities are apparent at birth. Untreated children with classic phenylketonuria fail to attain early developmental milestones and demonstrate progressive impairment of cerebral function with IQ scores usually less than 50. Most require chronic institutionalization within a few years of birth because of the hyperactivity and seizures that accompany the severe mental retardation. Electroencephalogram abnormalities, "mousy" odor of skin, hair, and urine (due to phenylacetate accumulation), and a tendency to hypopigmentation and eczema complete the devastating clinical picture. In contrast, children who are detected at birth and treated promptly show none of these abnormalities. Children with transient hyperphenylalaninemia or with the benign variant are not at risk for any of the clinical consequences seen in untreated classic phenylketonuria. Those few children with dihydropteridine reductase deficiency, however, are the most unfortunate. Seizures appear early, followed by progressive cerebral and basal ganglia dysfunction (rigidity, chorea, spasms, hypotonia). Each has succumbed to secondary infection within a few years despite early diagnosis and standard treatment.

Occasionally, women with untreated classic phenylketonuria have reached adulthood and had children. More than 90 percent of the offspring are markedly retarded, and many have exhibited other congenital anomalies such as microcephaly, growth retardation, and congenital heart defects. Since these children are heterozygous, not homozygous for the phenylketonuria mutation, their clinical manifestations must be attributed to intrauterine damage produced by the elevated maternal concentrations of phenylalanine to which they have been exposed.

DIAGNOSIS Plasma phenylalanine concentrations may be normal at birth in all the hyperphenylalaninemias but rise rapidly after institution of protein feedings and are usually markedly abnormal by day 4. Since diagnosis and initiation of dietary treatment of classic phenylketonuria must be completed before 30 days of age if developmental retardation is to be prevented, most newborns in North America and Europe are screened by determinations of blood phenylalanine concentration using the Guthrie bacterial inhibition assay. Infants with abnormal values are followed up with more quantitative fluorometric or chromatographic assays. In classic phenylketonuria and in dihydropteridine reductase deficiency, values greater than 20 mg per 100 ml are regularly observed. In transient or benign hyperphenylalaninemia concentrations are usually lower but still above control values of less than 1 mg per 100 ml. Distinction of classic phenylketonuria from its benign variants depends on following serial plasma phenylalanine concentrations as a function of age and dietary restriction. In transient hyperphenylalaninemia plasma values return to normal within 3 to 4 months. In benign hyperphenylalaninemia dietary restriction produces a more profound fall in plasma phenylalanine than that observed in classic phenylketonuria. Deficiency of dihydropteridine reductase deficiency must be considered in any child with hyperphenylalaninemia who develops progressive neurological impairment despite prompt diagnosis and dietary treatment. Diagnostic confirmation of this variant can be achieved by enzyme assay on extracts of cultured fibroblasts.

TREATMENT Classic phenylketonuria was the first inherited metabolic disease in which it was demonstrated that mitigating the accumulation of the offending metabolite prevented the clinical abnormalities. This is accomplished by a special diet in which the bulk of protein is replaced by an artificial amino acid mixture low in phenylalanine. By supplementing this formula with a small amount of natural foods, an amount of dietary phenylalanine is provided that is sufficient for normal growth but is insufficient to produce markedly increased quantities of phenylalanine in blood. Ordinarily, plasma phenylalanine concentrations are maintained between 3 and 12 mg per 100 ml.

Until it is determined whether dietary treatment can be terminated safely after 6 to 8 years, dietary restriction in classic phenylketonuria should be continued indefinitely. The transient and benign forms of hyperphenylalaninemia do not require long-term dietary restriction. As mentioned earlier, children with dihydropteridine reductase deficiency deteriorate despite dietary phenylalanine restriction; attempts at pteridine cofactor replacement have been unrewarding.

THE HOMOCYSTINURIAS

The homocystinurias are three biochemically and clinically distinct disorders (Table 88-1), each characterized by increased concentration of the sulfur-containing amino acid, homocystine, in blood and urine. The most common form results from markedly reduced activity of cystathionine β-synthase, an enzyme catalyzing a key step in the transsulfuration pathway by which methionine is converted to cysteine. The two other forms are the result of impaired conversion of homocysteine to methionine, a reaction catalyzed by homocysteine: methyltetrahydrofolate methyltransferase and two essential cofactors methyltetrahydrofolate and methylcobalamin (methyl-vitamin B_{12}). Depending on the underlying disorder, some patients with each of the homocystinurias show chemical and, in some instances, clinical improvement following administration of specific vitamin supplements (pyridoxine, folate, or cobalamin).

CYSTATHIONINE β-SYNTHASE DEFICIENCY **Definition** Deficiency of this enzyme leads to increased concentrations of methionine and homocystine in body fluids and to decreased concentrations of cysteine and cystine. The clinical hallmark is dislocated optic lenses. Mental retardation, osteoporosis, and thrombotic vascular disease are frequent.

Etiology and pathogenesis The sulfur atom of the essential amino acid methionine is transferred ultimately to cysteine by a series of reactions designated as the transsulfuration pathway. In one of these steps, homocysteine condenses with serine to form cystathionine. This reaction is catalyzed by the pyridoxal phosphate-dependent enzyme, cystathionine β-synthase. Since 1964 more than 200 patients have been described with deficiency of this enzyme. The condition is common in Ireland (1 in 40,000 births) but rare elsewhere (less than 1 in 200,000 births).

Homocysteine and methionine accumulate in cells and body fluids; cysteine synthesis is impaired, resulting in reduced concentrations of this amino acid and its disulfide form, cystine. In approximately half of patients synthase activity in liver, brain, leukocytes, and cultured fibroblasts is absent. In the remaining patients, tissues retain 1 to 5 percent of normal activity. Heterozygous carriers of this autosomal recessive trait show no chemical abnormalities in body fluids but have reduced tissue synthase activity.

Homocysteine interferes with the normal cross-linking of collagen, an effect that likely plays an important role in the ocular, skeletal, and vascular complications.

Altered collagen in the suspensory ligament of the optic lens and in bone matrix may account for the dislocated lenses and osteoporosis. Similarly, interference with normal ground substance metabolism in vascular walls may predispose to the arterial and venous thrombotic diathesis. Recurrent cerebrovascular accidents secondary to thrombotic disease may account for the mental retardation, but direct chemical effects on cerebral cell metabolism have not been excluded.

Clinical manifestations More than 95 percent of patients have dislocated optic lenses. This abnormality usually appears by 3 to 4 years of age and often results in acute glaucoma as well as impaired visual acuity. Mental retardation occurs in less than 50 percent, often accompanied by ill-defined behavioral disturbances. Osteoporosis is a common radiological finding but rarely causes clinical disease. Life-threatening vascular complications, probably initiated by damage to vascular endothelium, are the major cause of morbidity and mortality. Occlusion of coronary, renal, and cerebral arteries with attendant tissue infarction can occur during the first decade of life. Many patients die of vascular disease before age 30. These vascular complications seem to be exacerbated by angiographic procedures.

TABLE 88-1
Inherited disorders of amino acid catabolism

Amino acid(s) affected	Disorder or condition	Enzyme defect
AROMATIC—HETEROCYCLIC		
Phenylalanine	Classic phenylketonuria	Phenylalanine hydroxylase
	Benign hyperphenylalaninemia	Phenylalanine hydroxylase
	Transient hyperphenylalaninemia	Phenylalanine hydroxylase
	Variant phenylketonuria	Dihydropteridine reductase
Tyrosine	Hypertyrosinemia	Tyrosine aminotransferase (cytosol)
	Tyrosinosis	Tyrosine aminotransferase (?)
	Hereditary tyrosinemia	Hydroxyphenylpyruvate oxidase (?)
	Alkaptonuria	Homogentisic acid oxidase
	Albinism (oculocutaneous)	Tyrosinase
	Albinism (ocular)	Unknown
Tryptophan	Tryptophanuria	Tryptophan pyrrolase
	Xanthurenic aciduria	Kynureninase
Histidine	Histidinemia	Histidine-ammonia lyase
	Urocanic aciduria	Urocanase
	Formiminoglutamic aciduria	Formiminotransferase
GLYCINE-IMINO ACIDS		
Glycine	Hyperglycinemia	Glycine cleavage
	Sarcosinemia	Sarcosine dehydrogenase
	Hyperoxaluria (type I)	α-Ketoglutarate: glyoxylate carboligase
	Hyperoxaluria (type II)	D-Glyceric acid dehydrogenase
Imino acids	Hyperprolinemia (type I)	proline oxidase
	Hyperprolinemia (type II)	Δ'-Pyrroline dehydrogenase
	Hyperhydroxyprolinemia	Hydroxyproline reductase
	Iminopeptiduria	Prolidase
SULFUR-CONTAINING		
Methionine	Hypermethioninemia	Methionine adenosyltransferase
Homocystine	Homocystinuria	Cystathione β-synthase
	Homocystinuria	5,10-Methylenetetrahydrofolate reductase
	Homocystinuria and methylmalonic acidemia (cbl C, D)‡	Cobalamin (vitamin B_{12}) reductase (cytosol) (?)
Cystathionine	Cystathioninuria	Cystathionase
Cystine	Cystinosis	Unknown
S-Sulfo-L-cysteine	S-Sulfo-L-cysteine, sulfite, and thiosulfaturia	Sulfite oxidase
CATIONIC		
Lysine	Hyperlysinemia (type I)	Lysine dehydrogenase
	Hyperlysinemia (type II)	Lysine: α-ketoglutarate reductase
	Saccharopinuria	Saccharopine dehydrogenase
	Hydroxylysinemia	Unknown
	Pipecolic acidemia	Unknown
	α-Ketoadipic aciduria	α-Ketoadipic acid decarboxylase

Clinical manifestations*

Mental retardation	Neuropsychiatric dysfunction	Protein intolerance	Metabolic ketoacidosis	Ammonia intoxication	Other	Inheritance pattern†
+	+	−	−	−	Hypopigmented skin and hair, eczema	AR
−	−	−	−	−		AR
−	−	−	−	−		(AR)
+	+	−	−	−		(AR)
+	−	−	−	−	Palmar keratosis, corneal dystrophy	(AR)
−	−	−	−	−	Myasthenia gravis	?
−	−	−	−	−	Cirrhosis, hepatic failure, renal tubular dysfunction	AR
−	−	−	−	−	Ochronosis, arthritis	AR
−	−	−	−	−	Hypopigmentation of hair, skin, and optic fundus	AR
−	−	−	−	−	Hypopigmentation of optic fundus	XL
+	+	−	−	−	Photosensitive skin rash	AR
?	−	−	−	−		?
±	±	−	−	−	Hearing and speech deficit	AR
+	+	−	−	−		?
?	+	−	−	−		(AR)
+	+	−	−	−		AR
−	−	−	−	−		AR
−	−	−	−	−	Renal failure	AR
−	−	−	−	−	Calcium oxalate nephrolithiasis, renal failure	AR
−	−	−	−	−		AR
−	−	−	−	−		AR
−	−	−	−	−		AR
+	−	−	−	−	Crusting, erythematous, ecchymotic dermatitis	AR
−	−	−	−	−		?
±	±	−	−	−	Dislocated lenses, osteoporosis, thrombotic vascular disease	AR
±	±	−	−	−		(AR)
±	±	−	−	−	Megalobastic anemia	(AR)
±	−	−	−	−		AR
−	−	−	−	−	Fanconi syndrome, renal failure, photophobia	AR
+	+	−	−	−	Dislocated lenses	AR
−	+	+	−	+		?
±	±	−	−	−		AR
−	−	−	−	−		?
+	−	−	−	−		(AR)
+	+	−	−	−	Hepatomegaly, dysplastic optic disks	?
±	±	−	−	−		?

* +, regularly present; ±, sometimes present; −, absent; ?, uncertain; all designations refer to manifestations in untreated disorder.
† AR, autosomal recessive; XL, X-linked; (AR), probably autosomal recessive.
‡ Designations in parentheses refer to complementation groups assigned by genetic analysis with cultured cells.

Diagnosis The cyanide-nitroprusside test is a simple way of demonstrating increased excretion of sulfhydryl-containing compounds in urine. Since cystine and *S*-sulfocysteine also give a positive test, other disorders of sulfur metabolism must be excluded, but this is usually simple on clinical grounds. Distinction of cystathionine β-synthase deficiency from other causes of homocystinuria can usually be accomplished by measurements of plasma methionine, which tend to be markedly increased in synthase-deficient patients and normal or low in those with impaired methionine formation (see below). Diagnostic confirmation depends on measurements of synthase activity in tissue extracts.

Treatment As with classic phenylketonuria, effective treatment depends on early diagnosis. A few infants diagnosed in the newborn period have been treated successfully with methionine-restricted, cystine-supplemented diets. Their clinical course has, thus far, been benign compared with that of untreated affected siblings. In approximately half of patients, oral supplements of pyridoxine (25 to 500 mg per day) produce a marked fall in plasma and urinary methionine and homocystine and an increase in cystine concentration in body fluids. This effect probably reflects a modest increase in synthase activity in cells of patients in whom the enzymatic defect is characterized by either reduced affinity for cofactor or accelerated degradation of mutant enzyme. Since such vitamin supplementation is simple and apparently harmless, it should be tried in all patients. There are no reports of the effect of pyridoxine supplementation therapy that has been initiated soon after birth.

5,10-METHYLENETETRAHYDROFOLATE REDUCTASE DEFICIENCY **Definition** In this form of homocystinuria, methionine concentrations in body fluids are normal or decreased because deficiency of 5,10-methylenetetrahydrofolate reductase leads to impaired synthesis of 5-methyltetrahydrofolate, a cofactor in the enzymatic formation of methionine from homocysteine. Central nervous system dysfunction occurs in most patients.

Etiology and pathogenesis 5-Methyltetrahydrofolate:homocysteine methyltransferase catalyzes the conversion of homocysteine to methionine. The methyl group transferred in this reaction comes from 5-methyltetrahydrofolate, which is converted to tetrahydrofolate in the process. 5-Methyltetrahydrofolate, in turn, is synthesized enzymatically from 5,10-methylenetetrahydrofolate by another folate cycle enzyme, 5,10-methylenetetrahydrofolate reductase. Thus, reductase activity controls both methionine synthesis and tetrahydrofolate generation. This series of reactions is critical to normal DNA and RNA synthesis. A primary defect in the reductase activity results, secondarily, in deficient methyltransferase activity and impaired conversion of homocysteine to methionine. Although the mechanism of the central nervous system dysfunction is unknown, methionine deficiency and impaired nucleic acid synthesis are likely explanations. The disorder appears to be inherited as an autosomal recessive trait.

Clinical manifestations Fewer than 10 children with homocystinuria due to reductase deficiency have been reported. The most severely affected have presented with profound developmental retardation and cerebral atrophy early in life. Others manifested prominent behavioral disturbances (catatonia) during the second decade. In the remainder, mild retardation has

TABLE 88-1 *(continued)*
Inherited disorders of amino acid catabolism

Amino acid(s) affected	Disorder or condition	Enzyme defect
CATIONIC *(continued)*		
	Glutaric aciduria (type I)	Glutaryl CoA dehydrogenase
	Glutaric aciduria (type II)	Medium-chain acyl CoA dehydrogenase (?)
Ornithine	Hyperornithinemia (type I)	Ornithine decarboxylase
	Hyperornithinemia (type II)	Ornithine aminotransferase
UREA CYCLE		
Carbamyl-phosphate	Hyperammonemia (type I)	Carbamylphosphate synthetase I
Ornithine	Hyperammonemia (type II)	Ornithine transcarbamylase
Citrulline	Citrullinemia	Argininosuccinate synthetase
Arginino-succinic acid	Argininosuccinic aciduria	Argininosuccinase
Arginine	Argininemia	Arginase
BRANCHED-CHAIN		
Valine	Hypervalinemia	Valine aminotransferase
Leucine, isoleucine	Hyperleucine-isoleucinemia	Leucine-isoleucine aminotransferase
Valine, leucine, isoleucine	Classic branched-chain ketoaciduria	Branched-chain ketoacid dehydrogenase
	Intermittent branched-chain ketoaciduria	Branched-chain ketoacid dehydrogenase
Leucine	Isovaleric acidemia	Isovaleryl CoA dehydrogenase
	β-Methylcrotonyl glycinuria	β-Methylcrotonyl CoA carboxylase
	β-Hydroxy-β-methylglutaric aciduria	β-Hydroxy-β-methylglutaryl CoA lyase
Isoleucine, valine	α-Methylacetoacetic aciduria	β-Ketothiolase
	Propionic acidemia (pcc A, B, C)‡	Propionyl CoA carboxylase
	Propionic acidemia (bio)‡	Holocarboxylase synthetase (?)
	Methylmalonic acidemia (mut)‡	Methylmalonyl CoA mutase
	Methylmalonic acidemia (cbl A)‡	Cobalamin (vitamin B_{12}) reductase (mitochondrial) (?)
	Methylmalonic acidemia (cbl B)‡	Cobalamin (vitamin B_{12}): ATP adenosyltransferase
DICARBOXYLIC		
Glutamic acid	Glutathionemia	γ-Glutamyl-transpeptidase
	5-Oxoprolinuria	Glutathione synthetase

been observed. Presumably the severity of the clinical manifestations reflects the severity of the reductase deficiency.

Diagnosis and treatment The combination of increased concentrations of homocystine in body fluids with normal or decreased concentrations of methionine should suggest this entity. Serum folate concentrations are low in some patients. Confirmation requires direct reductase assays in tissue extracts (brain, liver, cultured fibroblasts). Although therapeutic experience is limited, one teen-age girl with a catatonic psychosis responded dramatically, both chemically and clinically, to fo-

Clinical manifestations*						Inheritance pattern†
Mental retardation	Neuropsychiatric dysfunction	Protein intolerance	Metabolic ketoacidosis	Ammonia intoxication	Other	
−	+	−	−	−		AR
−	+	−	−	−	Hypoglycemia	?
+	+	+	−	+		(AR)
−	−	−	−	−	Gyrate atrophy of choroid and retina	AR
+	+	+	−	+		AR
±	+	+	−	+		XL
+	+	+	−	+		AR
+	+	+	−	+		AR
+	+	+	−	+		AR
+	+	+	−	−		?
+	+	+	−	−		?
+	+	+	+	−	"Maple syrup" odor	AR
±	−	+	+	−		AR
±	±	+	+	−	"Sweaty feet" odor	AR
+	+	−	+	−	"Cat's urine" odor	AR
−	+	+	+	−		?
±	±	+	+	+		AR
±	±	+	+	+		AR
+	±	+	+	−		?
±	±	+	+	+		AR
±	±	+	+	+		AR
±	±	+	+	+		AR
+	−	−	−	−		(?)
±	±	±	+	−		AR

late supplements (5 to 10 mg per day). When the folate was withdrawn, behavior worsened. This observation suggests that early diagnosis followed by folate supplementation may forestall neurological or psychiatric disturbances.

DEFICIENCY OF COBALAMIN (VITAMIN B$_{12}$) COENZYME SYNTHESIS **Definition** This form of homocystinuria also reflects impaired conversion of homocysteine to methionine. The primary defect is in the synthesis of methylcobalamin, a cobalamin (vitamin B$_{12}$) coenzyme required by methyltetrahydrofolate:homocysteine methyltransferase. Methylmalonic acid accumulates in body fluids as well because synthesis of a second coenzyme, adenosylcobalamin, required for isomerization of methylmalonyl coenzyme A (CoA) to succinyl CoA is also impaired.

Etiology and pathogenesis As with 5,10-methylenetetrahydrofolate reductase deficiency, this disorder involves remethylation of homocysteine. The primary defect concerns deficient synthesis of cobalamin coenzymes from precursor vitamin. Since methylcobalamin is required for methyl-group transfer from methyltetrahydrofolate to homocysteine, impaired cobalamin metabolism leads to deficient methyltransferase activity. The precise defect responsible for impaired synthesis of methylcobalamin is unknown but involves some early step in lysosomal or cytosolic activation of the vitamin precursor. Somatic cell genetic studies indicate that two distinct lesions underlie deficient coenzyme formation, each of which appears to be inherited as an autosomal recessive trait.

Clinical manifestations The first reported patient died of infection at age 6 weeks following severely arrested development. Clinical manifestations in the other affected children vary: two had megaloblastic anemia and pancytopenia; three had significant spinocerebellar neurological impairment; one exhibited little clinical abnormality.

Diagnosis and treatment Homocystinuria, hypomethioninemia, and methylmalonic aciduria are the chemical hallmarks. These findings may also be present in juvenile or adult onset pernicious anemia in which intestinal cobalamin absorption is impaired. Measurement of serum cobalamin concentrations, low in pernicious anemia and normal in patients with defective conversion of cobalamin vitamin to coenzymes, helps in the differential diagnosis. Definitive diagnosis depends on demonstrating impaired coenzyme synthesis in cultured cells. Treatment of affected children with cobalamin supplements (1 to 2 mg per day) shows promise: Homocystine and methylmalonate excretion fall to near normal values; the hematologic and neurological deficits have also lessened to a more variable degree.

REFERENCES

KNOX WE: Phenylketonuria, in *The Metabolic Basis of Inherited Disease,* 3d ed, JB Stanbury et al (eds). New York, McGraw-Hill, 1972, pp 266–295

KOCH R et al: Phenylalaninemia and phenylketonuria, in *Heritable Disorders of Amino Acid Metabolism,* WL Nyhan (ed). New York, Wiley, 1974, pp 109–140

MCKUSICK VA: Homocystinuria, in *Heritable Disorders of Connective Tissue,* 4th ed. St. Louis, Mosby, 1972, pp 224–281

MUDD SH, LEVY HL: Disorders of transsulfuration, in *The Metabolic Basis of Inherited Disease,* 4th ed, JB Stanbury et al (eds). New York, McGraw-Hill, 1978, pp 458–503

NYHAN WL (ed): *Heritable Disorders of Amino Acid Metabolism.* New York, Wiley, 1974

ROSENBERG LE, SCRIVER CR: Disorders of amino acid metabolism, in *Metabolic Control and Disease,* 8th ed, PK Bondy, LE Rosenberg (eds). Philadelphia, Saunders (in press)

———, TANAKA K: Disorders of amino acid and organic acid metabolism, in *The Year in Metabolism 1977,* N Freinkel (ed). New York, Plenum, 1978, pp 219–246

89
STORAGE DISEASES OF AMINO ACID METABOLISM

LEON E. ROSENBERG

A number of inherited metabolic disorders are characterized by deposition or storage of particular metabolites in tissues. In most, storage reflects impaired degradation of the substance in question; in others, the mechanism is unknown. Many storage diseases involve large molecules such as glycogen, sphingolipids, mucolipids, cholesterol esters, and mucopolysaccharides (see Chaps. 97, 100, and 101); in others, metals such as iron and copper are deposited (see Chaps. 94 and 95). Finally, there is a group of storage diseases in which relatively small organic molecules are deposited. These include gout (see Chap. 92) and a group of disorders of amino acid metabolism.

ALKAPTONURIA

DEFINITION Alkaptonuria is a rare disorder of tyrosine catabolism. Deficiency of the enzyme homogentisic acid oxidase leads to excretion of large amounts of homogentisic acid in urine and to accumulation of oxidized homogentisic acid pigment in connective tissues (ochronosis). After many years ochronosis produces a distinctive form of degenerative arthritis.

ETIOLOGY AND PATHOGENESIS Homogentisic acid is a normal intermediate formed during the catabolism of tyrosine to fumarate and acetoacetate. Activity of homogentisic acid oxidase, the enzyme that catalyzes the opening of the phenolic ring yielding maleylacetoacetic acid, is virtually absent in liver and kidney of patients with alkaptonuria, and homogentisic acid accumulates in cells and body fluids. Patients have minimally increased concentrations of homogentisic acid in blood because it is rapidly cleared by the kidney. As much as 3 to 7 g homogentisic acid may be excreted in the urine per day, but this is of little pathophysiologic significance. However, homogentisic acid and its oxidized polymers bind to collagen, leading to the progressive deposition of a grey to bluish black pigment. The mechanism(s) by which degenerative changes develop in cartilage, intervertebral disk, and other connective tissues is unknown but may involve direct chemical irritation or inhibition of one or more enzyme systems involved in normal connective tissue metabolism.

Alkaptonuria was the first human disease shown to be inherited as an autosomal recessive trait. Affected homozygotes occur with a frequency no greater than 1 in 200,000. Heterozygous carriers are clinically well and excrete no homogentisic acid in urine, even after loading doses of tyrosine.

CLINICAL MANIFESTATIONS Alkaptonuria often goes unrecognized until middle life when degenerative joint disease appears in the majority. Prior to this time the tendency of the patient's urine to darken on standing may go unnoticed, as may slight discoloration of the sclerae and external ears. The latter manifestations of homogentisic acid deposition in tissue are generally the earliest external evidence of the disorder with appearance after age 20 to 30. Foci of grey-brown scleral pigment and generalized darkening of the concha, antihelix, and, finally, helix of the ear are typical. Ear cartilages may feel irregular and thickened. *Ochronotic arthritis* is heralded by pain, stiffness, and some limitation of motion of the hips, knees, and shoulders. Intermittent periods of acute arthritis, which may resemble rheumatoid arthritis, occur, but small joints are usually spared. Limitation of motion and ankylosis of the lumbosacral spine are common late manifestations. Pigmentation of heart valves, larynx, tympanic membranes, and skin occurs, and occasional patients develop pigmented renal or prostatic calculi. An increased incidence of degenerative cardiovascular disease has been reported in older patients, but a clear relationship between these findings and ochronosis has not been established.

DIAGNOSIS A patient whose urine darkens to blackness on standing must be suspected of having alkaptonuria, but because of modern plumbing conditions this finding is not often observed. The diagnosis is usually made from the triad of degenerative arthritis, ochronotic pigmentation, and urine which turns black upon alkalinization. Homogentisic acid in urine may be identified presumptively by other tests: upon addition of ferric chloride, a purple-black color is observed; treatment with Benedict's reagent yields a brown color; and addition of a saturated silver nitrate solution produces an immediate black color. These screening tests can be confirmed by chromatographic, enzymatic, or spectrophotometric determinations of homogentisic acid. X-rays of the lumbar spine are virtually pathognomonic. They show degeneration and dense calcification of the intervertebral disks and narrowing of the intervertebral spaces.

TREATMENT There is no specific treatment for ochronotic arthritis. It is conceivable that joint manifestations could be mitigated if homogentisic acid accumulation and deposition could be curbed by dietary restriction of phenylalanine and tyrosine, but the long course of the disease has discouraged such therapeutic attempts. Since ascorbic acid impedes oxidation and polymerization of homogentisic acid in vitro, its use has been suggested as a possible means of decreasing pigment formation and deposition. The efficacy of this form of treatment has not been established. Symptomatic treatment is similar to that for osteoarthritis (Chap. 361).

CYSTINOSIS

DEFINITION Cystinosis is a rare disorder characterized by the intralysosomal accumulation of free cystine in body tissues. This results in the appearance of cystine crystals in the cornea, conjunctiva, bone marrow, lymph nodes, leukocytes, and internal organs. Three clinical forms have been identified: an infantile (nephropathic) form leading to the Fanconi syndrome and renal insufficiency in the first decade; a juvenile (intermediate) form in which renal disease becomes manifest during the second decade; and an adult (benign) form characterized by deposition of cystine in the cornea but not in the kidney.

ETIOLOGY AND PATHOGENESIS The basic defect has not been identified. Numerous studies of enzymes concerned with cystine metabolism have not yielded any consistent abnormality, nor have investigations of cystine or cysteine transport. The cystine content of tissues in the infantile form may be more than 100 times normal, that in the adult form more than 30 times normal. Intracellular cystine appears to be located only in lysosomes and does not exchange with other intracellular or extracellular pools of this amino acid. Neither plasma nor urinary concentrations of cystine are particularly elevated.

The extent of cystine crystal deposition varies considerably from patient to patient, depending on both the form of the disease and the methods used to prepare pathological specimens. In the kidney cystine accumulation causes renal insufficiency in the infantile and juvenile forms. The kidneys are pale and shrunken, the capsule is adherent, and the corticomedullary junction is obscured. Microscopically, nephron organization is interrupted, glomeruli are hyalinized, connective tissue is increased, and the normal epithelium of the tubules is replaced by cuboidal cells. Narrowing and shortening of the proximal tubule produces the so-called "swan neck deformity" now known not to be specific for cystinosis. Patchy depigmentation of the peripheral retina occurs in the infantile and juvenile forms. This retinal degeneration is to be distinguished from the deposition of cystine crystals in the ocular conjunctiva or uvea.

Each form of cystinosis appears to be inherited as an autosomal recessive trait. Obligate heterozygotes have intracellular cystine contents intermediate between those of normal persons and affected patients but are free of clinical abnormalities.

CLINICAL MANIFESTATIONS In the infantile form abnormalities are usually apparent by 4 to 6 months of age. Growth retardation, vomiting, fever, vitamin D–resistant rickets, polyuria, dehydration, and metabolic acidosis are prominent. Generalized proximal tubular dysfunction (the Fanconi syndrome)

leads to hyperphosphaturia and hypophosphatemia, renal glycosuria, generalized aminoaciduria, hypouricemia, and often hypokalemia. Pyelonephritis is common and may contribute, along with interstitial fibrosis, to progressive glomerular insufficiency. Death due to uremia or intercurrent infection usually occurs before age 10. Ocular manifestations are also prominent. Photophobia is usually demonstrable within the first few years of life due to cystine deposits in the cornea, and retinal degeneration may appear even earlier.

In contrast, patients with the adult form manifest only ocular abnormalities. Photophobia, headache, and burning or itching of the eyes are major complaints. Glomerular and tubular function and the integrity of the retina are preserved. The findings in the juvenile variant fall between these extremes. These patients have both ocular and renal manifestations, but the latter do not become significant until the second decade. The renal lesion, albeit milder than that seen in the infantile form, eventually leads to renal insufficiency.

DIAGNOSIS Cystinosis must be considered in any child with vitamin D–resistant rickets, the Fanconi syndrome, or glomerular insufficiency. Hexagonal or rectangular cystine crystals are most easily detected in the cornea (by slit-lamp examination), in unstained preparations of leukocytes from peripheral blood or bone marrow, or in biopsies of rectal mucosa. Diagnosis can be confirmed by quantitative determination of cystine in extracts of peripheral blood leukocytes or cultured fibroblasts. The infantile form of cystinosis has been diagnosed prenatally by the demonstration of vastly increased cystine content in cultured amniotic fluid cells.

TREATMENT The adult form of cystinosis is benign and requires no treatment. Symptomatic treatment of renal disease in patients with the infantile or juvenile form of cystinosis does not differ from that of other forms of chronic renal insufficiency: maintenance of adequate fluid intake to prevent dehydration; administration of sodium citrate or sodium bicarbonate to correct the metabolic acidosis; and ingestion of supplementary calcium, phosphate, and vitamin D to heal the rickets. Such measures are critical in maintaining growth, development, and well-being in affected children for a time. Two types of more specific therapy have been attempted without much success. Cystine-restricted diets are difficult to prepare and have not prevented progression of renal disease. Likewise, the use of sulfhydryl reagents (D-penicillamine, dimercaprol) and reducing agents (vitamin C) have yielded no long-term benefit.

The most promising form of therapy for nephropathic cystinosis is renal transplantation. More than 20 affected children with end-stage renal disease have been so treated. Those patients who tolerated the procedure and did not develop immunologic problems have shown return of kidney function toward normal. Several patients have been followed for 3 or more years after transplantation. The transplanted kidneys have not developed the functional abnormalities typical of cystinosis (i.e., the Fanconi syndrome or glomerular insufficiency). They may, however, reaccumulate some cystine, apparently owing to migration of interstitial or mesangial cells from the host. This experience justifies offering renal transplantation to patients with terminal renal failure.

PRIMARY HYPEROXALURIA

DEFINITION Primary hyperoxaluria is the designation for two rare disorders characterized by chronic excessive urinary excretion of oxalic acid and by calcium oxalate nephrolithiasis and nephrocalcinosis. Typically, patients with either form develop renal insufficiency early in life and die of uremia. At postmortem examination, calcium oxalate deposits are generally widespread in renal and extrarenal tissues, a condition referred to as *oxalosis*.

ETIOLOGY AND PATHOGENESIS Since both types of primary hyperoxaluria result from increased oxalate synthesis and since glyoxylate is the only significant precursor of oxalate in humans, the metabolic basis for the primary hyperoxalurias logically involves pathways of glyoxylate metabolism. In type I hyperoxaluria, urinary excretion of oxalate, the oxidized form of glyoxylate, and glycolic acid, the reduced form, is increased. The excessive synthesis of these substances in this condition results from a block in one of the routes of metabolism of glyoxylate. Activity of the cytosolic enzyme α-ketoglutarate:glyoxylate carboligase, which catalyzes the formation of α-hydroxy-β-ketoadipic acid, is markedly reduced in extracts of liver, kidney, and spleen. The resulting expansion of the glyoxylate pool behind this metabolic block leads to oxidation of glyoxylate to oxalate and to reduction of glyoxylate to glycolate. Each of these 2-carbon acids is then excreted in excess in the urine. In type II hyperoxaluria, L-glyceric acid is excreted in excess along with oxalate. In this condition, activity of D-glyceric acid dehydrogenase, an enzyme that catalyzes the reduction of hydroxypyruvate to D-glyceric acid in the catabolic pathway of serine metabolism, is absent in leukocytes (and presumably other tissues). The accumulated hydroxypyruvate is instead reduced by lactic dehydrogenase to the L-isomer of glycerate, which is excreted in the urine. Apparently the reduction of hydroxypyruvate is coupled in some way to the oxidation of glyoxylate to oxalate, thus causing the formation of increased oxalate.

Both disorders appear to be inherited as autosomal recessive traits. Heterozygotes are asymptomatic. Partial enzyme deficiency has been observed in heterozygotes for type II hyperoxaluria, but no studies with type I heterozygotes have been reported.

The pathogenesis of stone formation, nephrocalcinosis, and oxalosis relates directly to the insolubility of calcium oxalate. Extrarenal deposits of oxalate have been most widely reported in the heart, walls of arteries and veins, male urogenital tract, and bone.

CLINICAL MANIFESTATIONS Nephrolithiasis and oxalosis may become manifest during the first year of life. Most patients experience initial symptoms of renal colic or hematuria between ages 2 and 10 and succumb to uremia before age 20. With the onset of uremia, patients may develop severe peripheral arterial spasm and necrosis with resulting vascular insufficiency. In patients with delayed onset of symptoms, survival to age 50 or 60 has been reported, despite recurrent attacks of nephrolithiasis.

DIAGNOSIS Oxalate excretion in normal children or adults is less than 60 mg per 1.73 m² per day. Patients with type I or type II hyperoxaluria generally excrete two to four times this amount. Distinction between the two types of primary hyperoxaluria depends on measurements of the other organic acids that identify them: glycolic acid in type I and L-glyceric acid in type II. Since patients with pyridoxine deficiency or chronic ileal disease may excrete excessive amounts of oxalate, these conditions must be excluded.

TREATMENT There is no satisfactory treatment for primary hyperoxaluria. Urinary oxalate concentration can be reduced by increasing the urinary flow rate, but success is transient. Large doses of pyridoxine (100 mg per day) may reduce urinary oxalate in some patients, but long-term effects are not dramatic. A diet high in phosphate content seems to reduce the frequency of attacks of renal colic, but oxalate excretion is unaffected. Finally, renal transplantation has been attempted several times, but in each instance renal function was lost because of calcium oxalate deposition in the transplanted kidney.

REFERENCES

BOQUIST L et al: Primary oxalosis. Am J Med 54:673, 1973

LADU NB: Alcaptonuria, in *The Metabolic Basis of Inherited Disease*, 4th ed, JB Stanbury et al (eds). New York, McGraw-Hill, 1978, pp 268–282

O'BRIEN W et al: Biochemical, pathologic and clinical aspects of alcaptonuria, ochronosis and ochronotic arthropathy. Am J Med 34:813, 1963

SCHNEIDER JA et al: Cystinosis and the Fanconi syndrome, in *The Metabolic Basis of Inherited Disease*, 4th ed, JB Stanbury et al (eds). New York, McGraw-Hill, 1978, pp 1660–1682

SCHULMAN JD (ed): *Cystinosis*, US Department of Health, Education, and Welfare Publication (NIH) 72–249, 1972

WILLIAMS HE, SMITH LH JR: Primary hyperoxaluria, in *The Metabolic Basis of Inherited Disease*, 4th ed, JB Stanbury et al (eds). New York, McGraw-Hill, 1978, pp 182–204

90

INHERITED DEFECTS OF MEMBRANE TRANSPORT

LEON E. ROSENBERG
ELIZABETH M. SHORT

The passage of certain large and small molecules across mammalian plasma cell membranes depends on the existence of specific transport systems that owe their specificity to a variety of membrane receptor and "carrier" proteins. These specific membrane constituents recognize individual substrates or a group of structurally related ones and catalyze their transmembrane movement by mechanisms poorly understood. The disorders considered in this chapter have three features in common: each is characterized by a specific defect in the transport of one or more compounds; each is inherited as a dominant or recessive, implying that a single genetic locus is involved; and each is presumed to reflect a primary alteration in a specific membrane protein. Many of these defects have been well characterized physiologically, but in none has the putative mutant transport protein been isolated.

More than 20 inherited disorders of membrane transport have been described in humans (Table 90-1). Most affect the gut and/or kidney only. Numerous classes of substrates are represented, including amino acids, hexoses, cations, anions, vitamins, and water. Some are discussed elsewhere in this text. Those impairing the transport of amino acids, hexoses, urate, and chloride are discussed here as examples of the range and significance of the abnormalities encountered.

DISORDERS OF AMINO ACID TRANSPORT

As noted in Table 90-1, 10 distinct disorders of amino acid transport have been described. Five of these (cystinuria, dibasicaminoaciduria, Hartnup disease, iminoglycinuria, and dicarboxylicaminoaciduria) show transport abnormalities for groups of structurally related amino acids, thereby implying the existence of group-specific membrane receptors or carriers. With the exception of iminoglycinuria and dicarboxylicaminoaciduria, these defects have important clinical consequences. The remaining five disorders affect the transport of only one amino acid, implying the existence of substrate-specific as well as group-specific transport systems. Each of these conditions affects transport in the kidney, gut, or both; none has been shown to alter transport in other tissues.

CYSTINURIA **Definition** Cystinuria is the most common inborn error of amino acid transport. It is characterized by excessive urinary excretion of the dibasic amino acids: lysine, arginine, ornithine, and cystine. This aminoaciduria results from impaired tubular reabsorption of these amino acids. A similar transport defect exists in the intestinal mucosa. Because cystine is the least soluble of the naturally occurring amino acids, its overexcretion predisposes to the formation of renal, ureteral, and bladder calculi. Such calculi are responsible for the signs and symptoms in affected patients.

Etiology and pathogenesis Massive excretion of cystine and the other dibasic amino acids occurs only in classic cystinuria. The disorder, inherited as an autosomal recessive trait, is believed to result from alterations in a membrane carrier protein essential for transport of this group of amino acids in the apical brush border of proximal renal tubule and small intestinal cells. Renal clearance studies indicate that the putative protein has a greater affinity for ornithine and arginine than for lysine and cystine. Although the endogenous renal clearance of all four amino acids is increased in homozygotes, the presence of some residual transport capacity for these compounds plus the existence of three other disorders marked by selective excretion of members of this group (dibasicaminoaciduria, hypercystinuria, lysinuria) argues for the existence of at least three discrete renal transport systems for these amino acids: one for each amino acid alone; one shared by lysine, arginine, and ornithine; and one for all four amino acids.

Whereas urinary excretion patterns and renal clearance abnormalities in all homozygotes are similar, evidence for three allelic variants has come from studies of intestinal transport in homozygotes and of urinary excretion in obligate heterozygotes. These variants have been designated types I, II, and III. Type I homozygotes lack mediated intestinal transport of cystine, lysine, arginine, and ornithine; their heterozygous relatives have normal urinary amino acid excretion patterns. Type II homozygotes lack mediated lysine transport in the gut but retain some capacity for cystine transport; heterozygotes have moderately increased urinary excretion of each of the four amino acids. Type III homozygotes retain some capacity for mediated intestinal transport of the four involved substrates; heterozygotes have modestly increased urinary lysine and cystine.

Clinical manifestations Cystinuria is among the most common inborn errors, homozygotes occurring with a frequency of 1 in 10,000 to 1 in 15,000 in many ethnic groups. Cystine stones account for 1 to 2 percent of all urinary tract calculi. The maximum solubility of cystine in the physiological urinary pH range of 4.5 to 7.0 is about 300 mg per liter. Since affected homozygotes regularly excrete 600 to 1800 mg per day, crystalluria and calculus formation are a constant threat. Cystine stone formation usually becomes manifest in the second or third decade but has been reported as early as the first year of life. Symptoms and signs are those typical of urolithiasis regardless of etiology: hematuria, flank pain, renal colic, obstructive uropathy, and infection. Recurrent episodes of urolithiasis may lead to progressive renal insufficiency.

Diagnosis The presence of cystine in a urinary tract stone is pathognomonic of cystinuria. However, since 50 percent of the stones excreted by cystinuric subjects are of mixed composition and since as many as 10 percent may contain *no* detectable cystine, a urinary nitroprusside test should be done on all patients with urolithiasis to exclude this diagnosis. The nitroprusside test is also positive (appearance of a cherry red color) in some heterozygotes for cystinuria, in patients with hypercystinuria, homocystinuria, and cysteine β-mercaptolactate disulfiduria, and in the presence of acetone in the urine. When cystine content exceeds 250 mg per liter, cystine crystals may be seen in the sediment of acidified, concentrated, chilled urine. These crystals, in the form of hexagonal plates, are pathognomonic of cystine overexcretion in patients not taking sulfonamides.

Diagnostic confirmation of cystinuria depends upon the demonstration of the characteristic amino acid excretion pattern in the urine. Selective excretion of cystine, lysine, arginine, and ornithine can be demonstrated by paper chromatography or electrophoresis, and quantitative determinations can be made by column chromatography. Quantitation becomes important in differentiating some heterozygotes from homozygotes and in documenting the reduction of free cystine excretion during therapy.

Treatment Medical management of cystinuria is aimed at reducing the concentration of cystine in urine. The single most important aspect of this treatment is maintenance of a large urine volume. Fluid ingestion in excess of 4 liters per day is essential, and 5 to 7 liters per day is optimal. Stones can be prevented and even dissolved by such vigorous hydration. It must be made clear to the cystinuric subject that water is a drug. Solubility of cystine rises sharply in urine above pH 7.5, and various regimens of urinary alkalinization have been used therapeutically. Vigorous administration of sodium bicarbonate, Diamox, and polycitrates is required to maintain a persistently alkaline pH, but this measure introduces the danger of inducing formation of other "alkaline" stones (calcium oxalate, calcium phosphate, magnesium ammonium phosphate) and even of producing nephrocalcinosis.

Another medical approach to treatment involves administration of D-penicillamine (β,β-dimethylcysteine) which undergoes sulfhydryl-disulfide exchange with cystine to form the mixed disulfide of penicillamine and cysteine. Since this disulfide is more than 50 times as soluble as cystine, D-penicillamine (in doses of 1 to 3 g per day) has the capacity to reduce free cystine excretion markedly, thereby preventing new stone formation and promoting dissolution of existing calculi. Unfortunately D-penicillamine is immunogenic, and allergic manifestations include acute serum sickness, agranulocytosis, pancytopenia, immune glomerulitis, and the Goodpasture syndrome. Thus, its use should be reserved for patients who fail to respond to hydration alone or who are in a particularly high-risk category (one remaining kidney, renal insufficiency). When medical management fails, urologic surgery is required. An occasional patient may require renal transplantation because of renal failure.

DIBASICAMINOACIDURIA A number of families have been described in which affected members have a defect in renal tubular reabsorption of lysine, arginine, and ornithine but *not* of cystine. The disorder almost surely reflects mutations in the genes coding for a renal transport protein used by the three dibasic amino acids only. Two clinically distinct variants have been observed, each apparently inherited as an autosomal re-

TABLE 90-1
Genetic disorders of membrane transport

Class of substance and disorder	Individual substrates	Tissues manifesting transport defect	Proposed molecular basis of defect	Major clinical manifestations	Mode of inheritance	Location of discussion
AMINO ACIDS						
Classic cystinuria	Cystine, lysine, arginine, ornithine	Proximal renal tubule, jejunal mucosa	Mutation of shared dibasic-cystine transport protein	Cystine nephrolithiasis	Autosomal recessive	Chap. 90
Dibasicamino-aciduria	Lysine, arginine, ornithine	Proximal renal tubule, jejunal mucosa	Mutation of dibasic transport protein	Type I: Moderate retardation Type II: Protein intolerance, hyperammonemia, retardation	Autosomal recessive	Chap. 90
Hypercystinuria	Cystine	Proximal renal tubule	Mutation of cystine transport protein	Some risk of cystine nephrolithiasis	Autosomal recessive	Chap. 90
Lysinuria	Lysine	Proximal renal tubule, jejunal mucosa	Mutation of lysine transport protein	Seizures, physical and mental retardation	Possible autosomal recessive	Chap. 90
Hartnup disease	Neutral amino acids	Proximal renal tubule, jejunal mucosa	Mutation of neutral amino acid-shared transport protein	Constant neutral aminoaciduria, intermittent symptoms of pellagra	Autosomal recessive	Chap. 90
Tryptophan malabsorption	Tryptophan	Jejunal mucosa	Mutation of tryptophan transport protein	Indoluria, ?hypercalcemia, ?nephrocalcinosis	Probable autosomal recessive	Chap. 90
Methionine malabsorption	Methionine	Jejunal mucosa	Mutation of methionine transport protein	α-Hydroxybutyricaciduria, white hair, mental retardation, convulsions, hyperneic attacks, edema	Probable autosomal recessive	Chap. 90
Histidinuria	Histidine	Proximal renal tubule, jejunal mucosa	Mutation of histidine transport protein	Mental retardation	Autosomal recessive	Chap. 90
Iminoglycinuria	Glycine, proline, hydroxyproline	Proximal renal tubule, jejunal mucosa	Mutation of shared glycine-imino acid transport protein	None	Autosomal recessive	Chap. 90
Dicarboxylica-minoaciduria	Glutamic acid, aspartic acid	Proximal renal tubule, jejunal mucosa	Mutation of shared dicarboxylic amino acid transport protein	None	Probable autosomal recessive	Chap. 90
HEXOSES						
Renal glycosuria	D-Glucose	Proximal renal tubule	Mutation of D-glucose transport protein	Glycosuria with normal blood glucose	Autosomal recessive	Chap. 90
Glucose-galactose malabsorption	D-Gluose D-Galactose	Jejunal mucosa, proximal renal tubule	Mutation of shared glucose-galactose transport protein	Watery diarrhea on feeding glucose, lactose, sucrose, or galactose	Autosomal recessive	Chaps. 90, 292
LIPIDS						
Familial hyper-cholesterolemia	Cholesterol	Fibroblasts, lymphoid lines, leukocytes	Mutation of membrane LDL-cholesterol receptor protein	Hypercholesterolemia, tendon xanthomas, arcus corneae, coronary artery atherosclerosis	Autosomal dominant	Chap. 100
URATE						
Hypouricemia	Uric acid	Proximal renal tubule	Mutation of urate transport protein	Hypouricemia, hyperuricosuria, ?hypercalcinuria	Autosomal recessive	Chap. 90
ANIONS						
Familial hypophosphatemic rickets	Inorganic phosphate	Proximal renal tubule, jejunal mucosa	Mutation of inorganic phosphate transport protein	Hypophosphatemia, phosphaturia, phosphatopenic rickets/osteomalacia	X-linked dominant	Chap. 352

TABLE 90-1 *(continued)*
Genetic disorders of membrane transport

Class of substance and disorder	Individual substrates	Tissues manifesting transport defect	Proposed molecular basis of defect	Major clinical manifestations	Mode of inheritance	Location of discussion
ANIONS *(continued)*						
Congenital chloridorrhea	Chloride	Ileal and colonic mucosa	Mutation of Cl^-/HCO_3^- exchange pump carrier protein	Hydramnios, watery diarrhea, elevated fecal chloride, achloriduria, metabolic alkalosis with volume depletion, hyperaldosteronism	Autosomal recessive	Chaps. 90, 292
Familial goiter	Inorganic iodide	Thyroid gland, salivary gland, gastric mucosa	Mutation of iodide transport protein	Congenital hypothyroidism (cretinism), goiter	Probable autosomal recessive	Chap. 335
CATIONS						
Distal renal tubular acidosis (type I—gradient)	Hydrogen ion	Distal renal tubule	Mutation of distal tubule H^+ pump carrier protein	Hyperchloremic acidosis, hypokalemia, acquired nephrocalcinosis, and hypercalcinuria	Autosomal dominant	Chap. 283
Proximal renal tubular acidosis (type II—HCO_3 wasting)	Hydrogen ion	Proximal renal tubule	Mutation of proximal tubule H^+ pump carrier protein	Hyperchloremic acidosis, bicarbonate wasting	Probable autosomal recessive	Chap. 283
Menkes' disease	Copper	Duodenal and jejunal intestinal cells	Possible serosal transport protein or intracellular transport defect	Severe mental retardation, pili torti (kinky hair), typical facies, arterial tortuosity, excess Wormian bones, thermal instability	X-linked recessive	Chap. 83
Hereditary: Spherocytosis Elliptocytosis Ovalocytosis Stomatocytosis	Sodium	Red blood cell (RBC) membranes	Mutation of membrane structure (? lipid or protein) resulting in increased sodium permeability	Increased RBC fragility resulting in variable degrees of hemolytic anemia, splenomegaly, and jaundice; RBC shape respectively spherocytic, elliptocytic, ovalocytic, or stomatocytic (target-shaped)	Each of these diseases of RBC morphology is a separately inherited autosomal dominant	Chap. 314
WATER						
Nephrogenic diabetes insipidus (ADH-resistant)	Water	Distal renal tubule	Lack of activation of ADH-responsive luminal membrane adenylate cyclase, possible defect in receptor or enzyme protein	Polyuria, polydipsia, hyposthenuria	X-linked recessive	Chap. 283

cessive trait. Clinical manifestations appear to be related to the significant losses of ornithine, arginine, and perhaps lysine.

In the common form of dibasicaminoaciduria (type II), homozygotes show defective intestinal transport of dibasic amino acids as well as exaggerated renal losses. A defect in hepatic cell uptake of these substances has also been proposed. Affected patients present in childhood with hepatosplenomegaly, protein intolerance, and episodic ammonia intoxication. Plasma concentrations of lysine, arginine, and ornithine are reduced. The clinical findings have been attributed to hyperammonemia resulting from insufficient amounts of arginine

and ornithine to maintain proper function of the Krebs-Henseleit urea cycle. Treatment includes dietary protein restriction and supplementation with arginine and ornithine. Obligate heterozygotes are clinically well and show no excess urinary loss of dibasic amino acids.

Type I dibasicaminoaciduria has been described in only one homozygote. She was moderately mentally retarded but had no clear history of protein intolerance or hyperammonemia. Her urinary losses of dibasic amino acids were not as great as those seen in type II homozygotes. The condition was distinguished from type I by the presence of modest excesses of dibasic amino acids in urine of both asymptomatic parents. Other pedigrees containing asymptomatic heterozygotes have been identified by urinary screening programs.

HARTNUP DISEASE Pellagra-like skin lesions, variable neurological manifestations, and a constant renal aminoaciduria for the monoaminomonocarboxylic amino acids with neutral or aromatic side chains characterize Hartnup disease. Alanine, serine, threonine, valine, leucine, isoleucine, phenylalanine, tyrosine, tryptophan, glutamine, asparagine, and histidine are excreted in urine in quantities from five to ten times normal, and an intestinal transport defect for these same amino acids has been demonstrated. The clinical spectrum appears to relate solely to nutritional deficiency of the essential amino acid tryptophan, caused by the combination of intestinal malabsorption and renal loss. Disease manifestations are episodic, related, at least in part, to metabolic demands for tryptophan.

The major catabolic pathway of tryptophan metabolism leads to the synthesis of niacin and nicotinamide-adenine dinucleotide (NAD). This pathway supplies about 50 percent of daily niacin needs. In patients with Hartnup disease, the renal and intestinal transport defect for neutral and aromatic amino acids, including tryptophan, leads to niacin deficiency. The transport defect likely reflects abnormalities of a group-specific system for neutral amino acids. Renal clearance studies show some residual reabsorptive capacity for each involved amino acid. This suggests that they are transported by other carrier systems as well, a conclusion supported by the subsequent description of patients with substrate-specific transport errors for tryptophan, methionine, and histidine.

Hartnup disease is inherited as an autosomal recessive trait. Homozygotes occur with a frequency of about 1 in 16,000 births. Heterozygotes exhibit no clinical or chemical abnormalities.

Pellagra is the clinical syndrome produced by dietary niacin deficiency, and its clinical features of diarrhea, dementia, and dermatitis are those which characterize Hartnup disease (see Chap. 79). The diagnosis should be suspected in any patient with pellagra without a history of severe dietary niacin deficiency. The neurological and psychiatric manifestations range from attacks of cerebellar ataxia to mild emotional lability to frank delirium and usually accompany exacerbations of the erythematous, eczematoid skin rash. Fever, sunlight, stress, and sulfonamide therapy provoke clinical relapses. Diagnosis is made by detection of the pathological neutral aminoaciduria which does not occur in dietary niacin deficiency. Treatment is directed at niacin repletion and includes a high-protein diet and daily nicotinamide supplementation (50 to 250 mg).

IMINOGLYCINURIA This trait is characterized by excessive urinary excretion of glycine and the imino acids proline and hydroxyproline. Homozygotes for this autosomal recessive disorder occur with a frequency of about 1 in 16,000. The exaggerated renal clearance of glycine, proline, and hydroxyproline reflects a defect in the tubular transport system shared by these three compounds. An intestinal transport defect has been demonstrated in some. This suggests that more than one mutation may lead to persistent iminoglycinuria, a thesis corroborated by studies of urinary amino acid excretion in obligate heterozygotes from different families. No consistent clinical abnormalities have been reported in homozygotes, who are usually detected by urinary amino acid screening programs. Individuals with iminoglycinuria should be reassured as to the benign nature of the disturbance.

DICARBOXYLICAMINOACIDURIA Selective urinary loss and exaggerated endogenous renal clearance of glutamic and aspartic acids have been described in two unrelated children. Intestinal absorption of these dicarboxylic amino acids was impaired in one but not in the other. The former suffered from recurrent hypoglycemia; the latter was asymptomatic. It remains to be determined whether this defect is of clinical significance.

SUBSTRATE-SPECIFIC DEFECTS IN AMINO ACID TRANSPORT
Rare pedigrees exist in which individuals have defective renal tubular reabsorption and/or impaired intestinal absorption of a single free amino acid. These disorders, each apparently inherited as an autosomal recessive trait, provide the strongest evidence that transmembrane transport of amino acids is catalyzed by substrate-specific as well as group-specific transport mechanisms.

Hypercystinuria Two siblings exhibited modest cystinuria without excessive urinary excretion of lysine, arginine, or ornithine. Fractional tubular reabsorption of cystine was reduced to about 80 percent of the filtered load, and up to 250 mg per day was excreted in the urine. Neither showed any abnormality in intestinal absorption of cystine. Both were clinically well, although their cystine excretion would appear to place them at some risk for cystine urolithiasis. Urinary cystine excretion by both parents was unremarkable.

Lysinuria Only a single child with selective impairment of renal tubular reabsorption of lysine has been described. Endogenous lysine clearance was increased; intestinal transport was impaired; plasma lysine was reduced. Severe mental and growth retardation and seizures were present. A lysine-supplemented diet appeared to stimulate growth. Urinary excretion of lysine was normal in the parents.

Histidinuria Two siblings, each with moderate mental retardation, exhibited a renal transport defect for histidine only. Urinary loss of histidine approached 40 to 50 percent of the filtered load, and an intestinal transport defect for histidine was also present. The clinically normal parents had normal urinary excretion but a modest defect in intestinal absorption of histidine.

Methionine malabsorption Single children from two pedigrees have shown an intestinal transport defect for methionine. One may have had a renal transport defect as well. This disorder was detected because of urinary excretion of α-hydroxybutyric acid, a distinctive by-product of the intestinal bacterial breakdown of the unabsorbed methionine. This compound, which gives an unusual odor resembling malt or dried celery to the urine, appears to be responsible for the white hair, attacks of hyperpnea, convulsions, edema, and mental retardation. Treatment of one of these children with a methionine-restricted diet was followed by improvement in all clinical manifestations.

Tryptophan malabsorption An isolated defect in intestinal absorption of tryptophan has been described in two siblings. The renal tubular reabsorption of tryptophan was normal. A variety of indoles were excreted in stool and urine. These compounds result from chemical degradation of unabsorbed tryptophan by intestinal bacteria and have been described in patients with Hartnup disease as well. Because of concomitant renal parenchymal disease, hydrolytic enzymes were released into the urine, acted upon the indoles found there, and led to the formation of a blue pigment, indigotin. This sequence of events earned this condition the sobriquet "blue-diaper syndrome." No pellagra-like symptoms were described. The patients' mother also excreted modest excesses of indole compounds, suggesting that she is a carrier of this trait.

DISORDERS OF HEXOSE TRANSPORT

Nondiabetic melituria occurs in a number of conditions. Pentoses, hexoses, heptoses, and disaccharides have been identified in the urine; all except sucrose yield a positive test for reducing substances. Some meliturias result from diffuse renal injury, others from ingestion of nonmetabolizable sugars. In still others the sugars accumulate in blood due to deficient activity of catabolizing enzyme systems and "spill" into the urine. Only among the hexoses have specific inherited disorders of sugar transport been identified. The existence of renal glycosuria and intestinal glucose-galactose malabsorption as heritable, autosomal recessive disorders points to the existence of at least two specific carrier proteins for hexoses in human jejunal and renal brush border membranes: one for glucose and one shared by glucose and galactose.

RENAL GLYCOSURIA To avoid confusion with diabetes mellitus, Marble's criteria for the diagnosis of renal glycosuria should be followed: (1) glycosuria in the absence of hyperglycemia, (2) constant glycosuria with little fluctuation related to diet, (3) normal (or slightly flat) oral glucose tolerance test, (4) identification of urinary reducing substance as glucose, and (5) normal storage and utilization of carbohydrates. The Fanconi syndrome, in which renal glycosuria occurs as part of generalized proximal tubular dysfunction, should also be excluded. The incidence is less than 1 in 500. The condition is benign, but occasionally glycosuria may be great enough to cause polyuria and polydipsia. Even more rarely, dehydration or ketosis may develop under conditions of stress such as pregnancy or starvation.

In normal persons glucose is present in the glomerular filtrate at a concentration equal to that in plasma water and is actively reabsorbed throughout the proximal renal tubule by a sodium-dependent, phlorizin-inhibitable transport process. Reabsorptive capacity exceeds normal plasma glucose concentration. Thus, glucose does not appear in the urine until the threshold for reabsorption is reached. Titration studies suggest that the plasma concentration at which some filtered glucose begins to escape proximal tubular reabsorption is 200 to 240 mg per 100 ml. Maximal renal reabsorptive capacity is exceeded at a filtered load of 325 ± 36 mg/min per 1.73 m^2, and this value is defined as the tubular maximum for glucose (TmG).

Titration studies in subjects with renal glycosuria have shown two patterns of glycosuria: type A characterized by a reduced tubular maximum reabsorptive capacity and type B showing a reduced threshold for glycosuria, an increased "splay" in the titration curve, and a normal TmG. Marked renal glycosuria occurs in individuals homozygous for either of these recessively inherited mutations of the specific membrane transport process for glucose and in genetic compounds for these presumably allelic mutations. Modest reduction in renal threshold or TmG has been demonstrated in obligate heterozygotes in some pedigrees; modest glycosuria can be expected in such family members when plasma glucose is elevated.

GLUCOSE-GALACTOSE MALABSORPTION In this condition, infants develop a profuse, watery diarrhea when fed milk or foods containing lactose, sucrose, glucose, or galactose. Fructose or carbohydrate-free formulas are well tolerated. A specific defect in intestinal absorption of glucose and galactose can be demonstrated by oral tolerance tests that produce little or no increase in plasma glucose or galactose. Treatment with a glucose- and galactose-free diet leads to resolution of symptoms in childhood. Although the basic transport defect can be demonstrated throughout life, most patients show an improved tolerance for glucose and galactose as they get older.

Intestinal transport studies performed in vitro on small biopsy specimens of jejunal mucosa have shown a complete absence of active D-glucose and D-galactose transport in affected children and intermediate transport capacity in their parents. These findings confirm the specificity of the mutation for these two sugars and the autosomal recessive inheritance of this transport disorder.

A number of these patients have renal glycosuria at normal plasma glucose concentrations. Renal titration studies generally demonstrate a reduced threshold for glucose reabsorption (type B renal glycosuria) with a normal TmG. Urinary glucose loss is not as severe as in isolated renal glycosuria. This finding suggests the presence of multiple glucose transport proteins in the kidney. One, responsible for the bulk of glucose reabsorption and specific for glucose only, is affected in renal glycosuria; another, shared by glucose and galactose and responsible for transporting less of the filtered load of glucose, is affected in glucose-galactose malabsorption. Either the former is not present in intestinal mucosa or the shared system is more important in that tissue. In both disorders transport of sugars in all other tested tissues is normal, reflecting the multiplicity and tissue specificity of membrane transport proteins.

DEFECTIVE URATE TRANSPORT: HYPOURICEMIA

A small number of pedigrees have been described containing individuals with a selective defect in renal tubular reabsorption of sodium urate. These subjects are identified by the presence of marked hypouricemia. Since little serum urate is bound to plasma proteins, failure to reabsorb filtered urate results in a serum urate ranging from 0.2 to 1.8 mg per 100 ml. No disease is associated with this isolated defect, although the risk of uric acid nephrolithiasis is theoretically present.

Renal urate clearance normally averages 15 percent of glomerular filtration rate, and the excreted urate is composed both of filtered urate that has escaped reabsorption and secreted urate. Subjects with isolated hypouricemia have urate clearances averaging from 33 to 85 percent of the filtration rate; in some, urate clearance exceeds the glomerular filtration rate. Studies with probenecid, which blocks tubular reabsorption of urate, and pyrazinamide, which blocks tubular secretion, suggest that the disorder is due to a partial defect in proximal tubular reabsorption. In two families hypercalcinuria due to enhanced intestinal calcium absorption was also present, but in all others only uricosuria has been demonstrated. The defect is inherited as an autosomal recessive. Urate transport has not been studied in nonrenal tissue or in obligate heterozygotes. The defect is presumed to reflect mutation of a proximal renal tubular membrane protein that selectively transports sodium urate.

DEFECTIVE ANION TRANSPORT: CHLORIDORRHEA

This rare, autosomal recessive disease results from impairment of active transport of chloride in the ileum and colon. Absence of the chloride-bicarbonate ion exchange "pump" causes profound symptoms even before birth (polyhydramnios and absence of meconium). Massive watery diarrhea is apparent from the first days of life. This fluid loss, with its attendant impairment of electrolyte homeostasis, is life-threatening. A hypokalemic, hypochloremic, hyponatremic metabolic alkalosis develops with dehydration and secondary hyperaldosteronism. Fecal fluid contains an excess of chloride ion over the sum of the accompanying cations, sodium and potassium. Fecal chloride concentration always exceeds 90 mmol per liter when volume and serum electrolyte disturbances are corrected, and this chloridorrhea is diagnostic. Renal chloride transport is normal. Decreased urine chloride results from the kidney's attempts to conserve salt and water.

Treatment necessitates adequate, life-long repletion of electrolyte and fluid losses, since no way has yet been found to mitigate the transport disorder. Exact replacement of water, sodium chloride, and potassium chloride can prevent the growth and psychomotor retardation and the development of progressive renal damage. The renal lesion, with hyalinized glomeruli, juxtaglomerular hyperplasia, calcifications, and arteriolar changes, is probably a result of chronic volume depletion.

REFERENCES

ELSAS LJ, ROSENBERG LE: Renal glycosuria, in *Strauss and Welt's Diseases of the Kidney,* 3d ed, LE Earley, CW Gottschalk (eds). Boston, Little, Brown, 1979 (in press)

GORDEN P, LEVITIN H: Congenital alkalosis with diarrhea; a sequel to Darrow's original description. Ann Intern Med 87:876, 1973

HOLMBERG C et al: Congenital chloride diarrhoea. Arch Dis Child 52:255, 1977

KRANE SM: Renal glycosuria, in *The Metabolic Basis of Inherited Disease,* 4th ed, JB Stanbury et al (eds). New York, McGraw-Hill, 1978, pp 1607–1617

ROSENBERG LE: Intestinal hexose transport in familial glucose-galactose malabsorption, in *Membranes and Disease,* L Bolis et al (eds). New York, Raven Press, 1976

———, SCRIVER CR: Disorders of amino acid metabolism, in *Metabolic Control and Disease,* 8th ed, PK Bondy, LE Rosenberg (eds). Philadelphia, Saunders, 1979 (in press)

SHORT EM, ROSENBERG LE: Renal aminoaciduria, in *Strauss and Welt's Diseases of the Kidney,* 3d ed, LE Earley, CW Gottschalk (eds). Boston, Little, Brown, 1979 (in press)

THIER SO, SEGAL S: Cystinuria, in *The Metabolic Basis of Inherited Disease,* 4th ed, JB Stanbury et al (eds). New York, McGraw-Hill, 1978, pp 1578–1592

WYNGAARDEN JB, KELLEY WN: *Gout and Hyperuricemia.* New York, Grune & Stratton, 1976, pp 411–420

91
CARCINOID SYNDROME

JOHN A. OATES

The association of carcinoid tumors with cutaneous flushes, telangiectasia, diarrhea, cardiac valvular lesions, and bronchial constriction eluded recognition until 1953. Once this connection was established by Thorson, Biörk, Björkman, and Waldenström, and independently by Isler and Hedinger, it was clear that the syndrome was mediated by release of one or more biologically active agents by the tumor. Serotonin was the first such agent to be discovered, and overproduction of this amine is the most consistent biochemical indicator of the carcinoid syndrome. Serotonin, however, is not the sole mediator of the clinical syndrome. These tumors vary in their synthesis of indoles and may elaborate chemically unrelated agents such as bradykinin, histamine, and adrenocorticotropic hormone (ACTH). Furthermore, evidence suggests that an additional unidentified substance participates in the production of flushing. Within the broad classification of carcinoid tumors there is great diversity in the production of biologically active substances and in the mechanisms for their storage and release.

Accordingly, there is a varied spectrum of clinical manifestations.

PATHOLOGICAL ANATOMY OF THE TUMOR Carcinoid tumors are slowly growing neoplasms of enterochromaffin cells. The metastatic tumors associated with carcinoid syndrome usually arise from small primary tumors in the ileum. The syndrome is also produced by neoplasms arising from the remainder of the small intestine, from organs derived from the embryonic foregut (e.g., bronchus, stomach, pancreas, and thyroid), and from ovarian or testicular teratomas.

Carcinoid tumors have an unusual proclivity for metastasis to the liver and may involve this organ extensively, with minimal metastatic disease elsewhere. Extrahepatic metastases occur in bone, where they are often osteoblastic, and in lung, pancreas, spleen, ovaries, adrenals, and other organs.

Primary carcinoid tumors of the appendix are common, but they rarely metastasize. Those from the large intestine may metastasize but almost never exhibit endocrine effects.

The usual carcinoid tumor arising from the ileum has the classic histological pattern of dense nests of cells with uniform size and nuclear appearance. Histochemically, they typically exhibit an argentaffin reaction in which the cells convert a silver salt to metallic silver. A positive argentaffin reaction is not required for the diagnosis, however, and carcinoid tumors arising from organs of the embryonic foregut are usually argyrophyllic, containing few if any argentaffin cells. Tumors from these organs also have a broad histological spectrum, which in the lung ranges from typical bronchial carcinoid to a form indistinguishable from oat-cell carcinoma.

Neoplasms of foregut origin with histological features resembling carcinoids may produce excessive amounts of polypeptide hormones such as gastrin, insulin, calcitonin, glucagon, corticotropin, and vasoactive intestinal polypeptide without exhibiting the usual features of carcinoid syndrome. These carcinoid tumors probably share a common embryologic origin with those producing carcinoid syndrome, arising from the neuroectodermal cells of the neural crest.

CLINICAL FEATURES Unlike most metastatic neoplasms, carcinoid tumors have an unusually slow rate of growth; most patients survive for 5 to 10 years after the disease is recognized. For much of the duration of the illness, morbidity may result largely from the endocrine function of the tumor. Death results from cardiac or hepatic failure and from complications associated with tumor growth.

Vasomotor paroxysms The most common clinical feature is cutaneous *flushing.* The typical flush is erythematous and involves the head and neck (blush area). Some patients exhibit vivid color changes from red to violaceous to pallor during its course. Prolonged flushing attacks may be associated with lacrimation and periorbital edema. The systemic effects of the flush are variable. It may be accompanied by tachycardia, and the blood pressure usually falls or does not change. A rise in blood pressure during flushing is rare, and carcinoid syndrome is not a cause of sustained hypertension.

Flushing may be provoked by excitement, exertion, eating, and ethanol ingestion. In addition, the administration of pentagastrin and beta-adrenoceptor agonists such as epinephrine can trigger episodes of vasodilatation; as the hemodynamic changes associated with such pharmacologically induced attacks may be severe, these drugs should be administered with great caution.

Telangiectasia In addition to paroxysms of cutaneous vasodilatation, some patients also develop purple telangiectasia, primarily on the face and neck and most marked in the malar area.

Gastrointestinal symptoms Intestinal hypermotility with borborygmi, cramping, and explosive diarrhea may accompany the episodic flushes. Chronic hypermotility with diarrhea is more common. When this is severe, malabsorption may occur.

Cardiac manifestations There is a unique deposition of fibrous tissue on the endocardium of the valvular cusps and cardiac chambers. It occurs primarily in the right side of the heart, but may involve the left side to a minimal degree. The fibrous deposition does not penetrate the internal elastic membrane. Distortion of the valve cusps, chordae tendineae, and papillary muscles interferes with valvular function in the right side of the heart and may lead to regurgitation, stenosis, or combined functional lesions. There is, however, a tendency for the fibrosing process to produce incompetence at the tricuspid valve and stenosis of the smaller pulmonary orifice, a deleterious hemodynamic combination. A high cardiac output, with its attendant imposition on cardiac function, may be found in some patients with carcinoid syndrome; this is due either to a continuing release of a vasodilator or to excessive flow in the metastatic tumors.

Pulmonary symptoms Bronchoconstriction is a less common feature of the syndrome, but it may be severe. It is usually most pronounced during flushing attacks.

General In addition to the endocrine effects, the tumors themselves may cause intestinal obstruction or bleeding. Necrosis of intestinal or hepatic tumor masses may produce abdominal pain, tenderness, fever, and leukocytosis. Hepatomegaly from the metastatic disease is usually present with the syndrome. Extensive metastatic involvement of the liver by these slowly growing tumors may occur before the liver function test results become abnormal.

ENDOCRINE FUNCTION OF THE TUMORS **Serotonin** The most constant biochemical characteristic of carcinoid tumors is the presence of tryptophan hydroxylase, which catalyzes the formation of 5-hydroxytryptophan (5-HTP) from tryptophan (Fig. 91-1). Most tumors also contain the enzyme aromatic L-amino acid decarboxylase, which catalyzes the formation of 5-hydroxytryptamine (serotonin). Carcinoids from the stomach and from other organs derived from the embryonic foregut, however, are frequently deficient in this decarboxylase and release 5-HTP from the tumor.

Following its release from the tumor, serotonin is inactivated primarily by the enzyme monoamine oxidase; uptake into platelets also contributes to removal of free serotonin from blood. Monoamine oxidase oxidizes serotonin to 5-hydroxyindoleacetaldehyde, which is rapidly converted to 5-hydroxyindoleacetic acid (5-HIAA) by aldehyde dehydrogenase. This acid is rapidly excreted in the urine, and almost all circulating serotonin can be accounted for as urinary 5-HIAA.

Carcinoid tumors vary widely in their capacity to store serotonin, with concentrations of the amine in tumors ranging from a few micrograms per gram to 3 mg/g. The concentration in the tumor appears unrelated to the rate of synthesis of serotonin as reflected by urinary 5-HIAA. Generally, tumors from the ileum have a much higher storage capacity for serotonin than do tumors from organs of the embryonic foregut.

Bradykinin A potent vasodilator peptide, bradykinin is released during flushes in some cases of carcinoid syndrome. In a few of these, excessive amounts continue to be released between flushes. Bradykinin and related kinins are formed by the action of a group of enzymes (kallikreins) which split these peptides from kininogen, a plasma globulin. It is thought that catecholamines and other stimuli initiate bradykinin formation, either by release of kallikrein from the tumor or by initi-

ation of a sequence that leads to activation of the kallikrein normally present in plasma.

Other biologically active substances Some carcinoid tumors, particularly those of gastric origin, produce and release excessive amounts of histamine. This can be detected by an increased excretion of this amine in the urine. In such patients, the release of histamine from the tumors is responsible for the episodic vasodilatation with flushing, tachycardia, and hypotension.

Carcinoid syndrome has been associated with hyperadrenocorticism in a number of instances. This results from ectopic production of an adrenocorticotropic hormone by the tumors, which usually originate from sites other than the ileum (bronchus, pancreas, ovary, and stomach). (See Chap. 347.)

In a few cases, "multiple endocrine adenomas" have been seen in conjunction with carcinoids arising from organs of the embryonic foregut. The associated tumors have included parathyroid adenomas and pancreatic tumors, producing Zollinger-Ellison syndrome. (See Chap. 348.)

FIGURE 91-1
Metabolic pathway of serotonin.

Tryptophan

Tryptophan
hydroxylase

5-Hydroxytryptophan

Aromatic-L-amino
acid decarboxylase

5-Hydroxytryptamine (Serotonin)

Monoamine
oxidase

5-Hydroxyindoleacetaldehyde

Aldehyde
dehydrogenase

5-Hydroxyindoleacetic acid
(5-HIAA)

PATHOPHYSIOLOGY Serotonin contributes to those aspects of the syndrome related to intestinal hypermotility, and there is evidence that the fibrous deposits on the endocardium also result from increased levels of circulating serotonin.

A secondary effect of serotonin overproduction occurs when a large fraction of dietary tryptophan is shunted into the hydroxylation pathway, leaving less tryptophan available for the formation of nicotinic acid and protein. When urinary excretion of 5-HIAA exceeds 200 to 300 mg daily, low levels of plasma tryptophan and evidence of nicotinamide deficiency are seen. (See Chap. 79.)

Mechanism of the flush Although the flushes of patients with gastric carcinoids that secrete histamine can be attributed to this amine, the mechanism of the flush in the more typical carcinoid syndrome has not yet been elucidated. Release of the flush-provoking substance(s) can be triggered by the catecholamines, and this probably accounts for the association of flushing with excitement and emotional stimuli. For experimental induction of flushing, injection of isoproterenol in amounts of as little as 0.5 μg may be effective. Pentagastrin in doses of as small as 0.25 μg also can trigger flushing, an action that may explain the provocation of flushes by eating in some patients. Serotonin was originally thought to be the mediator of flushes, but injection of this amine does not produce a mimicking of the carcinoid flush, and patients may exhibit flushes without increased levels of plasma serotonin. Bradykinin is a potent vasodilator, and its injection will simulate one type of carcinoid flush which is characterized by erythema in association with tachycardia and hypotension. Release of this peptide, however, could not be detected in a number of patients during flushing. While bradykinin, serotonin, and histamine may contribute to the varied types of flushes observed in the carcinoid syndrome, there appears to be an additional flush substance which has not yet been identified.

DIAGNOSIS With its full constellation of clinical features, carcinoid syndrome is easily recognized. The diagnosis also must be considered when any one of its features is present.

The diagnostic hallmark of carcinoid syndrome is *overproduction of 5-hydroxyindoles* with *increased urinary excretion of 5-hydroxyindoleacetic acid.* Normally, excretion of 5-HIAA does not exceed 9 mg daily. Ingestion of foods containing serotonin may complicate the biochemical diagnosis of carcinoid syndrome; both walnuts and bananas contain enough serotonin to produce abnormally elevated urinary excretion of 5-HIAA after their ingestion. Some drugs also interfere with the analysis of urinary 5-HIAA; cough syrups containing guaiacolate cause falsely elevated values, and phenothiazines interfere with the colorimetric test. When dietary 5-hydroxyindoles are excluded, a urinary excretion of more than 25 mg 5-HIAA daily is diagnostic of carcinoid. Elevations in the range of 9 to 25 mg may be seen with carcinoid syndrome, nontropical sprue, or acute intestinal obstruction.

Measurement of *serotonin in blood or platelets* is of interest but has less diagnostic value than assay of the major metabolite of serotonin in the urine.

Measurement of an increased concentration of *serotonin in tumor tissue* is a useful and sometimes necessary supplement to histological examination. A portion of suspected tumor should always be frozen for serotonin analysis (see Table 91-1).

VARIANTS OF THE SYNDROME: RELATION TO SITE OF TUMOR ORIGIN The origin of the tumor influences the biologically active substances produced and their storage and release. Carcinoid tumors arising from organs derived from the embryonic foregut (bronchus, stomach, and pancreas) tend to differ from those arising distal to the midduodenum (midgut). The typical carcinoid syndrome usually results from tumors of midgut origin, which almost invariably secrete serotonin with little or no 5-HTP. Tumor serotonin content is likely to be high, and the tumor usually contains dense nests of argentaffin-positive cells. Metastasis to bone and skin is infrequent.

In contrast, tumors arising from the embryonic foregut contain fewer argentaffin cells, have lower serotonin content, and may secrete 5-HTP. Hyperadrenocorticism and multiple endocrine adenomas are more likely to be associated with this group, and metastasis to bone and skin is more frequent.

In addition to the general characteristics of the foregut group, certain clinical and biochemical features have been associated with gastric and bronchial carcinoids. Patients with gastric carcinoids frequently exhibit unique flushing which begins as a bright red patchy erythema with sharply delineated serpentine borders; these patches tend to coalesce as the blush heightens. Food ingestion is especially likely to produce flushes. The tumors usually are deficient in decarboxylase enzyme and secrete 5-HTP; histamine secretion is also common, as is a high incidence of peptic ulceration. Diarrhea and heart lesions are not prominent features in the patients who secrete largely 5-HTP from the tumor without much preformed serotonin.

When the carcinoid tumor arises from the bronchus, attacks of flushing tend to be prolonged and severe and may be associated with periorbital edema, excessive lacrimation and salivation, hypotension, tachycardia, anxiety, and tremulousness. Nausea, vomiting, explosive diarrhea, and bronchoconstriction may progress to a severe degree. This group is therapeutically unique in that the severe flushes often can be prevented by corticosteroids, and chlorpromazine may be helpful in relieving the symptoms.

TREATMENT Recognition of the carcinoid syndrome has led to complete surgical cure of a few patients with tumors arising in ovarian or testicular teratomas or in the bronchus; by releasing their secretions directly into the systemic circulation, tumors from these locations can produce the syndrome before metastatic disease occurs. As the humoral substances released by tumors draining into the portal circulation are largely metabolized by the liver, tumors arising in this location produce the syndrome only after hepatic metastasis. Because of the relatively slow growth of carcinoid tumors, palliative resection of hepatic metastases is beneficial in carefully selected cases. Resection of large isolated hepatic metastases has led to relief of the symptoms of carcinoid syndrome and marked reductions in urinary 5-HIAA excretion for periods of several years. In some cases with multiple metastases, removal of as much as a hepatic lobe may be considered when the metastases are located primarily in the portion of the liver to be resected, as determined by arteriography, scintillation scanning of gamma-emitting colloidal particles taken up by the liver, and inspection of the hepatic surface at surgical exploration.

TABLE 91-1
Outline of diagnostic approach to a patient with suspected carcinoid syndrome

I Quantitative determination of 24-h urinary excretion of 5-HIAA (5-hydroxyindoleacetic acid).
II When elevated 5-HIAA confirms clinical evidence for carcinoid syndrome, curable ovarian, testicular, or bronchial primary tumors should be sought.
III Consideration of possible treatment of the syndrome by surgical resection of hepatic metastases requires:
   A Assessment of the location and character of hepatic metastases with arteriography and scintillation scanning of the liver.
   B Evaluation of hepatic and cardiac function.
   C A search for extrahepatic metastases in bone and other sites.
IV In patients with substantial diarrhea, possible malabsorption of nutrients should be investigated.

Chemotherapy of carcinoid tumors has not yielded the extent or duration of palliation achieved with selective removal of hepatic metastases. Radiation treatment has been effective in some patients.

Pharmacological therapy directed at the humoral mediators of the syndrome is useful in some cases. When the flush is associated with release of histamine, as may be the case with gastric carcinoids, combined treatment with an H_1 antagonist (e.g., diphenhydramine) and an H_2 antagonist (cimetidine) will block the vasodilator action of histamine. Methysergide, a serotonin antagonist, will improve the diarrhea, but prolonged therapy with this agent can produce retroperitoneal fibrosis. Blockade of serotonin synthesis with the tryptophan hydroxylase inhibitor p-chlorophenylalanine also ameliorates the diarrhea. The prevention of severe flushing by corticosteroids and amelioration of the syndrome by phenothiazines are limited largely to patients with tumors arising from the bronchus and other organs derived from the embryonic foregut.

Nicotinamide should be given to those patients who shunt a large fraction of dietary tryptophan into the hydroxyindole pathway.

Hypotensive episodes should not be treated with catecholamines; by stimulating the release of vasoactive substances from the tumor, norepinephrine, epinephrine, and other agents with adrenergic activity can exaggerate and prolong the circulatory disturbance. If hypotension requires therapy, volume expansion or methoxamine infusion is the preferred approach.

REFERENCES

OATES JA, BUTLER TC: Pharmacologic and endocrine aspects of carcinoid syndrome. Adv Pharmacol 5:109, 1967

ROBERTSON JIS et al: The mechanism of facial flushing in the carcinoid syndrome. Q J Med 31:103, 1962

SJOERDSMA A et al: A clinical, physiologic and biochemical study of patients with malignant carcinoid. Am J Med 20:520, 1956

VAN SICKLE DG: Carcinoid tumors; analysis of 61 cases, including 11 cases of carcinoid syndrome. Cleveland Clin Q 39:79, 1972

Disorders of nucleic acid metabolism

92

GOUT AND OTHER DISORDERS OF PURINE METABOLISM

WILLIAM N. KELLEY

Gout is a term representing a heterogeneous group of diseases found exclusively in humans, which in their full development are manifested by (1) an increase in the serum urate concentration; (2) recurrent attacks of a characteristic type of acute arthritis, in which crystals of monosodium urate monohydrate are demonstrable in leukocytes of synovial fluid; (3) aggregated deposits of monosodium urate monohydrate (tophi) chiefly in and around the joints of the extremities and sometimes leading to severe crippling and deformity; (4) renal disease involving interstitial tissues and blood vessels; and (5) uric acid nephrolithiasis. These may occur singly or in combination.

PREVALENCE AND EPIDEMIOLOGY The serum urate value is elevated in an absolute sense when it exceeds the limit of solubility of monosodium urate in serum. At 37°C the saturation value of urate in plasma is about 7.0 mg per 100 ml; a value above this represents supersaturation in a physicochemical sense. The serum urate concentration is relatively elevated when it exceeds the upper limit of an arbitrary normal range, usually defined as the mean serum urate value plus two standard deviations in a healthy population matched for age and sex. In most epidemiological studies the upper limit is about 7.0 mg per 100 ml in men and 6.0 mg per 100 ml in women. In epidemiological terms a serum urate value in excess of 7.0 mg

per 100 ml carries an increased risk of gouty arthritis or renal stones.

Sex and age have an important influence on the serum urate. The serum urate concentration before puberty in both boys and girls averages approximately 3.6 mg per 100 ml. After the onset of puberty levels increase in boys more than in girls. Values in men reach a plateau in the early twenties and are essentially stable thereafter. Values in women are constant from age 20 through 40, but with menopause the values rise and approach or equal those in men. Age and sex differences in the serum urate are thought to be related to differences in the renal clearance of urate, perhaps determined in turn by the levels of estrogens and androgens. Other factors, including warm ambient temperature, obesity, high social status, and achievement or intelligence appear to correlate with a higher serum urate concentration.

Hyperuricemia by one or more of the above definitions is present in 2 to 18 percent of the populations studied. In one hospitalized population, 13 percent of adult men exhibited a serum urate concentration in excess of 7.0 mg per 100 ml.

The prevalence of gout is substantially less than that of hyperuricemia and is widely different around the world. In most of the Western world it ranges from 0.13 to 0.37 percent of the population. Gout is primarily a disease of adult men, and only about 5 percent of cases occur in women; it occurs rarely in the prepubertal child of either sex. The usual form of gout is uncommon before the third decade, and the peak incidence is in the fifth decade.

INHERITANCE In the United States a family history of gout is obtained in 6 to 18 percent of gouty subjects, and figures as high as 75 percent are noted after persistent questioning. A more precise definition of the inheritance of gout is complicated by the numerous environmental factors capable of altering the serum urate concentration. In addition, the identification of several specific genetic causes of gout has established that gout is merely the common clinical manifestation of a heterogeneous group of diseases. Accordingly, study of the inheritance of hyperuricemia and gout in the population or even within families is difficult. Two specific enzymatic causes of gout, hypoxanthine-guanine phosphoribosyltransferase deficiency and 5-phosphoribosyl-1-pyrophosphate (PRPP) synthetase overactivity, are X-linked. Pedigrees have been reported in which the inheritance pattern is consistent with an autosomal dominant mode. More commonly genetic studies suggest multifactorial inheritance patterns.

CLINICAL FEATURES In the full development of its natural history, gout passes through four stages: asymptomatic hyperuricemia, acute gouty arthritis, intercritical gout, and chronic tophaceous gout. Nephrolithiasis may occur in any stage but the first.

Asymptomatic hyperuricemia Asymptomatic hyperuricemia is that stage in which the serum urate level is raised but arthritic symptoms, tophi, or uric acid stones have not yet appeared. In men vulnerable to classic gout hyperuricemia begins at puberty, whereas in women at risk hyperuricemia is usually delayed until menopause. In contrast, patients with certain of the enzyme defects to be described later may be hyperuricemic from birth. While asymptomatic hyperuricemia may last throughout the lifetime with no recognizable consequences, the tendency toward acute gouty arthritis increases as a function of serum urate concentration and the duration of hyperuricemia. The risk of nephrolithiasis also increases as serum urate values increase and correlates with the magnitude of uric acid excretion. While virtually all gouty subjects are hyperuricemic, perhaps no more than 5 percent of hyperuricemics ever develop gout.

The phase of asymptomatic hyperuricemia ends with the first attack of gouty arthritis or nephrolithiasis. In most, gout comes before stone, usually after at least 20 to 30 years of sustained hyperuricemia. However, between 10 and 40 percent of gouty subjects have renal colic prior to the first episode of arthritis.

Acute gouty arthritis The primary manifestation of acute gout is exquisitely painful arthritis, at first usually monoarticular and associated with few constitutional symptoms, but later often polyarticular and accompanied by fever. Attacks last a variable but limited period of time and are separated by intervals of freedom from all symptoms. About 90 percent of first attacks occur in a single joint, and in at least half the initial attack occurs in the first metatarsal phalangeal joint. Ultimately, 90 percent of patients experience an acute attack in the great toe (podagra).

Acute gouty arthritis is predominantly a disease of the lower extremities. The more distal the site of involvement the more typical are the attacks. Following the toe in order of frequency as sites of initial involvement are the insteps, ankles, heels, knees, wrists, fingers, and elbows. While acute attacks may occur in other joints, such as shoulder, hips, spine, sacroiliac, sternoclavicular, and mandibular joints, these sites are rare except in patients with established, severe disease. The patient may report trivial episodes of pain preceding the first dramatic gouty attack. Commonly, the major attack begins at night, is exquisitely painful with inflamed joints, and may be triggered by a specific event such as trauma, alcohol ingestion, certain drugs, dietary excess, or surgery. It is difficult to improve upon Syndenham's classical description:

The victim goes to bed and sleeps in good health. About two o'clock in the morning he is awakened by a severe pain in the great toe; more rarely in the heel, ankle or instep. This pain is like that of a dislocation, and yet the parts feel as if cold water were poured over them. Then follow chills and shivers, and a little fever. The pain, which was at first moderate, becomes more intense. With its intensity the chills and shivers increase. After a time this comes to its height, accommodating itself to the bones and ligaments of the tarsus and metatarsus. Now it is a violent stretching and tearing of the ligaments—now it is a gnawing pain and now a pressure and tightening. So exquisite and lively meanwhile is the feeling of the part affected, that it cannot bear the weight of bedclothes nor the jar of a person walking in the room. The night is passed in torture, sleeplessness, turning of the part affected, and perpetual change of posture; the tossing about of the body being as incessant as the pain of the tortured joint, and being worse as the fit comes on. Hence the vain effort by change of posture, both in the body and the limb affected, to obtain an abatement of the pain.

Intercritical period The attack of gout may last only a day or two or up to several weeks but characteristically subsides spontaneously. An asymptomatic phase termed the *intercritical period* then commences. The patient will be totally free of symptoms during this stage, a feature that is diagnostically important. While approximately 7 percent of patients never have a second attack, most experience a recurrence within 1 year. However, the intercritical period may last up to 10 years. Later attacks tend to be polyarticular, more severe, more prolonged, and associated with fever. In this stage gout may be difficult to differentiate from other types of polyarticular arthritis such as rheumatoid arthritis. While most patients experience the intermittent course just described, rare patients progress directly from the initial acute attack to chronic polyarticular disease with no remissions.

Tophi and chronic gouty arthritis In the untreated patient the urate pool expands and crystal deposits of monosodium urate eventually appear in cartilage, synovial membranes, tendons, and soft tissues. The rate of formation of these tophaceous deposits appears to be a direct function of the degree and duration of hyperuricemia and of the severity of renal disease. The classic location of a tophus is the helix or antihelix of the ear (Fig. 92-1). Tophi also commonly occur along the ulnar surface of the forearm, as saccular distensions of the olecranon bursae (Fig. 92-2), as enlargements of the Achilles tendon, or at other pressure points. Patients with the most severe tophi, interestingly, often have sparing of the helix and antihelix of the ear.

FIGURE 92-1
Tophus of the helix of the ear adjacent to the auricular tubercle.

FIGURE 92-2
Effusions of olecranon bursae of patient with gout. Note also the cutaneous deposits of urate and the minimal inflammatory response.

Tophi are difficult to differentiate from rheumatoid nodules and other types of subcutaneous nodules. They may ulcerate and exude chalky or pasty material rich in monosodium urate crystals. In contrast to other subcutaneous nodules, tophi are rarely transient although they may resolve slowly in response to effective treatment of hyperuricemia. For reasons that are unclear, it is rare for a tophus to become infected. Patients with severe tophaceous disease appear to have milder and less frequent attacks of acute gouty arthritis than nontophaceous subjects. Chronic tophaceous gout rarely occurs prior to the onset of gouty arthritis.

Since the advent of effective antihyperuricemic therapy, only a minority of patients develop visible tophi, permanent joint changes, or chronic symptoms. Thus, effective therapy has altered the natural history of the disease.

Nephropathy   Some renal dysfunction is present in up to 90 percent of subjects with a history of gouty arthritis. Prior to the advent of chronic hemodialysis, renal failure accounted for 17 to 25 percent of deaths in the gouty population. The initial manifestation of renal involvement may be albuminuria or isosthenuria. If the patient presents in an advanced stage of renal failure it may be difficult to determine whether renal failure is a consequence of hyperuricemia or hyperuricemia is the result of renal disease.

Several types of parenchymal renal damage have been described. The first, urate nephropathy, has been attributed to the deposition of monosodium urate crystals in the renal interstitial tissue. The second, obstructive uropathy, is due to the formation of uric acid crystals in the collecting tubules, renal pelvis, or ureter, with resulting blockage of urine flow.

There is considerable controversy over the pathogenesis of urate nephropathy. While crystals of monosodium urate have been demonstrated in the interstitium of kidneys from gouty subjects, such crystals are not demonstrable in the kidneys of most people with gout. Further, there is a close correlation between the development of renal disease and the presence of hypertension in patients with gout. It is not clear, therefore, whether the hypertension causes the renal disease or the gouty renal disease is the cause of the hypertension.

Acute obstructive uropathy is a severe form of acute renal failure due to the precipitation of uric acid crystals in collecting ducts and ureters. This condition occurs most commonly in (1) patients with profound overproduction of uric acid, particularly subjects with leukemia or lymphoma who are subjected to aggressive chemotherapy, (2) patients with gout and marked

hyperuricaciduria, and (3) (possibly) in patients following severe exercise or convulsions. Postmortem studies reveal intraluminal precipitates of uric acid with dilatation of proximal tubules. Therapy designed to decrease the formation of uric acid, accelerate urine flow, and increase the fraction of uric acid present as the more soluble ionized form, monosodium urate, is effective in the reversal of this process.

Nephrolithiasis   While the overall prevalence of uric acid stones in the population of the United States is about 0.01 percent, the prevalence in gouty subjects ranges from 10 to 25 percent. The major factor favoring formation of uric acid stones is the increased urinary excretion of uric acid. When the urinary uric acid exceeds 1100 mg per day the incidence reaches 50 percent. There is also correlation with increasing serum urate concentrations, the prevalence reaching approximately 50 percent at a serum urate value of 13 mg per 100 ml or above. Other factors contributing to the formation of uric acid stones include (1) undue acidity of the urine, (2) increased urine concentration, and (3) (perhaps) abnormalities of urinary constituents that affect the solubility of uric acid itself.

Gouty subjects also have an increased frequency of calcium-containing stones; the occurrence in gout is 1 to 3 percent, while that in the general population is about 0.1 percent. While the mechanisms for this association are unclear, there is a high frequency of hyperuricemia and hyperuricaciduria in patients seen because of calcium stones. It is possible that uric acid crystals serve as a nidus for calcium stone formation.

Associated conditions   Obesity, hypertriglyceridemia, and hypertension are common. The hypertriglyceridemia of primary gout is strongly associated with obesity or alcohol ingestion and not with hyperuricemia itself. The incidence of hypertension in the nongouty population is correlated with age, sex, and obesity; when these factors are appropriately scored there appears to be little or no direct relationship between hyperuricemia and hypertension. The increased frequency of diabetes is also probably related to factors such as age and obesity and not to hyperuricemia itself. Finally, the increased incidence of atherosclerosis has been attributed to the concomitant obesity, hypertension, diabetes, and hypertriglyceridemia.

Independent analysis of these variables suggests that obesity is most important. Hyperuricemia in the obese subject appears to be related to both increased production and reduced excretion of uric acid.

DIAGNOSIS AND DIFFERENTIAL DIAGNOSIS   The diagnosis of acute gouty arthritis can be established by demonstration of monosodium urate crystals in white cells of synovial fluid obtained from the inflamed joint by compensated polarized light microscopy (Fig. 92-3). Such crystals can be identified in synovial fluid from virtually every patient with acute gouty arthritis. Failure to demonstrate urate crystals in synovial fluid after careful search under appropriate conditions makes the diagnosis unlikely.

Demonstration of intracellular urate crystals establishes the diagnosis but does not exclude the possibility that another type of arthropathy is present concurrently.

Synovial fluid analysis may also be helpful in other ways. The total leukocyte count may range from 1000 to more than 70,000 per milliliter. The predominant cell type is the polymorphonuclear leukocyte. As with other inflammatory fluids, the mucin clot is fair to poor. The concentrations of glucose and uric acid are the same as in serum.

FIGURE 92-3
Crystals of monosodium urate monohydrate in joint aspirate.

In the patient in whom synovial fluid cannot be obtained or in whom intracellular crystals cannot be demonstrated, a presumptive diagnosis of gout can be seriously entertained if the patient has (1) hyperuricemia, (2) the classical clinical features described above, and (3) a dramatic response to colchicine. In the absence of crystals or this highly suggestive triad, the diagnosis of gout should be considered tentative. While a dramatic therapeutic response to colchicine is strongly suggestive of the diagnosis of gouty arthritis, it is not pathognomonic by itself.

Acute gouty arthritis must be differentiated from other conditions in which monoarticular or polyarticular arthritis occurs. The most common initial presentation in the gouty patient is podagra, but many conditions mimic the painful, swollen big toe characteristic of the disease. These include soft tissue infection, inflamed bunions, local trauma, rheumatoid arthritis, degenerative arthritis with acute inflammation, acute sarcoidosis, psoriatic arthritis, pseudogout, acute calcific tendonitis, palindromic rheumatism, Reiter's disease, and sporotrichosis. Rarely, confusion may be caused by cellulitis, gonor-

rhea, fibrosis of the sole and heel, hematoma, and subacute bacterial endocarditis with embolization or suppurative arthritis. Gouty involvement of other joints such as the knee must also be differentiated from acute rheumatic fever, serum sickness, hemarthrosis, and the peripheral joint involvement of ankylosing spondylitis or inflammatory bowel disease.

PATHOPHYSIOLOGY OF HYPERURICEMIA Classification

The biochemical hallmark and prerequisite of gout is hyperuricemia. The concentration of uric acid in body fluids is determined by the balance between rates of production and elimination. Uric acid is formed by oxidation of purine bases, which may be exogenous or endogenous in origin. About two-thirds of uric acid is excreted into the urine (300 to 600 mg per day), and approximately one-third is excreted into the gastrointestinal tract, where it is ultimately destroyed by bacteria. Hyperuricemia may be due to an excessive rate of uric acid production, a decrease in the renal excretion of uric acid, or a combination of both events.

Hyperuricemia and gout may be classified as primary, secondary, or idiopathic (Table 92-1). In the classification used here *primary* refers to those cases in which gout or hyperuricemia is the central manifestation of the disease, namely, gout that is neither secondary to another acquired disorder nor a subordinate manifestation of an inborn error that leads initially to a major disease unlike gout. While some cases of primary gout have a defined genetic basis, others do not. *Secondary* hyperuricemia or gout refers to those cases which develop in the course of another disease or as a consequence of drugs. Finally, the term *idiopathic* is used to describe those cases in which the underlying defect has not been defined and a more precise classification (overproduction or underexcretion) cannot be made. Further subdivisions within each of the three major categories are based on the identification of overproduction or underexcretion or both as responsible for the hyperuricemia.

Overproduction of uric acid Overproducers of uric acid by definition excrete in excess of 600 mg per day after a 5-day period of dietary purine restriction; such patients probably represent less than 10 percent of the gouty population. In these patients there is an acceleration in the rate of purine biosynthesis de novo. Overproduction of uric acid can occur either as the result of a specific enzyme defect, as the secondary consequence of a proliferative disorder, or in idiopathic gout. Understanding the basic mechanisms responsible for these abnor-

TABLE 92-1
Classification of hyperuricemia and gout

Type	Metabolic disturbance	Inheritance
Primary:		
Molecular defects undefined:		
Underexcretion (90% of primary gout)	Not established	Polygenic
Overproduction (10% of primary gout)	Not established	Polygenic
Associated with specific enzyme defects:		
P-ribose-PP synthetase variants; increased activity	Overproduction of PP-ribose-P and of uric acid	X-linked
Hypoxanthine-guanine phosphoribosyltransferase deficiency, partial	Overproduction of uric acid; increased purine biosynthesis de novo driven by surplus P-ribose-PP	X-linked
Secondary:		
Associated with increased purine biosynthesis de novo:		
Glucose 6-phosphatase deficiency or absence	Overproduction plus underexcretion of uric acid; glycogen storage disease, type I (von Gierke)	Autosomal recessive
Hypoxanthine-guanine phosphoribosyltransferase deficiency "virtually complete"	Overproduction of uric acid; Lesch-Nyhan syndrome	X-linked
Associated with increased nucleic acid turnover	Overproduction of uric acid	
Associated with decreased renal excretion of uric acid	Decreased filtration of uric acid Inhibited tubular secretion of uric acid, or enhanced tubular reabsorption of uric acid	
Idiopathic		Unknown

SOURCE: *After Wyngaarden and Kelley, 1976.*

malities requires a brief review of purine metabolism (Fig. 92-4).

The purine nucleotides, adenylic acid (AMP), inosinic acid (IMP), and guanylic acid (GMP), are the end products of purine biosynthesis. They can be synthesized in one of two ways: either directly from the purine bases, e.g., guanine to GMP, hypoxanthine to IMP, and adenine to AMP; or they may be synthesized de novo, beginning with nonpurine precursors and progressing through a series of steps to the formation of IMP, which is the common intermediate purine nucleotide. IMP can be converted either to AMP or to GMP. Once the purine nucleotides are formed, they are utilized for the synthesis of nucleic acids, cyclic AMP, cyclic GMP, ATP, and certain cofactors.

The various purine components are degraded to the purine nucleotide monophosphates. GMP is degraded via guanosine, guanine, and xanthine to uric acid. IMP is degraded through inosine, hypoxanthine, and xanthine to uric acid. AMP can be deaminated to IMP and further catabolized through inosine to uric acid, or it may be degraded to inosine by an alternate pathway with the intermediate formation of adenosine.

While the purine pathway is regulated in a complex manner, the intracellular concentration of 5-phosphoribosyl-1-pyrophosphate (PRPP) appears to be a major determinant of the rate of synthesis of uric acid in humans. Generally, when the concentration of PRPP in the cell is elevated, uric acid synthesis is elevated; when the concentration of PRPP is reduced, the synthesis of uric acid is also reduced. Although exceptions are recognized, this concept is applicable to most situations.

From 5 to 10 percent of adult gouty subjects with overproduction of uric acid have a partial deficiency of hypoxanthine-guanine phosphoribosyltransferase, the enzyme that catalyzes the conversion of hypoxanthine to inosinic acid and guanine to guanylic acid (reaction 2, Fig. 92-4). The deficiency of hypoxanthine-guanine phosphoribosyltransferase leads to a decreased consumption and increased accumulation of PRPP, thus accelerating purine biosynthesis and the production of uric acid. These patients typically have the onset of gouty arthritis at a young age (15 to 30 years), a high incidence of uric acid stones (75 percent), and the occasional occurrence of mild neurologic dysfunction characterized by dysarthria, hyperreflexia, incoordination, and/or mental retardation. This disease

is inherited in an X-linked manner so that males are affected through carrier females. A more severe deficiency of the same enzyme leads to the development of the Lesch-Nyhan syndrome.

Several families are described in which there is increased activity of the enzyme PRPP synthetase (reaction 3, Fig. 92-4). The mutant enzymes, of which three different types are recognized, all exhibit increased activity, resulting in increased intracellular concentrations of PRPP, accelerated purine biosynthesis, and elevated excretion of uric acid. The inheritance pattern in this disease is also X-linked. These patients, like those with partial hypoxanthine-guanine phosphoribosyltransferase deficiency, generally develop gout in the second or third decade and have a high incidence of uric acid stones.

These two inborn errors of purine metabolism, hypoxanthine-guanine phosphoribosyltransferase deficiency and PRPP synthetase overactivity, account for less than 15 percent of all patients with what is now considered to be primary hyperuricemia associated with an overproduction of uric acid. The cause of the overproduction in the majority of patients has not been defined (idiopathic).

There are numerous causes of secondary hyperuricemia associated with an increased production of uric acid. In some, the increased excretion of uric acid is related, as it is in primary gout, to an accelerated rate of purine biosynthesis de novo. Patients with glucose 6-phosphatase deficiency (type I glycogen storage disease) uniformly exhibit an increased production of uric acid as well as an accelerated rate of purine biosynthesis de novo (see Chap. 97). It is postulated that patients with this enzyme defect also have an increased concentration of PRPP, which in turn is responsible for the accelerated rate of purine biosynthesis and uric acid overproduction. Patients with the Lesch-Nyhan syndrome, which is due to a virtually complete deficiency of hypoxanthine-guanine phosphoribosyltransferase, also uniformly exhibit a profound overproduction of uric acid and an accelerated rate of purine biosynthesis de novo. In these patients, as in those with gout due to a partial deficiency of hypoxanthine-guanine phosphoribosyltransfer-

FIGURE 92-4

Outline of purine metabolism: (1) amidophosphoribosyltransferase; (2) hypoxanthine-guanine phosphoribosyltransferase; (3) PRPP synthetase; (4) adenine phosphoribosyltransferase; (5) adenosine deaminase; (6) purine nucleoside phosphorylase; (7) 5'-nucleotidase; (8) xanthine oxidase.

484

ase, the basic mechanism is thought to be related to a decreased consumption of PRPP.

In the majority of patients with secondary hyperuricemia due to an overproduction of uric acid, the predominant abnormality appears to be an increased turnover of nucleic acids. A number of diseases, including the myeloproliferative and lymphoproliferative disorders, multiple myeloma, secondary polycythemia, pernicious anemia, certain hemoglobinopathies, thalassemia, other hemolytic anemias, infectious mononucleosis, and some carcinomas may be associated with increased marrow activity or increased cell turnover at other sites and an associated increased turnover of nucleic acids. The increased turnover in nucleic acids leads in turn to hyperuricemia, hyperuricaciduria, and a compensatory increase in the rate of purine biosynthesis de novo.

Reduced excretion A large proportion of gouty subjects require a plasma urate value of 1 to 2 mg per 100 ml higher than normal subjects to achieve a given rate of uric acid excretion (Fig. 92-5). This abnormality is most prominent in the gouty subject with a normal production of uric acid and is not present in most subjects with overproduction of uric acid.

The excretion of urate is dependent on glomerular filtration, tubular reabsorption, and tubular secretion. Uric acid appears to be completely filtered at the glomerulus and reabsorbed in the proximal tubule (i.e., presecretory reabsorption). Uric acid secretion then occurs in a subsequent segment of the proximal tubule, and partial reabsorption takes place at a second reabsorptive site in the distal portion of the proximal tubule (i.e., postsecretory reabsorption). While some uric acid reabsorption may also occur in the ascending limb of the loop of Henle and in the collecting duct, these latter two sites are

FIGURE 92-5

Rate of uric acid excretion at various plasma urate levels in nongouty (solid symbols) and gouty (open symbols) subjects. Large symbols represent mean values; small symbols represent individual data of a few mean values selected to illustrate the degree of scatter within groups. Studies were conducted under basal conditions, after RNA feeding, and after infusions of lithium urate. (From Wyngaarden. Reproduced by permission of Academic Press.)

thought to be quantitatively less important. Attempts to define further the location and nature of these latter sites and to quantify their contribution to uric acid transport in normal humans or in various disease states have been largely unrewarding.

Theoretically, the altered renal excretion of uric acid exhibited by most patients with gout could be due to (1) reduced filtration of uric acid, (2) enhanced reabsorption, or (3) decreased secretion. While there are no unequivocal data to establish any one of these three mechanisms as the basic defect, it seems likely that all three types of abnormalities will be found to be operative within the gouty population.

Numerous secondary causes of hyperuricemia and gout can also be attributed to a decrease in the renal excretion of uric acid. A reduction in the glomerular filtration rate leads to a decrease in the filtered load of uric acid and thus to hyperuricemia; patients with renal disease are hyperuricemic on this basis. Other factors, such as decreased secretion of uric acid, have been postulated in patients with some types of renal disease (e.g., polycystic kidney disease and lead nephropathy). Gout is a rare complication of the secondary hyperuricemia due to renal disease.

Diuretic therapy is one of the most important causes of secondary hyperuricemia. Diuretic-induced volume depletion leads to enhanced tubular reabsorption of uric acid as well as decreased uric acid filtration. Decreased secretion of uric acid has also been postulated as a possible mechanism in diuretic-induced hyperuricemia. A number of other drugs lead to hyperuricemia by undefined renal mechanisms; these agents include low-dose aspirin, pyrazinamide, nicotinic acid, ethambutol, and ethanol.

Impaired renal excretion of uric acid is thought to be an important mechanism for the hyperuricemia associated with several disease states. Volume depletion may be important in patients with hyperuricemia associated with adrenal insufficiency and nephrogenic diabetes insipidus. In some situations hyperuricemia has been attributed to competitive inhibition of uric acid secretion by excess organic acids thought to be secreted by the same renal tubular mechanism responsible for uric acid secretion. Examples include starvation (ketosis and free fatty acids), alcoholic ketosis, diabetic ketoacidosis, maple syrup urine disease, and lactic acidosis of any cause. Hyperuricemia in conditions such as hyperparathyroidism, hypoparathyroidism, pseudohypoparathyroidism, and hypothyroidism may also have a renal basis, but the mechanism is unclear.

PATHOGENESIS OF ACUTE GOUTY ARTHRITIS The events leading to the initial crystallization of monosodium urate in a joint after an average of 30 years of asymptomatic hyperuricemia are not completely understood. Sustained hyperuricemia leads eventually to the development of microtophi in the synovial lining cells and perhaps to an accumulation of monosodium urate in cartilage on proteoglycans that have a high affinity for urate. By one of several mechanisms, probably including trauma with disruption of the microtophi and increased turnover of the cartilage proteoglycans, there is an episodic release of urate crystals into the synovial fluid. Other factors, such as a lower temperature in the joint space or an unequal reabsorption of water and urate from the synovial fluid, may accelerate urate precipitation.

A sufficient number of crystals in the joint space triggers the acute attack by a process that appears to include (1) phagocytosis of the crystals by leukocytes with the rapid release of a chemotactic protein from the leukocytes, (2) activation of the kallikrein system, (3) activation of complement with the consequent formation of the chemotactic complement components, and (4) the ultimate urate-mediated disruption of lysosomes within the leukocytes, leading to destruction of white blood cells and release of lysosomal products into the synovial fluid.

While progress in the understanding of acute gouty arthritis has occurred, questions about factors responsible for spontaneous resolution of the acute attack and the effect of colchicine remain to be completely answered.

TREATMENT The therapeutic aims in gout are (1) to terminate the acute attack as promptly and gently as possible; (2) to prevent recurrences of acute gouty arthritis; (3) to prevent or reverse complications of the disease resulting from deposition of monosodium urate crystals in joints, kidneys, and other sites; (4) to prevent or reverse associated features such as obesity, hypertriglyceridemia, or hypertension; and (5) to prevent formation of uric acid kidney stones.

Treatment of the acute gouty attack Acute gouty arthritis is treated with an anti-inflammatory agent. Colchicine is the drug most frequently employed. Standard therapy involves administration of 0.5 mg each hour or 1.0 mg every 2 hours by mouth until one of three things occurs: (1) the patient improves, (2) gastrointestinal side effects develop, or (3) a maximum of 6 mg is taken without relief. Colchicine is most effective if therapy is begun shortly after the onset of symptoms. Over 75 percent of patients with gout show major improvement in symptoms within the first 12 h of treatment. However, as many as 80 percent of patients are unable to tolerate an optimal dose because of gastrointestinal side effects, which may precede or coincide with clinical improvement. Intravenous administration of colchicine eliminates the gastrointestinal side effects for the majority and also provides a more rapid response.

Colchicine levels become high in leukocytes, remain constant for 24 h, and are detectable for over 10 days after a single intravenous infusion. As an initial dose 2 mg should be given intravenously, followed by two additional doses of 1 mg at 6-h intervals if needed. Special care must be taken in the intravenous administration of colchicine. The drug is irritative and can lead to severe pain and necrosis if allowed to extravasate to surrounding tissues. It is important to make certain that the intravenous route is secure and that the drug is diluted with 5 to 10 volumes of normal saline and infused over a period of no less than 5 min. Colchicine by either oral or parenteral route may cause bone marrow depression, alopecia, hepatocellular failure, mental depression, seizures, ascending paralysis, respiratory depression, and death. Toxic effects are more likely in patients with significant hepatic, bone marrow, or renal disease and in those subjects on prophylactic maintenance colchicine. The dosage should be reduced for these individuals, and the drug should not be used in neutropenic patients.

Other anti-inflammatory agents, including indomethacin, phenylbutazone, naproxen, and fenoprofen, are also effective in the treatment of acute gouty arthritis. Indomethacin may be given at a dose of 75 mg orally, followed by 50 mg every 6 h and continued at that dose for 24 h after relief is obtained. The drug is then tapered to 50 mg every 8 h for three doses, and then to 25 mg every 8 h for three doses. Side effects of indomethacin include gastrointestinal toxicity, sodium retention, and complaints referable to the central nervous system. While the incidence of side effects may be as high as 60 percent in patients taking the doses described above, the drug is generally better tolerated than colchicine and probably is the treatment of choice in the patient with a well-established diagnosis of acute gouty arthritis. To improve the therapeutic response and thus diminish morbidity of the disease, the patient may be instructed to begin therapy with an anti-inflammatory agent at the first twinge of an acute attack.

Prophylaxis Once the acute episode has resolved, a number of measures can reduce the likelihood of recurrence. These include (1) the institution of prophylactic daily colchicine or indomethacin, (2) controlled weight reduction for the obese patient, (3) avoidance of known precipitating factors such as heavy alcohol consumption or a diet rich in purines, and (4) the institution of antihyperuricemic therapy.

The administration of small daily doses of colchicine for prophylaxis against further acute attacks is effective. A program of 1 to 2 mg colchicine a day is completely successful in about three-fourths of patients with gout and fails completely in only about 5 percent. In addition, this program is safe and essentially free of side effects. However, unless serum urate is maintained at normal levels, the patient is spared only acute arthritis and may well proceed to develop other manifestations of gout. Maintenance colchicine therapy is particularly helpful during the first year or two after institution of antihyperuricemic drugs.

Prevention or reversal of the deposition of monosodium urate in tissues Antihyperuricemic agents are effective in reducing serum urate concentration and should be used in patients with (1) one or more attacks of acute gouty arthritis, (2) one or more tophi, and (3) uric acid nephrolithiasis. The aim of antihyperuricemic therapy is to maintain the serum urate below 7.0 mg per 100 ml, the minimal concentration at which urate saturates the extracellular fluid. Reduction to these levels may be achieved by use of drugs that increase the renal excretion of uric acid or decrease uric acid production. Antihyperuricemic drugs generally do not have anti-inflammatory properties. Uricosuric agents reduce serum urate by enhancing the renal excretion. While a large number of drugs exhibit this property, the most effective agents available in the United States are probenecid and sulfinpyrazone. Probenecid is usually started in doses of 250 mg twice a day; it is increased over a period of several weeks to the dose necessary to achieve effective reversal of the hyperuricemia. A total dose of 1 g per day is appropriate for half of patients; the maximum dose should not exceed 3.0 g per day. Because the half-life is 6 to 12 h, it should be given in two to four evenly spaced doses per day. Hypersensitivity, skin rash, and gastrointestinal complaints are the major side effects. Although serious toxicity is rare, side effects may cause up to a third of the patients to discontinue probenecid.

Sulfinpyrazone is a metabolite of phenylbutazone with no anti-inflammatory activity. The drug is usually started at a dose of 50 mg twice a day and gradually increased to a maintenance level of 300 to 400 mg per day given in three or four divided doses. The maximum effective daily dose is 800 mg. Side effects are similar to those with probenecid, although the incidence of bone marrow toxicity may be higher. Approximately a fourth of patients stop the drug for one reason or another.

Probenecid and sulfinpyrazone are effective in 75 to 80 percent of patients with hyperuricemia and gout. In addition to intolerance, failures can result from poor patient compliance, concomitant salicylate ingestion, or impaired renal function. Aspirin at any dose blocks the uricosuric effect of probenecid and sulfinpyrazone. These agents begin to lose effectiveness as the creatinine clearance falls below 80 ml/min and are completely ineffective when clearance reaches 30 ml/min.

During the negative urate balance that commences upon initiation of uricosuric therapy, the serum urate value drops, and urinary uric acid excretion is elevated above pretreatment levels. With continuation of therapy excess urate is mobilized and eliminated, the serum urate falls, and uric acid excretion returns essentially to pretreatment levels. The transient increase in uric acid excretion, which usually lasts for only a few days, may lead to the development of renal calculi in as many as 9 percent of patients so treated. To avoid this complication uricosuric agents should be started at low doses and gradually increased as described. Maintaining an ample urine flow with adequate hydration and alkalinizing the urine with oral sodium bicarbonate alone or in combination with acetazolamide reduce the likelihood of stone formation. The ideal candidate for uricosuric agents is under 60 years old and has normal renal function (creatinine clearance greater than 80 ml/min), uric acid excretion of less than 700 mg per day on a general diet, and no history of renal stones.

Hyperuricemia may also be controlled by allopurinol, a drug that decreases uric acid synthesis. Allopurinol inhibits xanthine oxidase (reaction 8, Fig. 92-4), the enzyme that catalyzes the oxidation of hypoxanthine to xanthine and xanthine to uric acid. While allopurinol has a half-life in vivo of only 2 to 3 h, it is metabolized largely to oxipurinol, which also is an effective inhibitor of xanthine oxidase and has a half-life ranging from 18 to 30 h. In most patients 300 mg per day represents an effective antihyperuricemic dose. Because of the long half-life of the major metabolite the drug may be administered once a day with no loss of effectiveness. Since oxipurinol is largely excreted in the urine, its half-life is prolonged in patients with renal insufficiency. The dose of allopurinol should, therefore, be reduced by one-half in patients with significant renal dysfunction.

The significant side affects of allopurinol include gastrointestinal distress, skin rashes, fever, toxic epidermal necrolysis, alopecia, bone marrow suppression, hepatitis, jaundice, and vasculitis. The overall incidence of side effects is about 20 percent. Toxic effects appear to be more common in the presence of renal insufficiency. In only 5 percent of patients are the side effects sufficiently distressing to force discontinuation of the medication. Important drug-drug interactions involving allopurinol include prolongation of the half-lives of 6-mercaptopurine and azathioprine and enhancement of the toxicity of cyclophosphamide.

Specific indications for choosing allopurinol over a uricosuric drug include (1) an increased urinary uric acid excretion (greater than 700 mg per day on a general diet), (2) impairment of renal function with a creatinine clearance less than 80 ml/min, (3) tophaceous gout regardless of renal function, (4) uric acid nephrolithiasis, and (5) gout not controlled by uricosuric agents because of ineffectiveness or intolerance. Allopurinol and a uricosuric drug may be used simultaneously in the rare hyperuricemic patient who cannot be controlled by a single medication. The addition of allopurinol to a program that includes a uricosuric drug usually results in further lowering of the serum urate concentration. No modification in the dosage of either agent is required with combination therapy.

Acute gouty arthritis may occur whenever there is a rapid and substantial change in the serum urate concentration. Thus, the initiation of antihyperuricemic therapy with any agent may precipitate an acute attack of gouty arthritis. In addition, recurrent attacks may occur for a year or longer when large tophaceous deposits are present, even if hyperuricemia is controlled. For these reasons, it is prudent to begin prophylactic therapy with colchicine just prior to initiation of antihyperuricemic drugs, and to continue it until the serum urate is controlled for at least a year or until all tophi have resolved. Patients should be warned of the possibility of flare-up during the early phase of therapy. While it is usually not necessary to limit purine intake in most gouty patients, strict dietary purine restriction should be instituted in patients with severe tophaceous gout and/or renal failure.

Prevention and treatment of acute uric acid nephropathy Immediate and vigorous therapy is essential for acute uric acid nephropathy. The first step is to increase urine flow by vigorous hydration coupled with administration of a potent diuretic such as furosemide. The urine should be alkalinized to achieve conversion of uric acid to the more soluble monosodium urate. Alkalinization can be accomplished by the administration of sodium bicarbonate alone or by the simultaneous administration of sodium bicarbonate and acetazolamide. Allopurinol therapy should also be employed to reduce uric acid formation. The initial dose in this setting should be 8 mg/kg per day given as a single daily dose. The dose should be decreased after 3 or 4 days to 100 to 200 mg per day if renal insufficiency persists. Principles of treatment for uric acid kidney stones are similar to those described for acute uric acid nephropathy. In most cases of uric acid nephrolithiasis allopurinol therapy combined only with high fluid intake is effective.

WORKUP OF THE HYPERURICEMIC PATIENT Evaluation of the patient with hyperuricemia is directed toward (1) defining the cause of the hyperuricemia (which may disclose an important disease other than gout), (2) assessing the presence and extent of damage to tissues and organs, and (3) identifying associated abnormalities. From a practical standpoint these inquiries are pursued simultaneously, since decisions about the significance of hyperuricemia and about therapy depend on the answers to all of these.

History Is the hyperuricemia primary or secondary? Is the patient asymptomatic? Has there been hypertension or a history of cardiovascular disease? Is there a family history of hyperuricemia, gout, kidney stones, or renal disease? Is there a history of lead exposure?

Physical examination Are the joints normal? Are tophi present? Is there evidence of atherosclerosis? Are there features suggestive of a secondary cause of hyperuricemia, such as lymphadenopathy, splenomegaly, or hepatomegaly? Is the patient obese?

Initial laboratory test data The most important single test in the hyperuricemic patient is analysis of the urine for uric acid. If a history of stone disease is present, a flat plate of the abdomen and intravenous pyelogram may be indicated. If a renal stone is recovered, analysis for uric acid and other constituents is useful. If joint disease is present, synovial fluid analysis and x-rays of the involved joints are helpful. If there is a history of exposure to lead, measurement of urinary lead excretion after an infusion of calcium EDTA may be useful in documenting the presence of gout due to lead exposure. In cases where the patient appears to be an overproducer, measurement of erythrocyte hypoxanthine-guanine phosphoribosyltransferase and PRPP synthetase levels may be indicated.

Management of asymptomatic hyperuricemia There is considerable controversy about the indications for therapy of the patient with asymptomatic hyperuricemia. Generally, treatment should be withheld unless the patient (1) becomes symptomatic; (2) has a strong family history of gout, nephrolithiasis, or renal failure; or (3) is excreting large quantities of uric acid (greater than 1100 mg per day).

OTHER DISORDERS OF PURINE METABOLISM **Lesch-Nyhan syndrome** The Lesch-Nyhan syndrome is an X-linked disorder, which was described in 1964. Affected patients have hyperuricemia and a profound overproduction of uric acid. In addition, they have a bizarre neurologic disorder characterized by self-mutilation, choreoathetosis, spasticity, and retardation of growth and mental function. The incidence is estimated at 1:100,000 births. The characteristic biochemical abnormality is a profound deficiency of the enzyme hypoxanthine-guanine phosphoribosyltransferase (reaction 2, Fig. 92-4).

Adenine phosphoribosyltransferase deficiency Adenine phosphoribosyltransferase catalyzes the conversion of adenine to AMP (reaction 4, Fig. 92-4). The first family with a deficiency of adenine phosphoribosyltransferase was discovered in 1968. These subjects were heterozygous for deficiency of the enzyme and had no associated disease. It subsequently became apparent that heterozygosity for this deficiency is common, perhaps as frequent as 1:100. A homozygous deficiency of adenine phosphoribosyltransferase has now been described in three patients with a history of renal stones composed of 2,8-dioxyadenine. Because of chemical similarity, 2,8-dioxyadenine may be confused with uric acid, and in each of these patients an incorrect diagnosis of uric acid nephrolithiasis was made initially.

Adenosine deaminase deficiency and purine nucleoside phosphorylase deficiency Adenosine deaminase catalyzes the deamination of adenosine to inosine (reaction 5, Fig. 92-4). Patients with adenosine deaminase deficiency have severe combined immunodeficiency disease, i.e., a severe abnormality in T-cell function and somewhat milder B-cell dysfunction.

Deficiency of purine nucleoside phosphorylase (reaction 6, Fig. 92-4), the enzyme that catalyzes the conversion of inosine to hypoxanthine and guanosine to guanine also causes combined immunodeficiency disease. These two inborn errors of purine metabolism represent the first enzyme defects to be associated with immune dysfunction.

Xanthine oxidase deficiency Xanthine oxidase catalyzes the oxidation of hypoxanthine to xanthine, xanthine to uric acid, and adenine to 2,8-dioxyadenine (reaction 8, Fig. 92-4). Xanthinuria, the first inborn error of purine metabolism to be defined at the enzyme level, is due to a deficiency of xanthine oxidase. As a result, affected patients with xanthinuria have hypouricemia and hypouricaciduria as well as an increased urinary excretion of the oxypurines, hypoxanthine, and xanthine. Half are asymptomatic and a third have urinary xanthine stones. Several patients have been noted to have a myopathy and one patient with polyarthritis has been reported. Precipitation of xanthine is thought to be the important factor in the development of each of these clinical manifestations.

REFERENCES

GIBLETT ER et al: Adenosine deaminase deficiency in two patients with severely impaired cellular immunity. Lancet 2:1067, 1972
——— et al: Nucleoside-phosphorylase deficiency in a child with severely defective T-cell immunity and normal B-cell immunity. Lancet 1:1010, 1975
KELLEY WN: Crystal-induced arthropathies, in *The Clinics in Rheumatic Diseases.* Philadelphia, Saunders, 1977, vol 3, pp 1–171
——— et al: Hypoxanthine-guanine phosphoribosyltransferase deficiency in gout. Ann Intern Med, 70:155, 1969
SEEGMILLER JE: Diseases of purine and pyrimidine metabolism, in *Duncan's Diseases of Metabolism,* 7th ed, PK Bondy, LE Rosenberg (eds). Philadelphia, Saunders, 1974
TALBOTT JH, YU TF: *Gout and Uric Acid Metabolism.* New York, Stratton, 1976
WYNGAARDEN JB: Gout, in *Advances in Metabolic Disorders,* R Levine, and R Luft (eds). New York, Academic, 1965, vol 2, pp 2–78
———, Kelley WN: *Gout and Hyperuricemia.* New York, Grune & Stratton, 1976
———, ———: Gout, in *The Metabolic Basis of Inherited Diseases,* 4th ed, JB Stanbury et al (eds). New York, McGraw-Hill, 1978, pp 916–1010

93
HEREDITARY OROTIC ACIDURIA

WILLIAM N. KELLEY

Hereditary orotic aciduria is a rare disorder of pyrimidine metabolism usually characterized by retarded growth and development, hypochromic anemia associated with a megaloblastic marrow unresponsive to usual hematinic therapy, and excessive urinary excretion of orotic acid. The first patient with orotic aciduria was recognized and reported by Huguley and coworkers in 1959. Since that time eight additional cases have been described.

PATHOGENESIS The synthesis of pyrimidine nucleotides de novo is outlined in Fig. 93-1. Orotic aciduria occurs when the rate of synthesis of orotic acid exceeds the rate at which it is converted to orotidine 5′-monophosphate in the reaction catalyzed by orotate phosphoribosyltransferase. Patients with hereditary orotic aciduria have a genetically determined deficiency of orotate phosphoribosyltransferase and orotidine 5′-phosphate decarboxylase (type 1) or of orotidine 5′-phosphate decarboxylase alone (type 2). In the former the capacity of the cell to convert orotic acid to orotidine 5′-monophosphate is reduced. In the latter it is assumed that orotidine 5′-phosphate accumulates and thus inhibits orotate phosphoribosyltransferase activity. The two enzymes, orotate phosphoribosyltransferase and orotidine 5′-phosphate decarboxylase, are intimately associated in a complex. In patients with the double enzyme defect, it has been proposed that a mutation affecting the structure of orotate phosphoribosyltransferase destabilizes the complex, leading to the concomitant loss of orotidine 5′-phosphate decarboxylase activity.

Patients with both types of hereditary orotic aciduria excrete 600 to 1500 mg orotic acid in the urine per day, 3000 to 5000 times normal. In addition, patients excrete 15 to 30 mg orotidine per day, 20 to 40 times normal.

The clinical manifestations of hereditary orotic aciduria are due to (1) increased excretion of orotic acid and (2) pyrimidine nucleotide deficiency. Accumulation of orotic acid per se is harmful in that it may crystallize in the urine and obstruct urine flow. Orotidine is more soluble than orotic acid and does not form stones. The remaining clinical features of hereditary orotic aciduria are due to deficiency of nucleic acid precursors.

CLINICAL FEATURES The most specific early finding in patients with hereditary orotic aciduria is severe hypochromic anemia with marked anisocytosis and poikilocytosis, associated with erythroid hyperplasia and atypical megaloblastic changes in the bone marrow. Leukopenia but not thrombocytopenia is also a consistent finding. The megaloblastosis probably results from a selective defect of DNA synthesis which interferes with mitosis. The megaloblasts in hereditary orotic aciduria are not as large as in pernicious anemia or folic acid deficiency, but the cellular abnormalities in orotic aciduria are more pronounced in the more mature red blood cell precursors. The degree of microcytosis and hypochromia in circulating erythrocytes also differentiates this from other megaloblastic anemias. Typically, poor growth and development are evident during the first few months of life with lassitude, pallor, and nonspecific failure to thrive. While no characteristic neurological picture exists, most patients appear to have some mental retardation. Orotic acid crystalluria is uniformly present, and urinary tract obstruction occurs in about half.

GENETICS Orotic aciduria is transmitted as an autosomal recessive disease. Heterozygotes are asymptomatic and excrete only slightly increased amounts of orotic acid in the urine.

FIGURE 93-1

Pyrimidine biosynthesis de novo. (1) Carbamyl phosphate synthetase, (2) aspartate transcarbamylase, (3) dihydroorotase, (4) dihydroorotic acid dehydrogenase, (5) orotate phosphoribosyltransferase, and (6) orotidine 5′-monophosphate decarboxylase.

TREATMENT The hematologic abnormalities and the retardation of growth and development respond promptly and completely to doses of uridine in the range of 100 to 150 mg/kg per day. Uridine is converted directly to uridine 5′-phosphate in the reaction catalyzed by the enzyme uridine kinase, thus bypassing the enzymatic defect and correcting the pyrimidine nucleotide deficiency and the deficiency in nucleic acid synthesis. Uridine therapy also produces a substantial decrease in the urinary excretion of orotic acid, probably by virtue of the increased levels of pyrimidine nucleotides and the consequent inhibition of pyrimidine biosynthesis de novo. The fatal outcome of untreated hereditary orotic aciduria as well as the residual impairment of mental function that may occur serves to emphasize the importance of early diagnosis and treatment.

Glucocorticoid therapy causes partial hematologic remission without reversal of the megaloblastic changes in the bone marrow. Oral administration of a mixture of yeast nucleotides has also been associated with rapid improvement in the general clinical state with hematologic remission and a decrease in urinary orotic acid. This preparation, however, is not well tolerated because of gastrointestinal side effects.

OTHER CAUSES OF OROTIC ACIDURIA Drugs such as allopurinol, oxipurinol, and azauridine produce modest orotic aciduria and orotidinuria. In each case one or more nucleotide derivatives of the drug are potent inhibitors of orotidine 5′-phosphate decarboxylase. There is no evidence that patients develop a significant deficiency of pyrimidine nucleotides.

5-Phosphoribosyl-1-pyrophosphate (PRPP) is an essential and rate-limiting substrate for the orotate phosphoribosyltransferase reaction. A low intracellular level of PRPP as, for example, in a patient unable to synthesize PRPP due to PRPP synthetase deficiency is also associated with orotic aciduria, megaloblastic anemia, and mental retardation.

Several disorders of the urea cycle, including ornithine transcarbamylase deficiency, argininosuccinic aciduria, and citrullinemia, lead to orotic aciduria. In each of these diseases, carbamyl phosphate utilization in the urea cycle is reduced, and its availability for pyrimidine biosynthesis is enhanced. This shift in carbamyl phosphate utilization to the pyrimidine pathway appears to enhance the rate of pyrimidine biosynthesis de novo up to at least the step of orotic acid formation.

REFERENCES

HUGULEY CM et al: Refractory megaloblastic anemia associated with excretion of orotic acid. Blood 14:615, 1959

KELLEY WN, SMITH LH: Hereditary orotic aciduria, in *The Metabolic Basis of Inherited Diseases*, 4th ed, JB Stanbury et al (eds). New York, McGraw-Hill, 1978, pp 1045–1071

Disorders of metals and metallo proteins

94
HEMOCHROMATOSIS

LAWRIE W. POWELL
KURT J. ISSELBACHER

DEFINITION Hemochromatosis (bronze diabetes) is an iron-storage disorder in which an excessive iron absorption and/or parenteral iron loading results in parenchymal deposition of iron with eventual tissue damage and functional insufficiency of the organs involved, especially the liver, pancreas, heart, and pituitary. The increased iron stores may result from one or more different mechanisms (see below). The inherited form of the disease known as *idiopathic hemochromatosis* is now increasingly recognized during its early stages when the iron overload is of lesser degree and organ damage minimal. At this stage the disease is referred to as *latent* or *precirrhotic hemochromatosis*. The first clinical description of the disease was given by Trousseau in 1865; in 1889 von Recklinghausen named the disease *hemochromatosis* and the iron-storage pigment *hemosiderin* because he believed it was derived from the blood.

INCIDENCE Hemochromatosis is a rare disease. Estimates of its prevalence have ranged from 1 in 20,000 hospital admissions to 2.5 per 10,000 necropsies and 1 in 10,000 of the white Anglo-Saxon population. It is observed five to ten times more frequently in males than in females. Nearly 70 percent of all patients develop their first symptoms between age 40 and 60. The disease is rarely clinically evident below age 20.

PATHOGENESIS The disease is observed in the following types of patients: (1) those with idiopathic (primary, familial, hereditary) hemochromatosis; (2) those with a defect in hemoglobin synthesis associated with ineffective erythropoiesis (erythropoietic hemochromatosis); (3) those with excessive oral iron intake over many years, usually from an alcoholic beverage, for example, in certain South African Negroes.

Idiopathic hemochromatosis is the consequence of an abnormality in the regulatory mechanism for iron absorption, the nature of which is unknown. The resulting progressive accumulation of iron is reflected in an early increase in the plasma iron and percentage saturation of transferrin. In advanced disease, the tissues contain over 20 g iron; total body iron normally is in the range of 3 to 5 g. The excess iron is deposited mainly in parenchymal cells of the liver, pancreas, and heart. Iron in the liver and pancreas increases 50- to 100-fold; in the heart, 5- to 25-fold; in the spleen, kidney, and skin, about 5-fold. Tissue injury may result from disruption of iron-laden lysosomes. The recent demonstration of an increased incidence of certain histocompatability antigens (viz., HLA-A3, HLA-B14, and HLA-B7) has confirmed the genetic basis for the disease. The mode of inheritance is autosomal recessive although more than one form of the disease may exist. It has been suggested that homozygotes have large iron stores and manifest the disease; heterozygotes tend to have normal or slightly elevated iron stores and develop the disease only when added factors such as alcohol, anemia, or increased oral iron intake contribute to an accumulation of iron in excess of their usual stores.

Erythropoietic hemochromatosis is observed in association with chronic disorders or erythropoiesis, particularly in those with a defect in hemoglobin synthesis and ineffective erythropoiesis. Also in this group of disorders the absorption of iron is increased, and such patients are frequently treated with medicinal iron and transfusions. Erythropoietic hemochromatosis has been observed primarily in patients with sideroblastic anemia and thalassemia. Porphyria cutanea tarda, a disorder characterized by a defect in porphyrin biosynthesis, is also associated with excessive parenchymal iron deposits; however, the magnitude of the iron load is usually insufficient to produce tissue damage.

Alcoholic subjects with chronic liver disease may show evidence of hemochromatosis. Such patients are probably heterozygotes in whom iron accumulation has been accentuated by alcohol. There is evidence that alcohol may enhance iron absorption. Ineffective erythropoiesis in association with folate deficiency or an abnormality in pyridoxal phosphate metabolism may be a complicating factor in some patients. In addition, alcoholic beverages, particularly red wine, may contain appreciable quantities of iron.

Excessive iron ingestion over many years may, in certain circumstances, result in the syndrome of hemochromatosis. This occurs, for example, in certain South African Negroes (Bantu) in whom the intake of excessive iron in an alcoholic beverage results from the practice of brewing fermented beverages in vessels made of iron. There are a few isolated reports of the development of hemochromatosis in normal subjects taking medicinal iron over many years, but it is possible that such subjects have been heterozygous for the inherited trait.

The common denominator in all patients with hemochromatosis is the presence of *excessive amounts of iron in parenchymal tissues* with resultant tissue damage. Parenteral administration of iron in the form of transfusions or iron preparations results in *reticuloendothelial cell* iron overload. Only in patients with an abnormality in erythropoiesis does the parenteral administration of iron result in deposition of iron in parenchymal tissues.

PATHOLOGY At autopsy the enlarged, nodular liver and pancreas present a striking ochre color. Histologically iron is found in increased amounts in many organs, particularly in the liver and pancreas and to a lesser extent in the endocrine glands and the heart. A notable exception is the testis, the iron content of which is relatively low despite the fact that gonadal failure is a characteristic and early feature of the disease. In contrast, the pituitary gland is almost always involved. The epidermis of the skin is thin, and increased *melanin* is found in the cells of the basal layer. Deposits of iron are observed around the synovial lining cells of the joints, and calcium pyrophosphate crystals may be seen to lie within deposits of calcium embedded in the synovial tissue.

As indicated above, iron deposition in the liver of patients with idiopathic hemochromatosis occurs predominantly in the parenchymal cells in the form of hemosiderin. In the early stages, hemosiderin is deposited in the periportal parenchyma being found within lysosomes in the pericanalicular cytoplasm of the hepatocytes. This stage progresses to perilobular fibrosis and deposition of iron in bile duct epithelium, Kupffer cells, and fibrous septa. Inflammatory cells are few in contrast to prominent proliferation of bile ductules. Wedge biopsy specimens show a characteristic pattern of fibrosis with dense fibrous septa surrounding groups of lobules somewhat analogous to the pattern seen in chronic biliary disease. In the advanced stage, an irregular multilobular cirrhosis of postnecrotic type develops.

CLINICAL MANIFESTATIONS The symptoms and signs of hemochromatosis are related to skin pigmentation, diabetes, liver and cardiac impairment, arthropathy, and hypogonadism. The initial symptoms most frequently encountered are weakness, lassitude, weight loss, change in skin color, abdominal pain, loss of libido, and symptoms related to the onset of diabetes. Hepatomegaly, pigmentation, spider angiomas, splenomegaly, arthropathy, ascites, cardiac arrhythmias, congestive heart failure, loss of body hair, testicular atrophy, and jaundice are the most prominent physical signs.

The *liver* is usually the first organ to be damaged, and hepatomegaly is present in more than 95 percent of symptomatic cases. Hepatic enlargement may exist in the absence of symptoms or in the presence of normal liver function tests. Indeed, over half the patients with symptomatic hemochromatosis have little or no laboratory evidence of functional impairment of the liver, in spite of hepatomegaly and fibrosis. Loss of body hair, palmar erythema, testicular atrophy, and gynecomastia are often seen. Manifestations of portal hypertension and esophageal varices may occur but are less commonly observed than in Laennec's cirrhosis. Splenomegaly is present in approximately half the cases. Hepatocellular carcinoma develops in about 35 percent. The incidence of this last complication increases with age and is now the most common cause of death in treated patients.

Excessive *skin pigmentation* is present in about 90 percent of the patients at the time the diagnosis is established. Pigmentation is largely due to *melanin* deposition, and in some instances there may also be some increase in iron. Melanin deposition usually gives rise to bronzing. The characteristic metallic gray hue is believed to result from the presence of increased melanin or both melanin and iron in the dermis. Pigmentation usually is diffuse and generalized, but frequently it is deeper on the face, neck, extensor aspects of the lower forearms, dorsa of the hands, lower legs, genital regions, and in scars. In only 10 to 15 percent of cases is there demonstrable pigmentation of the oral mucosa. Pigmentation of the hard palate and retina has been described.

Diabetes and symptoms therefrom develop in about 65 percent of patients. Diabetes is more likely to develop in patients with a family history of diabetes. The presence of a family history of diabetes, the existence of liver disease, and direct damage to the pancreas by iron deposition may all contribute to the development of diabetes in hemochromatosis. The management of the diabetes is similar to that of diabetes mellitus except for a higher incidence of insulin resistance and of insulin fat atrophy. Late degenerative sequelae are the same as in diabetes mellitus.

Arthropathy, which differs from osteoarthritis and rheumatoid arthritis, develops in 25 to 50 percent of patients. It most commonly occurs after the age of 50 but may occur at any time in the course of the disease, even as a first manifestation or long after therapy. The small joints of the hands, especially the second and third metacarpophalangeal joints, are usually the first joints to be involved. A progressive polyarthritis involving wrists, hips, and knees may ensue. Acute brief attacks of synovitis may occur, associated with deposition of calcium pyrophosphate (chondrocalcinosis or pseudogout), chiefly in the knees. Roentgenologic manifestations consist of cystic changes of sclerosis of the subchondral bones, loss of articular cartilage with narrowing of the joint space, diffuse demineralization, and hypertrophic bone proliferation. The mechanism of these abnormalities and their relationship to iron metabolism is not known.

Cardiac involvement is the presenting manifestation in about 15 percent of patients. The most common cardiac manifestation is congestive heart failure. It is observed not infrequently in young adults, and symptoms of congestive failure may develop suddenly, with rapid progression to death if untreated. The heart is diffusely enlarged, and such cases may be misdiagnosed as idiopathic cardiomyopathy if other overt manifestations are absent. A great variety of cardiac arrhythmias may be present, particularly supraventricular beats and paroxysmal tachyarrhythmias. Atrial flutter, atrial fibrillation, and varying degrees of atrioventricular block have also been described.

Loss of libido and *testicular atrophy* are common in hemochromatosis. The former may antedate the other clinical manifestations of the disease. Testicular atrophy is probably due to the decreased production of gonadotropins associated with impaired hypothalamic pituitary function due to iron deposition. Addison's disease, hypothyroidism, and hypoparathyroidism have been described but are exceedingly rare.

DIAGNOSIS The association of (1) hepatomegaly, (2) skin pigmentation, (3) diabetes mellitus, (4) heart disease, (5) arthritis, and (6) evidence of hypogonadism should suggest the diagnosis of hemochromatosis. However, a parenchymal iron overload of insufficient duration or modest degree may exist without any of these clinical manifestations, or with only some of them. Therefore, the diagnosis should be considered in any patient with unexplained hepatomegaly, idiopathic cardiomyopathy, abnormal skin pigmentation, or loss of libido.

The history should be particularly detailed in regard to disease in other members of the family, alcohol ingestion, and iron intake. The blood should be examined for evidence of anemia and abnormal erythropoiesis to rule out iron loading secondary to a hematologic disorder, such as thalassemia or sideroblastic anemia. Confirmation of the presence of liver, pancreatic, cardiac, and joint disease should be obtained by physical examination, roentgenologic examination, and routine function tests of these organs. It then remains to be demonstrated that there is an increase in total body iron stores and, in particular, an increased parenchymal iron concentration associated with tissue damage.

The methods available for the demonstration of excessive parenchymal iron stores include (1) measurement of serum iron, (2) determination of percent saturation of transferrin, (3) estimation of chelatable iron stores using the agent desferrioxamine, (4) measurement of serum ferritin concentration, and (5) liver biopsy (Table 94-1). Each has its inherent advantages and limitations. The serum iron level and percent saturation of transferrin are elevated early in the course of the disease, but their specificity is reduced by relatively high false-positive and false-negative rates. In particular, an increased serum iron concentration may be present is patients with alcoholic liver disease without iron overload; in this situation, however, the iron-binding capacity is usually not decreased as in hemochromatosis.

There has been considerable focus on the serum ferritin concentration as an estimate of body iron stores. In untreated patients with hemochromatosis, the serum ferritin level is greatly increased (Table 94-1). This test is useful as a noninvasive screening test for the diagnosis of early disease, since it is usually abnormal before there is any morphological evidence of liver damage and the ferritin concentration correlates with the magnitude of body iron stores. It will probably, therefore, replace the more cumbersome screening tests involving urinary iron excretion. However, it should be noted that in patients with infection and hepatocellular necrosis serum ferritin levels may be elevated out of proportion to body iron stores. Also, at least three families have been reported in whom serum ferritin levels in relatives have been normal despite increased iron stores; the reason for the latter finding is unclear but would appear to be an exceptional situation. In clinical practice, the *combined measurements* of the (1) serum iron concentration, (2) percent transferrin saturation, and (3) serum ferritin level provide the simplest and most reliable screening test for hemochromatosis, including the precirrhotic phase of the disease. If any of these tests are abnormal, liver biopsy should be performed since it is the *definitive* test for the diagnosis of hemochromatosis. It permits histochemical estimation of tissue iron, measurement of hepatic iron concentration, and assessment of the extent of tissue damage.

TABLE 94-1
Representative iron values in normal subjects and in patients with idiopathic hemochromatosis

Determination	Normal subjects	Patients with idiopathic hemochromatosis
Plasma iron, $\mu g/100$ ml	50–150	180–300
Total iron-binding capacity, $\mu g/100$ ml	250–370	200–300
Percent transferrin saturation, $\mu g/100$ ml	22–46	80–100
Serum ferritin, ng/ml	10–200	900–6000
Urinary iron,* mg/24 h	0–2	9–23
Liver iron, $\mu g/100$ mg dry wt	30–140	600–1800

* *After intramuscular administration of 0.5 g desferrioxamine.*

It is of particular importance to examine family members when the diagnosis of idiopathic hemochromatosis is established. Asymptomatic as well as symptomatic family members with the disease will usually have an increase in plasma iron, a decrease in total iron-binding capacity, an increased saturation of transferrin, and an increased serum ferritin concentration. These changes occur even before the iron stores are greatly increased. A liver biopsy should then be performed, since it is imperative to establish the diagnosis and begin therapy before tissue damage occurs. Preliminary studies suggest that affected relatives usually have an HLA haplotype identical with that of the proband.

The differential diagnosis between parenchymal iron overload and reticuloendothelial iron overload is usually not difficult. Reticuloendothelial iron overload is not associated with tissue damage, the plasma iron is not increased, and the urinary excretion of iron after desferrioxamine administration does not exceed 4 mg. The relative degrees of parenchymal iron overload and reticuloendothelial iron overload can be determined definitively by liver biopsy.

The distinction between idiopathic hemochromatosis and alcoholic cirrhosis associated with iron overload is sometimes difficult. In general, patients with alcoholic cirrhosis of the liver have a lesser degree of iron overload, as determined by the plasma iron concentration, serum ferritin concentration, and urinary iron excretion after desferrioxamine administration. The degree of parenchymal iron deposition in liver biopsy specimens from patients with alcoholic cirrhosis is usually mild in comparison with the degree of fibrosis. Reticuloendothelial (RE) iron deposition is often considerable. In idiopathic hemochromatosis there is very little RE iron, and the amount of parenchymal iron is out of proportion to the degree of fibrosis. Family studies will often resolve the problem, particularly if nonalcoholic relatives are affected and HLA antigen typing may be useful.

TREATMENT The therapy of idiopathic hemochromatosis involves the removal of the excess body iron and supportive treatment of damaged organs.

Iron is best removed from the body by weekly or twice weekly phlebotomy of 500 ml. Although there is an initial modest decline in the volume of packed red blood cells to about 35 ml per 100 ml, the anemia stabilizes after several weeks. The plasma iron concentration remains increased until the available iron stores are depleted. Since one 500-ml unit of blood contains from 200 to 250 mg iron and about 25 g iron must be removed, 2 or 3 years of weekly phlebotomy are usually required. When the plasma iron level becomes normal, phlebotomies are performed at such time intervals as are required to maintain a plasma iron concentration of less than 150 μg per 100 ml. Usually one phlebotomy every 3 months will suffice. The adequacy of the therapy may be evaluated at any time by measuring the plasma iron, the percentage of saturation of transferrin with iron, or the urinary iron excretion after desferrioxamine administration. These measurements become abnormal promptly with iron reaccumulation and precede the increase in serum ferritin concentration.

Chelating agents such as desferrioxamine, when given parenterally, remove 10 to 20 mg iron per day, less than half that mobilized by one weekly phlebotomy. Phlebotomy is not only a more effective but also a less expensive, more convenient, and safer treatment for patients with idiopathic hemochromatosis. Chelating agents may be used as a substitute method for iron removal when anemia or hypoproteinemia is severe enough to preclude phlebotomy.

The management of the hepatic failure, cardiac failure, and diabetes differs little from conventional management of these conditions. Loss of libido and change in secondary sex characteristics are partially relieved by testosterone therapy or gonadotropin therapy.

PROGNOSIS The life expectancy of *untreated* patients with idiopathic hemochromatosis after the disease has become clinically manifest averages 4.4 years, but several instances have been recorded of patients living up to 20 or 30 years. The principal causes of death in *untreated* patients are cardiac failure (30 percent), hepatic coma (15 percent), hematemesis (14 percent), hepatocellular carcinoma (14 percent), and pneumonia (12 percent).

Life expectancy is extended to an average of more than 8 years by removal of the excessive stores of iron and maintenance of these stores at near-normal levels. The 5-year survival rate with therapy is increased from 33 to 89 percent. With removal of iron by repeated phlebotomy, the liver and spleen decrease in size, liver function studies return to normal, pigmentation of skin decreases, and cardiac failure is reversed. Carbohydrate tolerance improves in about 40 percent of cases. The fibrosis in the liver may decrease, but cirrhosis is irreversible. Removal of excess iron has little or no effect on hypogonadism or arthropathy. Hepatocellular carcinoma occurs as a late sequela in about one-third of the patients despite adequate iron removal; the apparent increase in its incidence in treated patients is probably related to their increased life span. This complication does not appear to develop if the disease is treated in the precirrhotic stage. Hence, the importance of family screening and early therapy cannot be emphasized too strongly.

REFERENCES

EDWARDS CQ et al: Hereditary hemochromatosis. N Engl J Med 297:7, 1977

HALLIDAY JW et al: Serum ferritin in the diagnosis of early haemochromatosis: A study of 43 families. Lancet 2:621, 1977

PETERS TJ, SEYMOUR CA: Acid hydrolase activities and lysosomal integrity in liver biopsies from patients with iron overload. Clin Sci Mol Med 50:75, 1976

POWELL LW, KERR JFR: The pathology of liver in hemochromatosis, in *Pathobiology Annual,* H Joacim (ed). New York, Appleton Century Crofts, 1975

SIMON M et al: Idiopathic hemochromatosis and iron overload in alcoholic liver disease: Differentiation by HLA phenotype. Gastroenterology 73:655, 1977

95
WILSON'S DISEASE

I. HERBERT SCHEINBERG

Wilson's disease is an inherited autosomal recessive abnormality in the hepatic excretion of copper that results in toxic accumulations of the metal in liver, brain, and other organs. Deficiency of the plasma copper-protein ceruloplasmin is a characteristic feature.

NATURAL HISTORY Normal babies have low plasma concentrations of ceruloplasmin and high concentrations of hepatic copper. During the first year of life ceruloplasmin values rise, and hepatic copper concentrations fall to normal adult levels.

In contrast, serum ceruloplasmin changes very little in Wilson homozygotes, and the concentration of hepatic copper increases steadily with age. However, clinical manifestations of copper excess are rare before age 6, and half of untreated patients remain asymptomatic to age 16.

Wilson's disease presents with hepatic involvement in somewhat less than half of patients. The toxic effects of copper in the liver may be manifest as acute hepatitis, cirrhosis of the liver, or asymptomatic hepatosplenomegaly. The acute hepatitis is similar to viral hepatitis, can be mistaken for infectious mononucleosis, and may evolve in three different ways. The first is a fulminant, sometimes lethal disease characterized by jaundice, malaise, and at times ascites, hypoalbuminemia, and elevated levels of liver enzymes in plasma. In the acute phase sufficient copper may be released into plasma to cause a hemolytic anemia. The disease may not be diagnosed until autopsy or until the diagnosis in a younger sibling leads to retrospective analysis of preserved tissues. Second, there may be insidious development of parenchymal liver disease resulting in a clinical and histological picture indistinguishable from chronic active hepatitis. Third, patients may apparently recover from the hepatitis. Years or decades may elapse with no sign or symptom of disease. In these patients the past history of an episode of hepatitis can be overlooked unless they are questioned carefully.

More frequently, the copper-induced hepatic disease evolves to cirrhosis without any recognized overt indication of hepatitis. In these patients the initial manifestations are extrahepatic. Neurological or psychiatric disturbances are the first clinical signs in most of this group and are always accompanied by Kayser-Fleischer rings (Plate 8-8). These green or golden deposits of copper in Descemet's membrane of the cornea never interfere with vision but indicate that hepatic copper has been released and caused the brain damage. Rarely Kayser-Fleischer rings may be accompanied by sunflower cataracts. If a patient with frank neurological or psychiatric disease does not have Kayser-Fleischer rings when examined by a trained observer using a slit-lamp, the diagnosis of Wilson's disease can be excluded.

The primary neurological manifestation is that of a movement disorder, particularly resting and intention tremors. Spasticity, rigidity, chorea, drooling, dysphagia, and dysarthria are common. Babinski responses and absent abdominal reflexes are occasionally noted; sensory changes are rare. Psychiatric disturbances, in part due to the toxic effects of copper on the brain and in part to the reactions to a life-threatening disease, are evident in most patients with symptomatic disease. Syndromes indistinguishable from schizophrenia, manic-depressive psychoses, and classic neuroses have been observed, and some bizarre behavioral disturbances defy classification. Improvement in the psychiatric state can occur with pharmacological reduction of the copper excess, but psychotherapy is often also required.

In occasional patients the clinical onset reflects neither a hepatic nor a central nervous system disturbance. For example, primary or secondary amenorrhea may be the first evidence of disease in some young women; in others, repeated spontaneous abortions may result from excess free copper in intrauterine secretions. Routine ophthalmologic examination in patients without symptomatic liver or neurological disease occasionally reveals Kayser-Fleischer rings, leading to the diagnosis. Cirrhosis may be observed incidentally at surgery.

PATHOGENESIS The metabolic defect in Wilson's disease is an inability to maintain a near-zero balance of copper. Excess copper accumulates possibly because hepatic lysosomes lack the normal mechanism to excrete into bile the copper that has been catabolically cleaved from ceruloplasmin. This may cause deficiency of ceruloplasmin since a stoichiometric excess of copper inhibits the formation of ceruloplasmin from apoceruloplasmin and copper. The capacity of hepatocytes to store copper is eventually exceeded, and release into blood and uptake in extrahepatic sites occur (Table 95-1).

Under normal circumstances essentially all tissue copper is present as the prosthetic element of copper proteins such as cytochrome oxidase, tyrosinase, superoxide dismutase, and ceruloplasmin. There is normally little or no free (non-protein-bound) copper. In Wilson's disease more copper is present than can be bound by specific copper proteins; such copper is as toxic as excess iron, zinc, mercury, or lead. Toxicity of these cations is probably effected in large degree by pathological combinations with proteins that ordinarily do not contain metal.

The pathological consequences of the accumulated copper occur first in the liver. Abnormal fat and glycogen deposits are the earliest findings by light microscopy (Fig. 95-1). With electron microscopy mitochondrial abnormalities are observed early and appear to be specific for Wilson's disease (Fig. 95-2). Later, necrosis, inflammation, fibrosis, bile duct proliferation, and cirrhosis are seen. Abnormalities in liver function tests develop later than the histological changes.

Death can occur from copper damage to the central nervous system with little or no evidence of liver dysfunction, but in most subjects significant liver disease becomes apparent sometime during the course. Patients with prolonged survival always show hepatic cirrhosis.

In the brain the excess copper is distributed ubiquitously. Necrosis of neurons with cavitation may be preceded by the appearance of Opalski and Alzheimer type II cells; however neither is specific for Wilson's disease.

Increased copper in the kidney produces little if any structural change and commonly does not alter renal function. He-

TABLE 95-1
Summary of analytical data in patients with Wilson's disease, heterozygous carriers, and control subjects

Group	Serum ceruloplasmin			Hepatic copper concentration		
	No. of patients	Range, mg/100 ml	Mean ± SD, mg/100 ml	No. of patients	Range, μg/g dry weight	Mean ± SD, μg/g dry weight
Wilson's disease:						
Asymptomatic	31	0–19.5	3.6 ± 5.3	36	152–1828	983.5 ± 368
Symptomatic	84	0–43.0	5.9 ± 7.1	33	94–1360	588.3 ± 304
Heterozygous carriers	95*	1–50.1	28.4 ± 8.5	14	39–213	117.0 ± 51
Normal subjects	180	18.5–65.9	30.7 ± 3.5	16	20–45	31.5 ± 6.8

* 71 parents of patients with Wilson's disease and 24 children, each of whom had one parent with Wilson's disease.
SOURCE: Sternlieb and Scheinberg, 1968.

FIGURE 95-1
Fatty changes, glycogen deposits, and cellular infiltrates in a hematoxylin and eosin–stained section of liver from an asymptomatic boy with Wilson's disease.

The drug of choice is D-penicillamine. It is administered orally in an average dose of 1 g daily, usually in divided doses before meals and at bedtime. Since penicillamine has an antipyridoxine effect in animals, 25 mg per day of vitamin B$_6$ is also given. Effectiveness of therapy should be assayed chemically and clinically. Initially, the patient's 24-h urinary excretion of copper should increase fivefold or more over the pretreatment level, and 1 to 3 mg copper per day may be excreted during the first months of therapy.

White blood cell and platelet counts, urinalysis, and body temperature should be monitored several times weekly for the first month of therapy and at intervals thereafter. Sensitivity to penicillamine usually appears within the first 14 days of treatment and may cause rash, fever, leukopenia, thrombocytopenia, lymphadenopathy, or proteinuria. Discontinuation of treatment is required if sensitivity develops. Therapy can often be resumed if the drug is reinstituted in small and gradually increasing dosage; alternatively, 20 mg prednisone can be given daily for the first 2 weeks of penicillamine treatment and subsequently gradually discontinued. Reactions requiring a desensitizing regimen may recur several times before penicillamine can be administered without a steroid.

Lifelong treatment is required. Inadequate treatment or in-

maturia, proteinuria, the Fanconi syndrome, and renal tubular acidosis occur rarely. Pathological effects in other organs and tissues are minor.

DIAGNOSIS The diagnosis is easy *provided it is suspected.* Wilson's disease should be considered in any patient under the age of 40 with an unexplained disorder of the central nervous system, signs or symptoms of chronic active hepatitis, unexplained persistent elevations of serum transaminase, acquired hemolytic anemia (particularly in the presence of hepatitis), or unexplained cirrhosis, or in any patient who has a relative with Wilson's disease.

The diagnosis is confirmed in suspected cases by the demonstration either of (1) a serum concentration of ceruloplasmin less than 20 mg per 100 ml and Kayser-Fleischer rings, or (2) a serum ceruloplasmin less than 20 mg per 100 ml and a concentration of copper in a liver biopsy sample greater than 250 μg per gram of dry weight. Most patients also excrete more than 100 μg copper per day in urine and exhibit histological abnormalities on liver biopsy.

About 5 percent of patients have a serum concentration of ceruloplasmin greater than 20 mg per 100 ml, and some patients with other hepatic disorders have elevated hepatic copper and Kayser-Fleischer rings. In either circumstance measurement of the ability to incorporate radioactive copper into ceruloplasmin is useful as a discriminating test. Even in the presence of a normal concentration of ceruloplasmin, patients with Wilson's disease incorporate little or no isotope into the protein, while patients with other liver disorders and elevated hepatic copper incorporate the isotope normally.

TREATMENT Treatment consists of removing the deposits of copper as rapidly as possible and should be instituted once the diagnosis is secure whether the patient is ill or asymptomatic.

FIGURE 95-2
Electron micrograph showing portions of two hepatocytes from the liver biopsy of a young asymptomatic woman with Wilson's disease. There are lipid droplets (L) and grossly abnormal mitochondria (M) in the cytoplasm. N, nucleus; P, peroxisome.

terruption of therapy causes relapse that may be irreversible. Reinstitution of penicillamine after temporary interruption of therapy may be accompanied by the appearance or reappearance of sensitivity reactions. At any time—even after years of uneventful administration—granulocytopenia (or agranulocytosis), thrombocytopenia, the nephrotic syndrome, the Goodpasture syndrome, systemic lupus erythematosus, severe arthralgias, or myasthenia gravis may supervene. Toxicity is sometimes dose-related, and reduction of the dose to a level that is therapeutically effective but nontoxic may be possible. Continued low dosage of steroids may control penicillamine-associated lupus or arthralgias. After temporary interruption of the drug in patients with the nephrotic syndrome, it is sometimes possible to reinstitute therapy without recurrence of proteinuria. However, although irreversible intolerance to D-penicillamine is rare, the toxicity may be such that the drug must be withdrawn permanently. The lifelong administration of dimercaprol by injection is impractical, and the only other alternative mode of therapy is an investigational drug, triethylene tetramine.

After therapy with penicillamine has been successfully instituted, the patient should be seen indefinitely at 1- to 3-month intervals to detect drug toxicity and manage the disease. Physical examination, including relevant neurological assessment and inspection of the corneas with a slit-lamp, together with the patient's own evaluation, provides the best indicator of the efficacy of treatment. Serial determinations of serum transaminase levels, albumin, and bilirubin are useful in following the course of liver function. Lack of clinical improvement or worsening of the disease may be due to irreversible damage present before therapy was begun, to poor patient compliance, or to inadequate dosage of penicillamine. Quantitative determinations of urinary copper excretion and of free copper in serum (total serum copper minus ceruloplasmin-bound copper) can help determine which is the case. After treatment for long periods, urinary copper should be lower than at the onset of therapy and rarely exceeds 1.5 mg per day. Even more helpful, an adequately treated patient generally has a concentration of free serum copper less than 10 μg per 100 ml. After a patient has remained asymptomatic with no laboratory evidence of liver dysfunction for a year and in patients with minimal residual disease that has not changed, the dose of penicillamine may be reduced to 0.75 g per day.

Treatment of more than 100 asymptomatic patients with a confirmed diagnosis over the past 15 years has established that continued administration of D-penicillamine can prevent virtually every manifestation of this disease.

REFERENCES

CARTWRIGHT GE: The diagnosis of treatable Wilson's disease. N Engl J Med 298:1347, 1978

Copper: Report of the Committee on Medical and Biologic Effects of Environmental Pollutants. Washington, DC, National Academy of Sciences, 1977

STERNLIEB I: Evolution of the hepatic lesion in Wilson's disease (hepatolenticular degeneration), in *Progress in Liver Diseases,* vol IV, H Popper et al (eds). New York, Grune & Stratton, 1972

———, SCHEINBERG IH: Prevention of Wilson's disease in asymptomatic patients. N Engl J Med 278:352, 1968

———, ———: Chronic hepatitis as a first manifestation of Wilson's disease. Ann Intern Med 76:59, 1972

WALSHE JM: Wilson's disease (hepatolenticular degeneration), in *Handbook of Clinical Neurology,* vol 27, PJ Vinken et al (eds). New York, American Elsevier, 1976

96
PORPHYRIAS

URS A. MEYER

The porphyrias are a group of clinically heterogeneous diseases associated with inherited or acquired disturbances in heme biosynthesis. Porphyrins are tetrapyrrole pigments that serve as intermediates in this pathway. They are formed from the precursors δ-aminolevulinic acid (ALA) and porphobilinogen. Heme, the ferrous iron complex of protoporphyrin IX, functions as a prosthetic group for hemoproteins such as hemoglobin, microsomal and mitochondrial cytochromes, catalase, tryptophan oxygenase, and others. Disturbances of heme biosynthesis differ from most other metabolic diseases by involving a pathway essential to life and operative in all aerobic cells.

Each of the porphyrias is characterized by a unique pattern of overproduction, accumulation, and excretion of intermediates of heme biosynthesis. These patterns are the metabolic expression of genetically determined deficiencies of specific enzymes of the heme biosynthetic pathway (Table 96-1).

The main clinical manifestations are intermittent attacks of nervous system dysfunction and sensitivity of the skin to sunlight. The *neurological syndrome* is characteristically precipitated by drugs such as barbiturates and results in abdominal pain, peripheral neuropathy, and mental disturbance. These neuropsychiatric symptoms occur only in those porphyrias in which there is great overproduction of the porphyrin precursors ALA and porphobilinogen. The pathogenesis of the neurological lesion is unclear. The *skin photosensitivity* is related directly to increased porphyrin accumulation, although the lesions differ among diseases. The photosensitivity is due to the photodynamic action of porphyrins and is probably mediated through the formation of singlet-oxygen with consequent destructive processes such as the peroxidation of lipids in the membranes of lysosomes. The dominantly inherited human porphyrias exhibit variable expressivity. In many patients only the biochemical or enzymatic abnormalities are apparent. Exacerbations in ordinarily asymptomatic patients can be precipitated by factors such as drugs, hormones, or liver disease. Clinically or chemically latent disease may occur as a phase or persist throughout life.

CLASSIFICATION The porphyrias are usually divided into two main groups, erythropoietic and hepatic, according to the two major sites of heme synthesis where the error of metabolism is expressed (Table 96-1). The only pure erythropoietic form of porphyria is the rare *congenital erythropoietic porphyria* (CEP). In *protoporphyria* (PP) porphyrins accumulate in both erythropoietic and hepatic tissue. In *intermittent acute porphyria* (IAP), *hereditary coproporphyria* (HCP), and *variegate porphyria* (VP), dominantly inherited enzyme deficiencies impair heme biosynthesis predominantly in the liver, apparently without affecting hemoglobin formation. *Porphyria cutanea tarda* (PCT) was previously considered to be an acquired hepatic porphyria. However most if not all patients with this disease have been found to have hereditary deficiency of uroporphyrinogen decarboxylase. Toxic acquired porphyria resembling PCT occurs in individuals accidentally exposed to polychlorinated hydrocarbons and in association with hepatic tumors. Poisoning with lead produces well-recognized abnormalities in porphyrin and heme synthesis (see Chap. 225). Increased urinary excretion of porphyrins or precursors and accumulation of porphyrins in erythrocytes may also occur in numerous clinical conditions; these are secondary phenomena which do not produce symptoms or signs of porphyria.

TABLE 96-1
Characteristics of the porphyrias

	Erythropoietic porphyria	Hepatic porphyrias				Erythrohepatic porphyria
	Congenital erythropoietic porphyria (CEP)	Intermittent acute porphyria (IAP)	Hereditary coproporphyria (HCP)	Variegate porphyria (VP)	Porphyria cutanea tarda (PCT)	Protoporphyria (PP)
Enzyme deficiency	Uroporphyrinogen I synthetase and/or uroporphyrinogen III cosynthetase (?)	Uroporphyrinogen I synthetase	Coproporphyrinogen oxidase	Protoporphyrinogen oxidase or ferrochelatase (?)	Uroporphyrinogen decarboxylase	Ferrochelatase
Inheritance	Autosomal recessive	Autosomal dominant	Autosomal dominant	Autosomal dominant	Autosomal dominant	Autosomal dominant
Metabolic expression	Erythroid cells	Liver	Liver	Liver	Liver	Erythroid cells and liver
Signs and symptoms:						
Photosensitive cutaneous lesions	Yes	No	Infrequent	Yes	Yes	Yes
Attacks of abdominal pain, neuropsychiatric syndrome	No	Yes	Yes	Yes	No	No
Laboratory abnormalities:						
Red blood cells:						
Uroporphyrin	+ + +	N	N	N	N	N
Coproporphyrin	+ +	N	N	N	N	+
Protoporphyrin	(+)	N	N	N	N	+ + +
Urine:						
δ-Aminolevulinic acid	N	(+ + +)	(+ + +)	(+ + +)	N	N
Porphobilinogen	N	(+ + +)	(+ + +)	(+ + +)	N	N
Uroporphyrin	+ + +	+ +	+	+	+ + +	N
Coproporphyrin	+ +	N	+ +	+ +	+	(+)
Feces:						
Coproporphyrin	+	N	+ + +	+	(+)	(+)
Protoporphyrin	+	N	+	+ + +	N	+ +

NOTE: *N, normal; +, increased levels or excretion; + +, moderately increased; + + +, markedly increased; (+), increased in some patients only; (+ + +), frequently increased only during acute attacks.*

BIOCHEMICAL CONSIDERATIONS A schematic outline of heme biosynthesis is presented in Fig. 96-1. The sequence of reactions that leads from the simple substrates glycine and succinyl coenzyme A to ALA, porphobilinogen (PBG), and finally heme is composed of four mitochondrial and four cytosolic enzymes. Differences exist in the regulation of heme biosynthesis among tissues.

In the liver ALA synthetase catalyzes the rate-limiting reaction for heme formation under physiological conditions. The enzymes subsequent to ALA synthetase are present in excess. The principal regulation of ALA synthetase is feedback repression by heme, the end product of the pathway. Increased demands for heme are met by the synthesis of ALA synthetase. Hepatic ALA synthetase can be induced by a large number of lipid-soluble drugs, naturally occurring steroids, and chemicals that are substrates and inducers of cytochrome P_{450}, the terminal oxidase in microsomal drug metabolism. This induction is modulated by multiple genetic, metabolic, and environmental factors. The interdependence of heme synthesis and microsomal drug oxidation is important in some hepatic porphyrias where clinical symptoms are produced by certain drugs.

In the bone marrow ALA synthetase is also rate-limiting in certain cells, but little is known of the role of the enzyme in overall heme synthesis during division, differentiation, and maturation of erythroid cells. With maturation of erythroid cells the nuclei and mitochondria are extruded, and the mitochondrial enzymes of heme synthesis disappear, while the cytosolic enzymes catalyzing the reactions between ALA and coproporphyrinogen persist. Therefore, erythrocytes can be used for the diagnosis and study of porphyrias provided the deficiency is in a cytosolic enzyme.

Bone marrow and liver differ in the role of specific enzymes in control of heme synthesis. The level of ALA synthetase is the major determinant of heme formation in the liver, while heme synthesis in the bone marrow is triggered by the complex process of erythroid differentiation. These considerations probably explain the different phenotypic expression of specific enzyme defects of heme synthesis in erythroid cells and liver.

The porphyrinogens, reduced forms of porphyrins, serve as intermediates between porphobilinogen and protoporphyrin. Porphyrinogens are colorless and nonfluorescent. Porphyrins are by-products that have escaped from the biosynthetic path by irreversible oxidation of the corresponding porphyrinogen. Porphyrins do not possess physiological function but are responsible, through their pigment and fluorescent properties, for the spectacular appearance of urine and erythrocytes in some patients.

The arrangement of two substituent side chains on the pyrrole ring of porphyrins determines the structural isomer types, numbered I to IV. In nature only types I and III have been identified, and only type III serves as substrate for the terminal steps of the pathway leading to protoporphyrin IX and heme. The catabolism of heme does not lead to porphyrins but to noncyclic tetrapyrroles referred to as *bile pigments*.

CONGENITAL ERYTHROPOIETIC PORPHYRIA

DEFINITION Congenital erythropoietic porphyria (CEP; Günther's disease, congenital photosensitive porphyria, erythropoietic uroporphyria) is a rare, recessively inherited defect that causes chronic photosensitivity with severe, mutilating skin lesions and hemolytic anemia.

GENETICS, INCIDENCE, AND PATHOGENESIS Only about 80 cases have been reported. Affected individuals are homozygous

FIGURE 96-1

Outline of heme biosynthesis. (ALA, δ-aminolevulinic acid; PBG, porphobilinogen; URO, uroporphyrin; UROgen, uroporphyrinogen; COPRO- *gen, coproporphyrinogen; PROTOgen, protoporphyrinogen; PROTO, protoporphyrin; X, postulated intermediate.)*

for an autosomal recessive gene; heterozygotes rarely have demonstrable abnormalities in porphyrin metabolism and appear normal. The underlying enzyme abnormality has not been entirely elucidated, but there appears to be a functional imbalance between the activities of uroporphyrinogen I synthetase and uroporphyrinogen III cosynthetase. The defect is expressed solely in maturing erythroid cells and results in massive overproduction of uroporphyrinogen I while the overall production of uroporphyrinogen III is normal or slightly increased. Uroporphyrinogen I cannot be used for heme synthesis but is converted to coproporphyrinogen I which cannot be metabolized further. Uroporphyrin I, coproporphyrinogen I, and coproporphyrin I accumulate in tissues and are excreted in excess amounts in urine and feces.

CLINICAL PRESENTATION AND DIAGNOSIS Porphyrins accumulate within the body of affected individuals during fetal development. Excretion of pink or red urine usually begins at or shortly after birth, whereas cutaneous photosensitivity, intermittent hemolysis, and splenomegaly may not be detected until later. Hypertrichosis and red discoloration of the teeth and bones are common. Death may occur in childhood. With longer survival, severe scarring and mutilation occur, mostly affecting fingers, nose, and ears. The urine contains high concentrations of uroporphyrin I and increased amounts of coproporphyrin as well as porphyrins with seven, six, five, and three

carboxyl groups, whereas the excretion of ALA and PBG is normal. Large amounts of coproporphyrin I are found in the feces. Normoblasts, reticulocytes, and erythrocytes contain large quantities of uroporphyrin I and lower concentrations of coproporphyrinogen I. Normoblasts and reticulocytes exhibit intense red fluorescence. In accordance with the normal excretion of ALA and PBG, neurological disturbance does not occur in CEP.

TREATMENT Exposure to sunlight should be avoided. In some cases, splenectomy has ameliorated hemolytic anemia, porphyrin excretion, and photosensitivity. The use of hematin infusions and oral beta-carotene remains experimental.

HEPATIC PORPHYRIAS

Three hepatic porphyrias, intermittent acute porphyria (IAP), hereditary coproporphyria (HCP), and variegate porphyria (VP), have many features in common. All are genetically transmitted as autosomal dominants. Acute attacks of a life-threatening neurological syndrome are precipitated by a variety of drugs as well as by hormones and other agents. During acute attacks excessive urinary excretion of the porphyrin precursors ALA and PBG occurs in all, but the patterns of porphyrins excreted in urine and feces differ (Fig. 96-2).

INTERMITTENT ACUTE PORPHYRIA **Definition** Intermittent acute porphyria [IAP, acute intermittent porphyria (AIP), pyrroloporphyria] is characterized by recurrent attacks of neurological and psychiatric dysfunction. Photosensitivity does not occur. The primary defect is in uroporphyrinogen I synthetase.

Genetics, incidence, and pathogenesis IAP is inherited as an autosomal dominant trait with variable expressivity. The overall frequency of the abnormal gene is estimated to be between 1 in 10,000 and 1 in 50,000, but in certain regions the incidence may be higher. Homozygous cases of IAP have not been observed. The defect consists of a partial (50 percent) deficiency of uroporphyrinogen I synthetase, the enzyme that converts PBG to uroporphyrinogen I. In the liver this leads to increased activity and/or inducibility of ALA synthetase by drugs and other factors and, consequently, to increased formation and urinary excretion of ALA and PBG. Preformed porphyrins do not accumulate, and, therefore, cutaneous photosensitivity does not occur. Decreased uroporphyrinogen I synthetase activity has been demonstrated in liver, erythrocytes, cultured skin fibroblasts, lymphocytes, and amniotic cells of patients with IAP. Thus, the enzymatic defect of IAP is present, albeit metabolically unexpressed, in tissues other than liver. Deficiency of uroporphyrinogen I synthetase does not necessarily result in clinical manifestations of acute porphyria without additional acquired factors, and families with large numbers of phenotypically normal carriers of the genetic defect have been found (latent porphyria). The relation between the genetic defect and the neurological lesions is unknown.

Clinical presentation and diagnosis Symptoms rarely occur before puberty. Abdominal pain is frequently the initial or most prominent symptom of the porphyric attack. It may be moderate or severe, colicky, localized or generalized; radiation to the back or loins may occur. The pain probably results from autonomic neuropathy causing disturbed gastrointestinal motility with alternate areas of spasm and dilatation. The abdomen is usually soft, and tenderness is not marked. Because it is often accompanied by fever and leukocytosis, the abdominal pain of the acute porphyric attack can mimic any inflammatory abdominal disease. Severe vomiting and persistent constipation are commonly associated. Neurological manifestations

and signs of mental disturbance are variable. Peripheral nerves, the autonomic nervous system, brainstem, cranial nerves, or cerebral function may be involved. Sinus tachycardia and labile hypertension with postural hypotension, urinary retention, and excessive sweating are frequent during the acute attack. The pulse rate is a good index of the activity of the disease. Hypertension and tachycardia correlate with increased excretion of catecholamines. Peripheral neuropathy is usually predominantly motor, but sensory components may be present. Deep tendon reflexes are diminished or absent. Neuritic pain in the extremities, areas of hypesthesia and paresthesia, and foot and wrist drop are typical. Paraplegia or complete flaccid quadriplegia may ensue. In the past, complications due to respiratory paralysis were a leading cause of death. Cranial nerve involvement may lead to optic nerve atrophy, ophthalmoplegia, and dysphagia. With more severe CNS involvement, delirium, coma, and seizures occur. Although the neuropathy is reversible to a surprising degree, residual paresis may last for several years following an acute attack. Many patients have a long history of vague nervousness, emotional instability, and functional disturbances. Significant signs of mental disturbance occur in one-third, and an organic brain syndrome with restlessness, disorientation, and visual hallucinations may supervene. During attacks hyponatremia can be severe. Multiple mechanisms (including gastrointestinal loss of sodium, imprudent fluid therapy, and a sodium-losing nephropathy related to a toxic effect of ALA) have been implicated, but the major mechanism appears to be inappropriate release of antidiuretic hormone.

Acute attacks may last from several days to several months and vary considerably in frequency and severity. In periods of remission symptoms may be slight or completely absent. Clinical (and biochemical) manifestations are frequently precipitated by usual therapeutic doses of several drugs including barbiturates, anticonvulsants, estrogens, contraceptives, and alcohol. All these drugs are oxidized by hepatic microsomes and thus involve the hemoproteins of the cytochrome P_{450} system. Impaired hepatic metabolism of some of these drugs has

FIGURE 96-2
Patterns of urinary porphyrin and porphyrin precursor excretion in the hepatic porphyrias in relation to the pathway of heme biosynthesis. Intermediates of the pathway excessively excreted during the acute phase of   *each of the hepatic porphyrias are within the respective brackets. (ALA, δ-aminolevulinic acid; PBG, porphobilinogen; UROgen, uroporphyrinogen; COPROgen, coproporphyrinogen; PROTOgen, protoporphyrinogen.)*

been demonstrated during acute attacks of IAP. In some women, exacerbations are correlated with the menstrual cycle, and latent porphyria may become clinically manifest late in pregnancy or shortly after delivery. Prolonged periods of decreased caloric intake (deliberate fasting) and infections may also provoke attacks.

LABORATORY FINDINGS   Excessive excretion of ALA and PBG in the urine is characteristic during acute attacks. It does not differentiate IAP from HCP and VP, and the levels do not correlate with the severity of the symptoms. The qualitative determination of porphobilinogen in the urine by the Watson-Schwartz or the Hoesch test is a simple and valuable screening aid for the diagnosis of an acute attack in IAP, HCP, and VP. These tests are almost always positive during episodes of neuropsychiatric dysfunction. However, both screening tests become positive only when the concentration of PBG in the urine is three to five times the upper limit of normal; as a consequence, they may be negative in latent cases and in patients in whom urinary excretion of PBG becomes normal following recovery from an acute attack. In these instances urinary ALA and PBG excretion should be measured quantitatively by chromatographic methods. In latent IAP with normal excretion of ALA and PBG, diagnosis is possible only by measuring the activity of uroporphyrinogen I synthetase in erythrocytes, lymphocytes, or cultured skin fibroblasts.

In IAP only the porphyrin precursors ALA and PBG are excreted in increased amounts, consistent with the enzymatic defect. Freshly passed urine is, therefore, colorless and contains little preformed uro- or coproporphyrin. The urine may darken on standing because PBG polymerizes spontaneously to uroporphyrin and porphobilin, a dark brown pigment of unknown structure. The fecal porphyrin concentration in IAP is usually normal. In the other two hepatic porphyrias associated with acute neuropsychiatric attacks, increased amounts of preformed porphyrins are excreted in urine and feces.

Conventional liver function tests are normal except for increased Bromsulphalein (BSP) retention. A moderate reduction in red blood cell mass and blood volume or a transient normochromic, normocytic anemia are the only hematologic disturbances. Numerous metabolic abnormalities may be associated with acute attacks including hypercholesterolemia with increased low-density lipoprotein levels, increased serum thyroxine (without hyperthyroidism), abnormal glucose tolerance, and defective 5α reduction of testosterone in liver. The relationship of these abnormalities to the genetic defect is unknown.

Treatment   The treatment of the acute attack is identical in IAP, HCP, and VP. Some acute attacks seemingly can be aborted by administration of large quantities of carbohydrates (glucose effect), although no objective study of the efficacy of this therapy has been performed. Intravenous administration of glucose at a rate of 10 to 20 g/h is recommended. If the patient does not improve within 48 h of continued glucose infusion or if neuropsychiatric symptoms progress, intravenous infusion of hematin (4 mg per kilogram of body weight infused over 10 to 12 min every 12 h) should be tried. Both hematin and glucose effectively prevent the induction of hepatic ALA-synthetase in experimental animals, and both procedures appear to reverse the biochemical abnormalities and cause clinical improvement within 48 h in many patients. Supportive treatment with careful monitoring of fluid and electrolytes is important because hyponatremia, hypomagnesemia, and azotemia commonly occur. Tachycardia and hypertension should be treated with beta-adrenergic blocking drugs. A list of agents considered to be "safe" or "probably safe" in patients with

TABLE 96-2
Drugs considered to be safe (or probably safe) in patients with intermittent acute porphyria, hereditary coproporphyria, and variegate porphyria

Analgesics:
   Salicylates
   Morphine and related opiates (pethidine)
Antibiotics:
   Penicillins
Psychoactive drugs:
   Phenothiazines (chlorpromazine)
Antihistamines:
   Diphenhydramine
Antihypertensives:
   Guanethidine
   Propranolol
   Reserpine
Miscellaneous:
   Atropine
   Neostigmine
   Propanidid
   Procaine
   Succinylcholine
   Ether
   Nitrous oxide

latent and acute IAP, HCP, and VP is given in Table 96-2. The most important measure in the management is prevention of acute attacks by instructing the carrier of the abnormal gene about the avoidance of provocative factors, namely drugs, steroids, and deliberate fasting. With early recognition of the condition, immediate withdrawal of provocative agents, careful fluid and electrolyte therapy, and the use of glucose and/or hematin infusions most attacks are reversible, and fatalities are rare.

HEREDITARY COPROPORPHYRIA Definition and genetics
Hereditary coproporphyria (HCP) is a hepatic porphyria characterized by acute attacks of neuropsychiatric dysfunction identical to those of IAP and VP. In addition, photosensitivity occurs in some. The primary genetic defect is a deficiency of coproporphyrinogen oxidase. The disease is inherited as an autosomal dominant trait. Accurate assessment of the incidence of HCP is difficult since over half of affected individuals remain asymptomatic.

Pathogenesis and clinical picture   Biochemically, HCP is characterized by the excretion of large amounts of coproporphyrin III, mainly in feces but also in urine. Excretion of ALA and PBG is increased during acute attacks (positive Watson-Schwartz or Hoesch test) but usually returns to normal during remission. Acute attacks are indistinguishable from those of IAP and VP and are precipitated by the same factors. Skin photosensitivity occurs in approximately one-third of patients with overt HCP. Its onset is frequently associated with intercurrent hepatic disease. A partial deficiency of coproporphyrinogen oxidase can be demonstrated in leukocytes and cultured skin fibroblasts.

Treatment   Treatment is identical to that described for IAP.

VARIEGATE PORPHYRIA Definition   Variegate porphyria (VP; South African genetic porphyria) is characterized by both acute attacks of neuropsychiatric dysfunction and chronic skin sensitivity to sunlight and to mechanical trauma. The primary enzymatic lesion in heme biosynthesis has not been identified.

Genetics, incidence, and pathogenesis   VP is inherited as an autosomal dominant trait. The disease is particularly common among the white population of South Africa, where its incidence is estimated at 1 in 400, and many cases can be identified as descendants of a woman who emigrated to Cape Town from the Netherlands in 1688. Elsewhere the disease is less frequent, but VP has been recognized in many countries. The defect leads to the excretion of large amounts of protoporphyrin in bile and feces (with lesser increases in the fecal excretion of coproporphyrin) and to markedly increased urinary excretion of ALA, PBG, and coproporphyrin during acute attacks. The excretion pattern suggests a deficiency either of protoporphyrinogen oxidase or ferrochelatase, but a defect of these enzymes has not been demonstrated.

Clinical presentation and diagnosis   Overt cases with VP usually present in the second or third decade. The clinical picture includes acute attacks of abdominal pain and neuropsychiatric symptoms, coupled with photocutaneous lesions. Neurological and cutaneous manifestations may occur simultaneously or at different times. More than 80 percent of the South African patients have signs of cutaneous involvement, consisting of dermal abrasions, superficial erosions, and blister formation after trivial mechanical trauma. The mechanical fragility usually is limited to light-exposed parts of the skin. The lesions often leave depigmented or pigmented scars. Secondary infection frequently delays healing. Hyperpigmentation of the face and hands is common, and women often have hypertrichosis. The skin lesions are indistinguishable from those of porphyria cutanea tarda (PCT). Severe exacerbations of the cutaneous lesions sometimes are associated with intercurrent hepatic disease, presumably related to diminution of fecal excretion and a concomitant increase in the urinary excretion of porphyrins. Acute attacks of neuropsychiatric dysfunction are indistinguishable from those of IAP and HCP and are precipitated by the same factors. The characteristic chemical finding in VP is the continuous excretion of large amounts of proto- and coproporphyrin, even when clinical manifestations are minimal or absent. The levels of protoporphyrin exceed those of coproporphyrin, the reverse of the situation in HCP. Urinary excretion of ALA, PBG, and porphyrins is either normal or moderately increased in asymptomatic patients or those who have only skin symptoms. During acute attacks the urinary excretion of ALA and PBG is increased (positive Watson-Schwartz or Hoesch test), and there also is increased urinary excretion of coproporphyrin and uroporphyrin. Erythrocyte porphyrins are normal, allowing distinction from protoporphyria.

Treatment   Prophylactic measures and treatment of the acute attack with glucose and possibly hematin infusions are the same as for IAP and HCP, although the experience with hematin in VP is limited. Avoidance of exposure to direct sunlight and use of protective clothing (gloves, hats) are advocated.

PORPHYRIA CUTANEA TARDA   Definition   Porphyria cutanea tarda (PCT; symptomatic cutaneous hepatic porphyria, symptomatic porphyria) is the most common form of porphyria. The disease is characterized by chronic skin lesions, the frequent presence of hepatic disease (and hepatic siderosis), and a distinct pattern of urinary excretion of porphyrins. The disorder is probably caused by an inherited deficiency of hepatic uroporphyrinogen decarboxylase. Neurological manifestations are absent.

Genetics, incidence, and pathogenesis   PCT was considered to be an acquired disorder because of its sporadic (and usually nonfamilial) occurrence late in life and its common association (in most series more than 70 percent of patients) with alcoholic liver disease and hepatic siderosis.

The true incidence of the disease has not been evaluated, but PCT is frequent where both alcoholism and iron overload are common, as among the Bantus in South Africa. Recent studies suggest that PCT can be a familial disease, inherited in an autosomal dominant fashion with variable expressivity. The inherited defect consists of a decrease in hepatic and erythrocyte uroporphyrinogen decarboxylase activity; clinically and chemically latent carriers of the defect have been identified. It is not clear whether in some patients PCT also may occur as a consequence of an acquired (or toxic) decrease in hepatic uroporphyrinogen decarboxylase activity. Deficiency (of whatever etiology) in uroporphyrinogen decarboxylase, which catalyzes the conversion of uroporphyrinogen to coproporphyrinogen, leads to a disturbance of hepatic heme synthesis and consequent skin photosensitivity only in the presence of additional factors such as iron overload, usually in association with liver disease. The mechanism by which iron overload causes clinical expression of latent PCT is unknown. In contrast to IAP, HCP, and VP, the enzymatic defect in PCT does not result in altered regulation of the hepatic heme synthetic pathway, and ALA synthetase activity remains normal or only minimally increased even in overt cases. This probably accounts for the absence of acute neuropsychiatric attacks, the usually normal urinary ALA and PBG, and the lack of sensitivity to drugs such as barbiturates.

Clinical presentation and diagnosis   Photosensitivity is the only major manifestation of PCT. The skin lesions are indistinguishable from those in VP. Skin symptoms usually begin insidiously, most often in men age 40 to 60, and consist of enhanced facial pigmentation, increased fragility to trauma, erythema, and vesicular and ulcerative lesions. Sclerodermatous changes and increased hair on the forehead, malar region, or forearms are common.

Chemical and histological evidence of liver disease, frequently related to alcohol, is common, and hepatic siderosis is an almost constant finding, although the degree of iron deposition is variable and rarely severe. Spontaneous remission may occur. Occasionally, estrogens (including contraceptive pills) or known hepatotoxic drugs precipitate the clinical disease. The incidence of diabetes mellitus is increased in PCT, and frequent association with systemic lupus erythematosus and other autoimmune syndromes has been noted.

The excretion of uroporphyrin and, to a lesser extent, coproporphyrin in the urine is increased. The urine may be pink or brown. The excretion of ALA and PBG in the urine is usually normal (negative Watson-Schwartz or Hoesch test). Although uroporphyrin is the major porphyrin in the urine, intermediary porphyrins (particularly heptacarboxylic porphyrin) are also found. Increases in fecal porphyrins are less striking and usually restricted to the coproporphyrin fraction. The diagnosis of PCT is established by the combined presence of skin photosensitivity, liver disease, increased urinary uroporphyrin excretion, the lack of an increase in porphyrin precursors (ALA, PBG), and absence of a history of neuropsychiatric attacks.

Toxic acquired porphyria resembling PCT has occurred in individuals accidentally exposed to hexachlorobenzene, polychlorinated biphenyls, tetrachlorodibenzo-*p*-dioxin (TCDD), and other polychlorinated hydrocarbons. Moreover, several instances of benign or malignant primary tumors of the liver have been observed in association with PCT.

Treatment   Abstinence in alcoholic patients usually leads to improvement of PCT. Removal of hepatic iron by repeated phlebotomy is effective and may lead to long-lasting remissions. Alternatively, chelation therapy with desferoxamine may be tried. The administration of small doses of chloroquine apparently removes uroporphyrins from the liver and has been employed successfully in some patients. However, its use is inadvisable because of the risk of hepatic necrosis.

PROTOPORPHYRIA

DEFINITION Protoporphyria (PP; erythropoietic protoporphyria, erythrohepatic protoporphyria) is a genetic disorder in which mild skin photosensitivity is associated with high concentrations of protoporphyrin in erythrocytes. It is due to a deficiency of ferrochelatase. Protoporphyrin also accumulates in the liver in some patients.

GENETICS, INCIDENCE, AND PATHOGENESIS PP is inherited as an autosomal dominant trait with variable expressivity. Several hundred cases have been reported. Deficient activity of ferrochelatase, the mitochondrial enzyme that catalyzes the incorporation of ferrous iron into protoporphyrin, can be demonstrated in bone marrow, peripheral blood, liver, and cultured skin fibroblasts of patients with PP. This generalized enzyme deficiency results in the excessive accumulation of protoporphyrin in late normoblasts, reticulocytes, and young erythrocytes; protoporphyrin leaks into the plasma from erythrocytes as they age. Photosensitivity is mediated by protoporphyrin in plasma and skin and is evoked by visible light (380 to 560 nm). The liver participates in excess porphyrin production in some patients or, alternatively, may take up protoporphyrin from plasma. Many carriers of the genetic defect remain clinically (and chemically) asymptomatic, and detection may be possible only through enzymatic studies. Skin photosensitivity in symptomatic patients shows seasonal variability.

CLINICAL PRESENTATION AND DIAGNOSIS Mild photosensitivity usually begins in childhood. Exposure to sunlight is rapidly followed by pruritus, erythema, and occasional edema (solar urticaria). The lesions subside over hours or days without scarring. In some patients, cutaneous manifestations occur only after prolonged exposure to sunlight; in others the initial skin lesions progress to a chronic eczematous phase (solar eczema). There is no abnormal mechanical fragility or blister formation as is characteristic for VP and PCT. Erythrodontia, hypertrichosis, and hyperpigmentation are absent. Attacks of neuropsychiatric dysfunction do not occur.

PP generally is a benign disease, but a number of patients have been reported who have associated abnormalities of liver, biliary tract, or blood. The incidence of cholelithiasis is increased, and the gallstones contain protoporphyrin. In rare cases, liver disease has developed owing to massive deposition of protoporphyrin; it may progress to fatal cirrhosis. Many patients with overt PP have mild anemia.

PP is diagnosed by the detection of high concentrations of protoporphyrin in erythrocytes. When a smear of blood from a patient is examined under the fluorescent microscope, large numbers of red-fluorescing erythrocytes are seen. Protoporphyrin may also be elevated in plasma and feces, while urinary porphyrins, ALA, and PBG usually are normal.

TREATMENT Topical sunscreens are ineffective. Orally administered β-carotene (usually as a mixture of β-carotene and canthaxanthine) substantially improves the tolerance to sunlight.

REFERENCES

DEAN G: *The Porphyrias*, 2d ed. London, Pitman Medical Publishing Company, 1972

DHAR GJ et al: Effects of hematin in hepatic porphyria. Further studies. Ann Intern Med 83:20, 1975

ELDER GH et al: The porphyrias: A review. J Clin Pathol 25:1013, 1972

MEYER UA, SCHMID R: The porphyrias, in *The Metabolic Basis of Inherited Disease*, 4th ed, JB Stanbury et al (eds). New York, McGraw-Hill, 1978, p 1166

TSCHUDY DP: Porphyrin metabolism and the porphyrias, in *Duncan's Diseases of Metabolism*, 7th ed, PK Bondy, LE Rosenberg (eds). Philadelphia, Saunders, 1974, p 775

Disorders of carbohydrate metabolism

97
DISEASES OF GLYCOGEN METABOLISM

JAMES B. FIELD

The diseases of glycogen metabolism are inherited conditions resulting from deficiencies of specific enzymes involved in glycogen synthesis or degradation. The clinical features and organ involvement depend upon the specific enzymatic defect and its tissue distribution. Although enzymatic defects have been identified in many patients, characteristic clinical features have been described in other subjects whose specific enzymatic defects have not been identified. Such patients complicate attempts at classification based solely on the enzymatic defect and the tissue involved. Furthermore, the same apparent enzymatic deficiency may be associated with different clinical presentations (e.g., the infantile and adult forms of type II, α-1,4-glucosidase deficiency). Although uncommon, the diseases of glycogen metabolism have been of major importance in elucidating pathways of glycogen synthesis and degradation. They were also the first diseases proved to be due to deficiency of a single enzyme. Table 97-1 presents a classification of these diseases. The location of the enzymatic defects in relation to the glycogen metabolism is detailed in Fig. 97-1.

TYPE I GLYCOGENOSIS

Type I glycogenosis (von Gierke's disease) is due to deficient glucose 6-phosphatase activity in the liver, kidney, and intestinal mucosa. While platelets and placenta may also be involved, patients with type 1 glycogenosis have had normal pregnancies. The disease is inherited in autosomal recessive fashion, and heterozygotes have been identified by the demonstration of diminished glucose 6-phosphatase in biopsies of small-bowel mucosa. Type I glycogenosis accounts for about 25 percent of all patients with glycogen storage disease.

PATHOLOGICAL PHYSIOLOGY The absence of hepatic glucose 6-phosphatase causes a profound deficiency in hepatic glucose production from either glycogenolysis or gluconeogenesis, although some glucose may be released from the liver by amylo-1,6-glucosidase (debrancher enzyme). That enzyme hydrolyzes the 6 to 8 percent of the glucose residues in the 1,6 linkage which forms the branch points of the glycogen molecule. Severe hypoglycemia is seen during fasting, with blood glucose values frequently in the range of 10 to 15 mg per 100 ml. Since glucose 6-phosphate cannot be converted to glucose, it traverses the Embden-Meyerhof pathway and significantly increases hepatic production of lactic acid. Chronic hypoglycemia is associated with accelerated lipid mobilization and ketonemia. Hypercholesterolemia and hypertriglyceridemia are seen during periods of inadequate carbohydrate intake. Chronic metabolic acidosis may be present due to increased lactic acid and ketone body production. Elevated uric acid levels are characteristic, but clinical gout is usually not a problem until the second decade of life. The hyperuricemia reflects impaired renal excretion secondary to elevated lactic and β-hydroxybutyric acids coupled with increased uric acid production. The mechanism of the latter is not known but might reflect increased production of phosphoribosylpyrophosphate, a precursor of uric acid or increased degradation of adenine nucleotides due to diminished hepatic inorganic phosphate or adenosine triphosphate (ATP) concentrations.

PATHOLOGY The liver is enlarged because of excess glycogen (>5 g per 100 g weight) and fat. Splenomegaly does not occur. Despite hepatomegaly and abnormal histology, liver function is unimpaired except for those parameters involving glycogen metabolism. With increasing age, a significant number of patients develop adenomas of the liver, some of which progress to hepatomas. Renal enlargement is usually not associated with abnormalities of kidney function, although occasional patients may develop Fanconi syndrome. Increased glycogen is present in the renal tubules. Deficient glucose 6-phosphatase in intestinal mucosa seems to be of little clinical consequence although steatorrhea has been reported.

CLINICAL MANIFESTATIONS Although hepatomegaly is usually present at birth, the child with type I glycogen storage disease may not attract medical attention for several months and then present with hypoglycemic seizures, hepatomegaly, or failure to thrive. Respiratory infections, which are common, may precipitate symptomatic hypoglycemia and accentuate the chronic hyperventilation that results from metabolic acidosis. A bleeding diathesis is common and appears to be due to abnormal platelet function. The child may exhibit a typical "doll-like" facies with increased adiposity in the cheeks and buttocks. Eruptive xanthomas on extensor surfaces reflect the hyperlipidemia, and lipemia retinalis is common. The abdomen is greatly enlarged producing a waddling gait. Retarded physical growth, characteristic of this type of glycogen storage disease, may be severe but is not associated with abnormalities in pituitary, thyroid, or adrenal function. It probably reflects hypoglycemia and chronic metabolic acidosis. The latter also causes osteoporosis and negative calcium balance. Adolescent maturation is almost always delayed.

The symptoms usually ameliorate as the patient grows older if death from severe hypoglycemia, overwhelming infections, or metabolic acidosis can be prevented. While brain damage may result from hypoglycemia, the discrepancy between the low blood glucose values and the symptoms of hypoglycemia is noteworthy. Blood sugar values as low as 10 mg per 100 ml appear to be well tolerated, presumably because the brain utilizes the elevated blood ketone bodies as alternative substrate. Symptomatic gout involving both the joints and the kidneys may be a problem in those patients reaching adulthood.

DIAGNOSIS The presence of hypoglycemia, chronic metabolic acidosis, and elevated plasma levels of lactate, free fatty acids, pyruvate, glycerol, triglycerides, phospholipids, cholesterol, ketones, and uric acid suggests the diagnosis of type I glycogen storage disease. Precise diagnosis requires the demonstration of absent glucose 6-phosphatase from properly obtained and processed biopsy material from liver, intestinal mucosa, or kidney. The enzyme assay should include a control for nonspecific phosphatase activity. Histological appearance of the liver is not diagnostic. Open liver biopsy is preferable to a needle biopsy since it provides more tissue for measurement of the structure and content of glycogen and the assay of relevant

TABLE 97-1
Diseases of glycogen metabolism

Type	Enzyme defect	Glycogen Amount	Glycogen Structure	Affected tissues	Alternate names
I	Glucose 6-phosphatase	Increased	Normal	Liver, kidney, small-bowel mucosa	von Gierke's disease, hepatorenal disease
II	Lysosomal α-1,4-glucosidase	Increased	Normal	Generalized	Pompe's generalized
III	Amylo-1,6-glucosidase (debrancher enzyme)	Increased	Short outer chains (limit dextrin)	Liver, muscle, white blood cells	Cori's limit dextrinosis, Forbes' disease, limit dextrinosis
IV	Amylo-1,4→1,6-transglucosidase (branching enzyme)	Normal or decreased	Long outer chains, few branch points (amylopectin)	Generalized	Andersen's disease, amylopectinosis
V*	Muscle phosphorylase	Increased	Normal	Muscle	McArdle's disease
VI	Liver phosphorylase	Increased	Normal	Liver	Hers' disease
VIa	Liver phosphorylase kinase	Increased	Normal	Liver, white blood cells	
O	Glycogen synthetase	Decreased	Normal	Liver	

* *A similar clinical picture results from a deficiency of phosphofructokinase, phosphoglucomutase, or phosphohexoseisomerase in muscle.*

FIGURE 97-1

Pathways of glycogen synthesis and degradation. The pathway of glycogen synthesis involves phosphorylation of glucose to glucose 6-phosphate which is then converted to glucose 1-phosphate. Glucose 1-phosphate plus uridine triphosphate (UTP) reacts to form uridine diphosphate glucose (UDP, •), the donor of glucose residues in glycogen synthesis. The glucose from UDP (•) is transferred to the nonreducing terminal unit of a glycogen molecule in a 1,4 glucosidic linkage (•) by the enzyme, glycogen synthetase (e) to form a glycogen molecule with an additional glucose residue. This is repeated until the chain length contains at least seven glucose residues. A branch point is formed by the enzyme amylo-1,4→1,6-transglucosidase (branching enzyme, f) which transfers a 7-glucose unit from a 1,4 linkage to a 1,6 linkage (O). The repeated action of glycogen synthetase then extends both of these terminal chains until they are the appropriate length to form new branch points.

Glycogen breakdown is initiated by the enzyme phosphorylase (g) which sequentially hydrolyzes terminal glucose residues in 1,4 linkage to form glucose 1-phosphate. Phosphorylase activity continues to within four glucose residues of a branch point. This molecule is known as a phosphorylase limit dextrin. The enzyme oligo-1,4→1,4-glucantransferase (h) then transfers a three-glucose unit from an outer side chain to an outer main chain of the phosphorylase limit dextrin. This then exposes a branch point glucose molecule in 1,6 linkage which is removed as free glucose by the enzyme amylo-1,6-glucosidase (i). These last two enzyme activities have not been separated and are known as the debranching enzyme. After removal of the branch point, the residual glycogen molecule is available to phosphorylase until another branch point is reached. The alternate action of phosphorylase and debranching enzyme is capable of completely degrading glycogen. Glucose 1-phosphate is converted to glucose 6-phosphate by the enzyme phosphoglucomutase (d). Glucose 6-phosphate can be converted to free glucose by glucose 6-phosphatase (a) or to fructose 6-phosphate by phosphohexoseisomerase (b). The latter compound is phosphorylated by phosphofructokinase (c) to form fructose 1,6-diphosphate, which is metabolized by the Embden-Meyerhof pathway to pyruvate and lactate. Another pathway of glycogen degradation involves the lysosomal enzyme acid α-glucosidase which is capable of breaking both 1,4 and 1,6 glucosidic bonds.

enzymes. It also allows adequate hemostasis in patients with a bleeding diathesis. If the appropriate enzyme assays are not available, advance arrangements should be made with a center where they can be done.

Functional tests are helpful in establishing the appropriate diagnosis. Patients with type I glycogenosis do not increase plasma glucose concentrations following administration of epinephrine or glucagon. Since glycogen degradation is normal but free glucose cannot be released, lactate production is augmented by these hormones, thus exaggerating the metabolic acidosis. Administration of fructose, galactose, or glycerol increases plasma lactate but not glucose. Currently the diagnosis of type I glycogen storage disease cannot be made prenatally.

THERAPY Specific therapy for patients with type I glycogenosis is not available. Treatment is aimed at amelioration of hypoglycemia which appears to be responsible for most of, if not all, the clinical abnormalities. Constant nocturnal infusion of a high glucose formula through a small plastic nasogastric tube has been reported to reverse all the metabolic aberrations and increase the growth rate of patients within 4 weeks of initiation. High-starch, low-fat feedings are given every 3 h during the day. This program has been utilized at home by some patients for over a year with good clinical results including reduction of hepatic size. Portacaval transposition and portacaval shunting have also caused improvement in some patients. The results are better when the patients receive hyperalimentation preoperatively. Continuous parenteral nutrition or continuous intragastric infusion is also beneficial during acute intercurrent problems.

TYPE II GLYCOGENOSIS

Type II glycogenosis is associated with deficiency of the lysosomal enzyme α-1,4-glucosidase or acid maltase. (For a discussion of the pathophysiology of lysosomal storage diseases, see Chap. 101.) Increased glycogen concentration has been found in all tissues. The disease occurs in severe infantile and milder adult forms. Different mutant alleles probably exist for α-1,4-glucosidase to account for this clinical heterogeneity. The infantile variety is inherited as an autosomal recessive condition, and the diagnosis can be established before birth by assay of α-1,4-glucosidase in amniotic fluid cells grown in tissue culture. A neutral glucosidase in amniotic fluid precludes its use for this purpose. Type II glycogenosis is present in 1 out of every 150,000 to 400,000 births.

PATHOLOGICAL PHYSIOLOGY Despite the generalized increase in tissue glycogen concentration (especially in lysosomes) the basis for the clinical symptoms and reasons for the differences between infantile and adult forms are not clear. Patients with the infantile form of the disease have no muscle α-1,4-glucosidase, while adult patients may have residual activity. Infantile patients also have decreased neutral maltase activity, whereas this enzyme is normal in the adult variant. Since the enzymes involved in the degradation and synthesis of glycogen are normal, except for the lysosomal α-1,4-glucosidase, hypoglycemia, hyperlipidemia, metabolic acidosis, and other systemic metabolic alterations are not present. Increased lysosomal glycogen concentration can be accounted for by the deficiency of α-1,4-glucosidase, but the explanation for the augmented extralysosomal cytoplasmic glycogen is unknown. In the infantile form, increased glycogen is present in cardiac and skeletal muscle as well as in liver, kidney, and central nervous system. The absent or minimal cardiac involvement in the adult patients may account for their longer survival. Accumulation of glycogen in the lysosomes of cardiac and skeletal muscle may impair their function, but the mechanism is unknown.

CLINICAL MANIFESTATIONS In the infantile form the characteristic clinical features result from myocardial and neuromuscular involvement. Classically symptoms of congestive heart failure with progressive cardiac enlargement begin within a few weeks after birth. Repeated respiratory infections are common. The patients fail to thrive and manifest anorexia, easy fatigability, generalized weakness, drooling, and shortness of breath. The tongue is frequently enlarged. The muscle mass is increased and has a firm, rubbery consistency, but the muscles are weak and hypotonic. The liver is usually firm and moderately enlarged. Neurological abnormalities may be present with retarded motor and intellectual development. The cardiac image is globular and markedly enlarged on chest x-ray. The electrocardiogram demonstrates left axis deviation, short PR interval, QRS complexes of large amplitude, depression of the ST segment, and inversion of the T waves. Death usually occurs within the first year or two of life due to intractable congestive heart failure. About 20 percent of the patients also have endocardial fibroelastosis.

The milder adult form presents with muscle weakness which is greater proximally than distally and involves the pelvic more than the pectoral muscles. Respiratory muscles may also be involved. Symptoms usually become prominent in the third to sixth decade. In the adult form there is no relationship between the clinical picture and the amount of residual α-1,4-glucosidase activity.

DIAGNOSIS Type II glycogen storage disease is diagnosed by demonstrating α-1,4-glucosidase deficiency in white blood cells, cultured skin fibroblasts, or skeletal muscle. The glycogen content of tissue is increased (liver, >5 percent; muscle, >1 percent), but its structure is normal. While the histological localization of increased glycogen in lysosomes is suggestive, the diagnosis should be confirmed by appropriate enzyme assay. It is important to distinguish between neutral and acid α-1,4-glucosidase activity in biopsy specimens.

THERAPY No effective treatment exists for the infantile form. Supportive measures such as digitalis, diuretics, and salt restriction are of little value in the treatment of the congestive heart failure. α-1,4-Glucosidase prepared from both *Aspergillus niger* and human placenta has been administered to infants with type II glycogenosis, but no beneficial effect on the clinical course of the disease was observed.

TYPE III GLYCOGEN STORAGE DISEASE

The enzyme amylo-1,6-glucosidase, the debrancher enzyme, is deficient in this form of glycogen storage disease. The enzyme deficiency in liver and muscle is responsible for the clinical disease, but white and red blood cells also share the defect. Several variants have been described on the basis of tissue distribution of the enzyme deficiency and the method of the enzyme assay. Type III glycogenosis is probably the commonest form of glycogen storage disease and appears to be inherited in autosomal recessive fashion.

PATHOLOGICAL PHYSIOLOGY The absence of amylo-1,6-glucosidase prevents further degradation of glycogen beyond a branch point and results in a molecule with very short outer chains (limit dextrin). Normal glycogen degradation involves removal of glucosyl units in 1,4 linkage in the outer chains by phosphorylase until four such residues remain on either side of the branch point, a glucose molecule which has both a 1,6 and a 1,4 linkage (Fig. 97-1). Three glucose residues on the branched chain are then transferred to the terminal position on the main chain by the enzyme oligo-1,4→1,4-glucantransferase. This enzyme activity has not been separated physically from the amylo-1,6-glucosidase which splits the glucosyl unit

in 1,6 linkage at the branch point to free glucose. Following removal of the branch point, phosphorylase then continues degradation of glycogen until the next branch point is approached. During fasting, the abnormal glycogen (limit dextrin) cannot be further degraded, leading to hypoglycemia. The hypoglycemia is less severe than in patients with type I glycogen storage disease because gluconeogenesis is still intact. Abnormalities in lipid metabolism are also less prominent than in type I glycogen storage disease. Plasma lactate and uric acid concentrations are usually normal. Since amylo-1,6-glucosidase may also be absent in skeletal muscle, the disorder may be associated with hypotonia, muscle weakness, and increased muscle glycogen content.

CLINICAL MANIFESTATIONS The clinical presentation is similar to that of patients with type I glycogenosis but less severe. Hypoglycemia tends to be mild, but growth retardation, hepatomegaly, and splenomegaly may be present. As the patient grows older, the symptoms ameliorate, and hepatomegaly diminishes.

DIAGNOSIS Diagnosis depends upon the demonstration of the enzyme defect in cultured skin fibroblasts or in muscle or liver obtained by biopsy. The finding of increased amounts of glycogen with abnormal structure (short outer-branch chains) is confirmatory. Assay of either white or red blood cells for amylo-1,6-glucosidase and glycogen structure can also be useful in genetic studies. Children with type III glycogenosis frequently have elevations of serum transaminase without other evidence of generalized hepatic dysfunction. Since glycogen cannot be degraded beyond the initial phosphorylase cleavages, administration of glucagon or epinephrine in the fasting state usually does not increase the blood glucose. However, administration of these substances several hours after a meal does cause an elevation in blood glucose since carbohydrate ingestion restores the outer chains of glycogen, rendering them available for degradation by phosphorylase. In contrast to patients with type I glycogen storage disease, glucagon administration does not increase plasma lactate concentration, and administration of fructose, galactose, glycerol, or alanine increases the blood glucose.

THERAPY Hypoglycemia can usually be prevented by frequent feedings, but in some patients the problem is severe enough to warrant portacaval shunting. Generally, constant nocturnal infusion of a high-carbohydrate formula is preferable to surgery, especially since the disease ameliorates with time. In contrast to patients with type I glycogen storage disease, there is no need to restrict the lactose or sucrose content of the diet.

TYPE IV GLYCOGENOSIS

This type of glycogen deposition disease is associated with deficiency of amylo-1,4→1,6-transglucosidase (branching enzyme). This enzyme initiates the branching of glycogen by transferring a 7-glucose unit from a 1,4 linkage to a 1,6 linkage. The enzyme is deficient in multiple tissues including liver, heart, smooth and skeletal muscle, kidney, spleen, central nervous system, and white blood cells. The glycogen content of these tissues may be normal or decreased but is abnormal in structure, resembling amylopectin with decreased branch points and long outer chains. The molecule has a high chromogenicity, and the absorption maximum is shifted. Only 13 cases have been reported, and it appears to be transmitted as an autosomal recessive. Heterozygotes may have diminished branching enzyme in white blood cells, but this has not been found uniformly. Assay of enzyme in amniotic fluid fibroblasts has been used for antenatal diagnosis.

PATHOLOGICAL PHYSIOLOGY This type of glycogenosis is not associated with any abnormality in carbohydrate metabolism since the enzymatic defect does not prevent glycogen degradation by phosphorylase and since gluconeogenesis is unimpaired. However, the disease is associated with progressive development of either cirrhosis or cardiac failure, of unknown mechanism.

CLINICAL MANIFESTATIONS At birth, patients appear normal but fail to thrive in the first few months of life. Hepatomegaly and abnormal liver function usually accompany clinical deterioration, and splenomegaly and ascites develop as the liver failure progresses. The muscles are hypotonic, and congestive heart failure may develop. This disease is uniformly fatal in the first few years of life.

DIAGNOSIS Type IV glycogenosis should be considered in all infants with cirrhosis or congestive heart failure. The diagnosis is established by finding deficient branching-enzyme activity in white blood cells or in tissue obtained by biopsy. The demonstration of glycogen structure resembling amylopectin is indicative of the disease, but the diagnosis should be confirmed by enzyme assay.

THERAPY No specific therapy is available. Cirrhosis and heart failure are treated symptomatically.

TYPE V GLYCOGEN STORAGE DISEASE

Muscle phosphorylase is absent in this form of glycogen storage disease. This enzyme is immunologically and genetically distinct from the liver enzyme. The disease is inherited as an autosomal recessive.

PATHOLOGICAL PHYSIOLOGY Glycogenolysis is an important source of energy for muscle contraction. Phosphorylase deficiency precludes this source of energy and accounts for the difficulty these patients have during sustained muscle activity. Normally during exercise the combination of increased glycogenolysis and inadequate oxygen elevates plasma lactic acid. This normal increase in lactic acid with exercise does not occur in patients with type V glycogenosis.

CLINICAL MANIFESTATIONS For unknown reasons affected patients have very few symptoms during the first or second decade of life. Thereafter, exercise causes weakness and cramping of the involved muscles. Myoglobinuria is common, especially with strenuous exercise, and muscle enzymes are characteristically elevated in the plasma. There are no definitive physical findings, but in later life some muscle atrophy may be present.

DIAGNOSIS The diagnosis is suggested by the lack of increase in plasma lactate after muscular exercise. However, demonstration of absent muscle phosphorylase is necessary to establish the diagnosis since a similar clinical picture with absent lactate elevation has been described in patients with normal phosphorylase activity but other enzyme deficiencies in their muscles. The latter include phosphofructokinase, phosphoglucomutase, and phosphohexoseisomerase, deficiencies of which would impede anaerobic glycolysis in muscle.

THERAPY Ingestion of glucose or fructose prior to and during exercise is frequently associated with improved exercise tolerance. Patients learn their exercise tolerance and avoid symptoms by not exceeding it. Within these limitations, the long-term prognosis is good.

TYPE VI GLYCOGEN STORAGE DISEASE

Abnormalities in the phosphorylase system of the liver are found in patients with type VI glycogen storage disease. A cyclic AMP–dependent protein kinase stimulated by glucagon activates the enzyme phosphorylase kinase which in turn converts inactive phosphorylase to the active enzyme. The product of phosphorylase degradation, glucose 1-phosphate, is then converted to glucose 6-phosphate. While absence of any of the enzymes in this cascade could produce the clinical picture, only deficiencies of phosphorylase kinase and phosphorylase have been adequately documented. The former deficiency is more common. Phosphorylase deficiency, considered as type VI glycogen storage disease, is inherited as an autosomal recessive trait. Type VIa glycogen storage disease is due to deficiency of phosphorylase kinase and exists in two forms. One is inherited as an autosomal recessive and the other as an X-linked recessive trait.

CLINICAL MANIFESTATIONS These patients are similar to those with type III glycogen storage disease and are less symptomatic than patients with the type I disorder. Types VI and VIa glycogen storage diseases are clinically indistinguishable. Hepatic enlargement is prominent during preadolescent years but often disappears with amelioration of symptoms as the child grows older. Fasting hypoglycemia, when present, is usually mild, and hyperlipidemia and metabolic acidosis are usually absent. Frequently the deficiency of phosphorylase is incomplete and, in addition, gluconeogenesis is unimpaired. Patients may have some retardation in physical and motor development initially but almost always ultimately attain normal adult height.

DIAGNOSIS This type of glycogen storage disease should be suspected in patients who present with a picture similar to type III disease. The specific diagnosis can be established by appropriate assay for the enzyme in either liver or leukocytes. Despite the reduction of activity of the phosphorylase system, these patients may have a normal blood glucose response to either epinephrine or glucagon. Several patients have been described who had other defects of the phosphorylase system. One patient with hepatomegaly, truncal ataxia, nystagmus, hypotonia and spasticity had normal total liver phosphorylase, but the enzyme was entirely in the inactive form. An additional patient with defective cyclic AMP–dependent protein kinase in muscle and liver has been reported.

THERAPY Since these patients, for the most part, have mild symptoms that diminish as they grow older, no specific treatment is necessary over and above prevention of hypoglycemia.

PATIENTS WITH MULTIPLE OR NO ENZYMATIC DEFECTS

Several patients with the clinical picture of type I glycogen storage disease have deficiency of another enzyme in addition to glucose 6-phosphatase. The second enzyme is most frequently amylo-1,6-glucosidase, but occasionally it may be phosphorylase. Children in the same family may have different enzymatic defects. It is conceivable that the second enzyme deficiency is an artifact due to inadequate tissue preservation or assay techniques. Patients with the clinical features of glycogen storage diseases have also been reported who have no detectable enzyme defect when the liver biopsy is assayed for all the enzymes involved in the recognized types of glycogen storage disease.

GLYCOGEN SYNTHETASE DEFICIENCY

This disease is caused by deficiency of hepatic glycogen synthetase, the enzyme responsible for adding glucosyl units to glycogen. Hypoglycemia is usually the presenting manifestation, although the infant may present because of failure to thrive. The liver is not enlarged. Fasting ketonuria is present, and a relationship to ketotic hypoglycemia has been suggested. Feeding is associated with elevated plasma lactic acid levels, and glycosuria may occur. Administration of glucagon in the fed state increases blood glucose somewhat but brings no response during a fast. Plasma alanine levels are low. The diagnosis is established by assay of liver for glycogen synthetase. Treatment should be aimed at prevention of hypoglycemia by utilizing a program of constant nocturnal infusion as outlined for type I glycogen storage disease.

REFERENCES

AYNSLEY-GREEN AW et al: Hepatic glycogen synthetase deficiency. Definition of syndrome from metabolic and enzyme studies on a 9-year old girl. Arch Dis Child 52:573, 1977

DRASH A, FIELD JB: The glycogen storage diseases. Dis Mon, October 1971

GREENE HL et al: Continuous nocturnal intragastric feeding for management of type 1 glycogen-storage disease. N Engl J Med 294:423, 1976

HOWELL RR: The glycogen storage diseases, in *The Metabolic Basis of Inherited Diseases,* 4th ed, JB Stanbury et al (eds). New York, McGraw-Hill, 1978, p 137

HUG G: Glycogen storage diseases. Birth Defects 12:145, 1976

HUIJING F: Glycogen metabolism and glycogen-storage disease. Physiol Rev 55:609, 1975

MAHLER RF: Disorders of glycogen metabolism. Clin Endocrinol Metab 5:579, 1976

SENIOR B, SADEGHI-NEJAD A: The glycogenoses and other inherited disorders of carbohydrate metabolism. Clin Perinatal 3:79, 1976

98
GALACTOSEMIA

KURT J. ISSELBACHER

DEFINITION Galactosemia refers to an inborn error of metabolism associated with an impairment in the metabolism of galactose. Two disorders are currently recognized. "Classic" galactosemia is due to the deficiency of the enzyme galactose 1-phosphate uridyl transferase; it is typically associated with cataract formation, mental retardation, and cirrhosis. The second disorder, first described in 1965, is due to galactokinase deficiency and leads primarily to cataract formation.

PATHOGENESIS Lactose, the main carbohydrate in milk, is a disaccharide containing galactose and glucose; when ingested it is hydrolyzed by intestinal lactase. Normally the absorbed galactose is converted in the liver to glucose. The first reaction in this pathway involves the phosphorylation of galactose to galactose 1-phosphate by galactokinase:

$$\text{Galactose} + \text{ATP} \xrightarrow{\text{galactokinase}} \text{galactose 1-phosphate}$$

The gene for galactokinase has been assigned to chromosome 17. The next step involves the conversion of galactose 1-phosphate to glucose 1-phosphate. This involves the participation of uridine diphosphate (UDP) sugars and the enzyme galactose 1-phosphate uridyl transferase as follows:

$$\text{Galactose 1-phosphate} + \text{UDP-glucose} \xrightarrow{\text{transferase}} \text{UDP-galactose} + \text{glucose 1-phosphate}$$

The UDP sugars can be reversibly interconverted by an epimerase reaction:

$$\text{UDP-galactose} \xrightleftharpoons{\text{epimerase}} \text{UDP-glucose}$$

Several alternate pathways of galactose metabolism appear to exist. Galactose can be converted (reduced) in the presence of NADPH (or NADH) to galactitol (dulcitol) by aldose reductase, an enzyme which occurs especially in the lens. Galactose can be oxidized to a limited extent by galactose dehydrogenase leading eventually to the formation of galactonic acid, xylulose, and CO_2. There is also a pyrophosphorylase reaction involving the interaction of galactose 1-phosphate with uridine triphosphate to form UDP-galactose. One or more of these pathways may account for a limited galactose metabolism in some patients with galactosemia.

In galactokinase deficiency, galactose accumulates in the blood and tissues. In the lens galactose is converted by aldose reductase to galactitol, a sugar to which the lens is impermeable. As a consequence, excessive hydration occurs which, together with a decrease in lenticular glutathione, leads to cataract formation.

In classic galactosemia, transferase deficiency leads to tissue accumulation of galactose 1-phosphate and galactose. As in galactokinase deficiency, cataracts develop secondary to galactitol accumulation in the lens. It is assumed but not proved that the cirrhosis and mental retardation of classic galactosemia are in some manner related to increased amounts of galactose 1-phosphate in these tissues. Elevated blood galactose levels may lead to a decreased hepatic output of glucose and hypoglycemia. In the kidney and intestine, accumulation of galactose and galactose 1-phosphate appears to lead to an inhibition of amino acid transport.

Both galactokinase- and transferase-deficiency galactosemia are transmitted as autosomal recessive traits. Heterozygotes for these disorders have half-normal enzyme levels but are asymptomatic. Maternal deficiency of galactokinase, together with a significant lactose intake during pregnancy, may contribute to cataract formation during fetal development. However, not all persons with half-normal transferase enzymes in their cells are carriers of galactosemia. Some individuals homozygous for another gene, called the Duarte variant, normally have only half-normal transferase levels. This group can be differentiated from galactosemia heterozygotes on the basis of the electrophoretic properties of the mutant enzyme. In both types of galactosemia, the disorder is due either to the functional deficiency or absence of the involved enzyme. In the classic type of galactosemia there is evidence that the disorder is due to a structural gene mutation and that the enzyme (transferase) protein is present but structurally altered and not functioning normally. Several other clinical variants with altered enzyme electrophoretic mobility have been described.

The exact incidence of classic galactosemia is still unclear. Estimates range from 1 in 18,000 to 1 in 100,000 births. Population studies indicate that 0.8 to 1.3 percent of the population are heterozygous for the galactosemia gene and about 10 percent carry the Duarte variant.

CLINICAL FEATURES Symptoms of classic galactosemia usually begin within days to several weeks after birth. The infant usually is reluctant to ingest breast milk or milk formulas, develops vomiting, shows poor nutrition, and fails to thrive. Jaundice, hepatomegaly, and evidence of liver disease may then develop. Cataracts are usually not present at birth but occur gradually over a period of weeks to months. Mental retardation may be difficult to detect but becomes evident after 6 or 12 months. Infants with classical galactosemia are subject to bacterial sepsis (especially with *Escherichia coli*), and this may be the primary cause of death in the neonatal period. The only recognized complication of galactokinase deficiency is cataract formation.

DIAGNOSIS Galactokinase deficiency should be suspected in infants or children with cataract formation who have non-glucose-reducing substances in their urine. The diagnosis is made by demonstrating the deficiency of galactokinase in red blood cells.

Classic galactosemia must be considered when one or more of the clinical features described above are found. If the patient is ingesting milk, reducing sugar may be found in the urine, which gives a negative glucose oxidase reaction (i.e., is not glucose) and is identified as galactose by other techniques, such as chromatography. If the child is vomiting, has a poor food intake, or is on intravenous glucose feedings, galactose may not be present in the urine. The definitive diagnosis consists of demonstrating a lack or deficiency of red cell galactose 1-phosphate uridyl transferase. A variety of assay techniques have been described. The disease can also be diagnosed prenatally by enzyme studies on cultured cells obtained by amniocentesis.

In the neonatal period galactosemia needs to be differentiated from primary liver disease. With liver damage, galactose removal from the blood is impaired, and elevated blood galactose levels as well as galactosuria may occur. However, in hepatitis or cirrhosis the transferase levels will be normal.

TREATMENT The treatment of galactosemia consists of the removal of galactose-containing foods from the diet, especially milk. In infants, milk substitutes such as DextriMaltose and Nutramigen are often used. Soybean preparations have also been used in the past, but their polysaccharides contain some galactose and they should be avoided.

The institution of a galactose-free diet usually leads to a dramatic improvement in the patient; in fact, all clinical features except for mental retardation may improve or disappear. In general, patients are kept on galactose-free diets indefinitely or at least until they have reached adequate physical and neurologic development.

REFERENCES

GITZELMANN R et al: Galactose metabolism in a patient with hereditary galactokinase deficiency. Eur J Clin Invest 4:79, 1974

LEVY HL et al: Sepsis due to *Escherichia coli* in neonates with galactosemia. N Engl J Med 297:737, 1975

SEGAL S: Disorders of galactose metabolism, in *The Metabolic Basis of Inherited Disease*, 4th ed, JB Stanbury et al (eds). New York, McGraw-Hill, 1978, p 160

TEDESCO TA et al: The genetic defect in galactosemia. N Engl J Med 292:737, 1975

99
HEREDITARY FRUCTOSE INTOLERANCE

DANIEL W. FOSTER

Hereditary fructose intolerance is an autosomal recessive disorder characterized by vomiting and hypoglycemia following the ingestion of fructose-containing foods. The underlying molecular defect is a deficiency of the enzyme fructose 1-phosphate aldolase.

CLINICAL PICTURE Clinical manifestations of fructose intolerance vary with age, the most severe form occurring in infants. Characteristically the baby is normal when breast fed but develops symptoms once fructose-containing formulas or foods are ingested. The primary response to fructose is severe vomiting and diarrhea with consequent failure to thrive. Hepatic disease is invariable; hepatomegaly is accompanied by hyperbilirubinemia, elevated levels of hepatic enzymes in plasma, hypoalbuminemia, and even ascites. Hemorrhage may be a major problem due to deficiencies of prothrombin, fibrinogen, and other clotting factors. Postprandial hypoglycemia may lead to loss of consciousness or convulsions. Albuminuria and renal tubular acidosis of the proximal type with aminoaciduria and bicarbonate wastage are common. The children are vulnerable to lactic acidosis.

Older children and adults have a less severe syndrome, often because they learn spontaneously to avoid sweets. The usual picture is that of abdominal pain, nausea, bloating, and diarrhea with or without signs of hypoglycemia following the ingestion of foods containing fructose, sucrose, or sorbitol (which is converted to fructose in the body). Hyperuricemia and uricosuria are common, and kidney stones may be present. Dental caries are unusual because of diminished sugar intake. Hepatic disease is less severe in the adult.

If the diagnosis is made early and effective treatment is initiated, all manifestations of the disease disappear; i.e., the renal and hepatic lesions are reversible. Prolonged exposure to fructose in infants may result in permanent liver damage with changes of portal or biliary cirrhosis evident on pathological examination.

PATHOPHYSIOLOGY The disorder is due to deficiency of fructose 1-phosphate aldolase. When fructose is ingested, the first step in its metabolism is the formation of fructose 1-phosphate, a reaction catalyzed by the enzyme fructokinase. Fructose 1-phosphate is then split to form the trioses glyceraldehyde and dihydroxyacetone phosphate by fructose 1-phosphate aldolase. A deficiency of the enzyme results in the accumulation of fructose 1-phosphate in the tissues following ingestion of fructose and sorbitol. This intermediate is presumably directly responsible for hepatic and renal tubular damage. Fructose 1-phosphate also secondarily inhibits other enzymes. Inhibition of fructokinase accounts for fructosemia and fructosuria, while postprandial hypoglycemia is presumably due to inhibition of hepatic glycogen phosphorylase activity, an impairment that also accounts for glucagon unresponsiveness in the syndrome. Fructose 1-phosphate also inhibits fructose 1,6-diphosphate aldolase, thereby blocking gluconeogenesis. While the block in glycogen breakdown is the primary reason for postprandial hypoglycemia, impairment of gluconeogenesis plays a contributing role. Sharp falls in tissue and plasma inorganic phosphate concentrations occur with fructose ingestion and presumably account for the depletion of tissue adenosine triphosphate that characteristically follows. The reason for hyperuricemia is not known but may be related to increased turnover of purine nucleotides.

DIAGNOSIS The diagnosis is usually suggested by history. In infants the differential lies between hereditary fructose intolerance, galactosemia, and tyrosinosis. The latter two syndromes are also associated with postprandial vomiting and failure to thrive and are due to the ingestion of galactose and tyrosine, respectively. If symptoms are immediately relieved by the intravenous infusion of glucose and do not return when a sucrose- and fructose-free diet is consumed, the diagnosis is clear. Confirmation requires testing with fructose. While normal persons develop hypoglycemia with large fructose loads, the administration of small doses of the hexose (0.25 g/kg in adults, 3 g per square meter of body surface area in children) produces symptoms and a fall in plasma glucose and phosphorus concentrations only in subjects with the disease.

TREATMENT Treatment consists of eliminating sucrose, fructose, and sorbitol from the diet.

REFERENCES

FROESCH ER: Essential fructosuria, hereditary fructose intolerance, and fructose-1,6-diphosphatase deficiency, in *The Metabolic Basis of Inherited Disease,* JB Stanbury et al (eds). New York, McGraw-Hill, 1978, pp 121–136

ODIÈVRE M et al: Hereditary fructose intolerance in childhood. Am J Dis Child 132:605, 1978

STEINER G et al: Studies of glucose turnover and renal function in an unusual case of hereditary fructose intolerance. Am J Med 62:150, 1977

Disorders of lipid metabolism

100
THE HYPERLIPOPROTEINEMIAS AND OTHER DISORDERS OF LIPID METABOLISM

MICHAEL S. BROWN
JOSEPH L. GOLDSTEIN

The *hyperlipoproteinemias* are disturbances of lipid transport that result from abnormalities in the synthesis or degradation of plasma lipoproteins. The clinical importance of the elevated plasma lipoprotein level derives from the ability of plasma lipoproteins to cause two life-threatening diseases: atherosclerosis and pancreatitis. Some hyperlipoproteinemias are the direct result of *primary* defects in the metabolism of lipoprotein particles. Other hyperlipoproteinemias are *secondary,* that is, the elevated plasma lipoprotein level occurs as part of a constellation of abnormalities caused by an underlying disorder in a related metabolic system, such as thyroid hormone deficiency or insulin deficiency. The primary hyperlipoproteinemias can be divided into two broad categories: (1) *single-gene disorders* that are transmitted by simple dominant or recessive mechanisms and (2) *multifactorial disorders* with complex inheritance patterns in which multiple variant genes interact with environmental factors to produce varying degrees of hyperlipoproteinemia in members of a family.

PHYSIOLOGIC ROLE OF LIPOPROTEINS IN LIPID TRANSPORT
The lipoproteins are globular particles of high molecular weight that transport nonpolar lipids (primarily *triglycerides* and *cholesteryl esters*) through the plasma. A general model for the structure of a lipoprotein particle is shown in Fig. 100-1. Each lipoprotein particle contains a nonpolar *core,* in which many molecules of hydrophobic lipid are packed to form an oil droplet. This hydrophobic core, which accounts for most of the mass of the particle, consists of triglycerides and cholesteryl esters in varying proportions. Surrounding the core is a polar *surface coat* of phospholipids that stabilize the lipoprotein particle so that it can remain in solution in the plasma. In addition to phospholipids, the polar coat contains small amounts of unesterified cholesterol. Each lipoprotein particle also contains specific proteins (termed *apoproteins*) that are partly exposed at the surface. The apoprotein binds to specific enzymes or transport proteins on cell membranes, thus directing the lipoprotein to its sites of metabolism.

Table 100-1 describes the characteristics of the five major classes of lipoproteins that normally circulate in human plasma. These lipoprotein classes differ in the composition of the nonpolar lipids in the core; in the composition of the apoproteins; and in density, size, and electrophoretic mobility.

Lipid transport: the exogenous pathway Figure 100-2 shows the pathways by which lipoproteins transport lipids in plasma. The largest amounts of lipoproteins are involved in the transport of dietary fat, which amounts to more than 100 g triglyceride and about 1 g cholesterol per day. Within intestinal epithelial cells, dietary triglycerides and cholesterol are incorporated into large lipoprotein particles called *chylomicrons*. The chylomicrons are secreted into the intestinal lymph and pass into the general circulation for transport to the capillaries of adipose tissue and skeletal muscle, where they adhere to binding sites on the capillary walls. While bound to these endothelial surfaces, the chylomicrons are exposed to the enzyme *lipoprotein lipase,* which hydrolyzes the triglycerides of the chylomicrons, releasing free fatty acids and monoglycerides. The fatty acids pass through the endothelial cells and enter the underlying adipocytes or muscle cells, where they are either reesterified to triglycerides or oxidized.

After the core triglycerides have been removed, the remainder of the chylomicron dissociates from the capillary endothe-

A. TYPICAL LIPOPROTEIN PARTICLE

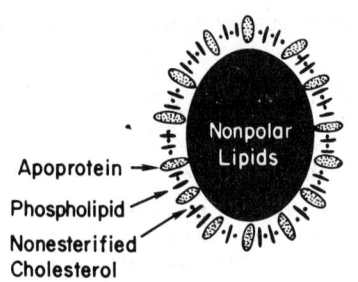

Apoprotein →

Phospholipid →

Nonesterified
Cholesterol →

Nonpolar
Lipids

B. NONPOLAR LIPIDS

Triglyceride

$$CH_2-\overset{\overset{O}{\|}}{C}-(CH_2)_n-CH_3$$

$$CH_2-\overset{\overset{O}{\|}}{C}-(CH_2)_n-CH_3$$

$$CH_2-\overset{\overset{O}{\|}}{C}-(CH_2)_n-CH_3$$

Cholesteryl
Ester

$$CH_3-(CH_2)_n-\overset{\overset{O}{\|}}{C}-O-$$

FIGURE 100-1

A. Diagrammatic representation of the structure of a typical plasma lipoprotein particle. The core *of the spherical lipoprotein particle is composed of two nonpolar lipids, triglyceride and cholesteryl ester, which are present in different lipoproteins in varying amounts. The nonpolar core is surrounded by a* surface coat *composed primarily of phospholipids. Apoproteins are exposed at the surface and extend into the core. Variable amounts of unesterified cholesterol are interdigitated with the phospholip-* *ids of the surface coat. The qualitative composition of each of the five major classes of lipoprotein particles in human plasma is summarized in Table 100-1. B. Structures of the two nonpolar lipids, triglyceride and cholesteryl ester. In order for these nonpolar lipids to be assimilated into tissues, the ester bonds between the fatty acids and either glycerol (triglycerides) or cholesterol (cholesteryl esters) must be broken by lipoprotein lipase and the lysosomal cholesterol esterase, respectively.*

lium and reenters the circulation. It has now been transformed into a particle that is relatively poor in triglyceride and enriched in cholesteryl esters. It has also undergone an exchange of apoproteins with other plasma lipoproteins. The net result is the conversion of the chylomicron to a *remnant particle,* enriched in cholesteryl esters and apoproteins B, CIII, and E. This remnant travels to the liver, where it is taken up with great efficiency. The overall result of the chylomicron transport process is to deliver dietary triglyceride to adipose tissue and cholesterol to the liver.

Some of the cholesterol that reaches the liver is converted to bile acids, which are excreted into the intestine to act as detergents and facilitate the absorption of dietary fat. In addition, some cholesterol is excreted into the bile without metabolism to bile acids. The liver also distributes cholesterol to other tissues (discussed below).

Lipid transport: the endogenous pathway Triglyceride synthesis in the liver is enhanced when the diet contains excess carbohydrates. The liver converts the carbohydrate to fatty acids, esterifies the fatty acids with glycerol to form triglycerides, and secretes the triglyceride into the bloodstream in the core of *very low density lipoproteins (VLDL).* The VLDL particles are relatively large, carry five to ten times more triglycerides than cholesteryl esters, and contain apoproteins that are similar to those of chylomicrons (Table 100-1).

The VLDL particles are transported to tissue capillaries, where they interact with the same lipoprotein lipase enzyme that catabolizes chylomicrons. The core triglycerides of the

VLDL are hydrolyzed, and the fatty acids are used for triglyceride synthesis within adipose tissue. The remnants generated from the action of lipoprotein lipase on VLDL are similar to those formed from chylomicrons. However, in contrast to chylomicron remnants, most of the VLDL remnants are not catabolized by the liver in humans. Rather, the VLDL remnants undergo a further transformation in which nearly all the residual triglycerides are removed and replaced with cholesteryl esters. During this conversion, all the apoproteins are removed from the particle with the exception of apoprotein B. The result is the transformation of the VLDL remnant particle into the cholesterol-rich *low-density lipoprotein* (LDL). The core of LDL is composed almost entirely of cholesteryl esters, and the surface coat contains only one apoprotein, apoprotein B. About three-fourths of the total cholesterol in normal human plasma is contained within LDL particles.

The function of LDL is to supply cholesterol to a variety of extrahepatic parenchymal cells, such as adrenal cortical cells, lymphocytes, muscle cells, and renal cells.

These cells have *LDL receptors* localized on the cell surface. LDL that binds to this receptor is taken up and digested by lysosomes within the cells. The cholesteryl esters of LDL are hydrolyzed by a lysosomal cholesteryl esterase (acid lipase), and the liberated cholesterol is used both for membrane synthesis and as a precursor for steroid hormone synthesis. This LDL receptor pathway serves as the major route for the degradation of LDL.

In addition to its degradation by the LDL pathway in extrahepatic parenchymal cells, some of the LDL is degraded by

TABLE 100-1
Characteristics of the major classes of lipoproteins in human plasma

Lipoprotein class	Major core lipids	Major apoproteins	Density, g/ml	Diameter, Å	Electrophoretic mobility
Chylomicrons	Dietary triglycerides	AI, AII, B, CI, CII, CIII	<1.006	800–5000	Remains at origin
VLDL	Endogenous triglycerides	B, CI, CII, CIII, E	<1.006	300–800	Pre-β
Remnants	Cholesteryl esters, triglycerides	B, CIII, E	<1.019	250–350	Slow pre-β
LDL	Cholesteryl esters	B	1.019–1.063	180–280	β
HDL	Cholesteryl esters	AI, AII	1.063–1.210	50–120	α

a scavenger cell system that consists of phagocytic cells in the reticuloendothelial system. In contrast to the receptor-mediated pathway for LDL degradation, the scavenger cell pathway is thought to function solely to degrade LDL when the lipoprotein reaches high concentrations in plasma rather than to supply cholesterol to cells.

As the membranes of parenchymal and scavenger cells undergo turnover and as cells die and are renewed, unesterified cholesterol is released into plasma, where it binds initially to *high-density lipoprotein (HDL)*. This unesterified cholesterol is then coupled to a fatty acid in an esterification reaction catalyzed by the plasma enzyme *lecithin:cholesterol acyltransferase (LCAT)*. The cholesteryl esters that are formed on the surface of HDL are transferred to VLDL and eventually appear in LDL. This establishes a cycle by which LDL delivers cholesterol to extrahepatic cells and by which cholesterol is returned to LDL from extrahepatic cells via HDL. Some of the cholesterol released from extrahepatic tissues is transported to the liver for excretion in the bile. The mechanism by which the liver takes up this cholesterol is unknown, but it is possible that hepatic LDL receptors are involved.

DIAGNOSIS OF HYPERLIPOPROTEINEMIA A variety of diseases cause elevations in the concentrations of one or more lipoprotein classes in plasma. In general, these abnormalities are detected by the finding of an elevated concentration of triglycerides or cholesterol in fasting plasma, a condition called *hyperlipidemia*. The value for plasma cholesterol represents the total cholesterol, which includes both cholesteryl esters and unesterified cholesterol. The absolute and relative values for the plasma cholesterol and triglyceride levels provide information regarding the nature of the lipoprotein particle that is increased. An isolated elevation in plasma triglycerides indicates that the concentrations of chylomicrons, VLDL, and/or remnants are increased. On the other hand, an isolated elevation of plasma cholesterol nearly always indicates that the concentration of LDL is increased. Frequently, both triglycerides and cholesterol are elevated. Such a combined abnormality may be produced by a marked elevation in chylomicrons or VLDL, in which case the ratio of triglyceride to cholesterol in plasma will be greater than 5:1. Alternatively, there may be an elevation of both VLDL and LDL, in which case the triglyceride/cholesterol ratio in plasma is less than 5:1.

The definition of hyperlipoproteinemia is arbitrary because plasma lipid and lipoprotein levels exhibit a bell-shaped distribution in the population, without clear separation between normal and abnormal values. Since lipoprotein concentrations

are influenced by diet and other environmental factors, standards must be established for the population under consideration. What is usually done is to set arbitrary statistical limits of normal concentrations based on the examination of a large number of healthy-appearing subjects of different ages. The cut-off limit that is usually used is the upper 5 to 10 percent of values found in apparently healthy individuals (i.e., the 90th to 95th percentile values). However, a vast amount of epidemiologic data from both industrialized and more agrarian cultures indicate that lipid and lipoprotein concentrations that are "normal" in a statistical sense are not necessarily healthy. As a working rule, clinically significant hyperlipoproteinemia is considered to be present in any individual below the age of 20 whose total plasma cholesterol level exceeds 200 mg per 100 ml or whose triglyceride level exceeds 140 mg per 100 ml. In individuals above the age of 20, significant hyperlipoproteinemia exists whenever the plasma cholesterol level exceeds 240 mg per 100 ml or the triglyceride level exceeds 200 mg per 100 ml.

The various combinations of elevated lipoproteins that occur in disease states have been divided into six lipoprotein types or patterns. These are summarized in Table 100-2. As shown in Table 100-3, most of the lipoprotein types can be caused by several different genetic diseases; conversely, some genetic diseases can produce more than one lipoprotein pattern. In addition, each of the abnormal lipoprotein types can occur as a secondary consequence of another metabolic disease (Table 100-4). Hence, the lipoprotein type is a shorthand notation to describe an abnormal lipoprotein pattern in plasma and not a designation of a specific disease state.

Ordinarily, the simple measurement of plasma lipid levels, coupled with a clinical assessment, is sufficient to classify the type of lipoprotein abnormality present (Table 100-2). Occasionally, paper electrophoresis of the plasma is useful either when an elevation in remnant particles is suspected (type 3 lipoprotein pattern giving a "broad beta" band on electrophoresis) or when chylomicronemia is a possibility (type 1 pattern). Recently, there has been interest in the measurement of HDL levels, since high levels of this lipoprotein class are statistically associated with a decreased risk of myocardial infarction (see Chap. 250). The level of HDL can be estimated in clinical laboratories using standardized lipoprotein separation techniques, but the value of such measurement for predicting

FIGURE 100-2

Model for plasma triglyceride and cholesterol transport in humans. The details of this model are discussed in the text. VLDL denotes very low density lipoprotein, LDL denotes low-density lipoprotein, HDL denotes high-density lipoprotein, and LCAT denotes lecithin:cholesterol acyltransferase.

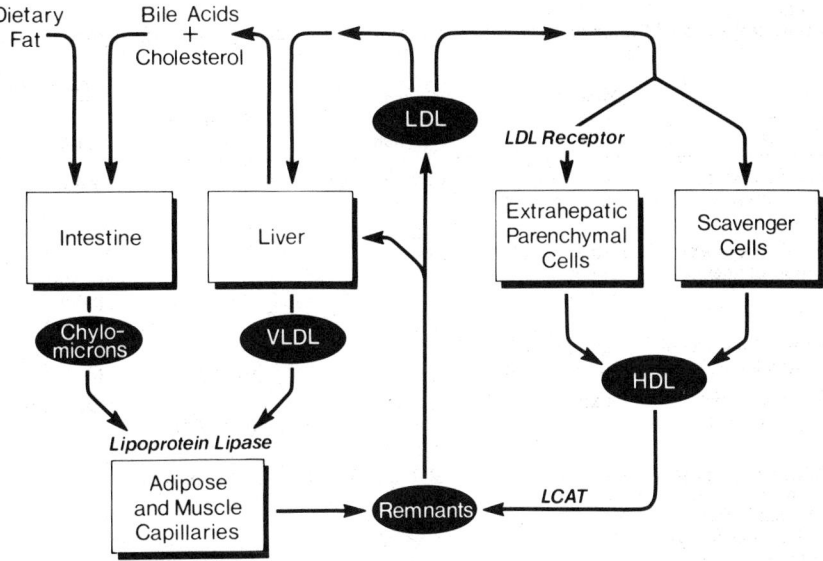

TABLE 100-2
Patterns of lipoprotein elevation in plasma (lipoprotein types)

Lipoprotein pattern	Major elevation in plasma	
	Lipoprotein	Lipid
Type 1	Chylomicrons	Triglycerides
Type 2a	LDL	Cholesterol
Type 2b	LDL and VLDL	Cholesterol and triglycerides
Type 3	Remnants	Triglycerides and cholesterol
Type 4	VLDL	Triglycerides
Type 5	VLDL and chylomicrons	Triglycerides and cholesterol

the occurrence of myocardial infarction in the individual patient has not been established.

PRIMARY HYPERLIPOPROTEINEMIAS RESULTING FROM SINGLE GENE MUTATIONS

FAMILIAL LIPOPROTEIN LIPASE DEFICIENCY This is a rare autosomal recessive disorder due to the absence or marked reduction in the activity of the enzyme lipoprotein lipase. This deficiency leads to a metabolic block in the metabolism of chylomicrons, causing these lipoproteins to accumulate to massive levels in plasma.

Clinical features The disease usually presents in infancy or childhood with recurrent attacks of abdominal pain. The pain is due to pancreatitis occurring as a consequence of the massive elevation of chylomicrons in plasma. Affected individuals intermittently develop eruptive xanthomas, small yellowish papules, frequently surrounded by an erythematous base, that appear predominantly on the buttocks and other pressure-sensitive surfaces. The xanthomas are caused by the deposition of large amounts of chylomicron triglycerides in cutaneous histiocytes. Triglycerides are also deposited at widespread sites in phagocytes of the reticuloendothelial system, producing hepatomegaly, splenomegaly, and foam-cell infiltration of the bone marrow. When the level of chylomicrons in the blood is massively elevated (i.e., plasma triglyceride level greater than 2000 mg per 100 ml), the blood appears pale and creamy and is said to be *lipemic*. When viewed with the ophthalmoscope, the retina appears pale, and the retinal vessels are white, producing the classic appearance of lipemia retinalis. Despite the massive

elevation of triglycerides in the bloodstream, accelerated atherosclerosis does not occur in this disorder.

Pathogenesis Affected individuals are homozygous for a mutation that prevents normal expression of lipoprotein lipase activity. The parents are obligate heterozygotes for this defect, but they are clinically normal. As a result of the deficiency of lipoprotein lipase, chylomicrons cannot be metabolized normally and the level of chylomicrons in the blood rises to high levels after a fat meal. In normal individuals chylomicrons disappear from the blood after a 12-h fast. However, in affected patients high levels of chylomicrons are found in the plasma even after several days of fasting or ingestion of a fat-free diet.

The circulating chylomicrons inflame the pancreas when they pass through its capillaries. Within the capillary lumen in the pancreas, chylomicrons are exposed to small amounts of pancreatic lipase that leaks from the tissue. Partial hydrolysis of the triglycerides and phospholipids of the chylomicron produces toxic products, including fatty acids and lysolecithin, that break down tissue membranes and cause further leakage of lipase from the pancreatic acinar cells. This produces a vicious cycle that eventually causes fulminant pancreatitis.

Diagnosis The diagnosis of familial lipoprotein lipase deficiency is suggested by the finding of lipemic plasma in a young individual who has been fasting for at least 12 h. This lipemic plasma, when collected in the presence of EDTA, has a characteristic appearance after it has incubated overnight in a refrigerator at 4°C. A white layer of cream (which consists of chylomicrons) appears at the top of the tube. The layer beneath the cream is clear. The diagnosis of familial lipoprotein lipase deficiency is supported by the finding of a type 1 pattern on lipoprotein electrophoresis. It is confirmed by the demonstration that lipoprotein lipase levels in plasma fail to increase following the infusion of heparin. In normal individuals, intravenous heparin releases lipoprotein lipase from its binding sites within the capillary endothelium, and increased amounts of enzyme can then be assayed in the plasma.

Treatment All the symptoms and signs of the disease recede when the patient is placed on a fat-free diet. Every attempt should be made to maintain the fasting plasma triglyceride level below 1000 mg per 100 ml to prevent pancreatitis. It has been found empirically that the chronic fat intake in affected adults must be less than 20 g per day to prevent symptomatic

TABLE 100-3
Characteristics of the primary hyperlipoproteinemias resulting from single gene mutations

Genetic disorder	Primary biochemical defect	Plasma lipoprotein elevation	Lipoprotein pattern	Typical clinical findings			Lipoprotein pattern in affected relatives
				Xanthomas	Pancreatitis	Premature atherosclerosis	
Familial lipoprotein lipase deficiency	Deficiency of lipoprotein lipase	Chylomicrons	1	Eruptive	+		1
Familial dysbetalipoproteinemia	Deficiency of apoprotein EIII of VLDL	Remnants	3	Xanthelasma; tuberous; palmar creases		+	3 or 4
Familial hypercholesterolemia	Deficiency of LDL receptor	LDL	2a (rarely 2b)	Xanthelasma; tendon		+	2a (rarely 2b)
Familial hypertriglyceridemia	Unknown	VLDL (rarely chylomicrons)	4 (rarely 5)	(Eruptive)	(+)	+	4 (rarely 5)
Multiple lipoprotein-type hyperlipidemia (familial combined hyperlipidemia)	Unknown	LDL and VLDL	2a, 2b, or 4 (rarely 5)			+	2a, 2b, or 4 (rarely 5)

TABLE 100-4
Clinical disorders associated with secondary hyperlipoproteinemia

Underlying disorder	Plasma lipoprotein elevation				Lipoprotein type	Proposed mechanism for hyperlipoproteinemia	Associated abnormality of carbohydrate metabolism
	Chylomicrons	Remnants	VLDL	LDL			
ENDOCRINE AND METABOLIC							
Diabetes mellitus	+		+ + +		4 (rarely 5)	Increased secretion of VLDL. Decreased catabolism of VLDL and chylomicrons due to reduced lipoprotein lipase activity	Insulin deficiency or resistance
von Gierke's disease (glycogenosis, type I)	+		+ + +		4 (rarely 5)	Increased secretion of VLDL. Decreased catabolism of VLDL and chylomicrons due to reduced lipoprotein lipase activity	Hypoglycemia with decreased insulin secretion
Lipodystrophies (congenital and acquired forms)			+ +		4	Increased secretion of VLDL	Insulin resistance
Cushing's syndrome			+	+ +	2a or 2b	Increased secretion of VLDL with conversion to LDL	Insulin resistance
Sexual ateliotic dwarfism (isolated growth hormone deficiency)			+ +	+ +	2b	Increased secretion of VLDL with conversion to LDL	Insulin deficiency or resistance
Acromegaly			+		4	Increased secretion of VLDL	Insulin resistance
Hypothyroidism		+		+ + +	2a (rarely 3)	Decreased catabolism of LDL and remnants	
Anorexia nervosa				+ +	2a	Reduced biliary excretion of cholesterol and bile acids	
Werner's syndrome				+ +	2a	Unknown	Insulin resistance
Acute intermittent porphyria				+ +	2a	Unknown	
DRUG-INDUCED							
Alcohol	+		+ + +		4 (rarely 5)	Increased secretion of VLDL in individuals genetically predisposed to hypertriglyceridemia	
Oral contraceptives	+		+ + +		4 (rarely 5)	Increased secretion of VLDL in individuals genetically predisposed to hypertriglyceridemia	Insulin resistance
Glucogenic corticosteroids			+	+ +	2a or 2b	Increased secretion of VLDL with conversion to LDL	Insulin resistance
RENAL							
Uremia			+ + +		4	Decreased catabolism of VLDL due to reduced lipoprotein lipase activity	Insulin resistance
Nephrotic syndrome			+ +	+ + +	2a or 2b	Increased secretion of VLDL. Direct secretion of LDL from liver. Decreased catabolism of VLDL and LDL	
HEPATIC							
Primary biliary cirrhosis and extrahepatic biliary obstruction					↑ Cholesterol ↑ Phospholipids ↑ Lipoprotein X	Diversion of biliary cholesterol and phospholipids into bloodstream	
Acute hepatitis (nonfulminant)			+ + +		4	Decreased hepatic secretion of lecithin: cholesterol acyltransferase (LCAT)	

TABLE 100-4 (continued)
Clinical disorders associated with secondary hyperlipoproteinemia

Underlying disorder	Plasma lipoprotein elevation				Lipoprotein type	Proposed mechanism for hyperlipoproteinemia	Associated abnormality of carbohydrate metabolism
	Chylo-microns	Remnants	VLDL	LDL			
HEPATIC (continued)							
Hepatoma				+ +	2a	Lack of feedback inhibition of hepatic cholesterol synthesis by dietary cholesterol	
IMMUNOLOGIC							
Systemic lupus erythematosis	+ +				1	Presence of IgG or IgM that binds heparin, thereby decreasing activity of lipoprotein lipase	
Monoclonal gammopathies (myeloma, macroglobulinemia, lymphoma)		+ +	+ +		3 or 4	Presence of IgG or IgM that forms immune complex with remnants and/or VLDL, thereby decreasing their catabolism	
STRESS-INDUCED							
Emotional stress, acute myocardial infarction, extensive burns, acute gram-negative sepsis			+ +		4	Increased secretion and decreased catabolism of VLDL	

hyperlipemia. Since medium chain triglycerides are not normally incorporated into chylomicrons, they have been employed to help achieve normal caloric intake. The diet should be supplemented with fat-soluble vitamins.

FAMILIAL DYSBETALIPOPROTEINEMIA This is an inherited disorder in which the plasma concentrations of cholesterol and triglycerides are both elevated owing to the accumulation in plasma of remnant-like particles derived from the partial catabolism of VLDL. Also called familial type 3 hyperlipidemia, the disorder is transmitted by a single-gene mechanism, but its expression appears to require the presence of contributory environmental and/or genetic factors (discussed below).

Clinical features Affected individuals characteristically do not manifest hyperlipidemia or any of the other clinical features of the disease until after age 20. A unique clinical feature of the disorder is the occurrence of two types of cutaneous xanthomas. These are xanthoma striata palmaris, which appear as orange or yellow discolorations of the palmar and digital creases, and tuberous or tuberoeruptive xanthomas, which are bulbous cutaneous xanthomas that may vary from pea to lemon size. These tuberous xanthomas are characteristically located over the elbows and knees. Xanthelasmas of the eyelids also occur, but these are not unique to this disorder (see "Familial Hypercholesterolemia," below).

Severe and fulminant atherosclerosis involving the coronary arteries, the internal carotids, and the abdominal aorta and its branches is also a prominent feature. The clinical sequelae include the occurrence of premature myocardial infarctions, strokes, intermittent claudication, and gangrene of the lower extremities. Patients who develop clinical manifestations of dysbetalipoproteinemia often have hypothyroidism, obesity, or diabetes mellitus.

Pathogenesis The hyperlipidemia is caused by the accumulation of relatively large lipoprotein particles that contain both triglycerides and cholesteryl esters. These particles resemble the remnants that are normally produced from the catabolism of VLDL through the action of lipoprotein lipase. In normal

subjects such remnant particles are rapidly taken up by the liver, and hence they are barely detectable in plasma. In patients with familial dysbetalipoproteinemia the uptake of VLDL remnants by the liver is blocked, and these lipoproteins accumulate to high levels in plasma and deposit in tissues, producing xanthomas and atherosclerosis.

The mutation responsible for this disease appears to involve the gene that encodes the structure of apoprotein E, a protein normally found in VLDL and its remnants. This protein is thought to play a role in the uptake of VLDL remnants by the liver. Apoprotein E is actually a family of proteins that can be resolved by isoelectric focusing into three components, designated EI, EII, and EIII. Patients with familial dysbetalipoproteinemia are homozygous for a mutant gene that results in a complete deficiency of EIII in their plasma.

Both parents of an EIII deficient subject and 50 percent of first-degree relatives have half-normal levels of EIII, suggesting that they have one normal allele and one mutant allele at the genetic locus that specifies the EIII apoprotein. Inasmuch as the occurrence of familial dysbetalipoproteinemia requires a complete EIII deficiency, the disease would be expected to behave like a simple autosomal recessive trait. However, several factors make the inheritance pattern atypical for an autosomal recessive disease. First, the frequency of the heterozygous state of EIII deficiency among the general population is high, involving 12 percent of asymptomatic individuals. Moreover, about 1 percent of unselected asymptomatic individuals are homozygous for the EIII deficiency, yet most of these latter subjects have normal lipid levels. Only about 1 in 100 individuals with complete EIII deficiency express the familial dysbetalipoproteinemia syndrome. Thus, all patients with symptomatic familial dysbetalipoproteinemia have homozygous EIII deficiency, but most patients with homozygous EIII deficiency never develop clinical signs of familial dysbetalipoproteinemia. Probably no more than 1 in 10,000 people among the general population show the typical clinical features of familial dysbetalipoproteinemia.

The high frequency of the heterozygous state for EIII deficiency gives rise to pedigrees in which symptomatic familial dysbetalipoproteinemia occurs in several generations of the same family. Such a pseudodominant inheritance pattern is caused by the fact that an individual homozygous for EIII deficiency has a 12 percent chance of marrying a heterozygote. In such a mating half the children have homozygous EIII deficiency, and thus a recessive trait occurs in a parent and a child. In the absence of consanguinity, this situation is rare in typical recessive syndromes where the heterozygous state has a lower frequency in the population.

Some of the factors that produce symptomatic dysbetalipoproteinemia in patients with homozygous EIII deficiency are now known. The disease is exacerbated by hypothyroidism, and many patients with EIII deficiency who develop symptomatic dysbetalipoproteinemia have hypothyroidism. Other factors that predispose to the expression of the disease in an EIII deficient individual include obesity and the independent inheritance of diabetes mellitus or multiple lipoprotein-type hyperlipidemia.

Diagnosis The diagnosis is suggested by the finding of palmar or tuberous xanthomas in a patient with elevated plasma levels of both cholesterol and triglyceride. Approximately 80 percent of symptomatic patients exhibit these xanthomas. The diagnosis is also suggested when a moderate elevation in the plasma concentration of both cholesterol and triglyceride occurs in such a way that the absolute concentrations of cholesterol and triglyceride are nearly equal (e.g., the plasma cholesterol and triglyceride level are both about 300 mg per 100 ml). However, this finding does not always hold true and becomes especially unreliable when the disease is in severe exacerbation, in which case the plasma triglyceride tends to rise higher than cholesterol.

The diagnosis is supported by the finding of a so-called "broad beta" band on lipoprotein electrophoresis (type 3 pattern). This appearance results from the presence of the remnant particles that migrate between β and pre-β lipoproteins and cause a distinctive smear of this region of the electrophoretogram. The diagnosis can be established in specialized laboratories by two procedures. First, the plasma can be subjected to ultracentrifugation, and the chemical composition of the VLDL fraction can be measured. In affected patients, the VLDL fraction contains the abnormal remnant particles and has a relatively high ratio of cholesterol to triglyceride. Second, the diagnosis can be confirmed by the finding of a complete deficiency of apoprotein EIII on isoelectric focusing of the proteins extracted from the remnant particles.

Treatment A vigorous search for occult hypothyroidism should be made, including measurement of plasma thyroid stimulating hormone levels. If hypothyroidism exists, L-thyroxine should be instituted. Patients who have hypothyroidism show a dramatic lowering of lipid levels with treatment. In addition, attempts should be made to control obesity and diabetes mellitus through diet and insulin treatment. If these measures are not successful, patients with familial dysbetalipoproteinemia should be treated with clofibrate. Affected patients usually show a dramatic and sustained reduction in plasma lipid levels when treated with this drug.

FAMILIAL HYPERCHOLESTEROLEMIA This common autosomal dominant disorder affects approximately 1 in 500 persons in the general population. Heterozygotes manifest a two- to three-fold elevation in the concentration of total plasma cholesterol which is attributable to an elevation in the level of LDL. Patients with the homozygous form have six- to eight-fold elevations in plasma LDL-cholesterol levels.

Clinical features Heterozygotes with familial hypercholesterolemia can often be diagnosed at birth because their umbilical cord blood contains a two- to three-fold increase in the concentration of LDL cholesterol. The elevated levels of plasma LDL persist throughout life, but symptoms typically do not develop until the third or fourth decade. The most important clinical feature is the occurrence of premature and accelerated coronary atherosclerosis. Myocardial infarctions begin to occur in affected men in the third decade and show a peak incidence in the fourth and fifth decades. By age 60, approximately 85 percent have experienced a myocardial infarction. In women the incidence of myocardial infarction is also elevated, but the mean age of onset is delayed 10 years as compared with males. Heterozygotes for this disorder constitute about 5 percent of all patients who have a myocardial infarction.

Xanthomas of the tendons constitute the second major clinical manifestation of the heterozygous state. These xanthomas are nodular swellings that typically involve the Achilles and other tendons about the knee, elbow, and dorsum of the hand. They are formed by the deposition of LDL-derived cholesteryl esters in tissue macrophages located in interstitial spaces. The macrophages are swollen with lipid droplets and form foam cells. Cholesterol is also deposited in the soft tissue of the eyelid, producing xanthelasma, and within the cornea, producing arcus corneae. Whereas tendon xanthomas are essentially diagnostic of familial hypercholesterolemia, xanthelasma and arcus corneae are not specific. The latter abnormalities also occur in many adults with normal plasma lipid levels. The incidence of tendon xanthomas in familial hypercholesterolemia increases with age, and up to 75 percent of affected heterozygotes display this sign.

Approximately 1 in 1 million persons in the general population inherits two copies of the familial hypercholesterolemia gene and is a homozygote for the disorder. These individuals have marked elevations in the plasma level of LDL from birth. A unique type of planar cutaneous xanthoma is often present at birth and always develops within the first six years of life. These characteristic xanthomas are raised, yellow, plaque-like lesions that occur at points of cutaneous trauma, such as over the knees, elbows, and buttocks. Xanthomas are almost always present in the interdigital webs of the hands, particularly between the thumb and index finger. Tendon xanthomas, arcus corneae, and xanthelasma are also characteristic. Coronary artery atherosclerosis frequently has its clinical onset in homozygotes before age 10, and myocardial infarction has been reported as early as 18 months of age. In addition to coronary atherosclerosis homozygotes frequently develop cholesterol deposition in the aortic valve, producing symptomatic aortic stenosis. Homozygotes usually succumb to the complications of myocardial infarction before age 20.

In contrast to the disorders causing hypertriglyceridemia, obesity and diabetes mellitus do not occur with increased frequency in familial hypercholesterolemia. A slender body habitus is the rule.

Pathogenesis The primary defect resides in the gene for the LDL receptor. Three types of mutant alleles have been described at this locus. The most common, designated receptor-negative or R^{b0}, specifies a gene product that is nonfunctional. The second most frequent mutant, designated receptor-defective or R^{b-}, produces a receptor that has 1 to 10 percent of normal LDL binding activity. The third type, designated $R^{b+,0}$, produces a receptor that binds LDL normally but is unable to transport the receptor-bound lipoprotein into the cell. This very rare allele produces the so-called "internalization defect."

Phenotypic homozygotes possess two mutant alleles at the

LDL receptor locus, and hence their cells show a total or near-total inability to bind or take up LDL. Heterozygotes have one normal allele and one of the three mutant alleles at the LDL receptor locus, and hence their cells are able to bind and take up LDL at approximately half the normal rate.

Because of the reduction in LDL receptor activity, LDL catabolism is blocked and the level of LDL in plasma rises in a manner that is inversely proportional to the reduction in LDL receptors. In addition to the impaired catabolism of LDL, an increased production of LDL has also been noted in homozygotes. Enhanced production of LDL has been attributed to the lack of an LDL receptor on liver cells such that the liver fails to sense the adequacy of the plasma LDL level. In contrast to normal individuals in whom all plasma LDL appears to be derived from VLDL, in FH homozygotes a large fraction of circulating LDL is secreted directly from the liver into the plasma. This overproduction of LDL, together with its reduced catabolism, accounts for the high concentrations seen in affected patients. The elevated LDL levels cause an increase in the uptake of LDL by scavenger cells, which accumulate at various sites in the body, producing xanthomas.

The accelerated coronary atherosclerosis in familial hypercholesterolemia also results from the high LDL levels, which lead to an enhanced infiltration of LDL into the artery wall following episodes of endothelial damage. The large amounts of LDL that penetrate the artery wall are greater than can be cleared from the interstitial space by the scavenger cells, and atherosclerosis ultimately results. Evidence also indicates that the high LDL levels may act to accelerate platelet aggregation at sites of endothelial injury, thereby enhancing the growth of the atherosclerotic plaque (see Chap. 250).

Diagnosis The diagnosis of heterozygous familial hypercholesterolemia is suggested by the finding of an isolated elevation of plasma cholesterol, with a normal concentration of plasma triglycerides. In nearly all cases, such an isolated elevation in plasma cholesterol is due to an elevation in the plasma concentration of LDL alone (type 2a pattern). However, most individuals in the general population with type 2a hyperlipoproteinemia do not have familial hypercholesterolemia. Rather, they have a form of polygenic hypercholesterolemia that puts them on the upper end of the bell-shaped curve for the general population (see "Polygenic Hypercholesterolemia" below). Type 2a hyperlipoproteinemia is also caused by multiple lipoprotein-type hyperlipidemia (discussed below). In addition, a variety of metabolic disorders, including hypothyroidism and nephrotic syndrome, can cause type 2a hyperlipoproteinemia (Table 100-4).

Among individuals who have a type 2a lipoprotein pattern, those with heterozygous familial hypercholesterolemia can be distinguished from those with polygenic hypercholesterolemia and multiple lipoprotein-type hyperlipidemia on several grounds. (1) In familial hypercholesterolemia the plasma cholesterol level tends to be higher. A plasma cholesterol level in the range of 350 to 400 mg per 100 ml is more suggestive of heterozygous familial hypercholesterolemia than of the other disorders. However, many patients with heterozygous familial hypercholesterolemia have cholesterol levels of 285 to 350 mg per 100 ml, a range in which the other disorders cannot be excluded. (2) The occurrence of tendon xanthomas virtually establishes the diagnosis of familial hypercholesterolemia, since such xanthomas usually do not occur in patients with other forms of hyperlipidemia. (3) In cases in which the diagnosis is in doubt, other family members should be surveyed. In familial hypercholesterolemia the expression of the gene is usually constant with half of first-degree relatives showing an elevated plasma cholesterol level. Hypercholesterolemia is partic-ularly informative when it occurs in children, since elevated levels of cholesterol in childhood are characteristic of familial hypercholesterolemia but not of any of the other aforementioned disorders.

Approximately 10 percent of heterozygotes with familial hypercholesterolemia have concomitant elevation in plasma triglyceride levels (type 2b pattern). In these cases, the disease is difficult to differentiate from multiple lipoprotein-type hyperlipidemia. The finding of a tendon xanthoma or a hypercholesterolemic child in the family favors the diagnosis of familial hypercholesterolemia.

The diagnosis of homozygous familial hypercholesterolemia ordinarily affords no problem, providing the physician is familiar with the clinical picture. Most patients are first seen by dermatologists in childhood because of the cutaneous xanthomas. Occasionally, the presentation is delayed until the onset of angina pectoris or until the child suffers a syncopal episode owing to the xanthomatous aortic stenosis. The finding of a cholesterol level greater than 600 mg per 100 ml with normal triglyceride values in a nonjaundiced child is highly suggestive of the diagnosis. Both parents should have moderately elevated cholesterol levels and other features of heterozygous familial hypercholesterolemia.

In specialized laboratories the diagnosis of both heterozygous and homozygous familial hypercholesterolemia can be made by direct measurement of the number of LDL receptors on cultured skin fibroblasts or freshly isolated blood lymphocytes. Homozygous familial hypercholesterolemia has been diagnosed in utero by the finding of absence of LDL receptors on cultured amniotic fluid cells.

Treatment Inasmuch as the atherosclerosis in this disorder is a consequence of the long-standing elevation in plasma LDL levels, every effort should be made to lower the plasma LDL level into the normal range. Patients should be placed on a diet that is low in cholesterol, low in saturated fats, and high in polyunsaturated fats. This generally means the avoidance of milk, butter, cheese, chocolate, shellfish, and fatty meats and the addition of polyunsaturated cooking oils such as corn oil and safflower oil. With such a diet heterozygotes usually show a 10 to 15 percent drop in plasma cholesterol level.

Bile acid–binding resins, such as cholestyramine, should be added to the regimen when dietary therapy fails to lower the cholesterol levels to the normal range. These resins trap the bile acids excreted by the liver into the intestine and carry them into the feces. Since the body responds to bile acid depletion by converting additional cholesterol into bile acids, the initial result is a dramatic loss of cholesterol from the body. However, affected subjects respond to bile acid depletion by enhancing cholesterol synthesis in the liver, and this compensatory response ultimately limits the long-term success of therapy. With the combination of diet and bile acid–binding resins, the extent of reduction in plasma cholesterol level usually is in the range of 25 percent in heterozygotes. The addition of nicotinic acid may help to block the compensatory increase in hepatic cholesterol synthesis, thus allowing a further lowering of the cholesterol. Major side effects of bile acid–binding resins include gastrointestinal bloating, cramps, and constipation. The major side effect of nicotinic acid is hepatotoxicity; it also produces flushing and headaches in most patients. Probucol has also been used for the treatment of familial hypercholesterolemia, but its efficacy has not been established.

Heterozygotes often show a moderate to marked lowering of plasma cholesterol level in response to the creation of an intestinal anastomosis that bypasses the ileum. This operation has the same functional effect as bile acid–binding resins, i.e., it accelerates the loss of bile acids in the stool. In certain patients in whom drug therapy is not tolerated, the creation of an ileal bypass may be indicated.

Homozygotes tend to be more resistant to treatment. In general, combination therapy consisting of diet, a bile acid–binding resin, and nicotinic acid has little effect. Ileal bypass is uniformly ineffective. Several children have responded to surgical creation of a portacaval anastomosis. However, this procedure is still experimental. The use of a continuous-flow blood cell centrifuge to perform plasma exchanges at monthly intervals is one treatment that will lower the cholesterol in all homozygotes. After each plasma exchange, the plasma cholesterol level drops to about 300 mg per 100 ml and then gradually rises over the ensuing 4 weeks to the pretreatment level. If facilities are available, plasma exchange is the treatment of choice for homozygotes.

FAMILIAL HYPERTRIGLYCERIDEMIA This is a common autosomal dominant disorder in which the concentration of VLDL is elevated in the plasma, causing hypertriglyceridemia.

Clinical features Affected individuals do not usually express hypertriglyceridemia until puberty or early adulthood. Thereafter, the fasting plasma triglyceride level tends to be moderately elevated in the range of 200 to 500 mg per 100 ml (type 4 lipoprotein pattern). The typical affected patient exhibits a clinical triad consisting of obesity, hyperglycemia, and hyperinsulinemia. In addition, hypertension and hyperuricemia are frequent.

The incidence of atherosclerosis is increased. In one study affected patients constituted 6 percent of all individuals with myocardial infarction. However, it has not been established that the hypertriglyceridemia per se causes the increased atherosclerosis. As discussed above, many patients with this disease have diabetes, obesity, and hypertension. Each of these disorders by itself may predispose to atherosclerosis. Xanthomas are not a characteristic feature of familial hypertriglyceridemia.

Affected patients ordinarily have mild to moderate hypertriglyceridemia but can develop a severe exacerbation when exposed to a variety of precipitating factors. These include poorly controlled diabetes mellitus, excessive consumption of alcohol, ingestion of birth control pills containing estrogen, and the development of hypothyroidism. In response to any of these stimuli, the plasma triglyceride level can rise to more than 1000 mg per 100 ml. Under these conditions, large triglyceride-laden particles with the characteristics of chylomicrons appear in plasma. During exacerbations such patients develop *mixed hyperlipemia;* that is, they show an elevation in the concentration of both VLDL and chylomicrons (type 5 lipoprotein pattern). Whenever the concentration of chylomicrons rises to high levels, patients are predisposed to the formation of eruptive xanthomas and the development of pancreatitis. With treatment of the exacerbating condition, the chylomicron-like particles disappear from plasma, and the concentration of triglycerides returns to the moderately elevated basal condition.

In certain families some patients exhibit a severe mixed hyperlipemia, even in the absence of known exacerbating factors. This is the so-called "familial type 5 hyperlipidemia." Other individuals in the same family may have only the mild form of the disease with moderate hypertriglyceridemia and no hyperchylomicronemia (type 4 pattern).

Pathogenesis The disease is transmitted as an autosomal dominant trait, implying a mutation in a single gene. However, the nature of the mutant gene and the mechanism by which it produces hypertriglyceridemia have not been identified. It is likely that the disorder is genetically heterogeneous; that is, the hypertriglyceridemia phenotype in different families may result from different mutations.

Some affected patients have an elevated production rate of VLDL, especially when they ingest diets high in carbohydrate.

However, many of these patients have obesity and diabetes mellitus. Other individuals with obesity and diabetes mellitus, who have normal plasma VLDL levels, also overproduce VLDL. Thus, patients with familial hypertriglyceridemia may have an underlying defect in the ability to catabolize the triglycerides of VLDL. When VLDL production rates become elevated due to obesity or diabetes, they are unable to increase the catabolism of VLDL proportionately and hypertriglyceridemia results. However, lipoprotein lipase activity increases normally in plasma after the administration of heparin, and no abnormalities of lipoprotein structure have been identified.

The increased prevalence of diabetes and obesity in this syndrome is believed to be fortuitous, owing to the fact that both conditions tend to increase VLDL production and hence to exacerbate hypertriglyceridemia. Thus, in family studies, one can find relatives who have diabetes without hypertriglyceridemia and relatives who have hypertriglyceridemia without diabetes, indicating that the two are inherited by independent mechanisms. When an individual inherits both the gene(s) for diabetes and the gene for hypertriglyceridemia, the hypertriglyceridemia is more severe, and such a person is more apt to come to medical attention. Similarly, an individual with familial hypertriglyceridemia who has a normal weight usually has mild hypertriglyceridemia and is less likely to come to medical attention. However, if obesity develops, the hypertriglyceridemia worsens, and a diagnosis is more likely to be made.

Diagnosis The finding of a moderate elevation in plasma triglyceride level, together with a normal cholesterol level, raises the possibility of familial hypertriglyceridemia. In most patients, the plasma is clear to somewhat cloudy on inspection. Chylomicrons typically are not found at the top of the plasma after overnight refrigeration. Electrophoresis of the plasma reveals an increase in the pre-β fraction (type 4 lipoprotein pattern). As mentioned above, an occasional patient exhibits severe hypertriglyceridemia with an elevation in both chylomicrons and VLDL. In this case, a cream layer develops on top (chylomicrons) and a cloudy infranatant (VLDL) is present after overnight storage of plasma in the refrigerator (type 5 lipoprotein pattern).

Given an individual who has an elevation in VLDL levels with or without an elevation in chylomicrons, no simple test exists to determine whether this subject has familial hypertriglyceridemia or hypertriglyceridemia due to some other genetic or acquired cause, such as multiple lipoprotein-type hyperlipidemia or sporadic hypertriglyceridemia. In a typical case of familial hypertriglyceridemia, half of the first-degree relatives have hypertriglyceridemia and no relatives with isolated hypercholesterolemia should be found. Measurement of plasma lipid levels in children is not helpful inasmuch as the disease is typically not manifest until the time of puberty.

Treatment Attempts should be made to control all the exacerbating conditions. Caloric restriction is required in the obese subject. The dietary content of saturated fat should also be limited. Alcohol and oral contraceptives should be avoided. Diabetes mellitus, if present, should be treated vigorously. Thyroid function should be checked, and hypothyroidism treated if found. If the above measures fail, patients respond to the administration of clofibrate, a drug whose mechanism of action is unknown.

MULTIPLE LIPOPROTEIN-TYPE HYPERLIPIDEMIA This common disorder, which is also called familial combined hyperlipidemia, is inherited as an autosomal dominant trait. Affected individuals in a single family characteristically show one of three different lipoprotein patterns: hypercholesterolemia (type 2a), hypertriglyceridemia (type 4), or both hypercholesterolemia and hypertriglyceridemia (type 2b).

Clinical features Hyperlipidemia is not ordinarily present in childhood. Elevations in the plasma cholesterol and/or triglyceride level begin to appear at puberty and continue throughout life. The lipid elevations tend to be mild and vary from time to time so that affected individuals may have a mildly elevated cholesterol level at one examination and/or a mildly elevated triglyceride level at another time. Xanthomas are not a feature. However, premature atherosclerosis occurs, and the incidence of myocardial infarction in middle age is elevated in affected women as well as men.

Patients usually have a strong family history of premature coronary artery disease. This disorder is found in about 10 percent of all patients who have a myocardial infarction. The frequency of obesity, hyperuricemia, and glucose intolerance is increased in affected individuals, especially those with hypertriglyceridemia. However, this association is not as striking as in familial hypertriglyceridemia.

Pathogenesis The disease is transmitted within families as an autosomal dominant trait, implying a mutation in a single gene. Family studies show that about half of the first-degree relatives of an affected individual have hyperlipidemia. However, blood lipid levels are variable among affected individuals in the same family as well as in the same individual at different times. About one-third of hyperlipidemic relatives have hypercholesterolemia (type 2a lipoprotein pattern), one-third hypertriglyceridemia (type 4), and one-third both hypercholesterolemia and hypertriglyceridemia (type 2b). In most affected relatives the plasma lipid levels tend to be just above the 95th percentile for the population and to dip into the normal range intermittently.

While the extent (if any) of the genetic heterogeneity and the nature of the underlying biochemical mechanisms are not known, it has been postulated that affected individuals have an elevated secretion rate of VLDL by the liver. Depending on the interplay of factors governing the efficiency of conversion of VLDL to LDL and the efficiency of catabolism of LDL, this overproduction of VLDL may manifest itself alternatively as an elevation in plasma VLDL levels (hypertriglyceridemia), an elevation in LDL levels (hypercholesterolemia), or both. The hyperlipidemia is worsened by diabetes, alcoholism, and hypothyroidism.

Diagnosis No clinical or laboratory methods exist by which to determine whether an individual with hyperlipidemia has the multiple lipoprotein-type disorder. The 2a, 2b, and 4 lipoprotein patterns can each occur in patients with several other diseases (see Tables 100-3 and 100-4). However, this disorder should be suspected in any individual whose hyperlipoproteinemia is mild and whose lipoprotein type changes with time. The diagnosis is supported by the finding of multiple abnormal lipoprotein types in relatives. The diagnosis can be ruled out by the finding of tendon xanthomas in the patient or his relatives or by the finding of hypercholesterolemia in a relative under the age of 10 years.

Treatment Therapy should be directed at the predominant lipid elevated at the time of examination. General measures such as weight reduction, restriction of dietary saturated fat and cholesterol, and avoidance of alcohol and oral contraceptives are useful. Triglyceride elevations may respond to clofi-

brate. When only the cholesterol level is elevated, a bile acid–binding resin should be given. However, in some individuals the lowering of cholesterol levels with such a drug is accompanied by an increase in triglyceride levels.

PRIMARY HYPERLIPOPROTEINEMIAS OF UNKNOWN ETIOLOGY

POLYGENIC HYPERCHOLESTEROLEMIA By definition, 5 percent of individuals in the general population have LDL-cholesterol levels that exceed the 95th percentile and therefore have hypercholesterolemia (type 2a or type 2b lipoprotein patterns). On the average, among every 20 such hypercholesterolemic persons, one person has the heterozygous form of familial hypercholesterolemia, and two have multiple lipoprotein-type hyperlipidemia. The remaining 17 have a form of hypercholesterolemia, designated polygenic hypercholesterolemia, that owes its origin not to a single mutant gene but rather to a complex interaction of multiple genetic and environmental factors.

Most of the factors that place an individual in the upper part of the bell-shaped curve for cholesterol levels are not known. It is likely that subtle genetic differences exist among people with regard to many processes governing cholesterol metabolism. For example, among normal people there may be genetic polymorphisms in the proteins that govern the rates of intestinal cholesterol absorption, bile acid synthesis, cholesterol synthesis, and LDL synthesis or catabolism. Certain unfavorable combinations of these mildly altered proteins, coupled with an environmental challenge, such as a diet high in cholesterol or saturated fat, may raise the plasma cholesterol level.

Clinically, polygenic hypercholesterolemia can be distinguished from familial hypercholesterolemia and multiple lipoprotein-type hyperlipidemia in two ways: (1) family studies (hyperlipidemia is present in no more than 10 percent of first-degree relatives in polygenic hypercholesterolemia in contrast to 50 percent in the other two disorders) and (2) examination for tendon xanthomas (absent in both polygenic hypercholesterolemia and multiple lipoprotein-type hyperlipidemia but present in about 75 percent of adult heterozygotes with familial hypercholesterolemia).

Certain patients with polygenic hypercholesterolemia respond well to dietary restriction of saturated fat and cholesterol. Other patients require drug therapy to achieve a significant lowering of plasma cholesterol levels. Clofibrate is sometimes effective in this latter group. Cholestyramine may also be used.

SPORADIC HYPERTRIGLYCERIDEMIA In addition to the forms of primary hypertriglyceridemia that show familial aggregation, endogenous hypertriglyceridemia with or without hyperchylomicronemia is sometimes seen in individuals whose relatives do not manifest hyperlipidemia. For purposes of classification, this disorder is called sporadic hypertriglyceridemia. Affected patients comprise a heterogeneous group. Some would undoubtedly be classified under one of the genetic disorders described above if a larger number of relatives were available for lipid measurements. Other than an absence of hyperlipidemic relatives, patients with sporadic hypertriglyceridemia cannot be distinguished clinically from patients with the single-gene forms of primary hypertriglyceridemia. Inasmuch as patients with sporadic hypertriglyceridemia may develop hyperchylomicronemia and pancreatitis, they should be treated with diet and drugs as in the familial disease.

FAMILIAL HYPERALPHALIPOPROTEINEMIA This entity is characterized by elevated plasma levels of HDL, also called alpha lipoprotein. The plasma levels of LDL, VLDL, and triglycerides are normal. The elevated HDL causes a slight elevation in the total plasma cholesterol level. Although a selective elevation in plasma HDL cholesterol can be observed in individuals after exposure to chlorinated hydrocarbon pesticides, in alcoholism and after administration of exogenous estrogen, most cases of hyperalphalipoproteinemia have a genetic basis. In some hyperalphalipoproteinemia is inherited as an autosomal dominant trait, while in others a multifactorial or polygenic basis is suspected.

Individual subjects with familial hyperalphalipoproteinemia show no distinctive clinical features.

Statistical studies suggest that the hyperalphalipoproteinemia is associated with a slightly increased longevity and an apparent protection against myocardial infarction. The mechanism for the increase in plasma HDL levels in this disorder has not been determined.

SECONDARY HYPERLIPOPROTEINEMIAS

A variety of clinical disorders produce secondary hyperlipoproteinemias. These are summarized in Table 100-4 (see references). The most frequently encountered forms of secondary hyperlipoproteinemia occur in association with diabetes mellitus, consumption of alcohol, and ingestion of oral contraceptives.

DIABETES MELLITUS Three distinct patterns of hypertriglyceridemia occur in patients with diabetes mellitus. Classical "diabetic hyperlipemia" consists of a massive elevation in the plasma triglyceride level that occurs in patients who have suffered from insulin deficiency or insulin resistance for many weeks or months. Such insulin-deprived patients develop a progressive increase in concentration of plasma VLDL and eventually of chylomicrons as well. Triglyceride levels as high as 25,000 mg per 100 ml are seen. Eruptive xanthomas, lipemia retinalis, and hepatomegaly can occur. Ketosis is frequently present, but severe acidosis is not characteristic. This form of massive hyperlipemia is only seen in partial insulin deficiency. Patients with this form of diabetic hyperlipemia usually respond to a fat-free diet and to the administration of insulin, although triglyceride levels may not return entirely to normal.

The second type of hypertriglyceridemia in diabetics is associated with acute ketoacidosis. Such patients usually exhibit a mild hyperlipidemia with elevations of VLDL but not chylomicrons. On occasion, however, marked elevations of triglyceride are seen with lipemia retinalis. In this case both VLDL and chylomicrons are present.

The third type of hypertriglyceridemia is a mild to moderate elevation in plasma VLDL that persists even when patients appear to be adequately treated for their diabetes. This chronic triglyceride elevation generally occurs in patients who are obese. Inasmuch as most patients with well-controlled diabetes have normal plasma triglyceride levels, the occasional patient with persistent hypertriglyceridemia is likely to have an underlying familial hyperlipoproteinemic disorder. Indeed, family studies indicate that many of these patients have inherited the trait for familial hypertriglyceridemia in a pattern independent of the inheritance of diabetes mellitus.

The insulin deficiency or insulin resistance of diabetes produces a high VLDL level by two mechanisms. With acute insulin deprivation there is an increase in VLDL secretion from the liver as a secondary response to the increased mobilization of free fatty acids from adipose tissue. As the state of insulin deprivation becomes prolonged, the rate of removal of VLDL and chylomicrons from the circulation declines because lipoprotein lipase activity becomes diminished.

ALCOHOL CONSUMPTION In any individual the daily consumption of large amounts of ethanol can produce a mild, asymptomatic elevation in the plasma triglyceride level due to an elevation of VLDL. However, in a subgroup ethanol ingestion regularly produces massive and clinically significant hyperlipemia with elevations in both VLDL and chylomicrons (type 5 lipoprotein pattern). In most of this group, the VLDL level remains mildly elevated (type 4 lipoprotein pattern), even in the basal state after recovery from the severe alcoholic hyperlipemia. This suggests that these individuals have a form of familial hypertriglyceridemia or multiple lipoprotein-type hyperlipidemia that is exacerbated and converted to a type 5 pattern by the ethanol ingestion.

Ethanol elevates the plasma triglyceride level primarily because it inhibits fatty acid oxidation and enhances fatty acid synthesis in the liver. The excess fatty acids are esterified to triglyceride. Some of this excess triglyceride accumulates in the liver, producing the characteristic enlarged fatty liver of alcoholics. The remainder of the newly formed triglyceride is secreted into plasma, resulting in an increased secretion of VLDL. In those who develop massive alcoholic hyperlipemia, there appears to be a partial defect in the catabolism of these VLDL particles. As the concentration of VLDL increases, the lipoprotein begins to compete with chylomicrons for hydrolysis by lipoprotein lipase, and the plasma concentration of chylomicrons also rises.

In severe alcoholic hyperlipemia, eruptive xanthomas and lipemia retinalis are frequently present. The most serious complication is pancreatitis. Pancreatitis may be difficult to diagnose, since elevated triglyceride levels can interfere with the estimation of serum amylase. There is no solid evidence to indicate that pancreatitis itself can cause hyperlipemia; rather the hyperlipemia is the cause of the pancreatitis.

Plasma from patients with alcoholic hyperlipemia is creamy in appearance. If a blood sample is drawn in EDTA and the plasma placed in the refrigerator at 4°C overnight, the chylomicrons float to the top, and the infranatant layer is turbid, owing to the combined elevation of VLDL and chylomicrons (type 5 pattern).

ORAL CONTRACEPTIVES The ingestion of estrogen-containing birth control pills is regularly associated with an increase in the VLDL secretion rate from the liver. In most women the catabolism of VLDL also increases, so that the overall increase in plasma triglyceride level is only modest. However, in women who have an underlying genetic disorder (such as familial hypertriglyceridemia or multiple lipoprotein-type hyperlipidemia) the plasma VLDL-triglyceride level can increase markedly, and hyperchylomicronemia can develop when estrogen-containing medications are taken. These women generally have mild to moderate hypertriglyceridemia prior to the institution of oral contraceptive therapy, and they presumably are unable to increase VLDL catabolism in response to the stimulation of VLDL production. As the plasma VLDL concentration rises, the elevated VLDL prevents the normal catabolism of chylomicrons by lipoprotein lipase, and secondary hyperchylomicronemia ensues. When the latter develops, severe pancreatitis can occur.

Ingestion of oral contraceptives has also been implicated as a risk factor in promoting thromboembolic disease in young women, especially those with preexisting hypercholesterolemia. Thus, it is important to measure the plasma cholesterol and triglyceride levels prior to the institution of birth control therapy. The finding of hyperlipidemia is a contraindication to the use of these drugs.

TABLE 100-5
Rare autosomal recessive disorders of lipid metabolism

Disorder	Typical age of onset	Plasma lipid abnormality	Major clinical manifestations	Pathogenesis	Treatment
Abetalipoproteinemia	Early childhood	Cholesterol, ~ 50 mg/100 ml; triglycerides, < 10 mg/100 ml	Malabsorption of fat, ataxia, neuropathy, retinitis pigmentosa, acanthocytosis	Defective synthesis of apoprotein B leads to absence of chylomicrons, VLDL, and LDL in plasma	Vitamin E
Tangier disease	Childhood	Cholesterol, 40 to 125 mg/100 ml; triglycerides, normal to slightly elevated	Large orange tonsils, corneal opacities, relapsing polyneuropathy No premature atherosclerosis	Absence of HDL from plasma leads to generation of abnormal chylomicron remnants, which are taken up and stored as cholesteryl esters in phagocytic cells	None
Lecithin:cholesterol acyltransferase (LCAT) deficiency	Young adult	Total plasma cholesterol level variable with marked decrease in esterified cholesterol and increase in unesterified cholesterol; elevated VLDL level Structure of all lipoproteins is abnormal	Hemolytic anemia, renal insufficiency, premature atherosclerosis	Decreased LCAT activity in plasma leads to accumulation of excess unesterified cholesterol in plasma and body tissues	Fat-restricted diet, kidney transplantation
Cerebrotendinous xanthomatosis	Young adult	None	Progressive cerebellar ataxia, dementia and spinal cord paresis, subnormal intelligence, tendon xanthomas, cataracts	Primary defect is unknown Cholesterol and cholestanol accumulate in brain, tendons, and other tissues Defective synthesis of primary bile acids in liver	None
β-sitosterolemia	Adult	Elevated levels of plant sterols in plasma; normal levels of cholesterol and triglycerides	Tendon xanthomas	Increased intestinal absorption of dietary β-sitosterol with accumulation in plasma and tendons	Diet low in plant sterols

RARE DISORDERS OF LIPID METABOLISM

Table 100-5 summarizes the clinical and pathophysiological features of five rare disorders of lipid metabolism, each of which is inherited as an autosomal recessive trait. In two—abetalipoproteinemia and Tangier disease—the major effect of the abnormality is to cause a decrease in lipid levels in plasma. In two—cerebrotendinous xanthomatosis and β-sitosterolemia—the major effect of the inborn error is to cause an accumulation of unusual sterols in tissues. In LCAT deficiency, the underlying mutation produces both an abnormal pattern of lipoproteins in plasma and an accumulation of unesterified cholesterol in tissues.

REFERENCES

EDER HA: Drugs used in the prevention and treatment of atherosclerosis, in *The Pharmacological Basis of Therapeutics*, 5th ed, LS Goodman, A Gilman (eds). New York, Macmillan, 1975, chap 35

FREDRICKSON DS et al: The familial hyperlipoproteinemias, in *The Metabolic Basis of Inherited Disease*, 4th ed, JB Stanbury et al (eds). New York, McGraw-Hill, 1978, chap 30

GOLDSTEIN JL, BROWN MS: The low density lipoprotein pathway and its relation to atherosclerosis. Annu Rev Biochem 46:897, 1977

HAVEL RJ et al: Lipoprotein and lipid transport, in *Diseases of Metabolism*, 8th ed, PK Bondy, LE Rosenberg (eds). Philadelphia, Saunders, 1980, chap 7

JACKSON RL et al: Lipoprotein structure and metabolism. Physiol Rev 56:259, 1976

MOTULSKY AG: The genetic hyperlipidemias. N Engl J Med 294:823, 1976

STANBURY JB et al (eds): *The Metabolic Basis of Inherited Disease*, 4th ed. New York, McGraw-Hill, 1978, chaps 28, 29, 31

UTERMANN G et al: Polymorphism of apolipoprotein E. Clin Genet 15:37, 63, 1979

101
LYSOSOMAL STORAGE DISEASES

ARTHUR L. BEAUDET

GENERAL FEATURES

DEFINITION Lysosomes are cytoplasmic organelles which enclose an acidic environment containing numerous enzymes capable of hydrolyzing most biological macromolecules. Primary lysosomes, the original bodies derived from the Golgi apparatus, may fuse with other membrane-bound vesicles to form secondary lysosomes. Secondary lysosomes contain material derived from outside the cell through endocytosis or material from within the cell through autophagy. The lysosome functions as an efficient recovery system for reutilization of components and disposition of used macromolecules. The continuous remodeling of tissues and turnover of macromolecules underline the importance of this degradative capacity. Recent studies of lipoprotein and vitamin B_{12} metabolism suggest that the lysosome is important not only in the processing of used macromolecules but also in the acquisition of essential compounds from the exterior of the cell through the process of endocytosis and degradation of carrier proteins.

The concept of lysosomal storage diseases arose from the studies of type II (Pompe) glycogen storage disease. The demonstration of lysosomal accumulation of glycogen as the result of α-glucosidase deficiency and data from other disorders led Hers to define an inborn lysosomal disease as one in which (1) a single lysosomal enzyme is deficient and (2) abnormal deposits (of substrate) lie within vacuoles related to lysosomes. This definition can be modified to include single gene defects affecting one or more lysosomal enzymes and thus encompass disorders such as the mucolipidoses and multiple sulfatase deficiency.

The lysosomal storage diseases include most of the lipid storage disorders, the mucopolysaccharidoses, the mucolipidoses, glycoprotein storage diseases, and others, as indicated in Table 101-1. The enzyme deficiencies have an autosomal recessive basis with the exception of Hunter mucopolysaccharidosis II (MPS II), which is X-linked recessive, and Fabry disease, which is X-linked with frequent manifestations in females. The target organs are determined by the usual sites of degradation for a macromolecule. For example, cerebral white matter is affected in patients with defects in degradation of myelin, hepatosplenomegaly develops in those with defects in degradation of glycolipids from red cell stroma, and generalized tissue involvement may occur in patients with defects in the degradation of ubiquitous mucopolysaccharides. The accumulated material often causes visceromegaly or macrocephaly, but secondary atrophy also can occur, particularly in brain or muscle. In simple terms, the symptoms appear to be due to damage from stored material, but exactly how this causes cell death or dysfunction often is unclear. All the disorders are progressive, and many are fatal in childhood or adolescence. Definitive diagnosis is accomplished best by specific enzyme assays on serum, leukocytes, or cultured skin fibroblasts, selecting the appropriate tests on clinical grounds. There is extensive phenotypic variation within disorders with infantile, juvenile, and adult forms of many entities. In addition, varying combinations of visceral, skeletal, and neurological involvement can occur within a single enzyme disorder.

DIAGNOSIS A lysosomal storage disease is usually suspected on the basis of progressive neurological dysfunction, visceromegaly, skeletal dysostosis, or some more specific finding, as outlined in Table 101-1. Progressive or degenerative disease is the hallmark of these disorders. The superimposition of degeneration upon normal childhood development results in a slowing of progress prior to loss of previously acquired abilities. The history should focus on the course of childhood development, neurological symptoms, including seizures and visual or auditory impairment, the course of physical growth, and more specific findings such as coarsening facies, corneal clouding, exaggerated startle response, abdominal distention, joint pain, joint stiffness, and recurrent infection. The family history may reveal similarly affected siblings or consanguinity in autosomal recessive disease or other affected male family members in X-linked disorders. Ethnic background may be helpful since several lipid storage diseases are more frequent in Ashkenazi Jews and since disorders such as mannosidosis and aspartylglucosaminuria may occur with increased frequency in Scandinavian populations.

On physical examination the head circumference may be enlarged. Gigantism occurs early in the course of some MPS disorders and glycoprotein storage diseases, while short stature is a later finding in many disorders. Ophthalmologic examination should include slit-lamp and careful funduscopic examination. Enlargement of the tongue, coarsening of the facies, and hepatosplenomegaly may occur. Skeletal findings may include gibbus deformity, broadening of the long bones, and joint stiffness. Cutaneous findings are rare except in fucosidosis, Fabry disease, and Hunter disease. Careful neurologic examination should attempt to distinguish the extent of involvement of gray matter, white matter, and peripheral nerves. Preliminary diagnostic studies should include examination of the peripheral blood smear for vacuolated or granulated leukocytes, urinary spot test for mucopolysaccharide, and radiological bone survey. The preferred method of diagnosis is to use the above information to select specific enzyme assays in serum, leukocytes, or cultured skin fibroblasts. If a mucopolysaccharide screening test is positive or if clinical findings are suggestive, quantitative mucopolysaccharide analysis can be carried out. If a specific diagnosis is not readily established, biopsy of skin, bone marrow, rectal mucosa, liver, peripheral nerve, or other tissue for light and electron microscopy can be helpful. Electron microscopic findings can direct one toward or away from the general category of lysosomal storage diseases based on the presence or absence of engorged lysosomes. When significant evidence favors a lysosomal storage disease but no enzyme deficiency is demonstrable, chemical analysis of biopsy tissue from liver or brain is an appropriate investigative starting point.

HETEROGENEITY There is extensive clinical and biochemical heterogeneity within the lysosomal storage diseases. The biochemical genetic principles underlying this heterogeneity are reviewed in Chaps. 58 and 87. In general, a structural gene for lysosomal enzyme produces a product which acts to degrade one or more macromolecules. Most or all of the lysosomal enzymes undergo posttranslational modification to become glycoproteins, often resulting in a series of electrophoretic variants or isozymes. These isozymes may hydrolyze one or a variety of substrates, and the substrate specificity of particular isozymes may vary. Differences in substrate specificity also arise from the occurrence of similar but genetically distinct enzymes, for example, the β-galactosidases. Mutations within a gene may totally eliminate or reduce enzyme activity, alter the ability of the enzyme to undergo posttranslational modification, or alter the activity of the enzyme for specific substrates.

Different mutations within the same gene probably account for varying degrees of severity from individual to individual as well as the diverse combinations of visceral, skeletal, neurological, ocular, and other manifestations. The heterogeneity is increased further by the recessive nature of most of the conditions in that each affected individual must have two mutant genes of the same allele. Except in the instance of consanguinity, the exact mutation within each gene may vary so that either one or both may encode some form of residual activity for one or more substrates (so-called "genetic compounds"). An excellent example of a genetic compound is MPS I, to be discussed below. Although it is useful to characterize clinical phenotypes as infantile, juvenile, adult, neuropathic, or nonneuropathic, the existence of different mutant alleles and of genetic compounds provides an explanation for those occasional patients who appear aberrant or intermediate as compared with the usual phenotype. Another type of heterogeneity is illustrated by MPS III A and B, which are virtually indistinguishable clinical disorders caused by different gene defects. Thus these genocopies demonstrate that biochemical heterogeneity can underlie apparent clinical homogeneity.

Further complexity results from the fact that certain enzyme activities are derived from complexes of nonidentical subunits. As a consequence, different mutations can cause deficiency of the same enzyme, as for example, hexosaminidase A deficiency in Tay-Sachs and Sandhoff diseases, and can explain multiple enzyme deficiencies due to a single gene defect as in Sandhoff disease. Genetic disorders involving the post-

TABLE 101-1
Summary of lysosomal storage diseases

Disorder	Heterogeneity (onset)	Enzyme deficiency	Stored material	Neurological
G_{MI} gangliosidosis	Infantile (birth)			
	Juvenile (6-20 mo) Adult	β-Galactosidase	G_{MI} ganglioside Glycoproteins Keratan sulfate	Mental retardation, seizures, blindness; later in juvenile form, variable in adults
Tay-Sachs and variants, G_{M2} gangliosidosis	Infantile (3-6 mo) Juvenile Adult forms	Hexosaminidase A	G_{M2} ganglioside	Mental retardation, seizures, blindness; later in juvenile form
Sandhoff, G_{M2} gangliosidosis	Infantile (3-6 mo)	Hexosaminidase A and B	G_{M2} ganglioside Globoside	Mental retardation, seizures, blindness
Krabbe, galactosylceramide lipidosis	Infantile (2-6 mo) Late onset	Galactosylceramide β-Galactosidase	↑ Galactoscerebroside/sulfatide ratio	Mental retardation, leukodystrophy; variable in late onset
Metachromatic leukodystrophy, sulfatide lipidosis	Late infantile (1-4 yr) Juvenile (4-20 yr) Adult	Arylsulfatase A (cerebroside sulfatase)	Galactosyl sulfatides	Mental retardation, leukodystrophy, psychosis and dementia in adults
Niemann-Pick, sphingomyelin lipidosis	Infantile neuropathic (1-4 mo) Late onset neuropathic Visceral	Sphingomyelinase ? Specific isozymes in some	Sphingomyelin	Mental retardation, ataxia, and seizures in neuropathic forms
Gaucher, glucosylceramide lipidosis	Infantile (1-12 mo) Juvenile (2-6 yr) Adult	β-Glucocerebrosidase	Glucosylceramide	Mental retardation; spastic, later flaccid, ataxia in juvenile; no neurologic symptoms in adult form
Fabry, trihexosyl ceramidosis	Hemizygous males Heterozygous females	α-Galactosidase A	Trihexosylceramide	Painful neuropathy
Acid lipase deficiency	Infantile Wolman disease (0-3 mo) Late onset cholesteryl ester storage disease	Acid lipase	Cholesteryl ester Triglyceride	Mental retardation but mild related to growth failure in Wolman; none in CESD
Farber, ceramide deficiency	Infantile (0-4 mo) Rare juvenile	Ceramidase	Ceramide	Occasional mental retardation, but may be secondary to somatic features
Lactosylceramidosis	May not exist; one report probably represented case of Niemann-Pick disease			
Pompe, glycogen storage type II	Infantile (0-6 mo) Juvenile Adult	Acid maltase (α-1,4- and 1,6-glucosidase)	Glycogen	Probably normal mentally
Acid phosphatase deficiency	Infantile (0-3 mo)	Acid phosphatase	Not characterized	Mental retardation

* *AR = autosomal recessive.*

Liver and/or spleen enlargement	Skeletal dysplasia	Ophthalmic	Hematologic	Genetics	Unique manifestations	References
+ + + + Less in juvenile, variable in adult	+ + + + Variable in juvenile and adult forms	Cherry red spot in 50% of infantile; corneal clouding variable but more in adults	Foam cells Vacuolated lymphocytes	AR*	Coarse facies, edema, macroglossia, mucopolysacchariduria; early blindness in infantile, milder in juvenile; in adults often spondyloepiphyseal dysplasia +/– mucopolysacchariduria	Hers and Van Hoof, chap 12 Stanbury et al, chap 40 Ho et al
0	0	Cherry red spot in infantile form, rare in juvenile	0	AR	Macrocephaly, hyperaucusis in infantile; increased in Ashkenazi Jews	Hers and Van Hoof, chap 13 Stanbury et al, chap 40 Ho et al
0	0	Cherry red spot	0	AR	Macrocephaly, hyperaucusis, visceral histiocytosis	Hers and Van Hoof, chap 14 Stanbury et al, chap 40 Ho et al
0	0	Optic atrophy	0	AR	Extreme irritability, ↑ CSF protein, fever, globoid cell neuropathology	Hers and Van Hoof, chap 17 Stanbury et al, chap 37 Ho et al
0	0	Optic atrophy, less in juvenile and adult forms	0	AR	↑ CSF protein and early gait abnormalities in late infantile; peripheral neuropathy	Hers and Van Hoof, chap 18 Stanbury et al, chap 38
+ + + + Less prominent in late onset forms	0	Macular degeneration and cherry red spot in neuropathic forms	Distinctive foam cell Vacuolated lymphocytes	AR	Pulmonary infiltrates, brownish skin, infantile neuronopathic form increased in Ashkenazi Jews, sea blue histiocytes	Hers and Van Hoof, chap 19 Stanbury et al, chap 35
+ + + + Hypersplenism common	+ +	Usually normal	Distinctive foam cell	AR	Adult form includes ↑ acid phosphatase, pathologic fractures; Ashkenazi Jewish predilection	Hers and Van Hoof, chap 16 Stanbury et al, chap 36 Ho et al
0	0	Corneal dystrophy, vascular lesions, cataracts	0	X-linked dominant	Cutaneous angiokeratoma, vascular thromboses, hypohidrosis	Hers and Van Hoof, chap 15 Stanbury et al, chap 39 Ho et al
+ + +	0	0	Foam cells Vacuolated lymphocytes	AR	Adrenal calcification, anemia, vomiting and poor growth in Wolman; hepatic fibrosis and ↑ blood cholesterol in CESO	Hers and Van Hoof, chap 20 Stanbury et al, chap 32
+/–	?	Mild macular degeneration	0	AR	Arthropathy—subcutaneous, periarticular and visceral nodules (lipogranulomatosis); ↑ CSF protein	Hers and Van Hoof, chap 24 Stanbury et al, chap 34 Ho et al
Mild hepatomegaly	0	0	0	AR	Lethal skeletal and cardiac myopathy in infantile; primarily skeletal myopathy in adults	See chap 97 Hers and Van Hoof, chap 7 Stanbury et al, chap 7
+ +	0	0	0	AR?	Lethal disorders described in two families	Hers and Van Hoof, chap 21 Hirschhorn and Weissmann

TABLE 101-1 (continued)
Summary of lysosomal storage diseases

Disorder	Heterogeneity (onset)	Enzyme deficiency	Stored material	Neurological
Fucosidosis	Infantile (3-12 mo) Juvenile	α-Fucosidase	Glycopeptides Glycolipids Oligosaccharides	Mental retardation
Mannosidosis	Infantile (6-18 mo) Milder form	α-Mannosidase	Oligosaccharides	Mental retardation
Aspartylglucosaminuria	Young adult onset	Aspartylglucosamine amidase	Aspartylglucosamine	Mental retardation
Mucopolysaccharidosis 1H and 1S	Infantile Hurler (6-12 mo) Intermediate Adult Scheie	α-Iduronidase	Dermatan sulfate Heparan sulfate	Mental retardation, absent in Scheie
Hunter, mucopolysaccharidosis II	Severe infantile (6-12 mo) Mild juvenile	Iduronosulfate sulfatase	Dermatan sulfate Heparan sulfate	Mental retardation, less in mild form
Sanfilippo A, mucopolysaccharidosis III A	Late infantile (1-4 yr)	Heparan N-sulfatase (sulfamidase)	Heparan sulfate	Severe mental retardation
Sanfilippo B, mucopolysaccharidosis III B	Late infantile (1-4 yr)	N-Acetyl-α-glucosaminidase	Heparan sulfate	Severe mental retardation
Morquio, mucopolysaccharidosis IV	Some variation	N-Acetylgalactosamine 6-sulfate sulfatase	Keratan sulfate	0
Maroteaux-Lamy, mucopolysaccharidosis VI	Variation in severity and cardiovascular involvement	N-Acetylhexosamine-4-sulfate sulfatase (arylsulfatase B)	Dermatan sulfate	0
β-Glucuronidase deficiency, mucopolysaccharidosis VII	Few patients; infantile to adult forms	β-Glucuronidase	Dermatan sulfate ? Heparan sulfate	Mental retardation ? absent in some adults
Mucopolysaccharidosis VIII	One patient	N-Acetylglucosamine 6-sulfate sulfatase	Heparan sulfate Keratan sulfate	Mental retardation
Multiple sulfatase deficiency	Late infantile (1-4 yr)	Arylsulfatases A, B and C Other sulfatases	Sulfatides Mucopolysaccharides	Mental retardation
Sialidase deficiency	Infantile mucolipidosis I Late myoclonus and cherry red spot	Sialidase (neuraminidase)	Glycoproteins Glycolipids Sialyloligosaccharides	Mental retardation, myoclonus
Mucolipidosis II, I cell disease	Infantile (0-3 mo)	Elevated serum enzymes Primary defect unknown	Glycoproteins Glycolipids	Mental retardation
Mucolipidosis III, pseudo-Hurler polydystrophy	Late infantile (>2 yr)	Elevated serum enzymes Primary defect unknown	Glycoproteins Glycolipids	Mild mental retardation
Mucolipidosis VI	Infantile	Unknown	? Multiple	Mental retardation
Neuronal ceroid lipofuscinoses	Late infantile Juvenile Adult	Unknown	"Ceroid" "Lipofuscin"	Mental retardation, dementia variable in adults, seizures

Liver and/or spleen enlargement	Skeletal dysplasia	Ophthalmic	Hematologic	Genetics	Unique manifestations	References
+ +	+ +	0	Vacuolated lymphocytes Foam cells	AR	Coarse facies, increased sweat electrolytes, nonfunctional gall bladder; angiokeratoma in juvenile	Hers and Van Hoof, chap 11 Ho et al
+ + +	+ +	Cataracts, corneal clouding	Vacuolated lymphocytes Granulated neutrophils	AR	Coarse facies, enlarged tongue	Hers and Van Hoof, chap 11 Hirschhorn and Weissmann
0	+ +	Lens opacities	Vacuolated lymphocytes	AR	Coarse facies, detectable by urine amino acid analysis; Finnish predilection	Hers and Van Hoof, chap 24
+ + +	+ + + +	Corneal clouding	Granulated lymphocytes	AR	Coarse facies, cardiovascular involvement, joint stiffness	Hers and Van Hoof, chaps 8 and 9 Stanbury et al, chap 53 McKusick
+ + +	+ + + +	Retinal degeneration, no significant corneal clouding	Granulated lymphocytes	X-linked	Coarse facies, cardiovascular involvement, joint stiffness	
+	+	0	Granulated lymphocytes	AR	Mild coarsening of facies	
+	+	0	Granulated lymphocytes	AR	Nearly indistinguishable from MPS IIIA	
+	Severe, distinctive	Corneal clouding	Granulated neutrophils	AR	Severe deformity, odontoid hypoplasia, aortic regurgitation	
+ +	+ + + +	Corneal clouding	Granulated neutrophils and lymphocytes	AR	Mild coarsening of facies, joint stiffness, valvular heart disease	
+ + +	+ + +	Corneal clouding	Granulated neutrophils	AR	Coarse facies, ↑ vascular involvement	
+ +	+ +	Normal at age 6	?	? AR	Coarse facies	
+	MPS features	Retinal degeneration	Vacuolated and granulated cells	AR	Icthyosis, combined MPS and metachromatic leukodystrophy phenotype	Hers and Van Hoof, chaps 8 and 18 Stanbury et al, chap 38
+ + Less in late form	+ + Less or absent in late form	Cherry red spot	Vacuolated lymphocytes	AR	ML I patients have MPS phenotype; unclear if all ML I patients have sialidase deficiency	Hers and Van Hoof, chap 8 O'Brien
0/ +	+ + + +	Corneal clouding	Vacuolated and granulated neutrophils	AR	Coarse facies, inclusions in cultured fibroblasts, normal mucopolysacchariduria	Hers and Van Hoof, chap 8 Stanbury et al, chap 38
0	+ + +	Corneal clouding	Vacuolated plasma cells	AR	Coarse facies, inclusions in cultured fibroblasts, joint contractures, valvular heart disease, normal mucopolysacchariduria	
0	0	Corneal clouding, retinal degeneration	0	AR	Diagnosis based on electron microscopy; ? Ashkenazi Jewish predilection	Stanbury et al, chap 38
0	0	Optic atrophy, macular degeneration, retinitis pigmentosa	Vacuolated lymphocytes Granulated neutrophils	AR AR	Electron microscopy helpful, degree of genetic heterogeneity unknown	Hers and Van Hoof, chap 23

translational modification of lysosomal enzymes and general defects in the integrity and function of the lysosome may also cause lysosomal storage diseases. The mucolipidoses II and III appear to represent situations in which a single gene defect alters the ability of a number of lysosomal enzymes to enter or be retained within the lysosome. Thus, mutations outside the structural genes for the enzymes themselves can account for further heterogeneity. Better biochemical understanding of the identity, subunit structure, posttranslational processing, and substrate specificities of lysosomal enzymes should provide further insight into phenotypic and genotypic heterogeneity.

Clinical diagnosis is facilitated but also somewhat complicated by the widespread use of synthetic substrates for measuring lysosomal enzyme activities. These substrates often measure a group of related activities attributable to different enzymes. Thus, the activity of β-galactosidase using an artificial substrate may represent the sum of various β-galactosidases encoded by different structural genes and having different substrate specificities. Clinical reliability generally is achieved by manipulating in vitro conditions to reflect that enzyme activity whose deficiency is characteristic of a clinical disorder. Genetic heterogeneity has, however, resulted in individuals with mutant enzyme that either hydrolyzes the natural substrate and not the artificial substrate, or vice versa. This is exemplified by the normal individuals who have hexosaminidase A deficiency using artificial substrate and by patients with Tay-Sachs disease who have substantial levels of hexosaminidase A activity with artificial substrates. The presence or absence of disease correlates with ability to hydrolyze the natural G_{M2} ganglioside substrate. These phenomena have considerable significance for identification of affected patients, for heterozygote screening and for prenatal diagnosis. They indicate the need to go beyond artificial substrate enzyme assays if normal results occur in the face of overwhelming clinical, electron microscopic, or chemical evidence of a storage disease.

MANAGEMENT AND PREVENTION Specific therapy is not effective in lysosomal storage diseases at present, and care is largely symptomatic. The relentless, progressive course in many instances represents a tragic burden. Transplantation is effective in reversing the renal failure that commonly occurs in Fabry disease, and splenectomy frequently is helpful in adult Gaucher disease. Considerable attention has been focused on enzyme replacement for lysosomal storage diseases using organ or fibroblast transplantation or the infusion of either plasma, leukocytes, purified enzyme itself, or enzyme trapped in erythrocytes or liposomes. Although these approaches offer promise for treatment of manifestations outside the central nervous system, they are not of proved efficacy.

The most distressing aspects of lysosomal storage diseases involve the central nervous system, where the blood-brain barrier and the lack of pinocytotic activity by neurons present additional obstacles to the development of effective enzyme replacement therapy.

Genetic counseling is an important aspect of the management of these disorders. All the lysosomal storage diseases in which the specific enzyme deficiency is known either have been or presumably could be diagnosed in utero, since lysosomal enzyme activities appear to be expressed in cultured amniotic fluid cells as well as in cultured skin fibroblasts. Artificial insemination is an alternative for couples who have children affected with an autosomal recessive disease. Heterozygote detection in close relatives is frequently possible with careful laboratory analysis. This is particularly important in the X-linked Fabry and Hunter disorders, since numerous female members of the family may be at risk for bearing affected children. More effective approaches to prevention require

identification of heterozygous couples prior to the birth of an affected offspring. The feasibility of this approach has been demonstrated by heterozygote testing programs for Tay-Sachs disease. Such programs could allow the elimination of these disorders through extensive testing and appropriate reproductive decisions on the part of the rare couples identified as being at risk for having affected offspring; the high frequency of the heterozygous state in Ashkenazi Jews and favorable biochemical aspects of carrier detection for Tay-Sachs disease have facilitated this program. Efficient and extremely accurate heterozygote detection methods are needed to apply this approach to other diseases and to populations with lower heterozygote frequencies. Even under optimal conditions genetic variants might cause false positive or false negative results in any screening process.

SPECIFIC DISORDERS

SPHINGOLIPIDOSES G_{M1} **gangliosidosis** G_{M1} gangliosidosis was recognized in 1965 in infants with features of Tay-Sachs disease and mucopolysaccharidosis and is due to deficiency of β-galactosidase. Prominent features of the infantile form are the presence of abnormalities at or near birth, developmental delay, seizures, coarse facies, edema, hepatosplenomegaly, macroglossia, ocular cherry red spot, and a distinctive mucopolysaccharidosis-like dysostosis multiplex. Death usually occurs in the first or second year of life. The juvenile form is characterized by a later onset, survival to the latter half of the first decade, neurological impairment and seizures, and milder skeletal and ocular findings. In the adult form of spondyloepiphyseal dysplasia similar to MPS IV, corneal clouding and normal intelligence are common. Joint pain and limitation of motion, particularly at the hips, can be disabling in these patients. Prominent spasticity and ataxia with mild bony abnormalities have occurred in other adult patients. A high index of suspicion is necessary to recognize the diverse phenotypes caused by β-galactosidase deficiency in juvenile and adult patients, since almost any combination of skeletal, ocular, neurologic, and visceral findings can occur. Isozymes of β-galactosidase occur, but evidence suggests that these derive from a single gene on chromosome 22. Thus, the diversity of phenotypes is due to different mutations in the structural gene. All forms of G_{M1} gangliosidosis have an autosomal recessive inheritance. There is no ethnic predilection. The frequency of the disease is low, with less than 50 patients reported for any given phenotype.

G_{M2} **gangliosidosis** Tay-Sachs disease, first recognized in 1881, is a relatively common inborn error of metabolism with thousands of documented cases. Although clinically indistinguishable from Sandhoff disease, the two are genetically distinct with deficiency of hexosaminidase A in the former and hexosaminidase A and B in the latter. The presenting features in both are a developmental delay beginning in the third to sixth month with subsequent rapidly progressive neurologic deterioration. Macrocephaly, seizures, retinal cherry-red spot, and an augmented startle response to sound suggest the diagnosis. The diagnosis is confirmed by enzyme assay. Most juvenile onset patients with hexosaminidase deficiency present with dementia, seizures and ocular findings, and some have an atypical spinocerebellar degeneration.

Sandhoff disease is nonallelic with Tay-Sachs disease, but the juvenile forms of hexosaminidase deficiency likely are allelic with Tay-Sachs disease. Tay-Sachs disease is the most frequent form of hexosaminidase deficiency, the risk being about 100-fold in Ashkenazi Jews compared with other ethnic groups. All forms of G_{M2} gangliosidosis are autosomal recessive. There is evidence that hexosaminidase B is composed of β subunits whose structural locus is on chromosome 5, while hexosaminidase A is composed of α and β subunits with the structural locus for the α subunit on chromosome 15.

Although no specific therapy is available, extensive programs for heterozyote detection in the prevention of Tay-Sachs disease have been carried out throughout the world. As of 1976, more than 150,000 people were tested with the identification of more than 6000 heterozygotes and more than 120 couples at risk for Tay-Sachs disease in their offspring. There had been 371 pregnancies monitored by prenatal diagnosis because of a previous affected child and 90 pregnancies monitored based on results of carrier screening.

LEUKODYSTROPHIES Krabbe galactosylceramide lipidosis or globoid cell leukodystrophy is an infantile disease due to deficiency of galactosylceramide β-galactosidase and characterized by onset at 2 to 6 months of age, with irritability, hyperesthesia, hypersensitivity to external stimuli, unexplained fever, optic atrophy, and sometimes seizures. Spinal fluid protein is usually increased. Initially there is hypertonicity and increased deep tendon reflexes with progression to a hypotonic state. Rapid neurologic deterioration, and death occur within 1 to 2 years of onset. Premortem diagnosis is accomplished by enzyme assay. The presence of globoid cells on neuropathologic examination is characteristic and possibly specific for this enzyme deficiency. Galactosylceramide β-galactosidase functions in the degradation of sulfatides derived from myelin. Myelin synthesis is so impaired by tissue damage that the absolute amount of the galactocerebroside substrate is usually not increased in postmortem tissue. Galactosylceramide β-galactosidase is genetically distinct from the β-galactosidase that is deficient in G_{M1} gangliosidosis.

Krabbe disease is relatively rare, with about 150 reported cases and numerous unreported cases. It has an autosomal recessive genetic basis and is present in all ethnic groups with a possible increased frequency in the Scandinavian countries. Although no specific therapy is available, prenatal diagnosis has been accomplished.

Deficiency of arylsulfatase A (cerebroside sulfatase) is the basis of metachromatic leukodystrophy, a lipid storage disease with a frequency of 1 in 40,000. The age of onset is later than that in Tay-Sachs disease or Krabbe disease. Patients develop the ability to walk and frequently present with gait abnormalities in the second to fourth year of life. Initially the patients may be hypotonic with decreased deep tendon reflexes, the latter reflecting peripheral nerve involvement. The disease progresses over the first decade to include ataxia, increased muscle tone, decorticate or decerebrate posturing, and eventual loss of all contact with surroundings. Duration of survival depends on nursing care and support such as nasogastric or gastrostomy feeding.

Diagnosis is accomplished using enzyme assay, originally in urine and more recently in leukocytes or fibroblasts. Changes demonstrable on metachromatic staining of nerve tissue are nonspecific and not an adequate substitute for enzyme assay. Rare patients with a juvenile form of metachromatic leukodystrophy are described with an onset between 4 and 20 years of age and a slower progression. The adult form of this disease deserves special mention as an example of the difficulties presented by subtle, slowly progressive forms of lysosomal storage diseases. The onset is in the second to fifth decade with a slowly progressive dementia. Emotional difficulties, motor dysfunction, and indistinct speech are often present. Even though conduction velocity in peripheral nerves is usually diminished, the deep tendon reflexes are often increased. Typical premortem diagnoses include organic dementia, schizophrenia, and multiple sclerosis; a correct premortem diagnosis has been made in only a minority.

Arylsulfatase A is routinely measured using artificial substrate, and complexities involving low levels of activity in nor-

mal individuals and moderate levels of residual activity in symptomatic patients have been described. Heterogeneity involving mutations in multiple components of the cerebroside sulfatase activity may exist, but the majority of patients probably have simple allelic disorders on an autosomal recessive basis. Arylsulfatase A deficiency also occurs in multiple sulfatase deficiency discussed below.

NIEMANN-PICK DISEASE Niemann-Pick disease is a lipidosis caused by deficiency of sphingomyelinase which hydrolyzes sphingomyelin ceramide and phosphorylcholine. The most common form is an infantile neuropathic disorder which begins shortly after birth with hepatosplenomegaly, failure to thrive, and neurologic impairment. Retinal cherry red spots occur, but seizures and functional hypersplenism are rare. The diagnosis can be made with considerable confidence by recognition of the distinctive Niemann-Pick cell in the bone marrow, but enzyme assay should be performed. Patients with later onset and slower progression have been described as well as a number of patients with visceral disease and no neurologic involvement. Many patients described with the sea blue histiocyte syndrome may have had sphingomyelinase deficiency; other patients with the sea blue histiocyte syndrome may represent unique disorders not yet biochemically characterized.

GAUCHER DISEASE Gaucher disease is a glucosylceramide lipidosis caused by deficiency of glucosylceramidase. An infantile form is characterized by early onset, marked hepatosplenomegaly, and severe neurological progression to early death. A juvenile form with milder neurologic involvement exists. The adult form of the disease may be the most commonly encountered lysosomal storage disease. Patients with juvenile and adult Gaucher disease have been observed within the same family but not within the same sibships, supporting the hypothesis that these are allelic disorders.

All forms of Gaucher disease have an autosomal recessive genetic basis. The disorder is about 30 times more frequent in Ashkenazi Jews, with an incidence in this ethnic group of about 1 in 2500 births. Although commonly termed "adult Gaucher disease," this variant frequently has its onset in childhood. Absence of neurologic involvement is the criterion for inclusion in this category. Manifestations include hepatosplenomegaly, hypersplenism, bleeding diathesis, bone pain, pathological fractures, and pulmonary involvement with associated pneumonia. Serum acid phosphatase is characteristically elevated. A distinctive storage cell occurs in the bone marrow in all forms of Gaucher disease, but enzyme assay should be performed because the Gaucher cell may also be found in patients with granulocytic leukemia and myeloma.

The clinical course is variable; pulmonary involvement may lead to early death, but in many patients life span is not shortened by the disease. Bleeding secondary to thrombocytopenia frequently responds to splenectomy with considerable benefit. Because of the frequency of the disease and the lack of neurologic involvement, the adult form of Gaucher disease is potentially amenable to enzyme replacement therapy.

FABRY DISEASE Fabry disease involves the accumulation of a trihexoside, galactosylgalactosylglucosylceramide due to deficiency of α-galactosidase A. The disorder is X-linked, and the most severe symptoms are seen in hemizygous males. Onset is in childhood with periodic crises of severe pain in the extremities, cutaneous angiokeratomas, a characteristic corneal dystrophy, hypohidrosis, vascular thromboses, and progressive renal impairment. Death most often results from renal failure, typically in the third to fifth decade. Heterozygous females are affected more mildly. Corneal dystrophy is the most frequent finding, but all other manifestations may also be seen. Life expectancy is greater in women, although fatal complications can rarely occur. Renal failure can be treated by chronic dialysis or transplantation. Enzyme replacement therapy has been attempted in this disease. In addition, patients undergoing transplantation presumably derive normal enzyme from the transplanted kidney. Administration of phenytoin sodium (Dilantin) has been used in treatment of the painful neuropathy.

There is evidence that the α galactosidase A structural gene resides on the X chromosome, although alternative explanations involving regulatory components have been suggested. Clinically the disorder should be considered as an X-linked dominant, since heterozygous females usually manifest the condition.

ACID LIPASE DEFICIENCY Acid lipase deficiency is the basis for two disorders with different phenotypic features. Wolman disease is a severe disorder of early onset, with prominent hepatosplenomegaly, anemia, vomiting, failure to thrive, and characteristic adrenal calcification. Neurologic involvement is minimal compared with the severe somatic handicap. Cholesteryl ester storage disease is a rare disorder with mild phenotypic features by comparison. The most constant features are hepatosplenomegaly and increased plasma cholesterol. Hepatic fibrosis, esophageal varices, and poor growth have occurred. One reported sibship may represent an intermediate phenotype, since two females died at 7 and 9 years of age with unexplained acute hepatic failure, and a third sibling developed adrenal calcification and pulmonary hypertension early in life. Tissues from patients with acid lipase deficiency demonstrate inability to hydrolyze triglycerides as well as cholesteryl esters. Possibly a single enzyme hydrolyzes multiple substrates, but the subunit structure and hydrolytic capacities of various lysosomal lipases are not well studied. Deficiency of acid lipase results in impairment of the LDL pathway as described in Chap. 100 and may be associated with premature atherosclerosis. Both Wolman and cholesteryl ester storage diseases have an autosomal recessive basis.

GLYCOPROTEIN STORAGE DISORDERS Fucosidosis, mannosidosis, and aspartylglucosaminuria are rare, autosomal recessive disorders involving hydrolases that degrade polysaccharide linkages. Glycolipids as well as glycoproteins are accumulated in fucosidosis. All are characterized by mental retardation and varying somatic involvements, as outlined in Table 101-1. Fucosidosis and mannosidosis are most often lethal disorders in childhood, while aspartylglucosaminuria presents as a late-onset lysosomal storage disease with prominent mental retardation and a prolonged course. Abnormal sweat electrolytes and cutaneous angiokeratomas are distinctive in fucosidosis, and an unusual cartwheel-type cataract occurs in mannosidosis. Aspartylglucosaminuria is remarkable in that urinary amino acid analysis is diagnostic with an increase of aspartylglucosamine; it is more frequent in the Finnish population. Each of the disorders can be diagnosed by appropriate enzyme assay.

MUCOPOLYSACCHARIDOSIS (MPS) The mucopolysaccharidoses represent a broad spectrum of disorders due to deficiencies of one of a group of enzymes which degrade three classes of mucopolysaccharides: heparan sulfate, dermatan sulfate, and keratan sulfate. The general MPS phenotype includes coarse facies, corneal clouding, hepatosplenomegaly, joint stiffness, hernias, dysostosis multiplex, mucopolysaccharide excretion in the urine, and metachromatic staining in peripheral

leukocytes and bone marrow. Various components of the MPS phenotype are also found in the mucolipidoses, glycoprotein storage disorders, and other lysosomal storage diseases. Detailed clinical and radiologic evaluation and identification of the type of MPS excreted in the urine help to narrow the diagnostic possibilities. Definitive diagnosis requires assay of specific enzymes in various tissues such as cultured skin fibroblasts.

The Hurler or MPS IH disorder is the prototype MPS. Virtually all the components of the phenotype mentioned above are present and expressed in a severe degree. Nasal congestion and grossly visible corneal clouding are early features. Excessive growth during the first year of life is followed by poor growth late in the course. Radiologic features include enlargement of the sella turcica with a distinctive "shoe-shaped" fossa, broadening and shortening of the long bones, and hypoplasia and beaking of the vertebrae in the lumbar area. The vertebral beaking gives rise to an accentuated kyphosis or gibbus deformity. Death occurs within the first decade; postmortem findings include hydrocephalus and cardiovascular disease due to occlusion of the coronary arteries. The biochemical hallmark is α-iduronidase deficiency with accumulation of heparan sulfate and dermatan sulfate.

MPS IS, or Scheie syndrome, is a clinically distinct disorder of adult onset characterized by joint stiffness, corneal clouding, aortic regurgitation, and usually normal intelligence. Surprisingly, this much milder disorder is also the result of α-iduronidase deficiency; it is allelic with the Hurler syndrome, as shown by lack of cross-correction of enzyme activity in cocultures of skin fibroblasts. Phenotypes occur that are clearly intermediate between Hurler and Scheie syndromes. It is believed that patients with an intermediate phenotype represent genetic compounds with one Hurler allele and one Scheie allele. Although genetic compounds must occur, their existence is difficult to distinguish in any one case from still other mutations of intermediate severity.

The Hunter or MPS II syndrome is distinguishable from the Hurler phenotype by the absence of gross corneal clouding and the X-linked recessive inheritance. The infantile form resembles the Hurler phenotype, and a milder form allows survival into adulthood. The severe and mild forms may be allelic, since both are sex-linked and share the same enzyme deficiency (iduronosulfate sulfatase).

The Sanfilippo mucopolysaccharidoses (MPS IIIA and IIIB) are distinguished by the accumulation of heparan sulfate without dermatan or keratan sulfate and by the marked central nervous system involvement with milder somatic involvement. Because the somatic features of this MPS are mild, the condition can be overlooked in the evaluation of an apparently isolated central nervous system problem. Death usually occurs during the second decade. MPS IIIA and MPS IIIB represent hallmark examples of genocopies. That is, two different enzyme deficiencies give rise to a virtually indistinguishable clinical phenotype with the same storage product. The two MPS III disorders can be diagnosed and distinguished by enzyme assay (Table 101-1).

The Morquio or MPS IV syndrome is distinguished by the absence of mental retardation and the presence of a distinctive bony dystrophy which can be classified as a spondyloepiphyseal dysplasia. Marked hypoplasia of the odontoid process can cause cervical dislocation and usually leads to some degree of spinal cord compression. Aortic regurgitation is frequent. The deficiency of N-acetylgalactosamine 6-sulfate sulfatase is the basis for this condition. This enzyme is distinct from an N-acetylglucosamine 6-sulfate sulfatase whose deficiency results in MPS VIII. Bone changes somewhat suggestive of the Morquio syndrome may also occur in MPS VIII, in β-galactosidase deficiency, and in other forms of spondyloepiphyseal dysplasia. The Maroteaux-Lamy or MPS VI disorder is characterized by prominent osseous involvement, corneal clouding, and normal intellect. Allelic forms with variable severity but the same deficiency of arylsulfatase B (*N*-acetylhexosamine 4-sulfate sulfatase) have been described. MPS VII, or β-glucuronidase deficiency has been described in less than 10 patients with a rather complete MPS phenotype. Extreme variability from a lethal infantile form to a mild adult disease has occurred. Two patients with MPS VIII were found to have *N*-acetylglucosamine 6-sulfate sulfatase deficiency with mucopolysacchariduria involving heparan sulfate and keratan sulfate. As might be expected, the patients had a phenotype combining features of MPS III and MPS IV.

MULTIPLE SULFATASE DEFICIENCY   Multiple sulfatase deficiency is a unique disorder, which, although autosomal recessive, is characterized by deficiency of five or more cellular sulfatases. Arylsulfatase A, arylsulfatase B, other mucopolysaccharide sulfatases, and a nonlysosomal placental sulfatase are deficient in this condition. The clinical picture combines features of metachromatic leukodystrophy, an MPS phenotype, and ichthyosis. The last feature presumably relates to the placental sulfatase deficiency which also occurs as an isolated X-linked enzyme deficiency characterized by abnormal parturition and ichthyosis. Biochemical studies of this condition should provide further insight into biochemical and clinical genetic heterogeneity.

MUCOLIPIDOSES   Mucolipidosis is a general term for lysosomal storage diseases involving some combination of MPS, glycoprotein, oligosaccharide, and glycolipids. Although G$_{M1}$ gangliosidosis, fucosidosis, mannosidosis, and other disorders might qualify as mucolipidoses, these can be considered more specifically since the biochemical basis is understood. Findings in mucolipidosis I include mental retardation, hepatosplenomegaly, an MPS phenotype, and ocular cherry red spot on an autosomal recessive basis. Some or most patients with mucolipidosis I have a deficiency of sialidase (neuraminidase). Another disorder described in the literature, the cherry red spot–myoclonus syndrome, also appears to be due to sialidase deficiency, suggesting that these may be allelic disorders.

Mucolipidosis II, or I-cell disease, is an early onset disorder with mental retardation and an MPS phenotype. The distinctive features are striking inclusions in cultured skin fibroblasts and markedly elevated serum levels of lysosomal enzymes. The disorder has an autosomal recessive basis and is thought to involve a defect in the processes for entry into, or maintenance of, lysosomal enzymes within that organelle. Mucolipidosis III or psuedo-Hurler polydystrophy is a milder disorder with many aspects of the MPS phenotype, particularly dysostosis multiplex. The disorder presents in the first decade with joint stiffness, the diagnosis of rheumatoid arthritis often being considered. The major handicaps are progressive physical disabilities, particularly claw hand deformity and hip dysplasia. Mild mental retardation is common. Aortic and/or mitral valvular disease is routinely present, although often not functionally significant. Survival into adult life with possible stabilization of the condition is characteristic, with greater disability in males than in females. Inclusions in cultured skin fibroblasts and elevation of serum lysosomal enzymes are essentially identical with the findings in mucolipidosis II, suggesting that these may be allelic disorders. Mucolipidosis IV is a disorder with mental retardation, corneal clouding, and retinal degeneration without other somatic features. Diagnosis has been based primarily on electron microscopic findings. A small number of patients, all of Ashkenazi Jewish origin, have been described.

NEURONAL CEROID LIPOFUSCINOSES   The neuronal ceroid lipofuscinosis group of disorders includes a wide clinical spectrum with onset in childhood, juvenile, or adult periods. It is unknown whether single or multiple biochemical genetic disorders are present in the patients reported. The clinical features include central nervous system deterioration with cerebral atrophy, usually commensurate with degree of impairment. Seizures, particularly myoclonic jerks, are a prominent feature. Ocular involvement with optic atrophy, retinitis pigmentosa, and macular degeneration is present in the infantile and juvenile disorders but often absent in adult forms. Autosomal recessive inheritance is likely in most instances. The neuropathologic findings form the basis of the descriptive term for the disease. Electron microscopy demonstrates abnormal inclusions within lysosomes throughout a wide variety of tissues, despite the rather isolated neurological clinical involvement. The presence of curvilinear bodies, electron-dense material, and fingerprint profiles on electron microscopy of white blood cells, liver biopsy, or muscle biopsy can be helpful diagnostically.

OTHER LYSOSOMAL STORAGE DISEASES   Glycogen storage disease type II (Pompe disease) is the prototype lysosomal storage disease. The predominant clinical features of skeletal and cardiac myopathy are described in Chap. 97. Acid phosphatase deficiency and Farber lipogranulomatosis are included in Table 101-1. Lactosyl ceramidosis appears to represent a variant of Niemann-Pick disease; in vitro hydrolysis of lactosyl ceramide is accomplished by those enzymes that are deficient in G$_{M1}$ gangliosidosis or in Krabbe disease, depending upon the in vitro conditions used. Adrenoleukodystrophy is identifiable as a distinct X-linked disorder with accumulation of long-chain fatty acid cholesteryl esters in tissues, but it is unclear whether this is a lysosomal storage disease. A Sanfilippo C or MPS III C disorder may occur with α-glucosaminidase as its basis. The recognition of females with the Hunter MPS II phenotype and identical enzyme deficiency has raised the possibility of an autosomal recessive form of the Hunter syndrome. Such could occur if the enzyme in question had nonidentical subunits coded for by one autosomal and one X-linked gene, or if regulatory genetic elements were invoked. On the other hand females with phenotypic manifestations could occur, owing to X-chromosome inactivation. One family has been described with G$_{M3}$ gangliosidosis. This is not a lysosomal storage disease but does possibly represent a defect in ganglioside synthesis. The clinical features are similar to those seen in lysosomal storage diseases, but inconsistencies between siblings leave question of whether this is a unique genetic disorder. Other neurodegenerative diseases may eventually become classifiable as lysosomal storage diseases. Disorders such as juvenile dystonic lipidosis, neuroaxonal dystrophy, Hallervorden-Spatz disease, Pelizaeus-Merzbacher disease, and other candidates exist. In addition, it is not unusual to identify patients with distinctive clinical features suggestive of lipidosis, mucolipidosis, or mucopolysaccharidosis, in which none of the present biochemically identifiable disorders can be identified. For these reasons, the number of distinct lysosomal storage diseases is likely to continue to increase.

REFERENCES

HERS HG, VAN HOOF F (eds): *Lysosomes and Storage Diseases.* New York, Academic, 1973

HIRSCHHORN R, WEISSMANN G: Genetic disorders of lysosomes, in *Progress in Medical Genetics,* AG Steinberg et al, (eds). Philadelphia, Saunders, 1976, vol 1

Ho MW et al: Glycosphingolipid hydrolases: Properties and molecular genetics. Mol Cell Biochem 17:125, 1977

McKusick VA: *Heritable Disorders of Connective Tissue,* 4th ed. St Louis, Mosby, 1972

O'Brien JS: Neuraminidase deficiency in the cherry red spot–myoclonus syndrome. Biochem Biophys Res Comm 79:1136, 1977

Stanbury JB et al (eds): *The Metabolic Basis of Inherited Disease,* 4th ed. New York, McGraw-Hill, 1978

102
RARE DISORDERS OF ADIPOSE TISSUE

DANIEL W. FOSTER

This chapter is concerned with syndromes characterized by abnormalities in adipose tissue. The disorders are rare, the pathophysiology is frequently not clear, and only clinical descriptions can be given.

THE LIPODYSTROPHIES

The lipodystrophies are characterized by generalized or partial loss of body fat and a series of metabolic disorders, including insulin resistance, hyperglycemia, and hypertriglyceridemia.

GENERALIZED LIPODYSTROPHY Generalized lipodystrophy (also called lipoatrophic diabetes) may be either congenital or acquired. The congenital form is transmitted as an autosomal recessive trait. Rates of parental consanguinity are high. Loss of fat is obvious at birth, but the rest of the clinical picture may not develop until later. The acquired disease often develops after some other illness. Infections such as measles, chicken pox, whooping cough, or infectious mononucleosis are common precipitating events, but hypothyroidism, hyperthyroidism, and pregnancy have also been implicated. Some cases begin with the appearance of painful nodular swellings of adipose tissue resembling acute panniculitis (see below). While certain differences exist, the congenital and acquired forms are basically similar in clinical manifestations (Table 102-1).

Fat atrophy Loss of body fat is the characteristic finding. In congenital cases the skin of the face is tightly drawn over the bony structures, and the entire body is devoid of adipose tissue. Rarely, a small amount of breast fat remains. In the acquired form the face may be spared, but all other fat disappears. Microscopically adipose tissue cells can be identified, but they contain no triglyceride stores. Paradoxically the liver is stuffed with fat, and the reticuloendothelial system contains lipid-laden macrophages (foam cells). The cause of the fat atrophy is not known. While many studies have attempted to

identify defects in triglyceride transport, triglyceride synthesis, or lipolysis, no uniform abnormality has been found. Small molecular weight fat-mobilizing polypeptides have been reported in the urine of patients with generalized lipodystrophy, but their role in the disease is uncertain. Release of free fatty acids into plasma following norepinephrine infusion is impaired, but this may simply reflect the depleted triglyceride stores. Adipose tissue from a dystrophic site in a patient with partial lipodystrophy accumulates fat when transplanted into a normal region of the body, while fat from an uninvolved region loses its triglyceride on transplantation to a dystrophic area, suggesting a localized (neuropathic?) cause for fat atrophy.

Growth and maturation Linear growth is accelerated in the first few years of life in the congenital disorder and in acquired disease that begins early in childhood. Epiphyses close early, however, so that the final height in most patients is normal. True muscular hypertrophy is present, and patients may have an acromegalic appearance with coarse facial features and large hands and feet. The ears tend to be prominent in the congenital form. Many viscera are enlarged, and generalized lymphadenopathy may be present.

Liver The liver is uniformly enlarged, and as a consequence the abdomen is protuberant. Fatty liver may progress to cirrhosis, especially in the acquired form. Several patients have died from bleeding esophageal varices. Splenomegaly probably does not occur in the absence of portal hypertension.

Kidneys The kidneys are usually enlarged. Subjects with the acquired disorder may have proteinuria and the nephrotic syndrome, although not as frequently as in partial lipodystrophy. Moderate hypertension is common.

Genitalia The external genitalia (penis and testes in males, clitoris in females) are usually hypertrophied in congenital disease. In girls polycystic ovaries are common, resulting in the clinical picture of Stein-Leventhal syndrome.

Skin Acanthosis nigricans is present in most. Hypertrichosis of face, neck, trunk, and limbs is frequent. Scalp hair is usually thick and curly, particularly early in life.

Central nervous system Mental retardation is present in about half the congenital cases. Dilatation of the third ventricle and basal cisterns has been demonstrated by pneumoencephalography. Central nervous system involvement appears to be less marked in the acquired disease, although two patients had astrocytomas arising in the floor of the third ventricle.

Endocrine and metabolic abnormalities Three major disturbances characterize the lipodystrophic patient: (1) Severe insu-

TABLE 102-1
Characteristics of the lipodystrophies

Finding	Congenital general	Acquired general	Acquired partial	Dominant partial
Inheritance	Autosomal recessive	Sporadic	Usually sporadic	Autosomal dominant
Age of onset	Infancy	Childhood to adult	Childhood to adult	Puberty
Sex incidence	Males and females equal	Female preponderance	Female preponderance	Female preponderance
Lipoatrophy	Face, trunk, limbs	Face, trunk, limbs	Face, upper trunk, upper limbs	Trunk and limbs
Liver involvement	+	+ +	Rare	0
Renal disease	+	+	+ +	0
Insulin resistance	+	+	+	+
Hyperglycemia	+	+	+	+
Hypertriglyceridemia	+	+	+	+
Acanthosis nigricans	+	+	Rare	+
Genital hypertrophy	+	+	Rare	+
Bone age	Accelerated	Normal to accelerated	Normal	Normal

lin resistance with hyperglycemia. Diminished affinity of insulin receptors for the hormone has been demonstrated utilizing monocytes from affected patients, and this receptor defect may account for the resistant state. Receptor number is probably normal. Despite insulin resistance, ketoacidosis does not develop, even with severe hyperglycemia. Muscle capillary basement membranes are not thickened, differentiating lipodystrophy from the common forms of diabetes mellitus. (2) Severe hypertriglyceridemia with the accumulation of both chylomicrons and very low density lipoproteins in the blood. The mechanism is not clear. (3) A hypermetabolic state with normal thyroid function. Basal metabolic rates are markedly elevated. Patients do not gain weight with excessive caloric intake, indicating a facile capacity to waste calories as heat. Thyroidectomy in one patient decreased but did not normalize the basal metabolic rate; symptoms and signs of hypothyroidism supervened in this patient, requiring treatment with thyroid hormone despite continued high metabolic rates, thus confirming that hypermetabolism was not due to hyperthyroidism.

ACQUIRED PARTIAL LIPODYSTROPHY This is the most common of the lipodystrophies and usually affects women. Fat atrophy occurs in the upper half of the body, including the face, but spares the lower extremities. Rarely the lower half of the body is affected, leaving the upper torso intact. Occasionally the lesion affects only one side. The other anatomic features of generalized lipodystrophy are usually absent, and liver disease appears to be rare. Proteinuria, with or without the nephrotic syndrome, occurs much more frequently than in other forms. The complement system is abnormal, and C_3 levels tend to be low. C_3 splitting factor ("nephritic factor") is present in the serum. Dermatomyositis and Sjögren's syndrome occur in some patients. Rarely partial lipodystrophy converts or progresses to the generalized form of the disease.

LIPODYSTROPHY WITH DOMINANT TRANSMISSION This syndrome was first described in 1974 and represents a variant characterized by fat atrophy of the limbs and trunk with sparing of the face, which may actually be rounded. The neck may also be exempt. The disease usually begins at puberty but may not appear until middle age. Males are rarely affected. Insulin resistance and hyperglycemia are usual, and severe hypertriglyceridemia with eruptive xanthoma may occur. The vaginal labia are hypertrophied and polycystic ovaries may be seen. Acanthosis nigricans is usually present. Liver and renal disease do not occur.

MULTIPLE SYMMETRIC LIPOMATOSIS

This disease is characterized by the formation of multiple, nonencapsulated lipomas in the nape of the neck, supraclavicular, and deltoid regions to produce an extraordinary bull-necked appearance (sometimes called "Madelung collar"). Lipomas can also appear elsewhere in the body. Expansion of the lipomas with infiltration between fascial planes can cause tracheal, laryngeal, and mediastinal compression. Most cases occur in alcoholics for reasons that are not clear. Hypertriglyceridemia, hyperuricemia, hyperinsulinemia, and renal tubular acidosis have been reported in some subjects.

The etiology is not known. Fat cells in the tumors have been reported to be small, suggesting new formation of adipocytes rather than a defect in triglyceride storage. Catecholamine-induced lipolysis is impaired in tumor tissue, but this may be a result rather than the cause of the lesion.

ADIPOSIS DOLOROSA

Adiposis dolorosa is a rare disease characterized by the presence of painful, circumscribed fatty deposits in the subcutaneous tissue of the extremities and occasionally elsewhere in the body. The face is not involved. Pain may occur spontaneously or upon pressure. Involved areas vary in size from 0.5 to 5.0 cm. Affected subjects are usually obese, postmenopausal women who have weakness and asthenia. Epilepsy has been noted in a number of cases, and emotional instability or frank dementia may be present. Most cases probably are sporadic, but familial inheritance in a dominant pattern has been noted. Microscopic examination of involved adipose tissue shows granulomas with giant-cell formation. Fat necrosis is unusual. The only reported biochemical defect is an inability to synthesize 18 carbon fatty acids despite the capacity for normal synthesis of 16 carbon fatty acids. Even if this defect is present, its relation to the clinical picture is uncertain.

Treatment is unsatisfactory, possibly because many of the complaints are functional. Oral analgesics and injection with local anesthetics have been tried. In one patient with extreme pain recalcitrant to all measures, the intravenous infusion of lidocaine (200 to 400 mg) over a 20-min period gave relief for 10 h. After the pain cycle was broken, lidocaine was given as a single infusion every other day. It is not known whether the effects were real or due to a placebo response.

ACUTE (RELAPSING) PANNICULITIS

The appearance of single or multiple crops of tender nodules in subcutaneous fat with a histologic picture of fat cell necrosis, infiltration of inflammatory cells, and development of fat-filled macrophages (foam cells) is the hallmark of panniculitis. The nodules range in size from 0.5 to 10 cm and may be firm or fluctuant. On occasion they drain an oily solution, and suppuration is sometimes seen. Individual lesions last from 1 to 8 weeks before disappearing. Often a pigmented depressed area is left at the involved site. While some patients have only nodular relapsing panniculitis, others develop a syndrome that includes fever, abnormal liver function, involvement of the bone marrow with leukemoid response or bleeding tendencies, nodular pulmonary lesions, evidence of pancreatic disease with elevated plasma amylase and lipase levels, and an unusual prevalence of collagen-vascular disease. This constellation of findings has been called Weber-Christian disease. It now seems clear that painful or nonpainful panniculitis occurs in several conditions and that Weber-Christian disease is not a specific entity. In a series of 34 patients with panniculitis studied at the Mayo Clinic, ultimate diagnoses included erythema nodosum, 15; local skin infections, 6; erythema enduratum, 5; Weber-Christian-like disease, 5; traumatic panniculitis, 2; and vasculitis, 1. Erythema enduratum is probably a localized hypersensitivity vasculitis. It is often found in association with tuberculosis but may develop in the absence of that disease. "Weber-Christian-like" referred to a picture of relapsing, febrile panniculitis with elevation of lipase and amylase activities in the plasma. Some of these patients could, in fact, have had metastatic fat necrosis (see below). Generalized vasculitis as a cause of acute panniculitis may be more common than indicated in the Mayo series, since in 57 autopsied cases presumed to have Weber-Christian disease there were 2 cases of dermatomyositis; 2 of scleroderma; and 6 with either lupus, polyarteritis, or rheumatoid arthritis. A fulminant downhill course in a patient with panniculitis can be assumed to be a collagen-vascular disease or metastatic fat necrosis.

The Weber-Christian notation should probably be abandoned. Patients with histologically proved panniculitis should be diagnosed as having acute (relapsing) panniculitis and a search made for the underlying etiology. Treatment is unsatisfactory, though glucocorticoids are usually tried.

METASTATIC FAT NECROSIS

Metastatic fat necrosis is a syndrome of extensive adipose tissue inflammation and cell death resembling or identical with acute nodular panniculitis. It is accompanied by fever, destructive polyarthritis (which may cause flail joints), lytic bone lesions, pleural and pericardial effusions, ascites, and elevation of lipase and amylase levels in the plasma. Eosinophilia occurs in some patients. Pancreatic disease is invariably present. About two-thirds of patients have pancreatitis, while the remainder have a carcinoma of the pancreas, usually acinar. The cause of the syndrome is unknown. Fat necrosis has been speculated to be due to pancreatic lipase acting at multiple sites in the body, but the entire picture may actually result from an autoimmune phenomenon. Complement levels are low, and involved tissues show immunofluorescent staining for IgG and the third component of complement. Prognosis is poor, and death often occurs within a few months whether or not the underlying cause is cancer.

REFERENCES

Lipodystrophy

Dunnigan MG et al: Familial lipoatrophic diabetes with dominant transmission. Q J Med 169:33, 1974

Oseid S et al: Decreased binding of insulin to its receptor in patients with congenital generalized lipodystrophy. N Engl J Med 296:245, 1977
Seip M: Generalized lipodystrophy. Ergeb Inn Med Kinderheilkd 31:59, 1971

Multiple symmetric lipomatosis

Enzi G et al: Multiple symmetric lipomatosis. A defect in adrenergic-stimulated lipolysis. J Clin Invest 60:1221, 1977

Adiposis dolorosa

Blomstrand R et al: Adiposis dolorosa associated with defects of lipid metabolism. Acta Derm Venereol 51:243, 1971
Cantu JM et al: Autosomal dominant inheritance in adiposis dolorosa (Dercum's disease). Humangenetik 18:89, 1973

Acute (relapsing) panniculitis

Förström L, RK Winkelmann: Acute panniculitis. A clinical and histopathologic study of 34 cases. Arch Dermatol 113:909, 1977
MacDonald A, M Feiwel: A review of the concept of Weber-Christian panniculitis with a report of five cases. Br J Dermatol 80:355, 1968

Metastatic fat necrosis

Good AE et al: Acinar pancreatic tumor with metastatic fat necrosis. Report of a case and review of rheumatic manifestations. Am J Dig Dis 21:978, 1976
Potts DE et al: Syndrome of pancreatic disease, subcutaneous fat necrosis and polyserositis. Case report and review of literature. Am J Med 58:417, 1975

Genetic disorders affecting multiple organ systems

103
DISORDERS OF CONNECTIVE TISSUE

PHILIP J. FIALKOW

Elastin, collagen, glycoproteins, and proteinpolysaccharides are the major extracellular macromolecules of connective tissue. An inherited abnormality in connective tissue may affect any one of the numerous steps in the biosynthesis and the metabolism of these substances or the processes by which the macromolecules are physically organized and oriented to one another.

Heritable, generalized disorders of connective tissue may be classified as primary or secondary. The former group includes those diseases caused by mutations in genes that directly involve the synthesis or metabolism of elements such as collagen or elastin. In secondary disorders, mutant genes affect metabolism exogenous to connective tissue pathways, resulting in the accumulation of a product that damages connective tissue (e.g., homocystinuria, Chap. 88).

The heritable disorders discussed in this chapter are thought to be primary and to involve collagen or elastic fibers. With some exceptions the basic defects are undefined, and it is not known whether the mutations affect connective tissue primarily or secondarily. In some cases it is not certain whether the abnormalities involve collagen, elastin, or other connective tissue components. All the disorders are genetically heterogeneous, i.e., two or more different mutations produce clinically similar diseases. Diseases primarily affecting mucopolysaccharides are described in Chap. 101.

THE EHLERS-DANLOS SYNDROME

The Ehlers-Danlos syndrome (EDS) constitutes a group of heritable, generalized disorders of connective tissue whose major features include fragile and hyperextensible skin (Fig. 103-1), easy bruising, and loose-jointedness. There are at least seven distinct types that vary in clinical manifestations from mild to severe. The patterns of inheritance include autosomal dominant and recessive and X-linked recessive. The prevalence is uncertain.

The EDS presumably involves collagen fibers. The basic building block of these fibers, the collagen monomer, is a triple helix of three α chains. Several different forms of collagen are known. The ubiquitous molecule (type I) is a triple helix containing two different α chains and is found in skin, tendon, ligament, bone, blood vessels, dentin, and other organs. EDS I,

II, and III are thought to involve this macromolecule. Type II collagen is found primarily in cartilage and consists of three α chains, similar to but not identical with, those found in type I. Type III collagen, the molecule thought to be involved in EDS IV, has three identical α chains which differ from those found in types I and II. It has a similar tissue distribution to type I but is not found in bone or dentin.

EDS I, GRAVIS TYPE This is the classical EDS, which, because of its severe clinical manifestations, is termed *gravis*.

Clinical manifestations SKIN The skin is soft, velvety, and hyperextensible. It can be pulled far away from the underlying structures, but upon release it promptly returns to its original position (Fig. 103-1). With advancing age focal losses of elasticity may cause the skin over some areas such as the palms to become lax. The skin is fragile and easily bruised. Minor trauma often produces a gaping, fish-mouth wound that is hard to suture but does not bleed extensively. Paper-thin scars develop with healing. Minor injury often results in purpura or hematomas which may organize, calcify, and resemble a neoplasm. Another type of pseudotumor develops over pressure points such as the knees and elbows. These smaller, subcutaneous pea-sized "spherules" occur on the extremities, calcify, and are visible on roentgenograms.

MUSCULOSKELETAL SYSTEM Hyperextensible joints may allow patients to perform unusual contortions (e.g., "India rubber man," "human pretzel"). Because of joint instability, these patients are prone to develop effusions or recurrent dislocations of the hip, patella, shoulder, and other joints. Hemarthroses sometimes occur. Backward curvature of the knees (genu recurvatum), flatfeet, kyphoscoliosis, and looseness of the clavicles at their sternal ends are common. Joint hyperextensibility may decrease somewhat with advancing age. High-arched palate, "pigeon breast," and spondylolisthesis may be seen. Muscle hypotonia, dental abnormalities, and nocturnal leg cramps are frequent.

BLEEDING This may occur into the skin and joints as described above. Severe gastrointestinal or respiratory tract

bleeding occasionally occurs. The gums may bleed with minor trauma (e.g., brushing of the teeth), and bleeding may complicate tooth extraction or tonsillectomy. Weakness of vessel walls or abnormal interactions of platelets with collagen apparently underlies the hemorrhagic diathesis; consistent abnormalities in clotting factors have not been described.

EYES Blue scleras are common. Epicanthal folds are frequent in younger patients. In older patients the eyes may appear widely spaced.

CARDIOVASCULAR SYSTEM Mitral valve prolapse occurs in this and other forms of EDS, especially types II and III. Right bundle branch block or other conduction abnormalities are found in some patients with EDS. Aortic valve regurgitation and dissecting aneurysm of the aorta are rare complications.

Congenital cardiac anomalies have also been reported, but their prevalence may not be higher in EDS than in the general population. Vascular complications such as spontaneous rupture of the large arteries and rupture of intracranial aneurysms leading to cerebral vascular accidents are rare and are more likely to be seen in EDS IV. Because the arteries may be friable, cerebral angiography and other diagnostic arterial invasions should be performed cautiously.

OTHER MANIFESTATIONS Generalized tissue fragility makes surgery and subsequent wound healing difficult and may lead to spontaneous rupture of the bowel or to pneumothorax. Premature birth due to early rupture of the fetal membranes is common. Diaphragmatic and other hernias and gastrointestinal tract diverticula occur with increased frequency.

Inheritance EDS I is inherited as an autosomal dominant and may itself be genetically heterogeneous.

Pathogenesis The basic defect in EDS I is unknown. Dermal collagen bundles often appear fragmented, and collagen fibrils are abnormal on electron microscopy. The abnormalities are presumed to involve type I collagen.

EDS II, MITIS TYPE Clinical manifestations are similar to those of EDS I but are less severe. Hence EDS II is also termed "mitis" type. Skin and joint changes are mild, and hyperextensibility may be limited to joints of the hands and feet. Tissue friability is not a problem, and internal manifestations are uncommon with the exception of mitral valve prolapse. As in EDS I, this form of EDS is inherited as an autosomal dominant and may be genetically heterogeneous. Ultrastructural studies suggest an abnormality in type I collagen.

EDS III, BENIGN HYPERMOBILE TYPE The striking features are generalized joint hypermobility with joint dislocations and effusions and eventual degenerative arthritis. Cutaneous manifestations are minimal. Mitral valve prolapse may occur. EDS III is transmitted as an autosomal dominant.

EDS IV, ECCHYMOTIC OR ARTERIAL TYPE In this rare form of EDS, the skin is fragile, thin, and translucent, allowing easy visualization of subcutaneous veins. In contrast to other types of the EDS, the skin is not hyperextensible and may even be tight. Severe bruising occurs easily. Joint hypermobility is usually found only in the digits. Severe complications which may lead to premature death are rupture of hollow viscera or of

FIGURE 103-1
Hyperextensible skin in a patient with an unclassified form of Ehlers-Danlos syndrome.

large arteries. This form of EDS is genetically heterogeneous, and families with autosomal dominant or recessive inheritance have been described. The recessive varieties are more severe and are associated with a decrease in life expectancy. The life expectancy in the dominant variety is only slightly reduced. Normal blood vessels are especially rich in type III collagen, and the tissue content of this type of collagen is decreased in many, if not all, varieties of EDS IV. The precise biochemical defects are unknown.

EDS V, X-LINKED TYPE The most striking feature is hyperextensible skin with moderate fragility, thin scars, and bruising. Joint hypermobility is mild. These features are similar to those of EDS II, and EDS V is distinguished more by its pattern of inheritance (X-linked recessive) than by its clinical manifestations. In some patients with apparently X-linked recessive EDS, short stature, and severe joint hypermobility occur. Such patients may have deficient activity of lysyl oxidase, an enzyme necessary for normal formation of interchain cross-links in collagen (see EDS VI). Deficiency of this enzyme activity is also found in the X-linked recessive form of cutis laxa.

EDS VI, OCULAR TYPE Hyperextensible skin and joints with the ensuing complications are present, but the distinctive features of this type of EDS are the ocular manifestations, severe scoliosis, and mild to moderate arachnodactyly. The cornea may be abnormal in size or shape and, like the sclera, is fragile and prone to rupture from even mild trauma. Glaucoma and retinal detachment also occur.

The primary abnormality in this autosomal recessive disorder is deficient activity of lysyl hydroxylase. The tensile strength of collagen fibrils in tissues depends upon the formation of interchain cross-links, which in large part result from interactions involving lysyl- or hydroxylysyl-derived aldehydes. With deficient lysyl hydroxylase activity, the hydroxylysine residue content of collagen is markedly decreased, hydroxylysine interchain cross-links are diminished, tensile strength is decreased, and the clinical manifestations ensue.

EDS VII, ARTHROCHALASIS MULTIPLEX CONGENITA This rare form of EDS is inherited as an autosomal recessive and is characterized by short stature and marked joint hypermobility with only mild skin hyperextensibility. The primary defect is deficient activity of a protease involved in the formation of collagen from its precursor, procollagen.

DIFFERENTIAL DIAGNOSIS Congenital joint hypermobility occurs as an isolated finding, sometimes in more than one relative, and is probably a distinct entity from the EDS. Loose-jointedness also occurs in the Marfan and Noonan syndromes and in osteogenesis imperfecta. In cutis laxa the skin is not only hyperextensible, but it is also lax, i.e., it has decreased elasticity and may hang in loose folds. Late in the course of EDS the skin in localized areas may resemble that seen in cutis laxa.

TREATMENT AND PROGNOSIS No specific therapy is known. Trauma to skin and joints should be avoided. In moderate and severe forms of the EDS, surgery should be undertaken with caution because of the fragility of skin, arteries, and internal organs. Wound dehiscence is frequent, and sutures should be left in place longer than usual.

Pregnancy may be accompanied by increased bruisability and exacerbation of joint manifestations and carries increased risk for development of abdominal herniae; leg and vulva varicosities; complications of episiotomy and cesarean section; and, in type I EDS, for premature delivery.

Death from arterial rupture is relatively frequent in patients with the severe variety of EDS IV. In other types of EDS death may occasionally occur from internal complications, but the prognosis for normal life expectancy is good. Some patients experience considerable morbidity from cutaneous and joint abnormalities.

MARFAN SYNDROME

The Marfan syndrome is an inherited, generalized disorder of connective tissue with ocular, skeletal, and cardiovascular manifestations. There is wide variability in clinical expression, and some patients have findings in only one or two systems. The prevalence of the disorder has been estimated to be more than 1 in 50,000, perhaps 1 in 10,000 persons.

Clinical manifestations These result from abnormalities in the supporting tissues of the ocular, cardiovascular, and skeletal systems. Although the diagnosis may be apparent during infancy, ordinarily it is not made until the second decade or later.

EYES Weakness and redundancy of the supporting tissues of the lens is the cause of the most characteristic finding in the Marfan syndrome, bilateral subluxation, or dislocation of the lens (ectopia lentis). This occurs in about 80 percent of patients, and its presence may be signaled by tremor of the iris (iridodenesis). The lens dislocation is most frequently upward. Complications of subluxated lens include uveitis, glaucoma, and cataracts. Minor dislocation is frequent and can be excluded only by careful slit-lamp examination. High-grade myopia is also common. Spontaneous retinal detachment may occur, and some patients have blue sclerae.

CARDIOVASCULAR SYSTEM About 90 percent of patients have cardiovascular abnormalities, some of which may be evident only with sensitive diagnostic modalities such as echocardiography. Weakness in the media of the aorta causes the most life-threatening abnormality in the Marfan syndrome, progressive dilatation, and dissecting aneurysm of the proximal portion of the ascending aorta. Clinical manifestations such as diastolic murmur or roentgenographic evidence of aortic dilatation may be detected in infancy or as late as in the fifth or sixth decades. The predilection for involvement of the ascending aorta is not surprising in view of the hemodynamic stresses that occur there.

Although *severe* mitral valve regurgitation is less common than *severe* aortic valve disease, echocardiographic studies in most patients reveal some abnormality of the mitral valve, including mitral valve prolapse (the "click murmur" syndrome, Chap. 242). Echocardiography may also be useful in following patients with aortic root and valve abnormalities. Bacterial endocarditis may involve heart valves with only minor antecedent alterations. Coarctation of the aorta and abnormalities in the conduction system are also found in the Marfan syndrome.

SKELETAL SYSTEM Increased length of the tubular bones is the most conspicuous external feature of the disease (Fig. 102-2). The extremities are long and thin (dolichostenomelia); almost all patients are tall, either absolutely or relatively when their heights are assessed against the background of their families.

Abnormal body proportions are even more specific. The distance from the top of the pubic symphysis to the sole of the foot ("lower segment") is increased in patients with the Marfan syndrome, causing a low ratio of the upper segment (pubic symphysis to crown) to the lower segment of the body. In normal postpubertal whites this ratio is 0.92 ± 0.04, and in normal blacks it is 0.85 ± 0.03. A significant decrease in these values is helpful in establishing the diagnosis of the Marfan syndrome. The arm span may be greater than the height.

Excessively long finger bones (arachnodactyly, "spider fingers") are found in most patients with the Marfan syndrome. When this is subtle, roentgenograms of the hands with calculation of the "metacarpal index" may be helpful. The length of each of the last four metacarpal bones is divided by the width at its midpoint, and the values are averaged. In patients with the Marfan syndrome the index is often greater than 8.4; in normal individuals it is usually less than 8. Sternal displacement upward causes "pigeon breast" (pectus carinatum), and sternal displacement inward causes pectus excavatum. The palate is often high and arched, and the facies, long and narrow.

Weakness and redundancy of the ligaments and other supporting tissues of the joints lead to loose- or "double-jointedness," flatfeet, backward curvature of the knees (genu recurvatum), kyphoscoliosis, and recurrent dislocations, especially of the hip and patella. Inguinal or femoral hernias are frequent.

OTHER MANIFESTATIONS Many patients have sparse subcutaneous fat and muscle hypotonia. Striae may be present, especially in the skin of the pectoral, deltoid, and thigh areas. Lung cysts with spontaneous pneumothorax occasionally occur.

Inheritance The Marfan syndrome is inherited as an autosomal dominant. There is wide variability in clinical expression

FIGURE 103-2

A 16-year-old boy with the Marfan syndrome. Manifestations include dislocated lens, long, thin face, long fingers (arachnodactyly) and extremities (dolichostenomelia), and inward displacement of the sternum (pectus excavatum). (Courtesy of JG Hall.)

("variable expressivity"), and an affected relative may have only mild manifestations confined to one system (e.g., dislocated lens detected only by slit-lamp examination). Rarely, an individual genetically proved to possess the Marfan gene (e.g., a person with an affected parent and offspring) does not have any detectable expression (lack of "penetrance"). Perhaps 15 percent of cases are sporadic and presumably the result of a fresh mutation in a parental germ cell. Fathers of sporadic cases are, on average, 7 years older than fathers of patients who have inherited the disease from an affected parent. Elevated paternal age is considered a factor in the occurrence of fresh mutations.

Pathology and pathogenesis The basic biochemical abnormality is unknown. Defective collagen cross-linking is possible, but unproved. The early aortic changes are those of cystic medial necrosis (Chap. 252). Later findings are loss of elastic fibers and scarring with irregular whorls of smooth muscle. No histological changes or electron microscopic abnormalities in collagen have been reported in ligaments or tendons.

Differential diagnosis Because the disorder displays wide variability in clinical expression and because there is no specific test for the Marfan syndrome, the diagnosis may be difficult to establish in patients without the classical triad of dislocated lens, aortic dilatation or aneurysm, and excessive length of tubular bones. In such cases careful examination of close relatives and exclusion of disorders resembling the Marfan syndrome can be helpful. It may be impossible to establish the diagnosis definitively in a patient with skeletal or cardiac abnormalities who does not have a dislocated lens or a clearly affected relative.

The homocystinurias, inborn errors of methionine metabolism with secondary effects on connective tissue (Chap. 88), are the principal diseases to be distinguished from the Marfan syndrome. The disorders have dislocated lens and skeletal deformities in common but differ in other clinical manifestations and in their pattern of inheritance (Table 103-1). As its name implies, there is a specific laboratory test for homocystinuria.

A "marfanoid hypermobility" syndrome is characterized by hyperextensible joints and skin changes similar to those seen in Ehlers-Danlos syndrome as well as by arachnodactyly, pectus deformity, and regurgitation of the aortic and mitral valves.

Congenital contractural arachnodactyly, an autosomal dominant disorder associated with severe kyphoscoliosis, generalized osteopenia, and arachnodactyly, is distinguished from the Marfan syndrome by the presence of congenital contractures of the fingers and abnormally shaped ears. It has been suggested that congenital contractural arachnodactyly and the marfanoid hypermobility disorder are forms of, and reflect genetic heterogeneity of, the Marfan syndrome and that the more typical cases of the Marfan syndrome can be subdivided into at least two types: asthenic, mainly in children, and nonasthenic.

Dislocation of the lens is a feature of another genetic disorder of connective tissue, the Weill-Marchesani syndrome, but the skeletal abnormalities in this autosomal recessive disorder are short stature and stiffness of joints.

Treatment and prognosis Estrogen therapy may reduce adult height in girls who are already tall in the prepubertal period and may also partially prevent severe kyphoscoliosis. The potential benefits of estrogens must be weighed against their possible complications, including the psychological and physical effects of inducing precocious puberty. Prophylactic administration of drugs like propranolol which decrease myocardial contractility and diminish the stress on the aorta have thus far not been documented to be beneficial in patients with early aortic changes. The risks of surgery for aortic or valvular disease are high, primarily because the abnormal connective tissue may not hold sutures well. However, therapy is often successful.

The major threats to life, severe cardiovascular complications, may occur anytime from infancy to the seventh decade. These complications include dilatation, dissection, or rupture of the aorta, and severe regurgitation of the aortic or mitral valve. In one series, the mean age at death was 43 for men and 46 for women. Pregnancy may be particularly hazardous for women with aortic disease.

Patients with the Marfan syndrome may be disabled by profound kyphoscoliosis; recurrent joint dislocations; recurrent pneumothorax; or serious visual impairment from myopia, retinal detachment, or the uveitis and glaucoma that result from subluxation of the lens.

OSTEOGENESIS IMPERFECTA

Osteogenesis imperfecta (OI; fragilitas ossium, maladie de Lobstein) is a group of heritable, generalized disorders of connective tissue with clinical manifestations in the skeleton, ear, joints and ligaments, teeth, sclera, and skin. The basic defect is unknown but presumably involves an abnormality in collagen. The frequency of OI has been estimated at more than 1 in every 20,000 births.

Clinical manifestations The cardinal features are blue sclerae, multiple fractures, loose-jointedness, and deafness; clinical expression is variable.

SKELETON Narrow bones with osteoporosis, thin cortices, and excessive fragility underlie the multiple fractures and skeletal deformities characteristic of the common types of OI. The fractures occur with minor trauma and frequently involve the long bones of the legs. Callus formed with healing may be large and on occasion may be mistaken for osteogenic sarcoma. In severe cases multiple fractures in utero allow antenatal diagnosis. Generally, susceptibility to fractures decreases after puberty, but may return later, especially with inactivity, pregnancy, or menopause. The extremities are often short, and associated deformities include saber shins, marked bowing of the legs, and pseudoarthroses. There is often lateral bulging of the calvarium with a characteristic triangular shape of the face. Chest deformities such as sternal displacement inward (pectus excavatum) or outward ("pigeon breast," pectus carinatum) are

frequent. Frequently, dome forehead and overhanging occiput are seen. Roentgenograms of the bones may show osteoporosis, basilar impression of the skull (platybasia), "codfish" or "hourglass" vertebrae, and wormian bones in the skull. This last finding may help establish the diagnosis.

EYES The scleras appear translucent, thin, and usually blue, owing to partial visualization of the underlying choroid. This is the most frequent manifestation of OI.

EARS Progressive hearing impairment from otosclerosis may begin in childhood, but deafness usually does not develop until adulthood. The tympanic membranes may appear blue.

JOINTS Abnormalities in the ligaments and tendons lead to loose-jointedness, which causes in turn the increased frequency of kyphoscoliosis, flatfeet, and recurrent joint dislocations. Tendons may rupture from minor stress.

TEETH Hypoplasia of dentine and pulp causes the characteristically small, misshapen, blue-yellow teeth (dentinogenesis imperfecta).

OTHER MANIFESTATIONS The skin tends to be thin, translucent, and easily bruised. Hernias occur frequently. Cardiovascular disorders, including mitral valve prolapse or aortic regurgitation, may occur.

Inheritance As in the other heritable disorders of connective tissue, clinical and genetic heterogeneity occurs in OI. The subdivision of OI on clinical grounds into congenita (features present at birth) and tarda (onset of fractures afterward) may also have genetic validity. Almost all cases of OI tarda are transmitted as autosomal dominants, but there appear to be two forms of OI congenita distinguishable by roentgenography: one, probably often dominant, with thin bones, and the other, recessive, with thick bones. There is also evidence for heterogeneity within the OI tarda patients.

Without knowledge of the basic defects and distinguishing biochemical tests, clinical classification of OI is difficult, in large part due to the variable gene expression, sometimes evident even within the same family. Furthermore, it is likely that additional types of OI will be recognized. For these reasons, the following classification must be regarded as preliminary. The designations tarda and congenita are not absolute but characterize the majority of patients within each category.

A few patients with what is called OI tarda first experience fractures early in infancy, and some patients designated as OI congenita may not experience fractures until 12 to 15 months of age. Furthermore, individuals with onset of fractures before birth and in infancy may be encountered in the same family.

TABLE 103-1
Comparison of the Marfan syndrome with homocystinuria

Disorder	Mode of inheritance	Basic biochemical defect	Clinical manifestations			Cutaneous and subcutaneous	Cardiovascular	Mental retardation
			Ectopia lentis	Skeletal				
				Arachnodactyly	Pectus deformities			
Marfan syndrome	Autosomal dominant	Unknown	+++ (usually upward)	++++	+++	Striae; sparse subcutaneous fat	Mitral valve prolapse Aorta: regurgitation/dissecting aneurysm	– –
Homocystinuria	Autosomal recessive	Usually decreased cystathionine synthase activity	++++ (usually downward)	++	++	Malar flush	Vascular thrombosis	++

OI TARDA This, the most common variety of OI, is characterized by osteoporosis, frequent fractures, dental abnormalities, blue sclerae, and deafness. Fractures, rare at birth, usually occur by age 3. The course is variable, but skeletal deformities are usually mild. Inheritance is autosomal dominant. There may be two distinct subtypes, one with and the other without dental abnormalities. There may also be a rarer, distinct disorder inherited as an autosomal dominant but without blue sclerae (and perhaps also without deafness). Occasionally, families are encountered in which OI tarda is apparently inherited as an autosomal recessive.

OI CONGENITA I (THIN BONE TYPE) This is a severe disease characterized by osteoporosis, fractures, progressive skeletal deformities with shortness of stature, and thin bones on roentgenograms. The majority of affected infants have fractures at or before birth. The scleras are blue in infancy, but, as in normal children, frequently become white. Deafness may not be an important feature. Live-born infants often survive but may be disabled by multiple fractures and bone deformities, or by complications of intracranial hemorrhage in the perinatal period. The pattern of inheritance is not well defined. Almost all cases occur sporadically. Some patients, however, have an autosomal recessive disease, others an autosomal dominant. The latter presumably result from a fresh mutation in a parental gamete.

OI CONGENITA II (THICK BONE TYPE) This very severe disease is generally lethal in infancy. The bones appear thick and crumpled on roentgenograms. Inheritance is autosomal recessive.

Pathology and pathogenesis The bone cortices and trabeculae are usually thin. Osteoid is diminished and replaced by basophilic, periodic acid-Schiff-staining material. In other tissues mature collagen is not seen. Biochemical studies suggest that the defects in OI involve aberrations in collagen, but the basic abnormalities are unknown.

Differential diagnosis The correct diagnosis is obvious in patients with the classical triad of blue scleras, pathologic fractures, and deafness. However, only 60 percent of affected subjects have clinical bone disease, and some patients manifest only blue scleras or otosclerosis. According to one survey, 60 percent of adult patients with blue scleras have multiple fractures, 60 percent have otosclerosis, and 44 percent have all three manifestations. It is likely that this variability reflects the fact that there are several distinct OI syndromes, i.e., genetic and clinical heterogeneity. However, variability in clinical manifestations can sometimes occur among relatives in the same family.

Without a clear family history, it may be difficult to distinguish OI early in its course from "idiopathic" osteoporosis. The same is true after the menopause in women with OI who have experienced few fractures earlier in life. When the legs are short and the head appears large, OI may resemble achondroplasia. OI congenita must also be distinguished from hypophosphatasia.

Treatment and prognosis No specific therapy is known. Careful orthopedic management is necessary, and immobilization should be avoided. Infants with severe OI congenita are often born dead or die in infancy. OI tarda is a more benign disease, but disability may occur from multiple fractures, skeletal deformities, or deafness. Nonetheless, many patients adjust to their disease and lead normal lives. The frequency of fractures generally decreases after puberty but may again increase later in life. Deafness is present in about 35 percent of patients in the fourth decade and in about 50 percent in the sixth decade.

PSEUDOXANTHOMA ELASTICUM

Pseudoxanthoma elasticum (PXE; Groenblad-Strandberg syndrome) is a genetically determined disorder with protean clinical manifestations most frequently involving the skin, eyes, and arteries. The basic pathogenetic abnormality is unknown but probably involves elastic fibers. Clinical changes usually first appear in the second or third decade and thereafter are progressive. The prevalence of PXE has been estimated at between 1 in 200,000 and 1 in 50,000 adults.

Clinical manifestations SKIN PXE derives its name from the characteristic yellow xanthoma-like papular and reticulated skin lesions. Skin changes are usually evident in the second or third decade and in later life are found in virtually all.

The changes are most notable in the neck and axillae, and the antecubital fossae, periumbilical area, groin, and penis may also be involved. The abnormalities range from a few yellow papules confined to one or two areas (usually the neck, axilla, or both) to confluent yellow papules and plaques that cause redundant folds of lax skin over flexural surfaces. The skin around the mouth, chin, and nasolabial folds may be thickened as well as lax.

The extent of changes detected histologically correlates with the severity of clinical cutaneous lesions, but occasionally changes of PXE may be seen in a biopsy from a patient without obvious clinical alterations.

EYES Angioid streaks are first noted during the second or third decade and found thereafter in all but a very few patients. The streaks are bilateral. They lie beneath the retinal vessels, are flat, are usually three to five times the diameter of retinal veins, and are red, brown, or gray. Angioid streaks are most numerous around the optic disks from which they appear to emanate. Later changes include hemorrhage and chorioretinal scarring; when these alterations are marked, the streaks may be obscured. Visual impairment may result in near blindness.

VASCULAR SYSTEM Most patients with PXE have some combination of peripheral, cardiac, or cerebrovascular abnormalities. Involvement of peripheral arteries results in weak or absent pulses and often in calcification. Easy fatigability of the limbs and intermittent claudication are common. Some patients develop early-onset hypertension or coronary artery disease that usually presents as angina or an altered ECG. Cerebrovascular symptoms are less frequent and may be rare in the absence of hypertension. Hypothyroidism, perhaps from altered thyroid vasculature may occur.

Upper gastrointestinal tract bleeding is frequent, often severe, and occasionally the presenting manifestation. The hemorrhage is probably from arterial disease in the gastrointestinal tract. Sometimes peptic ulcer or hiatus hernia is present, but in many the source of the bleeding is not detected. Uterine bleeding may be severe. Hemorrhage may also occur in the urinary and upper respiratory tracts.

Inheritance PXE is a genetically heterogeneous disorder. In most families it is autosomal recessive, but autosomal dominant inheritance also occurs. There may be at least two varieties of autosomal dominant PXE. Type I is characterized by classic orange-peel-like skin changes, severe vascular manifestations, and choroiditis. Patients with the more frequent type II have a much milder disease. The skin is hyperextensible, and the rash is macular (or focal). Other manifestations such as high-arched palate, blue sclerae, and loose-jointedness may also occur in patients with type II.

Pathology and pathogenesis The basic defect in PXE is unknown, but probably involves, either primarily or secondarily, elastic fibers in the skin, media of arteries, and elsewhere. Angioid streaks in the eyes represent breaks in the Bruch membrane behind the retina. Early skin changes are small patchy areas of swollen, fragmented, and irregularly clumped basophilic elastic fibers in the middermis.

These altered areas have affinity for calcium, and von Kossa staining (for calcium) may be valuable in confirming subtle lesions. Later in the disease all the elastic fibers of the mid and lower dermis are affected. Studies with the electron microscope indicate that the principal alterations are in the elastin moiety of the elastic fibers.

Differential diagnosis Virtually all patients with PXE have characteristic cutaneous changes, and the diagnosis can be confirmed with a skin biopsy. Actinic (or "senile") elastosis may cause confusion in some patients; however, the changes are limited to exposed sites, and the disorder is histologically distinguishable from PXE. Angioid streaks are present in the great majority of patients with PXE, and while their presence is very suggestive of the diagnosis, they are also found in other disorders, including sickle-cell anemia and Paget's disease.

Treatment and prognosis No specific treatment for PXE is known. Skin changes may be a cosmetic problem. Most patients with PXE have some visual impairment, but complete blindness is rare. Early death may occur from hemorrhage, cardiac disease, or cerebrovascular accidents, but some patients have a normal life span.

REFERENCES

BORNSTEIN P, BYERS PH: Disorders of collagen, in *Duncan's Diseases of Metabolism*, 8th ed, P Bondy et al (eds). Philadelphia, Saunders, 1979 (in press)

McKUSICK VA: *Heritable Disorders of Connective Tissue*, 4th ed. St Louis, Mosby, 1972

VITTO J, LICHTENSTEIN JR: Defects in the biochemistry of collagen in diseases of connective tissue. J Invest Dermatol 66:59, 1976

104
OTHER DISORDERS INVOLVING MULTIPLE ORGAN SYSTEMS

PHILIP J. FIALKOW

The pathophysiology of many clinically important genetic diseases is unknown. Most of these disorders are described under the principal organ systems affected. Some others involving multiple organ systems are discussed here.

NOONAN SYNDROME

The Noonan syndrome shows wide phenotypic variability and comprises multiple congenital anomalies of the skin, skeleton, heart, and gonads. Many patients have short stature and intellectual impairment. The prevalence, clinical spectrum, natural history, pathogenesis, and mode of inheritance are poorly delineated. The syndrome probably comprises several distinct

but, as yet, undefined disorders. Furthermore, only within the last 10 to 15 years has it been appreciated that the Noonan syndrome is separable from the Turner syndrome (gonadal dysgenesis), which is due to a partial or complete absence of one sex chromosome. It is likely that most patients previously described as Ullrich, male Turner or female pseudo-Turner syndromes and as Turner, Ullrich, or Bonnevie-Ullrich phenotype with normal chromosomes fall within the spectrum of the Noonan syndrome.

CLINICAL MANIFESTATIONS Since few family studies have been performed, the spectrum and prevalence of individual abnormalities given here cannot be regarded as definitive.

Facies Patients with the Noonan syndrome have a characteristic appearance, including a narrow maxilla and small mandible with triangular-shaped mouth, epicanthic eye folds, hypertelorism, ptosis, downward ("antimongoloid") slant of the eyes, and ears that are prominent, fleshy, low-set and posteriorly rotated (Fig. 104-1). Webbing of the neck and a low posterior hairline are found in about half of patients.

Skin Multiple pigmented nevi and dystrophic nails are frequent. Patients may have congenital lymphangiectatic edema of the hands and feet lasting until age 6 to 9 months or, in some patients, into adulthood. Keloid formation is frequent. The skin may be hyperelastic. Dermatoglyphic patterns may be abnormal but are nonspecific.

Skeletal system Most patients are short. Others have normal stature but are not as tall as would be expected for their genetic background. Skeletal abnormalities are common and include high-arched palate, dental malocclusion, increased car-

FIGURE 104-1
A 14-year-old boy with the Noonan syndrome. Manifestations include downward ("antimongoloid") slant of the eyes, epicanthic eye folds, midface hypoplasia, prominent ears, broad neck, and upturned nose. (Courtesy of JG Hall.)

rying angle of the arms (cubitus valgus), shield-shaped chest with wide-spaced nipples, pectus deformities, and kyphoscoliosis. Anomalies of the sternum, vertebrae, limbs, or skull may be seen radiographically. Often the pectus deformity is distinctive in that the upper portion of the sternum is displaced outward and the lower portion is displaced inward; that is, pectus carinatum and excavatum are both present in the same patient. The joints may be hyperextensible.

Intellectual development Intelligence ranges from superior to profoundly retarded, but most have mild or borderline mental retardation, as compared with nonaffected family members. From 25 to 50 percent of patients have normal intelligence.

Heart The true prevalence of congenital heart disease is unknown, but may be between 30 and 50 percent. The most frequent finding is valvular pulmonic stenosis, alone or in combination with septal defects (especially atrial), asymmetric septal hypertrophy, or pulmonary artery branch stenosis. The last three abnormalities are less frequent in the absence of valvular pulmonic stenosis. In contrast to the Turner syndrome coarctation of the aorta is rare.

Sexual development Penile size may be normal or decreased; more than half of the males have cryptorchidism. Fertility is rare in men with the Noonan syndrome. In contrast, most affected females apparently are fertile.

Other manifestations Hydronephrosis with pyeloureteral obstruction and other renal anomalies occur, but the prevalence is unknown. Other abnormalities include thyroiditis, hypothyroidism, and hepatosplenomegaly in the absence of cardiac failure.

INHERITANCE Clinical and genetic heterogeneity clearly occurs. There are likely to be several "cardiofacial" syndromes which have in common unusual facies and congenital cardiac abnormalities. Among these is the typical Noonan syndrome.

No chromosomal abnormality has been found in patients with the Noonan syndrome. Autosomal dominant inheritance, described in some families, may be the mode of transmission for most patients. The relatively high proportion of sporadic cases (theoretically representing new mutations) would not be unusual for an autosomal dominant disorder often accompanied by infertility. In some families "unaffected" relatives have mild signs of the disorder.

Genetic counseling should include a discussion not only of disease recurrence risks but also of the wide range of clinical expression, especially as it pertains to cardiac anomalies, intelligence, stature, and fertility. Until the presumed heterogeneity is better defined, prognosis and recurrence risks are difficult to estimate and should be based largely on individual findings in the patient and family. The risk of severe disease in a patient's sibling or child is higher if the patient is severely affected.

DIFFERENTIAL DIAGNOSIS Noonan syndrome must be distinguished from the Turner syndrome (gonadal dysgenesis) (Chap. 344). Shortness of stature and anomalies of the skeleton, skin, and integument are common in both disorders. Although the characteristic facies is seen to some extent in every Noonan patient, it alone may not be distinctive enough to exclude the Turner syndrome. Clinical features that help identify the Turner syndrome include normal intelligence, infertility, and negative family history for other affected individuals. Pulmonic stenosis is common in the Noonan but infrequent in the Turner syndrome, whereas the reverse is true for coarctation of the aorta. Finally, chromosome studies will usually allow the definitive diagnosis of the Turner syndrome.

The Aarskog syndrome (faciogenital dysplasia) is also associated with shortness of stature and facial anomalies but is further characterized by its X-linked recessive pattern of inheritance and by the fact that the scrotum overhangs the penis ("saddle-bag scrotum"). The fetal alcohol, fetal hydantoin, and Williams syndromes, all characterized by growth retardation, mild to moderate mental retardation and craniofacial abnormalities, must also be distinguished from the Noonan syndrome. In Noonan patients with hyperelastic skin and loose-jointedness, an erroneous diagnosis of Ehlers-Danlos syndrome may be made.

TREATMENT AND PROGNOSIS Therapy is directed toward correcting debilitating and life-threatening anomalies. Decisions to operate on patients for ptosis and webbing of the neck must be tempered by the reports of increased predilection to keloid formation. Surgical correction of valvular pulmonic stenosis should be performed when indicated, but results may be unsatisfactory because both the valve and contiguous tissue may be dysplastic. Orchiopexy for undescended testes should be attempted but is frequently unsuccessful. Although poorly defined, the life span in the Noonan syndrome, excluding cardiovascular problems and a possible increased frequency of neoplasia, is probably normal.

LAURENCE-MOON-BIEDL SYNDROME

The Laurence-Moon-Biedl (LMB) syndrome (Laurence-Moon-Biedl-Bardet syndrome, Bardet-Biedl syndrome, Biedl-Bardet syndrome) is a heritable disorder characterized by obesity, mental retardation, digital anomalies, hypogonadism, and retinal degeneration with pigmentary changes. The basic defect and the prevalence of the LMB syndrome are unknown. Over 400 cases have been recorded.

CLINICAL MANIFESTATIONS **Obesity** Usually truncal in location, obesity is present in at least 80 percent of patients with the LMB syndrome. It begins in childhood and increases in severity with advancing age.

Eyes Retinal degeneration occurs in over 90 percent, leading either to typical or atypical retinitis pigmentosa. The electroretinogram may be abnormal before clinical changes are evident. The earliest symptom often is night-blindness. Decreased visual acuity may be discovered at school age and is progressive, culminating in total blindness by age 30. Optic atrophy and congenital tapetoretinal blindness also occur in patients with the LMB syndrome.

Gonads Hypogonadism is present in at least 75 percent of males and 50 percent of females. In many instances gonadotropin levels are low, but primary gonadal failure also occurs.

Digits Anomalies are noted in about 80 percent. The most frequent finding is postaxial polydactyly in one or more extremities, but some have only syndactyly or brachydactyly.

Mental retardation Mild to moderate intellectual impairment is the usual finding. About a tenth of patients have severe retardation and another tenth have normal intelligence.

Kidney Kidney abnormalities ranging from mesangial tissue proliferation to glomerular sclerosis, interstitial scarring, and cyst formation with death from uremia may occur.

Other manifestations Congenital heart defects may occur. Brachycephaly or other skull anomalies have been described. In contrast to the Alstrom syndrome, diabetes mellitus and nerve deafness are infrequent in the LMB syndrome.

INHERITANCE The LMB syndrome is transmitted as an autosomal recessive disorder. There may be genetic heterogeneity.

DIFFERENTIAL DIAGNOSIS Since there is no specific test for the LMB syndrome, the diagnosis must be established clinically. This can be done with little difficulty in the presence of the five cardinal manifestations (obesity, mental retardation, polydactyly, retinal degeneration, and hypogonadism). However, the limits of the syndrome are poorly defined, and the diagnosis is often extended to patients with only some of these components. Variability in clinical expression occurs even among patients within the same family.

The patients originally described by Laurence and Moon had mental retardation, pigmentary retinal degeneration, hypogenitalism, and spastic paraplegia without obesity or digital anomalies. This is undoubtedly a different disorder from what is now usually called the LMB syndrome. (Thus, in a strict sense the LMB syndrome should be called the Bardet-Biedl syndrome.)

The LMB syndrome must be distinguished from syndromes bearing the eponyms Alstrom, Biemond, and Carpenter. Comparison with the Alstrom syndrome is discussed in the following section. The LMB, Biemond, and Carpenter syndromes are all characterized by hypogonadism, polydactyly, mental retardation, and autosomal recessive inheritance, but only LMB has been associated with retinal degeneration. The Biemond syndrome is distinguished by the presence of iris coloboma, and the Carpenter syndrome is characterized by acrocephalosyndactyly and peculiar facies.

ALSTROM SYNDROME

The Alstrom syndrome is a rare inherited disease with major involvement of the retina, ear, kidney, and endocrine glands. In childhood, the typical patient has obesity, moderately severe nerve deafness, and retinal degeneration with later pigmentary changes ("atypical retinitis pigmentosa") and blindness. In adulthood, carbohydrate intolerance and slowly progressive renal disease develop; obesity may disappear. Males often have an unusual form of primary hypogonadism in which normal secondary sex characteristics occur, despite small testes, low plasma testosterone, and elevated gonadotropin levels. Females lack evidence of hypogonadism, but menses are irregular. Other clinical manifestations include hyperuricemia, hypertriglyceridemia, acanthosis nigricans, baldness, scoliosis, and hyperostosis frontalis. Although signs and symptoms appear early in life, the correct diagnosis is usually not made until the third decade. Before that time cases may be classified as congenital blindness or deafness or the Laurence-Moon-Biedl syndrome.

Although the Alstrom and the Laurence-Moon-Biedl syndromes both have retinal degeneration, childhood obesity, and nephropathy, they can be distinguished clinically. Most noteworthy are the rarity of mental retardation and digital anomalies in the Alstrom syndrome and the rarity of nerve deafness and diabetes mellitus in the Laurence-Moon-Biedl syndrome. Furthermore, total blindness occurs in the Alstrom syndrome at about 7 years and in the Laurence-Moon-Biedl syndrome at about 30 years.

Although the Alstrom syndrome is inherited as an autosomal recessive, suggesting an abnormality in a single enzyme, the primary biochemical defect is unknown. Membrane thickening and hyalinization in the kidney, testes, and skin suggest that the basic abnormality involves an element in membranes common to these organs, the retina, neural apparatus of the ear, and perhaps, adipose tissue. Patients with the Alstrom syndrome are resistant to the action of at least three polypeptide hormones: insulin, vasopressin, and gonadotropins. This resistance may reflect membrane changes or degeneration of cells in the target organs.

REFERENCES

COLLINS E, TURNER G: The Noonan syndrome. J Pediatr 83:941, 1973
GOLDSTEIN J, FIALKOW PJ: The Alstrom syndrome. Medicine 52:53, 1973

PART FOUR | DISORDERS CAUSED BY BIOLOGICAL AND ENVIRONMENTAL AGENTS

section 1 | Important considerations in infectious disease

105

AN APPROACH TO INFECTIOUS DISEASES

ROBERT G. PETERSDORF

INTRODUCTION The vast majority of human and animal diseases of known etiology are produced by biologic agents: viruses, rickettsias, bacteria, mycoplasma, *Chlamydia,* fungi, protozoa, or nematodes. No small part of the past and present importance of infectious diseases in medical practice is attributable to their enormous frequency and the public health implications of their contagiousness. However, developments in sanitary engineering, vector control, immunization, and specific chemotherapy have modified the situation favorably. Although important exceptions remain, infectious diseases as a class are more easily prevented and more easily cured than any other major group of disorders. Despite the virtual elimination of certain infectious diseases such as smallpox and the profound reduction in the morbidity and mortality of many, humans are by no means free of infection. In fact, the total human load of disease produced by microbial parasites has decreased only modestly, primarily through smallpox and malaria control and better health care in developing countries. As certain specific microbial infections have been controlled, others have emerged as troublesome therapeutic and epidemiologic problems. With the introduction of cytotoxic drugs, massive irradiation in the treatment of malignant diseases, and immunosuppressive agents to control the rejection of transplanted organs, the insertion of prosthetic devices into the bloodstream, and the progressive longevity of people with chronic degenerative diseases, infections due to organisms previously considered saprophytic or commensal have increased. These infections have also been termed *opportunistic.* As Dubos has pointed out, microbial infections appear to form an inherent part of human life.

Because of better environmental sanitation and other measures that now prevent contact with many microbial agents, and the development of acquired immunity early in childhood, certain infections have been seen more frequently in adults. For example, as contact with poliomyelitis virus in childhood declined in many countries, paralytic poliomyelitis became more common in young adults. *Hemophilus influenzae* meningitis is being reported more frequently in adults than heretofore, and decreasing infection with the tubercle bacillus raises questions about the status of antituberculous immunity in adults. For reasons that are not clear, hepatitis A is predominantly a disease of young adults, while non-A, non-B hepatitis tends to occur in individuals over 35 years of age.

As antimicrobial agents reduce the mortality associated with certain common infections, other microbes emerge as important causes of human disease. If an infection occurs during or immediately following a course of chemotherapy, it is often caused by a microorganism that is resistant to the drug that was given; such an infection is termed a *superinfection.* While it is relatively unusual nowadays for patients to die of uncomplicated pneumococcal pneumonia, a disease readily handled with available antimicrobials, it is common to see serious disease produced by microorganisms which are much more resistant even though they are often part of the normal microbial flora in humans. These include staphylococci, gram-negative enteric bacilli, and a variety of anaerobes and fungi. One important mechanism by which resistance is conferred on gram-negative enteric bacteria is the action of R factors (Chap. 108).

THE PARASITE AND THE HOST The interaction between microorganism and humans that results in infection and disease is complex. Much has been learned about the way in which microbes enter the body, the ways in which they produce tissue injury, the influence of specific immunity and "nonspecific" resistance of the host, and the mechanisms of recovery. However, it is not yet possible to transfer in any specific way much of the information that has been acquired to the individual patient with an infection. In this and the subsequent chapter, those aspects of the host-parasite relationship that form the basis for diagnostic procedures, that are of importance in deriving therapeutic principles, or that help explain the epidemiology of infection are stressed.

INFECTION AND CLINICAL DISEASE It is well known that microorganisms of different species or different strains of the same species vary widely in their capacity to produce disease and that human beings are not equally susceptible to the disease caused by a given bacterium or virus. Furthermore, while a specific infectious disease will not occur in the absence of the causative organism, the mere presence of the organism in the body does not lead invariably to clinical illness. Indeed, the production of symptoms in humans by many parasites is the exception rather than the rule, and the *subclinical infection* or the "carrier state" is the usual host-parasite relationship. *Dis-*

ease in a clinical sense is not synonymous with the presence of the organism or *infection* in a microbiological sense. In fact, for most organisms the number of subclinical infections far exceeds that of clinical disease.

MECHANISMS OF INJURY It is customary to refer to bacteria or other microorganisms that are capable of producing disease as *pathogenic. Virulence,* the *degree* of pathogenicity, should be distinguished from *invasiveness,* the ability to spread and disseminate in the body. For example, *Clostridium tetani* is pathogenic and, by virtue of its exotoxin, highly virulent, but it is almost completely lacking in invasiveness. Moreover, in certain circumstances and in certain anatomic locations, mildly "pathogenic" organisms can produce fatal disease, or highly "pathogenic" species can multiply without producing any harmful effect.

A few parasites produce *toxins* that account for the tissue damage and physiological alterations of infection. *Hypersensitivity* to components of the parasite is demonstrable in several infections to account for the manifestations of disease. For many pathogenic agents, an explanation of their damaging effects upon the host is incomplete or wholly lacking. Generally, therefore, the aim of therapy is to stop multiplication or to kill the parasites with appropriate drugs; in diseases caused by toxin-producing organisms, the use of antiserum (as in tetanus or diphtheria) is the definitive procedure, and chemotherapy is of secondary importance.

The tendency of certain pathogenic organisms to *localize in certain cells or organs* and to produce disease in a specific anatomic site or evoke a combination of symptoms referable to certain organs often suggests the identity of the causative organism. For example, the pneumococcus usually causes infection in the lung but almost never in the kidney, and *H. influenzae* infections are confined almost solely to the respiratory tract and meninges. Similarly, in the presence of disease known to be caused by a given agent, complicating involvement of other tissues can be anticipated or predicted. Examples include the multiple lung abscesses which are so characteristic of hematogenously disseminated staphylococcal disease and the metastatic skin lesions which complicate *Pseudomonas* bacteremia.

Frequently, the proper management of infectious disease involves the use of techniques completely unrelated to microbiology or chemotherapy, in an effort to support the function of damaged organs. Survival in poliomyelitis may depend upon treatment of respiratory failure, the management of heart failure in endocarditis is sometimes a greater problem than the eradication of the causative organism, in cholera the repletion of the volume deficit and in Weil's disease the treatment of acute renal failure with peritoneal or hemodialysis are the important therapeutic objectives.

RESISTANCE AND SUSCEPTIBILITY Many so-called "host factors" are known to influence the likelihood that disease will occur if organisms enter the tissues, or to play a determining role in the outcome once the infection has become established. These include natural or acquired antibodies, interferon, properdin, phagocytic activity, and the level of the general inflammatory response, which is generally manifested by cellular activity such as chemotaxis, phagocytosis, and release of lysozomal enzymes.

In experimental animals, sex, microbial strain, age, route of infection, the presence of specific antibody, other diseases, nutritional state, and the use of such procedures as exposure to ionizing radiation or high environmental temperature or administration of mucin, nitrogen mustard, adrenal steroids, epinephrine, xerosin, and metabolic analogues can be shown to exert a profound effect on infection by bacteria, viruses, and other agents.

In humans, these factors are no less important, although controlled studies are lacking for many. Alcoholism; diabetes; deficiency or absence of immunoglobulins (Chap. 62); defects in cellular immunity (Chap. 65); malnutrition; chronic administration of adrenal hormones; chronic lymphedema; ischemia; the presence of foreign bodies such as bullets, calculi, or bone fragments; obstruction of a bronchus, the urethra, or any hollow tube; agranulocytosis or congenital defects in bactericidal or virucidal activity; various blood dyscrasias, and many other circumstances influence susceptibility to systemic or local infection. Furthermore, in those instances where the extenuating condition is remediable, the probability of recovery is enhanced.

Racial differences in susceptibility, such as the poor resistance of dark-skinned people to tuberculosis and their predilection for developing disseminated coccidioidomycosis, are well established. Resistance to infection may be determined genetically. The relation of sickle-cell trait to malaria is one example. The increased frequency and severity of some infections in children, of others in pregnant women, and still others in the aged are familiar.

Prior contact with an organism or its products, whether by active infection or by artificial immunization, increases resistance to some infections, such as measles, diphtheria, and pertussis by stimulating antibody production, but seems to have little influence on resistance to others, such as gonorrhea.

Knowledge of the factors involved in human resistance and susceptibility is incomplete. Explanations such as changes in physical or chemical activity of phagocytes; antibacterial substances such as lysozyme, phagocytin, or lysozomal enzymes; qualitative or quantitative alterations in serum proteins; disordered metabolism at the cellular level, "products of tissue injury" that influence vascular permeability, and the effects of tissue pressure remain to a considerable extent in the realm of hypothesis.

The profound influence of host factors upon the infectious process makes it clear, however, that their understanding is probably essential for the control of infections in predictable fashion.

PATHOGENESIS OF INFECTION With relatively minor variations, the development of an infectious disease follows a consistent pattern. The parasites enter the body through the skin, nasopharynx, lung, intestine, urethra, or other portal. A number of microorganisms adhere to their site of primary attack through fimbriae, pili, and surface antigens; the adherence of *Bordetella pertussis* to respiratory epithelium, the gonococcus to urethral epithelium, and possibly some gram-negative urinary pathogens to the epithelium of the renal pelvis are some examples. Once established in the host, the organisms can multiply and, in so doing, establish a local or primary lesion. From this site, there may be local spread along fascial planes or tubular structures, such as a bronchus or ureter. The next step may be systemic spread of the microorganisms via the circulating blood. Bacteria can enter the bloodstream by direct invasion of vessels, a relatively unusual occurrence, or more commonly by traversing peripheral lymph nodes to enter the thoracic duct lymph and thence the venous system. In the bloodstream, they spread to other tissues and can produce distant or secondary lesions. In infections such as tetanus and diphtheria, distant lesions are produced by toxins elaborated at the primary site without systemic spread of the parasites. The infectious process may terminate in recovery or death at any stage: the local lesion, systemic spread, or distant lesion.

The apparent inconsistency of this pattern in clinical medicine is attributable to the fact that the infection is recognized as a clinical entity only at the stage when symptoms are most likely to appear. For example, pneumococcal pneumonia is a local lesion, and the distant lesion, pneumococcal meningitis, is referred to clinically as a complication. In meningococcal infections, the local lesion, nasopharyngitis, is rarely symptomatic and has no status as a clinical entity, but the stage of spread, meningococcemia, and the commonest distant lesion, meningitis, are clinical entities. A rarer distant lesion, arthritis, is called a complication. In a patient who has osteomyelitis, a clinical entity, a recent furuncle may be referred to as a predisposing factor. In another patient with extensive furunculosis who develops osteomyelitis, the infection in bone may be regarded as a complication of the superficial infection. The stages mentioned are in no way limited to bacterial diseases; the primary lesion of poliomyelitis is intestinal, viremia may occur without neurological involvement, or a distant lesion manifested by symptomatic involvement of the central nervous system may be established.

Because clinical usage and terminology are based upon the symptomatic illness that leads patients to seek medical aid, the consistency of this general sequence in the pathogenesis of infection is often not recognized. However, the concept is useful and offers some basis for systematizing what may otherwise seem to be a miscellaneous collection of unrelated clinical signs and symptoms.

CLINICAL MANIFESTATIONS OF INFECTIONS So varied are the disorders attributable to infection or infestation of humans by lower organisms that generalizations about them are difficult. The clinical manifestations of infection can duplicate those of diseases of any other etiology. However, certain clinical features are highly suggestive of infection, including abrupt onset, fever, chills, myalgia, photophobia, pharyngitis, acute lymphadenopathy and splenomegaly, gastrointestinal upset, and leukocytosis or leukopenia. It is obvious that the presence of one, several, or all of these features does not constitute proof of the microbial origin of illness in a given patient. Conversely, serious, even fatal, infectious disease may exist in the absence of fever or other signs and symptoms.

Although there is no infallible clinical criterion of infection, it it still possible to recognize accurately many specific infectious diseases from information obtained by *history, physical examination, blood count, and urinalysis.* The importance of interrogation about past illness, predisposing factors such as alcoholism, familial disease, exposure to ill persons, contact with animals or insects, ingestion of contaminated food, type and order of onset of symptoms, and recent or remote residence in endemic areas is discussed in the subsequent chapters that deal with specific diseases and etiologic agents. Cardinal physical signs are also described for each entity.

The mechanisms that produce most of the signs and symptoms of human infection are unknown. The pathogenesis of fever is discussed in Chap. 9. The physiological alterations underlying "malaise," "postinfectious asthenia," "toxicity," and other common complaints are completely mysterious. The factors responsible for leukocytosis or leukopenia are only partially understood (Chap. 56). Why the rash of typhus begins on the trunk while that of another rickettsiosis, Rocky Mountain spotted fever, begins on the extremities is unanswered. Failure to understand these manifestations does not impair their clinical usefulness, although it is probable that understanding them might lead to more accurate diagnosis and better management.

DIAGNOSTIC PROCEDURES The specific procedures for the diagnosis of infectious disease have become sufficiently complex to warrant separate discussion. This is provided in Chap. 106.

Importance of specific diagnosis in infectious diseases The diagnostic procedures employed for infectious diseases are no more absolute than those in other diseases; they cannot be blindly equated with the science of microbiology. The responsibility for interpreting the facts supplied by the bacteriologist, immunologist, and virologist in the total context of a patient's illness remains that of the physician. A positive tuberculin skin test certainly does not indicate that a patient has active tuberculosis. The finding of *Candida albicans* in a stool culture does not necessarily mean that a patient's diarrhea is caused by intestinal candidiasis. The presence of staphylococci in nasal cultures from a patient with headaches does not establish a diagnosis of staphylococcal sinusitis. A throat culture containing group A beta-hemolytic streptococci does not rule out diphtheria, nor does such a culture establish that a febrile illness in a patient with mitral stenosis is a recurrence of acute rheumatic fever rather than bacterial endocarditis. A positive serologic test for syphilis may be the first sign of lupus erythematosus.

The etiologic agent From a practical point of view, two important steps are vital to the correct diagnosis of infection: (1) the organ(s) or organ systems involved must be found, and (2) the etiologic agents causing the infections must be identified precisely. Chapter 106 deals with the diagnostic approaches that are available. Most of the remaining chapters in this part take up the specific bacteria, spirochetes, fungi, rickettsias, viruses, *Mycoplasma,* and Protozoa which cause infections. The common syndromes caused by these agents are described either in chapters dealing with specific organisms or in chapters dealing with infections in individual organ systems such as pneumonia (Chap. 260), bacterial endocarditis (Chap. 243), urinary tract infections (Chap. 280), osteomyelitis (Chap. 360), and meningitis (Chap. 368).

When confronted with specific organ involvement, it is important to know the most common pathogens which cause disease in the involved organ. Table 105-1 provides a listing of those pathogens. Used in conjunction with the individual chapters dealing with specific agents and the summary of chemotherapy (Chap. 111), the table should provide a rational guide to treatment which often must be instituted before the results of antimicrobial sensitivity tests are available.

CHEMOTHERAPY The impact of chemotherapy upon mortality and morbidity from infection and upon epidemic disease is a matter of record. These therapeutic agents, however, have in no way lessened the importance of specific diagnosis; indeed, their availability has increased the need for obtaining exact etiologic information. It requires but a moment's reflection to realize that the substitution of a prescription for a broad-spectrum antibiotic or a quick injection of penicillin for the systematic collection of facts and thoughtful consideration of diagnostic possibilities is a fallacious, unwise, and dangerous practice. Numerous antibiotics with overlapping spectra are now available, dosages for different infections vary widely, the drugs themselves are potentially dangerous, and their administration entails considerable expense. They should never be prescribed as placebos, antipyretics, or substitutes for diagnosis. In the vast majority of instances in which this is done, patients recover just as they would if no "therapy" had been given, and the drugs are wasted. More importantly, an inadequate dosage of a drug or the wrong agent may suppress symptoms temporarily without achieving cure and may make isolation of the etiologic agent difficult, delay recognition of the true nature of an illness, and postpone the institution of curative treatment. Furthermore, antibiotics may select out resistant variants or facilitate the transfer of R factors between pathogenic and commensal enterobacteria. Resistant variants can then replace sensitive strains and pose the additional hazard of spread to others. Finally, to expose a patient to the risk of a drug reaction without proper indication is inexcusable, whether the drug is an antibiotic, a sedative, a laxative, or a narcotic.

EPIDEMIOLOGIC AND OTHER CONSIDERATIONS Just as the decision to administer antibiotics to a patient with a febrile illness of presumed infectious etiology must be made on an individual basis, the selection of cases in which extensive cultural and serologic testing is required is a matter of judgment. The majority of common grippe-like illnesses subside spontaneously, and symptomatic treatment is sufficient. However, because of this tendency toward spontaneous recovery and also because the results of serologic tests may not be available until after recovery has taken place, the effort to determine the specific etiology of illness is often considered an impractical, "academic" procedure. Such an attitude fails to recognize that in addition to the individual patient, the welfare of the community must be considered. For example, a clinical diagnosis of "virus pneumonia" may turn out, following serologic tests, to be psittacosis. Although the "index" patient may have recovered completely, others in the community may be at risk until the "pet parakeet" which was the source of the illness has been eliminated.

Pursuing the diagnosis of obscure, often self-limited, illnesses may be academic, but this approach has led to clarification of some important etiologic relations. For example, the syndrome of infectious mononucleosis has been linked with development of antibody to a herpes-like virus, the EB virus (Chap. 195); some cases of erythema multiforme may be due to herpes simplex virus; several patients with encephalitis have been found to have central nervous system infections with myxoviruses. Some congenital anomalies have been related to prenatal viral infections; this relationship is well known for rubella (Chap. 182), but a number of other viruses (CMV, varicella, herpes simplex) have been implicated, although with less certainty. The finding of bacteria-like bodies in the intestinal mucosa of patients with Whipple's disease and the improvement of these patients with tetracycline therapy provides another example of an entity of unknown etiology entering the realm of infectious diseases. Patients with sarcoidosis have been shown to have high titers against herpes-like virus, similar to patients with infectious mononucleosis, Burkitt's lymphoma, and carcinoma of the posterior nasal space. The relation of these viruses to these diseases is not clear; suffice it to say, these associations raise some interesting possibilities concerning the lymphocytic system and virus infections. Along the same vein, the possibility has been raised that the Chédiak-Higashi syndrome, a rare familial disorder characterized by albinism, photophobia, nystagmus, anomalous cellular granules, marked susceptibility to infection, and development of lymphoma, is caused by a virus.

TABLE 105-1
The syndromic approach to treatable infections

Type of infection	Etiologic agents		
	Common	Relatively common	Unusual but important
Skin and subcutaneous tissue	*Staphylococcus aureus*	*Streptococcus pyogenes, Candida,* and superficial fungi	Gram-negative bacilli (burns, wounds)
Sinusitis	*Streptococcus pneumoniae S. aureus*	*S. pyogenes, Hemophilus influenzae*	Mucorales
Pharyngitis	Respiratory viruses, *S. pyogenes*	Gonococcus	*Corynebacterium diphtheriae*
Epiglottitis	*H. influenzae*		
Otitis, mastoiditis	*S. pneumoniae, H. influenzae* (children)	*S. aureus, S. pyogenes*	*Pseudomonas, Proteus*
Pneumonitis	*S. pneumoniae, Mycoplasma pneumoniae, Mycobacterium tuberculosis*	*S. aureus, Klebsiella-Enterobacter,* respiratory viruses, *Legionella pneumophilia*	*S. pyogenes,* gram-negative enteric bacilli, psittacosis, systemic fungi, *Pneumocystis, H. influenzae, Pasteurella multocida*
Empyema and lung abscess	*S. aureus,* anaerobic streptococcus, *Bacteroides, Fusobacterium*	*Klebsiella* (abscess)	
Bacterial endocarditis	*Streptococcus viridans, S. aureus,* enterococcus	*S. pneumoniae,* anaerobic streptococci	*Pseudomonas, Candida, Staphylococcus epidermidis*
Gastroenteritis	*Salmonella, Shigella,* enteric viruses	*S. aureus, Escherichia coli* (enterotoxic), clostridia, *Giardia*	*Pseudomonas, Entamoeba histolytica, Vibrio cholerae, V. parahemolyticus*
Peritonitis, cholangitis, intraabdominal abscess	*E. coli,* enterococcus, *Bacteroides,* anaerobic streptococcus, *Fusobacterium*	*Klebsiella-Enterobacter, Proteus* species	Clostridia, *S. aureus*
Urinary infection (cystitis, pyelonephritis)	*E. coli, Klebsiella-Enterobacter,* paracolon, *Proteus,* enterococcus	*Pseudomonas*	*S. aureus*
Urethritis	Gonococcus, ?*Mycoplasma, Chlamydia,* ?*Acinetobacter* (*Mima-herellea*)	*Treponema pallidum*	
Pelvic inflammatory disease	Gonococcus, *E. coli Bacteroides,* anaerobic streptococci, *Chlamydia*	*Klebsiella-Enterobacter,* enterococcus, *Fusobacterium*	Clostridia, *S. aureus*
Bones (osteomyelitis)	*S. aureus*	*Salmonella*	*S. pyogenes*
Joints	*S. aureus,* gonococcus, *S. pneumoniae, H. influenzae*	*S. pyogenes, Neisseria meningitidis*	
Meninges	*S. pneumoniae, H. influenzae, N. meningitidis*	*E. coli, Klebsiella-Enterobacter, Proteus, Pseudomonas*	*S. pyogenes, M. tuberculosis, Cryptococcus, S. aureus, Listeria monocytogenes*

This association, among others, relates the field of infection to that of oncogenesis.

Legionnaires' disease (Chap. 138) is the most striking example, demonstrating the importance of identifying the causative organism of an infection definitively. By dint of hard "shoe leather" epidemiology and by application of the most advanced microbiologic techniques available, an important new organism has been identified and steps to contain it have been instituted.

Similar results can be expected from other "academic procedures" which may have little immediate applicability to infection in a particular patient. Yet, just as was the case with Legionnaires' disease, organisms that seem to have little biological significance at present may assume practical importance in the future.

REFERENCES

BURNET M: *Natural History of Infectious Disease,* 4th ed. New York, Cambridge, 1972

CLUFF LE, JOHNSON JE III: *Clinical Concepts of Infectious Diseases,* 2d ed. Baltimore, Williams & Wilkins, 1978

DAVIS BD et al: *Microbiology,* 2d ed. New York, Harper & Row, 1972

DUBOS RJ: *Biochemical Determinants of Microbial Disease.* Cambridge, Harvard, 1954

————: *The Evolution of Microbial Diseases: Bacterial and Mycotic Diseases of Man,* 4th ed. Philadelphia, Lippincott, 1965, p 20

HORSFALL FL, TAMM I: *Viral and Rickettsial Infections of Man,* 4th ed. Philadelphia, Lippincott, 1965

WILSON GA, MILES AA: *Topley and Wilson's Principles of Bacteriology and Immunity,* 6th ed. Baltimore, Williams & Wilkens, 1975

106
THE DIAGNOSIS OF INFECTIOUS DISEASES

JAMES J. PLORDE
ROBERT G. PETERSDORF

The diagnosis of an infectious disease requires the direct or indirect demonstration of a pathogenic microbe on or within the tissues of the afflicted host. This is accomplished in four steps:

1 *Test selection.* The selection of appropriate laboratory tests begins with the performance of a careful history and physical examination. This is followed by the establishment of a provisional etiologic diagnosis based on that examination and consultation with the laboratory concerning the most efficient methods available for confirming the diagnosis.
2 *Specimen collection and transportation.* Detailed written instructions on the appropriate methods for the collection, transportation, and labeling of biological specimens must be available, and these instructions must be followed explicitly by the clinical staff. Failure to do so may result in the contamination of the specimen with normal flora during the process of collection, death of pathogenic microbes during delayed or defective transportation, and/or specimen mix-up during laboratory processing.
3 *Testing.* The clinical microbiology laboratory has a large number of testing procedures available for demonstrating the presence of pathogens within clinical specimens. These include visualization of the organisms by direct microscopic examination of exudates, body fluids, and tissues; cultivation of the organisms in artificial media, tissues, or experimental animals; demonstration of microbial antigens or

their by-products and the demonstration of characteristic host responses to the invading organism such as specific antibody formation or histological reactions.
4 *Data interpretation.* The mere demonstration of a potential pathogen is not prima facie evidence of its etiologic significance. It may represent a member of the patient's normal microbial flora or a contaminant introduced at the time the specimen was collected or processed. Similarly, high titers of specific antibody in the serum may represent a serologic response to resident flora or past exposure to a pathogenic microbe rather than evidence of a current infection.

SPECIMEN COLLECTION

SPECIMEN TYPES The diagnostic value of a culture specimen depends to a large extent on the likelihood that it has been collected free of contamination with either the transient or resident microbial flora. Specimens can be divided into three major categories based on the site from which they are collected.

Deep closed body areas Specimens obtained from closed, normally sterile, body areas are the most satisfactory for bacteriologic examination. Examples include the deep tissues, the vascular and subarachnoid spaces, pleura, peritoneum, and joints. If the specimen is collected by surgical excision or closed needle aspiration following careful disinfection of the overlying skin surface, the likelihood of contamination is small. The recovery of either aerobic or anaerobic organisms under such conditions is strong evidence that they are of pathogenic significance.

Deep communicating body areas As with the areas just mentioned, the lower respiratory tract, bladder, endometrium, and bone are normally devoid of a resident bacterial flora. Usually, however, specimens from these areas are collected only after they have been spontaneously ejected through a communicating pathway such as the oropharynx, urethra, cervix, or a sinus tract. These are invariably heavily contaminated with bacterial flora, including large concentrations of anaerobes. For this reason, these specimens are generally not suitable for anaerobic culture, and even the growth of aerobic or facultative organisms must be interpreted with caution. In many instances the degree of contamination can be lessened by disinfecting the area around the orifice (e.g., periurethra, cervix), cleansing the pathway (e.g., midstream urine), or aspirating through a sterile tube inserted into the pathway. Moreover, true pathogens can, at times, be distinguished from contaminants by their number (e.g., quantitative urine culture) or species (*Staphylococcus aureus* vs. *S. epidermidis*). Nevertheless, areas of confusion cannot be totally eliminated. As a result, cultures from these areas are seldom as reliable as those from deep closed areas unless collection techniques which bypass the colonized pathway, such as transtracheal or suprapubic aspiration, are employed.

Skin and mucous membranes The mouth, throat, gastrointestinal stomata, fissures, and fistulas, and superficial wounds such as decubitus ulcers are heavily contaminated with both transient and permanent organisms. Culture of these areas is unlikely to be helpful unless:

1 There is gross pus.
2 A specific bacterial pathogen that strongly suggests disease is being sought, such as *Salmonella* or *Shigella* from the stool, or *Neisseria gonorrhoeae* from the urethra or vagina.

3 The base of the lesion can be aspirated through normal adjoining skin or biopsied after disinfection of the lesion's surface. The use of swabs is much less satisfactory. The resulting sample size is small, and organisms are exposed to the drying environment of the air. Moreover, the unsaturated fatty acids present in cotton swabs are often toxic to microbes. If swabs are to be used, this inhibitory activity may be minimized by treating the swab with serum or charcoal. Alternatively, the cotton may be replaced with a synthetic fiber such as calcium alginate which is less toxic and is soluble in salt solutions. If the swab is to be used on a dry surface, it should first be moistened in a sterile fluid such as saline or broth. Swab cultures are not satisfactory for recovery of anaerobic bacteria or fungi.

DISINFECTION When specimens from deep closed lesions are collected, the site of percutaneous needle aspiration should be cleansed first by using 70% isopropyl or ethyl alcohol and then disinfected with a 2% tincture of iodine or an appropriate iodophor. The iodine is applied in a concentric fashion beginning at the site of aspiration and allowed to act for 1 to 2 min before the aspiration is performed. The area should not be probed or manipulated unless sterile gloves are worn or the involved fingers have also been disinfected. If the initial attempt at collection fails, subsequent efforts should be carried out with a new needle through a freshly disinfected site. At the completion of the procedure the iodine should be removed with alcohol to avoid the danger of sensitization. If the specimen for culture is drawn through an indwelling cannula, the site of withdrawal must be disinfected in the same fashion.

When specimens are to be collected from the uterus, a draining wound, or sinus tract, the orifice must be thoroughly cleansed and disinfected as described above, a sterile intravenous catheter or multilumen tube is introduced as deeply as possible through the orifice, and the specimen aspirated into a sterile syringe. Culture from an open lesion may be collected by biopsy, aspiration from the margin, or by swabbing the surface. In the first two situations the wound is prepared as for a deep closed lesion. For swab cultures, the wound surface is cleansed only with sterile saline to remove debris and saprophytic flora.

TRANSPORTATION All specimens submitted for microbial culture should be transported to the laboratory as rapidly as possible, preferably within 1 h. Delay beyond this time may result in death of fastidious organisms, overgrowth of contaminants, and/or change in the number of bacteria unless special procedures are employed to overcome these problems. Rapid transportation is particularly important when dealing with blood, body fluid, and exudates which may harbor pathogenic *Neisseria* or anaerobes. The container should be clean, sterile (stool specimens excepted), and appropriately labeled. Respiratory secretions, urine, large pieces of tissue, and large volumes of fluid can be safely transmitted in plastic containers with leakproof lids. Aspirates are conveniently and safely transported in the same syringe used in the collection procedure, providing all air is expressed from the syringe and the needle is capped with a sterile holder. Alternatively, such fluid may be injected into a sealed gassed-out vial suitable for transport of anaerobic specimens. If such vials are used, it is important that the indicator in the vial be checked to ascertain whether it is still colorless. A pink or blue color indicates the presence of oxygen and suggests that the vial is no longer adequate for the transport of specimens for anaerobic culture. Small pieces of tissue (less than 1 cm²) are transported best in sterile rubber-stoppered gassed-out tubes. After the anaerobic

indicator is checked, the tube is held upright to minimize the loss of the heavy inert gas, the stopper removed, specimen inserted, and the tube recapped.

Swabs submitted for the culture of group A beta-hemolytic streptococci can be transported in dry sterile test tubes. All other swabs should be submitted in one of several commercially available transport media. These prevent both the desiccation of organisms implanted on the swab and the overgrowth of hardy organisms at the expense of more fastidious ones. Although special anaerobic transport materials are available, use of swab cultures for the recovery of such organisms is not encouraged.

SEROLOGIC STUDIES Although blood is the specimen most commonly examined for the presence of antibody, a variety of other fluids including cerebrospinal, pleural, peritoneal, and joint fluids may be examined under appropriate conditions. Because a rise or fall in antibody titer is more significant than the absolute level, it is usually helpful, and often necessary, to obtain a specimen during both the acute and convalescent phases of illness. The optimum interval between these two specimens averages 10 to 14 days but varies with both the type of antibody being measured and the etiologic agent. The volume should approximate 5 ml whenever possible; much smaller specimens are sufficient for certain types of procedures. The testing laboratory should be consulted for details. Whenever possible the blood should be collected aseptically; if whole blood is required for the test, the specimen should be drawn into a tube containing anticoagulant. When the specimen is to be transported to another institution for testing, a preservative which does not influence the outcome of the serologic test should be added to inhibit bacterial contamination. Alternatively the specimen can be lyophilized or, in some cases, simply dried on filter paper before it is dispatched.

VIROLOGIC SPECIMENS The selection of specimens for the diagnosis of viral illness depends on both the stage of the disease and its clinical presentation. If the patient is seen early in the course of illness, frequently it is possible to demonstrate viral antigen in body tissue or fluids and/or to recover the virus by appropriate culture techniques. If the patient is seen later, during the recovery or convalescent stages, the diagnosis is often best established by serologic means. The type of specimen submitted for culture and the method of specimen transport depend to some extent on the nature of the illness. Throat swabs are helpful in the diagnosis of most viral infections. Because respiratory viruses are extremely labile, the swabs are placed in a buffered, high-protein transport medium containing antibiotic agents. If the specimen is to be transported to another institution, the specimen should be stored at −60°C and shipped on dry ice.

Cerebrospinal fluid from patients presenting with meningitis or encephalitis can also be submitted for culture. As with throat swabs, these specimens should be stored at low temperatures and shipped on dry ice. Stool should be collected in patients with respiratory illnesses, meningitis, or encephalitis, if either adenoviruses or enteroviruses are thought to be involved. Since these organisms are hardy, the feces can be collected in any sterile screw-top bottle and dispatched without refrigeration. Urine cultures are seldom helpful except in the diagnosis of cytomegalovirus infections. Vesicular fluid is a rich source of virus and viral antigen in patients presenting with exanthems. Pericardial fluid may be of help in patients with myocarditis or pericarditis. Viral blood cultures are seldom useful except in the diagnosis of arboviral infections. Isolation techniques for these viruses are highly specialized and are not available in most virus laboratories. Buffy coat cultures for cytomegalovirus and herpesvirus may be of help in immunosuppressed patients. Brain biopsy is the best single method for diagnosing *Herpes simplex* encephalitis (Chap. 193). The biopsy specimen should be placed in a sterile screw-top bottle and stored and dispatched in the frozen state.

LABORATORY PROCEDURES

DIRECT MICROSCOPIC EXAMINATION The direct microscopic examination of body fluids, exudates, and tissues is both the simplest and one of the most helpful laboratory procedures available for the diagnosis of infectious diseases. In many situations the examination allows an accurate, highly specific identification of the causative agent. Examples include the recognition of *Borrelia* or *Plasmodium* species in blood smears taken from patients with relapsing fever or malaria. At times only a tentative identification can be made on the basis of microbial morphology. Nevertheless, this is often sufficiently precise to allow the selection of an appropriate chemotherapeutic agent pending the results of more definitive investigations. A variety of techniques are used in direct microscopy. If the agent being sought is sufficiently large or characteristic, the specimen can be prepared as an unstained wet mount and examined by light-field, dark-field, or phase contrast microscopy. More commonly, a dried smear is made; this allows the application of a variety of stains which assist the visualization and identification of the microbe in question. The smear is prepared in a way that spreads tissue and inflammatory cells evenly in an undamaged monolayer over the glass slide. After drying, the smears are fixed, stained, and examined with a light, fluorescent, or electron microscope.

Wet mounts Dark-field examination of fluid from genital lesions for the spirochete of syphilis is a well-known, but neglected, procedure. More often, wet mounts are used for the diagnosis of fungal and parasitic infections. The examination of hair fragments, skin scrapings, or nail clippings is useful in establishing the presence of superficial mycoses. The specimens are placed in a drop of 10% KOH, a cover slip added, the preparation cleared by heating, and the mount examined under low-power magnification for the presence of hyphae and arthrospores. At times, as for tinea versicolor infections, the fungous elements will be sufficiently characteristic to allow the specific identification of the causative agent. Occasionally a presumptive diagnosis of a systemic fungous infection can also be established with this procedure. Two examples are cryptococcal meningitis by demonstrating the encapsulated organism in an India ink preparation of cerebrospinal fluid, and coccidiodomycosis by finding characteristic spherules in expectorated sputum.

Examination of saline or iodine mounts of stool or duodenal drainage is also the initial first step in establishing the diagnosis of intestinal protozoal infections such as amebiasis and giardiasis. Moreover, it is the definitive procedure diagnosing intestinal helminthic infections including ascariasis, trichuriasis, strongyloidiasis, and hookworm. Finally, filariasis and sleeping sickness can be recognized by demonstrating the characteristic motility of microfilariae and trypanosomes in blood or other body fluids.

Stain-enhanced microscopy Despite many recent technical advances in the field of microbiology, Gram's stain remains, after 90 years of use, the best single technique available for the rapid diagnosis of bacterial infections. It can be applied to virtually all clinical specimens and is of particular value in the examination of exudates, aspirates, body fluids, including cerebrospinal fluid, and urine. Gram's stains should be examined first under the lower-power objective to demonstrate the presence of pink-staining inflammatory cells. The paucity of such cells in the presence of many squamous epithelial cells suggests that the specimen was contaminated during the process of collection and may not be representative of the inflammatory process. After the evaluation under low-power objective, the smear is then examined for the presence of bacteria using the oil immersion lens; bacteria will appear either as dark blue (gram-positive) or pink (gram-negative) bodies. Their color and morphological appearance often make possible a presumptive identification of the genus and occasionally the species with a significant degree of accuracy. The demonstration of pneumococci in the sputum, Enterobacteriaceae in the urine, staphylococci in localized abscesses, gonococci in urethral exudates, clostridia in foul-smelling discharge, and pneumococci, meningococci, or *Hemophilus influenzae* in stained smears of the cerebrospinal fluid permits the initiation of specific chemotherapy with the assurance that the regimen is the proper one. In some immunosuppressed patients *Candida* blastospores and pseudohyphae can be found in blood smears several days before candidemia is demonstrable by culture.

A variety of other stains are available for the demonstration of specific microbes. Mycobacteria have the unique capacity to resist the decolorization by strong mineral acid alcohol solutions once they have been stained with basic carbol-fuchsin or one of the fluorochromes. This allows their immediate recognition in body tissues and fluids. The presence of a large number of acid-fast bacilli in the expectorated sputum establishes the presumptive diagnosis of respiratory tuberculosis and is sufficient evidence for initiating isolation procedures and antituberculosis therapy once additional specimens are collected for culture. Subsequent examination of the sputum with acid-fast stains is an important element in monitoring the success of therapy. The traditional Ziehl-Neelsen and Kinyoun stains are now being supplanted by the fluorochromes which allow a much more rapid scanning of smears using relatively low magnification.

Acid-fast smears can also be used to identify pathogenic strains of *Nocardia* if mineral acid rather than acid-alcohol is used for decolorization. When an even weaker decolorizing agent such as organic acid is used, organisms such as *Actinomyces* may also be visualized.

Both Giemsa's and iodine stains may be used to diagnose chlamydial infections involving the eye, urethra, or cervix. When epithelial cells obtained by scraping these areas are stained with Giemsa's stain, a typical semilunar dense inclusion body composed of many blue- or purplish-staining particles is seen adjoining the nucleus of the cell. Iodine stains reveal a similar reddish brown mass in scrapings from the eye but are not useful in cervical specimens.

A number of stains are available for the definitive identification of parasites. *Pneumocystis carinii* can be recognized in transbronchial brush biopsies using a modified Wright's stain, toluidine blue, or methenamine silver. The latter produces a very distinctive black-stained cyst. Blood and tissue protozoa such as plasmodia and *Leishmania* can be demonstrated best with Romanowsky-type mixtures containing methyline blue and eosin. These render the nuclei red to violet and the cytoplasm blue. The identification of intestinal protozoa, on the other hand, requires the use of stains such as iron hematoxyline or trichome to demonstrate the taxonomically important nuclear detail.

Immune microscopy This method combines the specificity of immunologic procedures with the speed of direct microscopy. In the immunofluorescent technique, smears thought to contain viral, bacterial, fungal, or parasitic organisms are stained with specific antibody preparations labeled with fluorescent compounds and examined with a fluorescent microscope. At present, the most useful application of this technique is the examination of brain tissue for Herpes simplex or rabies virus; lung tissue, pleural fluid, and sputum for the Legionnaires' disease bacillus; and cervical, urethral, and conjunctival scrapings for trachoma-inclusion conjunctivitis agent.

Direct fluorescent antibody staining of nasal epithelial cells may also be used for the rapid diagnosis of influenza, parainfluenza, and respiratory syncytial virus infections.

Finally, the direct immunofluorescence technique for detecting antibody-coated bacteria in the urinary sediment has been useful in distinguishing kidney from bladder infection in females.

Unfortunately, the need for expensive fluorescent microscopes, the poor quality of many of the commercially available conjugated antiserums, and the need for well-trained technologists restrict the routine use of these procedures to reference laboratories.

Enzyme-linked immunoabsorbent assay (ELISA) tests are similar to the immunofluorescence test except that the antiserum is reacted with a peroxidase-labeled antispecies conjugate. After treatment with appropriate reagents, the peroxidase assumes a dark-brown color that can be visualized with the ordinary light microscope, obviating the need for expensive equipment. Its potential application in the diagnosis of a wide variety of infectious diseases is obvious, but its final role in clinical microbiology remains to be established.

Electron microscopy The electron microscopic examination of vesicular fluid or scabs of patients with febrile exanthems allows a very rapid differentiation of varicella-zoster infections from smallpox. This technique also has been useful in the identification of certain viral infections which do not produce cytopathic effects in cell cultures. It has been particularly valuable in the detection of rotaviruses in the stool specimens of infants and small children suffering from gastroenteritis. The large number and characteristic appearance of these virus particles allow specific identification to be made on morphological grounds alone. Electron microscopy has also been used in the diagnosis of the so-called "winter vomiting disease" caused by the Norwalk and Hawaii agents. These agents are morphologically similar to those of the picornavirus group, and specific identification requires aggregation of the virus particles with immune serum. This technique of immune electron microscopy may have wide application in virology and has been used to identify virus-like particles associated with non-A, non-B hepatitis in experimental animals.

CULTURE Despite the time and complexity, the isolation of the etiologic agent by cultivation in artificial media, tissue cultures, or animals is generally the most definitive diagnostic procedure available. When laboratory confirmation of the presence or absence of a specific microorganism such as *Streptococcus pyogenes, Corynebacterium diphtheriae, Salmonella,* or *Shigella* is needed, artificial media specifically designed to recover these organisms are employed. More commonly, however, the laboratory is asked to screen for the presence of any potential bacterial pathogen. In that situation, the specimen is inoculated on a variety of artificial media designed to recover the most commonly encountered pathogens. Differential media, which allow demonstration of certain biochemical characteristics of isolated organisms, and selective media, which inhibit the growth of resident microbes, are commonly included in this initial battery. Special media may be required to recover rare or unusually fastidious microbes, such as *Listeria, Leptospira,* and *Brucella.* The appropriate selection of such media

requires close and constant communication between the clinical and laboratory staffs.

For most purposes, the specimen is inoculated onto a small area of solid medium contained in a petri dish and then is distributed over the remainder of the medium's surface with a sterile bacteriologic loop. If this procedure is performed appropriately, the bacterial growth will appear as isolated colonies. These can then be characterized morphologically, subcultured in pure form, identified biochemically, and tested for their sensitivity to antimicrobial agents. In addition, this inoculation procedure allows an estimate to be made of the quantity of organisms present in the original specimen. This is usually recorded in the semiquantitative fashion, but in the case of urine, blood, and occasionally other specimens, the inoculum size can be measured precisely and the total number of colonies enumerated. The clinical significance of bacterial growth must be evaluated both qualitatively and quantitatively. The isolation of certain bacterial pathogens such as *N. gonorrhoeae, Salmonella,* and *Shigella* almost always indicates disease. The isolation of most bacterial pathogens, however, is of questionable significance unless (1) the gross and microscopic appearance of the specimen suggests that it was adequately collected, (2) the bacterial species in question is present in large numbers on both the Gram's stain and culture media, and (3) the organism represents the predominant bacterial species grown.

Although it is often necessary to initiate chemotherapy prior to the availability of culture results, it is mandatory that treatment not be started until the culture specimens have been collected.

There are new developments in identification of a wide variety of viruses in tissue culture, and refinements of these techniques are increasing the value of tissue culture in clinical diagnosis. Many viruses can also be isolated by the inoculation of appropriate animals. This is rarely feasible for ordinary clinical diagnosis, and for several agents it is hazardous. Animal inoculation has also been used for several nonviral infections, including rat-bite fever, certain mycoses, tuberculosis, and some rickettsioses. Although this is a cumbersome procedure for routine use, it may need to be employed with appropriate precautions in selected instances.

DETECTION OF MICROBIAL ANTIGENS AND THEIR BY-PRODUCTS The relative nonspecificity of many direct microscopic methods and the delay inherent in culture procedures have resulted in the introduction of a variety of techniques aimed at the rapid detection of microbial antigens or their by-products.

Counterimmunoelectrophoresis The most widely used of these techniques is counterimmunoelectrophoresis (CIE). In this variation of the agar gel diffusion test, the specimen being tested for antigen is placed in an agar well and specific antiserum in a second apposed well. An electric current is then passed through the agar resulting in rapid confluence of antigen and antibody with the formation of a precipitant within a matter of minutes. CIE has proved most useful for the rapid diagnosis of bacterial meningitis in childhood where the cerebrospinal fluid is checked for the presence of pneumococcal, meningococcal, group B streptococcal, or *H. influenzae* antigens. The technique has approximately the same order of sensitivity as Gram's stain but has the advantage of heightened specificity. CIE has also been used for the detection of the above-mentioned bacterial antigens in serum, pneumococcal capsular antigens in sputum, and the detection of rotavirus and enterovirus in stool.

Latex agglutination This test has been utilized in many of the same situations as CIE. Although greater sensitivity has been claimed for latex agglutination, the test is plagued by false-positive reactions from heat labile serum components and rheumatoid factor. Perhaps its greatest usefulness has been in the detection of cryptococcal antigen in the spinal fluid of patients with chronic meningoencephalitis.

Radioimmunoassay The most spectacular application of this technique is in the detection of hepatitis B surface antigen–associated (HBsAg-associated) infection and in the prevention of such infections by the screening of blood and blood products for the presence of the antigen. This procedure is highly sensitive, and results can be obtained within a few hours with commercially available test kits. In this method HBsAg-labeled ^{125}I competes with antigen in a test serum for a specific antibody in the test mixture. Free and bound antigens are separated by washing. The reactivity of the antigen-antibody complex is then analyzed with a gamma counter.

Gas chromatography This method involves the direct examination of clinical specimens by gas liquid chromatography for the detection of characteristic microbial by-products. It has been thought helpful in differentiating aerobic from anaerobic organisms in pus and blood. It has also been used to differentiate staphylococcal, streptococcal, and gonococcal from traumatic arthritis and to detect *Candida* in the blood of patients with fungemia. Although the role of gas chromatography in the identification of anaerobic bacteria is established, its usefulness in the direct analysis of clinical specimens remains to be determined.

IMMUNOLOGIC METHODS These diagnostic methods are intended to supply evidence of past or present infection by demonstrating antibodies in serum or other body fluids, by indicating changed reactivity of the host (hypersensitivity, allergy) to products of the organism, or, rarely, to detect components of the causative organism in the body.

Serologic tests The finding on a single occasion that a patient's serum contains antibody which reacts with a certain antigen merely indicates that the patient has had previous contact with the antigen or a closely related substance. For this reason, with rare exceptions, the clinical interpretation of serologic tests depends on serial determinations. If the antibody titer is found to *rise or fall significantly,* the response likely is a result of recent contact with the antigen. In subsequent chapters, the need for serologic testing of acute phase and convalescent serum is emphasized repeatedly. *In any patient with a puzzling illness, a sterile specimen of serum should be preserved in a frozen state so that it can, if necessary, be studied and compared with serum collected at a later date.*

Prior contact with an antigen may be the result of past immunization with vaccines; interpretation of serum agglutinin titers for typhoid bacilli is often made difficult by prior immunization. The so-called "anamnestic reaction," a nonspecific stimulation of antibody formation by an acute illness (e.g., a rise in *Brucella* agglutinins in a patient with acute tularemia), occurs only when the two organisms are antigenically related, and rarely presents a serious problem.

The methods employed for detecting antibody rises in various infections have been selected empirically on the basis of the ease with which the test can be performed and careful study to correlate the results of the test with other diagnostic criteria in patients. Therefore, the fact that antibodies against one agent are detected by a precipitin technique, another by agglutination of whole organisms or the production of capsular swelling, another by indirect fluorescent-antibody methods, and still another by complement fixation is a practical matter and bears no necessary relation to the agent, the type of infection, or its pathogenesis. By coating some particulate material, such as erythrocytes or latex, with antigen derived from a cer-

tain organism, antibody can sometimes be demonstrated by an agglutination test rather than by some more complex method.

Particular properties of the causative organism can sometimes be utilized to devise a simplified clinical test for antibody. Two striking instances of this are widely used. The ability of influenza and related viruses to clump erythrocytes makes possible the demonstration of antibody to virus by merely testing the capacity of a patient's serum to prevent the agglutination of red blood cells by suspensions of virus, the so-called "hemagglutination-inhibition" reaction. Similarly, because many microorganisms possess hemolytic components or toxins, the assay of a patient's serum for capacity to prevent lysis of red blood cells is a convenient and simple clinical test for antibody. The antistreptolysin O test in group A *S. pyogenes* infections is an example of this.

In a few infections, predominantly those caused by viruses, the only reliable serologic test is a *neutralization or protection* test, an assay of the protection afforded by the patient's serum against active infection in tissue culture or in experimental animals. This technique is time-consuming and is usually performed only in diagnostic virology laboratories.

Some mention of "nonspecific" serologic changes may serve to emphasize again that clinical laboratory tests have come into use *only because they have been found to correlate reasonably well with clinical findings.* In several diseases it has been found, often accidentally, that serum antibody develops which will react with antigens derived from sources other than the etiologic agent (which may actually be unknown). Common examples are heterophil agglutinins in infectious mononucleosis, cold agglutinins in mycoplasma pneumonia, and the agglutination of certain strains of *Proteus* bacilli by serum of patients with rickettsial diseases. The VDRL test for syphilis and related flocculation tests are performed with antigens derived from sources completely unrelated to *Treponema pallidum.*

The results of serologic tests must be interpreted in the light of other information about the patient, including such factors as previous immunizations and illnesses, the possibility of exposure to chemically but etiologically unrelated antigens, and the importance of a changing titer in serial tests as opposed to a single isolated observation.

Skin tests Exposure to antigens of certain types, by various routes, and under circumstances not completely understood often results in the development of immediate (anaphylactic, atopic) hypersensitivity or delayed (bacterial, tuberculin) hypersensitivity.

Active infection with some, but not all, bacteria and viruses results in delayed hypersensitivity to the infecting agent in some, but not all, individuals. Clinically, this allergic state is detected by intradermal injection of the organism or one of its components; in a sensitive individual, induration and erythema will appear at the local site within 24 to 48 h. If an individual is highly "sensitive" or if the amount of antigen injected is excessive, there may be extensive local inflammation with necrosis, vesicle formation, edema, regional lymphadenopathy, and even malaise and fever. Antigens prepared in concentrations unlikely to provoke severe reactions are generally available for intradermal testing for tuberculosis, leprosy, mumps, lymphogranuloma venereum, cat-scratch disease, chancroid, brucellosis, tularemia, glanders, toxoplasmosis, blastomycosis, histoplasmosis, coccidioidomycosis, and many other infections. The immune reaction to vaccination (Chap. 184) is also an example of delayed dermal hypersensitivity.

The reliability, specificity, and usefulness of the individual tests differ and are discussed in the chapters on specific infections. However, certain general principles apply to their use and interpretation:

1 They are highly useful in epidemiologic surveys as indicators of the incidence of infection in a population.
2 In most individuals, dermal reactivity persists for many years or for life. A single positive test means only that at some past time the individual was infected with the organism (or a closely related one). Unless supplementary information in the form of clinical findings, cultural studies, or more specific serologic data bear out the presence of active infection, a diagnosis of the disease is not justified.
3 The appearance of a positive dermal reaction in an individual known to have been nonreactive a short time before is good evidence of recent infection; this is a useful method for detecting tuberculosis.
4 *A negative intradermal test does not rule out past or present infection.* For unknown reasons, patients with measles, Hodgkin's disease, or sarcoidosis often develop a state of *anergy,* or inability to react to intradermally injected antigens. In several diseases, dermal sensitivity develops after weeks or months of infection; an important example is acute histoplasmosis, in which patients can be ill for many weeks without showing a positive skin test. The skin test to coccidiodin is always negative in disseminated coccidioidomycosis; in far-advanced or miliary tuberculosis in elderly patients, failure to react to intradermal tuberculin in the usual amounts employed for testing occurs in as many as 10 to 15 percent of the cases.

Intradermal injection of antigens derived from sources other than microorganisms usually produces an immediate *wheal and erythema* reaction which subsides promptly. The greatest clinical usefulness of this type of reaction is in the detection of allergy to foreign serums, pollens, and animal dander (Chap. 65). The skin tests for demonstrating infestation with helminths (trichinosis, filariasis) produce reactions of the immediate type in allergic individuals, but many of the antigens employed are so nonspecific that they are of little use in diagnosis.

INTERPRETATION AND REPORTING

As the number, cost, and complexity of laboratory procedures increase, so does the need for the clinical laboratory to assist the physician in the selection of tests and in the interpretation of their results. Such consultations can decrease unnecessary testing, avoid inappropriate antimicrobial therapy, and increase the speed and effectiveness of therapy when it is indicated. One important aspect of such consultation is the immediate interpretation of Gram's stain smears because this can be helpful in selecting appropriate antimicrobial agents or in suggesting the need to collect a second more satisfactory specimen prior to the beginning of therapy.

The laboratory should provide the physician with information on the results of all cultures within 24 h and the significance of both positive and negative results for each specimen. Failure of the culture to grow within this time interval may result in recommendations for further testing or occasionally for discontinuation of therapy. Polymicrobial growth on aerobic cultures can also lead to further testing using better collection techniques. Finally, the identification of the organism and its likely susceptibility to antimicrobial agents often can be surmised accurately on the basis of colonial morphology and rapid biochemical testing.

The clinical laboratory may choose not to report certain data if they are likely to be misleading. For example, the laboratory may choose not to report the susceptibility of an orga

nism to a given antimicrobial agent if there is a contraindication to the use of that agent for treatment of the infection in question.

MANAGEMENT OF SPECIFIC SPECIMENS

UPPER RESPIRATORY TRACT Because the throat and nasopharynx are normally heavily colonized by both saprophytic and potentially pathogenic bacteria, culture of this area is seldom useful except when a particular bacterial pathogen is being sought, e.g., *S. pyogenes, Bordetella pertussis, C. diphtheriae,* meningococci, or gonococci.

Throat cultures When throat cultures are submitted to the laboratory without specifying the pathogen being sought, the laboratory will generally report only the presence or absence of *S. pyogenes.* Since a single properly obtained throat swab will detect at least 90 percent of patients with streptococcal pharyngitis, a negative culture is very helpful in excluding the possibility of this disease. Similarly, a heavy or predominant growth of group A beta-hemolytic streptococci in patients presenting with the signs and symptoms of streptococcal pharyngitis is highly predictive of an antibody response to streptococcal antigens and, therefore, presumably disease. It is far more difficult to interpret cultures with a light or nonpredominant growth of *S. pyogenes.* A large proportion of these patients do not mount an appreciable immunologic response, suggesting that bacterial growth represents a carrier state.

Throat cultures may not be indicated in adults presenting with sore throat if they lack fever, cervical lymphadenopathy, or recent exposure to another patient with streptococcal pharyngitis since fewer than 5 percent of this population have positive cultures. Conversely, adults with temperatures of 38°C or higher, tender cervical lymphadenopathy, or pharyngeal exudate are so frequently culture positive that immediate antibiotic therapy is more cost effective than waiting for the result of culture.

Mouth cultures Usually massively mixed flora of aerobic and anaerobic bacteria is present in mouth cultures, and they are not clinically useful except when a careful attempt to avoid contamination with indigenous flora has been made. This is particularly true for the isolation of *Actinomyces israelii.* This organism is part of the normal oropharyngeal flora, and the time and effort required for its isolation is not justified unless an uncontaminated specimen can be provided.

LOWER RESPIRATORY TRACT Although culture of expectorated sputum is the most frequently employed technique for the diagnosis of lower respiratory tract infections, both its sensitivity and specificity are open to question. Studies of patients with bacteremic pneumococcal pneumonia have shown the etiologic agent to be present in the sputum in only 50 to 94 percent of cases. Moreover, expectorated sputum is almost always contaminated with oropharyngeal flora including, in many cases, bacterial species commonly associated with pulmonary infections. Even when a potential pathogen is recovered, its role in the causation of a lower respiratory tract infection is uncertain. Attempts to remove saliva and nasal secretions from the sputum by repeated washing or to differentiate upper and lower tract organisms on the basis of quantitative sputum culture have been ineffective or unacceptably tedious. Some confusion can be avoided if the specimen is collected appropriately and screened carefully for both gross and microscopic characteristics prior to inoculation of the culture. Ideally, sputum specimens should be collected early in the morning under direct supervision of a physician or respiratory therapist. If the patient is unable to produce sputum, coughing may be stimu lated by lowering the head of the patient's bed for a few minutes or exposing the patient to an aerosol of warm hypertonic saline.

Because sputum is rarely homogeneous, it should be examined carefully for bits of pus and blood. These should then be used to prepare a Gram's stain smear which is examined for the presence of squamous epithelial cells (SEC) and leukocytes under the low-power objective (10×) of the microscope. If there are fewer than 10 SEC and greater than 25 leukocytes per field, the results of the culture are more likely to represent lower tract flora. This is particularly true if a single or clearly predominant bacterial type grows, or, in the case of chronic obstructive pulmonary disease, if both pneumococci and *H. influenzae* are isolated. If squamous epithelial cells number more than 10 per low-power field, the specimen can be considered heavily contaminated with oropharyngeal flora and should be discarded. In most cases a second carefully collected expectorated sputum will yield a satisfactory specimen.

Direct endotracheal or endobronchial aspiration may be employed when a satisfactory expectorated sputum cannot be produced. However, such specimens are subject to contamination by oropharyngeal flora which is introduced during the passage of the aspiration instrument. Fiberoptic bronchoscopy, which allows the direct visualization and aspiration of bronchial secretions, is a relatively inocuous procedure and may result in a somewhat better specimen. When possible, however, bronchial brushings or biopsy material should be obtained, because they are less likely to be diluted with topical anesthetics or saliva.

Alternatively, the specimen may be collected by a technique that totally bypasses the oropharynx. The most widely used is transtracheal aspiration. This method entails a definite risk of hemoptysis, subcutaneous and mediastinal emphysema, vagal discharge, or respiratory embarrassment and is contraindicated in the presence of a bleeding diathesis. It should be used only when results from expectorated sputum are unsatisfactory and the infection is severe enough to merit the attendant risks. The technique produces a more reliable sputum specimen than either expectoration or bronchoscopy and is probably the only satisfactory method for collecting specimens for anaerobic culture. However, some 20 percent of specimens from patients without clinical evidence of pneumonia yield potential respiratory pathogens. These "false positive" specimens are primarily from patients who have chronic pulmonary disease, who have recently suffered minor bouts of aspiration, or in whom the tip of the catheter was coughed into the hypopharynx during the collection procedure.

Needle aspiration of a pulmonary infiltrate under fluoroscopic control also produces specimens of excellent quality. The percutaneous method gives both a high yield and accurate results but has at least a 5 percent chance of complications, particularly pneumothorax. The morbidity risk is greater than with transtracheal aspiration biopsy, but the diagnostic yield may be superior.

Whatever technique is used to sample the lower respiratory tract, the physician should always obtain a concomitant blood culture. If a pleural effusion is present, it should also be aspirated and cultured.

In addition to bacterial pathogens, pneumonia can be caused by viruses, *Rickettsia, Chlamydia, Mycoplasma pneumoniae,* and Legionnaires' disease bacillus. Techniques for the recovery of these agents from the sputum are generally not available in a routine clinical microbiology laboratory, and the diagnosis is most frequently made by clinical and/or serologic methods. Legionnaires' disease bacillus can be cultured from lung tissue or empyema fluid. In addition, it can be demonstrated by direct fluorescent antibody staining in both of these specimen types and in transtracheal aspirates. This allows early diagnosis and rapid institution of appropriate therapy. For discussion of the techniques used for the recovery of mycobacteria and fungi from the lower respiratory tract, the sections devoted to these organisms should be consulted.

URINE CULTURES Voided urine, like expectorated sputum, is usually contaminated with the normal microbial flora, in this case from the urethra and external genitalia. Urine cultures, however, are more reliable than those of expectorated sputum, because the periurethral area can be disinfected and the urethra itself flushed with the first portion of the urine stream before a sample is taken. In addition, quantitation of the bacterial growth is helpful in separating contaminated specimens from true infection. In general, bacterial counts exceeding 100,000 organisms per milliliter of urine indicate true bacteriuria while those less than 10,000 organisms per milliliter reflect contamination with perineal or urethral flora. Before a high bacterial count can be accepted as evidence of infection, however, the following factors need to be considered: (1) the adequacy of the disinfection procedures, (2) the sex of the patient, (3) the interval between specimen collection and plating, and (4) the number of bacterial species isolated. It is important that patients be carefully instructed in the techniques of collecting clean voided specimens or that the collection be supervised by a trained attendant. In brief, the foreskin of males must be retracted completely; in females the labia must be separated widely. The periurethral area is repeatedly cleansed with an appropriate disinfectant and then rinsed with warm sterile water. Following this, the patient voids. After the first 20 to 25 ml is discarded, the specimen is caught directly in a sterile container without interrupting the stream. The cup should be held in a way to avoid contact with the legs or perineal area. When this procedure is followed conscientiously, a single specimen from a male which yields a colony count in excess of 100,000 organisms per milliliter is highly indicative of bacteriuria. In women, the colony count must exceed 100,000 organisms per milliliter in two consecutive urine specimens before infection can be considered to be present. Because urine is a good culture medium, contaminating organisms will multiply to large numbers if the urine is allowed to stand at room temperature for prolonged periods of time. For this reason, specimens which cannot be dispatched to the laboratory within an hour should be refrigerated. They can be held at 4°C for 4 to 6 h without an appreciable change in the bacterial colony count. In most instances, urinary tract infections are caused by a single bacterial species. The isolation of three or more species in a urine culture usually reflects contamination even when the colony count is high. True polymicrobial bacteriuria does occur but is generally restricted to patients with chronic indwelling urethral catheters. In contrast, colony counts of less than 100,000 organisms per milliliter may sometimes represent true bacteriuria. In fact, up to one-third of urinary tract infections are associated with counts in the range of 10,000 to 100,000 organisms per milliliter. This is particularly true of specimens from male patients or patients receiving antimicrobial therapy, and of specimens obtained by ureteral or urethral catheterization and by suprapubic aspiration.

When an adequate clean-voided urine specimen cannot be obtained, or when anaerobic cultures are desired, suprapubic aspiration may be employed. Specimens obtained in this manner are unlikely to be contaminated, and even slight growth may be significant. When an indwelling catheter is in place, a specimen should be collected directly from the catheter by means of a sterile needle and syringe after careful disinfection of the exterior surface. Urine should not be taken from the drainage tube or bag, because these are frequently contaminated. Occasionally Foley catheter tips are submitted to the laboratory for culture when a catheterized patient shows signs or symptoms of urinary tract infection. Statistical analysis has shown this practice to be both futile and potentially misleading.

Examination of a Gram's stain smear of uncentrifuged urine is often helpful in the rapid diagnosis of urinary tract infection. The presence of many squamous epithelial cells and mixed bacterial flora indicates contamination and the need for another specimen. In the absence of the epithelial cells, the presence of one or more bacterial cells per oil immersion field usually indicates true bacteriuria especially when accompanied by one or more leukocytes.

BLOOD CULTURES Because of the peculiar clinical importance of demonstrating bacteria in the bloodstream and because there are varying opinions about optimal timing and sites of sampling for blood cultures, it is of practical importance to understand something about the mechanisms of bacteremia.

Excepting intravascular infections (bacterial endocarditis or endarteritis, mycotic aneurysm, suppurative thrombophlebitis), bacteria usually enter the circulation through the lymphatic system. Consequently, when bacteria multiply at a site of local infection in the tissues, the likelihood of bacteremia parallels the occurrence of local conditions that favor drainage of lymph from the infected area to the thoracic duct and eventually to the venous blood. These factors include the number and anatomic arrangement of local lymph vessels, accumulation of fluid, increase in tissue pressure, and manipulation of the part.

Once bacteria enter the blood, they are removed rapidly by the fixed phagocytes of the reticuloendothelial system in the liver, spleen, and bone marrow and by engulfment in polymorphonuclear leukocytes in capillaries, especially those of the lung.

Clinically, bacteremia can be transient, intermittent, or continuous. Many transient bacteremias result from manipulation of infected or contaminated tissues, common examples being instrumentation of the genitourinary tract, tonsillectomy, dental procedures, and massage or surgical incision of furuncles or abscesses. In the vast majority of instances, the sudden discharge of bacteria into the blood produces no symptoms or, at most, a rigor and brief fever, and the organisms are promptly removed. The great danger of these "man-made" bacteremias is their role in producing bacterial endocarditis in patients with endocardial damage or intracardiac prostheses.

Transient bacteremia accompanies the early phase of many infections. In pneumococcal pneumonia, the typical rigor at the onset is a result of transient bacteremia. In most cases, with localization of the pulmonary lesion, blood cultures rapidly revert to negative. The poor prognosis of patients with pneumonia who continue to have positive blood cultures is not due to the presence of organisms in the blood but reflects spreading infection in the lung itself.

A sudden single influx of microorganisms into the bloodstream may be followed by a shaking chill and fever. However, there is a "lag period" of 30 to 90 min before the febrile response. During this delay, the bacteria are usually promptly removed from the circulation by phagocytosis; consequently, a blood culture taken at the time of the rigor may be negative.

Continuous bacteremia is a feature of the first several days of typhoid fever, of brucellosis, and of intravascular infections such as endocarditis or endarteritis.

Blood cultures should be obtained from all febrile patients who have rigors, are seriously ill, are thought to have endocar-

ditis or intravascular infection, or are immunosuppressed. If viremia, fungemia, brucellosis, tularemia, leptospirosis, or an infection with cell wall–deficient bacteria is suspected, the laboratory should be contacted for special instructions. In general, three blood cultures taken at intervals of no less than 60 min are adequate to document the presence of bacteremia in an adult. In emergent situations, two cultures taken simultaneously from different anatomic sites will usually suffice. In patients who have received antimicrobial agents within the previous 2 weeks or in whom endocarditis is suspected, a total of six cultures taken over a 2-day period may be useful. If the patient is receiving antimicrobial agents, the cultures should be taken immediately prior to the next dose, and the laboratory should be notified to allow the addition of penicillinase and/or extensive dilution of the blood specimen. The collection of specimens over and above the number listed above is seldom helpful in detecting occult bacteremia unless the culture procedures, media, or conditions of incubation are altered to allow detection of fastidious organisms.

Specimens are best collected by percutaneous venipuncture. If possible, aspirations from the femoral vein should be avoided since disinfecting the skin of the groin is often difficult. The increasingly common practice of drawing blood for culture through an indwelling intravascular cannula often results in a higher level of contamination without substantially improving the detection of bacteremia. Similarly there is no evidence that arterial blood cultures possess any advantage over venous cultures. Bone marrow cultures may reveal the etiologic agent when it cannot be obtained by other means in occasional patients with disseminated salmonellosis, tuberculosis, and deep mycoses.

To minimize the chance of contamination with skin flora, the site of aspiration should be carefully disinfected as described in "Management of Specific Specimens" above. Following aspiration, the blood should be inoculated into both aerobic and anaerobic broths immediately. The dilution ratio of blood to broth should be at least 1:10 to minimize the normal bactericidal activity of serum and the activity of any antimicrobial agents that may be present. If direct inoculation into broth is not feasible, the blood may be drawn into a sterile Vacutainer tube containing sodium polyethanol sulfanate (SPS). This anticoagulant is anticomplementary and inactivates leukocytes and certain aminoglycoside and polypeptide antibiotics. Nevertheless, it will not delay bacterial death indefinitely, and Vacutainer specimens should be sent to the laboratory for dilution in broth within 30 min of the time the blood is drawn. If fungemia is suspected, the laboratory should be notified since the standard techniques described above are less satisfactory for the isolation of fungi. The yield can be improved by the use of a large inoculum of blood in a Castaneda-type biphasic medium of brain-heart infusion agar and broth which is incubated for up to 4 weeks.

Gram's stain examination of buffy coat smears is seldom indicated. Although a number of microorganisms, particularly meningococci and staphylococci, can be detected within granulocytes in approximately 4 percent of submitted blood culture specimens, the procedure is time-consuming and seldom of therapeutic value. It may be justified if fungemia is suspected. The toxicity of amphotericin B therapy precludes initiation of treatment without strong evidence of systemic fungal infection. Because these organisms often require 4 to 5 days to grow, a positive buffy coat smear would be of obvious therapeutic importance.

Approximately two-thirds of blood cultures from bacteremic patients are found to be positive within 24 h and 90 percent within 3 days. Despite strict adherence to disinfectant procedures on the ward and sterile technique in the laboratory, contamination occasionally occurs. The following are characteristics of "false-positive" blood cultures: (1) pour plates are seldom positive, (2) repeat cultures are seldom positive for the same organism, (3) bacterial growth in broth generally occurs after 3 days of incubation, and (4) the organisms are often identified as diphtheroids, *Bacillus*, or *S. epidermidis*. However, any of these species can occasionally be responsible for true bacteremia, particularly in immunosuppressed patients.

CEREBROSPINAL FLUID   Examination of the CSF from patients suspected of having meningitis represents one of the major emergency procedures faced by the clinical microbiology laboratory. Bacterial meningitis can be rapidly fatal if treatment is delayed or inadequate, and appropriate therapy often requires specific identification of the etiologic agent. Because of the clinical urgency, CSF specimens should be collected as soon as the diagnosis is considered, and the specimen promptly transported to the laboratory. The laboratory should be notified if the specimen has been collected from an abscess within the CNS to ensure that it is cultured both aerobically and anaerobically. If possible, at least 2 ml CSF should be obtained and the specimen sent for glucose, quantitative protein level, and cell count in addition to microbiologic studies. A simultaneous blood sugar also should be drawn for correlation with the CSF glucose level. Fastidious organisms, particularly *N. meningitidis,* may not survive prolonged storage at temperatures below that of the body. If a delay in CSF examination cannot be avoided, specimens should be held at 37°C.

After receipt, the specimen is concentrated by centrifugation or filtration, Gram stained, and cultured aerobically. The inflammatory response in the CSF is helpful in distinguishing acute bacterial meningitis from nonbacterial forms of the disease. In bacterial meningitis, polymorphonuclear leukocytes predominate, while in tuberculous, fungal, or protozoal meningitis, the inflammatory cells usually consist of lymphocytes, and the response is less intense. Although polymorphonuclear leukocytes may dominate early in the course of aseptic meningitis, there is usually a clear shift to mononuclear cells within 8 h. Cytologic changes in the CSF may also be seen in patients with brain abscess. However, smears and cultures are generally negative in these cases unless the abscess ruptures into the subarachnoid space or into the ventricles. The Gram's stain smear of the CSF should be examined carefully for stainable organisms, particularly meningococci, pneumococci, *Enterobacteriaceae, Listeria,* and staphylococci in patients with atrioventricular shunts. Stainable, but nonviable, organisms in the CSF are fairly common and may result in a "false-positive" Gram's stain. In addition, in cases of partially treated bacterial meningitis there is a tendency for gram-positive organisms to stain gram-negative.

When a large number of organisms is present and specific antiserums are available, the etiologic agent can often be rapidly identified by the quellung reaction or a precipitin test. Counterimmunoelectrophoresis is even more sensitive and may be positive when the Gram's stain is not. Moreover, detection of microbial antigens in the CSF by CIE is often the only method of identification of an infectious agent from a patient with partially treated meningitis. In the presence of a significant number of mononuclear cells without stainable bacteria, encapsulated cryptococci or cryptococcal antigen can be identified with the India ink preparation or latex agglutination tests, respectively.

Regardless of the results of these studies, the CSF must be cultured and any resulting growth identified to the species level. Mycobacterial and fungal cultures should be set up on patients who present with chronic meningitis and a mononuclear inflammatory response in the CSF.

Naegleria filaria, the cause of amoebic meningoencephalitis, can often be recognized by its amoeboid movements in wet-mount preparations of cerebrospinal fluid. This organism

should be looked for in patients who develop hemorrhagic meningoencephalitis during the summer months (Chap. 199).

GASTROINTESTINAL INFECTIONS   Cultures of the mouth, periodontal lesions, or saliva usually yield a mixed flora of aerobic and anaerobic organisms including *A. israelli* and *Candida* spp. The isolation of these organisms is without significance unless the specimen was collected in a way which avoided contamination with indigenous flora. If actinomycosis is suspected, the laboratory should be contacted for special instructions. The diagnosis of oral thrush and Vincent's infection can be made with stained smears from scrapings of the suspected lesion.

Cultures of ileostomy or colostomy stomata, gastrointestinal fistulas, and rectal fissures invariably grow both aerobic and anaerobic intestinal flora. They are seldom helpful, therefore, unless a search is made for specific intestinal pathogens.

Fecal cultures are helpful in determining the etiology of diarrhea and in detecting carrier states. Such specimens are routinely cultured for species of *Salmonella, Shigella,* and *Arizona.* Many laboratories are now also looking for *Vibrio parahemolyticus, Yersinia enterocolitica,* and *Camphylobacter fetus.* There is at present no convenient and reliable method of identifying enterotoxogenic strains of *E. coli* in the clinical laboratory. The physician should indicate whether any of these, or any other unusual infection such as antibiotic-associated pseudomembranous enterocolitis, candidiasis, clostridial food poisoning, or cholera, are suspected.

Although rectal swabs are adequate for the diagnosis of bacterial diarrhea, they are less satisfactory for the detection of carrier states. If swabs are used, they should show obvious soiling and be sent to the laboratory in appropriate transport media. Whole stool should be collected free of urine, placed in clean waxed cardboard cartons, and promptly dispatched to the laboratory. If delivery cannot be made within 1 h, the stool should be preserved in phosphate-buffered glycerol to prevent death of fastidious organisms such as *Shigella* spp. It is seldom necessary to submit more than three consecutive daily specimens. Isolated pathogens should be identified both serologically and biochemically before the final report is issued. It is important, however, that the physician be notified as soon as a potential pathogen has been isolated.

GENITAL TRACT   Genital specimens are submitted primarily for the diagnosis of venereal disease including gonorrhea, syphilis, chancroid, trichomoniasis, and chlamydial infections. Instructions for the collection of specimens should be sought in the sections of the text dealing with these specific diseases. In addition to the venereal pathogens, a number of organisms may infect the endometrium, tuboovarian tissues, and vagina. Endometrial cultures must be collected through a double or triple lumen tube inserted through a decontaminated cervical os if contamination with vaginal and cervical flora is to be avoided. The specimens should be delivered to the laboratory in either a gassed-out vial or a sealed syringe to ensure recovery of anaerobic organisms. When a patient presents with vaginitis, a specimen is collected by swabbing the vaginal fornix under direct visualization. If trichomoniasis is suspected, the swab should be placed in a small amount of sterile saline and sent to the laboratory immediately. If the swab is received within 10 to 15 min, the organism can be identified without difficulty by its characteristic motility in a wet-mount preparation. Cultural examination should focus on the recovery of agents thought capable of causing vaginitis such as *H. vaginalis,* group B beta-hemolytic streptococci, and *Candida albicans.*

EXUDATES AND BODY FLUIDS Pus from undrained abscesses as well as pericardial, pleural, peritoneal and synovial fluids is best collected by syringe and needle aspiration through disinfected skin. Prior rinsing of the syringe with a sterile anticoagulant such as heparin or SPS will help prevent formation of clots. Because anaerobic organisms are commonly involved in infection of these areas, the syringe should be sealed and sent immediately to the microbiology laboratory. Alternatively, the aspirate may be injected into a gassed-out anaerobic transport vial. The use of swabs is not encouraged since the sample size is small and fastidious organisms including anaerobes are unusually susceptible to desiccation and oxidation. Deep suppurative lesions which communicate with the surface of the body through fistulas or sinus tracts present a difficult problem in specimen collection. The communicating pathway is generally colonized by a wide variety of bacterial flora which contaminate drainage being ejected through the fistula opening. The degree of contamination can be lessened in many instances by carefully disinfecting the orifice and aspirating material via a sterile plastic catheter inserted deep into the sinus. Even when these precautions are taken, however, sinus tract cultures often fail to correlate well with pathogens isolated from operative specimens. For this reason, a bacteriologic diagnosis of draining suppurative lesions should be based on a culture of currettings or biopsy rather than sinus drainage. If actinomycosis is suspected, the draining sinus tract may be covered with gauze which is left in place until it is thoroughly saturated. The gauze is then submitted to the laboratory where it is carefully examined for the presence of granules which can be picked out and then identified.

SKIN, SOFT TISSUE, AND SUPERFICIAL WOUNDS Specimens collected from these areas are usually heavily contaminated with the normal flora of their respective sites. Swab cultures should be obtained only if gross pus is present or if the physician wishes to confirm the presence or absence of only a single bacterial pathogen, such as *C. diphtheriae;* in this case, the wound should first be cleansed mechanically with saline to remove as much exudate as possible. Material from bullae and areas of cellulitis is best obtained with a syringe. Successful aspiration of an area of cellulitis may require initial injection of a small amount of sterile saline. It is important that this solution not contain a preservative which may affect the viability of some bacteria. Alternatively, a punch biopsy may be obtained of the area after appropriate disinfection. Similarly, cultures from open lesions may be obtained by biopsy or by aspirating from the margins of these lesions using a syringe and needle. Semiquantitative cultures of burn eschars are useful in identifying patients at risk of bacteremia.

Intravenous and intraarterial catheter tips are best collected by disinfecting the area of the skin penetrated by the catheter, carefully withdrawing the catheter, and aseptically cutting off its tip into a sterile container. The tip is then delivered to the microbiology laboratory where semiquantitative cultures are done. In general, catheter tips which are contaminated during removal will have only a few colonies on agar plates, while infected catheter tips will show heavy growth.

REFERENCES

BARRY AL: Clinical specimens for microbiologic examinations, in *Infectious Diseases*, 2d ed, PD Hoeprich (ed). Hagerstown, Md, Harper & Row, 1977

———— et al: Microscopic examinations in infection, in *Infectious Diseases*, 2d ed, PD Hoeprich (ed). Hagerstown, Md, Harper & Row, 1977

BARTLETT RC: Control of cost and medical relevance in clinical microbiology. Am J Clin Path 64:518, 1975

DOLAN CT et al: *Proceedings of the 1975 Aspen Conference on Clinical Relevance in Microbiology.* Chicago, College of American Pathologists, 1977

EISENBERG HD et al: Collection, handling and processing of specimens, in *Manual of Clinical Microbiology*, 2d ed, EH Lennette et al (eds). Washington, DC, American Society for Microbiology, 1974

NEU HC: What should the clinic expect from the microbiology laboratory? Ann Intern Med 89:781, 1978

107
INFECTIONS IN THE COMPROMISED HOST

DAVID C. DALE

DEFINITION An individual who is abnormally susceptible to infections is called a *compromised host.* This heightened susceptibility often is attributable to specific abnormalities in host defense mechanisms (e.g., leukocytes, immunoglobulins, complement, mucosal and epithelial barriers, tissue vascular supply), alterations in normal surface bacteria caused by antibiotics, or the insertion of a foreign body (e.g., endotracheal tube, artificial heart valve, shunt, or catheter) (Table 107-1).

HOST DEFENSE MECHANISMS The skin and mucous membranes are the principal barriers which prevent invasion of the body by microorganisms. A variety of bacteria, including *Staphylococcus epidermidis, Streptococcus pyogenes,* and *Corynebacterium acnes,* inhabit the superficial layers of the normal skin. The mucosal surfaces of the upper respiratory tract, the lower gastrointestinal tract, and lower urinary tract are also in constant contact with bacteria, whereas the lower respiratory and upper urinary tracts are normally free of microorganisms. The subcutaneous tissues are protected from infection by the tough stratum corneum and antimicrobial substances derived from the sweat and sebaceous glands. Mucus in the respiratory and gastrointestinal tracts, together with secretory immunoglobulin (IgA), lysozyme, lactoferrin, α-antitrypsin, and bacteriocins produced by the normal bacterial flora serve to prevent colonization of the mucosal surfaces by new organisms. Bacteria and foreign debris are constantly swept toward the body orifices by the ciliated epithelial cells lining the mucosal surfaces. Normally a constant, low-grade exudation of leukocytes to these surfaces provides added protection.

If an organism penetrates a body surface and enters the tissues, a series of host responses occurs. An inflammatory exudate containing immunoglobulins, complement components, and other plasma proteins quickly appears. If the immunoglobulin is specific for the invading organism, it attaches to the bacterial cell wall, opsonizes the organism, and activates the complement system via the classic pathway. If specific immunoglobulin is lacking, the C3 component of complement will serve to opsonize the organism and facilitate phagocytosis. Complement activation also generates chemotactic factors which attract neutrophils, monocytes, and eosinophils to the inflammatory site (Chap. 56).

Normally within 1 to 3 h, neutrophils have begun to accumulate at a site of inflammation anywhere in the body, and they continue to arrive until the invading microbes are killed and eliminated, or a chronic inflammatory reaction consisting of monocytes, lymphocytes, and macrophages has developed. When infection spreads from the tissues to the blood, the circulating organisms ordinarily are removed by cells of the fixed mononuclear phagocytic system in the lungs, liver, spleen, and bone marrow.

TABLE 107-1
Infections in the compromised host

	Disease	Infection	Etiologic agents
HUMORAL DEFECTS			
Antibody deficiency	Bruton's X-linked agamma-globulinemia, multiple myeloma, chronic lymphocytic leukemia, Waldenstrom's macroglobulinemia, Wiskott-Aldrich syndrome, ataxia telangiectasia, isolated IgA deficiency	Sinusitis, bacterial pneumonia, bacteremia	*S. pneumoniae, H. influenzae, G. lamblia*
Complement deficiency	C3 deficiency, C5 deficiency, other isolated complement factor deficiencies, systemic lupus erythematosus, sickle-cell anemia	Otitis, sinusitis, pneumonia, bacteremia	*S. aureus, E. coli, Pseudomonas, N. gonorrhoeae*
PHAGOCYTIC DEFECTS			
Neutropenia	Agranulocytosis, acute leukemia, aplastic anemia, cyclic neutropenia, cytotoxic drug therapy, Chédiak-Higashi syndrome	Cellulitis, pharyngitis, perirectal abscess, pneumonia, bacteremia	*S. aureus, E. coli, Pseudomonas, Candida, Aspergillus*
Chemotactic defects	Chédiak-Higashi syndrome, diabetes mellitus, rheumatoid arthritis	Cellulitis, abscesses, septic arthritis, skin ulcers	*S. aureus, S. pyogenes*
Phagocytic defects	Acute leukemia	Pharyngitis, perirectal abscess, pneumonia, bacteremia	*E. coli, Pseudomonas, Candida*
Microbicidal defects	Chronic granulomatous disease of childhood, myeloperoxidase deficiency, Chédiak-Higashi syndrome, lysosomal granule deficiency	Recurrent skin abscesses, lymphadenitis, osteomyelitis, liver abscess, lung abscess, pneumonia	*S. aureus, Salmonella, Serratia*
DEFECTS OF CELLULAR IMMUNITY			
T-cell deficit, with intact B cells	Hodgkin's disease, chronic mucocutaneous candidiasis, thymic dysplasia (Nezelof's syndrome), thymic-parathyroid hypoplasia (Di George's syndrome), sarcoidosis, lepromatous leprosy	Superficial skin infections (especially with *Candida*), hepatitis, tuberculosis, fungal pneumonia, chronic meningitis, meningoencephalitis	*Candida, Cryptococcus, M. tuberculosis, Listeria, Toxoplasma,* herpes zoster
Combined B-cell and T-cell defects	Severe combined immunodeficiency (adenosine deaminase deficiency), ataxia telangiectasia, Wiskott-Aldrich syndrome, cartilage-hair hypoplasia, thymoma with immunodeficiency, intestinal lymphangiectasia secondary to Whipple's disease, Crohn's disease, pericarditis, tricuspid regurgitation, chronic lymphocytic leukemia	Disseminated skin infection (especially viral), otitis, sinusitis, bronchitis, pneumonia, bacteremias, abscesses	*Staph. aureus, gram-negative bacilli,* herpes zoster, herpes simplex, *cytomegalovirus*
OTHER DEFECTS			
Impaired tissue perfusion	Diabetes mellitus, nephrotic syndrome, sickle-cell anemia, severe atherosclerosis	Skin ulcers, cellulitis, wet gangrene, osteomyelitis	*S. aureus, E. coli,* and other gram-negative enteric bacilli
Abnormal drainage	Cystic fibrosis, bronchogenic carcinoma, ureteral and urethral obstruction, obstruction tumors at any site	Bronchitis, bronchiectasis, pneumonia with atelectasis, urinary tract infection, ascending cholangitis	*S. aureus, E. coli,* and other gram-negative bacilli
Integumental damage	Burns, eczema, compound fractures	Cellulitis, pneumonia, bacteremia, osteomyelitis	*S. aureus, S. pyogenes, Pseudomonas*
Antibiotics	Superinfection	Pneumonia, bacteremia	*S. aureus,* resistant gram-negative bacilli, especially *Pseudomonas, Serratia, Mima-Herellea, Candida*
Prosthetic devices and foreign bodies		Abscesses, bacteremia, osteomyelitis	*S. aureus, S. epidermidis,* gram-negative enteric bacilli, *Candida*

Certain pathogens, such as mycobacteria, DNA virus, and fungi, which are not readily killed by neutrophils, tend to persist intracellularly; they require a different host response for their containment. This mechanism, commonly referred to as *cellular immunity*, involves the interaction of monocytes and sensitized lymphocytes, the transformation of monocytes to activated macrophages, and the killing of organisms by macrophages and lymphocytes by both intracellular and extracellular mechanisms. The mediators of cellular immunity include migration inhibitory factor, transfer factor, chemotactic factor, and other lymphokines which are produced by T lymphocytes (Chap. 61).

SPECIFIC DEFECTS IN HOST DEFENSES Defects in skin and mucous membranes Burns and extensive trauma which leave patients with raw skin exposed to endogenous and environmental organisms rapidly become infected. *Pseudomonas* infections are frequently encountered in these patients, particularly those who have received antibiotics (Chap. 121). Atherosclerosis and neuropathy commonly predispose diabetic individuals to cutaneous infections of the lower extremities, particularly with staphylococci. Decubitus ulcers which become secondarily infected occur in severely ill patients who are not repositioned regularly. Burns, inhalation of toxic materials, and viral infections, e.g., influenza, can damage the respiratory tract epithelium predisposing to secondary infection by upper respiratory tract flora, especially pneumococci and staphylococci. Obtundation, intubation, and mechanical ventilation also enhance the risk of pneumonia because these factors interfere with the clearance of debris and bacteria from the lower respiratory tract. Urinary tract catheters, intravenous catheters, and other devices which connect the integument to any internal organ provide a route for microbial invasion from the skin. This problem is compounded by the fact that the porous surfaces of these foreign bodies provide crevices where bacteria can grow protected from the host's phagocytic cells.

Defects in the humoral system Immunoglobulin deficiency due to B-lymphocyte deficiency or dysfunction occurs in agammaglobulinemia (Chap. 62), multiple myeloma (Chap. 63), and chronic lymphocytic leukemia (Chap. 326) and with intensive immunosuppressive therapies. It results in decreased bacterial opsonization and inefficient function of the phagocytic system. Patients with these disorders are prone to infections by encapsulated bacteria, particularly pneumococci and *Hemophilus influenzae*. Patients with reduced or absent immunoglobulins and patients with defects of complement components C1, C2, or C4 are able to utilize the alternate complement pathway to activate C3 and the later complement components, i.e., C5 through C9. Patients with early complement component defects have fewer problems with infections than patients with deficiencies of complement components C3 through C9. These complement-related host defense defects are, in general, quite uncommon (Chap. 61).

Defects in the phagocytic system The most frequently encountered problem in phagocytic defenses is neutropenia. Blood neutrophil counts below 500 cells per cubic millimeter, and particularly counts below 100 cells per cubic millimeter, are associated with a greatly increased frequency of fever and infections. This is especially true in idiopathic or drug-induced agranulocytosis, leukemia, and aplastic anemia. Far less commonly, patients are encountered with specific defects in the granulocyte bactericidal mechanisms, e.g., chronic granulomatous disease and the Chédiak-Higashi syndrome (Chap. 56). In some patients with diabetes, uremia, lupus erythematosus, and rheumatoid arthritis, defects in neutrophils have been recognized which are attributed to abnormalities in the environment (excess glucose, uremic toxins, immune complexes) in which the cells function. When these patients' cells are suspended in normal serum or plasma they generally function normally.

Defects in cell-mediated immunity Patients with Hodgkin's disease, sarcoidosis, lepromatous leprosy, chronic mucocutaneous candidiasis, and certain congenital syndromes, e.g., Nezelof's syndrome, Di George's syndrome, Wiskott-Aldrich syndrome, and combined immunodeficiency, have defective lymphocyte-monocyte function most easily identified by reduced or absent cutaneous, delayed hypersensitivity responses

(Chap. 62). Tuberculosis, candidiasis, and disseminated viral infections, particularly herpes zoster infections, seem to occur with increased frequency in these patients.

Splenectomy The magnitude of the risk of overwhelming infection in the splenectomized patient is related to the underlying disease which called for removal of the spleen. However, even splenectomy for trauma in an otherwise normal individual appears to increase the risk of severe bacteremic infections. There is an impressive predominance of pneumococcal infections in splenectomized individuals; other organisms encountered frequently have included *Neisseria meningitidis*, *Escherichia coli*, and *Pseudomonas*. Malaria and other intracellular parasitic infections such as *Toxoplasma* and *Babesia* also may occur with increased frequency.

Defects induced by drugs *Antibiotics*, particularly when taken orally, regularly alter the normal host bacterial flora and predispose patients to superinfections, i.e., infections occurring specifically as a consequence of antibiotic treatment. Characteristically, these infections are caused by organisms resistant to the antibiotic being administered. These infections occur more commonly when antimicrobials are given in large doses, when several antimicrobials are administered concurrently, or when broad-spectrum agents are used.

It is often difficult to distinguish between superinfections and simple surface colonization by new organisms. Usually superinfections are identified by the occurrence of new symptoms, e.g., fever, cough, dysuria, or diarrhea, and the finding of resistant organisms in an area of new inflammation during the course of treating a defined infection (Chap. 114). Most of the time, antimicrobial therapy does not promote superinfection. However, when the concentration of organisms replacing the normal flora is high and when anatomic conditions are favorable, superinfection is likely. Certain circumstances, such as the tendency for *Pseudomonas* to infect patients treated with the cephalosporins and for *Candida* to infect patients treated with broad-spectrum combinations of antibiotics, are well recognized. Superinfections are also common during treatment of pneumonia in patients with severe, chronic, obstructive pulmonary disease where intubation is necessary, and when urinary tract infections are treated in patients with urinary stones or catheters.

Glucocorticosteroid therapy, particularly when given for long periods and in high doses, is thought to increase the risk of infections in humans. Although this risk is well documented in animal experiments, properly controlled human studies have been difficult to conduct. In the laboratory, steroids decrease mobilization of neutrophils to the sites of inflammation, decrease the killing of microbes by monocytes, and interfere with cell-mediated immune responses, possibly by altering the responsiveness of monocytes and macrophages to lymphokines. Because steroids induce such a broad defect in host defense mechanisms, both common and unusual pathogens must be considered in the steroid-treated patient with a presumed infection.

Immunosuppressive drugs, e.g., cyclophosphamide, chlorambucil, methotrexate, and many others, are now widely used for nonmalignant and malignant diseases. Nearly all of these agents cause neutropenia, lymphopenia, and monocytopenia through suppression of cell production. They also impair the rates of cell renewal in other tissues vital for host defenses including the epithelial cells lining the mucosal surfaces. Most of the infectious complications of these agents occur concomitant with the drug-induced neutropenia. Especially when used with corticosteroids in high doses, patients treated with these agents are severely compromised both in their ability to resist new infections and to handle established ones.

Defects with transplantation Immunosuppressive drugs, anti-lymphocyte globulin, and corticosteroids are generally used to prolong and to prevent rejection of kidney, heart, and other homografts. Because these agents are used in high doses during periods of impending graft rejection and because cellular resistance to infections may be impaired by the graft rejection process itself, at times these patients are inordinately susceptible to infections, particularly to severe fungal and viral infections (Chap. 69).

Bone marrow transplant patients have marked susceptibility to infection at the time of marrow grafting because of neutropenia and bone marrow ablation. After transplantation and marrow engraftment, despite the rise in their neutrophil counts, their host defenses remain severely compromised for 1 to 3 months because of a persisting impairment in cellular immunity. During this period, they frequently develop catastrophic pulmonary infections due to fungi, viruses, and parasites (Chaps. 69 and 312).

RECOGNIZING THE COMPROMISED HOST Most disease states associated with increased susceptibility to infections are easily identified. Examples include patients with leukemia, lymphoma, or aplastic anemia; therapy with steroids, immunosuppressive drugs, and broad-spectrum antibiotics; and specific anatomic defects such as bronchiectasis, chronic obstructive lung disease, or obstructive uropathy. Not infrequently the occurrence of fever and infection leads to the diagnosis of certain diseases associated with defects in host defenses. For example, a diabetic may be recognized because of recurrent abscesses or candidiasis in the perineal region. A severely granulocytopenic patient may be recognized because of fever, sore throat, or sepsis. Recurrent pneumococcal meningitis may lead to recognition of a small skull fracture with chronic CSF leakage. Recurrent fever and lymphadenitis usually precede recognition of chronic granulamatous disease.

Several reasonably reliable associations of specific organisms and certain host defense defects have been recognized and may be helpful in identifying or caring for the compromised host. These include *Staphylococcus aureus* with foreign bodies; *S. aureus, Serratia,* and *Salmonella* with chronic granulomatous disease; *Streptococcus pneumoniae* with agammaglobulinemia and splenectomy; mucoid *Pseudomonas* strains with cystic fibrosis; *Salmonella* with sickle-cell disease; *Nocardia* with alveolar proteinosis; *Mycobacterium tuberculosis, Cryptococcus,* and herpes zoster with Hodgkin's disease; and *Candida* with hypoparathyroidism.

The evaluation of a patient to identify a defect in host defenses should proceed systematically. After a complete history and physical examination, complete blood cell counts, blood glucose, liver and renal function tests, and chest and other appropriate x-ray examinations are obtained. Serum protein electrophoresis, quantitative immunoglobulins, and isohemagglutinins or selective febrile agglutinins are then measured to evaluate B-lymphocyte function. T-lymphocyte functions are evaluated with a panel of delayed hypersensitivity skin tests, generally including PPD, mumps, *Candida,* trichophytin, and streptokinase-streptodornase. Contact sensitization with dinitrochlorobenzene (DNCB) or keyhole hemocyanin (KLH) may also be performed. Complement defects usually can be recognized by obtaining total hemolytic complement levels (CH_{50}) or C3 assays. The principal screening test for recognizing the various forms of chronic granulomatous disease is the nitroblue tetrazolium (NBT) test. At this point in any patient's evaluation, consultation with an individual engaged in studying host defense defects is usually necessary.

Useful clues for persisting in a patient's evaluation to try to define a specific abnormality are: repetitive episodes of proven bacterial infections with the same organism; infections which do not respond to treatment that is usually considered to be effective or which relapse when therapy is discontinued, and repeated infections caused by unusual organisms.

THERAPEUTIC CONSIDERATIONS Successful treatment of infections in the compromised host depends upon early diagnosis, prompt intervention, and avoidance of certain pitfalls in patient management. Because infections in the compromised host tend to be chronic, long-term care by a concerned physician who understands the patient's host defense deficiency is vitally important. Laboratory facilities for accurate culture and sensitivity testing also are essential. In the febrile compromised host, the clinician must collect blood, body fluids, and exudate for cultures as quickly as possible. When these materials do not yield a diagnosis promptly, aspiration or biopsy of sites of presumed infection is often necessary and should not be delayed.

Often it is necessary to initiate antibiotic treatment before results of cultures and sensitivity tests are available. This is particularly true in patients with shock and presumed bacteremia, patients with fever and severe neutropenia, and those with severe respiratory tract infections where sputum or transtracheal washings are difficult or impossible to obtain. In these instances broad-spectrum coverage with a combination of antibiotics should be used initially (Chap. 111), but the coverage should be narrowed as quickly as possible to avoid superinfections. Often patients with neutropenia, corticosteroid treatment, and certain specific host defense defects fail to mount an inflammatory response as rapidly as normal individuals. Consequently, when these patients have pneumonia, cellulitis, or abscesses, the diagnosis may not be apparent when the patient is first seen. Repeated careful examinations are the only way to establish the diagnosis.

Although sometimes essential, indwelling catheters should be avoided in the compromised host whenever possible (Chap. 108). The prophylactic use of antibiotics in these patients has rarely been successful (Chap. 114). With time, the patients simply become colonized by microbes resistant to the prophylactic agents chosen. Oral nonabsorbable antibiotics can delay infections briefly in the highly susceptible neutropenic host, but patients' acceptance of this form of therapy is poor. Gamma globulin therapy can be helpful in patients with agammaglobulinemia (Chap. 62), but is of no benefit to most patients with multiple myeloma or other hypogammaglobulinemic states in which there is low, but detectable, serum IgG. Active and passive immunization to prevent specific infections and the use of prophylactic granulocyte transfusions are under investigation. Protective isolation with laminar airflow rooms, sterile food, and antibiotic treatment will prevent or delay infection and probably is useful when the duration of maximum susceptibility to the infection is no longer than a few days to a few weeks.

SPECIFIC INFECTIONS Certain organisms are encountered as pathogens almost exclusively in the compromised host, e.g., *Pneumocystis carinii, Phycomyces,* and *Aspergillus.* Others, e.g., *Candida, Histoplasma,* herpes simplex, and cytomegalovirus, are common pathogens for both the normal and compromised host. The following organisms are encountered frequently or present special problems. Separate chapters in the text deal with each of these and their treatment in greater detail.

Staphylococcus In general, staphylococcal infections are not inordinately difficult to manage in the compromised host. Staphylococcal infections related to intravenous catheters present a special problem. Although it is always best to remove the catheter, it may be possible, on occasion, to cure infections caused by antibiotic-sensitive staphylococci at the site of arteriovenous shunts and at the tips of chronic parenteral nutrition catheters (Chap. 116).

Listeria Bacteremia, peritonitis, and meningitis are encountered particularly in newborns, alcoholics, diabetics, and patients with lymphoreticular malignancies. The diagnosis may be missed initially because relatively few organisms are found in exudate (e.g., peritoneal fluid or cerebrospinal fluid) or the organism is confused with other gram-positive rods, such as diphtheroids, and regarded as a contaminant (Chap. 132).

Corynebacterium Diphtheroids are among the most common organisms encountered as contaminants of blood cultures. With increasing frequency, however, they are being found as the cause of significant bacteremias, particularly in severely ill patients with intravenous catheters and cerebrospinal fluid reservoirs and shunts.

Gram-negative bacilli *E. coli, Pseudomonas, Proteus,* and other Enterobacteriaceae remain the major pathogens for patients with compromised host defenses. The portal for entry is generally the gastrointestinal tract. Gram-negative bacteremia, pneumonia, and meningitis are well recognized. *Ecthyma gangrenosum* is an important clue to early recognition of *Pseudomonas* sepsis (Chaps. 120 and 121).

Mycobacterium With the declining frequency of pulmonary tuberculosis in the United States, an increasing proportion of cases involve patients with compromised host defenses who often present with unusual manifestations of the disease. For this reason it is important to know the tuberculin status of every patient with a chronic debilitating disease which may predispose the patient to infections or which may require treatment with corticosteroids or immunosuppressive drugs. The practice of treating all tuberculin-positive patients receiving steroids with isoniazid is becoming less frequent with recognition of the toxicity of the drug and the relatively small risk of activation of latent disease, at least in certain conditions such as asthma and rheumatoid arthritis. However, this approach necessitates careful follow-up of every tuberculin reactor (Chap. 143).

Candida This organism has emerged as a major cause for superinfection in the compromised host. *Candida* pharyngitis, laryngitis, esophagitis, pneumonia, and candidemia are common in patients with reduced host defenses who are receiving broad-spectrum antibiotics. The diagnosis of disseminated candidiasis often poses considerable difficulty (Chap. 158).

Histoplasma Disseminated histoplasmosis is becoming an increasingly important problem, particularly among patients with Hodgkin's disease, chronic lymphocytic leukemia, acute lymphocytic leukemia, and those undergoing intensive immunosuppressive therapy. Both reactivation of latent infections and inordinately severe initial infections have been documented. It is important to establish because the infection responds well to amphotericin in many instances (Chap. 155).

Nocardia See Chap. 152.

Aspergillus See Chap. 159.

Phycomyces See Chap. 160.

Herpes zoster Disseminated Herpes zoster infections occur with increased frequency in disorders of cellular immunity, es-

pecially Hodgkin's disease and chronic lymphocytic leukemia, and in patients receiving corticosteroids and immunosuppressive drugs (Chap. 185).

Herpes simplex Disseminated infections with diffuse skin lesions, pneumonitis, encephalitis, and hepatitis have been increasing, especially in renal transplant patients and in others receiving intensive immunosuppression (Chap. 193).

Cytomegalovirus See Chap. 194.

Toxoplasmosis See Chap. 203.

Pneumocystis See Chap. 204.

REFERENCES

ALLEN JC: *Infections and the Compromised Host.* Baltimore, Williams & Wilkens, 1976

CLIFT RA et al: Granulocyte transfusions for prevention of infection in patients receiving bone marrow transplants. N Engl J Med 298:1052, 1978

CLINE MJ: *The White Cell.* Cambridge, Mass, Harvard University Press, 1975

CODISH SD, TOBIAS JS: Managing systemic mycoses in the compromised host. JAMA 235:2132, 1976

EDITORIAL: Infective hazards of splenectomy. Lancet 1:1167, 1976

FAUCI AS et al: Glucocorticosteroid therapy: Mechanisms of action and clinical considerations. Ann Intern Med 84:304, 1976

FEIGIN RD, SHEARER WT: Opportunistic infection in children. J Pediatr 87:507, 677, 852, 1975

GREENMAN RL et al: Lung biopsy in the immunocompromised host. Am J Med 59:488, 1975

GURWITH MJ et al: Granulocytopenia in hospitalized patients: I. Prognostic factors and etiology of fever. Am J Med 64:121, 1978

LEVINE AS et al: Hematologic malignances and other marrow failure states: Progress in management of complicating infections. Semin Hematol 11:141, 1974

NIEMAN PE et al: A prospective analysis of interstitial pneumonia and opportunistic viral infection among recipients of allogeneic bone marrow graft. J Infect Dis 136:754, 1977

RODRIQUEZ V et al: Randomized trial of protected environment–prophylactic antibiotics in 145 adults with acute leukemia. Medicine 57:253, 1978

SCHIMPF SC et al: Three antibiotic regimens in the treatment of infections in febrile granulocytopenic patients with cancer. J Infect Dis 137:14, 1978

SMITH FG, PALMER DL: Alcoholism, infection and altered host defenses: A review of clinical and experimental observations. J Chron Dis 29:35, 1976

VALDIVIESO M et al: Gram-negative bacillary pneumonia in the compromised host. Medicine 56:241, 1977

108
HOSPITAL-ACQUIRED INFECTIONS

PIERCE GARDNER
WILLIAM A. CAUSEY

DEFINITION Hospital-acquired infections (also called *nosocomial infections*) are significant causes of human morbidity and mortality. They may be defined as clinical infections occurring in patients after admission to the hospital that were neither present nor in a period of incubation at the time of admission. Also included are infections that are contracted in the hospital but do not become clinically evident until after the patient is discharged. Although many of these infections can be prevented, some cannot, and the term *hospital-acquired infection* should not be equated with *iatrogenic infection*, which is usually defined as an infection caused by a diagnostic or therapeutic maneuver such as insertion of an urethral or intravenous catheter. Infections caused by organisms in the patient's own flora are termed *autochthonous infections* and are often unavoidable because they are related to defects in mucosal barriers or other host defenses rather than being preventable environmental risks.

EPIDEMIOLOGY Incidence and cost Hospital-acquired infections occur in from 2 to 15 percent of patients admitted to general hospitals. The highest infection rates are recorded in municipal hospitals and tertiary care centers such as university hospitals, while the prevalence of these infections is much lower in community hospitals. Hospital-acquired infections have a mortality rate of approximately 1 percent and contribute to death in an additional 3 percent of cases. Estimates for the United States indicate that 1.5 million hospital-acquired infections occur annually, cause 15,000 deaths, and contribute to mortality in an additional 45,000 patients. The prolongation in hospital stays and additional diagnostic tests, medications, and physicians' fees contribute significantly to the high cost of hospital care.

ETIOLOGY Causative pathogens Gram-negative bacilli dominate the list of nosocomial pathogens, although *Staphylococcus aureus*, the scourge of the 1950s and early 1960s, remains an important pathogen in all sites except the urinary tract (Table 108-1). During the past decade antibiotic susceptibility patterns of the gram-positive cocci have remained relatively stable. However, the isolation of strains of pneumococci resistant to penicillins and cephalosporins in South Africa and the possible significance of bacterial tolerance (organisms are inhibited but not killed by bactericidal drugs) among isolates of *S. aureus* to β-lactamase–resistant penicillins suggest that important problems with antimicrobial resistance may lie ahead. The

gram-negative bacilli have tended to develop resistance to many of the antimicrobial agents in common use. In large part, this resistance is due to the acquisition of plasmids called *resistance factors* (R factors). R-factor plasmids consist of extra-chromosomal circular deoxyribonucleic acid (DNA) which mediates antibiotic resistance by coding for enzymes that inactivate the drug or by conferring properties altering the permeability of the bacterial cell wall to the drug. Two properties of R factors are of major public health concern: (1) resistance to several antibiotics is often linked on the same R factor, and (2) R-factor transfer can occur across species lines from one gram-negative organism to another. Under the appropriate selective conditions these properties make possible the rapid dissemination of multiple antibiotic resistance among a wide variety of gram-negative pathogens.

Whatever the mechanism, the major reason for the development of antimicrobial-resistant bacteria in the hospital setting is the use of antibiotics. These drugs tend to eliminate susceptible bacteria in the host's own flora, leading to replacement by antibiotic-resistant organisms. Once colonized by these organisms, susceptible individuals may develop clinical infections. The importance of antibiotics as a selective force favoring the emergence of resistant bacteria is emphasized by the observation that a number of hospital epidemics have been aborted by limiting the use of some of these drugs and by interdicting others altogether (Chap. 114).

Opportunistic infections (Chap. 107) may be defined as infections occurring in patients with impaired host defenses which would not ordinarily occur in normal hosts. Commonly they are due to pathogens that do not ordinarily cause disease in healthy persons but colonize and invade individuals whose host defenses are faulty. These infections have become so frequent that *Candida* spp. appears among the list of most com-

TABLE 108-1
Incidence* and relative frequency† of selected pathogens causing nosocomial infections, by site of infection, January to December 1976

	Primary bacteremia	Surgical wound	Lower respiratory	Urinary tract	Cutaneous	Other	All sites
Staphylococcus aureus	2.1 (12.8%)	18.9 (15.5%)	7.4 (10.4%)	2.9 (1.7%)	8.7 (33.7%)	5.8 (12.7%)	45.8 (10.0%)
Staphylococcus epidermidis	1.3 (7.7%)	5.5 (4.5%)	0.4 (0.5%)	5.1 (2.9%)	1.1 (4.3%)	1.6 (3.5%)	15.0 (3.3%)
Streptococcus, group D	1.2 (7.4%)	12.7 (10.3%)	0.9 (1.2%)	24.4 (13.9%)	1.6 (6.1%)	2.7 (5.9%)	43.5 (9.6%)
Escherichia coli	2.4 (14.3%)	19.1 (15.7%)	5.2 (7.2%)	55.3 (31.7%)	2.2 (8.5%)	4.2 (9.2%)	88.4 (19.4%)
Klebsiella spp.	1.8 (10.6%)	6.4 (5.2%)	7.9 (11.1%)	15.3 (8.8%)	1.1 (4.3%)	2.1 (4.6%)	34.6 (7.6%)
Enterobacter spp.	0.9 (5.2%)	4.9 (4.0%)	4.7 (6.5%)	7.2 (4.1%)	0.8 (3.1%)	1.1 (2.4%)	19.6 (4.3%)
Proteus-Providencia spp.	0.6 (3.6%)	8.6 (7.1%)	4.0 (5.6%)	18.2 (10.4%)	1.4 (5.5%)	2.6 (5.7%)	35.4 (7.8%)
Pseudomonas aeruginosa	0.9 (5.2%)	5.0 (4.1%)	5.2 (7.3%)	15.5 (8.9%)	1.2 (4.7%)	2.2 (4.8%)	30.0 (6.6%)
Candida spp.	0.5 (3.3%)	1.0 (0.8%)	2.5 (3.5%)	7.3 (4.2%)	0.7 (2.9%)	3.8 (8.3%)	15.8 (3.5%)
All pathogens	16.6 (100.0%)	121.9 (100.0%)	71.4 (100.0%)	174.6 (100.0%)	25.7 (100.0%)	45.9 (100.0%)	456.1 (100.0%)
Secondary bacteremia	NA	3.8 (3.1%)	3.0 (4.1%)	4.5 (2.6%)	1.3 (5.0%)	3.7 (7.9%)	16.3 (3.7%)

* *Incidence is number of isolates reported per 100,000 discharges; up to four isolates may be reported per infection.*
† *Relative frequency is expressed as percent of all isolates from each site.*
SOURCE: *Center for Disease Control, National Nosocomial Infections Study Report, Annual Summary 1976, Washington, DC, US Government Printing Office, 1978.*

mon nosocomial pathogens. Although surveillance and reporting of opportunistic viral and protozoan infections are variable, cytomegalovirus, *Pneumocystis carinii*, and *Toxoplasma gondii* have gained increased recognition as causes of hospital-acquired infection.

Transmission of nosocomial pathogens Even before the recognition of bacteria as causative agents of disease, Ignaz Semmelweis, by simple epidemiologic methods, identified the contaminated hands of physicians and medical students as the major transmitters of puerperal sepsis, the most significant hospital-acquired infection of his day. Although the major sites and pathogens of hospital-acquired infection have changed during the past century, contact with hospital personnel remains the principal mode of spread of nosocomial pathogens. Usually, transmission occurs via the hands of hospital personnel, but other skin surfaces and respiratory droplets may also be important. Inanimate sources of hospital-associated microorganisms include food and drinking water, sinks and bath water, ventilation systems, contaminated horizontal surfaces, and the catheters and equipment needed for life-support systems and diagnostic procedures.

A *common-source epidemic* occurs when a single contaminating source is responsible for multiple infections. In this situation, patients commonly become colonized with hospital-associated bacteria following exposure to a particular procedure or area of the hospital. The epidemiologic steps in the evaluation of a common-source epidemic include recognition of a clustering of infections in both time and place, use of antibiotic susceptibility patterns or other biologic markers to allow more precise definition of the epidemic strain, and analysis of the geographic distribution and diagnostic experiences which are common to the infected patients but absent in the noninfected patients.

Host factors The age and underlying disease of patients, the integrity of their mucosal and integumentary surfaces, and the status of their immunological defenses are among the major determinants of both the incidence and outcome of hospital-acquired infections (Chap. 107).

COMMON HOSPITAL-ACQUIRED INFECTIONS Urinary tract infections These infections account for approximately 40 percent of hospital-acquired infections and are usually a consequence of instrumentation of the urethra, bladder, or kidneys. The most common predisposing factor is the insertion of an indwelling urethral catheter which permits bacteria to ascend from the external environment to the bladder. Hospital surveys show that 10 to 15 percent of all adult patients have indwelling catheters, a number of which appear to be unnecessary. Because the urinary tract is the most common site of infection resulting in secondary bacteremia, preventive measures involving urethral catheters should be a major focus of efforts to reduce the frequency of gram-negative sepsis in hospitalized patients. Several principles should be followed in managing urethral catheters in hospitalized patients:

1 Indwelling catheters should not be used unless they are required for management of bladder outlet obstruction or for close monitoring of fluid and electrolyte balance in severely ill patients.
2 There should be rigorous adherence to sterile technique during insertion of the catheter.
3 Maintaining a system of closed drainage is essential and can usually keep the urine sterile for 5 to 7 days. After that, the risk of infection increases with time, 5 to 10 percent for each day of catheterization.

4 In catheterized patients, specimens of urine for laboratory tests should be aspirated from the catheter by use of a sterile syringe, and the collecting tubing and bag must be unobstructed and in a dependent position.
5 Daily perineal care including the application of antibacterial ointment at the meatal-catheter junction may also be of benefit.
6 Occasionally, intermittent straight catheterization for patients with anticipated short-term needs for bladder drainage may avoid an indwelling catheter altogether.

Wound infections Most surgical wound infections are due to organisms introduced into the tissues at the time of the operative procedures. Most infecting organisms originate from the resident skin flora of the patient, and airborne bacteria are of little consequence in the etiology of wound infections. The major factors affecting the incidence of wound infection include the type of operation, its duration, the skill of the surgeon, and the basic health of the patient. Operations involving contaminated sites such as the bowel or a previously infected area are more likely to be complicated by infection than sites which are clean prior to surgery. Operations of long duration or in which devitalized tissue, foreign bodies, or hematomas are left behind are associated with a high rate of wound infection. Other factors predisposing to wound infection include advanced age, poor nutritional status, the presence of distant foci of infection, diabetes mellitus, renal failure, and corticosteroid therapy.

Most wound infections appear from 3 to 7 days following surgery. Early postoperative wound infections (those occurring within 24 to 48 h of surgery) are commonly caused by group A *Streptococcus* or *Clostridium* spp. Gram-stained smears of wound exudate, followed by culture, may provide valuable early clues to the bacterial etiology in wound infections. Staphylococcal wound infections characteristically become evident 4 to 6 days after surgery, and those caused by gram-negative bacilli and anaerobic bacteria may not appear for a week or more. If perioperative antibiotics are used, the manifestations of infection may be delayed.

In addition to emphasis on maintaining sterility in the operating room and insistence on operative techniques that minimize tissue trauma and blood loss, increased attention is being given to preventing postoperative wound infections with short prophylactic courses of systemic antibiotics during the perioperative period. The principles that should govern this use of antibiotics include (1) beginning the drug during the immediate preoperative period but not earlier, (2) assuring adequate tissue levels throughout surgery by giving intraoperative doses of antibiotics if necessary, and (3) discontinuing antibiotic prophylaxis within 24 to 48 h of surgery. This use of antibiotics does not appear to significantly alter the flora or promote colonization with resistant strains. Prolonged pre- and postoperative courses are unnecessary, expensive, and potentially harmful because of toxicity or superinfection. Antibiotic prophylaxis administered according to these principles has been reported to reduce infectious morbidity in a variety of orthopedic, gynecologic, and abdominal operations. The antibiotics used for surgical prophylaxis should be aimed at the most likely causative organisms (Chap. 111). Examples are *Escherichia coli* in biliary tree and gynecologic surgery and staphylococci in vascular and cardiac surgery.

Nonsurgical wounds that are common sites of nosocomial infection include burns, injection sites, decubitus ulcers, and cutaneous ulcers resulting from venous or arterial occlusive disease. In general, the offending pathogens are similar to those found in wound infections, with the exception that burn wound infections and soft tissue infections in neutropenic patients frequently are caused by *Pseudomonas aeruginosa*. Bacteremic *Pseudomonas* infections may result in bacterial arteritis and cutaneous infarction manifested by hemorrhagic bullae (ecthyma gangrenosum, Chap. 121).

Pneumonia Lower respiratory tract infections are the leading cause of mortality among hospital-acquired infections, although they rank third in incidence behind urinary tract infections and wound infections. The major pathogens are the gram-negative bacilli and *S. aureus,* all of which are invasive and characteristically cause a necrotizing bronchopneumonia. These organisms reach the lower respiratory tract by inhalation or aspiration rather than by hematogenous spread. The observation that the pharyngeal flora of seriously ill patients consists predominantly of gram-negative bacilli is consistent with the pathogenesis of this infection. The three settings in which nosocomial pneumonias most commonly occur are (1) in obtunded patients whose gag reflex and cough are ineffective, (2) in patients with underlying pulmonary disease or congestive heart failure whose pulmonary clearance mechanisms are impaired, and (3) in patients who require respiratory tract instrumentation or ventilatory assistance.

Positioning the patient in a swimmer's or Gatch position is the cornerstone of preventing aspiration by obtunded patients. Frequent suctioning of secretions using sterile technique, particularly from intubated or tracheostomized patients, is also an important prophylactic measure. Treatment of congestive failure will improve the effectiveness of the lung's defenses and will also reduce pulmonary edema fluid which serves as an excellent culture medium. Respiratory assistance apparatus must be maintained in the most nearly sterile state possible. Moreover, intermittent positive pressure breathing as part of routine perioperative care is often unnecessary and subjects the patients to the infectious risk inherent in exposure to ventilatory equipment. Finally, regular monitoring of the respiratory flora, particularly in intubated patients, with gram-stained smears and cultures provides useful information in choosing appropriate early therapy for pulmonary superinfections, should they occur.

Hospital transmission of viral respiratory pathogens is common especially on pediatric services but, except for influenza and respiratory syncytial virus (in infants), rarely results in severe disease. When influenza A is widespread in the community, amantadine prophylaxis, as well as immunization, should be considered for unimmunized hospital patients identified as being at high risk for complications of influenza.

Bacteremia Although bacterial invasion of the bloodstream can occur in any nosocomial infection, the infected intravenous cannula is one of the most common and also most remediable causes of hospital-acquired bacteremia. Annually in the United States more than 10 million persons (more than one in four hospitalized patients) receive intravenous therapy, and even a low rate of complications will involve a large number of patients. Intravenous devices account for about 5 percent of all nosocomial infections and 10 percent of all positive blood cultures. The most common isolates from catheter tips are *S. epidermidis, S. aureus,* gram-negative bacilli (especially *Klebsiella, Enterobacter, Serratia*), and enterococci. Although microorganisms can enter at any point, the intravenous system most commonly is contaminated at the site of cannula entry during insertion and subsequent manipulation, and at the connecting points of the intravenous set to the cannula and to the intravenous fluid bag. Intravenous fluids also may become contaminated in the process of manufacture or as a result of addition of medications. The type of intravenous cannula, the choice of intravenous site, the adequacy of skin preparation, and the length of time during which the cannula is in use are important determinants of the risk of septic complications. Steel needles, especially scalp vein needles, are preferable to plastic cannulae which have greater risks of local phlebitis, contamination, and

sepsis. For example, suppurative phlebitis, the most feared complication of cannula-related infections, is virtually unknown with steel needles. Arms are better intravenous sites than legs owing to the lower rate of phlebitis and sepsis. The risk of bacteremia increases with time and is unacceptably high when cannulas are left in place longer than 48 to 72 h. Prolonged use of an intravenous site and failure to remove the cannula at the earliest sign of inflammation or cannula malfunction are common errors. Preventive measures designed to reduce the incidence of intravenous-associated infections are listed in Table 108-2. With meticulous care, catheters used for parenteral hyperalimentation can be maintained free of infection for prolonged periods. However, infectious complications, particularly *Candida* sepsis, are not uncommon in this setting.

Transient bacteremias frequently follow diagnostic or therapeutic manipulations of the mouth or the respiratory, gastrointestinal, or genitourinary tract and are usually well tolerated by the normal host. However, the patient with valvular or congenital heart disease (or a valve prosthesis) may be at risk of developing endocarditis and should receive antibiotic prophylaxis when undergoing procedures associated with significant risk of bacteremia (Chap. 243). These procedures include dental manipulations, urinary tract instrumentation, abdominal surgery, and other surgery involving infected tissue. For patients with prosthetic heart valves, these recommendations have been extended. Detailed programs of prophylaxis are given in the chapter on infective endocarditis (Chap. 243).

Hepatitis B (see also Chap. 302) The risk of hospital-acquired hepatitis B is significant not only for patients, especially those who receive blood products or undergo renal dialysis, but also for hospital personnel who work with patients or handle their blood specimens. The widespread practice of screening blood products for hepatitis B surface antigen (HBsAg) has reduced markedly the incidence of posttransfusion hepatitis B. Currently most posttransfusion hepatitis is caused by unidentified agents (non-A, non-B hepatitis). However, hepatitis B remains an endemic problem on many renal dialysis and oncology services. Moreover, for unknown reasons, infections often are more severe in clinical and laboratory staff than in patients. Meticulous attention to precautions designed to limit spread of pathogens by direct contact is the major focus in the prevention of hepatitis B in dialysis units. Other important control measures include active serologic surveillance of patients and staff, attention to environmental cleanliness, and needle-blood precautions. Hepatitis B immunoglobulin (HBIG) contains high levels of antibodies to hepatitis B (anti-HBs) and is recommended for personnel directly exposed to HBsAg-positive

TABLE 108-2
Guidelines to reduce the incidence of intravenous-associated infections

1 Establish strict indications for use of intravenous fluid therapy.
2 Avoid high-risk sites, such as the leg.
3 Use stainless steel needles in preference to plastic catheters.
4 Adequately disinfect the skin over the intravenous site.
5 Use sterile technique in insertion of cannulas, including careful handwashing, sterile gloves, and, when possible, sterile drapes.
6 Securely anchor cannula to prevent to-and-fro motion.
7 Apply sterile dressing over intravenous site (topical antibiotic ointment optional).
8 Inspect the infusion site daily and remove cannula if inflammation, phlebitis, or cannula malfunction is present.
9 Change the cannula at frequent (~48 h) intervals.

SOURCE: *After Goldmann et al.*

material by accidental needle stick, mucous membrane contact, or oral ingestion.

Standard immunoglobulin (IG) usually contains some anti-HBs and may be effective for pre- and postexposure prophylaxis of hepatitis B. Prophylaxis with HBIG or standard IG for patients and personnel with continuing exposure to hepatitis B virus is not routinely recommended, but may be indicated in epidemic situations.

Considerable concern has been generated about the infectivity of the approximately 1 percent of physicians and dentists who are asymptomatic carriers of HBsAg. Although several instances of physician-to-patient transmission have been identified, the great majority of HBsAg-positive health care personnel do not appear to present a hazard to patients. While they have been encouraged to pay particular attention to handwashing and other measures to prevent contact spread, their patient-related activities need not necessarily be restricted.

CONTROL MEASURES Infection control team The goals of those concerned with infection control are (1) to reduce the risk of patients acquiring infections in the hospital, (2) to provide adequate care for patients with a potentially communicable infection, and (3) to minimize risks related to infections to employees, visitors, and community contacts. The functions of the infection control team include (1) development of enforceable policies necessary for appropriate management of patients with communicable infections; (2) development of a surveillance system which identifies patients with communicable infections, quantitates the incidence and prevalence of hospital-acquired infection, and investigates problems that are likely to be remediable; (3) liaison with personnel from nursing, central supply, housekeeping, maintenance, pharmacy, and other services to ensure that appropriate cleaning and sterilization techniques and materials are employed, and to permit evaluation of new germicides and other products as they become available; (4) education of employees in appropriate techniques to prevent spread of infectious agents within the hospital; (5) communication with employee health services to ensure adequate immunizations and to provide whatever care is necessary for susceptible personnel exposed to a communicable disease; and (6) monitoring of antibiotic utilization and the susceptibility patterns of common nosocomial pathogens. Most large hospitals employ full-time nurse(s) and/or physician(s), called *infection control officers,* to lead the multidisciplinary team effort that is necessary to carry out these functions.

Prevention Sir William Osler once remarked, "Soap, water and common sense are the best disinfectants." The basic principles of handwashing between patient contacts, appropriate isolation of patients harboring communicable organisms, and application of epidemiologic methods to identify and correct potential sources of infection remain the cornerstones of preventing nosocomial infections. Specific preventive measures related to particular hazards such as catheters and respirators have been mentioned in preceding sections.

EMPLOYEE HEALTH SERVICE Preventive medicine applies not only to patients but also to hospital personnel, and the employee health service should be encouraged to maintain surveillance for tuberculosis by tuberculin skin tests and/or chest x-rays and to immunize personnel who are susceptible to measles, mumps, poliomyelitis, diphtheria, or tetanus. The availability of improved influenza vaccines makes it rational to recommend annual immunization for all hospital personnel. Premenopausal women should be tested for antibodies to rubella, and rubella immunization should be offered to nonpreg-

nant susceptible women who are practicing effective contraception. Routine smallpox immunization of employees is no longer indicated. Hospital personnel who develop significant infections should be removed from patient contact during the period of communicability. Paronychias and other pustular lesions due to *S. aureus* or group A streptococci are often underrated by staff, and it is commonly forgotten that herpes zoster lesions may cause chickenpox in susceptible contacts.

ADMISSION SCREENING A patient scheduled for elective admission who has, or is thought to be incubating, a communicable disease should be sent home until the period of potential communicability has passed. Admission screening for communicable infections is particularly important for patients being admitted to oncology or dialysis services, which tend to have a high percentage of immunocompromised patients. Infections such as chickenpox and measles can be devastating in such patients, and their spread among them must be avoided at all costs.

CONTAINMENT Microorganisms can be spread from one person to another by several routes, including (1) contact, either directly from person to person or indirectly via contaminated equipment, linens, etc. (including contaminated hands); (2) airborne, via droplet nuclei reaching respiratory tract or wound surfaces; (3) vehicles, such as contaminated food, water, parenteral drugs, or blood; and (4) vectors, such as insects or arthropods.

Each pathogen has its characteristic mode(s) of spread, and, on the basis of this knowledge, isolation precautions can be tailored to fit the situation. Isolation procedures are time-consuming and expensive and can hinder needed patient care if applied too rigidly. They should be used only when necessary and for the shortest period consistent with good practice.

The following are the types of isolation and precautions in common use:

1 *Strict isolation,* where both airborne and contact transmission of an organism are possible, e.g., staphylococcal pneumonia.
2 *Respiratory isolation,* where the infectious agent is contained in airborne droplets of respiratory secretions, e.g., tuberculosis.
3 *Wound and skin isolation,* where direct or indirect contact with skin lesions or dressings may transmit the organism, e.g., a staphylococcal furuncle.
4 *Enteric precautions,* where transmission usually occurs via the fecal-oral route and contact with articles contaminated by feces is to be avoided, e.g., *Salmonella* gastroenteritis.
5 *Protective (reverse) isolation,* where the precautions are designed to protect the patient with impaired host defenses from organisms in the environment or carried by personnel, e.g., patients with total neutropenia or burns.
6 *Blood precautions,* where the transmission is by accidental inoculation or ingestion of blood or blood products, e.g., hepatitis B.

If preventive measures fail and a communicable infection develops in an inpatient, the following principles of containment should be observed:

1 Prevent further transmission of disease by the index case. This is usually accomplished by initiating appropriate isolation procedures or, if the patient's condition allows, arranging discharge home.
2 In cases of contagious disease, identify all contacts of the index case and determine their susceptibility and degree of exposure.
3 Give indicated prophylaxis to exposed susceptibles. The indications for passive immunization, active immunization,

and prophylaxis with antimicrobial agents vary with the pathogen (Chap. 114). The most common nosocomial infections requiring treatment of exposed susceptibles are hepatitis A and B.

4 Design a plan to prevent the spread of the infectious agent from the exposed susceptibles to other patients and personnel. This plan must take cognizance of the epidemiology of the communicable disease, the efficacy and feasibility of various control measures, and the potential consequences of further disease transmission.

The methods commonly employed to limit the tertiary spread of communicable diseases by exposed susceptibles are (1) early discharge of patients when feasible, (2) rearranging personnel assignments to avoid patient contact during the period of communicability, and (3) cohorting—grouping exposed susceptible patients (and personnel) together and treating them as an epidemiologic unit with appropriate precautions during the period of communicability. Cohorting is cumbersome but remains a major control measure for hospital outbreaks of chickenpox and epidemic diarrhea.

PROGNOSIS Most nosocomial infections are diseases of medical progress, and the ever-increasing orientation of modern medicine to technologically sophisticated procedures makes it likely that the risk of patients acquiring infections in the hospital will continue to increase. On the other hand, many of the factors that promote infections in the hospital have been identified, and measures for their control have been developed. Influencing hospital personnel to carry out these control measures, such as handwashing, catheter care, and restraint in the use of antibiotics, remains a major challenge.

REFERENCES

AMERICAN COLLEGE OF SURGEONS: *Manual in Control of Infections in Surgical Patients.* Philadelphia, Lippincott, 1976

BENENSON AS (ed): *Control of Communicable Diseases in Man,* 12th ed. Washington, DC, American Public Health Association, 1975

BENNETT JV, BRACHMAN PS: *Nosocomial Infections.* Boston, Little, Brown, 1978

CAMERON JL, ZUIDEMA GD: Aspiration pneumonia. JAMA 219:1194, 1972

CENTER FOR DISEASE CONTROL: *Isolation Techniques for Use in Hospitals,* 2d ed. Washington, DC, US Government Printing Office, 1975

EVERETT ED, HIRSCHMANN JV: Transient bacteremia and endocarditis prophylaxis. A review. Medicine 56:61, 1977

GARDNER P et al: Hospital isolation and precaution guidelines. Pediatrics 53:663, 1974

——— et al: Hospital management of patients and personnel exposed to communicable diseases. Pediatrics 56:700, 1975

GOLDMANN DA et al: Guidelines for infection control in intravenous therapy. Ann Intern Med 79:848, 1973

JOHANSON WG et al: Nosocomial respiratory infections with gram-negative bacilli. Ann Intern Med 77:701, 1972

SNYDMAN DR et al: Prevention of nosocomial viral hepatitis, type B. Ann Intern Med 83:838, 1975

STAMM WE: Guidelines for prevention of catheter-associated urinary tract infections. Ann Intern Med 82:386, 1975

STEERE AC, MALLISON GF: Handwashing practices for the prevention of nosocomial infections. Ann Intern Med 83:683, 1975

109

GRAM-NEGATIVE BACTEREMIA AND SEPTIC SHOCK

ROBERT G. PETERSDORF
DAVID C. DALE

DEFINITION Septic shock is characterized by inadequate tissue perfusion, usually following bacteremia with gram-negative enteric bacilli. Hypotension, oliguria, tachycardia, tachypnea, and fever are observed in most patients. The circulatory insufficiency is due principally to cell and tissue injury initiated by endotoxin and to the resultant pooling of blood in the microcirculation.

ETIOLOGY Septic shock may be associated with gram-positive infections, notably those due to pneumococci and streptococci, although it is more common following bacteremia, with gram-negative bacilli: the Enterobacteriaceae (Chap. 120) and *Pseudomonas* and related organisms (Chap. 121). Gram-negative anaerobic bacteremia with *Bacteroides* species is also a precursor of septic shock, although in this situation the syndrome is less fulminating than with aerobic gram-negative bacilli. The shock syndrome is not due to bloodstream invasion with bacteria per se, but is related to release of endotoxin, the lipopolysaccharide moiety of the organisms' cell walls, into the circulation.

EPIDEMIOLOGY Gram-negative bacteremia and septic shock occur primarily in hospitalized patients who usually have underlying diseases which render them susceptible to bloodstream invasion. Predisposing factors include diabetes mellitus; cirrhosis; leukemia, lymphoma, or disseminated carcinoma; transplantation and its associated immunosuppression; childbirth; and a variety of surgical procedures and antecedent infections in the urinary, biliary, or gastrointestinal tracts. Most adults with gram-negative sepsis are elderly males, but neonates and child-bearing women are also prone to develop this syndrome. There has been an appreciable increase in the prevalence of serious gram-negative infections among hospitalized patients since 1935. The current incidence of gram-negative bacteremic sepsis is about 6 cases per 1000 hospital admissions. In addition to the predisposing factors mentioned above, the widespread use of antibiotics, immunosuppressive and cytotoxic agents, adrenal steroids, intravenous catheters, humidifiers, and other hospital equipment (Chaps. 107 and 108) and the increasing longevity of patients with chronic diseases contribute to this serious problem.

PATHOGENESIS AND PATHOLOGY With the exception of *Pseudomonas* and *Acinetobacter,* which are ubiquitous in the hospital environment, most of the bacteria causing gram-negative sepsis are normal commensals in the gastrointestinal tract. From there they may spread to contiguous structures, as in peritonitis after appendiceal perforation, or they may migrate from the perineum into the urethra or bladder. Gram-negative bacteremia follows infection in a primary focus, usually the genitourinary tract; biliary tree; gastrointestinal tract and adjoining structures or lungs; and, less commonly, the skin, bones, and joints. In patients with leukemia, the skin and subcutaneous tissues or the lungs are often portals of entry, as is also the case in burn patients. In many instances, however, notably in patients with debilitating diseases, cirrhosis, and cancer, no primary focus is apparent. When bacteremia is followed by metastatic lesions in distant sites, classic abscess formation occurs. More often, however, the autopsy findings in gram-negative sepsis reflect primarily the infection at the primary locus and show involvement of target organs: pulmonary edema, hemorrhage and hyaline membrane formation in the lungs; tubular or cortical necrosis in the kidney; patchy necrosis in the myocardium; superficial ulceration in the gastrointestinal tract; and generalized thrombi in the capillaries.

PATHOPHYSIOLOGY Cellular injury in shock Exposure of mammalian cells to endotoxin results in cell injury by several mechanisms: (1) direct cell membrane damage by endotoxin, (2) extracellular release of lysosomal enzymes from leukocytes, (3) activation of the complement cascade, and (4) metabolic injury due to tissue anoxia. The toxic component of endotoxin is principally lipid A. When endotoxin is administered to experimental animals, diffuse endothelial cell damage occurs. The cells show vacuolization and other cytoplasmic and nuclear abnormalities. There is diffuse desquamation of the endothelial cells, and the damaged cells often can be seen in the circulating blood. Endotoxin administration also causes an abrupt thrombocytopenia and granulocytopenia; in both instances this is attributed to endotoxin injury to these circulating blood elements. The damaged endothelial cells, leukocytes, and platelets all release substances activating blood coagulation, which leads to fibrin deposition in many tissues. The damaged platelets release the vasoactive substances serotonin and epinephrine. Polymorphonuclear leukocyte injury releases a variety of lysosomal enzymes as well as substances activating the complement system; the complement system is also activated directly by endotoxin, chiefly through the alternate complement pathway (Chap. 61).

Animal studies suggest a number of interactions between the complement system and the changes in platelets and leukocytes. Animals depleted of complement by pretreatment with cobra venom factor, which depletes C3 and later complement components, are less prone to develop thrombocytopenia and granulocytopenia after endotoxin than normal animals. Activation of complement in the circulation by endotoxin, specifically the component C5a, appears to increase granulocyte margination and may enhance the extracellular release of granulocyte enzymes. However, animals depleted of platelets or granulocytes and animals with congenital deficiencies in complement, e.g., C4 deficiency in guinea pigs and C6 deficiency in rabbits, are as susceptible to the lethal effects of endotoxin as normal animals are. These observations suggest that the critical initial event in septic shock is probably direct endothelial cell injury by endotoxin.

Cells in many tissues are also injured by the hypoxia that results from reduced tissue perfusion in endotoxic shock. The tissue injury closely resembles that occurring in hemorrhagic and cardiogenic shock. The result of hypoxia is uncoupling of oxidative phosphorylation and lactic acidosis.

Hemodynamic alterations Endotoxin exerts its major effects on small blood vessels with sympathetic (alpha-receptor) innervation. The toxin causes intense arteriolar and venospasm leading to significant immobilization of blood in the pulmonary, splanchnic, and renal capillaries, and to stagnant anoxia in these tissues. Through the activation of Hageman factor (factor XII), endotoxin activates bradykinin, a potent vasodilator which may be the humoral substance principally responsible for the pooling of blood in the peripheral tissues. It also increases capillary permeability. As a result, blood pools in the capillary bed and plasma proteins leak into the interstitial fluid. This, in turn, results in a sharp decrease in effective circulating blood volume and lowered cardiac output and systemic arterial hypotension, which stimulates the baroreceptors and results in further sympathetic activity, vasoconstriction, and selective reduction of blood flow to visceral organs and skin. If ineffective perfusion of vital organs is permitted to

continue, metabolic acidosis and severe parenchymal damage ensue, and shock is then irreversible. In man, the kidneys and lungs are the organs particularly susceptible to endotoxin; oliguria as well as tachypnea and, in some instances, pulmonary edema develop early. In general, the heart and brain are spared early in shock, and myocardial failure and coma are late and often terminal manifestations of the shock syndrome. There is also experimental evidence that, after the administration of live gram-negative bacteria, significant arteriovenous shunting occurs around the capillary beds of susceptible organs. This intensifies tissue anoxia. Finally, in some instances the cells seem unable to utilize available oxygen. The net result of defective tissue perfusion is a sharp decrease in arteriovenous (AV) oxygen difference and lactic acidemia.

Many of the observations dealing with the pathophysiology of endotoxin shock were made in animals, and the hemodynamic data often varied according to the species studied and the dose of endotoxin administered. The establishment of centers for the study of shock has permitted detailed pathophysiologic studies in man. The results of these studies may vary with the time at which they are performed. For example, early in septic shock, the picture is one primarily of vasodilatation with an increase in cardiac output, a decrease in systemic vascular resistance, a decrease in central venous pressure, and an increase in stroke volume. In contrast, later in septic shock, the predominant picture is one of vasoconstriction with an increase in systemic vascular resistance, a decrease in cardiac output, a decrease in central venous pressure, and a decrease in stroke volume. Despite these differences, certain patterns of septic shock have emerged when large groups of patients have been studied. These may be summarized as follows:

1 Shock characterized by a normal cardiac output, normal blood volume, normal circulation time, normal or high central venous pressure, normal or high pH, and *reduced* peripheral resistance. These patients have warm, dry skin. While hypotension, oliguria, and lactic acidemia are present, the prognosis is generally good. Shock in this group has been attributed to shunting of blood through arteriovenous communications, making it unavailable for perfusion of vital organs.

2 Patients with low blood volume, low central venous pressure, high hematocrit, increased peripheral resistance, low cardiac output, hypotension, oliguria, but only a moderate elevation of blood lactate and normal or slightly high pH. These patients may be hypovolemic before bacteremia, and their prognosis is reasonably good, provided intravascular volume is restored, bacteremia is treated with appropriate antibiotics, septic foci are removed or drained, and vasoactive drugs are given.

3 Shock characterized by normal blood volume, high central venous pressure, normal or high cardiac output, reduced peripheral resistance but *marked metabolic acidosis*, oliguria, and very high blood lactate, indicating ineffective tissue perfusion or impaired oxygen utilization. Despite the presence of warm, dry extremities in these patients, the prognosis is unfavorable.

4 Shock characterized by low blood volume, low central venous pressure, low cardiac output, marked decompensated metabolic acidosis, and severe lactic acidemia. In these patients the extremities are cool and cyanotic. The prognosis is extremely poor.

These observations suggest that there are various stages of septic shock, from hyperventilation, respiratory alkalosis, vasodilatation, and high or normal cardiac output in early shock, to perfusion failure characterized by high-grade lactic acidemia, metabolic acidosis, low cardiac output, and small AV oxygen difference in irreversible, late shock. Moreover, in some patients there is little correlation between the outcome and the hemodynamic abnormalities.

COMPLICATIONS Coagulation defects In most patients with septic shock there is a deficiency in several clotting factors, due to consumption of these factors, a syndrome termed *disseminated intravascular coagulation* (DIC). The pathogenesis of this syndrome involves the activation of the intrinsic clotting system by factor XII (Hageman factor) followed by deposition of fibrin-platelet aggregates on the capillary thrombi that have formed as a result of the generalized Shwartzman reaction. The fibrin-platelet aggregates are typical of DIC, which is characterized by a decrease in factors II, V, and VIII, fibrinogen, and platelets. There may be some degree of fibrinolysis, with appearance of split products. These clotting abnormalities are present to some degree in most patients with septic shock, but usually there is no clinical bleeding, although hemorrhagic phenomena due to thrombocytopenia or deficiency in clotting factors occur occasionally. A more important effect of further disseminated intravascular coagulation is development of capillary thrombi, particularly in the lung. Unless there is bleeding, the coagulopathy requires no therapy and disappears spontaneously as shock is treated.

Respiratory failure Respiratory failure is the most important cause of death in patients with shock, particularly after the hemodynamic aberrations have been corrected. The respiratory lesion has been called the "shock lung," and is characterized by pulmonary edema, hemorrhage, atelectasis, hyaline membrane formation, and formation of capillary thrombi. The severe pulmonary edema may be a consequence of a marked increase in capillary permeability, resulting in a "pulmonary leak." It may occur in the absence of heart failure. Respiratory failure may develop and progress even as other abnormalities return to normal. Pulmonary surfactant decreases, and pulmonary compliance becomes progressively compromised.

Renal failure Oliguria occurs early in shock and is probably due to low intravascular volume and inadequate renal perfusion. If renal perfusion remains inadequate, acute tubular necrosis develops. In an occasional patient, renal cortical necrosis, as occurs in the generalized Shwartzman reaction, is seen.

Cardiac failure Many patients with septic shock develop myocardial failure even though they were free of heart disease before development of shock. On the basis of experimental data, heart failure has been attributed to a product of lysosomal enzyme activity in the ischemic splanchnic region. This product has been termed myocardial depressant factor (MDF). Functionally, there is left ventricular failure as indicated by an increase in left ventricular end-diastolic pressure.

Other organs Superficial ulcerations of the gastrointestinal tract manifested by hemorrhage are common, as are abnormalities in liver function, characterized by hypoprothrombinemia, hypoalbuminemia, and mild jaundice.

CLINICAL MANIFESTATIONS Usually gram-negative bacteremia begins abruptly with chills, fever, nausea, vomiting, diarrhea, and prostration. When septic shock develops, there are, in addition, tachycardia; tachypnea; hypotension; cool, pale extremities, often with peripheral cyanosis; mental obtundation; and oliguria. When present in its full-blown form, gram-negative shock is detected readily, but occasionally the findings are quite subtle, particularly in old, debilitated patients or in infants. Unexplained hypotension, increasing confusion, and disorientation or hyperventilation may be the only clues to septic shock. Some patients are hypothermic, and in the absence of fever the diagnosis is often missed. Jaundice occurs

occasionally and signifies infection in the biliary tree, intravascular hemolysis, or "toxic" hepatitis. As shock progresses, oliguria persists, and heart failure, respiratory insufficiency, and coma supervene. Death usually occurs from pulmonary edema, generalized anoxemia secondary to respiratory insufficiency, cardiac arrhythmias, disseminated intravascular coagulation with bleeding, cerebral anoxia, or a combination of these factors.

LABORATORY FINDINGS The laboratory data in septic shock vary greatly and depend in many instances on the cause of the shock syndrome and on the stage of shock. The hematocrit is often elevated and falls to below normal as the volume deficit is repaired. There usually is *leukocytosis* with a white blood cell count between 15,000 and 30,000 per cubic millimeter with a shift to the left. However, the white blood cell count may be normal, and some patients have leukopenia. The *platelet count* is usually decreased, and the prothrombin time and partial thromboplastin times may be abnormal, reflecting a consumption of *clotting factors*.

The *urinalysis* shows no specific abnormalities. Initially, the specific gravity is high; as oliguria persists, isosthenuria develops. The *blood urea nitrogen* and *creatinine* are elevated, and creatinine clearance is reduced.

Simultaneous measurements of urine and plasma osmolalities are a useful clue to impending renal failure. If the urinary osmolality is greater than 400 mosmol and the ratio of urine to plasma osmolality is greater than 1.5, renal function is preserved and oliguria is probably due to volume depletion. On the other hand, a urine osmolality of less than 400 mosmol and a urine/plasma ratio less than 1.5 signify renal failure. Other useful clues to suggest prerenal azotemia are urine sodium less than 20 meq per liter, a urine creatinine/serum creatinine ratio greater than 40, or a BUN/serum creatinine ratio greater than 20. Electrolyte patterns vary considerably, but there is a tendency to *hyponatremia* and hypochloremia. The serum potassium may be high, low, or normal. The *bicarbonate concentration* is usually low and *blood lactate* is elevated. A high level of blood lactate is the most reliable clue to poor tissue perfusion.

Early in endotoxin shock there is *respiratory alkalosis* manifested by a low P_{CO_2} and high arterial pH, probably because of progressive anoxemia and an attempt to blow off CO_2 to compensate for developing lactic acidemia. As shock progresses, *metabolic acidosis* develops. There often is striking *anoxemia*, and P_{O_2} values below 70 mmHg are common. The *electrocardiogram* generally shows depression of the ST segment, inversion of the T waves, and a variety of arrhythmias, and may mistakenly suggest the diagnosis of myocardial infarction.

In untreated septic shock, the blood cultures should reveal the causative pathogens, but bacteremia may be intermittent and the blood cultures may be negative. Furthermore, many patients will have received antimicrobial agents when they are first seen, masking the bacteriologic diagnosis. *A negative blood culture does not exclude the diagnosis of septic shock.* Culture of the primary septic focus may aid in the diagnosis, but the bacteriology may have been altered by prior chemotherapy. The ability of endotoxin to coagulate the blood of the horseshoe crab *Limulus* is the basis of a test for endotoxemia, but this test is not widely available and is of limited clinical usefulness.

DIAGNOSIS The diagnosis of septic shock is not difficult in the presence of chills, fever, and an overt focus of infection. However, none of the obvious clues may be present. Elderly, debilitated patients, in particular, may have severe infections in the absence of fever. Unexplained confusion and disorientation and hyperventilation without abnormal chest x-rays should call the diagnosis to mind. Pulmonary embolism, myocardial infarction, cardiac tamponade, aortic dissection, and silent hemorrhage are entities often confused with septic shock.

COURSE The rational treatment of septic shock depends upon careful monitoring of patients. A flow sheet for recording clinical data is very helpful. Specifically four parameters need to be followed at the bedside:

1 The status of the *pulmonary circulation* and, to a lesser extent, of left ventricular function should be monitored by insertion of a Swan-Ganz catheter. A pulmonary wedge pressure in excess of 15 to 18 cmH$_2$O signifies fluid overload. When a Swan-Ganz catheter is not available, the *central venous pressure* (CVP) should be measured. Insertion of a catheter into the great veins or right atrium provides an accurate index of the relation between right ventricular competence and effective blood volume and should be used as a guide to fluid replacement therapy. When the CVP exceeds 12 to 14 cmH$_2$O, there is some danger of overloading the circulation and precipitating pulmonary edema. It is important to be sure that the flow through the catheter is free and that the catheter is not in the right ventricle. Either a Swan-Ganz catheter or a CVP line should be placed in every patient with septic shock.

2 The *pulse pressure* serves as an estimate of stroke volume.

3 *Cutaneous vasoconstriction* provides a clue to peripheral resistance, although it does not reflect accurately blood flow to kidney, brain, or gut.

4 Hourly *urine output* should be used to monitor splanchnic blood flow and visceral perfusion. Usually this requires placement of an indwelling urethral catheter.

By means of these four measurements the patient with shock can be followed carefully and managed intelligently. Indirect arterial blood pressure does not provide an accurate picture of the hemodynamic situation, and perfusion of vital organs may be adequate in patients with hypotension; conversely, some patients with normal blood pressures may have marked pooling and inadequate visceral blood flow. Direct measurement of arterial pressure is helpful but usually not necessary.

Where possible, these patients should be treated in intensive care units in hospitals that have laboratories available for measurement of arterial pH, blood gases, blood lactate, renal function, and electrolytes.

TREATMENT Support of respiration In many patients with septic shock arterial P_{O_2} is markedly depressed. It is essential to establish an airway at the outset and to administer oxygen nasally or by mask. Tracheal intubation usually suffices; tracheostomy is rarely necessary. However, a positive pressure–volume-cycled respirator should be employed early to achieve proper ventilation and to overcome the severe hypoxia.

Volume replacement With the CVP or pulmonary wedge pressure as a guide, blood volume should be replaced with blood (if anemia is present), plasma, or other colloids, especially human serum albumin, and appropriate electrolyte solutions, primarily dextrose-saline and bicarbonate (which is preferable to lactate for treating the acidosis). Bicarbonate should be given to increase the blood pH to about 7.2 to 7.3 but not higher under most circumstances. The quantity of fluid required may be considerably in excess of "normal" blood volume and may amount to 8 to 12 liters in only a few hours. Large quantities may be required even when the cardiac index

is normal. *Oliguria in the presence of hypotension is not a contraindication to continued vigorous fluid therapy.* In order to guard against pulmonary edema, diuresis with furosemide should be attempted when the CVP reaches a level of approximately 10 to 12 cmH$_2$O and the pulmonary artery pressure 16 to 18 cmH$_2$O.

Antibiotics Blood cultures and cultures of relevant body fluids or exudates should be taken before instituting antimicrobial therapy. Drugs should be given intravenously, and bactericidal agents used when possible. When the results of blood cultures and sensitivities are known, one of the appropriate drugs recommended in the chapters dealing with the specific infections and discussed in Chap. 111 should be given. Usually cultures and sensitivities are not at hand at the onset of shock, and the etiologic diagnosis entails an educated guess based upon culture from the primary focus—urine, bile, pus, or sputum, or on the setting in which the infection occurs. For example, a young woman with dysuria, chills, and flank pain and septic shock is likely to have *Escherichia coli* bacteremia, while gram-negative sepsis in a burn patient is probably caused by *Pseudomonas*. The drugs of choice for gram-negative bacteremia are:

E. coli	Ampicillin or a parenteral cephalosporin
Klebsiella-Enterobacter	Gentamicin
Proteus mirabilis	Ampicillin or a parenteral cephalosporin
P. rettgeri, morganii, or *vulgaris*	Gentamicin and/or carbenicillin
Acinetobacter	Gentamicin and/or carbenicillin
Pseudomonas	Gentamicin and/or carbenicillin

The dosages and routes of administration for these agents are detailed in Chap. 111. A cephalosporin can be substituted for ampicillin in patients with a history of penicillin allergy. Because of its toxic effect on the vestibular portion of the eighth nerve, gentamicin must be given cautiously to oliguric patients; a single dose of 80 mg achieves blood levels which should suffice throughout the period of oliguria. Similar precautions should be taken with kanamycin, where the loading dose is 1.0 g.

When the cause of septic shock is unknown, therapy should be initiated with both gentamicin and a cephalosporin or a penicillinase-resistant penicillin; many physicians add carbenicillin to this regimen. If *Bacteroides* is suspected, chloramphenicol, 7-chlorlincomycin (clindamycin), or carbenicillin can be added. As soon as culture results become available, the unnecessary drugs can be deleted.

Surgical intervention Many patients with septic shock have an abscess, infarcted or necrotic bowel, inflamed gallbladder, infected uterus, pyonephrosis, or other local situations which lend themselves to surgical drainage or excision. As a rule, successful treatment of shock requires surgical intervention even if the patient is desperately ill. Operations should not be postponed "to get the patient in shape" because these patients' condition will continue to deteriorate unless the septic focus is removed or drained.

Vasoactive drugs Usually, septic shock is accompanied by maximal stimulation of alpha-adrenergic receptors, and pressor agents which act by stimulating these receptors, such as norepinephrine, levarterenol, and metaraminol are generally not indicated. The two groups of drugs which have been of value in septic shock are beta-receptor stimulants (notably isoproterenol and dopamine) and alpha-receptor blocking agents (phenoxybenzamine and phentolamine).

Dopamine hydrochloride is used widely for treatment of

shock. Unlike other vasoactive agents, this drug increases renal blood flow and with it glomerular filtration, sodium excretion, and urine flow. This effect is seen at low doses [1 to 2 (μg/kg)/min]. At a dose of 2 to 10 (μg/kg)/min, the beta receptors in the heart are stimulated with a resulting increase in cardiac output but without increase in heart rate or blood pressure. Between 10 and 20 (μg/kg)/min there is some effect on the alpha receptors with a rise in blood pressure. Above 20 (μg/kg)/min, alpha stimulation predominates, and vasoconstriction may reverse the dopaminergic effects on the renal and splanchnic circulations. Treatment should be started at 2 to 5 (μg/kg)/min and the dose increased until urine flow and blood pressure respond. Most patients respond to doses of 20 (μg/kg)/min or less. Side effects include ectopic rhythms, nausea and vomiting, and occasionally tachyarrhythmias. They usually disappear with reduction in dosage.

Isoproterenol (Isuprel) counteracts arteriolar and venous constriction in the microcirculation by its direct vasodilating effect. In addition, the drug exerts a direct inotropic effect on the heart. Cardiac output is increased by stimulation of the myocardium and by reduction of cardiac work as peripheral resistance decreases. The dose of isoproterenol is 2 to 8 μg/min for the average adult. Ventricular arrhythmias may result from this drug, and shock may be made worse if fluid administration does not keep pace with relieved vasoconstriction.

Phenoxybenzamine (Dibenzyline), an adrenolytic agent, effects a central phlebotomy by reducing resistance and increasing intravascular capacity. Hence there is a redistribution of blood. Blood leaves the lungs, relieving pulmonary edema and enhancing gas exchange. Central venous pressure and left ventricular end-diastolic pressure fall, cardiac output rises, and peripheral venous constriction regresses. The recommended dose is 0.2 to 2.0 mg/kg intravenously. Small doses can be injected instantaneously and large doses over a period of 40 to 60 min. Fluids must be given simultaneously to compensate for the increment in venous capacitance; failure to do so aggravates shock. Dibenzyline is not available for general use, and experience with phentolamine has not been great enough to recommend it.

Chlorpromazine in multiple small doses of 2.5 to 5 mg also relieves vasoconstriction through its direct adrenolytic effect and by ganglionic blockage.

Diuretics and digitalis It is important to maintain urine flow to try to prevent the development of renal tubular necrosis. Once the volume status of the patient is repaired, a diuretic, preferably furosemide, should be given to keep the hourly urine output up to greater than 30 to 40 ml/h. In patients who remain hypotensive despite an elevated CVP or pulmonary wedge pressure, digitalization with digoxin or Cedilanid may be beneficial. Therapy with digitalis preparations should be undertaken with caution in patients with impaired renal function, elevated serum potassium, and severe acid-base abnormalities.

Glucocorticosteroids Numerous experimental studies provide a rationale for the use of corticosteroid therapy to ameliorate the effects of endotoxemia and septic shock. Steroids appear to protect cell membranes from endotoxin-mediated injury and to decrease platelet aggregation and the extracellular release of leukocyte enzymes. Some studies suggest that steroids also may have a direct effect on reducing peripheral vascular resistance. Because of the complexity of the clinical circumstances surrounding the patient with endotoxic shock, it has been difficult to prove that steroid therapy is clearly helpful. One controlled study has demonstrated a substantial benefit for treating patients with methylprednisolone (30 mg/kg) or dexamethasone (3 mg/kg) as soon as shock was recognized. Therapy was repeated in 4 h in the most severely ill patients. This

study and experience in many shock centers supports the early use of steroids in high doses for relatively brief periods (24 to 48 h). Prolonged steroid therapy substantially increases the problems of hyperglycemia, gastrointestinal bleeding, and other steroid side effects and should be avoided.

Other measures Hemorrhage must be controlled with whole blood, fresh frozen plasma, cryoprecipitate, or platelet transfusion, depending on the clotting abnormality. Treatment of disseminated intravascular coagulation with heparin remains a controversial and hazardous procedure. Hyperbaric oxygen has been tried in gram-negative bacteremia with indifferent results.

PROGNOSIS The measures described above usually will resuscitate most patients, at least temporarily. Indicators of a favorable response are:

1 Improved sensorium and general appearance
2 Decreased peripheral cyanosis
3 Warming of the skin over the extremities
4 Urine output of 40 to 50 ml/h
5 Increased pulse pressure
6 Return of CVP and pulmonary artery pressure to normal
7 Increased blood pressure

The ultimate outcome, however, is dependent upon several other factors:

1 Ability to eliminate the source of infection with surgery or antibiotics. The prognosis of urinary tract infections, septic abortions, abdominal abscesses, gastrointestinal or biliary fistulas, and subcutaneous or anorectal abscesses is better than that of primary foci in the skin or lungs. However, extensive abdominal surgery, even if necessary, is associated with a poor prognosis.
2 Previous contact with the organism. Patients with chronic urinary tract infections who develop bacteremia rarely have severe gram-negative shock, perhaps because they have become tolerant to the endotoxin.
3 Underlying disease. Patients with lymphoma or leukemia who develop septic shock while their hematologic disease is out of control rarely recover; conversely, if hematologic remission is achieved, the shock is more likely to respond to therapy. Patients with antecedent heart disease and with diabetes mellitus also have a poor prognosis.
4 Metabolic status. The development of severe metabolic acidosis and lactic acidemia—irrespective of cardiac output—is associated with a poor prognosis.
5 Development of pulmonary insufficiency even after the hemodynamic abnormalities have been corrected is associated with an unfavorable outcome.

The overall mortality rate of septic shock remains 50 percent; however, with better monitoring and more physiologic treatment, the outcome should improve.

PREVENTION The poor results in the treatment of septic shock are not due to lack of potent antibiotics or vasoactive agents. Rather, failure to institute therapy sufficiently early is a major roadblock to success. Septic shock usually is recognized too late, all too often after irreversible changes have taken place. Because 70 percent of patients who are likely to develop septic shock are in the hospital *before* signs and symptoms of shock appear, it is essential to watch patients who are candidates for development of shock assiduously, to treat their infections vigorously and early, and to perform appropriate surgery before catastrophic complications occur. It is particularly important to watch for infected venous and urinary catheters which may act as portals of entry for the organisms that cause gram-negative sepsis and to remove them from all patients as soon as feasible. There is some preliminary evidence that early therapy of septic shock improves the ultimate outcome. Finally, the protective effect of antiserum in experimental animals may, at some time in the future, be applicable to humans.

REFERENCES

BRYANT RD et al: Factors affecting mortality of gram-negative rod bacteremia. Arch Intern Med 127:120, 1971

CAVANAGH D et al: Septic shock in obstetrics and gynecology. Major Probl Obstet Gynecol 11:1, 1977

CORRIGAN JJ JR et al: Changes in the blood coagulation system associated with septicemia. N Engl J Med 279:851, 1968

FEARON DT et al: Activation of properdin pathway of complement in patients with gram-negative bacteremia. N Engl J Med 292:937, 1975

GOLDBERG LI: Dopamine: Clinical uses of an endogenous catecholamine. N Engl J Med 291:707, 1974

HARDAWAY RM et al: Intensive study and treatment of shock in man. JAMA 199:799, 1967.

JONES LW, WEIL MH: Water, creatinine and sodium excretion following circulatory shock with renal failure. Am J Med 41:314, 1971

MACLEAN LD et al: Patterns of septic shock in man: A detailed study of 56 patients. Ann Surg 166:543, 1967

MCHENRY MC, HANK WA: Bacteremia caused by gram-negative bacilli. Med Clin North Am 58:623, 1974

MILLER RI: Biochemical mechanisms of generation of bradykinin by endotoxin. J Infect Dis 128:S144, 1973

NISHIJIMA H et al: Hemodynamic and metabolic studies in shock associated with gram-negative bacteremia. Medicine 42:287, 1973

ROBIN ED et al: Capillary leak syndrome with pulmonary edema. Arch Intern Med 130:66, 1972

ROBINSON JA et al: Endotoxin, prekallikrein, complement and systemic vascular resistance. Am J Med 49:61, 1975

SCHUMER W: Steroids in the treatment of clinical septic shock. Ann Surg 184:333, 1976

TARAZI RC: Sympathomimetic agents in the treatment of shock. Ann Intern Med 81:364, 1974

ULEVITCH RJ et al: Role of complement in lethal bacterial lipopolysaccharide-induced hypotensive and coagulative changes. Infect Immun 19:204, 1978

WINSLOW EJ et al: Hemodynamic studies and results of therapy in 50 patients with bacteremic shock. Am J Med 54:421, 1973

110
LOCALIZED INFECTIONS AND ABSCESSES

ROBERT G. PETERSDORF
JAN V. HIRSCHMANN

GENERAL CONSIDERATIONS

In contrast to many bacterial diseases, which can be conveniently described in terms of their specific etiologic pathogens, there are some in which the clinical picture is determined primarily by their location. Examples of such infections include abscesses, soft-tissue infections, bacterial endocarditis (Chap. 243), pyogenic infections of the central nervous system (Chap. 368), urinary tract infections (Chap. 280), lung abscess (Chap. 260), mediastinitis (Chap. 269), appendicitis and appendiceal abscess (Chap. 296), diverticulitis (Chap. 294), osteomyelitis (Chap. 360), and infections of the pericardium (Chap. 249). Infections in these sites can be caused by many pathogens, and although their bacteriologic identification may be time-consuming, knowledge of the usual flora causing infection in certain anatomic loci should permit institution of therapy before the results of cultures are available. Although treatment of these infections is usually surgical, the internist may be the first one to see these patients and may also be the one to prescribe chemotherapy on the basis of the presumed pathogen.

ETIOLOGY Localized pyogenic infection can develop in any region or organ of the body, and may be initiated by *trauma* and secondary bacterial contamination, by some *alteration in local conditions* that renders a tissue susceptible to infection with organisms already present as part of the "normal flora" to which it is ordinarily resistant, by *contiguous spread* from a nearby lesion, or by *metastatic implantation* of microorganisms carried in blood or lymph.

Under appropriate conditions of lowered tissue resistance, almost any of the common bacteria can initiate an infectious process. Cultures from open lesions such as those of the skin or from intraabdominal foci arising from perforations of the gastrointestinal tract frequently contain several bacterial species; as might be expected, the organisms found most frequently are the "normal flora" of these regions.

Infection in some areas is more likely to be caused by certain organisms, staphylococci in the skin and coliform bacteria in the urinary tract, and special features of the tissue reaction produced by some bacterial species make it possible to recognize infection by them with considerable accuracy. The *staphylococci* produce rapid necrosis and early suppuration with large amounts of creamy yellow pus (Chap. 116). Group A beta-hemolytic streptococcal infections (Chap. 117) tend to spread rapidly through tissues, causing intense edema and erythema but relatively little necrosis and thin, serumlike exudate; anaerobic bacteria (Chap. 142) produce necrosis and profuse, brownish, foul-smelling pus.

The identification of infecting organisms is important in the choice of local or systemic chemotherapy. However, when infection occurs in certain areas, as in paranasal sinuses or cutaneous ulcers, or shows up in sputum, it is unlikely that cultured specimens can ever be rendered sterile. In these locations, serial cultures during antimicrobial administration must be interpreted in this light, and therapy should be guided largely by the clinical response.

PATHOGENESIS Factors predisposing to the initiation and persistence of infection in a tissue include trauma, obstruction of normal drainage (sweat glands, biliary tract, bronchial tree, urinary tract), ischemia (infarction, gangrene), chemical irritation (by gastric contents, bile, or intramuscularly injected drugs), hematoma formation, accumulation of fluid (lymphatic obstruction, cardiac edema), foreign bodies (bullets, splinters, sutures), and others such as the occurrence of stasis or turbulence in the vascular system.

Infection in soft tissue usually begins as a *cellulitis,* a diffuse acute inflammation with hyperemia, edema, and leukocytic infiltration but little or no necrosis and suppuration. With some organisms, this is followed by necrosis, liquefaction, accumulation of leukocytes and debris, suppuration, loculation of the pus, and formation of one or more *abscesses.* Abscess formation is particularly likely to follow infection in a preexisting space or cavity, examples being the fallopian tubes or lung cysts.

The local spread of infection generally follows the path of least resistance along fascial planes; proper surgical treatment is based upon a knowledge of these routes, which will be described for specific infections later in this chapter. Lymphatic spread may lead to lymphangitis, lymphadenitis, or, if the regional nodes suppurate, to the formation of a *bubo.* Involvement of local venules or large veins may lead to infective thrombophlebitis with resulting bacteremia, septic embolization, and systemic dissemination of infection. Staphylococci, streptococci, and *Bacteroides* are notorious for the frequency with which they produce vascular lesions of this type.

Depending upon the infecting organism and the anatomy of the affected region, a small abscess may subside completely; there may be gradual encapsulation of the accumulated pus and persistence of the focus in a quiescent state; or the lesion may "point" and rupture into adjacent tissues or to the outside surface of the body, as usually happens with furuncles. Spontaneous drainage ordinarily leads to subsidence and healing of a superficially situated suppurative focus. However, if the abscess is deeply situated and well encapsulated, there are often persistence of a fistulous tract and the formation of a chronic, draining sinus. *The development of persistent sinuses over an area of suppuration produced by ordinary pyogenic bacteria should always suggest involvement of underlying bone or the presence of a foreign body.* Fistulas that open onto the skin are, of course, soon colonized by microorganisms from the external environment. Ordinary bacterial cultures of drainage fluid almost invariably show a mixed flora and should not be relied upon for the etiologic diagnosis of the underlying disease. This is particularly important in disorders that characteristically lead to persistent sinus formation: tuberculosis, actinomycosis, blastomycosis, melioidosis and glanders, and, rarely, amebic abscess of the liver or cecum. In these situations, superficial organisms about the opening of the sinus tract may mask the true nature of the lesion by obscuring the real pathogen.

MANIFESTATIONS Secondary infection of wounds and cutaneous ulcers is usually recognizable by inspection. Infections of the skin and subcutaneous tissues almost invariably produce the classic manifestations: *redness, tenderness, heat,* and *swelling.* Reddish streaks extending proximally and associated with tender enlargement of regional lymph nodes indicate lymphangitis. Systemic symptoms may be absent or mild, or there may be fever, malaise, prostration, and leukocytosis.

Infection and suppuration in deeper tissues or in body cavities are often manifested by local pain and tenderness, but the task of locating and determining the exact nature of the lesion may be difficult. The palpation of a tender mass is helpful, but muscle spasm and intervening structures often interfere. Abdominal or pelvic examination under anesthesia is sometimes useful in these circumstances.

Auscultation may reveal a friction rub over an abdominal viscus, the pleura, or the pericardium. The rapid development of an effusion in the pericardium, pleura, abdomen, or a joint should suggest infection. Similarly, fluid detected by transillumination of paranasal sinuses or inspection of the tympanic membrane may be the first sign of infection.

Depending on the location of an abscess, symptoms and signs referable to encroachment upon adjacent structures may dominate the picture. Respiratory obstruction may be the first sign of mediastinal abscess; dysphagia often first calls attention to peritonsillar or retropharyngeal abscesses; and tamponade is sometimes the initial clue to pericardial infection. Localizing signs of dysfunction are especially striking and important with brain and spinal cord abscesses, although brain abscesses may be clinically silent (Chap. 368). In some patients local pain and tenderness or signs of dysfunction are mild or equivocal, and fever, prostration, and weight loss dominate the picture. The fever may be low-grade but is often hectic, with repeated rigors and drenching night sweats. Fatigue and anemia are frequent, and weight loss may be so rapid as to result in emaciation within a few weeks. A patient with these symptoms and signs may have chronic subphrenic, perinephric, or other abscess in the complete absence of any detectable physical sign pointing to the location of a large accumulation of pus. With the advent of antibiotics some deep-seated abscesses present the picture of a chronic illness manifested by no more than malaise, easy fatigability, low-grade fever, mild anemia, and an elevated sedimentation rate because of prior treatment with antimicrobials.

Fluctuation of a mass on palpation is a reliable sign that it contains fluid, perhaps pus, but failure to detect this sign when deeper structures are examined is no guarantee that suppuration is absent and should not be taken by itself to indicate that the mass is noninfectious in origin or that drainage is not required.

LABORATORY FINDINGS Peripheral polymorphonuclear leukocytosis is frequent with abscesses, and significant unexplained elevation of the white blood cell count in any patient should lead to a search for localized suppuration. Depending on the severity and duration of infection, there may be a chronic normocytic, normochromic anemia. The sedimentation rate is almost always rapid. Mild albuminuria, occasionally noted in febrile patients, has no diagnostic import.

Pus or fluid obtained by needle aspiration or incision of a suspected lesion should *always* be stained and examined directly in addition to being cultured aerobically and anaerobically. Pus is a poor metabolic substrate, and bacteria may fail to grow in cultures from an abscess of long standing. In such instances, the findings on microscopic examination may be the only guide in choosing proper chemotherapy. *Failure to examine exudates with Gram's stain is the single greatest deterrent to appropriate antimicrobial therapy;* it is the responsibility of the internist as well as the surgeon to see that this procedure is performed.

Blood cultures are often positive in intravascular infections such as septic thrombophlebitis and endocarditis and in pyogenic infections in which localized abscesses are metastatic, as in staphylococcal, streptococcal, and *Salmonella* bacteremias. Moreover, manipulation, including surgical incision, of any localized infection may be followed by transient bacteremia.

Noninvasive techniques are often helpful in the diagnosis of abscess. X-ray examinations may be of considerable help in detecting localized collections of pus when they show atypical collections of gas, displacement of organs, and tissue densities in abnormal locations. Radionuclide scans may demonstrate abscesses in brain, liver, spleen, and thyroid. The isotope [^{67}Ga] gallium citrate is selectively concentrated in abscesses, but in noninfectious inflammation and neoplasms as well, and many have found gallium scans of limited value in locating abscesses. Of even more potential value is the technique of diagnostic ultrasound, which is not only useful in localizing abscess but also may provide clues to the size of the abscess and to the presence of multiple abscesses or loculation. Angiography is useful in detecting abscesses in highly vascular organs such as the spleen. Computerized tomography (CT scan) may be helpful in demonstrating abscesses, especially in the brain and in areas not easily evaluated by other methods, such as the retroperitoneum.

THERAPEUTIC CONSIDERATIONS Recognition of the striking symptomatic improvement that follows spontaneous evacuation of a suppurative focus led long ago to the adoption of *surgical incision* for the treatment of abscesses. The exact reasons for the amelioration of local and constitutional manifestations that results from drainage of pus are unknown, but, clinically, the benefits of adequate incision and drainage are unequivocal.

Incision of infected tissue before the stage of liquefaction and accumulation of pus is often deleterious and fails to relieve discomfort. Premature incision may even at times facilitate spread of infection. For this reason, it is sometimes necessary to wait until an abscess "ripens," i.e., localizes and "comes to a head." The *application of heat* to an area of inflammation will relieve pain and often speed the subsidence of cellulitis without suppuration. If necrosis of tissue is already under way, hot applications appear to facilitate localization of the process and accumulation of pus, making incision and drainage feasible at an earlier time. Another procedure that aids in reduction of swelling and relief of pain is *elevation of the affected part.*

The availability of specific chemotherapeutic drugs has modified the need for heat, elevation, and incision surprisingly little. The early administration of chemotherapeutics has reduced the incidence of suppurative complications in many disorders, but once suppuration has appeared, antimicrobial drugs become remarkably incapable of eradicating the infecting organisms, although they may mask the classic clinical features of abscess formation.

Some antimicrobials, notably the penicillins, appear to retain their antibacterial activity in the presence of pus, while others, exemplified by the aminoglycosides and the polymyxins, are at least partially inactivated in purulent exudates. However, inability of the drug to penetrate into an area of suppuration is rarely the reason for therapeutic failure. Although this possibility exists in some infections, such as osteomyelitis, it is usually overcome by increasing dosage. Because direct instillation of the antibiotic into an infected area is not, by itself, a curative procedure, other factors are probably more important than faulty diffusion of the agent into the purulent focus.

An established inflammatory exudate is a relatively poor environment for bacterial multiplication. Because the bactericidal action of the penicillins and the cephalosporins is exerted only against multiplying organisms, failure of these antibiotics to eradicate bacteria in an abscess may be related to the organisms' inactive metabolic state. Although the mechanism of their antibacterial action differs from that of the penicillins, bacteriostatic agents such as tetracycline or chloramphenicol also are incapable of eradicating bacteria in the static phase of growth. Furthermore, by definition, these drugs only inhibit multiplication of bacteria and usually exert no direct lethal action; the death of organisms in any infection treated with bacteriostatic agents depends on other mechanisms. For most pyogenic bacteria, phagocytosis is one of the most important of these mechanisms (although there must be others that have not been studied so carefully), and, in the absence of phagocytes or in circumstances which inhibit their activity, bacteriostatic drugs are relatively ineffective. In fluid-filled cavities, particularly in the metabolically unfavorable milieu of an abscess, phagocytosis is greatly reduced. Consequently, despite inhibition of bacterial multiplication, organisms can remain dormant and survive for long periods of time. It is probably a combination of these two circumstances, decreased multiplication of bacteria and decreased phagocytosis, that makes infection in the heart valves, in the kidney, or in the meninges so relatively resistant to antimicrobial therapy. Relatively large doses of bactericidal drugs for long periods are needed to achieve cure.

Antimicrobial drugs may be expected to prevent suppuration if given early or to prevent spread of an existing abscess, but cannot be substituted for surgical drainage. Indeed, their use in the face of a lesion requiring evacuation of pus is one of the most common serious errors in treating pyogenic infections.

In empyema, suppurative pericarditis, or pyarthrosis, excellent therapeutic results are sometimes achieved by aspiration of pus and systemic antimicrobial therapy. The success of this procedure, however, fully depends on the adequacy of drainage as it is upon the instillation of the antibiotic, and if there is loculation or if the exudate becomes too viscid to allow removal, surgical incision and drainage through a large-bore tube become mandatory.

In the presence of infective thrombophlebitis, surgical interruption of the veins by ligation or, in some cases, by total excision of an infected segment is sometimes indicated to prevent seeding of other organs by infected emboli.

CLINICAL FEATURES OF INFECTIONS IN VARIOUS REGIONS

SUPERFICIAL ABSCESSES Skin and subcutaneous tissues
Impetigo is a superficial infection caused by group A hemolytic streptococci, sometimes combined with *Staphylococcus aureus*. It is primarily a disease of children, common in warm weather, characterized by multiple erythematous lesions which vesiculate and are intensely pruritic. Local spread occurs through scratching and release of infected vesicle fluid. Serious complications are metastatic abscesses and hemorrhagic nephritis. Treatment consists of local and general cleansing of the skin and appropriate systemic antibiotics.

Deeper infections of the skin are almost invariably staphylococcal in origin and are described in Chap. 116. Erysipelas, a characteristic dermal lesion produced by group A streptococci, is described in Chap. 117.

Lymphadenitis with or without suppuration may complicate any pyogenic skin lesion and is often striking with superficial streptococcal infections. Specific diseases characterized by suppurative regional lymphadenitis include lymphogranuloma venereum (Chap. 174), cat-scratch disease (Chap. 197), tularemia (Chap. 128), and bubonic plague (Chap. 129).

Infections of the hand   These are almost invariably secondary to trauma and are very common. Because of the rapidity with which infection can spread through the complex fascial spaces of the hand, wrist, and forearm, with the production of irreparable functional damage, *any deep infection in this area should receive expert surgical attention immediately.* The importance of such care has in no way been lessened by the availability of antibiotics.

The ordinary *paronychia,* or "run-around," is a superficial infection of the epithelium lateral to a nail, usually a result of tearing a hangnail and most frequently caused by staphylococcus. Hot applications will lead to subsidence of paronychial cellulitis, but often a superficial blister of pus appears. A small incision or simply separation of the nail fold from the nail will promote adequate drainage. If the infection burrows beneath the nail to form a painful *subungual abscess,* incision and drainage with partial or complete removal of the nail are necessary. Recurrence is common, especially in nail biters, and this seemingly trivial infection can cause painful disability. Chronic paronychial inflammation produced by various fungi occurs in diabetics, and a similar lesion is seen in psoriasis and some types of pemphigus.

What appears to be a small furuncle of the webs of the fingers sometimes produces a *collar-button abscess,* consisting of a superficial and deep compartment connected by a narrow tract. Evacuation of the shallow pocket without emptying the deeper abscess can lead to puzzling persistence of infection. Sometimes a foreign-body granuloma forms in the skin of the digital webs. This is most common in barbers, in whom a hair is the core of the foreign-body granuloma, the "barber's interdigital pilonidal sinus."

Infection of the distal phalanx of a finger, usually acquired by pinprick, thorn prick, etc., may lead to the formation of a *felon,* or *whitlow.* This is a suppurative infection in the tightly enclosed fibrous compartments of the finger pulp, the "anterior closed space," which can compromise the distal blood supply by compression of the digital arteries, with consequent necrosis of bone and the development of osteomyelitis. The manifestations are swelling, extreme pain, and tenderness of the palmar surface of the finger tip. The treatment is immediate incision directly over the lesion, sometimes by the use of a trephine, and cutting all the fibrous septa that radiate from the periosteum to the subcutaneous fascia.

Suppurative tenosynovitis, usually a complication of a puncture wound, is an even more serious infection of the hand from the point of view of functional damage; early diagnosis and treatment are mandatory to prevent permanent disability from destruction of the tendon or its sheath. The three cardinal manifestations of tenosynovitis are (1) exquisite tenderness limited to the course of the sheath, (2) flexion of the fingers, and (3) excruciating pain, most marked at the base of the digit, on extension of the involved finger. *Immediate incision* of the sheath is indicated, not only to prevent damage to the tendon itself but to avoid proximal extension of the process into the major fascial spaces of the hand or forearm. Vigorous antibiotic treatment should accompany surgery. The definitive treatment of any serious infection of the hand is a matter for a skilled surgeon, but the early recognition of the need for surgery often falls to other physicians.

Human bites lead to very important hand infections, which, if neglected, almost invariably produce a highly destructive, necrotizing lesion contaminated by a mixture of aerobic and anaerobic organisms. A deliberately inflicted bite on the hand or elsewhere is usually recognized as dangerously contaminated, but wounds on the knuckles produced by striking an opponent's teeth with the fists may not be recognized as potentially dangerous. In general, bite wounds should be cleaned thoroughly and not sutured. Patients should be given prophylaxis for tetanus and antibiotics, preferably both a penicillinase-resistant penicillin and ampicillin.

Chronic cutaneous ulcers A partial list of the causes of chronic ulcers of the skin includes circulatory disturbances, such as varicose veins and obliterative arterial disease, extensive injury from frostbite or burns, trophic changes accompanying many neurological disorders, bedsores or decubiti, systemic diseases such as sickle-cell disease and myxedema, neoplasms, and various infections. No matter what the underlying disease, secondary infection is very likely to occur and to interfere with healing, complicate grafting or other restorative procedures, or produce extension of the process.

The management of secondary bacterial infection in skin ulcers associated with obliterative arterial disease, a common problem in diabetics, is especially important, because infection is frequently the factor that precipitates spreading gangrene and makes amputation necessary.

Studies of the microflora of chronic cutaneous ulcers have almost invariably shown bacteria of many species, including staphylococci, aerobic and anaerobic streptococci, coliform bacilli, and members of the *Proteus* and *Pseudomonas* groups. Depending on the patient's environment and on systemically or locally administered antimicrobial drugs, the predominating bacterial species show great variation when lesions are cultured serially. Particularly noteworthy is the replacement of sensitive organisms by resistant strains or species during the course of chemotherapy.

Treatment of chronic dermal ulcers should be directed toward the underlying disorder but should also include *local debridement* and *chemotherapy.* Debridement by surgical excision is often needed, but the local application of wet-to-dry dressings or other forms of "medical debridement" frequently suffice. Intensive systemic administration of antibiotics should be carried out only in conjunction with definitive surgical procedures or when infection can be controlled in no other way. The prevention of infection by "prophylactic" administration of antimicrobial drugs is futile because it results in the development of a flora resistant to the drugs being used. The *local application of antibiotics* is sometimes highly effective, and it is in the management of chronic mixed infections of this type that several potent but toxic antibiotics have great value. An ointment or solution containing neomycin, bacitracin, and polymyxin exerts a bactericidal effect against a wide variety of organisms and will sometimes temporarily sterilize a chronic lesion. Other useful topical medications are furacin and 3 percent acetic acid, which is especially helpful in *Pseudomonas* infections.

Diphtheritic ulcer of the skin is discussed in Chap. 133.

INFECTIONS OF THE HEAD AND NECK Pustules of the nose and upper lip may be particularly dangerous, because they are likely to extend intracranially through the angular vein to the cavernous sinus. These lesions should be treated conservatively, manipulation or incision should be avoided if possible, and systemic antibiotics should be used if local swelling or redness appears.

Suppurative parotitis Typically, suppurative parotitis occurs in elderly and chronically ill patients who have a dry mouth from decreased oral intake, often following general anesthesia and surgery, or from medications with atropine-like effects, such as antihistamines or phenothiazines. In most patients, it is an ascending infection due to *S. aureus,* which normally colonizes the opening to Stensen's duct. Occasionally, there is an obstructing calculus. Its onset, usually sudden, is heralded by unilateral local pain and swelling, frequently with fever and chills. Frank pus can often be expressed from the duct and may show gram-positive cocci in clumps. The gland itself is firm and tender and often shows redness and edema of the overlying skin. Treatment consists of systemic antimicrobial therapy with a penicillinase-resistant penicillin or another agent effective against *S. aureus,* combined with improved hydration and oral hygiene. Massage of the gland and sialagogues, like lemon drops, help promote drainage through the duct. Surgery is usually unnecessary and should be reserved for patients failing to improve after 4 to 5 days of medical management.

Rare complications include fistula formation, facial nerve palsy, or extension of the infection to involve the mediastinum. The mortality rate is about 20 to 30 percent, probably because this infection occurs in severely debilitated patients.

The use of penicillin and other antibiotics has reduced the incidence of many formerly common suppurative complications of streptococcal pharyngitis. However, as a result of streptococcal sore throat, *Bacteroides* infections of the pharynx, or introduction of infection by trauma to the floor of the mouth or the pharyngeal wall, abscesses of the deep cervical structures still occur. *Suppurative cervical adenitis,* once an all-too-common sequel to streptococcal pharyngitis in children, is now rare. *Peritonsillar abscess* (*quinsy*) is manifested by fever, sore throat, cervical lymphadenopathy, unilateral pain radiating to the ear on swallowing, and enlargement of the tonsil with redness and swelling of the adjacent soft palate. Treatment with penicillin and irrigations of warm saline solution sometimes lead to subsidence of the process, but if digital palpation reveals fluctuation, surgical drainage with or without tonsillectomy is indicated. Organisms associated with peritonsillar abscess include *Streptococcus pyogenes* and oral anaerobic bacteria.

The course of *deep cervical infections* is fully as dependent upon the anatomic arrangement of fascial planes as is that of infections of the hand. Infection in this area is serious and is attended by fever, prostration, and leukocytosis. A tender mass may be palpated, but *surgical evacuation of such an infection should not be delayed because of failure to detect fluctuation,* which is usually absent because of the dense fascial layers.

Infection of the *sublingual* and submandibular spaces, so-called "Ludwig's angina," is characterized by brawny induration of the submaxillary region, edema of the floor of the mouth, and elevation of the tongue. It usually originates from apical abscesses of the second and third mandibular molars. There are severe pain, dysphagia, and, within hours, dyspnea from respiratory obstruction. The causative organisms of this and other neck abscesses are mainly streptococci and oral anaerobes. Mortality was formerly about 50 percent. *Treatment* consists of large doses of penicillin and careful observation. With significant airway obstruction, tracheostomy is necessary. Since the infection is largely a cellulitis, incision and drainage are reserved for evidence of fluctuation.

The retropharyngeal space lies between the muscles anterior to the cervical vertebrae and the pharyngeal mucosa. *Retropharyngeal abscess,* formerly common in children, is manifested by dysphagia, progressive stridor, pain, and fever. The bulging mass is easily seen and can completely occlude the airway within hours. Incision and drainage are mandatory; spontaneous rupture may lead to death by aspiration. Esophageal perforation during endoscopy may result in abscess as a late complication. Tuberculous abscess, secondary to spinal disease, occasionally appears in the retropharyngeal space; it is painless, and relief of obstruction follows surgical incision.

Submastoid abscess, or suppuration in the submastoid space, known as *Bezold's abscess,* is usually secondary to otitis and produces nuchal rigidity, which may lead to a mistaken diagnosis of otogenous meningitis. Infection can extend down the carotid sheath to the mediastinum. A suppurative thrombophlebitis of the jugular vein usually accompanies this infection, and the vessel is easily felt as a tender cord. Bacteremia and systemic spread of infection are common, and the involved venous segment may need to be excised. Spontaneous rupture of the carotid artery with rapid death from exsanguination is a rare complication.

Therapy of head and neck abscesses includes surgical incision and drainage, open treatment of infected wounds, and systemic antibiotics, which should include agents active against anaerobic organisms, particularly if there is foul-smelling pus. Penicillin is usually the drug of choice.

DEEP-SEATED INFECTIONS **Hepatic abscess** These abscesses are usually amebic (Chap. 199) or bacterial (pyogenic). Bacterial abscesses usually develop by one of five mechanisms: (1) portal vein bacteremia arising from an infected intraabdominal site, such as appendicitis, diverticulitis, or perforated bowel; (2) systemic bacteremia originating from a distant site, in which bacteria reach the liver via the hepatic artery; (3) ascending cholangitis in a biliary tract completely or partially obstructed by stone, malignancy, or stricture; (4) direct extension from a contiguous focus of infection outside the biliary tract, such as a subphrenic abscess; or (5) trauma, either penetrating, with direct introduction of organisms into the liver, or

blunt, causing a hematoma that becomes secondarily infected. In most cases the cause is apparent, but in some the pathogenesis of the abscess is unexplained ("cryptogenic"). Most abscesses are single; multiple abscesses are typically microscopic and associated with systemic bacteremia or complete biliary tract obstruction. In these cases, the onset is acute, and the clinical features of the predisposing disease predominate.

Most other cases of hepatic abscess have a subacute onset, and an illness lasting several weeks is the rule. Fever is nearly always present and is accompanied by such nonspecific symptoms as chills, nausea, vomiting, anorexia, weight loss, and weakness. Right upper quadrant abdominal pain or tenderness is present in about one-half of patients, as is hepatomegaly. Some complain of right pleuritic chest pain. Jaundice is usually evident only when there is biliary tract obstruction.

Laboratory findings in most patients include one or more of the following: anemia, leukocytosis, increased erythrocyte sedimentation rate, increased alkaline phosphatase, decreased serum albumin, and usually mildly increased serum bilirubin. The chest roentgenogram is abnormal in about one-half of patients and shows right-sided basilar atelectasis, pneumonia, pleural effusion, or an elevated hemidiaphragm.

The radionuclide liver scan demonstrates filling defects for most abscesses greater than 2 cm in diameter. Ultrasound scans are usually positive and can distinguish fluid-filled from solid masses, helping to discriminate between infectious and neoplastic lesions. Computerized tomography and hepatic arteriography may also demonstrate the abscesses but generally provide no additional useful information.

The bacteriology of liver abscesses depends upon the cause. With systemic bacteremia staphylococci or streptococci are common. Abscesses originating from an intraabdominal infection, however, usually contain aerobic gram-negative rods, especially *Escherichia coli* and *Klebsiella-Enterobacter;* anaerobic bacteria, especially anaerobic gram-positive cocci, *Fusobacterium nucleatum,* and *B. fragilis;* or a mixture of aerobes and anaerobes. Blood cultures are positive in a substantial minority of patients.

Treatment consists of surgical drainage supplemented by appropriate antibiotic therapy. When the bacteriology is unknown, chloramphenicol or a combination of clindamycin and an aminoglycoside should be effective. Antibiotics are usually continued for several weeks following drainage.

Complications of hepatic abscesses include formation of a subphrenic abscess, bleeding into the abscess, and rupture into the lung, pleural cavity, or peritoneum. In correctly diagnosed and treated patients the mortality rate is about 20 to 40 percent, and is higher in those with multiple rather than single abscesses.

In patients with a clinical picture suggesting a liver abscess and an abnormal hepatic radionuclide or ultrasound scan, it is important to distinguish between a bacterial and an amebic abscess, since the latter usually requires no surgical drainage. Features suggesting an amebic etiology are: age under 50; single rather than multiple abscesses; a history of diarrhea, especially if bloody; the presence of *Entamoeba histolytica* in the stool; and the absence of a condition predisposing to bacterial liver abscess. The most helpful differential point is that nearly all patients with amebic liver abscesses have a positive serology for *E. histolytica.*

Splenic abscess Most splenic abscesses are multiple, small, and clinically silent lesions found incidentally at autopsy and occurring as a terminal manifestation of uncontrolled infection elsewhere. Clinically important splenic abscesses are generally solitary and arise from (1) systemic bacteremia originating in another site, such as endocarditis or salmonellosis; (2) infection, probably by the hematogenous route, of a spleen damaged by bland infarction (as occurs in hemoglobinopathies, especially sickle-cell trait or sickle-cell disease), trauma, penetrating or blunt (with superinfection of a subcapsular hematoma), or other diseases (malaria, hydatid cysts); or (3) extension from a contiguous focus of infection, such as a subphrenic abscess. The most common organisms are staphylococci, streptococci, anaerobes, and aerobic gram-negative rods, including *Salmonella.*

The onset is typically subacute, and the major features are fever and left-sided pain which is often pleuritic and located in the upper abdomen, lower chest, or flank. The pain may radiate to the left shoulder. Left upper quadrant abdominal tenderness and splenomegaly are common, but an audible splenic friction rub is rare. Leukocytosis is usually present.

Radiographic findings may include (1) a left upper quadrant soft-tissue abdominal mass, (2) extraintestinal gas from gas-forming organisms in the abscess, (3) displacement of other organs, including the colon, kidney, and stomach, (4) elevation of the left hemidiaphragm, and (5) left pleural effusion. A liver-spleen radionuclide scan is valuable in detecting abscesses larger than 2 or 3 cm. A combined spleen-lung scan may provide clues to perisplenic (or left subdiaphragmatic) abscesses. An ultrasound scan may be positive for macroscopic splenic abscesses. Arteriography, which may reveal an avascular mass and mycotic aneurysms, or CT scan may be helpful when these other tests fail to demonstrate a suspected lesion.

Treatment consists of appropriate systemic antibiotics and splenectomy. Complications of untreated splenic abscesses include hemorrhage into the abscess cavity or rupture into the peritoneum, bowel, bronchus, or pleural space. Splenic abscesses should be considered a possible, although rare, cause of continued bacteremia in acute endocarditis despite appropriate chemotherapy, and splenectomy may be necessary to achieve final eradication of the infection.

Subphrenic abscess Peritoneal infections show a striking tendency to localize in the upper part of the abdomen between the transverse colon and the diaphragm. True subphrenic abscesses form between the liver and diaphragm on the left or right, and many so-called "subphrenic infections" are, in fact, subhepatic. Most of these infections are related to perforations in the gastrointestinal or biliary tracts, and over half of them follow operations on the gallbladder, duodenum, or stomach. Subphrenic abscesses following perforated appendicitis occur rarely nowadays. Closed blunt trauma is an important cause. A few abscesses occur without predisposing neighborhood infection. The most common organisms are *E. coli,* non-group A streptococci, staphylococci, *Klebsiella-Enterobacter,* and anaerobes, especially *Bacteroides* spp.; mixed infections are common. About 60 percent of abscesses occur on the right, 25 percent on the left, and 15 percent are bilateral. They are more common in males and elderly patients, who often have a debilitating disease such as cancer. *Any patient with persistent fever and a history of a recent abdominal operation or recent intraabdominal sepsis should be suspected of having a subphrenic abscess.*

Manifestations include fever, upper abdominal pain, and tenderness, usually along the costal margin. Shoulder pain, dyspnea, dullness, and rales at the lung base are more common than abdominal signs and symptoms, and emphasize the location of a true abscess between the liver and the diaphragm. Foul sputum connotes perforation of the abscess into the lung. The localizing signs are by no means striking in all cases, however. The widespread practice of "covering" postoperative patients with antibiotics prophylactically can attenuate subphrenic infection without eradicating it and may result in an insidiously progressive illness with weight loss, malaise, fatigue, and low-grade fever beginning weeks or months after a laparotomy, a syndrome termed *chronic subphrenic abscess.* Roentgenograms may show gas, sometimes with an air-fluid

level beneath the diaphragm. The gas may be from a perforated viscus or the result of bacterial multiplication.

Other radiographic findings include pleural effusion, which is usually sterile, basilar infiltrates, and elevation—but not necessarily fixation—of the diaphragm. Barium meal with the patient in the head-down position may show indentation of the gastric fundus in left subphrenic abscess, a lesion that is often notoriously difficult to localize. Combined lung-liver scintiscan may show a widened subphrenic space. Ultrasound scans are useful in detecting subphrenic abscesses, and CT scan will usually demonstrate extraintestinal gas or fluid.

Treatment includes adequate surgical drainage and appropriate systemic antibiotics. Chloramphenicol or clindamycin and an aminoglycoside are good choices pending culture results. The outlook in subphrenic abscesses is often poor because of delayed diagnosis, the debilitated state of the patient, and failure to attain complete drainage. Even with proper surgery, the mortality rate is about 30 percent.

Retroperitoneal infections Strictly speaking, all perinephric, most pancreatic, and many subphrenic abscesses are located outside the peritoneum, but the term *retroperitoneal abscess* usually refers to infection in the lumbar and iliac regions. Suppuration in these areas is relatively rare, but the importance of recognizing its existence in patients with fever and pain in the lower part of the back is great. In one series, the average duration of illness in 65 patients before diagnosis was approximately 1 month.

Infection in the retroperitoneal space usually reflects extension from posterior perforations of the appendix, small bowel or colon, pancreatic, renal, or spinal infections, and occasionally suppurative lymphadenitis in the iliac area, usually secondary to streptococcal infections of the lower extremities in children. Sometimes, the infection is apparently spread hematogenously.

Lumbar abscess is characterized by tenderness and spasm of the back muscles on the affected side, and a mass is usually palpable in the lumbar region; or there may be a prominent, tender abdominal mass without lumbar pain or spasm. Infection in the wall of the abdominal aneurysm, often with *Salmonella,* may present as a lumbar abscess. Flexion of the hip (psoas sign) occurs in a few cases but is more often present with infections lower in the retroperitoneal area. *Fever, leukocytosis,* and *lumbar spasm* should suggest the diagnosis. The absence of a palpable mass may lead to protracted observation, and it is in these instances that palpation under anesthesia is often helpful.

Psoas (iliac) abscess is typically attended by abdominal pain in the iliac or inguinal region, and, particularly when the psoas muscle is involved, severe pain may be referred to the hip, thigh, or knee. Careful palpation of the lower part of the abdomen or groin usually reveals a mass, and fullness and tenderness on rectal examination are common. Hip spasm (psoas sign) is often present. Although psoas abscesses characteristically occur in association with tuberculosis of the spine, the acute bacterial form has been reported in perforation or fistula formation of the bowel in appendicitis, diverticulitis, colonic carcinoma, and Crohn's disease (regional enteritis). Roentgenograms may delineate the inflammatory mass; pyelography shows displacement of the kidney or ureter in some cases, scoliosis with concavity on the side of the infection, and blurring of the psoas shadow. Barium studies of the small and large bowel may demonstrate an intestinal site of origin. Computerized tomography may be useful in revealing a suspected abscess when other studies are negative. Treatment consists of surgical drainage and appropriate antibiotic therapy.

Pancreatic abscess These abscesses usually occur in a site of pancreatic necrosis following acute pancreatitis. Typically, the patient improves after the attack of pancreatitis, but about 10 to 21 days later fever, abdominal pain and tenderness, nausea, vomiting, and sometimes persistent ileus begin; in those cases, persistent fever, leukocytosis, and abdominal findings beyond 7 to 10 days should suggest an abscess. A mass is palpable in about half of cases. The serum amylase is irregularly elevated, but leukocytosis is usually present. The serum alkaline phosphatase may be increased and the albumin decreased.

Chest roentgenograms often show a left pleural effusion, basilar atelectasis or pneumonia, or a raised hemidiaphragm. Plain films of the abdomen or barium studies of the intestinal tract may show extraintestinal gas in the pancreatic area from gas-forming organisms in the abscess or may demonstrate displacement of adjacent structures. Ultrasound is very useful in revealing fluid-filled pancreatic masses. Computerized tomography is also a sensitive test.

Treatment is surgical drainage and appropriate antibiotic therapy. Since the usual organisms are coliforms and anaerobes, chloramphenicol or clindamycin and an aminoglycoside are reasonable choices until culture results return. Complications of undrained abscess include perforation into adjacent structures; erosion of the left gastric, splenic, and gastroduodenal arteries with exsanguination; and the development of further abscesses in the pancreas or peritoneal and retroperitoneal spaces. Even with surgical drainage the mortality rate is about 40 percent, and recurrent abscesses requiring reoperation are common.

Renal abscess Single or multiple abscesses of the renal *cortex* are almost invariably the result of metastatic implantation of staphylococci from another focus. There is no relationship to previous renal disease; the infection occurs in younger individuals, is usually unilateral, and occurs on the right side oftener than on the left. Many patients give a history of recent skin infection such as furuncle. Although acute pyelonephritis is a diffuse disease with foci of cellular infiltrates in the interstitium of the renal medulla, these inflammatory foci may coalesce to form a distinct abscess cavity in the medulla. This situation probably ensues more frequently than is generally appreciated.

The onset of renal abscess is abrupt, with chills and fever, followed by costovertebral pain and tenderness. If the abscess is cortical, the urine contains *no white blood cells;* medullary abscesses are usually accompanied by pyuria. The stained urinary sediment may show myriads of gram-positive cocci in cortical abscesses and gram-negative organisms in medullary abscesses. Transient gross or microscopic hematuria may occur at the onset. The white blood cell count is usually elevated and may exceed 30,000 cells per cubic millimeter. Physical signs are usually localized to the region of the kidney, but abdominal spasm may lead to confusion with appendicitis, cholecystitis, or pancreatitis. Early in the disease, ureteral calculus or acute hydronephrosis may be considered as possible diagnoses. Sudden onset of *fever, leukocytosis, and renal pain in the absence of pyuria* should suggest the diagnosis of renal abscess, especially in a patient with infection elsewhere. Obstruction of the ureter by pus or cellular debris may also yield a urine sediment sparse in white blood cells and bacteria. Excretory urograms typically reveal an intrarenal mass, and ultrasound scans usually demonstrate the abscess as a fluid-filled defect. *Treatment* consists of appropriate antibiotics, adequate fluids, and relief of pain. An abscess may suddenly discharge into the renal pelvis, with relief of pain and the passage of cloudy urine

containing enormous numbers of leukocytes and bacteria. *Complications* include formation of a thick-walled chronic renal "carbuncle," requiring surgical removal, rupture into the perirenal space, and secondary pyelonephritis, usually produced by coliform bacilli. Recovery is ordinarily prompt, and chronic sequelae are rare. Failure to achieve rapid defervescence following treatment suggests an incorrect diagnosis or the necessity of drainage, either by needle aspiration or by surgery.

Perinephric abscess Rupture of a renal parenchymal abscess into the perinephric space can cause a perinephric abscess. Such an abscess may be staphylococcal following hematogenous dissemination from another site, usually the skin, but more commonly it arises from pyelonephritis which is usually associated with renal calculus disease. The causative organisms, therefore, are those responsible for acute pyelonephritis: *E. coli, Proteus* sp., and *Klebsiella-Enterobacter.* The main symptoms are fever, chills, and unilateral flank pain. Dysuria is frequently present. Most patients are febrile and have unilateral flank or abdominal tenderness, often with a palpable mass. Leukocytosis, pyuria, and a positive urine culture are typical. Blood cultures are positive in 20 to 40 percent of patients. Perinephric abscess generally can be distinguished clinically from uncomplicated acute pyelonephritis by the longer duration of symptoms before hospitalization (usually more than 5 days) and the failure of patients to become afebrile within 5 days following the institution of antimicrobial therapy.

The chest roentgenograms often show ipsilateral pneumonia or atelectasis, pleural effusion, or a raised hemidiaphragm. An abdominal plain film may reveal the loss of the psoas shadow, a mass, calculi, or extraintestinal gas in the perinephric area secondary to gas-forming organisms. Findings on excretory urogram may include: a nonvisualizing or a poorly visualizing kidney, distorted calyces, anterior displacement of the kidney on lateral views, and unilateral fixation of the kidney that is demonstrated best by fluoroscopy or inspiration-expiration films. Ultrasound scans are very sensitive in detecting perinephric abscesses. Treatment is surgical drainage and relief of any urinary obstruction; occasionally, nephrectomy is necessary. Appropriate systemic antibiotics (not urinary antiseptics) should be administered along with surgical measures.

Rectal abscess Most of these infections are superficial and involve the perirectal region, and many are associated with fistulas. Infection in the apocrine glands (hidradenitis) or folliculitis in the perianal region, extension of cryptitis or obstructions in the "anal glands" which open into the crypts of Morgagni, and contamination of submucosal hematomas, sclerosed hemorrhoids, or anal fissures may lead to abscess formation. In most patients, the cause of infection is not apparent. These are usually painful, easily palpable, often visible on inspection. Treatment is incision and drainage. Antibiotics may be indicated in some instances.

Difficulties in diagnosis are likely to arise with infections higher in the rectum. Most are in the ischiorectal area, but those above the pelvic diaphragm, the so-called "supralevator abscess," are particularly elusive. Patients with this type of infection often have fever, malaise, and leukocytosis for several days or even weeks before any symptoms referable to the rectum develop. There is vague pelvic discomfort, relieved by defecation, and constipation punctuated by short episodes of diarrhea is common. In males, the inflammation often involves the base of the bladder, and urinary urgency or retention may occur, falsely centering attention on the urinary tract as the source of fever and malaise. Eventually, the abscess produces severe pain, chills, and fever; palpation and instrumentation will reveal the swelling in the rectal ampulla. Such an abscess may surround the rectum and produce narrowing that is differentiated from neoplasm by the fact that the mucosa remains intact. A useful sign of deep rectal abscess is severe pain with pressure in the region between the anus and the coccyx. The supralevator space is continuous with the ischiorectal space, with both the gluteal and obturator regions, and with the retroperitoneal space. In neglected cases, the abscess may drain through the skin of the perineum, the groin, or the buttock or may extend as high as the perirenal areas. Rectal abscesses are not uncommon in patients with preexisting anorectal disease, diabetes, alcoholism, and neurological disease; infections in this area are also peculiarly frequent in patients with acute leukemia, especially when neutropenia is present. Because the clinical picture may be that of "fever of unknown origin" for a long period, it is important that thorough digital and endoscopic examination of the rectum be carried out in patients with unexplained fever. Patients with diabetic ketoacidosis should receive a careful rectal examination because a rectal abscess may be the infection responsible for precipitating the ketoacidosis.

A rectal abscess may be a forerunner of both ulcerative colitis and regional enteritis, and may occur months and even years before other overt manifestations of these diseases. For this reason, proctosigmoidoscopy, colonoscopy, barium enema, and, often, upper gastrointestinal roentgenograms are indicated in nonhealing or recurrent rectal lesions.

Treatment of high rectal abscesses consists of incision and drainage, analgesics, and antibiotics directed at *E. coli, Klebsiella-Enterobacter, Bacteroides,* and a variety of streptococci, which constitute the polymicrobial flora of these lesions.

REFERENCES

BARTLETT JG et al: Anaerobic infections of the head and neck. Otolaryngol Clin North Am 9:655, 1976

CHOW AW et al: Orofacial odontogenic infections. Ann Intern Med 88:392, 1978

CHULAY JD et al: Splenic abscess: Report of 10 cases and review of the literature. Am J Med 61:513, 1976

DOUST BD et al: Ultrasonic diagnosis of abdominal abscess. Am J Dig Dis 21:569, 1976

GOLIGHER JC: *Surgery of the Anus, Rectum, and Colon,* 3d ed. Springfield, Ill, Charles C Thomas, 1975

HARDCASTLE JD: Acute nontuberculous psoas abscess. Report of 10 cases and review of the literature. Br J Surg 57:103, 1970

KONVOLINKA CW et al: Subphrenic abscess. Curr Probl Surg, January 1972

LAZARCHICK J et al: Pyogenic liver abscess. Mayo Clin Proc 48:349, 1973

LINSCHEID RL et al: Common and uncommon infections of the hand. Orthop Clin North Am 6:1063, 1975

RUBIN RH et al: Hepatic abscess: Changes in clinical, bacteriologic and therapeutic aspects. Am J Med 57:601, 1974

SABBAJ J et al: Anaerobic pyogenic liver abscess. Ann Intern Med 77:629, 1972

SPEIRS CF et al: Acute septic parotitis: Incidence, aetiology, and management. Scott Med J 17:62, 1972

THORLEY JD et al: Perinephric abscess. Medicine 53:441, 1974

WARSHAW AL: Inflammatory masses following acute pancreatitis: Phlegmon, pseudocyst, and abscess. Surg Clin North Am 54:621, 1974

111
CHEMOTHERAPY OF INFECTION

WILLIAM M. M. KIRBY

INTRODUCTION From the standpoint of overall reduction in morbidity and mortality rates, the greatest impact of drug therapy has been in the field of infectious diseases. Modern chemotherapy of infectious diseases dates from the mid-1930s when the sulfonamides were introduced. Penicillin G, the first of the antibiotics to be used systemically, came into widespread use in the early 1940s, and since then several dozen chemotherapeutic agents have appeared that are effective in a wide variety of bacterial, rickettsial, fungal, and parasitic infections. The efficacy of antimicrobial agents is due to their action in inhibiting growth of the parasite rather than to an enhancement of defense mechanisms, and it is remarkable that such a large number of substances can interfere effectively with multiplication of invading organisms without seriously damaging the cells of the host. Effective new agents continue to appear in surprising numbers, both from large-scale screening programs in which samples of organic matter are tested for antimicrobial activity and from chemical modifications of the known chemotherapeutic drugs. Specific recommendations for therapy are made in chapters dealing with individual diseases; this section is devoted to general principles of chemotherapy and to a consideration of individual therapeutic agents.

FACTORS INFLUENCING SELECTION OF ANTIMICROBIAL AGENTS AND THE OUTCOME OF THERAPY

SUSCEPTIBILITY OF THE INFECTING MICROORGANISMS No antimicrobial agent is effective against all pathogenic microorganisms; each has its own spectrum of activity against one or a variety of species, within which the majority of strains have been found to be susceptible. There are a few instances, such as the susceptibility of group A streptococci to penicillin G, in which resistant strains occur rarely if at all, and where treatment with penicillin can be given without concern about resistance. With the majority of chemotherapeutic agents, however, a variable percentage of strains of each susceptible species is resistant, i.e., they are not inhibited by concentrations of the drug attainable in the patient's blood and tissues with the usual dosage schedules. It is customary, therefore, in serious infections to determine the susceptibility of most pathogens to a variety of chemotherapeutic agents, and this has become one of the most important functions of clinical microbiology laboratories. *Dilution methods* of susceptibility testing, considered to be the most accurate, involve making serial dilutions of each agent to be tested in agar or broth, adding a standardized inoculum of the infecting organisms, and determining the smallest amount (the minimal inhibitory concentration, MIC) of the drug that inhibits growth after overnight incubation. *Agar dilution tests* are used routinely in some laboratories with sufficient volume to justify them, and mechanized or preprepared *broth dilution methods* are available. Automated methods are also being developed commercially. Although expensive, they are becoming simpler and more accurate, and at least one provides a result within 3 h. For the majority of laboratories, however, the simpler *agar diffusion method,* which is accurate and reliable when properly performed, remains the one usually used. With this technique, zones of inhibition of growth of a standardized inoculum of the infecting organism around filter paper disks impregnated with antibiotics are measured, and the zone sizes are inversely proportional to inhibitory concentrations (MICs) of drug, which are in turn related to the blood levels usually attained. Susceptibility of 8 to 10 chemotherapeutic agents can be tested on a single large agar plate, and a report of *susceptible, intermediate,* or *resistant* can be made. Intermediate sensitivity indicates the organisms' possible susceptibility with increased doses, or in urinary tract infections where high concentrations of drug can be attained in the urine. Disk testing has a number of limitations; it is applicable chiefly to rapidly growing pathogens, and the results are usually not reported until 24 h after the pathogen is isolated.

BACTERICIDAL VERSUS BACTERIOSTATIC AGENTS Although these are relative terms, some chemotherapeutic drugs can be clearly shown to have a killing (bactericidal) action at or near the minimal inhibitory concentration, while others simply inhibit bacterial growth (bacteriostatic), leaving the host to strike the *coup de grâce.* Bactericidal agents include the penicillins, cephalosporins, aminoglycosides, polymyxins, and vancomycin, while examples of bacteriostatic agents are the tetracyclines, sulfonamides, chloramphenicol, erythromycin, and clindamycin. Bactericidal agents give definitely superior results in diseases such as bacterial endocarditis and are more likely to give a favorable response in life-threatening infections, particularly when there is impairment of the host's defense mechanisms. In mild infections in otherwise healthy individuals, on the other hand, there is little to choose between "-cidal" and "-static" agents. In uncomplicated urinary tract infections, due to *Escherichia coli,* for example, the clinical results are as good with sulfonamides as with broad-spectrum penicillins or cephalosporins.

CLINICAL PHARMACOLOGY Knowledge of the clinical pharmacology of antimicrobial agents is helpful in prescribing therapy that is both safe and effective. Important information includes details of absorption and excretion, blood and urine levels with various routes of administration, protein binding, renal clearance, half-lives of drugs, stability in solutions and within the body, and the conversion to metabolic breakdown products. With some agents, such as ampicillin, much higher blood levels are obtained with the same doses given parenterally than orally, whereas with others such as doxycycline, where there is complete absorption from the intestinal tract, the oral and parenteral doses are the same. Because of possible incompatibilities, *it is advisable never to administer more than one agent at a time by the intravenous route.* Absorption from the intestinal tract is impaired by a variety of foods and chemicals, and, in general, antimicrobials should be administered temporally as far removed from food and other drugs, such as antacids, as possible.

Antimicrobials are bound to a varying extent to serum proteins, especially albumin. Although the significance of protein binding is uncertain and controversial, it is clear that the bound antibiotic has no antimicrobial activity, and it is probable that the concentration of free, unbound antibiotic in the tissues, at any one time, is no greater than the peak level of free antibiotic in the blood. All other features being equal, antimicrobials with relatively low binding should be preferable to those with a high degree of binding. In general, this point of view is reflected in the dosages of antimicrobial agents that are commonly recommended.

Renal clearance is one of the most important determinants of antibiotic blood levels and is mainly responsible, for example, for the much higher levels attained with the same dose of cephaloridine than of cephalothin, and of carbenicillin than of ampicillin. Antibiotics with a high renal clearance such as penicillin G and cephalothin have a large component of tubular secretion, and their blood levels are elevated to a greater degree by probenecid than those of ampicillin and cephaloridine, where the tubular contribution is less important. Plasma half-life, the time required for a blood level to fall by one-half,

is also determined primarily by renal clearance mechanisms and is much shorter for those penicillins and cephalosporins that are secreted by the renal tubules than for antibiotics such as the aminoglycosides with little or no tubular component. Protein binding also has an important influence on the half-life of antibiotics, particularly those that are excreted mainly or entirely by glomerular filtration. For example, the plasma half-life of gentamicin, which is not bound by proteins, is 2 h, whereas that of doxycycline, which is over 90 percent protein-bound, is about 16 h. Antibiotics with little or no protein binding have a much larger apparent volume of distribution (AVD) than those with a high degree of binding, i.e., the AVD of gentamicin is 30 percent of body weight compared with 14 percent for cefazolin. Cephalothin has a high plasma clearance with a high rate of nonrenal clearance due to its partial conversion in the body to a less active metabolic breakdown product. These are a few examples of the pharmacologic features of individual antimicrobial agents; others will be mentioned as the individual drugs are considered.

DOSE, ROUTE, AND DURATION OF THERAPY In prescribing dosages of antimicrobial agents, the objective is to deliver a concentration in excess of that needed to inhibit and/or kill the infecting organism at the site of infection. Since it is difficult to measure tissue concentrations, a blood level that exceeds the MIC two- to eightfold is a commonly accepted guideline. This is an arbitrary concentration of drug and obviously does not take into account all the variations in penetration into different tissues, or the role of host defense mechanisms. These variations may be very important because, in many instances, infections have been cured with antibiotics such as the tetracyclines where the concentration of free, active drug in the blood is not much greater than the MIC. The relation between blood levels and MIC does not hold in urinary tract infection, where the concentration of drug cleared by the kidney usually far exceeds the MIC. In this situation, an excess of drug in the urine is obviously important.

The route of administration, as well as the dose, is important in achieving appropriate drug levels. In general, parenteral therapy should usually be given in severe infections to be certain that high, effective blood levels are attained. The *intravenous route* is especially indicated initially in meningitis, endocarditis, and osteomyelitis, where barriers to penetration of the antimicrobial agent can be overcome by high blood levels. Intravenous therapy is also indicated when there is hypotension, and when bleeding diatheses are present. For milder infections, *intramuscular administration* is often an acceptable or preferable alternative, particularly with antibiotics such as procaine penicillin that cause relatively little pain and produce prolonged, effective blood levels. With gentamicin, blood levels are the same with an intramuscular injection as with an intravenous infusion given over a period of 60 min, so that the route can be chosen on the basis of comfort for the patient and the need for other intravenous medications. The *oral route* is used chiefly for mild to moderate infections, and for completion of therapy of severe infections after they have been brought under control with parenteral therapy. Absorption from the intestinal tract is variable even in the fasting state, and all oral antibiotics should be taken at least 1 h before and 3 h after food and other medications. This presents difficulties with drugs such as antacids that need to be taken frequently and that are especially likely to interfere with absorption of antimicrobial agents. Parenteral administration is often the only solution to this problem.

The optimal duration of antimicrobial treatment is unknown for many infections, and there is considerable variation from one medical center to another in the length of time antimicrobial therapy is given. In bacterial endocarditis, for example, the usual course of parenteral therapy may vary from 2 to

8 weeks with an average of about four weeks. For most acute infections a good general rule is to continue therapy for 2 to 3 days after the temperature has returned to normal and all signs of infection have subsided. However, fever can continue for weeks from sterile effusions complicating pneumonia, and cerebrospinal fluid abnormalities can persist for considerable periods in bacterial meningitis, leading to a continuation of chemotherapy for much longer than is necessary. Empiricism needs to be tempered with reason and experience, and in actual practice the guidelines for duration of therapy must be sufficiently flexible to be appropriate for the patient being treated.

ALLERGY AND TOXICITY The patient's allergic history should always be explored before prescribing antimicrobial agents. In addition to allergic manifestations in general, a report of previous drug allergies is of particular importance, and agents that have caused clear-cut reactions should be avoided. Unfortunately, no reliable test is available to determine the presence of allergy to the penicillins, and they may or may not be well tolerated by patients with a history of a previous reaction. The possibility of a severe anaphylactic reaction can be reliably excluded by skin tests containing major and minor determinant mixtures, but only the major mixture is commercially available. When administration of a penicillin is considered essential, one approach is to begin with a very small dose intravenously and increase the amount every few minutes until it is learned whether the patient can tolerate the antibiotic. Specifically, with an intravenous infusion running 1 unit penicillin diluted in 3 to 5 ml saline or glucose solution is injected slowly into the tubing, and 5 min is allowed to elapse to see if an untoward reaction occurs. A solution of epinephrine is available in another syringe to be injected if needed. If no reaction occurs, 2, 5, 10, 25, and 50 units, etc., are injected at 5-min intervals, and within an hour or so it either becomes apparent that the patient can tolerate a full therapeutic dose, or he develops a reaction that is readily controlled by epinephrine. If a reaction occurs, administering another antibiotic is usually best, although in mild reactions, continuing the penicillin along with antihistamines and/or steroids is possible in some instances. Such a program can be quite troublesome as well as risky, requiring frequent adjustments to suppress urticaria and itching. The number of alternative antibiotics available is large enough that switching to another agent is usually the best course to follow.

Drug toxicity related to renal function is of particular importance. Some antimicrobials, such as the penicillins, cephalothin, chloramphenicol, erythromycin, and lincomycin, are relatively safe at normal or only slightly reduced dosage in the presence of impaired renal function. Other agents, such as the aminoglycosides, are potentially quite toxic but can be administered safely at reduced dosage if proper guidelines, based on serial determinations of the serum creatinine, are followed, and particularly if blood levels can be monitored. Certain toxic agents should be avoided if at all possible in the presence of renal insufficiency. These include most of the tetracyclines, streptomycin, cephaloridine, the sulfonamides, the nitrofurans, and nalidixic acid. One of the long-acting tetracyclines, doxycycline, has the same half-life in healthy and uremic subjects, and can be administered to patients with impaired renal function either orally or intravenously. Many patients with chronic renal failure are being maintained on dialysis programs and may require antimicrobials for a variety of infections. Table 111-1 summarizes adult dosage schedules for various antibiotics for patients with renal failure, on or off dialysis.

SITE OF INFECTION Soft-tissue infections in sites with a good blood supply and a minimum of tissue necrosis are, in general,

easily treated. In meningitis and endocarditis, on the other hand, penetration into the site of the infection presents formidable problems and is not infrequently responsible for treatment failures. Penetration across the blood-brain barrier is a complex phenomenon involving protein binding, lipid solubility, and ionization of the drug being administered. In addition, the permeability of this barrier to drugs depends on the degree of inflammation. Because of their low toxicity the penicillins can be administered in doses large enough to provide therapeutic concentrations in the spinal fluid, whereas more toxic drugs such as the aminoglycosides and polymyxins must be injected intrathecally to be effective clinically in meningitis. On the other hand, agents such as the sulfonamides, chloramphenicol, and the tetracyclines appear in the spinal fluid in amounts adequate for the treatment of some types of meningitis when they are given in doses appropriate for the treatment of systemic infections.

Other examples of problems of penetration, and of the influence of localized physiologic conditions, may be cited. The sulfonamides are excreted in the saliva in amounts adequate to eradicate the meningococcal carrier state, whereas most penicillins and tetracyclines are not. However, most of the strains of meningococci encountered at the present time are sulfonamide-resistant. In urinary infections, erythromycin and the aminoglycosides are relatively ineffective at an acid pH, whereas a pH at less than 5.5 is essential for the activity of methenamine mandelate (Mandelamine). The lack of efficacy of sulfonamides in the presence of pus, due to the competition for binding sites by the large amounts of p-aminobenzoic acid present, greatly limits the usefulness of this class of drugs.

Foreign bodies, abscesses, and obstruction to normal pathways of drainage almost always interfere with the response to chemotherapy and usually prevent cure until they are removed, drained, or relieved. Suture materials, prostheses, sequestrations, and calculi are examples of foreign bodies that interfere with drug therapy and usually, but not always, need to be removed. In many abscesses, bacteria tend to be in a metabolically inactive state in which they are not actively synthesizing cell wall and are not susceptible to the damaging effects of some antimicrobial drugs; hence drainage plus chemotherapy is necessary to eradicate the infection. Obstruction to bronchial, biliary, and renal drainage interferes seriously with the response of bacterial infections to antibiotics, and these infections generally cannot be cured with drugs until the obstruction is relieved. A thorough knowledge of the mechanical, metabolic, and physiologic factors is essential in planning therapy that will bring about optimal results in infections located in different parts of the body.

COMBINATION THERAPY, SYNERGISM, ANTAGONISM Once the etiologic agent is known or can be anticipated, most bacterial infections can be treated successfully with a *single* antimicrobial agent. Combination therapy is used frequently, however, to broaden the antibacterial spectrum while awaiting the results of cultures, and also to cover the possibility that a polymicrobial infection might be present. For example, in a hospitalized patient who suddenly becomes ill with presumed sepsis, cephalothin and gentamicin may be given empirically to provide antibacterial activity against a variety of gram-positive and -negative pathogens that might be fatal if therapy were delayed (Chap. 109). Over 100 fixed-dose combinations were once available commercially in the United States for oral or parenteral therapy, but virtually all have been ordered off the market by the Food and Drug Administration on the grounds that it has not been shown in controlled studies that both agents contribute to the claimed therapeutic effects, that the amounts of each agent present were often not appropriate, and that patients were often being exposed to the potential hazards of two drugs when only one was needed. When combination therapy is indicated, it is most rational to prescribe separately the indicated drugs in doses that take into the account the patient's age, weight, and physiologic status.

A clinically significant enhancement of antibacterial activity from exposing microorganisms to two or more drugs is rare. Usually, the drugs have an indifferent effect in vitro; sometimes an additive action is observed, but this is difficult to demonstrate in patients.

True synergism occurs between penicillins and aminoglycosides with a number of gram-positive and gram-negative pathogens. The classic example is enterococcal endocarditis; penicillins (G, V, ampicillin, carbenicillin) disrupt the cell wall, permitting streptomycin to gain access to the ribosomes where their action is lethal. About one-third of enterococci are ribosomally resistant to streptomycin, but few if any strains are

resistant to gentamicin and tobramycin, and so these aminoglycosides are replacing streptomycin in treating this disease. Of the penicillinase-resistant penicillins, only nafcillin is synergistic against most strains of enterococci. In contrast, with viridans streptococci streptomycin is synergistic with penicillins against virtually all strains, and it is probable that, in bacterial endocarditis due to viridans streptococci, there are fewer relapses with combined therapy than with penicillin G alone (Chap. 243).

Gentamicin and tobramycin are synergistic with carbenicillin against *Pseudomonas* and some other gram-negative bacilli. Theoretically, it would be possible to reduce doses of the antibiotics, but in severe *Pseudomonas* infections full doses are usually given so as not to risk compromising the therapeutic result.

Trimethoprim-sulfamethoxazole, another synergistic combination, will be described below.

Clinically, significant antagonism between antimicrobial agents is also rare, a prime example being a higher mortality rate in pneumococcal meningitis with penicillin and tetracycline than with penicillin alone. The rate of killing by penicillin

TABLE 111-1
Dosages of antimicrobials in renal failure

Drug	Normal dose	Normal dose interval	Mild (C_{cr}* 50–80 ml/min)	Moderate (C_{cr}* 10–50 ml/min)	Severe (C_{cr}* 10 ml/min)	Significant dialysis of drug	Add at end of each dialysis	Significant dialysis of drug	Add parenterally during dialysis	Alternative, add to dialysate after the regular parenteral loading dose
			Dose interval for degree of renal failure			Hemodialysis		Peritoneal dialysis		
Ampicillin	0.5–3 g	Every 6 h	6 h	9 h	12–15 h (1 g)	Yes	0.5–1 g	No		50 µg/ml
Amoxicillin	0.25–1 g PO	Every 8 h	8 h	12 h	16 h (0.5 g)	Yes	0.5 g	No		
Penicillin G	0.25–4 million U	4 h	4 h (2 million U)	4 h (1.5 million U)	6 h (1 million U)	No		No		
Methicillin, oxacillin, nafcillin	1–2 g	4 h	4 h	4 h	8–12 h (1 g)	No		No		
Cloxacillin, dicloxacillin	0.5–1 g PO	6 h	6 h	6 h	6 h	No		No		
Carbenicillin	4–5 g	4 h	4 h	6–8 h (2 g)	12 h (2 g)	Yes	1–2 g	No	1 g every 6 h	200 µg/ml
Cephalexin, cephradine	0.25–1 g	4 h	4 h	6 h	Every 6 h (0.25 g)	Yes	0.25–0.5 g	Yes	0.25 g PO every 6 h	
Cephalothin, cephapirin	1–2 g	4 h	4 h	6 h	8–12 h (1 g)	Yes	1 g	Yes	1 g every 6 h	50 µg/ml
Cefazolin	0.5–1 g	8 h	12 h	12 h (0.5 g)	24 h (0.5 g)	No	0.5 g	No		75 µg/ml
Cefamandole, cefoxitin	0.5–2 g	6 h	8 h	12 h (1 g)	12 h (1 g)	No	0.5 g	No		50 µg/ml
Gentamicin,†,‡ tobramycin	1–1.7 mg/kg	8 h	8–12 h	12–24 h	48–72 h	Yes	1.5 mg/kg	No		8 µg/ml
Amikacin,†,‡ kanamycin	7.5 mg/kg	12 h	24 h	24–72 h	72–96 h	Yes	3.5 mg/kg	No		20 µg/ml
Streptomycin	0.5 g	12 h	24 h	24–72 h	72–96 h	Yes	0.25 g	Yes	?	
Chloramphenicol	0.25–1 g	6 h	6 h	8 h	8 h	No		No		
Erythromcyin	0.25–1 g	6 h	6 h	8 h	8–12 h	?		?		
Clindamycin	0.3–0.6 g	6–8 h	8 h	8 h	12 h (0.3 g)	No		No		
Vancomycin	0.25–0.5 g	6 h	24 h	48–72 h	7 days	No		No		15 µg/ml
Tetracycline	0.25–0.5 g	6 h	8–12 h	Avoid	Avoid	No		No		
Doxycycline	0.1–0.2 g	12–24 h	12–24 h	24 h	24 h	No		No		
Sulfisoxazole	1 g	6 h	6 h	8–12 h	Avoid	Yes	?			

* C_{cr} = creatinine clearance rate.
† Frequency of the dose can be estimated more accurately by multiplying the serum creatinine by 8 (for gentamicin and tobramycin) or by 9 (for amikacin and kanamycin).
‡ An alternate method is to give smaller doses at 8- to 12-h intervals by relating the elimination constants of the drugs to the patient's creatinine clearance. A dosing chart applicable to all the aminoglycosides has been described by Sarubbi and Hull.

is slowed by the bacteriostatic agent, tetracycline, and this can alter the outcome when survival depends on rapid killing of the pneumococci.

SUPERINFECTION AND RESISTANCE DURING ANTIMICROBIAL THERAPY A number of microorganisms are genetically resistant to clinically feasible levels of one or more antimicrobials, and they obviously will not be affected by antibiotic therapy. Most antibiotics will alter the host's normal flora by removing those organisms which are sensitive to the drug. In most cases this ecologic change is of little consequence, but occasionally the commensal bacteria of the host set up infection in the same location as the original infection, a state termed *superinfection* (Chap. 107). The superinfecting organism is resistant to the drug being administered, and determining its susceptibility is helpful in selecting the most appropriate antimicrobial drug. Some superinfecting organisms, particularly gram-negatives, acquire resistance to multiple drugs by an episomal transfer mechanism (R factors). For example, multiple-resistant *E. coli* and *Klebsiella-Enterobacter* pose a particular hazard to hospitalized patients.

Comparatively few organisms become resistant to the antibiotic being given during therapy. Some that do develop resistance are *E. coli* to streptomycin and nalidixic acid, occasional strains of staphylococci to erythromycin, and *Pseudomonas* to carbenicillin. In general, however, sensitive organisms are supplanted by resistant ones, rather than acquiring resistance themselves. From a practical point of view, it is important to know which agents are likely to induce resistance, and to look for this phenomenon clinically.

SPECIFIC ANTIMICROBIALS

PENICILLINS Penicillinase-susceptible The prototype, *Penicillin G* (benzyl penicillin), is still widely used, especially parenterally, when high blood levels are desirable as in meningitis and endocarditis. Large doses are necessary either continuously or at 3- to 4-h intervals because of problems of penetration into vegetations and across the blood-brain barrier, and also because of its high renal clearance, which is due chiefly to rapid tubular secretion. Blood levels can be doubled by the concomitant administration of probenecid, 0.5 g every 6 h, but since penicillin G is now quite inexpensive and the optimal blood levels are not known precisely, it is customary in most instances simply to give more penicillin. *Procaine penicillin* is well tolerated intramuscularly and is absorbed quite slowly so that injections need to be given only every 12 h for the treatment of many infections due to susceptible bacteria. In dosage of 300,000 to 600,000 units every 12 h, it is the drug of choice for most patients with pneumococcal pneumonia. *Benzathine penicillin* provides a depot in the muscle that releases penicillin so slowly that low blood levels are present for 2 to 3 weeks. These low levels are adequate for the therapy and prevention of streptococcal pharyngitis, for the treatment of some forms of syphilis, and for the prevention of recurrences of rheumatic fever.

Penicillin G given orally in doses of 250,000 units once or twice daily is also effective in preventing streptococcal sore throats, but less so than benzathine penicillin (Chap. 241). Because of its instability in the presence of acid, however, it is less reliable for therapy than the acid-stable penicillin V (phenoxymethyl penicillin), and attempts to overcome this disadvantage by giving larger amounts of penicillin G are associated with an increased incidence of nausea and diarrhea. This has resulted in the development of a number of penicillin G analogs which continue to have some usefulness because very little resistance has developed to them. An exception are the pneumococci

where a small number of resistant strains have been isolated in various parts of the world.

Broad-spectrum penicillins *Ampicillin* differs from penicillin G only in the presence of an amino group in the side chain, but this minor chemical difference is responsible for some unique features that have led to the widespread use of this antibiotic. Ampicillin is active in low concentrations against a number of gram-negative bacteria causing respiratory (*Hemophilus influenzae*), intestinal (*Shigella, Salmonella*), and urinary (*E. coli, Proteus mirabilis*) infections. When it is given orally, the peak blood level occurs later (2 to 3 h versus ½ to 1 h) and is lower than with penicillin V, and the ampicillin blood level then declines more slowly. This more prolonged blood level, along with its greater in vitro activity, is probably responsible for the greater efficacy of ampicillin, compared with penicillin V, in the oral therapy of gonococcal urethritis.

When given in an intravenous infusion, blood levels are more than 80 percent higher with ampicillin than with penicillin G chiefly because of the much higher rate of renal clearance of penicillin G (390 versus 210 ml/min per 1.73 m^2). When the in vitro activity of the infecting organisms is the same for the two antibiotics, this difference can mean equal efficacy with smaller doses of ampicillin, or higher blood levels with the same dose when maximum serum concentrations are considered necessary. Ampicillin is also more stable in the body, with a serum half-life twice as long as penicillin G, due chiefly to slower breakdown by the liver. Serum protein binding of ampicillin is approximately 20 percent compared with 60 percent for penicillin G and 80 percent for penicillin V; this may mean that with ampicillin there is a higher concentration of free, active antibiotic at the site of infection. All these features contribute to the efficacy and widespread use of ampicillin, and in the United States, competition has led to a marked decrease in the cost in the last few years. Although ampicillin has remained an effective drug against most organisms, increasing resistance has developed among a significant number of strains of *E. coli, Salmonella, Shigella,* and *H. influenzae.*

Hypersensitivity reactions occur with about the same frequency with ampicillin as with penicillin G and V, and with all three are much more frequent and severe when the drug is given parenterally and topically than by the oral route. About 5 to 10 percent of patients develop skin rashes with oral ampicillin, but the incidence is as high as 90 percent when patients with infectious mononucleosis take this drug. This remarkably high incidence, which does not occur with penicillins G and V, does not represent true penicillin allergy, and its exact nature is not known. Maculopapular (as opposed to urticarial) rashes beginning 4 days or more after initiating treatment with ampicillin do not indicate a need to discontinue therapy, or to avoid subsequent courses of the antibiotic. Although acid-stable, ampicillin is not very well absorbed when taken orally, giving peak blood levels only one-sixth as high as dicloxacillin and cephalexin. *Amoxicillin,* a derivative with a hydroxyl group on the benzene ring, is much better absorbed orally, with blood levels and urinary excretion more than twice as great on the average as ampicillin. Blood levels are roughly equivalent to those of ampicillin given intramuscularly, and amoxicillin has a lower incidence of intestinal side effects when given in half the dose orally. Bacampicillin, a rapidly hydrolyzed ester with much better intestinal absorption, provides peak blood levels and urinary excretion of ampicillin more than twice as great as does ampicillin alone. It is not yet available commercially. *Hetacillin,* a penicillin with a complex side chain, is hydrolyzed rapidly in the body to ampicillin, and for practical therapeutic purposes can be regarded as the same as ampicillin.

Carbenicillin is a broad-spectrum penicillin similar chemically to ampicillin, except that the amino group in the side chain is replaced by a carboxyl group. As a result, carbenicillin is active in vitro against *Pseudomonas,* indole-positive *Proteus,* and some strains of *Enterobacter,* in addition to the other gram-negatives that are susceptible to ampicillin. Like ampicillin, it is not active against *Klebsiella.* The MIC for *Pseudomonas* is much higher than that usually considered within the therapeutic range for other antibiotics, i.e., about 75 to 100 $\mu g/ml$ for most strains and as high as 500 $\mu g/ml$ for a few. However, extraordinarily high blood levels can be readily attained, in the range of 200 to 400 $\mu g/ml$, so that carbenicillin provides the safety and bactericidal activity of a penicillin for some organisms that have been notably refractory to most other antibiotics. The much higher blood levels that can be readily attained with carbenicillin compared to ampicillin are due chiefly to its much lower renal clearance (100 versus 210 ml/min per 1.73 m^2). In addition, carbenicillin is much more stable in the body, so that blood levels obtained with 30 g a day in patients with normal renal function can be achieved with only 3 or 4 g a day in patients with no renal function. Since many patients with severe gram-negative infections have considerable renal impairment, reduced doses can be administered with the knowledge that full therapeutic blood levels will be achieved. To give 30 g daily for the therapy of severe *Pseudomonas* infections in patients with normal renal function, it is customary to administer 5 g intravenously every 4 h, diluting each dose in 100 to 200 ml fluid and allowing it to drip into the vein within 1 to 2 h. Except for severe *Pseudomonas* infections, 30 g daily is not necessary, and much smaller doses, 10 or 15 g daily, are adequate for the therapy of other gram-negative infections, including those caused by indole-positive *Proteus* and *Enterobacter.* Urinary concentrations in excess of 1000 $\mu g/ml$ are attained with 0.5- or 1.0-g doses intramuscularly, so that doses comparable with those used with ampicillin are appropriate for urinary tract infections, including those due to *Pseudomonas.* An oral form of carbenicillin, the indanyl salt of the sodium ester, has become available, and one or two 0.5-g tablets (each equivalent to 382 mg carbenicillin) every 6 h produce urinary concentrations well in excess of MICs for susceptible gram-negative bacilli, including *Pseudomonas.*

An increase in bacterial resistance has been noted in some patients with severe gram-negative infections treated with carbenicillin, but the frequency and extent of the resistance has varied in different reports. The concomitant administration of aminoglycosides has tended to delay the development of resistance to carbenicillin, and in addition a synergistic action has been found to occur with these two antibiotics against many gram-negative bacilli. It has therefore become customary in severe infections to give both these antibiotics, to enhance antibacterial activity, and to delay the emergence of resistance as well. Since there is inactivation of the antibiotics, especially gentamicin, when the two are present in the same solution for several hours, it is preferable to administer them separately, either intramuscularly or intravenously, and under these circumstances the blood levels of each are the same as if they were being given alone. *Ticarcillin,* a newer semisynthetic penicillin, has pharmacokinetic properties very similar to those of carbenicillin but is two to four times as active in vitro against *Pseudomonas.* A daily dose of 18 g is considered equal to 30 g carbenicillin for *Pseudomonas* infections and provides a lower sodium load (both antibiotics contain about 5.5 meq sodium per gram). Disadvantages of the lower dose are that the greater activity of ticarcillin is found only against *Pseudomonas,* and that 18 g ticarcillin is more expensive than 30 g carbenicillin.

Piperacillin, another new penicillin even more active against *Pseudomonas* and other gram-negative organisms, has been quite promising in extensive clinical trials.

Penicillinase-resistant penicillins   The advent of these antibiotics in the early 1960s greatly enhanced the ability to cope with severe staphylococcal infections, because at that time over three-fourths of strains causing infections in hospitals were penicillinase producers, and this high incidence has persisted. Furthermore, the number of strains resistant to these new penicillins has remained small, especially in the United States. This is probably due to the low incidence of naturally occurring methicillin-resistant strains, and the fact that only a small proportion of the cells in a "resistant" culture are actually lacking in susceptibility. In contrast, certain European hospitals now report that over 20 percent of strains of *Staphylococcus aureus* are methicillin-resistant; the reason for the difference is unknown.

Five penicillinase-resistant penicillins are currently marketed in the United States: *methicillin, oxacillin, nafcillin, cloxacillin,* and *dicloxacillin.* The first three are available for parenteral administration. Methicillin is less active when tested in broth cultures than are oxacillin and nafcillin, but this is probably offset by its much lower protein binding, 40 percent compared with 90 percent or more for the other two. Clinical studies do not provide convincing evidence of superiority of any of these three penicillins for the parenteral therapy of severe staphylococcal infections. Methicillin is given in the same dose as, or in twice the dose of, the other two because of its lower in vitro activity, i.e., 1 or 2 g every 4 to 6 h in adults. For intravenous administration, each dose is diluted in 50 to 100 ml fluid, and is infused over a period of 30 min to minimize phlebitis. Intramuscular injections are painful and are poorly tolerated for more than a few days. Methicillin nephritis, an uncommon but important allergic reaction, has been reported rarely with oxacillin and nafcillin; it is not known whether this is due simply to the fact that methicillin is more widely used. Nafcillin has been found by many observers to give lower blood levels than equal doses of oxacillin; this appears to be due to sequestration of nafcillin in the liver and possibly in other tissues so that less is available to circulate in the blood. The therapeutic implications of this phenomenon are unknown.

With oral administration, both nafcillin and oxacillin give low blood levels, but cloxacillin gives blood levels twice as high and dicloxacillin four times as high as oxacillin when the same doses are given orally. However, there is also a progressive increase in serum protein binding (92 percent for oxacillin, 94 percent for cloxacillin, and 96 percent for dicloxacillin), so that the differences in free, active antibiotic may offset the blood level differences. In general, cloxacillin or dicloxacillin in doses of 0.25 or 0.5 g four times daily is preferred for oral administration. The efficacy of these antibiotics, either initially in mild to moderate soft-tissue infections, or for completion of therapy following administration of one of the three parenteral preparations described above, is well established.

The chief indication for the penicillinase-resistant penicillins is the therapy of infections caused by penicillinase-producing staphylococci, but they are often administered empirically before the etiologic organism is known. Pneumococci and most streptococci are more susceptible to penicillin G and ampicillin, but blood levels are sufficiently high with the penicillinase-resistant penicillins, especially when given parenterally, so that it is not necessary to give both types of penicillins to provide coverage for these organisms. However, infections caused by enterococci and *Neisseria* cannot be expected to respond to therapy with a penicillinase-resistant penicillin given alone, and if these organisms are suspected, penicillin G or ampicillin should be used.

In addition to the various allergic manifestations mentioned above, reactions to penicillins include myoclonus, seizures, potassium intoxication, hemolysis, leukopenia, thrombocytopenia, and neuropathy, usually with very high blood levels. Mental disturbances occur in a small percentage of patients following large doses of procaine penicillin.

CEPHALOSPORINS The cephalosporins differ from the penicillins in having a six-membered dihydrothiazine ring, instead of a five-membered thiazolidine ring, fused to the beta-lactam ring. As a result of this chemical difference there is no true cross-allergenicity, and most patients who are allergic to penicillins can be treated with cephalosporins without hypersensitivity reactions. The small number in whom this is not possible seem to be highly allergic individuals who react separately to the two groups of antibiotics.

Most bacteria susceptible to the penicillins are also susceptible to the cephalosporins, including group A and viridans streptococci, pneumococci, penicillin G-sensitive and resistant *S. aureus, Neisseria, Clostridia, Actinomyces,* and *Corynebacterium diphtheriae.* Among the gram-negatives most strains of *E. coli, P. mirabilis, Klebsiella* but not *Enterobacter, Shigella, Salmonella,* and most strains of *H. influenzae,* are susceptible. The spectrum has been extended appreciably by the addition of cefamandole and cefoxitin (see below). The cephalosporins act on the cell wall in a manner similar to the penicillins, and are bactericidal. As with the penicillins, there has been little tendency for susceptible species to become resistant despite widespread use of the cephalosporins for more than a decade.

Nine cephalosporins are now marketed in the United States, and at least that many more are under investigation. Orally, *cephalexin* and *cephradine* are very similar and can be considered interchangeable. They are well absorbed, a 0.5 g dose giving an average peak blood level in adults of about 18 μg/ml, six times as high as with the same dose of ampicillin. Serum protein binding is low and comparable with that of ampicillin (about 15 percent), and over 90 percent of these drugs are excreted in the urine, without nephrotoxicity. These two antibiotics are less active in vitro against gram-positive bacteria, especially staphylococci, than the injectable cephalosporins, but, because of the high blood levels, clinical results have been good, particularly after initial parenteral therapy. There is considerable variability in the susceptibility of *H. influenzae,* and twice the usual dose is recommended in the official labeling for otitis media. *Cephaloglycin,* a drug that is poorly absorbed orally and that gives low blood levels, has gradually been abandoned in the treatment of urinary infections because of the superior characteristics of the other two compounds.

Parenteral preparations of seven cephalosporins are commercially available. Both for therapy and prophylaxis *cephalothin* has had the longest and most extensive use. It is usually administered intravenously, 1 or 2 g every 4 or 6 h in at least 50 ml fluid to minimize phlebitis. It is partially converted in the body to a metabolic breakdown product, desacetylcephalothin, which is less active, particularly against gram-negative bacteria. This appears to have no clinical significance because of the large amount of the parent compound present. Cephalothin may cause some nephrotoxicity, especially when given in conjunction with aminoglycosides, but establishing this point clearly has been difficult. *Cephapirin* is very similar to cephalothin in its in vitro activity and pharmacological characteristics and may be interchangeable clinically, although fewer reports of its efficacy are available. *Cephaloridine,* another early cephalosporin, has low serum protein binding and is well tolerated intramuscularly, but clearly causes renal tubular damage in large doses and, because of its potential nephrotoxicity, should not be used. Cephradine is available parenterally as well as orally, but published documentation of efficacy with parenteral administration is not extensive.

Cefazolin has had increasing use parenterally because of its high and prolonged blood levels, which are due to high serum protein binding (85 percent) and low renal clearance. Its serum half-life is 1.8 h compared with 0.5 h for cephalothin. Cefazolin 0.5 g is probably equivalent to 1.0 g cephalothin therapeutically, taking into consideration the differences in blood levels and protein binding. Cefazolin is also well tolerated intramuscularly, whereas cephalothin and cephapirin are not. Also cefazolin is inactivated by large inocula of some strains of *S. aureus* while cephalothin is not; whether the inactivation is of any clinical significance has not been established.

Cefoxitin and *cefamandole* are the latest parenteral cephalosporins that have become available, and their relative usefulness is still being tested. Both agents have similar pharmacological characteristics that are superior to those of cephalothin, and a broader antibacterial spectrum that includes greater activity against indole-positive *Proteus* and *H. influenzae.* Cefamandole also has increased activity against *Enterobacter, Citrobacter,* and *Providencia,* and cefoxitin is active against *Serratia* and *Bacteroides fragilis.* Because of the importance of *B. fragilis* as a pathogen in abdominal and pelvic infections, cefoxitin might replace cephalothin and cefazolin as the antibiotic that is widely used in surgery.

Although cephalosporins penetrate most body fluids quite well, none can be clearly recommended for parenteral therapy of bacterial meningitis. Good results have been observed with cephaloridine in pneumococcal meningitis, but intrathecal therapy has been necessary when the antibiotic is given in recommended doses. Cefamandole has been reported to give a high cure rate in meningococcal meningitis, but, in cases of *H. influenzae* meningitis, the results have been equivocal. Further studies are needed before parenteral therapy can be given routinely, particularly in cases where the causative organism is not known.

Most patients who are thought to be allergic to penicillins can tolerate cephalosporins without adverse reactions. There is probably not true cross-reactivity, but a small number of highly allergic individuals do react to both drugs. In patients with previous penicillin anaphylaxis, or with positive immediate-type skin reactions to penicillin, therapy with cephalosporins should be instituted in small doses that are increased gradually. Rashes, urticaria, and anaphylaxis have been reported with cephalosporins, as have neutropenia, hemolytic anemia, thrombocytopenia, positive Coombs' tests, and transient rise in serum glutamic oxaloacetic transaminase and alkaline phosphatase.

AMINOGLYCOSIDES *Streptomycin,* one of the first antibiotics available for systemic administration, was widely used during the late 1940s and the 1950s. For a number of years it was given almost routinely in conjunction with penicillin in surgical cases for the prophylaxis and treatment of postoperative infections. Because of the tendency for highly resistant organisms to appear within 2 or 3 days, and its potential for causing vestibular damage and deafness, streptomycin has been largely supplanted by kanamycin, gentamicin, tobramycin, and amikacin, although it is still in use for certain specific purposes. Tuberculosis is still treated with streptomycin, particularly when triple drug regimens are used for the first few weeks. Streptomycin is also used in conjunction with penicillin to treat *Strep. viridans* endocarditis and some enterococcal infections and for the treatment of certain less common infections such as brucellosis and tularemia. In addition to vestibular nerve toxicity, other adverse reactions of streptomycin include rashes, fever, contact dermatitis, pancytopenia, anaphylaxis, and renal irritation.

Neomycin, another aminoglycoside that appeared in the 1940s, is no longer used parenterally because of its nephro- and neurotoxicity. Respiratory arrest is a serious adverse reaction that has occurred when neomycin is instilled topically in the peritoneal cavity in anesthetized patients, and deafness has resulted from the topical application of neomycin soaks injudiciously in burns and wounds. Neomycin is useful and relatively safe when given orally in doses of 4 to 6 g daily to "prepare" the bowel preoperatively, and in patients with hepatic insufficiency where inhibition of bacterial growth in the intestine is necessary to reduce the absorption of nitrogenous substances. However, the amount of neomycin absorbed from the intestine is variable, and toxic levels have been demonstrated in some patients. Neomycin is also used as a spray and an ointment to decrease the bacterial count in individuals who are nasal carriers of staphylococci.

Kanamycin is similar in structure to neomycin but less toxic and has been widely used parenterally for infections caused by most commonly encountered gram-negative bacilli except *Pseudomonas. Amikacin,* a semisynthetic derivative of kanamycin, has almost identical characteristics except that it is active against *Pseudomonas.* Both are active in vitro against staphylococci but are not used to treat severe staphylococcal infections because much higher blood levels can be attained safely with penicillins and cephalosporins. These aminoglycosides are not active against common gram-positive pathogens such as streptococci and pneumococci. They should be administered intramuscularly or by slow intravenous infusion in doses not larger than 7.5 mg/kg every 12 h, with the total dose not exceeding 15 g. Excretion is by glomerular filtration, the serum half-life is 2 h, and the drugs are not protein-bound.

Gentamicin and *tobramycin* are widely used aminoglycosides that are very similar except that tobramycin is two to four times more active against most strains of *Pseudomonas.* Smaller doses are used than for amikacin (3 to 5 versus 15 mg/kg per day), giving peak blood levels following intramuscular injections of 4 to 5 μg/ml for gentamicin and tobramycin versus about 20 μg/ml for amikacin. However, minimal inhibitory concentrations are also higher with amikacin, and it has not been shown that the higher blood levels are associated with a better clinical response.

Bacterial resistance, transmitted by plasmids and due to enzymatic transformations, is a potential threat with the aminoglycosides but has been relatively uncommon in most hospitals. Since amikacin has the least potential for resistance by this mechanism, many hospitals have established the policy of holding it in reserve. However, in some hospitals where gentamicin resistance has become a significant problem (25 to 30 percent of resistant strains), amikacin is the drug of choice for seriously ill patients requiring an aminoglycoside.

To minimize ototoxicity and nephrotoxicity, both significant problems with the aminoglycosides, it is important to reduce the dosage in patients with impaired renal function, and this is done in one of two ways. With the first, the full dose is given at an interval determined by multiplying the patient's serum creatinine by 8. This can result in a long interval between doses, when the serum concentration is at a low level. Therefore, the second method, giving a reduced dose at 8- or 12-h intervals, is used more widely. The serum creatinine, or preferably the creatinine clearance, is applied to a nomogram, and blood levels are monitored. The peak level is determined 30 min after an intramuscular, or 5 to 10 min after an intravenous, dose, and is more important than the trough. Serum concentrations can be determined by bioassay or radioimmuno-

assay within 2 to 4 h. The latter method is more expensive unless at least six or eight specimens are run every day.

With the ever-increasing occurrence of infections due to gram-negative bacteria the aminoglycosides are among the most widely used antibiotics in hospitals. Tobramycin and gentamicin have, to a great extent, replaced kanamycin, because of the adverse effects and bacterial resistance associated with its use. The role of amikacin remains in flux because its relative efficacy, toxicity, and potential for resistance have not been determined with certainty, particularly in relation to gentamicin and tobramycin. *Sisomicin* and *netilmicin* are new aminoglycosides that are being tested clinically and may have some advantages over drugs presently available.

TETRACYCLINES Since they first appeared in the late 1940s, the tetracycline antibiotics have been used widely because of their broad spectrum of activity against many gram-positive and gram-negative bacteria, and also other microorganisms such as *Mycoplasma, Rickettsia,* and *Chlamydia.* They have been effective, although not necessarily the drugs of choice, in the treatment of common venereal diseases including gonorrhea, syphilis, lymphogranuloma venereum, and granuloma inguinale. Their use has become more restricted during the last decade because of the advent of bactericidal antibiotics such as the cephalosporins, the penicillinase-resistant penicillins, and the aminoglycosides, together with an increasing awareness of the limitations of the tetracyclines. These limitations include the appearance of resistant strains among commonly encountered pathogens such as group A streptococci and pneumococci, the primarily bacteriostatic action of the tetracyclines, the occurrence of hepatotoxicity with high blood levels, the relatively high incidence of superinfections, and the common occurrence of side effects such as nausea, diarrhea, and photosensitivity reactions. Despite these limitations, the tetracyclines are still widely used for respiratory, urinary, soft tissue, and venereal infections.

Chlortetracycline (Aureomycin) and *oxytetracycline* (Terramycin), the two original compounds, have been largely replaced by *tetracycline,* which is marketed by a number of companies, and competition has led to a marked reduction in its price. The usual adult dose is 1 to 2 g daily in two to four equally divided doses. Intramuscular preparations are not very satisfactory, but the intravenous form is well-tolerated and gives relatively high blood levels with doses of 0.5 g every 12 h. Excessive blood levels occur with renal insufficiency unless the dose is decreased, and can cause fatty degeneration of the liver which may be fatal. Tetracycline persists in the body for many days when its normal route of excretion through the kidneys is blocked.

Four long-acting tetracyclines are available: *demeclocycline, methacycline, doxycycline,* and *minocycline.* They have high protein binding (over 90 versus 70 percent for tetracycline) and a prolonged plasma half-life, so that blood levels are well maintained when they are administered orally only every 12 to 24 h. However, the half-life of tetracycline is sufficiently prolonged so that blood levels with administration only every 12 h are similar to those of the smaller doses recommended for the long-acting tetracyclines. Unfortunately, the reduction in dose is not matched by a proportional decrease in price. The potential advantages for the long-active tetracyclines, i.e., greater convenience from less frequent administration and decreased cost from lower doses, have not been realized fully. Doxycycline does not give excessive blood levels in the presence of renal insufficiency following either oral or intravenous administration, and this provides a safety feature when the exact status of the patient's renal function is uncertain or unknown. Doxycycline is also active against the majority of strains of *B. fragilis,* and its efficacy in abdominal and pelvic infections has received considerable attention.

Untoward effects of the tetracyclines include staining of the teeth in children under 10, photosensitivity, intestinal irritation, increased urinary nitrogen loss, potential nephrotoxicity especially when given with other nephrotoxic drugs or with outdated supplies, vertigo (with minocycline), fatty hepatic changes in pregnancy, and increased intracranial pressure in children.

ERYTHROMYCIN, LINCOMYCIN, CLINDAMYCIN *Erythromycin* is primarily a bacteriostatic antibiotic that is active against the commonly encountered gram-positive bacteria, and is used chiefly for the oral therapy of respiratory and soft-tissue infections, particularly in patients thought to be allergic to penicillin. The susceptibility of *Mycoplasma pneumoniae* to erythromycin enhances its usefulness in respiratory infections. Erythromycin base is absorbed in an erratic manner, but some enteric-coated preparations now available give good and reliable serum concentrations. Erythromycin estolate has been thought to give much higher blood levels than erythromycin stearate, but the difference may be not as great as was once postulated because the estolate needs to be hydrolyzed in the body to the active form, and the hydrolysis is not as complete as during the blood level assay procedure. The estolate salt is associated with a low incidence of cholestatic hepatitis, which is readily reversible and rarely serious. Clinical results with the estolate, stearate, and the newer enteric-coated preparations appear to be comparable. The usual oral dose is 1 or 2 g daily. Intramuscular preparations are irritating, and intravenous administration is not used widely, partly because the preparations are not entirely satisfactory but chiefly because oral therapy is adequate for most infections treated with erythromycin.

Lincomycin and *clindamycin* are similar in antibacterial activity and clinical usefulness to erythromycin. Clindamycin gives higher blood levels, is more potent, and may cause less gastrointestinal side effects than lincomycin. The usual oral dose is 150 to 300 mg every 6 h. An excellent parenteral preparation of both is available, and 300 to 600 mg is given every 6 or 8 h. Clindamycin is considerably more active against *B. fragilis,* and intravenous administration of this antibiotic in abdominal and pelvic infections is widely advocated for this reason. However, pseudomembranous colitis is a fairly frequent and at times serious side effect which has led to recommendations that these antibiotics be used chiefly for hospitalized patients with significant infections, and that they be discontinued at once if diarrhea occurs. The colitis is probably due to toxin-producing strains of clostridia that are resistant to clindamycin.

CHLORAMPHENICOL This antibiotic has a broad spectrum of activity similar to the tetracyclines and during the 1950s was used widely. However, the occurrence of aplastic anemia, even though quite uncommon (about 1 in 25,000 persons exposed) has led to a restriction of chloramphenicol to those serious infections in which it is quite clearly the drug of choice. Typhoid fever is the principal example, and there are occasionally other severe gram-negative infections where the etiologic agent is susceptible only to chloramphenicol. With increasing interest in anaerobic infections, it is now realized that *B. fragilis* is the commonest of the anaerobic pathogens and that over half the strains are resistant to the penicillins and tetracyclines. This has led to an increase in the use of chloramphenicol since almost all *Bacteroides* strains are susceptible to it. However, clindamycin is also very active against *B. fragilis,* and it has partially replaced chloramphenicol for the treatment of patients with proved or presumed *Bacteroides* infections. Clindamycin lacks the broad gram-negative spectrum of chloramphenicol, and for this reason, the latter may be preferred under certain circumstances. In addition, clindamycin's propensity to producing colitis should restrict its use. Chloramphenicol is also used frequently in bacterial meningitis when the causative organism is not clearly recognizable on Gram's stain of the spinal fluid, since a number of strains of *H. influenzae* are now resistant to ampicillin.

Chloramphenicol is well absorbed by the oral route, and the usual adult dose is 0.5 g every 6 h. The parenteral preparation, chloramphenicol succinate, is hydrolyzed in the body to the active form, and this conversion is incomplete so that the blood levels with intravenous administration are not much higher than when the antibiotic is taken by mouth. With intramuscular administration, blood levels are considerably lower than with the oral route, and although the drug was widely used by this route for a number of years, the present labeling does not authorize intramuscular injections.

In addition to aplastic anemia, which may be an allergic or "idiosyncratic" reaction that usually occurs with prolonged and repeated administration, chloramphenicol inhibits protein synthesis, especially with doses larger than 2 g a day, an effect that is reversible. Clinically this is manifested by leukopenia, inadequate erythropoiesis (anemia), and thrombocytopenia as well as absence of reticulocytosis, high serum iron, and full saturation of transferrin. To monitor toxicity, blood counts should be performed at least twice weekly, and treatment with the antibiotic should be discontinued if there is significant hematologic toxicity. The gray syndrome, consisting of pallor, listlessness, and often death, occurs in neonates who have inadequately developed hepatic and renal mechanisms for metabolizing chloramphenicol; this can be prevented by restricting the dose to 25 mg/kg per day.

POLYMYXINS Polymyxin B and E (colistin) are polypeptide antibiotics that are active against most gram-negative bacteria except for the *Proteus* group. They have been of importance chiefly because of their action against *Pseudomonas aeruginosa*. However, their use systemically has decreased markedly since the advent of the aminoglycosides and carbenicillin which are clearly superior.

Polymyxin B is administered intramuscularly every 8 h, or as a continuous intravenous infusion, in doses no larger than 2.0 mg/kg per day. It is effective in treating urinary infections, but its efficacy in systemic infections is uncertain. Polymyxin B is also administered topically for eye and ear infections, and intrathecally for *Pseudomonas* meningitis. Colistin is available as the sodium salt of colistimethate and is administered in doses of 3.0 to 5.0 mg/kg per day intramuscularly or intravenously as described for polymyxin B.

Polymyxin B and colistimethate both cause perioral paresthesias and other neurotoxic manifestations with excessive blood levels; of these, apnea is the most life-threatening. Renal irritation and azotemia, which are usually reversible, may also occur. It is important to monitor renal function and to decrease the dose in the presence of renal insufficiency.

VANCOMYCIN Vancomycin is a relatively toxic but highly effective antibiotic that warrants special consideration because of its usefulness in treating certain specific infections. Vancomycin is bactericidal and is effective against gram-positive bacteria including penicillinase-producing staphylococci and enterococci. It is particularly useful in treating severe staphylococcal infections when penicillins and cephalosporins cannot be given, and in the treatment of *S. viridans* and enterococcal endocarditis under the same circumstances. It can be given only by the intravenous route, and 0.5 g every 6 h for 2 or 3 weeks is the usual dose. Thrombophlebitis is the principal side effect; it can be minimized by diluting each dose in 100 ml fluid and administering it over a period of at least 1 h. Chills, fever, renal irritation, and deafness are other adverse reactions that have been described, and these can be minimized by slow administration and by reduction of the dose if renal function is impaired. Vancomycin has had a considerable revival. One special indication is infections in patients with renal failure requiring dialysis, where a single dose of 1 g every 7 to 10 days gives adequate blood levels.

SULFONAMIDES The sulfonamides have been used clinically since 1937 and were the principal drugs administered for systemic antibacterial chemotherapy before penicillin and the other antibiotics became generally available. Their role has declined steadily, and they now occupy an important although relatively small place in clinical therapy since they are less active than the antibiotics, they are primarily bacteriostatic, resistant organisms occur frequently, and adverse reactions are common. Uncomplicated urinary tract infections due to *E. coli* are the principal indication for sulfonamides because of their efficacy, relative safety, and low cost. In addition, sulfonamides are the drugs of choice for the therapy of nocardiosis. They are no longer the preferred agents for the treatment of bacillary dysentery, meningococcal infections, and *H. influenzae* meningitis. Sulfonamides are still prescribed on a large scale for upper respiratory infections, but their efficacy in these situations is highly questionable since the majority of such infections is caused by viruses.

Sulfadiazine, once widely used as an all-purpose sulfonamide, tends to produce crystalluria and has been largely replaced by the more soluble *sulfisoxazole* (Gantrisin) and its close congener, *sulfamethoxazole* (Gantanol) which is also used widely now in a fixed-dose combination with trimethoprim (see "Miscellaneous Antibacterial Agents" below). Mixtures of three sulfonamides (trisulfapyrimidines) are also widely used because they are associated with a low incidence of crystalluria. The sulfonamides are usually administered orally, although very satisfactory intravenous preparations of the sodium salts are available. Orally, an initial dose of 2 to 4 g is followed by 1 g every 4 to 6 h.

Long-acting sulfonamides have also been used widely, and their only advantage is that they can be administered orally only once or twice daily. Examples are sulfamethoxypyridazine and sulfadimethoxine. The primary clinical indication for these long-acting compounds has been urinary tract infections, in instances where the convenience of taking only one dose a day has been considered important. However, it is undesirable to use a drug that leaves the body slowly, because this may prolong adverse reactions. Moreover, certain severe toxic reactions such as erythema multiforme or myocarditis have been reported to occur more commonly with long-acting sulfonamides. It is probably best not to use this class of compounds at all.

There are also some poorly absorbed sulfonamides, succinylsulfathiazole (Sulfasuxidine) and phthalysulfathiazole (Sulfathalidine), that are used principally to decrease the number of bacteria in the colon prior to certain types of abdominal surgery. These agents are of doubtful value. The drug Azulfidine (Chap. 294) is of value in ulcerative colitis.

Adverse reactions caused by the sulfonamides include erythema multiforme, serum sickness, hemolytic (in patients with glucose 6-phosphate dehydrogenase deficiency) and aplastic anemias, arthralgias, hepatitis, nausea, vertigo, lesions resembling those of polyarteritis nodosa, and kernicterus.

ANTIFUNGAL AGENTS *Amphotericin B* is a highly toxic antibiotic that is effective in the treatment of deep-seated mycotic infections. It produces marked improvement and occasional cures in cryptococcosis, histoplasmosis, blastomycosis, disseminated candidiasis, and coccidioidomycosis, and has a beneficial effect in at least some cases of aspergillosis and mucormycosis. It is administered intravenously in 5% dextrose solution over a period of 5 or 6 h. The safest procedure is to administer 1 mg on the first day, 5 mg on the second, and 10 mg on the third. The dose is then increased by 5 to 10 mg each day until 1 mg/kg is being administered daily. The dose may then be changed to 1.5 mg/kg every other day; treatment is continued for 2 to 4 months, depending on the severity of the infection and upon the patient's response. In patients with severe infections where intensive therapy is considered essential, it may be necessary to assume the risk of administering 15 mg very cautiously as the initial dose, with the addition of antihistamines and/or steroids to help ameliorate the chills and fever, which are quite variable from patient to patient. In some debilitated patients who develop *Candida* infections with oral or esophageal lesions, or bacteremias secondary to intravenous catheters, 10 or 15 mg amphotericin B daily for only 3 or 4 days may be adequate to bring the infection under control.

Some degree of renal impairment invariably occurs when amphotericin B is administered for several weeks; this is manifested during therapy by a rise in the blood urea nitrogen (BUN) and serum creatinine. Renal function may return to normal following therapy if attention is devoted to giving the minimum amount of drug that is compatible with a satisfactory therapeutic response, and if particular care is exercised in lowering the dose and frequency of administration when the creatinine becomes markedly elevated. Many patients have permanent renal damage; this poses special problems when relapses occur and subsequent courses of therapy are needed. Other adverse effects of amphotericin B include anemia, hypokalemia, thrombocytopenia, and hepatitis.

Nystatin (Mycostatin) is another antifungal antibiotic that is less potent than amphotericin B and is too toxic for systemic administration. It is applied topically in ointments, tablets, and suspension. It is used particularly for oral, intestinal, skin, and vaginal lesions due to *Candida,* and the best results are obtained when applications are made several times a day. The individual dose varies from 100,000 to 1 million units, depending on the location of the lesion.

Flucytosine is an oral antifungal agent that is relatively nontoxic and has been used successfully in cryptococcal, *Candida,* and *Torulopsis* infections. The dose is 150 mg/kg per day administered in divided doses at 6-h intervals. Some cases of cryptococcal meningitis and pulmonary disease have seemed to respond as well as to amphotericin B, but flucytosine is, in general, less potent than amphotericin. An appreciable percentage of initial isolates of *Candida* are resistant to the drug, and resistance also occurs during therapy. Adverse effects have consisted chiefly of nausea, vomiting, diarrhea, and rashes, but pancytopenia and abnormal liver function tests have also been reported. The drug is excreted in the urine, and the dose needs to be decreased in uremia in accordance with the package insert.

Flucytosine is not effective in histoplasmosis, blastomycosis, and coccidioidomycosis. It is indicated chiefly in patients with severe cryptococcal, *Candida,* and *Torulopsis* infections who cannot tolerate amphotericin B. It can also be used for *Candida* infections of the bladder and for superficial lesions that do not respond to topical therapy. There is in vitro evidence of synergism between flucytosine and amphotericin B, and clinical results in some severe systemic infections appear to have been improved by administering these two antifungal agents together.

Miconazole, an investigational synthetic imidazole derivative, has been used intravenously in systemic cryptococcal, *Candida,* and *coccidioides* infections with at least moderate effectiveness. It causes little or no nephrotoxicity. Itching and nausea have been significant side effects.

ANTITUBERCULOSIS DRUGS *Isoniazid* remains the most important single agent for the treatment of tuberculosis. After years of being considered virtually free from adverse reactions, hepatotoxicity has been reported on a number of occasions. Individuals receiving this drug should be monitored with liver function tests (Chap. 143). *Ethambutol* has largely replaced *p*-aminosalicylic acid (PAS) as the usual companion drug for isoniazid because it avoids the necessity of taking large numbers of tablets and also avoids the gastrointestinal side effects associated with PAS. *Rifampin* is another important drug that is comparable to isoniazid in activity against tuberculosis; it should be used in combination with other drugs to prevent the emergence of rifampin-resistant tubercle bacilli. Streptomycin is still used to some extent, particularly for triple drug therapy in seriously ill, hospitalized patients. The secondary drugs, used chiefly in cases that have failed to respond to initial therapy, are cycloserine, pyrazinamide, ethionamide, and viomycin. These drugs are all associated with significant toxic side effects and should be administered and monitored by experts who are familiar with their use. A more detailed consideration of the antituberculosis drugs and the present treatment regimens are given in Chap. 143.

MISCELLANEOUS ANTIBACTERIAL AGENTS *Spectinomycin* is an antibiotic that is effective in single 2- to 4-g doses intramuscularly for the treatment of gonorrhea. Side effects are minimal, and it is useful to have an agent similar in effectiveness to penicillin available for the treatment of patients who are allergic to penicillin or who have failed to be cured by penicillin.

Nitrofurantoin is an antibacterial agent that is effective in treating urinary tract infections although susceptibility of the *Proteus* group is variable and *Pseudomonas* is resistant. It is usually administered orally in doses of 100 mg four times a day. In addition to treating acute uncomplicated urinary tract infections, it is widely used to suppress symptoms of infection in patients with prostatism and other chronic obstructive uropathies. Nausea is sometimes troublesome, and pulmonary hypersensitivity and peripheral neuropathy may occur. The latter is especially likely to occur with renal insufficiency, and nitrofurantoin should be used very cautiously in the presence of uremia.

Nalidixic acid is another drug used orally for urinary tract infections. Its principal defect lies in the rapidity with which bacteria become resistant to it. This means that cultures should be made during, as well as following, therapy to be sure that bacteria are being cleared from the urinary tract. The usual dose is 4 g daily in divided doses for 1 to 2 weeks. Nausea, vomiting, and rashes are the chief adverse reactions.

Co-trimoxazole, a fixed-dose combination of trimethoprim (80 mg) and sulfamethoxazole (400 mg), is synergistic in this ratio against most gram-negatives causing urinary tract infections except for *Pseudomonas.* It is also active in vitro against a variety of other pathogens and is used in other countries for many types of infections. In the United States it is approved so far for urinary infections, otitis media, and pneumonia due to *Pneumocystis carinii.* Its use prophylactically in immunosuppressed patients appears promising for preventing severe *Pneumocystis* infestations. Because of its cost it should be used chiefly when the infecting organisms are not susceptible to other antimicrobials. It may be of particular value, however, in preventing recurrent bouts of bacteriuria.

Troleandomycin (TAO) is an antibiotic similar to, although less active than, the erythromycins. It is an ester and occasionally causes cholestatic jaundice. In general, erythromycin, lincomycin, and clindamycin are preferable to troleandomycin because of their greater antibacterial activity.

DRUGS OF CHOICE

It is quite clear from reading about the pharmacology of individual agents, as well as about their indications and uses in individual diseases, that many agents are available for the treatment of these diseases. Table 111-2 presents a summary of drugs, indications, dosage schedules, routes of administration, and duration of therapy. The table presents only a limited number of drugs, and many equally acceptable regimens are available. Moreover, while these treatment programs are appropriate for the present, changes in them should be expected as new drugs come on the market and as more experience with the newer agents is gathered.

REASONS FOR FAILURE OF CHEMOTHERAPY

This chapter as well as others dealing with specific disease entities has documented that there are few organisms not sensitive to some antibiotic. Despite this seemingly salutary observation, a large number of patients develop infections and many continue to die from them. In these patients antibiotics appear to have failed. Often this failure of chemotherapy is more apparent than real and may be attributed to one of several causes.

FAILURE TO ADJUST THE DOSE OF THE ANTIBIOTIC Different doses of antibiotics are required in different locations. For example, 600,000 units penicillin G is more than adequate to cure pneumococcal pneumonia, but as much as 20 million units may be required to cure pneumococcal meningitis and more than 50 million units to treat pneumococcal endocarditis. The pneumococcus in each of these locations remains exquisitely sensitive to penicillin, nor is the penetration of the drug inadequate. However, the host's environment is such that higher doses are required to cure the infections in different locations. Failure to appreciate this phenomenon may lead to inadequate doses.

TREATMENT OF NONBACTERIAL INFECTIONS Viral infections do not respond to the drugs generally considered as antibiotic agents, and these drugs must not be expected to exact a therapeutic effect in these situations. Similarly, antibiotics do not prevent bacterial complications of viral infections.

FAILURE TO DRAIN PURULENT MATERIAL OR TO REMOVE OBSTRUCTION Antimicrobial drugs work well only in an environment free of obstruction. Infections will not respond optimally unless obstructions such as a plug of mucus or an enlarged prostate, or a foreign body such as a suture or splinter, are removed, or unless purulent material is drained. It is particularly important to drain an abscess cavity because antibiotics do not kill bacteria enmeshed in pus.

SUPERINFECTIONS The role of antibiotics in promoting superinfections is discussed in Chaps. 107 and 108. In 2 to 3 percent of patients seeming failure of antimicrobials is a consequence of superinfection.

DRUG REACTION The development of drug fever without rash or any other manifestation of hypersensitivity may make it appear as if the infection were not responding to therapy, when instead the fever is due to the very drug being given to cure the infection. Drug fever is extremely common with certain antimicrobials, particularly penicillin. The best way to

TABLE 111-2
Conventional antibiotic regimens for adults with normal renal and hepatic function

Organism	Disease	Drug	Dosage	Route	Duration
Pneumococcus	Lung	Penicillin G (procaine)	600,000 U q 12 h	IM	5–10 days[a]
	Meningitis	Penicillin G	20 million U/day	IV	7–10 days
	Joints	Penicillin G } (aqueous)	20 million U/day	IV	7–10 days
	Endocarditis	Penicillin G	20 million U/day	IV	4–6 weeks[b]
Group A *Streptococcus*	Pharyngitis	Penicillin G } (procaine)	600,000 U/day	IM	10 days[c]
	Erysipelas	Penicillin G	600,000 U/day	IM	10 days[c]
	Other sites	See pneumococcus			
Coagulase-positive *Staphylococcus*[d]	Furunculosis, cellulitis, abscess	Erythromycin	500 mg q 6 h	PO	7–10 days
		or cloxacillin	500 mg q 6 h	PO	7–10 days
		or cephalexin	500 mg q 6 h	PO	7–10 days
	Pneumonia	Methicillin	1.0 g q 4 h	IM, IV	10–14 days
		or cloxacillin	500 mg q 6 h	PO	10–14 days
		or dicloxacillin	250 mg q 6 h	PO	10–14 days
		or cephalothin	1.0 g q 4 h	IV	10–14 days
	Arthritis	Methicillin	1.0 g q 4 h	IV	10–14 days
		or cephalothin	1.0 g q 4 h	IV	10–14 days
	Meningitis, endocarditis	Methicillin	1.0 g q 2 h	IV	4 weeks
		or cephalothin	1.0 g q 2 h	IV	4 weeks
	Enterocolitis	Vancomycin	500 mg q 6 h	PO	Until diarrhea ceases
Streptococcus viridans	Endocarditis	Penicillin G,	6–12 million U/day	IV	14 days
		then penicillin V	500 mg q 4 h	PO	14 days
		Penicillin G	6–12 million U/day	IV	14 days
		plus streptomycin	500 mg q 12 h	IM	14 days
Streptococcus fecalis (enterococcus)	Genitourinary infection	Ampicillin	500 mg q 6 h	PO	10–14 days
		plus gentamicin	3 mg/kg/day	IM, IV	10–14 days
	Surgical wound	Ampicillin	1 g q 6 h	IM or IV	7–10 days
		plus gentamicin	3–5 mg/kg/day	IM, IV	7–10 days
	Endocarditis	Ampicillin	8–12 g/day	IV	4 weeks
		or penicillin G	20 million U/day	IV	4 weeks
		plus gentamicin,	3–5 mg/kg/day	IM, IV	2 weeks
		or kanamycin	7.5 mg/kg q 12 h	IM	2 weeks
		or streptomycin	500 mg q 12 h	IM, IV	2 weeks
Streptococcus bovis	Endocarditis	Penicillin G	6–12 million U/day	IV	14 days
		then penicillin V	500 mg q 4 h	PO	14 days
		Penicillin G	6–12 million U/day	IV	14 days
		plus streptomycin	500 mg q 12 h	IM	14 days
Neisseria meningitidis	Meningitis, meningococcemia	Penicillin G	20 million U/day	IV	7–10 days
		or chloramphenicol	50–100 mg/kg/day (given q 6 h)	IV	7–10 days
N. gonorrheae	Urethritis	Penicillin G	4.8 million U/day	IM	1 dose
		plus probenecid	1 g	PO	1 dose
		or spectinomycin[e]	2 g/day	IM	1 dose
	Arthritis	Penicillin G (aqueous)	6 million U/day	IV	7–10 days
Hemophilus influenzae	Bronchitis and pneumonia	Ampicillin	500 mg q 4 h	PO	5–7 days
		or tetracycline	500 mg q 6 h	PO	5–7 days
	Meningitis	Ampicillin	8–12 g/day	IV	7–10 days
		plus chloramphenicol	50–100 mg/kg/day (given q 6 h)	IV	7–10 days
Brucella	Brucellosis	Tetracycline	500 mg q 6 h	PO	14 days
		and streptomycin	500 mg q 12 h	IM	14 days
Salmonella typhosa	Typhoid fever	Chloramphenicol[f]	1.0 g q 8 h	IV, PO	14 days
		or ampicillin[f]	1.0 g q 6 h	PO, IM IV	14 days
Salmonella	Abscess, bacteremia	Ampicillin	1.0 g q 4 h	IV	2–4 weeks
Shigella	Shigellosis	Ampicillin	500 mg q 4–6 h	PO, IM IV	7 days
Klebsiella	Genitourinary infection	Gentamicin	3 mg/kg q 8 h	IM, IV	10–14 days
		or cephalothin	500 mg q 6 h	IM, IV	10–14 days
		or cefazolin	500 mg q 6 h	IM, IV	10–14 days
		or kanamycin	7.5 mg/kg q 12 h	IM	10–14 days
K. pneumoniae	Pneumonia, bacteremia	Cephalothin	1.0 g q 4 h	IV	7 days
		or cefazolin	1.0 g q 4 h	IV	7 days
		or kanamycin	7.5 mg/kg q 12 h	IM	7 days
		or gentamicin	5 mg/kg/day	IM, IV	7 days

[a] *Last 3–4 days can be given orally as penicillin V 2 g/day in many cases.*
[b] *Last 2 weeks can be given as penicillin V 4–6 g/day orally.*
[c] *Penicillin V 1–2 g/day for 10 days, or a single shot of 1.2 × 10⁶ U benzathine penicillin is an acceptable alternate.*
[d] *Appropriate doses (see Pneumococcus and Streptococcus) of penicillin G (parenteral) or penicillin V (oral) if organism is sensitive to penicillin G.*
[e] *For patients allergic to penicillin.*
[f] *Start with parenteral but switch to oral as soon as possible.*

TABLE 111-2 *(continued)*
Conventional antibiotic regimens for adults with normal renal and hepatic function

Organism	Disease	Drug	Dosage	Route	Duration
Pasturella tularensis	Tularemia	Streptomycin	1.0 g q 12 h	IM	10–14 days
Enterobacter aerogenes	Genitourinary infection	Nalidixic acid[g]	1.0 mg q 6 h	PO	10–14 days
		or kanamycin	7.5 mg/kg q 12 h	IM	7 days
		or gentamicin	3 mg/kg/day	IM, IV	7 days
	Bacteremia	Kanamycin	7.5 mg/kg q 12 h	IM	7 days
		or gentamicin	3–5 mg/kg/day	IM, IV	7 days
		and/or carbenicillin	30 g/day	IV	7 days
Escherichia coli	Genitourinary infection	Sulfisoxazole[h]	1 g q 6 h	PO	10–14 days
		or tetracycline	500 mg q 6 h	PO	10–14 days
		or ampicillin	500 mg q 6 h	PO	10–14 days
		or nitrofurantoin	100 mg q 6 h	PO	10–14 days
	Bacteremia, arthritis, peritonitis	Ampicillin	6–12 g/day	IV	7–10 days
		or kanamycin	7.5 mg/kg q 12 h	IM	7–10 days
		or gentamicin	3–5 mg/kg/day	IM, IV	7–10 days
		or cephalothin	1–2 g q 4 h	IV	7–10 days
	Meningitis	Ampicillin	8–12 g q 4 h	IV	7–10 days
		or chloramphenicol	50–100 mg/kg/day (q 6 h)	IV	7–10 days
Proteus mirabilis	Urine	Ampicillin	500 mg q 6 h	PO	10–14 days
		or cephalexin	500 mg q 6 h	PO	10–14 days
	Blood	Ampicillin	6.0 g/day	IV	7–10 days
		or kanamycin	7.5 mg/kg q 12 h	IM	7–10 days
		or cephalothin	6.0 g/day	IV	7–10 days
		or gentamicin	5 mg/kg/day	IM, IV	7–10 days
Indole-positive *Proteus*	Urine	Kanamycin	7.5 mg/kg q 12 h	IM	10–14 days
		or carbenicillin[i]	1 g q 6 h	IV	10–14 days
		or nalidixic acid	1 g q 6 h	PO	10–14 days
		or gentamicin	3–5 mg/kg/day	IM, IV	10–14 days
	Blood	Kanamycin	7.5 mg/kg q 12 h	IM	7–10 days
		or carbenicillin	4 g q 4 h	IV	7–10 days
		or gentamicin	5 mg/kg/day	IM	7–10 days
Pseudomonas	Blood, joint	Gentamicin	5 mg/kg/day	IM, IV	7 days
		plus carbenicillin	5–6 g q 4 h	IV	7 days
	Meningitis, brain abscess	Gentamicin	5 mg/kg/day	IV, IM	7–14 days
		plus carbenicillin	5–6 g q 4 h	IV	7–14 days
		and gentamicin	4 mg q 12–18 h	Intrathecally	7 days
	Urine	Gentamicin	3 mg/kg/day	IM, IV	10–14 days
		or carbenicillin	2 g q 6 h	IM, IV	10–14 days
		or colistin	75 mg q 6 h	IM	10–14 days
		or polymyxin B	30 mg q 6 h	IM, IV	10–14 days
		or oxytetracycline	500 mg q 6 h	PO	10–14 days
Bacteroides	Abscess, bacteremia	Chloramphenicol	0.5 g q 4 h	IV, PO	10–14 days
		or Clindamycin	0.6 g q 6–8 h *then* 0.3 g q 6 h	IV / PO	10–14 days / As long as necessary
Mycoplasma	Sputum	Erythromycin	250–500 mg q 6 h	PO	7 days
		or tetracycline	500 mg q 6 h	PO	7 days

[g] Early follow-up cultures are essential to be sure resistance has not developed.
[h] Uncomplicated infections only.
[i] The indanyl ester of carbenicillin 1 g q 6 h may be given orally.

make the diagnosis is simply to discontinue therapy. If fever disappears, the diagnosis is established. A second challenge with the suspected drug is neither necessary nor safe.

INCORRECT DRUG Only rarely does chemotherapy fail because the incorrect drug has been administered. Most drugs have a sufficiently broad spectrum, and combinations of drugs are administered with sufficient frequency, whether indicated or not, to make it highly unlikely that the patient is not given an agent active against the etiologic pathogen. One of the most common errors, when the patient is not responding, is to add more antimicrobials indiscriminately, when the correct course should be to discontinue therapy and to watch the patient.

DEFECTS IN HOST RESISTANCE The type of patient requiring antimicrobial therapy has changed from a young or middle-aged individual to an elderly one with degenerative and debilitating disease or one whose host defenses have been compromised by neoplastic disease, large doses of antimicrobials, antineoplastic or immunosuppressive drugs, x-ray therapy, major surgical procedures, or transplants. For a variety of reasons, this type of patient does not, and should not be expected to, respond to antimicrobials as does a normal individual. This factor is often ignored in gauging the results of chemotherapy. It does not mean that antibiotics should not be used when indicated; rather, no miraculous results should be expected in patients with severe associated disease of noninfectious origin.

REFERENCES

APPEL GB, NEU HC: The nephrotoxicity of antimicrobial agents. N Engl J Med 296:663, 1977

BENNETT WM et al: A guide to drug therapy in renal failure. JAMA 230:1544, 1974

CLUFF LE, JOHNSON JE (eds): *Clinical Concepts of the Infectious Diseases,* 2d ed. Baltimore, Williams & Wilkins, 1978

Handbook of Antimicrobial Therapy, rev ed. New Rochelle, NY, Medical Letter, 1978

HOEPRICH PD: *Infectious Diseases,* 2d ed. New York, Harper & Row, 1977

KUNIN CM: Audits of antimicrobial usage. JAMA 237:1003, 1134, 1241, 1243, 1366, 1376, 1481, 1482, 1605, 1607, 1723, 1724, 1725, 1859, 1880, 1967, 1968, 1969; 1977

PRATT WB: *Chemotherapy of Infection.* New York, Oxford University Press, 1977

SARUBBI FA, HULL JH: Amikacin serum concentrations. Ann Intern Med 89:612, 1978

Symposium on Amikacin. Am J Med 62:799, 1977

Symposium on Cefamandole. J Infect Dis 137:S1–194, 1978

112
ACUTE INFECTIOUS DIARRHEAL DISEASE AND BACTERIAL FOOD POISONING

CHARLES C. J. CARPENTER

Acute diarrheal illnesses caused by bacterial, viral, or protozoal pathogens vary from slightly annoying bowel dysfunction to fulminant, life-threatening diseases. Until recent years, a specific etiologic agent could not be isolated from most patients with acute diarrhea. During the past decade, however, largely because of the recognition of enterotoxigenic *E. coli* as a major cause of acute diarrheal disease in adults and the identification of rotavirus as a frequent cause in young children, specific etiologic agents have been isolated from 80 to 85 percent of patients with acute diarrheal illnesses. Those illnesses caused by bacterial pathogens are more serious, although numerically fewer than those due to viruses, at least among adults, and for that reason, they will be addressed first. This chapter is aimed at presenting an overview of these diseases and, in most instances, the entities are discussed in more detail in the chapters dealing with the specific etiologic agent.

In considering the bacterial diarrheas, it is useful to divide them into two groups, those caused by invasive and those caused by noninvasive microorganisms. The invasive pathogens, of which *Shigella* (Chap. 124) may be considered the prototype, generally cause abdominal pain, fever, and other systemic symptoms, often including headache and myalgia. Illness caused by the noninvasive pathogens, of which cholera (Chap. 134) is the prototype, is generally characterized by the absence of fever and few systemic symptoms (except those directly related to intestinal fluid loss). The invasive pathogens characteristically destroy gut mucosal cells, typically involving the terminal ileum and colon, so that both leukocytes and erythrocytes are present, to a variable degree, in the stool. Inflammatory cells are generally absent from the stool in acute diarrheal disease caused by noninvasive bacterial pathogens.

NONINVASIVE BACTERIAL PATHOGENS

ENTEROTOXIGENIC *ESCHERICHIA COLI* **Etiology and epidemiology** Enterotoxin-producing *E. coli,* which has the dual capacity to adhere to small-bowel epithelial cells and to produce one or more diarrheagenic toxins, is now recognized as a major cause of acute diarrheal disease in the adult population throughout most of the world. Largely because current techniques for demonstrating toxigenicity remain cumbersome, the epidemiology of *E. coli* diarrhea is poorly understood. It has been demonstrated that enterotoxigenic *E. coli* is responsible for many cases of "traveler's diarrhea" in visitors to Mexico and in Peace Corps volunteers in East Africa, and that it is also the etiologic agent in most cases of acute diarrheal disease in adolescents and adults in rural Bangladesh. *Escherichia coli* plays a far less important role in episodic diarrheal illness in the United States. There is, as yet, no satisfactory explanation

for the observation that *E. coli* has been implicated as a major cause of fulminant, cholera-like diarrheal disease in adult patients only in South and Southeast Asia.

Pathogenesis The ability to cause diarrheal disease is not restricted to any one *E. coli* serotype, but appears to be dependent upon the presence of both a plasmid-mediated colonization factor, which allows the *E. coli* to adhere to small-bowel mucosal cells, and either one or both of two plasmids which code for the production of the two diarrheagenic toxins which may be produced by *E. coli.* The kinetics and mode of action of one of the toxins, which is heat labile (LT) and of relatively high molecular weight ($> 70,000$), are similar to those of cholera enterotoxin (Chap. 134); the diarrheagenic effect results from stimulation of adenylate cyclase in the gut epithelial cells. The other toxin, which is heat stable (ST) and of a lower molecular weight (< 5000), has a more rapid onset of action and probably exerts its effect through stimulation of guanylate cyclase in the gut mucosal cells. Either or both toxins may be produced by enterotoxigenic *E. coli.* Most isolates from patients with diarrheal disease in Bangladesh produce both LT and ST, whereas isolates from patients in other developing nations have shown widely varying capacities for the production of LT, ST, or both. The wide clinical spectrum may be, in part, related to the predominant production of either LT or ST by the culpable microorganisms.

Manifestations Both clinical observations and volunteer studies indicate that the incubation period is generally between 24 and 72 h. The illness which follows is quite variable, ranging from the fulminant, cholera-like disease often seen on the Indian subcontinent to the much milder Mexican "turista," in which the symptoms of mild, watery diarrhea, abdominal cramps, and occasional low-grade fever are more troublesome than life-threatening. Vomiting occurs in fewer than half the adults with *E. coli* diarrhea and is seldom responsible for major fluid losses.

In fulminant cases, the severe diarrhea seldom lasts longer than 24 to 36 h, and the response to either oral or intravenous electrolyte repletion is predictable and dramatic. With milder disease, the symptoms subside more gradually, occasionally persisting for a week or longer.

Laboratory findings As with cholera, no erythrocytes and few, if any, polymorphonuclear leukocytes are seen in a stool preparation stained by Loeffler's methylene blue. Because *E. coli* occurs normally among stool flora, and because its ability to produce enterotoxin is not restricted to any specific serotype, there is no rapid and simple means of laboratory diagnosis of enterotoxigenic *E. coli.* Bioassays for LT, based on the ability of *E. coli* isolates to produce fluid in isolated intestinal loops of experimental animals, or to stimulate adenyl cyclase in cells in tissue culture, as well as the suckling mouse bioassay for ST, are reliable but of little practical value.

Treatment The intestinal fluid losses are qualitatively identical to those in cholera. Therefore, in those patients who develop clinically significant saline depletion, the principles of fluid administration are identical to those described for cholera (Chap. 134). Oral solutions containing electrolytes plus glucose or sucrose are quite effective in correcting the saline depletion. Antimicrobials have not been shown to be effective in the *treatment* of diarrhea due to enterotoxigenic *E. coli,* although tetracyclines like doxycycline, 100 mg per day, may be of significant short-term *prophylactic* value in preventing *E. coli* diarrhea in travelers. Bismuth subsalicylate, 60 ml hourly for 4 doses, provides symptomatic relief (less frequent stools, less severe abdominal cramps) but has no effect on the total stool volume. Antiperistaltic agents such as anticholinergics or Lomotil are of no demonstrable value in enterotoxigenic *E. coli* diarrhea.

Prognosis With even the more fulminant cases of disease caused by enterotoxigenic *E. coli,* the prognosis is excellent with adequate fluid replacement.

Prevention Careful hygienic practices, with special attention to ingestion of clean water and adequately cooked foods when living in a generally unsanitary environment, provide the most certain protection against enterotoxigenic *E. coli.* Antibiotic prophylaxis is detailed above and is likely to be effective.

CHOLERA See Chap. 134.

OTHER ENTEROTOXIGENIC ENTEROBACTERIACEAE Noninvasive strains of *Klebsiella* and *Enterobacter* occasionally have been incriminated in acute diarrheal disease in the developing areas of the world. The culpable microorganisms have been shown to produce both heat labile (LT) and heat stable (ST) enterotoxins; the LT associated with these microorganisms is immunologically related to *E. coli* LT. The clinical illness produced is indistinguishable from the milder cases of diarrhea caused by enterotoxigenic *E. coli,* and treatment is the same.

CLOSTRIDIUM PERFRINGENS (Chap. 141) This organism remains a significant cause of diarrheal disease and was, in 1973, implicated in more cases of acute food poisoning in the United States than any other single microorganism. Both the epidemiologic background and the clinical picture of *C. perfringens* diarrhea differ strikingly from that caused by *E. coli.* *Clostridium perfringens* diarrhea tends to occur in a microepidemic pattern following ingestion of contaminated meat, poultry products, or legumes. The relatively short incubation period of 6 to 12 h is an important diagnostic clue. Typically, two or more patients who have ingested the same meat dish for dinner become ill at roughly the same time during the early morning hours. The production of a specific enterotoxin by the actively sporulating microorganisms in the intestinal tract appears to be responsible for all the symptoms.

The clinical picture of diarrhea caused by *C. perfringens* is different from that caused by enterotoxigenic *E. coli* in one important respect, namely, that moderately severe, cramping abdominal pain, which is usually not prominent with *E. coli,* is a major presenting symptom.

Treatment consists of symptomatic therapy with codeine to alleviate the cramping abdominal pain, and intravenous fluid therapy in the small proportion of patients in whom there is clinical evidence of saline depletion. The illness is self-limited and rarely lasts for more than 24 h. Because of the relatively short natural course of the illness, antimicrobial therapy is of no value. Because *C. perfringens* normally inhibits mammalian and avian intestinal tracts, prevention is dependent upon adequate cooking and handling of meat and poultry products. The practice of allowing cooked meat products to cool slowly toward room temperature over 12 to 24 h permits germination of contaminating clostridial spores; this practice must be avoided.

STAPHYLOCOCCUS AUREUS (Chap. 116) Acute staphylococcal diarrhea, classical "food poisoning," is due entirely to ingestion of preformed enterotoxin, and the causative organisms are often absent from stool during the acute illness. This form of diarrhea often occurs in institutional outbreaks, and is characterized by a short incubation period (1 to 6 h), relatively short duration (usually less less than 10 h), and very high attack rates (often greater than 75 percent of the population at risk). In addition to its distinctive epidemiologic features, acute staphylococcal diarrhea differs from other noninvasive bacterial diarrheas by the prominence of vomiting. Vomiting is an almost constant feature, and is apparently mediated by a direct effect of the absorbed toxin on the central nervous system.

Treatment is directed toward correction of the saline depletion (intravenous fluids are required in 10 to 20 percent of patients) and, when necessary, toward symptomatic relief of vomiting. Because staphylococcal food poisoning is caused by preformed enterotoxin and is not perpetuated by viable microorganisms, antimicrobials are of no value.

A good example of the explosive nature of staphylococcal food poisoning was provided by an outbreak on a jet liner flying from Anchorage to Copenhagen. In this episode, 57 percent of 343 passengers developed an acute illness characterized by vomiting, diarrhea, and cramping abdominal pain. Thirty of the 200 affected individuals required intravenous fluids, but none had serious sequelae. The food, contaminated by a pustule on the hand of a food handler, had not been adequately refrigerated aboard the plane, allowing abundant growth of the staphylococcus, with production of enterotoxin. Since staphylococci are ubiquitous, the prevention of massive contamination is dependent largely on control of growth conditions, primarily temperature. *Staphylococcus aureus* can multiply at temperatures from 4 to 46°C and if contaminated food is allowed to remain at ambient temperatures after cooking, these organisms have ample opportunity to multiply, especially in such items as cream pastries, potato salad, and mayonnaise.

BACILLUS CEREUS *Bacillus cereus* is a cause of acute diarrheal disease which, although uncommon, has been identified with increasing frequency in the past decade, especially in Europe. The illness results from gross contamination of food with this gram-positive rod, which is capable of producing at least two discrete enterotoxins, one of which has characteristics similar to those of the labile enterotoxin of *E. coli,* and the other of which has effects similar to that of staphylococcal enterotoxin. *Bacillus cereus* may therefore cause two distinct clinical syndromes, a diarrheal form resulting from the *E. coli* LT type of enterotoxin and an emetic form caused by the staphylococcal type of enterotoxin. The diarrheal syndrome caused by *B. cereus* is generally similar to that caused by enterotoxin-producing *E. coli,* with the exceptions that abdominal cramps are more common (75 percent of cases) and both the incubation period (6 to 14 h) and median duration of illness (20 h) are shorter. The emetic syndrome is clinically indistinguishable from that caused by staphylococcal enterotoxin, with a short incubation period (median 2 h), short duration (median 9 h), and prominent vomiting (100 percent compared with less than 25 percent in the diarrheal syndrome).

Because both syndromes are self-limited and generally mild, no specific therapy is indicated. When *B. cereus* food poisoning is suspected clinically, the diagnosis can be confirmed by demonstration of 10^5 or more *B. cereus* organisms in epidemiologically incriminated food. *Bacillus cereus* grows readily on simple laboratory media, including blood agar, but will not generally be identified as a pathogen unless such identification is specifically requested. Isolation of *B. cereus* from stool alone does not establish it as the etiologic agent. *Bacillus cereus* is frequently found in the fecal flora of normal individuals.

Since *B. cereus* is ubiquitous in soil, as well as in many raw, dried, and processed foods, proper food handling is the only practical means of preventing this form of food poisoning. The emetic form of *B. cereus* food poisoning has almost invariably been associated with ingestion of contaminated fried rice. *Bacillus cereus* is commonly present in uncooked rice, and its spores survive boiling and germinate, with production of the enterotoxin, when boiled rice is left unrefrigerated. Brief rewarming before serving is not adequate to destroy the relatively heat-stable toxin. Prompt refrigeration of boiled rice will prevent transmission of the disease.

INVASIVE ENTERIC PATHOGENS

Shigellae characteristically invade the colon and terminal ileum, destroy segments of intestinal mucosa, cause extensive inflammatory changes in the lamina propria, and are the prototype of the invasive enteric bacterial pathogens. Other important invasive bacterial enteric pathogens include *Salmonella, Yersinia enterocolitica,* invasive *E. coli,* and *Vibrio parahemolyticus,* which may have the capacity both to damage intestinal mucosa and to produce an enterotoxin. As opposed to the noninvasive pathogens, the invasive enteric organisms frequently cause systemic symptoms, including headache, myalgias, chills, and fever. As a general rule, antiperistaltic agents such as opiates, diphenoxylate, and atropine are contraindicated in diarrheal disease caused by invasive enteric pathogens because they clearly worsen the clinical course in human shigellosis, as well as salmonellosis and shigellosis in animal models.

The major therapeutic challenge in invasive bacterial diarrheas is that of distinguishing between (1) shigellosis and yersiniosis, in which antimicrobial therapy is usually indicated because of the severity of diarrhea and the frequency of rectal bleeding, dysentery, and systemic symptoms, (2) infections caused by salmonella, which are characterized primarily by watery diarrhea and few systemic symptoms and in which antimicrobial therapy may cause prolonged excretion of the pathogen, and (3) invasive *E. coli* infections, in which antimicrobials are of no demonstrable value.

SHIGELLOSIS See Chap. 124.

SALMONELLOSIS See Chap. 123.

YERSINIA ENTEROCOLITICA See Chap. 129.

VIBRIO PARAHEMOLYTICUS See Chap. 134.

INVASIVE *ESCHERICHIA COLI* Invasive *E. coli,* which are far less common pathogens than enterotoxigenic *E. coli,* may cause a clinical syndrome quite similar to shigellosis with the exceptions that vomiting seldom occurs with the invasive *E. coli* and the illness is of shorter duration. Diarrhea caused by invasive *E. coli* is rare in the United States but has been a significant cause of short-term disability in Southeast Asia and South America. Since the illness caused by invasive *E. coli* is relatively short-lived antimicrobial therapy has not been shown to be helpful.

ACUTE VIRAL DIARRHEAS

Acute viral gastroenteritis is discussed in detail in Chap. 187. These illnesses are both more common and more life-threatening in small children than adults. In the United States, rotaviruses account for a large proportion of diarrheal illnesses during the first 2 years of life and usually occur during the winter. They have seldom been implicated in adult illness. In rural Bangladesh, infection with rotavirus accounts for roughly 60 percent of episodes of diarrhea in children under the age of 2, for about 5 percent in the 2- to 5-year-old age group, and

seldom occurs in adolescents and adults. The illness usually presents gradually with vomiting, watery diarrhea, and low-grade fever with little or no associated abdominal pain. Vomiting is a prominent and almost constant early manifestation of rotavirus enteritis but rarely persists beyond the first 36 h. Diarrhea often persists for 4 to 6 days. Although the illness is generally not life-threatening, many patients require fluid and electrolyte repletion. Following subsidence of vomiting, this can generally be achieved by the oral route, using the same fluids that are effective in the treatment of cholera (Chap. 134).

The diagnosis can be confirmed by a variety of tests including demonstration of the virus in stool by electron microscopy, a rise in complement-fixing antibody titers, radioimmunoassay, etc. The most useful and reliable test for rapid diagnosis under field conditions consists of direct demonstration of the antigen in stool by the enzyme-linked immunosorbent assay (ELISA).

Other viruses (e.g., Norwalk virus, Hawaii virus), although implicated in occasional common-source outbreaks involving adults, usually cause relatively mild, short (< 36 h), and self-limited disease, for which neither fluid nor antimicrobial therapy is necessary (Chap. 187).

ACUTE PROTOZOAL DIARRHEAS

Over the past decade, *Giardia lamblia* has emerged as a major cause of acute diarrheal disease (Chap. 210). Although formerly thought to be a pathogen only in children and later considered to be a significant cause of diarrheal disease only in developing nations, this organism was the pathogen most commonly incriminated in outbreaks of waterborne diarrheal disease in the United States in 1976. In North America, it occurs most commonly in the Rocky Mountain states, and more frequently causes disease in visitors than in the indigenous population. The illness characteristically presents with the sudden onset of watery diarrhea and malabsorption, accompanied by mild to moderate abdominal discomfort, bloating, and flatulence, and may persist unless appropriate antimicrobials are administered. Prolonged disease with malabsorption occurs from time to time in previously normal individuals but is particularly common in patients with IgA deficiency, who tend to have the most severe form of giardiasis.

The attack rate may be quite high ($>$ 50 percent) in individuals exposed to contaminated water sources. In certain groups of North American travelers returning from Leningrad, where the water supply appears to be heavily contaminated with giardia cysts, up to 60 percent of individuals have developed clinical giardiasis. The usual incubation period is 10 to 20 days. The illness, therefore, frequently develops after a traveler returns home, and the travel history is a critical element in suspecting the diagnosis. Occasionally the disease occurs endemically in individuals who have not traveled. The diagnosis can be confirmed in approximately half the cases by examining the stool for cysts; if the stool examination is negative in a patient with characteristic clinical features, duodenal aspirates or biopsies will usually yield the characteristic trophozoites. Treatment with quinacrine, 100 mg tid for 5 to 7 days, is generally curative; metronidazole, 250 mg tid for 7 days, is an acceptable alternative regimen.

REFERENCES

CENTER FOR DISEASE CONTROL: *Foodborne Outbreaks: Annual Summary 1973.* 1974

DUPONT HL et al: Pathogenesis of *Escherichia coli* diarrhea. N Engl J Med 285:1, 1971

——— et al: Symptomatic treatment of diarrhea with bismuth subsalicylate among students attending a Mexican university. Gastroenterology 73:715, 1977

Evans DG et al: Plasmid-controlled colonization factor associated with virulence in *Escherichia coli* enterotoxigenic for humans. Infect Immunol 12:656, 1975

Gorbach SL et al: Traveller's diarrhea and toxigenic *Escherichia coli.* N Engl J Med 292:933, 1975

Guerrant RL et al: Role of toxigenic and invasive bacteria in acute diarrhea of childhood. N Engl J Med 293:576, 1974

Merson MH et al: Traveller's diarrhea in Mexico. A prospective study of physicians and family members attending a Congress. N Engl J Med 294:1299, 1976

Sack RB et al: Enterotoxigenic *Escherichia coli* isolated from patients with severe cholera-like disease. J Infect Dis 123:378, 1971

——— et al: Human diarrheal disease caused by enterotoxigenic *Escherichia coli.* Ann Rev Microbiol 29:333, 1975

———: Prophylactic doxycycline for traveller's diarrhea. N Engl J Med 298:758, 1978

Terranova W et al: Current concepts: *Bacillus cereus* food poisoning. N Engl J Med 298:143, 1978

113
SEXUALLY TRANSMITTED DISEASES

KING K. HOLMES

INTRODUCTION Venereology today encompasses not only the five "venerable" venereal diseases (gonorrhea, syphilis, chancroid, lymphogranuloma venereum, and granuloma inguinale), but also a growing number of other diseases which might be considered the "new generation" of sexually transmitted diseases (STDs). Many of these newer STDs, like gonorrhea, have become epidemic in nearly all countries of the world during the past two decades. With increasing interest in these diseases and improved methods for diagnosis has come awareness of the growing consequences of STD in areas of health and society which extend beyond the traditional sphere of venereology. In particular, major impact of the newer STDs has been noted on maternal and infant morbidity and on human reproduction and infertility.

CLASSIFICATION OF SEXUALLY TRANSMITTED DISEASES
These diseases can be classified on the basis of either their etiology or their clinical manifestations. Table 113-1 gives an etiologic classification of STD. Sexual transmission has been implicated as a major factor in the propagation of each of the pathogens listed in this table although evidence for sexual transmission of some, such as group B streptococcal infection and cytomegalovirus infection, is quite preliminary. There have been sporadic case reports of sexual transmission of many other pathogenic agents. However, the diseases caused by these other agents are not generally considered sexually transmitted diseases, since sexual transmission seems to be a minor factor in their propagation. For each of the agents listed in Table 113-1, there are one or more diseases or syndromes known to be caused by the agent, and others (indicated by a question mark) for which a causal association is suspected but not proved.

APPROACH TO SEXUALLY TRANSMITTED DISEASE
It is necessary for the clinician to consider the approach to STD syndromes before an etiologic diagnosis is established. Table 113-2 lists some of the most common clinical syndromes and complications caused by sexually transmitted pathogens. Strategies for the management of the three most common syndromes seen in venereology are outlined below.

MALE URETHRITIS Urethritis in the male is classified as gonococcal or nongonococcal. The incidence of gonococcal urethritis has stabilized in many Western countries, while that

TABLE 113-1
Twenty-one sexually transmitted pathogens and the diseases they cause

Agent	Disease or syndrome
BACTERIAL	
Neisseria gonorrhoeae	Urethritis, cervicitis, proctitis, pharyngitis, conjunctivitis, endometritis, pelvic inflammatory disease, perihepatitis, bartholinitis, amniotic infection syndrome, disseminated gonococcal infection, ?premature rupture of membranes and premature delivery
Chlamydia trachomatis	Nongonococcal urethritis, epididymitis, cervicitis, salpingitis, inclusion conjunctivitis, infant pneumonia, trachoma, and lymphogranuloma venereum, ?perihepatitis, ?bartholinitis, ?proctitis, ?otitis media
Mycoplasma hominis	Postpartum fever, ?salpingitis
Ureaplasma urealyticum	?Nongonococcal urethritis, ?premature rupture of membranes and premature delivery
Treponema pallidum	Syphilis
Hemophilus vaginalis	?Nonspecific vaginitis
Hemophilus ducreyi	Chancroid
Calymmatobacterium granulomatis	Granuloma inguinale
Shigella spp.	Shigellosis in homosexual men
?Group B streptococcus	Neonatal sepsis, neonatal meningitis
VIRAL	
Herpes simplex virus	Initial and recurrent genital herpes, aseptic meningitis, neonatal herpes, ?carcinoma of the uterine cervix
Hepatitis B virus	Acute hepatitis, chronic active hepatitis, persistent (unresolved) hepatitis, polyarteritis nodosa, chronic membranous glomerulonephritis, ?mixed cryoglobulinemia, ?polymyalgia rheumatica, ?hepatoma
?Cytomegalovirus	Heterophile-negative infectious mononucleosis; congenital infection: gross birth defects and infant mortality; cognitive impairment (e.g., mental retardation, sensorineural deafness); ?cervicitis; protean manifestations in the immunosuppressed host
Genital wart virus	Condyloma accuminata, ?laryngeal papilloma in infants
Molluscum contagiosum virus	Genital molluscum contagiosum
PROTOZOAN	
Trichomonas vaginalis	Trichomonal vaginitis
Entamoeba histolytica	Amebiasis in homosexual men
Giardia lamblia	Giardiasis in homosexual men
FUNGAL	
Candida albicans	Vulvovaginitis, balanitis, and balanoposthitis
ECTOPARASITICAL	
Phthirius pubis	Pubic lice infestation
Sarcoptes scabiei	Scabies

of nongonococcal urethritis (NGU) continues to rise, suggesting that current measures for control of NGU are relatively ineffective. In general, gonorrhea and NGU are equally common among men seen in STD clinics in the United States, whereas NGU is approximately three times as common as gonorrhea among men seen by physicians in private practice and 10 times as common as gonorrhea among college students.

About 40 to 50 percent of NGU is caused by *Chlamydia trachomatis*. Herpes simplex virus and trichomonal vaginitis each cause a small additional proportion of NGU cases in the United States, but about 50 percent of cases cannot be attributed to any of these three pathogens. *Ureaplasma urealyticum* has been implicated in case-control studies as a probable cause of most of the *Chlamydia*-negative cases. Since facilities for isolation of *C. trachomatis* are not widely available, and the role of *U. urealyticum* is not certain, the diagnosis of male urethritis usually does not include cultures for *C. trachomatis* or *U. urealyticum*. The following steps should be taken in evaluating sexually active men with symptoms of urethral discharge and/or dysuria.

1 *Establish the presence of urethritis.* Urethral discharge should be demonstrated. Commonly in NGU, and less often in gonorrhea, discharge can be demonstrated only by milking the urethra after the patient has gone several hours, preferably overnight, without voiding. If no overt discharge is demonstrable, urethral exudate can be demonstrated by inserting a small urethrogenital swab 1 to 2 cm into the urethra and examining the Gram-stained direct smear prepared from this swab for leukocytes. Five or more leukocytes per $1000\times$ field in areas containing cells suggest urethritis. Patients with symptoms of urethritis who lack objective confirmatory evidence of urethritis may have functional problems and generally do not benefit from repeated courses of antibiotics.

2 *Exclude complications or alternative diagnosis.* Epididymitis and systemic complications, such as the gonococcal arthritis-dermatitis syndrome, and *Reiter's* syndrome, should be excluded by brief history and examination. Rectal examination for prostatitis is seldom informative in patients with overt urethritis, unless concomitant symptoms such as perineal, suprapubic, or rectal discomfort are present. Bacterial prostatitis and cystitis should, of course, be excluded by appropriate tests in men with dysuria who lack signs of urethritis.

3 *Gram's stain examination of urethral exudate.* The diagnosis of gonorrhea is confirmed by demonstrating typical gram-negative diplococci within neutrophils. The diagnosis of NGU is warranted if no gram-negative *Neisseria gonorrhoeae* are found in such cases. Smears containing only extracellular or atypical gram-negative diplococci are equivocal and should lead to attempts to isolate *N. gonorrhoeae* by culture. The above approach is illustrated in Fig. 113-1. The treatment of gonorrhea and NGU is discussed in Chaps. 119 and 174, respectively.

LOWER GENITOURINARY INFECTION IN WOMEN Infections of the female urinary tract, vulva, and vagina produce certain overlapping symptoms in women such as burning on urination, vulvar irritation, and dyspareunia. Infections of the cervix and vagina produce other symptoms such as altered quality or increased quantity of vaginal discharge. There is insufficient consensus on clinical or laboratory guidelines for differentiating among these various categories on the basis of symptomatology, and they are often referred to in vague terms such as "nonspecific genital infection." Lack of nosologic precision is attributable not only to overlapping symptomatology, but also to uncertainty about the etiology of the inflammatory conditions of the urinary tract, vulva, vagina, and cervix in women; to the lack of consistent application of available laboratory testing where the etiology is known; and to the difficulty clinicians experience in differentiating true inflammatory conditions from functional, psychosomatic genitourinary complaints.

Although the etiology of certain genitourinary inflammatory conditions in women remains uncertain, some data allow improved diagnostic precision, which in turn should lead to improved management. One estimate of the relative frequency of diagnostic entities that produce lower urogenital symptoms (unusual vaginal discharge, vulvar itching or irritation, dysuria, frequency, etc.) was provided in a study of 821 young women (mean age 24) examined in a primary care clinic. Vaginitis was found to be more than five times as common as cystitis or urethritis (UTI). Two steps are required in the evaluation of lower genitourinary symptoms in women: (1) differentiation among cystitis, urethritis, vaginitis, cervicitis, and cervical ectopy, and (2) exclusion of associated upper tract disease (e.g., pyelonephritis, salpingitis).

Cystitis/urethritis Although dysuria is more common in UTI than in vaginitis, in young women dysuria is attributable to vaginitis more often than UTI, because vaginitis is so much more common than UTI. However, when women were asked to localize the dysuria as "internal" (felt inside the body) or "external" (felt on the vaginal labia when the stream of urine passed), "internal" dysuria correlated with UTI. Among women considered to have UTI without vaginal infection, about half have bacterial cystitis, with 10^5 bacteria per millili-

TABLE 113-2
Selected syndromes and complications with corresponding sexually transmitted etiologic agents*

Syndrome	Agent
Male urethritis	*N. gonorrhoeae, C. trachomatis,* herpes simplex virus, *?U. urealyticum*
Lower genitourinary infection in women	Vulvitis: *C. albicans,* herpes simplex virus
	Vaginitis: *T. vaginalis, C. albicans, H. vaginalis*
	Cervicitis: *N. gonorrhoeae, C. trachomatis,* herpes simplex virus
	Female urethritis: *N. gonorrhoeae, C. trachomatis*
Genital ulceration	Herpes simplex virus, *Treponema pallidum, H. ducreyi, Cal. granulomatis, C. trachomatis* (LGV)
Pelvic inflammatory disease	*N. gonorrhoeae, C. trachomatis*
Proctitis	*N. gonorrhoeae,* herpes simplex virus, *?C. trachomatis*
Acute arthritis with genital infection	*N. gonorrhoeae, ?C. trachomatis*
Neonate and infant: "TORCHES" syndrome	Cytomegalovirus, herpes simplex virus, *T. pallidum*
Other infant and childhood morbidity	Conjunctivitis: *C. trachomatis, N. gonorrhoeae*
	Pneumonia: *C. trachomatis*
	Otitis media: *C. trachomatis*
	Sepsis, death: Group B streptococcus
	Cognitive impairment: Cytomegalovirus, herpes simplex virus, *T. pallidum*
Infertility: Postsalpingitis, postobstetric, postabortion	*N. gonorrhoeae, C. trachomatis, M. hominis*
Spontaneous abortion	Herpes simplex virus, *?N. gonorrhoeae, ?C. trachomatis,* fetal wastage

* For each of the above syndromes and complications, a variable proportion cannot yet be ascribed to any cause and must currently be considered idiopathic.

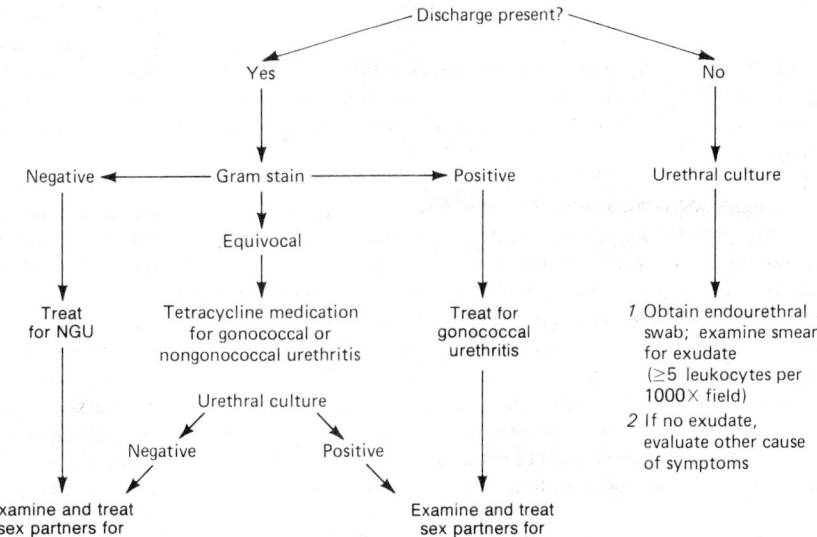

FIGURE 113-1

Diagnosis and management of suspected urethritis in males.

ter of urine, while half have urethritis—often termed the *urethral syndrome*. Both sexual intercourse and oral contraception have been identified as risk factors predisposing to bacterial UTI in women. The role of sexual intercourse in predisposing to the urethral syndrome is uncertain. However, in populations having a high risk of gonorrhea, *N. gonorrhoeae* clearly is a common cause of urethritis among women without significant bacteriuria. *Chlamydia trachomatis* has also been implicated as a cause of urethritis among women (Chap. 174).

DIAGNOSIS AND THERAPY   The diagnosis of UTI in young women involves first the differentiation of UTI from vaginitis by history and examination. Among women with suspected UTI, bacterial UTI must then be differentiated from the urethral syndrome. The absence of bacteriuria in women with suspected UTI suggests the diagnosis of the urethral syndrome. Gonorrhea should be excluded by appropriate culture of the cervix and urethra. The value of antimicrobial therapy for the urethral syndrome, if gonorrhea is not present, has not been studied in controlled fashion.

VAGINITIS   In self-referred female STD clinic patients, vaginitis is the most common diagnosis. The relative frequency of *Candida albicans, Hemophilus vaginalis,* and *Trichomonas vaginalis* as causes of vaginitis varies, with *T. vaginalis* being relatively more common among those of low socioeconomic status.

Vaginitis, without UTI, is characterized by one or more of the following symptoms: Increased volume of discharge; abnormal yellow or green color of discharge, caused by increased concentration of polymorphonuclear leukocytes, which contain myeloperoxidase pigment; vulvar itching, irritation, or burning; introital dyspareunia; and malodor. *Trichomonas vaginalis* produces a profuse, yellow or green purulent discharge which is often malodorous. In contrast, the predominant symptom in *C. albicans* vaginitis is usually vulvar itching, often with signs of vulvitis as well as vaginitis, but without odor. The discharge in *Candida* vaginitis is typically white and may resemble curds of cottage cheese. The vagina occasionally contains adherent thrush-like plaques of matted mycelia, polymorphonuclear leukocytes, and epithelial cells. Nonspecific vaginitis, associated with *H. vaginalis* infection, is associated with moderately increased malodorous vaginal discharge. The discharge is homogeneous, low in viscosity, contains fewer leukocytes than are usually found in *T. vaginalis* or *C. albicans* infection, and is uniformally adherent to the vaginal walls. Colposcopy may show abnormally dilated vessels and/or in-

creased density of vessels on the vaginal or cervical wall in *Candida* and *Trichomonas* vaginitis, but not in nonspecific vaginitis (NSV). While the symptomatology and examination may suggest an etiologic diagnosis, several studies have shown poor correlation between clinical and microbiological findings in determining the etiology of vaginitis. A most important contribution of the clinical evaluation of vaginal discharge is ascertaining by speculum examination whether the discharge emanates from the vagina or cervix, and whether the discharge is, in fact, abnormal. Occasionally, subjective symptoms of vaginitis are not associated with objective signs of vaginitis. Psychological testing is normal in most such cases. The diagnosis and therapy of the three types of vaginitis are summarized in Table 113-3.

***Trichomonas vaginalis* vaginitis**   Sexual transmission of *T. vaginalis* is well established, although the age distribution of *T. vaginalis* infection in women is skewed toward the older age group more than for other STDs, suggesting that nonsexual transmission of *T. vaginalis* may be important. Routine sampling indicates that many women and most men with infection are asymptomatic. Among patients with asymptomatic infections, the potential for development of symptoms is high.

TABLE 113-3
Diagnostic features and therapy of infectious vaginitis

Etiology	Diagnostic features	Therapy
Trichomonas vaginalis	Motile trichomonads pH = 5.5–6.0 Amine odor volatilized by adding 10% KOH	Metronidazole 2.0 g single oral dose Metronidazole 250 mg three times daily for 10 days
Candida albicans	Yeast, pseudomycelia pH < 4.5 No odor with 10% KOH Isolation of *C. albicans*	Nystatin vaginal tablet twice daily for 7 days Imidazole (clotrimazole or miconazole) intravaginally once daily for 7 days
Hemophilus vaginalis	Clue cells pH > 4.5 Amine odor with 10% KOH Isolation of *H. vaginalis*	Ampicillin 500 mg four times daily for 7 days Metronidazole 500 mg twice daily for 7 days
Uninfected	Normal vaginal secretions pH < 4.5 No odor with 10% KOH	No medication

Treatment of symptomatic as well as asymptomatic cases is recommended to reduce the reservoir of infection and the possible risk of transmission and to prevent the future development of symptoms.

DIAGNOSIS AND THERAPY The diagnosis in women is confirmed by demonstration of motile trichomonads in vaginal secretions mixed with normal saline and examined promptly under a low-power or high dry (400×) microscopic field. Wet-mount examination is at least 80 to 90 percent as sensitive as culture in symptomatic cases. The diagnosis of *T. vaginalis* infection in men is difficult.

The pH of vaginal secretions is usually greater than 5.0 in symptomatic *T. vaginalis* infections, and the addition of 10% potassium hydroxide (KOH) to vaginal secretions may liberate an amine-like fishy odor in trichomonal vaginitis as well as in NSV.

Nitroimidazoles are the only consistently effective drugs for treating trichomoniasis. Several studies show that a single 2.0-g oral dose is as effective as the former higher dosage schedules. Tinidazole, a structurally related 5-nitroimidazole, has a longer half-life than metronidazole (12.5 h vs. 7.3 h after a single oral 2.0-g dose) which might conceivably be of benefit in single-dose therapy, but this drug has not been shown to give better results than metronidazole in single-dose therapy of trichomoniasis.

Several studies have demonstrated *T. vaginalis* infection in one-third to two-thirds of male sex partners of women with *T. vaginalis* infections. On the basis of these data, and in view of

FIGURE 113-2
A. Vaginal epithelial "clue cells." Note granular appearance due to adherent H. vaginalis *and indistinct cell margins. 400×. B. Normal vaginal epithelial cells. The cell margins are distinct and lack granularity.*

A

B

the difficulty in demonstrating *T. vaginalis* in men, routine treatment of sex partners of either sex seems advisable to reduce the risk of reinfection and to reduce the reservoir of infection. However, caution is warranted in using nitroimidazoles. It is recommended that metronidazole not be given to women during the first trimester of pregnancy because of teratogenicity in animals, and that alcohol be avoided for 24 h after treatment because of the Antabuse-like effect of the drug. Metronidazole is also mutagenic, and massive doses cause several types of tumors in rodents.

Nonspecific vaginitis Vaginal discharge not associated with *T. vaginalis, C. albicans,* or uterine infection is usually attributed to nonspecific vaginitis (NSV). *Hemophilus vaginalis* has been associated with NSV, and although this association has been challenged, it was supported by finding *H. vaginalis* in vaginal secretions from 17 (96 percent) of 18 women with NSV and only 1 (4 percent) of 18 normal matching women. The concentration of anaerobic bacteria in vaginal washings from women with NSV has also been found to be increased, though no specific anaerobe has been implicated.

The evidence linking *H. vaginalis* to NSV is somewhat similar to that linking *U. urealyticum* to *Chlamydia*-negative NGU. That is, *H. vaginalis* is recovered more often and in higher quantity from women with NSV than from those with other forms of vaginitis or from normal women, and improvement of clinical signs of NSV correlates with eradication of *H. vaginalis*. It is clear that *H. vaginalis* is frequently present in vaginal secretions of asymptomatic women who may or may not have signs of an increased malodorous vaginal discharge. The factors responsible for the presence or absence of symptoms in women infected by *H. vaginalis* require further study. Evidence for sexual transmission of *H. vaginalis* is also circumstantial, although recurrence of *H. vaginalis*–associated NSV after initially successful treatment has been demonstrated after sexual reexposure.

DIAGNOSIS AND TREATMENT In a patient with symptoms and/or signs of abnormal vaginal discharge the diagnosis of NSV can be made with reasonable certainty by the following:

1 Exclusion of *C. albicans, T. vaginalis,* cervicitis, and cervical ectopy.
2 Demonstration of the presence of "clue cells" by microscopic examination of vaginal secretions diluted 1:1 in normal saline (wet-mount examination) (Fig. 113-2). Clue cells are vaginal epithelial cells coated with coccobaccillary forms of *H. vaginalis,* to the extent that the borders of the cells are completely obscured. Several media are available for isolation of *H. vaginalis;* the addition of colistin and nalidixic acid selectively inhibits other organisms, and addition of 5 percent human blood permits rapid detection of beta-hemolytic colonies of *H. vaginalis* on primary isolation.
3 Liberation of an amine-like fishy odor immediately after mixing vaginal secretion with 10% KOH (for microscopic identification of yeasts). Vaginal secretions in NSV contain several amines, including putrescine, cadaverine, methylamine, isobutylamine, histamine, tyramine, and phenethylamine. Amines are not produced by *H. vaginalis* per se. They may also be released from vaginal secretions from women with *T. vaginalis* infection when KOH is added, but not from secretions from women with *Candida* vaginitis or from normal women.
4 Demonstration of pH of vaginal secretions greater than 4.5. The elevated pH may be partly due to the presence of amines.

Treatment of *H. vaginalis*–associated NSV generally has been frustrating. Sulfonamide-containing vaginal creams are ineffective, perhaps because sulfonamides are uniformly inactive against *H. vaginalis* in vitro. Tetracycline therapy is also usually ineffective, partly because many strains of *H. vaginalis* are resistant to tetracyclines in vitro. Ampicillin, 500 mg four times daily for 7 days, has been effective in 33 to 100 percent of cases of NSV. The most consistently effective therapy consists of metronidazole 500 mg twice daily for 7 days, which eradicated *H. vaginalis* and cleared symptoms in 80 of 81 women with NSV. The efficacy of this regimen, which is not approved for use for NSV in the United States, should be weighed against its potential toxicity. Asymptomatic urethral colonization of *H. vaginalis* is demonstrable in most male sex partners of women with NSV and may contribute to reinfection of the female. The need for treatment of male partners of women with NSV and the efficacy of various antimicrobials in men require further study.

Candidal vaginitis *Candida albicans* and *Torulopsis glabrata* were detected in 21 and 4 percent of female STD clinic patients, respectively. Other yeasts were rare. Pruritus and vulvovaginitis were more common among those with *C. albicans* than among those with *T. glabrata*. Other species found with varying frequency in the vagina include *C. tropicalis, C. stellatoidea, C. krusei, C. parakrusei, C. pseudotropicalis, C. parapsilosis,* and *C. guillermondi*. These other species are generally not associated with vaginitis. Sexual transmission from the male and spread of infection from the anus may account for vaginal yeast infection or for reinfection of the vagina following therapy.

DIAGNOSIS AND THERAPY The diagnosis of *Candida* vaginitis involves demonstration of yeast by microscopic examination of vaginal secretions in saline or 10% KOH, or by Gram's stain. Demonstration of hyphae or pseudohyphae strengthens the diagnosis of *C. albicans* vaginitis. Microscopic examination is less sensitive than culture. The pH of vaginal secretions is less than 4.5 in yeast vaginitis, and the vaginal odor is normal. Vulvitis often accompanies vaginitis and may result in excoriations which must be differentiated from HSV infection. Most clinicians recommend therapy for *C. albicans* vaginal infection only if the patient is symptomatic.

Therapy of yeast vaginitis involves the use of the polyene antifungal agent, nystatin, or one of the imidazoles, clotrimazole or miconazole. Many trials suggest that the imidazoles are more effective than the polyenes. Imidazoles have the apparent additional advantage of requiring only once nightly vaginal application, as opposed to twice daily application currently recommended for nystatin, but imidazoles have the disadvantage of costing more. The recommended duration of therapy for clinical as well as mycologic cure is 7 days for both mycostatin and the imidazoles. The need for simultaneous oral therapy to attempt to eradicate gut infections and for treatment of the male sex partner has not been determined.

MUCOPURULENT CERVICITIS Cervicitis may accompany vaginitis due to *C. albicans* or *T. vaginalis*. Cervicitis without vaginitis can be caused by *N. gonorrhoeae, C. trachomatis,* or herpes simplex virus. *Neisseria gonorrhoeae* and *C. trachomatis* both produce endocervicitis, with mucopurulent exudate emanating from the cervical os.

Mucopurulent cervicitis requires antimicrobial therapy, and nongonococcal endocervicitis should probably be regarded as being caused by *C. trachomatis* unless infection by that agent can be specifically excluded by culture. The diagnosis of gonococcal cervicitis is made by Gram's stain and culture. If a specimen is properly collected from the endocervical os, after first wiping the cervix clean to remove vaginal flora, then the sensitivity of the Gram's stain showing intracellular gramnegative diplococci, in comparison with culture is about 60 percent, and the specificity approaches 100 percent. The sensi-

tivity of a single endocervical culture is estimated to be 80 to 90 percent.

Chlamydia trachomatis infection of the cervix can be demonstrated reliably only by isolation of the organisms in tissue cell culture, since direct stains and even immunofluorescent stains of exfoliated cervical cells are insensitive. If tissue cell isolate capabilities are lacking, and cultures for *N. gonorrhoeae* are negative, consideration should be given to tetracycline therapy for nongonococcal mucopurulent cervicitis, as is recommended for nongonococcal urethritis in men. The recommended regimen consists of 1 to 2 g tetracycline hydrochloride orally for 1 to 3 weeks. For pregnant women, comparable doses of erythromycin base can be used.

Genital herpes simplex virus (HSV) infection produces ulcerative inflammation of the exocervix, as well as of the endocervix. HSV can be isolated from the cervix in 80 percent of women with an initial attack of genital herpes simplex virus infection, and these patients often have *true* ulcerative erosions of the cervix. In contrast, only 5 percent or less of women with recurrent vulvar HSV infection shed HSV from cervical lesions. If laboratory capabilities for isolation of HSV are not available, HSV can be demonstrated by Papanicolaou smear in about 50 percent of women with HSV cervicitis. In the absence of vaginitis, no infectious cause of cervicitis other than *N. gonorrhoeae, C. trachomatis,* and HSV has been identified.

Cervical ectopy True cervicitis must be differentiated from cervical ectopy, which is often mislabeled "cervical erosion." Ectopy represents movement of the one-cell thick columnar endocervical epithelium into an exposed visible position on the cervix, where it appears redder than the 20-cell-thick stratified squamous vaginal epithelium. The cervical os contains clear or slightly cloudy mucous in ectopy, but not mucopus. Colposcopy shows that the epithelium is intact and not eroded. The mechanism by which ectopy occurs is uncertain, but oral contraceptive usage favors its development. Ectopy may cause increased vaginal discharge which may be symptomatic but which does not require therapy. The use of traumatic cauterizing procedures to eliminate ectopy is no longer recommended.

ULCERATIVE LESIONS OF THE GENITALIA Genital skin lesions can be classified as ulcerative or nonulcerative. Patients seen in an STD clinic for nonulcerative genital lesions often have a sexually transmitted infection, such as scabies, genital warts, *Candida* balanoposthitis or vulvitis, and genital molluscum contagiosium, but the differential diagnosis involves a broad spectrum of dermatologic conditions.

The incidence and etiology of ulcerative lesions of the genitalia vary greatly in different areas of the world. In Asia and Africa, genital ulcers are seen as frequently as gonorrhea in some STD clinics, and limited studies suggest chancroid is the commonest form of genital ulceration. In the industrialized Western countries, genital ulcers are considerably less common than urethritis or vaginitis, and genital herpes simplex virus infection is the commonest form of ulceration. Syphilis is less common, chancroid is rare, and lymphogranuloma venereum (LGV) and granuloma inguinale are almost never seen.

Diagnosis and therapy In industrialized countries, the differential diagnosis of genital ulceration, when trauma and excoriated lesions are excluded, usually rests among genital herpes simplex virus infection, syphilis, and, rarely, chancroid. Epidemiologic factors such as acquisition of infection in a developing country or from a prostitute or homosexual contact,

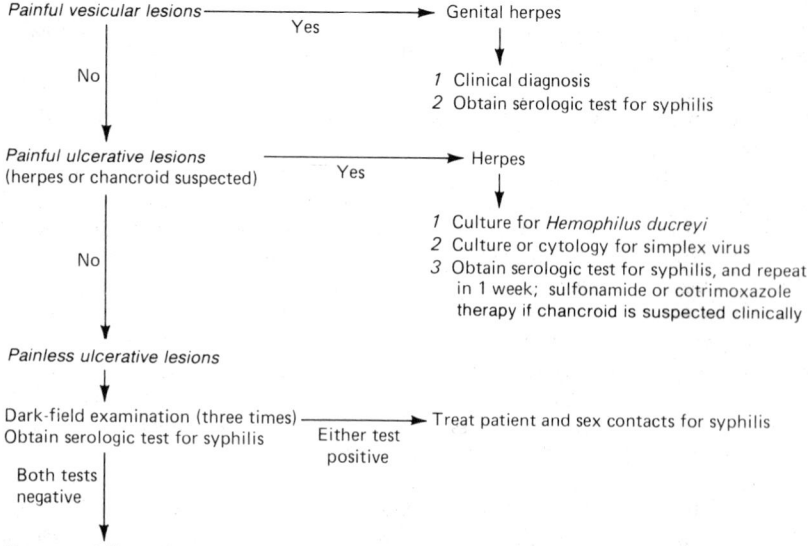

FIGURE 113-3

Management of ulcerative genital lesions.

prostitution, or very low socioeconomic status increase the likelihood of chancroid, LGV, or granuloma inguinale. Although the clinical findings are occasionally diagnostic (e.g., presence of herpetic vesicles) and clinical findings plus epidemiologic considerations help dictate the initial therapy pending further studies, most genital ulcerations cannot be diagnosed on clinical grounds. It is axiomatic to exclude syphilis by appropriate serology in all cases. Dark-field examination should also be performed, by experienced technicians when possible, on lesions suggesting primary or secondary syphilis. Chancroid should not be used as a "wastebasket" diagnosis for all ulcerative lesions not attributable to syphilis or genital herpes, since few such lesions are confirmed as chancroid. Newer selective enrichment media for isolation of *H. ducreyi* should be used for the etiologic evaluation of genital ulcers. However, even when all available diagnostic tests are used by an experienced dermatovenereologist, many ulcerative genital lesions are still classified as idiopathic.

The following general guidelines are recommended for management of ulcerative genital lesions (Fig. 113-3):

1 *If typical painful herpetic vesicopustules are present:* In this case the clinical diagnosis of herpes is warranted, although a reaginic serologic test for syphilis should be performed. The diagnosis can be confirmed by isolation of herpes simplex virus in 90 percent of patients and by cytology (Papanicolaou) smear in about two-thirds.

2 *If painful nonvesicular ulcer(s) raise the suspicion of herpes or chancroid:* If the lesion(s) or inguinal node(s) are painful or have other features suggestive of herpes or chancroid, attempts to demonstrate herpes simplex virus or *H. ducreyi* are indicated. Cytology for demonstrating herpes virus is slightly less sensitive in the ulcerative stage than in the vesicular stage. Syphilis should be excluded by reaginic serologic testing, which should be repeated 1 to 2 weeks later if negative initially and if other diagnoses cannot be confirmed.

Topical antimicrobial therapy is not indicated for ulcerative genital lesions. In settings where genital herpes is much commoner than chancroid, as in the United States, antimicrobial therapy for painful genital ulcers can generally be deferred, pending the results of initial studies. Initial attacks of genital herpes generally begin to improve spontaneously 10 to 14 days after onset, and recurrent episodes 4 to 7 days after onset. The value of antimicrobial therapy for idiopathic ulcerative lesions of the genitalia is uncertain, but a course

of sulfonamide, cotrimoxazole, or tetracycline therapy, as recommended for chancroid (Chap. 126) seems reasonable for lesions of recent onset that persist or progress during several days of observation and that cannot be attributed to herpes, chancroid, or syphilis. Sulfonamides will not interfere with subsequent dark-field examination and should be given promptly for ulcerative lesions considered "typical" of chancroid, especially if regional lymph node suppuration is present or appears imminent.

3 *If painless ulcerative lesions suggest the diagnosis of syphilis:* If lesions are at all suggestive of syphilis, or there are reasons to suspect syphilis, such as recent exposure, then dark-field examination and/or a rapid reagin test should be performed for prompt diagnosis. If these are negative, two more dark-field examinations on successive days are recommended, and a serologic test for syphilis should be repeated 1 week and 6 weeks later.

If patients do not improve or worsen during 1 or 2 weeks of observation and the diagnosis remains obscure, attempts to isolate *H. ducreyi* should be made or repeated, and other infectious (e.g., granuloma inguinale) and noninfectious etiologies should be considered.

REFERENCES

CHAPEL TA et al: How reliable is the morphologic diagnosis of penile ulcerations? Sex Trans Dis 4:150, 1977

ESCHENBACH, DA, HOLMES KK: Acute pelvic inflammatory disease: Current concepts of pathogenesis, etiology and management. Clin Obstet Gynecol 18:35, 1975

HART G: *Chancroid, Donovanosis, Lymphogranuloma Venereum*, US Department of Health, Education, and Welfare Publication (CDC) 75-8302

HOLMES KK, KIVIAT MD: Urethritis, in *Campbell's Urology*, HH Harrison et al (eds). Philadelphia, Saunders, 1978, p 538

KAWAMURA N: Metronidazole and tinidazole in a single large dose for treating urogenital infections with *Trichomonas vaginalis* in men. Br J Vener Dis 54:81, 1978

KOMAROFF AL et al: Management strategies for urinary and vaginal infections. Arch Intern Med 138:1069, 1978

ORIEL JD et al: Genital yeast infections. Br Med J 4:761, 1972

PHEIFER TA et al: Nonspecific vaginitis: Role of *Hemophilus vaginalis* and treatment with metronidazole. N Engl J Med 298:1429, 1978

REES E et al: Chlamydia in relation to cervical infection and pelvic inflammatory disease, in *Nongonococcal Urethritis and Related Infections*, D Hobson, KK Holmes (eds). Washington, DC, American Society of Microbiology, 1977, p 67

PREVENTION OF INFECTION: IMMUNIZATION AND ANTIMICROBIAL PROPHYLAXIS

LAWRENCE COREY
ROBERT G. PETERSDORF

There are three major ways to prevent infections: (1) by reducing exposure, (2) by acquiring or inducing immunity, and (3) by using antimicrobial agents to prevent colonization and infection. Exposure can be reduced by diminishing the prevalence of the infecting agent, by community-wide vaccination programs, and by cohorting of infected patients. On an individual basis, however, the most reliable way to prevent infectious disease is to provide effective immunization and, less commonly, chemoprophylaxis against the causative agent. This chapter summarizes current immunization practices and principles of antimicrobial prophylaxis. Additional details are provided in the chapters dealing with individual diseases.

IMMUNIZATION

Immunity may be defined as the ability of the individual to resist or overcome infection; it may be innate or acquired. For many infectious diseases, immunity is acquired during recovery from an infection or induced by the administration of vaccines prepared from inactivated or live microorganisms of modified disease-producing potential, or from specific antigen(s) derived from these organisms. The purpose of immunization, therefore, is to provoke a specific immunologic response to a selected microbial agent or its antigens with the expectation that this will result in humoral, and/or secretory, and/or cell-mediated immunity. While this protection may diminish over time, future exposures to the same stimulus will result in a rapid return of the immune response because of heightened reactivity of antibody-forming, phagocytic, and other cells that mediate immune mechanisms (Chap. 61).

Certain infectious diseases present special situations that impede the development of vaccines. For example, *Salmonella* organisms and rhinoviruses consist of several hundred antigenically unique strains, making production of a vaccine unfeasible. Secondly, the portal of entry of an organism and the role of local immunity are important in determining whether a vaccine given parenterally will offer protection from either infection or disease. Finally, even when effective immunizing agents are available, difficulties in delivering them to the susceptible population may preclude their use.

GENERAL PRINCIPLES OF IMMUNIZATION
Infections can be prevented or controlled by active and/or passive immunization. Active immunization with live attenuated vaccines generally results in subclinical or mild clinical illness which duplicates, to a limited extent, the disease that is marked for prevention; generally, it provides both local and durable humoral immunity. "Killed" or inactivated vaccines, such as influenza, rabies, typhoid, and cholera vaccines, maintain immunogenicity, without infectivity, but have several disadvantages including the large amount of antigen that must be administered by the parenteral route and the greater time period between administration of the antigen and the appearance of a protective effect. Table 114-1 summarizes active immunizing agents.

The use of any biological substance requires balancing its benefits and risks, and each vaccine must be evaluated accordingly. While some immunizations are recommended for all individuals, for example, diphtheria, tetanus, and poliomyelitis, others should be used only in those who have an increased risk of either acquiring the disease or developing complications. Pneumococcal polysaccharide vaccine, influenza vaccine, bacillus Calmette-Guérin (BCG) vaccine, and meningococcal vaccine are some examples.

Inactivated vaccines can be administered simultaneously at separate sites, although vaccines known to be associated with severe side effects should generally be given on separate occasions. Some vaccines contain trace amounts of preservatives or antibiotics to which patients may be sensitive, and, although reactions to them are unusual, reviewing the manufacturers' package insert prior to use of these agents may be helpful. Live virus vaccines prepared by growing viruses in cell culture are usually devoid of potential allergic substances. Many live virus vaccinations can be given simultaneously; measles, mumps, and rubella are some examples. However, when more than one dose of live viral vaccine is required, repeated administration should be separated by at least 1 month.

Contraindications to vaccination Virus replication following administration of live attenuated virus vaccines can be accentuated in immune deficiency diseases and in patients whose immune responses have been suppressed as in leukemia, lymphoma, or generalized malignancy or following therapy with corticosteroids, alkylating drugs, antimetabolites, and radiation. Such patients should not be given live attenuated virus vaccines. Vaccination of persons with severe febrile disease should be deferred to avoid superimposing the adverse effects of the vaccine on the underlying illness. Occasionally, viral interference, as might occur with concurrent enterovirus infection in the gut, may affect the efficacy of vaccines adversely. Because of a theoretical risk to the developing fetus, live attenuated virus vaccines generally should not be given to pregnant women. For some vaccines, particularly live attenuated rubella vaccine, pregnancy is an absolute contraindication to vaccination. Passively acquired antibody can interfere with the response to live attenuated virus vaccines; therefore, administration of live vaccine should be postponed until approximately 3 months after passive immunization.

IMMUNIZATION IN ADULTS   Diphtheria The myocardial and peripheral nervous system involvement associated with *Corynebacterium diphtheriae* is due to elaboration of an exotoxin (Chap. 133). Diphtheria toxoid is a cell-free preparation of diphtheria toxin treated with formaldehyde. When administered intramuscularly, it produces a specific immune response to the toxin. While detailed controlled studies have not been undertaken, extensive experience in many countries indicates that the use of diphtheria toxoid has been associated with a steady reduction in the incidence of diphtheria. Moreover, although clinical diphtheria occurs occasionally in immunized individuals, the disease appears milder. Diphtheria toxoid provides protection against only the toxin and not the somatic components of *C. diphtheriae,* and local infection, either in the respiratory tract or skin, occurs occasionally in immune individuals. Nontoxigenic strains also may cause mild, focal infections.

All children less than 7 years of age should receive routine immunization against diphtheria in the form of absorbed diphtheria and tetanus toxoids and pertussis vaccine (DPT). Absorbed toxoids are produced by the addition of aluminum compounds to the formaldehyde-inactivated toxoid and are more antigenic than the fluid (plain) preparation. A preparation without pertussis vaccine is available for primary immunization of children who are unable to tolerate the pertussis vac-

TABLE 114-1
Active immunization in adults

	Type of vaccine	Administration and frequency*	Comments
ALL ADULTS			
Tetanus and diphtheria	Adsorbed toxoid	IM at least every 10 years	Usually administered together as Td vaccine
Poliomyelitis	Live attenuated	Oral polio vaccine (OPV)	Preferred for routine use and during epidemics
	Formalin-inactivated	Inactivated polio vaccine (IPV)	Selective use in unimmunized adults
WOMEN OF CHILD-BEARING AGE			
Rubella vaccine	Live attenuated	SC once	Only to women who are antibody (HI) negative and if pregnancy can be prevented for 3 months post-vaccination
POSTPUBERTAL MALES			
Mumps	Live attenuated	SC once	Prevention of orchitis in susceptible seronegative males
PERSONS AT HIGH RISK OF COMPLICATIONS OF DISEASE (CHRONIC HEART AND PULMONARY DISEASE)			
Influenza vaccine	Inactivated	SC yearly	Directed at reducing morbidity and mortality in those at risk of complications of influenza including those over 65 years
Pneumococcal polysaccharide vaccine	Purified dodecavalent polysaccharide vaccine	SC once	Also useful in patients with functional or surgical asplenia, agammaglobulinemia, cirrhosis, multiple myeloma, and nephrotic syndrome
POPULATIONS EXPOSED TO LOCALIZED OUTBREAKS			
Meningococcal vaccine A, C, AC	Purified capsular polysaccharide	SC once	Control of localized epidemics and adjunct to chemoprophylaxis in household contacts
Measles vaccine	Live attenuated	SC once	Control of outbreaks usually among adolescents or young adults
BCG vaccine	Live attenuated	SC or intradermally, once	Use in groups with excessive risk of new infection with tuberculosis or individuals persistently exposed to sputum-positive tuberculosis
Adenovirus vaccine	Live attenuated bivalent (types 4 and 7)	PO once	Only used for military recruits
Typhoid vaccine	Inactivated bacilli	SC in two doses	Household contact of documented *Salmonella typhi* carrier
Rubella vaccine	Live attenuated	SC once	Control of outbreaks among adolescents and young adults (must screen pubertal females with HI test prior to vaccination)
TRAVELERS TO FOREIGN COUNTRIES			
Smallpox	Live vaccinia virus	Intradermally, every 3–5 years	Presently recommended only for travel to endemic areas
Yellow fever	Live attenuated	SC once per 10 years	Administered at yellow fever vaccination centers
Cholera	Phenol-inactivated suspension of *Vibrio cholerae*	SC approximately every 6 months	Only 50% effective and not effective in decreasing transmission of disease
Typhoid	Inactivated bacilli	SC in half doses 4 weeks apart	70–90% efficacy in "normal" exposure
Typhus	Formaldehyde-inactivated *Rickettsia prowazekii*	SC in two doses 4 weeks apart	Only to persons in close contact to those where disease is indigenous
Plague	Formaldehyde-inactivated *Yersinia pestis*	SC in three injections of 0.5 ml at least 1 week apart, booster approximately every 2 years	Agricultural workers who reside in plague-endemic areas
Poliomyelitis	Oral or inactivated polio vaccine	See text	Most adults already immune
Hepatitis A	Immune serum globulin	IM every 3 months	See "Passive Immunization" in this chapter

* *PO, orally; SC, subcutaneously; IM, intramuscularly.*

cine (DT). To avoid the febrile reactions that may accompany repeated exposure to diphtheria toxoid among patients with prior exposure to diphtheria antigens, the preparation recommended for use in adults is a combination of tetanus and diphtheria toxoid in which the diphtheria toxoid is reduced to a maximum of two flocculating units per dose. This vaccine (Td) is recommended for primary immunization of adults and children older than 6 years of age and is also routinely used for booster immunization, both for the prevention of tetanus at the time of injury and for diphtheria prophylaxis.

Tetanus (see also Chap. 139) Tetanus toxoid is a formaldehyde-detoxified bacteria-free filtrate of *Clostridium tetani*. The antibody response to toxoid is often variable. However, two doses of the absorbed toxoid or three doses of fluid toxoid generally result in a protective level of antibody, 0.01 units per milliliter tetanus antitoxin toxoid. Tetanus toxoid may be used singly or in combination with diphtheria toxoid (DT or Td), or with both diphtheria toxoid and pertussis vaccine (DPT). When used singly, primary immunization with the fluid toxoid is given in three doses at least 1 month apart with a booster 8 to 12 months later and then at 10-year intervals. The absorbed form should be given in two doses, 1 month apart.

Poliomyelitis (see also Chap. 187) While routine polio vaccination of adults residing in the United States is generally not necessary because most are immune and the risk of exposure is small, susceptible adults at increased risk by virtue of travel or exposure to wild or vaccine polio virus should receive primary immunization with either inactivated or wild attenuated polio vaccines. Both a live attenuated oral polio vaccine (OPV) and an inactivated polio vaccine (IPV) are licensed in the United States. OPV has been favored over IPV because it is easier to administer, orally versus injection, confers more resistance in the alimentary tract to reinfection, and interferes with simultaneous infection by wild polioviruses. These properties are of special value during epidemics of poliomyelitis. Vaccination with OPV results in shedding of virus contained in the vaccine, and spread of virus to unvaccinated persons occurs. Rarely, recipients of oral vaccine or people in contact with them have contracted paralytic polio. Between 1969 and 1976, 132 cases of paralytic poliomyelitis were reported in the United States; 44 were classified as vaccine-associated. The risk of vaccine-associated polio has been estimated to be one case per recipient for every 11.5 million persons vaccinated with OPV, one case in a household contact for every 3.9 million persons vaccinated, and one case in a community contact for every 22.9 million persons vaccinated. The relative risk of paralytic disease is slightly higher in susceptible adults than in children. Such a risk seems acceptable. On the other hand, no serious complications have been reported with IPV. While oral trivalent polio vaccine is the principal vaccine in the United States, use of inactivated polio vaccine may be beneficial in selective circumstances such as primary immunization of susceptible adults.

For infants and children, the primary series of vaccination with OPV consists of three doses. The first two should be given not less than 6 and preferably 8 weeks apart. The third dose should follow 8 to 12 months after the second dose.

A booster dose of trivalent OPV should be given when the child enters kindergarten or first grade. Additional preadolescent immunization (at age 11 to 12) has been recommended by an expert committee of the National Academy of Sciences to provide additional protection during adulthood. The rationale for this recommendation is twofold: (1) vaccine-associated paralytic disease is rare under age 20; and (2) most vaccine-associated cases have occured in young adults following contact with vaccinated infants.

Inactivated polio vaccine should be considered for persons with heightened susceptibility to infection, including immunodeficient children and their siblings, and immunosuppressed persons and adults undergoing initial vaccination when traveling to areas where the incidence of polio is high or whose household contacts are undergoing OPV vaccination. Live attenuated oral polio vaccine is acceptable for adults who have been vaccinated previously or whose circumstances do not allow adequate time for administration of IVP and who are not in a category in which oral vaccine is contraindicated. Primary immunization with IPV consists of four doses: three at 1- to 2-month intervals and a booster 6 to 12 months after the third. Booster doses at 2- to 3-year intervals either with IPV or with one dose of OPV after primary immunization with IPV will sustain long-lasting immunity.

IMMUNIZATION IN WOMEN OF CHILDBEARING AGE Rubella (see also Chap. 182) The purpose of rubella vaccination is to prevent rubella embryopathy in the fetus. The direct approach to this goal would be to immunize all women before they become pregnant. However, the difficulty is being sure that a woman is not pregnant at the time of vaccination, and the increased risk of joint symptoms associated with vaccination in women has rendered this approach impractical. Because children are a major source of spread of rubella to pregnant famales, rubella vaccination has been routinely recommended for all children older than 12 months. When given in combination with measles antigen, rubella vaccine should be administered when a child is about 15 months of age to achieve the maximum rate of measles seroconversion.

Since 1969 when rubella vaccine was first licensed, the incidence of rubella has declined steadily, and the lack of a rubella epidemic during the early 1970s suggests that the vaccine is effective in interrupting the 7- to 9-year epidemiologic cycle that has characterized nationwide rubella outbreaks. However, the congenital rubella syndrome still occurs in the United States, and increased emphasis should be placed on vaccinating unimmunized prepubertal girls and susceptible adolescent and adult women who are not pregnant and who agree to prevent pregnancy for 3 months after receiving vaccine. In addition, testing for rubella antibody by hemagglutination inhibition during the perinatal or antepartum period, and vaccination of susceptible women in the immediate postpartum period, are warranted. Routine premarital rubella antibody determinations by either hemagglutination inhibition or enzyme-linked immunoabsorbent assay would enhance effects to identify susceptible females before their first pregnancy. Rubella immunization of medical personnel having frequent contact with pregnant women is also advisable.

Rubella vaccine is prepared in cell cultures and is administered by subcutaneous injection. A single dose induces antibodies in approximately 95 percent of susceptible persons.

Rubella vaccine virus has been demonstrated to cross the placenta and infect the fetus. Infants born to more than 60 susceptible women, who inadvertently received rubella vaccine during early pregnancy and continued their pregnancies to term, did not have any recognizable malformations attributable to rubella. However, fetal infection with vaccine-like rubella virus may produce pathological changes in developing organs. While the risk of teratogenicity is felt to be much lower from the vaccine virus than from the wild virus, if a pregnant woman is inadvertently vaccinated or if she becomes pregnant within 3 months of vaccination, she should be advised of the theoretical risk to the fetus.

VACCINATION OF SUSCEPTIBLE POSTPUBERTAL MALES
Mumps (see also Chap. 188) Mumps is a relatively benign disease of childhood with a low case fatality rate. Meningoencephalitis associated with mumps is usually uncomplicated, self-limited, and, therefore, the stimulus for prevention of mumps by vaccination is due to the occurrence of orchitis in postpubertal males. While this has been documented to occur as frequently as 20 percent of the time in epidemic mumps, the incidence of subsequent sterility is low. Both a live attenuated mumps vaccine (Jeryl-Lynn strain) grown in chick embryo cell cultures and a killed vaccine have been developed, but only live mumps vaccine clearly has demonstrated safety and efficacy. Mumps vaccination is recommended for all children older than 1 year and especially in children approaching puberty, adolescents, and adults, particularly males, who have not had mumps or who have no serologic evidence of mumps immunity. A single dose is given subcutaneously; protective antibodies have been shown to persist for at least 8 years after vaccination. Patients with severe febrile illness or hypersensitivity to egg products, with malignancy who are receiving immunosuppressive therapy, or who are pregnant should not be vaccinated.

VACCINATION OF PERSONS WITH CHRONIC HEART, PULMONARY, AND METABOLIC DISEASE **Influenza** (see also Chap. 179) Influenza occurs every year in the United States but with variation in incidence and geographic distribution. Epidemics occur periodically; more are caused by influenza A viruses than by influenza B. More importantly, influenza A epidemics are notable for causing mortality in excess of what is usually expected. In the 1957 to 1958 Asian influenza epidemic, nearly 70,000 excess deaths were reported in the United States during the 12-week epidemic period. Most nationwide influenza epidemics have resulted in 10,000 to 20,000 excess deaths. Repeated observations have indicated that during influenza epidemics deaths occur primarily among children and chronically ill adults, especially those over age 65. These high-risk persons should be vaccinated annually. Vaccination of the entire population has not been considered a reasonable public health policy because protection is of limited duration owing both to the antigenic drift of the virus, as well as the short-lived antibody response to the inactivated vaccine, and the low incidence of serious infections in healthy persons.

Influenza vaccines are inactivated products of the prevalent circulating types of influenza virus. The vaccine is usually bivalent and contains an influenza A as well as an influenza B prototype antigen. Two types of vaccines are available, whole virus vaccines and "split-product" or subunit vaccines. Generally, whole virus vaccines are more immunogenic but have a slightly higher reaction rate than split-product vaccines. Studies with both preparations indicate a 60 to 95 percent protection rate, depending upon the population group studied and the relationship between the "epidemic" strain and the vaccine strain. In adults either form of vaccine can be used, but because of the high frequency of febrile reactions, children under 12 should receive two doses of split-product vaccine at approximately 3 to 6-week intervals. Vaccine is generally administered during the fall of the year and is given subcutaneously. While intradermal vaccination may elicit a good humoral antibody response, the clinical efficacy of this route of administration has not been well documented. Because even the zonally centrifuged inactivated influenza vaccines contain trace amounts of egg protein, patients who are allergic to egg or egg protein should not receive this vaccine. Severe adverse reactions to influenza vaccine are uncommon. The relationship between influenza vaccination and the Landry-Guillain-Barré syndrome is discussed in Chap. 179.

While influenza vaccine is the preferred form of prophylaxis, because of its low cost, greater efficacy, and slight toxicity, amantadine hydrochloride has been effective in preventing influenza infection especially during interepidemic intervals. Patients at risk of developing the complications of influenza who failed to receive their annual influenza vaccination should be placed on 100 mg amantadine hydrochloride twice daily during the period in which influenza A virus is identified in the community.

Pneumococcal vaccine (see also Chap. 115) Despite antibiotic therapy, the morbidity and mortality of pneumococcal disease remains a problem. Bacteremic pneumococcal disease appears to be unusually common in persons with sickle-cell anemia, anatomic or functional asplenia, agammaglobulinemia, multiple myeloma, nephrotic syndrome, cirrhosis, alcoholism, diabetes mellitus, and chronic cardiorespiratory disease; in these situations vaccination is generally indicated. Other situations in which pneumococcal vaccine may be of benefit include closed populations in which systemic pneumococcal disease has been identified as an epidemic or endemic problem, or where an antibiotic-resistant strain of pneumococcus has emerged.

The dodecavalent polysaccharide vaccine licensed for use in the United States is composed of purified capsular material extracted separately from the 14 types of pneumococcal organisms in the vaccine. These 14 types, 1 to 4, 6, 8, 12, 14, 19, 23, 25, 51, and 56, are responsible for at least 80 percent of all bacteremic pneumococcal disease in the United States. One dose of vaccine contains 50 μg of each polysaccharide. The majority of adults and most children over 2 years of age respond with development of measurable humoral antibody. Immunity exists only against the pneumococcal types contained in the vaccine, although theoretically there may be some degree of cross-protection among immunologically similar types. The duration of protection is unknown, but elevated antibody levels appear to persist for at least 2 years after immunization. Booster doses do not seem to increase the levels of antibody, and children under 2 develop lower levels of antibody than adults. Vaccination reduces the likelihood of acquiring the pneumococcal types in the vaccine in the nasopharynx. There has been no evidence of a relative increase in disease caused by other microbial pathogens among vaccine recipients. Vaccination has reduced the incidence of pneumococcal pneumonia and bacteremia due to types in the vaccine by 80 percent. Local erythema and pain at the injection site occur in approximately half the recipients, but serious adverse reactions are rare.

VACCINES USEFUL IN LOCALIZED OUTBREAKS **Meningococcal vaccine** (see also Chap. 118) Meningococcal disease is endemic in the United States and throughout the world. In recent years meningococcal disease in civilians has occurred primarily in single isolated cases, usually due to groups B or C or, infrequently, in small localized clusters. Secondary cases occur more frequently in household contacts than in the general population, and appropriate antibiotic prophylaxis has been the principal method of reducing the risk for immediate contacts. Vaccines have been used to curtail recent outbreaks of group A disease in several cities in the Pacific Northwest (Chap. 118) as well as extensive outbreaks in Brazil of groups A and C meningococcal disease. When epidemic meningococcal disease due to groups A or C occurs, the population at risk should be identified and vaccinated. Vaccination also should be considered as an adjunct to antibiotic prophylaxis for household contacts of cases of meningococcal disease. The reason for this is that one-half of the secondary cases in families occurs more than 5 days after the primary case; this is long enough to yield potential benefits from vaccination if antibiotic chemoprophylaxis should not be successful.

Three meningococcal polysaccharide vaccines, monovalent A, monovalent C, and bivalent AC vaccine, are licensed for selective use in the United States. These vaccines are chemically defined antigens consisting of purified capsular polysaccharides and induce specific immunity to the serologic groups. The vaccine is administered parenterally as a single dose. Adverse reactions consist principally of localized erythema lasting 1 to 2 days. The vaccine appears effective in all age groups beyond the first year of life, and there is suggestive evidence of efficacy in children as young as 3 months of age.

Measles (see also Chap. 181) Two categories of live measles vaccine exist: (1) vaccine made from attenuated Edmonston strain and (2) further-attenuated measles vaccine (Schwarz strain) derived from passage of the Edmonston strain in chick cell culture. The further-attenuated vaccines are associated with fewer reactions, can be administered without the concomitant use of gamma globulin, and are the preferable mode of vaccination.

While measles vaccination is highly effective, the number of cases of measles reported in the United States in 1976 and 1977 has increased over that reported in the early 1970s. Much of this increase is due to localized outbreaks among patients 10 to 19 years old, often among populations thought to be highly immunized. It has been suggested that these cases have occurred in children who were vaccinated prior to age 12 months or who received measles vaccine concomitantly with immune serum globulin (ISG). Both of these circumstances may not provide adequate immunity against infection.

Measles vaccination has been recommended for all children older than 12 months. During measles outbreaks, it is recommended that all susceptible children, as well as adolescents and adults at risk, be immunized. Individuals can be defined as susceptible to measles when they lack a certificate of adequate immunization with live measles vaccine at age of at least 12 months or who lack adequate evidence of having had measles. Persons who should not be considered adequately protected and who should be revaccinated include (1) children vaccinated with live vaccine before they were 12 months old (these children should be revaccinated at 15 months of age or older); (2) children who received live vaccine with immune serum globulin, regardless of their age at vaccination; and (3) persons previously vaccinated with killed measles virus vaccine. Repeat vaccination with live measles vaccine poses no increased risk for individuals who have previously had natural measles or who have been vaccinated.

Up to 15 percent of vaccinated children will have fever beginning the sixth day after vaccination and lasting up to 5 days. Local induration and edema at the injection site may occur in persons who previously received killed measles vaccine.

BCG vaccine Efforts to control tuberculosis in the United States are directed toward the early identification and treatment of active cases and preventive therapy with isoniazid. Use of BCG vaccine should be considered for uninfected persons who are exposed repeatedly to infected cases and who cannot or will not obtain or accept treatment. In selected circumstances, where multiple-drug-resistant *Mycobacterium tuberculosis* is the "epidemic" strain, vaccination with BCG may also be useful. In the United States, BCG vaccination should be reserved for persons who are skin test negative to 5 tuberculin units (TU) of tuberculin purified protein derivative (PPD). BCG recipients should have repeat skin tests 2 to 3 months later; if they are negative, vaccination should be repeated. The World Health Organization (WHO) recommends that BCG vaccine be administered by the intradermal route, but vaccine

for percutaneous administration is also available. BCG should not be given to persons with impaired immune responses, and although no harmful effects of BCG on the fetus have been observed, it is best to avoid vaccination during pregnancy.

Adenovirus vaccine The epidemiologic syndrome of epidemic acute respiratory disease due to adenovirus 4 or 7 is almost exclusively a problem of military recruits. While an effective oral attenuated adenovirus vaccine has been manufactured, clinical illness caused by these adenoviruses has not been associated with significant morbidity or mortality in the civilian population, and hence use of this vaccine outside the military is not recommended.

Typhoid vaccine Routine typhoid vaccination is no longer recommended in the United States, but selective immunization is indicated for persons who are household contacts of a documented typhoid carrier. Typhoid vaccine is generally not necessary among persons affected by flooding or other natural disasters or for those utilizing rural summer camps. Typhoid vaccine consists of whole typhoid bacilli that have been killed, concentrated, and preserved by various methods. The vaccine should be given in two doses of 0.5 ml subcutaneously or 0.1 ml intradermally, according to the manufacturers' recommendations. Local reactions such as erythema, induration, and moderate fever for about 24 h are not uncommon. Controlled trials indicate a 70 to 90 percent protection rate, although immunity may be overcome by exposure to high inocula of *Salmonella.*

VACCINATION OF TRAVELERS TO FOREIGN COUNTRIES There are two objectives for immunization of foreign travelers: (1) to satisfy a country's requirements, as modified by international regulations, regarding prevention of the introduction and spread of disease (e.g., smallpox, yellow fever, and cholera), and (2) to protect the traveler.

Smallpox vaccination (see also Chap. 184) The success of the WHO smallpox eradication program, the concomitant decrease of worldwide smallpox, and the low risk of importation of smallpox make the morbidity of smallpox vaccination greater than the risk of exposure to smallpox itself. For this reason, routine use of smallpox vaccine is no longer recommended in the United States. Only travelers going to endemic areas should be vaccinated before departing the United States. The complications and contraindications to vaccination are outlined in Chap. 184.

Yellow fever vaccine Many countries require a current international certificate of vaccination against yellow fever from persons older than 6 months who have been in the countries reporting yellow fever (South America and the African subcontinent) in the preceding 6 days. Because these requirements change and often vary with the length of stay in the country, all travelers to areas where yellow fever is endemic should seek current information from health departments or international airlines before departing. Yellow fever vaccine must be administered at a designated yellow fever center. Vaccination certificates are valid for a period of 10 years, beginning 10 days after vaccination. The only yellow fever vaccine licensed in the United States is a live attenuated vaccine produced in chick embryos which must be administered subcutaneously in 0.5-ml amounts. Fever and malaise occur in 10 percent of recipients, but major reactions such as encephalitis are fortunately very rare. While pregnant females should generally not be vaccinated with live attenuated virus, the risk to the fetus is felt to be small, and pregnant women who must travel to areas where the risk of yellow fever is high should be vaccinated. Yellow fever virus vaccine should not be given to patients with severe underlying diseases such as leukemia or those receiving immunosuppressive therapy.

Cholera (see also Chap. 134) Travelers to the Middle East, Asia, and Africa may require evidence of cholera vaccination. Ideally, travelers to these countries should be vaccinated 1 month prior to their departure. A single primary series or booster dose of vaccine is generally sufficient. The risk of cholera for travelers who use ordinary tourist accommodations is very slight, and currently available cholera vaccines are only about 50 percent effective in reducing the incidence of clinical illness for a period of only 3 to 6 months. They do not prevent transmission of disease.

Typhoid Travelers going to regions where food and water sanitation is poor may wish to receive typhoid vaccine. However, care in selecting food and water is the best protection.

Typhus (see also Chap. 168) Vaccination against typhus is not required by any country as a condition for entry, and typhus has not occurred in American travelers in recent years. Typhus vaccination is, therefore, suggested only for persons who work in close contact with the organisms in the laboratory or who live in or visit areas where the disease actually occurs and who will be in close contact with the population in such areas. Typhus vaccine is prepared from formaldehyde-inactivated *Rickettsia prowazekii* grown in embryonated eggs. This vaccine provides protection only against louse-borne (epidemic) typhus, not against murine or scrub typhus. Two subcutaneous injections of the vaccine 4 or more weeks apart are recommended. Boosters at yearly intervals may be necessary.

Plague (see also Chap. 129) Immunization against *Yersinia pestis* is recommended only for laboratory workers and for individuals such as Peace Corps volunteers or agricultural advisors who reside in plague-enzootic or plague-epidemic rural areas where avoidance of rodents and fleas is difficult. Travelers to countries or areas reporting endemic plague do not need to receive vaccine.

UNUSUAL OCCUPATIONAL EXPOSURES In general, vaccination of personnel such as laboratory or field workers whose vocation or avocation puts them at particular risk of developing an immunizable disease should receive preexposure immunization. For example, laboratory workers involved with rabies, *Y. pestis*, smallpox, *R. prowazekii*, *R. rickettsii*, yellow fever virus, or Venezuelan or Eastern equine encephalitis viruses, anthrax bacillus, or tularemia should be vaccinated against the appropriate agent. Occupational exposure requiring vaccination includes preexposure immunization against rabies for veterinarians, spelunkers, and other animal handlers exposed to potentially rabid dogs, cats, skunks, foxes, and bats; *Yersinia* vaccination for field workers in endemic areas; and anthrax vaccination for industrial workers who process hides, hair, bone meal, and wool of potentially infected animals.

PASSIVE IMMUNIZATION (See Table 114-2) Prophylaxis or therapy of infection can also be accomplished in some instances by passive immunization which involves the administration of preformed antibody obtained from humans or other animals who have been actively immunized. Because animal antiserum can induce a hypersensitivity response in the recipient, antiserums from humans are preferable. The duration of immunity provided by passive immunization is brief. Intracellular virus generally is not affected by antibody, and once infection has been initiated, the role of antibody is limited to resisting the spread of the virus.

Hepatitis A (see also Chap. 302) Immune serum globulin administered before exposure and during the incubation period of hepatitis A is 80 to 90 percent effective in preventing or modifying the disease. The prophylactic effect of ISG is greatest when given early in the incubation period, and the use of ISG more than 2 weeks after exposure or after onset of clinical illness is not indicated. Immune serum globulin is recommended for household contacts of patients with hepatitis A but not for contacts at school, hospital, or work. In institutional settings where periodic epidemics of hepatitis A are common, the administration of ISG to residents and staff may limit the spread of the disease. The dose of ISG for postexposure prophylaxis is 0.02 ml per kilogram of body weight.

The risk of hepatitis A for residents of the United States traveling abroad is small. Travelers to tropical areas or to developing countries who bypass the usual tourist routes should probably be given ISG. In addition, travelers staying in developing countries or in tropical areas longer than 3 months should receive a single injection of ISG, 0.05 ml per kilogram of body weight. This dose should be repeated every 4 to 6 months.

Hepatitis B (see also Chaps. 108 and 302) Much information remains to be acquired before definite recommendations concerning the passive immunization of hepatitis B can be made. Most studies, however, indicate that either ISG-containing antibody to hepatitis B surface antigen (anti-HBs) or hyperimmune globulin containing a high titer of anti-HBs hepatitis B immunoglobulin (HBI) should be given to susceptible health care personnel who are anti-HBs negative and who have been exposed to needle sticks with blood from documented HBsAg-positive donors. Because of its lower cost, ISG may be used in susceptible persons with needle exposures from unknown sources. The role of passive immunization in the prophylaxis of hepatitis B in dialysis units, or among household contacts, requires further definition. HBI has been partially effective in protecting spouses of patients with acute hepatitis B. However, in endemic environments, like dialysis units, or among persons continuously exposed to chronic HBsAg carriers, passive immunization may only delay the incubation period of the disease. Although data concerning prophylaxis of infants born to mothers with HBsAg-positive hepatitis at the time of delivery are insufficient to form firm recommendations, the information available suggests that administration of either HBI or standard ISG-containing anti-HBs appears warranted.

Zoster serum immune globulin (ZIG) Within 72 h after exposure, ZIG may prevent or ameliorate varicella-zoster among immunosuppressed susceptible patients. Indications for the use of ZIG are listed in Chap. 185. A list of regional ZIG consultants may be obtained from the Center for Disease Control, Atlanta, Georgia.

Diphtheria antitoxin (see also Chap. 133) Diphtheria antitoxin may be useful in the prophylaxis of asymptomatic unimmunized household contacts along with (1) chemoprophylaxis with either oral erythromycin or intramuscular benzathine penicillin or (2) immunization with diphtheria toxoid. The risk of diphtheria among household contacts, which was approximately 20 percent before the antibiotic era but is negligible now, versus that of serum sickness from equine antiserum must be weighed before using this product.

TABLE 114-2
Passive immunization

Disease	Preparation	Route and dose*	Comments
Hepatitis A	ISG, human	IM (0.02–0.06 ml/kg)	Household contacts
Hepatitis B	Human, hepatitis B immunoglobulin	IM (0.06 ml/kg; two doses 4 weeks apart)	Prophylaxis of direct parenteral exposure (needle stick) or mucous-membrane contact in susceptibles; both HBIG and ISG with anti-HBs may be useful in preventing nonparenteral transmission of hepatitis B
	ISG, human	IM (0.05 ml/kg; two doses 4 weeks apart)	
Vaccinia immunoglobulin	Human VIG	IM (0.3 ml/kg)	Use in eczema vaccinatum, disseminated vaccinia, vaccinia in pregnancy
Herpes zoster	Human ZIG	IM (1.2 ml/10 kg up to 5 ml)	Prevention and amelioration of varicella in susceptible immunosuppressed patients
Diphtheria	Diphtheria antitoxin, horse	IM or IV (10,000–100,000 units)	Dose dependent on extent of membrane and degree of toxicity; may also be used in unimmunized household contacts
Tetanus	Human tetanus immunoglobulin (TIG)	IM (250 units)	When given with tetanus toxoid, use separate syringes and sites
Rabies	Human rabies immunoglobulin	One-half locally and one-half IM (20 IU/kg)	Used for postexposure prophylaxis with 21-dose primary series and two booster doses of duck embryo rabies vaccine
	Equine antirabies globulin	One-half locally and one-half IM (40 IU/kg)	Same as above
Pertussis	Pertussis immunoglobulin, human	IM (1.5 ml, repeat in 5–7 days)	No studies suggest efficacy in susceptible infants
Measles	ISG, human	IM (0.05–0.1 ml/kg)	Susceptible household contacts less than 1 year old, exposed susceptible pregnant females, or immunodeficient persons
Rubella	ISG, human	IM (20–30 ml)	Exposed susceptible pregnant females who will not consider termination
Botulism (Chap. 140)	Horse serum, trivalent AB	One-half IM and one-half IV (8–32 ml)	Use only therapeutically: greatest efficacy in type E
Snake bite (Chap. 215)	Polyvalent crotaline antivenom (pit vipers)	IV (dose function of severity of bite)	See Chap. 215
Spider bite (Chap. 215)	Equine	IM (2.5 ml)	*Latrodectus* (black widow spider) poisoning

* IM, intramuscularly; IV, intravenously.

Tetanus immune globulin (TIG) (see also Chap. 139) The product of choice when contaminated wounds are present in persons whose history of previous tetanus immunization is uncertain or inadequate is TIG. The current recommended prophylactic dose of TIG is 250 to 1000 units given intramuscularly.

Rabies (see also Chap. 189) Postexposure prophylaxis for rabies consists of both passive and active immunization. Although more expensive, human rabies immune globulin is the preferred immunizing agent. The dose is 20 IU per kilogram of body weight given half intramuscularly and half intravenously.

Pertussis (see also Chap. 125) Hyperimmune pertussis globulin does not appear effective in preventing disease among unvaccinated susceptible neonates.

Measles (see also Chap. 181) Immune serum globulin should not be used to control measles outbreaks. Live measles vaccination can usually prevent development of disease if administered within 2 days of exposure. Immune serum globulin should be reserved for susceptible household contacts of measles patients, particularly for those under 1 year of age, exposed pregnant females, or for persons in whom measles vaccine is contraindicated, such as immune deficient hosts. The usual dose is 10 to 20 ml intramuscularly.

Rubella (see also Chap. 182) After exposure to rubella, ISG will not prevent infection or viremia with rubella virus but may modify or suppress symptoms. The routine use of ISG for postexposure prophylaxis of rubella in early pregnancy is not recommended, and infants with congenital rubella have been born to women who were given ISG shortly after exposure.

CHEMOPROPHYLAXIS OF INFECTION

USE OF A SINGLE DRUG Antibiotics have been used prophylactically to (1) prevent the acquisition of an exogenous organism, (2) prevent a resident organism from infecting a normally sterile site, and (3) prevent a dormant pathogenic organism from causing disease. In general, antimicrobial prophylaxis with a single drug, administered over a moderate period of time and directed at a single pathogen, has been successful. Examples of this type of prophylaxis employing low doses of "narrow-spectrum" antimicrobials include the prevention of recurrent episodes of rheumatic fever secondary to group A streptococcal disease with benzathine penicillin, of malaria with chloroquine, and of influenza A with amantadine. Table 114-3 lists some clinical situations where prolonged chemoprophylaxis either to prevent exposure to an exogenous organism or to reactivate a dormant organism in a uniquely susceptible host has been useful.

There are also situations in which the short-term use of antibiotics may prevent bacteremia, as in prophylaxis of bacterial endocarditis in individuals with acquired or congenital heart disease, or may abort localized mucosal infections. Here the use of antibiotics is based on the rationale that brief, low-dose exposure to an antimicrobial, early in the disease before

TABLE 114-3
Drugs that may be administered prophylactically for prolonged exposure or for extended periods of time

Disease/organism	Drug
Group A streptococcus (rheumatic fever)	Penicillin G, sulfonamide
Influenza A infection*	Amantadine
Malaria	Chloroquine
Tuberculosis contacts	Isoniazid
*Pneumocystis carinii** in cancer patients receiving cytotoxic agents	Trimethoprim-sulfamethoxazole
Recurrent urinary tract infection in females	Trimethoprim-sulfamethoxazole, nitrofurantoin

* May require only short courses.

bacterial multiplication has led to established infection, may prevent full-blown disease. Some examples of short-term prophylaxis are given in Table 114–4.

ANTIBIOTIC PROPHYLAXIS IN SURGERY Controlled evaluations of short courses of prophylactic antimicrobials have indicated that the selective use of antibiotics, particularly in operative procedures involving potentially contaminated surgical sites, will lower the rate of postoperative infections. The following principles should be applied in using antimicrobial prophylaxis in surgery (Table 114-5): (1) there must be a high prevalence of postoperative infections that are potentially severe before employing antimicrobial drugs; (2) the prophylactic antimicrobial must be effective against the most frequent postoperative pathogens; (3) the drug should be administered from immediately before and during the operation, and for only a short period thereafter; and (4) where possible, prophylaxis should be carried out with a single drug. This topic is also discussed in Chap. 118. For choice of the appropriate agent, Chap. 111 should be consulted.

TABLE 114-4
Short-term antimicrobial prophylaxis

Disease	Antibiotic
USUALLY EFFECTIVE	
Subacute bacterial endocarditis:	
Streptococcus viridans	Penicillin V, procaine penicillin G plus streptomycin
Enterococcus	Ampicillin or penicillin G plus gentamicin or streptomycin
Neisseria gonorrheae (ophthalmia)	Penicillin, silver nitrate
Neisseria gonorrheae (genital infection)	Tetracycline
Nongonococcal urethritis	Tetracycline
Congenital or incubating syphilis	Penicillin
Toxigenic *Escherichia coli* ("tourista")	Tetracycline
Enteropathogenic *E. coli* diarrhea	Neomycin or kanamycin
Neisseria meningitidis	Sulfonamides (sensitive strains only), rifampin, minocycline
Corynebacterium diphtheriae	Erythromycin, clindamycin, penicillin
SOMETIMES EFFECTIVE	
Shigellosis	Ampicillin, neomycin
Chronic bronchitis*	Ampicillin, tetracycline
Short-term urethral catheterization (<24 h)	Ampicillin, tetracycline, nitrofurantoin, trimethoprim-sulfamethoxazole

* Prophylaxis may require prolonged administration.

TABLE 114-5
Systemic antimicrobial prophylaxis in surgery

PROPHYLAXIS INDICATED

Obstetric-gynecologic surgery:
   Vaginal and abdominal hysterectomy
   Caesarean section after prolonged rupture of membranes
Colorectal surgery
Cardiac surgery
Valvular, noncardiac thoracic surgery
Orthopedic surgery (joint replacement, prosthesis, compound fractures)
Peripheral artery surgery with graft replacement
Contaminated surgical wounds

PROPHYLAXIS OF UNCERTAIN VALUE

Gastroduodenal surgery
Biliary tract surgery
Microsurgical craniotomy
Extensive ear, nose, or throat surgery

PROPHYLAXIS UNLIKELY TO BE OF VALUE

Clean abdominal surgery
Gynecologic surgery (other than mentioned above)
Coronary artery bypass surgery
Prophylaxis of wound infections

ANTIBIOTICS IN SUSCEPTIBLE HOSTS In contrast to short-term antimicrobial prophylaxis with a single drug which, while at times not effective, is unlikely to be deleterious, attempts to prevent infection with multiple drugs administered in high doses for relatively prolonged periods are much more likely to be harmful. Adverse effects of "prolonged" antimicrobial prophylaxis include (1) superinfection (defined as an infection with a resistant organism that has developed during antibiotic therapy), (2) increased incidence of toxic or allergic reactions to drugs, (3) increased cost, and last but not least, (4) a sense of false security on the part of many physicians, resulting in less stringent observation of the patient. However, many of the patients who are given antibiotics prophylactically are precisely the ones who are susceptible to complicating infections, and particular care must be taken to watch assiduously for the development of infection and to treat it promptly when it occurs. Such policy is often superior to the use of antimicrobial prophylaxis.

Prophylactic antibiotics have not been useful in preventing bacterial complications of antecedent viral respiratory illness such as influenza or in preventing colonization of pathogenic organisms in intensive care units. Indeed, in these and many other clinical situations the risk of superinfection with resistant, difficult-to-treat organisms outweighs the unlikely effectiveness of prophylactic antibiotics (Table 114-6).

There are a number of situations in which the use of antimicrobial prophylaxis remains controversial but where these drugs seem to have decreased the frequency of overt infection. One of these is patients with severe neutropenia—less than 200

TABLE 114-6
Antibiotic prophylaxis in susceptible hosts in whom its use is not indicated

OUTPATIENT USE

Viral respiratory disease
Viral exanthems
Preventing acute exacerbations of asthma

HOSPITALIZED PATIENTS

Preventing pneumonia in comatose patients
Preventing tracheal colonization with pathogenic organisms
Preventing infections in patients with congestive heart failure
Prolonged urethral catheterization (>24 h)
Prolonged intravenous catheterization (>48 h)
High-dose steroid therapy
Prematurity
Shock

white blood cells per cubic millimeter in whom fever is often suppressed as long as the patient is receiving antibiotics (Chaps. 107 and 220). The use of antibiotics in burn patients presents the enigma of prophylaxis versus therapy. Most of these patients receive topical antibiotics from the outset and for this and other reasons may have a lower incidence of infection. A textbook of surgery should be consulted for a more detailed treatment of this subject.

REFERENCES

AMMAN AJ et al: Polyvalent pneumococcal polysaccharide immunization of patients with sickle-cell anemia and patients with splenectomy. N Engl J Med 297:897, 1977

BARRETT-CONNER E: Chemoprophylaxis of malaria for travelers. Ann Intern Med 81:219, 1974

GLASSO GJ et al: Overview of clinical trials of influenza vaccines 1976. J Infect Dis S136:S4-25, 1977

KRUGMAN S: Effect of human immune serum globulin on infectivity of hepatitis A virus. J Infect Dis 134:70, 1976

MAYNARD JE et al: Passive immunization against hepatitis B. A review of recent studies and comment on current aspects of control. Am J Epidemiol 107:77, 1978

MODLIN JF et al: Risk of congenital abnormality after inadvertent rubella vaccination of pregnant women. N Engl J Med 294:972, 1976

NIGHTINGALE EO: Recommendations for a national policy on poliomyelitis vaccination. N Engl J Med 297:249, 1977

PELTOLA H et al: Clinical efficacy of meningococcus Group A capsular polysaccharide vaccine in children 3 months to 5 years of age. N Engl J Med 297:686, 1977

RUBEN FL: Antitoxin responses in the elderly to tetanus-diphtheria (Td) immunization. Am J Epidemiol 108:145, 1978

SHASBY DM et al: Epidemic measles in a highly vaccinated population. N Engl J Med 296:585, 1977

section 2 | Infections caused by gram-positive cocci

115
PNEUMOCOCCAL INFECTIONS

ROBERT AUSTRIAN

ETIOLOGY

The pneumococcus *(Streptococcus pneumoniae)* is a gram-positive encapsulated coccus that usually grows in pairs or short chains. In the diplococcal form, the adjacent margins are rounded and the opposite ends slightly pointed, giving the organisms a lancet shape. In stained preparations of exudate, gram-negative forms are sometimes present. Pneumococcal colonies are surrounded by greenish discoloration on or in blood agar and are confused at times with other alpha-hemolytic streptococci to which they are closely related. Their isolation from respiratory secretions may be facilitated by inclusion of 5 μg gentamicin per milliliter in the medium. Pneumococci can be distinguished by their bile solubility and mouse virulence or by serologic typing. Another method, utilizing inhibition of pneumococci by Optochin-impregnated paper disks, is less cumbersome and very effective, but standard zones of inhibition determined for aerobic cultures cannot be applied to cultures grown in 5% carbon dioxide for the presumptive identification of pneumococcus.

The capsular substances are complex polysaccharides and are the basis for dividing pneumococci into serotypes. Organisms exposed to type-specific antiserum show a positive capsular precipitin reaction, the *Neufeld quellung reaction;* by this means, 84 serotypes have been identified. All are pathogenic for human beings, but types 1, 3, 4, 7, 8, and 12 are encountered most frequently in clinical practice. Types 6, 14, 19, and 23 often cause pneumonia and otitis media in children but are less common in adults.

Specific typing of pneumococci remains of great clinical importance if pneumococcus is to be identified with regularity, but it has largely been abandoned since the introduction of sulfonamides and antibiotics, which are effective against pneumococci of all types. Recognition of pneumococcus has decreased significantly since the abandonment of capsular typing by most clinical laboratories. The detection of pneumococcal capsular polysaccharides in sputum and in other body fluids by counterimmunoelectrophoresis provides an alternative to bacteriologic techniques for the presumptive diagnosis of pneumococcal infection. Because of cross reactions between the polysaccharides of pneumococci and of other bacterial species, immunologic diagnosis is somewhat less specific than bacteriologic diagnosis.

PATHOGENESIS

The mechanism by which pneumococci damage the mammalian host is obscure. It is conceivable that toxic substances may be elaborated, but no such toxin has been shown to play a major pathogenic role in pneumococcal infection. The capsular polysaccharides, though nontoxic, are known to be necessary factors in virulence and to protect the organism to a certain extent from engulfment by phagocytes.

Although "pneumococcal pharyngitis" is a doubtful entity, invasion of the tissue of the nasopharynx may occur in the infant and occasionally in the nonimmune adult and be followed by spread to the circulation via the cervical lymphatics. At times, secondary infection of serous cavities in the absence of demonstrable focal infection of the upper or lower respiratory tract may occur. The organisms multiply readily in vivo and may produce acute inflammation of the lungs, serous cavities, and endocardium.

The normal human respiratory tract is provided with a variety of mechanisms which act to guard the lungs from infection. The lower respiratory tract is protected by the glottis and larynx, and material passing these barriers stimulates the expulsive cough reflex. Removal of small particles impinging on the walls of the trachea and bronchi is facilitated by their mucociliary lining; and growth of bacteria reaching normal alveoli is inhibited by their relative dryness and by the phagocytic activity of alveolar macrophages. Any anatomic or physiologic derangement of these coordinated defenses tends to augment the susceptibility of the lungs to infection. Anesthesia, alcoholic intoxication, convulsions, and disturbed innervation of the larynx depress the cough reflex and may permit aspiration of infected material. Alterations in the tracheobronchial tree leading to anatomic changes in the epithelial lining or to localized obstruction increase the vulnerability of the lungs to infection. Pulmonary edema, local or generalized, resulting from viral infection, inhalation of irritant gases, cardiac failure, or contusion of the chest wall, provides a fluid menstruum in the alveoli for the growth of bacteria and their spread to adjacent areas of the lung. Viral infection of the respiratory epithelium with concomitant disruption of its component cells interferes significantly with the clearance of bacteria from the lungs, an observation in accord with the high incidence of pneumococcal pneumonia during epidemics of viral influenza and its frequent clinical association with sporadic viral respiratory infections.

Pneumonia begins usually in the right lower, right middle, or left lower lobe, those areas to which gravity is most likely to carry upper respiratory secretions aspirated during sleep. Bronchial embolization with infected mucinous secretions during the course of an upper respiratory infection appears to be the initiating factor in many cases of pneumococcal pneumonia. Protected initially from phagocytosis by mucinous material, the bacteria multiply and, in infected alveoli, evoke the outpouring of proteinaceous fluid, which serves both as a nutrient and as a vehicle for spread to adjacent alveoli. Soon thereafter, polymorphonuclear leukocytes migrate from the pulmonary capillaries to phagocytize a part of the pneumococcal population before the appearance of detectable antibody. Delay in the polymorphonuclear leukocytic response occurs during alcoholic intoxication and certain forms of anesthesia, permitting spread of infection. Adrenocortical steroids and their congeners may also interfere with leukocyte migration. Later, as the pneumonic lesion evolves, macrophages appear in the exudate and remove the debris of fibrin and cells. It is probable that antibody to the capsular polysaccharide of the invading pneumococcus makes its appearance locally in the lung before being detectable in the circulation. Such antibody increases the efficiency of phagocytosis approximately twofold and causes agglutination of the organisms and their adherence to alveolar walls, thereby slowing their dissemination in the lung. The outcome of infection depends, therefore, on the rate at which bacteria can multiply in the edema fluid and spread, and on the host's ability to immobilize and destroy them by phagocytosis. Individuals with hypogammaglobulinemia and patients with multiple myeloma incapable of producing anticapsular antibody are liable to recurrent attacks of pneumococcal pneumonia. Repeated infection with the same pneumococcal type should always prompt a search for dysgammaglobulinemia.

Failure of local defense mechanisms in the lung results in lymphatic spread of pneumococci to the hilar lymph nodes. In the sinusoids of these organs, a sequence of events not unlike that in the lung ensues. If infection is not checked in this secondary line of defense, organisms find their way into the thoracic duct and then into the circulation. Although transient bacteremia may occur at the onset of many cases of pneumococcal pneumonia, it is detectable in only 25 to 30 percent of cases. Bacteremia, which reflects the body's inability to localize the pulmonary infection, is a poor prognostic sign and carries with it the danger of metastatic infection. The mortality of treated or untreated bacteremic pneumococcal pneumonia is four times that resulting from comparably managed nonbacteremic infections. Metastatic infection secondary to bacteremia may occur in the meninges, joints, or peritoneum or on the endocardium. Direct spread from the infected lung may give rise to pleural empyema or to pericarditis.

Natural recovery from pneumococcal infection coincides usually, but not invariably, with the appearance of detectable type-specific antibody in the circulation and is often accompanied by a dramatic and abrupt fall in temperature, the so-called "crisis." Antibody aids recovery by increasing the efficiency of phagocytosis and by limiting dissemination of the organisms. Bacteriostatic drugs, such as sulfonamides, facilitate control of the infection by limiting the size of the pneumococcal population, but the host's defense mechanisms are still required for the elimination of the bacteria. Bactericidal agents, such as penicillin, cause the death of pneumococci in the lung and are effective when some of the host's defense mechanisms are compromised. With the arrest of infection, the alveolar exudate undergoes liquefaction, the inflammatory debris is removed by expectoration and via the lymphatic channels, and the lung is restored to its normal state. Necrosis of pulmonary tissue as a result of pneumococcal infection is distinctly uncommon. Primary pneumococcal lung abscess is a rare clinical entity, although the diagnosis is mistakenly made at times when pneumococcal infection complicates lung abscess of other origins.

In addition to causing pneumonia and its metastatic sequelae, pneumococcus can extend from the nasopharynx to its adjacent structures, giving rise to otitis media, mastoiditis, paranasal sinusitis, or conjunctivitis. Soft-tissue abscesses are rare but may occur.

PNEUMOCOCCAL PNEUMONIA

Pneumococcal pneumonia is a disease remarkable for its uniformity, in contrast to other infections such as typhoid fever and tuberculosis. The diseases produced by different pneumococcal serotypes show little variation in severity or in clinical manifestations. The prognosis in type 3 pneumococcal pneumonia is usually regarded as poor, probably because type 3 infections occur frequently in the aged and in patients with other debilitating diseases, such as diabetes and congestive heart failure. The usual lesion in adults is segmental or lobar in distribution, but in children and the aged, bronchopneumonia, characterized by patchy involvement, is frequent.

MANIFESTATIONS Pneumonia is often preceded for a few days by coryza or some other form of common respiratory disease. The onset is usually so abrupt that patients frequently can state the exact hour that illness began. There is a sudden *shaking chill* in more than 80 percent of the cases and a rapid rise in temperature, with corresponding tachycardia and an increase in respiratory rate (tachypnea). Most patients with pneumococcal pneumonia have a single rigor unless antipyretic drugs are administered, and repeated chills should suggest another etiologic agent.

About 75 percent of patients develop severe *pleuritic pain* and *cough,* productive of pinkish or "rusty" mucoid sputum within a few hours. The chest pain is agonizing, and respirations become rapid, shallow, and grunting as the patient tries to splint the affected side. Many patients are mildly cyanotic as a result of hypoxia caused by V/Q abnormality or shunt, which accompanies altered respiration, and show dilatation of the alae nasi when first seen. Patients appear acutely ill; but nausea, headache, and malaise are not prominent, and most individuals are alert. Pleuritic pain and dyspnea are the dominant complaints.

In the untreated disease, there are sustained fever of 102.5 to 105°F, continued pleuritic pain, cough, and expectoration; and *abdominal distention* is frequent. *Herpes labialis* is a common complication. After 7 to 10 days, there are diaphoresis, abrupt defervescence, and dramatic improvement in well-being, the "crisis."

In cases which terminate fatally, there is usually extensive pulmonary involvement, and dyspnea, cyanosis, and tachycardia are prominent. Circulatory collapse or a picture resembling heart failure is common. Death in a few patients is associated with empyema or some other suppurative complication such as meningitis or endocarditis.

Physical examination reveals restricted motion of the affected hemithorax. Tactile fremitus may be decreased during the initial day of illness but is usually increased when consolidation is fully established. Deviation of the trachea away from the affected lung suggests pleural effusion or empyema. The percussion note is dull, and if the lesion is in an upper lobe, impaired motion of the diaphragm can be detected on the affected side. Very early in the course of infection, breath sounds are diminished, but as the lesion evolves, they become tubular or bronchial in quality, and bronchophony and whispered pectoriloquy can be elicited. These findings are accompanied by fine crepitant rales.

EFFECT OF SPECIFIC CHEMOTHERAPY Pneumococcal pneumonia usually improves promptly when an appropriate antimicrobial drug is given. Within 12 to 36 h after initiation of treatment with penicillin, temperature, pulse, and respiration begin to fall and may reach normal values, pleuritic pain subsides, and the spread of the inflammatory process is halted. The temperature of approximately half the patients, however, requires 4 days or longer to become normal, and failure of the patient's temperature to reach normal in 24 to 48 h should not prompt a change in antibacterial therapy in the absence of other indications.

COMPLICATIONS The typical course of pneumococcal pneumonia can be modified by the development of one or more local or distant complications:

In the lung ATELECTASIS Atelectasis of all or part of a lobe may occur during the active stage of pneumonia or after treatment has been instituted. The patient may complain of sudden recurrence of pleuritic pain and show rapid respirations. Small areas of atelectasis are often detected by x-ray in the absence of symptoms. These areas usually clear with coughing and deep breathing, but bronchoscopic aspiration is occasionally necessary. If atelectasis is allowed to persist, the affected area becomes fibrotic and functionless.

DELAYED RESOLUTION Return to normal of physical findings in the lung after pneumococcal pneumonia is usually complete within 2 to 4 weeks. X-ray evidence of residual pulmonary consolidation, however, may persist as long as 8 weeks, and other radiologic manifestations of the infection (volume loss, stranding and pleural disease) may persist for up to 18 weeks. The process of resolution may require a longer time in those over 50 years of age and in those with chronic obstructive airway disease or alcoholism.

ABSCESS Lung abscess is a rare sequel to pneumococcal infection, although pneumococcal pneumonia is a not uncommon complication of lung abscess of other origins. It is manifested by continued fever and profuse expectoration of purulent sputum. X-ray shows one or more cavities. This complication is exceedingly rare in patients who receive penicillin therapy and is most likely to follow infection with pneumococcus type 3.

In adjacent structures PLEURAL EFFUSION Pleural effusion occurs in about 5 percent of patients with pneumococcal pneumonia, even with specific therapy. The amount of fluid is usually not sufficient to cause obvious displacement of mediastinal structures. Usually the effusion is sterile and is reabsorbed spontaneously within a week or two. Sometimes, however, the effusion is large and requires aspiration.

EMPYEMA Before the introduction of effective chemotherapy, empyema occurred in 5 to 8 percent of patients with pneumococcal pneumonia; it is now observed in less than 1 percent of treated cases. It is manifested by persistent fever or pleuritic pain, together with signs of pleural effusion. In the early stages, the gross appearance of infected fluid may not differ from that of a sterile pleural effusion; later, there is a profuse outpouring of polymorphonuclear leukocytes and fibrin, resulting in an exudate of thick greenish pus containing large clots of fibrin. The quantity of exudate may become large enough to displace mediastinal structures. In neglected cases, this process leads to extensive pleural scarring, with limitation of thoracic movement. Rupture and drainage through the chest wall (*empyema necessitatis*) occurs, but is rare. Metastatic *brain abscess* is an occasional complication of chronic empyema.

PERICARDITIS A particularly serious complication is spread of infection to the pericardial sac. This lesion is characterized by pain in the precordial region, a friction rub synchronous with the heartbeat, and distention of cervical veins, although one or all of these findings may be absent. The possibility of coexisting purulent pericarditis should be considered whenever a very ill patient with pneumonia develops empyema.

Metastatic infections *Arthritis* occurs more often in children than in adults. The affected joint is swollen, red, and painful, with a purulent effusion. It usually subsides promptly with systemic administration of penicillin, although aspiration and intraarticular injection of penicillin may be necessary in adults.

Acute bacterial endocarditis complicates pneumococcal pneumonia in fewer than 0.5 percent of cases. Its manifestations and treatment are discussed below. Meningitis, another complication of pneumococcal pneumonia, is also discussed subsequently.

Paralytic ileus Gaseous abdominal distention is commonly present and in severely ill patients may assume such serious proportions that the term *paralytic ileus* is justified. This complication further impairs respiratory movement by elevation of the diaphragm and constitutes a difficult problem in management. A rarer and more serious gastrointestinal complication is acute gastric dilatation.

Impaired liver function Alterations in hepatic function are common during the course of pneumococcal pneumonia, and mild jaundice is not at all rare. The pathogenesis of the jaundice is not entirely clear, although in some patients it appears to be related to glucose 6-phosphate dehydrogenase deficiency.

LABORATORY FINDINGS *Sputum* should be obtained by the physician in his or her presence before the administration of antimicrobial drugs to ensure its quality. Although re̲____ transtracheal aspiration or lung puncture may be̲____ occasion to establish the cause of pneu̲____ these invasive techniques is not re̲____ attendant, albeit infrequen̲____

Gram's method, the sputum shows polymorphonuclear leukocytes and variable numbers of gram-positive cocci, singly and in pairs. These can be typed directly by the Neufeld quellung or capsular precipitin technique, and this procedure should be followed to facilitate diagnosis whenever possible. The *blood culture* is positive for pneumococci during the first days of untreated illness in 20 to 25 percent of cases. The white blood count usually shows a polymorphonuclear *leukocytosis* ranging from 12,000 to 25,000 cells per cubic millimeter. A normal white count or leukopenia is sometimes observed in patients with overwhelming infection and bacteremia. Occasionally, pneumococci may be seen directly in granulocytes of patients with bacteremia by examining the buffy coat after staining with Wright's stain. These patients often have asplenia. *X-ray of the chest* usually reveals a homogenous density in the affected area of the lung. In well-established cases, the density may occupy one or more entire lobes. Atypical patterns of consolidation may be seen in those with underlying chronic pulmonary disease.

EXTRAPULMONARY PNEUMOCOCCAL INFECTION

PNEUMOCOCCAL MENINGITIS The pneumococcus is second only to the meningococcus as a cause of purulent meningitis in adults; in children, meningitis caused by *Hemophilus influenzae* is also more frequent than pneumococcal infection.

Pneumococcal meningitis can develop as a "primary" disease without preceding signs of infection elsewhere; as a complication of pneumococcal pneumonia; by extension from otitis, mastoiditis, or sinusitis; or following a skull fracture which creates an opening between the subarachnoid space and the nasal cavity or paranasal sinuses. Patients with pneumococcal endocarditis frequently develop meningeal infection. Patients with multiple myeloma and with sickle-cell disease seem to be liable to pneumococcal infection of the meninges, just as they are to pneumonia.

The *manifestations* are of those of any acute pyogenic meningitis (Chap. 368) and include chills, fever, headache, nuchal rigidity, Kernig's and Brudzinski's signs, delirium, and cranial nerve palsies. Evidence of otitis, sinusitis, or pneumonia should be carefully sought by physical and roentgenographic examination in all patients.

The *spinal fluid* is under increased pressure, appears cloudy, often with a greenish tint, and shows a high protein and low glucose content. Stained smears usually reveal gram-positive diplococci and polymorphonuclear leukocytes; in some patients, the number of cells in the spinal fluid is surprisingly small, and much of the cloudiness is produced by the bacterial content. The diagnosis can be established rapidly by identification of pneumococci in the spinal fluid by Gram's stain and by direct typing with the Neufeld quellung reaction.

With appropriate chemotherapy, recovery can be expected in 70 percent of cases; the prognosis is better in children than in ____ or in adults. Relapse may occur but is unusual if ____ ____atment is carried out. Subarachnoid block, the re-____ ____lation of large amounts of thick exudate in the ____ ____nd at the base of the brain, is now an un-

____DITIS Endocarditis is usually a ____meningitis. The clinical picture ____itis (Chap. 243), with remit-____ic infection of the lungs, ____Petechiae are uncom-____ and is particular-

ly likely to occur in the aortic valve. The valvular infection is destructive, and loud murmurs and heart failure develop rapidly. Rupture or perforation of cusps or even rupture of the aorta may occur. The blood culture is consistently positive for the pneumococcus in the absence of treatment with antimicrobial drugs; yet at the same time antibodies to the infecting organism may be demonstrable in the blood, a combination of findings seldom observed except in endocarditis or brucellosis. Although the infection is relatively easy to cure with penicillin, damage to valve leaflets, especially to the cusps of the aortic valve, may be followed by rapidly progressive heart failure. Surgical repair or replacement of damaged valvular structures should be carried out early, before heart failure becomes intractable.

PNEUMOCOCCAL PERITONITIS Pneumococcal peritonitis is a rare disease and is probably the sequela to transient pneumococcal bacteremia, although, because of its somewhat greater frequency in young girls, it has been hypothesized that the organism may gain entry to the peritoneum via the vagina and fallopian tubes. Peritonitis was formerly a common complication of the nephrotic syndrome, particularly in children, but it occurs now with a frequency of approximately 2 percent. In adults, the disease is seen in association with cirrhosis or with carcinoma of the liver. The diagnosis is made by examination of the ascitic fluid; blood cultures are often positive, and a polymorphonuclear leukocytosis is the rule.

TREATMENT

SPECIFIC ANTIMICROBIAL THERAPY Although resistance of pneumococci to antimicrobial drugs has not been regarded as a significant problem in the past, some strains have been found to be resistant to one or the other of the following agents: penicillins, cephalosporins, tetracyclines, chloramphenicol, erythromycin, clindamycin, cotrimoxazole, and aminoglycosides. For this reason sensitivity of the infecting organism to the infecting drug should be determined, particularly in extrapulmonary infection. In the absence of resistance or of hypersensitivity to it, penicillin G (benzyl penicillin) is the drug of choice for all manifestations of pneumococcal infection. Strains of pneumococcus manifesting a modest increase in resistance to penicillin have been recovered infrequently from humans; and although the level of such resistance does not preclude treatment with this antibiotic, awareness of the phenomenon is necessary. The minimum curative dose for *pneumonia* caused by strains of usual sensitivity to penicillin G is less than 60,000 units daily, and a total dose of 600,000 units daily provides a good margin of safety for bacteremic and nonbacteremic pulmonary infection in adults in the absence of an extrapulmonary focus. Treatment may be administered at 12-h intervals in doses of 300,000 units aqueous crystalline penicillin G or procaine penicillin. Therapy should be continued until the patient has been afebrile for 48 to 72 h. The response is usually dramatic, and relapse is extremely uncommon. Pneumococcal pneumonia can be treated adequately with oral penicillin, preferably one of the drugs resistant to gastric acid (Chap. 111), in dosage of 1.2 to 2.4 million units daily. *Peritonitis* usually responds within 36 to 48 h to 2 to 4 million units of penicillin daily.

Pneumococcal *meningitis* should be treated with 12 to 20 million units aqueous penicillin G daily intravenously in adults. In many clinics, even larger amounts are used, though care must be taken to avoid neurotoxicity from excessive dosage. Intrathecal administration of penicillin is not necessary. The addition of sulfadiazine to this regimen affords no advantage, and supplementary administration of chlortetracycline (and presumably, of other broad-spectrum drugs) may exert a deleterious effect. In the presence of sinusitis, otitis, or mastoiditis, surgical drainage should be carried out as soon as is feasible. The response of meningitis is usually less dramatic than that of pneumonia; patients often remain febrile and disoriented, and signs of meningeal irritation may persist for several days, but improvement becomes gradually evident with continued treatment.

Large doses are required in pneumococcal endocarditis also—12 to 20 million units daily by intravenous infusion. Rapidly developing heart failure in these patients and the tendency to form myocardial abscess, however, often lead to a fatal outcome despite large doses of antibiotics. Surgical repair or replacement of damaged heart valves should be considered when cardiac failure develops.

Cephalosporins in parenteral doses of 1 to 2 g daily are effective in pneumococcal pneumonia but must be administered with caution to those hypersensitive to penicillin. These drugs should *not* be used to treat pneumococcal meningitis because of their poor ability to penetrate the blood-cerebrospinal fluid barrier. The *tetracyclines* in doses 1 to 2 g daily, *erythromycin* in doses of 1.6 g daily, or *clindamycin* in doses of 1.2 g daily are effective treatment for pneumococcal pneumonia if it is caused by a sensitive strain, but they are recommended only for patients who have had untoward reactions to penicillins or cephalosporins. Despite its efficacy, *chloramphenicol* should not be used to treat pneumococcal infections other than meningitis in patients hypersensitive to penicillin who are infected with a drug-sensitive strain. For patients with illness caused by multiple drug-resistant pneumococci, *vancomycin* in doses of 2 g daily is the drug of choice. Sulfonamides have little place in the present-day treatment of pneumococcal pneumonia and are useless in endocarditis and meningitis. Aminoglycosides, such as gentamicin, tobramycin, and amikacin, should not be employed to treat pneumococcal infection.

Pneumococcal arthritis responds to systemic penicillin, but aspiration and intraarticular instillation of the drug may be necessary.

Empyema should be detected and treated as early as possible. When an effusion is found, the fluid should be examined for organisms; and if they are present, 50,000 to 200,000 units of penicillin G should be injected intrapleurally. In addition the same antibiotic should be administered systemically in doses of 6 to 8 million units a day. Aspiration of fluid and instillation of penicillin should be carried out at 1- to 2-day intervals until cultures are persistently negative and fever disappears. Fluoroscopic guidance may be needed for aspiration of small empyema pockets. If the exudate is especially thick or viscid, streptokinase-streptodornase (Varidase) may facilitate its withdrawal. When definite improvement is not evident in 4 to 6 days or when the empyema is of long duration, a large-lumen intercostal tube should be placed in the pleural cavity to facilitate drainage. Failure to effect prompt cure of empyema may be followed by pleural fibrosis and necessitate subsequent surgical decortication of the lung to restore pulmonary function.

OTHER MEASURES Oxygen administered through a face mask should be used to treat significant cyanosis, cardiac failure, and delirium. Codeine, 32 to 64 mg every 4 h, will usually control pleuritic pain. When pain is severe, it may require intercostal nerve block with 1 to 2 percent procaine for relief.

PROGNOSIS AND PREVENTION

Although the mortality from pneumococcal pneumonia has diminished significantly since the advent of antimicrobial drugs, available evidence indicates that the incidence of the disease has changed little, if at all. The fatality rate in patients over the age of 12 years with bacteremic pneumococcal pneumonia treated with an antibiotic is 18 percent, and in patients over the age of 50 and in those with underlying systemic illness, it is significantly higher.

Signs of poor prognosis in pneumonia include leukopenia, bacteremia, multilobar involvement, any extrapulmonary focus of pneumococcal infection, presence of preexisting systemic disease, circulatory collapse, and occurrence of the infection in the first year of life or after the age of 55. Infection with pneumococcus type 3 has a higher mortality rate than that caused by other pneumococcal types. Death is most likely to occur in individuals sustaining irreversible physiologic damage early in the course which is unaltered by antimicrobial therapy. Until the nature of the injury produced by pneumococcus is understood and ways devised to repair it, vaccination will remain the only means of protecting those at high risk of a fatal outcome.

A tetradecavalent vaccine containing the capsular polysaccharides of pneumococcal types 1, 2, 3, 4, 6, 8, 9, 12, 14, 19, 23, 25, 51, and 56, which are responsible for 80 percent of bacteremic infections in the United States, is available for prevention of pneumococcal infection caused by these types in individuals at high risk of a fatal outcome. Those at higher than average risk are individuals over the age of 55 and patients with a variety of chronic systemic illnesses including heart disease, chronic bronchopulmonary disease, hepatic disease, renal insufficiency, diabetes, and a variety of malignancies. Persons with sicklaemia of all ages have an increased risk of developing pneumococcal infection, and the vaccine is recommended for those with this disorder over the age of 2 years. Since anatomic or functional asplenia is associated with fulminant overwhelming pneumococcal septicemia with disseminated intravascular coagulation, giving rise to a clinical picture resembling the Waterhouse-Friderichsen syndrome, such individuals should also be immunized. It should be recognized, however, that the vaccine contains a limited number of pneumococcal antigens, and that infection caused by other pneumococcal types may occur occasionally in the immunized subject. Reactions to the vaccine are usually absent or mild, although in the occasional individual they may resemble those following immunization with typhoid vaccine: local pain, erythema, and elevation of temperature. The most severe local and systemic reactions to the vaccine appear to be associated with preexisting high levels of antibody to one or more of the antigens in the vaccine. Because of the persistence of pneumococcal antibodies after a single injection of vaccine, reimmunization in less than 3 years after the initial injection is not recommended. The vaccine is 80 to 90 percent effective in adults. The efficacy of the vaccine in infants and in children under 2 years is currently under investigation, and its efficacy in preventing pneumococcal otitis media, pneumonia, and meningitis in individuals in this age group remains to be determined. Further data are needed to assess the efficacy of pneumococcal vaccine in immunosuppressed individuals.

REFERENCES

AMMANN AJ et al: Polyvalent pneumococcal-polysaccharide immunization of patients with sickle-cell anemia and patients with splenectomy. N Engl J Med 297:897, 1977

APPELBAUM PC et al: Multiple-antibiotic resistance of pneumococci—South Africa. Morb Mort Week Rep 26:285, 1977

AUSTRIAN R: Pneumococcal endocarditis, meningitis and rupture of the aortic valve. Arch Intern Med 99:539, 1957

———, GOLD J: Pneumococcal bacteremia with especial reference to bacteremic pneumococcal pneumonia. Ann Intern Med 60:759, 1964

——— et al: Prevention of pneumococcal pneumonia by vaccination. Trans Assoc Am Phys 89:184, 1976

GOPAL V, BISNO AL: Fulminant pneumococcal infections in "normal" asplenic hosts. Arch Intern Med 137:1526, 1977

HEFFRON R: *Pneumonia with Special Reference to Pneumococcus Lobar Pneumonia.* New York, Commonwealth Fund, 1939

KAUFFMAN CA et al: Purulent pneumococcic pericarditis: Continuing problem in antibiotic era. Am J Med 54:743, 1973

LEACH RP, COONROD JD: Detection of pneumococcal antigens in sputum in pneumococcal pneumonia. Am Rev Respir Dis 116:847, 1977

LEPPER MH, DOWLING HF: Treatment of pneumococcal meningitis with penicillin compared with penicillin plus aureomycin. Arch Intern Med 88:489, 1951

MERRILL CW et al: Rapid identification of pneumococci: Gram stain vs. quellung reaction. N Engl J Med 288:510, 1973

SHULMAN JA et al: Errors and hazards in the diagnosis and treatment of bacterial pneumonias. Ann Intern Med 62:41, 1965

STEPHEN JJ et al: The radiographic resolution of *Streptococcus pneumoniae* pneumonia. N Engl J Med 293:798, 1975

TUGWELL P, WILLIAMS AO: Jaundice associated with lobar pneumonia. Q J Med 46:97, 1977

WOOD WB JR: Studies on the cellular immunology of acute bacterial infections. Harvey Lect 42:72, 1951-1952

ZINNEMAN HW, HALL WH: Recurrent pneumonia in multiple myeloma. Ann Intern Med 41:1152, 1954

116
STAPHYLOCOCCAL INFECTIONS

MARVIN TURCK
WALTER STAMM

INTRODUCTION Staphylococci most commonly produce relatively harmless superficial suppurative infections in human beings. They also produce serious infections of the lungs, pleural space, endocardium, myocardium, long bones, kidneys, and surgical wounds.

The majority of life-threatening staphylococcal infections arise within hospitals, and are among the "diseases of medical progress." Staphylococcal cross infection in hospitals may be less frequent now than it was 10 to 15 years ago, and gram-negative rods are now the most common nosocomial pathogens; nevertheless staphylococci still account for 20 percent of all hospital-acquired infections.

ETIOLOGY Staphylococci are members of the genus *Micrococcus,* which includes many morphologically similar saprophytic microorganisms that do not cause human infection. The parasitic micrococci of primary concern in medicine are grouped in the species *M. pyogenes.* Through established usage these pathogenic micrococci are termed *staphylococci.*

Staphylococci are spherical gram-positive cells. On solid agar media, staphylococcal colonies develop characteristic pigmentation: *M. pyogenes* var. *aureus (Staphylococcus aureus),* golden yellow; *M. pyogenes* var. *albus (S. albus),* ivory white; and *M. citreus,* lemon yellow. Most human infections are caused by *S. aureus,* and a few are caused by *S. albus (S. epidermidis).* The name *staphylococcus* derives from the characteristic grape-like clusters of organisms seen in stained smears prepared from colonies on solid media. In stained smears obtained from pus, smaller clusters, diploids, and short chains resembling streptococci are seen. In such preparations, staphylococci characteristically retain their uniform round shape, in contrast to the boat-like forms assumed by pneumococci. Staphylococci may be seen within the cytoplasm of polymorphonuclear cells in pus, a rare finding in other gram-positive coccal infections. They can be readily differentiated from streptococci by their positive catalase reaction.

Staphylococci that are coagulase-positive and that ferment mannitol are classified as *S. aureus.* Most laboratories label all coagulase-negative strains as *S. epidermidis,* although other micrococci share this characteristic. Other methods to differentiate *S. aureus* from *S. epidermidis* (pigment production, pattern of hemolysis, and antibiotic susceptibility) are unreliable. In general, *S. aureus* strains possess a broader complement of biochemical activity (production of coagulase, hemolysins, and several toxins) than *S. epidermidis.*

Different strains of *S. aureus* can be recognized by the patterns of lysis produced by staphylococcal bacteriophages. Although it is cumbersome, phage typing has allowed more precise strain characterization and is commonly used in studies of intrahospital disease and epidemics of staphylococcal infection. It provides no information that is useful clinically in treating an individual patient. Methods for subtyping *S. epidermidis* (phage lysis and biotyping) have also been developed.

PATHOGENESIS Little is known of the events which allow staphylococci to invade host tissues. Though strains of staphylococci are common skin and mucous membrane inhabitants, an enormous number of bacteria must be used to establish experimental infections in animals or humans, and more than a million organisms are necessary to produce serious infection in most laboratory animals. The inoculum required to produce infection is greatly reduced in the presence of a foreign body. More than 50 percent of serious staphylococcal infections of deep tissues arise from cutaneous foci, and a smaller number originate in the respiratory or genitourinary tract. Direct inoculation of staphylococci into the bloodstream is also an important route of infection in hospitalized patients with intravenous catheters and in drug addicts. The integument and mucous membranes of heroin addicts and insulin-using diabetics appear to have a unique susceptibility to colonization by *S. aureus.*

Staphylococcal disease is more common in patients with *diabetes, liver disease, renal failure,* and severe *debilitation* and/or *malnutrition.* When skin continuity is broken through *abrasions, wounds, insect bites, burns, exfoliative dermatitis,* or *chronic skin diseases,* the areas affected are commonly infected with staphylococci. *Influenza, measles,* and *mucoviscidosis* appear to predispose to primary staphylococcal invasion of the lung. Patients receiving *broad-spectrum antimicrobial therapy* also appear to have a higher incidence of staphylococcal disease.

Staphylococci often invade the integument via hair follicles and sebaceous glands. When skin continuity has been breached, local microbial multiplication is accompanied by inflammation and tissue necrosis at the site of infection. Polymorphonuclear leukocytes rapidly enter the area and ingest large numbers of staphylococci. Thrombosis of surrounding capillaries occurs; fibrin is deposited about the periphery; and, later, fibroblasts create a relatively avascular wall about the area. The fully developed staphylococcal lesion consists of a central core of dead and dying leukocytes and bacteria which gradually liquefies to form characteristic thick, creamy pus, surrounded by a fibroblastic wall.

When host mechanisms fail to contain the cutaneous or subcutaneous infection, staphylococci may enter the bloodstream. Common sites of metastatic seeding are the diaphyseal ends of long bones in children, lungs, kidneys, endocardium, myocardium, liver, spleen, and brain.

Certain biologic properties of staphylococci appear to contribute to pathogenicity. Many *S. aureus* strains elaborate an *exotoxin* (alpha toxin) capable of causing dermal necrosis in animals. Fever, tachycardia, cyanosis, shock, and death ensue when exotoxin is administered to experimental animals, a picture similar to that seen occasionally in certain fulminating cases of staphylococcal bacteremia in human beings. A delta toxin also has been incriminated in the pathogenesis of severe staphylococcal infection. However, the exact role played by both of these toxins remains uncertain. About 40 percent of *S. aureus* lysed by phages in group II produce an exotoxin that causes intraepidermal cleavage and bulla formation.

The high correlation between *coagulase* production and virulence suggests that this substance is important in the pathogenesis of staphylococcal infections. Coagulase has been said to protect staphylococci from phagocytosis by polymorphonuclear leukocytes, to promote abscess formation in humans and in animal species which have coagulable plasmas, or to protect staphylococci from bacteriostatic substances present in normal serum. However, the precise role of coagulase as a determinant of pathogenicity has not been established.

Some *S. aureus* strains produce a *leukocidin* which destroys human and rabbit leukocytes in vitro. Some strains elaborate *hyaluronidase*. Many staphylococci produce an *enterotoxin* which produces nausea, vomiting, and diarrhea in certain experimental animals and in humans.

In vitro and in vivo studies have indicated that pathogenic staphylococci can survive within human leukocytes, whereas nonpathogenic strains do not. Such intracellular survival may be a means of transporting staphylococci and spreading them to distant tissues. This intracellular survival may also account for the relative refractoriness of staphylococcal infection to antibiotic treatment.

Staphylococcus epidermidis strains appear particularly likely to cause infections in the presence of certain foreign bodies: prosthetic heart valves, CSF shunts, and orthopedic prostheses. The unique ability of some *S. epidermidis* strains to adhere to these foreign surfaces seems to at least partly explain this propensity.

IMMUNITY Some degree of resistance to staphylococcal infections develops with age. For example, primary staphylococcal pneumonia is common in infants but rare in adults. Acute staphylococcal osteomyelitis is almost exclusively a disease of children. Both superficial staphylococcal pyoderma and staphylococcal bacteremia are more frequent in infants, while actual abscess formation occurs more often in adults.

Intact polymorphonuclear leukocytes capable of normal chemotaxis, ingestion, and killing appear to be the major protective mechanism against staphylococcal infections. Persons with inherited or acquired defects in any of these leukocyte functions are particularly susceptible to staphylococcal infections (Chap. 56). Coagulase-positive staphylococci have a characteristic cell wall teichoic acid, which may be antiphagocytic. Certain unusual strains possess a definite mucopolysaccharide capsular structure which impedes phagocytosis, and specific opsonizing antibody is required for the ingestion of these unusual strains. A number of antistaphylococcal antibodies have been shown to pass from mother to fetus, and the incidence of a variety of antibodies rapidly rises with age. Virtually 100 percent of adults possess antibodies to several staphylococcal antigens in their serum. Nevertheless, the role of humoral immunity in modifying or protecting against staphylococcal infection is uncertain. Immunization of animals with alpha toxin, toxoids, coagulase, or whole staphylococci may prolong experimental staphylococcal infection, but does not protect against eventual death. There has been no satisfactory demonstration that human staphylococcal disease is followed by immunity or that infection can be modified significantly by vaccination.

EPIDEMIOLOGY *Staphylococcus aureus* transiently colonizes the nasopharynx of 70 to 90 percent of individuals, and resides relatively permanently in the anterior nares of 20 to 30 percent. Nasal carriage often leads to skin colonization as well. Hospital patients and personnel have significantly higher staphylococcal carrier rates than the general population.

While staphylococci remain viable for long periods in dust, blankets, or clothing, and viable staphylococci are often demonstrable in the environment by air-sampling techniques, the significance of airborne transmission remains uncertain, and the best evidence suggests that direct person-to-person contact is the most important means of transmission of staphylococci. Most often, staphylococci are carried from patient to patient on the hands of hospital workers who neglect handwashing. Patients or hospital employees with active staphylococcal infections are probably a more serious source of cross infection than the simple carrier state. However, in some circumstances asymptomatic nasal carriers have been the source of staphylococcal infections. The factors which cause some staphylococcal carriers to become dangerous disseminators remain poorly understood. Discontinuation of the use of hexachlorophene in hospital nurseries has been associated with an increase in infection in some hospitals, and it is apparent that continued surveillance is necessary to thwart the development of epidemics of staphylococcal infection.

Certain phage types of staphylococci have been associated with intrahospital infections. Some strains, particularly antibiotic-resistant strains in phage group III, appear to have greater "epidemic virulence" than other staphylococci. In specific hospitals, one phage type often emerges and may cause most of the serious intrahospital infections. Such "epidemic strains" have shifted from time to time and vary from hospital to hospital. In other hospitals, multiple phage types cause infection. The high incidence of active staphylococcal disease in carriers of certain strains (e.g., the 80/81 strains) suggests that some staphylococci may possess higher virulence for humans than others. Some of the decrease in the frequency of staphylococcal infection in hospitals has been attributed to the disappearance of 80/81 strains.

ANTIMICROBIAL RESISTANCE In the past, the introduction of new antibiotics active against staphylococci has generally been followed by the appearance of staphylococci specifically resistant to that agent. When penicillin was first introduced, fewer than 10 percent of staphylococcal strains isolated from patients or carriers were resistant. Now 60 to 90 percent of staphylococci isolated from hospitalized patients throughout the Western world are resistant to penicillin G, and the incidence of infection due to penicillinase-producing strains in nonhospitalized individuals is almost as high. The prevalence of resistance to a specific antimicrobial has correlated closely with the frequency of its administration, and the emergence of resistant strains has followed the use of most antibiotics. Vancomycin, first employed in 1958, and the penicillinase-resistant penicillins and the cephalosporins, both introduced in the 1960s, have been exceptions to this rule. In general, these agents have retained a high degree of activity against both penicillin-sensitive and penicillin-resistant staphylococci. However, methicillin-resistant strains have become increasingly common in England and France, and in this country, epidemics of methicillin-resistant staphylococci have occurred in several hospitals and burn treatment centers. Gentamicin-resistant staphylococci have also been isolated with greater frequency in recent years.

Most observations on the prevalence of antimicrobial-resistant strains have been made within hospitals where antimicrobial use is heaviest. It has been shown that drug-susceptible strains carried by patients may be replaced by drug-resistant phage group III staphylococci present in the hospital environment during antimicrobial treatment. These strains are in turn acquired by hospital personnel who serve as reservoirs of potentially pathogenic, antimicrobial-resistant strains. Staphylococci isolated from population groups outside the hospital have shown a slower increase in the percentage of antimicrobial-resistant strains, but in some communities the incidence of extrahospital infections caused by penicillin-resistant strains is similar to that found in hospitalized patients.

MANIFESTATIONS Superficial infections Simple infection of hair follicles manifested by a minute erythematous nodule without involvement of the surrounding skin or deeper tissues is termed *folliculitis.* A more extensive and invasive follicular or sebaceous gland infection with some involvement of subcutaneous tissues is termed a *furuncle, or boil.* Itching and mild pain are followed by progressive local swelling and erythema, and the overlying skin becomes exquisitely painful on pressure or motion. Relief of pain occurs promptly after spontaneous or surgical drainage.

Furuncles occur most commonly on the face, neck, axillas, forearms, buttocks, thighs, breast, upper back, and labia. The acne of adolescence is frequently complicated by secondary furunculosis. Staphylococcal infection may involve the sweat glands in the axillas *(hidradenitis suppurativa).* These infections may be deep-seated, slow to localize and drain, and are liable to recurrence and scarring.

Staphylococcal infections within the thick, fibrous, inelastic skin of the back of the neck and upper part of the back lead to formation of a *carbuncle.* The relative thickness and impermeability of the overlying skin lead to lateral extension and loculation, and a large, indurated, painful lesion with multiple ineffective drainage sites results. These extensive lesions appear more frequently among diabetics. Carbuncles produce fever, leukocytosis, extreme pain, and prostration. Bacteremia is common.

Staphylococci frequently colonize impetiginous lesions, but most impetigo in children and adults is due to group A streptococci. However, staphylococcal impetigo does occur, and while it cannot be clearly differentiated from streptococcal impetigo clinically, it tends to produce more localized disease, has a grayish rather than golden yellow crust, and less often produces high fever and lymphadenitis.

One form of impetigo characteristically caused by *S. aureus* is bullous impetigo. This disease represents one of several exfoliative staphylococcal pyodermas. *Staphylococcus aureus* strains lysed by group II phages, usually type 71, cause this group of diseases through production of an exotoxin (exfoliatin), which produces separation of the epidermis at the granular cell layer. Production of this exotoxin is plasmid-mediated.

Several clinical syndromes have been associated with exfoliative toxin-producing strains. Local pyoderma may be followed by a tender, scarlatiniform, finely desquamative rash that can be localized or generalized (staphylococcal scarlet fever). Bullous impetigo is the more severe form of this disease. Characteristically, local pyoderma precedes the sudden onset of generalized erythema, fever, and leukocytosis. Several days later large flaccid bullae form and then burst, resulting in red, denuded skin resembling a burn. The syndrom may be localized or rarely generalized (toxic epidermal necrolysis, Ritter's

syndrome, Lyell's disease, or scalded skin syndrome). In the localized form, staphylococci can usually be recovered from the bullous lesions, while in the generalized form they usually cannot be.

Osteomyelitis Staphylococci are responsible for the majority of cases of *acute osteomyelitis.* This infection occurs most commonly in children under the age of 12, but adults also are susceptible to acute osteomyelitis, especially of the spine. There appears to have been a sharp decrease in the incidence of acute osteomyelitis since the introduction of antibiotics. Approximately 50 percent of patients give a history of a furuncle or superficial staphylococcal infection preceding osteomyelitis. Bone involvement follows hematogenous dissemination of bacteria. The frequent localization in the diaphyseal end of long bones is thought to be due to the endarterial circulation of the diaphysis. Many patients give a history of preceding trauma to the involved area. Recently cases of clavicular osteomyelitis secondary to infected subclavian catheters have been reported.

Once established, infection spreads through the newly formed juxtaepiphyseal bone to the periosteum or along the marrow cavity. If the infection reaches the subperiosteal space, the periosteum is lifted, a subperiosteal abscess forms, and rupture with infection of the subcutaneous tissues may occur. Rarely, the joint capsule is penetrated, producing a pyogenic arthritis. There is death of bone, producing a *sequestrum,* followed by new bone formation, the *involucrum.*

Occasionally indolent staphylococcal infections of bone remain localized within dense granulation tissue about a central necrotic cavity. Such a local infection may persist for years as a so-called "Brodie's abscess."

Osteomyelitis in children usually begins abruptly with chills, high fever, nausea, vomiting, and progressive pain at the site of bony involvement. Muscle spasm about the affected bone is a common early sign of osteomyelitis, and the child may refuse to move the affected limb. Leukocytosis is the rule. Blood cultures are positive for staphylococci in 50 to 60 percent of cases early in the disease. The tissues overlying the involved bone become edematous and warm, and the skin become erythematous and shiny. Anemia develops during the course of untreated disease. Roentgenograms are usually normal during the first week, but radionucleide scans may be abnormal. Bony rarefaction, local periosteal elevation, and new bone formation can frequently be seen during the second week.

Staphylococcal spinal infection in the adult differs considerably from acute osteomyelitis in the child. The onset is less abrupt, and there is a greater tendency for bony fusion with obliteration of the disk space (Chap. 360).

DIAGNOSIS Osteomyelitis should be suspected in any child with fever, limb pain, and leukocytosis. Similarly, neck or back pain in an adult, when accompanied by fever, should raise the possibility of acute osteomyelitis or a disk space infection. History of a preceding cutaneous infection, local tenderness over the bone, and the finding of *S. aureus* in blood cultures are confirmatory. In early stages, osteomyelitis must be differentiated from acute rheumatic fever and pyogenic arthritis.

PROGNOSIS Before the advent of antimicrobials, the overall mortality was approximately 25 percent. Death was more common in individuals with demonstrable bacteremia. Chronic osteomyelitis with recurrent activation and metastatic foci in other bones was common. However, acute staphylococcal osteomyelitis is declining in incidence, death is rare, and chronic osteomyelitis is also becoming less frequent.

Staphylococcal pneumonia Staphylococci are the cause of approximately 1 percent of bacterial pneumonias acquired outside hospitals. This disease occurs sporadically except during epidemics of influenza, when staphylococcal pneumonia is more common, although even then it is not as frequent as pneumococcal infection.

Primary staphylococcal pneumonia in infants and young children frequently causes pyopneumothorax, and pneumatoceles occur early and should suggest *S. aureus* infection. In older children and healthy adults staphylococcal pneumonia is generally preceded by an influenza-like respiratory infection (influenza, measles, or other viruses). Onset of staphylococcal involvement is abrupt, with chills, high fever, progressive dyspnea, cyanosis, cough, and pleural pain. Early peripheral vascular collapse is common, and examination frequently reveals a patient who seems sicker than his physical findings would suggest. Sputum in the early phases is not characteristic, but may be bloody or frankly purulent. Admixture with blood may produce a thick, creamy pink sputum.

Staphylococci are one of the causes of pneumonia occurring in hospitalized patients. These infections usually begin insidiously. Increasing fever, tachycardia, and an elevated respiratory rate may be the only indications of infection. Typical pneumonic symptoms may be absent. The disease is also less abrupt when pulmonary involvement occurs during the course of staphylococcal bacteremia, as may be the case in drug addicts or in patients with endocarditis. Staphylococci generally produce patchy, centrally located areas of pneumonia. Pleural involvement and empyema are common. Many of these patients developing nosocomial staphylococcal pneumonia have chronic lung disease, leukemia, mucoviscidosis, or other debilitating diseases.

Because of the central pulmonary involvement, chest findings are variable. Signs of frank consolidation are rare. Scattered fine to coarse rales and rhonchi may be heard over the involved areas. Empyema produces typical signs of pleural fluid. Signs of abscess may appear late in the course of the disease. Bacteremia is not common in primary staphylococcal pneumonia (less than 20 percent of patients), and *its presence should suggest that the pneumonic involvement is metastatic and secondary to foci of infection elsewhere.*

The course of staphylococcal pneumonia may be stormy despite adequate antimicrobial therapy. Gradual defervescence starting 48 to 72 h after the initiation of therapy is the rule. Pulmonary abscesses or empyema cavities may require surgical treatment.

DIAGNOSIS Staphylococcal pneumonia must be differentiated from other pneumonias. The preceding influenza-like illness, rapid onset of pleural pain, cyanosis, and prostration out of proportion to physical findings should suggest primary staphylococcal pneumonia. The finding of masses of polymorphonuclear leukocytes and gram-positive intraleukocytic cocci strongly suggests the diagnosis. The blood leukocyte count is generally above 15,000 per cubic millimeter. When pneumonia develops suddenly or insidiously, with higher fever, tachycardia, and leukocytosis, in debilitated hospitalized patients receiving antimicrobials staphylococci should be strongly considered as the etiologic agent.

PROGNOSIS Before 1942, mortality ranged from 50 to 95 percent. The presence of bacteremia was almost invariably associated with a fatal outcome. The prognosis has improved with the use of antimicrobials, but some patients continue to die with staphylococcal pneumonia, especially debilitated individuals acquiring staphylococcal pneumonia in the hospital. Abscess formation and pleural involvement often prolong convalescence.

Staphylococcal bacteremia Staphylococcal bacteremia may arise from any local staphylococcal infection. Infections of the skin (including infections about inlying venous cutdowns or catheters), respiratory tract, bones, or genitourinary tract precede bacteremia. Trauma to local lesions, such as pinching, or surgical drainage before adequte localization may precipitate bacteremia.

Rarely, patients with bacteremia die in 12 to 24 h, with high fever, tachycardia, cyanosis, gastrointestinal symptoms, and vascular collapse. Commonly, the disease progresses more slowly, with hectic fever and metastatic abscess formation in the skin, bones, kidneys, brain, lungs, myocardium, spleen, or other tissues. *Meningitis* is an occasional complication.

Endocarditis (Chap. 243) may occur in patients with protracted bacteremia. Normal heart valves are frequently involved, the aortic being the most frequent. Typically, staphylococcal endocarditis runs an acute course with high fever, progressive anemia, and metastatic abscesses in the skin and deeper structures. Rupture of the valve leaflets and valve ring abscesses are common. Specific diagnosis of endocardial involvement is difficult; because of its frequency, it should be assumed to be present in patients with staphylococcal bacteremia with demonstrable cutaneous lesions (petechiae or cutaneous pustules) and a significant heart murmur. Echocardiography may facilitate diagnosis if valvular vegetations can be demonstrated. At times, especially among addicts with right-sided valvular lesions, a significant heart murmur may not be demonstrable. In these patients, septic pulmonary emboli often produce chest pain, hemoptysis, and multiple small pulmonary infiltrates. Both coagulase-positive and coagulase-negative staphylococci have been a major cause of endocarditis in patients undergoing cardiac surgical procedures, particularly valve replacement, and both coagulase-positive and coagulase-negative staphylococci occasionally produce a subacute endocarditis indistinguishable from that produced by *Streptococcus viridans.* Persistent *Staphylococcus epidermidis* bacteremia has also been common after ventriculoatriostomy.

Staphylococcal bacteremia is generally accompanied by a polymorphonuclear leukocytosis of 12,000 to 20,000 but a normal leukocyte count or leukopenia is occasionally seen. Diagnosis of bacteremia can be facilitated by doing a Gram's stain of the buffy coat, which may show staphylococci within the cytoplasm of polymorphonuclear cells. Anemia develops rapidly during the course of the illness. Cyanosis and hypoxemia may be seen with staphylococcal bacteremia, even in the absence of significant pulmonary lesions on chest roentgenogram. Demonstration of antibodies to the staphylococcal cell wall component teichoic acid by counterimmunoelectrophoresis has been useful in the diagnosis of culture-negative endocarditis.

PROGNOSIS Staphylococcal bacteremia is an extremely serious disease. Before the development of antimicrobials, over 80 percent of individuals died, the majority within 10 days of the onset of illness. The development of endocarditis or meningitis during bacteremia was almost invariably fatal. The sulfonamides produced little alteration in this mortality rate. With the administration of effective antibiotics and appropriate surgical treatment of local sites of infection, 50 to 70 percent of patients survive. With left-sided endocarditis, the fatality/case ratio is 30 percent. The prognosis for drug addicts with right-sided endocarditis appears particularly good; only 10 percent die. However, when staphylococcal endocarditis has occurred on a prosthetic cardiac valve, the outcome has been almost invariably fatal unless reconstructive surgery can be performed. Early surgical intervention is indicated in such cases.

Staphylococcal food poisoning See Chap. 112.

Genitourinary infections *Staphylococcus aureus* rarely causes urinary tract infections by retrograde spread from the bladder. Hence, the isolation of *S. aureus* from a well-collected urine specimen should prompt a search for renal, perinephric, or prostatic abscesses secondary to bacteremic staphylococcal infection elsewhere. Diabetics, drug addicts, and patients with valve protheses are particularly prone to this complication. *Staphylococcus epidermidis* has been increasingly recognized as a cause of acute lower urinary tract infection in young women. Many of these strains have the unique characteristic of being novobiocin and nalidixic acid–resistant and may have a specific species designation *(S. saphrophyticus).*

Miscellaneous infections Staphylococci may cause conjunctivitis, otitis, sinusitis, or mastoid infections as well as infection in and around the orbit. Epidemics of staphylococcal pyoderma in newborn infants and maternal breast abscesses are a recurring problem in maternity units.

TREATMENT Features of staphylococcal infection which influence therapy While the development of penicillinase-resistant penicillins and cephalosporins has simplified treatment, certain characteristics of staphylococcal disease should be borne in mind in designing therapy.

1 The host setting in which infection occurs. Acute staphylococcal infections arising outside the hospital in otherwise healthy adults have a better prognosis than intrahospital infections arising in sick individuals with compromised host defense mechanisms.
2 The rapid necrosis of tissues produced by staphylococci. Delays in effective therapy may allow a progressing infection to advance to frank abscess formation. While many antimicrobials reach abscess cavities in adequate concentrations, the physiologic insusceptibility of microorganisms residing in the areas of extensive necrosis or suppuration renders antibiotic therapy quite ineffective in this situation. Surgical drainage of such lesions is often required.
3 The sluggish response to therapy. Staphylococci are killed slowly by antimicrobials, and relapses are frequent. Hence antimicrobial therapy must be continued longer than in many bacterial infections.
4 The problem of antimicrobial resistance. While treatment must be initiated empirically when serious staphylococcal infection is suspected, rational therapy requires that the antibiotic susceptibility of the infecting strain be known.

Treatment of serious staphylococcal infections The effectiveness of the penicillinase-resistant penicillins has simplified the approach to life-threatening staphylococcal disease. Since nearly all strains of staphylococci are susceptible to penicillinase-resistant penicillins, and because of the high incidence of penicillinase-producing staphylococci as causes of infection, most authorities initiate treatment with methicillin, oxacillin, or nafcillin alone, shifting to aqueous penicillin G if the strain is subsequently proved to be susceptible to that drug. Methicillin is rapidly eliminated from the body, and initial doses of 2 g every 4 h are indicated. Parenteral oxacillin or nafcillin in doses of 1 or 2 g every 4 h can be substituted for methicillin. For penicillin-sensitive strains, adults should be given aqueous penicillin, 20 million units, by continuous infusion.

Despite differences in structure, the major allergenic properties of the penicillins reside in the 6-aminopenicillanic acid molecule. There is significant cross allergenicity between penicillins, and patients who have had well-established allergic reactions to penicillin G should not receive penicillinase-resistant penicillins. Further, there is increasing evidence that a signifi-

cant number of these individuals may react to the cephalosporin derivatives as well. These agents, which are good antistaphylococcal drugs, have a 7-aminocephalosporanic acid nucleus quite similar to that of penicillins and should be used with caution in patients with prior reactions to penicillin.

Several cephalosporins can be given parenterally for treatment of serious staphylococcal infections. Cephalothin is highly active against both penicillin-sensitive and penicillin-resistant strains; intramuscular or intravenous doses of 1 to 2 g every 4 h are recommended. The usual dose of cefazolin for severe staphylococcal infection is 1 g every 6 h intramuscularly or intravenously and the dose and route of administration for cephapirin are similar. Nephrotoxicity and an increased susceptibility to penicillinase limit the usefulness of cephaloridine. Cephalosporins should not be used in the treatment of serious staphylococcal infections caused by methicillin-resistant strains of *S. aureus* or *S. epidermidis.* Such strains are generally resistant to cephalosporins despite disk-diffusion results that may indicate sensitivity.

Vancomycin is uniformly active against coagulase-positive staphylococci regardless of their sensitivity to penicillin. It should be given intravenously in doses of 1 to 1.5 g over a 30- to 40-min period every 12 h.

The development of these new agents has relegated several antibiotics formerly used in treatment to minor or secondary roles. Lincomycin, clindamycin, and erythromycin are still useful in certain circumstances, but are not front-line agents in staphylococcal bacteremia. They are used primarily in patients allergic to penicillin.

Changes in therapy Established staphylococcal infections repond slowly even to the most effective antimicrobial regimens, making it difficult to know when therapy should be considered inadequate. Characteristically, 24 to 48 h elapse before a decline in fever is noted, and recovery is accompanied by slow return of the temperature to normal in 7 to 10 days.

Special therapeutic situations ASYMPTOMATIC NASAL CARRIER STATE The role of asymptomatic carriers in hospital transmission of infection remains controversial. Many hospital personnel carry *S. aureus* in their anterior nares but do not appear to disseminate the strain. However, some persons readily disseminate their strain and are a cause of nosocomial infections. Unfortunately, simple methods for recognition of such "dangerous disseminators" are not available, and they are most often detected when increased numbers of *S. aureus* infections prompt an epidemiologic investigation. It is generally agreed that disseminators must be removed from nursery units, operating theaters, delivery rooms, and surgical floors. Although no method of treatment has been uniformly satisfactory, the following regimens have had limited success in treatment of nasal carriers.

1 Simple removal from the hospital environment for 3 to 4 weeks
2 Frequent baths with vermicidal soaps
3 The use of topical antibiotics of low sensitizing potential in a water-soluble base (i.e., bacitracin, neomycin, gentamicin, or a combination of these agents) four to five times daily for 2 weeks

If the carrier state returns, a second course of treatment is indicated.

SUPERFICIAL INFECTIONS Superficial infections frequently do not require the use of antibiotics. There is no adequate therapy for recurrent furunculosis, but if the disease is severe, antimicrobial treatment may be attempted. Antibiotics to which the strain is susceptible should be administered systemically for a minimum of 10 to 14 days. Cloxacillin (2 g per day divided into four doses) or dicloxacillin (2 g per day divided into four doses) can usually be used. Local moist heat, immobilization of the infected part, and incision and drainage should be utilized. The surrounding skin should be protected with a coating of zinc oxide to prevent maceration. Treatment of the nasal carrier state by the local application of topical antibiotics (see above) may be advisable. Careful daily baths with germicidal soaps, attention to personal and family hygiene, and the passage of time appear to be measures most likely to interrupt the process. Attempts to prevent recurrence by autogenous or other vaccines have not been effective.

EMPYEMA Empyema should be treated by aspiration, generally with a large-bore tube since loculation and thick exudate may prevent adequate needle drainage. Intravenous antibiotics as already outlined for serious infections should be given. Direct instillation of penicillin or methicillin into the pleural space may be beneficial in some instances. Similarly, while the local instillation of proteolytic enzymes may occasionally aid in liquefying the exudate, surgical drainage is generally necessary and should be performed promptly.

OSTEOMYELITIS The initial regimen already outlined for other serious infections is recommended, and treatment should be continued for 14 to 28 days in acute osteomyelitis. Local drainage of abscess cavities in soft tissues or bones should be considered in all patients in whom severe pain persists or when response to antimicrobials is inadequate. If sequestration occurs, devitalized bone should be removed. Lincomycin has been reported to be superior to other agents in the treatment of chronic osteomyelitis, but the evidence for this is not convincing. The optimal duration of treatment in established chronic infection is not known, but frequently several months of antimicrobial therapy are recommended.

BACTEREMIA AND ENDOCARDITIS Most authorities recommend 4 to 6 weeks of parenteral antibiotic therapy in proved or suspected staphylococcal endocarditis. However, shorter courses of therapy may be successful, especially in drug addicts with tricuspid endocarditis. In some centers, gentamicin is given with a penicillinase-resistant penicillin in an attempt to kill staphylococci more rapidly. When staphylococcal bacteremia occurs secondary to a removable focus of localized infection (an abscess or an infected intravenous catheter), 10 to 14 days of parenteral therapy is probably sufficient provided the patient has no clinical evidence of endocarditis and demonstrates prompt clinical improvement.

REFERENCES

EICKHOFF TE: Hospital infections. Dis Mon, September 1972

JANNINI PB, CROSSLEY K: Therapy of S. aureus bacteremia associated with a removable focus of infection. Ann Intern Med 84:558, 1976

JESSEN O et al: Changing staphylococci and staphylococcal infections. N Engl J Med 281:627, 1969

KOENIG MG: Staphylococcal infections: Treatment and control. Dis Mon, April 1968

MUSHER DM, MCKENZIE SO: Infections due to Staphylococcus aureus. Medicine 56:383, 1977

NAHMIAS AJ, EICKHOFF TC: Staphylococcal infections in hospitals. N Engl J Med 265:74, 120, 177, 1962

NOLAN CM, BEATY HN: S. Aureus bacteremia: Current clinical patterns. Am J Med 60:495, 1976

WATANAKUNAKORN C et al: Some salient features of Staphylococcus aureus endocarditis. Am J Med 54:473, 1973

WISE RI: Modern management of severe staphylococcal disease. Medicine 52:295, 1973

117

STREPTOCOCCAL INFECTIONS

ALAN L. BISNO

Streptococci are among the commonest bacterial pathogens of humans. They are responsible for a diverse spectrum of diseases including pharyngitis and tonsillitis, scarlet fever, erysipelas, impetigo, lymphangitis, and perinatal infections of mother and child. Certain representatives of this genus are prominent causes of endocarditis and urinary tract infections. In addition to their role in causing acute pyogenic infections, strains of *Streptococcus pyogenes* are capable of giving rise to the delayed nonsuppurative sequels of acute rheumatic fever and acute glomerulonephritis.

ETIOLOGY AND CLASSIFICATION Streptococci are spherical or ovoid bacterial cells which grow in pairs or chains of varying lengths. Most are facultative anaerobes, although some are strict anaerobes. The organisms are gram-positive, usually nonmotile, non-spore-forming, and catalase-negative. No single system of classification suffices to differentiate this heterogeneous group of organisms. Instead, classification depends upon a combination of features, including patterns of hemolysis observed on blood agar plates, antigenic composition, growth characteristics, and biochemical reactions.

When cultivated on blood agar plates, streptococci may produce one of three different patterns of hemolysis. Alpha-hemolytic colonies are surrounded by a zone of partial hemolysis; in addition, such organisms usually produce a greenish discoloration in the medium due to the presence of an unidentified reductant of hemoglobin. This greening reaction gives rise to the term *S. viridans,* which is often applied to alpha-hemolytic strains. Strains of *S. pneumoniae* are alpha-hemolytic, as are many other streptococci which normally inhabit the upper respiratory and gastrointestinal tracts. Beta-hemolytic colonies are surrounded by clear colorless zones within which the red blood cells in the medium have been completely lysed. This pattern of complete hemolysis is exhibited by *S. pyogenes* and many of the other streptococci pathogenic for humans. Gamma streptococci are those which fail to produce hemolysis upon blood agar plates.

Although classification of streptococci on the basis of hemolytic reactions is quite useful in certain clinical situations, more precise identification of beta-hemolytic streptococci is accomplished by differentiation into serogroups, as originally described by Lancefield, on the basis of antigenic differences in cell wall carbohydrates. These antigens are readily extracted from streptococcal cell walls and identified by precipitin reactions using specific antiserums. Groups A to H and K to T are recognized. The vast majority of beta-hemolytic streptococci isolated from human sources belongs to groups A to D, F, and G. Although the Lancefield grouping system was initially devised for identification of beta-hemolytic streptococci, certain alpha-hemolytic and nonhemolytic strains also contain group-specific antigens. The most important of these are the group D streptococci, including the so-called "enterococci," among which many strains fail to show beta hemolysis. There are 21 recognized species of streptococci. Species designation is based upon growth characteristics under varying conditions of temperature, pH, and media composition. Five species do not possess group antigens, and, conversely, a number of serogroups do not encompass any of the recognized species.

Anaerobic and microaerophilic streptococci include members of the family Peptococceae, genus *Peptostreptococcus*; five species are recognized. Hemolytic reactions of these organisms are variable, and no satisfactory method of classifying them has been devised.

GROUP A STREPTOCOCCAL INFECTIONS

Streptococci of Lancefield's group A (*S. pyogenes*) are responsible for the great majority of human streptococcal infections and are uniquely important because of their role as precursors of rheumatic fever and glomerulonephritis.

ETIOLOGY The *group-specific carbohydrate* of group A streptococci is a polymer of rhamnose and *N*-acetylglucosamine. There are more than 60 recognized group A serotypes. The typing system is based upon antigenic differences in a cell wall constituent known as *M protein,* which is the principal virulence factor of group A organisms. Strains rich in M protein are highly resistant to phagocytosis by polymorphonuclear leukocytes in vitro and are capable of initiating disease in humans and experimental animals. Strains lacking M protein are avirulent. Acquired human immunity to streptococcal infection is based upon development of opsonic antibodies directed against the antiphagocytic moiety of M protein. This immunity is type-specific and lasts for many years, perhaps indefinitely. M protein is a macromolecule which contains, in addition to the type-specific determinant, a variety of non-type-specific antigens which are widely shared by strains of differing serotypes. *T protein* serves as the basis of a subsidiary typing system which has been useful in classifying strains not typable by the M systems; unlike M protein, the T antigen plays no role in virulence. *Lipoteichoic acid,* a substance which has a marked affinity for biological membranes, has been found to play a crucial role in colonization by binding group A streptococci to specific receptor sites on human epithelial cells. *Opacity factor,* an α-lipoproteinase closely associated with the M-protein molecule, is produced by certain serotypes only. Strains positive for opacity factor may be somewhat attenuated in their virulence, or at least in their ability to elicit antibody response to type-specific and non-type-specific antigens of M protein. The streptococcal *cell membrane* contains a number of antigenic structures, certain of which have been reported to share determinants with constituents of human heart and with basement membrane of the renal glomerulus. Group A streptococci are enveloped in a slimy *hyaluronic acid capsule* which serves to retard phagocytosis and, therefore, represents an accessory virulence factor. Streptococcal hyaluronate is nonantigenic in humans, presumably because it is identical to that found in human connective tissue.

As streptococci grow in vitro or in vivo, they elaborate a number of extracellular products, a few of which require mention. *Erythrogenic toxin,* which is induced by lysogeny with a temperature bacteriophage, is responsible for the rash of scarlet fever. There are three serologically distinct toxins, the effects of which may be neutralized by antibody. Two distinct hemolysins are elaborated. *Streptolysin O* is reversibly inhibited by oxygen (hence exerting its effect primarily on subsurface colonies) and irreversibly inhibited by cholesterol. It is produced by almost all group A strains as well as by many group C and G organisms. Titration of antistreptolysin O (ASO) antibodies in human serums is the most widely used serologic procedure to detect group A streptococcal infection in clinical practice. Hemolysis on the surface of blood agar plates is due primarily to the action of *streptolysin S.* Although streptolysin S differs from streptolysin O in being oxygen-stable and nonantigenic, both hemolysins possess the capacity to damage membranes of polymorphonuclear leukocytes, platelets, and subcellular organelles. A number of other extracellular products exert effects which might serve to facilitate the organisms' survival in vivo by liquefying pus [streptokinase and deoxyribonucleases (DNases) A to D] or by allowing spread through tissue planes (*hyaluronidase* and *proteinase*).

The role of these substances in streptococcal virulence remains unproved.

The two most frequent types of group A streptococcal infection are pharyngitis and pyoderma. They differ markedly in their epidemiologic, clinical, and bacteriologic characteristics.

STREPTOCOCCAL PHARYNGITIS **Epidemiology** This is one of the commonest bacterial infections of humans. The incidence is highest in children aged 5 to 15 years; males and females are affected equally. The great majority of such infections are due to group A streptococci, but strains of other serogroups, particularly group C or G, are involved occasionally. The organism is ordinarily transmitted directly from person to person, most likely by droplet spread, and crowding markedly facilitates interpersonal transmission. This may account for the increased incidence of streptococcal pharyngitis in northern latitudes during the colder months of the year, as well as for the explosive outbreaks which occur in military recruit camps and other crowded institutional settings. Common-source epidemics of streptococcal sore throat with high attack rates occasionally occur following contamination of a food item with beta-hemolytic streptococci. Environmental reservoirs of streptococci, such as viable organisms in room dust or on blankets, are not important in spread of disease.

Patients with acute streptococcal pharyngitis harbor large numbers of organisms in the anterior nares and throat. If antibiotics are not administered, the organisms may persist in the upper respiratory tract for weeks to months after symptoms have subsided. However, as the length of the carrier state increases, the organisms decrease in number, disappear from the anterior nasal secretions, and lose detectable M protein. Therefore, convalescent carriers are less likely than acutely ill patients to transmit group A streptococci to exposed individuals. Group A pharyngeal carriage rates vary with geographic location, season of the year, and age group. Among school-aged children, rates of 15 to 20 percent have been reported; the carriage rate among adults is considerably lower.

Symptoms The usual incubation period of streptococcal pharyngitis is between 2 and 4 days. The classic syndrome, as observed in older children and adults, is ushered in by the rather abrupt onset of sore throat, manifested particularly by pain on swallowing. Associated symptoms include headache, malaise, feverishness, and anorexia. Chilliness is a frequent symptom, but true rigors are rare. Nausea, vomiting, and abdominal pain are common in children.

Physical signs The patient appears moderately ill with tachycardia and fever which frequently exceeds 38.3°C (101°F). There is diffuse erythema, edema, and lymphoid hyperplasia of the posterior pharynx. The uvula is edematous. The tonsils, if present, are enlarged, reddened, and covered by a punctate or coalescent exudate which may be yellow, gray, or white. Discrete areas of pinhead-size exudate are frequently present on the posterior pharynx but may be concealed by mucopurulent nasal secretions. The anterior cervical lymph nodes at the angles of the jaw are enlarged and tender. Cough and hoarseness, if present, are mild and, in the absence of the signs and symptoms indicated above, do not in themselves suggest the diagnosis of streptococcal pharyngitis. Laryngeal involvement with loss of voice is not a feature of streptococcal infection.

The full-blown clinical syndrome of acute exudative tonsillopharyngitis is seen frequently during explosive epidemics of streptococcal disease, particularly those occurring in institutional settings such as military recruit camps. In endemically occurring infections among civilian populations, however, the illness is frequently much milder. Indeed, in such circumstances, only about half the children with sore throats and positive cultures for group A streptococci will have tonsillar exudate, and a third or less may have fever greater than 38.3°C (101°F) or marked leukocytosis. Patients who have undergone tonsillectomy tend to experience a milder clinical syndrome. In infants, streptococcal upper respiratory infections tend to be less sharply localized to the lymphoid tissue of the faucial and posterior pharyngeal areas. Infections at this age are characterized by rhinorrhea with excoriation of the nares, low-grade fever, anorexia, and a protracted clinical course. Exudative pharyngitis in children less than 3 years of age is rarely streptococcal in etiology.

Course The course of streptococcal pharyngitis is usually brief and self-limited. Fever abates within a week, usually within 3 to 5 days. Constitutional symptoms and sore throat disappear with defervescence or shortly thereafter. Several weeks may be required, however, for the tonsils and lymph nodes to return to normal size.

Scarlet fever When streptococcal pharyngitis is due to a lysogenic strain producing erythrogenic toxin, and when the host is not immune to the toxin, scarlet fever ensues. The rash usually appears within 2 days after onset of sore throat, involves first the neck, upper chest, and back, then spreads over the remainder of the trunk and the extremities, and spares the palms and soles. The rash may be difficult to appreciate in black patients. It consists of a diffuse erythema, which blanches on pressure, with numerous 1- to 2-mm punctate elevations that impart a "sandpaper" texture to the skin. Discrete lesions are absent from the face, but there is a generalized facial flush which contrasts with the prominent circumoral pallor. The rash is more intense along skin folds, such as those of the antecubital fossae and axillary folds, and in these locations often produces linear striations of confluent petachiae known as *Pastia's lines*. Increased capillary fragility, which contributes to the formation of Pastia's lines, is confirmed by a positive Rumpel-Leede's test.

The exanthem of scarlet fever is accompanied by an enanthem, consisting of punctate erythema and petechiae on the soft palate. Early in the disease, the tongue is covered with a white coat through which hypertrophied papillae protrude as islands of red (strawberry tongue). By the fourth or fifth day the coating is gone and the entire tongue appears beefy red (raspberry tongue). In rare cases, scarlet fever may be complicated by hepatic involvement with jaundice, pleural effusion, and arthralgia. It is unclear how often arthralgia is a manifestation of scarlet fever or how often it presages the development of rheumatic fever.

The rash usually lasts 4 to 5 days and is followed by extensive desquamation which begins as early as a few days or as late as 3 to 4 weeks after onset of the disease and is often a striking feature of the convalescent phase of scarlet fever.

Although scarlet fever usually follows upper respiratory infection due to group A streptococci, rarely other erythrogenic toxins are produced by streptococci of groups C and G and by certain strains of staphylococci. Moreover, scarlet fever may follow streptococcal impetigo or secondary streptococcal infection of superficial wounds. The disease must be differentiated from various of the childhood exanthems, infectious mononucleosis when the latter is associated with rash, and drug eruptions. The management of scarlet fever consists of adequate treatment of the causative infection.

Two tests previously employed in assessment of scarlet fever are no longer in clinical use. The *Dick test* is performed by inoculating erythrogenic toxin intracutaneously. Individuals who are susceptible to the toxin will experience local erythema (positive Dick test), while individuals with antitoxin immunity will have no reaction (negative Dick test). Conversion from a positive to a negative Dick test during the course of a rash illness strongly suggests the diagnosis of scarlet fever. Another test consists of injection of scarlatinal antitoxin into an area of cutaneous rash, which produces blanching if the eruption is due to erythrogenic toxin. This test, previously used for diagnosis of scarlet fever, is known as the Schultz-Charlton reaction.

Complications Streptococcal pharyngitis may give rise to suppurative complications, among which acute otitis media and acute sinusitis are the most frequent. Suppurative cervical lymphadenitis may also occur. Inflammation of the faucial area induced by streptococcal infection may give rise to peritonsillar cellulitis, peritonsillar abscess, or retropharyngeal abscess. The abscesses themselves, however, usually contain a variety of oropharyngeal flora, including anaerobic bacteria, rather than group A streptococci. A variety of other complications, common in the past, are almost never seen in the antibiotic era: (1) extension up the cribriform plate of the ethmoid or via the mastoid, giving rise to meningitis, brain abscess, or thrombosis of cerebral venous sinuses; and (2) bacteremia with metastatic foci of infection such as suppurative arthritis, osteomyelitis, or liver abscess. Much of the intense clinical and investigative interest focused upon streptococcal pharyngitis is due to its association with two delayed nonsuppurative sequels: acute rheumatic fever (ARF) and acute glomerulonephritis (AGN). These are discussed in Chaps. 241 and 278, respectively.

Diagnosis Sore throat due to group A streptococci must be differentiated from that caused by a number of other agents. *Diphtheria* is rare in immunized populations. It is characterized by the presence of an extensive diphtheritic membrane, respiratory embarrassment due to laryngeal involvement, myocarditis, cranial nerve palsies, and positive cultures for *Corynebacterium diphtheriae*. *Gonococcal* tonsillopharyngitis should be suggested by a history of homosexuality or fellatio. *Vincent's angina* is characterized by sore throat and tonsillopharyngeal exudate. Unlike streptococcal sore throat, however, there is an insidious onset without constitutional symptoms, pharyngeal ulcerations are frequent, and the disease is usually unilateral.

The major differential diagnostic confusion is with viral upper respiratory infections, which occur more frequently than does streptococcal infection. In many cases, the viral etiology may be suspected because of the more prominent catarrhal, "common cold-like" quality of these viral infections. *Adenoviruses* may cause an exudative pharyngitis which is virtually indistinguishable clinically from that due to group A streptococci. *Infectious mononucleosis* also produces severe exudative pharyngitis with fever and toxicity and at times is accompanied by a rash which may be confused with scarlet fever. The generalized lymphadenopathy, splenomegaly, prolonged fever, and presence of abnormal lymphocytes and heterophile antibodies in the peripheral blood serve to differentiate this entity. Pharyngitis due to group A coxsackie viruses (*herpangina*) or to primary infection with *herpes simplex* is characterized by formation of vesicles, which rupture and leave shallow ulcers. *Influenza* virus infections frequently occur in epidemics; they are accompanied by severe myalgias, bronchitis is a frequent clinical feature, and all age groups are affected. *Mycoplasma pneumonia* infections may cause pharyngitis that at times may be exudative. Bullous myringitis, if present, should suggest this diagnosis.

Despite the differential features set forth above, in many instances it is impossible to differentiate streptococcal from nonstreptococcal sore throat on clinical grounds alone. Even experienced observers are able to predict the presence of streptococcal pharyngeal infection in no more than 50 to 75 percent of cases. For this reason, precise diagnosis requires performance of a throat culture. In obtaining the culture, it is important to rub the cotton swab over both tonsils or tonsillar fossae, the oropharynx, and the nasopharynx posterior to the uvula. The swab should be inoculated onto a sheep blood agar plate to allow evaluation of patterns of hemolysis after overnight incubation. If beta-hemolytic streptococci are isolated, they may be presumed to be group A by sensitivity to a low-potency bacitracin disk or may be identified definitively by fluorescent antibody, coagglutination, or precipitin techniques. A number of the positive cultures obtained, particularly those with few organisms on the culture plate, will represent streptococcal carriers rather than cases of acute infection. It is not possible to differentiate cases from carriers confidently on the basis of culture results, but culture does serve to exclude from antimicrobial therapy the bulk of patients with sore throat (approximately 70 percent) who have negative cultures for beta-hemolytic streptococci. Assay of serum antibodies to streptococcal extracellular products (e.g., ASO) provides confirmatory evidence of recent streptococcal infection in patients suspected of having acute rheumatic fever or acute glomerulonephritis, but such tests are of no value in the diagnosis of acute streptococcal infection.

Treatment Therapy of streptococcal pharyngitis is directed primarily toward prevention of suppurative sequelae and of ARF. It is unclear whether treatment of the antecedent streptococcal infection will prevent development of AGN. Prevention of ARF depends upon eradication of the infecting organism from the pharynx, and attainment of this objective requires prolonged antibiotic treatment. Penicillin is the drug of choice because it is inexpensive and nontoxic and because all group A streptococci have remained exquisitely sensitive to this agent. A single intramuscular injection of benzathine penicillin G, 600,000 units for children less than 60 lb and 1.2 million units for all others, ensures a prolonged penicillinemia and is the most effective form of therapy. If oral therapy is elected, penicillin G, 250,000 units, or penicillin V, 250 mg, three or four times daily, is the treatment of choice. Penicillin-allergic individuals may be treated with erythromycin, 20 mg/lb per day (not to exceed 1 g per day). Nearly all group A streptococci in the United States have remained susceptible to erythromycin, but extensive resistance has been reported in certain areas of the world such as Japan. On the other hand, tetracycline-resistant strains are encountered with some frequency in the United States, and this drug is not recommended. Sulfonamides are ineffective in eradication of established streptococcal infection, although they are useful prophylactically in preventing new pharyngeal acquisitions of group A streptococci and in preventing recurrences of ARF (Chap. 241). All oral regimens are less effective than intramuscular benzathine penicillin G in eradicating the infecting streptococcus, a fact that is due at least in part to the difficulty of ensuring faithful compliance once the acute symptoms have subsided. It is advisable to reculture the throat within 48 h of completion of oral therapy. If group A streptococci persist, as they may in 15 percent of cases, retreatment, preferably with benzathine penicillin G, is indicated. Multiple repetitive courses of antibiotics are not of further value and should be avoided.

Appropriate antibiotic therapy is effective in preventing ARF, even when initiated as long as 9 days after the onset of acute pharyngitis. Therefore, in the patient seen early after the course of his illness, the delay in initiating therapy occasioned by obtaining a positive throat culture is not ordinarily a matter of concern. In patients who are severely ill or in whom development of suppurative complications is apparent, therapy may be instituted at the time of the initial visit after a throat culture has been obtained. If oral antibiotic therapy is elected, the throat culture serves as a guide to the necessity of completion of a full 10-day course or, alternatively, of recalling the patient for definitive therapy with an injection of benzathine penicillin G.

Patients with more severe suppurative complications, such as infections involving the mastoid or ethmoids, require larger doses of penicillin than those used for treatment of uncomplicated sore throat. When streptococcal upper respiratory infection is complicated by the development of abscesses associated with suppurative cervical adenitis or in the peritonsillar or retrophyaryngeal soft tissues, incision and drainage are usually required.

The role of tonsillectomy, if any, in the management of patients with frequent recurrences of acute pharyngitis or in the prevention of ARF remains undefined. Clinical episodes of pharyngitis occur less frequently and tend to be milder following tonsillectomy, but this may possibly make detection and appropriate treatment of immunologically significant streptococcal infections more difficult.

Family contacts of patients with streptococcal sore throat frequently develop symptomatic infections or become asymptomatic pharyngeal carriers. Secondary cases in families should, of course, be treated appropriately. Asymptomatic family contacts should also be cultured in high-risk circumstances. These include the presence of a rheumatic subject in the family, known cases of ARF occurring in the general area, and families in a lower socioeconomic group with a large number of children living in crowded circumstances. In situations where the risk is lower, the decision to culture and treat asymptomatic family contacts must be made for each involved individual and should be based upon factors such as the geographic and socioeconomic setting, and the current prevalence of streptococcal disease and its sequels.

STREPTOCOCCAL SKIN INFECTIONS **Erysipelas** Also known as Saint Anthony's fire, erysipelas is an acute infection of the skin and subcutaneous tissues caused by group A streptococci. Other streptococci, and even staphylococci and pneumococci, have been implicated on rare occasions. The disease most frequently affects infants, young children, and elderly individuals. The commonest site of involvement is the face, where cutaneous infection originates from an upper respiratory source, presumably by way of small or inapparent breaks in the skin. Erysipelas may also result from streptococcal infection of wounds, surgical incisions, or even areas of dermatophytosis, in which case any portion of the body may be involved.

The onset is usually abrupt; initial symptoms include malaise, chilliness, feverishness, headache, and vomiting. The skin lesion may begin with itching and mild discomfort at the site of infection and is followed shortly thereafter by a small area of erythema which enlarges during the ensuing hours. The lesion spreads rapidly, reaching its maximum extent in 3 to 6 days. It is warm, pink to deep red in color, and has an advancing elevated margin which protrudes irregularly into the surrounding areas of normal skin. Vesicles and bullae may appear; these rupture leaving crusts on the surface. While the advancing margin remains inflamed, central clearing may be evident with a return of the skin to normal appearance or with residual pigmentation. The eruption may be less well demarcated in areas where the skin is loose, but edema and erythema are constant features. Facial erysipelas commonly involves the bridge of the nose and one or more cheeks in a "butterfly" distribution (Fig. 117-1).

FIGURE 117-1
This patient with facial erysipelas exhibits the characteristic "butterfly" distribution of the lesion. The picture was obtained after 48 h of penicillin therapy when the acute inflammation and systemic toxicity had abated slightly.

The disease process may be accompanied by high fever and bacteremia. Recovery is usually apparent by the end of a week, but this varies with the severity of the infection. The substantial mortality attending bacteremic cases of erysipelas in the preantibiotic era has been markedly reduced by penicillin. Fatalities still occur among children within the first few months of life and elderly, debilitated, immunosuppressed individuals. The disease is noted for its propensity to recur, especially in the areas of chronic lymphatic obstruction.

The diagnosis of erysipelas is primarily clinical. Group A streptococci may at times be isolated from the respiratory tract or the bloodstream. Culture of edema fluid or of saline injected intracutaneously and then withdrawn from the advancing margin may yield streptococci, but this maneuver is rarely successful.

Pyoderma This term is used collectively to denote localized purulent streptococcal skin infections. Some pyoderma lesions represent obvious secondary infections of wounds or burns. For the most part, however, the term is used synonymously with streptococcal impetigo or impetigo contagiosa and refers to discrete purulent lesions which appear to be primary infections of the skin. Streptococcal impetigo differs from streptococcal pharyngitis in a number of particulars (Table 117-1). Epidemiologically, impetigo is more prevalent among underprivileged children residing in warm, humid climates such as the southeastern United States or the tropics. However, the disease may also occur during the summer in northern settings, such as the American Indian reservations of Minnesota. The peak incidence is in young children (2 to 6 years), and there is no definite sex or racial predisposition.

The mode of spread of streptococcal pyoderma is unknown, but personal contact and insect vectors such as *Hippelates* flies are probably both important. "Skin strains" of group A streptococci (i.e., strains of M and T types usually associated with pyoderma) are capable of contaminating unbroken skin, from where they may be inoculated intradermally by local scratches, abrasions, or insect bites. A number of interesting epidemiologic relationships have been observed; they include secondary streptococcal infection in the lesions of scabies and the co-

existence of *S. pyogenes* and *C. diphtheriae* in impetiginous lesions in Mississippi and Trinidad. Nasal and pharyngeal carriage of skin strains is frequent in children with impetigo, but such carriage does not ordinarily occur until after establishment of cutaneous carriage or overt infection.

The pattern of immunologic responses to streptococcal impetigo differs from that associated with upper respiratory infection. In particular, the ASO response to impetigo is weak, perhaps because streptolysin O is inactivated by lipids present in the skin. Brisk antibody responses to anti-DNAse B and anti-hyaluronidase, as well as to the Streptozyme slide hemagglutination reagent, are observed, however. Type-specific anti-M responses are variable, depending in part upon the antigenicity of the infecting strain, but in general such responses are weaker than in pharyngeal infections. The role of type-specific antibodies in protection against reinfection in pyoderma has not been adequately studied.

Streptococcal impetigo occurs on exposed areas of the body, most frequently on the lower extremities. The lesions remain well-localized but are frequently multiple. They begin as papules but rapidly evolve into vesicles surrounded by an area of erythema. The vesicular lesions are rarely recognized clinically; they give rise to papules which gradually enlarge, then break down over 4 to 6 days to form characteristic thick crusts. The lesions heal slowly, leaving depigmented areas. A deeply ulcerated form of impetigo is known as *echthyma*. Although regional lymphadenitis often occurs, systemic symptoms are not ordinarily present.

In addition to the indolent, impetiginous skin infections of young children, a more severe and extensive form of pyoderma has been observed in combat troops serving in hot, wet environments such as the jungles of Southeast Asia. During the Vietnam conflict, such "jungle sores" became a major medical problem among infantry personnel. In their most common form, they consist of multiple echthymatous ulcers located on the ankle or dorsum of the foot. The ulcers are usually circular, punched-out lesions 0.5 to 3.0 cm in diameter, have borders, and are surrounded by a zone of erythema. They are filled with purulent material and covered with grayish yellow adherent crusts. Secondary cellulitis or lymphadenitis may be present.

TABLE 117-1
Comparative features of pharyngitis and pyoderma due to group A streptococci

	Pharyngitis	*Pyoderma*
Predominant geographic distribution	Temperate	Subtropic-tropic
Season (temperate zone)	Winter-spring	Summer-fall
Peak age group	5–15 years	2–5 years
Mode of spread	Direct contact (droplet)	Unknown (?insects)
Clinical illness	Acute	Indolent
Streptococcal types	Generally lower-numbered M types	Generally higher-numbered M types
ASO responses	Good	Weak
Type-specific antibody responses	Generally good	Variable, often poor
Nonsuppurative sequels	Acute rheumatic fever, acute glomerulonephritis	Acute glomerulonephritis

SOURCE: *After Wannamaker.*

The diagnosis of streptococcal pyoderma is made by bacteriologic culture. Adequate cultures require removal of the surface crusts in order to obtain specimens from the base of the lesions. Although both *S. pyogenes* and *Staphylococcus aureus* may be isolated from the lesions, the former is the major pathogen. Morphologically characteristic lesions respond well to penicillin therapy, even when penicillinase-resistant staphylococci are recovered. These lesions contrast with bullous impetigo, which is ordinarily due to *S. aureus* and not to streptococci. Antibiotic regimens are the same as those for pharyngitis, and benzathine penicillin G, oral penicillin V, or oral erythromycin all result in cure rates in excess of 95 percent. Topical antiseptics and antibiotics are of little, if any, value. Prevention of pyoderma depends primarily upon adherence to good personal hygiene, with special attention to frequent scrubbing with soap and water.

Streptococcal pyoderma does not give rise to ARF. This observation remains unexplained, but may indicate a requirement for infection at the pharyngeal site, with its rich endowment of lymphoid tissue, in order to initiate the immunologic events leading to ARF. On the other hand, studies of populations in which ARF and AGN occur simultaneously indicate that the streptococcal strains responsible for each sequel are distinct and suggest that "pyoderma strains" of group A streptococci may be nonrheumatogenic. When pyoderma is due to a nephritogenic strain of group A streptococcus, AGN may ensue. Indeed, pyoderma is by far the commonest antecedent of poststreptococcal glomerulonephritis in subtropical and tropical regions of the world. Strains of a number of M types (49, 55, 57, and others) have been associated both with sporadic cases and large epidemics of pyoderma-associated nephritis in diverse geographic areas. There are no conclusive data to indicate that treatment of an individual case of pyoderma will prevent the subsequent occurrence of AGN in that patient. Such treatment is important, however, in eradicating nephritogenic streptococci from the environment in epidemiologic settings in which these strains are prevalent.

Cellulitis Streptococcal cellulitis may occur in areas of tissue damage due to trauma, operative wounds, or stasis ulceration. It is an acute inflammation of the skin and subcutaneous tissues marked by pain, tenderness, erythema, fever, and often regional lymphadenopathy. In contrast to erysipelas, the margins of the lesions are neither elevated nor sharply demarcated from the surrounding uninvolved tissue. Rarely such lesions may progress to frank gangrene. Cellulitis of the perianal area may be manifested by painful defecation or by pruritus; asymptomatic anal colonization has been the source of several outbreaks of hospital-acquired streptococcal infection. Vaginal colonization by group A streptococci has a number of features in common with perianal involvement. In both instances there is a close epidemiologic association with streptococcal upper respiratory infection. Anal and vaginal streptococcal infection may be either symptomatic or asymptomatic. At least one outbreak of nosocomial streptococcal infection has been attributed to an asymptomatic vaginal carrier.

LYMPHANGITIS AND PUERPERAL SEPSIS Local trauma, whether or not complicated by frank cellulitis, may give rise to *acute lymphangitis*. This entity is characterized by the appearance of red linear streaks extending from the portal of entry to the draining regional lymph nodes, which are enlarged and tender. Systemic symptoms, including chills, fever, malaise, and headache, are prominent, and the process may be accompanied by demonstrable bacteremia. Streptococcal bacteremia, from whatever cause, may give rise to metastatic foci of infection, such as suppurative arthritis, osteomyelitis, peritonitis, endocarditis, meningitis, or visceral abscesses. The clinical course of streptococcal bacteremia may at times be fulminant and lead rapidly to prostration, shock, purpura fulminans, disseminated intravascular coagulation, and death.

Puerperal sepsis follows abortion or childbirth when streptococci invade the endometrium and surrounding structures and then the lymphatics and bloodstream. The pathological process may be further complicated by pelvic cellulitis, septic pelvic thrombophlebitis, peritonitis, or pelvic abscess. The causative organism may be transmitted to the pregnant woman directly by medical personnel or attendants, as was demonstrated by Semmelweiss in the mid-nineteenth century. In recent years, group B streptococci have supplanted other organisms as the most frequent cause of perinatal streptococcal infections of mother and child (see below). Anaerobic streptococci, along with other anaerobic organisms, have also been implicated.

PNEUMONIA AND EMPYEMA Pneumonia due to group A streptococci is uncommon and usually occurs following viral infections such as influenza, measles, pertussis, or varicella. The illness occurs in epidemic form in military recruit camps and is characterized by abrupt onset of fever, chills, myalgia, dyspnea, cough, pleuritic chest pain, and hemoptysis. Patients are severely ill and often cyanotic. Pathologically and radiologically, this is usually a bronchopneumonia, and lobar consolidation is uncommon. A characteristic feature of streptococcal pneumonia is the early and rapid accumulation of copious amounts of thin, serosanguinous empyema fluid. Bacteremia occurs in 10 to 15 percent of cases. Extension of the pneumonic process to the pericardium may give rise to a purulent pericarditis. Other potential complications include mediastinitis, pneumothorax, and bronchiectasis. Therapy consists of 4 to 6 million units parenteral penicillin in the form of aqueous procaine penicillin G, given every 6 to 12 h intramuscularly, or intravenous aqueous crystalline penicillin G, and adequate drainage of empyema fluid, which usually requires insertion of a chest tube.

GROUP B STREPTOCOCCAL INFECTIONS

Streptococci belonging to serogroup B have long been of interest to veterinarians because of their association with bovine mastitis, an association which led to their species designation as *S. agalactiae*. The organisms are beta-hemolytic and usually, but not uniformly, resistant to bacitracin. In addition to the presence of group B carbohydrate in their cell walls, *S. agalactiae* may be identified by biochemical means, including their production of hippuricase and so-called "cyclic AMP factor." Group B streptococci may be subdivided by means of surface polysaccharides and protein antigens into five serotypes: Ia, Ib, Ic, II, and III.

Human strains of group B streptococci, which appear to be biologically distinct from bovine strains, frequently colonize the female genital tract as well as the throat and rectum. Asymptomatic vaginal carriage rates in postpubertal women generally have ranged between 6 and 25 percent, depending on the bacteriologic methods employed and on the socioeconomic status and geographic residence of the women sampled. The majority of serious group B infections occur as perinatal events. Maternal infections include chorioamnionitis, septic abortion, and puerperal sepsis. *Streptococcus agalactiae* now ranks with *Escherichia coli* as one of the two most frequent causes of neonatal sepsis and meningitis. Neonatal disease takes one of two forms. Early-onset disease, occurring within the first 10 days of life, is usually due to organisms acquired from the maternal genital tract. It involves primarily the lungs, probably as a result of aspiration of infected amniotic fluid, but the organism can be cultured from many sites such as the blood, nasopharynx, skin, and myocardium. Early-onset group B streptococcal infection occurs in approximately two of every thousand live births (the incidence is higher following prolonged or complicated delivery) and is attended by a high mortality rate. Late-onset disease occurs in infants over 10 days old, may be due to nosocomial transmission of group B streptococci, is manifested primarily by meningitis and bacteremia, and has a lower mortality rate than early-onset disease. Although the serotypes involved in early-onset illness are variable, type III organisms predominate as the cause of late-onset meningeal infection. Transplacentally acquired antibodies to type III organisms may protect against late-onset disease: they are reported to be present in serums of most women delivering healthy babies but are usually lacking in serums of mothers whose offspring develop late-onset meningitis due to type III group B streptococci.

Group B streptococci also cause a group of adult infections not associated with the puerperium. These include urinary tract infections in both sexes; the infections in men often occur in elderly individuals, perhaps due to associated prostatism. A second syndrome occurs in patients with adult-onset, insulin-dependent diabetes mellitus, peripheral vascular insufficiency, and suppurative gangrenous lesions, infected with *S. agalactiae.* Bacteremia may accompany this syndrome. Other adult infections due to group B organisms include endocarditis, pneumonia, empyema, meningitis, peritonitis, and terminal bacteremia in patients with malignancy. Although recovered from a small proportion of throat cultures, group B streptococci are rarely, if ever, the cause of clinically significant pharyngitis. All strains are susceptible to penicillin, which is the drug of choice, although group B organisms have slightly higher minimal inhibitory concentrations for penicillin than do group A strains. Only occasional strains are resistant to erythromycin. Tetracyclines should not be used without prior susceptibility testing because resistance to them is quite common.

OTHER STREPTOCOCCAL INFECTIONS

Streptococci of groups C and G are capable of causing exudative pharyngitis, and epidemics of upper respiratory disease due to these organisms have been reported, particularly following ingestion of contaminated food items. Strains of both serogroups produce streptolysin O, and pharyngeal infections with groups C and G elicit rises in ASO titer. However, most reported instances of human disease due to these two serogroups have been skin and wound infections or puerperal infections. Associated bacteremia may result in endocarditis.

Lancefield's group D streptococci consist of enterococcal species (*S. faecalis, S. faecium, S. durans*) and nonenterococci (*S. bovis, S. equinus*). Group D streptococci are frequent causes of urinary tract infection in patients with structural abnormalities of the urinary tract and frequently are associated with bacterial endocarditis. These microorganisms are usually alpha-hemolytic or nonhemolytic but may be beta-hemolytic. The treatment of severe enterococcal infections, particularly bacterial endocarditis, is complicated by the fact that the organisms are frequently resistant to many antibiotics, including the penicillins. In the therapy of enterococcal endocarditis, a combination of intravenous penicillin G or ampicillin in high doses plus an aminoglycoside antibiotic should be used, because this combination exerts a synergistic effect in the killing of enterococci (Chap. 243). While formerly streptomycin was the aminoglycoside of choice, high-level resistance (>2000 µg/ml) to streptomycin and kanamycin has been found in a significant number of enterococcal isolates. This is due to a plasmid which is transferable, by conjugation under laboratory conditions, from resistant to sensitive strains. For this reason, aminoglycosides such as gentamicin or tobramycin should be used along with penicillin or ampicillin in treatment of serious enterococcal infections.

In contrast, nonenterococcal group D streptococci, of which *S. bovis* is the only known pathogen, remain extremely sensitive to penicillin and are amenable to therapy with this agent alone. Laboratory differentiation of *S. bovis* from enterococci is sometimes difficult. Likewise, *S. mutans,* a penicillin-sensitive viridans streptococcus which is normally found in the mouth and occasionally causes endocarditis, may be confused with group D streptococci. A series of precise biochemical tests is required to identify the various species correctly. In particular, enterococci grow in 6.5% sodium chloride broth, while *S. bovis* and *S. mutans* do not. Treatment of life-threatening enterococcal infections in patients who cannot tolerate penicillin is difficult. Cephalothin and clindamycin are of no value, but vancomycin, often in combination with gentamicin, is likely to be effective.

Streptococci of most groups have been isolated at least occasionally from infected heart valves, soft tissues, or visceral abscesses. Such infections may occur as "opportunists" following surgical manipulation or in patients with malignant disease. Danish and Dutch investigators have reported a number of instances of meningitis and bacteremia in humans due to streptococci of serogroup R, a group of organisms well-known as pathogens of swine. In nearly all human cases there had been a history of contact with pigs.

Viridans streptococci are normal inhabitants of the oropharynx and gastrointestinal tract. They remain the most frequent causative agents of subacute bacterial endocarditis (Chap. 243). The taxonomy of these organisms is confused, but one classification scheme recognizes five species (in addition to *S. pneumoniae*): *salivarius, mitior, milleri, sanguis,* and *mutans.* Although viridans streptococci are not usually considered to be highly invasive, *S. milleri* is capable of causing serious pyogenic infections such as liver and brain abscesses, peritonitis, and empyema. Cases of endocarditis due to *S. milleri* are more likely to be complicated by abscess formation in peripheral tissues than are similar infections due to other species of viridans streptococci. *Streptococcus milleri* is usually considered "microaerophilic," and its clinical behavior is similar to that of the anaerobic streptococci. All the viridans species, including *S. milleri,* are susceptible to penicillin. Modest increases in the minimal inhibitory concentrations of oral streptococci to penicillin occur following prolonged oral therapy with this antibiotic.

Anaerobic streptococci (see also Chap. 142) abound in the mouth, intestinal tract, and vagina. They may be found, either alone or in combination with other anaerobic and aerobic microorganisms, in abscess cavities throughout the body. In the head and neck, anaerobic streptococci may be found in infected paranasal sinuses, brain abscess, dental abscess, infections of the retropharyngeal or lateral pharyngeal spaces, and in cases of Ludwig's angina. In the chest, these organisms occur in lung abscesses and empyema fluids. Abscesses of the liver and other intraabdominal viscera, as well as perirectal abscesses and pelvic abscesses in women, may be due in part to peptostreptococci. Finally, these organisms may thrive in dead or devitalized muscle, skin, or subcutaneous tissue. *Streptococcal myositis* is characterized by marked edema, crepitant myositis, pain, and the presence of chains of gram-positive cocci in a seropurulent exudate. *Progressive synergistic gangrene* usually develops about a surgical incision and consists of an ulcerated lesion surrounded by gangrenous skin. The infection is associated particularly with the use of through-and-through sutures after abdominal surgery, and is thought most often to be due to the synergistic action of *S. aureus* and microaerophilic streptococci. *Chronic burrowing ulcer* is a deep soft-tissue infection caused by microaerophilic streptococci which erodes through subcutaneous tissue to emerge as an ulcer at a distant site. Management of anaerobic streptococcal infections consists of drainage of abscesses, debridement of devitalized tissues, and high-dose intravenous penicillin therapy.

REFERENCES

BAKER CJ, DENNIS KL: Immunological investigation of infants with septicemia and meningitis due to group B streptococcus. J Infect Dis 136:598, 1977

BISNO AL et al: Factors influencing serum antibody responses in streptococcal pyoderma. J Lab Clin Med 81:410, 1973

DUMA RJ et al: Streptococcal infections: A bacteriologic and clinical study of streptococcal bacteremia. Medicine 48:87, 1969

KAPLAN EL et al: Diagnosis of streptococcal pharyngitis: Differentiation of active infection from the carrier state in the symptomatic child. J Infect Dis 123:490, 1971

KROGSTAD DJ: Plasmid-mediated resistance to antibiotic synergism to enterococci. J Clin Invest 61:1645, 1978

LERNER PI et al: Group B streptococcus (*S. agalactiae*) bacteremia in adults: Analysis of 32 cases and review of the literature. Medicine 56:457, 1977

MURRAY HW et al: Serious infections caused by *Streptococcus milleri.* Am J Med 64:759, 1978

STOLLERMAN GH: *Rheumatic Fever and Streptococcal Infection.* New York, Grune & Stratton, 1975

WANNAMAKER LW: Differences between streptococcal infections of the throat and the skin. N Engl J Med 282:23, 1970

section 3 | Diseases caused by gram-negative cocci

118
MENINGOCOCCAL INFECTIONS

HARRY N. BEATY

DEFINITION *Neisseria meningitidis* is the causative organism of a variety of infections, notably meningitis and bacteremia.

ETIOLOGY The organism responsible for "cerebrospinal fever" was first described by Weichselbaum in 1887. It was subsequently assigned to the genus *Neisseria,* and is now designated by the binominal *Neisseria meningitidis* and the common name meningococcus. In stained smears, meningococci are gram-negative and characteristically appear as single cocci or diplococci with flattened adjacent sides. They grow well on solid or semisolid media containing blood, serum, or ascitic fluid, and thrive best at temperatures between 35 and 37°C in an atmosphere reduced in oxygen and containing 5 to 10 percent CO_2. The organism is recovered readily from biologic fluids when fresh specimens are inoculated on warm chocolate agar plates which are incubated 18 to 24 h in a candle jar or in a more sophisticated apparatus that provides a suitable environment.

The biochemical reactions of the *Neisseria* are relatively limited, but they contain cytochrome oxidase, which is responsible for the positive "oxidase" test; the clinically significant species usually are differentiated by their ability to produce acid in glucose, maltose, or sucrose. Typically the meningococcus ferments both glucose and maltose, but on occasion maltose-negative strains have been isolated.

Meningococci can be divided into serologic groups on the basis of agglutination reactions with immune serum. The present classification into groups A, B, C, and D was agreed upon in 1950, but since 1960, new groups including X, Y, and Z have been identified. The major groups are remarkably heterogeneous, but subclassification with bacteriocin typing or additional serologic markers has been possible. Subcapsular antigens, some of which are proteins, have provided the basis for serological typing schemes, which have been used to divide strains of groups A, B, C, and Y into distinct types that are independent of their capsular serogroup.

EPIDEMIOLOGY The natural habitat of meningococci is the nasopharynx of humans, and no other reservoir or vector has been recognized. The principal means of spread is through inhalation of droplets of infected nasopharyngeal secretions. It is unlikely that the disease is spread by contact with contaminated fomites. Meningococci cause either epidemic or sporadic disease, and there is a cyclic variation in the prevalence of meningococcal infection with peaks of increased frequency occurring every 8 to 12 years and lasting 4 to 6 years. A minor upward trend in this cycle began in the United States in 1962 and reached a peak in 1965. For the epidemic years 1967 through 1971, the attack rate of meningococcal disease was lower and constant, but subsequently it has declined further. The prevalence of meningococcal infection is also subject to seasonal influences; the lowest attack rate occurs in midsummer and the highest in late winter and early spring. This seasonal variation follows that of other bacterial and viral respiratory infections.

The attack rate of meningococcal disease is highest for children between 6 months and 1 year of age. A second, much lower, peak in incidence occurs among adolescents, and the lowest attack rate occurs in individuals over 25. There is no clear-cut tendency for racial or sexual predominance, but presumably because of an increased opportunity to acquire infection, males develop meningitis and meningococcemia more frequently than females. The attack rate in household contacts of sporadic cases of meningococcal disease is 1000 times the overall endemic rate; in epidemic periods, the attack rate among household contacts may be as much as 15,000 times that of the general population. Experience with recent group A outbreaks in Alaska and the northwestern part of the United States indicates that alcoholics and Alaska natives are at increased risk for infection. Military recruits also are particularly susceptible to meningococcal disease, although outbreaks that appear to be restricted to the military usually parallel less apparent trends in the civilian population.

Since 1915, most epidemics of meningococcal disease have been caused by group A meningococci, and strains of groups B and C have been associated with sporadic, interepidemic infections. However, in the United States outbreaks of 1963 and 1964 a major shift in the pattern of meningococcal infection became apparent as group B meningococci were isolated from the majority of clinical infections in both civilian and military populations. In 1967, over 70 percent of meningococci isolated were group B. However, early in 1968, another shift began, and in the epidemic years 1969 through 1972, the majority of meningococcal strains submitted to the Center for Disease Control were group C. More recently, group B has again become the most prevalent serogroup isolated in the United States, and group Y is increasing in importance. This organism is more likely to cause respiratory disease and pneumonia than meningococcemia and meningitis.

Only a small proportion of the meningococci isolated in this country are group A. However, in Alaska and the Pacific Northwest, group A organisms are isolated from 30 to 60 percent of patients with meningococcal disease.

Studies using a serotyping system have allowed identification of a few strains that possess unique epidemic potential. Isolates from group B, C, and Y outbreaks are almost exclusively representatives of two serotypes, with type CII predominating. These observations may have great significance in future vaccine development, because in the case of group B organisms, it is the type-specific antigen which induces bactericidal antibody formation.

Coincident with these epidemiologic shifts has been a waxing and waning of the proportion of isolates which are resistant to sulfadiazine. When the majority of meningococci causing disease were group B, most strains were resistant to sulfadiazine. Today, approximately 95 percent are sensitive. Similarly, as group C emerged as the predominant serogroup, sulfadiazine resistance was the rule, but in the epidemic year 1974, about one-third of group C isolates were sensitive. Sulfadiazine resistance has been recognized among isolates of all major serogroups, and future major shifts may occur.

The potential for the meningococcus to produce serious outbreaks of disease has been reemphasized by recent events in Brazil and Finland. A large urban epidemic was first recognized in São Paulo in 1971, and it increased in intensity over the next several years. In 1974, the predominant strain of meningococcus producing disease there changed abruptly from group C to group A, and the epidemic spread to other major cities in Brazil. In July and August, 1974, about 13,000 cases of meningococcal disease occurred in São Paulo alone. An epidemic of group A meningococcal disease began in Finland early in 1973. It peaked in 1974 when the incidence of infection rose to 15 per 100,000 population (in the same year, there were 0.6 cases per 100,000 population in the United States). Massive immunization programs apparently have curtailed both of these major epidemics.

Carriers Between epidemics, 2 to 15 percent of the individuals in urban centers harbor meningococci in the nasopharynx. When sporadic cases of meningococcal disease occur, the carrier rate in close contacts may rise to 40 percent, and in closed populations or during epidemics, may approach 100 percent. Although some individuals harbor meningococci for years, nasopharyngeal infection is usually transient, and in 75 percent of carriers the organism disappears within a few weeks to a few months. The relation between the proportion of carriers in a population and the occurrence of meningococcal disease is unclear. Case-to-case transmission of infection is documented rarely, and carriers, not patients, are the foci from which disease is spread. It appears that the prevalence of meningococcal disease can be attributed to the prevailing carrier rate only in a general way, and that the occurrence of clinical disease is most dependent on unknown circumstances within the host which lead to spread of infection beyond the nasopharynx.

Immunity The fact that meningococcal meningitis is primarily a disease of childhood has suggested that natural immunity develops in most individuals within the first two decades of life. There is a correlation between susceptibility to meningococcal disease and absence of bactericidal antibody in the serum, and the serum of most adults contains antibodies to pathogenic strains of meningococci. Natural immunization appears to result from asymptomatic carriage of meningococci in the nasopharynx. Not only does the carrier state produce antibodies to the infecting strain, but cross-reacting antibodies may develop, even after colonization with avirulent nongroupable organisms. Nasopharyngeal carriage of a closely related species, *N. lactamica,* also may play a role in the development of natural immunity to meningococcal disease.

The immunity conferred by meningococcal meningitis or meningococcemia is usually group-specific, and second episodes of meningococcal disease have been encountered only infrequently.

PATHOGENESIS The primary focus of meningococcal infection is the nasopharynx. In most instances, this infection is subclinical, but occasionally localized inflammation occurs and mild symptoms develop. Dissemination of meningococci from the nasopharynx occurs via the bloodstream, and generally is followed by clinical manifestations of meningococcal disease. *Purulent meningitis* is the most common form of metastatic infection encountered and is either associated with signs and symptoms of meningococcemia or constitutes the predominant clinical expression of illness. Organisms in the meninges induce an acute inflammatory reaction, and purulent exudate spreads across the surface of the brain. Rarely, a more extensive inflammatory reaction is responsible for an acute diffuse encephalitis.

Although the mechanisms responsible for the pathologic changes associated with meningococcal infection have not been explained entirely, the tissue injury observed in laboratory animals appears to be caused by an endotoxin which is biochemically and biologically similar to endotoxins of enteric bacilli. It may be responsible for hypotension and vascular collapse observed in fulminant meningococcemia and may also play a role in the pathogenesis of the purpura and visceral hemorrhages associated with meningococcal bacteremia. Thrombosis of dermal venules, adrenal sinusoids, and renal glomerular capillaries is most commonly seen in patients who die of fulminant meningococcemia and is strikingly similar to the pathologic changes observed in the experimental Shwartzman reaction. It is postulated that endotoxin either induces a Shwartzman reaction directly or effects the release of clotting factors which initiate intravascular coagulation and produce these characteristic pathologic changes.

CLINICAL MANIFESTATIONS Ninety to ninety-five percent of patients with meningococcal disease have meningococcemia and/or meningitis.

Meningococcemia Thirty to fifty percent of patients who develop overt disease have meningococcemia without meningitis.

The onset of clinical illness may be abrupt, but patients usually have nonspecific prodromal symptoms of cough, headache, and sore throat followed by the sudden development of spiking fever, chills, arthralgia, and muscle pains which may be particularly severe in the lower extremities and back. Patients usually appear acutely ill with an inordinate degree of prostration. In addition to high fever, tachycardia, and tachypnea, mild hypotension may be present. However, clinical shock does not occur unless fulminant meningococcemia supervenes. In the course of meningococcal bacteremia, about three-fourths of the patients develop a characteristic petechial rash. Lesions are frequently sparse, and the axillae, flanks, wrists, and ankles are the most commonly involved sites. Often petechiae are located in the center of lighter-colored macules, and they may become nodular as the disease progresses. The diagnosis of meningococcemia occasionally can be established by demonstrating gram-negative diplococci in scrapings from these nodular lesions. In severe cases, purpuric spots or large ecchymoses develop, and a widespread petechial or purpuric eruption suggests fulminating disease. However, the absence of rash does not necessarily indicate that the illness will be mild.

Fulminant meningococcemia, or the Waterhouse-Friderichsen syndrome, is meningococcemia associated with vasomotor collapse and shock. It occurs in 10 to 20 percent of patients with generalized meningococcal infection, and is associated with a high fatality rate. The onset is abrupt, and profound prostration frequently occurs within a few hours. Petechiae and purpuric lesions enlarge rapidly, and hemorrhage into the skin may be extensive. Early in the preshock stage, there is generalized vasoconstriction; patients are alert and pale, with circumoral cyanosis and cold extremities. Upon entering the shock stage, however, coma develops, the cardiac output decreases, and the blood pressure drops. Unless incipient shock is recognized and appropriate therapy instituted early, death from cardiac and/or respiratory failure almost invariably occurs. Patients who recover may have extensive sloughing of skin lesions and even loss of digits because of gangrene.

Chronic meningococcemia is a rare form of meningococcal infection which lasts for weeks or months and is characterized by fever, rash, and arthritis or arthralgia. Typically, the fever is intermittent, and during afebrile periods, which may last several days, patients appear remarkably well. The usual rash is a maculopapular or polymorphous eruption which waxes and wanes with the fever, but petechial or nodular lesions may be seen. Joint involvement is present in two-thirds of the patients, and splenomegaly is detected in about 20 percent. If the diagnosis is not suspected or treatment is otherwise delayed, complications such as meningitis, carditis, or nephritis may occur.

Meningitis Meningitis is a common form of meningococcal disease which occurs primarily in children over 6 months of age and in adolescents. Fever, vomiting, headache, and confusion or lethargy are the commonest symptoms; in about one-fourth of the patients, symptoms begin abruptly and rapidly increase in severity. The more typical patient, however, has symptoms of an upper respiratory tract infection followed by an illness which progresses over several days. Twenty to forty percent of patients have meningitis without clinical evidence of meningococcemia, and the diagnosis depends upon bacteriologic examination of the cerebrospinal fluid. However, when meningitis occurs in association with a petechial or purpuric rash, a presumptive diagnosis of meningococcal disease is warranted, because this pattern of illness is seen only rarely in other infections.

Barer manifestations The meningococcus is a rare cause of purulent conjunctivitis or sinusitis. Primary pneumonia previously was considered a rare manifestation of meningococcal infection, but increasing numbers of cases are being reported. In one study of military recruits, 68 cases of clinical pneumonia due to group Y meningococci were reported. Bacterial endocarditis, primary pericarditis, and osteomyelitis have also been reported. On rare occasion, meningococci have produced genital infections clinically indistinguishable from gonococcal disease. *Neisseria meningitidis* has been isolated with increasing frequency from the genitourinary tract and anal canal of symptomatic and asymptomatic patients of both sexes.

LABORATORY FINDINGS Aside from bacteriologic data, laboratory studies are of little value in establishing the diagnosis of meningococcal infection. Polymorphonuclear leukocyte counts usually range from 12,000 to 40,000 cells per cubic millimeter, but in meningococcemia, normal or low leukocyte counts may be encountered. Anemia is uncommon, and levels of serum electrolytes and blood urea nitrogen are normal unless shock develops. Patients with prominent hemorrhagic manifestations may have low platelet counts and decreased levels of circulating clotting factors as a result of intravascular coagulation. In meningitis, the cerebrospinal fluid pressure is increased, and the fluid usually contains from 100 to 40,000 polymorphonuclear leukocytes per cubic millimeter. The protein content is increased, and the concentration of glucose is almost always less than 35 mg per 100 ml and often is between 0 and 10 mg per 100 ml.

Meningococci can be recovered readily from cultures of blood or spinal fluid, and, on occasion, material aspirated from skin lesions or joints yields the organism. In addition, gram-negative diplococci may be seen in stains of nodular petechiae or the buffy coat of blood from patients with meningococcemia. In meningococcal meningitis, a smear of the spinal fluid is diagnostic in about half the patients but often shows only a few intracellular bacteria which are located with difficulty.

COMPLICATIONS Herpes labialis occurs in 5 to 20 percent of patients with meningococcal disease. Other complications, which result from neurologic damage or secondary foci of infection, are uncommon following appropriate treatment and are often transient. Seizures or deafness occur in 10 to 20 percent of patients during the acute stages of meningitis, but postmeningitic epilepsy is rare, and the frequency of permanent eighth nerve damage is probably less than 5 percent. Peripheral neuropathy, cranial nerve palsies, and hemiplegia are seen occasionally, but usually clear completely within 2 to 4 months. Hydrocephalus and thrombosis of venous sinuses, once frequent sequelae of meningococcal meningitis, are encountered rarely. A number of patients complain of recurrent headache, emotional lability, insomnia, backache, memory loss, and difficulty in concentrating for months after an episode of meningitis. The organic basis for these symptoms is obscure, but they usually disappear a year or two after the infection.

Arthritis is a common metastatic complication of meningococcemia and occurs in 2 to 10 percent of patients. As a rule, multiple joints are involved, and signs and symptoms may not appear until after treatment of meningitis or meningococcemia has been instituted. Joint fluid usually contains many granulocytes, but meningococci are recovered infrequently. Antibiotic therapy does not appear to influence the course of the arthritis, and permanent joint changes are rare. Other purulent complications have become extremely uncommon since antibiotics have gained widespread use. Pneumonia occurs occasionally, but it is uncertain whether it is caused by the meningococcus or coincident infection with other bacteria. Bacterial endocarditis is quite rare, but *a high proportion of patients who die of meningococcal infection have myocarditis*. The etiology of these myocardial changes is uncertain, but cardiac failure may be an important factor in the pathogenesis of the shock syndrome in meningococcemia. A pericardial friction rub or electrocardiographic change of pericarditis is seen in about 5 percent of patients, and rarely purulent pericarditis may develop.

DIAGNOSIS The diagnosis of meningococcal disease depends upon recovering *N. meningitidis* from cultures of blood, spinal fluid, or petechial scrapings from patients with a typical clinical picture. Where available, counterimmunoelectrophoresis of biological fluids to detect meningococcal antigen may be helpful. Recovery of meningococci from the nasopharynx does not, in itself, establish the diagnosis.

Few diseases need to be considered seriously in the differential diagnosis of meningococcal disease. If meningococcal meningitis is not accompanied by manifestations of bacteremia, it is indistinguishable from meningitis caused by other common pathogens. Occasionally, the common viral exanthems, Rocky Mountain spotted fever (Chap. 164), and vascular purpuras may be confused with meningococcemia, and their differentiation depends upon demonstration of the organism and knowledge of the epidemiology and clinical manifestations of each disease.

TREATMENT Antimicrobial therapy of suspected or documented meningococcal disease should be instituted as early as possible. Penicillin G is the drug of choice, and should be administered intravenously. The dosage for treatment of meningitis in adults is 12 to 24 million units per day, and in the pediatric age group, 16 million units per square meter (day). Meningococcemia can be treated with 5 to 10 million units per day, because it is not necessary to achieve high levels of antibiotic in the spinal fluid. If treatment with these doses is continued for a minimum of 7 days, or 4 to 5 days after the patient becomes afebrile, relapse is extremely rare. Ampicillin in doses of 200 to 400 mg/kg per day is as effective as penicillin G. When bacteriologic confirmation of meningococcal disease is available, however, treatment should be switched to penicillin G because it is less costly. Meningococci are susceptible to other antimicrobial agents such as chloramphenicol and tetracycline, but they should not be used unless a patient is allergic to penicillin. Under these circumstances, chloramphenicol hemisuccinate 4.0 to 6.0 g per day in divided doses (in adults) is an acceptable alternate. Sensitivity tests usually indicate that cephalothin could be a suitable alternative to penicillin, but treatment failures with this drug have been reported. *Because a significant proportion of meningococci isolated are resistant to sulfonamides, these drugs should not be used alone in the treatment of meningococcal infections,* and their use in combination with penicillin offers no advantage.

Patients with meningococcal infections require supportive treatment as well as antimicrobial therapy. Maintenance of fluid and electrolyte balance and prevention of respiratory complications in comatose patients are of primary concern. When shock occurs, visceral perfusion must be improved by maintenance of an adequate intravascular volume, treatment of heart failure, and support of the blood pressure. Vasoactive drugs should be employed according to the pathophysiologic derangement in each individual case. These derangements can be determined best by carefully monitoring the blood pressure, pulse, arterial blood gases, cardiac output, peripheral resistance, pulmonary artery wedge pressures, and arteriovenous oxygen differences. When blood pressure must be raised immediately, norepinephrine may be indicated. However, if improved tissue perfusion is the primary goal, an agent such as dopamine is likely to be more effective. When heart failure is present, diuretics and digitalis should be given. When intravas-

cular coagulation is recognized, treatment with heparin, whole blood, or fibrinogen can be tried, but dramatic results should not be expected. Massive doses of adrenal cortical steroids as used in the treatment of septic shock (Chap. 109) may be helpful, but lower "replacement" doses are of uncertain value.

PREVENTION With the widespread emergence of sulfonamide-resistant meningococci, alternate methods of preventing meningococcal disease in closed populations were sought. High-molecular-weight polysaccharide antigens from organisms of serogroups A and C have been shown to induce a group-specific bactericidal antibody response after subcutaneous injection. Large-scale field trials with the group C vaccine led to a 90 percent reduction in group C disease among vaccinated recruits. Similar results have been observed with group A vaccine in the Brazilian and Finnish epidemics. An effective group B vaccine has not yet been developed.

For intimate contacts of sporadic cases of meningococcal disease, chemoprophylaxis should be administered. If the organism isolated from the patient is sensitive to sulfonamides, these drugs are preferred for prophylaxis. When sensitivities are not known or the organism is resistant to sulfonamides, rifampin in dosage of 600 mg a day for 4 days or minocycline in dosage of 100 mg every 12 h for 5 days can be expected to temporarily eradicate the carrier state and minimize spread of meningococci. Because of some reports of a high incidence of vestibular symptoms with minocycline, rifampin is considered by some to be the drug of choice. However, in large populations, rifampin may not be effective because of rapid appearance of rifampin resistance.

With increased availability of group A and C vaccines, their use as adjuncts to chemoprophylaxis for household or other intimate contacts of sporadic cases of group A or C meningococcal disease has been recommended. The rationale behind this recommendation is sound, and this approach to prevention of secondary cases deserves consideration.

PROGNOSIS Before the introduction of antibiotics, meningococcal meningitis, and meningococcemia were almost invariably fatal. With prompt and appropriate chemotherapy, the mortality rate of meningitis without fulminant meningococcemia has dropped to less than 10 percent in the United States, and neurologic sequelae are rare. The mortality of fulminant infection remains high primarily because patients are often in irreversible shock when treatment is instituted. Most deaths occur within 24 to 48 h of admission, and the capacity of the meningococcus to kill a perfectly healthy individual within a few hours remains one of the most awesome characteristics of this disease.

REFERENCES

Davis CE, Arnold K: Role of meningococcal endotoxin in meningococcal purpura. J Exp Med 140:158, 1974

Jacobson JA et al: Trends in meningococcal disease, 1974. J Infect Dis 132:480, 1975

Koppes, GM et al: Group Y meningococcal disease in United States Air Force recruits. Am J Med 62:661, 1977

McCormick JB, Bennett JV: Public health considerations in the management of meningococcal disease. Ann Intern Med 83:883, 1975

Meningococcal Disease Surveillance Group: Analysis of endemic meningococcal disease by serogroup and evaluation of chemoprophylaxis. J Infect Dis 134:201, 1976

PELTOLA H et al: Vaccination against meningococcal group A disease in Finland 1974–75. Scand J Infect Dis 8:169, 1976

—— et al: Clinical efficacy of meningococcus Group A capsular polysaccharide vaccine in children three months to five years of age. N Engl J Med 297:686, 1977

SMILACK JD: Group Y meningococcal disease. Ann Intern Med 81:740, 1974

119
GONOCOCCAL INFECTIONS

KING K. HOLMES

DEFINITION Gonorrhea, an infection of columnar and transitional epithelium caused by *Neisseria gonorrhoeae,* is the most common reportable communicable disease in the United States. Anatomic sites which can be infected directly by the gonococcus include the urethra, anal canal, conjunctivas, pharynx, and endocervix. Local complications include endometritis, salpingitis, peritonitis, and bartholinitis in the female, and periurethral abscess and epididymitis in the male. Systemic manifestations of gonococcemia include arthritis, dermatitis, endocarditis, and meningitis as well as myopericarditis and hepatitis.

ETIOLOGY *Neisseria gonorrhoeae* is a gram-negative diplococcus which forms oxidase-positive colonies and is differentiated from other *Neisseria* by its ability to dissimilate glucose, but not maltose, sucrose, or lactose, or by specific immunofluorescent staining.

At least four morphologically distinct forms of colonies occur when gonococci are passed in vitro. Colony forms T_1 and T_2 retain virulence during repeated selective subculture in vitro and are covered by surface projections called *pili,* which are visible on electron microscopy. Spontaneous transition to colony forms T_3 and T_4 results in some loss of virulence, together with disappearance of pili. Gonococcal strains cannot be differentiated by colonial morphology since each strain gives rise to all colony forms. However, gonococcal strains now can be typed on the basis of nutritional auxotrophic requirements (auxotyping) or surface antigenic variation.

EPIDEMIOLOGY The only natural hosts for *N. gonorrhoeae* are humans. One million cases of gonorrhea were reported in the United States in 1977, and an estimated 2 million cases went unreported. The annual incidence rates quadrupled from 1960 to 1975 and then leveled off. The peak incidence rates occur from ages 20 to 24 (2 cases per 100 population per year); 85 percent of the cases are age 30 or younger. The reported incidence rate in the United States is now three times higher than in England and Wales. The true incidence rate is probably nearly 10 times higher in the United States, since reporting of gonorrhea is far more complete in the United Kingdom, where most patients with gonorrhea are seen in public clinics for sexually transmitted diseases. Suboptimal clinical practice, including use of subcurative therapy and especially failure to trace infected contacts, probably contributes to the higher incidence rate in the United States.

Gonorrhea incidence and prevalence rates are known to be related to age, sex, race, socioeconomic status, and marital status—risk factors which influence sexual behavior, illness behavior, and accessibility of health care. The highest rates occur at ages 18 to 19, in noncaucasians, in the poor, in large cities, and in unmarried persons—particularly those who live alone.

The incidence is perceived as highest in men, while the prevalence is perceived as highest in women. The prevalence rate is so high among women in the United States that endocervical cultures are advocated for gonorrhea case detection in sexually active asymptomatic women age 30 or under. Approximately 2 percent of women tested by private physicians have gonorrhea. Unfortunately, there is now greater reliance in the United States upon routine endocervical culturing than upon contact tracing, which is far more efficient for control of gonorrhea. The single most important axiom about the epidemiology of this disease is that *gonorrhea is usually spread by carriers who have no symptoms or have ignored symptoms.* Symptomatic patients, male or female, have usually been recently infected by such carriers, who must in turn be traced and treated to prevent reinfection. *Men and women with symptomatic gonorrhea should always be interviewed to identify their recent sex contacts, who should be examined and treated if infected.*

There are interesting regional differences in the antibiotic resistance of *N. gonorrhoeae.* Resistance is greatest in Southeast Asia and Africa where prophylactic or low-dose therapy is common; intermediate in the United States and Australia; and least in Scandinavia, the United Kingdom, and Western Europe. Increasing levels of gonococcal resistance to penicillin G and tetracycline were noted during the 1960s in the United States, where subcurative therapy was common and importation of resistant strains occurred during the Vietnam war. From 1970 through 1975, no further increase in resistance to these antibiotics was noted in the United States. However, in 1976, β-lactamase–producing strains of *N. gonorrhoeae,* completely resistant to penicillin and ampicillin, appeared almost simultaneously in two areas of the world: in England, where they had probably been imported from West Africa, and in the United States where they had clearly been imported from the Philippines. Infections with these penicillin-resistant gonococci are not cured by penicillin therapy. The β-lactamase enzymes produced by these strains are coded on small plasmids which have DNA sequences homologous with the β-lactamase plasmid that first appeared in *Hemophilus influenzae* just 4 years earlier. Such plasmids were not present in gonococci prior to 1976. The African and Asian β-lactamase–producing gonococci show intriguing differences. The African plasmid has a molecular weight of 3.2 million Daltons and has been found in only one particular gonococcal auxotype. The Asian plasmid, which can be found in 20 to 50 percent of gonococci isolated in some cities in the Philippine island of Luzon, is slightly larger and has entered several different auxotypes and serotypes of gonococci. This is probably because the Asian β-lactamase frequently coexists with a larger, conjugative plasmid which is capable of transferring the β-lactamase plasmid to other bacterial cells such as other types of gonococci. This type of molecular epidemiology is instructive—both β-lactamase–producing plasmids apparently enter gonococci and persist in gonococci in areas of the world where prostitution is exceptionally common and where access to subcurative antimicrobial therapy is unrestricted. Fortunately, β-lactamase–producing gonococci have not become established in any of the industrialized countries. Although localized outbreaks have occurred in several cities in the United States and England, they have been contained by rapid use of epidemiologic measures (Fig. 119-1).

CLINICAL MANIFESTATIONS The clinical spectrum of gonococcal infections depends upon the site of inoculation, the duration of infection, and the presence or absence of local or systemic spread of the organism.

Gonorrhea in the male The usual incubation period of gonococcal urethritis ("clap") in the male is 2 to 6 days following exposure, although longer intervals are not infrequent, and

FIGURE 119-1

Penicillinase-producing Neisseria gonorrhoeae (PPNG). The number of cases occurring by month in the United States (including outlying areas) from March 1976 to September 1978. (Courtesy of P Perine.)

some men never develop symptoms. In one study, one fastidious auxotype, which has distinctive nutritional requirements, was associated with 96 percent of asymptomatic infections and only 40 percent of symptomatic infections. Symptoms include a purulent urethral discharge, usually associated with dysuria and frequent urination. Although approximately 90 to 95 percent of men who acquire urethral gonococcal infection develop urethral discharge, most symptomatic men seek treatment and are removed from the infectious pool. The remaining men who never develop symptoms or who ignore their symptoms constitute about two-thirds of the infected men at any point in time, and they serve as the source of spread of infection to women. Before antibiotic treatment became available, symptoms of urethritis persisted for an average of 8 weeks, and unilateral epididymitis occurred in 5 to 10 percent of untreated men. Epididymitis is now an uncommon complication (see below), and gonococcal prostatitis occurs rarely, if at all. Other local complications of gonorrhea which are now unusual include inguinal lymphadenitis, edema of the penis due to dorsal lymphangitis or thrombophlebitis, submucous inflammatory "soft" infiltration of the urethral wall, periurethral abscess or fistula, unilateral inflammation or abscess of Cowper's gland (which lies between the thumb and forefinger when the forefinger is in the anal canal and the thumb is positioned anteriorly on the perineum), abscess of Tyson's gland(s) (which open on either side of the frenulum), and, rarely, seminal vesiculitis.

In homosexual men, anorectal and pharyngeal gonococcal infection are common. Anorectal infection may be asymptomatic from the outset or may produce anorectal burning or pruritus, tenesmus, and a bloody, mucopurulent rectal discharge. Proctoscopy is essential to exclude syphilis, lymphogranuloma venereum, granuloma inguinale, and other conditions which cause similar symptoms. These symptoms may subside without treatment, leaving a chronic asymptomatic carrier state. Pharyngeal gonococcal infection occurs in approximately 20 percent of homosexual men or heterosexual women who engage in fellatio with men who have urethral infection. Pharyngeal infection may produce exudative tonsillitis but frequently is asymptomatic.

Gonorrhea in the female Acute uncomplicated gonorrhea in the female often causes dysuria, frequent urination, increased vaginal discharge due to exudative endocervicitis, abnormal menstrual bleeding, and anorectal discomfort. While dysuria and frequency in young men arouse the suspicion of gonococcal urethritis, the same symptoms in a young woman are often automatically attributed to "cystitis." Actually, only about one-half of young women with these symptoms are found to

have at least 10^5 coliform bacteria per ml of clean voided midstream urine, while many of those without significant bacteriuria have gonococcal infection of the urethra and of Skene's glands. Young women with dysuria should have a pelvic examination and endocervical culture for gonorrhea. Compression of the urethra through the anterior vaginal wall against the symphysis pubis may express urethral exudate which can be examined by Gram's stain and culture. Acute symptoms of gonococcal urethritis in the female may subside spontaneously or following subcurative therapy with sulfonamides or urinary antiseptics. The proportion of women with gonorrhea who never develop symptoms is undefined.

Asymptomatic gonococcal infection in the female involves the endocervix, urethra, anal canal, and pharynx, in decreasing order of frequency. Extension of infection from the endocervix to the fallopian tubes occurs in at least 15 percent of women with gonorrhea. This tends to occur soon after acquisition of infection or during menstruation and results in *acute salpingitis,* the major complication of gonorrhea. Extension of infection to the pelvis may produce signs of pelvic peritonitis, accompanied by nausea and vomiting, and may lead to pelvic abscess. Early antibiotic treatment, before development of adnexal masses, restores normal tubal function and fertility in nearly all cases of salpingitis. However, if prominent adnexal swelling has occurred before treatment is begun, bilateral tubal dysfunction occurs in 15 to 25 percent.

Spread of gonococci into the upper abdomen may cause *gonococcal perihepatitis* (Fitz-Hugh–Curtis syndrome) manifested by right upper quadrant or bilateral upper abdominal pain and tenderness, and occasionally by a hepatic friction rub.

Acute inflammation of Bartholin's gland is usually unilateral and frequently is due to gonococcal infection. The acutely infected duct is surrounded by a red halo and exudes pus at the posterior third of the labium majus. Occlusion of the duct results in formation of a Bartholin's abscess. Chronic Bartholin cysts are rarely caused by active gonococcal infection.

There is suggestive evidence that endocervical gonococcal infection is associated with prematurity and prolonged labor following rupture of membranes, both of which may produce increased perinatal morbidity.

Gonorrhea in children During childbirth, the gonococcus may infect the conjunctivas, pharynx, respiratory tract, or anal canal of the newborn. The risk of contamination increases with prolonged rupture of membranes. Prevention of gonococcal ophthalmia by prophylactic use of 1% silver nitrate eyedrops has led to the emergence of inclusion conjunctivitis caused by *Chlamydia* as a more common form of ophthalmia neonatorum. During the first year of life, infection of the infant usually results from accidental contamination of the eye or vagina by an adult. Between 1 year of age and puberty, most cases of gonorrhea involve vulvovaginitis in females who have been molested by a relative, and medicolegal considerations necessitate a complete bacteriologic diagnosis.

Disseminated gonococcal infection In some areas of the world, from 1 to 3 percent of adults with gonococcal infection develop gonococcemia. Approximately two-thirds of such patients are women. The majority of men and women with gonococcemia do not have symptoms of urogenital, anorectal, or pharyngeal gonococcal infection. Gonococcemia may occur soon after acquisition of new infection or later, during menstruation. There is suggestive evidence that gonococci which cause disseminated infection are uniquely resistant to the complement-mediated bactericidal activity of normal human serum. These organisms tend to be fastidious strains with the same distinctive auxotype that is correlated with asymptomatic urethral infection in men. Patients with deficiency in the sixth, seventh, and eighth components of complement have increased susceptibility to gonococcemia and meningococcemia, but not to other infections. Nine of the first seventeen patients reported to have a deficiency of C6, C7, and C8 had at least one episode of documented bacteremia with *N. gonorrhoeae* or *N. meningitidis*. Serum bactericidal activity, rather than opsonic activity, appears essential for protection against gonococcal bacteremia.

The onset of gonococcemia is characterized by fever, polyarthralgias, and papular, petechial, pustular, hemorrhagic, or necrotic skin lesions. Approximately 3 to 20 such lesions appear, usually on the distal extremities. Gonococci are demonstrable by immunofluorescent staining in about two-thirds of gonococcal skin lesions. The initial joint involvement is characteristically limited to tenosynovitis involving several joints asymmetrically. The wrists, fingers, knees, and ankles are most often involved. Circulating immune complexes have been demonstrated at this stage of infection. Without treatment, the duration of gonococcemia is variable; the systemic manifestations of bacteremia may subside spontaneously within a week. (It is possible that many such cases go undiagnosed and the actual risk of gonococcemia exceeds current estimates.) Alternatively, septic arthritis ensues, often without prior symptoms of bacteremia. Pain and swelling then increase in one or, very occasionally, more joints, with accumulation of purulent synovial fluid, leading to progressive destruction of the joint if treatment is delayed. A continuum exists from the manifestations of bacteremia (polyarthralgias, new skin lesions) to septic arthritis, but the probability of positive blood cultures decreases after 48 h of illness, and the probability of recovery of gonococci from synovial fluid increases with increasing duration of illness. Gonococci are infrequently recovered from early effusions containing less than 20,000 leukocytes per cubic millimeter, but are usually recovered from effusions containing more than 80,000 leukocytes per cubic millimeter. In the individual patient, gonococci are seldom recovered from blood and synovial fluid simultaneously.

Other common manifestations of disseminated gonococcal infection include mild myopericarditis and "toxic" hepatitis. Endocarditis and meningitis are infrequent but severe complications. Endocarditis is suggested by pathological or changing heart murmurs, major embolic phenomena, severe myocarditis, deterioration of renal function, or an unusually large number of skin lesions.

DIFFERENTIAL DIAGNOSIS Gonococcal infection produces several common clinical syndromes which have multiple etiologies or which mimic other conditions. The differential diagnosis of urethritis in men and of vaginitis and cervicitis is discussed in Chap. 113. Three additional complications of gonorrhea are discussed below.

Pelvic inflammatory disease (PID) The incidence of acute, spontaneous PID, unrelated to obstetrical complications or surgery, can be estimated as about a half-million cases per year in the United States. About 50 percent of these are caused by *N. gonorrhoeae,* alone or in combination with cervicovaginal commensal bacteria. Nongonococcal PID is usually caused by cervicovaginal bacteria, including *Bacteroides fragilis* and anaerobic gram-positive cocci. The peak incidence of gonorrhea occurs in the late summer and autumn each year, and the proportion of cases of PID which are associated with gonococcal infection is also highest during these months.

PID should always be considered in young women with lower abdominal pain and tenderness. Pelvic examination discloses maximal tenderness in the adnexal area, which is usually bilateral and is reproduced by cervical motion. Recent onset of abnormal vaginal discharge or abnormal menstrual bleeding in a patient with abdominal pain strongly suggests PID. Fever, chills, nausea, vomiting, adnexal mass, leukocytosis, and elevation of the erythroctye sedimentation rate are common but are *not always* present. Purulent cervical exudate, onset of pain during menstruation, dysuria, proctitis, and history of recent exposure to a male with urethritis all are more common in gonococcal PID than in nongonococcal PID. The risk of PID is increased two- to ninefold in women wearing an intrauterine contraceptive device (IUD). The risk is maximal during the first 2 months after insertion, but persists as long as the device is in place. IUD-associated salpingitis usually is nongonococcal. There is no fever, and the major manifestation is indolent progression of minimally symptomatic adnexal masses.

Gonococcal perihepatitis may mimic acute cholecystitis, with transient nonvisualization of the gallbladder and mild liver function abnormalities. Perihepatitis should be distinguished from the hepatitis which occurs during gonococcemia. Perihepatitis also occurs as a complication of nongonococcal PID, presumably resulting from spread of other bacteria from the pelvis to the upper abdomen. Bacteremia and suppurative pelvic thrombophlebitis are unusual in acute spontaneously occurring PID.

The clinical diagnosis of PID is imprecise, and failure to respond to appropriate antibiotic therapy should always lead to reevaluation of the diagnosis before consideration of a change in antibiotics. Laparoscopy may disclose other diagnoses, such as ectopic pregnancy, acute appendicitis, pelvic endometriosis, corpus luteum hematoma, ovarian tumor, mesenteric lymphadenitis, or occasional complications such as tuboovarian abscess.

Epididymitis Acute epididymitis is almost always unilateral and must be differentiated from testicular torsion, tumor, and trauma. Torsion, a surgical emergency, occurs predominantly in teen-agers and is suggested by the acuteness of the pain, elevation of the testicle within the scrotal sac, and abscess of blood flow on Doppler-flow examination. In men under 35, acute epididymitis is usually caused by *N. gonorrhoeae* or *Chlamydia trachomatis* and is usually, but not always, associated with urethral exudate, demonstrable by milking the urethra. The recommended treatment includes bed rest, scrotal elevation, and antimicrobial therapy. Treatment of gonococcal epididymitis is the same as for gonococcal pelvic inflammatory disease. Optimal treatment for nongonococcal epididymitis (presumably caused by *C. trachomatis* in men under 35) is tetracycline hydrochloride, 500 mg four times daily by mouth for 10 days.

Acute epididymitis in older men is usually caused by urinary pathogens such as *Escherichia coli* or *Pseudomonas aeruginosa*. Urethritis is usually absent, but bacteriuria is present. Treatment should be with the appropriate antibiotics as determined by sensitivity tests.

Acute arthritis The gonococcal arthritis-dermatitis syndrome is probably the commonest form of acute arthritis in young adults, and must be differentiated in particular from Reiter's syndrome, other forms of septic arthritis, acute rheumatoid arthritis, and systemic lupus erythematosus. Gonococcemia may be complicated by myocarditis, which mimics acute rheumatic fever or bacterial endocarditis, and by "toxic" hepatitis, which must be differentiated from hepatitis B viremia. Meningococcemia, *Yersinia* infection, and sarcoidosis are less common causes of acute polyarthritis.

Demonstration of *N. gonorrhoeae* by culture or specific immunofluorescent antibody stain in synovial fluid, blood, cerebrospinal fluid, or skin lesions is diagnostic of acute gonococcal arthritis. Failing this, the diagnosis of gonococcal arthritis is virtually certain if (1) *N. gonorrhoeae* is recovered from the urethra, cervix, pharynx, anal canal, or conjunctiva, or from the patient's sex partner; (2) pustular, hemorrhagic, or necrotic skin lesions are distributed on the extremities; and (3) a therapeutic antibiotic trial produces subjective improvement and normal temperature within 48 h, and loss of all objective signs of arthritis within 2 weeks. Patients with gonococcal arthritis who have highly purulent synovial effusions may, however, have persistent fever and progressive arthritis despite adequate antimicrobial therapy, and may require repeated closed joint irrigations with saline before improvement occurs.

If only two of the above three criteria are met, the diagnosis of gonococcal arthritis remains probable, particularly if other diagnoses listed above are excluded. Conjunctivitis rarely occurs in gonococcal arthritis and suggests the diagnosis of Reiter's syndrome in men with acute arthritis. HLA histocompatibility haplotype B27 is associated with Reiter's syndrome but not with gonococcal arthritis. Gonococcal arthritis has been reported in several women with active lupus erythematosus, in whom hypocomplementemia may predispose to gonococcemia.

LABORATORY DIAGNOSIS The Gram's stain of urethral or endocervical exudate is considered diagnostic of gonorrhea when typical gram-negative diplococci are seen within leukocytes, is equivocal if only extracellular or atypical gram-negative diplococci are seen, and is negative if no gram-negative diplococci are seen. When these criteria are employed by experienced microbiologists, the sensitivity and specificity of Gram's stain of the urethral exudate approach 100 percent. The specificity of Gram's stain of purulent cervical exudate also is high, but the sensitivity is only 60 percent or less. Thayer-Martin (TM) medium, which contains antibiotics to inhibit most other organisms selectively, is most useful for recovering the gonococcus from the endocervix, anal canal, and pharynx, which are colonized by a mixed bacterial flora. After inoculation, the TM medium should be placed in an atmosphere containing 3 to 10 percent carbon dioxide to permit growth of the gonococcus. This can be accomplished in a candle jar, by packaging the TM medium in sealed vials to which carbon dioxide was added before sealing (Transgrow medium), or by generation of carbon dioxide chemically within packets which are sealed after inoculation. Inoculated media should be incubated at 36°C for 48 h, and putative gonococcal colonies should be confirmed by oxidase reaction, Gram's stain, and sugar fermentation tests. The latter are especially important for isolates from the pharynx and anal canal and for cultures obtained from populations which have a low prevalence of gonorrhea, such as prenatal patients. Anal canal cultures are most important as a test of cure in women, since about one-quarter of all treatment failures in women involve only that site.

In men with incubating or chronic asymptomatic urethral infection without exudate, or as a test of cure following treatment, a very thin cotton swab or wire bacteriologic loop should be inserted 2 cm into the anterior urethra and used to inoculate TM medium. Cultures of the pharynx and anal canal should be obtained from all homosexual men with suspected gonorrhea.

The most efficient test for gonorrhea in women is the endocervical culture, which is positive on a single examination in approximately 80 percent of those with gonorrhea. This diagnostic yield can be increased by performing a second endocervical culture on enriched chocolate agar medium which does not contain antibiotics and by performing cultures of the anal canal, urethra, and pharynx.

Standard blood culture broth medium containing 3 to 10 percent carbon dioxide should be used in culturing blood and is also recommended for culturing synovial fluid. In pus from skin lesions, *N. gonorrhoeae* is more often demonstrable by Gram's stain or immunofluorescent staining than by culture. A fourfold or greater rise in gonococcal antibody can be demonstrated in paired serums from many patients with gonococcal arthritis, using complement fixation, immunofluorescent, or gonococcal pili antigen-binding assays, but such tests are not generally available. Techniques designed to detect gonococcal infection by testing of a single serum have been limited thus far by inability to differentiate antibody due to past gonorrhea from antibody due to current infection, and by false-positive tests caused by cross-reactive meningococci in the pharynx.

TREATMENT The preferred drugs for gonococcal infection are penicillin G, ampicillin, or amoxicillin, tetracycline hydrochloride, and spectinomycin. As shown in Table 119-1, the Communicable Disease Center (CDC) recommended treatment schedules now list three regimens as coequal choices for uncomplicated gonorrhea in men and women. Single-dose treatment is preferred in patients who are unlikely to complete the multiple-dose tetracycline regimen. The aqueous procaine penicillin G (APPG) regimen is preferred for men with anorectal infection and for pharyngeal infection in men and women. With parenteral penicillin G, the risk of anaphylaxis in patients who deny previous penicillin allergy has been shown to be 0.04 percent. The risk of procaine reaction due to transient neurotoxic serum concentrations of procaine is probably between 0.1 and 1 percent with the currently recommended dosage. Ampicillin 3.5 g (or amoxicillin 3.0 g) can be given orally with probenecid with nearly equal efficacy and less toxicity. A single intramuscular dose of 2 g spectinomycin is adequate for gonorrhea in both sexes and is recommended for treatment failures, because gonococci which demonstrate increased resistance to penicillin, ampicillin, or tetracycline show no cross-resistance to spectinomycin. Most recurrent infections after treatment with the recommended schedules are due to *reinfection* and indicate a need for improved contact tracing and patient education. Since infection by β-lactamase–producing gonococci is a cause of treatment failure, posttreatment isolates should be tested for β-lactamase production. Spectinomycin is the treatment of choice for β-lactamase–producing *N. gonorrhoeae*.

Either spectinomycin or tetracycline can be used for penicillin-allergic patients. Tetracycline is no longer effective for gonorrhea as a single dose. Other tetracyclines are not more effective than tetracycline hydrochloride. Tetracycline has the significant advantage of curing simultaneously acquired *Chlamydia* and *Ureaplasma* infections, thus preventing postgonococcal urethritis (PGU). Usually appearing 2 or 3 weeks after treatment, PGU occurs in from 20 to 50 percent of men treated for gonorrhea with penicillin, ampicillin, or spectinomycin.

About half of the cases of PGU appear to be caused by *Chlamydia trachomatis* which was probably acquired at the same time as gonorrhea but did not become clinically apparent until later because of the longer incubation period of chlamydial infection. When PGU occurs, it can be managed, like nongonococcal urethritis, with tetracycline, 0.5 g four times a day for at least 7 days. Men and women exposed to gonorrhea should be examined, cultured, and treated with one of the recommended treatment schedules.

All patients with gonorrhea should have a serologic test for syphilis at the time of diagnosis. Patients with incubating seronegative syphilis, without clinical signs of syphilis, are likely to be cured by any of the recommended regimens (except spectinomycin) and need not have later follow-up tests for syphilis. However, patients with gonorrhea who also have syphilis or who are established contacts of someone with syphilis should be given additional treatment appropriate to the stage of syphilis. As a test of cure of gonorrhea, follow-up cervical, anal canal, and other appropriate cultures should be obtained from women, and urethral and other appropriate cultures from men,

7 to 14 days after completion of therapy. Because true treatment failure is uncommon with the recommended regimen, some authorities advocate one reexamination approximately 6 weeks after treatment, at which time approximately 15 percent of individuals are again infected, presumably because of reinfection.

Hospitalization is recommended for women with suspected salpingitis if the diagnosis is uncertain and surgical emergencies, such as appendicitis or ectopic pregnancy, must be excluded, if there is suspicion of pelvic abscess, if the patient is pregnant or unable to follow an outpatient regimen of oral medication because of nausea and vomiting, if she is severely ill, or if she is not responding to outpatient therapy. Failure to improve on recommended therapy does not indicate a need for stepwise additional antibiotics but requires clinical reassessment. Most authorities recommend removal of an intrauterine device, if present in a woman with acute PID, although the effect of an IUD on response to therapy and risk of recurrence has not been studied. The treatment schedules recommended in Table 119-1 for PID have given satisfactory short-term results in both gonococcal and nongonococcal PID in limited trials, but additional data are needed. It is clear, however, that the single-dose procaine penicillin G-probenecid regimen recommended for uncomplicated gonorrhea is inadequate for the treatment of PID, even for gonococcal PID. For ambulatory patients with nongonococcal PID, tetracycline is the preferred drug. In severe cases of PID, especially when pelvic abscess is suspected, treatment must be individualized, and alternative antibiotics and surgical drainage may be needed. Adequate treatment of women with acute salpingitis must include examination and appropriate treatment of their sex partners because of their high prevalence of nonsympatomatic urethral infection. Failure to treat sex partners is a major cause of recurrent gonococcal salpingitis.

Treatment of gonococcal arthritis can be accomplished satisfactorily with several regimens. Gonococci recovered from patients with gonococcal arthritis have been significantly less resistant to penicillin or tetracycline than isolates from patients with uncomplicated gonorrhea. However, because of the threat of endocarditis, meningitis, and joint sepsis, all patients with disseminated infection should preferably be hospitalized and treated with aqueous crystalline penicillin G intravenously, 10 million units per day until clinical improvement occurs. Treatment can then be completed on an outpatient basis with ampicillin, 2 g per day orally to complete a 7- to 10-day course of therapy. As summarized in the CDC recommendation, a 3-day course of high-dose intravenous penicillin therapy alone, or treatment with ampicillin, 3.5 g daily orally with 1 g probenecid, followed by 0.5 g four times a day for 7 days, also probably represents adequate therapy for disseminated gonococcal infection. Failure to improve with one of these regimens strongly suggests a diagnosis other than disseminated gonococcal infection. Repeated joint aspiration or closed irrigation of the joint with sterile saline may be required to reduce inflammation in patients with high synovial fluid leukocyte counts. Open drainage is seldom, if ever, required for gonococcal arthritis, except in infants with hip infection. Temporary immobilization of the joint may reduce discomfort for the patient and may be useful during initial ambulation in patients with persistent effusions of the knee or ankle. Antibiotics should not be injected directly into the joint.

Gonococcal conjunctivitis in the adult or newborn should be managed as a medical emergency by irrigation of the conjunctiva with saline, together with penicillin G given intravenously.

PREVENTION AND CONTROL There is probably no more striking illustration than gonorrhea of the failure of a specific

TABLE 119-1
Recommended treatment for gonococcal infection

Diagnosis	Treatment of choice
Uncomplicated gonococcal infection in men and women	Aqueous procaine penicillin G (APPG), 4.8 million units injected intramuscularly, at two sites with 1.0 g probenecid by mouth *or* tetracycline 0.5 g by mouth four times a day for 5 days (total dosage 10.0 g) *or* ampicillin 3.5 g (or amoxicillin 3.0 g) single oral dose, given with 1.0 g probenecid by mouth
Anorectal infection in men	APPG, 4.8 million units, with 1.0 g probenecid
Pharyngeal infection, either sex	APPG, 4.8 million units, with 1.0 g probenecid
Treatment failures	Spectinomycin, 2.0 g intramuscularly
Penicillinase-producing *N. gonorrhoeae*	Spectinomycin, 2.0 g intramuscularly
Gonorrhea in pregnancy	APPG, 4.8 million units intramuscularly with 1.0 g probenecid by mouth (if pregnant patient is allergic to penicillin, spectinomycin 2.0 g intramuscularly is recommended)
Acute PID, outpatient	Tetracycline 0.5 g orally four times a day for 10 days *or* APPG 4.8 million units intramuscularly plus 1.0 g probenecid orally, followed by ampicillin 0.5 g orally four times a day for 10 days
Acute PID, hospitalized	Aqueous crystalline penicillin G, 20 million units intravenously each day until improvement occurs, followed by ampicillin 0.5 g orally four times a day to complete 10 days of therapy. Since optimal therapy for hospitalized patients has not been established, alternative regimens, such as gentamicin plus clindamycin, or chloramphenicol, are often used for severe PID in hospitalized patients.
Acute epididymitis	Tetracycline 0.5 g orally four times a day for 10 days
Disseminated gonococcal infection	Aqueous crystalline penicillin G, 10 million units intravenously per day until improvement occurs, followed by ampicillin 0.5 g four times daily to complete 7 days of therapy *or* ampicillin 3.5 g orally with probenecid 1.0 g, followed by ampicillin 0.5 g orally four times a day for 7 days *Penicillin allergy:* Tetracycline 0.5 g orally four times daily for 7 days
Pediatric gonococcal infection	See "Gonorrhea—CDC recommended treatment schedules" in References

treatment alone to eradicate a communicable disease. Vaccination is not available, and there is some doubt as to whether any resistance to reinfection occurs during natural infection, although humoral, local, and cellular immune responses have all been demonstrated during acute or recurrent gonococcal infection. Use of the condom can prevent transmission. Prophylactic antibiotics (e.g., 200 mg minocycline or doxycycline taken soon after sexual exposure) have been shown to be effective but are not recommended for general use or for individuals with known exposure to gonorrhea, who should receive one of the regimens recommended for established gonorrhea. The efficacy of local vaginal antiseptic and spermicidal preparations for prevention of venereal disease requires further study. The most effective additional measure now available for control of gonorrhea is tracing sexual contacts of infected patients. Experienced interviewers are able to identify and bring to treatment an average of one additional case for every patient interviewed.

REFERENCES

BROOKS GF et al: Immunobiology of *Neisseria gonorrhaeae.* Washington, DC, American Society of Microbiology, 1978

CUNNINGHAM FG et al: Evaluation of tetracycline or penicillin-ampicillin for treatment of acute pelvic inflammatory disease. N Engl J Med 296:1380, 1977

ESCHENBACH DA et al: Polymicrobial etiology of acute pelvic inflammatory disease. N Engl J Med 293:166, 1975

FALK V: Treatment of acute nontuberculous salpingitis alone and in combination with glucocorticoids. Acta Obstet Gynecol Scand, vol 44, suppl 6, 1965

Gonorrhea—CDC recommended treatment schedules. Morb Mort Week Rep 28:1, 1978

HANDSFIELD HH et al: Treatment of the gonococcal arthritis-dermatitis syndrome. Ann Intern Med 84:661, 1976

HOLMES KK et al: Disseminated gonococcal infection. Ann Intern Med 74:979, 1971

JACOBSEN L, WESTROM L: Objectivized diagnosis of acute pelvic inflammatory disease. Am J Obstet Gynecol 105:1088, 1969

KARNEY WW et al: Spectinomycin vs tetracycline for the treatment of gonorrhea. N Engl J Med 296:889, 1977

KAUFMAN RE et al: National gonorrhea therapy monitoring study: Treatment results. N Engl J Med 294:1, 1976

ROBERTS M et al: Molecular characterization of two beta-lactamase specifying plasmids isolated from *Neisseria gonorrhoeae.* J Bacteriol 131:557, 1977

———, FALKOW S: Conjugal transfer of R plasmids in *Neisseria gonorrhoeae.* Nature 266:630, 1977

ROBERTS RB: *The Gonococcus.* New York, Wiley, 1977

SCHOOLNIK GK et al: Gonococci causing disseminated gonococcal infection are resistant to the bactericidal action of normal human sera. J Clin Invest 58:1163, 1976

SIEGEL MS et al: Penicillinase producing *Neisseria gonorrhoeae:* Results of surveillance in the United States. J Infect Dis 137:170, 1978

section 4 | Diseases caused by enteric gram-negative bacilli

120
INFECTIONS DUE TO ENTEROBACTERIACEAE

MARVIN TURCK
DENNIS SCHABERG

ESCHERICHIA COLI INFECTIONS

ETIOLOGY *Escherichia coli* is a group of gram-negative non-sporing rods which belong to the tribe Enterobacteriaceae. They generally ferment lactose, as opposed to the medically significant non-lactose-fermenting organisms, such as *Salmonella, Shigella,* and *Proteus.* The so-called "paracolon" bacilli are organisms which ferment lactose late, irregularly, or not at all, and on more careful biochemical and antigenic testing are found to belong to one or another of the genera of the Enterobacteriaceae, which comprise *Salmonella, Arizona, Citrobacter, Shigella, Escherichia, Klebsiella, Enterobacter, Hafnia, Serratia, Proteus,* and *Providencia.* All these organisms are readily culturable on ordinary media and are aerobic and facultatively anaerobic. All species ferment glucose, reduce nitrates to nitrites, and are oxidase-negative and catalase-positive. They are differentiated among members of their own tribe by biochemical and serologic tests. It is important to make this differentiation, not only taxonomically, but also because of epidemiologic and therapeutic implications.

PATHOGENESIS *Escherichia coli* is regarded generally as a normal commensal in the gastrointestinal tract, from which it may spread to infect contiguous structures if normal anatomic barriers are interrupted, as occurs in appendiceal perforation. It is believed that the urinary tract is infected from without via urethral contamination, but direct hematogenous spread may also account for renal infection. Once infection has occurred in a primary focus, further spread to distant organs may occur via the bloodstream. There is experimental and clinical evidence that *E. coli* tends to settle in avascular or necrotic tissue. In more than 50 percent of *E. coli* infections the urinary tract is the portal of entry; infections of the hepatobiliary tree, peritoneal cavity, skin, and lung are not uncommon. A number of patients with *E. coli* bacteremia have no demonstrable portal of entry; they often have neoplastic and hematologic diseases, and *E. coli* is considered an "opportunistic" invader. There may be other defects in host resistance, including diabetes mellitus, cirrhosis, and sickle-cell anemia, or recent administration of irradiation, cytotoxic drugs, adrenal steroids, or antibiotics. There also is epidemiologic evidence that *E. coli* and other

Enterobacteriaceae tend to colonize the skin and mucous membranes of debilitated patients, possibly accounting for the increased frequency of these infections in patients with advanced illness. Morphologically the lesions produced in various tissues show typical acute inflammation with pus and abscess formation. There is a common misconception that *E. coli* bacterial infections are characterized by a foul-smelling, feculent exudate. Such an odor is caused by anaerobic streptococci or *Bacteroides* species, which are often associated with coliform bacteria in mixed infection. In fact, organisms of the genus *Bacteroides* frequently far outnumber *E. coli* as the most prevalent gram-negative flora in the intestine.

EPIDEMIOLOGY Strains of *E. coli* are characterized by their somatic (O), flagellar (H), and capsular (K or B) antigens, and there are hundreds of different serologic varieties. Any of the strains is capable of causing disease. Clinical and epidemiologic studies have demonstrated that certain specific *E. coli* serotypes are more frequently incriminated in diarrheal disease of the infant and newborn. Strains incriminated in infantile diarrhea probably are disseminated within nurseries by symptomatic or asymptomatic infant carriers, mothers, and nurses. Although fecal contamination is the usual mode of spread, airborne contamination and fomite spread may also occur.

Some epidemiologic studies have suggested that *E. coli* 04, 06, and 075 are responsible for most *E. coli* infections other than infantile diarrhea. It is unclear whether these strains actually are more virulent or merely are more prevalent than other somatic types. In fact, virulence factors may be associated more closely with the K than with the somatic antigen, and may account for the frequency with which certain strains cause parenchymal infection.

MANIFESTATIONS **Urinary tract infections** *Escherichia coli* accounts for well over 75 percent of urinary tract infections, including cystitis, pyelitis, pyelonephritis, and asymptomatic bacteriuria. Strains cultured from patients with acute, uncomplicated urinary tract infections are almost invariably *E. coli*, whereas other Enterobacteriaceae and strains of *Pseudomonas* become prevalent among patients with chronic infection. Urinary tract infections are discussed in Chap. 280.

Peritoneal and biliary infections *Escherichia coli* can usually be cultured from a perforated or inflamed appendix or from abscesses secondary to perforated diverticula, peptic ulcers, subphrenic or lesser sac abscesses, or mesenteric infarction. Often, other organisms, including anaerobic streptococci, clostridia, and *Bacteroides*, are found along with *E. coli*. Acute cholecystitis with gangrene and perforation is often associated with *E. coli* infection. An air-fluid level associated with stones or a circumferential layer of gas in the wall of the gallbladder may be detectable by x-ray and is characteristic of acute emphysematous cholecystitis. From the gallbladder, infection may ascend via the biliary tree to produce cholangitis and multiple liver abscesses. More rarely *E. coli* infection in the peritoneal cavity may produce a septic thrombophlebitis of the portal vein (pylephlebitis), which in turn is followed by liver abscesses.

Bacteremia Invasion of the bloodstream is the most serious manifestation of *E. coli* infection; it is characterized usually by the sudden onset of fever and chills, but sometimes only by mental confusion, dyspnea, or unexplained hypotension. It is most common in patients with urinary tract infection and biliary or intraperitoneal sepsis, and following abortions or pelvic surgery. In some patients no portal of entry is evident. Most

cases occur in elderly males, presumably because of the high incidence of urethral instrumentation and catheterization in this group. Fever ranges between 100 and 106°F and is higher in younger patients. Hyperventilation may be an early sign. Hypotension may be present from the onset but usually occurs within 12 to 16 h after bacteremia; if it is persistent, it is accompanied by oliguria and often by mental confusion, stupor, and coma. The skin is warm and dry initially, but most patients develop some evidence of peripheral vasoconstriction characterized by cold and cyanotic extremities. Fortunately hypotension is transient and self-limited in most patients with *E. coli* bacteremia and is absent altogether in some. However, about 25 percent of patients with bacteremia develop more prolonged hypotension, a syndrome known as *gram-negative* or *endotoxin shock,* which is discussed in Chap. 109.

Occasionally *E. coli* bacteremia develops in patients with cirrhosis without an overt portal of entry. This has been variably attributed to portosystemic shunts both in and around the liver, impaired reticuloendothelial function, and diminution in humoral and cellular defense mechanisms.

Other manifestations *Escherichia coli* may produce abscesses anywhere in the body. Subcutaneous infections are found at the site of insulin administration in diabetics, in extremities with ischemic gangrene, or in surgical wounds. Perirectal phlegmons are not uncommon in patients with leukemia. Subcutaneous abscesses are often characterized by formation of gas in tissue, especially among diabetics, which may be detected by crepitation or by x-ray and which must be differentiated from clostridial infection. From 5 to 10 percent of patients with *E. coli* bacteremia develop metastatic infection in bone, brain, liver, and lung. *Escherichia coli* may cause pneumonia de novo; also, *E. coli* are often cultured from sputum in pulmonary superinfections.

Neonatal infection Neonates, particularly premature infants, often develop *E. coli* bacteremia associated with meningitis and bloodborne pyelonephritis. Fecal soiling and absence of maternal gamma-G globulin (IgM) antibody are two of the factors which render this group particularly susceptible to *E. coli* infections.

Gastroenteritis Children under 2 years of age develop gastroenteritis, typified by nausea, vomiting, and diarrhea. Most outbreaks have occurred in nurseries and have been due to specific strains of enteropathogenic *E. coli* (EPEC). These particular strains produce a toxin similar to the toxin elaborated by *Vibrio cholerae.* Fluorescent antibody techniques have been useful in the rapid identification of organisms with serotypes frequently implicated in this syndrome. Although theoretically any *E. coli* strain might be cultured, since the genetic information coding for toxin production is found on a plasmid and can be transferred between *E. coli* strains, the number of different serotypes involved remains restricted. Although diarrhea is usually mediated through production of enterotoxins, occasionally *E. coli* may be enteroinvasive, involving the mucosa and causing disease akin to *Shigella* dysentery. The rapid dehydration, with its attendant high mortality, demands prompt recognition of this condition, isolation of the infants, and treatment of both patients and contacts with the appropriate antibiotic. *Escherichia coli* is also being recognized as a cause of acute diarrheal disease in adults, especially foreign travelers.

LABORATORY FINDINGS There are no characteristic laboratory abnormalities. The white blood cell count is usually elevated, and there is a preponderance of granulocytes. At times, however, the white count is normal or low. When *E. coli* infection occurs in previously healthy individuals, anemia is absent, but more commonly there is anemia which is usually related to the patient's underlying disease. *Escherichia coli* grows readily in a variety of bacteriologic media and should be cultured from appropriate secretions and blood. In the presence of gram-negative shock, there are often profound metabolic derangements, including azotemia, metabolic acidosis, hypokalemia, and hyperkalemia, as well as variety of coagulation defects (Chap. 109).

DIAGNOSIS *Escherichia coli* cannot be differentiated from most other gram-negative bacteria on Gram's stain, and culture followed by appropriate biochemical characterization is necessary to identify the organism precisely. Fluorescent antibody techniques have been used for identifying EPEC. In addition, serologic typing of *E. coli* may be useful in individual patients with recurrent urinary tract infections in order to help differentiate between relapse and reinfection.

TREATMENT As with other infections, drainage of pus and removal of foreign bodies are essential. If *E. coli* is suspected as the etiologic agent in a particular infection, choice of an appropriate antimicrobial will depend upon the site and type of infection as well as upon its severity. Often the outcome of the infection depends upon the status of the associated disease, rather than on eradication of bacteria. For example, in acute, uncomplicated urinary tract infection in females, the disease is frequently self-limited even without antimicrobial therapy, and there is no evidence that antibiotics are superior to sulfonamides. Conversely, *E. coli* bacteremia in a patient with leukemia may not respond to antimicrobials unless a hematologic remission is achieved simultaneously.

In most situations, antibiotics should be selected, when possible, on the basis of their in vitro sensitivity tests. Although no drug is uniformly active against all strains of *E. coli*, a number of agents are effective against the majority of clinical isolates. If average obtainable plasma concentrations become the criteria for in vitro susceptibility, approximately 75 percent of *E. coli* strains are likely to be sensitive to the tetracyclines, 85 to 90 percent to chloramphenicol or ampicillin, and 90 percent to gentamicin, kanamycin, polymyxin B, or colistin; 50 percent of *E. coli* isolated from hospitalized patients will be inhibited by streptomycin, and 75 to 90 percent by one of the cephalosporin antibiotics. Many strains of *E. coli* are sensitive to high concentrations of penicillin G (50 to 100 $\mu g/ml$), and this drug may be used in dosage of 10 to 40 million units intravenously daily, particularly if probenecid is given concomitantly. This regimen has been largely superseded by ampicillin, 2 to 4 g per day intravenously or intramuscularly; for severe infections the dose can be raised to 6 to 12 g per day. The antibacterial spectrum of ampicillin against *E. coli* is probably identical with that achieved with very high concentrations of penicillin G, and with the spectrum covered by the tetracyclines or chloramphenicol. However, the bactericidal properties of ampicillin may be a distinct advantage over these two drugs, particularly in deep-seated infections. Gentamicin has been employed effectively in the initial treatment of severe *E. coli* infections in doses of 5 mg/kg per day in divided doses every 8 h. This drug has superseded kanamycin in the treatment of many patients although kanamycin remains effective against most *E. coli* in doses of 15 mg/kg per day given intramuscularly in divided doses every 8 to 12 h. Cephalosporins in concentration of 25 $\mu g/ml$ or less are effective against many *E. coli* strains. This serum concentration can be obtained only with 1.5- to 2.0-g dosages at 3- to 4-h intervals with cephalothin. Newer cephalosporins have been developed which give slightly higher peak serum concentrations and in some instances have lower MICs for *E. coli* (Chap. 111). Tetracyclines and chloramphenicol are

still widely used in the treatment of *E. coli* infection, but better drugs are now available. Polymyxin B and colistin are also effective in vitro against the majority of *E. coli*. However, it is difficult to obtain adequate tissue and serum concentrations with these agents, and they should probably not be used for treatment of systemic *E. coli* infections. Although combinations of antimicrobials, i.e., streptomycin and tetracycline or streptomycin and chloramphenicol, have been recommended, there is little need to employ more than one agent in most situations. Nitrofurantoin (400 mg) and nalidixic acid (2 to 4 g) are reserved for treating patients with *E. coli* bacteriuria, and should not be employed when infection is suspected outside the urinary tract. Trimethroprim sulfa is also useful in urinary tract infections (Chap. 280).

PREVENTION Isolation and antimicrobial therapy of infants and contacts are essential to abort epidemic infantile diarrhea. In adults, many *E. coli* infections are hospital-associated, and their incidence can be reduced by limiting use of indwelling urinary and intravenous catheters, by careful surgical aseptic technique, by appropriate isolation of infection-prone patients, and by judicious use of antibiotics, steroids, and cytotoxic agents. There is mounting evidence that the promiscuous use of antibiotics may propagate the transfer of resistance factors among intestinal *E. coli*. These organisms may in turn transmit their resistance to other virulent Enterobacteriaceae, such as *Salmonella*.

KLEBSIELLA-ENTEROBACTER-SERRATIA INFECTIONS

ETIOLOGY Next to *E. coli*, strains of *Klebsiella, Enterobacter,* and *Serratia* are the most important enteric organisms infecting man. In many laboratories *Klebsiella* are, in general, more resistant to antibiotics than *E. coli*, and their isolation from blood, purulent exudates, and urine is of more serious epidemiologic and prognostic significance. The Friedländer bacilli (*K. pneumoniae*) are encapsulated gram-negative bacilli, found among the normal flora of the mouth and intestinal tracts. *Klebsiella pneumoniae* has been considered to be a virulent respiratory pathogen since first described by Friedländer in 1882. *Klebsiella* is closely related to the genera *Enterobacter* and *Serratia* and may be differentiated only by certain amino acid decarboxylase tests. In addition to differentiation by these biochemical tests, which group *Klebsiella, Enterobacter,* and *Serratia,* strains of *Klebsiella* usually are nonmotile and form large mucoid colonies on solid media, whereas the other species are typically motile. Klebsiellas also are usually sensitive to concentrations of cephalosporin antibiotics, to which *Enterobacter* and *Serratia* are resistant. These characteristics, however, are not invariable enough to differentiate various isolates from clinical sources. Strains of *Klebsiella* can be further distinguished on the basis of type-specific capsular antigens; more than 75 known capsular types have been identified. There is little evidence that certain types are more virulent than others, and the main role of capsular typing of *Klebsiella* is as an epidemiologic tool in nosocomial outbreaks of infection.

Klebsiella rhinoscleromatis is probably the causative agent of rhinoscleroma, and *K. ozenae* has been isolated occasionally from the nose of patients with ozena, a chronic severe rhinitis associated with turbinate atrophy and progressive anosmia.

PATHOGENESIS *Klebsiella, Enterobacter,* and *Serratia* are all capable of causing disease in diverse anatomic sites. However, results of clinical and epidemiologic studies suggest that differences in pathogenicity may exist among these genera and that precise taxonomic identification is of value. Although infections of the respiratory tract with *K. pneumoniae* have been emphasized most in the past, the urinary tract presently accounts for the majority of clinical isolates. In this site clinical manifestations and pathogenesis are similar to infections produced by *E. coli*, but klebsiellas are more frequently found in patients with complicated and obstructive urinary tract disease. Infections of the biliary tract, the peritoneal cavity, the middle ear, mastoids, paranasal sinuses, and meninges also are not uncommon. In these locations, *Klebsiella* is more frequent than either *Enterobacter* or *Serratia* and is more likely to produce an illness of greater severity. The apparent increased frequency of infection by *Serratia* represents an increase primarily due to nosocomial spread of this organism.

MANIFESTATIONS Symptoms and signs of common infections caused by *Klebsiella*—namely, those involving the urinary tract, biliary tree, and peritoneal cavity—are indistinguishable from those caused by *E. coli*. These infections commonly occur in diabetics and in the form of superinfections in patients who have received antimicrobials to which these organisms are resistant. *Klebsiella* infection is also an important etiologic factor in septic shock. *Serratia* and *Enterobacter* are almost exclusively nosocomial pathogens. These organisms have been implicated as pathogens in a wide variety of infections, most frequently pneumonia, urinary tract infections and bacteremia.

Pneumonia *Klebsiella* is well recognized as a pulmonary pathogen, but probably accounts for less than 1 percent of all cases of bacterial pneumonia. The disease is most common in men over 40 years of age and is most frequently found in alcoholics. Other factors associated with increased susceptibility include diabetes mellitus and chronic bronchopulmonary disease. Aspiration of oropharyngeal secretions containing *Klebsiella* organisms is the likely inciting factor among alcoholic patients. The clinical manifestations are indistinguishable from those of pneumococcal pneumonia (Chap. 115), with sudden onset of chills, fever, productive cough, and severe pleuritic chest pain. Patients are frequently delirious and prostrated, but this may also occur with pneumococcal infection. A "characteristic" clinical feature, which occurs in only 25 to 50 percent of patients, is the dark-brown or red-currant-jelly sputum which may be so tenacious that the patient has difficulty in expelling it from his mouth and lips. The pulmonary lesion is most frequent in the right upper lobe but often rapidly progresses and, if untreated, may spread from lobe to lobe. Cyanosis and dyspnea develop rapidly, and jaundice, vomiting, and diarrhea may be present. Physical findings consist primarily of signs of consolidation unless pleural effusion or necrotizing pneumonitis with rapid cavitation has intervened. The blood leukocyte count may be elevated but is often low, which probably is merely a reflection of severe infection in an alcoholic patient with poor bone marrow reserve and folate deficiency. Lung abscess and empyema are much more frequent than in pneumococcal pneumonia and are related to the destructive capabilities of this organism. So-called "characteristic" and radiographic features such as bulging fissures and loss of lung volume occur only occasionally, and also may be found in pneumococcal infection, as well as in necrotizing pneumonia caused by other gram-negative species.

Klebsiella, Serratia, and *Enterobacter* are frequently seen in nosocomial pneumonia. Older patients become colonized with gram-negative bacilli in the oropharynx and these organisms can then gain access to the respiratory tract and cause pneumonia or purulent bronchitis. Common-source outbreaks, with contamination of a variety of respiratory therapy devices have been implicated in infections with these pathogens, especially *Serratia*.

Chronic infection of the lung Rarely, infection with *Klebsiella* may progress, often in indolent fashion, to a chronic necrotizing pneumonitis resembling tuberculosis. It may follow acute *Klebsiella* pneumonia but is also seen in patients who give no history of an acute onset. The principal symptoms are productive cough, weakness, and anemia. Hemoptysis, chronic empyema, or sterile serous effusions are also encountered. Cavitation, frequently with thin walls, occurs primarily in the upper lobes.

DIAGNOSIS Diagnosis of community-acquired pneumonia is established by an awareness of the clinical setting in which *Klebsiella* infections occur and by isolation of the organism. A presumptive diagnosis of *Klebsiella* pneumonia should be made on the basis of a Gram stain of the sputum which shows a predominance of short, plump, gram-negative bacilli, frequently surrounded by a clear space because of the capsule. Often these gram-negative organisms occur together with gram-positive cocci, and because the gram-positives are easier to see, the gram-negative bacteria may be ignored and the diagnosis may be missed, which, in turn, may lead to potentially serious delays in instituting therapy. Additional proof of *Klebsiella* infection in the lung is afforded by isolation of the organisms from blood and pleural exudate. In extrapulmonary infections, the organisms are readily seen in, and cultured from, pus or secretions of involved organs.

The diagnosis of nosocomial respiratory infection with these organisms may be more difficult, mainly because colonization has to be distinguished from infection. Careful evaluation of the clinical course is necessary in establishing a diagnosis. Transtracheal aspiration of sputum for culture and Gram's stain may be useful in difficult cases.

TREATMENT *Klebsiella, Enterobacter,* and *Serratia* have variable suceptiblity to antimicrobial drugs, and cultures of these organisms need to be tested in vitro. Frequently, however, antimicrobial therapy needs to be insituted before results of antibiotic susceptibility tests become available. In general, the majority of strains of *Klebsiella* is susceptible to gentamicin, kanamycin, cephalosporins, chloramphenicol, and polymyxin B or colistin. *Klebsiella* isolates do not respond to penicillin and its analogues, although many isolates of *Enterobacter* are inhibited by 25 µg/ml carbenicillin. *Serratia* isolates are frequently resistant to many antimicrobials, and resistance to gentamicin and tobramycin is being encountered with increasing frequency. Amikacin has been used effectively in these drug-resistant infections. The antimicrobial regimen of choice in the treatment of *Klebsiella, Enterobacter,* and *Serratia* infection will vary from one institution to another depending on the resistance patterns as well as upon the degree of clinical severity of infection. In severely ill patients, the combination of an aminoglycoside such as tobramycin or gentamicin (3 to 5 mg/ kg per day) or kanamycin (15 mg/kg per day) with cephalothin, cephapirin, or cefazolin (4 to 12 g per day) is usually preferred. Amikacin, a newer aminoglycoside, in a dose of 15 mg/kg per day, may be effective when the organisms are resistant to either gentamicin or tobramycin. Because of the relatively poor blood and tissue levels obtained with the polymyxins, they should not be employed as first-line agents in the treatment of severe *Klebsiella* infections despite apparent in vitro susceptibility. Regardless of the antimicrobial regimen employed, treatment should be continued for a minimum of 10 to 14 days and prolonged if there is extensive cavitation. Pleural effusions must be drained; antibiotic therapy alone is not sufficient treatment for closed-space infections of the pleural cavity. At times, rib resection with open drainage may be necessary, and should be considered if effusions recur.

PROGNOSIS Before the introduction of antimicrobials, the fatality rate from these infections varied from 50 to 80 percent, and death within 48 h was not infrequent. Even with antimicrobial treatment the course of these infections is quite variable and the prognosis must be guarded. For the most part, this prognosis reflects the age group involved and the frequent association of *Klebsiella* infections with alcoholism, malnutrition, and severe underlying disease.

PROTEUS INFECTIONS

ETIOLOGY The genus *Proteus* consists of gram-negative bacilli which do not ferment lactose and are characterized by their active motility and spreading growth on solid media. There are four pathogenic species: *P. mirabilis, P. vulgaris, P. morganii,* and *P. rettgeri. Proteus mirabilis* causes 75 to 90 percent of human infections and is distinguishable from the other three species by its inability to form indole. All four split urea, with production of ammonia. Some strains of *P. vulgaris* share a common antigen with certain rickettsia, accounting for the appearance of antibodies against *Proteus* organisms (Weil-Felix reaction) in typhus, scrub typhus, and Rocky Mountain spotted fever. The *Providence* group of organisms resembles those of the genus *Proteus* closely except that it fails to produce a urease.

EPIDEMIOLOGY AND PATHOGENESIS Members of the genus *Proteus* are normally found in soil, water, and sewage and are part of the normal fecal flora. Occasionally, they have been implicated as a cause of epidemic diarrhea in infants, but the evidence for this is inconclusive. The organism is frequently cultured from superficial wounds, draining ears, and sputum, particularly in patients who have received antibiotics, and replaces the more susceptible flora eradicated by these drugs. *Proteus* organisms often localize in already damaged tissues, where they produce a typical exudative inflammatory reaction.

MANIFESTATIONS *Proteus* organisms are rarely primary invaders but produce disease in locations previously infected by other organisms. These locations include the skin, ears and mastoid, sinuses, eyes, peritoneal cavity, bone, urinary tract, meninges, lung, and bloodstream.

Cutaneous infections *Proteus* organisms are frequently isolated from surgical wounds, particularly following antimicrobial therapy, but they do not interfere with normal wound healing provided that the tissues are viable and foreign bodies are not present. Burns, varicose ulcers, and decubiti may become contaminated with *Proteus* organisms, often in company with other gram-negative organisms or staphylococci.

Infections of the ears and mastoid sinuses Otitis media and mastoiditis in which *Proteus* organisms are present can result in extensive destruction of the middle ear and mastoid sinuses. Fetid otorrhea, cholesteatoma, and granulation tissue constitute a chronic focus of infection in the middle and inner ears and mastoid, and deafness ensues. Paralysis of the facial nerve

is an occasional complication. The great danger of these infections lies in intracranial extension, leading to thrombosis of the lateral sinus, meningitis, brain abscess, and bacteremia.

Ocular infections *Proteus* infection may cause corneal ulcers, usually following trauma to the eye, which occasionally terminate in panophthalmitis and destruction of the eyeball.

Peritonitis Being part of the normal intestinal flora, *Proteus* organisms may be isolated from the peritoneal cavity following perforation of viscera or mesenteric infarction.

Urinary tract infections *Proteus* organisms are a common cause of urinary tract infections, usually in patients with chronic bacteriuria, many of whom have had obstructive uropathy, a history of instrumentation of the bladder, and repeated courses of chemotherapy. The organism is rarely a pathogen in anatomically normal urinary tracts except occasionally in patients with diabetes mellitus. *Proteus* organisms are also often cultured from bacteriuric patients with renal or bladder calculi. This fact may be related to the urease activity of this organism, which renders the urine alkaline and provides a fertile medium for formation of ammonium-magnesium-phosphate stones.

Bacteremia Bloodstream invasion is the most serious manifestation of infection with this organism. In 75 percent of cases, the urinary tract serves as the portal of entry; in the remainder, the biliary tree, gastrointestinal tract, ears and sinuses, and skin are the primary foci. *Proteus* bacteremia is frequently preceded by cystoscopy, urethral catheterization, transurethral prostatic resection, or other operative procedures. Clinically, the signs, symptoms, and laboratory findings of *Proteus* sepsis—high fever, chills, shock, metastatic abscesses, leukocytosis, and rarely thrombocytopenia—are indistinguishable from those of bloodstream infections with other gram-negative bacteria.

DIAGNOSIS The diagnosis of *Proteus* infection depends on culture of the organism from blood, urine, or exudate and its identification by appropriate biochemical tests. It is especially important to separate *P. mirabilis,* the indole-negative species, from *P. morganii, rettgeri,* and *vulgaris,* which are indole-positive, because only *P. mirabilis* is susceptible to the action of penicillin and many other antibiotics. *Proteus* organisms are often present in mixed infections with other pathogens. Particular care should be exercised in the isolation of other organisms growing in the same medium with members of the genus *Proteus* lest they be masked by its spreading growth. The spreading character of this organism may also make antibiotic sensitivity tests difficult to interpret.

TREATMENT Most strains of *P. mirabilis* are sensitive to penicillin in high concentration (10 units per milliliter or greater), ampicillin, carbenicillin, kanamycin, gentamicin or tobramycin, the cephalosporin antibiotics, and chloramphenicol. *Proteus* bacteriuria can be readily eradicated with any of these drugs during treatment; ampicillin in dosage of 0.5 g every 4 to 6 h is highly effective. In severe infection, therapy should be parenteral: 6 to 12 g ampicillin or 20 million units of penicillin G plus kanamycin or gentamicin in divided doses of 15 mg/kg per day and 5 mg/kg per day, respectively, if renal function is adequate. There is good evidence that kanamycin is synergistic with ampicillin and penicillin G in *Proteus* infections, and that chloramphenicol may be ineffective despite the results of in vitro tests. In view of the numerous more effective agents, there is no reason to use chloramphenicol in *Proteus* infections. In general, all strains of *P. mirabilis* are resistant to tetracycline. Most strains other than *P. mirabilis* and *Providence* bacilli are sensitive only to kanamycin, gentamicin, tobramycin or amikacin. Gentamicin, tobramycin and amikacin in particular appear to be effective against indole-positive *Proteus*. In addition, although ampicillin and penicillin G alone are ineffective against indole-positive *Proteus,* a combination of either drug and an aminoglycoside may be synergistic. Carbenicillin and ticarcillin, semisynthetic penicillins, are also effective against the majority of indole-positive *Proteus* species. As with all other gram-negative infections, appropriate attention must be given to drainage of pus, maintenance of fluid and electrolyte status, and treatment of circulatory collapse.

REFERENCES

Enterobacteriaceae: General

PIERCE AK, SANFORD JP: Aerobic gram-negative bacillary pneumonias. Am Rev Respir Dis 110:647, 1974

SCHABERG DR et al: Epidemics of nosocomial urinary tract infection caused by multiply-resistant gram-negative bacilli: Epidemiology and control. J Infect Dis 133:363, 1976

STAMM WE: Guidelines for prevention of catheter-associated urinary tract infections. Ann Intern Med 82:386, 1975

Escherichia coli infections

CONN HO, FESSEL JM: Spontaneous bacterial peritonitis in cirrhosis. Medicine 50:161, 1971

GORBACH SL et al: Travelers' diarrhea and toxigenic *Escherichia coli.* N Engl J Med 292:933, 1975

TILLOTSON JR, LERNER AM: Characteristics of pneumonia caused by *Escherichia coli.* N Engl J Med 277:115, 1967

TULLOCH EF JR et al: Invasive enteropathic *Escherichia coli* dysentery: Outbreak in 28 adults. Ann Intern Med 79:13, 1973

TURCK M et al: Studies on the epidemiology of *Escherichia coli* 1960–1968. J Infect Dis 120:13, 1969

Klebsiella-Enterobacter-Serratia infections

EDMONDSON EG, SANFORD JP: The *Klebsiella-Enterobacter (Aerobacter)-Serratia* group. Medicine 46:323, 1967

MAKI DG et al: Noscomial urinary tract infection with *Serratia marcescens:* An epidemiologic study. J Infect Dis 128:579, 1973

MANFREDI F et al: Clinical observations of acute Friedländer pneumonia. Ann Intern Med 58:642, 1963

MELTZ DJ, GRIECO MH: Characteristics of *Serratia marcescens* pneumonia. Arch Intern Med 132:359, 1973

PRICE DJE, SLEIGH JD: Control of infection due to *Klebsiella* aerogenes in neurosurgical unit by withdrawal of all antibiotics. Lancet 2:213, 1970

Proteus infections

LEWIS J, FEKETY FR: *Proteus* bacteremia. Johns Hopkins Med J 124:151, 1969

MUSHER DM et al: Role of urease in pyelonephritis resulting from urinary tract infection with *Proteus.* J Infect Dis 131:177, 1975

SERIFF NS: Lobar pneumonia due to *Proteus* infection in a previously healthy adult. Am J Med 46:480, 1969

TILLOTSON JR, LERNER AM: Characteristics of pneumonia caused by bacillus *Proteus.* Ann Intern Med 68:287, 1968

TURCK M et al: The role of carbenicillin in treatment of infections of the urinary tract. J Infect Dis 122:529, 1970

121

PSEUDOMONAS, ACINETOBACTER, AND EIKENELLA INFECTIONS

MARVIN TURCK
DENNIS SCHABERG

PSEUDOMONAS INFECTIONS

ETIOLOGY *Pseudomonas aeruginosa* is a gram-negative motile rod which generally is not encapsulated and forms no spores. It grows readily in all ordinary culture media, and on agar it forms irregular, soft, iridescent colonies which usually have a fluorescent yellow-green color because of diffusion into the medium of two pigments, pyocyanin and fluorescin. *Pseudomonas* produces acid but no gas in glucose, and it is proteolytic. It is oxidase-positive and produces ammonia from arginine. A number of different strains have been identified by immunofluorescent techniques or bacteriophage typing. There is no evidence that these strains vary in their virulence for man. Other *Pseudomonas* species (*P. maltophilia, P. cepacia, P. fluorescens, P. testosteroni,* and *P. putida*) also may cause infection in man. For the most part, these organisms have been associated with common-source nosocomial outbreaks; in addition, they have been incriminated in bacteremia, endocarditis, and osteomyelitis in narcotic addicts.

EPIDEMIOLOGY *Pseudomonas* organisms are present on the skin of some normal persons, particularly in the axilla and anogenital regions. They are uncommon in the stools of adults not receiving antibiotics. In the majority of instances, *Pseudomonas* organisms are cultured as avirulent secondary contaminants in superficial wounds, or from the sputum of patients treated with antibiotics. Ordinarily this is of little consequence because the organisms merely fill the bacteriologic vacuum left by the elimination of more sensitive bacteria. Occasionally, however, infections with *Pseudomonas* organisms occur in the ear, lung, skin, or urinary tract of patients, often when a primary pathogen has been eradicated by antibiotics. Serious infections are almost invariably associated with damage to local tissue or with diminished host resistance. Premature infants; children with congenital anomalies and patients with leukemia, usually receiving antibiotics, adrenal steroids, or antineoplastic drugs; patients with burns; and geriatric patients with debilitating diseases are likely to develop *Pseudomonas* infections. Most often these infections occur in the hospital environment and generally are exogenous infections with the organism acquired from sources other than the patient's normal flora. The organisms have been cultured from a variety of sources in hospitals, sharing in common an aqueous environment including such items as sinks, antiseptic solutions, and aqueous medications. The organism is prevalent in urine receptacles and catheters, and on the hands of orderlies, nurses, and physicians; in several outbreaks, *Pseudomonas* urinary tract infections appeared to have been transmitted from patient to patient by human carriers. Similar epidemics have been reported in nurseries among premature infants, and cross infection on burn wards is also common.

PATHOGENESIS The portal of entry of *Pseudomonas* organisms varies with the patient's age and underlying disease. In infancy and childhood, the skin, umbilical cord, and gastrointestinal tract predominate; in old age, the urinary tract is more often the primary focus. Often the infections remain localized in the skin or subcutaneous tissues. In burns the region below the eschar may become massively infiltrated with bacteria and inflammatory cells, and usually serves as the focus for bacteremia, the single most lethal complication. Hematogenous dissemination is characterized by hemorrhagic nodules in many areas, including the skin, heart, lungs, kidneys, and meninges. The histologic picture is one of necrosis and hemorrhage. Typically the walls of arterioles are heavily infiltrated with bacteria, and the vessels are partially or wholly thrombosed.

MANIFESTATIONS *Pseudomonas* infections occur in many locations, including the skin, subcutaneous tissue, bone and joints, eyes, ears, mastoid and paranasal sinuses, meninges, and heart valves. Bacteremia without a detectable primary focus may also occur and should raise the question of contamination of intravenous medications, intravenous solutions, or antiseptics used for preparing the intravenous site, especially when non-*aeruginosa Pseudmonas* species are isolated.

Infections of the skin and subcutaneous tissues *Pseudomonas* organisms are frequently cultured from surgical wounds, varicose and decubitus ulcers, and burns, particularly following antibiotic therapy. Draining tuberculous or osteomyelitic sinuses may become secondarily infected. The mere presence of *Pseudomonas* in these sites is of little significance provided that bacterial multiplication deep in subcutaneous tissues does not occur and bacteremia does not ensue. Cutaneous infections usually heal after removal or slough of devitalized tissue. *Pseudomonas* organisms may be responsible for green nails in persons whose hands are excessively exposed to water, soap, and detergents, who have onychomycosis, or whose hands are subject to mechanical trauma. The organism can usually be cultured from the nail plate.

Osteomyelitis Osteomyelitis is unusual with *Pseudomonas* except as a complication of bacteremia and puncture wounds. If a puncture wound, especially a nail puncture of the foot in children, fails to respond to standard therapy within 3 to 4 days, complicating *Pseudomonas* osteomyelitis must be considered.

Infections of the ear, mastoid, and paranasal sinuses Otitis externa is the most common form of *Pseudomonas* infection which involves the ear. It is particularly troublesome in tropical climates and is characterized by chronic serosanguineous and purulent drainage from the external auditory canal. Otitis media or mastoiditis usually occurs as a superinfection following eradication of pneumococci, streptococci, or staphylococci by antimicrobial agents. Frequently *Pseudomonas* organisms are present in association with other gram-negative or gram-positive organisms.

Infection of the eye Corneal ulceration is the most severe form of ocular *Pseudomonas* infection. It usually follows a traumatic abrasion and may terminate in panophthalmitis and destruction of the globe. Purulent conjuncitivitis occurs as a manifestation of *Pseudomonas* infection in premature infants. Contamination of contact lenses or lens fluid may be an important means of infecting the eyes with *Pseudomonas* organisms.

Urinary tract infections *Pseudomonas* organisms are common pathogens in the urinary tract and are usually found in patients with obstructive uropathy who have been subjected to repeated urethral manipulations or to urologic surgery. At times *Pseudomonas* is one of several pathogenic bacteria in the urine, the others being *Escherichia coli, Klebsiella, Proteus,* and enterococci. *Pseudomonas* bacteriuria is in no way unique and cannot be distinguished from infection with other organisms on clinical grounds.

Gastrointestinal tract *Pseudomonas* organisms have been implicated as a cause of epidemic diarrhea of infancy. In addition, a number of infants dying from neonatal sepsis have the classic necrotic, avascular ulcers of *Pseudomonas* bacteremia in the bowel at autopsy. A "typhoidal" form of *Pseudomonas* infection characterized by fever, myalgia, and diarrhea occurs predominantly in the tropics. This illness, also called 13-day fever or Shanghai fever, is self-limited, and the prognosis is good.

Respiratory tract Primary *Pseudomonas* pneumonia is infrequent, and culture of this organism from the sputum usually is indicative of aspiration of oropharyngeal contents with secondary infection or of superinfection following eradication of a more sensitive flora with antibiotics. The normal oropharyngeal flora of hospitalized patients is frequently replaced by gram-negative rods, including *Pseudomonas,* early in hospitalization. A variety of nosocomial events, most notably administration of sedative medications, endotracheal intubation, and intermittent positive pressure breathing treatments, can predispose to respiratory infection with *Pseudomonas.* Pulmonary infection is often associated with microabscesses. The organism is often isolated from the sputum of patients with bronchiectasis, chronic bronchitis, or cystic fibrosis who have lingering infections punctuated by multiple courses of chemotherapy and is recovered frequently from the stomata of tracheostomy sites. *Pseudomonas* bronchitis and bronchiolitis may be the terminal event in cystic fibrosis and the isolates from these patients often are found to have a characteristic mucoid colonial morphology when cultured on agar.

Meningitis Spontaneous *Pseudomonas* meningitis is most unusual, but the bacilli may be introduced into the subarachnoid space by lumbar puncture, spinal anesthesia, intrathecal medication, or head trauma. Ventriculomastoid or ventriculoatrial shunts performed for hydrocephalus may become contaminated with *Pseudomonas* organisms. Usually revision or removal of the shunt offers the best hope of cure. Meningitis may be a terminal phenomenon in *Pseudomonas* bacteremia and in this instance represents a metastatic infection in the meninges.

Bacteremia Bloodstream invasion tends to occur in debilitated patients, premature infants, children with congenital defects, patients with lymphomas, leukemias, or other malignant tumors, and elderly patients who have undergone surgery or instrumentation of the biliary or urinary tract. *Pseudomonas* bacteremia is an important cause of death in patients with severe burns. In adults, *Pseudomonas* bacteremia is indistinguishable from bloodstream infection with other bacterial species except for two findings: (1) ecthyma gangrenosum, the classic skin lesion, often located in the anogenital or axillary region as a round, indurated, purple-black area about 1 cm in diameter with an ulcerated center and a surrounding zone of erythema; and (2) the passage rarely of green urine, presumably due to the hemoglobin pigment, verdoglobin. Other features of *Pseudomonas* sepsis include hectic fever, shaking chills, hyperventilation, confusion, delirium, and circulatory collapse. Hypothermia, leukopenia, and thrombocytopenia are more common in *Pseudomonas* bacteremia than in other gram-negative bacteremias but are often related to an underlying blood dyscrasia. In addition to ecthyma gangrenosum, other skin lesions consist of hemorrhagic cellulitis and macular lesions on the trunk similar to "rose spots." Organisms usually can be cultured from cutaneous lesions and may provide an early clue to the diagnosis. *Pseudomonas* organisms may be in the bloodstream concomitantly with other organisms, notably Enterobacteriaceae or staphylococci. More often, however, *Pseudomonas* bacteremia follows staphylococcal sepsis in patients with burns.

Bacterial endocarditis A number of cases of *Pseudomonas* subacute bacterial endocarditis have followed open-heart surgery. Usually the organisms become implanted on a silk suture or a synthetic patch employed for closure of septal defects. Reoperation with removal of the vegetation and foreign bodies offers the best hope of cure. *Pseudomonas* endocarditis has been found on normal heart valves in patients with burns or in drug addicts; it has been postulated that staphylococcal endocarditis develops first and that the vegetation is secondarily infected with *Pseudomonas* organisms. Metastatic abscesses in bone, joints, brain, adrenal glands, and lungs are frequent consequences of *Pseudomonas* endocarditis.

TREATMENT Localized *Pseudomonas* infection can be treated by irrigation with 1% acetic acid or topical therapy with colistin or polymyxin B. Debridement and drainage of purulent material is essential when deeper tissues are involved. For deep-seated tissue infections and life-threatening infection, such as pneumonia or bacteremia, parenteral therapy must be employed. The aminoglycoside antibiotics, tobramycin and gentamicin, inhibit most strains of *Pseudomonas*. In patients with normal renal function, 5 mg/kg per day in divided doses will provide inhibitory levels. Amikacin, a newer aminoglycoside, is also active against *Pseudomonas*. It is especially useful against strains which have developed enzyme-mediated drug resistance to tobramycin and gentamicin. It should be given in doses of 15 mg/kg per day in divided doses. Ticarcillin and carbenicillin are also active against many strains of *Pseudomonas* in doses of 24 to 30 g per day for carbenicillin and 16 to 20 g per day for ticarcillin. The combination of an aminoglycoside active against *Pseudomonas* plus carbenicillin or ticarcillin is frequently employed to delay emergence of resistance during therapy and provides some enhanced activity, especially in the granulocytopenic patient with *Pseudomonas* infection. Asymptomatic bacteriuria, particularly when confined to the bladder, should be treated with the least toxic agent, which at times may be a sulfonamide or tetracycline. The antimicrobial susceptiblity of *Pseudomonas,* other than *P. aeruginosa,* is variable and many of these isolates may be sensitive to chloramphenicol and resistant to aminoglycoside antibiotics.

PROPHYLAXIS *Pseudomonas* cross infections in hospitals can be reduced by careful attention to aseptic techniques, particularly in nurseries for premature infants, operating rooms, and urologic wards; avoidance of cold sterilization procedures wherever possible; and scrupulous attention to clean plumbing fixtures, humidifying equipment, etc. Judicious use of antibiotics, steroids, and cytotoxic agents should also diminish the incidence of *Pseudomonas* infections. Systemic antibiotic prophylaxis aimed at preventing colonization and infection with *Pseudomonas* organisms has been notoriously unsuccessful and should be interdicted. A polyvalent vaccine for *Pseudomonas* has been developed as well as hyperimmune λ globulin. The vaccine has proved useful in prophylaxis against *Pseudomonas* infection in patients with thermal injury and may be useful in other selected populations such as those with solid tumors undergoing cancer chemotherapy.

PROGNOSIS The mortality rate in *Pseudomonas* bacteremia is 75 percent and is highest in patients with shock or severe associated disease such as massive third-degree burns, leukemia, or prematurity. When bacteremia originates in the urinary tract and is not accompanied by shock, the prognosis is considerably better. Localized *Pseudomonas* infections do not present a threat to life unless hematogenous dissemination occurs.

ACINETOBACTER INFECTIONS

DEFINITION Organisms of the genus *Acinetobacter* are pleomorphic, gram-negative bacilli which are easily confused with members of the genus *Neisseria*. Severe infections with these organisms, including meningitis, bacterial endocarditis, pneumonia, and bacteremia, have been described with increasing frequency.

ETIOLOGY *Acinetobacter calcoaceticus* var. *lwoffi* was described by DeBord as *Mima polymorpha* in 1939. It is one of two well-characterized varieties of *Acinetobacter,* the other being *Acinetobacter calcoaceticus* var. *anitratus,* formerly called *Herellea vaginicola.* Organisms described as *Bacterium anitratum* and B5W are synonymous with *Acinetobacter.* These organisms are pleomorphic, gram-negative, encapsulated, and nonmotile. They grow well on ordinary media, forming white, convex, smooth colonies. Diplococcal forms predominate in colonies grown on solid media; rods and filamentous forms are more common in liquid media. The species can be differentiated from the Enterobacteriaceae by their negative nitrate reaction and from members of the genus *Neisseria,* which they may resemble morphologically, by their simple growth requirements, their bacillary form in liquid media, and their usually negative oxidase reaction.

EPIDEMIOLOGY AND PATHOGENESIS *Acinetobacter* organisms are ubiquitous and have been cultured from a variety of human sources, including urethral, vaginal, and conjunctival secretions, sputum, pleural fluid, blood, cerebrospinal fluid, feces, cutaneous ulcers, abscesses, chancroid lesions, joint fluid, ascitic fluid, and bone marrow. In addition, these organisms have been found in river water, humidifiers, and oxygen tents. Twenty-five percent of normal subjects are skin carriers of *Acinetobacter.* The striking association of *Acinetobacter* bacteremia with cutdowns or indwelling intravenous catheters favors the skin as a major portal of entry in man. The increasing incidence of *Acinetobacter* pneumonia, both as a primary infection and as a superinfection, also points to the respiratory tract as an important portal of entry. It appears that *Acinetobacter* organisms are normal human commensals of relatively low virulence with colonization much more frequent than infection. Infections seem to occur in patients subjected to the same epidemiologic pressures encountered with nosocomial, gram-negative bacilli producing serious infections under conditions of decreased host resistance, or in the presence of instrumentation and with prior broad-spectrum antimicrobial therapy. The role of these organisms as a cause of conjunctivitis, vaginitis, and urethritis requires further documentation.

MANIFESTATIONS Serious infections caused by *Acinetobacter* include (1) meningitis, (2) subacute and acute bacterial endocarditis, (3) pneumonia, (4) urinary tract infections, and (5) bacteremia. Usually, the signs and symptoms associated with infections in these sites are no different from those produced by other pathogens. For example, subacute bacterial endocarditis has usually been reported in patients with congenital or rheumatic heart disease and pursues an indolent course, while urinary tract infections may be manifested by asymptomatic bacteriuria, cystitis, or pyelonephritis. Pneumonia often occurs in the form of a superinfection in patients who have received antibiotics and who have either a tracheostomy or endotracheal intubation. Bronchopneumonia is the most common roentgenographic finding. Occasionally, *Acinetobacter* may be the cause of a fulminating bacteremia, with high fever, vascular collapse, petechiae, and ecchymoses, indistinguishable from fulminant meningococcemia. More often, however, bacteremia is associated with an overt portal of entry, such as infected cutdowns or indwelling intravenous catheters, surgical wounds, or burns, or it may follow urethral or other surgical instrumentation. These patients usually have severe debilitating disease or have undergone surgery. Many times they have received antibiotics, adrenal cortical hormones, irradiation, or tumor chemotherapy and have had infections with other organisms prior to development of sepsis with *Acinetobacter*. The clinical picture presented by these patients is dominated by endotoxemia, and the prognosis is poor.

DIAGNOSIS The diagnosis of *Acinetobacter* infection can be missed because the clinical bacteriology laboratory is unfamiliar with these organisms and reports them incorrectly or because they are considered contaminant. The confusion attending the taxonomic classification of these organisms has not simplified matters. For practical purposes, isolation of *Acinetobacter* or synonyms (*Mimae herelleae, B. anitratum*, B5W, *Diplococcus mucosus*, or *Neisseria winogradskyi*) from blood, spinal fluid, sputum, urine, or pus should be considered significant unless there is no evidence of infection on clinical grounds. Since *Acinetobacter* isolates are resistant to penicillin and members of the genus *Neisseria* are sensitive, differentiation of these organisms is of obvious importance.

TREATMENT Antibiotic sensitivites of *Acinetobacter* strains vary, but most strains are inhibited by kanamycin, gentamicin, tobramycin, colistin, or polymyxin B. Sensitivity to the tetracyclines is unpredictable, and most strains are resistant to penicillin, ampicillin, cephalothin, erythromycin, and chloramphenicol. For serious systemic infections, the appropriate antibiotic, generally an aminoglycoside, should be administered, and since these organisms may produce localized abscesses, surgical drainage may be necessary.

EIKENELLA INFECTIONS

ETIOLOGY *Eikenella corrodens* is a facultatively anaerobic or capnophilic gram-negative rod which is oxidase-positive. As colonies develop on blood agar, characteristic "pitting" or "corroding" of the agar is seen with many strains and generally requires 48 to 72 h of growth to develop.

EPIDEMIOLOGY *Eikenella corrodens* is an inhabitant of the mouth, upper respiratory tract, and gastrointestinal tract of man. Infections frequently involve bowel or oral contamination. A striking association between *Eikenella* infections and methylphenidate (Ritalin) abuse has been noted, perhaps related to the low redox potential created by "skin popping" of this agent as well as a tendency for needles to become contaminated with oral secretions through needle licking.

MANIFESTATIONS The most common infection caused by *Eikenella* is that of skin or soft tissue. Endocarditis, osteomyelitis, and meningitis are reported but are rare. *Eikenella* infections frequently mimic infections caused by strict anaerobes such as *Bacteroides fragilis* or *Peptostreptococcus*. The infections are indolent, frequently mixed with aerobic gram-positive cocci, and drainage is often foul smelling. Abscess formation is common.

TREATMENT *Eikenella corrodens* is susceptible to penicillin, ampicillin, carbenicillin, and tetracycline. Adequate drainage of purulent material is essential in the management of these infections. Ampicillin or penicillin coupled with surgical drainage generally provides a good response. Of note is the marked resistance of *Eikenella* to clindamycin, making the differentiation of *Eikenella* infections from those caused by mixed anaerobes even more important.

REFERENCES

Acinetobacter infections

GLEW RH et al: Infections with *Acinetobacter calcoaceticus:* Clinical and laboratory studies. Medicine 56:79, 1977
INCLAN AP et al: Organisms of the tribe Mimae: Incidence of isolation and clinical correlation. South Med J 58:1261, 1965
REYNOLDS RC, CLUFF LE: Infections of man with Mimae. Ann Intern Med 58:759, 1963

Eikenella infections

BROOKS GF et al: *Eikenella corrodens*, a recently recognized pathogen. Medicine 53:325, 1974
DORFF GJ et al: Infections with *Eikenella corrodens*. Ann Intern Med 80:305, 1974

Pseudomonas infections

ALEXANDER JW et al: Immunologic control of *Pseudomonas* infection in burn patients: Clinical evaluation. Arch Surg 102:31, 1971
ARTENSTEIN MS, SANFORD JP (eds): Symposium on *Pseudomonas aeruginosa*. J Infect Dis 130:S1, November 1974
BODEY GP: Epidemiologic studies of *Pseudomonas* species in patients with leukemia. Am J Med Sci 260:82, 1970
FLICK MR, CLUFF LE: *Pseudomonas* bacteremia: Review of 108 cases. Am J Med 60:501, 1976
PENNINGTON JE et al: *Pseudomona pneumonia:* A retrospective study of 36 cases. Am J Med 55:155, 1973
PHILLIPS I et al: Control of respirator-associated infection due to *Pseudomonas aeruginosa*. Lancet 2:871, 1974
STONE HH: Review of *Pseudomonas* sepsis in thermal injury. Ann Surg 163:297, 1966

122
MELIOIDOSIS AND GLANDERS

JAY P. SANFORD

MELIOIDOSIS

DEFINITION Melioidosis is a glanders-like infection of human beings and animals with a protean clinical spectrum. Melioidosis, which means "a resemblance to distemper of asses," bears a striking resemblance to glanders both clinically and pathologically, but is epidemiologically dissimilar.

ETIOLOGY Melioidosis is caused by a gram-negative motile bacillus, *Pseudomonas pseudomallei*, which can be differentiated from *Pseudomonas mallei* by bacteriologic and serologic means. *Pseudomonas pseudomallei* (also known as Whitmore's bacillus) is a small, gram-negative, motile, aerobic bacillus. When it is stained with methylene blue, Wayson's, or Wright's stain, marked irregularities with a bipolar "safety pin" pattern are observed. It grows well on standard bacteriologic media, with a characteristic wrinkling of colony surfaces after 48 to 72 h of incubation.

EPIDEMIOLOGY The disease is endemic in Southeast Asia, with the greatest concentration of cases reported from Vietnam, Cambodia, Laos, Thailand, Malaysia, and Burma. Cases in human beings have also been reported from adjacent areas including India, Borneo, the Philippines, Guam, Indonesia, Ceylon, New Guinea, and North Queensland. Cases in humans or animals have been reported from Madagascar, Chad, Central West Africa, and Turkey. Human melioidosis has been described only rarely in the Western Hemisphere (Panama, Ecuador)—a neonatal case in Hawaii and a possible case in Oklahoma. With these exceptions, confirmed melioidosis has occurred in United States or European residents only when they have traveled in endemic areas. As of January 1973, when all American forces had been withdrawn from Vietnam, there had been 343 cases with 36 deaths reported in United States Army personnel who were or had been in Vietnam. The majority of these cases occurred in individuals without intercurrent illness, although patients who sustained burn injuries in Vietnam accounted for a disproportionately high number of the cases.

Pseudomonas pseudomallei is a saprophyte which can be isolated from soil, stagnant streams, ponds, rice paddies, and market produce in endemic areas. Its ubiquitous nature is illustrated by its isolation as a laboratory contaminant. *Pseudomonas pseudomallei* is capable of causing disease in epizootic form among sheep, goats, swine, and horses. Occasional isolates have also been reported from cows, rodents, dogs, and cats. Although animals are susceptible to the disease, they apparently do not represent a reservoir for human disease. Attempts to culture *P. pseudomallei* from the urine and feces of a large variety of healthy animals have been unsuccessful. Arthropod-borne infection does not occur naturally. Human beings contract melioidosis by soil contamination of skin abrasions. Ingestion, nasal instillation, and inhalation are other probable methods of spread. In contrast to glanders, infections have been uncommon in laboratory workers. Person-to-person transmission of melioidosis is rare. Venereal transmission from a patient with chronic prostatitis with *P. pseudomallei* isolated from prostatic secretions to his wife, who had never been in an endemic area and who had a hemagglutination titer of 1:10,240, has been recorded. Also, the development of melioidosis in a 2-day-old newborn in Hawaii and demonstration of a significant antibody titer in a nurse who had never been in an endemic area but who had worked on wards with melioidosis patients raise the question of spread from person-to-person within a hospital.

PATHOLOGY In acute infections, the majority of lesions occur in the lungs, with occasional abscesses in other organs. In subacute infections, lung abscesses tend to be more extensive, and lesions are found throughout the body, in the skin, subcutaneous tissue, meninges, brain, eye, heart, liver, kidney, spleen, bone, prostate, synovial membranes, and lymph nodes. The acute abscesses are characterized by an outer border of hemorrhage, a medial zone heavily infiltrated with polymorphonuclear leukocytes, and an inner core of necrotic debris containing large histiocytes with two or three nuclei that have been termed *giant cells*. A striking histological feature has been the marked karyorrhexis. In chronic infections, the lesion consists of a central area of caseation necrosis, mononuclear and plasma cells, and granulation tissue. Calcification does not occur.

CLINICAL MANIFESTATIONS The clinical manifestations of melioidosis are variable. The illness can present as an acute, subacute, or chronic process. The incubation period has not been defined; however, judging by the lapse of time between injury and the development of infection, it may be as short as 2 days. Following a laboratory accident, an incubation period of 3 days ensued. Clinically inapparent infections may remain latent for a number of years after an individual leaves an endemic area, with an interval of 26 years reported in one patient. Men are more often affected than women, a finding which is thought to represent occupational exposure. Melioidosis may be recognized as inapparent infection, asymptomatic pulmonary infiltration, acute localized suppurative infection, acute pulmonary infection, acute septicemic infection, or chronic suppurative infection.

Inapparent infection In Thailand, Vietnam, and Malaysia, 6 to 8 percent of healthy adult men have significant antibody titers against *P. pseudomallei,* with the prevalence reaching 20 percent in a group of Army recruits from the rice-growing states of Western Malaysia. Only 1 percent of Thai women had positive reactions. None of the serums from a control group from the United States was positive. The prevalence of significant antibody titers has been reported as 2 percent for Europeans living in Vietnam and 1 to 9 percent in unselected patients in United States Army hospitals and in a group of normal uninjured soldiers who had served in Vietnam. Occasionally, asymptomatic infections have been discovered by routine chest x-ray.

Acute localized suppurative infection Infection by inoculation of a break in the skin usually results in a nodule with an area of acute lymphangitis and regional lymphadenitis. There are usually fever and generalized malaise. This form of infection may rapidly progress to the acute septicemic form.

Acute pulmonary infection The most common form of the disease has been pulmonary infection, which may represent a primary pneumonitis or hematogenous spread. The acute pulmonary infection can vary in severity from a mild bronchitis to overwhelming necrotizing pneumonia. The onset may be abrupt without prodromal symptoms or more gradual, with headache, anorexia, and generalized myalgia. Fever occurs in almost all patients, is often in excess of 38.9°C (102°F) and may be associated with rigors. Dull or pleuritic chest pain is common. Cough, with or without sputum, occurs. There may be mild pharyngitis. Tachypnea may be out of proportion to the fever and findings on physical or x-ray examination. Chest findings may be minimal but usually consist of rales in the area of pneumonitis. In the absence of dissemination, the spleen and liver are not palpable. Laboratory findings include total leukocyte counts ranging from normal to 20,000 cells per cubic millimeter. Mild normochromic, normocytic anemia may appear during the illness. The pneumonia usually involves the upper lobes with the radiographic appearance of consolidation. Thin-walled cavities, usually 2 to 7 cm in diameter, frequently occur. Without specific therapy, the temperature may become normal within a few days; however, the upper lobe cavitation persists, resulting in a radiographic appearance of tuberculosis. While uncommon, pleural effusions and a pleural mass have been reported. Progressive pulmonary spread or hematogenous dissemination with the development of septicemic manifestations may ensue.

Acute septicemic infection This is the form originally described primarily among narcotic addicts. Subsequent reports, however, have not shown a predilection for debilitated patients. The onset may be abrupt, with the dominant symptoms depending upon site of major involvement. In individuals with bacteremia complicating pneumonitis, symptoms may include disorientation, extreme dyspnea, severe headache, pharyngitis, watery diarrhea, and development of cutaneous pustular lesions on the head, trunk, or extremities. There is high fever, extreme tachypnea, a flushed skin, and cyanosis. Muscle tenderness may be striking. On examination of the chest, signs may be absent, or rales, rhonchi, and pleural rubs may be heard. The liver and spleen may be palpable. Signs of arthritis or meningitis may appear. Patients with the septicemic form usually have a rapidly progressive fatal course, which in some instances may be too fulminant to be altered by therapy. The leukocyte count may be normal or slightly increased. Chest radiographs most commonly show irregular nodular densities 4 to 10 mm in diameter disseminated throughout the lungs. These enlarge, coalesce, and often undergo cavitation as the disease progresses. Pleural effusion is rare. Other radiographic patterns include unilateral irregular mottled densities which become confluent.

Chronic suppurative infection In some patients secondary abscesses develop which dominate the clinical picture. Organs involved include skin, brain, lung, myocardium, liver, spleen, bones, joints, lymph nodes, and even the eye. These patients may be afebrile.

Recrudescent infection Disease may present as acute localized suppurative, acute pulmonary, acute septicemic, or chronic suppurative infection remote from the probable time of exposure (up to 26 years having been reported). In 11 of 15 reported cases, surgery, trauma, or intercurrent illness appeared to act as triggering events.

DIAGNOSIS Melioidosis should be considered in the differential diagnosis of any febrile illness in an individual who has been in an endemic area, especially if the presenting features are those of fulminant respiratory failure, if multiple pustular or necrotic skin or subcutaneous lesions develop, or if there is a radiographic pattern of tuberculosis in a patient from whom tubercle bacilli cannot be isolated.

Microscopic examination of exudates will reveal poorly staining, small, gram-negative bacilli which show the characteristic staining irregularities and "safety pin" bipolar staining with methylene blue. *Pseudomonas pseudomallei* will grow on most laboratory media, including eosinmethylene blue agar (EMB) or MacConkey's agar, in 24 to 48 h. The organisms can be readily differentiated from *P. mallei* and *P. aeruginosa* by standard bacteriologic procedures. The characteristic wrinkling of the colonies may require 72 h or longer. The hemagglutination, direct agglutination test, and complement fixation test are aids in diagnosis if a fourfold or greater rise in titer is demonstrated in paired serums. Single low titers are difficult to interpret because of nonspecific responses. The complement fixation test is said to be specific with titers above 1:8 during the acute illness, but may cross-react with *P. mallei*. A negative complement fixation test does not exclude disease. The hemagglutination and agglutination tests show more cross-reactions. Titers of 1:40 or more suggest infection.

TREATMENT The treatment regimen should vary with the form of the disease. Individuals with low-titer positive serologic tests but with no clinical evidence of infection do not require therapy. The choice of antibiotics in active infection should be based upon sensitivity studies, and therapy should be given for a minimum of 30 days. *Pseudomonas pseudomallei* is usually sensitive in vitro to the tetracyclines, chloramphenicol, novobiocin, kanamycin, sulfadiazine or sulfisoxazole, and trimethoprimsulfamethoxazole, and in most instances is resistant to penicillin G, ampicillin, carbenicillin, dicloxacillin, streptomycin, gentamicin, tobramycin, cephalosporins, vancomycin, lincomycin, rifampin, nalidixic acid, and colistin. In patients with pneumonitis who are not too ill, effective therapy has included tetracycline, 2 to 3 g daily (40 mg/kg); chloramphenicol, 3 g daily (40 mg/kg); sulfisoxazole, 4 g daily (70 mg/kg); or trimethoprim-sulfamethoxazole (4 mg/kg trimethoprim, 20 mg/kg sulfamethoxazole) for 60 to 150 days. If the patient is severely ill, two of these antimicrobials in combination have been recommended for 30 days followed by another 30 to 120 days of tetracycline alone. The mean interval for sputum cultures to become negative has been 6 weeks. If sputum cultures remain positive for 6 months, surgery with lobectomy should be considered. In patients with extrapulmonary suppurative lesions, therapy should be continued for 6 months to 1 year. The usual principles of surgical drainage should be followed. In desperately ill patients with severe pneumonitis or the septicemic form, multiple antibiotics should be administered by the parenteral route. One such regimen has included the use of chloramphenicol, 12 g per day; novobiocin, 6 g per day; and kanamycin, 4 g per day. In view of the severe potential toxicity of this regimen, its use should be considered only in extremely ill patients, and then only on a short-term basis. Current recommendations for antibiotics in the septicemic form of melioidosis are tetracycline, 4 to 6 g per day (80 mg/kg); chloramphenicol, 4 to 6 g per day (80 mg/kg); and one of the following: trimethoprim-sulfamethoxazole (9 mg/kg trimethoprim, 45 mg/kg sulfamethoxazole), sulfisoxazole (140 mg/kg), kanamycin (30 mg/kg), or novobiocin (60 mg/kg). In vitro studies have revealed antagonism between the following pairs of drugs: chloramphenicol-kanamycin, tetracycline-kanamycin, and sulfadiazine-chloramphenicol. Though the significance of such antagonism in clinical therapy has not been assessed, the data would favor selection of trimethoprim-sulfamethoxazole or novobiocin as the third drug. The dosage should be tapered rapidly as clinical improvement occurs.

PROGNOSIS Prior to antimicrobials, the mortality rate of apparent infection was 95 percent. With better diagnosis and more prolonged appropriate therapy, the mortality rate in all except the septicemic form is low. Even with vigorous appropriate antibiotics and supportive therapy, the mortality rate in patients with melioidosis septicemia is greater than 50 percent. Very few patients have had long-term follow-up, and the incidence of late relapses cannot be predicted.

PREVENTION There is no means of active immunization. In endemic areas, vigorous cleansing of abrasions and lacerations is recommended.

GLANDERS

DEFINITION Glanders is a serious infection of equine animals caused by *P. mallei*, which is transmitted occasionally to other domestic animals and to human beings.

ETIOLOGY *Pseudomonas mallei* is a small, slender, nonmotile, gram-negative bacillus. When it is stained with methylene blue, marked irregularities in staining are observed. Organisms grow on most common meat infusion media but require glycerol for optimum growth.

EPIDEMIOLOGY Glanders was at one time widespread throughout Europe, but owing to the introduction of control measures, its incidence has decreased steadily in most countries. The disease still occurs in Asia, Africa, and South America, but not in the United States. Glanders has never been common in human beings; the occasional infection, however, may be very serious. There have been no naturally acquired infections in the United States since 1938.

Glanders is primarily a disease of horses, mules, and donkeys, although goats, sheep, cats, and dogs sometimes naturally contract the disease. Pigs and cattle are resistant. In horses, the disease may be systemic, with prominent pulmonary involvement (*glanders*) or may be characterized by subcutaneous ulcerative lesions, and lymphatic thickening with nodules (*farcy*). Inhalation, ingestion, and inoculation through breaks in the skin have been suggested as routes of infection in animals. In human beings, the disease occurs primarily in individuals with close contact with horses, mules, or donkeys through inoculation of or a break in the skin or by exposing the nasal mucosa to contaminated discharges. A number of instances of airborne infection have been reported in laboratory workers.

PATHOLOGY   The acute lesion is characterized by nodules consisting of polymorphonuclear leukocytes surrounded by a zone of congestion. A characteristic histological feature is a peculiar nuclear degeneration known as *chromatotexis* which occurs early and is extensive. Small foci of deeply staining detritus within the abscess result from this degeneration. In older nodules, the reaction is characterized by epitheloid cells surrounding an area of central necrosis. Giant cells may be present. Virtually any organ may be involved.

CLINICAL MANIFESTATIONS   The manifestations which frequently overlap may be categorized as (1) acute localized suppurative infection, (2) acute pulmonary infection, (3) acute septicemic infection, and (4) chronic suppurative infection. Nearly 60 percent of patients have been between the ages of 20 and 40 years. The disease has been rare in women, probably because of less opportunity for contact.

Infection acquired by inoculation through an abrasion in the skin usually results in a nodule with an area of acute lymphangitis. The incubation period is probably 1 to 5 days. In all types of acute glanders, there are usually fever, generalized malaise, and prostration.

Infection of the mucous membranes may result in a mucopurulent discharge involving the eye, nose, or lips followed by extensive ulcerating granulomatous lesions which may or may not be associated with systemic reactions. With systemic invasion, a generalized papular eruption which may become pustular is frequent. This septicemic form of disease is usually fatal in 7 to 10 days.

Infection by inhalation is followed by an incubation period of 10 to 14 days. The more common symptoms include fever, occasionally associated with rigors, generalized myalgia, fatigue, headache, and pleuritic chest pain. Other symptoms consist of photophobia, lacrimation, and diarrhea. Findings on physical examination are usually normal except for fever and occasional lymphadenopathy, especially in the cervical chain, and splenomegaly. Laboratory findings include mild leukocytosis with 60 to 80 percent neutrophilic leukocytes, but leukopenia with relative lymphocytosis has been recorded. In the acute pulmonary form, chest radiographs characteristically reveal circumscribed densities which suggest early lung abscesses. Other findings may include lobar or bronchopneumonia. In the chronic suppurative form of the disease, the most frequent finding consists of multiple subcutaneous and intramuscular abscesses which most often involve the arms or legs. Approximately one-half the patients will have associated fever, lymphadenopathy, and nasal discharge or ulceration. Visceral involvement including pulmonary or pleural, ocular, skeletal,

hepatic, splenic, and meningeal or intracranial involvement occurs in some patients.

DIAGNOSIS   Microscopic examination of exudates may reveal small gram-negative bacilli which stain irregularly with methylene blue; however, organisms generally are very scanty, and it is often difficult to find them even in acute abscesses. Giemsa or other modifications of the Romanowski stain may be the best way to identify organisms. *Pseudomonas mallei* and *P. pseudomallei* cannot be distinguished morphologically. Culturing is often avoided because of the hazard to laboratory personnel; however, if cultures are made, growth occurs on most meat infusion nutrient media. The material is often contaminated with other microorganisms, and incubation with penicillin G (1000 units per milliliter) prior to culturing may be helpful. Subcutaneous inoculation of material into a guinea pig or hamster affords an alternative means of isolation. Blood cultures are usually negative except in the terminal stages of disease. Serologic tests show a rapidly rising agglutination titer, which reaches levels of 1:640 within 2 weeks. Serum from normal persons has been reported to show agglutination titers in dilutions up to 1:320. The complement fixation test is less sensitive but more specific and usually becomes positive during the third week; it is considered positive in dilutions of 1:20 or greater.

TREATMENT   The limited number of recent infections in human beings has precluded evaluation of most of the antibiotic agents. Sulfadiazine has been found to be an effective agent in experimental animals and in humans. The dosage utilized has been approximately 100 mg/kg administered in divided doses. In experimental infections, 3 weeks of therapy gave better results than 1 week. Benzyl penicillin is ineffective in vitro and in experimental infections. Streptomycin is bacteriostatic in vitro but was ineffective in experimental infections in hamsters. Antibiotics such as tetracycline, chloramphenicol, the antipseudomonal aminoglycosides, carbenicillin, the polymyxins, and trimethoprim have not been evaluated. In the absence of clinical experience and pending in vitro susceptibility studies, it would seem most reasonable to utilize the regimens appropriate for patients with various manifestations of melioidosis. In the acute infections, appropriate supportive measures are essential, and in chronic suppurative infections, the usual principles of surgical drainage should be followed.

PROGNOSIS   The prognosis depends upon the type of infection. The acute septicemic form has been uniformly fatal. The localized or chronic forms have a much better prognosis.

PREVENTION   Next to acquisition from diseased horses, the commonest source of natural disease in human beings has been contact with human glanders. Isolation is indicated.

REFERENCES

EICKHOFF TC et al: *Pseudomonas pseudomallei:* Susceptibility to chemotherapeutic agents. J Infect Dis 121:95, 1970

EVERETT ED, NELSON R: Pulmonary melioidosis, observations in 39 cases. Am Rev Resp Dis 112:331, 1975

HOWE C, MILLER WR: Human glanders: Report of six cases. Ann Intern Med 26:93, 1947

—— et al: The pseudomallei: A review. J Infect Dis 124:598, 1971

JACKSON AE et al: Recrudescent melioidosis associated with diabetic ketoacidosis. Arch Intern Med 130:268, 1972

MAYS EE, RICKETS EA: Melioidosis: Recrudescence associated with bronchogenic carcinoma twenty-six years following initial geographic exposure. Chest 68:261, 1975

McCORMICK JB et al: Human to human transmission of *Pseudomonas pseudomallei.* Ann Intern Med 83:512, 1975

SANFORD JP: Melioidosis: Another great imitator, in *Infectious Diseases: Current Topics in Diagnosis and Treatment,* DN Gilbert, JP Sanford (eds). New York, Grune & Stratton, 1978

ZAJTCHUK R et al: Surgical treatment of melioidosis. J Thorac Cardiovasc Surg 66:838, 1973

123
SALMONELLA INFECTIONS

EDWARD W. HOOK
RICHARD L. GUERRANT

INTRODUCTION The genus *Salmonella* consists of three species which include more than 1700 different serologic types. Striking variation in pathogenicity of serotypes occurs, but almost all are pathogenic for animals and humans. Specific host preferences characterize certain serotypes, such as *S. typhi,* which under natural conditions of transmission produces disease only in humans. *Salmonella* infections in humans present a spectrum of clinical syndromes, which sometimes overlap. The syndromes are (1) enteric fever (typhoid or paratyphoid fever), (2) acute gastroenteritis, (3) bacteremia, and (4) localized infection which may occur at almost any site. In addition, *asymptomatic intestinal infections* and *transient convalescent intestinal carrier* states are common. Occasionally, a focus of infection persists in the gallbladder or urinary tract to produce a *chronic carrier* state.

ETIOLOGY Salmonellae are motile gram-negative bacilli that do not ferment lactose or sucrose but ferment glucose. Almost all serotypes produce gas, although *S. typhi* is a notable exception. Salmonellae are divided into three species by biochemical means: *S. typhi, S. cholerae-suis,* and *S. enteritidis.* The species are further subdivided into serotypes, which are identified by highly specific O (somatic) and H (flagellar) antigens. A given serotype will contain a specific combination of multiple O and H antigens. Identification by serotype is accomplished routinely only in large salmonella typing centers, which have the necessary collection of antiserums required for such work. Salmonellae are also divided into groups on the basis of O antigen composition. Most isolates from natural sources fall into five groups, A to E.

The species *S. typhi* and *S. cholerae-suis* consist of only one serotype each (in groups D and C, respectively), whereas the species *S. enteritidis* comprises over 1700 serotypes (in all groups, including C and D). Considerable overlap in antigenic composition is responsible for the cross-reactivity which is commonly seen in serologic tests with salmonellae.

The Salmonella Surveillance Unit of the Center for Disease Control reports 20,000 to 25,000 isolations of salmonellae annually from human beings in the United States. This number has been consistent over the decade from 1967 to 1976. In descending order, the most frequently isolated serotypes in 1976 were *S. typhimurium, S. heidelberg, S. agona, S. newport, S. enteritidis, S. infantis, S. saint-paul, S. typhi, S. oranienburg,* and *S. muenchen.* The 10 most frequently isolated serotypes account for about 70 percent of the total isolates from man over this period. *Salmonella typhimurium* perennially accounts for 25 to 35 percent of the isolates. A significant recent change in serotypes isolated from human sources in the United States is the rapidly increasing rate of isolation each year of *S. agona,* an organism apparently introduced indirectly via animals fed Peruvian fish meal in 1971. Concern has also arisen over the multiple-drug-resistant *S. wein,* which was the most frequent *Salmonella* isolate in France in 1974 and which is now being isolated in the United States; *S. wein* is resistant to chloramphenicol, ampicillin, sulfonamides, and tetracyclines.

In the subsequent section, typhoid fever, the classic example of enteric fever, is considered separately from other *Salmonella* infections because of its historical importance, the host specificity of *S. typhi,* and the extensive clinical experience with the disease.

TYPHOID FEVER

DEFINITION Typhoid fever is an acute systemic disease resulting from infection with *S. typhi.* The disease is unique to humans. It is characterized by malaise, fever, abdominal discomfort, transient rash, splenomegaly, and leukopenia. The most prominent major complications are intestinal hemorrhage and perforation. The disease is the classic example of enteric fever caused by salmonellas. However, enteric fever, similar to typhoid, can also be caused by other *Salmonella* serotypes and is termed *paratyphoid fever.*

EPIDEMIOLOGY *Salmonella typhi* gains access to the body by the oral route in almost all cases as a consequence of the ingestion of contaminated food, water, or milk. Humans are the only true reservoir of *S. typhi* in nature, and persons with typhoid fever or convalescent or chronic carriers always serve as the ultimate source of infection. Infected individuals can excrete millions of viable typhoid bacilli in the feces, which are the usual source of contamination of food or drink. Patients with active disease also occasionally have organisms in respiratory secretions, vomitus, or other body fluids. Flies or other insects can carry organisms from feces or other infected material to food or drink and have been implicated in a few outbreaks. The fact that *S. typhi* may survive freezing or drying enhances the possibility of spread by contaminated ice, dust, foods, and sewage. Oysters or other shellfish are contaminated at times in polluted waters and occasionally serve as sources of typhoid.

The incidence of typhoid fever has steadily decreased in the United States during the past century to the present relatively low level of less than 400 cases per annum. The decrease in incidence has been coincident with improvement in socioeconomic conditions and is specifically related to development of pure water supplies, effective sewage disposal, pasteurization of milk, and methods to detect and control spread of organisms from persons with active disease or from carriers. Typhoid continues to occur on a large scale in countries where sanitation is suboptimal. About 40 percent of the patients with typhoid fever in the United States appear to have acquired the infection in another area of the world.

Typhoid can be eradicated ultimately because the infection is confined to humans and both the disease and the carrier state can be controlled by appropriate therapy. The importance of sewage disposal, a pure water supply, and control of carriers is highlighted repeatedly by the occurrence of outbreaks which develop when defects in sanitation occur during natural disasters such as flood.

The sex distribution of patients with typhoid fever in the United States shows no significant predilection. In recent years, about 75 percent of cases have occurred in persons less than 30 years of age. In contrast, the chronic carrier state is much more common in females than males (the female/male ratio is 3:1) and in older individuals (88 percent over 50 years of age).

There is no seasonal variation in incidence of typhoid fever in the United States. However, in areas of the world where the disease is endemic, the incidence increases in the summer months.

PATHOGENESIS The outcome of the interaction between the typhoid bacillus and humans is determined during the early hours after ingestion of the organisms. Typhoid bacilli reach the small intestine shortly after ingestion and may multiply there. The organisms may then penetrate the mucosa with minimal epithelial destruction and enter intestinal lymphatics, perhaps via the Peyer's patches, to be carried to the bloodstream. This initial early bacteremia apparently occurs within 24 to 72 h after ingestion of organisms and is rarely detected in natural infections because patients are usually asymptomatic at this early stage. The bacteremia is transient and is rapidly terminated as bacilli are phagocytized by cells of the reticuloendothelial system. Nevertheless, viable bacilli are disseminated throughout the body and apparently persist within reticuloendothelial cells. If multiplication at the intracellular site takes place, organisms reenter the bloodstream, producing a continuous bacteremia for days or weeks. The reappearance of bacteremia corresponds with the onset of manifestations of the disease. The intracellular organisms are eventually destroyed as manifestations of disease subside and recovery ensues. Enhanced intracellular killing and recovery appear to be related to the onset of delayed hypersensitivity. Recovery is unrelated to the appearance, even in high titer, of agglutinins against the somatic, flagellar, or Vi antigens of the typhoid bacillus.

The number of organisms ingested is of obvious importance in determining whether typhoid fever results from exposure to *S. typhi*. Studies in volunteers have shown that about 10^7 typhoid bacilli of the Quailes strain must be taken orally to produce typhoid fever in 50 percent of normal volunteers. The number of organisms ingested also influences the incubation period, and short incubation periods, in general, correspond to large doses of organisms. The volunteer studies have also demonstrated that different strains of typhoid bacilli vary considerably in their capacity to produce disease in humans.

The normal flora of the upper intestinal tract is an important protective mechanism against invasion by *S. typhi*. Volunteer studies have demonstrated that antimicrobial therapy a day or so before oral challenge with *S. typhi* markedly decreases the number of viable bacilli required to produce disease. It is possible that certain factors known to be associated with typhoid outbreaks, such as malnutrition, enhance susceptibility to typhoid infection by alterations in the intestinal flora.

During the phase of persistent bacteremia, all organs are repeatedly exposed to typhoid bacilli. Abscess formation may occur but is unusual. However, localization does occur in the gallbladder in almost all cases. Organisms multiply in the bile to high titer, usually without manifestations of cholecystitis, and are excreted with bile into the intestinal tract. Stool cultures, which are usually negative for *S. typhi* during the incubation period and early phases of the disease, become positive in a large proportion of cases during the third or fourth week of the disease, when excretion of organisms multiplying in the bile reaches a peak.

The factors responsible for the fever, leukopenia, and other manifestations of typhoid fever have been inadequately defined. Typhoid bacilli contain biologically active lipopolysaccharides or endotoxins which produce fever, leukopenia, thrombocytopenia, and hyperplasia of reticuloendothelial cells when injected into animals or humans. It has been assumed for years that these materials play an important role in the patho-

genesis of the signs and symptoms of typhoid fever. However, the evidence regarding the role of endotoxin in the genesis of the manifestations of typhoid is inconclusive. For example, tolerance to the pyrogenic effects of endotoxins can be demonstrated during convalescence from typhoid fever, which suggests release of endotoxins during infection. While laboratory evidence for low-grade, subclinical disseminated intravascular coagulation can often be demonstrated in patients with typhoid fever, endotoxemia is usually not detectable. Other studies show that typhoid fever follows a normal course in volunteers rendered tolerant to endotoxins prior to challenge, indicating that more complex mechanisms than endotoxemia alone are responsible for the sustained fever and toxemia.

PATHOLOGY The most prominent microscopic lesion in typhoid fever is proliferation of large mononuclear cells in many different tissues. Mononuclear hyperplasia leads to lymphadenopathy, splenomegaly, and impressive enlargement of lymphoid tissues in the intestines, especially in the terminal ileum (Peyer's patches). Proliferating mononuclear cells may also be observed in bone marrow, liver, and lung. Studies in volunteers using ^{131}I-tagged aggregated albumin have shown increased phagocytic activity of the reticuloendothelial system by the third to fifth days after onset of symptoms. Necrosis in hyperplastic Peyer's patches may be associated with erosion of blood vessels in the lesions in the intestinal tract, which leads to oozing of blood or massive hemorrhage. Lesions may extend deep into the intestinal wall and cause perforation of the bowel, an event which characteristically occurs late in the disease, most often in the third febrile week. The site of perforation is usually in the distal 24 in of the ileum.

The gallbladder and bile ducts are routinely infected during the disease. As a rule, this biliary infection is asymptomatic, although acute cholecystitis may occur occasionally. Biliary infection terminates spontaneously during convalescence in the vast majority of patients within 12 months, but about 3 percent of adults continue to harbor organisms in the gallbladder and become chronic carriers of the typhoid bacillus.

MANIFESTATIONS The incubation period averages about 10 days but may vary from extremes of 3 to 60 days depending on the infecting dose.

The clinical manifestations and duration of illness vary markedly from one patient to another. Mild forms of the disease, characterized primarily by fever, may last only a week, or illness may be prolonged, lasting 8 weeks or more if untreated.

In a typical patient not treated with antimicrobials, the illness lasts about 4 weeks. The onset is insidious with headache, malaise, anorexia, and fever. Headache may be the first manifestation of disease and is usually generalized and severe. Chilly sensations are common, and frank chills may be observed. The fever is remittent, frequently increasing in a steplike manner from day to day as the illness develops. Abdominal discomfort, bloating, and constipation are common during the early phase of illness. A dry cough is observed in about two-thirds of the patients and occasionally may be so prominent as to direct attention away from the generalized nature of the infectious process. Nosebleeds may occur during the early phase of illness.

The temperature gradually increases for 5 to 7 days and then plateaus as a continuous or mildly remittent fever in the range of 39 to 40°C. The temperature may be sustained at these levels with little variation for 2 or 3 weeks. A relative bradycardia occurs in 30 to 40 percent of the patients. The prolonged persistent fever leads to general debility; patients are weak and anorectic. Mental dullness is common and delirium may occur. Abdominal pain and marked distention are usual. Constipation, relatively common during the early phase of illness, may give way to diarrhea later in the course of the disease.

The characteristic rash (rose spots) is most often observed during the second week of the disease. The lesions are small, 2- to 4-mm, erythematous macules which occur in small numbers on the upper abdomen and anterior thorax. The lesions blanch on pressure and last only 2 to 3 days. Some reports describe rose spots in as many as 90 percent of patients, whereas other reports indicate a frequency of only 10 percent or even less. The evasive nature of the rash and the difficulties encountered in detecting lesions in highly pigmented individuals probably account for the marked variation in incidence reported in the literature.

The liver and spleen are frequently enlarged and palpable from the end of the first week of illness. The spleen is palpable in about three-quarters of the patients. The liver may be tender, and occasionally a friction rub is audible over the spleen.

Abdominal tenderness is frequent and distention occurs in the majority of cases. Marked abdominal pain with signs of peritonitis should call attention to the possibility of perforation of the bowel.

After the third week, the symptoms slowly abate, and the temperature returns to normal over a period of days.

Jaundice secondary to extensive mononuclear cell infiltration in the liver and hepatic cell necrosis is a rare complication of typhoid. Acute renal failure also is observed rarely; the pathogenesis of this so-called "typhoid nephritis" has not been adequately defined. Disseminated intravascular coagulation may develop in severe typhoid and lead to additional clinical manifestations secondary to thrombosis or hemorrhage.

Complications Prior to the introduction of chloramphenicol, the prolonged febrile course of typhoid often led to profound debility, weight loss, and multiple nutritional deficiencies. Intestinal hemorrhage and bowel perforation, the most feared complications, were common causes of death. The frequency of complications in typhoid fever has been reduced since the advent of effective chemotherapy.

INTESTINAL HEMORRHAGE Erosion of blood vessels in hyperplastic and necrotic Peyer's patches or in other mononuclear cell accumulations in the wall of the intestine leads to bleeding into the intestinal tract. Occult blood in feces is quite common during the course of the disease, occurring in 20 percent or more of patients. Gross blood is present in feces in about 10 percent of patients, and massive hemorrhage occurs occasionally. Major hemorrhage is usually a late complication, occurring most often during the second or third week of disease. A sudden drop in blood pressure or temperature may be the first manifestation of hemorrhage.

INTESTINAL PERFORATION The pathological process in the lymphoid tissues of the intestine may also involve the muscular and serosal layers of the bowel and lead to perforation. Prior to the advent of chloramphenicol, perforation occurred in about 3 percent of patients with typhoid. The incidence has been reduced by antimicrobial therapy to about 1 percent. Perforation is most common in the distal 24 in of ileum and is observed most frequently during the third week of the disease. The onset of perforation may be quite unexpected during an otherwise uncomplicated convalescence. Pain in the right lower quadrant of the abdomen is the most frequent initial manifestation, but signs of localized or generalized peritonitis develop rapidly.

OTHER COMPLICATIONS Typhoid bacilli may localize in any tissue in the body with the production of localized suppurative infection. Meningitis, chondritis, periostitis, osteomyelitis, ar-

thritis, and pyelonephritis are examples of localized infections that may be observed occasionally. Pneumonia is not unusual and may be related to the typhoid bacillus or to a secondary bacterial invader, such as the pneumococcus. Severe deep thrombophlebitis may occur during the febrile period. Late complications also include peripheral neuritis, deafness, and alopecia. Hemolytic anemia may be observed, especially in infected individuals deficient in glucose 6-phosphate dehydrogenase.

Relapse After illness has subsided for a variable period, usually about 2 weeks, all the manifestations which characterized the initial infection may recur. Blood cultures, negative during convalescence, may become positive again. Although relapse may be severe, it is usually milder and of shorter duration than the original illness. The incidence of relapse was about 5 to 10 percent prior to the introduction of effective chemotherapy. Chloramphenicol has not decreased the frequency of relapse; in fact, the relapse rate in chloramphenicol-treated patients is higher than in patients not receiving the drug. Periods of antimicrobial therapy longer than 2 weeks do not seem to alter the incidence of relapse. Relapse cannot be correlated with the titer of agglutinins against the flagellar, somatic, or Vi antigens of the typhoid bacillus.

Chronic carriers Although the vast majority of patients with typhoid fever eradicate the site of infection in the gallbladder during convalescence, about 3 percent of adults do not, and these individuals become chronic typhoid carriers who continue to excrete organisms in feces for years, usually for life. A chronic carrier is defined as a person documented to have been excreting typhoid bacilli in the stool for a period of at least 1 year. In the United States, almost all chronic carriers have a persistent site of infection in the gallbladder from which organisms reach the intestinal tract in bile. Chronic carriers may be detected by follow-up of patients with typhoid fever, but many carriers give no history of typhoid. In these patients, it is assumed that the initial illness was so mild as to go unrecognized or undiagnosed. Once organisms have been demonstrated in the stools for as long as a year, it is quite unlikely that the focus of infection in the gallbladder will terminate spontaneously. The chronic carrier state is rare in children and occurs more commonly with increasing age and is about three times more common in women than men. It is possible that these age and sex characteristics are related to the greater prevalence of gallbladder disease in older women, a factor which would favor persistence of organisms in the biliary tract.

The chronic biliary carrier is usually asymptomatic. Despite millions of organisms entering the intestine in each milliliter of bile, patients show no systemic manifestations. Gallstones and dysfunction of the gallbladder on cholecystogram can be demonstrated in a large proportion of chronic carriers, and carriers occasionally develop acute cholecystitis.

In areas of the world where *Schistosoma haematobium* infections are common, a chronic urinary carrier state results from localization of typhoid bacilli or other *Salmonella* serotypes in the obstructed urinary tract or adjacent lesions resulting from the schistosomiasis. These chronic urinary carriers not only excrete *Salmonella* in the urine but also may have intermittent bacteremic episodes which are not necessarily accompanied by fever.

LABORATORY FINDINGS Leukopenia of 3000 to 4000 cells per cubic millimeter is characteristic of the febrile phase of typhoid fever. A sudden increase in leukocyte count to 10,000 cells per cubic millimeter or higher should suggest the possibility of intestinal perforation, hemorrhage, or a pyogenic complication, but these complications may occur in the absence of leukocytosis. A normocytic normochromic anemia develops during the course of the disease and may be aggravated by blood loss from intestinal lesions. Occult blood and a mononuclear leukocytosis in feces is common from the second week of disease. Urine is usually normal except for transient albuminuria during the febrile period.

The most dependable way to establish a definitive diagnosis of typhoid fever is by blood culture. Organisms can be recovered by culture of blood in 70 to 90 percent of patients during the first week of disease. Bacteremia is continuous and prolonged. Positive blood cultures are obtained in as many as 30 or 40 percent of patients during the third week of disease, but the incidence of bacteremia rapidly decreases after this time. Blood cultures frequently are positive during relapse. Recent evidence in partially treated cases suggests that culture of bone marrow may yield the organism when other cultures are negative.

Only about 10 to 15 percent of patients have positive stool cultures during the first week of disease. However, the frequency of positive stool cultures increases as the disease progresses, reaching a maximum of about 75 percent during the third or fourth week of illness. The frequency of positive cultures then begins to decline so that only about 10 percent of patients have positive stool cultures 8 weeks after onset of illness. Most of these patients' cultures become negative over the next several weeks or months, but about 3 percent of adults continue to excrete organisms even after 1 year. Persistent excretion in these chronic carriers is secondary to infection in the gallbladder and biliary tract.

The incidence of positive urine cultures varies markedly during the course of typhoid fever and parallels the frequency of positive stool cultures. At least some of the positive cultures represent contamination of urine with feces harboring typhoid bacilli.

The majority of patients, but by no means all, develop a fourfold or greater rise in agglutinins against the somatic or O antigens of the typhoid bacillus during the course of the disease. A fourfold or greater increase in titer in the absence of recent typhoid immunization is compatible with infection with *S. typhi* but is by no means specific. All the group D organisms, one of which is *S. typhi*, as well as organisms in groups A and B, have certain common antigens which can evoke the formation of antibodies reactive with the O antigen used in the Widal test. Agglutinins against flagellar or H antigens also appear, frequently in higher titer than agglutinins against the O antigens. However, the H agglutinins are even more subject to nonspecific variation than O agglutinins and are of no value in diagnosis. Agglutinins begin to appear after about 1 week of illness and reach a peak titer during the fifth or sixth week. Early antimicrobial therapy may dampen the immunologic response in patients with typhoid fever. Relapse bears no relation to agglutinin titer. Rheumatoid factor activity in high titer can be detected in a large proportion of patients with typhoid or paratyphoid fever.

DIFFERENTIAL DIAGNOSIS The clinical features of typhoid fever, while characteristic and suggestive of the diagnosis, are certainly not pathognomonic. Many other diseases give a clinical picture which may be confused with typhoid; these include the rickettsioses, brucellosis, tularemia, leptospirosis, psittacosis, infectious hepatitis, infectious mononucleosis, primary atypical pneumonia, miliary tuberculosis, malaria, lymphoma, and rheumatic fever. Typhoid should be considered in any patient with unexplained fever, especially if there is a history of recent foreign travel to endemic areas.

TREATMENT   Antimicrobial therapy   Chloramphenicol is the antibiotic of choice for the treatment of typhoid fever. Despite the fact that a number of antimicrobial agents show excellent in vitro activity against *S. typhi*, chloramphenicol has consistently been shown to be more effective in terminating the febrile toxic course of the disease in the greatest proportion of patients in the shortest period of time. Nevertheless, the response to chloramphenicol is not dramatic or rapid. Subjective improvement usually occurs within about 48 h after beginning therapy, but the temperature usually does not return to normal for 2 to 5 days after initiating treatment. Bacteremia usually clears within hours after therapy is instituted, but occasionally organisms can be recovered from the blood 24 to 48 h after beginning treatment. The dose of chloramphenicol should be 50 mg per kilogram of body weight per day divided into three or four equal doses given orally at intervals of 6 to 8 h. After the patient has become afebrile, the dose may be reduced to 30 mg/kg per day. Therapy should be continued for 2 weeks. If chloramphenicol cannot be given by the oral route, comparable doses should be given parenterally.

Ampicillin in doses of 80 mg/kg per day or 6 g per day for adults divided into four or six doses given parenterally or a combination of trimethoprim and sulfamethoxazole is effective in the treatment of typhoid, but the response is not as predictable or as prompt as with chloramphenicol. If there is a contraindication to therapy with chloramphenicol, ampicillin, amoxicillin, or trimethoprim-sulfamethoxazole is recommended.

Occasional patients with typhoid without evidence of suppurative complications do not respond clinically even after 4 or 5 days of antimicrobial therapy, even though blood cultures become negative. Delayed responses of this type occur in only about 1 percent of patients treated with chloramphenicol, in contrast to 5 or 10 percent of patients treated with ampicillin.

Chloramphenicol-resistant strains have been reported since 1972 from Mexico, Southeast Asia, and India. Resistance is due to a transferable R factor which also codes for resistance to sulfonamides, tetracycline, and streptomycin. *Salmonella typhi* resistant to both chloramphenicol and ampicillin have been isolated from a few patients. If chloramphenicol resistance is encountered, then ampicillin, amoxicillin, or trimethoprim and sulfamethoxazole should be used.

Adrenal hormones   The administration of prednisone or steroids with similar activity can terminate within a matter of hours the severe febrile toxemic state seen in some patients. Because of the lag in time between institution of antimicrobial therapy and evidence of response, patients with life-threatening toxemia should be treated with a brief course of adrenal corticosteroids in addition to chloramphenicol. An appropriate regimen is 60 mg prednisone the first day; no additional steroid therapy should be administered. Hypothermia and hypotension occasionally occur within hours after initiation of steroids.

Supportive treatment   Nursing care and attention to nutritional requirements are important. Laxatives and enemas should be avoided despite constipation because of the danger of precipitating hemorrhage or perforation. Salicylates should not be used, because in addition to their effects on blood platelets and irritating action on the bowel, these compounds can induce wide swings in temperature with very uncomfortable chills and sweats. Hypothermia and hypotension occur in some patients after administration of salicylates.

Hemorrhage and perforation Patients should be observed carefully to detect these complications at an early stage. Typing and cross matching should be carried out at the time of initial diagnosis of typhoid, and transfusion is indicated in the event of significant hemorrhage. Patients with typhoid are poor surgical risks. If perforation is suspected, emphasis should be placed on efforts to combat shock and decompress the bowel. Additional antimicrobials may have to be added to control peritonitis. Small perforations may localize and can be managed without surgical intervention. However, if evidence of localization does not develop, surgical intervention may be required.

Relapse The therapy of relapse is identical to that for the primary episode.

Chronic carriers Chronic carriers should be investigated for the presence of gallstones or a nonfunctioning gallbladder. Carriers without evidence of gallstones or gallbladder disease on cholecystogram usually can be cured with a prolonged course of ampicillin. One program which has been found to be effective consists of 6 g ampicillin divided into four equal oral doses each day with probenecid for a period of 6 weeks. If gallstones or a nonfunctioning gallbladder are demonstrated on cholecystogram, antimicrobial therapy is unlikely to be effective in terminating the carrier state. These patients should have cholecystectomy, which cures the chronic carrier state in about 85 percent of patients. Ampicillin may be used in conjunction with cholecystectomy. Therapy should be started a few days prior to the procedure and continued for 2 or 3 weeks.

PREVENTION AND CONTROL Although immunization with typhoid vaccine affords significant protection against typhoid infection, the degree of immunity is not great and can be readily overcome with a large dose of organisms. Nevertheless, immunization is recommended for individuals living or traveling in areas where the disease is endemic and for persons working with the organism in laboratories. Adults should receive 0.5 ml vaccine on two occasions separated by a period of 1 or 2 weeks. A yearly booster is required to maintain immunity. Immunization with typhoid vaccine causes a transient elevation for several months in titer of agglutinins against typhoid O antigens and a persistently elevated titer for H antigens.

All typhoid patients should be reported to local health authorities, and stool specimens should be cultured during convalescence. Three consecutively negative stool cultures obtained at weekly intervals indicate that a carrier state has not developed.

Caution should be observed to prevent spread of infection from persons with active disease or from carriers. Chronic or convalescent carriers should not be allowed to prepare food until clear documentation shows that at least three or more stool cultures are negative for typhoid bacilli. Carriers should be cautioned regarding routine sanitary techniques.

PROGNOSIS The mortality rate of typhoid fever prior to the introduction of chloramphenicol was about 12 percent. Death was associated with toxemia, inanition, pneumonia, bowel perforation, and intestinal hemorrhage. The mortality rate is still 2 or 3 percent; deaths are observed primarily in infants, the aged, or individuals with malnutrition or other underlying diseases.

OTHER *SALMONELLA* INFECTIONS

DEFINITION Bacteria of the genus *Salmonella* may produce asymptomatic infection of the intestinal tract in humans or several different clinical syndromes including acute gastroenteritis (or enterocolitis), bacteremia, paratyphoid fever, or localized infections ranging from osteomyelitis to endocarditis. The clinical syndromes resulting from infection with *Salmonella* cannot always be sharply differentiated and sometimes overlap.

Salmonella infections are among the most prevalent communicable diseases caused by bacteria in the United States today. These infections are transmitted in the vast majority of cases from animals to humans and occasionally from person to person and are usually brief, self-limited, and mild.

EPIDEMIOLOGY Salmonellas can be isolated from the intestinal tracts of humans and many lower animals. The prevalence of asymptomatic excretors of these organisms in the general population is about 0.2 percent, but the most important reservoir of salmonellas is in domestic and wild animal species in which infection rates vary from less than 1 to more than 20 percent. An incomplete list of animals from which *Salmonella* species have been isolated includes chickens, turkeys, ducks, pigs, cows, dogs, cats, rats, parakeets, as well as certain cold-blooded animals and insects. Animals sold as pets, especially baby chicks, ducks, and turtles, may also harbor *Salmonella* and serve as sources of infection.

Salmonella infection is almost always acquired by the oral route, usually by ingestion of contaminated food or drink. Any food product is a potential source of human infection. The source of contamination of food or drink may be asymptomatic human carriers or persons with active clinical disease, but the greatest single source of human infection in the United States is the vast reservoir of *Salmonella* in lower animals. The high incidence of infection in domestic animals used as a source of food for humans and present methods of processing foods and food products in bulk result in the availability of foods for human consumption with a potentially high incidence of contamination with *Salmonella*. For example, a significant proportion varying from 1 to more than 50 percent of raw meats purchased in retail markets is contaminated with *Salmonella*. Meat is contaminated by many routes, but the most common are natural infection of the animal used as a source of meat and contamination of the carcass during slaughter and processing. Eggs or egg products, including dried or frozen eggs, are also common sources of *Salmonella* infection. Of the various animal species, domestic fowl, including chickens, turkeys, ducks, and eggs and egg products, constitute the single largest reservoir of infection and the source most often responsible for infection of humans. Adequate cooking of food prior to human consumption serves to decrease the possibility of infection. However, salmonellas may survive cooking at low temperature, or food may be recontaminated after cooking by organisms from kitchen equipment or personnel.

Food or drink may also be contaminated by rats, mice, insects, or other vermin harboring these organisms. Cross infection occurs occasionally by the airborne route from dried foods such as egg whites or dust which contain viable *Salmonella*. *Salmonella* contamination of a large variety of processed foods has also been documented. Some of these foods contain ingredients of animal origin such as eggs, whereas others contain contaminated products of vegetable origin such as coconut or yeast. A variety of pharmaceutical products of animal origin have been shown to be responsible for *Salmonella* infections of humans; these products include carmine dye, pancreatin, bile salts, and extracts of various organs such as thyroid, adrenal, and stomach.

Pet turtles may be an important source of *Salmonella* infection in humans, especially in children, accounting for perhaps as many as 10 to 20 percent of reported *Salmonella* infections in certain areas. Turtles are infected on breeding farms and continue to excrete organisms in feces into tank water for long periods of time. Although knowledge of the manner of transmission to humans is incomplete, it is likely that turtle feces or tank water harboring salmonellas contaminate hands of handlers, from which organisms are passed to the mouth or to food or drink.

Salmonella species may also be transmitted directly or via fomites from humans to humans or from animals to humans without the intervention of contaminated food or drink, but this method of spread is not common. However, cross infection of this type has been shown to be responsible for a number of outbreaks of salmonellosis among patients in nurseries and hospitals. Nosocomial salmonellosis poses a particular threat to newborns, immunosuppressed patients, patients in burn units, and those receiving multiple broad-spectrum antibiotics, who may be infected by relatively few organisms. Multiple-drug-resistant salmonellas are often found in this setting. Nursery outbreaks have been traced to newborn infants from mothers with recent *Salmonella* infections.

Fish meal, meat meal, bone meal, and other by-products of the meat-packing industry are often contaminated with *Salmonella* organisms. These products are incorporated in animal and poultry feeds and apparently play an important role in the perpetuation of infection among domestic animals that can be spread to humans.

The true incidence of *Salmonella* infection is difficult to determine. The reported isolations of salmonellas from humans in the United States represent about 10 cases per 100,000 population per annum. However, reported cases represent only a small proportion of the actual number because bacteriologic studies are usually performed only on patients with severe or protracted diarrhea, and many outbreaks are not investigated. Although *Salmonella* infection occurs throughout the year, the Salmonella Surveillance Unit of the National Communicable Disease Center has observed a distinct seasonal pattern with the greatest number of isolations reported from July through October for each year.

A close correlation exists between the *Salmonella* serotypes most often responsible for human infection and those isolated from animals in any specific geographic area. The similarities document the importance of nonhuman reservoirs of *Salmonella* in the epidemiology of *Salmonella* infection in man.

PATHOGENESIS The course of events after salmonellas have gained access to the gastrointestinal tract is determined by the dose, serotype, and invasive potential of the organism, and by the resistance of the host. Different *Salmonella* serotypes show marked variation in invasive potential and capacity to produce disease in man. For example, *S. anatum* characteristically produces asymptomatic intestinal infection and rarely invades the bloodstream. In contrast, *S. cholerae-suis*, the most invasive serotype, frequently produces bacteremia and metastatic infection. Bloodstream invasion may occur as a complication of gastroenteritis but usually develops without preceding intestinal symptoms. Bacteremia with any serotype may be transient or prolonged, and may be accompanied by recurrent chills and fever or manifestations of paratyphoid fever. Bloodborne bacteria may localize at any site and lead to suppuration in bone, joints, meninges, pleura, or other tissues.

Multiplication of ingested organisms in the intestinal tract may be followed by symptoms of gastroenteritis. The intestinal irritation and inflammation are produced by a true infection deep in the mucosa as evidenced by polymorphonuclear leukocytes typically found in the diarrheal stool. However, studies in animals have shown that mucosal invasion alone is not sufficient to account for the intestinal fluid observed in experimental infections. The secretory effects of certain strains of *S. typhimurium* can be abolished in animals by indomethicin without altering the invasive process. This has led to the hypothesis of a possible enterotoxin-like effect on upper intestinal transport. An enterotoxin-like effect has also been shown in animals and tissue culture models used to study *Escherichia coli* and cholera enterotoxins.

Studies in human volunteers indicate that large numbers of viable organisms must be ingested to produce clinically apparent disease. However, a transient carrier state can be produced with doses 10 or 100 times smaller than those required to evoke symptoms of infection. The minimal infectious dose varies markedly among different serotypes.

Many host factors influence the frequency and nature of *Salmonella* infections. The minimal infectious dose varies considerably among different individual hosts and can be reduced by antacids, antimotility drugs, or antimicrobial agents in experimental animals. Some have reported the precipitation of severe systemic disease following antimotility therapy for mild gastroenteritis.

The bacterial flora of the intestine is important in determining the fate of ingested salmonellas. Administration of certain antibiotics by the oral route to mice results in a 10,000-fold increase in susceptibility to infection with *S. enteritidis*. Somewhat similar observations have been made in experimental typhoid fever in volunteers. In these studies the dose of *S. typhi* required to initiate infection by the oral route in humans can be reduced sharply by giving certain antimicrobials orally prior to challenge. Epidemiologic studies have also shown that prior antimicrobial therapy alters the capacity of the human intestinal tract to eradicate *Salmonella* acquired naturally. The effect of antibiotic therapy may be related to a marked diminution in number of *Bacteroides* or other organisms which produce antimicrobial substances such as short-chain fatty acids that are active against *Salmonella*. Alteration in intestinal flora also has been suggested as a mechanism of the increased susceptibility of patients with previous major gastric surgery, especially gastrectomy and gastroenterostomy, to intestinal infection with salmonellas. However, reduced acidity or rapid emptying time consequent to gastric surgery also appear to play a role by increasing the number of viable organisms reaching the small intestine.

Cell-mediated immune mechanisms appear to be important in host resistance to infection with salmonellas. About one-third of patients who are hospitalized because of salmonellosis have some type of major underlying disease, such as leukemia, lymphoma, lupus erythematosus, or aplastic anemia. This may be coincidence but more often reflects a decrease in resistance to bacterial infection in general. In a few diseases there is evidence to indicate an almost specific predisposition to infection by salmonellas that exceeds susceptibility to other bacterial species. Patients with sickle-cell anemia and other hemolytic processes are unusually susceptible to bloodstream invasion by salmonellas. In patients with sickle hemoglobinopathies there is a strong tendency for localization in bone, and salmonellas, not staphylococci, are the most common cause of osteomyelitis in patients with sickle-cell diseases. *Salmonella* bacteremia is also an unusually frequent complication of the acute hemolytic phase of bartonellosis (Chap. 136).

Infants are more susceptible to *Salmonella* infection and remain convalescent carriers for a longer period of time than adults. The mortality rate from the disease is also higher in infants and in the elderly than in young adults.

CLINICAL MANIFESTATIONS Gastroenteritis Although gastroenteritis often occurs in large epidemics among individuals who have eaten the same contaminated food, family outbreaks and sporadic cases are even more common. After an incubation period of 8 to 48 h, there is sudden onset of colicky abdominal pain and loose, watery diarrhea, occasionally with mucus or blood. Nausea and vomiting are frequent but are rarely severe or protracted. Fever of 38 to 39°C is common, and there may be an initial chill. Patients usually have mild to moderate abdominal tenderness on palpation, but severe tenderness, even with rebound, occurs in occasional patients. Peristalsis is usually hyperactive. Abdominal findings may be prominent in some patients and lead to confusion with certain intraabdominal emergencies, such as acute appendicitis or acute cholecystitis. Symptoms usually subside promptly within 2 to 5 days and recovery is uneventful. However, the illness is occasionally more protracted, with persistence of diarrhea and low-grade fever for 10 to 14 days. Fatalities rarely exceed 1 percent of the affected population and are limited almost entirely to infants, the aged, and debilitated patients.

The causative organism can often be isolated from the suspected food and from feces during the acute illness. Stool cultures usually become negative for salmonellas within 1 to 4 weeks, but occasional patients continue to excrete organisms for months. Organisms tend to persist in the stools of infants and young children for longer periods than in older children or adults. The blood leukocyte count is usually normal. The blood culture is usually negative.

Enteric or paratyphoid fever Certain species can produce an illness clinically indistinguishable from typhoid fever, with prolonged fever, rose spots, splenomegaly, leukopenia, gastrointestinal symptoms, and positive blood and stool cultures. The organisms most likely to produce this picture are *S. choleraesuis* and *S. enteritidis*, serotypes *paratyphi A* and *paratyphi B*. Occasionally a typical attack of food poisoning is followed in a few days by manifestations of paratyphoid fever. Generally, paratyphoid fevers tend to be milder than *S. typhi* infections, but differentiation on clinical grounds is not possible in the individual case. Recovery may be followed by continued excretion of the causative organism in the stools for several months, but the chronic carrier state is less frequent than in typhoid fever.

Bacteremia *Salmonella* species may produce a syndrome characterized primarily by prolonged fever and positive blood cultures. Although symptoms of gastroenteritis can precede bacteremia, they are usually lacking, and most cases arise sporadically. In many instances, the only manifestations are prolonged fever, which is usually spiking and is accompanied by repeated rigors, sweats, aching, anorexia, and weight loss. The characteristic features of typhoid and paratyphoid fever, such as rose spots, persistent leukopenia, and sustained fever, are absent. Stool cultures are usually negative. In contrast to the constant bacteremia of typhoid fever, discharge of organisms into the bloodstream is intermittent, and repeated blood cultures may be required to demonstrate the causative organism. At some time in the course of the illness, localizing signs of infection appear in about one-fourth of the cases. Pulmonary infection in the form of bronchopneumonia or abscess, pleurisy, empyema, pericarditis, endocarditis, pyelonephritis, meningitis, osteomyelitis, and arthritis are relatively common. The blood leukocyte count is usually normal, but with the development of focal lesions, polymorphonuclear leukocytosis as high as 20,000 to 25,000 cells per cubic millimeter occurs. *Salmonella* bacteremia can be a very puzzling disorder, especially before localization takes place, and should be considered in cases of fever of unknown origin.

A prolonged febrile illness lasting weeks or months and characterized by weight loss, marked anemia, hepatosplenomegaly, and bacteremia with *Salmonella* has been described in Brazil and other areas of the world in patients with hepatosplenic schistosomiasis due to *Schistosoma mansoni*. Intermittent bacteremia with *Salmonella* also occurs in patients with *Schistosoma haematobium* infection who are also urinary carriers of *Salmonella*.

Local pyogenic infections *Salmonella* organisms can produce abscesses in almost any anatomic site, and these can occur independently of previous symptoms of gastroenteritis or other systemic illness, or as complications of bacteremias. There is nothing characteristic about the suppurative lesions, and the correct etiologic diagnosis is rarely made on the basis of clinical findings alone. There is a strong tendency for salmonellas to localize in tissues that are the site of preexisting disease. Localization has been described in aneurysms, bone adjacent to aortic aneurysms, hematomas, and many different tumors, including hypernephroma, ovarian cyst, and pheochromocytoma. Meningeal localization of infection is common in newborns and infants, and occasional small outbreaks of *Salmonella* infection in nurseries have consisted almost entirely of meningitis. In addition to suppurative joint disease, a chronic aseptic polyarthritis has been described.

DIAGNOSIS Febrile gastroenteritis produced by presumed viral agents and shigellosis can be distinguished from *Salmonella* gastroenteritis only by appropriate stool cultures, especially in sporadic cases. Polymorphonuclear fecal leukocytes are frequently present in *Salmonella* gastroenteritis and in bacillary dysentery (shigellosis), but not in viral, giardial, or enterotoxin-induced gastroenteritis. Staphylococcal food poisoning usually is not associated with fever, and vomiting is a more prominent feature than in most *Salmonella* infections. Systemic manifestations are usually absent in patients with gastroenteritis caused by enterotoxigenic *E. coli* and *Clostridium perfringens*. Many toxic agents and drugs can produce diarrhea, nausea, and abdominal pain, but fever is rarely a feature of these disorders, and the diagnosis depends upon a history of exposure or ingestion. The diagnosis of paratyphoid fever or *Salmonella* bacteremia depends upon isolation of the causative organism. Agglutination tests with acute and convalescent serums as performed in the usual clinical laboratory are not very helpful. The possibility of an underlying disease should be considered in every patient with a severe *Salmonella* infection.

TREATMENT The treatment of *Salmonella* gastroenteritis is supportive. Dehydration should be corrected by parenteral administration of fluids and electrolytes. Abdominal cramps and diarrhea often are much improved if the patient takes nothing by mouth for 8 to 12 h. Antimicrobial therapy, irrespective of type, does not appear to exert a beneficial effect on the clinical course of *Salmonella* gastroenteritis or decrease the duration of excretion of organisms in the stool. In fact, recent studies show that the period of excretion of *Salmonella* in stools during convalescence is actually longer in patients who have been treated with antimicrobial drugs during the acute illness than in patients who received no antimicrobial therapy. Unless there is documented bacteremia or a protracted febrile course suggesting the diagnosis of enteric fever, antibiotics are *not* indicated in uncomplicated *Salmonella* gastroenteritis.

Chloramphenicol in doses of 3 g daily in adults is the antibiotic of choice in systemic infections including *Salmonella*

648

bacteremia, metastatic infection, and paratyphoid fever. The response is characteristically slow, and the temperature rarely returns to normal until 3 to 4 days after beginning therapy. Therapy should be continued for at least 2 weeks, but in certain infections, such as osteomyelitis or meningitis, the duration may have to be extended. Resistance to multiple antibiotics, including chloramphenicol and ampicillin, occurs, particularly in salmonellas acquired outside the United States. Therefore, antibiotic sensitivity of the organism should be tested in cases of bacteremia, metastatic infection, or enteric fever.

Ampicillin is also effective in systemic infections caused by *Salmonella* strains sensitive to the action of this antibiotic. However, a significant proportion of *Salmonella* strains are highly resistant to ampicillin in vitro. For this reason, ampicillin should not be used in therapy of serious infections unless it is known that the causative organism is sensitive. As in cases of typhoid fever, the combination of trimethoprim and sulfamethoxazole may hold promise in the therapy of salmonella infection when the organism is resistant to chloramphenicol and ampicillin. The tetracycline derivatives have sometimes appeared to exert a beneficial effect, but streptomycin, polymyxin, neomycin, kanamycin, and the sulfonamides are generally ineffective. Antimicrobial resistance is usually related to transferable resistance factors.

Antimicrobial therapy is usually not indicated in convalescent or asymptomatic transient carriers of *Salmonella* species. The carrier state will cease spontaneously in 1 to 3 months in the vast majority of individuals.

The chronic carrier state with localization of infection in the gallbladder and positive stool cultures for a period of time exceeding 1 year is rarely caused by *Salmonella* serotypes other than *S. typhi* and *S. paratyphi* A and B. Its treatment has been discussed. Surgically accessible suppurative lesions should be drained.

PREVENTION AND CONTROL Continuous surveillance and careful reporting of all *Salmonella* isolates improve awareness of new strains, common sources, antibiotic resistance, and the carrier state. Because of the great number of specific serotypes, surveillance and serotyping have occasionally brought attention to widespread occurrence of relatively rare serotypes traced to single sources. Central surveillance of all reported serotypes led to the discovery of an international outbreak in 1974 of *S. eastbourne,* an otherwise rare serotype that was traced to Canadian chocolates. Adequate cooking of meat and egg products and careful surveillance of poultry products and persons who handle food have been only moderately successful in controlling salmonellosis. Probably most important, besides food surveillance, is personal hygiene, including handwashing. Transient or permanent carriers should be warned to take these precautions and, as much as possible, to avoid food preparation. Minimizing the time that foods are allowed to stand at room temperature (as between cooking and refrigeration) should reduce the chances of bacterial growth to infectious inocula.

Careful obstetrical histories for any diarrheal illness at the time a woman enters for delivery should always be obtained, and mothers and infants so affected should be isolated until cultures rule out *Salmonella* carriage. Finally, because of the increasing antibiotic resistance and the enhanced susceptibility of patients receiving antibiotics, the indiscriminate use of unnecessary or "prophylactic" antimicrobial agents should be avoided.

REFERENCES

BAINE WB et al: Institutional salmonellosis, J Infect Dis 128:357, 1973

BENNETT IL JR, HOOK EW: Some aspects of salmonellosis. Ann Rev Med 10:1, 1959

BUTLER T et al: Typhoid fever: Studies of blood coagulation, bacteremia and endotoxemia. Arch Intern Med 138:407, 1978

CLARK GM et al: Epidemiology of an international outbreak of *Salmonella agona.* Lancet 2:490, 1973

DINBAR A et al: The treatment of chronic biliary salmonella carriers. Am J Med 47:236, 1969

FELDMAN RE et al: Epidemiology of *Salmonella typhi* infection in a migrant labor camp in Dade County, Florida. J Infect Dis 130:354, 1974

FREITAG JL: Treatment of chronic typhoid carriers by cholecystectomy. Public Health Rept US 79:7, 1964

GIANNELLA RA et al: Pathogenesis of salmonellosis: Studies of fluid secretion, mucosal invasion, and morphologic reaction in the rabbit ileum. J Clin Invest 52:441, 1973

HORNICK RB et al: Typhoid fever: Pathogenesis and immunologic control. N Engl J Med 283:686, 739, 1970

KAYE D et al: Treatment of chronic enteric carriers of Salmonella typhosa with ampicillin. Ann NY Acad Sci 145:429, 1967

MCHUGH GL et al: Salmonella typhimurium resistant to silver nitrate, chloramphenicol, and ampicillin: A new threat to burn units? Lancet 1:235, 1975

OLARTE J, GALINDO E: *Salmonella typhi* resistant to chloramphenicol, ampicillin, and other antimicrobial agents: Strains isolated during an extensive typhoid fever epidemic in Mexico. Antimicrob Agents Chemother 4:597, 1973

REYNOLDS EW et al: Diagnostic specificity of Widal's reaction for typhoid fever. JAMA 214:2192, 1970

RICE PA et al: *Salmonella typhi* infections in the United States, 1967-1972: Increasing importance of international travelers. Am J Epidemiol 106:160, 1977

ROBERTSON RP et al: Chloramphenicol and ampicillin in salmonella enteric fever. N Engl J Med 278:171, 1968

Salmonella surveillance: Annual Summary 1976. Atlanta, Center for Disease Control, 1977

SCHROEDER SA et al: Epidemic salmonellosis in hospitals and institutions: A five-year review. N Engl J Med 279:674, 1968

124
SHIGELLOSIS

HARRY N. BEATY

DEFINITION Shigellosis is an acute, self-limited infection of the intestinal tract of humans which is characterized by diarrhea, fever, and abdominal pain. The disease is frequently called *bacillary dysentery,* but the term *shigellosis* is preferred.

ETIOLOGY The genus *Shigella* of the family Enterobacteriaceae includes a group of closely related species which are nonmotile, nonencapsulated, slender, gram-negative rods. They are aerobes or facultative anaerobes and grow best at 37°C. Nutritional requirements are relatively simple, and the ability of these organisms to grow in the presence of bile salts is used in devising selective media which facilitate their isolation. However, *S. dysenteriae* type 1 may be inhibited by these media, and growth may not be apparent for several days. Fermentation of carbohydrates differs according to species, but all strains produce acid in glucose and either fail to ferment lactose or do so only slowly. The shigellas are classified into subgroups A, B, C, or D on the basis of biochemical and antigenic characteristics. The clinically important species within the respective groups are *S. dysenteriae, S. flexneri, S. boydii,* and *S.*

sonnei. While these shigellas share antigens among themselves and with other enteric bacilli, serologic classification is not difficult, and with the exception of *S. sonnei* a number of serotypes of each species has been recognized.

The somatic antigen of the shigellas is an endotoxin which is chemically and biologically similar to the endotoxins of other gram-negative bacilli. *Shigella dysenteriae* type 1 (Shiga bacillus) also produces an exotoxin(s) which has cytotoxic, neurotoxic, and enterotoxic properties. The role of this exotoxin in the pathogenesis of shigellosis is unknown, but a biologically and antigenically similar toxin is elaborated by certain strains of *S. flexneri* and *S. sonnei,* and there is increasing speculation that toxin may be a virulence factor.

EPIDEMIOLOGY The principal habitat of the shigellas is the gastrointestinal tract of higher primates. Natural disease occurs in humans, gorillas, and some species of monkey. The convalescent or asymptomatic carrier is the only recognized reservoir. In 1972 a family outbreak of the disease was attributed to a pet monkey. Spread of infection from person to person occurs primarily when organisms on hands and inanimate objects contaminated with infected feces are ingested. In the United States, common source outbreaks usually involve food which has been contaminated by careless handlers. Outbreaks associated with drinking water have been reported, and swimming in contaminated rivers or pools can be a cause of infection. In regions where sanitation is poor, flies which have been in contact with infected human feces may serve as an important vector in the transmission of this disease.

Shigellosis is worldwide in distribution, and is particularly common in countries where effective sanitation is lacking. Around 10,000 cases are reported annually in the United States, but many more undoubtedly occur. *Shigella sonnei* is responsible for about three-fourths of the infections encountered in this country; *S. flexneri* is isolated from all but a small percentage of the rest. *Shigella dysenteriae* type 1, which formerly produced disease predominantly in Asia, has been responsible for large outbreaks of diarrhea in Central America. In the United States, infections with this species occur almost exclusively among foreign travelers or their contacts.

Major epidemics of shigellosis are uncommon in this country, but high-risk groups exist in the inner cities, in mental or penal institutions, and on Indian reservations. Poor sanitation, low standards of personal hygiene, crowded conditions, and a high proportion of children in a population favor spread of the infection. Infected persons may excrete organisms intermittently during convalescence, but the carrier state infrequently persists longer than 3 months.

Humoral antibodies to somatic antigens and toxins frequently develop in response to clinical infection, but there is no evidence that they influence the course of the disease or protect against reinfection. Nevertheless, persons living in endemic areas seem to develop immunity to recurrent episodes of clinical disease, and volunteers infected with a specific strain are resistant to rechallenge with that strain for weeks to months. This immunity may be mediated by coproantibody, which has been identified in the stool of patients with shigellosis, or by cellular defense mechanisms in the wall of the bowel. In any event, it has led to the development of live, attenuated vaccines which, given orally, induce the same degree of immunity as natural infection. Parenteral vaccines are of no value.

PATHOGENESIS AND PATHOLOGY The pathogenesis of shigellosis is complex, but reasonably well understood. In order to produce disease, viable organisms must first adhere to the mucosal surface and then penetrate the epithelial cell lining. These virulence properties are genetically controlled by at least three separate regions of the chromosome; loss of any one through mutation renders a strain avirulent. Unlike members of the genus *Salmonella,* which require a large inoculum to produce infection, as few as 10 to 100 virulent *Shigella* can cause disease.

Once organisms penetrate the mucosal surface, they multiply within epithelial cells and rarely extend beyond the limits of the intestinal mucous membrane. Although superficial, the inflammatory reaction is severe and usually involves the entire colon. A fibrinous exudate often develops, and necrosis of the mucosa produces shallow ulcers that bleed readily. Microscopic examination shows that the submucosa and muscularis mucosa are infiltrated with bacteria and polymorphonuclear leukocytes. Ulcers are sharply demarcated and are not undermined. The question of whether toxins are important in the pathogenesis of shigellosis is unsettled. However, there is mounting evidence that species other than *S. dysenteriae* are toxigenic, and the hypothesis has been proposed that toxin produced in the lumen of the jejunum binds to specific receptors on epithelial cells, leading to activation of adenylate cyclase and production of cholera-like diarrhea in the early stages of shigellosis. It has long been proposed that systemic manifestations of this disease are due to absorbed toxins, because bacteremia is extremely rare except when infection is due to the Shiga bacillus.

CLINICAL MANIFESTATIONS *Shigella* infections are characterized by fever, abdominal pain, and diarrhea. However, mild diarrhea alone or asymptomatic infection occurs in a significant proportion of individuals infected. The incubation period is usually 24 to 48 h, and the first symptom is often colicky abdominal pain which is followed within an hour by high fever and diarrhea, often accompanied by tenesmus. Other symptoms include nausea, vomiting, headache, myalgia, and convulsions in children. The stools are liquid, greenish in color, contain shreds of mucus, and in 20 to 30 percent of cases various amounts of gross blood. Depending upon the severity of diarrhea and the height of fever, patients may become profoundly dehydrated, and circulatory collapse can occur. Lower abdominal tenderness and hyperactive bowel sounds are common, but there is no peritoneal irritation. Splenomegaly has been reported, but is rare. Sigmoidoscopic examination reveals diffuse mucosal inflammation, often with multiple ulcerations.

LABORATORY FINDINGS Blood leukocyte counts usually range between 5000 and 15,000 per cubic millimeter, but a leukemoid reaction with counts in the range of 30,000 to 50,000 per cubic millimeter is seen occasionally with *S. dysenteriae* infections. Anemia is uncommon. Microscopic examination of stool reveals shreds of mucus and erythrocytes. A methylene blue wet mount preparation shows many polymorphonuclear leukocytes, which helps to distinguish diarrhea caused by *Shigella* from that caused by *Salmonella typhosa* or nonbacterial infections. Stool cultures usually are positive, but blood cultures rarely are. Electrolyte abnormalities depend on the degree of vomiting and diarrhea.

COURSE Shigellosis is generally a self-limited disease, and patients usually become afebrile in about 4 days. Diarrhea and abdominal cramps may continue a few days longer, but within a week most patients have recovered. However, a significant proportion of untreated patients continue to shed organisms in the stool for 2 or more weeks. In about 10 percent of cases a clinical or bacteriologic relapse occurs unless antibiotics are given. In the United States, the overall mortality rate associated with shigellosis is less than 0.1 percent. However, among young children and elderly patients, the illness is often more severe and the prognosis poorer. *Shigella dysenteriae* type 1 produces particularly severe infections, and mortality rates of 25 to 50 percent have been recorded in epidemics produced by this species.

Complications of *Shigella* infections are encountered infrequently. An uncommon but significant problem is perforation of the colon. Hematogenous dissemination of the shigellas is also rare, but these organisms have been encountered in metastatic foci of infection such as abscesses and meningitis. In some series, bacteremia due to other gram-negative bacilli has been seen in association with shigellosis. Reiter's syndrome has been reported following shigellosis and is particularly likely to occur in patients who have the histocompatibility antigen B27. Likewise, the hemolytic-uremic syndrome has been recognized as an infrequent complication of shigellosis. Conjunctivitis, iritis, and peripheral neuropathy accompany shigellosis on rare occasions.

DIAGNOSIS A definitive diagnosis can be established when pathogenic members of the genus *Shigella* are isolated from cultures. Stool cultures are positive in over 90 percent of cases if they are obtained in the first 3 days of illness; but only about 75 percent are positive if they are obtained more than 1 week after the onset of diarrhea. The organisms survive for only a short time in feces, and fresh stool specimens or rectal swabs should be cultured promptly. Recovery of the shigellas is facilitated if saline suspensions of stool are streaked directly onto selective media such as SS agar or desoxycholate citrate agar. Antibodies can be detected in the serum of the majority of patients with positive cultures and may occasionally be of value in establishing the diagnosis of shigellosis. Immunofluorescent techniques which allow rapid detection of organisms in the stool have been developed.

Shigellosis infection should be considered in every febrile illness associated with diarrhea. Occasionally, children with infections such as tonsillitis or otitis have diarrhea, but the major differential diagnosis of shigellosis includes acute ulcerative colitis, viral enteritis, amebic dysentery, salmonellosis, and clostridial or staphylococcal food poisoning. Shigellosis can closely mimic acute ulcerative colitis, and should be excluded with cultures in patients thought to have this disease. In viral infections, fever is uncommon, and the stool usually does not contain gross blood or pus. The onset of amebic colitis is gradual, and the diarrhea is relatively mild. Staphylococcal food poisoning is associated with more nausea and vomiting, and usually is not associated with fever. *Salmonella* infections can be differentiated with certainty only by bacteriologic studies.

TREATMENT The treatment of shigellosis is primarily supportive, and the major goal is correction of fluid and electrolyte abnormalities. Antibiotics are of secondary importance, and are used chiefly to shorten the duration of illness and to prevent relapse. Sulfonamides formerly were effective in the treatment of bacillary dysentery, but almost 90 percent of *S. sonnei* isolated in the United States are resistant to these drugs. More significantly, since 1955 epidemics of shigellosis in various parts of the world, including the United States, have been caused by organisms resistant to multiple antibiotics. The molecular basis for multiple drug resistance involves the episomal transfer (R factor) of drug-resistant determinants between enteric bacilli.

Currently, increasing numbers of isolates in the United States are resistant to a number of antimicrobials. Ampicillin and tetracycline were the drugs of choice for shigellosis, but widespread resistance to these agents makes it advisable to determine the antibiotic susceptibility of all *Shigella* isolates before chemotherapy with these drugs is instituted. Cotrimoxazole, which has proven to be as effective as ampicillin, is preferred by many for the treatment of these infections. The decision whether to treat patients with antimicrobials should be based on several factors such as the nature of the organism (e.g., *S. dysenteriae* infections should be treated), the severity of the illness, the availability of safe and effective drugs, and the patient's social and physical environment.

Lomotil and antispasmodics such as paregoric should not be used in individuals with shigellosis, because these agents have an adverse effect on the course of infection caused by invasive pathogens.

PREVENTION The most important prophylactic measures are the maintenance of proper sanitation and adequate sewage disposal. The detection and elimination of carriers are difficult and rarely practical. Methods for increasing resistance with oral vaccines may be useful in preventing outbreaks among susceptible populations.

REFERENCES

DuPont HL, Hornick RB: Clinical approach to infectious diarrheas. Medicine 52:265, 1973

Gemski P Jr, Formal SB: Shigellosis: An invasive infection of the gastrointestinal tract, in *Microbiology 1975*, D Schlessinger (ed). Washington, DC, American Society for Microbiology, 1975, p 165

Keusch GT, Jacewicz M: Pathogenesis of *Shigella* diarrhea: VII. Evidence for a cell membrane toxin receptor involving β-1,4 linked *N*-acetyl-*d*-glucosamine oligomers. J Exp Med 146:535, 1977

Nelson JD et al: Trimethoprim-sulfamethoxazole therapy for shigellosis. JAMA 235:1239, 1976

125
HEMOPHILUS INFECTIONS

DAVID W. SMITH

Hemophilus influenzae was isolated by Pfeiffer in 1892 from the sputum of individuals afflicted during an influenza pandemic. The requirement of blood for in vitro growth and its presumptive role in the pandemic prompted the designation of this genus. Other species have since been classified as members of the *Hemophilus* genus on the basis of morphology and physiology: small, pleomorphic, facultatively aerobic, nonmotile, nonspore-forming, gram-negative bacilli that require enriched media containing blood or certain derivatives and that are strict parasites of humans. Certain of these species are closely related genetically.

Hemophilus influenzae and *H. pertussis* are the most important cause of human disease among this genus; other pathogenic species include *H. aegyptius*, *H. aphrophilus*, *H. ducreyi*, *H. parapertussis*, and *H. vaginalis*. *Hemophilus hemolyticus*, *H. parainfluenzae*, and *H. bronchiseptica* infect the upper respiratory tract but rarely cause disease.

HEMOPHILUS INFLUENZAE

ETIOLOGY *Hemophilus influenzae* is distinguished by its growth requirement of a heat-labile V factor and a heat-stable

X factor found in erythrocytes and by its inability to hemolyze erythrocytes during growth. V factor can be replaced by coenzyme I (DPN), coenzyme II (TPN), or nicotinamide nucleoside, and X factor by hematin. X factor is not required for anaerobic growth. Fermentation reactions and tests of other metabolic activities are not useful in identification but may help in "biotyping" individual isolates.

Hemophilus influenzae will grow in any enriched supplemented medium, but optimal growth occurs on media in which erythrocytes are disrupted to release the growth factors, e.g., chocolate or Levinthal agar. "Satellitism" around colonies of hemolytic *Staphylococcus aureus* growing on solid blood agar is often used to identify *H. influenzae*. Some strains grow best in 5 to 10 percent carbon dioxide; many laboratories therefore incubate specimens suspected of containing *H. influenzae* in a candle jar or an incubator purged with carbon dioxide. Since viability of this bacterium is lost rapidly on drying or heating, clinical specimens should be inoculated without delay.

The organism exists with or without a polysaccharide capsule. Colonies of nonencapsulated isolates are usually 0.5 to 1.5 mm in diameter and appear granular after overnight incubation on solid agar; those of encapsulated isolates are usually 3 to 4 mm in diameter and initially appear mucoid or glistening. *Hemophilus influenzae* grown on enriched media appear microscopically as relatively uniform, small coccobacilli (1 by 0.3 μm); under less than optimal growth conditions, long filaments or short chains are common. The morphology of *H. influenzae* in clinical specimens is generally variable. Moreover, the organism does not always react optimally with safranin dye. *Hemophilus influenzae* is, therefore, not infrequently misdiagnosed in gram-stained smears of infected material.

The outer membrane of *H. influenzae*, like that of other gram-negative bacilli, is composed of a lipopolysaccharide (endotoxin)-containing cell wall and a number of immunogenic proteins. The antigenic composition of *H. influenzae* endotoxin and the outer-membrane proteins is poorly defined. Only a small percentage of isolates recovered from the respiratory tract are encapsulated. Six antigenically distinguishable capsular types, designated a to f, have been identified. Each is a complex carbohydrate. Type a, b, and c capsules share antigenic determinants with certain pneumococci, while that of type b, polyribose ribitol phosphate (PRP), cross-reacts immunologically with the capsules or cell walls of several species of gram-positive cocci and rods, and with enteric bacilli.

Strains with decreased or absent capsular antigen arise spontaneously from encapsulated strains. This variation most likely proceeds from M (fully encapsulated) → S (partially encapsulated) → R (nonencapsulated). The genetic basis of this variation and the natural existence of its converse, that is, R→S→M, are not well described. Alexander demonstrated that DNA purified from an M strain could transform an R strain to the serotype of the donor M strain. Transformation of *H. influenzae* in the host has not been studied, but the demonstration of pneumococcal transformation in experimentally infected mice supports that possibility. Transformations between *H. aegyptius* and *H. influenzae* and between *H. influenzae* and *H. parainfluenzae* demonstrate the close genetic relation of these species.

Hemophilus influenzae type b releases its capsular antigen (PRP) during growth in vitro and in vivo. PRP can be identified immunologically by countercurrent immunoelectrophoresis or agglutination of latex particles to which antibody is absorbed.

Hemophilus influenzae was previously susceptible to many antibiotics, but resistance to tetracycline has been increasing, and up to 10 percent of type b and a higher percentage of nonencapsulated strains isolated in the United States are now resistant to ampicillin. Chloramphenicol-resistant and multiply

resistant (chloramphenicol, tetracycline, and/or ampicillin) strains have been isolated in Europe. Resistant strains are widely but variably distributed and are as pathogenic and transmissible as antibiotic-sensitive strains.

EPIDEMIOLOGY *Hemophilus influenzae* infects only humans, primarily their upper respiratory tracts. It can be recovered from the nasopharynx of up to 80 percent of healthy individuals, with the frequency of infection related inversely to age, being greatest with young persons. Asymptomatic nasopharyngeal infection lasts days to a few months, is not eradicated by systemic antibody, and often is not eliminated by antibiotic therapy adequate to cure type b meningitis. Of the isolated strains, up to 25 percent are encapsulated, one-half of which are type b.

Hemophilus influenzae diseases occur worldwide and for the most part are endemic. Unusually high attack rates of systemic type b diseases occur in certain communities and within closed populations of susceptible persons. A 10-year review of patients with systemic type b disease revealed multiple cases in 3 percent of affected families. Systemic *H. influenzae* b diseases occur more commonly among impoverished and rural populations and blacks. Persons with sickle-cell disease, splenectomy, agammaglobulinemia, and treated Hodgkin's disease are unusually susceptible. Alcoholic adults appear to be at increased risk of *H. influenzae* pneumonia. Systemic *H. influenzae* diseases have a marked age relationship: newborns, older children, and adults are uncommonly affected. In temperate climates. these diseases occur most commonly during the winter months.

The incidence of systemic *H. influenzae* b diseases seems to have increased during the past 30 to 40 years, and more adults are being affected. The basis for this increased attack rate is not understood. Improved diagnostic laboratories and diminution in the prevalence of protective antibody due to excessive use of antibiotics have been implicated. The possibility that the organism has changed its antigenic composition and/or virulence also deserves evaluation.

PATHOGENICITY The relatively common asymptomatic nasopharyngeal infection occasionally develops into symptomatic disease which may spread contiguously to involve the sinuses, middle ear, or bronchi. Nonencapsulated strains produce luminal diseases. Encapsulated strains may invade local tissues, causing epiglottitis, pneumonia, pericarditis, or facial cellulitis, or they may enter the bloodstream and produce metastatic disease in the meninges or joints.

Virtually all *H. influenzae* causing systemic disease are encapsulated, and at least 90 percent are type b. The pathogenicity of invasive strains is related directly to the inhibition of phagocytosis produced by the capsule. The basis for the disproportionate virulence of type b strains is unknown. The role of outer membrane proteins and other constitutents in pathogenicity is also ill-defined. Synergy between *H. influenzae* and certain respiratory viruses has been demonstrated in studies of human disease and in experimental models.

IMMUNITY Susceptibility to *H. influenzae* b meningitis was always correlated inversely to the presence of anticapsular antibody. The role of anti-PRP has been questioned recently, however, because of its apparent variable distribution among adults who have no increased incidence of *H. influenzae* b disease. The interpretation of these data remain in question because of the lack of standard methods in performing the classic bactericidal assay for antibody. Moreover, the limits of sensitivity of the bactericidal assay (about 200 ng antibody per milliliter) exceed by tenfold the antibody concentration needed to protect animals from lethal, experimental disease. Radioimmunoassays which detect 10 ng anti-PRP per milliliter should provide important insights into this question.

Although recent evidence suggests that immunity to *H. influenzae* is mediated by antibody of multiple specificity, anti-PRP antibody is a potent resistance factor. It promotes phagocytosis and bacteriolysis in vitro, protects animals from a lethal concentration of *H. influenzae,* and was responsible for the beneficial effects of rabbit anti-*H. influenzae* serum in human disease. Moreover, recent field trials with a purified PRP vaccine have demonstrated protection of young children from systemic diseases when an antibody response is mounted.

Antibody to PRP can be stimulated by infection with bacteria bearing cross-reactive surface antigens. Such antibody is bacteriolytic in vitro and protective in experimental disease. Antibody to *H. influenzae* outer membrane (OM) antigens also promotes phagocytosis and bacteriolysis in vitro and protects experimentally infected animals. Antibody to OM antigens has been found in high titers in certain adults and older children clinically resistant to *H. influenzae* but deficient in anti-PRP antibody. This observation suggests that natural resistance to this pathogen appears to result from a composite of antibody activities stimulated by each of several antigens.

Studies of patients recovering from systemic *H. influenzae* b disease and of those immunized with PRP have revealed a marked age relation to anti-PRP antibody: infants respond infrequently and poorly; younger children have intermediate reactivity; all older children and adults develop marked, nonboostable responses. The level of detectable antibody activity following disease is further complicated by antigenemia, which may last days to weeks, and which is more common and prolonged in infants. A few children have failed to produce anti-PRP antibody (measured by radioimmunoassay) following systemic disease and subsequently developed a second distinct episode of type b invasive disease. Although these children appear to have been "immunologically nonreactive" for periods up to months, all those studied to date have subsequently raised anti-PRP antibody activity. These observations indicate the need for further study and close follow-up of young children recuperating from invasive *H. influenzae* b disease. Likewise, survivors of intensive radio- and/or chemotherapy for Hodgkin's disease, many of whom have also had a splenectomy, are incapable of an appropriate anti-PRP antibody response, even following systemic disease.

Children recuperating from certain *H. influenzae* b diseases were found in one study to have lower anti-PRP titers and significant differences in the composition of certain erythrocyte and/or lymphocyte antigens compared with healthy blood donors. These data support the concept of a genetic basis for the production of anti-PRP antibody and/or development of certain *H. influenzae* b diseases, and deserve further evaluation.

CLINICAL MANIFESTATIONS *Hemophilus influenzae* can cause local respiratory tract or invasive diseases. A 1-year survey of children hospitalized in Denver, Colorado, revealed that *H. influenzae* b was the most common cause of bacteremic disease and that 54 percent of children with *H. influenzae* disease had meningitis; 14 percent, pneumonia (4 percent with pericarditis); 11 percent, bacteremia without a primary focus; 11 percent, facial cellulitis; 10 percent, epiglottitis; and 1 percent, pyarthrosis. Adults may develop *H. influenzae* bacteremia, meningitis, and, less commonly, epiglottitis; however, in them bronchitis, due to nonencapsulated strains, and pneumonia are more common.

Hemophilus influenzae diseases are generally acute with symptoms reflecting the pyogenic process; however, the clinical course of certain of these diseases may be surprisingly prolonged and subacute.

Meningitis (see also Chap. 368) *Hemophilus influenzae* is the most common cause of bacterial meningitis, primarily affecting children 9 months to 4 years of age. The signs and symptoms depend on the patient's age and the time in the course of the disease when medical care is sought. Young children and those early in the disease generally have a nonspecific clinical picture: preceding upper respiratory tract symptoms, fever, anorexia, lethargy, vomiting, and, in older children and adults, headache. A history of stiff neck or back may be elicited. Confusion, paresis of one or another cranial nerve, coma, convulsions, opisthotonus, and shock occur with more prolonged and serious disease. The clinical findings are indistinguishable from other bacterial meningitides. Age and certain concurrent manifestations, such as cellulitis, pyarthrosis, or epiglottitis, suggest *H. influenzae,* but the diagnosis depends on bacteriologic studies.

Pneumonia *Hemophilus influenzae* may cause either a broncho- or lobar pneumonia. Approximately one-half of the children with lobar pneumonia have an associated empyema. The pneumonic disease sometimes spreads to produce a purulent pericarditis. Lobar disease, particularly with pleural involvement, is most often confused with pneumococcal or *S. aureus* pneumonia, but the course may be prolonged enough to suggest tuberculosis. Elderly adults, particularly those with chronic obstructive lung disease and/or alcoholism, are being affected increasingly with *H. influenzae* pneumonia (Chap. 260).

Bacteremia without local disease Children, particularly those between 6 months and 3 years of age, may develop bacteremia without evidence of local disease. The diagnosis is made most often in those with a temperature greater than 38.9°C (102°F) and an elevated circulating neutrophil count. Persons with sickle-cell disease, previous splenectomy, and chemotherapy for Hodgkin's disease are at increased risk of bacteremia without local disease. Although pneumococci are the most common cause of this syndrome, *H. influenzae* b is the second most common etiologic agent. Fever, chills, anxiety, anorexia, and lethargy dominate the clinical picture. Among highly susceptible hosts, the disease may be fulminating with rapid progress to shock and death within a few hours.

Cellulitis *Hemophilus influenzae* causes a cellulitis, particularly among children 6 to 24 months of age, which is characterized as a raised, warm, tender area with a distinctive reddish blue hue, usually located on one cheek or, less commonly, in the periorbital area. The child is moderately febrile and has a history of preceding rhinorrhea, fever, and, at times, ipsilateral otitis media. The cellulitis develops and spreads within a few hours. *Hemophilus influenzae* cellulitis involving the limbs and hands is seen rarely, usually in older children. The distinctive color, location, and clinical course suggest the etiology. A significant percentage of the involved infants develops sepsis and metastatic disease, notably meningitis.

Epiglottitis *Hemophilus influenzae* b is the leading cause of this potentially lethal, septic disease with a dramatically rapid course that primarily affects preschool-age children. Acute onset of high fever, dysphagia, and an aura of not feeling well are followed by puddling of oropharyngeal secretions and tachypnea with inspiratory retractions. Increasing airway obstruction is accompanied by increasing hypoxia and anxiety. Over one-half of these patients require hospitalization and airway intubation within 12 h after the onset of initial symptoms. The diagnostic examination can provoke further edema of the markedly swollen, inflamed epiglottis and should, therefore, be conducted only in a locale in which an airway can be inserted.

Pyarthrosis *Hemophilus influenzae* b joint disease occurs during a septic invasion with or without other systemic disease. Although an uncommon manifestation of *H. influenzae* sepsis, pyarthrosis in children under 2 years of age is most commonly caused by *H. influenzae.* Single, large weight-bearing joints are usually involved without osteomyelitis (Chap. 360). Response to systemic antibiotics without surgical drainage is dramatic and curative, but long-term follow-up reveals some joint dysfunction in a significant percentage of children.

Pericarditis *Hemophilus influenzae* b causes purulent pericarditis usually as a part of a bout of pneumonia. The clinical signs and symptoms are similar to those of pyogenic pericarditis of other etiology, although the course is often less acute (Chap. 249).

Other respiratory tract diseases *Hemophilus influenzae* is the second leading cause of childhood otitis media and often causes sinusitis. Nearly all the etiologic strains are nonencapsulated. These diseases cannot be distinguished clinically from those produced by other microbial agents (Chap. 267), nor can the disease caused by encapsulated or nonencapsulated *H. influenzae* be differentiated clinically. Fever, local pain, irritability, and, in sinusitis, foul breath, postnasal drip, and cough predominate. Chronic bronchitis, particularly among adults and those with agamma- or hypogammaglobulinemia, is often caused by nonencapsulated *H. influenzae* or mixed bacterial species among which *H. influenzae* predominates. Cough productive of purulent sputum, dyspnea with prolonged expiration, and anorexia dominate this process which is aggravated by smoking and other respiratory pollutants.

Other diseases *Hemophilus influenzae* can cause endocarditis and brain abscess, but such cases are very rare and are usually associated with a primary underlying disease. *Hemophilus influenzae* endophthalmitis, renal disease, and osteomyelitis have been reported. Pharyngitis is only rarely caused by *H. influenzae,* and the role of this organism in bronchiolitis has been dismissed.

DIAGNOSIS The etiology of many *H. influenzae* diseases, i.e., pyarthrosis in a child under 2 years, facial cellulitis, and epiglottitis, can generally be suspected on the basis of the history and clinical findings. Chemical analysis of infected fluids is consistent with any pyogenic etiology. A leukocytosis is common, and children often have a significant anemia. Gram's stains of infected body fluids, e.g., spinal fluid, correlate with culture results in 70 percent of cases. Of the rest of culture-positive specimens, 15 percent have negative smears, while another 15 percent have misinterpreted smears. Staining such specimens with methylene blue generally does not improve these results. Quellung reactions are usually even less accurate.

PRP can be detected by countercurrent electrophoresis in the serum, CSF, or concentrated urine of 90 percent of children with meningitis. Despite the apparent widespread distribution of immunologically cross-reactive antigens among bacteria in nature, false-positive reactions are unusual. False-positive reactions due to antibodies to serum constituents may occur in some acutely infected patients. PRP is generally detected in infected pericardial fluid or joint fluid but is found infrequently in the serum of children with epiglottitis, presumably because the fulminant course of this disease does not en-

tail the time required for antigen to be released from the invasive bacteria. Detection of antigen in the supernatant of liquid cultures can expedite the laboratory diagnosis. Antigen, and nonviable bacteria, often persist in serum and other body fluids following antibiotic therapy. This makes antigen detection very helpful in the diagnosis of patients with *H. influenzae* meningitis who have received prior antibiotics.

Positive nasopharyngeal cultures are not meaningful because of the high carriage rate of *H. influenzae* by healthy individuals. Needle aspiration of the edge of the site of cellulitis or of diseased lung markedly increases the rate of bacterial isolation and may be necessary, particularly in sick patients. Cultures of empyema, pericardial, and joint fluid and an inflamed epiglottis are usually diagnostic. Blood cultures are positive in up to 80 percent of patients with *H. influenzae* septic arthritis, facial cellulitis, epiglottitis, and meningitis prior to the onset of antibiotic therapy. Even if antibiotic therapy has been initiated, the yield is sufficiently great to recommend that blood cultures be taken. It has been suggested that *H. influenzae* pneumonia, in which 30 percent of persons have a positive blood culture, is underdiagnosed. The role of antigen detection in the diagnosis of this disease deserves further evaluation.

TREATMENT Without treatment, systemic *H. influenzae* disease, particularly meningitis and epiglottitis, has a very high, if not uniform, mortality. Therapy with intrathecal streptomycin and a systemic sulfonamide was one of the earliest therapeutic regimens for meningitis. It produced reasonably satisfactory results but is no longer advocated. Chloramphenicol yields very high concentrations of antibiotic in the joint and cerebrospinal fluids relative to serum and produces excellent clinical results. However, the potential toxicity of chloramphenicol and the highly satisfactory results obtained with ampicillin for many years made ampicillin the antibiotic of choice for *H. influenzae* diseases. The current prevalence of ampicillin-resistant strains requires that all systemic diseases potentially due to *H. influenzae* be treated with chloramphenicol, 100 mg/kg per day for children, or 4 g per day for adults, given intravenously at 6-h intervals until the etiologic agent is proved to be sensitive to ampicillin. Some, including the American Academy of Pediatrics, also recommend that ampicillin be used along with chloramphenicol. If the etiologic strain is sensitive, ampicillin is given intravenously in dosage of 200 to 400 mg/kg per day for children and 4 g per day for adults divided into six infusions given at 4-h intervals. Other antibiotics are also useful in *H. influenzae* infections. Carbenicillin is thought to be particularly sensitive to the β-lactamase of *H. influenzae,* and high concentrations of bacteria, as found in clinical disease, are resistant to carbenicillin. Moreover, carbenicillin is no more effective than ampicillin in therapy of experimental *H. influenzae* b meningitis caused by ampicillin-resistant strains. Amoxicillin is useful in ambulatory therapy of ampicillin-sensitive *H. influenzae* infections. Tetracycline can be used to treat bronchitis and other respiratory diseases caused by sensitive strains. Cephamandole appears promising in the therapy of non-life-threatening ampicillin-sensitive or resistant *H. influenzae* diseases. Trimethoprim-sulfa therapy has recently been approved for *H. influenzae* upper respiratory tract disease.

The duration of chemotherapy for *H. influenzae* disease depends on the disease and the status of the individual patient. All systemic diseases are treated intravenously at least until cultures of the infected area are sterile and the patient is afebrile and without clinical and laboratory evidence of active infection for 3 to 5 days. Patients with meningitis are usually treated for 10 to 14 days. Occasionally, ampicillin does not clear the bacteria from the CSF, and clinical relapses follow the cessation of therapy. Such therapeutic failures have often been associated with antibiotic courses that were too brief, dosages too low, or administration of the drug by a route other than the intravenous one. In a few instances, treatment failures could be attributed to loculated disease that was not completely eradicated by acceptable therapy. Treatment failures require retreatment with ampicillin or chloramphenicol.

Children with endocarditis or pericarditis should receive 6 weeks of intravenous therapy. Ampicillin or chloramphenicol diffuse well into inflamed joint spaces, and there is no indication for local instillation of antibiotics in septic arthritis. Children with otitis media may be treated orally with amoxicillin in dosage of 50 mg/kg per day, adults with 2 g per day, in four divided doses until their symptoms are alleviated or for a total course of 7 to 10 days. Sinusitis requires therapy for 3 or more weeks; therapy of bronchitis may be prolonged even further, depending upon the symptoms.

Only a few *H. influenzae* isolates resistant to chloramphenicol have been recovered in the United States, but their isolation in European centers strongly suggests the need to test invasive organisms for chloramphenicol sensitivity routinely, particularly when the results of chloramphenicol therapy are disappointing.

Antibiotic therapy is only one facet of the management of the patient with a systemic *H. influenzae* disease. Careful evaluation of the airway, consideration of oxygen therapy and transfusion, vigorous treatment of shock and defects in coagulation, conservative fluid replacement, anticonvulsant therapy, and medical management of cerebral edema are often critical. Repeated aspirations of an infected joint or an empyema or placements of a pericardial "window" for drainage may be needed.

PREVENTION Although secondary cases of invasive *H. influenzae* diseases occur at significantly increased rates among young, close contacts of primary cases, no successful antibiotic prophylactic regimen currently exists. The increased attack rate, constant mortality (5 to 10 percent), and significant neurological morbidity during the past two decades for *H. influenzae* meninigitis in children and the prevalence of ampicillin-resistant strains has promoted attempts to produce a vaccine to prevent *H. influenzae* diseases. Because of the primacy of the type b capsule in pathogenicity and the efficacy of anticapsular serum, attention was focused initially on a vaccine composed of purified capsular PRP. Such a vaccine has been prepared and found nontoxic and immunogenic for older children and adults. Recent data indicate that a single dose of this vaccine protects children older than 18 months from meningitis and sepsis for at least 2 years; however, the vaccine is not immunogenic or protective for younger children. New approaches have, therefore, been initiated to develop an effective agent for younger children.

A less purified, systemically administered vaccine in which the native outer membrane complex of lipopolysaccharide-protein-PRP of *H. influenzae* b is conserved is currently being evaluated. Protective antibiotics directed to PRP and to the OM proteins are generated in adults and children; the efficacy of this vaccine in infants is under study.

HEMOPHILUS AEGYPTIUS

Often known as the Koch-Weeks bacillus, *H. aegyptius* causes conjunctivitis in humans. Morphologically and biochemically, this organism closely resembles an unencapsulated *H. influ-*

enzae. Moreover, *H. aegyptius* and *H. influenzae* share certain antigens, and each can be transformed by DNA of the other species.

The conjunctivitis primarily affects children and occurs throughout the world often in epidemics and, in some areas, seasonally. This organism must be distinguished from trachoma-inclusion conjunctivitis (TRIC) agents, adenoviruses, and other bacterial agents, e.g., pneumococcus, *Staphylococcus aureus*, *Neisseria gonorroheae*. Therapy consists of local instillation of antibiotic drops or ointment, sulfonamide, polymyxin B, or gentamicin five or six times daily and moist soaks to keep the eyelids clean.

HEMOPHILUS APHROPHILUS

Hemophilus aphrophilus is an uncommon cause of bacteremia, bacterial endocarditis, acute and chronic sinusitis, pneumonia, and deep tissue abscesses, such as brain abscess. This organism requires X but not V factor and extra carbon dioxide for aerobic growth; it grows anaerobically without X factor. Most strains are sensitive to most families of antibiotics: penicillin, cephalosporins, aminoglycosides, and chloramphenicol.

HEMOPHILUS DUCREYI

See Chap. 126.

HEMOPHILUS PARAINFLUENZAE

This species differs from *H. influenzae* by requiring V but not X factor for growth. Since *H. influenzae* does not require X factor for anaerobic growth, diagnostic confusion can arise, particularly in stabbed cultures. This phenomenon may have played a role in certain instances of systemic disease allegedly caused by *H. parainfluenzae* which, on further testing, were found to be caused by *H. influenzae*.

Acute upper respiratory disease, including otitis media, and less commonly meningitis, pneumonia, endocarditis, and brain abscess have been ascribed to *H. parainfluenzae*. A small but significant percentage of *H. parainfluenzae* carry plasmids mediating β-lactamase production and ampicillin resistance.

HEMOPHILUS VAGINALIS (See Chap. 113)

Hemophilus vaginalis (sometimes called *Corynebacterium vaginale*) appears to cause vaginitis, and less commonly septic abortion and puerperal fever, and asymptomatic urethal infection in men. The growth requirements are not precisely defined but include factor V and probably X; incubation in increased carbon dioxide is important.

The pathogenic role of *H. vaginalis* is disputed because of its recovery from asymptomatic persons. However, recent data have revealed a significant correlation between isolation of *H. vaginalis* and nonspecific vaginitis. The results of therapy support the causal relationship. The clinical diagnosis is suggested by the presence of "clue" cells—vaginal epithelial cells to which multiple gram-negative bacilli are attached—in a vaginal discharge with a pH $\geq$ 5.0 which releases an amine-like odor upon alkalinization. *Hemophilus vaginalis* is not eradicated by oral tetracycline, ampicillin, or sulfonamide vaginal cream. Oral metronidazole is effective, but its use must be weighed against the drug's potential toxicity and the high potential of reinfection from sexual partners.

HEMOPHILUS PERTUSSIS

This bacterium causes an acute bronchitis, primarily in infants and young children, that is characterized by a repetitious, paroxysmal cough and prolonged, inspiratory stridor, "whooping cough."

ETIOLOGY *Hemophilus pertussis* is a minute, aerobic nonmotile, gram-negative coccobacillus that grows slowly and, as a primary isolate, only on a complex medium. The classic Bordet-Gengou medium, which contains blood, is used for primary culture. Charcoal, ion-exchange resin, or starch can be substituted for the blood which apparently binds toxic lipids rather than providing essential growth factors. The absence of an antigenic relationship and inability to transform *H. pertussis* with *H. influenzae* DNA, or vice versa, also suggest that these species are not closely related. *Hemophilus pertussis* is closely related to *H. parapertussis*, which can cause a milder, similar disease in humans, and *H. bronchiseptica,* which causes such a disease in animals but rarely in humans.

Primary isolates, phase I cells, change morphology and antigenic content and lose pathogenicity on in vitro culture; this conversion to phase IV cells is a type of S→R conversion. Killed phase I cells provoke several physiological changes when injected into experimental animals: increased sensitivity to histamine and serotonin, increased susceptibility to experimental allergic encephalomyelitis, a heightened antibody response to heterologous antigens, and lymphocytosis. Factors responsible for these phemonena as well as human pathogenicity of *H. pertussis* are subjects of considerable study and include O antigen (endotoxin), six different K antigens (agglutinogens), which are probably outer-membrane proteins, a heat-labile and a heat-stabile toxin, a hemagglutinin, and a histamine-sensitizing factor. Recent studies suggest that the pilus of *H. pertussis* is identical to the previously identified lymphocytosis-promoting factor. This protein can apparently attach to certain lymphocytes and inhibit their sequestration in lymphoid tissues. The characteristic lymphocytosis in *H. pertussis* disease may result from the prolonged circulation of these lymphocytes. The presence of a capsule on *H. pertussis* is reported only irregularly. The surface antigen content, including the K antigens, can shift phenotypically and genotypically. Such shifts are reflected in changes of vaccine potency. This plethora of antigens also has provoked the development of multiple serologic methods.

EPIDEMIOLOGY *Hemophilus pertussis* exists worldwide and in nature affects only humans; however, primates and mice can be experimentally infected. Pertussis is one of the most contagious of infectious diseases because it is transmitted by aerosolized droplets. The infectivity of respiratory secretions and contact transmission has not been well studied. Up to 90 percent of exposed, susceptible persons develop disease. Asymptomatic infection is rare. Although pertussis may occur endemically, it produces epidemics in a susceptible population. The incidence is greater in the winter in temperate climates. Although adults were earlier thought resistant, recent studies have revealed that neither disease nor active immunization provides life-long immunity. Hospital personnel are at increased risk, as evidenced by reports of epidemics involving hospital staff and patients. The level of maternal immunity and the lack of transplacental transfer of bacteriolytic antibody (which is an IgM globulin) leave the infant particularly susceptible; not surprisingly, more than 50 percent of *H. pertussis* disease occurs in infants.

About 3000 cases of pertussis are officially reported each year in the United States. Most observers think this number is falsely low owing to the difficulty in bacteriologic confirmation. Pertussis remains a very significant health problem in developing countries, particularly in areas of poor nutrition and immunization. The recent decline (1978) in the rate of immunization to pertussis in Great Britain to 30 percent of children has been accompanied by an epidemic affecting as many persons as in the prevaccine era. Certain adenoviruses can cause an identical clinical picture, but there is little doubt that *H. pertussis* can be a primary pathogen.

PATHOGENICITY Inhaled *H. pertussis* attaches to the respiratory epithelium by a specialized pilus; the organisms multiply on the surface of the airway lumen but do not invade the lung or the bloodstream. Acute inflammation results; epithelial cell ciliary action is inhibited, and mucous secretion is stimulated. The subsequent necrosis results in patchy ulceration of the epithelium. The bronchi and bronchioles are primarily affected; the trachea, larynx, and nasophyarynx may be involved, but less severely. The mucopurulent exudate can compromise the diminutive airway of the infant or small child. Focal atelectasis and emphysema are common; peribronchial infiltration by inflammatory cells, particularly lymphocytes, occurs, but the alveoli are spared. The basis for the neurological symptoms—whether from the primary action of a bacterial neurotoxin or secondary hypoxia—remains undefined.

CLINICAL MANIFESTATIONS Following an incubation period of 7 to 10 days, sneezing, mild fever, rhinorrhea, anorexia, and a mild cough become evident (catarrhal period). After 1 to 2 weeks the cough increases in frequency and intensity. Paroxysms are followed, particularly in infants, by a prolonged, often distressing gasp (the whoop). The cough occurs at variable intervals, often every few minutes, for 2 to 3 weeks (paroxysmal period). The disease is much more severe in the infant. The cough inhibits oral intake, and swallowed mucus provokes vomiting. Dehydration and weight loss can be significant. The cough can provoke venous congestion with hemoptysis, epistaxis, and hemorrhage from small blood vessels. Hypoxia may be more common and severe than is commonly appreciated. Apprehension is a major symptom in infants; convulsions and cerebral dysfunction are very rare. Adults and older children are less ill but have the symptoms of a severe, prolonged bronchitis. A recovery period of 1 to 6 weeks follows. During this period the cough decreases, but spasms can be provoked, particularly by smoke or irritating inhalants.

Death results primarily from dehydration and electrolyte imbalance, cerebral anoxia or hemorrhage, or secondary bacterial pneumonia. Mortality is now less than 5 percent among children hospitalized in the United States, but it is significant in developing countries. Up to 90 percent of deaths occur in children under 1 year of age, up to 70 percent in those of 6 months or younger. Among survivors, transient atelectasis is frequent, but bronchiectasis, reported commonly a few decades ago, is now uncommon. Permanent cerebral dysfunction is also unusual among children provided with optimal therapy.

DIAGNOSIS Pertussis is exceedingly difficult to diagnose clinically in the catarrhal state without a history of contact but should be considered in any nonimmune person with a repetitious cough. The differential diagnosis includes viral tracheobronchitis, *Mycoplasma pneumoniae* pneumonia, particularly in adults, and, in infants, *Chlamydia* infection (Chap. 174).

A marked absolute and relative lymphocytosis is characteristic. The organism is isolated from a deep nasopharyngeal (NP) culture; the recovery rate on "cough plates" is too low to recommend this technique. NP swabs must be plated immediately because *H. pertussis* loses viability rapidly with drying. Optimal results occur with fresh medium that contains an antibiotic, such as penicillin, to prevent the growth of NP flora. *Hemophilus pertussis* can be isolated from as many as 90 percent of patients during the catarrhal stage of the disease, but from no greater than 50 percent during the paroxysmal stage. Fluorescent-labeled antibody can detect *H. pertussis* in NP smears; the positive identification rate is generally up to twice that of NP cultures, but false-positive results may be 30 to 40 percent. Serologic studies are of little value. Blood cultures are sterile and should not be done; a chest x-ray, which may show peribronchial thickening, is not diagnostic. Dual infection with adenoviruses occurs, and positive viral cultures do not exclude *H. pertussis* as an etiologic agent.

TREATMENT General supportive care is critical: careful nursing, avoidance of stimuli that provoke paroxysms, oxygen, suctioning of respiratory secretions, and attention to caloric needs and fluid and electrolyte balance. A recent single controlled study reported beneficial effects of steroids for severely ill infants.

Hemophilus pertussis is sensitive to many antibiotics in vitro. Antibiotics can eliminate infection and, if given in the catarrhal phase, prevent disease. Since the pathological process is well developed by the time paroxysms occur, antibiotic therapy given thereafter does not affect the clinical course. Erythromycin is the preferred drug and should be used to prevent interpersonal transmission. Tetracycline and chloramphenicol are nearly as effective but are not recommended because of potential toxicity, particularly for infants. Ampicillin appears to be relatively ineffective in eradicating nasopharyngeal infection. Hyperimmune, antibacterial rabbit serum has no proved effect on bacterial shedding or clinical manifestations and is not recommended.

PREVENTION Patients suspected of having pertussis should be isolated until the diagnosis is disproved or infection eradicated by antibiotics. Exposed susceptibles should be vaccinated to prevent disease (see below) and treated with erythromycin to prevent infection and retransmission.

Prior to the availability of a vaccine, pertussis caused as many deaths in the United States as all other contagious diseases of children *combined!* In order to prevent the disease, a vaccine composed of a chemical extract of bacterial cells was developed. Because of the risk of pertussis to infants, start of immunization as early in life as possible was proposed. Unfortunately, pertussis immunization at 7 days of age produces a limited antibody response in only a small percentage of infants, and it results in reduced booster responses at 1 year. This vaccine is now mixed with diphtheria and tetanus toxoids, for convenience and because pertussis enhances the antibody responses to the toxoids, and is given five times through the first 6 years of life, with three doses being given at 2-month intervals starting at 8 weeks of age.

Although the vaccine was 70 to 80 percent effective in preventing disease among intimately exposed children, its effectiveness and toxicity have been questioned. Completely immunized children may develop pertussis, although the disease is milder than among the unimmunized. Furthermore, the protection provided by the vaccine is transient with only minimal resistance being evident a decade following the last immunization. Indeed, improved housing, hygiene, and nutrition are cited by some as responsible for the dramatic decline in pertussis during the past several decades. However, available data indicate that the degree of decline in the attack rate of pertussis in the United States has been positively affected by the vaccine. The association of an epidemic of pertussis in Great Britain, with a decline in pertussis immunization, also strongly supports the efficacy of the vaccine.

Pertussis vaccine provokes local reactions in up to 50 percent of recipients; neurological complications, including uncontrollable screaming fits, convulsions, and encephalopathy, are a rare but real risk. Neurological complications of pertussis vaccine are more common in families with neurological disease, such as epilepsy. Unfortunately, pertussis vaccine preparations are not uniform in composition, and the risk of any given inoculation is hard to calculate. Any neurological response to pertussis vaccine precludes reimmunization. Vaccine is rarely recommended for persons older than 6 years because of the potential neurotoxicity and decreased risk of pertussis as a life-threatening disease. However, pertussis vaccine (not diphtheria-pertussis-tetanus vaccine) has been used in reduced dosages successfully and without complications among hospital personnel involved in an epidemic. Patients with active pertussis or convalescent from it may have a very severe reaction to the vaccine and should not be immunized.

REFERENCES

Hemophilus aphrophilus

ELSTER SK et al: *Hemophilus aphrophilus* endocarditis: A review of 23 cases. Am J Cardiol 35:72, 1975

SUTTER VL, FINEGOLD SM: *Hemophilus aphrophilus* infections: Clinical and bacteriologic studies. Ann NY Acad Sci 174:468, 1970

Hemophilus influenzae

ALEXANDER HE: Treatment of type b *Hemophilus influenzae* meningitis. J Pediatr 25:517, 1975

AMERICAN ACADEMY OF PEDIATRICS COMMITTEE ON INFECTIOUS DISEASES: Ampicillin-resistant strains of *Hemophilus influenzae* type b. Pediatrics 55:145, 1975

BRADSHAW MW et al: Bacterial antigens cross-reactive with the capsular polysaccharide of *Hemophilus influenzae* b. Lancet 1:1095, 1971

FOTHERGILL LD, WRIGHT J: Influenzal meningitis: Relation of age incidence to bactericidal power of blood against causal organism. J Immunol 24:273, 1933

JACOBSEN JA et al: Epidemiologic characteristics of infections caused by ampicillin-resistant *Hemophilus influenzae*. Pediatrics 58:388, 1976

LEVIN DC et al: Bacteremic *Hemophilus influenzae* pneumonia in adults: Report of 24 cases and review of the literature. Am J Med 62:219, 1977

PELTDA H et al: *Haemophilus influenzae* type b capsular polysaccharide vaccine in children: A double-blind field study of 100,000 vaccines 3 months to 5 years of age in Finland. Pediatrics 60:730, 1977

ROBBINS JB et al: *Haemophilus influenzae* type b: Disease and immunity in humans. Ann Intern Med 78:259, 1973

SMITH DH et al: Responses of children immunized with the capsular polysaccharide of *Hemophilus influenzae* type b. Pediatrics 52:637, 1973

SMITH EWP JR, HAYNES RE: Changing incidence of *Hemophilus influenzae* meningitis. Pediatrics 50:723, 1972

TODD JK, BRUHN FW: Severe *Haemophilus influenzae* infections. Am J Dis Child 129:607, 1975

vanKLINGEREN B et al: Plasmid-mediated chloramphenicol resistance in *Haemophilus influenzae*. Antimicrob Agents Chemother 11:383, 1977

Hemophilus parainfluenzae

CHUNN CJ et al: *Haemophilus parainfluenzae* infective endocarditis. Medicine 56:99, 1977

HABLE KA et al: Three *Hemophilus* species. Am J Dis Child 121:35, 1971

Hemophilus pertussis

BASSILI WR, STEWART GT: Epidemiological evaluation of immunisation and other factors in the control of whooping cough. Lancet 1:471, 1976

BRADFORD WL, SLAVIN B: Nasopharyngeal cultures in pertussis. Proc Soc Exp Biol Med 43:590, 1940

BYERS RK, MOLL FC: Encephalopathies following prophylactic pertussis vaccine. Pediatrics 1:437, 1948

DONALDSON P, WHITAKER J: Diagnoses of pertussis by fluorescent antibody staining of nasopharyngeal smears. Am J Dis Child 99:423, 1960

KURT TL et al: Spread of pertussis by hospital staff. JAMA 221:264, 1972

LAMBERT HJ: Epidemiology of a small pertussis outbreak in Kent County, Michigan. Public Health Rep 80:365, 1965

MEDICAL RESEARCH COUNCIL INVESTIGATION: The prevention of whooping cough by vaccination. Br Med J 1:1463, 1951

OLSON LC: Pertussis. Medicine 54:427, 1975

Report of the Committee on Infectious Diseases, 17th ed. Evanston, Ill, American Academy of Pediatrics, 1974

Hemophilus vaginalis

GARDNER HL, DUKES CD: Haemophilus vaginalis vaginitis: A newly defined specific infection previously classified "non-specific vaginitis." Am J Obstet Gynecol 69:962, 1955

PHEIFER TA et al: Non-specific vaginitis. Role of Haemophilus vaginitis and treatment with metroindazole. N Engl J Med 298:1429, 1978

REGAMEY C, SCHOENKNECHT FD: Puerperal fever with Haemophilus vaginalis septicemia. JAMA 225:1621, 1973

126
CHANCROID

KING K. HOLMES
ALAN R. RONALD

DEFINITION Chancroid, or soft chancre, is an acute, sexually transmitted infection characterized by painful genital ulcerations usually associated with inflammatory, inguinal adenopathy which often progresses to suppuration. A presumptive diagnosis is supported by exclusion of syphilis, genital herpes, and other specific causes of genital ulceration, together with improvement following sulfonamide therapy. A specific diagnosis is proved only when *Hemophilus ducreyi* is isolated from the lesion or suppurative node.

ETIOLOGY The specific microbial etiology of chancroid has repeatedly been supported by isolation of Ducrey's bacterium, *H. ducreyi*, in mixed culture from chancroidal ulcers and rarely in pure culture from buboes. However, *Bacteroides fragilis, B. melaninogenicus,* and gram-positive cocci are often present in genital ulcers, and anaerobic spirochetes which can be confused with *Treponema pallidum* are occasionally seen as well. The role of such organisms as synergistic or independent pathogens remains undefined. The reported frequency of recovery of *H. ducreyi* from typical chancroid ulcers ranges from 15 to 90 percent. *Hemophilus ducreyi* is a poorly characterized gram-negative aerobe which requires hemin (X factor) but not nicotinamide adenine dinucleotide (V factor) for growth. No unique colonial, biochemical, or immunologic characterizations have been demonstrated, and isolates are identified principally by their streptobacillary "chaining" appearance on Gram's stain.

EPIDEMIOLOGY The incidence of chancroid is unknown, since bacteriologic diagnosis is difficult, clinical diagnosis inaccurate, and reporting incomplete. However, chancroid on a worldwide basis is estimated to be more prevalent than syphilis. Chancroid is most common in Southeast Asia, Africa, and South and Central America but is rare in developed countries. Less than 1000 cases of chancroid are reported annually in the

United States. Localized outbreaks of disease do occur. The sex ratio of reported cases in the United States is five males to one female. Uncircumcised men are more susceptible to chancroid than circumcised men. Prostitution plays a significant role in transmission, and among merchant seamen and military troops whose sexual contacts are prostitutes, chancroid appears to be far more common than syphilis. The extent of the organism's reservoir and the role of carriers in the spread of chancroid are undetermined. Commonly female contacts of infected males will not have genital ulcers. It is presumed that they are carriers of *H. ducreyi*, and organisms resembling *H. ducreyi* have been recovered from smegma of normal men and the vagina of normal women.

CLINICAL MANIFESTATIONS After an incubation period of 3 to 5 days, a small inflammatory papule appears, which becomes pustular or occasionally vesiculopustular and ulcerative within 2 to 3 days. The classic chancroid (Fig. 126-1) is superficial and shallow, ranging from a few millimeters to 2 cm in diameter. The edge usually appears ragged or scalloped and is surrounded by an inflammatory red halo. The base is covered by a necrotic exudate and bleeds easily when the exudate is removed. In contrast with syphilitic chancre, the chancroidal ulcer is extremely painful and tender and is not indurated. In men, the most frequent locations are the preputial orifice or internal surface of the prepuce and the frenulum; in women, the labia, fourchette, and perianal region. The lesions in females tend to be more superficial and less painful. Multiple ulcers are more common than single ulcers. Extragenital ulcers can occur but are rare.

FIGURE 126-1
The classic chancroid.

Acute, painful, tender, inflammatory inguinal adenopathy accompanies over 50 percent of cases and is unilateral in about two-thirds. In untreated patients, the involved nodes become matted, forming a unilocular suppurative bubo. The overlying skin becomes erythematous, tense, and thinned and finally ruptures, forming a single ulcer.

DIAGNOSIS Other diseases which may be confused with chancroid in decreasing order of frequency are genital herpes, primary syphilis, and lymphogranuloma venereum (LGV). One United States study of 100 consecutive men with penile ulceration disclosed genital herpes in 22, syphilis in 17, and traumatic lesions in 8. Classic chancroid ulcers were noted in 12, only 2 of which yielded *H. ducreyi* on culture. Most of the remaining ulcers were of uncertain etiology. The morphological diagnosis of genital lesions is fraught with error, and the majority of lesions diagnosed as chancroid in clinical practice probably are actually genital herpes, syphilis, or traumatic lesions. Careful repeated dark-field search for *T. pallidum* are serial serology for syphilis should be carried out even in patients with clinical features of chancroid.

Primary genital infection with herpes simplex virus produces tender inguinal adenopathy in approximately 50 percent of cases, but primary genital herpes can usually be readily distinguished by the history of onset with vesicular lesions. Primary genital herpes often produces dysuria and symptoms suggestive of viremia, such as fever, myalgia, and arthralgia, whereas chancroid rarely causes systemic symptoms. Over 80 percent of women with primary herpes have transient cervical ulcerations. A localized cluster of vesicles and a past history of similar lesions characterize recurrent genital herpes.

If viral isolation cannot be attempted, a simple means for diagnosing genital herpes is by cytology (Papanicolaou) smear obtained from the base of the genital lesion. Multinucleated cells and/or intranuclear inclusions can be seen in about two-thirds of vesicular or pustular herpetic lesions and about 50 percent of ulcerative lesions. In primary syphilis, the chancre is indurated, and the associated adenopathy is bilateral, nontender, and nonsuppurative. However, at least three dark-field examinations should be performed on separate days together with monthly serologic tests for syphilis for 3 months, to exclude syphilis.

The inguinal adenopathy of LGV differs from that of chancroid. The adenopathy of LGV develops after the genital lesion is healed, is indolent, often bilateral and nontender, and develops multilocular suppuration and fistulas. Chancroidal adenopathy appears rapidly, nearly always before the ulcer has healed, is more often unilateral, is more painful, and develops suppuration. A negative LGV complement fixation test provides evidence against LGV.

The only reliable method for laboratory diagnosis of chancroid consists of isolation of *H. ducreyi* from the ulcer or bubo. Inoculation of pus into rabbit blood has been the standard culture technique. Overgrowth of concomitant flora has usually precluded successful isolation. Direct plating onto chocolate agar containing 1% Isovitalex plus 3 μg/ml vancomycin is more likely to yield the organism. Incubation in 5% CO_2 with 100 percent humidity for 3 to 5 days is necessary for discernible colonial growth. Immunodiagnostic tests for chancroid are needed urgently.

TREATMENT Comparisons of various antibiotics for treatment of chancroid have been inconclusive, because treated cases seldom have been confirmed by isolation of *H. ducreyi*. Small genital lesions, treated only with good hygiene and saline soaks, may heal in 2 to 4 weeks without antibacterial ther-

apy. Genital herpes usually begins to improve spontaneously about 10 days after onset of primary lesions and 4 days after onset of recurrent lesions, while primary syphilis usually heals 4 to 6 weeks after onset. Sulfonamides are considered more effective than tetracycline or streptomycin for chancroid. Also sulfonamide therapy will not interfere with dark-field examination for *T. pallidum* or with development of a positive serologic test for syphilis. If initial dark-field examination of a chancroidal lesion is negative, sulfonamide therapy can be started, and the dark-field examination can be repeated on subsequent days. Sulfisoxazole (Gantrisin) is usually effective in a dose of 4 g daily and should be continued until the lesion and adenopathy have healed, which usually requires about 2 weeks. Fluctuant lymph nodes should be aspirated to prevent rupture, since suppuration may progress despite therapy. Buboes larger than 5 cm in diameter almost always require drainage. After three successive dark-field examinations have been negative, if the response to sulfisoxazole is unsatisfactory, tetracycline hydrochloride should be added in a dose of 2 g daily. *Hemophilus ducreyi* is susceptible to a number of antibiotics including streptomycin, chloramphenicol, erythromycin, and usually penicillin. Plasmid-mediated resistance to one or multiple antibiotics is present in some strains.

REFERENCES

CHAPEL T et al: The microbiological flora of penile ulcerations. J Infect Dis 137:50, 1978

HAMMOND GW et al: Antimicrobial susceptibility of *Haemophilus ducreyi*. Antimicrob Agents Chemother 13:608, 1978

——— et al: Comparison of specimen collection and laboratory techniques for isolation of *Haemophilus ducreyi*. J Clin Microbiol 7:39, 1978

——— et al: Determination of the hemin requirement of *Haemophilus ducreyi*: Evaluation of the porphyrin test and media used in the satellite growth test. J. Clin Microbiol 7:243, 1978

KERFER RE et al: Treatment of chancroid. A comparison of tetracycline and sulfisoxazole. Arch Dermatol 100:604, 1979

SULLIVAN M: Chancroid. Am J Syph Gonorrhea Vener Dis 24:482, 1940

127
BRUCELLOSIS

WESLEY W. SPINK

DEFINITION Brucellosis (undulant fever) is caused by microorganisms belonging to the genus *Brucella* and is transmitted to human beings from lower animals. The acute illness is frequently characterized by fever without localized findings, while the chronic form consists of fever, weakness, and vague complaints, which may persist for months and years.

HISTORY The first clear-cut picture of the disease was presented in 1863 by Marston, and the etiologic agent (*Brucella melitensis*) was discovered by Bruce in 1886. In 1897, Bang reported that *B. abortus* was the cause of contagious abortion in cattle in Denmark. Traum first identified *Brucella* organisms (*B. suis*) from aborting sows in 1914. New species include *B. canis,* which causes abortions in dogs, especially the beagle breed, and *B. ovis,* which causes epidemics that result in sterility in rams.

ETIOLOGY Human brucellosis is primarily due to one of three species: *B. melitensis* (goats), *B. suis* (hogs), and *B. abortus* (cattle). Several subtypes have been described under each of these three main categories. *Brucella suis,* subtype II (*B. rangiferi tarandi*), is a serious disease of reindeer in Alaska and Siberia, and a common cause of human illness. *Brucella canis* has caused illness in few humans, and no human disease has been ascribed to *B. ovis.* Brucellae are small, nonmotile, non-spore-forming, gram-negative rods. Growth is best at 37°C in trypticase soy broth or tryptose phosphate broth having a pH of 6.6 to 6.8, under conditions in which 10 percent of the air is displaced by carbon dioxide. The differentiation of the three species is dependent upon biochemical and serologic reaction. Strain 19, *B. abortus,* is a viable attenuated strain used widely for vaccinating cattle. Accidental injection through the skin in veterinarians causes an acute febrile illness, which should be treated with tetracycline.

EPIDEMIOLOGY The natural reservoir of brucellosis is in domestic animals, particularly cattle, swine, goats, and sheep. The disease is very rarely transmitted from person to person.

Studies in the United States and elsewhere indicate that the majority of cases are acquired through contact, and fewer cases are caused by the ingestion of milk or milk products. This trend is due to the enactment of local and state ordinances requiring all milk sold for human consumption to be pasteurized. There is some evidence that brucellosis may be airborne, the disease resulting from the inhalation of *Brucella.* Infections caused by *B. abortus* are spread through cow's milk or through dermal contact with *Brucella.* Contact with infected porcine tissue is a common cause of infections due to *B. suis.* Thus, brucellosis is primarily an occupational disease of rural areas, involving primarily meat-packing plant employees, farmers, veterinarians, and livestock producers. Disease due to *B. melitensis* is the most common type of brucellosis on a worldwide basis. It occurs in local areas in the United States and is due to the ingestion of goat's milk cheese.

PATHOGENESIS Following invasion of the body by brucellae through the oropharynx or through the skin, the organisms tend to localize in tissues of the reticuloendothelial system, such as the bone marrow, lymph nodes, liver, spleen, and also the kidneys. A characteristic but nonspecific reaction of these tissues to the brucellae is the appearance of epithelioid cells, giant cells of the foreign body and Langhans' types, and lymphocytes and plasma cells. Necrosis and caseation rarely occur in these granulomatous areas. When caseation is encountered, it is usually caused by *B. suis.* The granulomas are similar to those of sarcoidosis and tuberculosis. Other, less frequent, sites of localization of *Brucella* organisms are the bones (especially the spine), the endocardium, and the testes. Although the central nervous system and peripheral nerves are commonly affected deleteriously by brucellae, the mechanism whereby this takes place is not known. Like other blood-borne bacilli, brucellae may on occasion localize in any tissue or organ in the body. Though brucellosis is a common cause of abortions in cattle, swine, and goats, authentic human abortions occur no more frequently with this disease than with other bacteremias. Orchitis in the male is rarely the cause of subsequent sterility.

MANIFESTATIONS The incubation period varies between 5 and 21 days, though many months may elapse between the time of infection and the first appearance of symptoms. The onset in many instances may be insidious; patients have a low-grade fever with no localized findings and complain of headache, weakness, insomnia, sweats, anorexia, constipation, pain over the spine, and generalized aches and pains. Less frequently, the disease may be ushered in by chills, high fever, and prostration, but, again, localizing abnormal physical findings may be absent. An enlarged and tender spleen is usually associated with the more severe cases. Pain on pressure over

the vertebrae occurs occasionally, and pain along the course of peripheral nerves, particularly the sciatic nerve, is encountered. Orchitis appears after several days of illness and, like the orchitis of mumps, is ushered in with a chill or chilliness, high fever, and tender and enlarged testes. Painful and swollen joints are seen occasionally, but persistent and deforming arthritis is rare. Signs and symptoms referable to the lungs and pleurae are uncommon. A rare but serious complication is subacute bacterial endocarditis. Ocular disorders are associated with the more chronic forms of the disease.

The initial febrile stage of the illness may last from a few days up to several weeks. The persistence of fever and symptoms is definitely related to physical activity. Rest in bed during the acute illness is frequently associated with prompt improvement. The natural course of the disease in the majority of patients is marked by a permanent remission of fever and symptoms within 3 to 6 months or sooner. A small number of patients with bacteriologically proved cases may have an illness that persists for a year or more.

The status of *chronic brucellosis* is extremely difficult to assess. There is no doubt that the infection may persist in a relatively small number of individuals for months and years. Such patients are in a state of ill health manifested by weakness, fatigue, mental depression, vague aches and pains, and no abnormal physical findings. Intermittent fever may occur. Of considerable importance in the suspected chronic case is the investigation of possible sites of chronic suppuration manifested by calcified caseating areas in the liver and spleen that can be detected by careful x-ray films of the abdomen or by liver or spleen scan. Abacteriuric pyuria should suggest, among other causes, renal suppuration due to brucellae.

LABORATORY FINDINGS A precise diagnosis of brucellosis is dependent upon the results of laboratory procedures.

Blood The total leukocyte count is usually normal, or slightly reduced, but is rarely over 10,000 cells per cubic millimeter. The differential count reveals a relative lymphocytosis. The erythrocyte sedimentation rate is of no specific diagnostic aid, being normal or accelerated.

The most practical method for screening suspected cases of brucellosis is the agglutination reaction. Agglutinins usually appear during the second or third week of illness. If proper techniques and antigens are employed, agglutinins are demonstrated in the vast majority of bacteriologically proved cases. Active brucellosis is usually associated with titers of 1:100 or above. On rare occasions, the titer may be depressed by "blocking antibodies" in chronic illness. Only very rarely are agglutinins absent in patients with bacteriologically proved disease. Agglutinins for brucellosis are not always specific, since cross reactions occur with the cholera vibrio and with *Pasteurella tularensis.* Agglutinins may persist in the blood long after the patient has recovered. One of the most critical diagnostic problems in the sporadic case of brucellosis is the interpretation of an agglutination titer of 1 to 100 or lower in the absence of definitive bacteriologic data and localizing signs. *Brucella*-agglutinating immunoglobulins in serum consist of both 7S and 19S globulins, but only 7S globulins have been associated with active disease in acute and chronic cases, providing a stimulating dose of antigen (skin test) has not been given before obtaining blood from the patient. The absence of 7S agglutinating antibody in the serum of a suspected case of brucellosis strongly militates against the presence of active disease as the cause of illness.

At least one, and preferably more, cultures of blood should be carried out in every suspected case of brucellosis and kept for 6 weeks before being discarded as negative. Brucellae have been isolated from aspirated sternal bone marrow when simultaneous blood cultures were sterile. It is too impractical for routine purposes to attempt to isolate brucellae from the urine, bile, or feces.

Intradermal tests A positive reaction to *Brucella* antigen has no more significance than that obtained with tuberculin in suspected cases of tuberculosis. A positive reaction indicates previous invasion of the body by brucellae and does not mean that active disease is present. When agglutinins are absent and cultures remain sterile, considerable caution must be exercised before making a diagnosis of brucellosis, even though the skin test is positive.

DIFFERENTIAL DIAGNOSIS Brucellosis must be differentiated from other acute febrile illnesses such as influenza and other upper respiratory diseases of doubtful etiology. Other diseases from which it must be differentiated include malaria and typhoid fever. Brucellosis may be confused with infectious mononucleosis.

Chronic brucellosis simulates psychoneurosis, anxiety states, and chronic nervous exhaustion. Indeed, a patient with brucellosis may also have these nervous disorders.

TREATMENT Patients with acute brucellosis should be reassured that a large majority of those with the disease recover spontaneously. Rest and psychotherapy are important during the febrile illness.

The course of acute brucellosis can be shortened and complications prevented by the prompt use of tetracycline, in dosage of 0.5 g four times daily orally for at least 3 weeks. In case of a relapse, this dose schedule can be repeated. Except in rare instances there is no advantage in more than two courses of tetracycline therapy. For more seriously ill patients streptomycin in dosage of 0.5 g twice daily may be used in addition to tetracycline. Tetracycline therapy, with and without streptomycin, is also effective in proved chronic brucellosis.

Febrile patients with either acute or chronic brucellosis sometimes have severe anorexia, depression, and generalized debilitation. Such individuals should receive an adrenocorticoid steroid preparation in addition to antibiotic therapy. Prednisone in oral dosage of 20 mg can be given twice daily for 72 to 96 h, or 100 mg hydrocortisone can be administered intravenously, followed by 50 mg orally twice daily.

The therapeutic use of brucella vaccine in chronic brucellosis is of questionable value and is not recommended.

For the relief of headache and the generalized aches and pains, salicylates may be prescribed; the occasional use of barbiturates is desirable for the insomnia which is so commonly a part of the disease.

PROGNOSIS Although brucellosis may be a chronic and disabling disease, the overall mortality rate is low. Even without the aid of effective drug therapy, only 15 percent of patients have an illness exceeding 3 months.

Cases of bacteriologically proved brucellosis in which the disease has continued for up to 25 years have been studied at the University of Minnesota Hospitals, but such cases are rare. So-called "chronic brucellosis" is diagnosed all too often on the basis of procedures of doubtful value, especially the intradermal test with *Brucella* antigen.

Relapses occur in some chronic cases of brucellosis. These recurrences are not common and are manifested by fever, men-

tal and physical disability, and generalized aches and pains. Too little attention has been given to the problem of reinfections. Clinical observations in meat-packing plant employees have confirmed studies made in experimentally infected animals, showing that the immunity induced by one attack of brucellosis is only relative and that second and third infections do take place. In individuals who continue to be exposed to the disease, it may be quite difficult to differentiate between relapses and reinfections. Furthermore, patients who have recovered from brucellosis have an acquired *Brucella* hypersensitivity that may render them extremely susceptible to the effects of contact with *Brucella* antigen. This is particularly applicable to veterinarians who have accidentally injected viable *Brucella* antigen into their skin while immunizing animals. Violent local and systemic febrile reactions follow such an incident within a few hours.

PREVENTION As long as a reservoir of brucellosis persists in domestic animals, human brucellosis will occur. The only practical means of eliminating the disease in human beings is to eradicate the disease from cattle, hogs, sheep, and goats. Control measures in animals have been worked out in the United States, especially for cattle, and considerable progress is being made in eliminating *B. suis* from herds of swine. Since human brucellosis may be contracted through the ingestion of contaminated milk and milk products, it is essential that only properly pasteurized milk be utilized for human consumption. Brucellosis is an occupational disease involving farmers, livestock workers, veterinarians, and those working in meat-packing plants, and there is no entirely safe means for immunizing these groups against the disease.

REFERENCES

BUCHANAN TM et al: Brucellosis in the United States, 1960-1972. An abattoir-associated disease. Medicine 53:403, 1974

CENTER FOR DISEASE CONTROL: *Brucellosis Surveillance: Annual Summary 1976.* October 1977

MEYER ME: Advances in research on brucellosis, 1957-1972, in *Advances in Veterinary Science and Comparative Medicine,* vol 18, CA Brandly, CE Cornelius (eds). New York, Academic, 1974, pp 231-249

SAEGUSA J et al: A survey of *Brucella canis* infection in dogs from Tokyo area. Jpn J Vet Sci 40:75, 1978

SPINK WW: *The Nature of Brucellosis.* Minneapolis, University of Minnesota Press, 1956

————: The significance of bacterial hypersensitivity in human brucellosis: Studies on infections due to strain 19, *Brucella abortus.* Ann Intern Med 47:861, 1957.

128
TULAREMIA

LEIGHTON E. CLUFF

DEFINITION Tularemia (rabbit fever, deer-fly fever, Ohara's disease) is an infectious disease of animals transmitted to human beings by direct contact or by insect vectors. A cutaneous or mucous membrane lesion at the site of inoculation and regional lymph node enlargement are the characteristic manifestations of the disease in humans. Pneumonia or fever without regional manifestations also is a feature of tularemia.

HISTORY The microorganism responsible for tularemia was identified by McCoy and Chapin in 1912 among infected ground squirrels in Tulare County, California. The first description of tularemia in man was by Wherry and Lamb in 1914.

ETIOLOGY *Francisella* (*Pasteurella*) *tularensis* is a pleomorphic, nonsporulating, gram-negative bacillus. It can be cultured only on media containing glucose, cystine, and serum. Thorough cooking renders meat from infected animals safe for eating, but tularemia can develop in persons handling carcasses that have been frozen for many days. *Francisella tularensis* is related antigenically to the causative organisms of brucellosis and plague and possesses an endotoxin similar to those of many other gram-negative bacteria.

EPIDEMIOLOGY AND PATHOGENESIS Contact with infected animals is the commonest source of tularemia in humans, but the disease also may be acquired from insects or by exposure to the organism in the laboratory. A variety of rodents, carnivores, ungulates, birds, and arthropods are naturally infected by *F. tularensis,* including rabbits, squirrels, woodchucks, muskrats, skunks, coyotes, foxes, cats, opossums, mice, rats, quail, chickens, pheasants, snakes, ticks, and flies. The Rocky Mountain tick, western wood tick, eastern dog tick, and the Lone Star tick (*Dermacentor andersoni, D. variabilis, D. occidentalis,* and *Amblyomma americanum*) may act as reservoirs of infection. One species of deerfly (*Chrysops discalis*) and, in Sweden, a mosquito (*Aedes cinereus*) can transmit tularemia to humans. Ticks are an important reservoir of the disease because the microorganism is transferred transovarially from the female to her progeny. Sporadic episodes and epidemic tularemia have occurred among humans after contact with water and fish contaminated by infected animal carcasses. However, human-to-human transmission of infection does not occur. Wild cottontail rabbits are the principal source of tularemia in the United States. A large-scale epidemic, presumably transmitted by infected muskrats, occurred in Vermont in 1968. A case of human infection has been reported after a cat bite.

Human beings are highly susceptible to tularemia; the organism usually invades through the skin, mucous membrane, gastrointestinal tract, or respiratory tract. Hunters, butchers, and housewives are most often affected.

PATHOLOGY Microscopically, the primary cutaneous lesion shows neutrophilic infiltration, granulomatous reaction, and necrosis. The regional lymph nodes develop similar changes and often suppurate. The granulomatous reaction in tularemia resembles tubercles in liver, spleen, lung, and kidney. *Francisella tularensis* has been recovered from lymph nodes many days after apparent subsidence of the disease.

MANIFESTATIONS The incubation period is 3 to 7 days. The typical lesion of skin or mucous membranes begins as a reddened papule that may be pruritic and soon ulcerates. The primary lesion in this *ulceroglandular* form of the disease is rarely very painful, is usually present before onset of systemic symptoms, and may not heal until convalescence is well under way. Frequently it is overlooked, or its relation to severe systemic symptoms is not recognized. Regional lymph node enlargement is usually more prominent than that accompanying infections of similar severity produced by other microorganisms. The involved nodes are often exquisitely tender, fluctuant, hot, and reddened. Drainage can occur spontaneously. Generalized lymphadenopathy is present in some cases, but the regional nodes are most prominently involved. There is considerable variation in the intensity of the systemic symptoms of ulceroglandular tularemia; the patient may be almost asymptomatic or severely ill. Clinical and roentgenographic evidence of pneumonitis may accompany this form of the disease, illustrating its disseminated character, but bacteremia is rarely demonstrable.

Localized lymph node enlargement without a detectable skin lesion is referred to as *glandular* tularemia. The pathogenesis of this form of the disease is probably identical with that of ulceroglandular tularemia, and the features of the illness are also the same.

Rarely, the portal of entry of the organism is the conjunctiva, where there develops an ulcer, with edema, congestion, lacrimation, photophobia, and pain. In this *oculoglandular* type of tularemia the preauricular, submaxillary, and anterior cervical lymph nodes may enlarge. Corneal ulceration and scarring or perforation of the globe may occur.

Ingestion of contaminated meat or water may result in primary lesions in the *gastrointestinal tract.* This rare form of the disease produces diarrhea, abdominal pain, nausea, vomiting, melena, and hematemesis, but otherwise differs little from tularemia introduced through other portals. Ulcerative lesions are often found in the buccal mucosa, pharynx, or intestine, and the mesenteric or cervical lymph nodes are involved early in the disease.

Tularemia without obvious primary ulcer or localized lymphadenitis is referred to as *typhoidal.* Constitutional symptoms in typhoidal tularemia differ in no way from those in other types of the disease, although there is usually more prostration. In the absence of localized manifestations, the diagnosis of tularemia is more difficult and depends on serologic tests, isolation of the organism, or a strong epidemiologic history.

Pneumonia may accompany tularemia. Involvement of the lung is secondary to hematogenous dissemination, even when infection is acquired by inhalation of the organism (as in bacteriology laboratories). Pneumonitis in tularemia may cause cough, mucoid sputum, hemoptysis, pleuritic pain, dyspnea, and cyanosis; but extensive x-ray evidence of pneumonitis is sometimes present in the absence of any symptoms of pulmonary disease. Physical findings often correlate poorly with the roentgenologic changes, which consist of diffuse patchy or lobar infiltrations and inconstant hilar adenopathy. Pleural effusion may occur, but lung abscess is rare.

Rarely *F. tularensis* causes endocarditis, pericarditis, peritonitis, appendicitis, osteomyelitis, or meningitis.

Fever in tularemia develops abruptly, often with rigors, and in untreated patients may persist with temperatures of 104 to 106°F for as long as 4 weeks. The fever is sustained or mildly remittent, and defervescence is by lysis.

Splenomegaly is detectable in many patients. An evanescent macular or papular rash is sometimes present on the trunk and extremities early in the disease.

Convalescence in untreated tularemia is prolonged; and fever, lassitude, fatigability, myalgia, irritability, or anorexia may persist or recur for many months. Recovery is usually prompt if acute tularemia is treated with antibiotics. When therapy is delayed, however, patients are more likely to be left with mild debilitation that is unresponsive to further administration of antimicrobial drugs.

Recovery from tularemia is usually followed by immunity to recurrence of disease. However, immunity is not complete, and several instances of second, even third, attacks of tularemia have been recorded. Almost invariably, they have consisted of the development of a local lesion and mild regional adenopathy without systemic symptoms and with little or no fever.

LABORATORY FINDINGS Serum agglutinins for *F. tularensis* are present after the second week of illness. Cross-agglutination may occur with antigens of *Brucella,* but this is not a constant finding. The procedure of choice is a microagglutination method, although the standard tube agglutination test is equally sensitive.

Francisella tularensis can be recovered by appropriate cultures or animal inoculation. It is rarely found in blood but can be isolated from the mucocutaneous ulcer or regional lymph nodes with regularity. The organism has been cultured from the sputum and gastric washings, even in patients without roentgenographic evidence of pneumonitis. Accidental infection of personnel in diagnostic laboratories may occur.

The skin test with a diluted suspension of killed *F. tularensis,* or purified antigen, becomes positive during the first week of disease. The cutaneous hypersensitivity response is "delayed" and resembles the tuberculin reaction. The skin test may become positive earlier and may remain so longer than the agglutination test.

The total blood leukocyte count is usually normal. The erythrocyte sedimentation rate is normal in ulceroglandular or mild disease but is frequently elevated in severe typhoidal tularemia.

DIFFERENTIAL DIAGNOSIS Brucellosis, typhoid fever, disseminated tuberculosis, the early stage of several rickettsial diseases, and infectious mononucleosis may closely resemble typhoidal tularemia. History of possible contacts is important, and appropriate serologic and cultural studies are usually successful in differentiating these infections. Pneumonic tularemia must be distinguished from viral, mycotic, and other bacterial infections of the lung. The differential diagnosis of pneumonia is discussed in Chap. 260. Oculoglandular syndromes likely to be confused with tularemia are described in Chap. 197.

Ulceroglandular tularemia must be distinguished from a variety of infections in which a *local cutaneous ulcer with regional lymphadenopathy* may occur. Besides pyoderma caused by streptococci or staphylococci, these infections include lymphogranuloma venereum, cat-scratch fever, rat-bite fever, bubonic plague, anthrax, glanders, several rickettsioses of which the important one in this country is rickettsialpox, several viral infections of the skin such as orf and cowpox, and inoculation syphilis or tuberculosis. In all these, with the exception of lymphogranuloma venereum and cat-scratch fever, the regional lymph node involvement is usually proportional to the size of the cutaneous ulcer. Extragenital lymphogranuloma is rare; fever and systemic symptoms in cat-scratch fever are rarely severe for more than a few days.

TREATMENT Streptomycin is the antibiotic of choice for tularemia. The dosage is 0.5 to 1 g every 12 h for 10 days. *Francisella tularensis* cannot be recovered from lymph nodes or skin lesions after 24 to 48 h of therapy. However, the regional lymph nodes may continue to enlarge and suppurate for several days. Pulmonary lesions usually subside rapidly, although the evolution of the cutaneous lesion is not interrupted. The tetracycline antibiotics and chloramphenicol also are effective, although fever and other manifestations may recur 7 to 14 days after cessation of therapy. Recrudescent illness, however, responds rapidly to readministration of the antibiotic. Aspiration of pus from suppurating nodes rarely is necessary; but if fistulas persist, total surgical removal of the involved tissue can be carried out. Surgery may be followed by transient recurrence of fever despite failure to demonstrate the organism in excised tissues.

PROPHYLAXIS A killed bacterial vaccine developed by Foshay has been shown to stimulate serum agglutinins and induces positive skin reactions to the bacterial antigens, but it produces little immunity to infection with *F. tularensis.* An attenuated live bacterial vaccine has been developed, however, and is effective in inducing protection against infection, particularly the typhoidal form.

Antibiotic prophylaxis with streptomycin after exposure to tularemia will protect against infection. Chloramphenicol and tetracycline, however, only prolong the incubation period of the disease and do not prevent its occurrence.

Avoidance of contact with possible sources of infection is important in prevention, and the incidence of tularemia in several localities has fallen sharply with the introduction of laws prohibiting the sale of wild rabbits by butchers.

PROGNOSIS The mortality rate in untreated tularemia is 6 to 7 percent. With antimicrobial therapy, death is rare.

REFERENCES

BUCHANAN TM et al: The tularemia skin test: 325 skin tests in 210 persons: Serologic correlation and review of the literature. Ann Intern Med 74:336, 1971

BURKE DS: Immunization against tularemia: Analysis of the effectiveness of live *Francisella tularensis* vaccine in the prevention of laboratory-acquired tularemia. J Infect Dis 135:55, 1977

MASSEY ED, MANGIAFICO JA: Microagglutination test for detecting and measuring serum agglutinins of *Francisella tularensis.* Applied Microbiol 27:25, 1974

STUART BM, PULLEN RL: Tularemic pneumonia: Review of American literature and report of fifteen additional cases. Am J Med Sci 210:233, 1945

YOUNG LS et al: Tularemia epidemic: Vermont 1968. Forty-seven cases linked to contact with muskrats. N Engl J Med 280:1253, 1969

129
YERSINIA (PASTEURELLA) INFECTIONS, INCLUDING PLAGUE

JOSEPH E. JOHNSON III

Gram-negative bacilli of the genus *Pasteurella* have been reclassified recently in accordance with increasing knowledge about the characteristics of the bacteria. *Pasteurella pestis* (the plague bacillus) and *P. pseudotuberculosis* are now included in the genus *Yersinia* along with a third closely related organism, *Y. enterocolitica. Pasteurella multocida* (formerly *P. septica*) initially included a group of several closely related species producing hemorrhagic septicemia in animals and man. Related species with at least potential pathogenicity for humans include *P. urae, P. haemolytica,* and *P. pneumotropica.*

PLAGUE Definition Plague is an infectious disease of animals (principally wild and domestic rodents) which is transmitted to humans through the bite of infected ectoparasites (especially the rat flea). Disease in humans is usually characterized by the abrupt onset of high fever, lymphadenopathy with painful enlargement of regional lymph nodes draining the exposure site, bacteremia, and prostration. This clinical form of the disease is known as *bubonic* plague because of the presence of enlarged lymph nodes, or *buboes.* Secondary pneumonia may occur and lead to direct respiratory transmission by infectious aerosols from person to person. This primary *pneumonic* type of human disease is highly fatal.

History Plague was known and feared in ancient times and has been the subject of dread as well as a source of literary stimulation to authors from Dionysius in the third century to Camus in the present. At least three major pandemics have occurred in which large segments of the population were destroyed. The first authentic pandemic was recorded in the sixth century A.D.; the second great pandemic occurred in the fourteenth century and was known as the "Black Death," and the last major pandemic originated in China in 1894, spread eventually to all continents, and was first recognized in the United States in 1900. It is likely, however, that the disease was present in the wild rodent population (sylvatic plague) in California long before this. The disease is now well established in wild rodents in many parts of the world, including the western United States. It is present on every continent except Australia. Human disease is endemic in parts of Asia, Africa, and South America, and sporadic human cases still occur in the United States.

Etiology The causative agent, *Yersinia pestis,* is a gram-negative, nonmotile, and non-spore-forming bacillus which grows both aerobically and anaerobically. It is pleomorphic in exudate or sputum and may appear bacillary, ovoid, or coccal. When stained with Giemsa's or Wayson's stain, it displays a bipolar "safety pin" structure. *Yersinia pestis* grows readily although somewhat slowly on ordinary culture media, forming small, round, transparent colonies which assume a "beaten-copper" appearance after 48 h. At least two types of toxins have been identified, including a soluble exotoxin-like protein and an insoluble endotoxic lipopolysaccharide. Although readily killed by sunlight, organisms have been shown to survive in sterile soil for 16 months and in nonsterile soil for as long as 7 months, and it is likely that organisms may be present in rodent burrows in the absence of fleas and rats for long periods.

Epidemiology Plague is firmly entrenched as an enzootic among approximately 200 species of rodents in many parts of the world. While the disease in wild rodents (sylvatic plague) is not usually a direct threat to man, it nevertheless serves as a vast reservoir for infection of domestic rats (murine or rat plague) which, along with their ectoparasites, live in close association with man. The endemic reservoir of sylvatic plague includes wild rats, ground squirrels, rock squirrels, mice, marmots, gophers, rabbits, prairie dogs, and chipmunks. Other animal species which are not reservoir hosts are important potential transmitters of the disease. Sick domesticated cats have been implicated in human cases. Dogs are relatively resistant to plague, showing seroconversion following exposure but usually without clinical illness. In the Western Hemisphere the disease is firmly entrenched in the wild rodent population of California, Oregon, Washington, Utah, Idaho, Nevada, New Mexico, Texas, Arizona, Colorado, Montana, Wyoming, and in wide areas in South America. The principal murine hosts are the domestic rats, *Rattus rattus* and *R. norvegicus,* which are found throughout the world. Although ticks, lice, and bedbugs may occasionally serve as vectors, the principal ectoparasite vectors are the oriental rat fleas, *Xenopsylla cheopis* and *Diamanus montanus.*

Between epidemics the infection persists as a chronic disease of wild rodents which is maintained by the insect vector. Although occasionally acquired through contact with wild rodents and their parasites, in major outbreaks of human disease infection has usually resulted from association with domestic rats and occurs in urban areas in the wake of rat epizootics. When the concentration of people and of rats under circumstances of poor sanitation provides opportunity for the migration of fleas from rats to man, an outbreak is likely to occur. Because sylvatic plague appears virtually impossible to eradicate, it will continue to pose a constant threat of extension into urban rat populations and thence to man. Infection of the flea takes place through ingestion of blood of a bacteremic animal. After multiplication in the intestinal tract of the flea, the organisms are regurgitated when the flea attempts to ingest another blood meal. Because rat fleas will attack man if rats are not immediately available, the infection is likely to be transmitted as the rat population decreases and the fleas transfer from dead hosts to human beings. Plague can be acquired by direct contact with the tissues of an infected animal, by its bite, or by scratching of infected material into the skin.

The bubonic form of the disease rarely results in transmission from person to person because bacteremia in human disease is rarely of a level sufficient to allow infection of fleas. The principal mode of spread from person to person is by the pulmonary route, which occurs when a patient with bubonic disease develops secondary plague pneumonia and thereafter excretes large quantities of organisms in the sputum. Airborne infection by droplet nuclei is highly contagious, and primary pneumonic plague is common among those attending such a patient. Although asymptomatic oropharyngeal carriers have been identified among healthy family contacts of bubonic plague patients in Vietnam, the role of these carriers in the transmission of the disease has not been determined.

Pathogenesis In the more common bubonic form of disease, *Y. pestis* gains entry into the human host through the bite of an infected flea. Organisms are carried to the local lymphatics, then to the bloodstream and finally are disseminated. The prominent clinical manifestations are usually in the lymphatic system. In bubonic plague, a hemorrhagic zone of edema surrounds an inflamed and suppurating group of regional lymph nodes. The glands are hyperplastic and show multiple areas of necrosis, in which there are swarms of organisms. Metastatic lesions sometimes develop in other lymphatics or in the viscera. Particularly likely is the occurrence of secondary pneumonia, which constitutes a potential source of pneumonic spread. Hemorrhages are numerous, probably as a result of a toxin produced by *Y. pestis* and it is not unusual for individuals given chemotherapy late in the disease to die of toxemia when plague bacilli can no longer be cultured from any organ. Primary pneumonic spread occurs through the inhalation of infectious aerosols emanating from another case or, rarely, from infected fomites. It is apparent that the tonsils and/or oropharyngeal mucous membranes may occasionally serve as portals of entry resulting in a cervical bubonic-septicemic form of the disease. Rarely a skin papule forms at the site of entry of the bacillus and may develop into a pustule or a carbuncle.

Bacteremia is a constant feature of bubonic and pneumonic plague. The precise mechanisms by which the plague bacillus and its toxic factors produce severe tissue injury are not understood completely.

Manifestations After an incubation period of 1 to 12 days (usually 2 to 4 days), the patient develops an acute and often fulminant illness. In the more common *bubonic* variety, symptoms begin abruptly with chills, a rise in temperature to 38.9 to 40.6°C (102 to 105°F), tachycardia, headache, vomiting, uncertain gait, marked prostration, and delirium. The spleen is sometimes palpable. The fleabite at the portal of entry rarely can be seen; if present, it is marked by a papule or vesicle which ultimately becomes pustular. Pain and tenderness are present in the infected regional lymph nodes. Of the buboes, 60 to 75 percent are in the inguinal or femoral regions because the lower extremities are more commonly the site of the initial fleabite. Less often, especially in children, buboes are found in the axillary or cervical regions. Infection may extend to other superficial or deeply situated groups of glands. The bubo consists of a firm, matted group of glands measuring 2 to 5 cm in diameter and is surrounded by a boggy and frequently hemorrhagic zone of edema. It may occasionally suppurate and drain spontaneously after 1 or 2 weeks, although in some instances there is complete resorption.

There is a marked hemorrhagic tendency, presumably because of the effect of plague toxin on blood vessels, and the development of an intravascular coagulopathy (DIC). Petechiae or ecchymoses occur often. Bleeding may occur into a viscus or a serous cavity, or from the nose and alimentary, respiratory, or urinary tracts.

The course of bubonic plague is marked by an irregular or remittent fever, which often drops at the time of appearance of the bubo, only to rise again. In favorable cases, the temperature falls gradually during the second week concomitant with improvement in the general clinical condition. A rise to hyperpyrexic levels or a precipitous fall to normal or to subnormal frequently heralds approaching death. Most fatalities occur during the first week of illness. Although bubonic plague is usually severe, mild cases called *pestis minor* are sometimes seen during epidemics.

The "primary septicemic" form of plague is actually a variant of bubonic disease. The patient experiences a sudden and overwhelming systemic illness. There is a marked constitutional reaction, with chills, fever, rapid pulse, severe headache, nausea, vomiting, and delirium. Death ensues within a few days, before localizing lesions become clinically apparent. Nevertheless, autopsy usually reveals inflammation in some part of the lymphatic system.

Plague also may take the form of pneumonia. The initial cases appear in patients with bubonic plague, of whom as many as 5 percent develop secondary lesions in the lungs. These individuals may provide the starting point for a person-to-person epidemiologic cycle of airborne primary pneumonic plague. It is a fulminating infection accompanied by great prostration, cough, dyspnea, and, in the later stages, cyanosis. The sputum is abundant, blood-stained, and teeming with *Y. pestis*. Often there are no clear-cut pulmonary signs, though scattered rales or areas of dullness may be found. In the absence of specific therapy, plague pneumonia invariably ends fatally within 1 to 5 days.

Infection may localize in other regions of the body. Subcutaneous abscesses and cutaneous ulcerations sometimes occur, and occasionally the meninges are involved.

Laboratory findings Laboratory confirmation of plague is relatively simple, although the disease is often misdiagnosed in the United States because of its rarity. Consideration of epidemiologic and clinical features provides highly characteristic leads, and once a suspicion of plague is entertained, it can readily be verified by smear, culture, or animal inoculation of appropriate specimens. The technique of staining a suspected specimen with fluorescent specific antiserum provides an elegant method for rapid identification of *Y. pestis*. If a bubo is present, a small quantity of interstitial fluid should be aspirated from its center. Large numbers of morphologically characteristic bacilli are usually seen in a stained smear. Infected sputum likewise contains many organisms. Bacteremia of varying degrees occurs at some time during the course of the disease in nearly all cases, and methylene-blue staining of venous blood may be useful. Pus and sputum should be cultured on blood agar plates, while blood is inoculated into nutrient broth. Organisms are identified by their morphologic and colonial characteristics, by agglutination with specific antiserum, fluorescent antibody staining, and biochemical reactions. The phage lysis test is relatively simple and helpful in distinguishing *Y. pestis* from other *Yersinia*. Caution should be observed in handling infected materials or animals, because of the great danger of infection to laboratory workers.

Specific antibodies appear in the serum of patients convalescing from the disease and can usually be detected early in the second week by complement fixation, agglutination, passive hemagglutination, or immunoelectrophoretic agar-gel precipitation methods. A passive mouse-protective test serves to indicate the immune status of a convalescent or vaccinated individual.

The white blood cell count is elevated to levels often above 20,000 cells per cubic millimeter, and there is a predominance of polymorphonuclear leukocytes. The red blood cell count usually is normal.

Diagnosis Early in the acute phase of illness, before the appearance of localizing signs, plague may be confused with severe systemic illnesses such as typhoid, typhus, or malaria. The presence of buboes may suggest other forms of infectious lymphadenitis, including tularemia, syphilis, and lymphogranuloma venereum, as well as lymphadenitis of staphylococcal or streptococcal origin. Pneumonic plague must be distinguished from tularemic, pneumococcal, and other gram-negative pneumonias as well as from anthrax, psittacosis, and mycoplasma pneumonia. The consideration of epidemiologic factors, plus bacteriologic studies, will aid in the differentiation. Serologic diagnosis is important for retrospective confirmation. When plague is suspected, it is imperative to begin treatment as soon as adequate specimens have been taken for culture because early institution of therapy is essential to ensure recovery. To delay treatment may risk toxemic death in the face of a bacteriologic cure.

Treatment When antibiotic treatment is instituted early in the course of the disease, the response is usually dramatic and complete. Early treatment in pneumonic and septicemic disease is particularly urgent since irreversible progression may occur within 15 h after onset. Streptomycin and tetracycline are the drugs of choice. Streptomycin is given intramuscularly in doses of 0.5 g every 4 h for 48 h followed by 0.5 g every 6 h for a total of 7 to 10 days or until the patient has been afebrile at least 3 days. Kanamycin is also effective and may be particularly useful if streptomycin resistance increases. Tetracyclines are given in initial doses of 2 to 3 g daily intravenously, and the dose is reduced to 2 g daily orally when improvement occurs. Chloramphenicol is also a potent antiplague agent and should be given in initial doses of 6 to 8 g daily intravenously (100 mg/kg) and the dose reduced to 3 g (50 to 75 mg/kg) daily orally for a total dose of 20 to 25 g. Sulfonamides are less effective, especially in pneumonic plague, and should be used only when the other agents are not available. Trimethoprim-sulfamethoxazole (co-trimoxazole) has been used successfully. Buboes are treated with hot, moist applications. Incision and drainage is not indicated unless the lesion becomes clearly fluctuant and the patient has been treated with antibiotics.

Control Prevention of plague must be directed toward elimination of endemic rodent foci, and in endemic urban areas constant vigilance is required in detecting and combating rodent epizootics. Prevention includes eradication of ectoparasite vectors, extermination of rats, and sometimes the immunization of the human population. Rats are attacked by poisoning and trapping, by elimination of harborage areas, and by separating them from their food supplies. Unfortunately, rodent control has proved to be most difficult in the endemic areas because of generally poor living standards. Vector control with DDT has been used with brilliant success in diminishing the flea population infecting both rodents and human beings, but studies in Southeast Asia show a significant incidence of DDT-resistant fleas; however, these may yield to other insecticides such as aldrin, dieldrin, and chlordane. The complete elimination of sylvatic plague appears to be impossible in the foreseeable future, and the control program must be aimed at eradicating foci of wild rodent infection around areas of human habitation. In these peripheral zones, the wild and the domestic rodents live commensally, exchange fleas, and threaten the human community.

Patients must be disinfested and carefully isolated, while other intimately exposed persons should be quarantined. Prophylaxis has been achieved effectively in the past by administering sulfadiazine in a dose of 3 g per day for 1 week. However, there is now significant in vitro resistance to sulfadiazine. Alternatively, prophylaxis with streptomycin in a dose of 1 g per day or with tetracycline is often effective.

Vaccines have been used for many years and apparently provide limited and transitory immunity. Several types of vaccines have been available. A formalin-killed vaccine approved for use in the United States has been advised for all persons traveling to plague-enzootic areas such as Southeast Asia, for those whose vocations bring them into frequent and regular contact with wild rodents in plague enzootic areas, such as Peace Corps volunteers and agricultural workers, and for all laboratory personnel working with *Y. pestis* or with plague-infected rodents. Although the precise effectiveness of this vaccine has not been measured satisfactorily, it appears to reduce the incidence and severity of the disease. A second promising vaccine is a living attenuated strain of the organism which may be particularly suitable for endemic areas in Asia. Studies in the U.S.S.R. indicate that the attenuated vaccine administered by the aerosol route may be especially valuable in prevention of pneumonic plague. A third vaccine consisting of a chemical extract has been effective in experimental laboratory infections. Immunity is relative, and protection is not always conferred by the active disease, since a number of reinfections have been described. Although general vaccination may be worthwhile in an area threatened by an epidemic, the results are too slow for immediate prophylaxis. In such epidemic situations, combined use of all available control measures is indicated.

Prognosis The availability of effective antibiotic therapy has improved the prognosis in this formerly highly fatal disease. In the past the mortality rate of bubonic plague varied from 50 to 90 percent, and the pneumonic, septicemic, and meningitic forms were almost invariably fatal. In treated cases the mortality is 5 to 10 percent, and even the gravest varieties of infection respond to chemotherapy if treated early enough.

OTHER *YERSINIA* INFECTIONS (*Y. PSEUDOTUBERCULOSIS* AND *Y. ENTEROCOLITICA*) **Etiology** *Yersinia pseudotuberculosis* is a gram-negative, aerobic, facultatively anaerobic, non-spore-forming bacillus, which is coccobacillary when virulent and bacillary when avirulent. It is easily confused with other non-lactose-fermenting Enterobacteriaceae. It is nonmotile at 37°C (98.6°F) but usually motile at 22°C (71.6°F). *Yersinia enterocolitica*, a closely related organism, has similar characteristics but is distinguished on the basis of biochemical reactions.

Manifestations *Yersinia pseudotuberculosis* is a ubiquitous animal pathogen, worldwide in distribution but identified only in the last decade as a potentially significant human pathogen. Several hundred cases of human infection have now been identified in Europe (especially Scandinavia) and increasingly from Canada and the United States. *Yersinia enterocolitica*, isolated less frequently from animals in the United States, has also now been recognized as a potential cause of a variety of human disease syndromes. Both organisms have been associated with diarrheal diseases, both acute and chronic, and also a usually benign and self-limited form of mesenteric adenitis, clinically simulating appendicitis. Cervical adenitis has also been seen. Rarely, potentially fatal typhoidal and septicemic forms of infection have been described, especially in patients with underlying debilitating diseases. Increasingly, polyarthritis with and without associated erythema nodosum has been associated with *Yersinia* infection.

Reported cases have indicated a 3:1 male predominance especially in older children and young adults infected with *Y. pseudotuberculosis*, while equal sex distribution and a greater incidence in young children and infants has been observed with *Y. enterocolitica*. In addition, *Y. enterocolitica* has been incriminated in institutional and multiple-family outbreaks.

Transmission has usually been traced to contact with infected animals or contaminated food or water, although person-to-person, hand-to-mouth transmission appears also to be a significant possibility.

Diagnosis Diagnosis may be confirmed by culture of lymph nodes, occasionally of stools, or by serologic titers. Cross reactions with *Salmonella, Brucella,* and *Escherichia coli* antigens occur, and serums must be cross-absorbed. With use of both agglutination and hemagglutination methods, titers up to 1:10,240 have been found. Titers lower than 1:160 are not considered significant. The highest antibody titers usually occur during the acute phase of illness, rapidly disappearing by the fourth or fifth month of convalescence, probably reflecting the elicitation of IgM-type antibodies.

Although both species are easily grown on standard laboratory media, identification is more difficult, and routine methods for pathogenic Enterobacteriaceae are inadequate.

The variety of clinical syndromes which have been observed in association with *Y. pseudotuberculosis* and *Y. enterocolitica* may also be confusing. Acute or subacute yersinial enteritis may mimic salmonellosis, shigellosis, and other common enteropathogenic syndromes. Fever, diarrhea, and vomiting are the most common findings in infants and younger children. Fecal leukocytosis has been found in yersinial enteritis indicating ulceration of the intestinal mucosa. Ulcerative colitis may be simulated. Acute septicemic yersiniosis may resemble systemic salmonellosis and other "typhoidal" syndromes. Subacute localizing yersiniosis with hepatic or splenic abscesses may resemble amebic hepatitis. Patients with mesenteric adenitis (usually children) may present the clinical picture of acute appendicitis with mid- or right-lower quadrant abdominal pain, fever, and leukocytosis. At laparotomy the appendix is usually normal, but large inflamed mesenteric lymph nodes are found, sometimes with associated terminal ileitis. Histologic examination of inflamed nodes has revealed reticulogranulocytic infiltration with or without small abscess formation. Polyarthritis of varying severity and duration has been observed and most often mimics rheumatic fever or juvenile rheumatoid arthritis. Reiter's syndrome may also be simulated. Erythema nodosum has also been increasingly identified in patients with agglutinin rises to *Yersinia,* with or without associated arthritis. Common features in adults have been abdominal pain and fever, with or without arthritis or erythema nodosum. Possible associations of *Yersinia* infection with glomerulonephritis, thyroid disease, and pulmonary lesions have been reported but need further clarification.

Treatment Antibiotic treatment is indicated in the more severe cases, especially the septicemic and subacute localizing forms of disease. *Yersinia pseudotuberculosis* is usually susceptible to the aminoglycoside antibiotics (gentamicin, streptomycin, or kanamycin) as well as to tetracycline, chloramphenicol, ampicillin, and the cephalosporins. *Yersinia enterocolitica* is resistant to penicillin G and only variably sensitive to ampicillin and the cephalosporins. In vitro studies indicate a potential role for trimethoprim-sulfamethoxazole.

PASTEURELLA MULTOCIDA INFECTION   Definition   *Pasteurella multocida* (formerly *P. septica*) is a gram-negative nonsporulating bacillus which differs from *Yersinia* organisms in cultural characteristics, antibiotic sensitivity, and pattern of animal parasitism. For example, all strains of *P. multocida* are sensitive to penicillin. *Pasteurella multocida* is frequently identified as a commensal in cattle, horses, swine, sheep, fowl, dogs, cats, and rats, and on occasion causes hemorrhagic septicemia, or chronic pulmonary infiltrates, in these species. Human infection with *P. multocida* is uncommon and usually related to animal contact. Related species which have occasionally been identified as human pathogens include *P. urae, P. haemolytica,* and *P. pneumotropica.*

Manifestations   Human disease due to *P. multocida* is usually a consequence of a dog or cat bite and appears as a localized wound infection with cellulitis, suppuration, and adenitis. Osteomyelitis sometimes ensues. Rarely, in patients with bronchiectasis, *P. multocida* is isolated from sputum, and animal handlers are sometimes identified as asymptomatic respiratory carriers. Empyema has occasionally been associated with the organisms. Bacteremia with fever and chills may develop after an animal bite, occasionally without an apparent local lesion. Meningitis, brain abscess, pyogenic arthritis, endocarditis, and pyelonephritis may occasionally complicate the bacteremia.

Not all *P. multocida* infections follow documented animal bites or animal contact.

Diagnosis   Except for the association with animal (especially cat) bites, local infections with *P. multocida* show no unique characteristics, and may resemble cat-scratch fever, tularemia, or staphylococcal or streptococcal infection. Leukocytosis, uncommon in tularemia and cat-scratch fever, is the rule in *P. multocida* infection.

Gram's stain of infected material shows pleomorphic gram-negative bacilli which are usually extracellular. The bacteria may have bipolar staining and may be mistaken for gram-negative diplococci prior to cultural identification.

Treatment   Penicillin in a dosage of 600,000 to 1.2 million units daily is the preferred antibiotic, but a variety of other antibiotics may be effective.

REFERENCES

Plague

CANTEY JR: Plague in Vietnam, clinical observations and treatment with kanamycin. Arch Intern Med 133:280, 1974

GIRARD G: Plague. Annu Rev Microbiol 69:253, 1955

HIRST LF: *The Conquest of Plague: A Study of the Evolution of Epidemiology.* Fair Lawn, NJ, Oxford University Press, 1953

MEYER KF et al: Plague immunization. I. Past and present trends. J Infect Dis 129:S13, 1974

POLAND JD et al: Human bubonic plague from exposure to a naturally infected wild carnivore. Am J Epidemiol 97:332, 1973

POLLITZER R: *Plague.* Geneva, World Health Organization, 1954

REED WB et al: Bubonic plague in the southwestern United States. Medicine 49:465, 1970

RUST JD et al: The role of domestic animals in the epidemiology of plague. I. Experimental infection of dogs and cats. J Infect Dis 124:522, 1971

VON REYN CF et al: Epidemiologic and clinical features of an outbreak of bubonic plague in New Mexico. J Infect Dis 136:489, 1977

WHO EXPERT COMMITTEE ON PLAGUE: Fourth report. Tech Rep Ser 447, Geneva, 1970

P. Multocida

BEARN AG et al: *Pasteurella multocida* septicemia in man. Am J Med 18:167, 1955

MORRIS AJ et al: *Pasteurella multocida* and bronchiectasis. Bull Johns Hopkins Hosp 91:174, 1952

SWARTZ MN, KUNZ LJ: *Pasteurella multocida* infections in man: Report of two cases—meningitis and infected cat bite. N Engl J Med 261:888, 1959

Yersinia

ARVASTON B et al: Clinical symptoms of infection with *Yersinia enterocolitica.* Scand J Infect Dis 3:37, 1971

GUTMAN LT et al: An inter-familial outbreak of *Yersinia entercolitica* enteritis. N Engl J Med 288:1372, 1974

HUBERT WT et al: *Yersinia pseudotuberculosis* infection in the United States: Septicemia, appendicitis and mesenteric lymphadenitis. Am J Trop Med 20:679, 1971

JEPSEN OB et al: *Yersinia enterocolitica* infection in patients with acute surgical abdominal disease: A prospective study. Scand J Infect Dis 8:189, 1976

LEINO R, KALLIOMAKI JL: Yersiniosis as an internal disease. Ann Intern Med 81:458, 1974

RABSON AR et al: Generalized *Yersinia enterocolitica* infection. J Infect Dis 131:447, 1975

SAARI TN, TRIPLETT DA: *Yersinia pseudotuberculosis* mesenteric adenitis. J Pediatr 85:656, 1974

SHENKMAN L, BOTTONE EJ: Antibodies in *Yersinia enterocolitica* in thyroid disease. Ann Intern Med 85:735, 1976

SPIRA TJ, KABINS SA: *Yersinia enterocolitica* septicemia with septic arthritis. Arch Intern Med 136:1305, 1976

130
RAT-BITE FEVER (*STREPTOBACILLUS MONILIFORMIS* AND *SPIRILLUM MINUS* INFECTIONS)

JAN V. HIRSCHMANN

DEFINITION   *Rat-bite fever* refers to infection by either *Streptobacillus moniliformis* or *Spirillum minus.* The latter infection is also known by its Japanese name *sodoku.*

ETIOLOGY AND EPIDEMIOLOGY   *Streptobacillus moniliformis* is an aerobic nonmotile gram-negative bacterium that may grow in chains of fusiform bacilli. In blood cultures the typical puffball colonies generally appear in 2 to 7 days. Stable L forms frequently develop spontaneously.

The nasopharynx of rats is the natural reservoir of *S. moniliformis,* which grows from as many as half those studied. Human infection usually follows bites from wild rats, but bites from laboratory rats and occasionally other rodents have caused disease. Infection may also occur from ingestion of contaminated food. An epidemic in Haverhill, Massachusetts, in 1926 involving 86 people and caused by contaminated milk or ice cream has led to the term *Haverhill fever* when infection is food-borne.

Spirillum minus is a short, thick spiral gram-negative spiral organism 2 to 5 μm with two to five curves and terminal flagellae that increase its total length to 6 to 10 μm. On dark-field microscopy the organism has characteristic spasmodic motions of the body and darting movements of the flagella. Although it may be visible on Wright's stains of blood from infected patients or animals, it does not grow on artificial media and requires animal inoculation for isolation from patients.

Carrier rates in wild rats, the natural reservoir, are as high as 25 percent in some locations. In them it may cause interstitial keratitis and conjunctivitis. Human infections with *S. minus* almost always follow rat bites.

CLINICAL MANIFESTATIONS Although up to 22 days may elapse, the incubation period for *S. moniliformis* infection is generally short, typically less than 10 days, usually 1 to 3 days. The onset is sudden, with fever, chills, headache, and myalgias the initial symptoms. The bite site is usually unimpressive; occasionally swelling, ulceration, and regional lymphadenopathy are present. A macular rash develops in about 75 percent of cases, usually 1 to 3 days after the onset of symptoms, and is most prominent on the extremities, where it may involve palms and soles. Sometimes it may be generalized, petechial, purpuric, or pustular. Arthralgias or arthritis occurs in about half the cases within the first week, usually with multiple, asymmetric large joint involvement. Without treatment the course of disease may be prolonged for several weeks with persistent or recurrent fever and arthritis. Complications of *S. moniliformis* infection include endocarditis and localized abscesses in soft tissues or brain.

In *Spirillum minus* infections the incubation period is typically longer, usually 1 to 4 weeks, with a range of 1 to 36 days. Usually the bite site, after initial prompt healing, becomes swollen, painful, and red at the onset of fever and chills. There is often lymphangitis and regional lymphadenopathy as well. The fever is usually relapsing, with febrile periods of 2 to 4 days alternating with afebrile periods of about the same duration. During the fever, headache, photophobia, nausea, and vomiting may occur. Joint complaints are rare. A rash develops in more than half the patients that is usually macular and reddish brown or purple-red and occurs typically on the extremities. When untreated, this relapsing illness may persist for months. Rarely, bacterial endocarditis occurs.

LABORATORY FINDINGS In *S. moniliformis* infections the leukocyte count is typically elevated, with neutrophilia and increased immature forms. The organism can be isolated from blood, joint fluid, or pus. Serologic response can be demonstrated during the second week by agglutination tests.

In *S. minus* infections the leukocyte count may be normal or elevated. The organism may be visible on Wright's stained smears or dark-field examination of the patient's blood. In suspected cases the blood should be injected into the peritoneum of mice or guinea pigs; 5 to 15 days later the organism will be visible on dark-field examination of the animals' blood or peritoneal fluid. In about one-half of patients there are biological false-positive tests for syphilis.

DIFFERENTIAL DIAGNOSIS With a history of a rat bite, the major clinical features distinguishing *S. moniliformis* from *S. minus* infection are the differences in the incubation period, the condition of the bite site, the nature of the fever, and the presence or absence of joint symptoms.

TREATMENT AND PROGNOSIS Before effective chemotherapy was available, the mortality rate from *S. moniliformis* infections was about 10 percent; for *S. minus* it was about 6 percent. The treatment of choice is the same for both organisms: 7 to 10 days of procaine penicillin, 600,000 units twice daily intramuscularly, or oral penicillin V, 2 g daily in four divided doses. For penicillin-allergic patients oral erythromycin or tetracycline, 2 g daily in four divided doses, are alternatives. Patients with endocarditis should receive a 4-week course of intravenous penicillin G in a daily dose of 12 to 16 million units.

REFERENCES

COLE JS et al: Rat-bite fever. Ann Intern Med 71:979, 1969

McCORMACK RC et al: Endocarditis due to *Streptobacillus moniliformis*. JAMA 200:77, 1967

ROUGHGARDEN JW: Antimicrobial therapy of rat-bite fever: A review. Arch Intern Med 116:39, 1965

section 5 | Other aerobic bacterial infections

131
ANTHRAX

LEIGHTON E. CLUFF

DEFINITION Anthrax (also called malignant pustule, charbon, splenic fever, milzbrand, woolsorter's disease) is a disease of wild and domesticated animals that is transmitted to human beings by contact with infected animals or their products and, rarely, by insect vectors which act as mechanical carriers of the etiologic organism. The characteristic lesion of human anthrax is a necrotic cutaneous ulcer, the *malignant pustule.* The disease also may be associated with disseminated infection and medi-

astinitis without mucous membrane involvement or cutaneous ulcer.

HISTORY The classic studies of Robert Koch in 1877, showing that *Bacillus anthracis* was the cause of anthrax, serve as the prototype for the establishment of causation of infectious diseases.

ETIOLOGY *Bacillus anthracis* is a large, encapsulated, gram-positive, aerobic, spore-forming microorganism that grows well in most nutrient media. Its pathogenicity for laboratory animals differentiates it from *Bacillus subtilis,* which it closely resembles. The spores are killed by boiling for 10 min, but can survive for many years in soil and animal products, an important factor in the persistence and spread of the disease. The anthrax bacillus possesses a capsule of glutamyl polypeptide, which interferes with phagocytosis of the microorganism. In addition, it contains an anticomplementary substance and elaborates a "protective" antigen and a toxin which is probably of importance in determining virulence.

EPIDEMIOLOGY Anthrax is worldwide; repeated outbreaks have occurred in Southern Europe, Africa, Australia, Asia, and on both American continents.

Cattle, horses, sheep, goats, and swine are most commonly infected. There have been outbreaks of anthrax among animals in the United States, centering mostly in South Dakota, Nebraska, Arkansas, Mississippi, Louisiana, Texas, and California. The disease tends to occur in animals in late summer and early fall. An outbreak of anthrax, acquired from goatskin bongo drum heads and goatskin rugs, occurred in Haiti in 1973, and though importation from Haiti of goatskins or products made in whole or part from them has been restricted since 1974, commercial importation of potentially contaminated raw goatskin for tanning is not restricted in the United States. In 1974, an epidemic of anthrax developed in cattle in Texas, and in the state of Washington in horses infected from contaminated saddle packs containing goat hair imported from Pakistan.

The disease in human beings is acquired by butchering, skinning, or dissecting infected carcasses or by handling contaminated hides, wool, hair, or other materials. It is seen principally in agricultural and industrial employees. The majority of cases of human anthrax involve workers handling imported and unprocessed wool, hair, or hides. The disease usually follows inoculation of bacilli or spores into the skin, often through a wound or abrasion. Intestinal infection has followed ingestion of contaminated meat, and anthrax may develop after inhalation of spores.

PATHOGENESIS The malignant pustule which follows cutaneous inoculation of anthrax organisms is characterized by vesiculation, neutrophilic infiltration, gelatinous edema, and necrosis. Suppuration is rare in the absence of secondary pyogenic infection. Spread of the bacilli to the regional lymph nodes may be followed by systemic dissemination. Examination of tissues from fatal human cases reveals masses of the bacteria in blood vessels, lymph nodes, and the parenchyma of various organs. There is scanty or no cellular exudation at these foci, but hemorrhage and edema are widespread. So-called "anthrax pneumonia" and "anthrax meningitis" are, in all probability, an expression of this generalized hemorrhage and edema.

The blood of fatally infected experimental animals contains a lethal toxin, which can be neutralized by specific antiserum. This toxin has been isolated in vitro and is important in the pathogenesis of some of the manifestations of the disease.

MANIFESTATIONS The malignant pustule of human anthrax begins usually on an exposed body surface, as a painless, pruritic, erythematous papule which vesiculates and ulcerates to form a black eschar. Tiny satellite vesicles are frequent. The ulcer may be surrounded by extensive edematous swelling, which is nontender, nonpitting, and so characteristic of anthrax that it is a valuable diagnostic sign. After about 5 days the ulcer begins to subside, but edema may persist for many days or weeks. Mild tenderness and enlargement of regional lymph nodes are frequently present. Constitutional symptoms are often absent despite extensive local changes, but there may be mild fever, headache, and malaise. In disseminated anthrax,

high fever, prostration, and a rapidly fatal course are seen. So-called "woolsorter's disease," a highly fatal disseminated infection, is characterized by cyanosis, dyspnea, mediastinitis, and hemoptysis and is probably dependent on the pulmonary route of inoculation. Human infection may occur from ingestion of poorly cooked meat of infected animals. This form of the disease is called *intestinal anthrax*. Clinically, it resembles an acute abdomen; massive diarrhea similar to cholera may be present. The disease is usually eventually fatal.

LABORATORY FINDINGS The fluid from the cutaneous lesion frequently contains many bacilli, demonstrable by Gram's stain and culture. Bacilli may be found on direct examination or culture of the blood of patients with bacteremia. The blood leukocyte count is normal in mild cases, but there is polymorphonuclear leukocytosis in severe disease. Similarly, the erythrocyte sedimentation rate may be increased. Patients with meningeal involvement show bloody spinal fluid, in which the organisms are easily found by direct examination or culture.

DIAGNOSIS An indirect microhemagglutination test (IMH test) has supplanted the agar-gel precipitation (AGPI) test because it is more sensitive and less time consuming. The IMH test has detected antibodies in 93 percent of patients, 98 percent of vaccinees, and none of the controls. It is useful in confirming the diagnosis, which can, of course, also be established by isolation of the organism in culture. A history of occupational exposure and characteristic eschar and edema should suggest the proper diagnosis. Pyogenic infections of the skin are usually painful; the malignant pustule is not. In addition, cutaneous anthrax is rarely purulent. The differential diagnosis of other diseases characterized by local ulceration at the portal of entry is discussed in Chap. 128.

TREATMENT AND PROPHYLAXIS Many antibiotics are effective in the treatment of human anthrax, including penicillin, chloramphenicol, tetracycline, erythromycin, and streptomycin. A dose of 600,000 units penicillin should be given twice daily until the local edema subsides. The eschar goes through its natural evolution in spite of treatment, and lymph node enlargement may persist for several days. *Bacillus anthracis* cannot be recovered from the skin lesion after 24 to 48 h of penicillin therapy, but it may persist for a longer period when chloramphenicol or tetracycline is used.

Infection of personnel in industrial plants where contaminated animal products are handled still occurs. An outbreak of inhalation anthrax with a high mortality rate was reported in a goat hair processing mill in the United States in the late 1950s. Sterilization of all raw wool, mohair, etc., would probably remove the hazard but has had only limited use. A vaccine prepared from the "protective" antigen of *B. anthracis* is available and is effective in reducing the incidence of infection in an exposed population. Spore vaccines of various types are used with good effect in domestic animals in endemic areas but are not suitable for use in human beings.

Transmission of anthrax from one human being to another has never been recognized. The cutaneous disease was fatal in 20 to 30 percent of cases before antimicrobial drugs were available. The mortality rate now is less than 1 percent with proper treatment.

REFERENCES

BRACHMAN PS: Anthrax, in *Tice's Practice of Medicine,* vol 3. Hagerstown, Md, Harper & Row, 1970

BUCHANAN TM et al: Anthrax indirect microagglutination test. J Immunol 107:1631, 1971

CENTER FOR DISEASE CONTROL: Morb Mort Week Rep, February 4, 1977

GOLD H: Anthrax: Report of 117 cases. Arch Intern Med 96:387, 1955

NALIN DR et al: Survival of a patient with intestinal anthrax. Am J Med 62:130, 1977

132

INFECTIONS CAUSED BY *LISTERIA MONOCYTOGENES* AND *ERYSIPELOTHRIX RHUSIOPATHIAE*

PAUL D. HOEPRICH

LISTERIA MONOCYTOGENES INFECTIONS

DEFINITION Listeriosis, a disease caused by *L. monocytogenes*, consists of many clinical syndromes. Perinatal infection, acquired either transplacentally or during parturition, is the most nearly unique form of listeriosis.

ETIOLOGY *Listeria monocytogenes* are gram-positive, non-acid-fast, microaerophilic, motile bacilli that form smooth colonies, but do not produce either capsules or spores. Several serotypes have been defined on the basis of O and H antigens. The epidemiologically essential aid of typing is available from the Center for Disease Control in Atlanta, Georgia. Types 4b, 1b, and 1a account for most of the cases in the United States. Weakly hemolytic gram-positive bacilli are presumed to be listerias if they are motile (when grown at 20 to 25°C), reduce 2,3,5-triphenyltetrazolium chloride, and display characteristic animal pathogenicity. The Anton test is classical: 3 to 5 days after inoculation into the conjunctival sac of a rabbit or a guinea pig, *L. monocytogenes* causes a keratoconjunctivitis. Also, general listeriosis in the rabbit typically provokes a monocytosis, and focal hepatic necrosis is usual in lethal murine listeriosis.

EPIDEMIOLOGY AND PATHOGENESIS Found on every continent save the Antarctic, *L. monocytogenes* may be primarily saprophytic on decaying organic matter in nature. They are distinct from the nonhemolytic, nonpathogenic, nonmonocytogenic, and serologically different bacilli (found mainly in soil, decaying matter, and feces) which have been variously assigned either to the genus *Listeria* or to a new genus *Murrayi*. Although typical *L. monocytogenes* have been isolated from silage, other vegetative sources, and 1 to 5 percent of specimens of human feces, listeriosis is uncommon and occurs sporadically; moreover, listeriosis is actually more common in urban than rural dwellers, occurring most frequently in July and August (Northern Hemisphere). The reservoir from which human beings become infected is frequently occult and the mode of transmission often obscure. Direct transmission from an infected nonhuman animal via contaminated secretions has been documented only rarely. On the other hand, transmission from the infected pregnant female to her offspring is well established as a route of infection.

Transplacental perinatal infection results in disseminated fetal listeriosis. The fetus is usually stillborn or is prematurely ejected, virtually always with lethal listeriosis. Fetal listeriosis acquired during delivery is typically not clinically evident for 1 or 2 weeks postpartum and usually presents as a meningitis.

Listeriosis is preponderantly a disease of persons under 1 month (about 27 percent) and over 40 years (about 56 percent) in age.

Persons in apparent good health may develop listeriosis. However, other diseases, particularly those with diminished cell-mediated immunity (listerias are cytophilic), facilitate the occurrence of listeriosis: for example, neoplasias (especially of the lymphoreticular system) and any conditions requiring treatment with pharmacologic doses of glucosteroids, irradiation, or cytotoxic agents; alcoholism; cardiovascular disease; diabetes mellitus; and tuberculosis.

MANIFESTATIONS *Meningitis* accounts for about three-fourths of the cases verified by culture and is the predominant clinical form of listeriosis in the United States. Clinically, meningitis caused by *L. monocytogenes* cannot be distinguished from meningitis caused by other kinds of bacteria.

Listeriosis of the newborn, the most nearly unique clinical form of listeriosis, ranges from meningitis that is clinically apparent within 1 month postpartum to diffuse disseminated disease in aborted, premature, stillborn infants, and neonates, who die within minutes to days after birth. If clinical disease is delayed to 1 to 4 weeks postpartum, it is generally localized to the central nervous system, as is the rule when children 1 month to 6 years of age are afflicted.

Infants born alive with listeriosis may or may not have fever; yet these babies are critically ill, with cardiorespiratory distress, vomiting, and diarrhea. Dark-red skin papules are frequent, particularly on the lower extremities. Hepatosplenomegaly may be present. This form of listeriosis is also known as septic or miliary granulomatosis, granulomatosis infantiseptica, argentophil-rod infection, or pseudotuberculosis. The findings at postmortem examination are characteristic and mimic those seen in listeriosis of rodents: widely disseminated abscesses varying in size from grossly visible to microscopic, involving, in order of decreasing frequency, liver, spleen, adrenal glands, lungs, pharynx, gastrointestinal tract, central nervous system, and skin. Typically, the lesions are abscesses, but classic granulomas may be seen, depending principally on the duration of infection before death. Microscopic examination of a Gram's stained smear of meconium from the normal newborn infant does not disclose bacteria; fetal listeriosis results in meconium laden with gram-positive bacilli. For this reason, examination of meconium by Gram's stain and by culture should be carried out whenever there is gross soiling of the amniotic liquid with meconium, prematurity, or unexplained fever in the mother before or at the onset of labor. This is particularly important because listeriosis in the pregnant woman may be asymptomatic or may cause a nonspecific illness. Thus, a week to a month prepartum, there may have been malaise, a chill, diarrhea, pain in the back or flanks, and itching. Even when symptomatic, the disease is benign and self-limited in the mother; however, as symptoms subside, a decrease or cessation of fetal movement may be noted. Infection of the fetus may occur as early as the fifth month of gestation. Following delivery of infants with proved fetal listeriosis, cervical cultures are, or soon become, negative for *L. monocytogenes;* subsequent conception, gestation, and delivery of normal offspring are usual.

Oculoglandular listeriosis is the rare human analog of the illness initiated in the rabbit by conjunctival inoculation of *L. monocytogenes*. There is a purulent conjunctivitis, which may lead to corneal ulceration. Regional-node involvement usually limits the spread from the eye. However, listerial meningitis has been reported as a complication of oculoglandular listeriosis.

Other rare syndromes caused by *L. monocytogenes* include general illness with bacteremia and high fever, endocarditis, polyserositis, and cutaneous infection.

LABORATORY FINDINGS Although *L. monocytogenes* bacilli grow well on the usual culture media, etiologic diagnosis by isolation and identification may be hampered by failure of differentiation from *Corynebacterium* spp. *Erysipelothrix rhusiopathiae,* and *Streptococcus* spp. Recognition of listerial colonies in a mixed culture, as may result with vaginal or cervical specimens, is difficult and may be aided by using selective media and/or enrichment procedures.

Serodiagnosis by assay for agglutinins has not been useful because of the common finding of so-called "natural antibodies." Such nonspecific reactions may reflect the known antigenic relationship between *Staphylococcus aureus* and several listerial serotypes. The humoral antibody response to listeriosis in humans is almost exclusively IgM throughout the disease, whereas staphylococci elicit IgG as well as IgM; i.e., treatment of serums with 2-mercaptoethanol may not eliminate nonspecific reactivity.

Monocytosis is not common in human listeriosis. Leukocytosis with neutrophilia, as in any acute bacterial infection, is seen in listerial meningitis, oculoglandular infection, bacteremia, and endocarditis. The cerebrospinal fluid in meningitis is compatible with that in other purulent meningitides.

DIFFERENTIAL DIAGNOSIS Abortion, premature delivery, stillbirth, and neonatal death are more often due to causes other than listeriosis: Rh incompatibility, syphilis, or toxoplasmosis.

In patients with leptomeningitis, conjunctivitis, endocarditis, bacteremia, or polyserositis, reports of isolation of "diphtheroids" or "nonpathogens" must always be challenged. A statement that *L. monocytogenes* has been excluded should be required.

TREATMENT *Listeria monocytogenes* are susceptible to several antimicrobals in vitro, including penicillin G, tetracyclines, and erythromycin. Dosage and duration of therapy should vary according to the kind of listerial infection under treatment.

In fetal listeriosis, therapy must be rapidly effective and should be bactericidal. Penicillin G [100 to 150 mg (160,000 to 240,000 units) per kilogram of body weight per day given intravenously in six equal portions, one every 4 h] along with either gentamicin (4 to 5 mg/kg per day given intravenously in four equal portions, one every 6 h) or erythromycin (25 to 30 mg/kg per day given intravenously in four equal portions, one every 6 h) should be given.

Listerial meningitis will usually respond to treatment with penicillin G in a dose of 150 mg (240,000 units) per kilogram of body weight per day, given intravenously in six equal portions, one every 4 h. Cephalothin is not an acceptable alternative. Erythromycin as the gluceptate or lactobionate can be given in a dose of 60 to 75 mg/kg per day in four equal portions given intravenously, one every 6 h. Tetracycline is effective—15 mg/kg per day in four equal portions given intravenously, one every 6 h. Treatment should be continued in full dosage by intravenous injection for 7 days after defervescence.

Listeriosis in the pregnant female and oculoglandular listeriosis can be treated with a 2-week course of erythromycin (25 to 30 mg/kg per day given as four equal portions, one every 6 h by mouth).

Endocarditis and bacteremia from an unknown site require vigorous therapy: penicillin G 150 mg (240,000 units) per kilogram of body weight per day by continuous intravenous injection. The addition of erythromycin or gentamicin (doses as given for meningitis) should be evaluated by assay of serum bactericidal activity against the patient's isolate.

PROGNOSIS Prompt, vigorous antimicrobial treatment of the acute forms of listeriosis, excepting fetal listeriosis, is usually curative. On the basis of agglutinin titers, specific antibody disappears during the months following cure. However, reinfection has not been reported.

ERYSIPELOTHRIX RHUSIOPATHIAE INFECTIONS

DEFINITION Erysipeloid is the commonest and most nearly unique form of infection in humans caused by *Erysipelothrix rhusiopathiae.* Infective endocarditis and arthritis are rare forms of erysipelothricosis in human beings.

ETIOLOGY As gram-positive, microaerophilic bacilli, *E. rhusiopathiae* may be confused with nontoxinogenic *Corynebacterium* spp. and *Listeria monocytogenes.* However, *E. rhusiopathiae* is nonmotile and fails to grow on media selective for *Corynebacterium* spp. Also, unlike *L. monocytogenes, E. rhusiopathiae* only rarely causes conjunctivitis, following conjunctival inoculation, or monocytosis, after intravenous inoculation, in the rabbit. Because alpha hemolysis is commonly evident after 48 h of incubation of *E. rhusiopathiae,* confusion with streptococci may also occur. Isolates of *E. rhusiopathiae* appear to be serologically homogeneous. Although serodifferentiation from other gram-positive bacilli is possible, few laboratories are capable of definitive serodiagnosis.

EPIDEMIOLOGY AND PATHOGENESIS Primarily a saprophyte, *E. rhusiopathiae* is worldwide in distribution. Human beings are virtually always infected by traumatic dermal inoculation; erysipeloid is the usual result. The disease is almost wholly restricted to persons who in their occupations handle edible or nonedible dead animal products. If the bacilli are not successfully confined to the skin, bacteremia may result and may lead to infective endocarditis; in about half the reported cases, there was no evidence of preexisting valvular heart disease.

The seasonal incidence of erysipeloid parallels that of swine erysipelas, being highest in summer and early fall. Yet persons who tend pigs, even pigs ill with porcine erysipelas, do not commonly develop erysipeloid.

MANIFESTATIONS Erysipeloid begins 2 to 7 days after injury, often after the initial lesion has healed. An itching, burning, painful irritation may precede and always accompanies the appearance of the maculopapular, nonvesiculated, sharply defined, raised, purplish red zone surrounding the site of entry. There is local swelling, and when, as is usual, a finger or the hand is involved, nearby joints may become stiff and painful. Centrifugal spread from the site of inoculation is apparent in a day or so. Movement is slow, 1 to 2 cm per 24 h maximally, and more rapid proximally than distally; involvement of the terminal phalanx of a finger is rare, while spread to other fingers and the hand below the wrist is common. With extension, the original center subsides without desquamation or suppuration. There are usually no systemic signs or symptoms; regional lymphangitis and lymphadenitis are rare. Untreated, the disease heals within 3 weeks in most patients, although relapse has been observed.

The manifestations of erysipelothrical endocarditis may be either acute or chronic, depending on the virulence of the infecting strain and on the state of resistance of the host. Usually, there are no classic erysipeloid skin lesions to suggest the disease at the time that endocarditis is clinically evident. However, a history of recent erysipeloid may be helpful.

Erysipelothrical arthritis is not clinically characteristic but usually can be related to erysipeloid or erysipelothrical bacteremia. Isolation of *E. rhusiopathiae* from synovial fluid has not been reported.

LABORATORY FINDINGS The usual culture media are adequate for the growth of *E. rhusiopathiae*. However, differentiation from diphtheroids, listerias, and streptococci depends primarily on the clinician's alerting the laboratory to the possibility of erysipelothricosis.

In erysipeloid, *E. rhusiopathiae* are best recovered by incubating, in broth containing glucose, a full-thickness biopsy of skin removed from the advancing edge of a lesion. Culture of an aspirate obtained after injection of sterile, bacteriostat-free 0.9% NaCl solution into the periphery of a lesion is less likely to yield *E. rhusiopathiae*.

With endocarditis and arthritis, the findings are in keeping with the respective clinical syndromes and are in no way characteristic for *E. rhusiopathiae*.

DIFFERENTIAL DIAGNOSIS The appearance and location of erysipeloid, its slow and limited spread, the lack of constitutional reaction, the history of occupation and injury, all serve to identify this disease. The afflicted skin in *erysipelas* is very erythematous, and the face and scalp are affected; there are regional lymphangitis and lymphadenitis, leukocytosis, fever, and malaise. Eczematous lesions may itch, but they display vesicles and little abnormal color. The various erythemas have a different location and do not usually itch or burn; they are more apt to be chronic and nonmigratory.

TREATMENT The penicillins, the cephalosporins, erythromycin, clindamycin, the tetracyclines, and chloramphenicol inhibit *E. rhusiopathiae* in vitro at concentrations practical in therapy. Penicillin G is the agent of choice. Erysipeloid is adequately treated by injection of 1.2 million units of benzathine penicillin G. Erythromycin (15 mg/kg per day in four equal portions taken orally for 5 to 7 days) is an alternative. Cure of erysipelothrical endocarditis has been effected by the daily injection of 2 to 20 million units of penicillin per day for 4 to 6 weeks; the dose should be monitored by determination of the bactericidal activity of serum from the patient against his infecting strain. Intractable cardiac failure may oblige surgical excision of an infected valve and insertion of a prosthesis.

PROGNOSIS Penicillin therapy is highly effective in curing erysipelothrical infections. As with infective endocarditis from any cause, the prognosis is primarily a function of the severity of the valvular damage. Of reported cases, approximately half have been fatal; earlier diagnosis, and, perhaps, earlier resort to surgical excision and replacement of infected valves, may improve the outcome.

REFERENCES

Bojsen-Moller J: Human listeriosis. Diagnostic, epidemiological and clinical studies. Acta Pathol Microbiol Scand B 229:13, 1972

Hoeprich PD: Listeriosis, in *Infectious Diseases,* 2d ed, PD Hoeprich (ed). New York, Harper & Row, 1977, chap 48

———: Erysipeloid, in *Infectious Diseases,* 2d ed, PD Hoeprich (ed). New York, Harper & Row, 1977, chap 99

Moore RM, Zehmer RB: Listeriosis in the United States—1971. J Infect Dis 127:610, 1973

Nelson E: Five hundred cases of erysipeloid. Rocky Mt Med J 52:40, 1955

Seeliger HPR: *Listeriosis.* Basel, Karger, 1961

Wiggins GL et al: Antibiotic susceptibility of clinical isolates *Listeria monocytogenes.* Antimicrob Agents Chemother 13:854, 1978

133
DIPHTHERIA

JAMES P. HARNISCH

DEFINITION Diphtheria is an acute infectious disease produced by *Corynebacterium diphtheriae*. It is characterized by a local inflammatory lesion, usually in the upper part of the respiratory tract, and by remote effects resulting from toxin, which affects particularly the heart and peripheral nerves.

ETIOLOGY *Corynebacterium diphtheriae* is a gram-positive, nonsporulating, nonmotile rod. There is a characteristic swelling at one end of the bacillus, which gives it a club shape. A Chinese letter configuration is usually seen in stained smears owing to the alignment of the bacilli at sharp angles with each other. Diphtheria bacilli have been classified into *mitis, gravis*, and *intermedius* groups on the basis of colonial morphology, appearance on tellurite medium, fermentation reactions, and ability to produce hemolysis. European workers have suggested that there is a significant difference in the clinical manifestations and in the severity of disease related to the strain; gravis and intermedius infections are thought to be accompanied by more severe toxic manifestations and a higher death rate. In the United States, the gravis strain is comparatively uncommon, and less significance is attached to the relationship of the type of organism and the clinical form of the disease.

Corynebacterium diphtheriae produces a protein exotoxin which is responsible for many of the clinical manifestations; as little as 0.0001 mg is lethal for guinea pigs. Strains of diphtheria bacilli which elaborate exotoxin are lysogenic. Absence of lysogeny generally is associated with lack of toxin formation and virulence. However, symptomatic diphtheria may also follow invasion by strains of *C. diphtheriae* that cannot be shown to produce toxin.

EPIDEMIOLOGY Diphtheria occurs primarily in the Temperate Zone and is still very common in some parts of the world. Since 1966, there has been an irregular increase in the number of cases of diphtheria in the United States. Two outbreaks in Texas early in this decade accounted for most of the cases. However, since 1973, more than 75 percent of the cases were reported from the Pacific Northwest and the Southwest. The western provinces of Canada experienced a similar increase in diphtheria. Until this geographic trend was recognized, the highest frequency had been in children between 1 and 9 years of age. The attack rate for unimmunized children was 70 times higher than the rate for children who had received primary immunization. In the Pacific Northwest, 77 percent of isolates have been obtained from adults with symptomatic skin lesions. Another striking change has been a decrease in the incidence of laryngeal involvement. In general, diphtheria is acquired by droplet transmission from active cases or carriers, but fomites may play a role in the spread of cutaneous infection. Each diphtheria infection must be classified as either a case or a carrier. A *case* is an individual who is colonized in the respiratory tract with *C. diphtheriae* and is symptomatic. The concomitant presence of other organisms, such as beta-hemolytic streptococci, does not change the definition or prognosis of a diphtheria case. A *carrier* is colonized with *C. diphtheriae* but lacks symptoms. No attempt should be made to classify an instance of cutaneous diphtheria as a case or a carrier.

PATHOGENESIS AND PATHOLOGY The commonest portal of entry for the diphtheria bacillus is the upper respiratory tract. The skin, genitalia, eye, and middle ear may also be sites of invasion. Growth of the organism is superficial in most cases, and there is little tendency to invade the lymphatics or bloodstream except in the terminal stages. The exotoxin elaborated in the local lesion is absorbed and carried by the blood to all parts of the body. The intensity of the toxic effects is greatest when the primary lesion is in the pharynx, less when it is in the larynx, and least when it is on the nasal mucosa or skin. Simultaneous involvement of the pharynx, larynx, trachea, and bronchial tree is associated with most severe intoxication.

The *membrane,* the primary lesion of diphtheria, is thick, leathery, and blue-white and is composed of bacteria, necrotic epithelium, phagocytes, and fibrin. It is surrounded by a narrow zone of inflammation and is firmly adherent to the underlying tissues; bleeding follows its forcible removal. Ulceration is not a regular feature. Regional lymphadenitis is frequent.

The *toxic manifestations* involve primarily the heart, kidneys, and peripheral nerves. The brain is rarely affected. Cardiac enlargement is frequent; this appears to be related to myocarditis rather than hypertrophy. The kidneys may be enlarged and reveal cloudy swelling and interstitial changes. Bronchopneumonia due to *C. diphtheriae* or to secondary invading organisms occurs in some patients, especially those with laryngeal involvement. Membrane is present throughout the bronchial tree when the diphtheria bacillus is responsible for the pulmonary infection. The peripheral nerves may reveal fatty degeneration, disintegration of the medullary sheaths, and involvement of the axis cylinder. Both motor and sensory fibers are affected, but the main impact is on motor innervation. The anterior horn cells and the posterior columns of the spinal cord may be damaged. Other central nervous system involvement includes cerebral hemorrhage, meningitis, and encephalitis. Petechial and purpuric lesions are occasionally present in the kidneys, skin, or adrenals. Endocarditis due to *C. diphtheriae* is rare.

Death results from respiratory obstruction by membrane or edema, or from the effects of toxin on the heart, nervous system, or other organs.

IMMUNITY Susceptibility to the complications of diphtheria is related to the presence or absence of circulating antibody to exotoxin. The Schick test yields a rough estimate of the quantity of antitoxin in the circulation. This test is carried out in the following manner: 0.1 ml purified diphtheria toxin (one-fiftieth the minimum lethal dose) dissolved in buffered human serum albumin is injected intradermally on the volar surface of the forearm; 0.1 ml purified diphtheria toxoid is injected into the other arm as a control. These areas are examined at 24 and 48 h and between the fourth and seventh days and interpreted in the following way:

1 *Positive reaction:* The site of injection of toxin begins to redden in 24 h; the reddening increases and reaches a maximum in about a week, at which time the lesion may be as large as 3 cm in diameter and moderately swollen and tender. There is usually a small (1 to 1.5 cm) dark red central zone which gradually turns brown, desquamates, and leaves a pigmented area. The area of toxoid injection shows no reaction. A positive test indicates little or no circulating antitoxin and no immunity.
2 *Negative reaction:* There is no reaction at the site of injection of either toxoid or toxin. This is consistent with a blood antitoxin level of 1/30 to 1/100 unit and immunity to ordinary exposure.
3 *Pseudoreaction:* Inflammation at both sites of injection within 12 to 14 h, which reaches a maximum in 48 to 72 h and then fades. This usually indicates immunity plus hypersensitivity to the toxin or other materials in the solution.

4 *Combined reaction:* This begins like the pseudoreaction, but the inflammatory response at the toxin site persists after that in the area of toxoid injection has faded. It indicates delayed sensitivity to toxin or other proteins and either low levels or no antitoxin. The incidence of combined reactions increases with age and is highest in unimmunized groups living in areas where diphtheria is prevalent.

Individuals with negative Schick tests occasionally contract diphtheria, and some persons with positive Schick reactions do not develop the disease after exposure. In some parts of the United States fewer than 50 percent of adults have "protective" levels of circulating antitoxin. The Schick test is not used routinely in the United States, and the lack of ability to perform it should not delay the treatment of asymptomatic contacts of diphtheria.

Second attacks of respiratory diphtheria are rare despite the fact that about 10 percent of patients who have had the disease remain Schick-positive. This suggests that factors other than antitoxin may play a role in protection against infection. In general, immunized patients have a milder illness than unimmunized ones when the initial clinical picture and level of circulating antitoxin are the same. Early therapy of diphtheria with antibiotics may lead to recurrence of the disease if exposure to fresh infections occurs shortly after discontinuation of treatment, suggesting that the development of antitoxic immunity is suppressed in these cases. Full immunization with diphtheria toxoid does not prevent nasopharyngeal carriage of the organism but significantly reduces the case fatality ratio. It also ameliorates the symptoms of active disease.

CLINICAL MANIFESTATIONS The incubation period of diphtheria is 1 to 7 days. The local symptoms vary with the site of the primary lesion. A membrane is not always present. The constitutional reaction usually is of only minor to moderate severity in uncomplicated disease. Fever is usually low [37.8 to 38.3°C (100 to 101°F)], unless infection with another organism (often group A *Streptococcus pyogenes*) supervenes. When toxic manifestations are absent, patients feel well except for a varying degree of discomfort at the site of the local lesion. Pallor, listlessness, tachycardia, and weakness are common in more severe cases. Nausea or vomiting is more frequent in young children. Peripheral vascular collapse often develops in the terminal stages of the disease.

Nasal diphtheria Diphtheria is occasionally restricted to the nasal mucosa. It is usually localized to the septum or turbinates in the anterior portion of one side of the nose, does not extend, and may persist for a long time. A foreign body is frequently present. A unilateral serosanguineous discharge is characteristic. When the disease is located in the posterior nasal areas, it commonly extends to the pharynx, from which toxin is absorbed.

Pharyngeal diphtheria The early diphtheritic membrane in the pharynx consists of small areas of soft exudate which wipe off easily and leave no bleeding points. As the disease progresses, the discrete exudate coalesces to form an easily removable thin sheet which spreads to cover tonsils or pharynx, or both. Later, it becomes thicker, bluish white, gray, or black, depending on the degree of hemorrhage, and is so firmly attached to the underlying tissues that attempts to remove it result in bleeding. If infection with group A *Streptococcus pyogenes* is superimposed, the pharynx is diffusely red and edematous. Sore throat is the most common complaint. Pain on swallowing may occur in over 25 percent of the cases and in some patients may be severe. There is a moderate leukocytosis with 15,000 or fewer white blood cells per cubic millimeter.

Local spread of the pharyngeal membrane may occur, and the throat, tonsils, and soft and hard palates become completely covered. Patients with severe disease may develop so-called "malignant" diphtheria, characterized by marked edema of the submandibular areas and the anterior neck, giving the characteristic "bullneck" appearance. Respiration is noisy, the tongue protrudes, the breath is foul, and the speech thick. The pharyngeal tissues are red and edematous, and the cervical lymph nodes are enlarged. The skin is pale and cool. The patient complains of overwhelming weakness. Purpuric eruptions of the skin, particularly on the neck and anterior chest wall, may appear occasionally. Drowsiness and delirium are common.

Laryngeal diphtheria Involvement of the larynx is usually the result of extension of the diphtheritic membrane from the pharynx. The infection may rarely be limited to the larynx or trachea. This possibility must be considered in the differential diagnosis of all cases of "croup"; it can be ruled out only by direct examination of the airway. The clinical features of this type of disease are described below.

Cutaneous diphtheria Until recently, diphtheria of the skin was a problem primarily in tropical areas where it is responsible for some cases of "jungle sore." However, since 1972, there has been a significant increase in skin diphtheria in the Pacific Northwest and the Southwest. A high attack rate has occurred in native Americans and in indigent males living in "skid row" areas where crowding and poor personal and community hygiene abound. *Corynebacterium diphtheriae,* being unable to penetrate unbroken skin, invades wounds, burns, or abrasions. Any break in the skin may be colonized with *C. diphtheriae.* Coagulase-positive *Staphylococcus aureus* and/or beta-hemolytic streptococci frequently are recovered concomitantly. Although the lesions develop most often on the extremities, they may appear at any site including the perianal area. In tropical zones, the typical lesion appears as a round, deep "punched-out" ulcer, 0.5 cm to several centimeters in diameter. In the early stages, it is covered by a gray-yellow or gray-brown membrane which strips off easily to reveal a clean hemorrhagic base that dries quickly and becomes covered by a thin, leathery, dark-brown or black, adherent membrane. In the untreated case, this separates spontaneously 1 to 3 weeks after infection. The margin of the fully developed ulcer is usually slightly undermined, purple, rolled, and sharply defined. When lesions are infected with a toxigenic strain, anesthesia over the lesion develops within a few weeks. In temperate climates, the lesions are not sufficiently specific to permit visual diagnosis. Cutaneous diphtheria should be suspected in any adult with skin lesions, particularly in the proper epidemiologic setting. Antibiotic therapy will change the character of the skin lesions. Twenty percent of patients with cutaneous diphtheria also have infections in the nasopharynx with the same biotype. Myocarditis or neuropathy occurs in about 3 to 5 percent of patients with cutaneous diphtheria. The Landry-Guillain-Barré syndrome develops occasionally.

Diphtheritic lesions in other areas Diphtheria may involve the uterine cervix, vagina, vulva, bladder, urethra, or penis (after circumcision). Toxic manifestations are common. The tongue, buccal mucous membrane, gums, and esophagus may also be affected. Infection of the conjunctiva occurs rarely. Otitis media may occur as an isolated syndrome or secondary to diphtheria in the upper part of the respiratory tract; the aural infection may become chronic; virulent organisms may be isolated from the discharge for many months.

COMPLICATIONS OF DIPHTHERIA The complications of diphtheria are of two types: (1) those that result from spread of the membrane in the respiratory tract, and (2) those due to the effects of the toxin.

Extension and spread of membrane The membrane of diphtheria may spread from the fauces over the posterior pharyngeal wall into the larynx, trachea, and, uncommonly, the bronchial tree, leading to severe illness and a high incidence of toxic manifestations. Occlusion of the airway is manifested by tachypnea and, as obstruction increases, restlessness, use of accessory muscles of respiration, cyanosis, and finally death. In some cases, the membrane extends diffusely into the bronchial tree and produces clinical manifestations of pneumonia. Hoarseness and a croup-like cough are seen with laryngeal involvement. Bronchopulmonary diphtheria is very serious, not only because of obstruction but also because of the large surface from which toxin can be absorbed; the death rate is very high. When the pulmonary lesion regresses, pieces of membrane may break off and produce sudden occlusion of the airway; a cast of the bronchial tree may be coughed up. Occasionally, pharyngeal membrane has extended into the esophagus and cardia of the stomach.

Toxic complications of diphtheria Diphtheria toxin is produced only by isolates of *C. diphtheriae* lysogenic for corynephages that carry the tox structural gene. Nontoxigenic strains can be converted to toxin-producing organisms through transference of this phage. The bacterial host regulates expression of the tox structural gene. The toxin is a single polypeptide chain composed of two fragments. Fragment B recognizes specific surface receptors on sensitive cell membranes, and fragment A crosses the plasma membrane. In the cytoplasm, protein synthesis is inhibited by fragment A through the inactivation of the eukaryotic translocating enzyme, elongation factor 2. A cofactor, nicotinamideadenine dinucleotide, is required for activity of the toxin. The effects of the toxin on the myocardium are thought to result from its ability to decrease the rate of oxidation of long-chain fatty acids by interfering with the metabolism of carnitine. Because of this action, triglycerides accumulate in the myocardium and cause fatty degeneration of muscle.

Myocarditis develops in about two-thirds of patients with diphtheria. However, it is clinically evident in only about 10 percent of cases; alterations in the intensity of the heart sounds, systolic murmurs, bundle branch block, incomplete or complete heart block, atrial fibrillation, and ventricular premature beats or tachycardia, or both, are common. Ventricular fibrillation is a constant threat and is frequently responsible for sudden death. Ninety percent of patients with atrial fibrillation, ventricular tachycardia, or complete heart block die. Overt congestive cardiac failure is uncommon. Evidence of decompensation of the right side of the heart usually develops first; the most common symptom is pain in the right upper quadrant of the abdomen due to rapid engorgement of the liver. Failure of the left side of the heart may appear later. Diphtheritic heart disease is not necessarily "benign" in survivors of the disease; permanent cardiac damage may occur. Fibrosis of the myocardium has been observed in patients who have expired several weeks after "mild" myocarditis was detected electrocardiographically. The degree and extent of fibrotic change have often been greater than could have been predicted on the basis of the type of abnormality present in the ECG.

Peripheral neuritis may occur in the course of diphtheria. Paralysis of the soft palate and posterior pharyngeal wall occasionally appears very early in the disease (2 to 3 days). A more common neuritis (10 percent of cases) usually develops 2 to 6 weeks after onset of the disease. It is characterized by cranial nerve dysfunction; the third, sixth, seventh, ninth, and tenth nerves are most commonly involved. Loss of accommodation, nasal voice, and difficulty in swallowing are the most frequent manifestations. However, any of the peripheral nerves may be affected, with resulting paralysis of the extremities, diaphragm, or intercostal muscles; death may occur from failure of respiration. The peripheral neuritides which appear in the second to the sixth week of the disease are characterized primarily by motor loss; sensory changes are uncommon and, when present, are minor. Peripheral neuritis may not appear until 2 to 3 months after the onset of diphtheria. In these cases, the clinical picture and course resemble infectious polyneuritis. The outstanding findings are loss of sensation in the "glove-and-stocking" distribution and albuminocytological dissociation in the cerebrospinal fluid identical with that observed in the Landry-Guillain-Barré syndrome. Motor weakness and areflexia may develop with progression of involvement. Facial diplegia may accompany the other neurological manifestations. A fatal, rapidly ascending paralysis of the Landry type may develop rarely. Complete recovery is the rule in this late peripheral neuritis, although it may require as long as a year. Encephalitis is a rare toxic complication of diphtheria.

Shock, which develops suddenly and without warning, is an occasional cause of sudden death in this disease. In some instances, this may be a consequence of myocarditis; in others, no cause can be discovered.

Other complications Cerebral infarction with hemiplegia occurs rarely; it is probably due to embolization from atrial thrombi in patients with myocarditis and cardiac dilatation. Superinfection of the lungs is a risk in all patients with diphtheria who are given antimicrobial agents. Purpuric skin eruptions may be seen in severe, malignant cases; thrombocytopenia occurs rarely. A mild morbilliform rash may be present during the early stage of diphtheria. Secondary invasion of the pharynx by group A *S. pyogenes* may take place in patients who have not received an antibiotic. Serum sickness occasionally follows the use of antitoxin. Relapses of diphtheria may occur when patients given antimicrobial agents are exposed to fresh cases soon after therapy has been discontinued. Bacteremia, endocarditis, and meningitis are rare complications.

COURSE AND PROGNOSIS The diphtheritic membrane may be present for only 3 to 4 days in mild cases, even when no antitoxin is given; it usually lasts for about a week in cases of moderate severity. Commonly, the pharyngeal lesion increases in extent and thickness during the first 24 h after the administration of antitoxin. As the disease begins to recede, the exudate softens, wipes off easily, leaving no bleeding areas, becomes patchy so that it resembles the picture of "follicular" tonsillitis, and finally disappears, leaving normal underlying mucous membrane.

The fatality rate of diphtheria prior to the use of specific antitoxin was about 35 percent in average cases and 90 percent in those with laryngeal involvement. Since specific serotherapy has been employed, this rate has been reduced to a range of 3.5 to 22 percent, but it is still highest when the larynx is affected. The overall death rate in the United States is about 10 percent. Death is most frequent in the very young and the old. Immunization is a factor of great importance in prognosis. The fatality rate in immunized individuals is one-tenth that in the unimmunized population. Paralysis is five times and "malignant" disease 15 times less common in immune than in nonimmune

individuals. As a rule, the longer the delay in the administration of antitoxin, the greater the incidence of complications and death. However, antitoxin is ineffective in reducing risks of complications and death if it is given much later than 48 h after diphtheria begins.

A white blood cell count higher than 25,000 per cubic millimeter is associated with a higher risk of complications and death.

DIAGNOSIS The clinical features of the fully developed diphtheritic membrane, especially in the pharynx, are sufficiently characteristic to suggest the possibility of the disease in most instances. However, the appearance of the pharyngeal exudate alone does not clinch the diagnosis. There are a number of other infections in which pseudomembranes resembling those of diphtheria are present; among those are infectious mononucleosis, streptococcal pharyngitis, viral exudative pharyngitis, fusospirochetal infection, and acute pharyngeal candidiasis.

The specific diagnosis of diphtheria depends completely on demonstration of the organism in stained smears and their recovery by culture. Methylene blue–stained preparations are positive, in experienced hands, in 75 to 85 percent of cases. Diphtheria bacilli can be recovered by culture on Loeffler's medium in 8 to 12 h if patients have not been receiving antimicrobial agents. *Corynebacterium diphtheriae* also multiplies, but more slowly, on ordinary blood agar. If an antibiotic, especially penicillin or erythromycin, has been administered prior to obtaining cultures, the organisms may not grow for as long as 5 days or may fail to grow at all.

Staining of suspected material with fluorescein-labeled diphtheria antitoxin may allow rapid diagnosis. Toxigenicity of *C. diphtheriae* isolates should be determined by passive agar diffusion (Elek plate method), guinea pig inoculation, or counterimmunoelectrophoresis.

TREATMENT Patients with diphtheria should be isolated and kept at strict bed rest; physical effort should be reduced during the early convalescent stages. Local therapy of the diphtheritic pharyngeal lesion is useless. The only specific treatment for diphtheria is antitoxin. Antiserum must never be given until the patient's sensitivity to horse serum, using the eye and skin tests, has been determined. There are several regimens for the administration of antitoxin, and the amount given is often based on an empiric decision. In general, the more severe the disease or the more extensive the membrane formation, the greater is the amount of antitoxin required. Mildly symptomatic cases may be treated with 10,000 to 20,000 units. Moderately severe cases, such as those with a pharyngeal membrane, should be given 20,000 to 40,000 units. Severe diphtheria, as with laryngeal involvement, requires 50,000 to 100,000 units. The total dose should be given at one time rather than in split doses over a long period. For doses less than 20,000 units, the intramuscular route is convenient. When this method is used, only one-half the dose should be given intramuscularly and the remainder intravenously in order to expedite delivery of the antitoxin. Alternatively, after appropriate testing for sensitivity, the entire amount of antitoxin may be given intravenously in 100 to 200 ml isotonic saline over a 30-min period. Desensitization should be attempted if the initial skin or eye test is positive. A rare patient may be sensitive to such a high degree that the antiserum cannot be administered without the risk of death.

Antitoxin should be given as early in the course of diphtheria as possible. It is capable of binding or inactivating only the toxin present in blood or extracellular fluid. Once the toxin has entered the cell, the effect cannot be reversed or prevented. Antitoxin must be given when diphtheria is suspected clinically; laboratory confirmation prior to administration of the antitoxin is not necessary. Since mortality increases directly with delay in use of antitoxin, it is better to treat clinically suspect but culture-negative cases than to withhold specific therapy.

The history of military service is not reliable proof of adequate immunization. From World War II until 1956, immunization for diphtheria in the United States military was inconsistent. Since 1957, all branches of the Armed Forces have routinely immunized their personnel. When the immunization history is not clear, it is best to provide antitoxin promptly. Antimicrobial agents do not alter the course, incidence of complications, or outcome of diphtheria.

Patients with laryngeal obstruction should be watched very carefully. In mild cases, inhalation of warm or cool steam may be beneficial. If advancing signs of airway obstruction develop, intubation or tracheostomy is indicated. These procedures must never be delayed until cyanosis appears, because, at this point, stimulation of the pharynx or trachea may produce cardiac standstill and death. Sedative or hypnotic agents should never be given because they may obscure increasing respiratory difficulty.

The pulse and blood pressure should be measured frequently. Little can be done to alter the course of the myocarditis. Quinidine has been tried to prevent and treat arrhythmias but appears to be of no value; there is some suspicion that it may produce deleterious effects. The use of procainamide when ventricular premature beats or tachycardia supervene has been suggested, but no documented observations of its effect have been recorded. The administration of digitalis for cardiac failure in diphtheria is controversial. Some consider this drug to be completely contraindicated; others feel, however, that, used carefully, digitalis may be given safely and with beneficial effects. Shock should be treated according to its etiology (Chaps. 30 and 109). There is no evidence that corticosteroids or corticotropin are of any value in the treatment of diphtheria or any of its complications. Antibiotics should be used to treat symptomatic cases only after antitoxin is administered. Circulating exotoxin is not affected by antibiotics, and their prompt use may give false assurance to the clinician. Patients with diphtheria should be quarantined until two successive cultures of the nose, throat, or other infected areas, taken at 24-h intervals, are negative. If antibiotics have been given, cultural studies should not be initiated until at least 24 h after cessation of therapy.

Treatment of carriers *Corynebacterium diphtheriae* usually disappears from the upper part of the respiratory tract after 2 to 4 weeks in patients who do not receive antimicrobial drugs; in a small number of individuals the organism may persist for a long time or be present permanently. The most effective treatment of the acute and chronic carrier state is erythromycin. A dose of 2 g per day orally in divided doses for 7 days appears to be adequate. Alternative antimicrobials include procaine penicillin G, 600,000 units intramuscularly every 12 h for 10 days; clindamycin, 150 mg four times a day orally for 7 days; and rifampin, 600 mg as a single oral dose for 7 days. Tetracyclines, semisynthetic penicillins, aminoglycosides, and oral cephalosporins are inadequate for the eradication of *C. diphtheriae*. Parenteral cephalosporins such as cephalothin or cephamandole are effective. In some areas of the United States endemic for cutaneous diphtheria, resistance of *C. diphtheriae* to erythromycin has been recognized. Retreatment is indicated for carriers whose organisms do not disappear on the first trial. This is preferable to tonsillectomy, which may be considered as a last resort should the carrier state persist despite repeated courses of antibiotic. Persistence of the organism after appropriate antimicrobial therapy may represent a lack of compliance rather than drug resistance.

PREVENTION Diphtheria is, for the most part, a preventable disease. Immunization at the age of 3 months should be routine. Diphtheria toxoid is best given together with tetanus toxoid and pertussis vaccine (DPT), because antibody titers are higher with combined immunization than with either agent alone. Booster doses should be administered at the age of 1 year and again just before a child goes to school. Although it has been suggested that Schick testing is not necessary in those who have been immunized, many physicians still carry this out to determine the status of antitoxic immunity. A Schick test acts as a booster. A negative reaction does not indicate absolute protection. The development of highly purified toxoid has made it possible to protect adults with little or no risk of untoward sequelae. In this situation, a combination of adult tetanus-diphtheria (Td) toxoid containing 1 to 2 flocculation (Lf) units per milliliter should be used. With this preparation, severe reactions can be avoided. The Moloney test need not be carried out. Adults should receive booster doses at least every 10 years.

Treatment of unimmunized persons exposed to an active case of diphtheria remains controversial. One approach has been to administer 3000 units of antitoxin intramuscularly, after appropriate skin and eye tests. Alternatively, cultures for *C. diphtheriae* can be taken, and a primary series of immunizations initiated. The exposed individual then can be observed closely for signs of active disease. If symptoms occur, antitoxin can be given immediately. In those who have been previously immunized, a booster dose of toxoid is usually sufficient. Cultures from the nasopharynx or open wounds should be obtained from close contacts or family members of a diphtheria case or carrier.

REFERENCES

BELSEY MA, LeBLANC DR: Skin infections and the epidemiology of diphtheria: Acquisition and persistence of *C. diphtheriae* infections. Am J Epidemiol 102:179, 1975

BROOKS GR et al: Diphtheria in the United States 1959–1970. J Infect Dis 129:172, 1974

GOOD I: Myocardial changes in fatal diphtheria: A summary of observations in 221 cases. Am J Med Sci 219:257, 1948

GOOR RS, PAPPENHEIMER AM JR: Studies on the mode of action of diphtheria toxin. J Exp Med 126:899, 913, 923, 1967

IPSEN J: Circulating antitoxin at the onset of diphtheria in 425 patients. J Immunol 54:325, 1946

———: Immunization of adults against diphtheria and tetanus. N Engl J Med 251:459, 1954

LIVINGOOD CS et al: Cutaneous diphtheria: A report of 140 cases. J Invest Dermatol 7:341, 1946

McCLOSKEY RV et al: The 1970 epidemic of diphtheria in San Antonio. Ann Intern Med 75:495, 1971

NAIDITCH MJ, BOWER AG: Diphtheria: A study of 1,433 cases observed during a ten-year period at the Los Angeles County Hospital. Am J Med 17:229, 1954

PAPPENHEIMER AM JR: Diphtheria toxin. Annu Rev Biochem 46:69, 1977

SCHEID W: Diphtherial paralysis: An analysis of 2,292 cases of diphtheria in adults which include 174 cases of polyneuritis. J Nerv Ment Dis 116:1095, 1952

THOMPSON NL, ELLNER PD: Rapid determination of *Corynebacterium diphtheriae* toxigenicity by counterimmunoelectrophoresis. J Clin Microbiol 7:493, 1978

WITTELS B, BRESSLER R: Biochemical lesion of diphtheria toxin on the heart. J Clin Invest 43:630, 1964

134

CHOLERA AND *VIBRIO PARAHEMOLYTICUS* INFECTIONS

CHARLES C. J. CARPENTER

CHOLERA

DEFINITION Cholera is an acute illness which results from colonization of the small intestine by *Vibrio cholerae.* The disease is characterized by its epidemic occurrence and the production in the more severe cases of massive diarrhea with rapid depletion of extracellular fluid and electrolytes.

ETIOLOGY AND EPIDEMIOLOGY *Vibrio cholerae* is a curved, aerobic, gram-negative bacillus with a single polar flagellum. It is rapidly motile and possesses both O and H antigens. Serologic identification is based on differences in the polysaccharide O antigens.

Cholera has been endemic for a century and a half in the Gangetic Delta of West Bengal and Bangladesh and is often epidemic throughout South and Southeast Asia. The seventh and most recent pandemic spread of this disease, from 1961 to 1975, extended from the Celebes northward to Korea and westward to the whole of Africa and Southern Europe. The last major epidemic of cholera in the Western Hemisphere occurred during 1866 to 1867. However, in August and September 1978, at least 11 persons developed cholera, serotype Inaba, after ingestion of inadequately cooked crabs caught in lakes or coastal waters of Louisiana.

The majority of major epidemics have clearly been waterborne, but direct contamination of food by infected feces probably contributes to spread during major outbreaks. Poor sanitation appears to be primarily responsible for the continuing presence of cholera, but host factors, such as relative or absolute achlorhydria, also play an important role in the susceptibility of the individual to infection. In endemic areas, cholera is predominantly a disease of children; in rural Bangladesh attack rates are 10 times greater in the 1- to 5-year-old age group than in those above 14 years of age. However, when the disease spreads to previously uninvolved areas, the attack rates are initially at least as high in adults as in children.

A chronic gallbladder carrier state has been observed in a small percentage of elderly convalescent cholera patients. These chronic *V. cholerae* carriers may provide a vehicle for spread outside of endemic areas. The basis for the annual cholera epidemics throughout the Gangetic Delta, for the periodic outbreaks throughout the remainder of South and Southeast Asia, and for the occasional global pandemics has, however, not been clearly delineated.

PATHOGENESIS *Vibrio cholerae* produces a protein enterotoxin which appears to be responsible for all known pathophysiologic aberrations in cholera. This enterotoxin, which has a molecular weight of 84,000, stimulates adenyl cyclase in the intestine epithelial cells, and the resultant increase in intracellular cyclic adenosine $3',5'$-monophosphate leads to secretion of isotonic fluid by all segments of the small intestine. The enterotoxin-induced electrolyte secretion occurs in the absence of any demonstrable histologic damage to intestine epithelial cells or to the capillary endothelial cells of the lamina propria. Precise studies have demonstrated that the stool of the adult cholera patient is nearly isotonic, with sodium and chloride concentrations slightly less than those of plasma, a bicarbonate concentration approximately twice that of plasma, and a potassium concentration three to five times that of plasma. Disease caused by all known strains of *V. cholerae* results in the same stool electrolyte pattern. The pathophysiologic defect in cholera is extracellular fluid depletion with resultant hypovolemic shock, base-deficit acidosis, and progressive potassium depletion. There is no evidence that the cholera *Vibrio* invades any tissue, nor has the enterotoxin been shown, in human disease, to have any direct effect on any organ other than the small intestine.

MANIFESTATIONS The incubation period is generally from 6 to 48 h. This is followed by the abrupt onset of watery, generally painless diarrhea. In the more severe cases, the initial diarrheal stool may be in excess of 1000 ml, and several liters of isotonic fluid may be lost within hours, leading rapidly to profound shock. Vomiting generally follows, but occasionally precedes, the onset of diarrhea; the vomiting is characteristically effortless and not preceded by nausea. As saline depletion progresses, severe muscle cramps, commonly involving the calves, occur.

When first seen, the typical severely ill cholera patient is cyanotic, with pinched facies, scaphoid abdomen, poor skin turgor, and thready or absent peripheral pulses. The voice is faint, high-pitched, and often inaudible, and there are tachycardia, hypotension, and varying degrees of tachypnea. In all epidemics there are many subclinical or mild cases in which gastrointestinal fluid loss is not severe enough to require hospitalization. With the *el tor* strain of *V. cholerae,* which has been responsible for the most recent pandemic, the ratio of subclinical infections to clinical cholera cases is greater than 10:1.

The disease runs its course in 2 to 7 days, and subsequent manifestations depend on the adequacy of electrolyte repletion therapy. With prompt fluid and electrolyte repletion, physiologic recovery is remarkably rapid, and mortality exceptionally rare. The important causes of death, in inadequately treated patients, are hypovolemic shock, metabolic acidosis, and uremia resulting from acute tubular necrosis.

LABORATORY FINDINGS In epidemics or in endemic areas, the clinical picture should arouse strong suspicion immediately. The most reliable technique for identification of *V. cholerae* consists of direct plating of a sample of cholera stool on bile salt, gelatin-tellurite-taurocholate (GTT), or thiosulfate-citrate-bile salt-sucrose (TCBS) agar. On bile salt or GTT agar the organisms appear as typical translucent colonies within 24 h. On TCBS agar, *V. cholerae* appear at 24 h as distinct, large, yellow colonies. Further classification requires agglutination with type-specific antiserums. In mild or convalescent cases, recovery of vibrios may be enhanced by initial enrichment for 6 h in alkaline peptone water followed by subculture on bile salt, GTT, or TCBS agar. Rapid diagnosis is possible either by directly observing immobilization of vibrios by type-specific antiserums, using dark-field or phase microscopy, or identifying the organisms by immunofluorescent methods.

TREATMENT Successful therapy requires only prompt and adequate replacement of gastrointestinal losses of saline and alkali. A uniformly satisfactory solution for intravenous fluid therapy can be simply prepared by the addition of 5 g sodium chloride, 4 g sodium bicarbonate, and 1 g potassium chloride to 1 liter of pyrogen-free distilled water. If commercially prepared fluids are available, a combination of isotonic sodium bicarbonate (or acetate or lactate) and isotonic sodium chloride, infused in a 2:1 ratio, may be employed. The intravenous fluids are initially infused at 50 to 100 ml/min, until a strong pulse has been restored. The same fluids should subsequently be infused in quantities equal to the gastrointestinal losses. If losses cannot be measured accurately, intravenous fluids should be given at a rate sufficient to maintain a normal radial pulse and normal skin turgor. Overhydration can be avoided by careful observation of neck venous filling and auscultation of the lungs. Close observation is mandatory during the acute phase of the illness, because the cholera patient can lose as much as 1 liter of isotonic fluid per hour during the first 24 h of the disease. Inadequate or delayed restoration of fecal fluid losses may result in a high incidence of acute renal failure. Serious hypokalemic symptoms are rare in adults, and potassium repletion can be carried out orally if potassium-containing intravenous fluids are not available. Hypokalemia contributes significantly, however, to the morbidity in inadequately treated pediatric cholera, and potassium, 10 to 13 meq per liter, should be included in the intravenous fluids administered to pediatric patients.

Although adequate intravenous saline and alkali repletion alone results in rapid recovery of virtually all cholera patients, a dramatic reduction in the duration and volume of the diarrhea and early eradication of vibrios from the stool may be effected by antibiotic therapy. Oral tetracycline, 500 mg every 6 h for the first 48 h of treatment, has been most successful. Other antibiotics, including chloramphenicol and furazolidone, are also of value, but both appear to be slightly less effective than tetracycline.

Oral therapy   Since the cholera enterotoxin does not alter glucose-facilitated sodium absorption, fluid repletion can be effected by the oral administration of glucose-containing electrolyte solutions. Since the limiting factor in treatment of cholera in both epidemic and endemic situations is often the lack of adequate quantities of intravenous fluids, the availability of an oral treatment regimen has greatly reduced the mortality from cholera outbreaks during the most recent pandemic spread of this disease. A solution containing glucose 20 g per liter (or sucrose 40 g per liter), sodium bicarbonate 2.5 g per liter, sodium chloride 3.5 g per liter, and potassium chloride 15 g per liter can be readily prepared and should be satisfactory for treatment of all age groups. This solution, administered orally at a rate equal to the stool losses, can be given to patients with milder cholera throughout the course of illness and is satisfactory in the more severe cases, once the hypovolemic shock has been corrected by intravenous fluid therapy. Oral therapy does not decrease the rate of intestinal fluid loss but provides an electrolyte solution which can be absorbed at a rate sufficient, in most cases, to counterbalance the continuing fluid losses. Therefore, successful management of the cholera patient with oral therapy requires just as close supervision, with careful monitoring of pulse volume, skin turgor, and neck veins, as does management with intravenous solutions. Supplemental intravenous fluids must be administered whenever clinical signs of saline depletion recur.

PROGNOSIS   Under ideal conditions and with prompt and adequate fluid replacement, mortality approaches zero, and significant sequelae are rare. Unfortunately, death rates as high as 60 percent still occur, especially during the initial phases of certain outbreaks. This high mortality reflects lack of pyrogen-free intravenous fluids in remote areas, the difficulties of initiating treatment promptly when large numbers of cases are occurring in poverty-stricken populations, and the compromises which may have to be made under emergency conditions.

PREVENTION   Immunization by standard commercial vaccine, containing 10 billion killed organisms per milliliter, provides only limited (40 to 60 percent) protection for a relatively short (4- to 6-month) period. Vaccination, therefore, is not recommended for Americans who are traveling abroad. Careful hygiene provides the only sure protection against cholera.

VIBRIO PARAHEMOLYTICUS INFECTION

ETIOLOGY AND EPIDEMIOLOGY   *Vibrio parahemolyticus* is a curved, aerobic, nonmotile, gram-negative bacillus. Although present in coastal waters throughout the temperate zone, it has most commonly been associated with acute diarrheal illness in Japan, presumably because of the frequency of ingestion of raw seafood. It has been implicated in several outbreaks of acute diarrheal disease in the coastal United States, always as a common-source outbreak related to ingestion of inadequately cooked seafood, usually shrimp. Secondary cases caused by person-to-person transmission occur rarely, if at all. Several epidemics of *V. parahemolyticus* infections on cruise ships have been reported.

PATHOGENESIS   Although *V. parahemolyticus* produces a toxin capable of causing intestinal fluid accumulation in the experimental animal, the role of this toxin in human disease is less clear-cut than is that of the cholera enterotoxin. The volume of fluid lost with *V. parahemolyticus* infection is relatively small, and intravenous fluids are seldom required. Unlike *V. cholerae, V. parahemolyticus* causes an inflammatory response in the intestinal mucosa: stools usually contain numerous polymorphonuclear leukocytes and are occasionally grossly bloody. The illness is almost always self-limited, with a median duration of just under 24 h.

MANIFESTATIONS   Within 6 to 48 h after ingestion of raw or inadequately cooked seafood, the patient develops an acute diarrheal illness. The volume of fluid lost is generally not great, moderately severe abdominal cramps may be a prominent feature, and chills and fever are observed in roughly half the cases. Vomiting is generally not a prominent feature and occurs in no more than one-third of patients. The illness is almost invariably self-limited, and no deaths have been reported in outbreaks involving over a thousand patients in the United States.

LABORATORY FINDINGS   When a common-source outbreak of acute diarrheal disease occurs in a group exposed to fresh or frozen seafood, the index of suspicion should be high and the diagnosis should be confirmed by plating a rectal swab on thiosulfate–citrate–bile salt–sucrose (TCBS) agar, on which typical colonies of *V. parahemolyticus* appear at 24 h. (This organism grows poorly and is therefore easily overlooked on deoxycholate culture plates). The stool generally has numerous polymorphonuclear leukocytes and smaller numbers of erythrocytes, but these findings are generally less prominent than in shigellosis.

TREATMENT   No therapy is required by the large majority of patients. The disease is self-limited, and antimicrobial therapy shortens neither the course nor the duration of pathogen excretion. Antiperistaltic agents are not of clear-cut benefit. An occasional patient may lose sufficient quantities of intestinal fluid to require oral or intravenous therapy, guided by the same principles employed in the treatment of cholera.

PROGNOSIS   The outcome is almost always good. Fatal cases, occasionally reported from Japan, appear to have occurred in rare instances in patients with serious underlying disease.

PREVENTION Since *V. parahemolyticus* is widely distributed in coastal waters, the only effective preventive measure is avoidance of ingestion of inadequately cooked shellfish.

REFERENCES

Cholera

CARPENTER CCJ et al: Clinical studies in Asiatic cholera, I-VI. Bull Johns Hopkins Hosp 118:165, 1966

GANGAROSA EF et al: The nature of the gastrointestinal lesion in Asiatic cholera and its relation to pathogenesis: A biopsy study. Am J Trop Med Hyg 9:125, 1960

HIRSCHHORN N et al: The treatment of cholera, in *Cholera*, D Barua, W Burrows (eds). Philadelphia, Saunders, 1974, p 235

MAHALANOBIS D et al: Oral fluid therapy of cholera among Bangladesh refugees, Johns Hopkins Med J 132:197, 1973

WALLACE CK et al: Optimal antibiotic therapy in cholera. Bull WHO 39:239, 1968

WATTEN RH et al: Water and electrolyte studies in cholera. J Clin Invest 38:1879, 1959

Vibrio parahemolyticus

BARKER WH JR et al: *Vibrio parahemolyticus* outbreak in Covington, Louisiana in August, 1972. Am J Epidemiol 100:316, 1974

THATCHER FS, CLARK DS (eds): *Microorganisms in Foods: Their Significance and Methods of Enumeration.* Toronto, University of Toronto Press, 1968, p 14

ZEN-YOJI H et al: Epidemiology, enteropathogenicity and classification of *Vibrio parahemolyticus.* J Infect Dis 115:436, 1965

135
CAMPYLOBACTER FETUS AND NONCHOLERAIC VIBRIO INFECTIONS

MARVIN TURCK
DENNIS SCHABERG

CAMPYLOBACTER FETUS INFECTIONS

DEFINITION *Campylobacter fetus* (formerly *Vibrio fetus*) infection is economically the most important cause of infectious abortion in cattle. In human beings, this organism may be associated with obscure febrile illnesses, subacute bacterial endocarditis, meningoencephalitis, and perhaps abortion.

ETIOLOGY *Campylobacter fetus* is a motile, comma-shaped or spirillar, gram-negative rod with a single unipolar flagellum. It is best identified by its appearance in smears made from cultured material. The organism is slow-growing and microaerophilic, and grows best in liquid media incubated under increased CO_2 tension. Several serotypes have been isolated by agglutination with antiserums from human and bovine strains. Cross-agglutination reactions occur with other bacterial species, particularly *Brucella abortus.*

EPIDEMIOLOGY AND PATHOGENESIS *Campylobacter* causes a venereal infection of cattle, sheep, and goats; when transmitted to gravid heifers or ewes, it results in abortion. The male acts as an asymptomatic carrier of the infection, and the organism has been isolated from the genitalia and semen of bulls. Although *Campylobacter* infection has been thought to occur only rarely in humans, reports of this disease are appearing with increasing frequency. *Campylobacter* infection in human beings may result from direct contact with the organism,

as happens in laboratory-acquired infection, or from direct contact with infected cattle. Food and water have been implicated, without convincing evidence, as vehicles for infection. The mouth has been postulated as a portal of entry because cases of *C. fetus* endocarditis have followed dental extractions. Because *C. fetus* has been isolated from several aborted fetuses and has been the cause of neonatal meningitis, a venereal route of infection has been postulated. It is presumed that, as in cattle, the male acts as an asymptomatic carrier who transmits the infection to a pregnant partner. The relation of *C. fetus* to prematurity, abortion, and neonatal meningitis requires further documentation. In most instances of *Campylobacter* infection, the portal of entry is not known.

MANIFESTATIONS Fever is the only characteristic sign of *Campylobacter* infection in adults, and may be relapsing in character. Thrombophlebitis involving both arms and legs is not uncommon. The disease may also present as classic subacute bacterial endocarditis; septic arthritis or osteomyelitis; chronic, indolent meningoencephalitis; and fever and abortion in pregnant women. A number of patients have had coexisting disease, including cirrhosis, cardiac amyloidosis, and chronic lymphatic leukemia, or antecedent gastric surgery. Several neonates with fulminating, lethal meningoencephalitis have been reported. It has been postulated that infection was transmitted to these infants via the placenta. *Campylobacter* has also been implicated in the etiology of outbreaks of acute gastroenteritis.

DIAGNOSIS Lack of awareness of *Campylobacter* infection by both the bacteriologist and the clinician has resulted in mistaken diagnosis in most instances. The organisms have been erroneously described as "fastidious strains of *Hemophilus.*" Recovery of spirillar organisms in blood cultures should suggest the diagnosis because other spirochetes causing relapsing fever usually do not grow in artificial media. Failure to incubate blood cultures under increased CO_2 tensions may delay growth. Identification of the organisms in smears of cultures is the only definitive method of making the diagnosis, which should then be confirmed by agglutinating the vibrios with specific antiserums. Complement-fixing antibody may be present in high titers in the active phase of the disease. Clinically, *Campylobacter* infection should be suspected in obscure febrile illnesses associated with thrombophlebitis or abortion and premature delivery in pregnant women.

TREATMENT There are few reports of antibiotic sensitivity of the organisms, and various antibiotics, alone or in combination, have been used. A 10-day course of tetracycline or chloramphenicol in dosage of 2 g per day, alone or coupled with streptomycin, 1 g per day, should eradicate the organisms in most instances. In cases of endocarditis, antimicrobial therapy should be extended to 6 weeks. Kanamycin and erythromycin have also been effective in vitro. Penicillin, novobiocin, vancomycin, and polymyxin B are ineffective.

NONCHOLERAIC VIBRIO INFECTIONS

DEFINITION *Vibrio parahemolyticus, V. alginolyticus,* and an unnamed lactose-positive *Vibrio* species are halophilic marine vibrios associated with wound infections, septicemia and, in the case of *V. parahemolyticus,* food-borne gastroenteritis (Chaps. 112 and 134). Nonagglutinating *V. cholerae* is biochemically identical with, but serologically distinct from, true *V. cholerae* and has been implicated in gastroenteritis as well as sepsis and wound infection.

EPIDEMIOLOGY AND PATHOGENESIS These marine vibrios are ubiquitous organisms found in oceans worldwide. Infection appears to result from direct contact of wounds with seawater or from handling or ingesting seafood. In the United States the majority of infections are acquired in the coastal states. Acquisition of the organism also occurs in travelers outside the United States.

MANIFESTATIONS Illness can begin as a wound infection or can present as a systemic illness without antecedent wound infection. Rapidly developing swelling, erythema, and bullae formation at the site of a wound exposed to seawater should raise the possibility of *Vibrio* infection. Secondary bloodstream invasion can develop.

Presentation as a systemic illness typically involves fever and chills. Hypotension and leukopenia are not uncommon findings. A history of recent seafood ingestion, especially raw oysters, is often obtained in those patients who have preexisting hepatic disease. Progression to a full-blown syndrome of gram-negative sepsis with shock, disseminated intravascular coagulation, and mortality has been noted in up to one-third of cases.

DIAGNOSIS Clinically, noncholeraic *Vibrio* infection should be suspected when patients present with wound infection and seawater exposure or present with a systemic febrile illness, preexisting hepatic disease, and a history of seafood ingestion. These marine vibrios grow well in artificial media, although when *Vibrio* infection is suspected, the use of thiosulfate-citrate-bile salts-sucrose (TCBS) agar may facilitate isolation. Cultures of wound drainage and blood will yield the causative agent within 24 to 48 h of incubation.

TREATMENT A wide variety of antimicrobial agents has been used in the therapy of noncholeraic *Vibrio* infections. Limited clinical experience and in vitro studies would suggest that tetracycline or chloramphenicol in doses of 2 g per day should be effective. In vitro studies also show that cephalothin or aminoglycoside antibiotics should be effective, but clinical experience with these agents is lacking.

REFERENCES

Campylobacter infections

FRANKLIN B et al: Human infection with *Vibrio fetus.* West J Med 120:200, 1974

LAWRENCE GD et al: Infection caused by *Vibrio fetus.* Arch Intern Med 120:459, 1967

SKIRROW MB: *Campylobacter* enteritis: A "new" disease. Br Med J 2:9, 1977

Noncholeraic *Vibrio* infections

BLAKE PA et al: Disease caused by a marine *Vibrio:* Clinical characteristics and epidemiology. N Engl J Med 300:1, 1979

HOLLIS DG et al: Halophilic *Vibrio* species isolated from blood cultures. J Clin Microbiol 3:425, 1976

HUGHES JM et al: Non-cholera *Vibrio* infections in the United States: Clinical, epidemiologic, and laboratory features. Ann Intern Med 88:602, 1978

136
BARTONELLOSIS

JAMES J. PLORDE

DEFINITION Bartonellosis (Carrión's disease) is an infection with *Bartonella bacilliformis.* Two well-defined clinical stages occur: an acute febrile anemia of rapid onset and high mortal-

ity, designated *Oroya fever,* and a benign eruptive form with chronic cutaneous lesions, called *verruga peruana.* Either of these types may be mild, and asymptomatic cases constitute the greatest epidemiologic hazard.

ETIOLOGY *Bartonella bacilliformis* is a small, motile, aerobic, pleomorphic, gram-negative bacillus which stains reddish violet with Giemsa's stain. It can be cultured on enriched media and does not produce a hemolysin. The organisms are sensitive to several antibiotics in vitro.

EPIDEMIOLOGY The disease is limited to certain valleys in the Andes Mountains comprising parts of Peru, Ecuador, and Colombia. It occurs in regions between the altitudes of 2400 and 8000 ft where the sandfly vector, *Phlebotomus,* propagates. Although only *P. verrucarum* has been shown to transmit the disease, other species are undoubtedly involved. Asymptomatic cases and convalescent carriers are the only known reservoir of infection. A low-grade bacteremia may persist for years following resolution of symptoms, and *B. bacilliformis* can be recovered from the blood of 5 to 10 percent of the apparently normal population in an endemic area. Epidemics often coincide with immigration of workers from uninfected areas.

PATHOLOGY AND PATHOGENESIS The manifestations of the disease are thought to reflect the immune status of the host. In nonimmune individuals Oroya fever develops. Large numbers of the *Bartonella* bacteria enter the bloodstream, adhere to erythrocytes, and invade the endothelial cells of the capillaries and lymphatics. The presence of the organisms on the surface of the red blood cell results in their phagocytosis and destruction by the liver and spleen. The red blood cell life span is greatly shortened, and anemia develops. This is accentuated by a defective erythropoietic response early in the course of infection. The pathogenesis of the hemolytic anemia remains unknown. Agglutinins and hemolysins have not been found, and tests for mechanical fragility of red blood cells have given variable results. Invasion and swelling of capillary endothelial cells may lead to vascular occlusion and tissue infarcts. It is possible that an impairment of reticuloendothelial function secondary to massive phagocytosis of red blood cells is responsible for the frequency with which *Salmonella* and other coliform bacteremias are seen in Oroya fever.

With developing immunity, the bacteria nearly disappear from the peripheral blood and capillary endothelium. After a latent period they reappear in the skin and subcutaneous tissue where they are apparently responsible for the development of the hemangioid lesions of verruga peruana. Second attacks of Carrión's disease are unusual. When they occur, they almost invariably present as verruga.

CLINICAL MANIFESTATIONS The incubation period is approximately 3 weeks but may be longer. The initial symptoms are fever and pains in the bones, joints, and muscles. At this point the disease often resembles influenza or malaria, but blood cultures are positive. After these prodromes, the patient usually develops one of the two classic forms of the infection.

Oroya fever This form is characterized by sudden onset of high fever, extreme pallor, weakness, and a precipitous drop in the number of red blood cells. The count may fall from normal to 1 million per cubic millimeter within 4 or 5 days. The anemia is characterized by normochromic macrocytes in the peripheral blood, striking polychromasia and polychromatophilia, nucleated red blood cells, Howell-Jolly bodies, Cabot rings, and basophilic stippling. There may also be a mild leukocytosis with a shift to the left. Organisms are numerous in the blood, and stained smears may show 90 percent of the erythrocytes heavily invaded. Salmonellosis, malaria, amebiasis, tuberculosis, and other intercurrent infections may occur and are an important factor in fatal cases.

Muscle and joint pain and headache are severe, and insomnia, delirium, and coma are the terminal manifestations. In untreated patients, the mortality rate may exceed 50 percent; death occurs within 10 days to 4 weeks. With treatment, or sometimes spontaneously, recovery results if the organisms decrease and fever abates. The red blood cell count stabilizes and approaches normal values in about 6 weeks, when convalescence begins.

Verruga peruana This form of the disease, characterized by a profuse skin eruption, may follow the anemic form or may occur in patients without previous symptoms. The verrugas vary in color from red to purple. They may be miliary, nodular, or eroding, and they range in size from 2 to 10 mm up to 3 or 4 cm in diameter. The three types of verruga may occur together; since eruption takes place in successive crops, verrugas of all types and in all stages of development may be found on the same patient. The chief sites involved are the limbs and face, and less frequently the genitalia, scalp, and mucosa of the mouth and pharynx. They may persist for 1 month to 2 years. The eruption is accompanied by pain, fever, and moderate anemia. Bartonellas may be demonstrated in the lesions and cultured from the blood.

DIAGNOSIS A clinical diagnosis can be made with accuracy in endemic areas. During Oroya fever the organism is easily seen on peripheral blood smears. It may be recovered from blood cultures in all stages of the disease.

TREATMENT Oroya fever responds dramatically to a number of antibiotics including tetracycline and chloramphenicol. The latter in a dose of 2 g per day for 7 days is often preferred because of the frequency with which *Salmonella* infections complicate this disease. Fever disappears within 48 h, and the patient recovers rapidly. Transfusions may be required when the anemia is severe. Antibiotic therapy of the verrugal stage may hasten the involution of these lesions. The use of DDT in both the interior and exterior of human dwellings is highly effective in controlling the night-biting sandflies. Insect repellents and bed netting afford personal protection.

REFERENCES

Cuadra MC: Salmonellosis complication in human bartonellosis. Tex Rep Biol Med 14:97, 1956

Kaye D et al: Factors influencing host resistance to *Salmonella* infections: The effects of hemolysis and erythrophagocytosis. Am J Med Sci 254:205, 1967

Ricketts WE: Clinical manifestations of Carrión's disease. AMA Arch Intern Med 84:751, 1949

Schultz MG: Daniel Carrión's experiment. N Engl J Med 278:1323, 1968

Ureteaga OB, Payne EH: Treatment of the acute febrile phase of Carrión's disease with chloramphenicol. Am J Trop Med 4:507, 1955

Weinman D: The bartonella group, in *Bacterial and Mycotic Infections of Man*, 4th ed, RJ Dubos, JG Hirsch (eds). Philadelphia, Lippincott, 1965, p 775

137

GRANULOMA INGUINALE

KING K. HOLMES

DEFINITION Granuloma inguinale is a mildly contagious, chronic, indolent, progressive, autoinoculable, ulcerative disease involving the skin and lymphatics of the genital or perianal areas. The disease may be sexually transmitted and is associated with the presence in affected tissues of an intracellular microorganism, identified morphologically as the Donovan body.

ETIOLOGY Granuloma inguinale was described by McLeod in India in 1882, and in 1905 Donovan described the intracellular bodies which are thought to cause the disease. Granuloma inguinale has been reproduced in humans by inoculation of pus containing Donovan bodies. Similar attempts to reproduce the disease in experimental animals have been unsuccessful. Encapsulated bacteria resembling Donovan bodies have been recovered from lesions and pseudobuboes of granuloma inguinale by inoculation of chick embryo yolk sacs or yolk-agar medium. These bacteria, which are known as *Calymmatobacterium granulomatis*, are antigenically related to *Klebsiella* species but do not reproduce the disease when inoculated intradermally in humans. It is uncertain whether these isolates are responsible for the disease. Similar bacteria have been isolated from feces. Electron microscopic studies of Donovan bodies confirm their morphological resemblance to gram-negative bacteria.

EPIDEMIOLOGY Granuloma inguinale is endemic in the tropics, particularly in New Guinea and among Hindus in India. In the United States the disease is rare. Most cases occur in the southeastern states and involve male homosexuals. In reported cases the sex ratio of males to females is nearly 10:1. The disease is uncommon in Caucasians. The reported frequency of granuloma inguinale in conjugal partners of chronically infected patients ranges from 1 to 64 percent. Evidence for sexual transmission includes the age-specific incidence, which corresponds to that of other sexually transmitted diseases, the frequent concomitant presence of syphilis, and the predilection for genital involvement in heterosexuals and for anorectal infection in male homosexuals.

CLINICAL MANIFESTATIONS The incubation period ranges from 8 days to 12 weeks, but most lesions appear within 30 days after sexual exposure.

Granuloma inguinale begins as a papule, which ulcerates and develops into a painless elevated zone of clean, beefy-red, friable granulation tissue. The edges are irregular and spread by continuity or by autoinoculation of approximated skin surfaces. Secondary anaerobic infection may produce pain and a foul-smelling exudate. Less common complications of the disease include deep ulcerations, chronic cicatricial lesions, and exuberant epithelial proliferation which grossly resembles carcinoma. In men, the lesions are usually located on the glans, prepuce, or shaft of the penis (Fig. 137-1*A*) or the perianal area, while infection of the labia is most common in women. Lesions in women often arise at the fourchette and progress anteriorly in a V shape along the vulva. Extragenital lesions may occur, involving the face, neck, mouth, and other sites. The chronicity of the disease is of diagnostic importance, since several months often elapse before patients seek treatment. Extension to the inguinal region by autoinoculation or via the

A

B

FIGURE 137-1

A. Extensive granuloma inguinale, extending along the scrotum and involving both inguinal areas, with elevated, clean, exuberant granulation tissue. B. Same patient, following treatment. (Courtesy of A Brathwaite.)

lymphatics results in diffuse intradermal and subcutaneous swelling or suppuration, known as "pseudobubo," because involvement of the underlying lymph nodes is minimal. Locally destructive lesions and secondary infection may produce severe morbidity or death. Fatal disseminated disease, involving the bones or joints, has been reported after several years of chronic local infection. The relationship of granuloma inguinale to subsequent carcinoma of the genitalia is uncertain.

DIAGNOSIS Early granuloma inguinale may be mistaken for the primary chancre or condyloma latum of syphilis. Epithelial proliferation resembling neoplasia in the genital or perianal region in a young subject should always raise the suspicion of granuloma inguinale if unnecessary destructive surgery is to be avoided. Chronic ulcerative or cicatricial changes may resemble lymphogranuloma venereum. Histological studies in granuloma inguinale reveal marked acanthosis and pseudoepitheli-

omatous hyperplasia. Because Donovan bodies are seldom detectable in sections stained with hematoxylin and eosin, these changes may lead to an erroneous diagnosis of carcinoma and to unnecessary, destructive surgery. Although silver impregnation techniques are useful for demonstration of Donovan bodies in sections, the diagnosis is best made by examination of impression smears prepared from specimens obtained by punch biopsy from the periphery of a lesion; the deep portion of the specimen is removed, crushed between two slides which are air-dried and fixed in methanol, and stained with Wright-Giemsa stain. With this method, Donovan bodies appear as very rounded coccobacilli, 1 by 2 μm in size, which lie within cystic spaces in the cytoplasm of large mononuclear

FIGURE 137-2

Biopsy from granuloma inguinale ulcer, showing mononuclear cells containing Donovan bodies. Wright-Giemsa stain.

cells (Fig. 137-2). The capsule stains as a dense acidophilic zone surrounding the bipolar basophilic bacterium, which resembles a closed safety pin. The pathognomonic mononuclear cell is 25 to 90 μm in diameter and has many cystic areas containing Donovan bodies.

Perianal granuloma inguinale may resemble condylomata lata of secondary syphilis. Other venereal diseases, particularly syphilis, very frequently coexist with granuloma inguinale. Repeated dark-field examinations of lesions before treatment and a serologic test for syphilis should therefore be performed.

TREATMENT The treatment of choice is tetracycline, 2 g daily, continued for at least 10 days. The risk of relapse is reduced if treatment is continued until healing is complete. Healing is usually apparent within 3 weeks, as the lesions become pale, flatter, and develop peripheral reepithelialization (Fig. 137-1B). Donovan bodies disappear from lesions within a few days after onset of therapy. If tetracycline cannot be given, streptomycin may be used in a dose of 1 g intramuscularly every 12 h for 10 to 15 days. In New Guinea, chloramphenicol or gentamicin is used for cases which appear resistant to tetracycline.

REFERENCES

BEERMAN H, SONCK CE: The epithelial changes in granuloma inguinale. Am J Syph Gonorrhea Vener Dis 36:501, 1952

DAVIS CM: Granuloma inguinale. A clinical, histological, and ultrastructural study. JAMA 211:632, 1970

GOLDBERG J: Studies on granuloma inguinale. Br J Vener Dis 40:140, 1964

LAL S: Continued efficacy of streptomycin in the treatment of granuloma inguinale. Br J Vener Dis 47:454, 1971

———, NICHOLAS C: Epidemiological and clinical features in 165 cases of granuloma inguinale. Br J Vener Dis 46:461, 1970

Management of chancroid, granuloma inguinale, lymphogranuloma verereum in general practice. US Public Health Serv Publ 255:15, 1964

RIBEIRO J: Granuloma inguinale. Practitioner 209:628, 1972

138
LEGIONNAIRES' DISEASE

HARRY N. BEATY

DEFINITION Legionnaires' disease is an acute respiratory infection caused by a newly recognized, distinctive gram-negative bacterium that was first isolated from fatal cases of pneumonia among individuals attending an American Legion Convention in Philadelphia.

HISTORY In July of 1976, an explosive outbreak of severe respiratory illness occurred in Philadelphia—chiefly among delegates of an American Legion Convention. Initial investigation failed to document a familiar infective or toxic etiology, and so a comprehensive, coordinated effort was undertaken to define the epidemiology and cause of the outbreak. As the ensuing saga unfolded, it became apparent that at least 182 cases of pneumonia—29 of which were fatal—resulted from a common source of airborne infection that was present for several days inside and in the immediate vicinity outside one of the convention hotels. The infective agent was proved to be a previously unknown gram-negative bacterium.

Using serologic techniques, it has been shown that the same organism, or antigenically related species, has caused at least eight other outbreaks of respiratory illness. The earliest of these occurred in 1965 when 80 patients in a psychiatric hospital in Washington, D.C., developed an unexplained pneumonic illness; 12 of these patients died. Other clusters of cases with additional deaths have occurred in Spain (1973) and England (1977). One outbreak of particular significance involved visitors and employees in an office of the county health department in Pontiac, Michigan (1968). Pneumonia was not seen among the 144 persons who developed an influenza-like illness, and there were no deaths. The agent responsible for Legionnaires' disease has been directly linked to this outbreak, because it has been isolated from environmental samples and tissues of experimental animals, which were stored in the frozen state after they were studied unsuccessfully during the initial investigation.

ETIOLOGY The bacterium responsible for Legionnaires' disease was first isolated by inoculating suspensions of lung tissue from four of the fatal Philadelphia cases intraperitoneally into guinea pigs. Suspensions of spleen and other organs from animals with a progressive febrile illness produced infection in embryonated eggs. From infected eggs, the organism was isolated in pure culture on an artificial medium. An inoculum from this medium was used to induce infection in guinea pigs, fulfilling Koch's postulate.

The bacterium is a gram-negative bacillus which is 0.3 to 0.4 μm in width and usually 2 to 3 μm long. However, bacilli from 10 to 50 μm have been seen. Pleomorphism is affected by the medium on which the organism is grown; in tissue, the filamentous forms are not encountered. Electron microscopy reveals a structure typical of gram-negative rods, but gas-liquid chromatography shows a distinctive branched-chain fatty acid profile that is more characteristic of gram-positive bacteria.

With the use of the direct fluorescent-antibody technique, no antigenic cross-reactivity was found with 374 strains including 25 bacterial genera and 59 species. One strain each of *Pseudomonas fluorescens* and *P. alcaligenes* has shown some reaction with anti-Legionnaires' agent conjugate, but numerous other strains of the same species have been tested without additional evidence of cross-reactivity. Studies of DNA relatedness also have failed to show that the bacterium responsible for Legionnaires' disease is related to any other organism. As a consequence of all of these studies, the organism has been named *Legionella pneumophilia* to establish it as the first isolate of a previously unrecognized genus and species.

Legionella pneumophilia is fastidious, and either does not grow or grows rather poorly on most artificial media. For this reason it is infrequently isolated directly from patients. Mueller-Hinton agar containing 1 percent hemoglobin and 1 percent IsoVitale X was the medium used in early studies, but more recently a yeast extract agar containing activated charcoal has produced better growth of the organisms. Inoculated plates should be incubated at 35°C in 5% CO_2 or in candle jars. On clear media, a soluble brown pigment that fluoresces under a Wood's lamp can be seen. The organism is catalase-positive and causes a weakly positive oxidase reaction.

Several distinct serogroups of *L. pneumophilia* have been identified; some were isolated from patients with Legionnaires' disease and others from soil and/or water. Serologic cross-reactions between groups may be absent or weak, which necessitates the use of multiple diagnostic conjugates to detect all strains of *L. pneumophila*.

EPIDEMIOLOGY Knowledge of the distribution of *L. pneumophilia* in nature is incomplete, but it has been isolated from soil and water. Several outbreaks of Legionnaires' disease have been linked to contaminated condensates from air-conditioning cooling towers, and prolonged survival in drinking water has been documented experimentally. The possibility that organisms in soil became airborne during excavation was raised as a possible cause of disease early in the epidemiologic studies of the Philadelphia outbreak.

Infection appears to be acquired by the respiratory route with a usual incubation period of 2 to 10 days. By use of the direct fluorescent-antibody technique, organisms have been identified in the sputum of patients with Legionnaires' disease, but person-to-person spread has not been documented. Common-source outbreaks have received the greatest public attention, but hundreds of sporadic cases of Legionnaires' disease occur each year. Incidence may increase in the summer and early fall, but the disease occurs year-round.

Although this infection has been reported in children, most patients are middle-aged or older. Cigarette smokers and individuals with serious underlying diseases such as chronic renal failure, malignancy, and immunosuppression have increased susceptibility to infection. The mortality rate of Legionnaires' pneumonia that is serious enough to require hospitalization is around 15 percent; among immunocompromised patients it may exceed 50 percent.

Serologic surveys using the indirect fluorescent-antibody technique have shown that less than 5 percent of healthy individuals from around the United States have reciprocal antibody titers to *L. pneumophilia* of 128 or higher. However, some more geographically restricted surveys have shown that 15 to 25 percent of the population have similar serologic evidence of significant exposure to *L. pneumophilia* or antigenically related organisms. This suggests that the infection may be endemic in some regions.

Most cases of Legionnaires' disease are diagnosed by demonstration of at least a fourfold rise in serum antibody titer to *L. pneumophilia*. A significant proportion of patients maintain high titers for years. It is not known whether these individuals are immune to reinfection with the same or closely related organisms.

PATHOLOGY AND PATHOGENESIS Pathologic features of Legionnaires' disease are limited to the lungs. Apparent lobar involvement almost always represents confluent bronchopneumonia. Prominent microscopic features include extensive exudation of proteinaceous fluid and inflammatory cells into alveoli. In most cases, the cellular component of the exudate is a mixture of polymorphonuclear neutrophils and macrophages. Extensive lysis of inflammatory cells, with accumulations of nuclear debris and fibrin, is a distinctive feature of this pneumonia. Alveolar septa usually are edematous and infiltrated with inflammatory cells; hyalin membranes are seen in about half the cases. Terminal bronchioles are routinely involved, but larger bronchioles and bronchi are unaffected. None of these changes is unique to Legionnaires' pneumonia, but the histopathologic alterations are sufficiently distinctive to suggest the diagnosis.

Bacteria usually can be demonstrated in the inflammatory exudate with the Dieterle stain or by direct fluorescent-antibody techniques. Other stains are less reliable. Many bacilli appear to be intracellular, and an increase in the number of organisms is associated with lysis of inflammatory cells.

Little is known about the pathogenesis of Legionnaires' pneumonia. The fact that cigarette smokers are more susceptible to infection than nonsmokers suggests that the defective alveolar macrophage function plays a role in development of disease. The extensive lysis of inflammatory cells and the edema of the interstitium raise the possibility that a toxin is produced by the Legionnaires' disease bacterium. Such a toxin might be responsible for some of the clinical features seen with this infection.

CLINICAL MANIFESTATIONS The total spectrum of clinical manifestations of Legionnaires' disease is not known. Mild respiratory illness has been recognized, and asymptomatic infection has not been excluded as a possible explanation for elevated antibody titers among healthy individuals. The outbreak in Pontiac, Michigan, was characterized by the acute onset and short duration of a moderately severe influenza-like syndrome of fever, myalgia, and headache.

The more typical patient with Legionnaires' disease has pneumonia. In the Philadelphia outbreak over 80 percent of the recognized cases were severe enough to require hospitalization. Some patients have a constellation of symptoms that strongly suggest the diagnosis, particularly in a setting of known Legionnaires' disease activity. These patients have malaise and a slight headache, which precedes a rapidly rising fever by less than a day. Within 24 to 48 h, temperatures reach 40°C in about half the patients, and shaking chills are common. A modest, nonproductive cough frequently is present early; it progresses in severity over the first few days of illness and usually becomes productive of variable amounts of mucoid to mucopurulent sputum. Minimal hemoptysis is seen in about 20 percent of patients. Additional symptoms that occur less frequently include dyspnea, pleuritic chest pain, and myalgia. About 25 percent of patients have various combinations of gastrointestinal symptoms which include nausea and vomiting, diarrhea, and abdominal pain. In a few patients, these manifestations predominate despite the presence of pneumonia. In some individuals, the onset of Legionnaires' disease is more protracted and the clinical expression less distinctive. These cases are likely to be missed unless the epidemiologic setting or subtle clinical clues stimulate physicians to suspect the diagnosis. The findings on physical examination are not specific for Legionnaires' disease, and they are affected by patients' associated diseases. High fever, tachypnea, and tachycardia are common. Patients frequently are flushed, mildly diaphoretic, and appear moderately to severely prostrated. Examination of the chest shows moist rales, but signs of consolidation usually are absent. Chest roentgenograms characteristically show more involvement of the lungs than is suspected on clinical grounds.

During the first 4 to 6 days, the disease becomes progressively worse. An additional 4 to 5 days may pass before definite clinical improvement begins. The average duration of fever in one large series was 13 days. Clearing of pulmonary infiltrates lags significantly behind improvement of other manifestations of infection, and minor residual scarring is not uncommon. Many patients experience weakness and easy fatigability for weeks after the acute stages of the illness.

The major complication of Legionnaires' disease is respiratory failure. Twenty to thirty percent of patients sick enough to require hospitalization have hyperventilation and hypoxemia. In about half of these patients, progression of disease leads to intubation and mechanical ventilation. The mortality rate among patients with respiratory failure is high. Hypotension and shock, with secondary acute renal failure, are additional complications that may be encountered. Whether these are caused by undetected bacteremia or toxemia has not been determined.

LABORATORY FINDINGS Most patients have a modest granulocytosis, but about 20 percent have leukocyte counts in excess of 20,000 per cubic millimeter. The erythrocyte sedimentation rate is elevated, and there is moderate proteinuria. Transient renal insufficiency and mild changes in liver function have been reported, but it is not always possible to attribute these abnormalities to the infection.

Chest roentgenograms show unilateral pulmonary parenchymal infiltrates in about 65 percent of cases early in the illness. By the time of maximal involvement, the pneumonia has progressed to involve both sides in most cases. Nonspecific poorly marginated rounded opacities or diffuse patchy lobar shadows predominate. Small pleural effusions are seen in about a third of cases.

Routine bacteriologic studies including blood and sputum cultures are negative. Lower respiratory tract secretions obtained by transtracheal aspiration or other suitable techniques show many granulocytes and alveolar macrophages but are sterile on Gram's stain and currently available culture media.

DIAGNOSIS The diagnosis of Legionnaires' disease has been made in a very few instances by isolation of the causative organism from lung tissue or pleural field. As bacteriologic techniques improve, this may become more common. For the moment, the diagnosis depends on demonstration of a significant rise in antibody in paired serum specimens or by identifying organisms in fresh or Formalin-fixed lung tissue by the direct fluorescent-antibody technique. Serum antibody can be measured in a number of ways, but the indirect fluorescent-antibody method is the most specific and sensitive one available. Because antibody titers rise slowly in some patients, the first serum specimen should be obtained during the first week of illness, and the second at least 21 days after the onset of symptoms.

In some cases, *L. pneumophilia* has been demonstrated in sputum by the direct fluorescent-antibody technique. When this is accomplished in a patient with pneumonia and a single reciprocal antibody titer of 256 or greater, a presumptive diagnosis of Legionnaires' disease can be made. Because antibody titers are known to remain elevated for years in some patients, simple demonstration of a high titer without supporting evidence does not establish the diagnosis with certainty.

Legionnaires' disease may be difficult to differentiate from "atypical" pneumonias. When patients have a constellation of findings which include temperature elevations to 40°C, granulocytosis, and sterile lower respiratory tract secretions that contain many granulocytes and alveolar macrophages, Legionnaires' disease should be suspected. In immunocompromised patients, *Pneumocystis* or fungal infection enters into the differential diagnosis. Rarely, pulmonary embolism can be confused with early Legionnaires' disease.

TREATMENT Although in vitro sensitivity tests indicate that a number of antibiotics might be effective in the treatment of Legionnaires' disease, clinical experience has shown that the lowest case-fatality ratio is achieved with erythromycin in a dose of 0.5 to 1 g every 6 h for adults and 15 mg/kg every 6 h for children. Erythromycin also has been shown to be highly efficacious in treatment of experimental infections in embryonated eggs and guinea pigs. Tetracycline is less effective in all these settings. Rifampin has shown promise in laboratory testing, but its propensity to induce resistance may limit its potential usefulness.

Although the case-fatality ratio of patients treated with erythromycin is low, response to treatment frequently is not dramatic. If therapy is continued for at least 14 days, relapses are uncommon. When they occur, they usually respond to a second course of erythromycin. Because Legionnaires' disease can cause pneumonia in patients not sick enough to be hospitalized and who are assumed to have either *Mycoplasma* infection or early pneumococcal infection, erythromycin should be considered the drug of choice for the treatment of pneumonia in an ambulatory care setting.

There is more to treatment of Legionnaires' disease than administration of antibiotics. High fever, diaphoresis, and tachypnea produce excessive fluid loss, and volume replacement with intravenous fluids may be needed. Hypoxic patients should receive supplemental oxygen.

PROGNOSIS The overall mortality rate of Legionnaires' disease is unknown. Among patients with pneumonia who are sick enough to require hospitalization, the mortality rate is around 15 percent. The presence of complicating associated illnesses may raise that figure two- or threefold. Individuals who recover from Legionnaires' pneumonia usually have no significant residua of their infection. It is not known whether they are immune to reinfection with the same or related organisms.

REFERENCES

BEATY HN et al: Legionnaires' disease in Vermont, May to October 1977. JAMA 240:127, 1978

FRASER DW et al: Legionnaires' disease—description of an epidemic of pneumonia. N Engl J Med 297:1189, 1977

KIRBY, BD et al: Legionnaires' disease: Clinical features of 24 cases. Ann Intern Med 89:297, 1978

MCDADE JE et al: Legionnaires' disease—isolation of a bacterium and demonstration of its role in other respiratory disease. N Engl J Med 297:1197, 1977

WINN WC et al: The pathology of Legionnaires' disease—fourteen fatal cases from the 1977 outbreak in Vermont. Arch Pathol Lab Med 102:344, 1978

139
TETANUS

HARRY N. BEATY

DEFINITION Tetanus is an acute, often fatal, disease caused by an exotoxin produced in a wound by *Clostridium tetani*. It is characterized by generalized increased rigidity and convulsive spasms of skeletal muscles.

ETIOLOGY *Clostridium tetani* is a strictly anaerobic, gram-positive rod which is motile and readily forms endospores. In stained preparations, organisms may occur singly, in pairs, or in long chains. Spore-bearing bacilli usually contain a single, spheric, terminal endospore which swells the end of the organism and produces a characteristic "clubbed" appearance.

The organism grows well on blood agar at 37°C under anaerobic conditions. Slight hemolysis is usually apparent, but isolated colonies are rare because the organism tends to swarm. *Clostridium tetani* is relatively inert biochemically, with no proteolytic activity and no fermentation of carbohydrates. Vegetative forms of the tetanus bacillus are no more resistant to adverse conditions than other bacteria are, but spores are highly resistant to antiseptics and moderately resistant to heat.

Ten distinct types of *C. tetani* can be distinguished on the basis of flagellar antigens. All these types have one or more common somatic antigens, and are capable of producing at least two exotoxins. One, a hemolysin, is relatively unimportant clinically. The other, tetanospasmin, generally referred to as tetanus toxin, is a protein with a molecular weight of approximately 145,000 in its dimer form, and is responsible for the clinical manifestations of tetanus. The tetanospasmins produced by the various types of *C. tetani* are nearly identical antigenically, and only one antitoxin is needed to neutralize the tetanus toxins produced by all strains.

EPIDEMIOLOGY The tetanus bacillus is found in the superficial layers of soil and as a saprophyte in the intestinal tract of man and certain animals. It is most frequently encountered in densely populated regions in hot, damp climates and in soil rich in organic matter. This explains, in part, why the disease is rare in the polar regions and relatively uncommon in the U.S.S.R., North America, and most of Europe. Urbanization, mechanization of agriculture, and socioeconomic factors such as poverty and lack of availability of health services also significantly influence the occurrence of this disease.

Worldwide, there are probably 300,000 to 500,000 cases of tetanus each year, with a mortality rate of roughly 45 percent. There is no racial predilection, but the male-to-female ratio is 2.5:1, even among neonates, in which the opportunity for infection is presumably equal. In the United States, there are less than 200 reported cases each year, and these occur almost exclusively in nonimmunized or only partially immunized individuals. The highest incidence of disease is among nonwhites in the southern states. However, spores of *C. tetani* are distributed widely throughout urban centers and rural areas of the entire country, and are found commonly on clothing and in house dust, placing the nonimmune individual at risk after relatively minor household injuries. Tetanus has been known to follow surgery and innocuous procedures such as skin testing or intramuscular injection of medication. The disease is inordinately common in narcotic addicts, perhaps because heroin is frequently "cut" with quinine, which drastically lowers the redox potential at the site of injection and favors the growth of *C. tetani*.

Tetanus neonatorum is a major cause of infant mortality in developing countries and is directly related to poor obstetric conditions and lack of maternal immunization programs.

PATHOGENESIS AND PATHOLOGY *Clostridium tetani* is a noninvasive organism. Therefore, tetanus can occur only after spore or vegetative bacteria gain access to tissues and produce toxin locally. The usual mode of entry is through a puncture wound or laceration on the hand, foot, or leg. However, tetanus may follow elective surgery, burn wounds, otitis media, dental infection, abortion, and pregnancy. Neonatal tetanus usually follows infection of the umbilical stump. The disease not infrequently follows injuries too trivial to be seen by a physician, and in 20 to 40 percent of cases there is neither a history of injury nor a detectable lesion.

Wounds are undoubtedly contaminated frequently with spores of *C. tetani*, but tetanus develops rarely because germination of spores occurs only when the oxygen tension is much lower than that of normal tissue. Spores may survive in the body for months to years and finally produce disease at some later date after minor trauma which alters local conditions. Toxin production in wounds is favored by necrotic tissue, foreign bodies, calcium salts, and associated infections which establish low oxidation-reduction potentials. Infection caused by the tetanus bacillus remains strictly localized, but the toxin produced is transported to the central nervous system via neural pathways. Toxin entering the circulation persists for days, and probably must enter peripheral nerves to spread centrally and cause disease.

The typical clinical manifestations of tetanus are caused by the effect of tetanospasmin on the central nervous system. The toxin attacks synaptic functions to produce disinhibition of both the alpha and gamma motor systems. Generalized muscle rigidity arises from uninhibited afferent stimuli entering the central nervous system from the periphery. When the stimuli become more vigorous, spasms occur. Emotional and, to a lesser extent, visual stimuli can also cause muscle spasm. Tetanus toxin also has other effects. Peripherally it produces neuromuscular blockade similar to that of botulinum toxin, and it acts directly on muscle to produce contraction which is unaccompanied by an action potential in nerves. Certain clinical observations have raised the possibility that tetanus toxin also has an effect on the sympathetic nervous system.

All the effects of tetanus toxin appear to be self-limited and completely reversible, because patients who recover from the disease have no residual defect. Although there are no distinguishable pathologic changes which are characteristic of tetanus, brainstem lesions have been reported in patients dying from tetanus, and toxic myocarditis has been recognized.

CLINICAL MANIFESTATIONS The *incubation period* of tetanus, i.e., the time between injury and the appearance of unmistakable symptoms, ranges from 2 to 56 days. However, over 80 percent of patients become symptomatic within 14 days. A short incubation period indicates severe disease, and when symptoms occur within 2 or 3 days of injury, the mortality rate approaches 100 percent.

Nonspecific premonitory symptoms such as restlessness, irritability, and headache are encountered occasionally, but the commonest presenting complaints are pain and stiffness in the jaw, abdomen, or back and difficulty in swallowing. As the disease progresses, stiffness gives way to rigidity, and patients often complain of difficulty in opening their mouths. In fact, trismus is the commonest manifestation of tetanus and is responsible for the familiar descriptive name of *lockjaw*. As more muscles are involved, rigidity becomes generalized, and sustained contractions of facial muscles produce a characteristic expression called *risus sardonicus*. The intensity and sequence of muscle involvement is quite variable. In a small proportion of patients, only local signs and symptoms develop in the region of the injury. In the vast majority, however, most muscles are involved to some degree, and the signs and symptoms encountered depend upon the major muscle groups affected.

Reflex spasms usually occur within 24 to 72 h of the first symptoms, an interval referred to as the *onset time*. As in the case of the incubation period, a short onset time is associated with a poor prognosis. Spasms are caused by sudden intensification of afferent stimuli arising in the periphery, which increases rigidity and causes simultaneous and excessive contraction of muscles and their antagonists. Spasms may be both painful and dangerous. As the disease progresses, minimal or inapparent stimuli produce more intense and longer-lasting spasms with increasing frequency. Respiration may be impaired by laryngospasm or tonic contraction of respiratory muscles which prevents adequate ventilation. Hypoxia may then lead to irreversible central nervous system damage and death.

Patients are almost invariably conscious and mentally alert at the time of admission. Low-grade fever, profuse sweating, and tachycardia are common. Deep tendon reflexes are hyperactive, and there may be labile hypertension. The physical examination should be undertaken with care, because reflex convulsive spasms may be precipitated easily. The wound through which *C. tetani* was introduced should be evaluated, and the examination should determine the extent of rigidity; the severity of trismus; the presence or absence of dysphagia and respiratory embarrassment; the frequency, intensity, and duration of convulsive spasms; and the presence of complications such as respiratory infection.

Characteristically, the manifestations of tetanus increase in severity for about 3 days after the first sign, and then remain stable for the next 5 to 7 days. After about 10 days, spasms begin to occur less frequently, and by the end of 2 weeks, they disappear altogether. Although residual stiffness may persist for a prolonged period, most survivors recover completely in 4 weeks.

Tetanus neonatorum is a severe form of the disease which usually occurs within 10 days of birth. Early signs include difficulty in sucking, irritability, and excessive crying, associated with peculiar grimacing. Intense rigidity characteristically produces opisthotonus, flexion of the arms, clenched fists, extension of the legs, and plantar flexion of the toes. Typical spasms occur with minimal stimuli.

Complications Complications contribute significantly to the morbidity and mortality of tetanus. Some result from overly vigorous therapy and prolonged bed rest, while others are attributed to the action of tetanus toxin. Inadequate ventilation, either from laryngospasm or spasm of respiratory muscles, is a constant threat. In addition to hypoxia, atelectasis is a common consequence of impaired respiration. Difficulty in swallowing leads to aspiration of secretions, which may also cause atelectasis and initiate pulmonary infection. Thrombophlebitis is occasionally encountered, but bland venous thrombosis is more common and may lead to pulmonary embolization. Cardiovascular complications thought to be due to hyperactivity of the sympathetic nervous system include vasomotor instability, hypertension, tachycardia, arrhythmias, and severe vasoconstriction. Pulmonary edema and hypotension may occur as a consequence of myocarditis. High fever usually signifies secondary infection. Pneumonia is a common late complication of tetanus, and is found in 50 to 70 percent of autopsied cases. Other frequent sites of secondary infections include the original wound, decubitus ulcers, and the urinary tract of patients with indwelling bladder catheters. Fractures of midthoracic vertebrae are probably due to severe spasms, and are particularly common among children and adolescents. Gastrointestinal complications include acute peptic ulceration, paralytic ileus, and constipation. Hemolysis is seen in a small proportion of patients.

Pneumonia is a major cause of death. Other autopsy findings in early deaths include intense congestion of viscera and, occasionally, intracranial hemorrhage or thrombosis. In about 20 percent of cases, no obvious pathology is identified, and death is attributed to the direct effects of tetanus toxin.

LABORATORY FINDINGS There are no laboratory findings characteristic of tetanus. Granulocytosis is seen in about one-third of patients, but anemia is rare. Blood chemistries are almost always normal initially, but various fluid and electrolyte disturbances may arise in the course of the disease. The electrocardiogram usually shows only sinus tachycardia, but occasionally T-wave inversion is seen. Roentgenograms are not helpful except in the evaluation of complications.

The diagnosis of tetanus is entirely clinical and does not depend upon bacteriologic confirmation. *Clostridium tetani* is recovered from the wound in only 30 percent of cases, and not infrequently it is isolated from patients who do not have tetanus. Laboratory identification depends on cultural and morphologic characteristics, absence of fermentative activity, and, most importantly, demonstration of toxin production in mice.

DIFFERENTIAL DIAGNOSIS No disease resembles fully developed tetanus. However, strychnine poisoning and dystonic reactions due to phenothiazines and metoclopramide produce a syndrome that has been referred to as pseudotetanus. These rare reactions usually follow brief exposure to drugs, and subside 24 to 48 h after their administration is discontinued. Early in the course of true tetanus, exclusion of local causes of jaw pain may be difficult, and the combination of neck stiffness and fever may suggest meningitis. However, this can be excluded by lumbar puncture, because in tetanus the spinal fluid is normal. When there is doubt about the diagnosis, clinical observation usually settles the issue within a matter of hours.

TREATMENT In order to formulate a rational plan of therapy, it is useful to assess the severity of tetanus. *Mild tetanus* is characterized by an incubation period of at least 14 days and an onset time of more than 6 days. Trismus is usually present, but dysphagia is absent, and generalized spasms are brief and mild. *Moderately severe tetanus* has a somewhat shorter incubation period and onset time; trismus is marked, dysphagia and generalized rigidity are present, but ventilation remains adequate even during spasms. The criteria for *severe tetanus* include a short incubation time, an onset time of 72 h or less, severe trismus, dysphagia and rigidity, and frequent, prolonged, generalized convulsive spasms. Because of the poor prognosis of tetanus in older individuals, the disease should be considered moderate to severe in all patients over 50.

General measures Patients should be hospitalized in an intensive care unit. After initial evaluation, necrotic tissue and foreign bodies should be removed from the infected wound, and abscesses should be drained. Patients should be placed in a quiet room and observed closely for development of complications or unexpected changes in the course of the disease. While it is a good general principle to disturb patients as little as possible, vital signs must be monitored and aspiration must be averted by positioning the patient carefully and by aspirating nasopharyngeal secretions frequently. Care must be taken to prevent development of decubitus ulcers or contractures, but many routine nursing procedures should be omitted because they may precipitate uncomfortable or dangerous spasms. Initially, nutrition is not a major consideration, and fluid and electrolyte balance should be maintained over the first several days by administration of appropriate solutions intravenously, accompanied by careful recording of intake and output. Patients with severe tetanus are in an intense catabolic state, and may have tremendous fluid losses. Early consideration should be given to intravenous hyperalimentation as a means of meeting the nutritional requirements of these patients.

Antiserum Antiserum does not neutralize tetanus toxin fixed in the central nervous system, and does little to ameliorate symptoms already present at the time of admission. However, the case/fatality ratio in mild to moderately severe disease is reduced significantly when antiserum is administered early. Human tetanus immune globulin (TIG) is generally available in the United States, and is far superior to equine antiserum. Because its half-life is about 25 days, only one dose of 3000 to 10,000 units intramuscularly is recommended, even though as little as 500 units may be equally effective. Local infiltration at the site of the wound is of no proved value, but intrathecal injections may prove to be effective after more careful study. Hypersensitivity reactions do not occur with TIG, obviating the need for pretreatment testing.

If human antitoxin is not available, a single dose of equine antiserum should be given after the patient has been tested for hypersensitivity to horse serum. Although the dosage of heterologous antitoxin often recommended for adults is 100,000 to 200,000 units, 10,000 units is probably optimal. Anaphylaxis can occur despite negative sensitivity tests, and patients must be observed carefully to institute treatment at the first sign of an anaphylactic reaction. Up to 25 percent of patients develop delayed reactions including serum sickness after equine antitoxin. Occasionally, serious neurologic complications accompany other manifestations of serum sickness.

Active immunization of patients with tetanus is necessary, because the disease does not confer natural immunity. However, there is no need to begin primary immunization until the patient has recovered.

Management of muscle spasms Muscle relaxation is the key to therapy, but mild sedation is desirable also because it reduces the effect of sensory stimuli. Ideally, this should be accomplished without significantly affecting respiration. Although a variety of agents have been used in the treatment of tetanus, none has achieved universal acceptance. Among the barbiturates, phenobarbital, in adult doses of 50 to 100 mg every 3 to 6 h, produces adequate sedation which may suffice in the management of mild tetanus. When rapid action is required, amylbarbital or pentobarbital, 50 to 200 mg intravenously, may be used. Frequent and severe spasms cannot be managed with barbiturates alone, because the dosage required

for control leads to unconsciousness and suppressed respiration. For this reason, muscle relaxants usually are used, either alone or in combination with barbiturates, in the treatment of moderate or severe tetanus. Electromyographic studies have shown that the phenothiazines effectively produce relaxation while sparing the sensorium and respirations. Chlorpromazine, in doses of 200 to 300 mg a day, minimizes rigidity and decreases the frequency of spasms. Diazepam, in adult doses of 40 to 120 mg a day, is very effective in the treatment of tetanus; it acts quickly, relieves rigidity, and has significant sedative effect without depressing respiration. Given alone to patients with moderately severe disease, diazepam has been shown to lower oxygen consumption from levels that are three to five times normal to near normal. In combination with other drugs, diazepam may significantly reduce mortality in nonneonates with severe tetanus. Other drugs which have been employed extensively include mephenesin, meprobamate, paraldehyde, and chloral hydrate.

Another approach to the management of muscle spasms involves the use of neuromuscular blocking agents such as tubocurare or pancuronium. This method can be used only where facilities and personnel are available to provide controlled mechanical ventilation for the paralyzed patient. It should be reserved for treatment of severe tetanus that is not adequately controlled by other measures. In centers with a team experienced in handling these patients, this approach, in conjunction with meticulous attention to other details of care, has produced encouraging results.

Tracheostomy Tracheostomy has an important role in the management of tetanus. It protects against suffocation due to laryngospasm, reduces the risk of aspiration, and facilitates mechanical assistance of ventilation. While most patients with mild tetanus and some with more severe disease can be managed without it, all patients should be considered candidates for tracheostomy, and the necessary equipment should be at the bedside. Where secretions are copious or respiration has been compromised, the need for tracheostomy should be recognized early, and whenever possible it should be performed electively rather than as an emergency.

Other measures Although antibiotics are frequently prescribed to treat the infected wound and prevent toxin production, there is no indication that they influence the disease favorably. If antibiotics are used, penicillin G is the drug of choice because it is highly effective against the tetanus bacillus, and its limited spectrum is less likely to predispose patients to superinfections. Appropriate cultures to detect complicating infections should be obtained periodically throughout the course of the disease, and specific antibiotics prescribed when indicated. Adrenocortical steroids have been used empirically in the treatment of tetanus, but there is no experimental or clinical evidence to support their effectiveness. Likewise, beneficial results have been claimed for hyperbaric oxygen, but insufficient information is available to evaluate its potential.

PREVENTION *Clostridium tetani* is so ubiquitous in nature that the only hope for prevention of tetanus lies in massive immunization programs. Effective active immunization is possible, and if applied universally, according to recommendations, tetanus could be virtually eliminated. Even tetanus neonatorum could be prevented, because infants are protected by antibody which passes the placental barrier. Two types of tetanus toxoids are available for immunization, a fluid and an adsorbed form. The adsorbed toxoid is preferred because it produces higher antitoxin titers and longer-lasting immunity. Immunization failures are exceedingly rare.

According to current recommendations, children 2 months to 6 years of age should be immunized with diphtheria and tetanus toxoids and pertussis vaccine (DPT). Ideally, the first dose should be administered within 2 or 3 months of birth, the second and third should follow at 4- to 6-week intervals, and the fourth dose should be given 1 year after the third. Schoolchildren and adults should be immunized with three doses of adult-type tetanus and diphtheria toxoids (Td). The second dose should be given 4 to 6 weeks after the first, and the third 6 months to 1 year after the second. A booster of DPT is recommended for children at the time of entrance into kindergarten or elementary school. Thereafter and for everyone else who has received a primary immunization series, routine boosters of Td should be given every 10 years. Side effects are uncommon after the primary series, but occur more frequently in persons who have received an excessive number of booster injections. Reactions usually take the form of local swelling, erythema, lymphadenopathy, and fever, but on rare occasions more severe hypersensitivity reactions occur.

In the management of wounds, the question of prophylaxis against tetanus frequently arises. Because active immunization is so effective, a reliable immunization history can greatly simplify the problem. If a patient has received three or more doses of toxoid, antiserum need not be given, and a toxoid booster is required only if more than 5 to 10 years has elapsed since the last dose. The shorter interval pertains for all but clean, minor wounds. In all other instances, the decision must be made on an individual basis, taking into consideration the characteristics of the wound, the conditions under which it was incurred, its age, and the patient's previous active immunization against tetanus. Table 139-1 provides guidelines which may be useful in making appropriate decisions about tetanus prophylaxis. For patients who have received fewer than two doses of toxoid, the primary immunization series should be completed in the succeeding weeks to months.

When passive immunization is contemplated, TIG is preferred to horse serum because it offers longer protection and freedom from serious reactions. The currently recommended prophylactic dose for adults is 250 units intramuscularly, which ensures a protective level of antitoxin in the plasma ($>$ 0.01 unit per milliliter) for as long as 4 weeks. If TIG is not available, equine antitoxin in doses of 3000 to 6000 units should be administered after careful screening for sensitivity to horse serum. When both toxoid and antitoxin are indicated, they can be given simultaneously, but separate syringes and separate injection sites should be used.

Prompt and adequate care of wounds is also important in preventing tetanus. They should be cleaned carefully, and foreign bodies or necrotic, devitalized tissue should be removed. Administration of tetracycline or penicillin is advocated by some to prevent multiplication of *C. tetani*, but tetanus may

occur in spite of prophylactic antibiotics, and their role in the prevention of tetanus has not been established. However, severe wounds should be examined regularly and treated promptly with antimicrobials if infection develops.

PROGNOSIS The overall case/fatality ratio of tetanus is variable, but in the United States it ranges between 40 and 60 percent. This reflects the fact that the incidence of tetanus is eight to ten times greater among people over 60 compared with people 10 to 20 years of age, and the mortality rate is 25 to 50 times greater in the elderly. Neonatal tetanus is uncommon in this country but is fatal in more than 60 percent of cases. The shorter the incubation period and onset time, the poorer the prognosis in tetanus. Three-fourths of the deaths occur within the first week, primarily from pulmonary infection, aspiration, or pulmonary embolization. Survivors recover completely, but remain susceptible to the disease unless actively immunized with tetanus toxoid.

REFERENCES

BLAKE PA et al: Serologic therapy of tetanus in the United States. JAMA 235:42, 1976

COCHLIN DL: Dystonic reactions due to metoclopramide and phenothiazines resembling tetanus. Br J Clin Pract 28:201, 1974

FURSTE W: Four keys to 100 percent success in tetanus prophylaxis. Am J Surg 128:616, 1974

———, WHEELER W: Tetanus: A team disease, in *Current Problems in Surgery.* Chicago, Year Book, 1972

TSUEDA K et al: Cardiovascular manifestations of tetanus. Anesthesiology 40:588, 1974

140
BOTULISM

HARRY N. BEATY
ROBERT W. GRAEBNER

DEFINITION Botulism is an acute form of poisoning which results from ingestion of a toxin produced by *Clostridium botulinum*. The illness is characterized by progressive descending muscle paralysis, and is often fatal.

HISTORY AND EPIDEMIOLOGY The disease was first recognized over 200 years ago by South German physicians who adopted the term *botulismus* for the often fatal syndrome which sometimes followed the consumption of spoiled sausage (*botulus* is Latin for sausage). Botulism was rare in the United States before World War I. The growth of commercial and home canning at this time led to a great increase in cases. A series of studies by K. F. Meyer and his associates in the early 1920s defined the habitat of *C. botulinum,* the foods often incriminated, and the conditions necessary for the destruction of *C. botulinum* spores. This knowledge led to the virtual elimination of botulism from the commercial canning industry, and most cases of clinical botulism now follow consumption of improperly canned, home-preserved foods. However, the need for constant surveillance is emphasized by periodic outbreaks of botulism caused by commercially processed foods. For example, in 1977, 59 people developed botulism after eating home-canned peppers in a restaurant in Pontiac, Michigan; and in 1978, 32 people manifested the disease after dining at a country club in Clovis, New Mexico. These are the largest outbreaks ever reported in the United States, and contrast sharply with the usual situation in which fewer than three individuals are affected after eating home-canned foods.

TABLE 139-1
Guidelines for tetanus prophylaxis

Active immunization	Toxoid	Antitoxin	
		Minor wound*	Other wounds
Uncertain	Yes	No	Yes
None	Yes	No	Yes
< 3 doses	Yes	No	Yes‡
≥ 3 doses	No†	No	No

* *Fresh, clean, minor wounds incurred in a setting unlikely to cause tetanus.*
† *Unless more than 10 years since last dose.*
‡ *Except in patients who have received at least two previous doses of toxoid and have fresh non-tetanus-prone wounds.*

ETIOLOGY *Clostridium botulinum* is a strictly anaerobic, spore-forming, gram-positive rod which elaborates a potent exotoxin during growth and autolysis. Morphologically and culturally similar strains are differentiated into types A, B, C, D, E, or F on the basis of antigenic characteristics of the toxin each produces. Type A, B, and E toxins have been implicated most frequently in human disease in the United States. Only two outbreaks of type F botulism have been reported. Types C and D produce disease almost exclusively in animals, including wild waterfowl, cattle, horses, and mink.

Type A and B spores are widely distributed in soil throughout the world. Type A spores are most common in the United States, especially along the Pacific Coast and the Rocky Mountain states. Type B spores have been found more frequently in the Eastern states and in Europe. Type E spores have been demonstrated in lakeshore mud, coastal sand, and sea-bottom silt in northern latitudes. Fish apparently contaminate their intestinal tracts with these spores, which accounts for the high incidence of type E strains in fish-borne botulism. Type F spores have been found in marine sediments collected off the coast of California and Oregon and in salmon taken from the Columbia River.

Botulinus toxins are the most potent poisons known. Types A through F have been purified and identified as simple proteins. Although they differ in terms of antigenicity, molecular size, electrophoretic mobility, and amino acid content, they appear to have a similar effect on neuromuscular transmission. Pharmacologic differences are manifested by the variable susceptibility of specific animal species to the different toxins.

Spores of *C. botulinum* can withstand 100°C for several hours. Moist heat at 120°C for 30 min will destroy spores of all types, but the toxins are considerably more heat-labile. All varieties of toxin are destroyed by boiling for 10 min, or by temperatures of 80°C for 30 min.

PATHOGENESIS Most human botulism follows the ingestion of foodstuffs contaminated with preformed botulinus toxin. Rarely, wounds infected with *C. botulinum* have been the portal of entry of the toxin. Until recently, there was convincing evidence that the botulinus bacillus produces toxin in the human gastrointestinal tract. That is still the case in adults, but the newly recognized syndrome of infant botulism results from ingestion of *C. botulinum* followed by sporulation and toxin production. Symptoms are slowly progressive because toxin is absorbed as it is produced rather than all at once, which is the case when toxin is ingested in contaminated food. Clinical botulism can occur when the following conditions are met: (1) a food product is contaminated with viable *C. botulinum* bacilli or spores; (2) proper conditions for germination of the spores exist; (3) time and conditions permit production of toxin before eating; (4) the food is not heated or is heated insufficiently to destroy botulinus toxin; and (5) the toxin-containing food is ingested by a susceptible host (Table 140-1). Though a relatively anaerobic environment and temperatures above 30°C (86°F) are optimal for toxin production, strict anaerobic conditions are not necessary and toxin production by some type E strains has been observed at temperatures as low as 6°C (42.8°F).

Although a variety of home-processed foods have been sources of botulism in the United States, certain foods seem to be safer than others. This may be because low pH (acidity) inhibits germination of spores and, therefore, toxin production. Commercially processed smoked fish, tuna, peppers, and soup (vichyssoise) have been implicated in outbreaks of botulism. Contaminated foods may appear putrefied, but frequently look and taste perfectly normal, regardless of toxin type. Honey has been proved to be the source of *C. botulinum* in a number of cases of infant botulism. This and the finding of botulinal organisms in a number of random samples of honey tested have led to the recommendation that honey not be fed to children less than 1 year old. None of the samples tested contained botulinus toxin, so honey remains a safe food for older children and adults.

Botulinus toxins are absorbed primarily in the stomach and upper part of the small intestine. The toxins are large protein molecules which are absorbed after they have been reduced in size by proteolytic enzymes which do not destroy activity. In fact, the toxicity of type E toxin may be enhanced by tryptic digestion. Either absorption is incomplete or toxins are inactivated partially by digestion, because the amount of toxin which appears in the bloodstream is variable, and in animals the lethal dose orally is 1000 times greater than the lethal dose intravenously. Toxin which reaches the lower part of the small intestine and colon may be absorbed slowly, which probably accounts for the delayed onset and the prolonged symptoms observed in many patients.

Botulinus toxins exert their major effect by blocking neuromuscular transmission in cholinergic nerve fibers. They either inhibit the release of acetylcholine or bind with it at or near its site of release within presynaptic clefts. Muscle reactivity to acetylcholine applied directly to the motor end plate is unimpaired. Central nervous system cholinergic pathways do not appear to be affected significantly in human beings.

CLINICAL MANIFESTATIONS Botulism may vary from a mild illness for which patients seek no medical advice to a fulminant disease which ends in death within 24 h. Symptoms usually begin 12 to 36 h after ingestion of toxin, although the extremes of 3 h to 14 days are recorded. In general, the earlier the symptoms appear, the more serious the disease.

The commonest symptoms are ocular; diplopia, blurred vision, and photophobia are frequently the first to appear. Bulbar weakness is manifested by dysphonia, dysarthria, dysphagia, and weakness of the tongue. Symmetric paralysis of the extremities appears, and may progress rapidly in a descending or ascending manner. Weakness of the respiratory muscles may occur early, but this is often asymptomatic until function is moderately impaired.

Impairment of cholinergic autonomic transmission may result in constipation, urinary retention, and reduced salivation and lacrimation. Nausea and vomiting are early symptoms in half the patients, but the absence of these symptoms does not rule out botulism. Gastrointestinal symptoms are more common in type B and E disease than in type A. Some patients with type B disease may have minimal weakness but marked constipation and decreased secretions.

TABLE 140-1
Important factors in the pathogenesis of botulism

SPORES

1 Survive at 6°C (42.8°F) for several months
2 Can withstand boiling for several hours
3 Destroyed at 120°C (248°F) after 30 min

TOXIN PRODUCTION

1 Strict anaerobic conditions not always required
2 Can occur at 6°C (42.8°F)
3 Optimal temperature 30°C (86°F)
4 Reduced at low pH

TOXIN

1 Destroyed at 80°C (176°F) after 30 min or 100°C for 10 min
2 Unstable at high pH
3 Type E toxin activated by trypsin

On examination patients are usually alert, oriented, and afebrile, even with severe disease. Ocular signs include ptosis, weakness of extraocular motion, and in some patients failure of accommodation. The pupils are normal in many patients, but in some cases may react sluggishly or may be dilated and unreactive to light. Widespread neuromuscular block results in symmetric flaccid weakness of the palate, tongue, larynx, respiratory muscles, and extremities. Severe paralytic ileus and bladder distention may be present. Deep-tendon reflexes are intact in milder cases, but if significant paralysis is present they are reduced or absent. No pathologic reflexes are detectable. Findings on sensory examination are always entirely normal. Some patients have apparent gait disturbances and incoordination, but this is due to generalized weakness.

Once symptoms are noted, the disease may progress rapidly over several days, with significant changes in status occurring at hourly intervals. A period of stabilization is then followed by gradual recovery over a period of days to months, depending on the severity of intoxication. The mechanism of recovery is not well understood. In wound botulism the patient may be febrile, but the clinical manifestations are otherwise similar. A 10- to 14-day incubation period is common from the time of infection to the onset of toxic symptoms. In the infant form of botulism, constipation is usually the first manifestation; slowly progressive weakness of skeletal muscles, poor feeding, and "floppiness" follow.

LABORATORY FINDINGS Routine laboratory studies do not aid in diagnosing botulism. When botulism is suspected, public health authorities should be consulted to assist in special studies to confirm the diagnosis. Specimens of blood, feces, and gastric contents, as well as suspected foods and their containers, should be obtained. Because of the extreme potency of botulinus toxin, careful collection and laboratory precautions should be used. The food, stool, and serum should be studied for the presence of toxin by injecting extracts intraperitoneally into mice. If toxin is present, the animals will develop botulism and die within 24 h. Mice protected by specific antiserum will survive. The food and stool should be submitted for special anaerobic culture. This battery of tests will result in an overall case recognition rate of about 85 percent. Immunofluorescent techniques are useful for the early recognition of the organisms. If wound botulism is suspected, the exudate should be submitted for culture and toxin analysis.

The spinal fluid is always normal. Electrocardiographic abnormalities, including minor disturbances in conduction, nonspecific T-wave and ST-segment changes, and various disorders of rhythm, have been described. Electrodiagnostic studies have been shown to be of value in differentiating botulism from other paralytic diseases. The evoked motor action potential may be of low voltage, but will facilitate with tetanic stimulation in a manner similar to the myasthenic syndrome (Eaton-Lambert syndrome). Electromyography may show small, short-duration, overly abundant motor units. In severe cases, denervation can occur, resulting in fibrillation activity after several weeks.

DIFFERENTIAL DIAGNOSIS Botulism must be differentiated from other conditions that produce generalized paralysis. In the Guillain-Barré syndrome, mild sensory abnormalities are nearly always present, and the spinal fluid protein is often elevated. The variant of the Guillain-Barré syndrome with ophthalmoplegia, areflexia, and ataxia (Fisher's syndrome) may prove particularly confusing. The course of myasthenia gravis is seldom so acute, and the deep tendon reflexes and pupils are normal. Some patients with botulism may show mild improvement after injection of edrophonium (Tensilon), but this im-

provement is not of the magnitude seen in myasthenia gravis. In tick paralysis the weakness is generally of an ascending pattern, patients may have paresthesias, and a tick is found. In diphtheria, palatal weakness is frequently the first symptom, and a history of prior pharyngitis may be obtained. Cutaneous diphtheria can be differentiated from wound botulism by appropriate cultures. In poliomyelitis the spinal fluid is abnormal and the weakness is often asymmetric and spares the ocular muscles. Vascular accidents of the brainstem can be recognized by associated neurologic signs. Belladonna poisoning presents with markedly dilated pupils and delirium. In organophosphate poisoning the pupils are markedly miotic. Shellfish poisoning, aminoglycoside antibiotic paralysis, and familial periodic paralysis might also prove confusing.

Patients with marked dry mouth may develop a picture simulating pharyngitis. Patients with gastrointestinal complaints and ileus may appear to have other forms of food poisoning or intestinal obstruction.

TREATMENT The most immediate threat to the survival of patients with botulism is respiratory failure. Patients with symptoms or known exposure should be hospitalized. Close observation is essential, and vital capacity should be measured frequently. If respiratory insufficiency develops, the patient may require assisted ventilation with a respirator. Respiratory difficulties may develop rapidly; elective tracheostomy should be performed before onset of respiratory failure, and may be needed to manage secretions even if ventilation is otherwise adequate. Some milder cases may be managed with endotracheal intubation.

If there is no ileus, cathartics and enemas should be given to remove unabsorbed toxin from the intestine, but magnesium citrate and magnesium sulfate should not be given, as the magnesium may potentiate the neuromuscular block produced by botulinus toxin. Nasogastric suction and intravenous hyperalimentation may be needed if ileus is severe. If the bladder is atonic a catheter will be required. Meticulous nursing care and physical therapy are essential to prevent complications.

As soon as the diagnosis of botulism is suspected, the patient should be tested for hypersensitivity to horse serum and treated with trivalent ABE antitoxin (Connaught), which is available from public health authorities. Type-specific antitoxin has been shown to be of benefit in several outbreaks of type E intoxication, but the value in type A and B outbreaks is less certain, particularly when paralysis has already occurred. Nonfatal hypersensitivity reactions occur in 15 to 20 percent of patients receiving the equine antitoxin, and those that react to a test dose must be desensitized prior to further treatment.

Because there is little evidence that *C. botulinum* can multiply in the gastrointestinal tract of adults, antibiotics should be reserved for specific infectious complications. In infant botulism, where multiplication of ingested organisms may be a factor, antibiotics have been ineffective in eradicating the organism, though this eventually may occur spontaneously. The value of antibiotic therapy in wound botulism has not been determined. It is essential that public health officials be notified so that toxin-containing foods can be confiscated and so that those with possible exposure can be notified.

A number of reports have appeared since 1967 describing the use of guanidine hydrochloride in the treatment of botulism. This drug presumably acts by enhancing the release of acetylcholine from terminal nerve fibers. About two-thirds of the reported cases have shown some improvement with oral doses of 15 to 50 mg/kg per day, but the drug seems ineffective in those patients with severe respiratory impairment, and probably has no effect on mortality rate. Dose-related side effects include gastrointestinal upset, paresthesias, and fasciculations. Idiosyncratic reactions include cardiac arrhythmias and blood dyscrasias.

PROGNOSIS The current mortality rate of botulism in the United States is about 10 percent, with type A outbreaks having somewhat higher mortality than types B and E. Death is due to complications such as respiratory failure and pneumonia. With rapid diagnosis and aggressive supportive care, even severely involved patients can recover fully. Some patients may have mild residual weakness due to denervation atrophy. Artificial respiratory support may be required for many months, and clinical weakness and autonomic symptoms may be noted for as long as 1 year after the onset of disease.

REFERENCES

ARNON SS et al: Infant botulism: Epidemiological, clinical, and laboratory aspects. JAMA 237:1946, 1977

BLACK RE, ARNON SS: Botulism in the United States, 1976. J Infect Dis 135:829, 1977

CENTER FOR DISEASE CONTROL: *Botulism in the United States, 1899-1973. Handbook for Epidemiologists, Clinicians, and Laboratory Workers.* June 1974

CHERINGTON M: Botulism: Ten-year experience. Arch Neurol 30:432, 1974

DOWELL VR et al: Coproexamination for botulinal toxin and *Clostridium botulinum:* A new procedure for laboratory diagnosis of botulism. JAMA 238:1829, 1977

FAICH GA et al: Failure of guanidine therapy in botulism A. N Engl J Med 285:773, 1971

KOENIG MC et al: Type B botulism in man. Am J Med 42:208, 1967

MERSON MH, DOWELL VR: Epidemiologic, clinical and laboratory aspects of wound botulism. N Engl J Med 289:1005, 1973

WERNER SB, CHIN J: Botulism—diagnosis, management and public health considerations. Calif Med 118:84, 1973

141
OTHER CLOSTRIDIAL INFECTIONS

EDWARD W. HOOK
MERLE A. SANDE

INTRODUCTION Bacteria of the genus *Clostridium* are normal inhabitants of soil and the gastrointestinal tracts of humans and animals. Most of the species that have been described are saprophytic, but some are pathogenic for humans and animals, usually under conditions of lowered host and tissue resistance. Infections with these organisms are often associated with profound systemic manifestations, and all pathogenic clostridia, except *C. tetani* and *C. botulinum,* are capable of causing extensive tissue destruction. Diseases caused by these other clostridia are gas gangrene, cellulitis, postabortal and puerperal sepsis, and, on occasion, pneumonia, empyema, peritonitis, meningitis, endocarditis, osteomyelitis, and arthritis. Ingestion of food contaminated with *C. perfringens* type A is a common cause of enterocolitis, and *C. difficile* has recently been implicated in antibiotic-induced (clindamycin) pseudomembranous colitis.

ETIOLOGY Wounds complicated by gas gangrene usually contain a mixture of pathogenic and saprophytic clostridia, often including *C. tetani,* as well as a variety of other bacteria. *Clostridium perfringens,* the most common, *C. novyi,* or *C. septicum* can be cultured from most cases of gas gangrene and clostridial cellulitis, and *C. perfringens* causes virtually all clostridial infections of the uterus. *Clostridium bifermentans, C. histolyticum,* and *C. fallax* are less virulent organisms that occasionally cause gas gangrene but are more commonly associated with localized cellulitis. Proliferation of *C. botulinum* in wounds occasionally leads to clinical manifestations of botulism (Chap. 140).

The clostridia of gas gangrene and related infections are anaerobic or microaerophilic gram-positive bacilli that produce abundant gas in artificial media and form subterminal endospores. *Clostridium perfringens* is encapsulated and nonmotile, rarely sporulates in artificial media, and produces spores that can usually be destroyed by boiling.

Clostridium difficile has been isolated in large numbers from stools of patients with antibiotic-associated pseudomembranous colitis. This organism produces a toxin that is destructive to the intestinal mucosa and is usually resistant to clindamycin, the antibiotic most commonly implicated in enterocolitis.

EPIDEMIOLOGY AND PATHOGENESIS Clostridia can be cultured from one-third to two-thirds of severe traumatic wounds, but gas gangrene develops in only an occasional case. The most important prerequisite for the conversion of clostridial contamination of a wound to a progressive infection is an environment with low oxidation-reduction potential, which permits spore germination and anaerobic growth. Local oxidation-reduction potential can be reduced by failure of the blood supply to a contaminated area, by the presence of foreign bodies such as clothing, soil, or fragments of metal or wood, or by the multiplication of other bacteria in the wound. Once multiplication and toxin production are established, rapid invasion and destruction of healthy tissue follow.

The pathogenicity of clostridia is related to the capacity of these organisms to form exotoxins which destroy tissue cells. The nature and amount of toxins vary considerably for different species and strains. For example, at least 12 different extracellular *toxins* are produced by *C. perfringens.* Alpha toxin, a lecithinase, is clearly the most important and is the principal tissue-destroying, hemolytic, and lethal toxin. Other *C. perfringens* products include collagenase, hyaluronidase, hemolytic theta toxin, leukocidin, deoxyribonuclease, and fibrinolysin.

Gas gangrene is characterized by marked systemic symptoms and a local reaction with extensive necrotizing myositis, edema, thrombosis of small vessels, interstitial gas bubbles, and minimal infiltration by leukocytes. The local reaction in infected tissue can be explained by the action of clostridial toxins, especially alpha toxin, but the factors responsible for the systemic reaction are unknown. Alpha toxin, or other clostridial toxins, have not been demonstrated in circulating blood during the course of severe clostridial myonecrosis.

The toxin responsible for antibiotic-associated pseudomembranous colitis has not been completely characterized. It is found in high titer in cell-free filtrates of feces from patients with this disease. The toxin is produced by *C. difficile* which is usually resistant to clindamycin and proliferates in the colon when the antibiotic-sensitive flora is suppressed. The toxin is heat-labile and cytopathic for certain cells in culture, and it produces an increase in vascular permeability and hemorrhage after injection intradermally in rabbits. Pseudomembranous colitis can be produced by introducing the toxin or the organism into the cecum of hamsters or by treating hamsters with clindamycin. The toxic effects can be blocked by either gas-gangrene equine antitoxin or *C. sordellii* antitoxin; the latter has been shown to cross-react with toxin produced by *C. difficile.*

CLINICAL MANIFESTATIONS Clostridial myonecrosis (gas gangrene, clostridial myositis) Gas gangrene develops in anoxic devitalized tissues in which the arterial circulation has been compromised by trauma, constricting tourniquets or casts, or obliterative arterial disease. Infection is most frequent after extensive injury to skeletal muscle, particularly of the thigh and buttock, and is more common in wounds complicated by compound fractures or lodgment of foreign bodies. It may also follow surgical procedures, especially those involving the large bowel and rectum; amputation of ischemic limbs; and reconstructive surgery of the hip. Gas gangrene has also been described following intramuscular injection, especially injection of epinephrine. Minor trauma also occasionally activates clostridial spores dormant in scar tissue and leads to development of myonecrosis years after original injury. Once infection is established, it rapidly spreads to involve healthy muscle undamaged by previous trauma or ischemia.

The incubation period is usually 1 to 4 days but may vary from 3 h to 6 weeks or longer. The earliest symptom is sudden, severe pain in the injured part which may develop an intense "woody hard" edema. The distal portion of an involved limb becomes cold and edematous within a few hours, and eventually pulseless and gangrenous. The wound drains a watery, brown, or hemorrhagic material which may have a peculiar sweet odor. The appearance of the wound is usually not that of a pyogenic inflammatory lesion. Depending on the duration of the process, the surrounding skin may be normal, white, and tense, or dusky brown and reddish. Vesicles or hemorrhagic bullae may develop, particularly in *C. septicum* infections. Gas is usually not detectable in the tissues by palpation except in advanced lesions, although it may be visible easily by x-ray. Occasionally, tiny bubbles may be seen in the discharge from the wound; rarely, crepitation can be detected at an early stage by auscultation. The involved muscle appears dark red or black, may herniate through the wound, and is noncontractile when stimulated.

Systemic manifestations developing shortly after onset of severe pain and swelling of an injured extremity strongly suggest gas gangrene. The patient is prostrated, pale, and motionless but is usually well oriented, alert, and extremely apprehensive. The temperature usually does not exceed 38.3°C (101°F) and may be normal. As the illness progresses, there may be anorexia, vomiting, profuse watery or bloody diarrhea, and eventually circulatory collapse. The pulse rate usually exceeds 120 beats per minute and is elevated out of proportion to the temperature. Massive intravascular hemolysis is rare in patients with clostridial myositis. Pericardial effusion is sometimes noted. Delirium and coma may precede death, but more commonly the patient dies suddenly several days after onset of illness, often during surgery or anesthesia. Acute renal failure is occasionally a late complication.

Gas gangrene must be differentiated from nonclostridial infections of gangrenous limbs caused by anaerobic streptococci, aerobic gas-forming coliform bacilli (most commonly *Escherichia coli*), *Bacteroides* species, and group A streptococci.

Clostridial cellulitis This is a relatively benign infection of skin and subcutaneous tissues that occurs in a small proportion of wounds contaminated with pathogenic clostridia. The disease is characterized by spreading necrosis of superficial tissues and a profuse, foul-smelling, brown, seropurulent exudate. Gas, which crepitates on palpation, invariably forms in the subcutaneous tissues and may involve an entire limb or form a localized gas pocket. In clostridial cellulitis, the underlying skeletal muscle is not involved, pain is not severe, and the only systemic manifestations are slight fever and moderate tachycardia. It can usually be differentiated from group A streptococcal cellulitis by the presence of subcutaneous gas and the absence of erythema.

Postabortal and puerperal sepsis Uterine infections with *C. perfringens* usually occur after incomplete abortions induced under unsterile conditions and occasionally after spontaneous abortions, prolonged labor at term, ruptured membranes, or operative interference with pregnancy. The organisms presumably invade the damaged endometrium through the retained products of conception. The earliest symptoms may be related to instrumentation and consist of metrorrhagia, suprapubic and back pain, chills, and fever. Fever of 37.8 to 39.4°C (100 to 103°F), often with chills, usually recurs several days after abortion, but the incubation period can be as short as 6 h. Vaginal bleeding is almost invariably present, and there is often a brown, foul-smelling, vaginal discharge containing necrotic tissue. The cervix is soft and patulous, and the uterus and adnexae are usually very tender. The lower abdominal wall is often tense, or signs of generalized peritonitis may be present, secondary to perforation of the uterus or parametrial extension of infection. Nausea, vomiting, and profuse diarrhea are often prominent.

Systemic manifestations may appear with dramatic suddenness. Massive intravascular hemolysis, accompanied by hemoglobinemia, hemoglobinuria, and jaundice, may be the most striking feature of the disease. Icterus may appear within hours after onset of illness. As in gas gangrene, the clinical picture may be dominated by circulatory collapse with hypotension, extreme tachycardia, cyanosis, hyperpnea, and pulmonary edema. Despite severe prostration, the patient is frequently well oriented, alert, and apprehensive. The mortality rate in postabortal or puerperal sepsis caused by *C. perfringens* and associated with intense hemolysis is 40 to 70 percent. Death may occur a few hours after onset or may be delayed for days. Acute renal failure secondary to shock, dehydration, or hemolysis occurs frequently.

Unusual local complications of uterine infection are gas gangrene of the vagina and rectum and clostridial cellulitis of the anterior abdominal wall following cesarean section or hysterectomy. At times, the infectious process is confined to the endometrium and myometrium with intrauterine gas formation (physometra).

Septic abortion with *C. perfringens* bacteremia without overt hemolysis is a more common occurrence than bacteremia with gross hemolysis, as described above. Death is unusual in the absence of hemolysis.

Diseases to be considered in the *differential diagnosis* include perforated uterus, ruptured ectopic pregnancy, ingestion of toxic abortifacients, septic endometritis caused by aerobic or anaerobic streptococci, enteric bacilli or other microorganisms, pelvic thrombophlebitis with septic pulmonary emboli, acute hepatic necrosis of pregnancy, and sickle-cell crisis.

***Clostridium perfringens* food poisoning** Meat and meat products contaminated with *C. perfringens* type A are frequently responsible for outbreaks of acute gastroenteritis. In 1976 in the United States, *C. perfringens* accounted for 14.2 percent of cases in reported foodborne outbreaks.

Most outbreaks of *C. perfringens* food poisoning have been associated with the ingestion of meat or poultry dishes. Most market meats and poultry are heavily contaminated, and the organism can be isolated with ease from soil, water, air, and human or animal feces. The usual story is that the food has been prepared and cooked 24 h or more before consumption, allowed to cool slowly at room temperature, and then served either cold or warmed. During this period of incubation, contaminating spores which have survived cooking germinate, and clostridia grow to large numbers sufficient to constitute an infectious inoculum. *Clostridium perfringens* food poisoning can be reproduced experimentally in humans by feeding the actively growing organisms which apparently multiply and sporulate in the small intestine. Sporulation is associated with the production of an enterotoxin in situ.

Typical symptoms of diarrhea with abdominal pain and cramps develop 6 to 24 h after ingestion of meat (especially beef and poultry), stew, or soup which has been stored at a warm temperature for several hours after cooking. Nausea occurs occasionally, but vomiting is rare. Systemic manifestations are usually absent, and recovery is uneventful after 12 to 24 h.

A severe form of clostridial infection termed *enteritis necrotans* was observed in Germany after World War II. This disease was characterized by hemorrhagic necrosis of the small intestine, bloody diarrhea, severe dehydration, shock, and death. A similar infection termed *necrotizing jejunitis* has been described in natives of New Guinea who had eaten inadequately cooked pork.

Antibiotic-associated colitis Diarrhea has been reported in up to 20 percent of patients receiving clindamycin. In one study up to one-half of these patients were found to have evidence of pseudomembranous colitis on proctoscopic examination although the usual rate is much less. *Clostridium difficile* has been implicated as the etiologic agent, but whether this organism accounts for all or only a portion of the cases has not been established. Symptoms of cramping, lower abdominal pain, fever, and diarrhea are common. Fever and cramps precede or coincide with the onset of diarrhea which usually develops between the fourth and ninth days of clindamycin therapy. In some cases, colitis develops within 5 days after discontinuation of the drug. The diarrhea is usually watery but rarely bloody. The symptoms usually subside within a week after administration of clindamycin is discontinued; however, the diarrhea may become protracted, lasting up to 2 to 4 weeks especially if administration of the drug is continued. In patients with severe protracted diarrhea, electrolyte imbalance, protein loss, and death may occur, especially in patients with significant underlying disease. Patients with pseudomembranous colitis occasionally will have associated abdominal tenderness with rebound and leukocytosis. Toxic megacolon is a rare complication. Although clindamycin has received the most attention, other antibiotics such as lincomycin, ampicillin, cephalexin, tetracyclines, and chloramphenicol also produce diarrhea and have been implicated as a cause of pseudomembranous colitis. The role of clostridia in diarrheal disease associated with these agents has not been completely defined, although the *C. difficile* toxin has been found in ampicillin-associated colitis.

Miscellaneous clostridial infections Clostridia can be isolated from bile obtained at elective cholecystectomy in patients without symptoms of clostridial infection. Clostridial cellulitis or myonecrosis may occasionally follow surgical procedures, particularly surgery on the gastrointestinal tract or gallbladder. Pathogenic clostridia are occasionally introduced into the abdomen, thoracic cavity, or cranium through penetrating wounds. Primary pneumonia in the absence of a penetrating wound or distant focus has been described. Clostridial pleurisy may involve the underlying lung but is usually an indolent localized infection with minimal systemic manifestations. Meningitis is usually secondary to a puncture wound of the skull and is often associated with a necrotizing cerebritis. Clostridial peritonitis may occur spontaneously but usually follows perforation of the gallbladder, appendix, or other viscus and is usually rapidly fatal.

Clostridial septicemia also develops occasionally in patients with aplastic anemia or far-advanced neoplastic disease, including leukemias, lymphomas, and metastatic solid tumors. Over two-thirds of these patients have been receiving antineo-

plastic chemotherapy or radiation therapy. The primary site of invasion is usually the gastrointestinal tract which is frequently extensively involved by the neoplastic process. Abdominal surgical procedures, endoscopy, small-bowel series, and paracentesis have been reported to predispose to sepsis in these patients. The course of the disease is rapid, death often occurring within 24 h after onset of recognizable infection. Hypotension, hyperpyrexia, and dyspnea are the most common clinical manifestations. Jaundice and hemolysis occur occasionally. Cellulitis, with or without crepitation, may appear in the flanks and should suggest the diagnosis, especially in patients with leukemia or lymphoma.

Cystitis with pneumaturia, gaseous cholecystitis, endocarditis, osteomyelitis, arthritis, and bursitis after needle aspiration are other examples of rare clostridial infections.

LABORATORY FINDINGS The diagnosis of gas gangrene, clostridial cellulitis, postabortal sepsis, or other clostridial infections is based primarily on clinical criteria. Smears of wound exudate, uterine scrapings, or cervical discharge may show abundant large gram-positive rods, as well as other organisms. Spores are rarely observed in smears of exudates. Thioglycollate broth, deep meat broth, and blood-agar plates incubated in an anaerobic jar should be inoculated for definitive identification of specific clostridia. However, interpretation of positive wound cultures is difficult because clostridia are frequent contaminants. *Clostridium perfringens* bacteremia is common in postabortal infections but rare in gas gangrene.

Polymorphonuclear leukocytosis occurs frequently in gas gangrene and invariably in postabortal sepsis; total blood leukocyte counts range from 15,000 to 40,000 cells per cubic millimeter and occasionally exceed 60,000 cells per cubic millimeter. Marked thrombocytopenia develops in about 50 percent of patients with clostridial sepsis. The urine frequently contains protein and casts. Renal insufficiency may lead to severe uremia.

X-ray examination sometimes provides the first clue leading to the correct diagnosis by revealing the presence of gas in muscle, subcutaneous tissue, or uterus; however, demonstration of gas in tissues is not diagnostic of clostridial infection. Other bacteria, especially *Enterobacter* and *Escherichia*, may be responsible for gas production, and occasionally air is sucked into a wound at the time of penetrating injury.

Profound alterations of circulating erythrocytes are common in postabortal sepsis but are much less frequent in other clostridial infection. Hemolytic anemia may develop with almost unbelievable rapidity; the red blood cell count occasionally decreases by 2 million cells per cubic millimeter in less than 24 h and is associated with hemoglobinemia, hemoglobinuria, and elevated levels of serum bilirubin. Spherocytosis, increased osmotic and mechanical red blood cell fragility, erythrophagocytosis, and methemoglobinemia have also been described. Abnormalities of the clotting mechanism characteristic of intravascular coagulation may be observed in patients with severe clostridial infections.

The diagnosis of antibiotic-associated pseudomembranous colitis is established by proctoscopy, which shows raised yellow-whitish plaques that cover an erythematous edematous base. The membrane is composed of mucus, fibrin, desquamated epithelial cells, and polymorphonuclear leukocytes. The radiographic findings on plain films of the abdomen are of thickened and distorted haustra, generalized thickening of the colonic wall, "thumbprinting," small marginal irregularities (representing the pseudomembranous plaque), and total colonic involvement. The small bowel is usually not involved. Barium enema is not recommended in patients suspected to have colitis because of the possible association with toxic megacolon.

TREATMENT The traditional therapeutic approach to serious clostridial infection, such as diffuse, spreading myositis, is immediate surgical intervention with wide radical debridement followed by open drainage without closure or open amputation when necessary. Early surgery not only aids diagnosis, but permits decompression of fascial compartments and excision of devitalized muscle and may obviate amputation. A number of authorities feel that hyperbaric oxygen therapy has modified this traditional approach to gas gangrene by assuming priority over radical surgical debridement. Proponents report that hyperbaric oxygenation produces impressive, almost immediate improvement in patients with gas gangrene, with rapid disappearance of systemic toxicity and prompt arrest of local spread of the gangrenous infection. Opinions differ about whether conservative debridement should be carried out before or after hyperbaric oxygen therapy. Advocates emphasize that a single 90-min compression treatment frequently results in a clear-cut demarcation between healthy and devitalized tissue and aids in the surgical debridement. Hyperbaric oxygen alone is not adequate therapy for gas gangrene. Oxygen toxicity consequent to hyperbaric oxygenation has lead to convulsions in some patients.

Curettage of the uterus should be performed for diagnosis and treatment of postabortal clostridial infections. In the absence of hemolysis, standard therapy for septic abortion with antibiotics and uterine curettage usually produces rapid improvement, even in patients with bacteremia. The mortality rate in patients with abortion, *C. perfringens* bacteremia, and intense hemolysis is high irrespective of the therapeutic approach. The role of hysterectomy is controversial and ill-defined; some surgeons strongly advocate hysterectomy, whereas others feel that the potential benefits of the procedure do not outweigh the risks. Heparinization, exchange transfusion, and hyperbaric oxygen have been utilized but are not of established benefit.

Simple excision and adequate drainage usually suffice for treating clostridial cellulitis.

Penicillin is the antibiotic of choice for most clostridial infections and should be administered in doses of 20 million units a day by continuous intravenous infusion. Cephalosporins and chloramphenicol are also active against most strains of *Clostridium,* and either may be used as an alternative to penicillin in patients with hypersensitivity. Clostridial myonecrosis has developed while patients were receiving cephalothin (2 to 6 g intravenously daily) for prophylaxis, and only high doses (8 to 12 g intravenously daily) are recommended for treatment. Clostridia are also generally, but not universally, susceptible in vitro to carbenicillin, clindamycin, doxycycline, minocycline, and tetracycline.

The efficacy of polyvalent gas gangrene antitoxin is controversial. Most centers have discontinued the use of antitoxin in the management of patients with suspected gas gangrene or clostridial postabortal sepsis because of questionable efficacy and the risk of hypersensitivity reactions. At the present time this antitoxin is not being produced in the United States.

Intravenous infusions of blood, plasma volume expanders, fluids, and electrolytes are required to combat shock, anemia, and dehydration. Renal insufficiency should be treated in the same manner as acute tubular necrosis from other causes.

The most reliable protection against gas gangrene is early and adequate wound debridement. Antitoxin is ineffective as a prophylactic agent. The use of clostridial toxoids for prophylactic immunization of individuals in hazardous occupations awaits evaluation.

Therapy of antibiotic-associated pseudomembranous colitis includes immediate discontinuation of the antibiotic, and intravenous fluid to maintain an adequate intravascular volume and electrolyte balance. Vancomycin by the oral route has been effective in eradicating the experimental infection in hamsters. Treatment with vancomycin 500 mg orally every 6 h also appears to be beneficial in stopping the diarrhea in humans.

REFERENCES

BARTLETT JG et al: Antibiotic-associated pseudomembranous colitis due to toxin-producing clostridia. N Engl J Med 298:531, 1978

DARKE SG et al: Gas gangrene and related infection. Br J Surg 64:104, 1977

HOLLAND JA et al: Experimental and clinical experience with hyperbaric oxygen in the treatment of clostridial myonecrosis. Surgery 77:75, 1975

MACLENNAN JD: The histotoxic clostridial infections of man. Bacteriol Rev 26:177, 1962

MAHN E, DANTUONO LM: Postabortal septicotoxemia due to *Clostridium welchii:* Seventy-five cases from the maternity hospital, Santiago, Chile. 1948-1952. Am J Obstet Gynecol 70:604, 1955

MURREL TGC et al: Pig-bel: Enteritis necroticans: A study in diagnosis and management. Lancet 1:217, 1966

NAKAMURA M, SCHULZE JA: *Clostridium perfringens* food poisoning. Annu Rev Microbiol 24:359, 1970

PRITCHARD JA, WHALLEY PJ: Abortion complicated by *Clostridium perfringens* infection. Am J Obstet Gynecol 111:484, 1971

RIFKIN GD et al: Antibiotic-induced colitis: Implication of a toxin neutralized by *Clostridium sordellii* antitoxin. Lancet 2:1103, 1977

TEDESCO RJ: Clindamycin and colitis: A review. J Infect Dis 135S:S95, 1977

WEINSTEIN L, BARZA MA: Gas gangrene. N Engl J Med 289:1129, 1973

WYNE JW, ARMSTRONG D: Clostridial septicemia. Cancer 29:215, 1972

142
INFECTIONS DUE TO MIXED ANAEROBIC ORGANISMS

LAWRENCE L. PELLETIER, JR.

Anaerobic bacteria require conditions of reduced oxygen tension and low redox potential for growth. Anaerobes constitute the predominant normal flora on the skin and mucous membranes of humans and outnumber aerobic bacteria 1000 to 1 in the colon and 10 to 1 on the skin, mouth, and vagina. On body surfaces, anaerobic bacteria often coexist with other anaerobic species and aerobic and facultative organisms in poorly understood symbiotic relationships. Any site in the body is susceptible to infection by these endogenous organisms when skin and mucous membrane barriers are compromised by surgery, trauma, or tumor, and when local tissue redox potentials are reduced by ischemia, necrosis, or infection. Multiple species of anaerobic, facultative, or aerobic organisms are often present in infection, and their synergistic interaction is required for pathogenicity. Mixed anaerobic infections frequently cause dental abscess, chronic otitis media and sinusitis, brain abscess, subdural empyema, otogenic meningitis, necrotizing gingivitis, Ludwig's angina, aspiration pneumonia, lung abscess, thoracic empyema, liver abscess, pylephlebitis, peritonitis, intraabdominal abscesses, endometritis, tuboovarian abscess, pelvic cellulitis, gangrene, postsurgical wound infection, perirectal abscess, and human bite infections.

Botulism (Chap. 140), tetanus (Chap. 139), clostridial myonecrosis (Chap. 141), and actinomycosis (Chap. 151) are discussed elsewhere.

ETIOLOGY Because most mixed anaerobic infections develop from normal host flora associated with adjacent mucosal membranes, knowledge of the predominant bacteria at different sites and the pathogenicity of these organisms may permit the selection of appropriate therapy before the results of cultures are available. Advances in culture techniques and methods of microbial identification have clarified the taxonomic classification of anaerobic organisms and the relative pathogenicity of some species in mixed anaerobic infection, but the relative importance of many organisms that participate in mixed infections needs to be established. Certain organisms such as *Vibrio* spp., spirochetes, anaerobic gram-negative cocci, or very oxygen-labile anaerobes that may be seen in stains of clinical material or isolated from culture are not virulent in experimental infections. Formerly, many mixed anaerobic infections of the pharynx, lung, and genital tract were classified as fusospirochetal infections because fusobacteria and spirochetes were seen on stains of material from the lesions. Since spirochetes are not pathogenic and many other species of anaerobes and aerobes have been isolated from infected sites, it is more appropriate to term these infections as mixed anaerobic infections.

Lest normal flora be discounted as undesirable, it should be recognized that normal anaerobic flora play critical roles in protecting against both colonization and infection with pathogenic microorganisms and overgrowth of potentially pathogenic endogenous organisms. Administration of clindamycin or other antimicrobials that suppress the majority of anaerobic colon bacteria may be complicated by the overgrowth of clindamycin-resistant *Clostridia difficile*, which produces toxins that may damage colonic mucosa and cause pseudomembranous colitis (Chap. 141). Likewise, antibiotic suppression of normal flora may predispose to oropharyngeal or perianal symptomatic *Candida* spp. infection (thrush) (Chap. 158) or prolonged carriage of *Salmonella* spp. in the gut.

The functions of anaerobic gastrointestinal flora in health and disease are poorly understood, but it is known that vitamin K synthesis by *Escherichia coli* and *Bacteroides fragilis* in the gut represent important sources of this essential vitamin. *Bacteroides fragilis* and other organisms deconjugate bile acids in the intestine, permitting their reabsorption in the distal ileum and maintaining the bile acid pool. Alterations in the microbial flora in relation to diet may predispose to the development of carcinoma of the colon and to altered metabolism of dietary chemicals and orally administered drugs. Because of both the complexity of the flora and problems in sampling it, knowledge of this area of normal bacterial physiology is scanty, and it is a fertile area for future investigation.

The major anaerobic pathogens from clinical material include (1) gram-negative bacilli (*B. fragilis, B. melaninogenicus, Fusobacterium nucleatum, F. varium, F. necrophorum,* and *F. mortiferum*), (2) gram-positive cocci (*Peptostreptococcus* spp., *Peptococcus* spp., microaerophilic cocci, and streptococci), (3) gram-positive spore-forming bacilli (*Clostridia* spp.), and (4) gram-positive nonsporulating bacilli (*Actinomyces* spp., *Arachina* spp., *Eubacterium* spp., and *Bifidobacterium eriksonii*).

Anaerobic gram-negative bacilli and anaerobic gram-positive cocci are the most commonly isolated anaerobes from clinical infections; *B. fragilis* is the most frequently isolated species. Microaerophilic cocci and streptococci that require reduced oxygen tension and the presence of carbon dioxide for growth are facultative rather than true anaerobic bacteria. *Clostridia* spp. or *Actinomyces* spp. may produce disease as single pathogens or as one organism among many in mixed infections. Anaerobes should be considered significant pathogens when isolated from body fluids or tissues that are normally sterile, or from infected sites where they are repeatedly isolated in high concentrations when measures have been taken to reduce or eliminate contamination by normal flora.

Table 142-1 lists aerobic and anaerobic organisms constituting normal skin and mucosal flora that are potential pathogens. Normal skin flora include anaerobic *Propionibacterium acnes*, a common blood culture contaminant that produces significant infections only in association with a foreign body such as a prosthetic heart valve or cerebral spinal fluid shunts. Anaerobic gram-negative bacilli, e.g., *C. perfringens,* and other anaerobes may be transient skin flora of the perineum and lower extremities and may cause mixed anaerobic infection of decubitus, ischemic, or diabetic ulcers.

Organisms in the oropharynx may play a role in local disease or be involved in pleuropulmonary infections following aspiration of oropharyngeal secretions. Hospitalized patients have a higher frequency of colonization with aerobic coliform bacilli or *S. aureus*, and anaerobes play a greater role in aspiration pneumonias occurring outside the hospital.

Multiple aerobic and anaerobic pathogens are encountered in infections of the abdomen and female genital tract. All potential pathogens isolated from abdominal and genital tract infections should be considered significant with the possible exception of enterococci encountered in abscesses and soft tissue infections.

EPIDEMIOLOGY Mixed anaerobic infections are frequently encountered in hospitals with active surgical, trauma, and obstetrics and gynecologic services. No reliable data are available to establish the true incidence and prevalence of mixed anaer-

TABLE 142-1
Potential pathogens that constitute normal flora at different body sites

	Anaerobes	Aerobes
Skin	Gram-positive cocci *Eubacterium* spp.	*S. epidermidis* *S. aureus* *C. albicans* *S. pyogenes*
Pharynx	*B. melaninogenicus* *Fusobacterium* spp. Gram-positive cocci *Actinomyces* spp. *Bifidobacterium* spp. *Eubacterium* spp.	*Pneumococcus* *S. aureus* *S. pyogenes* *H. influenzae* *S. viridans* *K. pneumoniae* *Meningococcus* Gram-negative coliform bacilli *C. albicans*
Colon	*B. fragilis* *B. melaninogenicus* Gram-positive cocci *Clostridium* spp. *Bifidobacterium* spp. *Eubacterium* spp. *Fusobacterium* spp.	Gram-negative coliform bacilli *Achromobacter* spp. *Enterococcus* *P. aeruginosa* *S. viridans* *S. aureus*
Vagina	*B. fragilis* *B. melaninogenicus* Gram-positive cocci *Bifidobacterium* spp. *Clostridium* spp. *Eubacterium* spp. *Fusobacterium* spp.	Gram-negative coliform bacilli *Enterococcus* spp. *C. vaginalis* *Mycoplasma* spp. *C. albicans* *S. viridans*

obic infections. The lack of appropriate cultures, the submission of cultures contaminated by anaerobes from normal flora, and the lack, until recently, of reliable culture techniques have made accurate sampling of infectious anaerobes impossible. Anaerobic bacteria, predominately *B. fragilis* and anaerobic cocci, constitute 8 to 11 percent of blood culture isolates in many centers, and anaerobes have been isolated from 10 to 54 percent of clinical cultures.

PATHOGENESIS Anaerobes generally are not highly invasive; infection is usually secondary to an underlying disease, surgical procedure, or therapy which impairs the normal defenses of the host. These organisms utilize substances other than oxygen as the final electron acceptor in reactions which generate energy, and will grow only in an environment with a low redox potential. Healthy, well-vascularized tissue has a relatively high redox potential and will not support growth of anaerobes. Conditions that significantly lower redox potential, such as impairment of blood supply, tissue necrosis, or growth of aerobic bacteria, are necessary to create an environment conducive to proliferation of anaerobes. Infections, therefore, frequently occur secondary to vascular disease, trauma, surgery, a perforated viscus, shock, aspiration, intramuscular epinephrine injections, or malignancy.

Obligate anaerobes generally do not possess catalase or superoxide dismutase enzymes to protect them from peroxides that form in oxygenated surroundings. However, if the redox potential is low, many species can exist in sites that are well oxygenated, such as the mouth. Pathogenic anaerobic species tend to be more resistant to oxygen exposure than nonpathogenic strains.

Anaerobes involved in local infections originating from mucosal surfaces in the mouth, intestinal tract, or vagina may form pseudomembranes on mucosal surfaces. spreading gangrene from a site of trauma or a localized abscess. The characteristic foul odor of anaerobic lesions is caused by certain metabolic end products of bacterial origin, primarily short-chain fatty acids and volatile amines. Many species of anaerobes produce collagenases and proteinases that account for the propensity for abscess formation. Some bacteroides species produce a heparinase which may frequently lead to localized septic thrombophlebitis seen adjacent to areas of infection. Many bacteroides species also possess a capsule that may interfere with phagocytosis by granulocytes. Infection characteristically remains localized, but bloodstream invasion or direct extension to other areas may occur. Localization of bloodborne organisms at distant sites is not unusual and may result in abscess formation in brain, lung, liver, joints, kidneys, or other organs.

CLINICAL MANIFESTATIONS Anaerobic infection should be suspected when a foul odor emanates from lesions or pus; when infection is situated near a mucosal surface; when necrotic tissue or neoplasm is present; when a spreading gangrene involves skin, subcutaneous tissue, fascia, or muscle; when pseudomembranes or abscesses are formed; when gas in tissues is indicated by roentgenogram or crepitance; when septic thrombophlebitis or pulmonary embolus occurs following intraabdominal or pelvic infections; or when infection progresses despite aminoglycoside therapy.

Dental-periodontal infections Root canal infection caused by mixed anaerobic and aerobic oral flora may result from dental caries and produce dental pulp necrosis with periapical destruction of bone. Without drainage of the root canal, mandibular osteomyelitis or extension of the infection into the maxillary sinus, buccal tissues, and submandibular or submental spaces may occur depending upon the teeth involved. Periodontitis with purulent gingival pockets or abscesses may result in spreading anaerobic infection that involves adjacent bone or soft tissues. Secondary pulmonary anaerobic infection may occur from aspiration of purulent material. Mandibular osteomyelitis may also result from infection complicating tooth extraction, from open fractures, or in association with debilitation, diabetes mellitus, radiation therapy, and malnutrition.

Acute necrotizing ulcerative gingivitis (trench mouth, Vincent's stomatitis) The onset of disease is usually sudden and is associated with tender, bleeding gums, fetid breath, and a bad taste. The gingival mucosa, especially the papillae between the teeth, becomes ulcerated and may be covered by a gray exudate which is removable with gentle pressure. Although involvement of the gums is usually patchy, the process may extend to most of the gingival tissue. If the ulceration is extensive, fever, cervical lymphadenopathy, and leukocytosis are present. The disease may spread to involve other tissues of the oropharynx; it may become less severe and chronic; or it may subside spontaneously. Recurrent ulceration has been described. Most patients who develop ulcerative gingivitis are young adults with poor oral hygiene. Tartar deposits and eruption or extraction of teeth may damage the gums and allow bacterial invasion. Edentulous persons develop the disease infrequently. Ulcerative gingivitis is prevalent in wartime when nutritional deficiency, crowding, and emotional upsets are common. The role of these factors in pathogenesis is not known.

Acute necrotizing ulcerative mucositis (cancrum oris, noma) Occasionally, ulcerative gingivitis spreads to the buccal mucosa, the cheek, and the mandible or maxilla, resulting in widespread destruction of bone and soft tissue. The first indication of cancrum oris is usually slight inflammation of the skin of the cheek. The destruction of tissue proceeds very rapidly. The teeth may fall out, and large areas of bone, even the whole mandible, may be sloughed. A strong, putrid odor is present. The lesions are not usually painful. The gangrenous lesions eventually heal, but large disfiguring defects are left. Cancrum oris is seen most commonly following a debilitating illness in severely malnourished children in underdeveloped areas of the world. Cancrum oris may complicate acute leukemia or develop in individuals with a genetic deficiency of catalase.

Gangrenous pharyngitis (Vincent's angina) Necrotizing infections of the pharynx may occur alone or in association with ulcerative gingivitis. The main complaints are an extremely sore throat, foul breath, bad taste in the mouth, sensation of choking, and fever. The pharynx in the area of the tonsillar pillars is swollen, red, and ulcerated and is covered with a grayish membrane that peels easily. Lymphadenopathy and leukocytosis are common. The disease may last for only a few days or may persist for weeks if not treated. The lesion begins unilaterally but may spread to the other side of the pharynx or to the larynx. Aspiration of infected material may result in lung abscess.

Sinusitis Acute sinusitis is seldom caused by anaerobic organisms unless it is associated with a dental abscess. However, gram-positive anaerobic cocci and bacteroides are isolated from about one-half of patients undergoing surgery for chronic or recurrent maxillary sinusitis. Anaerobic organisms are also associated with chronic otitis media and mastoiditis. Chronic anaerobic sinusitis, otitis, or mastoiditis may lead to subdural or extradural empyemas, brain abscess, or anaerobic meningitis (Chap. 368).

Ludwig's angina Mandibular dental or periodontal infections, particularly of the third molar, may produce submandibular cellulitis that results in marked local swelling of tissues with pain, trismus, and superior-posterior displacement of the tongue. Submandibular swelling of the neck also develops. Inability to swallow and respiratory obstruction may result; tracheostomy may be lifesaving. Anaerobes and aerobes originating from oral flora have been implicated in this dramatic clinical syndrome.

Brain abscess Anaerobic bacteria, particularly bacteroides and anaerobic streptococci, have been isolated from 30 to 80 percent of brain abscesses in adults. In one study, 16 of 18 nontraumatic brain abscesses contained anaerobes, and half of these were bacteroides, including both *B. fragilis* and *B. melaninogenicus*. These lesions may result from either direct extension of suppurative infection involving the sinuses, middle ear, or mastoids, or from hematogenous dissemination from infections elsewhere, particularly the lungs. There is an increased incidence of brain abscess in patients with cyanotic heart disease. Signs and symptoms are mainly those of a space-occupying intracranial lesion with headache followed by changes in mentation, focal neurologic signs, and papilledema. The course may be indolent, and fever is frequently absent. Cerebrospinal fluid findings are variable but may mimic those of purulent or aseptic meningitis. Focal defects are usually present on computerized tomographic or radionucleotide scans of the brain and may need to be differentiated from neoplasms by cerebral angiography.

Pleuropulmonary infection Aspiration of oral secretions leads to production of mixed anaerobic infection of the lungs and pleura. The likelihood of anaerobic pulmonary infection is increased in the presence of poor dental hygiene, periodontal disease, and gingivitis. Bacteroides, fusobacteria, and anaerobic streptococci are isolated alone or in combination in a majority of cases of lung abscess and necrotizing pneumonia. Pneumonitis without necrosis or abscess formation may also occur. These anaerobes are second only to the pneumococcus as a cause of acute bacterial infection of the lungs. Although *B. melaninogenicus* is the most frequent *Bacteroides* species isolated in anaerobic pulmonary infections, *B. fragilis* can be found in 15 to 25 percent of cases. These infections occur primarily in patients with conditions that predispose to aspiration, such as oral surgical procedures, esophageal dysfunction, and altered consciousness due to alcoholism, major motor seizure disorders, general anesthesia, and drug abuse. Anaerobes may also produce infection distal to obstructive lesions of the bronchus. These infections are characterized by tissue necrosis, abscess formation, and the production of foul-smelling and foul-tasting sputum. Empyema is not an unusual complication of lung abscess or necrotizing pneumonia. Empyema with anaerobes may also occur as an extension from subdiaphragmatic infection. Septic pulmonary emboli may originate from abdominal or female genital tract infections. The bacterial flora of bronchiectatic cavities frequently includes bacteroides and other anaerobes.

Abdominal infection Intraabdominal abscesses and generalized peritonitis almost always contain anaerobes, especially when they are secondary to perforation or leakage from the gastrointestinal tract. These infections are uniformly polymicrobial, with an average of five anaerobic and aerobic pathogens that originate from bowel flora. Symptoms include fever with chills, localized or generalized abdominal pain with peritoneal signs, nausea, and vomiting. The abscess cavity will rarely be large enough to be palpable on abdominal or pelvic examination. *Bacteroides fragilis* is isolated from approximately 50 percent of abdominal surgical wounds after trauma involving perforation of the gut and in greater than 50 percent of wound infections following elective colon resection. Anaerobic wound infections may occur following appendectomy or may follow surgery on the small bowel, stomach, gallbladder, and biliary tract. Polymicrobial bacteremia may complicate local infection and frequently is due to facultative gram-negative bacilli or *B. fragilis*. Abdominal ultrasound, combined liver-spleen scans, and gallium scans may be helpful in localizing intraabdominal abscesses, but often surgical exploration may be necessary to establish the site of intraabdominal infection.

Intrahepatic infection Anaerobic bacteria have rarely been implicated in infections of the gallbladder, but they may produce ascending cholangitis and are isolated from 20 to 45 percent of pyogenic intrahepatic abscesses. Bacteroides account for approximately half the bacterial isolates from liver abscess. They may reach the intrahepatic tissue by direct extension from an ascending infection or by embolization from septic portal vein thrombosis. In most cases, the disease is manifested by fever, chills, abdominal pain—particularly in the right upper quadrant—hepatomegaly, and liver tenderness. The presence of jaundice and marked elevation of serum alkaline phosphatase usually indicates multiple abscesses. Hepatic abscesses may be detected by hepatic ultrasound or radionucleotide scanning of the liver.

Pelvic infection The predominant organisms isolated in greater than 75 percent of nongonococcal gynecologic infections are anaerobic species found in normal vaginal flora. Anaerobic species are the major cause of Bartholin's abscess, endometritis, parametritis, parametrial abscess, pelvic peritonitis, and nongonococcal tuboovarian abscesses. These infections often complicate malignancy or recent surgery and commonly develop within necrotic tissue or products of conception. They are characterized by drainage of foul-smelling pus or blood from the uterus, generalized uterine or localized pelvic tenderness, and continued fever and chills. Suppurative thrombophlebitis of the pelvic veins may complicate these infections and lead to repeated episodes of small septic pulmonary emboli.

Nonclostridial anaerobes, principally bacteroides and anaerobic streptococci, are also the major invasive pathogens in septic abortions. Bacteremia is often transient, frequently polymicrobic, and can be demonstrated in 50 to 60 percent of these patients.

Cutaneous infections Following operation or injury associated with contamination of the subcutaneous tissues, an *anaerobic cellulitis* may develop consisting of a spreading necrosis of skin and subcutaneous tissues with associated subcutaneous gas. This infection is frequently due to a mixed infection from which clostridia, anaerobic gram-positive cocci and gram-negative bacilli, and facultative coliform bacilli, streptococci, and staphylococci may be isolated. The onset of anaerobic cellulitis is usually gradual, with erythema, tenderness, and edema of involved tissues followed by the development of necrosis, crepitation, pus, and foul odor over a 2- to 5-day period. Local pain is not marked, and the deep fascia and muscle are spared. Once established, the infection may be associated with high fever, toxemia, and positive blood cultures. In diabetics, an identical syndrome may be produced by gas forming facultative coliform bacilli or *Staphylococcus aureus*. On occasion, intraabdominal abscesses may present as an anaerobic cellulitis or abscess of the thigh. Areas of involvement should be opened surgically with debridement of necrotic tissue and drainage of pus and gas. At surgery, the status of the underlying fascia and muscle should be ascertained.

Necrotizing fascitis caused mainly by group A streptococci, *S. aureus,* or facultative gram-negative rods is associated with separation of the skin from necrotic fascia. A surgical probe may be passed without obstruction in a plane superficial to the deep fascia into areas of undermined skin. Gas gangrene caused by clostridia is usually associated with a more rapid onset and progression than anaerobic cellulitis, with severe pain in the involved areas, tense white overlying skin, and severe systemic toxicity. At surgical exploration, the involved muscle is nonviable.

Bacterial synergistic gangrene occurs 1 to 2 weeks after abdominal or thoracic surgery and is caused by microaerophilic or anaerobic streptococci combined with *S. aureus* or aerobic coliform bacilli. The margin of the surgical wound becomes red, swollen, and tender; central necrosis of skin and subcutaneous tissues occurs; and the margin slowly expands to involve adjacent skin. Systemic toxicity is usually minimal, and treatment consists of local debridement and systemic antibiotics. *Meleney's chronic undermining ulcer* is also a slowly progressive gangrene that occurs following surgery without marked systemic toxicity. It differs from bacterial synergistic gangrene because cutaneous fissures and sinus tracts form and are separated from the leading margin of the ulcer by undermined but intact skin. Anaerobic and microaerophilic streptococci are the usual causative organisms.

Fournier's gangrene is an anaerobic cellulitis involving the scrotum, perineum, and anterior abdominal wall in which mixed anaerobic organisms spread along deep external fascial planes and cause extensive loss of skin. Diabetics are susceptible to a necrotizing infection of skin and subcutaneous tissues that also may involve fascia and muscle. These infections have a foul discharge, marked local pain, gas in tissues, and severe systemic toxemia; they are caused by mixed anaerobic and aerobic organisms, and are associated with bacteremia in one-third of patients.

Mixed anaerobic infection may complicate decubitus ulcers, diabetic ulcers, pilonidal cysts, hidradenitis suppurativa, and vascular gangrene.

Other local infections Anaerobic urinary tract infections are rare and are usually the result of invasion from adjacent foci of infection or from bacteremia. Usually, osteomyelitis also results from adjacent ischemic or diabetic ulcers or abscess, but an increasing number of hematogenous bone and joint infections are being reported. Gangrenous lesions resulting from human bites commonly contain mixed oral anaerobic flora. Gangrenous balanitis and ulcers and gangrene of the vulva have been associated with a mixed anaerobic flora.

Bacteremia Invasion of the bloodstream by anaerobes is usually secondary to local infection, particularly those involving the abdominal cavity and pelvis. The initial manifestations are determined by the portal of entry and may be those of endometritis, appendicitis, intraabdominal abscess, or others. When bloodstream invasion occurs, the patient may become extremely ill with chills and hectic fevers ranging from 101 to 106°F. Shock and disseminated intravascular coagulation may develop. The clinical picture may be quite similar to that seen in sepsis with gram-negative bacilli (Chap. 109), except for the occasional association of thrombophlebitis. When bacteremia complicates facial or oral infection, the internal jugular vein

may be the site of suppurative thrombophlebitis; and in pelvic infections, the iliac and femoral veins may be involved. Palpation along the course of the involved veins may disclose a firm, tender cord, indicating the presence of a thrombus. Emboli may be dislodged from peripheral sites of thrombophlebitis, resulting in multiple septic pulmonary infarcts. The pulmonary abscesses or empyema then become the main focus of clinical attention rather than the initial site of infection.

Transient anaerobic bacteremias may occur following dental manipulation, extraction, peridontal procedures, nasotracheal intubation, percutaneous liver biopsy, barium enema, gastrointestinal surgery, and urinary tract catheterization but usually are not symptomatic. From 8 to 11 percent of clinically significant bacteremias are caused by anaerobes, most commonly by *B. fragilis* originating in abdominal or female genital tract infections. Anaerobic streptococcal bacteremias usually originate from the female genital tract, and fusobacteria from the oropharynx. Anaerobes cause less than 10 percent of infective endocarditis and are predominately microaerophilic or anaerobic streptococci. *Bacteroides fragilis* is a rare cause of endocarditis. Routine anaerobic cultures should be performed in all cases of suspected bacteremia.

DIAGNOSIS Correct specimen collection and transport are critical for the isolation of anaerobic organisms. Even brief exposure to oxygen may kill the pathogens in clinical specimens. Abscess cavities should be aspirated directly with a syringe, the air expelled, and the needle capped with a sterile rubber stopper. The specimen can then be injected into a carrier bottle containing a reduced environment or transported immediately for direct culture on anaerobic media. Such a technique is preferred over the use of cotton swabs. If swabs must be used, then a swab from a gassed-out container should be placed in a reduced semisolid carrying medium before transport to the laboratory. Delays in transport may lead to failure to isolate anaerobes due to exposure to oxygen or overgrowth with facultative organisms which may eliminate or obscure the anaerobes that are present.

Only certain specimens should be cultured for anaerobic bacteria. Since all mucosal surfaces contain anaerobes, culturing them is of no value, and in fact, may lead to erroneous labeling of culture specimens as "contaminated" with mucosal bacteria, such as occurs in expectorated sputum, nasotracheal aspirates, bronchoscopic aspirates, feces, voided urine, vaginal secretions, or secretions from mucosal surfaces which normally harbor anaerobes. Acceptable materials for culture include blood, pleural fluid, transtracheal aspirates, pus obtained by direct aspiration from abscess cavity, culdocentesis, suprapubic bladder aspirates, and other tissues or fluids that are sterile under normal conditions.

All clinical specimens from suspected anaerobic infections should be Gram stained and examined diligently for organisms with characteristic morphology. Organisms may be seen on Gram's stain that are not isolated in culture. Purulent materials that are "sterile" or that demonstrate organisms on Gram's stain but do not grow on culture should be viewed with suspicion, and the method of collection, transport, and handling in the laboratory reviewed to assure that all reasonable precautions have been taken to permit isolation of fastidious anaerobes. Repeat cultures with immediate inoculation of freshly prepared media and prolonged anaerobic incubation may be required in special circumstances. Promising new techniques for rapid anaerobic diagnosis include fluorescent antibody staining of clinical materials with species specific antisera and direct gas-liquid chromatographic analysis of clinical specimens. However, definitive diagnosis depends upon the isolation and identification of pathogenic organisms.

TREATMENT Due to the association of anaerobic infections with abscess formation, tissue necrosis, and compression, appropriate surgical management is often essential for the control and elimination of infection. Drainage of abscess cavities should be carried out as soon as fluctuation and localization occur; perforations must be closed promptly; devitalized tissues or foreign bodies removed; closed space infections drained; tissue compartments decompressed; and an adequate blood supply established. Drainage of local suppurative lesions may be all that is required for cure in many cases. However, antimicrobial therapy is indicated in infections involving vital organs; to check the spread of infection into healthy tissues; or when bacteremia or systemic manifestations are present. Surgery also may be indicated to obtain appropriate material for culture by biopsy or excision. Thrombophlebitis not controlled by anticoagulation or recurrent septic pulmonary emboli may require surgical removal of thrombi or vein ligation.

It is often necessary to begin antimicrobial treatment of anaerobic infections before culture and susceptibility data are available. The type and location of infection combined with Gram's stain findings should suggest the likelihood of certain bacterial species and serve as a guide to antibiotic therapy. Chloramphenicol is the preferred drug for seriously ill patients with suspected anaerobic infection before susceptibility data are available. Generally, anaerobic infections above the diaphragm caused by oral or upper respiratory tract flora are susceptible to penicillin G. However, if *B. fragilis* is isolated, treatment with clindamycin or chloramphenicol is usually indicated. Mixed abdominal or pelvic infections necessitate multiple drug therapy due to the likelihood of penicillin-resistant strains of *B. fragilis* and facultative or aerobic gram-negative rods. A regimen for serious intraabdominal infection includes penicillin G, 24 to 30 million units a day, combined with chloramphenicol, 4 g per day, or combined with clindamycin, 300 to 600 mg every 6 h, and gentamicin, 1.6 to 2.0 mg/kg every 8 h. Chloramphenicol is the drug of choice for central nervous system anaerobic infections as well, although penicillin G and metronidazole also pass the blood-brain barrier. Bactericidal agents such as penicillin G, ampicillin, carbenicillin, and metronidazole have a definite advantage over bacteriostatic agents only in the presence of endocarditis or in patients with profound neutropenia.

Penicillin G and ampicillin have a wide range of activity against anaerobic bacteria. However, over 90 percent of *B. fragilis* strains, and some strains of fusobacteria, non-*C. perfringens* clostridia, and *B. melaninogenicus*, are resistant. Carbenicillin (25 to 30 g per day) or ticarcillin combine the antimicrobial spectrum of penicillin G with activity against 95 percent of *B. fragilis* strains and may be selected for mixed infections associated with resistant aerobic or facultative gram-negative rods such as *Pseudomonas aeruginosa* or *Proteus* organisms. Semisynthetic penicillinase-resistant penicillins are not active against anaerobes. Many anaerobes are susceptible to cephalothin or cephapirin, but *B. fragilis* is resistant to the cephalosporins. However, cefoxitin possesses activity against *B. fragilis.*

Chloramphenicol or clindamycin remain the drugs of choice for *B. fragilis* infections. Both drugs should be reserved for serious infections and should be administered intravenously. Chloramphenicol produces fatal aplastic anemia in 1 of 40,000 to 100,000 patients who receive the drug. The development of aplastic anemia is independent of a dose-related bone marrow suppression that is common with prolonged high dose regimens. Clindamycin produces pseudomembranous colitis in 0.1 to 10 percent of patients and diarrhea in as many as 20 percent of patients. Since diarrhea may precede pseudo-

membranous colitis, the administration of drug should be stopped if diarrhea develops during therapy. Resistance to chloramphenicol is rare, but clindamycin resistance is common for *F. varium* and for clostridia other than *C. perfringens;* rarely *B. fragilis* or peptococci are resistant.

Metronidazole has bactericidal activity against many anaerobes and is clinically effective in *B. fragilis* infections. However, actinomyces, eubacteria, and microaerophilic streptococci are resistant to this agent. Metronidazole has not been approved by the Food and Drug Administration for use in anaerobic infections, and a parenteral form is not yet available.

Tetracycline is not reliable due to widespread resistance among anaerobes. The role of doxycycline and minocycline, newer tetracycline derivatives with increased activity against anaerobes, is unclear. Erythromycin may be used in minor soft tissue infections above the diaphragm or in bowel preparation for colon surgery, but is less effective than clindamycin. Anaerobes are almost uniformly resistant to the aminoglycosides. Vancomycin is active against most gram-positive anaerobes and is administered orally to treat clostridia-induced pseudomembranous colitis.

Anaerobic lesions that fail to respond to treatment or relapse after responding initially should be recultured, and the need for surgical drainage or debridement should be reassessed. Superinfection with resistant gram-negative facultative or aerobic bacteria may necessitate changes in antimicrobial therapy. During treatment with broad-spectrum antibiotics, superinfection with *Candida* or *Torulopsis* may lead to systemic fungemia.

Additional supportive measures in the management of anaerobic infections include careful attention to fluid and electrolyte balance since extensive local edema formation may lead to hypovolemia; immobilization of infected extremities; therapy for septic shock (Chap. 109); maintenance of adequate nutrition during chronic infections by central or peripheral intravenous hyperalimentation if oral intake is inadequate; relief of pain; and anticoagulation with heparin for thrombophlebitis. Hyperbaric oxygen therapy is of unproven value.

OUTCOME Mortality rates may be substantial for serious anaerobic infections and approach 50 percent for brain abscess, 30 percent for necrotizing pneumonia, 25 percent for liver abscess, and 16 to 43 percent for *B. fragilis* sepsis.

PREVENTION Preventive measures include proper therapy of localized infection to prevent metastatic disease; effective debridement, cleansing, removal of foreign bodies, reestablishment of circulation, and early antimicrobial therapy of open traumatic wounds; early exploration and antibiotic therapy for penetrating abdominal wounds associated with bowel perforation; good dental and periodontal hygiene; prophylactic antibiotics for amputation of ischemic lower extremities, vaginal hysterectomy, radical pelvic surgery, and cesarean section with ruptured membranes; measures to prevent pulmonary aspiration; and possibly neomycin-erythromycin bowel preparation for colon surgery.

REFERENCES

BALOWS A et al: *Anaerobic Bacteria: Role in Disease.* Springfield, Thomas, 1974

BARTLETT JG, FINEGOLD SM: Anaerobic pleuropulmonary infections. Medicine 51:413, 1972

———— et al: Percutaneous transtracheal aspiration in the diagnosis of anaerobic pulmonary infection. Ann Intern Med 79:535, 1973

BUSCH DF et al: Activity of combinations of antimicrobial agents against *Bacteroides fragilis*. J Infect Dis 133:321, 1976

CHOW AW et al: Orofacial odontogenic infections. Ann Intern Med 88:392, 1978

————, GUZE LB: Bacteroidaceae bacteremia: Clinical experience with 112 patients. Medicine 53:93, 1974

FINEGOLD SM: *Anaerobic Bacteria in Human Disease.* New York, Academic, 1977

GORBACH SL, BARTLETT JG: Anaerobic infections. N Engl J Med 290:1177, 1237, 1289, 1974

LEDGER WJ: *Infection in the Female.* Philadelphia, Lea & Febiger, 1977

LENNETTE EH et al: *Manual of Clinical Microbiology,* 2d ed. Washington, DC, American Society for Microbiology, 1974

RAFF MJ, MELO JC: Anaerobic osteomyelitis, Medicine 57:83, 1978

SALAKI JS et al: *Bacteroides fragilis* resistant to the administration of clindamycin. Am J Med 60:426, 1976

SMITH LDS: *The Pathogenic Anaerobic Bacteria.* Springfield, Thomas, 1974

SUTTER VL et al: *Wadsworth Anaerobic Bacteriology Manual,* 2d ed. Los Angeles, UCLA Press, 1975

section 7 | Mycobacterial diseases

143
TUBERCULOSIS

WILLIAM W. STEAD
JOSEPH H. BATES

DEFINITION

Tuberculosis is a necrotizing bacterial infection with protean manifestations and wide distribution. The lungs are most commonly affected, but lesions may occur also in the kidneys, bones, lymph nodes, or meninges or be disseminated throughout the body. The infection may cause clinical disease either (1) shortly after inoculation (sometimes called "primary" tuberculosis) or (2) after a period of months or decades of dormancy (still sometimes erroneously referred to as "reinfection" tuberculosis). In the Western world where bovine tuberculosis has been controlled, the portal of entry in humans is almost exclusively the lung.

HISTORY

Some human races (Caucasian, Mongolian) have lived with tubercle bacilli throughout much of their history, and in them the infection produces a more chronic disease, only rarely being fulminant. On the other hand, African, American Indian, and Eskimo peoples have had contact with tuberculosis over a much shorter period, and in them the infection is more prone to produce fulminant disease. Tuberculosis was named to indicate its formation of firm nodules, or *tubercles.* For many years the chronic form (then often called *phthisis* or *consumption*) was considered a degenerative or hereditary disease, quite unrelated to the tuberculosis of childhood which was obviously infectious. Laennec (1819) was the first to recognize the chronic form as merely a later development in the same infection. Koch (1882) identified the causative organism. There has been a great drop in prevalence of tuberculosis in the economically developed countries. The death rate from tuberculosis had already begun to fall by 1900, coincident with improvement in nutrition and standard of living. For the person with clinical tuberculosis, however, the most important development occurred in 1944 with the discovery of streptomycin. With the introduction of *p*-aminosalicylic acid (PAS) in 1947, isoniazid (INH) in 1952, ethambutol in 1967, and rifampin in 1971, specific therapy became progressively better and easier to administer.

ETIOLOGY

Mycobacterium tuberculosis is a rod 2 to 4 μm in length and 0.3 μm in thickness. Its distinguishing staining property, i.e., resistance to decolorization by acid alcohol when stained with basic fuchsin, is related to the waxy component of the cell wall. This "acid fastness" is dependent in some way upon the structural integrity of the bacillus; it is lost when the organisms are damaged by grinding but is not affected by prolonged extraction with fat solvents.

Tubercle bacilli are strict aerobes and thrive best at a P_{O_2} of about 140 mmHg. The organs most commonly affected by tuberculosis are those with relatively high oxygen tension; metastatic foci are most common in the apexes of the lungs where the P_{O_2} is in the range of 120 to 130 mmHg in the upright position, followed by the kidney and the growing ends of bones, where P_{O_2} approaches 100 mmHg. The liver and spleen, where the P_{O_2} is quite low, are rarely affected, except in overwhelming disseminated infection.

Two species of tubercle bacilli affect humans: *M. tuberculosis* and *M. bovis.* By far the greatest number of cases in the United States are caused by the former strain. Programs for eradication of bovine tuberculosis have been so effective that the disease now appears only sporadically in this country.

Several other species of mycobacteria have been noted to cause chronic pulmonary infection (Chap. 145). The most common are *M. avium-intracellulare* and *M. kansasii.* Clinical infection due to other atypical mycobacteria is rare. These mycobacteria appear not to be transmissible, and the epidemiology of the infections they cause remains obscure. They tend to infect lungs that have been damaged by silicosis or chronic obstructive lung disease. *Mycobacterium kansasii* responds well to antituberculous drugs in high dosage, but *M. avium-intracellulare* is resistant to nearly all drugs presently in use, and a favorable clinical response is less common.

TRANSMISSION

Most cases of communicable tuberculosis among adults develop because of a late recrudescence of dormant infection with no history of recent exposure. The liquid caseum from a cavity in such a case abounds in tubercle bacilli which are excreted in aerosolized droplets during coughing, sneezing, and speaking. When inhaled, droplets larger than 10 μm are usually caught on the mucociliary blanket and cleared from the lung without harm, but droplets of smaller size may reach the respiratory bronchiole and deposit bacilli beyond the protective mucous blanket. There, in a susceptible host, the organisms may invade tissue and establish an infection. Persons who have been infected previously are largely protected from reinfection by specific immunity, which is mediated by T lymphocytes. Teachers, school bus drivers, and nursery workers with infectious tuberculosis are of particular epidemiologic significance because of the great susceptibility of children.

Infection in a susceptible host is caused by inhalation of tubercle bacilli in *fresh* droplet nuclei expelled by a person with cavitary tuberculosis. Transmission can be blocked effectively by irradiation of the upper air of the room with ultraviolet light and adequate ventilation and by chemotherapy of the infectious case. Even though tubercle bacilli can be cultured from dust in a room of a tuberculous person, they constitute no hazard to others in this state because the irregular shape and electrostatic charge of the attached dust particles prevent them from being carried beyond the mucociliary protective mechanism. Early in the course of tuberculous infection, persons are rarely infectious because they expel very few organisms. Tuberculosis cannot be spread on hands, dishes, glasses, utensils, or fomites.

Patients who are on an effective regimen of chemotherapy lose their ability to transmit infection within a short time (probably 2 weeks or less), despite the continued presence of tubercle bacilli on smear and culture of the sputum.

PREVALENCE AND INCIDENCE

There has been a great fall in prevalence of tuberculosis in the United States since 1900. Early in this century over 80 percent of the population was infected *before* the age of 20 years. In an autopsy study in 1946, there was evidence of tuberculosis in 80 percent of the persons over the age of 50. In 1978, only 2 to 5 percent of young adults reacted to tuberculin (except in some urban areas), whereas about 25 percent of persons over the age of 50 reacted. The decline in incidence of the infection is most apparent among children and young adults and is due to a reduction in the number of infectious cases, which in turn is attributable to an improved standard of living, reduced risk of late progression of infection, and more prompt recognition and treatment of infectious cases.

The great majority of persons who harbor tubercle bacilli have latent or dormant ("healed") tuberculosis. Apical scars containing viable organisms may remain dormant for many years and then reactivate and produce clinical tuberculosis. Other sites in which tubercle bacilli may lie dormant for years and then recrudesce include the kidney (from which bacilli may spread to the genital tract in the male), spine, long bones, fallopian tubes, brain, and lymph nodes in the hilum and in the neck.

In 1976 there were about 32,000 new cases of clinical tuberculosis in the United States, an incidence of 15 per 100,000, down from 24 in 1966 and 53 in 1953. There were about 15 million tuberculin reactors, indicating a prevalence of infection of 7000 per 100,000. Of these, 60,000 were under therapy for tuberculosis and 500,000 had healed or dormant tuberculosis. The remainder had never developed clinical tuberculosis but simply harbored foci of latent infection. It is toward the latter group that programs of prophylactic therapy with INH are directed.

Of new tuberculous infections revealed by conversion of tuberculin reaction from negative to positive, 5 to 15 percent progress to serious disease within 5 years if left untreated. The risk of direct progression varies with age: it is greatest when infection begins in the first years of life and next greatest in young adults and adolescents. Among those remaining well for 5 years, a further 3 to 5 percent may develop late recrudescence at some time during life. Thus, the total morbidity rate in persons infected with *M. tuberculosis* is 8 to 20 percent. Both the early and late appearance of tuberculosis can be prevented in 80 percent of individuals if prompt treatment with INH is given when tuberculin "conversion" is discovered.

Mortality has fallen steadily over the past 70 years. Tuberculosis has ceased being the leading cause of death, with over 200 deaths per 100,000 in 1906 but only 1.5 per 100,000 in 1976. This figure may be somewhat low, because residual pulmonary scarring may lead to cor pulmonale and cause death secondarily.

IMMUNITY

NATURAL RESISTANCE The Caucasian and Mongolian races have a distinct natural resistance to tuberculosis consisting of an ability to develop an immune response to the infection which permits spontaneous recovery from initial infection. However, late recrudescence may result in chronic disease characterized by cavitation and scarring. Africans, American Indians, and Eskimos were generally spared tuberculous infection until extensive contact began with personnel of European heritage. The former group shows a decreased ability to develop an effective immune response to new infection, and in them the infection tends to be more rapidly progressive.

SPECIFIC (ACQUIRED) IMMUNITY Immunity to tuberculosis is mediated largely by T lymphocytes, which, in response to specific antigenic stimulation, liberate several lymphokines which facilitate the killing of mycobacteria and may actually block the effect of sensitized T lymphocytes. The role of immunoglobulins in the process is less clear, although IgA is often increased in patients with active tuberculosis and drops as the infection is controlled by therapy.

The mechanism by which latent infection recrudesces is not completely understood. From the fact that it occurs more commonly in old age and during other forms of illness, recrudescence appears likely to be due to reduced immunologic surveillance by T lymphocytes.

TUBERCULIN HYPERSENSITIVITY The most readily obtained evidence of a past or present infection with tubercle bacilli is the finding of hypersensitivity to tuberculin, a protein derivative of the broth in which tubercle bacilli have been grown. Epidemiologic evidence strongly suggests that tuberculin hypersensitivity indicates the presence of living tubercle bacilli. The larger the skin reaction, the greater the chance that the infection is of clinical significance.

PATHOGENESIS AND PATHOLOGIC ANATOMY

INITIAL INFECTION ("PRIMARY" TUBERCULOSIS) In the nonimmune subject tubercle bacilli can gain entrance to the body by several routes: lung, gastrointestinal tract, and direct cutaneous or percutaneous inoculation (as in an accident at the autopsy table). For practical purposes, the only route that is of importance in the United States is the lung. The majority of lesions in the early phase of infection are in the lower two-thirds of the lungs, where ventilation is best and deposition of droplet nuclei more likely. Because they produce no toxins and no tissue reaction, tubercle bacilli initially are free to multiply without deterrence. After phagocytosis in the nonimmune host, they remain viable within macrophages for an extended period. Prolonged intracellular survival, which is the key to virulence and persistence, is associated with failure of the bacilli-containing phagosomes to fuse with lysosomes. This defect of fusion protects the bacilli from the killing effect of the digestive enzymes. The organisms reach regional (hilar) nodes and even the bloodstream before their progress is inhibited by the gradual development of specific immunity over a period of several weeks. At this time, the characteristic tissue reaction develops, with epithelioid cell granulomas and caseation necrosis in the pulmonary lesion, regional lymph nodes, and any site to which the bacilli have spread. The number of bacilli drops drastically with the appearance of caseation necrosis, indicating that caseation is associated with the release of lymphokines from T lymphocytes which, in turn, release lysosomal enzymes from macrophages and destroy host tissues as well as tubercle bacilli. Thereafter, the infection in the primary site usually heals by a combination of resolution, fibrosis, and calcification. Occasionally defenses fail, and the infection may overwhelm the host or proceed directly to a chronic stage.

SILENT DISSEMINATION Early in the course of a new infection tubercle bacilli reach the general circulation in varying numbers. This event is marked only by fever and mild symptoms and is recognized as tuberculosis only when a patient is being observed closely because of recent exposure to tuberculosis. This stage is important in the pathogenesis of tuberculosis, because it is the time when bacilli reach distant sites to establish metastatic foci of infection that are the seeds from which clinical tuberculosis may develop much later.

While bacilli presumably reach all organs during this silent bacillemia, they establish lesions with frequency in only a limited number of sites, which have one feature in common: high tissue oxygen tension. Despite a paucity of ventilation, the apexes of the lungs in the upright position have the highest oxygen tension in the body (130 mmHg) due to a high ventilation-perfusion ratio. Probably for this reason they are the most frequent sites in which viable bacilli persist in a dormant state in metastatic (Simon's) foci and produce clinical disease at a later time.

LATENT (DORMANT) INFECTION When a tuberculous lesion regresses and heals, the infection enters a latent phase in which it may persist without producing illness. Though the infection may remain dormant for life, it may develop into clinical tuberculosis at any time if the persisting intracellular organisms begin to multiply rapidly.

CLINICAL TUBERCULOSIS Fibrocaseous tuberculosis may develop from either direct progression of the initial infection or recrudescence of a dormant lesion, most commonly in the apical portion of the lung. An old caseous hilar lymph node occasionally liquefies and spills its contents into a bronchus, to produce a segmental or lobar tuberculous pneumonia. Massive bloodstream invasion (miliary tuberculosis) may also occur at any stage. Tuberculosis is characterized by localized nodular infiltrations, fibrosis, and cavitation.

MANIFESTATIONS

RECENT INFECTION Uncomplicated initial tuberculous infection often produces no significant clinical illness. It is usu-

ally diagnosed only when contacts of an infectious case are examined or when it progresses to a serious form of disease. The incubation period is 4 to 8 weeks from inoculation to appearance of mild fever, malaise, and tuberculin hypersensitivity. Symptoms usually subside without specific therapy because of the appearance of adequate specific immunity. Occasionally, however, the infection progresses, either in the lung or by dissemination through the bloodstream. This turn of events is extremely serious unless detected promptly and treated adequately.

Massive hematogenous dissemination is most likely to occur in a recently infected child of 3 years or younger. In older children infection only rarely progresses to a fatal form and often passes completely unnoticed. The principal danger arises later during adolescence or early adulthood when the infection may undergo late progression.

Initial tuberculous infection occasionally produces pleurisy with effusion, cervical lymphadenitis, miliary tuberculosis, or meningitis. In addition, allergic manifestations occasionally develop, e.g., erythema nodosum and phlyctenular conjunctivitis.

In the United States, 90 to 98 percent of young adults have never been infected with tuberculosis. There have been several "epidemics" of tuberculosis among such susceptible young persons. For example, when infectious tuberculosis develops aboard ship or in prison, many persons may be infected and some secondary cases may develop. Persons working in the Peace Corps, Armed Forces, or State Department who are assigned to countries where the prevalence of tuberculosis is high may be heavily exposed to the disease. As in children, recent tuberculous infection usually produces only mild and nonspecific symptoms, but in the young adult it has a greater tendency to progress to clinical disease. There may be an area of pneumonitis in any portion of the lung, but obvious hilar adenopathy is not common. When a young adult has a pleural effusion or a parenchymal infiltrate in the lung, a tuberculin test should be performed. If the skin test is positive, the possibility of tuberculosis should be considered strongly. The source of infection is usually an adult with cavitary tuberculosis.

PULMONARY TUBERCULOSIS Pulmonary tuberculosis may follow the initial infection directly or after a short or long period of dormancy. Progressive disease has been observed to develop after 60 years of clinical dormancy. The most striking features of late recrudescent tuberculosis are (1) absence of recent exposure to tuberculosis, (2) tendency to chronicity and cavitation, and (3) production of fibrous tissue of repair. The last two phenomena are characteristic of the responses in persons sensitized to tubercle bacilli. While the solid caseation necrosis of the initial stage contains few bacilli, the *liquid* caseum in a tuberculous cavity contains abundant bacilli and may spread infection via bronchi to other portions of the lungs and into the environment.

Symptoms In most instances, the onset of pulmonary tuberculosis is insidious, and the patient may be entirely asymptomatic. Many cases are discovered because a routine roentgenogram is taken upon admission of an elderly person to a hospital for some other illness.

The earliest symptoms are constitutional and probably result chiefly from liberation of lymphokines stimulated by absorption of tuberculoprotein from numerous bacilli in a hypersensitive host. Abdominal symptoms may dominate the clinical picture. It is common for a patient with tuberculosis to be unaware of a fever as high as 40°C. General malaise may be present, but often there is nothing more than irritability, depression, and excessive fatigue at the end of the day. Defervescence during sleep gives rise to profuse sweating which may soak the patient's pajamas (night sweat).

Weight loss may precede symptoms but is often passed off
as being due to overwork or to voluntary caloric restriction.
Often weight is well maintained until late in the course of the
illness. When abdominal symptoms predominate, loss of
weight may be rapid.

Headache may be noted occasionally, especially in the evening. Palpitation may occur during mild exertion. Menstruation is usually not disturbed until the disease is advanced,
when amenorrhea may develop.

Cough is frequent but not invariable and is often passed off
as a "cigarette cough." When sputum is produced, it is usually
odorless, green or yellow in color, and raised principally upon
arising in the morning. Hemoptysis may accompany the cough
and usually consists of streaking of the sputum with small
amounts of blood. In some patients the onset of pulmonary
tuberculosis is relatively sudden, with fever, productive cough,
or pleuritic pain suggestive of bacterial pneumonia.

Physical and roentgen examinations   Early asymptomatic infiltrations due to tuberculosis are usually undetectable by physical examination, even though obvious by x-ray. Crepitant
rales may be present, especially when inspiration is preceded
by full expiration and a small cough (posttussive rales).

Long-standing tuberculosis with extensive fibrosis causes
contraction and distortion of pulmonary tissue and of bronchi.
In such instances, a wide variety of physical signs may be present, such as apical dullness and bronchial breath sounds,
coarse rales, deviation of the trachea, and diminished mobility
of one hemithorax.

Because findings on examination of the lungs in the early
stages are so frequently unremarkable, the importance of the
chest roentgenogram in the diagnosis of tuberculosis cannot be
overemphasized. Of particular importance is the comparison of
the x-ray film with one made months or years earlier, so that
subtle changes can be detected in clinically dormant lesions.
Because fibrous tissue does not change appreciably with time,
any change in the lesions on serial films must be interpreted as
indicating pathologic activity of some disease. Among 90 patients over the age of 50 with recently developed pulmonary
tuberculosis, over 70 percent showed evidence of preexisting
tuberculous scars. Comparison of abnormal films with those
taken in previous examinations makes it possible to detect and
treat tuberculosis before liquefaction has occurred with spread
of bacilli to other portions of the lungs or to other persons.

Complications of pulmonary tuberculosis   CAVITATION   When
defense mechanisms fail, tuberculosis produces liquefaction
necrosis and cavitation. The liquid material abounds with tubercle bacilli, making the disease highly infectious.

HEMOPTYSIS   In the majority of instances of bleeding from the
lungs in tuberculosis, the blood arises from ulceration of the
bronchial mucosa and presents as streaks of bright red blood
on the sputum. Bleeding usually subsides spontaneously if the
patient lies quietly. Bleeding from the pulmonary artery is
much more serious. While the branches of the pulmonary artery within a tuberculous lesion usually thrombose, occasionally one may remain open, may be eroded by the liquefaction,
and form a mycotic (Rasmussen's) aneurysm. This may rupture and cause death from exsanguination or obstruction of
airways. The blood expectorated is copious and dark because
of deoxygenated hemoglobin in the pulmonary artery.

PLEURISY WITH EFFUSION   A superficial tuberculous lesion
may involve the overlying pleura and give rise to "dry" pleurisy, attended by localized pleuritic pain on deep inspiration.
Or a small caseous pulmonary focus may actually erode
through the visceral pleura and extrude a small amount of

liquid caseum. The immune response to such pleural contamination is a vigorous inflammatory reaction with formation of
considerable pleural exudate. Although a pleural effusion may
develop at any stage of tuberculosis, it is most common within
a few months of the initial infection, particularly in young
adults (age 15 to 35 years). The fluid is usually clear and light
yellow. Its exudative nature is identified by a high protein content ($>$ 3 g per 100 ml), an elevated lactic dehydrogenase
(LDH) level, a lymphocytic-cell response, and pH $<$ 7.20.

The importance of recognizing the tuberculous nature of
such a pleural exudate in a young adult is reinforced by the
finding that 65 percent of untreated patients sooner or later
develop active tuberculosis. The diagnosis must often be clinical, because smears of the pleural fluid rarely reveal tubercle
bacilli, and even the culture is positive in only 20 to 25 percent
of cases. Percutaneous needle biopsy may reveal granulomatous pleuritis, but organisms are often not demonstrable. In
most instances, proof of tuberculosis is lacking at the time the
antituberculous treatment must be given if development of
manifest tuberculosis is to be prevented. Fortunately, the intermediate tuberculin skin test is so regularly negative in healthy
young adults that a positive reaction in a patient with a lymphocytic pleural exudate constitutes adequate evidence of tuberculous etiology to warrant initiation of two-drug therapy.
However, it is not uncommon for the intermediate-strength
purified protein derivative (PPD) test to be negative in patients
with large tuberculous effusions, perhaps because the circulating tuberculin-specific T lymphocytes are rendered inactive by
suppressor-adherent cells. A second-strength PPD will almost
always be positive if the effusion is of tuberculous etiology.

TUBERCULOUS PNEUMONIA   The onset of tuberculosis occasionally is quite acute, resembling that of bacterial pneumonia.
This picture is seen most often in blacks, persons with diabetes,
children with overwhelming infection, and elderly persons
whose lungs are flooded with bacilli discharged from an area of
liquid necrosis in the lung or hilar nodes. Chills, fever, productive cough, pleuritic chest pain, and leukocytosis may be
noted. A stained smear of the sputum usually reveals numerous tubercle bacilli.

BRONCHOPLEURAL FISTULA AND EMPYEMA   Though minimal
pleural contamination from a small superficial caseous focus
produces only a clear exudate, massive contamination from
rupture of a large caseous lesion produces pneumothorax
(bronchopleural fistula) and tuberculous empyema. This is one
of the most dreaded complications of pulmonary tuberculosis.
Tubercle bacilli are usually easily found in the purulent exudate. Management is largely surgical and consists of establishing adequate drainage, in combination with the administration
of effective antituberculosis drugs.

TUBERCULOSIS OF BRONCHI, TRACHEA, AND LARYNX   These organs are all protected from implantation of *M. tuberculosis* by
a covering of secreted mucus but may become involved in advanced cavitary pulmonary tuberculosis with excretion of numerous tubercle bacilli. Bronchial ulceration may result in hemoptysis and a localized wheeze during respiration. The
bronchial lumen also may be compromised by pressure of enlarged hilar lymph nodes early in the course of infection.

In a patient with cavitary pulmonary tuberculosis, hoarseness and pain in the throat accentuated by swallowing suggest
tuberculous laryngitis. The diagnosis can be confirmed by indirect laryngoscopy. It is important to exclude cavitary tuberculosis before a laryngectomy is performed for carcinoma of

the larynx, because tuberculous laryngitis is occasionally mistaken for carcinoma, even on histologic examination. Antituberculous chemotherapy is highly effective for tuberculosis of the mucous membranes.

Bronchi which lie within tuberculous lesions are regularly weakened by the inflammatory process and dilated by contraction of fibrous tissue in healing. In the upper lobes this is rarely clinically significant, but in portions of the lung which are dependent when the patient is upright, it may lead to secondary infection, producing chronic productive cough and sporadic hemoptysis (see "Bronchiectasis," below).

GASTROINTESTINAL TUBERCULOSIS   The normal gastrointestinal tract is resistant to penetration by tubercle bacilli, but in cavitary pulmonary tuberculosis associated with excretion of large numbers of bacilli, the mucosa may be penetrated in the ileocecal region. The symptoms consist chiefly of intermittent abdominal pain, cramping, and diarrhea. Occasionally the infection spreads through the wall of the intestine, to produce tuberculous peritonitis (see "Peritoneum," below).

Differential diagnosis   The clinical picture presented by pulmonary tuberculosis varies widely and may simulate a great number of other diseases.

CARCINOMA OF THE LUNG (Chap. 268)   Tuberculosis is commonly confused with carcinoma of the lung because the highest incidence of both diseases is in the upper lobes and in older men. Both cause loss of weight, chronic cough, blood-streaked sputum, and mild fever. In addition to bacteriologic studies for tubercle bacilli, sputum cytology, bronchial brushing, and bronchoscopy should be employed to aid in the differentiation. Comparison of prior roentgenograms may be of considerable help, but in many instances nothing short of a diagnostic thoracotomy will serve to make the distinction. When tuberculosis is considered among the diagnostic possibilities, therapy with two antituberculous drugs should be instituted a few days before thoracotomy in order to minimize complications in the event the lesion is tuberculous.

MYCOTIC INFECTIONS (Chaps. 151 to 161)   When tubercle bacilli cannot be isolated from a patient suspected of having tuberculosis, appropriate tests should be made for the various fungus infections, which may present with a clinical picture indistinguishable from pulmonary tuberculosis. Helpful skin and serologic tests are available for coccidioidomycosis, histoplasmosis and aspergillosis, but blastomycosis, mucormycosis, cryptococcosis, and sporotrichosis can be diagnosed only by demonstrating the organisms in a biopsy specimen or on culture.

ACTINOMYCOSIS AND NOCARDIOSIS   Although usually referred to as fungus diseases, these infections are actually caused by bacteria. Diagnosis is made by culture.

SARCOIDOSIS (Chap. 216)   The typical patient with sarcoidosis is afebrile and has a negative tuberculin test and a roentgen picture of diffuse pulmonary infiltrations and hilar adenopathy, but the disease is protean in its manifestations and may mimic tuberculosis. Mediastinoscopy with biopsy of lymph nodes or lung biopsy is of greatest value in establishing this diagnosis. The Kveim test may be helpful when the antigen can be obtained.

ASPIRATION PNEUMONIA, LUNG ABSCESS (Chap. 260)   Pulmonary infection which is introduced by the drainage of contaminated saliva during sleep from a focus of pyorrhea occurs predominantly in the upper and midposterior portions of the lung and can mimic tuberculosis. The distinction can usually be made eventually, but much valuable time may be lost while the patient is treated for the wrong disease. The presence of putrid sputum, hemoptysis, fever, and leukocytosis in a patient who has pyorrhea and has recently undergone surgery or who drinks alcohol to excess strongly suggests a pyogenic abscess. If the differentiation cannot be made readily, it may be advisable to treat with antimicrobials in addition to antituberculosis medications.

OTHER FORMS OF PNEUMONIA   Bacterial or mycoplasma infection (Chap. 172) may present with clinical and roentgen appearances which at first may be indistinguishable from pulmonary tuberculosis. Cultures, cold agglutinins, precipitin, and complement fixation tests often establish the correct diagnosis. Cavitation is rare, and sputum examination does not yield tubercle bacilli. Early in the course of infection, tuberculosis may present with a localized infiltrate in the lung and slowly subside spontaneously or coincidentally with tetracycline therapy, similar to mycoplasma pneumonia. If clearing is incomplete, tuberculosis should be strongly considered. A tuberculin skin test should be performed in all patients with "viral pneumonia," particularly if a significant pleural effusion is present, since this is rare in viral pneumonia. A positive tuberculin skin test in an adolescent or young adult with pneumonitis strongly suggests tuberculosis because of the rarity of dormant infection in this age group.

PNEUMOCONIOSIS   Pulmonary infiltrations associated with exposure to silicon dioxide, asbestos, ferrous oxide, and beryllium as well as hypersensitivity reactions to various organic inhalants may present a roentgenographic appearance suggestive of tuberculosis (Chap. 258). Silicosis may present great difficulty in diagnosis because it may produce conglomerate masses and even cavitation that mimic tuberculosis. Silicosis impairs the pulmonary defense against tubercle bacilli. When the tuberculin skin test is positive in a patient with silicosis, smoldering tuberculosis is so likely that two-drug therapy is indicated if activity is suggested by x-ray, and prophylaxis with isoniazid is justified if there is no evidence of activity.

BRONCHIECTASIS (Chap. 261)   A productive cough due to chronic infection in dilated bronchi occurs much less frequently than formerly because of more effective antibiotic therapy for necrotizing pneumonias of childhood and the reduction in the number of children whose bronchi have been damaged by tuberculosis. The lower and middle lobes (or lingula on the left) are most often involved, and a bronchogram effectively demonstrates the pathologic condition. If the tuberculin skin test is positive, isoniazid should be administered prophylactically to prevent late progression of tuberculosis from coexistent foci in apexes, whether or not they are visible radiographically.

CONFUSION CAUSED BY SYSTEMIC EFFECTS OF TUBERCULOUS INFECTION   Because of the insidious nature of tuberculosis, the clinical picture may be mistaken for that produced by several other disorders. Malaise, easy fatigability, inability to concentrate, anorexia, and loss of weight may be mistaken for psychoneurosis. The symptoms may suggest hyperthyroidism or diabetes mellitus, but with a little care the distinction can be made. Tuberculosis should always be considered in the differential diagnosis of fever of unknown origin (Chap. 10). If the roentgenogram reveals a pulmonary infiltrate, the possibility of tuberculosis is increased, but in cases of disseminated or extrapulmonary tuberculosis, the chest roentgenogram may be normal. In these cases biopsy of an enlarged lymph node, bone marrow, or liver may be of help. Formerly, tuberculosis was overdiagnosed in patients presenting with general systemic symptoms. Today, however, because of a lessening awareness of tuberculosis, the principal danger is that tuberculosis will be overlooked. Furthermore, tuberculosis may appear by recrudescence without recent reexposure, in anyone who has ever been infected in the past.

TUBERCULOSIS OF OTHER ORGANS Localized tuberculous infection may occur in a number of other organs, notably, the lymph nodes, kidney, long bones, genital tract, brain, and meninges. Organisms reach these sites during the silent bacillemia which often occurs early in the infection.

Lymph nodes The most common involvement of lymph nodes occurs in the hilus draining the pulmonary site of initial infection. The enlargement is usually modest but may be massive and give rise to obstruction and even ulceration of a major bronchus. The prognosis is good with proper chemotherapy, but the nodes may continue to enlarge for a few weeks after therapy is started and then resolve slowly.

Cervical adenitis (scrofula) This disease has become uncommon in the United States as a result of the elimination of tuberculous cattle and pasteurization of milk, but it occasionally occurs early in the course of infection. Cervical lymphadenitis may also appear as a late manifestation, especially in blacks. The nodes may be large (several centimeters in diameter) and matted together in a mass with an area of soft fluctuation. Signs of acute inflammation are rarely present. Swelling begins insidiously without systemic symptoms. Spontaneous rupture may occur, with drainage of caseous material. In some cases the offending organism is *M. scrofulaceum* or *M. kansasii*, and for this reason culture of the pus is necessary for accurate diagnosis.

Kidney Second to the upper lobes of the lungs, the kidney is the most common site for the late appearance of localized tuberculous infection. The mechanism of implantation is the same as that in the pulmonary apexes, namely, by hematogenous spread early in the infection. The oxygen tension in the cortical portion of the kidney approaches that in arterial blood, which enhances the growth and persistence of tubercle bacilli. As in the lungs, foci of tuberculosis may remain dormant for many years and produce clinical disease late in life. The pathologic process is the same as in the lung: inflammation, followed by caseation, liquefaction, and discharge of contaminated material into the collecting system and down the ureter to the bladder and, in men, to the genital tract.

Symptoms of renal tuberculosis are usually insidious and may be overlooked completely until the appearance of cystitis or epididymitis. Gross or microscopic hematuria and pyuria with a "sterile" urine on culture for bacteria should always call tuberculosis to mind and lead to the performance of a tuberculin skin test and culture of urine for tubercle bacilli. Intravenous pyelography may reveal a cortical cavity communicating with the calyceal system. Symptoms usually subside promptly with chemotherapy. Resection of residual areas of destruction is only rarely necessary.

Male genitals Infection of the genital tract in the male is secondary to renal tuberculosis. Bacilli discharged from a caseous lesion in the kidney may reach the seminal vesicles, prostate gland, and epididymis through their connections with the excretory tract. Symptoms begin insidiously, most commonly with scrotal pain due to inflammation of the epididymis and vas deferens. Tenderness and swelling may be found in the vas, seminal vesicles, and/or the prostate gland.

Female genitals When tuberculosis infection occurs after puberty, tuberculosis occasionally spreads hematogenously to the highly vascular fallopian tube. Infection may then spread into

the uterus and give rise to endometritis. Symptoms are usually mild and of insidious onset, with abdominal pain, white vaginal discharge, metromenorrhagia, and dyspareunia. Systemic symptoms and signs are uncommon, probably because the infection is indolent and localized. The most common manifestation is sterility, but tubal scarring may cause pregnancy to be ectopic. Tuberculosis of the fallopian tube may also spread to the peritoneum and produce either a tuberculous pelvic abscess or generalized peritonitis.

Osseous tuberculosis Hematogenous spread of tuberculosis to the long bones and vertebrae is most common when infection occurs in childhood, because of the high P_{O_2} associated with the vascularity at the epiphyseal plates during active bone growth. It usually occurs within 3 years of infection, but dormant lesions may be reactivated by trauma years later. Infection begins in the ends of the long bones but becomes obvious when it involves the adjacent joint: hip, knee, elbow, or wrist. Tenosynovitis is most common at the wrist.

Tuberculous spondylitis (Pott's disease) This disease may result from hematogenous seeding or from spread of infection from paravertebral lymph nodes draining a tuberculous pleurisy. Spondylitis may develop in childhood or be delayed until later in life. Localized pain in the back may be present for months before x-rays reveal an abnormality. Though infection begins in the body of a vertebra, the first radiographic sign is usually destruction and narrowing of an intervertebral disk. A paravertebral abscess may be seen as a fusiform density extending the length of several vertebrae and occasionally dissects downward to the inguinal area. Therapy with two bactericidal drugs is the keystone of management, although some patients may require surgical drainage. Extensive orthopedic procedures are no longer necessary.

Peritoneum The peritoneum may be implanted with tubercle bacilli when they spread by any of at least four routes: (1) through the wall of infected intestine, (2) from a mesenteric lymph node, (3) from an infected fallopian tube, or (4) from hematogenous seeding in the course of disseminated tuberculosis. Symptoms are insidious, with increasing abdominal girth, but ultimately the patient has fever, night sweats, weakness, diarrhea, and abdominal pain. As with other forms of tuberculosis, there is an increased frequency among alcoholics. Tuberculosis should be strongly considered whenever ascitic fluid contains protein in excess of 3 g per 100 ml, when LDH is elevated, and when the white blood cells are mostly lymphocytes. Diagnosis may be made by open or percutaneous needle biopsy.

Pericardium Tuberculous infection may spread from the mediastinal lymph nodes or contiguous segments of lung to the pericardium in the same manner as to the pleura. The pathologic process is the same as in tuberculous pleurisy, with outpouring of a clear exudate, formation of granulomas, and subsequent fibrosis. The clinical picture may be that of chronic pericardial tamponade, with hepatomegaly, edema, friction rub, and enlargement of the cardiac shadow during the active phase, and constriction during the phase of fibrosis. When such an illness is acccompanied by afternoon fever or night sweats and a positive tuberculin reaction, tuberculosis should be strongly considered. The diagnosis is made best by open pericardial biopsy. A tuberculous pericardial effusion contains more than 3 g protein per 100 ml, an elevated LDH, and lymphocytes. Early in the disease, multiple-drug chemotherapy accompanied by corticosteroids is usually sufficient, but surgical resection of the pericardium is occasionally necessary when the process is well established before therapy is begun.

If tuberculous pericarditis has undergone spontaneous healing, the patient may present years later with the picture of constrictive pericarditis (Chap. 249). Pericardiectomy at this stage may improve cardiac function but may be technically difficult because of extensive calcification extending into the myocardium. The procedure may be complicated by marked impairment of cardiac output postoperatively due to cardiac dilatation and myocardial atrophy.

Adrenals Occasionally hematogenous tuberculosis localizes in the adrenal glands and may result in their total destruction, giving rise to adrenal cortical insufficiency (Addison's disease, Chap. 336). This must be differentiated from adrenal cortical atrophy, which is more common, and from other causes of adrenal destruction, such as histoplasmosis. Therapy consists of prolonged administration of antituberculosis agents plus physiologic doses of adrenal steroids.

Meninges Tuberculosis may involve the meninges, either as a part of miliary tuberculosis or as extension of infection from a focus within the brain. In areas with a high incidence of tuberculosis, tuberculous meningitis is seen most commonly in young children during the first year of infection. In areas of low incidence such as the United States, meningitis is more common among older adults as a result of late reactivation of dormant infection. Pathologically, the meninges contain small tubercles and a fibrinous exudate over the base of the brain.

Symptoms consist of headache, restlessness, and irritability, usually accompanied by fever, malaise, night sweats, and loss of weight. Nausea and vomiting may be prominent. Stiffness of the neck and Brudzinski's sign are usually present. Spinal puncture usually reveals increased pressure, clear fluid containing an increased amount of protein, reduced glucose (less than half the blood glucose), and 100 to 1000 white blood cells per milliliter, 80 to 95 percent of which are lymphocytes. Demonstration of tryptophan in the spinal fluid provides a presumptive diagnosis of tuberculous meningitis upon which to institute chemotherapy.

The differential diagnosis includes partially treated pyogenic meningitis, fungal meningitis, carcinomatosis or sarcoidosis of the meninges, and subarachnoid hemorrhage. There is considerable urgency in establishing the correct diagnosis because specific therapy is most effective when instituted early in the course of the illness. Irreversible brain damage may result from waiting 6 to 8 weeks for cultural proof of diagnosis. For this reason it is frequently necessary to begin therapy for tuberculosis on the basis of a presumptive clinical diagnosis while awaiting results of bacteriologic studies. Therapy should include isoniazid and rifampin, both of which cross the blood-brain barrier. Steroids are indicated only when there is an impending subarachnoid block or cerebral edema. Intrathecal therapy is not indicated.

Inappropriate secretion of antidiuretic hormone (ADH) Older persons with tuberculous meningitis or overwhelming pulmonary tuberculosis occasionally present with somnolence or coma associated with a very low serum sodium concentration (110 to 125 meq per liter), because of inappropriate secretion of ADH. This must be distinguished from adrenal insufficiency, in which the sodium serum concentration is also depressed in concert with an elevated serum potassium level. In addition to antituberculosis agents, adequate sodium chloride should be administered and water intake restricted.

DISSEMINATED TUBERCULOSIS Silent bacillemia Hematogenous dissemination of a small number of tubercle bacilli is common early in the course of infection but usually produces little clinical illness. The principal importance of the event is the seeding of bacilli in sites far removed from the pulmonary site of inoculation.

Massive dissemination (miliary tuberculosis) When a liquid caseous focus empties its contents into a vein, there is a massive dissemination of tubercle bacilli throughout the body. Defense mechanisms are overwhelmed, and tubercles become established in all organs of the body. Without specific therapy, death is almost a certainty.

Miliary tuberculosis is the most dreaded manifestation of tuberculosis. It may arise shortly after infection or from recrudescence of a dormant focus years or decades later. Because the resistance of the body is overwhelmed, lesions are not limited to those organs with an elevated P_{O_2} but are often found in the liver, spleen, bone marrow, and meninges. The best way to make the diagnosis of miliary tuberculosis is to perform a biopsy of the liver, lymph node, or bone marrow in search of caseating granulomas and tubercle bacilli.

Symptoms are usually nonspecific and consist of weight loss, weakness, gastrointestinal disturbance, fever, and sweats. The patient has usually had a course of penicillin or broad-spectrum antibiotics without control of the fever before the diagnosis comes to mind. Cough is not a prominent feature, but dyspnea may be. The correct diagnosis is often not suspected until the typical "miliary" pattern is noted on the chest roentgenogram. The white cell count may be normal or low, or may show a leukemoid pattern suggesting leukemia. There may be a monocytosis. An identical clinical picture can be presented by histoplasmosis, coccidioidomycosis, blastomycosis, cryptococcosis, and other chronic infections. Therefore, it is imperative to obtain any material possible by biopsy or aspiration to establish a correct diagnosis on which to base therapy.

Subacute and chronic dissemination Instead of a single massive invasion of the bloodstream, smaller numbers of tubercle bacilli may escape into the circulation intermittently and give rise to a variety of clinical manifestations, including myelophthisic anemia, low-grade fever, lymphadenopathy, effusion into pleural and peritoneal cavities, and plenomegaly. There may be destructive lesions of bones, kidneys, subcutaneous tissue, or skin. Such a clinical picture is most common in elderly persons with recrudescent infection.

The protean manifestations and bizarre clinical picture caused by subacute and chronic forms of hematogenous tuberculosis provide a tremendous diagnostic challenge. To add to the confusion, the tuberculin reaction is often suppressed in persons with overwhelming infection. The intermediate-strength tuberculin test is often negative, and the PPD no. 2 (see "Diagnosis," below) occasionally so. The solution to the clinical problem most commonly comes when the possibility of tuberculosis is belatedly considered. Confirmation must be sought from appropriate histologic and bacteriologic studies. The prognosis is uniformly bad without treatment but good with appropriate chemotherapy.

DIAGNOSIS

TUBERCULIN SKIN TEST Tuberculin is a protein fraction of tubercle bacilli. When introduced into the skin of a person with tuberculous infection, whether clinically apparent or dormant, it triggers release of several lymphokines which over the next 24 to 72 h cause a localized thickening of the skin due to edema and accumulation of sensitized lymphocytes. Although there are several methods for testing healthy populations with tuberculin for evidence of unsuspected infection, the method preferred in clinical practice is to inject 0.1 ml of a solution containing 5 tuberculin units (TU) of purified protein derivative stabilized with Tween 80 (5 TU of PPD-T) into the skin of the volar aspect of the forearm with a small needle—an "intermediate-strength tuberculin test." The test is read 48 to 72 h later and is considered positive if the diameter of skin thickening measures 10 mm or more, doubtful if it is 5 to 10 mm, and negative if it is less than 5 mm.

Intermediate-strength PPD produces a positive reaction in the majority of persons infected with tubercle bacilli. However, it is a biologic test which is dependent upon the presence of an adequate number of circulating sensitized T lymphocytes. False-negative results may occur in 15 to 20 percent of persons with clinical tuberculosis if sensitized T lymphocytes are temporarily nonfunctional, as in persons who are clinically ill, febrile, or have a large pleural effusion. If the intermediate PPD is negative in a patient in whom tuberculosis is suspected, the test should be repeated using "second-strength" PPD (100 or 250 TU). If this is also negative, tuberculosis can be dismissed with considerable certainty, although persons who are moribund from tuberculosis may fail to react even to PPD no. 2.

A positive reaction to intermediate-strength PPD indicates the presence of a tuberculous infection but does not help in distinguishing clinical from dormant infection. This distinction must be made on clinical, bacteriologic, and radiographic grounds. A positive reaction which is elicited only by PPD no. 2 in a patient who is clinically ill means that active tuberculosis cannot be dismissed as a diagnostic possibility. In healthy persons, however, it usually signifies only healed tuberculosis or infection with mycobacteria other than *M. tuberculosis*.

RADIOGRAPHY While never providing an etiologic diagnosis, x-rays of the chest provide extremely valuable information. The abnormality which is most suggestive of tuberculosis is a multinodular infiltrate with cavitation in one or both of the upper lobes of the lung. Because of the propensity of tuberculosis to spread via bronchi to other parts of the lungs, the basilar areas may also be involved. Occasionally, especially in the elderly, the lesions are limited to the lower lobe(s). Multiple infiltrates, especially if bilateral, are most suggestive of tuberculosis, because pyogenic pneumonia and primary carcinoma are much more likely to produce single lesions. Carcinoma usually produces a solid lesion, in contrast to the multinodular infiltrate of tuberculosis. Planigrams (laminagrams) are particularly valuable in making such distinctions and in detecting cavitation. Lateral, lordotic, and oblique films are also of value in defining the location and character of lesions. Initially tuberculous infection is not usually apical in location but may involve any other segment of the lungs. Hilar adenopathy is common early in the course of infection in children, but may not be obvious by x-ray in adults. Large pleural effusions are easily detected, but for small or infrapulmonary effusion it may be necessary to place the patient on the *involved* side to permit the fluid to be seen along the lateral chest wall (lateral decubitus film).

BACTERIOLOGIC DIAGNOSIS The only absolute proof of active tuberculosis is the cultural identification of *M. tuberculosis* from tissue or body fluid: sputum, gastric washing, urine, cerebrospinal fluid (CSF), serous effusion, or pus from an abscess or sinus. A useful preliminary examination, however, is to make a smear of the material and stain it for standard microscopy or to apply auromine-rhodamine stain for easier detection by fluorescence microscopy. The smear is not a very sensitive method, but it has the virtue of quickly identifying the patient who is discharging great numbers of organisms into the environment. For positive identification, cultures must be made either on solid egg medium (Löwenstein-Jensen) or Middlebrook 7H-11 medium using 20 to 40 mmHg CO_2 in the incubator.

The most commonly examined material is sputum. When it can be produced spontaneously (usually in the early morning), it makes the most satisfactory material for both smear and culture. If none can be produced spontaneously, the patient may be asked to inhale aerosolized heated saline to stimulate production of bronchial secretions. Bacteriologic specimens may also be collected by bronchial washing, bronchial brushing, or tracheal aspiration. Sputum should never be collected over a 24-h period because this increases the frequency of contamination.

When no sputum can be collected, as in young children or senile or psychotic persons, fasting morning gastric contents may be aspirated and cultured. Diagnosis by smear of this material is less reliable than examination of sputum because of the frequency of saprophytic acid-fast bacteria in the stomach, but the presence of large numbers of acid-fast bacilli strongly suggests that they are significant.

Multiple specimens may be needed before the organisms are recovered. This is particularly true early in the course of tuberculous infection, tuberculous pleurisy with effusion, and when the pulmonary lesions are small and noncavitary. Patients with old chronic tuberculous lesions may shed organisms only intermittently.

HEMATOLOGY The white blood cell count is usually not significantly elevated, except in tuberculous pneumonia (when it may suggest a pyogenic infection) and in miliary tuberculosis (when a leukemoid reaction may be mistaken for leukemia). Hemoglobin and hematocrit are usually normal unless a prolonged period of illness has produced anemia of infection.

URINALYSIS There are no specific changes except when a urinary tract lesion is present. Renal tuberculosis is not rare in older persons; it most often presents with microscopic hematuria and pyuria with negative cultures for pyogens. Two or three early morning specimens should be submitted for culture. About 10 percent of persons with pulmonary tuberculosis excrete bacilli in their urine, even without detectable urinary tract lesions.

OTHER TESTS Despite great efforts to develop one, there is no specific serologic test to distinguish clinical from dormant tuberculosis. Biopsy of the liver, bone marrow, or lymph node can be of great aid in reaching a presumptive diagnosis of disseminated tuberculosis by revealing caseating granulomas containing acid-fast bacilli. Such a finding may be lifesaving by permitting initiation of specific therapy without allowing the disease to progress while awaiting culture confirmation.

TREATMENT

Treatment of tuberculosis is based upon intensive and prolonged exposure of the organisms to bacterial antagonists. With proper management tuberculosis can be cured in 95 percent of patients, even though return to health may be limited by an associated disease. Heretofore conventional therapy has required 18 to 24 months, but by using a regimen of two bactericidal drugs treatment can now be completed in 9 months. Either form of therapy can be accomplished while the patient is ambulatory and even at work.

PRINCIPLES OF CHEMOTHERAPY To be effective in therapy, a drug must interfere with a vital function of the tubercle bacillus without harming the host. The choice of therapy should be guided by several well-established principles:

1 Drugs should be chosen to which the bacilli are likely to be susceptible. Fortunately, in the United States this presents little difficulty in most newly discovered cases because most strains are susceptible to the major drugs. If a patient has been treated previously or contracted the infection in an area where drug resistance is common (e.g., Southeast Asia, Phillippines, Mexico), it must be assumed that the bacilli will be resistant to isoniazid (INH) and the regimen should include at least two other drugs until the results of susceptibility studies are known.

2 Even in a generally susceptible population of bacilli, a naturally resistant mutant occurs about once in 10^5 to 10^6 organisms. For this reason at least two effective drugs should always be given to patients with clinical tuberculosis to avoid multiplication of drug-resistant mutants.

3 Bactericidal drugs are always preferred. Both rifampin and isoniazid are bactericidal for both extra- and intracellular bacilli. For this reason these two drugs are effective both for immediate reduction in the large extracellular population of bacilli and for ultimate eradication of the smaller intracellular population.

4 When treatment appears to be failing (bacteriology fails to become negative within 3 to 4 months), the addition of a single drug is an invitation to disaster. Therapy should always be changed to an entirely new regimen of at least two new drugs, and great care should be taken to ensure that the patient takes the medication regularly.

5 Therapy must be continued long enough to eradicate the bacilli from the body. When two bactericidal drugs are used, this can be accomplished in 9 months, but when one of the drugs is bacteriostatic, a treatment period of 18 to 24 months is required.

6 All medications should be given before breakfast and in a single dose, if possible, in order to achieve a single combined peak concentration for maximum effect on the bacilli.

MAJOR DRUGS Isoniazid (INH) Isoniazid interferes with DNA synthesis and intermediary metabolism of the tubercle bacillus. It is the keystone of antituberculous chemotherapy. It is acetylated in the liver and excreted by the kidney.

DOSE The usual dose for adults is 5 mg/kg per day, usually 300 mg, given in a single dose. In children the dosage is higher because of more rapid excretion: 10 to 15 mg/kg per day. It is a safe drug for use in pregnancy, although elective chemoprophylaxis should be deferred until after delivery. Although some persons acetylate INH more rapidly than others, this has proved to be of little clinical significance unless the interval between doses is 5 days or more. When used in "pulse" therapy, the dose is about 15 mg/kg given twice weekly or 10 mg/kg given three times per week. A matrix form of INH for slower release is under investigation as a means of reducing the frequency of doses. In renal failure, the standard dose is usually tolerated well.

TOXICITY Although not common, three types of toxicity from INH occur: (1) Direct toxicity consists of peripheral neuropathy and anemia due to competition of INH with pyridoxine. Pyridoxine in a dose of 30 to 50 mg per day effectively combats this problem, which is most common when a large dose is used and in alcoholics whose nutrition is impaired. (2) Allergic reac-

tions consist of skin rash, swelling of the tongue, arthralgia, and fever and may require withdrawal of the drug. (3) Hepatocellular toxicity is the most serious toxic effect of INH. Contrary to earlier thought, hepatitis is not due to allergy but may be due to a reaction to a metabolic product of INH degradation in the liver. Symptoms consist of malaise and anorexia followed by nausea, vomiting, fever, and finally, jaundice. The best way to detect INH hepatitis is to acquaint each patient with the symptoms for which to be alert (anorexia, nausea, vomiting) with the request that they be reported without delay. No more than a 1-month supply of INH should be given, and inquiry about symptoms should be made each time the patient is seen. A suspected reaction must be confirmed by the following procedure: discontinue INH at once and draw blood for determination of SGOT, alkaline phosphatase, and serum bilirubin. If these tests are normal or SGOT is only mildly elevated, INH therapy may be reinstituted cautiously. If any of the tests show a threefold elevation, INH hepatitis is very likely and the drug should not be given. For minor elevations, one should repeat the studies; if they are normal, restart treatment with INH, beginning with 50 mg (one-sixth of a 300-mg tablet), and recheck the laboratory results. If symptoms recur and the SGOT shows a sharp rise, INH toxicity exists and the drug should be discontinued. The only therapy required is the withdrawal of the drug, but if INH is continued in the face of symptoms of hepatitis, it may prove fatal.

Rifampin (RIF) Rifampin acts by inhibition of RNA polymerase of both extra- and intracellular bacilli. The dose is about 10 mg/kg per day, or 450 to 600 mg per day, for adults and about 15 mg/kg per day for children. Although RIF has not been cleared for use during pregnancy, wide experience has produced no evidence of teratogenicity. Toxicity consists of jaundice (about 1 percent), gastrointestinal symptoms, and fever. Hypersensitivity reactions such as "flu syndrome," renal failure, and thrombocytopenia may occur when a large dose (900 to 1200 mg) is administered intermittently, but are uncommon when smaller doses (450 to 600 mg) are administered two or three times per week. Hypersensitivity reactions may occur when RIF is resumed after a longer interruption. While there is some laboratory evidence of suppression of immunity, there appears to be no clinical effect.

Streptomycin (SM) and capreomycin (CM) These drugs inhibit protein synthesis and are bactericidal for extracellular bacilli. They do not penetrate the cell walls of macrophages to reach the intracellular organisms. Dosage for each is 1 g per day for adults, reduced to 0.5 g per day in persons over age 60, of small stature, or with renal impairment. Dosage in children is 20 mg/kg per day. Actually, daily medication can be given 5 days per week with no apparent loss of effectiveness, which facilitates administration of medication by visiting nurses. Toxicity may be allergic in type with fever, rash, malaise, etc., or related to the eighth cranial nerve or the renal tubule. The latter two are total-dose related; therefore, medication is best given daily (five times per week) for only about 2 months and then two or three times per week for an additional 4 to 6 weeks to minimize the total amount of the drug used. Streptomycin is safe during pregnancy, although it may exert a toxic effect upon the eighth cranial nerve of the fetus in late pregnancy. Slight dizziness and circumoral paresthesias are common immediately after injections, but are generally harmless.

Pyrazinamide (PZA) A very effective drug whose mode of action remains obscure, PZA penetrates the cell wall of the macrophage and is bactericidal in the acid intracellular milieu. When used with SM or CM, a very effective bactericidal combination results against organisms in both locations. Dosage is 30 mg/kg per day given in a single daily dose. PZA can also be given twice a week in a dose of 50 mg/kg. It regularly causes a striking increase in serum uric acid, due to interference with renal excretion of uric acid, but this is harmless except in persons with gout. Toxicity consists of jaundice (rare), fever, or rash.

Ethambutol (EMB)   Ethambutol inhibits RNA synthesis and is bacteriostatic against extracellular tubercle bacilli. Its principal value is inhibition of the growth of mutants which are resistant to INH or RIF. It was the second most commonly used drug in the United States until it was realized that the combination of RIF and INH makes it possible to administer two bactericidal drugs and thus reduce the total duration of therapy. Its principal use now is as a substitute drug used when toxicity precludes the use of a more effective one. EMB is well tolerated in a dose of 15 mg/kg per day with only rare instances of ocular toxicity (optic neuritis). In the more effective dose of 25 mg/kg per day which is necessary as a substitute drug, the incidence of optic neuritis approaches 1 percent and requires careful surveillance. It is not recommended in pregnancy or in children too young to cooperate in the testing of vision. In addition to periodic examination of visual acuity, color vision, and visual fields, patients should be asked to report any reduction in acuity noted in reading newsprint with their usual glasses. This drug can be used in supervised twice weekly treatment for which the dosage is 50 mg/kg.

OTHER DRUGS Ethionamide (ETA)   Ethionamide inhibits protein synthesis and is of value in re-treatment of patients who harbor organisms that show multiple drug resistance. Dosage is 750 to 1000 mg per day for adults. Because gastric irritation is so common, this drug must be given in divided doses after meals.

Cycloserine (CS)   This drug inhibits cell wall synthesis and is of use in re-treatment cases. Dosage is 750 to 1500 mg per day for adults, divided into two doses, each accompanied by pyridoxine, 100 mg. CS should not be used in epileptics or persons with a history of psychosis.

_p_-Aminosalicylic acid (PAS)   _p_-Aminosalicylic acid interferes with intermediary metabolism and is bacteriostatic for the tubercle bacillus. Because of a high incidence of gastrointestinal intolerance, it is infrequently used today. It should not be used with RIF because PAS interferes with its absorption. Dosage is 200 mg/kg per day in divided doses.

Kanamycin   An aminoglycoside, kanamycin interferes with protein synthesis and can be used in selected re-treatment of resistant cases. Eighth nerve toxicity is so common and severe that it greatly limits its usefulness.

Thiacetazone and isoxyl   These are inexpensive drugs in common use in developing countries. They are not available for clinical use in the United States, however, because of a high incidence of toxic side effects.

Viomycin   This drug is no longer manufactured in the United States.

CHOICE OF THERAPY FOR CLINICAL TUBERCULOSIS   The immediate goal of chemotherapy is to kill the organisms without permitting the selection of resistant mutants. It is very important to adhere to the principles of therapy outlined above in choosing and carrying out a therapeutic regimen. Chemo-

therapy of tuberculosis is so effective that such modalities as bed rest, collapse therapy, surgical resection, etc., need no longer be discussed.

Initial treatment   It is now apparent that therapy for tuberculosis, regardless of the organ involved, can be completed in 9 months _provided two bactericidal drugs are given together for the full period._ If the regimen consists of only one bactericidal drug and one bacteriostatic drug, therapy must be given for 18 to 24 months to achieve comparable success.

Preferred regimens   When there is no reason to suspect resistance to INH (see the first principle of therapy), the regimen should consist of INH and RIF from the start and usually no other drug is needed. Where the possibility of INH and/or SM resistance is recognized, additional drugs should be given to ensure that at least two effective agents are included pending the report of drug susceptibilities.

Several safe and effective short-course regimens of therapy for tuberculosis have been described. INH 300 mg and RIF 600 mg daily for 9 months is curative in 95 percent of cases with a relapse rate of less than 2 percent. A 9-month regimen has been in use in Arkansas for over 3 years that has been equally effective and requires only one-third as much RIF. In the Arkansas regimen, INH and RIF are given daily for 4 to 6 weeks. At that time RIF is given in the same dose of 600 mg, but the INH dose is increased to 15 mg/kg (usually 900 mg for adults) twice a week (e.g., on Tuesdays and Fridays) for the remainder of the 9 months. We have had no serious allergic reactions in giving RIF in this manner to over 600 patients, many of whom were quite elderly. Another advantage of this regimen is that it lends itself to total supervision of drug ingestion when necessary to ensure compliance.

The regimen used in Great Britain consists of RIF 450 to 600 mg and INH 300 mg for 9 months with the addition of either SM 0.75 g or EMB 25 mg/kg daily for the first 2 months. The third drug adds little if the organisms are sensitive to INH, but can be good insurance against failure if the organisms should be resistant to INH.

In recent studies four bactericidal drugs have been given at the outset to reduce the population of organisms as quickly as possible in an effort to shorten therapy still further. For the moment, however, this appears to have little advantage to offset the disadvantage of increased drug toxicity, except when drug resistance is known or suspected.

About 4 to 6 percent of patients are unable to take RIF and INH because of toxicity, forcing the discontinuance of the offending drug(s) and substitution of others (e.g., SM, PZA, EMB). Hepatic toxicity is uncommon, i.e., less than 2 percent in our experience. Whenever the advantage of giving two bactericidal drugs together is lost, therapy then must be prolonged to 18 to 24 months to achieve success.

Prior to the introduction of the bactericidal therapy described above, the most widely used regimen was a combination of INH 300 mg per day combined with EMB in a dose of 15 to 25 mg/kg per day. When a large population of organisms was indicated by a positive sputum smear, it was common practice to add SM 1 g per day for the first 2 months in order to reduce further the risk of selection of INH-resistant mutants. The total period of therapy with this regimen must be 18 to 24 months in order to ensure lasting success. This form of therapy is now used principally when toxicity secondary to a bactericidal drug forces substitution of a bacteriostatic one.

With the bactericidal combination of RIF and INH, conversion of cultures to negative is quite prompt, i.e., 89 percent in 2 months and 96 percent in 3 months. This is appreciably better than what could be achieved with earlier regimens. Relapse after successful therapy with RIF and INH has been less than 2 percent, largely within the first 6 months following completion of 9 months of therapy. If the full course of 18 to 24 months of the formerly used regimen is followed, relapses should be uncommon (about 3 to 4 percent), but this is often difficult to achieve. When relapse occurs following treatment with RIF and INH, the organisms almost always remain sensitive to both drugs and further treatment with the same regimen given for a longer period of time is usually successful. When relapse occurs following other forms of therapy, the chance of INH-resistant organisms is greater and a multiple-drug retreatment regimen is often necessary to achieve ultimate success.

The two most important tasks during treatment are (1) careful bacteriologic monitoring to be certain of the effectiveness of the medications and to provide samples of the bacilli to test for susceptibility in the event of failure and (2) careful monitoring for the toxic side effects of the drugs being given. To achieve both these ends, the patient should be seen no less frequently than every week or two at the outset and then at monthly intervals when the patient appears stable and recovery is going smoothly. To detect the occasional relapse, sputum specimens should be collected at monthly intervals for the first 6 months after completion of therapy and then every 3 months for an additional year.

When the patient's clinical condition requires hospitalization, it should be brief. Effective chemotherapy reduces infectiousness promptly even while the sputum smear is still positive for tubercle bacilli. For home therapy to be successful, the patient must comprehend enough of the nature of the disease and chemotherapy to ensure cooperation. Irregularity of medication or premature discontinuation are the major causes of failure and relapse. The booklet *Understanding Tuberculosis Today* by W. W. Stead (Central Press, Milwaukee, 1979) is available from many local affiliates of the American Lung Association. It explains tuberculosis and its therapy in terms most patients can comprehend and is helpful in achieving compliance.

Re-treatment of "resistant cases" Need for a regimen for re-treatment may arise from inadequate use of drugs at the outset, from premature discontinuation of medication, or from relapse after apparently successful therapy. The skill required to manage a re-treatment case is greater than for initial therapy, and advice should be sought from a physician experienced in this field. Re-treatment must always involve a completely *new regimen of drugs*. When the patient has received several drugs in the past, it is usually desirable to await results of susceptibility tests before selecting therapy. When INH resistance is suspected but not yet proved, an excellent regimen is SM, PZA, RIF, and INH. The drugs should be given daily for 6 to 8 weeks or until drug susceptibilities are known. CM may be substituted if SM resistance is suspected. If the bacilli are later found to be susceptible to RIF and INH, daily or twice weekly therapy with only these medications for another 7 months is adequate. If INH resistance is confirmed, RIF, SM, and PZA should be continued either daily or twice weekly for a total of 9 months. For poorly compliant patients whose ingestion of medication must be supervised, the twice weekly regimen is preferable. When EMB must be substituted for any of the drugs, therapy must be continued for at least 12 to 15 months *after conversion* of sputum to negative.

Corticosteroids The use of cortisone and its derivatives has been shown to increase the chance of recrudescence of dormant tuberculosis. Despite this, in patients who are very seriously ill with tuberculosis, these agents may be lifesaving. They should be used only when there is an immediate threat to life, such as hypotension, debilitating fever, dyspnea, or an impending blockage of the subarachnoid space in tuberculous meningitis. Prednisone may be used in a dosage of 40 mg per day for 1 to 2 weeks, then 20 mg for another 8 weeks, and then gradually withdrawn over a period of 3 to 4 weeks in order to prevent a "steroid rebound." The effect upon the temperature and the general well-being of the patient may be dramatic, but there is no decrease in residual fibrosis. In general, the frequency of side effects makes the routine use of steroids in conjunction with chemotherapy unwise.

PREVENTION

Chemoprophylaxis Clinically inapparent tuberculous infection can be prevented from developing into tuberculosis by judicious use of isoniazid therapy both in recently infected persons and in those with a dormant infection.

Recently infected persons Close contacts of an infectious case of tuberculosis should be tested with tuberculin. Hospital and nursing home personnel should be tested at the time of employment and then annually. Any reactor with detectable disease or symptoms should be examined bacteriologically and given treatment with two drugs as outlined earlier. Newly infected persons with normal chest x-rays should be given preventive treatment with isoniazid. The risk of development of clinical tuberculosis in such persons is appreciable (see "Prevalence and Incidence," above) and greatly exceeds the risk of toxicity from isoniazid.

Close contacts of an infectious case who are under the age of 4 years are at special risk and should be started on therapy even though the tuberculin test is negative and they appear well. If in 3 months the skin test is still negative, therapy may be discontinued; if positive, treatment should be given for a full year.

Persons with dormant infections Dormant tuberculous infection may be prevented from developing into clinical disease by treatment with isoniazid. Treatment is generally recommended for reactors under the age of 35 years and especially for those under 25. Over the age of 35 the risk of hepatitis from isoniazid increases somewhat, and preventive therapy is recommended for reactors of unknown duration only if one of the following factors that increases the risk of tuberculosis is present: (1) radiographically detectable apical scars (Simon's foci) suggestive of healed tuberculosis, (2) diabetes mellitus, (3) prolonged steroid therapy, (4) history of gastrectomy, (5) silicosis, or (6) any chronic malignancy, such as Hodgkin's disease.

Preventive therapy consists of isoniazid, 300 mg for adults and 5 to 10 mg/kg for children given in a single daily dose for 9 to 12 months. Preventive therapy reduces the risk of clinical tuberculosis by about 80 percent, and protection appears to be lasting. When the apparent source case excretes tubercle bacilli which are resistant to isoniazid, rifampin should be given for a year as prophylaxis.

Toxic reactions to isoniazid are uncommon below age 35, but thereafter may be as high as 2 to 3 percent. They need not be serious if early symptoms are heeded and the medication stopped promptly, as outlined earlier. The booklet *Understanding Tuberculosis Today*, mentioned above, can help patients understand the risk of tuberculosis and the rationale for prophylactic chemotherapy.

BIOLOGIC PROPHYLAXIS BCG vaccine BCG, or bacillus Calmette-Guerin, is a live, attenuated strain of bovine tubercle bacilli which has been used widely in many countries to induce specific immunity against tuberculosis. Although it does not reduce the chance of natural infection, it does prevent the development of serious forms of tuberculosis when natural infection occurs. There has been controversy on the effectiveness of BCG, but most authorities agree that it affords about 80 percent protection against the development of clinical tuberculosis. Its greatest value is in infants in countries with high prevalence where exposure of children is common. In the United States vaccination is indicated only for nonreactors who cannot avoid exposure, as when assigned to countries of high prevalence in the Peace Corps, State Department, Armed Forces, etc.

ERADICATION OF TUBERCULOSIS The decline in mortality rates from tuberculosis early in the century led some to predict the eradication of the disease in the United States by 1945. This prediction was based on the idea that infection with tubercle bacilli was harmless and that only reinfections were dangerous. It was reasoned that tuberculosis would disappear when reinfections could be prevented by isolating all infectious cases. It is now clear, however, that clinical tuberculosis developed largely from reactivation of dormant infections and that eradication must await the natural disappearance of tubercle bacilli from the population. It is hoped that this process can be accelerated by the judicious use of INH as prophylactic therapy, but clinical tuberculosis will continue to occur for many years.

IMPLICATIONS OF A POSITIVE TUBERCULIN REACTION In the United States, the chance of a tuberculin reactor developing clinical tuberculosis from a dormant infection is greater than that of a nonreactor acquiring an infection. Therefore, it is preferable to be tuberculin-negative, unless the positive reaction is induced by vaccination. On the other hand, living in a country of high prevalence a nonreactor would be more likely to become infected than a healthy reactor. Under these circumstances, it would be preferable to be tuberculin-positive and to have the immunologic protection against acquiring a new infection.

REFERENCES

BATES JH: Treatment of tuberculosis. Adv Intern Med 20:1, 1975
———, STEAD WW: Effect of chemotherapy on infectiousness of tuberculosis. N Engl J Med 290:459, 1974
DUTT AK, STEAD WW: Short-course chemotherapy for tuberculosis with largely twice-weekly isoniazid-rifampin: Results up to 30 months. Chest 75:441, 1979
FOX W, MITCHISON DA: State of the art "short-course chemotherapy for pulmonary tuberculosis." Am Rev Respir Dis 111:325, 1975
JOHNSTON RF, WILDRICK KH: The impact of chemotherapy on the care of patients with tuberculosis. Am Rev Respir Dis 109:636, 1974
STEAD WW: Pathogenesis of the sporadic case of tuberculosis. N Engl J Med 277:1008, 1967
———, BATES JH: Evidence of "silent" bacillemia in primary tuberculosis. Ann Intern Med 74:559, 1971
———, TEXTER EC: Isoniazid hepatitis. A backlash of progress. Ann Intern Med 79:125, 1973
——— et al: The clinical spectrum of primary tuberculosis in adults: Confusion with reinfection in the pathogenesis of chronic tuberculosis. Ann Intern Med 68:731, 1968
YOUMANS GP: Relationship between delayed hypersensitivity and immunity in tuberculosis. Am Rev Respir Dis 111:109, 1975

144
LEPROSY

CHARLES C. SHEPARD

DEFINITION Leprosy (Hansen's disease) is a chronic granulomatous infection of man, which, in its various clinical forms, attacks superficial tissues, especially the skin, peripheral nerves, and nasal mucosa. The two major clinical types are *lepromatous* and *tuberculoid;* when the disease has features of both these types, it is called *borderline.* In addition, an early indeterminate form is seen, which may later develop into one of the three types mentioned.

ETIOLOGY *Mycobacterium leprae,* or Hansen's bacillus, is the causal agent of leprosy. It is an acid-fast rod, found in enormous numbers in lepromatous lesions. Although it has not been cultivated in artificial media, nor convincingly in tissue cultures, it can be propagated in cooler tissues of small rodents, very consistently in the foot pads of mice. The bacillus will also produce heavy systemic infections in a proportion of nine-banded armadillos; armadillos have a lower body temperature. The bacillus multiplies very slowly, so mouse experiments take 6 to 12 months and armadillo experiments take several years. The mouse model has been used much for the study of antileprosy drugs, and the high bacterial yield from armadillos is making many immunologic studies possible. Estimates of bacillary viability can be made microscopically by determination of the "solid ratio" or "morphologic index"; only viable bacilli are thought to stain solidly.

Lepromin is a suspension of killed *M. leprae* prepared from the tissues of lepromatous patients. Intradermal injection elicits, somewhat irregularly, a tuberculin-like reaction at 48 h (Fernandez' reaction) and more consistently, a papular reaction at 4 weeks (Mitsuda's reaction). The Mitsuda reaction is usually positive in tuberculoid patients and negative in lepromatous patients and is therefore an aid in clinical classification. However, because it is also positive in nearly all normal adults, it has no diagnostic value.

EPIDEMIOLOGY At present, there are probably 10 to 20 million persons affected with leprosy in the world. The disease is more common in tropical countries, in many of which 1 to 2 percent or more of the population is affected. It is also common in certain regions with cooler climates, such as Korea, China, and central Mexico. In the United States the chief leprosy areas are Texas, California, Hawaii, Louisiana, Florida, and New York. Some of the cases are acquired domestically, some are acquired abroad.

Leprosy is frequently a family infection. Many patients give a history of prolonged exposure, and in close family contacts (spouse-spouse) of untreated lepromatous patients the attack rate is 5 to 10 percent. Among young children of untreated lepromatous parents, 30 to 50 percent develop a mild, single-lesion type of leprosy which heals spontaneously. After the index case is under treatment, spread within the family does not occur. Transmission from patients with tuberculoid leprosy is uncommon. The portal of entry is a matter of conjecture, but is probably either the skin or the nasal mucosa. The chief portal of exit is thought to be the nasal mucosa of lepromatous patients.

The incubation period is frequently 3 to 5 years, but it has been reported to range from 6 months to several decades.

CLINICOPATHOLOGIC CLASSIFICATION As is true of other chronic infections, such as syphilis and tuberculosis, the manifestations of leprosy are many and variable. The classification now in general use is based on clinical findings, histopathologic changes, and the lepromin test.

Lepromatous leprosy is one of the polar forms. The involvement is extensive, diffuse, and bilaterally symmetrical. Histologically, there is a diffuse granulomatous reaction with macrophages, large foam (Virchow's) cells, and many intracellular bacilli, frequently in spheroidal masses (globi). The lepromin reaction is negative.

Tuberculoid leprosy is the other polar type. Skin lesions are single or few and are sharply demarcated. Neurologic involvement is relatively pronounced and may be severe. The histologic picture consists of lymphocytes, epithelioid cells, and perhaps giant cells; bacilli are few and sometimes difficult to demonstrate. The lepromin reaction is usually positive.

Borderline, or *dimorphous*, leprosy is a form in which the clinical features and histologic changes are a combination of the two polar types. The disease may shift toward the lepromatous form in the untreated patient or toward the tuberculoid form in the treated patient. Change of either polar type to the other is exceedingly rare.

In all forms of leprosy peripheral nerve involvement is a constant feature. In any histologic section involvement of nerves will tend to be more severe than involvement of other tissues, and in some sections the nerves may be the only tissues involved.

PATHOGENESIS *Mycobacterium leprae* probably enters the body through the skin or nasal mucosa. The early stages of infection have not been described accurately. In lepromatous leprosy bacillemia is frequent and often so profuse that the organisms can be seen in stained smears of peripheral blood. Even in the most advanced lepromatous cases, destructive lesions are limited to the skin, peripheral nerves, anterior portion of the eye, upper respiratory passages above the larynx, testes, and structures of the hands and feet. The probable reason for the predilection of the disease for these tissues is that they are all usually several degrees cooler than 37°C. Two sites of preferential involvement are the ulnar nerves near the elbow and the peroneal nerves where they pass around the head of the fibula; above and below these levels where these nerves take deeper courses, they are much less severely involved. In mice that have been experimentally infected in the foot pads, bacillary multiplication is maximal when the mice are kept at air temperatures at which the foot pad tissues are about 30°C; this is also the usual temperature of the most severely involved tissues of human beings. In patients with lepromatous leprosy, collections of bacilli are also found in the liver, spleen, and bone marrow, but these are probably scavenged from the blood.

A profound lack of cellular immunity for *M. leprae* in lepromatous leprosy is indicated by the histology and by the negative lepromin reaction. Further evidence comes from observations that lepromatous patients' lymphocytes fail to react in vitro to *M. leprae* antigens either with a mitogenic response or by the formation of migration inhibitory factor (MIF). Under the same in vitro conditions the lymphocytes of tuberculoid patients react positively. Moreover, many normal persons exposed to leprosy give positive reactions, indicating the presence of subclinical infections. In addition to this depressed specific cellular immunity for *M. leprae*, lepromatous patients frequently have a partial depression of cellular immunity in general. They have been shown to be deficient in the ability to develop delayed hypersensitivity, their lymphocyte transformation response to plant mitogen may be weak, and the paracortical areas of their lymph nodes are deficient in lymphocytes. Furthermore, mice that have been rendered T-cell

deficient by thymectomy and irradiation followed by bone marrow replacement respond to inoculations of *M. leprae* by developing heavier infections. For these reasons, lepromatous leprosy is thought to be the result of a poor immune response, and tuberculoid leprosy the result of a stronger immune response, but whether these differences in immune state precede the infection or are caused by it is not clear.

CLINICAL MANIFESTATIONS   Early leprosy The first signs of leprosy are usually cutaneous. One or more hypopigmented or hyperpigmented macules or plaques may be seen. Often an anesthetic or paresthetic patch is the first symptom noted by the patient, but on careful examination skin involvement can also be found. When contacts are being examined, a single skin lesion is often noted, especially in children; usually, this is a hypesthetic macule that may clear in a year or two without treatment, but specific treatment is usually recommended.

Tuberculoid leprosy Early tuberculoid leprosy is frequently manifested by a hypopigmented macule, sharply demarcated and hypesthetic. Later the lesions are larger, and the margins are elevated and circinate or gyrate. There is peripheral spread and central healing. The lesions appear singly or are few in number and are not symmetrical. Nerve involvement occurs early, and the nerves leading from the lesions may be enlarged. The larger peripheral nerves may be palpably and visibly enlarged, especially the ulnar, peroneal, and greater auricular nerves. There may be severe neuritic pain. Neural involvement leads to muscle atrophy, especially of the small muscles of the hand. Contractures of the hand and foot are frequent. Trauma, especially from burns and splinters from excessive pressure, leads to secondary infection of the hands and to plantar ulcers. Later, resorption and loss of phalanges is frequent. When the facial nerves are involved, there may be lagophthalmos, exposure keratitis, and corneal ulceration leading to blindness.

Lepromatous leprosy The skin lesions are macules, nodules, or papules. The macules are often hypopigmented. The borders of the lesions are not sharp, and the centers of raised lesions are convex (rather than concave as in tuberculoid disease). There is also diffuse infiltration between the lesions. The sites of predilection are the face (cheeks, nose, brows), ears, wrists, elbows, buttocks, and knees. Involvement with infiltration and little or no nodulation may progress so subtly that the disease goes unnoticed. Loss of the eyebrows, especially the lateral portions, is common. Much later the skin of the face and forehead becomes thickened and corrugated (leonine facies), and the earlobes become pendulous.

Nasal symptoms (nasal "stuffiness," epistaxis, and obstructed breathing) are common early symptoms. Complete nasal obstruction, then laryngitis and hoarseness, are also frequent. Septal perforation and nasal collapse lead to saddle-nose.

In adult males infiltration and scarring of the testes lead to sterility. Gynecomastia is common. Invasion of the anterior portion of the eye leads to keratitis and iridocyclitis. Painless inguinal and axillary lymphadenopathy occurs.

Neurologic involvement, of the same type as that seen in tuberculoid disease, is less prominent in the lepromatous form. A diffuse hypesthesia involving the peripheral portions of the extremities is common in advanced lepromatous disease.

Reactional states The general course of leprosy is indolent, but it may be interrupted by two types of reaction, which tend to complicate chemotherapy.

Erythema nodosum leprosum (ENL) occurs in lepromatous patients, most frequently toward the end of the first year of treatment. Tender, inflamed subcutaneous nodules develop, usually in crops. Each nodule lasts a week or two, but more develop. ENL may last only a week or two, or it may continue for long periods. Low-grade fever accompanies severe ENL, and lymphadenopathy and arthralgias may appear. Even in untreated patients with ENL the bacilli have greatly reduced viability, as indicated by low infectivity for mice and by low "solid ratios." Histologically, ENL is characterized by polymorphonuclear infiltration and deposits of IgG and complement; hence, it resembles an Arthus reaction.

Borderline reaction is seen in borderline patients, more often during treatment. Existing skin lesions develop erythema and swelling, and new lesions may appear. An early influx of lymphocytes is followed by edema and a shift toward tuberculoid histology. Cellular immunity increases. Borderline reactions can be differentiated from frank progression, such as occurs when drug-resistant bacilli appear, by mouse inoculations to test bacillary viability and by histologic studies.

The *Lucio phenomenon* is limited to patients with a diffuse nonnodular lepromatous disease; it is seen more often in Mexico and Central America. Arteritis leads to ulceration of the skin, in a characteristic angular shape, and subsequently to angular thin scars.

COMPLICATIONS The crippling that follows involvement of the peripheral nerves has been mentioned. Leprosy is probably the most frequent cause of crippling of the hand in the world. Blindness also is common.

Amyloidosis is a complication of severe lepromatous disease in the United States but is less common in many other countries.

Patients with leprosy are said to be likely to develop other chronic infections. Tuberculosis is the chief cause of death in many leprosariums.

DIAGNOSIS The demonstration of acid-fast bacilli in the skin smears made by the scraped-incision method is strong evidence for leprosy, but in tuberculoid disease bacilli may be too few for demonstration. Wherever possible, a skin biopsy specimen confined to the affected area should be sent to a pathologist knowledgeable in leprosy. The histologic involvement of peripheral nerves is pathognomonic.

The lepromin reaction has no diagnostic value. No diagnostic blood changes occur. Lepromatous patients frequently have mild anemia, elevated erythrocyte sedimentation rate, and hyperglobulinemia. From 10 to 40 percent of lepromatous patients have false-positive serologic tests for syphilis.

The combination of a chronic skin disease and peripheral nerve involvement should always lead to the consideration of leprosy.

The differential diagnosis includes conditions such as lupus erythematosus, lupus vulgaris, sarcoidosis, yaws, dermal leishmaniasis, and a host of banal skin diseases. The skin lesions of leprosy, especially of tuberculoid disease, are characterized by hyperesthesia, however, and peripheral nerve involvement can always be demonstrated. Peripheral neuropathy from other causes and syringomyelia may be confused with leprosy.

TREATMENT The treatment of leprosy is largely in the hands of specialists, and hospitalization is advantageous for the first few months while the treatment is being established.

Specific chemotherapy Dapsone (4,4'-diaminodiphenylsulfone, DDS, diaphenylsulfone) is the principal drug. The daily dosage is 50 to 100 mg in adults, often raised gradually to that level during the first few weeks. In a few months in lepromatous disease enough bacilli are killed to render mouse inoculations negative. However, in this form of the disease nonviable

bacilli disappear only slowly and may be found in the tissues for 5 to 10 years. Moreover, a few viable bacilli (persisters) may persist in the tissues for many years and may cause a relapse if treatment is discontinued. Consequently in lepromatous disease, treatment should be continued at least 6 to 10 years after bacilli are no longer demonstrable in skin smears, or perhaps for life.

Sulfone resistance occurs in some patients. After 5 to 20 or more years, during which the response is favorable, such a patient will develop clinical and bacteriologic relapse in spite of regular therapy, and sulfone resistance can be proved on isolates in mice. The frequency of this secondary resistance has been 2 to 8 percent in different countries, depending on the sulfone used and regularity of administration. Recently, primary resistance in previously untreated patients has been described.

Because of the problems of drug-resistant bacilli and of persister bacilli, multiple-drug therapy is now recommended for lepromatous disease. The additional drugs most commonly used are clofazimine (B663) and rifampin (rifampicin). Because clofazimine results in cutaneous pigmentation, light-skinned patients often object to the drug. It is also moderately expensive. As rifampin is even more expensive, regimens combining two or three of these drugs in various schedules are under study. In infections with dapsone-resistant *M. leprae,* clofazimine and rifampin are given in combination. Rifampin-resistant *M. leprae* has been demonstrated in patients relapsing after treatment with this drug alone. Other drugs such as prothionamide, ethionamide, thiambutosine, and thiacetazone, thought to be unsuitable for single-drug therapy, are now being studied in combination with dapsone.

Other sulfones, such as sulfoxone or Sulphetrone, are not used much. Acedapsone (DADDS), a repository sulfone, which releases dapsone slowly and is given only five times a year, is under extensive study; in lepromatous leprosy, it has been found necessary to add a 90-day course of rifampin to the continued acedapsone.

In tuberculoid and indeterminate leprosy, persistent and drug-resistant bacilli have not been a problem, and treatment with dapsone or acedapsone alone has been sufficient. Treatment is continued until all signs of activity have been absent for 3 years. The treatment of borderline leprosy depends upon the severity of the disease.

The clinical response to adequate therapy may be confused by the reactional conditions, but the disease stops progressing and the skin lesions gradually improve. Recovery from neurological impairment is limited.

Treatment of reactional states Moderate ENL is managed by antipyretics and analgesics. If severe, it can be treated with corticosteroids; the dosage is adjusted to alleviate severe distress but not to eliminate all signs of reaction. Sulfone therapy should be continued, if necessary, in reduced dosage. In the past some leprologists have discontinued sulfone therapy at the first signs of ENL, but most now feel that such action is not warranted because it allows bacillary multiplication. Corticosteroid therapy promotes the viability of *M. leprae* in mice not given antileprosy drugs. Thalidomide is the most effective drug and in appropriate dosage can completely suppress ENL. Because of its teratogenicity, however, its use is severely restricted, and it can be used only when its administration can be strictly controlled.

Borderline reactions, if severe, can be controlled with corticosteroids. They do not respond to thalidomide.

Other measures Many of the deformities and disabilities of leprosy are preventable through proper attention from the beginning of treatment. Plantar ulcers, which are very common, may be prevented by rigid-soled footwear or walking plaster casts and contractures of the hand may be prevented by physical therapy and application of casts. Reconstructive surgery is sometimes helpful. Nerve and tendon transplants and release of contractures can give patients more functional ability. Vocational retraining is often necessary for those with permanent disability. Plastic repair of facial deformities assists acceptance of patients in society. The psychologic trauma which results from prolonged segregation is now minimized by permitting patients to continue therapy at home as soon as possible.

CONTROL Early detection and treatment of the disease, which prevent the further development of deformities and simplify sulfone therapy, can be aided by education of physicians and laity in endemic areas. Because the disease is best treated by specialists, the establishment of clinics is helpful. Regular and complete skin examination of family contacts is essential. Field trials of BCG vaccination in endemic areas have shown contradictory results. Chemoprophylaxis with low dosages of dapsone or with acedapsone injections should be considered for family contacts and groups with high attack rates. Removal of patients from their families and normal environment is not necessary, unless the patient fails to cooperate with his therapeutic program.

REFERENCES

Cochrane RG, Davey TF (eds): *Leprosy in Theory and Practice*, 2d ed. Baltimore, Williams & Wilkins, 1964

Fasal P: A primer in leprosy. Cutis 7:525, 1971

Immunological problems in leprosy research. 1. Bull WHO 48:345, 483, 1973

Leprosy—United States, Puerto Rico. Morb Mort Week Rep, May 28, 1976

Ridley DS: Histological classification and the immunolgical spectrum in leprosy. Bull WHO 51:451, 1974

Shepard CC: The first decade in experimental leprosy. Bull WHO 44:821, 1971

WHO Expert Committee on Leprosy: Fifth Report. WHO Technical Report Series 607, 1977

145
OTHER MYCOBACTERIAL INFECTIONS

CHARLES C. SHEPARD

The two most important human mycobacterial pathogens are *Mycobacterium tuberculosis* and *M. leprae,* but morphologically similar acid-fast bacteria are widely distributed in nature as saprophytes and as pathogens of lower animals. In addition, a number of other mycobacteria are known to cause human disease, chiefly chronic cutaneous disease, pulmonary disease, or lymphadenitis. Sometimes in the past, these other human mycobacterial pathogens have been called "atypical mycobacteria" or other confusing terms. An early, tentative classification by Runyon was an important step. In it the slowly growing cultures were placed in three groups: group I, photochromogens; group II, scotochromogens; and group III, nonchromogens. Rapidly growing cultures formed a group IV.

As numerical taxonomic studies have now allowed identification of the several pathogenic and nonpathogenic species contained in the groups, the species names should be used. As is the case with other microbial pathogens, individual species cause particular diseases and sometimes several species cause very similar diseases (Table 145-1).

SKIN INFECTIONS *Mycobacterium marinum* **(M. balnei, "swimming pool" or "fishtank" bacillus)** This acid-fast organism inhabits swimming pools, aquaria (saltwater and freshwater), and natural bodies of water that are usually brackish or saline. From contaminated swimming pools, it gains entry through human epidermis through cutaneous abrasions from rough concrete; from aquaria, through cuts; and from fish, through cuts and wounds. A few weeks later nodules develop at the site; they may become verrucous, or they may ulcerate and enlarge to form superficial granulation tissue. The involved area is usually not extensive. In another form, new lesions form centrally from the initial site. The lesions usually remain minor and regress after a year or two, but they may last for years. *Mycobacterium marinum* grows optimally at 25 to 35°C and poorly, if at all, at 37°C. This temperature range probably accounts for the lack of systemic spread; regional lymph nodes remain uninvolved unless secondary pyogenic infection occurs.

The diagnosis is made by culturing the organism, usually from biopsy material, at appropriate temperatures. Although it grows slowly on primary isolation, on transfer it grows more rapidly. Histologically, a chronic granuloma with epithelioid and giant cells and sometimes with caseous necrosis is seen. Acid-fast bacteria may be difficult to observe. Many, but not all, patients become tuberculin-positive.

If chemotherapy is needed, ethambutol and rifampin are indicated. Tests for antibiotic sensitivity are helpful.

Prevention of swimming pool outbreaks requires disinfection of the pool. The pool may need to be reconstructed to eliminate rough concrete surfaces.

Mycobacterium ulcerans The ulcers caused by the organism are known by several local names, such as Bairnsdale, Kaferiku, and Buruli, but they are best designated by the name of the organism, since local differences are trivial. The characteristic disease is extensive granulomatous ulceration that destroys subcutaneous tissue down to the muscle or fascia and extends peripherally under an undermined edge. The extensor surfaces of arms or legs are most often affected, but the trunk may be involved. Histologically, necrosis is prominent, and epithelialization extends under the overhanging margins. Systemic invasion does not occur, although new lesions may develop at distant sites. In its natural course, the lesion starts as a local swelling which then ulcerates; it may heal spontaneously or persist for many years with extensive ulceration and contractures. Originally observed in Southern Australia, the disease has since been described in Central Africa, Southeast Asia, and tropical America. Recently, large outbreaks have been described near swamps in Uganda. While a soil habitat is the suspected source, the organism has not been isolated from soil.

Mycobacterium ulcerans grows optimally at 30 to 33°C and poorly, if at all, at 37°C. It grows very slowly even at optimal temperature, and colonies require 7 weeks to grow. Inoculation of mouse foot pads may be helpful in isolation.

Treatment is best carried out with surgical extirpation of necrotic tissue and overlapping margins of the ulcer, followed by skin grafting. Although experimental results indicate that clofazimine and rifampin are active against the organism, chemotherapy seems not to be beneficial in human disease.

Other mycobacteria Mycobacterial skin infection caused by an unidentified mycobacterium occurs in a geographically limited area centered on Minnesota and southern Manitoba. A single red raised area enlarges over a period of weeks to a papule, which often breaks down in 1 to 2 months with some drainage. Most patients have enlarged regional lymph nodes. Recovery is prompt after surgery or chemotherapy. Most infections occur in fall or winter and involve people of all ages. Only a few cases have been described in adult males.

Mycobacterium avium-intracellulare, M. scrofulaceum, M. kansasii, and *M. fortuitum* occasionally cause infections that involve skin.

PULMONARY INFECTIONS Several mycobacterial species other than *M. tuberculosis* can cause chronic progressive pulmonary disease with cavitation and fibrosis closely resembling pulmonary tuberculosis.

Etiology The species are listed in Table 145-1. *Mycobacterium avium* and *M. intracellulare* are closely related organisms, sometimes difficult to differentiate, and best spoken of as a complex. Cultures have been isolated from soil and from animals, especially chickens, but the source of infection is not established. Cultures of *M. kansasii* have been isolated from the environment. *Mycobacterium xenopi* was first isolated from a toad. *Mycobacterium szulgai* is the most recently recognized species, and all cultures have originated from human disease. *Mycobacterium scrofulaceum* needs to be differentiated from *M. gordonae,* also scotochromogenic and commonly found in soil and water. The *M. fortuitum-chelonei* complex includes *M. abscessus* as a subspecies of *M. chelonei.*

Since similar species may be isolated from normal sputum and the identification of the several species is often carried out in reference laboratories, the etiologic diagnosis may be delayed. However, isolation of the suspect culture from repeated specimens and the presence of multiple (more than 10) colonies in the primary cultures are strong evidence that the organism has an etiologic role.

Epidemiology The mode of transmission of all these pulmonary infections is unsettled. There is cross-sensitization between antigens of the tubercle bacillus and other mycobacteria, but sensitization to the etiologic organism is greater. Comparative tests with antigens from *M. avium-intracellulare* and the tuberculin indicate that many healthy individuals in the southeastern United States have been infected by organisms of this group, and in this area, chronic pulmonary disease that is not caused by *M. tuberculosis* is often caused by *M. avium-intracellulare.* In Texas, Oklahoma, and Chicago *M. kansasii* is a more frequent causative agent than *M. avium-intracellulare.* The proportion of new cases caused by myco-

bacteria other than *M. tuberculosis* varies from 2 to 15 percent and is expected to increase as the number of infections due to *M. tuberculosis* decreases. In contrast to tuberculosis, multiple cases in the same family are very rare, and isolation of the patient is not necessary. In terms of frequency *M. avium-intracellulare* and *M. kansasii* are much the most important, followed by *M. scrofulaceum.* Infections with other species are rare.

Manifestations The symptoms and signs are those of pulmonary tuberculosis (Chap. 143), although there is some tendency for most of the infections to be more indolent. Infections with *M. avium-intracellulare* are more frequent in older adults and in men. Underlying chronic obstructive pulmonary disease is often present in infections due to *M. avium-intracellulare, M. scrofulaceum,* and *M. fortuitum-chelonei,* and is sometimes present with the other mycobacteria. Extrapulmonary lesions are rare.

Treatment Rational chemotherapy depends upon identification of the etiologic mycobacterium and determination of its drug sensitivity. *Mycobacterium kansasii* infections usually respond well to intensive triple-drug therapy with rifampin and a pair selected from isoniazid, ethambutol, and streptomycin. *Mycobacterium avium-intracellulare* infections are often resistant to chemotherapy. Treatment with four drugs chosen from isoniazid, rifampin, ethambutol, ethionamide, and streptomycin (or capreomycin or kanamycin) is recommended, along with appropriate surgery for unclosed cavities. Infections with *M. scrofulaceum* also are often resistant to drugs, and therapy is the same as for *M. avium-intracellulare.* Infections with *M. szulgai* have responded well to chemotherapy, but the others have been difficult to treat.

OTHER INFECTIONS *Mycobacterium avium-intracellulare* and *M. scrofulaceum* cause lymphadenitis in children, especially of the nodes draining the buccal mucous membrane. Excision of the node before it has ruptured or drained is the treatment of choice. The *M. fortuitum* and *M. chelonei* cause local abscesses, particularly from injections given with contaminated needles or syringes; cervical lymphadenitis and cellulitis also occur, with the site of entry probably the mouth. *Mycobacterium chelonei* has caused two recent outbreaks of infection of sternal incisions after cardiac surgery (coronary bypass and valve replacement). The source of the organism could not be determined. In addition, contamination of porcine cardiac valve prostheses by *M. chelonei* has occasionally been detected, but

TABLE 145-1
Human mycobacterial pathogens other than *M. tuberculosis* and *M. leprae*

Mycobacterium	Pigmentation of culture*	Usual site of disease	Usual source of infection	Response to drugs
M. marinum	P	Skin	Swimming pools, aquaria, fish	Good
M. ulcerans	N	Skin	Tropical environment	Variable
M. avium-intracellulare	N	Lungs	Environment, animals?	Poor
M. kansasii	P	Lungs	Environment?	Good
M. xenopi	S	Lungs	Water, animals?	Variable
M. szulgai	S†	Lungs	?	Good
M. scrofulaceum	S	Lungs, lymph nodes	Water, soil	Poor
M. fortuitum	N	Skin (abscesses), lungs	Soil, dirt	Poor
M. chelonei	N	Skin (abscesses), lungs	Soil, dirt	Poor

* P = photochromogenic (develops yellow-orange pigment only when exposed to light). N = nonpigmented. S = scotochromogenic (develops yellow-orange pigment in dark light).
† Scotochromogenic at 37°C, photochromogenic at 25°C.

infection following the implantation of the contaminated valves has been rare. *Mycobacterium kansasii* and *M. scrofulaceum* can cause disease of bones and joints. Widely disseminated, usually fatal infections with any of these mycobacteria can occur, especially in immunosuppressed patients.

REFERENCES

BARKER DJP: Epidemiology of *Mycobacterium ulcerans* infections. Trans R Soc Trop Med Hyg 67:43, 1973

FELDMAN RA, HERSHFIELD E: Mycobacterial skin infection by an unidentified species. A report of 29 patients. Ann Intern Med 80:445, 1974

JOLLY HW JR, SEABURY JH: Infections with *Mycobacterium marinum.* Arch Dermatol 106:32, 1972

KUBICA GP: Differential identification of mycobacteria. VII. Key features for identification of clinically significant mycobacteria. Am Rev Respir Dis 107:9, 1973

LINCOLN EM, GILBERT LA: Disease in children due to mycobacteria other than *Mycobacterium tuberculosis.* Am Rev Respir Dis 105:683, 1972

WOLINSKY E: Nontuberculous mycobacterial infections of man. Med Clin North Am 58:639, 1974

section 8 | Spirochetal diseases

146
SYPHILIS

KING K. HOLMES

The great ailment of modern syphilological practice is a lack of comprehension of the why and wherefore, rather than the what to do.

J. H. Stokes

DEFINITION Syphilis is a chronic systemic infection caused by *Treponema pallidum,* is usually sexually transmitted, and is characterized by an incubation period averaging 3 weeks, followed by a primary lesion associated with regional lymphadenopathy; a secondary bacteremic stage associated with generalized mucocutaneous lesions and generalized lymphadenopathy; a latent period of subclinical infection lasting many years; and, in about one-third of untreated cases, a tertiary stage characterized by progressive destructive mucocutaneous musculoskeletal or parenchymal lesions, aortitis, or central nervous system disease.

ETIOLOGY The discovery of *Treponema pallidum* in syphilitic material was made by Schaudinn and Hoffman in 1905. *Treponema pallidum* is one of the many spiral-shaped microorganisms which propel themselves by spinning around their longitudinal axis. The spiral organisms of medical significance, the Treponemataceae, include three groups which are pathogenic for humans and for a variety of other animals: the *Leptospira,* which cause human leptospirosis; the *Borrelia,* including *B. recurrentis* and *B. vincentii,* which cause relapsing fever and Vincent's angina, respectively; and the *Treponema,* responsible for the diseases known as treponematoses. The *Treponema* include *T. pallidum; T. pertenue,* and *T. carateum,* the organisms which cause yaws and pinta (Chap. 147); and *T. cuniculi,* the cause of rabbit syphilis. Other treponema include nonpathogenic species found in the human mouth and several species of anaerobic saprophytic genital treponemes of low pathogenicity which often coexist with anaerobic gram-negative rods in ulcerative genital lesions (so-called "fusospirochetal" infections). These can also be confused with *T. pallidum* on dark-field examination by inexperienced individuals.

Treponema pallidum is a thin, delicate organism with 6 to 14 spirals and tapered ends, measuring 6 to 15 μm in total length and 0.2 μm in width. The cytoplasm is surrounded by a trilaminar cytoplasmic membrane, which in turn is surrounded by a delicate inner mucopeptide layer, the periplast, thought to be composed of alternating molecules of *N*-acetyl glucosamine and *N*-acetyl muramic acid, and which provides some structural rigidity, while an outer lipoprotein membrane is selectively permeable and osmotically sensitive. The unique spiral structure of *T. pallidum* is maintained by six fibrils, three arising at each end of the organism, which wind around the cell body in a groove between the inner cell wall and the outer cell membrane, and may be the contractile elements responsible for motility. None of the four pathogenic treponemes has yet been cultured in vitro, and no convincing morphological, serologic, or metabolic differences between them have been discerned. They are distinguished primarily according to the clinical syndrome they produce. Limited animal inoculation studies also indicate some differences in host range and virulence, even among different strains of *T. pallidum.* The only known natural host for *T. pallidum* is the human being. Most mammals can be infected with *T. pallidum,* but only humans, higher apes, and a few laboratory animals regularly develop syphilitic lesions. Virulent strains of *T. pallidum* are maintained in rabbits.

HISTORY The first clear descriptions of syphilis were recorded at the end of the fifteenth century, when a pandemic known as the great pox, as distinguished from smallpox, swept over Europe and Asia. Severe morbidity or death often occurred during the secondary stage, indicating an unexplained virulence then which is almost unknown today, except in congenital syphilis. The source of the European pandemic 500 years ago is controversial. The sudden appearance and high morbidity of syphilis in 1494 led to the theory of the importation of a highly virulent strain of *Treponema pallidum* from America. However, many historians discern earlier references to syphilis in various writings dating from Hippocrates.

The sexual mode of transmission of syphilis was recognized early during the European pandemic, and description of the primary and secondary stages of the disease followed. The major cardiovascular and neurological complications of late syphilis were recognized during the eighteenth and nineteenth centuries. However, the erroneous concept that gonorrhea, chancroid, and syphilis were the same disease was strengthened by John Hunter, who developed syphilis following self-inoculation with gonorrheal pus in 1767. These three diseases were finally distinguished by Ricord and his students in the mid-1800s, although their etiologies were not established until the turn of this century. Gummas were not recognized as being syphilitic in origin until this century.

A rapid series of important advances began in 1903 with the successful inoculation of syphilis into primates by Metchnikoff and Rowe. The discovery of *Treponema pallidum* in serum from secondary lesions was made by Schaudinn in 1905 and was confirmed by Landsteiner by dark-field microscopy in 1906. In 1910, Wasserman introduced the complement fixation test for the diagnosis of syphilis, and in the same year, Ehrlich and Hata introduced an arsenic derivative, arsphenamine (Compound 606, Salvarsan), which was effective in treatment. More importantly, arsphenamine was the first specific antimicrobial drug.

EPIDEMIOLOGY Nearly all cases of syphilis are now acquired by sexual contact with infectious lesions (i.e., the chancre, mucous patch, or condyloma latum). Uncommon modes of transmission include nonsexual personal contact, contact with contaminated fomites, or infection in utero or following blood transfusions.

In the United States, infant deaths due to syphilis, and new admissions of patients with syphilitic psychoses, have fallen by 99 percent since 1940. The total reported number of cases of late and late latent syphilis has fallen almost every year since 1943. The 10.4 cases per 100,000 population reported in 1977 represent a decrease of 91 percent since 1943. Only 463 cases of congenital syphilis were reported in 1977, a decrease of 97 percent since 1941. The number of new cases of infectious syphilis reached a peak in 1947, then fell steadily to about 6000 in 1957, but then began to increase again.

Although the reported incidence of syphilis appears higher in nonwhites than in whites, and is higher in urban than in rural areas, these differences partly reflect the fact that indigent urban racial groups are treated at public clinics, where case reporting is complete. The case rates of early syphilis are highest in the South and Southwest, and in those states with large urban populations. The peak incidence of syphilis occurs in the age group 20 to 24. In the United States, the male/female ratio of reported early cases (<1 year) has increased from 0.8:1 in 1950 to over 2:1 in 1977. In England the ratio is 6:1.

Of all men with primary, secondary, or early latent syphilis interviewed in the United States during 1977–1978, one-half were homosexual or bisexual. Primary syphilis is usually not diagnosed in women or in homosexual men. For example, during 1974 in the United States, 42 percent of cases of early syphilis in heterosexual men were detected in the primary stage, whereas only 23 percent of early cases in homosexual men and 11 percent of early cases in women were detected in the primary stage. Anorectal chancres make up over 50 percent of primary syphilis among homosexuals examined in venereology clinics in the United Kingdom, but only 15 percent of primary syphilis among homosexuals examined in the United States. This remarkable difference suggests either a greater reticence of physicians in the United States to examine the anal canal or failure to consider syphilis in the evaluation of anal lesions in men.

In 1977, there were 20,362 cases of primary and secondary syphilis and 21,297 cases of early latent syphilis reported, and the number of unreported cases was estimated to be two to three times greater. Comparison of reported case rates of primary and secondary syphilis in the United States with those in England for 1975 shows that the rates per 100,000 persons between ages 20 and 24 were 3.6 times higher for males and 6.1 times higher for females in the United States than in England. The actual difference in case rates between the United States and England is undoubtedly greater, because most cases of syphilis in England are treated by venereologists and reported, whereas most cases in the United States are seen by physicians in private practice and many are not reported. The higher case rates in the United States may be partly attributable to inadequate tracing of sexual contacts of unreported cases.

Interviews of patients with early syphilis disclose an average of 2.8 sexual contacts at risk per patient, and "cluster" tracing of additional associates of the patient or his or her contacts discloses an average of 0.7 others who are also at risk. Approximately one of two individuals named as contacts of infectious syphilis becomes infected. Many contacts will have already developed manifestations of syphilis when they are first seen, and about 30 percent of apparently uninfected contacts of infectious syphilis who are examined within 30 days of exposure will actually be in the incubation stage and will themselves develop infectious syphilis if not treated. Because of this, the identification and "epidemiologic" treatment of all recently exposed contacts has become an important aspect of syphilis control. Also important is the identification of syphilitics by serologic testing of pregnant women, hospital admissions, military inductees, and persons undergoing examination in physicians' offices. Of 43 million blood specimens examined during 1977 in the United States, 1.5 million tests were reactive, representing untreated syphilis, previously treated syphilis, or false-positive tests. Over one-half of all reported early syphilis cases of less than 1 year's duration were detected as a direct result of either contact tracing or serologic testing. More controversial are laws and regulations requiring routine premarital serologic testing for syphilis. This program, which drains approximately 10 percent of all public funds for control of sexually transmitted diseases, yields very few cases of early syphilis. Syphilis is under control in some states in which new cases are limited to sporadic outbreaks which tend to involve homosexual men and are contained by aggressive contact tracing.

NATURAL COURSE AND PATHOGENESIS OF UNTREATED SYPHILIS *Treponema pallidum* can rapidly penetrate intact mucous membranes or abraded skin and within a few hours enters the lymphatics and blood to produce systemic infection and metastatic foci long before and after the appearance of a primary lesion. Thus, blood from a patient with incubating syphilis is infectious. The generation time of *T. pallidum* in humans is 30 to 33 h, and the incubation period of syphilis is inversely proportional to the number of organisms inoculated. The concentration of treponemes generally reaches at least 10^7 per gram of tissue before the appearance of a clinical lesion. In experimental infection in rabbits or humans, a single treponeme can initiate infection which leads to a discernible lesion only after 6 weeks, although histopathologic changes are evident earlier, while intradermal injection of 10^7 organisms usually produces a lesion within 72 h. The median incubation period in humans is about 21 days. Although the incubation period is traditionally stated as ranging from 9 to 90 days, experimental inoculations of humans and rabbits show that the period from inoculation until the primary lesion is discernible rarely exceeds 6 weeks. Subcurative therapy during the incubation period may delay the onset of the primary lesion but does not seem to prevent ultimate development of symptomatic disease.

The primary lesion appears at the site of inoculation, persists for 2 to 6 weeks, and then heals spontaneously. Histopathology of primary lesions shows perivascular infiltration, chiefly by plasma cells and histiocytes, capillary proliferation, and eventually obliteration of small blood vessels. At this time

T. pallidum is demonstrable in the chancre in spaces between epithelial cells as well as within invaginations or phagosomes of epithelial cells, fibroblasts, plasma cells, and the endothelial cells of small capillaries, within lymphatic channels, and in the regional lymph nodes. Macrophages and polymorphonuclear leukocytes can be seen taking up treponemes into phagocytic vacuoles where the organisms are destroyed.

The generalized parenchymal, constitutional, and mucocutaneous manifestations of secondary syphilis usually appear about 6 weeks after healing of the chancre, although secondary lesions may appear while the chancre is still present, or only after several months have passed. Secondary maculopapular skin lesions show histopathologic features of hyperkeratosis of the epidermis, capillary proliferation with endothelial swelling in the superficial corium, and dermal papillae with transmigration of polymorphonuclear leukocytes, and in the deeper corium, perivascular infiltration by plasma cells. Treponemes are found in many tissues including the aqueous humor of the eye and the cerebrospinal fluid. Cerebrospinal fluid abnormalities are detected in as many as 17 to 33 percent of patients during the secondary stage. Immune complex–induced glomerulonephritis occurs. Generalized lymphadenopathy is present and is characterized by marked follicular hyperplasia, with histiocytic infiltration and lymphocyte depletion of the paracortical areas, where treponema are present in greatest numbers. The reason for the paradoxical appearance of secondary manifestations in the face of high titers of humoral antibody (including immobilizing antibody) to *T. pallidum* is unknown. The secondary lesions subside within 2 to 6 weeks, and the patient enters the latent stage, which is detectable only by serologic testing. Approximately 25 percent of untreated patients experience one or more subsequent generalized or localized mucocutaneous relapses at some time during the first 2 to 4 years after infection. Since 90 percent of such infectious relapses occur during the first year, identification and examination of sexual contacts are most important for patients with syphilis of less than 1 year's duration. However, in the International Classification of Diseases, latent syphilis is arbitrarily divided into early latent (less than 2 years' duration) and late latent (over 2 years' duration) stages. About one-third of patients with untreated latent syphilis develop clinically apparent tertiary disease. In the past, the most common type of tertiary disease was the gumma, a usually benign granulomatous lesion. Today, gummas are very uncommon, perhaps because they respond to very low doses of antitreponemal drugs. The remaining tertiary lesions are caused by obliterative small-vessel endarteritis which usually involves the vasa vasorum of the ascending aorta and less often the central nervous system. Factors which determine development of tertiary disease are unknown, except that trauma may predispose to gumma.

The course of untreated syphilis has been studied retrospectively in a group of nearly 2000 patients with primary or secondary syphilis diagnosed clinically, before the dark-field and Wasserman tests came into use (the *Oslo Study*, 1891–1951); prospectively in 431 Negro men with seropositive latent syphilis of 3 or more years' duration (the *Tuskegee Study*, 1932–1972); and retrospectively in a review of 198 autopsies of patients with untreated syphilis.

In the Oslo Study, 24 percent of the patients developed relapsing secondary lesions within 4 years, and 28 percent eventually developed one or more manifestations of late syphilis. Cardiovascular syphilis, including aortitis, was detected in 10.4 percent, with no cases occurring in those infected before age 15; symptomatic neurosyphilis occurred in 6.5 percent, and 16 percent developed benign tertiary syphilis (gumma of the skin, mucous membranes, and skeleton). Syphilis was the primary cause of death in 15.1 percent of males and 8.3 percent of the females. However, many patients alive when the Oslo Study was completed remained at risk for developing complications, while tuberculosis and other infections prematurely eliminated others before complications of syphilis occurred, so the Oslo figures probably represent minimum estimates of the risk of late complications. Cardiovascular syphilis was found in 35 percent of men and 22 percent of women who eventually underwent autopsy. In general, serious late complications were nearly twice as common in men as in women.

The Tuskegee Study showed that the death rate of syphilitic Negro men, 25 to 50 years of age, was 17 percent greater than in nonsyphilitics, and 30 percent of all deaths were attributable to cardiovascular or central nervous system syphilis. By far the most important factor in increased mortality was cardiovascular syphilis. Anatomic evidence of aortitis was found in 40 to 60 percent of autopsied syphilitics (versus 15 percent of controls), while central nervous system lues was found in only 4 percent. Hypertension was also increased in the syphilitics. Thus, the incidence of cardiovascular syphilis was higher and central nervous system syphilis lower in the prospective Tuskegee Study, as compared with the Oslo Study. These studies each show that about one-third of patients with untreated syphilis develop clinical or pathological evidence of tertiary syphilis; about one-fourth die as a direct result of tertiary syphilis; and additional excess mortality not directly attributable to tertiary syphilis is also seen. Untreated syphilis may make people more susceptible to other diseases, or individuals who get syphilis coincidentally may be more susceptible to other diseases, perhaps because of socioeconomic factors.

MANIFESTATIONS **Primary syphilis** The typical primary chancre usually begins as a single painless papule which rapidly becomes eroded and usually, but not always, is indurated, with a characteristic cartilaginous consistency on palpation of the edge and base of the ulcer. Histological examination of the ulcer shows mononuclear and histiocytic infiltrates with obliterative endarteritis and periarteritis of small vessels. *Treponema pallidum* is seen by electron microscopy to lie in interstitial perivascular spaces and within invaginations or phagosomes of neutrophils, macrophages, endothelial cells, and plasma cells.

In heterosexual men, the chancre is usually located on the penis. In homosexual men, the chancre is often found in the anal canal, usually within view if the buttocks are spread, within the mouth, or on the external genitalia. It may occur on any site of the body. In women, primary sites which are commonly overlooked include the cervix and labia. Regional lymphadenopathy accompanies the primary lesion, appearing within 1 week of the onset of the lesion. The nodes are firm, nonsuppurative, and painless. Inguinal lymphadenopathy is bilateral. The chancre heals within 4 to 6 weeks (range 2 to 12 weeks), but the lymphadenopathy may persist for months.

Atypical primary lesions are common. The clinical appearance depends upon the number of treponemes inoculated and upon the preinfection immune status of the patient. A large inoculum produces a dark-field positive ulcerative lesion in nonimmune human volunteers, but in individuals with a previous history of syphilis produces either a small dark-field negative papule, an asymptomatic but seropositive latent infection, or no response at all. A small inoculum usually produces only a papular lesion, even in nonimmune humans. Thus, syphilis should be considered even in the evaluation of trivial or atypical, dark-field negative, genital lesions. The most common genital lesions which must be differentiated from primary syphilis include traumatic, superinfected lesions, genital herpes simplex virus infection (Chap. 193), and chancroid (Chap. 126). *Primary genital herpes* may produce inguinal adenopathy but is initially characterized by multiple painful vesicles which later ulcerate, and with systemic symptoms including fever; *recurrent genital herpes* typically begins with a cluster of painful vesicles without associated adenopathy. *Chancroid* produces painful, superficial exudative, nonindurated, usually multiple ulcers; adenopathy is either unilateral or bilateral, tender, and may suppurate.

Secondary syphilis The manifestations of the secondary stage are protean but usually include localized or diffuse symmetric mucocutaneous lesions and generalized nontender lymphadenopathy. The remnant of the healing primary chancre is still present in many cases. The skin rash consists of macular, papular, papulosquamous, and occasionally pustular syphilides, often with one or more forms present simultaneously. Initial lesions are bilaterally symmetric, pale red or pink, nonpruritic, discrete, round macules, 5 to 10 mm in diameter, distributed on the trunk and proximal extremities. After 1 to 2 months, red, papular lesions 3 to 10 mm in diameter also appear. These may progress to necrotic (pustular) lesions in association with increasing endarteritis and perivascular mononuclear infiltration. These lesions are distributed widely and may occur on the palms, soles, face, and scalp. Tiny papular *follicular syphilides* involving hair follicles may result in patchy alopecia and loss of eyebrows or beard. Progressive endarteritis obliterans and ischemia result in superficial scaling of papules (*papulosquamous syphilides*) and eventually may lead to central necrosis (*pustular syphilide*). In warm, moist, intertriginous areas, including the perianal area, vulva, scrotum, and inner thighs, axillas, and the skin under pendulous breasts, papules enlarge and become eroded, to produce broad, moist, pink or gray-white highly infectious lesions called *condyloma lata*. Superficial mucosal erosions, called *mucous patches,* occur in about a third of patients and may involve lips, oral mucosa, tongue, palate, pharynx, vulva and vagina, glans penis, or inner prepuce. The typical mucous patch is a silver-gray erosion surrounded by a red periphery and is usually painless.

During relapses of secondary syphilis, condyloma lata are particularly common, and skin lesions tend to be asymmetrically distributed and more infiltrated, resembling skin lesions of late syphilis, perhaps reflecting increasing cellular immunity.

Constitutional symptoms which may accompany secondary syphilis include fever, weight loss, malaise, and anorexia. Headache and meningismus are common. Acute meningitis occurs in only 1 to 2 percent of patients, but increased cells and protein have been found in the cerebrospinal fluid in 30 percent or more of patients. *Treponema pallidum* has also been recovered by rabbit inoculation from cerebrospinal fluid during secondary syphilis even in the absence of other cerebrospinal fluid abnormalities.

Other less common complications described in secondary syphilis include hepatitis, nephropathy, arthritis and periostitis, and iridocyclitis. It is uncertain whether the association between secondary syphilis and hepatitis is causal or coincidental. *Syphilitic hepatitis* is distinguished by an unusually high serum alkaline phosphatase and by a nonspecific histological appearance which is unlike viral hepatitis and includes moderate inflammation with polymorphonuclear leukocytes and lymphocytes, some hepatocellular damage, and no cholestasis. The *renal involvement* is associated with proteinuria, an acute nephrotic syndrome, or rarely with hemorrhagic glomerulonephritis, and which is characterized by subepithelial electron-dense deposits and glomerular immune complexes, suggesting that this complication is a form of immune complex glomerulonephritis. Anterior uveitis has been reported in 5 to 10 percent of patients with secondary syphilis, and *T. pallidum* can be demonstrated in the aqueous humor in such cases. Posterior uveitis occurs rarely.

Latent syphilis A diagnosis of latent syphilis is established by the finding of a positive specific treponemal antibody test for syphilis, together with a normal cerebrospinal fluid examination, the absence of clinical manifestations of syphilis on physical examination and chest films, and a history of primary or secondary lesions, history of exposure to syphilis, or delivery of an infant with congenital syphilis. *Early latent* syphilis encompasses the first 2 years after infection, during which relapse of mucocutaneous lesions may occur, while *late latent* syphilis, beginning 2 years after infection, in the untreated patient, is associated with immunity to infectious relapse and with resistance to reinfection. *Treponema pallidum* may still intermittently seed the bloodstream during this stage, pregnant women with latent syphilis may infect the fetus in utero, and transfusion syphilis has been transmitted from patients with latent syphilis of many years' duration. Until recently it was thought that untreated late latent syphilis had three possible outcomes: (1) it could persist throughout the life of the infected individual; (2) it could end in development of late syphilis; or (3) it could end with spontaneous cure of infection, with reversion of serologic tests to negative. It is now apparent, however, that the more sensitive treponemal antibody tests rarely if ever become negative. Thus, 50 to 70 percent of untreated patients with latent syphilis never develop clinically evident late syphilis, but the occurrence of spontaneous cure is in doubt.

Late syphilis The onset of slowly progressive inflammatory disease of the aorta or central nervous system begins early during latent syphilis. Pathogenic studies have shown evidence of early syphilitic aortitis soon after the secondary lesions subside, while asymptomatic neurosyphilis can be detected readily during life by cerebrospinal fluid (CSF) examination.

ASYMPTOMATIC NEUROSYPHILIS In patients with untreated latent syphilis, if the CSF is normal 2 years or more after infection, there is probably no future risk of subsequent development of neurosyphilis, except for the purely vascular type. The diagnosis of asymptomatic neurosyphilis is made in patients with no clinical manifestations of neurosyphilis who have cerebrospinal fluid abnormalities, including pleocytosis, elevated protein, or positive cerebrospinal fluid Wasserman or Venereal Disease Research Laboratory (VDRL) test. One or more of these findings are present in 20 to 30 percent of patients with untreated syphilis after 2 years. The risk of progression to symptomatic neurosyphilis is two or three times greater in Caucasians than in Negroes and is twice as common in men as in women. The risk of parenchymal neurosyphilis (tabes dorsalis or general paresis) is five times greater in men than in women, supposedly because pregnancy after the initial infection somehow protects women from parenchymal neurosyphilis. In patients with untreated asymptomatic neurosyphilis, the overall cumulative probability of progression to clinical neurosyphilis is about 20 percent in the first 10 years, but increases with passing time, and is highest in those who show the greatest degree of pleocytosis or protein elevation. The fluorescent treponemal antibody (FTA) test on undiluted cerebrospinal fluid has been found to be reactive far more often than the VDRL test in cases of latent syphilis. The prognosis of patients with a positive CSF-FTA test without other cerebrospinal fluid abnormalities is not known, but very likely this finding merely represents passive transfer of serum antibody into the CSF, not asymptomatic neurosyphilis. Similarly, the finding of a positive CSF-FTA test without other cerebrospinal fluid abnormalities in patients with a positive serum FTA-ABS (fluorescent treponemal antibody-absorption) associated with nonspecific neurological findings does not necessarily prove a diagnosis of "atypical" neurosyphilis. However, a therapeutic trial of penicillin in doses adequate for neurosyphilis is warranted in any patient with a positive serum treponemal antibody test who also has unexplained neurological findings.

SYMPTOMATIC NEUROSYPHILIS The risk of neurosyphilis is two or three times greater in Caucasians than in Negroes, and is twice as common in men as in women. Although mixed features are common, the major clinical categories of symptomatic neurosyphilis include meningovascular and parenchymatous syphilis. The latter category includes general paresis and tabes dorsalis. The average interval from infection to onset of symptoms is 5 to 10 years for meningovascular syphilis, 20 years for general paresis, and 25 to 30 years for tabes dorsalis. However, many patients with symptomatic neurosyphilis do not present a classic picture, but have mixed or incomplete syndromes. *Meningovascular syphilis* is associated with inflammation of the pia and arachnoid, together with evidence of focal or widespread cerebrovascular disease or often only with pupillary or reflex changes. The manifestations of *general paresis* reflect widespread parenchymal damage and include abnormalities corresponding to the mnemonic *paresis* [*p*ersonality, *a*ffect, *r*eflexes (hyperactive), *e*ye (e.g., Argyll Robertson pupils), *s*ensorium (illusions, delusions, hallucinations), *i*ntellect (decreased recent memory orientation, calculations, judgment, insight), and *s*peech]. *Tabes dorsalis* presents symptoms and signs of demyelinization of the posterior columns, dorsal roots, and dorsal root ganglia. Symptoms include ataxic, wide-based gait and footslap, paresthesias, bladder disturbances, impotence, and signs including areflexia, loss of position, deep pain, and temperature sensation. Trophic joint degeneration (Charcot's joints) and perforating ulceration of the feet may result from loss of pain sensation. The Argyll Robertson pupil, seen in both tabes dorsalis and paresis, is a small, irregular pupil which reacts to accommodation but not to light. *Optic atrophy* also occurs frequently in association with tabes.

CARDIOVASCULAR SYPHILIS Cardiovascular manifestations are limited to the large vessels in which the blood supply is provided by vasa vasorum. Endarteritis obliterans of the vasa vasorum produces medial necrosis with destruction of elastic tissue, particularly in the ascending and transverse segments of the aortic arch, resulting in uncomplicated aortitis, aortic regurgitation, saccular aneurysm, or coronary ostial stenosis. Until recently, these complications had not been described following congenital syphilis or syphilis acquired before age 14, suggesting some unexplained resistance of the large blood vessels in youth to invasion by *T. pallidum*. The onset of symptoms occurs from 10 to 40 years after infection. Cardiovascular complications are commoner and occur at an earlier age in men than in women, and in Negroes than in Caucasians. The incidence of symptomatic cardiovascular complications in late untreated syphilis is approximately 10 percent, with aortic regurgitation being two to four times as common as aneurysm. However, syphilitic aortitis can be demonstrated at autopsy in about one-half of Negro males with untreated syphilis.

Asymptomatic syphilitic aortitis may be suspected in life if linear calcification of the ascending aorta is demonstrated on chest x-ray films, since arteriosclerotic disease seldom produces this sign. Aortic dilatation and a tambour quality of the sound of aortic closure are unreliable signs of aortitis. Syphilitic aneurysms are usually saccular, occasionally fusiform, and do not lead to dissection. Approximately 1 in 10 aortic aneurysms of syphilitic origin may involve the abdominal aorta, but tend to occur above the renal arteries, whereas arteriosclerotic abdominal aneurysms usually are found below the renal arteries. With increasing age, the nervous system is also affected in up to 40 percent of patients with cardiovascular syphilis.

LATE LESIONS OF THE EYES Iritis associated with pain, photophobia, and dimness of vision or chorioretinitis occurs not only during secondary syphilis, but also as a relatively common manifestation of late syphilis. Adhesions of the iris to the anterior lens may produce a fixed pupil, not to be confused with Argyll Robertson pupil.

LATE BENIGN SYPHILIS (GUMMA) Gummas may be multiple or diffuse, but are usually solitary lesions which range from microscopic size to several centimeters in diameter, and histologically consist of nonspecific granulomatous inflammation with central necrosis surrounded by mononuclear, epithelioid, and fibroblastic cells, occasional giant cells, and perivasculitis. Although *T. pallidum* cannot be demonstrated microscopically, it can be recovered from the lesions by rabbit inoculation. The most commonly involved sites are the skin and skeletal systems, mouth and upper respiratory tract, larynx, liver, and stomach. Virtually any organ may be involved. Gummas of skin produce painless nodular, papulosquamous, or ulcerative lesions, which are indurated, and form characteristic circles or arcs, with peripheral hyperpigmentation. The lesions are usually indolent, and may heal spontaneously with scarring, but may also be explosive in onset and are often destructive. These lesions may resemble many other chronic granulomatous conditions, including *tuberculosis* and *sarcoidosis* of skin, leprosy, and *deep fungal infections*. Skeletal gummas involve long bones of the legs with greatest frequency, although any bone may be affected. Trauma may predispose to involvement of a specific site. Presenting symptoms usually include focal pain and tenderness. When sufficiently advanced to produce radiographic abnormalities, the findings may include periostitis or destructive or sclerosing osteitis. Gummas of the upper respiratory tract can lead to perforation of the nasal septum or palate. Gummatous hepatitis may produce epigastric pain and tenderness and low-grade fever, and may be associated with splenomegaly and anemia.

The histopathology and extensive tissue necrosis associated with gummas suggest that delayed hypersensitivity to *T. pallidum* produces these lesions. Certain individuals appear to develop an exaggerated delayed hypersensitivity response to *T. pallidum*, presumably mediated by sensitized T lymphocytes and macrophages. In areas where syphilis is endemic in childhood, reinfection may result in gummas; when one member of a household acquires a fresh infection, other members of the household who then become reinfected develop gummas. Experimental inoculation of *T. pallidum* into individuals with latent or late syphilis also sometimes results in gumma formation at the site of inoculation.

Since the histological changes may be suggestive but are nonspecific, the diagnosis of late benign syphilis is confirmed by serologic testing and by therapeutic trial. Treatment with penicillin results in rapid healing of active gummatous lesions.

Congenital syphilis Transmission of *T. pallidum* from a syphilitic mother to her fetus across the placenta may occur at any stage of pregnancy, but the lesions of congenital syphilis develop only after the fourth month of gestation, when immunologic competence begins to develop. This suggests that the pathogenesis of congenital syphilis may depend upon the immune response of the host rather than upon a direct toxic effect of *T. pallidum*. The risk of infection of the fetus during untreated early maternal syphilis is estimated to be 80 to 95 percent, decreases to about 70 percent at 4 years, and is still lower during late latent maternal syphilis. Adequate treatment of the mother before the sixteenth week of pregnancy should prevent fetal damage. During the past decade, the number of reported cases of congenital syphilis in the United States has remained steady at about 5 cases per 100 reported cases of primary and secondary syphilis in women. A study of cases reported in 1972 showed that 37 percent of the mothers of infected children had not sought prenatal examination, while 44 percent had had a nonreactive serologic test during the first trimester, presumably due either to false-negative first trimester tests or to acquisition of syphilis during pregnancy. Syphilis acquired during pregnancy is likely to remain subclinical in the mother while nearly always causing serious fetal infection. Untreated early maternal infection may result in up to 40 percent fetal loss (stillbirth is more common than abortion, because of the late onset of fetal infection), prematurity, neonatal death, or nonfatal congenital syphilis. Therefore, routine serologic testing in early pregnancy as well as at delivery and repeat serologic testing of "high risk" pregnant women in the third trimester are fully justified.

Only fulminant cases of congenital syphilis are clinically apparent in live infants at birth, and these babies have a very poor prognosis. The most common clinical problem is the healthy appearing baby born to a mother who has a positive serologic test.

The manifestations of congenital syphilis can be divided into (1) early manifestations, which appear within the first 2 years of life, often between 2 and 10 weeks of age, are infectious, and resemble severe secondary syphilis in the adult; (2) late manifestations, which appear after 2 years, and are noninfectious; and (3) the residual stigmata of congenital syphilis. Only about 25 percent of cases of congenital syphilis are diagnosed during the first year of life.

The earliest sign of congenital syphilis is usually rhinitis ("snuffles") soon followed by other mucocutaneous lesions. These may include bullae (syphilitic pemphigus), vesicles, superficial desquamation, petechial, and later, papulosquamous lesions, mucous patches, and condyloma latum. The most common early manifestations are osteochondritis and osteitis, particularly involving the metaphyses of long bones, progressing in severity during the first 6 months of life, then spontaneously subsiding; and periostitis, which continues to progress after the first 6 months. Hepatosplenomegaly, lymphadenopathy, anemia, jaundice, thrombocytopenia, and leukocytosis are common. The anemia is usually hypoproliferative but may be hemolytic (paroxysmal cold hemoglobinuria). The nephrotic syndrome in early congenital syphilis, as in adult secondary syphilis, represents an immune complex–induced glomerulonephritis.

Neonatal congenital syphilis must be differentiated from other generalized congenital infections, including rubella, cytomegalovirus infection, and toxoplasmosis, and also from erythroblastosis fetalis. Neonatal death is usually due to pulmonary hemorrhage, secondary bacterial infection, or severe hepatitis. Pathological findings include interstitial and perivascular inflammation followed by variable fibroblastic proliferation, involving skin, bones, liver, kidneys, pancreas, spleen, lungs, and intestines, and extramedullary hematopoiesis.

Late congenital syphilis is defined as congenital syphilis which remains untreated after 2 years of age. In perhaps 60 percent of cases, the infection remains latent, while the clinical spectrum in the remainder differs in certain respects from that of acquired late syphilis in the adult. For example, cardiovascular syphilis rarely develops in late congenital syphilis, whereas interstitial keratitis is much more common and occurs between ages 5 and 25. The onset is acute with photophobia, pain, and circumcorneal injection, followed by superficial and deep vascularization of the cornea, which progresses despite antibiotic therapy, and eventually becomes bilateral. The symptoms and signs may be suppressed with corticosteroid therapy. Although treponemes have occasionally been demonstrated in aqueous humor in interstitial keratitis, the pathogenesis is obscure and is ascribed to "hypersensitivity." Other manifestations associated with interstitial keratitis are eighth-nerve deafness and recurrent arthropathy. Bilateral knee effusions are known as *Clutton's joints*. Examination of CSF discloses asymptomatic neurosyphilis in about one-third of untreated patients without other late clinical manifestations, and clinical neurosyphilis occurs in a quarter of untreated individuals with congenital syphilis over 6 years of age. The clinical manifestations of congenital neurosyphilis correspond to those seen in adult neurosyphilis. Gummatous periostitis occurs between ages 5 and 20 and, as in endemic nonvenereal childhood syphilis, tends to cause destructive lesions of the palate and nasal septum.

Characteristic stigmata include Hutchinson's teeth, the centrally notched, widely spaced, peg-shaped upper central incisors, and "mulberry" molars, sixth-year molars which have multiple, poorly developed cusps, rather than the usual four. The abnormal facies, which includes frontal bossing, saddle-nose, and poorly developed maxilla, may also be seen in congenital ectodermal dysplasia. Saber shins, or anterior tibial bowing, are rare but were probably more common in the past when syphilitic periostitis of the anterior tibia was associated with vitamin D deficiency. *Rhagades* are linear scars at the angles of the mouth and nose caused by secondary bacterial infection of the early facial eruption. Other stigmata include unexplained nerve deafness, old chorioretinitis, optic atrophy, and corneal opacities due to past interstitial keratitis.

LABORATORY EXAMINATIONS Dark-field examination technique Dark-field examination is essential in evaluating cutaneous lesions, such as the chancre of primary syphilis, or condyloma lata of secondary syphilis. Although it is difficult to demonstrate *T. pallidum* in dry maculopapular lesions in secondary syphilis by dark-field examination, the organism may be demonstrated by saline aspiration of lymph nodes during this stage. The surface of the suspected ulcerated lesion should be cleaned with saline and gauze, then gently abraded further with dry gauze, without production of bleeding. The lesion is then squeezed to express a serous transudate, and a drop of the transudate is picked up on the surface of a glass slide. A drop of saline (without bacteriostatic additives) may be mixed with the transudate if necessary, and this is then covered with a coverslip and examined immediately for *T. pallidum* with a dark-field or phase contrast microscope by an experienced individual. A single negative examination does not exclude syphilis, since at least 10^4 treponemes per milliliter transudate must be present to be detected, and prior use of topical antiseptic or cleansing by the patient may obfuscate the examination. Cleansing or use of topical medication should, therefore, be avoided, and the dark-field examination should be repeated on three successive days before being considered negative.

Serologic tests for syphilis The profusion of serologic tests for syphilis causes much unnecessary confusion. Syphilitic infection produces two types of antibodies, the *nonspecific reaginic antibody* and *specific antitreponemal* antibody.

The term *reagin* is unfortunate, since the unrelated gamma-E globulin (IgE) antibody involved in certain allergic phenomena is also known as *reagin*. The nontreponemal reaginic antibodies produced in syphilis contain both IgG and IgM immunoglobulins directed against a lipoidal antigen that results from the interaction of *T. pallidum* with host tissues, and possibly against a lipoidal antigen of *T. pallidum* itself. The cardiolipin antigens initially used in the detection of reaginic antibody are relatively crude extracts of beef heart, and it is not surprising that false-positive reactions were extremely common in many conditions other than syphilis. The cardiolipin-cholesterol-lecithin antigen now in use in a variety of tests for reaginic antibody (Table 146-1) is more purified and gives fewer false-positive reactions than did earlier antigens. The tests for treponemal antibody employ antigens derived from *T. pallidum*, rather than from tissues, and detect antibody related only to past or present treponemal infections.

The most widely used reagin antibody tests are the sensitive rapid plasma reagin (RPR) tests, which can be automated and are used to screen large numbers of serums, and the VDRL slide flocculation test, which is used to determine quantitatively the exact titer of serum reagin antibody. The reagin titer reflects the activity of the disease: false-positive VDRL titers usually do not exceed 1:8; a fourfold or greater rise in titer may be seen during the evolution of primary syphilis; VDRL titers usually reach 1:32 or higher in secondary syphilis; a persistent fall in titer following treatment of early syphilis provides essential evidence of an adequate response to therapy.

The standard antitreponemal antibody test is the FTA-ABS test. The patient's serum is first absorbed with a nonpathogenic treponemal antigen (sorbent) to remove group-specific antibody which may be produced against saprophytic oral and genital treponemes. The patient's absorbed serum is then placed on a slide which contains dried *T. pallidum*. If specific antibody to *T. pallidum* remains in the patient's serum after the absorption step, it is fixed to the dried treponemes, and then is detected by the addition of fluorescein-labeled antihuman gamma-globulin and subsequent examination of the slide by fluorescence microscopy. The *T. pallidum* immobilization (TPI) test, in which immobilization of live *T. pallidum* is produced by immune serum plus complement, is more laborious and in the United States is available only in research laboratories. The *T. pallidum* hemagglutination tests (MHA-TP and TPHA) are convenient tests for treponemal antibody but less sensitive than the FTA-ABS test for detection of early primary syphilis. Both the MHA-TP and FTA-ABS tests are very specific when used for confirmation of positive reaginic antibody tests but give false-positive rates as high as 1 to 2 percent when used for screening normal populations. The relative sensitivities of the VDRL, FTA-ABS, TPI, and MHA-TP tests in the various stages of syphilis are shown in Table 146-2.

The VDRL is negative in nearly one-third of patients with primary or late syphilis. Obtaining a reagin antibody test alone is not sufficient in evaluating late symptomatic syphilis; the more sensitive FTA-ABS test should be routinely obtained in suspected late syphilis. In early primary syphilis, the detection of antibody can be maximized either by performing an FTA-ABS test or simply by repeating a VDRL test after 1 to 2 weeks if the initial VDRL was negative. However, both tests are always positive during secondary syphilis, and a negative

VDRL or FTA-ABS virtually excludes syphilis in a patient with otherwise compatible mucocutaneous lesions. (An estimated 1 percent of patients with secondary syphilis have a negative VDRL test with undiluted serum which becomes positive in higher dilutions—the *prozone* phenomenon.)

False-positive serologic tests for syphilis An estimated 20 to 40 percent of all positive reagin tests are false-positive tests, but the percentages vary widely depending upon the population being examined. False-positive reagin tests are classified as acute if they become negative within 6 months. Acute false-positive reagin tests occur during mycoplasma pneumonia, malaria, and various acute bacterial or viral infections, and following smallpox vaccinations. Chronic reactions, which persist 6 months or longer, occur in addiction, autoimmune diseases, and aging. False-positive reagin tests occur in 25 percent of narcotics addicts, and in 10 to 20 percent of patients with active systemic lupus erythematosus. Other antibodies which have been found with great frequency in serums from chronic false-positive reactors include antinuclear, antithyroid, and antimitochondrial antibodies, as well as rheumatoid factor and cryoglobulins. The Donath-Landsteiner antibody responsible for paroxysmal cold hemoglobinuria is a hemolysin which appears in syphilis. The autoimmune nature of the false-positive reagin test is further suggested by the occurrence of systemic lupus erythematosus or other connective tissue diseases in 15 to 45 percent of chronic false-positive reactors. The prevalence of false-positive reagin tests increases with advancing age, and 10 percent of people over 70 years of age have false-positive reactions. Other diseases associated with hyperglobulinemia, such as leprosy, may also produce chronic false-positive reactions.

In the patient with a false-positive reagin test, syphilis is excluded by obtaining a negative FTA-ABS or MHA-TP test. The results of the FTA-ABS test are reported as negative, borderline, or positive. *Borderline* results are more common in patients who are pregnant or have diseases associated with abnormal or increased globulins, and are frequently not associated with either clinical, historical, or other serologic evidence of syphilis. Borderline results should, therefore, always be repeated in questionable cases and interpreted with caution. A typical "positive" FTA-ABS occurs infrequently in conditions other than syphilis. Although false-positive FTA-ABS tests have been reported in 15 percent of patients with active systemic lupus erythematosus, the fluorescent staining is "borderline" or has an atypical "beaded" appearance in most cases (thought to be due to attachment of antinuclear antibody to treponemal DNA or nucleoprotein leaked through breaks in the outer treponemal membranes). However, because of the occasional occurrence of false-positive FTA-ABS tests, only a positive TPI provides conclusive proof of past or present treponemal infection. Both the FTA-ABS and TPI tests are positive in patients who have had yaws or pinta.

For practical purposes, most clinicians need to be familiar with the three uses of serologic tests for syphilis: (1) for screen-

TABLE 146-1
Common serologic tests for syphilis

NONSPECIFIC (REAGIN) ANTIBODY TESTS

Flocculation: VDRL
Complement fixation: Kolmer
Agglutination: rapid plasma reagin (RPR)

SPECIFIC TREPONEMAL ANTIBODY TESTS

Immunofluorescence: fluorescent treponemal antibody-absorption (FTA-ABS)
Immobilization: *Treponema pallidum* immobilization (TPI)
Hemagglutination: *T. pallidum* hemagglutination assay (MHA-TP, TPHA)

TABLE 146-2
Reactivity of serodiagnostic tests in untreated syphilis

Test	Stage of disease,* % positive			
	Primary	Secondary	Latent	Tertiary
VDRL	72	100	73	77
FTA-ABS	91	100	97	100
TPI	46	98	95	95
MHA-TP	69	100	98	100

* *Percentage figures provided should not be interpreted as absolute values because there are small numbers in certain categories and test results vary from study to study.*
SOURCE: *Data compiled by the Center for Disease Control.*

ing large numbers of serums for reaginic antibody (e.g., RPR); (2) for quantitative measurement of reaginic antibody titer in order to assess the clinical activity of syphilis, and to follow the reagin titer in response to therapy (e.g., VDRL); and (3) to confirm the diagnosis of syphilis in a patient with a positive reagin antibody test or with a suspected clinical diagnosis of syphilis (e.g., FTA-ABS).

IgM-FTA-ABS test for active congenital syphilis in the newborn
All newborn infants of mothers with reactive VDRL or FTA-ABS tests will themselves have reactive tests whether or not they have become infected, because of passive transplacental transfer of maternal IgG immunoglobulins which are reactive in these tests. However, if IgM antitreponemal antibody is present in the infant's serum, it reflects fetal antibody production in response to intrauterine infection, particularly if there is a rise in titer, since maternal IgM antibody does not cross the intact placental barrier. Neonatal IgM antibody is detected in cord or neonatal serums in a modified FTA-ABS test, employing fluorescein-labeled antihuman IgM to detect antitreponemal IgM antibody. Similar tests have been developed for detection of congenital toxoplasmosis, rubella, and cytomegalovirus infections. The IgM-FTA-ABS test is sensitive and is positive in infants with active congenital syphilis. When the mother and fetus become infected very late during pregnancy, this test may be negative in the neonatal period. However, the specificity of this test is in doubt because of evidence that infants with a variety of congenital infections may produce IgM antibody to maternal allotypes of IgG. Thus, IgM antibody detected in the IgM-FTA-ABS test may be directed against maternal IgG antibody bound specifically to *T. pallidum*, rather than against *T. pallidum* itself.

TREATMENT AND FOLLOW-UP MANAGEMENT Penicillin G is the drug of choice for all stages of syphilis. *Treponema pallidum* is killed by very low concentrations of penicillin G, although a long period of exposure to penicillin is required for treatment because of the unusually slow rate of multiplication of the organism. The efficacy of penicillin for syphilis remains undiminished after 30 years of use. Other antibiotics which are effective in syphilis include the tetracyclines, erythromycin, and the cephalosporins. Streptomycin inhibits *T. pallidum* only in very large doses, and the sulfonamides are inactive. The optimal dose and duration of therapy have not been established for any antimicrobial for any stage of syphilis. The United States Public Health Service recommendations are based on limited therapeutic trials and should be interpreted in light of the considerations noted below.

Recurrence rates for a given regimen increase as infection progresses from incubating syphilis to seronegative primary to seropositive primary to secondary to late syphilis. Therefore it is probable, but unproved, that a longer duration of therapy is required to effect cure as the lesion progresses. For these reasons some authorities use more prolonged penicillin therapy than that recommended by the United States Public Health Service when treating secondary, latent, or late syphilis.

The optimal dose and duration of therapy have not been carefully evaluated in well-controlled studies. A variety of data suggest that it is necessary to achieve serum levels of penicillin G of 0.03 μg/ml or more for at least 7 days to effect cure of early syphilis. Other tentative conclusions which can be gleaned from published studies include the following: (1) extending therapy with aqueous procaine penicillin G beyond 2 weeks does not improve cure rates for primary or secondary syphilis; (2) studies of experimental syphilis show that *T. pallidum* begins to regenerate if penicillinemia is allowed to fall to subinhibitory levels for periods of 18 to 24 h; (3) in humans, increases in the dosage of crystalline penicillin G administered over 9 h from 0.03 to 0.6 mg/kg progressively increased the rate of disappearance of *T. pallidum* from chancres, but further increases in dosage did not further speed the disappearance of treponemes; and (4) the serum concentration of penicillin G achieved after one injection of 2.4 million units of benzathine penicillin G probably does not kill *T. pallidum* at the maximum rate.

The treatment regimens currently recommended for syphilis by the Center for Disease Control are summarized in Table 146-3 and described below.

TABLE 146-3
Recommended therapy for syphilis

Stage of syphilis	Patients without penicillin allergy	Patients with penicillin allergy
Primary, secondary, or early latent	Benzathine penicillin G, 2.4 million units single dose (1.2 million units in each hip) *or* aqueous procaine penicillin G, 600,000 units daily for 8 days	Erythromycin base, stearate, or ethyl succinate, 2 g daily for 15 days *or* tetracycline hydrochloride, 2 g daily for 15 days
Late latent or latent or uncertain duration	*CSF normal:* Treat as primary *CSF abnormal:* Treat as neurosyphilis	Lumbar puncture *CSF normal:* Treat as primary *CSF abnormal:* Treat as neurosyphilis
Late neurosyphilis* (asymptomatic or symptomatic)	Aqueous procaine penicillin G, 600,000 units daily for 14 days *or* aqueous penicillin G, 12 to 24 million units per day intravenously for at least 10 days	Erythromycin base, stearate, or ethyl succinate, 2 g daily for 30 days *or* tetracycline hydrochloride, 2 g daily for 30 days
Late cardiovascular or benign tertiary	Benzathine penicillin G, 2.4 million units weekly for 3 weeks *or* aqueous procaine penicillin G, 600,000 units weekly for 10 days	Treat as for neurosyphilis
Congenital (treat *all* neonates with either proved *or* suspected congenital syphilis)	Aqueous penicillin G, 50,000 units/kg per day for at least 10 days *or* aqueous penicillin G, 50,000 units/kg per day in two divided daily doses for at least 10 days *or, only if CSF normal:* Benzathine penicillin G, 50,000 units/kg in a single dose	Antibiotics other than penicillin should not be used

* *Benzathine penicillin G has given inferior results for treatment of symptomatic neurosyphilis. Although only erythromycin or tetracycline was recommended by the CDC Syphilis Therapy Advisory Committee for CNS Syphilis, chloramphenicol may be theoretically preferable, since it reaches higher concentrations in the CSF.*
SOURCE: *From CDC recommendations, revised 1976.*

Early syphilis In very early incubating syphilis, treatment of concurrently acquired gonorrhea with 4.8 million units of procaine penicillin G (plus 1.0 g probenecid) aborts the syphilis. The ampicillin-probenecid and tetracycline regimens recommended for gonorrhea are probably also effective against incubating syphilis, although proof is not available. Follow-up serologic testing for syphilis is considered unnecessary in patients treated for gonorrhea with the recommended dose of procaine penicillin G, ampicillin, or tetracycline. Preventive (abortive, "epidemiologic") treatment is recommended for seronegative individuals without signs of syphilis who were exposed to syphilis when the contact was infectious and the exposure occurred within the previous 6 weeks. Before treatment is given, every effort should be made to establish a diagnosis by examination and serologic testing. The regimens recommended for preventive treatment are the same as those recommended for early syphilis.

Benzathine penicillin G is the most widely used form of treatment for early syphilis, although it is more painful on injection than procaine penicillin G. A single dose of 2.4 million units cures over 95 percent of cases of primary syphilis. Because efficacy for secondary syphilis may be slightly lower, some physicians administer a second dose of 2.4 million units 1 week after the initial dose for secondary syphilis.

Pregnant patients with early syphilis should receive penicillin in the same doses used for nonpregnant patients. If they have well-documented penicillin allergy, no satisfactory alternative is available. Erythromycin, the leading alternative in penicillin-allergic nonpregnant patients, crosses the placenta poorly, with total blood levels varying from 0 to 20 percent of maternal levels. Erythromycin estolate is associated with frequent liver toxicity in pregnancy. Doxycycline 100 mg twice daily for 15 days, or a cephalosporin, may be preferable alternatives, although doxycycline has potential toxicity in pregnancy and cephalosporins may be cross-allergenic in penicillin-allergic patients. After treatment, a quantitative reagin test should be repeated monthly throughout pregnancy, and if a fourfold rise in titer occurs, treatment should be repeated.

If adequate treatment of the mother is accomplished during pregnancy, the risk of congenital syphilis in the newborn is minimal; the child should then be examined monthly after delivery until his or her reaginic antibody test becomes negative. However, if the seropositive mother received inadequate penicillin treatment or treatment other than penicillin, or her treatment status is unknown, or if the infant may be difficult to follow, treatment should be given promptly. It is unwise to require proof of diagnosis before treatment in such cases. Similarly, every infant with suspected or proved congenital syphilis should be treated promptly. The CSF should be examined as a base line before treatment of such infants. The calculation of penicillin dosage for treatment of late congenital syphilis is the same as for that used in the infant, until dosage based upon body weight reaches that used for adult neurosyphilis.

The response of early syphilis to treatment should be determined by following the quantitative VDRL titer 1, 3, 6, and 12 months after treatment. Because the FTA-ABS and TPHA tests remain positive after 2 years in nearly all patients treated for seropositive early syphilis, this test is not useful in following the response to therapy. However, IgM antibody detected in the FTA-ABS test is uniformly present in untreated syphilis in all stages, but disappears over a period of several months after successful treatment. After successful treatment of seropositive primary or secondary syphilis, the VDRL titer progressively declines, becoming negative within 3 to 12 months in about 75 percent of seropositive primary cases and 40 percent of second-

ary cases. After 2 years, nearly all patients with primary syphilis have a negative VDRL, although 25 percent of secondary cases and a higher proportion of those treated for early latent syphilis still maintain low titers of reagin. If the VDRL becomes negative or reaches a fixed low titer within 1 or 2 years, performing a lumbar puncture is unnecessary at that time, since the spinal fluid examination is invariably normal and there is no risk of subsequent neurosyphilis. However, if a VDRL titer of 1:8 or more fails to fall at least fourfold within 12 months, the VDRL titer rises fourfold, or clinical symptoms persist or recur, re-treatment is indicated. Every effort should be made to differentiate treatment failure from reinfection. If signs of secondary syphilis recur, the CSF should be examined. Suspected treatment failures, especially those with abnormal CSF, should be treated as described for neurosyphilis. If the patient remains seropositive but asymptomatic after such re-treatment, no further therapy is necessary.

Asymptomatic neurosyphilis The activity of asymptomatic neurosyphilis correlates best with the degree of cerebrospinal fluid pleocytosis. Changes in the cerebrospinal fluid cell count, and to a lesser extent, in cerebrospinal fluid protein concentration, provide the most sensitive index of response to treatment. Spinal fluid examination should be performed every 3 to 6 months for 3 years after treatment of asymptomatic neurosyphilis. An elevated cerebrospinal fluid cell count falls to 10 or less per cubic millimeter within 3 to 12 months in 95 percent of adequately treated cases, and becomes normal in all cases within 2 to 4 years. Elevated levels of cerebrospinal fluid protein fall more slowly, and the cerebrospinal fluid reagin titer declines slowly over a period of several years. Since benzathine penicillin G given in single doses of 2.4 million units to adults or 50,000 units per kilogram to infants does not produce detectable concentrations of penicillin G in cerebrospinal fluid, this form of penicillin is unreliable for the treatment of neurosyphilis in the adult, or for congenital syphilis, and asymptomatic neurosyphilis has been found to relapse in up to one-quarter of patients treated with 2.4 million units of benzathine penicillin. Symptomatic neurosyphilis has rarely, if ever, occurred in patients who received a total dose of 6 million units or more of other forms of penicillin G for asymptomatic neurosyphilis.

Late syphilis Lumbar puncture should be performed even in the evaluation of late complications other than symptomatic neurosyphilis, since asymptomatic neurosyphilis may coexist with other late complications, and abnormal cerebrospinal fluid findings can then be followed serially as a guide to therapy. No studies of benzathine penicillin G for cardiovascular syphilis have ever been reported, and the efficacy of penicillin therapy in any form for cardiovascular syphilis has not been proved. The response of cardiovascular syphilis to penicillin is seldom dramatic because aortic aneurysm and aortic regurgitation cannot be reversed by antibiotic treatment, although further progression of these lesions may be arrested by treatment.

In contrast, the response of benign tertiary syphilis and of meningovascular syphilis to penicillin G is usually impressive. The response of parenchymal neurosyphilis has been variable. In a cooperative study of the treatment of 1086 general paretics with penicillin, the frequency of clinical improvement or termination of progression ranged from 38 percent of those with severe involvement to 81 percent of those with mild involvement. All patients who relapsed following initial improvement in cerebrospinal fluid pleocytosis had received less than 6 million units of penicillin, and all improved with subsequent therapy. Tabes dorsalis or optic atrophy responds less often. In general, treatment of inactive neurosyphilis in which permanent neurological damage has already occurred may not produce any clinical change, and re-treatment of such cases is not warranted. However, persistence of cerebrospinal fluid pleocytosis, or recurrence following initial response to treatment, indicates continuing active infection, which should respond to additional treatment. The optimal dose and duration of penicillin for neurosyphilis has not been determined, but administration of 600,000 to 900,000 units of procaine penicillin G daily for 10 days has been about 90 percent effective. Some physicians advocate administration of intravenous penicillin G in doses of 12 million units per day or more for 10 days or longer, to ensure maximally treponemacidal concentrations of penicillin G in cerobrospinal fluid. Such therapy has occasionally cured patients who failed to respond to conventional therapy. There are no data to support the use of antibiotics other than penicillin G for the treatment of neurosyphilis. Therefore follow-up for at least 3 years, with reexamination of spinal fluid every 3 to 6 months, is especially important if antibiotics other than penicillin were used.

Jarish-Herxheimer reaction A dramatic reaction consisting of fever (average temperature elevation, 1.5°C), chills, myalgias, headache, tachycardia, increased respiratory rate, increased circulating neutrophil count (average total white blood cell count, 12,500 per cubic millimeter), and vasodilatation with mild hypotension, may occur following initiation of treatment of syphilis. This reaction occurs in approximately 50 percent of patients with primary syphilis, 90 percent with secondary, and 25 percent with early latent syphilis. The onset occurs within 2 h of treatment, the peak temperature occurs at about 7 h, and defervescence takes place within 12 to 24 h. In patients with secondary syphilis, an increase in erythema and edema of the mucocutaneous lesions occurs; occasionally subclinical or early mucocutaneous lesions may first become apparent during the reaction. The pathogenesis of this reaction may involve release of endotoxin in tissues. Patients should be warned to expect such symptoms, which can be managed by bed rest and aspirin. The Jarisch-Herxheimer reaction in neurosyphilis or cardiovascular syphilis has, on very rare occasions, been associated with acute progression of irreversible organ damage.

Persistence of treponemal forms The persistence of *T. pallidum* in the aqueous humor, cerebrospinal fluid, lymph nodes, brain, inflamed temporal arteries, and other tissues following "adequate" penicillin treatment of latent or late syphilis has been suggested by dark-field microscopy and by immunofluorescent antibody and silver staining techniques. Treponemal forms have also been demonstrated in patients with various clinical findings suggestive of syphilis, but in whom serologic tests, including the FTA-ABS test, were negative. Although many of these findings could be explained by artifact or by the coincidental presence of nonpathogenic treponemes, in a few cases the persistence of pathogenic *T. pallidum* after antibiotic treatment was proved by rabbit inoculation experiments. The question has been raised as to whether the lifelong persistence of antitreponemal antibody measured in the TPI and FTA-ABS tests following treatment of latent or late syphilis represents prolonged immunologic memory or continued antigenic stimulation by persisting treponemes in lymph nodes and other tissues.

It is not surprising that *T. pallidum* might persist in the aqueous humor or cerebrospinal fluid despite penicillin treatment, because of poor penetration of the antibiotic, but persistence in lymph nodes and other sites remains unexplained. Limited evidence indicates no increase in resistance to penicillin of such persistent treponemes. Since the data on persisting treponemes are scanty, no modification of the treatment recommendations for latent or late syphilis seems warranted.

IMMUNITY AND PREVENTION OF SYPHILIS Only about 50 percent of the named contacts of primary and secondary syphilis become infected. The actual risk of infection from a single exposure is probably much lower. The relative importance of variations in sexual and hygienic practices, inoculum size, body and environmental temperature, and other local and systemic factors affecting transmissibility of syphilis remains undefined. There is some interest in the possible efficacy of intravaginal contraceptive gels as prophylactics against venereal diseases including syphilis, since many available preparations have bacteriostatic as well as spermicidal properties.

Humans have no natural resistance to infection by pathogenic treponemes. The rate of development of acquired resistance to *T. pallidum* following natural or experimental infection is quantitatively related to the amount of the antigenic stimulus, which depends upon both the size of the infecting inoculum and the duration of infection prior to treatment.

Resistance to reinfection or superinfection by challenge inoculation develops about three months after the primary (immunizing) infection in animals with experimental syphilis. Resistance of human beings to reinfection by intradermal inoculation of *T. pallidum* was studied in volunteers. Those who had previously been treated for *early* syphilis developed a primary lesion and a serologic response, while the majority of those who had previously been treated for *late latent* syphilis and all those with *untreated latent* syphilis developed neither primary lesions nor serologic response following inoculation. Two patients treated for late latent or late congenital syphilis developed gummas at the site of inoculation.

The role of serum antibody in conferring immunity to syphilis remains controversial. Reagin antibody is not protective, and the evidence is equivocal that antibody directed against specific treponemal antigens confers immunity. Nonetheless, passive transfer of serum antibody from rabbits recovering from experimental syphilis partially protects antibody-recipient rabbits from experimental infection with *T. pallidum*. Delayed hypersensitivity to *T. pallidum* has been demonstrated by skin test in late syphilis, and lymphocytes from patients with syphilis have been demonstrated to undergo blast transformation when exposed to treponemal or cardiolipin antigen. The histopathology of gummas suggests that the cellular immune response is somehow involved in the pathogenesis of these lesions.

Inability to cultivate pathogenic treponemes in vitro has hindered analysis, purification, and concentration of treponemal antigens, and attempts to induce immunity to syphilis by vaccination have shown limited promise. Injection of rabbits with motile strains irradiated with x-rays or with strains of *T. pallidum* inactivated during cold storage has conferred limited immunity, but many injections over long periods of time were required. Attempts to provide cross-resistance by immunization of rabbits with cultivated nonpathogenic treponemas have been unsuccessful. Experiments in humans have shown that varying degrees of cross-immunity exist in patients infected with *T. pallidum*, *T. pertenue*, and *T. carateum*, but chimpanzees with experimental pinta have not developed cross-resistance to syphilis. These findings indicate that the prospects for a syphilis vaccine remain remote, and that the prevention of syphilis depends upon use of mechanical or antiseptic prophylactic agents, and upon detection and treatment of infectious cases.

REFERENCES

CLARK EG, DANBOLT N: The Oslo study of the natural course of untreated syphilis. Med Clin North Am 48:613, 1964

IDSOE O et al: Penicillin in the treatment of syphilis. Bull WHO 47(suppl):1, 1972

JAFFE HW: The laboratory diagnosis of syphilis: New concepts. Ann Intern Med 83:846, 1975

JOHNSON RC (ed): *The Biology of the Parasitic Spirochetes.* New York, Academic, 1976

MAGNUSON HG et al: Inoculation syphilis in human volunteers. Medicine 35:33, 1956

MERRITT HH et al (eds): *Neurosyphilis.* New York, Oxford, 1946

O'NEILL P, NICOL CS: IgM class antitreponemal antibody in treated and untreated syphilis. Br J Vener Dis 48:460, 1972

REIMER CB et al: The specificity of fetal IgM: Antibody or anti-antibody? NY Acad Sci 254:77, 1975

ROSAHN PD: *Autopsy Studies in Syphilis,* CDC Publication no 433. US Department of Health, Education, and Welfare, 1960

SCHROETER AL et al: Treatment for early syphilis and reactivity of serologic tests. JAMA 221:471, 1972

Sexually Transmitted Disease (STD) Statistical Letter, CDC Publication no 127. US Department of Health, Education, and Welfare, 1978

SHERLOCK S: The liver in secondary (early) syphilis. N Engl J Med 284:1437, 1971

SHORT DH et al: Neurosyphilis, the search for adequate treatment: A review and report of a study using benzathine penicillin G. Arch Dermatol 93:87, 1966

Syphilotherapy 1976. Position paper for the current USPHS recommendations. J Am Vener Dis Assoc 3:98, 1976

TURNER TB: *Syphilis and the Treponematoses, Infectious Agents and Host Reaction,* S Mudd (ed). Philadelphia, Saunders, 1970, p 346

WORLD HEALTH ORGANIZATION: Treponematosis research: Report of a WHO scientific group. WHO Tech Rep Ser 455, 1970

147
NONVENEREAL TREPONEMATOSES: YAWS, PINTA, AND ENDEMIC SYPHILIS

KING K. HOLMES
PETER L. PERINE

GENERAL CONSIDERATIONS Nonvenereal treponematoses occur in remote, impoverished areas of the world. Yaws, pinta, and endemic syphilis are distinguished from venereal syphilis solely by clinical and epidemiologic features. Yaws and pinta are caused by treponemes which are conventionally designated as unique species (*Treponema pertenue* causes yaws, and *T. carateum* pinta), but no convincing morphologic or antigenic differences have yet been demonstrated among *T. pertenue, T. carateum,* and *T. pallidum.* The etiologic agent of endemic syphilis is generally held to be identical with *T. pallidum* and is sometimes designated as *T. pallidum endemicum.* Pinta involves the skin alone; yaws affects skin and bones; and endemic syphilis involves the skin, bone, and mucous membranes. Congenital infections and cardiovascular and central nervous system involvement occur rarely if ever in the nonvenereal treponematoses but are common in syphilis. It remains unclear whether the clinical and epidemiologic differences among yaws, pinta, endemic syphilis, and venereal syphilis are solely determined by environmental and host factors or are attributable to undefined biological differences among the causal treponemes. The relationship of the treponematoses is summarized in Table 147-1.

EPIDEMIOLOGY Treponemal antibodies are demonstrable in a high proportion of nonhuman primates in regions of Africa where human yaws and endemic syphilis are common, and pathogenic treponemes have been found in skin lesions and lymph nodes of seropositive animals. These treponemes have produced yaws-like lesions in susceptible monkeys and hamsters. Treponemes related to or identical with *T. pertenue* thus may antedate *Homo sapiens.*

Yaws and endemic syphilis are diseases of young children. Yaws occurs throughout the world between the Tropics of Cancer and Capricorn, in humid, warm environments. Transmission of yaws among children is favored by scanty clothing, poor hygiene, and frequent skin trauma. Spread occurs by direct contact with infected lesions and perhaps by passive transfer of treponemes by insects. Endemic syphilis occurs in arid subtropical or temperate climates in Africa, the eastern Mediterranean, the Arabian Peninsula, Central Asia, and Australia. It is not observed in the Western Hemisphere. Skin-to-skin transmission is less important than in yaws; instead, infection of mucous membranes results from direct mouth-to-mouth contact or from contaminated fomites, such as shared drinking or eating utensils. Household outbreaks of endemic childhood syphilis still occur in modern cities when crowding and poverty favor childhood transmission of *T. pallidum.*

Although cutaneous pigmentary changes resembling pinta occur in yaws or endemic syphilis, most authorities believe pinta is a separate, more benign disease which occurs only in the Western Hemisphere. The onset is typically later than in yaws or endemic syphilis, usually when the person is between 10 and 20 years of age. The method of transmission is not well defined.

The WHO/UNICEF-assisted mass campaign for eradication of endemic nonvenereal treponematosis from 1948 to 1965 was an unusually successful public health campaign. Over 160 million people were examined in 46 countries, and approximately 50 million cases, contacts, and latent infections were treated. The impact of this program was remarkable. The prevalence of active yaws lesions was reduced from over 20 percent to less than 1 percent in many rural areas. In Bosnia, Yugoslavia, endemic syphilis was eradicated—the only example of eradication of endemic treponematosis.

Unfortunately, relaxation of active surveillance activities after the mass campaigns has led to a resurgence of yaws, particularly in Africa. Yaws has not been eradicated in any large area. For example, in Ghana reported cases of yaws increased fivefold from 1970 to 1974, and recrudescences have been reported in Senegal, the Congo, and the Ivory Coast. Among pygmies in Cameroon and Zaire surveyed from 1969 to 1978, the prevalence of clinical yaws was 10 percent, and the prevalence of FTA-ABS antibody ranged from 75 percent for children under 5 years to 90 percent or more for those over 20. Similarly, WHO surveys during the early 1970s showed that the prevalence of active endemic syphilis, though lower than before the eradication program, ranged from 1 to 5 percent in remote poor populations of Senegal, Mauritania, Mali, Chad, Niger, Upper Volta, Kenya, Ethiopia, and Somalia.

Antitreponemal and reaginic seroreactivity has been detected in a small percentage of children without clinical disease born after the mass campaigns in some areas (e.g., Nigeria, New Guinea, and Bosnia). This may represent asymptomatic infection or may simply reflect the decreased predictive value of serologic tests (probability that disease is present if the test is positive) when the prevalence of disease is sharply reduced.

In the Americas, the major residual foci of yaws are Haiti; Dominica, St. Lucia, and St. Vincent; Peru, Colombia, and Ecuador; a few areas of Brazil; and possibly Guyana and Surinam. Pinta is confined to Central America and Northern South America, where it appears to have regressed to remote Indian villages.

TABLE 147-1
Etiology, epidemiology, and clinical manifestations of the treponematoses

	Venereal syphilis	*Endemic syphilis*	*Yaws*	*Pinta*
Organism	*Treponema pallidum*	*T. pallidum endemicum*	*T. pertenue*	*T. carateum*
Transmission	Sexual, transplacental*	Household contacts: mouth-to-mouth or via drinking, eating utensils	Skin-to-skin ? Insect vector	Skin-to-skin ? Insect vector
Usual age	Adult	Early childhood	Early childhood	Adolescent
Primary lesion	Cutaneous ulcer (chancre)	Rarely seen	Framboise (raspberry), or "mother yaw"	Nonulcerating papule with satellites
Secondary lesion	Mucocutaneous; occasional periostitis	Florid mucocutaneous lesions (mucous patch, split papule, condyloma latum); osteoperiostitis	Cutaneous papulosquamous lesions	Pintides
Tertiary	Gumma, cardiovascular, and CNS lues	Destructive cutaneous osteoarticular gummas	Destructive cutaneous osteoarticular gummas	Dyschromic, achromic macules

* *Since the nonvenereal treponematoses are usually acquired in childhood and treponemal bacteremia ceases with time, only in adult-onset venereal syphilis is there any likelihood of a mother giving birth to an infected child.*

BIOLOGICAL RELATIONSHIPS Specific humoral antibodies to *T. pallidum* are produced in individuals with yaws, pinta, or endemic syphilis, but the time of appearance of antibodies after onset of infections is variable. The fluorescent treponemal antibody absorption (FTA-ABS) test, the *T. pallidum* hemagglutination test (TPHA), and the *T. pallidum* immobilization (TPI) test cannot differentiate among the treponematoses.

In addition to the clinical and epidemiologic differences among the treponematoses in humans, the range of susceptible animal hosts and some manifestations of experimental infection are also different. In particular, *T. carateum* has produced an infection in chimpanzees which resembles pinta, but attempts to infect other experimental animals have usually been unsuccessful. Turner and Hollander reported differences between *T. pallidum* and *T. pertenue* in infections produced in the rabbit and golden hamster, and also found that experimental rabbit infection with one species conferred greater immunity to reinfection with the homologous species than with the heterologous species. However, these interspecies differences in superinfection immunity are no greater than intraspecies differences which exist among different strains of *T. pallidum*. Individuals who have had yaws or pinta are considered relatively immune to syphilis, and the extensive studies of Medina in Caracas show that persons with active pinta or syphilis cannot be superinfected with *T. pertenue* by experimental inoculation.

CLINICAL MANIFESTATIONS Yaws Also known as pian, framboesia, buba, or bouba, yaws is a chronic infectious disease of childhood caused by *T. pertenue*. The disease is characterized by an initial skin lesion followed by relapsing, nondestructive, secondary lesions of skin and bone. In the late stages, destructive lesions of skin, bone, and joints occur.

The incubation period following experimental inoculation of susceptible human beings is 3 to 4 weeks. Disruption of the skin by insect bites, abrasions, or injuries promotes acquisition of natural infection from infected contacts. The initial early lesion is a single papule which is usually located on a leg. The lesion enlarges and becomes papillomatous. This lesion is known as a framboise (raspberry) or "mother yaw." It becomes superficially eroded and covered by a thin yellow crust of serous exudate containing *T. pertenue*. Erythema and induration are not common. The lesion is pruritic, and regional lymphadenopathy occurs. The initial lesion usually heals in 6 months. As a result of treponemal bacteremia, a generalized secondary eruption of similar lesions appears either before or after the initial lesion has healed and is most extensive on the exposed surfaces of the body. These early cutaneous lesions of yaws have a variety of forms including desquamative macular

and papular as well as papillomatous types. Painful papules on the soles of the feet result in a crab-like gait referred to as *crab yaws*. Early lesions are infectious and heal slowly; they may result in scarring, hyperpigmentation, or depigmentation, resembling the pigmentary changes seen in pinta. Histological findings are mononuclear-cell infiltration, acanthosis, hyperkeratosis, and the presence of many treponemes. Other manifestations of early yaws include lymphadenopathy and nocturnal bone pain and polydactylitis due to periostitis. Fever and other constitutional symptoms may occur. Infectious cutaneous relapses may occur any time during the first 5 years after infection. Late yaws lesions occur 5 years or more after infection and differ histologically from early lesions in showing endarteritis. Late lesions include gummas of the skin and long bones, particularly of the legs, hyperkeratoses of the soles and palms, osteitis, periostitis, juxtaarticular fibromatous nodes, and hydrarthrosis.

Late lesions of yaws are characteristically extensive and usually destructive. Destruction of the nose, maxilla, palate, and pharynx, termed *gangosa*, or *rhinopharyngitis mutilans*, occurs in late yaws, as well as in leprosy and leishmaniasis. Hypertrophic paranasal maxillary osteitis produces distinctive facies known as *goundou*.

The clinical features of yaws have become less reliable for diagnosis as the prevalence of yaws has decreased, necessitating the use of easily performed serologic tests, such as the rapid plasma reagin (RPR) card test, by paramedical field workers engaged in the consolidation phase of yaws surveillance.

Treponema pertenue can be demonstrated by dark-field examination in early cutaneous lesions but should not be confused with other spirochetes found in tropical ulcers. The serum reagin antibody tests become positive after 1 month, and the FTA-ABS test is also positive.

Endemic syphilis Synonyms for endemic syphilis are Bejel, Siti, Dichuchwa, Njovera, Belesh, and Skerljevo. It is a chronic nonvenereal, treponemal infection of childhood characterized by early mucous membrane or mucocutaneous lesions, a latent period of indeterminate duration, and late complications including gummas of bone and skin. The causative organism is indistinguishable from *T. pallidum*. Endemic syphilis differs from congenital syphilis in that dental changes, interstitial keratitis, and neurosyphilis rarely occur. Cardiovascular complications are considered rare in both endemic and congenital syphilis.

Primary cutaneous lesions are infrequent and when present are extragenital. The earliest manifestation of endemic syphilis is usually an intraoral mucous patch or mucocutaneous lesion resembling the split papules or condylomata of secondary syphilis. Periostitis is common. Regional lymphadenopathy occurs, but generalized lymphadenopathy is unusual. Treponemes are abundant in the moist early lesions and in aspirates from regional lymph nodes. After a variable latent period, late lesions may develop and are the most frequent clinical manifestations. These resemble the lesions of late benign syphilis and include osseous or cutaneous gummas. Destructive gummas, osteitis, and periostitis of nasopharyngeal structures are more common than in late yaws. Gummas occur on the nipples of mothers who have themselves previously had endemic syphilis who breastfeed infants with oral lesions. Both early and late forms of endemic syphilis thus may coexist in the same family. The tertiary lesions of endemic syphilis sometimes may be a consequence of repeated reexposure of a previously sensitized host to reinfection.

Pinta Also known as mal del pinto, carate, azul, or purupuru, pinta is an infectious disease of the skin caused by *T. carateum*. This disease has three cutaneous stages characterized by marked changes in the skin color, does not involve the viscera, and causes no disability other than that associated with cosmetic disfigurement.

The initial lesion is a small papule which appears 7 to 30 days after exposure and is located most often on the extremities, face, neck, or buttocks. It increases in size slowly by peripheral extension and by coalescing with smaller satellite papules. Regional lymphadenopathy occurs. A secondary eruption not associated with generalized lymphadenopathy appears 1 month to 1 year after the appearance of the initial lesion. The secondary lesions are termed *pintides,* may be numerous, and evolve into a psoriatic or circinate configuration. Pintides are initially red but become deeply pigmented, reaching a slate-blue color after a period of time which is related to exposure to sun. Pigmentation occurs most rapidly on the exposed parts of the body. These pigmented lesions are known as dyschromic macules and contain treponemes which are located principally in the epidermis in older lesions. Histologically there is deposition of pigment in the dermis with decreased melanin pigment in the basal-cell layer. Within 3 months to a year, most of the pintides show varying degrees of depigmentation, becoming brown and finally white and giving the skin a mottled appearance. The porcelain-white achromic lesions represent the "late" stage of the disease in which the epidermis is atrophic and melanocytes and melanin are absent. *Treponema carateum* can be demonstrated in transudates from initial, early secondary, or dyschromic lesions. Serologic reaginic and antitreponemal antibody tests are positive, but may take four times longer to become positive in pinta than in venereal syphilis.

TREATMENT Treatment is similar for all the treponematoses. Intramuscular injection of 2.4 million units of benzathine penicillin G in adults and half this dose in children results in rapid resolution of lesions and prevents recurrence. Procaine penicillin G in oil and 2% aluminum monostearate (PAM) has been used extensively. In persons who are allergic to penicillin, tetracycline hydrochloride in a dose similar to that used for infectious syphilis (Chap. 146) is effective. In areas where less than 5 percent of the population has active disease, cases are managed on an individual basis, and all contacts of infected persons are treated with antibiotics.

PREVENTION Although the nonvenereal treponematoses are less amenable to eradication than smallpox, the resurgence of yaws has led some authorities to suggest that the application of *selective epidemiologic control* as used in smallpox eradication be applied to yaws control. This strategy would emphasize ongoing active surveillance, investigation of outbreaks, and treatment of active cases and their contacts rather than mass treatment.

REFERENCES

Bibliography on Yaws 1905–1962. Geneva, WHO, 1963
FURTADO T: Some problems of late yaws. Int J Dermatol 12:123, 1973
GRIN EI, GUTHE T: Evaluation of a previous mass campaign against endemic syphilis in Bosnia and Herzogovina. Br J Vener Dis 49:1, 1973
GUTHE T: Clinical, serological and epidemiological features of framboesia tropica (yaws) and its control in rural communities. Acta Derm Venereol 49:343, 1969
HACKETT CJ: An international nomenclature of yaws lesions. Geneva, WHO, 1957
HOPKINS DR: After smallpox eradication: Yaws? Am J Trop Med Hyg 25:860, 1976
———: Yaws in the Americas, 1950–1975. J Infect Dis 136:548, 1977
HUDSON EH: *Nonvenereal Syphilis.* Edinburgh, E and S Livingstone, 1958
MARQUEZ F et al: Mal del pinto in Mexico. Bull WHO 13:299, 1955
PAMPIGLIONE S, WILKINSON AE: A study of yaws among pygmies in Cameroon and Zaire. Br J Vener Dis 51:165, 1975
TANEJA BL: Yaws: Clinical manifestations and criteria for diagnosis. Indian J Med Res 56:100, 1968
Treponematoses Research: Report of a WHO Scientific Group, WHO Technical Report Series 455, 1970
TURNER TB, HOLLANDER DH: *Biology of the Treponematoses,* WHO Monograph Series 35, 1957
WILLCOX RR: Changing patterns of treponemal disease. Br J Vener Dis 50:169, 1974

148
LEPTOSPIROSIS

JAY P. SANFORD

DEFINITION *Leptospirosis* is a term applied to disease caused by all leptospiras regardless of specific serotype. Correlation of clinical syndromes with infection by differing serotypes leads to the conclusion that a single serotype of *Leptospira* may be responsible for a variety of clinical features; conversely, a single syndrome, e.g., aseptic meningitis, may be caused by multiple serotypes. Hence there is a preference for the general term leptospirosis rather than the synonyms such as Weil's disease and canicola fever.

ETIOLOGY The genus *Leptospira* contains only one species, *L. interrogans,* which may be subdivided into two complexes, interrogans and biflexa. The interrogans complex includes the pathogenic strains, while the biflexa complex includes saprophytic strains. Within each complex the organisms show antigenic variations that are stable and allow them to be classed as serotypes (serovars). Serotypes with common antigens are arranged in serogroups. Despite contrary common usage, an example of the correct designation of *Leptospira* is as follows: Pomona serogroup of *L. interrogans* or *L. interrogans* serovar pomona, not *L. pomona.* The interrogans complex now contains about 130 serotypes arranged in 16 serogroups (the number in parentheses refers to number of serotypes within the serogroup): Icterohemorrhagiae (13), Hebdomadis (28), Autumnalis (13), Canicola (11), Australis (10), Tarassovi or Hyos (10), Pyrogenes (9), Bataviae (8), Javanica (6), Pomona (6), Ballum (3), Cynopteri (3), Celledoni (2), Grippotyphosa (2), Panama (2), and Shermani (1). At least 22 serotypes of *Leptospira* occur naturally in the United States.

EPIDEMIOLOGY Although leptospirosis is not a common disease, it has been reported from all regions of the United States. Between 1964 and 1976, approximately 50 to 150 cases were reported annually. Occasional upswings in number of cases have been the result of common-source outbreaks. Infection in human beings is an incidental occurrence and is not essential to the maintenance of leptospirosis. The disease occurs in a wide range of domestic and wild animal hosts. In many species, such as opossums, skunks, raccoons, and foxes, infectivity ratios in the range of 10 to 50 percent are not unusual. Interspecies spread of specific serotypes of leptospiras between animal hosts is frequent, e.g., Pomona, a serotype principally associated with livestock, has been demonstrated in dogs. Infection in animals may vary from inapparent illness to severe fatal disease. The carrier state, in which the host may shed leptospiras in its urine for months to years, may develop in many animals. Immunization of dogs may not prevent the carrier, or shedder, state.

Survival of pathogenic leptospiras in nature is governed by factors including pH of the urine of the host, pH of soil or water into which they are shed, and ambient temperature. Acid urine permits only limited survival; however, if the urine is neutral or alkaline and is shed into a similar moist environment which has low salinity, is not badly polluted with microorganisms or detergents, and has a temperature above 22°C, leptospiras may survive for several weeks. Human infections can occur either by direct contact with urine or tissue of an infected animal or indirectly through contaminated water, soil, or vegetation. The usual portals of entry in humans are abraded skin, particularly about the feet, and exposed conjunctival, nasal, and oral mucous membranes. The previously held concept that organisms could penetrate intact skin has been questioned. While leptospiras have been isolated from ticks, these arthropods appear to be unimportant in transmission.

With the ubiquitous infection of animals, leptospirosis in human beings can occur in all age groups, at all seasons, and in both sexes. However, it is primarily a disease of teen-age children and young adults (about one-half of patients are between the ages of 10 and 39), occurs predominantly in males (80 percent), and develops most frequently in hot weather (in the United States one-half of infections occur from July to October). The wide spectrum of animal hosts results in both urban and rural human disease. Leptospirosis has been considered an occupational disease; however, improved methods of rat control and better standards of hygiene have reduced the incidence among occupational groups such as coal miners and people who work in sewers. Currently less than 20 percent of patients have direct contact with animals; they are mostly farmers, trappers, or abattoir workers. In the majority of patients exposure is incidental; two-thirds of cases occur in children, students, or housewives. Swimming or partial immersion in contaminated water, e.g., riding motorcycles through contaminated pools of water, has been implicated in one-fifth of patients and has accounted for most of the recognized common-source outbreaks.

PATHOLOGY In patients who have died with either hepatic involvement (Weil's syndrome), renal involvement, or both, the significant gross changes include hemorrhages and bile staining of tissues. The hemorrhages, which vary from petechial to ecchymotic, are widespread and are most prominent in skeletal muscle, kidneys, adrenals, liver, stomach, spleen, and lungs.

In skeletal muscle, focal, necrotic, and necrobiotic changes thought to be typical of leptospirosis occur. Biopsies early in the illness demonstrate swelling and vacuolation. Leptospiral antigen has been demonstrated in these lesions by the fluorescent antibody technique. Healing ensues by the formation of new myofibrils with minimal fibrosis. The renal lesions in the acute phase involve predominantly the tubules and vary from simple dilatation of distal convoluted tubules to degeneration, necrosis, and basement membrane rupture. Interstitial edema and cellular infiltrates consisting of lymphocytes, neutrophilic leukocytes, histiocytes, and plasma cells are uniformly present. Glomerular lesions either are absent or consist of mesangial hyperplasia and focal foot process fusion which are interpreted as representing nonspecific changes associated with acute inflammation and protein filtration. Microscopic alterations in the liver are not diagnostic and correlate poorly with the degree of functional impairment. The changes include cloudy swelling of parenchymal cells, disruption of liver cords, enlargement of Kupffer cells, and bile stasis in biliary canaliculi. The changes in the brain and meninges are also minimal and are not diagnostic. Microscopic evidence of myocarditis has been recorded. Pulmonary findings consist of a patchy, localized hemorrhagic pneumonitis. Special staining techniques utilizing silver impregnation methods have demonstrated organisms in the lumina of renal tubules but rarely in other organs.

CLINICAL MANIFESTATIONS **General features** The incubation period following immersion or accidental laboratory exposure has shown extremes of 2 to 26 days, the usual range being 7 to 13 days and the average 10 days.

Leptospirosis is a typically biphasic illness. *During the leptospiremic* or *first phase,* leptospiras are present in the blood and cerebrospinal fluid. The onset is typically abrupt, and initial symptoms include headache, which is usually frontal, less often retroorbital, but occasionally may be bitemporal or occipital. Severe muscle aching occurs in most patients, the muscles of the thighs and lumbar areas being most prominently involved, and often is accompanied by severe pain on palpation. The myalgia may be accompanied by extreme cutaneous hyperesthesia (causalgia). Chills followed by a rapidly rising temperature are prominent. Following the abrupt onset, the leptospiremic phase typically lasts 4 to 9 days. Features during this interval include recurrent chills, high spiking temperatures [usually 38.9°C (102°F) or greater], headache, and continued severe myalgia. Anorexia, nausea, and vomiting are encountered in one-half or more of the patients. Occasional patients have diarrhea. Pulmonary manifestations, usually either cough or chest pain, have varied in frequency of occurrence from less than 25 percent to 86 percent. Hemoptysis occurs but is rare. Examination during this phase reveals an acutely ill, febrile patient, with a relative bradycardia and normal blood pressure, although European authors comment on early hypotension. Disturbances in sensorium may be encountered in up to 25 percent of patients. The most characteristic physical sign is conjunctival suffusion, which usually first appears on the third or fourth day. It may be lacking in some patients but more often is overlooked. This may be associated with photophobia, but serous or purulent secretion is unusual. Less common findings may include pharyngeal injection, cutaneous hemorrhages, and skin rashes that are usually macular, maculopapular, or urticarial and usually occur on the trunk. Uncommon findings are splenomegaly, hepatomegaly, lymphadenopathy, or jaundice. The first phase terminates after 4 to 9 days, usually with defervescence and improvement in symptoms. This coincides with the disappearance of leptospiras from the blood and cerebrospinal fluid.

The second phase has been characterized as the "immune" phase and correlates with the appearance of circulating IgM antibodies. The concentration of C3 in serum has remained within normal range during this phase. The clinical manifestations of this phase show greater variability than those during the first phase. After a relatively asymptomatic period of 1 to 3 days, the fever and earlier symptoms recur and meningismus may develop. The fever rarely exceeds 38.9°C (102°F) and is usually of 1 to 3 days' duration. It is not uncommon for fever to be absent or quite transient. Even when symptoms or signs of meningeal irritation are absent, routine examination of cerebrospinal fluid after the seventh day has revealed pleocytosis in 50 to 90 percent of patients. Less common features include iridocyclitis, optic neuritis, and other nervous system manifestations, including encephalitis, myelitis, and peripheral neuropathy.

Some clinicians recognize a third or convalescent phase, usually between the second and fourth weeks, when both fever and aching may recur. The pathogenesis of this stage is not understood.

Leptospirosis during pregnancy may be associated with an increased risk of fetal loss.

Specific features WEIL'S SYNDROME Weil's syndrome, which may be due to serotypes other than Icterohemorrhagiae, is defined as severe leptospirosis with jaundice, usually accompanied by azotemia, hemorrhages, anemia, disturbances in consciousness, and continued fever. There is uncertainty as to the pathogenesis of the syndrome, i.e., whether it represents direct toxic damage due to leptospiras or whether it is the consequence of immune response to leptospiral antigens. The consensus favors toxic damage.

The onset and first stage are identical with the less severe forms of leptospirosis. The distinctive features of Weil's syndrome appear from the third to the sixth days but do not reach their peak until well into the second stage. As in milder forms of leptospirosis, there is a tendency for defervescence about the seventh day; however, with recurrence, fever is marked and may persist for several weeks. Either renal or hepatic manifestations may predominate. Hepatic disturbances include tenderness in the right upper quadrant and hepatic enlargement, both of which are common when jaundice is present. Serum glutamic oxaloacetic transaminase (SGOT) values are rarely increased more than fivefold regardless of the degree of hyperbilirubinemia, which is predominantly conjugated (direct): e.g., serum bilirubin, 40 mg per 100 ml; SGOT, 170 IU. The predominant mechanism appears to be an intracellular block to bilirubin excretion.

Renal manifestations consist primarily of proteinuria, pyuria, hematuria, and azotemia. Dysuria is rare. Serious renal damage usually occurs in the form of acute tubular necrosis associated with oliguria. The peak elevation of blood urea nitrogen usually is seen on the fifth to seventh day. Hemorrhagic manifestations are most prevalent in this group of patients and include epistaxis, hemoptysis, gastrointestinal bleeding, hemorrhage into the adrenal glands, hemorrhagic pneumonitis, and subarachnoid hemorrhage. These have been explained on the basis of diffuse vasculitis with capillary injury. In addition, in some patients hypoprothrombinemia and thrombocytopenia have been observed.

ASEPTIC MENINGITIS A leptospiral etiology has been incriminated in 5 to 13 percent of sporadic cases of aseptic meningitis. The pleocytosis is not present before the immune phase, when it develops rapidly. There are usually tens to hundreds of leukocytes, occasionally 1000, per cubic milliliter, among which neutrophils or mononuclear cells may predominate. The cerebrospinal fluid glucose concentration is almost always normal, but occasional instances of lowered glucose levels (hypoglycorrhachia) have been recorded. In contrast to the observations with many viral causes of aseptic meningitis, with leptospirosis

the cerebrospinal fluid protein may exceed 100 mg per 100 ml early in the course. Xanthochromic cerebrospinal fluid has been observed in the presence of jaundice. Each of the serotypes of leptospiras that are pathogenic for human beings is probably capable of causing aseptic meningitis. The most prevalent serotypes have been Canicola, Icterohemorrhagiae, and Pomona.

PRETIBIAL (FORT BRAGG) FEVER An illness was observed in the summer of 1942 that had an onset identical with that of the first phase of leptospirosis. The most distinctive feature was the development on about the fourth day of a rash, characterized by 2- to 5-cm, slightly raised, erythematous lesions that were usually symmetrically distributed over the pretibial areas. In contrast to other leptospiral syndromes, splenomegaly occurred in 95 percent of these patients. This outbreak was shown to be due to the Autumnalis serogroup. Subsequently, Pomona has been observed in association with rashes, which are usually truncal but which have also been pretibial.

MYOCARDITIS Cardiac arrhythmias including paroxysmal atrial fibrillation, atrial flutter, ventricular tachycardia, and premature ventricular contractions have been described but are usually of little clinical significance. However, on rare occasions definite cardiac dilatation with acute left ventricular failure has been observed. Associated manifestations have included jaundice, pulmonary infiltrates, arthritis, and skin rashes. The serotypes thus far incriminated have included Icterohemorrhagiae, Pomona, and Grippotyphosa.

CHILDREN Several clinical features occur in children which are not seen or are very rare in adults: hypertension, acalculous cholecystitis (five of nine children in one series), pancreatitis, abdominal causalgia, and peripheral desquamation of a rash which may be associated with gangrene and cardiopulmonary arrest. The features of desquamation, myocardial involvement, and hydrops of the gallbladder suggest mucocutaneous lymph node syndrome (Chap. 180).

LABORATORY FEATURES Leukocyte counts vary from leukopenic levels to mild elevations in the anicteric patients. In patients with jaundice, leukocytosis as high as 70,000 cells per cubic millimeter may be present. However, regardless of the total leukocyte count, neutrophilia of greater than 70 percent is very frequently encountered during the first stage.

Hemolytic substances have been demonstrated in cultures of pathogenic leptospiras. In contrast to many hemolysins of bacterial origin which are not hemolytic in vivo, the leptospiral hemolysins appear to be active in vivo. In patients with jaundice, anemia may be severe and is most characteristically due to intravascular hemolysis. Other mechanisms of anemia include azotemia and blood loss secondary to hemorrhage. Anemia due to leptospirosis is unusual in anicteric patients.

Rarely thrombocytopenia sufficient to be associated with bleeding is encountered. Additional hematologic abnormalities include elevation of the erythrocyte sedimentation rate in over one-half of patients, but it is usually less than 50 mm/h.

Urinalysis during the leptospiremic phase reveals mild proteinuria, casts, and an increase in cellular elements. In anicteric infections, these abnormalities rapidly disappear after the first week. Proteinuria and abnormalities in the urine sediment usually are not associated with elevations in blood urea nitrogen. Since the anicteric form of the disease often has gone undiagnosed, estimates of the frequency of azotemia and jaundice are probably high. Azotemia has been reported in approximately one-fourth of patients. In three-fourths of these patients, the blood urea nitrogen is less than 100 mg per 100 ml. Azotemia is usually associated with jaundice. The serum bilirubin levels may reach 65 mg per 100 ml; however, in two-thirds of patients the levels are less than 20 mg per 100 ml. During the first phase, one-half of the patients have increased serum creatine phosphokinase (CPK) levels, with mean values of five times normal. Such increases are not seen in viral hepatitis, and a slight increase in transaminase with a definite increase in CPK suggests leptospirosis rather than viral hepatitis.

DIAGNOSIS Diagnosis is based upon culture of the organism or serologic proof of its existence. The most common initial diagnostic impressions in patients with leptospirosis are meningitis, hepatitis, nephritis, fever of undetermined origin (FUO), and influenza. Leptospiras may be isolated quite readily during the first phase from blood and cerebrospinal fluid or during the second phase from the urine. Leptospiras may be excreted in the urine for up to 11 months after the onset of illness and may persist despite antimicrobial therapy. Whole blood should be inoculated immediately into tubes containing semisolid medium, such as Fletcher's medium. If culture medium is not available, leptospiras reportedly will remain viable up to 11 days in blood to which anticoagulants, preferably sodium oxalate, have been added. Animal inoculation (preferably either suckling hamsters or guinea pigs) may be used and is of particular value if specimens are contaminated. Direct examination of blood or urine by dark-field methods has been employed; *however, this method so frequently results in failure or misdiagnosis that it should not be employed.* Serologic methods are applicable during the second phase; antibodies appear from the sixth to the twelfth days of illness. Two serologic methods are commonly used: a macroscopic or slide agglutination test which is easy to perform but lacks specificity and sensitivity, and hence is suitable for screening only, and the microscopic agglutination test which is more complicated but also more specific. Serologic criteria for diagnosis include a fourfold or greater rise in titer during the course of illness. Cross-agglutination reactions between various serotypes commonly occur so that the infection serotype often cannot be determined with certainty without isolation of leptospiras.

PROGNOSIS The prognosis is dependent upon both the virulence of the organism and the general condition of the patient. In 1976, there were six deaths (7 percent) in the 81 patients reported in the United States. Age is the most significant host factor related to increased mortality. In a representative series, the mortality rose from 10 percent in men less than 50 years of age to 56 percent in those over 51 years of age. The virulence of the infecting leptospiras correlates best with the development of jaundice. In anicteric patients, mortality does not occur, but with the development of jaundice, mortality in various series has ranged from 15 to 40 percent. The long-term prognosis following the acute renal lesion of leptospirosis is good. Glomerular filtration rates have returned to normal; however, a few patients show residual tubular dysfunction such as a defect in renal concentrating capacity.

TREATMENT A variety of antimicrobial drugs, including penicillin, streptomycin, the tetracycline congeners, chloramphenicol, and erythromycin, have been effective in vitro and in experimental leptospiral infections. Data concerning the efficacy of antibiotics in human beings are conflicting. If antimicrobial drugs are to have any beneficial effect, they must be administered within 4 days, and preferably within 2 days, of the onset of illness. Large doses of penicillin G (usually 600,000 units intramuscularly every 4 h) are considered the preferred treatment, although the tetracyclines are also effective. Within 4 to 6 h after initiation of penicillin G therapy, a Jarisch-Herxheimer type of reaction, which suggests antileptospiral activity, may occur. There is general agreement that antimicrobials administered after the fifth day of illness have no beneficial effect. There exists the clinical impression that early bedrest may minimize subsequent morbidity. Azotemia and jaundice require meticulous attention to fluid and electrolyte therapy. Since the renal damage is reversible, patients with azotemia should be considered for peritoneal dialysis or hemodialysis. From case reports exchange transfusion has been suggested to be beneficial in the management of patients with extreme hyperbilirubinemia.

REFERENCES

ALSTON JM, BROOM JC: *Leptospirosis in Man and Animals.* Edinburgh, E & S Livingstone, 1958

CENTER FOR DISEASE CONTROL: *Leptospirosis Surveillance: Annual Summary 1976.* April 1978

EDWARDS GA, DOMM M: Human leptospirosis. Medicine 39:117, 1960

FEIGIN RD, ANDERSON DC: Human leptospirosis. CRC Crit Rev Clin Lab Sci 5:413, 1975

HEATH CW JR, ALEXANDER AD: Leptospirosis in the United States: Analysis of 483 cases in man, 1949–1961. N Engl J Med 273:857, 915, 1965

JOHNSON ND JR et al: Serum creatine phosphokinase in leptospirosis. JAMA 233:981, 1975

JOHNSON RC: *The Biology of Parasitic Spirochetes.* New York, Academic, 1976

TURNER LH: Leptospirosis. Br Med J 1:537, 1973

WONG ML et al: Leptospirosis: A childhood disease. J Pediatr 90:532, 1977

149
RELAPSING FEVER

JAMES J. PLORDE

DEFINITION Relapsing fever refers to a group of acute infectious diseases that are characterized clinically by cyclic periods of fever and apyrexia. They are caused by spirochetes of the genus *Borrelia* and occur in two epidemiologic varieties, louseborne and tick-borne.

ETIOLOGY Borreliae are slender helical organisms which measure 10 to 20 μm in length. They have 3 to 10 irregular coils, move in a corkscrew fashion, and divide by transverse fission. Unlike other spirochetes, they readily stain with aniline dyes. *Borrelia recurrentis* is the causative agent of louse-borne relapsing fever. Many strains of *Borrelia* have been found in tick-borne disease; *B. turicatae*, *B. parkeri*, and *B. hermsii* are responsible for the disease seen in this country. The organisms grow poorly on artificial media and readily in developing chick embryos.

EPIDEMIOLOGY Louse-borne relapsing fever is transmitted from person to person by the human body louse. Spirochetes that are ingested by the vector during feeding penetrate the wall of the intestine and multiply in the body cavity. Human infection occurs when the louse is crushed against an abrasion or wound. There is no known animal reservoir. The disease persists in endemic focuses in Ethiopia, the Sudan, South America, and the Far East. Like typhus, it occurs in epidemic form during war and famine. Major epidemics involving millions of people occurred in Europe and Africa after both the

First and Second World Wars. A third, much smaller, outbreak was seen at the time of the Korean conflict. An occasional case of louse-borne relapsing fever has been imported into the United States.

The tick vectors of relapsing fever belong to several species of the genus *Ornithodoros*. These soft ticks are reclusive night feeders whose bites are quick and painless. They then detach themselves, leaving their host with a 2- to 3-mm pruritic eschar. Like lice, they ingest the borreliae during feeding. The organisms may remain viable in the ticks for several years and can be passed transovarily to the next generation, making the tick a major reservoir of the disease. It is likely that rodents and other small animals act as vertebrate reservoirs in some locales. Human beings are involved when they come into contact with an infected tick in its natural habitat. Transmission occurs if the tick's saliva or coxal fluid contaminates the feeding site. The tick-borne disease is found in localized areas throughout the world. In the United States it occurs primarily in Western mountain states, from Texas in the South to Washington, Montana, and Idaho in the Northwest. Outbreaks have occurred among Boy Scouts in northeastern Washington and tourists visiting the north rim of the Grand Canyon. In both outbreaks, the patients contracted the disease while sleeping overnight in tick-infested cabins. The disease has also been carried to other parts of the country, where it usually does not occur, by western travelers.

PATHOGENESIS AND PATHOLOGY After inoculation into a human being, the borreliae reach the bloodstream, producing spirochetemia and a febrile illness. After several days, immobilizing and borrelicidal antibodies appear, the organisms are cleared from the peripheral blood, and the fever resolves. Following a latent period of approximately 1 week, during which the spirochetes are sequestered in the body, a new antigenic variant of the organism arises. There is reinvasion of the bloodstream, causing a second paroxysm of fever and eventually, with the formation of specific antibodies, a second defervescence by crisis. The continued sequential production of new antigenic variants and specific antibodies results in the characteristic relapsing febrile course. Endotoxin has been detected in the blood of febrile patients with louse-borne disease. Whether the toxin is released by dying spirochetes or is liberated from anoxic gutwall is not known. However, decreased blood levels of Hageman factors and prekaillekrein as well as hypocomplementemia all suggest a role for endotoxin in the pathogenesis of this disease (Chap. 109).

At autopsy follicular splenic abscesses, histiocytic interstitial myocarditis, intracranial hemorrhage, and hepatitis with focal necrosis may be seen. Spontaneous splenic rupture and hemorrhagic gastrointestinal lesions have been noted occasionally. Borreliae have been recovered from the brain, heart, spleen, liver, and skin.

MANIFESTATIONS Clinical manifestations vary from outbreak to outbreak and between the tick- and louse-borne varieties of the disease. Generally, patients with louse-borne relapsing fever are more seriously ill but have fewer relapses than those with tick-borne illnesses. After an incubation period of 4 to 18 days, the disease begins abruptly with rigors, headache, anorexia, nausea, vomiting, photophobia, and pain in the muscles and joints. The temperature rises rapidly, reaching 39 to 40°C (102.2 to 104°F), where it remains until the time of the crisis. The patient appears dull, apathetic, and is uncomplaining. He may have conjunctival suffusion and a macular or petechial rash. Cough, tachypnea, and rhonchi are common. A gallop rhythm and premature ventricular beats may occur in

the louse-borne variety. Cardiac enlargement and heart failure are more uncommon. Upper abdominal tenderness is frequent. The liver and spleen are palpable and tender in 20 to 80 percent of cases, and may enlarge 6 to 10 cm during the course of fever. Jaundice secondary to hepatocellular destruction is present in 7 to 36 percent of patients. It is usually seen in louse-borne disease, occurs relatively late in the illness, and if severe, is often associated with purpura.

Bleeding is common in louse-borne relapsing fever. Petechiae develop in the skin and serous membranes, apparently as a result of damage to the capillary endothelium by clumps of spirochetes. Mild epistaxes and microscopic hematuria are present in many patients early in the disease. Later, with the development of liver disease, severe prolonged epistaxes and widespread ecchymoses occur. Infrequently, there may be massive gastrointestinal, urinary, or intracranial hemorrhage. Disseminated intravascular coagulation has been described. Neck stiffness, confusion, and transient focal neurologic signs may be seen even without intracranial bleeding. Patients with tick-borne disease with repeated relapses may develop iritis or iridocyclitis with permanent visual impairment. Pregnant women with relapsing fever often abort.

Three to six days after the onset of illness, the attack ends in a crisis. Clinically this is characterized by a chill and an abrupt but transient rise in temperature, heart rate, respiratory rate, and arterial blood pressure. As the spirochetes disappear, the patient becomes flushed, diaphoretic, and hypotensive. Occasionally, cardiovascular collapse and death may occur at this point. More frequently the blood pressure and temperature return to normal over several hours, leaving the patient comfortable but exhausted. After 7 to 10 afebrile days, a relapse occurs which mimics the original illness. In the louse-borne disease there is usually only a single relapse, but in tick-borne relapsing fever there may be several, each somewhat briefer and milder than the preceding one.

LABORATORY FINDINGS A moderate anemia is common. The leukocyte count is usually normal or slightly elevated. During the crisis, a marked leukopenia occurs which may be followed by a transient rebound leukocytosis. A consumptive thrombocytopenia is seen in most cases, and the prothrombin and partial thromboplastin times may be prolonged. Fibrinogen levels are increased. Liver function tests reveal disturbed hepatocellular function. In severe cases, the total serum bilirubin level may reach 16 mg per 100 ml. Azotemia unrelated to extracellular fluid depletion is common among jaundiced patients. Electrocardiogram abnormalities, including a prolonged QTc interval and ST-T wave changes, may occur. Reagin tests for syphilis are positive in 5 to 10 percent of cases, and experimental data suggest that false-positive FTA-ABS tests may also occur. Patients with louse-borne relapsing fever frequently develop agglutinins to *Proteus* OXK antigens.

The definitive diagnosis is made by demonstrating borreliae in the peripheral blood during a febrile episode. This is most easily accomplished by examining thick and thin films stained with Giemsa's and Wright's stains. Repeated examinations may be required, especially in tick-borne disease. Blood spun in a microhematocrit tube and examined microscopically may reveal organisms when thin and thick smears are negative. Spirochetes may also be seen in wet mounts with phase-contrast microscopy. When the direct methods are negative, blood may be injected into mice or rats and their blood examined frequently for the presence of borreliae.

DIFFERENTIAL DIAGNOSIS Many acute febrile illnesses, including malaria, salmonellosis, typhus, dengue, rat-bite fever, and Weil's disease, must be considered. Practically, there is seldom confusion if blood films are examined carefully.

TREATMENT The peripheral blood is quickly cleared of spirochetes by a variety of drugs, including penicillin, tetracycline, and chloramphenicol. Treatment with these antimicrobial agents, however, is accompanied by a Jarisch-Herxheimer-like reaction which contributes to the morbidity, and perhaps mortality, of the disease. The reaction appears both clinically and pathophysiologically to be an exaggeration of the spontaneously occurring crisis. Its mechanism is unknown, but it may be related to an accelerated release of endotoxin liberated during destruction of spirochetes. It is certainly related temporally to disappearance of spirochetes from the blood, and its severity appears to depend upon the speed with which they are removed.

In louse-borne relapsing fever, where the spirochetemia is often intense and the Jarisch-Herxheimer reaction severe, the drug of choice is a repository penicillin such as penicillin aluminum monostearate (PAM). Unlike tetracycline, this drug achieves a very gradual clearing of the spirochetes and a correspondingly mild reaction. The drug is given intramuscularly in a dose of 600,000 units. If the shorter-acting procaine penicillin is used, the dose should be repeated in 12 to 24 h to prevent relapse. In epidemics, a single 0.5-g oral dose of tetracycline, erythromycin, or chloramphenicol can be used with good results.

In tick-borne disease where penicillin is not effective in terminating relapses, tetracycline is most rapidly borrelicidal. This drug should be given in a dose of 0.5 g four times a day for 5 to 10 days. Doxycycline, 100 mg twice daily, is also effective. The Jarisch-Herxheimer reaction tends to be less severe in this form of the disease.

PROGNOSIS When epidemics strike a nonimmune population, the high mortality rate due to the louse-borne disease shows the potential menace of this disease. Most patients, however, recover quickly and completely; relapses do not occur if antibiotic therapy is adequate. Adverse signs are deep jaundice, uncontrolled bleeding, and a grossly prolonged QTc interval.

Typhus and enteric fever may occur simultaneously with louse-borne relapsing fever, and they probably contribute to the mortality rate, particularly during epidemics.

REFERENCES

BOYER KM et al: Tick-borne relapsing fever: An interstate outbreak originating at Grand Canyon National Park. Am J Epidemiol 105:469, 1977

BRYCESON ADM et al: Louse-borne relapsing fever: A clinical and laboratory study of 62 cases in Ethiopia and a reconsideration of the literature. Q J Med 39:139, 1970

BUTLER T et al: *Borrelia recurrentis* infection: Single dose antibiotic regimens and management of the Jarisch-Herxheimer reaction. J Infect Dis 137:573, 1978

GALLOWAY RE et al: Activation of protein mediators of inflammation and evidence of endotoxemia in *Borrelia recurrentis* infection. Am J Med 63:933, 1977

JOHNSON RC: The spirochetes. Annu Rev Microbiol 31:89, 1977

JUDGE DM et al: Louse-borne relapsing fever in man. Arch Pathol 97:136, 1974

SOUTHERN PM JR, SANFORD JP: Relapsing fever. Medicine 48:129, 1969

section 9 | Infections caused by higher bacteria and fungi

150 GENERAL CONSIDERATIONS

JOHN E. BENNETT

Actinomycetes and fungi are being considered together in this section, but this should not obscure profound differences between these two groups of organisms. The agents of actinomycosis, nocardiosis, and actinomycetoma are actinomycetes. These organisms are gram-positive higher bacteria which branch but have the diameter, antibiotic susceptibility, and ability to induce a neutrophilic inflammatory response in common with other bacteria. Actinomycetes resemble fungi in causing infections which may be extremely chronic and which are poorly transmissible from person to person. *Actinomyces israelii* and *Candida albicans* colonize the gastrointestinal tract early in life, presumably by person-to-person spread. Infection results in later life when specialized conditions permit entry of normal flora into deeper tissue. The largest number of actinomycetes and fungi enter the body from a source in nature, where the microbe grows as a saprophyte. The two major means of entry into the body are by inhalation into the lungs (histoplasmosis, coccidioidomycosis, blastomycosis, cryptococcosis, nocardiosis, mucormycosis, aspergillosis, paracoccidioidomycosis) and by cutaneous inoculation (sporotrichosis, mycetoma, chromomycosis, dermatophytosis).

Certain problems with names of actinomycetes and fungi need to be recognized. The taxonomy of agents causing actinomycetoma and chromomycosis has been unstable, resulting in a disconcerting number of name changes. The discovery of a perfect state for several fungi has created an additional name for these species. *Perfect state* or *sexual state* refers to a part of the fungal life cycle in which meiosis occurs. This part of the life cycle usually is not encountered in a routine diagnostic laboratory so the report ordinarily should give the name of the species in the imperfect state, generally a more familiar name.

Several facts common to the diagnosis and treatment of many mycoses are most economically dealt with in this section. Fungi are not detected reliably in histological sections stained with hematoxylin and eosin. Gomori methenamine silver stain with a homogeneous counterstain is the most sensitive procedure. Periodic acid–Schiff will stain many fungi, but the lesser contrast makes a small number of organisms more difficult to detect.

Therapy with intravenous amphotericin B is best initiated with a test dose of 1 mg. Patients with profound febrile reactions to this dose will require gradual increments in dose. Patients with fulminant mycoses should have their doses advanced rapidly to at least 0.3 mg/kg per day. Hydrocortisone hemisuccinate added to the infusion may help control febrile reactions. Double-dose alternate-day therapy has the same toxicity and efficacy as single-dose daily therapy, with the following exceptions. Alternate-day double-dose therapy causes more fever, but the patient has fewer infusions and therefore less phlebitis. Appetite and ambulation may be improved on the days-off therapy. The final dose will depend on nephrotoxicity and the specific mycosis. Intrathecal amphotericin B is used in coccidioidal and sometimes other mycotic meningitides. In experienced hands, intracisternal injections are preferable. Triweekly doses are increased from 0.05 to 0.5 mg over six doses. Addition of hydrocortisone 15 mg to the intrathecal injection decreases side effects. As the meningitis is controlled, the frequency of injection can be decreased to once or twice a week. The same schedule may be used for lumbar hyperbaric intrathecal injections or for intraventricular injections via a subcutaneous reservoir. These routes encounter more complications.

REFERENCES

AL-DOORY Y (ed): *The Epidemiology of Human Mycotic Diseases.* Springfield, Ill, Charles C Thomas, 1975

BAKER RD (ed): *Human Infections with Fungi, Actinomycetes and Algae.* New York, Springer-Verlag, 1971

BENNETT JE: Chemotherapy of systemic mycoses. New Engl J Med 290:30, 320, 1974

BUECHNER HA (ed): *Management of Fungus Diseases of the Lungs.* Springfield, Ill, Charles C Thomas, 1971

EMMONS CW: *Medical Mycology.* Philadelphia, Lea & Febiger, 1977

FETTER BF et al: *Mycoses of the Central Nervous System.* Baltimore, Williams & Wilkins, 1967

RIPPON JW: *Medical Mycology.* Philadelphia, Saunders, 1974

151
ACTINOMYCOSIS

JOHN E. BENNETT

DEFINITION Actinomycosis is an indolent suppurative infection caused by certain anaerobic actinomycetes. The microorganisms grow within the tissue as grossly visible tightly knit clusters, called *grains*.

ETIOLOGY *Actinomyces israelii* is the usual causative agent but *A. naeslundi* and *Arachnia propionica* are occasional causes. These gram-positive branching, anaerobic or microaerophilic organisms are the same width as bacteria. When they are cultured on blood agar, small colonies appear after 2 to 4 days of incubation at 37°C under anaerobic conditions. Catalase and other biochemical tests distinguish these organisms from the common skin contaminant *Propionibacterium acnes.* Final identification is best left to a reference laboratory.

PATHOLOGY AND PATHOGENESIS All agents of actinomycosis are commensals in the mouth and gastrointestinal tract of humans. The portal of entry appears to be either a break in the integrity of the mucosa or aspiration into the lung. Poor dental hygiene and dental abscess predispose to oral lesions. Within the gastrointestinal tract, the appendiceal area is the most common site. Infection presents as a chronic suppurative inflammation, usually in the cervicofacial, thoracic, or abdominal area. In histopathologic section, each grain is typically surrounded by polymorphonuclear neutrophils. Adjacent tissue shows subacute or chronic inflammation with extensive fibrosis and formation of sinus tracts. Giant cells are infrequent. The grain stains variably with hematoxylin and eosin. Grains may have an eosinophilic coating composed of human proteins. Hyphal filaments cannot be seen on hematoxylin and eosin stain but may be demonstrated in the periphery of the grain by tissue Gram's stain (such as Brown and Brenn) or by a heavily stained Gomori methenamine silver. These stains may be useful if there is chance for confusion with the grains of eumycetoma or staphylococcal botryomycosis. Grains are a few millimeters in diameter, making them difficult to miss if they are present in the histological section being examined. Several sections may have to be searched to find a grain. Grains may be observed grossly in pus or on bandages covering draining sinuses. These pale yellow, cheese-like particles can be crushed on a microscope slide, and the gram-positive branching filaments demonstrated on Gram's stain.

Infection spreads by direct extension and hematogenously. Direct extension through the skin causes one or more chronic draining sinuses to appear in the abdomen, chest, or cervicofacial area. Hematogenous foci may appear in bone, brain, liver, or other organs.

CLINICAL MANIFESTATIONS Cervicofacial actinomycosis presents as a red or purplish firmly indurated subcutaneous mass, typically in the submandibular area or in the anterior cervical triangle near the angle of the mandible. One or more draining sinuses may be present. Tenderness is slight or absent. Lethargy, weight loss, variable low-grade fever, anemia, and leukocytosis are infrequent in cervicofacial actinomycosis but common in thoracic and abdominal actinomycosis. Localizing findings in the latter forms include draining sinuses and, in thoracic actinomycosis, cough and purulent sputum. Pain or a palpable mass may appear in abdominal actinomycosis. Pelvic actinomycosis, once rare, is now being seen in women with an implanted intrauterine device for contraception. The indolent onset, variable low-grade fever, abdominal pain, and adnexal mass may lead to an erroneous diagnosis of pelvic inflammatory disease or tumor. In all forms of actinomycosis, disease typically has been present for weeks or months at time of diagnosis.

Chest x-ray may reveal an area of dense pneumonitis. Fibrosis, empyema, or cavitation may be seen. Periappendiceal abscess may appear as an extrinsic mass on barium enema.

DIAGNOSIS Laboratory tests other than culture or histological section are not helpful. Blood cultures are rarely positive. Isolation of *Actinomyces* or *Arachnia* species from the mouth, sputum, stool, or feculent draining sinuses is not diagnostic. Demonstration of a grain in pus or deep tissue is diagnostic, if botryomycosis and mycetoma can be excluded. Nocardiosis can be distinguished by the absence of grains, identification of the organism in culture, and, usually, by the weak acid-fast staining of *Nocardia.*

TREATMENT Milder cases of actinomycosis, including most cervicofacial infections, respond well to oral tetracycline or penicillin V, an adult dose being 500 mg qid of either drug. Oral erythromycin would be second choice. More severe cases, including many thoracic and abdominal infections, should receive parenteral penicillin G for roughly 6 weeks (adults receive 2 to 5 million units per day) followed by prolonged therapy with oral penicillin V or tetracycline. The likelihood of relapse is reduced if the total duration of therapy is 2 to 4 months in mild cases and up to 6 to 12 months in severe forms. Drug resistance has not been encountered in relapsed cases. Curettage of bone lesions and surgical drainage of empyema, brain abscess, or other large collections of pus appear to facilitate recovery but are usually not curative by themselves.

It is common in actinomycosis to isolate microbes other than actinomycetes from pus. In general, the antibiotic susceptibility of these secondary organisms does not have to be considered in the selection of therapeutic agents.

REFERENCES

Davies M, Keddie NC: Abdominal actinomycosis. Br J Surg 60:18, 1973

Eastridge CE et al: Actinomycosis. A 24 year experience. South Med J 65:839, 1972

Fradis M et al: Actinomycosis of the face and neck. Arch Otolaryngol 102:87, 1976

Seabury J: Actinomycosis and nocardiosis, in *Management of Fungus Disease of the Lungs,* HA Buechner (ed). Springfield, Ill, Charles C Thomas, 1971, pp 197–211

Seligman P et al: Tubo-ovarian actinomycosis. NY State J Med 76:278, 1976

Slade PR et al: Thoracic actinomycosis. Thorax 28:73, 1973

152
NOCARDIOSIS

JOHN E. BENNETT

DEFINITION Nocardiosis is an acute, subacute, or chronic infection, most often beginning in the lung.

ETIOLOGY *Nocardia asteroides, N. brasiliensis,* and *N. caviae* are the etiologic agents of two different diseases, nocardiosis and mycetoma. In the latter infection, the organism enters the skin by trauma, forms grains within tissue, and spreads slowly to contiguous tissue (see Chap. 161). In nocardiosis, the organism usually enters via the lung, does not form grains, and is prone to hematogenous spread. Even though the etiologic agents of these diseases do overlap, *N. asteroides* causes most cases of nocardiosis and *N. brasiliensis* is the species usually isolated from mycetoma. *Nocardia caviae* is a rare cause of either disease. *Nocardia brasiliensis* can also cause a lymphocutaneous disease closely resembling sporotrichosis; this infection differs from mycetoma by its lymphangitic spread and by the absence of grains.

Nocardia species are aerobic actinomycetes with branching hyphae the same width as bacteria. Hyphae are weakly gram-positive and weakly acid-fast. Growth appears in 2 to 5 days on blood agar, Sabouraud's agar, or other simple media. Incorporation of antibiotics into the media to inhibit bacterial growth usually inhibits *Nocardia* as well. Colonies become rough and chalky with an orange or yellow hue. Identification of *Nocardia* species, including distinction between *Streptomyces, Actinomadura,* and *Nocardia,* is difficult and best assigned to a reference laboratory.

PATHOGENESIS AND PATHOLOGY *Nocardia* is a soil saprophyte widely distributed throughout the world. Infection is acquired from sites in nature, never from infected persons or animals. Males are infected two to three times more commonly than females. No age or exposure is known to predispose to

nocardiosis. Many patients have serious preexisting conditions, such as adrenal corticosteroid therapy, cancer, pulmonary alveolar proteinosis, or chronic granulomatous disease of childhood.

Lesions of nocardiosis show suppuration, necrosis, and abscess formation. Neutrophils are the predominant inflammatory cell. Hyphae are scattered throughout the lesion without formation of grains. Tissue Gram's stain or overstained methenamine silver best demonstrate the hyphae. A modified Fite-Faraco stain of histological sections can be used to demonstrate acid-fastness, but this property is not always demonstrable.

CLINICAL MANIFESTATIONS *Nocardia* pneumonia presents with fever and productive cough of several days' or up to several months' duration. The initial illness may resemble a bacterial pneumonia, but slow radiologic progression continues despite antibiotic therapy often with cavitation of radiodense central areas. Hematogenous dissemination to brain and subcutaneous tissue is frequent in nocardiosis. A pulmonary portal is usually but not always detectable clinically. Brain lesions are typically multiple thin-walled abscesses. Purulent meningitis may result from rupture of an abscess into the ventricle. The subcutaneous lesion typically consists of one or a few indolent abscesses. Hematogenous dissemination to other organs occurs but is rarely detectable clinically.

DIAGNOSIS *Nocardia* is difficult enough to detect in sputum culture, Gram's stain, or histological section so that the diagnosis is readily missed. A progressive pneumonia with purulent sputum should suggest the diagnosis, particularly if cavitation or spread to brain or subcutaneous tissue occurs. Sputum, pus, bronchial brushing, or bronchial washing specimens should be examined by Gram's stain and modified acid-fast stain. On Gram's stain the hyphae are usually branching, beaded, and refractile. They are not strongly gram-positive but take the red counterstain even less well. Conventional acid-fast staining procedures such as Ziehl-Neelsen or a fluorochrome do not stain *Nocardia.* Identification of branching, weakly acid-fast organisms in histological section or smear of pus or sputum is sufficient to establish the diagnosis of nocardiosis. Cultural confirmation is highly desirable, but isolation of *Nocardia* from heavily contaminated specimens is difficult. Isolation of *Nocardia* from otherwise sterile pus is readily accomplished. *Nocardia* is rarely isolated from blood, but diphasic culture media are said to facilitate isolation.

When *Nocardia* is isolated from sputum, the diagnosis of nocardiosis should be suspected, but occasionally no disease can be detected. Rarely, *Nocardia* is an airborne contaminant.

TREATMENT Surgical drainage of empyema and abscesses in brain or subcutaneous tissue is helpful but not sufficient therapy. Virtually all patients should receive prolonged chemotherapy. The treatment of choice is a sulfonamide, given in sufficient dose to maintain a blood concentration of 10 to 15 mg per 100 ml. Sulfadiazine is preferred because of its penetration into the cerebrospinal fluid and other tissues. Also, more experience is available with sulfadiazine than other sulfonamides. The danger of crystalluria and oliguria requires copious fluid intake and urine alkalinization during high-dose sulfadiazine. A reasonable starting regimen is sulfadiazine 100 mg/kg per day and sodium bicarbonate 50 mg/kg per day, both in four divided doses. Patients who show progressive improvement may be changed to sulfisoxazole or trisulfapyrimidines,

60 mg/kg per day after 4 to 6 weeks. Therapy is continued for a total of 12 to 18 months.

Sulfisoxazole is a reasonable starting drug when fluid loading and urine alkalinization are difficult. Trimethoprim-sulfamethoxazole has been used successfully in a few cases, but the contribution of trimethoprim is unclear. Addition of other antibiotics to sulfa drugs may be indicated in patients who show continued deterioration. Ampicillin 150 mg/kg per day is preferred. High doses of minocycline or erythromycin also have been advocated. Parsimonious use of other drugs during sulfa therapy of nocardiosis minimizes the probability that a drug allergy will necessitate discontinuance of sulfa. Antimicrobial susceptibility tests are used to guide therapy of patients with serious allergic reactions to sulfa drugs, but such regimens are not of proved efficacy.

Pulmonary nocardiosis in a previously normal host has a 50 to 60 percent chance of cure with appropriate therapy, and cerebral nocardiosis a 13 percent chance. Continued use of immunosuppressive therapy seems to impair therapeutic response in nocardiosis.

REFERENCES

FRAZIER AR et al: Nocardiosis. A review of 25 cases occurring during 24 months. Mayo Clin Proc 50:657, 1975

KRICK JA et al: Nocardia infection in heart transplant patients. Ann Intern Med 82:18, 1975

PADRON S et al: Lymphocutaneous *Nocardia brasiliensis* infection mimicking sporotrichosis. South Med J 66:609, 1973

PALMER DL et al: Diagnostic and therapeutic considerations in *Nocardia asteroides* infection. Medicine 53:391, 1974

153
CRYPTOCOCCOSIS

JOHN E. BENNETT

DEFINITION Cryptococcosis is an infection caused by the yeast-like fungus *Cryptococcus neoformans*. The most common presentation is as a subacute or chronic meningoencephalitis.

ETIOLOGY *Cryptococcus neoformans* should be divided into two different species, one of which would retain the name *C. neoformans* and the other species would be called *C. bacillisporus*. Mating of compatible strains within these two species yields a perfect state called *Filobasidiella neoformans* and *Filobasidiella bacillispora*. There are biochemical, epidemiological, and serotypic differences between *C. neoformans* and *C. bacillisporus*, but the clinical disease and response to therapy appear to be the same. Therefore, the remainder of this chapter will follow the older practice of calling the two species simply *C. neoformans*.

Cryptococcus neoformans reproduces by budding and forms round, yeast-like cells 4 to 6 μm in diameter. Within the host and on certain culture media, a large polysaccharide capsule surrounds each yeast cell. The fungus grows well as smooth, creamy white colonies on Sabouraud's or other simple media at 20 to 37°C. Certain culture media for ringworm contain cycloheximide, which inhibits *C. neoformans*. Identification is based on gross and microscopic appearance, biochemical tests, and growth at 37°C.

PATHOGENESIS AND PATHOLOGY Infection is thought to be acquired by inhalation of fungus into the lungs. Pulmonary infection has a tendency toward spontaneous resolution and is frequently asymptomatic. Silent hematogenous spread to the brain leads to clusters of cryptococci in the perivascular areas of cortical gray matter, basal ganglia, and, to a lesser extent, other areas of the central nervous system. Inflammatory response around these foci is usually scant. In the more chronic cases, a dense basilar arachnoiditis occurs. Lung lesions exhibit an intense granulomatous inflammation. Cryptococci are best seen in tissue by staining with methenamine silver or periodic acid–Schiff. A strongly positive mucicarmine stain of the organism in tissue is diagnostic, but staining varies from intense to absent.

Cryptococcus neoformans has been isolated from several sites in nature, particularly weathered pigeon droppings. Patients are usually unaware of any unusual exposure to pigeon droppings. No significant case clustering, highly endemic areas, or racial or occupational predisposition is known. Infection before puberty is uncommon. The male/female ratio is about 2:1. Approximately half the patients have a predisposing condition, such as lymphoma, sarcoidosis, or supraphysiological doses of adrenal corticosteroids. Cryptococcosis occurs in animals, especially the cat family. Transmission from animals to humans or from person to person has never been documented.

CLINICAL MANIFESTATIONS The majority of patients has meningoencephalitis at time of diagnosis. This form of the infection is invariably fatal without appropriate therapy, and death occurs anywhere from 2 weeks to several years from onset of symptoms. Early manifestations include headache, nausea, staggering gait, dementia, irritability, confusion, and blurred vision. Both fever and nuchal rigidity are usually mild or absent. Papilledema is present in one-third of the patients at time of diagnosis. Cranial nerve palsies, typically asymmetric, occur in about one-fourth of the patients. Other lateralizing signs are rare. With progression of the infection, deepening coma and signs of brainstem compression appear. Autopsy often reveals cerebral edema in the more acute cases or hydrocephalus in more chronic cases.

Pulmonary cryptococcosis is asymptomatic or associated with dry cough or mild, dull chest ache. Chest x-ray shows one or more dense infiltrates, which are often well circumscribed. Cavitation, pleural effusions, or hilar adenopathy are infrequent. Calcification is not present, and fibrotic stranding is rarely noticeable.

Skin lesions are present in 10 percent of patients with cryptococcosis. These appear to be hematogenously disseminated because the vast majority of patients will be found to have disseminated infection. One or a few asymptomatic tiny papular lesions appear, slowly enlarge, and tend to show central softening leading to ulceration. Osteolytic bone lesions occur in 4 percent of patients and usually present as a cold abscess. Rare manifestations of cryptococcosis include prostatitis, endophthalmitis, hepatitis, pericarditis, endocarditis, and renal abscess.

DIAGNOSIS Cryptococcal meningoencephalitis must be distinguished from tuberculosis, neoplasm, coccidioidomycosis, histoplasmosis, candidiasis, viral aseptic meningitis, and sarcoidosis. Focal lesions are virtually never demonstrable in cryptococcosis by technetium brain scan, cerebral angiography, or electroencephalogram. Computerized tomography (CT) scan will occasionally show one or two sharply demarcated radiodense masses with a central area of lesser density. Lumbar puncture is the single most useful test. An India ink smear of centrifuged spinal fluid sediment reveals encapsulated yeast in one-half the cases, but artifacts resembling cryptococci may cause confusion. Cerebrospinal fluid glucose is reduced in half the cases, protein concentration is usually increased, and

20 to 600 leukocytes per cubic millimeter are typically present and consist predominantly of lymphocytes. Approximately 90 percent of patients with cryptococcal meningoencephalitis, including all those with a positive cerebrospinal fluid smear, will have capsular antigen detectable in cerebrospinal fluid or serum by latex agglutination. False-positive tests occur occasionally, making culture the definitive diagnostic test. *Cryptococcus neoformans* is often present in urine in patients with meningoencephalitis. Fungemia occurs in only 10 percent of patients and portends a lethal outcome.

Pulmonary cryptococcosis mimics malignancy by x-ray and symptoms. Sputum culture is positive in only 10 percent, and serum antigen tests are positive in only a third. Occasionally, *C. neoformans* appears in one or multiple sputum specimens as an endobronchial saprophyte. Biopsy is usually required for diagnosis of pulmonary cryptococcosis. Cutaneous cryptococcosis may be mistaken for a comedone, basal-cell carcinoma, or sarcoidosis. Biopsy reveals a myriad of cyptococci. Osseous cryptococcosis resembles tuberculosis.

TREATMENT Patients with meningoencephalitis and previously normal kidney and bone marrow function should be treated with oral flucytosine 150 mg/kg per day in four divided doses and intravenous amphotericin B 0.3 mg/kg per day. Flucytosine toxicity may be minimized by careful observation for leukopenia, thrombocytopenia, and enterocolitis, as well as appropriate reduction in dose if azotemia is present. As a rough guide, the total daily dose should be:

$$\text{Total daily dose (mg/kg)} = \frac{150}{\text{serum creatinine}}$$

Flucytosine in patients with unstable, moderate, or severe azotemia is hazardous without frequent serum flucytosine assays. Intravenous amphotericin B used alone in dosage of 0.5 to 0.6 mg/kg once daily or 1.0 to 1.2 mg/kg every other day cures 50 to 70 percent of patients with cryptococcal meningoencephalitis and has the advantage that azotemia and hemodialysis do not alter drug clearance. Treatment with either regimen is continued for at least 6 weeks and until at least four weekly cultures of 2 to 4 ml cerebrospinal fluid are sterile. Intrathecal amphotericin B is usually reserved for treatment of severely azotemic patients not receiving dialysis or for patients who have relapsed. Permanent sequelae include dementia, personality change, hydrocephalus, and blindness.

Patients with extraneural cryptococcosis most often require intravenous amphotericin B, with or without flucytosine. Observation or excision of lesions may suffice for some patients who are previously normal, who have a single focus in lung, skin, or bone, and who have no cryptococci in the cerebrospinal fluid, urine, or blood. All too often, however, patients who present with a presumed single focus of extracranial cryptococcosis are discovered to have early asymptomatic meningoencephalitis or dissemination to other organs.

REFERENCES

Bennett JE: Flucytosine. Ann Intern Med 86:319, 1977

Diamond RD, Bennett JE: Prognostic factors in cryptococcal meningitis. Ann Intern Med 80:176, 1974

Gordonson J et al: Pulmonary cryptococcosis. Radiology 112:557, 1974

Littman ML, Zimmerman LE: *Cryptococcosis.* New York, Grune & Stratton, 1956

Schupbach CW et al: Cutaneous manifestations of disseminated cryptococcosis. Arch Dermatol 112:1734, 1976

Tunes B et al: Variant forms of pulmonary cryptococcosis. Ann Intern Med 69:1117, 1968

154
BLASTOMYCOSIS

JOHN E. BENNETT

DEFINITION Blastomycosis (North American blastomycosis) is the infection caused by the fungus *Blastomyces dermatitidis.* Illness most often presents as a chronic pneumonia, chronic skin lesions, or both.

ETIOLOGY *Blastomyces dermatitidis* is a dimorphic fungus, growing at room temperature as a white or tan mold but growing within the host or at 37°C as budding, round yeast-like cells. The fungus is identified by its appearance, its dimorphism, and by the appearance of small spores borne on hyphae of the mold form. When isolates of the two opposite mating types are grown closely together on specialized culture media, sporulating structures appear which characterize the perfect form, *Ajellomyces dermatitidis.*

PATHOGENESIS AND PATHOLOGY The infection is restricted by geography and age. Blastomycosis is uncommon in any locality, but the majority of cases have occurred in the Southeast, Central and Midatlantic areas of the United States, with occasional cases in other localities in the United States and Canada. Cases have also been encountered in Africa, Mexico, Central America, and, rarely, South America. Infection is most common between the ages of 25 and 65 years. The male/female ratio is about 10:1. There is no occupational predisposition.

Infection appears to be acquired by inhalation of the fungus from nature, but the reservoir remains unknown. To date, the fungus has been isolated only from infected humans or animals. No carrier state or transmission from animal to human or from person to person has been observed. Patients presenting with infection in other sites but no detectable lung lesion appear to represent the self-healing that is seen, albeit rarely, in documented lung lesions. Infection has a marked propensity to spread to skin, subcutaneous tissue, and bone, but infection of mucous membranes, genitourinary tract, central nervous system, liver, and spleen is not rare. The inflammatory response includes lymphocytes, giant cells, and neutrophils. Pseudoepitheliomatous hyperplasia may be striking and lead to a mistaken diagnosis of squamous-cell carcinoma.

CLINICAL MANIFESTATIONS One-third of patients present with detectable infection in only one organ, usually the lung or skin. In multiorgan disease, the lung and skin remain the two most common sites so that, overall, about two-thirds of the patients have lung disease and an equal portion skin disease. Pulmonary blastomycosis may present subacutely with pulmonary consolidation resembling bacterial pneumonia on chest x-ray. More commonly, the onset is indolent and the infiltrate on chest x-ray is more likely to be fibronodular, contracted, and, in about one-fourth of patients, cavitary. Calcification, hilar adenopathy, and large pleural effusions are rare. Skin lesions may be single or multiple from the head and extremities and enlarge over weeks or months. Each lesion tends to be painless, well circumscribed, and verrucous or ulcerated. A dark eschar may cover the ulcer. Large chronic lesions may show central healing with scarring and contracture. Mucous membrane lesions in the mouth, nose, and larynx resemble squamous-cell carcinoma. Subcutaneous lesions form draining abscesses. Blastomycosis of bone, joint, prostate, and epididymis resembles tuberculosis. Fatal cases show lesions in many viscera. In contrast to paracoccidioidomycosis (South American blastomycosis), gastrointestinal lesions are very rare. If all forms of blastomycosis are considered together, the most prominent symptoms are cough, weight loss, malaise, skin or subcutaneous lesions, chest pain, and fever.

DIAGNOSIS   The diagnosis is made best by demonstrating the fungus in culture of sputum, pus, or urine. In experienced hands, diagnosis by appearance of the organism in wet smear or histopathologic section is adequate. Skin tests and serologic tests lack sufficient sensitivity and specificity to be useful.

TREATMENT   A few patients have been observed with transitory lung lesions, but no guidelines are known to distinguish these patients from those who will progress locally or disseminate. Therefore, every patient should receive intravenous amphotericin B. Skin and noncavitary lung lesions should be treated for about 8 to 10 weeks. Cavitary lung disease or infection beyond the lung and skin should be treated for about 10 to 12 weeks. Hydroxystilbamidine is less effective and rarely indicated. Iodide therapy is ineffective. The mortality rate in appropriately treated cases is 15 percent or less.

REFERENCES

Blastomycosis Cooperative Study of the Veterans Administration: Blastomycosis. I. A review of 198 collected cases in Veterans Administration Hospitals. Am Rev Resp Dis 89:659, 1964

Busey JF: Blastomycosis. III. A cooperative study of 2-hydroxystilbamidine and amphotericin B therapy. Am Rev Resp Dis 105:812, 1972

Cush R et al: Clinical and roentgenographic manifestations of acute and chronic blastomycosis. Chest 69:345, 1976

Witorsch P, Utz JP: North American blastomycosis: A study of 40 patients. Medicine 47:169, 1968

155
HISTOPLASMOSIS

JOHN E. BENNETT

DEFINITION   Histoplasmosis is the mycosis acquired by inhalation of spores from *Histoplasma capsulatum*.

ETIOLOGY   *Histoplasma capsulatum* is a dimorphic fungus that grows in nature or on Sabouraud's agar at room temperature as a mold. Hyphae bear both large and small spores that are used for identification. *Histoplasma capsulatum* grows as a small budding yeast in host tissue and on enriched agar, such as blood cysteine glucose, at 37°C. Despite the name, the fungus is unencapsulated. When two isolates of the opposite mating type, both in mold form, are grown closely together on an appropriate culture medium, specialized spore-bearing structures are formed which characterize the perfect state, *Emmonsiella capsulata*.

PATHOGENESIS AND PATHOLOGY   Infection with *H. capsulatum* has been encountered in many areas of the world but is much more frequent in certain areas. Within the United States infection is more common in the Southeastern, Midatlantic, and Central states than in other areas. Endemic areas are probably determined by the availability of proper conditions in nature for growth of the fungus. *Histoplasma capsulatum* prefers moist surface soil, particularly when it is enriched by droppings of certain birds and bats. The fungus has not only been isolated repeatedly from such sites but many case clusters have occurred 5 to 18 days after groups were exposed to such dust, for example, by raking, cleaning dirt floored chicken coops, bulldozing, or cave exploring. In many endemic areas, 80 percent or more of residents over age 16 have been exposed, judging by skin test reactivity.

Microconidia, or small spores, of *H. capsulatum* are small enough to reach the alveoli on inhalation and are transformed to budding forms. With time, an intense granulomatous reaction occurs. Caseation necrosis or calcification may mimic tuberculosis. The primary infection in children usually heals completely but may leave spotty calcification in the hilar nodes or lung. Transient dissemination may leave calcified granulomas in the spleen. In adults, a rounded mass of scar tissue, with or without central calcification, may remain in the lung. This has been called a *histoplasmoma*. Previous exposure is thought to confer some protection against reinfection, but infection of persons with prior positive skin tests clearly has occurred.

In a small proportion of patients, histoplasmosis becomes a progressive, potentially fatal infection. The disease occurs either as chronic fibrocavitary pneumonia or, less commonly, as disseminated infection. Patients with either form lack a history of acute primary pulmonary histoplasmosis. Chronic pulmonary infection favors otherwise healthy males over the age of 40 years. A history of cigarette use seems unusually common. An acute, rapidly fatal course is most likely to be encountered in young children and immunosuppressed patients. A more chronic but equally lethal disseminated infection is more common in previously healthy adults.

CLINICAL MANIFESTATIONS   The vast majority of infections are either asymptomatic or mild, and the diagnosis is elusive. Cough, fever, malaise, and chest x-ray findings of hilar adenopathy with or without one or more areas of pneumonitis occur. Erythema nodosum and erythema multiforme have been reported in a few outbreaks. Hilar adenopathy may cause temporary compression of the right middle lobe bronchus in children and young adults. Subacute pericarditis may occur, probably by extension from contiguous lymph nodes. Rarely, many hilar nodes undergo a caseous, granulomatous reaction with perinodal fibrosis. Mediastinal structures become encased by progressive fibrosis, and, over many years, compression of the pulmonary veins, superior vena cava, pulmonary arteries, and esophagus may occur. Late in mediastinal disease only rare nonviable histoplasma can be found in caseous residua of lymph nodes.

Patients with chronic pulmonary histoplasmosis have a gradual onset over weeks or months of increasing productive cough, weight loss, and sometimes nightsweats. Chest x-ray reveals uni- or bilateral fibronodular apical infiltrates. Approximately one-third of cases will stabilize or improve spontaneously early in the course. The remainder have insidious progression. Retraction and cavitation of the upper lobes occur with spread to the apex of the lower lobes and other areas of the lung. Emphysema and bullae formation further compromise pulmonary function. Death from cor pulmonale, bacterial pneumonia, or histoplasmosis occurs after months or years.

Acute disseminated histoplasmosis may be mistaken for miliary tuberculosis. Common findings include fever, emaciation, hepatosplenomegaly, lymphadenopathy, jaundice, anemia, leukopenia, and thrombocytopenia. All these features may occur in chronic dissemination, but the disease tends to be more localized. Indurated ulcers of the mouth, tongue, nose, or larynx occur in about a fourth of patients. Other focal findings include granulomatous hepatitis, Addison's disease, gastrointestinal ulceration, endocarditis, and chronic meningitis. Chest x-ray abnormalities occur in half the cases and show discrete nodules or a miliary pattern.

The presumed ocular histoplasmosis syndrome is a distinct clinical form of uveitis. Although a positive histoplasmin skin test is a requisite for diagnosis, none of these patients has had active histoplasmosis, despite the frequent use of adrenal corticosteroid therapy.

DIAGNOSIS Histoplasmosis may be suspected by serologic tests and clinical manifestations, but definitive diagnosis requires demonstration of the organism by culture or histology. Serologic tests are performed with either histoplasmin, a culture filtrate, or whole yeast form cells. The results are interchangeable. Complement fixation is quantifiable and is the best test. Agar gel diffusion with histoplasmin is a useful but not quantifiable test. Frequent false negatives and false positives limit all current serologic tests. Serologic conversion is helpful but occurs rarely except in acute pulmonary histoplasmosis. Higher complement fixation titers, such as 1:32 or greater, are most suggestive of the diagnosis, but no titer is diagnostic. Cross-reactions with serologic tests for blastomycosis are very common. A 5-mm or more diameter area of induration 24 to 48 h after skin testing with histoplasmin has been very helpful in identifying prior exposure to histoplasma, but false negatives and false positives are so frequent that skin testing has little value in the study of ill patients. Further, approximately one-fourth of normal volunteers with a positive skin test will convert their histoplasmin serology from negative to positive after skin testing.

Culture of *H. capsulatum* from sputum is difficult but is the procedure of choice in chronic pulmonary histoplasmosis. Digestion by proteolytic enzymes and centrifugation of sputum are helpful. In disseminated histoplasmosis, cultures of bone marrow, blood, centrifuged urine, and biopsy specimens are most often positive. Cultures should be performed on agar surfaces of enriched media at room temperature. Growth occurs in 2 to 6 weeks. Histological sections of bone marrow, liver, lymph node, lung, and mucosal lesions may yield the diagnosis.

TREATMENT Acute pulmonary histoplasmosis requires no therapy. Mediastinal fibrosis may benefit by surgery, but the ultimate progress is poor. All patients with disseminated or chronic fibronodular pulmonary histoplasmosis should receive intravenous amphotericin B. Rapid culture conversion and a cure rate in excess of 50 percent can be achieved in both forms, but a formidable relapse rate after short courses has led to use of a 10- to 12-week course of 0.4 to 0.6 mg/kg per day. In chronic pulmonary histoplasmosis, chest x-ray abnormalities improve somewhat, but pulmonary function improves very little. Successful therapy prevents progression. Addisonian crisis is a preventable cause of death in disseminated histoplasmosis.

AFRICAN HISTOPLASMOSIS Patients have been encountered in Africa who seem to be infected with *H. capsulatum* except that the yeast form is larger. Clinical manifestations resemble blastomycosis more than histoplasmosis, because skin and bone lesions are very common.

REFERENCES

GOODWIN RA et al: Mediastinal fibrosis complicating healed primary histoplasmosis and tuberculosis. Medicine 51:227, 1972

PARKER JD et al: Treatment of chronic pulmonary histoplasmosis. N Engl J Med 283:225, 1970

SAROSI GA et al: Disseminated histoplasmosis: Results of long term follow-up. Ann Intern Med 75:511, 1971

SMITH JW, UTZ JP: Progressive disseminated histoplasmosis. Ann Intern Med 76:557, 1972

SUTLIFF WD: Histoplasmosis cooperative study. V. Amphotericin B dosage for chronic pulmonary histoplasmosis. Am Rev Resp Dis 105:60, 1972

COCCIDIOIDOMYCOSIS

JOHN E. BENNETT

DEFINITION Coccidioidomycosis is the mycosis acquired by inhalation of *Coccidioides immitis.*

ETIOLOGY *Coccidioides immitis* is a dimorphic fungus, growing as a white fluffy mold on most culture media but as a nonbudding spherical form, a spherule, in host tissue or under specialized conditions. Reproduction in the host tissue is by formation of small endospores within mature spherules. After rupture of the spherule, the released endospores enlarge, become spherules, and repeat the cycle. The fungus is identified by its appearance and by formation of thick-walled, barrel-shaped spores, called *arthrospores,* in the hyphae of the mold form.

PATHOGENESIS AND PATHOLOGY *Coccidioides immitis* is a soil saprophyte in certain arid regions of the United States, Mexico, Central America, and South America. Within the United States, most cases are acquired in California, Arizona, West Texas, and New Mexico. A few cases are acquired in bordering areas and by exposure to fomites from endemic areas, such as cotton bales.

Infection in humans and animals results from inhalation of windborne arthrospores arising from soil sites. This primary pulmonary infection is symptomatic in only 40 percent of individuals, with symptoms ranging from a mild, influenza-like illness to severe pneumonia. Mild, self-limited infections may come to medical attention because of case clusters or hypersensitivity reactions: erythema nodosum, erythema multiforme, toxic erythema, arthralgia, arthritis, conjunctivitis, or episcleritis. Case clusters occur 10 to 14 days after a group of susceptible individuals is exposed to dust in an endemic area through such activities as unearthing Indian relics, rock hunting, military maneuvers, or construction. The usual course of primary pulmonary infection is complete healing, though an area of pneumonitis on x-ray may heal by forming a coin-like lesion, or coccidioidoma. Less commonly, a single thin-walled cavity remains as a chronic sequela in the area of consolidation. Also, the consolidation may persist as a chronic pneumonia or progress to fibronodular, cavitary disease.

Pleural effusion may be the only manifestation of primary infection. Self-healing of this form is common.

An uncommon but dreaded complication of coccidioidomycosis is dissemination beyond the lung and hilar lymph nodes. Dissemination is more frequent in blacks, Filipinos, native Americans, Mexican-Americans, and pregnant or immunosuppressed patients.

Coccidioides immitis incites a chronic granulomatous reaction in host tissue, often with caseation necrosis. Lung and hilar node lesions may show calcification. Both IgM and IgG antibodies against *C. immitis* are induced by infection but neither appears protective. The amount of specific IgG antibody is a rough measure of the antigenic mass, i.e., of the amount of infection, making a high titer a poor prognostic sign. Appearance of delayed hypersensitivity to antigens of *C. immitis* is most common in those clinical forms of disease with a good prognosis, such as self-limited primary pulmonary disease. Negative skin tests to *Coccidioides* antigens in roughly half the patients with disseminated disease has led to therapeutic trials of "transfer factor." Conversion of skin tests and in vitro tests correlating with delayed hypersensitivity has been achieved with transfer factor, but whether the infection has improved remains unclear.

CLINICAL MANIFESTATIONS Symptomatic primary pulmonary infection is manifested by fever, cough, chest pain, malaise, and sometimes hypersensitivity reactions. Chest x-ray may show an infiltrate, hilar adenopathy, or pleural effusion. Peripheral blood may show a mild eosinophilia. Spontaneous improvement begins after several days to 2 weeks of illness and usually culminates in complete recovery.

The symptoms of a chronic thin-walled cavity include cough or hemoptysis in half the cases; the other patients are asymptomatic. Chronic progressive pulmonary coccidioidomycosis produces cough, sputum, variable degrees of fever, and weight loss. The first indications of dissemination usually appear during the primary infection. Reactivation with dissemination in later years occurs occasionally, especially if Hodgkin's disease, non-Hodgkin's lymphoma, renal transplantation, or other immunosuppression has supervened. Dissemination should be suspected when fever, malaise, hilar or paratracheal lymphadenopathy, and elevated sedimentation rate show abnormal persistence in patients with primary pulmonary coccidioidomycosis. High complement fixation titers support this concern. With time, lesions appear in the bone, skin, subcutaneous tissue, meninges, joints, and other sites. Without therapy, dissemination may progress rapidly to death or wax and wane for years.

DIAGNOSIS When coccidioidomycosis is suspected, sputum, urine, and pus should be examined for *C. immitis* by wet smear and culture. The laboratory request should indicate clearly that coccidioidomycosis is suspected because the mold form must be handled with extreme care to prevent infection of laboratory personnel. On biopsy, smaller spherules must be distinguished from nonbudding forms of *Blastomyces* and *Cryptococcus,* but appearance of the mature spherule is diagnostic.

Serologic tests are very helpful in coccidioidomycosis. Latex agglutination and agar gel diffusion tests are useful in screening serums for antibody to coccidioides. The complement fixation test is used on cerebrospinal fluid and to confirm and quantitate serum antibody detected by screening tests. The number of cases with a positive complement fixation test will depend upon the severity of disease and upon the laboratory performing the test. Positive tests are least common in patients with solitary pulmonary cavities or primary pulmonary infection, while serums from patients with multiorgan disseminated disease are nearly all positive. Seroconversion is helpful in primary pulmonary coccidioidomycosis but may not occur for up to 8 weeks after onset. A positive complement fixation test in unconcentrated cerebrospinal fluid is diagnostic of meningitis.

Conversion of skin test from negative to positive (≥ 5 mm induration at 24 or 48 h) with either coccidioidin or spherulin, the two commercially available antigens, may be observed between the third and twenty-first days of symptoms in primary pulmonary coccidioidomycosis. Skin testing can also be helpful in epidemiologic studies, such as investigation of case clusters or definition of endemic areas. The utility of skin testing as a diagnostic tool is limited by the presence of persistent positive tests resulting from remote exposures to coccidioides and by the frequency of negative skin tests in many patients with either thin-walled cavities or disseminated coccidioidomycosis.

TREATMENT Primary pulmonary coccidioidomycosis usually resolves spontaneously. Some physicians give a few weeks of intravenous amphotericin B when patients show an unusually severe or protracted primary infection, hoping to abort disseminated or chronic pulmonary disease. There is no solid evidence to support this practice, but the stronger the suspicion of dissemination becomes in any given patient, the more logical this approach appears. Once evidence for dissemination becomes incontrovertible, amphotericin B may be palliative rather than curative. Nevertheless, every patient with disseminated coccidioidomycosis should receive sufficient amphotericin B to attempt cure, usually 0.5 to 0.7 mg/kg per day or a double dose every other day for 10 to 12 weeks. Surgical curettage of bone lesions, drainage of abscesses, and resection of lung lesions contribute to cure. Unfortunately, intravenous amphotericin B is not curative in coccidioidal meningitis, and all such patients should receive prolonged therapy with intrathecal amphotericin B. In all forms of disseminated coccidioidomycosis, relapse after months or years of therapy is frequent. Intravenous miconazole has resulted in improvement of disseminated coccidioidomycosis, but its efficacy compared with amphotericin B is unknown.

Patients with a thin-walled solitary pulmonary cavity will close the cavity spontaneously in 25 to 50 percent of cases. Lobectomy with perioperative amphotericin B may be indicated for hemoptysis, superinfection, or progressive enlargement of such cavities.

REFERENCES

DERESINSKI SC, STEVENS DA: Coccidioidomycosis in compromised hosts. Medicine 54:377, 1974

DRUTZ DJ, CATANZARO A: Coccidioidomycosis. Am Rev Resp Dis 117:559, 727, 1978

FIESE MJ: *Coccidioidomycosis.* Springfield, Ill, Charles C Thomas, 1958

LONKY SA et al: Acute coccidioidal pleural effusion. Am Rev Resp Dis 114:681, 1976

WERIN WA: A long term study of 300 patients with cavitary-abscess lesions of the lung of coccidioidal origin. Dis Chest 54 (suppl 1):12, 1968

157
SPOROTRICHOSIS

JOHN E. BENNETT

DEFINITION Sporotrichosis is the mycosis caused by *Sporothrix schenckii.*

ETIOLOGY *Sporothrix schenckii* lives as a saprophyte on plants in many areas of the world. In nature and on culture at room temperature the fungus grows as a mold, but within host tissue or at 37°C on enriched media it grows as a budding yeast. Identification is by appearance of the fungus in mold and yeast forms. Small spores with a hair-like attachment to hyphae give the fungus the name, *Sporothrix.*

PATHOGENESIS AND PATHOLOGY Infection results when minor trauma inoculates the fungus into subcutaneous tissue. Nursery workers, florists, and gardeners acquire the illness from roses, sphagnum moss, and other plants. Infection may be limited to the site of inoculation (plaque sporotrichosis) or extend along proximal lymphatic channels (lymphangitic sporotrichosis). Spread on an extremity, the usual site, even as far as inguinal or axillary nodes is rare, and hematogenous dissemination from the skin remains unproved. The portal for osteoarticular, pulmonary, and other extracutaneous forms of sporotrichosis is unknown but is likely the lung.

Untreated sporotrichosis shows little evidence of self-healing and is capable of extreme chronicity. The inflammatory response contains both clusters of neutrophils and a marked granulomatous response with epithelioid cells and giant cells.

CLINICAL MANIFESTATIONS Lymphangitic sporotrichosis, by far the most common manifestation, forms a nearly painless red papule at the site of inoculation. Over the next several weeks, similar nodules form along proximal lymphatic channels. Nodules intermittently discharge small amounts of pus. Ulceration may occur. The proximal extension of these lesions, often with skip areas, is quite distinctive but may be mimicked by lesions of *Nocardia brasiliensis, Mycobacterium marinum,* or, on rare occasions, by *Leishmania brasiliensis* or *M. kansasii.*

Plaque sporotrichosis is a nontender red maculopapular granuloma confined to the site of inoculation. Osteoarticular sporotrichosis presents as mono- or polyarticular arthritis of indolent onset and progression over months or years, involving the elbows, knees, wrists, ankles, and, rarely, smaller joints of the extremities. Periarticular bone gradually appears "motheaten," and draining sinuses may appear over joints and bursas. Hematogenous spread to the skin may be observed during polyarticular disease, but none of the skin lesions shows lymphangitic spread. Immunosuppression predisposes to such spread. Pulmonary sporotrichosis usually presents as a single chronic cavitary upper-lobe lung lesion.

DIAGNOSIS Culture of pus, joint fluid, sputum, or skin biopsy specimen is the preferred method of diagnosis. Appearance of *S. schenckii* in tissue is quite variable. In skin lesions, organisms are hard to find.

TREATMENT Cutaneous sporotrichosis can be cured with oral administration of a saturated solution of potassium iodide, given in increasing divided daily doses up to 9 to 12 ml per day for adults. Gastrointestinal disturbance or acneform rash over the cape area and face are common, but therapy should be continued for 1 month after resolution of all lesions. Patients with serious allergic reactions to iodides may respond to local heat, particularly when plaque sporotrichosis is the only form of disease. Extracutaneous sporotrichosis does not respond to iodides, but cures have been obtained in over half such patients with prolonged courses of intravenous amphotericin B.

REFERENCES

Crout JE et al: Sporotrichosis arthritis. Clinical features of seven patients. Ann Intern Med 86:294, 1977

Lynch PJ et al: Systemic sporotrichosis. Ann Intern Med 73:23, 1970

Orr ER, Riley HD: Sporotrichosis in childhood, report of ten cases. J Pediatr 78:951, 1971

Wilson DE et al: Clinical features of extracutaneous sporotrichosis. Medicine 46:265, 1967

158
CANDIDIASIS

JOHN E. BENNETT

DEFINITION Candidiasis (moniliasis, candidosis) is infection caused by any of several species of the yeast-like fungus, *Candida.* Candidiasis of mucous membranes is also called *thrush.*

ETIOLOGY *Candida albicans* is the most common cause of candidiasis, but *C. tropicalis, C. parapsilosis, C. guilliermondii, C. krusei,* and a few other species can cause candidiasis and may even be fatal. *Candida parapsilosis* is particularly notable for its ability to cause endocarditis. All *Candida* species pathogenic for humans are also encountered as commensals of humans, particularly in the mouth, stool, and vagina. These species grow rapidly at 25 to 37°C on simple media as oval budding cells. In specialized agar media, hyphae or elongated branching structures called pseudohyphae are formed. *Candida albicans* can be identified presumptively by its ability to form germ tubes in serum or by the formation of thick-walled large spores, called *chlamydospores.* Final identification of all species requires biochemical tests.

PATHOGENESIS AND PATHOLOGY Either local or systemic factors may lead to tissue invasion by *Candida.* Chronic maceration predisposes to cutaneous candidiasis, as in diaper rash, intertrigo in obese patients, or paronychia in bartenders or cannery workers. Age is important because neonatal colonization often leads to oral thrush. Women in the third trimester of pregnancy are prone to vulvovaginal thrush. Patients with diabetes mellitus or hematologic malignancy, or who are receiving broad-spectrum antibiotics or supraphysiologic doses of adrenal corticosteroids, are especially susceptible to candidiasis. Breaks in the integrity of the skin or mucous membranes may provide access to deeper tissues. Examples include: perforation of the gastrointestinal tract by trauma, surgery, and peptic ulceration; indwelling catheters for intravenous alimentation, peritoneal dialysis, and urinary tract drainage; severe burns and intravenous drug abuse.

Candida grows within tissues in both yeast and pseudohyphal forms. Rarely, only one form is present. Visceral lesions are characterized by necrosis and a neutrophilic inflammatory response. Neutrophils kill *Candida* yeast cells and damage segments of pseudohyphae in vitro, suggesting a major role for the neutrophil in host defense against this fungus. Visceral lesions show a preference for kidney, brain, spleen, heart, and liver.

CLINICAL MANIFESTATIONS Oral thrush presents as discrete and confluent adherent white plaques on the oral and pharyngeal mucosa, particularly in the mouth and tongue. These lesions are usually painless, but fissuring at the corners of the mouth can be painful. Cutaneous candidiasis presents as red, macerated intertriginous areas, paronychia, balanitis, or pruritus ani. Candidiasis of the perineal and scrotal skin may be accompanied by discrete pustular lesions on the inner aspects of the thighs. Chronic mucocutaneous candidiasis or *Candida* granuloma typically presents as circumscribed hyperkeratotic skin lesions, crumbling dystrophic nails, partial alopecia in areas of scalp lesions, and both oral and vaginal thrush. Systemic infection is very rare, but disfigurement of the face and hands can be severe. Other findings may include chronic epidermophytosis, dental dysplasia, and hypofunction of the parathyroid, adrenal, or thyroid glands. A variety of defects in T-cell function have been described in these patients. Vulvovaginal thrush causes pruritus, discharge, and sometimes pain on intercourse or urination. Speculum examination reveals an inflamed mucosa and a thin exudate, often with white curds.

From one to multiple small shallow ulcerations due to *Candida* may appear in the esophagus or gastrointestinal tract. Esophageal lesions favor the distal third and may cause dysphagia or substernal pain. Other such lesions tend to be asymptomatic but assume importance in the leukemic patient as a portal for disseminated candidiasis. Within the urinary tract, the most common lesions are either hematogenously disseminated renal abscesses, which can cause azotemia, or bladder thrush. Bladder invasion usually follows catheterization or instrumentation of a patient with diabetes mellitus or who is receiving broad-spectrum antibiotics. This lesion generally is asymptomatic and benign. Rarely, retrograde invasion of the renal pelvis leads to renal papillary necrosis.

Hematogenous dissemination of *Candida* presents with fever and toxicity but with few localizing findings. One or more retinal abscesses may appear and extend slowly into the vitreous humor. The patient may note orbital pain, blurred vision, scotoma, or opacities floating across the visual field. Pulmonary candidiasis is almost always hematogenous and is visible on chest x-ray only when the abscesses are numerous enough to cause a diffuse, vaguely nodular infiltrate. Candidiasis of the endocardium or around intracardiac prostheses resembles bacterial infection of these sites. Chronic *Candida* meningitis or arthritis may occur, from either disseminated disease or insertion of a plastic prosthesis in the case of arthritis. Rare focal manifestations of disseminated disease include osteomyelitis, pustular skin lesions, myositis, and brain abscess.

DIAGNOSIS Demonstration of pseudohyphae on wet smear with confirmation by culture is the procedure of choice for diagnosing superficial candidiasis. Scrapings for the smear may be obtained from skin, nails, and oral and vaginal mucosa. Culture alone is not diagnostic.

Deeper lesions of *Candida* may be diagnosed by histological section of biopsy specimens or by culture of cerebrospinal fluid, blood, joint fluid, or surgical specimens. Blood culture in vented bottles is very useful in *Candida* endocarditis but is positive less often in other forms of disseminated disease. The utility of serodiagnosis remains controversial.

TREATMENT Cutaneous candidiasis of macerated areas responds to measures which reduce moisture and chafing plus a topically applied antifungal agent in a nonocclusive base. Nystatin, clotrimazole, miconazole, and amphotericin B appear roughly equivalent. The first three of these are available also for vaginal application. Oral candidiasis should be treated with nystatin suspension. Swallowing nystatin suspension or sucking on the tablets compounded for vaginal use may improve symptoms of esophageal candidiasis. When esophageal symptoms are pronounced, a 5- to 10-day course of intravenous amphotericin B, 0.3 mg/kg per day, may be beneficial. Bladder thrush responds to bladder irrigations with amphotericin B, 50 μg/ml for 5 days. In all forms of skin and mucosal candidiasis, relapse after successful treatment is common.

Intravenous amphotericin B is the drug of choice in disseminated candidiasis. The drug is usually given as 0.4 to 0.5 mg/kg every day or as a double dose on alternate days for several weeks. In patients with no contraindication to the use of flucytosine, administration of that drug in dosage of 100 to 150 mg/kg per day plus amphotericin B, 0.3 mg/kg per day, is an effective alternative.

Candida isolated from a properly obtained blood culture should be considered significant, for true false positives are rare. Whether a patient with candidiasis should receive antifungal therapy will depend on the degree of illness and the likelihood of spontaneous recovery. For example, a febrile, severely immunosuppressed patient with one positive blood culture should receive prompt therapy because a rapidly fatal course is common. A nonimmunosuppressed patient acquiring candidiasis from an indwelling intravenous plastic catheter may recover spontaneously if the catheter is removed promptly. The species of *Candida* is irrelevant to this decision. Patients with candidiasis in whom antifungal therapy is withheld should be observed carefully for the development of endophthalmitis, endocarditis, arthritis, osteomyelitis, or other visceral lesions that require therapy.

REFERENCES

EDWARDS JE et al: Ocular manifestations of Candida septicemia. Review of 76 cases of haematogenous candida endophthalmitis. Medicine 53:47, 1974

ERAS P et al: Candida infection of the gastrointestinal tract. Medicine 51:367, 1972

GAINES JD, REMINGTON JS: Disseminated candidiasis in the surgical patient. Surgery 72:730, 1972

ROSE HD, SHETH NK: Pulmonary candidiasis. A clinical and pathological correlation. Arch Intern Med 138:964, 1978

YOUNG RC et al: Fungemia with compromised host resistance. Ann Intern Med 80:605, 1974

159
ASPERGILLOSIS

JOHN E. BENNETT

DEFINITION The name *aspergillosis* embraces a variety of widely differing diseases having in common only some pathogenetic relationship to the fungus *Aspergillus*. In these diseases the fungus either elicits an allergic reaction, invades tissue, or grows within air spaces, such as a bronchus, pulmonary cavity, or paranasal sinus.

ETIOLOGY *Aspergillus fumigatus* is the most common pathogen, but *A. flavus, A. niger,* and several other species can cause disease. *Aspergillus* is a mold with septate hyphae about 4 μm in diameter. Sporulating structures, called *conidial heads,* may be seen when the fungus is growing in nature, on an artificial medium, or within air-containing spaces of the body. The appearance of the colonies and of conidial heads is used for identification.

PATHOGENESIS AND PATHOLOGY All the common species of *Aspergillus* which cause disease in humans are ubiquitous in the environment, growing on dead leaves, stored grain, compost piles, hay, and other decaying vegetation. Inhalation of *Aspergillus* spores must be extremely common, but disease is rare. Invasion of lung tissue is almost entirely confined to immunosuppressed patients. Roughly 90 percent will have two of these three conditions: less than 500 granulocytes per cubic millimeter of peripheral blood, supraphysiological doses of adrenal corticosteroids, and a history of taking cytotoxic drugs such as azathioprine. Infection in such patients is characterized by hyphal invasion of blood vessels, thrombosis, necrosis, and hemorrhagic infarction. Chronic granulomatous disease of childhood also predisposes to invasive pulmonary aspergillosis, but here the inflammatory response is granulomatous. Blood vessel invasion is rare.

Massive inhalation of *Aspergillus* spores by normal persons can lead to an acute, diffuse, self-limited pneumonitis. Epithelioid granulomas with giant cells and central pyogenic areas containing hyphae are seen. Spontaneous recovery taking several weeks is the usual course.

Aspergillus can colonize the damaged bronchial tree, pulmonary cysts, or cavities of patients with underlying lung disease. Balls of hyphae within cysts or cavities may reach several centimeters in diameter and be visible on chest x-ray. Tissue invasion does not occur. The term *allergic bronchial aspergillosis* denotes the condition of patients with preexisting asthma who have eosinophilia, IgE antibody to *Aspergillus*, and fleeting pulmonary infiltrates from bronchial plugging. Some of these asthmatic patients also have endobronchial colonization with *Aspergillus*. It is not clear what role *Aspergillus* plays in noninvasive lung disease. Plugs of hyphae may obstruct bronchi. Perhaps allergic or toxic reactions to *Aspergillus* antigens cause bronchial constriction and damage.

CLINICAL MANIFESTATIONS Endobronchial pulmonary aspergillosis presents as chronic productive cough and often hemoptysis in a patient with prior chronic lung disease, such as tuberculosis, sarcoidosis, bronchiectasis, or histoplasmosis. *Aspergilloma* refers to a ball of hyphae within a lung cyst or cavity, usually in the upper lobe. *Aspergillus* may be spread from its endocavitary or endobronchial site to the pleura during the course of bacterial lung abscess or surgery.

Invasive aspergillosis in the immunosuppressed host presents as an acute pneumonia. Infection progresses by hematogenous spread as well as extension to surrounding lung and other contiguous structures. Occasionally the portal of infection in the immunosuppressed host is the paranasal sinus, gastrointestinal tract, skin, palate, or epiglottis.

Aspergillus sinusitis in nonimmunosuppressed patients may take two forms. A ball of hyphae may form in a chronically obstructed paranasal sinus, without tissue invasion. A chronic, fibrosing granulomatous inflammation with scanty *Aspergillus* hyphae within tissue may begin in the sinus and spread slowly to the orbit and brain.

Growth of *Aspergillus* on cerumen and detritus within the external auditory canal is termed *otomycosis*. Trauma to the cornea may cause chronic *Aspergillus* keratitis. Endophthalmitis follows introduction of *Aspergillus* into the globe by trauma or surgery. *Aspergillus* may infect intracardiac or intravascular prostheses.

DIAGNOSIS Culture of *Aspergillus* from sputum usually has no diagnostic significance. Repeated isolation of *Aspergillus* from sputum or demonstration of hyphae in the sputum smear suggests endobronchial colonization. Fungus ball of the lung is usually detectable by chest x-ray. Antibody of the IgG class to *Aspergillus* antigens is demonstrable in the serum of many colonized patients and of virtually all patients with fungus ball.

Biopsy is usually required to diagnose invasive aspergillosis of the lung, paranasal sinus, or sites of dissemination. Blood cultures are rarely positive, even in patients with infected cardiac prosthetic valves. *Aspergillus* hyphae can be identified presumptively by histology, but culture is required for confirmation and determination of species. Serologic and skin tests have not proved helpful in invasive aspergillosis.

TREATMENT Patients with severe hemoptysis due to fungus ball of the lung may benefit by lobectomy. Poor pulmonary function in residual lung and dense pleural adhesions around the lesion can complicate the resection. Systemic chemotherapy is of no value in endobronchial or endocavitary aspergillosis.

Intravenous amphotericin B has resulted in arrest or cure of invasive aspergillosis when immunosuppression is not severe. Combined flucytosine–amphotericin B may be useful in nonneutropenic patients with invasive aspergillosis, but current information to evaluate this regimen is inadequate.

REFERENCES

AISNER J et al: Treatment of invasive aspergillosis: Relation of early diagnosis and treatment to response. Ann Intern Med 86:539, 1977

GREEN WF et al: Aspergillosis of the orbit. Arch Ophthalmol 82:302, 1969

KILMAN JW et al: Surgery for pulmonary aspergillosis. J Thorac Cardiovasc Surg 57:642, 1969

MEYER RD et al: Aspergillosis complicating neoplastic disease. Am J Med 54:6, 1973

YOUNG RC et al: Aspergillosis: Spectrum of the disease in 98 patients. Medicine 49:149, 1970

MUCORMYCOSIS

JOHN E. BENNETT

DEFINITION Mucormycosis is an acute infection caused by fungi of the order Mucorales. *Zygomycosis* and *phycomycosis* are synonymous terms which encompass mucormycosis and several entirely different diseases.

ETIOLOGY *Rhizopus* and *Mucor* species are the principal pathogens. These molds have broad, rarely septate hyphae of uneven diameter, ranging from 6 to 50 μm. The fungus is inexplicably difficult to grow from infected tissue. When it occurs, growth is rapid and profuse on most media at room temperature. Identification is based upon gross and microscopic appearance of the mold.

PATHOGENESIS AND PATHOLOGY *Rhizopus* and *Mucor* species are ubiquitous, appearing on decaying vegetation, dung, and foods of high sugar content. Infection is uncommon and largely confined to patients with serious preexisting diseases. Mucormycosis originating in the paranasal sinuses and nose occurs predominantly in patients with poorly controlled diabetes mellitus. Mucormycosis in patients with hematologic malignancy or organ transplantation more often originates in the lung than in the nose and paranasal sinuses. Gastrointestinal mucormycosis occurs in a variety of conditions, including uremia, severe malnutrition, and diarrheal diseases. Infection is acquired from nature, with no person-to-person spread.

In all forms of mucormycosis, vascular invasion by hyphae is prominent. Ischemic or hemorrhagic necrosis is the predominant histological finding.

CLINICAL MANIFESTATIONS Mucormycosis originating in the nose and paranasal sinuses produces a characteristic clinical picture. Low-grade fever, dull sinus pain, and sometimes nasal congestion or a thin, bloody nasal discharge are followed in a few days by double vision, increasing fever and obtundation. Examination reveals a unilateral generalized reduction of ocular motion, chemosis, and proptosis. The nasal turbinates on the involved side may be dusky red or necrotic. A sharply delineated area of necrosis, strictly respecting the midline, may appear in the hard palate. The skin of the cheek may become inflamed. Fungal invasion of the globe or ophthalmic artery leads to blindness. Opacification of one or more sinuses is found on x-ray. Carotid arteriogram may show invasion or obstruction of the carotid siphon. Coma is due to direct invasion of the frontal lobe. Early symptoms mimic bacterial sinusitis. Clouding of the sensorium may be attributed to diabetic acidosis. Cavernous sinus thrombosis may be considered when orbital invasion occurs. Without treatment, death may occur in a few days to a few weeks.

Pulmonary mucormycosis is a progressive severe pneumonia, accompanied by high fever and toxicity. The necrotic center of large infiltrates may cavitate. Hematogenous spread to other areas of the lung, as well as to brain and other organs is common. Survival beyond 2 weeks is unusual. Gastrointestinal invasion presents as one or more ulcers which tend to perforate. Hematogenous dissemination can originate from the gastrointestinal tract, lung, or paranasal sinuses. Sometimes no portal of entry can be found.

DIAGNOSIS Lesions of the lung and craniofacial structures are best diagnosed by biopsy and histological section. Cultural confirmation should be attempted. Wet smear of crushed tissue can provide rapid diagnosis. Cultures of blood and cerebrospinal fluid are negative. Smear and culture of sputum may be positive during cavitation of a lung lesion. Serologic tests are under investigation but are unlikely to aid diagnosis of rapidly fatal cases.

TREATMENT Regulation of diabetes mellitus and decreasing immunosuppressive drugs aid in the treatment. Extensive debridement of craniofacial lesions appears to be very important. Orbital exenteration may be required. Intravenous amphotericin B is clearly of value in craniofacial mucormycosis and should be employed in the other forms of mucormycosis as well. Maximum tolerated doses are given until progression is halted. The drug is continued for a total of 10 to 12 weeks. Appropriate management results in cure of about half of the craniofacial infections. Survival of patients with pulmonary, gastrointestinal, or disseminated mucormycosis is rare.

REFERENCES

ADDLESTONE RB, BAYLIN CJ: Rhinocerebral mucormycosis. Radiology 115:113, 1975

BARTRUM RJ et al: Roentgenographic findings in pulmonary mucormycosis. Am J Roentgenol 117:810, 1973

LOWE JT, HUDSON WR: Rhinocerebral phycomycosis and internal carotid artery thrombosis. Arch Otolaryngol 101:100, 1975

MEYER RD, ARMSTRONG D: Mucormycosis—changing status. CRC Crit Rev Clin Lab Sci 4:421, 1973

161
OTHER DEEP MYCOSES
Paracoccidioidomycosis, petriellidiosis, torulopsosis, mycetoma, and chromomycosis

JOHN E. BENNETT

PARACOCCIDIOIDOMYCOSIS

DEFINITION Paracoccidioidomycosis, formerly called *South American blastomycosis,* is the mycosis caused by *Paracoccidioides brasiliensis.*

ETIOLOGY A dimorphic fungus, *P. brasiliensis* grows as a budding yeast but may be grown as either yeast or mold on a culture medium. Identification is by gross and microscopic appearance. A superficial resemblance to *Blastomyces dermatitidis* may cause misdiagnosis.

PATHOGENESIS AND PATHOLOGY Infection is thought to be acquired by inhalation of spores from environmental sources, but the reservoir in nature remains obscure. Pulmonary infection produces few symptoms initially. Hematogenous spread to the mucous membranes of the mouth and nose, the lymph nodes, and other sites brings the patient to medical attention. Fatal cases show spread to the adrenal, the gastrointestinal tract, and many other viscera.

CLINICAL MANIFESTATIONS Common symptoms include indurated ulcers of the mouth, oropharynx, larynx, and nose, enlarged and draining lymph nodes, lesions of the skin and genitalia, productive cough, weight loss, dyspnea, and sometimes fever. Acquisition of infection is restricted to South America, Central America, and Mexico, but the extreme indolence of this infection may lead to recognition many years after the patient has left the endemic area. Chest x-ray most often shows a bilateral patchy pneumonia.

DIAGNOSIS Cultures of sputum, pus, and mucosal lesions are often diagnostic. The diagnosis can be made by smear or histological section, though confirmation by culture is preferable. Serologic tests are useful in suggesting the diagnosis and monitoring therapy.

TREATMENT Milder cases may be cured by several years of treatment with oral sulfonamide therapy. More advanced cases are given intravenous amphotericin B, followed by prolonged oral sulfa drugs.

PETRIELLIDIOSIS

DEFINITION Petriellidiosis refers to all mycoses caused by *Petriellidium boydii* other than mycetoma.

ETIOLOGY Also called *Allescheria boydii, P. boydii* is a mold frequently found in soil. When the fungus is isolated in the imperfect state, it is called *Monosporium apiospermum.*

PATHOGENESIS AND PATHOLOGY Wind-borne spores of *P. boydii,* arising in soil, are the presumed source of infection. The fungus grows as a mold within tissue, causing necrosis and abscess formation.

CLINICAL MANIFESTATIONS *Petriellidium boydii* resembles *Aspergillus* in its ability to colonize the endobronchial tree, to form fungus balls in the lung or paranasal sinuses, to invade the cornea or globe following trauma or surgery, and by its propensity to invade the immunosuppressed host. Hyphae of *P. boydii* in tissue may be difficult to distinguish from *Aspergillus.* Infection with *P. boydii* is much less common than with *Aspergillus. Petriellidium boydii* is the single most common cause in the United States of mycetoma. Intravascular hyphae, a hallmark of invasive aspergillosis, are less prominent in petriellidiosis. Occasional normal patients have developed necrotizing pneumonia or abscesses in brain or other organs due to *P. boydii.*

DIAGNOSIS Demonstration of hyphae in tissue and culture confirmation are required for diagnosis.

TREATMENT Intravenous miconazole has been recommended, but therapeutic response to all drugs has been poor.

TORULOPSOSIS

DEFINITION Torulopsosis is the infection caused by *Torulopsis glabrata.*

ETIOLOGY *Torulopsis glabrata* is a small yeast-like fungus, the same size as the yeast form of *Histoplasma capsulatum. Torulopsis glabrata* does not form hyphae or pseudohyphae. Identification is by biochemical tests.

PATHOGENESIS AND PATHOLOGY *Torulopsis glabrata* is a normal inhabitant of the human gastrointestinal tract and vagina. Within tissue, *T. glabrata* causes abscess formation with a neutrophilic inflammatory response. In immunosuppressed patients, a scanty or mononuclear inflammatory response may be seen.

CLINICAL MANIFESTATIONS Torulopsosis mimics many of the manifestations of candidiasis, but infection is less common and often less severe. Clinical entities include intravenous catheter–induced sepsis or endocarditis, gastrointestinal and disseminated infection in immunosuppressed patients, and retrograde infection of the urinary tract.

DIAGNOSIS Torulopsis may be difficult to distinguish from yeast cells of *Candida* in histological section. Culture is the most reliable diagnostic tool.

TREATMENT Therapeutic measures used in candidiasis appear appropriate for torulopsosis.

MYCETOMA

DEFINITION *Mycetoma* is a chronic suppurative infection originating in subcutaneous tissue and characterized by the presence of grains, which are tightly clumped colonies of the causative agent.

ETIOLOGY *Actinomycetoma* refers to infection by actinomycetes of the genus *Nocardia, Streptomyces,* and *Actinomadura. Eumycetoma* is caused by true fungi of many different genera. The most common agent varies with the locality.

PATHOGENESIS AND PATHOLOGY The pathogens live in the soil and enter the skin through minor trauma. The most common site of infection is the foot. Infection runs a relentless course over many years, with destruction of contiguous bone and fascia. Grains are found in purulent foci, surrounded by fibrosis and a mononuclear cell inflammatory response.

CLINICAL MANIFESTATIONS The infected site shows painless swelling, woody induration, and sinus tracts which discharge pus intermittently. Systemic symptoms and spread to distant sites in the body are not seen.

DIAGNOSIS The clinical picture is characteristic, but confusion with chronic osteomyelitis or botryomycosis may occur. The diagnosis requires demonstration of grains in pus from the draining sinus or in biopsy sections. Many histological sections may need to be examined to locate a grain.

TREATMENT Actinomycetoma may respond to prolonged therapy with sulfonamides, trimethoprim-sulfamethoxazole, or other antibacterial agents. Eumycetoma does not respond reliably to any drug. Amputation may be required.

CHROMOMYCOSIS

DEFINITION *Chromomycosis* is a clinical syndrome characterized by chronic verrucoid, ulcerated, or crusted skin lesions.

ETIOLOGY The five species of fungi currently recognized as causing this syndrome have received a bewildering number of different names. Using Emmons' classification, these fungi are called *Phialophora verrucosa, P. pedrosoi, P. compacta, P. dermatitidis,* and *Cladosporium carrionii.*

PATHOGENESIS AND PATHOLOGY Infection occurs in tropical and subtropical areas where workers acquire many small puncture wounds from thorns or splinters. Histopathologic section of the skin lesion shows pseudoepitheliomatous hyperplasia and a granulomatous dermal infiltrate. Microabscesses with neutrophils also occur. Clumps of the pathogenic organism are found in these abscesses or elsewhere in the dermis as rounded, thick-walled brown cells. The epidermis and superficial crusts may contain branching brown hyphae.

CLINICAL MANIFESTATIONS The site of the lesion depends upon the area of trauma but is usually the foot or leg. The lesion begins as a pimple, pustule, or ulcer with slow progression over many years. Lesions may remain flat or become pe-

dunculated. Pain is minimal, but itching is common. Infection usually remains confined to the same extremity, but a few cases have spread hematogenously to cause brain abscess.

DIAGNOSIS Demonstration of the characteristic organisms in histological sections of skin biopsy is the best diagnostic method. Positive cultures are obtained readily, but accurate identification may require the service of a reference laboratory.

TREATMENT Prolonged therapy with oral flucytosine appears to be the regimen of choice. Relapse with secondary drug resistance has been encountered, but no reliable alternative treatment is known.

REFERENCES

Chromomycosis

MAUCERI AA et al: Flucytosine. An effective oral treatment for chromomycosis. Arch Dermatol 109:873, 1974

Mycetoma

GREEN WO, ADAMS TE: Mycetoma in the United States. Am J Clin Pathol 42:75, 1964

MAHGOUB ES, MURRAY IG: *Mycetoma.* London, Heinemann, 1973, pp 1–97

Paracoccidioidomycosis

LONDERO AT, RAMOS CD: Paracoccidioidomycosis. A clinical and mycologic study of forty-one cases observed in Santa Maria, RS, Brazil. Am J Med 52:771, 1972

MURRAY HW et al: Disseminated paracoccidioidomycosis (South American blastomycosis) in the United States. Am J Med 56:209, 1974

RESTREPO A et al: Paracoccidioidomycosis (South American blastomycosis). A study of 39 cases observed in Medellin, Columbia. Am J Trop Med Hyg 19:68, 1970

Petriellidiosis

ARNETT JC, HATCH HB: Pulmonary allescheriasis. Report of a case and review of the literature. Arch Intern Med 135:1250, 1975

LUTWICK LI et al: Visceral fungal infections due to *Petrillidium boydii (Allescheria boydii).* Am J Med 61:632, 1976

WINSTON DJ et al: *Allescheria boydii* infections in the immunosuppressed host. Am J Med 63:830, 1977

Torulopsosis

KAUFFMAN CA, TAN JS: *Torulopsis glabrata* renal infection. Am J Med 57:217, 1974

PANKEY GA, DALOVISO JR: Fungemia caused by *Torulopsis glabrata.* Medicine 52:395, 1973

VALDIVIESO M et al: Fungemia due to *Torulopsis glabrata* in the compromised host. Cancer 38:1750, 1976

162
DERMATOPHYTOSIS

JOHN E. BENNETT

DEFINITION Dermatophytosis, also known as ringworm or tinea, is a chronic fungal infection of the skin, hair, or nails.

ETIOLOGY Species of *Trichophyton, Microsporum,* and *Epidermophyton* are called *dermatophytes.* They grow in and remain confined to the keratinous structures of the body. Other mycoses can show fungal invasion of keratinous structures, such as candidiasis, pityriasis versicolor, and tinea nigra, but are traditionally not termed *dermatophytoses*.

PATHOLOGY AND PATHOGENESIS Dermatophyte species are called anthropophilic, zoophilic, or geophilic, depending on whether their usual reservoir within nature appears to be humans, animals, or soil. Infectivity of all those sources is low and group outbreaks are largely confined to an occasional case clustering of scalp infections in children. Acquisition of a dermatophytosis appears to be favored by minor trauma, maceration, and poor hygiene of the skin. Infection does not seem to confer solid immunity. Repeated infection with the same species is commonplace, particularly with anthropophilic species. Infrequency of scalp infection in adults has been attributed to local factors rather than immunity.

Invasion of the stratum corneum by dermatophytes may cause little inflammation, or, particularly with zoophilic fungi, inflammation can be intense. Shedding of the stratum corneum is increased by inflammation. To the extent that fungal growth cannot keep up with shedding, inflammation may help terminate infection. Conversely, infection is probably favored when shedding is reduced by corticosteroids and cytotoxic drugs. Antifungal drugs interfere with the ability of fungal growth to keep up with shedding.

CLINICAL MANIFESTATIONS The disease varies with the site of infection and fungal species. Foot infection (athlete's foot, tinea pedis) may present as fissuring of the toe webs, scaling of the plantar surfaces, or vesicles around the toe webs and soles. Interdigital lesions may be pruritic or, when bacterial superinfection occurs, may be painful. Hand infection is less common but resembles foot infection. Scalp dermatophytosis (tinea capitis) is characterized by areas of alopecia and scaling. In so-called "endothrix infection," the hair shaft breaks off at the skin surface, leaving the hairs visible as black dots in the scalp. With some forms of scalp infection an intense boggy suppuration occurs, called a *kerion*. Dermatophytosis of the glabrous skin (tinea corporis) presents as circumscribed lesions with a wide variety of appearances. Scales, vesicles, or pustules may appear. Inflammation may be minimal or intense. Central healing of less inflamed lesions may be seen. The serpiginous border of inflammation is the source of the name *ringworm*. Dermatophytosis of the bearded area (tinea barbae) appears as a pustular folliculitis. Onychomycosis (tinea unguium) presents as white discolored nails or thickened, chalky crumbling nails. Peeling and fissuring of the perinychia or keratotic debris under the nail edge may also be seen.

DIAGNOSIS Discolored hairs, scales, and keratotic debris under infected nails should be collected for KOH smear and culture. In the scraping of skin lesions, a drop of water on the skin site may keep the removed scales from flying off and aid in their collection. Culture is important in distinguishing dermatophytes from *Candida* and fungal saprophytes growing in keratinaceous debris.

TREATMENT Skin lesions should be treated topically if the lesions are few and small or located on the feet. Miconazole or clotrimazole cream should be applied twice daily until the lesion disappears and smears are negative. Undecylenic acid, haloprogin, or tolnaftate can also be used. Extensive skin lesions and infection of hair or nails should be treated with oral griseofulvin. The recommended dose for adults is 500 mg bid. Treatment must be continued until all infected keratin is gone. Cutting of infected hair, epilating nails, and cleansing interdigital webs can expedite cure. Secondary bacterial infection of the foot may require soaks or antibacterial agents. Relapse of dermatophyte foot infections may be decreased by measures to keep the feet clean and dry.

section 10 | The rickettsioses

163
GENERAL CONSIDERATIONS

THEODORE E. WOODWARD

The rickettsial diseases of humans consist of a variety of clinical entities caused by microorganisms of the family Rickettsiaceae. The rickettsias are obligate intracellular parasites about the size of bacteria and are usually seen microscopically as pleomorphic coccobacilli. Each of the rickettsias pathogenic for human beings is capable of multiplying in one or more species of arthropod as well as in animals and humans. Indeed, the majority of the rickettsias are maintained in nature by a cycle which involves an insect vector and an animal reservoir, and infection of humans is unimportant in the cycle. Epidemic typhus presents a number of points of dissimilarity to most of the other rickettsioses, because the natural cycle of the infection involves only humans and the louse.

A compendium of information of the rickettsial diseases is given in Table 163-1. Because each of the rickettsioses responds therapeutically to tetracyclines or chloramphenicol, the table mentions no therapy. Procedures for diagnostic isolation of the rickettsias are omitted because they generally are less useful than serologic methods, and the techniques which they require are highly specialized and hazardous. Information on isolation may be found in textbooks devoted to viral and rickettsial diseases.

HISTORY OF THE RICKETTSIAL DISEASES Of all the afflictions of the human race the rickettsial diseases, particularly epidemic typhus, rank among the foremost as a cause of suffering and death.

The record of deaths from epidemic typhus in this century in the Balkan countries and in Poland and Russia reached astounding figures. Typhus ravaged Russia and eastern Poland from 1915 to 1922, infecting 30 million of the inhabitants and causing an estimated 3 million deaths.

The past two decades have seen the development of excellent methods for the prevention and treatment of rickettsioses. In fact, these measures have been so successful that the rickettsioses have become of minor importance in the United States and in many other countries. Although conquered, the rickettsioses have not been eliminated, and they could again become rampant if the will to control them, the present high standards of sanitation, and the necessary industrial capacities for production of effective insecticides and therapeutic agents should be decreased through war or disaster.

Gerhard in 1836 differentiated typhoid fever from louse-borne typhus fever. In 1899, Maxcy described the clinical manifestations of Rocky Mountain spotted fever. In a series of studies from 1906 to 1909, Ricketts, for whom the rickettsial microorganisms are named, successfully transmitted this disease to guinea pigs, incriminated the wood tick as a vector, and observed rickettsias in smears prepared from tick tissues.

Nicolle in 1909 reproduced typhus fever in monkeys and demonstrated transmission by the body louse. Von Prowazek in 1914 and Da Rocha-Lima in 1916 demonstrated small microorganisms in the tissues of lice taken from typhus patients.

Brill in 1910 recognized a febrile disease in patients in New York City as an example of mild epidemic typhus unassociated with lousiness. Zinsser in 1934 postulated that this disease was a recurrent form of typhus occurring in patients during periods of stress or waning immunity. Subsequent studies have confirmed Zinsser's hypothesis. This entity is now called Brill-Zinsser disease.

Weil and Felix, working with typhus patients in Poland in 1915, recognized that agglutinins for certain *Proteus* organisms appeared in the serum of convalescent patients. The Weil-Felix reaction, although nonspecific, affords a simple and valuable screening method for several rickettsioses.

In 1926, Maxcy, on purely epidemiologic evidence, surmised that typhus in the United States had its reservoir in rodents and was transmitted to humans by ticks or fleas. Confirmation of Maxcy's hypothesis was obtained in Baltimore in 1930 by Dyer and others when they isolated rickettsias from

TABLE 163-1
Rickettsial diseases

Disease Type	Agent	Geographic distribution	Natural cycle Arthropod	Natural cycle Mammal	Principal means of transmission to humans	Serologic diagnosis Weil-Felix reaction	Serologic diagnosis CF, MA, and IFA reactions*
SPOTTED FEVER GROUP							
Rocky Mountain spotted fever	R. rickettsii	Western Hemisphere	Ticks	Wild rodents; dogs	Tick bite	Positive OX-19 OX-2	Positive group- and type-specific
Boutonneuse fever	R. conorii	Africa, Europe, Middle East, India					
Queensland tick typhus	R. australis	Australia		Marsupials, wild rodents			
North Asian tick-borne rickettsiosis	R. sibirica	Siberia, Mongolia		Wild rodents			
Rickettsial-pox	R. akari	United States, Russia, Africa(?)	Blood-sucking mite	House mouse, other rodents	Mite bite	Negative	
TYPHUS GROUP							
Endemic (murine)	R. mooseri	Worldwide	Flea	Small rodents	Infected flea feces into broken skin	Positive OX-19	Positive group- and type-specific
Epidemic	R. prowazekii	Worldwide	Body louse	Humans	Infected louse feces into broken skin	Positive OX-19	
	R. Canada	North America	Ticks	?Flying squirrels		Positive OX-19	
Brill-Zinsser disease	R. prowazekii	Worldwide	Recurrence years after original attack of epidemic typhus			Usually negative	
Scrub	R. tsutsuga-mushi	Asia, Australia, Pacific islands	Trombiculid mites	Wild rodents	Mite bite	Positive OX-K	Positive in about 50% of patients
OTHER RICKETTSIAL DISEASES							
Q fever	R. burnetii	Worldwide	Ticks	Small mammals, cattle, sheep, goats	Inhalation of dried infected material	Negative	Positive
Trench fever	R. quintana†	Europe, Africa, North America	Body louse	Humans	Infected louse feces into broken skin	Negative	None available

* CF = complement fixation; MA = microscopic agglutination; IFA = immunofluoresent antibody.
† Some authorities no longer place the agent in the genus Rickettsia because it can be cultured on artificial media.

the brains of rats and shortly thereafter incriminated the flea as a vector. This disease, caused by *Rickettsia mooseri* and now designated endemic or murine typhus, is distinct from epidemic typhus and Brill-Zinsser disease. There is increasing evidence of the presence of *R. prowazekii* in flying squirrels as well as infection of its ectoparasites. This poses a potential human threat. *Rickettsia canada* is a member of the typhus group of rickettsias isolated from *Haemphysalis leporis-palustris* ticks in Canada in 1967. Human infections resemble mild Rocky Mountain spotted fever.

The development of suitable vaccines and specific diagnostic antigens was impeded until it was possible to prepare appreciable quantities of highly infectious rickettsial material in the laboratory. The most important steps were (1) the Weigl vaccine (1930), a phenolized suspension of gut tissue obtained from body lice which had been injected intrarectally with the rickettsias of epidemic typhus; (2) the killed murine typhus prepared by Casteneda (1939) from lung tissues of rats, injected intranasally; and (3) the inactivated Rocky Mountain spotted fever vaccine obtained by Cox (1941) from infected yolk sacs of embryonated hen eggs. The low cost and relative simplicity of the egg techniques have led to their general use for preparation of vaccines and diagnostic antigens. A new formalin-inactivated vaccine prepared by sucrose density-gradient centrifugation of *R. rickettsii* grown in chick embryo cell tissue is under development.

The years of World War II saw many strides in the conquest of the rickettsioses; perhaps greatest among these were the highly successful attacks on the arthropod vectors. The lousicide DDT proved to be ideal for control when dusted on the clothes of infested persons. The epidemic at Naples during the winter of 1943 to 1944 established a milestone, because it was the first to be suppressed by the use of insecticides. Scrub typhus (mite-borne typhus) was creating a major problem in the Pacific area. Here, too, the major contributions to successful control were concerned with application of miticidal chemicals to persons and their clothes.

The advent of broad-spectrum antibiotics—first chloramphenicol, then chlortetracycline, and later oxytetracycline—provided dramatic therapeutic results in each of the rickettsioses.

PATHOGENESIS Rickettsial diseases develop after infection through the skin or the respiratory track. Agents of the typhus and spotted fever group are introduced through the bite of the infected arthropod vector. Ticks and mites, which transmit the agents of spotted fever and scrub typhus, inoculate the rickettsias directly into the dermis during feeding. The louse and flea, which transmit epidemic and murine typhus, respectively, deposit infected feces on the skin; infection occurs when organisms are rubbed into the puncture wound made by the arthropod. The rickettsias of Q fever gain entry through the respiratory tract when infected dust is inhaled; moreover, the respiratory route is occasionally implicated in epidemic typhus when infection results from inhalation of dried infected louse feces.

Although organisms probably multiply at the original site of entry in all instances, local lesions appear with regularity only in certain diseases, namely, the initial cutaneous lesions of scrub typhus, rickettsialpox, and boutonneuse fever, and the pneumonitis which develops in about half the persons infected with Q fever.

Volunteers infected with either scrub typhus or Q fever develop rickettsemia late in the incubation period, often some hours before the onset of fever. Similar events probably occur in all the rickettsial diseases; circulating rickettsias can be detected during the early febrile period in practically all patients.

Little is known about the pathogenesis of infection during the midportion of the incubation period. However, it is reasonable to assume that during this time, in patients with typhus or spotted fever, a transient low-grade rickettsemia results from release of organisms multiplying at the initial site of infection and that this seeds infection in the endothelial cells of the vascular tree. Vascular lesions developing at such sites account for the pathologic changes, including the rash.

Rickettsias apparently invade and proliferate in the endothelial cells of small blood vessels. Endothelial cell destruction occurs from the proliferation of organisms and eventual disruption. Rickettsias may exert a cytotoxic effect on endothelial cells; in mice the rickettsial toxin causes remarkable increase in capillary permeability, independent of proliferation. Later manifestations in rickettsial diseases may result from immunopathologic mechanisms, since humoral antibodies are present during the second febrile week, when increases in capillary permeability and vascular thrombosis and ecchymoses are greatest. Also, a delayed type of hypersensitivity occurs during infection.

The underlying cause of the toxic-febrile state which characterizes the rickettsial diseases remains unknown. Several rickettsial species contain type-specific toxins which are lethal for mice; these may play a role.

PATHOLOGIC PHYSIOLOGY Peripheral vascular collapse results in death in fulminating cases during the first week, with capillary dilatation and pooling of blood without increased capillary permeability or loss of fluid into extravascular spaces. As proliferative and thrombotic lesions develop in small vessels, anoxia occurs in the areas supplied, resulting in necrosis and increased capillary permeability, with loss of water, electrolytes, proteins, and erythrocytes. This in turn results in a decrease in blood volume, together with an increase in extravascular space and clinical edema. Edema, anoxia of the myocardium, and histologic evidence of myocarditis are disclosed by electrocardiographic abnormalities, including serious arrhythmias. Liver function is impaired. The azotemia which develops in seriously ill patients appears to be prerenal. Clinical manifestations resulting from the peripheral vascular collapse are oliguria and anuria, azotemia, anemia, hypoproteinemia, hyponatremia, edema, and coma. In spotted fever and typhus patients with hemorrhagic skin lesions, consumptive coagulopathy is present. All these alterations are absent or minimal in mild cases or in those who are given specific treatment early.

PATHOLOGY The basic changes in the spotted and typhus fever groups are vascular, with resultant widespread lesions in adjacent parenchymatous tissues throughout the body. They are most common in the skin, muscles, heart, lung, and brain. The most conspicuous and diverse are found in Rocky Mountain spotted fever. Here swelling, proliferation, and degeneration of the endothelial cells occur, frequently with thrombus formation which partially or completely occludes the lumen. The muscle cells of the arterioles undergo swelling and fibrinoid changes. The adventitial tissues are infiltrated with mononuclear leukocytes, lymphocytes, and plasma cells. The vascular damage is scattered along the arteries, veins and capillaries, with normal architecture prevailing throughout most of the vascular bed. The changes in murine, epidemic, and scrub typhus fevers resemble those in Rocky Mountain spotted fever, but thrombosis is uncommon and involvement of the musculature is rare.

Interstitial myocarditis occurs in each of these diseases but is usually most extensive in Rocky Mountain spotted fever and in scrub typhus. In the brain glial nodules are found in all members of the group, but microinfarcts in the brain tissue or in the myocardium are most often observed in spotted fever.

A rickettsial pneumonitis occurs, at least to some extent, in many patients with spotted or typhus fever and is the characteristic pathologic change in patients with Q fever. The process is patchy and consists microscopically of areas of congestion and edema. Within the consolidated areas the alveoli are filled with compact fibrinocellular exudate containing lymphocytes, plasma cells, large mononuclear cells, and erythrocytes but few, if any, polymorphonuclear leukocytes.

Rickettsias can occasionally be observed microscopically in sections of tissue. Failure to demonstrate them is of no diagnostic significance.

LABORATORY DIAGNOSIS Diagnostic procedures which depend on isolation of the etiologic agent from blood or other clinical material are expensive, time-consuming, and hazardous to laboratory personnel. Primary isolation of rickettsias by inoculation in the yolk sac of the chick embryo or tissue cells usually fails because of the small number of organisms in the patient's blood. Rickettsias have been identified in stained cultured monocytes of infected monkeys and by direct or indirect immunofluorescence of tissues of animals infected with *R. rickettsii*. Except in unusual circumstances, however, currently available serologic tests are adequate for laboratory confirmation of the clinical diagnosis in each of the rickettsial diseases. The demonstration of a rise in titer of specific antibody during convalescence is of prime importance in establishing the laboratory confirmation. Table 163-2 summarizes the serologic results usually encountered in persons who have rickettsial diseases in the United States. The Weil-Felix test employing *Proteus* strains OX-19 and OX-2 gives positive results in patients with spotted fever and murine typhus and negative results in those with rickettsialpox and Q fever. It is useful as a screening procedure but cannot be relied upon to differentiate spotted fever from murine typhus. In patients with Brill-Zinsser disease the *Proteus* OX-19 reaction is usually negative or low in titer.

Serologic tests employing group-specific rickettsial antigens provide data which clearly differentiate the most common infections, i.e., murine typhus, Rocky Mountain spotted fever, and Q fever. Moreover, if type-specific rickettsial antigens are employed, it is generally possible to distinguish rickettsialpox from spotted fever and Brill-Zinsser disease from murine typhus.

Antibodies during response to a primary infection of epidemic typhus or Rocky Mountain spotted fever are usually 19S globulins. In patients with Brill Zinsser disease, which is a recrudescence, antibodies occur more quickly (within several days after onset of illness), rise to a higher titer, and are 7S globulins.

Utilizing better antigens, other serologic procedures for rickettsial diseases not only distinguish between specific rickettsioses but help to determine the type of immunoglobulin in acute (IgM) and late or recurrent (IgG) illness, such as in recrudescent typhus (Brill-Zinsser disease). The Weil-Felix and complement fixation tests are useful for routine diagnosis; microscopic agglutination, immunofluorescent antibody, and hemagglutination reactions are valuable for specific identification.

Specific antibiotic therapy has little effect on the time of appearance of antibodies or on their ultimate titer, provided treatment is instituted some days after onset of the illness. However, if the illness is cut short by early and vigorous treatment, antibody production may be delayed for a week or so, and also the maximal titers attained may be below those illustrated in Table 163-2. Under these circumstances a sample of blood taken 4 to 6 weeks after onset of illness should also be tested.

The immunofluorescent antibody test is a very useful procedure for detecting rickettsia in the tissues of patients with the typhus group of rickettsioses, the spotted fevers, and Q fever. Identifiable rickettsias have been visualized in skin lesions of patients with Rocky Mountain spotted fever as early as the fourth day of illness and as late as the tenth day. The technique also visualizes rickettsias in ticks and the tissues of animals.

Normochromic anemia occurs in patients severely ill with rickettsial diseases. The white blood cell count in Rocky Mountain spotted fever, rickettsialpox, murine and epidemic typhus, Brill-Zinsser disease, Q fever, and other rickettsial diseases is usually within the normal range; 6000 to 10,000 cells per cubic millimeter. Leukopenia is occasionally observed, and in the presence of complications, such as superimposed infections and extensive vascular lesions, moderate leukocytosis occurs. The differential blood cell count is usually normal.

Thrombocytopenia occurs in severely ill spotted and scrub typhus fever patients with extensive vascular lesions; hypofibrinogenemia, prolonged prothrombin and partial thromboplastin times, and other clotting abnormalties occur. In primates showing peripheral gangrenous ecchymoses caused by *R. rickettsii* there are decreases in complement fractions C2 and C3.

REFERENCES

See Chap. 171.

TABLE 163-2
Serologic diagnosis of rickettsial diseases of the United States

Group	Disease	Weil-Felix reaction				Complement fixation tests with type-specific antigen				
			Illustrative titer		Cases with diagnostic titer		Illustrative titer			Cases with diagnostic titer
		Proteus	10th day	20th day		Rickettsial antigen	10th day	20th day	30th day	
Spotted fever	Rocky Mountain spotted fever	OX-19	40	320	Most	R. rickettsii	20	160	80	Most
		OX-2	20	160						
	Rickettsialpox	OX-19	0	0	None	R. akari	0	64	128	Most
		OX-2	0	0						
Typhus	Murine typhus	OX-19	160	640	Most	R. mooseri	0	160	160	Most
		OX-2	10	40						
	Brill-Zinsser disease	OX-19	160	20	Infrequent	R. prowazekii	1280	640	320	Most
		OX-2	0	0						
	Q fever	OX-19	0	0	None	R. burnetii	10	80	160	Most
		OX-2	0	0						

164

ROCKY MOUNTAIN SPOTTED FEVER

THEODORE E. WOODWARD

DEFINITION Rocky Mountain spotted fever is an acute febrile illness caused by *Rickettsia rickettsii*. It is transmitted to humans by ticks. The disease is characterized by sudden onset with headache and chills and by fever which persists for 2 to 3 weeks. A characteristic exanthem appears on the extremities and trunk about the fourth day of illness. Delerium, shock, and renal failure occur in the severely ill.

ETIOLOGY AND EPIDEMIOLOGY The causative microbe *R. rickettsii* is the prototype for the rickettsial group of agents. The minute organisms are purple when stained by Giemsa's method or red by Macchiavello's technique; most of them are gram-negative. These organisms often occur in pairs and possess a cell wall similar in structure and chemical composition to that of gram-negative bacteria; one finds a cell membrane, cytoplasmic granules corresponding to ribosomes, and prokaryotic organization of nuclear material. The cell membrane is selectively permeable; the cell wall is the focus of important antigens and an endotoxin-like substance.

The rickettsias grow in the nucleus and the cytoplasm of infected cells of ticks, mammals, and embryonated eggs; the intranuclear situation of the organisms is shared by the other members of the spotted fever group, but not by rickettsias of the typhus group. *Rickettsia rickettsii* is readily distinguishable from the agents of the typhus fevers by cross-immunity tests in guinea pigs and by complement fixation tests employing antigens prepared from infected yolk sac tissues. The differentiation of *R. rickettsii* from closely related members of the spotted fever group frequently requires elaborate procedures. Strains of the agent of Rocky Mountain spotted fever vary considerably in their virulence for humans and animals.

The first reports of spotted fever in Idaho and Montana during the final decade of the last century led to the name Rocky Mountain spotted fever. However, the disease has been reported from almost all states, as well as from Canada, Mexico, Colombia, and Brazil. Although related diseases are found on other continents, this particular infection is limited to the Western Hemisphere. In the years 1976 and 1977, 937 and 1115 cases respectively were reported. The mortality rate was about 20 percent in the days before specific therapy but has decreased to about 7 percent. More than half the cases occur in the South Atlantic and South Central states, with the greatest number of these in North Carolina, Virginia, Georgia, Maryland, Tennessee, and Oklahoma.

A number of species of ticks are found infected with *R. rickettsii* in nature, but only two are important in transmitting spotted fever to humans. These are *Dermacentor andersoni*, the wood tick, which is the principal vector in the West, and *D. variabilis*, the dog tick, which assumes this role in the East. Infected female ticks transmit the agent transovarially to at least some of their offspring. Ticks which become infected, either through the egg or at one of the stages during their development cycle by feeding on an infected mammal, harbor the rickettsias throughout their lifetime, which may be several years. Thus, the tick serves as a reservoir in addition to being a vector. Small wild mammals are suspected of playing an important role in spreading the rickettsias in nature by infecting ticks which feed on them during rickettsemia.

Disease in humans is generally acquired from the bite of an infected tick. Transmission is unlikely unless the tick remains attached for a number of hours. Infection may also be acquired through abrasions in the skin which become contaminated with infected tick feces or tissue juices; hence, the hazard associated with crushing ticks between the fingers when removing them from persons or animals. The agent of Rocky Mountain spotted fever has been transmitted accidentally to humans by transfusion of blood taken from a donor just before onset of illness.

There are seasonal variations in the incidence of cases of spotted fever, as well as differences in age and sex distribution of cases. In each instance these differences are related to exposure to ticks. Most cases are seen during the period of maximal tick activity, i.e., late spring and early summer, and 60 percent of cases occur in individuals under 20 years of age. This age distribution is undoubtedly influenced by propinquity to the wood and dog ticks, respectively. The mortality rate increases with the age of the patient.

Rocky Mountain spotted fever has been acquired by laboratory workers via aerosol transmission, and special precautions are necessary when the agent is handled in the laboratory.

CLINICAL MANIFESTATIONS **Incubation period and prodromata** A history of tick bite is elicited in approximately 80 percent of patients. The incubation period varies between 3 and 12 days with a mean of 7 days. A short incubation period usually indicates a more serious infection.

Onset In nonvaccinated persons, the onset is usually abrupt, with severe headache, a sudden shaking rigor, prostration, generalized myalgia, especially in the back and leg muscles, nausea with occasional vomiting, and fever which reaches 103 to 104°F within the first 2 days. Pain in the abdominal muscles may be severe, and arthralgia is not uncommon. Deep muscle palpation often elicits tenderness. Occasionally the debut of illness in children and adults is mild, accompanied by lethargy, anorexia, headache, and low-grade fever. These symptoms are similar to those of many acute infectious diseases, making specific diagnosis difficult during the first few days.

Pyrexia Fever continues for approximately 15 to 20 days in untreated cases. The febrile course in children may be shorter. Hyperthermia of 105°F or greater is of unfavorable prognostic significance, although fatalities may occur when the patient is hypothermic, with concurrent vasomotor collapse. Fever generally terminates by lysis over a period of several days, but rarely does so by crisis. Recurrent fever is uncommon except in the presence of secondary pyogenic complications.

The *headache* is generalized and excruciating, and frequently more intense over the frontal area. It persists throughout the first and second weeks of illness in untreated cases. Occasionally headache is mild. Malaise continues for the first week; irritability is notable, and the patient shuns distractions such as questioning and examination.

Cutaneous manifestations The rash which is present in practically all cases is the most characteristic and helpful diagnostic sign. It usually appears on the fourth febrile day; the range is 2 to 6 days. The initial lesions are on the wrists, ankles, palms, soles, and forearms. The first lesions are macular, nonfixed, pink, irregularly defined, and measure 2 to 6 mm. A warm compress applied to the extremity accentuates the rash in the early stages. The exanthem is most prominent when the temperature is elevated. After 6 to 12 h, the rash extends centripetally to the axilla, buttocks, trunk, neck, and face. (This is in contrast to the eruption of typhus fever, which begins on the trunk and spreads centrifugally, rarely involving the face, palms, or soles.) The rash becomes maculopapular after 2 to 3 days (it may be felt by light palpation) and assumes a deeper red hue. By about the fourth day it is petechial and fails to fade on pressure. Not uncommonly, the hemorrhagic lesions coalesce to form large ecchymotic blemishes; these lesions tend to form over bony prominences and may ultimately slough to form indolent, slow-healing ulcers. Patients who have had the typical rash show brownish discolorations at the site for several weeks during convalescence. In milder cases, the rash does not become purpuric and may disappear within a few days. Antibiotic therapy may abort the early exanthem; the later fixed lesion fades less rapidly with specific therapy. Occasionally, a rash does not occur or is unnoticed, particularly in dark-skinned patients.

The application of tourniquets for several minutes, or the occasional taking of the blood pressure may provoke additional petechiae (Rumpel-Leede phenomenon), further evidence of capillary abnormalities.

Cardiovascular and respiratory features During the early stages, the pulse is full and regular but accelerated in proportion to the height of the temperature, and the blood pressure is well sustained. During the peak of illness in seriously ill patients, the pulse is rapid and feeble, and hypotension of 90 mmHg is common. If circulatory failure is sustained, the resultant hypoxia and shock lead to agitation and delirium and contribute to the formation of ecchymoses and gangrene of fingers, toes, genitalia, buttocks, earlobes, and nose. Cyanosis of the peripheral parts of the body is common. Venous pressure determinations show no elevation. A reduction of the total blood volume is occasionally found, as is myocardial impairment as shown by low voltage of ventricular complexes, minor ST-segment deflections, and occasionally delay in atrioventricular conduction on the electrocardiogram. These changes are transient and nonspecific. Severely ill patients have a puffy appearance of the face, hands, ankles, feet, and lower parts of the sacrum.

Respirations are either normal or slightly accelerated. Cough may be harassing and nonproductive, and localized pneumonitis may occur, but pulmonary consolidation is extremely rare. Pulmonary edema may develop after injudicious use of intravenous fluids.

Hepatic and renal manifestations In the majority of patients, there is little alteration in renal or hepatic function. The liver may be enlarged, but jaundice is unusual. Oliguria commonly occurs in the seriously ill, and anuria may mark the critically ill patient. Azotemia is common; when marked, it is a very unfavorable sign. Abnormalities in liver function are probably responsible for the hypoproteinemia, with reduction in the albumin fraction.

Neurologic manifestations The principal neurologic manifestations are headache, restlessness, and varying degrees of insomnia. Stiffness of the back is common. The cerebrospinal fluid is clear, with normal dynamics and normal chemical constituents. Coma and muscular rigidity may occur. Athetoid movements, convulsive seizures, and hemiplegia are grave manifestations. Deafness during the active stages of the disease is not uncommon. As a rule, all neurologic signs abate without residua. Findings based upon follow-up examinations and electroencephalograms may be interpreted as indicative of minor residual brain damage for a year or more following recovery of certain patients from Rocky Mountain spotted fever.

Other physical manifestations Patients become dehydrated, with extreme dryness of lips, gums, tongue, and pharynx. The skin is hot and dry, the conjunctivas are frequently injected, and the eyes suffused. Photophobia is common in the early stages of illness. Petechial hemorrhages may be noted in the conjunctivas or in the retina. The spleen is enlarged in approximately one-half the cases and is firm and nontender. Abdominal distention is frequent, and occasionally some degree of intestinal ileus is observed. Constipation is usual.

COURSE In patients with mild and moderately severe cases who are given no specific antibiotic therapy, the disease abates within 2 weeks, and convalescence is rapid. In fatal cases death usually occurs during the latter part of the second week as a result of toxemia, vasomotor weakness, and shock or renal failure. In a few patients, the course is fulminant with death occurring as early as the sixth day of illness.

In vaccinated individuals who contract the disease, the illness is mild, with a short febrile course and an atypical rash.

COMPLICATIONS AND PROGNOSIS If the serious manifestations of spotted fever mentioned above are regarded as intrinsic parts of the disease, then complications are uncommon and consist mainly of secondary bacterial infections, namely, bronchopneumonia, otitis media, and parotitis. Thrombosis of major blood vessels may result in gangrene of a portion of an extremity. Hemiplegia and peripheral neuritis are rare sequelae.

The overall mortality rate for spotted fever was formerly about 20 percent. Death occurred in more than half of persons over 40 years of age, but the mortality rate was much lower in children and young adults. Since the introduction of the broad-spectrum antibiotics and the development of more precise knowledge regarding correction of the physiologic abnormalities which develop during the disease, fewer deaths occur from this infection. Some of the fatalities can be attributed to failure to consider spotted fever in the differential diagnosis.

DIFFERENTIAL DIAGNOSIS During the early stages of infection before the rash has appeared, differentiation from other acute infections is difficult. History of tick bite while living or traveling in a highly endemic area is helpful. The rash of meningococcemia (Chap. 118) resembles Rocky Mountain spotted fever in certain aspects, because it is macular, maculopapular, or petechial in the chronic form, and petechial, confluent, or ecchymotic in the fulminant type. The meningococcal skin lesion is tender and develops with extreme rapidity in the fulminant form, whereas the rickettsial rash occurs on about the fourth day of disease and gradually becomes petechial. *Spotted fever is often confused with measles.* The exanthem of rubeola rapidly becomes confluent, while that of rubella *usually remains discrete.*

Murine typhus is a milder disease than Rocky Mountain spotted fever; the rash is less extensive, nonpurpuric, and nonconfluent, and renal and vascular complications are uncommon. Not infrequently differentiation of these two rickettsial infections must await the results of specific serologic tests. Epidemic typhus fever is capable of causing all the pronounced clinical, physiologic, and anatomic alterations seen in patients with Rocky Mountain spotted fever, i.e., hypotension, peripheral vascular collapse, cyanosis, skin necrosis and gangrene of digits, renal failure and azotemia, and neurologic manifestations. However, the rash of classical typhus is noted initially in the axillary folds of the trunk and later extends peripherally, rarely involving the palms, soles, or face. The serologic patterns in these two diseases are distinctive when specific rickettsial antigens are employed. Moreover, louse-borne typhus is not recognized in the United States except in the form of Brill-Zinsser disease (recurrent typhus fever). Rickettsialpox, although caused by a member of the spotted fever group of organisms, is usually readily differentiated from Rocky Mountain spotted fever by the initial lesion, the relative mildness of the illness, and the early vesiculation of the maculopapular rash. The Weil-Felix reaction is positive in Rocky Mountain spotted fever and in murine and epidemic typhus, but is negative in rickettsialpox. Agglutinins against *Proteus* OX-19 and OX-2 appear in the serum of patients with spotted fever, but only those against OX-19 are generally found in murine and epidemic typhus.

THERAPY Certain physiochemical changes occurring in the patient seriously ill with one of the diseases of the typhus–spotted fever group should be understood before a therapeutic regimen is outlined. These changes are circulatory collapse, coma, oliguria and anuria, azotemia, anemia, hypoproteinemia, hypochloremia and hyponatremia, and edema. These alterations are often absent in the mildly ill, and in them management is much less complicated. The therapeutic principles necessary for treatment of all rickettsioses are (1) specific chemotherapy and (2) supportive care. Attention to both is mandatory for the seriously ill patient first recognized late in the disease. During the first week in the moderately ill patient, supportive therapy may be less energetic, because specific chemotherapy usually suffices. The early mild case may be successfully treated at home; later in the course of the disease patients should receive hospital care.

Therapeutic measures advisable for the management of Rocky Mountain spotted fever will be described in detail. Variations of this regimen which apply to the other rickettsioses are described in subsections dealing with other diseases of the typhus–spotted fever group and Q fever.

Specific therapy Specific therapy is most effective when initiated during the early stages of disease coincident with the appearance of the rash. When therapy is delayed until the rash has become hemorrhagic and widespread, the response is less dramatic. The antibiotics of choice are chloramphenicol and the tetracyclines, which are effective because of their rickettsiostatic properties. They are not rickettsiocidal.

The following antibiotic regimen is considered optimal: for chloramphenicol, an initial dose of 50 mg per kilogram of body weight, and for tetracycline, 25 mg/kg. Subsequent daily doses are the same as the initial loading dose, with the requirement divided equally and given at 6- to 8-h intervals. Antibiotic treatment is continued until the patient has improved and has been afebrile approximately 24 h. In patients too ill to take oral medication, an intravenous preparation of one of the antimicrobials should be employed.

Adrenal cortical hormones may need to be utilized for their antitoxemic effects, in patients first observed late in the course of severe illness. Large doses for brief periods of about 3 to 5 days, in combination with specific antibiotics, are recommended in critically ill patients.

Therapy with antibiotics is continued until the toxemia has abated, the general condition has markedly improved, and the temperature has remained at normal levels for 24 h. In uncomplicated cases of spotted fever, there is symptomatic improvement within 24 h and the temperature becomes normal in 60 to 72 h.

Supportive care Frequent turning of the patient relieves pressure from prominent bony parts and also militates against the development of aspiration pneumonia. Proper mouth care, with frequent swabbing of the oral cavity, may avert the development of parotitis and gingivitis. Sucking of the juice of a lemon or the oral use of glycerin or mineral oil is helpful.

A generous intake of protein should be provided by frequent feedings as soon as the disease is suspected, in order to avoid subsequent protein deficiency. Usually food is well toler-

ated by patients with rickettsial disease, and the daily diet should provide 3 to 5 g protein per kilogram of normal body weight, with adequate carbohydrate and fat to make it palatable. When the patient is uncooperative, the diet may be supplemented by hourly liquid protein feedings via stomach tube, provided that there is no abdominal distention.

At the critical stage, when hypoproteinemia is present and changes in capillary permeability lead to edema and vascular embarrassment, careful attention must be given to parenteral hyperalimentation with high concentration of glucose and amino acids. When indicated by hematologic studies, whole-blood transfusions given slowly are helpful. The judicious administration of one of the plasma expanders at this stage may have a definite favorable effect upon impending circulatory collapse. If the patient is anuric and azotemia is pronounced, overloading the circulation with fluids should be governed by clinical judgment and very careful laboratory studies. Frequent determinations of hemoglobin, hematocrit, electrolytes, and protein, sometimes at intervals of a few hours during crucial periods are necessary in order to ascertain abnormalities and to permit institution of corrective measures. Dialysis is indicated when there is clear-cut evidence of acute tubular necrosis (Chap. 275).

Complications *Pyogenic complications,* including otitis media and parotitis, are encountered in patients severely ill with Rocky Mountain spotted fever and other rickettsioses. These localized infections respond to therapy with appropriate antibiotics combined with surgical measures.

Pneumonitis usually develops as a result of specific rickettsial action. The sputum is scant but should be examined to determine whether superimposed bacterial infection is present. Specific therapy is guided by the results of these laboratory studies. The pneumonitis generally responds to the antibiotic therapy the patient is receiving, but if staphylococcal pneumonia is suspected, a penicillinase-resistant penicillin should be added to the broad-spectrum drug.

Circulatory failure of peripheral or central origin is combated by careful administration of plasma expanders and fluids. Heart failure may develop from the disease or as a result of overzealous intravenous therapy and is recognized by rapid pulse, gallop rhythm, and increase in venous pressure. When the clinical signs reveal unmistakable evidence of cardiac failure, digitalis should be employed. Oxygen therapy improves the cardiac and circulatory status and is helpful in hypoxemic patients with involvement of the central nervous system.

PREVENTION Prevention is attained primarily by avoidance of tick-infested areas. When this is impractical, prophylactic measures include (1) spraying the ground with dieldrin or chlordane for area control of ticks (though there are environmental objections to the use of residual insecticides in area control of ticks, under special conditions, such procedures may be warranted); (2) application of repellents such as diethyltoluamide or dimethylphthalate to clothing and exposed parts of the body, or in very heavily infested areas the wearing of clothing which interferes with the attachment of ticks, i.e., boots and a one-piece outer garment, preferably impregnated with repellent; and (3) daily inspection of the entire body, including the hairy parts, to detect and remove attached ticks. In removing attached ticks great care should be taken to avoid crushing the arthropod with resultant contamination of the bite wound; touching the tick with gasoline or whisky encourages detachment but gentle traction with tweezers applied close to the mouth parts may be necessary; the skin area should be disinfected with soap and water or other antiseptics. Similarly, precautions should be employed in removing engorged ticks from dogs and other animals, because infection through minor abrasions on the hands is possible. Improved vaccines containing inactivated *R. rickettsii* are under development and should be available commercially for those at great risk, namely, persons frequenting highly endemic areas and laboratory workers exposed to the agent. Because the broad-spectrum antibiotics are such excellent therapeutic agents in spotted fever, there has been less impetus for vaccination of persons who run only a minor risk of infection.

After tick bite in a known endemic area an exposed person should be observed for signs of fever, headache, prostration and rash; therapy is very effective at the early stage of illness.

REFERENCES

See Chap. 171.

165

OTHER TICK-BORNE RICKETTSIAL DISEASES

THEODORE E. WOODWARD

DEFINITION Boutonneuse fever, North Asian tick-borne rickettsiosis, and Queensland tick typhus, three diseases occurring in the Eastern Hemisphere, are caused by rickettsias closely related to one another and to the agent of Rocky Mountain spotted fever. Each is transmitted by the bite of an ixodid tick. These mild to moderately severe illnesses are characterized by an initial lesion (called *tache noire* in boutonneuse fever), a fever of several days to 2 weeks, and a generalized maculopapular erythematous rash which appears on about the fifth day and usually involves the palms and soles. Specific complement-fixing antibodies appear in the patients' serums during convalescence, but agglutinins to *Proteus* OX-19 (Weil-Felix reaction) are frequently found only in low titer.

ETIOLOGY AND EPIDEMIOLOGY The etiologic agents of these three diseases are all members of the spotted fever group of rickettsias. Together with *Rickettsia rickettsii* and *R. akari* they possess common group antigens which are readily demonstrated by agglutination, complement fixation, microscopic agglutination, and immunofluorescent antibody reactions.

Boutonneuse fever, which may be regarded as the prototype of the three, is caused by *R. conorii*. Modern serologic methods employing specific rickettsial antigens have shown this rickettsia to be the causative agent for a single widely disseminated disease known by various local names. Information on the distribution and etiology of the various tick-borne rickettsial diseases is contained in Table 163-1.

In general, the epidemiology of these tick-borne rickettsioses resembles that of spotted fever in the Western Hemisphere. Ixodid ticks and small wild animals maintain the rickettsias in nature; if humans intrude accidentally into the cycle, they become a dead end in the transmission chain. In certain areas, the cycle of boutonneuse fever involves domiciliary environments, with the brown dog tick *Rhipicephalus sanguineus* as the dominant vector.

CLINICAL MANIFESTATIONS These three tick-borne rickettsioses, which occur in different parts of the Eastern Hemisphere, resemble one another closely. The clinical course is usually milder than that of spotted fever, with a shorter febrile period and fewer severe complications; fatalities are rare and generally limited to the aged and debilitated. The initial lesion, which is present in most cases at the onset of fever, heals slowly; the regional lymph nodes are enlarged. The rash usually remains papular and only in severe cases becomes hemorrhagic.

The clinical picture (including the primary lesion), the geographic location, and epidemiologic considerations are helpful in establishing the diagnosis. The typhus fevers, meningococcal infections, and measles must be considered in the differential diagnosis; the serologic reactions, i.e., Weil-Felix and complement fixation tests, are of value here.

TREATMENT AND PREVENTION Chloramphenicol and the tetracyclines are effective therapeutic agents for boutonneuse fever. Patients generally become afebrile after 2 to 3 days of treatment, and recovery is rapid. The therapeutic procedures are comparable to those used in spotted fever. Presumably these measures are also applicable to North Asian tick-borne rickettsiosis and Queensland tick typhus.

The major effective methods of control are concerned with avoidance of tick bites; these include application of new repellents and prompt removal of attached ticks. Effective vaccines are not available commercially.

REFERENCES

See Chap. 171.

166

RICKETTSIALPOX

THEODORE E. WOODWARD

DEFINITION Rickettsialpox is a mild, nonfatal self-limited, febrile illness caused by *Rickettsia akari,* which is transmitted from mouse to humans by mites. It is characterized by an initial skin lesion at the site of the mite bite, a week's febrile course, and a papulovesicular rash.

ETIOLOGY AND EPIDEMIOLOGY Rickettsialpox was first recognized in New York City in 1946, and about 180 cases were reported annually for several years thereafter. It has been diagnosed in several other areas of the United States, and outbreaks have been reported in European Russia. The vector is a small, colorless mite, *Allodermanyssus sanguineus* (Hirst), which infests small mice and rodents. House mice serve as the reservoir of infection.

Rickettsia akari is morphologically and biologically similar to other rickettsias and is antigenically related to, but distinct from, *R. rickettsii,* the cause of Rocky Mountain spotted fever. Mice, guinea pigs, and fertile hen eggs are susceptible to experimental infection. Diagnostic antigens prepared from infected yolk sacs and tissue culture cells are used in serologic reactions.

CLINICAL MANIFESTATIONS The initial skin lesion appears about 7 to 10 days after the mite bite as a firm red papule 1 to 1.5 cm in diameter. In a few days, the center vesiculates, and the papule is surrounded by an area of erythema. The regional lymph glands are moderately enlarged. The primary lesion, which is never painful, becomes covered with a black scab; it heals slowly, and a small scar is visible on separation of the crust.

The febrile phase begins 3 to 7 days after the initial lesion, and exanthem may accompany the fever or begin several days later. The onset of fever is sudden, with chilly sensations or frank chills, headache, sweats, myalgia, anorexia, and photophobia. The pyrexia ranges from 103 to 104°F and continues for about a week, occasionally with morning remisssions.

The exanthem is maculopapular-vesicular, generalized in distribution, and may be abundant or scant. The lesions may involve the oral cavity but not the palms or soles. In a week, the vesicles dry and form scabs which eventually scale but leave no scar.

The constitutional symptoms are generally mild, and the course of illness is uncomplicated. No fatal cases have been reported.

The disease may be confused with chickenpox, which is different because it occurs usually in childhood and has no initial lesion and the papular cutaneous lesion is entirely transformed into a vesicle. Variola (smallpox) is accompanied by a more severe constitutional reaction, and the vesicles become pustules. The skin lesions of the other rickettsioses differ in their lack of vesiculation. The Weil-Felix reaction is usually negative in this rickettsial disease but specific complement fixation, microscopic agglutination, and immunofluorescent antibody reactions are useful diagnostic aids even though there is considerable crossing with materials from Rocky Mountain spotted fever.

TREATMENT AND PREVENTION Chloramphenicol and the tetracycline antibiotics are all effective for treating patients with rickettsialpox. The temperature reaches normal levels in about 2 days, and recovery is rapid.

Control measures should be directed toward elimination of house mice and the vector mites responsible for transmitting the disease.

REFERENCES

See Chap. 171.

167
MURINE (ENDEMIC) TYPHUS FEVER

THEODORE E. WOODWARD

DEFINITION Murine typhus fever is an acute febrile disease caused by *Rickettsia mooseri* and transmitted to humans by fleas. The clinical illness is characterized by fever of 9 to 14 days, headache, a maculopapular rash appearing on the third to fifth day, and myalgia.

ETIOLOGY AND EPIDEMIOLOGY *Rickettsia mooseri* resembles other rickettsias in morphologic properties, staining characteristics, and intracellular parasitism. Under the electron microscope *R. mooseri* is seen to contain dense masses of nuclear material in a less dense homogeneous protoplasmic substance, the whole of which is surrounded by a limiting membrane. It differs from *R. rickettsii* in that it always multiplies within the cytoplasm of cells, in contrast to the intranuclear and cytoplasmic positions of spotted fever rickettsias.

Invasion of the body by *R. mooseri* provokes specific and nonspecific immunologic responses. Utilizing highly purified antigens, specific antibodies may be demonstrated readily by complement fixation, microscopic agglutination, and immuno-fluorescent antibody reactions. The positive Weil-Felix reaction which occurs in this disease is nonspecific, because it is attributable to the presence of a common carbohydrate antigen in *Proteus* OX-19 and *R. mooseri* and because the reaction is also positive in epidemic typhus and spotted fever. Group-specific rickettsial antigens are common to both *R. mooseri and R. prowazekii*. Furthermore, both murine and epidemic rickettsias possess toxic factors which are lethal to mice and rats and can be neutralized by convalescent serum from humans or lower animals.

The common vector of *R. mooseri* for rats and humans is the rat flea (*Xenopsylla cheopis*). In nature, the rat louse (*Polypax spinulosis*) may transmit the agent among rodents. Customarily, rat fleas become infected on ingestion of blood from diseased rats; the rickettsias multiply within the intestinal cells of the arthropod and are excreted in the feces. Infection in humans occurs after the flea bite and contamination of the broken skin by rickettsia-laden feces. Dried flea feces may also infect via the conjuntivas or the upper part of the respiratory tract.

Rats and mice are naturally infected with murine typhus, and although the rodent disease is nonfatal, viable rickettsias persist in the brain for variable periods.

Murine typhus is one of the most benign and widespread of the rickettsioses in the United States. Prevalent in the Southeastern and Gulf Coast states, it has been identified in most of the other states and in harbor centers throughout the world wherever rats and fleas abound. Through control of rats and their fleas a sharp decline in incidence has occurred since 1951, particularly in the Southern United States. In urban areas the disease is more prevalent during the summer and fall months and occurs predominantly among persons working in proximity to granaries or food depots. There has been an extension to certain rural areas when changing agricultural practices have provided rats with ready access to adequate food supplies. Three cases of endemic typhus were reported in laboratory workers in 1978. This emphasizes the importance of taking special precautions when working with rickettsial organisms in the laboratory.

CLINICAL MANIFESTATIONS Incubation period and prodromata The incubation period ranges from 8 to 16 days, with a mean of 10. Common prodromata are headache, backache, arthralgia, and chilly sensations. Nausea, malaise, and transient temperature rises may precede the true onset of disease.

Onset and general symptoms A frank shaking chill and repeated rigors are present at the onset, associated with a severe frontal headache and fever. This triad of headache, chill, and pyrexia is usually followed within a few hours by nausea and vomiting. Prostration, malaise, and weakness are sufficient to enforce cessation of activity in adults, in contrast to children, whose illness is less severe. Occasionally, mild symptoms make it difficult to define the actual onset.

Pyrexia The usual febrile course in murine typhus lasts for about 12 days in adults; the temperature ranges from 102 to 104°F but may reach 105 to 106°F in children. The temperature may reach high levels abruptly after onset or ascend in a stepwise manner during the first few days. With the appearance of the rash, fever is usually sustained, with partial daily remissions which occasionally reach normal levels in the morning. Defervescence is generally by lysis over several days but sometimes occurs by crisis. Transient mild fever of 100°F is not uncommon during early convalescence. A few patients experience only low-grade fever throughout, but this does not necessarily connote a mild illness.

Cutaneous manifestations The early lesions, which are sparse and discrete, are hidden in the axillae and inner surface of the arm. Most patients then develop with surprising suddenness a generalized, dull red macular rash of the upper part of the abdomen, shoulders, chest, arms, and thighs. The individual lesions are discrete and pea size, with an ill-defined border, and fade on pressure during the first 24 h. They later become maculopapular, in contrast to the exanthem of epidemic typhus, which is persistently macular. The distribution over the trunk with sparse involvement of the extremities, palms, soles, and face differs from the peripheral distribution and facial involvement of Rocky Mountain spotted fever. The murine rash generally appears initially on the fifth febrile day, but rarely it is seen concurrently with the onset of fever or develops as late as the seventh day.

Eighty percent of patients develop a rash which persists for 4 to 8 days and fades before defervescence. The cutaneous manifestations vary greatly in intensity and duration and may be fleeting. They are readily overlooked in dark-skinned patients, in whom they should be sought by light palpation and indirect lighting.

Cardiovascular and respiratory features An irritating, nonproductive cough is frequent and is occasionally associated with moderate hemoptysis. Early in the second week, rales may be detected in the basilar lung areas. These changes are generally rickettsial rather than bacterial in origin and respond to the broad-spectrum antibiotics. Pulmonary congestion occurs in extremely ill and elderly patients.

Accelerated pulse, hypotension, and general circulatory weakness occur in this disease, although less frequently than in patients with epidemic typhus or Rocky Mountain spotted fever.

Neurologic manifestations Headache is the most common neurologic manifestation of murine typhus and may dominate the clinical picture. It is frontal and continues into the second week of illness. Stupor and prostration may occur in the second week, and in severe cases, there may be muttering delirium, extreme agitation, or coma. Coma in elderly patients after 2 weeks of illness presages death. Nuchal rigidity and general spasticity often suggest meningitis, although the spinal fluid is normal except for slight increases in pressure and lymphocytes (5 to 30 per cubic millimeter). Transient partial deafness occurs occasionally, but rarely is there localized neuritis or hemiplegia. Neurologic sequelae are unusual. Children experience minimal neurologic changes.

Other physical manifestations During the first 2 days of illness the patient may be nauseated and vomit, but vomiting later in the illness should arouse suspicion of an intercurrent complication. Abdominal pain is bothersome; when associated with diarrhea it responds to intravenous alimentation. Hepatomegaly and jaundice are unusual. There is splenomegaly in approximately 25 percent of patients.

Photophobia, retroocular pain, suffusion of the eyes, and congestion of the conjunctivas are common but are less severe than in the other typhus and spotted fevers.

Renal function is usually unaltered except in elderly patients with prolonged hypotension. Under these circumstances, azotemia may develop to the degree observed in epidemic typhus. In severe murine typhus, as in the epidemic typhus, hyponatremia and hypoalbuminemia are encountered.

COURSE After defervescence, murine typhus patients recover rapidly. Fatalities occur between the ninth and twelfth days in elderly or debilitated patients, usually as a result of circulatory and renal failure or intercurrent bacterial infection.

PROGNOSIS The mortality rate in murine typhus was low even before the introduction of modern specific therapy. Only 1 death occurred in 114 cases studied by Maxcy and none in the 180 reported by Stuart and Pullen.

DIFFERENTIAL DIAGNOSIS Because murine typhus and Rocky Mountain spotted fever occur in many of the same states, the problem of differential diagnosis often arises. Flea-borne murine typhus, which is predominantly an urban disease, is more likely to occur in late summer and autumn. In contrast, spotted fever is a rural and suburban disease in which exposure to ticks is important. Most cases occur in the spring and summer.

TREATMENT AND PREVENTION The therapeutic procedures are comparable to those used in spotted fever. Both chloramphenicol and the tetracycline antibiotics have controlled the disease.

Prevention of murine typhus in humans is attained by reducing the natural reservoir and vector by applying measures for eliminating rodents and employing appropriate insecticides in rat-infested areas to control fleas. Spraying of rat burrows with DDT effectively reduces the population of the vector.

REFERENCES

See Chap. 171.

168
EPIDEMIC TYPHUS FEVER AND BRILL-ZINSSER DISEASE

THEODORE E. WOODWARD

EPIDEMIC (LOUSE-BORNE) TYPHUS FEVER

DEFINITION The classical epidemic form of typhus is a severe, febrile disease caused by *Rickettsia prowazekii* and transmitted to humans by the body louse. Intense headache, continuous pyrexia of about 2 weeks, a macular skin eruption appearing on about the fifth febrile day, malaise, and vascular and neurologic disturbances represent the principal clinical features. Confirmation of the diagnosis is made by demonstration of *Proteus* OX-19 agglutinins and of specific complement-fixing antibodies in convalescence. The broad-spectrum antibiotics are specific therapeutic agents.

ETIOLOGY AND EPIDEMIOLOGY The causative microbe, *R. prowazekii,* is closely related to *R. mooseri,* which causes murine typhus; indeed, the two have a number of common antigens.

Human beings generally are infected when rickettsia-laden louse feces are rubbed into the broken skin; scratching the louse bite facilitates this process. *Pediculus humanus corporis,* which is peculiarly adapted to humans, is the only important vector of epidemic typhus. It dies of its infection and fails to transmit rickettsias to its offspring. *Rickettsia prowazekii* has been isolated from flying squirrels, and the organism probably infests their ectoparasites. Generally, however, the organism is maintained by a cycle involving human-louse-human. New epidemics apparently originate from patients with Brill-Zinsser disease (recurrent epidemic typhus). Pathogenic rickettsias reside for long periods in patients with epidemic typhus as well as Rocky Mountain spotted fever and scrub typhus. Lice readily become infected when fed on patients with recurrent typhus. Inhalation of dust containing dried louse feces may cause infection. An established nonhuman reservoir would pose a serious threat.

Epidemic typhus, if uncontrolled, behaves as a cyclic disease in a susceptible population, extending over a 3-year period. During the first year there is a gradual seeding of cases throughout the group; during the second there is epidemic spread; and during the third the epidemic tapers off, because the majority of persons have become immune. Outbreaks of epidemic typhus last occurred in the United States in the nineteenth century, and its presence is now recognized only in the form of Brill-Zinsser disease.

CLINICAL MANIFESTATIONS Epidemic typhus resembles murine typhus but is more severe. After an incubation period of about 7 days an abrupt onset of headache, chill, and rapidly mounting fever ushers in the illness. Headache, malaise, and prostration continue unabated until the rash appears on the fifth febrile day. It is initially macular in the axillary folds but ultimately invades the trunk and extremities as a pink, irregular macular lesion, which becomes fixed, petechial, and confluent in the later stages.

Neurologic features range from headache and general spasticity to extreme agitation, stupor, and coma. Circulatory disturbances consisting of tachycardia, hypotension, and cyanosis are more profound than those observed in murine typhus and are almost as severe as in Rocky Mountain spotted fever. Ultimately, in untreated cases azotemia often reaches high levels as a result of vascular and renal failure, and death occurs late in the second week of illness. Furthermore, thrombosis of major blood vessels and cutaneous gangrene develop in a manner similar to that seen in the virulent form of Rocky Mountain spotted fever.

The complications and sequelae of epidemic typhus are more severe than those in murine typhus, but not as severe as those in Rocky Mountain spotted fever. However, during certain outbreaks, epidemic typhus was fatal in 60 percent of those infected, and convalescence in survivors was prolonged. Broad-spectrum antibiotics have almost eradicated mortality in this dread disease, provided therapy is instituted before irreversible changes have been established in the tissues.

DIFFERENTIAL DIAGNOSIS Differentiation of epidemic typhus from the various rickettsioses and other diseases with which it may be confused is described in Chap. 164. The disease in epidemic form never occurs in the absence of lousiness in the general population. Under the conditions in which typhus epidemics are likely to occur, other diseases which may cause confusion include malaria, relapsing fever, pneumonia, and tuberculosis. Classic typhus contracted by a previously vaccinated person is usually mild and may be clinically indistinguishable from murine typhus except by serologic methods. An illness simulating Rocky Mountain spotted fever is caused by *R. canada,* a member of the typhus group.

TREATMENT AND PREVENTION Both chloramphenicol and the tetracycline antibiotics have been found to be highly efficient therapeutic agents in epidemic typhus. Usually the patient becomes afebrile after 2 days of treatment. The therapeutic procedures are comparable to those used in spotted fever. Under field conditions, 100 mg doxycycline in a single oral dose resulted in abatement of clinical manifestations and defervescence in epidemic typhus.

The most effective measures for controlling epidemic typhus are those which eliminate lousiness. DDT or lindane powder when dusted into clothing is suitable for this purpose. If resistant lice are found, malathion or carbaryl may prove effective.

A commercially available vaccine prepared from formalin-treated suspensions of infected yolk sac tissue is an effective immunizing agent. A viable vaccine utilizing an attenuated strain of *R. prowazekii* is under development.

BRILL-ZINSSER DISEASE (RECRUDESCENT TYPHUS)

DEFINITION Brill-Zinsser disease is a recrudescent episode of epidemic typhus fever which occurs years after the initial attack, in persons who had recovered from the epidemic disease acquired while residing in countries where it was prevalent. *Rickettsia prowazekii* have been isolated from lice fed on patients during the active stages of illness.

CLINICAL MANIFESTATIONS The clinical entity, not always mild, resembles epidemic typhus in the character of the rash, circulatory disturbances, and hepatic, renal, and nervous system changes. Recovery is the rule. The Weil-Felix reaction with the various *Proteus* antigens is usually negative, or positive in very low titer. The specific complement fixation, microscopic agglutination, and immunofluorescent antibody reactions are valuable in establishing the diagnosis. In Brill-Zinsser disease the specific complement-fixing antibodies appear as early as the fourth day after the onset of illness; the peak response is attained by the eighth to tenth days. Specific antibody titers in the primary attack of epidemic typhus begin later, about the eighth to twelfth day, with maximum titers on about the sixteenth day after onset. Antibodies in Brill-Zinsser disease and the primary attack are associated with 7S and 19S globulins, respectively. Therapy is like that used in spotted fever.

REFERENCES

See Chap. 171.

169
SCRUB TYPHUS

THEODORE E. WOODWARD

DEFINITION Scrub typhus is limited to eastern and southeastern Asia, India, northern Australia, and the adjacent islands. It is caused by *Rickettsia tsutsugamushi* and characterized by a primary lesion at the site of the bite of an infected mite, a fever of about 2 weeks' duration, a cutaneous rash which develops about the fifth day, and the appearance late in the second week of agglutinins against the OX-K strain of *Proteus* bacillus. The broad-spectrum antibiotics are specific therapeutic agents.

ETIOLOGY The agent of scrub typhus resembles other rickettsias in its physical properties but differs from them in antigenic structure, vector, and reservoir. The disease is transmitted by larvae of several species of mites, especially

Leptotrobidium (Trombicula) akamushi and *L. deliense.* These tiny chiggers attach themselves to the skin and during the process of obtaining a meal of tissue juice may acquire infection from the host or transmit rickettsias to the vertebrate. The infection is maintained in nature by a cycle involving mites and small rodents and by transovarial transmission in mites; human infection represents an accident attributable to propinquity.

CLINICAL MANIFESTATIONS About 10 to 12 days after infection, illness begins abruptly with chilliness, severe headache, fever, conjunctival injection, and moderate generalized lymphadenopathy, which is most prominent in the nodes draining the area of the primary lesion. The initial lesion at the beginning of fever is evidenced by an erythematous indurated area 1 cm in diameter, surmounted by a multiloculated vesicle; within a few days the vesicle ulcerates and becomes covered with a black crust.

Fever increases progressively during the first week, generally reaching 104 to 105°F, but the pulse remains relatively slow, 70 to 100 beats per minute. The red macular rash, which begins on the trunk about the fifth day and spreads to the extremities, sometimes becomes maculopapular but usually fades in a few days. The course of the disease and the complications resemble those of endemic and epidemic typhus; however, interstitial myocarditis is more prominent than in the other typhus fevers.

PROGNOSIS Before the introduction of the broad-spectrum antibiotics the mortality rate varied from 1 to 60 percent, depending on the geographic area and the virulence of the local strains of *R. tsutsugamushi,* and convalescence was prolonged. With modern therapeutic methods, deaths are rare and convalescence is short.

DIFFERENTIAL DIAGNOSIS Scrub typhus is to be differentiated from the other members of the typhus and the spotted fever group of diseases as well as from measles, typhoid fever, and the meningococcal infections. The geographic localization of scrub typhus, the primary lesion, and the occurrence of OX-K agglutinins are especially useful in establishing the diagnosis.

TREATMENT AND PREVENTION Chloramphenicol and the tetracycline antibiotics are valuable specific therapeutic agents in scrub typhus. The therapeutic procedures are comparable to those used in spotted fever. In fact, scrub typhus is more amenable to drugs than are the other rickettsial infections, and patients with this disease regularly become afebrile and are decidedly improved within 24 to 36 h after beginning treatment, irrespective of the stage of disease. Antibiotic treatment may be discontinued after several afebrile days.

Relapse of clinical illness is unusual unless specific treatment is initiated early, such as before the fifth febrile day. Under these circumstances, recrudescence is obviated by giving the antibiotic for several days and resuming treatment about 5 days after cessation of the initial course of therapy.

Prevention of disease in the individual is accomplished by the application of miticidal chemicals (dibutyl phthalate, benzyl benzoate, diethyltoluamide, and others) to clothing and the skin. There is no satisfactory vaccine.

REFERENCES

See Chap. 171.

170
Q FEVER

THEODORE E. WOODWARD

DEFINITION Q fever is an acute infectious disease caused by *Coxiella burnetii* and characterized by a sudden onset of fever, malaise, headache, weakness, anorexia, and interstitial pneumonitis. Rickettsemia occurs during the febrile period, and specific complement-fixing antibodies are present during convalescence. In contrast to the other rickettsioses, the disease is not associated with a cutaneous exanthem or agglutinins for the *Proteus* bacteria (Weil-Felix reaction).

ETIOLOGY AND EPIDEMIOLOGY *Coxiella burnetii* possesses the general properties of other rickettsias but is somewhat more resistant to inactivation in unfavorable environments and more pleomorphic than the others. Its infectivity after drying under natural conditions is of importance in the spread of infection to humans. *Coxiella burnetii* has a wide host range in nature, but guinea pigs and embryonated eggs are the common laboratory hosts employed for its propagation.

Human cases of Q fever are contracted by inhalation of infected dusts, by handling infected materials, possibly by drinking milk contaminated with *C. burnetii* and, in one instance, by blood transfusion. The disease in Australia is enzootic in animals, especially bandicoots, and is transmitted in nature by ticks. Rickettsia-laden tick feces may contaminate cattle hides, and inhalation of this material has caused infection in humans. In the United States, a number of species of ticks are naturally infected, among them *Dermacentor andersoni* and *Amblyomma americanum,* and in North Africa transovarial transmission of the agent in indigenous ticks has been demonstrated. Sheep, goats, and cows have been found to be naturally infected in North America and in Europe, and *C. burnetii* has been recovered from the milk of such animals. Milk, as well as infected excretions from livestock, probably accounts for certain outbreaks of human disease following inhalation by cows of infected dust from barns and pens. The airborne route of dried contaminated material is the most likely method of spread. A number of epidemics have occurred among laboratory workers engaged in studies on *C. burnetii.* The disease is not transmitted between humans.

CLINICAL MANIFESTATIONS After incubation of approximately 19 days (the range is 14 to 26 days), the disease begins with headache, chilly sensations, fever, malaise, myalgia, and anorexia. For several days, the temperature ranges from 101 to 104°F; the entire course rarely exceeds 2 weeks and usually ranges from 3 to 6 days. There may be wide fluctuations in the fever. Respiratory and gastrointestinal symptoms are not conspicuous in the early stages. Headache and fever predominate. A dry cough and chest pain occur after about 5 days, when rales are usually audible. Roentgenographic findings indistinguishable from those of primary atypical pneumonia are present usually by the third to fourth day of disease, first as patchy areas of consolidation involving a portion of one lobe, giving a homogeneous ground-glass appearance. These manifestations persist beyond the febrile period and may appear in patients who are unaware of pulmonary involvement. Complications are rare, and coincident with defervescence the appetite begins to return. Convalescence progresses slowly for several weeks, during which time the principal disability is weakness. It is not uncommon for patients to lose 15 to 20 lb during the active stages of disease. The disease may be protracted in approximately 20 percent of cases, with fever persisting for longer than

4 weeks, particularly in elderly patients. Occasionally relapse occurs, especially in patients treated with antibiotics during the first several days of disease.

Hepatitis, with the development of clinically detectable icterus, occurs in approximately one-third of patients with the protracted form. This form of Q fever is characterized by fever, malaise, absence of headache or respiratory signs, and hepatomegaly with right upper quadrant pain. Liver biopsy specimens show diffuse granulomatous changes with multinucleated giant cells and scattered infiltrations of polymorphonuclear leukocytes, lymphocytes, and macrophages. *Coxiella burnetii* may be demonstrated in such specimens with the fluorescent antibody technique. Therefore, Q fever must be included in the differential diagnosis of liver granulomas such as tuberculosis, sarcoidosis, histoplasmosis, brucellosis, tularemia, syphilis, and others.

Endocarditis also has been reported, and *C. burnetii* has been identified by smear and isolation in vegetations on the heart valves obtained at operation or autopsy. The aortic valve is most commonly involved, often with large vegetations. It is important, therefore, to suspect the possibility of Q fever in cases of apparent subacute bacterial endocarditis with persistently negative blood cultures. Operative intervention with replacement of damaged valves is usually necessary for recovery because the available antibiotics are not rickettsicidal.

A high complement-fixing antibody titer to phase I antigen is present in patients with endocarditis and granulomatous hepatitis.

PROGNOSIS Few fatalities have been recorded and, except for the patient with protracted illness and hepatic involvement or endocarditis, the course of disease is generally uncomplicated and benign.

TREATMENT AND CONTROL The tetracycline antibiotics and chloramphenicol are effective in the treatment of patients with Q fever. Most patients, when treated early in the course of disease, respond promptly and recover without relapses. The therapeutic procedures are comparable to those used in spotted fever.

Control of Q fever depends primarily on immunization of susceptible persons with specific vaccines. Vaccines made from phase I rickettsias are potent and afford considerable protection to slaughterhouse and dairy workers, herders, rendering-plant workers, woolsorters, tanners, laboratory workers, and others at risk. Measures should be taken to avoid exposure to infected aerosols; milk from infected domestic livestock must be pasteurized or boiled.

REFERENCES

See Chap. 171.

171
TRENCH FEVER

THEODORE E. WOODWARD

DEFINITION Trench fever is a febrile disease transmitted between humans by the body louse, *Pediculus humanus corporis.* It is characterized by a sudden onset with headache and severe pain in the muscles, bones, and joints. In most cases, the fever and other symptoms assume a relapsing character. Fatalities are rare. The disease is also known as shin bone fever, Volhynia fever, His-Werner disease, and Quintan fever.

ETIOLOGY AND EPIDEMIOLOGY *Rickettsia quintana,* the etiologic agent, grows extracellularly in the louse gut, in contrast to other pathogenic rickettsias which can multiply only within cells. A European strain of *R. quintana* has been cultivated on blood agar, and typical trench fever has been induced in volunteers.

Humans are the only known reservoir of infection. The louse does not transmit the organism transovarially but acquires its infection by ingesting the blood of a person with rickettsemia. The organisms multiply extracellularly in the louse gut, without injury to this host, and are excreted in large numbers with the feces. Humans become infected by the inoculation of the contaminated feces into abraded skin or conjunctivas. *Rickettsia quintana* may be recovered periodically from human blood for several years after convalescence from an acute attack. Trench fever is known to exist in Mexico, Tunisia, Eritrea, Poland, the U.S.S.R., and possibly China, and there is serologic evidence for its occurrence in Bolivia, Burundi, and Ethiopia.

PATHOLOGY Since there have been no recorded fatalities, histologic examination has been confined to excised macules of the skin, which have shown nonspecific perivascular infiltrates without the involvement of the vessel walls that is seen in typhus fever.

CLINICAL MANIFESTATIONS A variety of clinical manifestations is displayed in trench fever, ranging from a mild afebrile disease to a debilitating illness with a protracted clinical course involving numerous relapses. Following an incubation period of 10 to 30 days the onset may be insidious or dramatically abrupt. The acute disease is characterized by malaise, headache, fever, and bone and body pain, especially severe in the shins. In some cases only one fever peak occurs; in others the fever continues for 5 to 7 days; and in others there is an initial febrile episode lasting 1 to 3 days followed by relapses which characteristically occur at 4- to 5-day intervals. In some cases the fever and symptoms are continuous for 2 or 3 weeks. Enlargement of the spleen and a red macular rash occur in 70 to 80 percent of the cases. Pain and soreness in the muscles usually recur with each febrile relapse.

The disease is marked by a persistent rickettsemia, which is present during the initial attack and which continues during the relapses, throughout the asymptomatic periods between relapses, and for months or even years after cessation of physical symptoms. A relapse has been reported 10 years after the original attack.

PROGNOSIS The disease causes no known deaths, but its duration is variable. About 85 percent of patients are able to return to work within 2 months of onset, but about 5 percent of all cases become chronic. Recovery is even more delayed in the aged and debilitated.

DIFFERENTIAL DIAGNOSIS During epidemics, typical cases are easily diagnosed on the basis of symptoms. The disease may be differentiated from influenza, typhoid, typhus, dengue, and relapsing fever by the specific laboratory tests available for the diagnosis of each of these diseases.

TREATMENT AND PREVENTION *Rickettsia quintana* is highly sensitive in vitro to the broad-spectrum antibiotics but no reliable information has been obtained about the value of these drugs in treating trench fever. The treatment is symptomatic. Aspirin is used to control pain and discomfort, but codeine may be necessary. The patient should remain in bed for a week or more after complete cessation of subjective and objective evidence of infection. He should be kept under observation for several months and returned to bed at the first sign of relapse.

The methods employed to control epidemic typhus should be equally efficacious in controlling trench fever. These are based on the elimination of lousiness and the improvement of living conditons with provision for frequent bathing and washing of clothing. DDT or lindane powder should be applied by hand or power duster at appropriate intervals to clothes and persons of populations living under conditions favoring lousiness. If resistant lice are found, malathion or other effective lousicides may be substituted as a dusting powder.

REFERENCES

ANDREW R et al: Tick typhus in North Queensland. Med J Aust 2:253, 1946

BOZEMAN FM et al: Serologic evidence of *Rickettsia canada* infection in man. J Infect Dis 121:367, 1970

—— et al: Epidemic typhus rickettsiae isolated from flying squirrels. Nature 255:545, 1975

DERRICK EH: The epidemiology of Q fever: A review. Med J Aust 1:245, 1953

DeSHAZO RD et al: Early diagnosis of Rocky Mountain spotted fever. Use of primary monocyte culture technique. JAMA 235:1353, 1976

FERGUSON IC et al: Clinical, virological and pathological findings in a fatal case of Q fever endocarditis. Br J Clin Pathol 15:235, 1962

GAMBRILL MR, WISSEMAN CL JR: Mechanisms of immunity in typhus infections. Infect Immun 8:519, 1973

HARRELL GT: Rickettsial involvement of the nervous system. Med Clin North Am 37:395, 1953

HATTWICK MAW et al: Rocky Mountain spotted fever: Epidemiology of an increasing problem. Ann Intern Med 84:732, 1976

HAZARD GW et al: Rocky Mountain spotted fever in the Eastern United States. N Engl J Med 280:57, 1969

MARMION BP, STOKER MGP: The epidemiology of Q fever in Great Britian: An analysis of the findings and some conclusions. Br Med J 2:809, 1958

McKIEL JA et al: *Rickettsia canada:* A new member of the typhus group of rickettsiae isolated from *Haemaphysalis leporis-palustris* ticks in Canada. J Microbiol 12:503, 1967

MOHR CO, SMITH WW: Eradication of murine typhus fever in a rural area. Bull WHO 16:255, 1957

MOULTON FR (ed): *The Rickettsial Diseases of Man.* Washington, DC, American Association for the Advancement of Science, 1948

MURRAY ES et al: Brill's disease: I. Clinical and laboratory diagnosis. JAMA 142:1059, 1950

——, SNYDER JC: Brill's disease: II. Etiology. Am J Hyg 53:22, 1951

ORMSBEE RA et al: The influence of phase on the protective potency of Q fever vaccine. J Immunol 92:404, 1964

—— et al: Serologic diagnosis of epidemic typhus fever. Am J Epidemiol 105:261, 1977

OSTER CN et al: Laboratory acquired Rocky Mountain spotted fever: The hazard of aerosol transmision. N Engl J Med 297:859, 1977

PEDERSEN CE et al: Demonstration of *Rickettsia rickettsii* in Rhesus monkeys by immune fluorescence microscopy. J Clin Microbiol 2:121, 1975

PHILIP RN et al: A comparison of serologic methods for diagnosis of Rocky Mountain spotted fever. Am J Epidemiol 105:56, 1977

PRATT HD: The changing picture of murine typhus in the United States. Ann NY Acad Sci 70:516, 1958

ROSE HM: The clinical manifestations and laboratory diagnosis of rickettsialpox. Ann Intern Med 31:871, 1949

SCHACHTER J et al: Potential danger of Q fever in a university hospital environment. J Infect Dis 123:301, 1971

SCHAFFNER W, KOENIG MG: Thrombocytopenic Rocky Mountain spotted fever. Arch Intern Med 116:857, 1965

SMADEL JE: Influence of antibiotics on immunologic responses in scrub typhus. Am J Med 17:246, 1954

—— (ed): *Symposium on Q Fever,* Medical Science Publication 6. Washington, DC, Walter Reed Army Institute of Research, 1959

——, JACKSON EB: Rickettsial infections, in *Diagnostic Procedures of Viral and Rickettsial Diseases,* 3d ed. New York, American Public Health Association, 1964, p 743

SOMENSHINE DE et al: Epizootiology of epidemic typhus (*Rickettsia prowazekii*) in flying squirrels. Am J Trop Med Hyg 27:339, 1978

VINSON JW: Etiology of trench fever in Mexico, in *Industry and Tropical Health,* vol V. Boston, Harvard School of Public Health, 1964, p 109

WOODWARD TE: Rickettsial diseases in the United States. Med Clin North Am 43:1507, 1959

——: A historical account of the rickettsial diseases with a discussion of unsolved problems. The First Maxwell Finland Lecture. J Infect Dis 127:583, 1973

——: Identification of *Rickettsia* in skin tissues. J Infect Dis 134:297, 1976

section 11 | Mycoplasmal diseases

172
RESPIRATORY INFECTION WITH *MYCOPLASMA PNEUMONIAE*

VERNON KNIGHT

INTRODUCTION The mycoplasmas, formerly called pleuropneumonia-like organisms (PPLO) after the organism that caused a highly contagious form of bovine pneumonia and pleurisy in Europe in the eighteenth century, are now designated class Mollicutes, family Mycoplasmataceae, genus *My-*

coplasma. There are 37 species, 8 of which have been isolated from human beings (Table 172-1).

The only mycoplasma of importance in respiratory disease is *M. pneumoniae. Mycoplasma pneumoniae* grows on peptone-enriched beef-heart infusion broth as small round colonies partially buried in the agar without the "fried egg" periphery characteristic of growth of other mycoplasmas. *Mycoplasma pneumoniae* grows aerobically and anaerobically.

Mycoplasma pneumoniae is resistant to penicillin and antibiotics known to interfere with polymerization of cell wall precursors, and it does not retain the dye-iodine complex of Gram's stain. It is inhibited by tetracyclines, erythromycin, chloramphenicol, and some other antibiotics. Like bacteria, it

TABLE 172-1
The human mycoplasmas

Species	Usual site of occurrence
M. pneumoniae	Respiratory tract
M. salivarium	Oropharynx
M. orale 1	Oropharynx
M. orale 2	Oropharynx
M. orale 3	Oropharynx
M. fermentans	Oropharynx and genital tract (rarely detected)
M. hominis	Genital tract
T-strain mycoplasmas (ureaplasma urealyticum)	

grows outside the cell, possesses ribonucleic and deoxyribonucleic acids, reproduces by fission, and generates metabolic energy.

PNEUMONIA AND RESPIRATORY TRACT DISEASE CAUSED BY *MYCOPLASMA PNEUMONIAE*

Synonyms are primary atypical pneumonia, Eaton's agent pneumonia, cold agglutinin-positive pneumonia, and "virus" pneumonia.

Definition Pneumonia caused by *M. pneumoniae* is characterized by fever, pharyngitis, cough, and pulmonary infiltration, often multilobular, in which roentgenographic signs are more extensive than indicated by physical examination. This organism also causes upper respiratory illness without pneumonia and asymptomatic infection.

Etiology *Mycoplasma pneumoniae* is distinguished from other mycoplasmas by rapid hemolysis of guinea pig erythrocytes and utilization of glucose and other sugars. It also hemolyzes human and rat erythrocytes. It may also be distinguished from other mycoplasmas by fluorescent antibody, complement fixation, growth inhibition, and indirect hemagglutination tests, all of which are useful for serologic diagnosis of human infection. In addition to growing on agar, the organism grows on the surface of cells of embryonated eggs and monkey kidney cell culture with little evidence of cytopathic effect. In human cell cultures, however, there is intracellular growth with cytopathic effects.

Epidemiology In the general population *M. pneumoniae* infection is characterized by intrafamily spread. In most cases the infection is introduced into the family by a schoolchild. Once it is introduced, most family members become infected. In family outbreaks, pneumonia occurs with greatest frequency among school-age children, with a predominance in males. The disease is rare above age forty. *Mycoplasma pneumoniae* pneumonia occurs throughout the year, although prolonged wintertime outbreaks may occur in college groups or communities. The total incidence of *M. pneumoniae* pneumonia in a study in Seattle was 1.3 per 1000 per year, which constituted about 15 to 20 percent of pneumonia from all causes. At intervals of several years, epidemics of *M. pneumoniae* pneumonia may occur with about double the usual incidence of disease.

In the military, *M. pneumoniae* infections account for a small proportion of upper respiratory illness in recruits—in one study, 6.3 percent. However, it accounted for almost one-half of cases of pneumonia in the same military population. No more than 10 percent of infected military personnel develop pneumonia; the rest are asymptomatic. The disease appears to be endemic at military bases.

Mycoplasma pneumoniae is probably spread by means of infected respiratory secretions. The organisms can be cultured from sputum of naturally occurring cases and from volunteers inoculated artificially. Primary atypical pneumonia has been induced in volunteers both by nasopharyngeal inoculation and by inhalation of a small-particle aerosol containing the agent. In volunteers naturally acquired antibody is associated with a high degree of resistance to infection.

Clinical manifestations The incubation period is from 9 to 12 days, but the interval between cases in families is approximately 3 weeks. Illness usually begins with symptoms of upper respiratory infection, which in some patients progresses to bronchitis and pneumonia. Four syndromes of respiratory disease have been identified: pneumonia, tracheobronchitis, pharyngitis, and bullous myringitis. About one-third of cases in family members will develop pneumonia, up to one-half will have tracheobronchitis, 10 percent exhibit only pharyngitis, and 10 percent will be asymptomatic. Children 5 to 10 years old, especially boys, have the greatest incidence of disease. Ear involvement consisting of congestion of the tympanic membrane and of bullous and, rarely, hemorrhagic myringitis may occur in as many as 10 percent of cases of pneumonia, most often in children. Cough is almost universal in pneumonia and is frequent in cases without pulmonary involvement. Blood-flecked sputum may occur in the more severe cases, but gross hemoptysis is rare. A variety of other respiratory and systemic complaints may occur. Fever, nasal congestion, and sore throat are common. In pneumonia, harsh or diminished sounds are frequent but bronchial breathing is uncommon. Fine inspiratory rales are found in most patients but are not impressive. Pleural rubs and pleural effusion are infrequent. Studies on the distribution of pneumonia in one large series showed that more than one-half of cases were multilobular and slightly less than one-half were bilateral. Lower-lobe pneumonia was appreciably more frequent than upper-lobe pneumonia. Pulmonary infiltrates may occur as an isolated area in the lung periphery but more often spread from the hilum.

The disease is variable in severity, but high fever may persist for 1 to 2 weeks in untreated cases. X-ray changes last for as long as 3 weeks in untreated cases, but for 7 to 10 days in treated cases. Even in untreated cases, complications are rare and consist of occasional purulent sinusitis, persistent cough, and, rarely, pleurisy. Prolonged weakness and malaise follow the untreated illness in adults.

Rare complications include meningoencephalitis, polyneuritis, monoarticular arthritis, Stevens-Johnson syndrome, pericarditis, myocarditis, hepatitis, diffuse intravascular coagulation, and hemolytic anemia. Stevens-Johnson syndrome and other mucocutaneous reactions occur in patients with *M. pneumoniae* pneumonia in the absence of treatment, but the frequency is greatly increased in patients who have received antimicrobial drugs.

Laboratory findings During acute illness leukocytosis in the range of 10,000 to 15,000 leukocytes per cubic millimeter occurs in about 25 percent of cases. Increase in sedimentation rate above 40 mm/h occurs in at least two-thirds of cases. Urinalysis, electrocardiograms, and fluid and electrolyte and liver function studies show no characteristic changes. The complement fixation, fluorescent antibody, indirect hemagglutination, and growth inhibition tests all yield highly specific diagnostic information. The simplicity of the complement fixation text recommends it for general use. Fourfold rises in titer often occur within 2 weeks, and maximum rise is achieved in 4 weeks. A nonspecific test for *M. pneumoniae* infection in use for many years is the detection of cold agglutinins. The end point is the dilution of the patient's serum, which agglutinates human type O red blood cells at 4°C. The test depends on the presence of a macroglobulin antibody to phase I antigen of red blood cells. In *M. pneumoniae* infection, cold agglutinins appear at the end of the first week of illness and disappear in a week or so. The test is positive in a majority of patients, more commonly in those who are severely ill. The cold agglutinin reaction is nonspecific, however, and occurs with other red blood cell antigens in infectious mononucleosis, lymphoproliferative diseases and in several respiratory infections, particularly in children.

Differential diagnosis Pneumonia due to *M. pneumoniae* needs to be distinguished from pneumonia of all other types. It is usually less severe, is associated with less dense pulmonary infiltration than pneumococcal and other bacterial pneumonias, and occurs throughout the year. Pulmonary infiltrate in the absence of symptoms or physical signs may initially suggest acute pulmonary tuberculosis. In military populations adenoviral pneumonia must be excluded. Pneumonic involvement as a direct result of influenza viral infection or its complication by pneumococcal, streptococcal, staphylococcal, or *H. influenzae* infection may cause difficulty in diagnosis. Q fever, psittacosis, and tularemia are less frequent causes of pneumonia that may be difficult to distinguish from *M. pneumoniae* infection. In children, especially young infants, pneumonia due to respiratory syncytial, parainfluenza, adenovirus, and influenza viruses may resemble *M. pneumoniae* infection. Legionnaires' disease (Chap. 138) resembles severe cases of *M. pneumoniae* pneumonia.

Treatment Tetracycline derivatives and erythromycin are effective in treatment of pneumonia due to *M. pneumoniae*. Demethylchlortetracycline may be given to adults in daily doses of 0.9 g; tetracycline, 1.5 g; erythromycin stearate, 1.5 g. Response to treatment is characterized by prompt defervescence, rapid clearing of x-ray signs of pneumonia, and disappearance of malaise and weakness. Persistent cough, despite treatment, is a relatively common finding, especially in women.

Treatment temporarily reduces the frequency of positive cultures from the respiratory tract, but shedding may continue for several weeks after treatment, a finding similar to that in psittacosis pneumonia. Relapse of *M. pneumoniae* pneumonia occurs occasionally, but such cases respond to re-treatment. In cases in which there is doubt between the diagnosis of *M. pneumoniae* and pneumococcal infection, erythromycin should be used in preference to a tetracycline.

Prevention Although antibody is apparently highly protective, effective vaccines are not available. Acutely ill patients should be isolated from very young children and persons in whom a complicating respiratory illness would constitute a special hazard.

REFERENCES

CHERRY JD et al: *Mycoplasma pneumoniae* infections and exanthems. J Pediatr 87:369, 1975

COUCH RB: *Mycoplasma pneumoniae*, in *Viral and Mycoplasmal Infections of the Respiratory Tract*, V Knight (ed). Philadelphia, Lea & Febiger, 1973

FOY HM et al: Viral and mycoplasmal pneumonia in a prepaid medical care group during an eight year period. Am J Epidemiol 97:93, 1973

MCDADE JE et al: Legionnaires' disease. Isolation of a bacterium and demonstration of its role in other respiratory disease. N Engl J Med 297:1197, 1978

section 12 | Chlamydial infections

173
GENERAL CONSIDERATIONS

J. THOMAS GRAYSTON
KING K. HOLMES

The genus *Chlamydia* has two species, *C. trachomatis* and *C. psittaci*. The *C. trachomatis* species includes the two important exclusively human pathogens causing trachoma and lymphogranuloma venereum (LGV). The finding that the trachoma organisms are a major cause of venereal disease has led to a broadening of interest in these organisms in the past decade. The *C. psittaci* species contains a number of strains whose primary hosts are animals and birds. They infect humans as accidental hosts. All organisms in the *Chlamydia* genus have a common heat-stable lipopolysaccharide antigen. The species can be differentiated by inclusion type. The *C. trachomatis* inclusions stain with iodine and are compact, while the *C. psittaci* inclusions fail to stain with iodine and are diffuse. *Chlamydia trachomatis* is sensitive to sulfanomides, while *C. psittaci* is not.

NOMENCLATURE In the past the *Chlamydia* organisms have been known by a variety of names: *Miyagawanella*, *Bedsonia*, and psittacosis-LGV-trachoma (PLT). The trachoma organisms of *C. trachomatis* have also been referred to as *TRIC* (trachoma-inclusion conjunctivitis) *agents*. This terminology is being discarded because of confusion with *Trichomonas*. It is the non-LGV, *C. trachomatis* organisms that cause classic trachoma, nonendemic trachoma, and paratrachoma, inclusion conjunctivitis of both the newborn and the adult, nongonococcal urethritis (NGU), epididymitis, various diseases of the female genital tract (Chap. 174), and a distinctive pneumonia syndrome in infants.

MICROBIOLOGY Until recent years, the *Chlamydia* were considered large viruses because they are obligate, intracellular parasites. While remaining a unique group of microorganisms, they are now considered to be bacterial. They have a discrete cell wall quite similar to those of the gram-negative bacteria, contain both RNA and DNA, multiply by binary fission, and are susceptible to a variety of antimicrobials. Their intracellular parasitism is due to their inability to synthesize adenosine triphosphate (ATP), making them energy parasites.

The complex development cycle of the *Chlamydia* is not fully understood. There are two forms of the organisms: the reticulate (initial) body which is a metabolically active intracellular growth form and the elementary body which is the infectious extracellular form. The elementary body attaches to the surface of the host cell and is actively ingested by endocytosis. *Chlamydia* appears to induce its own phagocytosis. Within 6 to 8 h the elementary body is reorganized into the metabolically active reticulate body which divides continuously by binary fission within the phagosome for 18 to 24 h after infection, after which reticulate bodies reorganize into elementary bodies. The mature intracellular inclusion of *C. trachomatis* is shown in Fig. 173-1, just prior to rupture and dissemination of elementary bodies extracellularly.

IMMUNOTYPES The *C. trachomatis* strains of human origin have been classified immunologically. A total of 15 immunotypes have been identified, using a microimmunofluorescence (micro-IF) test. There are 12 types of trachoma organisms—A, B, Ba, C, D, E, F, G, H, I, J, and K—and three types of LGV organisms—L_1, L_2, and L_3. The three LGV types are closely related to the trachoma types. L_1 and L_2 to B, E, and D, and L_3 to K. Other relationships have been shown among the 15 serotypes. By use of the analogy of senior-junior relationship among influenza viruses, existence of similar associations can be shown among the *C. trachomatis* organisms. The LGV strains are all junior, while the types most often associated with endemic trachoma (B and C) are senior.

BIOLOGICAL CHARACTERISTICS OF LGV VERSUS TRACHOMA Despite the close immunologic relationship of LGV to trachoma organisms, the former have clearly different biological characteristics. They are lethal when inoculated into mice intracerebrally, while the trachoma agents are not. The LGV agents will grow by cell-to-cell serial transmission in tissue culture, while the trachoma agents require mechanical assistance for good growth.

FIGURE 173-1

Giemsa-stained human conjunctival cells. Three cells have cytoplasmic inclusions of trachoma organisms. Each inclusion is in the late stage of development prior to release of elementary bodies (1000×).

LATENCY OF CHLAMYDIA Latency has been recognized as an important part of the pathogenesis of chlamydial infection in both humans and animals. Psittacosis, LGV, and trachoma are all known to be capable of causing relapsing disease many years after the original infection. Because the organisms are obligate intracellular parasites, they do not simply persist in the body in some nonreplicating form; rather, they remain viable through low levels of multiplication which are held in check by the host's defense mechanisms. An example of this phenomenon is the ability of cortisone eye ointment to precipitate acute trachoma disease in patients with long-dormant eye infection.

PATHOGENESIS Trachoma organisms grow primarily in the columnar epithelium of the conjunctiva, urethra, and cervix. The role of serum and local antibody in *C. trachomatis* infections is uncertain. Similarly, the role of cellular immunity in limiting chlamydial infections or in contributing to its immunopathology remains undefined. The first eye infection with *C. trachomatis* organisms usually results in a self-limited acute papillary and follicular conjunctivitis. The chronic eye pathology of trachoma is thought to be related to an immunopathological response to reinfection. Primates are the only laboratory animals susceptible to eye infection with trachoma organisms.

DIAGNOSIS All diseases caused by *C. trachomatis*, except classic trachoma, require laboratory confirmation for diagnosis. The laboratory procedures include direct microscopic examination for typical intracytoplasmic inclusions or specific antigen, isolation of the organism, and detection of antibody in the serum or in local secretions. Direct microscopic examination of Giemsa- or iodine-stained cell scrapings is inefficient and has a low yield except in neonatal inclusion conjunctivitis. Nevertheless, it may be the only laboratory method available in many areas of the world. Unfortunately, false-positive interpretations by inexperienced observers are common. Direct fluorescent antibody staining of cell smears is more sensitive but is also inefficient and requires as much sophistication as cell culture isolation and serology. Cell culture techniques have replaced the yolk sac of embryonated eggs for isolation of *C. trachomatis*. The cell cultures are much more convenient and are more sensitive, particularly for strains from the genital tract. While LGV strains grow well in many cell lines, the trachoma strains are much more difficult to culture. The most common cell lines used are McCoy cells and HeLa 229 cells. Both cell lines require special pretreatment and centrifugation of the inoculum onto the monolayer for efficient isolation of trachoma strains. Positive cultures are determined by identifying typical intracytoplasmic inclusions stained by Giemsa's, iodine, or immunofluorescent techniques. Isolates may be immunotyped in the micro-IF test.

A complement fixation (CF) test with the heat-stable group-reactive antigen has been used for a long time to diagnose psittacosis and LGV with limited success. It is too insensitive to be useful with non-LGV *C. trachomatis* (trachoma organisms) infections. The micro-IF test with *C. trachomatis* antigens is sensitive and strain-specific. While it has been greatly simplified for diagnostic purposes, it remains available only in research laboratories. The test measures antibodies by immunotype specificity and by immunoglobulin class (IgM, IgG, IgA, secretory IgA) in both serum and local secretions.

ANTIBIOTIC SUSCEPTIBILITY *Chlamydia*, like other bacteria, is susceptible to certain antibiotics. In laboratory tests, death of inoculated mice and chick embryos, as well as growth in cell cultures, is prevented or inhibited by tetracyclines, erythromycin, rosarimicin, choramphenicol, and rifampin; sulfonamides and cycloserine are active against *C. trachomatis* but not *C. psittaci;* bacitracin and polymyxin B are less effective; penicillin and ampicillin suppress *Chlamydia* multiplication but do not eradicate the organisms in vitro. Streptomycin, gentamicin, neomycin, kanamycin, vancomycin, ristocetin, spectinomycin, and nystatin are not effective at concentrations inhibitory for most bacteria and fungi. For treatment of human infection, the tetracyclines and erythromycin are the most useful. The sulfonamides are also effective clinically against *C. trachomatis.*

REFERENCES

GRAYSTON JT, WANG SP: New knowledge of *Chlamydiae* and the diseases they cause. J Infect Dis 132:87, 1975
SCHACHTER J: Medical progress. Chlamydial infections. N Engl J Med 298:428, 490, 540, 1973

174
DISEASES DUE TO *CHLAMYDIA TRACHOMATIS*

KING K. HOLMES
J. THOMAS GRAYSTON
CHANDLER R. DAWSON
PETER L. PERINE

TRACHOMA AND INCLUSION CONJUNCTIVITIS

DEFINITION Trachoma is a chronic conjunctivitis. It is still the most important cause of preventable visual loss, having produced an estimated 20 million cases of blindness throughout the world. Inclusion conjunctivitis is an acute ocular inflammation caused by sexually transmitted chlamydial agents in adults exposed to infected genital secretions and in their newborn offspring.

EPIDEMIOLOGY Epidemiologically, two types of eye disease are caused by the trachoma organisms of the *Chlamydia trachomatis* species. In trachoma-endemic areas where the classic eye disease is seen, transmission is from eye to eye, via hands, towels, flies, etc. In nonendemic areas, the organisms are transmitted from the genital tract to the eye, usually causing only the inclusion conjunctivitis syndrome with or without keratitis. Rarely the eye disease progresses with the development of pannus and scars similar to endemic trachoma. These cases are referred to as *paratrachoma* to differentiate them from eye-to-eye transmitted endemic trachoma.

The worldwide incidence and severity of trachoma have decreased dramatically during the past 30 years in areas with improving hygienic and economic conditions. Endemic trachoma is still the major cause of preventable blindness in North Africa, sub-Saharan Africa, the Middle East, Australia, and parts of Asia. Transmission of the endemic disease occurs primarily through close personal contact, particularly among young children in the affected rural communities. In endemic areas, trachoma is usually associated with repeated exposure, but the infection can also be latent. In the United States a mild form of endemic trachoma still occurs in American Indians and in Mexican Americans as well as in immigrants from areas where trachoma is endemic. Acute relapse of old trachoma may be seen occasionally following treatment with cortisone eye ointment or in very old persons exposed in their youth.

Chlamydia trachomatis eye infection in nonendemic areas is a complication of what is now recognized as one of the most common venereal infections (see "Nongonococcal Urethritis" below). Adult inclusion conjunctivitis and paratrachoma are

uncommon complications of genital infections, usually in sexually promiscuous young adults. These sporadic, infrequent eye infections occur following transfer of infected genital discharges to the eye, either on the fingers or by orogenital sexual activities. Newborns become infected by exposure in the infected birth canal of their mothers during delivery.

CLINICAL MANIFESTATIONS Both endemic trachoma and adult inclusion conjunctivitis present initially as a conjunctivitis characterized by small lymphoid follicles in the conjunctiva. In regions with hyperendemic classic blinding trachoma, the disease usually starts insidiously before the age of 2 years. Reinfection is common. The cornea becomes involved with inflammatory leukocytic infiltration and superficial vascularization (pannus formation). As the inflammation continues, there is conjunctival scarring that eventually distorts the eyelids, causing them to turn inward so that the inturned lashes constantly abrade the eyeball (trichiasis and entropion); eventually the corneal epithelium is abraded and may then develop a bacterial corneal ulcer with subsequent corneal scarring and blindness. Destruction of the conjunctival goblet cells, lacrimal ducts, and lacrimal gland may produce a "dry-eye" syndrome with resultant corneal opacity due to drying (xerosis) or secondary bacterial corneal ulcers. Communities with blinding trachoma often experience seasonal epidemics of bacterial conjunctivitis with *Hemophilus influenza* (biotype III or the Koch-Weeks bacillus) and rarely with *Neisseria gonorrhoeae,* which contribute to the intensity of the inflammatory process. In such areas the active infectious process usually resolves spontaneously in affected persons between 10 and 15 years of age, but the conjunctival scars continue to shrink, producing trichiasis and entropion and subsequent corneal scarring in adult life. In areas with milder and less prevalent disease the process may be much slower, with active disease continuing into adulthood; blindness is rare in these cases.

Eye infection with genital *C. trachomatis* strains, usually in sexually active young adults, presents with acute onset of unilateral follicular conjunctivitis and preauricular lymphadenopathy similar to acute adenovirus or herpes virus conjunctivitis. If untreated, the disease may persist for 6 weeks to 2 years. It is frequently associated with corneal inflammation in the form of discrete opacities ("infiltrates"), punctate epithelial erosions, and minor degrees of superficial corneal vascularization. Very rarely conjunctival scarring and eyelid distortion occur, particularly in patients treated for many months with topical corticosteroids. Recurrent eye infections occur most often in patients whose sexual consorts are not treated with antibiotics.

DIAGNOSIS The clinical diagnosis of classic trachoma can be made if two of the following signs are present:

1 Lymphoid follicles on the upper tarsal conjunctiva
2 Typical conjunctival scarring
3 Vascular pannus
4 Limbal follicles or their sequelae, Herbert's pits

For public health purposes, it is necessary to determine whether a substantial proportion of the population has these minimal signs. Public health intervention will depend on the intensity of active inflammatory disease and on the prevalence of blinding or potentially blinding sequelae. In endemic trachoma, laboratory tests to support the clinical diagnosis should be obtained from children with more marked degrees of inflammation. Intracytoplasmic chlamydial inclusions occur in 10 to 60 percent of Giemsa-stained conjunctival smears in such populations, but isolation in cell cultures is more sensitive. Follicular conjunctivitis in adult Europeans or Americans living in trachomatous regions is rarely trachoma, although their children may acquire mild, nonblinding trachoma.

Sporadic cases of adult inclusion conjunctivitis must be differentiated from adenovirus and herpes simplex virus keratoconjunctivitis during the first 15 days after onset, and later from other forms of chronic follicular conjunctivitis. Laboratory demonstration of chlamydial infection by Giemsa- or immunofluorescent-stained smears or by isolation in cell cultures constitutes definitive evidence of infection, but only a few laboratories carry out these procedures. Serologic demonstration of antibody in serum cannot be taken as evidence of eye infection with chlamydial agents, since so many sexually active young adults have serum antibody titers. A practical diagnostic procedure in cases with chronic follicular conjunctivitis is treatment for 6 days with an oral tetracycline or erythromycin; a marked symptomatic response within 3 to 4 days is highly suggestive of inclusion conjunctivitis, and treatment should be continued for at least 3 weeks.

DIFFERENTIAL DIAGNOSIS Several viral eye infections should be considered in the differential diagnosis of trachoma and inclusion conjunctivitis. The eye and its adnexa may be infected during the course of many cutaneous and systemic viral diseases. Sometimes these ocular infections produce minor manifestations, such as the transient loss of accommodation of dengue and the milder forms of conjunctivitis in systemic adenovirus infections. Other virus infections, however, such as herpes simplex (Chap. 193), herpes zoster (Chap. 185), measles (Chap. 181), and vaccinia or smallpox (Chap. 184), occasionally produce serious and permanent visual loss. In addition, congenital viral infections are an important cause of blindness, particularly rubella, which leads to cataracts, microphthalmus, and cytomegalic inclusion disease with retinal involvement.

Among the viral infections limited to the outer eye and manifested as a follicular conjunctivitis are epidemic keratoconjunctivitis, herpes simplex keratoconjunctivitis, Newcastle disease virus (NDV) conjunctivitis, and acute hemorrhagic conjunctivitis.

Epidemic keratoconjunctivitis (EKC) Adenovirus types 8 and 19 are the usual cause of epidemics of EKC, although milder cases may be associated with other adenovirus types. The most common method for transmission of EKC is through manipulation of the eye by medical personnel, e.g., for foreign-body removal in industrial dispensaries (thus the name "shipyard eye") or during an ophthalmologic examination. The virus, which is unusually resistant to inactivation, is transmitted on the fingers, by instruments, or in solutions. Medical personnel not infrequently contract the disease and may act as a source of infection for patients.

Following an incubation period of 5 to 12 days, EKC presents a moderate to very severe follicular conjunctivitis with preauricular lymphadenopathy that is usually unilateral at onset. Severe cases may have subconjunctival hemorrhages and conjunctival membrane formation with subsequent conjunctival scarring. In adults, the associated systemic manifestations are minimal with little if any fever, headache, or malaise, but in children adenovirus type 8 infections may present as febrile upper respiratory disease, or otitis media, with only a minor conjunctivitis; such children may be a source of infection for adults. In EKC, the usual onset of focal corneal involvement is 7 days after onset of conjunctivitis when there is a severe foreign-body sensation, photophobia, and lacrimation. As the conjunctivitis subsides during the second week of the disease,

subepithelial corneal opacities 1 to 2 mm in diameter appear, and these opacities may persist for 2 years or longer.

There is no specific treatment for the acute stage of EKC, but the late opacities can be suppressed temporarily with topical corticosteroids if vision is impaired. Explosive epidemics in industrial dispensaries and ophthalmologists' offices can be prevented or controlled by scrupulous hand washing, adequate cleansing of instruments, and replacement of eye drops to break the chain of infection. Medical personnel with conjunctivitis should not come into contact with patients.

Herpes simplex virus (HSV) keratoconjunctivitis Occasionally HSV produces an acute follicular conjunctivitis that is usually accompanied by one or multiple herpetic skin vesicles on the eyelids. In children this may be the primary herpetic infection, but in adults the conjunctivitis is often a recurrent herpetic infection at a new site. The skin lesions may be inconspicuous, misdiagnosed as a sty, or even not present, so that the disease is indistinguishable from early EKC. The cornea may have focal epithelial lesions, a typical linear, branching (dendritic) ulcer, or no involvement at all. The conjunctivitis usually resolves in 2 weeks. If definite herpetic lid lesions are present or if HSV is isolated, treatment with a topical antiviral (idoxuridine, adenine arabinoside, or trifluorothymidine) should be given three to four times daily to prevent corneal involvement. Overt dendritic ulcerations or other corneal involvement should be treated more vigorously as described in Chap. 193. Topical corticosteroids should not be used in acute HSV infections of the eye except in rare instances and then under frequent supervision by an ophthalmologist.

Newcastle disease virus conjunctivitis Human infection with this avian virus, which is related to influenza, occurs mainly in poultry workers, veterinarians, and virologists. In humans, accidental introduction of contaminated material from naturally infected animals or from live virus (e.g., vaccines) is followed in 24 to 72 h by conjunctivitis, edema of the lids, and tearing. Systemic symptoms occur very rarely, and recovery is complete in 10 to 14 days. The diagnosis may be confirmed by virus isolation in embryonated eggs.

Acute hemorrhagic conjunctivitis (AHC) This disease was first described in 1969 in epidemics in Africa and Asia. It presents as an acute conjunctivitis with numerous punctate hemorrhages on the bulbar conjunctiva which become confluent within 24 h. There is also minor involvement of the cornea. The inflammation subsides in 4 to 5 days, but the hemorrhages do not resolve for 7 to 10 days. The only reported complication has been the rare occurrence of lumbar radiculomyelitis with resultant flaccid paralysis like poliomyelitis. Enterovirus 70 (a member of the picornavirus group) has been identified as the etiologic agent in most epidemics, but some outbreaks have been caused by coxsackievirus A24, another picornavirus. Epidemics of AHC have occurred in the crowded urban populations of developing countries, affecting all age groups and social classes. Occasional outbreaks in Europe have been centered around eye clinics. The disease has not been reported in the Western Hemisphere.

TREATMENT *Chlamydia trachomatis* strains are susceptible to the sulfonamides, tetracyclines, and erythromycin. Public health control programs for endemic trachoma consist of the mass application of tetracycline or erythromycin ointment to the eyes of all children in affected communities for 21 to 60 days or on an intermittent schedule. These programs also include surgical correction of inturned eyelids by a mobile surgical team that visits each locality. At one time systemic sulfonamides for 3 weeks were utilized, but the rate of untoward reactions was unacceptably high. Oral erythromycin, but not oral tetracyclines, offers a useful alternative method of mass antibiotic treatment for trachoma of young children and pregnant women.

Adult inclusion conjunctivitis responds well to treatment with full doses of systemic tetracycline or erythromycin for 3 weeks. Treating all sexual consorts of the patient simultaneously is also necessary to prevent ocular reinfection and to avoid the genital diseases due to chlamydial infection. Topical antibiotic treatment is not required in patients treated with systemic antibiotics.

PREVENTION Efforts to develop a practical trachoma vaccine have not been successful. General hygienic measures associated with improved living standards are effective in the elimination of trachoma. Adequate water supply for personal cleanliness may be a key factor. In some areas the reduction of flies in the household is important. In order to prevent spread of trachoma to uninfected family members, treatment of healthy contacts with antibiotic ointment may be effective.

NONGONOCOCCAL URETHRITIS AND OTHER GENITAL INFECTIONS

SPECTRUM OF *C. TRACHOMATIS* GENITAL INFECTIONS In adults the newly defined clinical spectrum of sexually transmitted *C. trachomatis* infections is easily understood because it parallels exactly the spectrum of gonococcal infections (Table 174-1). Although the causal role of *C. trachomatis* is not firmly established, both agents have been associated with urethritis, epididymitis, mucopurulent cervicitis, acute salpingitis, bartholinitis, and the Fitz-Hugh–Curtis syndrome (perihepatitis), and both can be associated with systemic complications, particularly with arthritis. The etiologic significance of *C. trachomatis* infection in certain of these syndromes, such as the Fitz-Hugh–Curtis syndrome and Reiter's syndrome, requires further study. The possible role of *C. trachomatis* in idiopathic proctitis in homosexual men and in women remains to be defined.

EPIDEMIOLOGY Genital infections other than LGV are caused by *C. trachomatis* immunotypes D through K. Although data are lacking, the incidence of genital *C. trachomatis* infection is probably increasing, since the incidence of nongonococcal urethritis (NGU) has risen dramatically over the last two decades, and *C. trachomatis* has consistently been isolated from 30 to 50 percent of men with NGU. The peak age incidence of genital *C. trachomatis* infections is in the late teens and early twenties, resembling other sexually transmitted infections. Further evidence for sexual transmission is the rising prevalence of serum antibody to *C. trachomatis* in proportion to an increasing number of sex partners of infected individuals. In the United States, the prevalence of *C. trachomatis* in the cervix of pregnant women is five to ten times higher than that of *N. gonorrhoeae*. The prevalence of genital infection with either agent is highest in individuals who are indigent, nonwhite, unmarried, and between ages 18 and 24. The ratio of chlamydial to gonococcal urethritis is highest for heterosexual men and those with high socioeconomic status, and lowest for homosexual men and indigent populations. The ratio of symptomatic to asymptomatic infections appears to be lower for *C. trachomatis* than for *N. gonorrhoeae*, as does the clinical severity of symptomatic infections. However, because the total number of *C. trachomatis* infections exceeds that of *N. gonorrhoeae* infections in industrialized countries, the total morbidity caused by *C. trachomatis* genital infections is comparable with that caused by *N. gonorrhoeae*. The prevalence of *C. trachomatis* is higher than that of *N. gonorrhoeae* in industrialized countries, in part because measures such as treatment of sex partners and routine cultures for case detection in asymptomatic individuals are being applied much more effectively for gonorrhea control than for control of *C. trachomatis* infection.

Nongonococcal and postgonococcal urethritis Nongonococcal urethritis is a diagnosis of exclusion that is applied to men with symptoms and/or signs of urethritis who do not have gonorrhea. Postgonococcal urethritis (PGU) refers to nongonococcal urethritis which develops 2 to 3 weeks after treatment of gonococcal urethritis in men. *Chlamydia trachomatis* causes 30 to 50 percent of the cases of NGU and PGU. The cause of the remainder is uncertain, although considerable evidence suggests that *Ureaplasma urealyticum* causes an additional 30 to 40 percent.

DIAGNOSIS The most suitable method for diagnosis of *C. trachomatis* urethritis is isolation of the agent in tissue cell culture. It is necessary to insert an endourethral swab 1 to 2 cm into the urethra to obtain an adequate specimen, since cultures of expressed exudate lack sensitivity, as do direct Giemsa-stained or immunofluorescent smears. Serologic techniques are as difficult to perform as culture, and serologic diagnosis by microimmunofluorescence (micro-IF) testing of serum requires demonstration of IgM antibody (lacking in the many patients who have previously experienced infection with the same immunotype) or a fourfold rise in antibody titer in paired serums. Because *C. trachomatis* infections are often mild, many patients do not seek therapy until it is too late to demonstrate a rise in antibody titer. Serologic techniques, therefore, often cannot differentiate current from past infections.

Where culture is not available, current practice is to diagnose NGU by documentation of a leukocytic urethral exudate and by exclusion of gonorrhea by Gram's stain or culture, rather than to pursue a specific etiologic diagnosis of NGU. *Chlamydia trachomatis* urethritis is generally less severe than gonococcal urethritis, although in an individual patient these two forms of urethritis cannot be differentiated solely on clinical grounds. Symptoms include urethral discharge, dysuria, and urethral itching, and there are meatal erythema and tenderness and a urethral exudate which is often demonstrable only by stripping the urethra in the morning before voiding. A substantial proportion of men with *C. trachomatis* urethral infection have no demonstrable signs and may or may not have symptoms of urethritis. An estimated 5 to 10 percent of male STD clinic patients have asymptomatic *C. trachomatis* urethral infection. Such patients frequently have first glass pyuria (15 leukocytes per 400× microscopic field in the sediment of first-

TABLE 174-1
Similarity of clinical manifestations of sexually transmitted infections caused by *Neisseria gonorrhoeae* and *Chlamydia trachomatis*

Site of infection	N. gonorrhoeae	C. trachomatis
MALE		
Urethra	Urethritis	Urethritis
Epididymis	Epididymitis	Epididymitis
Systemic	Disseminated gonococcal infection	Reiter's syndrome
FEMALE		
Cervix	Cervicitis	Cervicitis
Salpinx	Salpingitis	Salpingitis
Urethra	Urethritis	Urethral syndrome
Bartholin's gland	Bartholin's gland abscess	Bartholin's gland abscess

voided early morning urine) or an increased number of leukocytes on gram-stained smear prepared from a urogenital swab inserted 1 to 2 cm into the anterior urethra. The smear is first scanned at low power to identify areas of the slide containing the highest concentrations of leukocytes. These areas are then examined under oil immersion (1000×). An average of four leukocytes in five 1000× (oil immersion) fields is indicative of urethritis and correlates with recovery of *C. trachomatis.* To differentiate between true urethritis and functional symptoms among symptomatic patients, or to make a presumptive diagnosis of *C. trachomatis* infection in asymptomatic men [e.g., male patients in sexually transmitted disease (STD) clinics, sex partners of women with nongonococcal salpingitis or mucopurulent cervicitis, fathers of children with inclusion conjunctivitis], the examination of an endourethral specimen for increased leukocytes is useful.

Epididymitis *Chlamydia trachomatis* is also a cause of epididymitis in sexually active males. In one study, *C. trachomatis* infection was found by cultures of the urethra, urine, semen, or epididymal aspirate or by serology in 11 of 13 men under 35, but in 1 of 10 over 35 who presented with epididymitis. Coliform bacteria and *Pseudomonas aeruginosa* are the most common causes of epididymitis in men over 35. The presence of a urethral discharge in association with epididymitis suggests the diagnosis of chlamydial or gonococcal epididymitis, whereas the presence of midstream pyuria and bacteriuria in an older patient without urethral discharge suggests coliform or *Pseudomonas* infection.

Reiter's syndrome In recent studies, *C. trachomatis* has been recovered from the urethra from up to 70 percent of men with untreated Reiter's syndrome who have associated urethritis. This striking association is unexplained.

Genital *C. trachomatis* infection in women As with gonococcal infection, in recent studies *C. trachomatis* has been isolated from the cervix of 30 to 60 percent of women with gonorrhea, or contact with gonorrhea, from 10 to 20 percent of women attending sexually transmitted disease clinics who do not have a history of contact with a partner with urethritis, and from about 5 percent of United States college students, or young women attending gynecology clinics or prenatal clinics.

CERVICITIS Although many women with *C. trachomatis* cervical infection have a normal cervix or only nonspecific changes, there is a significant correlation of this infection with endocervicitis, manifested by mucopurulent exudate in the cervical os. A distinctive pattern of hypertrophic (edematous and congested) cervical erythema and increased friability also may be seen. Herpes simplex virus causes inflammation and ulceration of the exocervix, rather than of the endocervix alone, but can be confused with gonococcal or chlamydial cervicitis. The presence of mucopurulent endocervicitis suggests the presence of *C. trachomatis* or *N. gonorrhoeae* infection. If tests for gonorrhea are negative, nongonococcal endocervicitis should be treated with tetracycline, just as nongonococcal urethritis is treated, and male sex partners should be examined for NGU.

SALPINGITIS AND PERIHEPATITIS *Chlamydia trachomatis* has recently been implicated as a cause of acute salpingitis. In one study, it was isolated from the cervix of 19 of 53 women with acute salpingitis verified by laparoscopy, and it was recovered from the fallopian tube in the absence of other pathogens from six of seven who had *C. trachomatis* in the cervix.

A related development is the demonstration of IgM antibody to *C. trachomatis,* suggestive of recent *C. trachomatis* in-

fection, in 7 of 11 women with acute peritonitis and or perihepatitis (Fitz-Hugh–Curtis syndrome).

OTHER MANIFESTATIONS *Chlamydia trachomatis* has also been isolated from the rectum of 10 percent of women with genital chlamydial infection and from pus expressed from Bartholin's gland in association with bartholinitis. Other data suggest that *C. trachomatis* is a cause of some cases of the urethral syndrome in women.

CHLAMYDIA TRACHOMATIS INFECTION IN PREGNANCY *Chlamydia trachomatis* infection in pregnant women entails a risk of transmitting infection to the neonate. *Chlamydia trachomatis* in pregnancy also has been associated with fetal wastage and with a high risk of postpartum endometritis and salpingitis. Whether these complications are attributable to *C. trachomatis* remains to be determined. If so, detection and treatment of *C. trachomatis* in the mother and father early during pregnancy may be particularly important.

THERAPY OF GENITAL *C. TRACHOMATIS* INFECTION Therapy of *C. trachomatis* urethritis is more effective than therapy of other forms of NGU. *Chlamydia trachomatis* is eradicated from the urethra by treatment with tetracycline hydrochloride, 500 mg four times daily for 7 days. Alternative regimens which are also effective include erythromycin, 500 mg four times daily for 14 days, and sulfisoxazole, 500 mg four times daily for 10 days. However, sulfonamides are not effective for *Chlamydia*-negative NGU. Minocycline and doxycycline are more active than tetracycline against *C. trachomatis* in vitro and are effective clinically in a dose of 100 mg daily for 7 days. *Chlamydia trachomatis* is not reliably eradicated by single-dose therapy with any antimicrobial.

Eradication of *C. trachomatis* from the cervix has been demonstrated with similar doses of tetracycline and erythromycin. Erythromycin base, 500 mg four times daily for 7 to 10 days, is the regimen of choice for pregnant women with *C. trachomatis* infection. Tetracycline hydrochloride, 500 mg four times daily for 10 days, produces clinical and microbiological cure of epididymitis or salpingitis associated with *C. trachomatis* infection.

Treatment of sex partners The increase in genital *C. trachomatis* infections is related in part to changes in sexual behavior, but probably is also due to failure of the medical profession to diagnose and treat *C. trachomatis* infections in symptomatic patients or their sexual partners. Cases of NGU, epididymitis, Reiter's syndrome, and mucopurulent endocervicitis are frequently not treated with antimicrobials, and sex partners are treated even less often. Furthermore, even though 20 percent of men and 30 to 60 percent of women with gonorrhea have concurrent *C. trachomatis* infection, only one of the four treatment regimens recommended by the Center for Disease Control for gonorrhea (tetracycline, but not single-dose procaine penicillin G, ampicillin, or spectinomycin) eradicates *C. trachomatis. Chlamydia trachomatis* urethral or cervical infection has been well documented in the sex partners of patients with NGU, epididymitis, Reiter's syndrome, salpingitis, or endocervicitis. This is analogous to the problem of asymptomatic gonococcal infection in sex partners of patients with gonorrhea. In the absence of facilities for specific diagnosis of *C. trachomatis* infection, sex partners of patients with symptoms that are attributable to *C. trachomatis* infection should be examined and counseled. Those partners who themselves have clinical evidence of *C. trachomatis* infection clearly should be treated with an effective antimicrobial. Even those without evidence of clinical disease, who have been recently exposed to possible chlamydial infection (e.g., NGU), should probably also be offered therapy.

NEONATAL INCLUSION CONJUNCTIVITIS AND PNEUMONIA

EPIDEMIOLOGY Several studies in the United States have found *C. trachomatis* infections of the cervix in from 5 to 13 percent of pregnant women. In these studies from 3 to 6 percent of the newborn children showed laboratory evidence of *C. trachomatis* infection. Roughly half of the infants born to mothers with cervical infection developed laboratory evidence of infection, and half of these (or 25 percent of the group exposed) developed clinical inclusion conjunctivitis. In addition to eye infection, the *C. trachomatis* organisms were isolated frequently and persistently from the nasopharynx and even the rectum. Pneumonia and otitis media have also been shown to result from these birth canal infections.

INCLUSION CONJUNCTIVITIS OF THE NEWBORN (INCLUSION BLENNORRHEA) In the newborn, inclusion conjunctivitis can be differentiated from gonococcal ophthalmia by its longer incubation period (5 to 14 days versus 1 to 3 days). The other common causes of conjunctivitis in newborns include *Staphylococcus aureus, Hemophilus influenza,* and herpes simplex virus. Neonatal inclusion conjunctivitis has an acute onset and produces a profuse mucopurulent discharge with membrane formation and occasional scar formation on the conjunctiva. Inclusions within epithelial cells usually can be demonstrated in Giemsa-stained conjunctival smears. Relapses of the eye disease are frequent following treatment with topical tetracycline ophthalmic ointment. The therapy recommended is oral erythromycin (40 to 50 mg per kilogram of body weight) for 2 to 3 weeks. Rarely a trachoma-like eye disease with chlamydial infection occurs in children living in nonendemic areas and probably is the late result of neonatally acquired infection.

INFANT PNEUMONIA There is a distinctive pneumonia syndrome in infants infected with *C. trachomatis,* which appears to occur in two to six cases per 1000 live births. This pneumonia has been found in infants from 1 to 4 months of age. The onset is gradual and the course protracted, but the child is usually afebrile. There is diffuse interstitial involvement of the lungs. Most of the infants have a distinctive cough (a series of closely spaced staccato coughs, each separated by a brief inspiration), tachypnea, rales, hyperinflation, slight eosinophilia, and elevated serum immunoglobulins. Clinical illness lasts several weeks, while inspiratory rales and radiological signs may persist for months. About half of the infants with pneumonia also have conjunctivitis. While many of the pneumonia cases have recovered without therapy, a few have been severe. The diagnosis of *C. trachomatis* pneumonia has been confirmed by isolation of the organisms from lung biopsy. A probable diagnosis can be made by isolation of organisms from the nasopharynx, eye, or rectum, and by demonstration of a rising titer of IgG antibody (passively acquired maternal antibody will decrease) or by the presence of specific IgM antibody. Specific treatment with oral systemic erythromycin should be accompanied by supportive measures. Because *C. trachomatis* causes disease in adults, both parents should be treated with systemic erythromycin (especially nursing mothers) or tetracyclines.

LYMPHOGRANULOMA VENEREUM

DEFINITION Lymphogranuloma venereum (LGV) is a sexually transmitted infection caused by *C. trachomatis.* The acute disease in men is characterized by a transient primary genital lesion followed by multilocular suppurative regional lymphadenopathy. Women, homosexual men, and occasionally, heterosexual men may develop hemorrhagic proctocolitis with regional lymphadenitis. Acute LGV is almost always associated with nonspecific systemic symptoms, usually with fever and leukocytosis, and rarely with systemic complications such as meningoencephalitis. After a latent period of years, late complications include genital elephantiasis, strictures, and fistulas of the penis, urethra, and rectum.

ETIOLOGY Only three immunotypes of *C. trachomatis,* designated L_1, L_2, and L_3, cause LGV, with L_2 being most common. LGV immunotypes also have other distinguishing biological characteristics: they are more invasive than the other immunotypes of *C. trachomatis,* cause disease primarily in lymphatic tissue, grow more readily in tissue culture, and are pathogenic when inoculated intracerebrally into mice and monkeys.

EPIDEMIOLOGY Lymphogranuloma venereum usually is sexually transmitted, but occasional transmission by nonsexual personal contact, fomites, or laboratory accidents has been documented. The peak incidence corresponds to the age of greatest sexual activity, the second and third decades of life. The worldwide incidence of LGV is falling, for unexplained reasons, but the disease is still endemic and a major cause of morbidity in certain countries of Asia, Africa, and South America. In the United States, only 348 cases were reported during 1977, of which about one-third were from Washington, D.C.

Prevalence studies of LGV are difficult to interpret. Most have employed the Frei skin test or LGV complement fixation (CF) serologic test. Since the antigens used in these tests cross-react with other strains of *C. trachomatis* which are much more widely prevalent in developed countries than the three LGV strains, the specificity of the Frei and LGV CF tests is open to question. For example, 18 percent of patients attending a STD clinic had positive skin tests and 2 percent had high LGV titers, but only 1 percent had signs of LGV. Of the cases reported to the Center for Disease Control in 1977, many were based on the LGV CF test and could not be confirmed by the more specific microimmunofluorescence test.

The frequency of infection following exposure is believed to be much less than that associated with gonorrhea and syphilis. Early manifestations are recognized far more often in men than in women, who usually present with late complications. In the United States, where the reported sex ratio is 3.4 males to 1 female, most cases involve travelers, seamen, and military personnel returning from abroad; male homosexuals; and individuals of low socioeconomic status living in areas of low endemicity in the Southeast. The main reservoir of infection in the United States is presumed to be asymptomatically infected individuals, but attempts to isolate LGV strains from the urethra or cervix of sexually active persons without clinical LGV have been unsuccessful.

CLINICAL MANIFESTATIONS A *primary genital lesion* occurs from 3 days to 3 weeks after exposure. It is a small, painless vesicle or nonindurated ulcer or papule located on the penis in men or on the labia, posterior vagina, or fourchette in women. The primary lesion is noticed by less than one-third of men with LGV and only rarely by women. It heals in a few days without scarring and even when noticed is not recognized as LGV except in retrospect when it is followed by or merges with lymphadenitis. LGV strains of *C. trachomatis* have occasionally been recovered from the male urethra and the endocervix of patients who present with inguinal adenopathy, suggesting that these areas may be the primary site of infection in some cases.

In women and homosexual men, *primary anorectal infection* occurs following rectal intercourse. In women, this may also occur by spread via the pelvic lymphatics, or by direct spread of infection from the genitalia along the perineum to the anal canal. Anorectal colonization also occurs in women with cervical infections and in homosexual men. After an incubation period of unknown length, multiplication within intestinal epithelial cells leads to symptoms which include mucopurulent or bloody anal discharge, tenesmus, and diarrhea. Sigmoidoscopy reveals diffuse proctitis or discrete ulcerations limited to the rectosigmoid colon.

From the site of the primary infection, the organism spreads via the regional lymphatics. Penile, vulvar, and, occasionally, anal infection can lead to inguinal and femoral lymphadenitis. Anorectal infection produces hypogastric and deep iliac lymphadenitis. Upper vaginal or cervical infection results in enlargement of the obturator and iliac nodes. The most common presenting picture in heterosexual men is the *inguinal syndrome*. This also occurs in about 10 percent of men with anorectal infection. It is characterized by painful inguinal lymphadenopathy beginning 2 to 6 weeks after presumed exposure; rarely the onset occurs after a few months. The inguinal adenopathy is unilateral in two-thirds of cases, and palpable enlargement of the iliac and femoral nodes is often present on the same side as the enlarged inguinal nodes. The nodes are initially discrete, but progressive periadenitis results in a matted mass of nodes which become fluctuant and suppurative. The overlying skin becomes fixed, inflamed, and thinned and finally develops multiple draining fistulas. Extensive enlargement of chains of inguinal nodes above and below the inguinal ligament ("the sign of the groove") is characteristic but is present in only a minority of cases (Fig. 174-1). Histological involvement of nodes initially shows characteristic small stellate abscesses surrounded by histiocytes. These abscesses coalesce to cause large, necrotic, suppurative foci. Spontaneous healing usually occurs after several months, leaving inguinal scars or granulomatous masses of varying size which persist for life. Massive pelvic lymphadenopathy in women or homosexual men may lead to exploratory laparotomy.

Constitutional symptoms are common during the state of regional lymphadenopathy and include fever, chills, headache, meningismus, anorexia, myalgias, and arthralgias. These findings in the presence of lymphadenopathy are often mistaken

FIGURE 174-1

Lymphogranuloma venereum. Bilateral inguinal buboes, with the "sign of the groove," caused by adenopathy above and below Poupart's ligament. (Courtesy of A Brathwaite.)

for malignant lymphoma. Other systemic complications are infrequent but include arthritis with sterile effusion, aseptic meningitis, meningoencephalitis, conjunctivitis, hepatitis, and erythema nodosum. Chlamydiae have been recovered from the cerebrospinal fluid, and in one case from the blood in a patient with severe constitutional symptoms, indicating the occurrence of disseminated infection. Associated laboratory findings during the acute stage of infection include leukocytosis and mild elevation of the sedimentation rate. Abnormal liver function tests, hyperglobulinemia, mixed cryoglobulinemia, rheumatoid factor activity, and elevated IgG, IgA, and IgM have been reported in subacute and chronic LGV. False-positive serologic tests for syphilis are rare, and syphilis should be suspected if these tests are positive, as is often the case.

Complications of anorectal infection include perirectal abscess, fistula in ano, and rectovaginal, rectovesical, and ischiorectal fistulas. Secondary bacterial infection probably contributes to these complications. Rectal stricture is a late complication of anorectal infection and usually occurs 2 to 6 cm from the anal orifice, within reach on digital rectal examination. The stricture may extend proximally for several centimeters, leading to a mistaken clinical and radiographic diagnosis of carcinoma.

Approximately 5 percent of cases of LGV in men present with chronic progressive infiltrative, ulcerative, or fistular lesions of the penis, urethra, or scrotum. Urethral stricture may occur and usually involves the posterior urethra, causing incontinence or difficulty with micturition.

An uncommon late complication of LGV is *genital elephantiasis*, a chronic induration and edema of the penis or vulva caused by lymphatic obstruction. Polypoid swelling of the skin and large stellate hyperplastic keloidal scars of the genitalia may be associated with vulvar induration or lymphedema and are difficult to distinguish clinically from granuloma inguinale and genital tuberculosis. Chronic ulcerations of the vulva (esthiomene) and smooth pedunculated perianal growths (lymphorrhoids) also occur. The significance of reports of malignant changes associated with chronic anorectal or genital LGV is uncertain.

DIAGNOSIS Although LGV is uncommon, it frequently enters the differential diagnosis of common conditions such as inguinal lymphadenopathy; vesicular, papular, or ulcerative genital lesions; and perirectal abscess, fistula in ano, or proctocolitis. When methods for culture and serodiagnosis become more available, diagnostic testing for LGV in these conditions should increase.

The most reliable method of diagnosis is isolation of an LGV strain of *Chlamydia* from aspirated bubo pus or from the urethra, endocervix, or infected tissue. Isolation has been possible from bubo pus in about 30 percent of cases with both clinical and serologic evidence of LGV. The methods needed for isolation in tissue cell culture are widely available but seldom used. The most widely used immunodiagnostic tests have been the LGV complement fixation test and the Frei skin tests. The LGV complement fixation test becomes positive (serum titer $\geq$ 1:32) shortly after the bubo first appears and is positive in 80 to 90 percent of patients with the inguinal syndrome. The titer may not increase in paired serums since most patients have already been infected for several weeks when first seen. The Frei skin test is less sensitive than the LGV complement fixation test. It is performed by intradermal inoculation of 0.1 ml of a crude antigen prepared from infected yolk sac into the flexor surface of the forearm. The test is read at 72 h and is positive ($\geq$ 6 mm induration and erythema at the site of antigen inoculation, with no induration at the site of normal yolk sac control inoculation) in less than 50 percent of patients who present with the inguinal syndrome. The frequency of positive skin tests increases with the duration of untreated infection, and positive tests remain positive for life. *A negative Frei test does not exclude the diagnosis of LGV.* Conversely, a positive LGV complement fixation test or Frei skin test may not be specific for LGV. When other causes of inguinal or pelvic lymphadenopathy are suspected clinically, a positive Frei or LGV CF result should not unduly delay definitive diagnostic testing, which often means lymph node aspiration or excisional biopsy.

However, two serologic tests for LGV have been developed which appear to be both sensitive and specific. Limited experience indicates that the microimmunofluorescent antibody test developed by Wang detects antibody to *C. trachomatis* in nearly all patients with culture-proved LGV. Serum microimmunofluorescent antibody titers from patients with LGV exceed the highest titers that occur in chlamydial NGU and can usually be shown to be directed against immunotypes L_1, L_2, or L_3. A counterimmunoelectrophoresis test has also been developed using the soluble *C. trachomatis*-specific antigen extracted from the LGV strain. This test is positive in over 95 percent of patients whose microimmunofluorescent test shows antibody to LGV strain, but is negative in patients with chlamydial NGU. The histopathology of excised nodes or of rectal biopsy specimens is seldom definitive, but suggestive findings may raise the question of LGV and lead to more specific tests.

TREATMENT LGV chlamydiae are susceptible in vitro to the tetracyclines, sulfonamides, erythromycin, rifampin, and chloramphenicol and are slightly sensitive to the penicillins. They are resistant to the aminoglycosides such as streptomycin, as well as to bacitracin, vancomycin, and the polymyxins. Occasional isolates have been resistant to sulfonamides. Despite their in vitro activity, antibiotics do not have a dramatic effect on the duration and healing of inguinal buboes. However, acute constitutional symptoms are often terminated abruptly. Antibiotics are usually not helpful in improving late complications such as rectal stricture or genital elephantiasis unless secondary infection is also present. Genital elephantiasis and rectal, penile, and urethral strictures and fistulas require surgical correction, although sometimes urethral and even rectal strictures can be managed by repeated mechanical dilation.

The recommended treatment regimen is tetracycline hydrochloride, 0.5 g four times a day for 3 or 4 weeks. A sulfonamide preparation, 4 g per day for 3 or 4 weeks, can also be used, but occasional isolates have been resistant to sulfonamides in vitro. Fluctuant buboes should be aspirated through normal skin with a syringe and 18-gauge needle as often as necessary to prevent spontaneous rupture. It is not unusual for buboes to increase in size or to develop at another site after initiation of treatment. Although these seldom progress to fistula formation, they should be aspirated if fluctuant. A fourfold or greater fall in complement fixation titer occurs in most treated patients, and LGV *Chlamydia* cannot be isolated from lesions after the initiation of antibiotic treatment.

REFERENCES

General

SCHACHTER J, DAWSON CR: *Human Chlamydial Infections.* Littleton, Mass, PSG Medical Books, 1978

Lymphogranuloma venereum

ABRAMS AJ: Lymphogranuloma venereum. JAMA 205:199, 1968
CALDWELL HD, KUO CC: Serologic diagnosis of lymphogranuloma venereum by counterimmunoelectrophoresis with a *Chlamydia trachomatis* antigen. J Immunol 118:442, 1977
GREAVES AB: The frequency of lymphogranuloma venereum in persons with perirectal abscesses, fistula-in-ano, or both. Bull WHO 29:797, 1963
HOPSU-HAVU VK, SONCK CE: Infiltrative, ulcerative, and fistular le-

sions of the penis due to lymphogranuloma venereum. Br J Vener Dis 49:193, 1972
KING AF et al: Intradermal tests in the diagnosis of lymphogranuloma. Br J Vener Dis 32:208, 1956
SCHACHTER J et al: Lymphogranuloma venereum: I. Comparison of the Frei test, complement fixation test, and isolating the agent. J Infect Dis 120:372, 1969

Neonatal inclusion conjunctivitis and pneumonia

BEEM MO, SAXON EM: Respiratory tract colonization and a distinctive pneumonia syndrome in infants infected with *Chlamydia trachomatis.* N Engl J Med 296:306, 1977
HARRISON JR et al: *Chlamydia trachomatis* infants pneumonitis. N Engl J Med 298:702, 1978

Nongonococcal urethritis

BERGER RE et al: *Chlamydia trachomatis* as a cause of acute "idiopathic" epididymitis. N Engl J Med 298:301, 1978
BOWIE WR et al: Etiology of nongonococcal urethritis: Evidence for *Chlamydia trachomatis* and *Ureaplasma urealyticum.* J Clin Invest 59:735, 1977
HOLMES KK et al: Etiology of nongonococcal urethritis. N Engl J Med 292:1199, 1975
MARDH PA et al: *Chlamydia trachomatis* infection in patients with acute salpingitis. N Engl J Med 296:1377, 1977
REES E et al: Chlamydia in relation to cervical infection and pelvic inflammatory disease, in *Nongonococcal Urethritis and Related Infections,* D Hobson, KK Holmes (eds). Washington, DC, American Society for Microbiology, 1977, pp 67–76

Trachoma and inclusion conjunctivitis

DAWSON CR et al: Infections due to adenovirus type 8 in the United States: III. Epidemiological, clinical and microbiological features of epidemic keratoconjunctivitis. Am J Ophthalmol 69:473, 1970
────── et al: Blinding and nonblinding trachoma. Bull WHO 52(3):279, 1975
──────, TOGNI B: Herpes simplex eye infections: Clinical manifestations, pathogenesis and management. Surv Ophthalmol 21:121, 1976
GRAYSTON JT et al: Epidemic keratoconjunctivitis on Taiwan. Am J Trop Med 13:492, 1964
HALES RH, OSTLER HB: Newcastle disease conjunctivitis with subepithelial infiltrates. Br J Ophthalmol 57(9):694, 1973
MORDHORST CH et al: Childhood trachoma in a nonendemic area. JAMA 283:1765, 1978
O'DAY DM et al: Clinical and laboratory evaluation of epidemic keratoconjunctivitis due to adenovirus types 8 and 19. Am J Ophthalmol 81(2):207, 1976
WHITCHE JP et al: Acute hemorrhagic conjunctivitis in Tunisia: Report of viral isolations. Arch Ophthalmol, January 1976

175
PSITTACOSIS

VERNON KNIGHT

DEFINITION Psittacosis is an infectious disease of birds caused by an organism that has a number of properties in common with gram-negative bacteria. Transmission of infection from birds to humans results in a febrile illness characterized by pneumonitis and systemic manifestations. Inapparent infections or mild influenza-like illnesses may also occur. The term *ornithosis* is sometimes applied to infections contracted from birds other than parrots or parakeets, but *psittacosis* is the preferred generic term for all forms of the disease.

ETIOLOGY The causative agent *Chlamydia psittaci* is a gram-negative obligate intracellular parasite, formerly classified as a virus. Now chlamydias, along with the rickettsias, may be considered specialized bacteria. Both synthesize ribonucleic acid (RNA) and deoxyribonucleic acid (DNA), reproduce by binary fission, and are susceptible to antimicrobial drugs. In contrast to rickettsias, the chlamydias are dependent on their hosts for metabolic energy. Slight but definite homology of the DNA of members of the *Chlamydia* genus with the DNA of *Neisseria meningitidis* has been shown. The psittacosis agent is the prototype of a biologically and antigenically homogeneous class of microorganisms that includes the causative agents of lymphogranuloma venereum, trachoma, and 30 or more mammalian parasites which rarely produce human disease.

EPIDEMIOLOGY Psittacosis is widely distributed throughout the world, and almost any avian species can harbor the agent. Psittacine birds are most commonly infected, but human cases have been traced to contact with pigeons, ducks, turkeys, chickens, and many other birds. Psittacosis may be considered an occupational disease of pet-shop owners, poultry raisers, pigeon fanciers, taxidermists, and zoo attendants. The incidence of human infection in the United States rose steadily from 1930, owing in large measure to the increasing popularity of parrots and parakeets as pets and, as subsequently recognized, transmission of infection by barnyard fowl and pigeons. The number of reported cases reached a peak in 1956 and gradually declined thereafter. By 1963, with acceptance of control measures such as incorporation of tetracyclines in poultry feed, the disease had again become relatively uncommon. However, in recent years the disease has increased with cases occurring primarily among employees of poultry processing plants. In 1976 a plant in Nebraska experienced an outbreak involving 28 of 98 employees, whose disease was contracted from turkeys shipped from Texas. Other outbreaks of this type have occurred. In 1975 and 1976, 58 and 80 cases of psittacosis, respectively, were reported to the Center for Disease Control. The disease appears to be more common in England, where budgerigars are common household pets and where restrictions on the importation of these birds have been eased.

The agent is present in nasal secretions, excreta, tissues, and feathers of infected birds. Although the disease can be fatal, infected birds frequently show only minor evidence of illness, such as ruffled feathers, lethargy, and anorexia. Asymptomatic avian carriers are common, and complete recovery may be followed by continued shedding of the organism for many months.

Psittacosis is almost always transmitted to humans by the respiratory route and one-half or more of patients infected in fowl-processing plants may have pneumonia indicative of aerosol transmission of the infection. On rare occasions the disease may be acquired from the bite of a pet bird. Intimate and prolonged contact is not essential for transmission of the disease; a few minutes spent in an environment previously occupied by an infected bird has resulted in human infection. The severity of the disease in humans bears no apparent relationship to closeness or duration of contact, although sick birds are more likely to transmit infection than healthy ones. Transmission of a psittacosis-like agent between humans has occurred among hospital personnel, with severe and sometimes fatal infections. There is evidence that these "human" strains are more virulent than native avian organisms. There is no record of infection acquired by eating poultry products.

PATHOGENESIS The psittacosis agent gains entrance to the body through the upper part of the respiratory tract and eventually localizes in the pulmonary alveoli and in the reticuloendothelial cells of the spleen and liver. Invasion of the lung probably takes place by way of the bloodstream rather than by direct extension from the upper air passages. A lymphocytic inflammatory response occurs on both the interstitial and respiratory surfaces of the alveoli as well as in the perivascular spaces. The alveolar walls and interstitial tissues of the lung are thickened, edematous, necrotic, and occasionally hemorrhagic. Histologically, the affected areas show alveolar spaces filled with fluid, erythrocytes, and lymphocytes. The picture is not pathognomonic of psittacosis unless macrophages containing characteristic cytoplasmic inclusion bodies (LCL bodies) can be identified. The respiratory epithelium of the bronchi and bronchioles usually remains intact.

MANIFESTATIONS The clinical manifestations and course of psittacosis are extremely variable. After an incubation period of 7 to 14 days, or longer, the disease may start abruptly with shaking chills and fever ranging as high as 105°F, but the onset is often gradual with increasing fever over a 3- to 4-day period. Headache is almost always a prominent symptom; it is usually diffuse and excruciating and often the patient's chief complaint.

Many patients present with a dry hacking cough which is usually nonproductive, but small amounts of mucoid or bloody sputum may be raised as the disease progresses. Cough may appear early in the course of the disease or as late as 5 days after the onset of fever. Chest pain, pleurisy with effusion, or a friction rub may all occur but are rare. Pericarditis and myocarditis have been reported. Most patients have a normal or slightly increased respiratory rate; marked dyspnea with cyanosis occurs only in severe psittacosis with extensive pulmonary involvement. In psittacosis, as in most nonbacterial pneumonias, the physical signs of pneumonitis tend to be less prominent than symptoms and x-ray findings would suggest. The initial examination may reveal fine, sibilant rales, or clinical evidence of pneumonia may be completely lacking. Rales usually become audible and more numerous as the illness progresses. Signs of frank pulmonary consolidation are usually absent. Symptoms of upper respiratory tract infection are not prominent, although mild sore throat, pharyngeal infection, and cervical adenopathy are often present; on occasion they may be the only manifestations of illness. Epistaxis is encountered early in the course of nearly one-fourth of the cases. Photophobia is also a common complaint.

There is commonly a complaint of generalized myalgia, and spasm and stiffness of the muscles of the back and neck may lead to an erroneous diagnosis of meningitis. Lethargy, mental depression, agitation, insomnia, and disorientation have been prominent features of the illness in some epidemics, but not in others; delirium and stupor occur near the end of the first week in severe cases. Occasional patients are comatose when first seen, and the diagnosis of psittacosis may be missed. Gastrointestinal complaints such as abdominal pain, nausea, vomiting, or diarrhea are present in some cases; constipation and abdominal distention sometimes occur as late complications. Icterus, the result of severe hepatic involvement, is a rare and ominous finding. A faint, macular rash (Horder's spots) simulating the rose spots of typhoid fever has been described.

Patients without cough or other clinical evidence of respiratory involvement come to the physician with fever of unknown origin. The pulse rate is slow in relation to the fever. When splenomegaly is present in a patient with acute pneumonitis, psittacosis should be considered; the reported incidence of splenomegaly ranges from 10 to 70 percent. Nontender hepatic enlargement also occurs, but jaundice is rare. Thrombophlebitis is not unusual during convalescence; indeed, pulmonary infarction is sometimes a late complication and may be fatal.

In untreated cases of psittacosis, sustained or mildly remittent fever persists for 10 days to 3 weeks, or occasionally as long as 3 months. Defervescence is by lysis and is accompanied by abatement of respiratory manifestations. Psittacosis contracted from parrots or parakeets is more likely to be a severe, prolonged illness than infections acquired from pigeons or barnyard fowl. Relapses occur but are rare. Secondary bacterial infections are uncommon. Immunity to reinfection is probably permanent.

Laboratory findings The x-ray of the lungs in psittacosis mimics that in a great variety of pulmonary diseases. The pneumonic lesions are usually patchy in appearance but can be hazy, diffuse, homogeneous, lobar, atelectatic, wedge-shaped, nodular, or miliary. The white blood cell count is normal or moderately decreased in the acute phase of the disease but may rise in convalescence. The erythrocyte sedimentation rate is frequently not elevated. Transient proteinuria is common. The cerebrospinal fluid sometimes contains a few mononuclear cells but is otherwise normal. Cold agglutinins are rarely present.

The diagnosis can be confirmed only by isolation of the causative microorganism or serologic studies. The agent is present in the blood during the acute phase of the disease and in the bronchial secretions for weeks or sometimes years after infection, but it is difficult to isolate. Psittacosis is most readily diagnosed by the demonstration of a rising titer of complement-fixing antibody in the patient's blood. An acute and convalescent specimen should always be tested. Even a low titer of antibody during the acute febrile phase constitutes presumptive evidence of psittacosis. The prompt initiation of treatment with tetracycline has been shown to delay antibody rise in convalescence for several weeks or months. Interpretation of a single complement fixation test may sometimes be difficult because of the antigenic cross reaction between the agent of psittacosis and that of lymphogranuloma venereum.

Differential diagnosis A history of exposure to birds may be the only clinical basis for differentiating psittacosis from a great variety of infectious and noninfectious febrile disorders. A partial list of pneumonic disease that may be confused with psittacosis includes *Mycoplasma* pneumonia, Q fever, coccidioidomycosis, tuberculosis, carcinoma of the lung with bronchial obstruction, and bacterial pneumonias. In the early stages, before pneumonitis appears, psittacosis may be mistaken for influenza, typhoid fever, miliary tuberculosis, and infectious mononucleosis. A newly described entity, Legionnaires' disease (Chap. 138), caused by a difficult-to-cultivate gram-negative bacillus, causes pneumonia similar to psittacosis.

Treatment The tetracyclines are consistently effective in the treatment of psittacosis. Defervescence and alleviation of symptoms usually occur in 24 to 48 h after instituting therapy with 2 g daily in four divided doses. To avoid relapse, treatment should probably be continued for at least 7 days after defervescence. In severe cases, oxygen and other supportive measures are indicated.

REFERENCES

CENTER FOR DISEASE CONTROL: Morb Mort Week Rep 25:301, October 1, 1976
————: *Psittacosis Annual Summary, 1974,* June 1975.

section 13 | Viral diseases

176
INTRODUCTION TO VIRUS INFECTIONS: CLASSIFICATION, PATHOGENESIS, EPIDEMIOLOGY, DIAGNOSIS, AND CONTROL

A. MARTIN LERNER

Clinical virology has passed from the unitary realm of the research physician. Knowledge of the clinical syndromes associated with specific viruses, understanding of appropriate diagnostic tests, and utilization of available means for prevention and therapy are required of all internists. Common virus infections vary from inapparent to life threatening. Rapid progress continues. Of particular note have been (1) recognition of the causes of viral gastroenteritis, (2) further definitions of immunopathologic mechanisms of hepatitis viruses, and (3) definitive evidence for therapeutic efficacy of intravenous adenine arabinoside (ara-A) in disseminated varicella-zoster and herpes simplex virus encephalitis.

GENERAL PROPERTIES AND CLASSIFICATION OF VIRUSES
Viruses are grouped according to their biophysical characteristics: (1) presence of nucleic acid, (2) size, (3) sensitivity to

ether, (4) presence of an envelope, and (5) symmetry (cubic or helical). They contain macromolecular cores of ribonucleic acid (RNA) or deoxyribonucleic acid (DNA), but not both. (On the other hand, chlamydiae, *Mycoplasma,* and Rickettsiae contain both RNA and DNA.) Viruses have marked species and organ specificities, and on the whole, viruses infecting plants, insects, rickettsiae, bacteria, and other animals are distinct from their human counterparts.

Human viruses range in size from 17 nm (picornavirus) to 300 nm (poxvirus). They may be naked and contain only nucleic acid (genome) which is protected by a closed shell or tubing, the capsid. Other viruses have, in addition, a lipid envelope, acquired during maturation as virus evaginates from the nucleus (herpes simplex virus) or cytoplasm (influenza, herpes simplex virus). The lipid coat of these viruses surrounds the capsid. The capsid consists of protein and is composed of repeating subunits, capsomeres. Mature virus particles are called *virions* (Fig. 176-1). Specific antigens of the capsid may penetrate the lipid envelope.

The nucleic acid contains all the genetic material necessary to reproduce itself (transcription) and code for structural proteins and enzymes (translation) important in synthesis and attachment to susceptible cells. The nucleic acid core plus the capsid is known as the *nucleocapsid.* When the virion is stripped of its capsid, nucleic acid may enter a host of foreign

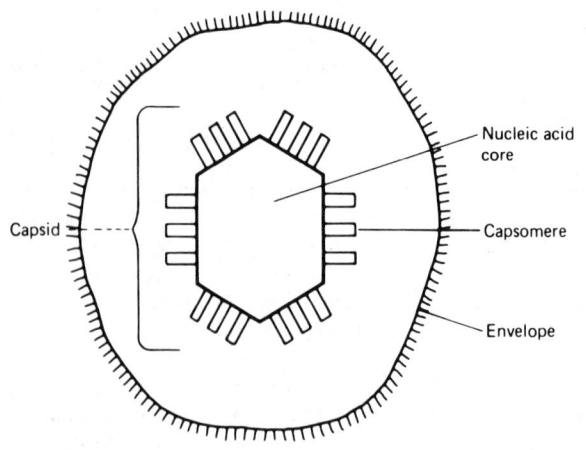

FIGURE 176-1

Components of a complete virus particle (virion).

species and produce a single cycle of mature virus (e.g., poliovirus in mouse renal cells). Species and organ specificities of virus-cell union are functions first of complementary physical characteristics and then of covalent union between proteins of the virus and susceptible cell membranes. For instance, molecules of neuraminic acid act as receptors on human red blood cells, allowing hemagglutination by influenza virus. Within several hours after virus adsorption, neuraminidase, one of the proteins of the influenza capsid, digests the neuraminic acid. Elution of influenza virus from red blood cells follows. Cells which allow virus multiplication are termed *permissive*, while those which do not are termed *nonpermissive*. The membrane fit may be HLA dependent and change with aging of the host. Some virus-cell unions may be permissive at one temperature

(37°C) but not at the lower temperatures of the upper respiratory tract (~30°C).

At present, there are seven known groups of RNA viruses (picornavirus, reovirus, arbovirus, myxovirus, rhabdovirus, coronavirus, arenavirus) and four groups of DNA viruses (papovavirus, adenovirus, herpesvirus, poxvirus) (Table 176-1). Nucleic acids of infectious and serum hepatitis viruses have not been absolutely identified. However, the agents of hepatitis A and non-A, non-B resemble RNA-containing enteroviruses, while hepatitis B has a herpesvirus-like lipid coat and contains a DNA genome. Rotaviruses (reovirus-like) and parvoviruses are recently discovered causative agents of viral gastroenteritis.

VIRUS MULTIPLICATION Virus adsorption is a specific physical and then chemical reaction. After absorption, virus enters the cell by pinocytosis and is uncoated; i.e., nucleic acid is stripped from the capsid. With DNA viruses, specific virus DNA strands are transcribed into specific messenger RNA (mRNA) which is then translated to synthesize virus-specific proteins and enzymes necessary for biosynthesis of virus DNA. In the case of virus RNA, single-stranded RNA serves as its own messenger. The mRNA is translated, resulting in the formation of an RNA polymerase. Synthesis of host cell protein and nucleic acid is suppressed to variable degrees. Assembly of protein subunits around virus DNA results in formation of complete virions which may be released by cell lysis or budding from the cytoplasm. Virions of RNA tumor viruses contain an enzyme which is capable of catalyzing synthesis of DNA. The product consists of small fragments of DNA, most of which are complementary in base sequence to 70S RNA of the virion. Thus, information can travel not only from DNA to RNA but also, at least in certain cases, in the reverse direction.

Virus multiplication may lead to a cytolytic infection with release of virus with necrosis of the infected cell, but other infections are persistent or latent and may reactivate at a later

Major groups of viruses infecting human beings

Generic name, nucleic acid, and prototype virus	Size, nm	Ether sensitive	Envelope	Symmetry
Picornavirus (RNA) Coxsackieviruses A and B; echo-, rhino-, and polioviruses	17–30	No	No	Cubic
Reovirus (RNA)	74	No	No	Cubic

Arbovirus (RNA)
  Group A (equine encephalitis, Semliki Forest)
  Group B (Japanese B, Russian tick-borne, yellow fever, dengue)
  Group C (Morituba, Oriboca)
  Ungrouped (Rift Valley, Colorado tick fever, sandfly)
	20–100	Yes	?	

Myxovirus and paramyxovirus (RNA) Influenza A, B, and C: parainfluenza, mumps, rubeola; respiratory syncytial	80–200	Yes	Yes	Helical
Rhabdovirus: rabies (RNA)	65–180	Yes	Yes	
Coronavirus (RNA)		Yes	Yes	

Arenavirus (RNA)
  Togavirus: rubella (most arboviruses of groups A and B)
  Tacaribe-LCM: lymphocytic choriomeningitis, South American hemorrhagic fevers (Lassa, Machupo)
	50
	50–300
		Yes
		Yes
			Yes
			Yes	

Papovavirus (DNA) Warts, simian virus 40	45–55	No	No	Cubic
Adenovirus (DNA)	65–85	No	No	Cubic
Herpesvirus (DNA) Herpes simplex, monkey B, varicella-herpes zoster, cytomegalovirus, Epstein-Barr	120–180	Yes	Yes	Cubic
Poxvirus (DNA) Variola, vaccinia, molluscum contagiosum, orf (milker's nodules)	150–300	Yes or no	Yes	Cubic

Classifications incomplete
  Hepatitis A: "Enterovirus-like"
  Hepatitis, non-A, non-B: "Enterovirus-like"
  Hepatitis B: Nucleic acid is DNA, contains lipid coat
  Rotavirus (arbovirus, duovirus): "Reovirus-like"
  Parvovirus (Norwalk, Hawaii, Montgomery County agents)				

time. In turn, the virus nucleic acid may become incorporated into the genome of the cell leading to malignant transformation. Virus infection may also lead to fusion of cellular membranes (giant cells) or demyelinization.

PATHOGENESIS OF VIRUS INFECTIONS The primary site of virus multiplication depends upon the route of acquisition and the special receptor-site complementarity of the host (Table 176-2). The modes of transmission of human virus infections

773

CHAPTER 176
INTRODUCTION TO VIRUS INFECTIONS: CLASSIFICATION, PATHOGENESIS, EPIDEMIOLOGY, DIAGNOSIS, AND CONTROL

are: respiratory, alimentary, contact (mucosal, bite, injection), or transplacental. Respiratory viruses are also exchanged by kissing or by the hands. The hands are also vital in fecal virus transfers.

Virus-specific structures (inclusion bodies) may be present within the cytoplasm (variola), nucleus (herpes simplex virus, varicella-zoster, adenovirus), or both (measles) of infected cells. Viremia may or may not occur. In many virus infections, in distinct contrast to bacteremias, viremia occurs during the incubation period when the patient is well. Viremia is usual with the exanthems of enteroviruses, rubeola, and varicella-zoster. Herpesviruses may multiply within lymphocytes sequestered from antibodies and phagocytes when there is no viremia. During coxsackievirus B3 viremia in mice, virus is present in the plasma, but erythrocytes, polymorphonuclear leukocytes, and platelets do not contain virus. On the third day of this plasma viremia infectious T and B lymphocyte-virus complexes circulate. Secondary sites of infection may be heart, liver, pancreas, kidneys, or brain.

RESPONSES OF THE HOST At sites of virus multiplication extracellular virus often abounds. Macrophages and a few polymorphonuclear leukocytes migrate to the area producing inflammation. Interferon (see below) is produced locally, and B and T lymphocytes appear. Macrophages attach to antigen markedly augmenting the efficiency of virus inactivation by specific neutralizing antibodies or sensitized T lymphocytes. During the first days of many virus infections there is a circulating lymphopenia of both B and T cells. Lymphocytes migrate to sites of infection and to the liver, spleen, or other organs of the mononuclear phagocytic system.

Interferon Viruses, endotoxin, certain parasites, and double-stranded RNA synthetic polyribonucleotide complexes such as polyinosinic polycytidilic ribonucleic acid (poly rI:rC) stimulate interferon, an antiviral protein. Within several hours after onset of virus infection, and days before humoral antibodies can be measured by ordinary methods, interferon is found in tissues where virus is synthesized and in the blood. Interferon is probably most effective as an antiviral substance early in infection when viral titers are low. Later, interferon's effect on virus in tissues is small. Interferon also has an important function as an immunoregulatory substance, either stimulator or depressor, depending upon the time during infection.

A delay in the appearance of interferon in vesicular fluid has been associated with viremic dissemination in herpes zoster. Likewise, decreased in vitro responsiveness of the patient's lymphocytes after stimulation by herpes simplex virus in the production of interferon has been correlated with recurrences of herpes labialis. Severe repetitive and exhausting exercise in mice infected with coxsackievirus B3 results in a delay in the appearance of circulating interferon and, later, in both a delay and a depression in the quantity of type-specific neutralizing antibody in serum. A marked increase in the quantity of myocardial virus and mortality follows. Exercise augmentation of coxsackievirus B3 virulence is also associated with thymic atrophy. Rest may be a very important factor in recovery from virus infections.

Interferons of two classes are produced. The first, a high-molecular-weight protein (8.5×10^4 daltons), is preformed and released within 2 h after infection. At 18 h, the serum contains proteins with biologic activity of interferon with molecular weights of 3 to 4×10^4 daltons. Interferon is acid-stable (pH 2), trypsin-sensitive, nondialyzable, and nonsedi-

TABLE 176-2
Modes of transmission of human viruses

Mode of transmission*	Symptoms/ other	Viruses
Respiratory (droplets or droplet-nuclei in air, bites, salivary transfer, mouth to hand or object)	Local	Adenoviruses (many serotypes) Rhinoviruses (many serotypes) Influenza viruses A, B, C Parainfluenza viruses (several serotypes) Coronaviruses (many serotypes)
	General	Varicella-zoster; Epstein-Barr (EB) virus Variola (smallpox) Rubella Mumps; rubeola (measles) Lymphocytic choriomeningitis; Lassa virus
Alimentary	Local	Adenoviruses (a few serotypes) Enteroviruses (a few serotypes) Parvoviruses (Norwalk agent) Reoviruses (including rotavirus)
	General	Enteroviruses (many serotypes, including polioviruses) Hepatitis viruses A, B, non-A, non-B
Contact (skin)		Papilloma (warts) Herpesviruses [herpes simplex viruses, type 1 (oral) and 2 (genital)]; EB virus Molluscum contagiosum; cowpox; milker's nodes
Arthropod bite	General	California encephalitis virus Western equine encephalitis virus Venezuelan equine encephalitis virus St. Louis encephalitis virus Colorado tick fever virus (reovirus-like orbivirus)
Animal bite	General	B virus Rabies virus
Infection by transfusion	General	Hepatitis B Cytomegalovirus (CMV); EB virus; hepatitis B; hepatitis, non-A, non-B
Transplacental	General	CMV Rubella
Instruments	Tonometer (examination for glaucoma)	Adenoviruses
	Corneal transplants	Jakob-Creutzfeldt "viroid"
	Neurosurgical or ophthalmologic procedures	
	Electrodes (electroencephalograms)	

* *Prevention and isolation/control are specifically directed by understanding the mode of transmission.*

mentable by ultracentrifugal forces sufficient to pellet viruses. Most cells tested produce interferon, but those of the reticuloendothelial system (especially the spleen) and lymphocytes are particularly important.

Interferon has no effect upon extracellular virus. Following entry of virus nucleic acid into a susceptible cell, the cell nucleus is stimulated to produce interferon. Interferon is released through the cytoplasm of the infected cell. Synthesis of virus-directed coat proteins and enzymes is prevented. New virus is not formed.

Interferons are not virus-specific and are active against a wide variety of viruses. However, interferon is an effective antiviral substance only in cells of the same species in which it is produced. For instance, anti-influenza A interferon produced in hamster tissue cultures is effective against influenza in hamsters but not in humans. Likewise, interferon produced in human leukocytes or human tissue cultures is effective in humans.

Viruses vary greatly in their sensitivity to interferon. Myxoviruses are quite sensitive, while herpesviruses are more resistant. The importance of interferon in recovery from virus infection probably varies. With coxsackievirus B3, interferon titers in tissues actually parallel virus titers. In animal models, interferon has been shown to have a prophylactic effect in a number of virus infections, but once the titers of virus are high, interferon is ineffective.

Antibodies Proteins of the virus capsid stimulate B lymphocytes (immunoglobulin-bearing, bone marrow-derived) to synthesize humoral antibodies (IgM, IgG, IgA, IgD) and secretory antibodies (IgA). Cell-associated antibodies (IgE) are also produced. Immunoglobulins are synthesized in local lymph nodes, at body surfaces (saliva, respiratory secretions, colostrum), and in inflammatory exudates within organs (kidney, brain, cervix). During the first 3 to 10 days after an initial exposure to a virus, IgM antibodies predominate. Later, IgG antibodies prevail. Immunoglobulin M is important in clearing viremias remaining within vascular spaces; IgG antibodies also enter interstitial spaces. On surfaces, IgA antibodies contain an added secretory piece, allowing their functional integrity in the presence of hydrolytic enzymes of the secretions. Many molecules of antibody combine with a single virion. Covering a critical number of essential sites on the virion renders an antigen-antibody complex noninfectious. Antigen-antibody complexes attract components of complement which are the mediators for chemotaxis of polymorphonuclear leukocytes. Immune complexes may be fixed in tissues, circulate or precipitate in the glomerulus, in the synovia of joints, or in the skin.

Secretory IgA antibodies in respiratory secretions are vital to the body's defenses against respiratory viruses. During viral respiratory infections viremia does not occur regularly. Humoral antibodies persist only for months. Immunity is transient and reinfections with the same virus occur. On the other hand, after systemic infections, humoral antibodies and immunity persist. After administration of killed virus vaccines immunity is also briefer than that which follows attenuated virus vaccines.

Circulating neutralizing antibody is effective protection against viremia, except possibly against very large inocula or in the presence of low antibody titers. Some viruses multiply and spread from cell to cell even in the presence of neutralizing antibodies. Herpes simplex virus, type 1, and rubeola in nervous tissues are examples. Cell-mediated immunity is the most important means of defense against herpesviruses, while antibody is vital to recovery from enteroviruses. In some cases antibodies or T lymphocytes (cytotoxic "killer" cells) may be

important in continuing the pathogenic process. Cytolytic T cells may be directed against neoantigens induced by, but biochemically different from, any structural component of the virus. This appears to be the pathogenetic mechanism in chronic murine coxsackievirus B3 myocardiopathy.

Antibodies to viruses are measured by neutralization of their cytopathic effects in tissue cultures, or by protection tests using embryonated eggs or animals. Complement fixation, precipitin, indirect hemagglutination, fluorescent antibody, immune hemadsorption, and radioimmunoassay are among the techniques used to measure viral antibodies. Early after infection, certain viruses such as herpes simplex virus, type 1, and cytomegalovirus induce complement-requiring neutralizing antibodies. Myxoviruses, some enteroviruses, and reoviruses hemagglutinate several species of red blood cells. In these cases antibodies can be measured by inhibition of hemagglutination. Virus capsids of nonhemagglutinating viruses may be absorbed to the surface of tanned sheep red blood cells. Antibodies are then assayed by indirect hemagglutination. Kinetics of rises and falls of the several antibodies suggest that different assays may test separate immunoglobulin responses to distinct proteins of the virus capsid.

Cell-mediated immunity Thymic-derived T lymphocytes are responsible for cellular immune functions. In most virus infections, both T and B lymphocytes participate in the containment of virus replication. After a latent period, usually lasting 3 to 4 days, stimulated T lymphocytes transform to lymphoblasts. They release a number of nonspecific, nondialyzable effector molecules which migrate with albumin on electrophoresis. Among these effector molecules are lymphocyte-transforming factor, migration-inhibitory factor, cytotoxin factor, and interferon. Components of complement react with the surface of sensitized lymphocytes, releasing a chemotactic factor to monocytes, which are the important phagocytes in cellular immunity. After stimulation by an antigen, evoking a potent T-lymphocyte response, macrophages are "activated," becoming more efficient phagocytes. This increased phagocytic ability of activated macrophages is not limited to the stimulating virus.

There are at least three subpopulations of T lymphocytes: T_o (cytolytic cells, antigen specific, without receptors for the F_c portion of immunoglobulin molecules); T_m (helper cells with F_c receptors on their surface for IgM); and T_g (suppressor cells with F_c receptors on their surface for IgG). T_m cells are necessary for a sustained IgG response. The elucidation of the functions of these T-cell subpopulations will clarify understanding of the pathogenesis of virus infections.

EPIDEMIOLOGY OF VIRUS INFECTIONS Virus infection occurs with disease, or it may be asymptomatic. Clinical illness is the rule with measles (rubeola virus), but inapparent infection is common with enteroviruses. The severity of disease may also be age-related. In adults, chickenpox and mumps are often severe with complications (varicella pneumonia, mumps orchitis, or encephalitis) which are rare during childhood.

The *incidence* of infection is the number of new cases of a disease occurring in a unit of time, while the *incidence rate* is the number of new cases occurring divided by the number of persons in the total population at risk in the area being studied. The incidence rate is usually calculated as the ratio of the number of new clinical cases divided by the population under surveillance in a given year. Incidence rates may also be calculated by measuring virus excretion or rises in antibody titers using acute and convalescent phase serums.

The *prevalence* is the number of cases of a disease existing at one time, while the *prevalence rate* is the number of cases of a given disease at one time divided by the population at risk. The *point prevalence* or *period prevalence* may be calculated.

Unlike most bacterial infections, isolation of virus from an ill patient and even demonstration of a fourfold rise in specific antibodies to that virus in temporally related acute and convalescent serums does not always prove a causative relation to the illness in question. Epidemiologic support is often required for firm etiologic associations. Age-matched, sex-matched, and time- and place-matched controls (compeer groups) must be studied in the same manner as the patients in question. The families of patients are an excellent group to examine. Inapparent simultaneous infection must be sought. Patients within the hospital as well as persons living in the immediate neighborhood of the patient are also often studied. Virus isolation and/or antibody rises in a patient group in significant excess over controls are strong evidence for an etiologic association. In this regard, *serologic epidemiology* is the systematic testing of blood specimens from a defined sample of a healthy population for the presence of antigens, antibodies, or other components.

Virus infections often occur in clusters of cases determined by the presence of the virus in the community and the susceptibility (antibody titers to the virus) of the population. An *epidemic* or outbreak is present when the number of cases is in excess of the expected number at that locality based upon past experience. For instance, an increased incidence of a mix of viral respiratory infections and pneumonias is expected each winter, but influenza epidemics occur over 4- to 6-week intervals only every several years. On the other hand, the occurrence of only a dozen cases of St. Louis encephalitis in Michigan during the late summer would constitute an epidemic.

Influenza A epidemics often affect several continents at the same time. When this occurs, *pandemic* influenza is present. Epidemic influenza B is rarely pandemic.

When an epidemic of echovirus type 9 aseptic meningitis occurs in the summer months, most cases of meningitis (often with rash) during mid- to late summer are due to this agent. However, each case must be studied individually so that discovery of the occasional case of bacterial meningitis or herpes simplex virus encephalitis is certain to be made.

The greater the number of persons immune to a given virus among the population of an area, the less is the likelihood of disease due to that agent among that population at that time. "Population immunity," or *herd immunity,* is usually measured by the presence of neutralizing or other protective antibodies. Susceptibles in the population are protected because of the high number of persons in the group who are immune.

The *incubation period* is the time period from first exposure to first symptom. With short incubation periods of 2 to 4 days (e.g., enteroviruses), multiple cases of illness occur at the same time. With longer incubation periods (e.g., several weeks as with chickenpox), illnesses occur sequentially. If common exposure to several persons occurs, illness may be simultaneous irrespective of the length of the incubation period.

An appropriate environment is necessary for the spread of human disease. Mosquito-borne St. Louis encephalitis ends with effective mosquito control or after the first frost. Respiratory contagion is facilitated by rebreathed air laden with aerosolized virus from coughs, sneezes, or speech. Droplets of water over 10 μm in size containing virus travel short distances through air, while droplet nuclei, minus moisture and less than 10 μm in size, waft over greater distances. Successful primary infection in a susceptible host depends upon (1) the number of virions circulating per cubic foot of air, and (2) the time of exposure which, in turn, determine the total size of the inoculum. For instance, if an aerosol contains four virions per liter of air and 30 virions are required for infection, then persons breathing this air will inspire an infectious dose within a half-hour. The smaller number of respiratory infections during summer may be due to the multiple exchanges of air that result from open windows. In hospitals, walls reaching to the ceilings

and closed doors are required for adequate respiratory isolation.

DIAGNOSIS OF VIRUS INFECTIONS   Isolation or recognition of viruses   Materials for virus isolation must be obtained as early during illness as possible. The earlier the specimen is taken, the higher is the titer of virus usually present, and the more likely that the specimen will be positive. Generally, specimens are collected in sterile screw-capped vials containing a balanced salt solution with antibiotics. Depending upon the pathogenesis of the particular infection, throat swab (or sputum), stool (or rectal swab), cerebrospinal fluid (CSF), urine, vesicular fluid, or tissues (biopsy or autopsy) should be obtained for inoculation into susceptible tissue cultures (or mice), prepared for electron microscopy, immunofluorescent radioimmunoassay, or enzyme-linked immunoassay (ELISA). These procedures can recognize viral antigens. If the specimen cannot be processed immediately, it should be frozen promptly to $-70°$C.

Vesicles should be opened and fluids or scrapings inoculated for virus. Scrapings and impression smears should be stained with Tzanck, Wright, and Gram's stains. Instructions relating to collection of specimens for various clinical syndromes are listed in Table 176-3.

Serologic tests   At the initial visit with a patient suspected of a viral illness a sample of 10 ml blood should be taken and allowed to clot. The serum should be separated to prevent hemolysis which can interfere with diagnostic tests. A second sample of blood should be obtained 2 to 3 weeks later. Both serums should be sent simultaneously to the virus diagnostic laboratory. Changes in antibody titers are most meaningful when paired serums are tested concomitantly.

Neutralization, complement fixation, hemagglutination inhibition, indirect hemagglutination, immunofluorescence, immune adherence hemagglutination, radioimmunoassay, and ELISA are procedures used to measure viral antibodies. After systemic viral infections neutralizing antibodies confer long-lasting immunity. Complement-fixing antibodies, on the other hand, often fall (or disappear) with convalescence. Particular tests are most appropriate for certain viruses (Table 176-4).

Isolation of virus coupled with a fourfold or greater rise in antibody titers between acute and convalescent-phase specimens is diagnostic of recent infection but is not necessarily diagnostic of the clinical syndrome in question. The most striking example of the possible disparity in isolation of virus and its etiologic relationship is herpes simplex virus (HSV), type 2, the cause of herpes labialis and HSV encephalitis. Biopsy of the brain is required for definitive diagnosis of HSV encephalitis. Rises in complement-fixing antibodies to HSV occur with herpes labialis which may accompany pneumococcal meningitis. Nevertheless, in most virus infections fourfold rises in specific antibodies strongly suggest the proper diagnosis. Cross-reactive antibodies among enteroviruses and among herpesviruses are possible and can be confusing. Isolation of virus from diseased tissues is definitive.

Group-specific antibody tests (e.g., group B arboviruses, influenza A, influenza B) often employ the complement-fixation method and are helpful, lessening the number of diagnostic antigens which must be available. If an initial serum is taken later in the illness, a high single titer or high constant titers in both acute and convalescent serums may be found. Single high titers are probably diagnostic if the disease is rare in the area, if the antibody is short-lived (e.g., complement fixing), or if the

TABLE 176-3
Appropriate specimens for virus isolation (or recognition)

Clinical syndrome	Viruses	Throat/ sputum*	Stool/ rectal swab*	CSF*	Urine*	Vesicular fluid*	Other
Meningitis-encephalitis	Mumps	+	−	+	+	None	Usually none
	Enteroviruses: Coxsackieviruses, group A or B	+	+	+	−‡	+†	Blood, brain, skeletal muscle, heart, pericardial fluid, testicle
	Echoviruses	+	+	+	−‡	+†	
	Polioviruses	+	+	−	−	None	Brain, spinal cord
	Herpes simplex: Type 1	+	−	−	−‡	+	Brain, buffy
	Type 2	+	−	+	−	+	coat of blood
	Arboviruses	−	−	+	−	None	Brain
Respiratory diseases	Influenza/parainfluenza viruses	+§	−	−	−	None	Lung, blood, heart
	Rhinoviruses	+	−	−	−	None	Usually none
	Adenoviruses	+	+	−	+	None	Conjunctiva
	Enteroviruses (see above)						
Exanthems	Rubeola (measles)	+	−	−	+	None	Brain
	Rubella	+	−	−	+	None	Brain
	Variola	+	−	−	−	+	
	Vaccinia	−	−	−	−	+	
	Varicella-zoster	−	−	−	−	+	Lung, heart
	Herpes simplex (see above)						
	Enteroviruses (see above)						
Myopericarditis	Enteroviruses (see above)						
Hepatitis	Hepatitis A and non-A, non-B	−	¶	−	−	None	
	Hepatitis B	−	−	−	−	None	Blood ¶
Virus diarrheas	Rotaviruses	−	¶	−	−	None	
	Parvoviruses	−	¶	−	−	None	
Other	Cytomegalovirus	−	−	−	+	None	Buffy coat of blood
	Progressive multifocal leukoencephalopathy	−	−	−	+	None	Brain
	Jakob-Creutzfeldt disease	−	−	?	−	None	Brain, eye

* +, present; −, absent.
† Vesicles are only occasionally present during coxsackievirus or echovirus infections.
‡ These viruses have occasionally been isolated from urine.
§ These viral antigens can also be promptly recognized in these specimens by immunofluorescent methods.
¶ Hepatitis A and non-A, non-B have been recognized by immune electron microscopy in feces. These viruses "appear" similar to enteroviruses. They have not yet been isolated in tissue cultures. Hepatitis B has been recognized by electron microscopy in blood and liver but has not yet been grown in tissue cultures. Diagnosis is usually made by immunochemical studies of blood (see Table 176-4). HBs, HBe, and DNA polymerase also identify this virus infection. Rotaviruses and parvoviruses have been recognized in feces of patients by immune electron microscopy, radioimmunoassay for virus antigen, and enzyme-linked immunoassay (ELISA) for virus antigen.

antibody is IgM. A fourfold fall in antibody titers is also suggestive. Similar paired serums may be tested from other members of the patient's family for they may be in different stages of apparent or inapparent infection with the same virus.

Nucleic acid hybridization using tumors may recognize viral nucleic acids implicating these viruses in the case of cancers. Herpes simplex virus, type 2, has been linked to cervical cancer and Epstein-Barr virus with Burkitt's lymphoma.

PREVENTION OF VIRUS DISEASES Prevention of virus disease has been achieved largely through the development of viral vaccines, either live attenuated and "killed" or inactivated. Inactivated vaccines are generally available for influenza A, influenza B, rabies, and polioviruses, and on a limited and/or experimental basis inactivated viral vaccines have been developed for adenovirus, Japanese-B, equine, and Russian spring-summer encephalitis. Vaccines derived from attenuated tissue cultures are available for rubella, mumps, measles, poliomyelitis, and yellow fever. Indications for use of these vaccines are discussed in Chap. 114.

Passive immunization with pooled human immune serum globulins or globulins with high titers to specific agents such as rabies, hepatitis B, or varicella has also been used in the prophylaxis of virus infections. These preparations generally are most useful when given early during the incubation period in order to prevent clinical illness. In selected instances, use of hyperimmune globulins may be useful in ameliorating illness once symptoms have developed. Lassa fever is an example. Specific indications for the use of passive immunization in the treatment and prevention of viral infections are discussed in Chap. 114.

Patients with slow virus infections of the central nervous

TABLE 176-4
Serologic tests employed in virus infections

Virus	Complement fixation	Neutralization	Hemagglutination inhibition	Indirect hemagglutination	Immunofluorescence	Immune adherence hemagglutination	Radioimmunoassay	ELISA	Immune electron microscopy
Mumps	+								
Enteroviruses		+							
Herpes simplex viruses	+			+	+	+		+	
Arboviruses	+		+						
Influenza/parainfluenza	+		+		+				
Rhinoviruses	+	+							
Adenoviruses	+								
Rubeola (measles)	+				+				
Rubella			+						
Variola	+				+				
Vaccinia	+				+				
Varicella-zoster	+			+		+			
Hepatitis A	+					+			
Hepatitis B							+		
Cytomegalovirus	+			+					
Rotavirus	+				+				+
Parvovirus	+				+				+

system (Jakob-Creutzfeldt disease) undergoing neurosurgical or ophthalmologic procedures are contagious by means of contaminated surgical equipment. Prolonged autoclaving (121°C, 15 psi, 60 min) and 5% hypochlorite or iodine soaks for 60 min will inactivate large infective doses of this unusual virus. Chemoprophylaxis against smallpox with oral N-methylisatin β-thiosemicarbazone (Marboran) is effective as is amantadine hydrochloride (Symmetrel) taken by mouth throughout the period of exposure to influenza A. Amantadine is not effective against strains of influenza B.

TREATMENT OF VIRUS INFECTIONS Two topical preparations, idoxuridine and adenine arabinoside, are effective, approved, and available therapeutic agents for herpes simplex virus keratitis. Intravenous adenine arabinoside (ara-A) is also an effective therapeutic agent for the treatment of herpes simplex virus encephalitis occurring after the perinatal period. This agent has its maximal effect when it is begun before the onset of paralysis or coma. Ara-A (IV) is also effective in promoting healing and in limiting dissemination of herpes zoster in immunosuppressed patients. These drugs have minimal toxicity and are available for general use.

Experimental testing of ara-A in other herpesvirus infections as well as in chronic active hepatitis (HBs positive) is underway. Controlled clinical trials have also proved that pharmacological megaunits of leukocytic-derived human interferon are effective therapy for disseminated herpes zoster in immunocompromised patients. Exogenous megaunit human interferon (with or without ara-A) will also suppress HBs antigenemia in chronic active hepatitis. Currently, clinical trials of exogenous human interferon are limited by its small supply and great expense. However, no other antiviral agents have proved efficacy or can be recommended. Corticosteroids suppress leukocyte chemotaxis and T and B lymphocytes; they should not be given during the period of active virus multiplication.

REFERENCES

Evans AS: *Viral Infections of Humans. Epidemiology and Control.* New York, Plenum, 1976

Horsfall FL Jr, Tamm I: *Viral and Rickettsial Infections of Man,* 4th ed. Philadelphia, Lippincott, 1965

Jawetz E et al: *Review of Medical Microbiology,* 11th ed. Los Altos, Lange, 1974

Notkins AL: *Viral Immunology and Immunopathology.* New York, Academic, 1975

Respiratory viruses

177
GENERAL CONSIDERATIONS OF VIRAL RESPIRATORY DISEASES

VERNON KNIGHT

The viral respiratory diseases as a group are responsible for one-half or more of all acute illnesses, and although influenza virus is the only agent among them which causes significant mortality in adults, several different viruses contribute to the 20 percent of childhood mortality due to respiratory disease. Respiratory disease morbidity, due primarily to virus infections, causes 30 to 50 percent of time lost from work by adults, and from 60 to 80 percent of time lost from school by children. These diseases are worldwide, and although studies in many areas are scanty, reports from Great Britain, Western Europe, U.S.S.R., Czechoslovakia, Latin America, and the Orient indicate many common denominators in cause, prevalence, and severity.

Viral respiratory diseases are associated with a spectrum of host responses ranging from asymptomatic carrier states to severe and sometimes fatal pneumonias. There is a recurring pattern of severe illness in infants and young children and of milder disease with increasing age. A few clinical and epidemiologic entities can be recognized without laboratory aids, such as acute respiratory disease (ARD) in military recruits, caused by adenovirus type 4 and rhinovirus coryza in adults. The causative agent in a large proportion of cases, however, cannot be identified with virologic study.

EPIDEMIOLOGY More than 150 serotypes, representing 12 groups of viruses, have been or may be associated with the majority of acute respiratory illness in humans. With the capacity to isolate this large group of agents and with the recognition of the role of *Mycoplasma pneumoniae* (Chap. 172) it is possible to define the cause of many respiratory illnesses. The recent identification of coronaviruses as a cause of respiratory illness increases the potential for diagnosis. Though some of the inability to identify agents is caused by lack of efficient application of known diagnostic methods, it is probable that additional viral and possibly other causes of respiratory illness remain to be discovered.

FREQUENCY AND SEVERITY Since 1957 the National Health Survey has made annual estimates from selected population samples of the incidence of acute respiratory illness in the United States. Since these estimates are designed to measure the socioeconomic impact of illness, cases are reported only if they caused restriction of daily activity or required medical care. There are in excess of 250 million cases of acute respiratory illness in the United States annually, an average of 1.4 illnesses per person per year. Loss of time from work or school averaged 4.2 days for the 80 percent of cases in which some restriction of activity was reported, and about 50 percent of individuals with respiratory disease sought medical attention. Analysis of these data indicates that two-thirds to three-fourths of the cases are caused by viruses; the remaining are divided

principally among infections with *M. pneumoniae,* streptococcal sore throat, bacterial pneumonia, and sinusitis.

In other studies, milder illness has been included, with a corresponding rise in annual frequency of reported cases. The Cleveland Family Study found an annual rate of illness of 6.2 per person per year, amounting to an estimated more than 1 billion cases annually in the United States. The greatest proportion of these illnesses were so mild that they constituted no hazard to health, but they are significant in the spread of infection. In addition, it is known that wholly asymptomatic virus infections occur.

Acute respiratory disease is a special problem in relation to older persons who have chronic bronchitis. It is a familiar finding that those with chronic pulmonary disease often undergo exacerbations of their disease as a consequence of acute respiratory infections. The question also arises whether individuals with chronic pulmonary disease experience more frequent acute respiratory illness than those without such involvement. Monto and Ross have shown that adults with mild or intermittent chronic cough and sputum production and diminished pulmonary function experience more frequent respiratory illness than those who are asymptomatic. The finding was present at different levels of smoking frequency, apparently excluding the role of smoking in the occurrences. There was no unusual concentration of cases among any of the several etiologic agents studied. The higher frequency of infection, the prolonged morbidity due to exacerbations of chronic bronchitis, and the large and increasing numbers of such patients in our aging population identify a major health problem for which there is no present solution.

Age, sex, and seasonal variation Infants and young children have the greatest number of viral respiratory infections; children under 6 may have twice as many illnesses per year as the average for the entire population. Females have more illness than males. This difference is most marked in adults, where the excess is 25 percent. In children respiratory viral infections appear to affect the sexes about equally, but boys have more lower respiratory tract disease with respiratory syncytial virus infection than girls.

There are prominent seasonal differences in the frequency of acute respiratory illnesses; the rates are highest in winter, with about 30 cases per 100 persons per quarter. Illness is least frequent during the summer—about one-third of the maximum. Epidemics of influenza cause pronounced increases in wintertime frequency of respiratory illness and are the most significant cause of mortality among the respiratory viruses. In pandemic years influenza may begin in summer or fall.

ETIOLOGY The known viral causes of acute respiratory disease and their estimated relative frequency in adults and older children in relation to their common patterns of illness are shown in Table 177-1. In younger or older persons the same agents may cause disease but the distribution of cases by etiology will vary.

Viruses, as a group, cause about three-fourths of acute respiratory illness, and nearly one-half of these illnesses are due to one of the rhinoviruses. The principal nonviral causes of respiratory illness are *M. pneumoniae* and hemolytic streptococci.

TABLE 177-1
Patterns of illness with respiratory viruses in older children and adults

Agent	Relative frequency per 100 cases	Manifestation				
		Rhinitis	Pharyngitis	Tracheo-bronchitis	Pneumonia	Constitutional
Rhinovirus*	40	+ +	±	+	Rare	± (usually afebrile)
Herpesvirus*	10	+	+ +	Rare	Rare	+
Influenza A and B viruses	10	+	+	+ +	Severe when present	+ + (high fever common)
Parainfluenza viruses†	8	+	+ +	+ +	Rare except in infants	+
Coronaviruses	8	+	+	+	In infants, also bronchiolitis	+
Respiratory syncytial virus	6	+ +	+	+	As above	+
Adenoviruses	1	+	+ +	+ +	Infants and recruits	+ + (high fever)
Coxsackievirus and echoviruses	<1	±	+	+	No	+ + (fever, visceral, and CNS complications)
Other	13 +	?	?	?	?	?

* College students; lower socioeconomic groups have primary infection earlier.
† Laryngeal involvement common.
NOTE: + + = *severe;* + = *moderately severe;* ± = *mild; ? = unknown or uncommon.*

Table 176-1 shows a current classification of the respiratory viruses based on size, structure, and biochemical and other properties. Adenoviruses and herpesvirus are DNA viruses, while the remainder possess RNA cores. Respiratory tract disease is not known to be associated with particular properties of the viruses except that the long incubation period of adenovirus infection may be related to its longer cycle of replication. The relatively nonspecific response of the respiratory tract to virus infection probably indicates that the target cells of the respiratory tract (i.e., the respiratory epithelium), when damaged by infection, have a limited variability of pathologic response. Classification of viruses will certainly assume greater importance, however, as new chemotherapeutic agents are developed, since many of them will act on specialized viral functions unique to single or related groups of viruses.

CLINICAL MANIFESTATIONS The descriptive term "common cold" was coined to describe the coryzal syndrome before its diverse causes were known. It refers to illness characterized by nasal obstruction and discharge, sneezing, moderate sore throat, and mild constitutional reaction, usually without fever. Patterns of illness shown in Table 177-1 demonstrate that most respiratory viral infections may produce this picture. However, in adults and older children, syndromes more or less restricted to these manifestations are caused by infection with rhinoviruses, respiratory syncytial virus, and coronaviruses. These three groups of viruses may account for as much as two-thirds of cases of acute respiratory viral disease. Herpesvirus causes disease usually localized to the pharynx and tonsils in this age group. The other agents listed, while causing coryzal syndrome, also cause varying degrees of involvement of the lower part of the respiratory tract, with additional symptoms.

The following chapter (Chap. 178) considers six of the seven groups of viruses chiefly responsible for respiratory disease, i.e., rhinoviruses, herpesviruses, parainfluenza viruses, coronaviruses, respiratory syncytial virus, and adenoviruses. Included also is a description of the small contribution to respiratory illness of the enteroviruses, coxsackieviruses A and B, and echoviruses, which are discussed in detail in Chap. 187. Influenza is described in Chap. 179. Respiratory diseases cased by *M. pneumoniae* and the psittacosis agent, both of which resemble viral respiratory diseases, are considered in Chaps. 172 and 175.

REFERENCES

KNIGHT V (ed): *Viral and Mycoplasmal Infections of the Respiratory Tract.* Philadelphia, Lea & Febiger, 1973

MONTO AS, ROSS HW: The Tecumseh study of respiratory illness: X. Relation of acute infections to smoking, lung function and chronic symptoms. Am J Epidemiol 107:47, 1978

178
COMMON VIRAL RESPIRATORY ILLNESSES
Rhinoviruses, herpesviruses, parainfluenza viruses, coronaviruses, respiratory syncytial virus, adenoviruses, coxsackieviruses, and echoviruses

VERNON KNIGHT

RHINOVIRUS INFECTIONS

ETIOLOGY More than 100 types of rhinovirus are known, and others are certain to be found. Some of the clinical properties of rhinoviruses are shown in Table 178-1. They resemble the other picornaviruses in being small (15 to 30 nm), non-lipid-enveloped, relatively stable agents. Rhinoviruses can be distinguished from enteroviruses, the other subgroup of picornaviruses, by their loss of infectivity when exposed to an acid medium for 1 to 3 h.

EPIDEMIOLOGY Rhinovirus infection is the cause of approximately 40 percent of respiratory illness in children and adults. While it occurs throughout the year, there are peaks of high incidence in spring and fall. Infection with rhinoviruses, as with other respiratory viruses, is much more frequent in infants and children than was previously thought. Children may develop second episodes of rhinovirus infection and illness with different serotypes within a few weeks. The disease is also more severe in children, especially those under two years of age. In the young, fever, cough, croup, and occasionally pneumonia occur.

Family infections are most often initiated by children, and up to three-fourths of family outbreaks may be introduced by children of preschool age; however, at all ages spread is much greater from ill than from well primary cases. Large families have more episodes of infection than small families. Family secondary attack rates are high at all ages, but highest in infants, of whom almost two-thirds of susceptibles may become infected. Infection occurs in about two-thirds or more of exposed persons without antibody, and about 60 percent of these develop illness. In persons with preexisting homotypic anti-

TABLE 178-1
Illness associated with rhinovirus infection

Diagnosis	Adults (n = 61)	Children (n = 32)	Adult volunteers with nasopharyngeal inoculation (n = 31)
Common cold	58 (92)*	14 (44)	26 (84)
Croup		1 (3)	
Bronchitis	1 (2)	7 (23)	2 (6)
Bronchiolitis		3 (9)	
Bronchopneumonia		3 (9)	
No disease	2 (3)	4 (12)	3 (10)

* Values in parentheses are given as percentages.
SOURCES: *Hamparian et al, Proc Soc Exp Biol Med 117:469, 1964; and Cate et al, J Clin Invest 43:56, 1964.*

body, rates of infection and illness are about half that of those without antibody. However, studies in volunteers indicate that high titers of homotypic antibody are uniformly protective. Before 1970 a majority of infections were caused by lower-numbered serotypes; more recently the proportion of infections caused by higher-numbered (and also more recently identified) serotypes has increased. Virus is shed in a high percentage of patients from the day before to 6 days after onset of illness. In general, about one-half of individuals whose infection is associated with virus shedding develop a significant serologic response.

CLINICAL MANIFESTATIONS The incubation period for rhinovirus infections is 1 to 2 days. The first signs of disease are scratchy throat, nasal congestion and discharge, malaise, and mild headache. There is usually no fever. Nasal secretions increase sharply between days 1 and 2 and then as promptly return to pre-illness values. Recovery is rapid and complete. Virus shedding begins a few hours after inoculation and continues for a week or more.

Table 178-2 summarizes clinical experience with naturally occurring rhinovirus infections in adults and children and artificial infection in volunteers. Most adults have only a common cold syndrome, with a rare case of bronchitis the only other form of illness. In contrast, more than one-half of children develop bronchitis, bronchiolitis, or bronchopneumonia. Although these findings resemble those of respiratory syncytial (RS) virus infection, rhinovirus disease is generally milder than that due to RS virus.

LABORATORY FINDINGS In illness with rhinovirus there is usually slight neutrophilia. About one-third of volunteers develop moderate elevations in sedimentation rate.

COMPLICATIONS No serious complications have been reported with rhinovirus infections.

DIFFERENTIAL DIAGNOSIS Among the respiratory viruses, rhinovirus infection most consistently causes coryzal illness. In

TABLE 178-2
Illness associated with adenovirus infection

Disease	Occurrence	Order of association (serotypes) Common	Less common	Respiratory tract involvement Common cold	Pharyngitis	Bronchitis	Pneumonia
Acute respiratory disease (ARD)	Epidemic in winter and spring in military recruits	4, 7	3, 14, 21	Often present	Most frequent, usually with fever, often with laryngitis	Frequent, usually with fever and laryngitis	Infrequent complication of ARD, but adenovirus pneumonia is an important type of pneumonia in recruits
Pharyngoconjunctival fever	Summer epidemics in civilians, often in school-age children, related to swimming pools. Sporadic cases of conjunctivitis may occur without pharyngitis	3, 7	4, 14	Often present	Most frequent, usually with fever and cervical lymphadenopathy, hoarseness	Uncommon	Rare
Febrile pharyngitis	Sporadic or epidemic, resembles ARD, often in children	3, 7	1, 2, 5	Often present	Most frequent, usually with fever	Frequent, especially in older children	Infrequent but severe complication
Pneumonia in children	Highly fatal illness in infants, sporadic or epidemic	3, 7		Sometimes present	Very frequent	Very frequent	Primary, with acidophilic necrosis of tracheal and bronchial mucosa resembling tissue culture cytopathogenic effect
Keratoconjunctivitis (EKC)	Epidemic disease in shipyard workers; also spread from infected eye solutions	8	11	Unusual	Uncommon	Not reported	Not reported
Acute hemorrhagic cystitis	Year-round sporadic disease	11	21	No respiratory disease syndrome; acute hematuria with dysuria, frequency, bladder pain, more common in boys			
Pertussis syndrome	Infrequent sporadic disease	1, 2, 3, 5		Often inconspicuous		Tracheobronchitis common	Bronchiolitis and bronchopneumonia described

any one case, however, the illness cannot be distinguished from coryza due to other agents. Except for rare confusion with an atypical case of streptococcal sore throat, only respiratory viral diseases and *Mycoplasma pneumoniae* infection need be considered in differential diagnosis.

TREATMENT AND PREVENTION There is no specific treatment, and no vaccines are currently available for rhinovirus infections. Analgesics, antihistamines, and nose drops may be beneficial.

HERPESVIRUS INFECTIONS

The purpose of this section is to consider the role of herpesviruses in acute respiratory disease. Other aspects of herpesvirus infection are discussed in Chap. 193.

EPIDEMIOLOGY Several studies have shown that about 10 percent of acute respiratory illness in college populations is due to herpesvirus hominis infection. The disease consists almost uniformly of acute ulcerative pharyngitis and tonsillitis, and illness is associated with a significant rise in herpesvirus-neutralizing and complement-fixing antibody, usually from initially immeasurable levels. In one study the early antibody response was predominantly in the IgM fraction, supporting the concept that the disease resulted from a primary infection. Moreover, lesions in the anterior mouth or on the lips were

uncommon, suggesting that a superficial recurrent herpetic infection (fever blisters) did not mask disease of another etiology in the pharynx.

The high prevalence of primary disease does not occur at college age in low socioeconomic groups, probably because members of this group experience their primary herpesvirus infections at a much younger age.

The disease occurs predominantly in the fall and winter. The route of transmission is not known, but virus can be readily isolated from respiratory secretions of patients with pharyngitis, or from vesicle fluid of fever blisters and is occasionally present in the saliva of asymptomatic persons.

CLINICAL MANIFESTATIONS Herpesvirus infections are characterized by pharyngitis similar to that caused by beta-hemolytic streptococci. There are shallow ulcers on the tonsils and posterior pharynx, and in about one-half of patients there is a grayish pharyngeal exudate. Streptococcal infections produce a creamy exudate. Anterior cervical or submandibular glands are enlarged, and tender lymph nodes occur in about one-half of cases. Fever rarely exceeds 102°F and disappears in a day or so. Recovery is rapid without complications.

LABORATORY FINDINGS Leukocyte counts are normal. Herpesvirus can usually be isolated from throat swabs taken early in infection, and neutralizing-antibody titers rise from unmeasurable levels to 1:16 to 1:64 in convalescence. Complement-fixing antibody also shows significant rises in titer.

COMPLICATIONS No significant sequelae have been observed.

DIFFERENTIAL DIAGNOSIS The disease most resembles acute β-hemolytic streptococcal pharyngitis. However, the systemic response is less severe and acute. Adenovirus pharyngitis is similar to herpesvirus pharyngitis. Pharyngitis that accompanies other respiratory viral and *Mycoplasma pneumoniae* infections is usually less severe and does not show ulcerations.

PREVENTION AND TREATMENT The disease does not appear to be highly contagious, but isolation of patients acutely ill with pharyngitis and tonsillitis is probably indicated.

No specific treatment is recommended for this relatively benign, self-limited disease, although potent chemotherapeutic agents are used for other forms of herpesvirus infection. Analgesics are recommended for pain and discomfort, and hot saline gargles may decrease throat symptoms.

PARAINFLUENZA VIRUS INFECTIONS

ETIOLOGY On the basis of antigenic differences, parainfluenza viruses are divided into four types, of which type 4 is divided into two subtypes. They agglutinate avian and mammalian erythroctyes and grow slowly in tissue culture; only type 2 produces readily visible cytopathic effects. Growth of these agents in tissue cultures is detected by addition of guinea pig erythrocytes, which absorb on the surface of infected cells to form rosettes, a process known as hemadsorption. Parainfluenza viruses have antigens common to Newcastle disease and mumps viruses, but influenza virus does not share these. Parainfluenza serotypes are distinguished in complement fixation, hemagglutination inhibition, or tissue culture neutralization tests. The serotypes can also be identified and differentiated from one another by immunofluorescence.

Constitutional reaction	Other
Headache, malaise, often high fever for several days	Usually no other involvement
Headache, malaise, high fever for several days	Acute follicular conjunctivitis, usually unilateral, occurs with varying frequency. Preauricular lymphadenopathy common with conjunctivitis
High fever, malaise, headache	Nausea, vomiting and diarrhea may occur, especially in infants
High fever, prostration	Conjunctivitis, skin rash, diarrhea, intussusception, and CNS invasion in some cases
Usually afebrile	Usually unilateral severe, acute conjunctivitis followed by corneal subepithelial keratosis; preauricular lymphadenopathy common
Slight	Causes 19 to 91% of cases of hemorrhagic cystitis in children
Prostration, vomiting with coughing spells	Usually no other involvement

Parainfluenza virus can be isolated in primary monkey or primary embryonic kidney cell cultures, but grows slowly or not at all in embryonated eggs.

EPIDEMIOLOGY The first three types of parainfluenza viruses have been found in many parts of the world; type 4 has so far been isolated only in the United States. Infection with parainfluenza viruses occurs early in life. By the age of 8 years, a majority of children show antibody to types 1 to 3, and it appears that most adults have antibody to all four types.

In children, illness with parainfluenza viruses occurs throughout the year, with seasonal increases in different years in the fall, winter, or spring. Type 3 virus spreads more rapidly than types 1 and 2 and may occur endemically throughout the year. Heterotypic antibody rises are frequent, with antibody to type 3 developing in half the cases with type 1 infection. In both children and adults, reinfection is frequent. In one outbreak, 96 percent of children without antibody, 67 percent with low levels, and 33 percent with high levels of antibody became infected. In adults, the disease is almost invariably a reinfection and is much milder than in children.

The total contribution of parainfluenza infections to respiratory illness is variable; its frequency is increasing in institutions in which general health status is lower than average and levels of sanitation and personal hygiene are less than optimum. In studies in the United States parainfluenza infections accounted for 4.3 to 17 percent of respiratory illness in children. The milder illness of adults constituted less than 5 percent of respiratory illnesses.

CLINICAL MANIFESTATIONS In all age groups, the incubation period appears to be 5 to 6 days. The disease is most serious in infants and children, and fever is a constant feature of the disease. The characteristic syndrome with type 1 parainfluenza is laryngotracheobronchitis or croup. Type 2 disease is less frequent but resembles that caused by type 1. Type 3 parainfluenza infections are about equally distributed as causes of croup, tracheobronchitis, bronchiolitis, and bronchopneumonia in infants and children. In older children, the disease is less serious, usually without evidence of pulmonary involvement, and in adults the virus produces a common cold syndrome with hoarseness and cough. Occasionally, adults may experience severe tracheobronchitis with fever with parainfluenza infection.

Physical findings are not distinctive. The throat is reddened, with little or no exudate. There may be tender submandibular lymphadenopathy.

LABORATORY FINDINGS In adult volunteers given type 2 virus, leukocyte counts were not abnormal. In children there is a considerable variation in leukocyte counts early in illness, making it difficult to distinguish this disease from pneumococcal and other bacterial infections. No characteristic alterations have been reported in other laboratory indexes such as liver or renal function tests, electrocardiograms, and urinalyses.

COURSE AND COMPLICATIONS In children, *otitis media* has occurred as a complication more often with parainfluenza than with the other respiratory viral infections. It is more often caused by pneumococci, streptococci, or *Hemophilus influenzae*.

Parainfluenza virus infection is characterized by slow resolution of pulmonary involvement and long persistence of cough and other symptoms. In very young or debilitated children, the outcome can be fatal. In adults, bacterial sinusitis may occur, and in persons with chronic bronchitis, emphysema, or bronchiectasis, the possibility of pulmonary bacterial superinfections should be considered.

TREATMENT There is no specific treatment. Therapy is limited to symptomatic measures and efforts aimed at early detection and treatment of bacterial complications such as otitis media or pneumonia. Nursing care is important in pediatric cases, especially children with croup. In adults, analgesics, antihistamines, and small doses of codeine for cough are generally sufficient.

PREVENTION Vaccines against parainfluenza virus infections are not available. In hospitals, respiratory precautions should be carried out. At home, bed rest or room isolation during acute illness is advised, with special effort to avoid contact with very young or aged persons.

CORONAVIRUS INFECTIONS

ETIOLOGY The disease in humans is caused by an antigenically heterogeneous group of lipid-enveloped RNA viruses sharing morphologic and other properties with mouse hepatitis virus (MHV) and avian infectious bronchitis virus (IBV). A few serotypes of human coronaviruses recovered in tracheal organ culture share antigens with the murine agent.

EPIDEMIOLOGY The disease, characteristically a common cold syndrome, occurs in winter and spring outbreaks that vary from year to year, with greatest incidence in the 15- to 19-year-old age group, but it may involve adults of 40 years of age and older. The incubation period is 3 to 5 days. One study showed lower respiratory tract disease in young children probably caused by coronaviruses ranking in frequency only behind respiratory syncytial virus and parainfluenza 3 infection.

CLINICAL FEATURES The disease resembles rhinovirus common cold with profuse watery and later mucopurulent nasal discharge, sore throat, moderate cough, and mild constitutional symptoms. It is of short duration. In young children, pneumonia and bronchiolitis with coronavirus infection is clinically like that with other respiratory viruses. About one-half of infants may require oxygen because of respiratory distress. Diagnosis is based on isolation of the agent in organ culture or human embryo kidney culture or by antibody rise. The neutralizing antibody test is more sensitive than the complement fixation test, and rises in titer persist for a longer time. Both tests, however, will provide adequate diagnostic information.

TREATMENT AND PREVENTION Treatment is symptomatic; no preventive measures are available.

RESPIRATORY SYNCYTIAL VIRUS INFECTION

ETIOLOGY Respiratory syncytial virus (RS) is classified as a subgroup of the myxoviruses. In tissue culture, it causes formation of giant cells, or syncytia, from which its name was derived. It grows well in several human primary and continuous cell lines and in primary rhesus monkey kidney culture. There is a soluble complement-fixing antigen which, with the neutralization test, permits virus identification and serologic studies. Viral antigen can also be detected by immunofluorescence of exudates from infected patients or in infected cell cultures. Respiratory syncytial virus contrasts with other myxoviruses because it does not grow in mice, guinea pigs, rabbits, or chick embryos and does not cause hemagglutination or hemadsorption.

EPIDEMIOLOGY Epidemiologic studies have delineated a very substantial role of this agent in acute respiratory disease in children. Illness in young children occurs most commonly in epidemics in the late winter and early spring. Attack rates are nearly 100 percent among susceptibles, who are mostly children under 4 years of age, but the peak occurrence of bronchiolitis and bronchopneumonia is observed at 2 to 3 months of age. In older children and adults, the disease appears in nonepidemic patterns. The limitation of epidemic disease to the younger age group is also evidence for unchanging antigenicity of the agent, in contrast to the situation with influenza virus, in which antigenic shifts are associated with recurrent epidemics in persons of all ages. In serologic surveys of volunteers, all were found to possess a measurable titer of neutralizing antibody to RS virus. Despite this finding, a report described the occurrence of febrile tracheobronchitis with increased airway resistance lasting several weeks among medical personnel caring for children with RS disease. Mild upper respiratory illness appears to be the usual form of the disease in adults, but the virus has been isolated from cases of acute tracheobronchitis in older persons with chronic pulmonary disease.

It is probable that RS virus is transmitted by means of infected respiratory secretions. The incubation period of naturally occurring disease in children is about 4 days, and in adult volunteers approximately 5 days. Virus was generally recovered from volunteers a day or so before the onset of illness, and throat swabs yielded a higher proportion of positive cultures than nasal swabs. Virus shedding continues for 3 to 4 days after onset of illness.

CLINICAL MANIFESTATIONS Somewhat less than one-half of infected children have symptoms defined as a common cold; the remainder have bronchiolitis or bronchopneumonia. Fever occurs in about 90 percent of ill children, with an average elevation to 102°F. Cough is almost invariably present, and severe malaise is frequent. Pharyngitis is not usually severe. Fatalities have been reported in infants.

LABORATORY FINDINGS In children, leukocytosis occurs with some frequency, but no significant hematologic changes were observed in adult volunteers. Bacterial flora of the nasopharynx and other laboratory indexes show no significant alterations in either age group.

COMPLICATIONS Except for progression to overwhelming lower respiratory tract disease in a few young children, no special complications are known. There is no evidence of secondary bacterial infection or systemic invasion by the virus in children. In adults, bacterial sinusitis occasionally complicates the virus infection.

DIFFERENTIAL DIAGNOSIS The resemblance of this disease in children to influenza has been suggested. In adults, the differential diagnosis should include rhinovirus and parainfluenza infection and, less often, other respiratory viral disease and *M. pneumoniae* infection.

TREATMENT As with other respiratory viral diseases, treatment should include rest and palliative medications such as aspirin, nose drops, and medication for sleep when restlessness occurs. The possibility of bacterial sinusitis in adults should be kept in mind and antimicrobial treatment, drainage procedures, or other therapy instituted when necessary.

PREVENTION A Formalin-inactivated RS vaccine elicited a high frequency of antibody, but a few months later vaccinated children experienced more severe illness than nonvaccinated children in the same population. This paradoxical effect of vaccination is a major contraindication to further attempts to develop a vaccine. The infection spreads rapidly among children in institutions and poses a threat to debilitated or very young children.

ADENOVIRUS INFECTIONS

ETIOLOGY The adenovirus group contains 31 human and 17 animal serotypes. Strains of types 3, 7, 11, 12, 14, 16, 18, 21, and 31 have been shown to cause sarcomas when injected into newborn hamsters.

Adenoviruses share a common antigenic determinant on a surface structure of the virus called a hexon, designated α. This antigen is the basis for an adenovirus group-diagnostic complement fixation test. It is not exposed on the intact virus and is not associated with immunity. A type-specific antigen ε, exposed on the hexon of the intact virus, gives rise to neutralizing antibody and is associated with immunity. An antigen γ, exposed on the fiber portion of a surface structure called the penton, is type-specific and elicits neutralizing and hemagglutination inhibiting antibody. Serotypes 12 and 18 do not hemagglutinate. An immunofluorescent test is also available that uses antihexon antibody to detect adenoviral group antigen present in exudates from patients or in infected cell cultures. Human adenoviruses grow well in continuous cell lines of epithelial origin.

EPIDEMIOLOGY Adenoviruses are most prevalent in infants and children; they are found in the throat and rectum of both sick and well children. Adenovirus-associated illness occurs throughout the year and accounts for about 2 to 10 percent of all respiratory illness in infants and children, but the highest frequency is in the period from the fall through the spring. Isolations of virus from well children show a similar pattern of seasonal prevalence but a lower frequency of occurrence. Adenovirus types most commonly associated with illness in children are 1, 2, 3, and 5.

The second most frequent occurrence of adenovirus disease is among military recruits. In the general adult population the disease is sporadic. An appreciable prevalence of infection with many adenovirus serotypes is suggested by serologic surveys, but definite virus-associated illness is limited to about 10. These serotypes produce five major patterns of illness, all of which occur in epidemics. A summary of these is presented in Table 178-2.

Acute respiratory disease (ARD) is a respiratory illness of military recruits caused principally by adenoviruses types 4 and 7 that occur in winter and spring outbreaks. Adenoviruses account for 15 to 50 percent of ARD in military groups, but only for about 2 percent of respiratory illness in civilian adults.

Febrile pharyngitis due to adenoviruses usually occurs sporadically or in small outbreaks in children. Its manifestations are summarized in Table 178-2. *Pharyngoconjunctival fever* is febrile pharyngitis associated with acute follicular conjunctivitis. This disease occurs as summer epidemics, frequently among children in relation to exposure in swimming pools. Although it is not limited to swimming pool exposure, it is believed that eye irritation from water, sun, or chlorine may be a factor in its initiation. Conjunctivitis may occur without pharyngitis.

Pneumonia due to adenovirus infection is rare in civilian adults, but occurs in military recruits, usually as an extension of ARD. In infants and children, sporadic and epidemic occurrence of highly fatal adenoviral pneumonia has been described in several parts of the world. Such outbreaks have been principally caused by types 3 and 7. The severity of disease in this

TABLE 178-3
Respiratory illness associated with coxsackieviruses A and B and echoviruses

Diagnosis	Description	Associated viruses
Herpangina	Febrile pharyngitis, anorexia, and discrete vesicular eruption on anterior faucial pillars. Occurs chiefly in children in summer and early fall outbreaks. Similar illnesses without eruption caused by the same viruses probably occur. An illness with nonulcerating nodules on anterior pillars caused by coxsackievirus A10 has also been described	Coxsackieviruses A1 through A6, A8, A10, and A12
Febrile respiratory illness ("summer grippe")	Undifferentiated febrile illness marked by headache, sore throat, and anorexia occurring in summer or early fall. Includes epidemics in recruits with coxsackievirus A21 infection, in which illness patterns have been confirmed by experimental inoculation of volunteers	Coxsackieviruses A21, A24, B2, B3, B5, (?), and echoviruses 1, 3, 6, 19, 20
Upper respiratory illness associated with gastroenteritis	Cases occurring largely in infants and exposed mothers	Echoviruses 1, 11, 19, 20
Acute laryngotracheobronchitis (croup)	Winter outbreaks in nurseries and institutions. Association less definite than with other syndromes	Coxsackieviruses A9, B5, and echoviruses 11
Pneumonitis and pleuritis	Largely confined to young infants and children; uncommon	Coxsackieviruses A9, B4, B5, and echoviruses 9, 19, 20

young age group may reflect the lack of prior experience with these agents, but other factors such as size and route of inoculation, general health, or greater susceptibility due to immaturity may be important.

Acute hemorrhagic cystitis and *pertussis syndrome* are summarized in Table 178-2.

Incubation period The period of incubation for pharyngoconjunctival fever and ARD is 5 to 10 days, and is probably similar for other syndromes, since induced disease in volunteers has a similar period of incubation.

PATHOGENESIS When the conjunctival sac is swabbed with suspensions of adenovirus, conjunctivitis occurs and there is sometimes respiratory involvement. The initiation of illness appears to require a significant degree of conjunctival irritation. Administration of virus aerosol by inhalation also produces illness. Volunteers inoculated in this way have developed ARD and mild pneumonia.

These observations suggest the existence of at least two routes of inoculation for naturally occurring respiratory illness with adenoviruses: (1) ocular inoculation associated with eye irritation such as may occur in outbreaks around swimming pools, with the development of *pharyngoconjunctival fever*; (2) inoculation through inhalation of infectious aerosol generated by sneezing and coughing of ill recruits under the crowded circumstances incidental to recruit training. The route of inoculation of infants is less likely to be limited to aerosolized virus, and whatever the route of inoculation, the occurrence of pneumonia may represent primarily a lack of resistance in this young age group.

Nasopharyngeal inoculation in volunteers often produces virus infection without illness, suggesting that the high frequency of antibody to many serotypes in the population may result from asymptomatic infections. Antibody may also result from intragroup cross reactions among serotypes in the three broad immunologic groups of adenovirus.

CLINICAL MANIFESTATIONS *Acute respiratory disease* is an acute febrile illness lasting about 1 week and characterized by fever, cough, hoarseness, and sore throat. Fever has gradual onset and reaches a maximum of 103 to 104°F on the second or third day. There are associated malaise and often headache. Pharyngitis, the most prominent localized manifestation of the disease, reaches maximum severity after about 3 days. There may also be regional lymphadenopathy, pharyngeal injection, some edema, frequent lymphoid follicular hyperplasia, but little or no faucial exudate. Nasal obstruction and discharge oc-

cur in almost one-half of cases, but these abnormalities are not usually conspicuous. Cough is almost always present, and hoarseness is frequent.

Pharyngoconjunctival fever is usually a milder respiratory illness than ARD, although fever may be high for 5 or 6 days. Nontender submandibular lymphadenopathy is common even in the absence of sore throat. Lower respiratory tract involvement has not been described. Conjunctivitis is mild to moderate but may last longer than respiratory symptoms. It is an acute, nonpurulent, follicular conjunctivitis. In some cases, unilateral preauricular lymphadenopathy occurs. There is usually no involvement of the cornea or uveal tract.

Febrile pharyngitis without conjunctivitis resembles the foregoing illness, except for the absence of conjunctivitis.

Adenoviral pneumonia in children occurs as a primary illness and is associated with as much as 15 percent mortality. Pediatric texts should be consulted for further details.

For further details about *hemorrhagic cystitis* and *pertussis-like syndrome,* pediatric texts should be consulted.

DIFFERENTIAL DIAGNOSIS The differential diagnosis of ARD should include the respiratory viral diseases described in the present chapter and influenza (Chap. 179), nonpneumonic forms of *M. pneumoniae* infection (Chap. 172), streptococcal sore throat, and purulent sinusitis. Pharyngitis and upper respiratory illness may also accompany the onset of infectious hepatitis and infectious mononucleosis.

Differential diagnosis of *pharyngoconjunctival fever,* when conjunctivitis is prominent, includes leptospirosis, influenza, measles, herpangina, and the nonpurulent conjunctivitides, such as inclusion conjunctivitis and physical or chemical trauma to the eye.

TREATMENT There is no specific treatment for adenovirus infection. Treatment is limited to alleviation of general discomfort, headache, and coughing, with analgesics, cough syrup containing terpin hydrate, codeine, antihistamines, or other antitussives.

PREVENTION The communicability of adenovirus infection probably extends from a day or so before onset of illness to recovery, and conventional precautions against respiratory spread should be employed during acute illness for patients in the hospital and to the extent reasonably possible in care of patients at home. Avoidance of swimming pools during outbreaks of pharyngoconjunctival fever is recommended.

Formalin-treated vaccines against types 3, 4, and 7 afford significant protection against infection and illness, but these vaccines were withdrawn from civilian use when it was discovered that some serotypes of adenoviruses produced tumors in hamsters. A live adenovirus vaccine given orally in enteric-coated capsules is highly effective in preventing infection with adenovirus types 3, 4, and 7 in military recruits. More recently, a vaccine prepared from hexons and the fiber portion of penton demonstrated a high degree of protection against experimental infections in volunteers. No vaccine is now marketed for civilian use.

COXSACKIEVIRUS AND ECHOVIRUS INFECTIONS

Diseases produced by these agents are described in Chap. 187. Table 178-3 summarizes the respiratory illnesses sometimes seen with infections caused by these viruses.

REFERENCES

Adenoviruses

BRANDT CD et al: Infections in 18,000 infants and children in a study of respiratory disease: II. Variation in adenovirus infections by year and seasons. Am J Epidemiol 95:218, 1972

KASEL JA: Adenoviruses, in *Diagnostic Procedures for Viral, Rickettsiae and Chlamydiae Infections,* 5th ed, EH Lennette, NJ Schmidt (eds). New York, American Public Health Association, 1978

KNIGHT V, KASEL JA: Adenoviruses, in *Viral and Mycoplasmal Infections of the Respiratory Tract,* V Knight (ed). Philadelphia, Lea & Febiger, 1973

MUFSON MB, BELSHO RB: A review of adenoviruses in the etiology of acute hemorrhagic cystitis. J Urol 115:191, 1976

Coronaviruses

CAVALLARO JJ, MONTO AS: Community-wide outbreak of infection with 229E-like coronavirus in Tecumseh, Michigan. J Infect Dis 122:27, 1970

KNIGHT V, MAYOR HD: Coronaviruses, in *Viral and Mycoplasmal Infections of the Respiratory Tract,* V Knight (ed). Philadelphia, Lea & Febiger, 1973

MCINTOSH K et al: Coronavirus infection in lower respiratory tract disease of infants. J Infect Dis 130:502, 1974

WENZEL RP et al: Coronavirus infections in military recruits. Am Rev Resp Dis 109:621, 1974

Herpesviruses

EVANS AS, DICK FC: Acute pharyngitis and tonsillitis in University of Wisconsin students. JAMA 190:699, 1964

GLEZEN WP et al: Acute respiratory disease of university students with special reference to the etiologic role of *Herpesvirus hominis.* Am J Epidemiol 101:111, 1975

MOGABGAB WJ: Acute respiratory illness in university (1962–1966), military and industrial (1962–1963) populations. Am Rev Respir Dis 98:359, 1968

Parainfluenza virus

GLEZEN WP et al: The parainfluenza viruses, in *Viral Infections of Humans,* AS Evans (ed). New York, Plenum, 1976, chap 15

MONTO AS: The Tecumseh study: V. Patterns of infection with respiratory disease. N Engl J Med 258:207, 1978

Respiratory syncytial virus

HALL WJ et al: Respiratory syncytial virus infection in adults. Clinical, virologic, and serial pulmonary function studies. Ann Intern Med 88:203, 1978

KNIGHT V: Respiratory syncytial viruses, in *Viral and Mycoplasmal Infections of the Respiratory Tract,* V Knight (ed). Philadelphia, Lea & Febiger, 1973

PARROT RH et al: Epidemiology of respiratory syncytial virus infection in Washington D.C.: II. Infection and disease with respect to age, immunologic status, race and sex. Am J Epidemiol 98:289, 1973

Rhinoviruses

CATE TR: Rhinoviruses, in *Viral and Mycoplasmal Infections of the Respiratory Tract,* V Knight (ed). Philadelphia, Lea & Febiger, 1973

FOX JP et al: The Seattle virus watch: V. Epidemiologic observations of rhinovirus infections, 1965–1969, in families with young children. Am J Epidemiol 101:122, 1975

179
INFLUENZA

VERNON KNIGHT

DEFINITION Influenza is an acute respiratory infection of specific viral etiology characterized by sudden onset of headache, myalgia, fever, and prostration. The terms *influenza* and "flu" should be restricted to those cases with clear-cut epidemiologic or laboratory evidence of infection with influenza viruses.

HISTORY According to the best available records, influenza was uncommon in Europe during the nineteenth century until the pandemic of 1889. Subsequently, the frequency and severity of epidemics increased, culminating in the disastrous pandemic of 1918, which caused an estimated 20 to 40 million deaths. The mortality rate from the disease has decreased progressively since 1918 owing in part to the introduction of antibiotics and also to such factors as possible change in virulence of the virus and improved living standards.

ETIOLOGY There are three distinct antigenic types of influenza virus, designated A, B, and C. Infection with one type confers no immunity to the other two. On the basis of intrinsic properties, the three types are grouped in a virus family named Orthomyxoviridae. The influenza viruses contain a single, segmented, negative-strand RNA genome. They are spherical or filamentous enveloped particles, 80 to 120 nm in diameter, with glycoprotein structures termed *hemagglutinin (H)* and *neuraminidase (N),* which protrude from the envelope. The former are responsible for attachment of virus to cell receptors; the latter enzymatically degrades the active receptor substance, frees virus from attachment sites if cell penetration is unsuccessful, and functions in the release of infectious virus from cells during the replication cycle. The H and N are antigenic and elicit antibodies which correlate with the prevention of infection and disease. Antihemagglutinin antibodies are more potent than those elicited by the N antigen.

The three types of influenza viruses are biologically related by their infectivity for chick embryos, capacity to agglutinate erythrocytes in vitro, and affinity for respiratory epithelium of various mammals.

EPIDEMIOLOGY **Influenza A** Influenza A viruses are the cause of epidemics that occur every 2 to 4 years and of pandemics that occur every decade or so. Recent studies have also revealed milder annual interepidemic occurrences of influenza A.

Influenza, especially type A infection, is a recurring disease, because the virus undergoes continuous antigenic variation with time, involving the surface antigens H and N. This progressive, but not necessarily regular, change produces viruses to which segments of the population become susceptible in numbers somewhat in proportion to the extent of antigenic variation. Thus the annual interepidemic outbreaks are not as severe nor as extensive as the less frequent epidemics. The origin of pandemic viruses is unknown, but they appear to arise by a different mechanism. The segmented genome of type A influenza virus exhibits a high recombination frequency. Consequently, a recombinational event between human and nonhuman type A influenza viruses could possibly give rise to antigenically different subtypes. Table 179-1 shows subtypes of influenza that have appeared in this century.

The characteristics of the 1918 virus are inferred from retrospective serologic analyses. The H antigen is the most important, and each new subtype has had a different H antigen (Hsw, H0, H1, H2, H3). The less mobile N antigen has changed only once, N1 to N2 in 1957.

Pandemics accompanied the introduction of three new subtypes, and the absence of pandemics in 1933 and 1947 is probably due to a limited antigenic relationship that existed among the 1918, 1933, and 1947 subtypes, so that individuals who were ill with swine virus influenza in 1918 had some resistance to the 1933 subtype, and similarly, individuals ill in 1933 had some resistance to the 1947 agent.

It was also noted that many older people did not become ill during the 1968 epidemic, and it was found that many of them possessed antibody to this subtype that was probably acquired in the period 1889 to 1890, when the subtype then prevalent shared antigenic properties with the 1968 subtype. There is also evidence that the 1957 virus shared antigens with the subtype that was prevalent before 1890, although due to the time lapse there were too few older people with antibody to have a measurable effect on the pandemic.

Variants within subtypes are identified by the site of first isolation of the new strain and the year of its isolation. The four most recent variants that caused epidemic disease in the United States and elsewhere are A/England/72 (H3N2), A/Port Chalmers/73 (H3N2), A/Victoria/1975 (H3N2), and A/Texas/1976 (H3N2). Differentiation among variants is important because vaccines to one variant show a progressive loss of protective effect against later emerging variants, so that after about 3 years the vaccine will have little effect.

In 1976 what was first thought to be a new pandemic strain, a virus resembling the 1918 swine virus, was isolated from recruits at Fort Dix, New Jersey. In preparation for a possible pandemic, millions of doses of vaccine against the new virus were prepared and given in the United States. The swine agent did not, however, spread to the general population, but an unexpected occurrence of a syndrome of peripheral neuritis (Guillain-Barré syndrome) was observed in association with persons immunized in a ratio of 1 case per 100,000 immunized. About 1 in 1 million had some degree of residual neurologic damage, and 1 in 2 million died.

These rates are eight- to tenfold greater than in an age-matched, unvaccinated control population. Such an observation would probably not have been possible if a swine virus influenza epidemic or pandemic had occurred. Whether or not this low-frequency occurrence has accompanied the use of other influenza vaccines is not known.

TABLE 179-1
Subtypes of influenza A and associated disease occurrences in the twentieth century

Pandemic 1918	A/Swine/1931 (HswN1)-like
Epidemic 1933	A/Puerto Rico/1934 (H0N1)
Epidemic 1947	A/FM1/1947 (H1N1)
Pandemic 1957	A/Japan/1957 (H2N2)
Pandemic 1968	A/Hong Kong/1968 (H3N2)

In 1978 a strain of influenza A of the H1N1 subtype similar to strains that prevailed in the period 1947 to 1957, but mostly resembling the variant of 1951, caused epidemics in China and Russia. Persons born after 1957, having never been exposed, will be susceptible to infection with this agent. Since limited outbreaks of disease were caused by the new H1N1 variant in 1977 to 1978, preparations have been made to include it in the vaccine to be distributed in 1978 and 1979.

Influenza A viruses infect pigs, horses, and fowl, especially ducks and turkeys. H and N antigens of some of these viruses are related to H and N antigens of human influenza A viruses. Recently, it was shown that the internal matrix protein of the virus is an antigen common to all influenza A viruses. The name *swine influenza* was given to the agent that caused the 1918 pandemic because an epidemic of influenza that occurred among swine at that time was thought possibly to have spread to swine from infected people. The swine agent has continued to infect swine populations since that time. The outbreak of "swine virus influenza" among military recruits at Fort Dix in 1976 was presumably an example of swine-to-human transmission. The pandemic A(H3N2) strain of 1968 shared antigens with an agent isolated from horses in 1963. Despite these findings and considerable experimentation with induction of infection across species lines, there is no solid evidence that lower animals are involved in the natural history of human influenza.

Influenza A epidemics start abruptly, reach a peak in 2 to 3 months, and subside almost as rapidly. The attack rate is variable but was noted in 1957 to exceed 50 percent in urban populations. An additional 25 percent of individuals may show serologic evidence of infection without clinical manifestations. Experiences in 1957 proved conclusively that crowding, even in summer months or in tropical countries, is a major factor predisposing to epidemics. School children, in particular, appear to be the primary focus and disseminators of infection in the United States. If the general immunity of a population is at low levels, community-wide epidemics may occur within a short period after the introduction of new strains of virus. If, however, immune individuals predominate, the case rate will rise slowly and may not reach epidemic proportions.

The mortality rate from all causes always increases markedly during epidemics of influenza. In the fall and winter of 1957 to 1958 it was estimated that 40 million persons in the United States became ill with influenza and the total number of influenza-associated deaths was reported to be in excess of 8000. In addition, approximately 60,000 more deaths from various causes occurred during this period than would be expected under normal conditions. The greatest incidence of excessive mortality occurred among infants under 1 year of age and adults over 60 years of age. Data from a small series of cases clearly indicate that influenza is frequently fatal in individuals with preexisting pulmonary or cardiac disease, regardless of age. Chronic rheumatic heart disease with mitral stenosis, in particular, appears to predispose to fatal influenzal pneumonia.

Influenza B and C Influenza B virus infection occurs sporadically or in localized outbreaks, particularly in schools and military camps and every 4 to 6 years causes more discrete epidemics than influenza A. Although influenza B virus possesses H and N coat proteins, it undergoes less variation than influenza A viruses, and it is not now the practice to designate the virus by these antigens. Illness with influenza B infection is less serious than that caused by influenza A viruses. The most serious problem with influenza B infections is a complication, Reye's syndrome, characterized by encephalopathy and fatty changes in the liver and other organs (see "Complications"). Illness with influenza C is rarely detected, although antibody surveys indicate a wide prevalence of the infection.

PATHOGENESIS Influenza is primarily an infection of the respiratory epithelium that is produced by inoculation with virus from respiratory secretions of infected persons. Experimental studies show that a small number of virus particles inhaled in a small-particle aerosol or severalfold larger doses in liquid suspension dropped in the nose will produce the disease. Infection thus could result from transfer of infected secretions by personal contact or fomites or, probably much more frequently, by inhalation of aerosols generated by sneezes, coughs, and other expiratory discharges of infected individuals.

After inoculation, the virus multiplies to maximum titers in a few days. In studies in volunteers the incubation period was prolonged up to 7 days with small inocula but was only a day or so with large inocula. Cells lining the respiratory tract, including ciliated epithelium, alveolar cells, mucous gland cells, and macrophages may become infected. Neutrophil leukocytes and endothelial cells do not appear to become infected. Evidence of virus infection by specific immunofluorescence is most conspicuous in cells that show fewest morphologic changes. Infected ciliated cells undergo degeneration after a day or so and are characterized by swelling of nuclei with shift from a longitudinal to a transverse position in the cell. Cytoplasmic changes are granulation, vacuolation, and swelling. Ultimately cells become necrotic and slough, in some areas to be replaced by flattened and metaplastic epithelial regrowth.

Based on the finding of high titers of virus in nasal washes and from throat swabs and a generalized inflammatory reaction in the nasopharynx, the nasopharynx must usually be widely involved with viral infection. Since tracheobronchitis is regularly a part of uncomplicated influenza, it seems probable that viral lesions also occur in this area. The finding of abnormal pulmonary function in apparently uncomplicated cases suggests that viral infection may ordinarily penetrate more deeply into the lung than earlier supposed. When pulmonary involvement is clinically detectable, high titers of virus are recoverable from sputum and tracheal aspirates and autopsy studies show large areas of pulmonary virus infection.

Despite often severe systemic symptoms, direct evidence of influenza infection beyond the respiratory tract is limited to the isolation of virus in fatal cases from lung, spleen, lymph nodes, liver, kidney, and heart. It is also possible that rare cases of encephalitis with influenza may be associated with viral infection of the central nervous system. Finally, one report describes the isolation of influenza virus A from the feces of children ill with the disease.

MANIFESTATIONS The disease assumes its typical form during major epidemics of influenza A, but clinical differentiation between influenza A and B is not possible in localized outbreaks. Sporadic infections with either influenza A or B are likely to result in relatively minor illnesses, with predominantly respiratory symptoms, similar to those of common respiratory disease. Influenza C is particularly difficult to recognize because of its mildness. Although the manifestations and severity of influenza A vary from year to year, cases in a single epidemic often follow a remarkably similar pattern. The clinical description that follows is a composite picture of epidemic influenza A of the past three decades.

The *incubation period* is usually 18 to 36 h but may be as long as 3 days. Mild prodromal symptoms of cough, malaise, and chilliness are sometimes present, but extremely sudden onset is often such a characteristic feature that many patients can recall its exact time. The most common initial symptom is severe generalized or frontal *headache,* frequently accompanied by stabbing retroorbital pain that is accentuated by lateral or upward gaze. Diffuse *myalgia,* particularly marked in the legs and over the lumbosacral area, occurs in more than half the cases. Pain and spasm of the abdominal muscles may simulate

acute peritonitis, and incapacitating periarticular pains are sometimes confused with acute arthritis. *Feverishness* and *chilliness,* or occasionally true rigors, may be the first manifestations, but more often they are preceded by headache and myalgia. The temperature rises abruptly to a maximum of 100 to 103°F several hours after onset; rarely it may reach 106°F. Thereafter, the fever and pain usually subside over a 2- to 3-day period but may persist for as long as a week. A common variant in the temperature course is rapid defervescence after the initial peak, with a secondary rise to the original level on the following day. In general, severity of illness parallels the height and duration of the fever. The pulse rate is usually slow in relation to the fever, but marked tachycardia may occur in severely ill patients.

Respiratory symptoms may be present at the onset but become most prominent when the systemic manifestations and fever begin to subside. They are frequently less pronounced than in common respiratory disease and may be entirely absent. Sneezing, watery nasal discharge, and stuffy nose occur in most cases; hoarseness and epistaxis are less frequent. Conjunctival suffusion and burning, itching, watery eyes are often noted. The throat may feel dry, and the pharynx often appears slightly injected. *Cough* develops during the course of the illness in more than three-fourths of the cases, and in about a third of these it is productive of small amounts of tenacious, mucoid sputum. *Chest pain,* usually substernal in location and accentuated by coughing but not by breathing, is present in almost half the patients. Pleurisy and pleural effusion are uncommon. Slight hyperpnea is often noted, but the most ominous, although infrequent, signs are dyspnea and cyanosis, which signal bronchiolar or pneumonic involvement. Findings on physical examination of the lungs are often negative in uncomplicated influenza, but scattered rhonchi, wheezes, and showers of moist rales have been reported in 5 to 40 percent of cases in different epidemics. These changes may persist for several days after apparent recovery. Patients with uncomplicated influenza may have restrictive ventilatory defects and increased alveolar-capillary oxygen tension gradients, suggesting the regular occurrence of lower pulmonary tract involvement in the disease. Influenzal bronchiolitis should be suspected if rales persist in the absence of x-ray evidence of pneumonitis and if the patient raises mucopurulent or blood-tinged sputum.

Prostration of some degree is almost invariable and is often the most prominent and alarming manifestation. The face is flushed, and the skin is hot and dry; however, profuse sweating and cold, mottled extremities are sometimes noted. Anorexia, nausea, and constipation are frequent secondary symptoms, but vomiting is rare. Diarrhea occurs with some frequency in children but is rare in adults. Meningoencephalitis, polyneuritis, cranial nerve palsies, transient nerve deafness, aphasia, hemiplegia, psychoses, and other neurologic disorders have been described in association with influenza but are very unusual. Hypotension, heart block, peripheral vasoconstriction, and fatal myocarditis have also been reported in a few cases.

COMPLICATIONS The chief complication of influenza is pneumonia, which occurs as a primary infection with influenza virus or as influenza virus pneumonia with superimposed bacterial pneumonia. In recent years, about 20 percent of pneumonic complications have resulted from primary viral infection. In patients whose pneumonia is complicated by bacterial infection, *Staphylococcus aureus* and pneumococci are the most frequent etiologic agents. Less frequent bacterial etiologies are *Hemophilus influenzae,* hemolytic streptococcus, and various gram-negative bacilli. Staphylococci and gram-negative bacilli are often resistant to some antibiotics and these resistant strains may have been selected by prior treatment with these drugs. In addition, the incidence of bacterial pneumonias without an apparent viral concomitant is greatly increased during influenza epidemics.

Primary influenza virus pneumonia typically has its onset about 1 week after the onset of influenza, often following a period of apparent improvement. The disease is characterized by severe dyspnea and cyanosis, scanty sputum containing gross blood, leukopenia, few physical signs, and perihilar infiltrates by x-ray. The disease has a rapid course and fatality, when it occurs, results from acute respiratory failure.

Pathologic findings in fatal cases of primary viral pneumonia consist of large areas of inflammatory reaction within alveolar septa, with little exudate in alveolar spaces. Involved septa are edematous and infiltrated with lymphocytes, macrophages, and occasionally plasma cells. Some neutrophils may be present. In severe cases, fibrin thrombi may obstruct alveolar capillaries and cause necrosis and hemorrhage. An eosinophilic hyaline membrane may be found lining alveoli and alveolar ducts, presumably resulting from transudation of fibrin through affected alveolar septa. The pleura are not usually involved. This picture is not specific for influenza virus infection and must be differentiated from *Mycoplasma pneumoniae* pneumonia and from the common respiratory viruses that cause pneumonia, predominantly in children.

Secondary bacterial pneumonia is usually detected by onset of production of purulent sputum, fever, and other signs of bacterial pneumonia after the initial episode of influenzal illness. It may occur at variable intervals in relation to the associated viral pneumonia. The pathologic findings vary with the bacterial etiology. In general, the changes associated with pyogenic infection will obscure the less conspicuous viral lesions.

Staphylococcus aureus causes a necrotizing tracheobronchobronchiolitis associated with a neutrophil leukocytosis, tissue necrosis, masses of staphylococci in necrotic areas, thromboses of small blood vessels, and hemorrhage. Purulent exudate plugs the respiratory passages. This process may extend into the lung parenchyma and cause bronchopneumonia associated with large and small abscesses surrounded by areas of hemorrhage, capillary thrombosis, edema, and fibrin deposition.

Pneumococcal pneumonia shows its characteristic fibrinous leukocytic exudate within alveolar air spaces. Necrotizing inflammation as with staphylococcal infection is rare, and the alveolar architecture is preserved. As with staphylococcal infection, the pneumococcal infection may obscure the lesions of viral infection. *Hemophilus influenzae* and gram-negative bacilli produce necrotizing tracheobronchobronchiolitis with lobular pneumonia and sometimes abscess formation. Bacterial pneumonia occurring during influenza epidemics that is not associated with influenza virus pneumonia is a more benign disease with pathologic findings typical of the particular infection.

Many studies have shown that pneumonic complications are most frequent and severe in the aged; in patients with rheumatic valvular or other heart disease, chronic lung disease, and serious systemic illness; and in pregnant women.

Sinusitis and otitis media caused by the usual common pathogens sometimes complicate influenza.

A complication of influenza B and, less frequently, of influenza A and other viral infections that has been identified increasingly is a syndrome of encephalopathy with acute cerebral edema and fatty infiltration of the liver called *Reye's syndrome*. Reduced activity of one or two mitochondrial hepatic enzymes of the urea cycle is noted in these patients. The mortality rate is high. Treatment has consisted of dexamethasone administration under continuous monitoring to maintain intracranial pressure at tolerable levels. Peritoneal dialysis is also used to remove excess blood ammonia commonly present in these patients.

Recovery from uncomplicated influenza is often complete in a week, but convalescence may be prolonged by "postinfectious asthenia" and depression particularly in elderly persons. Minor relapses with fever may occur but are uncommon.

LABORATORY FINDINGS Virus is isolated most readily during the acute phase of the disease by inoculation of throat swab or broth garglings into the amniotic cavity of chick embryos or into tissue cultures of monkey kidney cells. Influenza virus types A, B, and C may be identified in complement fixation tests. These tests depend on the nucleocapsid antigen found in the viral core and in soluble form in infected cells. Antiserum to whole virions readily detects the same or closely related strains by immunofluorescence in infected cell culture and, on occasion, directly in exudates from patients with infection. This methodology is useful in rapid diagnosis. Serologic diagnosis can be made most reliably by the hemagglutination inhibition test, using paired serum samples obtained in both the acute and convalescent phases. Type-specific antibody against soluble complement-fixing antigens of influenza A virus also appears in the circulation of patients during the acute illness.

In uncomplicated influenza the lungs usually appear normal by x-ray but pulmonary involvement with viral infection is often marked by increased vascular markings, basilar streaking, small areas of patchy infiltration, atelectasis or nodular densities. The blood leukocyte count may be low 2 to 4 days after onset of illness, but is often normal or slightly elevated. Leukocytosis with counts above 15,000 cells per cubic millimeter indicates secondary bacterial infection, but leukopenia may occur in severe pneumonia. Slight proteinuria is common during the height of the febrile illness.

DIFFERENTIAL DIAGNOSIS Many bacterial and viral infections simulate influenza at their onset, but few febrile diseases have such a self-limited course. Noninfluenzal respiratory diseases are generally characterized by more gradual onset; milder systemic manifestations; and predominant symptoms of coryza, rhinorrhea, pharyngitis, and conjunctivitis.

TREATMENT Antibiotics do not affect the course of uncomplicated influenza, nor is there any evidence that they prevent complications. Antibiotics should be reserved for secondary bacterial infections. Clinical trials have shown limited effectiveness of amantadine, a symmetric amine that inhibits an early step in replication of influenza virus, as a chemoprophylactic and therapeutic agent. Codeine affords relief from incapacitating cough and is more effective than salicylates for symptomatic treatment of headache and myalgia; salicylates often increase discomfort by causing drenching sweats and chills. Bed rest during illness and gradual return to full activities are advisable.

PROPHYLAXIS Formalinized egg vaccines purified by zonal ultracentrifugation or other methods and containing a mixture of influenza A (H3N2) and B viruses in whole or split forms are available commercially in the United States. Current vaccines can be expected to be effective when given in suitable dosage at an interval of several weeks to several months before exposure, and when the antigens of the vaccine are still closely related to the epidemic strain.

The U.S. Public Health Service strongly recommends routine yearly immunization with polyvalent influenza vaccine for high-risk groups, including persons of all ages who suffer from chronic rheumatic heart disease, other cardiovascular diseases, chronic bronchopulmonary diseases, diabetes mellitus, or

Addison's disease, and persons 65 years of age or older, regardless of their previous state of health. Pregnant women should be immunized only if they fall into one of the high-risk categories. For initial immunization of adults it is advisable to administer the vaccine subcutaneously in two doses of 0.5 ml each, the first injection in September and the second several weeks or months later. A single subcutaneous dose of 0.5 ml given each autumn is satisfactory as a yearly booster. Intradermal injection of vaccine is far less satisfactory because a sufficient antigenic mass cannot be administered.

Influenza vaccination is generally safe but not completely innocuous. The recent occurrence of the Guilliain-Barré syndrome as a complication of the use of inactivated swine influenza virus vaccine requires further evaluation. Fatal anaphylactic reactions and purpura have been reported in individuals sensitive to egg proteins, and inactivated virus itself is pyrogenic and can sometimes produce an illness similar to active influenza. Infants and children have experienced severe febrile convulsions following vaccination, and vaccine should be avoided in children with a history of this syndrome. A decision to vaccinate children, especially the very young, should be made on an individual basis. The subject of influenza prevention is also discussed in Chap. 114.

REFERENCES

Glezen WP, Couch RB: Interpandemic influenza in the Houston area, 1974–1976. N Engl J Med 298:587, 1978

Hochberg FH et al: Influenza type B-related encephalopathy, the 1971 outbreak of Reye's syndrome in Chicago. JAMA 231:817, 1975

Monto AS, Kioumehr F: The Tecumseh study of respiratory illness: IX. Occurrence of influenza in the community, 1966–1971. Am J Epidemiol 102:553, 1975

Mulder J, Hers JFP: Influenza. Groningen, The Netherlands, Wolters-Noordhoff Publishing, 1972, pp 1–288

Price DA et al: Influenza virus A2 infections presenting with febrile convulsions and gastrointestinal symptoms in young children. Clin Pediatr 15:361, 1976

Exanthems and enanthems

180
APPROACH TO THE PATIENT WITH RASH AND FEVER

LAWRENCE COREY

Because many infectious and noninfectious diseases produce cutaneous lesions, specific diagnosis of an acutely ill febrile patient with a rash is a clinical skill with important therapeutic implications. The cutaneous manifestations of an infectious disease may result from direct innoculation of the organism into skin or indirectly from lymphogenous, hematogenous, or contiguous spread of the pathogen. Exanthems are cutaneous eruptions due to systemic or contiguous spread of an organism. These eruptions may be due to multiplication of the etiologic agent in the skin or dermal vasculature or to the host's immune responses to the organism. The cutaneous manifestations of infections may involve the epidermis or the vascular or extravascular structures of the dermis. Some exanthems are unique to a particular pathogen, others are common to numerous etiologic agents. Classification of exanthematous illness into (1) maculopapular, (2) vesicular, and (3) petechial eruptions is useful in determining the etiology and in understanding the pathogenesis of an exanthem.

PATHOGENESIS The pathogenesis of an exanthem may be caused by (1) multiplication of the pathogen in the skin, (2) carriage of the agent in plasma or in infected hematopoietic cells (leukocytes and/or lymphocytes) into integumentary blood vessels, and (3) antigen-antibody or delayed hypersensitivity reactions to antigens derived from the infecting microorganism. For example, in many viral diseases, such as rubella, rubeola, and the enterovirus infections, initial viral replication occurs in the infected mucosal surface and regional lymphatic tissue. Primary viremia then ensues, and "seeding" of the virus into target organs, such as liver, muscle, central nervous system, or heart, may occur. Continued viral replication and a secondary viremia with hematogenous spread of the virus to the skin may then follow. In this model, regional multiplication of the virus, primary viremia, and visceral dissemination of virus occur prior to the development of the exanthem and explain why the initial clinical manifestations of many viral illnesses occur prior to the development of the rash. Humoral and cellular immune responses which prevent or ameliorate secondary viremia may prevent the development of a rash. This may explain why exanthems associated with enteroviruses occur more frequently in younger children than adolescents or adults: young children do not possess cross-reacting antibodies or cannot mount an anamnestic immune response to the infecting agent.

While some maculopapular exanthems appear to be related to direct viral or bacterial invasion of the skin, other exanthems result from local or systemic immune responses to the microorganism. Rubella virus can be recovered from rubella maculopapules as well as from areas of the body not involved by the exanthem. Administration of pooled immune serum globulin after exposure to rubella may not eliminate rubella viremia but does prevent rash. Similarly, the exanthem of rubeola may be a manifestation of an Arthus reaction produced by the deposition of viral antigen in the endothelium of dermal capillaries. Local factors such as exposure to light or local irritation of the skin have also been shown to modify the distribution of some exanthems.

Vesicular exanthems are usually associated with active viral invasion of the infected area. Characteristically, herpes simplex virus, varicella-zoster virus, or poxviruses can be demonstrated in vesicular fluid by viral culture or by immunologic techniques. Local host and immune responses are important in the progression of varicella lesions, and their duration has been correlated with both local and "immune" interferon production.

Petechial eruptions may arise from direct invasion of the cutaneous vasculature by a microorganism, as occurs with septic emboli, or may result from immunologic injury to the vascular endothelium. In Rocky Mountain spotted fever, *Rickettsia rickettsiae* can be demonstrated in the smooth-muscle wall of arterioles. Vascular damage, microinfarction, and extravasation of red blood cells produce the characteristic petechial exanthem. Occasionally, a petechial eruption may complicate previous maculopapular or vesicular exanthems, usually coinciding with the development of diffuse intravascular coagulation. This may be seen in hemorrhagic dengue, measles, or varicella. In some petechial eruptions, direct evidence of viral or bacterial invasion can be obtained by direct aspiration and culture of the lesion, by demonstration of the agent with Gram's stain, or by immunofluorescent stain to detect microbial agents.

CLINICAL DIAGNOSIS OF MACULOPAPULAR ERUPTIONS

Table 180-1 lists the numerous viral, bacterial, rickettsial, and noninfectious agents that may be associated with maculopapular exanthems. One helpful approach to the physical examination of viral maculopapular (*not* vesicular) rashes is that these eruptions *relatively* spare the palms and soles in contrast to eruptions associated with drug reactions, bacteria, mycoplasma, and rickettsial and/or immunologic diseases. In the latter entities, a prominent palmar or plantar distribution is often present.

While some exanthematous diseases produce characteristic cutaneous patterns, e.g., measles or erythema infectiosum, overlap in the cutaneous manifestations of viral induced maculopapular exanthems is the rule. Therefore, the presence of associated signs or symptoms as well as the epidemiologic characteristics of the disease such as the season of the year, the patient's age, and history of exposure and previous immunization are useful in formulating a diagnostic impression. Because viral maculopapular exanthems are manifestations of the agent's systemic spread, evidence of mucosal viral replication in the form of an enanthem is often a valuable aid in determining the etiology of a viral rash. Koplik spots in rubeola, ulcerative lesions on the hard and soft palate with herpangina due to coxsackievirus A, and palatal petechiae in early infectious mononucleosis are all helpful clinical signs. Associated clinical findings such as coryza, conjunctivitis, and cough with rubeola, mild fever and posterior auricular lymphadenopathy in rubella, or localized mastitis or furunculosis in staphylococcal scalded-skin syndrome should be looked for. Concomitant arthritis, renal disease, and/or heart disease generally suggests immunologically mediated entities such as acute rheumatic fever, subacute bacterial endocarditis, serum sickness, or collagen vascular disease.

The distribution of the rash provides important information. Erythema infectiosum presents with a diffuse erythema of the cheeks ("slapped cheeks"). In addition, central clearing of the eruption on the extremities results in a lace-like appearance of the exanthem. Erythema marginatum occurs in 10 percent of patients with acute rheumatic fever and is characterized by a ringed eruption which rapidly spreads to the trunk and extremities. Scarlet fever due to erythrogenic toxin elaborated by a group A streptococcus produces a rash that starts on the neck and spreads to the trunk and extremities within 36 h. The rash consists of numerous punctate papular lesions at the site of hair follicles and feels like rough sandpaper. Circumoral

TABLE 180-1
Differential diagnosis of patients with rash and fever

Macules or papules	Vesicles	Petechiae-purpura
VIRAL		
Rubeola	Herpes simplex	Enteroviruses (echovirus)
Rubella	Varicella-zoster	Viral hemorrhagic fevers
Enteroviruses	Vaccinia	Dengue
Cytomegalovirus	Enteroviruses (herpangina)	Adenoviruses
Hepatitis B	Hand-foot-and-mouth disease (A16)	Yellow fever
Erythema infectiosum	Orf	Atypical measles
Exanthem subitum	Molluscum contagiosum	
Adenoviruses	Vesicular stomatitis virus	
Arboviruses		
Rhabdovirus group		
Reoviruses		
Live virus vaccines (measles, rubella)		
BACTERIAL		
Group A streptococci:	Staphylococcal scalded-skin syndrome	Severe sepsis with diffuse intravascular coagulation
Scarlet fever	Bullous impetigo	Meningococcemia
Erysipelas		Gonococcemia
Erythema marginatum		Pseudomonas sepsis
Staphylococcal scalded-skin syndrome		Subacute bacterial endocarditis
Subacute bacterial endocarditis		*Listeria monocytogenes*
Secondary syphilis		
Typhoid fever		
Erysipelothrix		
Mycobacterium leprae		
Rat bite fever		
Leptospirosis		
Chronic meningococcemia		
Pseudomonas sepsis		
RICKETTSIAL		
Rocky Mountain spotted fever (early)	Rickettsialpox	Rocky Mountain spotted fever
Murine typhus		Epidemic (louseborne) typhus
FUNGAL		
Candidiasis		
Sporotrichosis		
Cryptococcosis		
CHLAMYDIAL		
Psittacosis		
PROTOZOAL		
Toxoplasmosis		Trichinosis
Trichinosis		Plasmodia (blackwater fever)
UNKNOWN		
Mucocutaneous lymph node syndrome		
IMMUNOLOGIC		
Erythema multiforme	Stevens-Johnson syndrome	Henoch-Schönlein purpura
Erythema nodosum	Pemphigoid	
	Behçet's syndrome	
	Inflammatory bowel disease	
DRUGS		
Drug eruptions	Drug eruptions	Drug eruptions

pallor, large red fungiform papillae (strawberry tongue), extension of the rash into body folds including the antecubital fossae, concomitant tonsillitis and cervical lymphadenopathy, and the subsequent desquamation of the rash, especially on the palms and soles, confirm the clinical diagnosis. Erysipelas due to group A (uncommonly group G) streptococci and staphylococci is characterized by an edematous indurated superficial cellulitis. Characteristically, the rash is shiny with a sharply demarcated edge. Occasionally streptococci can be demonstrated on Gram's stain and culture of material aspirated from the advancing edge of the lesion.

Some strains of *Staphylococcus aureus* (phage group 2) can elaborate a toxin which produces a diffuse erythema of the skin (staphylococcal scalded-skin syndrome). The development of bullae resulting in the easy separation of the epidermis (Nikolsky's sign) may occur but is not specific for this entity.

The course of the eruption is also helpful in differentiating the etiology of viral exanthems. Rubeola usually starts in the hairline area and spreads downward until the involved areas coalesce into a diffuse morbilliform eruption. In contrast, the eruption of rubella tends to disappear from its original sites of involvement as it spreads.

The rash of Rocky Mountain spotted fever usually starts on the extremities and spreads centripetally to the trunk. In contrast, the rash of roseola subitum starts on the trunk and spreads centrifugally to the arms and legs. Pityriasis rosea is characterized by the development of papular lesions along the lines of cleavage of the trunk ("fir tree" effect). The development of the earlier appearing "herald patch" and the lack of fever characterize this exanthem.

While papular lesions may be a manifestation of viral disease, systemic bacterial and/or fungal disease may also produce these lesions. Chronic meningococcemia may be associated with pale rose colored maculopapular lesions that may be mistaken for erythema nodosum when located on the lower extremities. The cutaneous lesions tend to wax and wane with fever. Organisms usually are not demonstrated in Gram's stain or cultures of these lesions. However, blood cultures taken during febrile periods may be positive. The development of discrete papules on the trunk in a patient with a previous history of diarrhea should suggest the possibility of typhoid fever. These "rose spots" are 1- to 3-mm papules which disappear in 3 to 4 days. In the untreated patient new lesions will emerge over the next 2 to 3 weeks. Pseudomonas bacteremia can also produce small painless papules on the trunk. The papulosquamous lesions of secondary syphilis often involve the trunk, palms, soles, and mucous membranes and may be present for days to several weeks. The serology (VDRL) is invariably positive in secondary syphilis.

Papulonodular lesions can be identified in 10 to 15 percent of patients with disseminated candidiasis. The appearance of these lesions in febrile immunosuppressed patients who fail to respond to antimicrobials should suggest the possibility of disseminated candidiasis. Biopsy and culture of the lesions should demonstrate the blastospores and pseudohyphae of *Candida* species.

In all infectious diseases, knowledge of the epidemiologic milieu of the patient is of great aid in arriving at a presumptive diagnosis of a patient with fever and a maculopapular eruption. Erysipeloid should be considered in persons with exposure to swine or saltwater fish; rat bite fever in those with a history of rodent exposure; sporotrichosis in those with contact with roses or spaghnum; leptospirosis in those patients who have contact with potentially infected animals and who also have hepatitis, conjunctivitis, and/or meningitis; and Rocky Mountain spotted fever in individuals who live in areas endemic for tick bites.

Mucocutaneous lymph node syndrome Also termed *Kawasaki's disease* mucocutaneous lymph node syndrome is a multisystem disease that occurs in children and is being recognized more frequently in the United States.

This entity was first described in Japan in the 1960s. It affects children from 2 months to 9 years of age, with 50 percent of cases occurring in children under 2 years of age. Characteristically, the patient presents with a fever between 38.3 and 40°C (101 and 104°F) of 1 to 2 weeks' duration which is unresponsive to antimicrobials. Bilateral conjunctivitis; dryness, redness, and fissuring of the lips; diffuse erythema of the oral and pharyngeal mucosa; "strawberry tongue," and cervical adenopathy may be present. On the third to fifth day of illness, a macular erythematous eruption, usually starting on the extremities, appears. Pronounced reddening of the palms and soles is present, and the child's hands and feet may swell due to an indurative edema. Characteristically during the second week of the illness desquamation of the rash starts at the junction of the nails and skin of the fingers and toes. Myocardial involvement is common, with abnormal ECG findings in over 50 percent of patients. Coronary angiography may reveal aneurysms and pathological changes in the vessels similar to infantile periarteritis nodosa. In severe cases, myocardial infarction due to coronary thrombosis may occur. Arthritis, hepatitis, and "aseptic meningitis" may also be seen. Laboratory data include an abnormal sedimentation rate, normal antistreptolysin O (ASO) titers, presence of elevated C-reactive protein, and peripheral leukocytosis. The prognosis is usually good; death occurs in 1 to 2 percent of patients and is usually due to coronary thrombosis. In the United States, cases have been clustered geographically and temporally. The etiology of this entity is unknown.

CLINICAL DIAGNOSIS OF VESICULAR ERUPTIONS The distribution of the eruption is often helpful in determining a clinical and etiologic diagnosis of a vesicular exanthem. Varicella begins on the trunk, spreads centrifugally, and demonstrates lesions in all stages of healing, i.e., vesicles, ulcers, and crusts. Variola usually begins on the extremities, spreads centripetally, and is characterized by lesions in similar stages of development. The vesicular ulcerative pharyngeal lesions of herpangina are present only on the palate, whereas primary herpes simplex gingivostomatitis also involves the anterior gingival area and/or the lips. Hand, foot, and mouth disease due to coxsackievirus A16 presents as multiple linear vesicles or pustules on the palms and soles; this is an unusual distribution for either herpes simplex or varicella-zoster virus.

Primary herpes simplex virus (HSV) infection is clinically distinct from recrudescent disease. Initial oral or genital HSV infection is often accompanied by constitutional symptoms such as fever, malaise, and myalgias; numerous vesicles, bilateral, tender regional lymphadenopathy, and a 2- to 3-week course between the onset of lesions and their complete reepitheliazation are the rule. Contiguous spread of virus as evidenced by the appearance of new vesicles after onset of the initial lesions is common, and inoculation at distant sites such as the fingers, thighs, eyes, and buttocks may be seen in 10 to 20 percent of primary herpes simplex. In contrast, patients with recurrent HSV are usually afebrile and have only a few clustered unilateral lesions which last from 5 to 12 days. Patients will often complain of a "prodrome," a tingling sensation near or at the eventual site of lesion, from 2 to 48 h prior to the appearance of vesicles. Occasionally, HSV infection will present in a dermatomal distribution that is usually characteristic of herpes zoster. Because cytological techniques do not differentiate between these two agents, viral cultures or use of specific techniques such as immunofluorescence must be employed in order to differentiate these two viruses.

The appearance of the vesicles may be helpful. Herpes simplex and varicella lesions have a surrounding zone of erythema and a thin vesicular roof, and they are tender when irritated. The lesions of molluscum contagiosum are umbilicated, contain an expressible white core, and are usually not tender when scraped gently. The lack of surrounding erythema, the large size of the bullae, and the presence of Nikolsky's sign are helpful in differentiating pemphigus or toxic epidermal necrolysis from viral vesicular eruptions. The vesicular-ulcerative lesions associated with Behçet's syndrome or inflammatory bowel disease tend to be present for longer periods than those associated with herpes virus infection. The unremitting course, tendency of the lesions to produce a deep ulcer and the prevalence of associated clinical findings such as colitis, urethritis, arthritis, and neurological disease in Behçet's syndrome should suggest this entity.

PETECHIAL ERUPTIONS Many hematologic and immunologic entities produce thrombocytopenia as a result of defects in the production, maturation, sequestration, or destruction of platelets. A consequence is the development of petechiae. However, the physician who is presented with an acutely ill patient with a petechial exanthem must be concerned with systemic bacterial or rickettsial disease. The common microorganisms associated with petechial exanthems are listed in Table 180-1. However, any microorganism that is capable of initiating the cascade of hematologic events termed *disseminated intravascular coagulation* may produce a petechial exanthem.

Petechiae due to septic embolization are characteristic of subacute bacterial endocarditis. Lesions may occur anywhere on the skin and/or mucous membranes but are most common over the upper anterior trunk. Splinter hemorrhages under the nails are difficult to differentiate from traumatic lesions and may be seen in hematologic, malignant, and other infective disorders.

Petechial lesions associated with meningococcemia are small, irregularly shaped slightly raised pale grayish lesions with a vesicular-pustular center. The lesions are usually asymmetric and are seen most often on the trunk and extremities, although the conjunctivas and mucous membranes may also be affected. Fulminant meningococcal infection will produce coalescence of the petechiae into grossly ecchymotic areas (purpura fulminans).

Gonococcal infection usually produces lesions on the distal extremities, often over joints. The presence of these pustular, hemorrhagic skin lesions in a patient with asymmetric tenosynovitis or polyarthritis, involving the wrists, fingers, knees, or ankles, should suggest the gonococcal arthritis-dermatitis syndrome. The majority of patients with disseminated gonococcal infection do not have symptoms of urogenital, anorectal, or pharyngeal gonococcal disease.

The metastatic lesions of staphylococcal bacteremia include pustules, subcutaneous abscesses, and purulent petechiae. Aspiration of material from the purulent center of the lesion will often reveal gram-positive cocci in clumps. Pseudomonas septicemia may produce ecthyma gangrenosum, a round, indurated, painless, necrotic eschar usually located in the anogenital or axillary area. In addition, hemorrhagic lesions with surrounding erythema resembling erythema multiforme may be associated with pseudomonas sepsis.

Rickettsial disease may produce an arteriolar vasculitis that results in a petechial exanthem. The rash of Rocky Mountain spotted fever generally starts as a blanching maculopapular exanthem on the extremities, and after 2 to 4 days petechiae appear in the involved areas. The lesions no longer fade, and decreased capillary fragility, manifested by a positive Rumpel-Leede test, is often present. These cutaneous findings in a patient with the abrupt onset of fever, chills, headache, myalgias, and arthralgias should suggest this diagnosis. If the patient comes from an endemic area, and a tick bite or tick exposure is present, appropriate therapy should be instituted.

Summer febrile illness due to enteroviruses, especially the echovirus group, may occasionally produce a petechial eruption. While involvement of the face is common, the distribution of the exanthem is usually not distinctive, and because fever, headache, and meningismus may also be present, the clinical differentiation between *Neisseria meningitidis* infection and viral aseptic meningitis may be difficult.

Atypical measles is another viral exanthem that produces a petechial eruption. It begins on the arms and legs and spreads to the trunk and face. The rash differs from typical measles because it has features of raised papules, blisters, and pinpoint hemorrhages into the skin. Koplik's spots are not present, while high fever, cough, bilateral interstitial pulmonary infiltrates, and eosinophils usually are. Patients with this syndrome have a history of previous immunization with inactivated (killed) measles vaccine or of receiving live measles vaccine within 3 months after killed vaccine. The history of previous antigenic exposure to measles virus plus eosinophilia suggests a "hypersensitivity" reaction. A fourfold rise in measles complement fixation antibody titer between acute and convalescent specimens may be demonstrated.

Allergic vasculitis (Henoch-Schönlein purpura) is found most frequently in children less than 16 years of age. The presence of symmetrical red papules ("palpable purpura"), commonly occurring on the lower extremities, accompanied by abdominal pain, gastrointestinal bleeding and renal involvement (edema, hypoproteinemia, hematuria), and arthalgias characterizes this entity.

Petechial eruptions and profuse mucosal bleeding are often major manifestations of the viral hemorrhagic fevers. This syndrome is associated with a number of the arenaviruses (Lassa, Junin), arthropod-borne viruses (dengue), and rhabdoviruses (Ebolla, Marburg). Recent travel to endemic or epidemic areas, involvement of the liver, spleen, heart, kidneys, and lungs, and evidence of diffuse intravascular coagulation are usually present.

LABORATORY DIAGNOSIS The laboratory studies most useful in determining the etiology of an exanthem in an acutely febrile patient are directed at demonstrating the microorganism at the cutaneous site. Gram's stain and culture of the lesions, dark-field microscopy of putative spirochetal lesions, and the use of immunofluorescent miscroscopy of skin scrapings or skin biopsy specimens for the detection of microbial antigens should be employed. Because exanthems are generally manifestations of a systemic illness, blood cultures should be taken prior to antimicrobial therapy. The agent should also be isolated from other extravascular sites such as stool specimens in the case of *Salmonella* or enteroviruses or the throat or urethra in the case of gonococci. Histological identification of organism from skin biopsies of lesions may be of great help, especially with slowly growing agents such as fungi or mycobacteria.

Because local viral invasion is characteristic of vesicular exanthems, isolation of the agent from these lesions provides the diagnosis. The development of rapid viral diagnostic testing has been especially useful to the clinician in the differential diagnosis of vesicular lesions. Biopsies or scrapings of exfoliated cells from vesicular lesions of herpes group viruses (varicella-zoster, herpes simplex virus) contain multinucleated giant cells and/or intranuclear inclusions. However, because the Tzanck smear is only 40 to 70 percent as sensitive as viral isolation, the absence of giant cells does not rule out herpes infection. Herpes simplex and zoster can be differentiated by viral isolation as well as antigen detection techniques such as fluorescent microscopy or enzyme-linked immunoabsorbent assays (ELISA). Immunofluorescence may also be useful in confirming the diagnosis of immunologically related diseases such as pemphigus vulgaris.

Electron microscopy is useful in differentiating the distinct morphology of poxviruses, vaccinia, variola, and molluscum from herpes viruses. In addition, molluscum bodies can be demonstrated by light microscopy with use of a 10% KOH preparation.

In viral exanthems, demonstration of local viral replication in throat secretions or rectal swabs provides presumptive evidence of the etiology of the exanthem; an example is the demonstration of coxsackievirus A16 in throat secretions of patients with hand-foot-and-mouth syndrome. In Behçet's syndrome or in collagen vascular disease, the absence of viruses in an early vesicular or active ulcerative lesion is useful in relating these mucosal lesions to the underlying multisystem illness.

Serologic determinations of acute phase serums are helpful in the diagnosis of syphilis, leptospirosis, streptococcal disease, Epstein-Barr virus infection, hepatitis B, toxoplasmosis, typhoid fever, and occasionally rickettsial disease. Evidence of autoantibody fixation may be useful in diagnosing some collagen vascular diseases. Demonstration of a fourfold or greater rise in antibody titer between acute and convalescent serums will confirm the diagnosis in rubella, rubeola, cytomegalovirus, rickettsial, or chlamydial infection.

REFERENCES

FULGINITI VA et al: Altered reactivity to measles virus. JAMA 202:105, 1967

GILCHEST B, BARDEN HP: Photodistribution of viral exanthems. Pediatrics 54:136, 1974

HEGGIN AD: Pathogenesis of rubella exanthems. J Infect Dis 137:74, 1978

KAWASAKI T et al: A new infantile acute febrile mucocutaneous lymph node syndrome (MLNS) prevailing in Japan. Pediatrics 54:271, 1974

KIMURA A et al: Measles rash, light and electron microscopic study of measles skin eruptions. Arch Virol 47:295, 1975

MIMS CA: Pathogenesis of rashes in virus diseases. Bacteriol Rev 30:739, 1966

181
MEASLES (RUBEOLA)

C. GEORGE RAY

DEFINITION Measles, or rubeola, is an acute febrile eruption which has been one of the most common diseases of civilization. With the development of effective prophylactic measures it should become a rarity.

HISTORY Measles probably was not a significant problem before the building of large cities. Rhazes wrote about it in the tenth century, and Sydenham in the seventeenth century wrote a full account of the disease and differentiated it from other exanthems. In 1905 measles was transmitted by the blood of infected persons to human volunteers and in 1911 to monkeys by both blood and nasopharyngeal secretions that had previously been passed through bacteria-retaining filters. In 1954,

Enders and Peebles obtained an agent from patients with measles that produced cytopathic changes in cell cultures. This achievement allowed the investigation of the characteristics of the measles virus and of the pathogenesis of the disease, with subsequent development of diagnostic and prophylactic measures.

ETIOLOGY The measles virion is composed of a central core of ribonucleic acid with a helically arranged protein coat surrounded by a lipoprotein envelope with small, spike-like structures. The virion is 120 to 250 nm in diameter and is classified as a paramyxovirus.

The measles virus is isolated most easily from infected persons in the first 4 or 5 days of illness, by utilizing primary cell cultures of monkey or human kidney, although primary isolations have been accomplished by using cells from human amnion or chorion or dog kidney. After several passages, the virus can be propagated on a number of types of cell cultures, including chick embryo cells, upon which many of the vaccine strains are grown.

Measles virus infection of cells in culture results in the formation of multinucleated giant cells, many with eosinophilic intranuclear and intracytoplasmic inclusions.

EPIDEMIOLOGY Measles occurs naturally only in human beings, although infection with the virus can be demonstrated in laboratory colonies of monkeys exposed to infected individuals. Before active immunization was available, epidemics of measles occurred in 2- to 3-year cycles, usually during the spring months, and about 95 percent of town and city dwellers developed the disease before the age of 15 years. The virus is transmitted by transfer of nasopharyngeal secretions, either directly or in airborne droplets, to the respiratory mucous membranes or conjunctivas of susceptile individuals. Persons infected with the virus may transmit the disease during a period which extends from 5 days after exposure until 5 days after skin lesions have appeared. The virus is highly contagious, with secondary attack rates among susceptible household contacts usually exceeding 90 percent; asymptomatic primary infections are rare. Measles is typically a disease of childhood in populous areas, but may occur at any age in remote isolated communities if the disease is introduced. In recent years in the United States, there has been a distinct shift in age-specific attack rates, with outbreaks frequently occurring among teenagers and young adults. Infants are uncommonly affected under the age of 6 to 8 months, presumably because of the persistence of maternal antibody acquired by transplacental transmission.

PATHOGENESIS AND PATHOLOGY It is probable that, after infection, measles virus multiplies in the epithelium of the respiratory tract and is disseminated by way of the blood to distant sites. For a few days before the rash appears, and for 1 or 2 days after, the virus can be isolated from blood or washed white blood cells, conjunctiva, lymphoid tissue, and respiratory mucous membranes and secretions. The virus can be obtained from urine for as long as 4 days after the onset of the eruptions.

The mucous membrane lesions (Koplik's spots) consist of vesicle formation and epithelial necrosis. Histology of the Koplik's spots reveals cytoplasmic and intranuclear inclusions, giant cells, and intercellular edema. Electron microscopy of the Koplik's spots and skin lesions has demonstrated microtubular aggregates which are thought to be the measles virus, and suggests that both the exanthem and enanthem are associated with local viral replication. Large multinucleated epithelial giant cells can be found during the prodrome and acute stages of illness in the buccal mucosa, pharynx, tracheobronchial mucosa, and occasionally in the urine. In addition, reticuloendothelial giant cells (Warthin-Finkeldey cells) are found in hyperplastic lymphoid tissues, including lymph nodes, tonsils, spleen, and thymus. An unusually high number of white blood cells from patients with the disease contain broken chromosomes. The epithelium of the respiratory passages may become necrotic and slough, leading to secondary bacterial infection; in addition, interstitial pneumonia with giant-cell infiltration may be observed. Changes in the brain of patients with encephalitis resemble those seen in other postviral encephalitides and consist of focal hemorrhage, congestion, and perivenous demyelination.

MANIFESTATIONS The time from exposure to the development of the first symptoms of measles infection is usually 9 to 11 days, and from exposure to the appearance of rash is about 2 weeks. The initial manifestations of the disease are malaise, irritability, fever as high as 105°F, conjunctivitis with excessive lacrimation, edema of the eyelids and photophobia, moderately severe hacking cough, and nasal discharge. The prodromal period usually lasts 3 to 4 days, with a range of 1 to 8 days before the onset of a rash. Koplik's spots—small, red, irregular lesions with blue-white centers—appear 1 or 2 days before the onset of the rash on the mucous membranes of the mouth and occasionally on the conjunctiva or intestinal mucosa. The findings of the prodromal illness subside or disappear within 1 or 2 days after the appearance of skin lesions, although the cough may persist throughout the course of the disease.

The red maculopapular rash of measles breaks out first on the forehead, spreads downward over the face, neck, and trunk, and appears on the feet on the third day. The density of lesions is greatest on the forehead, face, and shoulders, where coalescence of individual spots usually occurs. The lesions in each area persist for about 3 days and disappear in the same order in which they appeared, resulting in total duration of rash of about 6 days. As the maculopapules fade, a brown discoloration of the skin may be noticed, and finely granular desquamation may occur. In adults the duration of fever may be longer, the rash more prominent, and the incidence of complications higher.

The course of measles can be altered by the administration of gamma globulin soon after exposure. The incubation period may be prolonged for as long as 20 days. The prodromal period of the modified disease may be shorter, the fever, respiratory symptoms, and conjunctivitis milder, and the rash less marked; Koplik's spots may not be present. An atypical, severe form of measles is seen in some persons who received inactivated measles vaccine several years before exposure. The prodromal period with prominent fever, headache, myalgias, and abdominal symptoms lasts for 2 or 3 days and is followed by an eruption of maculopapules, vesicles, and petechiae. In contrast to natural measles, the rash begins on the feet and progresses toward the head and is especially prominent on the legs and in the body creases. Peripheral edema and pneumonia have been prevalent in this form of atypical measles. The pneumonia is lobar or segmental; hilar lymphadenopathy and pleural effusion are frequent. Ill-defined nodular shadows may persist at the periphery of the lung for as long as 1 to 2 years.

COMPLICATIONS Measles, usually a benign self-limited disease, may be associated with a number of complicating illnesses. Viral involvement of the respiratory tract may lead to croup, bronchitis, bronchiolitis, or rarely to *interstitial giant-cell pneumonia,* which is seen most often in children suffering from severe systemic disease such as leukemia, congenital immunodeficiency, or severe malnutrition, and which is characterized by severe respiratory symptoms, pulmonary infiltrations, and the presence in the lungs of multinucleated giant cells. It may occur in the absence of the typical measles exanthem. *Conjunctivitis,* which is seen regularly in the course of uncomplicated measles, may occasionally progress to corneal ulceration, keratitis, and blindness. *Myocarditis,* characterized by transient changes in the electrocardiogram, occurs in about 20 percent of patients with measles, but clinical evidence of cardiac dysfunction is rare. Viral involvement of the mesenteric lymph nodes and appendix may result in abdominal pain and signs of peritoneal inflammation so severe that surgical exploration is considered. The situation is especially confusing if the evidence of appendiceal involvement becomes manifest during the preeruptive phase of the disease. Measles infection of pregnant women results in death of the fetus in about 20 percent of the cases; however, a teratogenic effect such as that observed in rubella has not been demonstrated.

Superimposed bacterial pneumonia caused by streptococci, pneumococci, staphylococci, or *Hemophilus influenzae* is considerably more common than giant-cell pneumonia and occasionally may progress to formation of empyema or lung abscess. Bacterial otitis media is a frequent sequel of measles infection in children. In tropical areas, stomatitis, probably of bacterial origin, progressing to cancrum oris may be encountered during the course of the disease.

In addition to conditions associated with the viral infection and the complications resulting from superimposed bacterial infection, several situations may arise after measles infection which are of uncertain pathogenesis. Clinically apparent *encephalomyelitis* occurs in 1 of 1000 patients with measles. It usually begins 4 to 7 days after the appearance of the eruption, but may precede the rash by 10 days or follow it by 24 days. It is characterized by high fever, headache, drowsiness, and coma, and in some patients by focal brain or spinal cord involvement. Death occurs in about 10 percent of affected individuals, and persistent signs of central nervous system damage, including mental changes, epilepsy, and paralysis, are encountered. Electroencephalographic abnormalities without other signs of central nervous system dysfunction may be demonstrated in 50 percent of patients with otherwise uncomplicated measles. Though it is generally postulated that the encephalomyelitis is "postinfectious" or allergic in origin, a report of isolation of the virus from the brain of a patient with a fatal case suggests direct viral invasion of the central nervous system. A progressive, fatal encephalitis has been described in children with lymphatic malignancies treated with immunosuppressive drugs, with onset 1 to 6 months after an episode of measles. Other, more unusual neurologic complications include transverse myelitis and ascending myelitis. An extremely rare condition, *subacute sclerosing panencephalitis* (Chap. 192), is now thought to be a late complication of measles. *Thrombocytopenia* may occur 3 to 15 days after the onset of symptoms and results in purpura as well as bleeding from mouth, intestine, and genitourinary tract. Measles is also associated with transient suppression of delayed hypersensitivity to tuberculin, exacerbation of existing tuberculosis, and an increased incidence of new tuberculous infections.

LABORATORY FINDINGS Leukopenia is frequent in the prodromal phase of measles, and the appearance of leukocytosis suggests bacterial superinfection or another complication. Extreme lymphopenia (less than 2000 lymphocytes per cubic millimeter) is considered to be a poor prognostic sign. During the prodrome and in the early eruptive phase, multinucleated giant cells can be identified in stained preparations of sputum, nasal secretions, or urine, and the measles virus can be isolated by inoculation of the same materials into appropriate cell cultures. Complement fixation, neutralization and hemagglutination inhibition tests are available for serologic confirmation of measles. Spinal fluid protein of patients with encephalomyelitis ranges from 48 to 240 mg/ml, and lymphocyte counts are usually in a range of 5 to 99 per cubic millimeter, although counts as high as 1000 per cubic millimeter have been reported. Bacterial infection can be identified by appropriate cultures.

DIFFERENTIAL DIAGNOSIS Measles, with its prodrome, Koplik's spots, and characteristic rash, is infrequently confused with other diseases. Rubella is a milder disease of shorter duration with mild respiratory complaints or none at all. Infectious mononucleosis and toxoplasmosis can be identified by the presence of atypical lymphocytes and by serologic tests. Secondary syphilis may display skin lesions similar to the measles rash. Other infections which can sometimes mimic measles include those caused by adenoviruses, enteroviruses, *Mycoplasma pneumoniae,* and *Streptococcus pyogenes,* e.g., scarlet fever. Drug reactions, particularly those associated with ampicillin and Dilantin, can also produce a morbilliform rash. The atypical form of measles in patients previously immunized with inactivated vaccine may suggest Rocky Mountain spotted fever.

PROPHYLAXIS Measles can be prevented by the administration of 0.25 ml/kg gamma globulin within 5 days of exposure. Passive immunization should be considered for any susceptible person exposed to the disease, but is especially important for children under 3 years of age, for pregnant women, for patients with tuberculosis, and for those patients in whom immune mechanisms are impaired. A modified, less severe form of the disease which results in some degree of active immunity may be observed if 0.04 ml/kg gamma globulin is given within 5 days of exposure (see "Manifestations," above). Prophylactic administration of antibiotics does not decrease the frequency or severity of bacterial superinfections.

Active immunity can be induced by the use of live, attenuated measles virus without spread to contacts of vaccinated individuals. Further attenuated vaccine strains (Schwarz, Attenuvax) derived from additional chick cell culture passages of the original Edmonston B strains are currently recommended and are associated with few local or systemic reactions. Vaccination with these preparations induces antibody formation in more than 95 percent of susceptible individuals. The vaccine can induce protection if given before, or within 2 days after, exposure. After this time, active immunization is less predictable in its ability to confer protection to the already exposed individual, although no ill effects have been noted when vaccination followed exposure by more than two days. Vaccination results in protection for at least 10 years, but the total duration of immunity is not known. Live measles vaccine should not be given to pregnant women, to patients with untreated tuberculosis, to patients with leukemia or lymphoma, or to those who are receiving therapy which depresses immune reponses. Hypersensitivity reactions have not been associated with the vaccine even among egg-sensitive individuals; however, the vaccine should not be given to persons known to be hypersensitive to vaccine components, such as trace amounts of antibiotics. Except in unusual circumstances, vaccination should not be given in the first 13 months of life. However, if epidemiologic circumstances suggest a risk to infants in the 6- to 13-month age group, the vaccine may be used, and a second dose administered at 15 to 18 months of age to ensure adequate seroconversion. The vaccine seems equally effective when administered alone or simultaneously in combination with rubella and mumps vaccines. Measles vaccination has been very effective in decreasing the incidence of measles in the United States without producing serious side effects. Measles occurs most commonly among the unvaccinated, who, for the most part, are members of low socioeconomic groups. The disease rarely

occurs in those who have been vaccinated, although there have been vaccine failures. These failures are related, in part, to early vaccination of infants who still have maternal neutralizing antibody or to the use of improperly stored vaccine.

There is no indication for the use of *inactivated* vaccine because of severe atypical measles which has been observed in persons immunized with it (see "Manifestations," above).

TREATMENT No therapy is indicated for uncomplicated measles. Gamma globulin, although effective in prophylaxis, is of no value once symptoms are evident. Patients should be monitored for the development of bacterial superinfections, with specific antibiotic selection based on clinical and bacteriologic findings.

REFERENCES

AICARDI J et al: Acute measles encephalitis in children with immunosuppression. Pediatrics 59:232, 1977

COOVADIA HM et al: Immunoparesis and outcome in measles. Lancet 1:619, 1977

ENDERS JF, PEEBLES T: Propagation in tissue cultures of cytopathogenic agents from patients with measles. Proc Soc Exp Biol Med 86:277, 1954

HORSTMANN DM: Problems in measles and rubella. Dis Mon, vol 24, no 6, 1978

KRUGMAN S: Present status of measles and rubella immunization in the United States: A medical progress report. J Pediatr 90:1, 1977

Measles prevention. Morb Mort Week Rep, vol 27, no 44, November 3, 1978

MEULEN V et al: Isolation of infectious measles virus in measles encephalitis. Lancet 2:1172, 1972

RAND KH et al: Measles in adults: Unforeseen consequences of immunization? JAMA 236:1028, 1976

RUUSKANEN O et al: Measles vaccination after exposure to natural measles. J Pediatr 93:43, 1978

WITTE JJ: The epidemiology and control of measles. Am J Epidemiol 100:77, 1974

182
RUBELLA ("GERMAN MEASLES")

C. GEORGE RAY

DEFINITION Rubella ("German measles," "3-day measles") is usually a benign febrile exanthem, but when it occurs in pregnant women, it may lead to serious chronic fetal infection and malformations.

ETIOLOGY In the late 1930s and 1940s rubella was transmitted to humans and monkeys, and in 1962 a viral agent was recovered in cell cultures inoculated with nasopharyngeal secretions of infected persons. Human primary amnion cells infected with rubella virus display rounding, clumping of nuclear chromatin, and eosinophilic intranuclear inclusions. Rabbit kidney and some other cell lines also display cytopathic effects. Rubella virus can be detected indirectly in African green monkey kidney cells by the interference or exclusion method. In this system, cells infected with rubella appear normal but are resistant to superinfection with viruses such as echovirus 11 or coxsackievirus A9 that ordinarily produce a cytopathic effect in these cells. Complement-fixing antigen and a hemagglutinin have been identified.

The rubella virion, 50 to 85 nm in diameter, is a somewhat spheroidal RNA virus which has been tentatively classified in the togavirus family.

PATHOGENESIS AND PATHOLOGY Rubella can be induced in susceptible persons by the instillation of virus into the nasopharynx, and natural infection is probably induced in the same way. Virus is present in blood, throat washings, and occasionally feces for several days before the exanthem becomes apparent. It can be detected in blood for 1 to 2 days, and in throat washings for as long as 7 days before appearance of rash, to 2 weeks after onset. Lymph nodes show edema and hyperplasia.

Congenital rubella results from transplacental transmission of virus to the fetus from an infected mother, and may be associated with growth retardation, infiltration of liver and spleen by hematopoietic tissue, interstitial pneumonia, a decreased number of megakaryocytes in the bone marrow, and various structural malformations of the cardiovascular and central nervous systems. The virus can persist in the fetus during intrauterine life and may be excreted for 6 to 31 months after birth.

EPIDEMIOLOGY Rubella is not as contagious as measles, and immunity to the disease is not so widespread. Estimates of susceptibility to rubella among women of childbearing age range from 10 to 25 percent. Before the routine introduction of vaccine in 1969, epidemics occurred at 6- to 9-year intervals; however, it is not known whether this cyclical pattern will continue in the future. In 1964 more than 1.8 million cases of rubella were reported in the United States; in 1976, 12,491 cases were reported in this country. Rubella was once most frequent among children 5 to 9 years of age, but with the advent of immunization programs often directed primarily at this age group as well as at preschoolers, a greater proportion of cases is now being reported among older school children and young adults. Sixty percent of the reported cases in 1976 occurred in persons 15 years of age or older.

MANIFESTATIONS The time from exposure to the appearance of the rash of rubella is 14 to 21 days, usually about 18 days. In adults there may be a prodromal illness preceding the exanthem by 1 to 7 days, consisting of malaise, headache, fever, mild conjunctivitis, and lymphadenopathy. In children the rash may be the first manifestation of disease. It is apparent from serologic studies that rubella infection may be associated with no signs or symptoms, or may result in lymph node enlargement without skin lesions; however, rash without lymphadenopathy is uncommon. Respiratory symptoms are mild or absent. Small, red lesions (Forchheimer's spots) occasionally may be seen on the soft palate but are not pathognomonic of the disease.

The rash begins on the forehead and face and spreads downward to the trunk and extremities. The small maculopapular lesions, of lighter hue than those of measles, are usually discrete but may coalesce to form a diffuse erythema suggestive of scarlet fever. The rash may last from 1 to 5 days, but is most commonly present for 3 days. Enlarged, tender lymph nodes appear before the rash, are most impressive during the early eruptive phase, and may persist several days after the rash has disappeared. Splenomegaly or generalized lymphadenopathy may occur, but the postauricular and suboccipital nodes are most strikingly involved. Arthralgias and slight joint swellings may be a complication of rubella, especially in young women. The pain and swelling, involving wrists, fingers, and knees, are most marked during the period of rash and may persist for 1 to 14 days after other manifestations of rubella

have disappeared. Recurring joint symptoms for a year or more have also been reported. Purpura with or without thrombocytopenia may occur and may be associated with hemorrhage. Encephalomyelitis following rubella resembles other postinfectious encephalitides and is much less common than encephalitis following measles. Testicular pain is also occasionally reported in young adults.

Congenital rubella The syndrome of congenital rubella has conventionally been thought to consist of heart malformations—patent ductus arteriosus, interventricular septal defect, or pulmonic stenosis; eye lesions—corneal clouding, cataracts, chorioretinitis, and microphthalmia; microcephaly, mental retardation, and deafness. In the American epidemic of 1964, thrombocytopenic purpura, hepatosplenomegaly, intrauterine growth retardation, interstitial pneumonia, myocarditis or myocardial necrosis, and metaphyseal bone lesions were encountered frequently in association with the previously recognized manifestations, leading to the term *expanded rubella syndrome*. Some infants have also been found to have significant humoral and/or cellular immunodeficiency, which generally resolves as chronic viral excretion diminishes and eventually ceases. Any combination of lesions may be seen in an individual infant, and the severity is highly variable.

Later complications include an apparent higher risk of subsequent development of diabetes mellitus. In addition, there are reports of patients with congenital rubella who develop a progressive, subacute panencephalitis, with onset in the second decade of life. This is characterized by intellectual deterioration, ataxia, seizures, and spasticity.

Congenital rubella is usually the result of maternal infection during the first trimester of pregnancy, although well-documented cases have resulted from infection several days before conception; deafness may occur as a result of infection in the fourth month. In the 1964 epidemic, about 10 percent of women with clinically recognized rubella during the first trimester gave birth to infants with the rubella syndrome. Serologically identified, asymptomatic maternal rubella can also result in severe fetal disease. It is therefore desirable to ascertain the immune status of every woman, either before conception or as early in the pregnancy as possible, by history of previous immunization or by serologic testing. If rubella antibodies are present before or within 10 days after exposure, the patient is considered immune, and the risk of fetal damage is virtually nil. If antibodies are not detectable and exposure has occurred, acute and convalescent antibody titers should be determined simultaneously on sera obtained 2 to 4 weeks apart, depending upon the time after exposure when the acute sample was drawn.

DIAGNOSIS Rubella is frequently confused with other diseases associated with maculopapular exanthems such as those described in Chaps. 180 and 183, and with infectious mononucleosis (Chap. 195), as well as with drug eruptions and scarlet fever. *A certain diagnosis of rubella can be made only by virus isolation and identification, or by changes in antibody titers.* Rubella hemagglutination-inhibiting antibodies may be present by the second day of rash and increase in quantity over the next 10 to 21 days. Patients with the congenital rubella syndrome may lose hemagglutination-inhibiting antibodies at age 3 or 4 years. Therefore a negative serologic test in a child over 3 years does not exclude the possibility of congenital rubella. There are no other laboratory findings helpful in the diagnosis of rubella, although lymphocytosis with atypical lymphocytes may occur. Congenital rubella should be differentiated by appropriate serologic tests from congenital syphilis (Chap. 146), toxoplasmosis (Chap. 203), and cytomegalic inclusion virus disease (Chap. 194).

PREVENTION In adults and children rubella is usually a mild disease with infrequent complications. However, the severity of congenital infection has prompted efforts to prevent the disease. Administration of gamma globulin to exposed persons can abort the clinical disease, but seroconversion and transmission of the disease from mother to fetus may occur despite the administration of large amounts of gamma globulin soon after exposure.

Active immunization with live attenuated rubella vaccines prepared in duck, dog, rabbit, or human diploid fibroblast cells has been practiced in this country since 1969, especially among young children. The aim has been to decrease the frequency of the infection in the population, thus decreasing the chance that susceptible pregnant women will be exposed. Because of concern for a possibly enlarging pool of susceptible adolescents and adults, there has been increasing enthusiasm for serologic screening of pubertal females with no history of immunization, followed by selective immunization of those who are seronegative. Such immunization must of course be done with appropriate precautions, as noted below.

The attenuated virus can be detected in the respiratory secretions of vaccines for as long as 4 weeks after immunization, but transmission to other susceptible individuals rarely, if ever, occurs. This has not been shown to be a problem, even in households where susceptible pregnant women are in contact with children who are being vaccinated. The vaccine induces antibodies in about 95 percent of recipients, but the degree and duration of protection are still being evaluated. After heavy exposure in closed populations, vaccinated individuals sometimes develop subclinical infections (diagnosed by antibody rises and virus isolation). However, viremia has not been demonstrated in immunized persons, which suggests that previously vaccinated pregnant women will not infect their fetuses even if they acquire subclinical rubella.

Side effects of fever, rash, lymphadenopathy, polyneuropathy, or arthralgias occur very seldom in vaccinated children, but joint pain and swelling or paresthesias were seen in more than 25 percent of women who were immunized with the earlier vaccines. The risk has been reduced to 2 to 9 percent with the advent of vaccines prepared in rabbit or human embryonic fibroblast cell cultures. The joint symptoms usually begin 2 to 10 weeks after vaccination, and they may be confused with other forms of arthritis. *Rubella vaccine must never be given to pregnant women or to those who may be pregnant within 2 months of immunization.* This precaution is necessary because the vaccine virus has the theoretical potential to damage the fetus of susceptible women.

REFERENCES

Fox JP et al: Rubella vaccine in postpubertal women. JAMA 236:837, 1976

Horstmann D: Problems in measles and rubella. Dis Mon, vol 24, no 6, 1978

Krugman S: Present status of measles and rubella immunization in the United States: A medical progress report. J Pediatr 90:1, 1977

Modlin JF et al: Risk of congenital abnormality after inadvertent rubella vaccination of pregnant women. N Engl J Med 294:972, 1976

Plotkin SA et al: Immunologic properties of RA 27/3 rubella virus vaccine. JAMA 225:585, 1973

Schlossberg D, Topolosky MK: Military rubella. JAMA 238:1273, 1977

Sever JL et al: Rubella epidemic, 1964: Effect on 6,000 pregnancies. Am J Dis Child 110:395,1965

Townsend JJ et al: Progressive rubella panencephalitis: Late onset after congenital rubella. N Engl J Med 292:990, 1975

Weil ML et al: Chronic progressive panencephalitis due to rubella virus stimulating SSPE. N Engl J Med 292:994, 1975

183
OTHER VIRAL EXANTHEMATOUS DISEASES

C. GEORGE RAY

In addition to the diseases such as measles, rubella and chickenpox, which historically have been associated with prominent skin lesions, there are other virus infections in which skin manifestations may occur. Table 183-1 lists the other most commonly recognized causes of maculopapular eruptions. Some of them, particularly the enteroviruses, can also occasionally cause papulovesicular or petechial rashes; others are capable of provoking erythema multiforme-like eruptions. One helpful aspect of the physical examination is the observation that viral-caused maculopapular (not vesicular) exanthems usually *relatively* spare the palms and soles. This is in contrast to eruptions associated with drug reactions, bacteria, *Mycoplasma,* and *Rickettsia,* in which a prominent palmar or plantar eruption is often noted.

EXANTHEM SUBITUM (ROSEOLA INFANTUM) Exanthem subitum is a benign disease of infants 6 to 24 months of age that is characterized by a high fever and rash. The disease can be transmitted to humans and monkeys by the transfer of blood obtained from a patient during the first few days of illness. The infectious agent is probably a virus, although it has not been isolated. The first manifestations of disease, after an estimated incubation period of 5 to 15 days, are the abrupt onset of irritability and fever, which lasts for 3 to 5 days; the temperature may be as high as 105°F. There may be mild pharyngitis and slight lymph node enlargement; convulsions may occur during the height of the fever. On the fourth to fifth day of illness, there is a sudden drop in temperature to normal or below normal; several hours before or after defervescence the rash suddenly and surprisingly appears. It is characterized by faint 2- to 3-mm macules or maculopapules over the neck and trunk and may extend to the thighs and buttocks; it may last for only a few hours or may be present for a day or two. Leukopenia is frequently noted later in the febrile period. The disease is benign and not associated with complications, although rarely an infant may show sequelae as a result of febrile convulsions. In the early, preeruptive phase, the disease may be difficult to differentiate from an acute, occult bacteremia, particularly from one associated with *Streptococcus pneumoniae.* Though a leukocytosis with an increase in band forms is often seen in occult bacteremias presenting in this fashion, blood cultures are necessary to aid in precise diagnosis.

ERYTHEMA INFECTIOSUM (FIFTH DISEASE) Erythema infectiosum is a mild febrile exanthematous disease with little or no prodrome. The incubation period is probably 5 to 10 days. The first manifestations are low-grade fever and the appearance of indurated, confluent erythema over the cheeks, giving a

TABLE 183-1
Causes of maculopapular eruptions

Viral	Other
Measles	*Mycoplasma pneumoniae*
Rubella	Syphilis
Exanthem subitum	Typhoid fever
Erythema infectiosum	Bacterial toxins:
Enteroviruses: coxsackievirus,	streptococci and staphylococci
echovirus	Rat-bite fever
Infectious mononucleosis	*Rickettsia*
Adenoviruses	Live-virus vaccines
Reoviruses	Drug eruptions
Arboviruses	

"slapped face" appearance. A day or so later, a bilaterally symmetric eruption is seen on the arms, legs, and trunk, but rarely on the palms or soles. The lesions are maculopapular and tend to be confluent, forming slightly raised blotchy areas and reticular or lacy patterns. The rash usually lasts about a week, and during this time it may disappear, only to reappear in the same areas a few hours later. The waxing and waning eruption may occasionally persist for several weeks, and can be brought on by fever, heat, exercise, sunlight exposure, or emotional stress. Mild joint pain and swelling have been observed in a large proportion of adults with the disease. Erythema infectiosum affects all ages but is most common in children of school age and may occur in epidemic form. The mode of transmission of the disease is not known, and an infectious agent has not been recovered. A clinical diagnosis of this disease must sometimes be made with caution, since rubella and some enteroviruses have also been shown at times to cause a nearly identical syndrome.

ENTEROVIRAL EXANTHEMS Many individual enteroviruses have been associated with rash. Of these, polioviruses are rarely implicated. More commonly, echovirus serotypes 1 through 7, 9, 11, 12, 14, 16, 18, 19, 20, 25, and 30, coxsackievirus serotypes A4, A5, A6, A9, A10, A16, and B2, B3, and B5 have all been implicated. With the exception of hand-foot-and-mouth disease, usually associated with coxsackievirus A16 infection (Chap. 187), there is no set of clinical or epidemiologic features that aid in differentiating the specific enteroviral agent involved in a specific case. All are capable of producing maculopapular rashes which vary in intensity and duration, and can also occasionally produce petechial or papulovesicular exanthems and enanthems. In community and household outbreaks, younger children and infants are usually more likely to manifest exanthems, while other features of enteroviral infection, such as fever, myalgia, and aseptic meningitis, are more prominent among older children and young adults. Two enterovirus infections which have been frequently associated with rashes and have been studied extensively are described here as examples of epidemic enteroviral infections.

Boston exanthem (infections with echovirus 16) Echovirus 16 infection was described first and most extensively during an epidemic in Boston in 1951. Children who were infected usually had a disease characterized by exanthem and low-grade fever, while adult family contacts often developed high fever, prostration, and signs of aseptic meningitis with absent or fleeting rash. The first manifestation of the disease in children was fever of 101 to 102°F, lasting for a day or two, pharyngitis with small ulcerated lesions resembling herpangina, and slight enlargement of the cervical and postauricular lymph nodes. The rash appeared during fever or after defervescence and consisted of small pink maculopapules on the face, upper part of the chest, and occasionally on the whole body, including the palms and soles. The rash lasted for 1 to 5 days, and there were no important complications or sequelae. The disease resembled exanthem subitum but occurred in children of all ages and in adults.

Infection with echovirus 9 Infection with this virus in children and adults has been characterized by a febrile illness with a high incidence of aseptic meningitis. The incubation period is 5 to 8 days. About 30 percent of patients have a rash, which may occur with or without meningitis. It is usually maculopapular, developing at the onset of fever. The exanthem appears first on the face and neck, spreads to the trunk and extremities, may involve the palms and soles, although slightly, and persists for 3 to 5 days. Petechiae with or without maculopapules have

been recognized; when they are seen in association with meningitis, there may be confusion with meningococcal meningitis. This can be a point of some concern, since concurrent outbreaks of echovirus 9 and meningococcal disease have been observed. A vesicular eruption with crusting lesions has been seen occasionally. An exanthem on the buccal mucosa and soft palate occurs in about 30 percent of patients and consists of small red areas with white centers which resemble Koplik's spots. The disease is usually benign but rarely has been associated with permanent central nervous system damage.

REFERENCES

BALFOUR HH: Erythema infectiosum: Clinical description of 91 cases seen in an epidemic. Clin Pediatr 8:721, 1969
———— et al: Erythema infectiosum: Recovery of rubella virus and echovirus 12. Pediatrics 50:285, 1972
HALL CB et al: The return of Boston exanthem. Echovirus 16 infections in 1974. Am J Dis Child 131:323, 1977
LAUER BA et al: Erythema infectiosum. Am J Dis Child 130:252, 1976
LERNER AM et al: New viral exanthems. N Engl J Med 269:678, 1963
NEVA FA et al: Clinical epidemiological features of unusual epidemic exanthem. JAMA 155:544, 1954
WENNER HA: Virus diseases associated with cutaneous eruptions. Prog Med Virol 16:269, 1973

184
SMALLPOX, VACCINIA, AND COWPOX

C. GEORGE RAY

Poxviruses are a group of large (200 to 320 nm), brick-shaped DNA-containing viruses that possess a common antigen and have a predilection for skin. Many of the poxviruses, such as myxoma and fowl pox agents, cause disease mainly in lower animals. Smallpox (variola major), alastrim (variola minor), vaccinia, and cowpox agents are closely related members of the poxvirus group that cause human disease. All these viruses grow and produce pox on the chorioallantoic membrane of chick embryos and can be cultivated in cells from various mammalian tissues with formation of intracytoplasmic inclusions, rounding fusion and heaping up of cells, and eventual degeneration of the infected area. The poxviruses responsible for human disease may be distinguished from one another by minor antigenic differences and by the type and severity of lesions they induce in experimental animals and humans. Smallpox and alastrim viruses produce smaller pox on the chorioallantoic membrane than vaccinia, and there are differences in incubation temperatures at which poxviruses produce lesions.

SMALLPOX (VARIOLA)

DEFINITION Smallpox is a severe, contagious, febrile disease characterized by a vesicular and pustular eruption. Alastrim is a similar but milder illness, with a lower mortality rate. Though the difference in severity between these diseases is apparent, the agents of smallpox and alastrim are biologically and immunologically indistinguishable from each other in the laboratory.

PATHOGENESIS AND PATHOLOGY The virus gains access to the body by the respiratory tract and multiplies in unidentified sites, probably in lymph nodes or liver. After several days, during which there is no evidence of infection, viremia ensues, with swelling of the endothelium of blood vessels in the corium and perivascular inflammation. Loculated vesicles are the result of cellular destruction and exudation of serum. The infected epithelial cells are swollen and contain intracytoplasmic inclusions surrounded by a halo (Guarnieri bodies). The extent of skin involvement is greater in smallpox than in chickenpox and reaches into the corium. Pitting, most commonly seen on the face, is said to result from destruction of sebaceous glands, which are abundant in this area. The liver, spleen, and lymph nodes may be enlarged and may show focal accumulations of large mononuclear cells.

EPIDEMIOLOGY Smallpox is not as contagious as measles or influenza, and ordinarily face-to-face contact with an infected person is required to transmit the disease; however, airborne dissemination from contaminated fomites has also been shown to occur. A patient with smallpox is infectious from a day before the rash appears until all lesions have healed and the scabs have fallen off. During the early phase of the illness, the virus is transmitted in nasopharyngeal secretions; when the eruption is fully formed, the lesions themselves are a major source of infectious material. Variola virus may contaminate clothing, bedding, dust, or other inanimate objects and remain infectious for months, necessitating disinfection of articles in the patient's environment. The World Health Organization's program to eradicate smallpox has resulted in marked decrease in the incidence of the disease since 1966, and the prospects for ultimate eradication seem bright. Two important epidemiologic factors which would suggest that this is possible are the absence of nonhuman reservoir for the virus, and the apparent nonexistence of completely asymptomatic human carriers. Control and the ultimate eradication of the disease, therefore, rely on complete reporting of cases and identification of even very mild ones, as a prelude to specific quarantine and selective immunization.

By April 1978 no new cases of smallpox had been reported from anywhere in the world since a case with onset of rash in October 1977 was identified in Somalia. That country is considered to be the last remaining endemic area, and, if a total of 2 years of effective surveillance elapses without further cases, it will be declared smallpox-free.

In August 1978 a case of laboratory-associated smallpox was reported from the medical school in Birmingham, England. Presumably the patient was infected by airborne transmission from a smallpox laboratory to her office area one floor removed.

MANIFESTATIONS The incubation period of smallpox, from the time of exposure to the onset of the prodrome, is about 12 days, with extremes of 7 to 17 days. The disease can be divided into a prodrome, an early eruptive phase, and a period of vesiculation and pustule formation. The prodrome is characterized by a temperature of 102 to 106°F, headache, myalgia especially in the back, abdominal pain, vomiting, and in some patients by a transient, blotchy, erythematous eruption. After 3 or 4 days the fever subsides, the symptoms decrease, and the patient seems to recover. It is at this time, when the patient is afebrile, that the focal eruption begins. Early manifestations are painful ulcers on the buccal mucosa and macules which appear first on the face and forearms, and rapidly become firm, shotty papules. The papules increase in number and spread from the face and distal extremities to involve the trunk. The individual lesions may remain discrete and scattered, or they may become confluent and involve most of the body. They are most concentrated on the face and distal extremities, including the palms and soles, and are relatively sparse in the axilla. On the third or fourth day after the appearance of the focal rash, the papules progress to vesicles containing clear fluid, which, over the next few days, becomes cloudy because of infiltration

by pus cells and desquamated epithelial cells; hemorrhage into the vesicles and surrounding skin may also be seen. During the course of smallpox, the lesions at any one time, in one area, are all at the same stage of evolution. At the time the vesicles become pustular, there is recurrence of fever, which may persist until healing occurs. The pustules umbilicate and form crusts and scabs which usually fall off 3 weeks after the beginning of illness, leaving small scars or deep pits.

The above description applies to disease of moderate severity. A milder illness may occur in previously immunized persons or in some who have no history of vaccination. It is characterized by the usual incubation period and prodrome, but is followed either by focal eruption of fewer than 100 papules, or by a rash resembling chickenpox. Smallpox with prodrome but with no eruption of any kind has been recognized (variola sine eruptione). The disease may also occur in a rapidly fulminating form ("sledgehammer" smallpox). After the usual incubation period, the patient develops an initial illness characterized by severe prostration, fever, bone marrow depression, hemorrhagic skin lesions, and bleeding. The disease progresses from inception to death within 3 or 4 days without evidence of the typical focal skin lesions.

Alastrim is similar to mild and moderate forms of variola major in that it has the same incubation period and prodromal illness, but the skin eruption is less extensive, and fatalities are rare and usually related to secondary bacterial infections.

COMPLICATIONS Bacterial superinfections of the lesions usually with *Staphylococcus aureus*, may occur in the late pustular stage. Bacterial pneumonia and sepsis may be seen in severe forms of smallpox. Mild conjunctivitis is quite common, and iritis and keratitis have been recognized. Encephalomyelitis may occur in the late stage of the disease and is similar to other postinfectious encephalitides. Osteomyelitis and joint effusions may complicate the disease, and orchitis has also been reported.

LABORATORY FINDINGS Leukopenia is present during the prodromal illness, and there is usually leukocytosis during the pustular stage. Rapid diagnosis of poxvirus infection can be made by the finding of characteristic brick-shaped particles in preparations of vesicle fluid examined by electron microscopy. Specific precipitation in agar by use of antigen prepared from lesions and antivariola or antivaccinia immune serum may also allow detection of poxvirus within a few hours. These tests do not distinguish variola from vaccinia or other poxviruses but do allow rapid differentiation from herpes simplex and varicella-zoster viruses. For definitive identification the virus must be grown in cell culture or on the chorioallantoic membrane and neutralized with specific antiserum.

DIFFERENTIAL DIAGNOSIS The major problem in differential diagnosis is in distinguishing smallpox from chickenpox. Smallpox is preceded by a longer prodrome than chickenpox, and the eruption vesiculates over a period of days instead of hours. The smallpox lesions are all characteristically in the same stage of development, whereas those of chickenpox may, in one area, display all stages of evolution. Electron microscopy and agar precipitation techniques (see above) are especially useful in distinguishing between smallpox and chickenpox. Cytologic examination of scrapings of the base of a vesicle can also be helpful in the differential diagnosis. The presence of multinucleated giant cells and/or intranuclear inclusions strongly suggests a herpes group infection (varicella-zoster or herpes simplex); such findings are not seen with poxvirus infections.

Other conditions which are sometimes confused with smallpox include eczema vaccinatum, eczema herpeticum, rickettsialpox, drug eruptions, some cases of contact dermatitis, and Stevens-Johnson syndrome. The fulminant, hemorrhagic smallpox may closely resemble meningococcemia, typhus, and hemorrhagic fevers.

PREVENTION Smallpox may be prevented among the patient's contacts by vaccination. Because this procedure is most successful if carried out during the early part of the incubation period, all exposed persons, regardless of previous immunization, should be vaccinated immediately upon recognition of exposure. Large, controlled, clinical trials have demonstrated that oral administration of *N*-methylisatin 3-thiosemicarbazone (methisazone), a drug which interferes with poxvirus multiplication, can prevent smallpox and alastrim in patients exposed to the diseases. The use of a drug together with prompt vaccination results in greater chance of protection than either measure alone. A drawback to the use of methisazone is its tendency to induce vomiting. The combined use of vaccination and parenteral administration of vaccinia immune globulin early in the incubation period is also effective in the prevention of smallpox in exposed individuals. It is now usual to apply these control measures selectively to the primary and secondary contacts of a patient rather than to all the inhabitants of a community.

In order to avoid laboratory-acquired smallpox, storage of the virus should be restricted to the five World Health Organization reference centers.

TREATMENT There is no specific therapy for smallpox. Thiosemicarbazone, although effective in prophylaxis, has not been shown to be of value in the treatment of established cases. Fluid deficits should be replaced by the administration of appropriate solutions. During the vesicular and pustular phases of the disease, an attempt should be made to prevent bacterial infection by the use of sterile sheets and aseptic nursing procedures. Antihistamines may be helpful in decreasing pruritus. Application of lotions or ointment should be avoided. Later in the course of the illness, when desquamation has begun, showers or baths may be helpful in removing desquamating tissue. If bacterial infection develops, an antibiotic active against the infecting organism should be given by the parenteral route. Topical antibiotics should be avoided.

VACCINIA

Vaccinia is a virus disease of the skin which is induced by inoculation for the prevention of smallpox. The exact origin of the vaccinia virus is obscure. The material first used by Jenner in 1796 was derived from cowpox lesions, and the infectious agent was propagated for many years by successive passage from person to person through use of exudate from fresh skin lesions. The original agent possibly became contaminated with variola virus during the period when transfer was being carried out without strict controls. It has been suggested that vaccinia virus is a hybrid of cowpox and variola agents, a contention supported by the finding that laboratory-induced hybrids of variola and cowpox viruses have many of the characteristics associated with vaccinia.

VACCINATION Live, lyophilized vaccinia virus prepared from vesicle fluid of infected calves is commercially available and maintains potency for 18 months at 46°F. It is dissolved in a diluent solution just prior to use. The usual method for vaccination is to apply a small drop of vaccine to the skin over the deltoid muscle and to press a sterile needle through the vaccine several times in such a way that only the superficial layer of skin is entered, or by simultaneous puncture utilizing a plastic tine device. Vaccination should always induce some form of skin reaction; complete absence of any kind of lesion indicates that the vaccine was not viable or was not administered properly. The reaction which occurs in nonimmune individuals is characterized by a red papule at the site of inoculation 3 to 5 days after vaccination. The papule becomes vesicular on about the fifth or sixth day and pustular by the ninth or eleventh day after inoculation. The vesicle and pustule may be surrounded by a large area of erythema. About 2 weeks after vaccination, the pustule dries and develops a crust which falls off by the end of the third week, leaving a scar. Fever, malaise, and irritability are common in children during the vesicular and pustular phases, and axillary lymphadenopathy may develop and persist for several months. In the partially immune person, a modified reaction develops without fever or constitutional symptoms. A papule appears on the skin within 3 days, vesiculates in 5 to 7 days, and heals without much scarring. The so-called "immune" reaction described by some, where a papule and/or erythema appears in a few days, then recedes without vesiculation, is an "equivocal" reaction, and may simply represent allergy to the components of an inadvertently inactivated vaccine. A successful vaccination is defined as the presence of a Jennerian vesicle (vesicular, pustular, or crusted) 7 days after inoculation. If the criterion is not met, the patient should be revaccinated, preferably with vaccine from a different lot.

Revaccination every 3 years is required to ensure protection, *but vaccination is currently indicated only for a few laboratory workers who might have contact with variola virus and for travelers to countries which still require vaccination as a condition for entry. Absolute contraindications* to vaccination include individuals with congenital or acquired immune deficiencies, lymphoma, leukemia or other blood dyscrasias, patients being treated with steroids, antimetabolites, alkylating agents, or ionizing irradiation, and individuals with a history of vaccinia encephalitis. *Relative contraindications* include patients or household contacts with eczema or a history of eczema, severe acne, or other similar dermatologic problems, pregnancy, and infants under twelve months of age. If the necessity to vaccinate any individual in this latter group is great, simultaneous administration of vaccinia immune globulin (VIG), 0.3 ml/kg, is suggested, to be given at a separate site intramuscularly at the time of immunization.

COMPLICATIONS Healing of the primary vaccinal lesion may not occur, and some patients go on to develop slowly progressive necrosis with destruction of large areas of skin, subcutaneous tissue, and underlying structures (*vaccinia gangrenosum*). In addition to the local destruction, there may be metastatic lesions on other parts of the skin surface and in bone and viscera. Vaccinia gangrenosum occurs most frequently in persons with disorders of immunity and, if untreated, is nearly always fatal. *Eczema vaccinatum* is a serious complication that is seen in persons with eczema or other types of chronic skin conditions. Widespread infection in the previously affected areas, as well as in normal skin, may result from direct vaccination of an eczematous patient or from exposure to a recently vaccinated individual. *Generalized vaccinia* in patients without preexisting skin disease is characterized by a few satellite lesions surrounding the inoculation site or by widely disseminated pox resembling the primary vaccination lesion. This condition is usually mild with generally complete recovery. Vaccinia virus may be transferred from the primary inoculation site to the eye or other sites by scratching. *Postvaccinal encephalomyelitis* appears from 2 to 25 days after vaccination. The patient suddenly becomes severely ill with nuchal rigidity, drowsiness, vomiting, convulsions, coma, and signs suggesting disease of the spinal cord. The period of coma lasts for a few days, and in those who recover there are usually no permanent sequelae. Death occurs in about 30 to 40 percent of the patients with encephalomyelitis. *Erythema multiforme bullosum, or diffuse blotchy erythema,* may occur in vaccinated patients 7 to 10 days after vaccination, and is thought to be an allergic reaction to the virus or other components of the vaccine.

The rates of adverse effects per million primarily vaccinated persons were vaccinia gangrenosum, 0.9; eczema vaccinatum, 10.4; generalized vaccinia, 23.4; vaccinal lesions resulting from accidental implantation of virus, 25.4; postvaccinal encephalitis, 2.9; other complications, 11.8; the death rate was 1 per million. In view of the current status of smallpox in the world, the risks of widespread routine immunization seem far greater than the risk of inadvertent introduction of disease in this country. Because of this, the sharp restriction of indications for vaccination appears to be justified.

Active treatment of vaccinia complications, aside from control of bacterial superinfection and treatment of any underlying defects, is limited. VIG is of possible value in accidental inoculation into secondary sites such as the eye, vaccinia gangrenosum, eczema vaccinatum, and generalized vaccinia. Dosage is usually 0.6 ml/kg intramuscularly, although much larger doses are sometimes used in severe cases. VIG is of no use in erythema multiforme or postvaccinal encephalitis. Thiosemicarbazone has apparently been of benefit in some cases of progressive vaccinia gangrenosum. 5-Iodo-2′-deoxyuridine, while not yet proved to be effective, is suggested for topical treatment of vaccinial keratitis and conjunctivitis.

COWPOX

Cowpox is primarily a disease of the teats and udders of cows. Humans are almost always infected by milking, but occasional spread to contacts may occur from an infected person. The human disease is characterized by low-grade fever and by small papules on the fingers and hand, which go through vesicular and pustular stages resembling the course of vaccinia infection. The lesions may be ruptured by trauma and spread to immediately adjacent areas on the hand and continue to ulcerate for several weeks. Edema, lymphangitis, and axillary lymph node enlargement are common. Very rare cases of postcowpox encephalitis and serious infections of eczematous persons have been reported. In general, the disease is benign, heals without scarring, and is usually uncomplicated.

PARAVACCINIA (MILKERS' NODULES)

Paravaccinia is a poxvirus which is antigenically unrelated to cowpox, but produces similar lesions in humans. It is primarily a disease of calves and milk cows, producing lesions on the teats of the cows and oral lesions in the suckling calf. Humans acquire infection through the skin by direct contact. The lesion is usually solitary, beginning as a macule on the finger, hand, or wrist, and progressing to a firm nodule, 1 to 2 cm in diameter, in 10 days. It then crusts and heals without scarring in 2 to 3 weeks. Occasionally, there is associated lymphadenitis. The lesion and its evolution are closely similar to ecthyma contagiosum (orf), a poxvirus of sheep, which can also infect humans by direct inoculation.

REFERENCES

BEDSON HS, DUMBELL K: Smallpox and vaccinia. Br Med Bull 23:119, 1967

BROWN GC (ed): Symposium: Is routine smallpox vaccination necessary in the United States? Am J Epidemiol 93:221, 1971

DIXON, CW: *Smallpox.* London, Churchill, 1962

DOUGLAS RG et al: Treatment of progressive vaccinia. Arch Intern Med 129:980, 1972

GOLDSTEIN JA et al: Smallpox vaccination reactions, prophylaxis, and therapy of complications. Pediatrics 55:342, 1975

JOKLIK WK: The poxviruses. Bacteriol Rev 30:33, 1966

Laboratory-associated smallpox—England. Morb Mort Week Rep, vol 27, no 35, September 1, 1978

LANE JM et al: Smallpox and smallpox vaccination policy. Annu Rev Med 22:251, 1971

RENNIE AGR et al: Ocular vaccinia. Lancet 2:273, 1974

WENNER HA: Virus diseases associated with cutaneous eruptions. Prog Med Virol 16:269, 1973

185
CHICKENPOX (VARICELLA) AND HERPES ZOSTER

C. GEORGE RAY

DEFINITION Chickenpox is a contagious disease characterized by fever and a disseminated vesicular eruption. Herpes zoster, or shingles, is characterized by segmental inflammation of the spinal or cranial nerves and their ganglions, and by a painful localized vesicular eruption of the skin along the distribution of the involved nerve. Chickenpox and herpes zoster are different manifestations of infection with the same viral agent.

ETIOLOGY In 1953 a virus was recovered from patients with chickenpox and herpes zoster that produced intranuclear, eosinophilic inclusions and multinucleated giant cells in lines of cells derived from various monkey and human tissues. The infectivity of varicella-zoster virus in culture is closely cell-associated, and ordinarily can be passed to other tissue cultures only by transfer of infected, intact cells. The structure of the varicella-zoster virion resembles that of herpes simplex and the other viruses of the herpes group.

PATHOGENESIS AND PATHOLOGY Varicella is presumably transmitted by the respiratory route, although the virus has only rarely been isolated from nasopharyngeal secretions of infected persons. Virus multiplication occurs at some unidentified site and probably results in intermittent viremia, as suggested by the successive crops of widely spaced lesions. Focal viral infection of blood vessels in the corium with intranuclear inclusions in endothelial cells, results in degeneration of the epidermis and formation of vesicles containing serum, polymorphonuclear leukocytes, and multinucleated giant cells. Virus can be isolated from vesicle fluid, but not usually from crusting lesions or scabs, for 3 to 4 days after eruption. In patients with varicella pneumonia, the tracheobronchial mucosa, the alveolar septa, and the interstitial areas of the lungs are edematous and contain monocytic inflammatory cells, cells with intranuclear inclusions and giant cells. The nodular areas of pneumonia may eventually become calcified. The changes in the central nervous system in patients with postinfectious varicella encephalomyelitis resemble those seen in measles. Rarely, encephalomyelitis with inclusion bodies resembling herpes simplex infection may occur, and varicella-zoster virus can be recovered from the central nervous system. In infants and children, acute encephalopathy with fatty infiltration of the viscera (Reye's syndrome) sometimes follows the acute phase of varicella; in this condition, only cerebral edema is found on pathologic examination of the brain.

The pathogenesis of herpes zoster is not clear (see "Epidemiology," below), but the tissue changes are well documented. The dorsal root ganglion of the affected nerve is swollen and hemorrhagic; the edema spreads along the peripheral nerve and may reach the spinal cord. The nerve tissue shows hemorrhagic infarction, inflammation, and necrosis of many of the ganglion cells, some of which contain intranuclear inclusions. The microscopic appearance of zoster skin lesions is almost identical with that described for chickenpox vesicles. Virus can be cultured from the lesions for as long as 8 days after onset.

EPIDEMIOLOGY Chickenpox is a highly contagious disease with attack rates of 80 percent or more among susceptible household contacts of an index case. The infectious period extends from a day or two before the rash until as long as 6 days after the appearance of new skin lesions, or until all vesicles have crusted over. Patients with herpes zoster may be the source of an outbreak of chickenpox among susceptible contacts. Children from 5 to 8 years of age are most commonly affected, but younger children, including newborn infants, and adults may develop chickenpox; an estimated 2 to 20 percent of cases occur in persons over the age of 15 years. Serologic surveys are limited, but indicate that as many as 9 percent of parturient women are susceptible to chickenpox. In the United States the disease is endemic, with superimposed epidemics every 2 to 5 years, usually in the winter or spring.

Herpes zoster is mainly a disease of adults who have previously had chickenpox. The epidemiologic evidence strongly suggests that herpes zoster results from reactivation of virus that has remained dormant in spinal ganglia since an episode of chickenpox. Exogenous acquisition of infection directly resulting in herpes zoster rarely, if ever, occurs. Most patients with zoster have had no recent exposure to patients with zoster or varicella, and the incidence of the disease does not increase during seasonal chickenpox epidemics.

Zoster occurs commonly in patients with neoplasms, most frequently in those with Hodgkin's disease, where the incidence may be as high as 25 percent. Advanced disease, cutaneous anergy, recent x-ray therapy to affected nodes, and possibly splenectomy predispose patients with Hodgkin's disease to zoster. The most significant common factor responsible for the development of zoster in these patients appears to be depressed cell-mediated immunity; there is no clear correlation with humoral immune status.

Recurrent herpes zoster is distinctly rare. If such a recurrence is documented, the likelihood of an underlying malignancy or immunodeficiency is great. When episodes of so-called recurrent zoster in healthy individuals have been carefully studied, herpes simplex virus has usually been found to be the causative agent. Like varicella-zoster virus, herpes simplex can cause zoster-like disease, but can also cause recurrent lesions.

MANIFESTATIONS Chickenpox The incubation period from the time of exposure to the appearance of varicella rash is 10 to 21 days, most often 14 to 17 days. There may be a 1- to 2-day prodrome with fever and malaise, but these symptoms usually begin when the rash appears. The first skin manifestations are pruritic maculopapules that evolve in a few hours to thin-walled vesicles which contain clear fluid and are surrounded by a red border. During the next day the erythema diminishes and the vesicles collapse in the center, forming annular or umbilicated lesions which dry further and form scabs that fall off, after several days, without scarring. New maculopapules continue to erupt during the first 3 or 4 days of illness and go through a similar evolution. The findings at one time, in one area, of skin lesions in all stages of development—maculopapules, vesicles, umbilicated lesions, and scabs—is characteristic of chickenpox. The rash is most concentrated on the trunk, but pox are frequently seen on the face and scalp, occasionally on the mucosal surface of the mouth or conjunctiva, and rarely on the palms and soles.

Chickenpox in adults is often more severe than in children, with more profuse rash, higher fever, and a greater incidence of pneumonia.

Herpes zoster Herpes zoster is a disease of nerves of the skin and other tissues that they supply. It most commonly affects the thoracic (55 percent of cases), cervical (20 percent), and lumbar and sacral nerves (15 percent), and the ophthalmic division of the trigeminal nerve.

Fever and pain that is localized to the areas served by the affected nerves may begin 4 or 5 days before or be concomitant with the appearance of the skin eruption. Rarely, characteristic pain and serologic evidence of zoster occur with no clinical involvement of the skin (zoster sine eruptione). The discomfort is mild to severe and can be sharp, burning, or dull. In addition to disorders of sensation, herpes zoster is occasionally associated with motor paralysis of arms, legs, intercostal muscles, or muscles innervated by cranial nerves. The skin lesion starts with local redness followed by red papules that progress over the next 2 weeks through vesicular, pustular, and crusting stages that resemble the evolution of individual pox of varicella. The lesions are arranged unilaterally in characteristic band-like clusters which follow radicular lines. They may run transversely along the hemithorax or vertically over the arm or leg.

Disease of the individual cranial nerves leads to characteristic groups of symptoms. If the trigeminal (Gasserian) ganglion is affected, there will usually be pain in the distribution of the nerve, headache, weakness of the eyelid muscles, and occasionally Argyll Robertson pupil. Lesions appear on the face, in the mouth, on the tongue, and frequently on the cornea. Iridocyclitis, anesthesia of the cornea, and scarring may result. If the geniculate ganglion is involved, there may be Bell's palsy, disorders of hearing, and vertigo, with unilateral herpetic lesions of the external ear and canal and of the anterior portion of the tongue. Central nervous system inflammation is prominent when herpes zoster attacks the cranial nerves, and meningeal signs and symptoms are frequent.

COMPLICATIONS Hemorrhage into vesicles and surrounding skin may be seen in adults with severe chickenpox or in children receiving adrenal steroids. Infection of the varicella lesions by bacteria, most commonly *Staphylococcus aureus,* results in delayed healing and scarring of skin, and occasionally in bacteremia.

Of adults with chickenpox, 15 percent develop primary *Varicella pneumonia.* Pneumonia is invariably associated with skin lesions and appears 1 to 6 days after onset of rash. The degree of pulmonary involvement correlates to some extent with the severity of the rash; patients may be virtually asymptomatic or may develop serious, life-threatening disease. Tachypnea, dyspnea, cough, and fever, with a temperature of 102°F or more, are present in most patients with symptomatic pneumonia; cyanosis, pleuritic chest pain, and hemoptysis each occur in 20 to 40 percent of the recorded cases. The physical examination may disclose no abnormalities, or there may be intercostal retractions, a few rhonchi, wheezes, scattered rales, and rarely, evidence of pleural effusion. In contrast to the paucity of physical signs, roentgenograms demonstrate widespread nodular infiltration of both lungs, most prominent at the hila and least evident at the apexes. Vital capacity is decreased, arterial oxygen saturation is diminished, and the airways may be blocked by tenacious bronchopulmonary secretions. Most patients with varicella pneumonia show symptomatic improvement when the rash begins to wane; however, seriously ill patients may remain febrile and dyspneic for as long as 2 weeks. Roentgenographic evidence of disease diminishes at the time of clinical improvement, but may persist for several weeks, followed in some cases by persistent miliary calcifications. Persistent abnormalities of pulmonary gas diffusion have been demonstrated several months after apparent recovery.

Central nervous system complications occur most frequently in children, with estimated rates as high as 1 in 200 cases. The most common manifestation is acute cerebellar ataxia, which usually begins 3 to 21 days after onset of rash and is usually benign. Other less common manifestations include acute encephalomyelitis, polyneuritis, ascending or transverse myelitis, optic neuritis, and Reye's syndrome.

Patients who contract *varicella while receiving steroids* may have recurrent crops of new skin lesions for as long as 3 weeks. They have a higher incidence of hemorrhagic and progressive gangrenous lesions and occasionally develop a fatal disseminated disease with viral infection in all the viscera. The fatal form of the disease has been encountered most frequently in children being treated with steroids for leukemia or other disease of the hematopoietic system, but it has also been seen in those receiving therapy for rheumatic fever and allergic disorders. Children with the rare syndrome of cartilage-hair hypoplasia may suffer from unusually severe and occasionally fatal chickenpox. *Other complications of chickenpox* such as myocarditis, corneal lesions, iritis, nephritis, nephrosis, monoarticular arthritis or polyarthritis, thrombocytopenic purpura, purpura fulminans, orchitis, and appendicitis have been recognized but are rare. Like measles, chickenpox can transiently produce anergy to tuberculin, and occasionally there may be reactivation of latent tuberculosis. Congenital infection with varicella can occur, and infants born of mothers with chickenpox may display the typical skin lesions. Congenital malformations as a result of infection in early pregnancy have been reported but are rare. The greatest mortality risk to the newborn infant appears to occur when onset of the maternal rash occurs in the 4-day period immediately before delivery or 48 h after delivery.

Postherpetic neuralgia may last for several months or years and become the most troublesome part of the disease. In nearly all patients with zoster, healing with loss of scab is complete within 2 to 3 weeks. In the young, pain persists for only a week or two after healing and then usually disappears, although hypo- or hyperesthesia may remain. However, in patients over 60 years of age, moderate to severe pain persists for more than 2 months in as many as 70 percent, even though the skin lesions have healed normally.

Zoster skin lesions do not always remain localized. *Generalized zoster* occurs in 5 percent of zoster patients with no underlying disease, and in as many as 70 percent of those with Hodgkin's disease, and is characterized by dissemination to all parts of the skin, producing a picture similar to that of chickenpox. The scattered lesions last 6 to 9 days in normal hosts, but they may persist for 3 to 4 weeks in those with serious underlying disease. In these patients dissemination may also involve the visceral organs (including the lungs) and occasionally results in death.

LABORATORY FINDINGS Multinucleated giant cells and epithelial cells with eosinophilic intranuclear inclusions can be identified in material scraped from the base of a vesicular lesion or in sputum from patients with varicella pneumonia. For specific diagnosis, virus can be isolated from vesicular fluid, and antigens can be demonstrated in vesicular fluid and in

crusts of lesions by the use of a simple gel-precipitin technique. Serologic confirmation is also possible, utilizing complement fixation or the more sensitive immune adherence hemagglutination or indirect immunofluorescent antibody tests. The white blood cell count in patients with uncomplicated chickenpox or zoster is normal. Mononuclear pleocytosis is present in the cerebrospinal fluid of patients with herpes zoster, especially those with involvement of the cranial nerves. The spinal fluid in varicella-zoster encephalomyelitis often contains increased protein, and cell counts may range from zero to 3000 lymphocytes per cubic millimeter.

DIFFERENTIAL DIAGNOSIS Chickenpox can usually be diagnosed by the history of recent exposure and the character of the rash. In situations where smallpox is a possibility, differentiation from chickenpox can be attempted by noting the distribution and evolution of the rash and by examining the cells from vesicles, but definitive diagnosis can be made only by identification of the virus or by serologic methods. Disseminated vaccinia lesions similar to chickenpox lesions may occur in patients, especially those with disorders of immunity or eczema, who have recently been vaccinated or exposed to a vaccinated person. Herpes simplex infection in patients with chronic eczema or neurodermatitis may present as a varicelliform eruption confined to previously involved areas of skin. The diagnosis can be confirmed by virus isolation. Rickettsialpox can be differentiated from chickenpox by the presence of an eschar in the area of mite bite, prominent headache, and specific complement-fixing antibodies to *Rickettsia akari*. Rarely, coxsackieviruses can produce a similar eruption in young children, although the lesions all tend to be in the same stage of development in one area. Stevens-Johnson syndrome has also been occasionally confused with chickenpox.

In the preeruptive stage, the diagnosis of herpes zoster is difficult, and the disease is usually confused with other causes of pain, such as pleurisy, appendicitis, pleurodynia, or collapsed intervertebral disk. After the unilateral eruption appears, the clinical features are so characteristic that the diagnosis is usually simple. Occasionally, localized herpes simplex along the distribution of a segmental nerve may simulate zoster, including the localized pain and tenderness. The diagnosis of herpes simplex infection can be confirmed in the laboratory by virus isolation.

PROPHYLAXIS Chickenpox can often be prevented or significantly modified by the administration of specific zoster immune globulin (ZIG) derived from the serum of patients recovering from herpes zoster, varicella-zoster immune globulin (VZIG) prepared from pooled plasma containing high titers of varicella antibody, or intravenous zoster immune plasma (ZIP). Both ZIG and VZIG should be given within 72 h of exposure to be effective, and limited data suggest some usefulness of ZIP if given within 6 days of exposure, in doses ranging from 3 to 14 ml/kg. Table 185-1 lists the current Center for Disease Control criteria which should be fulfilled before the use of VZIG in prophylaxis of chickenpox, and these also generally apply for ZIG and ZIP. Large doses of pooled human gamma globulin have also been shown to modify the disease if given shortly after exposure, but the quantity required to do so is so great (0.6 to 1.2 ml/kg) that this form of treatment is not generally recommended. There is no evidence that any of these preparations have any value in the prevention of herpes zoster, or the treatment of established infection of either type.

TABLE 185-1
Recommended criteria for the use of varicella-zoster immune globulin for prophylaxis of varicella

I One of the following underlying illnesses or conditions
  A Leukemia or lymphoma
  B Congenital or acquired immunodeficiency
  C Under immunosuppressive medication
  D Newly born of mother with varicella
II One of the following types of exposure to varicella or zoster patient
  A Household contact
  B Playmate contact (less than 1 h play indoors)
  C Hospital contact (in same two- to four-bed room or adjacent beds in a large ward)
  D Newborn contact (newborn whose mother contracted varicella within 4 days before delivery or within 48 h after delivery)
III Negative or unknown prior disease history
IV Age less than 15 years
V Request for treatment must be initiated within 72 h of exposure

Live, attenuated varicella-zoster virus vaccines have been tried as immunizing agents in high-risk children in Japan, but larger trials elsewhere have not yet been reported. Such vaccines are not available in the United States.

TREATMENT The patient with uncomplicated chickenpox seems to benefit most from cool, wet compresses or tepid water baths, rather than drying lotions, for the relief of itching. Secondary bacterial infections should be treated with appropriate antibacterial agents. Patients with varicella pneumonia require skillful nursing care, removal of excessive bronchial secretions, administration of oxygen, and on occasion assisted ventilation. Adrenal corticosteroids have been considered by some to be beneficial in the treatment of varicella pneumonia, but convincing evidence of their efficacy in this condition is not available. Patients suspected of having varicella-zoster infection of the eye should be promptly treated by an ophthalmologist. The therapy consists of analgesics for severe pain and the use of atropine to prevent synechiae. Some ophthalmologists recommend the use of steroids if uveitis is present. Topical 5-iodo-2′-deoxyuridine is of possible value for corneal or conjunctival ulcerative lesions.

Intravenous adenine arabinoside has been used in cases of severe zoster in patients on immunosuppressive therapy who are at high risk of dissemination, with encouraging results. Other studies, utilizing high doses of intramuscular human leukocyte interferon in similar patients, have also shown promise, but this form of treatment may be limited by the restricted availability of human interferon. However, further data are necessary before either mode of treatment can be more widely recommended. Moreover, there is no convincing evidence that such therapeutic modalities are effective in severe chickenpox or in herpes zoster after dissemination has already occurred.

It has been claimed that in older patients with herpes zoster and no underlying disease, the administration of a short course of adrenal steroids by mouth during the early eruptive phase of the disease reduces the incidence and duration of postherpetic neuralgia without inducing dissemination or other complications. Steroids should *not* be used for this purpose in patients with neoplasms or other underlying disease.

REFERENCES

ARVIN AM et al: Selective impairment of lymphocyte reactivity to varicella-zoster virus antigen among untreated patients with lymphoma. J Infect Dis 137:531, 1978

BABA K et al: Studies with live varicella vaccine and inactivated skin test antigen: Protective effect of the vaccine and clinical application of the skin test. Pediatrics 61:550, 1978

BALFOUR HH et al: Prevention or modification of varicella using zoster immune plasma. Am J Dis Child 131:693, 1977

BROOK I: Varicella arthritis in childhood. Clin Pediatr 16:1156, 1977

BRUNELL PA, GERSHON AA: Passive immunization against varicella-zoster infections and other modes of therapy. J Infect Dis 127:415, 1973

EAGLESTEIN WH et al: The effects of early corticosteroid therapy on the skin eruption and pain of herpes zoster. JAMA 211:1681, 1970

GERSHON AA et al: Antibody to varicella-zoster virus in parturient women and their offspring during the first year of life. Pediatrics 58:692, 1976

GROTH KE et al: Evaluation of zoster immune plasma. JAMA 239:1877, 1978

KREBS RA, BURVANT MU: Nephrotic syndrome in association with varicella. JAMA 222:325, 1972

MERIGAN RC et al: Interferon for the treatment of herpes zoster in patients with cancer. N Eng J Med 298:981, 1978

MINKOWITZ S et al: Acute glomerulonephritis associated with varicella infection. Am J Med 44:489, 1968

NORRIS FH et al: Herpes-zoster meningoencephalitis. J Infect Dis 122:335, 1970

RAIDER L: Calcification in chickenpox pneumonia. Chest 60:504, 1971

RUCKDESCHEL JC et al: Herpes zoster and impaired cell-associated immunity to the V-Z virus in patients with Hodgkin's disease. Am J Med 62:77, 1977

TRIEBWASSER JH et al: Varicella pneumonia in adults: Report of seven cases and a review of literature. Medicine 46:409, 1967

WEBSTER MH, SMITH CS: Congenital abnormalities and maternal herpes zoster. Br Med J 2:1193, 1977

WHITLEY RJ et al: Adenine arabinoside therapy of herpes zoster in the immunosuppressed. N Engl J Med 294:1193, 1976

Central nervous system viruses

186
APPROACH TO THE PATIENT WITH ASEPTIC MENINGITIS OR ENCEPHALITIS

LAWRENCE COREY

INTRODUCTION Viral infections of the central nervous system (CNS) can be classified into five clinical syndromes: (1) aseptic meningitis, (2) myelitis, (3) viral encephalitis, (4) postinfectious or "allergic" encephalitis, and (5) persistent or slow virus infections. While the predominant signs and symptoms of these syndromes differ, considerable overlap among them occurs. Aseptic meningitis, encephalitis, meningo-encephalitis, encephalomyelitis, and myelitis are descriptive terms; the choice of term depends upon whether the major impact of infection is upon the meninges, the brain, the spinal cord, or combinations of the three. Many viruses are associated with inflammation and infection of one anatomic site; for example, enteroviruses cause predominantly aseptic meningitis, arthropod-borne viruses produce encephalitis, while varicella-zoster is associated with postinfectious encephalitis. However, meningoencephalitis due to coxsackievirus or lymphocytic choriomeningitis virus, or aseptic meningitis due to St. Louis encephalitis, may occur. In addition, many nonviral infectious agents, focal inflammatory processes, and neoplastic and immunologic diseases may mimic viral CNS syndromes. These entities are listed in Table 186-1 and are discussed in detail in the referenced chapters. Despite these overlaps, definition of a clinical viral syndrome helps the physician both prognostically and therapeutically. In the adult, aseptic meningitis due to herpes simplex virus (usually type 2) is a benign self-limited disease, not requiring antiviral chemotherapy. In contrast, encephalitis caused by herpes simplex virus is a disease with a 75 percent mortality if left untreated.

ASEPTIC MENINGITIS The clinical syndrome of aseptic meningitis is manifested by fever, signs of meningeal irritation (nuchal rigidity, Kernig's or Brudzinski's signs), and a lymphocyte pleocytosis of the cerebrospinal fluid (CSF). The differentiation of viral meningitis from early or partially treated bacterial meningitis is a common diagnostic problem. In aseptic meningitis the CSF demonstrates a lymphocytic cellular response which may vary from 10 to over 1000 cells per cubic millimeter. Generally, a pleocytosis of more than 2500 cells per cubic millimeter is associated with bacterial, rather than viral, infection. Occasional cases of lymphocytic choriomeningitis may demonstrate CSF cell counts in the thousands, almost all of which are mononuclear, distinctly different from the polymorphonuclear response that occurs in bacterial meningitis. While lymphocytes are the usual CSF cell type in viral CNS infections, early in viral disease many patients will demonstrate a polymorphonuclear response in the CSF. In addition, a slight decrease in spinal fluid glucose (between 25 and 50 mg/ml) can occur in aseptic meningitis. Because of these overlaps in the

TABLE 186-1
Etiology and differential diagnosis of viral CNS disease

I Acute encephalitis or aseptic meningitis
  A Enteroviruses (Chap. 187)
    1 Poliovirus types 1 to 3
    2 Coxsackieviruses A1, A2, A4 to A11, A16 to A18, A22 to A24
    3 Coxsackieviruses B1 to B6
    4 Echovirus types 1 to 11, 25, 30 to 33
    5 Enterovirus types 68 to 70
  B Herpes simplex virus (Chap. 193)
    1 Type 2: Adult, aseptic meningitis; neonate, meningoencephalitis
    2 Type 1: Child or adult, focal encephalitis; neonate, meningo-encephalitis
  C Arboviruses (Chap. 190): In the United States: California, St. Louis, Western equine, and Eastern equine encephalitis
  D Mumps (Chap. 188)
  E Measles (Chap. 181)
  F Varicella-zoster (Chap. 185)
  G Rubella (Chap. 182)
  H Cytomegalovirus (Chap. 194)
  I Influenza (Chap. 179)
  J Adenovirus (Chap. 178)
  K Lymphocytic choriomeningitis (Chap. 191)
  L Epstein-Barr virus (Chap. 195)
  M Colorado tick fever (Chap. 190)
  N Encephalomyocarditis virus (Chap. 187)
  O Rhabdovirus (Chap. 189)
  P Cat-scratch disease (Chap. 197)
II Postinfectious agents
  A Measles (Chap. 181)
  B Varicella-zoster (Chap. 185)
  C Viral vaccines (rabies, vaccinia) (Chaps. 184, 189)
  D Mxyoviruses, including influenza (Chap. 179)
III Viral associated: Reye's syndrome (Chap. 369)
IV Nonviral infectious agents which may cause encephalitis-aseptic meningitis syndrome
  A Bacterial
    1 Bacterial meningitis (Chap. 368)
      a Early phase
      b Partially treated
    2 Mycobacteria (Chap. 143)
    3 Leptospirosis (Chap. 148)
    4 Syphilis (Chap. 113)
    5 Brain abscess (Chap. 368)
    6 Parameningeal focus (Chap. 368)
  B Mycotic: *Cryptococcus neoformans* (Chap. 153)
  C Rickettsial
    1 Rocky Mountain spotted fever (Chap. 164)
    2 Q fever (Chap. 170)
  D Chlamydial and mycoplasmal
    1 *Mycoplasma pneumoniae* (Chap. 172)
    2 Psittacosis (Chap. 175)
    3 Lymphogranuloma venereum (Chap. 174)
  E Parasitic
    1 Protozoa: Toxoplasmosis (Chap. 203), malaria (Chap. 200), trypanosomiasis (Chap. 202), *Naegleria* and other amoebas (Chap. 199)
    2 Nematodes (Chap. 207): *Toxocara, Trichinella* (Chap. 208), *Strongyloides stercoralis*, angiostronglyliasis cantonesis (eosinophilic meningitis) (Chap. 210), filariasis (Chap. 209)
  F Trematodes: Schistosomiasis (Chap. 211), cestodes, cysticercosis, echinococcosis (Chap. 213)
V Noninfectious causes of "encephalitis-like" syndromes
  A Toxic (lead, drug overdose, tick paralysis, botulism, tetanus)
  B Metabolic
  C Vascular (emboli, hemorrhagic)
  D Immune injury—"arteritis"
  E Carcinomatous
  F Mass lesions
  G Recurrent (Mollaret's) meningitis

CSF findings, the criteria which differentiate viral from bacterial infection cannot be interpreted too rigidly. Each patient must be evaluated both clinically and epidemiologically.

Aseptic meningitis occurs more frequently during the summer months and in patients under 40. In the summer, a child or young adult who presents with fever, headache, myalgias, a stiff neck, a mononuclear CSF pleocytosis, and a CSF Gram's stain lacking bacteria most likely has aseptic meningitis. Even if a polymorphonuclear pleocytosis is present, antibiotic therapy can be withheld and the lumbar puncture repeated in 8 to 12 h. A shift from a predominance of neutrophils to one of mononuclear cells, a stable or increasing CSF glucose, and the absence of organisms on a second CSF Gram's stain all suggest viral rather than bacterial infection. However, initial therapy with antimicrobial agents until bacterial culture results are complete is appropriate if the epidemiologic and clinical data do not suggest a viral etiology such as the occurrence of the illness in the winter months or in a patient over 40 years of age. If the patient has received antimicrobial therapy prior to CSF examination, the distinction between viral and bacterial infection may be very difficult. Laboratory techniques for the detection of viral or bacterial antigens or bacterial products may be helpful in this clinical situation.

Other causes of aseptic meningitis include leptospirosis, a nonviral pathogen which mimics aseptic meningitis. Exposure to animals (especially rodents), conjunctivitis, mild hepatitis, and/or renal abnormalities should suggest this diagnosis. Tuberculosis and cryptococcal meningitis may resemble aseptic meningitis. These infections are usually characterized by a more subacute course, a higher CSF protein concentration, and a lower CSF glucose concentration than are found in viral meningitis. In addition, evidence of cranial nerve palsies often occurs in tuberculous meningitis and is a helpful differential sign (Chap. 143).

Laboratory diagnosis Studies conducted in the 1950s and 1960s indicated that the enteroviruses, particularly poliomyelitis and mumps virus, were the most frequent cause of etiologically identified aseptic meningitis. Administration of mumps and poliomyelitis vaccines has decreased the incidence of these diseases and their neurological complications. In contrast, the sharp increase in genital herpes simplex virus infection has resulted in an increased recognition of the aseptic meningitis and sacral radiculitis syndromes associated with primary herpes virus infection. Echovirus and coxsackieviruses A and B account for the majority of cases of aseptic meningitis in the United States. However, the large number of serotypes of these agents (70 enteroviruses) preclude the use of routine "serologic batteries" for the evaluation of individual cases of aseptic meningitis. During localized outbreaks, consultation with regional viral diagnostic laboratories or public health officials may aid in the selection of appropriate serologic and/or culture techniques for isolating the virus.

In evaluating individual cases of sporadic viral CNS infection, viral isolation procedures are the most helpful laboratory tests in establishing an etiologic diagnosis. Isolation of a specific viral agent from the CSF or nervous tissue is diagnostic, while culture of an agent known to cause CNS disease from the throat, stool, or urine must be interpreted according to the patient's clinical syndrome and course. For example, isolation of mumps virus from saliva or urine in a young male with aseptic meningitis would be presumptive evidence of mumps meningoencephalitis. Similarly, the presence of clinical measles, the isolation of measles virus from nasopharyngeal secretions, or the demonstration of a fourfold or greater rise in anti-

body titer to measles virus in a patient with an acute encephalitis would also constitute presumptive evidence of CNS measles infection.

Nonpolio enteroviral excretion in feces occurs in up to 20 percent of the population, depending on the geography and season. Studies of coxsackie- or echovirus diseases indicate that the isolation of these agents from throat and rectal swabs occurs much more frequently in cases of aseptic meningitis and their household contacts than in well individuals.

Isolation of agents known to cause recurrent or persistent viral infection such as herpes simplex virus or adenovirus from throat washings, or cytomegalovirus from urine samples, should generally not be interpreted as having etiologic importance. On the other hand, many agents, including group A coxsackieviruses, flavovirus, many togaviruses, and lymphocytic choriomeningitis virus, will be detected only if specimens are inoculated into suckling or adult mice. Despite these shortcomings, the etiologic diagnosis of aseptic meningitis can be established with reasonable certainty in 60 to 75 percent of cases.

MYELITIS SYNDROMES Viral invasion of the CNS may also result in parenchymal spinal cord involvement. Poliomyelitis, with its devastating effect on motor neurons of the spinal cord and brainstem, was for many years one of the most feared of all infectious diseases. The advent of effective vaccines has markedly reduced but not eliminated this disease. To take its place, acute paralytic disease due to the nonpolio enteroviruses has become increasingly evident. Coxsackieviruses A4, A7, A9, A10, and B1 to B5 and echovirus types 1, 2, 4, 6, 9, 11, 16, and 30 have been associated with lower motor neuron involvement usually characterized by an asymmetric flaccid paralysis of the limbs. Generally, the illness associated with these agents is less severe and has a higher rate of recovery of neuromuscular function than poliomyelitis.

Acute transverse myelitis (Chap. 375) usually begins with the abrupt onset of bilateral weakness of the lower extremities with concomitant involvement of proprioceptive, pain, and touch pathways which may be due to noninfectious and infectious causes. Acute pyogenic spinal epidural abscess may present as an acute transverse myelopathy (Chap. 368). Similarly, transverse myelitis related to acute infection with mumps, measles, Epstein-Barr, herpes simplex, or varicella-zoster virus or echo-, polio-, or cytomegalovirus may occur. Occasionally, one of these agents may be isolated from the CSF or neural tissue. Because a slight lymphocytic pleocytosis may accompany the transverse myelopathy of noninfectious etiology, clinical differentiation may be difficult. In addition, antecedent viral infection or vaccination (smallpox, rabies, influenza) can initiate postinfectious transverse myelitis. The pathogenesis of the perivenous demyelination and perivascular cellular infiltration associated with postinfectious transverse myelitis is unknown but is thought to represent a form of "hypersensitivity." Corticosteroids have been used in the treatment of postinfectious myelitis, but their value in controlled studies has not been proved.

ENCEPHALITIS SYNDROMES When an acute febrile illness is associated with dysfunction of the cerebrum, brainstem, and/or cerebellum, then encephalitis must be considered. The distinction between viral encephalitis and an acute toxic (noninflammatory) encephalopathy may be difficult. Both entities present with the abrupt onset of disturbed consciousness. In addition, Reye's syndrome (acute encephalopathy with fatty degeneration of the viscera) usually is associated with a history of an antecedent febrile upper respiratory "viral" illness. An elevated blood ammonia level, a prolonged prothrombin time, and elevated serum aminotransferases in a patient with an acute encephalopathy are characteristic of Reye's syndrome. Cerebrospinal fluid examination is the best means of distinguishing between encephalopathy and an acute encephalitis. Cerebrospinal fluid pressures and protein concentrations may be increased in both entities; however, the presence of lymphocytic pleocytosis is characteristic of encephalitis.

Herpes simplex encephalitis (Chap. 193) The advent of successful antiviral chemotherapy for herpes simplex virus encephalitis has altered the traditionally laissez-faire attitude toward the etiologic diagnosis of acute viral encephalitis. The ability of herpes simplex virus to cause rapid necrosis of neuronal tissue, combined with the fact that patients treated with intravenously administered adenine arabinoside early in the course of illness have a better survival rate and less neurological deficits than patients treated late in the course of the disease, makes prompt and accurate diagnosis of this entity necessary. Clinically, the most distinctive aspect of herpes simplex virus encephalitis is its tendency to cause focal, especially temporoparietal lobe, destruction. For this reason, patients who present with focal neurological signs and symptoms should undergo immediate evaluation with electroencephalograms and/ or radionuclide scans, computerized axial tomography, or angiography to corroborate the presence of a focal or diffuse inflammatory process. If a focal defect is demonstrated, the diagnosis of herpes simplex encephalitis must be considered. Unfortunately, accurate, noninvasive techniques for differentiating herpes simplex virus (HSV) encephalitis from other focal encephalitides or focal pyogenic processes such as brain abscess are not available. Herpes simplex virus antigen in CSF by immunofluorescence is present in only 10 percent of confirmed cases. Moreover, HSV-specific CSF antibody usually cannot be detected early in the disease when accurate diagnosis and therapy are most needed. Brain biopsy remains the definitive procedure. This procedure is best performed in facilities that have the comprehensive virological support needed to diagnose HSV infections rapidly. The biopsy should be examined for HSV antigen by immunofluorescence or immunoperoxidase techniques, by electron microscopy for detection of herpes group virus in infected cells, and by histologic examination for evidence of intranuclear inclusions; then it should be submitted for viral isolation. Adenine arabinoside therapy may be initiated and, if no evidence of HSV infection is found, can be discontinued. Adenine arabinoside is not effective against RNA viruses and is not effective in suspected viral encephalitis. Moreover, its hepatic, hematopoietic, and neurological toxicity preclude its use in seriously ill patients with encephalitis who do not have HSV infection.

Diffuse encephalitis An attempt to make an etiologic diagnosis of a patient with diffuse encephalitis is often unrewarding; more than 50 percent of the cases reported to the Center for Disease Control are of undetermined origin. The number of potential pathogens is large, and, more importantly, the prognosis varies among viral pathogens. Some agents, such as rabies and Eastern equine encephalitis, are associated with a high case fatality rate. California or measles encephalitis infrequently causes death but may result in a neurological residua in as many as one-third of cases. In contrast, in adults, Western equine encephalitis is associated with severe neurological deficits only rarely.

Knowledge of the patient's age, the season, and the history of exposure is helpful in determining an etiologic diagnosis. During the summer months, arthropod-borne encephalitis, leptospirosis, and enteroviral disease may prevail. St. Louis encephalitis is more frequent in adults than children, while the converse is true for California and Western equine encephalitis. In the winter months, encephalitis associated with measles,

mumps, rubella, varicella-zoster virus, or, rarely, influenza is most common. Regional variations in the incidence of rickettsial infections and brucellosis may also affect the incidence of encephalitis. Herpes simplex virus encephalitis is endemic, but as the incidence of all other types of encephalitis increases during the summer months, the proportion of cases of herpes virus encephalitis falls to levels that are lower than in the winter.

Comparing levels of antibody in acute and convalescent serums is the most frequently used method of obtaining an etiologic diagnosis in diffuse viral encephalitis. Viral isolation procedures may be helpful, particularly in childhood exanthems, mumps, and encephalitis related to the respiratory viruses. If neural tissue is obtained, cultures for viral isolation, including mouse inoculation, should be performed.

The clinical distinction between acute encephalitis due to direct viral invasion versus postinfectious or "allergic" encephalitis is difficult. A previous illness or vaccination 1 to 6 weeks prior to the onset of CNS dysfunction, and demonstration of a demyelinating process affecting primarily "white" matter, suggest a postinfectious etiology.

Supportive care is the mainstay of therapy for diffuse viral encephalitis. Control of intracranial pressure and correction of the metabolic problems, disseminated intravascular coagulation, bleeding, renal failure, and pulmonary emboli or pneumonia associated with the illnesses are required.

CHRONIC VIRAL INFECTION Slow virus infections of the CNS can be divided into two categories: (1) diseases associated with persistent viral replication due to "conventional" viruses, and (2) the transmissible dementias or subacute spongiform encephalopathies associated with unconventional viruses (Table 186-2).

Chronic viral infection associated with persistent replication of measles, rubella or the papovavirus (Jakob-Creutzfeldt virus), involves both white and gray matter and shows histologic evidence of an inflammatory response. Isolation of virus from brain tissue, evidence of viral antigens in infected cells (immunofluorescence), or visualization of virions or viral byproducts by electron microscopy can be demonstrated. In subacute sclerosing panencephalitis associated with persistent measles virus and in progressive rubella panencephalitis, in-

TABLE 186-2
Chronic viral infections of the CNS (Chap. 192)

Disease	Agent
DUE TO CONVENTIONAL VIRUSES	
Subacute postmeasles leukoencephalitis	Measles
Subacute sclerosing panencephalitis	Measles
Subacute rubella panencephalitis	Rubella
Progressive rubella panencephalitis following congenital rubella	Rubella
Progressive multifocal leukoencephalopathy	Papovavirus Jakob-Creutzfeldt, SV40
DUE TO UNCONVENTIONAL VIRUSES	

In humans:
  Kuru
  Jakob-Creutzfeldt
  Familial Alzheimer's
In animals:
  Scrapie
  Transmissible mink encephalopathy	

creased antibody titers to these respective agents are present in serum and CSF. The serum and CSF of these patients should be examined for an increased concentration of gamma globulin, particularly that of monoclonal origin (oligoclonal banding), CSF hemagglutination inhibition (HI) antibody titers to measles and/or rubella virus should also be determined. The definitive diagnosis is made by isolation of the viral agent from neuronal tissue. These procedures are employed only in research laboratories.

In contrast, the transmissible viral dementias such as Jakob-Creutzfeldt disease are not associated with a prominent inflammatory response, nor can evidence of the etiologic agent(s) be identified by immunofluorescence or electron microscopy. A clinical history compatible with spongiform degeneration on brain biopsy provides a presumptive diagnosis. Propagation of the agent by inoculating it into a susceptible host is available only in a limited number of laboratories.

REFERENCES

Bell WE, McCormick WF: *Neurologic Infections in Children.* Philadelphia, Saunders, 1975

Feigen RD, Shakelford PG: Value of repeat lumbar puncture in the differential diagnosis of meningitis. N Engl J Med 289:571, 1973

Gajdusek DC: Unconventional viruses and the origin and disappearance of Kuru. Science 197, 4307:943, 1977

Whitley RS et al: Adenine arabinoside therapy of biopsy-proved herpes simplex encephalitis. N Engl J Med 297:289, 1977

Wilfert CM: Mumps meningoencephalitis with low cerebrospinal fluid glucose, prolonged pleocytosis and elevation of protein. N Engl J Med 280:855, 1969

187
ENTERIC VIRUSES
Coxsackieviruses, echoviruses, polioviruses, reoviruses, parvoviruses, and rotaviruses

A. MARTIN LERNER

GENERAL CONSIDERATIONS

It has been over 35 years since Dalldorf and Sickles isolated the first coxsackieviruses by inoculating suspensions of feces from two children with signs of clinical paralytic poliomyelitis into suckling mice. Subsequently, some 71 enteroviruses, including polioviruses and coxsackieviruses, and echoviruses, have been shown to multiply at various times in the gastrointestinal tracts of human beings. These viruses include four newly recognized members of the group which have been termed enterovirus, types 68 to 71 (Table 187-1). Enteroviruses have been recovered wherever attempts have been made; their distribution appears global. With notable exceptions such as coxsackievirus, type A21, and echovirus 28, which are predominantly respiratory pathogens and are only incidentally isolated from feces, enteroviruses like *Salmonella* periodically multiply within the human alimentary canal and sometimes concomitantly produce disease. Available information suggests that there is no normal enteric virus flora. In addition to enteroviruses, adenoviruses, reoviruses, and hepatitis A, non-A, and non-B, parvoviruses and rotaviruses are commonly recovered from stools. The latter two agents recently have been recognized as the cause of viral gastroenteritis.

Coxsackieviruses are named for their site of origin, the village of Coxsackie on the banks of the Hudson River in the state of New York. Echoviruses were descriptively named: *E,*

TABLE 187-1
Classification of human enteroviruses

I Enteroviruses
  A Polioviruses (3 types)*
  B Coxsackievirus A (24 types)
  C Coxsackievirus B (6 types)
  D Echoviruses (34 types)†
II Newly recognized enterovirus types
  A Enterovirus, type 68
  B Enterovirus, type 69
  C Enterovirus, type 70
  D Enterovirus, type 71

* *Typing is by neutralization of infectivity with immune serums either in suitable tissue cultures or in suckling mice.*
† *Echovirus, type 10, has been reclassified as belonging to another taxonomic group, now known as reoviruses.*

for their *enteric* residence; *C,* the filtrable agents produce *cytopathic* effects in tissue cultures of rhesus kidney; *H,* human; *O, orphan,* indicating that their relationship to disease remained to be established. They were viruses "in search of a disease." It is increasingly evident that a wide but definite variety of illnesses may result from enterovirus infections. As observations accumulate, these illnesses (Table 187-2) are continually being defined.

Etiologic associations are difficult to establish and usually require virologic, serologic, epidemiologic, and, when ethically possible, volunteer studies. These are especially useful if viruses are isolated only from the pharynx or anus, where they often multiply without causing significant injury to tissues. More meaningful are isolations from blood, vesicular fluids of patients with rashes, urine, cerebrospinal fluid, or from tissues at biopsy or autopsy. Coxsackieviruses and echoviruses have been recovered from lung, heart, pericardial fluid, liver, spleen, testicle, kidney, muscle, and brain. Dual virus infections and possible bacterial-virus synergisms occur. Until enteroviruses had been repeatedly documented in infants by isolations from pneumonic lungs, the prevalent opinion was that they did not produce pneumonias. The same skepticism exists concerning etiologic associations of enterovirus infections and chronic myocardiopathies, nonrheumatic valvular deformities, subendocardial fibroelastosis, and other congenital malformations. Firm evidence for an enterovirus cause of a chronic myocardiopathy, at least in a murine model, has now been established.

CHARACTERISTICS OF THE VIRUSES The enterovirus group is icosahedral-shaped, with a particle diameter of 17 to 30 nm and a ribonucleic acid core surrounded by a capsid of protein. Enteroviruses share about 20 percent of their nucleotide sequences, while within a grouping such as coxsackievirus B, there is 30 to 50 percent homology among types. The subunit structure of the outer protein capsid (capsomere) determines species, tissue, and age specificities for infection, as well as antigenicity. The RNA of the virus within infected cells transcribes and translates its own genetic information independent of the DNA (deoxyribonucleic acid) of the host. Enteroviruses are quite stable in acid and lipid solvents. They can be protected from thermal inactivation by certain cations.

When inoculated into suckling mice, group A coxsackieviruses induce primarily inflammation and necrosis of skeletal muscle, whereas group B viruses cause lesions of the central nervous system and other viscera, but only focal muscular involvement. Coxsackieviruses B and echoviruses are cytopathogenic for cultures of monkey kidney cells, but this is not the case for coxsackieviruses of group A. These distinctions are not without exception. Some strains of echoviruses, types 6 and 9, have been adapted to produce lesions in baby mice, the former in viscera and the latter in skeletal muscles. Some strains agglutinate human erythrocytes obtained from adults or umbili-

TABLE 187-2
Illnesses (or syndromes) associated with coxsackievirus, echovirus, or enterovirus infections

	Coxsackievirus types		Echovirus types	New enterovirus types
	Group A	Group B		
I No illness (probably 75% of cases)	1-24	1-6	1-8,* 11-34	69
II Mild or moderate illness				
A Undifferentiated mild febrile illness (nonspecific)	1-24	1-6	1-8, 11-34	
B Upper respiratory syndromes (rhinitis, pharyngitis, including herpangina and lymphonodular pharnygitis, conjunctivitis)	1-10, 16, 21, 22, 24†	1-5	1, 3, 6, 9, 16, 19, 20, 28	70
C Laryngotracheitis	9	5	11	
D Exanthems (various)	5, 9, 16	3, 5	2, 4, 5, 9, 11, 16	
E Lymphadenitis, with or without splenomegaly	5, 6, 9	5	4, 9, 16, 20	
F Pleurodynia (sometimes with pleural effusion)	4, 6, 10	1-5	1, 6, 9	
G Orchitis		1-5	9	
H Gastroenteritis	9	3, 4	2, 3, 6-9, 11-14, 18, 19, 22-24	
I Chronic myopathy				
III Severe or life-threatening illness				
A Hepatitis	4, 9	5	4, 9	
B Hemolytic-uremic syndrome	4	4		
C Pneumonia	9	1, 4	3, 8, 9, 19, 20	68
D Diabetes mellitus‡		4		
E Cardiac				
1 Myocarditis/pericarditis	1, 2, 4, 5, 8, 9, 16	1-6	1, 4, 6, 7, 9, 11, 14, 16, 19, 22, 25, 30	
2 Chronic myocardiopathy		2, 4, 5		
3 Subendocardial fibroelastosis‡		3		
4 Endocardial deformities		4		
5 Constrictive pericarditis		1, 2		
6 Congenital malformations‡	9	3, 4		
F Neurologic				
1 Aseptic meningitis/encephalitis including variants	7, 9, 16	1-5	1-9, 11-23, 25, 30-32	71
2 Acute cerebellar ataxia	3, 4			
3 Benign intracranial hypertension				
4 Transverse myelitis				
5 Postencephalitic parkinsonism				
6 Guillain-Barré syndrome‡				

* *Asymptomatic infection is common with echovirus, type 9. Variation in attack rates among types (and strains of a single type) occurs.*
† *Coxsackievirus A, type 21, is also known as Coe virus.*
‡ *Suggested (and probable), but cause not established.*

cal cords at the time of delivery. None of the coxsackieviruses or echoviruses has been adapted to grow in embryonated eggs.

EPIDEMIOLOGY Fecal-oral contact is the usual method of transmission. Personal hygiene (particularly hand washing) inhibits the infectious cycle. Toddlers often bring enteroviruses into a household. Insects, including flies and mosquitoes, may act as passive vectors. Echovirus, type 6, may multiply in the gastrointestinal tracts of dogs. This has not been noted with other coxsackieviruses or echoviruses, and with echovirus 6 canine-to-human transmission has not been demonstrated. Respiratory transmission by droplets or their nuclei also occurs.

The incubation period is 2 to 5 days. Multiple concurrent infections within a family are not unusual. Clinical manifestations of infection vary within the family and community. Thus a 2- to 3-year-old child may have a mild fever with rash, while an older sibling may have pleurodynia, myocarditis, or one of a number of syndromes heralding involvement of the central nervous system (Table 187-2). The mechanism of the varied expression of enterovirus disease is not well understood but may relate to developmental changes in the number or availability of specific receptors on the surfaces of susceptible cells.

Enterovirus infections are most common during the summer. Prevalence is mirrored by virus isolations from samples of sewage. Serotypes present in a community vary from year to year. The level of immunity of a population as reflected by the prevalence of type-specific neutralizing antibodies in serums apparently determines the likelihood of infection by a particular enterovirus. In an individual usually one enterovirus multi-plies within the intestine at any one time. Vaccination with attenuated polioviruses has virtually eliminated these interfering agents, and there may be a real increase in infections due to coxsackieviruses or echoviruses. Improved hygiene and urbanization have led to an "epidemiologic shift" from infants to adults. On the basis of intrahousehold spread, infectivity of coxsackieviruses is fairly high (76 percent of exposed susceptibles and 25 percent of immunes). For echoviruses, apparent infectivity is substantially lower (43 percent of susceptibles) and immune contacts are rarely infected. At least 49 percent of coxsackievirus and 55 percent of echovirus infections are subclinical.

An interesting correlate has been a seasonal incidence of new cases of insulin-dependent diabetes mellitus in patients under 30 years old. This autumn peak has been correlated with an annual prevalence for coxsackievirus B4, but does not relate to other virus infections. Recent epidemiologic studies show that there is no family history of diabetes mellitus in cases of juvenile onset. These cases show a predilection for certain HLA types, and pathologically, lymphocytes are found in their destroyed pancreatic islets. These data are consistent with, but do not prove, an infectious cause for juvenile diabetes. Adult-onset diabetes mellitus has a strong familial clustering and appears to be inherited.

VIRUS ISOLATION Primary multiplication occurs in epithelial and paraepithelial lymphatic cells of the pharynx. During this early period of infection the patient may be asymptomatic or have mild malaise, sore throat, or low-grade fever. Slightly later virus multiplies in the intestine. If a critical virus concentration within the pharynx results, viremia follows. During the viremic phase the patient is asymptomatic. Secondary foci of virus multiplication may occur in various tissues (skin, muscle, heart, nervous system, etc.). Major illness of moderate to serious severity sometimes results (Table 187-2). Occasionally (especially during infancy) aspiration of pharyngeal virus leads to lower respiratory infection.

Virus may be isolated from the throat during the minor illness and for as long as a week thereafter. Virus shedding persists in feces for a longer interval. Viremia can be documented during the incubation period until type-specific neutralizing antibodies appear.

PROTECTIVE RESPONSES AND SEROLOGIC DIAGNOSIS Intracellular virus multiplication stimulates interferon production within the infected cell (Chap. 176). About 3 days after the onset of infection specific antibodies appear in saliva and serum. These immunoglobulins combine with extracellular virus to limit spread of virus. Virus-antibody complexes are eliminated by phagocytosis.

Secretory immunoglobulins in saliva and succus entericus are in the IgA class, while the earliest antibodies to appear in serum are IgM. Both species of macromolecules have complement-fixing and neutralizing qualities. Within 3 to 4 weeks complement-fixing antibodies reach their peak and decline. Neutralizing antibodies of higher avidity (IgG) replace the IgM molecule about 2 weeks after the onset of infection. IgG antibodies persist and provide permanent type-specific immunity.

This information is important in diagnosis, because IgM molecules are susceptible to reduction and resultant biologic inactivation with sulfhydryl active compounds such as 2-mercaptoethanol (2-ME). IgG immunoglobulins are resistant to 2-ME.

IgG antibodies to coxsackieviruses and echoviruses traverse the placenta freely. IgM immunoglobulins do not. IgA antibodies in colostrum and milk are not absorbed, but apparently provide some local protection in the intestines of nursing babies. Passively acquired antibodies in serums protect the newborn from viremia for 3 to 6 months. Since the half-life of IgG immunoglobulins is about 3 weeks, duration of firm neonatal immunity depends upon initial titers of the transferred antibodies. Passively acquired antibodies inhibit active synthesis of immunoglobulins, and also may not protect the respiratory tract. Active synthesis of secretory antibody in saliva and nasal secretions is required. The role of cellular immunity in enterovirus infections remains to be fully defined. However, in coxsackievirus B3 murine cardiomyopathy, antibodies inhibit virus replication. Cytotoxic T lymphocytes augment the pathologic changes.

A fourfold rise in neutralizing antibodies or a titer which is similarly diminished by 2-ME indicates recent infection. When applicable, hemagglutination inhibition tests are simpler, and the results parallel those obtained in more cumbersome neutralization tests. Complement-fixing antibodies to enteroviruses are not type-specific. Many cross reactions render these tests less useful.

The neutralizing antibody response is highly type-specific in primary or initial enterovirus infections. In subsequent infections heterotypic responses occur with increasing frequency; they presumably arise from a booster effect of the current infecting virus on the level of antibodies to other types with which the individual has previously been infected. Levels of heterotypic antibody frequently exceed the level of homotypic antibody. Neutralizing antibodies to group B coxsackievirus,

types 1 to 5, are frequently found in titers of 1:64 to 1:512 in patients without evidence of current coxsackievirus infections (Table 176-4).

OTHER LABORATORY FINDINGS Enterovirus infections are usually acute processes, and persistent or chronic infections are unusual [e.g., chronic myopathy (coxsackievirus A9) or chronic myocardiopathy (coxsackievirus B3)]. Hence, changes in concentrations of hemoglobin, albumin, or globulins are unusual. Occasionally hemolysis occurs (see "Group A Coxsackievirus Infections" and "Echovirus Infections," further on in this chapter). White blood cell counts and the erythrocyte sedimentation rates are only mildly elevated. If there is necrosis (e.g., liver, lung), a neutrophilic leukemoid reaction may be noted. Hyperbilirubinemia and elevated transaminase and alkaline phosphatase levels may be seen in cases of hepatitis. Albuminuria often occurs transiently, but hematuria is rare.

PROPHYLAXIS AND TREATMENT Antiviral chemotherapy is not available. The 71 antigenic varieties of coxsackieviruses and echoviruses make prophylaxis with a single vaccine impractical. Pooled human globulin contains enterovirus antibodies, but during serious infections administration is not helpful. Most human enterovirus infections are mild, and globulin prophylaxis is not often warranted. As with poliomyelitis, tonsillectomy and other inoculations are probably best delayed during an outbreak of enterovirus disease. In a murine model of coxsackievirus B3 myocarditis, virus was isolated in higher titer from hearts of mice vigorously exercised daily by swimming, and a benign myocarditis was transformed into a lethal infection. Rest is the cornerstone of symptomatic therapy.

It has been repeatedly shown in experimental animals that during the acute phase of infection administration of steroids appreciably increases the quantity of virus in tissues and the degree of ensuing injury. Corticosteroids also depress cell-mediated immune functions, interferon and antibody synthesis, and leukocyte migration to the area of injury. Therefore at least during the acute phase of enterovirus infections, steroids are contraindicated. Pregnancy may be associated with enhanced susceptiblity to these and other infections. Alcohol, cold temperature, and chronic undernutrition are also associated with an increased virulence of coxsackievirus and perhaps other virus infections. Alcohol depresses phagocytic function. Malnutrition suppresses T and B lymphocytes, early mononuclear cell migration, and interferon production. In the presence of agammaglobulinemia, persistent enterovirus infections have been observed.

GROUP A COXSACKIEVIRUS INFECTIONS

Group A coxsackieviruses cause herpangina, lymphonodular pharyngitis, upper and lower respiratory disease, cutaneous eruptions, hepatitis, aseptic meningitis, paralytic disease, including acute infantile hemiplegia and unilateral oculomotor palsy, myopericarditis, and some sudden unexpected deaths in infancy. A chronic myopathy in an eleven-year-old girl has been associated with coxsackievirus A9. Picornavirus-like particles were seen on electron microscopy, and virus was isolated from the diaphragm at autopsy. Pharyngeal multiplication may induce infection of superficial vessels or diffuse moderate erythema. Purulent exudate is not seen. More characteristic is *herpangina,* a common febrile illness characterized by small papular, vesicular, or ulcerative lesions on the anterior pillars, soft palate, tonsils, pharyngeal mucous membrane, and posterior part of the buccal mucosa. Herpangina has been seen during infections with coxsackieviruses, group A, types 1 to 10, 16, and 22. Vesicular lesions of herpangina have also been described in patients with illnesses due to coxsackieviruses, group B, types 1 to 5, and echoviruses, types 9 and 17. Coxsackievirus

A10 may induce *acute lymphonodular pharyngitis*. Lesions here are raised, discrete, white to yellow 3- to 6-mm papules surrounded by a zone of erythema. All the papules appear at the same time; they do not ulcerate, and they occur on the uvula, anterior pillars, and posterior pharynx. Large outbreaks of mild to severe conjunctivitis have been caused by coxsackievirus A24. Typically, rapid onset of swelling of the eyelids, lacrimation, preauricular adenopathy and, in some cases, a mucopurulent discharge occur.

Coxsackievirus A21 (Coe virus) is predominantly a respiratory pathogen, being regularly isolated from the throat and occasionally from feces. It has been associated with several outbreaks of an illness resembling the common cold in military recruits.

The first enterovirus etiologically implicated in pneumonia was coxsackievirus A9. Subsequently, a number of other enteroviruses have been implicated (Table 187-2). Fatal cases have occurred in infants or young children. Hyperpnea, cyanosis, hyperpyrexia, leukocytosis (or leukemoid reactions), and subsequently coma have been characteristic. Interstitial diffuse polylobed bronchopneumonia with alternate areas of atelectasis and emphysema have been found. Microscopically mixed alveolar septal infiltration without necrosis or formation of giant cells is seen.

A striking cutaneous vesicular eruption, *hand-foot-and-mouth disease* has repeatedly been associated with infections due to coxsackievirus, group A, type 16. Infants and children with coxsackievirus, group A, type 4 (also coxsackievirus B14) infections have been described with respiratory or gastrointestinal symptoms, acute renal disease, thrombocytopenia, and hemolytic anemia. Reticulocytosis, albuminuria, and hematuria accompany this constellation of findings, which has been described as the *hemolytic-uremic syndrome*. Aseptic meningitis with occasional paralytic disease (especially with A7) also occurs. Acute myopericarditis has been associated with infections with coxsackievirus A, types 1, 2, 5, 8, 9, and 16; there are firmer etiologic data for coxsackievirus, types 4 and 16. One estimate suggests that 23 percent of acute virus cardiomyopathies may be caused by coxsackievirus A. A significantly greater incidence of infection with coxsackievirus, group A, type 9, has been reported in mothers of infants with congenital heart disease.

GROUP B COXSACKIEVIRUS INFECTIONS

Infections with group B coxsackieviruses cause a number of upper respiratory syndromes, exanthems, diarrheas, pleurodynia, orchitis (with subsequent atrophy), pneumonia, hemolytic-uremic syndrome, and cardiac and central nervous system disease. Pleurodynia and cardiac disease due to enteroviruses were first associated with this group of enteroviruses (Table 187-2). In 1965 the Public Health Service (Britain) reported 1160 coxsackievirus B5 infections. Gastroenteritis (90 percent), aseptic meningitis (31 percent), myalgia and Bornholm's disease (23 percent), respiratory disorders (15 percent), and cardiomyopathies (5 percent) were included. There were 41 patients with pericarditis and 5 with myocarditis. Of 6 deaths, 2 each were due to neurologic, respiratory, or cardiac cause. During infancy, the mortality rate of patients with acute infectious myocarditis approaches 50 percent.

PLEURODYNIA (EPIDEMIC MYALGIA, BORNHOLM'S DISEASE, DEVIL'S GRIP) Prodromal symptoms of malaise, sore throat, and anorexia are interrupted by increasing debility, fever, and sudden onset of muscle, pleuritic, and abdominal pain. Pain is sharp, severe, and paroxysmal over the lower ribs or substernal area. It is accentuated by moving, breathing, coughing, sneezing, and hiccuping, and may be referred to the shoulders, neck,

or scapulae. Pain and spasm of anterior abdominal muscles occur in about half the cases, often in combination with chest pain. Muscle tenderness is usually not prominent, but some patients complain of intense cutaneous hyperesthesia and paresthesia over the affected area. The illness usually lasts 3 to 7 days, but relapses may occur. Among differential diagnoses are myocardial infarction and acute surgical conditions of the abdomen. Coxsackieviruses B have been isolated from striated muscles of patients with pleurodynia during epidemics. Occasinally pleuritis is accompanied by effusion, and virus has been isolated from pleural fluid. Bornholm's disease may occur at any age but is most common in children and young adults.

Early in the course of illness meningitis, myocarditis, or hepatitis may ensue. Liver biopsy in patients with complicating jaundice shows subacute portal triaditis and intense cloudy swelling of central-zone hepatocytes. A late complication is orchitis, occurring in 3 to 5 percent of patients with pleurodynia during relapse.

CARDIAC DISEASE Acute myocarditis may be caused by coxsackieviruses of groups A and B as well as echoviruses. Infections with strains of coxsackievirus, group B, have been most frequent. When congenital or neonatal infection occurs, the course is often rapidly fatal, with concomitant myocarditis, encephalitis, hepatitis, and sometimes adrenal necrosis. Later in childhood or in adult life the heart and pericardium more frequently are involved as the single site of disease. Cardiac inflammation varies in intensity and degree of muscle necrosis. Pericarditis may dominate the clinical presentation, with myalgia, fever, precordial pain, friction rub, and even cardiac tamponade. There may be prominent signs of myocarditis, with myocardial failure or arrhythmias. Illnesses may be self-limited and recovery complete. However, of 22 episodes of acute virus cardiomyopathies associated with infections due to coxsackieviruses, group B, 12 patients developed chronic heart disease. Strict bed rest until all electrocardiographic changes have reverted to normal (or as stationary) is indicated. This may require 4 to 6 weeks. Since steroids increase virulence of coxsackievirus B myocarditis in mice, they are contraindicated. Some infections may heal with significant myocardial scarring.

Coxsackievirus particles have been localized along tubules of the sarcoplasmic reticulum in infected mice with myocarditis. There is epidemiologic evidence associating coxsackievirus B, types 3 and 4, with congenital heart disease. Most infections in pregnant mothers are subclinical and occur in the first trimester. Suggestive evidence indicates that the following conditions may be caused by infections with coxsackieviruses belonging to group B: chronic continuing cardiomyopathies (B2, B4, B5); congenital calcific pancarditis (B3); and constrictive pericarditis (B1 and B2), with or without superior or inferior vena caval obstruction.

The possible courses and pathogenesis of enterovirus cardiomyopathies have been extensively studied in mice. It is likely that the similarity to humans is great. Enteroviruses affect the myocardium and pericardium, but there is no conclusive evidence to support the occurrence of a murine virus valvulitis. Coxsackievirus A9 induces an interstitial myocarditis in adult mice healing without scar (Figure 187-1). On the other hand, coxsackievirus B4 produces a transmural necrotizing myocarditis in baby mice. Ventricular aneurysms, mural thrombi, and pulmonary emboli have followed. (There certainly is serologic evidence in humans that some "myocardial infarctions" may be, in reality, myocarditis.) In weanling mice

Benign virus (e.g., coxsackievirus A9) ⟶ Acute (infectious) phase ⟶ Complete recovery

Ventricular arrhythmia

Death

Ventricular arrhythmia +
congestive heart failure,
cardiac tamponade,
hemopericardium

Virulent virus (e.g., coxsackievirus B3) ⟶ Acute (infectious) phase

Chronic (noninfectious immunopathic) phase ⟶ Death

(Chronic cardiomyopathy),
ventricular aneurysm,
mural thrombi,
constrictive pericarditis,
endocardial fibroelastosis,
superior/inferior vena cava obstruction

Ventricular arrhythmia,
congestive heart failure,
cardiac tamponade,
pulmonary emboli

FIGURE 187-1

The possible courses of a benign (nonmyonecrotic) and virulent (myonecrotic) myocarditis are shown. [From GL Mandel et al (eds), Principles and Practice of Infectious Diseases, New York, Wiley, 1978, with permission.]

coxsackievirus B3 causes an immunopathic, cytolytic, T-lymphocyte–induced necrotizing myocarditis leading to a severe chronic cardiomyopathy. Constrictive pericarditis with or without superior or inferior vena caval obstruction, endocardial fibroelastosis, and congestive heart failure are other sequelae. The frequency of these illnesses in humans remains a major epidemiologic problem requiring resolution.

ECHOVIRUS INFECTIONS

Echovirus infections may be asymptomatic or mild, moderate, or life-threatening (Table 187-2). Mild to moderate are undifferentiated fevers, upper respiratory infections, various rashes, pleurodynia, and diarrheas. Pneumonia, myopericarditis, hemolytic-uremic syndromes, and neurologic involvement may be quite serious. They do not differ from similar illnesses caused by coxsackieviruses.

Enterovirus 70 is the most widespread of the new enterovirus types. It causes highly contagious infections which became pandemic in 1969 to 1971. After a 24-h incubation period, enterovirus 70 causes acute subconjunctival hemorrhagic conjunctivitis. The lesion may be discrete petechial to large and blotchy and covers the bulbar conjunctiva. Corneal involvement may occur but is transient.

ASEPTIC MENINGITIS (Chaps. 186 and 369) There may be a mild prodromal malaise, but major illness usually begins with fever, headache, and stiff neck. Papilledema and Kering's and Brudzinski's signs may be present. Localizing sensory or motor deficits are unusual. Confusion and delirium are common. These acute findings may persist for 4 to 7 days. Cerebrospinal pleocytosis is usually less than 500 cells per cubic millimeter. Early, there may be as many as 90 percent polymorphonuclear leukocytes, but within 48 h the cellular response becomes completely mononuclear. Persistence of polymorphonuclear leukocytes in the cerebrospinal fluid suggests pyogenic meningitis or intracerebral, subdural, or epidural abscess. Gram's stain and appropriate spinal fluid cultures must be done to exclude bacterial meningitis, tuberculosis, or mycotic meningitis. Protein concentration in the cerebrospinal fluid is moderately elevated, but glucose is normal. Early in the illness echoviruses may be isolated from spinal fluid. It usually takes several weeks before the cerebrospinal fluid reverts to normal.

For attempts at virus isolation, throat and rectal swabs, serum, and cerebrospinal fluid should be collected as early in the course as possible (Table 176-3). Acute and convalescent serums should be studied for rises in type-specific neutralizing antibodies.

It is not possible to distinguish clinically between aseptic meningitis due to various enteroviruses and mumps. Localizing findings, hemiplegia, prolonged fevers, oculogyric crises, coma, and bloody spinal fluid favor the diagnosis of herpes simplex virus encephalitis (Chap. 193). Although echovirus aseptic meningitis most often is self-limited and recovery in persons afflicted after the first year of life complete, about 10 percent of patients have more serious involvement of the central nervous system. Minor muscle weakness with reflex changes may persist for weeks to months, but over 90 percent of patients recover completely within a year. Occasionally, choreiform movements, ataxia, nystagmus, transverse myelitis, Guillain-Barré syndrome, coma, bulbar involvement, and death result.

As with coxsackieviruses, intact B lymphocytes are required for eradication of echovirus infections. Persistent echovirus infection of the central nervous system documented by the presence of echoviruses types 30, 19, 9, and 33 have been recovered for from 2 months to 3 years in five patients with congenital agammaglobulinemias. Additionally, three of the patients had a dermatitis-like syndrome.

POLIOVIRUS INFECTIONS

Enteric infection with the enteroviruses, poliovirus types 1, 2, or 3, is entirely analogous to other similar infections with coxsackieviruses or echoviruses. The unique aspect of poliomyelitis is the predilection of these three viruses for the anterior horn cells of the spinal cord and motor nuclei of the cranial nerves. Nervous tissues necessary for sensation are uninvolved.

ETIOLOGY Three distinct antigenic types have been defined: type 1 (Brunhilde), type 2 (Lansing), and type 3 (Leon). Natural infection leads to type-specific immunity with long-lasting neutralizing antibodies which can be measured in serum. The Nobel prize was awarded to Drs. John F. Enders, Thomas H. Weller, and Frederick C. Robbins in 1954 for their discovery that polioviruses multiply in nonneural tissue cultures producing easily recognizable cytopathic effects. It was this singular contribution which heralded the modern era of virology and allowed the preparation of effective vaccine prophylaxis.

EPIDEMIOLOGY AND PATHOGENESIS The occurrence, distribution, and pathogenesis (including incubation period) of polioviruses are similar to those of coxsackieviruses and echoviruses (see preceding portion of this chapter). Prior to vaccine prophylaxis with oral attenuated viruses, these were extraordinarily common agents with peaks in prevalence from July through September. Live attenuated vaccine eliminates polioviruses from feces and sewage, but the formalinized killed vaccine, which prevents viremia and neurologic illness, does not limit asymptomatic enteric infection. In countries with poor sanitation, infection and occasional disease occur early in life leading to the designation "infantile paralysis." Physical exertion increases the risk of clinically apparent or paralytic poliomyelitis.

VIRUS ISOLATION AND PROTECTIVE RESPONSES (See Chap. 176) Like coxsackieviruses and echoviruses, polioviruses can be recovered from the throat or feces during the first week of infection. In fatal cases polioviruses are easily recovered from affected brain or spinal cord. In aseptic meningitis (nonparalytic poliomyelitis) caused by polioviruses, virus is rarely recovered from cerebrospinal fluid (CSF). This is in contradistinction to the aseptic meningitis syndrome caused by coxsackieviruses or echoviruses in which these viruses are easily recovered from CSF. Long-lasting immunity is mirrored by the presence of serum-neutralizing antibody, which also follows natural infection with wild viruses.

CLINICAL MANIFESTATIONS Infections with polioviruses types 1, 2, or 3 may induce inapparent infection (95 percent of cases), undifferentiated febrile illness (minor illness), aseptic meningitis, or paralytic disease. Recovery is complete except in paralytic disease.

Necrosis and loss of motor nerve cells in any area of the spinal cord, brain, or cranial nerves causes various muscle paralyses. The precentral gyrus, reticular formation of the medulla, the cerebellum, Auerbach's and Meissner's plexuses, and sympathetic ganglia are frequently affected. Bulbospinal poliomyelitis is very serious.

Disease begins with fever and "minor illness." Classically, after several days, symptoms disappear. In 5 to 10 days fever recurs, and signs of meningeal irritation and paralysis ensue. Cramping muscle pain and spasm as well as coarse twitching in affected parts follows. In children younger than 5 years, paralysis of one leg is most common. In patients 5 to 15 years of age, weakness of one arm or paraplegia is most frequent, while in adults quadriplegia is common. Urinary bladder and respiratory muscle dysfunction are also frequent in adults. Inoculations of vaccines are associated with involvement of the muscles around the site of injection.

Tendon reflexes are diminished or absent. Sensation is intact, separating poliomyelitis from the Guillain-Barré syndrome. Paralysis due to heavy metal poisoning, on the other hand, may be more difficult to distinguish clinically from poliomyelitis.

Among paralytic cases, 6 to 25 percent may be bulbar. Tonsilloadenoidectomies should not be done during epidemics of poliomyelitis for 85 percent of patients under these circumstances develop bulbar disease. Myocarditis, hypertension, pulmonary edema, shock, nosocomial gram-negative or staphylococcal pneumonias, urinary tract infections, and emotional problems are among the complications of severe paralytic disease. Treatment is supportive. About 2 to 5 percent of children and 15 to 30 percent of adults with paralyzing infection die. Initially paralyzed muscles usually recover some function, gradually improving over 1 to 2 years.

PREVENTION Poliovirus vaccines, used widely since the introduction of inactivated poliovaccine (IPV) in 1955, have dramatically reduced the incidence of poliomyelitis in the United States. In 1954 there were more than 18,000 new cases, but

there were only 8 in 1976. The risk of poliomyelitis is generally very small in the United States today, but epidemics are certain to recur if the population's immunity is not sustained. Data from a national survey in 1976 indicated that 38 percent of 1- to 4-year-old children had not had primary vaccination against poliomyelitis! In disadvantaged urban and rural areas vaccination rates are even lower. It is essential to immunize all children beginning in infancy.

A Canadian product, inactivated poliovirus vaccine (IPV), is being marketed in the United States. It produces immunity in more than 90 percent of recipients. The vaccine is given by injection and can be administered simultaneously with diphtheria, tetanus, and pertussis antigens. Children or adults with immunodeficiency diseases or altered immune states who are at risk of exposure to poliomyelitis should receive IPV. An antibody response cannot be assured in these immunodepressed persons, but some protection probably results. Four doses are given, the first three at 1- to 2-month intervals and the fourth 6 to 12 months after the third injection. If adults are traveling to areas where poliomyelitis is present, or if they are exposed to vaccine virus following routine immunization of their children, IPV may be given. Except for the possibility of hypersensitivity reactions to the trace amounts of streptomycin and neomycin in IPV, there are no associated risks.

Trivalent oral poliovaccine (TOPV), licensed in 1963, combines all three strains of polioviruses. Full primary vaccination produces immunity in more than 90 percent of recipients. It is the preferred poliovirus vaccine in this country. In rare instances oral polio vaccine has been associated temporally with paralytic diseases in vaccine recipients or their close contacts. Of 193 million doses of TOPV, 55 "vaccine associated" cases have been reported. Primary immunization for infants (6 to 12 weeks old), children, and adolescents through age 18 is three doses, the first followed in 6 to 8 weeks by the second, and the third 8 to 12 months later. Routine polio vaccination for adults living in this country is not necessary. A susceptible adult at increased risk of exposure to infection because of travel to an area where poliomyelitis is common should receive complete primary immunization with IPV or TOPV. Supplementary single doses of TOPV should be given to children upon entering school and at the age of 11 or 12. There is no evidence that a pregnant woman or her fetus is at greater risk from TOPV than other persons. Persons with immunodeficiency or altered immune states should not receive TOPV because of the increased risk of vaccine-associated paralysis. These conditions include combined immunodeficiency, hypogammaglobulinemia, agammaglobulinemia, leukemia, lymphoma, generalized malignancy, or lowered resistance from therapy with corticosteroids, alkylating or antimetabolic drugs, or radiation.

REOVIRUS INFECTIONS

Reoviruses were discovered inadvertently in studies of the intestinal viral flora of healthy children and adults. They were initially classified as echovirus, type 10, but were later reclassified. They were named to emphasize their (1) *respiratory* or (2) *enteric* human origins, and their (3) *orphan* status.

Reoviruses are quite different from picornaviruses (Table 187-1). They are about 2½ times larger (70 nm in diameter) and show icosahedral symmetry. Their RNA is unique in that it consists of 10 discrete segments and is resistant to ribonuclease. The protein capsid consists of an inner core and 92 outer shell capsomeres. The capsid is composed of seven species of polypeptides. Unlike those of enteroviruses, reovirus cytopathic effects are nonlytic. Reoviruses multiply in primate and nonprimate tissue cultures. The particles hemagglutinate human or avian erythrocytes. On the basis of tests of hemagglutination inhibition antibodies (HIA) with type-specific serums, there are three serotypes.

Human infections with reoviruses are common, and their distribution is worldwide. Like coxsackieviruses and echoviruses, reoviruses spread by enteric and respiratory routes. Fifty to eighty percent of adults in the Western Hemisphere have had reovirus infections, as measured by the presence of persisting neutralizing or hemagglutinating antibodies. Infections are more frequent in winter but occur in every season. Reoviruses have been isolated from human nasal secretions, posterior pharyngeal and rectal swabs, spinal fluid, brain, and lung. In addition, reovirus isolations or serologic data indicate that natural infections occur in cattle, dogs, cats, mice, horses, swine, birds, and monkeys. Although animal-to-human transmission has never been demonstrated, its possibility is likely.

Widespread evidence of infection and few associations with disease indicate that most infections with reoviruses are asymptomatic. Isolations of virus and fourfold rises in HIA in individual patients with common colds, nonspecific febrile illness, exanthem, and diarrhea suggest an etiologic role in some instances. Provocative data came from three thoroughly studied fatal cases of encephalitis, myocarditis, hepatitis, or interstitial pneumonias. In these patients reoviruses and no other bacterial or viral pathogens have been isolated.

VIRAL GASTROENTERITIS

In 1929, Zahorsky first used the term *winter vomiting disease* to describe an epidemic gastrointestinal illness usually occurring in the winter and characterized by a short afebrile course, persistent vomiting, and the absence of an upper respiratory infection. Subsequently, a mild self-limited syndrome with more or less fever, nausea or vomiting, gripping abdominal pain, headache, malaise, and diarrhea or dysentery without identifiable bacterial or parasitic cause was repetitively described as "epidemic nonbacterial gastroenteritis," "epidemic diarrhea of the newborn," "winter-vomiting disease," or "viral dysentery." In 1947, this diarrheal disease was transmitted to human volunteers by the oral administration of fecal filtrates. However, it is only within the past 5 years with the use of electron microscopic examination of diarrheal specimens of feces that viral gastroenteritis in its epidemic and endemic forms could be effectively studied.

Viral gastroenteritis is the second leading cause of illness in the United States. In the chronically malnourished, the elderly, and in debilitated persons, death may result. Immune electron microscopic examination of virus particles isolated from fecal specimens has uncovered two major virus groups which cause viral gastroenteritis.

Parvoviruses are primarily responsible for disease in adults and older children, while reovirus-like agents cause diarrhea in infants and young children. The attack rates for both infections may reach 50 percent, and the incubation period is about 48 h, so that explosive outbreaks are common. Diarrhea may persist for 5 to 8 days and be followed by steatorrhea. A malabsorption syndrome with abnormal xylose and lactose absorption follows for another week. Other viruses (e.g., echoviruses, types 1 or 18, or coronaviruses) may from time to time be involved in sporadic outbreaks of gastroenteritis, but their overall importance seems minor.

The Norwalk, Hawaii, and Montgomery County agents are parvoviruses named after the sites of their original epidemics, and are distinctive in that immunity to one of the agents does not confer protection against the others. Parvoviruses contain

DNA genomes without lipid coats, have cubic symmetry with particle diameters of 27 nm, and are stable at pH 2.7 and 60°C (30 min.)

Human reovirus-like agents (HRLA) have also been described as *duoviruses, rotaviruses,* or *orbiviruses*. Their final nomenclature has not yet been decided. HRLA are responsible for worldwide sporadic and epidemic outbreaks of gastroenteritis, usually occurring in the winter or fall in infants and young children 6 to 24 months old. By the time children in the United States are 2 years old, 50 to 90 percent of them have antibodies to HRLA. Rotaviruses are easily recognized in duodenal biopsies by electron microscopy and are seen as 70-nm particles with double-shelled capsids completely similar to those of reoviruses. On biopsy, the proximal small intestine shows shortened villi, and crypts are hyperplastic. Polymorphonuclear leukocytes and mononuclear cells infiltrate the lamina propria. Normally, columnar surface cells are vacuolated and cuboidal. During acute illness, a transient peripheral lymphopenia involving all lymphocyte subpopulations ensues.

Parvoviruses and reovirus-like agents multiply in the small bowel to titers of 10^8 organisms per gram of feces. The viruses can be seen on electron microscopy or recognized for diagnosis by counterimmunoelectrophoresis of fecal filtrates. The Nebraska calf diarrhea virus can be used as antigen for HRLA (which has not yet been grown in tissue cultures) in complement fixation tests for antibody rises. Fluorescent antibody methods are also available. It is clear, however, that the presence of antibodies in serum does not confer absolute immunity for the bowel. The role of local coproantibodies needs to be explored.

REFERENCES

General

GELFAND HM: Occurrence in nature of coxsackie and ECHO viruses. Prog Med Virol 3:193, 1961

KOGON A et al: The virus watch program: A continuing surveillance of viral infections in metropolitan New York families. VII. Observations on viral excretion, seroimmunity, intrafamilial spread and illness association in Coxsackie and echovirus infections. Am J Epidemiol 89:51, 1969

MELNICK JL: Enterovirus, in *Viral Infections of Humans, Epidemiology and Control,* AS Evans (ed). New York, Plenum, 1976, p 163

PHILIPSON L et al: Structural model for picornaviruses as suggested from an analysis of urea-degraded virions and procapsids of coxsackie virus B-3. Virology 54:69, 1973

WOODRUFF JF, WOODRUFF JJ: Involvement of T-lymphocytes in the pathogenesis of coxsackie virus B-3 heart disease. J Immunol 113:1726, 1974

Coxsackievirus A infection

CHALHUB EG et al: Coxsackie A9 focal encephalitis associated with acute infantile hemiplegia and porencephaly. Neurology 27:574, 1977

HUEBNER RJ et al: Herpangina: Etiological studies of a specific infectious disease. JAMA 145:628, 1951

LERNER AM et al: Infections due to coxsackievirus, group A, type 9, in Boston, 1959, with special reference to exanthems and pneumonia. N Engl J Med 163:1265, 1960

TANG TT et al: Chronic myopathy associated with coxsackievirus A9. A combined electron microscopical and viral isolation study. N Engl J Med 292:608, 1975

Coxsackievirus B infection

BAIN HW et al: Epidemic pleurodynia (Bornholm's disease) due to coxsackie B 5 virus: The interrelationship of pleurodynia, benign pericarditis and aseptic meningitis. Pediatrics 27:889, 1961

BROWN GC, EVANS TN: Serologic evidence of coxsackievirus etiology of congenital heart disease. JAMA 199:151, 1967

EL-KHATIB MR et al: Coxsackievirus B4 myocarditis in mice: Valvular changes in virus infected and control animals. J Infect Dis 137:410, 1978

——— et al: Ventricular aneurysms complicating Coxsackievirus group B, types 1 and 4 murine myocarditis. Circulation, 1979 (in press)

JOHNSON RT et al: Acute benign pericarditis: Virologic study of 34 patients. Arch Intern Med 108:828, 1961

KIBRICK S: Viral infections of the fetus and newborn. Perspect Virol Symp NY 2:140, 1961

LERNER AM: Myocarditis and pericarditis, in *Principles and Practice of Infectious Diseases*, GL Mandel et al (eds). New York, Wiley, 1979, chaps 55, 56

———, WILSON FM: Virus myocardiopathy. Prog Med Virol 15:63, 1973

SAINANI GS et al: Adult heart disease due to Coxsackievirus B infection. Medicine 47:133, 1968

Echovirus infection

HORSTMANN DM, YAMADA N: Enterovirus infection of the central nervous system. Res Publ Assoc Res Nerv Ment Dis 44:236, 1968

WILFERT KM: Persistent and fatal central nervous system infections in patients with agammaglobulinemia. N Engl J Med 296:1485, 1977

Poliovirus infection

HENDERSON DA et al: Paralytic disease associated with oral polio vaccines. JAMA 190:41, 1964

Poliomyelitis prevention. Recommendation of the Public Health Service Advisory Committee on Immunization Practices. Morb Mort Week Rep 26:329, 335, 1977

WEINSTEIN L: Diagnosis and treatment of poliomyelitis. Med Clin North Am 32:1377, 1948

Reovirus infection

EL-EAI FM, EVANS AS: Reovirus infections in children and young adults. Arch Environ Health 7:700, 1963

JOKLIK WK: The molecular biology of reovirus. J Cell Physiol 76:289, 1970

ROSEN L: Serologic grouping of reoviruses by hemagglutination-inhibition. Am J Hyg 77:29, 1963

——— et al: Reovirus infections in human volunteers. Am J Hyg 77:29, 1963

TILLOTSON JR, LERNER AM: Reovirus, type 3, associated with fatal pneumonia. N Engl J Med 276:1060, 1967

Viral gastroenteritis

GORDON I et al: Transmission of epidemic gastroenteritis to human volunteers by oral administration of fecal filtrates. J Exp Med 86:409, 1947

SHREIBER DS et al: Recent advances in viral gastroenteritis. Gastroenterology 73:174, 1977

ZAHORSKY J: Hyperimmune hiemis or the winter vomiting disease. Arch Pediat 46:391, 1929

188
MUMPS

C. GEORGE RAY
ROBERT G. PETERSDORF

DEFINITION Mumps is an acute communicable disease of viral origin characterized by painful enlargement of the salivary glands and sometimes by involvement of the gonads, meninges, pancreas, and other organs.

ETIOLOGY The causative agent of mumps is a paramyxovirus of intermediate size (150 to 250 nm in diameter). It has a tight helical inner core (RNA) enclosed in an outer shell of lipid and protein. The virus of mumps causes in vitro agglutination of erythrocytes of fowl, human beings, and some other species, produces hemolysis, and has two components capable of fixing complement. These are the soluble, or S, antigens derived from the nucleocapsid, and the V antigen derived from the surface hemagglutinin. It elicits a delayed allergic reaction when used as an antigen in persons who have had mumps infection. The virus can be cultivated in chick embryos and in a variety of mammalian cell cultures, including HeLa, monkey kidney and human pancreatic beta cells.

EPIDEMIOLOGY Human beings are the only natural host for mumps. The disease is worldwide and is endemic in urban communities. Epidemics are relatively infrequent and are confined to closely associated groups who live in orphanages, army camps, or schools. The disease is most frequent in the spring, particularly during April and May. Although mumps is generally considered less "contagious" than measles and chickenpox, this difference may be more apparent than real because many mumps infections (at least 25 percent) tend to be inapparent clinically. In some surveys, 80 to 90 percent of an adult population had serologic evidence of previous infection with mumps. The incidence of mumps in the United States has reached its lowest point since reporting began in 1922; in 1977, there were 44.3 percent fewer cases than in 1976.

Infections are rare before the age of 2 years and then increase rapidly in frequency, reaching a peak at ages 6 to 10. Clinical mumps may be more common in males than in females. In North American cities, most infections are contracted from schoolmates and infected family members. The virus is transmitted in infected salivary secretions, although its isolation from urine suggests that the virus may also spread via this route. Mumps virus is rarely isolated from stools. The saliva is infectious for approximately 6 days prior to the onset of parotitis, and virus has been recovered from this site for as long as 2 weeks after onset of parotid swelling. Viruria also persists for 2 to 3 weeks in some patients. Despite this prolonged secretion of virus, the peak of infectivity occurs a day or two before onset of parotitis and subsides rapidly after the appearance of glandular enlargement.

One attack of clinical or subclinical mumps confers lasting immunity, and second attacks are most unusual. Unilateral parotitis affords protection just as effectively as does bilateral disease.

PATHOGENESIS The virus enters via the respiratory route; during the incubation period of 15 to 21 days it presumably replicates in the upper respiratory tract and cervical lymph nodes, from which it is disseminated via the bloodstream to other organs, including the meninges, gonads, pancreas, breasts, thyroid, heart, liver, kidneys, and cranial nerves. The salivary adenitis is thought by many to be secondary to viremia, but primary spread from the respiratory tract has not been ruled out as an alternative mechanism.

MANIFESTATIONS Salivary adenitis The onset of typical parotitis is usually sudden, although it may be preceded by a prodromal period of malaise, anorexia, chilly sensations, feverishness, sore throat, and tenderness at the angle of the jaw. In many cases, however, parotid swelling is the first indication of illness. The glands enlarge progressively over a period of 1 to 3 days, and the swelling resolves within a week after maximal enlargement. The swollen gland extends from the ear to the lower portion of the mandibular ramus and to the inferior portion of the zygomatic arch, often displacing the ear upward and outward. The skin over the gland is usually not warm or erythematous, in contrast to what happens in bacterial parotitis. There may be reddening and pouting of the orifice of Stensen's duct. Usually, pain and tenderness are marked, although at times they are absent. The edema of mumps has been described as "gelatinous," and when the involved gland is tweaked, it rolls like jelly. Swelling may involve only the submaxillary and sublingual glands and may extend over the anterior part of the chest, producing *presternal edema.* Involvement of submaxillary glands alone can cause difficulty in distinguishing mumps from acute cervical adenitis. Swelling of the glottis occurs rarely but may require tracheostomy. Parotitis is bilateral in two-thirds of cases and remains confined to one side in the remainder. The second gland tends to swell as the first is subsiding, usually 4 to 5 days after onset. In general, parotitis is accompanied by a temperature of 100 to 103°F, malaise, headache, and anorexia, but systemic symptoms may be virtually absent, particularly in children. In most patients, the chief complaints refer to difficulty in eating, swallowing, and talking.

Epididymoorchitis Mumps is complicated by orchitis in 20 to 35 percent of postpubertal males. Testicular involvement usually appears 7 to 10 days after onset of parotitis, although it may precede it or appear simultaneously. Occasionally, orchitis occurs in the absence of parotitis. Gonadal involvement is bilateral in 3 to 17 percent of patients. Orchitis is heralded by recrudescence of malaise and appearance of chilly sensations, headache, nausea, and vomiting. Shaking chills and high fevers, with temperatures between 103 and 106°F, are frequent. The testicle becomes greatly swollen and acutely painful. The epididymis is often palpable as a swollen tender cord. Occasionally there may be epididymitis without orchitis. Swelling, pain, and tenderness persist for 3 to 7 days and gradually subside; lysis of fever usually parallels abatement of swelling. Occasionally, the temperature falls by crisis. Mumps orchitis is followed by progressive atrophy of the testicle in one-half the cases. Even after bilateral orchitis, sterility is unusual, provided no significant atrophy has taken place. However, if bilateral testicular atrophy occurs after mumps, sterility or subnormal sperm counts are quite common. Plasma testosterone levels are depressed during acute orchitis but return to normal with recovery. *Pulmonary infarction* has been noted to follow mumps orchitis. This may be the result of thrombosis of the veins in the prostatic and pelvic plexuses in association with the testicular inflammation. Priapism is a rare but painful complication of mumps orchitis.

Pancreatitis Pancreatic involvement is a potentially serious manifestation of mumps, which may rarely be complicated by shock or pseudocyst formation. It should be suspected in patients with abdominal pain and tenderness together with clinical or epidemiologic evidence of mumps. It is difficult to document, since hyperamylasemia, the hallmark of pancreatitis, is also often present in parotitis. Many times the symptoms resemble those of gastroenteritis, and it is conceivable that the high incidence of gastrointestinal symptoms seen in association with the mumps epidemic in Great Britain in 1961 was due to involvement of the pancreas. Although diabetes or pancreatic insufficiency rarely follows mumps pancreatitis, several children have developed "brittle" diabetes a few weeks after mumps.

Central nervous system involvement Nearly half the patients with mumps have an increased number of cells, usually lymphocytes, in the cerebrospinal fluid (CSF), although symptoms

of meningitis, stiff neck, headache, and drowsiness are less common. In typical cases, the onset of overt central nervous system signs and symptoms occurs 3 to 10 days after the onset of parotitis; however, the onset has also been noted to develop prior to the parotitis or 2 to 3 weeks later. In approximately 30 to 40 percent of laboratory-proved cases, there is *no* associated salivary gland involvement at any time in the course of illness. The CSF protein is moderately elevated, and CSF glucose tends to be normal, although in as many as 10 percent of patients low CSF glucose concentrations, in the range of 20 to 50 mg per 100 ml, may be seen. True encephalitis is unusual, although it is responsible for most of the central nervous system sequelae, including behavioral disturbances, headaches, seizures, deafness (usually unilateral), and visual disturbances. At least two cases of aqueductal stenosis and hydrocephalus have been reported as possible late sequelae to mumps encephalitis, but the association remains unproved. Mumps should also be recognized as capable of presenting a picture of mild paralytic poliomyelitis; definition of the cause depends on isolation of virus or serologic confirmation of mumps in the absence of changing antibody titers to poliomyelitis viruses. Rarely, mumps may produce a transverse myelitis, cerebellar ataxia, or the Guillain-Barré syndrome. Mumps meningitis, without clinical encephalitis, is generally thought to be benign.

Other manifestations Mumps virus tends to involve glandular tissues; inflammation of the lacrimal glands, thymus, thyroid, breasts, and ovaries occurs occasionally. *Oophoritis* may be recognized by persistence of pain in the lower part of the abdomen and fever. It does not result in sterility. Mumps virus has been implicated in the causation of subacute thyroiditis; the diagnosis can be made serologically, and occasionally the virus can be isolated from the thyroid gland. A case of myxedema following mumps thyroiditis has been reported. Ocular manifestations of mumps include dacryadenitis, optic neuritis, keratitis, iritis, conjunctivitis, and episcleritis. Although these conditions may transiently interfere with vision, complete resolution is the rule. Mumps *myocarditis,* evidenced primarily by transient abnormalities in the electrocardiogram, is relatively common but does not usually produce symptomatic disease or impair cardiac function. Similarly, *hepatic* involvement may be manifested by mild abnormalities in liver function, but icterus and other clinical signs of hepatic damage are extremely rare. *Thrombocytopenic purpura* as a complication of mumps has been described, and an occasional patient has a leukemoid reaction involving predominantly lymphocytes. Tracheobronchitis and interstitial pneumonia have also been associated with mumps infection, particularly among young children.

A rare but interesting manifestation of mumps is *polyarthritis* which is often migratory. It is most common in males between the ages of 20 and 30. Joint symptoms begin 1 to 2 weeks after subsidence of parotitis; usually the large joints are involved. The illness lasts 1 to 6 weeks, and complete recovery is the rule. It is not clear whether arthritis is due to viremia or whether it is a "hypersensitivity reaction."

Acute hemorrhagic glomerulonephritis in the absence of streptococcosis has been reported after mumps. The relationship of these two diseases is not clear.

Late complications With the exception of the rare central nervous system sequelae, the most serious of which is nerve deafness, which follow mumps encephalitis, and the occasional patient who is sterile following bilateral testicular involvement, mumps leaves no sequelae. There is no firm evidence that stillbirths and offspring with congenital defects are more common among mothers who have mumps during pregnancy. Likewise, the causal relationship between intrauterine mumps infection and endocardial fibroelastosis has not been clearly established.

LABORATORY FINDINGS In uncomplicated parotitis, the blood leukocyte count is normal, although there may be mild leukopenia with relative lymphocytosis. Patients with mumps orchitis, however, may have a marked leukocytosis with a shift to the left. In meningoencephalitis, the white blood cell count is usually within normal limits. The erythrocyte sedimentation rate is usually normal but may rise with testicular or pancreatic involvement. The serum amylase level is elevated both in pancreatitis and in salivary adenitis. It may also be elevated in some patients in whom the sole evidence of mumps is meningoencephalitis, and probably reflects subclinical involvement of the salivary glands. In contrast to the amylase, the serum lipase level is elevated only in pancreatitis, in which hyperglycemia and glucosuria also may occur. The cerebrospinal fluid contains 0 to 2000 cells per cubic millimeter, almost all mononuclear, although occasionally polymorphonuclear cells will predominate in the early stages. The pleocytosis in mumps meningitis tends to be greater than in aseptic meningitides caused by the poliomyelitis, coxsackie-, and echoviruses. There is no relationship between the cell count and the severity of central nervous system involvement. Transient hematuria and mild reversible abnormalities in renal function, including inability maximally to concentrate the urine and to clear creatinine, occur in association with the viruria of mumps.

DIAGNOSIS The definitive diagnosis of mumps depends on isolation of the virus from blood, throat swabs, secretions from Stensen's duct, cerebrospinal fluid, or urine. Immunofluorescence methods can detect positive cell cultures in 2 to 3 days rather than the 6 days required with standard methods. However, even with the simplification of viral isolation by means of tissue culture techniques, culture of the virus is rarely necessary in the typical case with associated parotitis. When an etiologic diagnosis is needed, as in aseptic meningitis or in atypical cases of parotitis, the complement fixation test is most commonly employed. Antibodies to the S antigen develop rather rapidly, often reaching a peak within 1 week after the onset of symptoms, and usually disappearing in 6 to 12 months. Complement-fixing antibodies to the V antigen follow a more typical pattern, reaching a peak titer within 2 to 3 weeks after onset, remaining elevated for at least 6 weeks, then persisting at lower levels for years afterward. Paired serums obtained 2 to 3 weeks apart are recommended. A fourfold increase in titer confirms recent infection. In cases where an acute serum is not obtained until later in the course of illness, an elevation of antibodies to the S antigen which exceeds the V antibody titer also suggests recent infection. The hemagglutination inhibition reaction is demonstrable somewhat later and persists for several months. The serum neutralization test is the most sensitive indicator of previous mumps infection, although it is more complicated to perform. However, it is a much better indicator of previous mumps infection than the skin test, and individuals with detectable specific neutralizing antibody are highly unlikely to contract mumps. The *skin test* consists of intradermal injection of killed mumps virus; previous exposure will result in a delayed reaction of the tuberculin type and an anamnestic antibody titer rise to mumps. The skin test is unreliable when used alone in determining the immune status of an individual, is useless in the diagnosis of acute mumps, and is no longer commercially available in the United States.

The diagnosis of mumps during an epidemic is usually obvious. Sporadic cases, however, must be distinguished from other causes of parotid enlargement. Parotitis may be caused by other viruses, notably parainfluenza, influenza, and coxsackieviruses. *Bacterial parotitis* usually occurs in debilitated patients with severe underlying diseases, such as uncontrolled diabetes mellitus, cerebrovascular accidents, or uremia. It may also follow surgical operations. The parotid glands are swollen, warm, and tender, and pus can be expressed from the orifices

of Stensen's ducts. Marked polymorphonuclear leukocytosis is present. The disease is usually acquired in the hospital, and *Staphylococcus aureus* is the usual causative organism. Dehydration followed by inspissation of secretions in the salivary ducts is an important predisposing factor. *Calculus* in a salivary duct is usually detectable by palpation or by injection of radiopaque media into Stensen's duct. *Drug reactions* may produce tender swelling of the parotid and other salivary glands. "Iodine mumps" is the commonest type; it may follow such procedures as intravenous urography. Mercurialism and the antihypertensive agent guanethidine may also cause parotid enlargement and tenderness. A careful history usually serves to clarify the cause of these reactions. *Cervical adenitis* caused by streptococci, "bullneck" diphtheria, infectious mononucleosis, cat-scratch disease, sublingual cellulitis (Ludwig's angina), and cellulitis of the external auditory canal are usually easy to distinguish from mumps by careful examination. Parotid tumors and chronic infections such as actinomycosis tend to follow a more indolent course, with slowly progressive swelling. The common "mixed tumor" of the parotid is well circumscribed, nontender, and very firm, almost cartilaginous on palpation. Parotid swelling and fever, often accompanied by lacrimal adenitis and uveitis (Mikulicz's syndrome), may occur in tuberculosis, leukemia, Hodgkin's disease, and lupus erythematosus. The onset may be sudden, but the process is usually painless and of long duration. "Uveoparotid fever" of similar type may be the first manifestation of sarcoidosis; in this disease parotid swelling is frequently accompanied by single or multiple palsies of cranial nerves, particularly the facial nerve, and is referred to as Heerfordt's syndrome. Presternal edema may also be a manifestation of malignant lymphoma involving retrosternal lymph nodes. Bilateral painless parotid swelling unassociated with fever is found in patients with Laennec's cirrhosis, chronic alcoholism, malnutrition, diabetes mellitus, pregnancy and lactation, and hypertriglyceridemia.

Sjögren's syndrome (Chap. 363) is a chronic inflammation of the parotid and other salivary glands which is often associated with atrophy of the lacrimal glands and occurs most commonly in women past the menopause. With cessation of lacrimal and salivary function, there may be striking dryness of the conjunctiva and the cornea (keratoconjunctivitis sicca) and of the mouth (xerostomia). These patients may also have a variety of systemic manifestations, including arthritis of the rheumatoid type, splenomegaly, leukopenia, and hemolytic anemia. The chronicity of the process and its occurrence in elderly women make confusion with mumps unlikely. Finally, benign hypertrophy of both masseter muscles, presumably due to habitual clenching and grinding of teeth, may be confused with painless parotid swelling.

The causes of aseptic meningitis are discussed in Chaps. 186 and 369.

Orchitis occurring in the absence of parotitis is likely to remain undiagnosed. Serologic testing may later confirm the diagnosis of mumps. Orchitis may occur in association with acute bacterial prostatitis and seminal vesiculitis. It is a rare complication of gonorrhea. Occasionally testicular inflammation accompanies pleurodynia, leptospirosis, melioidosis, relapsing fever, chickenpox, brucellosis, and lymphocytic choriomeningitis.

TREATMENT There is no specific treatment for infections with the mumps virus. Patients with parotitis should receive mouth care, analgesics, and a bland diet. Bed rest is advisable only as long as the patient is febrile; contrary to popular belief, physical activity has no influence on the development of orchitis or other complications. Patients with epididymoorchitis may be acutely ill and in great pain. Many forms of treatment, including surgical decompression of the testicle, infiltration of the spermatic cord with local anesthetics, estrogens, convalescent serum, and broad-spectrum antibiotics, have not been regularly effective. Despite failure to document their effectiveness in controlled studies, adrenal steroids have been of considerable benefit in diminishing fever, as well as testicular pain and swelling, and in restoring the sense of well-being in a number of patients. It is important to give a single large dose corresponding to 300 mg cortisone or 60 mg prednisone, initially. During the ensuing 24 h the same quantity should be given in divided doses. Subsequently, administration of the hormone can be tapered off over 7 to 10 days. Adrenal steroids have not exerted an adverse effect on concomitant pancreatitis or meningitis, although they have not benefited patients with meningeal involvement, and their withdrawal has usually been accompanied by a recrudescence of symptoms. Adrenal steroids have not prevented the appearance of parotid involvement on the contralateral side. Mumps arthritis is usually mild and requires no treatment. Mumps thyroiditis may subside spontaneously, but excellent relief has been obtained with adrenal hormones.

PREVENTION A live attenuated mumps virus vaccine (Jeryl Lynn strain) has been highly effective in producing significant rises in mumps antibody in individuals who are seronegative prior to vaccination, and has afforded 95 percent protection to individuals subsequently exposed to mumps. The vaccine also has boosted antibody levels in vaccinated individuals who are seropositive. The vaccine produces an inapparent, noncommunicable infection which is not associated with fever or mumps-like symptoms. It has conferred excellent protection for at least 10 years and has not interfered with vaccines against measles, rubella, and poliomyelitis or with smallpox vaccination given simultaneously. Protection has been demonstrated in both children and adults.

Live mumps vaccine can be administered at any time after 1 year of age, and should be particularly considered for children approaching puberty, adolescents, and adult males who have not had clinical mumps or live mumps vaccine in the past. Individuals living in groups or in institutions should be vaccinated, particularly because it has been shown that physical isolation of mumps patients does not effectively prevent transmission of the infection.

Vaccination is contraindicated in babies under the age of 1 year because of the interfering effect of maternal antibody; in individuals with a history of hypersensitivity to vaccine components; in patients with febrile illnesses, leukemia, lymphoma, or generalized malignancies; in those receiving steroids, alkylating drugs, antimetabolites, or irradiation; and during pregnancy.

It is not known whether the vaccine will prevent infection when administered after exposure, but no contraindication to its use in this situation exists. Specific mumps-immune globulin in large quantity is of doubtful efficacy in aborting orchitis when given 1 to 2 days after exposure, and does not prevent parotitis. Ordinary gamma globulin is not at all effective.

REFERENCES

BEARD CM et al: The incidence and outcome of mumps orchitis in Rochester Minnesota 1935 to 1974. Mayo Clin Proc 52:3, 1977

BRAY PF: Mumps—a cause of hydrocephalus? Pediatrics 49:446, 1972

BRUNNELL PA et al: Ineffectiveness of isolation of patients as a method of preventing the spread of mumps. N Engl J Med 279:1357, 1968

CARANASOS GH, FELKER JR: Mumps arthritis. Arch Intern Med 119:394, 1967

KALTREIDER HA, TALAL N: Bilateral parotid gland enlargement and hyperlipoproteinemia. JAMA 210:2067, 1969

KARCHMER AW et al: Simultaneous administration to live virus vaccines. Am J Dis Child 121:382, 1971

KOCEN RS, CRITCHLEY E: Mumps epididymo-orchitis and its treatment with cortisone. Br Med J 2:20, 1961

LEVITT LP et al: Central nervous system mumps: A review of 64 cases. Neurology 20:829, 1970

MODLIN JF et al: Current status of mumps in the United States. J Infect Dis 132:106, 1975

Mumps vaccine. Morb Mort Week Rep 26:393, 1977

ST GEME JW JR et al: Immunologic significance of the mumps virus skin test in infants, children and adults. Am J Epidemiol 101:253, 1975

UTZ JP et al: Studies of mumps. IV. Viruria and abnormal renal function. N Engl J Med 270:1283, 1964

WILFERT CM: Mumps meningoencephalitis with low cerebrospinal fluid glucose, prolonged pleocytosis and elevation of protein. N Engl J Med 280:855, 1969

189
RABIES AND OTHER RHABDOVIRUSES

LAWRENCE COREY

RABIES

DEFINITION Rabies is an acute viral disease of the central nervous system that affects all mammals and that is transmitted by infected secretions, usually saliva. Most exposures to rabies are through the bite of an infected animal, but on occasion a virus aerosol or the ingestion or transplantation of infected tissues may initiate the disease process.

ETIOLOGY The rabies virus is a bullet-shaped ribonucleic acid (RNA) virus belonging to the rhabdovirus group. It has a diameter of 750 to 800 Å and varies in length. Excrescences, 60 to 70 Å long, each with a knob-like structure at the distal end, cover the surface of the virion. These surface structures elicit neutralizing and hemagglutination-inhibiting antibodies, while a nucleocapsid antigen induces a complement-fixing antibody. Following immunization or active infection, a third group of antibodies is elicited which, together with complement, reacts with surface membranes of infected cells to produce lysis and cell death. While the first two classes of antibody appear to correlate with protection against the disease, the third may have an important injurious effect. Isolates of rabies virus may exhibit different biologic properties, but little antigenic variation has been documented. Interferon is induced by rabies virus, particularly in those tissues with high virus concentrations, and may play some role in retarding progressive infection.

EPIDEMIOLOGY Rabies exists in two epidemiologic forms: *urban*, propagated chiefly by unimmunized domestic dogs and/or cats, and *sylvatic*, propagated by skunks, foxes, raccoons, mongooses, wolves, and bats. Infection in domestic animals usually represents a "spillover" from sylvatic reservoirs of infection, and human beings can be infected by either. Hence, human infection tends to occur in locales where rabies is enzootic or epizootic, where there is a large population of unimmunized domestic animals, and where human contact with the outdoors is common. While only about 800 rabies deaths are reported to the World Health Organization (WHO) each year, "guestimates" of the worldwide incidence of rabies is approximated at 15,000 cases per year. Southeast Asia, the Philippines, Africa, and the Indian subcontinent are areas where the disease is especially common. Imported rabies combined with the recent epizootic of fox rabies in Western Europe has increased the importance of this disease in Europe. In the United States human rabies is exceedingly rare.

In most areas of the world, the dog is the important vector of rabies virus, but the wolf (Eastern Europe, Arctic regions), the mongoose (South Africa, the Caribbean), the fox (Western Europe), and the vampire bat (Latin America) may also be prominent vectors of the disease. In the United States, the skunk and bat have been the most important recent sources of human disease, with raccoons, foxes, and unimmunized dogs and cats also playing a role. While in the United States rabies in wildlife accounts for over 75 percent of the reported animal rabies, over 50 percent of the reported cases of post-exposure prophylaxis are associated with dog bites.

PATHOGENESIS The first event is the introduction of live virus through the epidermis or onto a mucous membrane. Initial viral replication appears to occur within striated muscle cells at the site of inoculation. The peripheral nervous system is exposed at the neuromuscular and/or neurotendinal spindles. The virus then spreads centripetally up the nerve to the central nervous system, probably via peripheral nerve axoplasm. Experimentally, viremia has been shown to occur, but is not thought to play a role in naturally acquired disease. Once the virus reaches the central nervous system, it replicates almost exclusively within the gray matter and then passes centrifugally along autonomic nerves to reach other tissue—the salivary glands, adrenal medulla, kidney, lung, liver, skeletal muscle, skin, and heart. Passage into the salivary glands facilitates further transmission of the disease via infected saliva. The incubation period of rabies is exceedingly variable, ranging from 10 days to over 1 year (mean 1 to 2 months). The time period appears to depend upon the amount of virus introduced, the amount of tissue involved, host defense mechanisms, and the actual distance that the virus has to travel from the site of inoculation to the central nervous system.

The neuropathology of rabies resembles other viral diseases of the central nervous system: hyperemia, varying degrees of chromatolysis, nuclear pyknosis, and neuronophagia of the nerve cells; infiltration by lymphocytes and plasma cells of the Virchow-Robin space; microglial infiltration, and parenchymal areas of nerve cell destruction. The pathognomonic lesion of rabies is the Negri body. This eosinophilic mass, approximately 10 nm in size, is made up of a finely fibrillar matrix and rabies virus particles. Negri bodies are distributed throughout the brain, particularly in Ammon's horn, the cerebral cortex, the brainstem, the Purkinje cells of the cerebellum, and the dorsal spinal ganglia. Negri bodies are not demonstrated in at least 20 percent of rabies, and their absence in brain material does not rule out the diagnosis.

MANIFESTATIONS The clinical manifestations of rabies can be divided into four stages: (1) a nonspecific prodrome, (2) an acute encephalitis similar to other viral encephalitides, (3) a profound dysfunction of brainstem centers which produces the classic features of rabies encephalitis, and (4) rarely, recovery.

The prodromal period usually persists for 1 to 4 days and is marked by fever, headache, malaise, myalgias, increased fatigability, anorexia, nausea and vomiting, sore throat, and a nonproductive cough. The prodromal symptom suggestive of rabies is the complaint of parasthesias and/or fasciculations at or about the site of inoculation of virus. This symptom is present in 50 to 80 percent of patients.

The encephalitic phase is usually ushered in by periods of excessive motor activity, excitation, and agitation. Quickly, confusion, hallucinations, combativeness, bizarre aberrations

of thought, muscle spasms, meningismus, opisthotonic posturing, seizures, and focal paralysis appear. Characteristically, the periods of mental aberration are interspersed with completely lucid periods, but as the disease progresses, the lucid periods get shorter until the patient lapses into coma. Hyperesthesia, with excessive sensitivity to bright light, loud noise, touch, and even gentle breezes, is very common. On physical examination the temperature may be found to be as high as 40.6°C (105°F). Abnormalities of the autonomic nervous system include dilated, irregular pupils, increased lacrimation, salivation, perspiration, and postural hypotension. Evidence of upper motor neuron paralysis with weakness, increased deep tendon reflexes, and extensor plantar responses is the rule. Paralysis of the vocal cords is common.

The manifestations of brainstem dysfunction begin shortly after the onset of the encephalitic phase. Cranial nerve involvement causes diplopia, facial palsies, optic neuritis, and the characteristic difficulty with deglutition. The combination of excessive salivation and difficulty in swallowing produces the traditional picture of "foaming at the mouth." Hydrophobia, the painful, violent involuntary contraction of the diaphragm, accessory respiratory, pharyngeal and laryngeal muscles initiated by swallowing liquids, is seen in about 50 percent of cases. Involvement of the amygdaloid nucleus may result in priapism and spontaneous ejaculation. The patient lapses into coma, and involvement of the respiratory center produces an apneic death. The prominence of early brainstem dysfunction distinguishes rabies from other viral encephalitides and accounts for the rapid downhill course. The median survival after the onset of symptoms is 4 days, with a maximum of 20, unless artificial supporting measures are instituted.

If intensive respiratory support is used, a number of late complications may appear and include inappropriate secretion of antidiuretic hormone, diabetes insipidus, cardiac arrythmias, vascular instability, adult respiratory distress syndrome, gastrointestinal bleeding, thrombocytopenia, and paralytic ileus. Recovery is very rare and when it occurs has been gradual. There have been only three well-documented nonfatal cases of rabies in humans. Two of these survivors received partial postexposure prophylaxis and the third, a case of laboratory-associated rabies, probably from an aerosol exposure, had received preexposure prophylaxis.

Occasionally, rabies may present as an ascending paralysis resembling the Landry-Guillain-Barré syndrome (dumb rabies, *rage tranquile*). This clinical pattern occurs most frequently in those bitten by vampire bats or who have received postexposure rabies prophylaxis.

The difficulty of suspecting rabies when it is associated with ascending paralysis is illustrated by the documentation of person-to-person transmission of the virus by tissue transplantation. A corneal transplant from a donor who died of presumed Landry-Gullain-Barré syndrome resulted in death of the recipient 7 weeks later. Pathologic examination of the brain of both patients demonstrated Negri bodies, and rabies virus was subsequently isolated from the donor's frozen eye.

LABORATORY FINDINGS Early in the disease the hemoglobin and routine blood chemistries are normal, but abnormalities occur as hypothalamic dysfunction, gastrointestinal bleeding, and other complications ensue. The peripheral white blood cell count is usually slightly elevated (12,000 to 17,000 per cubic millimeter) but may be normal or as high as 30,000 per cubic millimeter.

As in any viral infection, the specific diagnosis of rabies depends upon (1) the isolation of virus from infected secretions [saliva, rarely cerebrospinal fluid (CSF), or tissue (brain)], (2) the serologic demonstration of acute infection, or (3) the demonstration of viral antigen in infected tissue, e.g., corneal impression smears, skin biopsies, or brain. Samples of brain obtained either on postmortem examination or from brain biopsy should be subjected to (1) mouse inoculation studies for virus isolation, (2) fluorescent-antibody (FA) staining for viral antigen, and (3) histologic and/or electron microscopic examination for Negri bodies. While the mouse inoculation studies for virus isolation and direct FA staining for viral antigen are quite reliable and sensitive, if the patient's life has been prolonged and high levels of neutralizing antibody are present in serum and CSF, "autosterilization" may occur, and these tests may be negative. The use of FA staining of skin biopsies, corneal impression smears, and saliva for evidence of rabies antigen has been helpful in diagnosing rabies during life. Confirmation of these findings either serologically or by demonstration of virus in brain should be sought.

If the patient has not received antirabies immunization, then a fourfold rise in neutralizing antibody to rabies virus in serial serum samples is diagnostic. If the patient has received rabies vaccination, then a clue to the diagnosis may be obtained from the absolute titers of serum-neutralizing antibody and the presence of neutralizing antibody to rabies in CSF. Postexposure rabies prophylaxis rarely produces CSF-neutralizing antibody to rabies. If present, it is usually in low titer, e.g., less than 1:64, whereas CSF titers in human rabies may vary from 1:200 to 1:160,000.

DIFFERENTIAL DIAGNOSIS There is little to distinguish rabies from other viral encephalitides, and the most helpful point in diagnosis is the history of exposure. Other problems to be considered include hysterical reactions to animal bites (pseudohydrophobia), Landry-Guillain-Barré syndrome, poliomyelitis, and allergic encephalomyelitis to rabies vaccine. The latter occurs most commonly after use of nerve tissue–derived vaccine and usually begins 1 to 4 weeks after vaccination.

PREVENTION AND TREATMENT Each year more than 1 million Americans are bitten by animals. In each instance, a decision must be made whether to initiate postexposure rabies prophylaxis. When deciding whether to institute rabies prophylaxis, the following considerations apply: (1) whether the individual came into physical contact with saliva or another substance likely to contain rabies virus; (2) whether rabies is known or suspected in the species and area associated with the exposure (e.g., all persons within the continental United States bitten by a bat that then escapes should receive postexposure prophylaxis); (3) the circumstances surrounding the exposure; and (4) the treatment alternative and complications. A guide for postexposure rabies prophylaxis is illustrated in Fig. 189-1.

If rabies is known to be present or suspected to be present in the animal species involved in a human exposure, the animal should be captured, if possible. Captured wild animals or any ill, unvaccinated, or stray domestic animal involved in a rabies exposure, particularly any animal involved in an unprovoked bite, exhibiting abnormal behavior, or suspected of being rabid, should be captured and killed, and the head should be sent immediately to an appropriate laboratory for rabies fluorescent antibody (FA) examination. If examination of the brain by the FA technique is negative for rabies, it can be assumed that the saliva contains no virus, and the exposed person need not be treated. Persons exposed to escaped wild animals capable of carrying rabies (bats, skunks, coyotes, foxes, raccoons, etc.) in an area where rabies is known or sus-

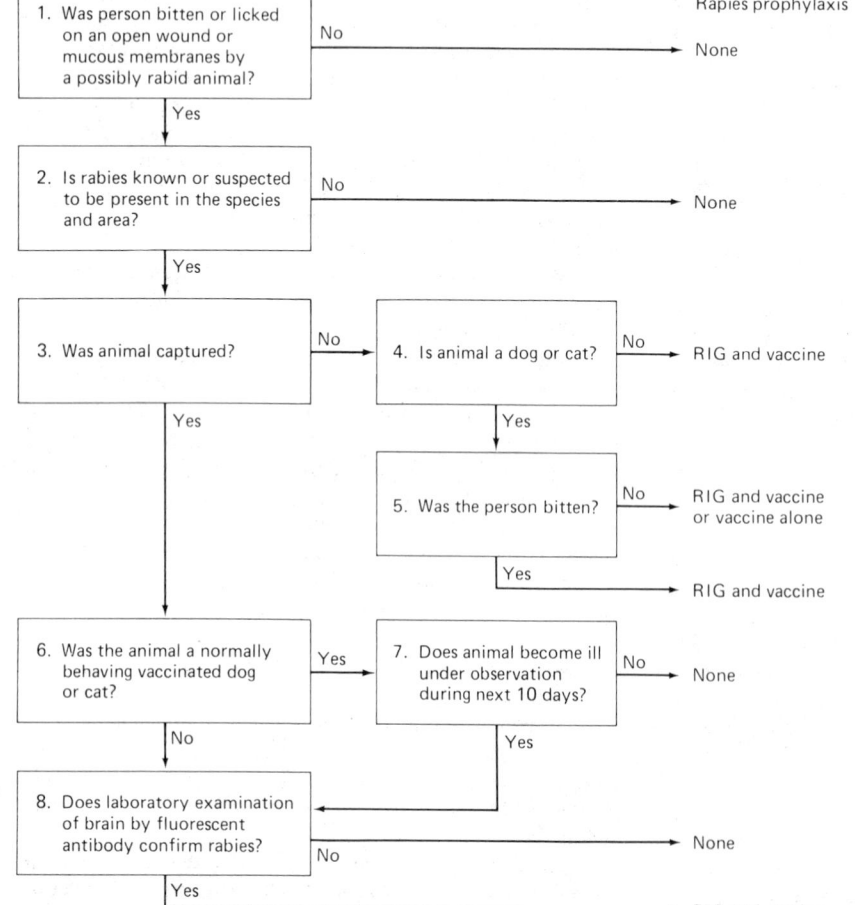

Rapies prophylaxis

FIGURE 189-1
Postexposure rabies prophylaxis algorithm. (Adapted from L Corey, MAW Hattwick, JAMA 232:272, 1975. Copyright 1975, American Medical Association.)

pected to be present should receive both passive and active immunization against rabies.

If a healthy vaccinated dog or cat bites a person, the animal should be captured, confined, and observed for 10 days. If any illness or abnormal behavior develops in the animal during the observation period, it should be killed for FA examination.

Postexposure prophylaxis Once a decision regarding the necessity to initiate postexposure rabies prophylaxis has been made, the general principle of postexposure therapy is to minimize the amount of virus at the site of inoculation with local treatment of the wound and to establish an early and long-lasting neutralizing antibody titer to rabies virus. The following therapeutic regimen is recommended:

1 *Local wound therapy* with generous scrubbing with soap and then flushing of the wound with water or ethyl alcohol, removing all vestiges of the soap. This is followed by a second scrubbing with a quaternary ammonium compound such as 1 to 2% benzalkonium chloride (Zephiran) or 1% cetrimonium bromide (Cetavlon). If indicated, tetanus toxoid and antibiotics (usually penicillin G) should be given.
2 *Active immunization* with antirabies vaccine. Duck embryo vaccine is the only currently licensed vaccine available in the United States. While major complications associated with duck embryo vaccine in postexposure prophylaxis are uncommon, local reactions, such as pain (100 percent), erythema (97 percent), and pruritus (13 percent) at the site of inoculation are common, and systemic symptoms, such as fever, malaise, or myalgia, occur in about 33 percent of postexposure recipients. Anaphylaxis is seen in less than 1 percent of recipients and usually occurs during administration of the first five doses. A history of hypersensitivity to avian products should be ruled out before initial therapy.

Central nervous system reactions to duck embryo vaccine are rare. Antihistamines will usually ameliorate local and systemic reactions to this vaccine. Corticosteroids interfere with the development of active immunity and may increase the likelihood of the development of clinical rabies; therefore use of these agents in treating adverse reactions is not recommended unless life-threatening complications to the vaccine occur.

A total of 23 doses of duck embryo vaccine should be given when it is used with hyperimmune serum. A primary series consisting of 21 doses of vaccine is given either as 21 daily doses or as two doses a day (separate injections or a double dose) for 7 days, followed by one dose daily for 7 days. This is followed by two booster doses on the tenth and twentieth days after completion of the primary series. Vaccine should be given subcutaneously in the abdomen or lateral aspect of the thigh, and rotation of injection sites is recommended. When vaccine is given alone, 14 daily doses are sufficient.
3 *Passive immunization* with antirabies antiserum of either equine or human origin. The latter is preferred when available, because of the high incidence of serum sickness (20 to 40 percent) with the equine product. Fifty percent of the total dose of 20 units/kg for human rabies immune globulin (RIG) and 40 units/kg for the equine antiserum is given by local infiltration of the wound, and the rest intramuscularly. Because many persons will not develop significant levels of neutralizing antibody [$>$1:5 by mouse inoculation or equivalent or 1:15 in the rapid fluorescent focus inhibition test (RFFIT)] after postexposure prophylaxis, a neutralizing antibody determination should be obtained after completion of therapy. "Nonresponders" may be candidates for the recently developed, more potent, tissue culture rabies vaccine.

An important development in rabies prophylaxis has been the development of several inactivated subunit human diploid cell strain rabies vaccines. These vaccines are licensed in Europe but are not yet available in the United States, except on a limited basis from the Viral Disease Division of the Center for Disease Control for those persons who (1) have a serious allergy to duck embryo vaccine, (2) do not show an adequate antibody response to duck embryo vaccine, or (3) have been bitten by an animal proved to be rabid. These tissue culture vaccines appear more immunogenic than duck embryo vaccine, and more than 95 percent of persons who received three doses of vaccines for preexposure immunization developed detectable antibody titers. While mild local reactions appear in 30 percent of recipients and febrile reactions in 5 to 10 percent, no serious neuroparalytic reactions have been identified. Data on the efficacy of these diploid vaccines in postexposure prophylaxis are still being accumulated, but published studies involving over 80 persons who have been bitten by animals proved to be rabid have indicated protection from clinical rabies. Treatment with a combination of human rabies immunoglobulin (20 ml/kg) on day 1 and six doses of tissue culture vaccine given on the first, third, seventh, fourteenth, thirtieth, and ninetieth days after exposure has been associated with an early, higher, and more sustained antibody response than that generally achieved with duck embryo vaccine. These vaccines require fewer doses, suggesting that morbidity associated with postexposure rabies prophylaxis will be diminished.

Preexposure prophylaxis The availability of the relatively safe duck embryo vaccine (DEV) has permitted the initiation of preexposure therapy for individuals with a high risk of contact with rabies virus: Veterinarians, spelunkers, laboratory workers, animal handlers, etc. Such preexposure therapy consists of two 1-ml subcutaneous injections of DEV given 1 month apart, followed by a 1-ml booster 7 months later. At the completion of the three-shot series, the neutralizing antibody titer should be checked.

Treatment While nonfatal human rabies has now been documented, once clinical symptoms develop, rabies is usually fatal. The basis for "therapy" of rabies must be prevention of acquisition of the disease through active domestic animal vaccination programs and postexposure prophylaxis. In the future, the availability of newly developed more immunogenic vaccines combined with the use of interferon or interferon-inducers may improve upon the efficacy and toxicity of the currently recommended regimens.

MARBURG VIRUS DISEASE

DEFINITION Marburg virus causes an acute systemic febrile illness characterized by the abrupt onset of headache, myalgias, pharyngitis, rash, and hemorrhagic manifestations. It was recognized first in 1967 when it caused simultaneous outbreaks in the Federal Republic of Germany and Yugoslavia among laboratory workers exposed to imported African green monkeys (*Cercopithecus aethiops*). The clinical manifestations are similar to other hemorrhagic fevers of the arenavirus class or flavovirus group (Argentina and Bolivian hemorrhagic fever, Chap. 191). The high case fatality rate and demonstrated ability for nosocomial spread has made recognition of this rare agent an important worldwide public health concern.

ETIOLOGY The Marburg virus has been isolated in guinea pig and various cell culture systems such as vervet monkey kidney. The virus particle contains lipid and RNA, and under the electron microscope the virus appears as an 80- to 100-nm elongated filamentous particle with occasional "blister-like excrescences." While the Marburg virus exhibits some morphologic relationship to other members of the rhabdoviruses (rabies, Ebola, and Mokola viruses), it appears antigenically distinct.

EPIDEMIOLOGY The initial outbreaks affected 31 patients in Marburg and Frankfurt, Germany, and Belgrade, Yugoslavia, and was epidemiologically linked to monkeys imported from the same source in Uganda. Virus was isolated from the blood and tissue of these monkeys. Of the 25 primary infections, there were seven deaths. Six secondary cases, involving two physicians, one nurse, a postmortem attendant, and the wife of a veterinarian occurred. Person-to-person transmission was felt to take place via accidental needle sticks or abrasions, although respiratory and conjunctival infection could not be ruled out. The wife of one patient developed Marburg virus disease at the onset of his illness; Marburg virus was demonstrated in semen of the original patient, despite the presence of circulating antibody, and this secondary case is believed to have been acquired through sexual intercourse. Subsequent investigations in the Lake Kyoga region of Uganda where the monkeys originated revealed no unusual illnesses or death among primates in the area. Complement fixation antibodies were demonstrated in 36 percent of *C. aethiops* trapped in the region, and antibody was detected in three monkey trappers.

PATHOLOGY Marburg virus appears "pantropic" and produces lesions in almost all organs including lymphoid tissue, liver, spleen, pancreas, adrenals, thyroid, kidney, testes, skin, and brain. In lymphoid tissue focal necrosis with degeneration of lymphoid tissue is apparent. In the liver, eosinophilic cytoplasmic bodies resembling the Councilman bodies of yellow fever have been noted. The lungs may show interstitial pneumonitis, as well as vascular lesions in small arterioles indicative of endarteritis. Neuropathologic changes consist of multiple small hemorrhagic infarcts with glial proliferation.

CLINICAL MANIFESTATIONS After an incubation period of 3 to 9 days, patients develop the abrupt onset of frontal and temporal headache, malaise, myalgias, especially in the lumbar area, nausea, and vomiting. Fever of 39.4 to 40°C (103 to 104°F) is characteristic, and about half the patients have conjunctivitis. Between 1 and 3 days after onset, watery diarrhea, which is often severe, lethargy, and a change in mentation are noted. An enanthem of the palate and tonsils, and cervical lymphadenopathy, may also be noted during the first week of illness. The most reliable clinical feature is the appearance of nonpruritic maculopapular rash which begins on the fifth to seventh day on the face and neck and spreads centrifugally to involve the extremities. A fine desquamation of the affected skin, especially the palms and soles, appears 4 to 5 days later. Hemorrhagic manifestations, including gastrointestinal, renal, vaginal, and/or conjunctival hemorrhages, generally develop between days 5 and 7 of disease.

During the first week, the temperature continues in the vicinity of 40°C (104°F), falling by lysis during the second week, to increase again between the twelfth and fourteenth days. Other clinical signs apparent in the second week of disease include splenomegaly, hepatomegaly, facial edema, and scrotal or labial reddening. Complications include orchitis, which may lead to testicular atrophy, myocarditis with irregular pulse and electrocardiographic abnormalities, and pancreatitis. The overall case fatality rate has been about 25 percent, with death usually occurring during the eighth to sixteenth days of illness. Recovery is often protracted over a 3- to 4-week period, and

during this period loss of hair, intermittent abdominal pain, poor appetite, and prolonged psychotic disturbances have been noted. Late sequelae including transverse myelitis and uveitis have been reported. Marburg virus has been isolated from the anterior eye chamber and semen nearly 3 months after onset of disease.

LABORATORY FINDINGS Abnormalities in granulocyte function are found, and leukopenia is detected as early as the first day, with leukocyte counts as low as 1000 per cubic millimeter and a neutrophilia by the fourth day. Subsequently, atypical lymphocytes, as well as neutrophils exhibiting the characteristic of the Pelger-Huet anomaly, may appear. Thrombocytopenia appears early and is most marked, often less than 10,000 cells per cubic millimeter, between the sixth and twelfth days. In fatal cases, evidence of disseminated intravascular coagulation can be demonstrated. Hypoproteinemia, proteinuria, and azotemia may occur. Elevations in serum glutamic oxaloacetic transaminase (SGOT) and alanine aminotransferase (SGPT) are usual. Lumbar puncture may be normal or reveal a minimal pleocytosis. The erythrocyte sedimentation rate is usually low.

DIAGNOSIS The characteristic clinical course and epidemiologic features are the basis of the diagnosis. Specific diagnosis requires isolation of the virus or serologic evidence of infection in paired serum samples. Viremia coincides with the febrile state of disease, and virus has been isolated from tissue as well as urine, semen, throat, and rectal swabs. Attempts to isolate virus must be carried out only in *specialized high-security laboratories.* All patients should be kept in strict isolation, and all specimens should be handled and shipped according to World Health Organization guidelines.

TREATMENT Patients have received a multiplicity of drugs without apparent influence on the course of the illness. Convalescent serum was administered to four patients, whose subsequent disease followed a mild course. However, similarly benign outcomes were observed in patients who did not receive serum.

EBOLA VIRUS

Between July and November 1976 simultaneous outbreaks of an acute febrile hemorrhagic disease occurred in Southern Sudan and Northern Zaire. "Secondary and tertiary" spread of infection, particularly among hospital staff, was noted. In the Sudan over 300 cases with 151 deaths and in Zaire 237 cases with 211 fatalities were reported. In one Sudanese hospital, 76 members of a staff of 230 were infected and 41 died. The virus isolated from patients in the Sudan and Zaire was morphologically similar to the Marburg agent but was antigenically distinct. The name Ebola virus, after the river in Zaire located near the epidemic, has been proposed.

Ebola virus has been propagated in tissue culture (Vero cells) and in suckling mice and guinea pigs. The source of the outbreak in both the Sudan and Zaire is unknown; however, as with other viral hemorrhagic fevers, peridomestic rodents are suspected as being a reservoir of the infection. Once established, nosocomial as well as community-acquired cases occur, especially among close and prolonged contact. Parenteral exposure to the virus through disinfected rather than sterilized needles may have played a role in transmission. Barrier nursing and strict isolation precautions using protective clothing appeared to decrease the number of nosocomial cases.

CLINICAL MANIFESTATIONS Clinically, the disease is similar to Marburg virus disease. The incubation period ranges from 4 to 6 days (mean is 7 days). Patients usually present on the fifth day of illness with a history of abrupt onset of headache, malaise, myalgias, high fever, diarrhea, abdominal pain, dehydration, and lethargy. Pleuritic chest pain, a dry hacking cough and a pronounced pharyngitis were also noted. A maculopapular eruption develops between days 5 to 7 of illness. On black skins the rash is often faint and not recognized until desquamation occurs. Hematemesis, melena, and bleeding from the nose, gums, and vagina are common. Abortion and massive metrorrhagia was a frequent complication among pregnant women. Death usually occurs in the second week of illness and is preceded by severe blood loss and shock.

TREATMENT Patients should be isolated until virological studies indicate they are free of virus, usually 21 days from onset of illness. Malaria parasites were frequently found in blood films of patients with Ebola virus infection in the Sudan indicating that the presence of parasitemia does not rule out concomitant viral illness. Treatment with plasma containing Ebola virus specific antibodies has resulted in diminished levels of viremia; however, further tests are required to establish the effectiveness of this form of therapy. Requests for viral isolation as well as convalescent plasma should be addressed to WHO Regional Centers in Atlanta or Geneva.

MOKOLA VIRUS

Mokola virus was first isolated from wild shrews captured in Nigeria and subsequently was shown to be related morphologically and serologically to rabies. However, neither of the two reported cases of human disease (both children) demonstrated classic clinical features of rabies. One patient had a nonfatal illness characterized by fever, pharyngitis, and convulsions. Mokola virus was recovered from her cerebrospinal fluid. The second patient initially had fever, cough, and vomiting, followed in several days by drowsiness, confusion, and generalized flaccid weakness. Her cerebrospinal fluid was normal. She progressed to deep coma and died within 10 days of onset. Mokola virus was isolated from her brain, and histopathologic sections revealed finely granular cytoplasmic inclusions that were distinguishable from Negri bodies in many neurons.

VESICULAR STOMATITIS VIRUS

Vesicular stomatitis is a viral illness of animals which can occasionally infect humans. It presents as an acute self-limited influenza-like disease. The disease in animals is found in the United States and South America and affects chiefly domestic cattle, horses, swine, and wild deer, raccoons, skunks, and bobcats.

In animals, vesicular stomatitis is characterized by the development of vesicles on the oral mucosa, particularly the tongue, udders, and heels. The mode of spread is probably by direct contact; however, epidemics tend to occur in warm weather, and the virus has been isolated from *Phlebotumus* sandflies in Panama and *Äedes* species in New Mexico, suggesting these as possible vectors. Two distinct serotypes, New Jersey and Indiana, have been recognized and most of the outbreaks in North America have been attributed to the New Jersey strain. The disease is most common in laboratory workers, and in one report three-fourths of laboratory personnel handling experimentally infected animals or manipulating the virus developed neutralizing antibodies. The disease is transmissible, however, under natural conditions among workers having direct contact with infected animals, especially cattle. The incubation period ranges from 1 to 6 days. This is followed by the sudden onset of fever, up to 40°C (104°F), chills, profuse sweating, myalgias, malaise, headache, and pain on ocular movement. One-third to one-half of patients have sore throat and cervical and/or submandibular adenopathy. Small

raised vesicular lesions may appear on the buccal mucosa. Conjunctivitis and coryza are present in about 20 percent of cases. Occasionally, small subcorneal, intraepithelial vesicles may appear on the fingers, usually associated with direct inoculation of the virus. Symptoms generally last 3 to 4 days, but occasionally a diphasic course may occur. Inapparent infection is common, and among laboratory workers with serologic evidence of infection, only about one-half reported clinical symptoms. In some areas of Panama, 17 to 35 percent of the population have neutralizing antibodies against vesicular stomatitis virus.

The differential diagnosis includes hand-foot-and-mouth disease, herpangina, primary herpetic pharyngitis and other mucocutaneous syndromes, and influenza. Viral isolation from patients is not common; however, a rise in complement fixation and/or neutralizing antibodies to vesicular stomatitis virus between acute and convalescent serums will help to confirm the diagnosis. Treatment is nonspecific.

REFERENCES

Marburg virus

GEAR JSS et al: Outbreak of Marburg virus disease in Johannesburg. Br Med J 4:489, 1975

MARTIN GA, SEIGERT R (eds): *Marburg Virus Disease*. New York, Springer-Verlag, 1971

SIMPSON DIH: Marburg and ebola virus infections: A guide for their diagnosis, management and control. WHO Offset Publication no 36, Geneva, 1977

Mokola virus

FAMILUSI JB: Fatal human infection with Mokola virus. Am J Trop Med Hyg. 21:959, 1972

Rabies

BAER GM: *The Natural History of Rabies*. New York, Academic, 1975

BAHMANYAR M: Successful protection of humans exposed to rabies. JAMA 236:2751, Dec. 13, 1976

COREY L, HATTWICK MA: Treatment of persons exposed to rabies. JAMA 232:272, 1975

HATTWICK MA et al: Recovery from rabies: A case report. Ann Intern Med 76:931, 1972

HOUGH SA et al: Human-to-human transmission of rabies virus by a corneal transplant. N Engl J Med 300:603, 1979

PLOTKIN SA, WIKTOR TJ: Rabies vaccination. Annu Rev Med 29:583, 1978

PUBLIC HEALTH SERVICE ADVISORY COMMITTEE ON IMMUNIZATION PRACTICES: Rabies prophylaxis. Morb Mort Week Rep 25(51):403, December 31, 1975

RUBIN RH et al: Adverse reactions to duck embryo vaccine. Ann Intern Med 78:643, 1973

190
ARBOVIRUS INFECTIONS

JAY P. SANFORD

Most viral infections in humans are either asymptomatic or present as undifferentiated illnesses characterized by fever, malaise, headache, and generalized myalgia. The similarities in clinical features between infections caused by viruses as dissimilar as the myxoviruses (e.g., influenza), the enteroviruses (e.g., poliovirus, coxsackievirus, echovirus), some of the herpesviruses (e.g., cytomegalovirus), and the arboviruses usually preclude an etiologic diagnosis based entirely on clinical manifestations without ancillary information regarding epidemiologic features and serologic findings. The purpose of this chapter is to direct attention to the ever-expanding list of viruses which produce febrile disease in humans. Because the number of agents is large, mention will be made of those which have been best documented, have demonstrated unusual features, or seem to be of greatest potential significance.

DEFINITION AND CLASSIFICATION It has not always been easy to determine that an agent is an arbovirus; hence with further characterization some agents which were initially registered as arboviruses have been reclassified, e.g., the zoonotic agents which have unique morphology on electron microscopy have been classified as arenaviruses (Chap. 191). Similarly, vesicular stomatitis virus, Mokola, and Lagos bat virus, provisionally registered as arboviruses, were found to be related to rabies virus and are now classified as rhabdoviruses (Chap. 189). The currently accepted definition of an arthropod-borne virus was published in 1967 by the World Health Organization:

Arboviruses are viruses which are maintained in nature principally, or to an important extent, through biological transmission between susceptible vertebrate hosts by hematophagous arthropods; they multiply and produce viremia in the vertebrates, multiply in the tissues of arthropods, and are passed on to new vertebrates by the bites of arthropods after a period of extrinsic incubation.

From this definition it can be appreciated that the term *arbovirus* is used in the ecological sense. Transmission by vectors is not correlated with virus architecture, which forms an important basis for current classification. Thus, the broad category arbovirus is being subdivided, and structurally related non-arthropod-borne agents may be classified with agents designated as arboviruses. Casal's serologic groups A and B arboviruses have been shown to be enveloped RNA agents with a spherical nucleocapsid forming the viral core, probably of icosohedral symmetry. Agents with these characteristics are now classified as togaviruses, with group A designated as alphaviruses and group B as flaviviruses. Other members of the togavirus group which are not transmitted by arthropods include rubella virus, equine arteritis virus, European swine fever/hog cholera virus, and viral disease of cattle agent.

There are more than 250 distinct arboviruses, which have been grouped into three families with some agents yet remaining unclassified. Within each family, the agents have been subdivided on the basis of antigenic differences (Table 190-1). The characteristics of individual members of this large group of viruses are not uniform; those in group A are 40 to 60 nm in diameter, and those in the Bunyamwera group are about 100 nm in diameter. The majority of agents contain single-stranded RNA, although some, such as Colorado tick fever, contain double-stranded RNA.

Arboviruses are of importance in both temperate and tropical zones. Representative viruses have been isolated in almost every geographic area outside the polar region.

Arbovirus infection of vertebrates is usually asymptomatic. The viremia stimulates an immune response which sharply limits the duration of the viremia. In arbovirus infections other than urban yellow fever, phlebotomus fever, chikungunya, o'nyong-nyong, mayaro, oropouche, and dengue, infection of humans represents an incidental occurrence which is tangential to the basic maintenance cycle of the virus. Hence, the isolation of virus from arthropod vectors or the detection of

TABLE 190-1
Classification of arboviruses

Family	Group	Specific agent	
Togaviruses	A (alpha-viruses)	Chikun-gunya* Eastern equine* Mayaro/ Semliki, Forest (Uruma)* Mucambo O'nyong-nyong*	Ross River* Sindbis* Venezuelan equine* Western equine*
	B (flavi-viruses)	Banzi Bat salivary gland* Bussuquara Central European encephalitis Dengue 1–4* Ilheus Japanese (B)* Kunjin Kyasanur Forest* Louping ill Murray Valley	Nataya Negishi Omsk hemor-rhagic* Powassan Rocio Russian spring-summer Spondwenii St. Louis* Uganda S Usutu Wesselbron West Nile* Yellow fever* Zika*
Bunyaviruses	C	Apeu* Caraparu* Itaqui* Madrid* Marituba*	Murutucui* Oriboca* Ossa* Restan*
	Bunyamwera	Bunyamwera Germiston Guaroa	Ilesha Wycomyia
	Bwamba	Bwamba	
	California	California LaCrosse*	Tahyna
	Ganjam	Dugbe	Ganjam
	Guama	Bimiti Catu	Guama
	Quaranfil	Quaranfil	
	Sandfly fever (Phleboto-mus)	Candiru* Chagres* Naples type*	Punta Toro* Sicilian type*
	Simbu	Shuni	Oropouche
	Thogoto	Thogoto	
	Ungrouped	Congo/ Crimean hemor-rhagic* Rift Valley fever* Nairobi sheep disease	Tataguine Zinga
Orbiviruses	Changuinola Kemerovo Ungrouped	Changuinola Kemerovo Colorado tick fever*	Tribec Lipovnik
Not classified		Nyando	

* *Discussed in the text.*

infection in the natural vertebrate host may provide a means for early detection and enable control of epizootic infection before significant spread to humans occurs.

As determined by serologic evidence of host responses, at least 80 immunologically distinct arboviruses are capable of infecting humans, while somewhat fewer have been incriminated as causing clinical disease. The spectrum of clinical illness produced by the arboviruses is varied both in predominant features and in severity. Five broad, often overlapping, and somewhat arbitrary clinical syndromes may be delineated (Table 190-2).

TABLE 190-2
Summary of clinical and epidemiologic features of arboviruses associated with infection in humans in the Western Hemisphere

Syndrome	Virus	Serologic group*	Vector	Known geographic range
Fever with malaise, *headaches,* and *myalgia*	Apeu	C	Mosquito	Brazil
	Anhembi	C	Mosquito	Brazil
	Candiru	Sandfly fever	Sandfly	Brazil
	Caraparu	C	Mosquito	Brazil, Panama, Trinidad
	Catu	Guama	Mosquito	Brazil, Trinidad
	Chagres	Sandfly fever	Sandfly	Panama
	Colorado tick fever	Ungrouped orbivirus	Tick	Western United States, Alberta, British Columbia
	Guama	Guama	Mosquito	Brazil, Trinidad
	Guaroa	Bunyamwera	Mosquito	Brazil, Colombia
	Itaqui	C	Mosquito	Brazil
	Madrid	C	?	Panama
	Marituba	C	Mosquito?	Brazil
	Mayaro	A	Mosquito	Brazil, Colombia, Central America, Trinidad
	Mucambo	A	Mosquito	Brazil
	Murutucui	C	Mosquito	Brazil
	Oropouche	Simbu	Mosquito	Brazil, Trinidad
	Ossa	C	?	Panama
	Punta Toro	Sandfly	Sandfly	Panama
	Quaranfil	Quaranfil	Tick	South America
	Restan	C	Mosquito	Trinidad
	Uruma	A	?	Bolivia
	U.S. Bat salivary gland	B	?	Southwestern United States
	Venezuelan equine encephalitis	A	Mosquito	Florida, Texas, Louisiana, Mexico, Central America, Ecuador, Peru, Colombia, Venezuela, Brazil, Trinidad, Surinam, Guyana
	Yellow fever	B	Mosquito	Central and South America
Fever with malaise, headaches, myalgia, *arthralgia,* and *rash*	Changuinola	Changuinola	*Phlebotomus*	Panama
	Mayaro	A	Mosquito	Brazil, Colombia, Central America, Trinidad
Fever with malaise, headaches, myalgia, rash, and *lymphadenopathy*	Dengue 1	B	Mosquito	Caribbean
	Dengue 2	B	Mosquito	Circumglobal
	Dengue 3	B	Mosquito	Caribbean
Fever with *central nervous system* involvement	California encephalitis	California	Mosquito	United States
	Eastern equine encephalitis	A	Mosquito	Eastern Canada, United States, Mexico, Dominican Republic, Jamaica, Panama, Trinidad, Brazil
	Ilheus	B	Mosquito	Northern South America, Trinidad, Central America, Florida
	Medoc		?	United States
	Powassan	B	Tick	Canada, New York
	Rocio	B	?	Brazil
	St. Louis encephalitis	B	Mosquito	Unites States, Caribbean, Panama, Brazil, Argentina
	Venezuelan equine encephalitis	A	Mosquito	Florida, Texas, Louisiana, Central America, Caribbean, Northern South America, Peru
	Western equine encephalitis	A	Mosquito	Canada, United States, Mexico, Brazil, Argentina
Fever with malaise, headaches, myalgia, and *hemorrhagic signs*	Dengue 1	B	Mosquito	Caribbean, including Puerto Rico
	Dengue 2	B	Mosquito	Caribbean, including Puerto Rico
	Dengue 3	B	Mosquito	Caribbean, including Puerto Rico
	Yellow fever	B	Mosquito	Central and South America

* *Antibody responses to viruses in the same serologic group often show cross-reactions with other members of the group.*

ARBOVIRUS INFECTIONS PRESENTING CHIEFLY WITH FEVER, MALAISE, HEADACHE, AND MYALGIA

PHLEBOTOMUS FEVER Phlebotomus (sandfly, pappataci, or 3-day) fever is an acute, relatively mild, self-limited infection caused by at least five immunologically distinct arboviruses (Naples, Sicilian, Punta Toro, Chagres, and Candiru). Serologic evidence of human infection has been demonstrated for four additional agents (Bujaru, Cacao, Karimabad, and Salehabad). Humans, the only known host, probably serve as a dead-end host. Voles are suspected of being an endemic host in the Middle East.

Prevalence The disease occurs throughout the Mediterranean Basin, the Balkans, the Near and Middle East, the eastern part of Africa, the Soviet republics of Central Asia, West Pakistan, and possibly certain parts of southern China. Recently, sandfly fever has been recognized in Panama and Brazil. In the Middle East and Central Asia native populations acquire the disease at an early age and develop and maintain high levels of immunity. Cases in Panama and Brazil are sporadic, occurring mainly in persons entering the forest. The apparent absence of phlebotomus fever in indigenous adult populations residing in areas where sandflies are abundant may present a deceptive picture of the actual risk to susceptible persons.

Epidemiology In the Middle East and Central Asia, the disease occurs during the hot, dry season (summer or autumn months) and is transmitted to human beings by the bite of infected sandflies (*Phlebotomus papatasi*). *Phlebotomus papatasi* is a small urban fly which can penetrate ordinary house screens. Only the female bites and usually does so during the night. In persons who are not sensitive, there is neither pain nor local irritation after the bite; hence only about 1 percent of patients will remember having been bitten. In contrast, most of the human-biting sandflies of tropical America are sylvan in their habits. Approximately 7 days after feeding on an infected individual, the fly acquires the capacity to transmit infection and remains infectious for its life span. Transovarial transmission of the virus to the next generation has been demonstrated and offers the best explanation for the mechanism of overwinter survival of the virus. In humans, the incubation period may be as short as 3 days. Viremia is present for at least 24 h before the onset of fever, but is not detectable for more than 2 days after the onset of illness.

Clinical manifestations The onset of symptoms is abrupt in over 90 percent of patients, with the temperature rapidly rising to its highest point, which may vary from 37.8 to 40.1°C (100 to 105°F). Headache is nearly always present and often is accompanied by pain on moving the eyes and by retroorbital pain. Myalgia is common and may be localized to the chest, resembling pleurodynia, or to the abdomen. Other symptoms may include vomiting, photophobia, giddiness, neck stiffness, alteration or loss of taste, and arthralgia. Conjunctival injection is present in approximately one-third of patients. Small vesicles may be seen on the palate, and macular or urticarial rashes occur. The spleen is rarely palpable, and lymphadenopathy is absent. The pulse rate may be elevated in proportion to the temperature on the first day; thereafter bradycardia is often present. The fever persists 3 days in most patients, with gradual defervescence. Giddiness, weakness, and feelings of depression are frequently encountered during convalescence. Second attacks 2 to 12 weeks after the first occur in 15 percent of cases.

In common with other arbovirus infections, phlebotomus fever may be associated with *aseptic meningitis*. In one series, 12 percent of patients had symptoms and signs sufficient to warrant a lumbar puncture. Findings in these patients included pleocytosis, with an average cell count of 90 per cubic millimeter and a predominance of either polymorphonuclear or mononuclear leukocytes. Spinal fluid protein concentration ranged from 20 to 130 mg per 100 ml. In another series mild papilledema was observed in a few patients with severe illness.

Laboratory findings The changes in leukocyte count constitute the only positive laboratory findings. Total leukocyte counts of less than 5000 per cubic millimeter are observed in 90 percent of patients if daily counts are done during the febrile period and convalescence. The leukopenia may not appear until the last day of fever or even after defervescence. The differential leukocyte count will reveal an absolute decrease in lymphocytes on the first day, accompanied by an increase in nonsegmented neutrophils. During the second or third day, the number of lymphocytes begins to return to normal and may constitute 40 to 65 percent of the total count. Concurrently, there is a reversal in proportion of segmented and band neutrophils. The differential count usually returns to normal within 5 to 8 days after defervescence. Erythrocyte values and urinalyses are usually normal.

Diagnosis In the absence of a specific serologic test, the diagnosis must be made on clinical and epidemiologic grounds.

Treatment The disease is self-limited, and no specific therapy is available. Symptomatic care, including bed rest, adequate fluid intake, and analgesia with aspirin, is recommended. Convalescence may require a week or longer.

Prognosis No fatalities have been recorded among the tens of thousands of cases.

COLORADO TICK FEVER Colorado tick fever is one of the two tick-transmitted virus diseases of human beings recognized in the United States and Canada, Powassan virus being the other. Though "mountain fever" had been described ever since the advent of immigrants to the Rocky Mountain region, Becker in 1930 differentiated it from mild Rocky Mountain spotted fever, established the clinical picture of disease, and renamed it Colorado tick fever.

Etiology Colorado tick fever virus is classified as an arbovirus because it replicates in ticks, but is a reovirus (orbivirus) on the basis of both its structure and its content of double-stranded RNA.

Prevalence The disease has been contracted in Colorado, Idaho, Nevada, Wyoming, Montana, Utah, the eastern portions of Oregon, Washington, California, and northern portions of Arizona and New Mexico, and Alberta and British Columbia. However, the virus of Colorado tick fever has been reported to have been isolated from the dog tick, *Dermacentor variabilis,* obtained from Long Island. This observation has not been confirmed, but suggests the possibility that Colorado tick fever may occur over a wider geographic area. The actual prevalence is difficult to assess, but the disease is relatively common. Mild and clinically inapparent forms of the disease occur, but its frequency has never been determined. The number of cases of Colorado tick fever reported in Colorado is 20 times greater than that of Rocky Mountain spotted fever. In fact, almost one-half of the patients diagnosed as having Rocky Mountain spotted fever in Utah were subsequently shown to have Colorado tick fever.

Epidemiology Colorado tick fever is transmitted to humans by the adult hard-shelled wood tick, *Dermacentor andersoni.* The virus has been found in as many as 14 percent of this species of ticks collected in endemic areas. Transovarial transmission of the virus in the tick has been established. Illness occurs from late March through September, with most cases in May and June. Virus can be recovered from blood for 2 weeks in most patients, for at least 1 month in nearly one-half, and from spinal fluid during the acute illness. The virus persists within erythrocytes of convalescent patients for as long as 120 days. Virus can be readily isolated from washed erythrocytes 100 days following infection. Transfusion-associated Colorado tick fever has been reported.

Clinical manifestations The incubation period is usually 3 to 6 days, and in 90 percent a history of tick contact within 10 days of onset of illness can be obtained. Failure to obtain such a history militates against the diagnosis. Persons affected usually are those whose occupational or recreational activities bring them in contact with ticks. The disease may occur at any age, although 40 percent in one series were 20 to 29 years of age. The clinical picture is characterized by the sudden onset of severe aching of the muscles of the back and legs, chilliness without true rigors, a rapid increase in temperature, which usually reaches 38.9 to 40°C (102 to 104°F), headache with pain on ocular movement, retroorbital pain, and photophobia. Abdominal pain and vomiting occur in one-fourth of patients; diarrhea is rare. The physical findings are not specific. Tachycardia in proportion to the temperature, flushed facies, and variable conjunctival injection may be present. Occasionally the spleen is palpable. Rash occurs in only 5 percent of patients, but on occasion a petechial rash involving primarily the arms and legs or a maculopapular rash over the entire body may occur. Rarely, punched-out ulcers may form at the site of tick bite. The fever with the associated symptoms lasts about 2 days, then abruptly lyses to normal or subnormal, leaving the patient very weak. After an afebrile period of about 2 days, the fever recurs, may be higher than in the first phase, and may last as long as 3 days. One-half of patients show this saddleback pattern of temperature. Rarely there may be three febrile phases. Convalescence of more than 3 weeks is reported in 70 percent of patients over age 30, while symptoms last less than 1 week in 60 percent of patients under 20. Prolonged convalescence has no relationship to persistent viremia.

Evidence of central nervous system involvement has been recorded in a few patients. The findings are those of either an aseptic meningitis with stiffness of the neck or encephalitis with clouding of the sensorium, delirium, and coma. Single instances of reported complications include epididymoorchitis and patchy pneumonitis.

Laboratory findings   The most important laboratory feature is moderate to marked leukopenia, although in one-third of confirmed cases leukocyte counts remain about 4500 per cubic millimeter. On the first day of illness, the total leukocyte count may be at normal levels, but usually by the fifth or sixth day there has been a decrease to 2000 to 3000 per cubic millimeter. Characteristically there is a proportionate decrease in lymphocytes and granulocytes. Toxic changes in neutrophils are often conspicuous, and "virocyte" types of lymphocytes are frequently observed. Bone marrow examination reveals "maturation arrest" in the granulocytic series. Erythrocyte values remain normal. Thrombocytopenia has been recorded in an isolated case report. The blood picture returns to normal within a week after the fever subsides.

Diagnosis   The diagnosis of Colorado tick fever is suspected on the basis of the epidemiologic history and clinical findings. Because of the infrequency of rash, patients who develop fever and rash after tick bites should be suspected of having Rocky Mountain spotted fever. The usual methods of confirming Colorado tick fever are mouse inoculation and fluorescent antibody (FA) staining of patients' erythrocyte; a combination of the two is best. Special handling of blood is not necessary for the FA test which remains positive during as well as several weeks after clinical illness.

Treatment   Treatment is entirely symptomatic.

Prognosis   The prognosis is excellent.

Prevention   Only one patient has been reported as having the disease twice. Active immunity with an attenuated virus has been produced, but the immunization itself frequently produced mild disease. Colorado tick fever is best prevented by avoiding contact with the wood tick. Convalescent individuals should be excluded as blood donors for at least 6 months.

VENEZUELAN EQUINE ENCEPHALITIS   Venezuelan equine encephalitis (VEE) was first noted in equines in Colombia in 1935.

Etiology   Like other alphaviruses, the causative agent of VEE is a relatively small, 40 to 45 nm, RNA virus. On the basis of serologic tests, differing serotypes have been identified, IA to IE, II, III, and IV. Strains ID, IE, II, III, and IV have remained sylvatic in distribution. IA was the original epidemic strain which occurred in Venezuela, and IB, which was recognized in Ecuador in 1963, spread through Central America into Mexico and was responsible for the epidemic in Mexico in

1971 which spread into southern Texas, with the occurrence of at least 76 laboratory-confirmed human cases. In early 1973, almost 4000 cases occurred in Peru.

Epidemiology   VEE has been primarily a disease of equines and other mammals, although occasionally the agent has infected humans. Evidence of human infection (virus isolation or specific neutralizing antibodies) has been found in Colombia, Ecuador, Panama, Surinam, Guyana, French Guiana, Mexico, Brazil, Curacao, Trinidad, Argentina, Peru, Florida, and Texas. The VEE virus complex in nature has been associated with numerous mosquitoes (at least 9 genera and 37 species), including *Aëdes, Mansonia, Psorophora,* and *Culex.* In this respect it differs markedly from other mosquito-borne encephalitogenic arboviruses, which usually are associated with only one to three vector species. VEE apparently has different vectors for its endemic-epizootic and its epidemic-epizootic cycles. The virus has a wide host range in wild mammals, with at least 20 genera, including capuchin monkeys, rats, mice, opossum, jack-rabbit, fox, and bats being naturally infected. Domestic animals other than equines which have been shown to be infected include cattle and pigs in Mexico and goats and sheep in Venezuela. VEE appears to multiply well in mammals with high titers of virus in the blood; e.g., infected horses may have titers of up to $10^{7.5}$ mouse intraperitoneal lethal doses per milliliter of blood. Though 29 species of wild birds have been shown to be naturally infected with VEE (20 percent of which are colonial nestling herons and related species), whether the VEE-viremia levels in birds are high enough to infect vector mosquitoes is not yet known. During the initial 3 days of illness, viremia has been detected in approximately two-thirds of patients. The levels of viremia are sufficiently high that humans could serve as a reservoir. VEE virus also has been isolated by pharyngeal swab in a few patients, suggesting the potential for person-to-person transmission. The available observations make it reasonable to consider that the natural vector is a mosquito, with the primary reservoir being either wild or domestic terrestrial mammals. However, natural infection can probably take place without an arthropod vector. Laboratory infections have occurred and are probably due to inhalation of aerosols.

Clinical manifestations   In humans, infection with VEE virus usually results in a mild acute febrile illness without neurological complications. No age is spared, and there is no sex preponderance. The incubation period is 2 to 5 days, followed by the abrupt onset of headache, fever often associated with rigors, malaise, and myalgia. Other common symptoms may include nausea, vomiting, diarrhea, and sore throat. Uncommon features include seizures, mental confusion, coma, tremors, and diplopia. On laboratory examination the cerebrospinal fluid may reveal pleocytosis with modest increases in protein concentration and normal glucose concentration. Virus may be isolated both from blood and from cerebrospinal fluid. The symptoms usually last 3 to 5 days in mild cases and up to 8 days in more severe cases, although one patient reported from Florida was febrile for 3 weeks. A biphasic course of illness may be encountered, with recrudescence of symptoms at the sixth to the ninth day. In one case report, palatine petechiae were noted and the patient vomited "coffee-grounds" material. In an epidemic in Venezuela in 1962, almost 16,000 cases of acute disease were evaluated; 38 percent were classified as encephalitis, but only 3 to 4 percent had severe neurological abnormalities: convulsions, nystagmus, drowsiness, delirium, or meningitis. The mortality rate was estimated to be less than 0.5 percent, and nearly all deaths occurred in young children.

RIFT VALLEY FEVER Rift Valley fever is an acute disease principally of sheep and cattle which is widespread throughout East and South Africa. It was first described in humans during an extensive epizootic of hepatitis in sheep in the Rift Valley in East Africa. A major outbreak occurred in Egypt, northeast of Cairo, including the province of Giza, and in Aswan in October to November 1977. An estimated 20,000 human cases occurred with several hundred deaths. Cases again occurred in the summer of 1978. Rift Valley fever had not occurred in Egypt previously. During an epizootic in South Africa in 1950–1951, an estimated 20,000 human beings became infected.

Virus has been found in several species of mosquitoes: *Eretmapodites chrysogaster, Aëdes caballus, Aëdes circumluteolus,* and *Culex theileri.* While antibodies to Rift Valley fever have been found in wild field rats in Uganda, the reservoir is unknown. Humans appear to be incidentally infected during the course of an epizootic. Although humans presumably can be infected by arthropods, many infections occur as a result of handling infected animal tissues. In addition, laboratory-acquired infections have been common, which suggests a respiratory route.

The incubation period is usually 3 to 6 days. The onset is abrupt, with malaise, chilly sensation or rigors, headache, retroorbital pain, and generalized aching and backache. The temperature rises rapidly to 38.3 to 40°C (101 to 104°F). Later complaints include anorexia, loss of taste, epigastric pain, and photophobia. Findings on examination are usually unremarkable except for flushing of the face and conjunctival injection. The temperature curve is often saddleback in type, with an initial elevation lasting 2 to 3 days, followed by a remission and second febrile period. Convalescence is typically rapid. Prior to the outbreak in Egypt, Rift Valley fever was a benign illness with almost no fatalities. In Egypt, approximately one percent of patients developed severe complications, such as encephalitis or hemorrhagic manifestations. Encephalitis appeared as the acute infection waned and was severe with serious residua in survivors. Hemorrhagic manifestations appeared as the disease evolved with generalized hemorrhages and icterus. Deaths from massive hepatic necrosis occurred at 7 to 10 days after onset of illness. Macular exudates, with decreased vision, occur. A characteristic finding is an initial normal total leukocyte count followed by leukopenia with a decrease in neutrophils associated with an increase in band forms. The diagnosis is made by isolating the virus from the blood by inoculation of mice. Three-fourths of patients are viremic (up to 10^8 mouse intraperitoneal lethal doses per milliliter blood) when first seen. Neutralizing antibodies have been demonstrated as early as 4 days after onset. There is no specific treatment. A killed vaccine which had been stockpiled in the United States is being utilized.

MAYARO-SEMLIKI FOREST VIRUS DISEASE Outbreaks involving a number of persons have occurred in Brazil and Bolivia. Survey for antibodies in serums obtained from residents in Rio de Janeiro showed that almost one-third were positive. Mayaro virus has been isolated from a wild mosquito, *Mansonia venezuelensis,* and can be maintained serially in *Aëdes aegypti* and *Anopheles quadrimaculatus.* Semliki Forest virus has been isolated from *Aëdes abnormalis* mosquitoes in Uganda and from various *Eretmapodites* mosquitoes in West Africa. Serologic surveys in humans document widespread virus activity. Antigenically these two alphaviruses are very closely

related, suggesting that both may have been derived from one strain, with geographic separation having led to some antigenic variation. The mechanism of spread has not been determined, but the presence of viremia favors a biting arthropod vector. The predominance of illness and greater incidence of immunity in males suggest a forest infection.

Symptoms include fever of several days' duration, which may be marked during the first 1 to 2 days. Systemic complaints include severe frontal headache, epigastric pain, backache, nausea, photophobia, and vertigo. Signs have included conjunctival injection, mild icterus in a few patients, and arthritis in at least one patient. The leukocyte count is in the range of 5000 to 8000 per cubic millimeter. The fever lasts 3 to 5 days in most patients. Recovery is usually complete, although in Bolivia the illness was more severe, and several fatalities were reported.

BAT SALIVARY GLAND VIRUS During a survey of rabies infection in bats, a virus related to the St. Louis encephalitis complex was obtained from the salivary glands of Mexican free-tailed bats in Texas. It is not known how the virus is maintained in nature. Five laboratory-acquired infections have been recorded. The illnesses were characterized by fever associated with headache, myalgia, and a mild nonproductive cough. In two patients, there was evidence of central nervous system involvement with encephalitis and aseptic meningitis. One patient had oophoritis, and two developed orchitis. By the sixth to seventh day of illness, leukopenia in the range of 2000 to 3000 leukocytes per cubic millimeter was observed in two individuals.

ZIKA VIRUS Zika virus was first isolated from a captive rhesus monkey in Uganda and subsequently from wild mosquitoes. On the basis of serologic surveys, it is known to infect humans in Uganda and Nigeria. During investigation in eastern Nigeria of an outbreak of jaundice that was suspected of being yellow fever, physicians isolated Zika virus from one patient and noted that two others had a rise in neutralizing antibodies. The symptoms in these patients included fever, arthralgia, and headache with retroorbital pain. Jaundice was present in one, and bile was demonstrated in the urine of another. Albuminuria was noted in one patient. Prothrombin times were normal. The clinical syndrome appears to simulate mild yellow fever.

GROUP C ARBOVIRUSES Currently 11 viruses are classified as Bunyaviruses, group C, of which 9 have been isolated from blood obtained from humans. The geographic distribution includes Brazil (Apeu, Caraparu, Itaqui, Marituba, Murutucui, Oriboca), Trinidad (Caraparu, Restan), and Panama (Madrid, Ossa). Several of these viruses have been isolated from Culicine and Subethine mosquitoes, as well as from several species of rodents. Isolates have been obtained mostly from forest workers and laboratory technicians. Epidemics have not been recognized. The disease begins with headache, fever [with temperature up to 40.6°C (105°F)], and myalgia. Additional symptoms include malaise, photophobia, vertigo, and nausea. Illness is generally mild, lasting 2 to 4 days, and is occasionally followed by a relapse. No fatalities have been reported. Occasionally a prolonged period of convalescence ensues. Leukopenia, with total leukocyte counts as low as 2600 per cubic millimeter, is a common finding. Diagnosis has been established mainly by virus isolation.

BUNYAMWERA GROUP Representative viruses of this group are found in all inhabited continents except Australia. Only five viruses of the group—Bunyamwera itself, Germiston, Ilesha, Guaroa, and Wycomyia—have been associated with clinical disease. Serologic surveys give evidence of a high prevalence of inapparent infection in some areas. The clinical patterns of infection due to Germiston, Ilesha, and Guaroa viruses seem similar, while infection due to Bunyamwera virus is associated often with arthralgia and sometimes with a rash. The mild clinical illness is characterized by low-grade fever, headache, and myalgia which last several days, and it may be followed by weakness during convalescence.

ARBOVIRUS INFECTIONS PRESENTING CHIEFLY WITH FEVER, MALAISE, ARTHRALGIA, AND RASH

CHIKUNGUNYA In 1952 an epidemic of a disease occurred in Tanzania, which was given the name *chikungunya* ("that which bends up") because of the sudden onset of joint pains. A group A arbovirus was isolated in 1956 both from serum of patients ill with the disease and from a pool of *A. aegypti* mosquitoes.

Chikungunya virus is responsible for a dengue-like illness in Africa, India, Southeast Asia, New Guinea, and Guam, as well as for a rather mild form of hemorrhagic fever in Asiatic children. Outbreaks have been associated with high attack rates, with as many as 80 percent of inhabitants in some settlements becoming ill. The only known host is the human being. *Aëdes aegypti* is a vector. Because virus has been isolated from *A. africanus* and because antibodies against the virus can be detected in chimpanzees, they may play a role in the natural cycle in Africa.

After an incubation estimated at no less than 9 days, the onset is typically abrupt, with a rapid rise in temperature to 38.9 to 40.6°C (102 to 105°F), often associated with a rigor and headache. Pain in large joints occurs early, incapacitating some individuals within a few minutes of onset. The arthralgia is often associated with objective arthritis. Sites of involvement include knees, ankles, shoulders, wrists, or proximal interphalangeal joints. Myalgia, especially backache, and malaise occur frequently. In 60 to 80 percent of patients a maculopapular eruption, which may appear at any time during the febrile course, is noted on the trunk or on the extensor surfaces of the extremities. Mild lymphadenopathy, predominantly in the axillary or inguinal areas, may be evident. Pharyngitis and conjunctival suffusion may be observed in a few patients. Fever continues for 1 to 6 days, and in some patients an afebrile interval of 1 to 3 days is followed by a secondary rise in temperature. The joint pains may continue after the temperature has returned to normal. In a few individuals joint pains have persisted for up to 4 months. Hematocrit values remain normal. Total leukocyte counts may be less than 5000 per cubic millimeter in some patients, while in others they remain normal. Urinalyses are normal. There is no specific antiviral treatment. Anti-inflammatory agents such as aspirin or indomethacin have been utilized. No second attacks have been recognized, and in the absence of the hemorrhagic fever syndrome, no deaths have been described.

O'NYONG-NYONG FEVER O'nyong-nyong fever was first noted as an epidemic illness characterized by joint pains, rash, and lymphadenopathy in the northern province of Uganda in 1959. The agent is a group A arbovirus which shows close antigenic relationships with chikungunya and Semliki Forest viruses. The original outbreak was associated with an explosive epidemic which spread to Tanzania and other areas in East Africa. By 1961, 2 million cases were recorded. In some areas, 91 percent of the population had either clinical disease or inapparent infection. Local outbreaks extended over the entire year. All age groups were affected. The most likely vector is *Anopheles funestus*. The clinical features are similar to those of chikungunya virus infection.

SINDBIS VIRUS Sindbis virus infection in humans rarely presents as a clinical disease. Of five cases from Uganda, one patient gave a history of joint pain. In the only well-studied clinical illness, a South African woman had arthritis as a prominent finding. Two days after a headache she noted swelling in her hands and feet. Soon thereafter she developed a confluent macular rash, followed by vesicle formation. The small joints of the hands and feet were swollen at the time of examination. Slight swelling of the fingers was present at 10 weeks, although she had otherwise recovered.

ROSS RIVER VIRUS Epidemics of polyarthritis associated with rashes have been observed in Australia since 1928. Outbreaks occur almost entirely in the period December to June. There is a predilection for women, and children are seldom involved (an obvious similarity with rubella, another Togavirus). The onset is characterized by headache, mild catarrh, and occasionally tenderness of the palms and soles. Initially fever may be absent or minimal [highest 38°C (100.4°F)]. In about one-half of patients, arthritis, involving mainly the small joints, wrists, and ankles and sometimes associated with swelling, and paresthesias precede a rash by 1 to 15 days. In the other half, the rash precedes the arthralgia. The rash, which lasts 2 to 10 days, is usually maculopapular, appears on the cheeks and forehead, occasionally spreads to the trunk, or may be restricted to the limbs. The rash may be pruritic. Vesicles occur rarely. Tender lymphadenopathy occurs in one-fifth of the patients. Joint symptoms persist for 3 weeks to 3 months. Patients with this syndrome have shown serologic evidence of infection with Ross River virus, although virus has not been isolated from synovial fluid. Serologic evidence of infection is common in New Guinea.

OTHER ARBOVIRUSES Mayaro and Bunyamwera viruses occasionally have been associated with the syndrome of rash and arthralgia.

ARBOVIRUS INFECTIONS PRESENTING CHIEFLY WITH FEVER, MALAISE, LYMPHADENOPATHY, AND RASH

DENGUE FEVER Dengue is endemic over large areas of the tropics and subtropics. Outbreaks of dengue have occurred in the Caribbean including Puerto Rico and the U.S. Virgin Islands since 1969. A number of travelers return to the mainland United States with clinical illness (52 confirmed cases in 1978). Cases were also imported from Tahiti. Despite intensive surveillance no secondary cases have been found in the continental United States. It is now recognized that the dengue syndrome can be caused by other arboviruses; hence the exact etiology of some of the earlier epidemics is uncertain.

Etiology There are four distinct serogroups of dengue viruses, types 1, 2, 3, and 4, all of which are group B arboviruses. In the Caribbean, type 1 was associated with the 1977-1978 outbreak, type 2 in 1968-1969, and type 3 in 1963-1964.

Epidemiology So far as is known, dengue infections in nature involve only human beings and *Aëdes* mosquitoes. Attempts have been made to implicate lower vertebrates, especially monkeys, as reservoir sylvatic hosts, but the data are inconclusive. *Aëdes aegypti* is the most important worldwide vector species. This species, as well as the less common vector species, is peridomestic, biting humans readily or even preferentially and breeding in small collections of water such as cisterns and backyard litter. They fly during the day. Humans appear to be uniformly susceptible, and susceptibility is not influenced by age, sex, or race. The disappearance of dengue from an area may be the result either of elimination of the vector or of exhaustion of the susceptible population. During outbreaks, attack rates may be very high; in Puerto Rico and the U.S. Virgin Islands, the overall rate of clinical illness was 20 percent, with infection rates as determined by serologic survey as high as 79 per 100. Over 10,000 cases of dengue-like illness were reported from Puerto Rico in 1978. For the first time in nearly 40 years, dengue was confirmed in Central America (Honduras and El Salvador).

Clinical manifestations Dengue viruses frequently produce inapparent infections in humans. When symptoms develop, three broad clinical patterns may be encountered: classic dengue, hemorrhagic fever, and a mild atypical form. Classic dengue (breakbone fever) occurs primarily in nonimmune individuals, specifically nonindigenous adults and children. The usual incubation period is 5 to 8 days. Prodromal symptoms such as mild conjunctivitis or coryza may occur, followed in hours by the abrupt onset of a severe splitting headache, retroorbital pain, backache, especially in the lumbar area, and leg and joint pains. The headache is aggravated by movement. At least three-fourths of patients have ocular soreness, with pain on moving the eyes. A few have mild photophobia. Though true rigors are common during the course, they are usually not present at the onset. Additional symptoms include insomnia, anorexia with loss of taste or bitter taste, and weakness. Mild transient rhinopharyngitis occurs in as many as one-quarter of the individuals. Cough is almost never seen. Epistaxis has been observed. Examination reveals scleral injection (90 percent), tenderness upon pressure on the ocular globe, and nontender posterior cervical, epitrochlear, and inguinal lymphadenopathy. Over one-half of patients have an enanthem characterized initially by pinpoint-sized vesicles over the posterior half of the soft palate. The tongue is often coated. Skin rashes, varying from diffuse flushing to scarlatiniform and morbilliform, are frequently present over the thorax and inner aspects of the arms. These are transient and fade, only to be followed by a more definite maculopapular rash which appears on the trunk on the third to the fifth day and spreads peripherally. The rash may be pruritic and generally terminates with desquamation. Extreme bradycardia is not observed. Within 2 to 3 days after the onset, the temperature may decrease to nearly normal and other symptoms disappear. The remission typically lasts 2 days and is followed by return of fever and the other symptoms, although they are generally less severe than during the initial phase. This "saddleback" diphasic febrile course is considered characteristic, but often is not encountered. The febrile illness usually lasts 5 to 6 days and terminates abruptly. Complaints of fatigue for several weeks after infection are common.

In addition to this "classic" syndrome, an atypically mild illness may occur. Symptoms include fever, anorexia, headache, and myalgia. On examination, evanescent rashes may be seen, but lymphadenopathy is usually absent. The course is usually less than 72 h in duration.

At the onset both in classic and in mild dengue, the leukocyte counts may be low or normal; however, by the third to the fifth day, leukopenia, usually with counts of less than 5000 leukocytes per cubic millimeter, and neutropenia are usually seen. Occasionally albuminuria of moderate degree occurs.

Diagnosis Virus isolation by tissue culture of serum obtained during the first days of illness is definitive. Diagnosis can be made by serologic tests employing paired serums for hemag-glutination inhibition tests and complement fixation tests. Specific serologic diagnosis is complicated by cross reactions with other group B arbovirus antibodies such as those following immunization with yellow fever vaccine.

Treatment Treatment is entirely symptomatic.

Prognosis Mortality is nil.

Prevention An attenuated vaccine for dengue type 2 is undergoing early experimental evaluation. Control depends upon mosquito abatement.

WEST NILE FEVER West Nile virus is a group B arbovirus distributed from South Africa to southeastern India, but has been shown as a cause of significant disease only in the Near East, where it can produce a clinical picture closely resembling dengue. Outbreaks of disease involving several hundred patients occurred in Israel in 1950 to 1952. In one outbreak, over 60 percent of the population developed overt disease.

Epidemiology The disease is highly endemic in Egypt but goes largely unrecognized. Presumably most of the adult population is immune, and the infection in childhood is an undifferentiated mild febrile illness, whereas in Israel it mainly affects adults. The infection occurs in the summer both in Israel and in Egypt. The transmission cycle in Egypt is believed to be bird-to-mosquito-to-bird, with *Culex univittatus* as the principal vector. Although humans and a variety of other vertebrates are infected by the virus, their involvement is believed to be tangential. In Israel, the most probable vectors are *Culex molestus* and *C. univittatus.*

Clinical manifestations Most of the patients in Israel have been young adults, with neither sex predominating. The onset is usually abrupt and without prodromal symptoms. The temperature quickly rises to 38.3 to 40°C (101 to 104°F), with chills occurring in one-third of patients. Symptoms include drowsiness, severe frontal headache, ocular pain, and pain in the abdomen and back. A small number of patients have anorexia, nausea, and dryness of the throat. Cough is uncommon. Signs observed include flushing of the face, conjunctival injection, and coating of the tongue. The prominent finding is general enlargement of lymph nodes, which are of moderate size but are not hard and are only slightly tender. Occipital, axillary, and inguinal nodes are usually involved. The spleen and liver are slightly enlarged in a small proportion of patients. In one-half the patients a rash may appear from the second to the fifth day of illness and may persist for several hours or until defervescence. The rash occurs predominantly over the trunk and consists of pale roseolar maculopapular lesions. The illness is self-limited and lasts 3 to 5 days in 80 percent of patients.

In a few patients, transitory meningeal involvement may be encountered. Spinal fluid examinations may reveal a pleocytosis and some increase in protein concentration.

Leukopenia occurs in the majority of patients, and total leukocyte counts are lower than 4000 per cubic millimeter in one-third. Differential counts vary from a moderate shift to the left to a slight lymphocytosis.

Convalescence is often prolonged, lasting 1 to 2 weeks, with prominent symptoms of fatigue. Enlargement of lymph nodes subsides over several months. Only rarely have complications, sequelae, or fatalities been seen in natural infections, although in one outbreak in a group of elderly patients a high proportion of patients developed meningoencephalitis, and four fatalities ensued.

Accurate diagnosis rests on virus isolation, which can be accomplished because viremia persists for as long as 6 days, or the demonstration of a rising specific antibody titer.

The treatment is symptomatic.

ARBOVIRUS INFECTIONS PRESENTING CHIEFLY WITH CENTRAL NERVOUS SYSTEM INVOLVEMENT

Four arboviruses are presently recognized as numerically important causes of central nervous system disease in the United States: St. Louis encephalitis virus, Eastern equine encephalitis virus, Western equine encephalitis virus, and the California encephalitis group of viruses. The spectrum of infection caused by these agents includes inapparent infection, fever with headache, aseptic meningitis, and encephalitis. Of the 4308 patients reported with encephalitis during 1975, over 2000 cases (49 percent) were due to arboviruses. Widespread epidemics of St. Louis encephalitis were responsible for 86 percent of these cases. For 10 of the 21 years from 1955 through 1975, St. Louis encephalitis virus was the most common cause of arboviral encephalitis in the United States. In contrast, from 1967 through 1975, the California encephalitis group of viruses accounted for one-half or more of the reported cases of human arthropod-borne encephalitis in each year except 1971, 1974, and 1975.

Etiology Despite the diversity of specific viral etiologies (Table 190-2), in individual patients the clinical manifestations of aseptic meningitis and encephalitis are very similar, and preclude an etiologic diagnosis without ancillary information regarding epidemiologic and serologic features (Table 190-3). The clinical features of aseptic meningitis due to arboviruses are indistinguishable from those due to the more prevalent enteroviruses, which are discussed in Chap. 187. Since transmission to humans in the United States and Canada involves arthropods, specifically mosquitoes, except for Powassan and Colorado tick fever, indigenously acquired disease occurs at times when mosquitoes are prevalent, such as late spring through early fall. The broad clinical picture of arbovirus encephalitis will be discussed; then the specific epidemiologic and prognostic features which characterize the major types will be presented.

Clinical manifestations The clinical features of arbovirus encephalitis differ among age groups. In infants under 1 year of age, the only consistently noted symptoms are sudden onset of fever, which is often accompanied by convulsions. Convulsions may be either generalized or focal. Typically the fever ranges between 38.9 and 40°C (102 and 104°F). Other physical findings may include bulging of the fontanelle, rigidity of the extremities, and abnormalities in reflexes.

In children between 5 and 14 years of age, subjective symptoms are more easily elicited. Headache, fever, and drowsiness of 2 to 3 days' duration before medical attention is sought are common. The symptoms may then subside or become more intense and may be associated with nausea, vomiting, muscular pain, photophobia, and, less frequently, convulsions (less than 10 percent except in California encephalitis). On examination, the child is found to be acutely ill, febrile, and lethargic. Nuchal rigidity and intention tremors are often present, and on occasion muscular weakness can be demonstrated.

In adults, the initial symptoms commonly include the fairly abrupt onset of fever, nausea with vomiting, and severe headache. The headache is most often frontal but may be occipital or diffuse in location. Mental aberrations, represented by confusion and disorientation, usually appear within the subsequent 24 h. Other symptoms may include diffuse myalgia and photophobia. The abnormalities found on physical examination predominantly relate to the neurological examination, although conjunctival suffusion is frequently seen and skin rashes may occur. Disturbances in mentation are among the most outstanding clinical features. These range from coma through severe disorientation to subtle abnormalities detected only by cerebral function tests such as the subtraction of serial 7s. A small proportion of patients show only lethargy, lying quietly, apparently asleep unless stimulated. Tremor is common and is observed more frequently in individuals over 40 years of age. The tremors vary in location and may be continuous or intention in type. Cranial nerve abnormalities resulting in oculomotor muscle paresis and nystagmus, facial weakness, and difficulty in deglutition may occur, and are usually present within the initial several days. Objective sensory changes are unusual. Hemiparesis or monoparesis may occur. Reflex abnormalities are also common; these include exaggerated palmomental reflexes, and suck and snout reflexes. Superficial abdominal and cremasteric reflexes are usually absent. Changes in the tendon reflexes are variable and inconstant. The plantar response may be extensor and fluctuates almost hourly. Dysdiadochokinesia often exists.

The duration of the fever and neurological symptoms and signs varies from several days to a month but usually ranges from 4 to 14 days. Clinical improvement generally follows the subsidence of the fever within several days unless irreversible anatomic changes have occurred.

Laboratory findings Erythrocyte values are usually normal. Total leukocyte counts often reveal both a slight to moderate leukocytosis (occasionally greater than 20,000 leukocytes per cubic millimeter) and neutrophilia. Examination of the cerebrospinal fluid usually reveals several hundred cells per cubic millimeter, but on occasion cloudy cerebrospinal fluid with cells in excess of 1000 per cubic millimeter may be seen.

TABLE 190-3
Features of arboviral encephalitides common in the United States

Etiology	Geographic predominance in the United States	Urban/ rural	Age, years	Sex	Unique clinical features	Mortality, %	Residua
California encephalitis	Midwest	Rural	5–10	M	Seizures	2	Seizures (one-fourth who had them in acute phase), behavioral problems (15%)
Eastern equine encephalitis	Eastern seaboard	Both	<5 >55	=	CSF may have >1000 WBC/mm³	50	Children < 10 years have emotional lability, retardation, convulsions
St. Louis encephalitis	Eastern and Midwest	Both	>35	=	Dysuria	2–12	Ataxia, speech difficulties (5%)
Western equine encephalitis	Entire	Both	<1 >55	=	None	3	Children <3 months have behavioral problems, convulsions

Within the first several days of illness, polymorphonuclear neutrophils may predominate. The initial cerebrospinal fluid protein is usually only slightly elevated but on occasion may exceed 100 mg per 100 ml. The level of spinal fluid sugar is normal; a significant decrease should raise serious consideration of an alternative diagnosis. As the illness progresses, mononuclear cells in the cerebrospinal fluid tend to increase so that they predominate and the protein concentration may increase. Other laboratory studies have been performed only sporadically, but abnormalities may include hyponatremia, often due to the inappropriate secretion of antidiuretic hormone, and elevations in serum creatine phosphokinase.

Diagnosis Specific diagnosis requires the isolation of the virus or detection of antibodies with a rising titer between the acute phase of disease and convalescence. Antibodies can be detected by hemagglutination inhibition, complement fixation, or virus neutralization techniques.

Treatment Treatment is entirely supportive and requires meticulous attention in the comatose patient.

CALIFORNIA (LACROSSE) ENCEPHALITIS A previously undescribed virus was isolated in 1943 from mosquitoes in Kern County, California. Since 1963, a large number of agents now designated as the California group of viruses have been isolated. Almost all the isolates have been LaCrosse virus.

Since 1966 in the Midwest United States, California (La-Crosse) encephalitis has been incriminated in 5 to 6 percent of cases of acute central nervous system disease, ranking above all agents except the enteroviruses.

Epidemiology Infection has been demonstrated to occur in the Midwest, especially in Ohio, Indiana, and Wisconsin, in wooded areas of eastern Texas and Louisiana, and along the Eastern Seaboard. The principal animal reservoir is the squirrel. The mosquito vectors are primarily woodland mosquitoes belonging to *Aëdes* species, principally *A. triseriatus*. The LaCrosse virus appears to overwinter in eggs of *A. triseriatus*. Transovarial transmission of California group viruses then occurs. California encephalitis occurs during the summer months (June to October), most often involving boys (60 percent) 5 to 10 years of age (60 percent) who live in rural areas.

Clinical manifestations Two clinical patterns have been defined. One is a mild form with a 2- to 3-day prodrome of fever, headache, malaise, and gastrointestinal symptoms. About the third day the temperature increases to 40°C (104°F), and the patient becomes lethargic and develops meningeal signs. These findings abate gradually over a 7- to 8-day period without overt sequelae. The second pattern, a severe form which occurs in at least one-half of the patients, begins abruptly with fever, headache, and vomiting, followed shortly by lethargy and disorientation. During the first 2 to 4 days the course is rapidly progressive with the occurrence of seizures (50 to 60 percent), focal neurological signs (20 percent), pathological reflexes (10 percent), and coma (10 percent). Focal neurological signs may include asymmetrical flaccid paralysis. Uncommon findings have included arthralgia and rash. Clinical laboratory features include peripheral leukocyte counts ranging from 7000 to 30,000 per cubic millimeter (median 16,000 per cubic millimeter) with neutrophilia. Cerebrospinal fluid examination reveals 10 to 500 cells per cubic millimeter, usually with a predominance of mononuclear cells, protein concentrations of less than 100 mg per 100 ml, and normal sugar concentrations. Electroencephalograms are abnormal in at least 80 percent of patients, revealing slow deltawave activity. In one-half of the pa-

tients the abnormality is asymmetrical, suggesting focal destructive lesions. Brain scans using [99Tc]pertechnetate also may be abnormal, and localized asymmetrical increased uptake has been observed. Beginning about the fourth day and proceeding over the next 3 to 7 days, there is progressive improvement, with almost all patients becoming afebrile, seizure-free, and ready for discharge from the hospital within 2 weeks after onset.

Diagnosis Neutralizing and hemagglutination-inhibition antibodies usually are present a few days after the onset. Complement-fixing antibodies become detectable 10 to 12 days after onset.

Treatment Initial seizure activity is frequently prolonged and difficult to control. The most effective anticonvulsant medication has been parenteral diazepam. Patients with the severe form of disease should be discharged on anticonvulsants such as phenobarbital for 6 to 12 months.

Prognosis The case fatality ratio is low (2 percent or less); however, one-third of patients may have abnormal neurological findings at the time of discharge. During the early convalescent period, emotional lability and irritability are common. In one series, recurrent seizures occurred in one-quarter of the patients who had seizures during the acute phase. In this same series EEGs were abnormal in one-third of patients evaluated 1 to 8 years after their acute illness. In another series, 15 percent had sequelae, predominantly personality or behavioral problems.

EASTERN EQUINE ENCEPHALITIS Eastern equine encephalitis, a group A arbovirus, was first isolated in 1933 from the brain tissue of horses during an outbreak of equine illness in New Jersey. The first recognized human outbreak occurred in Massachusetts in 1938.

Epidemiology The virus is distributed along the eastern coast of the Americas from Northeastern United States to Argentina. Viral isolations also have been reported in the Philippines, Thailand, Czechoslovakia, Poland, and the U.S.S.R., but the question of type specificity has not been resolved. In the Northeastern United States, epidemics occur in the late summer and early fall. Epizootics in horses precede the occurrence of human cases by 1 to 2 weeks. The disease affects mainly infants, children, and adults over 55 years of age. There is no sex preponderance. Inapparent infection occurs in all age groups, suggesting that the decreased likelihood of developing overt infection in the 15- to 54-year age group is not the result of decreased exposure. The ratio of inapparent infection to overt encephalitis approximates 25:1.

The natural reservoir is unknown. Isolations have been made from numerous species of wild birds and also from amphibians, reptiles, and mammals. The natural vector is the mosquito, including *A. sollicitans* and *Culiseta melanura*. *Aëdes sollicitans*, a salt-marsh mosquito which is an avid human feeder, has been postulated as the epidemic vector, while *C. melanura* is important in bird-to-bird transmission. Equine animals and human beings are probably "dead ends" in the transmission cycle, and infection in them is accidental.

Clinical manifestations Though human infections have been thought usually to result in serious, if not fatal, central nervous system involvement, the detection of inapparent infection as well as relatively mild disease establishes the occurrence of milder forms. In many patients, the cerebrospinal fluid is cloudy and contains in excess of 1000 cells per cubic millimeter.

Diagnosis The hemagglutination-inhibition or neutralization tests are the serologic methods of choice. The complement fixation test may be negative in patients with confirmed infections.

Prognosis The mortality rate in clinical infection exceeds 50 percent. In the most severe cases, death occurs between the third and fifth days. Children under 10 years of age have a greater likelihood of surviving the acute illness, but they also have a greater likelihood of developing severe disabling residuals: mental retardation, convulsions, emotional lability, blindness, deafness, speech disorders, and hemiplegia.

ST. LOUIS ENCEPHALITIS St. Louis encephalitis (SLE) was first recognized as an entity during a major outbreak in St. Louis, Missouri, and the surrounding area in 1933. Sporadic, unpredictable outbreaks occurred, for example, in Houston, 1974, Dallas, 1966, Memphis, 1974, Northern Mississippi and Illinois, 1975. The attack rate in Greenville, Mississippi, in 1975 was the highest which has been encountered, 10 per 10,000 population.

Epidemiology In the United States, epidemics of SLE fall into two epidemiologic patterns. One pattern is found in the West, where mixed outbreaks of Western equine encephalitis and SLE have occurred primarily in irrigated rural areas. The vector has been *Culex tarsalis*. The second pattern occurred in the original St. Louis outbreak and the numerous subsequent epidemics in the Midwest, Texas, New Jersey, and Florida. These outbreaks have been more urban in location and are characterized by a marked tendency for the development of encephalitis in older persons. In such urban-suburban epidemics, the epidemic vectors have been mosquitoes of the *Culex pipiens-quinquefasciatus* complex with the exception of the Florida epidemic, in which *Culex nigripalpus* was incriminated. The presence of SLE virus outside the United States has been proved by isolations in Trinidad, Panama, Jamaica, Brazil, and Argentina. However, except for Jamaica, SLE has not been reported outside the United States. The basic transmission cycle is that of wild bird-mosquito-wild bird. The virus survives the winter in female mosquitoes which ingested a blood meal from a viremic bird before overwintering. The disease in humans usually appears in midsummer to early fall. There is no sex preponderance. The human represents an accidental host and plays no role in the basic transmission cycle. Serologic studies following most urban epidemics indicate that infection rates are similar in all age groups, and that the increasing age-specific attack rate for clinical encephalitis which is typical of urban St. Louis encephalitis is probably due to age differences in host susceptibility to overt disease rather than to a higher rate of infection.

Clinical manifestations Infection with SLE virus most commonly results in an inapparent infection. Of the patients with confirmed disease, approximately three-fourths have clinical encephalitis; the remainder present with aseptic meningitis, febrile headaches, or nonspecific illness. Virtually all patients over 40 years of age have encephalitic manifestations. Urinary frequency and dysuria have been symptoms in approximately 20 percent of patients despite sterile routine aerobic urine cultures. SLE virus has been isolated from urine; this may account for the occurrence of urinary tract symptoms.

Diagnosis The occurrence of either encephalitis or aseptic meningitis as manifested by febrile illness with cerebrospinal fluid pleocytosis in the months of June through September in an adult, especially over 35 years of age, should raise the suspicion of St. Louis encephalitis. Because approximately 40 percent of patients with SLE have antibodies detectable by hem-

agglutination inhibition at the onset of illness, acute serum for serologic studies should be submitted promptly to a competent laboratory.

Prognosis The case fatality ratio in the original St. Louis epidemic was 20 percent. In most subsequent outbreaks the mortality rate has varied from 2 to 12 percent. Subjective nervous complaints, including nervousness, headaches, and easy fatigability and excitability, appear to be the most common residuals. Late organic defects such as speech defects, difficulty in walking, and disturbances in vision were demonstrated in approximately 5 percent of patients 3 years following infection.

WESTERN EQUINE ENCEPHALITIS Western equine encephalitis (WEE) virus is a group A arbovirus which was isolated in 1930 in California from horses with encephalitis. In 1938 it was recovered from a fatal human infection.

Epidemiology WEE virus has been isolated in the United States, Canada, Brazil, Guyana, and Argentina. Human disease has been diagnosed in the United States, Canada, and Brazil. In the United States, the virus is found in virtually all geographic areas. The central valley of California represents an important endemic area. The disease occurs mainly in early summer and midsummer. Wild birds, which develop viremia of sufficiently high titer to be able to infect mosquitoes that feed on them, are the basic reservoir, although nonavian vertebrate hosts may be important. *Culex tarsalis* is the principal vector in the Western United States. In areas east of the Appalachian Mountains, another vector must be operative. The virus has been repeatedly isolated from *Culiseta melanura;* however, the importance of this species has been questioned, since it is not primarily a human-biting mosquito. The ratio of inapparent infection to disease, as evidenced by serologic survey studies, varies from 58:1 in children to 1150:1 in adults. Approximately one-fourth of patients are less than 1 year of age. The highest attack rates occur in persons 50 years or older. In the summer of 1975, following the flooding of the Red River in North Dakota, an increase in equine and human cases of WEE occurred; 41 cases were reported from this region.

Prognosis The fatality rate approximates 3 percent in laboratory-confirmed cases. The incidence and severity of sequelae are related to age. Sequelae among very young infants are frequent (appearing in 61 percent of a group of patients less than 3 months old) and severe; they consist of upper motor neuron impairment, involving the pyramidal tracts, extrapyramidal structures, and cerebellum, and result in behavioral problems and convulsions. Both the incidence and severity of sequelae diminish rapidly after 1 year of age. Adults may complain of nervousness, irritability, easy fatigability, and tremulousness for 6 months or longer after the acute illness. Probably not more than 5 percent of adults have sequelae which are sufficiently severe to be of practical significance. Postencephalitic seizures are rare.

JAPANESE ENCEPHALITIS The name Japanese B encephalitis was employed during an epidemic which occurred in 1924 to distinguish it from von Economo's disease, which was designated as type A encephalitis. The designation as Japanese B no longer seems useful, and the term Japanese encephalitis will be employed.

Epidemiology Japanese encephalitis virus infection is known to occur in eastern Siberia, China, Korea, Taiwan, Japan, Malaya, Vietnam, Thailand, Singapore, Guam, and India. In temperate climates, the disease shows a late-summer early-fall seasonal incidence. In tropical climates there is no seasonal variation. The mosquito *C. tritaeniorhynchus* is the major vector species. It is a rural mosquito which breeds in rich fields and preferentially bites large domestic animals, such as pigs, but also feeds on birds and humans. The human is an accidental host in the transmission cycle. In several outbreaks, a higher incidence of cases has been reported in children than in adults. The ratio of inapparent infection, as evidenced by a serologic survey study of Australian troops in Vietnam, was 210:1.

Clinical manifestations The occurrence of severe rigors at the onset has been noted in almost 90 percent of patients. On admission, most patients are alert, but deterioration of mental status occurs in about three-fourths of patients within 3 to 4 days. Localized paresis is found more often than with other arboviral encephalitides, e.g., in 31 percent of cases, with predominantly upper extremity involvement; however, it resolves rapidly with defervescence. Weight loss has been very striking. The failure of the temperature to lyse, appearance of diaphoresis, tachypnea, and the accumulation of bronchial secretions are grave prognostic signs.

Prognosis The immediate mortality rate has varied from 7 to 33 percent or higher. The rate of occurrence of sequelae varies inversely with the fatality rate; in those series with high fatality rates (33 percent), sequelae occurred in 3 to 14 percent. In another series with a fatality rate of 7.4 percent, the sequelae rate was 32 percent. Individuals who had neurologic abnormalities during the acute phase but survived have no more than an 80 percent chance for complete recovery. Sequelae consist of seizures, persistent paralysis, ataxia, mental retardation, and behavioral disorders.

OTHER ARBOVIRUSES WITH CENTRAL NERVOUS SYSTEM INVOLVEMENT A large group of additional arboviruses have been associated with encephalitis or aseptic meningitis. Some of these agents are listed in Table 190-2. Though the epidemiologic picture of each of these agents is unique, the general features are sufficiently similar to require laboratory support for their differentiation.

ARBOVIRUS DISEASES PRESENTING CHIEFLY WITH HEMORRHAGIC MANIFESTATIONS

For 300 years, yellow fever was the only epidemic viral disease known to be accompanied by grave hemorrhagic manifestations. Since the 1930s diverse viral etiologies of the hemorrhagic fever syndrome have been recognized and are now known to be responsible for the variety of epidemiologic situations in which this syndrome occurs (Table 190-2). Additional agents include: Central Asian hemorrhagic fever, Chikungunya, Congo-Crimean hemorrhagic fever, Kyasanur Forest disease, Omsk hemorrhagic fever, Rift Valley fever, and the arenaviruses (Chap. 191). Despite the diverse viral etiology, there are many similar clinical manifestations. The onset is usually sudden, with headache, backache, generalized myalgia, conjunctivitis, and prostration. From approximately the third day, the initial stage is followed by hypotension, and hemorrhagic manifestations may occur; these are characterized by bleeding gums, epistaxis, hemoptysis, hematemesis, melena, petechiae, ecchymoses, and hemorrhages into most visceral organs. Early mild leukopenia develops, but with the appearance of hemorrhagic manifestations, leukocytosis may occur. The pathophysiology of the cardinal signs is attributable to hematopoietic and capillary damage, with variable localization of lesions. On the basis of limited confirmatory observations, variable degrees of disseminated intravascular coagulation may be in part responsible for the pathophysiology of the hemorrhagic fever syndromes. Death usually occurs in the second week of disease, at which time a high titer of antibody has developed and the patient may have become afebrile. Death is usually associated with coma, which is due not to encephalitis but to an encephalopathy. The pathological changes may be similar despite diverse viral etiologies, with midzonal hepatic necrosis and acidophilic cytoplasmic inclusions similar to the Councilman bodies of yellow fever.

YELLOW FEVER Yellow fever is an acute infectious disease of short duration and extremely variable severity; it is caused by a group B arbovirus and is followed by lifelong immunity. The classic triad of symptoms—jaundice, hemorrhages, and intense albuminuria—is present only in severe infections, which now compose only a small proportion of the total.

Prevalence Yellow fever remains the most dramatically serious arbovirus disease of the tropics. For more than 200 years, after the first identifiable outbreak occurred in Yucatan in 1648, it was one of the great plagues of the world. As late as 1905, New Orleans and other Southern United States ports experienced at least 5000 cases and 1000 deaths. Because of the existence of the sylvatic form of the disease, protective measures must be maintained against human disease, as demonstrated by outbreaks in Central America in 1948 to 1957, the Congo in 1958, the Sudan and Ethiopia in 1959 to 1962, Senegal in 1965, central West Africa in 1969, Brazil in 1973, Panama and Colombia in 1974, and Ecuador in 1975.

Epidemiology Human infection results from two basically different cycles of virus transmission, urban and sylvatic. The urban cycle is human-mosquito-human, i.e., *Aëdes aegypti*-transmitted yellow fever. After a 2-week extrinsic incubation period, mosquitoes can transmit infection. Sylvan yellow fever differs under various ecologic circumstances. In the rain forests of South and Central America, species of treetop *Haemagogus* or *Sabethes* mosquitoes maintain transmission in wild primates. Once infected, the mosquito vector remains infectious for life; hence it may serve as a reservoir as well as a vector. When humans come into proximity with the forest-canopy mosquitoes, sporadic cases or focal outbreaks may occur. With sylvan yellow fever, males predominate. Focal outbreaks may be quite extensive; in Brazil in 1973 at least 21,000 persons out of 1.5 million (1.4 percent) were infected. In East Africa, the mosquito-primate cycle is maintained by the forest-canopy mosquito, *A. africanus*, which seldom feeds on humans. The peridomestic mosquito *A. simpsoni* feeds upon primates entering the village gardens and can then in turn transmit the virus to humans. Once yellow fever is reintroduced into urban areas, the urban cycle can be reinitiated, with the potential for epidemic disease. Why yellow fever has never invaded Asia despite widespread distribution of human-biting *A. aegypti* mosquitoes has never been satisfactorily explained.

Pathology The diagnosis of yellow fever may be suspected by the presence of necrobiosis and acidophilic necrosis of the parenchymal cells of the liver with the formation of Councilman bodies which occur in a characteristically discontinuous fashion in the midzones of the liver lobules. In the kidney, the virus produces necrosis of the tubular epithelium. Multiple minute hemorrhages occur in the gastrointestinal tract. In the brain, the chief lesion is perivascular hemorrhage, which is most frequently found in the subthalamic and periventricular regions at the level of the mammillary bodies.

Clinical manifestations   The incubation period is usually 3 to 6 days. In accidental laboratory- or hospital-acquired infections longer incubation periods (10 to 13 days) have been reported. In considering the clinical features, it is advantageous to classify the illness as to severity: inapparent, mild, moderately severe, and malignant. In mild yellow fever the only symptoms may be the abrupt onset of fever and headache. Additional symptoms may include nausea, epistaxis, relative bradycardia known as Faget's sign [e.g., with a temperature of 38.9°C (102°F) the pulse may be only 48 to 52 beats per minute], and slight albuminuria. The mild illness lasts only 1 to 3 days and resembles influenza except that coryzal symptoms are lacking.

Moderately severe and malignant attacks of yellow fever are characterized by three distinct clinical periods: the period of infection, the period of remission, and the period of intoxication. Prodromal symptoms are usually absent. The onset is characteristically sudden, with headache, dizziness, and temperature elevations to 40°C (104°F) without a relative bradycardia. Young children may have febrile convulsions. The headache is followed quickly by pains in the neck, back, and legs. Often there is nausea with vomiting and retching. Examination reveals a flushed face and injection of the conjunctiva. The congestion of the eyes persists until the third day. The tongue characteristically shows bright red margins and tip and a white furred center. Faget's sign appears by the second day. Epistaxis and gingival bleeding are common. On the third day of illness, the fever may fall by crisis and the patient enters remission, or, in the malignant form, copious hemorrhages, anuria, or delirium may occur. The stage of remission lasts from several hours to several days. In the third stage, the "classic" symptoms develop; the fever returns but the pulse remains slow. Jaundice becomes detectable about the third day; however, jaundice often is not prominent even in fatal illnesses. Increased epistaxis, melena, and uterine hemorrhages are common, but gross hematuria is rare. Of the classic signs, "black vomit" is more characteristic than is jaundice. Hematemesis usually does not occur before the fourth day and is often associated with a fatal outcome. Albuminuria, which rarely develops before the third day, occurs in 90 percent of patients and may be quite marked (3 to 20 g albumin per liter). In spite of this massive albuminuria, edema or ascites has not been reported. In malignant infections, coma frequently occurs 2 to 3 days before death. Shortly before death, which usually occurs between the fourth and the sixth days, it is not uncommon for the patient to become delirious and wildly agitated. Though the duration of fever in the third stage is usually 5 to 7 days, the period of intoxication is the most variable of the stages and may last up to 2 weeks. Clinical yellow fever is relatively free from complications, suppurative parotitis being the most striking of those which do occur. Clinical relapses are not characteristic of yellow fever.

Laboratory findings   Early in the disease, progressive leukopenia may occur. By the fifth day, total leukocyte counts of 1500 to 2500 per cubic millimeter often are found, the decrease being due mostly to a decrease in neutrophils. Total leukocyte counts return to normal by the tenth day, and in fatal cases there may be a marked terminal leukocytosis. Hemoglobin values remain normal except terminally, when hemoconcentration or bleeding may occur. Platelet counts are reported to be normal. Detailed coagulation studies have been performed only in rhesus monkeys experimentally infected with yellow fever. Within 72 h after viral inoculation and prior to apparent clinical illness, a coagulation defect was observed. This was characterized by a prolonged one-stage prothrombin time and a prolonged partial thromboplastin time, reflecting measured deficiencies in factors II, V, VII, VIII, IX, X, and XI. Both the euglobulin lysis time and the thrombin time were prolonged, suggesting a depression of plasminogen activation and accumulation of fibrinogen degradation products. At this time platelet counts and chemical measurements of fibrinogen were normal. During the subsequent 48 h, these coagulation defects worsened as the monkeys developed clinical illness; terminally, depression of platelet counts and fibrinogen levels occasionally was observed. The disturbances in coagulation occurred during the stage of viremia and existed before the stage of hepatic necrosis in liver biopsy specimens. These data suggest that the *hemorrhagic manifestations are primarily caused by a disseminated intravascular coagulation rather than by hepatic failure.* Also, in experimental infections in primates, modest increases in total bilirubin and alkaline phosphatase levels and marked increases in serum glutamic oxalacetic transaminase occur. In Brazil in 1973, 7 of 29 patients with a clinical diagnosis of viral hepatitis had serologies compatible with recent yellow fever and lacked hepatitis B surface antigen. Electrocardiograms may show T-wave changes. Clinical examinations of cerebrospinal fluid have not revealed abnormalities.

Diagnosis   There are three established procedures for the laboratory diagnosis of yellow fever:

1 Isolation of the virus from blood. This must be done early, preferably during the first 3 days. Caution must be exercised to avoid autoinoculation.
2 Demonstration of increase in neutralizing antibody.
3 Demonstration of the typical, although not completely specific, histopathologic lesions on liver biopsy.

Treatment   The management has been symptomatic and supportive and should be based upon assessment and correction of the circulatory abnormalities. If evidence of disseminated intravascular coagulation is present, the administration of heparin should be considered. Close attention to fluids and electrolytes is essential.

Prognosis   The overall fatality rate in yellow fever is between 5 and 10 percent of clinical cases; it may be even less since many infections are mild or inapparent.

Prevention   Effective control measures are available. Immunization has been effective in the prevention of outbreaks. With the occurrence of sylvatic outbreaks, work in the area of epizootic activity should be discontinued and intensive mosquito abatement measures should be instituted. These measures may provide the time necessary for a mass immunization program.

MOSQUITO-BORNE HEMORRHAGIC FEVERS   The term *hemorrhagic fever* was first applied to illness in Southeast Asia in the Philippines in 1953. Subsequently the hemorrhagic fevers have grown steadily as a disease problem. Initially they were classified on the basis of geography as Philippine, Thai, and Southeast Asian hemorrhagic fevers. With further study it appeared more rational to classify the syndromes as hemorrhagic dengue or chikungunya, depending upon the etiology. These diseases are caused by viruses transmitted by *A. aegypti.*

Etiology   At least four (dengue types 1, 2, 3, 4) and possibly six types of dengue and chikungunya virus have been isolated from arthropods and humans during outbreaks of hemorrhagic fever.

Prevalence   Once regarded as an inevitable but trivial infection, dengue is now both a feared killer and a pathogenetic enigma. The reasons for the apparent sudden "appearance" of the syndrome in the past 26 years are completely obscure. However, during the 1922 epidemic of dengue fever in Louisiana, hemorrhagic manifestations, including epistaxis, bleeding gums, melena, menorrhagia, and even "black vomit," were observed. Hemorrhagic disease with dengue also was seen in Durban in 1927, in Athens in 1928, and in Curacao in 1968. Yet no deaths were attributed directly to the dengue. During the past 15 years, dengue has resulted in 200,000 hospital admissions with 5 to 10 percent deaths, and involved every country in tropical Asia except Bangladesh. In Asia, hemorrhagic fever is a disease of children, with virtually all cases occurring in children under age 14 years. In 1962 in Bangkok and Thonburi, an estimated 10 to 20 percent of children under age 15 had illness due either to dengue or to chikungunya virus. Approximately 5 percent of children with dengue or chikungunya had hemorrhagic fever. Dengue hemorrhagic fever occurs almost exclusively in indigenous populations; it has been observed only rarely in Caucasians of European descent despite the frequent occurrence of classic dengue in this group. During the 1975 dengue-2 epidemic in Puerto Rico, three patients with hemorrhagic manifestations, but without shock, were reported. Elsewhere in the Western Hemisphere, since 1967, dengue hemorrhagic fever has occurred in Curacao and Jamaica.

Epidemiology *Aëdes aegypti* is the vector of both dengue and chikungunya viruses. It is an urban mosquito which breeds in artificial containers and receptacles. Outbreaks are confined to the rainy season, although in areas without marked seasonal rainfall cases may occur throughout the year. Human-mosquito-human transmission of dengue is responsible for urban epidemics. Recent isolates of chikungunya virus from *Culex tritaeniorhynchus* in Thailand where human population densities are low suggest a nonhuman reservoir for this virus.

Clinical manifestations The hemorrhagic dengue syndrome is almost exclusively a disease of children. There is no sex predominance. Illness begins abruptly with a minor stage characterized by fever, cough, pharyngitis, headache, anorexia, nausea, vomiting, and abdominal pain which is often severe. This continues for 2 to 4 days. In contrast to classic dengue, myalgia, arthralgia, and bone pain are unusual. Physical signs include fever varying from 38.3 to 40.6°C (101 to 105°F), injection of the tonsils and pharynx, and palpable lymph nodes and liver. The initial state is followed by abrupt deterioration, with the rapid onset of lassitude and weakness (Table 190-4). On examination the child is found to be restless and to have cold clammy extremities with a warm trunk and a pallid face with circumoral cyanosis. Petechiae, most frequently located on the forehead and distal extremities, are seen in half the cases. Occasionally there may be a macular or maculopapular rash. The extremities are frequently cyanotic. Hypotension, with narrowing of the pulse pressure, and tachycardia occur. Pathological reflexes may be observed. Most fatalities occur in the fourth or fifth day of illness, melena, hematemesis, coma, or unresponsive shock being poor prognostic signs. Cyanosis, dyspnea, and convulsions are terminal manifestations. Following this critical period, survivors show steady and quite rapid improvement.

Laboratory findings In one study, hemoconcentration was found in one-fifth of the children. The majority had leukocyte counts between 5000 and 10,000 per cubic millimeter, with one-third showing a leukocytosis. Only 10 percent of children had a true leukopenia. The most characteristic findings were thrombocytopenia, rarely with blood platelets under 75,000 per cubic millimeter, positive tourniquet test, and prolonged bleeding time. Prothrombin time and partial thromboplastin times were usually near normal values. Depression of clotting factors V, VII, IX, and X may be present. Bone marrow examination may reveal maturation arrest of megakaryocytes. In Manila or Bangkok, hematuria has been infrequent even with other serious bleeding manifestations; however, in Tahiti, gross hematuria was common. Cerebrospinal fluid examinations are usually normal. Other abnormal laboratory findings may include hyponatremia, acidosis, elevated blood urea nitrogen levels, elevation in serum glutamic oxalacetic transaminase levels, mild hyperbilirubinemia, and hypoproteinemia. Electrocardiograms may reveal diffuse myocardial abnormalities. Two-thirds of patients have radiological evidence of bronchopneumonia, with many showing pleural effusions.

Diagnosis Specific virological diagnosis of dengue virus infection by serologic means often is difficult because broad antibody responses to group B arboviruses occur. Virus isolation may provide the only means of identifying the specific agent. Chikungunya virus diagnosis poses less difficulty, since it can be isolated from acute serum in suckling mice or hamster kidney cells. Serologic responses can also be demonstrated.

Pathophysiology The pathophysiologic processes that occur in dengue hemorrhagic fever (DHF) and that distinguish it from unmodified dengue fever are increased vascular permeability in which an increased hematocrit is accompanied by a decrease in serum protein concentration due to selective extravasation of albumin, decreased plasma volume, hypotension, thrombocytopenia, and a hemorrhagic diathesis. The association of DHF with a secondary-type antibody response suggested that primary dengue infection "sensitizes" the host to a severe response accompanying infection with a second type. Anamnestic antibody responses with high titers of anti-dengue IgG antibody early in the course of DHF support this concept. Activation of both the classic and alternate complement pathways, with depression of C1q, C3, C4, C5 to C8, and C3 proactivator levels, has been shown in most patients. In dengue shock syndrome (DSS), the blood clotting and fibrinolytic systems are activated, and levels of factor XII (Hageman factor) are depressed. Presumably, dengue virus acting in the presence of complement-fixing IgG antibody is responsible for activation of this system. However, this does not explain the occasional cases of DSS which occur with initial infections. Moreover, there is a limit to the time period after primary infection in which a second infection can precipitate DSS. Halstead and associates have reported enhanced growth of dengue viruses in peripheral blood leukocytes obtained from immune, compared with nonimmune, donors. Circulating leukocytes capable of supporting replication of dengue virus in vitro disap-

TABLE 190-4
World Health Organization's clinical classification of dengue hemorrhagic fever

	Grade	Clinical features	Laboratory findings
DHF* { DSS* {	I	Fever, constitutional symptoms, positive tourniquet test	Hemoconcentration Thrombocytopenia
	II	Grade I plus spontaneous bleeding (e.g., skin, gums, gastrointestinal tract)	Hemoconcentration Thrombocytopenia
	III	Grade II plus circulatory failure, agitation	Hemoconcentration Thrombocytopenia
	IV	Grade II plus profound shock (blood pressure = 0)	Hemoconcentration Thrombocytopenia

* *DHF, dengue hemorrhagic fever; DSS, dengue shock syndrome.*

pear within months to a few years. These observations may relate the difference between benign and severe disease to the number of infected cells.

Treatment The mainstay is correction of circulatory collapse while avoiding fluid overload. Administration of 5% glucose in 0.5 *N* saline at a rate of 40 ml/kg restored blood pressure within 1 to 2 h in one-half of patients. When stable, the rate of administration of intravenous fluids was slowed to 10 (ml/kg)/h. If improvement did not occur, plasma or a plasma expander (20 ml/kg) was administered. Transfusion of whole blood is not recommended. Glucocorticosteroids have been used, but doses of 25 mg/kg have not resulted in significant improvement. Since the evidence for severe disseminated intravascular coagulation is questionable, use of heparin is not clear-cut, although in a group of Filipino children with type 3 dengue virus, administration of heparin (1 mg sodium heparin per kilogram) was associated with a dramatic rise in number of platelets and level of plasma fibrinogen. Antibiotics are not indicated, and sympathomimetic amines are contraindicated. Recovery from vascular collapse usually occurs within 24 to 48 h, at which time diuretics and digitalis may be necessary.

Prognosis Mortality has varied from 6 to 23 percent. Deaths have been most common in infants under 1 year of age.

Prevention At present, vector control is the only method available to prevent hemorrhagic fever.

TICK-BORNE HEMORRHAGIC FEVERS Crimean hemorrhagic fever At the close of World War II, a new disease entity was recognized in the Crimea region of the U.S.S.R. Retrospective studies demonstrated that an almost identical syndrome had been recognized in the south central Asian republics of the U.S.S.R. for many years. Soviet workers repeatedly isolated virus strains during 1967 to 1969.

ETIOLOGY The virus of Crimean hemorrhagic fever (CHF) has been shown to be antigenically identical with Congo virus, which has been isolated from patients, cattle, and ticks in Africa (Kenya, Uganda, Congo, and Nigeria). CHF-Congo isolates now have been made from an area extending from southwestern and central U.S.S.R. to Pakistan and across central Africa from Nigeria to Kenya.

EPIDEMIOLOGY Approximately 30 cases of CHF have been recorded annually in each of the known areas of occurrence in the U.S.S.R. The cases occur between April and September. The sex distribution of CHF is equal, and 80 percent of the cases occur in the 20- to 60-year age group, with the majority occurring in milkmaids and agricultural workers. The major arthropod vectors for transmission to humans are ticks which belong to the genus *Hyalomma*. Cattle and wild hares appear to be important reservoirs, and rooks and other birds have been implicated, although the detailed epidemiology has yet to be defined.

CLINICAL MANIFESTATIONS The onset is abrupt, with temperatures to 40°C (104°F), dizziness, headache, and diffuse myalgia. The course of fever is occasionally biphasic, with an average duration of 8 days. Physical signs include flushing of the face, conjunctival injection, vomiting, and, on occasion, epigastric pain. Hepatomegaly is found in half the patients. Splenomegaly has been reported in 2 to 25 percent of patients. Respiratory symptoms or signs are unusual. Hemorrhagic manifestations generally begin on the fourth day with petechiae on the oral mucosa and skin, epistaxis, gingival bleeding, hematemesis, and melena. Neurological abnormalities, seen in

10 to 25 percent of patients, include nuchal rigidity, excitation, and coma. Laboratory findings show leukopenia, with the number of white blood cells falling as low as 1000 per cubic millimeter, and thrombocytopenia, which is often severe. Proteinuria and microscopic hematuria are common, but azotemia and oliguria are not. Convalescence may be prolonged. Death is usually attributed to shock or intercurrent infection. Sequelae include transient alopecia and mononeuritis or polyneuritis. Although the clinical disease seen in Africa due to Congo virus generally has not been associated with hemorrhagic manifestations, one fatal case with gastrointestinal bleeding has been reported from Uganda.

TREATMENT The major approach to therapy has been transfusions of blood or plasma. The clinical similarities to other hemorrhagic fever syndromes in which the phenomenon of intravascular coagulation seems to occur are sufficient to suggest that appropriate studies should be done. If evidence of disseminated intravascular coagulation is demonstrated, treatment with heparin should be considered.

PROGNOSIS The reported mortality rate has shown variation between 9 and 50 percent.

Omsk hemorrhagic fever OHF is an acute febrile disease which occurs in the Omsk and Novosibirsk oblasts in the U.S.S.R. and is caused by a group B arbovirus of the Russian spring-summer complex.

EPIDEMIOLOGY The seasonal occurrence of OHF shows a biphasic pattern with peaks in May and August. OHF is transmitted to humans either by the bite of infected ticks of the genus *Dermacentor* or by the handling of infected muskrats. The natural reservoir includes muskrats, other rodents, and ticks. Epidemics occurred from 1945 to 1948, but recently the disease has been less prevalent.

CLINICAL MANIFESTATIONS Following an incubation interval of 3 to 8 days, illness begins abruptly with fever, headache, and hemorrhagic manifestations, which include epistaxis and gastrointestinal and uterine bleeding. Rarely, neurologic abnormalities may occur. Laboratory features include leukopenia. In contrast to many of the other hemorrhagic fevers, OHF has a low case fatality rate (0.5 to 3.0 percent).

Kyasanur Forest disease Kyasanur Forest disease was first recognized in south India in 1957 as a discrete clinical entity shown to be due to an arbovirus.

ETIOLOGY The virus is a group B arbovirus immunologically related to the Russian spring-summer complex.

EPIDEMIOLOGY Kyasanur Forest disease occurs following occupational exposure to *Haemaphysalis spinigera* ticks in the tropical forests of western Mysore in southern India. The silent reservoir cycle which infects the primate- and bird-feeding *Haemaphysalis* ticks is now believed to be *Ixodes* ticks transmitted among small forest mammals, especially the shrew. Laboratory-associated infections have been common.

CLINICAL MANIFESTATIONS The major symptoms include abrupt onset of fever, headache, fatigue, myalgia (especially of the lumbar area and calf muscles), and retroorbital pain. Cough and abdominal pain occur in half the patients. Additional symptoms may include photophobia and polyarthralgia. Epistaxis and hematemesis are observed in some patients. On examination, findings include relative bradycardia, conjunctival injection, and generalized lymphadenopathy. Fine and coarse rales are frequently heard. Hepatosplenomegaly has been encountered occasionally. During the initial phase, generalized hyperesthesia of the skin occurs occasionally. The fever usually lasts from 6 to 11 days. After an afebrile period of 9 to 21 days, approximately half the patients may develop a second phase, which lasts from 2 to 12 days. This is manifested by recurrence of fever, severe headache, neck stiffness, mental disturbance, coarse tremors, giddiness, and abnormalities in reflexes, as well as by recurrence of many of the initial symptoms. No sequelae have been observed, but convalescence is often prolonged.

Only limited laboratory studies have been performed. During the initial phase, leukopenia is a constant feature, with a total leukocyte count of fewer than 3000 per cubic millimeter by the fourth to sixth day. The leukopenia is associated with neutropenia. During the second phase there is a mild leukocytosis. Lumbar puncture during the second phase has shown a pattern of aseptic meningitis.

DIAGNOSIS Diagnosis is based upon virus isolation from blood; this is readily accomplished, since viremia is prolonged. Serologic tests of paired serums also can be performed.

TREATMENT The management is supportive.

PROGNOSIS The mortality rate is approximately 5 percent.

REFERENCES

Arboviruses: Definition and classification

HORZINCK MC: The structure of Togaviruses. Prog Med Virol 16:109, 1973

THE SUBCOMMITTEE ON INFORMATION EXCHANGE OF THE AMERICAN COMMITTEE ON ARTHROPOD-BORNE VIRUSES: Catalogue of arthropod-borne and selected vertebrate viruses of the world. Am J Trop Med 20:1018, 1971

WHO SCIENTIFIC GROUP: *Arbovirus and Human Disease,* WHO Tech Rept Ser 369. Geneva, 1967

WHO STUDY GROUP: *Arthropod-borne Viruses,* WHO Tech Rep Ser 219. Geneva, 1961

Arbovirus infections characterized by fever, malaise, headaches, and myalgia

BECKER FE: Tick-borne infections in Colorado. Col Med 27:36, 1930

BRICENO ROSSIE AL: Rural epidemic encephalitis in Venezuela caused by a group A arbovirus (VEE). Prog Med Virol 9:176, 1967

CENTER FOR DISEASE CONTROL: Rift Valley fever—Egypt. Morb Mort Week Rep 39:113, 1978

DAUBNEY R et al: Enzootic hepatitis or Rift Valley Fever. J Pathol Bacteriol 34:545, 1931

DIASIO JS, RICHARDSON, FM: Clinical observation on dengue fever. Milit Surg 94:365, 1944

FLEMING J et al: Sandfly fever. Review of 664 cases. Lancet 1:443, 1947

FLORIO L et al: The etiology of Colorado tick fever. J Exp Med 83:1, 1946

GOODPASTURE HC et al: Colorado tick fever: Clinical, epidemiologic and laboratory aspects of 228 cases in Colorado in 1973–1974. Ann Intern Med 88:303, 1978

HUGHES LE et al: Persistence of Colorado tick fever virus in red blood cells. Am J Trop Med Hyg 23:530, 1974

LENNETTE EH, KOPROWSKI H: Human infection with Venezuelan equine encephalomyelitis virus. JAMA 123:1088, 1943

SABIN AB: Research on dengue during World War II. Am J Trop Med 1:30, 1952

——— et al: Phlebotomus (Papataci or sandfly) fever; disease of military importance: Summary of existing knowledge and preliminary report of original observations. JAMA 125:603, 693, 1944

SCHERER WF et al: Ecologic studies of Venezuelan encephalitis virus in Southeastern Mexico: VII. Infection of man. Am J Trop Med 21:79, 1972

SIDWELL RW et al: Epidemiological aspects of Venezuelan equine encephalitis virus infections. Bacterial Rev 31:65, 1967

SMITHBURN KC et al: Rift Valley fever. J Immunol 62:213, 1949

SPRUANCE SL, BAILEY A: Colorado tick fever. A review of 115 laboratory confirmed cases. Arch Intern Med 131:288, 1973

SULKIN SE et al: Bat salivary gland virus: Infections of man and monkey. Tex Rep Biol Med 20:113, 1962

TESH RB et al: Antigenic relationships among Phlebotomus fever group arboviruses and their implications for the epidemiology of sandfly fever. Am J Trop Med Hyg 24:135, 1975

Arbovirus infections presenting chiefly with fever, malaise, arthralgia, and rash

CLARK JA et al: Annually recurrent epidemic polyarthritis and Ross River virus activity in a coastal area of New South Wales. I. Occurrence of the disease. Am J Trop Med Hyg 22:543, 1973

DELLER JJ JR, RUSSELL PK: Chikungunya disease. Am J Trop Med 17:107, 1968

DOHERTY RL et al: Studies of epidemic polyarthritis: The significance of three group A arboviruses, isolated from mosquitoes in Queensland. Aust Ann Med 13:322, 1964

MALHERBE H et al: Sindbis virus infection in man. Report of a case with recovery of virus from skin lesions. S Afr Med J 37:547, 1963

ROBINSON MC: An epidemic of virus disease in Southern Province, Tanganyika territory in 1952–53: I. Clinical features. Trans R Soc Trop Med Hyg 49:28, 1955

SHORE H: O'nyong-nyong fever: An epidemic virus disease in East Africa: III. Some clinical and epidemiological observations in the Northern Province of Uganda. Trans R Soc Trop Med Hyg 55:361, 1961

Arbovirus infections presenting chiefly with fever, malaise, lymphadenopathy, and rash

MARBERG K et al: The natural history of West Nile fever: I. Clinical observations during an epidemic in Israel. Am J Hyg 64:259, 1956

PERELMAN A, STERN J: Acute pancreatitis in West Nile fever. Am J Trop Med Hyg 23:1150, 1974

TAYLOR RM et al: A study of the ecology of West Nile virus in Egypt. Am J Trop Med 5:579, 1956

Arbovirus infections presenting chiefly with central nervous system involvement

ALTMAN R et al: The impact of vector-borne viral diseases in the middle Atlantic States. Med Clin North Am 51:661, 1967

BALFOUR HH JR et al: California arbovirus (LaCrosse) infections. Pediatrics 52:680, 1973

DICKERSON RB et al: Diagnosis and immediate prognosis of Japanese B encephalitis. Observations based on more than 200 patients with detailed analysis of 65 serologically confirmed cases. Am J Med 12:277, 1952

FEEMSTER RF, HAYMAKER W: Eastern equine encephalitis. Neurology 8:882, 1958

FINLEY KH et al: Western equine and St. Louis encephalitis. Preliminary report of a clinical follow-up study in California. Neurology 5:223, 1955

GRABOW JD et al: The electroencephalogram and clinical sequelae of California arbovirus encephalitis. Neurology 19:394, 1969

HILTY MD et al: California encephalitis in children. Am J Dis Child 124:530, 1972

KETEL WB, OGNIBENE AJ: Japanese B encephalitis in Vietnam. Am J Med Sci 261:271, 1971

LUBY JP et al: The epidemiology of St. Louis encephalitis (SLE): A review. Ann Rev Med 20:329, 1969

SCHNEIDER RJ et al: Clinical sequelae after Japanese encephalitis: One year followup study in Thailand. Southeast Asian J Trop Med Public Health 5:560, 1974

WEAVER OM et al: Japanese encephalitis: Sequelae. Neurology 8:887, 1958

Arbovirus diseases presenting primarily with hemorrhagic manifestations

BOKISCH VA et al: The potential pathogenic role of complement in dengue-hemorrhagic fever syndrome. N Engl J Med 289:996, 1973

CASALS J et al: A current appraisal of hemorrhagic fevers in the USSR. Am J Trop Med 15:751, 1966

Dengue. Lancet 2:239, 1976

DENNIS LH et al: The original hemorrhagic fever: Yellow fever. Blood 30:858, 1967

HALSTEAD SB: Mosquito-borne haemorrhagic fevers of South and Southeast Asia. Bull WHO 35:3, 1966

KERR JA: Clinical aspects and diagnosis of yellow fever, in *Yellow Fever*, GK Strode (ed). New York, McGraw-Hill, 1951, p 389

KIRK R: An epidemic of yellow fever in the Nuba Mountains, Anglo-Egyptian Sudan. Ann Trop Med Parasitol 35:67, 1941

LOPEZ-CORREA RH et al: Dengue fever with hemorrhagic manifestations: A report of three cases from Puerto Rico. Am J Trop Med Hyg 27:1216, 1978

LOW GC, FAIRLEY NH: Laboratory and hospital infections with yellow fever in England. Br Med J 1:125, 1931

NELSON ER: Hemorrhagic fever in children in Thailand: Report of 69 cases. J Pediatr 56:101, 1960

PINHEIRO FP et al: An epidemic of yellow fever in Central Brazil 1972–1973: I. Epidemiological studies. Am J Trop Med Hyg 27:125, 1978

PONGPANICH B et al: Management of shock associated with dengue hemorrhagic fever based on pathophysiological findings. Southeast Asian J Trop Med Public Health 6:115, 1975

Technical guides for diagnosis, treatment, surveillance, prevention and control of dengue hemorrhagic fever. World Health Organization, Geneva, 1975

191
ARENAVIRUS INFECTIONS

JAY P. SANFORD

DEFINITION AND CLASSIFICATION The term *arenavirus* is the proposed designation for a group of RNA viruses which have unique morphology (Table 191-1). The virions are round, oval, or pleomorphic, with diameters between 60 and 350 nm, and contain an electron-dense membrane with projections and 2 to 10 inclusion-like dense particles (resembling ribosomes) that give the virion an appearance of having been sprinkled with sand (Latin *arenaceus,* "sandy"). A special property of arenaviruses that causes disease in humans, especially Machupo and lymphocytic choriomeningitis, is their capacity to induce persistent infection in their reservoir hosts with no ill effects and in the absence of an immune response.

LYMPHOCYTIC CHORIOMENINGITIS The first-recognized arenavirus was lymphocytic choriomeningitis (LCM) virus, isolated in 1934 from a laboratory monkey in the course of studies of the 1933 St. Louis encephalitis outbreak. It was recognized early that LCM was carried by apparently healthy laboratory mice. Clinically LCM has been considered primarily in the context of aseptic meningitis; however, it is associated with at least two clinical syndromes in humans: central nervous system and influenza-like illness which may be associated with rash, arthritis, or orchitis. LCM virus has provided a valuable model for the study of chronic, persistent, and generally symptomless viral infections in laboratory animals.

Prevalence In the United States, at present, human infection with LCM virus is rare; however, seroepidemiologic studies on specimens obtained in 1935 to 1940 from persons with no history of central nervous system disease from all parts of the United States revealed neutralizing antibodies in 10 to 28 percent. In a study of aseptic meningitis, Meyer and associates incriminated LCM in 8.1 percent. In recent years, the prevalence of infection seems to have decreased markedly.

Epidemiology The virus of LCM is worldwide in distribution. Although infection can be induced in a variety of animals, mice are the major natural reservoir as well as the primary host in which latent, asymptomatic infection occurs. The latency of infection in the mouse depends upon immunologic tolerance. Animals infected in utero or shortly after birth excrete LCM virus for life without overt disease. Human infections are secondary to contact with an infected rodent. The mode of transmission is thought to be via airborne spread or contact with excrement from infected animals. In the past, most cases have arisen in persons living in rodent-infested houses, but lately outbreaks of LCM virus disease in humans have been reported from Germany and from the United States in which the source of infection was traced to laboratory animals and household pets, specifically hamsters which, like mice, can shed LCM virus in urine and stool. LCM occurs throughout the year but has been more frequent in the colder months when "the mice come in from the fields." Person-to-person transmission has not been demonstrated.

Pathogenesis In natural infection, the portal of entry of the LCM virus is probably through the respiratory tract. Virus multiplication occurs initially in the respiratory epithelium, and an influenza-like illness develops. Dissemination of virus to extrapulmonary sites, presumably to reticuloendothelial cells, with multiplication and viremia occurs. LCM virus crosses the blood-brain barrier. In mice, the resulting meningi-

TABLE 191-1
Classification of arenaviruses

Virus	Clinical disease	Reservoir	Known geographic range
Lymphocytic choriomeningitis	Aseptic meningitis, meningoencephalitis, influenzal syndrome, orchitis, arthritis	Mice, hamsters	Worldwide except Australia
Tacaribe		Bats	Trinidad
Junin	Argentinian hemorrhagic fever	*Calomys musculinus*	Argentina
Machupo	Bolivian hemorrhagic fever	*Calomys callosus*	Northeast Bolivia
Amapari			Brazil
Latino			Bolivia
Parana			Paraguay
Pichinde			Colombia
Tamiami			Florida
Lassa	Lassa fever	*Mastomys natalensis*	Nigeria, Liberia, Sierra Leone, Republic of Guinea, Central African Republic
?	Far Eastern hemorrhagic fever (Korean, nephropathica epidemica)	*Apodemus agrarius*	U.S.S.R., Manchuria, China, Korea, Scandinavia

tis is attributed to a cell-mediated immune reaction. Support for this hypothesis derives from observations that disease but not infection can be prevented in experimental animals by neonatal thymectomy, irradiation, or immunodepressant drugs such as cyclophosphamide. Similar pathogenetic mechanisms may operate in humans, although isolation of LCM virus from the CSF of patients with aseptic meningitis is quite common.

Clinical manifestations The exact incubation period is not known. Following experimental inoculation of LCM virus into volunteers, fever occurred in 1½ to 3 days, while an influenza-like constellation of symptoms developed 5 to 10 days after exposure. An influenza-like illness with many features of other arenavirus and arbovirus infections is the commonest clinical pattern. In some patients, up to one-half in some series, the illness may be biphasic with subsequent aseptic meningitis or encephalomyelitis. Fever, usually from 38.3 to 40°C (101 to 104°F), associated with rigors, is uniformly noted. Other symptoms which are encountered in over one-half of patients include malaise, weakness, myalgia (especially lumbar aching), retroorbital headache, photophobia, anorexia, nausea, and light-headedness. Other prominent symptoms which occur in one-fourth to one-half of patients include sore throat, vomiting, and dysesthesias. Later arthralgias, especially in the hands, occur. Less common complaints (up to one-quarter of patients) include aching pain in the chest, associated with pneumonitis; increased hair loss progressing to generalized alopecia of the scalp, 2 or 3 weeks after the onset of illness; testicular pain or frank orchitis, usually unilateral, again 1 to 3 weeks after onset; and parotid pain, which may lead to a misdiagnosis of mumps. Physical findings in the first week of illness are few. Patients often have a relative bradycardia. Pharyngeal injection without exudate is commonly seen (60 percent). Mild nontender cervical or axillary lymphadenopathy may occur. The initial phase lasts from 5 days to 3 weeks followed by improvement. After a remission of 1 to 2 days many patients relapse with recurrent fever and more prominent headache. Physical signs may include skin rashes, swelling of metacarpophalangeal and proximal interphalangeal joints, meningeal signs, orchitis, parotitis, and alopecia of the scalp. Convalescence generally is of 1 to 4 weeks' duration, characterized by easy fatigability, an excessive need for sleep, dysesthesias, and occasional dizziness. Patients with aseptic meningitis almost always recover without sequelae. With encephalitis, 25 to 30 percent of patients have neurological residua.

Laboratory findings Leukopenia and thrombocytopenia are almost uniform during the first week of illness. Although leukocyte counts usually vary between 2000 and 3000 per cubic millimeter, counts as low as 600 per cubic millimeter have been recorded. Differential counts generally show slight relative lymphocytosis. Platelet counts are usually between 50,000 and 100,000 per cubic millimeter. Anemia is not encountered. The erythrocyte sedimentation rate often is normal. Mild elevations of the serum enzymes, serum glutamic oxaloacetic transaminase (SGOT) and lactic dehydrogenase (LDH), may occur. Chest radiographs may suggest basilar pneumonitis. In patients with meningeal signs examination of the cerebrospinal fluid usually reveals several hundred cells per cubic millimeter, although cell counts in excess of 1000 per cubic millimeter are reported in one-half patients in some series. Lymphocytes predominate (greater than 80 percent) even early. The initial cerebrospinal fluid protein is usually slightly elevated, but on occasion levels may exceed 150 mg per 100 ml. Although a normal cerebrospinal fluid glucose level is considered the hallmark of viral meningitides, hypoglycorrhachia has been observed in up

to 27 percent of patients with LCM, glucose values as low as 15 mg per 100 ml with normal simultaneous blood sugar levels having been reported.

Diagnosis The diagnosis of LCM can be established with certainty by recovery of the virus from blood or spinal fluid. Complement-fixing antibodies are usually detectable 1 to 2 weeks after the onset of infection, peak at 5 to 8 weeks, and are gone by 6 months. Neutralizing antibodies appear after 6 to 8 weeks, increase in titer slowly, and remain high for years. Immunofluorescent studies have detected antibody to LCM virus earlier in the course of illness, and its appearance seems to parallel the development of the neurological phase. The clinical manifestations of LCM cannot be differentiated from those produced by numerous other viruses. A detailed discussion of aseptic meningitis appears in Chap. 186.

Treatment The management is supportive and symptomatic.

HEMORRHAGIC FEVER WITH RENAL SYNDROME Synonyms for this disease include Korean hemorrhagic fever, Far Eastern hemorrhagic fever, endemic or epidemic nephrosonephritis, Manchurian epidemic hemorrhagic fever, Songo fever, and Churilov's disease. The same disease in Scandinavia has been called *nephropathica epidemica*.

Epidemic hemorrhagic fever (EHF) is an acute febrile, often fatal, otherwise self-limited illness caused by an agent, most likely an arenavirus, which has been propagated in the rodent *Apodemus agrarius* and that is characterized by severe toxemia, widespread capillary damage, hemorrhagic phenomena, and renal insufficiency. In 1932, the Russians first observed the disease in southeastern Siberia along the Amur River. In April 1951, a previously unknown illness, subsequently recognized as EHF, broke out among the United Nations forces in Korea.

Etiology In 1978, Lee and associates reported a yet to be identified agent in the lungs of the rodent *A. agrarius* which reacted with serums from patients convalescing from Korean hemorrhagic fever. Diagnostic increases in immunofluorescent antibodies were demonstrated in 113 of 116 cases of severe EHF. The agent has not yet been cultivated in tissue culture or in laboratory animals, although it has been passed in *A. agrarius*.

Prevalence In Korea between April 1951 and January 1953, 2070 cases of EHF were reported among United Nations personnel. The disease usually occurs as an isolated event; hence, overall attack rates have relatively less meaning. With this reservation, attack rates in two United States Army divisions stationed in Korea varied between 1.9 and 2.9 cases per 1000 persons per epidemic season. Approximately 800 cases per year have continued to occur; however, most cases are now seen in Korean civilians and military with less than 10 cases per year in U.S. military personnel. The U.S.S.R. reports 500 to 2000 cases yearly.

Epidemiology In Korea the majority of cases occur in May to June and in October to November. These peaks coincide with the dry seasons. Geographically, EHF originally occurred among troops stationed in the vicinity of Seoul north of the 38th parallel. More recently cases have been encountered throughout the Korean peninsula. The epidemiology of EHF observed in Korea remains unknown. No vector is known or suspected although earlier, chiggers, especially *Trombicula pallida*, correlated closely with the epidemiology of EHF in Korea. Since World War II, rather remarkable outbreaks have occurred in northeast Asia between November and January.

In these outbreaks, the peak of the epidemic was preceded by a marked increase in forest rodent populations (usually the red-backed vole *Clethrionomys glariolus*), which migrated into the fields, barns, and even houses near the forest. Nephropathica epidemica, a disease encountered in Scandinavia and in Eastern Europe which is clinically similar to EHF, has been shown to be related to the agent causing Korean hemorrhagic fever. There may be a very narrow variety of rodent hosts which distribute virus in urine or by eating dead carcasses. Humans are probably an incidental host who may become infected by the aerosol route.

Clinical manifestations The incubation period in EHF is usually 10 to 25 days, with possible extremes of 7 and 36 days. Individuals who contract the disease in an endemic area may easily not develop illness until their return to the United States. Inapparent or mild disease is less common than typical EHF.

The clinical course of EHF may be divided into phases on the basis of the underlying physiological aberrations: febrile, hypotensive, oliguric, diuretic, and convalescent. There is considerable variation among patients in the severity of the illness. In one study two-thirds of the 264 cases studied were classified as mild, while 14 percent were termed severe. The illness in most patients was of comparable severity in each phase.

FEBRILE (INVASIVE) PHASE From 10 to 20 percent of patients describe vague prodromal symptoms resembling mild upper respiratory infections. The onset is then usually abrupt, often initiated by a chill and accompanied by fever, headache, backache, abdominal pain, and generalized myalgia. Anorexia and thirst are almost universal, while nausea and vomiting are common although not constant symptoms. The headache is most commonly frontal or retroorbital. Eye symptoms, especially mild photophobia and pain on movement of the eyes, are characteristic. Diarrhea is not a feature. Fever is present in almost all patients; the temperature ranges from 37.8 to 41.1°C (100 to 106°F), reaches a peak on the third or fourth day after onset, and falls by lysis on the fourth to seventh day. There is a relative bradycardia. Initially the blood pressure is normal. One of the most typical early findings is a diffuse reddening of the skin, most marked over the face and V area of the neck. It may resemble a severe sunburn. The erythema blanches on pressure. Dermographism can be demonstrated in over 90 percent of patients at the same time as the flush. Slight edema of the upper eyelids causes a bleary-eyed appearance. Bulbar and palpebral conjunctivas show injection. Conjunctival petechiae may develop by the third or fifth day of illness. Subconjunctival hemorrhages may be striking. Intense pharyngeal reddening without significant sore throat is typical. The first location for petechiae is usually the palate, where they occur in half the patients. Within 12 to 24 h, petechiae appear at pressure areas such as the axillary folds, lateral chest wall, belt line, hips, and thighs. Retinal hemorrhages occur rarely. Cervical, axillary, and inguinal nodes are moderately enlarged but nontender. Abdominal and costovertebral tenderness is almost a constant finding. Splenomegaly is unusual and in Korea was generally attributable to malaria with which EHF coexisted in about 1 percent of patients. The degree of flush, fever, and conjunctival injection and the number of petechiae correlate quite well with the overall severity of illness.

Laboratory studies during this phase are often not striking. Initial hemoglobin and hematocrit values are usually normal. Prior to the fourth day, leukocyte counts range from 3600 to 6000 per cubic millimeter but are associated with neutrophilia. Early in the course urine specific gravity may be high. Albuminuria, which is an almost universal finding, appears, often abruptly, between the second and fifth days of illness. The urinary sediment reveals microscopic hematuria and hyaline,

granular, red blood cell casts, and/or white blood cell casts. Erythrocyte sedimentation rates are normal during the first week. Capillary fragility tests are usually positive at the time of admission and become most abnormal by the ninth day. Electrocardiographic abnormalities may be seen in 15 to 30 percent of patients; these include sinus bradycardia and low or inverted T waves. Lumbar punctures may reveal gross blood in the spinal fluid.

HYPOTENSIVE PHASE On about the fifth day of illness, during the last 24 to 48 h of the febrile phase, hypotension or shock may occur. In mild cases, only a transient fall in blood pressure occurs; among moderately and severely ill patients shock may persist for 1 to 3 days. In 828 patients, 16.5 percent had clinical shock, and another 14 percent had hypotension without shock. Headache often diminishes, but thirst persists. In the beginning of the hypotensive phase, most patients have warm, dry skin and extremities. As the hypotensive phase progresses and the systolic blood pressure decreases and pulse pressure narrows, the skin becomes cool and moist. Tachycardia replaces the relative bradycardia.

At this stage, an increase in hematocrit with no change in total serum protein level is found. This is thought to reflect a loss of plasma through damaged capillaries. On about the fifth day, all patients develop marked proteinuria. The previously normal urine specific gravity begins to fall and in 2 to 3 days is usually around 1.010. Blood urea nitrogen concentrations begin to increase. Other laboratory findings include leukocytosis with white blood cell counts of 10,000 to 56,000 per cubic millimeter with neutrophilia and toxic granulation. The number of platelets often decreases to less than 70,000 per cubic millimeter. In a single patient who became ill 30 days after leaving Korea and who was studied on the fourth day of illness (i.e., in the hypotensive phase), there was marked thrombocytopenia, hypofibrinogenemia, and hypoprothrombinemia with a prolonged thrombin time. The deficiency of multiple blood coagulation factors suggests that the bleeding defect was due to disseminated intravascular coagulation.

OLIGURIC PHASE (HEMORRHAGIC OR TOXIC PHASE) About the eighth day of illness, blood pressure returns to the normal range and in some instances increases to hypertensive levels. While oliguria may have appeared during the shock phase, it now becomes a prominent feature. Oliguria develops even though hypotension was not recognized. Symptomatically patients continue to feel weak and thirsty and have more severe backache. Protracted vomiting and hiccups may ensue.

Blood urea nitrogen levels increase rapidly and are associated with hyperkalemia, hyperphosphatemia, and hypocalcemia. Metabolic acidosis is rarely severe. Although platelets begin to return to normal, hemorrhagic manifestations become more prominent and include petechiae, hematemesis (analogous to "black vomit" in yellow fever), melena, hemoptysis, gross hematuria, and hemorrhages into the central nervous system. The enlarged lymph nodes may now become tender.

With the onset of diuresis on about the seventh day in moderately ill patients and the ninth to eleventh day in severely ill patients, symptoms of fluid and electrolyte abnormalities and central nervous system or pulmonary complications may appear. Central nervous system symptoms include disorientation, extreme restlessness, lethargy, paranoid delusions, and hallucinations. Grand mal seizures, pulmonary edema, and pulmonary infection occur in some patients.

DIURETIC PHASE With the onset of diuresis, progressive improvement is the rule. Most patients begin to eat and regain their strength. In fatal cases the diuretic phase is associated with a daily urine output of less than 4 liters and often less than 2 liters, in contrast to larger volumes in surviving patients.

CONVALESCENT PHASE The convalescent phase lasts 3 to 6 weeks. Weight is regained slowly. Complaints include muscular weakness, intention tremor, and lack of stamina. Hyposthenuria and polyuria are present; however, within 2 months most patients are able to concentrate their urine to a specific gravity of 1.023 or greater after a 12-h period of water deprivation.

Diagnosis Serologic tests are not currently available; hence, diagnosis is based on clinical-epidemiologic features. The following criteria are necessary for diagnosis: the patient must have been in the endemic area within the limits of the incubation period, and there must be a characteristic history, hemorrhagic findings, and evidence of renal involvement. In addition, studies to exclude other forms of the hemorrhagic fever syndrome must be undertaken, particularly in the sporadic cases.

Pathology The most characteristic fundamental alteration is widespread capillary and endothelial damage, with all subsequent manifestations being the result of this damage. This is manifested by dilatation of all small vessels in tissues, congestion, plasma transudation, and multiple small hemorrhages. Three features are prominent and characteristic: hemorrhage, particularly in the renal medulla, right atrium, and gastrointestinal submucosa; a peculiar type of necrosis of the renal pyramids, anterior lobe of the pituitary body, and adrenal gland; and a mononuclear cellular infiltration of the myocardium, spleen, and liver. Moderate to severe retroperitoneal edema was present in three-fourths of patients who died in the hypotensive phase of EHF.

Pathophysiology The physiological changes correlate with the clinical features. During the early febrile phase, the cardiac index is normal. Late in the febrile phase widespread capillary dysfunction becomes evident. This is manifest by loss of protein-rich plasma through damaged capillaries and results in hemoconcentration and a progressive fall in cardiac output. Measured total peripheral resistance is low, a finding compatible with the observed capillary dilatation and refractoriness to *l*-norepinephrine. During the hypotensive phase, the increases in hematocrit values and decreases in plasma volume are accentuated. These findings have the pathological corollary of marked retroperitoneal edema. The hypotensive phase is associated with a reduction in cardiac output and an increase in peripheral vascular resistance. The reduced cardiac output is probably the result of reduction in circulating blood volume, inadequate vasoconstriction, and possibly myocardial damage. Although adrenal hemorrhages can be seen at necropsy, adrenal insufficiency does not seem to be a contributing cause of shock. The initial pathophysiologic changes may result in impairment of circulation through various organs, with the development of functional and morphologic changes secondary to inadequate perfusion with its attendant hypoxemia. The hemorrhagic manifestations appear to be the result of capillary damage, with diapedesis of erythrocytes and the development of disseminated intravascular coagulation.

The plasma loss and arteriolar dysfunction are limited in duration, and, for unknown reasons, the sequestered plasma rather abruptly returns to the vascular system at the time of oliguric phase. During this phase, examination of nail bed capillaries reveals increased vasomotor activity and vasoconstriction. When patients who became hypertensive were divided on the basis of the presence or absence of diuresis, the clinical and hemodynamic differences became more apparent. During the hypertensive phase in anuric or oliguric patients, some individuals presented with full veins, an exaggerated cardiac apical thrust, and wide pulse pressure. In this group the cardiac index was high, and the peripheral resistance and hematocrit were low. Hypertensive patients who had begun to have diuresis had normal cardiac outputs and significantly elevated values for peripheral vascular resistance.

Although diuresis is a harbinger of convalescence, a daily urine output of 3 to 8 liters contributes to further serious fluid and electrolyte imbalances. If fluid output exceeds intake, low cardiac indexes may be seen and shock may ensue. Conversely, if fluid intake exceeds output, hypertension and pulmonary edema may develop.

Treatment Clinical management primarily revolves around meticulous supportive care. Trials with a variety of agents including antibiotics, adrenocortical steroid hormones, antihistamines, and convalescent serum were without significant beneficial effect during the Korean epidemics. The treatment of shock is discussed in Chap. 109 and that of acute tubular necrosis in Chap. 275.

Prognosis The Soviet experience indicates a mortality rate of 3 to 32 percent; in other early reports the mortality has ranged from 10 to 15 percent. Between April 1951 and December 1976 the overall case fatality ratio in Korea was 6.6 percent.

Residua are uncommon. Of 783 surviving patients cared for at the Hemorrhagic Fever Center in Korea between April and December 1952, only 16 were unable to return to duty within a period of 4 months. Fifteen of these individuals still had hyposthenuria. Follow-up studies on former EHF patients 3 to 5 years later showed that they had many more subsequent hospital admissions for urologic problems than did a control group and that the relative frequency correlated with the severity of the acute episode of EHF. Asymptomatic residual renal tubular dysfunction may be more common than has been appreciated.

ARGENTINIAN AND BOLIVIAN HEMORRHAGIC FEVERS The first cases of a new American hemorrhagic disease were seen near the Argentinian town of Junin near Buenos Aires in 1953. A virus was isolated from patients' blood and from local rodents and their mites. In 1959, cases of a disease thought to resemble severe epidemic typhus were noted among rural workers in northeastern Bolivia. The similarity between these syndromes was recognized. In 1963, the causal virus was isolated from patients and rodents and named the Machupo virus. Machupo virus is serologically related to but distinct from Junin virus.

Prevalence Junin virus infections have occurred in epidemic form since 1958 with between 100 and 3500 cases reported annually. The hemorrhagic disease in Bolivia has been particularly severe. Of a total population of 4000 to 6000 in the endemic area, 750 persons were affected between 1959 and 1963.

Epidemiology Argentinian hemorrhagic fever occurs in sharply endemic seasonal form (February to August), mostly among male rural workers, especially those exposed to fields at the time of the maize harvest. Virus is transmitted in the urine of rodents with chronic infection and viruria. Humans acquire the virus through contact with items or foodstuffs which have been contaminated with infected rodent urine. The main reservoir is two species of cricetidae, *Calomys laucha* and *C. musculinus*.

Bolivian hemorrhagic fever is similarly transmitted by the urine of *C. callosus* (a mouse-like rodent) chronically infected with Machupo virus. Direct person-to-person transmission is possible and may have occurred in the outbreak in Cochabamba. Disease has not occurred in medical personnel attending infected patients.

Clinical features Argentinian hemorrhagic fever presents manifestations of renal, cardiovascular, and hematologic involvement. Inapparent infections are rare. The incubation period is estimated to be 7 to 16 days, followed by a gradual onset of chills, fever, headache, malaise, myalgia, anorexia, nausea, and vomiting. The temperature reaches 38.9 to 40°C (102 to 104°F), facial flushing may be prominent, and there is a painless enanthem of the pharynx. Lymphadenopathy and splenomegaly are not present. From 3 to 5 days after the onset, the signs and symptoms worsen, with the appearance of signs of dehydration, hypotension to 50 to 100 mmHg, oliguria, and relative bradycardia. In the more severe cases, hemorrhagic manifestations, including bleeding from the gums, hematemesis, hematuria, and melena, occur. Progressive oliguria and tremor of the tongue and extremities may develop. Some patients develop psychic manifestations, with agitation, delirium, or stupor. Progressive shock, hypothermia, gallop rhythm, or gastrointestinal bleeding may occur from the seventh to tenth days. In fatal cases, pulmonary edema usually is the cause of death. During convalescence a temporary alopecia has been noted. Erythrocyte counts are normal or elevated. The total leukocyte count drops to 1200 to 3400 blood cells per cubic millimeter. Thrombocytopenia may occur. Complement components C2, C3, and C5 are decreased. The urine is dark and may approach the color of mahogany, with intense albuminuria. Blood urea nitrogen levels rise rapidly.

The clinical picture of Bolivian hemorrhagic fever is similar to Argentinian, although epistaxis and hematemesis at the onset is more common.

Diagnosis Complement-fixing antibodies appear in 15 to 30 days in about 75 percent of the clinically diagnosed cases.

Treatment Available reports do not provide details as to therapy. Supportive measures, including peritoneal dialysis to correct both the azotemia and the pulmonary edema, would seem to offer the most reasonable approach.

Prognosis The mortality rate among patients with Argentinian hemorrhagic fever is usually 3 to 15 percent, while that in Bolivian hemorrhagic fever is 5 to 30 percent.

Prevention In Bolivia, rodent control measures directed primarily against *C. callosus* populations in the houses resulted in a prompt and dramatic cessation of human cases.

LASSA FEVER A new virus disease, which is both highly contagious and virulent, occurred in a missionary nurse in Lassa, a town in northeast Nigeria, in 1969.

Epidemiology Since the initial outbreak at Lassa in 1969, during which one of the patients was transferred to New York City, there have been other outbreaks near Jos in Northern Nigeria in 1970 (32 suspected cases with 10 deaths), in Zorzor, Liberia, in 1972 (11 cases with 4 deaths), and in the eastern province of Sierra Leone with 63 suspected cases admitted to two hospitals between 1970 and 1972. In Jos and Zorzor, outbreaks apparently resulted from person-to-person nosocomial spread from the index case to hospital workers or other patients. In Sierra Leone, the great majority of cases were acquired outside the hospital, although hospital workers were at high risk. *Mastomys natalensis,* a multimammate rat widespread in Africa, is known to be an animal reservoir of the virus, and primary human cases probably result from contamination of foodstuffs with rodent urine. Human-to-human transmission may occur through contact with urine, feces, vomitus, or saliva through droplets and aerosols, and particularly through wounds contaminated with blood. Intrafamilial outbreaks have occurred around several cases. There are a number of cases which have been acquired through accidental autoinoculation with needles while starting intravenous fluids. At least one laboratory-acquired infection has occurred. In Sierra Leone 6 percent of the population surveyed had complement-fixing antibody against Lassa virus, while only 0.2 percent had recognized disease, suggesting mild disease or inapparent infection. In Liberia 10 percent of hospital personnel had antibodies. Positive serums were also obtained from individuals in Cameroon and Benin (formerly Dahomey).

Clinical features The incubation period is 1 to 24 days, being 10 days following accidental inoculation. Patients have ranged from 5 months to 46 years of age; approximately two-thirds are women. Three of eight women in one series were 22 to 28 weeks pregnant during their illness. The apparent predilection for women may relate to exposure to contaminated food or work in hospitals rather than to differences in susceptibility. The onset of illness was described by most patients as insidious. The most frequent initial symptoms are fever (100 percent), chilliness and true rigors, headache (50 percent), malaise (100 percent), and myalgia (50 percent). Most patients did not seek medical attention for 4 to 9 days after onset. Symptoms of a systemic viral illness then developed with anorexia, nausea, vomiting, myalgia, and pain in the chest, epigastrium, and lumbar area. Headache was usually present. Early examination reveals fever and flushing of the face and V area of the neck. Pharyngitis developed early and became progressively more severe during the first week; examination may reveal raised patches of whitish exudate occurring on the palatine arches which occasionally coalesce into a pseudomembrane. Oral ulcerations have been noted in up to one-half of cases. Generalized nontender lymphadenopathy occurred in one-half of patients. During the second week severe lower abdominal pain and intractable vomiting are common, and facial and neck swelling with conjunctival edema and infection frequently develop. Occasionally patients have tinnitus, epistaxis, bleeding from the gums and venapuncture sites, maculopapular rashes, cough, and dizziness. During the acute stage, systolic blood pressures of less than 90 mmHg with pulse pressures of less than 20 mmHg occurred in 60 to 80 percent of patients. Initially, relative bradycardia was common. During the second week, the patients who recovered defervesced, while the patients who died often developed signs of shock, clouding of the sensorium, rales, signs of pleural effusion, agitation and, on occasion, grand mal seizures. The duration of illness in surviving patients ranged from 7 to 31 days (average 15 days), while that in fatal cases was 7 to 26 days (average 12 days). The mortality rates in Jos and Zorzor were 52 percent and 36 percent, respectively, while in Sierra Leone the rate was 8 percent. During convalescence occasional flurries of rapid involuntary eye movements (oculogyric crises) occurred. Late sequelae include deafness in a number of patients (two of six in one series) and alopecia in one patient.

Laboratory features The hematologic findings include relatively normal hematocrit values and early leukopenia (less than 4000 cells per cubic millimeter in 36 percent) with a relative neutrophilia and immature forms of leukocytes. In two

844

cases in which it was recorded, the erythrocyte sedimentation rate was normal. Urinalyses revealed proteinuria, which was often massive. Chest radiographs may suggest basilar pneumonitis and pleural effusions. Electrocardiographic abnormalities compatible with diffuse myocardial disease have been encountered. Levels of serum enzymes, serum glutamic oxaloacetic transaminase (SGOT), creatinine phosphokinase (CPK), and lactic dehydrogenase (LDH) have been elevated. Lassa virus has been recovered from cerebrospinal fluid in two patients.

Diagnosis Diagnosis may be made quickly by staining conjunctival scrapings with fluorescent labelled anti-Lassa antiserums. Confirmation involves growth of the virus in tissue culture and a complement fixation test; however, the latter is rarely positive before the fourteenth day of illness.

Treatment The management has been supportive. Infusion of immune plasma from convalescent patients resulted in a dramatic effect in three of four patients. Because of the self-limited nature of the disease, these results cannot be assessed easily. In view of the hospital association and the presence of virus in pharyngeal secretions and urine, strict isolation is required. Known contacts should be kept under medical surveillance for at least 3 weeks.

REFERENCES

BAUM SG et al: Epidemic non-meningitic lymphocytic-choriomeningitis virus infection. N Engl J Med 274:934, 1966

CASALS J: Arenaviruses. Yale J Biol Med 48:115, 1975

DENNIS LH, CONRAD ME: Accelerated intravascular coagulation in a patient with Korean hemorrhagic fever. Arch Intern Med 121:499, 1968

FARMER TW, JANEWAY CA: Infections with the virus of lymphocytic choriomeningitis. Medicine 21:1, 1942

FRAME JD et al: Lassa fever, a new virus disease of man from West Africa: I. Clinical description and pathological findings. Am J Trop Med Hyg 19:670, 1970

GREISMAN SE: Capillary observations in patients with hemorrhagic fever and other infectious illnesses. J Clin Invest 36:1688, 1957

HIRSCH MS et al: Lymphocytic choriomeningitis infection traced to a pet hamster. N Engl J Med 291:610, 1974

JOHNSON KM et al: Hemorrhagic fever of Southeast Asia and South America. A comparative approach. Prog Med Virol 9:105, 1967

LEE HW et al: Isolation of the etiologic agent of Korean Hemorrhagic Fever. J Infect Dis 137:298, 1978

MACKENZIE RB et al: Epidemic hemorrhagic fever in Bolivia: I. A preliminary report of the epidemiologic and clinical findings in a new epidemic area in South America. Am J Trop Med Hyg 13:620, 1964

MERTENS PE et al: Clinical presentation of Lassa fever cases during the hospital epidemic at Zorzor, Liberia, March–April 1972. Am J Trop Med Hyg 22:780, 1973

MEYER HM JR et al: Central nervous syndromes of "viral" etiology: Study of 713 cases. Am J Med 29:334, 1960

MONATH TP et al: Lassa fever in the Eastern Province of Sierra Leone, 1970–1972: II. Clinical observations and virological studies on selected hospital cases. Am J Trop Med Hyg 23:1140, 1974

POWELL GM: Hemorrhagic fever. A study of 300 cases. Medicine 33:97, 1954

RUBINI ME et al: Renal residuals of acute epidemic hemorrhagic fever. Arch Intern Med 106:378, 1960

SHEEDY JA et al: The clinical course of epidemic hemorrhagic fever. Am J Med 16:619, 1954

VANZEE BE et al: Lymphocytic choriomeningitis in University hospital personnel. Clinical features. Am J Med 58:803, 1975

ZWEIGHAFT RM et al: Lassa fever: Response to an imported case. N Engl J Med 297:803, 1977

192 DISEASES CAUSED BY SLOW VIRUSES

DONALD H. HARTER

Slow virus diseases are characterized by a long asymptomatic period, often on the order of months or years, between the introduction of the infectious agent and the appearance of clinical illness.

The factors responsible for this protracted incubation period have not been defined. Viruses causing slow infections do not appear to have any unique or common features, and the slowness of the disease may be due in large measure to the manner in which the host reacts or accommodates to the virus.

Some slow viruses provoke a conventional inflammatory response during the time they are clinically silent; others are able to reside within cells for long periods without causing detectable cytopathic changes. The role of immunity in slow virus infection is largely unknown. Some slow virus infections occur in the presence of elevated levels of circulating antibodies; in others, there may be no detectable immune response. Viruses such as poliovirus and echovirus, which ordinarily cause a rapidly evolving illness, cause persistent or chronic infections of the central nervous system in immunodeficient patients.

In animals, slow viruses are known to produce a variety of pulmonary, hepatic, renal, and neurologic disorders. In addition to viral hepatitis, there are five definitely identified slow virus infections of human beings. These are five infrequently encountered neurologic diseases: *kuru, Creutzfeldt-Jakob disease, progressive multifocal leukoencephalopathy, subacute sclerosing panencephalitis,* and *progressive rubella encephalitis.* Kuru and Creutzfeldt-Jakob disease share common neuropathologic features and are referred to as the *subacute spongiform virus encephalopathies.* Although these diseases have been shown to be of infectious etiology by the transmission of neurologic illness to higher primates, the causative agents are still incompletely characterized. Viruses have been recovered from the nervous system of patients with subacute sclerosing panencephalitis, progressive multifocal leukoencephalopathy, and progressive rubella encephalitis, but the pathogenesis of these disorders is still largely unknown. At present, there is no consistently effective therapy for any of the five diseases.

KURU Kuru, or "trembling with fear," is a progressive and fatal neurologic disorder which occurs exclusively among natives of the New Guinea Highland.

Difficulty in walking is usually the first sign of kuru. This usually progresses from a minor disturbance in gait rhythm to marked side-to-side lurching and staggering. Eventually, ambulation becomes incoordinated, and the patient is unable to use his or her limbs. As the disease progresses, cerebellar involvement (intention tremor, inability to perform rapid alternating movements, slurring of speech, hypotonia), abnormal involuntary movements resembling myoclonus, athetosis, or chorea, and convergent strabismus appear. There are no blood or cerebrospinal fluid abnormalities. Dementia develops in the later phases of the disease. The illness terminates fatally in 4 to 24 months, usually from decubitus ulcers or bronchopneumonia. Approximately 80 percent of adults afflicted with the disease are women. The incubation period may be more than 30 years in older patients.

Pathologic changes are limited to the central nervous system and include widespread neuronal loss, intense astrocytic and microglial proliferation, loss of myelinated fibers, and the presence of plaque-like bodies. Perivascular cuffing by lymphocytes and mononuclear cells has been observed occasionally.

It was the close similarity between the neuropathologic and clinical findings found in kuru and in scrapie, a slow infectious disease to sheep, that suggested the possibility that kuru was caused by a virus or other infectious agent. The infectious origin of kuru was confirmed subsequently by the appearance of a kuru-like syndrome in chimpanzees 10 to 82 months after intracerebral inoculation of suspensions of brain from human cases. Disease has also been produced in chimpanzees by inoculation of tissues other than brain. The clinical illness in chimpanzees lasts 3 to 11 months. The disease has also been successfully transmitted to a number of New World and Old World monkeys as well as to minks and ferrets. Although a number of known and novel viruses have been recovered from tissue explants prepared from chimpanzees with the kuru syndrome, the specific agent responsible for the disease has not been fully characterized.

Cannibalism has been considered as the probable mode of transmission of kuru. Native custom in New Guinea dictates that marrow, viscera, and brain be cooked and eaten. The agent may be introduced by conjunctival, nasal, or skin contamination during the practice of ritual cannibalism. The marked predilection of kuru for the adult female may be explained by the observation that cannibalism appears more prevalent among women and that males who practice cannibalism seldom eat the bodies of women. The recent influx of foreign settlers into the kuru area has led to increasing rejection of cannibalistic practices, and this, in turn, may be responsible for the progressive decline in the number of cases of kuru since 1960. Oral feeding of kuru brain to chimpanzees has not yet been reported to produce disease.

CREUTZFELDT-JAKOB DISEASE Creutzfeldt-Jakob disease is a fatal degenerative disease of the central nervous system which afflicts persons between 40 and 60 years of age and presents as a rapidly evolving dementia with myoclonic seizures. Unlike kuru, the disease is not geographically limited.

Although Creutzfeldt-Jakob disease may have a diverse clinical presentation, it is usually first manifested by organic mental changes similar to those seen in the presenile dementias. The earliest changes include impairment of reasoning and judgment, memory disturbances, and bizarre behavior. The patient may complain of headaches and distortions in the shape and appearance of objects. Hallucinations, delusional ideas, and confusion occur as the disease progresses, and myoclonic movements and convulsive episodes develop. Ataxia, dysarthria, muscular atrophy, and other signs of anterior horn cell damage may be noted in some cases. Spasticity and rigidity appear later. About 10 percent of cases show a familial pattern of inheritance. The disease progresses rapidly to death within 3 to 12 months, often from intercurrent infection. There are no abnormalities in the cerebrospinal fluid, but the electroencephalogram is usually abnormal.

The cerebrum and cerebellum are affected predominantly. Widespread status spongiosus in gray matter and intense gliosis are seen. Vacuoles are located within the neuropil, within and around neurons. There is a marked proliferation of astrocytes and disappearance of nerve cells. Inflammatory changes are absent. In the spinal cord, anterior horn cells may be damaged or lost, and there may be degeneration of the corticospinal tracts.

A neurologic disease with the clinical and pathologic features of Creutzfeldt-Jakob disease occurs in chimpanzees 11 to 71 months after inoculation with brain suspensions from patients with Creutzfeldt-Jakob disease. It is also possible to transmit the disease to monkeys, the domestic cat, and guinea pigs. The agent persists for many months in tissue cultures of human brain cells without loss of virulence. Neutralizing antibodies to the Creutzfeldt-Jakob agent have not yet been demonstrated in the serums of patients with the disease of primates with the experimental disease.

There is an unexpectedly high incidence of previous brain or eye operations among patients with Creutzfeldt-Jakob disease. Human-to-human transmission has occurred by corneal transplantation and by implantation of contaminated stereotactic electroencephalographic electrodes after an incubation period of 15 to 20 months.

The Creutzfeldt-Jakob agent has been found in lymph nodes, liver, kidney, spleen, lung, cornea, and cerebrospinal fluid of patients afflicted with the disorder. The agent is also present in leukocytes of infected guinea pigs.

Exposure to breath, saliva, nasopharyngeal secretions, urine, or feces of the Creutzfeldt-Jakob patient should not be of special concern, but the patient's blood or cerebrospinal fluid should be considered a potential source of infection. Maximum caution should be taken to avoid accidental percutaneous exposure to blood and cerebrospinal fluid or tissue. Guidelines for the handling of materials from patients with these disorders have been developed. These should be rigorously applied to all patients who have evidence of intellectual deterioration, particularly if it is associated with myoclonic activity, when no space-occupying lesion is demonstrated in the brain.

PROGRESSIVE MULTIFOCAL LEUKOENCEPHALOPATHY This rare neurologic condition, first described in 1958, usually occurs in patients who have leukemia, malignant lymphomas, carcinomatosis, immunosuppressive therapy, or a variety of other chronic disease processes. The disease is consistently associated with disorders of cell-mediated immunity in which deficits in humoral antibody response may or may not coexist.

The disease affects adults of both sexes, and its duration from onset of symptoms to death is 1 to 4 months. The neurologic signs and symptoms show diffuse, asymmetric involvement of the cerebral hemispheres. Hemiplegia, hemianopsia, aphasia or dysarthria, and organic mental changes are frequent; visual field abnormalities and complete or incomplete transverse myelitis may develop. Headache and convulsive seizures are rare, but electroencephalographic abnormalities consisting of diffuse or focal abnormalities are often present. White matter lesions may be recognized in computerized tomographic brain scans. Cerebrospinal fluid is normal in most cases.

The pathologic changes consist of multiple areas of demyelination with little or no perivascular infiltration. The presence of distinctive intranuclear inclusions in oligodendrocytes first suggested that the disease was of a viral etiology. Electron microscopic observations show the intranuclear inclusion bodies to be composed of closely packed spheres, which have the physical dimensions and properties of the polyomavirus genus of the papovaviruses.

By employing tissue cultures derived from human fetal brain it has been possible to recover a new human polyomavirus serotype (JC virus) from the brains of patients with progressive multifocal leukoencephalopathy. A variant of SV40 virus has been incriminated as the causative agent in a few cases. Abundant numbers of virus particles are present in brain. Rapid identification of the virus in brain is possible using fluorescence antibody staining or electron microscopic agglutination with monospecific hyperimmune rabbit serum. Serologic diagnosis using the patient's serum is unreliable.

The virus has not been demonstrated in tissues other than brain; the disease has not been transmitted to animals.

There are isolated reports of clinical remission with cytosine arabinoside, or adenine arabinoside, but viral infection may remain active despite clinical improvement.

Progressive multifocal leukoencephalopathy may result from the activation of a polyomavirus which has been latent in brain or other tissues since childhood infection. Alternatively, there may be certain individuals who fail to acquire immunity in childhood and have their first encounter with the virus when a disease which interferes with cell-mediated immunity develops. The demyelination which occurs may be related to virus-induced damage of oligodendroglia, cells which appear to be required for the normal maintenance of myelin.

SUBACUTE SCLEROSING PANENCEPHALITIS (INCLUSION-BODY ENCEPHALITIS) This progressively fatal disease of children and adolescents has been suspected to be of viral origin since its initial description by Dawson in 1932. Measles virus or a virus very closely related to measles virus has been recovered from the brains of patients with the disease. The disorder may be considered to be a "slow" form of measles encephalitis.

Subacute sclerosing panencephalitis occurs between 4 and 20 years of age; 80 percent of patients are under 11. The disease affects boys three to ten times as frequently as girls. The incidence of the disease has fallen recently. Most patients are from rural areas or small towns. They are entirely well until the disease begins. Onset is usually insidious, and mental deterioration, often expressed by a decline in the patient's schoolwork, is the presenting symptom. Incoordination, ataxia, and myoclonic jerks develop along with abnormalities of the pyramidal and extrapyramidal motor systems. Cortical blindness, papilledema, and optic atrophy may be present, and focal chorioretinitis has been described. A few cases have occurred in association with infectious mononucleosis.

The patient becomes bedridden within 6 to 9 months. Death occurs from superimposed pulmonary or urinary tract infections or from decubiti. Signs of meningeal irritation do not occur.

The cerebrospinal fluid gamma-globulin level, as determined by electrophoresis, quantitative immunochemical assay, or colloidal gold curve, is elevated, but the fluid is otherwise normal. The electroencephalogram typically shows a "burst suppression" pattern characterized by synchronous and symmetric spike and high-voltage slow wave activity. Elevated levels of measles antibody are found in serum and cerebrospinal fluid. Brain biopsy may be required to make a definitive antemortem diagnosis.

Pathologic findings include round-cell infiltration about small cerebral arteries and veins, intranuclear and intracytoplasmic inclusions in neurons and glial cells, and varying degrees of demyelination.

Measles virus is now considered to be the etiologic agent. Electron microscopic studies show that the intranuclear inclusions in brain cells are composed of hollow tubular filaments resembling paramyxovirus internal nucleocapsid component. Staining of brain tissue from patients with the disease demonstrates measles virus antigen in the inclusions. An agent serologically identical with measles virus and having measles virus properties has been recovered from brain by cocultivating cell cultures originated from brain tissue with established laboratory cell lines.

Attempts to transmit the disease to animals have met with variable results. Ferrets inoculated with suspensions of brain from patients with the disease develop a nonfatal neurologic disorder with electroencephalographic changes.

Subacute sclerosing panencephalitis appears many years after the patient's initial experience with rubeola. There is evidence that subacute sclerosing panencephalitis patients have clinical measles at an unusually early age. A few reported cases may have been related to measles vaccination. The risk of subacute sclerosing panencephalitis following measles vaccination appears to be less, however, than the risk following natural measles. The disorder appears to represent an unusual response of the nervous system to measles infection. It is possible that the virus is present in a defective form or that a carrier state is produced wherein cells may continue to elaborate intracellular viral antigen without producing detectable amounts of mature infective virus. Similar virus-cell interactions may be important in the development of other diseases of the central nervous system such as parkinsonism and multiple sclerosis.

PROGRESSIVE RUBELLA ENCEPHALITIS A chronic progressive encephalitis developing in the second decade of life and sharing some of the features of subacute sclerosing panencephalitis has been described in patients with congenital rubella.

Deterioration of mental and motor functions begins after a stable period of 10 or more years. The cerebrospinal fluid has an increased cell count and the protein and IgG levels are elevated. High titers of antibody to rubella virus can be detected in both serum and cerebrospinal fluid. Rubella virus has been recovered from the brain by use of the cocultivation technique.

Unlike subacute sclerosing panencephalitis, patients with rubella panencephalitis have the stigmata of congenital rubella before the onset of progressive disease. Myoclonus is less constant, and the electroencephalogram does not show the "burst suppression" observed in subacute sclerosing panencephalitis. Histologic examination of the brain shows mineralization, but not the inclusion bodies characteristically found in subacute sclerosing panencephalitis.

The progressive rubella encephalitis also resembles the rare cases of juvenile paresis which may occur in patients with congenital syphilis. The immune status of patients with this disorder has not been fully defined, and the pathogenesis of the disease remains obscure.

REFERENCES

AGNARSDÓTTIR G: Subacute sclerosing panencephalitis, in *Recent Advances in Clinical Virology,* AP Waterson (ed). Churchill Livingstone, Edinburgh, 1977, chap 2, p 21

FREEMAN JM: The clinical spectrum and early diagnosis of Dawson's encephalitis. J Pediatr 75:590, 1969

GAJDUSEK DC: Unconventional viruses and the origin and disappearance of Kuru. Science 197:943, 1977

——— et al: Precautions in medical care of, and in handling materials from, patients with transmissible virus dementia (Creutzfeldt-Jakob disease). N Engl J Med 297:1253, 1977

MEULEN V TER et al: Subacute sclerosing panencephalitis: A review. Curr Top Microbiol Immunol 57:1, 1972

MODLIN JF et al: Epidemiologic studies of measles, measles vaccine and subacute sclerosing panencephalitis. Pediatrics 59:505, 1977

PADGETT BL et al: JC papovavirus in progressive multifocal leukoencephalopathy. J Infect Dis 133:686, 1976

RICHARDSON EP: Progressive multifocal leukoencephalopathy. N Engl J Med 265:815, 1961

ROOS R et al: The clinical characteristic of transmissible Creutzfeldt-Jakob disease. Brain 96:1, 1973

WEIL ML et al: Chronic progressive panencephalitis due to rubella virus simulating subacute sclerosing panencephalitis. N Engl J Med 292:994, 1975

ZuRHEIN GM: Association of papova-virions with a human demyelinating disease (progressive multifocal leukoencephalopathy). Prog Med Virol 11:185, 1969

Herpesviruses

193

INFECTIONS WITH HERPES SIMPLEX VIRUS

A. MARTIN LERNER

Herpes simplex virus types 1 and 2 (HSV1, HSV2), sometimes known as *herpesvirus hominis,* establishes diverse relations with humans. Acute disseminated primary infection (gingivostomatitis), chronic infection with continued or intermittent virus shedding (herpes keratitis and herpes labialis), and clinical reactivation occur. Virus multiplies in many tissues, including lymphocytes, and by its intracellular locus is able to escape anti-HSV antibodies. Herpes simplex virus antibody complexes may be infectious, and when this is the case, are called "sensitized virus." Interactions with the complement system are important in neutralizing sensitized virus. Since the decline of poliomyelitis with the development of an effective vaccine, herpes simplex virus encephalitis is the most frequent endemic encephalitis in this country. Type 2 herpes simplex virus is the second most frequent sexually transmitted disease (after gonorrhea). It has been associated with carcinoma of the cervix, but the etiologic association has not been proved.

ETIOLOGY The virus particle consists of DNA, protein, lipid, and carbohydrate. On an average there are 100 parts DNA, 25 parts carbohydrate, and 320 parts phospholipid to 1000 parts protein. Virus DNA is double-stranded with densities of 1.727 (type 1) and 1.729 (type 2). The molecular weight of the virion is about 100×10^6 daltons. By phosphotungstic acid staining on electron microscopy the virion is seen to consist of a roughly spheric central area or "core" of DNA which measures 75 nm in diameter, and a stable "capsid" which measures 100 nm in diameter; it appears to be an icosahedron with a 5:3:2 axial symmetry consisting of 162 capsomeres (9 to 10 nm by 12 to 13.5 nm) of which 150 are hexagonal and 12 pentagonal in cross section, and a surrounding envelope derived from host cell membranes, 145 to 200 nm. Particles appear with or without envelopes [enveloped and/or with or without cores ("full" or "empty")].

Although complete virions are more efficient, both "enveloped" and "naked" particles can infect cells. Phagocytosis of virions by susceptible cells, viropexis, precedes the digestion of virus envelopes and proteins. After initiation of infection, virus absorption is complete in 3 h. New virus infectivity rises sharply from the sixth to the ninth hour, when it levels off. Viral DNA enters the nucleus where new virus DNA is synthesized. Virus proteins are synthesized in the cytoplasm and migrate to the nucleus. The complete virion has a triple-layered envelope. The inner envelope is made within the nucleus, while the second and third are formed by evagination processes at the nuclear and cytoplasmic membranes, respectively. Host materials make up major portions of the envelope. An infected cell may produce about 1000 virus particles, but only 5 to 10 percent are infectious.

BIOLOGIC CHARACTERISTICS By means of neutralization kinetics, hyperimmune unitypic serums in conventional neutralization tests or direct immunofluorescent methods, strains of herpes simplex virus can be readily typed. Type 1 strains are recovered from the eye, nasopharynx, skin (other than thigh or buttocks), and brain in cases of postnatal encephalitis. Type 2 strains are usually related to the adult genital tract. Isolates have been recovered from the penis, cervix, endocervix, vagina, vulva, skin (usually, but not always below the waist), and spinal fluid. In infections of the newborn, HSV2 has been recovered from brain, liver, adrenal, and lung.

Optimal virus isolation occurs in rabbit or baby hamster kidney and human foreskin tissue cultures. Cytopathic effects are usually evident within 72 h after inoculation. However, when isolation of virus by brain biopsy is attempted, trypsinized suspensions of cells, rather than ground tissue suspensions, should be planted, both for primary growth and for cocultivation with HSV-susceptible tissue cultures. Typical of in vitro and in vivo cytopathic effects is the type A inclusion of Cowdry, an eosinophilic mass surrounded by a halo in a nucleus with marginated chromatin (Fig. 193-1).

In addition to site of recovery, a number of other properties separate type 1 from type 2 herpes simplex virus: HSV2 produces (1) larger pocks on the chorioallantoic membrane of embryonated eggs, (2) greater virulence in female mice which have been infected by the genital route, and (3) greater tendency toward formation of giant cells in tissue cultures. These strains also exhibit (4) difference in density and base composition of DNA and (5) antigenic distinctiveness. Likewise, (6) minimal inhibitory concentrations (MIC) of idoxuridine (IDU; 5-iodo-2'-deoxyuridine) for type 1 strains are 6.25 μg/ml, while similar values for type 2 herpesviruses are 62.5 μg/ml.

IMMUNOLOGY Following primary exposure to herpes simplex virus, humoral antibodies appear. Different polypeptides of the virus capsid probably stimulate distinct antibodies which rise and fall, describing separate kinetic curves. In contrast to other antibodies, such as conventional neutralizing, complement-fixing, and passive hemagglutination antibodies, complement-requiring neutralizing antibodies peak during the acute phase of primary infections with HSV1 and fall during convalescence.

After initial exposure IgM antibodies appear in serum within 1 week. In respiratory secretions IgA antibodies form. In cases of encephalitis, antibodies which are produced locally can be measured in cerebrospinal fluid. Seven days after infection IgG antibodies appear in serum, and antiherpesvirus IgM synthesis decreases. Complement-fixing antibodies appear in 14 days. After an initial exposure, complement-fixing antibodies fall to low levels within several months, while neutralizing antibodies persist for many years. Reactivations of infection evoke variable rises in serums of conventional neutralizing or complement-fixing IgG antibodies. There are some low-titered cross-reactions when anti-HSV antibodies are measured against varicella-zoster or cytomegalovirus.

Cellular immunity is also stimulated and may be the more important factor in inhibiting virus multiplication and relapse. Techniques for quantitating cell-mediated responses are being developed but are not yet routinely available.

CLINICAL FINDINGS: HSV1 Primary infection with HSV1 causes *acute gingivostomatitis, rhinitis, keratoconjunctivitis, me-*

FIGURE 193-1

Cowdry type A ("owl-eye") intranuclear inclusions are seen in this hematoxylin-eosin section (600 ×) in the brain of a patient with encephalitis (arrow). [From ESE Hafez et al (eds), The Human Vagina in Health and Disease, Amsterdam, Elsevier/North-Holland, 1978, with permission.]

ningoencephalitis, eczema herpeticum (Kaposi's varicelliform eruption), and *traumatic herpes,* including *herpetic whitlow* and *generalized cutaneous herpes simplex* in burned patients or wrestlers (*herpes gladiatorum*). In immunosuppressed patients initial infection or clinical reactivation may induce esophageal ulceration or interstitial pneumonia.

The incubation period is 2 to 12 days, averaging 6 or 7 days. The route of infection is contact with infected skin or mucosal surfaces. There is little or no evidence to support respiratory contagion by droplets or their dehydrated nuclei. During acute herpetic gingivostomatitis there are fever, irritability, red swollen gums, a vesicular eruption on the mucous membranes of the mouth, oral fetor, and local submaxillary adenopathy. A visit to the dentist may precede an attack. Any portion of the oral mucosa may be affected. Viremia during which the virus is free in plasma or is limited to mononuclear cells may occur. A generalized vesicular eruption may follow and appear in crops. Lesions are generally smaller than those of varicella. In the eczematous infant or adult (Kaposi's varicelliform eruption), large quantities of fluid, electrolytes, and protein may be lost.

Within the tense vesicles is a clear fluid. An impression smear of an opened vesicle demonstrates syncytial giant cells undergoing ballooning degeneration (Fig. 193-2). Intranuclear inclusions are seen. Virus is readily isolated from the fluid; no bacteria are seen by Gram's stain, and none may be cultured. Later, vesicles collapse and ulcerate. Sometimes the nose is the site of primary infection. Tiny vesicles surrounding reddened areolae appear in the nostrils. Usually, there is fever and the anterior cervical lymph nodes enlarge.

Patients contaminate their fingers or those of hospital personnel by introducing infected secretions through unnoticed abrasions, producing *herpetic whitlow* in persons without previous experience with HSV. *Herpetic paronychia* may be caused by HSV1 or HSV2. Painful deep vesicles appear suddenly and spread locally for about a week. The nail may be separated from its matrix by a lesion at its base. Recrudescent relapses may occur at any time, but the initial infection seems to occur in immunologically "virgin" persons. The importance of wearing rubber gloves when working about the mouth and of handwashing in prevention of infection is obvious.

Follicular conjunctivitis (often unilateral) with chemosis, edema of the lids, and conjunctival ulcers may be seen. The cornea may be involved in primary or recurrent infections; most of these infections are due to HSV1. When the cornea is affected, a diffuse epitheliolitis develops with superficial punctate erosions which extend into small dendritic ulcers. If untreated, this ulcer increases in size to form a large, anesthetic "geographic" ulcer. Erosions of the cornea recur. *Deeper interstitial keratitis* with secondary bacterial invasion, hypopyon, iridocyclitis, synechia, and opacification of the lens follows.

Others with preexisting neutralizing antibodies in serums may suffer *recurrent attacks of herpes labialis* or trigeminal neuralgia. Pneumococcal and meningococcal, but not gram-negative infections; menstruation; emotional upset; and other little-understood events seem to trigger recurrent localized episodes. Quiescence and recurrences of herpes labialis may be associated with alternating low and higher titers of virus shedding, but reactivation of latent infection also occurs. In the prodromal and erythema stages of herpes labialis mean virus titers are $< 10^1$ PFU (plaque-forming unit), but when vesiculation occurs 24 h later, fluids contain $10^{4.7}$ PFU of HSV. Herpes simplex virus resides in a quiescent state within sacral or trigeminal ganglia for years, intermittently releasing virus along nerve fibers. After traversing the axon, HSV reaches the skin, and vesiculation occurs.

Encephalitis Occasionally, and for ill-defined reasons, HSV1 begins an ascent from the respiratory epithelium of the nose up the olfactory tract to reach the frontal and temporal areas of the brain. An often fatal or severely damaging necrotizing encephalitis results. The immediate mortality of patients with seizures and paralysis who are in coma is about 38 percent, but the majority of the survivors are severely impaired and unable to live productive lives.

Patients of any age, either sex, and of any socioeconomic status may be affected. About 15 percent of patients who develop herpes simplex virus encephalitis have histories of recurrent herpes labialis. Prodromal illnesses begin 3 to 4 days before admission to the hospital. Various combinations of headache, rhinorrhea, sore throat, fever, nausea, or vomiting are noted. Less frequently photophobia, vertigo, insomnia, or anorexia occurs. One-third of the patients develop concurrent fever blisters during the course of their illness. Personality changes, lethargy, or seizures necessitate hospitalization, but only a few (3 of 15 brain-biopsy-proved cases) have paralysis

FIGURE 193-2

Characteristic intranuclear inclusion bodies of herpes simplex virus infection along with exfoliated multi- and single nucleated cells are shown (high power magnification). Note "ground glass" appearance of nuclear inclusion with peripheral rim of nuclear chromatin (arrow) or scattered polymorphonuclear leukocytes seen in the background. This is a Tzanck impression smear which may be obtained from an opened cutaneous vesicle or from the cervix. (From J W Regan, SF Patten, Cytology of the Female Reproductive Tract, Chicago, American Society of Clinical Pathologists, 1966, with permission.)

or coma at the time of hospitalization. The occurrence of paralysis and coma indicates that irreparable neurologic injury has occurred. In order of frequency, disorientation, personality change, hallucinations, photophobia, ataxia, facial weakness, incontinence of stool or urine, tremors, and amnesia appear. Patients with proved herpes simplex virus encephalitis have been mistaken for inebriates or psychotics. Neurologic signs include stupor, seizures (Jacksonian or generalized), coma, extensor plantar reflexes, nuchal rigidity, motor deficit, cranial nerve palsies, sensory deficit, decorticate and decerebrate posture, abnormal conjugate deviation of eyes, frontal lobe signs (glabella, snout, sucking), asymmetric deep tendon reflexes, and dysphasia. Coma (absence of response to all stimuli) indicates an ominous prognosis.

Leukocyte counts average 13,000 per cubic millimeter with a shift to the left. Cerebrospinal fluid samples are completely normal or contain only a few to several hundred leukocytes which may be predominantly mononuclear or polymorphonuclear. Grossly bloody spinal fluid is an ominous sign of far-advanced disease. Cerebrospinal fluid protein is normal or elevated as high as 250 mg per 100 ml. Glucose in cerebrospinal fluid is usually normal but may be low. In every case electroencephalograms are diffusely abnormal, or show focal lesions in the temporal or frontal regions. The abnormal electroencephalogram is an especially important finding, particularly in cases in which the cerebrospinal fluid is normal. Computerized tomography (CT scans) or carotid angiograms are indicated to rule out an epidural, subdural, or intracerebral hematoma, abscess, or tumor. In a few cases of HSV1 encephalitis, the focal hemorrhagic necrotic mass deviates carotid vessels, and craniotomy may be necessary for differentiation and diagnosis. Significant rises in HSV antibodies in serum do not determine the diagnosis of encephalitis caused by this virus because rises in these antibodies occur nonspecifically with bacterial pneumonias or bacterial meningitis and in uncomplicated herpes labialis and other conditions. Cowdry type A ("owl-eye") intranuclear inclusions may be demonstrated in the brain (Fig. 193-1). Attempts at isolation of other (e.g., enteroviruses) viruses from throat or rectal swabs, urine, and cerebrospinal fluid as well as, when possible, from brain, spinal cord, and vesicular fluid should be made. Paired serums should be tested for high titers of antibody against mumps virus or other agents known to be prevalent at the time of infection.

Isolation of HSV by brain biopsy is the only definitive means of diagnosing HSV encephalitis. Brain biopsy must be done as soon after admission to the hospital as possible before the onset of irreversible paralysis or coma, because if intravenous therapy with adenine arabinoside (ara-A) is begun before the onset of coma, full recovery may occur. Efforts toward earlier definitive nonsurgical diagnosis of HSV encephalitis continue. For example, serial concomitant paired serums (S) and cerebrospinal fluids (CSF) were taken from 8 patients with biopsy-proved HSV encephalitis. These specimen pairs were compared to 28 others from patients with various neurologic conditions. Both before and after reduction with 2-mercaptoethanol, a ratio of S to CSF antibody titers of ≤ 20 with either the passive hemagglutinating (PHA) or immune adherence hemagglutinating (IAHA) antibody tests occurred in three patients prior to biopsy of the brain, and in four patients by the tenth day of neurologic disease. Among controls, a ratio of S to CSF titers >20 was observed in all but four patients, each of whom had easily distinguishable neurologic diagnoses (e.g., HSV2 meningitis, active multiple sclerosis, varicella zoster encephalitis). This work is promising, but it would be better if HSV antigen could be detected in CSF earlier in the course of the disease. Another, perhaps more promising approach, is the early detection of virus-specific glycoproteins in the CSF.

CLINICAL FINDINGS: HSV2 Infection with HSV, type 2, is usually sexually transmitted. In one study seven of eight female contacts of men with penile herpetic infection showed evidence of current HSV genital infection. Similarly, 63 out of 64 HSV isolates from male genitalia and 155 of 162 from the female genital tract were HSV2. This infection is the most common cause of genital vesicles and/or ulcers found in women, and is second only to primary syphilis as the cause of such lesions in males. Teenagers make up one-fourth to one-half of patients with genital herpetic infections.

Neutralizing antibodies to HSV2 are reported to be present in 35.7 percent of patients who subsequently develop carcinoma in situ of the cervix, and are found in only 7.1 percent of matched controls. However, an etiologic relation between carcinoma of the cervix and infection with HSV2 is not established.

During primary infections fever, malaise, and inguinal adenopathy may be seen and viremia may follow. A benign aseptic meningitis has resulted. In the male there may be tiny vesicles on the glans or shaft of the penis, burning, urgency, frequency, and watery discharge. Herpesvirus is easily cultivated from vesicular fluids.

Antibody surveys suggest that 30 to 100 percent of adults have been infected with one or both of the herpes simplex viruses with the greatest incidence being among lower socioeconomic groups. Prostitutes have the highest frequency of HSV2 antibodies. For genital HSV2 infections, there are roughly 300,000 reported episodes each year, an incidence making it second only to gonorrhea among venereal diseases. Case reporting in other than venereal disease clinics is poor, and herpes may indeed be the most frequent of all of the venereal diseases.

Recurring episodes are probably twice as common as initial attacks. The majority of primary cases occur in young adults between the ages of 19 and 27 (mean 26.5 years). The mean age for recurrences is also 26.5 years. During the acute primary or recurrent attacks of genital herpes, the lesions are painful and sexual contacts are generally avoided. Several days later symptoms abate, but virus may still be present, and this is likely the time of greatest contagion. The attack rate with sexual contact is one in three.

Following recovery from an original episode, no further attacks may occur, or recurrences may vary from occasional to frequent. The reasons for the variability in the clinical course are unknown. Viremia probably occurs only during initial episodes when serum antibody is absent. Following primary HSV2 infections, virus follows a retrograde course along sensory nerves to reach spinal dorsal, lumbar, or sacral ganglia. Here the virus remains in a latent stage until lapses in cell-mediated immunity allow retrograde release of virus along nerves to the previously involved sites upon the skin or mucous membrane. Recurrences frequently involve the same locus on skin or mucous membrane.

In women, within several days after sexual relations with an infected partner, paresthesia and burning of the vulva begin and dyspareunia, dysuria, and tenesmus set in. There may be fever, malaise, headache, neuralgia, and tender inguinal nodes as well.

On examination, the skin and mucous membranes of the vulva, genitocrural folds, perianal region, and cervix show crops of 0.5- to 1.5-cm reddened papules which progress to vesicles and then ulcers. The vagina and urethra are affected infrequently. The vesicles on the vaginal vestibule ulcerate within several days, while those on less traumatized or cornified surfaces progress more slowly. Lesions within the vagina consist of mucous patches with collapsed gray, slightly elevated epithelium. The cervix is eroded and may appear as a necrotizing mass with a clear profuse or irritating discharge. Following viremia, similar skin lesions appear at distant sites. A tender enlarged liver and nuchal rigidity attest to the mild hepatitis and benign aseptic meningitis which may accompany primary HSV2 infection in the postnatal period.

Over several days systemic signs resolve, but lesions may persist for weeks. Unless secondary bacterial infection follows, ultimately healing is complete without scarring. The subsequent course is variable: (1) some patients remain well and culture negative indefinitely; (2) others have recurring episodes of differing severity at varying intervals; and (3) still others become symptomatic or asymptomatic HSV2 carriers in their cervical secretions. These patients have an increased incidence of cervical dysplasia.

Approximately two of every three women with primary HSV2 genital infection suffer relapses. Fever, menstruation, and physical or emotional trauma seem important in some re-

currences, but often no obvious inciting cause is recognized. Between clinical episodes the virus remains latent in sensory ganglia. Exogenous reinfection has also been documented occasionally.

During recurrence, the clinical findings are usually milder. Malaise, fever, and adenopathy are often absent and the lesions are localized, less painful, and less numerous. Pain on urination and defecation is absent, and the entire episode subsides within 7 to 10 days. The milder course reflects a stimulated, but not completely effective, humoral and cellular immune response to latent HSV2.

The clinical and laboratory findings in initial and recurrent herpes have been studied carefully. The mean number of lesions at first visit for initial (primary) episodes is 6.3, while it is 4.7 in recurrent (secondary) attacks, but patients sought medical advice earlier in relapses (2.5 days in secondary cases versus 4.6 days in primary cases). All attacks were associated with pain (primary, 96 percent; secondary, 89 percent), which lasted longer in primary episodes (13.0 versus 8.6 days). Virus was usually (87 percent) present in cervical secretions in primary episodes but was found rarely during relapses (4 percent). Lesions persisted for 16.6 days in primary attacks opposed to 10.5 days in relapses. During episodes new vesicles appeared for 10.1 days in primary, but for only 4.7 days in secondary disease. Virus could be recovered from lesions for 8.0 days (primary) versus 4.5 days, (secondary) and from the cervix for 11.4 days (primary) versus 3 days (secondary).

Cytomegalovirus, varicella zoster virus, variola virus, Behçet's disease, drug or contact dermatitis, autoimmune disorders, or infections with herpes simplex viruses may cause clusters of vulvovaginal vesicles or ulcers on an erythematous base. Cytologic examinations from open vesicles, the bases of ulcers, or the cervix (Fig. 193-2) and appropriate attempts at isolation or recognition of virus are necessary for the diagnosis. Comparison of antibody titers in paired serums is also useful in establishing the presence of herpes infection.

Tzanck smears are positive in preparations from fresh lesions in two of three cases. Multinucleated giant cells with or without intranuclear inclusions, epithelial cells, and lymphocytes are present. These findings do not differentiate HSV from varicella zoster virus infection. To perform a Tzanck test, several fresh vesicles are cleansed with alcohol, opened with a no. 22 needle, and a sterile cotton swab or wooden applicator is pressed to the base of the lesion. The swab is smeared onto several clean glass slides. Slides are immersed in 95% alcohol fixed as in Papanicolaou staining. For immunofluorescent staining for HSV2 antigen, slides are dried in air and fixed with acetone. Hematoxylin-eosin, Giemsa's, Papanicolaou's, Wright's, or Leishman's stains (Tzanck test) may be used.

Herpes simplex virus may be transferred from the vagina or cervix by the hand of patient or attendant to other areas of the skin or to the cornea (herpetic keratitis). Patients must be instructed concerning the importance of hand washing; medical personnel must wear gloves and gowns.

When *venereus herpes* occurs in the pregnant mother before the thirty-second week of gestation, the risk of neonatal infection is 10 percent, but when HSV2 is present at the time of delivery, 40 to 80 percent of the offspring are affected. Pregnant women with cytologically proven genital herpes during the first 20 weeks of gestation have a threefold increase in abortions. After the 20th week there is a slight increase in prematurity. In every case, effects upon the woman and fetus are most severe when the infection is a primary exposure.

Within 2 to 12 days after delivery, affected newborns may show conjunctivitis, keratitis, papulovesicular rashes, jaundice, cyanosis, seizures, and gastrointestinal bleeding, reflecting disseminated infection to the skin, eye, liver, central nervous system, adrenal glands, lungs, spleen, and bone marrow. Mortality in disseminated infection approaches 67 percent, and another 18 percent of the neonates survive, albeit with significant morbidity. Only 15 percent survive to develop as healthy babies.

Intrauterine transplacental congenital infection has been proved occasionally. The usual outcome is fetal death. However, mental retardation, microcephaly, microphthalmia, intracranial calcification, retinal dysplasia, and vesicles on the skin have been observed at the time of delivery. If HSV2 infection at the time of delivery is suspected clinically by Papanicolaou smear from the cervix or by culture of HSV2, delivery by cesarean section prior to rupture of the fetal membranes is indicated.

TREATMENT Neither a killed nor attenuated vaccine has been shown to be effective. When there is a history of recurrent herpetic vulvovaginitis coupled with a clinical exacerbation at term, delivery by cesarean section must be considered. If primary herpetic vulvovaginitis is documented during gestation, the fetus may be infected during the mother's viremia, and the indication for cesarean section is less clear.

Idoxuridine (5-iodo-2'-deoxyuridine, IDU) and adenine arabinoside (9β-D-arabinofuranosyladenine, vidarabine, ara-A) are effective topically in herpes simplex virus keratitis. For herpetic keratitis topical IDU is applied in a 0.1% solution every hour during the day and every 2 h during the night. A simpler means of application is a 0.5% ointment four to five times a day. There are no controlled clinical trials to support the efficacy of any local preparation in the treatment of herpes labialis or genital herpes simplex virus infection.

Intravenous ara-A is being evaluated in disseminated perinatal infections and encephalitis. Therapy with intravenous ara-A (15 mg/kg per day for 7 days) should be instituted if a newborn has cutaneous evidence by positive Tzanck smear from a lesion of HSV infection, because such early treatment may prevent dissemination. Interferon, interferon inducers, transfer factor, and corticosteroids have not been shown to be useful in HSV infections. On account of the development of resistance of strains of herpes simplex virus to photoactive heterotricyclic dyes (proflavine, neutral red) and the possible induction of malignant transformation by these agents, this treatment is not recommended.

Adenine arabinoside is now an established antiherpesvirus agent. It has been effective in varicella zoster in immunosuppressed patients (Chap. 185), and when given before the onset of coma in biopsy-proved HSV1 encephalitis, has a good therapeutic index (efficacy/toxicity). Since 1971 it has been used extensively in several university centers. It is active in preventing cytopathic effects in tissue culture of HSV1, HSV2, varicella zoster (VZ) virus, cytomegalovirus, and herpes B and vaccinia viruses. It is much less depressive to the bone marrow than older and now obsolete systemic nucleoside antiviral agents such as idoxuridine or cytosine arabinoside. Ara-A is not an immunosuppressive agent; it is immediately converted within cells by the ubiquitous enzyme adenosine deaminase to hypoxanthine arabinoside (ara-Hx), which, in turn, also has antiviral activity, albeit less than the parent compound. Ara-A specifically inhibits HSV DNA polymerase without inhibiting similar normal enzymes. The mechanism of action of ara-Hx is unknown. Experience to date suggests, but does not prove, that ara-A is useful in disseminated cutaneous HSV1 but is of dubious value in recurrent cutaneous HSV2 or cytomegalovirus infections. Permission must be obtained prior to each experimental use of ara-A.

Ara-A is diluted in 5% dextrose solutions at a ratio of at least 2 ml for each milligram of antiviral compound. Adenine arabinoside is given by slow, continuous intravenous infusions in a dose of 15 mg/kg per day for 10 days. The National Institute of Allergy and Infectious Diseases Collaborative Antiviral Study Group suggests that in suspected cases of HSV encephalitis ara-A should not be given without a brain biopsy and that treatment should be discontinued after 5 days if brain biopsies are negative for HSV. With ara-A, slight depressions in hemoglobin have been noted, and megaloblasts have been seen in the bone marrow. When patients are receiving other immunosuppressive or cytotoxic treatments or have renal insufficiency, toxicity of ara-A may be greater. A transient reversible akinetic mutism has been observed in several patients. Approximately 40 percent of the daily dose of ara-A is excreted in the urine within 24 h.

Considerable effort is being expended in development of antiviral pharmacokinetics so that antiviral drugs may be used predictively. For instance, ara-A and ara-Hx singly exhibit in vitro anti-HSV inhibitory (MIC) and lethal (MLC) activity at concentrations of drug not inhibiting cellular DNA, RNA, or protein synthesis. This in vitro finding may account for the beneficial therapeutic index in humans. An assay for the combined antiviral activity (AVA) in micrograms per milliliter of ara-A equivalents in human body fluids has been developed which is unaffected by the concomitant presence of anti-HSV antibody or interferon. The combined AVA of ara-A plus ara-Hx (the antiviral drug in vivo) is greater than the predicted values of each drug measured individually by chemical methods. Moreover, sustained AVA in serums (approximately 10 μg/ml) persists throughout the period of treatment. It is clear that the true AVA of ara-A is expressed intracellularly, and concentrations of drug within cells have not yet been measured by microbiologic assay.

REFERENCES

BARINGER JR: Recovery of herpes simplex virus from human sacral ganglions. N Engl J Med 291:828, 1974

BRYSON T et al: Determination of plaque inhibitory activity of adenine arabinoside (9β-D-arabinofuranosyladenine) for herpesvirus using an adenosine deaminase inhibitor. Antimicrob Agents Chemother 6:98, 1974

CHAMPNEY KJ et al: Anti-herpesvirus activity in human sera and urines after administration of adenine arabinoside (in vitro and in vivo synergy of adenine arabinoside and arabinosylhypoxanthine in combination). J Clin Invest 62:1142, 1978

CRANE LR, LERNER AM: Herpetic whitlow: A manifestation of primary infection with herpes simplex virus type 1 or type 2. J Infect Dis 137:856, 1978

LAUTER CB et al: Microbiological assays and neurological toxicity during use of adenine arabinoside in humans. J Infect Dis 134:75, 1976

LEVINE DP et al: Simultaneous serum and CSF antibodies in herpes simplex virus encephalitis. JAMA 240:356, 1978

MARKOWITZ A, LERNER AM: Virus infections of the vagina, in The Human Vagina: In Health and Disease, ESE Hafez, TN Evans (eds). Amsterdam, Elsevier/North-Holland, 1978 p 451

NAHMIAS AJ, JOSEY WE: Epidemiology of herpes simplex viruses 1 and 2, in Viral Infections of Humans: Epidemiology and Control, AS Evans (ed). New York, Plenum, 1976 p 253

SHIPMAN C JR et al: Antiviral activity of arabinosyladenine and arabinosylhypoxanthine in herpes simplex virus infected KB cells: Selective inhibition of viral deoxyribonucleic acid synthesis in synchronized suspension cultures. Antimicrob Agents Chemother 9:120, 1976

SPRUANCE SL et al: The natural history of recurrent herpes simplex labialis. N Engl J Med 297:69, 1977

TERNI M et al: Aseptic meningitis in association with herpes progenitalis. N Engl J Med 285:503, 1971

WHITLEY RJ et al: Adenine arabinoside therapy of biopsy-proved herpes simplex encephalitis. NIAID Collaborative Antiviral Study. N Engl J Med 294:289, 1976

———— et al: Adenine arabinoside therapy of herpes zoster in the immunosuppressed. NIAID Collaborative Antiviral Study. N Engl J Med 294:1193, 1976

WILLIAMS BB et al: Inhibitory and lethal concentrations of 9β-D-arabinofuranosyladenine and its hypoxanthine derivative versus herpes simplex virus, type 1. J Lab Clin Med 89:687, 1977

————, LERNER AM: Some previously unrecognized features of herpes simplex virus encephalitis. Neurology 28:1193, 1978

194
CYTOMEGALIC INCLUSION DISEASE (SALIVARY GLAND VIRUS DISEASE)

C. GEORGE RAY

DEFINITION Cytomegalic inclusion disease (CID) is a viral infection which can affect human beings at all ages beginning with conception. The agent was initially called *salivary gland virus* and was thought to be primarily responsible for occasional cases of disseminated, fatal illness in newborn infants, or subclinical salivary gland involvement only. Since its initial cultivation in 1956, the virus has been demonstrated to cause a broad spectrum of disease in humans. In adults the manifestations are frequently those of an illness like infectious mononucleosis, or may constitute a terminal complication of chronic debilitating disease.

ETIOLOGY Cytomegalovirus (CMV) belongs to the herpesvirus group and produces large, intranuclear (10 to 15 nm), and inconspicuous cytoplasmic (2 to 4 nm) inclusions which occur in all types of normal and neoplastic tissues. The agent is affected by temperature and other environmental factors. Low temperatures ($-80°C$) with added stabilizers are needed for shipment and storage. Several antigenically heterogeneous, but closely interrelated, strains have been isolated which are largely species-specific for man and grow in human fibroblast cultures. Of the various immunologic procedures available for diagnosis, the complement fixation test is most widely used, since the different human strains share a common complement-fixing antigen. Species-specific CMV occurs in many different animals and animal models. The mouse CMV systems are particularly important in the experimental study of the infection.

EPIDEMIOLOGY The infection is worldwide and, in this country, highest prevalence rates are found among young, preschool children of low socioeconomic background. CMV infection may be congenital but is more often acquired during the first year of life. At birth 0.5 to 2 percent of infants have been found to be excreting virus in the urine, and by 12 months of age, between 9 and 60 percent of infants in various population groups have acquired infection, with viruria. Among healthy adults, asymptomatic excretion rates are usually less than 1 percent; in late pregnancy, urine and/or uterine cervical virus excretion increases to between 2 and 13 percent. Complement-fixing antibody is relatively infrequent in infancy, increases during childhood, and is present in about 35 to 80 percent of adults. The virus persists in the host for a long time, perhaps indefinitely, and is excreted in saliva, urine, and semen even

in the presence of antibody. Breast milk and feces may also transmit the infection. Close and prolonged contact appears necessary for efficient transmission of the infection. Venereal transmission appears to be common among young adults. Transplacental passage of the virus produces congenital infection, and perinatal infection may follow exposure to the virus in the infected cervix uteri during delivery. In adults CID may represent either activation of latent infection or may be newly acquired. It can also be transmitted by transfusion of whole blood; the risk of infection per unit of fresh blood transfused has been estimated as between 5 to 7 percent. The majority of these infections, however, are subclinical, and only detectable by serologic conversion.

PATHOGENESIS Localized or systemic CID which may be latent or active occurs in hematopoietic and lymphocytic-reticular disorders (various anemias, leukemias, lymphomas), other chronic debilitating disease, and often during immunosuppression. It is a potential complication of any therapy which results in an impairment of humoral and/or cellular immunity. Physiologic factors related to age or late pregnancy favor viral proliferation and dissemination. CID may be associated with stillborn, premature, or low-birth-weight infants. Self-limited forms with generally mild clinical manifestations are being recognized more frequently in apparently normal persons.

PATHOLOGY Enlarged cells, 25 to 40 nm in diameter, with the distinctive nuclear inclusions, are the morphologic hallmark of the infection, and are similar in all forms and sites of infection. Infected cells elicit an inflammatory cell response only after cell death. In adults localized infection most commonly consists of interstitial pneumonitis and gastrointestinal ulcers. Less frequently affected are the nasal mucosa, salivary glands, liver, and adrenals. Hepatitis with the distinctive inclusions has been related to CID by serologic studies. In the disseminated form nearly every tissue may be affected, including the central nervous system. Involvement of the latter, however, has been noted most often in the immunosuppressed adult. In infancy the localized form is largely confined to the salivary glands, hence the original designation of salivary gland virus disease. In disseminated disease the more common sites are salivary glands, kidney, liver, lung, pancreas, gastrointestinal tract, thyroid, adrenal, and central nervous system. Multiple infections are frequently associated with CID. Bacterial, fungal, and various forms of other herpesvirus infections are common. Concomitant infection with pertussis, toxoplasmosis, and *Pneumocystis carinii* are frequent. Interesting interactions between CMV and toxoplasmosis and Newcastle disease virus have been noted experimentally.

CLINICAL MANIFESTATIONS While the majority of CMV infections are occult, there are a variety of manifestations of active disease which mimic other conditions. The categories of clinical infection can be grouped as follows: (1) congenital CMV, (2) perinatally or postnatally acquired CMV, (3) acquired CMV in healthy children and adults (including the CMV mononucleosis syndrome), (4) disseminated CMV in immunosuppressed patients, and (5) acquired or reactivated CMV infection in organ or bone-marrow transplant recipients.

Congenital CMV infection This disease can be detected virologically in 0.5 to 2 percent of all newborns. Of these, an estimated 10 to 15 percent will incur some tissue damage, with a risk of permanent sequelae or death. The greatest risk appears to be among infants born to women who experienced a primary infection during that pregnancy and are actively shedding virus at parturition. The clinical manifestations range from mild jaundice, respiratory distress, and failure to thrive to a variable constellation of signs including hepatosplenomegaly with hepatitis and cirrhosis, purpura, maculopapular exanthems, encephalitis, microcephaly with microgyria, growth retardation, chorioretinitis, acute or chronic pneumonitis, hemolytic anemia, and pathological fractures of long bones. It has been estimated that 10 percent of newborns with virologically proved congenital infection will develop significant neurological impairment, usually in the form of sensorineural hearing loss and variable degrees of mental retardation. This risk also extends to some infants with asymptomatic or mild congenital CMV. The differential diagnosis includes congenital rubella, enteroviruses, syphilis, and toxoplasmosis; bacterial sepsis must also be considered in some cases.

Perinatally or postnatally acquired CMV infection in infants
This is usually a much more subtle disease, with little or no risk for neurological sequelae, and is usually asymptomatic. The signs may include poor weight gain, hepatomegaly with mild to moderate liver function abnormalities, atypical lymphocytosis, and anemia. Occasionally, chronic interstitial pneumonitis has been attributed to infantile-acquired CMV infection, but its primary role as a pathogen is not clear. Recent studies, for example, have shown that CMV may coexist in the pulmonary tissue with other candidate lung pathogens in infants, such as *Chlamydia* and *P. carinii*. Also, there have been rare cases of severe hepatitis and cirrhosis presumed to be related to infantile-acquired CMV infection.

Acquired CMV infection in otherwise healthy children and adults
This disease has been associated with a myriad of disorders. The most common of these is the *CMV mononucleosis syndrome,* an acute febrile illness with relative or absolute lymphocytosis and many atypical lymphocytes. The patient often complains of headache, back and abdominal pain, and sore throat. Rubellalike rashes, usually lasting only 1 or 2 days, have also been noted. The appearance of extensive rash and prolongation of its duration can be aggravated by inadvertent treatment with ampicillin, an event similar to that seen in infectious mononucleosis treated with the same agent. Other findings have included hepatitis with icterus, hemolytic anemia, thrombocytopenia, purpura, pneumonitis, conjunctivitis, myocarditis, pericarditis, arthralgias, and occasional splenomegaly. The heterophile test and ox cell hemolysins are negative, and specific serologies will not confirm an Epstein-Barr virus infection. Liver function tests are frequently abnormal, and elevated cold agglutinin titers are found in severe cases. The disease occurs spontaneously or after perfusion with fresh whole blood (the postperfusion syndrome) and usually resolves without residua in 3 to 6 weeks; however, some patients will continue to experience recurrent fevers and malaise with atypical lymphocytosis for periods as long as 1 year. On the basis of observations of the postperfusion syndrome, the incubation period has been estimated to be 20 to 50 days.

The *differential diagnosis* of acquired CMV mononucleosis most commonly includes Epstein-Barr virus infection and toxoplasmosis. In some patients, particularly those with a protracted illness, autoimmune diseases and hematopoietic malignancies can become a concern. Unlike infectious mononucleosis, CMV does not evoke a heterophile antibody titer, and exudative pharyngitis and significant lymphadenopathy are unusual. CMV mononucleosis is more commonly seen among young adults, while infectious mononucleosis typically affects a slightly younger, although overlapping age group. Acquired toxoplasmosis can usually be differentiated by appropriate serologic testing.

There are other recognized manifestations of acquired CMV infections which may or may not be found in association with the CMV mononucleosis syndrome. These include the Guillain-Barré syndrome, in which it is estimated that as many as one-third of cases may be CMV-related. Occasional cases of acute encephalitis, thyroiditis, ulcerative gastrointestinal disease and protein-losing enteropathies, acute thrombocytopenic purpura, chorioretinitis, and granulomatous hepatitis have also been reported to be associated with CMV. Despite the common occurrence of viruria and inclusion-bearing cells in the kidney, progressive renal disease has not been a problem at any age.

Disseminated CMV in immunosuppressed patients This disease can be manifested as a severe, sometimes fatal form of the CMV mononucleosis syndrome, but atypical lymphocytosis is variable. Major organs involved include the lungs, liver, gastrointestinal tract, central nervous system, and eyes. Signs vary, but frequently include severe pneumonitis, jaundice, diarrhea, fever, and retinitis. The retinitis in such patients is often punctate, exudative, and hemorrhagic, and raises such differential diagnostic considerations as sarcoid, cryptococcosis, toxoplasmosis, and disseminated candidiasis. The interstitial pneumonitis may be difficult to distinguish from opportunistic bacterial, fungal, or protozoon infections, such as *P. carinii;* in fact, it is not uncommon for CMV to coexist with one or more of these pathogens, and a lung biopsy may be required to resolve the diagnosis.

CMV infection in transplant recipients This has become increasingly recognized as a serious problem. The situation is analogous to that of other immunosuppressed patients, but is also complicated by the fact that graft-versus-host reactions can reactivate latent infections and intensify both primary and reactivation disease. For kidney or heart transplant recipients, those who are seronegative before transplantation appear to be at greatest risk for active infection; in the case of renal transplantation there appears to be an even greater risk if the donor is seropositive and the recipient is seronegative for CMV, suggesting transmission of the primary infection via the transplanted organ. On the other hand, bone marrow recipients appear to have a higher risk of serious disease if they possess preexisting CMV antibodies, and no clear relation regarding risk could be correlated with the antibody status of the donor. While the spectrum of clinical disease is similar to that described for immunosuppressed patients, the major problems of CMV infection in transplantation are most often related to progressive, often fatal, interstitial pneumonia, a significant predisposition to pulmonary bacterial superinfection, and an increased incidence of graft rejection.

DIAGNOSIS Virus isolation from blood, body fluids, or tissues establishes the presence of active infection but cannot always be equated with disease, particularly in groups in which high asymptomatic infection rates are known to occur. Demonstration of significantly rising antibody titers are of some help, particularly in cases of acquired disease. However, spontaneous, wide fluctuations of complement-fixing antibody titers in healthy individuals have been demonstrated in one longitudinal study, and this rather unique lability of specific antibody tests should also be kept in mind when interpreting results. In congenital infections, the finding of elevated IgM-specific CMV antibody in the newborn generally correlates with active disease. However, false-positive results due to circulating rheumatoid factor have been found in some infants, and this possibility must be considered when interpreting the data. Morphologic demonstration of CMV inclusions is a relatively insensitive method of diagnosis, compared with cultures and serology. Roentgenographic and laboratory findings are nonspecific except for the lymphocytosis and atypical lymphocytes in CMV mononucleosis.

TREATMENT No specific therapy is available. Trials of interferon, interferon inducers, immunopotentiators such as levamisole, and viral antagonists such as adenine arabinoside have been limited, and without clearly beneficial results. A live, attenuated CMV vaccine is also under investigation, but is not available for routine use. The first use for such vaccine in the future, if it is at all effective, may be in the pretransplantation immunization of seronegative organ recipients.

REFERENCES

DOWLING P et al: Cytomegalovirus complement fixation antibody in Guillain-Barré syndrome. Neurology 27:1153, 1977

HANSHAW JB: Congenital cytomegalovirus infection: A fifteen year perspective. J Infect Dis 123:555, 1972

JORDAN MC et al: Spontaneous cytomegalovirus mononucleosis: Clinical and laboratory observations in nine cases. Ann Intern Med 79:153, 1973

MURRAY HW et al: Cytomegalovirus retinitis in adults. Am J Med 63:574, 1977

NEIMAN PE et al: A prospective analysis of interstitial pneumonia and opportunistic viral infection among recipients of allogeneic bone marrow grafts. J Infect Dis 136:754, 1977

PASS RF et al: Productive infection with cytomegalovirus and herpes simplex virus in renal transplant recipients: Role of source of kidney. J Infect Dis 137:556, 1978

PHILLIPS CA et al: Cytomegalovirus encephalitis in immunologically normal adults. JAMA 238:2299, 1977

PLOTKIN SA et al: Clinical trials of immunization with the Towne 125 strain of human cytomegalovirus. J Infect Dis 134:470, 1976

RAND KH et al: Increased pulmonary superinfections in cardiac-transplant patients undergoing primary cytomegalovirus infection. N Engl J Med 298:951, 1978

REYNOLDS DW et al: Congenital cytomegalovirus infection: Relation to auditory and mental deficiency. N Engl J Med 290:291, 1974

SUWANSIRIKUL S et al: Primary and secondary cytomegalovirus infection. Arch Intern Med 137:1026, 1977

WANER JL et al: Patterns of cytomegaloviral complement-fixing antibody activity: A longitudinal study of blood donors. J Infect Dis 127:538, 1973

WELLER TH: The cytomegaloviruses: Ubiquitous agents with protean clinical manifestations. N Engl J Med 285:203, 269, 1971

195

EPSTEIN-BARR VIRUS INFECTIONS, INCLUDING INFECTIOUS MONONUCLEOSIS

JAMES C. NIEDERMAN

DEFINITION Epstein-Barr virus (EBV), a lymphotropic herpes virus, infects all human populations. Primary infection in childhood is usually asymptomatic, but in adolescence or early adulthood, clinical manifestations of infectious mononucleosis (IM) develop in approximately 50 percent of infections. The characteristic clinical picture consists of fever, pharyngitis, lymphadenopathy, an increase of peripheral lymphocytes with a high proportion of atypical cells, and the development of transient heterophile and persistent EBV antibody responses.

ETIOLOGY EBV, which has the structural and immunologic characteristics of a member of the herpes group, was originally discovered by electron microscopic studies of tumor cells from biopsies of Burkitt's lymphoma grown in tissue culture. EBV antibodies measured by immunofluorescence techniques, complement fixation, immunodiffusion, enzyme-linked immunosorbent assay (ELISA), and virus neutralization are consistently absent before infectious mononucleosis, regularly develop during the course of the disease, and persist with little change for many years thereafter. In addition to IgG, EBV-specific IgM antibody is present during acute infectious mononucleosis in serums obtained 7 to 70 days after onset, and usually persists for several months.

Further evidence of a causative relationship is the presence of EBV in leukocytes cultured from serums of patients with acute mononucleosis as well as from subjects with a past history of the disease. The classical heterophil antibody of infectious mononucleosis has been produced experimentally in squirrel monkeys inoculated with EBV-transformed autologous leukocytes. In addition, inadvertent transmission of EBV by transfusion has been reported and in several instances was associated with the development of clinical infectious mononucleosis, including heterophil antibody.

EPIDEMIOLOGY Infectious mononucleosis has been recognized in all parts of the world. Although no yearly or seasonal trends are present in the general population, early fall and spring are periods of high frequency among college students. The most characteristic epidemiologic feature of the disease is its occurrence among young adults, especially in the 15- to 25-year age group.

Seroepidemiologic studies have demonstrated that the absence of EBV antibody correlates with susceptibility to infectious mononucleosis and its presence indicates immunity. The age at which infection is acquired is related to socioeconomic factors and hygienic environment. Among disadvantaged groups such as children living in certain tropical countries, antibody is acquired early. In contrast, in middle and upper socioeconomic groups, only 50 to 60 percent have detectable antibody during adolescent years and at the time of entry into college. Among these individuals, infectious mononucleosis is a well-recognized disorder. Studies measuring both apparent and inapparent infections suggest a clinical/subclinical ratio of 1:2 to 1:3 in young adults.

When EBV infection develops in early childhood, a mild and nonspecific or an inapparent illness occurs, both of which are associated with the appearance and persistence of specific antibody. If primary infection is delayed until adolescence or young adulthood, the clinical response is frequently typical infectious mononucleosis with the development of both heterophil and EBV antibodies.

Epidemiologic and laboratory evidence has suggested that transmission of EBV occurs through the oropharyngeal route

TABLE 195-1

Recovery of EBV in pharyngeal excretions from 25 cases of infectious mononucleosis

Time after onset of symptoms, days	No. specimens tested	No. specimens positive	Percent positive
0–14	16	13	81.3
15–28	12	10	83.3
29–150	11	11	100.0
>150	3	2	66.7
Total	42	36	85.7

SOURCE: *Miller et al.*

during close personal contact. Table 195-1 indicates that EBV is present in small amounts in throat washings from 1 week to many months after clinical illness.

This prolonged carrier state following clinical infectious mononucleosis, and perhaps also after inapparent EBV infection, may serve as a principal source of transmission. Investigations utilizing the presence of EBV antibody as an index of immunity have confirmed the low contagiousness of both the infection and the disease among susceptible college roommates; secondary attack rates for EBV infection within family units have also been low.

PATHOLOGY Generalized involvement of lymphoid tissue with lymphadenopathy, nasopharyngeal lymphoid hyperplasia, and splenomegaly is the outstanding pathologic feature. Widespread focal and perivascular aggregates of mononuclear cells, including atypical lymphocytes, are found throughout the body. Nonspecific hyperplastic changes in lymph nodes are present without infiltration of the capsule or surrounding tissues. Nonlymphoid organs and tissues, including liver, heart, kidneys, and central nervous system, are also infiltrated, and changes in these organs may be associated with functional disturbances. Bone marrow hyperplasia develops, and occasionally small granulomas are present.

MANIFESTATIONS In young adults an incubation period of 30 to 50 days has been suggested on the basis of contact infection studies. Infectious mononucleosis associated with the development of heterophil and EBV antibody has occurred in several patients 5 weeks following blood transfusion. Children appear to have shorter incubation periods, in the range of 10 to 14 days, but there is relatively little information on this point.

During a prodromal period of 3 to 5 days, mild symptoms, including headache, malaise, and fatigue, are common. Frank clinical features usually present over the next 7 to 20 days; they are variable in severity, but in over 80 percent of cases include fever, sore throat, and cervical adenopathy. In adults, temperature elevations which peak at 101 to 103°F may persist for 7 to 10 days. In severe cases, a daily rise in temperature to 105°F may continue even longer. On the other hand, children often have little or no fever accompanying the infection.

Sore throat occurs in the first week and is the most common feature of infectious mononucleosis. Hyperplasia of pharyngeal lymphoid tissue with inflammation and edema develops. A grayish white exudative tonsillitis persisting for 7 to 10 days is present in approximately 50 percent of cases. The uvula and palatal arch frequently have a gelatinous appearance. *Palatine petechiae*, located near the border of the hard and soft palate, are observed in about one-third of patients toward the end of the first week of illness. Although highly suggestive, their presence is not pathognomonic of the disease.

Lymph node enlargement is a hallmark of infectious mononucleosis. The onset is gradual, and anterior and posterior cervical chains are most commonly involved. Generalized adenopathy, including axillary, epitrochlear, and inguinal nodes, may also develop during the course of the disease. The nodes are affected singly or in groups and may be small or grapesized; they are firm, discrete, and moderately tender on palpation.

Splenomegaly occurs in approximately one-half the patients, and enlargement is greatest during the second and third weeks of illness. Although extremely rare, splenic rupture is one of the few potentially fatal complications of the disease.

Percussion tenderness over the liver and hepatomegaly develop in only about 10 percent of patients, but the majority (90 percent) have abnormal liver function test results which persist for several weeks. Jaundice occurs in no more than 4 to 5 percent of cases and is usually mild and uncomplicated.

During early stages of the disease a transient faint erythematous maculopapular eruption on the trunk and extremities is present in about 10 percent of patients. The rash often resembles rubella, but may be urticarial, hemorrhagic, or scarlatiniform in nature. *Bilateral supraorbital edema* may also be a transient finding early in the course of disease.

A wide variety of neurologic manifestations has been described, but they occur only rarely. Aseptic meningitis, encephalitis, blurred vision, coma, acute cerebellar syndrome, and the Guillain-Barré syndrome may appear at any time during the illness. Most patients experience complete recovery from central nervous system involvement; however, severe paralysis and/or respiratory incapacity occur in rare instances and are potentially fatal complications.

LABORATORY FINDINGS **Blood picture** Essential to the diagnosis of infectious mononucleosis is an increase in relative and absolute numbers of lymphocytes and monocytes, including 10 to 20 percent atypical forms. Early in disease this is the result of increased numbers of both B and T cells, and later of a predominance of T lymphocytes. The atypical lymphocytes are large cells with oval, horseshoe-shaped, or indented nuclei and basophilic, vacuolated foamy cytoplasm. Nuclear chromatin is usually dense and irregular, and nucleoli are rarely seen. During the first week of illness, either the total leukocyte count is normal or there may be a leukopenia due to granulocytopenia. The total count then rises to between 10,000 and 20,000 leukocytes per cubic millimeter by the second or third week of illness; rarely, the number of leukocytes may range as high as 50,000 per cubic millimeter. Characteristic leukocyte changes often persist for 4 to 8 weeks or more. Anemia is rare in infectious mononucleosis, but hemolytic anemia has been reported as a complication. Slight to moderate thrombocytopenia, which is usually symptomless, has been recognized during the early weeks of disease. In a few reported cases, the clinical picture has suggested idiopathic thrombocytopenic purpura.

Serologic diagnosis The serum of IM patients characteristically contains heterophil antibodies, i.e., agglutinins against sheep red blood cells, in high titer. Heterophil antibody is associated with the IgM fraction of serum and usually declines over a period of 3 to 6 months. In general, the higher the titer developed during clinical illness, the longer the antibodies will remain detectable in convalescence. Though a nonspecific serologic response, the heterophil antibody of infectious mononucleosis differs from other antibodies in human serums that also agglutinate sheep red blood cells. The latter are found at low levels in normal human serums and in high titers in serum sickness. Differentiation is based on absorption techniques utilizing guinea pig kidney and beef erythrocytes. The sheep cell agglutinins of infectious mononucleosis are completely absorbed by beef red blood cells but not by guinea pig kidney. Serum sickness agglutinins are absorbed by both, whereas nonspecific Forssman agglutinins are absorbed only by guinea pig kidney. A high order of specificity has now been achieved with other qualitative heterophil antibody tests which utilize formalin-treated horse red blood cells, ox red blood cells, and enzyme-treated and -untreated sheep cells.

Usually sheep cell agglutinins are present in the first week of illness, but they may be delayed in appearance. During the first 2 weeks after onset of the illness, 60 percent of young adult patients develop a positive heterophil antibody test. This percentage increases to 80 to 90 percent by the end of 1 month.

The height of the titer is not related to severity of the disease or to the degree of lymphocytosis. In the presence of clinical and hematologic findings, a sheep cell agglutinin titer of 1:224 or higher before guinea pig kidney absorption and 1:28 after absorption has diagnostic significance. In the beef cell hemolysin test, a titer of 1:280 or higher may be considered significant. A rising titer in early stages of disease is the best criterion.

During acute infectious mononucleosis an increase in total serum IgM levels up to 100 percent over control values and a 50 percent increase in IgG levels has been observed. Other protein alterations associated with the IgM fraction which may be present in the disorder include cold agglutinating antibody and transiently positive serologic tests for syphilis and rheumatoid factor. In IM, the presence of EBV antibody is a regular feature. Prospective clinical studies have shown that the disease occurs only in individuals who lack antibodies to EBV; patients become seropositive in almost all cases by the time acute symptoms appear. As measured by immunofluorescence techniques, levels of 1:80 to 1:320 are often found during early illness, and in only 15 to 20 percent of cases are significant antibody rises demonstrable. Rarely, the development of both EBV and heterophil antibodies is delayed several weeks following onset of symptoms. The relationships between clinical features and antibody levels in typical heterophil positive cases are shown in Fig. 195-1. In addition to development of antibody to EB viral capsid antigen, which is the most widely used clinically, antibodies to early antigen and EBV-specific IgM occur in 75 to 90 percent of patients with acute mononucleosis. Antibodies to other EBV-associated antigen systems (membrane, nuclear, complement-fixing, neutralizing, and immunoprecipitating) are also absent before infection and appear during the course of disease.

No direct correlation has been found between the levels of EBV and heterophil antibodies, nor between the anti-EBV titer and severity of clinical symptoms or hematologic findings. Heterophil antibody levels are highest during the first 4 to 6 weeks after onset, and then decline or disappear after several months. EBV antibodies also reach peak titers within 3 to 4 weeks but persist at lower levels for many years thereafter, if not for life. Antibody titers of 1:20 to 1:40 have been demonstrated in serum collected 45 years after laboratory documentation of heterophil-positive IM.

The appearance of EBV antibody has also been demonstrated in cases which have the clinical and hematologic characteristics of IM but do not develop heterophil antibody. These EBV-positive, heterophil-negative cases are apparently frequent in infants and children but rare in adults.

Other laboratory abnormalities   These consist primarily of abnormal liver function tests and may include an elevation in alkaline phosphatase level, retention of bromsulphalein, mild abnormalities in serum glutamic oxaloacetic transaminase and serum glutamic pyruvic transaminase, and mild icterus. With recovery, all these values return to normal.

Acute infectious mononucleosis is associated with depressed cell-mediated immunity manifested by loss of skin hypersensitivity and lymphocyte hyporesponsiveness to in vitro stimulation by a variety of mitogens and specific antigens.

DIAGNOSIS   The main diagnostic features of infectious mononucleosis are (1) irregular fever, sore throat, and lymphadenopathy; (2) an absolute increase in lymphocytes and monocytes exceeding 50 percent and including more than 10 percent atypical lymphocytes in the peripheral blood; (3) the transient appearance of sheep cell agglutinins and beef cell hemolysins; (4) the development of persistent antibody against Epstein-Barr virus; and (5) abnormalities of liver function tests.

Since many of these features are also seen in other diseases, IM may resemble a number of febrile disorders, especially those associated with fever, sore throat, adenopathy, and leukocytosis. In early stages of the disease, it is often difficult to distinguish IM from other forms of febrile exudative pharyngotonsillitis such as *streptococcal infections, exudative tonsillitis of viral etiology, Vincent's angina,* and *diphtheria.* Differentia-

FIGURE 195-1

Scheme of symptoms, antibody responses, and EBV oropharyngeal shedding in typical cases of infectious mononucleosis.

tion depends on the results of throat cultures and the development of the hematologic and serologic features characteristic of infectious mononucleosis.

Diseases with some similarities in hematologic abnormalities such as *acute leukemia* and other lymphoproliferative disorders may be mistaken for IM. Demonstration of very immature leukocytes in blood or bone marrow and the presence of anemia, severe thrombocytopenia, and a negative heterophil antibody test distinguish these disorders from IM.

Cytomegalovirus (CMV) mononucleosis usually involves a slightly older age group, i.e., 20 to 30 years. Splenomegaly, hepatic involvement, and the presence of atypical lymphocytes in blood are common features of this disease, whereas sore throat and cervical adenopathy are usually absent. In transfusion-associated CMV infections, cytomegalovirus is excreted in the urine and a rise in complement-fixing antibody can be demonstrated.

Acute infectious lymphocytosis, a benign disorder of children, should be considered in the differential diagnosis among younger age groups. The majority of these cases are associated with signs of an upper respiratory tract infection; adenopathy is minimal, and splenomegaly is absent. The major feature is leukocytosis consisting of small mature lymphocytes; this abnormal blood picture may persist for 4 to 5 weeks, and occasionally for several months. The heterophil antibody test is negative, and no relationship to EBV antibody has been found.

The prodromal stage of *rubella,* associated with fever, malaise, postauricular and posterior cervical adenopathy, and lymphocytosis, may be indistinguishable from early infectious mononucleosis. A distinguishing feature of the rash of rubella is its invariable presence on the face, while that of IM is prominent on the trunk and usually spares the face; it is rarely as florid as in typical rubella. The appearance of large numbers of atypical lymphocytes in the blood and the development of heterophil and/or EB viral antibodies indicate infectious mononucleosis. Isolation of rubella virus from the throat and demonstration of a rising rubella antibody titer will confirm a diagnosis of rubella.

Acquired *toxoplasmosis* may be associated with fever, generalized adenopathy, splenomegaly, and lymphocytosis. A definitive diagnosis is based on direct isolation of *Toxoplasma gondii* and/or the demonstration of the development of specific serologic responses.

Infectious mononucleosis with jaundice can frequently be confused with *infectious hepatitis.* In hepatitis, fever is often lower and disappears when jaundice develops. Similarly, the presence of atypical lymphocytes is usually transitory during the preicteric phase of hepatitis, and the disease is less frequently associated with splenomegaly and leukocytosis.

TREATMENT Therapy is symptomatic. Antibiotics have no effect on uncomplicated cases of infectious mononucleosis. During the febrile period rest in bed is advisable. Salicylates or other analgesics are usually sufficient to control headache and discomfort from sore throat. Gargling and irrigation with saline solutions provide symptomatic relief of pharyngitis and stomatitis. As a rule, most patients recover uneventfully on this

regimen in 2 to 4 weeks, with gradual return to normal activities. Patients with splenomegaly should be cautioned against heavy lifting and strenuous athletics until splenic enlargement has disappeared.

In patients with severe toxic exudative pharyngotonsillitis associated with extensive pharyngeal edema, corticosteroids are useful to induce a prompt anti-inflammatory effect. A short course of prednisone may be administered, starting with 40 to 60 mg the first day and decreasing this total dose 5 mg daily over 7 to 10 days. Steroids are not necessary in treatment of the usual patient with IM. However, full dosages of steroids should be employed in the management of severe complications, including (1) airway obstruction, in which a tracheostomy may also be required, (2) neurologic complications, (3) hemolytic anemia and thrombocytopenic purpura, and (4) myocarditis and pericarditis.

Approximately 20 percent of patients with infectious mononucleosis experience concurrent beta hemolytic streptococcal pharyngotonsillitis and should receive antibiotic treatment; a full 10-day course of penicillin V 250 mg four times daily, erythromycin 250 mg four times daily, or procaine penicillin G 600,000 units every 12 h, should be administered. Ampicillin should be avoided because of the high frequency of erythematous macular or maculopapular skin rashes associated with the use of this drug in patients with infectious mononucleosis.

Severe abdominal pain is rare in IM except in association with splenic rupture. This serious complication requires massive transfusions and immediate splenectomy.

REFERENCES

CARTER RL, PENMAN HG: *Infectious Mononucleosis.* Oxford, Blackwell, 1969

EPSTEIN MA, ACHONG BG: Pathogenesis of infectious mononucleosis. Lancet 2:1270, 1977

EVANS AS et al: Seroepidemiologic studies of infectious mononucleosis with EB virus. N Engl J Med 279:1121, 1968

HENLE G et al: Relation of Burkitt's tumor associated herpes-type virus in infectious mononucleosis. Proc Nat Acad Sci USA 59:94, 1968

———: Observations on childhood infections with Epstein-Barr virus. J Infect Dis 121:303, 1970

———: Antibodies to Epstein-Barr virus-associated nuclear antigen in infectious mononucleosis. J Infect Dis 130:231, 1974

MANGI RJ et al: Depression of cell-mediated immunity during acute infectious mononucleosis. N Engl J Med 291:1149, 1974

MILLER G et al: Prolonged oropharyngeal excretion of Epstein-Barr virus following infectious mononucleosis. N Engl J Med 288:299, 1973

NIEDERMAN JC et al: Infectious mononucleosis: Clinical manifestations in relation to EB virus antibodies. JAMA 203:205, 1968

———: Prevalence, incidence and persistence of EB virus antibody in young adults. N Engl J Med 282:361, 1970

———: Infectious mononucleosis: Epstein-Barr virus shedding in saliva and the oropharynx. N Engl J Med 294:1355, 1976

Miscellaneous and presumptive viral infections

196

WARTS AND MOLLUSCUM CONTAGIOSUM

LAWRENCE COREY

WARTS

DEFINITION Warts are benign neoplasms of the skin and contiguous mucous membranes caused by a member of the papovavirus group.

ETIOLOGY Warts or papillomata of several different clinical types are caused by the human papovavirus. Papovaviruses are spherical, small, double-stranded, DNA-containing viruses which replicate in the nucleus of the cells. Viruses composing the papovavirus group of agents include (1) the papilloma viruses (human wart virus, Schope papilloma virus of rabbits), (2) the polyoma viruses of mice, and (3) the vacuolating viruses of monkeys (SV40). These agents have been shown to induce the transformation of cells in tissue culture as well as to cause tumors in experimental animals. Human wart virus has been demonstrated by electron microscopy in extracts and thin sections of warts, and it has been propagated in a human epithelial cell line. Experimentally, cell-free filtrates of human warts will induce the formation of these lesions at the inoculated skin sites of human volunteers. The incubation period based upon these experimental inoculation studies varies from 1 to 20 months (mean 3 to 4 months).

EPIDEMIOLOGY Warts are found in approximately 7 to 10 percent of the population, with the highest frequency in the early teen-age years. They occur mainly on the skin areas unprotected by clothing except for the feet. Person-to-person transmission by direct contact with wart tissue and indirectly by virus contamination through contaminated secretions or instruments may occur. Autoinoculation of virus to contiguous or distant sites is frequent. Although warts of several animal species are caused by similar viruses, convincing evidence of interspecies transmission is lacking.

PATHOLOGY AND PATHOGENESIS The skin lesions induced by the wart virus are due to an abnormal proliferation of epidermal cells. In normal epidermis, cell division occurs mainly in the basal layer; however, in the wart, mitotic figures are seen in cells several layers higher. In addition, there is thickening of the cell layers, elongation and broadening of the interpapillary processes with the development of long, thin papilli containing blood vessels extending high into the wart. These vessels cause bleeding points when the wart is trimmed and, if thrombosed, may appear as small dark spots. Hematoxylin and eosin staining of warty lesions may reveal cells that contain both nuclear and cytoplasmic inclusions. The nuclear inclusions tend to be basophilic and represent aggregates of virus particles, while the cytoplasmic inclusions appear eosinophilic and are felt to represent deranged development of keratohyalin.

Warts are skin colored, can be single or occur in multiple clusters, and are often widely dispersed over the body. While warts may persist and spread within the same person for several years, or may recur in an individual several years after a total remission, most studies indicate that two-thirds of warts will resolve spontaneously within a 2-year period of time. Whether this is related to a limited life span of infected cells or is due to the host's defenses is unclear. The development of antiwart antibodies has been correlated with clinical regression of the lesions. In addition, warts have been known to increase in size during pregnancy and to reappear and disseminate during immunosuppressive therapy; hence cellular immunity has been implicated as an important aspect of the host's defenses to human wart virus.

CLINICAL MANIFESTATIONS Although many clinical types of warts exist, the same virus is thought to cause most varieties of warts. The clinical manifestations of the lesions are determined by the host response and the location of the lesions. For convenience, lesions are classified according to location and morphology.

Common warts (verrucae vulgaris) may occur anywhere on the skin but are most common on the hands or around the fingernails. Most lesions appear as solid, rounded tumors with rough, horny projections which may vary considerably in size (1 mm to 2 cm). Lesions occur in both children and adults, either singly or in clusters, may be localized along a scratch (Köbner phenomenon), and are usually asymptomatic.

Plantar warts occur beneath pressure points on the soles of the feet, particularly in children and young adults. The surfaces of the lesions are firm and flat and may occur individually or in mosaic-like clusters. These warts possess a conical shape, probably due to the pressure induced by walking. The lesions are covered by hyperkeratotic epithelial tissue which, upon removal, reveals the papillary structure of the soft whitish core containing thrombosed capillaries that appear as small dark specks. With further paring, capillary bleeding, which is diagnostic of warts rather than a callous corn or scar, can be induced. Local pressure upon the plantar wart usually induces pain which can be severe upon walking.

Flat warts (verrucae planae) present as skin-colored, smooth, flat, or slightly elevated, round or polygonal papules that vary between 1 and 5 mm in diameter. The common sites are the face, neck, chest, dorsum of the hands, and the flexor surfaces of the forearms and shins. The mucous membranes are involved rarely. The surfaces of these lesions show a stippled appearance when examined under a magnifying glass. Flat warts are most frequently confused with the lesions of lichen planus. Multiple lesions on the dorsum of the hands may be mistaken for one of the inherited disorders known as acrokeratosis verruciformis, epidermodysplasia verruciformis, or Darier's disease.

Warts which project finger-like structures are termed *filiform warts;* when present on the scalp, they are called *digitate warts.* Filiform warts are most frequent in adult males, usually on the bearded area of the face. The lips and eyelids may also be involved. The lesions are either single or multiple, and they grow to considerable size when left unattended. The differential diagnosis includes cutaneous horns and epidermal nevi.

Condylomata acuminata, or venereal warts, generally appear as multiple, polymorphic lesions which may coalesce to large masses in the genital and/or anal area. In men, they are found most frequently in the coronal or frenum area of the penis. Urethral warts usually affect the anterior urinary meatus. In women, warts may occur on the fourchette, on the adjacent labia and/or vulva, the cervix, and the lower and upper one-third of the vagina. In about 20 percent of patients, the lesions spread to the perineum and anal area. Anal warts may, however, appear without concomitant penile or vulvar disease and may extend into the anal canal.

The clinical and virological relationship between skin and genital warts has excited controversy. Even though the viruses from these lesions appear structurally identical, there is some evidence that there are antigenic and biochemical differences between the viruses extracted from skin and genital warts. Moreover, both the epidemiology and clinical manifestations of these two entities appear distinctive. While there are a small number of patients with skin warts who develop flat warts in the genital area due to autoinoculation, most studies indicate that genital warts is a disease of sexual maturity, and patients with genital warts do not have more skin warts than controls. The data suggest that genital warts are sexually transmitted. In one study, 60 percent of patients who had sexual contact with partners having active genital warts subsequently developed the disease, usually after an incubation period of 2 to 3 months.

The differential diagnosis of genital warts includes condylomata lata of secondary syphilis (darkfield microscopy for *Treponema pallidum* and serologic testing will differentiate between these two entities), granuloma inguinale in tropical countries, and carcinoma of the penis. Vulvar warts must be differentiated from fibroepitheliomas, molluscum contagiosum, and, in older women, seborrheic keratosis.

COMPLICATIONS Occasionally, a giant condyloma may cause destruction of the affected areas, e.g., the penis in Buschke-Lowenstein tumor. Despite its benign histology, this lesion may cause extensive perforation and destruction of tissue and may simulate a malignant growth. Biopsy is recommended. Vulvar warts may enlarge enough during pregnancy to cause problems in the management of labor and delivery.

Laryngeal papillomatosis of childhood appears related to condyloma acuminatum. These lesions, which are usually multiple, develop within the first 6 months of life, and most mothers of children who develop these multiple lesions have been noted to have genital warts at parturition. This condition appears to be etiologically distinct from the solitary laryngeal papilloma of elderly patients which tends to become malignant. Malignant transmission of warts is rare. An example is epidermodysplasia verruciformis, a condition with a familial predisposition that begins with multiple lesions similar to common warts on the dorsum of the hands and feet and soon spreads over the entire body surface.

TREATMENT There is no specific treatment for warts, although a variety of physical and chemical methods are used for their removal. These methods include electrodesiccation and curettage, surgical excision, x-ray, and cryosurgery by applying liquid nitrogen or dry ice. Repeated paring of warts followed by the application of caustic agents, such as mono- or trichloracetic acid, calicylic acid, cantharidin, or silver nitrate, is helpful. Topical antimetabolites such as 5-fluorouracil have also been used.

Condylomata acuminata are treated effectively by repeated topical application of a 25% podophyllum resin and tincture of benzoin. This preparation is applied to the lesions, washed off after 3 to 4 h, and repeated once or twice a week, while the time of application is lengthened until the lesions have resolved. Large quantities of podophyllum are toxic, however, and may cause hypokalemia and neuropathy. It is also advisable to avoid podophyllum in pregnancy. Radical therapy of warts should be eschewed because most warts will disappear eventually spontaneously without leaving any scars.

MOLLUSCUM CONTAGIOSUM

Molluscum contagiosum is an infectious disease of the skin and mucous membranes caused by a member of the poxvirus group. The virus of molluscum contagiosum is the largest of the true viruses to cause human disease, and, because of its size, 240 to 320 nm in diameter, it can be demonstrated in direct touch preparations of lesions using oil immersion light microscopy. Molluscum contagiosum is a disease of worldwide distribution occurring in all races and is seen most frequently in children. Occasionally, epidemics of the disease are seen in closed populations as in boarding schools or among wrestlers. Infection can be transmitted experimentally by injecting material expressed from the lesions. Clinically, infection can be transmitted directly through sexual intercourse or, like other poxviruses, through fomites such as shared towels. The incubation period varies between 2 weeks and 2 months.

Proliferation, hyperplasia, thickening, and degeneration of the epidermis characterize the lesions. Infected epithelial cells become enlarged and develop large intracytoplasmic eosinophilic hyalin inclusion bodies which displace the nucleus to one side.

Molluscum contagiosum is characterized by single or multiple, rounded dome-shaped waxy, pearly white pustules with an umbilical central pore. A cheesy material that stains blue with Giemsa's stain can be expressed from the central core. Microscopically, the umbilicated central porous area is composed of horn lamellae, debris, dyskeratotic cells, and molluscum bodies.

These molluscum bodies appear as a mass of viral particles on electron microscopy. The lesions may vary in number and size and range from 1 mm up to 1 to 2 cm in diameter. The principal sites of involvement include the face, especially the eyelids, the trunk, and the anogenital areas. The conjunctiva, lips, and buccal mucosa are involved rarely. Molluscum lesions are frequently traumatized resulting in autoinoculation. Occasionally, secondary bacterial infection occurs. The lesions are usually present for 6 months to a year but may persist and spread for 3 to 4 years. Spontaneous regression without scarring occurs eventually. In contrast to warts, recurrences are rare. Patients with underlying immunologic defects may develop extensive involvement with an intractable course.

The diagnosis of molluscum contagiosum is easy, especially when multiple lesions are present. A single lesion may be confused with a keratoacanthoma, basal cell epithelioma, or pyogenic granuloma. The definitive diagnosis can be made histologically from smears of expressed material or by electron microscopy. Treatment by sharp curettage or by expression of the porous material with a curved forceps will help clear up the lesion with little if any scarring.

REFERENCES

EISINGER M et al: Propagation of human wart virus in tissue culture. Nature 256:432, 1975

ORIEL JD: Genital warts. Sexually Transmitted Dis 4:153, 1977

ROWSON KEK, MAHY BJW: Human papova virus. Bacteriol Rev 31:110, 1967

SANDERS BB, STRETCHER GS: Warts, diagnosis and treatment. JAMA 235:2859, 1976

197
CAT–SCRATCH DISEASE

ROBERT G. PETERSDORF

DEFINITION Cat-scratch disease is an infection characterized by indolent, occasionally suppurative, regional lymphadenitis, secondary to a primary cutaneous lesion at the site of inoculation, usually a cat scratch. Because more than 90 percent of the reported cases have originated from cat scratches and a history of close contact with cats is often elicited, the name *cat-scratch disease* has become popular. However, rarely a similar disorder has been acquired from injury due to splinters, thorns, beef-bone fragments, and dog and monkey scratches, and in some patients no inciting trauma is recalled.

ETIOLOGY A specific etiologic agent has not been identified. Among the agents that have been incriminated are atypical acid-fast bacteria, organisms of the psittacosis-lymphogranuloma group, herpes-like (EB) virus, and most recently chlamydia. The evidence for ascribing a definitive causative role to any of these is not convincing.

EPIDEMIOLOGY Cats act only as vectors for the diseases. They are not ill, and have negative skin tests. The disease occurs mostly in children (75 percent), and several cases have been described in siblings, because of contact with the same cat. The disease is most common in fall and winter. Cats may act as long-term carriers, a hypothesis supported by the familial occurrence of several infections interspersed by months or years.

PATHOLOGY The histopathologic appearance of lymph nodes is not specific. Three stages have been described: (1) early lesions show reticulum-cell hyperplasia; (2) intermediate lesions show granuloma formation; and (3) late lesions show microabscesses. These reactions are not readily distinguished from those induced by the tubercle bacillus. However, acid-fast bacilli are invariably absent.

MANIFESTATIONS The incubation period lasts a few days to several weeks, with an average of 3 to 10 days. In a typical case the primary lesion consists of a raised, slightly tender, nonpruritic papule crowned by a small vesicle or eschar; it often resembles an indolent furuncle or insect bite. Multiple primary lesions have been described. In some patients a primary lesion cannot be found.

Regional lymphadenopathy becomes evident in a few days or as long as 6 weeks after infection. Adenopathy is unilateral and asymmetric; in most instances only one node is involved. The axillary, cervical, preauricular, submandibular, epitrochlear, femoral, or inguinal nodes (in decreasing order of frequency) on one side become visibly swollen and tender, often with redness of the overlying skin. The nodes occasionally suppurate, soften, and drain spontaneously; fistulas heal completely with only slight scarring. Usually the tenderness subsides gradually, and nontender, firm, enlarged nodes remain palpable for some weeks or even months. With rare exceptions, there is no generalized glandular enlargement, and the spleen is not palpable.

Systemic symptoms are usually mild and consist of headache, fever, and malaise, which subside within a few days. Shaking chills and fever with temperatures as high as 104°F can occur but are unusual. Many patients are entirely symptom-free. A transient macular or vesicular rash which subsides within 48 h is rarely present during the early stages. Erythema nodosum and multiforme have been reported.

Clinical forms of this disease other than that described above may be delineated. These include (1) encephalitis characterized by fever, convulsions, alterations in consciousness, mild cerebrospinal fluid pleocytosis and elevation in protein, and complete recovery; (2) Parinaud's oculoglandular syndrome characterized by granulomatous conjunctivitis and enlargement of the homolateral preauricular node; (3) more rarely, mesenteric lymphadenitis; (4) osteolytic bone lesions, which subside spontaneously; and (5) thrombocytopenic as well as nonthrombocytopenic purpura. In all these syndromes the diagnostic criteria for cat-scratch disease must be present before the illness can be ascribed to cat-scratch disease.

DIAGNOSIS The following criteria should be fulfilled before a diagnosis of cat-scratch disease is established: (1) history of contact with cats, (2) finding of a primary lesion, (3) regional lymphadenopathy, (4) positive intradermal skin test, (5) biopsy of lymph node with demonstration of histopathologic changes consistent with cat-scratch disease (this may not be necessary if the skin test is positive), and (6) failure to demonstrate other causative agents.

The specific diagnosis is made by means of a skin test. Antigen for this is prepared by mixing one part pus aspirated from infected lymph nodes with three parts saline solution, and inactivating the mixture by heating or by irradiation. A positive reaction is of the delayed tuberculin type, consisting of 5-mm induration and 1-cm erythema, that appears in 24 to 48 h. Although batches of antigen vary in potency, in general, patients reacting to one batch react to another. Skin test material can be preserved by freezing. The test becomes positive within 30 days after infection and may persist for many years. Each batch of antigen must be tested against patients known to have had the disease. A well-standardized batch should provide highly reliable results. Approximately 10 percent of normal individuals have false positive reactions. The chance of carrying hepatitis virus in the antigen is remote.

Other laboratory abnormalities include mild leukocytosis (up to 15,000 cells per cubic millimeter), occasional mild eosinophilia, and an elevated sedimentation rate. The Frei test is negative.

Patients with cat-scratch disease show significantly depressed lymphocyte transformation responses to phytohemagglutinin and *Candida albicans*. These reactions revert to normal as the disease subsides.

Cat-scratch disease is a benign illness, and the prognosis is uniformly good. Its main clinical importance lies in its possible confusion with other more serious diseases of the lymphatics. Diseases to be considered are tularemia, lymphatic tuberculosis, sporotrichosis, histoplasmosis, coccidioidomycosis, toxoplasmosis, and bacterial adenitis. Because of the indolent character of the adenopathy, Hodgkin's disease or other lymphomas may be suspected. Neck masses may be confused with thyroglossal duct cysts, bronchial cleft cysts, dermoids, cystic hygromas, thyroid and parathyroid adenomas, salivary gland tumors, carotid body tumors, aneurysms, pharyngeal or esophageal diverticula, and mesodermal tumors, as well as lymphomas. Appropriate serologic and cultural tests serve to rule out other infections; biopsy may be needed to exclude tumor, but a positive skin test with cat-scratch antigen effectively rules out the necessity for biopsy. Cat-scratch disease must be differentiated from tularemia, which occasionally can be transmitted by cats.

TREATMENT In instances of node suppuration, aspiration of accumulated pus affords relief of pain (and incidentally, serves as a source of material for the preparation of skin-test antigen). Aspiration is required in only a few cases. Antibiotics and steroids are ineffective.

REFERENCES

CARITHERS HA et al: Cat-scratch disease: Its natural history. JAMA 207:312, 1969

EMMONS RW et al: Continuing search for the etiology of cat-scratch disease. J Clin Microbiol 4:112, 1976

FUTRELL JW et al: Unsuspected etiology of lateral neck masses. Arch Otolaryngol 95:277, 1972

LYON LW: Neurologic manifestations of cat-scratch disease. Arch Neurol 25:23, 1971

MARGILETH AM: Cat-scratch disease: Nonbacterial regional lymphadenitis. Study of 145 patients and a review of the literature. Pediatrics 42:803, 1968

SCHULKIND ML, AYOUB EM: Cell-mediated immunity in cat-scratch disease. J Pediatr 85:199, 1974

WARWICK WJ: The cat-scratch syndrome: Many diseases or one disease? Prog Med Virol 9:256, 1967

section 14 | Infections caused by protozoa

198
APPROACH TO THE PATIENT WITH PROTOZOAN INFECTION

JAMES J. PLORDE

Protozoan diseases such as *malaria, trypanosomiasis, leishmaniasis, amebiasis,* and *toxoplasmosis* remain among the major causes of human sickness and death in the world today. Over 500 million people still live in malarious areas, and it is estimated that 100 million of these are infected at any given time. Of those infected, 1 million die of the disease annually.

In Africa, from the Sahara in the North to the Kalahari Desert in the South, human strains of *Trypanosoma brucei* cause one of the most lethal of all human diseases, *sleeping sickness.* Animal strains of this species limit food supply in the same area through their impact on animal husbandry. In South America, a related organism, *T. cruzi,* infects several million people, leaving many with severe heart and gastrointestinal lesions (*Chagas' disease*).

Leishmaniasis is found in parts of Europe, Asia, Africa, and South and Central America where it may present as a chronic, highly lethal infection of the reticuloendothelial system (kala azar), a mutilating mucocutaneous infection (espundia), or a self-limiting skin ulcer (oriental sore).

Ten percent of the world population, including 2 to 5 percent in the United States, are infected with the intestinal protozoa *Entamoeba histolytica.* Invasive disease resulting in an ulcerative colitis and/or liver abscess is particularly common in Mexico, western South America, South Asia, and West and Southwest Africa.

Toxoplasmosis, giardiasis, and *trichomoniasis* are three cosmopolitan protozoan infections well known to American physicians. The first infects perhaps one-third of the world's population. Although it is usually asymptomatic, congenital toxoplasmosis may result in abortion, stillbirth, prematurity, or severe neurological defects. Even when there are no obvious signs at birth, chorioretinitis with visual impairment may occur years later. Asymptomatic infection may also result in fatal encephalitis during periods of immunosuppression later in life.

In contrast, giardiasis and trichomoniasis seldom result in severe disability; nevertheless their morbidity can be attested to by millions of otherwise healthy individuals.

The pathogens responsible for these diseases are unicellular and possess a true, or membrane-limited, nucleus. Morphological differences in the cytoplasmic organelles of locomotion are useful in separating the protozoa pathogenic for human beings into four major groups: *flagellates, ciliates, amebas,* and *sporozoa.* The structures concerned with the motility of the first two groups are self-evident. Amebas move by means of pseudopodia, while the sporozoa generally lack any specific locomotor structures. Nuclear morphology, particularly the distribution pattern of the chromatin and karyosome (nucleolus), is used in distinguishing the species of certain organisms in the above groups.

Characteristically, the flagellates, ciliates, and amebas reproduce by asexual binary fission, while the sporozoa have alternating cycles of asexual (*schizogony*) and sexual (*sporogony*) reproduction. In the process of asexual multiplication the nucleus of the intracellular trophozoite first divides into several portions to form a schizont. Cytoplasmic division then occurs, resulting in the formation of daughter cells, or *merozoites.* These invade new host cells in which they become trophozoites, thus completing the asexual cycle. After one or more such cycles some merozoites initiate the sexual phase of reproduction by differentiating into male and female gametocytes. These mature and effect fertilization; the fertilized zygote, upon encysting, becomes known as an *oocyst*. Sporozoites formed within the oocyst are released, penetrate tissue cells, and begin another asexual cycle as trophozoites. These alternating sexual and asexual cycles may occur within the same (*Toxoplasma* spp., *Isospora* spp.) or different hosts (*Plasmodium* spp.).

The mode of transmission of these protozoa depends upon whether they are luminal or tissue parasites. Those which inhabit human gastrointestinal or genitourinary tracts are passed from human to human either directly as in the case of *Trichomonas vaginalis* or indirectly by the ingestion of contaminated food or water (fecal-oral transmission), e.g., *E. histolytica* and *Giardia lamblia*. In the former situation the infecting agent is the vegetative form, or trophozoite; in the latter it is a cyst capable of survival in the external environment for prolonged periods. Blood and tissue parasites, on the other hand, are generally transmitted via an arthropod which functions as both a vector and a second host. In the case of *Plasmodium* spp. this alternation of human and arthropod host is associated with the alternation of asexual and sexual generations described above.

These differences in transmission have a profound effect on both the distribution and control of protozoan diseases. Those spread by the fecal-oral route are essentially diseases of poverty and are found throughout the world wherever there is inadequate hygiene and sanitation. Their control depends upon the improvements in these areas which invariably accompany economic development. In contrast, the geographic distribution of the blood and tissue parasites is determined by the ecologic factors, particularly climate, responsible for the persistence of the arthropod vector. Attempts at disease prevention are characteristically directed at the control or elimination of the specific vectors. However, malaria, trypanosomiasis, and leishmaniasis can also be passed from person to person via blood transfusion, and careful screening of donors from endemic areas is important.

Clinically, protozoa exert their effects in a number of ways. In diseases such as malaria, the primary pathogenic mechanism appears to be the invasion and subsequent alteration or destruction of erythrocytes by the parasite. *Entamoeba histolytica* destroys host cells via enzymes or toxins without actual cellular invasion. In still other diseases, clinical manifestations are the result of a host-mounted inflammatory reaction, and in several, immunologic mechanisms are responsible for clinical findings, e.g., nephrotic syndrome in quartan malaria. *Giardia lamblia*, on the other hand, is thought by some to produce

malabsorption by simply covering a significant proportion of the microvilli in the small bowel.

By themselves, the clinical manifestations of disease are not always specific enough to ensure prompt diagnosis. Furthermore, general laboratory findings are often of little diagnostic aid. Although eosinophilia has been recognized as an important clue to the diagnosis of parasitic diseases, this phenomenon is characteristic of helminthic, not protozoan, infections. A carefully elicited travel, transfusion, and socioeconomic history often first suggests to the physician the possibility of a protozoan infection.

Reliable serologic tests have become available in the United States for many of the protozoan infections including malaria, amebiasis, toxoplasmosis, leishmaniasis, and South American trypanosomiasis. Many of these tests are performed by local institutions. For the remainder, blood samples can be sent to the individual state health departments for forwarding to the Center for Disease Control in Atlanta, Georgia. However, the definitive diagnosis usually rests upon the recovery and morphologic identification of the parasite from the genitourinary tract, intestinal contents, tissue, or blood.

Most intestinal protozoan agents are passed in the feces intermittently or in fluctuating numbers, and the examination of a single normally passed stool will detect only one-third to one-half of involved patients. The testing of three such specimens collected at intervals of 2 or 3 days will improve this yield substantially. Alternatively, a saline cathartic is administered to evacuate the cecal area where many protozoa are concentrated, and the entire purge is then examined. The stool must be free of interfering substances such as antidiarrheal or contrast agents, antacids, and antibiotics. If the appropriate specimens can not be obtained prior to administration of such substances, testing should be delayed for 1 week or, in the case of antimicrobial agents, 3 weeks after their discontinuation. The results of antiprotozoal therapy should be monitored by checking specimens at 1, 3, and 6 months. Occasionally, specimens other than stool must be examined. In the case of small-bowel infections such as giardiasis and coccidiosis, the diagnosis at times can be established only by sampling the duodenal contents or by performing a jejunal biopsy. Similarly, the recovery of large-bowel pathogens such as *E. histolytica* may require sigmoidoscopic aspiration of colonic ulcers. Whenever intestinal aspirates or soft to watery fecal specimens are collected, they should be immediately placed in a preservative such as polyvinyl alcohol (PVA) to prevent rapid disintegration of fragile trophozoites and allow the preparation of permanently stained smears. Formed stools generally contain the most resistant cyst forms. These will survive for 1 to 2 days at room temperature and indefinitely if placed in 5% formaldehyde.

Direct examination of the blood is useful for the detection of malaria parasites, leishmania, and trypanosomes. Preferably, fresh capillary blood should be used to prepare thin and thick blood smears and, when appropriate, wet mounts. Only specially prepared glass slides should be used as traces of soda lime or potash on uncleaned slides may alter the pH of the stain, making recognition of parasites difficult. If an experienced technologist is not available to assist in the bedside preparation of smears, it is preferable to collect venous blood in an EDTA Vacutainer and send it to the laboratory. As the concentration of malaria parasites in the peripheral blood may fluctuate, specimens should be collected three to four times a day for 2 or 3 days.

Many of the drugs used to treat protozoan infection are either not generally available or have not yet been approved for use in the United States. Fortunately, many of these agents are available through the Parasitic Disease Drug Service of the Center for Disease Control, Atlanta, Georgia. These drugs are listed in Table 198-1.

TABLE 198-1
Antiprotozoal agents available through the Parasitic Disease Drug Service*

Infection	Therapeutic agent
Amebiasis	Dehydroemetine
	Diloxanide furoate
Chagas' disease (*Trypanosoma cruzi*)	Bayer 2502 (Lampit)
Leishmaniasis	Sodium antimony gluconate (Pentostam)
Malaria	Parenteral chloroquine hydrochloride
	Parenteral quinine dehydrochloride
Pneumocystosis	Pentamidine isothionate
Sleeping sickness (*Trypanosoma brucei*)	Melarsoprol (Mel B)
	Pentamidine isothionate
	Suramin (Antrypol)

* *Parasitic Disease Branch, Bureau of Epidemiology, Center for Disease Control, Atlanta, Ga. 30333. Day telephone: (404) 633-3311, ext. 3496; nights, weekends, and holidays: (404) 633-2176.*

REFERENCES

Brown HW: *Basic Clinical Parasitology,* 4th ed. New York, Appleton-Century-Crofts, 1975

Drugs for parasitic infections. Med Lett 20(4):17, 1978

Health information for international travel 1978, US Department of Health, Education, and Welfare Publication (CDC) 78–82. Morb Mort Week Rep, vol. 27, suppl, September 1978

Hunter GW III et al (eds): *Tropical Medicine,* 5th ed. Philadelphia, Saunders, 1976

199
AMEBIASIS

JAMES J. PLORDE

DEFINITION Amebiasis is an infection of the large intestine produced by *Entamoeba histolytica.* It is an asymptomatic carrier state in most individuals, but diseases ranging from chronic, mild diarrhea to fulminant dysentery may occur. Among extraintestinal complications, the commonest is hepatic abscess, which may rupture into peritoneum, pleura, lung, or pericardium.

ETIOLOGY There are seven species of ameba that naturally parasitize the human mouth and intestine, but of these only *E. histolytica* causes disease. *Entamoeba coli* and *E. hartmanni* are the two species with which it is most likely to be confused in examination of stools.

Entamoeba histolytica exists in two forms: the motile trophozoite and the cyst. The trophozoite is the parasitic form and dwells in the lumen and/or wall of the colon, divides by binary fission, grows best under anaerobic conditions, and requires the presence of either bacteria or tissue substrates to satisfy its nutritional requirements. When diarrhea occurs, the trophozoites are passed unchanged in the liquid stool, where they can be distinguished by their size (10 to 20 μm in diameter), directional motility, sharply demarcated clear ectoplasm with slender finger-like pseudopodia, and finely granular endoplasm. In dysentery, the trophozoites are larger (up to 50 μm in diameter), and often contain ingested erythrocytes. In the absence of diarrhea, the trophozoites usually encyst before leaving the gut. The cysts are highly resistant to environmental changes, chlorine concentrations found in water purification systems, and gastric acid. With rare exception they are responsible for transmission of disease. Young cysts have a single nucleus, a glycogen vacuole, and sausage-shaped chromatoid bodies. As the cyst matures, it absorbs its cytoplasmic vacuoles and becomes quadrinucleate. The cysts of *E. histolytica* can be distinguished from those of *Entamoeba coli* by the presence of one to four nuclei with small centric karyosomes and fine peripheral chromatin and by their thick chromatoid bodies with round ends.

Entamoeba histolytica had been classified into large and small races depending upon whether they form cysts measuring more or less than 10 μm in diameter. Strains of the small race, however, are not pathogenic for human beings and are now considered as a distinct species, *Entamoeba hartmanni.*

Entamoeba histolytica-like amebas are organisms isolated from humans that are morphologically indistinguishable from true *E. histolytica.* However, unlike *E. histolytica* they are nonpathogenic, grow best at 20°C, and can multiply indefinitely in hypotonic solutions.

Entamoeba histolytica can be cultivated in artificial media, a procedure that is useful in direct diagnosis and in the preparation of purified antigens for serologic testing.

EPIDEMIOLOGY Infection with *E. histolytica* is worldwide. Stool surveys indicate that the prevalence of infection in the United States is between 1 and 5 percent. Rates as high as 50 percent may occur in tropical areas where the level of sanitation is low. Symptomatic amebiasis is unusual below the age of 10 years in temperate climates, and both intestinal and hepatic lesions predominate in adult males to an extent that is not readily explainable on the basis of different rates of exposure to infection. Reports of amebic liver abscess suggest that invasive amebiasis is concentrated in comparatively few parts of the world, most notably Mexico, western South America, South Asia, and West and Southwestern Africa. In the United States, the incidence of amebiasis has decreased sharply in the past 20 years. Furthermore, an increasing proportion of reported cases are now acquired outside the United States. Cases of dysentery and liver abscess can still be found, however, in institutions for the mentally retarded, Indian reservations, and migrant labor camps.

Although the parasite can sometimes infect rats, cats, dogs, and primates, human beings are the principal host and reservoir. Because trophozoites die rapidly after leaving the intestine, asymptomatic cyst passers are the source of new infections. The cysts are usually spread through contaminated food or water. Direct fecal-oral spread occurs between sexual partners and in conditions of poor personal hygiene. Venereal transmission appears to be particularly common among male homosexuals. Cases of amebic dysentery are usually sporadic, but epidemics, which are sometimes waterborne, have occurred. Outbreaks of amebiasis are never explosive, as are those produced by pathogenic intestinal bacteria.

PATHOGENESIS AND ANATOMIC CHANGES After ingestion, cysts undergo further nuclear division. In the small intestine, the cyst wall disintegrates, and trophozoites are released. The immature amebas are carried to the large intestine, where they live in the lumen of the gut as commensals feeding on bacteria and debris. On occasion the amebas may invade the mucosa, causing ulcerations that are sufficiently extensive to produce symptoms. The factors responsible for this are not completely understood, but the state of the host and the virulence of the infecting organism both play roles. Epidemiologic evidence suggests that amebic strains indigenous to temperate climates are usually avirulent. It has also been shown, however, that invasiveness is not a stable strain characteristic. It can either be lost after continued cultivation in vitro or enhanced by rapid animal passage. The virulence of various strains of *E. histolytica* is dependent upon the association with living bacteria.

Amebic ulceration of the intestinal wall is characteristic. A small mucosal defect overlies a larger, burrowing area of necrosis in the submucosa and muscularis, producing a bottle-shaped lesion. There is little acute inflammatory response, and in contrast to the picture in bacillary dysentery, the mucosa between ulcers is normal. The sites of involvement in order of frequency are cecum and ascending colon, rectum, sigmoid, appendix, and terminal ileum. In the cecum and sigmoid, chronic infection may lead to the formation of large masses of granulation tissue or *amebomas.* Amebas can enter the portal circulation and lodge in venules; liquefaction necrosis of liver tissue leads to the formation of an abscess cavity. Rarely, embolization results in lung, brain, or splenic abscess.

CLINICAL MANIFESTATIONS **Asymptomatic cyst passer** In the majority of patients with this common form of amebiasis, *E. histolytica* probably lives as a commensal in the bowel lumen. Individuals infected in temperate climates are unlikely to develop significant tissue invasion. However, invasion does occur occasionally, and so treatment of cyst passers is warranted.

Symptomatic intestinal amebiasis In some patients there is intermittent diarrhea consisting of one to four foul-smelling loose or watery stools daily. The stools sometimes contain mucus and blood. Loose stools alternate with periods of relative normality and may persist for months or years. Flatulence and abnormal cramping are frequent. The only physical findings are occasional tender hepatomegaly and slight pain when the cecum and ascending colon are palpated. Sigmoidoscopy sometimes reveals typical ulcerations with areas of normal mucosa interspersed. The diagnosis depends upon finding the organism in the feces or in ulcers.

Fulminating attacks of amebic dysentery are less common. Waterborne outbreaks may occur, but fulminating dysentery is more likely to occur spontaneously in debilitated individuals. Attacks may be precipitated by pregnancy or corticosteroids. The onset in half the cases is abrupt with high fever, between 40 and 40.6°C (104 and 105°F), severe abdominal cramps, and profuse, bloody diarrhea with tenesmus. There is diffuse abdominal tenderness, often so severe that peritonitis is suspected. Hepatomegaly is very frequent, and sigmoidoscopy almost always demonstrates extensive rectosigmoid ulceration. Trophozoites are numerous in stools and in material obtained directly from the ulcers.

In some cases there may be extensive destruction of the colonic mucosa and submucosa, massive hemorrhage or perforation of the bowel wall, with resultant peritonitis. Repeated severe attacks of intestinal amebiasis can lead to an ulcerative postdysenteric colitis. Amebas can usually not be demonstrated in this condition, but serologic tests are strongly positive. Invasion of the appendix may lead to a clinical picture of *appendicitis*. Penetration of trophozoites through the muscle wall of the bowel may result in the development of large masses of granulation tissue. When the entire circumference of the intestine is involved, there may then be partial obstruction, and a movable, tender, sausage-shaped mass is often palpable. This lesion or ameboma is most frequently seen in the cecum where a palpable mass and radiologic demonstration of a ragged encroachment of the lumen may lead to a mistaken diagnosis of adenocarcinoma.

Hepatic amebiasis The parasites usually reach the liver through the portal vein; rarely, they may traverse the lymphatic vessels. It has been believed for a long time that amebas which lodged in the liver could produce a diffuse hepatitis. Careful postmortem and biopsy studies indicate that the syndrome of tender hepatomegaly, right upper quadrant pain, fever, and leukocytosis in patients with amebic colitis is not a result of amebas in hepatic tissues, is accompanied by nonspecific periportal inflammation, and is rarely, if ever, a prelude to hepatic abscess. It is evident, then, that these manifestations are best regarded as an accompaniment of colitis and do not merit a separate diagnosis of "diffuse amebic hepatitis."

Hepatic abscess may develop insidiously, with fever, sweats, weight loss, and no local signs other than painless or slightly tender hepatomegaly. In other patients, there is abrupt onset, with chills, fever to 40.6°C (105°F), nausea, vomiting, severe upper abdominal pain, and polymorphonuclear leukocytosis. Initially, cholecystitis, perforated ulcer, or acute pancreatitis may be suspected.

Most commonly, the abscess occurs singly and is localized in the posterior portion of the right lobe of the liver, because this lobe receives most of the blood draining the right colon through the "streaming" effect in portal vein flow. This loca-

tion is responsible for several features that aid in diagnosis. *Point tenderness* in the posterolateral portion of a lower right intercostal space is frequent even in the absence of diffuse liver pain. Most abscesses enlarge upward, producing a bulge in the diaphragmatic dome, obliteration of the costophrenic gutter, small hydrothorax, basilar atelectasis, and pain referred to the right shoulder. Liver function tests may be mildly to moderately disturbed but are of little diagnostic aid. Jaundice is uncommon. Radiologically, unruptured abscesses do not show a fluid level, and calcification of the liver parenchyma is very rare. Isotope liver scan utilizing two, or preferably three, projections is invaluable in confirming both the presence and location of a liver abscess. Ultrasonic scanning reveals a fluid-filled cavity often with scattered internal echoes. It has been reported that hepatic tomograms will visualize amebic abscesses following intravenous Hypaque infusion. Serologic tests are positive in over 90 percent of patients.

Needle puncture results in the withdrawal of "pus" which consists of liquefied, necrotic liver. Typically, it is thick and odorless, resembling "chocolate syrup" or "anchovy paste." It may, however, be thin in consistency and yellow or green in color. The pus contains no polymorphonuclear leukocytes (barring secondary bacterial infection) and, usually, no amebas. The parasites are localized in the cyst wall and may be demonstrated in the terminal portion of the aspirate or, at times, by a Vim-Silverman needle biopsy of the cyst wall following aspiration of the abscess.

Hepatic abscess complicates asymptomatic infection of the colon more often than symptomatic intestinal disease, another factor making recognition difficult. Trophozoites or cysts are demonstrable in the feces of only about one-third of patients with abscess, and fewer than one-half can recall significant diarrheal illness.

Pleuropulmonary amebiasis The right pleural cavity and lung are involved by direct extension from the liver in 10 to 20 percent of patients with liver abscess. Rarely, amebic lung abscess has resulted from embolization rather than direct extension.

Manifestations are those of a consolidating pneumonia or lung abscess. If perforation into a bronchus occurs, patients expectorate large amounts of the typical exudate, some patients even commenting that the sputum "tastes like liver." Cough, pleural pain, fever, and leukocytosis are the rule, and secondary bacterial infection is frequent. Rupture into the free pleural space results in a massive pleural effusion; aspiration of "chocolate" fluid is diagnostic.

Other extraintestinal lesions Extension of an abscess from the left lobe of the liver to the pericardium is the most dangerous complication of hepatic abscess. It may be mistaken for tuberculous pericarditis or congestive cardiomyopathy. Less frequently, rapid cardiac tamponade occurs with ensuing dyspnea, shock, and death. *Peritonitis* is a result of perforation of colonic ulcer or rupture of liver abscess. Painful ulcers or condylomata of the genitalia, perianal skin, or abdominal wall (draining sinuses) are unusual complications which may be mistaken for syphilitic, tuberculous, or neoplastic lesions. They usually result from direct extension of intestinal disease; some are thought to result from sexual transmission. Metastatic brain abscess is rare, and an etiologic diagnosis is seldom made clinically. Splenic abscess has been reported but is very unusual.

DIFFERENTIAL DIAGNOSIS Intestinal amebiasis Patients with nondysenteric amebiasis are often misdiagnosed as having irritable bowel syndrome, diverticulitis, or regional enteritis. Ameboma may mimic colonic carcinoma or granulomatous disease, while the clinical spectrum of amebic dysentery overlaps those of shigellosis, salmonellosis, ulcerative colitis, and, in endemic areas, schistosomiasis. The invasive bacterial infections are usually more acute, severe, and self-limited than amebiasis. Stools from patients with shigellosis, salmonellosis, and ulcerative colitis contain large numbers of polymorphonuclear leukocytes, while those in amebic infection do not. Nevertheless, amebiasis may closely resemble any of the above diseases both clinically and radiologically and must be considered in the differential diagnosis of any chronic diarrhea or dysentery.

The identification of *E. histolytica* in the stool, however, does not eliminate other diagnostic possibilities. Amebic infection is often superimposed on or exacerbated by other colonic disease including cecal carcinoma. For this reason, patients with intestinal amebiasis and abdominal complaints still require stool culture, sigmoidoscopy, and a barium enema.

Hepatic abscess Once a filling defect has been demonstrated by isotope liver scanning, the differential diagnosis includes hepatic neoplasm, hydatid cyst, and pyogenic abscess. Neoplasms can usually be differentiated on the basis of their ultrasonic scanning characteristics, while the lack of constitutional manifestations and presence of an appropriate epidemiologic history is helpful in recognizing echinococcosis. The most difficult problem lies in the exclusion of a pyogenic abscess. An insidious onset in an adult male, a history of chronic diarrhea, significant pleuritic chest pain, and a single right lobe lesion favors the diagnosis of amebiasis. High fever, hyperbilirubinemia, multiple hepatic filling defects, and foul-smelling hepatic aspirate are more suggestive of pyogenic disease. Ultimately, the separation of the two diseases rests upon laboratory procedures.

LABORATORY DIAGNOSIS The diagnosis of intestinal amebiasis depends upon *identification of the organism in the stool or tissues.* Formed stools are examined initially in saline and iodine mounts for amebic cysts; concentration methods such as the formalin-ether technique increase the yield two- to threefold. Liquid or semiformed stools should be examined immediately in saline solution for the presence of motile hematophagous trophozoites. The addition of a supravital stain such as buffered methylene blue to the saline enhances nuclear detail and minimizes the possibility of confusing fecal leukocytes with amebic trophozoites, an error common to inexperienced parasitologists. If there is any delay in examination of the stool, a portion of the specimen may be refrigerated for a few hours at 4°C, or placed in polyvinyl alcohol and 10% formalin. Definitive identification of *E. histolytica* requires the examination of permanently stained slides prepared from the material preserved with polyvinyl alcohol. An ocular micrometer is necessary to separate *E. hartmanni* from its larger relative. Four to six stool specimens may be required for diagnosis. If possible, the stool should be examined before the administration of antimicrobial, antidiarrheal, or antacid preparations, because all these agents may interfere with the recovery of amebas. Likewise, enemas and radiographic procedures utilizing barium sulfate are best postponed until after a thorough search for *E. histolytica* has been made.

Sigmoidoscopy is of value in symptomatic cases. The mucosal lesions should be aspirated and the material examined for trophozoites as described above. Biopsy material obtained from such lesions and stained with periodic acid–Schiff solution also will frequently reveal trophozoites.

The diagnosis of extraintestinal amebiasis is difficult. The parasite usually cannot be recovered from stool or tissue. Cultivation of amebas from feces or pus is possible but is not practical in most laboratories. The most important diagnostic procedure in suspected liver abscess is a *therapeutic trial of antiamebic drugs.* The response is often dramatic within 3 days.

In the event that demonstrating parasites is difficult, the therapeutic trial should be instituted without hesitation.

Serologic tests employing purified antigens are positive in nearly all patients with proved amebic liver abscess and in a great majority of those with acute amebic dysentery. They are generally negative in asymptomatic cyst passers, suggesting that tissue invasion is required for antibody production. The persistence of significant antibody titers for months to years after complete cure makes serology, particularly in endemic areas, of more value in excluding the diagnosis than in confirming it. Some authors recommend the routine screening of all patients thought to have inflammatory bowel disease for serologic evidence of amebiasis. Steroid therapy could then be withheld in patients with positive tests pending the outcome of parasitological examination. Of the available tests, the indirect hemagglutination appears to be the most sensitive. Indirect immunofluorescence, countercurrent electrophoresis, and agar gel diffusion are also highly reliable. A number of rapid tests such as latex agglutination and cellulose acetate diffusion have made serologic testing available to most laboratories. Intradermal tests have been shown to be helpful in epidemiologic surveys, but their value in the diagnosis of amebiasis remains to be determined.

TREATMENT Treatment should be aimed at relief of symptoms, replacement of fluid, electrolyte, and blood losses, and eradication of the organism. Amebas may be found in the lumen of the bowel, in the intestinal wall, or extraintestinally. Most amebicides are not effective at all sites or when used alone, and a combination of drugs is often necessary to achieve cure. The available drugs based on their site of action fall into several different categories, as described below.

Luminal amebicides These oral agents act by direct contact with trophozoites dwelling in the bowel lumen but are ineffective against amebas in tissue. Of the large number of available drugs, diloxanide furoate (Furamide) is one of the most effective and well tolerated but is presently available in the United States only through the Center for Disease Control. A response rate of 80 to 85 percent has been noted; flatulence appears to be the only major side effect.

Diiodohydroxyquin has been effective in 60 to 70 percent of cases. As with its analogue iodochlorhydroxyquin (Entero-Vioform), myelooptic neuropathy has been reported after long-term use. However, no such case has been noted when the dosage was limited to that given in Table 199-1. The drug should not be used in patients with thyroid disease or preexisting optic neuropathy.

Tissue amebicides *Chloroquine diphosphate* (Aralen) is a systemic amebicide which is useful in hepatic disease because of its high concentration in the liver. It has little activity elsewhere.

Emetine is an alkaloid derivative of ipecac. When given intramuscularly, it is highly effective in destroying trophozoites in tissue including those in the wall of the intestine. It is ineffective against luminal amebas. Emetine is relatively toxic and may produce vomiting, diarrhea, abdominal cramping, weakness, muscle pain, tachycardia, hypotension, precordial pain, and electrocardiographic abnormalities. The common ECG changes include T-wave inversion and prolongation of the QTc interval. Rarely arrhythmias and prolongation of the QRS complex are seen. A synthetic derivative, dehydroemetine, is thought to be less toxic by virtue of its more rapid excretion and lower concentration in myocardial tissue. It is not free of toxicity, however, and patients treated with either drug should be at bed rest with ECG monitoring. Neither drug should be used in patients with renal, cardiac, or muscle disease, during pregnancy, or in children unless other drugs fail.

Metronidazole (Flagyl) is unique because it is both safe and effective against trophozoites at all sites, intestinally and extraintestinally. It is the drug of choice in most forms of amebiasis. For intestinal amebiasis it is given in dosage of 750 mg three times daily for 5 to 10 days. Smaller doses are effective in hepatic amebiasis. Metronidazole has an Antabuse-like action, and alcohol should be avoided during its administration. The recent evidence that this drug is carcinogenic and possibly teratogenic in animals when given in large doses is disturbing. The potential risk in human beings must be weighed against the severity of the disease, particularly in pregnant women.

Management (see Table 199-1) A course of diiodohydroxyquin or diloxanide furoate should be given in asymptomatic or mildly symptomatic patients. Stools should be examined monthly for 6 months to detect relapse. If it occurs, retreatment can be carried out with the alternate drug or metronidazole.

Treatment of acute dysentery involves control of symptoms as well as eradication of the organism. A number of regimens can be used:

For both mild and moderate dysentery, metronidazole given in a dose of 750 mg three times daily for 5 to 10 days is the simplest and least toxic regimen. This drug will cure about 90 percent of patients. The addition of one of the luminal amebicides will raise the cure rate close to 100 percent. Of some concern is the occurrence of amebic liver abscess in a few patients treated for dysentery with metronidazole. It is probable that this results from failure of metronidazole to eliminate luminal organisms in a small proportion of cases. For this reason, the routine addition of diiodohydroxyquin or diloxanide furoate seems indicated.

In severe dysentery, emetine or dehydroemetine should be

TABLE 199-1
Drug therapy of amebiasis

Clinical form and drug	Dosage
ASYMPTOMATIC INTESTINAL CARRIER	
Diiodohydroxyquin	600 mg tid for 20 days
or diloxanide furoate*	500 mg tid for 10 days
or metronidazole	750 mg tid for 5-10 days
MILD TO MODERATE INTESTINAL DISEASE	
Metronidazole	As above
plus diiodohydroxyquin	As above
or diloxanide furoate	As above
SEVERE INTESTINAL DISEASE	
Above regimen	
plus dehydroemetine*	1.0-1.5 mg/kg IM per day (maximum 90 mg per day) for up to 5 days
or emetine	1 mg/kg IM per day (maximum 60 mg per day) for up to 5 days
EXTRAINTESTINAL DISEASE	
Metronidazole	As above
or chloroquine phosphate	1 g per day for 2 days, then 500 mg per day for 4 weeks
plus dehydroemetine*	As above for 10 days
or emetine	As above for 10 days

* *Investigational drug available through the Parasitic Drug Service, Center for Disease Control, Atlanta, Ga., (404) 633-3311, nights and weekends 633-2176.*

added to the above regimen. These intramuscular agents rapidly control the acute attack, but because of their toxicity administration should be discontinued as soon as symptoms abate.

In extraintestinal amebiasis including hepatic abscess, metronidazole would appear to be the drug of choice; it is less toxic and probably just as effective as the chloroquine-emetine combination. In cases of relapse or in situations where the patient is unable to take oral medication, therapy with dehydroemetine or emetine should be instituted, and oral chloroquine added as soon as possible. Diagnostic trials should employ the chloroquine-emetine regimen because pyogenic liver abscesses may temporarily respond to metronidazole. Many authors prefer to add luminal amebicides to both the metronidazole and chloroquine-emetine programs. Treatment failures have been reported for both emetine-chloroquine and metronidazole. They appear to be unrelated to the organism's resistance.

There is debate over the value of routine aspiration of amebic liver abscesses. Certainly, if there is localized swelling over the liver, marked elevation of the diaphragm, severe localized liver tenderness, and failure to respond to systemic amebicides, it should be done. Adequate drainage can usually be accomplished by needle alone, and surgical drainage is rarely necessary. The greatest hazard in needling an abscess is secondary bacterial infection.

PROGNOSIS Intestinal amebiasis usually responds readily and completely to appropriate drugs. Parasitologic relapses sometimes occur, and posttreatment stools should be checked monthly for 6 months. Repeated relapses, however, are usually a manifestation of reinfection, complicating illness, inadequate therapy, or incorrect diagnosis. The fatality rate is less than 5 percent.

Hepatic and pulmonary amebiasis are still accompanied by an appreciable mortality, but no reliable figures are available.

PREVENTION For the individual, avoidance of contaminated food and water, scalding of vegetables, and the use of iodine-releasing tablets in drinking water (chlorine, in the form of halazone, is ineffective) are important measures. Globaline tablets, containing tetraglycine hydroperiodide, are convenient and effective.

Improvements in general sanitation and the detection of cyst passers and their removal from food-handling duties are general measures in prophylaxis, but such segregation of carriers is rarely practiced. Community control of amebic disease by periodic mass treatment with metronidazole and diloxanide furoate has been successful in some areas. At the present time, however, personal chemoprophylaxis for travelers is not recommended.

PRIMARY AMEBIC MENINGOENCEPHALITIS

Primary amebic meningoencephalitis is caused by free-living amebas, usually of the genus *Naegleria*. It most often affects children and young adults, appears to be acquired by swimming in fresh warm water, and is almost invariably fatal.

Free-living amebas are ubiquitous in nature where they are commonly found in soil and water. Although generally considered harmless, some varieties are clearly pathogenic for the central nervous system of mammals. In those instances of human meningoencephalitis where the responsible organism has been isolated and cultured, it has, with few exceptions, been identified as an amoeboflagellate, *Naegleria fowleri*.

Over 80 cases have been reported from different parts of the world including Australia, Czechoslovakia, Great Britain, New Zealand, and the United States. Serologic studies suggest that inapparent infections are much more common. Most of the 35 cases recognized in the United States have occurred in the Southeastern states, particularly Florida, Georgia, and Virginia. Characteristically the patients have fallen ill during the summer months approximately 1 week after swimming in fresh or brackish water. The 16 Czechoslovakian cases followed swimming in an indoor pool with chlorinated water maintained at 24°C, and 6 cases have been acquired apparently after bathing in hot mineral water. Histological evidence suggests that the amebas reach the central nervous system directly via the nasal mucosa at the level of the cribriform plate. Clinically, the illness is rapid in onset, brief in duration, and inexorable in course. The initial symptom is a severe, persistent, frontal headache followed by nausea, vomiting, fever, and nuchal rigidity. Unusual tastes or smells may be noted. Later, drowsiness, confusion, convulsions, and coma appear. Focal neurological findings may occur late in the course of the illness.

A more benign, chronic form of amebic meningoencephalitis has been linked to organisms of the genus *Acanthamoeba*. Patients with this clinical syndrome frequently lack a history of freshwater swimming and may recover spontaneously. Pathologically, the disease can be distinguished from *Naegleria* infections by the granulomatous nature of the inflammatory reaction and the presence of both trophozoites and cysts in the tissues. Unfortunately, the identification of the responsible organisms remains in some doubt as they have never been recovered by culture techniques. It is possible that the free-living ameba of several species are involved.

A careful examination of the cerebrospinal fluid is the single most helpful diagnostic procedure. The fluid is usually bloody or sanguinopurulent and demonstrates an intense neutrophilic response. The protein is elevated and the glucose diminished. No organisms are demonstrated on Gram's stain or routine culture. Early examination of a wet preparation of unspun spinal fluid will usually reveal viable trophozoites. They are 10 to 20 μm in diameter, possess a granular cytoplasm, a distinct ectoplasm, and bulbous pseudopodia. If the specimen is allowed to cool, the trophozoites may become immobile and more difficult to recognize. Although the amebas may be easily grown on ordinary culture media which have been seeded with coliform bacteria, this is not helpful in clinical management, so rapidly progressive is the disease. Treatment with standard antiprotozoal agents seems completely ineffective. *Naegleria,* however, is highly sensitive to amphotericin B, miconazole, tetracycline, and rifampin. To date only two patients have survived a *Naegleria* infection. Both were diagnosed early and treated, one with amphotericin B and the other with amphotericin B, miconazole, and rifampin. Intracisternal, as well as intravenous, administration of amphotericin is probably essential to rapidly obtain effective levels in the cerebrospinal fluid. The intraventricular dose is 0.5 to 1 mg for the first few days. The intravenous dose is similar to that for cryptococcal meningitis (Chap. 153).

If the source of the infection can be determined, further cases might be prevented by closing the area to bathing.

REFERENCES

Amebiasis

ADAMS EB, MacLEOD IN: Invasive amebiasis. Medicine 56:315, 1977

BARBOUR GL, JUNIPER K JR: A clinical comparison of amebic and pyogenic abscess of the liver in sixty-six patients. Am J Med 53:323, 1972

COHEN HG, REYNOLDS TB: Comparison of metronidazole and chloroquine for the treatment of amebic liver abscess. Gastroenterology 69:35, 1975

ELSDON-DEW R: The epidemiology of amebiasis. Adv Parasitol 6:1, 1968

GRIFFIN FH JR: Failure of metronidazole to cure hepatic amebic abscess. N Engl J Med 288:1397, 1973

JUNIPER K JR: Amebiasis. Clin Gastroenterol 7:3, 1978

KROGSTAD DJ et al: Amebiasis: Epidemiologic studies in the United States, 1971–1974. Ann Intern Med 88:89, 1978

——— et al: Current concepts in parasitology—amebiasis. N Engl J Med 298:262, 1978

The Medical Letter. 20(4):17, 1978

NEAL RA: Pathogenesis of amebiasis. Bull NY Acad Med 47:462, 1971

POWELL SJ et al: Metronidazole combined with diloxanide furoate in amebic liver abscess. Ann Trop Med Parasitol 67:367, 1973

SCHMERIN MJ et al: Amebiasis—an increasing problem among homosexuals in New York City. JAMA 238:1386, 1977

SODEMAN WA JR, DOWDA MC: Rapid serologic methods for the demonstration of *Entamoeba histolytica* activity. Gastroenterology 65:604, 1973

Primary amebic meningoencephalitis

CARTER RF: Primary amoebic meningoencephalitis: An appraisal of present knowledge. Trans R Soc Trop Med Hyg 67:193, 1972

DUMA RJ et al: Primary amebic meningoencephalitis caused by *Naegleria*. Ann Intern Med 74:861, 1971

———: Meningoencephalitis and brain abscess due to a free-living amoeba. Ann Intern Med 88:468, 1978

ROBERT VB, RORKE LB: Primary amebic encephalitis, probably from *Acanthamoeba*. Ann Intern Med 79:174, 1973

200
MALARIA

JAMES J. PLORDE

DEFINITION Malaria is a protozoan disease transmitted to humans by the bite of *Anopheles* mosquitoes. It is characterized by *rigors, fever, splenomegaly, anemia* and a *chronic relapsing course*. Despite the impressive results of the World Health Organization–sponsored malaria eradication program begun in the year 1956, technical and socioeconomic difficulties have led to a recent resurgence of the disease in many areas of the world. Consequently, malaria remains today, as it has been for centuries, one of the most serious infectious disease problems in the world. In the United States and Europe, several hundred imported cases are seen annually in travelers from endemic areas.

ETIOLOGY *The causative organisms are protozoa of the genus Plasmodium.* The four species known to infect human beings are *P. vivax, P. ovale, P. malariae,* and *P. falciparum.* Human infection begins when a female anopheline inoculates plasmodial *sporozoites* into the lymphohematogenous system while feeding. After a brief passage in the peripheral blood, these organisms invade hepatocytes where they initiate the preclinical hepatic (exoerythrocytic) phase of disease. By a process of asexual multiplication referred to as *schizogony,* a single sporozoite eventually produces 2000 to 40,000 hepatic *merozoites.* In 1 to 6 weeks, these daughter cells rupture back into the circulatory system. In *P. falciparum,* and presumably *P. malariae,* infections, the hepatic phase terminates at this point. In the other species, liver forms persist and produce new episodes of bloodstream invasion months to years later.

The erythrocytic or clinical phase of malaria starts with the attachment of a released merozoite to a specific receptor site on the red blood cell surface. This site appears to differ for each species of malaria; in the case of *P. vivax*, it is related in some way to the Duffy blood group antigens (Fy^a or Fy^b). Duffy-negative (FyFy) individuals, who include the majority of people of West African extraction, are resistant to vivax malaria, presumably for this reason. Following attachment, the merozoite invaginates the cell surface and is slowly interiorized. The intracellular parasite first appears as a ring-shaped trophozoite which later enlarges and assumes an irregular or ameboid shape. Its nucleus then divides into several portions to form a multinucleated *schizont*. Eventually, cytoplasm condenses around each daughter nucleus to form a new generation of merozoites. Forty-eight hours after its original invasion (72 h in the case of *P. malariae*) the erythrocyte ruptures, releasing 6 to 24 organisms, each of which is capable of initiating a new red blood cell cycle. With repetition of this cycle, some of the red blood cells become filled with *sexual forms* (gametocytes); these do not induce cell lysis and are unable to undergo further development unless ingested by an appropriate mosquito during a blood meal. In the stomach of the mosquito fertilization occurs, and the resulting *ookinete* encysts on the outer surface of the stomach and releases myriads of *sporozoites*. These migrate to the salivary glands and are inoculated into a human subject at the next feeding.

EPIDEMIOLOGY Malaria survives only in areas of the world where both the anopheline and infected human population remain above certain *critical densities* required for the sustained transmission of disease. Control measures are directed toward reducing both populations to levels that are too low for the infection to survive. Important procedures include drainage or filling of breeding areas, use of residual insecticide sprays, screening, use of skin repellents, effective treatment of cases,

and large-scale suppressive drug programs in some human populations.

An active international cooperative program aimed at the eradication of malaria resulted in a significant decline in the incidence of the disease between 1956 and 1968. In over three-quarters of the original malarial areas of the world, the disease was eradicated, or active eradication programs were instituted. Presently, however, malaria still infects 125 million inhabitants of 104 countries throughout Africa, Latin America, South America, Asia, and Oceania (Fig. 200-1). Tropical Africa alone harbors 100 million of these afflicted individuals and contributes most of the 1 million deaths that occur annually from this terrible disease. The presence of mobile populations, outdoor-biting mosquitoes, and high levels of disease transmission make successful eradication in these remaining areas unlikely. Furthermore, the emergence of insecticide-resistant mosquitoes as well as a variety of administrative and socioeconomic problems has produced serious setbacks to several previously successful eradication programs, particularly those on the Indian subcontinent. Added to these difficulties has been the continuing spread of drug-resistant *P. falciparum* throughout Southern Asia, the Western Pacific, Central America, and South America. A limited number of resistant strains have now been discovered in Africa, an area previously free of this problem.

Endemic malaria did not disappear from the United States until the 1950s. Imported cases and occasional outbreaks of malaria acquired by mosquito transmission from imported infections (*introduced malaria*) have continued to occur, but until 1966 the total never exceeded 200 cases a year. This number rapidly increased with the return of infected military personnel from Southeast Asia, reaching a peak of over 4000 in 1970. Associated with this wave of imported malaria was a smaller increase in the number of infections induced by blood transfusion and intravenous heroin use. Although this epidemic has

FIGURE 200-1

Areas of risk for malaria transmission as of December 1974. (From WHO Weekly Epidemiologic Record no 45, 1975.)

waned, the incidence of malaria in the civilian population has not (Fig. 200-2). From 1970 to 1977, the number of cases reported annually among tourists, businessmen, teachers, students, and other civilians rose from 151 to 466. With rare exceptions, malaria was acquired abroad: approximately 50 percent in Asia, 30 percent in Africa, and 10 percent in the Caribbean or Latin America. Clinical manifestations usually developed within 6 months of arrival in the United States, but in one-third of the vivax cases they were delayed beyond that point. In 1977, one-fifth of the cases and two out of the three deaths were caused by the virulent *P. falciparum.* Tragically, most of these cases could have been prevented with appropriate chemoprophylaxis. Until travelers are more fully informed of dangers inherent in traveling unprotected to malarious areas, the number of cases seen in this country each year will continue to increase.

PATHOGENESIS AND PATHOLOGY The invasion, alteration, and destruction of red blood cells by malaria parasites, systemic and local circulatory changes, and immune phenomena are all important in the pathophysiology of malaria.

Red blood cell changes Malaria species differ significantly in their ability to invade red blood cells. *Plasmodium vivax* and *P. ovale* attack only immature erythrocytes; *P. malariae,* only senescent ones. During infection with these species, therefore, no more than 1 or 2 percent of cells are involved at any one time. *Plasmodium falciparum* invades red blood cells regardless of age and may cause extremely high levels of parasitemia. Only the presence of certain abnormal hemoglobins, notably S, is capable of limiting parasitemia produced by the species. The same protective effect may be exerted in hemoglobin C, D, E thalassemia, and glucose 6-phosphate (G6PD) or pyridoxal-kinase deficiency, since these abnormalities are found more commonly in malarious areas. In thalassemia and related hemoglobinopathies, the protection may be related in part to the persistent production of fetal hemoglobin since maturation of *P. falciparum* is retarded in cells containing hemoglobin F.

Once parasitized, the cells may be destroyed at the time of sporulation or in the presence of specific opsonizing antibody phagocytosed in the liver or spleen. In the spleen the parasites are also removed from some cells, and the intact erythrocytes

are returned into the circulation. However, anemia usually develops and, in the case of falciparum malaria, may be severe. This species also induces physical changes in parasitized cells resulting in intravascular agglutination and sludging.

Although paroxysms of fever coincide with sporulation and the destruction of red blood cells, the cause of the fever remains obscure and may be related to release of an endogenous pyrogen from injured cells.

Circulatory changes The circulatory changes in malaria are characterized by vasoconstriction during the "cold" stage followed by vasodilation during the "hot" stage. In falciparum malaria vasodilation in the skin is accompanied by hypotension, decreased central venous pressure, increased radioiodinated serum albumin space, and increased excretion of aldosterone, suggesting a decrease in effective circulating blood volume due to enhanced vascular permeability and/or capacitance. On the other hand, there may be localized vasospasm, kinin-induced capillary permeability with a resulting increase in blood viscosity, obstruction of capillaries with agglutinated red blood cells, and, occasionally, intravascular coagulation which may compromise perfusion to vital organs such as the kidney, brain, liver, and lung.

Immune phenomena Normal as well as parasitized red blood cells are destroyed in malaria. The explanation for this phenomenon is unknown, although immunologic mechanisms including autoantibody production and adherence of antigen-antibody complexes to uninfected red blood cells have been suggested. The destruction is most profound in blackwater fever where there is massive intravascular hemolysis. More commonly, however, the red blood cells are sequestered and destroyed in the reticuloendothelial system of the liver and spleen. Thrombocytopenia is related to splenic pooling and shortened platelet life span. Both direct parasitic invasion and immune mechanisms may be operative in platelet destruction. Host γ- and β-1C-globulin deposits have been noted along the glomerular capillary basement membrane of patients with the

FIGURE 200-2
Military and civilian cases of malaria, United States, 1959–1977. (From Malaria Surveillance: Annual Summary 1977, Atlanta, Center for Disease Control, 1978.)

acute transient glomerulonephritis of falciparum malaria and the progressive nephrosis of chronic quartan malaria, establishing these as immune complex nephropathies.

IMMUNITY Recovery from malaria occurs slowly, apparently the function of acquired immunity. In simian malaria, this appears to require the presence of both T and B cell lymphocytes. Although the role of the T cell is known to be vital, its mechanism of action is uncertain. Some authors have suggested that it stimulates effector cells, perhaps macrophages, to release a nonspecific factor capable of inhibiting intraerythrocytic multiplication; others feel it may have a helper effect on antibody formation.

Strain-specific antiplasmodial antibodies do occur early in the course of parasitemia and reach high levels coincident with a fall in the number of circulating organisms. The relative rarity of malaria in young infants has been attributed to transplacental passage of IgG antibodies. It is uncertain whether these are directly lethal, act as opsonizing agents or block merozoitic invasion of erythrocytes. In simian malaria, antigenic change in the parasite results in cycles of recrudescent parasitemia and production of variant-specific antibodies. It seems probable that similar changes occur in humans, leading to the eventual disappearance of erythrocytic forms. In falciparum malaria, this results in cure. In vivax and ovale infections, the intracellular hepatic forms escape the humoral immune defenses and may later discharge fresh merozoites into the bloodstream to maintain the infection for a period of 3 to 5 years. *Plasmodium malariae* produces chronic disease of extremely long duration, up to 53 years in one case, despite the lack of a persistent exoerythrocytic focus. This effect is presumably due to long-term survival of circulating parasites in concentrations too low to be detected on routine blood films. How these parasites escape immunologic destruction is unknown. In a closely related simian malaria, however, splenectomy rapidly leads to termination of infection, suggesting that suppressor T cells in the spleen may play a protective role.

MANIFESTATIONS General The incubation period between the bite of the mosquito and onset of symptoms is usually 10 to 14 days in vivax and falciparum malaria and 18 days to 6 weeks in malariae infections. This period may be prolonged in persons who have taken antimalarial suppressants. In the United States, the interval between entry into the country and onset of disease exceeds 6 months in one-quarter of the patients developing vivax infections; it exceeds 1 month in a similar proportion of falciparum cases. There is some variation in clinical manifestations produced by the different plasmodia, but in all, chills, fever, headache, muscle pains, splenomegaly, and anemia are common. Herpes labialis is frequent and usually appears after the infection is well established. Hepatomegaly, mild icterus, and edema are often observed, especially in falciparum infections. Urticaria is common in patients with chronic malaria.

The hallmark of the disease is the malarial *paroxysm*, which recurs regularly in all but falciparum infections. The typical paroxysm begins with a rigor that lasts 20 to 60 min—the "cold stage"—followed by a "hot stage" of 3 to 8 h with temperature of 40 to 41.7°C (104 to 107°F). The "wet stage" consists of defervescence with profuse diaphoresis and leaves the patient exhausted.

First attacks are often severe, but repeated episodes become milder, although debilitation may be progressive. In untreated cases, the attacks may persist for weeks. The paroxysms eventually become more irregular and less frequent and finally cease, corresponding with the disappearance of parasites from the blood and marking the end of the primary attack. Relapses occur when exoerythrocytic parasites persisting in the liver reinvade the bloodstream.

Tertian malaria (*P. vivax* or *P. ovale*) This infection is rarely fatal, although relapses are common, and it is the most difficult to cure. A prodrome of myalgia, headache, chilliness, and low-grade fever for 48 to 72 h heralds the onset of the acute illness. Initially, the fever may be irregular because the maturation cycle of the parasite is not synchronized. Synchronization usually occurs toward the end of the first week, and typical paroxysms then occur on alternate days. The spleen becomes palpable at the end of the second week. Infections with *P. ovale* tend to be milder, and primary attacks shorter than those caused by *P. vivax*.

Quartan malaria (*P. malariae*) Paroxysms occur every third day and tend to be regular. The disease is usually more disabling than tertian but responds well to treatment. Edema, albuminuria, and hematuria (*not* hemoglobinuria), a clinical state similar to acute hemorrhagic nephritis, occasionally appear during the course. This complication should not be confused with *blackwater fever*. Chronic *P. malariae* infection may be associated with a clinically and histologically unique nephrosis. The prolonged duration of asymptomatic parasitemia characteristic of the species helps to explain the frequency with which it is implicated in transfusion-induced malaria.

Falciparum malaria (*P. falciparum*) Because of an asynchronous cycle of multiplication, onset may be insidious and fever continuous, remittent, or irregular. Typical paroxysms occur in a minority of patients. Splenomegaly occurs rapidly, and mental confusion, postural hypotension, edema, and gastrointestinal symptoms are common. If the acute attack is treated rapidly, the disease is usually mild and recovery uneventful. If left untreated, anemia becomes severe, and the decreased effective circulating blood volume results in capillary blockage that can give rise to serious complications. This feature of *P. falciparum* infections accounts for the protean manifestations of this form of malaria, and the high morbidity and mortality associated with it. Depending upon the organ system involved, several so-called *pernicious syndromes* are seen. *Cerebral malaria* can lead to hemiplegia, convulsions, delirium, hyperpyrexia, coma, and rapid death. When the *pulmonary* circulation is involved, there may be cough and blood-streaked sputum, leading to confusion with many other diseases of the lung. Severe pulmonary insufficiency closely resembling the "shock lung" syndrome frequently accompanies cerebral malaria. The splanchnic capillaries can be obstructed, with consequent vomiting, abdominal pain, diarrhea, or melena. Such patients are sometimes thought to have bacillary dysentery or cholera. Fever in these disorders may be low or absent. Indeed, in patients with predominantly gastrointestinal manifestations, there are usually cold, clammy skin, hypotension, profound weakness, and repeated syncopal attacks, so-called *algid malaria*. Tender hepatomegaly, with or without jaundice, and acute renal failure are common. The pernicious syndromes should be anticipated if the intensity of parasitemia exceeds 100,000 organisms per cubic millimeter.

Blackwater fever This is a disorder that occurs in association with malaria, particularly and perhaps only with *P. falciparum* infections. The usual attack begins with a rigor and fever followed by massive intravascular hemolysis, icterus, hemoglobinuria, collapse, and often acute renal failure and uremia. The pathological findings in the kidney are necrosis of tubules and occasionally hemoglobin casts. The mortality is 20 to 30 percent, and survivors are very likely to experience hemolytic episodes with subsequent malarial infections.

Although blackwater fever is often classified as one of the "pernicious" complications of falciparum malaria, its cause is obscure. In many patients, parasitemia is absent at the time hemolysis occurs. Because blackwater fever has usually occurred in patients with chronic falciparum infections who were treated with quinine, it was suggested that the hemolysis results from an autoimmune reaction to the red blood cells that have been altered by the drug, parasite, or both. However, blackwater fever can occur in patients not given drugs. The institution of an appropriate regimen for acute renal failure (Chap. 275) will reduce the fatality rate considerably.

Complications In addition to the several complications already mentioned, others deserve comment. Rupture of the spleen is relatively rare, but malaria is by far the commonest cause of spontaneous rupture and predisposes to traumatic rupture of this organ. It is most commonly seen in vivax infections.

Chronic malaria or repeated infection in an endemic area leads to anemia, debility, cachexia, and suppression of humoral antibody response to a variety of antigens. These manifestations are particularly severe in children under the age of 3 and in pregnant women. Infection in the latter population is associated with low birth weight of the resulting child and high neonatal mortality. Congenital malaria, although rare, does occur; it is probably most common in the offspring of nonimmune individuals. Secondary bacterial infection is frequent and is often the immediate cause of death. Bacillary dysentery, cholera, and pyogenic pneumonia are common. Tuberculous foci often extend in malarial patients, and miliary tuberculosis is occasionally observed.

Patients living in endemic malarious areas commonly present with chronic hepatosplenomegaly of unknown cause. In some of these, there is infiltration of hepatic sinusoids by lymphocytes, very high levels of serum IgM, and high malaria antibody titers. This condition, which is known as the *tropical splenomegaly syndrome,* is seldom seen before the age of 8. It differs from the ordinary hepatosplenomegaly of malaria in that parasitemia is rare. It has been suggested that the condition results from defective T-cell control of immunoglobulin production, leading to excessive macroglobulin production and immune complex formation. Long-term antimalarial therapy leads to a decrease in spleen size and a disappearance of hepatic sinusoidal lymphocytosis. The epidemiologic evidence implicating malaria as a contributory factor in the etiology of Burkitt's lymphoma has increased. It has been suggested that continuous stimulation of the lymphoid system in chronic malaria makes it more susceptible to neoplastic transformation in the presence of EB virus.

LABORATORY FINDINGS The blood leukocyte count is low or normal. The platelet count is often reduced, especially in falciparum malaria. The erythrocyte sedimentation rate is elevated. Plasmodia are demonstrable in smears of peripheral blood from the vast majority of patients with symptomatic malaria. When the disease is suspected, appropriately stained blood films should be examined diligently. For the inexperienced examiner, a thin smear of fingertip blood on a clean glass slide should be stained with Wright's or Giemsa's stain. Parasitized erythrocytes are most frequent at the edges of a smear; extracellular parasites are not found. Thick smears should be thoroughly dried and stained with diluted Giemsa's or Field stain. This method has the advantage of concentrating the parasites, but artifacts are numerous, and correct interpre-

tations of these preparations require much experience. The value of buffy coat smears in the detection of low-grade parasitemia remains to be determined.

The morphology of the four species of plasmodia that infect humans is specific enough to allow identification in blood smears. The parasitized red blood cells in *P. vivax* infections are enlarged and pale and may contain diffuse bright red dots (Schaffner's dots), and the parasite presents in a wide variety of shapes and sizes; in *P. ovale* infections, the red blood cells containing parasites are oval but otherwise resemble those in *P. vivax;* in *P. malariae* the red blood cells are of normal size and do not contain dots. The parasites often present in "band" forms, and the merozoites are arranged in a rosette around central pigment; in *P. falciparum* infections the rings are very small, may contain two rather than one chromatin dot, and often are found lying flat against the margin of the cell. Only the ring stages of the asexual forms are found in the peripheral smear, and there may be more than one ring in a single red blood cell. The gametocytes are distinctively large and banana-shaped.

There is no advantage of blood over material obtained by splenic or sternal puncture. The administration of epinephrine with the idea of dislodging parasites by producing contraction of the spleen has been advocated, but results are irregular. Serologic tests are used primarily for epidemiologic rather than diagnostic purposes but are also helpful in speciation of the infecting organism and in detection of occult malaria in the bloodstream. The indirect immunofluorescent test seems to be the most sensitive and specific.

DIAGNOSIS The most important diagnostic test is a careful medical history. The diagnosis must be considered in any febrile patient who has resided in or traveled to the Caribbean, Latin America, Asia, or Africa within the previous 12 months. History of previous attacks of malaria, typical malarial paroxysms, or some artificial exposure (blood transfusion, narcotic injections in an addict) should also suggest the disease. Splenomegaly is an almost invariable finding during the second week of illness. Leukocytosis is *not* a feature of malaria. The diagnosis is confirmed by demonstrating the parasites in the peripheral blood. Because the intensity of parasitemia varies greatly from hour to hour, particularly in *P. falciparum* infections, blood smears should be examined every 8 h for 2 or 3 days before the diagnosis is abandoned.

While final cure of malaria may be difficult, particularly in *P. vivax* infections, almost all cases will respond symptomatically to quinine or one of the newer antimalarial drugs, and failure of response to a therapeutic trial argues strongly against the diagnosis.

TREATMENT The use of appropriate chemotherapy can suppress symptoms in individuals exposed in endemic areas or cure malarial infection completely. However, the emergence of drug-resistant falciparum malaria in Southeast Asia, including Burma, Indonesia, and the Philippines, in South America, and in adjacent areas of Central America necessitates the use of drug combinations in the treatment of this infection.

Treatment of acute attack Treatment of an acute attack can be accomplished with chloroquine for all types of malaria except drug-resistant falciparum infection (Table 200-1). The drug usually produces complete subsidence of symptoms and destruction of the erythrocytic forms of the parasite. If vomiting is present, chloroquine hydrochloride should be given intramuscularly or, in the case of shock, intravenously. Oral therapy should be resumed as soon as possible. Although side effects are uncommon, this agent may produce epigastric distress, itching, and neurotoxicity, including involuntary movements and convulsions.

If patients have transfusion-induced malaria or have contracted the disease in an area known to harbor drug-resistant *P. falciparum,* they should be treated with a combination of quinine, pyrimethamine, and one of the sulfonamides or sulfones. *Quinine sulfate,* 0.6 g orally three times a day, should be given for 14 days. If nausea and vomiting preclude oral therapy, quinine dihydrochloride diluted in saline solution or glucose can be given very slowly intravenously. During infusion the pulse and blood pressure should be monitored constantly to detect arrhythmia or hypotension. Oral therapy should be instituted as soon as possible. In the presence of renal or hepatic failure, the dose of quinine should be limited to 0.6 g a day. An overdose of quinine produces cinchonism of which tinnitus is an early manifestation. The drug may also cause mild hemolysis, allergic purpura, and drug fever. The appearance of a Coombs-positive hemolytic anemia requires the immediate withdrawal of the drug. Pyrimethamine should be given orally in dosage of 25 mg two times daily for 3 days. This is an antifolate agent and may cause megaloblastic anemia. Sulfisoxazole or sulfadiazine, 2.0 g initially and then 0.5 g every 6 h for 5 days, should be given concurrently with the other two drugs. A variety of other combinations of antifolate agents with sulfonamides or sulfones have also been used with quinine to good effect. Fansidar, a fixed-drug combination containing 25 mg pyrimethamine and 500 mg sulfadoxine, has been particularly effective. However, it is presently not available in the United States. The combination of tetracycline 2.0 g per day for 7 days plus quinine has been suggested for the treatment of drug-resistant malaria.

Patients should be followed for 1 month to detect recrudescence of the infection. If there are circulating asexual erythrocytic forms, retreatment with pyrimethamine and a sulfonamide should be instituted. The presence of circulating gametocytes is not, however, an indication for retreatment.

Radical cure *Plasmodium vivax* and *P. ovale* persist in the liver in the exoerythrocytic stage and in this form are not affected by drugs used in the treatment of the acute attack. Unless destroyed, they will eventually reinvade the bloodstream. Primaquine base, 15 mg by mouth daily for 14 days, will effect a radical cure in most cases. If relapse occurs after primaquine therapy, a second course of the drug at twice the dosage should be given. Alternatively, 45 mg primaquine base can be given in combination with 300 mg chloroquine once weekly for 8 weeks. Primaquine may cause hemolysis in patients with G6PD deficiency, but in the dosage recommended this is rare and usually mild.

Treatment of complications This includes careful attention to fluid and electrolyte balance, prevention of fluid overload in patients with oliguria, and early diagnosis and treatment of renal failure. In severe hemolysis large doses of steroids may be helpful. Transfusions should be given in severe hemolysis, care being taken to match the donor's cells and plasma with those of the recipient. Intravenous low-molecular-weight dextran may be helpful in increasing capillary blood flow in cerebral malaria. Dexamethasone is used in management of cerebral edema. The value of heparin in this syndrome, even when evidence suggestive of intravascular coagulation is present, remains controversial.

PREVENTION General In areas of the world such as Africa where eradication is presently impractical, limited residual insecticides plus chemoprophylaxis for pregnant women and children are recommended. The long-term hope for eradication now depends on the development of new technologies. Two new areas of research hold some promise—biological control of mosquitoes and a malaria vaccine. The latter has been made more feasible by two recent achievements: the continuous culture of *P. falciparum* in red blood cells and the demonstration that merozoites can serve as effective immunogens. Although merozoite vaccines have already been used successfully in test animals, the adjuvants required preclude present use in humans. It is hoped that effective human vaccines can be developed within the next decade.

Personal protection In endemic areas, mosquito contact should be minimized through the use of house screens, mosquito netting around beds, insect repellants, and insecticides. In addition, patients traveling to endemic areas should receive chemoprophylaxis.

Chemoprophylaxis (see Table 200-2) Although it is not possible to prevent infection with chemotherapeutic agents, it is possible to suppress symptoms while the patient is residing in an endemic area by the administration of chloroquine base in dosage of 300 mg weekly (2 tablets Aralen). If the medication

TABLE 200-1
Malaria treatment

Purpose	Drug	Dosage
Cure chloroquine-resistant *P. falciparum* infection	Quinine sulfate*	650 mg PO tid for 10–14 days
	or quinine dihydrochloride*,†	600 mg in 300 ml normal saline IV over 1 h; repeat in 6–8 h; maximum 1800 mg per day
	plus pyrimethamine	25 mg PO bid for 3 days
	plus sulfadiazine	500 mg PO bid for 5 days
Cure *P. malariae* and chloroquine-sensitive *P. falciparum* infection	Chloroquine phosphate	1 g (600 mg base) PO, then 500 mg in 6 h, then 500 mg per day for 2 days
	or chloroquine hydrochloride†	250 mg (200 mg base) IM or IV every 6 h; administer IV dose as for quinine dihydrochloride above; maximum 900 mg per day
Cure *P. vivax* and *P. ovale* infection	Same as for *P. malariae* *plus* primaquine phosphate	26.3 mg (15 mg base) PO qd for 14 days

* *If quinine is not immediately available, begin with chloroquine and switch when quinine arrives.*
† *For use when patient cannot take oral drug. Switch to oral therapy as soon as possible.*

TABLE 200-2
Malaria chemoprophylaxis

Purpose	Drug	Dosage
To suppress clinical malaria in areas *without* chloroquine-resistant strains	Chloroquine phosphate	500 mg (300 mg base) PO once weekly, continued 6 weeks after leaving malarious area
	or amodiaquine dehydrochloride	520 mg (400 mg base) PO once weekly, continued 6 weeks after leaving malarious area
To suppress clinical malaria in areas *with* chloroquine-resistant strains	Same as above	
	plus pyrimethamine-sulfadoxine* (Fansidar, Hoffmann-LaRoche)	25 mg pyrimethamine and 500 mg sulfadoxine PO once weekly, continued 6 weeks after leaving malarious area
To prevent relapses of *P. vivax* and *P. ovale* infection	Primaquine phosphate†	26.3 mg (15 mg base) PO daily for 14 days or 79 mg (45 mg base) for 8 weeks; start during last 2 weeks of suppressive therapy or immediately upon its completion

* Presently not available in the United States.
† Recommended only for travelers without G6PD deficiency who have had heavy exposure.

is continued for 6 weeks after the patient has left the area, *P. malariae* and sensitive strains of *P. falciparum* will be eradicated. *Plasmodium ovale* and *P. vivax* will produce clinical manifestations some weeks or months after chloroquine is discontinued because of their persistence outside red blood cells. This can be circumvented by administration of primaquine after chloroquine is discontinued. Chloroquine is not effective in suppressing drug-resistant *P. falciparum*. In areas of the world where this is a problem pyrimethamine, 25 mg, plus sulfadoxine, 500 mg, can be taken orally once weekly. These drugs are available in combination form in most endemic areas. Leukopenia occurs in approximately 10 percent of patients using this regimen. Mefloquine, a highly effective prophylactic agent for chloroquine-resistant malaria, is currently undergoing clinical trials in several areas of the world.

Transfusions Transfusion malaria continues to occur in the United States; recently *P. falciparum* has been the most common cause. Adherence to recommendations of the American Association of Blood Banking will prevent most of these cases.

REFERENCES

Brown HW: *Basic Clinical Pathology*, 4th ed. New York, Appleton-Century-Crofts, 1975
Bruce-Chawatt LJ: Transfusion malaria. Bull WHO 50:337, 1974
Chemoprophylaxis of malaria. Morb Mort Week Rep Suppl 27(10):81, March 10, 1978
Drugs for parasitic infections. Med Lett 20(4):17, 1978
Heineman HS: The clinical syndrome of malaria in the United States. Arch Intern Med 129:607, 1972
Hendrickse RG et al: Quartan malarial nephrotic syndrome. Lancet 1:1143, 1972
Jeffery GM: Malaria control in the twentieth century. Am J Trop Med Hyg 25:361, 1976
Kean BH, Reilly PC Jr: Malaria—the mime. Recent lessons from a group of civilian travelers. Am J Med 61:159, 1976
Laderman C: Malaria and progress: Some historical and ecological considerations. Soc Sci Med 9:587, 1975
Miller LH: Current prospects and problems for a malaria vaccine. J Infect Dis 135:855, 1977
———: Hypothesis on the mechanism of erythrocyte invasion by malaria merozoites. Bull WHO 55:157, 1977
Trager W: Cultivation of *Plasmodium falciparum*. Arch Pathol Lab Med 101:277, 1977
Tropical splenomegaly syndrome. Lancet 1:1058, 1976
Wilson M et al: Comparison of the complement fixation, indirect immunofluorescence and indirect hemagglutination tests for malaria. Am J Trop Med Hyg 24:755, 1975

201
LEISHMANIASIS

JAMES J. PLORDE

DEFINITION Leishmaniasis designates a human disorder produced by flagellated tissue protozoa of the genus *Leishmania*. It is transmitted from animal to human being or sometimes from human to human by the bite of phlebotomine sandflies. The infection may be either visceral or cutaneous. The former, or kala azar, is characterized by chronic recurrent fever, splenomegaly, pancytopenia, weight loss, and high mortality. Cutaneous leishmaniasis may present as single or multiple chronic skin ulcers, destructive mucocutaneous lesions, or a disseminated infection resembling leprosy.

ETIOLOGY AND PATHOGENESIS There is confusion over speciation of *Leishmania*. These organisms appear morphologically identical and must be differentiated on serologic, biochemical, cultural, nosologic, and behavioral grounds which are not entirely satisfactory. Four main groups are generally recognized: *L. donovani*, *L. tropica*, *L. mexicana*, and *L. brasiliensis*. Each group contains a variety of strains which have been accorded separate species or subspecies status by some workers.

Leishmania donovani is the cause of kala azar, the visceral form of leishmaniasis.

Leishmania tropica causes Old World cutaneous leishmaniasis, or oriental sore, also known as Delhi boil, Bagdad boil, Aleppo button, and Salek and Pendeh sore. A variety of this organism, *L. tropica aethiopica*, causes both oriental sore and diffuse cutaneous leishmaniasis in Ethiopia.

Leishmania mexicana produces a cutaneous leishmaniasis known as bay sore and *chiclero ulcer* as well as the South American form of disseminated cutaneous disease. *Leishmania brasiliensis* is the cause of American mucocutaneous leishmaniasis also known as *espundia*. *Leishmania brasiliensis peruviana* produces *uta*, another type of cutaneous leishmaniasis.

In the sandfly, the parasites assume the flagellated leptomonas form, but in humans the organisms lose their flagella, enter mononuclear phagocytes, and multiply as small, rounded leishmanial forms 2 to 3 μm in diameter, containing a nucleus and kinetoplast, the pathognomonic Leishman-Donovan bodies.

In humans continued intracellular multiplication of the parasite leads to rupture of the affected phagocyte and invasion of other cells, resulting in extensive histiocytic proliferation. The course of the disease from this point is apparently determined by the host's cellular immunity as well as the species of the parasite. In cutaneous leishmaniasis, there is a marked lymphocytic infiltration associated with a reduction in the number of parasites, the development of a delayed skin (leishmanin) reaction, and spontaneous cure. In the mucocutaneous form, the spontaneous disappearance of the primary lesion may be followed by metastatic mucocutaneous lesions at some later date. The destructiveness of the cutaneous lesions is attributed to the development of hypersensitivity to parasitic antigens. An interesting exception to the general pattern in cutaneous disease is disseminated cutaneous leishmaniasis in which there is no infiltration of lymphocytes and plasma cells or reduction in the number of parasites, the leishmanin reaction is negative, and the skin lesions become chronic, progressive, and disseminated. In visceral leishmaniasis, the cellular changes are similar but the parasites spread to reticuloendothelial cells throughout the body. This spread is associated with development of marked hyperglobulinemia. As in the mucocutaneous form of the disease, circulating antibodies are detectable but do not seem to have a protective function. They may, in fact, be responsible for the pancytopenia and glomerulonephritis seen in visceral disease. A positive skin test develops in the visceral form after successful treatment.

KALA AZAR

DISTRIBUTION AND EPIDEMIOLOGY Kala azar occurs in China, Russia, India, the Middle East, Egypt, Sudan, East Africa, several Mediterranean countries, including Greece, Crete, and Malta, and a few areas of South and Central America. Although the manifestations of the disease throughout this area, which touches all continents but Australia, are basically similar, certain definite peculiarities in its behavior justify classification of visceral leishmaniasis into at least three main types. These differences are attributed to variations in the strains of *L. donovani* in a given area and, perhaps more important, to the length of time that the disease has been endemic in a population. It is believed that kala azar (and also infection by *L. tropica*) is introduced into a new area from animal reservoirs and that this "primitive" or zoonotic infection is likely to result in many cases of acute, rapidly fatal illness among the population coming into contact with the parasites for the first time. After generations, kala azar becomes endemic, the disease assumes a more chronic form, and the domestic dog becomes an important reservoir.

Mediterranean, or *infantile*, *kala azar* is seen primarily in the Mediterranean area, China, Russia, and Latin America. An outbreak in Kenya also appears to be of this type. It is a disease of children under the age of 4, but adults, particularly travelers to endemic areas, are not spared. Dogs, jackals, and foxes serve as reservoirs, and human-to-human transmission is thought to be rare. The strains responsible for the Eurasian and American diseases are sometimes referred to as *L. infantum* and *L. chagasi* respectively.

Indian kala azar affects older children and young adults, and males are involved more commonly than females. The human being is the only known reservoir, and transmission is carried out by anthropophilic species of sandflies. This form of disease has become uncommon as a result of antimalarial spraying.

African kala azar is found in the Eastern half of Africa from the Sahara in the North to the equator in the South. Its age and sex distribution is similar to that of Indian kala azar. It is endemic in gerbils and other rodents in many areas and is more resistant to therapy with antimony compounds than that found in the rest of the world.

MANIFESTATIONS The incubation period varies from 10 days to 1 year but is usually about 3 months. No lesion appears at the site of the infecting bite in most cases, but a primary "chancre" which heals with scarring before the onset of systemic symptoms is commonly noted in the African disease. The organisms multiply extensively in the macrophages of spleen, liver, bone marrow, lymph nodes, skin, and small intestine, accounting for many of the manifestations of the disease. Organisms may be found in the blood for several months before the onset of symptoms.

Fever, which is characterized at times by two daily spikes, may be abrupt or gradual in onset. It persists for 1 to 6 weeks and then disappears, only to reappear at irregular intervals during the course of the illness. Although prostration is absent even during periods of high fever, there is progressive weakness, pallor, weight loss, and tachycardia. Gastrointestinal disturbances are frequent in Indian cases. Physical findings include enormous splenomegaly, lymphadenopathy, hepatomegaly with signs of portal hypertension, and often edema, which tends to conceal the extent of the wasting. Hyperpigmentation is noted in light-skinned individuals, and mucocutaneous lesions similar to those seen in espundia occur in the African form of the disease. Anemia is the rule, and thrombocytopenia with gingival and other mucosal bleeding is common. The peripheral leukocyte count is low (usually less than 4000 per cubic millimeter); in children, agranulocytosis with cancrum oris (noma) and secondary pulmonary or intestinal infections contribute to the high mortality. The presence of a short erythrocyte life span, anti-red blood cell antibodies, positive Coombs' test, and antibody against white blood cells and platelets suggests an autoimmune basis for the pancytopenia.

Hypergammaglobulinemia is universally present. Proteinuria and hematuria are frequent in the course of kala azar and are thought to be related to the glomerular deposition of poorly soluble immune complexes. Uremia due to renal amyloidosis and symptoms of heart failure can occur.

Post-kala azar dermal leishmaniasis Patients treated successfully with antimony compounds for kala azar may develop cutaneous lesions called *leishmanoids*, in which *Leishmania* organisms are demonstrable. These are rare in Mediterranean or Chinese kala azar but develop in 3 percent of African cases almost immediately after systemic symptoms subside. They occur after a latent period of 1 to 2 years in as many as 10 percent of Indian cases. The lesions range from patchy areas of depigmentation to erythematous papules and confluent nodules which may involve the ears and mucous membranes and have been mistaken for leprosy. They are short-lived in African kala azar but may persist for years in the Indian variety, creating a persistent reservoir of infection.

DIAGNOSIS The diagnosis is made by finding *Leishmania* organisms in stained preparations of blood (often possible in Indian but rarely so in other forms), bone marrow, lymph nodes, or material obtained by splenic puncture. The last is the best source of organisms, but the spleen should be needled only when it is firm and enlarged well below the left costal margin. The organisms will grow out as flagellated forms in Nicolle-Novy-MacNeal (NNN) medium containing defibrinated rabbit blood incubated at 22°C.

Serologic tests are not totally satisfactory. The complement fixation test is sensitive and readily available but lacks specificity. Immunoelectrophoresis, by contrast, is highly specific but has a low sensitivity. The indirect immunofluorescence antibody test would appear to offer the advantages of both but is only group specific. A new enzyme-linked immunoabsorbent assay (ELISA) may be even more satisfactory.

The leishmanin skin test is negative during active kala azar but becomes positive several months after successful treatment of the disease.

TREATMENT Rest, good diet, transfusions, and treatment of complicating infections, of which tuberculosis, bacterial pneumonia, amebiasis, and bacillary dysentery are more important, must supplement or precede specific therapy. Pentavalent antimony compounds are highly effective against the parasites. Owing to its lack of toxicity, Pentostam (sodium antimony gluconate) given intravenously or intramuscularly is the drug of choice. The adult dose is 0.6 g (6 ml) daily for 6 days in Indian kala azar and for 30 days is other forms.

More than 90 percent of cases respond promptly to antimony, except in Africa, where the cure rate is as low as 70 percent. Resistant cases can be treated with either one of the more toxic diamidines or with amphotericin B. Pentamidine is given intramuscularly in the dose of 4 mg base per kilogram of body weight dissolved in 3 to 4 ml water daily for 10 days. The course may be repeated twice after intervals of 10 days. Hypotension, renal damage, hypoglycemia, and diabetes mellitus can complicate therapy with this drug.

PROGNOSIS AND CONTROL The mortality in untreated kala azar is 95 percent in adults and 80 percent in children. This has been greatly reduced by treatment with antimony and the aromatic diamidines. Relapses, occasionally several in number, occur in 5 to 15 percent of African and Mediterranean cases up to 2 years after treatment. Both relapses and post-kala azar dermal leishmaniasis should be re-treated in the same fashion as the initial illness.

The treatment of the disease in humans, the elimination of diseased dogs, and the use of DDT residual sprays against sandflies are the important preventive measures. Incidence of the disease has diminished greatly in many areas where DDT has been used to eradicate malaria—an unexpected added benefit of this program. When the vectors are exophilic, control is difficult. Attempts at vaccination with avirulent strains of *L. donovani* have been unsuccessful.

AMERICAN CUTANEOUS LEISHMANIASIS

These diseases occur in every country of Central and South America except Chile. In some areas, 10 to 20 percent of the population is infected. Three autochthonous infections have been reported from Texas. There are four varieties of American cutaneous leishmaniasis. All begin with a local lesion at the site of the infecting sandfly bite after an incubation period of from 10 days to 3 months.

Chiclero ulcer, which is found in Mexico, Guatemala, British Honduras, and possibly other parts of Central America, is a zoonosis caused by *L. mexicana.* The disease occurs naturally in several arboreal rodents. It is occasionally transmitted to persons entering forests to harvest chicle. In immunocompetent individuals, it is a relatively mild infection characterized by a single cutaneous lesion on the ear, face, or hand which is chronic and shows little tendency to ulceration. The leishmanin skin test is positive. Spontaneous healing usually occurs within 6 months. The parasites are never numerous in the lesions. Mucosal ulceration does not occur. Ear lesions cause extensive destruction of the pinna and should be treated with a single 350 mg intramuscular dose of cycloguanil pamoate. Immunization with live cultures of *L. mexicana* has been effective in forest workers.

Diffuse cutaneous leishmaniasis is found in Venezuela. It apparently results from a specific deficiency of cell-mediated immunity to leishmanial antigen. In South America, it is caused by members of the *L. mexicana* complex, usually *L. mexicana amazonensis.* This remarkable disease is characterized by massive dissemination of skin lesions without visceral involvement. The clinical picture often bears a striking resemblance to lepromatous leprosy. The diagnosis is not difficult, because the lesions contain a large number of organisms. In contrast to all other types of cutaneous leishmaniasis, the leishmanin skin test is negative. The disease is progressive and very refractory to treatment. Amphotericin B and pentamidine have been used to produce remissions, but cure is rare.

Uta, which occurs in cooler climates and at altitudes of more than 2000 ft, consists of single or multiple skin ulcers of the nose and lips in which parasites are readily demonstrable. Spontaneous healing within 3 months to a year is the rule, and mucosal spread is unusual. The etiologic agent is *L. peruviana,* a member of the *L. brasiliensis* group, and the reservoir is the domestic dog. With widespread use of insecticides in Peru, the disease has almost disappeared.

In tropical Latin America, *L. brasiliensis* causes the better-known and more serious *espundia.* The organism causes a natural infection in large forest rodents and is transmitted to human beings by sandflies when new settlements are made in jungle areas. The initial skin lesion enlarges progressively, and secondary bacterial infection is frequent. The disease may spread by direct extension or by lymphatics to the mucosal surfaces of the mouth and nose, where, after the primary lesion has healed, painful, destructive, and mutilating erosions scar and distort the involved structures. Fever, anemia, and weight loss accompany these mucosal complications. Destruction of the nasal septum produces a characteristic deformity called *tapir nose* or *camel nose.* The hard palate may be destroyed, and laryngeal erosion can lead to aphonia. In blacks, the lesion is often hypertrophic, and large polypoid masses deform the lips and cheeks, perhaps representing a type of keloid reaction. This can be mistaken for South American blastomycosis (Chap. 154). Secondary bacterial infection, inanition, and respiratory obstruction lead to death.

The diagnosis is made by finding the organisms in scrapings or by culture. The leishmanin skin test is specific and highly useful. Treatment consists of antibiotics for bacterial infections and pentavalent antimonials used as in kala azar. Cases that fail to respond to antimonials should be treated with amphotericin B, 0.25 to 1 mg/kg by slow infusion daily or every other day for up to 8 weeks.

The early lesions respond well, but even with repeated courses of antimony the mucosal complications of the espundia type heal slowly. In advanced cases, the prognosis is very poor.

OLD WORLD CUTANEOUS LEISHMANIASIS: ORIENTAL SORE

This, the least serious form of human leishmaniasis, consists of localized cutaneous ulceration which heals spontaneously and is endemic in the European countries bordering the eastern Mediterranean, in Africa, in Asia Minor, in Southwest Asia, and in India. Two major strains of the causative organism, *L. tropica,* produce similar but distinctive clinical syndromes. Homologous immunity after recovery from infection by either strain is solid and lifelong. Infection with *L. tropica major* protects against *L. tropica minor,* but the opposite is not the case. The rural type, caused by *L. tropica major,* has its reservoir in gerbils and other small rodents; the ulcers usually appear on the extremities 2 to 6 weeks after the bite of the sandfly and are accompanied by regional lymphadenopathy in a majority of cases. Spontaneous healing occurs within 3 to 6 months, leaving a depigmented, pitted scar.

The incubation period in the *urban,* or *dry,* type ranges

from 2 months to more than a year. The lesion is usually facial and begins as a pruritic, purplish nodule (the Aleppo button), which slowly enlarges and finally breaks down after 3 or 4 months. Lymphatic involvement is uncommon. Healing of the indolent, granulomatous ulcer may require a year or more. Occasionally, healing fails to occur, which results in lesions closely resembling lupus vulgaris. This condition, known as *leishmaniasis recidiva,* is thought to be the result of an exaggerated delayed hypersensitivity to leishmanial antigens. Humans and the domestic dog serve as the reservoirs of infection.

The typical oriental sore is a sharply punched-out, ragged ulcer about 1 in in diameter, surrounded by an erythematous rim. Satellite lesions which fuse with the original are not rare. The center of the granulating base of the ulcer frequently contains a hard excrescence called the *Montpellier sign* or the *rake* beneath which the parasites are most likely to be found when scrapings are examined.

The rural and urban types occur together in Asia Minor; indeed, it is not rare to find simultaneous infections in the same patient. In Southeastern Europe, India, and North Africa, the urban type is prevalent, while in the remainder of Africa the disease is predominantly rural.

A form of diffuse cutaneous leishmaniasis is seen in Ethiopia. It closely resembles the disease in Venezuela and appears to have a sylvatic reservoir.

Diagnosis is usually made on clinical grounds and is confirmed by finding the parasites, which occur both intra- and extracellularly. Pyogenic infection makes direct visualization difficult, but *L. tropica* can be cultured in NNN medium at room temperature, and a skin test using *L. tropica* antigen becomes positive in the vast majority of patients with the disease.

Treatment should include vigorous measures for bacterial infection, such as hot soaks and appropriate systemic antibiotics. Infrared heat treatment has also been suggested, as the leishmanial organisms are very heat-sensitive. Systemic antimonials may be required where ulceration is extensive or multiple. Pentostam is used as in kala azar in a course of 10 daily injections totaling 6 g. It may be injected locally in dosage of 0.6 g three to four times on alternate days. In endemic areas the custom is to withhold treatment directed against the parasite until the initial nodule ulcerates, to assure the development of immunity against reinfection.

Prevention consists of use of insect repellents on exposed parts of the body, residual DDT sprays, and fine-mesh screening for dwellings. The lesions should be covered to prevent infection of vectors and, of course, contact with the lesion or its discharges should be avoided.

REFERENCES

BRAY RS: Leishmaniasis in the Old World. Br Med Bull 28:39, 1972
———: Leishmania. Ann Rev Microbiol 28:189, 1974
BRITO T et al: Glomerular involvement in human kala azar. Am J Trop Med Hyg 24:9, 1975
BRYCESON ADM: Diffuse cutaneous leishmaniasis in Ethiopia. Trans R Soc Trop Med Hyg 64:369, 1970
HUNTER GW et al: *Tropical Medicine,* 5th ed. Philadelphia, Saunders, 1976
KERN F, PEDERSEN JK: Leishmaniasis in the United States: Report of ten cases in military personnel. JAMA 226:872, 1973
LAISON R, SHAW JJ: Epidemiology and ecology of leishmaniasis in Latin America. Nature (Parasitol Suppl) 273:595, 1978
MARSDEN PD et al: Mucocutaneous leishmaniasis—an unsolved clinical problem. Trop Doctor 7:7, 1977
SHAW PH et al: Autochthonous cutaneous leishmaniasis in Texas. Am J Trop Med Hyg 25:788, 1976
WOODRUFF AW et al: The anemia of kala azar. Br J Haematol 22:319, 1972

202
TRYPANOSOMIASIS

JAMES J. PLORDE

SLEEPING SICKNESS

DEFINITION African trypanosomiasis, or sleeping sickness, is a disease caused by the hemoflagellate *Trypanosoma brucei,* which is transmitted to human beings by several species of tsetse fly belonging to the genus *Glossina.* Clinically, the untreated disease is characterized by an acute febrile lymphadenopathy followed, after a variable period, by a chronic lethal meningoencephalomyelitis. It occurs in two principal epidemiologic patterns: Gambian, or Mid- and West African, sleeping sickness, and Rhodesian, or East African, sleeping sickness.

ETIOLOGY Trypanosomes are fusiform protozoa recognized by an undulating membrane which extends along the length of the cell and terminates in an anterior flagellum. The morphological characteristics of many varieties are so nearly identical that they are distinguishable only by their pathogenicity for certain animals, differences in biochemical requirements, and ability to multiply in insects. *Trypanosoma brucei* strains are polymorphic organisms varying in shape from slender to stumpy and in length from 8 to 30 μm. The slender forms have a long flagellum that in the shorter types is rudimentary or absent. The Gambian and Rhodesian forms of sleeping sickness were previously thought to be caused by two distinct species of trypanosomes, *T. gambiense* and *T. rhodesiense.* It is felt now, however, that they, along with the animal trypanosome responsible for *nagana* in cattle, are all variants of a single species. The individual varieties are referred to as *T. brucei gambiense, T. brucei rhodesiense,* and *T. brucei brucei.*

Trypanosomiasis in animals is a great economic problem in many parts of the world. It is probable that an area of approximately 4 million square miles in Africa is not populated because of the impossibility of keeping animals in sites where tsetse flies are infected with trypanosomes.

EPIDEMIOLOGY Gambian sleeping sickness occurs in tropical, West, and Central Africa extending from the Sahara to the Kalahari Deserts and east to the Rift Valley. The incidence of disease is particularly high in Zaire. Rhodesian trypanosomiasis is found in tropical East Africa from Ethiopia in the north to Botswana in the south.

Transmission of the trypanosomes of sleeping sickness occurs by what is referred to as the "anterior station." After ingestion by a feeding tsetse, the parasites first develop in the intestine of the fly and then migrate to the salivary glands, where they are discharged when the host is bitten. In some situations it is possible that the trypanosomes can be mechanically transmitted from host to host by the tsetse and other hematophagous arthropods. This may be of importance during epidemics.

The Gambian strains of *T. brucei* are transmitted mainly by *G. palpalis* and *G. tachinoides.* These species live in shaded areas near water. Less than 5 percent of the flies are infected even in the most notorious endemic foci. Although *G. palpalis* and *G. tachinoides* are not exclusively anthropophilic, human beings are thought to be the only reservoir for Gambian sleeping sickness.

Rhodesian sleeping sickness, on the other hand, is primarily a zoonosis. It is transmitted to humans from the bushbuck, a small antelope, by the bite of *G. morsitans,* a savannah tsetse. It is seen typically in individuals who travel away from their villages to hunt or fish. Domestic cattle and sheep may also serve as reservoirs, and transmission from human to fly to human can occur.

PATHOLOGY AND PATHOGENESIS The tsetse fly inoculates the organism into the subcutaneous pool of blood that forms during its feeding. Some of the parasites may reach the bloodstream directly, but most remain at the site of inoculation, where they multiply to produce a local chancre. Following the appearance of this lesion, the trypanosomes spread through tissue spaces and lymphatics, eventually spilling over into the general circulation where they continue to multiply by longitudinal fission. The parasitemia is of low intensity and typically occurs in waves; each wave disappears coincidentally with the production of antibody to an exoantigen of the protozoan and reappears as a new antigenic variant arises. These waves of parasitemia, which are accompanied by fever and mononuclear leukocytosis, tend to become more infrequent and irregular in the later stages of the disease. At some time during this stage of dissemination, trypanosomes localize in the tissues of the central nervous system. This is first manifested as a diffuse leptomeningitis and later by a perivascular cerebritis. If untreated, this parenchymal inflammation gives rise to a demyelinating panencephalitis. Leishmanial or short forms have been demonstrated in experimental *T. brucei* infections, suggesting that this organism has an intracellular tissue phase in its developmental cycle. This could be of significance in occult infections.

The mechanism by which the trypanosome elicits tissue damage is unknown. It has been suggested that antigen-antibody reactions lead to the release of kinins. The release of proteolytic enzymes by degenerating phagocytes may be important. The parasitemia stimulates the production of large quantities of IgM immunoglobulin, perhaps in response to the rapid antigenic variation of the parasite. It is not known whether these antibodies are protective. They may, in fact, contribute to the pathogenesis of the anemia and thrombocytopenia sometimes seen in this disease. Cell-mediated immunity is probably important.

CLINICAL MANIFESTATIONS The Gambian and Rhodesian forms of sleeping sickness differ somewhat in symptoms, severity, and duration. Rhodesian trypanosomiasis is the more acute and severe of the two forms, usually terminating fatally within a year. Fever is higher, emaciation more rapid, and lymphatic involvement less evident. Death from intercurrent infections or myocarditis usually occurs before the typical sleeping sickness syndrome appears. In the Gambian variety there are often successive bouts of clinical activity with intervening latent periods that persist for a number of years. The early stages may be mild, and the disease may go unrecognized until the central nervous system is involved. In both forms of the disease, however, an entry lesion, a febrile period of dissemination, and a stage of central nervous system involvement are found to some degree. The *trypanosomal chancre* appears as an erythematous nodule at the site of inoculation 2 or 3 days after the bite of an infected fly. It may occur anywhere in the body but is most commonly seen on the head or limbs and is accompanied by regional lymphadenopathy. The lesion, which subsides spontaneously, is noted more frequently in Rhodesian sleeping sickness, perhaps because of the acute nature of the disease.

The incubation period is usually about 2 weeks, but in *T. brucei gambiense* infections may be several years. Systemic manifestations generally become apparent during the hematogenous dissemination of the trypanosomes. In the usual case the patient develops a high remittent fever, severe headache, insomnia, and inability to concentrate. In Caucasians a characteristic circinate erythema resembling erythema marginatum is frequent. Transient firm areas of painful subcutaneous ede-

ma localized to the hands, feet, and periorbital tissues may appear. All these signs and symptoms may disappear and reappear intermittently over a period of months to years. Tender lymphadenopathy with gradual induration of the nodes and splenomegaly are almost invariably present in Gambian sleeping sickness. The lymph nodes of the posterior cervical triangle are frequently prominent. This is referred to as *Winterbottom's sign*. Eventually the parasites enter the central nervous system. This may occur early in the course of the disease or may be delayed for as long as 8 years. Cerebral trypanosomiasis can be explosive, causing repeated convulsions or deep coma and death within a few days. Most patients show gradual progression to the classic picture of *sleeping sickness*. A vacant expression develops, the eyelids droop, the lower lip hangs loosely, and it becomes more and more difficult to gain the patient's attention or prod him or her to any activity. Patients will eat when offered food, but they never ask for it or engage in spontaneous conversation, and speech gradually becomes blurred and indistinct. Tremors of the hands and tongue, choreiform movements, seizures with transient paralysis, loss of sphincter control, ophthalmoplegia, extensor plantar responses, and finally death in coma, in status epilepticus, or from hyperpyrexia follows inexorably.

Death may also occur from intercurrent infection, of which bacillary and amebic dysentery, malaria, and bacterial (often pneumococcal) pneumonia are the most important.

DIAGNOSIS AND LABORATORY FINDINGS *Anemia* and *hypermacroglobulinemia* are invariably present, and spontaneous clumping of erythrocytes in blood specimens is grossly evident in many cases. The sedimentation rate is rapid, and peripheral monocytosis is frequent. When there has been invasion of the central nervous system, the *cerebrospinal fluid* shows mononuclear pleocytosis and increased protein concentration. The protein concentration is a better index of severity of disease and therapeutic response than the number of cells. The presence of IgM in the spinal fluid is almost pathognomonic of cerebral trypanosomiasis.

The definitive diagnosis depends upon finding the trypanosomes in the blood, aspirate of lymph node, or cerebrospinal fluid. These should be examined first in wet mounts; actively motile organisms are seen easily under high power. For final identification thin and thick blood films should be stained with Wright's or Giemsa's stain. If the blood smears are negative, citrated blood should be centrifuged at 1000 r/min for 10 min, the supernatant (including the leukocytes) recentrifuged at 2000 r/min for 15 min, and the sediment examined. Cerebrospinal fluid should be centrifuged at 2000 r/min for 15 min before examination. Alternatively the blood and spinal fluid may be centrifuged in a heparinized capillary tube at 12,000 r/min for 4 min and the tubes examined under a microscope using a 10-power objective. The trypanosomes are found at the junction of the plasma and buffy layer in centrifuged blood and near the sealed end of the tube in centrifuged spinal fluid. If these methods are negative, inoculation of rats or mice can be helpful in the diagnosis of Rhodesian disease. A severalfold increase in IgM globulins in the serum is of confirmatory value. Complement fixation and indirect fluorescent antibody tests utilizing stable antigens are useful in endemic areas.

TREATMENT *Suramin* (Bayer 205, Antrypol) is the most effective agent before central nervous system involvement has occurred. The initial dose should be limited to 0.2 g intravenously because of possible idiosyncrasy. If there is no evidence of sensitivity, a full course of therapy can be instituted the following day. One gram (10 ml fresh 10% solution) is given intravenously on the first, third, seventh, fourteenth, and twenty-first days for a total of 5 g. If red blood cells, casts, or significant amounts of protein occur in the urine, therapy should be discontinued. Pentamidine given in water intramuscularly each day for 10 injections is also effective in early disease. The dose is 3 to 4 mg pentamidine base per kilogram for each injection. When the agent is given too rapidly by the intravenous route, it may cause hypotension.

Lumbar puncture should always be performed in patients who are about to undergo therapy for trypanosomiasis. If the central nervous system is involved, agents that will penetrate the blood-brain barrier must be used; for this purpose the most effective agent is *melarsoprol* (Mel B). This drug, an arsenic derivative of British antilewisite (BAL), is effective at all stages of the disease but is more toxic than suramin. It is given intravenously in a 3.6% solution. The initial dose is 0.5 ml. Each subsequent dose is increased by 0.5 ml until the maximum single dose of 5 ml is reached. The first three doses are given at daily intervals followed by a 7-day rest. This schedule is repeated until a total of 37.5 ml has been given over a period of 1 month. If signs of arsenic toxicity occur, the drug should be discontinued. A reactive encephalopathy, probably due to the release of trypanosomal antigen, may occur early in the course of treatment. Pretreatment with suramin may help avert this complication. A hemorrhagic encephalopathy, a direct arsenic toxic reaction, may also occur and is usually fatal. BAL may be of some use in this situation.

Nitrofurazone can also be given for cerebral trypanosomiasis in an oral dose of 0.5 g three times a day for 7 days, but is more toxic than melarsoprol, and it should not be used unless the patients have failed to respond to this drug. The increasing incidence of drug-resistant parasites has limited the usefulness of *tryparsamide* in the treatment of certain *T. brucei gambiense* infections.

PROGNOSIS The disease is probably always fatal if untreated. If the infection is treated with suramin prior to central nervous system involvement, the cure rate is high and recovery is rapid and complete. When the nervous system becomes involved, the prognosis is less bright, and in far-advanced disease the survivors may suffer neurological damage. Relapses may occur, particularly following treatment with suramin, if the central nervous system was already involved at the time therapy was instituted. Less commonly they may be the result of drug resistance. Examination of the spinal fluid 6 and 12 months after therapy, or earlier if symptoms recur, is helpful in detecting relapse. Such patients must be re-treated with a second therapeutic agent.

PREVENTION Personal protection is best achieved by the use of repellents and protective clothing. A single intramuscular injection of pentamidine in dosage of 3 to 4 mg base per kilogram (maximum 300 mg) will protect against the Gambian form of disease for 6 months or more; its usefulness in Rhodesian trypanosomiasis is controversial. Because of the danger of cryptic infections occurring during chemoprophylaxis, it has been generally restricted to mass prophylactic campaigns. Other methods of disease control include clearing vegetation and the use of insecticides.

CHAGAS' DISEASE

DEFINITION American trypanosomiasis is an infection caused by *T. cruzi* that is characterized by an acute, often asymptomatic illness followed by chronic cardiac and gastrointestinal sequelae.

ETIOLOGY *Trypanosoma cruzi* circulates in the blood as a slender, fusiform hemoflagellate measuring 20 μm in length. In stained preparations, its narrow undulating membrane, large kinetoplast, and characteristic C shape are easily recognized. Unlike the trypanosomes of sleeping sickness, it does not multiply within the bloodstream. After invading tissue cells, it loses its undulating membrane and flagellum, assumes its leishmania form, and divides by binary fission. Eventually, new flagellated forms are produced which reenter the general circulation to initiate another cycle.

Strains of *T. cruzi* vary widely in both virulence and tissue tropism.

EPIDEMIOLOGY This infection is found from Chile and Argentina to Mexico, where it affects more than 7 million people. *Trypanosoma cruzi* has been found in insect vectors and wild animals in several areas of the Southern United States, and serologic studies have documented that acquisition of human infection occurs within this country. There are to date, however, only a handful of clinically apparent autochthonous cases reported from Texas.

The disease is transmitted to humans by reduviid ("assassin" or "kissing") bugs, primarily those of the genera *Triatoma, Panstrongylus,* and *Rhodnius.* These winged, hematophagous insects can be found in the burrows of animals and in the cracks and thatches of poorly constructed rural dwellings. The insect attacks human beings at night, usually biting the face at the mucocutaneous junction (most frequently the lip or outer canthus of the eye). The flagellated trypanosomes are ingested by the bug while feeding, and after multiplying and developing in the midgut of the insect for 8 to 10 days, are discharged in the feces; human infection occurs through contamination of the bite wound. This is referred to as transmission by the "posterior station." The reduviid may remain infected as long as 2 years.

Human beings, domestic animals (cats and dogs), and wild animals, especially the opossum and armadillo, may serve as reservoirs for the infection. The close association of human beings, domestic animals, and the vector within human dwellings is of prime epidemiologic importance, but the disease is occasionally transmitted by a blood transfusion and via the placenta to newborn infants.

PATHOGENESIS AND CLINICAL MANIFESTATIONS A local inflammatory reaction, manifested clinically as an erythematous nodule or *chagoma,* appears within 1 to 3 weeks at the site of inoculation of the protozoan. If, as is commonly the case, the portal of entry has been the conjunctiva, the presenting manifestations are a unilateral, painless conjunctivitis, palpebral edema, and preauricular lymphadenopathy (Romaña's sign). This primary complex may persist for 1 to 2 months during which parasites can be demonstrated in the lesion.

Following an incubation period of 2 weeks, trypanosomal forms reach the general circulation, producing a parasitemia and initiating the acute phase of the illness. After circulating in the blood for some time, the trypanosomes invade tissue cells, and, in the leishmanial form, multiply, producing intracellular pseudocysts. In 4 to 6 days these pseudocysts rupture, releasing both leishmanial and newly formed trypanosomal organisms. The leishmanial forms disintegrate, eliciting an intense inflammatory reaction, while the trypanosomal forms regain the bloodstream to maintain the infection and invade new tissues, particularly the heart, skeletal muscle, smooth muscle, and nervous system.

Clinically, the patient experiences a continuous or recurrent fever, generalized lymphadenopathy, hepatosplenomegaly, and in some cases extensive gelatinous edema of the face and trunk. A transient morbilliform or urticarial skin eruption may occur early in the acute phase. Although trypanosomes frequently can be demonstrated in the cerebrospinal fluid at this time, acute meningoencephalitis is relatively rare; newborn infants and young children are affected most commonly. Myocarditis characterized by tachycardia and electrocardiographic changes is very common. In severe cases, there may be conduction disturbances, cardiac dilatation, and heart failure. The duration of the acute illness is variable. In 5 to 10 percent of cases, meningoencephalitis or severe heart disease results in a fatal outcome within a few days or weeks. Most often it resolves slowly over a period of several weeks. Parasites become extremely scanty in both the tissues and blood, and the patient remains asymptomatic until the onset of the chronic phase 1 or 2 years later. Most patients presenting with late manifestations, however, deny a history of acute illness, suggesting that subclinical infections often result in chronic disease. It has been suggested that the basic pathogenetic mechanism is a hypersensitivity or autoimmune inflammatory reaction involving mesenchymal tissues, and recently antibodies reactive with endocardium, striated muscle, and vascular tissues have been described. On the other hand, lymphocyte-mediated destruction of myocardial tissue has been demonstrated in experimental animals, and lymphocytic infiltrates are commonly seen in patients dying of chagasic cardiopathy. Some authors have also suggested that the late manifestations of disease are primarily due to neuropathies caused by the destruction of ganglionic nerve cells during the acute phase of the disease and resulting in the dilatation and malfunction of the affected organs.

The most important late manifestation is heart disease which may affect as much as 10 percent of the rural population in endemic areas. Symptoms and signs range from arrhythmias and heart block to chronic congestive heart failure (predominantly right-sided). Thromboembolic phenomena and sudden cardiac arrest are relatively common. Echocardiography has been shown to be of value both in screening patients with infection for evidence of cardiac involvement and in following the progress of those with established cardiomyopathy. At autopsy the hearts of patients with Chagas' disease may show a peculiar herniation of the endocardium through the apical muscle bundles. Megacolon and megaesophagus are sequelae seen in southern South America, but they are less common in Central America and in northern South America. Neurological manifestations including mental deficiency and cerebellar symptoms also have been reported in the chronic state of disease.

DIAGNOSIS The diagnosis depends on the demonstration of *T. cruzi* in the patient or upon serologic tests. In the acute phase of the disease the parasite may be seen in the peripheral blood by means of the same direct methods described for African trypanosomiasis. If these are negative, blood may be cultured in Nicolle-Novy-MacNeal (NNN) or Warren's medium or inoculated into rats, mice, or guinea pigs.

Trypanosoma cruzi is easily grown in blood broth and incubated at 28°C; a more sensitive tissue culture method has been described recently. The technique of *xenodiagnosis* is often used in endemic areas; a laboratory-reared vector, known to be parasite-free, is allowed to feed on subjects with suspected cases, and 2 weeks later, the insect's intestinal contents are examined for parasites. Confusion sometimes arises from the finding of trypanosomes in blood. Many children in Venezuela and other South American countries are infected with a harmless species *T. rangeli*, which produces no symptoms but may be present in the blood for many months. By utilization of both culture and xenodiagnosis repeatedly, organisms can be recovered from most acute cases and from up to 40 percent of chronic ones. Biopsy of an involved lymph node or calf muscle may reveal the organism during the initial illness when the parasites cannot be recovered from the blood. The Machado-Guerreiro test (a complement fixation reaction) is most helpful

in the diagnosis of chronic cases and in survey work. Fluorescent antibody and hemagglutination inhibition tests appear more sensitive and less specific. Rapid slide flocculation tests and enzyme-linked immunosorbent assay are currently being evaluated.

TREATMENT AND PREVENTION There is still no satisfactory treatment for Chagas' disease, although several drugs, including primaquine given in dosage suggested for malaria, will clear the blood of trypanosomes, but they do not affect the intracellular parasites. Bayer 2502 (Lampit), a nitrofurazone derivative given in dosage of 10 mg/kg per day for 3 or 4 months, shows promise as a curative agent. Chronic organ damage, however, is generally thought irreversible. Prevention consists of using residual insecticide sprays—of which benzene hexachloride (BHC) is the most effective—on the walls of houses, the main habitat of the vectors. Reinfestation, however, may occur within a year or two of spraying. Preliminary work on vaccine development is underway. Transfusion infections can be prevented by serologic screening of blood donors in endemic areas and by adding gentian violet to the blood. Immunosuppression may reactivate Chagas' disease, and patients from endemic areas should be serologically screened before such treatment is instituted.

REFERENCES

BARRETT-CONNOR E: Chemoprophylaxis of amebiasis and African trypanosomiasis. Ann Intern Med 77:797, 1972

BROWN HW: *Basic Clinical Parasitology*, 4th ed. New York, Appleton-Century-Crofts, 1975

COSSIO PM et al: Chagasic cardiomyopathy. Am J Pathol 86:533, 1977

GOODWIN LG: The pathology of African trypanosomiasis. Trans R Soc Trop Med Hyg 64:797, 1970

HOFF R et al: *Trypanosoma cruzi* in the cerebrospinal fluid during the acute stage of Chagas' disease. N Engl J Med 298:604, 1978

KABERLE F: Chagas' disease and Chagas' syndromes: The pathology of American trypanosomiasis. Adv Parasitol 6:63, 1968

LUMSDEN WHR: Trypanosomiasis. Br Med Bull 28:34, 1972

MAEGRATH BG, GILES HM: *Management and Treatment of Tropical Diseases*. Oxford, Blackwell Scientific Publications, 1971

MARTINI-CAMPOS JV, TAFURI WL: Chagas' enteropathy. Gut 14:910, 1973

PUIGBO JJ et al: Diagnosis of Chagas' cardiomyopathy by noninvasive techniques. Postgrad Med J 53:527, 1977

SPENCER HC JR et al: Imported African trypanosomiasis in the United States. Ann Intern Med 82:633, 1975

WHO MEMORANDA: Immunology of Chagas' disease. Bull WHO 50:549, 1974

203
TOXOPLASMOSIS

RIMA McLEOD
JACK S. REMINGTON

DEFINITION The term *toxoplasmosis* refers to disease caused by the obligate intracellular protozoan, *Toxoplasma gondii*, and must be differentiated from the more common asymptomatic infection caused by this organism. The infection and disease in older children and adults are discussed below. The reader is referred to the reference by Remington and Desmonts for information on congenital toxoplasmosis.

ETIOLOGY *Toxoplasma gondii* is classified among the coccidia and exists in three forms: trophozoite, cyst, and oocyst.

Trophozoites Also termed tachyzoites, trophozoites are crescent or oval, approximately 3 by 7 μm in size, and stain well with either Wright's stain or Giemsa's stain. Trophozoites invade all mammalian cells except nonnucleated erythrocytes and are found in tissues during the acute stage of infection.

Cysts Tissue cysts are formed within host cells and may contain thousands of organisms. They are 10 to 100 μm in size and stain well with periodic acid–Schiff stain; the cyst wall stains with silver stain. Cysts are important in transmission, as they may be present in animal tissues ingested by carnivores. They may persist in virtually every organ, but skeletal and heart muscle and the central nervous system appear to be the most common sites of chronic (latent) infection.

Oocysts Oocysts are oval and 10 to 12 μm in diameter. They are formed only in the mucosal cells of the intestines of members of the cat family and are subsequently excreted in the feces. The cat is the only animal in which the organism has a sexual cycle in the intestine, and cats have systemic infection with *T. gondii* as well. The time of appearance of oocysts in the feces depends on the form of the organism with which the cat becomes infected and varies from 3 to 24 days. Excretion continues for 7 to 20 days, and as many as 10 million oocysts are shed in the feces in a single day. Except under unusual conditions, once a cat has been infected and has excreted oocysts, it will not shed oocysts again. When a cat becomes infected with *Isospora felis*, renewed oocyst excretion has been reported to occur. Sporulation, which occurs from 2 to 3 days (at 24°C) after the oocysts are excreted, is required for the oocysts to become infectious and does not occur below 4°C or above 37°C. Oocysts may remain infectious for more than 1 year under favorable conditions (e.g., in warm, moist soil). This form presumably plays a major role in transmission by the oral route since ingestion of oocysts has been shown to transmit infection.

EPIDEMIOLOGY *Toxoplasma gondii* is ubiquitous and infects herbivorous, omnivorous, and carnivorous animals, including mammals, birds, and reptiles. Prevalence of infection varies with locale; prevalence of positive serologic reaction increases with age. In the United States, approximately 5 to 30 percent of individuals 10 to 19 years old and 10 to 67 percent of individuals over 50 years old have serologic evidence of infection. Generally, less infection occurs in cold regions, in hot and arid areas, and at high elevations. No particular genetic susceptibility has been documented for humans.

The natural mechanism of infection is by ingestion of cysts or oocysts or by transplacental transmission. Infection may also be acquired through blood transfusion, leukocyte transfusion, organ transplantation, and laboratory accident. Clinical illness due to reinfection from an exogenous source has not been reported.

Oral transmission Cysts are present in approximately 10 percent of lamb and 25 percent of pork used for human consumption; cysts have been isolated from beef, but their prevalence in beef has not been defined. Direct contact with any material contaminated by infected cat feces may result in ingestion of oocysts, and this form can be transmitted to food by insects. When humans or other animals (including cats) eat infected tissues (from any animal) or mature oocysts (excreted only by cats), the life cycle is completed. Approximately 1 percent of cats have been found to be excreting oocysts in their feces.

Transplacental transmission Accumulated data overwhelmingly support the concept that *Toxoplasma* is transmitted to the fetus in utero only if the pregnant woman is infected during the current pregnancy. Most often, when a mother is infected during pregnancy the outcome is a normal uninfected infant, but spontaneous abortion, stillbirth, or delivery of a premature or full-term infected infant may result. Congenital infection will occur in approximately one-third of infants born to mothers who acquire their infection during the current pregnancy. In infants born to mothers infected during the first trimester, congenital infection is least common (approximately 17 percent) but disease is most severe; in infants born to mothers infected during the third trimester, congenital infection is most common (approximately 65 percent) but is usually asymptomatic. The fetus is at risk whether or not the infection is symptomatic in the mother.

The following are general guidelines for ascertaining the risk of transmission of the organism to the fetus of a woman who is known to have been infected *prior to the pregnancy in question*. If a woman acquires *Toxoplasma* infection any time before gestation, she will not deliver an infected infant. If a woman had the acute infection during one pregnancy, whether or not she delivered an infected infant, she will not give birth to a child infected with *T. gondii* in a subsequent pregnancy. Studies in which data to the contrary have been presented lacked appropriate controls. Risk to the fetus in these settings, if present, must be exceedingly low. *Toxoplasma* has, however, been isolated on rare occasions from abortuses of women with chronic (latent) infection. At present, the frequency of chronic *Toxoplasma* infection as a cause of abortion has not been defined and is the subject of considerable controversy.

Transmission by blood or leukocyte transfusion *Toxoplasma* may be transmitted by blood or leukocyte transfusion. The organism has been isolated from leukocytes of individuals without recognized clinical evidence of *Toxoplasma* infection, and parasitemia has been reported to persist in otherwise normal individuals for as long as 1 year after acquisition of infection. The high incidence of isolation of the organism from the blood of patients who have chronic myelogenous leukemia and high antibody titers to *Toxoplasma* is particularly noteworthy. The organism has survived for 50 days in whole citrated blood stored at 4°C. Immunodeficient patients who require multiple blood transfusions may be particularly at risk for transmission of infection by this route.

PATHOGENESIS Organisms released from cysts or oocysts enter cells of the gastrointestinal tract, multiply, cause cell disruption, and then infect neighboring cells. Extracellular organisms or organisms within leukocytes are transported throughout the body via the lymphatic system and bloodstream and are capable of invading every organ and tissue. Proliferation of trophozoites usually leads to death of invaded cells, resulting in foci of necrosis, surrounded by an intense cellular reaction. The immune response of the host primarily governs the outcome of the acute process. Both humoral and cell-mediated immunity are important. In some apparently normal individuals and in immunodeficient patients, the acute infection may progress with acute necrotizing encephalitis, pneumonitis, or myocarditis which may be fatal. Trophozoites disappear from the tissues with development of the normal immune response.

A unique aspect of the infection is that organisms persist in cysts in many organs during the life span of the host. Either persistence of viable trophozoites within cells of the reticuloendothelial system or disruption of cysts may be the source of the recurrent parasitemias that occur in some asymptomatic individuals with chronic infection. Cysts are the probable origin of the organisms that cause recrudescent disease in immunocompromised patients or chorioretinitis in older children and adults with congenital toxoplasmosis.

PATHOLOGY The histopathologic changes in toxoplasmic lymphadenitis are characteristic and consist of reactive follicular hyperplasia with irregular clusters of epithelioid histiocytes that have vesicular nuclei and abundant eosinophilic cytoplasm and that encroach upon and blur the margins of germinal centers; numerous mitoses in the germinal centers; many necrotic cells and an associated focal distention of subcapsular and trabecular sinuses with monocytoid cells. Trophozoites or cysts are only rarely observed in conventionally stained sections.

Single or multiple foci of necrosis occur as the earliest manifestations of involvement of the eye. Infiltrates are composed largely of lymphocytes, plasma cells, and mononuclear phagocytic cells. There are intra- and extracellular trophozoites and cysts in the retinal lesions. Granulomatous inflammation of the choroid occurs secondary to necrotizing retinitis. Iridocyclitis, glaucoma, and cataracts may be complications of the chorioretinitis.

In cases of acute central nervous system infection, there is a focal or diffuse meningoencephalitis with necrosis and microglial nodules. Margins of areas of necrosis may be infiltrated with monocytes, lymphocytes, and plasma cells. Perivascular mononuclear inflammation frequently is present contiguous to areas of necrosis, and occasionally there is necrosis of vessel walls. Intra- and extracellular trophozoites are usually found at the periphery of areas of necrosis, and these areas of necrosis may mimic mass lesions. Cysts may be present after the first week of infection. The size of lesions and extent and location of central nervous system involvement vary considerably.

In cases of disseminated infection, pathologic changes occur in the heart, lungs, kidney, and multiple other organs. They consist of necrosis and the presence of trophozoites, cysts, and inflammatory cells alone or in combination. Glomerulonephritis with deposits of gamma-M globulin (IgM), fibrinogen, and *Toxoplasma* antigen and antibody has been reported. Involvement of the pancreas has been a prominent finding in infection in immunocompromised patients. Findings in skeletal muscle vary from parasitized fibers without pathologic changes to focal areas of infiltration to widespread myositis with necrosis.

CLINICAL MANIFESTATIONS Lymphadenopathy and other manifestations in the immunocompetent individual Lymphadenopathy is the most commonly recognized clinical manifestation of acute acquired toxoplasmosis. Cervical nodes are involved most frequently. Nodes may be single or multiple, and involvement may be symptomatic or asymptomatic. Asymptomatic lymphadenopathy may mimic lymphoma, and involvement of a pectoral node has been suspected to be carcinoma of the breast when detected on physical examination. Suboccipital, supraclavicular, axillary, inguinal, and mediastinal nodes may be involved. When mesenteric or retroperitoneal nodes are involved, abdominal pain and significant temperature elevation (e.g., up to 40°C) may occur. Involved lymph nodes vary in firmness, may be tender, do not suppurate, and are usually discrete. Malaise, fever, myalgias, headache, sore throat, maculopapular rash (which spares the palms and soles), hepatosplenomegaly, or reactive (atypical) lymphocytes may occur. Lymphadenopathic toxoplasmosis is self-limited, but malaise and/or lymphadenopathy may persist or recur for months.

Individuals who appear to be normal immunologically rarely may present with any of the following, alone or in combination: pneumonitis, myocarditis, pericarditis, hepatitis, polymyositis, encephalitis, or meningoencephalitis. Signs or symptoms of involvement of these organs are nonspecific. Significant morbidity has occurred, and some of these patients have died of the infection.

Ocular involvement *Toxoplasma* has been estimated to be the cause of approximately 35 percent of cases of chorioretinitis in children and adults. Although chorioretinitis has been estimated to occur in approximately 1 percent of patients with the acute acquired infection, ocular disease is most often a consequence of congenital *Toxoplasma* infection. Blurred vision, scotomas, pain, photophobia, or epiphora may be due to active chorioretinitis. If the macula is involved, impairment or loss of central vision may occur. In children, strabismus may be an early sign of chorioretinitis. Associated signs of systemic infection occur only rarely. Vision improves, but frequently visual acuity recovers only partially as inflammation subsides. Commonly, episodic flares of chorioretinitis cause destruction of irreplaceable retinal tissue. These multiple recurrences may result in glaucoma or loss of vision and ultimately may necessitate enucleation. The acute lesions appear as yellowish white, cotton-like patches that have elevated, indistinct margins surrounded by a zone of hyperemia. Inflammatory exudate in the vitreous may obscure the fundus. Older lesions characteristically appear as atrophic, whitish gray plaques with distinct borders and black spots of choroidal pigment. Lesions usually are located near the posterior pole of the retina, although they may be peripheral. They may be single but are more commonly multiple, and lesions of varying age may be seen simultaneously. Panuveitis and papillitis with optic atrophy occur less commonly. Isolated anterior uveitis due to *Toxoplasma* infection has never been proved.

Toxoplasmosis in the immunocompromised patient All forms of toxoplasmosis that occur in normal individuals may also occur in immunocompromised individuals. Patients receiving immunosuppressive therapy for lymphoproliferative disorders (especially Hodgkin's disease), for hematologic malignancy, or for prevention of organ graft rejection have the greatest predilection for life-threatening toxoplasmosis. The untreated infection in these patients is frequently fulminant and rapidly fatal. Central nervous system involvement, present in greater than 50 percent of documented cases, is the most characteristic clinical feature of toxoplasmosis in immunocompromised patients. Therefore, the diagnosis of toxoplasmosis must be excluded in any immunosuppressed patient with symptoms or signs referable to the central nervous system. Symptoms and signs are manifestations of diffuse encephalopathy, meningoencephalitis, or cerebral mass lesions and include changes in mental status, headache, focal neurologic deficits, and seizures. Brain involvement has been established by demonstration of trophozoites in material from brain biopsy or in material aspirated from mass lesions that may have the characteristic appearance of a brain abscess on computerized tomography (CT) scan. Typically, the cerebrospinal fluid shows a nononuclear pleocytosis, a moderate elevation in protein, and a normal glucose. Immunocompromised patients also may have other nonspecific manifestations of the infection which are reflections of inflammation and necrosis of the organs involved, particularly heart and lungs.

Toxoplasmosis and *Toxoplasma* infection in the pregnant woman *Toxoplasma* infection acquired by the mother during pregnancy is symptomatic in only about 10 to 20 percent of cases. See also "Transplacental Transmission" above.

DIAGNOSIS Acute infection with *Toxoplasma* may be diagnosed by isolation of *T. gondii* from body fluids or blood (see qualification under "Isolation Procedures" below), demonstration of trophozoites in histologic sections or in impression smears of tissue or body fluids, demonstration of characteristic lymph node histology, and serologic tests.

Isolation procedures The organism can be isolated by inoculation of leukocytes, body fluids, or tissue specimens into tissue culture or by subcutaneous or intraperitoneal inoculation into mice. Body fluids should be processed and inoculated immediately, but blood and tissues may be stored at 4°C overnight. Freezing or treatment of specimens with Formalin kills the organism. Mice should be examined for the presence of organisms in their peritoneal fluid 6 to 10 days after inoculation, or earlier if they die. Mice that survive 6 weeks should be tested for *Toxoplasma* antibody in their serum. When antibody is present, visualization of *Toxoplasma* cysts in the mouse brain establishes the diagnosis. If cysts are not demonstrable in brains of mice with *Toxoplasma* antibody, portions of brain, liver, and spleen should be inoculated into other mice.

Isolation of *T. gondii* from body fluids reflects the acute stage of infection, as does isolation from blood in most patients. Although persistent parasitemia has been described in asymptomatic individuals with latent infection, this appears to be a rare occurrence, except, perhaps, in patients with chronic myelogenous leukemia. Isolation from tissues (e.g., skeletal muscle, lung, brain, or eye) obtained by biopsy or at autopsy may reflect the presence of tissue cysts and does not prove that infection is acute.

Histologic diagnosis Demonstration of trophozoites in tissue sections or smears (e.g., brain biopsy, bone marrow aspirate) or in body fluids (e.g., cerebrospinal fluid, amniotic fluid) establishes the diagnosis of the acute infection. It is difficult to identify trophozoites by ordinary staining methods; direct and indirect immunofluorescent antibody techniques have been used successfully for this purpose. Demonstration of tissue cysts does not differentiate between acute or chronic infection. When there are numerous cysts in any organ, infection is usually of recent onset. Characteristic histologic criteria establish toxoplasmic lymphadenitis (see "Pathology" above).

Serologic tests Methods most widely used to establish the diagnosis of acute *Toxoplasma* infection are the Sabin-Feldman dye test, indirect fluorescent antibody (IFA) test, and indirect hemagglutination (IHA) test. Methods that detect antigenemia, although presently experimental, are promising. Measurement of antibodies by enzyme-linked immunosorbent assay or radioimmunoassay is potentially valuable because these techniques may be automated.

The dye test, which measures primarily IgG antibodies, is sensitive and specific. The World Health Organization has recommended that dye test titers be expressed in international units (IU/ml) and will supply a standard reference serum.

The IFA test appears to measure the same antibodies as the dye test and is the most widely available procedure. In both tests, titers tend to be parallel. Dye test and IFA test antibodies usually appear 1 to 2 weeks after infection, reach high titers ($\geq$ 1:1000) in 6 to 8 weeks, and gradually decline over months to years; low titers (e.g., 1:4 to 1:64) commonly persist for life (Fig. 203-1). Magnitude of antibody titer does not correlate with severity of illness.

The IgM-fluorescent antibody (IgM-IFA) test is especially useful in establishing the diagnosis of acute infection with *T. gondii* because IgM antibodies appear early (as early as 5 days after infection) and disappear early as contrasted with gamma-G globulin (IgG) antibodies. In most cases, IgM-IFA test antibodies rise rapidly (to levels of 1:80 to $\geq$ 1:1000) and fall to low titers (1:10 or 1:20) or disappear within a few weeks or months (Fig. 203-1). However, in some patients they are present at low titer for as long as several years. Some immunodeficient patients with acute toxoplasmosis and most patients with only active ocular toxoplasmosis may not have IgM *Toxoplasma* antibodies. Rheumatoid factor may cause false-positive reactions in the IgM-IFA test. Removal of rheumatoid factor (e.g., by absorption) will eliminate false-positive test results in the IgM-IFA test. Antinuclear antibodies may cause false-positive reactions in both the IFA and IgM-IFA tests.

The antibodies measured in the IHA test may persist for years and are different than those measured in the IFA and dye tests. The IHA test may be helpful when titers in the IFA or dye test have stabilized since IHA test titers rise later. However, the rise in titer may occur so late that its demonstration is not helpful in diagnosis of the acute infection at a clinically pertinent time. Proper standardization of methodology for this and all other serologic tests is needed, as is quality control of commercial kits that are often employed by laboratories inexperienced in performing these serologic tests.

FIGURE 203-1

Antibody response in humans to Toxoplasma *infection. IgM antibodies (— —), detectable by the IgM-IFA test, reach maximum titer within the first few weeks after infection and may decline within a few weeks (----) or persist for months (——·——). IgG antibodies (——), detectable by either Sabin-Feldman dye test or conventional IFA test, reach maximum titer within 2 months, plateau for months or years, and then decline, but usually persist at a low titer for life. (After G Desmonts, Feuill Biol 16:61, 1975.)*

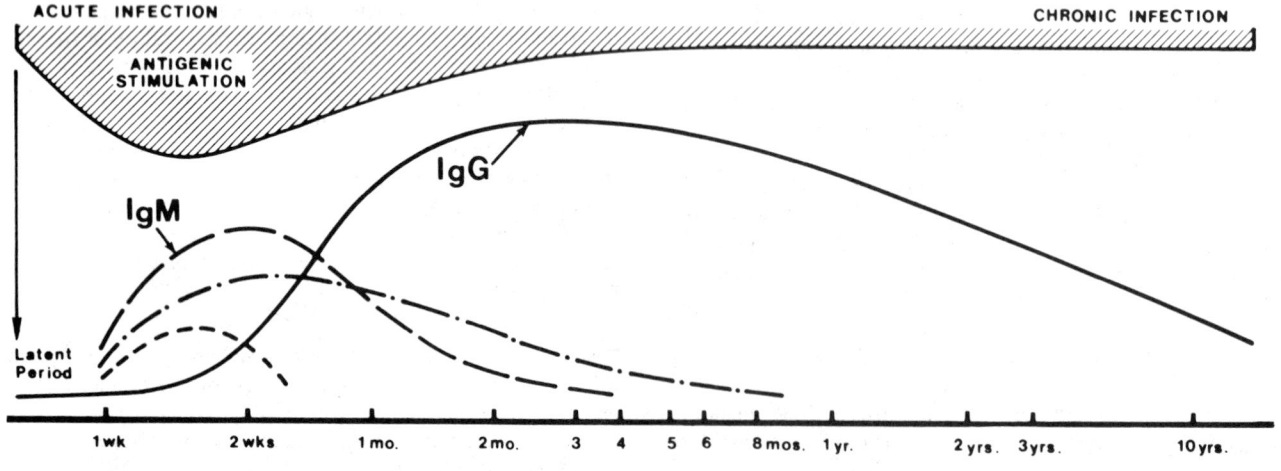

ACUTE INFECTION   CHRONIC INFECTION

Titers in the complement fixation (CF) test also may appear several weeks later than those measured in the IFA and dye tests and also may persist for years. A negative CF test titer does not exclude acute or chronic infection, and a single positive CF test titer does not prove acute infection. A significant rise in CF test titer (i.e., of two serial dilutions performed at the same time on serums obtained several weeks apart) establishes recent infection.

Local production of antibody in active ocular or central nervous system toxoplasmosis may be demonstrated by comparison of level of *Toxoplasma* antibody in cerebrospinal fluid or aqueous humor. Application of the following equation may be used to assess local antibody production:

$$C = \frac{\text{antibody titer in body fluid}}{\text{antibody titer in serum}}$$
$$\times \frac{\text{concentration of gamma globulin in serum}}{\text{concentration of gamma globulin in body fluid}}$$

A significant correlation coefficient *(C)* is ≥ 8 and reflects local antibody production that signifies active central nervous system or ocular infection. It is usually not possible to demonstrate significant local antibody production by application of this formula if the dye test or IFA test serum titer is $\geq 1:1000$.

Acute acquired *Toxoplasma* infection in the immunocompetent individual In settings in which acute acquired infection is suspected in an immunocompetent individual, a negative dye test or IFA test virtually excludes the diagnosis. The diagnosis of recent acute acquired infection is confirmed if there is a serial two-tube rise in titer when serums drawn at 3-week intervals are run at the same time or if there is seroconversion from a negative to a positive titer (in the absence of transfer of antibody by transfusion). A single high titer in any test does not prove the presence of active infection.

Guidelines for interpretation of test results are presented below and in Table 203-1. Exceptions to these generalizations may occur.

A dye test or IFA test titer of $\geq 1:1000$ and a high IgM-IFA test titer ($\geq 1:80$) are probably diagnostic of recent acute infection whether or not symptoms are present. In an individual with a positive titer in the dye test or IFA test, absence of

IgM-IFA test antibodies almost always excludes very recent acquisition of infection.

Ocular toxoplasmosis Diagnosis of ocular toxoplasmosis in older children and adults may be difficult because the level of antibody titer in serum does not necessarily correlate with presence of active lesions in the fundus. A patient with active *Toxoplasma* chorioretinitis usually has low serologic test titers (1:4 to 1:64). If a serologic test is negative when performed on undiluted serum, for practical purposes, toxoplasmic chorioretinitis is excluded. If retinal lesions are characteristic and serologic tests are positive (see also "Serologic Tests" above), the diagnosis can be made with a high degree of confidence. If retinal lesions are atypical and serologic tests are positive, diagnosis of toxoplasmosis is only presumptive; the high prevalence of *Toxoplasma* antibodies in the normal population precludes assumption of a causal relationship.

Active infection in the immunocompromised patient Because antibody formation may be deficient in immunocompromised patients, available serologic methods, including the IgM-IFA test, are at times insufficient for detection of active infection. Serologic tests to screen for *Toxoplasma* infection are useful in asymptomatic immunocompromised individuals in order to identify those patients who are at risk for primary infection or reactivation of latent infection (see also "Prevention" below).

Toxoplasmosis and *Toxoplasma* infection in the pregnant woman It seems advisable to perform serology in any woman considering becoming pregnant to determine whether she has *Toxoplasma* infection prior to pregnancy and to provide essential information when tests are performed during pregnancy (see "Transplacental Transmission" above).

In the absence of a routine screening program in which *Toxoplasma* serology is performed frequently during pregnancy, an IgM-IFA test should be performed if any other serologic test is found to be positive in any titer at any time during gestation. If the IgM-IFA test is not available, a repeat serologic test should be obtained in 3 weeks to determine if the

TABLE 203-1
Guidelines for interpretation of commonly employed serologic tests in the diagnosis of toxoplasmosis*

	Sabin-Feldman dye test	*Indirect fluorescent antibody (IFA) test*	*Indirect fluorescent antibody test for IgM Toxoplasma antibodies (IgM-IFA)*	*Indirect hemagglutination (IHA) test*	*Complement fixation (CF) test*
Positive titer	1:4, undiluted†	1:10‡	1:2 infants‡ 1:10 adults‡	1:16‡	1:4‡
Titer in acute infection	≥1:1000	≥1:1000	≥1:80	≥1:1000	Varies among laboratories
Titer in chronic (latent) infection	1:4–1:2000	1:8–1:2000	Negative to 1:20	1:16–1:256	Negative to 1:8
Duration of elevation of titer	Years	Years	Weeks to months; occasionally years	Years	Years
Special considerations	*1* No known cross reactions or false-positive results in humans.	*1* Antibody measured is same as that measured in dye test. *2* Antinuclear antibodies may cause false-positive results.	*1* Either antinuclear antibodies or rheumatoid factor (IgM) may cause false-positive results. Rheumatoid factor may be absorbed from serum.	*1* Not useful for diagnosis of congenital toxoplasmosis. *2* IHA antibodies rise later than in dye test and IFA. May be especially useful if rising IHA titer can be demonstrated.	*1* Antigen preparations have not been standardized. *2* CF antibodies also rise later than dye test and IFA; see special consideration 2 under IHA.

* *These guidelines are useful in the interpretation of test results, but exceptions to these generalizations may occur.*
† *In some cases of eye disease, the dye test may be positive only in undiluted serum.*
‡ *These values are representative, but normal values for each laboratory may differ significantly.*

titer is stable or rising. No further evaluation is necessary if the IgM-IFA test is negative and an IFA or dye test titer is stable and < 1:1000 (< 300 IU). If the dye test or IFA test is ≥ 1:1000 (≥ 300 IU) and stable (regardless of titer in the IgM-IFA test), the infection should be considered to have been acquired *at least* 4 weeks earlier and probably more than 8 weeks before the serum was obtained. Thus, for practical purposes, the fetus is not at risk if the dye test or IFA test titer is ≥ 1:1000 and stable in the first 2 months of pregnancy.

Whereas titers in the dye test or IFA test may have peaked and stabilized by 8 weeks after onset of infection, titers in the CF or IHA test may continue to rise for 4 to 6 months or longer after acquisition of infection. Therefore, rises in these latter two tests may not be helpful in defining when infection occurred relative to the time of conception and should not be used as the sole test for this purpose.

A common problem arises when an asymptomatic woman is tested for *Toxoplasma* antibody late in the first trimester or in the second trimester of pregnancy and her IFA or dye test titer is found to be in the vicinity of 1:2000, her IgM-IFA test titer is found to be negative, and no significant rise in titer in any test is demonstrable. It is not possible to establish whether infection occurred before, at, or after conception in this situation.

THERAPY **Therapy in specific clinical settings** The need for and duration of therapy are determined by the clinical severity of illness and by the underlying medical problem.

Most immunologically normal patients with lymphadenopathic toxoplasmosis do not require specific treatment. Indication for treatment in these cases is severe and persistent symptoms. Evidence of serious damage to vital organs is also an indication for therapy. Infections acquired via transfusions or in laboratory accidents may be more severe than naturally acquired infections and probably should be treated.

Patients with active chorioretinitis should be treated with specific therapy. When there is potential for serious visual impairment secondary to macular or optic nerve involvement, corticosteroids are added to the regimen.

Because of the high mortality rate associated with toxoplasmosis in patients whose resistance to infection is compromised by underlying disease or by therapy (e.g., corticosteroids or cytotoxic drugs), toxoplasmosis should be treated in all immunocompromised individuals. In immunocompromised patients, serologic evidence of acute infection (with or without signs and symptoms of infection) or demonstration of trophozoites in tissue (with or without serologic test titers or signs and symptoms) is an indication for therapy. Improvement has been reported to occur in the majority of patients to whom specific therapy was administered. Considering the diagnosis early enough to institute treatment is the major problem.

When a pregnant woman who acquired infection at any time during pregnancy is treated, the chance of congenital infection in her infant is decreased but not eliminated. In separate series reported from France and Germany, treatment decreased the incidence of infection significantly. The drugs employed were spiramycin in the study from France and pyrimethamine plus sulfonamide in the study from Germany. Spiramycin (not available in the United States) has been used safely for treatment in the first trimester. Pyrimethamine is a potential teratogen; therefore, sulfadiazine (which is highly effective in animal models when used alone) should be used alone if a decision is made to treat during the first trimester of pregnancy. When infection occurs during the first trimester, some authorities have recommended therapeutic abortion because of the high probability of severe damage when infection occurs early in fetal life. Other authorities recommend treat-

ment rather than abortion because the risk of transmission of the infection to the fetus is low (approximately 15 percent) in the first trimester and because the incidence of congenital toxoplasmosis can be reduced significantly by intrapartum therapy. They reason that drug therapy would result in saving a significant number of healthy fetuses. Decision about mode of therapy ultimately must be made by both the well-informed physician and the well-informed patient who must be aware of the risks. Carefully controlled studies are needed to define whether a pregnant woman who has *Toxoplasma* antibody and a history of habitual abortion will benefit from treatment.

Pyrimethamine plus sulfadiazine or trisulfapyrimidines In vivo, pyrimethamine and sulfadiazine act synergistically against *Toxoplasma*. Clinical experience confirms efficacy of this combination. Comparative tests have shown that sulfapyrazine, sulfamethazine, and sulfamerazine are about as effective as sulfadiazine. In general, other sulfonamides are much less effective.

Pyrimethamine In adults, a loading dose of 100 to 200 mg pyrimethamine is given orally in two divided doses on the first day of treatment. In young children, a loading dose of 2 mg per kilogram of body weight (not to exceed adult loading dose) is given for the first 2 to 3 days of treatment. Maintenance dose is 1 mg per kilogram of body weight (with a maximum of 25 mg) in a single dose. In view of the drug's half-life of 4 to 5 days, administration of the maintenance dose at 3- to 4-day intervals has been suggested. Daily administration is recommended for the patient who is very ill, since there are no data concerning absorption of the drug in this situation. Daily therapy is also recommended for active ocular infection. Pyrimethamine is available only in tablet form.

Pyrimethamine is a folic acid antagonist and produces a dose-related, usually gradual, and reversible depression of the bone marrow. Anemia, leukopenia, and thrombocytopenia may occur. Platelet and peripheral blood cell counts should be evaluated twice weekly in any patient receiving pyrimethamine.

Folinic acid To prevent suppression of the bone marrow, folinic acid (calcium leucovorin) is administered in conjunction with pyrimethamine therapy. Optimal frequency for administration of folinic acid has not been established. A single oral dose of 5 to 10 mg daily is recommended. If folinic acid is not available, bakers' yeast (3 to 4 cakes daily) may be used to prevent toxicity due to pyrimethamine. Neither folinic acid nor bakers' yeast inhibits the action of pyrimethamine on *T. gondii*, whereas folic acid does.

Sulfadiazine and trisulfapyrimidines The loading dose is 50 to 75 mg per kilogram of body weight; thereafter, a total daily dose of 75 to 100 mg per kilogram of body weight is administered in four divided doses at intervals of approximately 6 h. Tablet and liquid oral forms as well as an intravenous form of sulfadiazine are available. The potential toxicities of sulfonamides (e.g., crystalluria, hematuria, and rash) must be carefully monitored.

Other drugs Trimethoprim alone or in combination with a sulfonamide has not been proved to be effective in treatment of toxoplasmosis in humans, but the activity of this combination in vitro and in vivo in animal models warrants carefully designed and controlled clinical trials. This combination is significantly less active than the combination of pyrimethamine with sulfadiazine.

Duration of therapy Optimal duration of specific therapy has not been defined for any form of toxoplasmosis. Specific therapy should be continued for 4 to 6 weeks in a patient who appears to be immunologically normal but who requires treatment for severe and persistent symptoms or evidence of damage to vital organs (e.g., chorioretinitis, myocarditis). Longer treatment may be necessary.

It seems advisable to treat an immunocompromised patient for at least 4 to 6 weeks *beyond* complete resolution of all signs and symptoms of active disease. Careful follow-up of these patients is imperative because relapse may occur and requires prompt reinstitution of therapy. Although therapy may be effective against *T. gondii* trophozoites and may induce a beneficial clinical response, it does not eradicate cysts from the central nervous system.

Desmonts and Couvreur suggest that an acutely infected pregnant woman be treated with spiramycin and use a total dose of 2 to 3 daily, administered orally in four divided doses. A 3-week course of treatment is alternated with 2 weeks without treatment from the time of diagnosis until term. Another treatment regimen was used in Germany and consisted of a course of sulfonamide and pyrimethamine followed by one or two courses of sulfonamide administered alone or in combination with pyrimethamine. Each course of therapy was given for approximately 2 weeks and was alternated with a 3- to 4-week interval without treatment. Pyrimethamine was not administered during the first trimester of pregnancy.

PREVENTION Measures for prevention of infection involve intervention in the cycle of transmission and are most important for immunodeficient patients and seronegative pregnant women. To kill cysts, meat should be heated to 60°C or frozen at −20°C. (Freezers available commercially do not reach or maintain this temperature reliably.) Hands should be washed after touching uncooked meat, and fruits and vegetables that may be contaminated with oocysts should be washed. Dry heat (66°C) or boiling water renders oocysts noninfectious. Contact with cat feces should be avoided.

There are no definitive data to allow for a firm recommendation regarding the use of whole blood, leukocyte transfusions, or organ transplants when a donor is seropositive for *Toxoplasma* antibodies. It seems reasonable, however, that whenever feasible, blood or blood products donated by an individual with *Toxoplasma* antibody should not be used in an immunosuppressed individual, and an organ transplanted to a seronegative recipient should be from an individual without serologic evidence of *Toxoplasma* infection.

A nontoxic drug that eliminates the organism in the cyst as well as the trophozoite form is needed for prophylaxis against the devastating complications of recrudescent infection in immunocompromised individuals.

See "Therapy in Specific Clinical Settings" above for guidelines concerning prevention of transmission to the fetus.

At present, no effective vaccine to prevent infection with *Toxoplasma* has been developed. Development of a vaccine for use in nonimmune women of childbearing age should be explored since maternal immunity appears to prevent congenital transmission of *T. gondii*. Vaccines that prevent oocyst development in cats could prove valuable by interrupting the life cycle of *T. gondii*.

REFERENCES

DORFMAN RF, REMINGTON JS: Value of lymph node biopsy in the diagnosis of acute acquired toxoplasmosis. N Engl J Med 289:878, 1973

DUBEY JP et al: Characterization of the new fecal form of *Toxoplasma gondii*. J Parasitol 56:447, 1970

FELDMAN HA: Toxoplasmosis. N Engl J Med 279:1370, 1431, 1968

JONES TC et al: Toxoplasmic lymphadenitis. JAMA 192:87, 1965

KIMBALL AC et al: Congenital toxoplasmosis: A prospective study of 4048 obstetric patients. Am J Obstet Gynecol 111:211, 1971

O'CONNOR GR: Manifestations and management of ocular toxoplasmosis. Bull NY Acad Med 50:192, 1974

REMINGTON JS, DESMONTS G: Toxoplasmosis, in *Infectious Diseases of the Fetus and Newborn Infant*, JS Remington, JO Klein (eds). Philadelphia, Saunders, 1976, p 191

RUSKIN J, REMINGTON JS: Toxoplasmosis in the compromised host. Ann Intern Med 84:193, 1976

SIIM JC: Acquired toxoplasmosis. JAMA 147:1641, 1951

TOWNSEND JJ et al: Acquired toxoplasmosis. Arch Neurol 32:335, 1975

204
PNEUMOCYSTIS CARINII PNEUMONIA (PNEUMOCYSTOSIS, INTERSTITIAL PLASMA CELL PNEUMONIA)

C. GEORGE RAY

DEFINITION *Pneumocystis carinii* pneumonia occurs in patients with impaired antibody and/or cellular immune responses, or severe debility with protein-calorie malnutrition. Progressive pulmonary insufficiency is the cardinal clinical manifestation

ETIOLOGY In vitro cultivation of *P. carinii* has only recently been accomplished, using primary embryonic chick epithelial lung cells. Its taxonomic position now appears to be that of a protozoan. Histologically, 1- to 2-μm oval or crescentic "merozoite" forms with a single nucleus-like, chromatoid body can be seen. These are usually arranged in groups of two to eight within cysts measuring 5 to 10 μm. Cyst rupture permits release of mature trophozoites, measuring 2 to 4 μm, into alveoli. The crescentic appearance of the cysts is thought to be due to partial collapse after encystment of trophozoites. Electron microscopic studies reveal a complex structure and suggest the capacity for protein synthesis and oxidative metabolism, while structures usually associated with phagocytosis are lacking. The agent can be best visualized with special stains, particularly methenamine silver, toluidine blue 0, Gram-Weigert, or Giemsa's stain (but not with hematoxylin-eosin), with phase microscopy, and with fluorescent antibody. The organism seen in human beings is morphologically similar to that in animals, but species-specific antigenic differences may exist.

EPIDEMIOLOGY The incidence of *P. carinii* infection is uncertain, and epidemiologic data are based on indirect evidence. It appears that latent infection is not rare in humans and is frequent in many wild, domestic, and laboratory animals. Indirect fluorescent antibody studies suggest that 75 percent or more of children develop antibodies to the agent by 2 to 4 years of age. In humans the disease is worldwide and occurs in all age groups either as epidemics in nurseries or as isolated cases. Clinical observations suggest that the disease can be contagious. This is based on evidence suggesting aerosol transmission in nurseries with debilitated and malnourished infants under 6 months of age, possible spread among patients in cancer hospitals, and isolated reports of intrafamilial spread. However, while it is possible that person-to-person or even animal-to-person spread of infection may occur, the presence of an underlying immunologic or nutritional deficiency is usually required for the development of overt disease. Intrauterine *P. carinii* pneumonia probably acquired by transplacental transmission has also been reported. The incubation period is estimated to be 1 to 2 months.

PATHOGENESIS The organism is of low virulence, proliferates slowly, and may require the presence of another microbial agent for multiplication. When affecting persons in the first year of life, the disease is usually associated with congenital immunodeficiency syndromes or severe protein-calorie malnutrition; in patients over 1 year of age, it is most commonly a complication of neoplasia, particularly of malignant lymphoreticular disorders, cyclic neutropenia, various anemias, collagen vascular and autoimmune diseases, renal failure, and in patients with transplants who are receiving immunosuppressive drugs and adrenal steroids. Surprisingly, among patients with acute lymphocytic leukemia, the clinical manifestations of infection are most frequently found during periods of remission. *Pneumocystis carinii* pneumonia has also been reported occasionally in the absence of demonstrated underlying disease. Progressive *P. carinii* infection has been produced in various laboratory animals by corticosteroid-induced immunosuppression or malnutrition, both of which apparently activated latent infection.

The largest group of patients with *P. carinii* pneumonia in the past were premature or debilitated newborns in whom the disease, first described as interstitial plasma-cell pneumonia, occurred at about the age of 3 to 4 months, often in nursery epidemics. These epidemics are virtually unheard of in this country, and are becoming increasingly rare in other areas, presumably as a result of improved infant nutrition and less crowding. However, cases continue to be reported and often involve young infants from orphanages in southeast Asia.

Many infections occur together with *P. carinii* pneumonia, and these are often multiple. Acute and chronic bacterial infections are common, and a wide range of concurrent viral, fungal, and some protozoan infections has been observed. Localized and disseminated cytomegalic inclusion disease is a particularly frequent concomitant infection.

PATHOLOGY In widespread disease the lungs are massively consolidated. The consolidation may be focal and confined to the central or dorsal lung areas. The alveoli are distended by a foamy material which suggests the diagnosis, and, when stained appropriately, the organisms can be seen. Hyaline membranes may be present. The sparse cellular response consists of mononuclear cells. Alveolar septal infiltration with plasma cells (interstitial plasma-cell pneumonia) is prominent in many cases and absent in others. Septal fibrosis is generally slight. The changes appear reversible. Granuloma formation, calcification, and focal and diffuse persistent fibrosis have also been noted. In latent infection the lesions are few and minute, organisms are scanty, the foamy intraalveolar material is lacking, and the cellular response is sparse. The infection is generally confined to the lung, but organisms have been seen in the regional lymph nodes. Pleuritis is characteristically absent, and systemic dissemination with focal lesions in distant sites is extremely rare.

CLINICAL MANIFESTATIONS Generally the onset is insidious. The fully developed clinical picture includes severe dyspnea and tachypnea. The patient displays all signs of extreme air hunger and is anxious and cyanotic. There may be a dry cough which, together with the cyanosis, is aggravated by any movement. Fever is absent or slight. Pulmonary physical findings are scanty in contrast to the grave clinical state and the extensive lung involvement seen roentgenologically. Roent-

genograms show hazy alveolar infiltrates spreading from the hilum and eventually affecting most of the lung. Some patients may develop peripheral, somewhat nodular infiltrates, which can be confused with other infections or malignant processes and usually require biopsy for confirmation of the diagnosis. Focal emphysema may be present, but pleural effusions are rare. Blood gas studies indicate impaired diffusion, with severe hypoxemia and normal or only slightly elevated P_{CO_2} values. Other laboratory studies are generally nonrevealing, except for a frequently observed lymphopenia. In young infants with combined immunodeficiency and *P. carinii* infection, significant eosinophilia has been observed. Complications include pneumothorax from a ruptured emphysematous bleb and rib fractures from forced respiratory movements. Death occurs by progressive asphyxia or cardiac failure within 1 to 10 weeks in untreated cases.

The differential diagnosis usually includes viral infection, particularly cytomegalovirus, disseminated pulmonary aspergillosis, and occasionally other bacterial and mycotic infections. In addition, pulmonary alveolar proteinosis, desquamative interstitial pneumonia, pulmonary hemorrhage, and pulmonary fibrosis, either idiopathic or secondary to irradiation or drugs, such as bleomycin, methotrexate, busulfan, cyclophosphamide, or nitrofurantoin, must be considered. The best way to resolve this differential is to do open lung biopsy, whenever possible.

DIAGNOSIS The diagnosis depends on the morphologic demonstration of the organism. Bronchial secretion, tracheal lavage, and gastric aspirate examinations have been variably successful. Needle or open lung biopsy is often diagnostic but entails some risk, particularly in far-advanced cases. Endobronchial brush biopsy has been reported as a simple, frequently successful procedure as has percutaneous needle aspiration of the lung in some series in children.

Serological testing, using indirect immunofluorescence or complement fixation is of limited value in diagnosis, and cannot be relied upon as an alternative to direct identification of the organism. Newer methods being developed for the detection of circulating antigen during acute disease may be useful in the future.

PROGNOSIS Morbidity and mortality figures are uncertain. *Pneumocystis carinii* infection is not rare at any age, and it seems likely that it will be recognized more frequently. The prognosis of *P. carinii* pneumonia is grave since it is generally a complication of a severe underlying disorder. A mortality of 40 to 50 percent has been suggested. However, remissions and spontaneous cures have been reported. The outcome is heavily dependent on the course of the underlying disease.

TREATMENT The current treatment of choice of *P. carinii* infection is a combination of trimethoprim and sulfamethoxazole in doses of 20 mg trimethoprim per kilogram of body weight and 100 mg/kg sulfamethoxazole per day, given orally or intravenously in four divided doses for 14 to 16 days. In high-risk groups of cancer patients, particularly children with acute lymphocytic leukemia, long-term prophylaxis with low-dose trimethoprim-sulfamethoxazole (5 mg/kg trimethoprim and 20 mg/kg sulfamethoxazole, divided into two doses daily) has significantly decreased the incidence of *P. carinii* pneumonia, without serious adverse reactions.

Pentamidine isethionate was the previous drug of choice, but it is now considered a secondary agent for patients unable to tolerate standard therapy. The recommended daily dose is 4 mg/kg given as a single intramuscular injection for 12 to 14 days. Approximately 40 percent of patients develop systemic side effects including azotemia, hypoglycemia, changes in liver function, and pulmonary fibrosis.

In patients with malnutrition and the histopathology of interstitial plasma-cell pneumonia, response to either form of therapy is often very slow. It has been suggested that concomitant corticosteroid therapy might benefit these patients by suppressing the alveolar inflammatory response until the organisms are eradicated. Treatment with oxygen is usually indicated, with the objective of trying to maintain Pa_{O_2} levels at 70 mmHg or above. The inspired oxygen concentration should be kept at less than 50 percent, if possible, to avoid oxygen toxicity. Careful monitoring and assisted ventilation are often required to achieve these goals. Antibiotics, convalescent serum, and commercial immunoglobulin have no effect.

REFERENCES

BURKE BA, GOOD RA: *Pneumocystis carinii* infection. Medicine, 57:23, 1973

CROSS AS, STEIGBIGEL RT: *Pneumocystis carinii* pneumonia presenting as localized nodular densities. N Engl J Med 291:831, 1974

DUTZ W: *Pneumocystis carinii* pneumonia. Pathol Annu 5:309, 1971

HUGHES WT et al: Successful chemoprophylaxis for *Pneumocystis carinii* pneumonitis. N Engl J Med 297:1419, 1977

———— et al: Comparison of pentamidine isethionate and trimethoprim sulfamethoxazole in the treatment of *Pneumocystis carinii* pneumonia. J Pediatr 92:285, 1978

————: *Pneumocystis carinii* pneumonia. N Engl J Med 297:1381, 1977

LAU WK, YOUNG LS: Trimethoprim-sulfamethoxazole treatment of *Pneumocystis carinii* pneumonia in adults. N Engl J Med 295:716, 1976

PIFER LL et al: *Pneumocystis carinii* infection: Evidence for high prevalence in normal and immunosuppressed children. Pediatrics 61:35, 1978

WEBER WR et al: Lung biopsy in *Pneumocystis carinii* pneumonia. Am J Clin Pathol 67:11, 1977

205
MINOR PROTOZOAN DISEASES

JAMES J. PLORDE

TRICHOMONIASIS Trichomoniasis is a venereal infection caused by the protozoan *Trichomonas vaginalis.* Of the many members of the genus *Trichomonas,* three are parasites of human beings: *T. hominis* in the intestine, *T. tenax* in the oral cavity, and *T. vaginalis,* the only one capable of producing disease, in the vagina, urethra, and prostate. All three exist only in the trophozoite stage and resemble one another morphologically. *Trichomonas vaginalis* is the largest, however, and confusion in diagnosis is rare because of the anatomic specificity of their habits.

Trichomonas vaginalis is transmitted by sexual intercourse. Although the organism may survive on moist washcloths for a few hours, transmission of fomites has not been convincingly demonstrated and is probably rare. Newborn children of infected mothers have, on occasion, acquired the infection. The parasite is cosmopolitan in its distribution, and estimates hold that up to 25 percent of the sexually active population may be infected.

In the female, trichomoniasis usually presents as a persistent vaginitis. Initial manifestations include itching, burning, and profuse, creamy yellow, frothy leukorrhea. This acute stage may persist for a week or months, often fluctuating in intensity; it may worsen following menstruation. Eventually the discharge and other symptoms subside and may actually disappear completely, even though the patient still harbors trichomonads. Examination shows inflammation ranging from mild hyperemia of the vaginal vault to extensive erosion, petechial hemorrhages, and perianal intertrigo.

The prostate and urethra are the usual sites of infection in the male. It may present as persistent or recurring nonspecific urethritis, or, more commonly, it may be completely asymptomatic. Acute purulent urethritis occurs rarely.

The diagnosis is made by examining vaginal, prostatic, or urethral secretions for the presence of *Trichomonas.* The organism may also be found in the sedimented urine. A wet mount will usually reveal numerous motile organisms. A Giemsa-stained preparation is confirmatory. *Trichomonas vaginalis* may be grown in culture, but this technique is not generally available. A variety of serologic tests, including a complement fixation, an indirect hemagglutination, and an immunofluorescent reaction, have been described, but are not generally available or completely reliable.

Trichomonas is sometimes responsible for confusing changes in the cytologic pattern of exfoliated vaginal cells. Moreover, ordinary Papanicolaou preparations are not well suited to the diagnosis, and when trichomoniasis is suspected, fresh material should be looked at immediately.

Oral metronidazole (Flagyl), given either in dosage of 250 mg three times daily for 7 days or in a single 2-g dose, is an extremely effective therapeutic agent. Concurrent treatment of sexual partners will minimize recurrent infections.

The recent evidence that metronidazole is carcinogenic in rodents and mutagenic in bacteria has placed the role of this agent in trichomonas infections in doubt. The drug should not be used in pregnancy until further information on its teratogenicity is available. Some authorities suggest that the drug should not be used at all unless patients cannot be rendered asymptomatic by other means. Because of the agent's antabuse-like action, alcohol consumption is contraindicated during therapy and for 24 h following its completion.

GIARDIASIS *Giardia lamblia* is a pear-shaped multiflagellar protozoan that parasitizes the human duodenum and jejunum where it multiplies by longitudinal fission. Under a microscope, its two nuclei and central parabasal body give the organism the appearance of a face with two large eyes. It is actively motile but may attach itself to the intestinal mucosa by means of a large ventral sucker. Encystation occurs in transit through the colon. The resulting ovoid cysts are the infective form of the parasite and are transmitted by the fecal-oral route. Waterborne outbreaks involving well water, chlorinated community systems, and remote mountain streams have been reported. The latter episodes have been concentrated in the Rocky Mountains and suggest that wild animals may serve as alternate hosts. To date, only beavers have been implicated in an outbreak in Camas, Washington.

The infection is found worldwide and is particularly common in areas with poor sanitation and among populations unable to maintain adequate personal hygiene. In the United States, *G. lamblia* is isolated in 3.8 percent of examined stools, making it the single most frequently identified intestinal parasite. Children are three times more likely to be involved than adults and probably have more prominent clinical manifestations. Gastrectomy, decreased gastric acidity, and chronic pancreatitis in adults may increase their susceptibility. Giardiasis also has been reported frequently in patients with immunoglobulin deficiencies and may be a major cause of intestinal abnormalities in these patients. It has been suggested that this parasite is able to persist in such patients because of a relative deficiency in intestinal IgA. *Giardia lamblia* infections also appear to be a significant cause of travelers' diarrhea, particularly among visitors to the Caribbean, Latin America, India, Russia, and the Far East. Unlike the typical syndrome seen in travelers, however, the diarrhea usually begins late in the course of travels and may persist for several weeks. A study in New York demonstrated that all nontraveled immunocompetent males with giardiasis were homosexual. The actual prevalence of the disease in this population is unknown, but the opportunities for direct fecal-oral transmission suggest that it may be high.

Most often the infection is asymptomatic, but in some patients nausea, flatulence, epigastric pain, abdominal cramps, distention, and watery diarrhea occur. After a few days the stools may become semisolid, bulky, and malodorous. Symptoms and accompanying weight loss may persist for several weeks. These symptoms are more common in children and are usually self-limited. Rarely, fulminating and extensive duodenal ulceration has been described. Radiographically, asymptomatic carriers may show irritability of the duodenal bulb. Chronic giardiasis may lead to malabsorption of carbohydrate, fat, and vitamin B_{12}. Lactase intolerance and disaccharidase deficiencies have been described. The pathogenesis of these abnormalities is poorly understood. Mechanical blockage of microvilli or damage to their fuzzy coat by the parasite, organism-induced deconjugation of bile salts, altered motility, and mucosal invasion have been suggested as possible mechanisms. Patients with giardiasis and severe malabsorption had jejunal colonization with enterobacteria, suggesting that bacteria may potentiate the mucosal lesion and be responsible for the development of malabsorption. Jejunal biopsy of patients infested with *Giardia* sometimes shows flattening of the microvilli and an inflammatory infiltrate. Both malabsorption and the jejunal lesions have been reversed with specific treatment.

The diagnosis is made by identifying the cyst in formed feces or the trophozoite in diarrheal stools, duodenal secretions, or jejunal biopsies. In the majority of acute cases, the parasite can be easily demonstrated by the careful examination of one to three stool specimens. Excretion of the organism is often intermittent in chronic cases, however, making parasitological confirmation more difficult. Many of these patients can be diagnosed by examining specimens collected at weekly intervals for a period of 4 to 5 weeks. Alternatively, the duodenal contents can be sampled with a nylon string (Enterotest) or gastric tube and examined by direct wet-mount preparation. Occasionally, jejunal biopsy is required to establish the diagnosis in patients with typical clinical manifestations.

Treatment is usually carried out with quinacrine hydrochloride or metronidazole. Tinadazole, a third highly effective agent, is presently not available in the United States. Quinacrine, 0.1 g given three times daily for 5 days, eliminates the organisms in 70 to 95 percent of cases. Although the drug is usually well tolerated, it may produce gastrointestinal disturbances, exacerbate psoriasis, and, rarely, produce toxic psychosis. Metronidazole appears to be better tolerated and equally effective. However, it is not currently licensed for giardiasis, and there is concern over its mutagenicity. Household contacts and sexual partners of infected patients should be examined; individuals harboring the parasite should be treated even if asymptomatic to prevent the spread to others. Pregnant women, however, should receive therapy only if severely symptomatic.

COCCIDIOSIS This is an infrequently recognized disease characterized by fever, diarrhea, abdominal pain, and weight loss which results from ingestion of the oocysts of coccidia belonging to the genus *Isospora*. Coccidia are widespread in the animal kingdom; each vertebrate host harbors a specific species. *Isospora hominis* and *I. belli* are the two that most

commonly infect human beings. Parasitization is much more common in children and is worldwide in distribution, particularly in tropical areas.

Like the related plasmodia, there is both an asexual and sexual stage of multiplication in *I. belli* infections. However, both occur within a single host. Following the ingestion of an oocyst, *sporozoites* are released which invade the epithelial cells of the intestine to become trophozoites. These multiply asexually producing a large number of *merozoites,* which in turn invade other epithelial cells to continue the cycle. In some cells sexual gametocytes are produced. With the fertilization of the female gametocyte, an oocyst is formed which is then passed in the stool. Transmission is by the fecal-oral route. Volunteers develop symptoms about 1 week after the ingestion of viable oocysts. The illness usually has an acute onset with fever, headache, abdominal cramps, and diarrhea. Stools are often fatty and weight loss is common. Coccidiosis may be associated with a malabsorption syndrome and abnormalities of the mucosa in the small bowel. Symptoms, which presumably continue as long as the asexual cycle of multiplication continues, usually subside spontaneously within a few weeks. In some cases, however, they may persist for months or even years, eventually resulting in death.

Isospora hominis is probably identical to *Sarcocystis fusiformis.* Its oocysts are believed to be infectious only for pigs and cattle in which it produces tissue sarcocysts. Humans become infected by eating undercooked pork or beef containing the cysts. These liberate trophozoites which invade intestinal epithelial cells to undergo gametogony with the formation of new oocysts. The disease in humans is usually asymptomatic, but mild self-limited gastrointestinal manifestations have been described.

A peripheral eosinophilia occurs in approximately half of the infected patients. The diagnosis can be made by examination of stool for oocysts. These are often scanty, and concentration techniques such as zinc sulfate flotation or the formol-ether method must usually be employed. Incubation of the stool for 2 days at room temperature improves the recovery rate. Duodenal aspiration and jejunal biopsy are less cumbersome and more reliable.

Isospora belli infections have been successfully treated with combinations of pyrimethamine-sulfonamide and trimethoprim-sulfamethoxazole. *Isospora hominis* infections do not require specific therapy.

BALANTIDIASIS *Balantidium coli,* the largest protozoon of human beings, inhabits the large intestine. In addition to producing an asymptomatic carrier state, it elicits disease ranging from mild recurrent diarrhea to fulminant ulceration with perforation and death. In many respects the disease is similar to amebiasis in its range of manifestations, exclusive of spread to the liver.

The illness has been reproduced by feeding the organism to volunteers. The diagnosis is made by finding the trophozoite or cyst in the stool, but repeated examinations may be required because shedding of *Balantidium* is intermittent. The disease is more likely to occur in tropical areas, but at least 60 cases have been reported in the United States. Swine and rats are frequent carriers of *B. coli* and may play an important role in the spread of the disease to humans. Outbreaks have been noted in mental institutions where coprophagy implicated direct person-to-person transmission.

The tetracyclines in ordinary doses are highly effective in treatment, as is diiodohydroxyquin given in the dosage of 650 mg three times daily for 20 days.

BABESIOSIS Known since biblical times, babesiosis is a cosmopolitan infection of domestic and wild animals caused by protozoan agents of the genus *Babesia*. These organisms are transmitted by ticks, multiply in red blood cells, and produce an acute febrile illness characterized by hemolytic anemia and hemoglobinuria. The parasite was first described by Babes in 1888 and demonstrated to be tick-borne by Theobald Smith in 1893. This marked the first time a blood-feeding arthropod was implicated in the transmission of a pathogen to a vertebrate host, antedating Ross's description of malaria transmission by 5 years.

The first human case was described in Yugoslavia by Skrabalo in 1957. This and four other European cases were particularly severe with high fever, hemoglobinuria, jaundice, and renal failure. In both their clinical presentation and in the presence of small intraerythrocytic parasites they closely resembled falciparum malaria with which they were originally confused. All five occurred in splenectomized patients, and three ended fatally. The causative agent was presumably a bovine parasite *B. divergens*. Some 20 cases have now been documented in the United States. The first occurred in California and closely resembled the European infections; it was thought to have been caused by an equine parasite. The remaining cases have been seen on a number of offshore islands between New York and Massachusetts, including Nantucket, Shelter Island, and Martha's Vineyard. These patients all had intact spleens and experienced a prolonged illness characterized by the insidious onset of fever, chills, sweating, myalgia, and mild to moderate hemolytic anemia. The physical examination was usually negative except for occasional splenomegaly. Most patients were over 50 years of age and all recovered. The carrier state persisted for weeks to months in some. Serologic studies suggest that mild or asymptomatic cases occur with some frequency.

The cases were apparently all caused by *B. microti,* a parasite of rodents. This organism has been found in field moles and deer mice in New York State and California in addition to the offshore islands of New England. Hard ticks of the genus *Ixodes* serve as vectors. This arthropod does not have specific host preferences and may transmit the disease to humans in both the immature and mature stages. Since the engorged nymph measures only 2 mm in diameter, infested patients may be oblivious to its presence. Transovarial transmission of other *Babesia sp.* has been demonstrated.

The diagnosis depends on the demonstration of the intraerythrocytic parasite in Giemsa-stained peripheral blood smears. Like malaria parasites, these organisms measure 2 to 3 μm in diameter and demonstrate red-staining nuclear material with blue cytoplasm. In some cases band forms resembling *Plasmodium malariae* may be seen. In contrast to malaria parasites, however, neither gametocytes nor pigment can be demonstrated. Unique basket shapes and tetrads produced by budding are also helpful distinguishing characteristics. In heavy infections organisms can be seen outside the red blood cell. Serodiagnosis is helpful in epidemiologic studies. Active infections have been demonstrated in smear-negative, serology-positive infections by inducing infection in experimental animals.

There are presently no satisfactory drugs available for the treatment of this infection. Although chloroquine has been recommended, it appears to have little activity against this parasite. Antitrypanosomal agents may be more effective. In life-threatening disease in patients without spleens, pentamidine or Berenil, both available from the Center for Disease Control, should be considered. Therapy with these toxic drugs does not seem warranted in self-limited *B. microti* infections.

REFERENCES

Babesiosis

DAMMIN GJ: Babesiosis, in *Seminars in Infectious Diseases,* L Weinstein, J Fields (eds). New York, Stratton Intercontinental Medical Book Corp, 1978, pp 169–199

MILLER LH et al: Failure of chloroquine in human babesiosis (*Babesia microti*). Ann Intern Med 88:200, 1978

RUEBUSH TK II et al: Human babesiosis on Nantucket Island. N Engl J Med 297:825, 1977

WOLF RE et al: Intraerythrocytic parasitosis in humans with *Entopolypoides* species (family Babesiide). Ann Intern Med 88:769, 1978

Balantidiasis

WALZER PD et al: Balantidiasis outbreak in Truk Islands. Am J Trop Med Hyg 22:33, 1973

Coccidiosis

BRANDBORG LL et al: Human coccidiosis: A possible cause of malabsorption. N Engl J Med 283:1306, 1970

SMITSKAMP H, OEY-MULLER E: Geographical distribution and clinical significance of human coccidiosis. Trop Geogr Med 18:133, 1966

TRIER JS: Chronic intestinal coccidiosis in man: Intestinal morphology and response to treatment. Gastroenterology 66:923, 1974

Giardiasis

AMENT ME, RUBIN CE: Relation of giardiasis to abnormal intestinal structure and function in gastrointestinal immunodeficiency syndromes. Gastroenterology 62:216, 1972

BRADY PG, WOLFE JC: Waterborne giardiasis. Ann Intern Med 81:498, 1974

JOKIPII L, JOKIPII AMM: Giardiasis in travelers: A prospective study. J Infect Dis 130:295, 1974

KAMATH KR, MURUGASU R: A comparative study of four methods for detecting *Giardia lamblia* in children with diarrheal disease and malabsorption. Gastroenterology 66:16, 1974

KNIGHT R: Giardiasis, isosporiasis and balantidiosis. Clin Gastroenterol 7:31, 1978

WOLFE MS: Current concepts in parasitology—giardiasis, N Engl J Med 298:319, 1978

Trichomoniasis

JIROVEC O, PETRU M: *Trichomonas vaginalis* and trichomonas, in *Advances in Clinical Parasitology,* vol 6, B Dawes (ed). London, Academic, 1968, p 117

KEIGHLEY EE: Trichomonas in a closed community: Efficacy of metronidazole. Br Med J 1:207, 1971

206
APPROACH TO THE PATIENT WITH HELMINTHIC DISEASE

JAMES J. PLORDE

Helminths that parasitize humans can be divided into three major groups: roundworms (nematodes), tapeworms (cestodes), and flukes (trematodes). In contrast to the protozoa, helminths are large, multicellular organisms which have excretory, nervous, and reproductive systems. Of these, trematodes are the most highly differentiated, possessing fully developed male and female sexual organs capable of producing enormous numbers of offspring in the form of eggs, or larvae. With few exceptions these offspring must pass out of the *definitive host* harboring the sexually active adults before they can mature into forms capable of infecting their next host. The eggs of *Enterobius vermicularis* require only a few hours of embryonation on the perianal skin before they become infective. The eggs and larvae of most of the intestinal nematodes, however, require a prolonged period of incubation in soil under appropriate conditions of temperature and humidity, while those of the cestodes and trematodes must undergo developmental changes in one or more *intermediate hosts* before they are capable of completing their life cycle.

These differences in life cycle have a determinative influence on the epidemiology of helminthic parasites. *Enterobius vermicularis,* which can be spread directly from host to host because of its brief embryonation time in the external environment, has a cosmopolitan distribution. The remainder of the intestinal nematodes are spread via contamination of soil by eggs or larvae-containing human excrement. They are thus found in all areas of the world with poor sanitation where the appropriate conditions of temperature and humidity pertain. Finally, the distribution of trematodes such as the various species of *Schistosoma* are limited by the ecologic niches of their intermediate hosts.

Human disease can result when humans serve as either the definitive host, harboring the mature adults (e.g., *Taenia saginata*), or the intermediate host to the larval stages of the worm (e.g., echinococcosis). Occasionally a person may function as both the definitive (*T. solium*) and intermediate host (cysticercosis) for the same helminth. Since most adult helminths are incapable of multiplying within their definitive host, the manifestations of illness are related to the total number of worms acquired by the host. Most small worm load infections are, in fact, asymptomatic, and many need not even be treated. As helminths are usually long-lived, however, repeated infections can result from very high worm loads with disability typical of infections, particularly in endemic areas.

The pathogenesis of helminthic disease is variable. *Diphyllobothrium latum* competes with the host for nutrients, *Strongyloides stercoralis* and *Capillaria philippinensis* interfere with the absorption of food across the intestinal mucosa, and hookworm causes loss of iron, an essential mineral. Other parasites such as *Clonorchis sinensis* and *Schistosoma haematobium* compromise the function of important organs by obstruction and secondary bacterial infections. Long-term infections with both of the organisms can also be carcinogenic. Disease can result from simple mass effect as in the case of echinococcosis. Actual tissue invasion and destruction by larval forms occur in many infections. Immunologic mechanisms are undoubtedly responsible for tissue damage and clinical manifestations in many helminthic diseases.

Once the clinician thinks of the possibility of a helminthic infection, the diagnosis is usually straightforward. Although these infections are not common in the United States, the continuous arrival of travelers and immigrants and the importation of food from endemic areas of the world make it necessary to consider them in the differential diagnosis. Patients should be carefully questioned about their travels and food intake. Many helminths can survive within the host for a decade or more after he or she leaves an endemic area.

Although eosinophilia has long been recognized as a clue to the presence of helminthic infections, the failure to detect it does not preclude this diagnosis. The eosinophilia presumably reflects an immunologic response to the complex foreign proteins of the worm and is most marked during the early stages of tissue migration and invasion. Once migration ceases and the worm matures to adulthood, the eosinophilia may diminish or disappear.

The definitive diagnosis usually rests upon the recovery and morphological identification of the parasite in stool, urine, sputum, blood, or tissues. This process is facilitated by the large and relatively constant numbers of morphologically distinct progeny discharged by gravid worms. A simple wet mount of fresh or concentrated stool suffices for detection of most significant gastrointestinal infections. In strongyloidiasis where larvae are released into the duodenum and jejunum, aspirates of the upper intestine may reveal parasites when stool examination has been negative. Similarly, eggs of *Enterobius* (pinworm) and *Taenia* (tapeworm) can frequently be found on the perianal skin when absent from the feces. Biopsy of the rectal valves is the most reliable diagnostic procedure for intestinal schistosomiasis. Helminths dwelling within the tissues of the host are more difficult to identify. Some discharge their offspring into the bloodstream (filaria) or sputum (lung flukes) where they can be found with appropriate concentration procedures. In others, larvae can be recovered with skin (*Onchocerca volvulus*) or muscle (*Trichinella spiralis*) biopsies. In diseases such as toxocariasis, eosinophilic meningitis, and cysticercosis parasite recovery is uncommon. Immunodiagnostic tests, with the notable exceptions of those for trichinosis and ecchinococcosis, have been of limited help to date. However, introduction of purified homologous antigens and the adaption of the enzyme-linked immunosorbent and immunoelectrophoresis assays to helminthic infections are likely to improve this situation in the near future.

TABLE 206-1
Fecal egg counts associated with illness

Worm	Approximate egg output per female worm per day	Minimum egg output usually associated with illness
Necator americanus	25,000	>2000/ml
Trichuris trichiura	7500	>3000/g
Schistosoma mansoni	60–300	>200/g

SOURCE: *After DP Stevens, Clin Gastroenterol 7:236, 1978.*

TABLE 206-2
Antihelminthics available from the Parasitic Disease Drug Service*

Infection	Therapeutic agent
Dracunculosis	Niridazole (Ambilhar)
Fascioliasis	Bithionol
Onchocerciasis	Suramin (Antrypol)
Paragonimiasis	Bithionol
Schistosomiasis	Niridazole (Ambilhar) Sodium antimony dimercapto-succinate (Astiban)
Tapeworms *(T. saginata, T. solium, Hymenolepsis nana, H. diminuta, Diphyllobothrium latum, Dipylidium caninum)*	Niclosamide (Yomesan)

* *Center for Disease Control, Atlanta, Ga. 30333.*

The rational management of helminthic infections requires an estimation of the worm load. Since most worms do not multiply within the body and because disability is usually related to the intensity of infection, treatment is directed primarily at reducing the worm burden of moderately to heavily infected patients. Total eradication is often unnecessary and may be unwise considering the toxicity of many antihelminthics. Light infections should be treated only when (1) small numbers of worms may be dangerous as in the case of strongyloidiasis, (2) the chance of reinfection is slight, and/or (3) the antihelminthic agent in question is without serious side effects. The intensity of many intestinal infections can be determined by enumerating the eggs found in stool (Table 206-1). Multiplying the total seen on direct smear by 750 provides a rough estimate of the number present per gram of feces. The Stoll dilution and the various modifications of the Kato thick-smear technique provide more precise results.

Many antihelminthics are not generally available in the United States or have not yet been approved for use in that country. Fortunately, many of these are available through the Parasitic Disease Drug Service of the Center for Disease Control in Atlanta, Georgia (Table 206-2).

NEMATODE INFECTIONS

Nematodes are elongated, cylindrical, unsegmented organisms that vary in size from the tiny *Trichinella spiralis* and *Strongyloides stercoralis,* which are a few millimeters in length, to *Dracunculus medinensis,* which may measure more than a meter. They have a simple tubular digestive tract running from the mouth in the anterior end to the anus located ventrally near the tail. The sexes are separate, and the male, which is usually smaller than the female, generally has a curved posterior end. The life span varies from 1 to 2 months in the case of *T. spiralis* and *Enterobius vermicularis* to 10 years or more for hookworms. During this time the gravid female produces enormous numbers of progeny either as fertile eggs or larvae. With the sole exception of *Trichinella,* these offspring must undergo a period of development outside the definitive host.

Among the intestinal nematodes, this period of development occurs without the benefit of intermediate hosts. The eggs of *E. vermicularis,* or pinworm, are fully embryonated when laid and become infective within hours of being deposited on the perianal skin. After being ingested, these eggs mature into adult worms within the alimentary tract of humans. The life cycle of the whipworm, *Trichuris trichiura,* is similar except that the eggs must pass in the stool and incubate several weeks in soil before becoming infective for humans on ingestion. The external development of *Ascaris lumbricoides* eggs is identical. However, following ingestion, the embryonated eggs hatch, releasing larvae which penetrate the intestinal wall and are carried to the pulmonary capillaries via the bloodstream. Here they penetrate the alveoli, ascend the respiratory tract, and reach the glottis. Then, after completing their pulmonary migration, the larvae are swallowed, regain the intestinal lumen, and develop into mature adults.

The eggs of *Strongyloides* and of hookworm, in contrast to those of the above three, hatch shortly before (*Strongyloides*) or after (hookworm) being passed in the stool, producing rhabditiform soil larvae. Following several molts, these larvae are transformed into infective or filariform larvae, penetrate human skin, and after migrating through the lung in the manner described above for *Ascaris,* reach the intestine.

The life cycle of *Strongyloides* differs from that of hookworm in two important respects. First, rhabditiform larvae may, under certain conditions, develop into free-living adult male and female worms which reproduce in the soil. Second, rhabditiform larvae may develop into the infective filariform larvae while still within the human intestine. These may then reinfect the original host directly (autoinfection) without first going through a period of incubation in the external environment (Table 206-3).

The offspring of the tissue nematodes such as *Dracunculus* and the filarial worms undergo their development in a second

TABLE 206-3
Life cycle of intestinal nematodes

Species	Route of infection	Migration in body	Diagnostic form	Site of larval development	Infective form	Free-living stage
Enterobius vermicularis	Mouth	Intestinal	Egg	Perineum	Egg	No
Trichuris trichiura	Mouth	Intestinal	Egg	Soil	Egg	No
Ascaris lumbricoides	Mouth	Pulmonary	Egg	Soil	Egg	No
*Necator americanus**	Skin	Pulmonary	Egg	Soil	Filariform larvae	No
Strongyloides stercoralis	Skin	Pulmonary	Rhabditiform larvae	Soil, intestine†	Filariform larvae	Yes

* *Also* Ancylostoma duodenale.
† *Intestine only in cases of autoinfection.*

invertebrate host before they can complete their maturation in the human.

The nematodes infecting humans are usually divided into intestinal and tissue parasites. Those which produce clinical manifestations by virtue of the presence of the adult worm within the human alimentary tract are considered intestinal nematodes; they include *Enterobius, Trichuris, Ascaris,* the hookworms, and *Strongyloides.* A number of closely related nematodes infecting animals such as *Toxacara canis* and *Ancylostoma braziliense* which may infect, but usually fail to reach maturity within humans will also be included in this group in the following discussion. Listed among the tissue nematodes are those which produce disease by the migration of the adult and/or larval forms through tissues such as *Trichinella,* the filarial worms, and *Dracunculus.*

REFERENCES

Drugs for parasitic infections. Med Letter 20(4):17, 1978

Health information for international travel 1978, U.S. Department of Health, Education, and Welfare Publication (CDC) 78–82. Morb Mort Week Rep, vol 27, suppl, September 1978

HUNTER GW III et al (eds): *Tropical Medicine,* 5th ed. Philadelphia, Saunders, 1976

207
TISSUE NEMATODES

JAMES J. PLORDE

ANGIOSTRONGYLIASIS CANTONENSIS

DEFINITION *Angiostrongylus cantonensis,* the rat lungworm, is the etiologic agent of the common form of *eosinophilic meningitis* found in Southeast Asia in the tropical areas of the Pacific.

ETIOLOGY The delicate filariform adults (20 mm in length) reside and lay their eggs in the pulmonary arterioles of rats and certain other rodents. After hatching, the larvae break into the alveoli, migrate up the respiratory tract, are swallowed, and pass in the feces. They develop into infective third-stage larvae within snails and slugs, their natural intermediate host. Viable third-stage organisms may also be found in land planarians, crabs, and freshwater prawns. These carriers appear to acquire the larvae by feeding on the tissues of infected mollusks. Humans, like rodents, become parasitized when they ingest raw intermediate or carrier hosts containing the infective stage. In rodents the larvae migrate to the brain where they grow into young adults. After a period of further maturation, the worms travel to the lungs and begin to deposit eggs. The nematode does not complete its life cycle in humans and dies after reaching the central nervous system.

EPIDEMIOLOGY Human infections with *A. cantonensis* have been found in Thailand, Vietnam, Cambodia, Indonesia, the Philippines, Taiwan, Hawaii, and several smaller Pacific islands from Okinawa in the north to New Caledonia and Tahiti in the south. In addition, rodent infections have been found in the islands of East Africa, Sri Lanka, India, and China. The rat lungworm may have been spread from Madagascar to Asia and to the Pacific by the recent dispersal of the giant African land snail, *Achatina fulica.*

PATHOLOGY AND PATHOGENESIS The nematode can produce extensive tissue damage by moving through the brain when alive and provokes a marked inflammatory reaction when dead. The pathological lesions are characterized by (1) marked lymphocyte and eosinophilic infiltration of the meninges, (2) hemorrhagic and nonhemorrhagic worm tracts through the brainstem and spinal cord, (3) granuloma formation around dead parasites and necrotic debris which sheathes the worm, and (4) engorgement of almost all blood vessels, particularly the veins. Necrosis of vessel walls, aneurysmal dilatation of arteries, and perivascular hemorrhages have been noted. Living worms have been removed from the eyes of patients without central nervous system involvement.

CLINICAL MANIFESTATIONS The eosinophilic meningitis usually presents as an acute severe headache. Fever is usually mild or absent, and only 15 percent of patients show signs of meningeal irritation. Patients frequently complain of visual impairment and, in a majority of these, visual defects or blurring of the optic disk can be demonstrated. Paresthesias of the trunk and lower extremities are a common complaint, and paralysis of the sixth and seventh nerves is seen in 3 to 7 percent of cases. Paralysis of the limbs, convulsions, and loss of consciousness are rare. The disease usually ends in complete spontaneous recovery. The cerebrospinal fluid contains several hundred cells per cubic millimeter and many eosinophils, and the cerebrospinal fluid protein is elevated. There may or may not be an eosinophilia in the peripheral blood.

The second clinically distinct form of eosinophilic meningitis has been reported from Thailand. This presents as a radiculomyeloencephalitis with limb pain and paresis and is thought to be caused by the nematode *Gnathostoma spinigerum.* The cerebrospinal fluid eosinophilic leukocytosis is less marked than in *angiostrongylus* infections. The fluid is often xanthochromic. Death may occur from cerebral hemorrhage or destruction of vital centers.

DIAGNOSIS The diagnosis is made on the basis of the clinical manifestations in an endemic area. Angiostrongyliasis must be differentiated from other ectopic worm infections of the central nervous system including strongyloidiasis, filariasis, paragonimiasis, hydatid disease, schistosomiasis japonicum, trichinosis, cysticercosis, toxocariasis, and gnathostomiasis.

TREATMENT AND PREVENTION There is no known effective treatment. Anthelmintic therapy should not be given since the simultaneous death of many worms might produce a severe inflammatory reaction. Steroids may be beneficial in severe cases. Prevention depends upon avoidance or proper cooking of such foods as snails, prawns, and crabs. Raw vegetables should be carefully inspected for the presence of planarians and mollusks before they are eaten. Freezing of crustaceans and mollusks at −15°C for 12 h will destroy infective larvae of *A. cantonensis.*

ANGIOSTRONGYLIASIS COSTARICENSIS

Angiostrongylus costaricensis is a nematode that dwells in the mesenteric arteries of Central American rats. Larvae pass in the stool and develop in slugs, the intermediate hosts. Rats, and incidentally humans, are infected when they ingest slugs or vegetables contaminated with third-stage larvae. The larvae mature in the lymphatics and move to the mesenteric radicals of the cecum. Here they may cause arterial thrombosis, ischemic necrosis, ulceration, and eosinophilic granuloma formation. Infected patients present with fever, eosinophilic leukocytosis, abdominal pain, and a right lower quadrant mass.

Occasionally perforation of the bowel and generalized peritonitis occur. The fever may persist for up to 2 months. Children are more frequently involved than adults. Neither larvae nor eggs are seen in the stool of the human host. No specific therapy is available.

GNATHOSTOMIASIS

DEFINITION Gnathostomiasis is a tissue infection of humans caused by *Gnathostoma spinigerum,* an intestinal nematode of carnivores. Clinically it is manifest as migratory subcutaneous swellings, creeping eruption, or a lethal eosinophilic meningitis.

ETIOLOGY AND EPIDEMIOLOGY The parasite, which is found throughout the Far East, lives encysted in the gastric mucosa of dogs, cats, and wild felines. The ova are passed to the external environment via the feces, hatch in water, and are ingested by *Cyclops,* the first intermediate hosts. These in turn are eaten by freshwater fish, frogs, snakes, and eels in whose flesh the infective third-stage larvae develop. Ducks and chickens fed on these second intermediate hosts may also come to harbor infective larvae. Human infections, which are most commonly seen in Thailand and Japan, occur when humans ingest infected uncooked fish (somfak, sashimi), duck, or chicken.

PATHOGENESIS AND MANIFESTATIONS The parasite cannot complete its cycle in humans, and the immature worms migrate through the abdominal and thoracic organs producing localized areas of inflammation and hemorrhage. Clinically, this is manifest as fever, eosinophilic leukocytosis, urticaria, and pain. Typically, the systemic manifestations subside within a month as the worms make their way to the subcutaneous tissues. Here, their continued migration results in the production of transient serpiginous pruritic swellings, subcutaneous tunnels, and abscesses. If the worm invades the epidermis, the resulting lesions closely resemble those of cutanea larva migrans. Rarely the eye may be involved with orbital cellulitis, iritis, or uveitis. Migration into the central nervous system results in a lethal eosinophilic meningitis (see "Angiostrongyliasis cantonensis" above). This presents as a radiculomyeloencephalitis with limb pain and paresis. The cerebrospinal fluid eosinophilic leukocytosis is present but less marked than in *Angiostrongylus* infections. The fluid is often xanthochromic. Death may occur from cerebral hemorrhage or destruction of vital centers.

DIAGNOSIS AND TREATMENT Painless, recurrent migratory subcutaneous swellings and eosinophilic leukocytosis occurring in an endemic area make the diagnosis likely. It must be differentiated from cutanea larva migrans, however, and from angiostrongyliasis cantonensis when the central nervous system is involved. Definitive diagnosis depends upon the removal and identification of the worm. Other than excision, there is no specific therapy. The disease can be prevented by the adequate cooking of fish, chicken, and duck in endemic areas.

DRACUNCULIASIS

DEFINITION Dracunculiasis is an infection of human connective and subcutaneous tissues by the guinea worm, *Dracuncula medinensis.* The gravid female produces symptoms when she ruptures the skin to discharge her eggs.

ETIOLOGY AND EPIDEMIOLOGY Dracunculiasis affects about 50 million people in West, Central, and Northeast Africa, the Middle East, Iran, Pakistan, India, northeastern South America, and the Caribbean Islands. Humans acquire the parasite when they ingest raw drinking water containing infected copepods (*Cyclops* spp.) which serve as the intermediate host. Shallow ponds, cisterns, and wells are the usual habitat of these crustaceans. In the stomach the copepod is digested and the larvae are released. The larva penetrates the intestinal wall and matures in the connective tissue of the retroperitoneal space. The adult male is small, seldom seen, and presumably dies after mating. In contrast, the female *Dracunculus* is one of the largest nematodes known—1 to 2 mm in diameter and 300 to 800 mm in length. The female reaches gravidity in approximately one year and then migrates to the subcutaneous tissue of the lower extremities. When the anterior end of the worm approaches the skin, a blister forms. This breaks down in a few days, forming a superficial ulcer. When the protruding portion of the worm comes in contact with water, the uterus prolapses through the body and discharges large numbers of motile rhabditiform larvae. Following ingestion by one of several species of *Cyclops,* the larvae undergo further development, becoming infective in 10 to 12 days. Mammals other than humans may be infected, but their importance as a disease reservoir is uncertain.

PATHOGENESIS AND MANIFESTATIONS The infection is asymptomatic until the gravid female appears in the subcutaneous tissues where it may, on occasion, be palpable. A few days before the formation of the blister, the patient frequently has fever, generalized urticaria, periorbital edema, and wheezing. Blister formation is accompanied by intense local pain and pruritus; like the systemic manifestations, this is thought to represent an allergic reaction to prematurely liberated larvae. The local lesion is usually found over the feet and ankles but may occur on the trunk or the upper extremities. Multiple infections are common. With the rupture of the blister and the release of embryos, the systemic manifestations abate, and the worm is slowly extruded over a period of 4 to 5 weeks. Secondary infection and cellulitis are common, particularly if the worm is ruptured during the process of extraction. In Nigeria, guinea worm ulcers are a common portal of entry for the spores of *Clostridium tetani.* The female worm often fails to reach the surface and discharge her larvae. In most of these cases, it dies without producing symptoms. The calcified appearance on roentgenograms is characteristic. Occasionally the worm may invade the deep tissues, causing serious symptoms, and sterile abscesses may follow the release of embryos. Invasion of joint spaces by the adult worm or larvae results in arthritis.

DIAGNOSIS The clinical picture is characteristic. Placing a small amount of water on the worm results in discharge of larvae which can then be examined microscopically. A fluorescent antibody test may permit the diagnosis to be made prior to emergence of the gravid female.

TREATMENT AND PREVENTION If the outline of the worm can be clearly seen or palpated, it may sometimes be completely removed with a single incision. The gradual extraction of the worm can be accomplished by winding a few centimeters onto a stick each day. Administration of niridazole (Ambilhar) results in prompt remission of symptoms. The dose is 25 mg per kilogram of body weight given in three divided doses for 7 days. Thiabendazole in dosage of 25 mg/kg twice daily for 2 days or metronidazole 250 mg three times a day for

7 days is also effective in the relief of symptoms. At present, there is serious question whether any of the above agents hasten worm extrusion or death. Some authorities suggest the rapid symptomatic improvement induced by these agents is secondary to their antiinflammatory rather than anthelmintic properties. Dracunculiasis can be prevented by the chemical treatment of drinking water.

REFERENCES

ALICATA JE: Present status of *Angiostrongylus cantonensis* infection in man and animals in the tropics. J Trop Med Hyg 72:53, 1969

MORERA P, CESPEDES R: Abdominal angiostrongyliasis. A new human parasitic infection. Acta Med Costarric 14:159, 1971 (Spanish)

MULLER R: Dracunculus and dracunculiasis, in *Advances in Parasitology*, vol 9, B Dawes (ed). London, Academic, 1971, p 73

NYE SW et al: Lesions of the brain in eosinophilic meningitis. Arch Pathol 89:9, 1970

PUNYAGUPTA S et al: Eosinophilic meningitis in Thailand. Am J Trop Med 24:921, 1975

208
TRICHINOSIS

JAMES J. PLORDE

DEFINITION Trichinosis is an intestinal and tissue infection of humans and other mammals caused by the nematode *Trichinella spiralis*. The disease is characterized by diarrhea during the development of the adults in the intestine and by myositis, fever, prostration, periorbital edema, eosinophilic leukocytosis, and, occasionally, evidence of myocarditis or encephalitis during the stage of larval migration in tissue.

ETIOLOGY Trichinosis in humans is contracted by ingestion of meat containing the encysted larvae of *T. spiralis*. The meat has almost always been pork, but for the past several years about 10 percent of cases reported in this country have been attributed to bear meat. This has been particularly frequent in the Northern and Western states including Alaska, California, and Idaho. There are no intermediate hosts, and both the adult and larval stages develop in the same animal. Infection has been produced or observed in the bear, wild boar, wolf, coyote, fox, muskrat, horse, cow, dog, cat, rabbit, guinea pig, mouse, and marine mammals, in addition to the rat and the pig. Humans are particularly susceptible; most fowl are resistant. Among pigs, infection is contracted following feeding of the uncooked scraps, less often by eating infected rats. The incidence of infection in pigs has been reduced by laws requiring that garbage be cooked thoroughly before being fed. Rats also feed on uncooked pork scraps and, in addition, maintain a high incidence of infection by their cannibalism.

Soon after ingestion, the larvae are liberated from their cysts by gastric digestion and migrate into the intestinal mucosa, where copulation takes place. The male dies, and within a week, the viviparous female is discharging larvae (100 by 6 μm), which enter vascular channels and are distributed throughout the body. Larviposition continues for about 4 to 16 weeks, each female producing approximately 1500 offspring. The larvae enter skeletal muscle, grow, and begin encysting within 3 weeks; calcification of cysts begins in 6 to 18 months. The life span of the encysted organism has been estimated at 5 to 10 years. The muscles of the diaphragm, tongue, and eye, and the deltoid, pectoral, gastrocnemius, and intercostal mus-

cles are most often affected. Larvae carried to sites other than skeletal muscles do not encyst but disintegrate. The life cycle can be carried further only if a new host ingests the encysted larvae.

The description of a fatal case of trichinosis in an immunosuppressed patient emphasizes the importance of the immune response in limiting the intensity of infection. Apparently, it does so by acting directly on circulating larvae, inhibiting the reproduction of the female worms, and accelerating the expulsion of the adult parasites from the intestine. Eosinophils as well as B and T cell lymphocytes are involved in the response. The T cells appear to have a "helper" function in promoting the production of antibodies which, in collaboration with eosinophils, mediate the protective response.

EPIDEMIOLOGY Trichinosis is particularly common in Europe and North America, but with the exception of Australia and Asia it is found world-wide. In the United States its prevalence as measured by finding cysts in human diaphragms at autopsy has declined from 16.1 to 4.2 percent over the past 20 years. This decline has been accompanied by a similar reduction of trichinosis in pigs. The prevalence appears highest in the New England, Mid-Atlantic, and Pacific states. Currently, it is estimated that 1.5 million Americans carry live trichinae in their musculature and that somewhere between 150,000 and 300,000 acquire new infections annually. The overwhelming majority of these infections are asymptomatic, and many of those that become clinically manifest are never correctly diagnosed. In 1977 only 142 cases and no deaths were officially reported in the United States. Large outbreaks are usually caused by consumption of ready-to-eat pork sausage prepared in noninspected facilities or at home. The incidence appears highest among Americans of Italian, German, Polish, or Portuguese descent, presumably because of their inclination to make and eat pork sausage. Notable epidemics have followed the ingestion of trichinae-infected wild pig in Hawaii and California and walrus in Alaska. The latter is the first reported outbreak caused by this host in North America. Each year, a few cases are acquired from ground beef, attesting to the frequency with which this meat is adulterated with pork.

PATHOLOGY The most striking lesions are in the skeletal muscles, where there is a severe myositis with basophilic granular degeneration of the invaded muscle fiber. Adjacent fibers exhibit hyalin or hydropic degeneration, and the focus becomes infiltrated with neutrophilic and eosinophilic leukocytes, some lymphocytes, and mononuclear macrophages. Hyperemia, edema, and hemorrhages are constant features.

Larvae do not encyst in cardiac muscle, but an intense myocarditis has been observed in fatal cases.

In cases of central nervous system involvement, there may be granulomatous nodules, and vasculitis involving small arterioles and capillaries of the brain and meninges. Encystment of larvae in the brain is unusual.

CLINICAL MANIFESTATIONS The severity of the clinical manifestations is generally related to the number of larvae disseminated to the tissues of the host; patients with severe disease usually harbor 50 to 100 larvae per gram of muscle, while those with 10 or less are often asymptomatic. The first symptoms usually appear within 1 to 2 days after ingestion of the uncooked or undercooked meat containing encysted larvae. At that time diarrhea, abdominal pain, nausea, and sometimes prostration and fever develop. The next stage, that of muscular invasion, begins about the end of the first week and may last as long as 6 weeks. During this period, patients have fever, edema of the eyelids, conjunctivitis and subconjunctival hemorrhages, muscle pain and tenderness, and often severe weakness. There may be a maculopapular rash which lasts for several days and subungual "splinter hemorrhages." Central nervous system involvement may be evident as polyneuritis, poliomyelitis, myasthenia, meningitis, encephalitis, focal or diffuse pareses, delirium, psychosis, and coma. Despite the severity of central nervous system involvement in some patients, the cerebrospinal fluid remains normal.

Myocarditis is characterized by persistent tachycardia or development of congestive heart failure. There are marked electrocardiographic alterations, including ST-T wave changes and conduction abnormalities in 20 percent of patients.

LABORATORY FINDINGS The most constant finding, and one of significance early in the course of the disease, is the eosinophilic leukocytosis (over 500 eosinophilic leukocytes per cubic millimeter) which generally appears before the end of the second week. In cases of moderate severity, the proportion of eosinophilic leukocytes ranges between 15 and 50 percent. In severe cases, particularly terminally, the eosinophilic leukocytosis may disappear entirely.

The skin test to larval antigen becomes positive early in the third week of infection and may remain so for up to 20 years. The usual positive response is a wheal of 5 mm or more appearing within 30 min. Unfortunately, the commercially available skin test preparations are not reliable and their use is currently discouraged.

There are a variety of serologic tests for trichinosis, including the precipitin reaction, the complement fixation test, the indirect fluorescent antibody test, and the bentonite flocculation test, which is probably the best. A commercially available latex agglutination test appears to give comparable results. These serologic tests all become positive by about the third week of the disease and may remain positive for a few years. Since each may occasionally be falsely negative, two or more tests should be used. The serologic tests are most valuable if they are negative initially and then in turn positive or if there is a change in titer.

Muscle biopsy when carried out during the third or fourth week of infection remains the most useful test for demonstration of larvae or cysts. The deltoid or gastrocnemius muscles are the most useful sites for biopsy. A small portion of the excised muscle should be compressed between glass slides and examined under a low-power microscope for the presence of larvae. Calcified cysts or larvae represent an old infection. The remainder of the biopsy should be submitted for routine processing because myositis is a significant finding even in the absence of larvae or cysts.

In severe trichinosis there may be marked hypoalbuminemia, probably because of protein leakage from damaged capillaries. During the fourth, fifth, and sixth weeks of the disease, concomitant with a rise in antibody, diffuse hypergammaglobulinemia occurs. Elevated levels of circulating IgE have been reported. There may be moderate rises in serum glutamic oxaloacetic transaminase, serum aldolase, and creatine-phosphokinase, probably related to myositis; the sedimentation rate is characteristically slow.

DIFFERENTIAL DIAGNOSIS Trichinosis must be differentiated from diseases which are characterized by eosinophilia (such as Hodgkin's disease, eosinophilic leukemia, and periarteritis nodosa) and from entities which are characterized by myopathy, such as dermatomyositis. When the central nervous system is involved, the diagnosis may be very difficult.

TREATMENT Thiabendazole, in dosage of 25 mg/kg bid for 5 to 7 days, has resulted in apparent improvement in a number of patients, with relief of muscle pain and tenderness and with

lysis of fever. The results have not been uniform, however, and the use of this drug in trichinosis has been associated with nausea, vomiting, abdominal discomfort, dermatitis, and drug fever.

Patients with "allergic" manifestations of trichinosis, including angioedema and urticaria as well as myocardial or central nervous system involvement, should be treated with prednisone in dosage of 20 to 60 mg per day. Response to steroids usually has been prompt, particularly in central nervous system trichinosis. Not all focal lesions have resolved, however.

Other measures should be directed at relief of pain and maintenance of adequate caloric and fluid intake.

PROGNOSIS The prognosis in trichinosis has improved markedly, and even when the central nervous system is involved, the mortality rate has fallen to under 10 percent. The overall mortality rate is probably less than 2 percent.

PREVENTION The responsibility for control rests with the consumer. Adequate cooking of pork involves heating all portions of the meat to 60°C. Freezing procedures to kill the larvae require a temperature of −15°C for 20 days or −18°C for 24 h. Proper smoking and pickling will also destroy the larvae. Important in control is the cooking of garbage fed to hogs. There is no practical method of inspection which will detect trichinous pork.

REFERENCES

BARRETT-CONNER E et al: An epidemic of trichinosis after ingestion of wild pig in Hawaii. J Infect Dis 133:473, 1976

BROWN HW: *Basic Clinical Parasitology*, 4th ed. New York, Appleton-Century-Crofts, 1975

DALESSIO DJ, WOLFF HG: *Trichinella spiralis* infection of the central nervous system. Arch Neurol 4:407, 1961

DESPOMMIER D: Immunity to *Trichinella spiralis*. Am J Trop Med Hyg 26:68, 1977

GRAY DF et al: Trichinosis with neurologic and cardiac involvement. Ann Intern Med 57:230, 1962

METZLER MH et al: Second-degree atrioventricular block in acute trichinosis. Am J Dis Child 124:598, 1972

MOST H: Current concepts in parasitology. Trichinosis—preventable yet still with us. N Engl J Med 298:1178, 1978

ROSENBERG EB et al: Increased circulating IgE in trichinosis. Ann Intern Med 75:575, 1971

SULZER AJ, CHISHOLM ES: Comparison of the IFA and other tests for *Trichinella spiralis* antibodies. Pub Health Rep 81:729, 1966

WAND M, LYMAN D: Trichinosis from bear meat. JAMA 220:245, 1972

ZIMMERMAN WJ: Prevalence of *Trichinella spiralis* in commercial pork sausage. Pub Health Rep 85:717, 1970

——— et al: Trichinosis in the U.S. population 1966–70. Pub Health Rep 88:606, 1973

209
FILARIASIS

JAMES J. PLORDE

DEFINITION Filariasis is a group of disorders produced by infection with the threadlike nematodes of the superfamily Filarioidea. These worms invade the lymphatics and subcutaneous and deep tissues of humans producing reactions ranging from acute inflammation to chronic scarring. The viviparous female discharges microfilariae into the blood or subcutaneous tissues where they live for weeks or months until taken up by hematophagous arthropods. Within these vectors they are transformed into filariform larvae which then infect a new host when the arthropod takes another blood meal. The clinical pictures produced by various species in this group are more or less specific. The term *lymphatic filariasis* is commonly used to designate the disease produced by *Wuchereria bancrofti* and *Brugia malayi*, the organisms responsible for lymphatic blockade and elephantiasis. *Loa loa* causes loiasis, a disease characterized by transient subcutaneous (Calabar) swellings, and *Onchocerca volvulus* produces the blindness and pruritic skin rash typical of onchocerciasis. *Mansonella ozzardi, Dipetalonema perstans,* and *D. streptocerca* cause infections of questionable clinical significance to humans.

These parasites are identified by the location, periodicity, and morphological characteristics of their microfilariae. Those of *W. bancrofti, B. malayi, L. loa, D. perstans,* and *M. ozzardi* are all found in the blood, and, with the exception of the last, all display nocturnal or diurnal periodicity. *Onchocerca volvulus* and *D. streptocerca* are found in the subcutaneous tissues and are nonperiodic. Morphologically, the microfilariae are distinguished by the presence or absence of a sheath and by the distribution of their deeply staining column of nuclei. The sheath, which is an elongation of the original eggshell, can be seen extending beyond the head and tail only in the microfilariae of *W. bancrofti, B. malayi,* and *L. loa*. The nuclear column extends to the very tip of the microfilariae of *B. malayi, L. loa,* and the two species of *Dipetalonema*.

Skin and serologic tests are group-specific, lack sensitivity, and may be falsely negative in other nematode infections. In the absence of microfilariae and other helminthic infections, however, they may be helpful in establishing a diagnosis in clinically suspect cases.

LYMPHATIC FILARIASIS (BANCROFTIAN AND MALAYAN)

ETIOLOGY AND EPIDEMIOLOGY The threadlike adult worms live coiled together in human lymphatics. The male *W. bancrofti* measures 35 mm and the female 80 to 100 mm. The *B. malayi* adults are about one-half as long. Gravid females release microfilariae in large numbers into the lymphatics. These embryos, which are sheathed, measure approximately 200 to 300 μm. They eventually reach the peripheral blood, where further development depends on their ingestion by a proper mosquito vector. Species of *Culex, Aëdes,* and *Anopheles* transmit Bancroftian filariasis; *Mansonia* and *Anopheles* serve as vectors in Malayan disease. After further development in the vector, larvae migrate to the mouthparts. If the mosquito feeds on a human host, they penetrate the puncture site and reach maturity in about a year. In the absence of reinfection, humans harbor microfilariae for 5 to 10 years, the reproductive life of the adult worms. In most *W. bancrofti* and *B. malayi* infections, the microfilariae are found in the blood in greatest numbers between 9 P.M. and 2 A.M. During the day, apparently in response to changes in oxygen tension, they accumulate in the pulmonary vessels and disappear from the peripheral blood. However, in Polynesia and New Caledonia there is an *Aëdes*-transmitted variety of *W. bancrofti* (*W. pacifica*) that displays a diurnal periodicity in which the peak occurs in the early evenings (subperiodic form). Periodicity is of epidemiologic signif-

icance because it determines which species of mosquito serves as the vector. Furthermore, several subperiodic forms of *B. malayi* have been found in animals, suggesting the possibility that this disease has an animal reservoir. The human is the only known vertebrate host for *W. bancrofti*.

More than 250 million persons throughout the world are presently infected, and both the prevalence and distribution of the disease seem to be increasing in many parts of Africa and Asia.

Wuchereria bancrofti infection is endemic between latitudes 41°N and 30°S involving primarily Africa, the Pacific Islands, and Southeastern Asia from Korea on the north to India in the West. The West Indies, Central America, and the eastern coastal plains of South America are also involved. Distribution is irregular, and there are many peculiar "skip areas" in this geographic pattern, presumably because the endemic disease can be maintained only where human infection and mosquitoes are prevalent. *Brugia malayi* infection is much more restricted in its distribution and occurs in India, Burma, Thailand, Vietnam, China, South Korea, Japan, Malaysia, Indonesia, Borneo, New Guinea, and the Philippines. The parasite has recently disappeared from Sri Lanka.

Two new types of microfilaria have been described. One, found in Brazil, has been named *W. lewisi,* while the taxonomic status of the strain from Portuguese Timor has not been settled. It is provisionally called Brugia (Timor).

There were approximately 15,000 *W. bancrofti* infections among American military personnel in World War II. A small endemic focus of *W. bancrofti* once existed near Charleston, South Carolina, but no new cases have been observed since 1930.

PATHOGENESIS Pathological changes are caused primarily by the presence of the adult worm in the lymphatics and may be divided into inflammatory and obstructive. The inflammatory response, most marked around molting larvae and dead or dying adult worms, consists of infiltration with lymphocytes, plasma cells, and eosinophils. This is followed by a granulomatous reaction which may lead to lymphatic obstruction. There are hyperplasia of lymphatic endothelium, acute lymphangitis, and thrombosis. Repetition of this process over a period of years leads to permanent lymphatic obstruction. The tissues become edematous, thickened, and fibrotic. Secondary streptococcal infections are common and may contribute to lymphatic blockade. Dilated lymphatics may rupture into surrounding tissue. Elephantiasis is actually a relatively unusual complication of filarial infections. If repeated reinfections do not occur, the disease is self-limited.

MANIFESTATIONS The clinical manifestations vary with the geographic area, species of parasite, and intensity of infection. Light infections may be completely asymptomatic. Symptoms may occur within 3 months of infection, but ordinarily the incubation period is 8 to 12 months. The clinical findings closely reflect the pathological changes, with inflammation early in the disease followed by obstruction later. Inflammatory filariasis consists of a series of brief febrile attacks occurring over a period of weeks. Fever is usually low grade but may reach 40.6°C (105°F) and be accompanied by chills and sweats. Other symptoms include headache, nausea and vomiting, photophobia, and muscle pain. If the involved lymphatics lie close to the surface, the local symptoms dominate the clinical picture. Lymphangitis is very common, involving the legs more frequently than the arms. It often begins as a tender spot in the region of the malleoli or femoral area and spreads centrifugally. The involved vessels are palpably tender and painful. The overlying skin is red and swollen. When abdominal lymphatics are involved, the picture may simulate that of an acute abdomen. In Bancroftian filariasis the vessels of the spermatic cord and testes may be involved, resulting in painful orchitis, epididymitis, or funicultis. Lymphadenitis almost always accompanies and may sometimes precede lymphangitis. The inguinal, femoral, and epitrochlear nodes are involved. Abscesses which may form about involved lymphatics and lymph nodes may discharge to the surface, resulting in persistently draining sinus tracts. The acute manifestations last only a few days and then subside spontaneously, only to recur at irregular intervals over a period of weeks or months. Recovery finally ensues. With repeated infections, slowly progressive lymphatic obstruction may develop in areas where the inflammatory reactions have occurred previously. Edema, ascites, lymph scrotum, hydrocele, pleural effusion, or joint effusion may appear as a result of interference with lymphatic drainage. Lymphadenopathy persists. The lymphatic vessels become palpably enlarged as tense elastic masses beneath the skin, especially in the femoral, inguinal, and scrotal areas. They may rupture and form draining sinuses. Internal rupture of lymphatics may give rise to chylous ascites or chyluria. In a small percentage of cases elephantiasis develops. This complication is rare below the age of 20 even in natives of heavily infested areas. The chronic obstructive phase of the disease often is punctuated by acute inflammatory episodes.

Tropical eosinophilia Attention has been focused on an aberrant type of filariasis which is characterized by the presence of hypereosinophilia, circulating filarial antibodies, microfilariae in tissue but *not in the blood,* and a chronic, clinical course that can be terminated with specific antifilarial treatment. These amicrofilaremic forms were originally thought to be caused by zoonotic parasites, but it is more likely that they represent an atypical host response to various filariae including *W. bancrofti* and *B. malayi*. The syndrome is most commonly seen in India, Indonesia, Sri Lanka, Pakistan, and Southeast Asia, all areas of intense transmission for these organisms. Animal models suggest that hypersensitivity or immunity to microfilariae results in their being removed from the peripheral circulation and trapped in various tissue sites. Here, they incite an eosinophilic inflammatory reaction which, in time, progresses to granuloma formation and fibrosis. Clinically there may be marked enlargement of the lymph nodes and spleen (Meyers-Kouwenaar syndrome) and/or chronic cough, nocturnal bronchospasm, and miliary pulmonary infiltrates (Weingarten syndrome). The former syndrome is most frequently seen in children, and the latter in young male adults. Only one-quarter of the patients with pulmonary manifestations demonstrate obstructive defects on pulmonary function testing. All show restrictive disease, and irreversible pulmonary hypertension has been described in a few. A number of diseases characterized by pulmonary infiltration and eosinophilia (PIE) must be considered in the differential diagnosis of this disease. They include other helminthic infections, Loeffler's syndrome, chronic eosinophilic pneumonia, allergic aspergillosis, vasculitis, idiopathic hypereosinophilia, and drug allergies.

DIAGNOSIS A history of exposure, the long incubation period, the occurrence of typical inflammatory episodes, and the finding of regional lymphadenopathy, thickening of the spermatic cord, or swelling of an extremity should suggest the diagnosis. There is usually eosinophilia during acute episodes. Lymphangiography may reveal dilated afferent and small efferent lymphatics. The definitive diagnosis depends on demonstration of the parasite. Although adult worms can be demonstrated in biopsied lymph nodes, biopsy is not recommended because it may interfere further with lymphatic drainage. Microfilariae are found in the blood during intermediate stages but not early or late in the disease. As they are motile, they can often be seen in a wet mount or counting chamber. Definite identification, however, requires staining with Giemsa. As in malaria, they are demonstrated best in thick smears. Either the Knott concentration or membrane filtration technique should be employed if the parasite is not found in thick smears. Because the appearance of microfilariae in peripheral blood is periodic, it is essential to obtain blood at appropriate times. When this proves difficult, the oral administration of 100 mg diethylcarbamazine usually produces positive blood specimens within 30 to 60 min. Microfilariae may also be found in lymphatic fluid, hydrocele fluid, ascites, and pleural fluid. Skin tests as well as complement fixation, indirect hemagglutination, bentonite flocculation, and soluble antigen fluorescent antibody tests are available and, although not completely reliable, are helpful when microfilariae cannot be demonstrated. An indirect immunofluorescent test utilizing adult *B. malayi* as the source of antigen appears to be both more sensitive and specific than previously developed procedures.

The diagnosis of *tropical eosinophilia* is confirmed by (1) a history of prolonged residence in an endemic area, (2) lack of microfilariae in the peripheral blood despite examination of both day and night specimens by concentration techniques, (3) peripheral eosinophilia in excess of 300 cells per milliliter, (4) high titers of filarial antibodies, (5) IgE levels of at least 1000 units per milliliter, and (6) response to diethylcarbamazine within 7 to 10 days of initiating therapy. Recovery of microfilariae from the tissues is uncommon, and biopsy is not warranted.

TREATMENT Diethylcarbamazine (Hetrazan) rapidly eliminates microfilariae from the blood. It probably also kills or injures adult worms, impairing their ability to reproduce, and clears microfilariae permanently from the bloodstream of many patients. The drug is given in dosage of 2 mg/kg three times a day for 3 or 4 weeks. Treatment with this agent is often followed by allergic reactions to the dying parasite. These reactions may be quite severe, especially in Malayan filariasis. They can be controlled with aspirin, antihistamines, or steroid hormones. In heavy infections, it may be desirable to begin treatment with antihistamines before administration of Hetrazan.

Antimony compounds have no place in the treatment of filariasis.

Reassurance of the patient is very important in this disease. Vaccines and antiserums are valueless. Pressure bandages and surgery sometimes benefit elephantiasis. The prognosis for life is excellent, particularly if infected individuals leave endemic areas or otherwise avoid reinfections. Disease control is accomplished by combining mass treatment with mosquito control measures.

ONCHOCERCIASIS ("RIVER BLINDNESS")

DEFINITION Onchocerciasis is a cutaneous filariasis caused by *Onchocerca volvulus*. It is characterized by subcutaneous nodules, a pruritic skin rash, and ocular lesions.

ETIOLOGY AND EPIDEMIOLOGY The disease is found in focal areas within Mexico, Guatemala, Colombia, Venezuela,

Surinam, Brazil, and Yemen, and throughout tropical Africa. It is estimated that at least 40 million individuals are infected and that about 5 percent of these are blind as a result of the disease.

The infection is transmitted by black flies of the genus *Simulium,* which breed along fast-moving streams. An inoculated larva matures into a single male or female in approximately one year. Since larvae do not multiply within the human host, heavy parasite loads are the result of repeated infections. The adult worms are found coiled together in fibrous subcutaneous nodules. The gravid females, which may live as long as 15 years, release unsheathed microfilariae that are actively motile and migrate in the skin, subcutaneous tissue, and eye for up to 30 months or until they are ingested by a feeding *Simulium.*

PATHOGENESIS AND CLINICAL MANIFESTATIONS The subcutaneous nodules which enclose the adult worms are usually 2 to 3 cm in diameter when fully developed. They are firm, nontender, and freely movable, although occasionally they may be adherent to underlying tissue. Their location on the body is related to the biting habits of the vector. In Central America, where the fly bites on the upper part of the body, the nodules are frequently over the head; in Africa they are primarily on the trunk and thighs. They usually number less than 10, but more than 100 have been reported in a single patient.

The important pathological changes occur as a result of a hypersensitivity reaction to the dead or dying microfilariae. Pruritus is often severe and constant. The skin lesion may appear as an erysipelas-like reaction over the face or a papular rash over one extremity. In chronic cases thickening, lichenification, and depigmentation may be present. In Africa gross skin lesions are common and may be associated with large folds of skin called *hanging groins.* Some authors believe elephantiasis may occur. Children living in endemic areas may not demonstrate these changes for decades even though microfilariae are present. The most serious complications of onchocerciasis are eye lesions which are usually found in patients repeatedly infected on the upper part of the body. A punctate keratitis, iridocyclitis, or less commonly a chorioretinitis may eventually lead to blindness.

DIAGNOSIS The diagnosis is made by demonstrating microfilariae in a skin snip taken from an involved area. A thin sliver of superficial skin is removed with a razor or punch. Care must be taken to prevent bleeding and possible contamination with blood microfilariae. The skin is weighed and then is placed in saline, teased with a pair of sharp dissecting needles, and observed for emerging microfilariae over the next hour. The results should be expressed in microfilariae per milligram of tissue. Multiple skin snips may be necessary. In patients with eye lesions, microfilariae can sometimes be seen in the anterior chamber with a slit lamp. If organisms cannot be detected by the above methods, the patient may be given 50 mg diethylcarbamazine orally. The occurrence of a pruritic rash within 24 h strongly suggests the presence of cutaneous microfilariae (Mazzotti's test). One of the filarial serologic tests may also be helpful.

TREATMENT AND PREVENTION Diethylcarbamazine is effective in destroying microfilariae but has little effect on the adult worm. The drug must be used with great care as rapid destruction of the parasites may cause a severe allergic reaction. If the eye is involved, this can result in further ocular damage. The initial adult dose is 50 mg orally. It is increased to 50 mg three times daily on the second day, 100 mg three times daily on the third day, and finally 200 mg three times a day for an additional 7 days. Antihistamines, or in rare cases steroids, can be used to control allergic reactions. In ocular reactions, the pupil should be dilated and topical steroids applied.

The adult worms may be eliminated by excision of nodules on the head and neck, a procedure which is useful in preventing ocular complications, or by chemotherapy with suramin. Details of the administration and toxicity of this drug are given in Chap. 202. The dosage is 0.1 g given intravenously to detect drug idiosyncrasy, followed by 1.0 g intravenously once weekly for five to six doses.

Chemoprophylaxis is not practical, and personal protection depends upon the use of protective clothing. Insecticides, mass therapy, and nodulectomies have been used but have not been very satisfactory.

LOIASIS

This form of filariasis is produced by *Loa loa* and is prevalent in West and Central Africa. The infection is transmitted by deer flies of the genus *Chrysops.* The adult worms, which like the other filariae may live for 10 to 15 years, migrate continuously through the subcutaneous tissue. The resulting localized areas of allergic inflammation, *Calabar swellings,* are the hallmark of the disease. Occasionally the adult worms may be seen crossing the eye subconjunctivally. This usually results in intense lacrimation, pain, and anxiety. Infestation may, however, be completely asymptomatic. An association between loiasis and endomyocardial fibrosis has been reported. The diagnosis can be made by finding the adult worm or by demonstrating the distinctive sheathed microfilariae in contents of the Calabar swellings or in the bloodstream during the daytime. Microfilariae are often not found. In these cases, there are usually marked eosinophilia and a positive filarial complement fixation test. Diethylcarbamazine, administered for 2 to 3 weeks in the manner described for onchocerciasis, will kill both adult worms and microfilariae. This drug must be used with great care as it may induce an encephalopathy in this disease. It is taken in a dose of 200 mg twice daily for 3 days each month and is also effective as a chemoprophylactic agent.

DIPETALONEMIASIS

Dipetalonema perstans (Acanthocheilonema perstans) is a filarial parasite of humans and other primates inhabiting the tropical areas of Africa and Latin America. The adult worm lives encysted in the subserosal tissues of the pericardium, pleura, and peritoneum, particularly the mesentery. The unsheathed microfilariae, which can be found in the peripheral blood throughout the day, have four to six nuclei in their tail. They are transmitted from host to host by blood-sucking gnats of the genus *Culicoides.* Most infections are asymptomatic, and their principal significance lies in the fact that they may be confused with other, more serious, forms of filariasis. Nevertheless, some patients complain of fever, pruritus, Calabar swellings, erysipelas-like rashes, and abdominal pain. Peripheral eosinophilia is common, but filarial complement fixation tests are generally negative. Diagnosis is made by finding the characteristic microfilariae in the peripheral blood. Treatment with diethylcarbamazine is of doubtful benefit.

Dipetalonema streptocera is found in Equatorial Africa where it inhabits the dermis and subcutaneous tissues of chimpanzees and humans. Like *D. perstans,* it is transmitted by *Culicoides.* The microfilariae inhabit the dermal collagen where they elicit a lymphocytic and eosinophilic inflammatory response, fibrosis, lymphatic dilatation, pruritus, hypopigmented macules, and a papular rash. The diagnosis is made by recovering the nonperiodic microfilariae from skin snips as described for Onchocerciasis above. They are unsheathed and possess a sharply crooked tail with nuclei. Diethylcarbamazine, as described for Bancroftian filariasis above, is effective.

MANSONELLIASIS OZZARDI

Mansonella ozzardi are found as adult worms in the mesentery and visceral fat of people living in the tropical areas of Latin America. This species is thought to be transmitted by flies of the genus *Simulium* and gnats of the genus *Culicoides*. The nonperiodic microfilariae are released into the peripheral blood where they can be identified by their lack of a sheath or caudal nuclei. This common infection is thought to be asymptomatic, but reports of patients presenting with fever, lymphadenopathy, and hydroceles have been published. Diethylcarbamazine is ineffective.

DIROFILARIASIS

Dirofilaria immitis (canine heartworm) is a large, cosmopolitan filaria of dogs which lives in their right ventricle and pulmonary arteries and releases its microfilariae into the peripheral blood. It is transmitted by several types of mosquitoes. Human infections are occasionally reported, particularly from the southern United States. The worm does not mature in humans, and hence microfilaremia is not present. Although cardiac infections have been noted at autopsy, most human infections present as well-defined pulmonary nodules. The patients may complain of cough and chest pain or, less commonly, of hemoptysis, fever, chills, and myalgia. The diagnosis is usually made by the microscopic examination of excised pulmonary nodules.

Other *Dirofilariae* may rarely invade humans producing subcutaneous eosinophilic granulomas of the eyelid, trunk, or extremities. The nodules, which measure 1 to 2 cm in diameter, may be painful or completely asymptomatic. In the southern United States, the filaria most frequently involved is *D. tenuis,* a parasite of raccoons. The nodules are removed by surgical excision.

REFERENCES

AKISADA M, TANI S: Lymphangioadenopathy of filariasis. Trans R Soc Trop Med Hyg 64:885, 1970

ANDERSON J, FUGLSANG H: Ocular onchocerciasis. Trop Dis Bull 74:257, 1972

CHRISTIE RW: *Dirofilaria tenuis* in Vermont. N Engl J Med 297:706, 1977

CONNOR DH et al: Onchocerciasis, onchocercal dermatitis, lymphadenitis and elephantiasis in the Ubangi territory. Hum Pathol 1:553, 1970

DAYAL Y, NEAFIE RC: Human pulmonary dirofilariasis. A case report and review of the literature. Am Rev Resp Dis 112:437, 1975

EDESON JFB: Filariasis. Br Med Bull 28:60, 1972

HAWKING F: The 24-hour periodicity of microfilariae: Biological mechanisms responsible for its production and control. Proc R Soc Lond B 169:59, 1967

IVE FA et al: Endomyocardial fibrosis and filariasis. Q J Med 36:495, 1967

MEYERS WM et al: Human streptocerciasis. A clinico-pathological study of 40 Africans (Zaireans) including identification of the adult filaria. Am J Trop Med Hyg 21:528, 1972

NEVA FA, OTTESEN EA: Current concepts in parasitology. Tropical (filarial) eosinophilia. N Engl J Med 298:1129, 1978

ONKEL TC: Infections with *Dipetalonema perstans* and *Mansonella ozzardi* in the aboriginal Indians of Guyana. Am J Trop Med Hyg 16:628, 1967

PAK SC: The course of lung function in treated tropical pulmonary eosinophilia. Thorax 29:710, 1974

WHO EXPERT COMMITTEE ON FILARIASIS: Third Report. Tech Rept Ser 542, 1974

210
INTESTINAL NEMATODES

JAMES J. PLORDE

ENTEROBIASIS

DEFINITION Enterobiasis (pinworm, seatworm, or threadworm infection, oxyuriasis) is an intestinal infection of humans caused by *Enterobius vermicularis* and characterized by perianal pruritus. Eggs of this parasite have been found in a 100,000-year-old coprolith, making it the oldest demonstrated infection of humans. It has been estimated that the worm infects 200 million people, 30 to 40 million of them in the United States and Canada.

ETIOLOGY The female averages 10 mm in length, the male 3 mm. They live with their heads attached to the mucosa of the cecum, appendix, and adjacent parts of the bowel. The gravid female migrates through the anal canal at night, deposits her 10,000 eggs on the perianal skin, and dies. In female patients the worm may enter the vagina and occasionally gain access to the peritoneal cavity through the fallopian tubes. Each egg contains an embryo which, within a few hours, develops into an infective larva. After the egg has been ingested, the larva is released in the small intestine and migrates down the bowel lumen to the cecum. In less than 1 month from the time of ingestion, newly developed gravid females are again discharging eggs. They are planoconvex and measure approximately 20 by 50 μm. The shell is clear and doubly contoured.

EPIDEMIOLOGY Humans are usually infected by the direct transfer of eggs from the anus to the mouth by way of contaminated fingers. Retroinfection, which is seen primarily in adults, may occasionally take place when eggs hatch in the perianal area and the larvae migrate back into the bowel to mature. The eggs, which are relatively resistant to desiccation, also contaminate nightclothes and bed linen, where they remain viable and infective for 2 to 3 weeks. Airborne transmission is possible, and spread within family and children's groups occurs readily. Enterobiasis is found in all climates and is probably the most common helminthic infection of humans. Its low incidence in some tropical areas, however, is not fully explained.

CLINICAL MANIFESTATIONS The most common symptom is pruritus ani, which is most troublesome at night, being related to the migration of the gravid female worms. Irritability, insomnia, enuresis, and other minor complaints are probably secondary to the pruritus. Scratching may lead to perianal eczema or pyogenic infection. Vaginal discharge has been reported, and rarely a chronic granulomatous salpingitis or endometritis results from the presence of ectopic adults. An association between enterobiasis and cystitis in young females has been reported. This, it is suggested, results from the transport of enteric bacteria into the bladder by the migrating worm. Other rare ectopic locations include the lung, liver, and peritoneum. Probably the worms can penetrate the bowel wall only if its continuity has been compromised by some other disease.

LABORATORY FINDINGS Examination for ova of material obtained from the perianal skin by means of a Scotch brand cellophane tape swab is the preferable method for the detection of enterobiasis. The tape is folded sticky-side out over the end of a tongue blade, pressed firmly against the perianal area, and then spread on a glass slide and examined under the lower power of a microscope. The swab should be taken at home by the patient on three to five consecutive mornings prior to bathing and brought to the laboratory for examination. Searching for ova in the feces is rarely helpful, but scrapings from under the nails may reveal ova. The diagnosis is sometimes made by finding adult worms in the perianal area or in the feces following a laxative or an enema. Eosinophilic leukocytosis may occur but is not a typical finding.

TREATMENT All infected individuals in a family or communal group should be treated simultaneously. The frequently recommended sanitary measures aside from daily bathing and hand washing before meals and after stools are of dubious benefit. It is relatively easy to eradicate the worms, but reinfection is frequent. Retreatment does not appear necessary unless symptoms recur.

Two highly satisfactory drugs are available. Pyrantel pamoate (Banminth) given in a single oral dose of 11 mg/kg (maximum 1.0 g) is probably the drug of choice. Alternatively, a single 100-mg oral dose of mebendazole (Vermox) can be used. This drug is not recommended for infants or pregnant women. Pyrvinium pamoate (Povan) and piperazine citrate are equally effective but less convenient. The former is given orally as a single dose of 5 mg/kg in tablet or liquid form. This compound turns the stool red and may stain bedclothes or undergarments. Piperazine citrate is given in dosage of 65 mg/kg (maximum 2.5 g) once daily for 8 days. When renal insufficiency is present, the dose should be reduced to avoid neurotoxicity. In heavily contaminated environments, treatment with the above drugs may be repeated after an interval of 2 weeks to eliminate any new infections.

PREVENTION Methods of preventing autoinfection and dissemination within a group involving children are extremely difficult to enforce. Personal environmental hygiene should be stressed, and anthelmintic and symptomatic treatment of pruritus ani should be instituted. To control infection within a group, simultaneous treatment of all cases is mandatory.

TRICHURIASIS

DEFINITION Trichuriasis (whipworm infection, trichocephaliasis) is an intestinal infection of humans caused by *Trichuris trichiura* and is characterized by invasion of the colonic mucosa by the adult trichuris. Five hundred million persons are thought to be infected with this parasite including 2 million in the United States. It may be the most commonly encountered helminthic infection in Americans returning from tropical areas.

ETIOLOGY The adult whipworms are found in the large intestine with their anterior ends deeply embedded in the mu-

cosa. They are 30 to 50 mm in length and possess a threadlike anterior two-thirds with a stouter posterior third, giving them a whiplike structure. The female produces about 5000 eggs each day. They are characteristically barrel-shaped (20 to 50 μm), brown, thick-walled, and translucent with knoblike ends. The eggs, like those of *Ascaris,* must incubate at least 3 weeks in soil before they become infective. After ingestion, the eggs hatch in the small intestine and the larvae become embedded in the intestinal villi. After several days they migrate to the large intestine where they mature in about 3 months. The adult worms may live for 4 to 8 years. Occasionally, *T. vulpis,* the whipworm of dogs, may infect humans. The eggs are larger (35 by 75 μm) but otherwise identical to those of the human parasite.

EPIDEMIOLOGY Whipworm is a cosmopolitan parasite but is most commonly found in the tropics where the level of sanitation is low and environmental conditions necessary for the incubation of the eggs are optimal. In the United States, it is found throughout the rural areas of the Southeast. Its distribution is similar to that of *Ascaris* and hookworm, but the eggs are less resistant than those of *Ascaris* to sunlight and drying. Because of their general lack of sanitary habits, children and the mentally retarded have the highest incidence of infection. For example, 13 percent of patients confined to hospitals for the mentally subnormal were found to harbor *Trichuris.*

PATHOGENESIS AND CLINICAL MANIFESTATIONS Symptomatic infection generally requires the presence of large numbers of adult whipworms and may be correlated in part with the degree of mucosal involvement. Heavy infections usually occur only in children and may be accompanied by nausea, abdominal pain, diarrhea, and dysentery. It has been estimated that infected patients lose 0.005 ml blood per worm per day. Infections with more than 800 worms often results in anemia. In heavier infections, the distribution of worms throughout the colon and rectum may result in rectal prolapse while straining at stool. Some investigators also feel that *Trichuris* infections predispose to amebic dysentery and bacterial gastroenteritis.

LABORATORY FINDINGS In symptomatic infection, large numbers of eggs are present in the feces, and there may be eosinophilic leukocytosis and anemia. In light infections, concentration techniques may be necessary to recover the eggs. Quantitation of egg output is helpful since only counts above 3000 eggs per gram of feces are likely to be associated with symptoms. Stools should be cultured for bacterial pathogens and examined for the presence of *E. histolytica.*

TREATMENT Treatment is unsatisfactory. Mebendazole in the oral dose of 100 mg twice daily for 3 days is the drug of choice. Its cure rate is 60 to 70 percent, and it achieves a 90 percent reduction in egg burden. The dose may have to be repeated in patients with heavy infections. It is not recommended for children under the age of 2 or pregnant women.

PROGNOSIS Whipworm infection, unless characterized by severe diarrhea, blood loss, and systemic reaction, usually responds well to treatment. Serious infections may require supportive treatment as well as chemotherapy.

PREVENTION Measures recommended for ascariasis apply also to trichuriasis.

ASCARIASIS

DEFINITION Ascariasis is an infection of humans caused by *Ascaris lumbricoides* and characterized by an early pulmonary phase related to larval migration and a later, prolonged intestinal phase. It is estimated that 25 percent of the world's population, including 4 million Americans, are infected with this nematode.

ETIOLOGY The adult ascarids are large (15 to 40 cm in length), cylindric worms with blunt ends which maintain themselves in the lumen of the jejunum by virtue of their muscular activity. Despite a life span of only 6 to 18 months, the female releases millions of eggs, both fertile and infertile, into the fecal stream; the daily output is estimated to be 200,000 per worm. Fertilized eggs are elliptic (30 to 40 μm by 50 to 60 μm) with an irregular, dense outer shell and a regular, translucent inner shell. They require a period of soil incubation before they become infective. Under optimum conditions of warmth and moisture this occurs in 2 to 3 weeks. The eggs may then remain viable for up to 6 years in temperate climates. When an infective egg is ingested, the larva is liberated in the small intestine. It migrates through the wall and is carried by the bloodstream or lymphatics to the lung. After about 10 days in the pulmonary capillaries and alveoli, the larvae pass in turn up the bronchioles, bronchi, trachea, and epiglottis, are swallowed, and return to the jejunum. There they develop into mature adult worms within 2 to 3 months of ingestion. *Ascaris suum,* a roundworm of pigs, may occasionally complete a similar life cycle in humans.

EPIDEMIOLOGY Infection follows the ingestion of the embryonated eggs contained in contaminated food, or, more commonly, the introduction of the eggs into the mouth by the hands after contact with contaminated soil. Geophagia may produce massive infections. In endemic areas, the infection is maintained primarily by small children who defecate indiscriminately in the area of the home. In dry, windy climates, eggs may become airborne, get into the mouth, and be swallowed. Since the eggs are relatively resistant to desiccation and wide variations in temperature, the disease is worldwide. In the developing areas of the world where the lack of sanitary facilities exposes populations to the greatest risk, the prevalence of infection may be as high as 80 to 90 percent; children are almost universally infected in these areas. In temperate areas, the infection occurs in family clusters.

PATHOGENESIS AND CLINICAL MANIFESTATIONS Because of the extensive migration of which both the larvae and adults are capable, the manifestations may be diverse. Bronchopneumonia characterized by fever, cough, dyspnea, wheeze, eosinophilic leukocytosis, and migratory pulmonary infiltrates may occur during the passage of the larvae through the lung. This is most commonly seen in communities where *Ascaris* transmission is seasonal. The severity of symptoms is apparently related to both intensity of infection and the degree of sensitization resulting from previous exposures. Significant arterial oxygen desaturation and, rarely, death may occur. Adult worms may produce no symptoms if the infection is light and may be detected accidentally when the adult worm is vomited or passed in the stool. Heavier infections may cause abdominal pain, and occasionally a bolus of worms may result in volvulus, intussusception, or intestinal obstruction in the iliocecal area. Children are most likely to have these complications because of their anatomically smaller intestine and larger worm loads. Up to 2000 worms have been found in children, although the usual load is less than 50. In the United States where worm loads are usually modest, the incidence of obstruction is 2 per 1000 infected children per year. It often follows a febrile illness or drug therapy which stimulates the worms to increase motility. Rarely, an adult worm will migrate into the appendix, bile ducts, or pancreatic ducts, causing obstruction and inflammation of these organs. Biliary tract obstruction may be associated with bacterial cholangitis and liver abscess. Worms may also penetrate the intestinal wall, particularly at a site of surgical anastomosis, and patients should be dewormed prior to elective surgery. Migration of the worms into the oral pharynx and mouth may lead to acute respiratory distress.

Ascariasis has been associated with mild to moderate malabsorption of fat, protein, carbohydrate, and vitamins. It seems likely that large worm loads may interfere with the growth of marginally nourished children.

LABORATORY FINDINGS The diagnosis is usually made by finding the ova in the feces. The fertilized eggs are usually numerous, characteristic, and not easily confused with those of other helminths. The occasional unisexual infection may pose diagnostic problems. The male produces no eggs, and the unfertilized ova produced by a single female may be atypical and difficult to recognize. Occasionally the worms may be seen after a barium meal, either as negative images or after ingesting barium themselves. In biliary ascariasis an intravenous cholangiogram will often demonstrate dilatation of the common duct and/or the negative image of the parasite. Ascaris pneumonia may be diagnosed by finding larvae and eosinophils in the sputum or gastric aspirate. Eggs will usually not be found until after the larvae have matured in the intestine. Eosinophilic leukocytosis is usually noted during larval migration, but diminishes and often disappears during the chronic intestinal phase of infection.

TREATMENT Only symptomatic treatment can be used during the period of pulmonary involvement by the migrating larvae. For removal of the adult worms from the intestines, either pyrantel pamoate or mebendazole should be used. Pyrantel is given as a single oral dose of 11 mg/kg (maximum 1.0 g). Mebendazole is given as described for trichuriasis and is the preferred agent if both *Ascaris* and *Trichuris* are present. An older agent, piperazine citrate, is highly effective, less expensive, but slightly more toxic than the above two agents. It is given as a flavored syrup administered in a single dose after breakfast on two successive days and will cure the majority of cases. The drug acts by paralyzing the ascarids, which are then passed in the stool. The dose of piperazine is 75 mg/kg with a maximum of 4 g. No particular dietary regulation is necessary. The drug must be administered with caution to patients with renal insufficiency, because impaired elimination may produce neurotoxic signs. In intestinal obstruction, nasogastric suction should be initiated. After vomiting is controlled, piperazine should be given through the nasogastric tube every 12 to 24 h in dosage of 65 mg/kg (maximum 1.0 g) for six doses. Surgery usually is not required.

PROGNOSIS The prognosis in intestinal infection is generally good. When acute or chronic obstruction of ducts of hollow viscera has occurred, the immediate prognosis is determined by the promptness of diagnosis and treatment. The case fatality rate of intestinal obstruction in the United States is 3 percent.

PREVENTION Ascariasis is primarily a household infection of rural areas. All infections should be treated, personal hygiene stressed, and adequate toilet facilities provided.

TOXOCARIASIS (VISCERAL LARVA MIGRANS)

DEFINITION This is a human infection with *Toxocara canis* or *T. cati.* The animal ascarids are usually unable to complete their life cycle in humans, but they may be widely disseminated in the body, producing a variety of clinical manifestations, collectively referred to as *visceral larva migrans.*

ETIOLOGY AND EPIDEMIOLOGY The large adult toxocaral worms live in the intestine of cats and dogs. Their eggs must be passed in the stool and incubate in soil for 2 to 3 weeks before they become infective. If the ova are then ingested by a human, larvae are liberated in the intestine, penetrate the wall, and are carried in the blood to the liver, where most remain, and lung. At the time the larvae reach the pulmonary capillaries, they are still very small (approximately one-half the size of *A. lumbricoides*) and many pass through the lungs to reach the systemic circulation. Larvae penetrate the tissues where their gradually increasing size approaches the diameter of the vessel through which they are traveling. Rarely the organisms break into the alveoli, ascend the respiratory tract, and are swallowed to reach the small intestine where they mature into adult worms. *Toxocara* infections of cats and dogs are common and widespread. Transplacental transmission occurs in canines and accounts for infection rates of 80 percent or more in young puppies; they can shed a large number of ova within 4 weeks of birth. Viable ova were found in 25 percent of soil samples taken from public parks in Great Britain. Although most human infections have been reported from the United States and Europe, it seems likely that the disease is present in other areas of the world as well. Children from the age of 2 to 5 years, because of their sanitary habits and intimate association with domestic pets, are most frequently involved. In Great Britain, 4 percent of children who play in public parks have positive skin tests to *Toxocara* antigens.

PATHOGENESIS AND CLINICAL MANIFESTATIONS The larvae migrate freely in tissues, causing hemorrhage, necrosis, eosinophilic inflammatory reaction, and eventually granuloma formation. The most frequently involved organs are the liver, lungs, brain, eye, heart, and skeletal muscles. Symptoms and signs are related to the number and location of the granulomas as well as sensitization to the parasite antigen. Commonly, only asymptomatic eosinophilia marks the presence of infection. Symptomatic patients most frequently present with fever and tender hepatomegaly. Splenomegaly, skin rash, and recurrent pneumonitis with wheezing respirations may occur in more severe infections. Respiratory failure with death has been reported. Most fatalities, however, result from involvement of the myocardium or central nervous system; the latter may result in convulsions, behavior disorders, or focal neurological defects. There is often a history of dirt eating and contact with cats and dogs. Leukocytosis with eosinophilia to high levels (over 60 percent) and hypergammaglobulinemia with raised levels of IgG, IgM, and IgE are common. These manifestations may persist for months or years. At surgery or autopsy the liver may be studded with small granulomas. A granulomatous endophthalmitis, which may be mistaken for retinoblastoma, may be observed in older children and adults. Typically, this is unilateral and occurs in the absence of other clinical manifestations of visceral larva migrans.

DIAGNOSIS The diagnosis can usually be made on the basis of clinical findings. Infections with *A. lumbricoides,* hookworm, and *Strongyloides stercoralis,* as well as other nonhuman nematodes, may also on occasion present as visceral larva migrans, making the etiologic diagnosis difficult. Eosinophilic leukemia, trichinosis, trematode infections, and periarteritis nodosa must be ruled out. Isoagglutinin titers of 1:1024 or greater are often present. Antibodies to *Toxocara* and *Ascaris* antigens may be found, but, as with the isoagglutinins, these tests are neither very sensitive nor specific. The adaption of larval antigens to the enzyme-linked immunoabsorbent assay has, for the first time, provided clinicians with a serologic test of diagnostic value. In one study, the sensitivity and specificity were 78 and 92 percent, respectively. A definitive diagnosis depends on the identification of the larvae in sputum or tissue granuloma. Biopsy of the liver with serial sections of the specimen may reveal eosinophilic granulomas or a *Toxocara* larva.

TREATMENT No uniformly effective therapy is available. Diethylcarbamazine as used in bancroftian filariasis (Chap. 209) is probably the drug of choice. Thiabendazole in dosage of 25 to 50 mg/kg for 7 to 10 days may be helpful. Adrenocortical steroids may be beneficial when respiratory difficulty is pronounced. Control measures are directed toward preventing ingestion of eggs. Removal and repeated worming of infected cats and dogs must be considered. Animals less than 6 months of age should be wormed monthly; older ones every 2 or 3 months.

ANISAKIASIS

Ascarids belonging to family Anisakidae infect seals, dolphins, porpoises, whales, and other large sea mammals. Their larval stages are found in the flesh of squid and several marine fish including cod, salmon, and herring. Humans are infected by eating raw, pickled, or slightly salted fish delicacies such as "green herring," sashimi, sunomono, creviche, and gravlax which contain the third-stage larvae. The infection may be asymptomatic and noted only when the worm is coughed or vomited up. More characteristically, the larvae burrow into the mucosa of the stomach, small intestine, or more rarely the colon. Here they produce eosinophilic granulomatous tumors with edema, thickening, and induration of the bowel wall which may be mistaken for gastric carcinoma or regional enteritis. Occasionally, larvae may penetrate the intestinal wall to involve other abdominal organs. Perforations of the bowel with peritonitis have also been described. The pathological changes are thought to be the result of a hypersensitivity reaction. In the acute gastric syndrome common in Japan, the patient may develop epigastric pain, nausea, and vomiting within a few hours of ingesting infected fish. With a gastroscope 2- to 4-cm larvae can be seen penetrating the mucosa and can sometimes be removed. In Europeans, the small intestine has been the site most frequently involved. The clinical picture may be severe enough to simulate an acute surgical abdomen. More commonly, colicky pain, diffuse abdominal tenderness, fever, and leukocytosis develop a week or more after the ingestion of fish. Peripheral eosinophilia is not always present, and a definitive diagnosis can be made only by the identification of larvae in tissue. Serologic tests are being developed, but are neither highly reliable nor generally available. The disease usually subsides spontaneously with conservative therapy. Occasionally, a chronic illness develops which requires surgical resection of the lesion.

Hundreds of cases have been recognized in the Netherlands and Japan, and several cases have been reported from North America. The disease can be prevented by storing marine fish at −20°C for a single day or by cooking it at normal cooking temperatures.

HOOKWORM DISEASE

DEFINITION Hookworm disease is a symptomatic infection caused by *Ancylostoma duodenale* or *Necator americanus.* Asymptomatic infection may be termed simply *hookworm infection,* and the individual with such infection is called a *carrier.*

ETIOLOGY *Ancylostoma duodenale,* also known as the "Old World" hookworm, possesses four prominent hooklike teeth in its adult stage. The adults are about 1 cm long and inhabit the upper part of the human small intestine, where they attach to the mucosa by means of the mouth parts and suck blood. Each adult extracts approximately 0.20 ml blood daily. The adults migrate within the small intestine, and each site of attachment persists temporarily as a bleeding point. Following fertilization, the female liberates approximately 20,000 eggs per day. They measure about 40 to 60 μm and are usually in the two-to-four-celled stage when discharged in the feces.

Necator americanus, the "New World" hookworm, has a buccal capsule containing dorsal and ventral plates rather than teeth. It is slightly smaller, deposits fewer eggs, and causes much less blood loss than *A. duodenale* (0.03 ml per worm daily). *Ancylostoma cylonicum,* a hookworm of cats found in the Far East, may occasionally reach maturity in humans.

The life cycles of both hookworms are similar. Under appropriate conditions, the eggs hatch in 24 to 48 h, releasing free-living or rhabditiform larvae. Within a few days, these develop into infective or filariform larvae which may remain viable in the soil for several weeks. These, in turn, penetrate the skin to enter vessels which carry them to the lungs. The larvae leave the alveolar capillaries, enter the alveoli, ascend the respiratory tree, enter the pharynx, and are swallowed. They reach the intestine about 1 week after penetration of the skin and mature within 5 weeks. Larval development of *Ancylostoma* may be arrested or retarded in the human host. This may result in a prolonged latent period between the onset of infection and the appearance of gravid females in the intestine. Adults have been known to survive in the human intestine for as long as 14 years, but *A. duodenale* seldom persists beyond 6 to 8 years, and most *N. americanus* infections are eliminated within 2 to 4 years.

EPIDEMIOLOGY It has been estimated that hookworms infect 700 million people and cause the loss of 7 million liters of blood daily throughout the world from 45°N to 30°S latitude. *Necator americanus* is found predominantly in the tropical areas of Africa, Asia, and the Americas, while *A. duodenale* occurs in the Mediterranean Basin, the Middle East, northern India, China, and Japan. In many areas both species are found. In general, *Ancylostoma* presents a greater public health hazard than *N. americanus,* the species which is most prevalent in the southern United States, because it is more persistent in the environment, more harmful to the host, and less amenable to treatment. Conditions conducive to the development of the hookworm egg into infective filariform larvae are a mean temperature between 23 and 33°C, abundant rainfall, shade, and well-drained sandy soil. Hookworm infection occurs where there is opportunity for disease contact of the skin with soil contaminated by promiscuous defecation. The disease may also be acquired by oral ingestion of infective larvae, particularly those of *A. duodenale.* Lactogenic transmission may also occur with this species; presumably this results from the activation of larvae whose development within the tissues of the host has been arrested or retarded. Probably because of greater exposure, males show a higher incidence of infection than females. Infections are particularly common in closed, heavily populated communities such as coffee or tea plantations.

Repeated infections of hookworm in dogs result in immunity and elimination of the parasite. It seems probable that a similar phenomenon occurs in human infections. When the possibility of reinfection is eliminated, the majority of worms is eliminated spontaneously within 1 or 2 years.

PATHOGENESIS AND CLINICAL MANIFESTATIONS During the invasion of the exposed skin by the larvae, there may be an erythematous maculopapular skin rash and edema with severe pruritus. These manifestations, which may persist for several days, are more marked in *N. americanus* infection. The lesions are most common about the feet, particularly between the toes, and have been termed "ground itch."

During migration through the lungs, cough, pneumonia, and, in severe infections, fever may occur. Usually, however, pulmonary involvement does not give rise to clinical symptoms.

Various gastrointestinal symptoms, ranging from vague epigastric distress and pica to typical ulcer pain, have been reported in association with hookworm infection. Roentgenographic studies may reveal nonspecific changes such as excessive peristalsis and "puddling," particularly in the proximal jejunum. However, gross and microscopic examination of the bowel itself reveals conspicuously little damage. Previous reports of absorptive abnormalities in hookworm infection have not been supported.

The major clinical manifestations of hookworm disease clearly are those of iron-deficiency anemia and hypoalbuminemia consequent to chronic intestinal blood loss. Whether anemia develops and how severe it becomes depends on the balance between iron lost in the gut and iron absorbed from the diet. In many endemic areas, dietary iron is largely of vegetable origin and is absorbed poorly. General dietary deficiency also may lower resistance to parasitic infections. The severity of the disease and the prognosis depend on such factors as the age of the patient, the magnitude of the worm burden, the duration of the disease, and diet. Young children often have extreme anemia, with cardiac insufficiency and anasarca. These conditions may precipitate kwashiorkor. Those who survive to puberty show retarded physical, mental, and sexual development. Milder degrees of the disease, as seen in older children and adults, are characterized by lassitude, dyspnea, palpitation, tachycardia, constipation, and pallor of the skin and mucous membranes.

Asymptomatic infections outnumber symptomatic infections, considering all age groups, 20 to 40 times in endemic areas. The worm burden is small in asymptomatic infections, and the carrier state may be indicative of some degree of acquired host resistance.

LABORATORY FINDINGS In symptomatic infection, hookworm eggs are usually numerous enough to be detected by microscopic examination of a direct or concentrated fecal smear. A quantitative egg count, using the Stoll or Beaver technique, allows an estimation of the intensity of infection. If a stool specimen is allowed to stand for several hours before examination, the eggs may hatch, releasing larvae which are easily confused with those of *Strongyloides.* The eggs must be differentiated from those of *Trichostrongylus* and *Ternidens diminutus,* which are larger and in a later stage of maturation when observed in a fresh fecal specimen than are those of *Necator* or *Ancylostoma.* Abdominal and pulmonary symptoms appear before the eggs are discharged, although a presumptive diagnosis may be made on the basis of the clinical history and the eosinophilic leukocytosis. The feces seldom contain gross blood in hookworm disease, although tests for occult blood are usually positive.

Generally, the leukocyte count is normal. However, in some early cases, leukocytosis may be marked, with an eosinophilia as high as 70 or 80 percent. The anemia is characteristically hypochromic and microcytic.

The species of hookworm may be determined by the identification of the adult worm passed in the stool following treatment or by culturing the feces and identifying the third-stage larvae. This is seldom important in clinical practice.

DIFFERENTIAL DIAGNOSIS Since hookworm disease occurs in areas in which beriberi and malaria are also common, these diseases must be differentiated from hookworm disease, or their coexistence must be established.

TREATMENT Therapy specific for the infection and directed toward the improvement of nutrition and the anemia should be considered simultaneously. In areas where reinfection is likely, administration of anthelmintics to patients with light infections (less than 2000 eggs per milliliter of feces) is probably not beneficial. In most cases requiring specific therapy, anthelmintics may be administered immediately, followed by iron and a high-protein diet. A number of satisfactory anthelmintic agents are available, but two, pyrantel pamoate (see "Ascariasis" above) and mebendazole (see "Trichuriasis" above) are currently favored. Where expense remains a major consideration, the drug of choice is tetrachloroethylene (TCE). It is highly effective, nontoxic, inexpensive, and ideal for mass treatment. (The USP tetrachloroethylene available to veterinarians may be used.) In most instances a single dose of this agent will decrease the worm load substantially. Complete cure may require several courses of treatment but is not necessary in endemic areas; the aim of therapy is reduction of the worm load to an asymptomatic level. Tetrachloroethylene is administered as a single 5-ml oral dose. Children should receive 0.12 ml/kg (to a maximum of 5 ml) by the same route. The night before treatment, the patient is permitted a light fat-free meal. The following morning, breakfast is omitted and the drug is administered. No food is permitted for 4 h and no alcohol for 24 h. Treatment can be repeated in a week if complete cure is desired and has not been accomplished. If ascariasis is also present, it should be treated first with piperazine citrate (see "Ascariasis" above). Bitoscanate (Jonit) in oral dosage of 100 mg every 12 h for three doses is equally effective against *N. americanus* and *A. duodenale*. It is not available in the United States.

The anemia requires iron replacement. When anemia is severe and there is malnutrition with anasarca, blood transfusions and a high-protein diet should be given before drug treatment is begun. Blood should be given in an amount sufficient to raise the hemoglobin level to 10 g per 100 ml. In advanced cases it may be necessary to delay drug treatment for 2 to 3 weeks.

PROGNOSIS The immediate prognosis is good. When opportunity for reinfection persists and nutrition cannot be maintained, a state of chronic debility develops. Maturation of children is impaired, and intercurrent disease is a serious problem in adults.

PREVENTION Many of the measures required are obvious but difficult to apply on a large scale. Even if facilities for proper disposal of feces are provided, it is no simple matter to educate the population in their use. Soil pollution must be eliminated. Avoidance of direct skin contact with the soil (by wearing shoes) is often not practical in endemic areas. Periodic mass treatment of the population has been used in some hookworm control programs.

CUTANEOUS LARVA MIGRANS (CREEPING ERUPTION)

DEFINITION Creeping eruption is an infection of human skin caused by the larvae of the dog and cat hookworm, *A. brasil-*

iense. The other dog hookworms, *A. caninum* and *Uncinaria stenocephala,* as well as the human parasites, *Strongyloides stercoralis* and *Necator americanus,* may also produce the disease. The larvae of *Gnathostoma spinigerum,* a nematode found in the Orient, and *Gasterophilus,* the horse bat fly, may produce a similar cutaneous infection.

ETIOLOGY *Ancylostoma brasiliense* reaches adulthood regularly only in the dog and cat. The larvae emerging from eggs discharged in the feces develop to the filariform stage and then are capable of penetrating the skin. In humans, the larvae usually remain in the skin and migrate, producing an irregular erythematous tunnel visible on the skin surface.

EPIDEMIOLOGY AND DISTRIBUTION Transmission to humans requires environmental temperature and humidity appropriate for development of the egg to the infective filariform larva stage. Beaches and other moist, sandy areas are hazardous, because animals choose such areas for defecation, and the *A. brasiliense* eggs develop well in such soil. In the United States infection is found in the southern Atlantic and Gulf states.

PATHOGENESIS AND CLINICAL MANIFESTATIONS The site of penetration of the skin by the larvae becomes apparent in a few hours. The migration of the larvae in the skin is accompanied by severe itching. Scratching may lead to bacterial infection. In the course of 1 week, the initial red papule develops into an irregular, erythematous, linear lesion which may attain a length of 15 to 20 cm. The larvae may persist for weeks to months without treatment.

Loeffler's syndrome has been observed in 26 of 52 cases of creeping eruption. Transient, migratory pulmonary infiltrations associated with an increased number of eosinophils in the blood and sputum were interpreted as an allergic reaction to the helminthic infection.

LABORATORY FINDINGS Eosinophils occur in the lesion, but eosinophilic leukocytosis is slight, except when Loeffler's syndrome appears. The percentage of eosinophils in the blood may then rise to 50 percent and in the sputum to 90 percent. Only rarely are larvae found on skin biopsy.

TREATMENT Thiabendazole is the drug of choice; it should be given orally in the dosage suggested for hookworm. It may be repeated if necessary. Alternatively, it may be applied topically as a 10% aqueous suspension. Topical administration avoids systemic toxicity. Superficial bacterial infections are improved by the application of wet dressing and elevation of the extremity. For intense itching, oral antihistaminics may be of aid.

PROGNOSIS Untreated infections last several months. Treatment, which is usually sought because of severe pruritus, is usually successful.

PREVENTION Dogs and cats should be prevented from contaminating recreation areas and children's sandboxes.

TRICHOSTRONGYLIASIS

DEFINITION Trichostrongyliasis is an intestinal infection of herbivorous animals throughout the world. Humans are an intermediate host.

ETIOLOGY Almost a dozen species of *Trichostrongylus* are known to have infected humans. The disease is common in Asia, the Middle East, and South America, but few human infections have been reported in the United States. In view of the high frequency of animal infections here, the low incidence of human infections is difficult to understand. The possibility exists that some such infections are mistaken for hookworm infections.

The ova resemble those of the hookworm but are larger, have more pointed ends, and, when observed in a fresh fecal specimen, show a more advanced stage of segmentation (16- to 32-cell stage).

PATHOGENESIS Infection is acquired by ingestion of green leafy plants contaminated with third-stage larvae. On reaching the small intestine, they attach themselves to the mucosa and develop into adult worms within 4 weeks. The adult at that time sucks blood and maintains residence in the intestine for long periods. Sandground, who infected himself, observed infection to last more than 8 years.

MANIFESTATIONS Most infections are asymptomatic, but massive infections may result in epigastric distress and anemia. The parasite owes its importance primarily to the resemblance of its ova to those of the hookworms. Moreover, because the trichostrongylidae do not respond to anthelmintics effective in hookworm infection, it may be assumed incorrectly that refractory hookworm infection is present.

LABORATORY DIAGNOSIS The diagnosis depends on the finding of the ova in the feces. Since they are few, they are usually found only when a concentration method is used. In symptomatic infections, there may be leukocytosis with marked eosinophilia (for example, 80 percent).

TREATMENT These infections do not respond to tetrachloroethylene. Thiabendazole 25 mg/kg twice daily for 2 or 3 days, or pyrantel pamoate as used in hookworm infections, is effective in symptomatic infections. Both are considered investigational drugs for this condition by the U.S. Food and Drug Administration.

PREVENTION Leafy vegetables should be cooked before ingestion in endemic areas.

STRONGYLOIDIASIS

DEFINITION Strongyloidiasis is an intestinal infection of humans caused by *Strongyloides stercoralis*. Extraintestinal involvement may occur in severe cases.

ETIOLOGY The tiny (2 mm in length) adult female resides and lays her eggs in the mucosa of the upper part of the jejunum. In heavy infections, the biliary and pancreatic ducts, the entire small bowel, and the colon may be parasitized. The eggs quickly hatch, releasing rhabditiform larvae which enter the lumen of the bowel and are passed in the feces. On reaching the soil, the larvae develop into the infective filariform stage. There, as in the case of the filariform larvae of hookworm, they penetrate the skin and small blood vessels of humans. They are then carried to the lungs where they leave the alveolar capillaries, ascend the respiratory tree, enter the pharynx, and are swallowed. On reaching the small intestine, they mature and copulate. The fertilized female burrows into the jejunal mucosa, while the male is excreted in the stool. Oviposition begins 17 to 28 days after the initial infection. It is likely that the females also reproduce parthenogenetically. In addition to the *direct* host-soil-host cycle, *Strongyloides* has two alternative cycles. In the first, or *indirect,* cycle, the rhabditiform larvae, after passing from the host, develop into free-living adults which reside and reproduce in the soil, thus creating a reservoir of infection independent of the human host. Under certain environmental conditions, the free-living larvae are capable of

transforming back into filariform larvae which initiate a new cycle in humans. In the second, or *autoinfection,* cycle, the rhabditiform larvae develop into filariform larvae before they are passed in the stool. They may then invade the intestinal mucosa or perianal skin of the same host without first going through a soil phase. This may explain the long persistence (20 to 30 years) of strongyloidiasis in patients who have left endemic areas and may also account for the extremely heavy worm loads in some individuals. The early transformation of the filariform larvae is probably also responsible for the frequency with which strongyloidiasis is seen in crowded, unsanitary institutions for the mentally retarded. It appears to occur frequently in patients with achlorhydria, delayed intestinal transit time, and blind loops or diverticula.

EPIDEMIOLOGY The usual mode of infection is the penetration of the skin by larvae. Some infections may result from ingestion of contaminated food and drink, and some are believed to be transmitted by contact. This disease is endemic in the tropics, where the warmth, moisture, and lack of sanitation favor its spread. Sporadic cases appear among Puerto Ricans and throughout the rural south of the continental United States.

PATHOGENESIS AND CLINICAL MANIFESTATIONS The initial cutaneous penetration of the filariform larvae usually produces no symptoms. However, transitory skin eruptions characterized by blotchy erythema, serpiginous lesions, and urticaria may be seen. These may recur at irregular intervals thereafter and are particularly common following recovery from an acute febrile illness. In these situations the lesions are generally found over the lower back and buttocks and are related to episodes of autoinfection. Cough, dyspnea, gross hemoptysis, and bronchospasm may accompany migration through the lungs. Chest x-rays may show pulmonary infiltration at this time. The intestinal infestation is usually asymptomatic or productive only of vague abdominal complaints. In heavier infections, epigastric pain and tenderness, nausea, flatulence, vomiting, and diarrhea alternating with constipation may be observed. Peptic ulcer may be simulated, but food often aggravates the pain. The mucosal inflammation may be severe enough to produce subacute obstruction, segmental ileus, and impaired absorption. A severe form of ulcerative colitis, accompanied by intestinal perforation and peritonitis, has been encountered. In debilitated, immunodepressed, or steroid-treated patients massive autoinfection with widespread dissemination of larvae to the extraintestinal organs including the central nervous system may occur. This hyperinfection is often associated with severe enterocolitis, persistent gram-negative bacteremia, and occasionally gram-negative meningitis. Unrecognized, it usually leads to death. Disseminated strongyloidiasis should be considered in any compromised host with unexplained gram-negative bacteremia, abdominal complaints, and pulmonary infiltrates with or without eosinophilia.

LABORATORY FINDINGS Although clinical findings may be suggestive, the definitive diagnosis can be made only in the laboratory. Fresh fecal specimens should be examined to avoid confusion with hookworm infection; generally, fresh specimens contain *larvae* in strongyloidiasis infections, while in hookworm infection they contain *eggs.* Since the number of larvae in the stool is small and varies from day to day, several samples should be checked, using concentration and culture techniques. If pulmonary involvement is present, the sputum should be examined for larvae. Microscopic examination of the duodenal washings and jejunal biopsies may also establish the diagnosis. Alternatively, a weighted string can be passed into the duodenum, allowed to remain for a short time, and then withdrawn. The bile-stained section of the string is stripped of fluid which is then examined for the presence of larvae. The filarial complement fixation test is positive in approximately 75 percent of patients and may be helpful in the diagnosis of light infections.

Eosinophilic leukocytosis is common, except in very severe cases. When eosinophilia occurs in association with peptic ulcer symptoms, strongyloidiasis should be suspected.

TREATMENT All infected patients should be treated to prevent the occurrence of severe invasive disease. The drug of choice is thiabendazole, which should be given orally in dosage of 25 mg/kg twice a day for 2 or 3 days. In disseminated strongyloidiasis, treatment should be continued for 7 days or more. Lightheadedness, nausea, and vomiting are common accompaniments of therapy with this agent. Hypersensitivity reactions may occur but usually respond to treatment with antihistamines. The stools should be rechecked at intervals of 3 months because the parasite is not easily eradicated and retreatment may be necessary.

PROGNOSIS In the usual case, the prognosis is good. Since the occurrence of hyperinfection is unpredictable, every effort should be made to eradicate the infection in each case. In severe cases with hyperinfection, the prognosis is poor.

PREVENTION In general, the measures are those for the control of hookworm infection. In addition, it is well to remember that infection may be contracted by ingestion of contaminated food (especially uncooked vegetables) or of contaminated drinking water and by contact. Patients who have a history of residence in an endemic area should be carefully checked for the presence of the parasite prior to the initiation of steroid or immunosuppressive therapy. Because the larvae may not appear in the stool for several weeks after the initiation of such therapy, repeated examinations of stool and upper intestinal aspirates are indicated. Since sputum, vomitus, stool, and body fluids of patients with disseminated disease may contain infective filariform larvae, gloves and gowns should be worn by hospital personnel caring for such patients.

INTESTINAL CAPILLARIASIS

DEFINITION Intestinal capillariasis is an infection of humans caused by the roundworm Capillaria philippinensis. This species of Capillaria was first discovered in 1963 from a fatal human infection occurring in the Philippines. The infection results in intractable diarrhea with a high mortality rate. Clinical studies have shown a severe protein-losing enteropathy and malabsorption of fats and sugars.

ETIOLOGY Capillaria are nematodes of the family Trichuroidea and are closely related to comembers Trichuris and Trichinella. Adult C. philippinensis are small, measuring 2 to 4 mm in length. The peanut-shaped eggs have flattened bipolar plugs and an average size of 42 by 20 μm. The adults inhabit the mucosa of the small intestine, especially the jejunum. Adults, larval forms, and eggs are found in the stool.

EPIDEMIOLOGY The infection has been found almost exclusively in persons residing in the Ilocano ethnic region in Northwest Luzon, Philippines. Two cases from Thailand have also been reported. Since 1966 the disease has occurred in epidemic form, and more than 1000 cases and 100 deaths have been

reported. Males are infected more frequently than females, perhaps because of occupational exposure. Prior to the discovery of an effective chemotherapeutic agent, the mortality rate in untreated cases was about 30 percent. With chemotherapy, the case fatality rate has been reduced to 6 percent.

The mode of transmission and life cycle of the parasite are not established. The presence of many adult worms, larviparous females, embryonated eggs, and all larval stages in human intestinal contents suggests that autoinfection may be part of the life cycle. In addition, indirect evidence indicates that person-to-person transmission occurs. The mechanism by which humans originally became infected remains obscure. Because the Ilocano people of the region eat many animal foods raw or semicooked, numerous species of local fauna have been examined for Capillaria, and developing larvae have been recovered from three species of fish.

PATHOGENESIS AND MANIFESTATIONS Adult worms in large numbers invade the small-intestinal mucosa and cause a severe protein-losing enteropathy and malabsorption. Hypokalemia, hypocalcemia, and hypoproteinemia are the rule. Autopsy studies have failed to show extraintestinal spread of the parasite. Initial symptoms of intestinal "gurgling" (borborygmi) and recurrent vague abdominal pain are followed, usually within 2 to 3 weeks, by a voluminous watery diarrhea. Other findings, consistent with the basic pathophysiologic process, are anorexia, vomiting, weight loss, muscle wasting and weakness, hyporeflexia, and edema. Abdominal tenderness and distention may occur. The period between onset of symptoms and death is usually 2 to 3 months. Subclinical infection has not been noted.

DIAGNOSIS The diagnosis is made by finding ova in the stool. The ova of C. philippinensis must be differentiated from those of T. trichiura, which are similar. Care must be taken that capillaria are not overlooked in patients with Trichuris infections because in the endemic area most patients with capillariasis have coexistent Trichuris infection.

TREATMENT Administration of mebendazole combined with fluid and electrolyte replacement leads to dramatic improvement; 400 mg per day in divided dosage should be given for 20 days to prevent relapse.

REFERENCES

Aur RJA et al: Thiabendazole in visceral larva migrans. Am J Dis Child 121:226, 1971

Aziz MA, Seddiqui AR: Morphological and absorption studies of small intestine hookworm disease (ancyclostomiasis) in West Pakistan. Gastroenterology 55:242, 1968

Banwell JG, Schad GA: Hookworm. Clin Gastroenterol 7:129, 1978

Blumenthal DS: Current concepts—intestinal nematodes in the United States. N Engl J Med 297:1437, 1977

Brown HW: Basic Clinical Parasitology, 4th ed. New York, Appleton-Century-Crofts, 1975

Cross JH et al: Studies on the experimental transmission of Capillaria philippinensis in monkeys. Trans R Soc Trop Med Hyg 66:819, 1972

Davis CM, Israel RM: Treatment of creeping eruption with topical thiabendazole. Arch Dermatol 97:325, 1968

Kamath KR: Severe infection with Trichuris trichuria in Malaysian children. Am J Trop Med Hyg 22:600, 1973

Layrisse M et al: Blood loss due to infection with Trichuris trichuria. Am J Trop Med Hyg 16:613, 1967

Markett EK: Pseudohookworm infection—trichostrongyliasis: Treatment with thiabendazole. N Engl J Med 278:831, 1968

Marsen JM, Turner JA: Reinfection of enterobiasis (pinworm infection): Simultaneous treatment of family members. Am J Dis Child 118:576, 1969

MILLER MJ et al: Mebendazole. An effective anthelmintic for trichuriasis and enterobiasis. JAMA 230:1412, 1974

PAWLOWSKI Z: Ascariasis. Clin Gastroenterol 7:157, 1978

PHILLS JA et al: Pulmonary abnormalities and eosinophilia due to *Ascaris suum.* N Engl J Med 286:965, 1972

PINKUS GS et al: Intestinal anisakiasis. First case report from North America. Am J Med 59:114, 1975

SCHANTZ PM, GLICKMAN LT: Current concepts in parasitology—toxocaral visceral larva migrans. N Engl J Med 298:436, 1978

SCOWDEN EB et al: Overwhelming strongyloidiasis—an unappreciated opportunistic infection. Medicine 57:527, 1978

WOLFE MS: Oxyuris, trichostrongylus and trichiuris. Clin Gastroenterol 7:201, 1978

ZINKHAM WH: Visceral larva migrans—a review and reassessment indicating two forms of clinical expression: visceral and ocular. Am J Dis Child 132:627, 1978

211
SCHISTOSOMIASIS (BILHARZIASIS)

JAMES J. PLORDE

DEFINITION Schistosomiasis (biharziasis) designates a group of diseases caused by three closely related species of digenetic trematodes, or blood flukes, belonging to the family Schistosomatidae—*Schistosoma mansoni, S. haematobium,* and *S. japonicum.* These blood flukes inhabit the circulatory system of humans and animals living in tropical and subtropical countries. Here they deposit large numbers of eggs, many of which are retained within the body of the host with the production of inflammatory lesions. The organs and tissues most frequently affected are the colon, urinary bladder, liver, lungs, and central nervous system.

ETIOLOGY AND LIFE CYCLE The adult worms, which grow and mature within the portal venous system of the liver, measure 1 to 2 cm in length. The male has a central trough, the gynecophoral canal, that enfolds the longer, more slender female during most of their 4- to 30-year life span. After copulation the male carries the female against the flow of portal blood to the small mesenteric vessels. *Schistosoma japonicum* ascends the superior and *S. mansoni,* the inferior mesenteric vein. Both eventually reach the submucosal vessels of the intestine; *S. japonicum* settles in the small intestine and ascending colon and *S. mansoni,* in the descending colon and rectum. *Schistosoma haematobium* finds its way through the hemorrhoidal anastomoses to the systemic capillaries of the bladder and other pelvic organs. When they can travel no further, the female deposits her eggs in clusters (or one by one in the case of *S. mansoni),* slowly retreating down the vessel in front of them. The daily egg output of each worm pair varies from 300 for *S. mansoni* to over 3000 in *S. japonicum* infections. The eggs, which remain viable for 3 weeks, secrete an enzymatic substance which destroys the surrounding tissue. If the eggs lie close to the mucosal surface, they rupture into the lumen of the gut (or bladder in the case of *S. haematobium)* and are carried to the outside in the urine or feces. On reaching fresh water, the embryonated eggs quickly hatch, liberating ciliated *miracidia.* These miracidia have a life span of 6 to 8 h in which to search out and penetrate the specific snail host appropriate to the species. Within the snail the miracidia are transformed by a two-generation process of asexual reproduction into thousands of infective larvae called *cercariae.* When cercariae are released 1 to 2 months after the original penetration of the snail, they swim around vigorously, and if they contact human skin within 2 days, they penetrate it and become *schistosomula.* Within 24 h the schistosomula work their way into the peripheral venules and are carried to the right side of the heart and then to the pulmonary capillaries. After some delay, they enter the systemic circulation. Those parasites that survive the passage through the mesenteric capillary bed finally reach the portal venous system, where they mature into adult flukes in 5 to 12 weeks.

EPIDEMIOLOGY AND CONTROL Schistosomiasis is possibly the most important of the helminthic diseases because of its worldwide distribution and the extensive pathological changes produced by the parasites. It is believed that over 200 million people in 71 countries are affected by this condition, and it is likely that increasing use of land irrigation in endemic areas will increase this number substantially. Owing to the lack of appropriate snail hosts, schistosomiasis is not transmitted in the continental United States. Approximately 400,000 imported cases occur, however, particularly among the Puerto Rican, Filipino, and Yemenite populations.

Within endemic areas, there are wide variations in both the intensity and prevalence of infection. In most patients the worm load is small, probably less than 10 worm pairs, and disease manifestations are absent. Because adult worms do not multiply within the body of their human host, heavy infections are the result of repeated reinfections occurring over a period of years. It is among this population that serious morbidity and mortality occurs.

The continuing presence of schistosomiasis depends on the disposal of infected human excrement into fresh water, the presence of suitable snail hosts, and the exposure of persons to water infested with cercarias. Promiscuous defecation, latrine drainage, and unsanitary sewage disposal are the more important sources of pollution of streams and rivers. The disease is contracted by persons washing clothes, bathing, wading, or working in contaminated water. There is a close correlation between the degree of water contact and infection rates in endemic areas. The infection rates and intensity of infection both peak in the second decade of life and then decrease with advancing age. This might be explained in part by reduced exposure to contaminated water but also may reflect slowly developing immunity. In animal models, immunity arises in response to the presence of viable adults, depends upon the presence of antibody, and is mediated by eosinophils. It is directed only at newly invading immature parasites; the adults appear to protect themselves by incorporating host antigen into their tegument.

Of these three disease-producing blood flukes in humans, *S. mansoni* is the most widespread and the only one present in the Western Hemisphere. It was brought to the Caribbean area and South America by African slaves. It is present in Venezuela, Surinam, Brazil, Puerto Rico, Dominican Republic, St. Lucia, and several other islands in the Caribbean. In Africa, it occurs in the Nile Delta, limited areas of East and South Africa, tropical Africa, and the Middle East including Yemen, Saudi Arabia, and Israel.

Schistosoma japonicum affects the agricultural population in Japan, China, the Philippines, the Celebes, Thailand, and Laos. Men are more frequently infected than women. An important source of infection in the Orient is the use of human excreta as a fertilizer in vegetable gardens.

Schistosoma haematobium is distributed widely throughout the African continent and is found in several countries of the Middle East. In Africa, it is highly prevalent among the agricultural population of the Nile Valley.

The best attack on schistosomiasis is prevention. Public health measures, including proper disposal of human excrement, provision of pure water supplies for domestic and recreational purposes, and mass anthelmintic therapy, should be carried out in endemic areas. The effectiveness of these measures is diminished if there are significant animal reservoirs of the disease, as in *S. japonicum* and possibly in *S. mansoni* infections. Extermination of the mollusk intermediate host by chemical agents has been used in areas where infestation rates are high. Available molluscicides include *N*-tritylmorpholine, yurimin, and niclosamide (Bayluscid). This drug appears to be the most effective, but the selection of an agent is determined in large part by the nature of the habitat. Biologic snail control methods, although showing promise, have not yet been demonstrated to be effective in the field. Careful attention to the design of irrigation systems in endemic areas is important. The use of concrete-lined ditches and intermittent or fluctuant application of water can be very effective in control of the snail population. The most successful control programs have combined mass therapy with mollusciciding and/or environmental control. Unfortunately, this approach is extremely costly and beyond the means of many countries.

SCHISTOSOMIASIS MANSONI (INTESTINAL BILHARZIASIS, SCHISTOSOMAL DYSENTERY)

ETIOLOGY *Schistosoma mansoni* is distinguished from the two other major species by the structure of its eggs and the adult flukes. The eggs are bluntly oval, have a lateral spine, and measure about 140 by about 60 μm. They are passed in feces and, rarely, in the urine. The intermediate snail hosts belong to the genera *Biomphalaria* and *Tropicorbis*. Humans are thought to be the principal host, but baboons in Kenya have been found to be infected naturally. It is not known as yet whether they constitute an important reservoir of the disease independent of humans.

PATHOGENESIS AND CLINICAL MANIFESTATIONS Schistosomiasis *mansoni* infections are usually asymptomatic. Serious disease occurs only in those who, by virtue of repeated exposures, develop and maintain heavy worm loads over prolonged periods. Clinical manifestations can be divided into three phases: (1) an early stage in which cercariae penetrate the skin and the resulting schistosomula are carried by the blood to the liver and mature into adult parasites within the intrahepatic portal veins, (2) an intermediate stage which begins with and continues through the duration of oviposition and egg extrusion, and (3) a late stage characterized by tissue proliferation and fibrosis in response to eggs that have been retained in tissue. Within a few hours of penetrating the skin, most cercariae die, producing a dermatitis characterized by round-cell infiltration, pruritus, and papular eruption. This is the result of both an immediate and delayed type of sensitivity reaction to cercarial antigen and rarely occurs in primary infection. The rash is commonly followed by headache, myalgia, abdominal pain, and diarrhea, manifestations presumably related to the migration of the schistosomula. These symptoms may persist for 1 or 2 weeks, terminating with a modest fever.

An acute, febrile illness, resembling serum sickness and beginning 1 to 2 months after exposure, marks the onset of oviposition and the beginning of the intermediate stage of illness. This so-called *Katayama syndrome* apparently represents an allergic response to the growing antigenic mass of ova and parasites. The illness is characterized by high spiking fever, chills, cough, urticaria, abdominal pain, diarrhea, and occasionally melena. Physical examination shows lymphadenopathy, enlarged tender liver, and fine scattered rales. Sigmoidoscopy reveals an inflamed, engorged mucosa with small areas of ulceration and hemorrhage. Laboratory tests demonstrate the presence of circulating immune complexes, nonspecific liver function abnormalities, and a marked eosinophilic leukocytosis. Eggs may not be present in the stool initially, and the clinical manifestations, with the exception of the eosinophilia, can be mistaken for typhoid. The acute illness may last as long as 3 months and on rare occasions may result in death. The syndrome is seen in its full intensity only in previously unexposed individuals who suffer a massive cercarial exposure. In endemic areas, it is most commonly brief and mild.

The late stage of illness is caused by the reaction of local tissue to the deposited eggs. Those which are extruded into the bowel lumen elicit little damage. The 50 percent or more that are retained, however, stimulate an eosinophilic and mononuclear-cell infiltration followed by edema, granuloma formation, and vascular obstruction. This has been demonstrated to be a delayed hypersensitivity reaction to a soluble antigen secreted by the egg. Early in infection the host response is vigorous, producing lesions which exceed the volume of the inciting egg by a hundredfold. In the chronic phase, however, this response appears to be moderated, and the pathological consequences are proportionately less severe. Healing occurs by fibrosis, calcification, and resorption.

In the bowel, these changes produce congestion, thickening, and, in severe infections, ulcerations and sessile or pedunculated polyps. Clinically, abdominal pain, diarrhea with or without blood, and a mild protein-losing enteropathy may be seen. Intestinal obstruction and rectal prolapse are rare complications. These changes often regress with treatment.

Of more severe consequence is the passage of eggs back into the venous system. These are carried to portal radicles of the liver where they produce an endophlebitis, pseudotubercle formation, acute vascular obstruction, and hepatic enlargement. With time, collars of fibrosis develop around the larger portal veins resulting in shrinkage of the liver and severe presinusoidal portal hypertension. The patient presents with hepatosplenomegaly and esophageal varices. Occasionally the enlarged spleen becomes enormous, producing a visible abdominal mass and the anemia, leukopenia, and thrombocytopenia of hypersplenism. Neovascularization and arterialization maintain hepatic blood flow at normal levels. As a result, hepatocellular function is usually well preserved, and spider nevi, gynecomastia, jaundice, and ascites are uncommon. Repeated bouts of esophageal bleeding may occur. Hepatic encephalopathy rarely results, however, and the outcome is usually favorable. When death does occur, it is the result of exsanguination.

With the development of portacaval anastomoses, some eggs are carried past the liver to the vessels of the lung where they may produce a similar histopathological reaction in the pulmonary arterioles. Interstitial fibrosis, destruction of pulmonary capillaries, and eventually pulmonary hypertension with cor pulmonale and aneurysms of the pulmonary artery may occur. On roentgenogram the granulomas may resemble miliary tuberculosis.

Occasionally ova are carried to the spinal cord through anastomotic venous channels or are deposited there by ectopic adults resulting in a transverse myelitis.

There is impressive evidence that circulating antigen antibody complexes may produce an immune-complex nephropathy in schistosomiasis *mansoni*. This has been observed primarily in patients with the chronic hepatosplenic form of the disease and may present as asymptomatic albuminuria, the nephrotic syndrome, or progressive renal failure. There is little information on its incidence or public health significance.

Chronic *Salmonella* and *Escherichia coli* bacteremias have been noted in patients suffering from hepatosplenic schistosomiasis. The chronicity of these infections may be related to the

DIAGNOSIS AND LABORATORY FINDINGS Diagnosis depends on finding the ova in the stools or the rectal mucosa. Stool concentration techniques such as gravity sedimentation or formol-ether centrifugation are often required for the detection of ova. Quantitation of the egg output by the Kato thick smear or similar methods is useful in estimating the severity of infection and in following response to therapy.

Rectal biopsy is probably the single most reliable method of diagnosis and it is often positive when repeated stool examinations are negative. By means of biopsy forceps and a proctoscope, mucosal snips are obtained from the valves of Houston, compressed between two glass slides, and examined under the low-power lens of a microscope. Eggs, often numbering in the hundreds, are clearly visible. Because dead eggs may persist in tissue for a long time after the death of the adult worms, active infection is confirmed only if the eggs can be shown to be viable. This may be done by observing the eggs for movement under the high-power lens or by hatching them in water.

Eosinophilia is usually present in schistosomiasis. An intradermal test of the immediate type becomes positive within 1 to 2 months of exposure and remains so for years despite parasitological cure. Since it is neither highly sensitive nor specific, it is of value chiefly as an epidemiologic tool. Twenty-five percent of patients with a history of swimmer's itch give a positive test.

Complement fixation, precipitin, counterimmunoelectrophoresis, and indirect fluorescent antibody tests can be done, but like the intradermal test most lack sensitivity and specificity.

Two tests show demonstrable improvement in both areas. One is an indirect fluorescent antibody procedure that utilizes frozen-sectioned adult antigens; the other a radioimmunoassay using purified egg antigen. Serologic tests become positive early in the course of infection, often before eggs can be recovered. A positive result should lead to a vigorous search for eggs by concentration methods or rectal biopsy, but by itself is not an indication for treatment.

TREATMENT No specific therapy is available for the treatment of schistosomal dermatitis or the acute illness resembling serum sickness seen in the early months of infection. Antihistamines and steroids have been used to control the manifestations of these two symptoms. Because late schistosomiasis is caused by the continued deposition of eggs by the mature worm pairs, the aim of therapy in this stage of the disease is the sterilization and destruction of these parasites. Adult schistosomicides are available for the purpose, but in light of their considerable toxicity, therapy should not be initiated unless the presence of an active infection is first proved by the recovery of *viable eggs* from the stool or rectal mucosa. Moreover, since the severity of disease is related to the intensity of infection, some authorities believe light infections (fewer than 50 eggs per gram of stool) do not require therapy. In heavier infections therapy will usually reduce egg output by 90 percent or more, and attempts to achieve cure by repeated use of toxic agents are unwise.

Trivalent antimony compounds, including tartar emetic (antimony potassium tartrate), stibophen (Fuadin), and stibocaptate (Astiban), have been the traditional agents for this disease. Only stibocaptate is still widely used and is probably the preferred agent. It is given by intramuscular injection as a 10% solution for five doses for a total of 35 to 50 mg/kg (maximum 2.0 g). Toxic side effects are mitigated if injections are given at weekly intervals.

Temporary ECG changes are common during therapy; they consist primarily of repolarization abnormalities which disappear a few days after the drug is discontinued. However, arrhythmias, collapse, and sudden death have been reported. Antimonials also may cause hepatitis, acute nephritis, hemolytic anemia, and thrombocytopenic purpura. Any of these complications calls for immediate discontinuation of therapy. Nausea and joint pains can usually be controlled by decreasing the individual dose or increasing the intervals between doses. Heart, renal, or liver disease constitutes a contraindication to therapy with this group of agents.

Ambilhar (niridazole) can be taken orally, 25 mg/kg every day in divided doses for 7 days. Since it is less toxic than the antimonials and probably just as effective, this agent has become the drug of choice in *S. mansoni* infections. Although ECG changes occur with this drug also, they are less common than with antimonial therapy. However, there has been a high incidence of neurological abnormalities, and as many as 80 percent of patients receiving the drug show electroencephalographic changes. Psychotic episodes or convulsions, which disappear when the drug is discontinued, have also been reported, particularly in adults. The incidence of neurological reactions seems to increase if there is serious liver disease with portacaval shunting. Niridazole should not be used in patients with a prior history of seizures.

Hycanthone is a new thioxanthone preparation that can be administered in a single intramuscular injection. Its hepatotoxicity and mutagenic properties may limit its usefulness. It is not available in the United States.

Success of treatment is judged by the disappearance of eggs from the stool, reduction in eosinophils, and alleviation of symptoms. Patients should be examined monthly for 6 to 12 months to detect relapses. The decision to retreat is based on factors such as intensity of egg output, presence of potentially reversible clinical manifestations, and the likelihood of reinfection.

Treatment of the patient with severe hepatic or pulmonary disease is largely symptomatic. There is little enthusiasm for portacaval shunting in the presence of esophageal varices. These patients usually have good hepatocellular function and, if treated carefully, will probably survive longer with repeated bleeding episodes than with surgery. Additionally, splenectomy makes these patients more susceptible to the recrudescence of chronic malaria.

PROGNOSIS The prognosis is good. Many patients never develop symptoms, and early states of colonic, hepatic, pulmonary, and central nervous system disease are completely reversible with adequate therapy. In the late fibrotic stage, the prognosis is worse.

SCHISTOSOMIASIS JAPONICA (KATAYAMA DISEASE)

ETIOLOGY The oval eggs are shorter, wider, and smaller than those of the other two species, measuring about 90 by 70 μm. Mature eggs have a minute hook, or spine, laterally situated and smaller than that of *S. mansoni*. The ova are passed in the feces only. The life cycle is similar to that of *S. mansoni*, except that amphibious snails of the genus *Oncomelania*, which are capable of prolonged existence away from water, are utilized as intermediate hosts, and water buffalo, horses, cattle, pigs, dogs, and cats as well as humans may harbor the adult worms.

Both factors add to the difficulty in disease control. *Schistosoma japonicum* lives in the superior mesenteric venules and frequently migrates to those of the colon for oviposition.

PATHOGENESIS AND CLINICAL MANIFESTATIONS The early manifestations of infection such as the pruritic dermatitis, cough, angioneurotic edema, diarrhea, and fever produced by the penetration and migration of the schistosomula are seen less commonly than in schistosomiasis *mansoni*. However, because *S. japonicum* eggs are deposited in greater number and in closer proximity to the liver than are those of *S. mansoni*, the intermediate and late manifestations of disease are usually both more frequent and more severe.

The allergic manifestations accompanying oviposition are particularly impressive in japonicum infections. Four to six weeks after exposure the patient notes the onset of a high spiking fever, chills, cough, urticaria, generalized lymphadenopathy, tender hepatosplenomegaly, and eosinophilic leukocytosis. The deposition of large numbers of eggs in the intestinal wall results in ulcerations, bloody mucoid stools, and abdominal pain. The acute illness may persist for 1 to 2 months but usually subsides leaving the patient relatively well. Death may occur in severe cases.

With continued oviposition fibrosis of the small bowel and liver develops. These changes are seen earlier than in *mansoni* infections, and as a result the entire disease may run its course in 2 to 5 years, ending in death.

In advanced cases the gross postmortem findings are emaciation and pallor; a large or contracted liver with periportal fibrosis; splenomegaly, with fibrosis of pulp; ascites; fibrotic nodules over the colonic peritoneum; fibrous thickening and rigidity of the colon, with small polyps projecting from the mucosa; and thickening and fibrosis of the omentum.

Clinically, signs of portal obstruction such as engorgement of superficial abdominal veins and ascites appear. Some individuals present marked splenomegaly, a small contracted liver, profound anemia, leukopenia, and thrombocytopenia associated with severe malnutrition and hypoproteinemia. The majority of individuals suffering from schistosomiasis japonica die of cirrhosis and cachexia, massive hemorrhage from rupture of esophageal varices, or intercurrent infections.

Central nervous system lesions occur more frequently in the brain than in the spinal cord, appear clinically as epilepsy in an expanding tumor, and usually result from the presence of ectopic adults.

DIAGNOSIS AND LABORATORY FINDINGS The characteristic ova must be found in the stools in order to establish the diagnosis. In established cases, ova are more difficult to demonstrate in the stools or in rectal biopsy; positive intradermal and serologic tests in suspected cases should lead to an intensive search for the egg.

TREATMENT In general, *S. japonicum* infections are more difficult to treat, and relapses are more frequent. There is debate over the preferred method of therapy. Some authorities recommend niridazole because of its limited toxicity and ability to substantially reduce worm load in most patients. Others, bothered by the relatively poor cure rate seen with this agent, prefer the more toxic and effective potassium antimony tartrate. It is administered as a freshly prepared 0.5% solution. The drug must be given slowly. Extravasation into surrounding tissue leads to painful necrosis. The initial dose is 0.04 g; subsequent doses are given on alternate days and gradually increased to a maximum of 0.12 g by the fifth dose. A total of 2.2 g should be given. The patient should be hospitalized during treatment and remain at bed rest for a few hours after each injection. If a lesion is present in the brain, prompt treatment may forestall the need for surgical intervention.

PROGNOSIS If the condition is not treated early, prognosis is poor in the majority of cases encountered in endemic communities.

SCHISTOSOMIASIS HAEMATOBIA (GENITOURINARY SCHISTOSOMIASIS, ENDEMIC HEMATURIA)

ETIOLOGY AND LIFE CYCLE The eggs are compact, elongated spindles, dilated in the middle and measuring about 140 by 50 μm. At one pole they present a short terminal spine. The ova are passed in the urine, and occasionally in the feces. The life cycle is similar to that of *S. mansoni*. The adult worms live in the hemorrhoidal plexus of veins, some going to the rectum for oviposition but most of them passing on to the vesical plexus. The intermediate hosts are snails of the genera *Bulinus*, *Physopsis*, and *Biomphalaria*.

PATHOGENESIS AND CLINICAL MANIFESTATIONS Large numbers of ova are deposited in the submucosa of the bladder where they incite an eosinophilic granulomatous reaction. The trigone is involved at first, but soon the entire mucosa is thickened and ulcerated. In chronic infections, the other coats become scarred and the muscularis hypertrophies. Pedunculated papillomas often develop at the trigone and about the urethral orifices. The bladder capacity becomes greatly reduced as the organ loses its contractility. Lesions occur in the distal third of the ureters in many cases, causing vesicoureteral reflux, obstruction, and hydronephrosis. Bacterial pyelonephritis may occur. In about 10 percent of cases, calculi develop in the bladder, renal pelvis, or ureters, and occasionally the entire calcified bladder can be visualized on roentgenograms. Fistulas between the urogenital tract and intestines may develop. The prostate and seminal vesicles in men and the cervix and vagina in women may be affected; lymphatic blockade with elephantiasis of the genitalia occurs rarely. Carcinoma of the bladder is a frequent late complication in Egypt but not in other areas. Because the ova are deposited in the vesical plexus, ectopic eggs are carried to the lungs where they produce miliary granulomas. Although in endemic areas the egg output usually decreases in adolescence, the pathological changes continue to progress in untreated infection.

MANIFESTATIONS Painful micturition, frequency, and terminal hematuria are the leading symptoms. Secondary bacterial infection of the urinary tract is frequent, and repeated hemorrhages from the bladder produce severe anemia. Chronic *Salmonella* bacteriuria with recurrent bouts of bacteremia have been reported from Egypt. An associated nephrotic syndrome which responds to antibiotic and anthelmintic therapy also occurred. With progressive obstruction, renal failure and uremia ensue.

DIAGNOSIS AND LABORATORY FINDINGS As in the other types of schistosomiasis, diagnosis is made by finding the characteristic ova in the urinary sediment, in tissues obtained from vesical mucosa, or, less frequently, in the stools. Egg output is highest in midmorning. Cystoscopy and biopsy of the bladder are usually diagnostic. In long-standing infections, urine cultures and intravenous urograms should be obtained.

TREATMENT Chemotherapy is very effective early in the disease and often results in dramatic reversal of symptoms and obstructive phenomena. The drugs are the same as those recommended for *S. mansoni*. Niridazole (Ambilhar) is the drug of choice. Surgery may be required for abscesses, fistulas, strictures, papillomas, and various other complications involving the bladder, but it should not be undertaken until the extent to which the lesions will resolve with medical treatment is known. Chemotherapy is indicated for secondary bacterial infections of the urinary tract, especially those caused by *Salmonella*. The criteria for cure are the absence of ova in the urine and bladder wall and the disappearance of ulcerative granulomatous lesions, as revealed by cystoscopic examination.

PROGNOSIS Provided treatment is started without delay, prognosis is good in recent infection, and fair when damage to the bladder and urinary infection have already occurred. Prognosis is very poor in chronic, late infections. After age 45, the mortality rate increases fourfold. The frequent coexistence of infection with *S. mansoni* aggravates prognosis and the clinical picture.

SCHISTOSOME DERMATITIS

DEFINITION AND GEOGRAPHIC DISTRIBUTION Certain nonhuman schistosome cercariae are capable of penetrating human skin but are unable to develop further. This results in a schistosome dermatitis similar to that seen with the species pathogenic for humans. This condition is also known as "swimmer's itch" and is common in many parts of the world. It apparently does not develop after a single contact with cercariae, but it ensues following multiple exposures. Definitive hosts of some of the schistosomes producing dermatitis are the muskrat and migratory birds. Both fresh- and saltwater mollusks serve as intermediate hosts.

Schistosome dermatitis has been reported from the freshwater areas of North Central and Western United States, Alaska, Canada, Central and South America, Western Europe (particularly Switzerland), and the Far East.

A seawater dermatitis believed to be produced by nonhuman schistosome cercariae has been reported in clam diggers and bathers along the coasts of New York, Rhode Island, California, Hawaii, and Florida.

PATHOGENESIS AND CLINICAL MANIFESTATIONS Because the dermatitis develops only after multiple exposures, it is believed to represent an allergic reaction, the nonhuman cercariae being the sensitizing agents. Exposed individuals show a positive intradermal reaction when tested with cercarial antigen. The initial symptom is usually a prickling sensation; occasionally urticaria is noted as the water evaporates from the skin. These manifestations disappear within an hour, leaving only a few macules to mark the site of cercarial penetration. Several hours later an intense itching accompanied by a papular and occasionally a vesicular rash begins. This is most intense on the second or third day and gradually subsides.

TREATMENT Local application of antipruritic lotions such as calamine with menthol or phenol is used to allay itching and thereby reduce the likelihood of secondary infection. Treatment with antihistaminic drugs will relieve the pruritus.

PREVENTION Immediate drying of the skin after swimming has been recommended as a prophylactic measure. This will not completely prevent lesions, since some penetration occurs during immersion. Dimethylphthalate cream has been reported as an effective cercarial repellent.

In some areas, control has been effected by destruction of snails. Copper sulfate and copper carbonate have been used for this purpose. Treatment of shallow waters where snails are abundant has been moderately effective.

REFERENCES

CHEEVER AW: A quantitative post-mortem study of schistosomiasis mansoni in man. Am J Trop Med 17:38, 1968

CLARK WD et al: Acute schistosomiasis mansoni in 10 boys—an outbreak in Caguas, Puerto Rico. Ann Intern Med 73:379, 1970

FALCAO HA, GOULD DB: Immune complex nephropathy in schistosomiasis. Ann Intern Med 83:148, 1975

JORDAN P: Epidemiology and control of schistosomiasis. Br Med Bull 28:55, 1972

LEHMAN JS JR et al: Urinary schistosomiasis in Egypt: Clinical, radiological, bacteriological, and parasitological correlations. Trans R Soc Trop Med Hyg 67:384, 1973

MAHMOUD AA: Current concepts—schistosomiasis. N Engl J Med 297:1329, 1977

MARCIAL-ROJAS RA, FIAL RE: Neurologic complications of schistosomiasis: Review of the literature and report of two cases of transverse myelitis due to *S. mansoni*. Ann Intern Med 59:215, 1963

ORRIS L, COMBES FC: Clam digger's dermatitis: Schistosome dermatitis from sea water. AMA Arch Dermatol Syphilol 66:367, 1952

PRATA A: Schistosomiasis mansoni. Clin Gastroenterol 7:49, 1978

SMITHERS SR: Recent advances in the immunology of schistosomiasis. Br Med Bull 28:49, 1972

WARREN KS: The pathology, pathobiology and pathogenesis of schistosomiasis. Nature (Parasitol Suppl) 273:609, 1978

———: Schistosomiasis japonicum. Clin Gastroenterol 7:77, 1978

212
OTHER TREMATODES OR FLUKES

JAMES J. PLORDE

The trematodes of humans are long-lived parasites which produce progressive damage to the tissues of their hosts. With the exception of schistosomes, they are similar in morphology and life cycle. The adult flukes are flat, leaflike hermaphrodites that vary in length from a few millimeters to several centimeters. Their digestive tract, unlike that of the nematodes, ends blindly. As their name indicates, they have two "holes" in the form of oral and ventral suckers which are used as organs of attachment and locomotion. The operculated eggs, which are passed in the feces or sputum, hatch in the water to produce a ciliated, free-swimming *miracidium*. The miracidium reaches and penetrates the tissue of an intermediate snail host to undergo a period of development, eventuating in the release of thousands of swarms of free-living *cercariae* from the snail. These thousands of tail-bearing larvae must, in turn, reach a second intermediate host, usually an aquatic animal or vegetation, where they encyst forming *metacercariae*. The definitive host is infected when he or she ingests the parasitized second intermediate host. The distribution of flukes is usually limited by the location of their molluscan intermediate host. With the exception of *Opisthorchis* and *Fasciola,* most hermaphroditic flukes are found only in tropical or subtropical areas.

PARAGONIMIASIS

DEFINITION Paragonimiasis (endemic hemoptysis) is a chronic infection of the lung caused by trematodes of the genus *Paragonimus.* Clinically, the disease is characterized by cough and hemoptysis. Ectopic worms may cause a variety of other manifestations. Geographically, it is probably the most widely distributed disease caused by hermaphroditic flukes.

ETIOLOGY AND EPIDEMIOLOGY Although *P. westermani,* which is widely distributed in the Far East, is the most common cause of human paragonimiasis, a number of other species, including *P. skrjabini, P. heterotremus* (China), *P. africanus, P. uterobilateralis* (Cameroons, Nigeria, and Zaire), *P. mexicanus, P. peruvianus,* and *P. caliensis* (Central and South America), may cause the disease. The short, plump adults (7 to 12 mm in length, 4 to 6 mm in width) have a life span of 4 to 5 years which they typically spend encysted in the lung parenchyma of the host. Their golden-brown operculated eggs (50 by 90 μm) reach the bronchioles from where they are coughed up and excreted in the sputum or swallowed and passed in the feces. They must embryonate several weeks in fresh water before hatching to release the miracidia.

The infection is acquired by ingestion of cysts in the second intermediate host, a crab or crayfish. The metacercariae excyst in the duodenum, burrow through the intestinal wall into the peritoneal cavity, and then usually migrate through the diaphragm and into the lung. The worms also may be found in the intestinal wall, liver, pancreas, kidney, mesentery, skeletal muscle, subcutaneous tissues, and central nervous system, particularly the brain. The dog, cat, pig, rat, and wild carnivores are definitive hosts for the parasite in addition to humans. In some of these, very young adults can be found in their striated muscles. Human infection has been reported following the ingestion of this undercooked flesh.

The incidence of paragonimiasis is often affected by food shortages or local customs. The metacercariae survive in vinegar, and lightly pickled or inadequately cooked food usually serves as the source of infection in the Far East. Fresh crab juice used for the treatment of measles in Korea and for infertility in the Cameroons may also transmit the parasite. Children may acquire the disease in endemic areas while handling or eating raw crabs during play.

PATHOGENESIS AND CLINICAL MANIFESTATIONS An eosinophilic granuloma forms about the adult worm, eventually leading to the formation of a fibrous cyst. The pulmonary lesions which measure up to 1 cm in diameter frequently communicate with a bronchiole, resulting in secondary bacterial infection. Small, fibrous nodules representing reaction around deposited eggs also occur. Clinically the picture is one of chronic bronchitis and bronchiectasis with production of brownish sputum and hemoptysis. A poorly resolving pulmonary infiltrate, lung abscess, or pleural effusion may be present in heavy infections. The roentgenographic findings vary with the stage of infection. Initially one or more soft infiltrates may be seen anywhere in the lungs excepting the apexes. These are then gradually replaced by round nodules which not infrequently cavitate. Eventually, fibrosis and calcification occur, presenting a picture closely resembling tuberculosis, a disease which often coexists with paragonimiasis.

An abdominal mass, pain, and dysentery characterize intestinal or peritoneal infections. Various types of paralysis and epilepsy occur in cerebral involvement. Homonymous hemianopsia, optic atrophy, and papilledema are common. The cerebrospinal fluid usually shows an eosinophilic leukocytosis and elevated protein. Cerebral calcifications are seen on x-ray in 50 percent of cases. *Paragonimus skrjabini* infections are characterized by migratory subcutaneous nodules that contain adult flukes.

LABORATORY FINDINGS Eosinophilia is a constant finding. Definitive diagnosis depends upon finding the characteristic operculated ova in the sputum, stool, pleural fluid, or tissue. Eggs may be rare or totally absent from the sputum during the first 3 months of infection but are eventually found in 75 to 85 percent of infected patients. Even later, however, repeated examinations using concentration techniques may be required for their recovery. Ziehl-Neelsen staining, often carried out for suspected tuberculosis, usually will not demonstrate the eggs. In fact, the sputum concentration techniques for tuberculosis may destroy the eggs that are present. Stool examination is frequently helpful in children. A complement fixation test is available, and the results correlate well with active infection. It usually becomes negative within 6 months of successful therapy. The skin test does not distinguish present and past infections and is used primarily for epidemiologic purposes.

TREATMENT AND PREVENTION Bithionol is the drug of choice. From 30 to 40 mg/kg in divided doses should be given every other day for a total of 10 to 15 treatment days. The symptoms disappear rapidly, and most infiltrates resolve within 3 months. Side effects are minor and consist of nausea, vomiting, and urticaria. Concomitant bacterial infection must be treated. Prevention of superinfection by the same parasite is important, because the disease is self-limiting.

The most practical control measure is the adequate cooking of all shellfish before they are eaten.

CLONORCHIASIS

DEFINITION Clonorchiasis is an infection of the biliary passages caused by *Clonorchis sinensis,* the most important liver fluke of humans. Although the infection is usually asymptomatic, heavy worm loads may produce manifestations of biliary obstruction.

ETIOLOGY AND EPIDEMIOLOGY *Clonorchis sinensis* is a small fluke (5 by 15 mm) that lives as long as 50 years in the biliary tree of its host. Here the flukes feed on mucosal secretions and pass operculated eggs into the feces. On reaching fresh water, the eggs are ingested by the intermediate snail host. After multiplication and development within the snail, the cercariae are released and penetrate freshwater fish. Infections result from ingestion of the raw, dried, salted, or pickled flesh of freshwater fish containing encysted metacercariae. The larva is released in the duodenum. It enters the common bile duct and migrates to the second-order bile ducts, where it develops into the adult form in about 1 month. In addition to humans, dogs, cats, pigs, and rats serve as disease reservoirs. The main endemic areas are Korea, Japan, Taiwan, Hong Kong, Southern China, and Vietnam where clonorchiasis may be perpetuated by the practice of fertilizing fish ponds with manure and human feces. Twenty-five percent of the population of Hong Kong and a small proportion of Chinese immigrants to this country have been shown to be infected. The disease may also be acquired in the United States by the ingestion of infected, dried, frozen, or pickled fish imported from the Far East. Clinically, apparent cases are restricted to the adult population in whom the accumulated worm load eventually produces pathological effects.

PATHOGENESIS AND CLINICAL MANIFESTATIONS Light infections are usually asymptomatic, but worm loads of 500 to 1000 flukes often result in clinical manifestations. During the migration of the larvae, the patient may have fever, chills, tender hepatomegaly, mild jaundice, and eosinophilia. The mature worm causes proliferation of the biliary epithelium, increased mucin production, adenoma formation, chronic pericholangitis, and periductal fibrosis. Hepatic parenchymal damage and portal hypertension are not seen in uncomplicated infections. Recurrent attacks of suppurative cholangitis with or without intrahepatic choledocholithiasis may follow biliary obstruction with dead flukes. These occasionally present as hypoglycemic coma. The occurrence of biliary stones in clonorchiasis is associated with an increased incidence of chronic *Salmonella typhi* carriage. Cholangiocarcinoma may occur in patients with severe, long-standing infections. The adult worms may infest the pancreatic ducts, where they can cause squamous metaplasia, periductal fibrosis, and acute pancreatitis.

LABORATORY DIAGNOSIS Clinical and epidemiologic findings often suggest the diagnosis. There may be elevation of the alkaline phosphatase and hyperbilirubinemia. Eosinophilia is variable. Occasionally, a plain film of the abdomen will demonstrate intrahepatic calcification. Liver scan is usually negative in asymptomatic infections but may show multiple areas of diminished uptake in acute symptomatic disease. Percutaneous transhepatic cholangiography in such patients often reveals dilatation of the peripheral intrahepatic bile ducts. The adult worms appear as round filling defects several millimeters in diameter. Definitive diagnosis depends on the demonstration of the eggs in the feces or the duodenal contents. They measure 29 by 16 μm, possess a conspicuous opercular rim as well as a posterior knob, and can be distinguished from the eggs of *Metagonimus, Heterophyes,* and *Opisthorchis* only with difficulty. An antigen extracted from adult worms can be used in a complement fixation test for the detection of the host's antibody response. Skin tests are also useful.

TREATMENT AND PREVENTION No consistently effective treatment is known, but some success has been noted with chloroquine diphosphate. Chloroquine is prescribed in a dose of 0.25 g three times daily for 6 weeks. Disturbances of mentation, vision, and gastrointestinal function are common during such prolonged therapy and may require a decrease in the daily dosage of chloroquine. In the majority of cases, egg output returns to pretreatment levels within 6 months, suggesting that the treatment of asymptomatic infections is not warranted. A number of experimental drugs have shown more satisfactory results in both experimental animal infection and humans; none are presently available in the United States. Thorough cooking of freshwater fish will prevent infection.

OPISTHORCHIASIS

Opisthorchiasis is caused by *Opisthorchis felineus* or *O. viverrini* and is characterized by hepatic lesions produced by adult worms in the larger bile ducts. The life cycle resembles that of *C. sinensis.* The geographic distribution differs in that *O. felineus* is endemic in Eastern and Central Europe and in Siberia and occurs in some parts of Asia, while *O. viverrini* is found in Thailand and Laos. Cats and wild carnivores act as the principal reservoir hosts, and the infection is found most commonly along rivers and lakes which harbor an abundant fish life. Up to 25 percent of inhabitants of northeastern Thailand are purported to carry the parasite. The clinical lesions are similar to those seen in clonorchiasis except that gallstones are rare. The diagnosis usually is based on the finding of the eggs in the feces

or duodenal contents. Treatment as recommended for clonorchiasis may be used. Infection can be prevented by eating only well-cooked fish.

FASCIOLIASIS

Fascioliasis is caused by *Fasciola hepatica,* which like *Clonorchis,* inhabits the bile ducts of the definitive host. When fully matured, the adult measures about 3 by 1 cm and discharges large operculate eggs 140 by 70 μm which must embryonate in fresh water before hatching.

Fascioliasis produces so-called "liver rot" in sheep, the principal definitive host. The disease is most common in sheep and cattle-raising countries but has been reported from many parts of the world. In North America it occurs in the Southern and Western United States, Central America, and in the Caribbean Islands.

Infection is contracted by ingestion of the encysted forms of the fluke attached to edible aquatic plants such as watercress. The larvae excyst in the duodenum, migrate through the intestinal wall, pass into the peritoneal cavity, penetrate the liver capsule, and finally reach the bile ducts, where they mature. Occasionally larvae may migrate to and mature in ectopic locations including subcutaneous tissue, chest cavity, or brain.

Early clinical manifestations are related to the migration of the larval form to and within the liver. Epigastric pain, fever, diarrhea, jaundice, urticaria, pruritus, arthralgia, and eosinophilia may be observed during this stage. Fibrosis of the liver similar to that found in clonorchiasis appears only after prolonged residence of many adult worms in the bile ducts. Obstruction of the bile duct occurs frequently and may be the presenting manifestation of disease. A pharyngeal form of the disease, called *halzoun,* can result from eating infected raw liver, the young adults attaching themselves to the pharyngeal mucosa, occasionally interfering with respiration.

The diagnosis usually is based on the finding of the eggs in the feces or in the duodenal contents. It is difficult to distinguish the eggs from those of *Fasciolopsis buski.* Complement fixation, hemagglutination, and precipitin tests have been reported to be helpful. A skin test is also available.

Treatment is unsatisfactory. Dehydroemetine dehydrochloride, 1 mg/kg per day intramuscularly for 10 days, may be helpful and at times curative. The drug should not be given to patients with chronic cardiac or renal disease or to children. Bithionol in an oral dose of 50 mg/kg every other day for 10 to 15 doses has also been effective and may be less toxic.

To prevent infection, aquatic plants such as watercress should not be eaten, vegetables grown in fields irrigated with polluted water should be boiled, and safe drinking water should be provided.

FASCIOLOPSIASIS

Fasciolopsiasis is caused by the large intestinal fluke *F. buski,* which inhabits the upper part of the intestine of its definitive host. The principal definitive host is the pig. In parts of China, India, and other areas in the Far East, infection of humans occurs following ingestion, or peeling with the teeth, of water chestnuts and other edible aquatic plants. The large adults attach themselves to the intestinal mucosa, and these sites may later ulcerate. The infection is usually asymptomatic. In heavy infections, diarrhea, abdominal pain, gastrointestinal hemorrhage, and intestinal obstruction may appear early. Later, asthenia with ascites and anasarca occurs. Diagnosis is based upon the history and the finding of eggs in the feces. The eggs resemble those of *Fasciola hepatica*. The prognosis in untreated heavy infections, especially in children, is poor. Tetrachloroethylene as given for hookworm infections is effective. Hexylresorcinol can also be expected to cure or markedly reduce the worm burden in the majority of cases.

HETEROPHYIASIS AND METAGONIMIASIS

Heterophyes heterophyes and *Metagonimus yakagawa* are small intestinal flukes of humans and other fish-eating mammals. They are found in the Far East and, in the case of *Heterophyes*, in India, Egypt, and Tunisia. Both are acquired by ingesting the raw or undercooked flesh of metacercarial-infected freshwater fish. The 2- to 3-mm adults attach themselves to the mucosa of the small intestine. If present in sufficient numbers, they may cause abdominal pain and/or diarrhea. Rarely the eggs have been found in sites such as the brain, spinal cord, or heart where they produce granulomatous lesions. Most commonly, they are passed in the stool where they very closely resemble those of *Clonorchis*. Both species can be treated with tetrachloroethylene as outlined in Chap. 210 for hookworm. As the life span of these trematodes is limited to a year or less, treatment is not indicated unless the patient is symptomatic.

REFERENCES

CHAN PH, TEOH TB: The pathology of *Clonorchis sinensis* infestation of the pancreas. J Pathol Bacteriol 93:185, 1967

JONES EA et al: Massive infection with *Fasciola hepatica* in man. Am J Med 63:842, 1977

KOENIGSTEIN RP: Observations on the epidemiology of infections with *Clonorchis sinensis*. Trans R Soc Trop Med Hyg 42:503, 1949

McFADZEAN AJS, YEUNG RTT: Hypoglycemia in suppurative pancholangitis due to Clonorchis sinensis. Trans R Soc Trop Med Hyg 59:179, 1965

OKUNDA K et al: Clonorchiasis studied by percutaneous cholangiogram and a therapeutic trial of 2,4-diisothiocyanate. Gastroenterology 65:457, 1973

PLANT AG et al: A clinical study of *Fasciolopsis buski* in Thailand. Trans R Soc Trop Med Hyg 63:470, 1969

SADUN EH, BUCK AA: Paragonimiasis in South Korea—Immunodiagnostic, epidemiologic, clinical, roentgenologic and therapeutic studies. Am J Trop Med 9:562, 1960

SEAH SKK: Digenetic trematodes. Clin Gastroenterol 7:87, 1978

YOKOGAWA M: *Paragonimus* and paragonimiasis. Exp Parasitol 10:81, 139, 1960

————: *Paragonimus* and paragonimiasis, in *Advances in Parasitology*, vol 7, B Dawes (ed). London, Academic, 1969, p 375

213
CESTODE (TAPEWORM) INFECTIONS

JAMES J. PLORDE

The tapeworms, or cestodes, are segmented ribbon-shaped hermaphroditic worms which inhabit the intestinal tract of many vertebrates. Unlike other helminths, these parasites lack a digestive tract, and they absorb food through their entire surface. Attachment to the host's intestinal mucosa is effected by means of sucking cups or grooves located on the head, or *scolex*. In some species, the head is also armed with hooklets which aid in attachment. Behind the globular scolex lies a short, narrow neck from which segments or *proglottides* de-

velop one at a time to form the chainlike *strobila* of the worm. These proglottides progressively mature as they are displaced further and further from the neck by the formation of newer segments. As each section reaches gravidity, it releases its mass of eggs by passing them through a uterine pore, by splitting open, or by simply disintegrating. Because the eggs of many tapeworms appear identical, species identification depends on the morphological characteristics of the scolex or gravid proglottides.

Except for *Hymenolepis nana* the tapeworm parasites of humans require one or more intermediate hosts for larval development. Among the *Taenia* group, there is a single intermediate. The eggs or *onchospheres* are passed onto the soil and ingested by the intermediate host in whose tissues they develop into cystlike structures. If the cyst contains a single scolex, it is referred to as a *cysticercus*, or *cysticercoid* in the case of *H. nana*. If several scolices develop within the cyst, it is called a *coenurus* (see "Coenurosis" below). However, if daughter cysts, each containing several scolices are formed, the structure is referred to as a *hydatid* (see "Echinococciasis" below).

Organisms belonging to the *Diphyllobothrium* genus require two intermediate hosts. The eggs, unlike those of the *Taenia* group, are operculated and must be deposited in fresh water. Here they hatch, releasing a free-swimming larva or *coracidium*. This is ingested by a suitable crustacean, the first intermediate host, and is transformed into a procercoid larva. If the infected crustacean is then swallowed by a freshwater fish, the larva invades the tissues of this second intermediate and develops into a plerocercoid larvae or sparganum (see "Sparganosis" below). In both the *Taenia* and *Diphyllobothrium* groups the definitive host is infected after ingesting the flesh of an intermediate host containing the infective larval form.

Human tapeworm infections fall into one of two major clinical groups. In the first, represented by taeniasis *saginata*, humans act as the definitive host, harboring the adult tapeworm in their intestine. In the second, humans are an intermediate host, and harbor the larval forms in their tissues. This is exemplified by sparganosis, coenurosis, and echinococcosis. Taeniasis *solium* is unique because the human may act both as the definitive and intermediate host.

TAENIASIS SAGINATA

DEFINITION Taeniasis saginata is an intestinal infection of humans caused by the beef tapeworm.

ETIOLOGY AND PATHOGENESIS In its adult stage, *Taenia saginata* inhabits the upper jejunum where it may survive for as long as 25 years. The cestode is 5 to 10 m in length and possesses a small, unarmed scolex with four prominent suckers and between 1000 and 2000 proglottides. The gravid segments are longer than they are wide (5 by 20 mm) and have 15 to 30 lateral uterine branches, thus distinguishing it from *T. solium*, which has 8 to 12. The eggs, which are passed within the intact proglottid, measure 30 by 40 μm, have a thick brown radially striated shell, and contain a fully developed embryo with three pairs of hooklets. They are indistinguishable from those of *T. solium*. After the eggs are deposited on soil or vegetation, they are ingested by cattle or other herbivores. The embryo is released in the intestine, invades the intestinal wall, and is carried by vascular channels to striated muscle in the hind limbs, diaphragm, and tongue. Here it is filtered out and is transformed over a period of 3 or 4 months into an ovoid bladder worm, or cysticercus. This form, which may remain viable for 1 to 3 years, measures about 5 by 10 mm and consists of a scolex held in a cystlike structure. After ingestion of the cyst in raw or undercooked beef by humans, about 2 months is required for the adult worm to develop in the intestine.

EPIDEMIOLOGY   Taeniasis saginata occurs in all countries in which it is the custom to eat raw or undercooked beef. It is particularly prevalent in Ethiopia, Kenya, the Middle East, Yugoslavia, Mexico, and parts of South America and the U.S.S.R. Beef tapeworm transmission, although uncommon, continues to occur in the United States, particularly in the Northeastern and Western parts of the country.

CLINICAL MANIFESTATIONS   In probably the majority of cases the disease is asymptomatic. Epigastric discomfort, diarrhea, hunger sensations, weight loss, irritability, nausea, and rarely an increase in appetite have been reported in association with *T. saginata* infections.

Movements of the worm are sometimes apparent, and occasionally proglottides may crawl through the anus, appearing in the bed linen or underclothing of the distraught host. Rarely, segments become impacted in the appendix or cystic or pancreatic duct producing obstruction and inflammation of these organs.

LABORATORY FINDINGS   The diagnosis is usually made by the finding of proglottides in the feces. Several proglottides are shed daily, making their recovery relatively easy. Eggs may be distributed on the stool or perianal area if a proglottid ruptures during defecation, and should be looked for in the absence of segments. The perianal region may be examined as for pinworm infection, using the Scotch-brand tape swab. By this method 85 to 95 percent of infections may be detected, whereas by stool examination only 50 to 75 percent can be recognized. Since the eggs cannot be distinguished from those of *T. solium*, it is necessary to examine carefully either the proglottides or the scolex to identify the tapeworm species correctly.

TREATMENT   Niclosamide (Yomesan) is a highly effective taenicide which kills the scolex and immature segments of the worm on contact. This drug may be given without preparation or purge in a single 2-g dose. Four 0.5-g tablets are thoroughly chewed at one time and swallowed with a small amount of water. Few side effects have been reported. As the worm is digested before it is passed in the stool, no attempt should be made to recover the scolex. The stool should be checked at 3 and 6 months to be certain a cure has been obtained. Alternatively, paromomycin, 1.0 g orally every 15 min for four doses, may be given. Quinacrine hydrochloride (Atabrine), for many years the standard medication for tapeworm, has been largely supplanted by the above medications because of its inconvenience and side effects. The agent does possess the advantage that the entire worm including the scolex is excreted intact, allowing morphological identification.

PREVENTION   The only practical means of preventing infection is the thorough cooking of beef. Temperatures as low as 56°C for as little as 5 min will destroy cysticerci. Refrigeration and salting for prolonged periods or freezing at −10°C for 5 days also destroys the cysticercus. Adequate meat inspection and proper disposal of human excreta also aid in control.

TAENIASIS SOLIUM AND CYSTICERCOSIS

DEFINITION   *Taenia solium*, the pork tapeworm, inhabits the intestinal lumen of humans, its only definitive host. The usual intermediate host is the hog, but in some circumstances, the larval or intermediate stages may also develop in humans, resulting in a condition referred to as *cysticercosis*.

EPIDEMIOLOGY   Taeniasis solium is worldwide but is most common in the U.S.S.R., Eastern Europe, Asia, Africa, Mexico, and South America. At the present time the disease is practically nonexistent in the United States.

ETIOLOGY AND PATHOGENESIS   The hermaphroditic adult resides in the upper jejunum and like *T. saginata* may live for decades. It is about 3 m in length and possesses a globular scolex containing a rostellum with two rows of hooklets. There are seldom more than 1000 proglottides. The gravid proglottid measures about 6 by 12 mm and contains a uterus with 8 to 12 lateral branchings. The eggs resemble those of *T. saginata* but are infective for both human and hog. Although humans may be autoinfected when gravid segments are returned to the stomach by reverse peristalsis, the eggs are more commonly transmitted by the fecal-oral route. When ova are ingested by the intermediate host, the embryo is released from the egg, penetrates the intestinal wall, and is carried by vascular channels to all parts of the body. Localization with development over a period of 2 to 3 months to the encysted larval stage ("bladder worm") occurs predominantly in striated muscle of the tongue, neck, and trunk. The cysticerci are ovoid, gray-white opalescent structures about 1 cm in diameter. They may survive for up to 5 years. Humans become infected with the adult stage following ingestion of undercooked pork containing cysticerci. The scolex is freed and attaches itself to the intestinal mucosa; development to the adult stage begins at this time.

CLINICAL MANIFESTATIONS   Clinical manifestations of adult worm infestation resemble those associated with *T. saginata*. The clinical picture is entirely different when humans serve as the intermediate host. Cysticerci develop in the subcutaneous tissues, in muscles, in viscera, and—of most significance—in the eye and brain. Only a moderate tissue reaction occurs while the scolex is viable, but symptoms occur only in heavy infections. The dead larva, however, behaves as a foreign body and provokes a marked tissue response with muscular pains, weakness, fever, and eosinophilia. The involvement in the brain may be in the form of a meningoencephalitis when the cysticerci are widely distributed. However, epilepsy, brain tumor, encephalitis, and other types of neurological or psychiatric disorders may be simulated. Degenerated cysticerci ultimately calcify.

Infection with the adult worm can be detected by finding eggs in perianal scrapings or in the feces. However, to differentiate *T. solium* from *T. saginata* infection, proglottides or the scolex must be examined. Cysticercosis should be suspected in an individual who has lived in a hyperendemic area and who develops neurological findings. Biopsy of subcutaneous nodules may lead to the identification of typical encysted larvae. Roentgenograms of the soft tissues also often reveal calcified cysticerci. Cerebral arteriography, EEG, or computerized tomography (CT) or radioisotope scan will demonstrate the presence of several small space-occupying lesions. The cysticercosis hemagglutination or complement fixation test may be of help in the diagnosis. The prognosis is in large part determined by the stage and location of the parasite. Surgery may be necessary in cerebral and ocular cysticercosis.

TREATMENT   For removal of the worm in the adult, Niclosamide or paromomycin is given as for taeniasis saginata above. However, because these drugs result in the maceration of worms with release of ova, cysticercosis could theoretically occur. To prevent this, a saline purge should be administered 1 h after completion of therapy.

COENUROSIS

This is a rare infection of humans by the larval stage, or *coenurus,* of the dog tapeworm *Multiceps multiceps.* As in cysticercosis, the subcutaneous tissue, eye, and central nervous system may be involved. Over 60 cases have been reported from around the world. In tropical areas the brain has usually been involved and the cases have ended fatally. Clinically, the presentation is one of a slowly growing tumor. Diagnosis and treatment both rely on surgical excision of the lesion.

HYMENOLEPIASIS NANA

DEFINITION   Hymenolepiasis nana is an intestinal infection of humans, mice, and rats by *Hymenolepis nana,* the dwarf tapeworm. The infection is particularly common in children in whom it is usually asymptomatic.

ETIOLOGY   The life cycle is unique in that both the larval and adult phases occur in the same host. The small, 2-cm adult lives only a few weeks, during which time it can be found in the proximal ileum. Its proglottides are wider than they are long and may number 100 to 200. The gravid segments break apart in the fecal stream releasing their spherical eggs. These measure 30 by 44 μm in diameter and have a double membrane enclosing the embryo with six hooklets. The inner vitelline membrane has four to eight slender filaments arising from each pole. The eggs are immediately infective and when ingested by a new host, the freed oncospheres penetrate the intestinal villi, becoming cysticercoids. Approximately 2 weeks later, the larvae migrate back to the intestinal lumen, attach themselves to the mucosa, and mature into adult worms. In some situations, the eggs hatch before passing in the stool, causing internal autoinfection.

DISTRIBUTION   Dwarf tapeworm infection has been reported in temperate and tropical regions around the globe. It is the most common tapeworm found in the United States, most of the infections occurring in the Southern states. The infection is spread by the direct fecal-oral route and is most common in children and institutional populations.

CLINICAL MANIFESTATIONS   This tapeworm infection is characterized by the presence of many adult worms in the host's intestine. When infection is massive, diarrhea and abdominal pain occur.

TREATMENT   Niclosamide, as prescribed for taeniasis saginata above, is given each day for five consecutive doses. Children under 8 should receive one-half the adult daily dose and infants one-fourth the adult dose. Cure is obtained in 90 percent of patients. Paromomycin, 45 mg/kg daily for 5 to 7 days, may also be effective.

PREVENTION   This is a difficult problem, similar to that encountered in enterobiasis. Only a single host is involved, and the eggs are immediately infective. Personal hygiene should be stressed. The contamination of food by rats and mice should be prevented.

HYMENOLEPIASIS DIMINUTA

Hymenolepis diminuta is a short-lived cestode of rats and mice that occasionally infects small children. Larval development occurs in a wide variety of insect hosts including fleas and mealworms. Humans become infected with the adult tapeworm when they ingest uncooked cereal foods contaminated with these insects. Infection is usually asymptomatic, and the diagnosis is made only when the characteristic eggs are found in the stool. They resemble those of *H. nana,* but are longer (58 by 86 μm) and lack polar filaments. Niclosamide as prescribed for hymenolepiasis nana is the treatment of choice.

DIPYLIDIASIS

Dipylidium caninum is the common tapeworm of cats and dogs. The orange-brown proglottid, which resembles a pumpkin seed, is often passed intact in the stool or migrates through the anal canal. This may cause animals harboring this parasite to drag their buttocks across the floor. The characteristic egg packets are then expelled by the proglottides and ingested by fleas to develop into infective larval forms. The definitive host becomes infected by swallowing involved fleas. Human infections occur primarily in small children who ingest fleas in the process of playing with their pets. The diagnosis is made by recovering the characteristic proglottid or egg packet. Treatment is the same as for *T. saginata* above. Prevention consists of periodic deworming of pets.

DIPHYLLOBOTHRIASIS LATUM

DEFINITION   *Diphyllobothrium latum,* the fish tapeworm or broad tapeworm, produces a disease in its definitive host, including humans, characterized by the presence of the adult worm in the intestinal lumen.

ETIOLOGY AND PATHOGENESIS   The adult *Diphyllobothrium* lies attached to the mucosa of the ileum and occasionally jejunum by a pair of sucking grooves located on the scolex. It may live up to 20 years and achieve a length of 10 to 30 ft. The 3000 to 4000 proglottides are wider than they are long. Unlike *Taenia,* the gravid segments are retained by the worm, and each day a million operculated ova are passed directly in the stool. On reaching water, the egg hatches, releasing a free-swimming embryo. This is eaten by small freshwater crustaceans belonging to the species *Cyclops* or *Diaptomus,* in which it develops into a *procercoid.* When the infected crustacean is swallowed by a fish, the larva migrates into the flesh and grows into a *plerocercoid,* or *sparganum,* larva. Humans are infected by ingesting raw infected fish. The tapeworm matures in the intestine and after 3 weeks is an adult capable of discharging eggs.

EPIDEMIOLOGY   The infection is common in the Baltic and Scandinavian countries, Switzerland, Italy, Russia, Japan, Chile, and Central Africa. It also occurs in the north central United States, south central Canada, and Florida. The maintenance of infection in these areas depends upon the continued disposal of raw sewage into freshwater lakes and the ingestion of improperly prepared fish. Women who sample lutefish or gefilte fish as they prepare these dishes often become infected. Among Ontario Indians, the infection is acquired by the ingestion of salted fresh fish.

CLINICAL MANIFESTATIONS   Most infections are asymptomatic or produce slight, transient abdominal discomfort. Rarely, there may be severe cramping abdominal pain, vomiting, weakness, and loss of weight. Intestinal obstruction has been reported in multiple infections. In a small percentage of infected patients, a tapeworm anemia develops which has many features in common with Addisonian pernicious anemia including central nervous system involvement. The anemia appears to be related to the ability of the tapeworm to compete successfully with its host for vitamin B$_{12}$. A worm located high in the jejunum may take up 80 to 100 percent of labeled vitamin B$_{12}$ ingested by a patient with anemia. Approximately forty percent of fish tapeworm carriers have low serum vitamin B$_{12}$ levels, but only 0.1 to 2 percent develop anemia. These patients tend to be elderly, have diminished production of intrinsic factor, and have worms located in the proximal small bowel. Folate absorption may also be diminished and contribute to the anemia. It has been suggested that lysolecithin, a product of the tapeworm, contributes to the severity of the disease. Neurological manifestations of vitamin B$_{12}$ deficiency are more common than in pernicious anemia and may occur in the absence of hematologic findings. Typically, they include paresthesias, impaired vibration sense, numbness, weakness, and, less commonly, central scotomas secondary to optic atrophy. These findings are reversible with expulsion of the worm.

DIAGNOSIS The characteristic eggs are discharged into the stools in large numbers, making the diagnosis quite easy. They measure 55 to 76 by 41 to 56 μm and possess a single shell with an operculum at one end and a knob on the other. Eosinophilia is often present.

TREATMENT Treatment as prescribed for taeniasis saginata will cure most infections. In the presence of severe macrocytic anemia, parenteral vitamin B$_{12}$ should be given.

PREVENTION The most practical control measure is prohibiting the disposal of untreated sewage into freshwater lakes. Personal protection consists of thorough cooking of all freshwater fish. Freezing of fish at $-10°C$ for 24 to 48 h will also prevent transmission.

SPARGANOSIS

The *sparganum,* or plerocercoid larva, of *Diphyllobothrium*-related tapeworms belonging to the genus *Spirometra* will develop in humans following ingestion (usually in drinking water) of a *Cyclops* bearing the procercoid larva. Sparganosis also follows ingestion of infected frogs or application of infected fresh frog flesh as a poultice. The frog tissues contain the sparganum, which is capable of invading human tissues. The dog and cat are definitive hosts for *Spirometra*. The infection often presents as a painful subcutaneous swelling. The periorbital tissues may be involved with marked palpebral edema and destruction of the globe. A marked eosinophilia is usually present. The location of the larvae determines the prognosis of the infection in humans. Surgery and injection of ethyl alcohol with epinephrine-free procaine to kill the worms is the preferred method of treatment.

ECHINOCOCCIASIS

DEFINITION Echinococciasis is a tissue infection of humans caused by the larval stage of *Echinococcus granulosus* or *E. multilocularis*. These species of echinococcus are distinct morphologically and biologically. In humans, *E. granulosus* produces cystic, expanding lesions, involving the liver and lungs primarily, whereas the lesions of *E. multilocularis* are destructive because of their invasive character.

ETIOLOGY The adult *E. granulosus* is found in the jejunum of dogs, wolves, and other canines, where it may live for 5 to 20 months. It is a small worm measuring 5 mm in length. In addition to the scolex and neck, it has three proglottides, one immature, one mature, and one gravid. The gravid segment splits, either before or after passage in the stool, to release eggs, which appear identical to those of *T. saginata*. When ingested by an appropriate intermediate host such as sheep, cattle, hogs, deer, camels, or humans, the embryos escape from the eggs, penetrate the intestinal mucosa, and enter the portal circulation. Approximately 60 percent are filtered out by the liver; 25 percent lodge in the lung, and the rest are carried into the general circulation to involve the brain, kidney, bones, and other tissues. The larvae that are not phagocytosed and destroyed develop into hydatid cysts, reaching the diameter of 1 cm within 5 months. Most cysts are unilocular and consist of an external laminated cuticula and an inner germinal layer. Fluid fills and distends the cyst. Brood capsules and second- or third-generation daughter cysts develop from the germinal layer. "Hydatid sand" found in the cyst consists of scolices liberated from ruptured brood capsules. Occasionally, evagination of the cyst wall occurs, with the development of a multilocular or alveolar type of lesion. In bone, the cysts are semisolid, invade the medullary cavity and slowly erode bone, producing pathological fractures. The cycle is completed when the hydatid cyst is ingested by a carnivore. The enormous number of scolices are released in the intestine and develop into adult worms. The life cycle of *E. multilocularis* is similar except that small rodents serve as the natural intermediate hosts, and the hydatid cyst is always of the multilocular or alveolar type. Most of the cysts develop in the liver, and progressive invasion of that organ usually occurs. The lesions may metastasize when growth extends into blood vessels.

EPIDEMIOLOGY The dog is the principal definitive host of *E. granulosa*. Sheep, cattle, and, in the Middle East, camels are common intermediates. Human echinococciasis, which is often acquired in childhood, has its highest incidence in countries where sheep and cattle raising is carried out with the help of dogs, particularly in East and South Africa, the Middle East, Central Europe, South America, Australia, and New Zealand. It has been reported from 15 states in this country, but most of these infections were probably contracted outside the United States. Only about 7 percent of cases diagnosed in this country are thought to be autochthonus. Most of these involve well-defined population groups, including the Southwestern Indians, Basque sheep farmers in California, and sheep raisers in Utah. A "sylvatic" focus of *E. granulosa* (var. *canadensis*) exists in Alaska and western Canada, where wolves act as the definitive host and caribou and moose as the intermediate host. A second sylvatic cycle involving deer and coyotes has been reported from California. When humans kill these herbivores and feed their viscera to dogs, a domestic cycle is initiated.

In *E. multilocularis* infection, rodents and deer mice are the natural intermediate hosts, while wolves, foxes, and coyotes serve as definitive hosts. A domestic dog and cat may also harbor the adult worms, and an urban cycle involving the cat and common house mouse has been described. Human infections have been reported from Russia, Central Europe, Canada, and Alaska. An extensive sylvatic focus has been described in the north central United States.

CLINICAL MANIFESTATIONS Enlarging hydatid cysts usually produce tissue damage by mechanical means. The resulting symptoms depend upon the site, type, and rate of growth of the cystic lesions. Approximately one-third of infected patients are asymptomatic when the diagnosis is made by routine medical examination. Of the remainder, most present with the complaint of local discomfort or pain of insidious onset. In 15 percent, however, hydatid rupture initiates an acute emergent illness. Most patients harbor a single hydatid, but as many as 40 percent may have multiple cysts involving more than a single site. The hydatids of *E. granulosa* var. *canadensis,* which occur principally in the lung, are small, grow very slowly, seldom cause symptoms, and are usually discovered on routine chest x-ray. The unilocular hydatids produced by other strains of *E. granulosa* grow somewhat more rapidly (0.25 to 1 cm per year) and eventually may reach enormous size. One-fifth rupture to produce cough, chest pain, and hemoptysis. Hepatic lesions may remain asymptomatic for 5 to 20 years, finally presenting as a palpable abdominal mass or abdominal pain. Rupture through the diaphragm, into the peritoneal cavity, or, most commonly, into the biliary tree occurs in 7 percent of patients. Intrabiliary extrusion often mimics acute recurrent cholecystitis. Obstruction of the bile duct may result in jaundice. Bone lesions with pathological fractures occur, and central nervous system involvement may be manifested by epilepsy or blindness. Cardiac cysts may produce embolic metastases. Unilocular lesions may be secondarily infected, resulting in abscess formation and sterilization of the cyst. Rupture of a hydatid into the bile duct, peritoneal cavity, lung, pleura, or bronchus may produce fever, pruritus, urticarial rash, or an anaphylactoid reaction which is occasionally fatal. Release of the numerous scolices leads to dissemination of echinococcal infection. The multilocular or alveolar cyst of *E. multilocularis* usually presents as a slowly growing hepatic tumor, with jaundice and portal hypertension.

DIAGNOSIS AND TREATMENT The clinical picture is seldom sufficiently characteristic to suggest the diagnosis. When eosinophilia is present, it is helpful. Pulmonary lesions usually present as round, somewhat irregular, masses of uniform density. A smooth rim of calcification is seen on plane x-rays of the abdomen in half of those with hepatic involvement. A liver scan with radioactive isotopes is extremely helpful in detecting the presence of hepatic lesions and should always be done in suspected cases. Ultrasonic scanning will detect small lesions missed with radioisotopic scanning and will reveal the lesion to be fluid-filled. Liver hydatids often show a characteristic rim of opacification on celiac arteriography. The skin test (Casoni's test) is usually positive, but lack of a standard antigen and testing technique limits its usefulness. Moreover, patients with other helminthic diseases, particularly schistosomiasis, may give false positive results. Until a single highly sensitive and specific test is available, immunodiagnosis should be carried out using a battery of tests. The indirect hemagglutination and latex agglutination are most frequently used for screening; they are positive in 90 percent of patients with hepatic and 60 percent of those with pulmonary hydatids. The complement fixation test, although less sensitive, rapidly returns to normal after surgical extirpation of cysts, making it a valuable screening test for residual or recurrent disease. Currently, indirect fluorescent antibody, enzyme-linked immunoabsorbent assay, and counterimmunoelectrophoresis techniques are being evaluated. It appears that the presence of "arc 5" in the recently described immunoelectrophoresis test allows the specific diagnosis of *E. granulosus* infections; technical considerations limit its wide-scale use at this time. Occasionally scolices may be demonstrated in the sputum with the Ziehl-Neelsen stain. Because of serious reactions to the leakage of cyst fluid into the tissues and body cavities, diagnostic aspiration should not be attempted.

There is no established medical therapy. Experimentally, prolonged administration of mebendazole has been shown to be larvicidal, but this treatment cannot be recommended until more information has become available. BCG administration is effective in suppressing the growth and metastasis of experimental *E. multilocularis* infections raising the possibility that effective immunotherapeutic modalities may be available in the future. At the present time, surgical treatment offers the only hope of cure. Patients with small calcified hepatic cysts and pulmonary hydatids of the "canadensis" variety need to be operated on only if they are symptomatic or the lesion continues to enlarge over time. All others should have their cysts excised or sterilized and drained. The cyst should be widely exposed and the contents sterilized with 10 ml 10% Formalin, 1% iodine, or 30% sodium chloride before an attempt is made to open it. The entire endocyst should then be removed if possible, and all biliary or bronchial fistulas carefully closed. The residual space must be obliterated to prevent postoperative infection or prolonged drainage. Omentoplasty is the procedure of choice in abdominal cases.

PREVENTION In prevention, (1) contact with infected dogs should be avoided, particularly fecal contamination of the hands and food; (2) infected carcasses and offal should be burned or buried, in order to prevent access of dogs to material containing scolices; and (3) dogs should be treated if found to be infected. The reduction of the incidence of echinococciasis in Iceland is an example of the efficacy of control measures.

REFERENCES

BARBOUR AG et al: Hydatid disease screening. Sanpete County, Utah 1971–1976. Am J Trop Med Hyg 27:94, 1978

CALAMAI G et al: Hydatid disease of the heart: Report of 5 cases and review of the literature. Thorax 29:451, 1974

GELFAND M, JEFFREY C: Cerebral cysticercosis in Rhodesia. J Trop Med Hyg 76:87, 1973

HERMOS JA et al: Fatal human cerebral coenurosis. JAMA 213:1461, 1970

JONES TC: Cestodes. Clin Gastroenterol 7:105, 1978

LITTLE JM: Hydatid disease at Royal Prince Alfred Hospital, 1964 to 1974. Med J Aust 1:903, 1976

MATOSSIAN RM: The immunologic diagnosis of human hydatid disease. Trans Roy Soc Trop Med Hyg 71:101, 1977

MOST H: Drug therapy: Common parasitic infections of man. N Engl J Med 287:495, 1972

NEWMAN CM, ARON BS: Roentgen diagnosis of tapeworm infestation. J Mt Sinai Hosp NY 28:91, 1961

PAWLOWSKI Z, SCHULTZ MG: Taeniasis and cysticercosis *Taenia (Taenia saginata).* Adv Parasitol 10:269, 1972

PERERA DR et al: Niclosamide treatment of cestodiasis: Clinical trials in the United States. Am J Trop Med 19:610, 1970

PORAT S, JOSEPH KN: Hydatid disease of bone. Israel J Med Sci 14:223, 1978

SCHULTZ MG et al: Epidemiology of beef tapeworm infection in the United States. Public Health Rep 85:169, 1970

TAYLOR RL: Sparganosis in the United States. Report of a case. Am J Clin Pathol 66:560, 1976

VICARY FR et al: Ultrasound and abdominal hydatid disease. Trans Roy Soc Trop Med Hyg 71:29, 1977

VON BONSDORFF B et al: Vitamin B$_{12}$ deficiency in carriers of the fish tapeworm, *Diphyllobothrium latum.* Acta Haematol 24:15, 1960

WILLIAMS JF et al: Current prevalence and distribution of hydatidosis with special reference to the Americas. Am J Trop Med 20:224, 1971

WILSON JF et al: Cystic hydatid disease in Alaska. Am Rev Resp Dis 98:1, 1968

XANTHAKIS D et al: Hydatid disease of the chest. Report of 91 cases surgically treated. Thorax 27:517, 1972

214

SCABIES, CHIGGERS, AND OTHER ECTOPARASITES

JAMES J. PLORDE

SCABIES Scabies is a cosmopolitan skin infection commonly referred to as the "seven-year itch." It is caused by a burrowing mite, *Sarcoptes scabiei,* and is transmitted from person to person by close bodily contact, particularly among bed partners. Although the disease is more common in the poor and unclean, sporadic cases involve individuals of all socioeconomic groups. There has been a worldwide resurgence of this infection over the past 20 years, and in the United States it currently involves 2 to 4 percent of patients seen in dermatologists' offices.

The turtle-shaped female measures 0.4 mm in length and possesses four pairs of legs. With the help of the two anterior pair and her mouth, she burrows into the superficial layer of the epidermis. Here she deposits two or three enormous eggs daily until she dies 30 to 60 days later. The newly hatched larvae mature to adulthood within 2 weeks to continue the cycle of infection. Although an involved person may harbour thousands or occasionally millions of adult mites, the average number of adult females per infection is 11.

Two-thirds of the burrows are found in the upper extremities, particularly on the interdigital spaces of the hands and the flexor surface of the wrists. In heavy infections, other sites are typically involved. These include the dorsal surfaces of the elbows, anterior axillary folds, female breasts, periumbilical area, penis, and buttocks. In bedridden patients, lesions are often concentrated over pressure points. The face, head, palms, and soles are seldom involved in adults. Characteristically, a burrow appears as a short dark wavy line which may end in a small vesicle, the site of the adult female.

Sensitization to the mites and their products begins approximately one month after infection and results in a papular or eczematous reaction at the sites of involvement. Itching is often severe and tends to be more marked at night or after a hot bath. Scratching frequently leads to secondary infection with pustulation; acute glomerulonephritis has followed infection with nephrogenic strains of streptococci. Occasionally, reddish pruritic nodules are seen in the groin and axillary regions. Infected individuals with good personal hygiene usually have few lesions, and burrows may be difficult to identify. In mentally retarded, debilitated, or immunosuppressed patients, a particularly virulent infection known as *Norwegian scabies* is sometimes seen. Millions of mites may be present, producing a highly infectious exfoliative dermatitis; itching is often mild or absent. Scabies usually terminates spontaneously in a few months, but chronic cases do occur.

The diagnosis should be considered in any patient presenting with a pruritic eruption, particularly if it involves several members of a living group. The occurrence of symmetric lesions at the sites of predilection should initiate a search for the characteristic burrows. These should be vigorously scraped with a sterile needle or scalpel blade, and the scrapings transferred to a drop of 10% potassium hydroxide on a glass slide. A cover slip is placed over the top, and the preparation examined for adults, larvae, and eggs. The diagnosis can also be made on histological sections prepared from a punch biopsy. Considering the mode of disease transmission, individuals shown to have scabies should also be checked for venereal disease.

All sexual contacts and household members should be treated simultaneously with the patient to prevent the occurrence of "ping-pong infections." The therapeutic agents are applied topically, covering the skin thinly but completely from the neck down. Although the patient is rendered noninfectious within 24 h, up to 2 months may be required for the clinical manifestations of the disease to disappear completely. Needless retreatment during this period can lead to contact dermatitis.

A number of effective agents are available for use. Gamma benzene hexachloride (Gamene, Kwell) is left on for 12 h and then thoroughly washed off. Care must be taken to keep it away from eyes and mucous membranes. It should not be used in infants or pregnant adults. Benzyl benzoate (25%) is administered in a similar fashion. Crotamiton (Eurax) is massaged into the skin, and a second dose applied 24 h later. Antihistamines or salicylates are helpful in counteracting pruritus. Topical steroids may potentiate the infection and should not be used. Antibiotics are required occasionally when there is a significant bacterial superinfection.

CHIGGER MITES The term *chigger* is used to refer to larvae of harvest mites belonging to the family Trombiculidae. The cosmopolitan adults feed on vegetable matter and deposit their eggs upon the ground. The tiny (0.4 mm) emergent larvae crawl along the ground and upward onto vegetation. Here, they await the passage of a vertebrate host, upon which they must feed before again dropping to the ground and molting. In humans, the chigger usually attaches about the ankles, but some advance along the skin until they are stopped by tight-fitting clothing. It then pierces the skin, releases a digestant to liquefy tissue cells, and feeds for 3 or 4 days. Within a few hours, the chigger's secretions have produced an intensely pruritic papule 0.5 to 2 cm in diameter. This usually vesiculates, resulting in a chickenpox-like lesion. Occasionally, subcutaneous bleeding results in a surrounding area of ecchymosis. The lesion and itching may persist for several weeks. In the United States, most clinical cases are seen during the summer months; in warm climates, the seasonal pattern is missing. Treatment is directed at the relief of itching and the prevention of secondary infections. Insect repellants are highly effective prophylactic agents.

FLEAS Fleas are small wingless laterally compressed ectoparasites of humans and other warm-blooded animals. They tend to be found on the hairy portions of the host where they feed and deposit their eggs. The active larvae which hatch in 3 days can be found on the host, in its nest, or in dust. They eventually pupate and may remain dormant for weeks or months before completing their development to adults.

Medically, fleas serve as both vectors and agents of disease. Rodent fleas of the genus *Xenopsylla* are the most important. They are responsible for the transmission of both plague (*Pasteurella pestis*) and murine typhus (*Rickettsia mooseri*) from animal reservoirs to humans. Humans may also acquire the rat tapeworm *Hymenolepis diminuta* by swallowing fleas containing the cysticeroid. The dog tapeworm *Dipylidium caninum* may be transmitted in a similar fashion. The bites of these and other species of fleas belonging to the family Pulicidae can induce an irritating dermatitis. In addition, the tungidae (*Tunga penetrans*) may burrow into the subcutaneous tissues, producing a painful and debilitating disease.

Flea dermatitis   The fleas of humans (*Pulex irritans*), cats and dogs (*Cetenocephalides*), and rodents (*Xenopsylla*) may all induce dermatitis. In many individuals, the bites seem completely innocuous, but in sensitive persons, the saliva induces an erythematous raised pruritic papule. Repeated scratching may result in secondary infection with pustulation or ulceration. The intense pruritus, the ability of the flea to escape capture by virtue of its prodigious jumping ability, and the difficulty involved in crushing their hard chitinous bodies has led to many a frustrating nocturnal safari dedicated to the destruction of this unwanted bed partner. Control is effected by the use of frequent vacuuming to remove eggs, larvae, pupae, and adults from the environment. Insecticide sprays are also of help, but fleas have developed resistance to many of these. Dogs and cats should be washed, flea collars should be applied, and kennels should be dusted or sprayed with DDT or Malathion. If rat runs can be located, they should also be dusted.

Tunga penetrans, sometimes referred to as a *jigger* or *chigoe flea*, is a burrowing flea found in the tropical areas of South America and Africa. These small (1 mm) free-living insects reside in sandy soil. The fertilized female burrows into the skin of the first warm-blooded animal encountered. In humans, they usually embed on the sole of the foot or under a toenail with only their anal pore exposed to the outside. Multiple infections are common. As the female becomes engorged with blood and eggs, a painful and pruritic pea-sized swelling is produced. Eventually, the overlying skin ulcerates, the flea dies, and the eggs are extruded. Secondary bacterial infections including tetanus and gas gangrene occur commonly. Autoamputation of the toes has been reported from Africa. The intact flea can usually be extracted by gently enlarging the entrance hole with a sterile needle and then applying pressure from the side. Alternatively, the lesion can be soaked in Lysol, the flea penetrated with a needle, and the lesion resoaked to kill the eggs and sterilize the wound. Antibiotics may be required to treat secondary bacterial infections.

PEDICULOSIS   Lice are obligate human ectoparasites that complete their entire 30- to 40-day life cycle on the body of the host. *Pediculus humanis* var. *capitis* infests the head, *P. humanis* var. *corporis* the body and clothing, and *Phthirius pubis* (crab lice) the genital and occasionally other hairy areas of the body. All three are flattened dorsoventrally and measure 2 to 3 mm in length. The crab louse is broader and flatter than *Pediculus* and possesses powerful claws on its second and third legs with which it clings to the pubic hair. The females lay five or six eggs daily which they firmly attach to the hairs or, in the case of the body louse, the clothing of the host. These clearly visible tiny white nits hatch in 8 to 10 days. The resulting nymph

matures to adulthood in an additional 2 weeks. Both the larvae and adults take two blood meals daily, leaving behind a small purpuric puncture site. With repeated exposure, the host develops an inflammatory hypersensitivity reaction manifested as a small red papule at each new feeding site. Pruritus results in scratching, a weeping dermatitis, and secondary infection. Chronic infections of the scalp may result in a fetid mass of matted hair and exudate. On the body and genital areas, the lesions may become pigmented—so-called "vagabond disease." Heavy infections with *P. pubis* may involve the eyebrows and eyelids leading to blepharitis.

Lice can be transferred from person to person by direct contact or via discarded clothing in which the body louse can survive for up to a week. Migration is stimulated by fever, making *P. humanis* var. *corporis* an efficient vector of relapsing fever (*Borrelia recurrentis*), typhus (*R. prowazeki*), and trench fever (*R. quintana*). *Phthirius pubis* is not known to be a vector of human disease.

The diagnosis is suggested by the typical dermatitis and confirmed by finding the adults or nits on the hair or clothing of the patient. The treatment of choice is 1% gamma benzene hexachloride (lindane, Kwell). In head infections, the hair should first be shampooed with ordinary soap. Kwell shampoo is then rubbed in at least 4 min, the hair rinsed, dried, and combed with a fine-tooth comb to remove the nits. The process should be repeated in 7 days. The clothing and bedding of the patient with body lice are heat-sterilized. The patient's body should be lathered for 4 min with Kwell shampoo and then rinsed thoroughly. The therapy may be repeated in 7 days. In crab louse infestations, Kwell cream or lotion should be used on the involved areas and left for 24 h. In hirsute individuals, the treatment can be repeated in 1 week. If the eyelashes are involved, 0.25% physostigmine ophthalmic ointment is applied twice daily for 10 days. Lice and nits are carefully removed with a cotton-tipped applicator. Narrow-angle glaucoma should be ruled out before the physostigmine is used.

MYIASIS   Infections with maggots or fly larvae are seen worldwide in a variety of animals. Human involvement occurs most frequently where people live in close contact with domestic animals. Many different species of flies are involved. In some, an animal host is required for larval development; in these, the larvae are capable of invading normal tissue or enter the body through the nose, mouth, or ears. Others are opportunists, depositing their eggs or larvae in the open wounds of debilitated patients. The clinical manifestations vary with the species of fly and site of involvement. Four of the more common clinical syndromes are described below.

Localized cutaneous myiasis   In tropical America the lesions are produced by *Dermatobia hominis*, the human bot fly. This remarkable forest-dwelling diptera captures a mosquito or other blood-feeding insect on which to deposit its packet of eggs. When this unwilling vector then lands on a warm-blooded animal to feed, the eggs hatch and penetrate the feeding site. Within the skin of the host, the larva develops for 2 or 3 months. Finally, it emerges, drops to the ground, and pupates. The lesions are most frequently seen on unprotected areas of the body including the hands, feet, head, and neck. During the first week of infection, the pruritic lesion closely resembles a mosquito bite. As the larva grows and begins to move, it produces severe pain and itching. Tissue destruction and inflammation results in the development of a furuncle-like lesion. Generally, a central opening is present through which the posterior end of the larva protrudes. A dark serosanguinous discharge containing the feces of the insect may be noted.

In Africa, a similar lesion is produced by *Cordylobia anthropophaga* (Tumbu fly). These flies deposit their eggs on sandy soil or laundry laid out to dry. The larvae hatch and invade the unbroken skin of humans or wild rodents, where they mature in 8 or 9 days. In either case, the larvae can be surgically extracted without difficulty. In Tumbu fly infections, letting the larvae mature and drop off spontaneously may be appropriate. This process can occasionally be hastened by applying mineral oil to the central opening. This results in the suffocation of the larva and stimulates its early exodus.

Cutanea larva migrans This is usually caused by the large (1 to 2 cm) horse bot flies belonging to the genus *Gasterophilus*. When the larvae hatch on the skin, they penetrate to the lower epidermis. Because they do not mature in humans, they may migrate in the skin for several months. Clinically, the infection presents as a pruritic serpiginous band of erythema closely resembling cutanea larva migrans produced by *Ancylostoma braziliense*. The diagnosis can be made by placing a small drop of mineral oil on the skin just in advance of the worm tract. This allows visualization of black backward-directed spines on its body segments. The parasite can be easily removed with a sharp needle. Occasionally, the larvae may penetrate the eye. A similar clinical picture is sometimes produced by the larvae of *Hypoderma* spp. (cattle bot fly). These, however, often penetrate deeply into the subcutaneous tissue and produce more pain and less pruritus than *Gasterophilus* larvae.

Deep-tissue myiasis Screw flies of several genera can deposit large batches of eggs on unbroken skin or in wounds, ears, or the nose. After hatching, the larvae burrow into the tissues and develop for 2 or 3 weeks. The mature 1- to 2-cm larvae then drop to the ground and pupate. At times, they penetrate deep tissues, including the eye, nasal sinuses, and cranium, where they produce destructive foul-smelling lesions. Bacterial superinfection is common. In India and Africa, the flies are usually of genus *Chrysomyia*. In the Western Hemisphere, *Callitroga* spp. are involved. The occurrence of human cases in the United States often accompanies epizootics of screw worm activity. Flesh flies of the family Sarcophagidae have also been implicated in deep-tissue myiasis both in the United States and elsewhere. In all the above infections, the lesions should be surgically incised and debrided, the larvae removed, and secondary infections treated.

Intestinal myiasis When humans ingest food contaminated with the eggs or larvae of several genera of flies, some survive passage through the stomach and later mature in the intestine before they are extruded in the stool. In the United States, *Tubifera tenax* is the most frequently implicated species. Invasions of the intestinal mucosa may occur with *Sarcophaga* infections.

REFERENCES

ACKERMAN AB: Crabs—the resurgence of *Phthirius pubis*. N Engl J Med 278:950, 1968

FAUST EC et al: *Craig and Faust's Clinical Parasitology,* 8th ed. Philadelphia, Lea & Febiger, 1970

HUNTER GW et al: *Tropical Medicine,* 5th ed. Philadelphia, Saunders, 1976

MACIAS EG et al: Cutaneous myiasis in South Texas. N Engl J Med 289:1239, 1973

MAEGRAITH BC (ed): *Adams and Maegraith Clinical Tropical Diseases,* 5th ed. Oxford, Blackwell Scientific Publications, 1971

ORKIN M, MAIBACH MI: Current concepts in parasitology. The scabies pandemic. N Engl J Med 298:496, 1978

215
DISORDERS CAUSED BY VENOMS, BITES, AND STINGS

JAMES F. WALLACE

INTRODUCTION Humans have the propensity to come into contact with a great variety of venomous animals. These contacts occur with many zoologic classes including snakes, lizards, sea animals, spiders, scorpions, and numerous species of insects. In general two types of injuries result: those due to the direct effect of venom on the victim, as exemplified in snakebite, and those due to indirect effects of the poison, of which hypersensitivity reaction to bee stings is an example. Each year in the United States at least 50 persons die as the result of venomous injuries. Three groups of animals—hymenopterous insects, snakes, and spiders—account for over 90 percent of the fatalities. Of even greater public health significance is the loss in economic productivity and human potential resulting from the many serious, nonfatal envenomations which occur annually in otherwise healthy children or working adults.

SNAKE BITE **Epidemiology** Fewer than one-tenth of the nearly 3500 known species of snakes are venomous. These poisonous varieties belong to five families or subfamilies: Elapidae (cobras, kraits, mambas, and coral snakes) found in all parts of the world except Europe; Viperidae (true vipers) found in all parts of the world except the Americas; Hydrophidae (sea snakes); Crotalidae (pit vipers) found in Asia and the Americas; and Colubridae (boomslangs, bird snakes) of the African continent. The poisonous varieties of the United States, with the single exception of the coral snake, are pit vipers and include rattlesnakes, the water moccasin, and the copperhead. Although this discussion centers around these species, the therapeutic measures outlined are applicable to snakes in all parts of the world.

The number of individuals bitten by poisonous snakes in the United States is estimated to be about 8000 per year, with a relatively large number occurring in the Southeastern and Gulf states, particularly Texas. Deaths are not reported separately but are undoubtedly rare, numbering fewer than 20 per year, and most are due to bites of various species of rattlesnake. In many European countries deaths from snakebite have averaged only one every 3 to 5 years for the last half-century. In contrast, the estimate of annual deaths from snakebite throughout the world is between 30,000 and 40,000 with the largest number occurring in the countries of Burma and Brazil, where 2000 deaths are estimated to occur each year.

Etiology The *coral snake* is found in the Southern states from Florida to Arizona. It is usually marked by alternating red and black bands separated by yellow rings; however, black and albino forms exist. Coral snakes are generally nocturnal in their activities, shy and elusive, and rarely bite humans. Their fangs are short and permanently erect; the highly toxic venom is injected into multiple puncture wounds produced by a series of chewing movements.

The *pit vipers* are so named because of a small pit between the eye and the nostril. Large venom glands in the temporal regions give the head a triangular appearance. They are generally aggressive and likely to strike if disturbed. The fangs are long and hinged, folding posteriorly when the mouth is closed. Pit vipers strike suddenly with a forward thrust of the head. The instant that the erect fangs make contact, venom is expressed by sudden muscular contraction.

The *rattlesnakes,* recognized by the horny rattle on the tail, which buzzes when the snake is disturbed, are widely distributed. The diamondbacks (*Crotalus adamanteus* in the Southeast and *C. atrox* in the Southwest) are the largest and most dangerous snakes in this country. Others include the prairie rattler (*C. confluentus*), the timber rattler (*C. horridus*), and the pigmy rattlers.

The *water moccasin,* or cottonmouth (*Agkistrodon piscivorus*), is found in swampy areas or along the banks of streams. It is a strong swimmer and can bite under water. This snake is notorious for inflicting severe facial bites when disturbed in the branches of small trees. The copperhead, or highland moccasin (*A. mokasen*), is a closely related species. Its bite is painful but rarely fatal.

Pathogenesis SNAKE VENOMS The venoms of most species which have been analyzed have been found to be mixtures of several toxic proteins and enzymes with diversified and complicated pharmacological effects. An an example, the venom of the Indian cobra (*Naja naja*) contains these distinct and separate substances: a neurotoxin, a hemolysin, a cardiotoxin, a cholinesterase, at least three phosphatases, a nucleotidase, and a potent inhibitor of cytochrome oxidase. Several venoms, including those of the pit vipers, contain hyaluronidase and numerous proteolytic enzymes. Although the exact roles of these components in toxicity are incompletely understood, the venom of a given species is usually predominantly neurotoxic or necrotizing, and frequently associated with hemolysis, abnormalities of blood coagulation, changes in cardiac dynamics, and alterations in vascular resistance. The venom of elapids, including the coral snake, is neurotoxic, with death resulting from respiratory paralysis probably caused by damage to brain centers and a curariform interference with transmission at the neuromuscular junction. The venom of crotalid snakes produces local tissue injury, hemorrhage, and hemolysis; death is often preceded by circulatory collapse associated with a marked fall in circulating blood volume resulting from pooling of blood in the microcirculation, and loss of plasma due to increased capillary permeability. Systemic absorption of venom occurs through the lymphatics, and therapeutic measures designed to reduce lymphatic function are helpful in controlling symptoms.

FACTORS AFFECTING SEVERITY OF SNAKE BITE Several factors affect the outcome of snake bite:

1 The age, size, and health of the patient. Envenomation in children is usually serious, and a fatal outcome more likely, since a relatively large dose of poison is injected into a small victim.
2 Location of bite. Bites on extremities or into adipose tissue are less dangerous than those on the trunk, face, or directly into a blood vessel. A direct strike of the fangs is more dangerous than a scratch, a glancing blow, or one hitting a bone. The discharge orifice of a fang is well above its tip so that the point of the fang can penetrate the skin without envenomation; even a thin layer of clothing may afford great protection. Because of the superficial nature of the wound as many as one-fifth of patients bitten by venomous snakes will have no evidence of envenomation, even though the fangs have penetrated the skin.
3 The size of the snake (a large pit viper can inject over 1000 mg venom, six times a lethal dose for an adult), the extent of its anger or fear (if hurt it may inject a larger amount of venom), the condition of the fangs (broken or recently renewed), and the condition of the venom glands (recently

discharged or full). All these factors are important. Contrary to popular belief, the bite of a snake which has recently killed and fed is not necessarily less venomous for humans; the snake usually does not exhaust its venom in a single bite.
4 The presence of various bacteria, particularly clostridia and other anaerobic organisms, in the mouth of the snake or on the skin of the victim. This may lead to serious infection in the necrotic tissues at the local site.
5 Exercise or exertion, such as running, immediately after the bite. This speeds systemic absorption of toxin.

Manifestations Following the bite of a pit viper, severe burning pain develops within a few minutes at the site of the wound. Local swelling rapidly develops and spreads in all directions, accompanied by the appearance of ecchymoses and bullae over the involved area. As the edema spreads, serosanguinous fluid oozes from the puncture wounds. Later gangrene of the skin and subcutaneous tissues may develop. Systemic effects resulting from the absorption of venom and local tissue destruction may include fever, nausea and vomiting, circulatory collapse, bleeding into the skin and from all body orifices, low-grade jaundice, neuropathic muscle cramping, pupillary constriction, disorientation, delirium, and convulsions. Death may occur after 6 to 48 h. Survival may be attended by massive local tissue loss from gangrene or secondary infection, or may be complicated by acute renal failure, secondary to disseminated intravascular clotting and cortical necrosis, or by tubular necrosis following circulatory collapse.

The bite of the coral snake causes little pain and local swelling. There are usually multiple fang marks. Within 10 to 15 min numbness and weakness begin in the region of the bite followed by ataxia, ptosis, pupillary dilatation, palatal and pharyngeal paralysis, slurring of speech, salivation, and occasionally nausea and vomiting. The patient becomes comatose, develops respiratory paralysis and seizures, and dies within 8 to 72 h.

Cobra bites are painful and are often accompanied by severe hemolysis, local necrosis, and sloughing in addition to their neurotoxic effects. There is little pain and no edema at the site of a sea snake bite. Symptoms of systemic envenomation follow a latent period which may vary from 15 min to 8 h. Although the venom is both myotoxic and neurotoxic, the injury to skeletal muscle is most prominent and is characterized by generalized muscle pain, weakness, and myoglobinuria. Hemorrhagic manifestations predominate following envenomation by colubrids (boomslangs and bird snakes) and many pit vipers including certain species of rattlesnake.

Laboratory abnormalities In severe cases, laboratory abnormalities may include progressive anemia, polymorphonuclear leukocytosis of 20,000 to 30,000 cells per cubic millimeter, thrombocytopenia, hypofibrinogenemia, disordered tests of coagulation, proteinuria, and azotemia.

Treatment An attempt should be made to determine with certainty that the patient has been bitten by a poisonous snake. Absence of distinct fang punctures and failure of local pain, edema, numbness, or weakness to appear within 20 min are strong evidence against snake venom poisoning. If the species of snake is not known, the offending reptile should be killed for the purpose of identification.

FIRST AID This consists of reassuring and calming the victim and instituting measures to retard the absorption of venom and to remove it from the tissues as quickly as possible after the bite. The patient should be promptly placed at rest and the bitten extremity immobilized to reduce the rate of spread of the venom. If anatomically feasible, a wide tourniquet should be placed a few centimeters above the bite and made tight enough to allow one finger to pass beneath with difficulty. The purpose is to impede lymph flow; it is not necessary to obstruct venous return. The tourniquet should be loosened and moved proximally at hourly intervals when local swelling causes it to tighten. Unless the victim can be transported to a hospital within less than 15 min, incision and suction of the wound should be started prior to evacuation. By use of whatever antisepsis is available, 1.0 cm *linear* (not cruciate) incisions about 0.5 cm deep should be carefully made through each fang mark and suction applied. A rubber bulb, breast pump, or heated jar are all preferable to mouth suction, but if other means are not available and no oral lesions are present, this method may be employed. Suction should be continued for at least 1 h following the bite, or until antivenin has been administered. The practice of making multiple incisions along the advancing edge of edema as swelling progresses has not been found to be beneficial and is no longer advised. *Incision and suction are extremely important and should be diligently carried out in every poisonous snake bite.* When begun promptly, they may result in the removal of up to 50 percent of subcutaneously injected venom.

As soon as possible, the patient should be transferred to a hospital. Immobilization of the affected part during transportation is important in controlling lymph flow and is best achieved by splinting. Although ice packs relieve pain and slow lymphatic drainage, they do not neutralize venom, and even a small amount of cooling may result in irreparable damage to already injured tissues by causing ischemia. For this reason, it is recommended that no form of cryotherapy be used.

IMMEDIATE HOSPITAL CARE This should include appropriate treatment for shock and respiratory difficulty, antivenin, measures to combat infection, and general supportive care.

Antivenin is the only specific treatment of snake venom poisoning, and its use in severe bites is vital. In the United States polyvalent crotaline antivenin effective against all American pit vipers and antivenin for North American coral snake poisoning are commercially available. Both products are a lyophylized powder of refined horse serum. Kits are available containing antivenin powder (reconstituted by diluting with water to 10 ml per ampul), syringe, normal horse serum for prior sensitivity testing of the patient, and detailed instructions. Intravenously administered antivenin leads to the most rapid and effective response. It is not advisable to infiltrate antivenin at the local site. The initial dose should depend upon the amount of envenomation; for bites accompanied by local swelling but no systemic symptoms, 2 to 5 vials (20 to 50 ml) is usually sufficient. When swelling has progressed beyond the site of the bite, and mild systemic symptoms and/or hematologic abnormalities are present, moderate envenomation has occurred, and initial treatment should be 5 to 9 vials (50 to 90 ml). For severe bites, associated with marked local as well as systemic effects and evidence of hemolysis or coagulation abnormalities, 10 to 15 vials (100 to 150 ml) or more should be administered. Larger doses of antivenin should be given to children or small adults to neutralize the relatively higher venom concentrations. When progressive swelling in the bitten part ceases, an adequate dose has generally been achieved; improvement in the victim's clinical signs is often extremely rapid.

In the patient with severe envenomation who is allergic to horse serum, the relative risks of death from anaphylaxis rather than from venom poisoning should be carefully weighed before undertaking desensitization with small doses of diluted horse serum.

No antivenin for other snakes is manufactured in the United States, but antiserum for various types is usually kept on hand at large zoos all over the world. A national antivenin index is maintained by the Oklahoma City Zoo [(405) 271-5454], and telephone consultation service for physicians is also available at the Venom Poisoning Unit of the Los Angeles County/University of Southern California Medical Center.

Maintaining *respiration* by mechanical or other means is important. In patients bitten by elapid snakes, respiratory failure is usually reversible. *Tetanus toxoid* or *tetanus immune globulin* of human origin should be given. If wound infections appear, antibiotics should be used with the knowledge that the predominant microorganisms in the mouths of snakes are gram-negative pathogens. Treatment should be preceded by appropriate aerobic and anaerobic cultures. *Fasciotomy* may be necessary to prevent further ischemic injury to a massively swollen limb. *Surgical debridement* of vesicles and superficial necrotic tissue should be done near the end of the first week following the bite. *Relief of pain* with salicylates or meperidine, moderate sedation, maintenance of fluid balance, measures to combat shock and hemorrhagic diathesis, and appropriate management of coma or convulsions are all important.

The usefulness of corticosteroids to prevent tissue damage or systemic intoxication has not been convincingly demonstrated. However, these drugs may be of value in the management of severe shock associated with envenomation and for allergic reactions following the administration of antivenin.

Prevention In snake-infested regions long trousers, high shoes, boots or leggings, and gloves should be worn. Most important of all is to look where one steps or reaches. A sharp knife or lancet, tourniquet, suction bulb, and antiseptic suffice for an emergency kit, and in inaccessible areas, antivenin should also be carried.

POISONOUS LIZARD BITE Of the nearly 3000 species of lizard in the world, only two are venomous: the Gila monster (*Heloderma suspectum*) of the arid southwestern United States and the closely related Mexican beaded lizard (*H. horridum*) which inhabits the lowland forests of Western Mexico. These reptiles are not aggressive, and virtually every instance of their attacking a human has involved teasing or handling the animals in captivity. The venom is elaborated in eight glands in the floor of the mouth and secreted directly into the oral cavity, where it bathes the teeth, which are grooved posteriorly. The lizard clings tenaciously and is often dislodged only after considerable effort; envenomation occurs by contamination of the wound. The venom contains a potent neurotoxin which is undoubtedly responsible for its lethal effect on experimental animals. Death in humans following a bite is extremely rare. Most often, human envenomation results in tissue injury, excruciating pain, massive edema, and patchy erythema. Acute systemic symptoms may last for 3 to 4 days and include nausea, vomiting, hematemesis, blurred vision, dyspnea, dysphonia, and profound weakness. Intense hyperesthesia of the bitten extremity may persist for several weeks. There is no antivenin available. Treatment should consist of tourniquet, incision, suction, cooling of the bitten area, measures to prevent or combat infection, including tetanus, and supportive measures. Parenteral meperidine (Demerol) or infiltration of local anesthetic around the bite should be used to relieve pain.

SPIDER BITES The bite of many spiders is locally irritating, and several species can cause severe, even fatal systemic poisoning in man. The most numerous and important of the venomous spiders are members of the genus *Latrodectus,* widely distributed throughout the world. In the United States and Canada, *Latrodectus mactans,* the black widow or show-button spider, causes a majority of clinically significant arachnidism. In Florida, *Latrodectus bishopi,* the red-legged widow spider, has been reported to produce human poisoning resembling mild black widow bite. From the Southern and Midwestern states, there are increasing numbers of reports of poisoning from the bite of common brown spiders, including *Loxosceles reclusa* and *Loxosceles unicolor.* These bites are characterized by intense local pain and ischemic necrosis at the site, often followed by deep ulceration. Hemolysis occasionally is seen, and in severe cases hemoglobinuria and acute renal failure may occur.

The symptoms and mortality from bites of large, hairy spiders, the tarantulas, such as *Lycosa raptoria* and *Phoneutria fera* in Brazil or *Glyptocranium gastereanthoides* in Peru, and of such spiders as *Loxosceles laeta* in Chile are similar, with severe ulceration, necrosis, and hemolysis. Neurotoxic manifestations of the type produced by *Latrodectus* are sometimes admixed with local necrosis and hemolysis.

It is the female *L. mactans,* the black widow, that bites humans. She is glossy black with a body 1 cm in diameter, a leg span of 5 cm, and a characteristic red hourglass mark on her abdomen. She spins her web in woodpiles, sheds, basements, or outdoor privies, is very aggressive, and will bite on slight provocation. The venom produces diffuse central and peripheral nervous excitement, autonomic activity, muscle spasm, hypertension, and vasoconstriction.

In the United States, most black widow bites occur between April and October, and many patients are males bitten on the genitalia or buttocks while using a privy. After a momentary sharp pain at the site, there is cramping pain that begins locally within 15 to 60 min and gradually spreads. It may involve all extremities and the trunk. The abdomen is boardlike, and the waves of pain become excruciating, causing the patient to turn, toss, and cry out. Respirations are often labored and grunting. There are also nausea, vomiting, headache, sweating, salivation, hyperactive reflexes, twitching, tremor, paresthesias of hands and feet, and occasionally, systolic hypertension. A mild polymorphonuclear leukocytosis is usual, and many patients have slight fever. After several hours, the pains subside, although mild recurrences for 2 or 3 days are common. It may be a week before well-being is restored. Deaths due to cardiac or respiratory failure have occurred, mostly in children and the aged.

Because the bite itself is not prominent, patients are often thought to have some abdominal catastrophe such as perforated ulcer, pancreatitis, or volvulus. Renal colic, coronary occlusion, tetanus, strychnine poisoning, tabetic crisis, lead colic, and porphyria are other conditions to be ruled out. The abdomen is not tender to palpation in arachnidism, and pains in the extremities are not typical of most of these other disorders.

Treatment   For *Latrodectus* poisoning, treatment consists of measures to relieve pain and administration of antiserum. Initial treatment should include a hot tub bath which affords prompt, although temporary, relief. An intravenous injection of calcium gluconate or magnesium sulfate usually produces dramatic, but transient, cessation of cramps. Opiates are sometimes necessary. When available, a single intramuscular injection of 1 ampul (2.5 ml) reconstituted antiserum usually is quite effective within a few hours. If the cramps return, administration of antiserum can be repeated.

Treatment of *Loxosceles* bites consists mainly of local wound management and treatment of secondary infection if it occurs. The parenteral use of corticosteroids within the first 24 h following a bite has been advocated in order to prevent progression of the lesion, but convincing evidence that this is efficacious is lacking. The ulcer usually heals spontaneously, although skin grafting may be required on occasion. Renal failure should be treated as advised in Chap. 275.

SCORPION STING   Scorpions are eight-legged arthropods. Glands in the terminal segment produce venom, which is injected into the victim by a stinger located on the tip of the tail. Scorpions often enter dwellings. During the day they retreat into crevices; emerging at night, they often get into shoes and clothing and even into bedding. They do not deliberately attack humans, but accidental contact results in a sting.

Of about 650 species, roughly 40 occur in the United States, distributed over three-fourths of the nation. They are most numerous in the South from Florida to California, but the only two lethal species, *Centruroides sculpturatus* and *C. gertschi,* are limited to Arizona and portions of neighboring states. These two species reach a maximal length of about 7 cm. Their sting may be fatal to young children or old people, but seldom to a healthy adult.

Most of the nonlethal species of scorpions in the United States cause only minor reactions, like a bee sting. Some in the Southwest, however, produce local edema and ecchymosis, with burning pain. In contrast, many species whose venom has potentially dangerous systemic effects, including the Arizona *Centruroides,* evoke little or no visible reaction at the site of the sting. There is an immediate burning sensation followed by local paresthesia ("pins and needles"), hyperesthesia, or numbness. These sensations spread to involve the whole extremity, and within an hour or two, malaise, restlessness, lacrimation, rhinorrhea, salivation, perspiration, nausea, and vomiting appear.

The patient passes from an agitated state with hyperactive reflexes into coma; convulsions follow. In addition to these neurotoxic symptoms, cardiovascular effects due to myocarditis may be seen and include various arrhythmias and intractable heart failure. Death usually occurs within 12 h, but sometimes as late as 2 days after the sting.

Treatment   This consists of immediately placing a tourniquet on the extremity just proximal to the sting in order to delay the absorption of venom. If available, ice packs may be applied to the wound and to the affected limb, with care not to create additional tissue injury through freezing. The tourniquet must be removed in 5 to 10 min, but the limb is kept cool for at least 2 h. After this time, if treatment has been applied promptly, no serious effects are experienced following the sting of *C. sculpturatus* or *C. gertschi.* If the sting is on the head, trunk, or genitalia, of course, a tourniquet cannot be used, but the area may be cooled.

Although tourniquet, incision, and suction as in the treatment of snake bite have been recommended, the amount of venom is minute; it produces no local necrotizing effect and is absorbed very rapidly.

Specific antivenin, reconstituted from lyophilized cat serum, is available in some areas and should be employed if the victim develops signs of central nervous system or cardiac involvement. Supportive therapy is directed at combating shock and dehydration. Barbiturates in large doses are useful in reducing restlessness.

Prevention   This depends upon alertness in avoiding contact with scorpions in infested areas. Clothing and shoes should be well shaken before being put on in the morning. Towels and bedclothes should be inspected. A house infested with scorpions can in time be rid of them by closing all obvious ways of ingress; picking up debris in the environment, such as piles of brush, logs, stones; introducing a mixture of fuel oil or kerosene, containing a small amount of creosote, between the earth and the house foundation; and spraying with a mixture of 2% chlordane, 10% DDT, and 0.2% pyrethrins in an oil base.

HYMENOPTERA STINGS Each year in the United States, nearly twice as many people die as a result of bites by hymenopterous insects (including bees, wasps, hornets, yellow jackets and fire ants) as from poisonous snake bites. Occasionally, multiple stings in enormous numbers (500 to 1000) are the cause of death. However, the majority of systemic reactions and deaths are due to allergic reactions to the venoms of these insects.

Hymenopteran venoms contain histamine, various kinins, and other vasoactive substances, phospholipases, and hyaluronidase. They are hemolytic and neurotoxic in addition to being effective hypersensitizing agents. The usual reaction to a single wasp sting or bee sting is sharp pain, local wheal and erythema, intense itching, and in loose tissues, such as the eyelid or genitalia, considerable edema which subsides in a few hours. Only in the rare case when a bee is swallowed or inhaled and edema of the laryngopharynx or glottis develops is there danger. A sting directly into a peripheral nerve can destroy its function for a time, much as does an injection of alcohol. Bell's palsy has followed a sting into the trunk of the facial nerve. Unusual reactions such as optic neuritis, generalized polyneuropathy, and myasthenia gravis may follow a sting. The etiology of these reactions is unknown.

In hypersensitive individuals, a single sting may produce serious anaphylaxis with urticaria, nausea, abdominal or uterine cramps, bronchospasm, massive edema of the face and glottis, dyspnea, cyanosis, hypotension, coma, and death. Sensitization is usually the result of previous stings although most fatalities have occurred in individuals who experienced no apparent allergic reaction to the earlier envenomation. Beekeepers who develop allergic rhinitis followed by asthma when near bees or objects that have been in contact with bees are likely to have serious reactions to stings. It has been estimated that nearly 1 percent of the general population in this country has hymenoptera allergy.

Many species of ant can produce stinging bites with local redness and swelling. The most notorious of these is the fire ant (*Solenopsis saevissima*), whose bite may result in extensive vesiculation and skin necrosis similar to that caused by the brown recluse spider.

Treatment The wound site should be examined for a stinger which, if present, should be carefully removed in order to prevent further envenomation from the attached gland. The local reaction to the usual sting is treated by local cool application and antipruritic lotions or oral antihistamines. Epinephrine, 0.3 to 0.5 ml of a 1:1000 aqueous solution subcutaneously repeated every 20 to 30 min, may be lifesaving in patients with an anaphylactic reaction to a bee sting or wasp sting. A tourniquet to slow the absorption of venom and ice packs to relieve pain may be used. Oxygen, endotracheal intubation, vasopressors, and other supportive measures should be used as needed. In addition, corticosteroids should be employed in severe cases, although their maximum effect is not achieved until several hours after administration.

Prevention Allergic persons should make every effort to avoid contact with these insects, including wearing shoes when outside and not wearing perfumes or bright colors which may attract them. In addition, they should keep epinephrine readily available for immediate use in case of a sting, without waiting for symptoms to develop. Sting kits containing premeasured doses of 1:1000 epinephrine in disposable syringes, tourniquets, and antihistamine tablets are commercially available. Careful instruction in their use should be provided by the person's physician.

Immunotherapy Desensitization by injection of extracts of crushed whole bodies of bees, wasps, hornets, and yellow jackets has been recommended for any patient who has had a systemic or generalized reaction to hymenopterous insect stings. This practice is based on retrospective studies suggesting benefit from this form of immunotherapy. However, skin testing with whole-body extracts has been found unreliable in identifying persons at risk for systemic reactions, and immunization with these extracts has been shown not to increase IgG-blocking antibodies to venom proteins, a response felt to be essential for protection in insect allergy. In contrast, purified hymenopteran venoms, currently available only for investigational use in the United States, have been found highly accurate in diagnosing insect sting allergy by skin testing and have provided much better protection than whole body extracts for immunotherapy of high risk patients. It is likely that purified venom antigens will soon be the preferred materials for diagnosis and desensitization.

TICK BITE The local reaction to the bite of a tick may be nothing more than an itching papule which subsides within a few days unless there is secondary bacterial infection. However, incomplete removal of a tick, with retention of the mouthparts, may result in the local formation of a nodule which continues to grow and is sometimes annoyingly pruritic. The definitive treatment is surgical excision of the nodule. Histologically, the nodule is a granuloma, but the inflammatory response is sometimes so bizarre and changes in the overlying epithelium are so striking that, in the absence of a history of tick bite, a mistaken diagnosis of malignant tumor may be made.

Removal of a tick by steady pulling is preferable to crushing. Touching with a hot object such as a glowing cigarette, freezing, or applying a drop of oil or nail polish facilitates removal without leaving embedded remnants.

Tick paralysis A progressive, ascending, flaccid paralysis which is reversible sometimes develops in humans and certain other mammals while a tick is engorging upon them. Human cases have most frequently been reported from the northwestern United States and Western Canada, where the wood tick, *Dermacentor andersoni* Stiles, is responsible. The dog tick, *D. variabilis* Say, has been identified in a number of cases occurring in the Southeastern states. *Amblyomma americanum,* the Lone Star tick, *A. maculatum,* the Gulf Coast tick, and *Ixodes scapularis,* the black-legged deer tick, have also been incriminated.

This disorder is caused by a neurotoxin apparently injected by the engorging tick. This toxin acts upon spinal and bulbar nuclei, slowing motor nerve conduction without affecting neuromuscular transmission. The toxin appears to be destroyed or excreted rapidly, for when the tick is removed the nerve cells soon regain normal function.

The tick must feed for several days before symptoms develop. Paralysis is seen in experimental animals after 5 to 6 days of engorgement. Male ticks feed for a shorter period than female ticks, a fact which may explain why they are less likely to cause paralysis.

Most human cases occur in children, generally in young girls. The tick is usually attached to the scalp and hidden by the hair, but may be found on any part of the body, especially the ear, axilla, groin, vulva, or popliteal region.

The patient may be irritable and have mild diarrhea for 24 h before frank motor involvement appears. There are weakness and poor control of the legs, the tendon reflexes in the legs are diminished or absent, and the Romberg sign is positive. Temporary improvement may occur, and if the tick is removed at this stage, true paralysis may never develop. Otherwise the symptoms recur within 24 h, with flaccid paralysis which extends in 24 to 48 h to involve the trunk, arms, neck, tongue, and pharynx. Sensory changes are usually absent, but there may be paresthesia and hyperesthesia in the affected extremities. Nystagmus, strabismus, truncal ataxia, and facial paralysis are sometimes noted. There is little or no fever unless a secondary infection is present. The leukocyte count is usually not elevated, but moderate leukocytosis may occur. The spinal fluid is almost always normal.

Tick paralysis is apt to be confused with poliomyelitis, the more so because ticks are active in warm weather when poliomyelitis is most prevalent. Among other diseases which might be considered in differential diagnosis are polyneuritis, transverse myelitis, the Guillain-Barré syndrome, myasthenia gravis, the Eaton-Lambert myasthenic syndrome, and botulism.

Definitive treatment is removal of the tick. Mouthparts retained in the skin should be promptly excised. The patient's body should be searched for other ticks. There is striking improvement within a few hours after removal of ticks.

If the tick is removed before bulbar involvement develops, the paralysis subsides and recovery is complete in a few days, sometimes within 24 h. The patient should be observed until the recovery trend is established, because if other ticks or retained mouthparts have been overlooked, the paralysis may progress. When bulbar or respiratory paralysis is present, death may occur if the tick is not removed in time. Other treatment is supportive.

OTHER ARTHROPOD BITES Flea bite There are many fleas that attack humans, including *Pulex irritans* and chicken fleas. In sensitive individuals, the salivary secretion of these bloodsuckers produces large, itching papules. It is thought that much of the papular urticaria of children is probably due to flea bites. Treatment is symptomatic only. Elimination of fleas from the environment may be very difficult, but persistent treatment of animals and of premises with appropriate insecticides is usually successful.

Centipede bite Local irritation is the usual reaction to centipede venom, although extensive necrosis and systemic illness have followed severe poisoning by tropical species. Treatment is purely symptomatic.

Caterpillar urticaria Contact with hairy caterpillars of many species produces irritation of skin or mucous membranes. The type of venom involved is not known, but severe pain, erythema, urticaria, and even blister formation may come on rapidly after direct contact with caterpillars, after handling cocoons, or on being exposed to windblown fuzz. There are often a regional lymphangitis and transient eosinophilic leukocytosis. The discomfort subsides within 24 h, but local soaks, oral antihistaminics, and, when pain is severe, oral codeine are often indicated.

Bedbug bite Members of the genus *Cimex* inflict bites that leave reactions varying from a simple puncture to large urticarial lesions, apparently depending on the sensitivity of the bitten individual. There is no specific treatment.

Chiggers or redbugs These are tiny mites which are commonly found in foliage, grass, etc., in many parts of the world. In the United States, the larval form of *Eutrobicula alfreddugesi* attacks the skin by secreting a substance which digests tissue, creating a red papule that itches intensely. The tiny reddish larva can be seen in the center of the lesion. Treatment is palliative and consists of antipruritic applications. The use of insect repellents, appropriate protective clothing, and prompt bathing after exposure reduce the risk of infestation considerably.

Bloodsucking-fly bite Many species of flies, particularly the horsefly and the deerfly, viciously attack and feed upon warm-blooded animals, including humans. Occasionally, transmission of diseases such as anthrax, tularemia, loiasis, and trypanosomiasis has been attributed to horseflies and deerflies. More commonly in North America, however, their bites are responsible for painful, intensely pruritic cutaneous lesions which may be followed by delayed localized allergic reactions characterized by erythema, edema, and urticaria. Treatment should include thorough cleaning of the bite sites, topical corticosteroids, and oral antihistaminics for severe itching. Antibiotics may be necessary if the wounds become secondarily infected.

MARINE ANIMAL VENOM DISEASES The venoms of certain marine animals are known to cause illness in humans after injection or inoculation under naturally occurring conditions. Information concerning these toxins is limited; most appear to be composed of proteins and peptides as well as other substances that are pharmacologically active. Although probably less complex than the venoms of reptiles, many marine animal venoms are capable of causing several pathologic effects including neurotoxicity as well as local necrosis.

Portuguese man-of-war and jellyfish stings The burning discomfort induced by contact with sea nettles or jellyfish is familiar to most surf bathers. Contact with the tentacles of the colorful Portuguese man-of-war (*Physalia* species), which is found mainly in or near the Gulf of Mexico, or the more toxic jellyfish (*Chiropsalmus* of the Indian Ocean and *Rhizostoma* of the Atlantic) is followed by burning pain, swelling, and erythema. Severe, generalized muscular cramps, nausea, vomiting, and pulmonary edema may occur. Victims have died as a result of jellyfish stings, sometimes within minutes after contact. In nonfatal cases, systemic symptoms usually subside within several hours.

Treatment consists of removing any tentacles still clinging to the skin after first inactivating the toxins in their nematocysts with local application of alcohol, ammonia, or even dry sand. Analgesics should be used for pain control, and antihistaminics if there is an accompanying pruritic rash. Corticosteroids may be helpful in severe cases.

Sea anemone sting ("sponge diver's disease") Contact with certain sea anemones (especially *Sargatia elegans*) in Mediterranean and African waters produces extensive dermatitis with chronic ulceration. Occasionally, especially during August and September, systemic symptoms of headache, sneezing, nausea, chills, fever, and collapse are noted. Rare fatalities have occurred. No specific therapy is known; symptomatic treatment with topical steroids or oral antihistaminics may provide temporary relief.

Cone shell poisoning The colorful cone shells are highly prized by collectors. However, many species in the Pacific are venomous, a great danger to unwary hobbyists who pick them up. The poison, a neurotoxin, is delivered into a wound inflicted by pointed hollow teeth resembling darts in the long proboscis of the animal. Local manifestations include sudden intense pain, followed by swelling and numbness which may persist for several days. Symptoms of serious poisoning include muscular incoordination and weakness progressing to respiratory paralysis. Death may occur within 3 to 6 h, but recovery within 24 h is the rule. There is no specific therapy; recommended treatment is the use of tourniquet, incision, and suction (as for snake bite), and supportive measures which may include artificial respiration and administration of oxygen.

Sponge dermatitis Direct contact with several species of sponge results in a painful dermatitis, which may persist for several weeks. The lesions appear to be caused by mechanical irritation from the exoskeleton of the sponge as well as by toxins within its tissues. Delayed hypersensitivity reactions may also occur. Antihistaminics provide relief from the pruritus; dilute acetic acid ameliorates local pain strikingly, while alkali will intensify it. The lesions are self-limited.

Sea urchin sting Contact with the spines of some species of sea urchin results in painful erythema and ulceration, occasionally accompanied by neurotoxic symptoms of weakness and frank paralysis of lips, tongue, and face lasting for several hours. Treatment is purely symptomatic and supportive. The toxins isolated from sea urchins have produced paralysis in animals and are notably resistant to heat. Deaths from paralysis and drowning have been reported.

Paralytic and neurotoxic shellfish poisoning Certain dinoflagellates, which compose part of the marine phytoplankton, elaborate a potent neurotoxin. Occasionally, conditions in coastal waters become favorable for the growth of excessive numbers of these organisms, causing the water to develop an amber appearance termed the "red tide" and killing massive numbers of fish by exhausting their oxygen supply. When humans ingest shellfish which have themselves ingested toxic dinoflagellates, an illness occurs characterized by paresthesias of the face and extremities, dysphonia, and generalized muscular weakness, often accompanied by nausea, vomiting, and diarrhea and occasionally by paralysis and respiratory arrest. The more severe syndrome, known as paralytic shellfish poisoning, is encountered along the Pacific Northwest and New England coasts. A milder form, not associated with paralysis in humans, is seen along the Gulf and Atlantic coasts of Florida. Treatment should include induced emesis and purgation to remove unabsorbed toxin from the gastointestinal tract and whatever additional supportive measures are necessary. Spontaneous recovery usually takes place within 24 h. There is a standardized mouse bioassay procedure for demonstrating and quantitating toxin in shellfish but no diagnostic test for detecting toxin in clinical specimens.

Venomous fish stings The dorsal fins or spines of bullhead sharks, dogfish, and ratfish and the dorsal and other fins of the scorpion fish, weeverfish, toadfish, and catfish are grooved, and at their bases are found venom glands. Injury by these spines results in severe pain and swelling and, in some instances, neurotoxic manifestations. Local gangrene with extensive tissue loss is a complication of catfish stings that may prolong convalescence. Little or nothing is known of the venoms involved. Suction and hot application are advocated immediately after injury. Tetanus toxoid or antitoxin should be given also. Narcotics are often required to control the pain. Secondary pyogenic infection is a frequent complication.

Probably the most frequent type of venomous fish injury in the United States is that produced by the lashing tail of the stingray of the California coast (*Urobatis halleri*). The bony spine is encased in a sheath of epithelial cells containing venom which is expressed into the puncture wound. The wound may be several centimeters deep; portions of the bony spine may break off in it, or, more often, the integumentary sheath remains in the wound. The venom is a circulatory depressant in animals, but local injury predominates in humans. There are immediately severe pain and blanching followed by erythema and edema. Symptoms due to systemic absorption of venom are infrequent but may include salivation, muscle cramps and weakness, cardiac arrhythmias, seizures, and death. Treatment consists of application of a tourniquet (the vast majority of these injuries occur on the legs) and copious syringing of the wound with saltwater to remove fragments of sheath followed by immersion in water as hot as the patient can stand for 1 h. The venom is heat-labile, and extensive trials have indicated the usefulness of this last procedure. Tetanus toxoid or antiserum is indicated; as with other fish stings, pyogenic infection is a frequent complication.

REFERENCES

Hymenoptera stings

BARNARD JH: Studies of 400 hymenoptera sting deaths in the United States. J Allergy Clin Immunol 52:259, 1973

BROWN LL: Fire ant allergy. South Med J 65:273, 1972

BRUMLIK J: Myasthenia gravis associated with wasp sting. JAMA 235:2120, 1976

HUNT KJ et al: Diagnosis of allergy to stinging insects by skin testing with hymenoptera venoms. Ann Intern Med 85:56, 1976

——— et al: A controlled trial of immunotherapy in insect hypersensitivity. N Engl J Med 299:158, 1978

LIGHT WC, REISMAN RE: Stinging insect allergy: Changing concepts. Postgrad Med 59:153, 1976

Marine animal venoms

HALSTEAD BW: Poisonous and venomous marine animals of the world. Washington, DC, US Government Printing Office, 1965, vol I; 1970, vol III

HUGHES JM, MERSON MH: Fish and shellfish poisoning. N Engl J Med 295:1117, 1976

KEEGAN HL, MACFARLANE WV (eds): *Venomous and Poisonous Animals and Noxious Plants of the Pacific Region.* Oxford, Pergamon, 1965

RUSSELL FE: Marine toxins and venomous and poisonous marine animals. Adv Marine Biol 3:255, 1965

SCOGGIN CH: Catfish stings. JAMA 231:176, 1975

SOUTHCOTT RV: Notes on stings of some venomous Australian fishes. Med J Aust 2:722, 1970

Other arthropod bites

FRAZIER CA: *Insect Allergy: Allergic and Toxic Reactions to Insects and Other Arthropods.* St Louis, Warren H Green, 1969

HANEVELD GT: Centipede bites. Br Med J 2:592, 1952

KINGERY FAJ: Sorting out bug bites. Med Times 105:102, 1977

MCMILLAN CW, PURCELL WR: Health hazard from caterpillars. N Engl J Med 271:147, 1964

Scorpion stings

BARTHOLOMEW C: Acute scorpion pancreatitis in Trinidad. Br Med J 1:666, 1970

HOREN WP: Insect and scorpion sting. JAMA 221:894, 1972

SITA DEVI S et al: Defibrination syndrome due to scorpion venom poisoning. Br Med J 1:345, 1970

STAHNKE HL: Arizona's lethal scorpion. Ariz Med 29:490, 1972

Snake and lizard bites

ALBRITTON DC et al: Venination by the Mexican beaded lizard (*Heloderma horridum*). Report of a case. S Dak J Med 23:9, 1970

MINTON SA JR: *Venom Diseases*. Springfield, Ill, Charles C Thomas, 1974

RUSSELL FE: Pharmacology of animal venoms. Clin Pharmacol Ther 8:849, 1967

——— et al: Snake venom poisoning in the United States: Experience with 550 cases. JAMA 233:341, 1975

STAHNKE HL et al: Bite of the Gila monster. Rocky Mt Med J 67:25, 1970

WATT CH JR: Poisonous snakebite treatment in the United States. JAMA 240:654, 1978

Spider bites

BERGER RS: A critical look at therapy for the brown recluse spider. Arch Dermatol 107:288, 1973

GORHAM JR: The brown recluse spider, loxosceles reclusa and necrotic spider bite—a new public health problem in the United States. J Environ Health 31:138, 1968.

HOREN WP: Arachnidism in the United States. JAMA 185:839, 1963

Spider bites. Lancet 2:509, 1969

Tick paralysis

CHERINGTON M, SNYDER RD: Tick paralysis: Neurophysiologic studies. N Engl J Med 278:95, 1968

SCHMITT N et al: Tick paralysis in British Columbia. Can Med Assoc J 100:417, 1969

Tick paralysis. Br Med J 3:314, 1969

section 17 | Diseases of uncertain etiology

216
SARCOIDOSIS

CAROL J. JOHNS

INTRODUCTION At the 1975 Seventh International Conference on Sarcoidosis it was proposed that sarcoidosis be described as "a multisystem granulomatous disorder of unknown etiology most commonly affecting young adults and presenting most frequently with bilateral hilar lymphadenopathy, pulmonary infiltration, skin or eye lesions." Other organs commonly involved include peripheral lymph nodes, liver, spleen, mucous membranes, parotid glands, phalangeal bones, muscles, heart, and nervous system. The diagnosis is established most securely when there is involvement of more than one organ system with clinical and radiographic findings, supported by histological evidence of widespread noncaseating epithelioid-cell granulomas in one tissue, with the absence of known agents capable of inducing similar granulomatous lesions (beryllium, tubercle bacillus, fungi, etc.). The Kveim-Siltzbach reaction is frequently positive and lends support to the diagnosis. Impairment of cell-mediated immunity is manifest by depression of tuberculin-type delayed hypersensitivity but well-maintained or increased production of humoral antibodies (immunoglobulins). The clinical course varies from that of a self-limited one, with spontaneous resolution, to that of progressive widespread granulomatous inflammation and fibrosis. Corticosteroids produce clinical remissions and suppress inflammation and granuloma formation. Long-term treatment for many years may be required to prevent clinical relapse.

ETIOLOGY The cause of sarcoidosis remains unknown but most authorities agree it is a specific disease. Whether there is a single inciting infectious or other exogenous agent is unclear. The immunologic features and abnormalities have attracted increasing attention. Impaired regulation of the cell functions of thymus-derived lymphocytes (T cells) and bone-marrow-derived lymphocytes (B cells) is suspected. Such changes could be primary or secondary. A persistent antigen could stimulate release of an immunosuppressive lymphokine and the formation of epithelioid granulomas, probably derived from macrophages. Immune complexes may be implicated. There are other possible factors of genetic susceptibility, but no pattern of histocompatibility antigens has been identified in sarcoidosis. A possible role of the tubercle bacillus has been debated and may be significant in some cases. The disease may be a result of an interaction between an infective agent and a subject with unusual immunologic responses. It cannot be assumed that all cases of sarcoidosis are associated with the same inciting agent. Studies in mice suggest a transmissible agent from human sarcoid tissue, and the tubercle bacillus was identified in a few mice after serial passages through mice and a 0.2-μm filter.

EPIDEMIOLOGY Sarcoidosis has been observed in virtually every country in which it has been sought. Blacks are affected 10 times more frequently than Caucasians in the United States, and the incidence in females is usually double that in males. An increased incidence in relation to pregnancy and lactation has been noted, especially in patients with erythema nodosum. The disease is most frequent in the third and fourth decades of life, but the range begins in childhood, particularly around adolescence, and extends to the sixth and seventh decades. Familial associations are noted occasionally.

PATHOLOGY Granulomatous inflammatory changes of sarcoidosis may occur in almost any organ. Disseminated granulomas are probably often present even with clinically localized disease, i.e., hepatic granulomas with only asymptomatic hilar adenopathy. The hard tubercles are generally sharply demarcated from surrounding tissues but may coalesce. Some central fibrinoid or granular necrosis may occur, especially in association with systemic active febrile disease, but caseation is usually absent, and inflammatory reaction is minimal. Giant cells containing laminated calcific Schaumann bodies or stellate "asteroid" bodies are frequent, but neither of these inclusions is found solely in sarcoidosis.

Similar histological changes may be seen in tuberculosis, fungous infections, leprosy, tertiary syphilis, beryllium disease, "farmer's lung," foreign-body reactions, lymphomas, and lymph nodes draining malignant tumors. The histological picture in sarcoid is not specific for that disease alone, and the above-mentioned possibilities cannot be excluded in the absence of other data.

Adrenal corticosteroids cause a prompt reduction in the nonspecific cellular inflammatory reaction of an acute or subacute process and hasten involution and resorption of the "sarcoid" tubercles. It seems likely that these hormones prevent or lessen but do not erase progressive scarring.

Autopsy material on patients with long-standing sarcoidosis may reveal widespread tubercles in many organs, a few scattered tubercles or focal hyalin scarring, or, rarely, no residual changes.

MANIFESTATIONS Clinical manifestations of sarcoidosis generally depend on the activity, degree, and site of tissue involvement and vary from incidental radiographic findings without associated symptoms, to severe incapacity and death. Impaired function is caused both by active granulomatous disease and by secondary fibrosis. Symptoms are frequently mild or absent.

Constitutional symptoms Fever, weight loss, and fatigue are often nonspecific presenting complaints, occasionally without other localizing symptoms. Persistent daily spiking fever to 38.3°C (101°F) may be observed and necessitates careful exclusion of tuberculosis. This is most commonly observed in association with active granulomatous inflammation in the liver. Fever in association with erythema nodosum is another form in which sarcoidosis may become evident. This syndrome includes transient tender erythematous subcutaneous nodules over the pretibial areas, arthralgias, and pulmonary hilar adenopathy on x-ray. Hepatic tubercles and a positive Kveim reaction are frequent. This syndrome has been regarded as an early manifestation of sarcoidosis and noted frequently in young women in Scandinavia and Great Britain. It is also observed in the United States, may be overlooked easily, and has a favorable prognosis. Fever, hepatosplenomegaly, and hypercalcemia form another presenting syndrome, which is observed more commonly in Caucasian patients.

Lymph nodes Mediastinal and hilar nodes are most frequently involved. Vague substernal discomfort may be present. Readily palpable peripheral nodes which are discrete, firm, and nontender are often prominent. There may be generalized lymphadenopathy, or involvement may be localized to the cervical, axillary, and femoral nodes. Usually, the changes are symmetrical and the epitrochlear nodes are palpable.

Lungs Pulmonary involvement is the most common and, perhaps, the most important manifestation of sarcoidosis. Spontaneous permanent remissions are observed, but significant lung disease represents the most frequent indication for treatment. Serious parenchymal changes, with or without hilar adenopathy, are evident on x-ray in about 50 percent of all patients. Varying and impressive degrees of dyspnea and cough are noted. A discrepancy in which the radiographic changes exceed the symptoms and signs is a diagnostic clue in early sarcoidosis. In some patients, usually Caucasian, striking radiographic changes may be associated with no symptoms, and ventilatory and diffusion measurements are normal. In others, often blacks, pathological and physiological abnormalities may be present when the x-ray shows only hilar adenopathy. Dyspnea may be severe and is present in approximately half the patients with parenchymal disease. This results from extensive interstitial changes which impair oxygenation by disturbances of ventilation and perfusion ratios and loss of effective diffusing surface. Compensatory hyperventilation is often noted. Large rounded intrapulmonary masses which may resemble metastatic tumor are probably a result of primary involvement of lymphoid tissue or localized infiltrates producing minimal physiological disturbance and minimal symptoms despite their dramatic x-ray appearance. Pleural effusions are unusual and should lead to the suspicion that other disease is present.

Cough may be severe and incapacitating and may occur in paroxysms which can even lead to vomiting. Sputum is scanty; occasional blood streaking results from the strain of coughing or endobronchial granulomas or in association with a picture that resembles bronchiectasis. Wheezing is occasionally produced by localized bronchial lesions with stenosis. Pulmonary obstruction is noted in late fibrotic chronic sarcoidosis. Physical findings are variable and nonspecific. Respiratory excursion may be restricted, crackling rales may be heard diffusely or at the lung bases, and the P_2 may be accentuated or split if pulmonary hypertension develops, or in the presence of bundle branch block.

Bronchoscopy generally reveals normal mucosa, although in a few cases it shows granulomatous inflammatory changes with endobronchial narrowing. Granulomas may be demonstrated occasionally in grossly normal-appearing mucosa.

In some patients sarcoidosis is a chronic progressive disease, and pulmonary insufficiency and cor pulmonale occur as late features. Bronchiolostenosis, resulting from peribronchial fibrosis and mucosal changes, may result in localized emphysema, giving rise to cystic changes, usually in the upper lung fields. With superimposed bacterial infection, a bronchiectasis-like picture results. Large cavitary or bullous lesions are rare but may lead to large and repeated hemoptyses, which are occasionally fatal. Such lesions may also form the locus for an aspergilloma, with recurrent hemoptyses. However, these "fungous balls" are usually saprophytic and often multiple. They may vary spontaneously in size and number over periods of 10 or more years, without invasive disease, even when steroid maintenance treatment is required. Surgical management is rarely feasible because of the diffuse and restrictive nature of the disease. Spontaneous pneumothorax is an occasional complication of lung involvement.

Eyes Acute granulomatous uveitis may be the initial manifestation of sarcoidosis. Ocular disease may progress to severe visual impairment and blindness with corneal and lenticular opacities and secondary glaucoma. A careful slit-lamp examination is worthwhile in all patients with sarcoid to detect early evidence of anterior uveitis. Lacrimal gland enlargement, conjunctival infiltrations, and keratoconjunctivitis sicca of the type seen in Sjögren's syndrome (Chap. 363) are common. Exophthalmos has been observed, as have retinal lesions with vasculitis producing papillitis and periphlebitis.

Skin Lesions occur in about 30 percent of patients, most dramatically around the nose, eyes, and mouth, and vary from extensive erythematous, infiltrated, and raised lesions to small nondescript plaques and papules. Mucosal lesions are often associated, extending into the nose, sinuses, and the hard palate. Increased or decreased pigmentation is frequently noted. Sarcoid changes often occur at sites of old scars or tattoos or recent injury. Subcutaneous nodular infiltrations occur, and in rare instances calcification of such lesions has been observed. Alopecia occurs if the scalp is affected. Skin lesions are associated with chronicity but often with otherwise mild disease. Erythema nodosum in early sarcoidosis usually presents a histologic picture of a nonspecific vasculitis.

Liver   Clinical manifestations of hepatic sarcoidosis are present in only about 20 percent of cases. Nevertheless, hepatic tubercles can be found by biopsy in about 75 percent. Asymptomatic hepatomegaly is frequent. Severe jaundice is unusual, but mild increase in bilirubin and striking elevation of serum alkaline phosphatase level are observed. Intense pruritus may be the presenting manifestation. Intrahepatic cholestasis may occur with a picture resembling biliary cirrhosis. The spectrum of hepatic sarcoid includes the incidental tubercle, tubercles with surrounding nonspecific inflammatory reaction, chronic active granulomatous hepatitis, postnecrotic cirrhosis with or without portal hypertension, and portal hypertension without significant cirrhosis. Esophageal varices have been demonstrated in patients with portal hypertension, and shunt procedures occasionally have been required. Response to steroids has been disappointing in severe hepatic sarcoid, but steroids are indicated with a significant active inflammatory process. In some patients the granulomatous disease is limited to the liver, spleen, and abdominal nodes without other clinical or radiographic evidence of sarcoidosis.

Spleen   Mild splenomegaly occurs in 20 to 30 percent of cases and often regresses promptly with administration of corticosteroids. Enlargement may be striking and associated with "hypersplenism," anemia, leukopenia, and thrombocytopenia. It may persist for 10 to 20 years without undue complications, although splenectomy will result in hematologic improvement.

Kidneys   Impaired renal function may occur secondary to hypercalcemia and hypercalciuria, secondary to hyperuricemia, and, less commonly, because of direct granulomatous involvement. Nephrocalcinosis and renal calculi are observed.

Heart   Effects are usually secondary to lung disease, with pulmonary hypertension and cor pulmonale. Primary myocardial sarcoidosis often is not recognized and is most commonly manifested by conduction disturbances, paroxysmal arrhythmias and infiltrative cardiomyopathy. Sudden death may result, and an artificial pacemaker may be required.

Salivary glands   Asymptomatic enlargement of the parotid, sublingual, and submaxillary glands occurs in about 6 percent of cases. Spontaneous regression commonly occurs. A syndrome of fever, uveitis, and lacrimal and salivary gland enlargement is known as uveoparotid fever, or *Heerfordt's syndrome.* Facial nerve palsies may be associated with parotid disease.

Muscle   Sarcoid granulomas occur in muscles far more frequently than is clinically indicated by pain and weakness. In a few cases symptoms may be severe and incapacitating. Muscle biopsy is likely to be positive in such patients and also in those with polyarthralgias.

Joints   Arthralgias may occur independently as an early prominent feature and are common in association with erythema nodosum and fever. Sarcoid tubercles have been observed in biopsies of synovium. Transient knee effusions are occasionally noted. Chronic periarticular swelling and tenderness may be associated with bony changes in the fingers and toes and skin lesions. Monoarticular arthritis raises the suspicion of tuberculosis.

Bones   Asymptomatic, punched-out lesions in the distal phalanges of the hands and feet are visible in roentgenograms in about 10 percent of cases. Associated overlying skin changes are common. Radiolucent skull lesions have been noted in a few patients. "Routine" hand x-rays are not likely to be abnormal in the absence of overlying skin changes.

Nervous system   Neurological manifestations are variable. Cranial and peripheral nerves may be affected by direct involvement of the nerve sheaths or roots. Facial nerve palsies, which may be bilateral and sequential, are the commonest neurological finding and may undergo full remission. Swallowing disorders are observed. A granulomatous basilar meningitis can affect the cranial nerves and produce pleocytosis and elevation of the spinal fluid protein level. Pituitary involvement produces diabetes insipidus. Involvement of the choroid plexuses may obstruct the ventricles. Cortical changes may result in convulsive seizures.

Other tissues   Involvement of the tonsils and laryngeal, buccal, and nasal mucosa (often with associated sinusitis) has been encountered. Bilateral nasal obstruction may be a presenting complaint. Submucous resections are contraindicated as they frequently result in septal perforations. Sarcoid lesions have been found in thyroid, parathyroid, and pancreatic tissues, and gastric granulomas have resulted in bleeding and perforation. Sarcoid involving the adrenal, cervix, uterus, epididymis, or testis is very unusual.

LABORATORY FINDINGS   Mild anemia, leukopenia, eosinophilia, and elevated sedimentation rate are common in active disease. Thrombocytopenia is unusual but may be severe.

Delayed skin reactions   Tuberculin anergy is noted in about two-thirds of patients, but a positive tuberculin reaction occurs if active tuberculosis supervenes. A previously known positive tuberculin reaction may become less reactive with active sarcoidosis. Associated generalized cutaneous anergy to other commonly occurring antigens such as *Candida albicans, Trichophyton,* and mumps virus has been noted. This depression of delayed skin reactivity is considered to be an important feature of sarcoidosis, but it varies with the duration and activity of the disease.

Chemical studies   Hypergammaglobulinemia and reduction of serum albumin are common. Hypercalcemia and hypercalciuria are infrequent but apparently result from increased intestinal absorption of calcium, which is possibly related to increased sensitivity to vitamin D. Serum uric acid level may be elevated even in the absence of renal insufficiency. Elevation of serum alkaline phosphatase level is attributable to intrahepatic tubercles, rather than to bone lesions, and may reach very high levels.

Other studies   Serum lysozyme levels are elevated in sarcoidosis (also tuberculosis) and are thought to reflect active granuloma formation. Levels seem to return to normal with corticosteroid therapy and inactivity of the disease. Elevated levels of serum angiotensin-converting enzyme (ACE) are similarly reported to correlate with the presence of active sarcoidosis. The specificity and sensitivity of ACE appears potentially useful. Elevated levels also have been observed in Gaucher's disease and occasionally in other diseases.

Roentgenographic studies   Approximately 90 percent of patients show intrathoracic disease on chest x-ray. Bilateral hilar adenopathy, often with associated right paratracheal adenopathy, is a common feature. Unilateral hilar adenopathy is unusual and should initiate a search for other diseases. Patients may be grouped according to the apparent extent and chronicity of the radiographic picture as follows: group I, hilar adenopathy with no parenchymal changes; group II, hilar adenopathy and diffuse parenchymal changes; group III, diffuse parenchymal changes without hilar adenopathy; group IV, chronic parenchymal changes of more than 2 years' duration with pulmonary fibrosis. The pulmonary changes are generally symmetrical, and may present a diffuse ground-glass appearance, fine reticular or miliary lesions, large nodular lesions, or multiple large confluent infiltrates resembling metastatic tumors. Fine diffuse interstitial fibrosis may be present. Pulmonary fibrosis may produce contraction and distortion, and extensive cystic and bullous lesions are common in the late stages. Bony changes in the phalanges, skull, and vertebrae may occur.

Pulmonary function tests These tests commonly demonstrate restriction, decreased compliance, and loss of effective diffusing surface. Vital capacity is reduced. Measurements of carbon monoxide–diffusing capacity are frequently reduced even in the absence of demonstrable radiographic changes or clinical symptoms. Measurements of vital capacity and diffusing capacity may serve as indicators of progression of disease and response to treatment. In diffuse disease, arterial blood studies reveal with exercise a reduced P_{O_2} because of perfusion of poorly ventilated areas of the lung. The arterial P_{CO_2} is commonly below normal because of compensatory hyperventilation. Some abnormalities of airway function are frequently observed in severe, late stages of pulmonary fibrosis, but carbon dioxide retention with elevation of arterial P_{CO_2} is a late and unusual feature. Significant impairment of pulmonary function frequently remains even after radiographic clearing. Following steroid therapy or a spontaneous remission, the vital capacity tends to return toward normal, but may remain somewhat reduced. The diffusing capacity may improve significantly but usually stabilizes well below normal despite complete remission of all symptoms. Improvement in diffusing capacity is less frequent than is that of the vital capacity. Deterioration of pulmonary function may occur gradually and progressively.

DIAGNOSIS The diagnosis depends on the clinical features along with histological evidence of epitheloid tubercles from tissue biopsy or from a positive Kveim reaction. The amount of histological support required varies inversely with the certainty with which the pattern of clinical features is recognized. It is essential to exclude other recognized causes of granulomatous disease. To exclude local sarcoid tissue reaction, as in nodes draining a malignant tumor, clinical evidence of involvement of more than one site is desirable. Careful search for tubercle bacilli, fungi, and foreign bodies must be made in all histological sections. A positive Kveim reaction is a special feature and often helps to exclude other granulomatous processes, although the specificity and selectivity of this reaction are debated. Tissue biopsy for histological diagnosis is most readily and easily obtained from superficial or palpable lesions in skin, lymph nodes, conjunctiva, and nasal, buccal, and bronchial mucosa. Almost any palpable lymph node is likely to be positive. Liver biopsies reveal granulomas in 70 to 80 percent of cases even without clinical evidence of impaired hepatic function. Biopsy of the gastrocnemius muscle frequently reveals granulomatous changes in patients with arthralgias and erythema nodosum. In the absence of palpable peripheral lymph nodes or dermal or mucosal lesions, transbronchial lung biopsy or mediastinoscopy and node biopsy, or biopsy of liver or muscle is in order. Flexible fiberoptic bronchoscopy with transbronchial lung biopsy frequently provides a dependable histological diagnosis. Along with tissue showing granulomas provided by the biopsy, bronchoalveolar lavage reveals an increased number of lymphocytes but fewer than are seen in hypersensitivity pneumonitis. Open lung biopsy is generally reserved for patients in whom other diagnostic maneuvers have not been successful or in whom the exclusion of other diseases is urgent. The indicated tissue biopsy is that which combines the least risk with the greatest likelihood of diagnostic yield. With typical clinical features with asymptomatic bilateral hilar adenopathy, a presumptive diagnosis may be justified, without histological verification. In mild or asymptomatic disease, when reliable Kveim material is available, this test is often useful in the diagnosis.

Kveim reaction In 50 to 80 percent of patients with sarcoidosis, the intracutaneous injection of a heat-sterilized suspension of human sarcoid tissues (spleen or lymph nodes) produces a papulonodular lesion with epithelioid tubercles. The nodule must be biopsied in 4 to 6 weeks for routine histological study. This reveals a spectrum from positive to negative, and includes a middle equivocal group. A positive reaction is limited to those with well-formed *epithelioid tubercles*. Test material must be assayed in patients of known reactivity, and experienced interpretation is essential. The Kveim reaction is very likely to be positive in the presence of sarcoid lymphadenopathy, in association with erythema nodosum, and when sarcoid skin lesions are present. The reaction is less likely to be positive in the absence of lymph node involvement and during steroid therapy. Tests in patients with a variety of granulomatous and collagen vascular diseases have revealed only 2 to 5 percent false-positive reactions, but many false-negative results are encountered in patients later shown to have sarcoidosis. The nature of the Kveim reaction is not understood, and its selectivity must be interpreted in concert with the clinical findings and the demonstrated performance of the particular Kveim preparation. This simple outpatient procedure is often useful.

COURSE Sarcoidosis is frequently no more than an incidental radiographic finding on routine chest x-ray. The course is often one of spontaneous remission over a period of 6 to 24 months, with little or no evidence of residual disease and with normal life expectancy. However, there may be persistent abnormalities with varying disability or progressive deterioration. Death related to sarcoidosis may ensue in 5 to 10 percent of cases and is most frequently related to advanced pulmonary disease. There may be impressive clearing of radiographic lesions, especially when the disease seems limited to the thorax. Following a spontaneous remission, recurrence is most unusual. Remissions are most frequent in the syndrome of erythema nodosum and hilar adenopathy. This "benign" form is more common in Caucasians than in blacks where chronic progressive diffuse systemic disease is more frequently encountered. Systemic manifestations in skin, bone, eyes, and salivary glands and hepatosplenomegaly herald a less favorable prognosis. Severe uveitis may progress to glaucoma, cataract formation, and blindness.

Steroids probably exert a favorable influence only when there is significant incapacitating disease and an active inflammatory process.

TREATMENT Relatively asymptomatic patients usually require no treatment. *Adrenal corticosteroids* dramatically suppress the active inflammatory reaction and provide important symptomatic improvement. Indications for treatment are (1) active ocular disease, (2) persistent or progressive pulmonary involvement, (3) persistent hypercalcemia or hypercalcinuria, (4) central nervous system involvement with significant functional impairment, (5) significant evidence of myocardial disease, (6) persistent systemic evidence of illness such as fever and weight loss, and (7) significant and progressive involvement of a vital organ. The disease remains in remission in some patients after administration of steroids, but it commonly recurs as the dose is reduced, even when therapy has been continued for 2 or more years. It is thought that steroids prevent the progression of disease, but healing may occur with hyalin scarring. Steroids clearly cannot reverse a fibrotic process. Early steroid therapy offers more hope than that initiated after 1 or 2 years of disease.

Steroids are most frequently required and beneficial for symptomatic lung disease. Uncertainty as to the value of steroids may stem from attempted evaluation of benefits in patients with asymptomatic minimal disease which probably required no treatment. Even relatively asymptomatic but significant lung disease should be treated if there is no evidence of spontaneous regression in 12 months, or if there is progression in 3 to 6 months. One should not wait for the appearance of symptoms when lung function is persistently and significantly reduced. Asymptomatic hilar adenopathy without clinical evidence of pulmonary parenchymal disease does not require therapy.

Prednisone is administered in initial divided daily doses of 40 mg, with 2-week periods on daily doses of 40, 30, and 25 mg, and then in single 8 A.M. daily maintenance doses of 20 to 10 mg. Symptomatic improvement occurs in 1 to 2 weeks, and the disease regresses over a period of several months. Therapy probably should be continued for a minimum of 6 to 8 months, with periodic attempts thereafter to reduce dosage or eliminate the drug. Objective criteria such as x-rays and measurements of pulmonary function are important. Maintenance therapy for many years has proved necessary in many patients in whom relapses recur at a dose below 10 to 15 mg. Dosage must be tapered slowly, with decrements of 2.5 mg no oftener than at 2- to 4-week intervals if long-term treatment has been used. Lifelong therapy may be required. Careful documentation and observation during tapering are essential in planning treatment. Alternate-day dosage may be used for maintenance therapy. It is probably not advisable for initial management. Endocrine side effects, with weight gain of 20 to 50 lb, have been observed in some women. Diabetes has appeared in some patients, particularly in association with significant hepatic involvement. Local steroid therapy has been effective in ocular sarcoid with anterior uveitis or iritis, although there is the risk of glaucoma. Intradermal steroids have been used with some success for disfiguring cutaneous lesions. Such lesions are not usually considered justification for systemic steroids.

Chloroquine (Aralen), in doses of 250 mg daily, after an initial period of 2 weeks with 500 mg daily, has been observed to induce dramatic improvement in skin and mucosal lesions over periods of several weeks, but relapse is common when the drug is withdrawn. With periodic ocular examinations and intermittent treatment periods of 6 months, no irreversible retinal damage has been encountered. Remission may be maintained with as little as 125 mg daily. Response to hydroxychloroquine (Plaquenil) has been slower and less satisfactory. Hypercalcemia has also appeared to respond to chloroquine.

Antituberculous therapy is ineffective in sarcoidosis. However, prophylactic isoniazid in association with corticosteroids is often recommended for black patients with extensive pulmonary disease, in areas with high risks of exposure to tuberculosis, and always for patients who are tuberculin-positive. If tuberculosis is really suspected, two drugs should be employed, e.g., isoniazid and ethambutol, especially if corticosteroids are to be administered.

COMPLICATIONS The complications are related to the effects of severe and progressive disease in various organs, the side effects of therapy, and superimposed infection. An increased incidence (2 to 5 percent) of tuberculosis in association with

sarcoidosis has been recognized. Associated fungous infections seem to be increasing. Saprophytic *aspergillus* fungous balls (mycetomas) have been noted in pulmonary cysts. Candidiasis and cryptococcosis in association with sarcoidosis have also been noted. It is possible that long-term steroid and antimicrobial therapy predispose to these fungous infections, but the predisposing pulmonary anatomic changes represent the underlying problem.

REFERENCES

DELANEY P: Neurologic manifestations in sarcoidosis: Review of the literature, with a report of 23 cases. Ann Intern Med 87:366, 1977

DeRemee RA: The present status of treatment of pulmonary sarcoidosis: A house divided. Chest 71:388, 1977

GUPTA RC et al: Pulmonary and extrapulmonary sarcoidosis in relation to circulatory immune complexes. Am Rev Resp Dis 166:261, 1977

JAMES DG et al: Immunology of sarcoidosis. Am J Med 59:388, 1975
——— et al: Sarcoidosis and respiratory disorders. Mt Sinai J Med 44:698, 1977

JOHNS CJ et al: Extended experience in the long-term corticosteroid treatment of pulmonary sarcoid. Ann NY Acad Sci 278:722, 1976

KOERNER SK et al: Transbronchial lung biopsy for the diagnosis of sarcoidosis. N Engl J Med 293:268, 1975

LEVINSON RS et al: Airway function in sarcoidosis. Am J Med 62:51, 1977

LIEBERMAN J: Elevation of serum angiotensin-converting-enzyme (ACE) level in sarcoidosis. Am J Med 59:365, 1975

LONGCOPE WT et al: A study of sarcoidosis: Based on a combined investigation of 160 cases including 30 autopsies from the Johns Hopkins Hospital and Massachusetts General Hospital. Medicine 31:1, 1952

MADDREY WC et al: Sarcoidosis and chronic hepatic disease: A clinical and pathologic study of 20 patients. Medicine 49:375, 1970

MAYOCK RL et al: Manifestations of sarcoidosis: Analysis of 145 patients with a review of 9 series selected from the literature. Am J Med 35:67, 1963

MITCHELL DN et al: Sarcoidosis. Am Rev Resp Dis 110:774, 1974
——— et al: Transmissible agents from human sarcoid and Crohn's disease tissues. Lancet 2:761, 1976

PROCEEDINGS OF THE EIGHTH INTERNATIONAL SARCOIDOSIS CONFERENCE, September 1978, Cardiff, Wales (in press)

ROBERTS WC et al: Sarcoidosis of the heart. A clinicopathologic study of 35 necropsy patients (group I) and review of 78 previously described necropsy patients (group II). Am J Med 63:86, 1977

SHARMA OP: *Sarcoidosis—A Clinical Approach.* Springfield, Ill, Charles C Thomas, 1975

SILVERMAN KJ et al: Cardiac sarcoid: A clinicopathologic study of 84 unselected patients with systemic sarcoidosis. Circulation 58:1204, 1978

Transactions of the New York Academy of Sciences: Seventh International Conference on Sarcoidosis and other Granulomatous Disorders. Ann NY Acad Sci 278:1, 1975

WEINBERGER SE et al: Bronchoalveolar lavage in interstitial lung disease. Ann Intern Med 89:459, 1978

217
FAMILIAL MEDITERRANEAN FEVER (FAMILIAL PAROXYSMAL POLYSEROSITIS)

SHELDON M. WOLFF

DEFINITION Familial Mediterranean fever (FMF) is an inherited disorder of unknown etiology, characterized by recurrent episodes of fever, peritonitis, and/or pleuritis. Arthritis, skin lesions, and amyloidosis are seen in some patients.

HISTORY Although the first report of FMF was by Janeway and Mosenthal in 1908, it was not until the report of five cases by Siegal in 1945 that attention was focused on FMF as a distinct entity. Subsequently, some authors have not applied strict clinical criteria, and many patients with other diseases have been reported as having FMF. The detailed and extensive descriptions by Heller and Sohar have clarified many of the clinical aspects of FMF.

TERMINOLOGY The variety of names given to FMF has led to confusion concerning its clinical features. None of the names, including FMF, is completely satisfactory, but FMF has received the widest acceptance. Such terms as *periodic disease, periodic peritonitis, la maladie periodique* are inaccurate because the disease often is not cyclical. *Benign paroxysmal peritonitis* is inappropriate because many of the patients have involvement of serosal surfaces other than the peritoneum, and some die of amyloidosis. *Familial paroxysmal polyserositis* is an acceptable alternative for the term *familial Mediterranean fever*.

ETHNOLOGY AND GENETICS FMF occurs predominantly in patients of non-Ashkenazic (Sephardic) Jewish, Armenian, and Arabic ancestry. However, the disease is not restricted to these groups, and has been seen in patients of Italian, Ashkenazic Jewish, and Anglo-Saxon descent as well as others.

The best studies of the genetics of FMF have been done in Israel, where relatively homogeneous population groups exist. In Israel, the disease appears to be inherited as an autosomal recessive. Nevertheless, approximately 50 percent of patients give no family history of the disease. Consanguinity among the parents of FMF patients is as high as 20 percent, a figure which may be an underestimate because most patients came from very inbred ethnic groups. Approximately 60 percent of patients are male.

ETIOLOGY Although numerous pathogenetic mechanisms have been suggested, the etiology of FMF is unknown. Fever and inflammation are such prominent signs that frequent attempts have been made to implicate infectious agents and/or their products. It has been suggested that FMF is a form of brucellosis or tuberculosis. Suffice it to say that extensive studies utilizing modern microbiological and serologic techniques have failed to implicate these or any other specific infectious agents.

It has been reported that FMF is due to an allergy or to hypersensitivity, but such hypersensitive states have not been substantiated. There is no firm evidence favoring an autoimmune etiology.

Reimann has suggested that FMF, like many other recurring illnesses (periodic disease), may be a pathological exaggeration of normal periodic temperature rhythmicity. However, extensive studies of temperature and other circadian rhythms in FMF patients have failed to demonstrate alterations from normal.

Because many FMF patients note that certain emotional or environmental changes may have profound effects on the frequency with which episodes of their disease occur, a psychosomatic basis has been suggested for the illness. There is no question that most patients eventually have transient or even permanent psychological alterations, which probably reflect their reaction to a chronic recurring illness that is forever threatening their social, economic, and personal well-being, but there is no evidence for a functional etiology for FMF.

The demonstration that FMF is inherited as an autosomal recessive disorder has led to the thesis that it is another inborn error of metabolism. Originally it was thought that the disorder might be one of altered lipid metabolism. Despite extensive studies, no such error has been found. Reported instances of

excessive urinary excretion of porphyrins in FMF are probably examples of true porphyria and not FMF.

It has been reported that blood levels of unconjugated etiocholanolone were elevated during fever in six patients with FMF. Subsequent studies, however, showed no correlation between levels of etiocholanolone and fever.

PATHOLOGY Despite the striking clinical manifestations during an acute attack of FMF, no specific pathological alterations have been found. Most FMF patients undergo at least one laparotomy, and only acute peritoneal inflammation in which the exudate contains a predominance of polymorphonuclear leukocytes is found to be present. A disproportionately large number of male patients develop gallbladder disease with and without cholelithiasis, but extensive histopathologic examination has failed to reveal any specific pathological changes. Pleural and joint inflammation are also nonspecific.

In the amyloidosis which accompanies FMF, amyloid is deposited in the intima and media of the arterioles, the subendothelial region of venules, the glomeruli, and the spleen. Aside from their vessels, the heart and liver are uninvolved.

MANIFESTATIONS In the majority of patients, the symptoms of FMF begin between the ages of 5 and 15, although attacks sometimes commence during infancy, and onset has occurred as late as age 52. The duration and frequency of attacks vary greatly in the same patient, and there is no set rhythm or periodicity to their occurrence. The usual acute episode lasts 24 to 48 h, but some may be prolonged for 7 to 10 days. The attacks range in frequency from twice weekly to once a year, but 2 to 4 weeks is the commonest interval. Spontaneous remissions lasting years have been seen. In the majority of cases, pregnancy is associated with an absence of acute episodes and many patients note less frequent attacks in the summer than in the winter. There may be a decrease in the severity and frequency of the attacks with age or with development of amyloidosis.

Fever Fever is a cardinal manifestation of FMF and is present during most but not all attacks. Rarely, fever may be present without serositis. The temperature may be preceded by a chill, and will peak in 12 to 24 h. Defervescence is often accompanied by diaphoresis. The fever ranges from 38.5 to 40°C but is quite variable.

Abdominal pain Abdominal pain occurs in more than 95 percent of patients, and may vary in severity in the same patient. Minor premonitory discomfort may precede an acute episode by 24 to 48 h. The pain usually starts in one quadrant and then spreads to involve the whole abdomen. The initial site is usually very tender. Tenderness may remain localized with referred pain in other areas, and there may be radiation to the back. There may be splinting of the chest and pain in one or both shoulders, typical of diaphragmatic irritation. Nausea and vomiting sometimes occur. The abdomen is usually distended, and may become rigid with decreased or absent bowel sounds. On x-ray, the wall of the small intestine may appear edematous, transit of barium is slowed, and fluid levels may be seen. Because the manifestations of an acute abdominal attack can simulate those of a perforated viscus so closely, patients should be advised to have an elective appendectomy between attacks so that acute appendicitis will not obfuscate the picture at a later date. An abdominal operation may precipitate an acute attack of FMF which may be confused with other postoperative complications.

Chest pain Most patients with abdominal attacks have referred chest pain at one time or another, and 75 percent also develop acute pleuritic pain with or without abdominal symptoms. In 30 percent, the attacks of pleuritis precede the onset of abdominal attacks by varying periods of time, and a small number of patients never develop abdominal attacks. Chest pain is usually unilateral and is associated with diminished breath sounds, a friction rub, or a transient pleural effusion.

Joint pain In Israel, 75 percent of patients report at least one episode of acute arthritis. Arthritis can be distinct from abdominal or pleural attacks, can be acute or, rarely, chronic, and may involve one or several joints. Effusions are common and the large joints are involved most frequently. Radiologic findings are nonspecific. Despite careful search, frank arthritis rarely has been seen in the United States. Some patients have a history of rheumatic fever-like illness in childhood, but in a large series of patients, including 30 from the Middle East, acute arthritis was not observed. Mild arthralgia is common during acute attacks but is nonspecific and can be seen in many febrile illnesses, including experimentally induced hyperthermia.

Skin manifestations Skin involvement is reported by 25 to 35 percent of patients. These lesions consist of painful, erythematous areas of swelling from 5 to 20 cm in diameter, usually located on the lower legs, the medial malleolus, or the dorsum of the foot. They may occur without abdominal or pleural pain and subside within 24 to 48 h.

Other signs and symptoms Involvement of other serosal membranes has been reported, but pericarditis is rare, and it is probable that descriptions of recurrent meningitis have been diseases other than FMF. Hematuria, splenomegaly, and small white dots called *colloid bodies* in the ocular fundus are among the findings of questionable significance. Rarely migraine-like headaches accompany acute abdominal attacks, and some patients have become somewhat irrational or show extreme emotional lability during attacks. Whether these are primary manifestations of FMF or secondary effects of pain and fever is not known.

Complications The most serious complication of FMF in the United States is drug addiction or habituation, and obviously efforts should be made to avoid use of narcotics. Depression and lack of motivation are common, and patients with FMF require considerable encouragement and support. A striking number of patients in one American series have developed gallbladder disease.

Another major complication of FMF is *amyloidosis*. Some investigators believe that few patients in Israel escape this complication and that it is an expression of the same gene that is responsible for the other manifestations of FMF. If the attacks occur first, as they do in over 90 percent of the patients, the patients are classified as being of phenotype I. Amyloidosis also occurs in siblings of FMF patients or precedes the abdominal attacks (phenotype II). The infiltration by amyloid involves the kidneys, and death is often attributable to renal failure.

Amyloidosis has been reported in Israel and North Africa, but there have been only three reported instances of amyloidosis complicating FMF in the United States. These findings are even more striking because there are probably as many known FMF patients in the United States as in Israel. These differences are unexplained and suggest that environmental or nutritional, as well as genetic, factors may play a role in the development of amyloidosis in FMF.

LABORATORY FINDINGS There is no specific diagnostic test. Polymorphonuclear leukocytosis ranging from 15,000 to 30,000 cells per cubic millimeter is almost invariable during acute attacks. The erythrocyte sedimentation rate is elevated during attacks but returns to normal between attacks. Plasma fibrinogen, serum haptoglobin, ceruloplasmin, and C-reactive protein increase during the episodes. Plasma lipids are normal, and there are no consistent abnormalities of hepatic or renal function. When amyloidosis is present, laboratory findings are typical of a nephrotic syndrome followed by renal insufficiency. Electrocardiographic and electroencephalographic changes are inconstant and nonspecific.

DIAGNOSIS When the typical acute attacks of FMF occur in an individual of appropriate ethnic background who has a family history of FMF, the diagnosis is easy. On the other hand, if the disease has not been present in the family and the patient resides in a community where FMF is rare, the diagnosis can be very difficult.

Most patients with undiagnosed FMF have had one or more abdominal operations with no relief of symptoms. When a patient is seen for the first time, a variety of other febrile illnesses must be excluded by appropriate study or observation. These include acute appendicitis, acute pancreatitis, porphyria, cholecystitis, intestinal obstruction, and other major abdominal catastrophes.

Some of the inherited forms of the hyperlipidemias may mimic the clinical picture of FMF, but measurement of serum cholesterol and triglycerides will eliminate them from consideration. The patient with FMF is not immune to the other diseases, and when an attack differs from the usual pattern or is more prolonged, consideration should be given to other diagnostic possibilities. The pleural form of the disease is sometimes difficult to differentiate from acute pulmonary infection or infarction, but the rapid disappearance of signs and symptoms resolves the problem. The joint manifestations may be more prolonged than other forms of FMF, and differentiation from septic arthritis, gout, and acute rheumatoid disease may be necessary. The erythema is sometimes difficult to differentiate from superficial thrombophlebitis or cellulitis.

Whether or not the patient is of the appropriate ethnic group, the most difficult diagnostic problem in FMF is the patient who presents with fever alone. In this situation, an extensive diagnostic work-up for fever of unknown origin may be required. Fortunately, such patients are rare, and all eventually develop serosal involvement. Until specific diagnostic tests for FMF are available, patients with recurrent fever but without signs of inflammation of one of the serosal membranes should not be categorized as having FMF.

PROGNOSIS The prognosis of patients with FMF varies greatly according to the country in which they live. In the United States, the prognosis for long life is excellent. Despite the severity of the symptoms during some acute attacks, most patients are remarkably free of any debilitation during the intervals between attacks. With encouragement and an understanding of their disease, most FMF patients lead fairly normal lives. The greatest hazard to patients is prolonged periods of hospitalization due to erroneous diagnoses or failure to understand the disease. The liberal and injudicious use of narcotics for analgesia in these patients can lead to major psychological and health problems. Establishment of a reasonable doctor-patient relationship and education of the patient avoids this hazard. In the United States, the prognosis of patients with FMF does not seem to be different from that of patients with other chronic nonfatal illnesses. Death usually results from causes unrelated to the underlying disease.

The complication of amyloidosis in Israel, parts of North Africa, Turkey, and other parts of the Middle East makes the prognosis quite different from that in America. Approximately 25 percent of FMF patients in Israel are known to have amyloidosis, and this complication usually leads to death. Because a majority of patients under observation in Israel are under 40 years of age, it has been suggested that fatal amyloidosis may eventually occur in nearly all patients. This would explain the rarity of older patients in that area.

TREATMENT Many forms of therapy had been tried in FMF, but until recently, nothing was effective. Among the therapies tried have been antibiotics, hormones (including estrogens and adrenal corticosteroids), antipyretic drugs, immunotherapy, psychotherapy, elimination and low-fat diets, chloroquine, and phenylbutazone. When carefully studied and followed up, none of these therapies proved effective.

During the past 10 years, the outlook of patients with FMF has been altered dramatically. Goldfinger reported in 1972 that the prophylactic use of colchicine in five patients dramatically reduced the number of attacks. Subsequently, controlled trials in the United States and Israel have shown that chronic administration of colchicine will greatly reduce the number of acute attacks of FMF. It is recommended that 0.6 mg colchicine be taken by mouth three times a day. Patients often develop gastrointestinal side effects with this dose, however, in which case the dose should be reduced to 0.6 mg taken twice a day. Although an occasional patient will respond to 0.6 mg taken only once a day, this amount is less likely to be beneficial. Most but not all FMF patients will respond favorably to colchicine prophylaxis.

Since colchicine is known to result in nondisjunction of chromosomes and in azospermia in some patients, it should not be given to any patient, especially a young one, unless the disease is severe enough to warrant taking the risk. In addition, everyone who requires therapy should first be tried on a course of intermittent colchicine. The patient should take 0.6 mg colchicine by mouth every hour for 4 h, then every 2 h for 4 h, and every 12 h thereafter for 48 h. The colchicine should be given at the first premonitory sign of an attack. When colchicine is taken on such a schedule, many patients will experience aborted attacks or no symptoms at all. If both acute and prophylactic colchicine therapy fail, supportive therapy is all that can be offered. Except for unusual circumstances, narcotics should not be given to FMF patients.

The mechanism of colchicine's action against acute attacks of FMF is unknown. It is postulated that it may work by preventing the normal cellular response to inflammation.

A few reports have appeared in which FMF patients with amyloidosis have had successful renal transplants.

REFERENCES

DINARELLO CA et al: Colchicine therapy for familial Mediterranean fever. A double-blind trial. N Engl J Med 291:934, 1974
——— et al: Effect of prophylactic colchicine therapy on leukocyte function in patients with Familial Mediterranean Fever. Arthritis Rheum 19:618, 1976
SCHWABE AD, PETERS RS: Familial Mediterranean fever in Armenians. Analysis of 100 cases. Medicine 53:453, 1974
SOHAR E et al: Familial Mediterranean fever. Am J Med 43:227, 1967
WRIGHT DG et al: Efficiency of intermittent colchicine therapy in Familial Mediterranean Fever. Ann Intern Med 86:162, 1977

218

WEGENER'S GRANULOMATOSIS AND MIDLINE GRANULOMA

SHELDON M. WOLFF

WEGENER'S GRANULOMATOSIS

DEFINITION Wegener's granulomatosis is characterized by necrotizing vasculitis and granulomatous inflammation which affects primarily the upper and/or lower respiratory tract and the kidneys. However, small vessels anywhere can be involved. Rarely is the disease restricted to the respiratory tract (localized Wegener's granulomatosis). In the vast majority of cases the kidneys are involved and such patients have generalized Wegener's granulomatosis.

ETIOLOGY The cause of Wegener's granulomatosis is unknown, but most studies suggest a hypersensitivity reaction. The vasculitis, glomerulonephritis, the occasional ultrastructural findings of subepithelial glomerular deposits which look like immune complex deposition, and the reported presence of immune complexes in the serums of a few patients strongly implicate immune complex formation as the basis for the pathogenesis of this disease. On the other hand, the granulomas seen in many tissues suggest that cellular immune responses may also be involved. The antigen initiating the response(s) is unknown but may be microbial or tissue in origin and probably has as its site of origin the respiratory tract.

PATHOLOGY In order to make the diagnosis of Wegener's granulomatosis both granulomas and necrotizing vasculitis must be demonstrated. These lesions can occur anywhere but are most commonly found in the sinus mucosa, lungs, and skin. The necrotizing vasculitis and granulomatous inflammation are in and of themselves not distinctive, but the demonstration of both is required. In the kidney the most common lesion is a focal and segmental glomerulonephritis, although on occasion frank vasculitis or even a granuloma may be observed.

CLINICAL FEATURES Wegener's granulomatosis has been reported as early as the first and as late as the eighth decade of life, but the mean age of onset is approximately 40 years. The disease occurs twice as often in males as in females. The initial signs or symptoms can occur anywhere but usually are seen in the upper or lower respiratory tract. For example, patients may have headache, sinusitis, rhinorrhea, and otitis media with or without hearing loss. Other prominent presenting symptoms can include fever, arthralgias, and anorexia. Cough, pain in the chest, and hemoptysis may predominate in some patients. Associated with the respiratory findings may be signs or symptoms of any of the organ systems involved, and these can include all organ systems. It is rare for a patient to present initially with signs or symptoms of renal failure, but this occurs in about ten percent of patients.

In most patients Wegener's granulomatosis is a generalized disease associated with involvement of multiple organ systems, often with manifestations of acute inflammation. The respiratory tract (upper, lower, or both) is involved in all patients. The sinuses are affected in over 90 percent of patients. Saddle-nose deformities are common, as is mucosal ulceration, but mutilation does not occur. Very often the sinuses become secondarily infected with bacteria, and such infections require aggressive antibiotic therapy and often surgical intervention. Radiographs demonstrate the sinus involvement in this disease. The pulmonary manifestations are varied. Signs and symptoms suggestive of a pneumonitis may occur. Similarly, pleuritic manifestations are sometimes seen. Occasionally massive hemoptysis or pneumothorax develops. The typical x-ray features are those of nodular and cavitary infiltrates. These lesions can be evanescent and spontaneously disappear even without therapy. Lung biopsy is commonly performed in these patients and often leads to the diagnosis.

Renal involvement is present in over 90 percent of patients with Wegener's granulomatosis and is a prerequisite for a diagnosis of the generalized form of the disease. Prior to the availability of effective therapy, the mean survival of patients with renal involvement was 5 months. The urinary findings are consistent with acute glomerulonephritis, and an active sediment is common. About one-half the patients have glomerulonephritis, and on biopsy a focal glomerulitis is seen. Others also have a picture compatible with the nephrotic syndrome. Approximately 10 percent of patients have rapidly progressive glomerulonephritis and on biopsy have necrotizing and proliferative glomerulonephritis and marked crescent formation. Such patients should be treated as medical emergencies. Deposition of immunoglobulins and possible immune complex deposits have been noted in some patients.

Approximately 50 percent of patients with Wegener's granulomatosis have involvement of the eyes. Iritis, scleritis, and conjunctivitis are common. Proptosis due to retrobulbar granulomatous inflammation is occasionally seen. About one-third of patients have cardiac involvement, ranging from coronary arteritis to pericarditis. In approximately one-quarter of the patients the nervous system is involved. Most commonly, patients have mononeuritis multiplex while others have cranial neuritis.

In addition to serous otitis media, hearing loss is common in Wegener's granulomatosis. Almost one-half of patients have dermatologic manifestations including petechiae, vesicles, and necrotic ulcerations. Although frank arthritis is uncommon, about two-thirds of Wegener's granulomatous patients have arthralgias.

LABORATORY FINDINGS There are no specific laboratory abnormalities in Wegener's granulomatosis. A normochromic, normocytic anemia is sometimes present. Leukocytosis is present in some patients but is usually seen when a superimposed bacterial infection has occurred. Thrombocytosis is seen in approximately ten percent of patients with the generalized form of the disease. The sedimentation rate is increased in almost all patients with active disease and is the most useful parameter with which to follow therapeutic efficacy. About fifty percent of patients have a positive test for rheumatoid factor, and many patients have hyperglobulinemia, particularly IgA. When renal involvement occurs, there are changes in the urine consistent with an active glomerulonephritis, and as the disease progresses, renal insufficiency is reflected in the usual laboratory abnormalities of uremia.

DIFFERENTIAL DIAGNOSIS The diagnosis of Wegener's granulomatosis is made when histological evidence of vasculitis and granulomatous inflammation is present. The purely vasculitic diseases such as polyarteritis nodosa and systemic lupus erythematosus do not have granulomatous inflammation as a histological hallmark. Conversely, granulomatous diseases such as tuberculosis, fungal disease, and sarcoidosis do not show histological evidence of vasculitis. Certain diseases do present problems in differentiation from Wegener's granulomatosis. Occasional patients with Wegener's granulomatosis will present with hemoptysis, pulmonary hemorrhage, and rap-

idly progressive renal failure, and a clinical diagnosis of Goodpasture's syndrome is suspected. However, appropriate biopsies and immunofluorescent studies should differentiate these two conditions. Midline granuloma is restricted to the head and neck and not associated with vasculitis. Lymphomatoid granulomatosis can present with a clinical picture indistinguishable from Wegener's granulomatosis. However, biopsy of involved organs (e.g., lung, skin) should demonstrate the characteristic cellular infiltrates. Occasional malignant tumors, particularly malignant lymphomas, will result in granulomatous inflammation and even vasculitis, but histological demonstration of the malignant cells leads to differentiation from Wegener's granulomatosis.

TREATMENT The use of cytotoxic agents in Wegener's granulomatosis has resulted in one of the most striking examples of the way modern chemotherapeutic intervention can alter the course of a hitherto lethal illness. Properly treated, over 95 percent of patients will go into remission, and since some remissions have lasted up to 15 years, it is not inappropriate to talk of cures in this disease.

The treatment of choice is cyclophosphamide, although in many cases azathioprine is equally as effective. Other alkylating agents, such as chlorambucil, may be used. In those patients where the disease is progressing rapidly, intravenous cyclophosphamide therapy may be used, but in general the oral route is preferred. Therapy ordinarily begins at 2 mg/kg cyclophosphamide daily, and this dose is adjusted according to the peripheral white blood cell count. Generally, the dose will decrease with time owing to depression of the white blood cell count. Treatment should be carried on for 1 year after the patient goes into remission. In patients with irreversible renal failure, dialysis may have to be employed, but renal transplantation should be considered in such patients as well. Adrenal corticosteroids are often used as adjunctive therapy in patients whose disease shows active inflammation. The steroid regimen of these patients should be converted to an alternate-day schedule as early as possible.

MIDLINE GRANULOMA

DEFINITION Midline granuloma is an uncommon disease characterized by localized inflammation, destruction, and often mutilation of the tissues of the upper respiratory tract and face. This condition has also been referred to as *lethal midline granuloma, malignant granuloma,* and *granuloma gangrenescens,* none of which is an appropriate term.

ETIOLOGY The etiology of midline granuloma is unknown. In view of the intense granulomatous inflammation, the disease is thought to represent a localized hypersensitivity reaction which leads to tissue destruction and mutilation. However, the responsible antigen(s) is unknown, and there is no immunologic evidence supporting this hypothesis. A variety of microorganisms have been considered as possible causative agents, but detailed microbiologic investigations have failed to detect the consistent presence of pathogenic organisms. In view of the clinical and pathological features of the illness as well as the fact that some upper-airway tumors can elicit a similar intense inflammatory response, some authors have suggested a neoplastic basis for midline granuloma. However, when malignant tissue (usually of a lymphomatous nature) is found in the lesions, the diagnosis of midline granuloma is no longer tenable.

PATHOLOGY The most characteristic pathological finding is acute or chronic inflammation with necrosis. Superimposed pyogenic infection of the involved tissues, including the sinuses, may contribute to nonspecific histological findings. The pathological hallmark, noncaseating granulomas, with or without giant cells, may be obscured by the inflammatory reaction, but when present are strong evidence in favor of the diagnosis. Primary vasculitis is seen rarely, and when it occurs, a search for other causes, most notably Wegener's granulomatosis, should be made. The presence of malignant cells makes the diagnosis of midline granuloma unacceptable. Until an etiology is established, the diagnosis of midline granuloma will rest on the characteristic clinical features outlined below.

CLINICAL FEATURES The disease may occur at any age, but the majority of patients are in the fifth and sixth decades. It is more common in women than men and has been reported in all races. Many patients report recurrent "sinus" problems, and some have histories of allergic rhinitis, although the significance of these features is unknown.

The major symptoms are usually related to the nose. Patients frequently complain of nasal stuffiness and occasionally of discharge. The first symptom in a smaller percentage of patients relates to ulceration of the mucosa of the nose, the buccal mucosa, or the gums. This has led to loosening of the teeth, and dentists are often first consulted by these patients. Rarely, patients will present first with eye findings related to conjunctival inflammation or even ulceration. Although the progression of symptoms in some patients may be slow, all too often the disease steadily, and sometimes rapidly, progresses. The characteristic symptoms of nasal discharge, difficulty in breathing through the nose, and pain over the sinuses, nose, or eye become more prominent with time. Once ulceration begins, the disease often progresses rapidly. The ulcers frequently involve the nasal septum and will lead to the characteristic septal perforation and a saddlenose deformity. The majority of patients develop ulceration and eventually perforations of the soft and hard palates. Untreated, the disease can lead to massive destruction and mutilation of the tissues involved, including the skin of the face and the eyes. Frequently, the necrotic tissue becomes infected, and systemic symptoms such as fever and anorexia appear. The destructive lesions can become very malodorous. The disease extends to involve local tissues and does not progress below the neck; if this happens, other diseases should be considered. As the necrotic process progresses and involves vital organs, patients may lose sight in the affected eye, experience dysphagia, and have difficulty in speech. Although spontaneous temporary remissions have been reported, untreated midline granuloma is fatal. The progression of the disease can be rapidly accelerated by surgical procedures in the affected areas. The patient usually dies from secondary infection, although erosion by the process into a major blood vessel or penetration into the central nervous system with superimposed meningitis can also cause death.

Aside from the granulomatous inflammation, necrosis, and destruction, no other specific clinical or pathological findings are associated with midline granuloma. Occasionally, with superimposed infection, local lymphadenopathy may be noted, but it is not characteristic of the disease per se.

LABORATORY FINDINGS With progression of the disease, a variety of nonspecific abnormalities may be noted. These changes are characteristic of inflammatory processes in general or of secondary infections. For example, mild anemia, leukocytosis, elevated sedimentation rate, and hyperglobulinemia are common in these patients. Radiographic examination reveals pansinusitis, and as the disease advances, destruction of bone in the involved areas is characteristic.

DIFFERENTIAL DIAGNOSIS The diagnosis of midline granuloma is made by finding the characteristic histological lesions in biopsies of the affected tissues. When the specimens show only inflammatory tissue, a presumptive diagnosis of midline granuloma can be made only when the characteristic clinical picture is present and other diseases with similar presentation have been excluded. The diagnosis of Wegener's granulomatosis is ruled out by the absence of vasculitis in the biopsy specimens and the localized nature of midline granuloma (i.e., no pulmonary or renal involvement). In addition, Wegener's granulomatosis rarely, if ever, causes erosion through facial tissues. It is often difficult to differentiate true midline granuloma from neoplasms of the upper airways such as malignant reticulosis and certain lymphomas. These may be clinically similar to midline granuloma and are often associated with granulomatous inflammation. Careful examination of generous biopsy material as well as concomitant work-up for disseminated neoplasm often provides the clinicopathological distinction. Other diseases to be excluded by appropriate laboratory techniques are histoplasmosis, blastomycosis, coccidioidomycosis, leprosy, tuberculosis, syphilis, mucocutaneous leishmaniasis, rhinoscleroma, and pseudotumor of the orbit.

TREATMENT The complications of midline granuloma such as superimposed infections can be treated specifically. Although adrenal corticosteroids are often used in the therapy of midline granuloma, they are of no value and probably are contraindicated if infection is present. Sporadic reports of therapy with cytotoxic agents are difficult to interpret, since some of the patients reported clearly had lymphoma or Wegener's granulomatosis, diseases where such agents are of definite value. Surgical removal of the involved tissue has been attempted but is useless and may, in fact, cause rapid progression of the disease.

The treatment of choice is radiotherapy to the local lesion. Although low dosages (1000 rads and below) have been reported to be effective, many patients relapse after such therapy. Radiotherapy should be given in a dose of 5000 rads to the involved areas. Where such a regimen is employed, long-lasting (more than 15 years) remissions and possible cures have been achieved. Following irradiation and after an appropriate period to allow for tissue healing (usually 1 year), reconstructive and plastic surgery, which may be of enormous cosmetic and functional value, can be undertaken.

REFERENCES

Midline granuloma

FAUCI AS et al: Radiation therapy of midline granuloma. Ann Intern Med 84:140, 1976

FECHNER RE, LAMPPIN DW: Midline malignant reticulosis. Arch Otolaryngol 95:467, 1972

WALTON EW: Reticuloendothelial sarcoma arising in the nose and palate (granuloma gangrenescens). J Clin Pathol 13:279, 1960

Wegener's granulomatosis

BLATT IM et al: Fatal granulomatosis of the respiratory tract (lethal midline granuloma—Wegener's granulomatosis) AMA Arch Otolaryngol 70:707, 1959

FAUCI AS et al: Wegener's granulomatosis: Studies in eight patients and a review of the literature. Medicine 52:535, 1973

———— et al: Wegener's granulomatosis and related diseases. Dis Mon 23:7, 1977

WOLFF SM et al: Wegener's granulomatosis. Ann Intern Med 81:513, 1974

219
TOBACCO SMOKING

JOHN H. HOLBROOK

Tobacco smoke is a ubiquitous personal and environmental pollutant. Although tobacco has been used in Western culture for more than 400 years, human inhalation of cigarette smoke is a twentieth century phenomenon with major medical and economic consequences. In industrialized nations cigarette smoking is a principal cause of preventable disease and premature death.

Important changes in smoking trends are occurring in the United States. In general, the trend is downward. For example, in 1977 per capita cigarette consumption for adults stabilized while consumption of cigar and pipe tobacco continued to decrease. More importantly, between 1965 and 1975 the proportion of adult cigarette smokers in the United States declined from 53 to 39 percent of men and 32 to 29 percent of women; this represented a decrease of 2.8 million adult cigarette smokers which occurred in the face of the population growth of more than 20 million adults (Table 219-1). The decline in smoking prevalence is due largely to men who have given up cigarette smoking. Unfortunately, an increasing number of teen-agers have taken up the smoking habit.

CIGARETTE SMOKE Large prospective epidemiologic studies have shown a strong association between cigarette smoking and several diseases (Fig. 219-1). Identification of more than 2000 substances in cigarette smoke provides a framework for understanding these diverse biologic effects.

Cigarette smoke is a heterogeneous aerosol produced by incomplete combustion of the tobacco leaf. It is composed of gases and vapors in which droplets are dispersed. Mainstream smoke emerges from the mouthpiece during puffing. Sidestream smoke is emitted between puffs at the burning cone and from the mouthpiece. The composition of the smoke is influenced by several factors including type of tobacco, temperature of combustion, length of the cigarette, porosity of the paper, additives, and filters. The major constituents of tobacco are carbohydrates, nonfatty organic acids, nitrogen-containing compounds, and resins. Cigarette temperatures vary greatly from 30°C at the mouthpiece to 900°C at the burning cone. In the presence of intense heat some tobacco constituents undergo thermic decomposition (pyrolysis). Volatile substances are distilled directly into the smoke. Unstable molecules recombine to generate new compounds (pyrosynthesis). Concentration of smoke constituents occurs as the smoke is filtered by unburnt tobacco and is redistilled by the burning cone. Some substances found in tobacco pass unchanged into cigarette smoke.

Each cigarette generates approximately 500 mg mainstream smoke of which 92 percent is present in a gas phase and 8 percent is present in a particulate phase. Mainstream smoke contains 2 to 5 billion particles per milliliter, with the particle size ranging from 0.1 to 1.0 μm. Nitrogen, oxygen, and carbon dioxide account for 85 percent of the smoke's weight. The remaining gases, vapors, and particulate matter are the substances of medical importance. (Selected constituents of cigarette smoke are listed in Table 219-2.) Some smoke constituents are absorbed directly through the mucosa of the mouth, nose, pharynx, and upper airways, while others are inhaled into the lungs where they are absorbed and retained. Concentrations of toxic constituents in smoke often far exceed threshold limits of industrial toxins.

PHARMACOLOGY Tissue and organ system responses to cigarette smoke inhalation are multiple and complex. Most studies in humans have dealt with exposure to whole smoke or selected constituents which are thought to pose the greatest risk to health, for example, nicotine and carbon monoxide. Relatively little is known about the individual effects and interactions of other potentially toxic smoke constituents that are often present in low concentrations.

Nicotine, the component most characteristic of tobacco, is a highly toxic alkaloid that is both a ganglionic stimulant and depressant. The average cigarette smoker who inhales absorbs about 2 mg nicotine per cigarette. The estimated acutely fatal oral dose for an adult is 1 mg/kg. Many of its complex effects are mediated by catecholamine release. Acute cardiovascular responses to nicotine observed in normal smokers include increases in systolic and diastolic blood pressure, heart rate, force of myocardial contraction, myocardial oxygen consumption, coronary artery flow, myocardial irritability, and peripheral vasoconstriction. Nicotine has also been shown to increase platelet aggregation and serum concentrations of free fatty acid and antidiuretic hormone. Nicotine plays an important but not exclusive role in maintaining the smoking habit.

Carbon monoxide is a toxic gas which interferes with oxygen transport and utilization. Because cigarette smoke contains 2 to 6 percent carbon monoxide, smokers inhale concentrations as high as 400 parts per million (ppm) and develop elevated carboxyhemoglobin (COHB) levels. While the range of COHB for smokers is 2 to 15 percent, levels for nonsmokers are near 1 percent. The average COHB level for moderate cigarette

TABLE 219-1
Estimated number of cigarette smokers in the United States, 1955, 1965, 1975

	Year	Total population, millions	Cigarette smokers, millions	% smokers
AGE GROUP, YEARS				
13–19	1955	16.0	2.2	14
	1965	24.4	3.5	14
	1975	29.5	6.0	20
20 and over	1955	104.8	39.6	38
	1965	118.0	49.7	42
	1975	138.8	46.9	34
SEX				
Adult male	1955	50.9	26.5	52
	1965	65.8	30.0	53
	1975	66.1	25.9	39
Adult female	1955	53.9	13.1	24
	1965	61.2	19.7	32
	1975	72.7	21.0	29

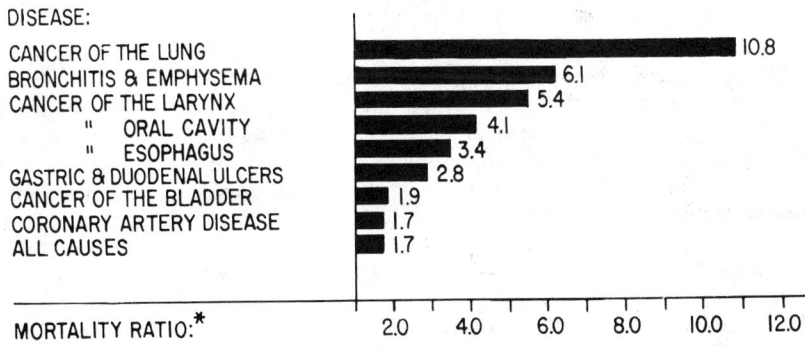

FIGURE 219-1

Mortality ratios for male cigarette smokers in seven prospective studies.

MORTALITY RATIO:*

* Death rate for current smokers divided by the death rate for those who never smoked regularly

smokers is 5 percent. Carbon monoxide produces its adverse effects by reducing the amount of available oxyhemoglobin and myoglobin, and displacing the oxygen-hemoglobin dissociation curve to the left. Chronic, mild elevations of COHB due to smoking are a common cause of polycythemia and may produce subtle impairment of central nervous system function.

Cigarette smoke and its condensate are carcinogenic in several species of animals. The major carcinogens in cigarette smoke are polynuclear aromatic hydrocarbons (Table 219-2). Tumor promoters and tumor accelerators present in cigarette smoke greatly enhance its carcinogenicity. Cigarette smoke condensate is also mutagenic in a microbial test system.

Potent pulmonary irritants and ciliotoxins are found in cigarette smoke (Table 219-2). These substances cause increased bronchial mucus secretion, and they mediate acute and chronic decreases in pulmonary and mucociliary function.

EPIDEMIOLOGY Data from large prospective studies of populations in several countries show that cigarette-smoking men, taken as a whole, have 30 to 80 percent higher death rates than nonsmokers. This excess male mortality is present in all groups over the age of 35, but it is proportionately greatest in the age group 45 to 54. In a study of British physicians it was shown that 40 percent of 35-year-old men who smoked more than 25 cigarettes per day died before the age of 65, compared with 15 percent of nonsmokers in the same category. The excess mortality of smoking women has been somewhat less than that of men, but recent trends suggest it is increasing. Coronary heart disease is the chief contributor to smoking-related excess mortality in men, accounting for more than twice as many deaths as the second leading cause, lung cancer. In the United States cigarette smokers experience more disability due to chronic illness and report 45 percent more days absent from work than do nonsmokers.

A strong dose-response relationship exists between tobacco exposure and excess mortality, as measured by age at onset of smoking, cigarette consumption, and smoke inhalation. Cessation of smoking is associated with a decrease in the excess mortality. These observations together with clinical, experimental, and pathological studies suggest that smoking, per se, causes the excess mortality.

CHARACTERISTICS OF SMOKERS Demographic, anthropometric, physiological, and laboratory features distinguish cigarette smokers from nonsmokers. Smokers drink more alcohol, coffee, and tea than do nonsmokers. Their weight and blood pressure are slightly less and their heart rate is slightly faster than those of nonsmokers. In women the menopause comes earlier in smokers than in nonsmokers. Smokers have impaired maximum exercise performance. A markedly increased number of pulmonary alveolar macrophages is present in smokers, and these cells contain high levels of aryl hydrocarbon hydroxylase. Serum thiocyanate levels are much higher in smokers. When compared with nonsmokers, smokers show small

increases in total white blood cell count and serum cholesterol, as well as small decreases in serum high-density lipoprotein, vitamin C, uric acid, and albumin. Other laboratory findings observed more commonly in smokers than in nonsmokers include proteinuria, increased levels of carcinoembryonic antigen, and an increased frequency of antinuclear autoantibodies.

CLINICAL CORRELATIONS **Cardiovascular disease** Premature coronary heart disease (CHD) is one of the most important consequences of cigarette smoking (Chap. 244). The risk of fatal or nonfatal CHD is 60 to 70 percent greater in male smokers than nonsmokers. Sudden death may be the first manifestation of CHD, and it is two to three times more likely in 35- to 54-year-old smoking males than in nonsmokers. Women who smoke cigarettes and use oral contraceptives increase their risk of suffering an acute myocardial infarction more than fivefold. Cigarette smoking acts both independently and synergistically with other factors to increase the risk of developing CHD. Cessation of smoking is associated with decreased CHD mortality, an effect which is measurable within 1 year. Those who continue to smoke after an acute myocardial infarction are more likely to die from CHD than are those who quit smoking. Cigarette smoking produces an imbalance be-

TABLE 219-2
Selected cigarette smoke constituents

Substance	Effect
PARTICULATE PHASE	
"Tar"*	Carcinogen
Polynuclear aromatic hydrocarbons	Carcinogen
Nicotine	Ganglionic stimulator and depressor
Phenol	Cocarcinogen and irritant
Cresol	Cocarcinogen and irritant
β-Naphthylamine	Carcinogen
N-Nitrosonornicotine	Carcinogen
Benzo[a]pyrene	Carcinogen
Benz[α]anthracene	Carcinogen
Trace metals (e.g., nickel, polonium 210)	Carcinogen
Indole	Tumor accelerator
Carbazole	Tumor accelerator
GAS PHASE	
Carbon monoxide	Impairs oxygen transport and utilization
Hydrocyanic acid	Ciliotoxin and irritant
Acetaldehyde	Ciliotoxin and irritant
Acrolein	Ciliotoxin and irritant
Ammonia	Ciliotoxin and irritant
Formaldehyde	Ciliotoxin and irritant
Oxides of nitrogen	Ciliotoxin and irritant
Nitrosamines	Carcinogen
Hydrazine	Carcinogen

* *The aggregate of particulate matter in cigarette smoke after subtracting nicotine and moisture.*

tween myocardial oxygen supply and demand, a decrease in the threshold for ventricular fibrillation, and an increase in platelet aggregation; avoidance of these effects may explain the rapid cardiac benefits of quitting smoking. Coronary atherosclerosis and intimal thickening of intramyocardial arteries and arterioles are more frequent in smokers than in nonsmokers.

Cigarette smoking is a major risk factor for arteriosclerosis obliterans (Chap. 250) and thromboangiitis obliterans (Chap. 253). It also aggravates peripheral ischemia and may adversely affect peripheral bypass grafts. The mortality rate for atherosclerotic aortic aneurysm is greater in male smokers than nonsmokers. Cigarette smoking may also exacerbate proliferative diabetic retinopathy. Because of the association with chronic obstructive lung disease, cigarette smoking is an important factor leading to cor pulmonale.

Cancer Although the cause and effect relationship between cigarette smoking and lung cancer is one of the best documented in medicine, the current epidemic continues (Chap. 268). In 1978 more persons in the United States, an estimated 92,000, died from lung cancer than from any other tumor. The risk of developing lung cancer is quantitatively related to cigarette smoke exposure. Men who smoke one pack a day increase their risk tenfold compared with nonsmokers; men who smoke two packs a day may increase their risk more than 25-fold compared with nonsmokers. Workers in the asbestos and uranium mining industries who smoke cigarettes are at especially high risk for developing lung cancer. In the past 25 years cigarette consumption in the United States declined in men under the age of 60, and lung cancer mortality is beginning to plateau in this group. Cigarette consumption by women increased in the United States during this period, and lung cancer mortality is currently increasing at a faster rate in women than in men. Because 5-year survival rates for lung cancer are less than 10 percent, emphasis must be placed on prevention. An estimated 80 percent of lung cancer deaths are attributable to cigarette smoking and are preventable. Giving up cigarettes is associated with a gradual decline in the risk of developing lung cancer. After 15 years the ex-smoker's risk approximates that of the nonsmoker. Squamous-cell and oat-cell carcinoma are the histological types of lung cancer most closely associated with cigarette smoking.

Cigarette, cigar, and pipe usage in men is associated with a fivefold increased risk of developing cancer of the oral cavity, larynx, and esophagus; alcohol consumption contributes to the increased risk. Carcinoma of the bladder is also associated with cigarette smoking in men.

Respiratory disease Cigarette smoking is the most important factor contributing to the development of chronic obstructive pulmonary disease (COPD), that is, chronic bronchitis and emphysema (Chap. 263). Of the estimated 25,000 deaths from COPD that occurred in the United States in 1978, approximately 70 percent were attributable to smoking, and many of these deaths were preceded by prolonged respiratory disability. Depending upon the extent of smoke exposure, male cigarette smokers experience from 4 to 25 times higher mortality secondary to COPD than do nonsmokers. Chronic cough, sputum production, and breathlessness are much more common in smokers. Tests of pulmonary function including measurements of large and small airway obstruction, loss of elastic recoil, ventilation-perfusion mismatching, and defects in diffusing capacity are abnormal in smokers compared with nonsmokers. Subtle pulmonary function abnormalities may be present even in teen-age smokers. When compared with continuing smokers, ex-smokers experience a decrease in mortality from

COPD, a decrease in prevalence of pulmonary symptoms, and improved pulmonary function. British studies suggest that regular measurement of the forced expiratory volume in middle age may identify individuals who are at high risk for developing symptomatic COPD. Cessation of smoking would be especially valuable for these patients. Chronic inhalation of pulmonary irritants and ciliotoxins (Table 219-2) may contribute to the development of COPD. Studies of the pathogenesis of emphysema suggest that smoking may lead to an excess of pulmonary proteases. The major site of obstruction in chronic bronchitis is the bronchiole measuring less than 2 mm in diameter, and cigarette smoking is associated with bronchiolitis and increased stickiness of bronchiolar mucus. For most people in the United States cigarette smoking is a more important cause of COPD than are occupational or environmental factors; however, several factors may act conjointly to increase morbidity and mortality from COPD. In a rare disorder, homozygous α_1-antitrypsin deficiency, smoking accelerates the tendency to panacinar emphysema; smoking may play an additive role in individuals heterozygous for this state.

Cigarette smoking has been associated with an increased incidence of respiratory infections and deaths from pneumonia and influenza. Postoperative respiratory complications and spontaneous pneumothorax are also more common in smokers. Because tobacco smoke may increase airway obstruction, asthmatics should be urged not to smoke. Nicotinic stomatitis and chronic laryngitis occur more frequently in smokers than in nonsmokers.

Pregnancy Smoking during pregnancy may affect the fetus adversely. Infants whose mothers smoked during pregnancy weigh, on an average, 170 g less than infants whose mothers did not smoke. Maternal smoking during pregnancy is related to an increase in early fetal and neonatal deaths. This increased risk may be much greater in pregnancies already at high risk due to other factors.

Gastrointestinal disorders Gastric and duodenal ulcer disease is more prevalent and causes more deaths in male cigarette smokers than in nonsmokers. Smoking impairs healing of peptic ulcers, inhibits pancreatic bicarbonate secretion, and decreases the pressure of esophageal and pyloric sphincters.

Involuntary smoke inhalation Indoor atmospheres and other confined spaces are often contaminated by tobacco smoke which is inhaled involuntarily by both smokers and nonsmokers. Most of the atmospheric pollutants arise from sidestream smoke. It contains greater concentrations of many smoke constituents than does mainstream smoke, but since sidestream smoke is diluted in a large volume of air, the smoke exposure and health hazards of involuntary inhalation are much less than those associated with smoking.

The maximum acceptable ambient carbon monoxide level in the United States is 9 ppm, and in the setting of poor ventilation and heavy smoking this level may exceed 50 ppm. Breathing smoke-polluted air may exacerbate symptomatic CHD and COPD. Ocular and upper respiratory tract irritation is common in nonsmokers exposed to smoke-contaminated air.

Drug metabolism Tobacco smoke constituents induce hepatic microsomal enzyme systems which are important in the metabolism of many drugs. For example, cigarette smoking appears to increase the metabolism of phenacetin, propoxyphene, and antipyrine. The theophylline half-life is shorter in heavy smokers than in nonsmokers, and consequently smokers may require higher maintenance doses of this drug. With cessation of smoking, adjustment of the dose may be necessary.

TYPES OF SMOKING During the past 20 years the amount of tar and nicotine delivered by cigarettes made in the United

States decreased by more than 50 percent. Currently, the average United States cigarette delivers about 1.1 mg nicotine and 17 mg tar. Filter cigarettes now account for about 90 percent of sales. Death rates for CHD and lung cancer are somewhat lower for smokers of "low" tar and nicotine cigarettes than for smokers of "high" tar and nicotine cigarettes; nonetheless, death rates of nonsmokers are still much lower than those of smokers of "low" tar and nicotine cigarettes.

Cigar and pipe smokers usually inhale less smoke than cigarette smokers. This is presumably related to the alkaline pH of cigar and pipe tobacco, which is irritating to the respiratory tract. The smoke exposure and overall mortality rates of pipe and cigar smokers in the United States are substantially less than those of cigarette smokers. Death rates of cigarette, cigar, and pipe smokers are approximately equal for carcinoma of the oral cavity, larynx, and esophagus, sites where exposures to cigarette, cigar, and pipe smoke are similar. The mortality rates of most cigar and pipe smokers for cancer at other sites, CHD, and COPD are not greatly elevated above the rates of nonsmokers, but cigar and pipe smokers who inhale consistently may experience adverse health effects comparable with those of cigarette smokers.

CESSATION OF SMOKING Psychosocial forces lead to the onset of smoking, especially among teen-agers. Later, drug dependency and psychological factors maintain the smoking habit. It is estimated that more than 30 million people in the United States have stopped smoking. Many long-term smokers quit because of smoking-related health problems. This seems to explain Hammond's observation that the death rate of men smoking more than 20 cigarettes a day was somewhat higher in the months immediately after quitting than that of continuing smokers. Thereafter, a gradual decline in death rates was observed in ex-smokers. Ten or more years after quitting, the death rate of smokers of more than 20 cigarettes a day had dropped about two-thirds, and the death rate of individuals smoking 20 cigarettes a day or less was about the same as that of nonsmokers (Fig. 219-2). Ex-smokers usually experience prompt symptomatic improvement. On the average they also gain about five pounds.

In the United States more than 80 percent of cigarette smokers would like to stop smoking. Many self-care and organized programs are available to assist these individuals. Organized programs employ several techniques including instruction, counseling, withdrawal clinics, behavioral modification, hypnosis, aversive conditioning, self-monitoring, and drug therapy. Even though individual successes result from these programs, their value is uncertain. One-year abstinence rates of 20 to 30 percent are common. Relapse usually occurs during the 3-month interval after quitting. Successful programs emphasize maintenance of the nonsmoking state during this critical period.

All smokers should be encouraged to quit, especially those in high-risk groups with chronic pulmonary disease, coronary artery disease, and pregnancy. Physicians can help their smoking patients in the following manner:

1 Obtain a quantitative smoking history.
2 Explain the health risks in a personally relevant fashion.
3 Emphasize the benefits associated with cessation.
4 Advise and assist the patient to quit smoking.
5 Support the patient in a maintenance program.

Patients who are unable to stop cigarette smoking should be assisted to reduce their smoke exposure by smoking low-tar and low-nicotine cigarettes, smoking fewer cigarettes, inhaling less, taking fewer puffs, and leaving a longer stub.

Ultimately, primary smoking prevention in the pediatric and adolescent age groups may be the most effective program. Young people who understand the consequences of smoking to their health and who appreciate the difficulty of quitting are less likely to start smoking.

REFERENCES

AMERICAN HEART ASSOCIATION: Report of the ad hoc committee on cigarette smoking and cardiovascular diseases. Circulation 57:404A, 1978

HAMMOND EC: Smoking in relation to the death rates of one million men and women, in *Epidemiological Approaches to the Study of Cancer and Other Chronic Diseases*, W Haenszel (ed). National Cancer Institute Monograph no 19, 1966, pp 127–204

ROYAL COLLEGE OF PHYSICIANS: *Smoking or Health*. Tunbridge Wells, Kent, Pitman Medical, 1977

SCHMELTZ I, HOFFMANN D: Chemical studies on tobacco smoke. XXXVIII. The physicochemical nature of cigarette smoke, in *Proceedings of the 3rd World Conference on Smoking and Health.* DHEW Publication no (NIH) 76–1221, 1976, pp 13–34

SCHWARTZ JL: Smoking cures: Ways to kick an unhealthy habit, in *Research on Smoking Behavior*. NIDA Research Monograph 17, DHEW Publication no (ADM) 78–581, 1977, pp 308–336

U.S. DEPARTMENT OF HEALTH, EDUCATION, AND WELFARE: *Smoking and Health*. PHS Publication no 1103, 1964

————: *The Health Consequences of Smoking: A Reference Edition*. DHEW Publication no (CDC) 78–8357, 1976

————: The effects of smoking on health. Morb Mort Week Rep 26:145, 1977

WORLD HEALTH ORGANIZATION: *Smoking and Its Effects on Health.* WHO Technical Report Series no 568, 1975

FIGURE 219-2
Male mortality ratios for current and past cigarette smokers.

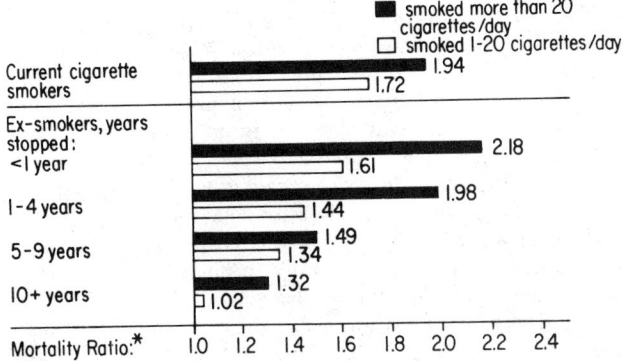

■ smoked more than 20 cigarettes/day
□ smoked 1-20 cigarettes/day

Current cigarette smokers	1.94 / 1.72
Ex-smokers, years stopped: <1 year	2.18 / 1.61
1-4 years	1.98 / 1.44
5-9 years	1.49 / 1.34
10+ years	1.32 / 1.02

Mortality Ratio:* 1.0 1.2 1.4 1.6 1.8 2.0 2.2 2.4

* Death rate for current or ex-smokers divided by the death rate for those who never smoked regularly

220
RADIATION INJURY

E. DONNALL THOMAS
EUGENE P. CRONKITE

TYPES OF RADIATION The types of ionizing radiation most often causing injury are x-rays, gamma rays, alpha rays, beta rays, protons, and neutrons. X-rays and gamma rays are photons. X-rays are produced by x-ray machines and as secondary emissions from particle accelerators or electron tubes. The energy spectrum of x-rays is continuous. Gamma rays are produced by radioactive decay. Beta rays are electrons. Alpha rays are composed of the nuclei of the helium atom with a mass of 4 and a charge of 2+. Protons are nuclei of hydrogen atoms with a mass of 1 and a charge of 1+. Protons are of interest because of their common use as primary particles in accelerators. They are also important because they are usually the secondary damaging particles produced by neutron interaction with tissue or other materials. Neutrons have a mass of 1 and a charge of 0. Biologic injury is produced primarily by ionization from secondary charged particles in diverse ways. Fast neutrons react principally with hydrogen atoms. As a result of collision, a portion of the energy is imparted to the hydrogen atom, and a proton is ejected causing the damage. With thermal or slow neutrons, damage is done by actual capture of the neutrons resulting in a secondary emission of ionizing radiation as the transmuted hydrogen, nitrogen, or other substance in tissue decays and emits radioactivity.

MECHANISM OF ACTION   The major biologic effects of radiation occur in three interlinked steps. First, photons penetrate the protoplasm, interacting to produce ion pairs. This reaction takes on the order of 10^{-13} s. The second step is a radiochemical reaction of these ions primarily with water, producing free radicals such as H and OH. These reactions take about 10^{-9} s. These free radicals produce a further chain of reactions with themselves and tissue water to produce additional reactive forms such as H_2O_2 and HO_2. These products persist for microseconds or at most a few seconds. The last reaction takes place between these products and critical protoplasmic molecules. The nature of this last reaction is not known, but, because the actual amount of energy imparted to the system is small, the damage is generally thought to involve substances of low concentration but major importance to the living system such as nucleic acids or enzymes.

DOSE UNITS   Two dose units are essential for the understanding of the quantitative effects of radiation. The *roentgen* (R), a measure of total exposure in air, is defined as the quantity of x-ray or gamma radiation such that the associated corpuscular emission per 0.001293 g air at standard conditions produces in air ions carrying one electrostatic unit of either sign. For energy to be deposited, there must be an interaction with matter. Hence, with x-rays passing through a vacuum, no radiation dose is delivered. In practice, the most important factor is the energy imparted to various tissues from a number of different types of radiation, and it is therefore essential to have a second unit of radiation which overcomes the limitation of the roentgen. This second unit, the *rad,* is a measure of absorbed dose equal to 100 ergs per gram of absorbed energy which applies to any type of radiation in any tissue. For small pieces of tissue in an x-ray beam of 1 R/min, the absorbed dose is very close to 1 rad/min. However, as irradiated objects become larger, the diminution in intensity due to the interaction of radiation and matter (buildup and then exponential attenuation) and the changing types of interaction (photoelectric effect, Compton effect, etc.) must be considered. In tissue of uniform density this leads to a decreasing absorbed dose in successive depth levels after equilibrium is attained. However, at interfaces such as soft tissue and bone, the absorbed dose may increase sharply. In addition to the exposure in roentgens and the absorbed dose in rads, attention must be given to the distribution of the absorbed dose in the anatomic area of interest.

The *density of ionization* in tissue varies with the energy and type of radiation as well as the composition of tissue. The density of ionization is referred to as *specific ionization* (ions per unit track length) or as *linear energy transfer* (LET) (kiloelectron volts deposited per unit track length). Among other factors, the density of ionization influences the biologic effect

for equivalent amount of energy deposited, with the effect being greater with more densely ionizing radiation. This leads to consideration of the relative biologic effectiveness (RBE), which is defined as the ratio of the dose in rads of standard radiation (usually x-ray or gamma radiation of 250 to 400 kV energy) to produce a given degree of biologic effect, to the dose in rads of an unknown radiation to produce the same degree of biologic effect. For example, if the median lethal dose (LD_{50}) of x-rays is 600 rads and for neutrons 300 rads, the RBE will be 2. The RBE may vary with the biologic response or the conditions of irradiation. For example, when the same radiations are used, a different value may be obtained for mortality, cataract, or tumor development. Another useful unit is the *rem,* which stands for *roentgen equivalent mammal.* Numerically, rem = rad × RBE.

Also of importance is the *dose rate.* In general, the lower the dose rate, the less will be the biologic effect. In a crude sense, dose rates in excess of approximately 5 rads/min give the same result. At lower dose rates the effect per unit of radiation becomes less as time becomes available for repair of radiation injury. In the past, genetic effects were believed to be independent of dose rate. This implies that all increments of radiation received by the gonads would add up directly as mutations. However, it is now known that there is a dose-rate dependence with respect to the production of mutations by irradiation of spermatogonia, and also for leukemogenesis in mice.

If the dose of radiation is sufficiently high, death of any living cell can be observed promptly as cell necrosis. However, after lower doses of radiation (precise values vary with the tissue) disturbances in cell proliferation are seen. These effects of radiation, other than the outright killing of cells, consist of interference with mitosis and DNA synthesis. DNA synthesis is impaired in two ways: (1) the rate of synthesis is slower, and (2) cells may continue DNA synthesis and become polyploid.

The diminution in the production of new cells in the tissues that are undergoing continual renewal (mucosa, bone marrow, gonads, etc.) results in a spectrum ranging from progressive hypoplasia to total atrophy, depending on the dose. Some cells still capable of mitosis that are not killed outright may be injured to such a degree that they will go through one or two generative cycles, producing abnormal progeny, such as giant metamyelocytes and hypersegmented neutrophils, before dying.

CLINICAL PHENOMENA IN RELATION TO DOSE AND TIME AFTER EXPOSURE   Experience with radiation exposure of the entire human body is based on the effects of atomic bombs, laboratory and reactor accidents, and total-body radiotherapy. After any radiation accident close cooperation of the physician and health physicist is essential to obtain the best estimate of the radiation dose and to evaluate its probable effect in terms of the likely distribution of the absorbed dose.

The acute radiation syndromes may be classified generally as cerebral, gastrointestinal, and hematopoietic.

The *cerebral* syndrome is produced by acute uniform exposure of the whole brain to several thousand rads and is usually fatal. It is characterized by nausea, vomiting, listlessness, and drowsiness followed by tremors, convulsions, ataxia, and death. This sequence was observed in an industrial accident with death occurring 36 h after exposure.

Therapeutic irradiation of the brain is usually spaced over a period of 2 to 4 weeks, and doses of 2400 rads [used for prophylaxis of central nervous system (CNS) leukemia] to 6000 rads, (used for brain cancer) result in no recognizable acute CNS toxicity. Late effects from demyelination may occur.

The *gastrointestinal* syndrome occurs when the dose of radiation is lower, in the range of 600 to 2000 rads, and is usually maximal 3 to 5 days after exposure. At the higher doses it is characterized by intractable nausea, vomiting, and diarrhea leading to severe dehydration and vascular collapse. Severe injury to the gastrointestinal tract is caused by direct killing of a fraction of the crypt cells and by inhibition of mitosis. The mature epithelial cells continue to migrate out onto the villi in an orderly fashion, eventually being lost from the tip of the villi, producing a progressive diminution in the number of cells covering the villi. The epithelial cells become progressively cuboidal and then squamous in appearance, and ultimately the intestinal villi become denuded. Death from the gastrointestinal syndrome can be prevented by plasma, fluid, and electrolyte replacement. If the patient can be supported, regeneration of the gastrointestinal epithelium begins about the sixth day and is remarkably complete within 2 weeks.

The *hematopoietic* syndrome which occurs following whole-body exposure may be preceded by anorexia, nausea, and vomiting that is maximal between 6 and 12 h after exposure to doses of radiation between 200 and 1000 rads. Within 24 to 36 h after exposure the subject is usually asymptomatic, and a period of relative well-being is experienced until the onset of bleeding and/or infection secondary to bone marrow failure.

Lymphopenia begins immediately and becomes maximal within 24 to 36 h as a result of a direct killing of these extremely radiosensitive cells. Thereafter the lymphocytes remain at low levels for weeks and recover over several months.

A neutrophilic leukocytosis appears within a few hours after irradiation as a result of an inflammatory release of granulocytes from the bone marrow. The granulocytes are not directly damaged by the radiation, and therefore peripheral blood neutropenia does not begin until the bone marrow reserves are depleted of the more mature granulocytes. The primary damage is to the radiosensitive precursor cells so that the marrow becomes extremely hypoplastic after a few days. After sublethal and low lethal doses the minimum values of granulocytes occur in 4 to 6 weeks. After high lethal doses granulocytes diminish more rapidly, and values approaching 0 appear within 7 to 10 days. Reticulocyte production is halted within a few days, but anemia due to failure of red blood cell production is slow in onset because of the long life span of the red blood cell.

Thrombocytopenia develops slowly over a period of approximately 30 days after doses of 200 to 400 rads. After doses of 600 to 1000 rads, which effectively stop new platelet production, the decline in the platelet count reflects the life span of the platelet, and levels below 20,000 per cubic millimeter develop in approximately 9 days. The bleeding component of the hematopoietic syndrome is due to the lack of platelets and can be corrected by platelet transfusions.

Studies of decreased resistance to infection following total-body exposure have disclosed many contributing factors including granulocytopenia, lymphopenia, impaired antibody production, impaired granulocyte function, decreased cellular ability to kill phagocytosed bacteria, and damage to skin and bowel which provides portals of entry for infectious agents. However, in the acute hematopoietic syndrome, the greatest factor by far is the quantitative reduction in circulating granulocytes, and there is a high probability of bacterial infection when the granulocyte level falls below 200 cells per cubic millimeter.

INHOMOGENOUS EXPOSURE TO RADIATION The preceding description of radiation injury was based primarily on human clinical experience and animal experimentation in which the distribution of the dose absorbed by tissues was relatively uniform. However, conditions of exposure may be such that there are marked inhomogeneities in the absorbed dose. For example, an exposure may result in almost no irradiation to the lower part of the body and very heavy exposure to the abdomen and hands, resulting in extensive necrosis of the skin of these areas in addition to the fatal injury of deeper tissues. In evaluating radiation accident, the physical conditions and the probable distribution of absorbed dose within the body must be considered. What may initially appear as a fatal accident in terms of air exposure may be sublethal when effects of distribution of the absorbed dose are calculated.

MANAGEMENT OF ACUTE HUMAN RADIATION INJURY Presumptive evidence of exposure to radiation and the onset of nausea and vomiting indicate a possible medical emergency. Therapy is directed toward the management of both the gastrointestinal and hematopoietic syndromes and should be instituted as if the exposure were in the lethal range. If subsequent evaluation indicates less irradiation, therapeutic efforts can be reduced. The following is an outline of the therapeutic regimen assuming a lethal exposure:

1 If the exposure involves radioactive materials or neutrons, the patient must be monitored for radioactivity and decontaminated if necessary.

2 History, physical examination, and laboratory studies, including a complete hematologic evaluation, should be completed as quickly as possible. Cytogenetic preparations of direct bone marrow and phytohemagglutinin-stimulated peripheral blood lymphocytes should be set up for later analysis as biological dosimeters useful in estimating the level of radiation exposure. Lymphocytes should be obtained immediately, while still available, for human lymphocyte antigen (HLA) typing and storage for later mixed leukocyte cultures. The results of the typing will be useful for matching for granulocyte and platelet transfusions and for identification of a possible bone marrow donor.

3 Fluid and electrolyte balance should be monitored closely and restored with appropriate replacement solutions.

4 Ultraisolation techniques have been shown to be effective in preventing infection in patients undergoing treatment for leukemia or subjected to bone marrow transplantation. By analogy, the victim of a radiation accident should, if at all possible, be admitted to a laminar airflow room with a complete regimen of skin sterilization, a sterile diet, and oral nonabsorbable antibiotics for gut sterilization. If this is not feasible, measures should be initiated to prevent endogenous or exogenous infection. Reduction of the gastrointestinal flora is essential, and this is usually accomplished with oral nonabsorbable broad-spectrum antibiotics and an antifungal agent. Particular attention should be paid to oral hygiene and dental care. The patient should be nursed in a single-bed room, and reverse isolation precautions should be enforced vigorously.

5 Platelet transfusions should be given when the platelet count falls below 20,000 per cubic millimeter and continued until values above that level can be sustained. If the patient becomes refractory to random donor platelets, use of HLA-matched platelets from unrelated donors may become necessary. Family member transfusions should not be administered until the possibility of bone marrow transplantation has been excluded because such transfusions might sensitize the patient to the transplantation antigens of a potential marrow donor.

6 Granulocyte transfusions are indicated to prevent infection in patients who are not in ultraisolation when the granulocyte count falls below 200 per cubic millimeter. Granulocyte transfusions are indicated for therapy of any significant infection in a granulocytopenic patient. Once initiated, granulocyte transfusions should be continued on

a daily basis until the patient can sustain a granulocyte count above 200 per cubic millimeter.

7 Infection is an ever-present danger, and bacteriologic cultures should be obtained frequently. The onset of significant fever (38.5°C) should arouse a strong suspicion of infection in the granulocytopenic patient. Fever with clinical signs of bacteremia or fever sustained more than 24 h is an indication for initiating systemic antibacterial therapy even though cultures are negative. Since the most likely bacterial agent is a gram-negative organism from the normal bowel flora, initial therapy usually includes an aminoglycoside and carbenicillin with additional antibiotics added as indicated by culture results. Subsequently, if cultures are negative but fever persists, therapy with a combination of trimethoprim and sulfamethoxazole or, more rarely, with amphotericin may be considered. Once broad-spectrum antibiotic therapy has been initiated, it should be continued until the granulocyte count rises above 200 per cubic millimeter.

8 Packed red blood cells should be given as indicated to keep the hematocrit above 25.

9 All blood products should be given 1500 rads before infusion into the patient in order to inactivate lymphocytes that might subsequently proliferate and cause a graft-versus-host reaction in the immunosuppressed patient.

10 Bone marrow transplantation only rarely will be of value in an irradiation accident victim because of uncertainties about the magnitude of the radiation dose, inhomogeneity of the dose, and the requirement that the dose be within the limits of rescue by marrow transplantation, approximately 600 to 2000 rads. If marrow transplantation is indicated, immediate efforts should be made to locate a donor who is HLAA, HLAB, and HLAD identical with the patient. A genetically identical twin is an ideal donor, and one irradiation victim exposed to approximately 600 rads showed a rapid hematopoietic recovery following the infusion of marrow from his twin. The patient's family members should be typed in an effort to identify an HLA-matched sibling. By use of an HLA-identical sibling donor, marrow transplantation has resulted in a number of long-term survivors for patients with acute leukemia given 1000 rads total body irradiation. It is now possible to identify unrelated individuals who are HLA matched, but, owing to the heterogeneity of the HLA genetic region, the magnitude of such an undertaking is formidable.

PREVENTION AND ANTICIPATION Nothing can substitute for prevention. Shielding, distance, and limiting the exposure time are the only effective preventive measures against exposure from radiation sources, whether in industry, medical practice, military action, or civil defense. A series of drugs containing sulfhydryl groups will protect against radiation by effectively reducing the toxicity of the dose by approximately 50 percent if administered within minutes preceding exposure. However, the toxic effects of these drugs prevent continuous prophylactic administration. Another anticipatory maneuver is to store bone marrow in the frozen state for long periods which enables it to retain the viability necessary for successful engraftment. It would seem reasonable to store marrow of individuals at high risk against the eventuality of an accident that might produce marrow-lethal exposure. Such a program would be expensive and requires that individuals whose risk of accidental exposure is high enough to justify the expense be identified.

LONG-TERM EFFECTS Radiation alters the "information system" of proliferating somatic and germ cells. These dividing cells of the blood, gastrointestinal tract, skin, lens, gonads, and other areas pass on either "bad" or "inadequate" information, presumably in the form of altered DNA, to their progeny, resulting in late somatic disease like cancer, cataracts, degenerative disorders, or nonspecific shortening of life. The survivors of the atomic bombs at Hiroshima and Nagasaki have been studied closely for 33 years. The most important finding has been an increased incidence of neoplasms in many organs, particularly leukemia and cancers of the thyroid, lung, and breast. The survivors continue to show increased posterior lenticular opacities and chromosome aberrations in peripheral blood lymphocytes. Impaired growth and development were observed following exposure during intrauterine life or childhood. To date no radiation-related genetic effects have been detected (see below).

In the course of radiation therapy of cancer, it is unavoidably necessary to expose normal tissues. Radiation injury results in a wide spectrum of tissue reaction depending upon injury to the tissue itself and to the small blood vessels supplying the tissue or organ. Rapidly dividing or growing tissues are most susceptible to injury, and the lag time for injury to appear is short. For example, irradiation of the scalp with 400 to 500 rads causes alopecia which is followed by prompt regrowth of hair, but irradiation of the testicle by 300 to 400 rads causes aspermia which persists for several years. Exposure of the kidney, liver, or lung results in injury that begins at about 1500 rads and increases progressively with increasing exposure. Radiation pneumonitis usually develops within 4 to 8 weeks after exposure, but fibrotic changes may occur over a period of months. Above 4000 rads, injury to the spinal cord is observed but may take 6 to 24 months to become apparent. Irradiation of muscle, bone, connective tissue, and the brain is usually well tolerated up to 6000 rads. Some late radiation effects, such as cancer of the skin, may take several decades to develop. Textbooks on radiation therapy should be consulted for details of these late effects of radiation injury.

Radiation can produce mutation of genes, the information and transmission centers for heredity. Not all mutations are harmful, but the chances are overwhelming that a change will be detrimental to the species. Not all mutations produce visible, immediately detectable effects. The concern is not only with an increase in the number of obvious malformations but with changes that will lead to such undesirable characteristics as lowered life expectancy, decreased fertility, a general increase in physical and mental disease, and an increase in fetal or neonatal death rates. The more obvious changes usually lead to early death of the individual and reduced fertility in those that survive. Therefore, the harmful mutant is relatively quickly deleted from the population. The more subtle changes, however, are propagated longer and may affect a larger number of individuals. The mutation may be dominant or recessive. Most dominant mutations are also lethal, and many such mutations may be missed because the fertilized egg never develops far enough to be recognized as a new individual. If the mutation is recessive, the mutant will not become evident unless both parents have the same mutant genes and transfer them to the child. If the mutation rate were increased by a single exposure of the population to radiation, the effects would be dispersed through many generations, and half the total damage produced would not be observed until some 30 to 50 generations had been born. For this reason, it is not possible to take negative evidence in populations that have been exposed to date as an indication that the genetic damage is small. If, for instance, an effect in the children born to individuals irradiated in Japan by the atom bombs were already obvious, it would mean that the total genetic effect would be great indeed. It has been hypothesized, but not proved, that radiation damage to the genetic material of the cell does not display a threshold effect. Therefore, the damage would be present, but not easily detected, even with very small doses, and would increase with increasing doses. Because exposure to irradiation cannot be avoided in modern industrial society and in the practice of modern medicine, and because of the uncertainty about its quantitative somatic or genetic effects, it is mandatory that exposure be minimal. Only by rigid control of radiation exposure can present generations be protected from its somatic effects, and future generations from its genetic consequences.

REFERENCES

ALAVI JB et al: A randomized clinical trial of granulocyte transfusions for infection in acute leukemia. N Engl J Med 296:706, 1977

BOND VP et al: *Mammalian Radiation Lethality.* New York, Academic, 1965

CASARETT AP: *Radiation Biology.* Englewood Cliffs, NJ, Prentice-Hall, 1968

CLIFT RA, BUCKNER CD: Supportive measures for patients with aplastic anaemia, in *Clinics in Haematology. Aplastic Anaemia.* Eastbourne, Saunders, 1978, chap 13.

——— et al: Granulocyte transfusions for the prevention of infection in patients receiving bone-marrow transplants. N Engl J Med 298:1052, 1978

CRONKITE EP, BOND VP: *Radiation Injury in Man.* Springfield, Ill, Charles C Thomas, 1960

HERZIG RH et al: Successful granulocyte transfusion therapy for gram-negative septicemia. A prospectively randomized controlled study. N Engl J Med 296:701, 1977

JABLON S, KATO H: Studies of the mortality of A-bomb survivors. 5. Radiation dose and mortality, 1950–1970. Radiat Res 50:649, 1972

LEVINE AS et al: Protected environments and prophylactic antibiotics. A prospective controlled study of their utility in the therapy of acute leukemia. N Engl J Med 228:477, 1973

RUBIN PR, CASARETT GW: *Clinical Radiation Pathology.* Philadelphia, Saunders, 1968

THOMAS ED et al: Bone-marrow transplantation. N Engl J Med 292:832, 895, 1975

221
ELECTRICAL INJURIES

JAMES F. WALLACE

EPIDEMIOLOGY Electrical injury has become progressively more common since the first human fatality from accidental electrocution was reported in 1879. In the United States, approximately 1000 deaths occur annually from electric current accidents, while another 200 persons die as a result of being struck by lightning. In addition, major electrical burns presently constitute nearly 5 percent of all admissions to burn centers in this country. Electrical injuries occur most commonly among utility pole linemen and construction workers who come into contact with high-tension current, but nearly a third result from accidents in the home or other settings including the hospital with its many electrically powered instruments and appliances.

PATHOGENESIS In understanding the fundamental aspects of electric current injury, it is helpful to consider some electrophysical principles. For an electric current to flow, there must be a closed pathway or circuit, and a difference in potential or voltage must exist between two points in this completed circuit. The flow of current is directly related to the voltage difference and inversely proportional to the electrical resistance between two points in the circuit (Ohm's law). High-resistance paths allow relatively small currents to flow, while low resistances permit large currents to flow. When the voltage is very high, the flow of current will likewise be relatively great, unless the resistance is increased proportionally to the voltage; however, if the potential difference between the two points can be minimized, the current flow can also be minimized regardless of resistance.

Although the end result of passage of an electric current through the human body is unpredictable in the individual case, many factors are known to influence the nature and severity of electrical injuries. Body tissues vary considerably in their *resistance* to the flow of current, with conductivity being roughly proportional to water content. Bone and skin offer relatively high resistance, while blood, muscle, and nerve are good conductors. The resistance of normal skin can be lowered by *moisture,* and this factor alone can convert what might ordinarily be a mild injury to a fatal shock. Of importance at the time of contact is *grounding* which, if effective, can minimize the voltage difference between two points in the electric circuit and lower the intensity of current passing through the body. The *pathway of the current through the body* is also crucial. An accident involving passage of a current between a point of contact on the leg and the ground is less likely to be injurious than one between the head and the foot, in which the heart lies between the two poles of the circuit. Similarly, a small current leak which would be innocuous when applied to the surface of the intact body may result in a fatal arrhythmia when conducted directly to the heart via a low-resistance intracardiac catheter. *Duration of contact* also influences the outcome of electrical injury. Alternating current is much more dangerous than direct current, partly because of its ability to produce tetanic muscular contractions which prevent the victim from being able to release contact with the circuit. This is usually accompanied by sweating, which lowers skin resistance, allowing current of still greater intensity to pass into the body until fatal cardiac arrhythmia results.

While the effects of electricity upon the body are incompletely understood, many pathophysiologic features of severe electrical injury have been described. In general, when sudden death occurs following low-voltage shock, it is due to the direct effect of relatively small amounts of current upon the myocardium resulting in ventricular fibrillation. With high-tension injury (greater than 1000 V) cardiac asystole and respiratory arrest occur probably as a result of injury to the medullary centers of the brain.

In addition, contact with high-intensity current may cause three types of thermal injuries. Current coursing externally to the body from the contact point to the ground may generate temperatures as high as 10,000°C and cause extensive carbonification of skin and immediately underlying tissues termed *arc* or *flash burns.* Such burns often ignite surrounding clothing or nearby objects which result in *flame burns.* Finally, there is injury due to the *direct heating* of tissues by electric current. As it traverses the skin, energy from current is converted into heat which produces coagulation necrosis at the points where it enters and exits from the skin as well as in striated muscle and blood vessels through which it passes. The associated vascular injury results in thromboses, often at sites distant from the body surface, and accounts for the observation that a greater amount of tissue destruction characteristically occurs in an electrical injury than is apparent on first inspection.

PATHOLOGY In patients who die immediately, autopsy findings are limited to burns and generalized petechial hemorrhages. If patients survive for a period of days or longer, postmortem examination reveals focal necrosis of bone, large blood vessels, muscle, peripheral nerves, spinal cord, or brain.

Renal tubular necrosis may also be seen when acute renal failure follows extensive tissue destruction.

CLINICAL MANIFESTATIONS Immediately after a severe electrical shock, patients are usually comatose, apneic, and in circulatory collapse from ventricular fibrillation or cardiac standstill. If they survive this stage, they often are disoriented, combative, and frequently may have seizures. Often they will be found to have fractures of bone caused either by convulsive muscular contractions accompanying the shock or from falls at the time of the accident. Hypovolemic shock often appears soon after high-tension electrical injury and is due to the rapid loss of fluid into areas of tissue damage, and from body surface burns. Hypotension, direct injury to the kidneys by the electric current, and renal tubular damage from myoglobin and hemoglobin pigments liberated during massive muscle necrosis and hemolysis may lead to acute renal failure.

Besides the extensive destruction of tissue occurring instantly in electrical burns, additional injury from ischemia produced by swelling of damaged tissues may appear later and is often accompanied by severe metabolic acidosis. Other serious complications which may be seen are gastrointestinal hemorrhage from preexisting or acute ulcers and both anaerobic and aerobic infections originating in inadequately debrided necrotic muscle masses.

Late effects include various neurological disabilities, visual disturbances, and the residual damage left by burns. Nervous system injuries are frequent and include peripheral neuropathies, incomplete transection of the spinal cord, and reflex sympathetic dystrophies, as well as late convulsive disorders and intractable headache. The development of cataracts of one or both eyes has been reported to occur up to 3 years following electrical injury.

LABORATORY FINDINGS Immediately following major electrical injury the hematocrit is elevated and the plasma volume reduced, reflecting sequestration of fluid in the wound. Unless extensive flame burns are also present, serial determinations of either of these parameters provide a good means of monitoring the adequacy of fluid replacement therapy. Myoglobinuria is seen frequently in association with severe shocks, and when it persists following establishment of urine flow, usually indicates massive muscle injury. In many patients arterial blood pH determinations will indicate the presence of metabolic acidosis. Lumbar puncture may show elevated pressure associated with cerebral edema or bloody spinal fluid as a result of intracerebral hemorrhage. The electrocardiogram not infrequently shows tachycardia and minor ST-segment alterations which can persist for several weeks following injury. Unexplained acute hypokalemia leading to respiratory arrest and cardiac arrhythmias has developed in some patients between the second and fourth weeks following injury.

TREATMENT Removal of victims from contact with the current should be accomplished immediately without touching them directly. Rescuers should use a rubber sheet, a leather belt applied as a sling, a wooden pole, or other nonconductive material to detach them, and this should be preceded by cutting off the source of current when possible. If the victim is not breathing, mouth-to-mouth ventilation should be instituted at once. Although most cases who survive develop spontaneous respiration within half an hour, complete recovery after longer periods occurs often enough so that respiratory support should be continued for at least 4 h. If there is no evidence of heartbeat, external cardiac massage should accompany ventilatory resuscitation. Persons struck by lightning frequently have cardiac asystole which responds to a manual blow to the chest, while victims of low-voltage shocks will usually require defibrillation to restore heart action. During cardiopulmonary resuscitation and evacuation to the hospital, attention should be paid to possible broken bones and spinal cord injuries incurred at the time of the accident.

Subsequent hospital management of patients with electrothermal injuries requires considerable specialized care; whenever feasible, they should be referred to an appropriate burn or trauma unit.

Rapid institution of fluid and electrolyte therapy for hypovolemic shock and acidosis is essential, with guidelines being the patient's urine output, hematocrit, osmolality, central venous pressure, and arterial blood gases. Standard burn formulas should not be used to estimate fluid therapy since these are based only upon extent of body surface area injury and do not take into account the extensive damage to muscle which is usually present. Instead, fluid replacement principles used in the treatment of crush injury, which electrical injury closely resembles, should be followed. Large volumes of fluid, preferably lactated Ringer's solution, should be administered in order to maintain urine output greater than 50 ml/h. If myoglobinuria persists after adequate urine flow has been established, the use of furosemide or an osmotic diuretic such as mannitol along with alkalinization of the urine is indicated. Management of the electrical wound should include adequate debridement of necrotic tissue and often will require fasciotomy to prevent further ischemic injury. Anticlostridial prophylaxis, including tetanus toxoid and high doses of penicillin, should be administered to all severely injured patients, while topical antimicrobial chemotherapy with mafenide (Sulfamylon) or silver sulfadiazine may be useful in preventing or delaying infections in extensive surface burns. Survivors of the acute episode often require extensive treatment for infection, cerebral edema, visceral injury, and delayed hemorrhage as devitalized tissues slough. If acute renal failure occurs, it should be managed as described in Chap. 275.

PREVENTION Proper installation of appliances, grounding of telephone lines and radio and television aerials, and the use of rubber gloves and dry shoes when working with electric circuits should be routine. Unused wall sockets should be kept plugged and live extension cords not left unattended, particularly in households where there are young children. During a severe thunderstorm, refuge near hilltops, riverbanks, hedges, telephone poles, and trees should be avoided. The safest shelter is the closed house, while a closed automobile, cave, ditch, or even lying on the ground curled up with hands close together is relatively secure. In hospitalized patients, the hazard of ventricular fibrillation precipitated by minute current leaks conducted directly to the myocardium from monitoring equipment via pacemakers or intravascular manometric catheters should be more widely appreciated. Hospital personnel should be aware that, in addition to medical instruments, patient contact with two or more other power line–operated devices such as television sets, radios, electric razors, lamps, and especially electric beds can also result in electrocution if the heart lies within the current path through the patient. These hazards can be minimized by proper grounding of equipment *before* a patient is connected to the instrument, periodic measurement for leakage of current supplied by each device, and by instruction in the principles of electrical safety for hospital personnel who use the complex and dangerous equipment that is so much a part of modern medical practice.

REFERENCES

APFELBERG DB et al: Pathophysiology and treatment of lightning injuries. J Trauma 14:453, 1974

ARTZ CP: Changing concepts of electrical injury. Am J Surg 128:600, 1974

BAXTER CR: Present concepts in the management of major electrical injury. Surg Clin North Am 50:1401, 1970

KAY NRM et al: The management of electrical injuries of the extremities. Surg Clin North Am 53:1459, 1973

KILPATRICK DG: The electrical environment. Med Clin North Am 55:1095, 1971

ROUSE RG, DIMICK AR: The treatment of electrical injury compared to burn injury. A review of pathophysiology and comparison of patient management protocols. J Trauma 18:43, 1978

TAUSSIG HB: Death from lightning—and the possibility of living again. Ann Intern Med 68:1345, 1968

222
DROWNING AND NEAR-DROWNING

JAMES F. WALLACE

EPIDEMIOLOGY In the United States, drowning accounts for approximately 7000 fatalities per year and is one of the three leading causes of accidental death. In addition, although no national statistics are available, it has been estimated that as many as 48,000 persons annually are near-drowning victims: those who live at least temporarily following an immersion incident. Children and young adults are most often the victims, and nearly 80 percent are males. However, with the increasing popularity of boating and water sports in this country nearly half the population is at risk of drowning each year, especially during the summer months.

PATHOPHYSIOLOGY Ten to twenty percent of drowning victims have no evidence of water aspiration in their lungs at autopsy ("dry drowning"). Death is due to asphyxia secondary to reflex laryngospasm and glottic closure. It is probable that a similar number of near-drowning victims also do not aspirate. If ventilation is reestablished before they sustain irreversible anoxic brain damage, prompt and complete recovery can be anticipated.

When aspiration accompanies drowning ("wet drowning"), the clinical situation is further complicated by the amount of surrounding water that is introduced into the respiratory tract as well as by the solutes and solids contained in it. A severe pulmonary injury often occurs, resulting in persistent arterial hypoxemia and metabolic acidosis even after ventilation has been restored.

In the past, an important distinction was made between the pathophysiology of saltwater and freshwater drowning with respect to changes in blood volume, serum electrolyte concentrations, and cardiovascular function. However, it has been established that the most important problem in human near-drowning is hypoxia and that the other disturbances are of considerably less significance in determining survival.

The mechanisms by which hypoxia develops in near-drowning with aspiration are often multiple: laryngospasm, bronchospasm, airway obstruction secondary to aspirated particulate matter, and pulmonary edema following prolonged hypoxia can take place regardless of the composition of the water aspirated, while other types of lung injury causing hypoxemia depend upon the osmolar and chemical characteristics of the immersion fluid. Aspiration of seawater, which is hypertonic compared with blood and chemically irritating to the pulmonary alveolocapillary membrane, causes a rapid shift of plasma proteins and water from the circulation into the alveolar lumen. Continued perfusion of these nonventilated, edema-filled alveoli results in an intrapulmonary right-to-left shunt and arterial hypoxemia. When hypotonic fresh water is aspirated, fluid is rapidly absorbed from the lung into the circulation.

Injury to alveolar lining cells takes place, altering or destroying the properties of pulmonary surfactant that maintains surface tension, and leading to alveolar collapse. Ventilation-perfusion ratios change in these atelectatic areas of lung, and hypoxemia is the result. Metabolic acidosis, which is present in as many as 70 percent of near-drowning victims, is a consequence of tissue hypoxia and may be severe.

Although changes in electrolyte concentrations occur, depending upon the type and volume of fluid aspirated, these disturbances are rarely life-threatening. Most persons who aspirate sufficient quantities to produce marked electrolyte abnormalities do not survive the immersion incident. Similarly, profound changes in circulating blood volume are unusual. However, hypovolemia requiring treatment may be seen in massive saltwater aspiration accompanied by shifts of fluid from the vascular space into the lung.

Although rarely of clinical significance, some hemolysis of red blood cells often takes place, especially with freshwater aspiration. Free hemoglobin may be found in the urine and blood, but the abnormality requires no specific therapy. Disseminated intravascular coagulation has been reported as a complication of freshwater near-drowning. It is thought that with extensive pulmonary injury "tissue factor" in lung parenchyma and plasminogen activator from pulmonary endothelium are released, triggering the extrinsic clotting and fibrinolytic systems. Other pathophysiologic events in near-drowning include the development of renal failure secondary to acute tubular necrosis, probably due to the combined effects of hypoxia and hypotension, and neurological deficits secondary to cerebral anoxia. Although the extent of the central nervous system injury tends to correlate with the duration of hypoxia, hypothermia accompanying the incident may be a moderating factor by reducing cerebral oxygen requirements. Complete neurological recovery has been reported in victims submerged as long as 40 min in water temperatures less than 20°C.

CLINICAL MANIFESTATIONS The clinical features in near-drowning are variable and depend upon many factors including the amount and type of water aspirated and the promptness and effectiveness of treatment. Pulmonary and neurological abnormalities usually predominate. Patients may present with mild cough and tachypnea, or with fulminant pulmonary edema. At least a third will require endotracheal intubation and some type of ventilatory therapy for the management of pulmonary injury. Instead of gradual recovery during the first 48 to 72 h of treatment, some patients will develop the adult respiratory distress syndrome, associated with progressive respiratory failure and reduction in lung compliance (Chap. 271). Other pulmonary complications often include regional atelectasis due to aspirated particulate matter; secondary bacterial pneumonia; lung abscess; empyema; and injuries such as pneumothorax or pneumomediastinum sustained during resuscitation or related to ventilator therapy.

Early neurological manifestations include seizures, especially during resuscitative efforts, and altered mental status, ranging from normal alertness to agitation, combativeness, or coma. Patients may present with speech, motor, or visual abnormalities or with more diffuse organic brain syndromes. Some of these neurological deficits will improve gradually and resolve over several months. However, 5 to 20 percent of patients will have permanent sequelae, many of which prove ultimately fatal. Neurological status usually does not continue to worsen after a near-drowning victim is admitted to the hospital unless there has been a preceding deterioration in pulmonary status. The possibility of unrecognized head trauma coincident with the drowning episode or a subdural hematoma should be considered as well.

Near-drowning victims often require treatment for cardiac as well as respiratory arrest during resuscitation. If this is successfully accomplished, most patients experience few additional cardiovascular problems. Supraventricular arrhythmias are common but usually resolve promptly when acidosis and hypoxia are treated. Heart failure secondary to myocardial ischemia or acutely expanded blood volume is unusual. Instead, pulmonary edema and low cardiac output states are usually due to the pulmonary injury from water aspiration with extravasation of fluid into the lung, resulting in hypovolemia.

Fever, frequently greater than 38°C, is seen in most patients within the first 24 h following significant aspiration. Its appearance later in the hospital course usually indicates a complicating infection. Vomiting is common during and after resuscitation. This often is associated with gastric distention by large quantities of fluid and air swallowed during the near-drowning episode and may result in additional aspiration. Other rare, but clinically important, features which may be encountered include acute renal failure and a severe hemorrhagic diathesis.

LABORATORY FINDINGS Arterial blood gas and pH determinations on admission reveal varying degrees of hypoxia and acidosis; follow-up values are the most reliable indicators of the effectiveness of ventilatory therapy. In 25 percent of near-drowning victims the initial chest x-ray film may be normal; however, this finding does not exclude the possibility that the patient has significant hypoxemia. In the remainder of cases, radiologic findings range from fine, symmetric, perihilar infiltrates with relative sparing of apexes, bases, and lateral lung fields to massive bilateral pulmonary edema with little or no areas of sparing. Marked clearing of these abnormalities usually takes place within 72 to 96 h.

Alterations in serum sodium and potassium may be noted, but these are generally mild and require no corrective treatment. Although leukocytosis up to 40,000 white blood cells per cubic millimeter is common during the first 24 to 48 h following near-drowning, significant changes in hematocrit and hemoglobin are rare, irrespective of the type of fluid aspirated. A *falling* hematocrit should raise the possibility of bleeding, not hemolysis, which, if it has occurred, should be apparent at the time of initial evaluation. Thrombocytopenia, prolonged prothrombin and partial thromboplastin times, hypofibrinogenemia, and elevated fibrin degradation products may be seen if disseminated intravascular coagulation takes place (Chap. 318).

THERAPY The primary objective of therapy is to correct hypoxemia and acidosis as rapidly as possible. On-the-scene efforts should include immediate institution of mouth-to-mouth breathing and, if necessary, closed-chest cardiac massage. Time should not be wasted with attempts to drain water from the victim's lungs. However, it is important to establish and maintain a clear airway at the onset of resuscitation in order to avoid accidental overdistention of the stomach which might result in regurgitation and aspiration. One hundred percent oxygen should be administered by inhalation as soon as possible, and other necessary resuscitative efforts continued during evacuation to the hospital. Even if spontaneous ventilation returns and the patient seems coherent, high concentrations of oxygen should be continued, since severe hypoxemia and acidosis may be present even in persons who are alert and without cyanosis.

All near-drowning victims should be taken to a hospital for further evaluation. Initial diagnostic studies should include arterial blood gas and pH determinations, hemogram, serum electrolytes, and chest x-ray. Patients who are alert, have normal chest x-rays, and show no evidence of hypoxemia or acidosis usually require no further therapy. Nevertheless they should be observed over several hours for evidence of deterioration in blood gas and acid-base status prior to discharge. Metabolic acidosis should be treated by intravenous administration of sodium bicarbonate ($NaHCO_3$), and hypoxemia with supplemental oxygen. If bronchospasm is present, aerosol inhalation of a bronchodilator may be given. Patients with pulmonary edema or hypoxemia which fails to respond to increasing inspired oxygen tensions up to 40 percent should be intubated endotracheally and have positive end-expiratory pressure (PEEP) applied to the airways. When respiratory failure is present, lung compliance is markedly reduced, or the patient is unable to breathe spontaneously, mechanical ventilatory support should be used in addition to PEEP. Arterial blood gas tensions and pH should be determined frequently to assess the adequacy of respiratory therapy. Treatment with PEEP should be continued long enough for the lung injury to stabilize before it is withdrawn. This may take 48 to 72 h or even longer. Monitoring the magnitude of the intrapulmonary shunt, the pulmonary wedge pressure, and cardiac output by means of a Swan-Ganz intraarterial catheter is often very helpful in weaning patients from PEEP as well as in managing cases complicated by low cardiac output and hypotension.

Other therapeutic measures are largely supportive. Patients should be observed closely for evidence of pulmonary infection and treated with appropriate antibiotics on the basis of results of cultures of respiratory secretions. Prophylactic use of antibiotics and corticosteroids has been of no benefit in near-drowning victims. Fluid and electrolyte balance should be carefully maintained. If hypovolemia is associated with low urinary output or hypotension, plasma expanders may be required. Transfusion with packed red blood cells or whole blood, depending upon circulating blood volume status, may be used for significant anemia. Acute renal failure should be managed as described in Chap. 275.

PROGNOSIS The prognosis depends largely upon the extent and duration of the hypoxic episode. In addition, such factors as the temperature of the submersion medium, the availability and appropriate application of specific treatment, and coexisting medical illness or trauma are often important in determining the outcome. In general, patients who are alert and have normal chest x-rays upon arrival at the hospital can be expected to survive, while those who present in coma or cardiopulmonary arrest usually die or are left with significant neurological deficits. Prediction of outcome on the basis of other presenting neurological features or laboratory abnormalities is unreliable. The fact that nearly 90 percent of victims who live long enough to receive definitive hospital care will survive should serve to emphasize that extensive resuscitative efforts are advisable in all cases of near-drowning.

REFERENCES

FULLER RH: Drowning and the postimmersion syndrome: A clinicopathologic study. Milit Med 128:22, 1963

GIAMMONA ST, MODELL JH: Drowning by total immersion: Effects on pulmonary surfactant of distilled water, isotonic saline and seawater. Am J Dis Child 114:612, 1967

MODELL JH: Biology of drowning. Annu Rev Med 29:1, 1978

——— et al: Clinical course of 91 consecutive near-drowning victims. Chest 70(2):231, 1976

PETERSON B: Morbidity of childhood near-drowning. Pediatrics 59(3):364, 1977

PORTS TA, DEVEL TF: Intravascular coagulation in fresh water submersion: Report of 3 cases. Ann Intern Med 87:60, 1977

SIEBKE H et al: Survival after 40 minutes' submersion without cerebral sequelae. Lancet 1:1275, 1975

223
GENERAL CONSIDERATIONS AND PRINCIPLES OF MANAGEMENT

PAUL A. FRIEDMAN

Poisoning by chemical agents is a common and serious medical problem. In the United States accidental poisonings cause about 5000 deaths each year. Suicides by chemical agents annually number more than 6000. Malicious poisoning has become less common since the development of scientific toxicology, but toxic chemicals administered by homicides and abortionists are responsible for more deaths than is generally appreciated. In addition to fatal poisonings there is a much greater number of persons who are made seriously ill by chemical agents but recover after appropriate therapy. Unfortunately, some such victims are left with permanent sequelae of their intoxication. Finally, chemical agents impair the health of very many people by mechanisms not generally thought of as intoxications. Chemical carcinogenesis and mutagenesis, chronic alcoholic liver disease, allergic reactions, and chemical addiction and withdrawal syndromes are the most important examples.

Accidental poisonings may occur in the home or through industrial exposure. The former are far more frequent and usually acute; industrial intoxication is ordinarily the result of chronic exposure. Accidental poisoning is most commonly due to ingestion of toxic substances and involves children in the majority of cases. Each year 1 to 2 million American children accidentally swallow toxic materials, and approximately 1 ingestion in 1000 is fatal. Aspirin is involved in 25 percent of all ingestions, other medicines in another 25 percent. Cleaning and polishing agents are ingested by 15 percent, while cosmetics, pesticides, petroleum products, and turpentine paints account for 6 percent each. Younger children tend to ingest household products, older children are more likely to choose drugs.

The frequency of accidental poisonings reflects the enormous number of toxic substances found in the American home. Many such accidents could be avoided by simple preventive measures. Physicians can play an effective role in safety education. All toxic substances must be kept out of the reach of small children. Household chemicals and medicines should be kept in the original containers, and all such containers should be labeled. Before taking or administering any medicine, one should check the label carefully.

Despite all precautions, accidental, suicidal, and criminal poisonings will remain an important problem which every physician must be prepared to treat promptly and effectively. Besides their immediate therapeutic responsibilities, physicians have legal obligations in cases of attempted suicide, homicide, criminal abortion, and industrial exposure. The physician should also obtain psychiatric care for any patient who has attempted suicide by poison.

DIAGNOSIS OF CHEMICAL POISONING

Optimal management of the poisoned patient requires a correct diagnosis. Unfortunately, in many such patients poisoning is initially not even considered as a possible cause of the clinical picture. The patient may be unaware of exposure to poison or, as after attempted suicide or abortion, may be unwilling to admit it. Although the toxic effects of some chemical substances are quite characteristic, most poisoning syndromes can simulate other diseases.

Poisoning is usually included in the differential diagnosis of coma, convulsions, acute psychosis, acute hepatic or renal insufficiency, and bone marrow depression. It may not be considered when the major manifestation is a mild psychiatric disturbance or neurological disorder, abdominal pain, bleeding, fever, hypotension, pulmonary congestion, or skin eruption. Chronic, insidious intoxications are much more frequently missed than acute poisonings whose symptoms appear suddenly and may be immediately related to a specific event. Physicians should always remember the variegated manifestations of poisoning and maintain a high index of suspicion.

In every case of poisoning, identification of the toxic agent should be attempted. Specific antidotal therapy is obviously impossible without such identification. In cases of homicide, suicide, or criminal abortion the identity of the poison may be of legal importance. When poisoning results from industrial exposure or therapeutic mishap, accurate knowledge of the responsible agents is essential for future prevention.

In acute accidental poisoning the offending substance may be known to the patient. In many other cases information can be obtained from relatives or acquaintances, by a search for containers at the scene of the poisoning, or by questioning the patient's physician or pharmacist. Frequently such procedures yield only the trade name of a product, which gives no clue to its component chemicals. A number of books which identify the active ingredients of household products, agricultural compounds, proprietary medicines, and poisonous plants are listed in the references to this chapter. A small handbook of this type should be carried in every physician's bag. Poison control centers and manufacturers' representatives are other useful sources of such information. When poisoning is chronic, rapid identification of the toxic agent from the history is frequently impossible. It is therefore fortunate that the lesser therapeutic urgency of such cases usually permits the required painstaking exploration of the patient's habits and environment.

Some poisons can produce clinical features characteristic enough to strongly suggest the diagnosis. Careful examination of the patient may reveal the unmistakable odor of cyanide; the cherry-colored flush of carboxyhemoglobin in skin and mucous membranes; the pupillary constriction, salivation, and gastrointestinal hyperactivity produced by cholinesterase-inhibitor insecticides; or the lead line and extensor paralyses of chronic lead poisoning. Unfortunately, these features are not always present, and in any case telltales are the exception in chemical poisonings.

Chemical analysis of body fluids provides the most definite identification of the intoxicating agent. Some common poisons, such as aspirin, bromides, and barbiturates, can be identified and even quantitated by relatively simple laboratory procedures. Others require more complex toxicologic techniques, such as gas chromatography or bioassay, which are performed only in specialized laboratories. Furthermore, the results of toxicologic determinations are rarely available in time to guide the initial treatment of acute poisoning. Nevertheless, specimens of vomitus, gastric aspirate, blood, urine, and feces should always be saved for toxicologic study if diagnostic or legal questions are likely to arise. Chemical analyses of body fluids or tissues are of particular value in the diagnosis and evaluation of chronic intoxications. Finally, they are useful in following the success of some forms of therapy.

TREATMENT OF CHEMICAL POISONING

Although the physician should always try to identify the poison, such attempts must never delay vital therapeutic measures. Most poisons do not have specific antidotes. Essential supportive care must be given as indicated by the patient's clinical state and does not require knowledge of the toxic agent. Symptomatic treatment of circulatory, respiratory, neurological, and renal function should be immediately administered as to any other seriously ill patient.

Correct treatment of the poisoned patients thus requires knowledge of both the general principles of management and the details of therapy for specific poisons. Treatment involves four steps: (1) prevention of further absorption of the poison, (2) removal of absorbed poison from the body, (3) symptomatic or supportive therapy, and (4) administration of systemic antidotes (Table 223-1). The first three are applicable to most types of poisoning. The fourth is most often used only when the toxic agent is known and a specific antidote is available. However, sometimes naloxone is given if the index of suspicion is high that the patient has had an overdose of an opiate. Success often depends upon speed of treatment, and, when indicated by the clinical situation, several approaches should be used simultaneously.

PREVENTION OF ABSORPTION OF INGESTED POISONS If appreciable amounts of a poison have been ingested, one should always attempt to minimize its absorption from the gastrointestinal tract. The success of such endeavors depends upon the time elapsed since ingestion and upon the site and

TABLE 223-1
Treatment of acute chemical poisoning

I Prevention of further absorption of poison
  A Poisoning by ingestion
    1 Emptying the stomach
      a Induction of vomiting
      b Gastric lavage
    2 Minimizing gastrointestinal absorption
      a Neutralization and precipitation
      b Adsorption
      c Catharsis
  B Poisoning by other routes
II Removal of absorbed poisons from body
  A Detoxification—enzyme induction?
  B Biliary excretion—interruption of enterohepatic circulation
  C Urinary excretion
    1 Forced diuresis
    2 Alteration of urinary pH
  D Dialysis
    1 Peritoneal dialysis
    2 Hemodialysis
  E Charcoal or resin hemoperfusion
  F Exchange transfusion
  G Chelation and chemical binding
III Supportive therapy
IV Administration of systemic antidotes
  A Chemical agents
  B Pharmacological antagonists

speed of absorption of the poison. Prompt action is essential, and it is better to proceed with makeshifts than to waste time while waiting for special equipment or drugs. Conversely, it is unwise to temporize with unpredictable remedies when reliable and effective methods for removal of poison from the gastrointestinal tract are available. When skillfully applied, these methods do not lead to such complications as pulmonary aspiration, gastrointestinal perforation, or convulsions.

Evacuation of the stomach Attempts to empty the stomach are always worthwhile unless specifically contraindicated. They may be highly successful if made soon after ingestion. Significant amounts of poison may be recovered from the stomach hours after ingestion because gastric emptying may be delayed by gastric atony or pylorospasm.

Emesis occurs spontaneously after the ingestion of many poisons. In a minority of instances it may be induced in the home by mechanical stimulation of the posterior pharynx. The emetic action of syrup of ipecac (not the 14 times more concentrated fluid extract) in 15- to 30-ml dosage is more effective and is safe enough for home use. Its action has an average latent period of 20 min and depends in part on gastrointestinal absorption, so that it cannot be used in conjunction with other measures intended to minimize absorption of the poison. A second dose of ipecac should be given if the patient fails to vomit after 20 min (90 to 95 percent of patients will vomit after two doses). If not available at home, every effort should be made to locate a source of ipecac even if this requires taking the patient to the hospital. Apomorphine, 0.06 mg/kg intramuscularly, acts within 5 min but may cause prolonged vomiting. When given intravenously in doses of 0.01 mg/kg, apomorphine tends to produce almost immediate vomiting which is not followed by any other central nervous system effects. On occasion it is impossible to induce vomiting, and valuable time should not be lost with hopeful waiting. Induction of vomiting should not be attempted in severely depressed or convulsing patients, or (because of the danger of gastroesophageal perforation or tracheal aspiration of vomitus) in patients who have ingested strong caustics or liquid hydrocarbons which are potent lung irritants (e.g., kerosene, furniture polish).

In comparison with emesis, *gastric lavage* is more predictably and immediately active but usually no more effective in removing poison from the stomach. It can be employed in unconscious patients, and removal of gastric contents reduces the risk of aspiration of vomitus in such patients. It is, however, contraindicated after the ingestion of strong corrosives because of danger of perforating injured tissues. When properly performed, gastric lavage carries little risk of aspiration of gastric contents into the lungs. The patient should be prone, with head and shoulders lowered. A mouth gag is placed, and a gastric tube of sufficient diameter to permit withdrawal of particulate matter (size 30) is passed into the stomach. If central nervous system function is depressed and introduction of the tube produces retching, or if pulmonary irritants have been ingested, it is wise to place a *cuffed endotracheal tube* before lavaging. Gastric contents are withdrawn with a large syringe and usually contain most of the poison that will be removed. Thereafter 200 ml (less in children) of warm water or other lavaging solution is alternately instilled and withdrawn until the aspirate becomes clear.

Interference with gastrointestinal absorption Since neither emesis nor gastric lavage empties the stomach completely, one should also minimize absorption by administering substances which trap ingested poisons. Some toxic alkaloids can be precipitated and rendered insoluble by the administration of sulfate. Many other poisons are effectively adsorbed by powdered, activated charcoal. A good grade of activated charcoal can rapidly adsorb as much as half its weight of many common poisons. It is more effective than the so-called "universal antidote," which should be relegated to oblivion. A slurry of activated charcoal (20 to 50 g in 100 to 200 ml) should be administered after evacuation of the stomach.

Adsorption by charcoal is reversible, and the effectiveness of adsorption of many poisons varies with the pH. Acidic substances are adsorbed better in acid solutions and may therefore be released in the small intestine. It is desirable to speed the charcoal with its adsorbed poison through the intestine as quickly as possible. This will also decrease intestinal absorption of any unabsorbed poison which has passed beyond the pylorus. In patients with good renal and cardiac function this is best accomplished by oral or gastric administration of an osmotic cathartic such as magnesium or sodium sulfate (10 to 30 g given in solution at a concentration of 10% or less).

PREVENTION OF ABSORPTION OF POISON FROM OTHER SITES Most topically applied poisons can be removed by copious flushing with water. In certain instances weak acids or bases or appropriate organic solvents are more effective, but rapid and voluminous washing with water should always proceed while they are being obtained. Chemical antidotes can be hazardous because tissue injury may result from the heat of the chemical reaction.

The systemic distribution of injected poisons can be slowed by the application of cold to the injection site or by the proximal application of a tourniquet. Cruciate incision and suction is generally ineffective except after poisonous bites.

Following inhalation of toxic gases, vapors, or dusts, the victim should be removed into clean air and adequate ventilation maintained. If the patient cannot be moved, a protective mask should be applied.

REMOVAL OF ABSORBED POISON FROM THE BODY Unlike prevention or retardation of absorption, measures to speed removal of the toxic agent from the body rarely have much influence on the peak poison concentration. However, they can significantly abbreviate the time during which the concentration of many poisons remains above any given level and may thereby reduce morbidity, avoid complications, and save lives. In judging the need for such measures one must consider the patient's clinical state, the properties and metabolic fate of the poison, and the amount absorbed as judged by the history and the blood level. Removal of some poisons can be accelerated by several methods; selection depends on the clinical urgency, the amount in the body, and the skills and equipment available.

Biliary excretion Certain organic acids and active drugs are secreted into the bile against large concentration gradients. However, this process takes time and cannot be accelerated. The intestinal resorption of substances already secreted into the bile, such as glutethimide, can be decreased by the administration of charcoal every 6 h. The organochlorine pesticide, chlordecone, is slowly eliminated from the body (blood half-time 165 days). Cholestyramine (16 g per day) significantly accelerates elimination (blood half-time 80 days).

Urinary excretion Acceleration of renal excretion is applicable to a much larger number of poisons. Renal excretion of toxic substances depends on glomerular filtration, active tubular secretion, and passive tubular resorption. The first two processes should be protected by maintenance of adequate circulation and renal function, but for practical purposes they cannot be accelerated. On the other hand, passive tubular resorption of many poisons plays an important role in the prolongation of their action and can frequently be decreased by readily available methods.

The effectiveness of forced diuresis by administration of large volumes of electrolyte solutions together with intravenous furosemide in increasing renal excretion has been demonstrated for many drugs such as salicylates, barbiturates, meprobamate, and glutethimide and is potentially applicable to all ultrafiltered poisons which are passively reabsorbed.

Alteration of the urinary pH can also inhibit passive back-diffusion of some poisons and increase their renal clearance. The renal tubular epithelium is more permeable to uncharged molecules than to ionized solutes. Weak organic acids and bases readily diffuse out of the tubular fluid in their un-ionized form but are trapped in it when ionized. Acidic poisons are largely ionized only at pHs above their pK_a. Alkalinization of the urine greatly increases the ionization in the tubular fluid of such organic acids as phenobarbital and salicylate. In contrast, the pK_a of pentobarbital (8.1) and secobarbital (8.0) is so high that renal clearance is not greatly increased by raising the urinary pH into the physiological alkaline range. Alkalinization of the urine is achieved by the infusion of sodium bicarbonate, sodium lactate, or tromethamine (which also acts as an osmotic diuretic) at a rate determined by the urinary and blood pH. Excessive systemic alkalosis or electrolyte disturbances must be carefully prevented. A combination of forced diuresis and alkalinization of the urine can raise the renal clearance of some acidic poisons tenfold or more and has been found highly effective in poisoning by salicylate and phenobarbital. The full range of its clinical applicability is undoubtedly much wider but remains to be established. Conversely, depression of the urinary pH beyond its usual range has been shown to augment significantly the clearance of amphetamines and phencyclidines.

Finally, the renal excretion of certain poisons can be increased in a highly specific fashion. An example is the removal of bromide by administration of chloride and chloriuretics. Such methods are discussed with the individual poisons.

Dialysis and hemoperfusion Dialysis has been found effective in the removal of many drugs including barbiturates, borate, bromide, chlorate, dimercaprol, diphenylhydantoin, ethanol, ethchlorvynol, ethinamate, glutethimide, glycols, isoniazid, methanol, salicylate, sulfonamides, and thiocyanate. Theoretically, it should accelerate the removal from the body of any dialyzable toxin which is not irreversibly bound to tissues. Obviously, its effectiveness does not extend to large-molecule, nondialyzable poisons and is decreased by a high degree of protein binding or lipid solubility of the toxic substance.

Peritoneal dialysis can be easily performed in any hospital and may be continued for long periods. It is valuable for the removal of poisons only if renal function is impaired, hemodialysis or hemoperfusion is not possible, or forced diuresis cannot be carried out.

Hemodialysis is unquestionably a more effective procedure for removing large amounts of dialyzable poisons. For barbiturates dialysance rates of 50 to 100 ml/min have been achieved, a removal rate two to ten times faster than during peritoneal dialysis or forced diuresis. Dialysis against solutions containing albumin or lipids can further speed removal of certain poisons. Perfusion of blood through activated charcoal or exchange resin achieves even higher clearance rates than hemodialysis for most poisons. Extracorporeal dialysis and hemoperfusion are clearly the procedures of choice for the rapid removal of poisons from patients who have absorbed amounts which make survival unlikely even under the best supportive care. Since the required equipment and skilled personnel are available only in a few hospitals, the possibility of transfer of such patients to one of these institutions should be considered.

Chelation and chemical binding The removal of some poisons is accelerated by chemical interaction with other substances followed by renal excretion. These substances are usually considered specific antidotes and are discussed with the individual poisons.

SUPPORTIVE THERAPY Most chemical poisonings are reversible, self-limited disease states. Skillful supportive therapy can keep many seriously poisoned patients alive and their detoxifying and excretory mechanisms functioning until the concentration of poison in the body has fallen to safe levels. Symptomatic measures are especially important when the poison is one of the many compounds for which no specific antidote is known. Even when an antidote is available, disturbances of vital functions must be prevented or controlled by appropriate supportive care.

The poisoned patient may suffer a variety of physiological disturbances. Most of these are not peculiar to chemical intoxications, and their therapeutic management is described elsewhere in this text. Only those aspects of supportive therapy specially relevant to poisonings are briefly discussed here.

Central nervous system depression Specific therapy directed against the depressant effects of poisons on the central nervous system is usually both unnecessary and difficult. Most poisoned patients will emerge from coma as from a prolonged anesthesia. During the period of unconsciousness meticulous nursing care and close observation are essential. If depression of medullary centers results in circulatory or respiratory failure, these vital functions must be immediately and vigorously supported by chemical or mechanical means.

The use of analeptics in the treatment of poison-induced central nervous system depression has been largely abandoned, for the following reasons: (1) Their effect is unpredictable, and their use in intoxicated patients produces an abnormal pattern of nervous activity in which paroxysmal excitation and convulsions may be superimposed on depression. (2) The availability of artificial ventilation and of effective measures to support the circulation has lessened the need for rapid restoration of normal medullary function. (3) It is doubtful that analeptics shorten the duration of coma sufficiently to justify their risks, and they have not been shown to improve prognosis. Certainly these agents should never be employed to restore consciousness, and it is doubtful whether their use to hasten the restoration of spontaneous breathing and active reflexes is ever justified. Naloxone, 0.4 mg administered intravenously, will generally reverse central nervous system depression secondary to narcotic overdosage.

Convulsions Many poisons (e.g., chlorinated hydrocarbons, insecticides, strychnine) cause convulsions by their specific excitatory effects. Poisoned patients may also have convulsions because of hypoxia, hypoglycemia, cerebral edema, or metabolic disturbances. In such cases these abnormalities should be corrected as far as possible. Regardless of the cause of the convulsions, anticonvulsant drugs are often required. Intravenously administered phenobarbital or one of the benzodiazepines, such as diazepam, is usually effective.

Cerebral edema Intracranial hypertension due to cerebral edema is also a characteristic effect of some poisons and a nonspecific result of other chemical intoxications. Cerebral edema is characteristically seen in poisoning by lead, carbon monoxide, and methanol. Symptomatic treatment consists of use of adrenocortical steroids and, when necessary, the intravenous administration of hypertonic solutions of mannitol or urea.

Hypotension The causes of hypotension and shock in the poisoned patient are legion, and often several of them coexist. Poisons can depress the medullary vasomotor centers, block autonomic ganglia or adrenergic receptors, directly depress the tone of arterial or venous smooth muscle, reduce myocardial contractility, or induce cardiac arrhythmias. Less specifically, the poisoned patient may be in shock because of tissue hypoxia, extensive tissue destruction from corrosives, loss of blood or fluids, or metabolic disturbances. When possible, these abnormalities should be promptly corrected. If the central venous pressure is low, fluid replacement should be the first therapeutic approach. Vasoactive drugs are often helpful and sometimes essential in the hypotensive poisoned patient, particularly in shock resulting from central depression. As in shock from other causes, choice of the most appropriate agent requires an analysis of the hemodynamic disturbance which goes beyond determination of the arterial pressure.

Cardiac arrhythmias Disturbances of cardiac impulse generation or conduction in the poisoned patient arise from the effects of certain poisons on the electrical properties of cardiac fibers or from myocardial hypoxia or metabolic disturbances. The latter should be corrected, and antiarrhythmic agents administered as indicated by the nature of the arrhythmia (Chap. 237).

Pulmonary edema The poisoned patient may develop pulmonary edema because of depressed myocardial contractility or because of alveolar injury from irritant gases or aspirated fluids. The latter type of edema is less responsive to treatment and may be associated with laryngeal edema. Therapeutic measures include suctioning, administration of high concentrations of oxygen under positive pressure, aerosols of surface-active agents, bronchodilators, and adrenocortical steroids.

Hypoxia Poisoning may cause tissue hypoxia by various mechanisms, and several of these may operate in one patient. Inadequate ventilation can result from central respiratory depression, from muscular paralysis, or from airway obstruction by retained secretions, laryngeal edema, or bronchospasm. Alveolar-capillary diffusion may be impaired by pulmonary edema. Anemia, methemoglobinemia, carboxyhemoglobinemia, or shock can interfere with oxygen transport. Cellular oxidation may be inhibited by cyanide, fluoroacetate, or general protoplasmic poisons. The highest priority in treatment must be given to maintenance of an adequate airway. The clinical situation and the site of obstruction may indicate frequent suctioning, insertion of an oropharyngeal airway or of an endotracheal tube, or a tracheotomy. If despite a clear airway ventilation remains inadequate, as judged by clinical appearance or by measurement of minute volume or blood gases, artificial ventilation by appropriate mechanical means is imperative. Administration of high concentrations of oxygen is indicated whenever tissue hypoxia occurs. When the central nervous system is severely depressed, oxygen administration often results in apnea and must be combined with artificial ventilation. Hyperbaric oxygen may be helpful in some situations. The treatment of methemoglobinemia, carboxyhemoglobinemia, and inhibition of cellular oxidation is discussed under the specific poisons which produce these changes.

Acute renal insufficiency Renal failure with oliguria or anuria may occur in the poisoned patient because of shock, dehydration, or electrolyte disturbances. More specifically, it may be due to the nephrotoxic potential of some poisons (e.g., mercury, phosphorus, carbon tetrachloride, bromate), many of which are concentrated and excreted by the kidney. Renal damage due to poisons is usually reversible. The management of acute renal insufficiency is outlined in Chap. 275.

Electrolyte and water disturbances Imbalances of fluid and electrolytes are common features of chemical poisoning. They may result from vomiting, diarrhea, renal insufficiency, or therapeutic maneuvers such as catharsis, forced diuresis, or dialysis. These disturbances are corrected or, ideally, prevented by appropriate therapy. Certain poisons produce more specific defects, such as metabolic acidosis (e.g., methanol, phenol, salicylate) or hypocalcemia (e.g., fluoride, oxalate). These abnormalities and any specific treatment are described under the individual poisons.

Acute hepatic insufficiency The primary manifestation of some poisonings (e.g., chlorinated hydrocarbons, phosphorus, cinchophen, certain mushrooms) is acute hepatic failure. Its management is described in Chap. 302.

ADMINISTRATION OF SYSTEMIC ANTIDOTES Specific antidotal therapy is available for only a few poisons. Some systemic antidotes are chemicals which exert their therapeutic effect by reducing the concentration of the toxic substance. They may do this by combining with the poison (e.g., ethylene diaminetetraacetate with lead, dimercaprol with mercury, sulfhydryl-containing reagents such as Mucomyst with a toxic metabolite of acetaminophen) or by increasing its excretion (e.g., chloride or mercurial diuretics in bromide poisoning). Other systemic antidotes compete with the poison for its receptor site (e.g., atropine with muscarine, naloxone with morphine, vitamin K_1 with coumadin anticoagulants; physostigmine reverses the anticholinergic effects of the tricyclic antidepressants, the antihistamines, and belladonna). Specific antidotes are discussed with the individual poisons.

REFERENCES

ARENA JM: *Poisoning,* 3d ed. Springfield, Ill, Charles C Thomas, 1974

ARLEFF AI et al: Coma following nonnarcotic drug overdosage—management of 208 adult patients. Am J Med Sci 266:405, 1973

BOURNE PG: *Acute Drug Abuse Emergencies.* New York, Academic, 1976

CASARETT LJ, DOULL J: *Toxicology: The Basic Science of Poisons.* New York, Macmillan, 1975

DREISBACH RH: *Handbook of Poisoning: Diagnosis and Treatment,* 9th ed. Los Altos, Calif, Lange, 1978

HAYDEN JW, COMSTOCK EG: Use of activated charcoal in acute poisoning. Clin Toxicol 8(5):515, 1975

LOOMIS TA: *Essentials of Toxicology,* 2d ed. Philadelphia, Lea & Febiger, 1974

LOVEJOY FH JR, ALPERT JH: Acute poisoning, in *Current Pediatric Therapy,* 8th ed, SS Gellis, BM Kegan (eds). Philadelphia, Saunders, pp 709–734, 1978

MOFENSON HC, GREENSHER J: The unknown poison. Pediatrics 54:336, 1974

Seminar on childhood poisoning. Paediatrician 6:3, 1977

SMITH RP, GOSSELIN RE: Current concepts about the treatment of selected poisonings. Annu Rev Pharmacol Toxicol 16:189, 1976

WINCHESTER JF et al: Dialysis and hemoperfusion of poisons and drugs—update. Trans Am Soc Artif Intern Organs 23:762, 1977

ZENZ C: *Occupational Medicine.* Chicago, Year Book, 1975

Toxic product information

Drug Identification Guide. Oradell, NJ, Medical Economics, 1975

GLEASON MN et al: *Clinical Toxicology of Commercial Products,* 4th ed. Baltimore, Williams & Wilkins, 1976

GOODMAN LS, GILMAN A: *The Pharmacological Basis of Therapeutics,* 5th ed. New York, Macmillan, 1975

HAYES WJ: *Toxicology of Pesticides.* Baltimore, Williams & Wilkins, 1975

The Merck Index, 9th ed. Rahway, NJ, Merck and Co, 1976

Poisindex. Englewood, Colo, Micromedex, 1974

Poisonous Plants and Fungi. Philadelphia, Rittenhouse, 1976

SCHERZ RG: The history of poison control centers in the United States. Clin Toxicol 12:291, 1978

WILSON CO, JONES TE: *American Drug Index.* Philadelphia, Lippincott, 1975

224
COMMON POISONS

PAUL A. FRIEDMAN

The poisons discussed in this chapter are some of those encountered by the general population such as commonly used drugs, household products, solvents, pesticides, and poisonous plants. It has been necessary to disregard many uncommon toxic materials as well as products to which exposure occurs only in specialized industrial environments. Details concerning poisoning by such compounds may be found in some of the references following Chap. 223. Toxic effects of many drugs are considered throughout this text in conjunction with their therapeutic use. Manifestations of hypersensitivity to chemicals are described in Chap. 71. The following discussions of specific poisons stress those details of their action which are pertinent to the recognition or treatment of clinical poisoning.

ACETAMINOPHEN Termed *paracetamol* in the United Kingdom, acetaminophen has become a popular alternative to salicylates as an analgesic and antipyretic. It is a frequent cause of poisoning. While the toxic and lethal doses of acetaminophen may vary from patient to patient, hepatic damage may be expected if an adult has taken more than 8 g as a single dose. A plasma concentration of greater than 200 µg/ml at 4 h after ingestion is also cause for concern. Clinical manifestations of acetaminophen poisoning are nonspecific. In the first few hours after ingestion lethargy, pallor, nausea, vomiting, and diaphoresis may occur; there are no acid-base derangements which may accompany aspirin overdose. Hepatic damage, the most important manifestation of acetaminophen toxicity, becomes evident 1 to 2 days after ingestion. While some patients show only elevation of serum transaminase and others show hepatic enlargement, tenderness, and jaundice, more severe damage can lead to hyperammonemia, asterixis, mental confusion, coma, bleeding, and death from acute liver failure. Acute tubular necrosis, pancreatitis, hypoglycemia, cardiac damage, and hypersensitivity reactions are sometimes seen.

There is good evidence that damage to tissue (especially liver) is caused by metabolites of acetaminophen and not the drug itself. At therapeutic doses acetaminophen is eliminated mainly conjugated to sulfate or glucuronic acid. A small amount of acetaminophen is activated by the cytochrome P_{450} system and conjugated with the sulfhydryl group of glutathione to yield a nontoxic mercapturic acid. After an overdose, the pathways of conjugation to the sulfate and glucuronic acid become saturated, an increasing fraction of the drug is activated by the P_{450} system, glutathione stores are depleted, and the reactive intermediates then become free to bind covalently to liver macromolecules and cause necrosis.

Treatment of acetaminophen poisoning should begin with induction of emesis or gastric lavage followed by administration of activated charcoal. Since endogenous glutathione appears to have a protective effect, the administration of several other sulfhydryl compounds has been studied for protection against acetaminophen hepatotoxicity. When administered orally within 10 h of ingestion, either *N*-acetylcysteine (Mucomyst) or cysteamine is effective in decreasing hepatotoxicity. A potentially toxic dose (>7.5 g) ingested within the previous 24 h is an indication for *N*-acetylcysteine therapy. Since early treatment is paramount, a patient suspected of having ingested a potentially hepatotoxic dose should be started on sulfhydryl therapy while awaiting the plasma acetaminophen level. A 5% solution of Mucomyst in a cola beverage or fruit juice is given with a loading dose of 140 mg/kg and a maintenance dose of 70 mg/kg every 4 h for 3 days. If sulfhydryl therapy is to be instituted, charcoal and osmotic cathartic administration are contraindicated since both may reduce absorption of the antidote. In a mixed poisoning, charcoal may be removed by lavage prior to administration of the antidote. The increment of acetaminophen clearance from forced diuresis is small compared with liver metabolism; both hemodialysis and charcoal hemoperfusion result in a greater clearance of drug, but as yet the effectiveness of these methods in reducing hepatotoxicity and mortality has not been demonstrated. Inducers of the cytochrome P_{450} enzyme system such as barbiturates should be avoided.

ACIDS Corrosive acids are used widely in industry and laboratories. Ingestion is almost always with suicidal intent. Death has occurred after an oral dose of 1 ml of a corrosive acid.

Toxic effects of corrosive acids are due to their direct chemical action. Ingestion of acids may produce irritation, bleeding, and sloughing in the mouth and esophagus with more severe burns occurring in the stomach, particularly in the pylorus. Perforations with peritonitis, though uncommon, may occur. Mouth and pharynx may be brownish black and may have a charred appearance. Yellow staining is seen after ingestion of nitric and picric acids. Severe pain in mouth, pharynx, chest, and abdomen is the rule and is soon followed by hematemesis and bloody diarrhea. Frequently profound shock develops. About half of those who ingest significant amounts of acid die from its immediate effects. Survivors can develop mediastinitis or peritonitis from esophageal or gastric perforation, and delayed perforation of the esophagus or stomach can also occur. Recovery from acid ingestion can be associated with stricture formation which most commonly involves the pylorus.

Ingested acid must be immediately diluted a hundredfold by water or milk. The danger of perforation contraindicates the use of emesis or gastric lavage except during the first 30 min after ingestion. Diagnostic esophagoscopy, if performed, should be done in the first 48 h after ingestion. Following the emergency measures, appropriate supportive therapy is administered for the relief of pain and the treatment of shock, perforation, and infection.

Certain gases found in industry (e.g., chlorine, phosgene) may combine with water in the lungs to form corrosive acids. During rapid decomposition of plant material in silos, oxides of nitrogen are released which form nitric acid in the lungs. Inhalation of such gases causes coughing and choking sensations which are followed after a latent period of 6 to 8 h by pulmonary edema. Treatment is supportive. Symptoms of dyspnea and hemoptysis may be prolonged, and frequent relapses may occur.

ALKALIES Strong alkalies such as ammonium hydroxide, potassium hydroxide (potash), potassium carbonate, sodium hydroxide (lye, Clinitest tablets), and sodium carbonate (washing soda) are widely used in industry and in cleansers and drain cleaners. Sodium and potassium phosphates find use as water softeners. Strong alkalies form soaps with fats and proteinates with proteins, resulting in penetrating necrosis of tissues. Fatalities have occurred from the ingestion of 5 to 30 g of such compounds.

The toxic effects of alkalies are due to irritation and destruction of local tissues. Ingestion is followed by severe pain in mouth, pharynx, chest, and abdomen. Vomiting of blood and sloughed mucosa and diarrhea are common. Reflex loss of vascular tone frequently leads to profound shock. Perforation of the esophagus or stomach may be immediate or delayed for several days. Mouth and pharynx show erythema and gelatinous necrotic areas. After ingestion of water softeners profound reduction in serum calcium may be seen and lead to tetany and hypotension. Survivors usually suffer from esophageal strictures.

Treatment consists of immediate administration of large amounts of water or milk. The volume of liquids should exceed that of the ingested alkali a hundredfold. Vomiting should be allowed to occur, and gastric lavage may be performed during the first half-hour after ingestion. Because of the danger of perforation, both are contraindicated thereafter. Esophagoscopy should be done within the first 48 h. With evidence of significant esophageal or gastric burns steroids are usually administered for about 3 weeks to decrease the incidence of stricture formation, although definitive evidence of efficacy is lacking. If steroids are given, a broad-spectrum antibiotic such as ampicillin or a cephalosporin should also be administered for prophylaxis. After the ingestion of water softeners (phosphates), calcium gluconate should be administered intravenously as needed. Treatment is otherwise symptomatic and directed at the relief of pain, respiratory obstruction due to edema of the hypopharynx, fluid loss, and shock.

Inhalation of ammonia, which is used as a refrigerant, results in irritation of the upper and lower parts of the respiratory tract. Laryngeal and pulmonary edema may occur and must be treated symptomatically.

ANILINE This substance is used in printing and clothmarking inks, paints, and paint removers. Both aniline and its derivatives, such as toluidine, nitroaniline, and nitrobenzene, are widely used in industrial synthesis. Aniline is absorbed from the gastrointestinal tract and through the lungs or skin. Ingestion of 1 g aniline has been fatal. Methemoglobinemia is the most important manifestation. Headache, dizziness, hypotension, convulsions, and coma may occur. If the acute period is survived, jaundice and anemia may appear. Treatment consists of correction of methemoglobinemia (see Chap. 315) and supportive measures.

ANTIHISTAMINES The common and unprescribed use of antihistamines makes them readily available for accidental overdosage and suicidal attempts. There is wide variation from patient to patient in tolerance to these drugs and in the manifestations of poisoning. A dose of 200 mg diphenhydramine has been fatal in one adult, whereas another tolerated 2 g. Manifestations of poisoning are central nervous system excitement or depression. In children the usual toxic manifestations are excitement, hyperthermia, hyperreflexia, tremors, and convulsions, followed by central nervous system depression. In adults depressive manifestations with drowsiness, stupor, and coma predominate, but convulsions followed by further depression may occur.

Treatment is supportive and directed toward removal of the unabsorbed drug and maintenance of vital functions. Convulsions may be controlled with phenobarbital or diazepam. Some antihistamines have prominent atropine-like properties. Patients poisoned with these drugs may show manifestations of atropine poisoning and are treated correspondingly.

ANTIMUSCARINIC COMPOUNDS Atropine, related belladonna alkaloids (hyoscyamine and scopolamine), and synthetic substitutes (e.g., benztropine, cyclopentolate, homatropine, methantheline, propantheline) are widely prescribed drugs and occur in many proprietary mixtures used in the treatment of gastrointestinal and upper respiratory diseases, asthma, and parkinsonism. Poisoning, especially in children, may also occur from the excessive use of ophthalmic solutions containing such compounds. Finally, children may be intoxicated by eating plants containing up to 0.5 percent of atropine or related alkaloids. Such plants are *Atropa belladonna* (deadly nightshade), *Hyoscyamus niger* (henbane), and *Datura stramonium* (Jamestown or Jimson weed).

Individual sensitivity to the toxic effects of belladonna alkaloids varies widely; fatalities have occurred from as little as 10 mg atropine, but doses of 500 mg have been survived. Young children are particularly susceptible to poisoning with belladonna alkaloids. Older persons appear to be more sensitive to the central nervous system effects of these drugs. Since atropine is both hydrolyzed in the liver and excreted unchanged in the urine, insufficiency of hepatic or renal function may lead to poisoning on therapeutic dosage.

The most characteristic manifestations of atropine poisoning are those of parasympathetic blockade: dryness of mucous membranes, thirst, dysphagia, hoarseness, xerophthalmia, dilated pupils, blurring of vision, rise in intraocular tension, flushing, dryness and increased temperature of the skin, fever, tachycardia, hypertension, urinary retention, and abdominal distention. This widespread parasympatholysis is almost diagnostic of belladonna poisoning, but the diagnosis can be further confirmed by the reversal of blockade by physostigmine (2 mg administered intravenously over several minutes).

Central nervous system symptoms are also very common during belladonna intoxication. Atropine and scopolamine produce similar toxic psychoses. Restlessness, excitation, confusion, and incoordination precede mania, hallucinations, and delirium. Patients intoxicated by scopolamine not infrequently show lethargy and somnolence rather than excitement. In severe intoxication with belladonna alkaloids, central nervous system depression and coma are the rule. When death results it is because of circulatory collapse and respiratory failure.

In the treatment of belladonna poisoning, emesis or gastric lavage should be followed by the administration of activated charcoal. Symptomatic treatment is directed at the reduction of body temperature, the moistening of mucous membranes, and, when necessary, urethral catheterization. Excitement or convulsions may require appropriate pharmacotherapy. Patients with deep coma, life-threatening cardiac arrhythmias, severe hallucinations, or severe hypertension have been treated with physostigmine with reversal of the effects. It has not been established whether physostigmine reduces mortality.

Death occurs in fewer than 1 percent of cases of atropine or scopolamine poisoning. No permanent sequelae have been observed, but manifestations may persist for several days.

BARIUM Poisoning may be due to the ingestion of rodenticides which contain soluble barium salts or of depilatories that contain barium sulfide. A soluble barium salt may be present as a contaminant in the insoluble barium sulfate used as a radiopaque contrast medium. Barium is extremely toxic, producing intense stimulation of muscles of all types. Its action on the gastrointestinal musculature causes vomiting, colic, and diarrhea. Skeletal muscle tremors and spasm are commonly seen. Arteriolar spasm results in marked hypertension. Cardiac arrhythmias may proceed to ventricular fibrillation. Anxiety, weakness, and convulsions may occur. Death is usually due to cardiac arrhythmia or respiratory arrest.

Treatment consists of the oral administration of 250 ml 10% sodium sulfate or 5% magnesium sulfate. This will precipitate and remove any unabsorbed barium in the gastrointestinal tract. A dose of 10 ml of a 10% solution of sodium sulfate should be slowly administered intravenously every 15 min until symptoms subside. Procainamide may be used to reduce the danger of fatal cardiac arrhythmias. Serum potassium may be reduced, in which case oral or intravenous supplementation is indicated. If necessary, pain should be relieved and artificial ventilation with oxygen administered.

BENZENE, TOLUENE These solvents are used in paint removers, dry-cleaning solutions, and rubber or plastic cements. Benzene is also present, to some extent, in most gasolines. Poisoning may result from ingestion or from the breathing of concentrated vapors. Toluene is the major ingredient in the cement used by teen-age glue sniffers.

Acute poisoning by these compounds causes central nervous system manifestations. With sufficient exposure, symptoms progress from an initial period of restlessness, excitement, euphoria, and dizziness to coma, convulsions, and respiratory failure. Ventricular arrhythmias may occur.

Chronic poisoning by benzene or toluene results from repeated exposure to their vapors in low concentration. Central nervous system symptoms include irritability, insomnia, headache, tremors, and paresthesias. Anorexia and nausea are also common. Fatty degeneration of the heart, liver, and kidneys may occur. By far the most important manifestation of chronic exposure to benzene is bone marrow depression, which may progress to aplastic anemia and complete aplasia of the bone marrow. Individual susceptibility to this effect varies greatly and may not become apparent for months after the initial exposure to the poison.

Treatment of both acute and chronic poisoning is symptomatic. After ingestion, emesis must not be induced, and gastric lavage should await placement of an endotracheal tube with an inflatable cuff. Neurological, pulmonary, or cardiovascular problems are treated as in poisoning by petroleum distillates.

BLEACHES Clorox, Purex, Sanichlor, and other bleaching solutions contain 3 to 6% sodium hypochlorite. The solution used for chlorinating swimming pools is 20%. Their corrosive action in mouth, pharynx, and esophagus is similar to that of sodium hydroxide. Acid gastric juice releases hypochlorous acid from such solutions. This compound is very irritating to mucous membranes, and inhalation of its fumes causes severe pulmonary irritation and pulmonary edema. However, the systemic toxicity of hypochlorous acid is low. Perforation and stricture formation are rare after the ingestion of bleaching solutions. The fatal dose is approximately 30 ml.

Treatment consists of dilution of the ingested bleach with water or milk. The usual bleaching solutions do not cause enough corrosive injury to the esophagus to preclude the induction of emesis or gastric lavage, but one should be wary of this possibility if a 20% solution has been ingested. Although sodium thiosulfate (100 ml of a 1 to 2.5% solution by lavage), which will reduce hypochlorite to nontoxic products, has been routinely administered to these patients, there is great doubt that it is of any use except in very large overdoses, very early after ingestion.

BORIC ACID This compound is a very weak germicide and has been widely employed in powders, lotions, solutions, and ointments. Though not highly toxic, boric acid is not nearly as benign as widely assumed. The lethal dose is approximately 15 g in adults and 5 g in infants. Such amounts can be absorbed through abraded skin, from serous cavities, and after ingestion.

Regardless of the route of administration, the first symptoms of poisoning are nausea, vomiting, and diarrhea. These are followed by headache, weakness, restlessness, and erythroderma which may progress to desquamation of skin and mucous membranes. Renal toxicity and shock are common, and more than 100 fatalities have occurred. Renal excretion of boric acid is slow, and clearance can be increased markedly by dialysis. Boric acid should always be labeled as poison, and since this substance has no therapeutic function which cannot be served equally well by less toxic preparations, it should be removed from home and hospital.

BROMATES These compounds are used as neutralizers in cold wave preparations. They produce widespread tissue injury, particularly in central nervous system and kidneys. The fatal oral dose of bromates is approximately 5 g. On contact of bromate with gastric acid, hydrogen bromate, an irritating acid, is formed. Ingestion of bromates is followed by vomiting, diarrhea, abdominal pain, drowsiness, coma, convulsions, hypotension, hematuria, oliguria, anuria, and hemolysis.

Treatment consists of emesis or gastric lavage with sodium bicarbonate solution followed by catharsis. A dose of 250 ml of a 1% sodium thiosulfate solution should be administered intravenously. Peritoneal dialysis or hemodialysis effectively removes bromate from the body. Appropriate supportive therapy should be given.

CARBON MONOXIDE Carbon monoxide is a colorless, odorless, tasteless, and nonirritating gas produced by the incomplete combustion of carbonaceous materials. Almost any flame or combustion device emits carbon monoxide. The gas is present in the exhaust of internal combustion engines in a concentration of 3 to 7 percent. Much higher concentrations are present in most illuminating and heating gases, but not in natural gas. Carbon monoxide is annually responsible for about 3500 accidental and suicidal deaths in the United States alone.

The toxic effects of carbon monoxide are the result of tissue hypoxia. Carbon monoxide combines with hemoglobin to form carboxyhemoglobin. Since carbon monoxide and oxygen react with the same group in the hemoglobin molecule, carboxyhemoglobin is incapable of carrying oxygen. The affinity of hemoglobin for carbon monoxide is two hundred times greater than for oxygen, and at equilibrium 1 part of carbon monoxide in 1500 parts of air will result in 50 percent conversion of hemoglobin to carboxyhemoglobin. Carboxyhemoglobin also interferes with the release of oxygen from oxyhemoglobin. This further reduces the amount of oxygen available to the tissues and explains why tissue anoxia appears in the carbon monoxide-poisoned person at levels of arterial oxyhemoglobin concentration well tolerated by the anemic patient.

The extent of saturation of hemoglobin with carbon monoxide depends on the concentration of the gas in inspired air and on the time of exposure. The severity of hypoxic symptoms depends further on an individual's state of activity, tissue oxygen needs, and hemoglobin concentration. As a general rule, no symptoms will develop at a concentration of 0.01 percent carbon monoxide in inspired air, since this will not raise blood saturation above 10 percent. Exposure to 0.05 percent for 1 h during light activity will produce a blood concentration of 20 percent carboxyhemoglobin and result in a mild or throbbing headache. Greater activity or longer exposure to the same concentration causes a blood saturation of 30 to 50 percent. At this point headache, irritability, confusion, dizziness, visual disturbances, nausea, vomiting, and fainting on exertion may be observed. After exposure for 1 h to concentrations of 0.1 percent in inspired air, the blood will contain 50 to 80 percent carboxyhemoglobin, which results in coma, convul-

sions, respiratory failure, and death. On inhalation of high concentrations of carbon monoxide, saturation of the blood proceeds so rapidly that unconsciousness may occur suddenly and without warning. When poisoning is more gradual, the individual may notice decreased exercise tolerance and dyspnea on exertion or even at rest. Excessive sweating, fever, hepatomegaly, skin lesions, leukocytosis, bleeding diathesis, albuminuria, and glycosuria have also been described. Cerebral edema and intracranial hypertension may result from the increased permeability of hypoxic capillaries. Myocardial hypoxia is reflected by electrocardiographic abnormalities.

The most characteristic sign of carbon monoxide poisoning is the cherry color of skin and mucous membranes, which is due to the bright red carboxyhemoglobin. If the characteristic flush is not present and carbon monoxide poisoning is suspected, 1 ml of the patient's blood can be diluted with 10 ml water; when 1 ml of 5% sodium hydroxide is added to this dilution, an oxyhemoglobin solution will turn brown. If significant amounts of carboxyhemoglobin are present, the solution will turn straw yellow (<20% carboxyhemoglobin) or will remain pink (>20% carboxyhemoglobin).

Treatment of carbon monoxide poisoning requires effective ventilation in the presence of high oxygen tensions and in the absence of carbon monoxide. If necessary, ventilation should be supported artificially. Pure oxygen should be administered. This will result not only in the replacement of carbon monoxide by oxygen in the hemoglobin molecule but also in the partial relief of tissue hypoxia by oxygen dissolved in the plasma. For the same reasons hyperbaric oxygen is helpful in seriously poisoned patients. Transfusion of blood or packed cells is also of value. In order to reduce tissue needs for oxygen, the patient must be kept absolutely quiet. Induction of hypothermia is not indicated. Cerebral edema should be treated with diuretics and steroids.

During the recovery from carbon monoxide poisoning symptoms regress gradually. If severe tissue hypoxia has obtained too long, neurological symptoms such as tremors, mental deterioration, and psychotic behavior may persist. Histological changes characteristic of hypoxia may be observed in cerebral cortex, medulla, myocardium, and other organs.

CASTOR BEANS The castor bean plant (*Ricinus communis*) is grown for commercial and ornamental purposes. The beans contain the protein ricin which is extremely toxic to mammalian cells. Like abrin, another toxic plant protein, ricin inhibits protein synthesis in eukaryotic cells. Both ricin and abrin consist of two polypeptide chains—one chain functions to bind the toxin to the cell surface while the second chain can then enter the cell and, in a specific and irreversible reaction, enzymatically inactivate the 60S ribosomal subunit, thus inhibiting protein synthesis. After a delay of several hours to 2 days following ingestion, abdominal pain, vomiting, and profuse diarrhea appear and produce severe dehydration. Extreme weakness, drowsiness, disorientation, stupor, coma, convulsions, respiratory depression, and circulatory collapse may develop. Intravascular clotting and hemolysis have been observed. If the patient survives the acute symptoms, oliguria may progress to anuria and uremia, with death after several days. Treatment consists of fluid replacement, alkalinization of the urine with sodium bicarbonate to prevent precipitation of hemoglobin in the kidneys, and supportive measures.

CHLORATES Sodium and potassium chlorates are strong oxidizing agents and are found in gargles, mouthwashes, matches, and weed killers. After oral ingestion, 2 g has been fatal for children and 10 g for adults. Chlorate ion acts as a catalyst in the production of methemoglobinemia, and absorption of a small amount can result in a high methemoglobin concentration. The symptoms of chlorate ingestion are those of local mucosal irritation and of methemoglobinemia (see Chaps. 53 and 315). Renal toxicity is common. Treatment is directed primarily at the methemoglobinemia. Absorbed chlorate can be removed effectively by dialysis.

CHLORINATED INSECTICIDES These compounds are ingredients of dusts, sprays, and solutions used as insecticides. The great majority of these compounds are chlorinated diphenyls (e.g., DDT, TDE, DFDT, DMC, Neotran) or chlorinated polycyclic compounds (e.g., aldrin, chlordane, dieldrin, endrin, heptachlor). Lindane is a hexachlorobenzene. Their toxicity has led to their greatly diminished use in recent years, and many are banned in certain locales, including the United States. The chlorinated insecticides are soluble in lipid and organic solvents but not in water. They are poorly absorbed unless dissolved in a vehicle such as kerosene, petroleum distillates, or other organic solvents. Under these circumstances they readily enter the body through the skin, lungs, or gastrointestinal tract. These compounds vary considerably in toxicity, and the toxicity of the dissolving vehicle must also be considered. The effects of the solvent may overshadow or modify those of the insecticide.

The initial symptoms of acute poisoning are nausea, vomiting, headache, dizziness, apprehension, excitement, and muscular tremors and weakness. These symptoms progress to generalized central nervous system hyperexcitability and delirium and clonic or tonic convulsions. This stage is in turn followed by progressive depression with paralysis, coma, and death. Except for endrin, which is strongly hepatotoxic, liver toxicity occurs only at extreme dosage levels. Treatment consists of induction of emesis or gastric lavage, activated charcoal administration, catharsis, anticonvulsive therapy, artificial ventilation, and other supportive measures. Sympathomimetic compounds should be avoided, since chlorinated insecticides apparently increase susceptibility to ventricular fibrillation. Cholestyramine accelerates the excretion of the chlorinated hydrocarbon kepone, and it may well have a similar effect on the excretion of pesticides such as DTT, dieldrin, chlordane, and heptachlor which remain in the body for prolonged periods.

CHOLINESTERASE INHIBITOR INSECTICIDES Many substances used in agriculture for control of soft-bodied insects are potent inhibitors of cholinesterase. Most of these compounds are organic phosphates (e.g., Parathion, Malathion, Systox, TEPP, HETP, OMPA), others are carbamates (e.g., Dimetan, Mactacil). The toxicity of these compounds varies widely. They are usually prepared for use by dilution with powders, organic solvents, or water. Formulations containing 1 to 95 percent of the active ingredient are available. The cholinesterase inhibitor insecticides are rapidly absorbed through the intact skin and after inhalation or ingestion.

The toxicity of these agents results from inactivation of acetylcholinesterase which allows accumulation of excessive amounts of acetylcholine at a number of sites: central nervous system, autonomic ganglia, parasympathetic nerve endings, and motor nerve endings. In the central nervous system coma and respiratory depression and less commonly seizures can occur. Toxic muscarinic effects include nausea, vomiting, diarrhea, involuntary defecation and urination, blurring of vision due to miosis, sweating, lacrimation, and salivation. Nicotinic effects include muscle twitching, fasciculations, weakness, and flaccid paralysis. Cardiac arrhythmias and pulmonary edema, as well as EEG abnormalities, also occur.

Management consists of emesis or lavage, charcoal instillation, catharsis, and washing of contaminated skin with soap and water. Atropine should be given immediately to block the parasympathetic and central nervous system effects. A dose of 2 mg is injected intramuscularly and repeated every 10 min until parasympathetic manifestations are controlled and signs of atropinization appear. The same dosage must be repeated frequently to maintain xerostomia and mild tachycardia. Fatal respiratory failure or pulmonary edema may occur quickly upon cessation of atropine therapy, and the drug should be judiciously withdrawn. Atropine is virtually ineffective against the autonomic ganglionic actions of acetycholine and against the peripheral neuromuscular paralysis. Relief of muscle weakness, in particular respiratory paralysis, can be achieved with certain oximes which can reactivate cholinesterase by reversing the phosphate ester bond formed by the organic phosphate at the enzyme active site. Pralidoxime is useful in the treatment of organic phosphate cholinesterase inhibition but should not be used if the inhibition is due to a carbamate. A dose of 1 g pralidoxime in aqueous solution is administered intravenously over a 5-min period, and this dose is repeated up to four times every 8 to 12 h. Supportive therapy includes administration of oxygen with artificial ventilation if necessary, removal of pulmonary secretions by suction, and treatment of convulsions with diazepam and phenobarbital. Energetic therapy with artificial ventilation, atropine, and pralidoxime allows survival after doses of organic phosphate esters vastly exceeding the usual fatal dose. In addition, charcoal hemoperfusion significantly increases the clearance of organophosphates and, when available, is indicated after large overdoses in which the patient cannot be supported with atropine and pralidoxime.

CYANIDE The cyanide ion is an exceedingly potent and rapid-acting poison, but one for which specific and effective antidotal therapy is available. Cyanide poisoning may result from the inhalation of hydrocyanic acid or from the ingestion of soluble inorganic cyanide salts or cyanide-releasing substances such as cyanamide, cyanogen chloride, and nitroprusside. Parts of many plants also contain substances such as amygdalin which release cyanide on digestion. Among these are the seeds of certain stone fruits (chokecherry, pin cherry, wild black cherry, peach, apricot, bitter almond), cassava roots, the berries of the jet berry bush, the leaves and shoots of elderberry, and all parts of hydrangea. The controversial drug laetrile, composed in part of an extract of apricot kernels, has been responsible for fatal cyanide poisoning. Cyanides are widely used in industry and for fumigation and may reach the home in photographic chemicals or silver polishes. As little as 300 mg potassium cyanide may cause death.

The extreme toxicity of cyanide is due to its ready reaction with the trivalent iron of cytochrome oxidase. The role of the enzyme in cellular oxygen utilization is inhibited by the formation of the cytochrome oxidase-cyanide complex. The resultant cytotoxic hypoxia leads to cellular dysfunction and death.

Inhalation of hydrogen cyanide may cause death within a minute. Oral doses act more slowly, requiring several minutes for the appearance of symptoms and up to several hours for death. The first effect is an increase in ventilation because of the blockade of oxidative metabolism in the chemoreceptor cells. As more cyanide is absorbed, there are headache, dizziness, nausea, drowsiness, hypotension, profound dyspnea, characteristic electrocardiographic changes, coma, and convulsions.

Cyanide poisoning is a true medical emergency. Treatment is highly effective if given rapidly. The chemical antidotes should be immediately available wherever emergency medical care is dispensed. The diagnosis may be made by the characteristic "bitter almond" odor on the breath of the victim, and physicians should familiarize themselves with this smell. Since the saturation of hemoglobin is not disturbed by cyanide, cyanosis is not seen until respiratory depression supervenes. The objective of treatment is the production of methemoglobin by the administration of nitrite. The trivalent iron of methemoglobin competes with cytochrome oxidase for the cyanide ion. The cytochrome oxidase-cyanide complex dissociates, and enzymatic function and cell respiration are restored. Further detoxification is then achieved by the administration of thiosulfate. The enzyme rhodanese catalyzes the reaction of thiosulfate with cyanide liberated by the dissociation of cyanmethemoglobin; thiocyanate, which is relatively nontoxic, is formed and readily excreted in the urine.

Since speed is of the essence, nitrite should be immediately administered by inhalation of amyl nitrite perles, one every 2 min unless blood pressure is below 80 mmHg. This is followed as soon as possible by the intravenous injection of 10 ml of 3% sodium nitrite over a 3-min period. An intravenous infusion of norepinephrine may be necessary to maintain blood pressure during this injection period. After the administration of sodium nitrite, 50 ml of 25% sodium thiosulfate should be administered intravenously over a 10-min period. Supportive measures, especially artificial respiration with 100% oxygen, should be instituted as soon as possible, but, unless methemoglobinemia is produced promptly, other forms of treatment are of no value. Administration of sodium nitrite and sodium thiosulfate may have to be repeated. Ideally, dosage should be based on methemoglobin determinations, and the methemoglobin should not exceed 40%. If the patient survives 4 h, recovery is likely but residual cerebral symptoms may persist.

DETERGENTS AND SOAPS These substances fall into the three groups of anionic, nonionic, and cationic detergents. The first group contains common soaps and household detergents. They may cause vomiting and diarrhea but have no serious effects, and no treatment is required. However, some laundry compounds contain phosphate water softeners whose ingestion may cause hypocalcemia. The ingestion of nonionic detergents is harmless and requires no treatment.

Cationic detergents, such as benzalkonium chloride (Zephiran) and many others, are commonly used for bactericidal purposes in hospitals and homes. These compounds are well absorbed from the gastrointestinal tract and interfere with cellular functions. The fatal oral dose is approximately 3 g. Concentrated preparations (>20% detergent) are corrosive to mouth and esophagus. Ingestion produces nausea and vomiting, and shock, coma, convulsions, and death may occur in a few hours. Treatment after ingestion of dilute preparations consists of minimizing gastrointestinal absorption by emesis and gastric lavage with ordinary soap solution, which rapidly inactivates cationic detergents. Emesis and lavage are contraindicated in the presence of esophageal injury which is unlikely to occur except after ingestion of concentrated preparations. Activated charcoal and an osmotic cathartic should be administered. If significant absorption has occurred, intensive supportive therapy may be required.

ERGOT This fungus (*Claviceps purpurea*) grows on rye and contains a number of highly toxic alkaloids (e.g., ergotamine, ergonovine) which are used in the treatment of migraine or as uterine stimulants. Poisoning may be due to therapeutic overdosage, particularly in patients with severe infections or liver disease, but more commonly results from the use of ergot as an abortifacient. The epidemic form of chronic ergot poisoning due to the ingestion of contaminated grain is now rarely seen. Ingestion of 1 g ergot has been fatal; ergotamine has caused gangrene in doses of 10 mg per day. Symptoms of acute or chronic ergot poisoning are vomiting, diarrhea, burning abdominal pain, severe muscle pains, ischemic peripheral gangrene, headache, psychotic behavior, muscle tremors, convul-

sions, and coma. Circulatory disturbances are due both to prolonged vasoconstriction and to intimal hyperplasia and thrombosis. Treatment of ergot poisoning is symptomatic. Vigorous vasodilator and analgesic therapy should be employed.

FLUORIDES Fluoride salts are widely used in insecticides. The gases fluorine and hydrogen fluoride are used in industry. The latter is a strong corrosive. Fluorine and fluorides are cellular poisons which inhibit a number of enzymatic reactions, probably the most important of which is to block the glycolytic degradation of glucose. Fluorides also form an insoluble precipitate with calcium and cause hypocalcemia. Finally, in an acid medium fluorides form the corrosive hydrofluoric acid. Ingestion of 1 to 2 g sodium fluoride may be fatal.

Inhalation of fluorine or hydrogen fluoride produces coughing and choking. After an asymptomatic period of a day or two, fever, cough, cyanosis, and pulmonary edema may develop. Ingestion of fluoride salts is followed by nausea, vomiting productive of corroded tissues, diarrhea, and abdominal pain. Consequent to the decrease in serum calcium the victim develops muscular hyperirritability, fasciculations, tremors, spasms, and convulsions. Death is due to respiratory paralysis or circulatory collapse. If the patient survives the acute period, jaundice and oliguria may appear. Chronic fluoride poisoning (fluorosis) is characterized by weight loss, weakness, anemia, brittle bones, and stiff joints. Mottling of teeth is seen when exposure occurs during enamel formation.

Acute fluoride poisoning is treated by immediate administration of milk, lime water, calcium gluconate, or calcium lactate solution to precipitate calcium fluoride. After lavage or emesis and charcoal instillation, calcium (e.g., calcium gluconate, 10 g) can be given again followed by an osmotic cathartic. Then 10% calcium gluconate or 1% calcium chloride should be slowly injected intravenously and repeated as needed to prevent a positive Chvostek's sign. Symptomatic and supportive therapy is administered as indicated.

FORMALDEHYDE This gas is available as 40% solution (Formalin) which is used as a disinfectant, fumigant, or deodorant. Poisoning by Formalin may be diagnosed by the characteristic odor of formaldehyde. Formaldehyde reacts chemically with cellular constituents, depresses cellular functions, and causes cell death. The fatal dose of Formalin is about 60 ml.

Ingestion of Formalin immediately causes severe abdominal pain, nausea, vomiting, and diarrhea. This may be followed by collapse, coma, severe metabolic acidosis, and anuria. Death is usually due to circulatory failure.

Since any organic material can inactivate formaldehyde, milk, bread, soup, etc., should be administered immediately unless activated charcoal is available. Formaldehyde is a corrosive, and emesis and lavage are not recommended.

Parenteral administration of sodium bicarbonate is indicated to combat acidosis. The treatment is otherwise supportive.

GLYCOLS Ethylene glycol and diethylene glycol are commonly used in antifreeze solutions. The more than 50 annual deaths from these compounds usually result from intentional drinking of antifreeze by alcoholics. The fatal dose of ethylene glycol is about 100 g, that of diethylene glycol somewhat lower. Glycols are metabolized by alcohol dehydrogenase to the aldehyde which is ultimately converted to oxalate. It is the metabolites of the glycols (particularly the aldehyde and oxalate) which are most responsible for toxicity after glycol ingestion.

The initial symptoms of acute poisoning by these glycols resemble those of alcoholic intoxication. They may progress to vomiting, stupor, coma with absent reflexes and anisocoria, and convulsions. Tachypnea, bradycardia, and hypothermia are commonly seen, as are metabolic acidosis and hypocalcemia. After massive ingestion death may occur from respiratory failure within a few hours or from pulmonary edema within a day or two. If the patient survives this stage, acute tubular necrosis often develops.

Intravenous infusion of ethanol to maintain a blood level of 100 mg per 100 ml is effective in competing for alcohol dehydrogenase, thus slowing the conversion of glycol to the more toxic aldehyde. Pyridoxine (100 mg daily administered intravenously) and thiamine (1 mg daily administered intravenously) are given to stimulate conversion of glyoxalate, the immediate metabolic precursor of oxalate, to the nontoxic metabolites, glycine and α-hydroxy-β-ketoadipate, respectively. However, the effectiveness of these latter procedures has not been definitely established. Dialysis is highly effective in the removal of ethylene and diethylene glycol from the body. Acidosis and hypocalcemia must be treated vigorously.

HALOGENATED HYDROCARBONS Halogenated hydrocarbons (carbon tetrachloride, ethylene chlorohydrin, ethylene dichloride, methyl halides, trichloroethane, trichloroethylene) find wide industrial use as solvents, refrigerants, fumigants, and in chemical synthesis. They enter the home in household cleaners, floor waxes, fire extinguishers, and rubber or plastic cements. These compounds are highly fat-soluble and produce cell damage either directly or after conversion in the body to other compounds. Individual halogenated hydrocarbons differ considerably in the degree and the exact manifestations of their toxicity, but in sufficient concentration all these compounds are capable of inducing central nervous system depression and varying amounts of hepatic and renal toxicity. Myocardial depression, vascular damage, and pulmonary edema may also occur.

The most important halogenated hydrocarbon is carbon tetrachloride, which is still widely employed as a nonflammable solvent and fire extinguisher fluid but which has largely been replaced in products intended for household use by the less toxic trichloroethane. Poisoning may occur from inhalation of the vapor, ingestion, or, rarely, percutaneous absorption. An oral dose of as little as 4 ml may be fatal. Absorption from the gastrointestinal tract is slow and unpredictable but is increased by the presence of fats and alcohol. Abdominal pain, hematemesis, and hepatic damage are more common and severe after ingestion than when the poison is inhaled. Inhalation may lead to irritation of the upper part of the respiratory tract.

Acute systemic absorption of carbon tetrachloride results in nausea, dizziness, confusion, and headache within a few minutes. Depending upon the quantity absorbed, the symptoms may quickly progress to stupor, coma, convulsions, respiratory failure, hypotension, or ventricular fibrillation. The patient may recover from these immediate manifestations until evidence of hepatic or renal toxicity appears several hours to several days after the exposure. Liver and kidney damage may also occur in the absence of any severe early central nervous system effects. Initially tender hepatomegaly may be present, jaundice may be rapidly progressive, and death due to severe centrilobular necrosis may occur within days. The renal lesion has the characteristics of acute tubular necrosis, and manifests itself by proteinuria, hematuria, oliguria, or anuria. Uremia, acidosis, hypertension, and pulmonary edema may develop as complications of renal failure. Optic neuritis, pancreatitis, and adrenal cortical necrosis are less common manifestations of carbon tetrachloride intoxication.

Chronic poisoning may occur after repeated exposures to low concentrations of carbon tetrachloride and may also lead to liver or kidney damage. Usually it manifests itself by vague symptoms of fatigue, weakness, mental confusion, abdominal pain, anorexia, nausea, blurring of vision, and paresthesias.

Treatment of acute poisoning by halogenated hydrocarbons includes vigorous effects at minimizing gastrointestinal absorption by lavage or emesis and catharsis. Treatment is otherwise symptomatic. Sympathomimetic drugs should be avoided because of the danger of inducing ventricular arrhythmias in the sensitized myocardium. Acute renal and hepatic failure must be carefully managed. Hemodialysis is often required and may be lifesaving until kidney function returns three or more weeks after poisoning. Both hemodialysis and hemoperfusion will effectively remove carbon tetrachloride and trichloroethane from the body but are potentially useful in preventing severe toxicity and death only when begun early in the postingestion period.

IODINE The traditional antiseptic iodine tincture is an alcoholic solution of 2% iodine and 2% sodium iodide. Strong iodine solution (Lugol's solution) is an aqueous solution of 5% iodine and 10% potassium iodide. The fatal dose of tincture of iodine is approximately 2 g. Iodides are very much less toxic, and no fatalities have been reported.

The diagnosis of iodine poisoning is suggested by the brown staining of the oral mucous membranes. The effects are largely due to the corrosive effects of the compound on the gastrointestinal tract. Burning abdominal pain, nausea, vomiting, and bloody diarrhea may occur soon after ingestion. If the stomach contained starch, the vomitus is blue or black. Tissue trauma from corrosive gastroenteritis and fluid loss by vomiting and diarrhea may result in shock. Severe edema of the glottis, fever, delirium, stupor, and anuria have also been observed.

Treatment consists of the immediate administration of milk, starch, bread, etc., or activated charcoal to provide a source other than human tissue with which the iodine can react. Catharsis should be induced. Sodium thiosulfate will reduce iodine to less toxic iodide; 100 ml of a 5% solution should be given orally and then an osmotic cathartic should be given. Ten milliliters of a 10% thiosulfate solution should also be given intravenously every 4 h. Induction of emesis and lavage should not be attempted if esophageal injury is suspected. With appropriate treatment most patients poisoned by iodine survive, but esophageal strictures may complicate their recovery.

IRON SALTS Ferrous or ferric salts produce gastrointestinal corrosive damage. Following mucosal damage, large amounts of iron may be absorbed, particularly in children. The fatal oral dose, calculated as elemental iron in the preparation, is about 300 mg/kg.

The potential toxic effects of iron ingestion can be divided conveniently into five phases: (1) within 30 min to 2 h there may be nausea, vomiting, abdominal pain, bloody diarrhea, lethargy, restlessness; (2) a period of apparent recovery may follow; (3) 2 to 12 h after ingestion the victim may develop shock, refractory acidosis, and fever; (4) 2 to 4 days after ingestion hepatic necrosis may occur; and (5) 2 to 4 weeks after ingestion gastrointestinal obstruction may develop—the end result of the initial corrosive effects of iron.

Treatment is initiated by emesis and lavage with a 5% sodium bicarbonate solution which will precipitate the ferrous ion. A dilution of Fleet's phosphate enema solution can also be used, but excessive lavage can cause hypernatremia, hyperphosphatemia, and hypocalcemia. When possible, at this point an abdominal roentgenogram should be obtained. If radiopaque tablets are still in the stomach, further lavage is indicated, and then an osmotic cathartic should be administered. Optimal management is aided by determination of the presence or absence of free serum iron. If free iron is present, if the total serum iron exceeds 350 meq per 100 ml, or if clinical symptoms are severe (coma, shock), the iron chelator deferoxamine methane sulfonate (Desferal) should be infused intravenously at no more than 10 (mg/kg)/h or given intramuscularly at a dose of 20 mg/kg every 4 to 6 h. The iron deferoxamine complex turns the urine pink to orange, and chelator therapy is continued until the urine loses this color. Treatment is otherwise supportive.

ISOPROPYL ALCOHOL This compound is used as a sterilizing agent or as rubbing alcohol. Ingestion produces gastric irritation and raises the danger of vomiting with aspiration. The systemic effects of isopropyl alcohol are similar to those of ethyl alcohol, but it is approximately twice as potent as the latter. Coma is readily produced but rarely lasts longer than 12 h. About 15% of an ingested dose of isopropanol is metabolized to acetone; transient acetonuria is common, but significant acidosis does not occur. Emesis should be induced, or gastric lavage should be performed. Supportive therapy is required only after ingestion of massive amounts, and there are no sequelae other than transient gastritis.

MAGNESIUM Magnesium sulfate is used intravenously as a hypotensive agent and orally as a cathartic. The magnesium ion is a profound depressant of the central nervous system and of neuromuscular transmission. Poisoning after oral or rectal administration is unlikely in the presence of normal renal function, because the kidney removes magnesium more rapidly than it is absorbed by the gastrointestinal tract. In the presence of impaired renal function an oral dose of 30 g may be fatal. Symptoms begin at a serum magnesium level of 4 meq per liter, and concentrations of over 12 meq per liter may be fatal. Oral ingestion of concentrated solutions may cause gastrointestinal irritation. Manifestations of systemic poisoning are depression of reflexes, flaccid paralysis, hypotension, hypothermia, coma, and respiratory failure. Respiratory death usually precedes significant myocardial depression. The actions of magnesium on neurological and neuromuscular function are antagonized by calcium. Treatment of magnesium poisoning therefore includes the intravenous administration of 10 ml of a 10% solution of calcium gluconate, which may be repeated as necessary.

METHYL ALCOHOL This simplest of alcohols, also called wood alcohol or methanol, is used as a solvent, antifreeze, paint remover, and as a denaturant in ethyl alcohol. Denatured ethyl alcohol preparations, such as Sterno or Solox, contain 5 to 15 percent methyl alcohol as well as other denaturants. Methyl alcohol poisoning is due almost entirely to its ingestion as a substitute for ethanol or to the drinking of denatured ethyl alcohol. The toxic dose is quite variable: death has occurred after a dose of 20 ml, but 250 ml has been ingested with survival. As little as 15 ml methanol has caused permanent blindness.

Methanol is less inebriating than ethyl alcohol, and inebriation is not a prominent symptom of methyl alcohol intoxication. Methanol is oxidized in the body by alcohol dehydrogenase first to formaldehyde and then to formic acid; these metabolites cause the toxic manifestations of methanol poisoning. The rate of its metabolism is only 15 percent that of ethanol for which alcohol dehydrogenase has a greater affinity and which can inhibit competitively the rate of metabolism of methanol. Formic acid and especially formaldehyde have toxic actions on many cells; the retina and optic nerve are specifically damaged. The toxic metabolites of methyl alcohol are also responsible for the severe acidosis, which is the most prominent feature of methyl alcohol poisoning. This acidosis is partly due to the accumulation of formic acid, but formate also appears to exert an inhibitory effect upon enzymes involved in the oxidation of carbohydrate with consequent accumulation of acid intermediates.

Symptoms of methanol poisoning usually do not appear until 12 to 24 h after ingestion, when sufficient toxic metabolites have accumulated. Manifestations include headache, dizziness, nausea, vomiting, vasomotor disturbances, central nervous system depression, and respiratory failure. Visual disturbance is almost universal and ranges from mild blurring of vision to total blindness. Impairment of vision may be transient, but permanent blindness may follow survival of the acute intoxication. The pupils are dilated and nonreactive, and there is hyperemia of the optic disk and retinal edema. Acidosis is commonly severe (plasma carbon dioxide-combining power below 20 meq per liter).

In the treatment of methyl alcohol intoxication emesis and gastric lavage are of use only within the first 2 h after ingestion. Intravenous administration of large amounts of sodium bicarbonate combats acidosis. Return of acidosis is frequent after initial correction, and additional alkali must be administered as indicated by close observation of the patient and laboratory determinations. It is most useful to obtain a blood methanol level as soon as possible. At any time after ingestion, levels between 20 and 50 mg per 100 ml are associated with acidosis and significant symptomatology and are an indication for intravenous ethanol therapy (1 ml absolute ethanol per kilogram of body weight in 5% dextrose in water over 15 min to load, then 7 to 10 ml/h in adults to maintain the blood ethanol level at about 100 mg per 100 ml). Severely symptomatic patients should be treated even if a methanol level cannot be obtained. A methanol level exceeding 50 mg per 100 ml is indication for hemodialysis as well as ethanol therapy; dialysis is also indicated in the presence of severe acidosis with lower blood levels.

MUSHROOMS There are many species of poisonous mushrooms, but in the United States most poisoning is due to *Amanita muscaria* (fly agaric) or *Amanita phalloides* (destroying angel). More than 100 deaths result each year from consumption of wild poisonous mushrooms, 90 percent being due to *A. phalloides*. Fatalities have occurred after ingestion of only part of one mushroom.

Amanita muscaria contains the parasympathomimetic alkaloid muscarine, as well as variable amounts of a substance active on the central nervous system and a parasympatholytic alkaloid. Symptoms are largely those of parasympathetic stimulation: lacrimation, pupillary constriction, perspiration, salivation, nausea, vomiting, diarrhea, abdominal pain, bronchorrhea, wheezing, dyspnea, bradycardia, and hypotension. Muscular tremors, confusion, excitement, and delirium are common in severe poisoning. Very rarely symptoms of atropine poisoning have predominated. After ingestion of *A. muscaria* symptoms appear within minutes to 2 h. The patient may die within a few hours, but with appropriate therapy complete recovery in 24 h is the rule.

Amanita phalloides, some other *Amanita* species, and *Galerina venenata* contain heat-stable cyclopeptide cytotoxins which are rapidly bound to tissues. The principal toxin is α-amanitin which binds to and inhibits specifically the mammalian RNA polymerase responsible for messenger RNA synthesis. Severe cell damage and fatty degeneration may occur in liver, kidneys, striated muscle, and brain. Ingestion of these dangerous mushrooms is followed by a latent period of 6 to 20 h. Manifestations of cytotoxicity may then appear suddenly and consist of severe nausea, violent abdominal pain, bloody vomiting and diarrhea, and cardiovascular collapse. Headache, mental confusion, coma, or convulsions are common. Painful and tender hepatomegaly, jaundice, hypoglycemia, dehydration, and oliguria or anuria frequently appear on the first or second day after ingestion. The victim may die from acute hepatic necrosis (yellow atrophy) within 4 days. About one-half of all poisonings with *A. phalloides* have a fatal outcome in 5 to 8 days. Recovery tends to be slow.

Ingestion of other poisonous mushrooms may cause gastrointestinal symptoms, visual disturbances, ataxia, disorientation, convulsions, coma, fever, hemolysis, and methemoglobinemia.

Treatment of mushroom poisoning depends upon the species ingested. If parasympathomimetic manifestations are prominent, atropine in doses of 1 to 2 mg is given intramuscularly and repeated every 30 min until symptoms are controlled. Poisoning by cytotoxic mushrooms is treated mainly symptomatically. Fluid and electrolyte balance must be carefully maintained. Hypoglycemia should be avoided; large quantities of carbohydrate may exert some protective effect on the liver. Excitement, convulsions, pain, hypotension, and fever may need symptomatic therapy. Early intensive hemoperfusion can remove α-amanitin from the body and is probably indicated in *A. phalloides* poisoning. Both thioctic acid (α-lipoic acid) and cytochrome c have been advocated as antidotes for α-amanitin poisoning, but convincing data as to their efficacy are lacking.

NAPHTHALENE Poisoning by this substance is almost always due to ingestion of moth repellents. An oral dose of 2 g has been fatal. Nausea, vomiting, and diarrhea are the initial symptoms. Larger doses may produce hepatic damage with jaundice and renal toxicity which may progress to hematuria, oliguria, or anuria. Depending upon the amount ingested, central nervous system manifestations may range from headache, mental confusion, and excitement to coma and convulsions. In persons with glucose 6-phosphate dehydrogenase–deficient red blood cells the ingestion of naphthalene will produce hemolysis. Treatment consists of emesis or gastric lavage, catharsis, and supportive measures.

NICOTINE This alkaloid is an exceedingly potent and rapidly acting poison. It is a component of many insecticides. Nicotine is readily absorbed from the oral and gastrointestinal mucosa, from the respiratory tract, and through the skin. The lethal dose for an adult is approximately 50 mg, the quantity contained in two cigarettes. However, tobacco is much less toxic than would be anticipated on the basis of its nicotine content. Nicotine is poorly absorbed from ingested tobacco, and on smoking, most of the nicotine is burned. Nicotine acts on chemoreceptors, on synapses in the central nervous system and in autonomic ganglia, on the adrenal medulla, and on neuroeffector junctions. Furthermore, its transient initial stimulant effects are followed by a more persistent depressant phase of action. It is not surprising that the manifestations of nicotine poisoning are highly complex and somewhat unpredictable.

Small doses of nicotine produce nausea, vomiting, diarrhea, headache, dizziness, and neurological stimulation manifested by tachycardia, hypertension, hyperpnea, tachypnea, sweating, and salivation. Larger doses also cause cortical irritability, progressing to convulsions, and myocardial arrhythmias. Finally coma, respiratory depression and arrest, and cardiac arrest or fibrillation may supervene. Severe poisoning may cause death from respiratory failure within a few minutes.

Treatment consists of induction of emesis or gastric lavage, followed by the instillation of activated charcoal and the administration of an osmotic cathartic. Potassium permanganate will oxidize nicotine, and a 1:10,000 solution can be used for lavage. Atropine, 2 mg, and phentolamine, 5 mg, may be given intramuscularly or intravenously and repeated as often as required to control signs and symptoms of parasympathetic or sympathetic hyperactivity. These compounds are ineffective in preventing paralysis of the respiratory muscles and distur-

bances in cardiac rhythm. Careful attention must be given to artificial ventilation with oxygen and to therapy of catecholamine-induced cardiac tachyarrhythmias. Propranolol is the drug of choice for the latter purpose. Nicotine is rapidly detoxified in the liver, and recovery will be prompt if the patient can be tided over the initial period.

NITRITES Poisoning by the nitrite ion may result from the ingestion of large amounts of drugs such as amyl nitrite or sodium nitrite. Nitrites are also used to preserve the color of meat, and amounts in excess of the allowable residue of 0.01 percent may appear in food. Ingested nitrates may be reduced to nitrite by intestinal bacteria, especially *Escherichia coli*. Except after the ingestion of very large amounts, adults usually absorb all nitrate before this reduction takes place. However, in children nitrite poisoning may result from the ingestion of nitrates or nitrate-containing well water. Fatalities have occurred from the oral ingestion of 2 to 4 g nitrites.

Acute nitrite poisoning may lead to severe headache, flushing, dizziness, hypotension, and syncope. Usually the patient need only be positioned to facilitate venous return to the heart. Pressor agents are seldom required. The most important toxic effect of the nitrite ion is its ability to oxidize hemoglobin to methemoglobin (Chaps. 53 and 315).

OXALIC ACID This acid is found in ink eradictors and stain removers. Ingestion causes irritation and corrosion of mouth, esophagus, and stomach, followed by vomiting and abdominal pain. After absorption it precipitates serum calcium as insoluble calcium oxalate, and the resultant hypocalcemia leads to muscular tremors, tetany, convulsions, and cardiovascular collapse. Ingestion of 5 g may cause death within minutes. Following recovery from the acute episode there may be renal failure due to blockage of renal tubules by calcium oxalate crystals.

Treatment consists of precipitating oxalate in the gastrointestinal tract by giving calcium in any form orally such as milk, limewater, chalk, or calcium salts. If tissue corrosion is suspected, neither emesis nor gastric lavage is indicated. A dose of 10 ml of 10% calcium gluconate should be given intravenously and repeated as required to maintain normal serum calcium and prevent tetany. In supportive therapy the maintenance of a high urine output is essential.

PARAQUAT Paraquat is a dipyridilium compound which is used in 5 to 20% aqueous solutions as a herbicide. An oral dose of 5 mg/kg may be fatal. Some victims die within 24 h in respiratory failure, often with refractive pulmonary edema. In others a serious toxic effect is the delayed (3 days to 2 weeks postingestion) development of progressive pulmonary fibrosis. The lungs selectively accumulate paraquat from the blood over several days until a critical concentration is reached, after which pulmonary edema and fibrosis ensue. Progressive respiratory failure is the usual cause of death. The metabolism of paraquat by lung tissue leads to the production of radical intermediates as well as the superoxide radical; the latter appears to be at least partly responsible for the toxicity of the compound.

Prolonged absorption (up to several days) of paraquat from the gastrointestinal tract is common. After gastric emptying, diluted bentonite (fuller's earth) or activated charcoal should be administered followed by an osmotic cathartic twice daily for 48 h. Forced diuresis, hemodialysis, and hemoperfusion significantly augment clearance of paraquat. Oxygen administration is associated with a higher mortality from paraquat poisoning in animals; it would seem prudent to avoid oxygen-enriched breathing mixtures in patients poisoned with paraquat if possible. Intravenous administration of superoxide dysmutase has been reported to decrease lung toxicity from paraquat in animals, but no beneficial effect has yet been demonstrated in humans.

PETROLEUM DISTILLATES Petroleum distillates (diesel oil, gasoline, kerosene, paint thinner, solvent distillate) are liquids with a boiling point between 50 and 325°C. They contain variable amounts of branched or straight-chain aliphatic and aromatic hydrocarbons. Kerosene is widely used as a fuel and as a vehicle for cleaning agents, furniture polishes, insecticides, and paint thinners. Not surprisingly, each year petroleum distillates cause about 100 accidental deaths in the United States, 90 percent of these in young children. Furthermore, these products are annually responsible for almost 20,000 hospitalizations. Ingestion of 10 ml kerosene has been fatal, but adults have recovered from as much as 250 ml. Petroleum distillates are central nervous system depressants; they damage cells by dissolving cellular lipids. Pulmonary damage manifested by pulmonary edema or pneumonitis is a common and serious complication.

Inhalation of gasoline or kerosene vapors induces a state resembling alcoholic intoxication. Headache, nausea, tinnitus, and a burning sensation in the chest may also be present. When aliphatic hydrocarbons are inhaled, these symptoms may progress to profound drowsiness or coma with absence of deep reflexes. If the distillate contains a high proportion of aromatic hydrocarbons, the coma is characterized by tremors, muscle jactitations, hyperactive reflexes, and convulsions. Death is usually due to respiratory depression, rarely to ventricular fibrillation.

The oral ingestion of petroleum distillates causes irritation of the mucous membranes of the upper part of the intestinal tract. When large amounts have been ingested, the same manifestations as after inhalation may appear. Frequently eructation or vomiting results in aspiration of petroleum distillates into the trachea. Because of their low surface tension, minute amounts of these substances may then spread widely throughout the lungs and produce pulmonary edema and pneumonitis. Pulmonary damage may also arise because of absorption of ingested petroleum distillates from the gastrointestinal tract. However, kerosene is at least one hundred times more toxic by the intratracheal route than when ingested.

In the treatment of poisoning by petroleum distillates extreme care must be used to prevent aspiration. If the patient is coughing when seen, aspiration is likely to have occurred already. When large amounts (>100 ml) have been ingested, gastric emptying is indicated. In the alert patient emesis may be induced; when vomiting occurs, the patient's head should be lower than his or her hips. Otherwise, gastric lavage should be performed but only after insertion of an endotracheal tube with an inflatable cuff. A saline cathartic may be administered. All victims of kerosene poisoning should be hospitalized for at least 24 h for observation. If signs or symptoms of pulmonary irritation appear, oxygen should be given. Steroids do not appear useful in treatment of this pulmonary lesion and may be detrimental. Prophylactic antibiotics are not indicated. Symptomatic therapy for central nervous system depression or treatment of convulsions may be necessary. Sympathomimetic amines should be avoided because of the danger of inducing ventricular fibrillation in the hydrocarbon-sensitized heart.

PHENCYCLIDINE Phencyclidine (PCP, "angel dust") has become a common and dangerous drug of abuse. It is structurally similar to ketamine hydrochloride and is used as a general anesthetic in veterinary medicine, but its powerful psychomimetic properties make it unsuitable for human use. The drug can be inhaled, smoked, swallowed, or injected; at doses as low as 1 to 5 mg euphoria, numbness, and emotional lability result. Higher doses cause disorientation, confusion, restlessness, and psychosis. Doses as high as 1 g have reportedly been taken and have resulted in prolonged comatose states, seizures, spasticity, opisthotonos, hypertension on occasion severe enough to cause intracranial hemorrhage, respiratory depression, and death.

Phencyclidine is metabolized by the liver, and the metabolites as well as some free drug are excreted in the urine. Treatment begins with emesis or lavage (even if the drug was not taken orally), charcoal instillation, and administration of an osmotic cathartic. The drug is a weak base, and its renal clearance can be increased as much as twentyfold by forced diuresis after acidification of the urine (pH<5). Oral ammonium chloride and intravenous ascorbic acid are used to achieve and maintain the urinary pH, and a diuretic is administered. In addition, a significant clearance of phencyclidine is obtained by a continuously draining nasogastric tube. Hypertension occasionally requires treatment, seizures should be controlled with diazepam, and psychosis is best treated with butyrophenones and not phenothiazines.

PHENOL Phenol and related compounds (creosote, cresols, hexachlorophene, hydroquinone, Lysol, resorcinol, tannic acid) are widely used as antiseptics, caustics, and preservatives. These substances poison all cells by denaturing and precipitating cellular proteins. The approximate fatal oral dose ranges from 2 ml for phenol and cresols to 20 ml for tannic acid.

Ingestion of phenolic compounds produces erosion of mucosa from mouth to stomach. The corroded areas may have a characteristic dead-white appearance. Hematemesis and bloody diarrhea may occur. After an initial phase of hyperpnea due to stimulation of the respiratory center, stupor, coma, convulsions, pulmonary edema, and shock are seen. The initial respiratory alkalosis is soon followed by a profound acidosis which results from the renal excretion of base during the alkalotic stage, from the acidic nature of phenol, and from disturbances in carbohydrate metabolism presumably due to defects in enzymatic function. If the patient survives the acute stage, acute tubular necrosis may lead to oliguria or anuria and hepatic toxicity to jaundice.

Poisoning by phenolic compounds may often be diagnosed by their characteristic odor. Development of a violet or blue color of the urine after addition of a few drops of ferric chloride indicates the presence of a phenolic compound.

Emesis and lavage are indicated for treatment in the absence of significant corrosive injury to the esophagus. Activated charcoal should be administered. Olive oil or castor oil, which dissolves phenol and retards its absorption, should be given, and followed with an osmotic cathartic. Supportive therapy consists of correction of the acidosis, the control of shock and convulsions, and the maintenance of a patent airway in the face of glottal edema by intubation or tracheotomy.

PHOSPHORUS Phosphorus occurs in two forms: a red, nonpoisonous form and a yellow, fat-soluble, highly toxic form. The latter is used in rodent and insect poisons and in fireworks. Yellow phosphorus and phosphides cause fatty degeneration and necrosis of tissues, particularly of the liver. The lethal ingested dose of yellow phosphorus is approximately 50 mg.

Ingestion of yellow phosphorus is followed within 1 h by burning pain in the upper part of the gastrointestinal tract, vomiting, diarrhea, and a garlic odor of the breath and excreta. The patient may die in coma during the first day or two, or symptoms may subside after a few hours. Then, 1 to 2 days later, the victim may develop tender hepatomegaly, jaundice, hypocalcemia, hypotension, and oliguria and may die following convulsions and coma. Death from acute hepatic necrosis may occur in a few days.

Treatment consists of induction of emesis or gastric lavage, instillation of activated charcoal, and administration of an osmotic cathartic. Calcium gluconate is given intravenously to maintain the serum calcium level. Treatment is otherwise supportive.

SALICYLATES Each year 30 million pounds of aspirin is consumed in the United States, and salicylates can probably be found in every American household. It is therefore not surprising that salicylates (aspirin, methyl salicylate, salicylic acid, sodium salicylate) are more commonly involved in poisonings than any other agent. Aspirin is found in almost all compound analgesic tablets. Methyl salicylate (oil of wintergreen) is present in most skin liniments, and salicylic acid is used in ointments and corn plasters. The ingestion of 10 to 30 g aspirin or sodium salicylate may be fatal to adults, but survival has been reported after an oral dose of 130 g aspirin. On the other hand 3 g salicylate in a teaspoon of methyl salicylate has been fatal in children.

Salicylate intoxication may result from the cumulative effect of therapeutic administration of high doses. There is considerable individual variation: toxic symptoms may begin at dosages of 3 g per day or may not appear when 10 g per day is given. Toxic symptoms are also poorly correlated with the serum salicylate concentration, but few patients become intoxicated at levels less than 15 mg per 100 ml and most at levels over 35 mg per 100 ml. Therapeutic salicylate intoxication is usually mild and is called "salicylism." The earliest symptoms are vertigo, tinnitus, and impairment of hearing. Further overdosage causes nausea, vomiting, sweating, diarrhea, fever, drowsiness, headache, dimness of vision, and mental aberrations. The latter may be characterized by confusion, excitement, restlessness, and talkativeness; this "salicylate jag" resembles alcoholic intoxication without the euphoria. The central nervous system effects may progress to hallucinations, convulsions, and coma. Toxic doses of salicylates also have a direct stimulant effect on the respiratory center, resulting in hyperventilation, loss of carbon dioxide, and respiratory alkalosis. Renal excretion of bicarbonate may partially compensate for this.

In acute salicylate poisoning due to accidental or suicidal ingestion of massive amounts, the same manifestations may be seen in more rapid succession. However, they are usually overshadowed by severe disturbances in the acid-base balance which follow a definite sequence. Early in the course of intoxication there may be only hyperpnea, and the seriousness of the poisoning may not be appreciated at that time. The hyperventilation causes a fall in blood P_{CO_2} and an increase in pH. Renal excretion of bicarbonate, sodium, and potassium will bring the pH back toward normal and produce a compensated respiratory alkalosis. At that point the buffering capacity of the extracellular fluid will have been significantly decreased. In young children and after large doses in adults further developments may then produce a combination of respiratory acidosis and metabolic acidosis which stems from a number of factors. High concentrations of salicylate depress the respiratory center and cause CO_2 retention. Renal function becomes impaired because of dehydration and hypotension, and inorganic, metabolic acids accumulate. Furthermore, salicylic acid derivatives may displace several milliequivalents of blood bicarbonate. Finally, salicylates impair carbohydrate metabolism and cause accumulation of acetoacetic, lactic, and pyruvic acids. Severe acidosis and disturbances in electrolyte balance are most commonly seen in febrile young children.

Blood salicylate levels are of value in the estimation of the severity of poisoning. Serious poisoning is rare at levels less than 50 mg per 100 ml but usual at levels between 50 and 100

mg per 100 ml. Levels above 100 mg per 100 ml during the first 6 h after poisoning signify severe intoxication and may be fatal. Excretion of salicylates is renal, and in the presence of normal renal function about 50 percent will be excreted in 24 h. Addition of a few drops of ferric chloride solution to 5 ml boiled acidified urine containing salicylate yields a violet color and may aid in diagnosis.

Treatment of salicylate poisoning consists of initially inducing emesis or of gastric lavage after which activated charcoal and then an osmotic cathartic are administered. Disturbances of acid-base or electrolyte balance and hypoglycemia are corrected by the intravenous administration of appropriate solutions. Respiratory depression may require artificial ventilation with oxygen. Convulsions may be treated with diazepam or phenobarbital. The renal clearance of salicylate is enhanced ten- to twentyfold if the pH of the urine can be kept between 7 and 8. In addition to intravenous bicarbonate and a diuretic it may be necessary to give potassium to prevent paradoxical aciduria to raise the urinary pH above 7. Peritoneal dialysis and hemodialysis are also highly effective in removing salicylate from seriously poisoned patients, but forced alkaline diuresis is so effective in clearing salicylate that these maneuvers are most often not required.

SMOKE Poisoning by smoke is usually due to carbon monoxide inhalation. However, burning material may also release irritant fumes. Many irritant gases combine with water to form corrosive acids or alkalies and cause chemical burns of exposed skin and of the upper part of the respiratory tract. Such gases (and the corrosives formed) are ammonia (ammonium hydroxide), nitrogen oxide (nitric acid), sulfur dioxide (sulfurous acid), and sulfur trioxide (sulfuric acid). These irritating gases as well as hydrogen sulfide may also be present in smog. Another highly toxic gas which may be inhaled by firefighters or victims is phosgene. This compound is formed by the high-temperature decomposition of chlorinated hydrocarbons and is released when carbon tetrachloride from fire extinguishers comes into contact with hot surfaces.

After inhalation of irritant gases the victim may notice burning pain in throat and chest and severe coughing. These symptoms may subside completely, but from several hours to a day after exposure dyspnea and cyanosis may appear and progress rapidly to severe pulmonary edema and death from respiratory and circulatory failure. Treatment consists of administration of oxygen and adrenal steroids and appropriate therapy of pulmonary edema, should that develop.

SULFIDES Hydrogen sulfide is a gas released by the decomposition of organic sulfur compounds and is widely used in industry. Carbon disulfide is an industrial solvent. Other sulfides have industrial uses and release hydrogen sulfide in contact with water or acids. Significant concentrations of hydrogen sulfide may be present in smoke or smog. Inhalation of hydrogen sulfide in concentrations above 50 ppm (50 times the minimum detectable by smell) causes conjunctivitis, headache, nausea, soreness of the upper respiratory passages, pulmonary edema, and drowsiness. Concentrations in excess of 300 ppm may cause coma, respiratory depression, and death. Ingestion of carbon disulfide or soluble sulfides is followed by vomiting, headache, hypotension, respiratory depression, tremors, coma, convulsions, and death. The fatal oral dose of carbon disulfide is approximately 1 g. Treatment of sulfide intoxication is supportive. Administration of sodium nitrite may promote the binding of sulfide in sulfmethemoglobin.

VOLATILE OILS The volatile or essential oils (citronella oil, eucalyptus oil, menthol, pine oil turpentine) are colorless liquids which irritate all tissues. Poisoning may result from occupational exposure (painters) and accidental or suicidal ingestion. Unfortunately, some volatile oils also have an undeserved reputation as abortifacients. Absorption occurs from skin, intestine, or lungs; the less volatile oils are more slowly absorbed. Ingestion of 15 g turpentine has been fatal.

Ingestion is rapidly followed by abdominal burning, nausea, vomiting, and diarrhea. Inhalation produces severe bronchial irritation and may be followed by delirium, coma, and convulsions. If the patient survives the acute stage of poisoning, evidence of renal damage may appear and progress to acute tubular necrosis with anuria.

Treatment is entirely supportive. When emesis is induced or gastric lavage is undertaken, aspiration must be prevented with extreme care. Hemodialysis may be required for renal failure.

REFERENCES

Acetaminophen

BARKER JD et al: Chronic excessive acetaminophen use and liver damage. Ann Intern Med 87:299, 1977

FARID NR et al: Hemodialysis in paracetamol self-poisoning. Lancet 2:396, 1972

GAZZARD BG et al: Charcoal hemoperfusion for paracetamol overdose. Br J Clin Pharmacol 1:271, 1974

LOVEJOY FJ, GOLDMAN P: Acetaminophen toxicity. J Pediatr 1979 (in press)

PETERSON RG, RUMACK BH: Toxicity of acetaminophen overdose. J Am Coll Emergency Physicians 7:202, 1978

PRESCOTT LF et al: Treatment of paracetamol poisoning with *N*-acetylcysteine. Lancet 2:432, 1977

Antimuscarinic compounds

GOWDY JM: Stromonium intoxication. JAMA 221:585, 1972

LEVY R: Jimson seed poisoning—a new hallucinogen on the horizon. J Am Coll Emergency Physicians 6:58, 1977

RUMACK BH: Anticholinergic poisoning: Treatment with physostigmine. Pediatrics 52:449, 1973

Barium

GOULD DB et al: Barium sulfide poisoning. Arch Intern Med 132:891, 1973

Benzene, toluene

BROWNING E: Toxic solvents: A review. Br J Ind Med 16:23, 1959

BROZOVSKY M, WINKLER EM: Glue sniffing in children and adolescents. NY State J Med 65:1984, 1965

GLASER HH, MASSENGALE ON: "Glue sniffing" in children. Deliberate inhalation of vaporized plastic cements. JAMA 181:300, 1962

HAYDEN JW: The clinical toxicology of solvent abuse. Clin Toxicol 9:169, 1976

Boric acid

VALDES-DAPENA MA, AREY JB: Boric acid poisoning. J Pediatr 61:531, 1962

WONG LC et al: Boric acid poisoning: Report of 11 cases. Can Med Assoc J 90:1018, 1964

Carbon monoxide

ANDERSON RF et al: Myocardial toxicity from carbon monoxide poisoning. Ann Intern Med 67:1172, 1967

COSBY RS, BERGERON M: Electrocardiographic changes in carbon monoxide poisoning. Am J Cardiol 11:93, 1963

MEIGS JW, HUGHES JPW: Acute carbon monoxide poisoning: An analysis of 105 cases. AMA Arch Ind Hyg 1:90, 1950

REMICK RA, MILES JE: Carbon monoxide poisoning: Neurologic and psychiatric sequelae. Can Med Assoc J 117:654, 1977

WINTER PM, MILLER JN: Carbon monoxide poisoning. JAMA 236:1502, 1976

Castor bean

BENSON S: On the mechanism of protein-synthesis inhibition by abrin and ricin. Eur J Biochem 59:573, 1975

BRUGHSCH HG: The castor bean. N Engl J Med 262:1039, 1960

Caustics

CAMPBELL GS et al: Treatment of corrosive burns of the esophagus. Arch Surg 112:495, 1977

RUMACK BH, BURLINGTON JD: Caustic ingestions: A rational look at diluents. Clin Toxicol 11(1):27, 1977

Chlorate

KNIGHT RK et al: Suicidal chlorate poisoning treated with peritoneal dialysis. Br Med J 3:601, 1967

Chlorinated insecticides

BOYLAN JJ et al: Cholestyramine: Use of a new therapeutic approach for chlordecone (Kepone) poisoning. Science 199:893, 1978

COBLE Y et al: Acute endrin poisoning. JAMA 202:489, 1967

ZAVON MR: Chlorinated hydrocarbon insecticides. JAMA 190:595, 1964

Cholinesterase inhibitor insecticides

LUZHNIKOR EA et al: Plasma perfusion through charcoal in methylparathion poisoning. Lancet 1:38, 1977

MANN JB: Diagnostic aids in organophosphate poisoning. Ann Intern Med 67:905, 1967

MILBY TH: Prevention and management of organophosphate poisoning. JAMA 216:2131, 1971

QUINBY GE: Further therapeutic experience with pralidoximes in organic phosphorus poisoning. JAMA 187:202, 1964

WYCKOFF W et al: Diagnostic and therapeutic problems of parathion poisonings. Ann Intern Med 68:875, 1968

Cyanide

BRAICO KT et al: Laetrile intoxication: Report of a fatal case. N Engl J Med 300:238, 1979

BURROWS GE et al: Effect of oxygen on cyanide intoxication. J Pharmacol Exp Ther 184:739, 1973

CHEN KK, ROSE CL: Treatment of acute cyanide poisoning. JAMA 162:1154, 1956

COPE C: The importance of oxygen in the treatment of cyanide poisoning. JAMA 175:1061, 1961

HUMBERT JR et al: Fatal cyanide poisoning: Accidental ingestion of amygdalin. JAMA 238:482, 1977

Detergents

ARENA JM: Poisonings and other health hazards associated with use of detergents. JAMA 190:56, 1964

WILSON, JT, BURR, IM: Benzalkonium chloride poisoning in infant twins. Am J Dis Child 129:1208, 1975

Fluorides

YOLKEN R et al: Acute fluoride poisoning. Pediatrics 58:90, 1976

Glycols

HAGSTAM KE et al: Ethylene glycol poisoning treated by haemodialysis. Acta Med Scand 178:599, 1965

MORIARTY RW, MCDONALD RH: The spectrum of ethylene glycol poisoning. Clin Toxicol 7:583, 1974

PARRY MF, WALLACH R: Ethylene glycol poisoning. Am J Med 57:143, 1974

Halogenated hydrocarbons

BAERG RD, KIMBERG DV: Centrilobular hepatic necrosis and acute renal failure in "solvent sniffers." Ann Intern Med 73:713, 1970

Oettingen WF von: *The Halogenated Hydrocarbons of Industrial and Toxicological Importance.* Amsterdam, Elsevier, 1964

Rechnagel RO: Carbon tetrachloride hepatotoxicity. Pharmacol Rev 19:145, 1967

Schwarzbeck A, Kosters W: Extracorporeal hemoperfusion in acute carbon tetrachloride intoxication. Arch Toxicol 35:207, 1976

Iron salts

Fischer DS et al: Acute iron poisoning in children. JAMA 218:1179, 1971

Jacobs J et al: Acute iron intoxication. N Engl J Med 273:1124, 1965

Leikin S: Deferoxamine as a chelating agent. J Pediatr 72:148, 1968

Isopropyl alcohol

Freireich AW et al: Hemodialysis for isopropanol poisoning. N Engl J Med 277:699, 1967

Methyl alcohol

Bennet H Jr et al: Acute methyl alcohol poisoning: A review based on experiences in an outbreak of 323 cases. Medicine 32:431, 1953

Cooper JR, Kini MM: Biochemical aspects of methanol poisoning. Biochem Pharmacol 11:405, 1962

Keyvan-Larijarni H, Tannenberg M: Methanol intoxication: Comparison of peritoneal and hemodialysis. Arch Intern Med 134:293, 1974

Smith ME: Interrelations in ethanol and methanol metabolism. J Pharmacol 134:233, 1961

Mushrooms

Litten W: The most poisonous mushrooms. Sci Am 232(3):90, 1975

Paaso B, Harrison DC: A new look at an old problem: Mushroom poisoning. Am J Med 58:505, 1975

Naphthalene

Haggerty RJ: Naphthalene poisoning. N Engl J Med 255:919, 1956

Nicotine

Gehlbach SH et al: Nicotine absorption by workers harvesting green tobacco. Lancet 1:478, 1975

Taylor WJR et al: Pesticide poisoning in children. Drug Ther 1(11):15, 1971

Nitrites

Keating JP et al: Infantile methemoglobinemia caused by carrot juice. N Engl J Med 288:824, 1973

Paraquat

Fairshter RD, Wilson RF: Paraquat poisoning: Manifestations and therapy. Am J Med 59:751, 1975

Okonabe S, Hofmann A: Efficacy of gut lavage, hemodialysis and hemoperfusion in the therapy of paraquat and diquat intoxication. Arch Toxikol 36:45, 1976

Petroleum distillates

Brown J et al: Experimental kerosene pneumonia: Evaluation of some therapeutic regimens. J Pediatr 84:396, 1974

Shirkey H: Treatment of petroleum distillate ingestion. Mod Treat 8:580, 1971

Taussig LN et al: Pulmonary function 8 to 10 years after hydrocarbon pneumonitis. Clin Pediatr 16:57, 1977

Phencyclidine

Aronow R, Done AK: Phencyclidine overdose: An emerging concept of managment. J Coll Emergency Physicians 7:56, 1978

Cohen S: Angel dust. JAMA 237:515, 1977

Liden CB et al: Phencyclidine: Nine cases of poisoning. JAMA 234:513, 1975

Phosphorus

Simon FA, Pickering LK: Acute yellow phosphorus poisoning. JAMA 235:1343, 1976

Talley RC et al: Acute elemental phosphorus poisoning in man: Cardiovascular toxicity. Am Heart J 84:139, 1972

Winek CL et al: Yellow phosphorus ingestions: Three fatal poisonings. Clin Toxicol 6:541, 1973

Salicylates

Anderson RJ et al: Unrecognized adult salicylate intoxication. Ann Intern Med 85:745, 1976

Buschanun N, Rabinowitz L: Infantile salicylism: A reappraisal. J Pediatr 84:391, 1974

Done AK: Salicylate intoxication; significance of measurements of salicylate in blood in cases of acute ingestions. Pediatrics 26:800, 1960

———: Salicylate poisoning. JAMA 192:770, 1965

———, Temple AR: Treatment of salicylate poisoning. Mod Treat 8:528, 1971

Hill JB: Salicylate intoxication. N Engl J Med 288:1110, 1973

Proudfoot AT, Brown SS: Acidaemia and salicylate poisoning in adults. Br Med J 2:537, 1969

Segar WE, Holliday MA: Physiologic abnormalities of salicylate intoxication. N Engl J Med 259:1191, 1958

225
HEAVY METALS

DAVID C. POSKANZER

Three highly effective chemicals, BAL, Versene, and penicillamine, are available for treatment of systemic poisoning with heavy metals by forming nontoxic, stable cyclic compounds with polyvalent metallic ions, thus permitting the offending material to be excreted safely in the urine.

The first to be developed was BAL (British antilewisite, 2,3-dimercaptopropanol, dimercaprol), which was originally intended as an antidote against the arsenical war gas, lewisite. Its tendency to combine with certain metallic ions such as arsenic, mercury, cobalt, nickel, antimony, and gold is so great that it can remove them from combination with the enzymes whose function they impair in the body. By itself BAL is not useful in treating lead poisoning. Because the effectiveness of BAL depends to some extent upon the speed with which its administration is begun, every attempt should be made to avoid delay in its use. For serious systemic intoxications, BAL should be given in doses of 5 mg per kilogram of body weight intramuscularly as a 10% solution in oil and 20% benzyl benzoate. No single dose should exceed 300 mg. This dose should be repeated every 4 h on the first day and every 6 h on the second day. Thereafter, it should be given three times daily for several days; doses should then be tapered and discontinued about 10 days after acute poisoning. When the dose of poison has been relatively small, the schedule of BAL administration may be reduced by one-third. Because BAL is excreted in part by the kidneys, it can accumulate to toxic concentrations in anuric patients. Overdosage results in nervousness, hyperactivity, muscle twitching, and hyperreflexia. Large doses may produce convulsions. The presence of the material in tears sometimes causes blepharospasm. In patients with anuria or oliguria, therefore, BAL should be administered with caution and at a lower dosage than outlined above. If symptoms of overdosage occur, sedatives should be administered.

The second antidote to metal poisons is the chelating agent Versene (ethylenediaminetetraacetate, EDTA), which forms cyclic, stable, soluble, nontoxic compounds with most metals.

Because Versene reacts with calcium in the same way as with other metals, it must be given as the calcium salt (Calcium Disodium Versenate, calcium disodium edetate) to avoid hypocalcemia. The material has been used with notable success in the treatment of lead poisoning. It is given in a dosage of 1.0 g in 250 ml of 5% glucose intravenously every 12 h for 5 days. After a pause to allow for further solution of metal from body stores, a second and even a third course may be given.

Penicillamine (Cuprimine, β,β-dimethylcysteine) is an excellent chelating agent for copper, mercury, and lead, promotes their excretion in the urine, and has the additional advantage of being well absorbed from the gastrointestinal tract. It may be given orally, while BAL and Versene require systemic injection. N-Acetyl-dl-penicillamine is even more effective than penicillamine in protecting against the effects of mercury, probably because it is more resistant to metabolic degradation, and it has the advantage of being less toxic. Penicillamine is administered orally in a dose of 1 to 4 g daily on an empty stomach to avoid chelation of dietary metals. It has much lower toxicity than BAL, the only other agent which is effective in the treatment of Wilson's disease (hepatolenticular degeneration), in which toxic amounts of copper are deposited in various tissues, but has the disadvantage of acute sensitivity reactions. It has also been shown to be useful in lead poisoning, but the excretion of urinary lead may not be as high after oral penicillamine as after intravenous Calcium Disodium Versenate.

N-Acetyl-dl-penicillamine, available as an investigational drug, has been demonstrated to be effective in mercury poisoning and has the advantage of allowing much higher doses with fewer toxic effects. It has less effect on copper levels than penicillamine and is, therefore, used in the treatment of mercury poisoning when one would wish to maintain copper levels. The administration of 1 to 2 g daily in divided doses for 10 days gives good results.

ANTIMONY Symptoms of poisoning after the ingestion of antimony may occur when an acid food is allowed to stand in cheap enamelware or "graniteware" for a sufficient time to allow solution of antimony, which is used in the manufacture of these products. Certain parasiticidal drugs also contain this metal. The symptoms are similar to those produced by arsenic, except that antimony causes a more rapid onset of gastrointestinal symptoms. Treatment is the same as for arsenic, including use of BAL. Circulatory collapse occurs early and requires vigorous supportive treatment.

ARSENIC Arsenic poisoning is usually the result of accidental or suicidal ingestion of insecticides or rodenticides containing paris green (copper acetoarsenate) or calcium or lead arsenate. Pesticides containing arsenic are a frequent source of poisoning in rural areas of the United States. Medications such as Fowler's solution (potassium arsenite) and the organic arsenicals (arsphenamines and arsenoxides) were once common causes of intoxication.

The toxic dose of inorganic arsenic varies considerably and seems to depend upon individual susceptibility. Orchardists have been found to ingest as much as 6.8 mg arsenic a day without any signs of intoxication. On the other hand, as little as 30 mg arsenic trioxide has been fatal. Arsenic has a predilection for keratin, and the concentration of arsenic in the hair and nails is higher than that in other tissues. Arsenic reacts with the —SH groups in certain tissue proteins and thus interferes with a number of enzyme systems essential to cellular metabolism. Pathological changes in fatal inorganic arsenical

poisoning are fatty degeneration of the liver, hyperemia and hemorrhages of the intestine, and renal tubular necrosis. The peripheral nerves often show fragmentation and resorption of myelin, with disintegration of axis cylinders (axonal neuropathy).

The symptoms of acute poisoning by the oral route are nausea, vomiting, diarrhea, severe burning of the mouth and throat, and agonizing abdominal pains. The vomitus often contains blood. Circulatory collapse is frequent, and death may ensue within a few hours. With chronic exposure, the first signs of poisoning are usually weakness, prostration, muscular aching, or nervous system involvement; gastrointestinal symptoms are minimal. In patients exposed to arsine gas (hydrogen arsenide), the outstanding features are hemolysis, chills, fever, and hemoglobinuria.

Patients who recover from acute poisoning and those with chronic intoxication usually develop skin and mucosal changes, peripheral neuropathy, and linear pigmentations in the fingernails (see Chap. 377). The cutaneous manifestations appear within 1 to 4 weeks and consist of a diffuse, dry, scaly desquamation, occasionally with hyperpigmentation, over the trunk and extremities. Hyperkeratoses of the palms and soles and edema of the face and extremities may also occur. The mucous membranes also show evidence of irritation, with conjunctivitis, photophobia, pharyngitis, or irritating cough. About 5 weeks after exposure to arsenic, a transverse white stria, 1 to 2 mm in width, appears above the lunula of each fingernail (Mees line). Patients with more than one exposure to arsenic may show double lines several millimeters apart.

Symptoms of headache, drowsiness, confusion, and convulsions are seen in both acute and chronic intoxication. Evidence of peripheral neuropathy usually appears 1 to 3 weeks after exposure. There are numbness, tingling, and burning of the feet and hands, followed by muscular weakness. The extremities show a decrease in touch, pain, and temperature sensations, in a symmetrical "stocking-glove" distribution, and distal weakness with inability to walk or stand, weakness of grip, and wrist drop. Tendon reflexes are absent or diminished, and atrophy of the affected muscles develops rapidly.

The laboratory findings usually consist of moderate anemia and a leukopenia of 2000 to 5000 white blood cells per cubic millimeter with mild eosinophilia. There is slight proteinuria, and liver function tests show mild abnormalities. The spinal fluid is normal.

None of the clinical or laboratory manifestations of arsenic poisoning is specific, and the diagnosis depends upon analysis of the urine for arsenic. Because arsenic is found widely in nature, and hence in water and food, its discovery in hair and nails may not be diagnostic. Normal persons have an average concentration of 0.05 mg arsenic per 100 g hair. Concentrations of arsenic greater than 0.1 mg per 100 g hair are considered indicative of poisoning. The minimal level of arsenic in the urine indicating intoxication is difficult to establish. Normal persons have been found to excrete between 0.01 and 0.06 mg arsenic per liter, and a few individuals as much as 0.2 mg per liter. Although there is considerable overlap, most patients with evidence of arsenic intoxication will be found to excrete more than 0.1 mg per liter; soon after acute exposure, many will show levels greater than 1 mg per liter.

The treatment for acute ingestion is gastric lavage (see Chap. 223). Replacement of lost fluids and elevation of blood pressure by vasopressor agents is often indicated. Immediate treatment with BAL should be instituted. Patients with peripheral neuropathy rarely show significant improvement with BAL and continue to have sensory disturbances and weakness for many months. Dramatic responses, however, have been observed with the use of BAL in the treatment of exfoliative dermatitis, bone marrow depression, and encephalopathy caused by the arsphenamines and the organic arsenicals. BAL is of little value in the treatment of the hemolysis caused by inhalation of arsine.

BISMUTH Poisoning by bismuth was formerly almost entirely a complication of antisyphilitic therapy. Now it rarely complicates bismuth salts taken for intestinal disorder. Toxic manifestations may appear in the mouth (gingivitis, followed by stomatitis), the kidneys (albuminuria and nephrotic syndrome), the skin (exfoliative dermatitis), and an acute confusional psychosis, requiring immediate interruption of bismuth injections or of the ingestion. The development of a bluish stippled line of pigmentation just at the margin of the gums is not dangerous but suggests that oral hygiene should be improved. Bismuth subnitrate occasionally gives rise to methemoglobinemia (Chap. 315).

CADMIUM Poisoning is likely to occur after ingestion of an acid food prepared in a cadmium-lined vessel. The classic example is lemonade served from metal cans. Symptoms of nausea, vomiting, diarrhea, and prostration usually develop within 10 min after ingestion. Treatment is symptomatic, and symptoms ordinarily subside within 24 h. The short length of time after ingestion and the typical circumstances suggest the diagnosis. Inhalation of cadmium fumes in industry produces an acute, extremely severe pneumonitis. The use of BAL is not recommended for cadmium intoxication, as the BAL-cadmium complex dissociates in the kidneys and cadmium is nephrotoxic.

COPPER See Chap. 83 for discussion of disturbances in trace element metabolism, including copper, zinc, cobalt, nickel, silicon, and fluorine.

GOLD Because practically all cases of poisoning by gold are associated with its use in the treatment of arthritis, diagnosis is usually easy. Manifestations are skin rashes of various types, bone marrow depression, icterus, oliguria, nausea, vomiting, and gastrointestinal bleeding. Treatment consists of symptomatic relief of discomfort and the use of BAL, an effective antidote.

LEAD Poisoning results from inhalation of fumes as from burning storage batteries, from solder, paint spraying, or processes requiring the remelting of metallic lead. Ingestion of lead-containing materials such as paint, or water which has stood in lead pipes, is less important in adults. Illicit whiskey contaminated by lead solder in the pipes of stills has been responsible for cases of poisoning. Bullets or buckshot containing lead can cause poisoning years after becoming embedded in a serous cavity. The most common form of lead poisoning today is that encountered in children who ingest lead-containing outdoor paint, often used indoors in older houses. It has a sweetish, apparently attractive taste. Absorption is slow by any route, and prolonged exposure is required for the development of symptoms. Lead is a cumulative poison, excreted slowly. Acute poisoning is virtually nonexistent. Symptoms may develop suddenly after chronic exposure. Most of the absorbed lead is deposited in the bones; blood, urine, and feces contain only small amounts.

Manifestations of poisoning are colic, encephalopathy, peripheral neuritis, and anemia.

Lead colic, or painter's cramps, is characterized by agonizing, wandering, poorly localized abdominal pain, often with spasm and rigidity of the musculature of the abdominal wall. There is no fever or leukocytosis. Needless surgery has been carried out in these patients for supposed perforation of peptic ulcer or other catastrophe. Morphine has surprisingly little effect upon the pain; intravenous injection of calcium salts affords relief within a short time, although pain may recur. Attacks of colic seem to be brought on by intercurrent infection or alcoholic overindulgence.

Encephalopathy occurs chiefly in children and is manifested by convulsions, somnolence, mania, confusion, or coma. The mortality rate is high when convulsive seizures and coma occur. In an unexplained acute encephalopathy of childhood, increased intracranial pressure associated with high protein and the absence of cells should suggest the possibility of lead poisoning.

Peripheral neuritis with paralysis, characteristically involving the muscles most used (e.g., wrist drop in painters, etc.), occurs in patients exposed to lead, often in the absence of other symptoms. It is rare in children. (See Chap. 375.)

Mild anemia, probably the result of increased brittleness of the erythrocytes as well as a defect in cell maturation, is common. Pallor is out of proportion to anemia in patients with chronic plumbism and is attributed to spasm of small vessels in the skin. Anemia is almost never severe and is characterized by the presence of large numbers of erythrocytes with basophilic stippling. This is seen in other hematologic disorders, but a smear showing stippling should arouse suspicion of lead poisoning. In patients with poor oral hygiene a "lead line" of black lead sulfide may develop along the gingival margins. This is not seen in edentulous persons and is rare in children.

Patients with lead poisoning excrete increased amounts of coproporphyrin III in the urine (see Chap. 96). This is so consistent that examination of a urine specimen for porphyrin is the best screening test in suspected cases. A few milliliters of urine should be acidified with acetic acid and shaken with an equal volume of ether. Exposure of a specimen prepared in this manner under a Wood's lamp will reveal reddish fluorescence of the ether layer if coproporphyrin is present. A positive test result is strongly in favor of lead intoxication. Urinary lead determinations are of aid in confirming the diagnosis; a level of 0.2 mg per liter or more is usually regarded as significant, although interpretations vary. Diagnosis can be confirmed by promoting lead excretion with three doses of Calcium Disodium Versenate (25 mg/kg) at 8-h intervals. Excretion of over 500 μg in 24 h is indicative of excessive lead burden. A single blood lead level is rarely of help in diagnosis in adults because blood is cleared promptly of circulating lead.

Lead encephalopathy occurs chiefly in children, has a significant mortality rate, and causes severe permanent brain damage in 25 percent of survivors. Encephalopathy in adults is rare and usually results from consumption of lead-contaminated illicit liquor. Once minor symptoms of poisoning are present, acute encephalopathy can develop with unpredictable rapidity. Any child with symptoms suggestive of lead poisoning should be considered to have a medical emergency and should be hospitalized immediately. The onset of encephalopathy is signaled by the development of gross ataxia, persistent vomiting, and intermittent lethargy and stupor. These symptoms are followed by convulsions, hyperactivity, and coma.

The most important single feature of treatment is removal of the patient from further exposure to lead. Once abnormal absorption is terminated, virtually all the lead in the body is shifted into bone. Chelating agents do not remove significant quantities of lead from bone. It takes approximately twice as long to excrete a given burden of lead as it does to accumulate it. As long as significant quantities of lead remain in bone, any intercurrent illness which causes demineralization can cause mobilization of toxic quantities of lead into soft tissues and exacerbate plumbism.

The treatment of lead encephalopathy is begun once adequate urine flow is established. A combination of BAL and Calcium Disodium Versenate is employed, and the Versene therapy continued for 5 to 7 days. If Calcium Disodium Versenate is given alone in the presence of very high tissue concentrations of lead, some of the toxic effects may be intensified. Acute symptoms usually subside within 48 to 72 h after Versene is begun. Within 2 weeks urinary excretion of coproporphyrin ceases, and there is sometimes a dramatic improvement in neuritis.

Symptoms of acute increased intracranial pressure are best treated with repeated doses of mannitol given intravenously. High-potency corticosteroids are also useful in relieving cerebral edema in patients with lead encephalopathy.

The problem of lead poisoning in children is so significant that many health departments are carrying out extensive programs for removal of lead-containing paints in old low-income housing areas.

In adults combined therapy with BAL and Calcium Disodium Versenate followed by oral penicillamine is probably indicated whenever blood levels exceed 100 mg lead per 100 g blood, even in the absence of symptoms. Evidence of lead toxicity is usually present at this level, and the risk of symptomatic episodes is considerable. The use of oral penicillamine alone in a dose of 1 to 1.5 g daily for 3 to 5 days in mildly symptomatic cases has been suggested and has the advantage of easy administration and the avoidance of painful injections.

MERCURY   Poisoning occurs chiefly as a result of the acute ingestion of a soluble salt, usually mercuric chloride (bichloride of mercury). Toxic symptoms may occur with 0.1 g, and 0.5 g is almost always fatal unless immediate treatment is instituted. The mercuric ion is corrosive and produces severe local inflammation. Oral, pharyngeal, and laryngeal pain are severe; abdominal cramps with nausea and vomiting occur within 15 min. As mercury is absorbed, it is concentrated in the kidneys, where it poisons the tubular cells, producing a tendency to diuresis within the first 2 to 3 h. The combination of vomiting, dehydration, shock, and progressive tubular damage, however, soon leads to anuria and uremia. The poison is also excreted into the colon and produces severe enteritis, with bloody diarrhea and tenesmus. Death is usually from uremia. The chief objectives of treatment are to prevent the shock of dehydration and to remove mercury from the body. Early in treatment, copious quantities of fluid should be infused intravenously to prevent dehydration and to reduce the concentration of mercuric ion in the renal tubules. That the patient is anuric early is often simply the result of dehydration and shock. In such instances, forcing fluids is advisable. However, the gradual development of oliguria and anuria in a hydrated patient indicates renal damage by mercury, and at this stage a regimen for acute renal shutdown should be instituted (Chap. 275).

Chronic poisoning from metallic mercury vapor occurs in persons exposed to large amounts of the metal in laboratories or in industry and occasionally as a result of prolonged therapeutic use, as in vaginal douches. Manifestations may be those of subacute poisoning, with salivation, stomatitis, and diarrhea or primary neurological signs, including tremors of the extremities, tongue, and lips, ataxia and dysarthria, erethism, a state of easy embarrassment, irritability, apprehension, withdrawal, and depression.

Methylmercuric salts were discovered to have a special effect, mainly on the nervous system. First it was observed that workers exposed in the manufacture of an insecticide containing this compound developed an acute cerebellar ataxia. Later in Minimata, Japan, an effluent from a factory was noted to cause cerebellar ataxia and cortical blindness. In some cases there was involvement of peripheral nerves and impairment of neuromuscular transmission (Rustam et al.). The damage to the central nervous system usually is permanent. Public health measures have been taken to eliminate such compounds from the environment.

Some poison can be removed from the body by gastric lavage, but more important in treatment is the binding of the mercuric ion in a harmless compound by BAL. The therapeutic usefulness of BAL depends on its immediate administration. In chronic mercury poisoning, N-acetyl-dl-penicillamine may well be the drug of choice. It can be administered orally and appears to chelate mercury selectively, with considerably less effect on copper, which is essential to many metabolic processes.

SILVER   Most poisoning by silver involves silver nitrate, a caustic salt. There are intense nausea, vomiting, and diarrhea after swallowing nitrate (lunar caustic), and death from shock may occur within a few hours. The mouth is usually deeply stained by silver nitrate. Treatment is entirely supportive, with fluid replacement and control of pain.

Chronic exposure (usually to nose drops) produces a peculiar bluish skin discoloration (argyria).

THALLIUM   Thallium is a component of certain rodenticides and depilatories, and clinical poisoning is usually a result of accidental ingestion of these materials. The fatal dose is approximately 1.0 g. Manifestations are vomiting, diarrhea, and leg pains, followed by a severe and sometimes fatal sensorimotor polyneuropathy. About 3 weeks after poisoning, the patient's hair falls out, providing a strong diagnostic clue if the cause has not previously been determined. Treatment is symptomatic. The alopecia is temporary if the patient recovers.

REFERENCES

ARENA JM: Treatment of mercury poisoning. Mod Treat 4:734, 1967

AUB JC et al: Lead poisoning. Medicine 4:1, 1925

BANK WJ et al: Thallium poisoning. Arch Neurol 26:456, 1974

CHISHOLM JJ JR: Poisoning due to heavy metals. Pediatr Clin North Am 17:591, 1970

DOOLAN PD et al: Acute renal insufficiency due to dichloride of mercury: Observations of gastrointestinal hemorrhage and BAL therapy. N Engl J Med 249:273, 1953

HAMILTON A, HARDY HL: Industrial Toxicology, 3d ed. Acton, Publishing Sciences Group, 1974

HEYMAN A: Systemic manifestations of bismuth toxicity: Observations on 4 patients with pre-existent kidney disease. Am J Syph Gonorrhea Vener Dis 28:721, 1944

JENKINS RB: Inorganic arsenic and the nervous system. Brain 89:479, 1966

KARK RAP et al: Mercury poisoning and its treatment with N-acetyl-d,l-penicillamine. N Engl J Med 285:10, 1971

KENDREY G, ROE FJC: Cadmium toxicology. Lancet 1:1206, 1969

KEUSLER CJ et al: Arsine poisoning, mode of action and treatment. J Pharmacol Exp Ther 88:99, 1946

LEVINE WG: Heavy-metal antagonists, in The Pharmacological Basis of Therapeutics, 5th ed, LS Goodman, A Gilman (eds). New York, Macmillan, 1975, p 912

LONGCOPE WT, LUETSCHER JA: The use of BAL (British antilewisite) in the treatment of the injurious effects of arsenic, mercury, and other metallic poisons. Ann Intern Med 31:545, 1949

RUSTAM H et al: Evidence for neuromuscular disorder in methyl mercury poisoning. Arch Environ Health 30:190, 1975

226
ALCOHOL

MAURICE VICTOR
RAYMOND D. ADAMS

Intemperance in the use of alcohol creates many problems in modern society, the importance of which can be judged by the repeated emphasis they receive in contemporary writings, both literary and scientific. These problems may be divided into three categories—psychological, medical, and sociologic. The main psychological problem is why individuals drink excessively, often with full knowledge that such action will result in physical injury to themselves and irreparable harm to their families. The medical problem embraces all aspects of the diseases which result from the abuse of alcohol. The sociologic problem comprises the effects of sustained inebriety on the family and community.

The various problems raised by excessive drinking cannot be separated from one another, and physicians must, therefore, be conversant with all parts of the subject. They may be asked to help patients conquer their alcoholic tendencies or to diagnose and to treat the numerous diseases to which they are subject; often they must admit or commit patients to a general or mental hospital, according to the nature of the presenting clinical disorder; and lastly, they may be required to enlist the aid of available social agencies when such services are needed by either patients or their families.

Alcoholism has been defined as both a chronic disease and a disorder of behavior, characterized in either context by drinking of alcohol to an extent that surpasses the social drinking customs of the community and that interferes with the drinker's health, interpersonal relations, or means of earning a livelihood. Reduced to pharmacologic terms, it is addiction to alcohol. Alcoholics are individuals who satisfy these medical, social, and pharmacologic criteria. The precise number of such persons in the United States is not known. In 1971, the Department of Health, Education, and Welfare estimated that about 9 million men and women (7 percent of the adult population) "manifested the behavior of alcohol abuse and alcoholism." It requires little projection of the imagination to conceive of the havoc wrought by alcohol in terms of decreased productivity, accidents, crime, mental and physical disease, and disruption of family life.

PHARMACOLOGY AND METABOLIC EFFECTS OF ALCOHOL

Ethyl alcohol, or ethanol, is the active ingredient in beer, wine, whiskey, gin, brandy, and other less common alcoholic beverages. In addition, the stronger spirits contain enanthic ethers, which give the flavor but have no important pharmacologic properties, and small amounts of impurities such as amyl alcohol and acetaldehyde, which act like alcohol but are more toxic. Contrary to prevailing opinion, the content of B vitamins in American beer and other liquors is so low as to have little nutritional value.

Alcohol is absorbed unaltered from both the stomach and the small intestine. Its presence may be detected in the blood within 5 min after ingestion, and the maximum concentration is reached in 30 to 90 min. The ingestion of milk and fatty foods impedes the absorption of alcohol, and water facilitates it. The rate of absorption increases after Billroth I and II gastrectomies, and in these individuals maximum blood alcohol concentrations are higher and attained faster than in subjects with intact stomachs.

After entering the bloodstream, alcohol enters the various organs of the body, as well as the spinal fluid, urine, and pulmonary alveolar air, in concentrations which bear a constant relationship to that in the blood. It is eliminated chiefly by oxidation to carbon dioxide, less than 10 percent being excreted chemically unchanged in the urine, sweat, and breath. The energy liberated by the oxidation of alcohol is equivalent to 7 kcal/g.

Alcohol is metabolized primarily in the liver, via the cytoplasmic enzyme alcohol dehydrogenase, to acetaldehyde. It can also be oxidized by catalase and a microsomal oxidase, but the physiological and quantitative roles of these pathways are not entirely clear. Acetaldehyde is converted by acetaldehyde dehydrogenase of liver mitochondria to acetylcoenzyme A and acetate, and the latter are metabolized further through well-established normal pathways to yield carbon dioxide and water.

For all practical purposes it may be accepted that once absorption is ended and an equilibrium established with the tissues, ethyl alcohol is oxidized at a constant rate, independent of its concentration in the blood (about 150 mg alcohol per kilogram of body weight per hour, or about 1 oz 90-proof whiskey or 10 to 12 oz beer per hour). Actually, more alcohol is burned per hour when the initial concentrations are very high, but this increment is of little clinical significance. On the other hand, the rate of oxidation of acetaldehyde does depend on its concentration in the tissues. This fact is of importance in connection with the drug disulfiram (Antabuse), which raises the tissue concentration necessary for the metabolism of a certain amount of acetaldehyde per unit of time. Patients taking both Antabuse and alcohol will accumulate an inordinate amount of acetaldehyde, resulting in nausea, vomiting, and hypotension, sometimes pronounced and even fatal in degree. This pharmacologic principle underlies the treatment of alcoholism with Antabuse.

Only a few factors are capable of increasing the rate of alcohol metabolism. It seems well established that chronic alcoholics metabolize alcohol somewhat faster than normal individuals. Amino acids (especially alanine), insulin, and fructose also enhance ethanol metabolism, but the clinical usefulness of these agents in speeding the oxidation of alcohol is limited. Alcohol also reduces the intestinal absorption of nutrients such as glucose, amino acids, calcium, folate and vitamin B_{12}. This impairment of absorption may contribute to the malnutrition frequently found in alcoholic subjects. On the other hand starvation slows the rate of alcohol metabolism in the liver.

Alcohol has a number of other metabolic effects. In the area of *lipid metabolism* it can cause hypertriglyceridemia as well as lead to a fatty liver. It interferes with *carbohydrate metabolism* and can produce hypoglycemia by impairing gluconeogenesis; however, a significant degree of hypoglycemia will occur only if hepatic glycogen stores are depleted. Under certain conditions alcohol can also interfere with the peripheral utilization of glucose and produce hyperglycemia. When ethanol is oxidized, there is a simultaneous generation of reduced nicotinamide adenine dinucleotide (NAD); as a result pyruvate is converted to lactate. Thus alcoholism may result in increased levels of serum lactate, occasionally *lactic acidosis*, and also *hyperuricemia*, which is secondary to the inhibitory action of lactic acid on the renal excretion of uric acid.

Other renal effects of alcohol ingestion are an increased urinary excretion of *phosphate and magnesium*, resulting in low serum levels of these ions, and an *increased urinary excretion of ammonium*. In addition to lactic acidosis, alcoholics may have other types of metabolic and respiratory acidosis. The metabolic acidosis is presumably due to an accumulation of acid metabolites, especially β-hydroxybutyrate. The respiratory acidosis is attributed to a direct action of alcohol on the respiratory center.

There are also well-recognized effects of alcohol on water excretion; thus the ingestion of 4 oz 100-proof bourbon whiskey may result in a diuresis comparable with that which follows the drinking of large amounts of water. This diuresis is most likely due to the transient suppression of the release of antidiuretic hormone (ADH) from the supraopticohypophyseal system, since a relatively small amount of alcohol injected directly into a carotid artery evokes a prompt diuresis without a detectable rise in the concentration of alcohol in the systemic blood. Alcohol does not alter the sensitivity of the kidney tubules to endogenous or exogenous ADH (pitressin) and has no discernible effect on renal hemodynamic function in normal persons. The degree of diuresis seems to be more closely related to the duration of the rising blood alcohol level than to the rate of increase or the absolute level attained if the period of alcohol intoxication is sustained. Diuresis occurs only during the initial phase of alcohol administration and does not persist during prolonged drinking.

Alcohol also appears to inhibit the hypothalamic and neurohypophyseal release of vasopressin and oxytocin. It has been demonstrated that the administration of alcohol to normal young men for periods up to 4 weeks decreased the rate of production and the plasma concentration of testosterone. These abnormalities in testosterone metabolism were traced to both a central (hypothalamus-pituitary) and gonadal effect of alcohol and were independent of nutritional deficiency and liver disease.

Alcohol has a direct effect on the excitability and contractility of heart muscle. With intoxicating doses there is a rise in cardiac rate and output and in systolic and pulse pressures, and a cutaneous vasodilatation at the expense of splanchnic constriction. Some authors have stated that prolonged intoxication may have a damaging effect on cardiac and skeletal muscle, a degeneration of fibers supposedly due to suppression of myophosphorylase activity. Increased sweating and vasodilatation cause a loss of body heat and a fall in body temperature.

In low concentrations, by whatever route it is administered, alcohol stimulates the parietal cells of the stomach mucosa to produce acid, apparently by antral activation of gastrin release, and possibly by causing the tissues to form or release histamine. With the ingestion of alcohol in concentrations of over 10 to 15 percent, the secretion of mucus is increased, the stomach mucosa becomes congested and hyperemic, and the secretion of acid may then become depressed. This is a state of acute gastritis, from which recovery may be relatively rapid. The increase in appetite following ingestion of alcohol is due to the stimulation of the end organs of taste and to a general sense of well-being. Similarly, the reviving effect of alcohol in fatigue states is a cerebral one, not due to a direct stimulating effect on muscle or other organs.

PSYCHOLOGICAL (BEHAVIORAL) EFFECTS OF ALCOHOL AND THE PHENOMENON OF TOLERANCE The most obvious actions of acute, nonlethal doses of alcohol are those exerted on the nervous system, constituting the characteristic symptoms and signs of alcohol intoxication. It is now accepted that alcohol is not a stimulant of the central nervous system but a depressant. Some of the early effects of alcohol, manifested by garrulousness, aggressiveness, excessive activity, and increased electrical excitability of the cerebral cortex, all of which suggest stimulation, are due probably to the inhibition of certain subcortical structures (probably the high brainstem reticular formation) which ordinarily modulate cerebral cortical activity. Similarly, the initial hyperactivity of tendon reflexes may represent a transitory escape of spinal motor neurons from higher inhibitory centers. With increasing amounts of alcohol, however, the depressant action spreads to involve the cerebral cortical neurons as well as other brainstem and spinal neurons.

The behavioral effects of acute ingestion of alcohol (1 to 6 ozs) in the nonaddicted person have been the subject of many studies. They have shown that all manner of motor performance, whether the simple maintenance of a standing posture, the control of speech and eye movements, or highly organized and complex motor skills, is adversely affected by alcohol. The movements involved in these acts are not only made slower than normal but also more inaccurate and random in character and therefore less adapted to the accomplishment of specific ends.

Alcohol also impairs the efficiency of mental function by interfering with the learning process, which is slowed and rendered less effective. The facility of forming associations, whether of words or of figures, tends to be hampered, and the power of attention and concentration is reduced. The person is not as versatile as usual in directing thought along new lines appropriate to the problems at hand. Finally, alcohol impairs the faculties of judgment and discrimination and, all in all, the ability to think and reason clearly.

A scale relating the various degrees of clinical intoxication to the blood alcohol levels in nonhabituated persons has been constructed. At blood alcohol levels of 30 mg per 100 ml, a mild euphoria is detectable, and at 50 mg per 100 ml, a mild incoordination. At 100 mg per 100 ml, ataxia is obvious; at 200 mg per 100 ml, the patient is drowsy and confused; at 300 mg per 100 ml, the patient is stuporous; and a level of 400 mg per 100 ml is accompanied by deep anesthesia and may prove fatal. These figures are valid provided that the alcohol content rises steadily over a 2-h period.

It should be emphasized that such a scale has little or no value in the chronic alcoholic patient since it does not take into account the adaptive changes that the organism makes to alcohol, which are an increased rate of alcohol metabolism by the liver and particularly the development of tolerance. These phenomena account for the large amounts of alcohol that can be consumed by the chronic drinker without significant signs of drunkenness. In the chronic alcoholic the ingestion of a given amount of alcohol will result in a lower blood alcohol level than in a nonalcoholic individual; furthermore, for a given blood alcohol level one will observe lesser degrees of "drunkenness" or inebriation. The organism is capable of adapting to alcohol after a very short exposure. If the alcohol concentration in the blood is raised very slowly, no symptoms may appear, even at quite high levels. It would seem that the important factor in this rapid adaptability is not so much the rate of increment or the height of the blood alcohol level, but the length of time the alcohol had been present in the body. It has also been shown that if the dosage of alcohol which causes blood levels to reach a certain height is held constant, the blood alcohol concentration falls and clinical evidence of intoxication disappears. The cause of this fall in alcohol concentration is not clear. It appears that ethanol has an important effect upon the neuronal membrane, but the nature of this effect or how it contributes to central nervous system (CNS) depression or to the development of tolerance is still an enigma. Removal of alcohol from the habituated CNS results in another disturbance in neuronal function, presumably an overactivity.

CLINICAL EFFECTS OF ALCOHOLISM The possible damaging effects of chronic alcohol ingestion on cardiac and skeletal muscle have already been mentioned. These are considered further on and in Chaps. 247 and 383.

That alcoholics are often anemic and thrombocytopenic is common clinical experience. Until recently these abnormalities were attributed to the malnutrition, infection, and liver disease that complicate severe alcoholism, but increasingly it has become apparent that the chronic ingestion of alcohol has a direct damaging effect upon cells of the bone marrow.

The most frequent and important clinical effects of alcoholism are on the digestive organs and on the nervous system.

Effect on digestive organs Symptoms of disordered gastrointestinal function are particularly common in alcoholics; of these the most distinctive are *morning nausea and vomiting*. Characteristically, patients can suppress these symptoms by taking a drink or two, after which they are able to consume large quantities of alcohol without their recurrence until the following morning. Since sufficient alcohol actually relieves these symptoms, they are probably not due to the local effects of alcohol on the stomach, but have a "central" origin and represent the mildest manifestations of the withdrawal syndrome (see below).

Other complaints referable to the gastrointestinal system are abdominal distention, epigastric distress, belching, typical or atypical ulcer symptoms, and hematemesis. The most common pathological basis for these symptoms is a superficial *gastritis,* which is an almost invariable sequel to prolonged drinking. Most instances of gastritis are benign, and the symptoms subside after a few days of abstinence, but more severe forms are associated with mucosal erosions or ulcerations and may be the source of serious bleeding. The incidence of *peptic ulcer* is exceptionally high in alcoholics. A serious cause of hematemesis is the *Mallory-Weiss syndrome,* which is characterized by lacerations of the mucosa at or just below the gastroesophageal junction. In many of these cases bleeding is preceded by an episode of forceful vomiting or protracted retching. The typical lesions appear to depend upon raising the intragastric pressure to 100 to 150 mmHg, i.e., to the range of pressure attained by normal subjects during a period of induced straining and retching.

Patients admitted to the hospital following a period of prolonged drinking and severe dietary depletion almost invariably show enlargement of the liver because of infiltration of the parenchymal cells with fat (see Chap. 299). This fatty liver is essentially reversible provided that patients remain abstinent and receive a nutritious diet. A form of hepatocellular necrosis or *alcoholic hepatitis* is observed frequently in chronic alcoholics, especially following a severe drinking bout. About 8 percent of patients with severe alcoholism develop a permanent form of liver disease, i.e., *cirrhosis,* in which a diffuse proliferation of fibrous tissue replaces the normal lobular architecture of the organ. The alcoholic forms of liver disease are discussed in Chap. 304.

The excessive use of alcohol is also a significant factor in the causation of pancreatitis. The mildest form of this disorder may be attributed to gastritis or may go unnoticed, unless discovered by elevations of the serum amylase level. In more severe form pancreatitis presents as an acute abdominal catastrophe, i.e., with epigastric pain, vomiting, and rigidity of the upper abdominal muscles. In these circumstances the pancreas appears tense and edematous, often with a serosanguineous exudation of fluid on its surface. The most severe form is that of hemorrhagic pancreatitis (Chap. 309). Alcoholics may also develop a chronic relapsing form of pancreatitis. This type is often associated with irregular calcification of the pancreas. Steatorrhea is a not infrequent complication and is probably related to abnormalities of pancreatic exocrine function, malnutrition, and interference with intestinal absorption of fat.

[The *management* of the various gastrointestinal complications of alcoholism is considered in the section dealing with these diseases (Chaps. 287 and 291).]

Effect on nervous system A large number of neurological disorders are associated with alcoholism. The factor common to

all of them is the abuse of alcohol, but the mechanism by which alcohol produces its effects varies from one group of disorders to another, a feature which serves as the basis for the following classification. For the most part, this classification is based on known mechanisms.

I Alcoholic intoxication—drunkenness, coma, excitement ("pathological intoxication," "blackouts")
II Abstinence or withdrawal syndrome—tremulousness, hallucinosis, "rum fits," delirium tremens
III Nutritional diseases of the nervous system secondary to alcoholism
  A Wernicke-Korsakoff syndrome
  B Polyneuropathy
  C Optic neuropathy ("tobacco-alcohol amblyopia")
  D Pellagra
IV Diseases of uncertain pathogenesis, associated with alcoholism
  A Cerebellar degeneration
  B Marchiafava-Bignami disease
  C Central pontine myelinolysis
  D Cerebral atrophy
  E "Alcoholic" cardiomyopathy and myopathy
  F Fetal alcohol syndrome
V Neurological disorders consequent upon Laennec's cirrhosis and portosystemic shunts
  A Hepatic stupor and coma
  B Chronic hepatocerebral degeneration

ALCOHOLIC INTOXICATION Drunkenness is such a common phenomenon that its clinical features require little elaboration. The signs consist of varying degrees of exhilaration and excitement, loss of restraint, irregularity of behavior, loquacity, slurred speech, incoordination of movement and gait, irritability, drowsiness, and, in advanced cases, stupor and coma. On rare occasions acute intoxication is characterized by an outburst of irrational, combative, and destructive behavior, which terminates when patients fall into a deep stupor and for which they may later have no memory. This state has been referred to as "pathological intoxication" or "acute alcoholic paranoid state." Allegedly this reaction may follow the ingestion of relatively small amounts of alcohol, and it has been variously ascribed to constitutional differences in susceptibility to alcohol, previous cerebral injury, and "an underlying epileptic predisposition." However, there are no critical data to support any of these contentions. An analogy may be drawn between this state of alcoholic excitement and a similar reaction which occasionally complicates the administration of barbiturates.

"Blackouts," in the language of alcoholics, refer to transient episodes of amnesia which accompany heavy intoxication. After patients become sober, they cannot recall events that had occurred over a period of several hours, even though the state of consciousness (as observed by others) was not importantly altered during this period. The significance of these episodes is not clear; they do not necessarily indicate progression of alcoholic addiction, as is generally assumed.

Alcohol acts on nerve cells in a manner akin to the general anesthetics. Unlike the latter, however, the margin between the dose of alcohol that produces surgical anesthesia and that which dangerously depresses respiration is a very narrow one, a fact which accounts for the occasional fatality in cases of alcoholic narcosis.

The signs of alcohol intoxication are distinctive, and most forms present no problem in diagnosis or management. On the other hand, coma due to alcohol may present difficulties in differential diagnosis. It should be stressed that the diagnosis of alcoholic coma is made not merely on the basis of a flushed face, stupor, and the odor of alcohol, but only after the careful exclusion of all other causes of coma (see Chap. 20).

Treatment of alcoholic intoxication   Mild to moderate degrees of intoxication require no special treatment. Certain time-honored remedies such as a cold shower, strong coffee, forced activity, or induction of vomiting may be helpful, but there is no evidence that any of these methods influences the rate of disappearance of alcohol from the blood. *Alcoholic stupor* is also a short, self-limited state, and if the vital signs are normal no special therapeutic measures are necessary. *Pathological intoxication* may require the use of restraints and the parenteral administration of phenobarbital sodium (200 mg subcutaneously) or amobarbital sodium (500 mg intramuscularly), repeated once in 30 to 40 min if necessary.

Coma due to alcoholic intoxication is a medical emergency. The main object of treatment is to prevent respiratory suppression and the complications which it engenders. The management of the comatose patient is described in Chap. 20. One should like to be able to lower the blood alcohol level as rapidly as possible. The administration of insulin and glucose or fructose for this purpose is of little practical value. Analeptic drugs such as amphetamine, pentylenetetrazole (Metrazol), and various mixtures of caffeine and picrotoxin are antagonistic to alcohol only insofar as they are powerful cerebral cortical stimulants and overall nervous system excitants; they do not hasten the combustion of alcohol.

ABSTINENCE OR WITHDRAWAL SYNDROME   A second category of alcoholic neurological disease comprises the tremulous, hallucinatory, epileptic, and delirious states. Although a sustained period of chronic intoxication is the underlying factor in each of these disorders, the symptoms become manifest only *after a period of relative or absolute abstinence* from alcohol—hence the designation *abstinence* or *withdrawal syndrome.* Each of the major manifestations of the withdrawal syndrome may occur distinct from the others and will be so described; more frequently, however, they occur in various combinations. The prototype of the patients afflicted with these symptoms is the spree or periodic drinker, although the steady drinker is not immune if, for some reason, he or she stops drinking.

Tremulousness   By far the most common manifestation of the abstinence syndrome is a state of tremulousness, commonly referred to as "the shakes" or "the jitters," combined with general irritability and gastrointestinal symptoms, particularly nausea and vomiting. The symptoms first show themselves after several days of drinking, usually in the morning, after the short period of abstinence that occurs during sleep. Patients then need to "quiet their nerves" with a few drinks. Indeed the symptoms are relieved by alcohol, only to return on successive mornings with increasing severity. The usual spree lasts about 2 weeks, but the duration varies greatly. It is terminated not only because of recurrent tremor and vomiting, but for one or more other reasons such as lack of funds, weakness, self-disgust, injury, illness, or collapse. The symptoms then become greatly augmented, reaching their peak intensity 24 to 36 h after the complete cessation of drinking.

At this stage, patients present a distinctive clinical picture. They are alert and startle easily. Their faces are deeply flushed, the conjunctivas are injected, and there is usually tachycardia, anorexia, nausea, and retching. They may complain of insomnia and crave rest and sleep. Preoccupied with their misery, they are inattentive and disinclined to answer questions, and may respond in a rude or perfunctory manner. Patients may be mildly disoriented in time and have a poor memory for events of the last few days of the drinking spree but show no serious confusion, being generally aware of their surroundings and the nature of their illness.

Generalized tremor is an outstanding feature of this illness. It is of fast frequency (6 to 8 oscillations per second), slightly irregular, and variable in its severity, tending to diminish when patients are in quiet surroundings and to increase with motor activity or emotional stress. The tremors may be so violent that patients cannot stand without help, speak clearly, or feed themselves. Sometimes there is little objective evidence of tremor, and patients complain only of being "shaky inside."

Although the flushed facies, anorexia, tachycardia, and tremor subside to a large extent within a few days, patients do not regain their full composure for a much longer time. The overalertness, tendency to startle easily, and jerkiness of movement may persist for a week or longer; the feeling of uneasiness may not leave patients completely for 10 to 14 days, and only at the end of this time are they able to sleep undisturbed, without sedation. An attempt should be made to keep patients in the hospital for this length of time. To discharge them after a few days increases the likelihood that they will turn to alcohol to suppress their still-present tenseness and sleeplessness.

Hallucinosis   Symptoms of disordered perception occur in about one-quarter of the tremulous patients. Patients may complain of "bad dreams"—nightmarish episodes associated with disturbed sleep, which are difficult to separate from real experience. Sounds and shadows may be misinterpreted, or familiar objects may appear distorted and assume unreal forms. Although these are not hallucinations in the strict sense of the term, they represent the most common forms of disordered sense perception in the alcoholic. Hallucinations may be purely visual or auditory in type, mixed visual and auditory, and occasionally tactile or olfactory. There is little evidence to support the popular belief that certain visual hallucinations are specific to alcoholism. They are more commonly animate than inanimate and may comprise various forms of human, animal, or insect life. They may occur singly or in panoramas; they may appear shrunken or enlarged; they may be natural in appearance or take distorted and hideous forms (see also Chap. 21).

ACUTE AND CHRONIC AUDITORY HALLUCINOSIS   This form of alcoholic psychosis, in which vivid auditory hallucinations are the major abnormality, merits separate consideration. Kraepelin referred to it as the *hallucinatory insanity of drunkards or alcoholic mania.* The central feature of the illness, in the beginning, is the occurrence of auditory hallucinations despite an otherwise clear sensorium; i.e., confusion, disorientation, and obtundation are minimal or absent, and memory is not significantly impaired. The hallucinations may be musical in nature, like a low-pitched hum or chant, or they may take the form of unstructured sounds such as buzzing, ringing, shots, or clicking. Usually vocal hallucinations are associated. When the voices can be identified, they are attributed to the family, friends, or neighbors of patients, rarely to God, radio, or radar. The voices may be addressed directly to patients, but more frequently they discuss them in the third person. In the majority of cases the voices are maligning, reproachful, or threatening in nature and are disturbing to patients; a significant proportion, however, are not unpleasant and leave patients undisturbed. The voices are intensely real and vivid, and they tend to be exteriorized; i.e., they come from behind the door, from the corridor, or through the floor. Another quality of these formed auditory hallucinations (and of visual ones) is the appropriateness of the emotional responses of patients to them. They may call on the police for protection or barricade themselves against invaders; they may even attempt suicide to avZAoid what the voices threaten. The hallucinations are most prominent during the night, and their duration varies greatly—they may last for a few minutes to an hour or two or for days, and they may recur intermittently for days on end and, in exceptional instances, for weeks or months.

Most patients, while hallucinating, have no appreciation of the unreality of their hallucinations. As improvement occurs, patients begin to doubt their reality, are reluctant to talk about them, and may even question whether they had been sane during the episode. Full recovery is characterized by the realization that the voices were imaginary and by the ability to recall, sometimes with remarkable clarity, the abnormal thought content of parts of the psychotic episode.

A unique feature of this psychosis is the evolution of a chronic auditory hallucinosis in a small proportion of the patients. Such patients become quiet and resigned, even though the hallucinations remain threatening and derogatory. Ideas of reference and influence and other poorly systematized paranoid delusions become prominent. At this stage these patients show many of the symptoms of schizophrenia—illogical thinking, vagueness, tangential associations, and a dissociation of affect and of thought content. There is some evidence that repeated attacks of acute auditory hallucinosis render the patient more vulnerable to this chronic schizophrenia-like syndrome (see Chap. 25).

Withdrawal seizures ("rum fits") In this particular setting (i.e., where relative or absolute abstinence follows a period of chronic inebriation) there is a marked tendency to develop convulsive seizures. Over 90 percent of seizures occur during the 7- to 48-h period following the cessation of drinking, with a peak incidence between 13 to 24 h. During the period of seizure activity electroencephalograms may be abnormal, but they revert to normal in a matter of days, even though patients may go on to develop delirium tremens. Also during the period of seizure activity patients are unusually sensitive to stroboscopic stimulation. About half of these patients respond to this activating procedure with generalized myoclonus (photomyoclonus) or a convulsive seizure (photoconvulsion). In contrast, patients with idiopathic epilepsy rarely show this type of response to photic stimulation.

Seizures occurring in the abstinence period have a number of other distinctive features. There may be only a single seizure, but, more often, a flurry of two to six seizures occurs over a span of several hours, and an occasional patient develops status epilepticus. The seizures are grand mal in type, i.e., major generalized convulsions with loss of consciousness. A focal seizure or seizures should always suggest the presence of a focal lesion (usually traumatic) in addition to the effects of alcohol. Almost one-third of the patients with generalized seizure activity go on to develop delirium tremens, in which case the seizures invariably precede the delirium. The postictal confusional state may blend imperceptibly with the onset of the delirium, or there may be a clearing of the postictal state, over several hours or even a day or two, before the delirium sets in. Seizures of this type occur in patients who have been drinking for many years, so that they have to be distinguished from other forms of epilepsy beginning in adult life.

It is suggested that the term *rum fits* be reserved for seizures which possess the attributes described above. It is the term used frequently by the alcoholic and serves to distinguish seizures that occur only in the immediate abstinence period from those which occur in the interdrinking period, long after withdrawal has been accomplished. It is important to note that the "idiopathic" or posttraumatic forms of epilepsy may be influenced by alcohol. In patients with these types of epilepsy, seizures may be precipitated by only a short period of drinking (e.g., a weekend, or even one evening of heavy social drinking); interestingly, in these circumstances, the seizures occur not

when patients are intoxicated, but usually the morning after, in the "sobering-up" period.

Electroencephalographic findings in patients with "rum fits" do not support the notion that the seizures merely represent latent epilepsy made manifest by alcohol. Instead, the electroencephalogram (EEG) reflects a sequence of changes induced by alcohol itself—a decrease in the frequency of brain waves during the period of chronic intoxication; a rapid return of the EEG to normal immediately after cessation of drinking; the occurrence of a brief period of dysrhythmia (sharp waves and paroxysmal changes) which coincides with the flurry of convulsive activity; and again, a rapid return of the EEG to normal. Except for the transient dysrhythmia in the withdrawal period, the incidence of EEG abnormalities in patients who have had "rum fits" is not greater than in the normal population, in sharp contrast to patients who are indeed subject to seizures (see Chap. 364).

Delirium tremens This is the most dramatic and serious form of the alcohol withdrawal syndrome. It is characterized by profound confusion, delusions, vivid hallucinations, tremor, agitation, and sleeplessness, as well as by increased activity of the autonomic nervous system, i.e., dilated pupils, fever, tachycardia, and profuse perspiration. The clinical features of delirium have been presented in detail in Chap. 21.

Delirium tremens develops in one of several settings. The patients, excessive and steady drinkers of many years' duration, may have been admitted to the hospital for an unrelated illness, accident, or operation, and 2 to 4 days later become delirious. Or, following a prolonged spree, they may have already experienced several days of tremulousness and hallucinosis, or one or more seizures, and may even be recovering from these symptoms, when they suddenly develop delirium tremens.

In the majority of cases delirium tremens is benign and short-lived, ending as abruptly as it begins. Consumed by the relentless activity and wakefulness of several days' duration, patients fall into a deep sleep; they awaken lucid, quiet, and exhausted, with virtually no memory for the events of the delirious period. Less commonly, the delirious state subsides gradually; more rarely still, there may be one or more relapses, with several discrete episodes of delirium separated by lucidity and the entire process lasting for as little as several days or as long as 4 to 5 weeks. When the delirium occurs as a single episode, the duration is 72 h or less in over 80 percent of the cases.

Five to fifteen percent of cases of delirium tremens, as defined above, end fatally. In many of these there is an associated infectious illness or injury, but in a few no complicating illness is discernible. Patients frequently die in a state of hyperthermia or peripheral circulatory collapse; in some, death comes so suddenly that the nature of the terminal events cannot be determined.

Closely related to typical delirium tremens and about as common are the *atypical delirious-hallucinatory* or *confusional states,* in which one facet of the delirium tremens complex assumes prominence to the practical exclusion of the other symptoms. Patients may simply exhibit a transient state of quiet confusion, agitation, and peculiar behavior lasting several days or weeks. Other patients present a vivid hallucinatory-delusional state and abnormal behavior, consistent with their false beliefs. Unlike typical delirium tremens, the atypical states always present as a single circumscribed episode without recurrences, are only rarely preceded by epilepsy, and do not end fatally. This may be another way of saying that they are a partial or less severe form of the disease.

Pathological examination is singularly unrevealing in patients with delirium tremens. Edema and brain swelling have been absent in the authors' pathological material except when there was shock or hypoxia terminally, and there have not been any significant microscopic changes in the brain. Abnormalities of the spinal fluid, blood nonprotein nitrogen, serum sodium, chloride, sugar, potassium, calcium, and phosphorus occur unpredictably. The electroencephalographic findings have been discussed in relation to alcoholic epilepsy.

The *pathogenesis* of the tremulous-hallucinatory-delirious state has been a matter of considerable controversy. The idea that it simply represents the most severe form of alcohol intoxication is not tenable. The symptoms of toxicity, consisting of slurred speech, uninhibited behavior, staggering gait, stupor, and coma, are distinctive and different from the symptom complex of tremor, hallucinations, fits, and delirium. The former symptoms are associated with an elevated blood alcohol level, whereas the latter become evident only when the blood alcohol is reduced. Finally, the toxic symptoms increase in severity as more alcohol is consumed, whereas tremor and hallucinosis and even full-blown delirium tremens may be nullified by the administration of alcohol. Although much discussed in the past, there is no evidence that endocrine abnormality or nutritional deficiency plays a role in the genesis of delirium tremens and related symptoms.

It is evident, from observations in both humans and experimental animals, that the one indispensable factor in the genesis of delirium tremens and related disorders is the withdrawal of alcohol, following a period of chronic intoxication. The emergence of withdrawal symptoms depends upon a decline in the blood alcohol level from a previously higher level and not necessarily upon the complete disappearance of alcohol from the blood. The mechanism(s) by which the withdrawal of alcohol produces symptoms is only beginning to be understood. It has been shown that the early phase of alcohol withdrawal (beginning 7 to 8 h after cessation of drinking) is regularly attended by a drop in serum magnesium levels and a rise in arterial pH values, on the basis of respiratory alkalosis. Indeed it is possible that the compounded effect of these two factors, both of which are associated with hyperexcitability of the nervous system, might be responsible for seizures and perhaps for other symptoms which characterize the early phase of withdrawal. The elevation in pH and drop in P_{CO_2} are explained as withdrawal release of the neurons of the "respiratory center," which had been previously rendered insensitive to circulating CO_2. In the "rebound" phase these cells become more sensitive than normal to CO_2, with resultant hyperventilation and respiratory alkalosis. But as an explanation of delirium tremens, hypomagnesemia is probably not important, since the serum magnesium level has frequently been restored to normal before the onset of the delirium.

Treatment of alcoholic withdrawal syndrome The general aspects of management of the delirious and confused patient have been described in Chap. 21.

More specifically the treatment of delirium tremens begins with a careful search, followed by appropriate treatment, for associated injuries (particularly head injury with cerebral lacerations or subdural hematoma), infections (pneumonia or meningitis), pancreatitis, and liver disease. Because of the frequency and seriousness of these complications, skull and chest roentgenograms should be obtained and lumbar puncture should be performed routinely. In severe forms of delirium tremens, the temperature, pulse, and blood pressure should be recorded at 30-min intervals in anticipation of peripheral circulatory collapse and hyperthermia, which, added to the effects of injury and infection, are the usual causes of death in this disease. In the case of shock, one must act quickly, utilizing whole-blood transfusions, fluids, and vasopressor drugs. The occurrence of hyperthermia demands the use of a cooling mattress in addition to specific treatment for any infection that may be present.

A very important element in treatment is the correction of fluid and electrolyte imbalance. Severe degrees of agitation and perspiration may require the administration of 6000 ml fluid daily, of which 1500 ml should be normal saline solution. The specific electrolytes and the amounts in which they are added are governed by the laboratory values for these electrolytes. Occasionally, the withdrawal syndrome is characterized by hypoglycemia, in which case the administration of glucose becomes of prime importance. Rarely, alcoholic patients present with severe ketoacidosis and normal or only slightly elevated blood glucose concentrations. Usually such patients recover promptly, without the use of insulin.

A special danger attends the use of glucose solutions in alcoholic patients. Usually these persons have subsisted on a diet disproportionately high in carbohydrate (alcohol is metabolized almost entirely as carbohydrate) and low in thiamine, and their reserves of B vitamins may have been further reduced by gastroenteritis and diarrhea. The administration of intravenous glucose may serve to consume the last available stores of thiamine and precipitate Wernicke's disease. For this reason it is good practice to add B vitamins in all cases requiring parenterally administered glucose, even though the alcoholic disorder under treatment, e.g., delirium tremens, is not primarily due to vitamin deficiency.

In respect to the use of drugs, it is important to distinguish between mild withdrawal symptoms, which are essentially benign and responsive to practically all sedative drugs, and delirium tremens, which has a serious mortality and is relatively unresponsive to drugs. In the case of minor withdrawal symptoms, the purpose of medication is to ensure rest and sleep. In delirium tremens, the object of drug therapy is to blunt agitation, prevent exhaustion, and facilitate the administration of parenteral fluid and nursing care; one does not attempt to suppress agitation at all costs, since to accomplish this requires an amount of drug that might seriously depress respiratory function.

A wide variety of drugs is effective in controlling withdrawal symptoms. Some of the more popular are prochlorperazine (Compazine), chlorpromazine (Thorazine), meprobamate, chlordiazepoxide (Librium), hydroxyzine (Vistaril), and diazepam (Valium). There is little difference in the therapeutic efficacy of these drugs, and it is not certain that any of them can prevent hallucinosis or delirium tremens or shorten the duration and decrease the mortality rate of the latter disorder. In general, phenothiazine drugs should be avoided because of their epileptogenic properties. Furthermore, the advantages of the oral administration of these drugs over paraldehyde have not been proved by controlled studies; in fact, there is some evidence that in the more severe forms of the withdrawal syndrome paraldehyde is superior to both chlorpromazine and promazine. Paraldehyde has the additional advantage of being extremely safe provided it is freshly prepared and kept in brown, tightly stoppered bottles to prevent deterioration and the accumulation of acetaldehyde. If the patient can take medication orally, doses of 8 to 12 ml in orange juice should be given. Paraldehyde may also be administered rectally, but the intramuscular route should be avoided if possible, since it may damage nerves, and it should be given intravenously only with great caution because of the danger of respiratory depression. If parenteral medication is necessary, sodium phenobarbital or sodium amytal in doses of 120 mg, repeated at 3- to 4-h intervals, may be given, provided there is no serious liver disease. Some physicians prefer to use intravenous diazepam, giving 10 mg initially and repeating this dose at 20- to 30-min intervals until the patient is calm but awake. Such treatment is effective but requires careful monitoring to avoid hypotension and hypoventilation. Adrenocorticotropic hormone and cortisone have no place in the treatment of the withdrawal syndrome.

Treatment of "rum fits"   In most cases the seizures that occur in the withdrawal period ("rum fits") do not require the use of anticonvulsant drugs. In this setting there may be only a single seizure or a brief flurry of seizures which usually have ceased by the time that certain medicines, such as phenytoin (Dilantin), become effective. The parenteral administration of sodium phenobarbital early in the withdrawal period could conceivably prevent "rum fits" in patients with a previous history of this disorder or in those who might be expected to develop seizures on withdrawal. Also, the long-term administration of anticonvulsants is not practical; if patients remain abstinent, they will be free of seizures, and if they resume drinking they usually abandon their medicines. Withdrawal seizures that take the form of status epilepticus should be managed like status of any other type (see Chap. 23). Alcoholics with a history of idiopathic or posttraumatic epilepsy should be urged to drink only in moderation or not at all, because of the deleterious effects of relatively short periods of drinking on their epilepsy, and they should be maintained on anticonvulsant drugs.

NUTRITIONAL DISEASES OF THE NERVOUS SYSTEM   These diseases compose a relatively small but serious group of illnesses in chronic alcoholics. In contrast to alcoholic intoxication and the abstinence syndromes, the role of alcohol in the genesis of nutritional diseases is secondary, serving mainly to displace food in the diet. These illnesses, the role of alcohol in their production, and their treatment, are discussed in Chap. 371, "Metabolic Diseases of the Nervous System," and Chap. 372, "Nutritional Diseases of the Nervous System."

ALCOHOLIC DISEASES OF UNCERTAIN PATHOGENESIS   Included under this heading is a group of diseases which have little in common except that they are either confined to or predominant in alcoholics. The relationship to alcohol is not understood in any one of these diseases and is probably not crucial, insofar as some of them also occur in nonalcoholics. There is indirect evidence that some of these disorders are nutritional in origin, but as yet this relationship must be regarded as unproved.

Alcoholic cerebellar degeneration   This term is applied to a nonfamilial type of cerebellar ataxia which occurs in adult life against a background of prolonged ingestion of alcohol. The symptoms may progress slowly over a long period, but more frequently they evolve in a subacute fashion (several weeks or months), after which they remain stationary for many years. Often they are present in mild form and worsen considerably after an attack of pneumonia or delirium tremens. The signs are those of cerebellar dysfunction, affecting stance and gait predominantly. The legs are involved more frequently and severely than the arms, and nystagmus and speech disturbances are rare. Once established, the signs change very little, although some improvement of gait (due mainly to recovery from complicating polyneuropathy) may follow cessation of drinking. The essential pathological changes consist of degeneration of varying severity of all the neurocellular elements of the cerebellar cortex, particularly of the Purkinje cells, with a striking topographic restriction to the anterior and superior aspects of the vermis and adjacent parts of the hemispheres.

The disorder of stance and gait seems to be related to the lesion in the vermis, and the ataxia of the limbs to involvement of the anterior lobe of the cerebellum. A similar clinical syndrome has been observed in a few nutritionally depleted nonalcoholic patients.

It is likely that the cerebellar lesions in this disorder and in Wernicke's disease represent the same disease process. The latter designation is used when the cerebellar abnormalities are associated with the characteristic ocular and mental disorders, and the term "alcoholic" cerebellar degeneration when only the cerebellar signs are clinically manifest.

Marchiafava-Bignami disease (primary degeneration of the corpus callosum)   This is a rare complication of alcoholism originally described in Italian men addicted to crude red wine. The symptoms are diverse and include psychic and emotional disorders, intellectual deterioration, convulsive seizures, and varying degrees of tremor, rigidity, paralysis, apraxia, aphasia, and sucking and grasping reflexes. The duration is variable, from several weeks to months, and recovery is possible. The pathological picture is more constant than the clinical one. It consists of symmetrical demyelination in the corpus callosum, particularly of the middle lamina, and less consistently of the anterior commissure and other parts of the white matter. Axis cylinders are better preserved than medullated fibers in these areas, and there are appropriate reactions in the macrophages and astrocytes. Various degrees of recovery may occur if abstinence from alcohol and good nutrition are established and maintained.

Central pontine myelinolysis (CPM)   This term refers to a unique pathological change affecting the center of the basis pontis, in which the medullated fibers are destroyed in a single symmetrical focus of varying size. In contrast, the axis cylinders, nerve cells, and blood vessels are relatively well preserved. Although the lesion is usually confined to the basis pontis, occasional cases also show symmetrically placed lesions of similar histological type in other parts of the brain. The disease may manifest itself clinically by pseudobulbar palsy, quadriplegia, and pseudocoma ("locked-in syndrome"), evolving over a period of several days, but usually the lesion is so small that it causes no symptoms and is found only at postmortem examination. Most cases of CPM have occurred in severely malnourished alcoholics, but the relationship of this condition to nutritional deficiency, alcohol, or other toxic factors is obscure. Recently, attention has been drawn to the frequent occurrence of *hyponatremia* in patients with CPM, but the significance of this finding is unclear also.

Cerebral atrophy   The pathological examination of relatively young alcoholic patients not infrequently discloses an unexpected degree of convolutional atrophy, most prominent in the frontal lobes, and a symmetrical enlargement of the lateral and third ventricles. In some of these cases the lesions of the Wernicke-Korsakoff syndrome, cerebral trauma, anoxic or hepatic encephalopathy, or communicating hydrocephalus are associated, but in others they are not. Ventricular enlargement and, less often, convolutional atrophy have also been found on pneumoencephalography, and more recently similar findings have been reported in chronic alcoholics examined by computerized tomography (CT) scan. The clinical correlates of these radiological findings have not been determined, however. Clinical examination may disclose various abnormalities of neurological and intellectual function, but many patients betray no symptoms or signs of neurological disease. Obviously, the nature of "alcoholic cerebral atrophy" remains to be defined, both clinically and pathologically.

"Alcoholic" myopathy Alcoholics as a group are particularly vulnerable to several disorders of cardiac and skeletal muscle, loosely referred to as alcoholic cardiomyopathy and alcoholic myopathy. Apart from their high incidence in alcoholics, these myopathies possess no unique features, and the same disorders may be observed in a variety of clinical settings in which alcohol plays no part.

One type of myopathic syndrome occurs acutely in the course of a prolonged bout of heavy drinking and is manifested by severe pain and tenderness and swelling of muscles, accompanied by cramps and muscle weakness. The muscular affection may be generalized or remarkably focal, and an affected limb may give the appearance of a deep phlebothrombosis or lymphatic obstruction. Some of the focal lesions are surely induced by trauma or pressure-ischemic injury during a period of alcoholic coma. Diffuse necrosis of muscle fibers, all in one stage of degeneration (rhabdomyolysis), is the underlying pathological change and is reflected by myoglobinuria (leading in some cases to fatal myoglobinuric nephrosis) and high serum levels of creatine phosphokinase (CPK). Some of these patients show a diminished rise in blood lactic acid in response to ischemic exercise, similar to that which occurs in McArdle's disease. In distinction to the latter, however, myophosphorylase levels are not consistently reduced in the alcoholic patients. How these biochemical abnormalities are related to muscle cramps and weakness is a matter of speculation. Most patients with this disorder recover, usually in a matter of weeks; in severe cases, complete restoration of motor power may take several months.

In other cases, a painless and predominantly proximal weakness develops over a period of several days or weeks in the course of a prolonged drinking bout and is associated with a severe degree of hypokalemia. The urinary excretion of potassium is not significantly increased. Usually the depletion of potassium is the result of vomiting and diarrhea, which precede the onset of muscular weakness, but sometimes the mechanism of depletion is unclear. In several reported cases with low serum phosphorus levels a bone tumor (e.g., an ossifying angioma) was found, and its removal restored muscle power to normal. The oral administration of phosphates has been beneficial in nontumorous cases. Some of the latter are accompanied by pain and stiffness.

From time to time, one observes in alcoholics the subacute or chronic evolution of painless weakness and atrophy of the proximal muscles of the limbs, especially of the legs, with only minimal signs of polyneuropathy in the distal segments of the legs and feet. Cases such as these have been referred to as *chronic alcoholic myopathy*, but the data are as yet insufficient to warrant this designation. Muscle biopsies that the authors have examined from such patients suggest that it may represent a proximal form of polyneuropathy. Treatment follows along the lines for alcoholic neuropathy, and complete recovery can be expected if the patient abstains from alcohol and improves his nutritional status.

Alcoholic cardiomyopathy is discussed in Chap. 247.

Fetal alcohol syndrome That maternal alcoholism may have an adverse effect on the offspring has been a recurrent theme in medical lore, but only in the past decade have the effects of alcohol abuse on the fetus been clearly documented. This congenital disorder has been termed the *fetal alcohol syndrome* (FAS). The affected infants are small in length in comparison

with weight, and most of them fall below the third percentile for head circumference. They are distinguished also by the presence of short palpebral fissures (probably a reflection of microphthalmia) and epicanthal folds; maxillary hypoplasia, thin vermillion of upper lip, micrognathia, and cleft palate; dislocation of the hips, flexion deformities of the fingers, and limited range of motion of other joints; cardiac anomalies (usually spontaneously closing septal defects); anomalous external genitalia; and capillary hemangiomata. The newborn infants suck and sleep poorly, and many of them are irritable, hyperactive and tremulous; the latter symptoms resemble those of alcohol withdrawal, except that they persist. In one series of such infants there was a neonatal mortality of 17 percent. Seriously affected infants who survive the neonatal period fail to achieve normal weight, length, and head circumference and remain backward mentally to a varying degree, even under optimal environmental conditions.

The anatomic basis of this syndrome, and the mechanism by which alcohol produces its effects, are not known; the limited evidence to date favors a toxic effect of alcohol or perhaps one of its metabolites or contaminants, rather than a nutritional or genetic factor. The critical degree of maternal alcoholism that is necessary to produce the FAS and the critical stage in gestation during which it occurs also need to be determined. Cases of the FAS observed to date have occurred only in children born to severely alcoholic mothers who continued to drink heavily (80 ml absolute alcohol per day) throughout their pregnancy. Studies of the effects on the fetus of lesser degrees of maternal alcoholism are in progress.

NEUROLOGICAL DISORDERS CONSEQUENT UPON CIRRHOSIS AND PORTAL-SYSTEM SHUNTS *Hepatic coma* refers to an episodic disorder of consciousness which frequently complicates (or terminates) advanced liver disease and/or portal-systemic shunts. This condition and the more chronic type of acquired hepatocerebral degeneration are described in Chaps. 304 and 371.

TREATMENT OF ALCOHOL ADDICTION Following recovery from the acute medical and neurological complications of alcoholism, the underlying problem—that of alcohol dependence—remains. To treat only the medical complications and to leave the management of the drinking problem to patients themselves is indeed shortsighted. Almost always drinking is resumed, with a predictable recurrence of medical illness. For this reason the physician must be prepared to deal with the addiction or at least to initiate treatment.

The problem of excessive drinking is formidable but not necessarily as hopeless as it is made out to be. A common misconception among physicians is that specialized training in psychiatry and an inordinately large amount of time are required to deal with the addictive drinker. Actually, a successful program of treatment can be initiated by any interested physician, using the standard techniques of history taking, establishing rapport with patients, and seeing them frequently, though not necessarily for prolonged periods. A useful point at which to undertake this task is during convalescence from a serious medical or neurological complication of alcoholism or in relation to loss of employment, arrest, or threatened divorce. Such crises may help convince patients, better than any argument presented by families or physicians, that their drinking has reached serious proportions.

The requisite for successful treatment is total abstinence from alcohol, and for all practical purposes, this represents the only permanent solution. It is generally agreed that any attempt to curb the drinking habit will fail if patients continue to drink. There are said to be cases in which patients have been able to reduce their intake of alcohol and eventually to drink in moderation, but they must be extremely rare. Also, it is frequently stated that patients must recognize that they are alcoholics, i.e., that their drinking is beyond their control, and they must express willingness to be helped. Undoubtedly there is truth in both these statements, but they should not be interpreted to mean that patients must gain this recognition and willingness entirely on their own initiative and that they will be helped only after they do so. Physicians can do a great deal to help patients understand the nature of their problem and thus to motivate them to accept treatment. Logic and reasoning must be used to convince them that abstinence is preferable to chronic inebriety. Patients must be made fully aware of the medical and social consequences of continued drinking and must also be made to understand that because of some constitutional peculiarity (like that of diabetics, who cannot handle sugar) they are incapable of drinking in moderation. These facts should be presented in much the same way as one would explain the essential features of any other disease. There is nothing to be gained from adopting a punitive or moralizing attitude; nor should patients be given the idea that they are in no way blameworthy for their illness. There appears to be an advantage in making patients feel that they are responsible for doing something about their drinking.

The prevalent belief that alcoholics will not stop drinking under duress also requires qualification. In fact, one of the few careful studies of this matter disclosed that relatively few patients would have sought help unless pressure had been exerted by family or employer; furthermore, patients who came to the clinic under duress of this sort did just as well as those who came voluntarily.

If earnest and sustained efforts by physicians fail to convince patients that alcohol offers a problem, it is usually impossible to modify their alcoholic tendencies. The only way to make such individuals discontinue drinking is to commit them to psychiatric hospitals or special institutions for the management of alcoholism in the hope that with forced abstinence and improvement in their physical state they will gain insight and later accept psychiatric or other forms of therapy.

On the other hand, if patients come to realize that their drinking is beyond their control and that they need to do something about it, their chances of being helped are raised considerably. Indeed, under these circumstances, many persons stop drinking of their own volition. Some of these patients, despite the best of intentions, will relapse. This should not serve as an excuse to abandon treatment; many patients have attained a state of prolonged sobriety after several false starts. A number of methods have proved valuable in the long-term management of patients. The most important of these are the use of Antabuse, psychotherapy, and the participation in social organizations for combating alcoholism.

Antabuse (tetraethylthiuram disulfide, disulfiram) interferes with the metabolism of alcohol, so that patients who take both alcohol and Antabuse accumulate an inordinate amount of acetaldehyde in the tissues, resulting in nausea, vomiting, and hypotension, sometimes pronounced in degree. It is no longer considered necessary to demonstrate these effects to patients; it is sufficient to warn them of the severe reactions that may result if they drink while they have the drug in their body. Treatment with Antabuse is instituted only after patients have been sober for several days, preferably longer. It should never be given to patients with cardiac or liver disease. The drug is taken each morning, or at another suitable time daily, in a dosage of 0.5 g, preferably under supervision. This form of treatment is of particular value in spree or periodic drinkers, in whom relapse from abstinence usually represents an impulsive rather than a carefully planned or premeditated act. Patients taking Antabuse, aware of the dangers of mixing liquor and the drug, are "protected" against the impulse to drink, and this protection may be renewed every 24 h by the simple expedient of taking a pill. The willingness with which patients accept this form of treatment also serves as a rough index of their motivation. Should patients drink when they are taking Antabuse, the ensuing reaction is usually severe enough to require medical attention, and a protracted spree can thus be prevented. Antabuse may in rare instances lead to a mild polyneuropathy if continued over a period of months or years. It must then be discontinued.

Alcoholics Anonymous (AA), an informal fellowship of former alcoholics, has proved to be the single most effective force in the rehabilitation of alcoholic patients. The philosophy of this organization is embodied in their so-called "twelve steps," a series of propositions about alcohol and alcoholism which guide the patient to recovery. The AA philosophy stresses in particular the practice of making restitution, the necessity to help other alcoholics, trust in God, the group confessional, and the belief that alcoholics are powerless over alcohol. AA philosophy also embodies the 24-h plan, in which alcoholics strive for just 24 h of abstinence (a concept inspired by the Sermon on the Mount) as a means of facilitating the maintenance of sobriety. Although accurate statistics are lacking, it is stated that about half the members who express more than a passing interest in the program have no relapses, and that a significant additional number relapse but eventually recover.

The methods used by AA are not suited to every patient; some prefer the more personalized approach offered by special clinics and centers for the treatment of alcoholism. The physician should, therefore, be fully aware of all the community resources which are available for the management of this problem and should be prepared to take advantage of them in appropriate cases.

Finally, it should be noted that alcoholism is frequently associated with psychiatric disease of some other type. There is among alcoholics an increased frequency of schizophrenia, psychoneurosis, sociopathy, and particularly manic-depressive disease. In the latter case, the prevailing mood is far more often one of depression than of mania, and is more often encountered in the female who is more apt to drink under these conditions than the male. The presence of concomitant psychiatric disease complicates the management of the alcoholism, and in these circumstances expert psychiatric help should be sought.

REFERENCES

Alcohol and Health. US Department of Health, Education, and Welfare Publication (HSM) 72-9099, 1971

CLARREN SK, SMITH DW: The fetal alcohol syndrome. N Engl J Med 298:1063, 1978

EPSTEIN PS et al: Alcoholism and cerebral atrophy. Alcoholism. Clin Exp Res 1:61, 1977

ISSELBACHER KJ: Metabolic and hepatic effects of alcohol. N Engl J Med 296:612, 1977

MENDELSON JH, MELLO NK: Behavioral and biochemical interrelationships in alcoholism. Annu Rev Med 27:321, 1976

THOMPSON WL et al: Diazepam and paraldehyde treatment of severe delirium tremens. A controlled trial. Ann Intern Med 82:175, 1975

VICTOR M: The pathophysiology of alcoholic epilepsy, in *The Addictive States.* Res Publ Assoc Res Nerv Ment Dis 46:431, 1968

———: Neurologic disorders due to alcoholism and malnutrition, in *Clinical Neurology,* AB Baker, LH Baker (eds). New York, Harper & Row, 1979

———, WOLFE SM: Causation and treatment of the alcohol withdrawal syndrome, in *Alcoholism: Progress in Research and Treatment,* PG Bourne, R Fox (eds). New York, Academic, 1973

227

OPIATES AND SYNTHETIC ANALGESICS

MAURICE VICTOR
RAYMOND D. ADAMS

The opiates, strictly speaking, include all the naturally occurring alkaloids in opium, which is prepared from the sap of the poppy *Papaver somniferum*. For clinical purposes, the term refers only to those alkaloids which have a high degree of analgesic activity, i.e., morphine and codeine (3-methoxymorphine). Thebaine, another opium alkaloid which, like morphine, possesses a phenanthrene nucleus, has few or no analgesic properties and is therefore not ordinarily considered an opiate. The terms *opioid* and *narcotic-analgesic* refer to any drug with actions similar to those of morphine. Compounds that are chemical modifications of morphine include heroin or diacetylmorphine (now the most commonly abused opioid), hydromorphone (Dilaudid), dihydrocodeinone (Hycodan), dihydroxycodeinone (Eucodal), oxymorphone (Numorphan), and oxycodone (Percodan). A second class of opioids comprises the *purely synthetic analgesics* pethidine or meperidine (Demerol), the merperidine derivatives anileridine and alphaprodine (Nisentil), methadone (Dolophine or amidone), metopon (6-methyldihydromorphinone), racemorphan (Dromoran), levorphan (*l*-Dromoran), *d*-propoxyphene (Darvon), diphenoxylate (the main component of Lomotil), and phenazocine (Prinadol). The latter drugs are similar to the opiates, both in their pharmacological effects and in the patterns of abuse, the differences being mainly quantitative. In fact, *d*-propoxyphene has such low addictive liabilities that it is not controlled by the federal narcotic laws. The same statement applies to the synthetic analgesic pentazocine (Talwin), and although its overall addictive quality is low, cases of physical dependency do occur.

As with alcohol and the barbiturates, the opioids will be considered from two points of view: (1) acute poisoning and (2) addiction.

OPIOID POISONING Because of the high incidence of addiction, which leads to irregular and nonmedical usage of opioids, poisoning is not an infrequent accident. This may happen as a result of ingestion with suicidal intent, errors in the calculation of dosage, variations in drug potency, or unusual sensitivity. Children may exhibit an increased susceptibility to opioids, so that relatively small doses prove toxic. This is true also in adults who have myxedema, Addison's disease, chronic liver disease, or pneumonia. Acute poisoning may also occur in addicts who are unaware that tolerance for opioids declines quickly after the withdrawal of the drug: upon resuming the habit a formerly well-tolerated dose can be fatal.

Varying degrees of unresponsiveness, shallow respirations, slow respiratory rate (e.g., two to four per minute), or periodic breathing, miosis, bradycardia, and hypothermia are the well-recognized clinical manifestations of acute poisoning. In the most advanced stage the pupils dilate, the skin and mucous membranes become cyanotic, and the circulation fails. The immediate cause of death is usually respiratory depression, with consequent asphyxia. Patients who have a cardiorespiratory arrest are sometimes left with a residuum of anoxic encephalopathy. Others who recover from coma may occasionally reveal a hemiplegia, presumably due to vascular occlusion. In the stage of mild intoxication, anorexia, nausea, vomiting, constipation, and loss of sexual interest are the only symptoms.

Treatment consists of gastric lavage (after oral ingestion), with a cuffed endotracheal tube in place should the patient be comatose. This procedure may be efficacious many hours after ingestion, since one of the toxic effects of opioids is severe pylorospasm, which may cause much of the drug to be retained in the stomach. Other measures must be directed toward the maintenance of an adequate airway and oxygenation, as described in Chap. 228, "Barbiturates," under "Management." If the patient does not respond rapidly to these measures, *naloxone* (Narcan) should be administered. This is a specific antidote to the opiates and also to the synthetic analgesics. It is now preferred to *N*-allylnormorphine (Nalline) because naloxone has no agonist properties; hence, naloxone will not depress respiration further if the diagnosis of opioid poisoning is mistaken. For such poisoning, the dose of naloxone is 0.7 mg per 70 kg *intravenously,* repeated once or twice if necessary at 5-min intervals for an adequate respiratory response. The improvement in circulation and respiration is usually dramatic. In fact, failure of naloxone to produce such a response should cast doubt on the diagnosis of opioid intoxication. If an adequate respiratory response to naloxone is obtained, the patient should be observed carefully for 24 h, and further doses of naloxone (50 percent higher than previously found effective) may be given *intramuscularly* as often as necessary. Naloxone has little direct effect on the impaired consciousness, however, and the patient may remain drowsy for many hours. This is not harmful, provided respiration is well maintained.

A new oxymorphone-derived antagonist, *naltrexone,* promises to be even more effective than naloxone. Naltrexone is relatively free of agonistic activity and has the additional advantage of being effective orally. It is about twice as potent as naloxone in precipitating abstinence phenomena in patients dependent upon opiates, and its half-life of antagonistic actions is at least twice as long as that of naloxone.

Once the patient regains consciousness, usually in about 8 h, other complaints such as severe pruritus, sneezing, persistent obstipation, and urinary retention may necessitate symptomatic treatment. Nausea and severe abdominal pain, due presumably to pancreatitis (from spasm of the sphincter of Oddi), are other troublesome symptoms. The antidote must be used with great caution in an addict who has taken an overdose of opioid, because in this circumstance it may precipitate withdrawal phenomena.

In addition to the toxic effects of the opioid itself, the addict is exposed to a variety of neurological and infectious complications, resulting mainly from the injection of crude adulterants (quinine, lactose, powdered milk, fruit sugars) and various infectious agents (injections often administered by unsterile methods). Amblyopia, due probably to the toxic effects of quinine in the heroin mixtures, has been reported, as well as transverse myelopathy and several types of peripheral neuropathy. The spinal cord disorder expresses itself clinically by the abrupt onset of paraplegia with a sensory level on the trunk. Pathologically, there is an acute necrotizing lesion involving both grey and white matter over a considerable vertical extent of the thoracic and occasionally the cervical region. In some cases the myelopathy has followed the first intravenous injection of heroin after a prolonged period of abstinence. Involvement of single peripheral nerves, particularly of the radial nerve, and painful affection of the brachial plexus, independent of compression and remote from the site of injection, have been observed.

An acute generalized myopathy with myoglobinuria and renal failure has been ascribed to the intravenous injection of adulterated heroin. Brawny edema and fibrosing myopathy are the sequelae common to venous obliteration resulting from the administration of heroin and its adulterants by the intramuscular and subcutaneous routes. Occasionally there may be an inexplicable swelling of an extremity (sometimes massive) into which heroin had been injected subcutaneously or intramuscularly. Infection and venous thrombosis appear to be involved in its causation.

The diagnosis of drug addiction or the suspicion of this diagnosis should always encourage surveillance for infectious complications, particularly abscesses and cellulitis at injection, sites, septic thrombophlebitis, serum hepatitis, septic arthritis, and periarteritis. Tetanus, endocarditis (due mainly to *Staphylococcus aureus*), spinal epidural abscess, meningitis, brain abscess, and tuberculosis are found less frequently.

OPIOID ADDICTION Between 15 and 20 years ago there were about 60,000 persons addicted to narcotic drugs in the United States, not including those who were receiving drugs because of hopeless medical diseases. This represented a relatively small public health problem, in comparison with alcoholism and barbiturate addiction; and the addiction problem was of serious proportions in only a few cities—New York, Chicago, Los Angeles, Washington, and Detroit. In the past 15 years a remarkable increase in opioid (principally heroin) addiction has taken place. The precise number of opioid addicts is not known but was estimated by the Drug Enforcement Administration, in 1970, to be more than 600,000. The peak incidence of heroin dependence occurred in 1972. The incidence declined between 1972 and 1974, then increased again, and has fluctuated at near peak levels over the past 4 years.

Etiology and pathogenesis A number of factors, socioeconomic, psychological, and pharmacological, all contribute to the genesis of opioid addiction. In our culture, the most susceptible subjects are young men or delinquent youths living in the economically depressed areas of large cities, but a significant number are now found in the suburbs, in small cities, and in rural areas in Southern states. The onset of opioid use is usually in adolescence, with a peak at 17 to 18 years. Fully two-thirds of addicts start using the drug before the age of 21. A disproportionately large number are American Negroes and persons of Puerto Rican or Mexican descent. In the Southern states, addicts are predominantly white. Almost 90 percent of addicts engage in criminal activity, often necessary to obtain their daily ration of drug, but most of these have had arrests or convictions prior to addiction. Also, many of them show psychiatric disorders, psychopathy and psychoneurosis being the most common. Monroe et al. examined a group of 837 opioid addicts, using the Lexington Personality Inventory, and found evidence of characterologic disorder (psychopathy or sociopathy) in 42 percent, emotional disturbance in 29 percent, and thinking disorder in 22 percent; only 7 percent were asymptomatic. Nevertheless, the precise "personality" factor which renders certain individuals vulnerable to addiction has not been defined.

Association with addicts is the chief reason for beginning addiction. One addict recruits another person into addiction, and the new recruit does likewise. In this sense opioid addiction is contagious, and as a result of this pattern of opioid abuse, heroin addiction, since the late 1960s, has attained virtually epidemic proportions. A small, almost insignificant, proportion of addicts are introduced to drugs by physicians in the course of an illness.

Opioid addiction evolves in three successive phases: (1) episodic intoxication, (2) pharmacogenic or physical dependence, or addiction, and (3) the propensity to "relapse after cure."

Some of the symptoms of opiate intoxication have already been considered. In persons who are distressed by pain or pain-anticipatory anxiety, the administration of opioid produces a sense of unusual well-being, a state that has been referred to in medical writings as "morphine euphoria." It should be emphasized that only a negligible proportion of such persons continue to use opioids habitually after the pain has subsided. The vast majority of potential addicts are not suffering from painful illnesses at the time they initiate opioid use, and in them the initial effects of the drug are not aptly described as euphoric. The latter persons are mainly teenagers who self-administer opioids (mainly heroin) under the tutelage of their peers and who learn, after several repetitions, to recognize what they refer to as a heroin "high," despite the recurrence of unpleasant symptoms (nausea, vomiting, faintness). The repeated self-administration of drug ("reinforcement," in the language of operant psychology) is the most important factor in the genesis of addiction. Regardless of how one characterizes the state of mind that is produced by episodic reinitiation of the drug, the individual quickly discovers the need to increase the dose in order to obtain the original effect. Although the initial effects may not be fully recaptured, the progressively increasing dose of drug does abate the discomforts which arise as the effects of each injection wear off. In this way a new *pharmacogenically induced need* is developed and the use of opioids becomes self-perpetuating. At the same time a marked degree of tolerance is produced, so that enormous amounts of drugs, e.g., 5000 mg morphine daily, have been administered without the development of toxic symptoms. The mechanism of tolerance is still not understood fully, although it is a subject of much interest and speculation. The various theories related to physical dependence have been discussed fully by Wikler (see "References").

The altered physiological state that develops with continued use of the drug is manifested in another dramatic way at the time of withdrawal. This constitutes a specific illness, termed the *abstinence syndrome*. Strictly speaking, addiction is defined as physical or pharmacological dependence. This definition distinguishes between *addicting drugs* (opiates, alcohol, barbiturates) and *habit-forming drugs* (bromides, cocaine, and marihuana), since no consistent abstinence symptoms follow the discontinuation of the latter group, even after prolonged exposure. Stated in another way, all addicting drugs are habit-forming, but the opposite is not true. The place of amphetamines in this scheme is uncertain. Undoubtedly they are habit-forming drugs. Withdrawal of *d*-amphetamine, following prolonged oral or intravenous use, is regularly followed by prolonged sleep [of which a high percentage is rapid eye movement (REM) sleep], from which the patient awakens with a ravenous appetite. The deep sleep can be reversed by administration of *d*-amphetamine.

The intensity of the opioid abstinence syndrome depends mainly on the dose of the drug and duration of addiction, but also on individual factors. In respect to morphine it has been found that the majority of individuals receiving 240 mg daily for 30 days or more will show moderately severe abstinence symptoms following withdrawal, whereas mild abstinence signs can be precipitated by narcotic antagonists in persons who have taken as little as 15 mg morphine, or an equivalent dose of methadone or heroin, three times daily for 3 days.

The abstinence syndrome which occurs in the morphine addict may be taken as the prototype of the opioid group. The first 8 to 16 h of abstinence usually pass asymptomatically. At the end of this period yawning, rhinorrhea, sweating, and lacrimation become manifest. At first mild, these symptoms increase in severity over a period of several hours and then remain constant for several days. The patient may be able to sleep during the early period but is restless, and thereafter insomnia remains a prominent feature. Dilatation of the pupils, recurring waves of gooseflesh, and twitchings of the muscles appear. The patient complains of severe aches in the back, abdomen, and legs and of hot and cold "flashes" so that he covers himself with blankets. By the end of about 36 h the restlessness becomes more extreme, and nausea, vomiting, and diarrhea usually develop. The temperature, respiration, and blood pressure are slightly elevated. All these symptoms reach their peak intensity 48 to 72 h after withdrawal, and then gradually decline. The abstinence syndrome is rarely fatal. After 7 to 10 days, all clinical signs of abstinence have disappeared, although the patient may complain of insomnia, nervousness, weakness, and muscle aches for several more weeks, and a small deviation of a number of physiological variables can be detected with refined techniques for up to 10 months (protracted abstinence).

Two types of abstinence changes have been recognized: *nonpurposive* and *purposive*. The former comprises the various autonomic and neuromuscular signs and are relatively transient in nature. That these symptoms represent an altered physiological state and are not psychic in origin has been clearly demonstrated experimentally. Physical dependence on morphine and other opioids develops even in the lower limbs of dogs whose spinal cords have been transected; the flexor and crossed extensor spinal reflexes that are depressed or abolished by the opioid become remarkably exaggerated when the drug is withdrawn. The purposive changes refer to the patient's craving for the drug and the manipulative activity directed toward obtaining it. These symptoms may persist indefinitely and are important in relation to that characteristic of addiction referred to as *habituation, emotional dependence,* or *psychic dependence.* These terms are used interchangeably and refer to the substitution of drug-seeking activities for all other aims and objects in life.

Psychic dependence is regarded as the most important quality of addiction, since it is this feature which governs the initial use of the drug and relapse following apparent cure of addiction. Relapse to the use of the drug may occur long after the nonpurposive abstinence changes seem to have disappeared. The cause of relapse is imperfectly understood. It has been theorized that fragments of the abstinence syndrome may remain as a conditioned response, and that these abstinence signs may be evoked by the appropriate environmental stimuli. Thus, when a "cured" addict finds himself in a situation where narcotic drugs are readily available, or in circumstances that were responsible for the initial use of drugs, the incompletely extinguished drug-seeking behavior reasserts itself.

The characteristics of addiction and of abstinence are qualitatively similar with all the drugs of the opiate group as well as the related synthetic analgesics. The differences are mainly quantitative and are related to the differences in dosage, potency, and length of action. Heroin is two to three times more potent than morphine but otherwise the same; nevertheless, the heroin withdrawal syndrome encountered in hospital practice is usually mild in degree because of the low dosage of this drug in the street product. Dilaudid and metopon are more potent than morphine and have a shorter duration of action; hence the addict requires more doses per day, and the abstinence syndrome comes on and subsides more rapidly. The length of action of racemorphan is somewhat longer than that of morphine, but withdrawal phenomena are similar to those of morphine in temporal course and intensity. Abstinence symptoms from codeine, while very definite, are less than those from morphine. The addiction liabilities of *d*-propoxyphene are even less than those of codeine. Abstinence symptoms from methadone are less intense than those from morphine and do not become evident until 3 to 4 days after withdrawal; furthermore, autonomic signs are less severe in the abstinence period. For these reasons methadone is used in the treatment of morphine addiction. Meperidine addiction is of particular importance because of the high incidence among physicians and nurses and because there is still a widespread belief that this drug is nonaddicting. Tolerance to the toxic effects of meperidine is not complete, so that the addict may show tremors, twitching of the muscles, confusion, hallucinations, and at times convulsions. Signs of abstinence appear 3 to 4 h after the last dose and reach maximum intensity between 8 and 12 h, at which time they may be worse than those of morphine abstinence.

Diagnosis of addiction This is usually made by the patient's statement that he is using and needs drugs. Should he decide to conceal this fact, one must rely on collateral evidence such as miosis, needle marks, emaciation, or abscess scars. Meperidine addicts are likely to have dilated pupils and twitching muscles. A method for the testing of the urine for opiates is now generally available. The finding of morphine or opiate derivatives (heroin is excreted as morphine) in the urine confirms the suspicion that the patient has taken or has been given a dose of such drugs within 24 h of the test.

Formerly it was necessary to isolate questionable cases and to observe the patient over a period of at least 2 days for signs of abstinence. Through use of the specific morphine antagonist *N*-allylnormorphine (nalorphine, Nalline) and naloxone (Narcan), a diagnosis of addiction to opiates and related analgesic drugs can be made within an hour. Naloxone, which is now preferred for this purpose, should be administered only in the presence of another physician or nurse, with the full understanding and permission of the patient. The drug is given intravenously, slowly, using a syringe containing 1 ampul (0.4 mg). The injection is stopped when pupillary dilatation, increased respiratory rate, lacrimation, rhinorrhea, sweating, and yawning appear. If, after 5 to 10 min, no such signs appear, a second injection may be given in the same way. If again the patient shows no abstinence signs, it may be assumed that he is not physically dependent upon opiates. Naloxone may be injected *subcutaneously,* in the same dosage as intravenously. Again, if the patient has taken more than occasional doses of the drug within a week of the test, the administration of naloxone will precipitate symptoms of abstinence. These become evident within 5 min of the first injection, reach their peak intensity in 20 min, begin to decline in 60 min, and disappear after 3 h. *N*-Allylnormorphine and naloxone do not precipitate abstinence symptoms in meperidine addiction, unless the patient has been taking more than 1600 mg daily.

Management and avoidance of addiction The ambulatory treatment of addiction never succeeds and should therefore not be undertaken, except in special settings, such as a carefully supervised methadone treatment program (see below). Addicts who are refused opiates may ask for methadone, meperidine, or racemorphine, on the ground that these drugs are synthetic and nonaddicting. These are addicting drugs and have been legally defined as such. Physicians should also be aware that they are breaking both the letter and the spirit of the regulations if they prescribe narcotics for an addict merely for the purpose of preventing abstinence changes. Occasional exceptions may be made in the case of seriously ill addicts who are awaiting treatment in a hospital or methadone program, or of patients who are suffering from incurable, painful disease.

An alternate method, and one that is used now almost exclusively, is to substitute methadone for opioid, in the ratio of 1 mg methadone for 3 mg morphine, 1 mg heroin, or 20 mg meperidine. Since methadone is long-acting and effective orally, it need be given only twice daily by mouth—10 to 20 mg per dose being sufficient to suppress abstinence symptoms. After a stabilization period of 3 to 5 days on this dosage of methadone alone, the drug may be reduced rapidly and withdrawn over a similar period of time. Regardless of the method of drug withdrawal employed, treatment is best carried out in an institution with proper facilities for postwithdrawal rehabilitation in a drug-free environment or where methadone or a morphine antagonist may be administered. Such institutions, private or municipal, are available in most large communities.

The physician must be constantly alert to the dangers of addiction, particularly in susceptible individuals, i.e., those with psychoneurosis, psychopathic personality, or alcoholism. The use of opioids should be limited to cases where pain is the chief problem; they should not be used primarily as sedatives, for the relief of asthma, or even in patients with chronic pain until all other measures have been exhausted. It follows that it is most important to make a precise diagnosis of the cause of pain, since in some cases measures other than opioids will suffice, while in others, such as hysteria and depression, narcotic analgesics are contraindicated.

If narcotics have to be used for the relief of pain, consideration should be given to the choice of the appropriate drug and to the mode of administration. Morphine is still the drug of choice for most patients requiring relief of severe pain for short periods. Demerol may be useful in patients who cannot tolerate morphine. Patients with chronic pain should be managed with the least potent and smallest dosage of drug that will relieve them; doses should be spaced as far apart as possible and discontinued as soon as the need for pain relief has passed. In general, the opioids should be administered orally whenever possible, and the intravenous route should be avoided, since this method produces maximum "euphoria" and, hence, the greatest danger of addiction. The oral administration of codeine and aspirin is a useful way to begin treatment of the patient with chronic pain. If these drugs fail to control the pain, the parenteral administration of codeine should be tried. If the more potent opioids are needed, methadone and levorphan should be used, because of their effectiveness by the oral route and the relatively slow development of tolerance. Should long-continued injections of morphine or meperidine become necessary, maximum analgesic effect is obtained with 10 mg morphine rather than with 15 mg, as is often prescribed, and with 60 to 70 mg rather than with 100 mg meperidine. In these cases, use of the narcotic antagonist pentazocine (Talwin) might be considered. It is claimed that this drug, administered parenterally in doses of 40 to 60 mg, has analgesic effects comparable with those of morphine and other opiates, but has less addicting properties. The respiratory depression produced by pentazocine, as by opiates, can be counteracted by naloxone.

Ambulatory treatment of opioid addiction The most significant development in the treatment of opioid (almost exclusively heroin) addiction has been the establishment and growth of ambulatory methadone maintenance clinics. The scope of this activity, like the incidence of addiction, cannot be stated precisely, but can be judged by the fact that in 1974, 135,000 addicts were participating in such programs nationwide.

The method of treatment consists of the oral administration of methadone, once daily, in doses sufficient to suppress the craving for heroin and to abolish the euphoria-producing effects of that drug given intravenously (heroin blockade). The daily dosage of methadone required to achieve these effects varies between 60 and 100 mg; some patients can be maintained on as little as 40 mg per day, and with higher dosage they need take the drug only once in 48 h. Recently a longer-acting form of methadone—*l*-acetylmethadol—has become available, which can be taken thrice or even twice weekly. In principle, these effects could be achieved by multiple daily injections of heroin or morphine, but the effectiveness of methadone orally, its prolonged duration of action, and the fact that it precludes the desire and need for taking other opioids make methadone far more practical.

Methadone is no longer dispensed in tablet form but only as a liquid (dissolved in fruit juice), which is taken under supervision. The collection of urine samples is also supervised, and these are analyzed for opiates and other drugs, to monitor the patient's adherence to the program. Once this has been established, the patient is allowed to take home a 1- to 3-day supply. These measures are designed to prevent the diversion of methadone into illicit channels. Various forms of individual psychotherapy, group psychotherapy, social service counseling, and vocational guidance are included in most programs. The use of former heroin addicts (who are themselves on methadone treatment) as counselors is considered to be a particularly important adjunct to methadone treatment.

The results of methadone treatment are difficult to assess and vary considerably from one program to another. Even the best programs suffer an attrition rate of about 25 percent after several years. In the patients who remain, heroin use is markedly reduced, and between 75 and 85 percent achieve a high degree of social rehabilitation, i.e., they are gainfully employed and no longer engage in criminal behavior or prostitution. These have been the most notable achievements of the methadone maintenance programs.

Although the effectiveness of methadone treatment in the social rehabilitation of many addicts cannot be doubted, a number of questions about this method remain. The usual practice of methadone programs is to accept only adult addicts with a history of heroin addiction for several years. This leaves unanswered the problem of the adolescent addict. Although some individuals have been withdrawn from methadone, this has been accomplished so far in a relatively small number, and their capacity to maintain a drug-free existence appears doubtful. This means that the large majority of addicts now enrolled in methadone programs are committed to an indefinite period of methadone maintenance, and the effects of such a regimen are uncertain.

An alternate method of ambulatory treatment of the opioid addict involves the use of narcotic antagonists. Cyclazocine is the best known of these. After withdrawal of the opiate, cyclazocine is administered orally, in increasing amounts over a period of 2 to 6 weeks, until a dosage of 2 mg per 70 kg is being taken twice daily. The cyclazocine-stabilized individual is highly refractory to the euphoria-producing and pharmacological effects of opiates. The idea of treatment is to continue the administration of cyclazocine until all drug-seeking behavior is extinguished, after which it is withdrawn. Good results have been achieved with this drug, but only in small numbers of highly motivated patients who chose cyclazocine maintenance in preference to other forms of treatment. More recently, interest has centered about the opiate antagonist naltrexone which is virtually devoid of agonistic activity and twice as potent as naloxone; it has the added advantages of being effective orally and in much smaller doses than naloxone. The value of this kind of "extinction therapy" has not yet been determined, but the results in some patients have been encouraging, and the search for improved methods of using opioid antagonists continues. One such agent, buprenorphine, presently under investigation, shows promise both as an analgesic of low abuse potential and as a maintenance drug in narcotic addiction (Jasinski et al.).

Obviously none of these methods promise lasting success unless combined with reeducation, vocational habilitation, and social adjustment.

REFERENCES

HOLLISTER LE: Effective use of analgesic drugs. Annu Rev Med 27:431, 1976

982

JASINSKI DR et al: Human pharmacology and abuse potential of the analgesic buprenorphine. Arch Gen Psychiatry 35:501, 1978

MARTIN WR: Realistic goals for antagonist therapy. Am J Drug Alcohol Abuse 2:353, 1975

—— et al: Naltrexone, an antagonist for the treatment of heroin dependence: Effects in man. Arch Gen Psychiatry 28:782, 1973

MONROE JJ et al: The decline of the addict as "psychopath": Implications for community care. Int J Addictions 6:601, 1971

RICHTER RW et al: Neurological complications of heroin addiction. Bull NY Acad Med 49:3, 1972

WIKLER A.: Theories related to physical dependence, in *The Chemical and Biological Aspects of Drug Dependence*, SJ Mule, H Brill (eds). Cleveland, Chemical Rubber Press, 1972, p 359

——: Drug dependence, in *Clinical Neurology*, AB Baker, LH Baker (eds). Hagerstown, Md, Harper & Row, 1975

——: Characteristics of opioid addiction, in *Psychopharmacology in the Practice of Medicine*, ME Jarvik (ed). New York, Appleton-Century-Crofts, 1977, p 417

ZINBERG NE: The crisis in methadone maintenance. N Engl J Med 296:1000, 1977

228
BARBITURATES

MAURICE VICTOR
RAYMOND D. ADAMS

The high incidence of addiction, suicides, and accidental deaths attributable to the improper use of the barbiturate drugs is a matter of continuing concern to the medical profession. The production of barbiturates greatly exceeds the amount needed for therapeutic purposes. It is estimated that barbiturates account for 20 percent of acute poisonings admitted to general hospitals and that they are responsible for 6 percent of suicides and 18 percent of accidental deaths, figures exceeded by no other single poison. More than 15,000 deaths secondary to barbiturate poisoning are reported annually in the United States, and this figure is undoubtedly an underestimation. The Domestic Council Drug Abuse Task Force (1975) estimated the total number of regular users of barbiturates who were "in trouble" (suicidal and accidental overdoses as well as medical complications of barbiturate abuse) to be 300,000.

About 50 barbiturates have been marketed for clinical use, but only the following are encountered with any frequency: pentobarbital (Nembutal), secobarbital (Seconal), amobarbital (Amytal), aprobarbital (Alurate), thiopental (Pentothal), barbital (Veronal), and phenobarbital (Luminal). In the United States, pentobarbital, secobarbital, and amobarbital are the most commonly abused barbiturates. All the barbiturates are similar pharmacologically and differ only in their speed of onset and duration of action. The clinical problems posed by the barbiturates vary, however, according to whether the intoxication is acute or chronic, and these two types will be considered separately.

ACUTE BARBITURATE INTOXICATION Acute barbiturate intoxication results from the ingestion of large amounts of the drug either accidentally or with suicidal intent. Another form of accidental poisoning occurs in individuals who are intoxicated with barbiturates or with alcohol and who, being confused, ingest more of the drug than was intended. This type of poisoning has been termed *drug automatism*.

The ingestion of barbiturates with suicidal intent is most frequently the act of a depressed person. The hysteric or psychopath may take an overdose as a suicidal gesture and sometimes become seriously intoxicated because of a miscalculation or ignorance of the toxic dosage. At times, no psychiatric disease is present, the drug being taken impulsively or while the individual is inebriated. The combination of alcohol and barbiturate intoxication is frequent and particularly dangerous, since these drugs have an additive effect.

Site and mode of action of barbiturates Barbiturates decrease the excitability of nerve cells, although the mechanism is not fully understood. Attempts have been made to localize the action of barbiturates to certain anatomic regions, or even to specific nuclei within the nervous system, but it would appear that all parts are to some extent sensitive to the drug. Nevertheless, the reticular formation of the thalami and midbrain are particularly susceptible. There is little experimental evidence to support the notion that the administration of barbiturates first depresses cerebral cortical activity and then sequentially affects the anatomically lower centers. Reflex and other activities of the nervous system are probably depressed simultaneously, although in some cases the spinal reflexes appear to be accentuated in the early stages of poisoning.

Symptoms and signs The symptoms and signs of acute barbiturate intoxication vary with the type and the amount of drug, as well as with the length of time that has elapsed since it was ingested. Pentobarbital and secobarbital produce their effects after a short delay, and recovery is relatively rapid. Phenobarbital induces coma more slowly, and its effects tend to be prolonged. The duration of action of these drugs can be judged by the hypnotic effect of an average oral dose. In the case of the long-acting barbiturates, such as phenobarbital, barbital, and diallylbarbituric acid, it lasts 6 h or more; with the intermediate-acting drugs, amobarbital and aprobarbital, 3 to 6 h; with the short-acting drugs, secobarbital and pentobarbital, less than 3 h.

In general, much larger doses of long-acting barbiturates are required to produce a depth of unconsciousness comparable with that produced by the short-acting ones. The ingestion by adults of more than 3.0 g secobarbital, pentobarbital, amobarbital, or diallylbarbituric acid at one time may be fatal unless intensive and skillful treatment is applied promptly; it has been estimated that to produce a comparable effect, the following amounts of long-acting barbiturates would have to be ingested: 6.0 to 9.0 g phenobarbital, 5.0 to 20.0 g barbital, and 15.0 g aprobarbital. Because of the serious complications of prolonged coma, the fatalities are greater with the long-acting than with the short-acting drugs.

Clinically, it is useful to recognize three grades of severity of acute barbiturate intoxication, particularly in regard to prognosis and treatment. Mild intoxication follows the ingestion of approximately 0.6 g pentobarbital or its equivalent. Patients are drowsy or asleep, a state from which they are readily roused by calling their name loudly or by shaking them. The symptoms resemble those of alcohol intoxication, except that the face is not flushed, the conjunctivas are not suffused, and there is no odor of alcohol. Patients think slowly, and there may be mild disorientation, lability of mood, impairment of judgment, slurred speech, drunken gait, and nystagmus. Reflex activity and vital signs are not affected.

Moderate intoxication follows the ingestion of five to ten times the oral hypnotic dose. Here the state of consciousness is more severely depressed and is usually accompanied by depressed or absent deep reflexes and slow but not shallow respiration. Corneal reflexes are retained, with occasional exceptions. At times patients can be roused by vigorous manual stimulation; when awakened, they are confused and dysarthric and, after a few moments, drift back into coma. At other times they cannot be roused by any means. In the latter case the depth of coma and seriousness of the respiratory depression may be roughly judged by the response of respiration to the inhalation of 10% carbon dioxide or to painful stimulation such as the application of firm pressure to the sternum or supraorbital ridge. If these stimuli cause an increase in the depth and rate of respiration, the outlook for recovery is good, and only symptomatic treatment is indicated.

Severe intoxication occurs with the ingestion of fifteen to twenty times the oral hypnotic dose. Patients cannot be roused by any of the means indicated. Respiration is slow and shallow or irregular, and pulmonary edema and cyanosis may be present. The deep tendon reflexes are usually but not invariably absent. Most often, patients show no response to plantar stimulation, but in those who do the plantar responses are extensor. In the most advanced cases the corneal and gag reflexes may also be abolished. Ordinarily the pupillary light reflex is retained in severe intoxication and is lost only if the patient is asphyxiated. In the early hours of coma, there may be a phase of rigidity of the limbs, hyperactive reflexes, ankle clonus, extensor plantar signs, and decerebrate posturing; persistence of these signs indicates a severe degree of anoxia. The temperature may be subnormal, the pulse thready and rapid, and the blood pressure at shock levels.

Diagnosis The diagnosis of barbiturate intoxication is made from the history and physical findings. If a reasonable suspicion of the diagnosis exists, a careful search for drugs or their containers may be rewarding. One should also examine the mouth and gastric contents for any characteristically colored capsules. Acute barbiturate intoxication which presents as a state of coma must be distinguished from other forms of coma by the methods outlined in Chap. 20, "Coma and Related Disturbances of Consciousness." Actually there are few conditions other than barbiturate intoxication which cause a flaccid coma with reactive pupils, hypothermia, and hypotension. Glutethimide poisoning may produce an identical clinical picture, excepting that the pupils are always fixed (a parasympathomimetic action). Laryngeal spasm and sudden apnea also characterize glutethimide intoxication. In the differential diagnosis, hysteria presents the main problem.

The use of gas chromatography has provided a reliable means of identifying the type and amount of barbiturate in the blood. The major virtue of this method is in determining the precise cause of coma when this is in question. The blood level also helps to identify the drug as long- or short-acting, thus giving information as to whether the therapeutic problem will be short or prolonged. A blood barbiturate level of 2 mg per 100 ml in a *comatose* patient is usually due to poisoning with secobarbital or pentobarbital; although the immediate mortality is high in such instances, the therapeutic problem will be short. A level of 11.5 to 12.0 mg per 100 ml is usually due to poisoning with barbital or phenobarbital, and the comatose state will be prolonged. Because of the additive effects of alcohol, a patient who has ingested both drugs may be comatose with relatively low blood barbiturate levels. For this reason, and also because of differences in individual tolerance, the correlation between blood barbiturate levels and depth of coma is not entirely dependable.

The *electroencephalogram* may also be useful in diagnosis, since characteristic patterns accompany barbiturate intoxication (Chap. 364). In mild intoxication, the normal activity is replaced by fast activity, in the range of 20 to 30 Hz, appearing first in the frontal regions and spreading to the parietal and occipital regions as intoxication worsens. In more severe intoxication, the fast waves become less regular and interspersed with 3- to 4-Hz slow activity. In still more advanced cases, there are short periods of suppression of all activity, separated by bursts of slow (delta) waves of variable frequency. In extreme overdosage, all electrical activity ceases. This is one instance in which a "flat" EEG cannot be equated with brain death, and the effects are fully reversible, unless anoxic damage has supervened.

MANAGEMENT The management of acute barbiturate intoxication depends on its severity. In mild or moderate intoxication, recovery is the rule, and no vigorous treatment is required. If the type and amount of ingested drug cannot be ascertained, it is important to empty the stomach and analyze its contents. In the responsive patient, gastric lavage with a large tube is difficult, and a simpler procedure is to induce vomiting with syrup of ipecac. Once this has been accomplished, the patient should be checked at frequent intervals for signs of deepening stupor and coma. If the patient is unresponsive, special attention should be given to maintaining respiration and urinary excretion and to the prevention of infection. It is most important to establish a patent airway by the insertion of an endotracheal tube; suctioning should be used when necessary, and the patient should be turned frequently. Tracheotomy and bronchoscopic suctioning usually become necessary if atelectasis becomes manifest, or if intubation must be maintained for longer than 48 h. If there is any risk of respiratory depression or underventilation, it is advisable to support respiration, so as to provide adequate oxygenation and minimize the risk of atelectasis. Also, early on, an intravenous fluid system should be established to promote the renal clearance of drug and permit rapid administration of drugs and electrolytes. In the unresponsive, intubated patient gastric lavage may be a useful therapeutic as well as a diagnostic measure. It must be performed within several hours of ingestion of the drug, since barbiturates are absorbed rapidly and completely.

Cases of severe respiratory depression, with cyanosis and pupillary dilatation, represent a serious medical emergency. A clear airway should be secured immediately, and some form of assisted respiration begun with an automatic intermittent positive-pressure respirator. If the patient is in shock, the foot of the bed should be elevated, and norepinephrine and whole blood or plasma administered. Catheterization is required to determine the adequacy of urinary output, to obtain samples for laboratory examination, and to prevent distention of the bladder. Since the amount of barbiturate cleared by the kidney is directly proportional to the amount of urine formed, 8 to 10 liters of 5% glucose in saline solution should be given daily. Forced diuresis is also important because toxic amounts of barbiturate have an antidiuretic effect. Coma of any significant duration requires the administration of other electrolytes as well, the amounts being governed by their serum and urinary values. The occurrence of pulmonary and urinary infections calls for the use of appropriate antibiotic treatment.

Hemodialysis has proved to be an effective form of therapy and should be used in all patients with profound coma who fail to respond to the measures outlined above. It is particularly useful in cases of coma due to long-acting barbiturates and is mandatory if anuria or uremia has developed.

The treatment of severe barbiturate intoxication with analeptic drugs (Metrazol, picrotoxin, Megimide), which enjoyed a brief period of popularity, has been generally abandoned. These drugs are antagonistic to barbiturates only insofar as they are powerful cortical stimulants as well as overall nervous system excitants; they do not affect the rate of metabolism or excretion of barbiturate. Alkalinization of the blood by the use of large amounts of bicarbonate solution, as a means of mobilizing the barbiturate and increasing its rate of excretion, seems to be a useful measure, particularly where phenobarbital is the responsible agent.

Occasionally, in the case of a barbiturate addict who has taken an overdose of the drug, recovery from acute intoxication is followed by the development of abstinence symptoms, which have to be managed by the methods outlined below.

CHRONIC BARBITURATE INTOXICATION Barbiturate addiction The problem of chronic barbiturate intoxication is quite different from that of acute intoxication, because of the phenomena of tolerance and addiction as well as the effects of withdrawal of drugs. In these respects there is a close similarity to the problems of opioid and alcohol addiction.

Chronic barbiturate intoxication, like other addictions, tends to develop on a background of some psychiatric disorder, most commonly depression or psychoneurosis with symptoms of anxiety and insomnia, or so-called "character disorder." The drug is usually prescribed for nervousness and insomnia; as the desired effects are lost, the patient increases the dose gradually until he is taking an amount sufficient to produce symptoms when it is withdrawn. Individuals with character disorders are usually introduced to the drug by associates; since the drug is taken for its intoxicating effect, the dose tends to be increased rapidly. Addiction to alcohol or to opiates may predispose to barbiturate addiction. Alcoholics find that barbiturates effectively relieve their nervousness and tremor (cross tolerance); then they may continue to take both alcohol and barbiturates, or the barbiturates may replace the alcohol. Heroin and morphine addicts may turn to barbiturates when they are unable to obtain opiates. As with other addicting drugs, the incidence of barbiturism is particularly high in individuals with ready access to drugs, such as physicians, pharmacists, and nurses.

The symptoms and signs of chronic barbiturate intoxication may be described in relation to (1) the toxic effects of the drug, (2) the development of tolerance, and (3) the effects of sudden withdrawal of the drug after a period of prolonged intoxication.

The toxic manifestations of chronic barbiturism are much the same as those of mild acute barbiturate or alcohol intoxication. The barbiturate addict thinks slowly, shows an increased emotional lability, and becomes untidy in his dress and personal habits. The neurological signs are quite characteristic and include dysarthria, nystagmus, and cerebellar incoordination. Both the mental and neurological signs fluctuate greatly, being more severe if the drug is taken in the fasting state and tending to increase during the day as more of the drug is ingested. If the dosage is elevated rapidly, the signs of moderate or severe intoxication become manifest.

A characteristic feature of chronic barbiturate intoxication is the development of tolerance, sometimes striking in degree. The average addict will ingest about 1.5 g daily of a potent barbiturate and will not develop signs of severe intoxication unless this amount is exceeded. Tolerance to barbiturates does not develop as rapidly as to opiates. Daily doses of 2 g have been reached, but this takes many months. Individual variations in the degree of tolerance make it difficult to state precisely the minimal amount of drug which must be ingested before the resulting condition is designated as chronic barbiturate intoxication. Most persons can ingest 0.4 g daily for as long as 3 months without developing major withdrawal signs (seizures or delirium). With a dosage of 0.8 g daily, the efficiency at all tasks is greatly reduced, and after the daily ingestion of this amount for a period of 2 months, abrupt withdrawal will result in serious symptoms in the majority of patients. Even after 2 weeks at this dosage, some patients will show mild withdrawal symptoms and paroxysmal electroencephalographic changes with photic stimulation. Individuals

taking 0.4 to 0.7 g daily fall into an intermediate category; practically all show some mental dulling, and episodes of forgetfulness and occasionally severe withdrawal symptoms may occur.

Abstinence or withdrawal syndrome Following the withdrawal of barbiturates from chronically intoxicated individuals, a characteristic sequence of symptoms occurs. Immediately following withdrawal patients seemingly improve over a period of 8 to 12 h as they lose the symptoms of intoxication. After this short period a new group of symptoms appears, consisting of nervousness, tremor, postural hypotension, weakness, and generalized seizures. With phenobarbital or barbital, the onset of withdrawal symptoms may not occur until 48 to 72 h after the final dose. Seizures usually occur between the second and fourth days of abstinence, occasionally as long as 6 or 7 days after withdrawal. There may be a single seizure, several, or rarely status epilepticus. The convulsive phase may be followed directly by a delusional-hallucinatory state or a full-blown delirium, indistinguishable from delirium tremens, or a varying degree of improvement may follow the seizures, before the delirium becomes manifest. Death has been reported under these circumstances. The abstinence or withdrawal syndrome may occur in varying degrees of completeness; some patients have seizures and recover without developing delirium, and others have a delirium without preceding seizures. The abrupt onset of seizures or an acute psychosis in adult life should always raise the suspicion of addiction to barbiturates or other sedative-hypnotic drugs and withdrawal effects.

The electroencephalogram (EEG) shows a number of changes during chronic barbiturate intoxication and following withdrawal. During chronic intoxication, the predominant pattern is that of fast activity of moderate voltage, interspersed with some 6- to 8-Hz activity chiefly in the frontal and parietal regions. The EEG findings do not correlate closely with the degree of intoxication, but some subjects do develop "EEG tolerance," i.e., a disappearance of the fast activity while receiving moderate doses of barbiturate (400 mg daily for 90 days). On withdrawal of barbiturates the fast activity diminishes. Also in the first few days of abstinence, paroxysmal bursts of mixed spike and slow waves or 4-Hz "spike and dome" paroxysmal discharges may occur, not necessarily associated with seizures. Characteristically, in the withdrawal period, there is a greatly heightened sensitivity to photic stimulation, to which the patient responds with myoclonus or a seizure, accompanied by paroxysmal changes in the EEG. Most of these abnormalities disappear after 4 or 5 days, and the EEG pattern is usually completely normal in 2 weeks.

TREATMENT OF CHRONIC BARBITURATE INTOXICATION This should always be carried out in the hospital. If the diagnosis of addiction is made before signs of abstinence have appeared, the first step in treatment should be the determination of the "stabilization dosage." This is the amount of short-acting barbiturate required to produce mild symptoms of intoxication (nystagmus, slight ataxia, and dysarthria). Usually 0.2 g pentobarbital given orally every 6 h is sufficient for this purpose. The patient is examined 1 h after each dose. If the signs of intoxication are severe, the next scheduled dose is reduced or omitted. If, instead, tremulousness and postural tachycardia appear, an additional 0.1 g pentobarbital is given and the next scheduled dose is increased. This method is preferable to a blind reduction of dosage, since patients frequently underestimate the amount of drug taken. In such patients, establishment of the "stabilization dosage" may have diagnostic as well as therapeutic value. A patient who can take 0.8 g or more pentobarbital daily, without developing signs of intoxication, is probably physically dependent on drugs of this type. Then a gradual withdrawal of the drug is undertaken, 0.1 g daily. The reduction is stopped for several days if abstinence symptoms appear.

An alternate method of managing barbiturate addiction is to stabilize the patient with phenobarbital rather than pentobarbital. The longer-acting barbiturate is safer than the shorter-acting ones and permits a withdrawal characterized by fewer fluctuations in blood levels (Wesson and Smith). The initial dosage of phenobarbital is calculated by substituting one sedative dose (30 mg) of phenobarbital for each hypnotic dose (100 mg) of the short-acting barbiturate which the patient had been using.

With either of these methods a severely addicted person can achieve abstinence in 14 to 21 days. Patients undergoing withdrawal treatment require careful observation for symptoms of abstinence, and special precautions have to be taken to prevent the smuggling or concealment of drugs.

If the patient presents with severe withdrawal symptoms, such as seizures, he should be given 0.3 to 0.5 g Luminal sodium intramuscularly and then enough to maintain a state of mild intoxication. Most anticonvulsant medicines have been shown to be ineffective against barbiturate withdrawal convulsions. Withdrawal should then be carried out as indicated above. If the abstinence symptoms are not severe, it is not necessary to reintoxicate the patient, but treatment can proceed along the lines laid down for the delirious and confused patient (Chap. 21).

After recovery has taken place, whether from symptoms of chronic intoxication or withdrawal or from acute intoxication due to attempted suicide, the psychiatric problem requires evaluation and an appropriate plan of therapy. Many of the considerations in the management of alcoholism are equally applicable to the patient addicted to barbiturate or nonbarbiturate hypnotic drugs (Chap. 226, "Alcohol").

BARBITURATE PROVOCATION OF OTHER DISEASES At times the administration of one of the barbiturates may induce an attack of another disease. The most striking example of this is in hereditary porphyria where a severe and sometimes fatal outbreak of abdominal pain, psychosis, and polyneuropathy may follow the ingestion of a few capsules of Seconal (see Chap. 96). With severe liver disease, detoxification of barbiturates may be impaired, as is discussed in Chap. 299.

REFERENCES

BLOOMER HA, MADDOCK RK JR: An assessment of diuresis and dialysis for treating acute barbiturate poisoning, in *Acute Barbiturate Poisoning*, H Mathew (ed). Amsterdam, Excerpta Medica, 1971, chap 15

CLEMMESEN C, NILSSON E: Therapeutic trends in the treatment of barbiturate poisoning: The Scandinavian method. Clin Pharmacol Ther 2:220, 1961

DOMESTIC COUNCIL DRUG ABUSE TASK FORCE: *White Paper on Drug Abuse.* Washington, DC, US Government Printing Office, September 1975

ESSIG C: Chronic abuse of sedative-hypnotic drugs, in *Drug Abuse,* CJD Zarafonetis (ed). Philadelphia, Lea & Febiger, 1972, p 205

HARVEY SC: Hypnotics and sedatives. The barbiturates, in *The Pharmacological Basis of Therapeutics*, 5th ed, LS Goodman, A Gilman (eds). New York, Macmillan, 1975, chap 9

ISBELL H et al: Chronic barbiturate intoxication: An experimental study. Arch Neurol Psychiatry 64:1, 1950

PLUM F, SWANSON AC: Barbiturate poisoning treated by physiological methods. JAMA 163:827, 1957

WESSON DR, SMITH DE: *Barbiturates: Their Use, Misuse and Abuse.* New York, Human Sciences Press, 1977

229

NONBARBITURATE SEDATIVE-HYPNOTICS; PSYCHOTHERAPEUTIC, STIMULANT, AND PSYCHOTOGENIC DRUGS

MAURICE VICTOR
RAYMOND D. ADAMS

SEDATIVE-HYPNOTIC DRUGS

This class of drugs, also referred to as *depressants,* may be divided into two main groups. The first includes the barbiturates (Chap. 228), the bromides, chloral hydrate, and paraldehyde. In the past 15 years these drugs have been largely displaced by a second group of sedative-hypnotics, comprising meprobamate and other glycerol derivates, and the benzodiazepines, the most important of which are chlordiazepoxide (Librium) and diazepam (Valium). Indeed, the benzodiazepines are the most commonly prescribed drugs in the world today. Their advantages over the older sedatives and hypnotics are their *relatively* low toxicity and addictive potential and their minimal interactions with other drugs.

BROMIDES Bromides are now seldom prescribed by physicians but are contained in certain "nerve tonics" and proprietary remedies (Nervine, Neurosine), so that cases of bromide intoxication are encountered with some regularity. Acute poisoning with bromide is rare because large doses of the drug are irritating to the gastric mucosa, and vomiting prevents the attainment of significant blood levels. Taken in smaller doses, however, bromide tends to accumulate in the body because of its slow excretion by the kidneys, and toxic symptoms may appear in a matter of weeks. These symptoms are caused by the bromide ion itself and are not simply a reflection of a decrease in chloride due to the displacement of the chloride by the bromide ion.

The symptoms of chronic bromide intoxication are predominantly in the mental sphere and range from dizziness, drowsiness, irritability, and emotional lability to a quiet confusional state, with impairment of thinking and memory and, in severe cases, to delirium and mania or stupor and coma. Skin manifestations are associated in many cases, taking the form usually of acne-like eruption and less frequently of proliferative nodular lesions, resembling those of tertiary syphilis. Headache, mild conjunctivitis, gastric distress, anorexia, and constipation may be associated. The blood bromide levels and the severity of toxic symptoms do not necessarily correspond. As a general rule, levels of 75 mg per 100 ml (9 meq per liter) or more are considered abnormal and diagnostic of bromism, if the clinical picture suggests it. However, higher levels are sometimes well tolerated, and symptoms of bromism may persist for some days even after the blood levels have been reduced to normal or near-normal levels.

Treatment consists of removing the source of bromide and administering sodium chloride (at least 6 g daily, in divided doses). Ammonium chloride may be substituted if an accumulation of sodium is to be avoided and if there is no danger of an uncompensated acidosis or hepatic failure. Confused or delirious patients require sedation, and anorectic and emaciated patients need careful nursing care and special attention to diet. The administration of a mercurial or thiazide diuretic serves to promote a bromide diuresis. Hemodialysis is an effective means of removing bromide and should be utilized in the most severe cases of intoxication.

CHLORAL HYDRATE This is the oldest and at the same time one of the safest, most effective, and cheapest of the sedative-hypnotic drugs. After oral administration, chloral hydrate is reduced rapidly to trichloroethanol, which is the agent responsible for the depressant effects on the central nervous system. A significant portion of the trichloroethanol is excreted in the urine as the glucuronide, which may give a false positive test for glucose.

In large doses, chloral hydrate is toxic to the heart, kidneys, and liver, but only in the presence of preexisting disease in these organs. Chloral hydrate is a strong gastric irritant, so that it requires dilution and should not be taken on an empty stomach. Tolerance and addiction to chloral hydrate develop only rarely, and for these reasons it is an appropriate medication for the management of insomnia, particularly the type which is associated with depression. Poisoning with chloral hydrate is a rare occurrence and resembles acute barbiturate intoxication, except for the finding of miosis, which is said to characterize the former. In combination with alcohol, the well-known "Mickey Finn" or "knockout drops," its effects are additive, leading to a rapid onset of coma. Death from poisoning is due to respiratory depression and hypotension; patients who survive these events may show signs of liver and kidney disease.

PARALDEHYDE This hypnotic is also effective and safe, providing that certain precautions are taken in its preparation and administration. On exposure to light, paraldehyde decomposes to acetaldehyde, which is very toxic, and oxidizes to acetic acid. It must be freshly prepared, therefore, and stored in tightly stoppered, amber-colored bottles. Paraldehyde is unique in that a significant proportion is excreted unchanged through the lungs; the remainder is detoxified in the liver, so that it should be used cautiously in patients with liver disease.

Paraldehyde has a wide margin of safety when administered orally (or rectally), and even three or four times the usual dose of 8 to 10 ml causes no more than prolonged sleep or mild stupor. Intramuscular use of the drug should be avoided because of its propensity to produce sterile abscesses and to damage the sciatic nerve if injected too close to it. Intravenous injections should be made with caution and only in a hospital, because of their unpredictable effects on respiration. The main objections to this drug are its bitter taste (this can be obviated by diluting in fruit juice) and its lingering, unpleasant odor.

Paraldehyde is very effective in suppressing the tremulousness, restlessness, and insomnia that characterize the early phase (6 to 60 h) of the alcohol withdrawal period. Patients with these symptoms make repeated demands for paraldehyde, which is not surprising in view of the pharmacological similarities between this drug and alcohol and the effectiveness of both drugs in suppressing withdrawal symptoms. This should not present a problem in management, however, if the need for the drug is determined before each dose is given and the drug is withdrawn as soon as the agitation and tremor are under control. Should a relapse from abstinence then occur, substitution of paraldehyde for alcohol rarely if ever occurs.

BENZODIAZEPINE GROUP The foregoing drugs have been replaced to a large extent by two drugs, chlordiazepoxide (Librium) and diazepam (Valium). These latter drugs have been used extensively to control anxiety, and they are probably more effective than the barbiturates in this respect. They have also been used to control overactivity and destructive behavior in children and the symptoms of alcohol withdrawal. Diazepam is particularly useful in the treatment of delirious patients who require parenteral medication. The benzodiazepines possess anticonvulsant properties, and the intravenous use of diazepam is an effective means of controlling status epilepticus, as indicated in Chap. 23. In addition, diazepam has been used with moderate success in the treatment of certain extrapyramidal movement disorders and dystonic spasms.

Other widely used benzodiazepine drugs are flurazepam (Dalmane), which is useful in the treatment of insomnia (see Chap 22), and carbamazepine (Tegretol), which now has a definite place in the treatment of seizures, especially those of temporal-lobe origin with behavioral abnormalities, and tic douloureux (Chap. 376). Two newer members of this group, clonazepam and nitrazepam, have also proved to be useful in the management of seizure disorders.

The benzodiazepine drugs, while comparatively safe in the recommended dosages, are far from ideal. They frequently cause unsteadiness of gait and drowsiness and at times hypotension and syncope, particularly in the elderly. In severely disturbed schizophrenic patients, rage, hostility, uncontrollable excitement, confusion, and depersonalization may develop. Nausea, diminished libido, headache, skin rashes, leukopenia, eosinophilia, agranulocytosis, and enhancement of the effects of alcohol have all been reported but are rare. Additional central nervous effects are slurred speech, dysphagia, ataxia, confusion, and faulty memory.

CARBONIC ACID DERIVATIVES These drugs are capable of modest depressant action and are appropriate for relieving mild degrees of nervousness, anxiety, and muscle tension, although they have no advantage over the barbiturates. Maximal action occurs with relatively small doses. Meprobamate (Equanil, Miltown) is the best-known member of this group. With typical doses (400 mg, three or four times a day) the patient is able to function quite effectively; large doses cause ataxia, drowsiness, stupor, coma, and vasomotor collapse. Hypersensitivity reactions in the form of fever, pruritis, and erythematous, maculopapular, and occasionally urticarial or bullous eruptions have been reported. Cutaneous petechiae or ecchymoses may also occur, without thrombocytopenia. Diplopia, syncope, menstrual irregularities, angioneurotic edema, peripheral edema, leukopenia, thrombocytopenia, and pancytopenia are other rare complications.

It should be emphasized that addiction to meprobamate, though reported infrequently, does occur, and if four or more times the daily recommended dose is taken over a period of weeks to months, withdrawal symptoms (including convulsions) may appear, resembling those which follow withdrawal of barbiturate in chronically intoxicated patients. Several other nonbarbiturate sedative-hypnotic drugs, when taken in increasingly large doses, have the same liability. These drugs are glutethimide (Doriden), ethinamate (Valmid), ethchlorvynol (Placidyl), methyprylon (Noludar), chlordiazepoxide (Librium), diazepam (Valium), methaqualone (Quaalude), and perhaps oxazepam (Serax). As with the barbiturates, the toxic effects consist of slurred speech, nystagmus, ataxic gait, drowsiness, confusion, and coma. Also upon withdrawal of these drugs, hallucinations, seizures, and delirium, symptoms indistinguishable from those of the barbiturate and alcohol withdrawal syndrome, may appear. There have been occasional reports of death following the withdrawal of meprobamate, methyprylon, and diazepam in persons who had been taking large doses of these drugs for protracted periods. In view of these observations, physicians must exercise caution in prescribing new sedative drugs which are continually being introduced and which are said to possess no addicting or habit-forming properties.

The management of patients addicted to nonbarbiturate sedative-hypnotics follows the lines indicated in Chap. 228 under "Barbiturate Addiction." Thus, if the drug and its dosage can be determined, it should be withdrawn at the rate of one therapeutic dose per day. Should abstinence symptoms appear, the reduction in dosage is stopped for several days. If the offending drug cannot be identified, a barbiturate such as Seconal should be administered to the point of mild intoxication and then withdrawn, in the manner indicated in Chap. 228. It should be noted that phenytoin (Dilantin) and phenothiazine derivatives are not effective against abstinence convulsions.

ANTIPSYCHOTIC DRUGS

Since the mid-1950s, a large series of pharmacological agents, loosely referred to as *tranquilizers* (because of their sedative properties), has come into prominent use. They are also referred to as *neuroleptics* because of their ability to increase motor activity in some patients. Mainly these drugs are used for the control of schizophrenia and to a lesser extent for psychotic states associated with organic brain syndromes, and certain instances of manic-depressive disease. The mechanism by which these drugs ameliorate disturbances of thought and affect in these psychotic states is poorly understood but has been attributed to their ability to inhibit or partially block transmission in dopaminergic pathways in the brain. Probably their parkinsonian side effects are attributable to blockade of the dopaminergic striatonigral pathways.

A large number of antipsychotic drugs are on the market (almost two hundred have been given generic names), and no attempt will be made here to describe or even list all. Some have had only an evanescent popularity, and others have yet to prove their value. Chemically these compounds form a heterogeneous group, but six categories are of particular clinical importance: (1) the phenothiazines, (2) the thioxanthines, (3) the butyrophenones, and (4) the *Rauwolfia* alkaloids; (5) an indole derivative, molindone (Moban), and (6) a dibenzoxazepine derivative, loxapine (Loxitane), have been introduced only recently. Experience to date indicates that in the management of schizophrenia, molindone and loxapine are about as effective as the phenothiazines, and their side effects are also the same. The main use of the newer antipsychotic drugs is in patients who are not responsive to the older ones or who suffer intolerable side effects from them. A new antipsychotic agent, clozapine (a dibenzodiazepine derivative), is of great current interest since it appears to be uniquely free of extrapyramidal side effects. Clozapine, metiapine, and timozide (a diphenylbutylpiperidine) are presently under investigation in the United States.

PHENOTHIAZINES This group comprises some of the most widely used tranquilizers such as chlorpromazine (Thorazine, Largactil), promazine (Sparine), triflupromazine (Vesprin), prochlorperazine (Compazine), perphenazine (Trilafon), fluphenazine (Permitil, Prolixin), thioridazine (Mellaril), and trifluoperazine (Stelazine). In addition to their psychotherapeutic effects, these drugs have a number of other actions, so that certain members of this group are used as antiemetics (prochlorperazine) and antihistaminics (promethazine).

The phenothiazines have had their widest application in the treatment of the psychoses (schizophrenia and to a lesser extent manic-depressive psychosis). Their use outside psychiatry should be discouraged. Under the influence of these drugs, many patients who would otherwise be hospitalized are able to live at home and even work productively. And the use of these drugs has greatly facilitated the hospital care of hyperactive and combative patients.

Side effects of the phenothiazines are frequent and often serious. All of them may cause a cholestatic type of jaundice, agranulocytosis, convulsive seizures, orthostatic hypotension, skin sensitivity reactions, mental depression, disorientation and hallucinations, and disorders of the extrapyramidal motor system. Jaundice and blood dyscrasias have occurred less often with prochlorperazine, perphenazine, and fluphenazine than with other members of the group, but the extrapyramidal side effects have been relatively more pronounced. Several types of extrapyramidal symptoms have been noted.

1 A parkinsonian syndrome—masked facies, tremor, generalized rigidity, shuffling gait, and slowness of movement; these symptoms appear after several weeks of drug therapy.
2 Muscle spasms and dystonia, taking the form of involuntary movements of facial muscles and protrusion of the tongue (so-called buccolingual or oral masticatory syndrome), dysphagia, torticollis and retrocollis, oculogyric crises, and tonic spasms of a limb (dyskinesias); these complications usually occur early in the administration of the drug, sometimes after the initial dose, and often can be improved dramatically by the intravenous administration of diphenhydramine hydrochloride (Benadryl).
3 An inability to sit still and an inner restlessness, so that the patient paces the floor constantly (akathisia).
4 Lingual-facial-buccal dyskinesia, restlessness, and choreoathetotic movements of the trunk and limbs may occur as late and persistent complications (tardive dyskinesia) of long-term therapy with phenothiazines or haloperidol.

These extrapyramidal reactions must be recognized at once and the medication discontinued, but even then the disorder may persist for weeks or months, and often permanently. Administration of antiparkinsonian drugs of the anticholinergic type (trihexyphenidyl, procyclidine, benztropine) may hasten the recovery from some of the symptoms. Oral, lingual, and laryngeal dyskinesias are affected relatively little by any of the antiparkinsonian drugs. Sometimes, however, one such medication has a better effect than another. Amantadine (Symmetrel) in doses of 50 to 100 mg tid has been useful in some cases of postphenothiazine dyskinesia. Chlorprothixene (Taractan), a *thioxanthene* drug with effects similar to the phenothiazines, and thioridazine (Mellaril), although not the best tranquilizing agents, are favored by some because of their lesser tendency to produce symptoms of extrapyramidal motor disorder. The latter drug, however, if given in large doses over a period of time, may cause deposits in the macula of the retina with resulting visual impairment.

BUTYROPHENONES These drugs (haloperidol, trifluperidol) have much the same antipsychotic effects as the phenothiazines, as well as the same side effects. Unlike the phenothiazines, they have little or no adrenergic blocking action. The butyrophenones are effective substitutes for the phenothiazines in patients who are intolerant to the latter drugs, particularly to their autonomic effects.

RESERPINE This is the prototype of the *Rauwolfia* alkaloids. It was in relation to the sedative effects of these drugs that the term *tranquilization* was used for the first time. These drugs, so effective in controlling hypertension, are no longer recommended for the treatment of mental disorders, except perhaps in patients who cannot tolerate phenothiazines. When given in therapeutic doses, the *Rauwolfia* alkaloids often provoke a parkinsonian syndrome or a serious depression of mood, which may prove more troublesome than the disorder for which they were prescribed.

Meprobamate, chlordiazepoxide, and diazepam are often referred to as "minor tranquilizers," the implication being that these drugs share the properties of the "major tranquilizers" or antipsychotic drugs. This is not the case. The so-called "minor tranquilizers" differ from the antipsychotics in both their chemical structure and pharmacologic effects. In fact, the minor tranquilizers more closely resemble the barbiturates in their pharmacologic (depressant) effects (including the ability to produce tolerance and physical dependence) and are more appropriately referred to as *antianxiety* drugs.

It hardly need be pointed out that the tranquilizing drugs have been much abused. This would be suspected just from the frequency with which they are being prescribed. It is stated that in the decade 1955 to 1965, 50 million patients in the United States received chlorpromazine alone. These powerful medications have specific indications, noted above, and the physician should be certain of the diagnosis before using them. The fact that these drugs can produce tardive dyskinesia in nonpsychotic patients is reason enough not to use them for nervousness, apprehension, anxiety, mild depression, and the many normal psychological reactions to trying environmental circumstances. These drugs are not curative, but only suppress or partially alleviate symptoms, and they should not serve as a substitute for, or divert the physician from, the use of other measures for the relief of the abnormal mental state.

ANTIDEPRESSANT DRUGS

Two classes of drugs—the monoamine oxidase (MAO) inhibitors and dibenzazepine derivatives—are particularly useful in the treatment of depression. The adjective *antidepressant* refers to their therapeutic effect and is used here in deference to common clinical practice. *Antidepressive* or *antidepression* drugs would be preferable terms since *depressant* still has a pharmacological connotation which does not necessarily equate with the therapeutic effect. For example, barbiturates and chloral hydrate, which may ameliorate the symptoms of depression, are in fact depressants in the pharmacological sense but act as mood elevators or antidepressants. The meaning of these terms must not be confused, for reference is made on the one hand to a drug that reduces nervous system excitability and on the other to the capacity of the drug to ameliorate the symptoms of mental depression.

MONOAMINE OXIDASE INHIBITORS The observation that iproniazid, an inhibitor of MAO, had a mood-elevating effect in tuberculous patients initiated a great deal of interest in compounds of this type and led quickly to their exploitation in the treatment of depression. Iproniazid (Marsilid) proved exceedingly toxic and was soon taken off the market, as have several more recently developed MAO inhibitors; but other drugs, much better tolerated, have become available. These include isocarboxizid (Marplan), nialamide (Niamid), phenelzine (Nardil), and tranylcypromine (Parnate), the latter two being the most frequently used. Tranylcypromine has proved to be the most potent of these agents, but it has also produced the most serious toxic effects.

The exact mode of action of the MAO inhibitors has not been determined. They have in common the ability to block the oxidative deamination of naturally occurring amines (norepinephrine, epinephrine, and serotonin), and it has been suggested that the accumulation of these neurohormonal substances is responsible for the antidepressant effect. However, these drugs inhibit many enzymes other than monoamine oxidases and have numerous actions unrelated to enzyme inhibition. Furthermore, many agents with antidepressant effects like those of the monoamine oxidase inhibitors do not inhibit this enzyme. At the present time, one cannot assume that the therapeutic effect of these drugs has a direct relation to the property of MAO inhibition.

These drugs must be dispensed with great caution and a constant awareness of their potentially serious side effects. They may at times cause excitement, restlessness, agitation, insomnia, and anxiety; occasionally, with the usual dose and more often with an overdose, mania and convulsions may occur (especially in epileptic patients). Other side effects are increased neuromuscular activity in the form of muscle twitching and involuntary movement of an extremity, urinary retention, skin rashes, tachycardia, hepatic disturbance, jaundice, visual impairment, enhancement of glaucoma, impotence, sweating, muscle spasms, and a variety of paresthesias. Orthostatic hypotension of a serious degree may develop.

Patients taking MAO inhibitors must be warned against the use of dibenzazepine derivatives (Tofranil and Elavil) and also sympathomimetic amines and tyramine, for they may induce a severe hypertensive episode and cerebral vascular accident, headache, atrial and ventricular arrhythmia, pulmonary edema, and even death. Sympathomimetic amines are contained in some of the commonly used nasal sprays, nose drops, and so-called "coryza tablets," and in tyramine-containing foods (cheeses, yogurt, beer, and wine).

The MAO inhibitors have the ability to potentiate the effect of many other drugs. In particular, phenothiazines and other powerful central nervous system stimulants should not be given with the MAO inhibitors, since severe reactions and occasional fatalities have followed their concomitant use. Exaggerated responses to the usual dose of meperidine (Demerol) and other narcotic drugs have also been observed; respiratory function may be depressed to a serious degree, and hyperpyrexia, agitation, and pronounced hypotension may occur as well, sometimes with fatal issue. Unpredictable side effects may also accompany the simultaneous administration of barbiturates and MAO inhibitors.

DIBENZAZEPINE DERIVATIVES (TRICYCLIC ANTIDEPRESSANTS) Soon after the first convincing successes in the treatment of depression with MAO inhibitors, a new class of tricyclic compounds appeared. The first of this group was imipramine (Tofranil), which was soon followed by amitriptyline (Elavil), and then by desipramine (Norpramin), nortriptyline (Aventyl), protriptyline (Vivactil, Triptil), and doxepin (Sinequan). The first two members of this group have proved to be the most popular.

The exact mode of action of these agents is unknown, but there is evidence that these agents inhibit re-uptake of norepinephrine by adrenergic nerve terminals, and their antidepressant effect has been attributed to this action. In the absence of other considerations, they are presently the most effective drugs for the treatment of patients with depressive illnesses, particularly those with retarded depressions, that are associated with insomnia (early morning awakening), decreased appetite, weight loss and decreased libido. Persistence of their pharmacological effects after the drug is stopped is very short in comparison with the MAO inhibitors, and their side effects are far less frequent and serious.

The tricyclic or dibenzazepine compounds are potent anticholinergic agents, and their most prominent and serious side effects (orthostatic hypotension, urinary bladder weakness) are due to peripheral anticholinergic action. They may also produce central nervous system excitement, leading to insomnia, agitation, and restlessness, but usually these effects are controlled readily by the use of phenothiazines or chlordiazepoxide given concurrently or in the evenings. Occasionally they may cause ataxia and blood dyscrasias. The dibenzazepine drugs should never be given with an MAO inhibitor, since the reactions which may occur are frequently serious; hypertensive crises and lethal hyperpyrexia have been reported. These reactions have allegedly occurred when small doses of imipramine were given to patients who had discontinued the MAO inhibitor 1 week previously.

STIMULANTS

These drugs, which act primarily as stimulants of the central nervous system, have a relatively limited therapeutic use but assume clinical importance for other reasons. Some members of the group, e.g., the amphetamines, are much abused, and others are not infrequent causes of poisoning.

AMPHETAMINES Amphetamine (Benzedrine) and its *d*-isomer, dextroamphetamine, are powerful analeptics and in addition have significant hypertensive, respiratory-stimulant, and appetite-depressant effects. These drugs are useful in the management of narcolepsy, but they are much more widely and indiscriminately used for the control of obesity and the abolition of fatigue. Undoubtedly, the initial effect of a moderate oral dose of amphetamine is to reverse fatigue, postpone the need for sleep, and elevate mood, but these effects are not entirely predictable and certainly not indefinite, and the user must pay for the period of wakefulness with even greater fatigue and often with depression. The intravenous use of a high dose of amphetamine produces an immediate ecstasy, "the flash." Because of the popularity of the amphetamines and ease with which they can be procured, instances of acute and chronic intoxication are observed frequently. Nonetheless, dextroamphetamine in doses of 5 mg morning and noon is a useful agent in the treatment of certain reactive depressions, such as the ones which follow myocardial infarction or stroke, and in suppressing overactivity of children who are impulsive and inattentive. The toxic signs are essentially an exaggeration of the analeptic effects—restlessness, excessive speech and motor activity, tremor, and insomnia. Occasionally grimacing, tic-like, choreoathetotic, and dystonic movements, similar to those produced by the phenothiazines, may develop as an acute idiosyncratic reaction to amphetamine. The chronic administration of large doses of amphetamine may give rise to hallucinations, delusions, and changes in affect and thought processes, a state that may be indistinguishable from paranoid schizophrenia (See Chap. 25). Treatment consists of removal of the offending drug and the administration of antipsychotic drugs. Nitrites may be useful if the blood pressure is markedly elevated.

METHYLPHENIDATE Having much the same type of action as amphetamine, this drug (Ritalin) is useful in the treatment of narcolepsy and, paradoxically, like dextroamphetamine, in the management of overactive children.

PICROTOXIN A powerful nervous system excitant, this drug exerts its main effects by producing convulsive seizures and reversing respiratory depression induced by drugs, particularly by barbiturates. However, the modern treatment of barbiturate intoxication does not include the use of picrotoxin or other analeptics, because of their epileptogenic properties and because barbiturate intoxication can be managed successfully by other means (see Chap. 228). It has been shown by Eccles and his colleagues that picrotoxin increases neuronal activity by blocking presynaptic inhibition, i.e., blocking the action of inhibitory fibers that synapse with the presynaptic terminals of excitatory fibers.

STRYCHNINE The action of strychnine is to increase neuronal excitability by interfering with postsynaptic inhibition; the therapeutic value is negligible. In children accidental poisoning may occur from ingestion of AS&B cathartic pills or "rat biscuits." Very rarely, strychnine is taken with suicidal intent. After a period of heightened irritability and muscle twitching, tonic seizures occur, characterized by opisthotonus, rigid extension of the legs, facial tetanus, and apnea due to spasm of the muscles of respiration. Death from anoxia may follow several seizures. The immediate need, in the treatment of strychnine poisoning, is to control the convulsions. This calls for the intravenous administration of a short-acting barbiturate or the application of inhalation anesthesia, if the appropriate drug is not immediately available; endotracheal intubation is an important safeguard. The patient must then be observed carefully, and if any signs of irritability recur, more sedative should be given. During this period, supportive care is indicated, as for any comatose patient. Morphine, which is principally a medullary depressant, is contraindicated.

PENTYLENETETRAZOL This drug (Metrazol, Cardiazol) is a potent stimulant of all parts of the nervous system. For a number of years it served as the convulsive agent in shock treatment of depression and schizophrenia but was abandoned in favor of less dangerous and more effective forms of convulsive therapy. The use of this drug to activate latent epileptogenic foci or to reproduce convulsions, with the purpose of studying the underlying cerebral mechanisms, although once a common procedure, has been virtually discontinued.

BEMEGRIDE, NIKETHAMIDE These two drugs, the latter with the trade name Coramine, act much like pentylenetetrazol. For many years common clinical practice was to administer nikethamide as a final therapeutic gesture in patients dying of cardiac and respiratory failure, but there is little evidence that the drug has a significant stimulant effect on either heart or respiration. Poisoning with these drugs, which is usually due to parenteral overdosage, is best treated with barbiturates.

CAFFEINE The therapeutic value of caffeine and other xanthine derivatives stems from their diuretic effects and their ability to stimulate the heart and nervous system. The major use of these agents is to abolish fatigue and maintain wakefulness, and the usual mode of administration is in coffee, a cup of which contains 100 to 150 mg caffeine. Overdosage leads to insomnia, tremulousness, mild delirium, tinnitus, tachycardia, prominent diuresis, and cardiac arrhythmias. The excitatory effects are easily controlled with barbiturates, and fatalities due to caffeine poisoning are extremely rare.

CAMPHOR Formerly a popular stimulant, camphor is now rarely used therapeutically; however, occasional cases of poisoning are still seen as a result of ingestion of liniment (camphorated oil) or moth flakes. The manifestations of poisoning are headache, sensation of warmth, confusion, clonic convulsions, and terminal respiratory depression; the characteristic odor of camphor facilitates the diagnosis. Treatment consists of supportive care and the cautious use of barbiturates to combat convulsions.

PSYCHOTOGENIC DRUGS

Included in this category are a heterogeneous group of drugs, the primary effect of which is to alter perception, mood, and thinking out of proportion to other aspects of cognitive function and consciousness. This group of drugs comprises lysergic acid derivatives, e.g., lysergic acid diethylamide (LSD); phenylethylamine derivatives (mescaline and peyote); psilocybin; certain indolic derivatives, *Cannabis* (marijuana), and a number of less important compounds. They are also referred to as psychotomimetic drugs, hallucinogens, illusinogens, and psychedelics, but none of these names is entirely suitable.

Tolerance to LSD, mescaline, psilocybin, and other psychotogenic drugs develops rapidly, even on a once-daily dosage. Furthermore, subjects tolerant to any one of these three specific drugs are cross-tolerant to the other two. Tolerance is lost rapidly when these drugs are discontinued abruptly, but no abstinence syndromes ensue. In this sense, addiction does not develop, although users may become dependent upon them for emotional support. In the case of marijuana, reverse tolerance (i.e., increasing sensitization) may be observed initially, but on continued use, tolerance to the euphoriant effects of the drug has been observed in one of the few chronic experimental studies that have been made, and the subjects reported jitteriness during the first 24 h after abrupt cessation of marijuana smoking, although no objective withdrawal signs could be detected.

LSD, MESCALINE, PSILOCYBIN These drugs produce much the same clinical effects if given in comparable amounts. The perceptual changes are the most dramatic—the user describes vivid visual hallucinations, alterations in the shape and color of objects, unusual dreams, and feelings of depersonalization. An increase in auditory acuity has been described, but auditory hallucinations are rare. Cognitive functions are difficult to assess because of inattention, drowsiness, and inability to concentrate and to cooperate in mental testing. The somatic symptoms consist of dizziness, nausea, drowsiness, paresthesias, and blurring of vision. Sympathomimetic effects—pupillary dilatation, piloerection, hyperthermia, and tachycardia—are prominent, and the user may also show hyperreflexia, incoordination of the limbs, and ataxia.

MARIJUANA When taken by inhaling the smoke from cigarettes, marijuana produces effects which are prompt in onset and evanescent. In low doses the symptoms are like those of mild intoxication with alcohol. With increasing amounts of the drug, the effects are similar to those of LSD, mescaline, and psilocybin, and they may be quite disabling for many hours. Very large doses result in severe depression and stupor, but death is unusual.

The fact that small quantities of these drugs can produce gross mental aberrations has stimulated the search for similar but endogenous substances that may be responsible for schizophrenia and other psychoses. The mechanisms involved in producing and antagonizing the psychotomimetic effects are also being studied intensively, in the hope of elucidating the mechanisms of the psychoses and finding improved psychotherapeutic agents. Doubtless these studies are adding greatly to our knowledge of abnormal behavior, but the fundamental problems remain to be solved.

Numerous claims have been made that LSD and related drugs are effective in the treatment of mental disease and a wide variety of social ills and that they have the capacity to increase one's intellectual performance, creativity, and self-understanding. At this time, there are no acceptable studies that validate any of these claims.

LSD is not yet an approved drug, and use of marijuana is governed by the federal narcotic laws. Nevertheless, these drugs are very widely used. They are taken by narcotic addicts as a temporary substitute for more potent drugs, by "drug heads," i.e., individuals who use literally any agent that alters consciousness, and by many troubled, unhappy college and high-school students, often for reasons that they cannot ascertain. The unsupervised use of these drugs is attended by a number of serious adverse reactions, taking the form of acute panic attacks, long-lasting psychotic states resembling paranoid schizophrenia, "flashbacks" (spontaneous recurrences of the original LSD experience, often precipitated by smoking marijuana and accompanied by panic attacks), or by serious physical injury, consequent upon impairment of the user's critical faculties. Whether prolonged usage leads to permanent damage to the nervous system is not certain; there are some data suggesting that this may happen. The reports claiming that LSD may cause chromosomal damage remain to be validated. A discussion of the legal implications of the illicit use of these drugs and their social impact is beyond the scope of this chapter but can be found in the references cited below.

REFERENCES

BYCK R: Drugs and the treatment of psychiatric disorders, in *The Pharmacological Basis of Therapeutics,* 5th ed, LS Goodman, A Gilman (eds). New York, Macmillan, 1975

DiMASCIO A, SHADER RI (eds): *Clinical Handbook of Psychopharmacology.* New York, Science House, 1970

DiPALMA JR (ed): *Drill's Pharmacology in Medicine.* New York, McGraw-Hill, 1971

HOLLISTER LE: Mental disorders—antianxiety and antidepressant drugs. N Engl J Med 286:1195, 1972

———: *The Clinical Use of Psychotherapeutic Drugs.* Springfield, Ill, Charles C Thomas, 1973

———: Antipsychotic medications and the treatment of schizophrenia, in *Psychopharmacology: From Theory to Practice,* JD Barchas et al (eds). New York, Oxford University Press, 1975, p 121

IVERSEN SD, IVERSEN LL: *Behavioral Pharmacology.* New York, Oxford, 1975

MARKS J: *The Benzodiazepines: Use, Overuse, Misuse, Abuse.* Baltimore, University Park Press, 1978

WIKLER A: The marijuana controversy, in *Marijuana: Effects on Human Behavior.* New York, Academic, 1974, p 25

———: Drug dependence, in *Clinical Neurology,* AB Baker, LH Baker (eds). New York, Harper & Row, 1975

VOLUME 2

PART FIVE
DISEASES OF THE ORGAN
SYSTEMS

Diagnostic methods

230
APPROACH TO THE PATIENT WITH HEART DISEASE

EUGENE BRAUNWALD

The initial symptoms of the patient with heart disease result most commonly from myocardial ischemia, from disturbance of the contractile activity of the myocardium, or from an abnormal cardiac rhythm or rate. Ischemia is manifest most frequently as chest pain, while reduction of the pumping ability of the heart commonly leads to weakness and fatigability or, when severe, produces cyanosis, hypotension, syncope, and elevated intravascular pressure upstream to a failing ventricle; the latter results in abnormal fluid accumulation, which in turn leads to dyspnea, orthopnea, and edema. Cardiac arrhythmias often develop suddenly, and the resulting signs and symptoms—palpitation, dyspnea, angina, hypotension, and syncope—generally occur abruptly and may disappear as rapidly as they develop.

A cardinal principle useful in the evaluation of the patient with suspected heart disease is that myocardial or coronary function which may be quite adequate at rest may be totally inadequate during exertion. Thus, a history of chest pain and/or dyspnea which appears only during activity is characteristic of heart disease, while the opposite pattern, i.e., the appearance of these symptoms at rest and their remission during exertion, is rarely observed in patients with organic heart disease.

Patients with cardiocirculatory disease may also be entirely asymptomatic, both at rest and during exertion, but may present an abnormal physical finding, such as a heart murmur, elevated systemic arterial pressure, or an abnormality of the electrocardiogram or of the cardiac silhouette on the chest roentgenogram.

Diseases of the heart and circulation are so common and the laity is so well acquainted with the major symptoms resulting from these disorders that patients, and occasionally physicians, erroneously attribute many complaints to organic cardiovascular disease. Furthermore, the combination of the widespread fear of heart disease in the Western world with the deep-seated emotional connotations concerning this organ's function results in the frequent development in persons with normal cardiovascular systems of symptoms which mimic those of organic disease. The correct interpretation of symptoms in patients with recognized organic cardiovascular distur-

bances is occasionally quite difficult. Such persons, in addition to having symptoms resulting from their disease, may also develop functional complaints referable to the cardiovascular system. The unraveling of symptoms and signs due to organic heart disease from those which are not directly related is an important and challenging task in these patients.

It must be recognized that dyspnea, one of the cardinal manifestations of diminished cardiac reserve, is not limited to disease of the heart, but is also characteristic of conditions as diverse as pulmonary disease, marked obesity, and anxiety (Chap. 27). Similarly, chest pain (Chap. 5) may result from a variety of causes other than myocardial ischemia. Whether heart disease is responsible for these symptoms can frequently be determined by carrying out a detailed clinical examination. The electrocardiogram and roentgenogram provide additional helpful information; more specialized examinations are often helpful but only occasionally essential.

In every branch of medicine the establishment of the prognosis and development of a rational plan of management are based on a correct diagnostic appraisal. However, in the case of patients with disorders of the cardiocirculatory system, particular care must be taken to establish not only a correct but also a *complete* diagnosis. As outlined by the New York Heart Association, the elements of a complete cardiac diagnosis include consideration of:

1 The underlying etiology. Is the disease congenital, rheumatic, hypertensive, or arteriosclerotic in origin?
2 The anatomic abnormalities. Which chambers are enlarged? Which valves are affected? Is there pericardial involvement? Has there been a myocardial infarction?
3 The physiologic disturbances. Is an arrhythmia present? Is there evidence of congestive heart failure or of myocardial ischemia?
4 The extent of functional disability. How strenuous is the physical activity required to elicit symptoms?

Two simple examples may serve to illustrate the importance of establishing a complete diagnosis. The identification of exertional chest pain caused by myocardial ischemia is of crucial significance. However, this diagnosis is insufficient to develop either a strategy of specific treatment or prognosis until the underlying disease process, e.g., coronary atherosclerosis, aortic stenosis, severe anemia, thyrotoxicosis, or atrial tachycardia, which is responsible for the myocardial ischemia, is identified. Similarly, determining that heart disease is congenital provides an important starting point, but the decision about whether surgical treatment is advisable generally depends upon the specific anatomic defect present and often upon the nature of the physiologic disturbance and the functional impairment.

The establishment of a correct and complete cardiac diagnosis often requires the use of six different methods of examination: (1) history, (2) physical examination (Chap. 231), (3) electrocardiogram (Chap. 232), (4) chest roentgenogram (Chap. 233), (5) noninvasive graphic examinations (echocardiogram, phonocardiogram, arterial and venous pulse tracings, Chap. 233), and occasionally (6) specialized examinations, such as cardiac catheterization or angiocardiography (Chap. 234). In order to be most effective, each of these six approaches should be employed independently of one another as well as with the information derived from the other methods clearly in mind. Only in this way can one avoid overlooking a subtle, though extremely significant, finding. For example, an electrocardiogram should be obtained in every patient suspected of having heart disease. It may provide the critical clue in establishing the correct diagnosis, e.g., the finding of an atrioventricular conduction disturbance in a patient with unexplained syncope, even when all other methods of examination reveal no abnormal findings. On the other hand, when combined intelligently with the results of other methods of examination, the electrocardiogram may provide essential confirmatory data. Thus, the knowledge that a patient has an apical diastolic rumbling murmur may direct particular attention to the P waves, and the recognition of left atrial enlargement electrocardiographically would support the suggestion that the murmur is caused by mitral stenosis. Under these circumstances the additional finding of right ventricular hypertrophy suggests that pulmonary hypertension is present. Although the electrocardiogram is an invaluable aspect of every cardiovascular examination, with the exception of the identification of arrhythmias it rarely permits establishment of a specific diagnosis. In the absence of any other abnormal findings, electrocardiographic changes must not be overinterpreted. The range of normal electrocardiographic findings is wide, and the tracing can be affected significantly by many noncardiac factors, such as age, body habitus, and serum electrolyte concentrations.

In obtaining the history of the patient with known or suspected cardiovascular disease, particular attention should be directed to the family history. Familial clustering is common in many forms of heart disease. Genetic transmission may occur, as in hypertrophic subaortic stenosis (Chap. 247) or Marfan's syndrome (Chap. 103). In patients with essential hypertension or coronary atherosclerosis the genetic component may be less obvious but is also of considerable importance. The nature of the response of the myocardium to an increased hemodynamic load, such as hypertension, or a valvular lesion may also be conditioned by hereditary factors. Familial clustering of cardiovascular diseases may not only occur on a genetic basis but may also be related to familial, dietary, or behavior patterns.

When an attempt is made to ascertain the severity of functional impairment in a patient with heart disease, it is essential to determine the precise extent of activity and the rate at which it is performed before symptoms develop. Thus, breathlessness which occurs after running up two long flights of stairs denotes far less functional impairment than similar symptoms occurring after taking a few steps on the level. Also, the degree of customary physical activity at work and during recreation should be considered. Similarly, the history must include a detailed consideration of the patient's therapeutic regimen. For example, the persistence or development of edema in a patient whose diet is rigidly restricted in sodium content and who is receiving optimum doses of digitalis and diuretics must be interpreted quite differently from the finding of edema in the absence of these measures.

The phonocardiogram and the graphic indirect recording of pulse tracings, such as the jugular venous pulse, the carotid arterial pulse, and the apex cardiogram (Chap. 233), may in some instances provide information of considerable diagnostic value by amplifying the physical findings. It must be appreciated, however, that these techniques are primarily of aid in the precise timing of specific events, such as heart sounds, murmurs, and pulsations, which are easily elicited on physical examination.

PITFALLS IN CARDIOVASCULAR MEDICINE Increasing subspecialization in internal medicine and the perfection of advanced diagnostic techniques in cardiology may sometimes be accompanied by several undesirable consequences, which can be summarized as follows:

1 Failure by the noncardiologist to recognize cardiac manifestations of systemic illnesses. The latter include: (*a*) mongolism (often associated with endocardial cushion defect); (*b*) gonadal dysgenesis, i.e., Turner's syndrome (associated with a variety of congenital defects, particularly coarctation of the aorta); (*c*) bony abnormalities of the upper extremities (associated with atrial septal defect); (*d*) muscular dystrophies (associated with cardiomyopathy); (*e*) hemochromatosis and glycogen storage disease (associated with myocardial infiltration); (*f*) congenital deafness (associated with serious cardiac arrhythmias); (*g*) Raynaud's disease (associated with primary pulmonary hypertension); (*h*) connective tissue disorders, i.e., Marfan's syndrome, Ehlers-Danlos syndrome, Hurler's syndrome, and related disorders of mucopolysaccharide metabolism (aortic dilatation, prolapsed mitral valve, a variety of arterial abnormalities); (*i*) chronic hemolytic anemia (cardiac dilatation); (*j*) Refsum's disease (myocardial failure and conduction defects); (*k*) acromegaly (accelerated coronary atherosclerosis, conduction defects, cardiomyopathy); (*l*) hyperthyroidism (heart failure, atrial fibrillation); (*m*) rheumatoid arthritis (pericarditis, aortic valve disease); (*n*) Whipple's disease (pericarditis and endocarditis); (*o*) scleroderma (cor pulmonale, myocardial fibrosis, pericarditis); (*p*) lupus erythematosus (valvulitis, myocarditis); (*q*) polymyositis (pericarditis, myocarditis); (*r*) sarcoidosis (arrhythmias, cardiomyopathy); (*s*) Fabry's disease (myocardial ischemia, heart failure); (*t*) exfoliative dermatitis (high-output heart failure). In patients in whom these and related systemic disorders with cardiovascular involvement are present or suspected, detailed cardiovascular examination should be carried out.
2 Failure by the cardiac specialist to recognize systemic illnesses in patients with cardiac disorders. Patients known or suspected of having heart disease require a detailed general assessment and a search for the frequent noncardiac manifestations of cardiac disorders. Indeed, the cardiovascular abnormality may provide the clue critical to the recognition of these disorders. Closely related is the failure to appreciate the profound effects of stress, such as that resulting from an intercurrent infection, of pregnancy, or from emotional disturbances, on cardiovascular performance and symptoms.
3 Overreliance on and overutilization of laboratory tests, particularly specialized invasive techniques.

The examinations noted above, such as catheterization of the right and left sides of the heart, selective angiography, and coronary arteriography (Chap. 234), provide precise diagnostic information under many circumstances. For example, they aid in establishing a specific anatomic diagnosis in patients with congenital heart disease, in patients with chest pain of uncertain etiology in whom coronary artery disease is suspected, and in determining the functional significance of valvular abnormalities in patients with rheumatic heart disease being considered for surgical treatment. Although a great deal of attention has been lavished on the newer specialized laboratory examinations, it should be recognized that they serve to *supplement*, not *supplant*, a careful clinical examination. There is an unfortunate tendency to carry out procedures such as coronary arteriography instead of taking a detailed and thoughtful history; the results often do not provide a definite answer to the question of whether a patient's complaint of chest pain is clearly attributable to coronary arteriosclerosis. Similarly, catheterization of the left side of the heart is all too frequently employed to determine whether operative treatment of valvular disease is indicated, even before the patient has had a trial of medical therapy. Despite their enormous value, it must not be overlooked that these specialized examinations entail some risk to the patient, involve discomfort and cost, and place a strain on existing medical facilities. Therefore, *they should be carried out only if there is a specific indication and if the results can be expected to modify or aid in the patient's management.*

REFERENCES

BRAUNWALD E (ed): *Heart Disease.* Philadelphia, Saunders, 1980

DRESSLER W: *Clinical Aids in Cardiac Diagnosis.* New York, Grune & Stratton, 1970

FOWLER NO: *Cardiac Diagnosis and Treatment,* 2d ed. Hagerstown, Harper & Row, 1976

GAZES PC: *Clinical Cardiology: A Bedside Approach.* Chicago, Year Book, 1975

HURST JW et al (ed): *The Heart,* 4th ed. New York, McGraw-Hill, 1978

NEW YORK HEART ASSOCIATION, INC, CRITERIA COMMITTEE: *Nomenclature and Criteria for Diagnosis of Diseases of the Heart and Great Vessels,* 7th ed. Boston, Little, Brown, 1973

SELZER A: *Principles of Clinical Cardiology: An Analytical Approach.* Philadelphia, Saunders, 1975

231
PHYSICAL EXAMINATION OF THE HEART

ROBERT A. O'ROURKE
EUGENE BRAUNWALD

The general examination of a patient with cardiac disease often provides important information concerning the status of the cardiovascular system at the time of evaluation. The patient may appear tired because of a persistently low cardiac output; the respiratory rate may be increased, indicating pulmonary venous congestion. Central cyanosis, often associated with clubbing of the fingers and toes, indicates right-to-left shunting of blood in the heart or great vessels or inadequate oxygenation of blood by the lungs. Cyanosis in the distal extremities, cool skin, and increased sweating result from vasoconstriction in patients with severe heart failure.

The blood pressure should be taken in both arms and with the patient supine and upright; the heart rate should be carefully timed for at least 1 min. Orthostatic hypotension and tachycardia may indicate a reduced blood volume, while resting tachycardia may be a clue to the presence of severe heart failure.

Careful examination of the optic fundi is essential, and the retinal vessels may show evidence of systemic hypertension, arteriosclerosis, or embolism. The latter may result from ath-

erosclerosis in larger vessels (e.g., carotid) or may represent a complication of valvular heart disease (e.g., endocarditis).

Palpation of the peripheral arterial pulses in the upper and lower extremities is necessary to define the adequacy of systemic blood flow and to detect the presence of occlusive arterial lesions. It is also important to examine both legs for evidence of edema, varicose veins, or thrombophlebitis.

The cardiovascular examination includes careful evaluation of both the arterial pressure pulse and the jugular venous pulse, as well as deliberate precordial palpation and attentive cardiac auscultation.

ARTERIAL PRESSURE PULSE The normal central aortic pulse wave is characterized by a fairly rapid rise to a somewhat rounded peak (Fig. 231-1). The anacrotic shoulder, present on the ascending limb, occurs at the time of peak rate of aortic flow just before maximum pressure is reached. The less steep descending limb is interrupted by a sharp downward deflection, synchronous with aortic valve closure, called the *incisura*. As the pulse wave is transmitted peripherally, the initial upstroke becomes steeper, the anacrotic shoulder becomes less apparent, and the incisura is replaced by the smoother dicrotic notch. Accordingly, palpation of a peripheral pulse (e.g., the brachial arterial) frequently gives less information than examination of a more central pulse (e.g., the carotid arterial) regarding alterations in left ventricular ejection or aortic valve function. However, certain findings such as the bounding pulses of aortic regurgitation or pulsus alternans are more readily evident in peripheral than in central arteries. In order to examine the carotid arteries, the sternocleidomastoid muscle should be relaxed and the head rotated slightly toward the examiner. The application of varying amounts of pressure with either the forefinger or the thumb may permit appreciation of the ascending limb, the systolic peak, and the descending limb of the pressure pulse. In most normal persons a dicrotic wave is not palpable.

A small weak pulse, *pulsus parvus*, is frequently present in conditions with a diminished left ventricular stroke volume, a narrow pulse pressure, and increased peripheral vascular re-

FIGURE 231-1

A. Simultaneous recordings of electrocardiogram, aortic pressure pulse (AOP), phonocardiogram recorded at the apex, and apex cardiogram (ACG). On the phonocardiogram, S_1, S_2, S_3, and S_4 represent the first through fourth heart sounds; OS represents the opening snap of the mitral valve, which occurs coincident with the O point of the apex cardiogram. S_3 occurs coincident with the termination of the rapid-filling wave (RFW) of the ACG, while S_4 occurs coincident with the a wave of the ACG. B. Simultaneous recording of electrocardiogram, indirect carotid pulse (CP), phonocardiogram along the left sternal border (LSB), and indirect jugular venous pulse (JVP). ES, ejection sound; SC, systolic click.

sistance. This may be due to hypovolemia, to left ventricular failure secondary to myocardial disease or myocardial infarction, to restrictive pericardial disease, or to mitral valve stenosis. In aortic valve stenosis the delayed systolic peak, *pulsus tardus,* is the result of mechanical obstruction to left ventricular ejection and is often accompanied by the transmission of a coarse systolic thrill. In contrast, a large bounding pulse is usually associated with an increased left ventricular stroke volume, a wide pulse pressure, and a decrease in peripheral vascular resistance. This occurs characteristically in patients with abnormally elevated stroke volumes as in complete heart block, hyperkinetic circulation due to anxiety, anemia, exercise, or fever, or in patients with an abnormally rapid run-off of blood from the arterial system (patent ductus arteriosus, peripheral arteriovenous fistula). Patients with mitral regurgitation or a ventricular septal defect may also have a bounding pulse, since vigorous left ventricular ejection produces a rapid upstroke in the arterial pulse even though the duration of systole and the forward stroke volume may be diminished. In aortic regurgitation the rapidly rising, bounding arterial pulse results from increased left ventricular stroke volume and the associated increased rate of ventricular ejection.

The *bisferiens pulse,* which consists of two systolic peaks, is characteristic of aortic regurgitation (with or without accompanying stenosis) and of idiopathic hypertrophic subaortic stenosis (Chap. 247). In the latter the pulse wave upstroke rises rapidly and forcefully, producing the first systolic peak ("percussion wave"). A brief decline in pressure follows, because of the sudden decrease in the rate of left ventricular ejection as severe obstruction develops during midsystole. This pressure trough is followed by a smaller and more slowly rising positive pulse wave ("tidal wave") produced by continued ventricular ejection and by reflected waves from the periphery. When the second positive wave is produced by an accentuated and palpable diastolic wave, the pulse is called *dicrotic.* It has been recorded in patients who have a low diastolic pressure and systemic vascular resistance such as those with fever or mild aortic regurgitation and in patients with a very low stroke volume, particularly those with diffuse myocardial disease.

Pulsus alternans refers to a pattern in which there is regular alteration of the pressure pulse amplitude, despite a regular rhythm. It is due to alternating left ventricular contractile force; it usually denotes severe left ventricular decompensation and commonly occurs in patients who also have a loud ventricular filling sound (S_3). Pulsus alternans may also occur during or following paroxysmal tachycardia or for several beats following a premature beat in patients without heart disease. In *pulsus bigeminus* there is also regular alteration of pressure pulse amplitude, but it is caused by a premature ventricular contraction that follows each regular beat; auscultation can reveal the cardiac irregularity. *Pulsus paradoxus* is an accentuation of the decrease in systolic arterial pressure accompanying the reduced amplitude of the arterial pulse which normally occurs during inspiration. In patients with pericardial tamponade, airway obstruction, or superior vena cava obstruction, the decrease in systolic arterial pressure frequently exceeds the normal of 10 mmHg and the peripheral pulse may disappear completely during inspiration.

Simultaneous palpation of the radial and femoral arterial pulses, which normally are virtually coincident, is important to rule out aortic coarctation, in which the latter is weaker and delayed (Chap. 240).

JUGULAR VENOUS PULSE (JVP) The two main objectives of the bedside examination of the neck veins are inspection of their waveform and estimation of the central venous pressure (CVP). In most patients, the right internal jugular vein is supe-

rior for both purposes, but occasionally examination of the left internal jugular vein, the external jugular veins, or the venous pulsations in the supraclavicular fossae may yield more information. In most normal subjects, maximum pulsation of the internal jugular vein is observed when the trunk is inclined by less than 30°. In patients with elevated venous pressure it may be necessary to elevate the trunk further, sometimes to as much as 90°. When the neck muscles are relaxed, shining a beam of light tangentially across the skin overlying the vein exposes the pulsations of the internal jugular vein. Simultaneous palpation of the left carotid artery aids the examiner in deciding which pulsations are venous and in relating the venous pulsations to their timing in the cardiac cycle.

The normal JVP reflects phasic pressure changes in the right atrium and consists of three positive waves and two negative troughs (Fig. 231-1). In considering this pulse, it is useful to refer to the events of the cardiac cycle (Fig. 233-2). The positive presystolic *a* wave is produced by venous distention consequent to right atrial contraction and is the dominant wave in the JVP, particularly during inspiration. Large *a* waves indicate that the right atrium is contracting against an increased resistance, such as occurs with obstruction at the tricuspid valve (tricuspid stenosis or right atrial myxoma) or more commonly with increased resistance to right ventricular filling (pulmonary hypertension or pulmonic stenosis). Large *a* waves also occur during arrhythmias whenever the right atrium contracts while the tricuspid valve is closed by right ventricular systole. Such "cannon" *a* waves may occur regularly (as during junctional rhythm) or irregularly (as in atrioventricular dissociation with ventricular tachycardia or complete heart block). The *a* wave is absent in patients with atrial fibrillation, and there is an increased temporal delay between the *a* wave and the carotid arterial pulse in patients with first-degree atrioventricular (AV) block.

The *c* wave, often observed in the JVP, is a positive wave produced by the bulging of the tricuspid valve into the right atrium during right ventricular isovolumetric systole and by the impact of the carotid artery adjacent to the jugular vein. The *x* descent is due to a combination of atrial relaxation and the downward displacement of the tricuspid valve during ventricular systole. In patients with constrictive pericarditis, there is often increased prominence of the *x* descent wave during systole, but this wave is reduced with right ventricular dilatation and may even be reversed in tricuspid regurgitation. The positive, late systolic *v* wave results from the increasing volume of blood in the venae cavae and right atrium during ventricular systole when the tricuspid valve is closed. After the peak of the *v* wave is reached, the right atrial pressure diminishes because of the decreased bulging of the tricuspid valve into the right atrium as right ventricular pressure declines and the tricuspid valve opens. With mild tricuspid regurgitation the *v* wave becomes more prominent, and when tricuspid regurgitation becomes severe, the prominent *v* wave and the obliteration of the *x* descent result in a single large positive systolic wave ("ventricularization").

Following the summit of the *v* wave there is a negative descending limb, referred to as the *y* descent or "diastolic collapse," which is produced mainly by tricuspid valve opening and the rapid inflow of blood into the right ventricle. A rapid, deep *y* descent in early diastole occurs with severe tricuspid regurgitation. A venous pulse characterized by a sharp *y* descent, a deep *y* trough, and a rapid ascent to the base line is seen in patients with constrictive pericarditis or with severe failure of the right side of the heart and a high venous pressure. A slow *y* descent in the JVP suggests an obstruction to right ventricular filling, as occurs with tricuspid stenosis or right atrial myxoma.

For accurate estimation of the CVP, the right internal jugular vein is best utilized, with the sternal angle as the reference point, since in the average patient the center of the right atrium lies approximately 5 cm below the sternal angle, regardless of body position. The patient is examined at the optimum degree of trunk elevation for visualization of venous pulsations. The vertical distance between the top of the oscillating venous column and the level of the sternal angle is determined and generally found to be less than 3 cm (3 cm + 5 cm = 8 cm blood). The most common cause of an elevated venous pressure is an elevated right ventricular diastolic pressure. In patients suspected of having right ventricular failure who have a normal CVP at rest, the hepatojugular reflux test may be helpful. The palm of the hand is placed over the right upper quadrant of the abdomen, and firm pressure is applied for 30 to 60 s. Normally, the jugular venous pressure is not significantly altered, but with impaired function of the right side of the heart the upper level of venous pulsation usually increases. The increased abdominal pressure most likely enhances systemic venous return, and the abnormal right ventricle is unable to accept this additional blood volume, causing pressure in the great veins to rise. Also, abdominal compression may elicit the typical JVP of tricuspid regurgitation when the resting pulse wave is normal.

PRECORDIAL PALPATION This is best accomplished while auscultating the heart in order to time the cardiac movements. The location, amplitude, duration, and direction of the impulse can usually be best appreciated by using the fingertips. The normal left ventricular apex impulse is located at or medial to the left midclavicular line in the fourth or fifth intercostal space and is a tapping, early systolic outward thrust localized to a point not more than 2 to 3 cm in diameter. It is due primarily to recoil of the heart as blood is ejected, and it is best evaluated with the patient lying supine. Left ventricular hypertrophy results in an exaggerated amplitude and duration of the normal left ventricular thrust. The impulse may be displaced laterally and downward into the sixth or seventh interspace, particularly in patients with a left ventricular volume load such as occurs in aortic regurgitation.

Additional abnormal features of the left ventricular apex impulse may become more obvious when the patient is turned on his left side. These include marked presystolic distention of the left ventricle, often accompanying a fourth heart sound in patients with an excessive left ventricular pressure load, and a prominent early diastolic rapid-filling wave, often accompanying a third heart sound in patients with left ventricular failure or mitral valve regurgitation (Fig. 231-1). A double systolic impulse is frequently palpable in patients with idiopathic hypertrophic subaortic stenosis.

Right ventricular hypertrophy results in a sustained systolic lift at the lower left parasternal area which starts in early systole and is synchronous with the left ventricular apical impulse. In patients with chronic obstructive pulmonary disease a right ventricular impulse may often be detected by sliding the fingers up under the rib cage just beneath the sternum. The enlarged right ventricle strikes the ends of the fingertips as an inferiorly directed movement.

Abnormal precordial pulsations occur in patients with motion disorders of the left ventricular wall due to coronary artery disease or to diffuse myocardial disease from some other cause. This is particularly true in patients with a recent transmural myocardial infarction, 70 percent of whom have abnormal left ventricular wall motion which is recordable by graphic methods. These ectopic impulses may occur in early, mid-, or late systole and may be present in some patients only during episodes of anginal pain. They are most commonly felt in the left midprecordium one or two interspaces above and/or 1 to 2 cm medial to the left ventricular apex. When a systolic bulge occurs in the region of the apex, it is difficult to distinguish it from the impulse of left ventricular hypertrophy.

A left parasternal lift is frequently present in patients with severe mitral regurgitation. This systolic lift occurs distinctly later than the left ventricular apical impulse, is synchronous with the *v* wave in the left atrial pressure curve, and is due to anterior displacement of the right ventricle by the large left atrium. A similar impulse occurring to the right of the sternum has been noted in some patients with severe tricuspid regurgitation and a giant right atrium. A vigorous pulsation of the right sternoclavicular joint may indicate a right-sided aortic arch or aneurysmal dilatation of the ascending aorta. Pulmonary artery pulsation is often visible and palpable in the second left intercostal space and may be normal in children or thin young adults. However, this pulsation usually denotes pulmonary hypertension, increased pulmonary blood flow, or poststenotic pulmonary artery dilatation.

Thrills are palpable low-frequency vibrations associated with heart murmurs. The diastolic rumble of mitral stenosis and the systolic murmur of mitral regurgitation may be palpated at the cardiac apex. When the palm of the hand is placed over the precordium, the thrill of aortic stenosis crosses the palm of the hand toward the right side of the neck, while the thrill of pulmonic stenosis tends to radiate more often to the left side of the neck. The thrill due to a ventricular septal defect is usually located in the third and fourth intercostal spaces near the left sternal border.

Percussion adds little to careful inspection and palpation in the recognition of cardiac enlargement. Occasionally, however, it is useful in detecting an abnormal rightward position of the heart, such as occurs in dextrocardia, dextroversion, right lung atelectasis, and left pneumothorax, as well as in demonstrating an increased area of dullness or flatness to the right of the sternum and at the upper left sternal border in a patient with a large pericardial effusion.

CARDIAC AUSCULTATION To obtain maximal information from cardiac auscultation, the observer should keep in mind several principles: (1) This portion of the examination should be carried out in a quiet room to avoid the distractions caused by the noises of normal activity. (2) In order to hear a faint heart sound or murmur, it is necessary to focus attention on that phase of the cardiac cycle during which the auscultatory event may be expected to occur. (3) The accurate timing of a heart sound or murmur necessarily involves ascertaining its relation to other observable events in the cardiac cycle—the carotid arterial pulse, the JVP, or the apical impulse. (4) To determine the significance of a cardiac sound or murmur, it is often necessary to observe alterations in its timing or intensity during various phases of the respiratory cycle, with changes in position, during and following a premature ventricular contraction, with handgrip exercise, and during the administration of vasoactive drugs such as amyl nitrite and phenylephrine.

HEART SOUNDS The major components of heart sounds are vibrations associated with the abrupt acceleration or deceleration of blood within the cardiovascular system, but there is continuing controversy regarding the relative significance of the vibrations of valves, muscles, vessels, and supporting structures in the production of the heart sounds. Recent studies using simultaneous echocardiographic-phonocardiographic recordings indicate that the first and second heart sounds are produced primarily by the closure of the AV and semilunar valves and the events that accompany these closures. The intensity of the *first heart sound* (S_1) is influenced by (1) the position of the mitral leaflets at the onset of ventricular systole, (2) the rate of rise of the left ventricular pressure pulse, (3) the presence or absence of structural disease of the mitral valve, and (4) the amount of tissue, air, or fluid between the heart and the stethoscope. The mitral valve is wide open at the end of diastole and S_1 is increased in intensity if diastole is shortened because of tachycardia, if atrioventricular flow is increased because of high cardiac output or prolonged because of mitral stenosis, or if atrial contraction precedes ventricular contractions by a short (PR) interval. The loud S_1 in mitral stenosis usually signifies that the valve is pliable and that the valve remains wide open at the onset of isovolumetric contraction because of the elevated left atrial pressure. A reduction in the intensity of S_1 may be due to poor conduction of sound through the chest wall, a slow rise of the left ventricular pressure pulse, a long PR interval, or imperfect closure due to reduced valve substance, as in mitral regurgitation. S_1 is also soft when the anterior mitral leaflet is immobile because of rigidity and calcification even in the presence of predominant mitral stenosis.

Splitting of the two high-pitched components of S_1 by 10 to 30 ms is a normal phenomenon (Fig. 231-1). The first component of S_1 normally is attributed to mitral valve closure and the second to tricuspid valve closure. A widened split of S_1 is most often due to complete right bundle branch block and the resulting delay in onset of the right ventricular pressure pulse. Reversed splitting of the S_1 with the mitral component following the tricuspid component has occasionally been noted in complete left bundle branch block and frequently is present in patients with severe mitral stenosis or a left atrial myxoma.

Splitting of S_2 into audibly distinct aortic (A_2) and pulmonic (P_2) components occurs normally during inspiration when augmented inflow into the right ventricle increases its stroke volume and ejection period and delays closure of the pulmonic valve. P_2 is coincident with the incisura of the pulmonary artery pressure curve, which is separated from the right ventricular pressure tracing by an interval termed the "hangout time." The absolute value of this interval reflects the resistance to pulmonary blood flow and the impedance characteristics of the pulmonary vascular bed. This interval is prolonged, and physiologic splitting of S_2 is accentuated in conditions associated with right ventricular volume overload and a distensible pulmonary vascular bed. However, in patients with an increase in pulmonary vascular resistance, the "hangout time" is markedly reduced and narrow splitting of S_2 is present. Audible expiratory splitting, heard best at the pulmonic area or left sternal border, is usually abnormal when the patient is in the upright position. Such splitting may be due to delayed activation of the right ventricle (right bundle branch block), to prolongation of right ventricular contraction with an increased right ventricular pressure load (pulmonary embolism or pulmonic stenosis), or to delayed pulmonic valve closure because of an increased right ventricular flow load associated with diminished impedance of the pulmonary vascular bed and a prolonged "hangout time" (atrial septal defect). In pulmonary hypertension, P_2 is increased in intensity and splitting of the second heart sound may be diminished, normal, or accentuated, depending on the cause of the pulmonary hypertension, the pulmonary vascular resistance, and the presence or absence of right ventricular decompensation. Early aortic valve closure, occurring with mitral regurgitation or a ventricular septal defect, may also produce audible expiratory splitting. In patients with large atrial septal defects the proportion of right atrial filling contributed by the left atrium and the venae cavae varies reciprocally during the respiratory cycle so that right atrial inflow remains relatively constant. Therefore, the volume and duration of the right ventricular ejection are not significantly increased by inspiration, and there is little inspiratory exaggeration of the splitting of S_2. This phenomenon, termed "fixed splitting" of the second heart sound, is of considerable diagnostic value. Fixed splitting of the second heart sound may also occur with impaired right ventricular function, when right ventricular stroke volume cannot rise even with augmented inspiratory inflow.

A delay in aortic valve closure causing P_2 to precede A_2 results in so-called "reversed" (paradoxic) splitting of S_2. Splitting is then maximal in expiration, and decreases during inspiration with the normal delay of pulmonic valve closure. The commonest causes of reversed (paradoxic) splitting of S_2 are left bundle branch block and delayed excitation of the left ventricle from a right ventricular ectopic beat. Mechanical prolongation of left ventricular systole, resulting in reversed splitting of S_2, may be caused by severe aortic outflow obstruction, a large aorta-to-pulmonary artery shunt, systolic hypertension, and ischemic heart disease or cardiomyopathy with left ventricular failure. P_2 is normally softer than A_2 in the second left intercostal space; when P_2 is greater than A_2 in this area, it suggests pulmonary hypertension, except in patients with atrial septal defect.

The *third heart sound* (ventricular or protodiastolic gallop) is a low-pitched sound produced in the ventricle 0.14 to 0.16 s after A_2, at the termination of rapid filling. This protodiastolic sound is frequent in normal children and in patients with high cardiac output. However, in patients over 40 years of age, an S_3 usually indicates ventricular decompensation, AV valve regurgitation, or other conditions which increase the rate or volume of ventricular filling. The left-sided S_3 is best heard with the bell piece of the stethoscope at the left ventricular apex during expiration and with the patient in the left lateral position. The right-sided S_3 is best heard at the left sternal border or just beneath the xiphoid and is increased with inspiration. Often it is accompanied by the systolic murmur of functional tricuspid regurgitation. Ventricular protodiastolic gallops often disappear with treatment of heart failure.

An earlier (0.10 to 0.12 s after A_2), higher-pitched third heart sound (pericardial knock) often occurs in patients with constrictive pericarditis; its presence is dependent upon the restrictive effect of the adherent pericardium, which halts diastolic filling abruptly.

The opening snap (OS) is a brief, high-pitched, early diastolic sound which is usually due to stenosis of an AV valve, more commonly the mitral valve. It is usually heard best at the lower left sternal border and radiates well to the base of the heart. The A_2-OS interval during exercise is inversely related to the height of the mean left atrial pressure, and ranges from 0.04 to 0.12 s. At the base an OS is often confused with P_2. However, careful auscultation at the upper left sternal border will reveal both components of the second heart sound, followed by the opening snap. The OS of tricuspid stenosis occurs later in diastole than the mitral OS. Since most patients with tricuspid stenosis also have severe mitral valve disease, the tricuspid OS is often overshadowed by the diastolic rumble and OS originating in the stenotic mitral valve. An OS also may occur when there is increased flow across an AV valve, such as exists with left-to-right intracardiac shunts and mitral or tricuspid regurgitation.

The *fourth heart sound* (atrial or presystolic gallop) is a low-pitched, presystolic sound produced in the ventricle during the ventricular filling associated with an effective atrial contraction, and is heard best with the bell piece of the stethoscope. The sound is absent in patients with atrial fibrillation. The atrial sound occurs when diminished ventricular compliance increases the resistance to ventricular filling, and it is frequently present in patients with systemic hypertension, aortic stenosis, hypertrophic cardiomyopathies, coronary artery disease, and acute mitral regurgitation. Most patients with an acute myocardial infarction and sinus rhythm have an audible

S4. The atrial sound is frequently accompanied by visible and palpable presystolic distention of the left ventricle. It is maximal in intensity at the left ventricular apex with the patient in the left lateral position, and is accentuated by mild supine exercise. The right-sided S_4 is present in patients with right ventricular hypertrophy, secondary to either pulmonary stenosis or pulmonary hypertension, and frequently accompanies a prominent presystolic *a* wave in the JVP.

Audible atrial sounds also may be present during increased ventricular filling and normal ventricular compliance such as occurs in patients with severe anemia, thyrotoxicosis, or a peripheral arteriovenous fistula. An S_4 frequently accompanies delayed AV conduction even in the absence of clinically detectable heart disease. The incidence of an audible atrial sound increases with increasing age. Whether an audible S_4 in adults without other evidence of cardiac disease is abnormal remains controversial.

The *systolic ejection sound* is a sharp, high-pitched event occurring in early systole closely following the first heart sound. Ejection sounds occur in the presence of semilunar valve stenosis, i.e., opening snaps of the aortic or pulmonic valves, and in conditions associated with dilatation of the aorta or pulmonary artery. The aortic ejection sound is usually heard best at the left ventricular apex and the second right interspace; the pulmonary ejection sound is of maximal intensity at the upper left sternal border. The latter, unlike most other right-sided acoustical events, is heard better during expiration.

Nonejection systolic clicks, occurring with or without a late systolic murmur, often denote mitral valve regurgitation due to prolapse of the posterior leaflet (Chap. 242). They probably result from functional unequal length of the chordae tendineae of the mitral valve and are heard best along the lower left sternal border and at the left ventricular apex. Systolic clicks may be single or multiple, and they may occur at any time in systole but usually later than the systolic ejection sound. Frequently the midsystolic click is misinterpreted as S_2, and the actual second heart sound is called an OS or S_3.

Heart murmurs Cardiac murmurs result from vibrations set up in the bloodstream and the surrounding heart and great vessels as a result of turbulent blood flow, the formation of eddies, and cavitation (bubble formation as a result of sudden decrease in pressure).

The intensity or loudness of murmurs may be graded from I to VI. A grade I murmur is so faint that it can be heard only with special effort, and a grade VI murmur is audible with the stethoscope removed from contact with the chest. The configuration of a murmur may be crescendo, decrescendo, crescendo-decrescendo (diamond-shaped), or plateau. The precise time of onset and time of cessation of a murmur depend on the instant in the cardiac cycle at which an adequate pressure difference between two chambers appears and disappears (Fig. 231-2).

The location on the chest wall where the murmur is best heard and the areas to which it radiates can be helpful in identifying the cardiac structure from which the murmur originates. For example, the murmur of aortic valve stenosis is usually loudest in the second right intercostal space and radiates to the carotid arteries. By contrast, the murmur of mitral regurgitation is most often loudest at the cardiac apex and may radiate to the left sternal border and base of the heart when the posterior mitral leaflet is predominantly involved or to the axilla and back when the anterior leaflet is more severely affected. In the former case, the regurgitant blood is directed toward the posterior left atrial wall.

Many times it is difficult to classify with certainty a cardiac murmur based on its timing, configuration, location, radiation, pitch, or intensity. However, by noting changes in the characteristics of the murmur during maneuvers which alter cardiac

hemodynamics, the auscultator often can identify its correct origin and significance.

Accentuation of a murmur during inspiration with the augmentation of systemic venous return implies that it originates on the right side of the circulation; expiratory exaggeration has less significance. Prolonged expiratory pressure against a closed glottis, the Valsalva maneuver, reduces intensity of most murmurs by diminishing both right and left ventricular filling. The systolic murmur associated with *idiopathic hypertrophic subaortic stenosis* and the late systolic murmur due to a *prolapse of the mitral valve* are exceptions and may be accentuated during the Valsalva maneuver. Murmurs due to flow across a normal or obstructed semilunar valve increase in intensity in the beat following a premature ventricular contraction or a long RR interval in atrial fibrillation. In contrast, murmurs due to AV valve regurgitation or a ventricular septal defect do not change appreciably during the beat following a prolonged diastole. Standing, which decreases heart size, accentuates the murmur of hypertrophic subaortic stenosis and occasionally the murmur due to a prolapse of the mitral valve. Squatting, which increases both venous return and systemic arterial resistance, increases most murmurs, except those due to idiopathic subaortic stenosis and mitral regurgitation due to a prolapsed mitral valve, which often decrease. Sustained handgrip exercise, which increases the systemic arterial pressure and heart rate, often accentuates the murmurs of mitral regurgitation, aortic regurgitation, and mitral stenosis but usually diminishes those due to aortic or subaortic stenosis.

Pansystolic (holosystolic) murmurs are generated when there is a flow between two chambers which have widely different pressures throughout systole, such as the left ventricle and either the left atrium or the right ventricle. The pressure gradient is established early in contraction and lasts until relaxation is almost complete. Therefore, holosystolic murmurs begin before aortic ejection, and at the area of maximal intensity they begin with S_1 and end after S_2. Pansystolic murmurs accompany mitral or tricuspid regurgitation, ventricular septal defect, and under certain circumstances, aorta-pulmonary

FIGURE 231-2

Simultaneous recordings of ECG, aortic pressure (AOP), left ventricular pressure (LVP), and left atrial pressure (LAP). HSM is a holosystolic murmur; PSM, a presystolic murmur; MDM, a middiastolic murmur; SEM, a systolic ejection murmur; EDM, an early diastolic murmur; LSM, a late systolic murmur; and CM, a continuous murmur.

shunts. Although the typical high-pitched murmur of mitral regurgitation usually continues throughout systole, the shape of the murmur may vary considerably. The pansystolic murmurs of mitral regurgitation and ventricular septal defect are augmented by raising the arterial pressure with intravenous phenylephrine and are diminished by lowering the left ventricular systolic pressure by inhalation of amyl nitrite. The murmur of tricuspid regurgitation associated with pulmonary hypertension is holosystolic and frequently increases during inspiration, a feature of diagnostic importance. Not all patients with mitral or tricuspid regurgitation or ventricular septal defect have pansystolic murmurs (Chap. 242).

Midsystolic murmurs occur when blood is ejected across the aortic or pulmonic outflow tracts. The murmur starts shortly after S_1 when the ventricular pressure rises sufficiently to open the semilunar valve. Ejection then begins and with it the onset of the murmur; as ejection increases, the murmur is augmented, and as ejection declines, it diminishes. The murmur ends before the ventricular pressure falls enough to permit closure of the aortic or pulmonic leaflets. In the presence of normal semilunar valves and increased flow rate, as may occur in states of elevated cardiac output, ejection into a dilated vessel beyond the valve, or increased transmission of sound through a thin chest wall, may be responsible for the production of this murmur. Most benign, functional murmurs are midsystolic and originate from the pulmonary outflow tract. Valvular or subvalvular obstruction to either ventricle may also cause such a midsystolic murmur, the intensity being related to the flow. Thus, the murmur of aortic stenosis may become faint ot disappear during heart failure and return when compensation has been restored.

The murmur of aortic stenosis is the prototype of the left-sided midsystolic murmur. The location and radiation of this murmur appear to be influenced by the direction of the high-velocity jet within the aortic root. In *valvular aortic stenosis* the murmur is usually maximal in the second right intercostal space, with radiation into the neck. In *supravalvular aortic stenosis* the murmur is occasionally loudest even higher, with disproportionate radiation into the right carotid artery. In idiopathic hypertrophic subaortic stenosis, the murmur originates within the left ventricular cavity, and is usually maximal at the lower left sternal edge and apex, with relatively little radiation to the carotids. When the aortic valve is immobile (calcified), the aortic closure sound (A_2) may be soft and inaudible so that the length and configuration of the murmur are difficult to determine.

The patient's age and the area of maximal intensity aid in determining the significance of midsystolic murmurs. Thus, in a young adult with a thin chest and high velocity of blood flow, a faint or moderate ejection murmur heard only in the pulmonic area is usually without clinical significance, while a somewhat louder murmur in the aortic area may indicate congenital aortic stenosis. In elderly patients pulmonary flow murmurs are rare, while aortic systolic murmurs are frequent and may be due to aortic dilatation, to a significant degree of valvular aortic stenosis, or to nonstenotic deformity of the aortic valve. Systolic ejection murmurs are intensified by amyl nitrite inhalation and during the cardiac cycle following a premature ventricular contraction. Aortic systolic murmurs are diminished by interventions which increase systemic arterial resistance such as intravenous phenylephrine. Cardiac catheterization may be necessary to separate a prominent and exaggerated functional murmur from one due to congenital semilunar valve stenosis.

Early systolic murmurs begin with the first heart sound and end in midsystole. They may be due to a very small *ventricular septal defect, a large defect with pulmonary hypertension,* or se-

vere acute mitral or *tricuspid regurgitation*. In large ventricular septal defects with pulmonary hypertension the shunting at the end of systole may be small or absent, resulting in an early systolic murmur. A similar murmur may occur with very small muscular ventricular septal defects, the shunt being interrupted in late systole. An early systolic murmur is a feature of tricuspid regurgitation occurring in the absence of pulmonary hypertension. This lesion is common in drug addicts with bacterial endocarditis, in whom a tall regurgitant right atrial *v* wave reaches the level of the normal right ventricular pressure in late systole, confining the murmur to early systole. In patients with acute mitral regurgitation and a large *v* wave in a noncompliant left atrium, a loud early systolic murmur is frequently heard which diminishes as the pressure gradient between left ventricle and left atrium decreases in late systole (Chap. 242).

Late systolic murmurs are faint or moderately loud high-pitched apical murmurs, which start well after ejection and do not mask either heart sound. They are probably related to papillary muscle dysfunction caused by infarction or ischemia of these muscles or to their distortion by left ventricular dilatation. They may appear only during angina but are common in patients with myocardial infarction or diffuse myocardial disease. Late systolic murmurs following midsystolic clicks are associated with late systolic mitral regurgitation caused by prolapse of the mitral valve into the left atrium (Chap. 242).

Early diastolic murmurs begin with or shortly after the second heart sound as soon as the corresponding ventricular pressure falls sufficiently below that in the aorta or pulmonary artery. The high-pitched murmurs of aortic regurgitation or pulmonic regurgitation due to pulmonary hypertension are generally decrescendo, since there is a progressive decline in the volume or rate of regurgitation during diastole. They may be musical when the regurgitation is associated with a flail, everted semilunar valve cusp. Faint, high-pitched murmurs of aortic regurgitation are difficult to hear unless they are specifically sought by applying firm pressure with the diaphragm over the left midsternal border while the patient sits, leans forward, and holds a breath in full expiration. The diastolic murmur of aortic regurgitation is enhanced by an acute elevation of the arterial pressure such as occurs with handgrip exercise; it diminishes with a decrease in arterial pressure such as occurs during amyl nitrite inhalation. The diastolic murmur of congenital pulmonic regurgitation in the absence of pulmonary hypertension is low to medium pitched. The onset of this murmur is delayed because at the onset of pulmonic valve closure the regurgitant flow is minimal, since the reverse pressure gradient responsible for the regurgitation is negligible at this time.

Middiastolic murmurs usually arise from the AV valves, occur during early ventricular filling, and like ejection murmurs, are due to disproportion between valve orifice size and flow rate. Such murmurs may be loud despite only slight AV valve stenosis when there is normal or increased blood flow. Conversely, the murmur may be soft or even absent despite severe obstruction if the cardiac output is markedly reduced. When stenosis is marked, the diastolic murmur is prolonged and the duration of the murmur is more reliable than its intensity as an index of the degree of valve obstruction.

The low-pitched, middiastolic murmur of mitral stenosis characteristically follows the opening snap. It should be specifically sought by placing the bell of the stethoscope at the site of the left ventricular impulse, which is best localized with the patient on the left side. Frequently the murmur of mitral stenosis is present only at the left ventricular apex, and it may be increased in intensity by mild supine exercise or by inhalation of amyl nitrite. In tricuspid stenosis the middiastolic murmur is localized to a relatively limited area along the left sternal edge and may increase in loudness during inspiration.

Middiastolic murmurs may be generated across the mitral valve in ventricular septal defect, patent ductus arteriosus, or mitral regurgitation, and across the tricuspid valve in atrial septal defect or tricuspid regurgitation. These murmurs are related to the torrential flow across an AV valve, usually follow a third heart sound, and tend to occur with large left-to-right shunts or severe AV valve regurgitation. A soft middiastolic murmur may sometimes be heard in patients with acute rheumatic fever (Carey-Coombs murmur). It has been attributed to inflammation of the mitral valve cusps or excessive left atrial blood flow as a consequence of mitral regurgitation.

In acute aortic regurgitation, the left ventricular diastolic pressure may exceed the left atrial pressure, resulting in a middiastolic murmur due to "diastolic mitral regurgitation." In severe chronic aortic regurgitation a murmur is frequently present which may be either middiastolic or presystolic (Austin Flint murmur). This murmur appears to originate at the anterior mitral valve leaflet when blood simultaneously enters the left ventricle from both the aortic root and the left atrium.

Presystolic murmurs begin during the period of ventricular filling that follows atrial contraction and therefore occur in sinus rhythm. They are usually due to AV valve stenosis and have the same quality as the middiastolic filling rumble but are usually crescendo, reaching peak intensity at the time of a loud S_1. The presystolic murmur corresponds to the AV valve gradient, which may be minimal until the moment of right or left atrial contraction. It is the presystolic rather than the middiastolic murmur which is most characteristic of tricuspid stenosis and sinus rhythm. A right or left *atrial myxoma* may occasionally cause either middiastolic or presystolic murmurs that resemble the murmurs of mitral or tricuspid stenosis.

Continuous murmurs begin in systole and persist through S_2 into all or part of diastole. These murmurs signify continuous flow due to communication between high- and low-pressure areas which persists through the end of systole and the beginning of diastole. A *patent ductus arteriosus* causes a continuous murmur as long as the pressure in the pulmonary artery is much below that in the aorta. The murmur is intensified by elevation of the systemic arterial pressure and is reduced by amyl nitrite inhalation. When pulmonary hypertension is present, the diastolic portion may disappear, leaving the murmur confined to systole. A continuous murmur is uncommon in aortopulmonary septal defects, since this malformation is generally associated with severe pulmonary hypertension. Surgically produced aortopulmonary connections and the subclavian–pulmonary artery anastomosis result in murmurs similar to that of a patent ductus.

Continuous murmurs may result from congenital or acquired *systemic arteriovenous fistula, coronary arterial fistula,* anomalous origin of the left coronary artery from the pulmonary artery, and communications between the *sinus of Valsalva and the right side of the heart.* Continuous murmurs may also occur when high left atrial pressure results in continuous flow across a small defect in the atrial septum. Murmurs associated with *pulmonary arteriovenous fistulas* may be continuous but are usually only systolic. Continuous murmurs may also be due to disturbances of flow pattern in constricted systemic (e.g., renal) or pulmonary arteries when marked pressure differences between the two sides of the narrow segment persist; a continuous murmur in the back may be present in *coarctation of the aorta; pulmonary embolism* may cause continuous murmurs in partially occluded vessels.

In nonconstricted arteries continuous murmurs may be due to rapid flow through a tortuous bed. Such murmurs typically occur within the bronchial arterial collateral circulation in cyanotic patients with severe pulmonary outflow obstruction. The "mammary souffle," an innocent murmur heard during late pregnancy and early postpartum, may be systolic or con-

tinuous. The innocent cervical venous hum is a continuous murmur usually heard over the medial aspect of the right supraclavicular fossa with the patient upright. The hum is usually louder during diastole and can be instantaneously abolished by digital compression of the ipsilateral internal jugular vein. Transmission of a loud venous hum to the area below the clavicles may result in a mistaken diagnosis of patent ductus arteriosus.

The *pericardial friction rub,* which may have presystolic, systolic, and early diastolic scratchy components, may be confused with a murmur or extracardiac sound when heard only in systole. It is best appreciated with the patient upright and leaning forward and may be accentuated during inspiration.

REFERENCES

BRAUNWALD E: Physical examination, in *Heart Disease,* E Braunwald (ed). Philadelphia, Saunders, 1980, chap 2

CRAWFORD MH, O'ROURKE RA: A systematic approach to the bedside differentiation of cardiac murmurs and abnormal sounds. Curr Probl Cardiol 1(11):1, 1977

FOWLER NO: Diagnostic methods in cardiology, in *Cardiovascular Clinics,* NO Fowler (ed). Philadelphia, Davis, 1975

————: Cardiac auscultation, in *Cardiac Diagnosis and Treatment,* 2d ed, NO Fowler (ed). Hagerstown, Harper & Row, 1976, chap 6, p 158

HURST JW et al (eds): Data to be collected on every patient, in *The Heart,* 4th ed. New York, McGraw-Hill, 1978, part IV, chaps 11–20

LEATHAM A: *Auscultation of the Heart and Phonocardiography,* 2d ed. New York, Churchill Livingstone, 1976

MILLS P, CRAIG E: Echophonocardiography. Prog Cardiovasc Dis 20:337, 1978

SHAVER JA, O'TOOLE JD: The second heart sound. New concepts. Mod Concepts Cardiovasc Dis 46:7, 1977

232
ELECTROCARDIOGRAPHY

ROBERT J. MYERBURG

CARDIAC ELECTROPHYSIOLOGY The electrocardiogram (ECG) is a graphic description of the electrical activity of the heart recorded from the body surface by a group of electrodes positioned to reflect activity from a variety of spatial perspectives. The source of cardiac electrical activity resides at a cellular level. Most cardiac cells maintain a *resting* membrane *polarization* of 90 mV, the inside of the cell negative with respect to the outside (that is, −90 mV); but the cells are electrically active, and a sufficient stimulus is able to initiate a *depolarization*. Cardiac tissue is unique among other electrically active tissues in the magnitude of the time delay between depolarization and the completion of recovery of excitability or *repolarization*. This results in refractory periods—the minimum intervals required for two successive responses to occur—which are relatively long. After repolarization and before the next depolarization, most cells maintain the state of resting polarization; but certain cardiac tissues undergo slow, *spontaneous depolarization*. If this continues to threshold potential, an impulse is initiated. It is this mechanism which permits the sinoatrial (SA) node to function as the pacemaker of the heart and other regions to provide normal backup pacemakers, or to usurp this function abnormally. Recently, another form of depolarization, which drives single cell membranes toward threshold potential, has been observed experimentally. This is referred to as *triggered activity* because it can be elicited or enhanced by premature stimulation or increasing rates of stimulation. In contrast to spontaneous depolarization, which usually spans diastole, triggered depolarization of single cells occurs relatively early in diastole and may establish sustained activity. The clinical significance of this form of activity has not yet been determined.

Under resting, steady-state conditions, ionic gradients are maintained across cardiac cell membranes. The extracellular concentration of Na^+ is about 10 to 15 times the intracellular concentration, and the intracellular concentration of K^+ is 30 to 35 times its extracellular concentration. The K^+ gradient is responsible for the resting transmembrane potential. During depolarization of most normal cardiac tissue, on the other hand, specific Na^+ channels in cell membranes open, permitting the rapid influx of Na^+ down its electrochemical gradient and very rapid depolarization, which is paralleled by rapid impulse conduction. Stimulation of partially depolarized tissue causes a slower rate of depolarization and a more slowly conducted impulse. The Na^+ channel is inactivated at membrane potentials less negative than -55 mV. Depolarization initiated at resting potentials less than -55 mV appears to result from ionic currents across a different channel—the so-called "slow channel"—carried primarily (but probably not solely) by Ca^{2+} ions. Such impulses are conducted more slowly. At levels of partial depolarization between -90 and -55 mV, slow depolarizations could probably result from either the partially inactivated fast (Na^+) channel or slow channel impulses.

In addition to the uniquely long delay between depolarization and repolarization in cardiac tissue, there is considerable variability in the electrical properties among the various cardiac tissues, including important variations in refractory periods. The electrically active tissues may be conveniently divided into two general types: (1) ordinary muscle and (2) specialized conducting tissue (SCT). The ordinary muscle of the atria and ventricles accounts for most of the cardiac mass. These tissues conduct impulses at a velocity much lower than the intraventricular SCT (the His-Purkinje system), but considerably faster than the atrioventricular (AV) node. The refractory periods of muscle are shorter in duration than SCT, and the SCT of the heart has a broader range of functional properties than does muscle. The primary function of the SA node is initiation of the cardiac impulse, and the cells are highly specialized for the purpose of impulse formation (automaticity). Spontaneous depolarization is the most prominent feature.

The AV node is a complex structure, in which the electrical activity may be predominantly or entirely dependent upon "slow channel," Ca^{2+}-dependent currents. Impulses propagating from the atria into the AV node undergo an abrupt and progressive decrease in conduction velocity, a phenomenon termed *decremental conduction;* i.e., the amplitude and velocity of the impulse diminish as it is conducted into an area which is less responsive, causing a still weaker response, which acts as a yet weaker stimulus for continued propagation. Should this sequence continue, the impulse would eventually be extinguished. However, at some point within the AV node the process reverses, responses to the weakly conducted impulse becoming stronger and propagating into more responsive tissue. After approximately 90 to 100 ms, propagation across the AV node is complete, and the impulse enters the next area of specialized conducting tissue, the bundle of His.

Propagation through the bundle of His is very rapid as this structure moves through the lower portion of the interatrial septum, giving off fibers which become the left bundle branch (LBB) as they pierce the membranous portion of the interventricular septum below the aortic ring. The rest of the bundle of His continues across the crest of the interventricular septum and courses down the right side of the septum as the right bundle branch (RBB). When the RBB reaches the apex of the right ventricle, it fans out onto the free wall as the Purkinje network.

The main LBB is a relatively short structure which bifurcates into two general collections of fibers on the upper portion of the interventricular septum, forming structures which have been referred to as the anterior (superior) and posterior (inferior) divisions of the LBB. The two divisions are not isolated end structures, there being numerous interconnections between them on the surface of the left ventricular septum. The cells of the RBB and LBB systems are highly specialized and conduct more rapidly than any other within the heart. Specialization for rapid conduction achieves an orderly and appropriately synchronous sequence of activation of the ventricles.

The magnitude and direction of the electrical activity on the body surface may be viewed conveniently as an average of the numerous cell depolarizations or repolarizations occurring at a given instant. Although much of the electrical activity from individual cells is canceled out at the body surface by opposing forces from other cells, the resultant recording is a reasonably reproducible and accurate approximation of net cardiac electrical activity.

Early in the development of the ECG, Einthoven popularized the concept that the human body represents a large volume conductor having the source of cardiac electrical activity at its center. While this theory is not strictly true, it still provides the clinician with a practical point from which to work. As an extension of this concept, the *net* electrical activity at any instant in the cardiac cycle may be viewed as originating from a polarized point source at a theoretical "electrical center" of the heart. Since this "equivalent dipole" would have direction and magnitude, one might then extend the pattern into a sequence of instantaneous vectors recordable from the body surface. The application of this concept to ECG analysis is discussed below.

LEAD SYSTEMS The ECG lead system is composed of five electrodes, one on each of the four limbs and one placed at various sites on the precordium. Each lead is a continuous recording of the change in electrical potential during the cardiac cycle between two of the electrodes, or between one electrode and a combination of the others. The right-leg electrode is an inactive ground electrode in all leads.

The original lead system developed by Einthoven is based on assumptions of (1) the homogeneity of the body volume conductor, (2) the symmetry of the leads, and (3) a single equivalent dipole at the center of the volume conductor. The *standard limb leads* (I, II, and III) are composed of three permutations of the right arm (RA), left arm (LA), and left leg (LL) electrodes [Fig. 232-1*A* (1)]. Lead I records the potential difference between the LA and the RA, the positive electrode on the LA, and the negative electrode on the RA [Fig. 232-1*A* (2)]. Lead II records the potential difference between the electrodes on the RA and the LL, the positive electrode on the LL. Lead III records the potential difference between the LA and the LL, with the positive electrode placed on the LL. It is likely that Einthoven arbitrarily selected the relationships between positive and negative electrodes in the three leads in order to have the major deflection of the QRS complex (see below) moving in an upward (positive) direction in most normal individuals.

The central terminal of Wilson (CTW) is constructed by connecting the RA, LA, and LL electrodes through 5000 Ω resistance, in order to cancel out the potentials from these three points. With the forces canceled out, the CTW theoreti-

FIGURE 232-1

Lead systems. A. Standard limb leads, showing (1) electrode positions, (2) the equilateral triangle of Einthoven, and (3) the conversion of the triangle to a triaxial reference system with positive (+) and negative (−) polarity. B. The unipolar check leads, showing (1) the central terminal of Wilson (CTW) (or the indifferent electrode −i) and the chest electrode (C) (or the exploring electrode − E). The 5000 Ω between CTW and each limb electrode is not shown. The relationship between CTW and V_1 to V_6 in the horizontal plane is shown in B (2). C. The augmented unipolar limb leads, using the modified CTW. D. The hexaxial frontal plane reference system. Normal ranges are described in the text, and applications are derived in Figs. 232-5 and 232-6. RA, right arm; LA, left arm; LL, left leg; RL, right leg.

cally remains inactive during the entire cardiac cycle, and an exploring electrode will function as a unipolar lead [Fig. 232-1B (1)]. The selection of the positions for the six *unipolar chest leads* [Figs. 232-1B (2) and 232-2] was based on the concept that the proximity of the heart to the anterior chest wall resulted in the unipolar chest leads functioning as semidirect leads, being influenced primarily by the tissue immediately beneath the electrode. While this concept does not have the quantitative significance originally assigned to it, and the recordings from such leads do reflect the activity of the total heart, there is weighting of the voltages recorded by the tissue closest to the exploring electrode. The six standard chest leads (V_1 to V_6) are recorded by positioning the exploring chest electrode as follows: V_1 in the fourth intercostal space (4ICS) at the right sternal border; V_2 in the 4ICS at the left sternal border; V_4 in the 5ICS at the midclavicular line; V_3 midway between V_2 and V_4; V_5 at the left anterior axillary line at the level of V_4 horizontally; and V_6 at the left midaxillary line at the level of V_4 horizontally (Fig. 232-2). The CTW is the indifferent electrode, and the exploring chest electrode is the active electrode.

Unipolar limb leads may be recorded by a system in which the CTW constitutes the indifferent electrode and the exploring is one of the three active limb electrodes. These leads are referred to as VR, VL, and VF. By disconnecting the input to

FIGURE 232-2

The unipolar chest leads. A. The position of the chest electrode for V_1 to V_6. B. The relationship between the CTW and the chest electrode (C) in the horizontal plane.

FIGURE 232-3

Standardization of the ECG. Standard time calibration is 1 mm = 0.04 s or 5 mm = 0.20 s. Standard voltage is 0.1 mV/mm. A repetitive event occurring every 5 mm (A) on time axis (0.20 s) is occurring at 300 per minute. A repetitive event occurring every 10 mm (B) (0.40 s) is occurring at 150 per minute. C, D, and E indicate that repetitive events at 0.60, 0.80, and 1.00 s are occurring at rates of 100, 75, and 60 per minute, respectively.

the CTW from the extremity being explored, an augmentation of the voltage of the unipolar limb leads by as much as 50 percent occurs. This modification is universally used for clinical ECGs, and the leads are labeled aVR, aVL, and aVF (Fig. 232-1C).

In recent years, the clinical value of chest wall mapping, using multiple electrodes (32 to 192) for simultaneous recording and computer processing for data reduction and display, has been studied by a number of investigators. This procedure yields information not available from the standard 12-lead ECG. New insights into normal and abnormal depolarization and repolarization patterns are evolving, and the value of sequential changes in ST segments during acute myocardial infarction is being studied.

FIGURE 232-4

The waves of the electrocardiogram—P, QRS, T, and U—are indicated. The measurements of the PR interval, QRS complex, ST segment, and QT interval are identified on the right.

ELECTROCARDIOGRAPHIC WAVEFORMS, DURATIONS, AND INTERVALS Clinical ECGs are recorded on paper having a graphic background (Fig. 232-3) to permit rapid measurement of standardized time intervals and voltages. Time lines are 1 mm apart, with every fifth line intensified. Standard paper speed is 25 mm/s. Thus, 1 mm = 0.04 s (lighter lines), and 5 mm = 0.20 s (heavier lines). The horizontal lines, 1 mm apart, permit calibration of the voltage deflections of the ECG. Normal standardization is ↑ 10 mm = + 1 mV (Fig. 232-3).

The P wave of atrial depolarization is normally the initial wave of activity during the cardiac cycle (Fig. 232-4). Ventricular muscle depolarization is represented by the *QRS complex*. A Q wave is an initial negative wave; an R wave is an initial positive wave or a positive wave following a Q wave; and an S wave is a negative deflection following an R wave (Fig. 232-4). A QRS complex having a Q wave which returns to the base line but does not produce a positive wave is labeled a QS complex, and the second R wave in a QRS complex having more than one R wave is labeled R′. The T wave represents ventricular muscle repolarization and is sometimes followed by a small wave, the U wave, the mechanism of which remains uncertain. Repolarization of atrial muscle is represented by the T_a (or T_p) wave, which occurs during the PR interval and QRS complex, and is usually difficult to identify. The interval between the end of the QRS complex and the onset of the T wave is the ST segment, representing the period of time between depolarization of the ventricles and the period of rapid repolarization of ventricular muscle.

The interval between the P wave and the QRS complex is the PR (or PQ) interval, measured from the *onset* of atrial depolarization (P) to the *onset* of ventricular depolarization (Q) (Fig. 232-4). The duration is 0.12 to 0.20 s in the adult. Since AV nodal activation begins before the end of depolarization of atrial muscle, the PR interval may be used as a rough approximation of AV conduction time.

The duration of the QRS complex (0.04 to 0.10 s) reflects the time required for depolarization of ventricular muscle. It may be slightly prolonged by regional block in a portion of the intraventricular SCT or by delayed conduction in a region of ventricular muscle. Block in a bundle branch prolongs it to a greater extent. An approximation of the refractory period of the ventricles may be obtained by measuring the QT interval (from the onset of the QRS to the end of the T wave) (Fig. 232-4). The QT interval is rate dependent, and may be affected by numerous pathophysiologic or pharmacologic influences.

THE VECTOR CONCEPT AND ELECTRICAL AXIS The representation of a force by a graphic description of its direction and magnitude is referred to as a *vector*. In specific reference to cardiac electrical activity, a vector may be projected onto a two-dimensional plane as a scalar vector (Fig. 232-5A to D), or considered in three dimensions as a spatial vector (Fig. 232-5E to H). It may be used to represent instantaneous forces in the sequence of the cardiac electrical cycle (Fig. 232-5A and E), or it may represent either the mean or maximum axis during the cardiac cycle (Fig. 232-5H). Mean, maximum, and instantaneous vectors are most commonly applied to the analysis of the QRS complex, but the same principles may be applied to the P wave, ST segment, or T wave.

When an instantaneous electrical force recorded from the body surface is oriented in a direction perpendicular (or nearly so) to one of the leads (Fig. 232-5C, vector 6), the potential recorded by that lead at that instant will be minimum or isoelectric (Fig. 232-5D, point 6). Conversely, if the lead system is oriented parallel to the direction of an instantaneous electrical force (Fig. 232-5C, vector 4), the potential recorded by that lead will be maximum (Fig. 232-5D, point 4). An intermediate direction will record an intermediate voltage (for example, Fig. 232-5C and D, vector 2). If the instantaneous electrical force is oriented to the positive side of the lead, the deflection will be positive (4 in Fig. 232-5C and D); if the direction is oriented to the negative side, the deflection will be negative (1 in Fig. 232-5C and D). These general considerations may be applied to either instantaneous vectors occurring at any point during the inscription of the QRS complex, or the mean vector produced by total ventricular depolarization (see below).

In Fig. 232-5E to H, seven instantaneous vectors are represented in three dimensions, indicating the spatial sequence of ventricular depolarization. In panel E, the mean spatial QRS vector, representing the net vector of all instantaneous forces, is shown. If the principles described above were applied, the QRS voltage would be large in lead I and small in aVF in the frontal plane (limb leads), and oriented posteriorly in the horizontal plane (chest leads).

When a triaxial system representing the augmented unipolar limb leads is superimposed on the triaxial system of Einthoven, a hexaxial system is obtained which is convenient for estimating the mean QRS axis, or any of the instantaneous vectors, in the frontal plane (Fig. 232-1D). When the appropriate positive and negative voltage orientations are assigned to each of the leads, the hexaxial reference system becomes a simple means of scalar vector analysis, requiring a minimum of two leads for estimation of the mean axis. An ECG which reveals a maximum positive QRS deflection in lead I and an isoelectric deflection in aVF would be oriented at 0°. Conversely, if the QRS voltage is positive and maximum in lead II and isoelectric in aVL, it would be oriented at +60°. The mean QRS axis in the frontal plane in normal adults ranges from −30 to +110°. Overlap between normal and abnormal occurs in the range of +90 to +110°. Generally, an axis > +90° is referred to as *right axis deviation*, and more negative than −30° as *abnormal left axis deviation*. The determination of the mean QRS axis in the horizontal plane (Fig. 232-2B) is similarly derived, normal orientation being to the left and posteriorly.

Three normal ECGs are shown in Fig. 232-6. Analysis of the mean QRS axis in the *frontal plane* (I, II, III, aVR, aVL, aVF) reveals the axis of A to be oriented horizontally, of C to be oriented vertically, and of B to be oriented in an intermediate range. In A the net voltage of the QRS complex is largest in lead I, almost isoelectric in lead III, and low in aVF, placing the mean axis in a direction almost perpendicular to lead III. In B, the voltages in lead I and aVF are almost identical, and maximum in lead II and aVR. The mean QRS axis is between lead II (+) and aVR (−). In C, net voltage is largest in leads II and aVF and almost isoelectric in lead I, placing the mean QRS axis almost perpendicular to lead I. A similar approach is applied to QRS axis determination in the *horizontal plane*. In C, the lead in which the net forces are isoelectric is V₃. Therefore, as shown in the axial representation of the horizontal

FIGURE 232-5

A. Frontal plane scalar projection of six instantaneous QRS vectors. B. Vectors originating from a point source at the electrical center of the heart. C. Projection of the vectors on the lead I axis. D. Lead I QRS produced by the instantaneous vectors in panel C (see text). E. Spatial representation of ventricular depolarization. Seven instantaneous vectors in the sequence of depolarization indicated in spatial orientations. F. Spatial vectors originating from the electrical center of the heart. G. A line drawn through the terminations of the spatial vectors produces a spatial QRS loop (vector loop). H. The mean spatial QRS vector, average of all the instantaneous vectors—to the left, slightly inferiorly, and posteriorly. (See text.) (From JW Hurst, RJ Myerburg, Introduction to Electrocardiography, 2d ed, New York, McGraw-Hill, 1973; modified and reproduced by permission of the publisher.)

FIGURE 232-6

Three normal ECGs demonstrating: (A) horizontal, (B) intermediate, and (C) vertical mean frontal plane QRS axes constructed on the hexaxial system. In addition, the horizontal plane vector in C is constructed on an axial system and is posteriorly oriented. T-wave vectors are similarly constructed.

plane of tracing *C,* the QRS is oriented to the left and posteriorly. If this information is added to that obtained from the frontal plane axis, it is apparent that the mean QRS vector of electrocardiogram *C* is oriented inferiorly, to the left, and posteriorly. Similar principles may be applied to the analysis of the mean T-wave axis, which is normally oriented in the same general direction as the QRS axis. An angle between the QRS and T axes >45° in the frontal plane, or >60° in the horizontal plane, is abnormal.

FIGURE 232-7

P waves of right atrial enlargement (RAE) and left atrial enlargement (LAE).

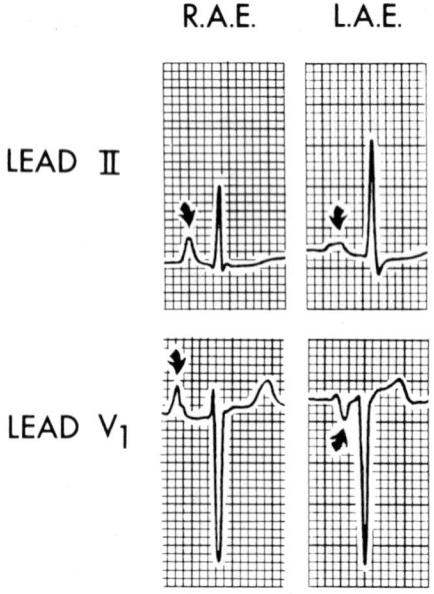

R.A.E.   L.A.E.

LEAD II

LEAD V₁

ELECTRICAL ACTIVITY OF THE ATRIA The mean P-wave vector is normally directed to the left, inferiorly, and slightly anteriorly; the frontal plane P axis is usually oriented between +30 and +60°. Right atrial enlargement causes tall, peaked P waves (≥ 0.25 mV), most prominent in standard leads II and V_1 (Fig. 232-7). Left atrial enlargement causes broad, notched P waves in lead II, and inverted or biphasic P waves (with the inverted portion of the biphasic P wave broader and deeper than the upright portion) in lead V_1. The criteria for left atrial enlargement are nonspecific, similar changes occurring in intraatrial conduction disturbances (Fig. 232-7).

ABNORMALITIES OF VENTRICULAR DEPOLARIZATION: QRS COMPLEX Since the QRS complex is the ECG representation of the sequence, time, and synchronization of total ventricular muscle depolarization, focal or diffuse abnormalities in ventricular muscle or in the SCT may cause changes in QRS form. Abnormalities may be confined to initial depolarization (Fig. 232-8*B*), terminal depolarization (Fig. 232-8*C*), or mid and late depolarization (Fig. 232-8*D*) or may be diffuse (Fig. 232-8*E* to *G*).

The normal earliest site of activation is in the midportion of the left side of the interventricular septum, followed closely by a site on the lower portion of the right side of the interventricular septum and the adjacent free wall endocardium. The dominant wavefront is that one arising on the left septum, which results in a small initial R wave in V_1 (anterior movement), and a small initial Q wave in I, aVL, and/or V_6 (rightward movement). Small initial Q waves in II, III, and aVF may be observed as an indication of a small superior movement of the initial wavefront. Normal septal Q waves are ≤ 0.02 s and of low amplitude. A normal R in V_1 is ≤ 0.4 mV.

After septal depolarization has been initiated, rapid endocardial propagation occurs through both ventricles. In the normal heart, the greater mass of the left ventricle predominates, and the magnitude and direction of the electrical vectors reflect this fact (Fig. 232-6). Most individuals will have maximum QRS duration (i.e., the lead having the longest measurable QRS) of 0.05 to 0.08 s (normal range is 0.04 to 0.10 s). In the range of 0.09 to 0.10 s, there is considerable overlap with abnormal patterns. During normal depolarization, the sequence of instantaneous vectors rotates from rightward and anterior to leftward, posterior, and superior, as illustrated in Fig. 232-5E to G. A QRS duration of 0.09 or 0.10 s may be a normal variant or may represent a conduction delay to limited regions of either ventricle. QRS durations ≥ 0.12 s represent left or right bundle branch block or severe degrees of diffuse intraventricular conduction delay (see below).

Abnormal initial Q waves or an abnormal initial R in V_1 usually represents (1) a loss of muscle mass; (2) abnormal sequence of depolarization; or (3) a change in the relative muscle mass in the two ventricles.

The *intrinsicoid deflection* of the QRS complex is the major deflection *returning* to the base line in a left (for example, $2 \rightarrow 3$ in Fig. 232-8D) or a right (S wave$\rightarrow 2$, Fig. 232-8E) precordial lead. Its *onset* does not exceed 0.035 s from the *onset* of the QRS complex in V_1, or 0.055 s from the *onset* of the QRS in V_5 or V_6. Delayed onset of the intrinsicoid deflection may indicate hypertrophy or conduction abnormalities (see below and Fig. 232-8).

ABNORMALITIES OF VENTRICULAR REPOLARIZATION: ST SEGMENT, T WAVE, AND U WAVE In the normal ECG, the ST segment is "isoelectric," resting at the same potential as the interval between the T wave and the next P wave. Deviations of the ST segment from the base line may occur as a result of injury to cardiac muscle, changes in the synchronization of ventricular muscle depolarization, or drug or electrolyte influences. Elevations of the ST segment, in association with an elevation of the takeoff point of the ST segment from the QRS complex (the J point), may occur as a normal variant, especially in young individuals (Fig. 232-9A). The most common

FIGURE 232-8

QRS complexes. The lead is indicated above each example. A. Normal. B. Prolongation due to initial QRS delay between arrows (1→2) in Wolff-Parkinson-White syndrome (see Chap. 237). C. Prolongation due to terminal delay (1→2) in right bundle branch block. D. Prolongation due to mid (1→2) and late (2→3) delay in left bundle branch block. E. Minor uniform prolongation (1→2) in left ventricular hypertrophy. F. Distortion of total QRS pattern (1→2) in a cardiomyopathy. G. Uniform prolongation (1→2) in an electrolyte abnormality. H. Pathologic Q wave (1→2) in myocardial infarction. Intrinsicoid deflection = 2→3 in D and S→2 in E.

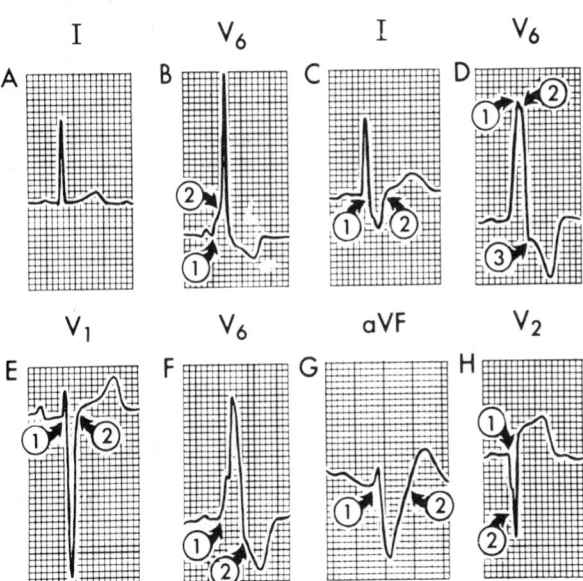

pathologic causes of ST-segment elevation are acute myocardial infarction and pericarditis (Fig. 232-9B to F), and the normal variant must be differentiated from these. Horizontal depression or a downsloping ST segment merging into the T wave occurs as a result of ischemia, ventricular strain, changes in the pattern of ventricular depolarization, or drug effects (Fig. 232-9H, I, M, N, Q, and R).

Since the sequence of ventricular muscle *de*polarization is from endocardium to epicardium, and *re*polarization represents an electrical current opposite in direction to depolarization, the T wave would be in the opposite direction to the QRS complex if the sequence of repolarization were in the same direction as depolarization. However, T waves generally assume the same direction as the major deflection of the QRS complex (see Fig. 232-6). It is assumed, therefore, that the direction of repolarization is opposite to the wave of depolarization—from epicardium to endocardium. T waves are generally considered abnormal when they are of low voltage, flat, or inverted in leads in which they are normally upright, or when they are abnormally tall and peaked. T-wave inversions are reflected vectorially by a widening of the angle between the QRS vector and the T vector (Fig. 232-6). Common causes of abnormalities of the T waves include ischemic heart disease, ventricular hypertrophy and strain, abnormal sequences of depolarization, electrolyte abnormalities, and drug influences (see Fig. 232-9C, D, F, I, K, L, and N to R). However, T-wave changes are often not specific.

The U wave is usually positive in leads in which the QRS complex is positive. The abnormal U wave is manifested as either an exaggeration of normal U-wave voltage, the appearance of a U wave in leads in which it is not normally seen, or inversion of a U wave. U-wave abnormalities occur in ischemic heart disease, left ventricular strain, and electrolyte disturbances.

ECG MANIFESTATIONS OF VENTRICULAR HYPERTROPHY The normal dominance of the left ventricle on the features of the QRS complex is decreased or reversed in right ventricular hypertrophy (RVH) and exaggerated in left ventricular hypertrophy (LVH) (Fig. 232-10). RVH causes a shift of the net forces of depolarization from the left and posterior toward the right and anteriorly. On the ECG, this produces tall R waves in V_1 (≥ 0.5 mV), with an abnormal S wave in V_5 or V_6 (≥ 0.7 mV). In the frontal plane, the mean QRS axis shifts to the right of vertical (usually $>110°$). Less extreme degrees of RVH may result in preservation of a moderately deep S wave in V_1, with an R-wave voltage exceeding the S-wave voltage, or a normal R wave with a shallow S wave and prominent terminal S waves in V_5 and V_6. The primary QRS manifestation of LVH is an increase in voltage in those leads which represent the electrical activity of the left ventricle. R waves in the standard limb leads may increase beyond the normal limit of 2.0 mV. Concomitantly, there is a tendency for a shift of the frontal plane QRS axis to the left. It is not likely that LVH alone will cause a shift in the QRS axis beyond $-30°$, but it commonly causes a shift in the range of 0 to $-30°$ (Fig. 232-10). LVH causes a deep S wave in lead V_1 or V_2 (>2.5 mV) or an abnormal R wave in lead V_5 or V_6 (>2.5 mV). When T waves are normal, the presence of voltage criteria for LVH must be interpreted in terms of body habitus of an individual. Young, healthy, thin-chested individuals will frequently exceed the voltage criteria for LVH in its absence. However, when the ST-segment and T-wave changes associated with "strain" are present (Figs. 232-9Q and 232-10), the voltage criteria must be

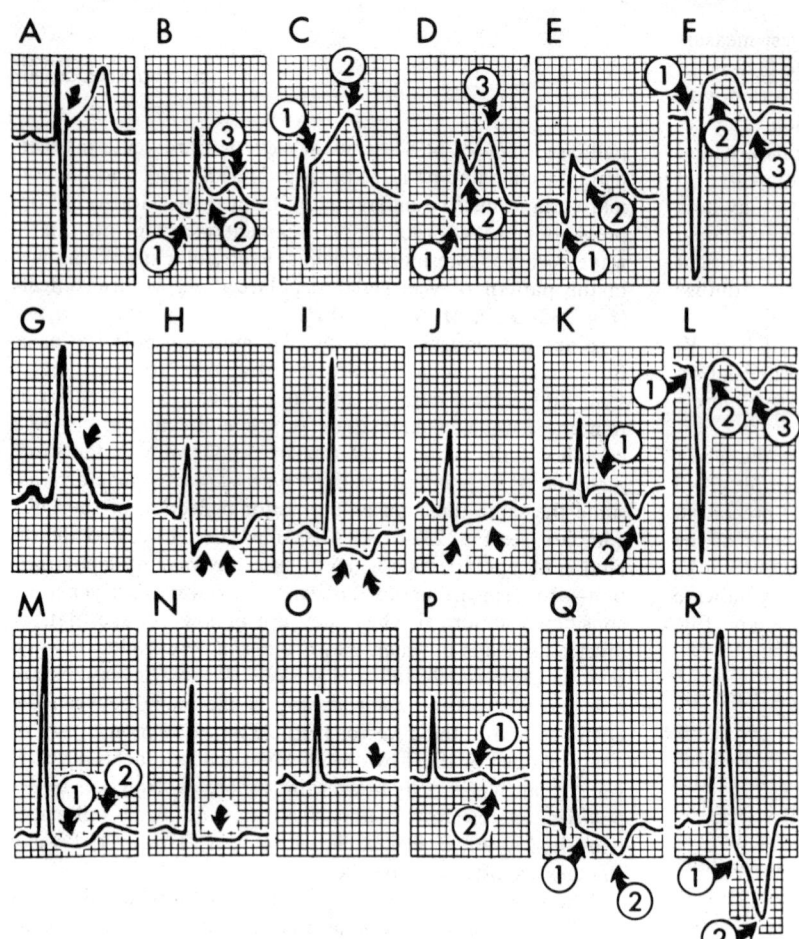

FIGURE 232-9

ST-segment and T-wave changes. Arrows in each panel indicate the major features of each complex. A. Early repolarization (J-point elevation), normal variant. B. Acute pericarditis: (1) depressed T_a; (2) elevated ST; (3) normal T. C. Early acute myocardial infarction (AMI): (1) elevated ST; (2) tall, peaked T wave; steep angle between 1 and 2. D. AMI: (1) small Q wave; (2) elevated ST segment; (3) tall, peaked T wave with steep 2→3 angle. E. AMI: (1) pathologic Q wave; (2) elevated ST segment. F. AMI: (1) Q wave; (2) elevated ST segment; (3) terminal T-wave inversion. G. Angina pectoris (Prinzmetal variant) with ST elevation during pain. H. and I. Angina pectoris (usual form) with horizontal or downward sloping ST segment during pain or exercise. J. J-point depression with upsloping ST segment during exercise, normal response. K. Primary T-wave inversion (2) in ischemia or primary muscle disease. L. Myocardial infarction (healed): (1) pathologic Q; (2) ST returning to base line; (3) symmetrically inverted T wave. M. Digitalis effect: (1) downward coving of ST segment, merging into (2) an upright T wave. N to P. Nonspecific ST-segment and T-wave changes often seen in chronic ischemic heart disease. Q. Left ventricular strain pattern with (1) downsloping ST segment and (2) asymmetrically inverted (secondary) T wave. R. Downsloping ST segment merging into a deeply inverted T wave in ventricular conduction abnormality.

accepted. Similarly, borderline voltage criteria carry more significance when associated with the ST-segment and T-wave changes of left ventricular strain.

ACUTE MYOCARDIAL INFARCTION Three pathophysiologic events occur, either in sequence or simultaneously, in an acute myocardial infarction—ischemia, injury, and infarction. The ECG manifestations of these processes involve changes in the T waves (ischemia), ST segments (injury), and QRS complexes (infarction). The earliest T-wave changes of acute myocardial ischemia are tall, peaked T waves ("hyperacute") (Fig. 232-9*C* and *D*), followed later by symmetrically inverted T waves (Fig. 232-9*F* and *K*). When the electrical integrity of the cell membranes is affected, currents of injury develop. The injury pattern on ECG during evolution of a transmural infarction is an elevation of the ST segments in the leads facing the infarcting

FIGURE 232-10

Ventricular hypertrophy. Left ventricular hypertrophy and strain with R wave >2.0 mV in limb leads; R >2.5 mV in V_5 and V_6, and S in V_1 >2.5 mV. The sum of S-V_1 or S-V_2 and R-V_5 or R-V_6 exceeds 3.5 mV. Strain is indicated by the downsloping ST segments and asymmetrically inverted T waves, especially in the lateral chest leads. The QRS-T vector angle is abnormally wide. Right ventricular hypertrophy is indicated by right axis deviation in the frontal plane and abnormal anterior forces in the horizontal plane. The former is indicated by a small R and deep S wave in lead I, and the latter by tall R waves in V_1 and V_2 with deep S waves in V_5 and V_6. The QRS-T angle is wide (strain).

FIGURE 232-11

Acute inferior wall myocardial infarction. The ECG of 11/29 shows minor nonspecific ST-segment and T-wave changes. On 12/5 an acute myocardial infarction occurred. There are pathologic Q waves (1), ST-segment elevation (2), and terminal T-wave inversion (3) in leads II, III, and aVF indicating the location of the infarct on the inferior wall (see text). Reciprocal changes in aVL (small arrow). Increasing R-wave voltage with ST depression and increased voltage of the T wave in V₂ is characteristic of true posterior wall extension of the inferior infarction.

area (Fig. 232-9*C* and *F*). The combination of ischemia and injury causes elevated ST segments, followed by either tall, peaked T waves (in the very early stages) or inverted T waves (Fig. 232-11). In leads opposite the region of the acute infarction, reciprocal changes occur: depressed ST segments and upright or isoelectric T waves (Figs. 232-11 and 232-12). As the period of active injury resolves, the ST segments return to the base line, but the inverted T waves may persist for months or years (Fig. 232-9*L*). Pathologic Q waves are the QRS manifestation of a transmural myocardial infarction. Q waves are pathologic when they appear in a lead in which Q waves were previously not present, or when the Q waves of normal septal depolarization become exaggerated (>20 ms; >0.2 mV).

The ECG in an acute inferior wall myocardial infarction is shown in Fig. 232-11. Leads II, III, and aVF, which face the inferior surface (see Fig. 232-1*D*), demonstrate the direct patterns of infarction (pathologic Q waves), injury (elevated ST segments), and ischemia (inversion of the T waves). Reciprocal changes (depressed ST, tall T) are demonstrated in aVL. The evolution of an acute anterior myocardial infarction is demonstrated in Fig. 232-12. The most obvious direct changes occur in aVL, V₂, and V₃, and reciprocal changes in II, III, and aVF. In the tracing of 4/11, ST elevations (most prominent in aVL, V₂, and V₃) are accompanied by "hyperacute" peaked T waves in V₂ and V₃. On 4/12, deeper Q waves are present in aVL and V₁ to V₃, and T waves have inverted in aVL and V₂ to V₅. ST elevations persist but less prominently. On 4/25, the pattern of a healing infarction—pathologic Q waves and ischemic T waves—is present. Eventually, the T waves might become partially or completely normal, with persistence of the Q waves. A nontransmural (subendocardial or subepicardial) myocardial infarction may cause ST-segment and T-wave evolutionary changes similar to those seen in transmural infarctions. How-

ever, pathologic Q waves do not appear on the QRS complex, although R-wave and/or S-wave voltages may change. The ST-segment and T-wave changes are common in leads I, II, III, aVL, aVF and/or V₄ to V₆. Similar, but transient, changes may occur during the pain of angina pectoris, in shock, after pulmonary embolism, and secondary to acute central nervous system lesions.

CHRONIC ISCHEMIC HEART DISEASE The ECG in chronic ischemic heart disease is often nonspecific. The patterns of chronic myocardial ischemia are intrinsically variable, and this is compounded by the problem of coexistent ECG changes related to pharmacologic interventions and/or LVH. Chronic ischemic heart disease causes a broad range of ST-segment and T-wave changes (Fig. 232-9*G* to *I, K, L, and N to P*). There may be moderate degrees of horizontal ST-segment depression or a downward sloping ST segment, flattening of inversion of T waves, and prominent U waves. It is difficult to define an abnormal ST-segment depression in precise quantiative terms. However, if the J point is more than 0.5 mm below the isoelectric line, the ST segment is horizontal or downsloping, and there is an associated T-wave abnormality, myocardial ischemia should be considered. The common clinical expression of chronic ischemic heart disease, angina pectoris, may be accompanied by a normal resting ECG or nonspecific ST-segment and T-wave changes. However, during spontaneous or exercise-induced pain, the ECG may demonstrate the horizontal or downward sloping ST-segment depressions shown in Fig. 232-9*H* and *I*, or rarely the variant pattern of spontaneous transient ST elevations (Prinzmetal variant) (Fig. 232-9*G*).

INTRAVENTRICULAR CONDUCTION DISTURBANCES The complex anatomy of the specialized conducting system of the

FIGURE 232-12

Acute anterior wall myocardial infarction. On 4/11, changes of a very early acute myocardial infarction in leads I, aVL, V₂, and V₃, with reciprocal changes in II, III, and aVF. On 4/12, ST segments remain elevated in the anterior leads, but T waves are inverted. On 4/25, a completed large anterior myocardial infarction is recorded—Q in I, aVL, V₁ to V₄.

ventricles, in conjunction with the focal nature of most cardiac diseases, is reflected in the multiplicity of ECG patterns which result from disorders of the sequence of activation of the ventricles. Disease of both the SCT and ventricular myocardium plays a role in the various patterns. The universal feature of ventricular conduction disturbances is a prolongation of the time required for depolarization of a portion of a ventricle, an entire ventricle, or both ventricles. Delayed or slow conduction may be diffuse or may be confined to a portion of the QRS complex (Fig. 232-8). Prolongation of the QRS may be modest as in left ventricular hypertrophy or extremely prolonged as in cardiomyopathies or metabolic abnormalities (Fig. 232-8).

The classic bundle branch block patterns are associated with specific lesions in the left or right bundle branch in the majority of cases. Complete right bundle branch block (RBBB) (Fig. 232-13) is characterized by prolongation of the QRS complex (≥ 0.12 s) with the delayed activation of the right ventricle accounting for a terminal delay on the ECG. Since septal activation from the left bundle branch system normally precedes right ventricular activation, the initial forces of ventricular depolarization are not disturbed in RBBB, and the ability to identify coexistent pathologic Q waves is not hindered. The delayed activation of the right ventricle is reflected by the presence of terminal forces directed anteriorly and to the right.

The rightward direction of the slow terminal forces are indicated by the broad terminal S wave in leads I, aVL, and V_6 (Fig. 232-13). The anterior orientation of these forces is indicated by a large terminal R wave (R′) in V_1. Since initial forces are not disturbed, the normal initial R wave in V_1, followed by an S wave, persists. Incomplete RBBB is present when the waveform criteria for RBBB (rSR′) are present, but the QRS duration is < 0.12 s.

Left bundle branch block (LBBB) is also characterized by a QRS duration ≥ 0.12 s. However, since normal initial ventricular depolarization is dependent upon the LBB to deliver the impulses of initial depolarization to the left septum, the patterns produced by LBBB are more complex. Normal septal depolarization is disturbed, and delay of the normally domi-

nant left ventricular forces produces a more generalized disturbance of QRS morphology. The septal Q wave in standard leads I, aVL, and V_6 is typically lost. In addition, the initial anterior force reflected by the small R wave in lead V_1 may be lost because of a less anterior orientation of the initial forces. The delay in left ventricular activation produces the greatest degree of slowing in the mid and late portion of the QRS complex. This often results in notching at the peak of the upstroke in leads I and V_6 (see Figs. 232-8D and 232-14), with a late intrinsicoid deflection (>0.055 s) in V_5 and V_6. Most cases of LBBB produce secondary T-wave abnormalities as demonstrated in Fig. 232-14. Because of the changes in the initial forces, and the secondary ST-segment and T-wave changes, it is usually difficult to evaluate the QRS-complex, ST-segment, and T-wave changes of coexistent ischemic heart disease. When the intrinsicoid deflection is delayed in leads V_5 or V_6, but the QRS duration is <0.12 s, incomplete LBBB may be present. LBBB may be associated with either a normal QRS axis (Fig. 232-13) or left axis deviation.

In recent years a great deal of attention has been given to the ECG patterns referred to as the *left* hemiblocks. As the name implies, *left anterior hemiblock* (LAH) has been proposed to result from disease in the anterior radiation of fibers referred to as the anterior division of the LBB. *Left posterior hemiblock* (LPH) has been assumed to result from disease in the left posterior radiation. The complex nature of the LBB system has thus far defied a determination of whether focal proximal disease or diffuse distal disease in the distribution of these portions of the LBB is the mechanism responsible for the hemiblock patterns, although it is known that the pathologic process tends to be diffuse in those cases studied at autopsy.

LAH results in a moderate delay of activation of the superior portion of the left ventricular free wall, causing a modest prolongation of the QRS complex and shift of the front plane axis to the left. Initial septal depolarization is undisturbed (Fig. 232-13), and the QRS complex rarely exceeds 0.09 to 0.10 s. The differentiation between LAH and left ventricular hypertrophy (LVH) may occasionally be difficult. In general, LVH alone will not produce a left axis shift beyond $-30°$, and LAH will often produce left axis deviation $\geq -60°$. The key QRS

FIGURE 232-13

Intraventricular conduction abnormalities. Illustrated are right bundle branch block (RBBB); left bundle branch block (LBBB): left anterior hemiblock (LAH); right bundle branch block with left anterior hemiblock (RBBB + LAH); and right bundle branch block with left posterior hemiblock (RBBB + LPH) (see text).

features in left anterior hemiblock include a small Q wave in leads I and aVL, with small initial R waves and deep S waves in leads II, III, and aVF.

LPH results in a moderate delay of activation of the posterior-inferior portion of the left ventricular free wall. Again, there is a modest prolongation of the QRS complex, but a shift of the frontal plane QRS axis to the *right*. Thus, the initial septal forces, though generally undisturbed, may be oriented more superiorly, producing small initial Q waves in leads II, III, and aVF. Since the specificity of the ECG manifestations of LPH is not very reliable, many clinicians will not make a diagnosis of isolated LPH without demonstrating a right axis shift on serial ECGs, plus positive exclusion of other causes of right axis shift. Of all the intraventricular conduction disturbances, isolated LPH is the most difficult to diagnose.

The hemiblocks frequently coexist with disease in the RBB system. The combination of RBB, plus LAH or LPH, is referred to as *bifascicular block*—the implication being that two fascicles of the trifascicular model of the intraventricular SCT are diseased. As stated earlier, this probably represents a pathophysiologic oversimplification, but it is useful for clinical purposes. Since RBBB alone does not produce abnormal axis deviation either to the left or to the right, the coexistence of RBBB with abnormal left axis deviation (Fig. 232-14) is usually interpreted as LAH plus RBBB. Similarly, abnormal right axis deviation in association with RBBB is usually interpreted as the coexistence of LPH with RBBB, when the QRS criteria for LPH are met (Fig. 232-13). As is the case in isolated LPH, the diagnosis of LPH plus RBBB is difficult because a number of clinical settings may cause abnormal right axis deviation in conjunction with RBBB.

Trifascicular block describes abnormal conduction in all three divisions of the intraventricular SCT. The ECG diagnosis can be made only by inference, when a patient has bifascicular block and a prolonged PR interval. Confirmation can be achieved only with His bundle electrocardiography (Chap. 237).

PERICARDITIS, MYOCARDITIS, AND THE CARDIOMYOPATHIES

Acute pericarditis causes elevation of the ST segments in many leads without the reciprocal changes seen in acute myocardial infarction (Fig. 232-14*A*). ST-segment elevation may occur in all leads except aVR and rarely involves V₁. After a period of days, the diffuse ST elevations return to the base line, and T-wave inversions may occur. Coexistent ST elevations and T-wave inversions do not occur as often as they do in myocardial

infarction (compare Figs. 232-11 and 232-14*A*). T-wave abnormalities may persist for weeks or months after the acute episode of pericarditis. If the pericarditis is accompanied by significant degrees of pericardial effusion, electrical alternans may occur. On alternate beats, ECG voltage shifts in magnitude. There also may be low voltage of the QRS complexes and T waves in all leads. Finally, the T_a waves may be transiently depressed because of atrial involvement by the inflammatory process [see Fig. 232-9*B* (1)].

The ECG changes of myocarditis and the cardiomyopathies may be either vague or dramatic, but are usually nonspecific (Chap. 247). It is often difficult to differentiate myocarditis (Fig. 232-14*B*) from the late phase of pericarditis in which symmetric T-wave inversions are present. However, myocarditis may occur in many other settings, and an appreciation of the range of the ECG changes is important. Almost all systemic infections may produce minor myocardial involvement. Measles, mumps, influenza, hepatitis, infectious mononucleosis, and scarlet fever, just to name a few diseases, may be associated with ECG abnormalities and with histopathologic evidence of myocardial inflammation. When the myocardial involvement is subclinical, the ECG changes are usually subtle and nonspecific. There are minor T-wave changes, manifested as flattening or perhaps shallow inversion of the T waves in multiple leads (Fig. 232-9*O* and *P*). The conducting system may be involved, and prolongation of the PR interval may be noted.

In more obvious myocarditis, the ECG demonstrates symmetrically inverted T waves in most of the standard limb leads and in the lateral precordial leads (Fig. 232-14*B*). When the specialized conducting system is involved, bundle branch block may occur, and patterns of diffuse nonspecific intraventricular conduction defects may occur.

The cardiomyopathies may be accompanied by striking ECG changes. The patterns observed may mimic the diffuse T-wave abnormalities which accompany myocarditis, there may be pathologic Q waves which are difficult to differentiate from the Q waves of healed myocardial infarctions, or there may be either bundle branch block patterns or patterns of nonspecific intraventricular conduction abnormalities (Fig. 232-14*C*). Certain specific cardiac muscle disorders produce specific ECG changes (Chap. 247).

FIGURE 232-14

A. Acute pericarditis with ST-segment elevations in all leads except III, aVR, and V₁. B. Myocarditis: diffuse ST-segment and T-wave changes, with low-voltage T waves in the limb leads and primary T-wave changes in the chest leads. C. Concentric cardiomyopathy: gross distortion of the QRS complex.

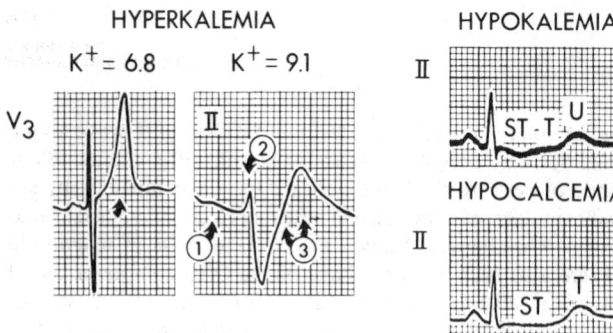

FIGURE 232-15

Electrolyte disturbances. Hyperkalemia (K⁺ = 6.8) with tall, peaked T waves. Severe hyperkalemia (K⁺ = 9.1) with (1) flattening of the P wave, and ↑PR interval (1→2), (2) marked widening of the QRS complex (2→3), and (3) merging of the S wave into the T wave. Hypokalemia produces flat or inverted T waves with prominent U waves, causing prolonged "QU" interval, while hypocalcemia produces true prolongation of the ST segment with marked QT prolongation.

ECG ABNORMALITIES IN METABOLIC AND ELECTROLYTE DISTURBANCES The electrically active tissues of the heart are particularly sensitive to changes in the extracellular concentration of K^+, and dramatic ECG changes may accompany abrupt changes in K^+. The initial effect of acute *hyper*kalemia is the appearance of tall, peaked T waves (Fig. 232-15). As the severity of hyperkalemia increases, the QRS complex blends into the tall, peaked T waves, P-wave voltage decreases and may disappear entirely, and the PR interval is prolonged. As these changes evolve, there is marked prolongation of the QRS complex (Fig. 232-15) with the evolution of continuity between the S wave and T wave, ultimately producing a sine wave configuration. This pattern is a very late and ominous manifestation of hyperkalemia. Equally dangerous is the occurrence of severe *hypo*kalemia, which also produces characteristic ECG changes. Instead of the tall, peaked T waves of hyperkalemia, hypokalemia produces a flattening or inversion of the T wave, but at the same time a prominence of the U wave. In its fully developed state, the ECG gives the appearance of a very long QT interval. Careful analysis reveals that the QT interval is not so prolonged, and the U wave has assumed the appearance of the T wave (Fig. 232-15). Thus, the major prolongation is a "QU" prolongation. This ECG manifestation of hypokalemia may forewarn of the occurrence of serious ventricular arrhythmias, especially in the presence of digitalis. One must be careful to differentiate the ECG effects of hypo*calcemia* from hypo*kalemia*. Whereas hypokalemia may produce the appearance of a long ST segment and late T wave because of flattening of the T wave and prominence of the U wave, hypocalcemia does, in fact, produce prolongation of the ST segment with a late T wave (Fig. 232-15). Hypocalcemia is not as immediately ominous as hypokalemia in regard to potentially serious ventricular arrhythmias. Most of the other electrolyte imbalances produce ECG changes too nonspecific to be clinically useful.

Abnormalities of metabolism, such as hyper- or hypothyroidism, Addison's disease, diabetic ketoacidosis, and the infiltrative diseases such as amyloidosis and hemachromatosis, all may produce ECG abnormalities which may be helpful in the recognition of the disease process but are often nonspecific.

VECTORCARDIOGRAPHY

A vectorcardiogram (VCG) is a continuous loop representing the sequence of instantaneous electrical vectors in a two-dimensional plane (shown diagrammatically in Fig. 232-5G). This form of recording, requiring simultaneous voltage infor-

mation from two leads, is achieved by recording one ECG lead on the vertical axis and replacing time by a second lead on the horizontal axis. The resulting loop is photographed on an oscilloscope screen. Most VCG systems today employ an XYZ lead system in which X is analogous to lead I (left-right), Y is analogous to lead aVF (superoinferior), and Z represents a lead in the anteroposterior orientation, most closely analogous to lead V_2. The XY plane records a vectorial loop in the frontal plane, projected on the hexaxial reference in Fig. 232-1D. The XZ plane records the horizontal loop in which the left-right orientation is plotted against the anteroposterior orientation on a reference system similar to that in Fig. 232-2B. In the YZ plane, the loop is in the sagittal orientation—the anteroposterior orientation (Z) plotted against the superoinferior orientation (Y). Recording in three planes provides reasonably precise information of spatial vectors, as in Fig. 232-5F. The loops are interrupted every 1 to 2.5 ms with intentional distortion of the interrupted display points. The result is a loop consisting of comma-shaped dots, the orientation of the comma indicating the direction of rotation, and the frequency of interruption providing a measurement of time. Closely grouped dots indicate a slow change in the magnitude and direction of the vector, while widely spread dots indicate rapid changes. Vectorial information of P waves, QRS complexes, ST segments, and T waves may be obtained, but the most valuable information is that derived from the QRS complexes.

The greatest value of the VCG today lies in the analysis of Q waves of uncertain significance and of certain intraventricular conduction abnormalities. When normal septal Q waves are absent in lead I or V_6, and no other evidence of septal infarction is present, the VCG may demonstrate either that the normal Q loop in the horizontal plane is absent, indicating a septal infarction or scarring, or conversely that the Q loop in the horizontal plane is morphologically normal but oriented directly anteriorly, accounting for the absence of the initial rightward forces. Similarly, the VCG can be helpful in assessing confusing initial forces or poor R-wave progression in the anterior precordial leads. Small Q waves, QS complexes, or poor R-wave progression may indicate anterior myocardial infarction (see above) but may also occur as a normal variant, as a consequence of chronic lung disease, or due to improperly positioned electrodes. The initial forces of the horizontal loop of the vectorcardiogram may be helpful when the VCG is either definitely normal or definitely abnormal.

The VCG is particularly useful in identifying inferior wall myocardial infarctions. When the ECG is equivocal, the VCG may show the superior displacement of initial forces in the frontal plane and the clockwise rotation that is characteristic of inferior wall myocardial infarction. Furthermore, the difficulty in differentiating inferior wall infarctions from left anterior hemiblock on ECG, or recognizing their coexistence, may be aided by a VCG. In left anterior hemiblock, the initial forces are often normal, but there is superior displacement of the major portion of the frontal plane loop. However, the rotation is counterclockwise, in contrast to the clockwise rotation of inferior wall myocardial infarction. When the combination of inferior wall myocardial infarction and left anterior hemiblock is present, the infarction may be masked on the ECG; but the VCG may show the distinctly abnormal superiorly displaced initial forces of inferior wall myocardial infarction plus the counterclockwise rotation in the frontal plane, characteristic of left anterior hemiblock.

In most other settings, the usefulness of VCG is limited, since much of the information can be obtained from the standard ECG. However, it may be helpful in patients with complex disease processes in which infarction and conduction disturbances are suspected, with chest wall deformities and unusual electrocardiographic patterns, and ECG abnormalities in the absence of clinical suspicion of heart disease.

REFERENCES

BERNE RM (ed): Electrophysiology of the heart, in *Handbook of Physiology*, sec 2: *The Cardiovascular System*, vol 1: *The Heart*. Washington, DC, American Physiological Society, 1979, pp 187–428

COOKSEY JD et al: *Clinical Vectorcardiography and Electrocardiography*, 2d ed. Chicago, Year Book, 1977

CRANEFIELD PF: Action potentials, afterpotentials, and arrhythmias. Circ Res 41:415, 1977

FISCH C (ed): *Cardiovascular Clinics*, vol 5, no 3: *Complex Electrocardiography I*. Philadelphia, Davis, 1973

———— (ed): *Cardiovascular Clinics*, vol 6, no 1: *Complex Electrocardiography II*. Philadelphia, Davis, 1974

HOFFMAN BF, CRANEFIELD PF: *Electrophysiology of the Heart*. New York, McGraw-Hill, 1960

HORAN L, FLOWERS NC: Echocardiography and vectorcardiography, in *Heart Disease*, E Braunwald (ed). Philadelphia, Saunders, 1980, chap 7

HURST JW, MYERBURG RJ: *Introduction to Electrocardiography*, 2d ed. New York, McGraw-Hill, 1973

LIPMAN BS et al: *Clinical Scalar Electrocardiography*, 6th ed. Chicago, Year Book, 1972

SCHLANT RC, HURST JW (eds): *Advances in Electrocardiography*, 2d ed. New York, Grune & Stratton, 1976

233

ECHOCARDIOGRAPHY AND OTHER NONINVASIVE METHODS OF CARDIAC EXAMINATION

ROBERT A. O'ROURKE
JOHN ROSS, JR.

The indirect methods for examination of the heart, which encompass special diagnostic approaches other than cardiac catheterization or injection of radiographic contrast medium into the circulation, include electrocardiography (Chap. 232); roentgenography, phonocardiography, external recordings of pulse waveforms, and the use of radioisotopes. Recently, there have been important advances in the use of reflected ultrasound to define cardiac anatomy and function in subjects with suspected or definite cardiac disease. As a result, echocardiography has become one of the most useful noninvasive techniques for examination of the heart.

ROENTGENOGRAPHY   Roentgenographic examination of the heart and lungs is one of the most valuable indirect tools available to the physician. Although standard 6-ft posteroanterior and lateral chest roentgenograms may provide adequate information, overpenetrated frontal, lateral, and oblique views obtained when the esophagus is filled with barium paste are essential for visualization of specific regions of the heart.

The cardiac silhouette   In the posteroanterior projection, left ventricular enlargement often causes convexity of the left cardiac border, and the cardiac apex is displaced downward, below the level of the diaphragm. Enlargement of the right ventricle, which has no representation in the frontal projection, may result in tipping upward of the cardiac apex. An enlarged left atrium may produce a round "double density" in the center of the cardiac silhouette and upward displacement of the left main bronchus.

In the right anterior oblique (RAO) projection, the barium-filled esophagus courses directly adjacent to the left atrium.

This projection is helpful for detecting right ventricular enlargement and is of particular value for recognizing compression or posterior displacement of the esophagus by an enlarged left atrium.

In the left anterior oblique (LAO) projection, the posterior aspect of the left ventricle normally clears the spine with the patient rotated to an angle of 60° or less in relation to the plane of the film. When the left ventricle is enlarged, it overlaps the spine when the patient is rotated 60° or more from the posteroanterior position, but it should be appreciated that marked right ventricular enlargement alone can cause posterior displacement of the left ventricle.

The dimensions of the cardiac silhouette relative to the bony thorax can be measured directly from the standard 6-ft chest roentgenogram. The measurement most commonly made is the cardiothoracic ratio, which is obtained by dividing the transverse diameter of the heart (defined as the distance from the outermost point of the right cardiac border to the midsternal line, plus the distance from the outermost point of the left cardiac border to the midsternal line) by the internal diameter of the thorax at its widest point above the diaphragm. Although the cardiothoracic ratio is dependent on the configuration of the chest, generally it is less than 0.5 in normal subjects.

Image-intensification fluroscopy may be employed to define further the size and the pulsations of the cardiac chambers and great vessels. It also is useful for detecting areas of calcification within the cardiac valves, coronary arteries, or pericardium. The characteristic motion of the cardiac valves observed on fluoroscopy aids considerably in identifying the site of a calcification.

The pulmonary vasculature   The size of the central and peripheral pulmonary blood vessels can be evaluated from the standard chest roentgenogram. Estimation of the degree of pulmonary vascularity may be of great diagnostic importance, particularly in patients suspected of having congenital heart disease, and a disproportion between the size of the central and peripheral pulmonary arteries (enlarged main vessels that taper sharply) suggests an elevated pulmonary vascular resistance.

An unusually prominent pulmonary vascular pattern is observed in lesions associated with left-to-right shunting of blood, and the main pulmonary artery segment often is enlarged. Examination of the heart for specific chamber enlargement often aids in determining the location of the shunt. For example, in patients with atrial septal defect there is right ventricular enlargement, but the left atrium and left ventricle are small because the defect allows decompression of those chambers. In contrast, in patients with ventricular septal defect both the left atrium and left ventricle are enlarged.

A selective increase in the caliber of the upper lobe pulmonary veins can be observed with lesions such as mitral stenosis that produce left atrial hypertension. In addition, the normal pattern in the upright subject, a more prominent vascular pattern at the lung bases than at the apexes, may be reversed in patients with an elevated left atrial pressure. Higher levels of pulmonary venous pressure (exceeding 15 to 20 mmHg) may also be associated with interstitial edema or fibrosis in the interlobular septa, resulting in the Kerley B lines, horizontal markings about 1 cm in length appearing above the diaphragm near the rib cage. Pulmonary edema (fluid within the alveoli) may be secondary to acute left atrial hypertension or left ventricular failure and is characterized by bilateral, confluent "butterfly" densities in the central lung fields.

Decreased pulmonary vascularity is observed most commonly with lesions that cause both obstruction to right ventricular outflow and right-to-left shunting of blood. The reduction in pulmonary blood flow results in diminished caliber of the pulmonary arteries and veins, and the left atrium also may be small; such findings are present in patients with tetralogy of Fallot. In patients with pure valvular pulmonic stenosis, the pulmonary vascularity often is not diminished, since the pulmonary blood flow may be normal.

RADIOISOTOPE EXAMINATION OF THE HEART The intravenous injection of macroaggregated ^{131}I-labeled albumin, with subsequent scanning of the lung fields for underperfused areas, is valuable in the detection of pulmonary emboli (Chap. 266). Another application of this approach is to scan the cardiac silhouette after intravenous injection of the radioisotope; the area of the cardiac silhouette occupied by the labeled intracardiac blood pool is then compared with the cardiac silhouette on the chest roentgenogram for the detection of pericardial effusion. The intravenous injection of a small bolus of a gamma emitter such as [^{99m}Tc]pertechnetate permits rapid, sequential visualization of the heart, great vessels, and pulmonary vasculature by use of an Anger scintillation camera. The image usually is recorded, stored on tape, replayed, and photographed. This technique is used in the diagnosis of a variety of congenital and acquired cardiac lesions as well as for detecting pulmonary emboli and pericardial effusion. Recently, several radionuclide techniques have attained wide usage for demonstrating myocardial ischemia in patients with angina pectoris, for diagnosing acute myocardial infarction, for the noninvasive

assessment of right and left ventricular performance, and for detecting ventricular wall motion abnormalities.

Myocardial perfusion imaging Thallium 201 (^{201}Tl), a radiopharmaceutical substance with biologic properties similar to those of potassium, is the most commonly used radionuclide for detecting myocardial ischemia in patients with coronary artery disease. When administered intravenously, the myocardial distribution of ^{201}Tl (half-life 72 h) is directly proportional to myocardial blood flow, and regions of the ventricle with low flow such as areas of acute ischemia, myocardial infarction, or scar will accumulate less radionuclide. Such regions appear as defects or "cold spots" on the myocardial image obtained by a scintillation camera positioned over the precordium (Fig. 233-1*A*).

Most patients with coronary artery disease but no infarction will have normal myocardial perfusion scans at rest; therefore, ^{201}Tl scans are commonly performed during stress when myocardial oxygen consumption is increased and relatively less tracer is delivered to ischemic myocardium distal to coronary lesions than to normal regions. Exercise myocardial perfusion imaging is performed in conjunction with the standard ECG exercise stress test with ^{201}Tl injected intravenously when the patient develops chest discomfort, ischemic ECG changes, or extreme fatigue. When possible, exercise is continued for 30 to 60 s to allow the radionuclide to distribute in the myocardium during exercise. Immediately following exercise, myocardial scintigrams are obtained in at least three projections. If a perfusion defect is present on the exercise scans, a second set of ^{201}Tl scans is taken at rest 4 h after exercise when the tracer has been redistributed in the myocardium, and/or

FIGURE 233-1

Examples of the use of three different scintigraphic techniques in patients with ischemic heart disease. Actual scintigrams at top and explanatory diagrams below. A. Thallium 201 scan immediately after exercise in the left anterior oblique (LAO) view shows an inferior wall perfusion defect (↑). RV = right ventricle and LV = left ventricle. B. A technetium
pyrophosphate (TcPYP) scan shows a localized region of heavy uptake (↑) in a patient with a recent inferior wall myocardial infarction. R = ribs and S = sternum. C. A gated blood pool scan in a postinfarction patient with septal and inferior wall akinesis (↑). ED = end-diastolic image and ES = end-systolic image. The posterior wall (far right) moves normally from ED to ES. (Courtesy of S Sorenson.)

A. Thallium 201 Scintiscan   B. 99m-Tc-PYP Scintiscan   C. 99m-Tc-Gated Blood Pool Scan

LAO   LAO   LAO

RV — LV   S — R   RV — LV — ED — ES

the myocardial imaging procedure is repeated a week later with the patient at rest. The comparison of scans obtained at rest to that following maximum stress permits the separation of patients into three groups: normal, those with transient ischemia, and those with infarction or scar in whom the scan is abnormal at rest.

Several recent studies indicate that exercise ^{201}Tl scintiscans are a useful adjunct to conventional exercise testing in detecting and localizing areas of myocardial ischemia, particularly when evaluating patients with abnormal resting ECGs, those who develop conduction defects or arrhythmias during exercise, and those who fail to achieve a predicted heart rate because of fatigue or breathlessness.

Acute infarct imaging   The bone-imaging radiopharmaceutical technetium 99m stannous pyrophosphate (^{99m}TcPYP) concentrates in acutely damaged myocardial tissue to produce a "hot spot" image in most patients 12 to 24 h after myocardial infarction and usually becomes increasingly positive over the next 24 to 72 h (Fig. 233-1*B*). ^{99m}TcPYP uptake is flow-dependent, and at least partial blood flow must continue to perfuse the area of myocardial damage in order for this increased uptake to occur. Imaging with ^{99m}TcPYP 24 to 48 h after the onset of pain will demonstrate the presence of infarction in most subjects with transmural infarction and in the majority of patients with nontransmural infarction; a totally normal scan occurs in less than 5 percent of patients with acute myocardial infarction. Infarct-avid imaging with ^{99m}TcPYP in several projections is useful for determining the presence or absence of infarction, its approximate location, and its relative size. An area of localized uptake with an intensity equal to or greater than that in the ribs is most specific for myocardial necrosis, but this pattern has also been observed in certain patients with calcified valves, unstable angina, or ventricular aneurysm. Diffusely positive scintiscans, commonly with a less intense uptake, may occur after acute myocardial infarction but also have been observed in patients with angina but no infarction and in some normal subjects.

In many patients, ^{99m}TcPYP myocardial scans fade or become negative approximately 6 days after acute myocardial infarction. However, in a subgroup of patients with acute infarction, the scans remain positive for weeks or months after infarction. The presence of a persistently positive scan following myocardial infarction has been associated with a poor prognosis and may be related to the presence of dystrophic cardiac calcification.

Ventricular performance   Utilizing a scintillation camera and a computer, measurements of ventricular performance which are independent of geometric assumptions can be made during the initial passage of a tracer (usually ^{99m}Tc) through the heart. Following intravenous injection of the isotope, the ejection fraction is measured by identifying a region of interest in the right or left ventricle from the computer display and asking the computer to generate an activity-vs.-time histogram as the bolus traverses the chamber. The time-activity curve contains peaks and valleys, each pair representing a cardiac cycle with the peak of maximal activity indicating end-diastole and minimal activity at end-systole. To obtain reliable data, several cardiac cycles are usually summed in phase and the ejection fraction and ejection rates determined. The images from these frames are usually converted by the computer into a film format resembling an angiogram and evaluated for wall motion abnormalities. With this "first pass technique," only one view is recorded with each injection, and multiple views require multiple injections.

Measurements of ventricular performance and assessment of segmental wall motion can also be made after a blood pool tracer equilibrates in the vasculature (Fig. 233-1*C*). Utilizing a computer, multiple gated acquisition (MUGA) images are usually recorded for a 10-min period at a temporal resolution of 20 to 30 frames per cardiac cycle following the intravenous administration of ^{99m}Tc-labeled albumin. That is, multiple "gates" or time windows at various times after the ECG QRS complex are used to gather data throughout many cardiac cycles. From MUGA data, the left ventricular ejection fraction, end-diastolic, and end-systolic volumes can be determined by either geometric means or from the changes in activity vs. time in the ventricle. The ability of these images to define segmental wall motion is greatly improved if the data are combined into a cine film with each frame representing a fraction of cardiac cycle. Gated blood pool studies of the ejection fraction and wall motion correlate well with cineangiographic results and have been valuable in the serial assessment of regional and global ventricular performance in patients with acute myocardial infarction. More recently, gated blood pool studies at rest and during exercise have been utilized to identify patients with significant coronary artery disease and to assess the effects of cardiac operations on resting and exercise ventricular performance and wall motion. Normally, the ejection fraction increases during exercise, but when myocardial ischemia develops it often shows no change or a fall.

PHONOCARDIOGRAPHY   The phonocardiogram provides a graphic display of heart sounds and murmurs, and enhances considerably the assessment of auscultatory events. The modern phonocardiograph is capable of recording sounds in a manner that resembles their detection by the ear. In order to simulate the relative insensitivity of the human ear to low-frequency vibrations and its great sensitivity to high-frequency signals, so-called "logarithmic" or high-frequency recordings are used to provide relatively greater amplification of high-frequency components. Filters also are employed to allow selective passage of low- and high-frequency sounds, perhaps the most satisfactory system consisting of a series of bandpass filters which encompass the frequency fields from 15 to 1000 Hz. The transducer of the phonocardiograph consists of a crystal (piezoelectric) microphone applied directly to the skin or attached indirectly through an air-coupled diaphragm or bell. The crystals within the microphone alter their electrical properties when stressed by sound pressure waves, and the resulting electrical signal is amplified and recorded on a high-frequency oscillograph.

Although the phonocardiogram is useful for determining the configuration and frequency composition of individual cardiac mumurs, its most important application is in the precise timing of cardiac sounds and murmurs (see Chap. 231). Thus, it allows clear definition of a sequence of events, such as the variation in the splitting of the second heart sound which occurs during respiration, or the differentiation of separate systolic and diastolic murmurs from a continuous murmur which continues throughout late systole and early diastole. The phonocardiogram also may provide important quantitative information, such as the precise duration of the interval between the aortic closure sound and the mitral valve opening snap in patients with mitral stenosis, an interval that correlates inversely with the atrioventricular pressure gradient (Chap. 242).

The electrocardiogram is recorded simultaneously with the phonocardiogram to provide a reference signal. Other externally recorded variables that are extremely helpful in timing auscultatory events are the venous pulse tracing (jugular phlebogram), the carotid pulse wave, and the apex cardiogram, each of which is discussed below.

In order to appreciate the significance of alterations in the timing of heart sounds which occur in various disease states and the relation that these sounds bear to external pulse tracings, it is essential to understand the normal temporal relations between the electrical and mechanical events of the cardiac cycle (Fig. 233-2). The normal cycle begins with the P wave of the electrocardiogram, which is followed by right atrial contraction, the initial mechanical event. Left atrial contraction occurs shortly thereafter. The QRS complex ensues, initiating the onset of isovolumetric left ventricular contraction 0.04 to 0.06 s after the onset of the QRS complex. Right ventricular contraction then starts, and the brief period of isovolumetric right ventricular contraction is followed by the onset of right ventricular ejection. The onset of left ventricular ejection is the next event, and since the duration of ejection is shorter on the left side than on the right, closure of the aortic valve precedes pulmonic valve closure. Isovolumetric relaxation of the ventricles terminates earlier on the right side than on the left (at the peak of the atrial v wave). A convenient way to remember this

FIGURE 233-2

Diagrammatic representation of pressure tracings recorded within the left and right ventricles correlated with the ECG and the phonocardiogram (Phono). The striped areas labeled IsoV represent the isovolumetric phases of left ventricular contraction and relaxation; isovolumetric right ventricular contraction and relaxation are shown as cross-hatched areas. M_1 and T_2, sounds produced by closure of the mitral and tricuspid valves, respectively; A_2 and P_2, sounds produced by the closure of the aortic and pulmonic valves, respectively; OT and OM, sounds produced by opening of the tricuspid and mitral valves, respectively. The QS_2 interval includes the preejection period (PEP) and the left ventricular ejection time (LVET), the latter being measured noninvasively from the delayed indirect carotid pulse tracing (see text).

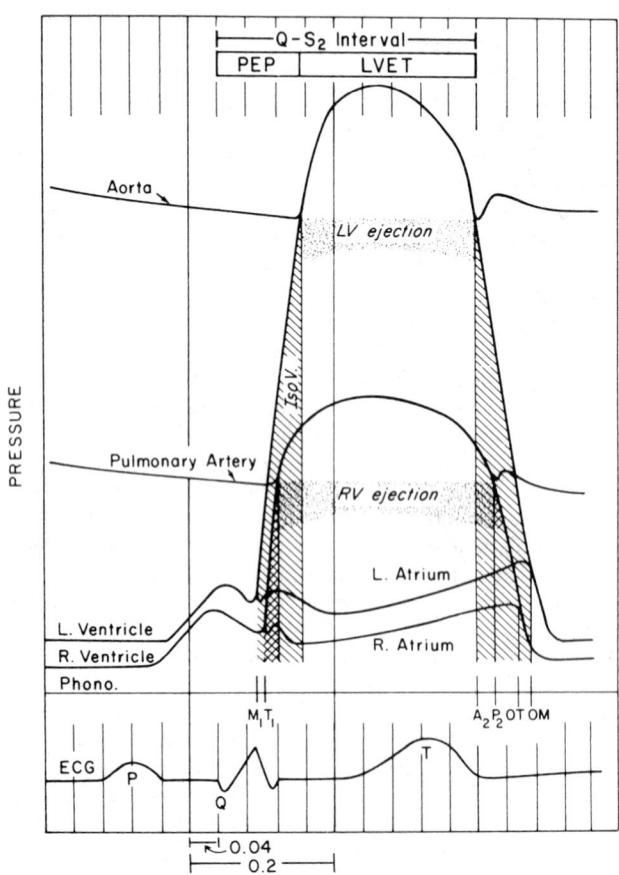

normal sequence of mechanical events in the two ventricles (onset of isovolumetric contraction, onset of ejection, end of ejection, end of isovolumetric relaxation) is to recall that isovolumetric phases of left ventricular contraction and relaxation completely encompass those of the right ventricle (Fig. 233-2).

The jugular venous pulse tracing is obtained by applying a cup transducer over the jugular bulb with slight suction; an inner chamber transmits the pressure changes induced by the venous pulsations to a crystal microphone. The nomenclature of the venous waves is the same as that employed in describing intraatrial pressure pulse contours recorded directly (Chaps. 231 and 234). Although some difficulty may be introduced by a variable delay in transmission of the venous waves to the neck (this delay generally averages 0.02 s), the venous tracing may be extremely helpful in studying the dynamics of the right side of the heart (see Chap. 231).

The indirect carotid arterial pulse wave is recorded with a transducer similar to that used for obtaining the jugular venous tracing. This signal provides an important means of analyzing the carotid pulse contours and for timing the sounds of aortic and pulmonic valve closure (Fig. 231-1). Alterations in the contour of the carotid arterial pulse are often helpful in the diagnosis of aortic valve disease, idiopathic hypertrophic subaortic stenosis, and left ventricular failure (see Chap. 231). Normally, the ascending limb of the systolic carotid wave is steeper than the descending limb; the upstroke time from onset to peak averages 100 ms (range, 60 to 140 ms),[1] and the normal duration of ejection averages 300 ms (range, 260 to 310 ms).

The aortic component of the second heart sound (A_2), generated at the closure of the aortic valve, can be identified by using the incisura of the carotid pulse wave as a reference point (Fig. 231-1). Since there is a slight delay in the transmission of the pulse wave to the neck, the recording of this sound precedes the incisura by approximately 0.02 s. In the normal person, closure of the pulmonic valve (P_2) always follows A_2 (Chap. 231). Although this interval is narrow during expiration (0.02 s) and the splitting may be inaudible, it may be recorded on the phonocardiogram.

Lesions that result in prolongation of left ventricular ejection may cause reversal of the normal sequence of aortic and pulmonic valve closure, termed *reversed splitting* of the second heart sound (Chap. 231). That A_2 follows P_2 may be verified on the phonocardiogram using the carotid pulse tracing for timing.

Systolic time intervals are calculated from the simultaneous recording at rapid paper speed of a high-frequency phonocardiogram, the indirect carotid arterial pulse wave, and the electrocardiogram. These measurements may be employed in the noninvasive evaluation of left ventricular performance. The intervals measured include electromechanical systole (QS_2), the period from the onset of the QRS complex to the first high-frequency deflection of S_2; the left ventricular ejection time (LVET), which begins with the upstroke of the carotid arterial pulse and ends with the incisura; and the preejection period (PEP), the difference between the duration of left ventricular electromechanical systole and LVET (PEP = QS_2 − LVET) (Fig. 233-2). Factors which affect the LVET include the heart rate, stroke volume, left ventricular afterload, the inotropic state of the myocardium, and the sex of the patient. Factors which influence the PEP include heart rate, aortic diastolic pressure, intraventricular conduction, and myocardial inotropic state. Systolic time intervals can be corrected both for heart rate and the patient's sex by using regression equations derived from data obtained in a large number of resting subjects without evidence of heart disease. However, the ratio of the PEP to

[1] *Corrected for heart rate by dividing the measured interval by the square root of the cycle length in seconds.*

the LVET (PEP/LVET) need not be corrected for heart rate or sex (normal = 0.345 ± 0.036 SD). In the presence of left ventricular failure, the PEP lengthens (reflecting primarily a decreased rate of ventricular pressure development) and the LVET diminishes (reflecting a decreased stroke volume), while the duration of electromechanical systole remains unchanged. These altered relationships during left ventricular failure may be expressed as an increase in the PEP/LVET ratio. An inverse linear correlation has been demonstrated between the PEP/LVET ratio and the ejection fraction (stroke volume/end-diastolic volume), the latter being obtained by left ventricular cineangiography in patients with a variety of cardiac diseases.

The apex cardiogram, a graphic recording of the left ventricular apical impulse, provides a reference signal that is of particular value in the analysis of diastolic events and heart sounds. The apex cardiogram is recorded using a bell-type, linear crystal microphone and a filter designed to pass only low frequencies (between 0.1 and 20 Hz). The O point on the apex cardiogram occurs at the end of isovolumetric left ventricular relaxation and at the onset of ventricular filling (Fig. 231-1). Thus, it corresponds closely in time to the opening of the mitral valve and is useful as a reference point for identifying the opening snap in patients with mitral stenosis. Normally, a rapid-filling wave of about 0.08 s follows the O point. In the presence of mitral stenosis this event is replaced by a slow-filling wave. On the other hand, in patients with myocardial failure, mitral regurgitation, or constrictive pericarditis, an exaggerated rapid-filling wave often is associated with a ventricular diastolic gallop or third heart sound (Chap. 231).

The *a* wave of the apex cardiogram is absent in patients with atrial fibrillation or mitral stenosis. This wave may be augmented and accompanied by a fourth heart sound in the presence of lesions, such as aortic stenosis, that produce left ventricular hypertrophy. In patients with hypertrophic subaortic stenosis, the apex cardiogram often exhibits a double systolic wave, or even a triple contour if the *a* wave is prominent as well.

ECHOCARDIOGRAPHY Single-probe unidirectional ultrasound is widely used in the noninvasive diagnosis of a variety of cardiac diseases such as pericardial effusion, mitral valve disease, idiopathic hypertrophic subaortic stenosis, left atrial myxoma, congestive cardiomyopathy, and a wide spectrum of congenital cardiac disorders. With the commonly used M-mode technique, a ceramic compound such as barium titanate is excited by short, high-frequency (1.6 to 2.5 mHz) electrical signals to provide inaudible ultrasonic pulses. Reflection of the ultrasonic pulses occurs at an interface between two media of different densities, only those interfaces which are relatively

perpendicular to the sound beam being sampled. The electromechanical transducer serves as both the emitter and the receiver of ultrasound at a repetition rate of 1000 impulses per second. The echoes are amplified and displayed on an oscilloscope. For recording the echoes, a "time-motion" presentation commonly is used which plots distance from chest wall against elapsed time and displays moving structures as undulating lines. Photographs of the echo display can be taken directly from the face of the oscilloscope, but more commonly the tracings are recorded on a strip chart recorder. The electrocardiogram and time-distance markers usually are displayed on the oscilloscope as well and are used as reference signals on the recorded tracing.

Tilting the ultrasound transducer cephalad or caudad in the fourth left intercostal space permits the echocardiographic demonstration of a number of cardiac structures between the aortic root and left atrium superiorly and the left ventricular apex inferiorly (Fig. 233-3). During the echocardiographic "sweep" the anterior aortic root is normally continuous with the interventricular septum inferiorly and the posterior aortic root with the anterior leaflet of the mitral valve. In position 1 (Fig. 233-3) the ultrasound beam traverses from anterior to posterior the right ventricular outflow tract, aortic root, and left atrium. Echoes from the right and noncoronary aortic cusps are often included in the ultrasound tracing; measurement of the width of the aortic root, the dimensions of the left atrium, and the excursion of aortic leaflets can be made from the echocardiographic recording. Marked dilatation of the aortic root can be demonstrated in Marfan's syndrome or aortic aneurysm; decreased excursion of aortic leaflets is evident when the stroke volume is low; thickening of the aortic leaflets can be seen in calcific aortic stenosis; and a large left atrium may accompany mitral stenosis and/or regurgitation. Furthermore, eccentric motion of aortic leaflets may be recorded in patients with bicuspid aortic valves, and thickened irregular systolic or diastolic echoes from aortic leaflets may occur in patients with aortic regurgitation due to endocarditis. Dense echoes within the left atrial cavity may be due to thrombus, tumor, vegetation, or ruptured mitral chordae.

In position 2 (Fig. 233-3) the echo beam passes through the right ventricle, interventricular septum, and left ventricle at the level of the anterior and posterior mitral valve leaflets, providing important information regarding the motion of both leaflets during systole and diastole (Figs. 233-3 and 233-4). The ultrasound tracing from the normal anterior mitral leaflet is easily recorded and has a characteristic M shape. Various

FIGURE 233-3

A schematic presentation of the cardiac structures traversed by three echo beams (A) is shown with a continuous echo "sweep" from a normal subject (B). T, transducer; CW, chest wall; RV, right ventricle; S, interventricular septum; Ao, aorta; LA, left atrium; and LV, left ventricle, AML, anterior mitral leaflet; PML, posterior mitral leaflet; AAR, anterior aortic root; PAR, posterior aortic root; CH, chordae tendineae; END, endocardium; and EPI, epicardium.

points on the echogram have been labeled A through F by convention and correspond to the positions of the anterior mitral leaflet at specific times in the cardiac cycle (Figs. 233-3 and 233-4). Following the onset of left ventricular diastole at point D, the mitral valve opens, and the anterior leaflet reaches its most anterior position (toward the chest wall) at point E. The initial opening of the mitral valve in diastole is normally followed by a partial closure of the valve which is recorded as a downward (posterior) deflection of the anterior leaflet on the ultrasound tracing. The end point of partial closure is the F point, and the speed of this semiclosure of the anterior leaflet during diastole can be measured by the slope (ratio of distance to time) of the EF segment (normally 80 to 150 mm/s). Subsequently, during left atrial contraction the mitral valve again opens farther, and this event is recorded as another anterior movement terminating in the A point on the echocardiogram. The valve leaflets then return to their intermediate position, and shortly after the onset of ventricular systole at B the anterior mitral leaflet reaches its most posterior (closed) position at point C. Depending upon the exact transducer position, various portions of the posterior mitral valve leaflet are also commonly detected. The normal movements of this leaflet are approximately opposite in direction to those of the anterior mitral valve leaflet during diastole. Shortly after the onset of systole (point C) both leaflets come together and stay in apposition until point D is reached, at which time valve opening begins. This anterior motion of the closed mitral leaflets from C to D is probably related to emptying of the left ventricle during ejection.

Echocardiographic recordings of the motion of the anterior leaflet of the mitral valve have been particularly valuable in evaluating the status of patients with mitral stenosis, idiopathic hypertrophic subaortic stenosis (Chap. 247), left atrial myxoma, or mitral regurgitation due to a prolapsing mitral leaflet;

characteristic movements of the mitral valve leaflet can be observed with each of these lesions (Fig. 233-4). *Mitral stenosis* frequently causes a decrease in the amplitude of anterior leaflet movement (normal = over 20 mm), a reduction of the EF slope (less than 40 mm/s), and a sustained anterior position during diastole (Fig. 233-4*A*). In addition, the posterior mitral valve leaflet usually maintains an anterior position during diastole instead of moving away from the transducer as it does normally. These phenomena result from the continued pressure gradient and sustained slow forward flow across the stenotic, domed valve, as well as from reduced mitral valve mobility consequent to thickening of the cusps and fusion of the commissures. Ultrasonic evaluation of mitral valve motion is particularly valuable in diagnosing patients with mitral stenosis in whom there is no audible diastolic murmur, despite evidence of severe pulmonary hypertension and a low cardiac output. It also is useful in distinguishing an Austin Flint murmur due to severe aortic regurgitation from the murmur of mitral stenosis. Fine high-frequency oscillations of the anterior mitral leaflet often occur with aortic regurgitation, and premature closure of the mitral valve can be demonstrated by ultrasound in patients with acute severe aortic regurgitation and a very high left ventricular diastolic pressure.

Abnormal anterior movement of the mitral valve leaflet during systole occurs in patients with *idiopathic hypertrophic subaortic stenosis* (IHSS) (Fig. 233-4*B*). The abnormal systolic movement begins with the onset of ventricular ejection and reaches a peak with the initial peak in the arterial pulse. The characteristic abnormality often can be provoked by maneuvers which increase ventricular contractility or decrease left ventricular volume (e.g., amyl nitrite, Valsalva maneuver). The systolic anterior movement of the mitral valve is probably related to abnormal papillary muscle position and pulling forward of the anterior leaflet into the left ventricular outflow tract as the obstruction to ejection develops. There is also a moderately reduced EF slope, reflecting a reduced rate of left ventricular filling due to diminished ventricular compliance.

FIGURE 233-4

A schematic presentation of the normal echocardiographic (ECHO) recording of anterior (AML) and posterior mitral leaflet (PML) motion is shown in the center with the simultaneous ECG. Abnormal mitral echocardiograms which occur in (A) mitral stenosis, (B) idiopathic hypertrophic subaortic stenosis, (C) left atrial myxoma, and (D) mitral valve prolapse are also depicted. In the ECHO, the A point represents the end of *anterior movement resulting from left atrial contraction, the CD segment represents the closed position of both mitral leaflets during ventricular systole, and point E ends the anterior movement as the leaflet opens. The slope EF results from posterior motion of the AML during rapid ventricular filling. In idiopathic hypertrophic subaortic stenosis, SAM represents systolic anterior movement.*

This finding may be present in other forms of left ventricular hypertrophy as well. An additional echocardiographic finding usually present in patients with IHSS is marked thickening of the interventricular septum which exceeds 12 mm in diastole and results in an increased septum to left ventricular posterior wall thickness ratio of >1.3:1 (see below). This finding of asymmetric hypertrophy has been reported as the only abnormal finding in relatives of patients with idiopathic hypertrophic subaortic stenosis, supporting the familial incidence of this syndrome. However, recent studies indicate that these echo criteria for asymmetric septal hypertrophy are also present, though rarely, in certain patients with systemic hypertension, valvular aortic stenosis, coronary artery disease, and right ventricular pressure loads.

Ultrasound is a useful technique in detecting left atrial tumors, particularly if the tumor advances partially into the mitral valve orifice at some time during the cardiac cycle. Either mitral valve obstruction or regurgitation may result. A *left atrial myxoma* may be recognized as an aggregation of multiple echoes behind the anterior leaflet (Fig. 233-4C), and there may be a diminished EF slope because of mitral valve obstruction.

Patients with a *prolapsing mitral valve,* in many of whom a midsystolic click and/or late systolic murmur is heard on auscultation, often have a characteristic echocardiogram. Normally, during diastole the posterior mitral valve leaflet echo moves in a direction exactly opposite to that of the anterior leaflet echo (away from the ultrasonic transducer), while during systole the two leaflets come together. In patients with billowing or prolapsing mitral valve leaflets, the echocardiogram may show displacement of the posterior mitral leaflet (Fig. 233-4D) or both leaflets during late systole, or there may be separation of the two leaflets during both early and late systole resulting in pansystolic bowing.

In ultrasound position 3 (Fig. 233-3) the beam traverses the right ventricle, interventricular septum, and left ventricle at the level of mitral valve chordae tendineae. With proper technique both sides of the septum can be recorded as well as the endocardial and epicardial surfaces of the posterior left ventricular wall. Measurements of right ventricular size, left ventricular end-diastolic and end-systolic dimensions, and septal and posterior wall thickness can be made from the echocardiographic tracing. The interventricular septum normally moves posteriorly, and the posterior wall moves anteriorly during systole as the left ventricle shortens in its transverse diameter. Paradoxical systolic septal motion (toward the transducer) occurs together with an enlarged right ventricle in disorders associated with right ventricular volume overload, such as atrial septal defect or tricuspid regurgitation. Diminished or paradoxical septal motion is often recorded by ultrasound in patients with anteroseptal myocardial infarction, congestive cardiomyopathy, or left bundle branch block. Increased thickness of the septum and posterior wall is frequently demonstrated in patients with a chronic left ventricular pressure overload (e.g., aortic stenosis, systemic hypertension), and enlarged left ventricular end-diastolic and end-systolic diameters may be recorded in patients with left ventricular volume overload (e.g., aortic or mitral regurgitation) or diffuse myocardial disease. From echocardiographic measurements of left ventricular end-diastolic and end-systolic dimensions, left ventricular performance can be estimated with a high degree of accuracy in subjects with normal or diffusely enlarged left ventricles, but this estimation is of lesser value in patients with segmental wall motion abnormalities.

Echocardiography also provides a simple, noninvasive method of reliably distinguishing *pericardial effusion* from a dilated heart (Chap. 249). In the presence of a pericardial effu-

sion, the prominent posterior echo from the pericardial-pleural surface is stationary, while a second, more anterior echo of lower amplitude originating from the posterior left ventricular wall moves with the heartbeat. The echo-free space between the two posterior echoes is roughly proportional to the amount of pericardial fluid present.

An echocardiographic tracing of the tricuspid valve can be recorded by angulating the ultrasound transducer medially. A reduced EF slope of the tricuspid leaflets occurs in tricuspid stenosis, an increased leaflet excursion and delayed valve closure in Ebstein's malformation, and systolic posterior displacement of the leaflet in tricuspid valve prolapse.

Movement of the posterior pulmonic valve leaflet away from the chest wall can often be recorded with the transducer positioned in the second or third left intercostal space. A reduced diastolic or reversed EF slope, a diminished presystolic *a* dip, and midsystolic notching during the posterior excursion of the pulmonic leaflet occur in pulmonary hypertension. A marked increase in the *a*-dip amplitude is an echocardiographic feature of moderate to severe valvular pulmonic stenosis.

Recent advances in echocardiography have been particularly helpful in defining the anatomic defects in infants with cyanotic heart disease (e.g., positions of the aorta and pulmonary artery), and the increasing availability of mechanically or electronically steered sector scanners for performing two-dimensional echocardiography should further enhance the value of reflected ultrasound in the diagnosis of various forms of congenital and acquired heart disease. This technique has proved valuable for determining the valve area in aortic and mitral stenosis, for demonstrating ventricular wall motion abnormalities (particularly aneurysms), and for detecting intracardiac tumors and thrombi.

REFERENCES

ASHBURN WL et al: Left ventricular ejection fraction—a review of several radionuclide angiographic approaches using the scintillation camera. Prog Cardiovasc Dis 20:267, 1978

CHUNG EK: *Non-invasive Cardiac Diagnosis.* Philadelphia, Lea & Febiger, 1976

CRAIG E: Phonocardiography, in *Heart Disease,* E Braunwald (ed). Philadelphia, Saunders, 1980, chap 3

FEIGENBAUM H: *Echocardiography,* 2d ed. Philadelphia, Lea & Febiger, 1976

FOWLER NO: Non-invasive methods of cardiac diagnosis, in *Cardiac Diagnosis and Treatment,* 2d ed, NO Fowler (ed). Hagerstown, Harper & Row, 1976, chap 11, p 214

HOLMAN LH: Radioisotopic examination of the cardiovascular system, in *Heart Disease,* E Braunwald (ed). Philadelphia, Saunders, 1980, chap 11

MARCUS MM, KERBER RE: Present status of the [99m]technetium pyrophosphate infarct scintigram. Circulation 56:335, 1977

MURPHY KF et al: Ultrasound in the diagnosis of congenital heart disease. Am Heart J 89:638, 1975

PARKEY RW et al: *Clinical Nuclear Cardiology.* New York, Appleton-Century-Crofts, 1979

SIEGEL W: Examination by external pulse recording and phonocardiography, in *The Heart,* 4th ed, JW Hurst et al (eds). New York, McGraw-Hill, chap 31, p 422

STRAUSS HW, PITT B: Gated cardiac blood-pool scan: Use in patients with coronary heart disease. Prog Cardiovasc Dis 20:207, 1977

234

CARDIAC CATHETERIZATION AND ANGIOGRAPHY

JOHN ROSS, JR.
KIRK L. PETERSON

In 1929, Werner Forssman described the insertion of a catheter through his own arm vein into the right atrium and proposed that the procedure might prove useful for physiologic studies. A little more than a decade later, Andre Cournand and his associates introduced the modern era of cardiac catheterization in man by showing that it was possible to advance the catheter with safety further into the right ventricle and pulmonary artery and to perform hemodynamic studies by measuring intracardiac pressures and cardiac output. The technique of angiography also was developed rapidly in the period between 1930 and 1940, as relatively nontoxic opaque organic iodide media were discovered, and their intravascular injection provided definition of a number of congenital and acquired cardiovascular malformations. Since then, the application of techniques for catheterizing both the left and right sides of the heart, and for selective injection of contrast media into the coronary arteries and cardiac chambers during the exposure of high-speed x-ray motion pictures (cineangiography), has provided precise information about the dynamic physiology and anatomy of the heart in the normal state and a variety of cardiac disorders (Table 234-1). By permitting accurate anatomic and functional diagnoses of complex cardiac lesions, these procedures have placed the selection of patients for surgical treatment on a firm, objective basis.

INDICATIONS

There are several types of problems for which hemodynamic or angiographic investigations commonly are performed, although other specific indications and contraindications may exist in the individual patient. These broad areas may be summarized as follows:

1 In patients with acquired valvular heart disease, hemodynamic assessment and angiographic studies often are required to determine whether the nature and severity of a mechanical valvular defect render it amenable to surgical treatment. In particular, cardiac catheterization studies may be indicated when both the mitral and aortic valves are involved, or when associated tricuspid valve disease is suspected to be of significance.
2 In patients with congenital heart disease, hemodynamic studies and angiography usually are necessary to characterize the primary defect and to determine whether associated lesions are present.
3 In patients with chest pain of undetermined cause, angiographic visualization of the coronary arteries may be indicated, and in patients with known coronary heart disease such studies may provide information that is useful prognos-

TABLE 234-1
Information that can be obtained by cardiac catheterization and angiography

1 Intracardiac and intravascular pressure measurements and determination of pressure gradients across the cardiac valves
2 Cardiac output and pulmonary vascular resistance
3 Radiographic anatomy of the cardiac chambers, great vessels (aorta, pulmonary artery), and coronary arteries
4 Detection and quantification of intracardiac shunts
5 Intracardiac electrograms, His bundle electrograms, and intracardiac phonocardiograms
6 Measurement of coronary blood flow
7 Endomyocardial biopsies

tically and helpful in determining whether operative treatment is feasible.
4 In patients who have undergone cardiac operations, cardiac catheterization studies may be indicated to evaluate the success of the operation, particularly when residual symptoms are present. Such studies may reveal malfunction of a prosthetic valve, loss of patency of a coronary artery bypass graft, inadequate correction of a congenital defect, or residual disease of the ventricular myocardium.
5 In patients with suspected myocardial or pericardial disease, cardiac catheterization may be undertaken in an effort to exclude lesions potentially amenable to surgical treatment, such as mitral regurgitation, coronary heart disease, constrictive pericarditis, and hypertrophic subaortic stenosis.
6 In patients with evidence of pulmonary hypertension, cardiac catheterization should be performed to search for such lesions as mitral stenosis, left-to-right shunts, multiple pulmonary emboli, or peripheral pulmonic stenosis.
7 In some patients in an intensive care setting (e.g., for hypotension or heart failure following acute myocardial infarction) catheterization of the right side of the heart by means of a balloon-tipped flotation catheter (Swan-Ganz catheter) often is employed to measure the pulmonary artery pressure, the pulmonary artery wedge pressure (as a measure of the left ventricular filling pressure), and the cardiac output. Such studies permit proper diagnosis, and repeated measurements allow accurate assessment of the effects of treatment.

GENERAL METHODS OF USE

CATHETERIZATION OF THE RIGHT SIDE OF THE HEART
Catheterization of the right side of the heart is now a safe and well-standardized procedure in the cardiac catheterization laboratory, as well as at the bedside in the intensive care unit. With the patient under local anesthesia, an antecubital or saphenous vein is isolated and a long, flexible radiopaque catheter is introduced. Alternatively, the percutaneous approach is employed, in which a needle is positioned in the vessel, a small, flexible wire passed through the needle, and with a vein dilator, a sheath is then passed over the dilator into the femoral or other vein. The guide wire is removed, leaving the sheath in place, and a catheter is introduced into the vein through it. Under fluoroscopic control, the cardiac catheter is guided into the right atrium, right ventricle, the pulmonary artery, and pulmonary arterial wedge position. At the bedside, when fluoroscopy is not available, a balloon-flotation catheter (often with a thermistor mounted near its tip) may be passed through the sheath, or directly into an exposed vein, and advanced blindly until it is considered to be near the right atrium. Then, while intracardiac pressure is being monitored, the balloon is inflated and the catheter advanced further, whereupon it is usually carried by the bloodstream directly into the right ventricle, the pulmonary artery, and into a third- or fourth-order pulmonary artery branch, from which a pulmonary arterial wedge tracing is obtained. When the balloon is deflated, the pulmonary artery pressure is recorded. Also, with a thermistor-tipped catheter, cardiac output can be measured serially by using the indicator dilution principle discussed subsequently in this chapter.

The course of the catheter alone in the right side of the heart on fluoroscopy or cineangiography may provide a clue to the diagnosis of certain congenital malformations. The catheter may enter an anomalous pulmonary vein or left superior vena cava; it may directly traverse a patent ductus arteriosus or an atrial septal defect; and inability to cross the tricuspid valve may indicate tricuspid atresia.

CATHETERIZATION OF THE LEFT SIDE OF THE HEART Various methods for catheterization of the left side of the heart

have been devised, and each has found application under certain circumstances. Currently, the retrograde arterial approach is used most widely for catheterization of the aorta and left ventricle. The catheter usually is inserted via the femoral artery by the percutaneous method, or through a small incision directly into the exposed brachial artery. The transseptal approach often is employed to gain access to the left atrium and left ventricle, particularly when disease of the mitral valve is suspected. With this method, a catheter is inserted via the right saphenous or femoral vein, and its tip is positioned in the right atrium. A long, curved needle is introduced through the catheter and employed to puncture the intact interatrial septum in the region of the fossa ovalis. Commonly, the catheter then is advanced over the needle into the left atrium and ventricle. Other methods of catheterization of the left side of the heart are used less commonly; e.g., with the anterior percutaneous approach a needle is introduced directly into the left ventricle in the region of the cardiac apex. This procedure sometimes is useful for measuring the left ventricular pressure in patients with valvular aortic stenosis or in postoperative patients with prosthetic valves in both the aortic and mitral positions.

CARDIAC ANGIOGRAPHY **Right side of heart** Selective injection of radiopaque contrast media at various sites within the right side of the heart also may be performed during cardiac catheterization. Injections into the superior or inferior vena cava are useful for detecting the thickened right atrial wall of constrictive pericarditis and for defining certain congenital lesions such as Ebstein's malformation of the tricuspid valve and tricuspid atresia. Selective right ventriculography is used commonly in the delineation of congenital cardiac lesions such as pulmonic stenosis and tetralogy of Fallot. Injection into the main pulmonary artery permits visualization of pulmonary thromboemboli, congenital pulmonary arterial branch stenosis, and anomalous pulmonary venous connections, and may be useful in the detection of tumor or thrombus within the left atrium.

Left side of heart Selective left ventriculography is employed generally to define congenital and acquired lesions affecting the mitral valve and the left ventricular outflow tract and to assess the adequacy of left ventricular function. Mitral stenosis may be detected by left ventriculography as thickening and/or

calcification of the valve leaflets, shortening of the chordal subvalvular apparatus, and reduced excursion and delayed closure of the leaflets. Mitral regurgitation may be detected and quantified subjectively by noting the amount and density of contrast agent which enters the left atrium (Fig. 234-1). In addition, systolic prolapse into the left atrium of one or both of the mitral valve leaflets, secondary to either chordal malfunction or primary myxomatous degeneration and redundancy of the leaflets themselves, may be identified. The site of discrete subvalvular, valvular, or supravalvular aortic stenosis may be visualized, and the abnormal apposition of the ventricular septum and the anterior mitral valve leaflet in hypertrophic subaortic stenosis can be defined. Congenital lesions such as the anomalous origin of the pulmonary artery from the left ventricle in D-transposition of the great vessels are also confirmed by left ventriculography.

Both regional as well as global left ventricular function can be determined from analysis of the left ventricular cavity silhouette on the left ventriculogram. Regions of absent contraction (akinesia), reduced contraction (hypokinesia), or paradoxical systolic expansion (dyskinesia), as well as frank aneurysm formation, can thereby be detected and assessed as to severity (Fig. 234-2). Mural thrombi also may be visualized within such areas of wall motion disorder. In addition, by determination of a magnification factor, the area of the left ventricular cavity can be measured accurately, and by assumption of a geometric model of an ellipse, the volume of the chamber at end-diastole and end-systole can be determined (Fig. 234-1), and the total stroke volume can be calculated. The total stroke volume minus the forward stroke volume (calculated by an independent method for determining cardiac output, as discussed below) can then be used to derive the amount of aortic or mitral regurgitation per beat.

Values for end-diastolic volume greater than 90 ml per square meter of body surface area (average normal, plus one standard deviation) generally indicate left ventricular dilatation due to heart failure, or to a volume overload such as occurs in aortic regurgitation. The ejection fraction, the ratio of stroke volume to end-diastolic volume, reflects the percent

FIGURE 234-1

Cineangiogram with injection of contrast medium into the left ventricle (LV). End-diastole is on the left and end-systole on the right. Study is performed in the right anterior oblique projection in a patient with severe mitral regurgitation in whom the left atrium (LA) is densely opacified simultaneously with the aorta (Ao) during ventricular systole.

Volume of LV is determined by planimetry of chamber area (enclosed by dashed line) and measurement of longest length (solid line between base and apex), using a geometric model of an ellipsoid. Thus, D = 4A/πL and V = π(D²L/6), where D = calculated diameter, L = long-

est measured length, A = area, and V = LV volume. Mean velocity of circumferential fiber shortening (mean V_{cf}, normalized to per unit circumference) can also be calculated by direct measurement of the minor axis (indicated by line with arrows) perpendicular to the midpoint of the long axis, and determination of the ejection time from cine frame rate and number of frames exposed from the beginning to the end of ejection.

$$\text{Mean } V_{cf} = \frac{\text{end-diastolic } D - \text{end-systolic } D}{\text{end-diastolic } D \times \text{ejection time}}$$

where D = minor axis diameter.

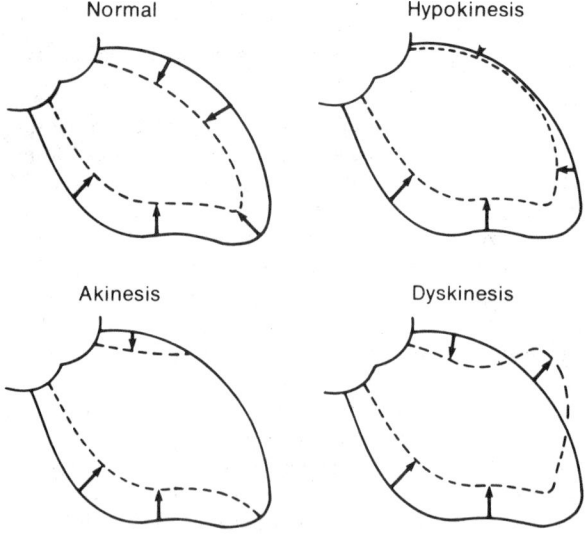

FIGURE 234-2

Diagrammatic representation of end-diastolic (solid line) and end-systolic (dashed line) silhouettes of left ventricular cineangiograms in various forms of localized wall motion disorders. Normal patient exhibits relatively symmetrical contraction; patient with hypokinesis exhibits reduced contraction over anterior and apical surfaces; patient with dyskinesis exhibits paradoxic, outward movement over anterior surface during systole.

shortening of the left ventricular myocardium (normal range 0.56 to 0.78). When the ejection fraction is reduced, the presence of depressed left ventricular contractile function is suggested. A further useful index of myocardial function is the mean velocity of circumferential fiber shortening (mean V_{cf}) or the fractional shortening per unit time of the minor axis of the left ventricular chamber (Fig. 234-1). Mean V_{cf} values below 1.2 end-diastolic circumferences per second in the basal state are considered indicative of depressed myocardial contractility. (Other measures of depressed contractility are discussed below under intravascular pressures.)

Selective ascending aortography is used for assessing the severity of aortic regurgitation, for determining the size and location of aortic aneurysms, and for the visualization of less common malformations such as sinus of Valsalva aneurysm. Direct injection into the left atrium has been used to study the movement of the mitral valve as well as to detect thrombi and tumors (myxoma) within that chamber.

Coronary arteriography Selective angiographic visualization of the coronary arterial tree was proved to be feasible and acceptably safe in the early 1960s, and it has since become one of the most commonly applied diagnostic procedures in the cardiac catheterization laboratory. Accurate visualization of coronary artery atherosclerotic lesions has significantly increased understanding of the pathogenesis and natural history of coronary heart disease. Moreover, this procedure has contributed in large measure to the advent of surgical procedures for bypassing obstructive lesions within the coronary arteries. Visualization of coronary artery anatomy is useful, likewise, for defining congenital abnormalities such as anomalous origin of the coronary arteries, or a coronary arteriovenous fistula.

Coronary arteriography is performed by selective injection of 5 to 10 ml of contrast medium directly into each coronary artery orifice with cinefilming at 30 to 60 frames per second and/or large film or photospot exposures at 4 to 6 per second, thereby obtaining dynamic as well as high-resolution images of the coronary arterial tree. Specially designed catheters are used: one type, which has an open, tapered tip and multiple side holes, is inserted via a brachial arteriotomy (Sones technique); another type is advanced over a guide wire inserted percutaneously via the femoral artery and is preshaped to allow ready access to the right or left coronary artery orifices (Judkins technique). Both techniques allow injections to be made with the patient in multiple oblique views and provide visualization of obstructive lesions within the main branches of the coronary vessels (Fig. 234-3*A* and *B*). In addition, collateral vessels, or new vascular pathways which serve to carry blood around a significant obstruction, can often be seen, and the vessel beyond a complete obstruction thereby visualized (Fig. 234-3*C*). The latter finding has obvious importance in determining the site for implantation of the distal end of a bypass graft.

COMPLICATIONS Catheterization of the right side of the heart is rarely associated with morbidity or mortality when performed under proper laboratory or bedside conditions.

FIGURE 234-3

Selective coronary arteriograms obtained in the right anterior oblique projection. A and B show a normal subject and C a patient with severe stenosis of the right coronary artery. LMCA, left main coronary artery; CCA, circumflex coronary artery; LADCA, left anterior descending coronary artery; RCA, right coronary artery. In C, arrow 1 indicates the area of narrowing in the right coronary artery, and arrow 2 shows retrograde filling of the anterior descending coronary artery via collateral vessels, indicating that a severe obstruction is present in that vessel as well. (Courtesy of MP Judkins.)

However, catheterization and angiography of the left side of the heart are procedures which unavoidably, although uncommonly, can lead to serious complications. Nevertheless, diagnostic cardiac catheterization procedures have been increasingly applied in recent years, primarily in response to the need for precise functional and anatomic information prior to carrying out cardiac operations. A comprehensive analysis of the incidence and types of complications of cardiac catheterization and angiography, a cooperative prospective 5-year study, was reported in 1968, and the incidence of important complications in patients of all ages (including cardiac perforation, major arrhythmias, hemorrhage, serious hypotension, vascular thrombosis, cerebral embolism, myocardial infarction, as well as death) was 3.6 percent. The mortality rate was 0.3 percent in patients over 60 years of age, but was 0.05 percent in patients between the ages of 5 and 14 years. Nearly 24 percent of all reported complications occurred in infants under 1 year of age, although they constituted only 9 percent of the total population, and mortality under age 60 days was 6 percent. In recent years, however, in the pediatric age group greater attention has been paid to preventing metabolic disorders (hypoxia and acidemia) and pulmonary difficulties, utilization of smaller amounts of contrast agents, and use of more flexible catheters; such precautions have significantly reduced the incidence of major complications and decreased the overall mortality rate in infants markedly. In adults, the advent of coronary artery bypass graft surgery has brought about a marked predominance in the application of coronary arteriography and left ventriculography by retrograde aortic catheterization, compared with other catheterization procedures. A nationwide survey of complications due to coronary arteriography reported in 1973 showed an overall mortality rate of 0.45 percent and a morbidity rate of 4.1 percent. However, both mortality and morbidity figures were significantly less in cardiac laboratories in which a large number of examinations were performed, and also varied with the approach employed, mortality with the percutaneous femoral artery approach being slightly higher than with brachial arteriotomy. For example, in institutions performing over 200 studies per year, mortality with the brachial approach averaged 0.13 percent, and with the femoral approach it averaged 0.47 percent. However, in recent years the routine use of prophylactic anticoagulation with heparin immediately before and during arterial catheterization has significantly diminished the complication rate of the percutaneous femoral approach. It seems clear that specialized invasive cardiac procedures in any age group should be performed only in well-equipped laboratories by highly experienced personnel, and the risks of cardiac catheterization and angiography should be weighed carefully in relation to the potential therapeutic benefits to be derived from an accurate anatomic and functional diagnosis.

MEASUREMENT OF INTRAVASCULAR PRESSURES

The pressures within the great vessels and chambers of the heart ordinarily are measured by means of a catheter-transducer system. The tip of the cardiac catheter is in communication with the transducer by means of the fluid column contained within the catheter lumen. A number of factors, such as movement of the catheter and the presence of air bubbles, can influence the dynamic accuracy of these catheter-transducer systems, and miniature pressure gauges attached directly to the tip of the cardiac catheter are finding increasing application. These microtransducers have frequency-response characteristics greatly superior to those of conventional catheter-transducer systems.

INTRACARDIAC PRESSURE PULSES The upper limits of normal for intracardiac pressures and certain other hemodynamic variables are shown in Table 234-2. In understanding the contours of the intracardiac pressure pulses, thorough knowledge of the temporal relations between the electrical and mechanical events of the cardiac cycle is important (see Fig. 233-2). Although detailed study of the contours of the atrial pressure pulses has proved less reliable in predicting relative degrees of mitral valve stenosis and regurgitation than once was anticipated, a general understanding of the atrial pressure pulses is useful in the hemodynamic evaluation of a number of cardiac lesions.

The *a* wave in the right atrium normally is larger than the *v* wave, whereas in the left atrium the *v* wave is dominant (Table 234-2). Therefore, when the *v* wave in the right atrial pressure pulse exceeds the *a* wave, abnormal filling of the right atrium during ventricular systole, as occurs in tricuspid regurgitation or atrial septal defect, should be suspected. A characteristic right atrial pressure pulse also may be seen in the presence of tricuspid stenosis, the contour resembling that of mitral stenosis (see below), as well as in constrictive pericarditis, when an early diastolic "dip" and "plateau" elevation of pressure in mid- and late diastole occur. In many patients, the *mean* level of pressure in the left atrium is reflected with reasonable accuracy by the pulmonary artery wedge pressure (also sometimes termed the pulmonary "capillary" pressure), although the excursions of the wedge tracing often do not coincide with those measured directly within the left atrium. The characteristic contours of the left atrial pressure pulse in a normal subject and in patients with several forms of mitral valve disease are shown in Fig. 234-4. In the normal pressure pulse, or in the presence of mitral regurgitation without stenosis, there is a rapid fall in pressure during early diastole (the *y* descent), and a slow rise in pressure occurs during late diastole (diastasis), reflecting equilibration between the atrial and ventricular pressures during this slow phase of ventricular filling (Fig. 234-4*A*). In contrast, in patients with mitral stenosis the *y* descent is slow and prolonged; pressure in the left atrium continues to fall throughout diastole, and evidence of diastasis on the left atrial pressure pulse is absent because of the persistent atrioventricular pressure gradient (Fig. 234-4*B*). When mitral stenosis is present with normal sinus rhythm (Fig. 234-4*C*), the *a* wave is present, and a large pressure gradient accompanies atrial contraction (often associated with a loud presystolic murmur in such patients). In patients with pure mitral regurgitation, the *v* wave is prominent and the descending limb of this wave (the *y* descent) is rapid (Fig. 234-4*D*).

TABLE 234-2
Normal hemodynamic values,* mmHg

	a wave	v wave	Mean	S/D
Right atrium	8	7	6	
Right ventricle				30/7
Left ventricle				145/12
Pulmonary artery			17	30/14
Pulmonary artery wedge or left atrium	10	15	12	

Cardiac index = 2.4–3.8 (liters/min)/m² body surface area.
AV O₂ difference = 3.5–5.0 ml per 100 ml.
Pulmonary vascular resistance = 250 (dyn·s)/cm⁵ (3 resistance units).

* The figures shown indicate the upper limits of pressure (mmHg) and resistance in normal adult subjects. The values for the pressure waves, the mean pressures, and the systolic and diastolic pressures (S/D) are shown; in the ventricles, D = end-diastolic pressure. The ranges for cardiac index and arterial–mixed venous (AV) O₂ differences are shown.

FIGURE 234-4

Simultaneously recorded left ventricular (LV) and left atrial (LA) pressure tracings in a normal subject (A) and in patients with various forms of mitral valve disease (B to D). The tracings are recorded at high sensitivity (0 to 40 mmHg), and therefore the top portion of the left ventricular pressure tracing is cut off. The electrocardiogram is recorded in the upper portion of each panel.

A. In the normal heart, diastole is initiated by a rapid-filling wave, which is followed by a period of slow ventricular filling or diastasis (bracket D), in which atrial and ventricular pressure rise together slowly. This period of diastasis is followed by the atrial contraction wave (a), which precedes the onset of isometric contraction in the ventricle, the end-diastolic pressure. The c wave occurs during the phase of isometric ventricular contraction and is followed by the x descent. The v wave occurs during late systole and the downslope of the v wave, constituting the y

descent, occurs immediately after opening of the mitral valve.

B. Tracings obtained in a patient with mitral stenosis and atrial fibrillation. The pressure gradient from left atrium to left ventricle during diastole is indicated by the diagonally shaded area. The a wave is absent, and the c-v wave is prominent.

C. Tracings from a patient with mitral stenosis and normal sinus rhythm. The pressure gradient is indicated by the diagonally shaded area. A large pressure gradient occurs at the time of atrial contraction. No pressure rise during the period of diastasis is evident in the left atrial pressure tracings of panels B and C.

D. Tracings from a patient with isolated, severe mitral regurgitation and atrial fibrillation. The c wave is not evident, and the giant v wave in the left atrial pressure pulse is nearly 70 mmHg. There is small pressure gradient during the phase of rapid ventricular filling, because of the large volume of antegrade flow across the mitral valve.

The left ventricular end-diastolic pressure immediately precedes the onset of isometric contraction in the left ventricular pressure pulse. This pressure point therefore follows the *a* wave and precedes the *c* wave, and the coincident pressure point in time in the left atrial tracing is termed the *z* point (Fig. 234-4*A*). The left ventricular end-diastolic pressure may be elevated in several situations: (1) in the presence of myocardial failure, (2) when the ventricle bears a high flow load (as in aortic or mitral regurgitation), (3) when the ventricle is hypertrophied and relatively noncompliant (restrictive myocardial disease), (4) in the presence of constrictive pericarditis, and (5) with cardiac tamponade secondary to a pericardial effusion.

The systolic pressure in the left ventricle is elevated over that in the aorta when any of the various forms of aortic stenosis obstruct outflow. In patients with valvular aortic stenosis, the left ventricular pressure pulse resembles that of an isometric contraction, the contour being more symmetric and the pressure peak more delayed than normal (a similar phenomenon is observed in the right ventricle in patients with pulmonic stenosis). The characteristics of the peripheral arterial pressure tracing also may be distinctive in patients with different types of aortic stenosis. Thus, when valvular stenosis is present, a slow and delayed rise of the peripheral arterial pulse

wave is seen, while in hypertrophic subaortic stenosis an initially sharp upstroke is followed first by a rapid decline in pressure and then by a secondary positive wave, which reflects the development of the obstruction during systole.

Derivatives of pressure pulses   The rate of change, or slope, of the isovolumetric phase of the right or left ventricular pressure pulse, called the first derivative or dp/dt, frequently is used in addition to ejection phase measures mentioned above (ejection fraction, mean V_{cf}) to characterize the contractile behavior of the ventricular myocardium. The dp/dt may be measured manually by determining the slope of the pressure rise, but it is recorded more accurately by means of an electronic circuit or by computer processing. The peak of this derivative tracing (maximum dp/dt) as well as the maximum value of the ratio of dp/dt to the corresponding instantaneous ventricular pressure [peak $(dp/dt)/p$] provide indexes of the speed of contraction of the ventricle and therefore can help to define the level of the inotropic or contractile state of the heart. These measures tend to be below 1200 mmHg/s and 32 per second, respectively, in the left ventricles of patients with disease of the left ventricular myocardium, and they may be augmented strikingly by agents which improve the contractility of the heart, such as digitalis or catecholamines.

The direct Fick and indicator-dilution methods presently are widely used in humans for the determination of volume blood flow, or the cardiac output. In general, the equations used with these techniques are derived from the principle proposed by Adolf Fick, which states that the rate at which a substance distributed in a fluid is delivered to an area by the moving fluid stream is equal to the product of the flow rate and the difference between the concentration of the substance at sites proximal and distal to the area. Thus,

$$q = F(C_a - C_v)$$

where q = the quantity of substance delivered per unit time
F = the flow rate
$C_a - C_v$ = the concentrations of the substance at proximal and distal sampling sites, respectively

(The same equation is applicable to the measurement of the removal rate, or clearance, of a substance.) When flow is the quantity to be derived, the equation is rearranged to

$$F = \frac{q}{C_a - C_v}$$

DIRECT FICK METHOD In this method for measuring the cardiac output it is assumed that at rest the oxygen uptake in the lungs is equal to that used by the tissues, and systemic flow, i.e., left ventricular output, therefore is equated with blood flow through the lungs. It is essential to this method that a sample of mixed venous blood be obtained, because blood samples in the venae cavae and the coronary sinus have widely differing oxygen concentrations, and therefore the venous blood sample generally is withdrawn from the right ventricular outflow tract or the pulmonary artery. In practice, arterial and venous blood samples ($C_a - C_v$) are obtained during the measurement of oxygen consumption q over a 3-min period by spirometry and subsequent chemical analysis of the expired gas. Flow F, or cardiac output, is then calculated. The subject must be in a steady state throughout the period of measurement to avoid transient changes in systemic blood flow or in the rate of ventilation that can negate the assumption that oxygen uptake in the lungs equals that taken up in the tissues.

INDICATOR-DILUTION METHOD This is a special application of Fick's principle. A variety of relatively nondiffusible indicators have been employed, the indicator substance being injected into the circulation and its concentration measured at a downstream sampling site by a suitable detector. For example, the dye indocyanine green is injected intravenously and blood is withdrawn from an artery at a constant rate through a calibrated densitometer, which provides direct measurement of the dye concentration. Generally, a single bolus of the indicator is injected rapidly and is thoroughly mixed in one of the vascular spaces, such as a ventricular chamber; the concentration versus time curve then provides a measure of the rate at which indicator was washed out of the mixing site. Prior to recirculation of the indicator, the downslope of this curve is exponential, and therefore extrapolation of the curve using semilog paper permits the elimination of recirculated indicator. The mean concentration $\bar{c}$ of the dye is determined from the area of this corrected curve and its duration. The rate of blood flow F then is directly related to the quantity of indicator injected i and is inversely related to the mean concentration of the indicator $\bar{c}$ and the duration of the curve t (in seconds) by the formula $F = 60i/\bar{c}t$. A simple example will serve to illustrate

this principle: if 8 mg dye is injected and a mean concentration of 2 mg per liter is recorded, and if the indicator takes 60 s to pass the sampling site, then the flow is 4 liters per minute.

Cold saline is another indicator which is used commonly when a thermodilution catheter is situated in the pulmonary artery. A standard amount of saline is injected at the junction of the superior or inferior vena cava with the right atrium, and the resultant change in temperature (analogous to concentration) is measured in the pulmonary artery by a small thermistor located 2 to 5 cm from the tip of the catheter. Although theoretically heat can be added or subtracted from the bolus during its passage between the injection and sampling sites, the thermodilution technique has demonstrated empirically an excellent correlation with other methods of measuring cardiac output. Cardiac output can also be computed by continuous infusion. Single thermodilution curves provide certain advantages: (1) no arterial entry is required, (2) the indicator is inexpensive, (3) recirculation is minimal, and (4) the analog signal is well suited to rapid calculation of the cardiac output by computer analysis.

MEASUREMENT OF PULMONARY VASCULAR RESISTANCE
In calculating the resistance offered by a vascular bed, blood flow is assumed to be laminar, and the general resistance formula then can be employed. This formula, in simplified form which omits consideration of vessel length and blood viscosity, states that resistance is directly proportional to the pressure drop or gradient across the bed and inversely proportional to the rate of blood flow. This ratio of mean pressure gradient to volume flow is expressed in dyne-seconds per cm^5 [$(dyn \cdot s)/cm^5$], the mean pressure gradient across the pulmonary bed being obtained by subtracting the mean left atrial or pulmonary artery wedge pressure from the mean pulmonary artery pressure.[1] The *resistance unit* (i.e., the pressure gradient in millimeters of mercury divided by the cardiac output in liters per minute and expressed in arbitrary units) also is commonly employed as an index of arteriolar resistance (Table 234-2). Estimation of the pulmonary vascular resistance, which normally is about 15 percent of that in the systemic vascular bed, is of importance in patients with congenital heart disease and circulatory shunts, as well as in certain forms of acquired cardiac and pulmonary diseases. Its calculation provides a useful means of interpreting the level of pulmonary arterial pressure relative to pulmonary blood flow, high pressure and high flow obviously bearing a different connotation than high pressure and low flow.

VALVE ORIFICE SIZE AND VALVULAR REGURGITATION
When the cardiac output is normal, the severity of a stenotic valve lesion may be estimated from the magnitude of the pressure gradient across the valve. When the cardiac output is elevated or reduced, however, reliance on the pressure gradient alone may lead to an erroneous estimate of the degree of mechanical obstruction. In addition, it is of importance to consider the heart rate in assessing the significance of a pressure gradient. When the heart rate is rapid, systole occupies a disproportionate amount of time in each cardiac cycle, diastole filling time is limited, and a large pressure gradient across the atrioventricular valve may exist in the face of relatively mild stenosis. The application of the hydraulic formula devised by

---

[1] $Resistance = \dfrac{[P_{PA}\ (mmHg) - P_{LA}\ (mmHg)] \times 1332\ dyn/cm^2}{cardiac\ output\ (ml/s)}$

where P_{PA} and P_{LA} = mean pulmonary artery and left atrial pressures, respectively. 1 mmHg = 1.36 cmH_2O; 1 cmH_2O = 980 dyn/cm^2 force.

Gorlin and Gorlin to the calculation of valve orifice size has proved helpful in analyzing the degree of valve stenosis in these situations. In simplest terms, this formula states that the area of a short-bore orifice is directly proportional to the rate of blood flow across the orifice and inversely proportional to the square root of the pressure gradient. For example, if the flow rate across a narrowed valve orifice of fixed size doubles, as may occur when the cardiac output increases during exertion, the pressure gradient will quadruple. Conversely, when the flow rate is reduced, as in patients with heart failure, a small pressure gradient may exist in the presence of a severe degree of valve stenosis. This relationship differs from the general resistance equation discussed above and reflects the fact that the kinetic energy losses across a stenotic valve are high, a large pressure head being expended in developing a rapid flow velocity across the narrowed orifice.

It should be pointed out that use of the orifice formula is not valid when significant valvular regurgitation is present and forward cardiac output alone is measured, since an unknown volume of blood is regurgitated and recrosses the valve during the subsequent cardiac cycle. Application of the formula under these circumstances leads to an underestimation of the valve orifice area, since forward flow across the valve is underestimated.

DIAGNOSIS OF CIRCULATORY SHUNTS

When a communication exists between the left and the right sides of the heart, and when pulmonary vascular resistance is lower than that in the systemic vascular bed, a left-to-right shunt of oxygenated blood will occur. Conversely, when the resistance in the pulmonary bed is higher than that in the systemic circulation, or an obstruction such as pulmonic stenosis exists distal to an intracardiac communication, a right-to-left shunt of venous blood may occur. These shunts can be readily visualized and localized by exposure of cineangiograms during selective injections of contrast medium.

Many types of indicators have been employed in the quantification and detection of circulatory shunts. The indicator may be the oxygen in room air, blood samples being withdrawn and analyzed for oxygen manometrically or by an oximeter. Foreign, inert gases such as hydrogen or krypton 85 may be employed; these, like oxygen, are "injected" into the pulmonary circulation by inhalation and sampled from the right side of the heart. They may be measured by a catheter-tip sensor (hydrogen) or by withdrawal of blood samples for analysis. In obtaining indicator-dilution curves, the substance most commonly injected is indocyanine green dye, detected by withdrawing blood through a densitometer.

The techniques used for localizing and quantifying shunts at cardiac catheterization may be divided into two basic categories: (1) Those methods in which an indicator is delivered distal to the site at which blood is sampled (the so-called "upstream" sampling method), e.g., indicator is injected into the pulmonary artery or is inhaled to enter the pulmonary veins and left side of the heart. Blood samples are then obtained upstream in the right side of the heart and analyzed for concentration of the indicator. (2) Those methods in which an indicator is delivered proximal to the sampling site (the so-called downstream sampling method), in which most frequently an indicator-dilution curve is obtained by intracardiac dye injection with sampling from a peripheral artery. This approach permits detection of right-to-left as well as left-to-right shunts.

UPSTREAM SAMPLING METHOD Blood samples are withdrawn in serial fashion from the pulmonary artery, right ven-

tricle, right atrium, and venae cavae, the indicator being introduced downstream (in the case of oxygen into the lungs). This approach permits localization of the site of a left-to-right shunt. With the oxygen sampling method, a step-up of 2.0 ml per 100 ml from the venae cavae to the right atrium, of 1.0 ml per 100 ml from the right atrium to the right ventricle, or of 0.5 ml per 100 ml from the right ventricle to the pulmonary artery is considered to be evidence of a left-to-right shunt. The use of a foreign gas improves the sensitivity of this approach, even a small left-to-right shunt being readily detected by appropriate sampling within the right side of the heart using a catheter-tip hydrogen electrode, for example.

For determination of the size of a left-to-right shunt, samples of venous blood proximal to the shunt and samples from the pulmonary artery and a systemic artery are obtained in close time sequence. The oxygen uptake at the lungs is measured simultaneously, or estimated, and the pulmonary and systemic blood flow rates (and hence the magnitude of the left-to-right shunt relative to systemic flow) can be calculated using Fick's equations. Generally a pulmonary to systemic flow ratio of 1.5:1 or greater is considered to indicate a left-to-right shunt of substantial magnitude.

DOWNSTREAM SAMPLING METHOD A needle is placed into a systemic artery and a time-concentration curve is recorded following upstream injection of the indicator. This technique is particularly useful for localizing the site of a right-to-left shunt. For example, when a right-to-left shunt exists at the ventricular level, an injection into the right ventricle and at all sites proximal to the right ventricle will result in an early appearance time of dye that has immediately traversed the defect (Fig. 234-5). However, an injection into the pulmonary artery, distal to the right-to-left shunt, shows a normal appearance

FIGURE 234-5

Diagrammatic representation of indicator-dilution curves using the downstream sampling method. The time of injection (Inj.) of an indicator, such as cardiogreen dye, is indicated by the arrow and by the square wave response on the recorded tracing. With right atrial (RA) injection and sampling at a peripheral artery, the normal appearance time is about 8 s, and the normal contour of the indicator-dilution curve is represented by the solid line. In a patient with a right-to-left (R-L) shunt at the atrial, ventricular, or pulmonary arterial levels, early appearance time of the dye is indicated by the dashed line. In a patient with a left-to-right (L-R) shunt, the appearance time need not be altered, but there is a reduced peak concentration of dye, and a break on the downslope, indicating early recirculation of the indicator.

time. A left-to-right shunt also may be detected, but not localized, by injection of indicator into the right side of the heart using peripheral arterial sampling. The indicator-dilution curve will show a reduced peak concentration of dye and a break on the downslope when compared with a normal indicator-dilution curve (Fig. 234-5). This contour occurs because a portion of the indicator traverses the left-to-right shunt during its initial passage to the left side of the heart, recirculates rapidly through the right side of the heart and lungs, and reappears at the peripheral artery before the downslope of the primary curve has been completely inscribed.

OTHER SPECIAL CARDIAC CATHETERIZATION TECHNIQUES

Miniaturization of electronics has permitted the construction and application of cardiac catheters with special measuring devices mounted on, or close to, the tip. For example, a catheter-tip micromanometer permits the measurement of intracardiac pressure free of the artifacts produced by fluid-filled manometer systems and catheter motion. Accurate high-fidelity pressure measurements are of particular utility in the assessment of the contractile and distensibility properties of the left ventricle. Micromanometer-tipped catheters also can be used for highly sensitive recordings of intracardiac sounds, murmurs, and clicks. In fact, an intracardiac phonocardiogram in the right ventricle is perhaps the most reliable method for documenting pulmonic insufficiency as the source of a diastolic, decrescendo murmur along the left sternal border. Other special catheters have been designed to record the intracardiac electrocardiogram and have made it possible to record selective potentials from the right atrium, right ventricle, and along the bundle of His. Recordings from the latter area are useful, for example, in determining whether a conduction delay or block on the surface electrocardiogram is located at or below the atrioventricular junction. His bundle recordings also have improved understanding of the mechanisms underlying paroxysmal atrial tachycardia and the preexcitation syndromes.

Electromagnetic or ultrasonic catheter-tip velocity probes also are available and have proved useful for study of phasic blood flow patterns in the venae cavae and pulmonary artery in patients with constrictive pericarditis and cardiac tamponade, and for analysis of the pattern and velocity of left ventricular ejection into the ascending aorta in patients with disorders of left ventricular function.

Transvascular intracardiac biopsy of the right and left ventricles by specially designed catheters also has been accomplished safely in a large number of patients. The specimens have proved to have some value from a diagnostic standpoint in uncommon varieties of infiltrative cardiomyopathy, e.g., those due to amyloid, iron, glycogen, granuloma, and neoplasm. Endomyocardial biopsy has also been used to detect early cardiac rejection following cardiac transplantation.

REFERENCES

ABRAMS HL: *Angiography,* 2d ed. Boston, Little, Brown, 1971

ADAMS D et al: The complications of coronary arteriography. Circulation 48:609, 1973

BARRY W, GROSSMAN W: Cardiac catheterization, in *Heart Disease,* E Braunwald (ed). Philadelphia, Saunders, 1980, chap 9

BRAUNWALD E, SWAN HJC: *Cooperative Study on Cardiac Catheterization* (monograph). New York, The American Heart Association, 1968

RACKLEY CE: Quantitative evaluation of left ventricular function by radiographic techniques. Circulation 54:862, 1976

SHABETAI R, ADOLPH RJ: Principles of cardiac catheterization, in *Cardiac Diagnosis and Treatment,* 2d ed, NO Fowler (ed). Hagerstown, Harper & Row, 1976, p 84

TAKARO T et al: An analysis of deaths occurring in association with coronary arteriography. Am Heart J 86:587, 1973

Functional abnormalities of the heart

235
DISORDERS OF MYOCARDIAL FUNCTION

EUGENE BRAUNWALD
JOHN ROSS, JR.
EDMUND H. SONNENBLICK

CELLULAR BASIS OF CARDIAC CONTRACTION

The myocardium is composed of individual striated muscle cells (fibers), normally 10 to 15 μm in diameter and 30 to 60 μm in length. Under the light microscope, each fiber is seen to contain multiple cross-banded strands (myofibrils), which run the length of the fiber and are composed of a serially repeating structure, the sarcomere. The remainder of the cytoplasm, lying between the myofibrils, contains other cell constituents, such as the single centrally located nucleus, numerous mitochondria, and intracellular membrane systems.

The sarcomere, the fundamental structural and functional unit of contraction, is delimited by two adjacent dark lines, the Z lines (Fig. 235-1). The distance between Z lines varies with the degree of contraction or stretch of the muscle and ranges between 1.5 and 2.2 μm. Within the confines of the sarcomere, alternating light and dark bands are seen, giving the myocardial fibers their striated appearance under the light microscope. At the center of the sarcomere is a broad dark band of constant width (1.5 μm), the A band, which is flanked by two lighter bands, the I bands, which are of variable width. The sarcomere of heart muscle, like that of skeletal muscle, is made up of two sets of myofilaments. Thicker filaments, composed principally of the protein myosin, traverse and are limited to the A band. They are about 100 Å in diameter, with tapered ends, and measure 1.5 to 1.6 μm in length. Thinner filaments, composed primarily of actin, course from the Z line through the I band into the A band. They are approximately 50 Å in diameter and 1.0 μm in length. Thus, there is overlapping of thick and thin filaments only within the A band, while the I

Intercalated disk

Nucleus

FIBER

A

10 μ

Fibrils

Sarcolemma

SARCOPLASMIC
RETICULUM

Longitudinal
System

'T' System

Terminal
cisternae

2 μ

Capillary N

N

FIBRIL

Mitochondria

Intercalated disk

B

SARCOMERE

Z   M L   Z

PSEUDO H ZONE   I BAND

A BAND 1.5 μ

C

CROSS SECTIONS

actin and myosin
myosin filaments   filaments   actin filaments

D

FIGURE 235-1

Microscopic structure of heart muscle. A. Myocardium as seen under the light microscope. Branching of fibers is evident. Each fiber, or cell, contains a centrally located nucleus. B. Myocardial cell, reconstructed from electron micrographs. Each cell is composed of multiple parallel fibrils. Each fibril is composed of serially connected sarcomeres (N, nucleus). C. Sarcomere from a myofibril, with diagrammatic representation of myofilaments. Thick filaments (1.5 μm long, composed of myosin) form the A band, and thin filaments (1 μm long, composed primarily of actin) extend from the Z line through the I band into the A band. The overlapping of thick and thin filaments is seen only in the A band. D. Cross sections of the sarcomere indicate the specific lattice arrangements of the myofilaments. In the center of the sarcomere only the thick, or myosin, filaments arranged in a hexagonal array are seen. In the distal portions of the A band, both thick and thin, or actin, filaments are found, with each thick filament surrounded by six thin filaments. In the I band only thin filaments are present. (From Braunwald et al, 1976.)

band contains only thin filaments (Fig. 235-1). On electromicroscopy, bridges may be seen to extend between the thick and thin filaments within the confines of the A band.

The "sliding" model for muscle rests on the fundamental observation that both the thick and thin filaments are constant in overall length, both at rest and during contraction. With activation of the sarcomere, repetitive interactions take place at the bridges between the actin and myosin filaments, and the actin filaments are propelled further into the A band. In the

process, the A band remains constant in width, whereas the I band become more narrow and the Z lines move toward one another.

The myosin molecule is a complex, asymmetric fibrous protein with a molecular weight of about 500,000; it has a rod-like portion that is about 1500 Å in length with a globular portion at its end. This globular portion contains the adenosine triphosphatase (ATPase) activity and forms the bridges. In forming the thick myofilament, the rod-like portions of the myosin molecules are laid down in an orderly, polarized manner, leaving the globular portions projecting outward so that they can interact with actin to generate force and shortening. Actin has a molecular weight of 47,000. The thin filament is composed of a double helix of two chains of actin molecules wound about each other, intimately associated with the protein tropomyosin, which appears to form the central core of this filament. Another protein complex, troponin, which can be separated into three components, is located periodically along the actin filament. In contrast to myosin, actin has no intrinsic enzymatic activity, but it has the ability to combine reversibly with myosin in the presence of ATP and Mg^{2+}, which activates the myosin ATPase. In relaxed muscle this interaction is inhibited by one of the components of troponin. During activation, Ca^{2+} becomes attached to another of the components and removes this inhibition. As a result, ATP is split, and linkages between actin and myosin filaments are made and broken cyclically. Mechanical forces are generated by these reactions, with resultant shortening of the sarcomere.

The sarcoplasmic reticulum, a complex network of anastomosing, membrane-lined intracellular channels, which invests the myofibrils, and which is less profuse in cardiac than in skeletal muscle, consists of a series of interconnecting longitudinally disposed membrane tubules closely applied to the surfaces of the individual sarcomeres; it has no direct continuity with the outside of the cell. Closely related, both functionally and structurally, are the transverse tubules or T system, formed by tubelike invaginations of the sarcolemma, which extend into the myocardial fiber, along the Z lines, i.e., the ends of the sarcomeres.

At rest, the cardiac cell is polarized; i.e., the interior has a negative charge relative to the outside of the cell, with a transmembrane potential of -80 to -100 mV (Chap. 232). The sarcolemma, which in the resting state is largely impermeable to Na^+ and has a Na^+- and K^+-stimulated pump requiring adenosine triphosphate (ATP) which extrudes Na^+ from the cell, plays a critical role in establishing this resting potential. Thus, the inside of the cell contains mainly K^+ with little Na^+, while the extracellular milieu is high in $[Na^+]$ and low in $[K^+]$. At the same time, in the resting state, the extracellular $[Ca^{2+}]$ greatly exceeds the free intracellular $[Ca^{2+}]$.

During the plateau of the action potential (phase 2) there is a slow inward current which reflects a movement of Ca^{2+} into the myoplasm. However, the absolute quantity of Ca^{2+} that crosses the surface membrane is relatively small and in and of itself appears to be incapable of bringing about full activation of the contractile apparatus. However, the depolarizing current not only extends across the surface of the cell but penetrates deeply into the cell by way of the ramifying T system. A flux of Ca^{2+} as well as Na^+ into the cell takes place, which may then lead to depolarization of the sarcoplasmic reticulum; this in turn leads to the release of much larger quantities of Ca^{2+} from the sarcoplasmic reticulum.

The Ca^{2+} then diffuses toward the sarcomere, combines with troponin, and, by repressing the inhibitor of contraction, activates the myofilaments to produce contraction, the strength and velocity of which are dependent on the quantity of Ca^{2+} that reaches the contractile sites. The sarcoplasmic reticulum then appears to reaccumulate Ca^{2+}, thereby lowering its concentration in the myofibril to a level that inhibits the actin-myosin interaction which is responsible for contraction, and in this manner leads to relaxation. Thus, the cell membrane, transverse tubules, and the sarcoplasmic reticulum, with their ability to transmit an action potential, to release and then reaccumulate Ca^{2+}, appear to play a fundamental role in the rhythmic contraction and relaxation of heart muscle.

The ATP formed from substrate oxidation is the principal source of energy for almost all the work performed by the myocardial cell. In the normally functioning heart the major fraction of energy is expended in the mechanical work of contraction. The high-energy phosphate stores in ATP are in equilibrium with those in the form of creatine phosphate.

In all forms of striated muscle, including cardiac muscle, the force of contraction depends on initial muscle length. The sarcomere length associated with the most forceful contraction is 2.2 μm. It is at this length that the two sets of myofilaments of the sarcomere are most ideally situated to provide the greatest area for their interaction. In support of the sliding-filament hypothesis, force development diminishes in direct proportion to the decrease in the overlap between thick and thin filaments, and the resultant decrease in the number of reactive sites. At a sarcomere length of 3.65 μm, developed tension falls to zero, and it is at this point that the thin filaments are entirely withdrawn from the A band. Similarly, when the sarcomeres are shorter than 2.0 μm, the thin filaments bypass one another, producing a double overlap of the thin filaments (Fig. 235-2), and force also falls. In addition to determining the number of interacting sites between actin and myosin myofilaments, the length of the sarcomere also appears to regulate the extent of activation of the contractile system, which is greatest at 2.2 μm.

The relation between the initial length of the muscle fibers and the developed force is of prime importance for the function of heart muscle. This forms the basis of the Frank-Starling relation (Starling's law of the heart), which states that, within limits, an augmentation of initial volume of the ventricle, which is a function of the initial length of the muscle, results in an increase in the force of ventricular contraction. It has been shown for heart muscle that sarcomere length is directly proportional to muscle length along the ascending limb of the length–active tension curve. As muscle length decreases to the point at which developed tension approaches zero and at which sarcomere length approaches 1.5 μm, the I bands at first narrow, then disappear while the A band remains constant in length. At this latter point, the Z line abuts on the edges of the A band. Thus, the sarcomere length–active tension curve forms the ultrastructural basis of Starling's law of the heart.

MYOCARDIAL MECHANICS

Extremely helpful methods for examining the behavior of muscle were provided by skeletal muscle physiologists early in this century. The mechanical activity of all muscle may be expressed externally in only two ways: shortening and the development of tension. Hill showed in skeletal muscle that the velocity of shortening is inversely related to the magnitude of tension development, an expression of the so-called "force-velocity relation," now acknowledged to be a fundamental property of muscle. Expressed simply, the greater the load the muscle is called upon to lift, the lower the velocity of shortening and vice versa. More recently, the concept of the force-velocity relation has been extended from skeletal to cardiac muscle. However, in this respect there is a basic difference between skeletal and cardiac muscle. Skeletal muscle has a single, essentially fixed, force-velocity curve; i.e., at any given muscle length, force and velocity are always related to each other in the same manner. The contractile activity of skeletal muscle is increased by the recruitment of additional muscle fibers, i.e., motor units, and by increasing the frequency of nerve impulses, while the contractility of each individual fiber remains constant. Although resting length also influences the characteristics of contraction, this variable remains essentially fixed in

A   **B**

FIGURE 235-2

Relation between sarcomere length and band patterns in skeletal muscle (frog sartorius). A. Band patterns as seen electromicroscopically. B. Disposition of the thick and thin filaments that create band patterns. The vertical arrows in both panels denote the ends of the thin filaments that insert at the Z line at the left. Line 3 represents the sarcomere at the apex of the length-tension curve, i.e., at L_{max}. In lines 1 and 2, sarcomere length has been progressively decreased, whereas in 4 and 5 it has been progressively elongated. Throughout, the A band remains constant in width. The placement of filaments to provide for maximum overlap is shown in B (3). Line 1 shows the sarcomere pattern in the contracted muscle; the I band has disappeared, and a secondary dark band has been formed at the center of the sarcomere, termed the C contraction band, which is due to the passage of thin filaments through this area as in B (1). In A (4 and 5), an expanding H zone has appeared, owing to the withdrawal of the thin filaments from the A band, as shown diagrammatically in B (4 and 5). (From Braunwald et al, 1976.)

vivo. In contrast, the number of cardiac cells activated remains constant during each contraction. However, the contractile activity of the myocardium may be readily altered under physiological conditions by changes in resting fiber length and by changes in the inotropic state, i.e., the contractility, both of which shift the myocardial force-velocity curve.

Variations in myocardial contractile activity may be expressed as displacements of the force-velocity curve. However, there are two fundamental ways in which the force-velocity curve can be shifted. Figure 235-3*A* shows a family of force-velocity curves obtained from an isolated cardiac muscle; each curve was obtained at a different preload, i.e., with a different degree of stretch on the muscle. Note that changing the preload alters the intercept of the force-velocity curve on the horizontal axis; i.e., it increases the isometric force developed by the muscle. However, within limits, these alterations in preload do not appear to alter the intrinsic velocity of shortening, since all the curves extrapolate to the same intercept on the vertical axis. Thus, a change in initial length of heart muscle shifts the force-velocity curve primarily by altering the total force which can be developed by the muscle, as illustrated by the isometric length-tension curve, shown in the insert of Fig. 235-3*A*.

This type of shift in the force-velocity curve may be contrasted with that obtained when a positive inotropic agent, such as Ca^{2+}, digitalis, or norepinephrine, is added to the muscle while the initial length is held constant (Fig. 235-3*B*). These agents not only increase the force which the muscle is capable of lifting, i.e., the intercept of the force-velocity curve on the horizontal axis, therefore shifting the isometric length-tension curve upward, but they also increase the velocity of shortening of the unloaded muscle, i.e., the extrapolated intercept on the vertical axis.

It has been postulated that an increase in initial muscle length up to an optimal length brings about an increase in the number of effective force-generating sites as a consequence of a more advantageous overlap of interdigitating contractile filaments within the sarcomere and in the extent of activation of the contractile sites. A change in the inotropic state, characterized by an increase in the velocity of shortening of the unloaded muscle, can also result from an increase in the rate of cyclic force-generating processes at the contractile sites, without a change in the number of these sites, i.e., at a constant muscle length. Increased contractility appears to be related to an increased availability of Ca^{2+} within the cell.

CONTRACTION OF THE INTACT VENTRICLE

Analysis of the heart as a pump has classically centered upon the relation between the filling pressure, or diastolic volume, of the ventricle (length of the muscle fibers) and its stroke volume (the Frank-Starling relation). It was shown clearly in the heart-lung preparation that the stroke volume is a function of diastolic fiber length, and that the failing heart delivers a smaller-than-normal stroke volume from a normal or elevated end-diastolic volume. Later, the concept of measuring stroke work (the product of stroke volume and mean aortic pressure) over a

FIGURE 235-3

A. Effects of increasing initial muscle length on the force-velocity relation of the cat papillary muscle. Initial velocity of shortening has been plotted as a function of load for five different muscle lengths. The maximum velocity of shortening is essentially unchanged, whereas the maximum force of contraction is augmented. The insert shows the places along the length-tension curves at which these force-velocity curves were determined. B. Effects of norepinephrine on the force-velocity relation of the cat papillary muscle. Both the maximum velocity of shortening and the force of contraction are increased. (From Braunwald et al, 1976.)

range of mean atrial or ventricular end-diastolic pressures, using one of these pressures as an index of diastolic volume, was expanded by Sarnoff and his collaborators. They concluded that this relation between the mean atrial or the ventricular end-diastolic pressure and the stroke work of the corresponding ventricle (the ventricular function curve) provided a definition of the level of the contractile, or inotropic, state of the ventricle. Significant increases in the level of ventricular contractility were accompanied by shifts of the ventricular function curve upward and to the left, while depression of contractility was identified by downward and rightward displacement of this relation.

Considerable effort also has been directed toward a study of the responses of the intact, unanesthetized animal, and it has been observed that during the adrenergic stimulation of the myocardium accompanying a stress such as exercise, relatively little change in ventricular end-diastolic size occurs, while minute cardiac output, aortic flow velocity, and the rate of ventricular pressure development are augmented. Thus, reflex and humorally mediated changes in myocardial contractility, heart rate, venous return, and peripheral vascular resistance may be more important in circulatory adaptation than changes in ventricular end-diastolic volume and the operation of the Frank-Starling mechanism.

The important influence of the neurotransmitter substance norepinephrine on the mechanical properties of the myocardium has long been recognized. Direct stimulation of the stellate ganglia has been shown to elevate the ventricular function curve, as a consequence of the release of norepinephrine from sympathetic nerve endings in the heart. In the intact animal, these adrenergic effects are evidenced by tachycardia, a reduc-

tion in cardiac dimensions, increased velocity of ejection, and an enhanced rate of tension development.

Surgically denervated hearts in situ, or isolated papillary muscles taken from such hearts, do not exhibit depression of their intrinsic inotropic state despite depletion of the norepinephrine stores within the sympathetic nerve endings of the muscle. The surgically or pharmacologically denervated heart of the intact organism, if otherwise normal, also appears capable of meeting many of the demands of muscular exercise. However, since it cannot be stimulated by neuronally released norepinephrine in the heart, the mechanisms by which the denervated heart increases its output differ from those of the intact animal. Thus, tachycardia is less marked, and the stroke volume and cardiac output rise more gradually than normal, and as a consequence of elevation of ventricular end-diastolic volume. In all these respects the activity of the heart muscle fiber differs from the activity of skeletal muscle fiber, the latter being totally dependent on its nerve supply and unable to contract effectively when denervated.

CONTROL OF CARDIAC PERFORMANCE AND OUTPUT

The extent of shortening of mammalian heart muscle and, therefore, the stroke volume of the intact ventricle are, in the final analysis, determined by four influences: (1) the length of the muscle at the start of contraction, i.e., the preload; (2) the inotropic state of the muscle, i.e., the position of its force-velocity-length relation or function curve; (3) the tension which the muscle is called upon to develop during contraction, i.e., the afterload; and (4) the heart rate, which determines the cardiac output at any stroke volume as long as ventricular filling is maintained.

VENTRICULAR END-DIASTOLIC VOLUME (PRELOAD) At any level of its inotropic state, the performance of the myocardium is influenced profoundly by ventricular end-diastolic fiber length and therefore by diastolic ventricular volume. The following are the major determinants of ventricular end-diastolic volume in the intact organism (see also Fig. 235-4):

I *Total blood volume.* When depleted, as in hemorrhage, venous return to the heart declines and ventricular end-diastolic volume falls, as does ventricular performance, as reflected in ventricular work.

II *Distribution of blood volume.* At any given total blood volume, the ventricular end-diastolic volume is influenced by the distribution of blood between the intra- and extrathoracic compartments. This distribution in turn is influenced by:

A *Body position.* Gravitational forces tend to pool blood in dependent portions. The upright posture augments extrathoracic at the expense of intrathoracic blood volume, and reduces ventricular work.

B *Intrathoracic pressure.* Normally, mean intrathoracic pressure is negative, a factor which acts to increase thoracic blood volume and ventricular end-diastolic volume, particularly during inspiration. Elevation of intrathoracic pressure, as occurs in a tension pneumothorax, during the Valsalva maneuver, or in prolonged bouts of coughing, tends to impede venous return to the heart, diminish intrathoracic blood volume, and ultimately reduce ventricular work.

C *Intrapericardial pressure.* When elevated, as in pericardial tamponade, there is interference with cardiac filling, and the resultant reduction in ventricular diastolic volume lowers ventricular work.

D *Venous tone.* The veins are not a simple system of passive conduits between the systemic capillary bed and the right atrium. Instead, the smooth muscle in venous walls responds to a variety of neural and humoral stimuli. Venoconstriction occurs during muscular exercise, deep respiration, fright, or marked hypotension, tending to diminish extrathoracic and to augment intrathoracic blood volume, venous return to the heart, and ventricular performance.

E *The pumping action of skeletal muscle.* During exercise the contracting skeletal muscles tend to squeeze blood out of the veins and, with the aid of the venous valves, to displace it centrally, thereby increasing intrathoracic blood volume, ventricular end-diastolic volume, and ventricular work.

III *Atrial contraction.* Vigorous, appropriately timed atrial contraction augments ventricular filling and end-diastolic volume. The atrial contribution to ventricular filling is of particular importance in patients with ventricular hypertrophy, in whom the loss of atrial systole (as in atrial fibrillation) tends to reduce ventricular end-diastolic pressure and volume, ultimately lowering myocardial performance.

INOTROPIC STATE (MYOCARDIAL CONTRACTILITY) A number of factors determine the level of ventricular performance at any given ventricular end-diastolic volume, i.e., the position of the ventricular function curve (Fig. 235-5). These influences may be considered to operate by modifying myocardial force-velocity-length relations.

Sympathetic nerve activity The quantity of norepinephrine released by sympathetic nerve endings in the heart is, under ordinary circumstances, dependent on the sympathetic nerve impulse traffic, and variations in the frequency of nerve impulses modify the quantity of norepinephrine released and acting upon the beta-adrenergic receptors in the myocardium. This mechanism is the most important one which acutely modifies the position of the force-velocity and ventricular function curves under physiological conditions.

Circulating catecholamines The adrenal medulla and other sympathetic ganglia outside the heart, when properly stimulated by sympathetic nerve impulses, release catecholamines, which augment the inotropic state of the myocardium.

The force-frequency relation The position of the myocardial force-velocity curve is influenced by the rate and rhythm of cardiac contraction; e.g., ventricular extrasystoles result in post-extrasystolic potentiation.

Exogenously administered inotropic agents The cardiac glycosides, isoproterenol and other sympathomimetic agents, cal-

FIGURE 235-4

Diagram of a Frank-Starling curve, relating ventricular end-diastolic volume (EDV) to ventricular performance (top right) and the major influences that determine the degree of stretching of the myocardium, i.e., the magnitude of the EDV (bottom left). (From Braunwald et al, 1976.)

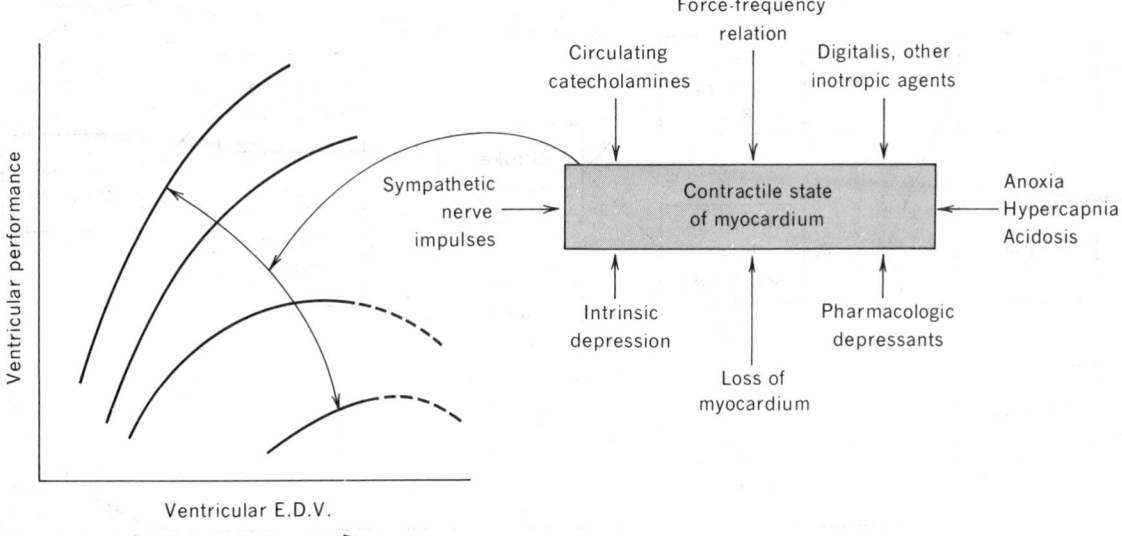

FIGURE 235-5

Diagram showing the major influences that elevate or depress the inotropic state of the myocardium (top right), and the manner in which alter- ations in the inotropic state of the myocardium affect the level of ventricular performance at any given level of ventricular end-diastolic volume (bottom left). (From Braunwald et al, 1976.)

cium, caffeine, theophylline, and their derivatives, all improve the myocardial force-velocity relation (Chap. 238) and therefore may be used therapeutically to augment ventricular performance at any given ventricular end-diastolic volume.

Physiological depressants Included among these are severe myocardial hypoxia, hypercapnea, and acidosis. Acting either singly or in combination, these influences exert a depressant effect on the myocardial force-velocity curve and lower the level of the left ventricular work at any given ventricular end-diastolic volume.

Pharmacological depressants These include quinidine, procainamide, barbiturates, and other local and general anesthetics (Chap. 238), as well as many other drugs.

Loss of ventricular substance When a portion of ventricular myocardium becomes nonfunctional or necrotic, as occurs temporarily in bouts of ischemia (Chap. 244), and permanently in myocardial infarction (Chap. 245), total ventricular performance at any given level of end-diastolic volume is depressed, even if the remaining myocardium functions normally.

Intrinsic myocardial depression Although the fundamental mechanisms responsible for depression of myocardial contractility in heart failure still remain to be elucidated, it is now apparent that in this condition the inotropic state of each unit of myocardium is depressed and that the level of ventricular performance at any ventricular end-diastolic volume is thereby lowered.

VENTRICULAR AFTERLOAD The stroke volume is ultimately a function of the extent of ventricular fiber shortening. As in isolated cardiac muscle, the velocity and extent of shortening at any given level of diastolic fiber length and myocardial inotropic state are inversely related to the afterload imposed on the muscle. The afterload on the intact heart is dependent on the level of aortic pressure, but it may be defined as the tension or stress developed in the wall of the ventricle during ejection. Therefore, the afterload on the ventricular muscle fibers also is dependent on the size of the heart, according to Laplace's law,

which indicates that the tension of the myocardial fiber is a function of the product of intracavitary ventricular pressure and the ventricular radius. Thus, at the same level of aortic pressure, the afterload faced by an enlarged left ventricle is higher than that encountered by a ventricle of normal size. The aortic pressure, in turn, is influenced largely by the peripheral vascular resistance, the physical characteristics of the arterial tree, and the volume of blood it contains at the onset of ejection. At any given ventricular end-diastolic volume and level of the myocardial state, the left ventricular stroke volume is a function of the afterload.

The critical role played by the ventricular afterload in cardiovascular regulation is summarized in Fig. 235-6. As already noted, increases in both preload and contractility increase myocardial fiber shortening, while increases in afterload reduce it. The extent of myocardial fiber shortening and left ventricular size are the determinants of stroke volume. Arterial pressure, in turn, is related to the product of cardiac output and systemic vascular resistance, while afterload is a function of left ventricular size and arterial pressure. An increase in arterial pressure induced by vasoconstriction, for example, augments afterload, which through a negative feedback depresses myocardial fiber shortening, stroke volume, and cardiac output; this in turn tends to restore arterial pressure to its previous level.

When left ventricular function becomes impaired, impedance to left ventricular ejection becomes increasingly important in determining cardiac performance. Increases in impedance may result from the influence on the arterial bed of neural, humoral, or structural changes which can occur in response to a fall in cardiac output. This increased impedance may further reduce cardiac output while myocardial oxygen requirements are increased. In this way, alterations in the peripheral vascular bed probably play an important role in the hemodynamic and metabolic events which usually are attributed to progressive impairment of the myocardium.

All the influences acting on cardiac performance enumerated above interact in a complex fashion to maintain cardiac output at a level appropriate to the requirements of the metabolizing tissues, and in a normal person interference with one of these mechanisms may not influence the cardiac output. For example, a moderate reduction of blood volume or the loss of

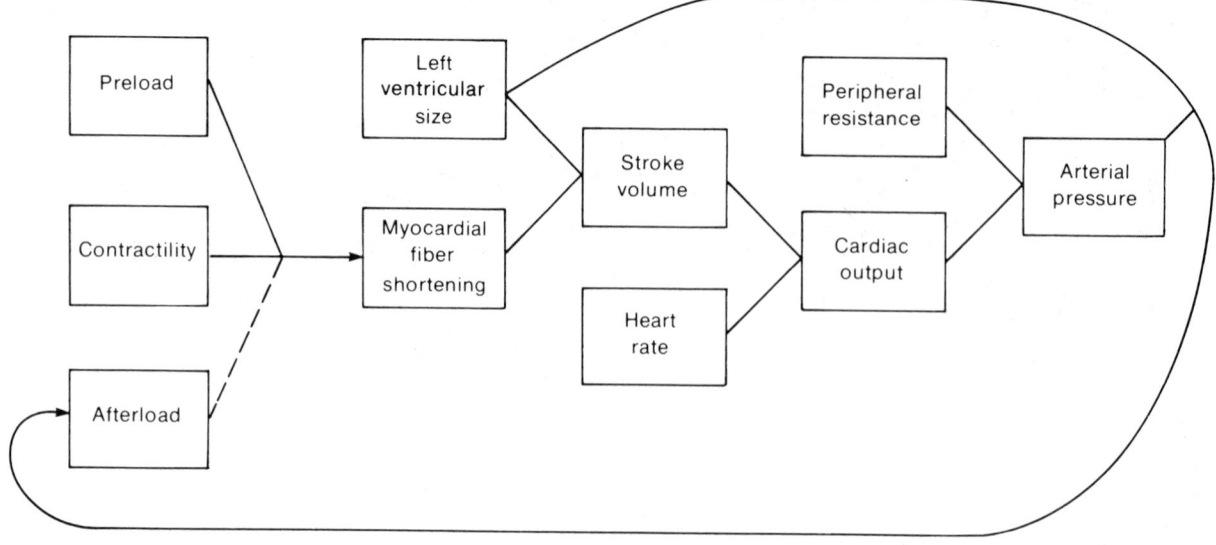

FIGURE 235-6

Scheme of interactions among various components that regulate cardiac activity. Solid lines indicate an augmenting effect; broken line represents an inhibiting effect. (From Braunwald, 1974.)

the atrial contribution to ventricular contraction can ordinarily be sustained without a reduction in the resting cardiac output. Presumably other factors, such as an increase in the frequency of sympathetic nerve impulses reaching the heart and an increase in heart rate, will, in the normal person, augment contractility and sustain output under these circumstances. Mechanisms are also available which prevent elevation of the cardiac output when there is no physiological demand for augmented flow. For example, expansion of blood volume or augmentation of myocardial contractility by means of cardiac glycosides does not increase the cardiac output in normal humans. Thus, in analyzing the effect of an intervention on cardiac output, it is important to recognize that it is the venous return, rather than the inotropic state, of the myocardium which limits cardiac output in the normal individual and that an improvement of myocardial contractility by a drug such as digitalis should not be expected to elevate the output in a normal subject. On the other hand, in the presence of congestive heart failure, the cardiac output usually is limited by the depressed contractile state of the myocardium, and a positive inotropic influence would be expected to raise cardiac output, and, indeed, does so.

EXERCISE The hemodynamic changes which normally occur during muscular exercise in the upright position are complex (Fig. 235-7). The hyperventilation of exercise, the pumping action of the exercising muscles, and the venoconstriction which occur all tend to augment venous return and hence ventricular filling. Simultaneously, the increase in the sympathetic nerve impulses to the myocardium, the increased concentration of circulating catecholamines, and the tachycardia which occur during exercise all result in an augmentation of the contractile state of the myocardium (Fig. 235-7, curves 1 and 2) and an elevation of stroke volume, with no change or even a decrease of end-diastolic pressure and volume (Fig. 235-7, points A and B). Vasodilatation occurs in the exercising muscles, thus reducing the afterload. This ultimately allows the achievement of a greatly elevated cardiac output during exercise, at an arterial pressure usually only slightly higher than in the resting state.

In heart failure, the fundamental abnormality resides in depressions of the myocardial force-velocity relationship and of

the length–active tension curve, reflecting reductions in the contractile state of the myocardium (Fig. 235-7, curves 1 to 3). In many instances, cardiac output and external ventricular performance at rest are within normal limits but are maintained at these levels only by an increased end-diastolic fiber length and an elevated ventricular end-diastolic volume, i.e., through the operation of the Frank-Starling mechanism (Fig. 235-7, points A to D). The elevations of left ventricular end-diastolic volume and pressure are associated with similar changes in the pulmonary capillary pressure, contributing to the dyspnea experienced by patients with heart failure. The normal improvement of contractility due to augmented sympathetic activity during exercise is attenuated or even prevented by norepinephrine depletion which occurs in heart failure (Fig. 235-7, curves 3 and 3′). The factors which tend to augment ventricular filling during exercise in the normal subject push the failing myocardium even farther along its flattened length–active tension curve, and although the left ventricle may perform somewhat better, this occurs only as a consequence of an inordinate elevation of ventricular end-diastolic volume and pressure and, therefore, of the pulmonary capillary pressure. The elevation of the latter intensifies dyspnea and therefore plays an important role in limiting the intensity of exercise which the patient can perform. Left ventricular failure becomes fatal when the myocardial length–active tension curve is depressed (Fig. 235-7, curve 4) to the point at which cardiac performance fails to satisfy the requirements of the peripheral tissues even at rest, and/or the left ventricular end-diastolic and pulmonary capillary pressures are elevated to levels which result in pulmonary edema (Fig. 235-7, point E).

THE FAILING HEART

Though heart failure may be readily described as a clinical syndrome, characterized by well-known symptoms and physical signs, a precise physiological or biochemical definition is far more difficult. However, from the clinical point of view, heart failure may be considered to be the disease state in which an abnormality of cardiac function is responsible for the inability of the heart to pump blood at a rate commensurate with the requirements of the metabolizing tissues. Though a defect in myocardial contraction is characteristic of heart failure, this defect may result from a primary abnormality in the heart muscle, or it may be secondary to a chronic excessive work load. It is important to distinguish heart failure from (1) states

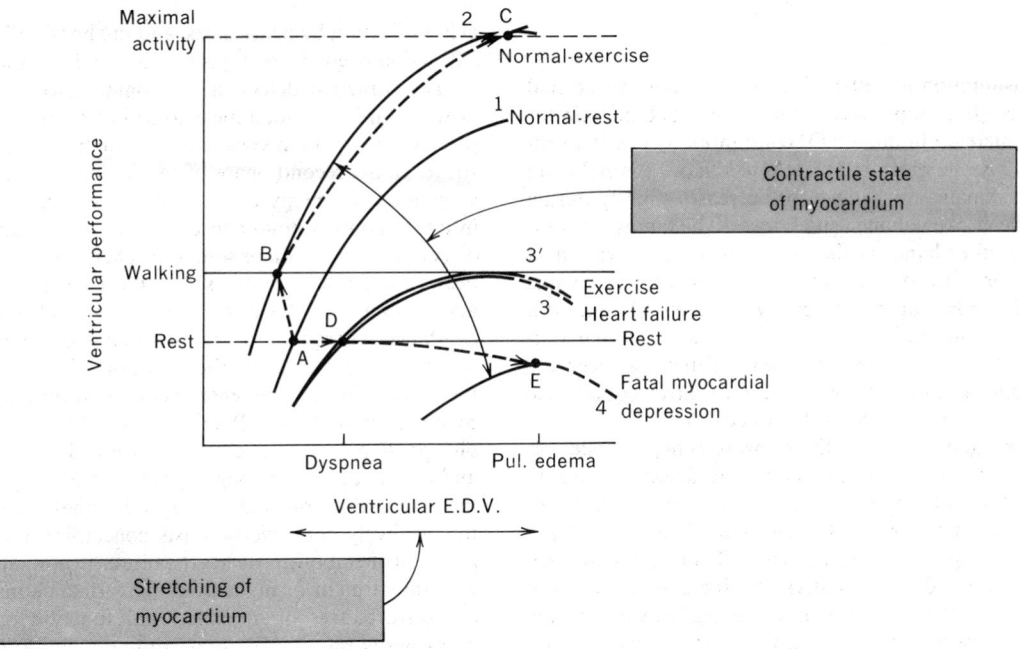

FIGURE 235-7

Diagram showing the interrelations among influences on ventricular end-diastolic volume (EDV) through stretching of the myocardium and the contractile state of the myocardium. Levels of ventricular EDV associated with filling pressures that result in dyspnea and pulmonary edema are shown on the abscissa. Levels of ventricular performance required when *the subject is at rest, while walking, and during maximal activity are designated on the ordinate. The dotted lines are the descending limbs of the ventricular-performance curves, which are rarely seen during life but which show the level of ventricular performance if end-diastolic volume could be elevated to very high levels. (From Braunwald et al, 1976.)*

of circulatory insufficiency in which myocardial function is not primarily impaired, such as cardiac tamponade, hemorrhagic shock, or tricuspid stenosis, (2) conditions in which there is circulatory congestion because of abnormal salt and water retention but in which there is no serious disturbance of myocardial function, and (3) conditions in which the normal heart is suddenly presented with a load which exceeds its capacity, e.g., accelerated hypertension or rupture of a valve cusp secondary to infective endocarditis.

Acute heart failure in the intact canine heart, studied in situ or in the heart-lung preparation, is characterized by a depression of ventricular stroke volume or stroke work at any given level of left ventricular end-diastolic volume or filling pressure. Further, as diastolic volume is augmented in the failing heart, an abnormally small increase or no change in stroke volume occurs. Thus, in order to maintain stroke volume at a normal level, the heart dilates and the Frank-Starling mechanism therefore might be considered one of the first lines of defense called upon to maintain cardiac output when myocardial contractility declines. An increase in the end-diastolic volume of the ventricle permits the ejection of a larger stroke volume, even when the extent of shortening of individual muscle fibers remains constant. The fact that when end-diastolic volume is augmented in the failing heart, stroke volume shows little change or is actually diminished clearly indicates that the relative degree of muscle fiber shortening must have decreased. Thus, an important mechanical defect which can be delineated in acute heart failure is a decrease in the extent of shortening of cardiac muscle fibers.

The intrinsic contractile state of myocardium removed from normal, hypertrophied, and failing animal hearts has been evaluated, and both ventricular hypertrophy and heart failure were shown to reduce the maximum isometric tension and velocity of shortening to subnormal levels; the changes were more marked in the myocardium of animals in which heart failure had been present than in those with hypertrophy alone. However, ventricular hypertrophy, in the absence of heart fail-

ure, also appears to be associated with a depression of the inotropic state per unit of myocardium, although the absolute increase of total muscle mass maintains overall cardiac compensation. Papillary muscles removed from the left ventricles of patients with heart failure have also shown a depression of the maximum degree of active tension which they can develop. Electronmicroscopic analysis of failing cat papillary muscles fixed at the apexes of the length–active tension curves revealed sarcomere lengths averaging 2.2 μm. Thus, the abnormalities of contractility do *not* appear to be produced by an alteration in the overlap of filaments within the sarcomere.

The failing ventricle may still eject a normal or nearly normal stroke volume despite considerable depression of function, when its end-diastolic volume increases, i.e., through the operation of the Frank-Starling mechanism. As outlined above, an increase in the initial volume of the ventricle is associated with stretching of the sarcomere, a process which augments the number of sites at which the actin and myosin filaments can interact. Furthermore, the development of ventricular hypertrophy may be considered to provide additional contractile units, and thereby constitutes an important compensatory mechanism when the intrinsic myocardial inotropic state is depressed.

Several techniques are available for defining impaired ventricular contractility in intact humans. With the patient at rest, the cardiac output and stroke volume may be depressed, but not uncommonly these variables are within normal limits. A more sensitive index is the ejection fraction, i.e., the ratio of stroke volume to end-diastolic volume, which may be estimated by biplane angiography (Chap. 234), and which is frequently depressed in heart failure even when the stroke volume itself is normal. An even more sensitive method for detecting impaired ventricular performance is based on the measurement of the circulatory changes occurring during stresses such as exercise or increased afterload. Thus, left ventricular performance may be estimated accurately by measuring the left ventricular end-diastolic pressure, cardiac output, and total body O_2 consumption at rest and during exercise. In normal persons, the cardiac output rises by more than 500 ml/min for each 100-ml increase in minute O_2 consumption. The left ventricular end-diastolic pressure at rest is less than 12 mmHg and rises slightly, remains unchanged, or decreases slightly during exercise, while stroke volume usually rises. The failing left ventricle, on the other hand, is characterized by an elevation of end-diastolic pressure during exercise, which reaches a value exceeding 12 mmHg, accompanied by either no change or a fall in stroke volume and a subnormal increase in cardiac output. Various degrees of impairment intermediate between the normal response and that of the failing left ventricle during the stress of exercise also have been described.

Another method consists of the measurement of stroke volume, arterial pressure, and ventricular end-diastolic pressure before and after ventricular afterload is increased by means of an infusion of a pressor agent such as angiotensin or by a sustained handgrip (isometric exercise). Though the normal left ventricle responds to this stress by increasing its stroke work and end-diastolic pressure, in the failing left ventricle the end-diastolic pressure rises markedly, but stroke work either remains constant or actually declines. Thus, as in the acutely failing experimental preparation, the failing human left ventricle appears to exhibit a depression of the relation between end-diastolic pressure and the stroke volume and stroke work which can be achieved. The potential value of stressing the left ventricle in some manner is emphasized by the fact that the basal values for left ventricular end-diastolic pressure, cardiac index, and ventricular stroke work may be in the same range in patients with depressed ventricular function as in normal persons. The response to these stresses may prove useful not only in the detection of the impairment of myocardial function, but also in expressing the severity of this impairment quantitatively.

The performance of the left ventricle in humans may also be characterized by examining the instantaneous myocardial force-velocity relations and the extent of shortening during individual cardiac cycles. Angiocardiographic studies and analyses of the rate of change of intraventricular pressure (dp/dt) as a function of the simultaneously recorded pressure during isovolumetric contraction have shown that depressions in the velocity of myocardial fiber shortening and of tension development exist in human heart failure. Further evidence for the decreases in the velocity of myocardial fiber shortening is provided by the finding of a reduced mean systolic ejection rate in patients with heart failure and a failure of the mean systolic ejection rate to rise normally during muscular exercise. Noninvasive, graphic techniques, particularly echocardiography and the determination of systolic time intervals, are of great value in the clinical assessment of myocardial function (Chap. 233).

CARDIAC METABOLISM IN HEART FAILURE

The common forms of low-output heart failure, secondary to arteriosclerosis, hypertension, and certain valvular and congenital lesions, are characterized by an absolute or a relative reduction in the useful external work delivered by the heart. Considerable attention has been directed to the question of whether cardiac failure is due to a defect in the production of energy, its conservation, or its utilization. Only in isolated instances of heart failure, such as those associated with beriberi, are there clear-cut disturbances of myocardial energy production. The major pathway by which pyruvate enters the citric acid cycle and some reactions within the cycle itself are dependent on the presence of adequate concentrations of thiamine (Chap. 80). Thiamine deficiency results in diminished pyruvic

acid utilization by heart slices, and in abnormally low pyruvate extraction coefficients in intact dogs and in humans.

The principal defect in the common forms of low-output heart failure does not appear to be in an impairment of energy production by the myocardium through the oxidation of substrate. In the second phase of cardiac metabolism, energy conservation, the energy of substrate oxidation is then converted into the terminal-bond energy of creatine phosphate (CP) and of ATP, the immediate source of chemical energy utilized by heart muscle. This process, known as oxidative phosphorylation, occurs in the mitochondria. The effectiveness of the combined energy production-conservation mechanisms may be studied by measuring the stores of ATP and CP existing in the myocardium, while energy conservation may be evaluated by determining (1) the P/O ratio, i.e., the ratio of high-energy phosphate produced to oxygen consumed in the mitochondria, and (2) the degree of coupling between electron transport and the generation of high-energy phosphate compounds. Although lively controversy exists concerning the status of this phase of metabolism in heart failure, it now appears that severe impairment of myocardial performance may occur without disturbances of mitochondrial function or reduction of high-energy phosphate stores, although abnormalities in these processes do occur in some forms of experimental heart failure.

In the absence of a definitive abnormality of energy liberation or conservation in the failing myocardium, attention has naturally been directed to the possibility that energy utilization is abnormal. An abnormality of energy liberation could certainly occur if the contractile proteins themselves were altered, and indeed this was once believed to be the basic biochemical abnormality occurring in congestive heart failure, a theory no longer supported. However, it has been shown that myofibrillar, actomyosin, and myosin ATPase activity are depressed in some forms of experimentally produced heart failure, and it is possible that this depression may be responsible for a defect in energy utilization, i.e., in the breakdown of ATP, the process which leads to the shortening and tension development by the contractile filaments. In addition, substantial evidence has been obtained that in heart failure there is an abnormality of excitation-contraction coupling, which alters the delivery of Ca^{2+} to the contractile sites, thereby impairing cardiac performance.

THE ADRENERGIC NERVOUS SYSTEM IN HEART FAILURE

In view of the importance of the adrenergic nervous system in stimulating the contractility of the normal myocardium, the activity of this system has also been studied intensively in patients with congestive heart failure. An index of the activity of this system, at rest and during exercise, is provided by measurements of the concentration of norepinephrine (NE) in arterial blood. No change or very little increase in the NE concentrations occurs during exercise in normal subjects; much greater increases are seen in patients with congestive heart failure, presumably because of an increased activity of the adrenergic nervous system during exercise in these patients. Marked elevations of a 24-h urinary NE excretion occur in patients with heart failure, indicating that the activity of their adrenergic nervous systems is also augmented at rest.

The importance of the increased activity of the adrenergic nervous system in maintaining ventricular contractility when the function of the myocardium is depressed in congestive heart failure also is shown by the effects of adrenergic blockade in patients with heart failure. Antiadrenergic drugs such as propranolol or guanethidine may cause sodium and water retention, as well as intensify heart failure. The adrenergic nervous system thus plays an important compensatory role in the circulatory adjustments of patients to congestive heart failure, and caution must be exercised in the use of antiadrenergic drugs, particularly beta-adrenergic blocking agents, in the treatment of patients with limited cardiac reserve (Chap. 236).

Both the concentration and content of the NE in atrial and ventricular tissue in patients with heart failure are reduced, sometimes to 10 percent of normal. This is a reduction in NE content in the heart and is not the result of a simple dilution of sympathetic nerve endings in a hypertrophied muscle mass.

The mechanism responsible for the depletion of cardiac NE stores is not entirely clear. A prolonged increase in cardiac sympathetic tone appears to play a critical role and to interfere in some manner with the biosynthesis of NE. Deficiencies in the activities of two of the enzymes involved in biosynthesis—tyrosine hydroxylase and dopamine oxidase—have been incriminated.

In view of the strongly positive inotropic effect exerted by the NE released from these nerves, the adrenergic nervous system may be considered to provide an important potential source of support to the failing myocardium. However, the increments of heart rate and contractile force which occur in animals with experimental heart failure and cardiac NE depletion are abolished or markedly reduced with stimulation of the cardiac sympathetic nerves. Thus, it is likely that when congestive heart failure is accompanied by depletion of cardiac NE stores, the quantity of NE released by the sympathetic nerve endings in the heart is deficient relative to the impulse traffic along these nerves.

Cardiac stores of NE are not fundamentally necessary for maintaining the intrinsic contractile state of the myocardium. However, since the reduction of NE stores in heart failure is associated with a diminished release of neurotransmitter, this depletion of NE may be responsible for loss of the much-needed adrenergic support in the failing heart. In the later stages of heart failure, when the levels of circulating catecholamines are elevated and the cardiac NE stores depleted, the myocardium is largely dependent on a more generalized adrenergic stimulation derived from extracardiac sources, presumably the adrenal medulla; this would explain the deterioration of cardiac performance which may occur in patients with heart failure who are treated with beta-adrenergic blocking drugs. This generalized adrenergic stimulation resulting from circulating catecholamines may, however, also exert undesirable side effects, because it elevates vascular resistance and may present the heart with an afterload which is higher than optimal.

REFERENCES

BRAUNWALD E: Regulation of the circulation. N Engl J Med 290:1124, 1420, 1974

———, ROSS JJ: Control of cardiac performance, in *Handbook of Physiology*, sec 2, vol 1, RM Berne (ed). Washington, DC, American Physiological Society, 1979, pp 553-580

——— et al: *Mechanisms of Contraction of the Normal and Failing Heart*, 2d ed. Boston, Little, Brown, 1976

FISHMAN AP (ed): *Heart Failure*. Washington DC, Hemisphere, McGraw-Hill, 1978

GUYTON AC et al: *Circulatory Physiology: Cardiac Output and Its Regulation*, 2d ed. Philadelphia, Saunders, 1973

JAMES TN, SHERF L: Ultrastructure of the myocardium, in *The Heart*, 4th ed, JW Hurst et al (eds). New York, McGraw-Hill, 1978, chap 6, p 57

JEWELL BR: A reexamination of the influence of muscle length on myocardial performance. Circ Res 40:814, 1977

KATZ AM: *Physiology of the Heart*. New York, Raven Press, 1977

SOLE MJ et al: A possible change in the rate-limiting step for cardiac norepinephrine synthesis in the cardiomyopathic Syrian hamster. Circ Res 41:814, 1977

THOMAS JA, MARKS BM: Plasma norepinephrine in congestive heart failure. Am J Cardiol 41:233, 1978

VASSALLE M (ed): *Cardiac Physiology for the Clinician*. New York, Academic, 1976

236
HEART FAILURE

EUGENE BRAUNWALD

Heart failure can be readily described as a clinical syndrome, characterized by well-known symptoms and physical signs, but it is more difficult to provide a precise physiological definition. However, for the purposes of this discussion, heart failure is considered to be the pathophysiologic state in which an abnormality of *cardiac* function is responsible for the failure of the heart to pump blood at a rate commensurate with the requirements of the metabolizing tissues. Heart failure is frequently, but not always, caused by a defect in myocardial contraction, and then the term *myocardial failure* is appropriate. The latter may result from a primary abnormality in the heart muscle, or it may be secondary to ischemia. Myocardial failure may also result from an extramyocardial abnormality, such as anatomic lesions of the heart valves or pericardium, which interferes with cardiac filling or emptying. For example, in many patients with rheumatic valvular disease and heart failure, the heart muscle has been damaged by the long-standing excessive hemodynamic burden imposed by the valvular abnormality, and/or by the rheumatic process (Chap. 242). In patients with chronic constrictive pericarditis, myocardial damage resulting from infiltration of the heart muscle by pericardial inflammation and calcification is common (Chap. 249).

In other patients with heart failure, however, a similar clinical syndrome is present, but without any detectable abnormality of *myocardial* function. These patients exhibit conditions in which the normal heart is suddenly presented with a load that exceeds its capacity, such as an acute hypertensive crisis, rupture of an aortic valve cusp, or massive pulmonary embolism, as well as chronic conditions in which there is impairment of filling of the ventricles due to tricuspid and/or mitral stenosis, constrictive pericarditis without myocardial involvement, and endocardial fibrosis. These are instances of *heart* failure, as opposed to *myocardial* failure.

Heart failure should be distinguished from conditions in which there is circulatory congestion consequent to abnormal salt and water retention but in which there is no disturbance of cardiac function per se. The latter syndrome, termed the *congested state*, may result from the abnormal salt and water retention of renal failure, or from excess parenteral administration of fluids and electrolytes.

CAUSES OF HEART FAILURE

It is important to identify not only the *underlying cause* of the heart disease but the *precipitating cause* of heart failure as well. The cardiac abnormality produced by a congenital or acquired lesion may exist for many years and produce no or only trivial disability. Frequently, however, serious manifestations of clinical heart failure appear for the first time in the course of some acute disturbance which places an additional load on a myocardium that chronically is excessively burdened, resulting in further deterioration of cardiac function. Identification of such precipitating causes is of critical importance because their prompt alleviation may be lifesaving. However, in the absence of underlying heart disease these acute disturbances do not usually, by themselves, lead to heart failure.

PRECIPITATING CAUSES

1 *Pulmonary embolism.* Patients with low cardiac output, circulatory stasis, and physical inactivity are likely to develop thrombi in the veins of the lower extremities or the pelvis. Pulmonary embolization may result in further acute elevation of pulmonary arterial pressure, which in turn may produce or intensify distention and failure of the right ventricle and may lower the cardiac output further. In the presence of pulmonary vascular congestion, such emboli may lead to infarction of the lung (Chap. 266).

2 *Infection.* Patients with pulmonary vascular congestion are particularly susceptible to pulmonary infections, but an infection anywhere in the body may precipitate heart failure. The resulting fever, tachycardia, hypoxemia, and the increased metabolic demands may place a further burden on the overloaded, but compensated, myocardium of a patient with chronic heart disease.

3 *Anemia.* The development of a significant reduction in the oxygen-carrying capacity of the blood may precipitate heart failure because in the presence of anemia the oxygen needs of the metabolizing tissues can be satisfied only by an increase in the cardiac output (Chap. 53). Though such an increase in the cardiac output might be sustained by a normal heart, a diseased, overloaded, but otherwise compensated heart may be unable to augment the volume of blood which it delivers to the periphery.

4 *Thyrotoxicosis and pregnancy.* As in anemia and fever, in these conditions adequate tissue perfusion requires an increased cardiac output. The development or intensification of heart failure may actually be one of the first clinical manifestations of hyperthyroidism in a patient with underlying heart disease (Chap. 335). Similarly, heart failure not infrequently occurs for the first time during pregnancy in women with rheumatic valvular disease; in such women cardiac compensation may return following delivery, after the excessive burden has been eliminated (Chap. 242).

5 *Arrhythmias.* Cardiac arrhythmias are among the most frequent precipitating causes of heart failure in patients with underlying but compensated heart disease for a variety of reasons: (*a*) tachyarrhythmias reduce the time period available for ventricular filling; (*b*) the dissociation between atrial and ventricular contractions characteristic of many supraventricular and ventricular arrhythmias result in the loss of the atrial booster pump mechanism, thereby tending to raise atrial pressures; (*c*) in ventricular tachycardia or any arrhythmia associated with abnormal intraventricular conduction, myocardial performance may become further impaired because of the loss of normal synchronicity of ventricular contraction; (*d*) the marked bradycardia associated with complete atrioventricular block requires a greatly elevated stroke volume if a marked reduction in cardiac output is to be prevented (Chap. 237).

6 *Rheumatic and other forms of myocarditis.* The development of acute rheumatic fever and a variety of allergic or infectious processes affecting the myocardium may further impair myocardial function in patients with preexisting heart disease (Chaps. 241 and 247).

7 *Infective endocarditis.* The anemia, fever, additional valvular damage, and myocarditis which often occur as a consequence of bacterial endocarditis may, singly or in concert, precipitate heart failure (Chap. 243).

8 *Physical, dietary, environmental, and emotional excesses.* The augmentation of sodium intake, the discontinuation of diuretics or digitalis glycosides, physical overexertion, excessive environmental heat or humidity, and emotional crises may all precipitate cardiac decompensation.

9 *Systemic hypertension.* Rapid elevation of arterial pressure, as may occur in some instances of hypertension of renal origin or upon discontinuation of antihypertensive medication, may result in cardiac decompensation (Chaps. 31 and 251).

10 *Myocardial infarction.* In patients with chronic but compensated ischemic heart disease, a fresh infarct, often silent clinically, may further impair ventricular function and precipitate heart failure (Chap. 245).

A careful and systematic search for one or more of these precipitating causes should be made in every patient with heart failure, particularly if it is refractory to the usual methods of therapy. If properly recognized, the precipitating cause of heart failure can usually be treated more effectively than the underlying cause. Furthermore, the prognosis in patients with heart failure in whom a precipitating cause can be identified and treated is more favorable than in patients in whom the underlying disease process has advanced to the point of producing heart failure.

FORMS OF HEART FAILURE

Heart failure may be described as *high-output* or *low-output*, *acute* or *chronic*, *right-sided* or *left-sided*, and *forward* or *backward*. Although these terms may be useful in a clinical setting, they are descriptive and do not signify fundamentally different disease states.

HIGH-OUTPUT VERSUS LOW-OUTPUT HEART FAILURE With the development of methods for the measurement of cardiac output, it became useful to classify patients with heart failure into those with a low cardiac output, i.e., *low-output heart failure*, and those with an elevated cardiac output, i.e., *high-output heart failure*. The cardiac output is often depressed in patients with heart failure secondary to coronary artery disease, hypertension, primary myocardial disease, valvular disease, and pericardial disease, but it tends to be elevated in patients with heart failure and hyperthyroidism, anemia, arteriovenous fistulas, beriberi, and Paget's disease. In clinical practice, however, it may be difficult to distinguish between low-output and high-output heart failure. The normal range of cardiac output is wide [2.5 to 4.0 (liters/min)/m²], and in many patients with so-called "low-output heart failure" the cardiac output may actually be within normal limits at rest, although it may fail to rise normally during exertion. On the other hand, in patients with so-called "high-output heart failure" the output may not be excessive but rather may be close to the upper limit of normal, particularly when heart failure is severe. Regardless of the absolute level of the cardiac output, however, cardiac failure may be said to be present when the characteristic clinical manifestations described below are accompanied by a depression of the curve relating ventricular end-diastolic volume to cardiac performance (Fig. 235-5).

An integral part of the heart failure syndrome is evidence that the heart does not deliver the quantity of oxygen required by the metabolizing tissues. In the absence of peripheral shunting of blood, such inadequate delivery of oxygen to the metabolizing tissues is reflected in an abnormal widening of the normal arterial-mixed venous oxygen difference (3.5 to 5.0 ml per 100 ml in the basal state), relative to the total body oxygen consumption. In mild cases, this abnormality may not be present at rest and may become evident only during exertion. In patients with the high-output cardiac states associated with conditions such as arteriovenous fistula, beriberi, thyrotoxicosis, and Paget's disease, the arterial-mixed venous oxygen difference is often abnormally low, because the mixed venous oxygen saturation is raised by the admixture of blood which has been shunted away from some of the metabolizing tissues, and it may be presumed that even in these patients the delivery of oxygen to the metabolizing tissues is reduced. When heart failure occurs in such patients, the arterial-mixed venous oxygen difference may be normal or even reduced, but it still exceeds the level which existed prior to the development of heart failure, and therefore the cardiac output, though normal or elevated, is lower than before heart failure occurred.

The mechanisms responsible for the development of heart failure in patients whose cardiac outputs are initially high are complex and depend on the underlying disease process. In most of these conditions the heart is called upon to pump abnormally large quantities of blood in order to deliver the normal quota of oxygen to the metabolizing tissues. The burden placed on the myocardium by the increased flow load resembles that produced by regurgitant valvular lesions. In addition, thyrotoxicosis and beriberi may impair myocardial metabolism directly, and severe anemia may interfere with myocardial function by producing myocardial anoxia.

ACUTE VERSUS CHRONIC HEART FAILURE The prototype of acute heart failure develops in patients with large myocardial infarctions or valve rupture, while chronic heart failure is typically observed in patients with multivalvular heart disease. Frequently, however, there is no fundamental distinction between these two conditions. For example, intensive efforts to prevent expansion of blood volume by means of dietary sodium restriction and the administration of diuretics will frequently delay the development of exertional dyspnea and ankle edema in patients with chronic valvular heart disease until an acute episode, such as an arrhythmia, or infection precipitates acute heart failure. Without intensive efforts to restrict blood volume the same patients would have been considered to have been suffering from chronic heart failure, even though their underlying myocardial disease were no further advanced.

RIGHT-SIDED VERSUS LEFT-SIDED HEART FAILURE Many of the clinical manifestations of heart failure result from the accumulation of excess fluid behind one or both ventricles (Chaps. 27 and 29). This fluid usually localizes upstream to the specific cardiac chamber which is initially affected. For example, patients in whom the abnormal load is placed on the left ventricle develop dyspnea and orthopnea as a result of pulmonary congestion, a condition referred to as *left-sided heart failure.* When heart failure has existed for months or years, such localization behind the failing ventricle may no longer exist. For example, patients with long-standing aortic valve disease or systemic hypertension may have ankle edema, congestive hepatomegaly, and systemic venous distention late in the course of their disease, even though the abnormal hemodynamic burden initially was placed on the left ventricle. In contrast, when the underlying abnormality affects the right ventricle primarily, e.g., valvular pulmonic stenosis or pulmonary hypertension secondary to pulmonary thromboembolism, symptoms resulting from pulmonary congestion such as orthopnea or paroxysmal nocturnal dyspnea are less common. However, severe exertional dyspnea may be observed in such patients.

Thus, although specific lesions may place an abnormal load on one or the other ventricle, when this load is excessive and applied for prolonged periods, failure of the heart as a whole occurs. Perhaps this is because the muscle bundles composing

both ventricles are continuous and both ventricles share a common wall, the interventricular septum. Also, biochemical changes which occur in heart failure and which may be involved in the impairment of myocardial function, such as norepinephrine depletion and alterations in the activity of myofibrillar ATPase, occur in the myocardium of both ventricles, regardless of the specific chamber on which the abnormal hemodynamic burden is placed.

BACKWARD VERSUS FORWARD HEART FAILURE For many years a controversy has revolved around the question of the mechanism of the clinical manifestations resulting from heart failure. The concept of *backward heart failure,* originated by James Hope in 1832, contends that when heart failure occurs, one or the other ventricle fails to discharge its contents normally, the end-diastolic volume of the ventricle rises, and the pressures and volumes in the atrium and venous system behind the failing ventricle become elevated. According to this concept, retention of sodium and water occurs as a consequence of the elevation of systemic venous and capillary pressures and the resultant transudation of fluid into the interstitial space, as well as from increased renal tubular reabsorption of sodium associated with an elevation of renal venous pressure (Chap. 29).

In contrast, the proponents of the *forward heart failure* hypothesis, expounded by MacKenzie in 1913, maintain that the clinical manifestations of heart failure result directly from an inadequate discharge of blood into the arterial system. Salt and water retention, according to this concept, is a consequence of diminished renal perfusion and/or excessive tubular sodium reabsorption through activation of the renin-angiotensin-aldosterone system.

A rigid distinction between *backward heart failure* and *forward heart failure* is artificial, since both mechanisms appear to operate to varying extents in most patients with chronic heart failure. However, the rate of onset of heart failure often influences the clinical manifestations. For example, when a large portion of the left ventricle is suddenly destroyed, as in myocardial infarction, acute pulmonary edema may develop rapidly, and although stroke volume is reduced, the patient may die of acute pulmonary edema before the reduced cardiac output can be responsible for the renal retention of salt and water. However, if the patient survives the acute insult, clinical manifestations resulting from the abnormal retention of fluid within the systemic vascular bed might develop. Similarly, the right ventricle may dilate and the systemic venous pressure may rise to high levels immediately following acute massive pulmonary embolism, but this state may have to be maintained for some days before sodium and water retention sufficient to produce edema occurs.

REDISTRIBUTION OF CARDIAC OUTPUT The redistribution of left ventricular output also serves as an important compensatory mechanism in the presence of severe impairment of cardiac function. This redistribution is most marked when a patient with heart failure exercises or an additional burden is imposed, such as fever or anemia, but as heart failure advances, redistribution occurs even in the basal state. Blood flow is redistributed so that the delivery of oxygen to vital organs, such as the brain and myocardium, is maintained at normal or near-normal levels, while blood flow to less critical areas, such as the cutaneous and muscular beds, is reduced. Vasoconstriction mediated by the sympathetic nervous system is largely responsible for this redistribution of peripheral blood flow.

SALT AND WATER RETENTION IN CHRONIC HEART FAILURE (See also Chap. 29)

When the volume of blood pumped by the left ventricle into the systemic vascular bed is chronically reduced, and when one or both of the ventricles fail to expel the normal fraction of their end-diastolic volume, a complex sequence of adjustments occurs which ultimately results in the abnormal accumulation of fluid. Though, on the one hand, many of the clinical manifestations of heart failure are secondary to this excessive retention of fluid, on the other hand, this abnormal fluid accumulation constitutes an important compensatory mechanism which tends to maintain cardiac output and therefore perfusion of the vital organs. Except in the terminal stages of heart failure, the ventricle operates on an ascending, albeit depressed and flattened function curve (Fig. 235-7), and the augmented ventricular end-diastolic volume and pressure characteristic of heart failure must be regarded as aiding the maintenance of cardiac output. The expansion of the intravascular blood volume, regardless of the mechanism responsible, tends to elevate ventricular end-diastolic volume, and, in accordance with the Frank-Starling principle, tends to augment ventricular performance. On the other hand, the maintenance of right ventricular end-diastolic volume and pressure at elevated levels raises systemic venous and capillary pressures, resulting ultimately in transudation of fluid from the vascular bed and edema formation. Similarly, the elevation of left ventricular end-diastolic volume and pressure will augment blood volume and, if the latter condition is severe, result in pulmonary edema.

In the presence of heart failure, effective filling of the systemic arterial tree is reduced, a condition which initiates the complex hemodynamic and hormonal adjustments that interact to promote reduced renal sodium and water excretion. Patients with very severe heart failure often exhibit a reduced capacity to excrete a water load, which may result in dilutional hyponatremia. These abnormalities may be caused, in part, by excess antidiuretic hormone activity and/or factors that prevent sodium reabsorption in the distal tubule, such as avid proximal tubular reabsorption of sodium or the action of a diuretic acting on the distal tubule.

The importance of elevated systemic venous pressure and of the alterations of renal and adrenal function characteristic of heart failure vary in their relative importance in the production of edema in different patients with heart failure. In patients with tricuspid valve disease or constrictive pericarditis the elevated venous pressure appears to play the dominant role. On the other hand, severe edema may be present in patients with ischemic or hypertensive heart disease, in whom systemic venous pressure is within normal limits or is only minimally elevated. In such patients, the fluid retention is probably due primarily to a redistribution of cardiac output and a concomitant reduction in renal perfusion. Regardless of the mechanisms involved in fluid retention, untreated patients with chronic congestive heart failure have elevations of total blood volume, interstitial fluid volume, and body sodium. These abnormalities diminish after clinical compensation has been achieved by treatment.

CLINICAL MANIFESTATIONS OF HEART FAILURE

DYSPNEA *Dyspnea,* or respiratory distress which occurs as the result of increased effort in breathing, is the most common symptom of heart failure (Chap. 27). It is at first observed only during activity, when it may simply represent an aggravation of the breathlessness which normally occurs under these circumstances. As heart failure advances, however, dyspnea appears with progressively less strenuous activity. Ultimately, breathlessness is present even when the patient is at rest. Thus, the chief difference between exertional dyspnea in normal persons and in cardiac patients is the degree of activity necessary to induce the symptom. Cardiac dyspnea is observed most frequently in patients with elevations of left atrial, pulmonary venous, and pulmonary capillary pressures. Such patients have engorged pulmonary vessels and interstitial pulmonary edema, which reduces the compliance of the lungs and thereby increases the work of the respiratory muscles required to inflate the lungs. The Hering-Breuer reflex, which inhibits inspiration, is enhanced, resulting in the rapid, shallow breathing of cardiac dyspnea. The oxygen cost of breathing is increased because of the excessive work of the respiratory muscles. This is coupled with the diminished delivery of oxygen to these muscles, which occurs as a consequence of the reduced cardiac output and which may contribute to the sensation of shortness of breath.

ORTHOPNEA The patient with orthopnea, i.e., dyspnea in the recumbent position, generally elevates his head on several pillows at night and frequently awakens short of breath if his head has slipped off the pillows. The sensation of breathlessness usually is relieved by sitting bolt upright, since this position reduces venous return and pulmonary capillary pressure, and many patients report that they find relief from sitting in front of an open window. As heart failure advances, orthopnea may be so severe that patients cannot lie down at all and must spend the entire night in a sitting position. On the other hand, in other patients with long-standing, severe heart failure, symptoms of pulmonary congestion may actually diminish with time as the function of the right ventricle becomes impaired.

PAROXYSMAL (NOCTURNAL) DYSPNEA This term refers to attacks of severe shortness of breath which generally occur at night and usually awaken the patient from sleep. Though simple orthopnea may be relieved by sitting upright at the side of the bed with legs dependent, in the patient with paroxysmal nocturnal dyspnea coughing and wheezing often persist even in this position. The depression of the respiratory center during sleep may reduce ventilation sufficiently to lower arterial oxygen tension, particularly in patients with interstitial lung edema and reduced pulmonary compliance. Also, ventricular function may be further impaired at night because of reduced adrenergic stimulation of myocardial function. Acute pulmonary edema (Chap. 27) is a severe form of cardiac asthma due to further elevation of pulmonary capillary pressure and associated with extreme shortness of breath, rales over both lung fields, and the transudation and expectoration of blood-tinged fluid. If not treated promptly (page 1044) acute pulmonary edema may be fatal.

CHEYNE-STOKES RESPIRATION Also known as *periodic* or *cyclic respiration,* Cheyne-Stokes respiration is characterized by diminished sensitivity of the respiratory center. In this form of respiration there is an apneic phase, during which the arterial P_{O_2} falls and the arterial P_{CO_2} rises. This combination of changes in the arterial blood stimulates the depressed respiratory center, resulting in hyperventilation and hypocapnia, followed in turn by apnea. Cheyne-Stokes respiration occurs most often in patients with cerebral atherosclerosis and other cerebral lesions, but the prolongation of the circulation time from the lung to the brain which occurs in heart failure, particularly in patients with hypertension and coronary artery disease and associated cerebral vascular disease, also appears to precipitate this form of breathing.

FATIGUE AND WEAKNESS These are nonspecific but common symptoms of heart failure and are related to the reduction of cardiac output. Anorexia and nausea associated with abdominal pain and fullness are frequent complaints in patients with severe heart failure; they may be related to the enlarged congested liver.

CEREBRAL SYMPTOMS In severe heart failure, particularly in elderly patients with accompanying cerebral arteriosclerosis and arterial hypoxemia, there may be alterations in the mental state characterized by confusion, difficulty in concentration, and impairment of memory, headache, insomnia, and anxiety.

PHYSICAL FINDINGS IN HEART FAILURE

In moderate heart failure the patient appears to be in no distress at rest except that he may become uncomfortable if asked to lie flat for more than a few minutes. In more severe heart failure the pulse pressure may be diminished, reflecting a reduction in stroke volume, and occasionally the diastolic arterial pressure may be elevated as a consequence of generalized vasoconstriction. There may be cyanosis of the lips and nail beds. Sinus tachycardia is common, as well as evidence of congested neck veins, which fill from below and which become distended with sustained pressure on the liver (positive hepatojugular reflux). *Systemic venous pressure* is often abnormally elevated in heart failure and may be recognized most readily by observing the extent of distention of the jugular veins. In the early stages of heart failure the venous pressure may be normal at rest but may become abnormally elevated during and immediately after exertion.

Early diastolic and presystolic gallop sounds (Chap. 231) are often audible but are not specific for heart failure, and *pulsus alternans*, i.e., a regular rhythm in which there is alternation of strong and weak cardiac contractions and therefore alternation in the strength of the peripheral pulses, may be present. Pulsus alternans may be detected by sphygmomanometry and in more severe instances by palpation; it frequently follows an extrasystole and is observed most commonly in patients with cardiomyopathy or with hypertensive or ischemic heart disease. It is caused by a reduction in the number of contractile units during weak contractions and/or by alternation in the ventricular end-diastolic volume.

BASAL PULMONARY RALES Moist, inspiratory, crepitant rales and dullness to percussion over the posterior lung bases are common in patients with heart failure and elevated pulmonary venous and capillary pressures. In patients with pulmonary edema, rales may be heard widely over both lung fields; they are frequently coarse and sibilant and may be accompanied by expiratory wheezing. Rales may, however, be caused by many other conditions.

CARDIAC EDEMA Cardiac edema is usually dependent, occurring in the legs symmetrically, particularly in the pretibial region and ankles in ambulatory patients, and in the sacral region of individuals at bed rest. Pitting edema of the arms and face occurs rarely and only late in the course of heart failure.

HYDROTHORAX Pleural effusion in congestive heart failure results from the elevation of pleural capillary pressure and transudation of fluid into the pleural cavities. Since the pleural veins drain into both the systemic and pulmonary veins, hydrothorax is observed most commonly in patients with marked elevation of pressure in both venous systems, but may also occur with marked elevation of pressure in either venous bed. It is noted more frequently in the right pleural cavity than the left.

ASCITES This also occurs as a consequence of transudation and results from increased pressure in the hepatic veins and the veins draining the peritoneum (Chap. 40). Ascites occurs most frequently in patients with tricuspid valve disease and with constrictive pericarditis.

CONGESTIVE HEPATOMEGALY An enlarged, tender, pulsating liver also accompanies systemic venous hypertension and is observed not only in the same conditions in which ascites occurs, but also in milder forms of heart failure from any cause. When systemic venous hypertension and hepatomegaly are prolonged and severe, enlargement of the spleen may also occur.

JAUNDICE This is a late finding in congestive heart failure and is associated with elevations of both the direct- and indirect-reacting bilirubin levels; it results from impairment of hepatic function secondary to hepatic congestion and the hepatocellular hypoxia associated with central lobular atrophy. Serum enzyme concentrations, particularly SGOT and SGPT, are frequently elevated. If hepatic congestion occurs acutely, the jaundice may be severe and the enzymes strikingly raised.

CARDIAC CACHEXIA With severe chronic heart failure there may be serious weight loss and cachexia because of (1) elevation of the metabolic rate, which results in part from the extra work performed by the respiratory muscles, the increased oxygen needs of the hypertrophied heart, and the discomfort associated with severe heart failure; (2) anorexia, nausea, and vomiting due to central causes or to congestive hepatomegaly and abdominal fullness; (3) some impairment of intestinal absorption due to congestion of the intestinal veins; and (4) rarely, in patients with particularly severe failure of the right side of the heart, a protein-losing enteropathy.

OTHER MANIFESTATIONS With reduction of blood flow the extremities may be cold, pale, and diaphoretic. Urine flow is depressed, and the urine contains protein and has a high specific gravity and a low concentration of sodium. In addition, there is prerenal azotemia.

ROENTGENOGRAPHIC FINDINGS IN HEART FAILURE

In addition to the enlargement of the particular chambers characteristic of the lesion responsible for heart failure, vascular changes in the lung fields are common in patients with heart failure and elevated pulmonary vascular pressures. Also, pleural effusions may be present and associated with interlobar effusions.

CLINICAL MANIFESTATIONS OF HIGH CARDIAC OUTPUT STATES ASSOCIATED WITH HEART FAILURE

THYROTOXICOSIS The characteristic clinical features of hyperthyroidism may be so conspicuous even after the development of heart failure that the diagnosis is simple on clinical grounds. In other cases, when eye phenomena and thyroid enlargement are not striking, the overactivity of the thyroid is hardly discernible. Thyrotoxicosis should be suspected as a contributing factor in patients with cardiac disease under the following circumstances: tachycardia that persists after prolonged rest and during sleep; any suggestion of heart failure with a high cardiac output in the absence of other recognizable causes; failure of the usual treatment measures to bring about a satisfactory response; attacks of paroxysmal atrial fibrillation or chronic atrial fibrillation in a person without obvious cause such as mitral valve disease and/or left atrial enlargement, particularly when the ventricular rate is resistant to the slowing effect of full doses of digitalis. The diagnosis is discussed fully in Chap. 335.

After treatment has restored the euthyroid state, remarkable improvement in a previously intractable form of heart disease usually follows. In about one-third of patients with atrial fibrillation the rhythm reverts spontaneously to a normal sinus mechanism; angina and congestive failure disappear or become easily controllable.

HEART FAILURE SECONDARY TO ANEMIA The clinical picture is that of high-output failure with anemia. One may find cardiac enlargement, occasionally with hypertrophy; systolic murmurs resulting from the combined effects of decreased viscosity, increased flow, or an aortic diastolic blowing murmur, presumably due to dilatation of the aortic ring. The latter may present a confusing problem of diagnosis. Furthermore, when slight fever is also present, infective endocarditis may be mimicked. In patients with sickle-cell anemia with fever and joint pains, acute rheumatic fever may be suspected.

When there is an organic obstruction in a coronary artery, the compensatory increase in coronary flow that would otherwise take place in anemia is prevented and angina may appear; alternatively, anemia may aggravate already existing angina.

HEART FAILURE SECONDARY TO THIAMINE DEFICIENCY (BERIBERI) Thiamine deficiency (Chap. 80) leads to a deficiency of cocarboxylase, resulting in impaired myocardial energy production. The defect in the peripheral tissues causes peripheral vasodilatation, increased venous return and cardiac output, and, consequently, an increased load on a heart already handicapped by the metabolic defect. Cardiac failure is more likely to occur in persons who have the least involvement of the nervous system and a greater capacity for work, i.e., who have a greater opportunity to develop an increased load on the heart.

The usual clinical picture of beriberi heart disease, as seen in the Orient, is characterized by enlargement of the heart, absence of arrhythmia, systemic venous hypertension, bounding arterial pulsations, and the classic phenomena of heart failure with a high cardiac output.

This picture is rarely encountered in the occidental countries; in these areas the more common description is that of a person who has been on a clearly deficient diet over a long period of time, who has had an excessive consumption of alcohol, who has heart disease of uncertain origin, heart failure that does not respond to the usual methods of treatment, signs of mild peripheral neuritis or other manifestations of dietary deficiency, and whose heart failure and cardiac enlargement disappear with the administration of thiamine.

The diagnosis depends mostly on securing a good dietary history and on observing the response to treatment. Beriberi heart disease should be suspected when heart failure with a normal or elevated cardiac output is observed in the absence of thyrotoxicosis or anemia. Furthermore, thiamine deficiency may contribute to the development of heart failure in alcoholics cardiomyopathy (Chap. 247).

DIFFERENTIAL DIAGNOSIS The diagnosis of congestive heart failure may be established by observing some combination of the clinical manifestations of heart failure, enumerated above, together with the findings characteristic of one of the etiologic forms of heart disease. Since heart failure is usually associated with an enlarged heart on physical examination and/or roentgenography, the diagnosis should be questioned, but is by no means excluded, when all chambers are normal in size. Heart failure may be difficult to distinguish from pulmonary disease, and the differential diagnosis is discussed in Chap. 27. Pulmonary embolism also presents many of the manifestations of heart failure, but fixed splitting of the second heart sound, a right ventricular lift, hemoptysis, pleuritic chest pain, and the characteristic mismatch between ventilation and perfusion on lung scan should point to this diagnosis (Chap. 266).

Ankle edema may be due to varicose veins, cyclic edema, or gravitational effects (Chap. 29), but in these patients there is no generalized systemic venous hypertension at rest, following exertion, or with pressure over the liver. Edema secondary to renal disease can usually be recognized by appropriate renal function tests and urinalysis and is rarely associated with elevation of the venous pressure. Enlargement of the liver and ascites occur in patients with hepatic cirrhosis, but may also be distinguished from heart failure by normal jugular antecubital venous pressures and absence of a positive hepatojugular reflux.

TREATMENT OF HEART FAILURE

The treatment of heart failure may be divided into three components: (1) removal of the precipitating cause, (2) correction of the underlying cause, and (3) control of the congestive heart failure state. The first two are discussed elsewhere, together with each specific disease entity or complication. The third component of the treatment of heart failure may, in turn, be divided into four categories: (1) reduction of physical activity, (2) enhancement of myocardial contractility, (3) control of excessive fluid retention, and (4) afterload reduction. The first two of these forms of therapy should be utilized simultaneously, and if abnormal fluid accumulation persists, the third should be applied. The vigor with which each of these measures is pursued in any individual patient should depend upon the severity of the heart failure state. Following effective treatment, recurrence of the clinical manifestations of heart failure may be prevented by continuing those measures that were originally effective.

REDUCTION OF PHYSICAL ACTIVITY Modest restriction of physical activity in mild cases and rest in bed or in a chair in severe failure remain cornerstones in the treatment of heart failure. Meals should be small in quantity, and every effort should be made to diminish the patient's anxiety. Physical and emotional rest tend to lower arterial pressure, and reduce the load on the myocardium by diminishing the requirements for cardiac output. These influences act in concert to diminish the need for redistribution of the cardiac output, and in many patients, particularly those with mild heart failure, simple bed rest and mild sedation often result in an effective diuresis.

Rest at home or in the hospital should be maintained for 1 to 2 weeks in patients with overt congestive failure and should be continued for several days after the patient's condition has stabilized. The hazards of phlebothrombosis and pulmonary embolism which occur with bed rest may be reduced with anticoagulants, leg exercises, and elastic stockings. Heavy sedation should be avoided, but small doses of barbiturates or tranquilizers may be helpful in calming the emotionally disturbed patient with heart failure through the first few days of therapy and in permitting much-needed sleep. In patients with chronic, mild heart failure, bed rest on weekends will frequently allow continuation of gainful employment. Following recovery from heart failure, the patient's activities must be carefully assessed, and often his or her responsibilities must be reduced. Intermittent rest during the day and the avoidance of strenuous exertion are often helpful once compensation has been restored. Weight reduction by restriction of caloric intake in the obese patient with heart failure also diminishes cardiac work load and is an essential component of the therapeutic program.

ENHANCEMENT OF MYOCARDIAL CONTRACTILITY The improvement of myocardial contractility by means of cardiac glycosides is the second of the four cornerstones in the control of the heart failure state. The pharmacology, indications, contraindications, and methods of administration of glycosides are considered in detail in Chap. 238. Digitalis is most effective in the common forms of heart failure associated with an excessive hemodynamic burden, such as hypertension and valvular heart disease, as well as in ischemic heart disease. It is particularly effective in the treatment of euthyroid patients with atrial fibrillation or atrial flutter and rapid ventricular rates associated with heart failure. In such patients the slowing of the ventricular rate, resulting from prolongation of the refractory period of the atrioventricular node combined with the improved inotropic state of the myocardium, results in striking and rapid clinical improvement. However, even in patients without these arrhythmias digitalis produces considerable clinical improvement as a consequence of its positive inotropic action.

Cardiac glycosides are less effective in diseases primarily affecting the myocardial cell, such as the toxic and infectious myocarditides, the various forms of cardiomyopathy, and in those forms of heart failure which are precipitated by infection, fever, anemia, thyrotoxicosis, beriberi, acute rheumatic fever, complete atrioventricular block, cor pulmonale, and constrictive pericarditis. Digitalis is contraindicated in patients with second-degree or unstable atrioventricular block, unless a pacemaker has been inserted, and in patients with idiopathic hypertrophic subaortic stenosis (Chap. 247).

Four sympathomimetic amines which act largely on beta-adrenergic receptors—epinephrine, isoproterenol, dopamine, and dobutamine—improve myocardial contractility in various forms of heart failure. The latter two agents (Chap. 238) appear to be most effective, since they increase cardiac output substantially, increase renal blood flow, and have little effect on peripheral resistance. They must be administered by constant intravenous infusion and are useful in intractable heart failure, particularly in patients who have undergone cardiac surgery, and in some instances of myocardial infarction and shock or pulmonary edema. While they improve the hemodynamics in that condition, it is not clear that they improve survival (Chap. 245).

CONTROL OF EXCESSIVE FLUID RETENTION Many of the clinical manifestations of heart failure are secondary to hypervolemia and expansion of the interstitial fluid volume. When fluid retention due to heart failure first becomes clinically evident, considerable expansion of the extracellular space has already occurred, and heart failure is already advanced. The quantity of extracellular fluid volume is largely dependent on the extracellular sodium content, and treatment aimed at reducing extracellular fluid volume is dependent primarily on lowering total body sodium stores, while fluid restriction, per se, is of less importance. A negative sodium balance can be achieved by reducing the dietary intake and increasing the urinary excretion of this ion with the aid of diuretics. In severe heart failure mechanical removal of extracellular fluid by means of thoracentesis, paracentesis, hemodialysis, or peritoneal dialysis may also be employed.

Diet In patients with mild heart failure, considerable improvement in symptoms may result from the simple reduction of sodium intake, particularly if this measure is accompanied by bed rest. In patients with more severe failure the sodium intake must be controlled more rigidly, even when other measures such as cardiac glycosides and diuretics are used, and following recovery from a bout of heart failure, at least moderate sodium restriction should be maintained. The normal diet contains approximately 6 to 10 g sodium chloride; this intake can be reduced by half simply by excluding salt-rich foods and salt which is added at the table. Reduction of the ordinary dietary intake to approximately one-fourth of normal may be achieved if, in addition, all salt is omitted from cooking. In patients with severe heart failure, in whom the daily sodium chloride intake is reduced to between 500 and 1000 mg, milk, cheese, bread, cereals, canned vegetables and soups, some salted cuts of meat, and fresh vegetables, including spinach, celery, and beets, must be eliminated. A variety of fresh fruit, green vegetables, specially processed breads and milk, and salt substitutes are permissible, but such diets are difficult to keep palatable outside the hospital. Water intake may be ad libitum in all but the most severe forms of congestive heart failure. However, late in the course of heart failure, dilutional hyponatremia may develop in patients who are unable to excrete a water load, sometimes because of excessive secretion of antidiuretic hormone. In such cases water intake as well as sodium intake must be restricted.

Attention must also be directed to the caloric content of the diet. Substantial improvement can result from caloric restriction in obese patients with heart failure, in whom weight loss will reduce the load placed on the myocardium. On the other hand, in individuals with severe heart failure and cardiac cachexia, an attempt must be made to maintain nutritional intake and to avoid caloric and vitamin deficiencies.

Diuretics A variety of diuretic agents is available, and in patients with mild heart failure almost all are effective. The choice of the particular diuretic to be employed depends to some extent on convenience. However, in the more severe forms of heart failure, the selection of diuretics is more difficult, and any existing abnormalities in the serum electrolytes must be taken into account. Overtreatment and resultant hypovolemia must be avoided, since excessive reduction of blood volume may reduce cardiac output, interfere with renal function, and produce profound weakness and lethargy.

THIAZIDE DIURETICS These agents are widely used in clinical practice because of their effectiveness when administered orally. In patients with chronic heart failure of mild or moderate severity the continued administration of chlorothiazide or one of its many analogues abolishes or diminishes the need for very rigid dietary sodium restriction, although salty foods and table salt should still be avoided. Thiazides are well absorbed following oral administration; chlorothiazide and hydrochlorothiazide reach their peak action in 4 h, and diuresis persists for approximately 12 h. Thiazide diuretics reduce the tubular reabsorption of sodium, and chloride and water follow the unreabsorbed sodium into the more distal tubule. Thiazides fail to increase free water clearance, and in some instances reduce it, supporting the hypothesis that these drugs inhibit selective sodium chloride reabsorption in the cortical diluting segment, at a site where the urine is normally diluted (Chap. 274). This results in the excretion of a hypertonic urine and may contribute to dilutional hyponatremia. As a consequence of the increased delivery of sodium to the distal nephron, sodium-potassium ion exchange is accelerated and kaliuresis results. The carbonic anhydrase-inhibiting properties of the thiazides are of limited importance and need not be invoked to account for most of the diuretic action. Chlorothiazide is administered in doses of up to 500 mg every 6 h. Many derivatives of this compound are available but differ principally in dosage and duration of action and therefore offer few, if any, significant advances over the parent compound. Potassium depletion is the chief adverse effect following prolonged administration of chlorothiazide, and may seriously enhance the dangers of digitalis intoxication and induce fatigue and lethargy. Hypokalemia may be prevented by the oral supplementation of potassium chloride solution. However, this is not palatable and may be hazardous in patients with renal failure. Therefore, to control potassium depletion produced by thiazides (as well as by ethacrynic acid and furosemide), intermittent dosage schedules, e.g., omitting the diuretic every third day, and the addition of a potassium-retaining diuretic, such as a spironolactone or triamterene, may be preferable. Other side effects of thiazides include reduction of the excretion of uric acid, which may lead to hyperuricemia, and a hyperglycemic effect, which is particularly troublesome in patients with overt or latent diabetes mellitus. Skin rashes, thrombocytopenia, and granulocytopenia have also been reported.

ETHACRYNIC ACID AND FUROSEMIDE These two diuretics are similar physiologically but differ chemically. Ethacrynic acid is an unsaturated ketone derivative of aryloxyacetic acid, while furosemide differs from the thiazides in that the thiadiasine ring has been replaced by a furfuryl group on the amino nitrogen of the anthranilic acid.

These are extremely powerful diuretics which reversibly inhibit the reabsorption throughout the nephron, but especially inhibit active chloride reabsorption in the thick ascending limb of the loop of Henle. These agents may induce renal cortical vasodilatation and can produce rates of urine formation which may be as high as one-third of the glomerular filtration rate. While other diuretics lose their effectiveness as blood volume is restored to normal levels, ethacrynic acid and furosemide remain effective despite the elimination of excessive extracellular fluid volume. The major side effects of these agents are due to this marked diuretic potency, which may result in circulatory collapse and in reductions in the renal blood flow and glomerular filtration rate. There is an inability to generate a dilute urine; alkalosis is produced by a large increase in the urinary excretion of chloride, hydrogen, and potassium ions. Hypokalemia and hyponatremia may occur, and hyperuricemia and hyperglycemia are observed occasionally, as with thiazide diuretics.

Both drugs are readily absorbed orally and are excreted in the bile and urine. They are usually effective by mouth, in doses of 25 to 100 mg two or four times daily, and intravenously in doses ranging from 10 to 100 mg. Both drugs can be given intravenously, and furosemide intramuscularly as well. Weakness, nausea, and dizziness may accompany both diuretics; ethacrynic acid has been associated with skin rash and granulocytopenia, as well as with transient or permanent deafness.

These extremely effective diuretics are useful in all forms of heart failure, particularly in otherwise refractory heart failure and pulmonary edema. Both agents have been shown to be effective in patients with hypoalbuminemia, hyponatremia, hypochloremia, hypokalemia, and reductions in the glomerular filtration rate, and to produce a diuresis in patients in whom thiazide diuretics and aldosterone antagonists are ineffective.

The effectiveness of ethacrynic acid or furosemide may be potentiated by spironolactone, triamterene, thiazide diuretics, carbonic anhydrase inhibitors, or osmotic diuretics, such as mannitol. In turn, when used in combination with these agents, ethacrynic acid or furosemide increases their effectiveness.

ALDOSTERONE ANTAGONISTS The 17-spironolactones resemble aldosterone structurally and act on the distal renal tubule by competitive inhibition of aldosterone, thereby blocking the exchange between sodium and both potassium and hydrogen in the distal tubules and collecting ducts. These agents produce a sodium diuresis, and, in contrast to the thiazides, ethacrynic acid, and furosemide, they tend to result in potassium retention. Although secondary hyperaldosteronism exists in some patients with congestive heart failure, the spironolactones are effective even in patients in whom the serum aldosterone concentration is within normal limits. Aldactone A may be administered in doses of 25 to 100 mg three to four times daily by mouth. The maximal effect of this regimen is not observed for approximately 4 days. Spironolactones are most effective when administered in combination with thiazide diuretics, ethacrynic acid, or furosemide. The opposing action of these drugs on urine and serum potassium makes possible a sodium diuresis without either hyper- or hypokalemia when spironolactone and one of these other agents are administered in combination. Also, since spironolactone (and triamterene) act on the distal tubule, they are particularly effective when used in combination with one of these other diuretics which acts more proximally.

Spironolactone should not be administered alone to patients with hyperkalemia, renal failure, or hyponatremia. Reported complications include nausea, epigastric distress, mental confusion, drowsiness, gynecomastia, and erythematous eruptions.

TRIAMTERENE AND AMILORIDE These two drugs exert renal effects similar to those of the spironolactones; i.e., they prevent sodium reabsorption and interfere with sodium-potassium exchange in the distal tubules. However, their fundamental mechanism of action differs from those of the spironolactones, since they are active in adrenalectomized animals. The effective dose of triamterene is 100 mg once or twice daily. Side effects include nausea, vomiting, diarrhea, headache, granulocytopenia, eosinophilia, and skin rash. Although both triamterene and the chemically unrelated diuretic amiloride resemble Aldactone A in that their diuretic potency is not great, they are extremely effective in preventing the hypokalemia characteristic of the administration of thiazides, furosemide, and ethacrynic acid.

ORGANOMERCURIALS Presumably these diuretics act by releasing inorganic mercury within the tubule cell, which then combines with sulfhydryl enzymes essential for active sodium transport in the ascending limb of Henle's loop. Mercurial diuretics reduce sodium reabsorption and make a greater quantity of sodium available for exchange with potassium in the distal tubule, thus tending to increase the excretion of potassium. Since these compounds produce a hypotonic diuresis, they may be useful in the treatment of patients with heart failure and dilutional hyponatremia. A serious disadvantage of mercurial diuretics is that they are not particularly effective when given by mouth and require parenteral administration. They are usually administered intramuscularly in doses of 0.5 or 1.0 ml, but may be given intravenously in patients with severe and refractory heart failure.

CHOICE OF A DIURETIC The thiazides, administered orally, are the agents of choice in the treatment of chronic cardiac edema of mild to moderate degree in patients without hyperglycemia or hyperuricemia. Spironolactones, triamterene, and amiloride are not potent diuretics when used alone, but they potentiate other diuretics, particularly the thiazides, ethacrynic acid, and furosemide. However, in patients with heart failure and severe secondary aldosteronism, spironolactone may be extremely effective. Ethacrynic acid or furosemide, given alone or with spironolactone or triamterene, are the agents of choice in patients with severe heart failure refractory to other diuretics. Mercurial diuretics are occasionally useful when a rapid diuresis is desired in patients with hyperglycemia or hyperuricemia.

VASODILATOR THERAPY In heart failure, left ventricular afterload is increased as a consequence of the many neural, humoral, and/or structural changes which constrict the peripheral vascular bed, and as the elevation of ventricular end-diastolic volume compensates for impaired cardiac function as a consequence of the operation of Laplace's law, myocardial wall tension (afterload) rises. The maintenance or even the elevation of arterial pressure is generally considered to be a useful compensatory mechanism that allows maintenance of blood flow to vital organs despite the marked inadequacy of total cardiac output, which occurs particularly during exertion. However, in the presence of severely impaired cardiac function, the increase in afterload may reduce cardiac output and elevate myocardial oxygen consumption further.

As pointed out in Chap. 235 (Fig. 235-6), afterload is a major determinant of cardiac function. A modest elevation in afterload will not necessarily alter stroke volume when cardiac function is normal, because the resultant small increase in left ventricular end-diastolic volume, i.e., preload, can be tolerated easily. However, when myocardial function is impaired, such an increase in preload evoked by an elevation of afterload may raise ventricular end-diastolic and pulmonary capillary pressures to levels that may produce pulmonary congestion and pulmonary edema. In many patients with heart failure, the ventricle is already operating at the peak, flat portion of its Frank-Starling curve (Fig. 235-7), and any additional increase in afterload will reduce stroke volume (page 1031). Conversely, a reduction of afterload will elevate the stroke volume of the failing ventricle.

The pharmacological reduction of impedance to left ventricular ejection, i.e., of afterload, with vasodilator drugs may be an important adjunct in the management of heart failure of diverse etiologies; this approach may be particularly helpful in patients with acute heart failure due to myocardial infarction (Chap. 245) and valvular regurgitation. The reduction of afterload by means of a variety of vasodilators, or mechanically by intraaortic balloon counterpulsation, reduces left ventricular end-diastolic pressure and oxygen consumption, while raising stroke volume and cardiac output and causing only modest reductions in aortic pressure.

In patients with both acute and chronic intractable heart failure secondary to coronary artery disease or cardiomyopathy who are treated with vasodilators, cardiac output increases substantially, the pulmonary wedge pressure falls, the signs and symptoms of heart failure are relieved, and a new steady state is generated in which cardiac output is higher and afterload lower with only mild reduction of arterial pressure. Furthermore, it has been proposed that the reduction of elevated left end-diastolic pressure might improve subendocardial perfusion. Afterload reduction should, therefore, be considered in the management of patients with intractable heart failure, but it requires careful hemodynamic monitoring.

Vasodilator therapy is particularly useful in the treatment of acute pulmonary edema, which, if not precipitated by myocardial infarction, is often associated with hypertension. Also, vasodilator therapy is often helpful in refractory congestive heart failure; when heart failure is acute, the addition of an inotropic agent such as dobutamine may be required, but the

use of oral vasodilators also appears to be helpful in the treatment of chronic heart failure.

The several available vasodilators vary in their hemodynamic effects, locus and duration of action, and mode of administration (Table 236-1). Some vasodilators, such as the alpha-adrenergic blocking agents and hydralazine, act predominantly on the arterial bed, while others, such as nitroglycerin, act exclusively, or almost so, on the venous side of the circulation. Some agents, such as sodium nitroprusside, must be administered by continuous intravenous infusion, nitroglycerin requires administration in ointment form when a prolonged effect is desired, while isosorbide dinitrate should be administered by the sublingual route to be effective.

The ideal vasodilator for the treatment of *acute* heart failure should have a rapid onset and brief duration of action when administered by intravenous infusion; sodium nitroprusside qualifies as such a drug. For the treatment of chronic congestive heart failure, the agent should be effective on oral administration, and its action should persist for at least 6 h. Both hydralazine and prazosin satisfy these requirements. Hydralazine acts on the arterial bed, while prazosin dilates both the arterial and venous beds.

In view of the spectrum of actions of available vasodilators, the selection of the specific agent or combinations of agents for any given patient should depend on the pathophysiologic state. For example, when the primary defect is a reduction of cardiac output and/or mitral regurgitation, an arterial vasodilator is the drug of choice; when pulmonary congestion is the principal defect, a venodilator would be preferable. When it is desired both to elevate cardiac output and to reduce pulmonary vascular pressures, an agent which acts both on the arterial and venous beds, such as prazosin, is indicated.

REFRACTORY HEART FAILURE When the response to treatment is inadequate, heart failure is considered to be refractory. Before assuming that this state simply reflects advanced, perhaps preterminal, myocardial depression, careful consideration must be given to several possibilities: (1) an underlying and overlooked cause of the heart disease that may be amenable to specific surgical or medical therapy, such as silent aortic or mitral stenosis, constrictive pericarditis, infective endocarditis, hypertension, or thyrotoxicosis; (2) one or a combination of the precipitating causes of heart failure, such as pulmonary or urinary tract infection, recurrent pulmonary emboli, arterial hypoxemia, anemia, or arrhythmia; and (3) complications of

TABLE 236-1
Spectrum of vasodilators used for the treatment of heart failure

	Primary site of action	Mode of administration	Duration of action
Phentolamine	Arterial	Continuous intravenous	Minutes
Phenoxybenzamine	Arterial	Oral	Hours
Hydralazine	Arterial	Oral	Hours
Minoxidil	Arterial	Oral	Hours
Nitroprusside	Arterial and venous	Continuous intravenous	Minutes
Trimethaphan	Arterial and venous	Continuous intravenous	Minutes
Prazosin	Arterial and venous	Oral	Hours
Nitroglycerin	Venous	Intravenous or sublingual	Minutes
		Ointment	Hours
Isosorbide dinitrate	Venous	Sublingual	Minutes to hours

overly vigorous therapy, such as digitalis intoxication, hypovolemia, or electrolyte imbalance.

Recognition and proper treatment of the aforementioned complications are likely to make the patient responsive to therapy again. Perhaps the most common complication results from overzealous treatment with diuretics. When they are administered too rapidly, sudden hypovolemia can occur before edema fluid can be mobilized to replace the loss, the result being a shock-like state with evidence of systemic hypoperfusion. The chronically excessively diuresed patient exchanges the hazards of pulmonary edema and the inconvenience of systemic edema for a persistently depressed cardiac output with its associated weakness, lethargy, prerenal azotemia, and sometimes cardiac cachexia. Temporarily easing up on salt restriction and diuretic administration may overcome this difficulty, but as heart failure worsens, this course of action may lead to increased pulmonary congestion which is equally unacceptable.

Hyponatremia is a late manifestation of refractory heart failure. It, too, may be a complication of overaggressive diuresis leading to reduced glomerular filtration rate and decreased delivery of NaCl to the diluting sites in the distal tubule. Hyponatremia may also result from nonosmotic stimuli for the continued secretion of antidiuretic hormone. Therapy involves improvement of the cardiovascular status, if possible, as well as temporary cessation of diuretic therapy and restriction of oral water intake.

TREATMENT OF ACUTE PULMONARY EDEMA Pulmonary edema secondary to left ventricular failure or mitral stenosis is described in Chap. 27. It is life-threatening and must be considered a medical emergency. As is the case for the more chronic forms of heart failure, in the treatment of pulmonary edema, attention must be directed to identifying and removing any precipitating causes of decompensation, such as an arrhythmia or infection. However, because of the acute nature of the problem, a number of additional nonspecific measures are necessary. When possible, and if it does not delay treatment unduly, recording pulmonary vascular pressures through a Swan-Ganz catheter and intraarterial pressure directly is advisable.

1 Morphine is administered by the subcutaneous, intramuscular, or intravenous routes in doses from 3 to 20 mg, depending upon the route chosen and the severity of the problem. This drug reduces anxiety, and thereby reduces adrenergic vasoconstrictor stimuli to the arteriolar and venous beds, and thereby breaks a vicious cycle. Naloxone should be available in case respiratory depression occurs.
2 High concentration of oxygen must be inhaled because the alveolar fluid interferes with oxygen diffusion, resulting in arterial hypoxemia. Therefore, 100 percent oxygen should be administered, preferably under positive pressure. The latter increases intraalveolar pressure and therefore reduces transudation of fluid from the alveolar capillaries and impedes venous return to the thorax, reducing pulmonary capillary pressure.
3 The patient should be maintained in the sitting position, which also tends to reduce venous return to the heart.
4 Rotating tourniquets should be applied to the extremities.
5 Intravenous diuretics, such as furosemide or ethacrynic acid (40 to 100 mg), will, by rapidly establishing a diuresis, reduce circulating blood volume and thereby hasten the relief of pulmonary edema. In addition when given intravenously, these drugs also exert a venodilator action, reduce venous return, and tend to reduce pulmonary edema even before the diuresis commences.

6 Afterload reduction is achieved with intravenous sodium nitroprusside at 20 to 30 μg/min in patients whose systolic arterial pressures exceed 100 mmHg.
7 If digitalis has not been administered previously, three-fourths of a full dose of a rapidly acting glycoside, such as ouabain, digoxin, or lanatoside C, should be administered intravenously (Chap. 238).
8 Aminophylline (theophylline ethylenediamine), 240 to 480 mg intravenously, is effective in diminishing bronchoconstriction, increasing renal blood flow and sodium excretion, and augmenting myocardial contractility.

After these emergency therapeutic measures have been instituted, and the precipitating factors treated, the diagnosis of the underlying cardiac disorder responsible for the pulmonary edema must be established if it is not already known. After stabilization of the patient's condition a long-range strategy for prevention of future episodes of pulmonary edema must be established, and this may require surgical treatment.

PROGNOSIS

The prognosis in heart failure depends primarily on the nature of the underlying heart disease and on the presence or absence of a precipitating factor which can be treated. Also, the long-term prognosis for heart failure is most favorable when the underlying forms of heart disease can be treated. When one of the latter can be identified and removed, the outlook for immediate survival is far better than if heart failure occurs without any obvious precipitating cause. The prognosis can also be estimated by observing the response to treatment. When clinical improvement occurs with only modest dietary sodium restriction and/or digitalis without the administration of diuretics, then the outlook is far better than if, in addition to these measures, intensive diuretic therapy is necessary.

REFERENCES

Braunwald E et al: Heart failure, in *Mechanisms of Contraction of the Normal and Failing Heart*, 2d ed. Boston, Little, Brown, 1976, chap 11

Brenner BM, Stein JH (eds): *Sodium and Homeostasis.* New York, Churchill Livingstone, 1978, p 250

Cherniack NS, Longobardo GS: Cheyne-Stokes breathing: An instability in physiologic control. N Engl J Med 288:952, 1973

Katz AM: Congestive heart failure: Role of altered myocardial cellular control. N Engl J Med 293:1184, 1975

Mason DT (ed): Symposium on vasodilator and inotropic therapy of heart failure. Am J Med 65:1, 1978

Smith TW, Braunwald E: Management of heart failure, in *Heart Disease*, E Braunwald (ed). Philadelphia, Saunders, 1980, chap 16

Stein J, Kunau R: Mechanisms of action and clinical use of diuretics, in *The Kidney*, BM Brenner, FC Rector (eds). Philadelphia, Saunders, 1980, chap 22

237
CARDIAC DYSRHYTHMIAS

BURTON E. SOBEL
EUGENE BRAUNWALD

The term *dysrhythmia* is not limited to irregularities of the heartbeat but is applied also to disturbances of rate and of conduction. We shall first present certain broad considerations and then deal with specific disorders. The mechanism of action of the most important drugs utilized in the treatment of dysrhythmias is considered in Chap. 238; treatment by electrical methods is the topic of Chap. 239.

GENERAL CONSIDERATIONS

ETIOLOGIC FACTORS Certain dysrhythmias are especially likely to occur in the absence of detectable structural disease of the heart. These include sinus arrhythmias, sinus bradycardia, and sinus tachycardia; atrial and ventricular premature beats; milder forms of first-degree atrioventricular (AV) block (that is, PR intervals of 0.21 to 0.25 s), paroxysmal atrial tachycardia, and on occasion atrial fibrillation or flutter. Only rarely can a specific agent such as tobacco, coffee, or ethanol be identified as an inciting cause of sinus or atrial tachycardia.

Other dysrhythmias are particularly likely to occur in persons with organic disease of the heart. These include ventricular tachycardia and fibrillation, atrial flutter and fibrillation, and second and third degrees of AV block. Although any type of structural cardiac disease may underlie any dysrhythmia, certain disturbances of rhythm are commonly associated with specifc underlying processes, for example, atrial fibrillation in patients with hypertension, thyrotoxicosis, mitral valve disease, and left atrial enlargement; and ventricular tachycardia in those with ischemic heart disease. Still other disturbances of rhythm should immediately arouse the suspicion that a drug is responsible. Ventricular bigeminy—a disorder in which a ventricular premature beat follows every supraventricular beat—and atrial tachycardia with atrioventricular block are often due to digitalis excess, especially when there is coexistent potassium deficiency induced by diuretics (Chap. 238). Bradycardia associated with suppression of sinus node and atrial activity and prolongation of AV and intraventricular conduction may reflect procainamide or quinidine toxicity or hyperkalemia.

A cardiac dysrhythmia may be a manifestation of a serious circulatory or metabolic disturbance and should result in a careful, deliberate search for the underlying abnormality, which may be (1) a pathologic process in the myocardium, e.g., a myocardial infarction or myocarditis; (2) a vascular event such as leakage from an aortic aneurysm, or pulmonary embolization; (3) a sudden drop in blood volume due to hemorrhage such as gastrointestinal bleeding; (4) an endocrine disturbance such as thyrotoxicosis or pheochromocytoma; (5) drug toxicity, especially evoked by cardioactive agents, including digitalis, glycosides, catecholamines, methyl xanthines, and antiarrhythmics (Chap. 238); (6) systemic infections; (7) a neoplasm with cardiac metastases such as carcinoma of the lung, lymphoma, or melanoma; or (8) the rapid development of sudden severe hypoxemia or hypercapnia.

Electrolyte disturbances are of particular importance in the genesis of cardiac dysrhythmias and deserve special consideration. They occur frequently in combination. Therefore, in practice it may be difficult to determine the specific ion abnormality responsible. *Hyperkalemia* leads to AV block, impairment of intraatrial and intraventricular conduction with prolonged P waves and QRS complexes, and rarely sinoventricular conduction. Death may occur from ventricular fibrillation or, less commonly, from ventricular asystole. *Hypokalemia* may produce atrial and ventricular extrasystoles, couplets, and tachycardias as well as mild atrioventricular and intraventricular conduction defects; severe hypokalemia may lead to multifocal premature ventricular contractions deteriorating into ventricular fibrillation. *Hypercalcemia* diminishes conduction velocity and shortens the refractory period, thereby facilitating reentry and the development of coupled ventricular beats, ventricular tachycardia, and ventricular fibrillation.

The treatment of dysrhythmias per se, without identification and management of the underlying abnormality, is often unrewarding. Also, often relatively little may be gained when treatment is directed toward a cardiac dysrhythmia which results from a structural abnormality, e.g., a greatly enlarged left atrium in a patient with mitral valvular disease. Effective control of atrial fibrillation under these circumstances might require surgical relief of the valvular abnormality.

MECHANISM OF DYSRHYTHMIAS Many cardiac dysrhythmias result from abnormalities in the automaticity of cardiac tissue. Increases in automaticity may result from (1) a more rapid rate of diastolic depolarization (Chap. 232); (2) a more negative threshold potential diminishing the change in potential required for excitation; (3) a less negative resting potential, which is therefore closer to the threshold potential; or (4) some combination of these abnormalities. Reductions in automaticity are produced by the opposite changes. Under physiologic conditions, the diastolic transmembrane potential of Purkinje fibers and ventricular myocardial cells is approximately -90 mV, and depolarization is attributable largely to rapid inward sodium flux (so-called primary, fast-current, or sodium-mediated depolarizations or responses). However, when the diastolic transmembrane potential is reduced, i.e., shifted in the direction of zero by the nature of depolarization changes. Under these conditions, depolarizations are mediated by transport of other ions, notably calcium, through a "slow channel" and are characterized by a diminished rate of rise of voltage, decreased amplitude, and abbreviation of the plateau phase of the action potential (secondary or slow-current depolarizations). Slow-current depolarizations are associated with repetitive depolarizations. Thus, conditions predisposing to slow responses such as regional acidosis or hyperkalemia accompanying ischemia may result in dysrhythmia due to increased automaticity reflecting repetitive depolarizations. Certain dysrhythmias, e.g., sinus tachycardia and some ectopic tachycardias, appear to result from increases in automaticity of the sinoatrial node or of pacemaker tissue elsewhere in the heart. Other disturbances, such as atrioventricular junctional rhythm or idioventricular rhythm, usually result from reduction in the automaticity of the sinoatrial node, with control of the cardiac rhythm assumed by a pacemaker which ordinarily exhibits a lower rate of automaticity.

Disturbances in the conduction of the action potential provide another important physiologic basis for cardiac dysrhythmias. Pathologic slowing or failure of propagation of the impulse from the atrium and AV junctional tissue to the ventricles results in various degrees of AV block. Under physiologic conditions, some cells in the heart, such as those in the sinus and AV nodes, exhibit slow-current responses and action potentials with low diastolic transmembrane potentials, low amplitude, slow rates of rise of voltage, and delayed recovery of excitability. Because the rate of rise of voltage and amplitude of slow-current responses are influenced by the nature of the stimulus initiating depolarization, in contrast to the case with fast-current depolarizations, conduction velocity through cells with slow-current responses is also affected. This phenomenon accounts for the decremental nature of conduction in AV nodal cells under physiologic conditions. Under pathologic conditions, decremental conduction may be accentuated accounting for unidirectional AV block. Analogous phenomena may occur when cells exhibiting fast responses under physiologic conditions are exposed to abnormal conditions, such as ischemia, resulting in slow-current depolarization. Slowed conduction or unidirectional block may occur and set the stage for development of tachyarrhythmias dependent on reentry.

Reentry is likely when an impulse leaves an area of reduced conduction velocity, finds the adjacent myocardium no longer refractory, and restimulates the adjacent tissue. Reentry can result also from either focal reexcitation due to the flow of current between adjacent portions of myocardium which are repolarized at different times (asynchronous recovery) or from circus current movement due to local impairment of conductivity. Reentry may occur within the AV or, rarely, sinus nodes, giving rise to supraventricular tachycardia. Reentry within accessory pathways occurs in some patients with preexcitation syndromes. In the arborizing fibers of the distal Purkinje system, reentry may be prominent at sites of "false-tendon" insertions of Purkinje fibers on ventricular myocardium. The action potential and effective refractory period are prolonged in these regions, which function as "gates" in prohibiting propagation of premature impulses. However, impulses blocked at a gate in one region may be conducted slowly through another gate into ventricular myocardium, and return in retrograde fashion through the first fiber, initiating a reentry rhythm.

Reentry is frequently responsible for coupled beats and some instances of bigeminal rhythm. Most reentrant beats or sustained reentry rhythms are characterized by both delayed conduction and unidirectional block. When these occur, reexcitation of normal tissue may be followed by retrograde repetitive excitation of the diseased area, and a self-sustaining tachycardia may result. Electrocardiographically, such rhythms appear to be initiated by a rapid ectopic pacemaker. In fact, however, although the dysrhythmia may be initiated by an ectopic impulse, it may be sustained by reentrant mechanisms. With recently available electrophysiologic techniques utilizing programmed electrical stimulation, several criteria of reentry rhythm have been established, including initiation and termination of tachyarrhythmia by appropriately timed premature beats and the appearance of a less than compensatory pause when interpolated beats are initiated during the tachycardia. Bigeminy due to digitalis, however, is probably due *not* to reentry but rather to increased automaticity associated with instability of Purkinje cells during repolarization, possibly due to slow-current, calcium-mediated depolarizations induced by the drug.

For a number of years considerable evidence supported the prevailing view that a *circus movement* is responsible for atrial flutter and fibrillation. However, some instances of these rhythms now appear to result from very rapid and irregular stimuli being discharged from a single focus. At the present time conflicting evidence favors and refutes both concepts; it is likely that each applies in different instances.

Concealed conduction is an additional important mechanism involved in complex dysrhythmias. This phenomenon usually affects the AV junction and occurs when an impulse penetrates the junction without traversing it. Thus, it may lead to apparent AV block or augmentation of the severity of block which actually is due to concealed conduction of ectopic impulses and "resetting" of the refractory period of the junction. Concealed conduction is probably responsbile for the nature of the irregularity of the ventricular response in the presence of atrial fibrillation.

Temporal dispersion of refractory periods in adjacent zones may lead to focal reexcitation, reentry with fragmentation of impulse transmission, and increased vulnerability of ventricular myocardium to fibrillation. Prolonged action potentials and refractory periods in the "false tendons" may serve to preclude conduction of premature impulses by serving as gates under physiologic conditions. Type I antiarrhythmic drugs, such as quinidine and procainamide (Chap. 238), prolong the refractory period at the gate and may thereby inhibit premature stimulation. However, the increased temporal dispersion may set the stage for reentry rhythms. Type II antiarrhythmics, such as lidocaine and phenytoin, reduce action potential duration at the gate and may diminish the likelihood of reentry rhythms by decreasing temporal dispersion. However, they may set the stage for premature stimulation of ventricular myocardium by impulses initiated in ectopic foci.

CIRCULATORY DERANGEMENTS ASSOCIATED WITH DYSRHYTHMIAS
Dysrhythmias alter cardiac function by a variety of mechanisms.

Effects of changes in heart rate In a resting person with a normal heart, because of compensatory changes in stroke volume, cardiac output remains constant, or almost so, despite variations in heart rate from approximately 40 to 160 contractions per minute; output decreases progressively at extremes beyond this range. However, in patients with significant myocardial, valvular, coronary arterial, or pericardial disease, such changes may seriously depress cardiac output because ventricular functional reserve mechanisms cannot compensate for altered stroke volume. The effect of bradycardia on cardiac output depends in part on its duration. Thus, in chronic longstanding AV block, cardiac output may be sustained even at rates as low as 35 beats per minute. When increased demands are placed on the normal heart, as during exertion, infection, or anemia, the acceleration of heart rate contributes substantially to the circulatory adjustment to the stress. However, when third-degree AV block is present with a fixed, slow ventricular rate, the cardiac output fails to rise normally, and the patient becomes especially symptomatic during the period of stress.

Loss of appropriately timed, vigorous atrial contraction The atria are not merely passive conduits for returning blood from the systemic and pulmonary venous beds to the ventricles. Rather, they should be considered as booster pumps which augment ventricular filling. In many dysrhythmias the normal temporal sequence between atrial and ventricular systole is lost. These include all degrees of AV block, AV junctional rhythms, ventricular tachycardia, and many instances of atrial tachycardia and flutter. In atrial fibrillation, effective atrial contraction does not occur.

Loss of atrial booster pump function will not usually lower the cardiac output in persons with otherwise normal cardiac function, since compensatory mechanisms such as augmented sympathetic stimulation of the myocardium help to maintain the output. However, loss of atrial function reduces the maximal cardiac output which can be achieved during marked exertion. On the other hand, in patients with impaired myocardial function (particularly those with overt or incipient chronic heart failure) or with acute myocardial infarction, atrial function is more critical, and loss of the atrial booster pump results in a lowering of cardiac output by as much as 40 percent, elevation of atrial pressures, or both. In patients with marked ventricular hypertrophy, such as occurs in hypertension, aortic stenosis, idiopathic hypertrophic subaortic stenosis, and the related cardiomyopathies characterized by ventricular hypertrophy, the atrial contribution to ventricular filling is particularly important, since the thickened ventricular wall impedes the inflow of blood. In patients with these lesions the sudden development of one of the aforementioned dysrhythmias may seriously impair cardiac performance and depress cardiac output and arterial pressure.

Effects on myocardial oxygen consumption and coronary blood flow The frequency of cardiac contraction is one of the major determinants of myocardial oxygen consumption (Chap. 5). Hence, when all other factors are constant, tachycardia increases and bradycardia reduces the need of the heart for oxygen. Coronary blood flow occurs predominantly during diastole, and since the total number of seconds of diastole per minute is reduced during tachycardia, a rapid heart rate may precipitate myocardial ischemia in the presence of coronary arterial narrowing. In turn, the ischemia may result in angina and in impairment of myocardial function. Thus, the development of AV block and a slow ventricular rate may diminish the severity of angina in patients with ischemic heart disease. On the other hand, excessive slowing of the heart rate associated with decreased cardiac output and impaired coronary perfusion may occasionally increase the severity of angina.

Effects on the ventricular contraction sequence Ventricular function depends on a synchronous, nearly simultaneous ventricular contraction. Though the ventricular myocardium contracts in ventricular fibrillation, the chaotic nature of the contraction prevents the development of sufficient intraventricular pressure to propel blood forward. Lesser degrees of asynchrony occur in dysrhythmias associated with intraventricular conduction abnormalities, such as ventricular tachycardia, ventricular extrasystoles, and supraventricular tachycardias with bundle branch block. Such asynchrony of contraction will not impair the cardiac output in an individual with an otherwise normal heart but may exert a significant depressant effect in patients with serious cardiac disease.

Effects on myocardial function Although the responsible mechanism has not been identified, prolonged severe tachycardia can depress myocardial function directly, and this depression may persist even after sinus rhythm has been restored.

METHODS OF EXAMINATION The most precise methods of diagnosis of the various dysrhythmias include electrocardiographic examination and recordings of His bundle electrograms. However, physicians who have regularly correlated their observations by simple physical examination with electrocardiographic tracings can usually recognize many dysrhythmias at the bedside.

The exact ventricular rate should be measured by auscultation for a full minute. Pulse rate may be misleading because of a pulse deficit. The presence or absence of irregularity should be noted. The intensity of the first heart sound and the amplitude of the peripheral pulse should be observed, and it should be especially noted whether they are constant, as in dysrhythmias in which the normal temporal relation between atrial and ventricular contraction is maintained (as in sinus, paroxysmal atrial, or junctional tachycardias), or variable, as in dysrhythmias in which the normal temporal relation between atrial and ventricular contraction is lost (e.g., in complete AV heart block, ventricular tachycardia, or atrial flutter). Atrial sounds independent of the first and second heart sounds are frequently audible in patients with third-degree AV block. If the rhythm is irregular, one should distinguish between a basic cadence that is predictable (regular irregularity, e.g., premature beats) and one that is entirely unpredictable (irregular irregularity, e.g., atrial fibrillation). In some instances the effect of mild exercise on the ventricular rate, and likewise on the degree of irregularity, should be observed; whether the deceleration immediately after exercise occurs in the normal gradual fashion (sinus tachycardia) or in one or more abrupt steps (atrial flutter) should also be noted.

Inspection of the jugular venous pulse is helpful, especially when, in a patient with a very slow or rapid rate, an occasional abrupt large venous excursion—"cannon wave"—is seen. This giant a wave occurs when the atria contract simultaneously with or after the ventricles and results from atrial contraction when the tricuspid valve is closed. Occasionally the jugular venous pulse will be of aid in the recognition of atrial flutter, with *a* waves perceptible at a frequency of 250 to 350 beats per minute.

Careful assessment of arterial blood pressure may be useful in suggesting the nature of tachycardias. When AV dissociation is present, phasic alterations of systolic blood pressure independent of respiration can be detected. Increased systemic arterial blood pressure accompanies those beats in which fortuitous physiologic sequencing of atrial and ventricular contraction is present because of the salutary effect of atrial transport on ventricular filling.

Observation of the effect of *carotid sinus massage* on the electrocardiogram may also be valuable. This maneuver elicits vagal efferent impulses which influence automaticity and conduction. After excluding occlusive carotid disease by examination, one may massage for a few seconds on one side. This may cause (1) no change in rate (ventricular tachycardia), (2) an abrupt slowing which persists after discontinuation of massage (atrial tachycardia), or (3) a temporary slowing which lasts only during the massage (atrial flutter or sinus tachycardia), with the rate returning to the previous level gradually (sinus tachycardia), at once, or following a brief period of irregular acceleration (atrial flutter). Carotid massage acts on the atrial mechanism (1) by gradually and temporarily slowing sinus rhythm or by abruptly interrupting a paroxysmal supraventricular tachycardia and/or (2) by increasing AV block.

The *electrocardiogram* should be studied systematically. The first and most important problem is to determine whether the dysrhythmia is ventricular or supraventricular in origin, a decision often made difficult by the presence of intraventricular conduction disturbances. The presence of P waves or flutter waves and their relation to the QRS complex in the tracing is especially important. P waves most often can be seen best in leads II, III, aVF, and/or those leads taken over the right precordium. Occasionally, other types of tracings may be necessary. For example, paroxysmal atrial tachycardia in the presence of a bundle branch block is exceedingly difficult to distinguish from ventricular tachycardia. Similarly, flutter impulses may be superimposed on the QRS complex or upon the T wave and make diagnosis difficult. In these instances, it may be necessary to employ esophageal electrodes or a bipolar anteroposterior lead. The right arm lead is placed over the right ventricle, the left arm lead on the back, and the electrocardiograph is set on lead I. Another bipolar chest lead may be used by placing the left arm lead at the cardiac apex and the right arm lead over the right ventricle. Intraatrial electrograms, esophageal, or surface electrocardiograms recorded during carotid sinus massage are often helpful in unraveling complex dysrhythmias.

Ambulatory electrocardiographic monitoring Compared to the standard electrocardiogram, results obtained with ambulatory monitoring (Holter recordings, dynamic electrocardiography) permit evaluation of a much larger number of cardiac cycles (exceeding 100,000 in 24 h) but less thorough delineation of each electrocardiographic complex because of the limited number of leads (one or two) employed. In addition to the longer interval for evaluation provided, it offers the advantage of detecting dysrhythmias occurring during sleep, of particular value in the recognition of paroxysmal supraventricular tachycardias, and during the course of normal activity and emotional stresses. Only approximately 20 percent of patients with ventricular dysrhythmia detectable by ambulatory monitoring will be identified on the basis of a single standard electrocardiogram, which provides only a 45-s sample. Exercise testing is somewhat less sensitive than 24-h ambulatory monitoring for detection of ventricular dysrhythmias. However, ventricular ectopic activity is elicited occasionally in patients subjected to exercise who fail to exhibit dysrhythmia during ambulatory monitoring.

Because of the considerable expense involved in obtaining and analyzing 24-h recordings, particularly when a large number are required because of the relative rarity of symptoms or episodes of dysrhythmia, devices activated by the patient have been developed to permit recording or storage of information during relatively brief intervals accompanying symptoms. Telemetry instruments, capable of transmitting analogue signals by telephone to a central recording and analysis station are particularly useful for monitoring the performance of artificial pacemakers or detecting and documenting rare dysrhythmia accompanied by signs or symptoms recognizable by the patient.

Recordings obtained during ambulatory monitoring are frequently analyzed at 1 to 120 times real time with the use of manual scanning devices. Technician or physician evaluation is required for each segment of the recording exhibiting variations in heart rate detectable by the device. More sophisticated automated analysis systems utilizing computers to characterize each QRS complex provide increased accuracy but still require operator interaction. Because of difficulties in establishing cause-and-effect relationships, interpretation requires correlation of electrocardiographically detectable events with a patient diary delineating activity and symptoms throughout the recording interval. For example, ventricular premature beats are extraordinarily common in elderly patients, many of whom may require evaluation for palpitations or syncope possibly related to complex ventricular dysrhythmia. The mere presence of dysrhythmia in Holter recordings is insufficient to establish a cause-and-effect relationship. Conversely, as many as 40 percent of patients with palpitations experience symptoms at times when ambulatory monitoring indicates no electrocardiographic disturbance, even though dysrhythmia may be present on different occasions during the recording interval.

Ambulatory monitoring is neither simple nor inexpensive, but its use has proliferated dramatically. Although it can be of unequivocal value in clarifying some clinical phenomena, its value in asymptomatic patients has not been established. Since the presence and severity of ventricular dysrhythmia are associated with increased risk of sudden death, ambulatory monitoring has been used to identify patients at high risk. Unfortunately, however, ventricular dysrhythmia may be simply a reflection of extensive coronary artery disease, and there is no objective evidence proving that suppression of premature ventricular complexes per se in ambulatory patients alters the risk of sudden death (Chap. 32). Since premature ventricular complexes are present in elderly normal subjects and in as many as 70 percent of patients who have recovered from acute myocardial infarction, routine screening by ambulatory monitoring often yields "positive" results, but the expense entailed in injudicious utilization of the procedure is certainly not justified.

Ambulatory monitoring has been proved to be of value for specific clinical indications in symptomatic patients, including evaluation of symptoms of suspected cardiac origin such as cerebral ischemia manifested by syncope, transient ischemic episodes, or seizures (Chap. 13); chest pain or palpitations of undefined origin despite conventional diagnostic procedures; and characterization of episodes of dysrhythmia such as paroxysmal supraventricular tachycardia, atrial fibrillation, or ventricular tachycardia. It is useful often for patients with known coronary artery disease, particularly as a guide to the effectiveness of drug therapy in suppressing complex ventricular dysrhythmias or dysrhythmia precipitating hemodynamic impairment and in assessing exercise tolerance and progress during formal rehabilitation programs. Occasionally, ambulatory monitoring is helpful in establishing the diagnosis of variant angina pectoris since ST-segment elevation may be detected during sleep or on other occasions during the recording interval associated with symptoms unrelated to exertion (Chap. 244).

Detection of disorders of the conduction system, including those due to idiopathic degeneration, cardiomyopathy, valvular disease with infiltrating calcification, inflammatory processes, or coronary artery disease is generally accomplished readily by standard electrocardiography. However, in some instances in which patients experience intermittent symptoms, ambulatory monitoring may help to establish the diagnosis. Similar considerations apply to patients with suspected preexcitation or prolonged QT-interval syndromes without manifestations on standard electrocardiograms but with symptoms related to dysrhythmias occurring intermittently.

Since diagnosis of the sick sinus syndrome (see below) is often an indication for treatment with an artificial pacemaker, and since manifestations of this syndrome are often evanescent, ambulatory monitoring is useful when this condition is suspected but not detectable with more conventional diagnostic procedures. Although ambulatory monitoring has been advocated for patients with mitral valve prolapse because of a high incidence of ventricular and supraventricular tachyarrhythmias and of bradycardia among symptomatic patients with this condition (Chap. 242), the rare patient with this disorder who is at high risk for sudden death cannot be identified definitively. Nevertheless, since sudden death among patients with mitral valve prolapse appears to be more common among young to middle-aged females with episodes of syncope and ST-segment deviation, ambulatory monitoring may be justified in occasional patients with this disorder to assess its apparent electrophysiologic severity.

Difficult diagnostic problems may necessitate evaluation with *His bundle electrograms,* recorded with the use of a transvenous electrode catheter positioned with its tip in the right ventricle adjacent to the tricuspid valve. Ordinarily, atrial depolarization (A), His bundle depolarization (H), ventricular depolarization (V), and ventricular repolarization produce well-defined characteristic waveforms on the electrogram (Fig. 237-1). Recognition of each is facilitated by reference to a simultaneously recorded standard surface electrocardiogram and by knowledge of the usual temporal relationships between components of the electrogram. Junctional beats with aberrant ventricular conduction are preceded by an H spike, and the HV interval is the same as in sinus beats. Ventricular premature beats are not preceded by an H spike, and in fact may be followed by an H depolarization and an A spike indicative of retrograde atrial depolarization. His bundle electrograms are useful in characterizing the nature of AV block. Prolonged A to H intervals are typical of AV junctional disease; prolonged HV intervals are typical of delayed conduction in more distal portions of the conduction system and hence of trifascicular block. The latter is far more common than the former, and since it is more likely to evolve into sudden third-degree block associated with syncope or sudden death, its recognition is of considerable importance.

His bundle electrocardiography This method may reveal concealed conduction of ectopic impulses originating in the His-Purkinje system which mimic AV block by depolarizing the AV node without spreading into ventricular myocardium. The differentiation is important because treatment requires suppression of ectopic foci rather than facilitation of conduction.

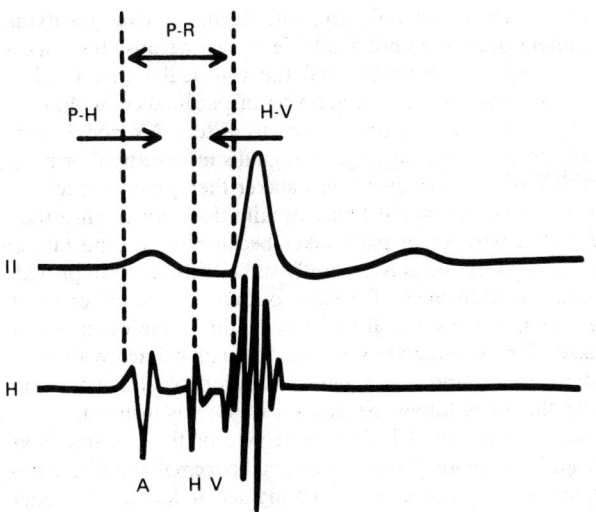

FIGURE 237-1

The relationship between deflections on the conventional electrocardiogram (II) and potentials evident on a simultaneously obtained His bundle recording (H). Three components are readily recognizable on the His bundle recording. The A spike follows the onset of the P wave and represents the atrial electrogram. The H spike represents depolarization of the His bundle. The V potential represents the recording of ventricular depolarization from the catheter electrode. The PR interval on the simultaneously recorded electrocardiogram is divided conveniently into two components on the basis of the time of occurrence of the H spike. Thus the PH component represents the time from the onset of atrial depolarization to His bundle depolarization and reflects the duration of conduction through atrial myocardium and the AV junction. The subsequent component of the PR interval, namely, the HV component, represents the time required for conduction of the impulse from the common His bundle to the ventricular myocardium. Normally, the PH interval is between 80 and 140 ms and the HV interval is between 35 and 55 ms. Prolongation of the PH interval is usually indicative of delay of conduction in the proximal AV junction and is often associated with Möbitz type I AV block. Prolongation of the HV interval is usually indicative of conduction delay in the His bundle, or in both bundle branches or all three fascicles of the distal conduction system, and is frequently associated with Möbitz type II AV block. Premature supraventricular beats with aberrant conduction are preceded by an H spike at the usual interval prior to the onset of QRS complex on the conventional electrocardiogram. On the other hand, premature ventricular beats are recognized by appearance of a V spike occurring prematurely after an H spike, prior to an H spike, or without any association with an H spike.

Intracardiac electrograms and characterization of the length of the refractory period in the AV junction and in accessory pathways in patients with preexcitation syndromes are useful in selection of pharmacologic agents to prevent or treat tachycardia. Diagnosis may be facilitated by unmasking delta waves indicative of preexcitation when atrial pacing or programmed electrical stimulation increases the A to H intervals, permitting expression of conduction through accessory pathways. Intra-atrial electrical stimulation is also useful for detection and evaluation of impaired sinus node function reflected by prolonged sinus node recovery time after atrial paced rhythm and for evaluation of sinoatrial conduction time, often prolonged in the sick sinus syndrome.

TREATMENT General measures The success or failure of specific treatment by drugs or by electric shock (Chap. 239) may be conditioned by appropriate systemic management. A precipitating cause of the dysrhythmia should be sought and treated. Obstruction of the air passages, hypoxia, and disturbances of pH and of electrolyte balance should be corrected. The coexistence of circulatory shock, whether of cardiac or

peripheral origin, may render the patient's heartbeat refractory to the usual antiarrhythmic drugs. Thus, it may be necessary first to improve hemodynamics by blood or fluid replacement, or to administer agents with positive inotropic effects when depressed contractility is a contributing factor. Since pressor amines tend to induce ectopic rhythms at elevated blood pressure levels, the arterial pressure as well as the electrocardiogram should be observed frequently.

Rapidly acting cardiac glycosides such as digoxin, ouabain, or lanatoside C are useful for the treatment of any of the supraventricular tachycardias except, of course, paroxysmal atrial tachycardia with block, which is frequently caused by digitalis intoxication (Chap. 238). The roles of antiarrhythmic drugs and of electrical reversion in the treatment of arrhythmias are discussed in Chaps. 238 and 239 and in this chapter in relation to individual arrhythmias. The management of dysrhythmias occurring with acute myocardial infarction is discussed in Chap. 245. In general, electrical reversion is most useful in the management of tachyarrhythmias which impair hemodynamics, while the antiarrhythmic drugs are indicated when tachyarrhythmias recur.

ARTIFICIAL CARDIAC PACEMAKERS The most common form of *direct* cardiac pacing is the endocardial, in which an electrode catheter is placed, generally in the right ventricle, through the venous route; it is employed with an external power supply for temporary pacing or one that is implanted subcutaneously for permanent pacing. Endocardial pacing of the atrium is more difficult to achieve on a long-term basis because of electrode instability but can sometimes be achieved with placement of the pacemaker within the coronary sinus. Epicardial pacing may be carried out by suturing wire leads to the atrial or ventricular myocardium at the time of thoracotomy, or by application of sutureless electrodes which screw into the myocardium. For permanent direct pacing the power supply is totally implanted.

Transvenous insertion of a permanent endocardial pacemaker entails minimal risk of postoperative fatality (1 to 3 percent) but a high incidence of displacement (5 to 20 percent), occurring mainly in the first month and especially in patients with a large right ventricle. Insertion at thoracotomy of an epicardial pacemaker entails a higher perioperative mortality rate (2 to 5 percent), virtually no incidence of displacement, but a high incidence of electrode breakage (approximately 20 percent) which may be diminished with newer sutureless electrodes. Increases in threshold with exit block occur more often with epicardial pacemakers, and perforation of the heart occurs (approximately 5 percent) more often with endocardial pacemakers. Infection (5 to 10 percent) is probably more common with epicardial devices. Transvenous endocardial pacing is still generally preferred except when atrial or sequential atrial and ventricular pacing are required.

Two principal modes of direct myocardial pacing may be employed. In *fixed-rate* pacing, cardiac stimulation is carried out continuously at a preset rate and is independent of the intrinsic electric activity of the heart. Consequently, if AV conduction is reestablished in patients with AV block, competition between the paced beats and the patient's intrinsic rhythm may occur. This competition may result in chaotic rhythms with an attendant, if small, hazard of the development of ventricular fibrillation. Although fixed-rate pacemakers are electronically relatively simple, they are now rarely used. Even among patients with long-established complete AV block, transitory return of conduction through the AV junction may occur, setting the stage for competitive dysrhythmia when a fixed-rate pacemaker is present.

Noncompetitive (demand) pacemakers fire only when the patient's ventricular rate falls below the preset rate of the pacemaker. In the ventricular-inhibited type the output of the pacemaker is inhibited when the frequency of spontaneous ventricular depolarizations is above this level. In the ventricular-activated type the pacemaker discharge is triggered by each spontaneous ventricular depolarization. In the absence of spontaneous depolarization the pacemaker discharges after a preset delay interval. These devices are designed with a refractory period in the range of 400 ms to preclude rapid repetitive pacemaker discharge triggered by the T wave. With triggered pacemakers evaluation of the sensing function is simplified because the stimulus artifact is present with each spontaneous ventricular depolarization.

The advantage of noncompetitive pacing is that if AV conduction returns, the hazards of competitive, fixed-rate pacing are eliminated. It is also useful in patients with paroxysms of symptomatic bradyarrhythmias other than AV block [including sinus bradycardia, sinoatrial (SA) block, and the so-called sick sinus syndrome] and in patients in whom bradycardia alternates with tachycardia. In patients with bradyarrhythmias the implantation of a demand pacemaker permits the administration of antiarrhythmic drugs to suppress the development of ventricular tachyarrhythmias.

Specific indications for implantation of artificial pacemakers
Artificial pacemakers should be utilized for treatment of persistent bradycardia of any origin if it compromises hemodynamics, or bradycardia documented to predispose to ventricular irritability manifested by premature beats or ventricular tachycardia. Although sinus bradycardia in a young, trained athlete is physiologic, comparable depression of heart rate in an elderly individual with limited ventricular function might compromise cardiac output and systemic arterial pressure, or predispose to ventricular dysrhythmia.

The most common indication for pacemaker therapy is AV block. Prior to the advent of reliable temporary and permanent ventricular transvenous pacing, pharmacologic approaches were utilized to facilitate AV conduction in patients with transitory or persistent AV block, but no pharmacologic approach rivals the efficacy or reliability of electrical pacing and none should be utilized as primary therapy.

Impaired conduction within the AV junction may be first-degree, manifested by a prolonged PR interval; second-degree, with occasional or periodically dropped beats; or third-degree, with complete AV block. AV block is often attributable to impaired conduction distal to the AV node itself, reflecting dysfunction of the His-Purkinje system. Second-degree block generally takes one of two electrocardiographic forms—Möbitz types I and II. Type I exhibits gradual and progressive prolongation of the PR interval prior to dropped beats and a narrow QRS complex. Type II exhibits dropped beats without preceding prolongation of the PR interval, frequently associated with wide QRS complexes of all beats. Based on results obtained with His bundle recordings, type I block has been found to be associated frequently with impairment of conduction within the AV node and type II has been associated with infranodal dysfunction, although exceptions are not infrequent.

Among patients with AV block unassociated with acute myocardial infarction in whom block is in the AV node, pacing is required when documentation of syncope or other symptoms resulting from the block can be obtained or when the block is third-degree. First- or second-degree block within the AV node

requires vigorous surveillance, but definitive data justifying permanent pacing are not available in part because the abnormality frequently regresses and the ventricular rate is often well maintained due to acceleration of pacemakers within the AV junction. For the same reason, transitory AV nodal block associated with cardiac surgery, digitalis intoxication, or myocarditis requires permanent pacemaker therapy only rarely.

Congenital AV nodal block usually does not require therapy with a permanent pacemaker because the escape rate of junctional pacemakers is generally sufficiently rapid to provide adequate maintenance of cardiac output. On the other hand, when complete AV nodal block is acquired, the degenerative disease of the conduction system is often associated with myocardial disease and consequent limitation of stroke volume. Under these conditions, pacemaker therapy is justified.

Acquired infranodal block of second or third degree is an indication for therapy with an artificial pacemaker because it is frequently progressive, even among asymptomatic patients. Despite the use of programmed electrical stimulation and His bundle electrocardiography, it is not possible to predict reliably which asymptomatic patients with unifascicular or bifascicular disease will develop high degrees of AV block. Thus, although the decision regarding each individual patient rests on several considerations, pacemaker therapy is generally warranted when bifascicular disease can be documented.

Indications for pacemaker therapy for AV block associated with acute myocardial infarction are somewhat different (Chap. 245). First-degree AV nodal block is common, particularly among patients with inferior infarction. It generally does not require specific therapy beyond inhibition of excess vagotonia with atropine. Vigorous surveillance is required because progression to higher degrees of block is common. Second-degree AV block associated with inferior infarction is generally Möbitz type I. Although it is associated with an increased overall early mortality rate, pacemaker therapy is not required unless it leads to ventricular irritability, congestive heart failure, or impaired hemodynamics. Möbitz type II block is relatively rare in the setting of acute myocardial infarction. However, temporary transvenous pacing should be implemented when it is detected because of its potential for progression to complete heart block.

Complete AV block in association with acute myocardial infarction occurs in less than 10 percent of patients. When it accompanies anterior infarction, it generally reflects extensive necrosis and is associated with an extremely high mortality rate. When it occurs with inferior infarction, it may reflect either AV nodal or infranodal disease. Overall, the survival rate among hospitalized patients with infarction complicated by complete heart block approximates only 50 percent. Because the poor outlook is a reflection not only of sequelae of AV block but also of the frequently associated extensive underlying infarction, definitive proof that implementation of temporary transvenous pacing reduces the mortality rate is lacking. Nevertheless, protection by pacing against transitory hemodynamic disturbances accompanying block is warranted.

Because of the high mortality rate for patients developing complete AV block with acute myocardial infarction, it has been difficult to determine whether permanent ventricular pacing reduces the mortality rate among survivors with persistent block at the time of discharge from the hospital. However, long-term pacing has been shown to reduce the risk for sudden death during the subsequent year among patients who develop transitory trifascicular block in association with acute infarction even if a conducted sinus rhythm is restored prior to discharge. Definitive data are not available regarding the implications of transitory bifascicular block, but permanent ventricular pacing may be justified in survivors with this complication as well.

Permanent ventricular pacing is justified among patients with the sick sinus syndrome since associated AV conduction system disease is so common. Asystole occurs frequently in this disorder, even among patients who have previously been asymptomatic. Although the natural history of the disorder is erratic and its recognition sometimes obscure, it should be suspected when relative or absolute sinus bradycardia is documented with or without sinus arrest or failure of AV junctional pacemakers to escape, or among patients with transitory or persistent atrial fibrillation without another obvious cause. When it is documented electrocardiographically or with the use of provocative tests including programmed atrial stimulation, permanent pacemaker therapy should be implemented.

Although cardiac arrest is due most often to ventricular fibrillation, occasionally it results from asystole (Chap. 32) requiring immediate implementation of ventricular pacing. For hospitalized patients who develop asystole, transthoracic insertion of the pacemaker provides the most expeditious approach.

Artificial pacemakers are sometimes useful in suppressing ventricular tachyarrhythmias resulting from enhanced automaticity. Recurrent ventricular tachyarrhythmias can be treated more effectively pharmacologically with concomitant permanent ventricular demand pacing because of the protection afforded by the artificial pacemaker against excessive suppression of endogenous automaticity or conduction.

SPECIFIC DISORDERS OF RATE AND RHYTHM

DERANGEMENTS ARISING IN THE SINUS NODE Sinus bradycardia This is characterized by a slow heart rate (below 60 beats per minute) with a normal spread of atrial excitation. It is frequent in athletes and is usually a sign of excellent physical fitness. However, in elderly subjects with symptoms attributable to failure of impulse formation or propagation, it may be one manifestation of sinus node dysfunction and may be associated with latent or overt AV conduction abnormalities as well. It occurs also in patients with increased intracerebral pressure, myxedema, or hypothermia.

Sinoatrial arrest This is due to a sporadic failure of the sinus impulse, and therefore, there is no sinus node–initiated ventricular excitation. The electrocardiogram shows a prolonged pause between two P waves. Sinoatrial arrest is most frequently due to digitalis or to some other cause of vagal stimulation but may result from myocardial disease. Aside from withholding digitalis and the occasional use of atropine, treatment is usually unnecessary.

Sinoatrial block In this dysrhythmia regular sinus impulse formation occurs but there are no atrial or ventricular depolarizations because the impulse is blocked from reaching these structures. The PP interval is prolonged, usually to some multiple of the regular intervals, but may progressively and periodically shorten, prior to a dropped P wave, when sinoatrial Wenckebach exit block is present. Sinoatrial block is infrequently accompanied by AV block; it may be precipitated by digitalis, quinidine, hyperkalemia, or acute myocardial infarction.

Sinus arrhythmia This dysrhythmia is present in most healthy young persons at rest; it consists of a quickening of the heart rate during inspiration and a slowing during expiration, tends to be intensified by deep breathing, and tends to disappear when the breath is held or when the heart rate is increased by exercise or fever. It has no pathologic significance.

Sinus tachycardia (Fig. 237-2*B*) Defined as a sinus-initiated heart rate faster than 100 beats per minute, this dysrhythmia must be distinguished from the various ectopic tachycardias.

The latter group will usually respond to therapy aimed directly at the heart; in sinus tachycardia, the treatment of the rapid rate depends on the management of the underlying condition. A reliable history of abrupt onset and cessation suggests that the attack represents an ectopic tachycardia rather than sinus tachycardia. However, the patient is often unable to make this differentiation with certainty. When the rate is less than 140 beats per minute, the odds favor sinus tachycardia, but a ventricular rate below 140 is also frequent in patients with digitalis-induced atrial tachycardia with AV block, some persons with atrial flutter or ventricular tachycardia, and some elderly patients with paroxysmal supraventricular tachycardia. Rates of 170 or more per minute are almost invariably the result of ectopic rhythms. Difficulty in distinguishing ectopic rhythms from sinus tachycardias occurs chiefly with heart rates between 140 and 170 beats per minute. In sinus tachycardia the rate is less constant than in ectopic tachycardia and is altered somewhat by changes in posture and activity. Anxiety, fever, blood loss, thyrotoxicosis, pregnancy, pheochromocytoma, or some other cause of the tachycardia is usually evident. The response to manual carotid sinus stimulation may help in the differentiation. As described above under "Methods of Examination," sinus tachycardia is usually slowed slightly but gradually by such massage.

Extremely rapid sinus tachycardia with heart rates exceeding 130 beats per minute is usually due to marked elevation of body temperature, severe thyrotoxicosis, profound circulatory collapse, or electrolyte imbalance. Frequently, patients with severe advanced chronic airway disease have a sustained tachycardia, usually not over 120 beats per minute; however, during episodes of respiratory decompensation initiated by intercurrent pulmonary infections, heart failure, or obstruction of the airways, the tachycardia may reach 160 beats per minute. Consequently, correcting the underlying systemic abnormality is paramount. A similar problem is often present in patients with chronic lung disease following a pneumonectomy or lobectomy. Maintaining airway patency, ventilation, and oxygenation is of great importance. Digitalis or other cardiac therapy is of no therapeutic value in patients with sinus tachycardia unless there are manifestations of congestive heart failure. Since the response of the sinus node to pharmacologic agents may reflect the dependence of its automaticity on slow-current, calcium-mediated depolarization, preferential sinus slowing may be possible with agents such as verapamil which may block calcium transport. On the other hand, the calcium dependence and sodium current independence of sinus node automaticity may account for its remarkable resistance to conventional antiarrhythmic agents such as lidocaine. However, effective management of sinus tachycardia generally requires discovering its basic cause and correcting it.

DERANGEMENTS ARISING IN THE ATRIUM Ectopic atrial beats (Fig. 237-2*A*) Also known as premature atrial beats, these originate from an abnormal focus in the atrium rather than the sinus node. Ectopic atrial beats have little clinical significance, but they may precede the onset of sustained atrial dysrhythmias, such as atrial tachycardia, flutter, or fibrillation. Also, their suppression may prevent the onset of these sustained tachyarrhythmias. Recognition of atrial ectopic beats is important, since they may be confused at the bedside with the often more serious ectopic ventricular beats; an electrocardiogram is usually necessary to distinguish between these two disorders. Ectopic atrial beats are best recognized on the electrocardiogram when a P wave can be detected preceding a QRS complex of normal duration and configuration. They usually occur prematurely after a normal beat and are followed by an incomplete compensatory pause; however, they are not always premature, and therefore the term *ectopic atrial beat* is preferred. Aberrant intraventricular conduction may alter the QRS complex in amplitude or configuration. Patterns resembling the QRS complex of right bundle branch block occur often. Aberrant conduction increases with prematurity. Definitive differentiation of supraventricular beats with aberrant conduction from ventricular ectopic beats may require His bundle electrograms.

Wandering atrial pacemaker Generally, this dysrhythmia is due to sinus bradycardia associated with escape of subsidiary

pacemakers within the atrium and the AV junction. Accordingly, it is characterized by *late* P waves of varying forms associated with varying PR intervals. Occasionally, there are atrial fusion complexes due to combined effects of depolarization initiated in the atria and sinus or AV nodes. In other instances, the sequential changes in P wave shape and PR interval suggest intermittent "wandering" of the pacemaker from the sinus node through the atrium to the AV node and back. Generally, this dysrhythmia occurs in subjects without heart disease and has no pathogenetic significance. On the other hand, it may be a manifestation of a more serious disorder such as the sick sinus syndrome, particularly in elderly patients.

Paroxysmal supraventricular tachycardia (Fig. 237-2*C*) This dysrhythmia has often been attributed to rapid discharges

FIGURE 237-2

Atrial rate / Ventric rate / Rhythm & rate disturbances

A. Ectopic atrial contraction

B. Sinus tachycardia

C. Paroxysmal supraventricular tachycardia

D. Paroxysmal atrial tachycardia with block (2:1)

E. Atrial flutter (2:1 block)

F. Atrial fibrillation

G. Ectopic ventricular contractions

H. Ventricular tachycardia

I. Ventricular fibrillation

Atrial rate / Ventric rate / Conduction disturbances

J. First degree heart block

K. Second degree heart block

L. Third degree heart block (complete H.B.)

M. Wenckebach

N. Wolff Parkinson White with delta waves

O. Wolff Parkinson White without delta waves

P. Right bundle branch block

Q. Left bundle branch block

from an abnormal atrial pacemaker and is therefore classically called *paroxysmal atrial tachycardia*. However, recent evidence suggests that many, if not all, instances of paroxysmal supraventricular tachycardia are the consequence of sustained reentry and are really manifestations of reciprocating rhythms. Initiation and termination of appropriately timed atrial extrastimuli induced by programmed electrical stimulation, the pattern of low to high atrial activation during tachycardia, and delineation of echo zones corresponding to intervals or "windows" between refractory periods of components of the reentry pathways support this interpretation. This concept is discussed in connection with the Wolff-Parkinson-White syndrome later in this chapter. When reentry occurs as the mechanism of sustained supraventricular tachycardia, it usually involves functional longitudinal stratification in the AV junction, with the reentry pathway encompassing the AV node (Fig. 237-3). In other cases reentry occurs in the sinus node or atrium. Sustained reciprocation may be initiated or terminated by an ectopic beat which precipitates or interrupts the circus current propagating the reentrant pathway. Tachycardia usually appears first in youth, and attacks may recur throughout life. Many patients with this disorder display no evidence of any other cardiac abnormality, and in the absence of structural disease, supraventricular tachycardia should be considered benign unless the rate is extremely rapid or the episodes unusually prolonged. Occasionally, the patient presents a history of precipitating events, such as emotional upset, nervousness, fatigue, indigestion, or alcohol ingestion; polyuria may occur after several hours of tachycardia. This arrhythmia may produce great anxiety on the part of the patient and the family. When a patient is seen during an attack, the heart is found to be perfectly regular and the rate ranges from 140 to 250 beats per minute. Carotid sinus pressure or other types of vagal stimulation either have no effect or will terminate the attack abruptly. Supraventricular tachycardia in the presence of intraventricular conduction disturbances may resemble ventricular tachycardia electrocardiographically, and the differentiation may be difficult. In these instances physical signs may be helpful. For example, varying intensity of the first heart sound, irregularly occurring cannon waves in the jugular venous pulse and nonrespiratory phasic alterations in systolic arterial blood pressure may be sufficient to establish the diagnosis of ventricular rather than atrial tachycardia. Esophageal, intraatrial leads or His bundle recordings may be required to demonstrate the sequence between atrial and ventricular depolarization and thereby differentiate between these two entities.

The causes of supraventricular tachycardia are not known, since most patients have no signs of organic disease. However, the possibility of underlying causes, such as atrial septal defect, mitral valve disease, and the Wolff-Parkinson-White syndrome, should be considered. Prognosis is excellent unless the attack brings on congestive failure or myocardial ischemia. The keystone of therapy is reasurance, coupled with attempts to prevent recurrences and to terminate the disorder when it occurs. For many patients digitalis is the most effective drug for the prevention of the attacks; in others, quinidine or propranolol alone or in combination with digitalis is more useful. Certain patients notice that the attacks are regularly precipitated by specific trigger factors, such as anxiety, digestive disturbances, or hypoglycemic episodes, and avoidance of these factors will have a salutary effect. In many, the attacks occur at such long intervals that the patient prefers to treat the disorder only when it transpires rather than to take a drug regularly to prevent the ectopic rhythm.

For the treatment of paroxysmal supraventricular tachycardia, the patient should assume the recumbent position and be given a sedative, such as sodium pentobarbital or secobarbital, 0.2 g intramuscularly. If significant hypotension is present (90 mmHg systolic or less, slightly higher if the patient has previ-

FIGURE 237-3

Diagrammatic representation of possible conduction pathways in a heart exhibiting functional bypass pathways under two conditions: sinus rhythm and reentrant tachycardia. Examples of the electrocardiogram that might be seen in each condition are included below the diagrams. AV, LBB, and RBB represent the AV junction, left bundle branch, and right bundle branch, respectively. During sinus rhythm, impulses are initiated at the SA node and propagated simultaneously through the functional bypass pathway and the AV junction. Because of the absence of delay in the bypass tract, the impulse reached the His bundle first by spread through the ventricular myocardium, accounting for the slurred upstroke in the conventional electrocardiogram as seen in V_6 and leading to both antegrade and retrograde conduction of the impulse in the His bundle. The subsequent portion of the ventricular depolarization occurs conventionally, since impulse transmission through the main branches of the conduction system is more rapid than that resulting from spread of the impulse from the bypass pathway. During reentry tachycardia, perhaps initiated by an appropriately timed supraventricular beat which might find the accessory pathway refractory but the proximal AV junction capable of transmitting the impulse, impulse transmission to the ventricle occurs via the main branches of the conduction system. However, each impulse fragments, with propagation occurring retrograde through the bypass pathway, reentering the atrium, and returning once again to the ventricle through the AV junction, His bundle, and bundle branches. Accordingly, a repetitive reentrant tachycardia results from each QRS complex showing normal morphology and failing to demonstrate the slurred upstroke which was present with sinus rhythm. The horizontal arrows in the conventional electrocardiographic representations indicate that in both sinus rhythm and reentrant tachycardia the "PJ" intervals (from the onset of atrial depolarization to the termination of ventricular depolarization) are identical because in each case the terminal portion of ventricular depolarization results from spread of the impulse through the main branches of the conducting system.

ously been hypertensive), elevation of the arterial pressure by intravenous phenylephrine or methoxamine to not more than 160 mmHg systolic may suffice to restore a normal rhythm or to make the heart more responsive to other measures. The carotid sinuses should be massaged, each one separately, for about 15 to 20 s, while the examiner listens to the heart and records the electrocardiogram; the massage is discontinued if the rate slows abruptly. Endrophonium hydrochloride, 10 mg intravenously, is often effective, particularly when combined with carotid sinus massage or the Valsalva maneuver. Usually, one of these procedures will be effective; if not, electrical countershock may be employed (Chap. 239). Electrical cardioversion is more likely to be successful when the atrial response is rapid. Failure of electrical cardioversion to interrupt the dysrhythmia except momentarily in approximately 30 percent of patients with this disorder may reflect the presence of enhanced atrial automaticity rather than the more common reentry mechanism in this subset. Thus, prompt recurrence of tachycardia may follow transient cardioversion. If the ectopic rhythm persists and electrical countershock is not available or is contraindicated, a rapidly acting cardiac glycoside, such as lanatoside C, 0.8 to 1.2 mg, may be given slowly intravenously, provided, of course, that the patient has not received digitalis during the preceding 2 weeks. The digitalis acts as a vagal stimulant. If after 1 h the tachycardia continues, carotid sinus pressure should again be attempted, and if this fails, cholinesterase inhibitors—neostigmine (Prostigmine), 0.5 to 1.0 mg intramuscularly, or edrophonium sulfate (Tensilon), 10 mg intravenously—may be administered, followed again by carotid sinus massage. Among the cholinesterase inhibitors, Tensilon is generally preferred because of its rapid onset and short duration of action. In patients with asthma, these agents must be used cautiously because they may exacerbate bronchoconstriction or increase bronchial secretions. If administration of cholinesterase inhibitors, maneuvers designed to increase vagal tone, or administration of digitalis fails to terminate the dysrhythmia, administration of propranolol may be effective in divided doses up to 0.15 mg/kg given intravenously at a rate of approximately 1 mg/min. Severe bronchoconstriction and marked depression of left ventricular function are contraindications. Although these measures are generally effective, on rare occasions refractory dysrhythmia will require synchronized electrical cardioversion, particularly when severe hemodynamic decomposition accompanies the tachycardia. Unfortunately, however, approximately 30 percent of episodes of supraventricular tachycardia are not reverted by electrical shock, perhaps reflecting the role of enhanced atrial automaticity in these cases rather than the usual underlying reentry mechanism.

Rapid atrial pacing is a useful alternative for termination of supraventricular tachycardia since it interrupts the reentry pathway by depolarizing a portion of it prematurely, thereby rendering it refractory to stimulation during the interval required to maintain the reentry circuit. This approach is of particular value among patients in whom occult or overt digitalis intoxication is present, since it avoids the risk of precipitating complex ventricular dysrhythmias that may accompany synchronized electrical cardioversion. If all these measures fail, morphine sulfate, 10 to 15 mg subcutaneously, may be given; during the ensuing sleep, the attack will often cease.

Quinidine, propranolol, or procainamide may be given by mouth to prevent recurrences. In patients with recurrent supraventricular tachycardia resistant to drugs, the insertion of a temporary or permanent pacemaker, which is activated when tachycardia occurs and which stimulates the right atrium or ventricle and thereby interrupts the reentrant pathway, has been found to be effective.

The treatment outlined above refers to the measures taken by the physician. Often, however, the patient has previously learned how to terminate the attack by utilizing carotid sinus pressure, or by inducing gagging and vomiting, or by the Valsalva maneuver (attempting to expire against a closed glottis). Naturally, these simple methods can also be employed by the physician before carotid sinus massage or drug therapy is instituted.

Atrial tachycardia with block (Fig. 237-2*D*) This form of tachyarrhythmia has certain characteristics resembling atrial flutter in that the responses to vagal stimulation are similar; it resembles supraventricular tachycardia in that the atrial rate is slower than flutter and usually is between 120 and 250 beats per minute. It is generally considered to be a variant of flutter, and the exact mechanism is not known. When tachycardia supervenes in the presence of established AV block, the P waves

are usually large, the atrial rate is precisely regular, the onset and offset are abrupt, and the response to carotid sinus pressure is typical of ordinary paroxysmal supraventricular tachycardia.

Digitalis intoxication is a common cause of atrial tachycardia with block (Chap. 238). It usually exhibits gradual onset and offset; small-amplitude P waves, often in a phasic pattern; and an unusual response to carotid sinus stimulation, in which AV block is dramatically accentuated in magnitude and degree and ventricular ectopic beats often become manifest. AV block in this rhythm may be latent and made overt only by carotid massage, which must be employed cautiously. Sensitivity to toxic effects of digitalis increases markedly with potassium depletion, apparently with the severity of heart failure, with hypoxia, decreased renal function, and possibly with age. Under these circumstances, serious digitalis intoxication may ensue with doses that would ordinarily be considered therapeutic.

Paroxysmal atrial tachycardia (PAT) with block should be sought in any digitalized patient who displays other symptoms of intoxication, such as nausea and vomiting, who has received vigorous diuretic treatment, who may otherwise have lost potassium as a result of vomiting or diarrhea, or whose heart rate increases after receiving full doses of digitalis. The electrocardiogram displays an atrial rate of 120 to 250 beats per minute, an isoelectric line between P waves of unusual configuration, and some degree of AV block.

The earliest stage is an alteration in the form of the P wave and an increase in the atrial rate, usually with a 1:1 ventricular response. Thus, the ventricular rate may increase to 120 to 140 beats per minute and still resemble normal sinus rhythm. At higher atrial rates, 2:1 block usually appears. However, the impaired AV conduction remains inapparent, except when carotid sinus pressure is applied, because every other P wave may be masked by the T deflections of the previous beat. The danger of this abnormal rhythm comes from the fact that although it may be a manifestation of serious digitalis intoxication, it is likely to be confused with sinus tachycardia or atrial flutter and, because of the frequent presence of congestive failure, may be treated with even larger doses of digitalis or with electrical shock. The serum potassium level must not be relied on as an absolute criterion of diagnosis; most patients with this form of disturbed heart action have little or no diminution in the level of serum potassium. The proper treatment is prompt cessation of digitalis and of potassium-wasting diuretic drugs and the administration of potassium by mouth or parenterally, depending on the urgency.

However, potassium must be administered with extreme caution and with continuous electrocardiographic monitoring for detection of signs of hyperkalemia as well as frequent determinations of plasma potassium because of the inhibitory effect of digitalis on the sodium-potassium ATPase system throughout the organism. Administration of phenytoin is a useful alternative that avoids the risk of precipitating hyperkalemia.

About one-fourth of patients with atrial tachycardia and block do not suffer from digitalis intoxication and/or potassium depletion. Typically digitalis-induced PAT with block responds to administration of potassium (not to be used if hyperkalemia is present) or phenytoin with slowing of the atrial rate and a decrease in AV block. If intravenous administration of 250 mg phenytoin over 5 min or 40 meq potassium over 2 to 4 h fails to elicit this response, the dysrhythmia is not likely to be digitalis-induced and can be treated similarly to atrial flutter.

Atrial flutter (Fig. 237-2*E*) This dysrhythmia is less common than atrial fibrillation. There is considerable controversy regarding its mechanism. A reciprocating rhythm or circus current movement is most likely. The atria contract at a rate of

250 to 350 beats per minute. AV block is almost always present, and its ratio is usually even-numbered (e.g., 2:1 or 4:1), with corresponding ventricular rates in the neighborhood of 150 or 75. In a common variation of flutter the ventricular rate is not a constant multiple of atrial rate. This occurs with two sites of block in the AV junction; high junctional 2:1 and low junctional 3:2 Wenckebach block. When the AV block is constant but the ratio is odd (3:1, 5:1, etc.), concealed retrograde conduction of ectopic ventricular beats with antegrade block should be suspected. When the block is constant and of high degree, atrial flutter is usually not suspected without an electrocardiogram. If it is suspected, its presence may be confirmed by the fact that exercise increases the rate suddenly and in a stepwise fashion rather than gradually, and in the postexercise period slowing occurs suddenly, not gradually. This occurs because exercise has no influence on the rate of the fluttering atrium, but the decrease in vagal tone during exercise reduces the degree of AV block, 4:1 giving way to 2:1 block, for example. Thus, the acceleration of ventricular rate occurs promptly, within one beat; the reverse takes place as vagal tone is restored in the postexercise period. Usually, 2:1 block is present when the ventricular rate is between 120 and 160 beats per minute. This fact alone would lead to the suspicion of flutter, because other types of tachycardias are likely to be associated with faster ventricular rates. Carotid sinus pressure slows the ventricular rate in flutter by increasing vagal tone and hence increasing the degree of AV block. The slowing is maintained only for the brief period of pressure, and both the slowing and quickening tend to occur in stepwise fashion rather than gradually, as would be the case with sinus tachycardia if there were any response at all. Occasionally, the block is so variable that the ventricular irregularity is virtually identical to that observed in atrial fibrillation. However, after exercise, the irregularity of flutter tends to disappear, whereas that seen with fibrillation is enhanced.

Careful auscultation frequently reveals an appreciable difference in the intensity of the first heart sound in atrial flutter, because of slight variations in timing of the ventricular contraction in relation to the preceding atrial contraction. The variation in the intensity of the first sound is never present in sinus tachycardia or paroxysmal atrial tachycardia (paroxysmal atrial tachycardia with variable block excepted), but it occurs frequently in ventricular tachycardia and thus serves to help limit the diagnostic possibilities. Atrial flutter is unlike paroxysmal atrial tachycardia without block, but resembles atrial fibrillation and atrial tachycardia with block because it usually occurs in patients with organic heart disease. It occurs most commonly with rheumatic mitral stenosis, but may also be seen with thyrotoxicosis, coronary disease, atrial septal defect, and chronic obstructive pulmonary disease.

The *usual treatment of atrial flutter is the administration of digitalis,* which slows the ventricular rate, by increasing the degree of AV block, and commonly converts flutter to fibrillation. When the drug is withdrawn, atrial flutter will frequently revert spontaneously to normal sinus rhythm; if this does not occur, quinidine may be employed to restore sinus rhythm; if this is unsuccessful, the patient may be maintained in chronic atrial fibrillation and treated appropriately (see below). Atrial flutter may be a difficult dysrhythmia to revert with drugs, but acute episodes frequently respond to intravenous propranolol (1 mg every 1 to 2 min with total dose generally not exceeding 0.15 mg/kg), with slowing of the ventricular response due to increased AV block often followed by reversion to sinus rhythm. Congestive heart failure or asthma are relative contraindications because of the possible cardiodepressant or bronchoconstrictive effects of the drug. Electrical reversion is often effective (Chap. 239). When flutter persists or recurs, increasing the AV block with digitalis (and when this is ineffective,

with propranolol as well) may be necessary for long-term therapy similar to that used to manage atrial fibrillation. Atrial flutter in patients with suspected or latent digitalis toxicity can often be converted to sinus rhythm by rapid atrial pacing, usually requiring stimulation at a rate exceeding 125 percent of the spontaneous atrial rate for at least 30 s after atrial capture has been accomplished. Abrupt cessation of pacing usually results in restoration of sinus rhythm, presumably because the reentrant flutter pathway has been interrupted. Occasionally, atrial fibrillation ensues, but generally the ventricular response can be managed more easily in this dysrhythmia than with flutter. Atrial fibrillation in this setting often reverts spontaneously to sinus rhythm.

In the presence of atrial flutter, quinidine may slow the atrial rate from about 300 to 200 beats per minute. Under these circumstances, the ventricular rate may suddenly increase paradoxically, as the previous 2:1 ratio is replaced by a 1:1 response. Furthermore, vagolytic effects of quinidine may lead to increased ventricular rates, because of enhanced AV conduction, even when the flutter rate remains constant. Accordingly, *quinidine should not be used in patients with flutter without prior or concomitant administration of digitalis or propranolol.*

Atrial fibrillation (Fig. 237-2*F*) This is a dysrhythmia in which the effective contraction of the atria is abolished and the AV node and the ventricles are bombarded with a very rapid and irregular series of stimuli. Many of these impulses are blocked at the AV node, but many are passed through, so that the ventricular contractions in the untreated patient are usually rapid and irregularly irregular.

The untoward effects of atrial fibrillation depend on the rapidity of the ventricular rate and the extent of the pulse deficit (i.e., on the proportion of the ineffective and wasted ventricular beats), on the prior state of the affected heart, on the duration of the dysrhythmia, and on the absence of effective atrial contraction. Cardiac output may be diminished, and heart failure may occur. Stagnation of blood in the atria tends to predispose to the development of thrombi and hence to embolism in both the pulmonary and systemic circulations. Finally, the cardiac irregularity may give an unpleasant consciousness of palpitation (Chap. 5).

When the ventricular rate is rapid, 120 beats or more per minute, the diagnosis is readily made by clinical examination, because atrial fibrillation is the only common condition in which one observes the combination of a marked tachycardia with a gross irregularity. When the rate is normal or only slightly increased, as in digitalized patients, the diagnosis is less apparent on clinical examination alone. The distinction from numerous extrasystoles can be made by noting that it is only in atrial fibrillation that abnormally long pauses occur, in groups of two or more. Moreover, exercise may abolish extrasystoles, whereas it exaggerates the irregularity of atrial fibrillation. More difficult, and frequently impossible, is the differentiation by physical examination of fibrillation from atrial flutter with varying block, and from a shifting pacemaker associated with multifocal atrial ectopic beats. Paroxysmal atrial tachycardia with block is also sometimes confused with atrial fibrillation.

Atrial fibrillation may be paroxysmal or persistent. Occasionally, the paroxysmal form occurs in healthy persons in whom no evidence of structural cardiac disease can be found. These patients (lone fibrillators) may have a variant of the preexcitation syndrome (page 1062), and their dysrhythmia may be due to functional AV junctional reentry pathways.

Atrial fibrillation is also encountered in persons who, otherwise normal, develop acute infections such as pneumonia, or in patients with rheumatic heart disease or acute myocardial infarction. Rarely, paroxysmal atrial fibrillation may be the consequence of the administration of anesthesia, surgical manipulation within the chest, potassium deficiency, digitalis intoxication, or other forms of poisoning. Most frequently, however, paroxysmal atrial fibrillation is seen in thyrotoxicosis, mitral stenosis, or in elderly persons, many but not all of whom have ischemic heart disease. The paroxysmal attacks frequently occur before the dysrhythmia is permanently established. The bouts may last for a few seconds to a few days, and, as in most types of paroxysmal rapid heart action, the onset and offset are sudden. Unless the patient happens to be observed during an attack, the physician must rely on the patient's observation that the onset was abrupt and that the heart action was highly irregular during the episode.

Permanent atrial fibrillation is confined almost exclusively to patients with myocardial disease, mitral stenosis, constrictive pericarditis, ischemic heart disease, hypertension, and thyrotoxicosis. In patients with thyrotoxicosis the clinical signs may be absent and the arrhythmia may be the only feature suggesting the possibility of thyroid disease. Rarely, chronic atrial fibrillation may be the sole cause of congestive failure that persists despite full digitalization, and in such instances reversion to normal rhythm improves ventricular performance markedly because of the reestablishment of the atrial transport function. When the ventricular rate fails to slow in the usual fashion after full doses of digitalis, fever may be present, or thyrotoxicosis, a recent silent coronary occlusion, multiple pulmonary infarcts, or acute rheumatic carditis. The onset of this dysrhythmia in a patient who has received therapeutic doses of digitalis and of diuretic drugs may be a manifestation of potassium deficiency and an indication for potassium therapy. Rarely, persistent atrial fibrillation occurs in individuals without other evidence of heart disease.

TREATMENT In a patient with atrial fibrillation, several choices of therapy are available: (1) allowing the rhythm to remain irregular but attempting to control the ventricular rate with digitalis; (2) abolishing the arrhythmia by quinidine or other antiarrhythmic drugs (Chap. 238); and (3) reverting the arrhythmia by electrical means (Chap. 239). In patients with mitral stenosis, or with marked cardiac enlargement with heart failure, it is rarely possible to restore normal sinus rhythm more than transiently. In other patients with chronic atrial fibrillation, normal sinus rhythm can be restored with large, nearly toxic doses of quinidine. Moreover, it can usually be maintained only with persistent large maintenance doses of quinidine, and even then, for only variable intervals before the dysrhythmia recurs. Quinidine frequently transforms atrial fibrillation into atrial flutter, with the risk of increased ventricular rate. Electrical reversion is usually the treatment of choice for atrial fibrillation (Chap. 239). However, the problem of maintaining sinus rhythm subsequently still remains. In some patients with chronic atrial fibrillation ventricular rate must be controlled with digitalis. Hence, reversion to sinus rhythm with electrical countershock or quinidine is likely to be of value in patients with fibrillation of recent development who are known to have had no evidence of congestive failure prior to the onset of the arrhythmia. Reversion to sinus rhythm should also be considered when the ventricular rate is not well controlled by digitalis, and it may be attempted in patients with intractable heart failure. In patients who cannot be maintained in sinus rhythm and in whom the ventricular rate cannot be slowed sufficiently with digitalis, small doses (5 to 10 mg qid) of propranolol will often control the ventricular rate. In all cases of atrial fibrillation, therapeutic doses of digitalis should be administered before quinidine is given, but reversion should not be attempted if occult or overt digitalis intoxication is suspected. When atrial fibrillation follows acute myocardial infarction, the first and most important objective is to slow the ventricular rate with digitalis. For the treatment of paroxysmal atrial fibrillation, a rapidly acting digitalis glycoside is preferable; for the control of established atrial fibrillation, one of the slower-acting digitalis preparations should be used.

In many instances of transient atrial fibrillation the administration of digitalis is followed by the disappearance of the dysrhythmia. This probably results from overall hemodynamic improvement, diminished sympathoadrenal myocardial stimulation, and diminution of atrial size, rather than from a direct pharmacologic effect of digitalis on the atria. When atrial fibrillation is of long duration, digitalis rarely abolishes it. Under these circumstances, the ventricular rate slows and becomes less obviously irregular unless complete AV block and a regular idioventricular or AV junctional rhythm develop; but electrocardiographic tracings reveal that the atria continue to fibrillate.

Thromboembolism is one of the dreaded complications in patients with atrial fibrillation (or less commonly with atrial flutter), particularly when the dysrhythmia is chronic and when mitral stenosis is present. Thromboembolism is responsible for about 20 percent of the deaths in patients with mitral stenosis. To prevent such catastrophes, long-term anticoagulant therapy is advocated in patients with atrial fibrillation, and is especially important in patients who have already experienced one or more episodes of embolism. When possible, anticoagulants should be administered for at least 2 weeks prior to attempts to reestablish sinus rhythm in order to minimize thromboembolic episodes associated with pharmacologic or electrical cardioversion.

Complex atrial dysrhythmias MULTIFOCAL ATRIAL TACHYCARDIA (MAT) This is a rapid, grossly irregular atrial dysrhythmia with a rapid ventricular response (from 120 to 200 beats per minute). Electrocardiographically it can be differentiated from atrial fibrillation by the presence of three or more types of morphologically distinct P waves, Numerous atrial premature complexes, AV block, and aberrant intraventricular conduction are generally present. Atrial flutter or fibrillation may supervene. MAT is generally a manifestation of advanced cardiac and/or pulmonary disease and hypoxemia. Specific antiarrhythmic therapy is generally ineffective; digitalis or theophylline may aggravate dysrhythmia further; and treatment should focus on the underlying disorder.

SICK SINUS SYNDROME The sick sinus syndrome, or sinoatrial dysfunction, generally results from arteriosclerotic, hypertensive, or rheumatic heart disease, although it may be idiopathic. Its manifestations include intermittent sinus arrest; sinus bradycardia which persists despite exercise, atropine, or isoproterenol; sinoatrial block; AV junctional escape rhythm; and ectopic atrial complexes. Marked carotid sinus sensitivity may trigger bradycardia. Paroxysmal supraventricular tachycardia, atrial fibrillation, atrial flutter, and episodes of alternating bradycardia and tachycardia (the bradycardia-tachycardia syndrome) are common concomitants. Asynchronous atrial repolarization favoring reentry may predispose to the episodes of paroxysmal tachycardia. On the other hand, tachycardia may precipitate asystole or severe bradycardia because of impaired sinus node recovery and the commonly associated atrioventricular and intraventricular conduction defects. Syncope and chest pain often accompany episodes of bradycardia and tachycardia. Long-term electrocardiographic monitoring, analysis of the response of heart rate to carotid sinus massage, stress testing, or drugs, and detection of abnormal sinus node suppression and measurement of sinoatrial conduction time by atrial pacing are most helpful diagnostically. The underlying mechanism is sometimes marked delay in sinoatrial conduction rather than sinus node suppression. Thus, diagnosis requires programmed atrial stimulation for assessment of sinoatrial conduction time as well as bursts of continuous atrial pacing followed by pauses for detection of sinus node recovery time. Permanent pacing is often required to treat bradycardia and permits safe suppression of tachycardia with agents such as digitalis and propranolol. Because of the high incidence of thromboembolic phenomena, long-term anticoagulation may be indicated.

REPETITIVE PAROXYSMAL TACHYCARDIA This dysrhythmia, frequently appearing in childhood (the Parkinson-Papp syndrome), comprises innumerable brief bursts of tachycardia, most frequently paroxysmal supraventricular tachycardia, atrial fibrillation, or atrial flutter, interspersed with brief episodes of sinus rhythm punctuated with multiple atrial premature complexes. Its etiology is often obscure, and it is generally not associated with obvious organic heart disease. Hundreds and even thousands of episodes may occur daily with disabling symptoms including chest discomfort, palpitations, and syncope. Numerous remissions and relapses are common. Overdrive suppression with pacing has not been helpful. Digitalis and conventional antiarrhythmic agents are often ineffective, but propranolol alone or in combination with digitalis or quinidine may be beneficial.

CHAOTIC ATRIAL MECHANISM This is a general term that has been used to refer to several complex atrial dysrhythmias including MAT, sick sinus syndrome, and repetitive paroxysmal tachycardia.

Sinoventricular conduction This unusual dysrhythmia, sometimes a manifestation of severe hyperkalemia, ischemia, or intoxication with type I antiarrhythmic drugs such as quinidine and procainamide, arises in the atria. It is characterized by impulse initiation in the sinoatrial node in a normal fashion and propagation via internodal pathways to the AV junction. However, spread of the impulse through atrial myocardium fails to occur, and hence no P wave is seen on the electrocardiogram, and atrial contraction is absent. Although the ventricular electrocardiographic complexes may be distorted because of aberrant conduction, ventricular rate varies, as it does in normal sinus rhythm when maneuvers such as carotid sinus stimulation are performed, with exercise, and following drug administration. The major significance of the dysrhythmia is loss of atrial transport function; also, when bizarre QRS complexes are present, there is the possibility of misdiagnosis as ventricular tachycardia.

DERANGEMENTS ARISING IN THE AV JUNCTION Ectopic junctional beats The AV junction refers to fibers adjacent to the node in the low right atrium, the AV node itself, and the His bundle. Cells in the N region, i.e., in the AV node itself, do not appear to initiate impulse formation spontaneously. Decremental conduction and the physiologic delay in AV impulse transmission occur in this region. The cephalad (AN) and caudad (NH) regions of the node appear to contain cells capable of spontaneous impulse formation, presumably dependent on slow-current, calcium-mediated depolarizations giving rise to ectopic beats. Other ectopic beats may originate in atrial and His bundle components of the AV junction. Ectopic beats originating in the low atrium or AN region exhibit a short PR interval and P waves of unusual configuration, unless there is aberrant ventricular conduction. When the impulse arises in the His bundle, retrograde atrial conduction causes impulse propagation into the atrium at about the same time that the impulse is propagated antegrade into the ventricular conduction system. Consequently, there is no visible electrocardiographic wave of atrial depolarization; again, the QRS complex is usually normal in configuration and duration, resembling a normal supraventricular beat but without a preceding visible P wave. Beats originating at a more distal site in the His-Purkinje system or those associated with delayed retrograde conduction into the atrium exhibit an abnormal P wave that regularly follows the QRS complex.

AV junctional tachycardias These are of two types: *idiojunctional tachycardia,* with a ventricular rate usually between 100 and 140 beats per minute; and *extrasystolic* (or paroxysmal) *AV junctional tachycardia,* with a ventricular rate generally between 140 and 200 beats per minute. In the former there is acceleration of the inherent idiojunctional rhythm, which becomes evident when its rate exceeds that of the SA pacemaker. It may be a manifestation of digitalis toxicity, and has also been noted in patients with acute myocardial infarction and acute rheumatic fever. When idiojunctional tachycardia is due to digitalis toxicity, it may be particularly grave, because it may degenerate into ventricular tachycardia and ventricular fibrillation. Reversion may occur after discontinuation of digitalis or administration of intravenous potassium. However, occasionally in critical situations, more vigorous therapy is required; in these instances lidocaine, procainamide, phenytoin, or propranolol may be effective. Paroxysmal AV junctional tachycardia resembles paroxysmal atrial tachycardia in its clinical significance and management, but is much less common.

AV junctional rhythm This is an escape rhythm which occurs when the sinus impulse fails to arrive at the AV junction because of sinoatrial depression, standstill, or block of the sinus impulse proximal to the AV junctional pacemaker. The ventricular rate is 40 to 60 beats per minute, and the rhythm is regular. The QRS complex is generally identical to that of the conducted sinus impulses. No treatment is necessary, as the circulation is usually adequate, but atropine or isoproterenol may be helpful to speed the sinus rate if the circulation is compromised by a ventricular rate below 50 beats per minute. The presence of AV junctional rhythm is generally a manifestation of a safety mechanism, rather than a primary derangement affecting the junctional pacemaker. However, it may be a manifestation of digitalis toxicity or inferior myocardial infarction with AV nodal block.

DERANGEMENTS ARISING IN THE VENTRICLES Ectopic ventricular beats (Fig. 237-2G) These are relatively more frequent in patients with structural cardiac disease than ectopic atrial beats, but they are so common in healthy individuals that their presence has no diagnostic significance unless they are unusually frequent, related to exercise, originate from the left ventricle, occur during the vulnerable period, or occur in pairs or salvos (Chap. 32). Their prevalence increases markedly with age. They are frequent concomitants of conditions with abnormal ventricular repolarization such as hereditary QT prolongation (syncope, sudden death, with or without congenital deafness), mitral valve prolapse, cerebrovascular accidents, and intoxication with drugs such as phenothiazines, tricyclic antidepressants, or quinidine. In the absence of organic heart disease, premature beats may be due to excessive use of tobacco, coffee, tea, and occasionally alcohol, bronchodilators such as catecholamines or theophylline, or reflexes from the gastrointestinal tract; often they are caused by emotional stress, but in many patients the cause cannot be ascertained.

Ventricular etopic beats are often easily recognized, as the ventricular depolarization and contraction occur before the next beat would ordinarily occur and are commonly followed by a compensatory pause. The patient may not be conscious of the premature beat but usually feels a skip followed by a thump accompanying the augmented stroke volume of the normal beat after the premature one. When extrasystoles are frequent, they may be confused with atrial fibrillation on clinical examination, an error that may sometimes be avoided by noting that the rhythm becomes regular when the heart rate is accelerated by exercise. There is still uncertainty whether ectopic ventricular beats are produced by an abnormal pacemaker or by reentry; probably each mechanism accounts for some instances of this disorder. In some patients ectopic ventricular beats and even ventricular tachycardia occur during episodes of severe bradycardia. When ectopic ventricular beats arise in an abnormal pacemaker, the latter is probably located in Purkinje cells rather than in myocardial cells per se. Ectopic beats may originate in a *parasystolic focus,* i.e., one "protected" from depolarization initiated elsewhere in the heart. The manifest rate of the parasystolic focus will depend on the degree of exit block from it, the refractoriness of surrounding myocardium, and the interplay between the rate of the focus and other pacemakers which are initiating impulses. Other ectopic beats originate in extrasystolic ventricular pacemakers which are not completely protected from depolarization by impulses arising in other pacemaker cells.

Bigeminal rhythm This is a state in which every alternate beat is premature; it may be caused by digitalis overdosage and disappears within a few days after the drug has been withheld. It should not be confused with *pulsus alternans* or with *paradoxic pulse,* conditions in which the rhythm remains regular. Bigeminy not due to digitalis is usually, though not always, associated with structural heart disease. Bigeminy probably results from several mechanisms, including electrical instability of the ectopic pacemaker during repolarization, reentry, and enhancement of spontaneous depolarization of the ectopic pacemaker by the preceding beat.

The *treatment of ectopic ventricular beats* depends on the clinical circumstances. When these beats occur occasionally, and evidence of cardiac disease is lacking, no treatment is necessary. If there is reason to believe that tobacco or coffee is a precipitating factor, its use should be discontinued or curtailed. In excitable patients, extrasystoles may disappear following the administration of a mild sedative, barbiturates, reserpine, or other tranquilizers. Ectopic ventricular beats, if caused by digitalis, will disappear if the drug is withdrawn; or if the irregularity occurs after the ingestion of a high-carbohydrate meal, it will be abolished by the administration of potassium. The occurrence of extrasystoles in undigitalized patients does not constitute a contraindication to the use of digitalis if the patient has congestive heart failure. Indeed, with the restoration of myocardial function, the irregularity will often disappear. Lidocaine, procainamide, phenytoin, quinidine, and disopyramide are all effective in the treatment, and the relative efficacy of each drug varies in different patients. In patients in whom the development of ventricular ectopic beats or ventricular tachycardia is precipitated by bradycardia, increasing the atrial rate with atropine or by pacing may be helpful.

Although ectopic ventricular beats may ordinarily be considered a benign form of irregularity, the occurrence of numerous such beats may diminish the efficiency of the heart with an impaired cardiac reserve. Moreover, the appearance of ventricular extrasystoles following an acute myocardial infarction should not be viewed with complacency, since they may herald the onset of ventricular tachycardia or fibrillation. An isolated ventricular beat may occur in the "vulnerable" period at the end of the previous systole (the time during ventricular repolarization when recovery is asynchronous, opportunity for reentry is maximized, and hence the ventricles are especially likely to develop ventricular fibrillation). Such beats are likely to initiate ventricular fibrillation and sudden death. It is for this reason that premature ventricular contractions occurring in patients with acute myocardial infarction should be treated vigorously, with intravenous lidocaine, procainamide, phenytoin, disopyramide, or quinidine (Chaps. 238 and 245). Propranolol, alone or in combination with other agents, may be particularly useful in suppressing premature ventricular contractions due to ischemia. Pharmacologic suppression of ventricular ectopic beats is less effective when the prevailing heart rate is high (greater than 120 beats per minute). Thus, concomitant therapy should be directed toward correction of factors responsible for the tachycardia or toward decreasing the sinus rate with beta-adrenergic blocking agents. The treatment of premature ventricular contractions in other patients is discussed in Chap. 32.

Ventricular tachycardia (Fig. 237-2*H*) This dysrhythmia is much less frequent and far more serious than paroxysmal atrial tachycardia. The most common causes are ischemic heart disease, myocarditis, cardiomyopathies, mitral valve prolapse, and syndromes associated with prolonged QT intervals. Ventricular tachycardia frequently occurs within a few days following the development of an acute myocardial infarction (Chap. 245). Less commonly, it is induced by digitalis or quinidine intoxication, and very rarely the arrhythmia appears spontaneously in otherwise healthy persons without any evidence of cardiac disease. The diagnosis should be suspected when the following clinical features are observed:

1. The patient has evidence of coronary disease, especially if accompanied by a ventricular aneurysm, or if he has been receiving digitalis or quinidine in large doses.
2. As a rule, there is no history of numerous previous attacks.
3. During the attack, the ventricular rate is usually between 150 and 210 beats per minute, and although the rhythm is essentially regular, there are often slight variations in it.
4. Carotid sinus stimulation has no effect on the rate.
5. An intermittent jugular cannon *a* wave is present.
6. The first heart sound varies in intensity, because the relationship between atrial and ventricular contractions is inconstant.
7. Systolic blood pressure varies because of inconsistent contributions to ventricular filling by fortuitously timed atrial contractions.

Although these clues are useful, the clinical impression should be confirmed by an electrocardiogram, but the interpretation even of the ECG may be rendered difficult because atrial tachycardia may be associated with intraventricular conduction defects (aberrant QRS complexes) which cause the tracing to resemble that of ventricular tachycardia. The diagnosis is supported by evidence that the P-wave rate is independent of the ventricular rate, by evidence that in the intervals between attacks ventricular premature beats occur which are identical in form with the complexes seen during the paroxysm, and by the presence of fusion beats comprising components of depolarization initiated by impulses arising in a supraventricular pacemaker and in the ectopic ventricular site. Nevertheless, the electrocardiographic diagnosis frequently cannot be made with certainty. Esophageal, atrial, or His bundle electrograms may be helpful. In ventricular tachycardia H spikes (originating from the bundle of His) may be shown to follow rather than precede the QRS complex. In as many as one-third of cases AV dissociation does not occur. Thus, atrial depolarization follows each ventricular depolarization. The dysrhythmia can be readily differentiated from junctional tachycardia, however, since the RP interval is consistently greater than 0.11 s.

Bidirectional ventricular tachycardia is a rare dysrhythmia with a grave prognosis associated with severe digitalis intoxication and advanced cardiac disease. The rapid, regular ventricular response at a rate of 120 to 220 beats per minute exhibits alternating electrocardiographic complexes with marked left and right axis deviation. Since all complexes generally exhibit a right bundle branch block pattern, the disturbance may reflect ectopic impulse formation in a left ventricular focus with alternating transmission along the posterior and anterior divisions of the left bundle. Treatment entails the discontinuation of digitalis and administration of phenytoin or lidocaine. Electrical cardioversion should not be attempted because of the risk that ventricular fibrillation will result.

Since it is but one step removed from the frequently fatal *ventricular fibrillation*, ventricular tachycardia is the most serious of the ectopic tachycardias. If the attack occurs during a bout of acute myocardial infarction, immediate electric countershock is utilized (Chap. 239), but there is a strong possibility that another episode will occur soon after the first. Hence, a maintenance dose of an antiarrhythmic drug (e.g., intravenous lidocaine, procainamide, phenytoin, or disopyramide, parenteral or oral) should be continued until cardiac electrical activity has become demonstrably stable. When heart failure occurs in an undigitalized patient with ventricular tachycardia, digitalis should be administered despite the dysrhythmia, since the drug is not necessarily more hazardous in such patients than in those without the disturbance.

The cardiac rhythm of patients with ventricular tachycardia who are receiving large doses of quinidine or of procainamide may fail to revert to the normal sinus mechanism, but the ventricular rate may still show marked slowing, to 120 beats per minute or less. Under these circumstances the administration of large doses of atropine (up to 2 mg intravenously) may increase the atrial rate to a level above that of the ectopic rhythm, which may permit the sinoatrial node to resume its normal role as pacemaker and restore the normal sinus mechanism; alternatively, atrial overdrive, i.e., electrical stimulation of the atria with an electrode catheter at a rate exceeding that of ventricular tachycardia, may exert a similar effect. However, the rate required for overdrive may be so high that ischemia is exacerbated with consequent intensification of ventricular ectopy. The extracardiac toxicities of procainamide and quinidine are not necessarily additive, and therefore it may be desirable to use the drugs simultaneously in patients who are especially liable to such side effects as diarrhea and tinnitus (quinidine) or hypotension, nausea, or a lupus-like syndrome (procainamide). Disopyramide and propranolol may also be useful alone or in combination with one or more other antiarrhythmic agents. Monitoring of serum levels of these agents to ensure adequate dosage and avoid toxicity is particularly important when vigorous treatment is required for refractory dysrhythmias.

Refractory, recurrent ventricular tachycardia has been successfully treated by surgical interruption of a reentry pathway documented by epicardial mapping studies at operation and identified preoperatively by electrophysiologic investigation utilizing programmed electrical cardiac stimulation and intracardiac electrograms. Occasionally, aneurysmectomy has led to cessation of recurrent ventricular tachycardia presumably by the same mechanism, although excision of an ectopic focus cannot be excluded.

Ventricular fibrillation (Fig. 237-2*I*) This chaotic rhythm may occur in very brief bursts, last for a few seconds, and then subside spontaneously, following which the rhythm previously present is resumed. These episodes are responsible for some of the Stokes-Adams attacks that occur in patients with prevailing slow rates due to high-grade AV block. Usually, however, unless it is recognized and treated immediately, ventricular fibrillation is synonymous with practically instantaneous death, since effective ventricular contraction and circulation cease (Chap. 32). Aside from AV block, ischemic heart disease is the most common cause of the dysrhythmia, particularly during attacks of acute myocardial infarction. It may also occur in patients with abnormal ventricular repolarization with QT prolongation associated with the hereditary QT prolongation syndrome, hypothermia, phenothiazine toxicity, mitral valve prolapse, or "quinidine syncope." Sympathetic nerve stimulation may provoke fibrillation, and stellate ganglion ablation or postganglionic sympathetic blockade with bretylium has been occasionally useful for prevention. Type I antiarrhythmic drugs (i.e., quinidine and procainamide) are contraindicated when ventricular fibrillation occurs as a manifestation of these unusual disorders because they slow repolarization further and probably increase temporal dispersion of recovery. There was no effective treatment for this calamitous disorder until introduction of externally applied electric shock (Chap. 239). Needless to say, this form of therapy must be applied promptly, because cessation of the circulation beyond 2 to 4 min leads to irreversible damage in the brain and heart. Thus, in individuals particularly susceptible to ventricular fibrillation, such as those with acute myocardial infarction or those with a history of Stokes-Adams attacks, the rhythm must be monitored constantly, and immediate availability and preparedness to apply external electric shock must be assured. Such precautions may be required for weeks, until cardiac electrical stability has been reestablished. In the absence of special equipment for delivering the countershock, closed-chest massage should be employed. This involves manual rhythmic compression of the sternum once per second, plus mouth-to-mouth respiration. Such maneuvers, described in Chap. 32 may be effective in sustaining life during the crucial time required to secure and apply the apparatus needed for countershock.

AV DISSOCIATION As its name implies, in this dysrhythmia the atria and ventricles are controlled by two independent pacemakers. Fundamentally, it may occur in two forms, with antegrade AV block and without it. In the first type, called AV dissociation with heart block, the ventricles are excited by a pacemaker in the AV junction, or the Purkinje system, because impulses arising in the sinoatrial node or atria are blocked in the AV conduction system. In the second type, called AV dissociation due to interference, AV dissociation occurs *without* antegrade block but the automaticity of the AV junction or ventricle exceeds that of the supraventricular pacemaker. Impulses from the atrium, while normally conducted to the ventricles, usually find these tissues refractory. Occasionally, the regular ventricular rhythm may be interrupted by a normally conducted impulse which arrives fortuitously, at an instant when the ventricle is not refractory. This dysrhythmia must be associated with some degree of retrograde block, or else the atria would be depolarized by the more rapidly firing AV junctional or ventricular pacemaker.

ABNORMALITIES OF CONDUCTION *Sinoatrial block*, which represents a disorder of excitation, has been considered above. The term *heart block* as herein employed refers to a condition in which the wave of excitation from the atria is delayed pathologically (or blocked) at the junctional tissues (AV node and His bundle). The PR interval represents the time required for the impulse to traverse the atrium, the AV node, His bundle, and the bundle branches. The generally accepted upper limit of normal in adults is 0.20 s; it is somewhat shorter in children. When the PR interval exceeds the normal duration and all the atrial beats are followed by ventricular beats, *first-degree AV block* exists. A more advanced disturbance in the conduction system, *second-degree block,* is present when from time to time the atrial impulses are incapable of penetrating the conduction system sufficiently to excite the ventricles. *Third-degree* or *complete AV block* describes the condition in which the conduction system is so altered that no atrial impulses reach the ventricles, and the atria and ventricles maintain separate and independent rhythms (atrioventricular dissociation due to third-degree antegrade AV block).

AV block is a general term referring to impaired conduction. The actual site(s) of impairment is not necessarily in the AV node itself. Block may exist because of impaired conduction in the atrial myocardium adjacent to the node (AN region); the node itself (N region); or the bundle of His adjacent to the node (NH region). Furthermore, block may exist only in more distal portions of the conduction system, i.e., the His bundle, the right or left bundle branches, or the anterior or posterior fascicles of the latter (Chap. 232). Proximal block is generally benign, and distal block more malignant. At each site block may be partial (first or second degree) or complete (third degree), and various sites of block may occur singly or in combination. As discussed below, bundle branch or fascicular block is generally associated with pathologic conditions other than those associated with AV junctional block proper, and it generally indicates a different prognosis. Congenital AV block generally exhibits impaired conduction high in the AV junction and narrow electrocardiographic QRS complexes. However, familial AV block may occur with trifascicular block with widened QRS complexes as well as proximal (high AV) block among individuals in the same family. Definitive differentiation between fascicular block and AV junctional block is possible with the aid of His bundle recordings (Fig. 237-1). In third-degree trifascicular block (involving the right bundle and both fascicles of the left bundle branch) ventricular depolarizations occur independently of His bundle depolarizations. However, when block occurs in the AV junction proximal to the His bundle, each ventricular depolarization is preceded by a His bundle depolarization separated from it by the normal interval of approximately 50 ms.

First-degree AV block (Fig. 237-2*J*) This is usually due to impaired conduction in the AV junction, i.e., proximal to the His bundle, but rarely, it may be a reflection of trifascicular block. It may be caused by digitalis or by any of the inflammatory, toxic, degenerative, or vascular processes that may affect the heart. Prolongation of the PR interval, for example, as seen in patients with acute rheumatic fever, may be suspected when the intensity of the first heart sound suddenly declines without any other change in the clinical picture and without evidence of fluid in the pericardium, or in patients with mitral stenosis when a presystolic murmur becomes middiastolic in the absence of atrial fibrillation. PR prolongation may be due to increased vagal tone in a healthy, normal person. In the absence of any other evidence of disease, this one electrocardiographic deviation from an arbitrary norm should not be construed as evidence of organic heart disease, and it requires no treatment.

Second-degree, or partial, AV block (Fig. 237-2*K*) This form may be divided into two groups. In the *Möbitz type I block*

(also called Wenckebach block) the PR interval increases progressively until finally a propagation of an impulse originating in the atrium is completely blocked, the corresponding ventricular beat dropping out (Wenckebach block, Fig. 237-2*M*). His bundle electrograms generally, but not always, reveal impaired conduction proximal to the His bundle. The ventricular rate generally increases prior to the dropped beat because the prolongation of AV conduction exhibits progressively smaller increments. The PR interval after the pause shortens to within the normal range. Accordingly, the pause resulting from the dropped beat is less than the duration of any two preceding cycles. After the resumption of conduction each successive PR interval lengthens, and the cycle is repeated periodically. The dropped beat may occur after six to eight conducted beats, or after every second atrial impulse, thus giving rise to 2:1 AV block and simulating the other type of 2:1 block (Möbitz type II), to be described below. With type I block the QRS duration is usually normal. Inhibition of vagal tone, as by intravenous injection of atropine (1 to 2 mg) or exercise, may help to differentiate these two types of block. In type I, the block often diminishes or disappears with such a procedure, whereas with Möbitz type II block it increases or it may temporarily change into a complete AV block. Möbitz type I second-degree block is often due to abnormal conduction in the AV junction proximal to the His bundle; it is frequently accentuated or precipitated by heightened vagal tone, occurring spontaneously or after carotid sinus pressure, following digitalis therapy, or after administration of morphine. It is usually a transitory phenomenon and requires no treatment unless hemodynamic disturbances result or the extent of block increases. It is a frequent complication of inferior myocardial infarction, presumably with ischemia of the junction.

Möbitz type II block is usually a more serious disorder. The PR interval is either normal or increased but fixed except when beats are dropped; QRS duration is often prolonged with complexes exhibiting a right bundle branch block pattern and associated hemiblock. The dysrhythmia exhibits dropped beats, that is, 2:1, 3:1, or 4:1 block or irregular ratios. This form of block usually results from block in the His bundle or trifascicular block and may be caused acutely by anterior myocardial infarction or myocarditis. Although it may be transient, it may progress suddenly to complete block. Idiopathic sclerosis producing damage of the conduction system (Lenegre's disease) and fibrocalcific degeneration of the myocardium involving the conduction system as well (Lev's disease) are perhaps the most common causes of chronic Möbitz type II block. It may also result from coronary narrowing in the absence of an acute episode of infarction; calcification of the mitral annulus; extension of the lesion of calcific aortic stenosis into the septum; any of the diffuse disorders of the myocardium such as cardiac amyloidosis; or congenital heart disease, usually an interventricular septal defect. This type of second-degree block is sometimes characterized by a unique phenomenon, a slowing of the ventricular rate during exercise as 2:1 block suddenly appears when the atrial rate increases.

Syncopal attacks (Stokes-Adams attacks) are common in type II block, and they have the characteristics of all such syncopal attacks that are due to a sudden cessation of the circulation (Chap. 13). The attacks occur suddenly and without warning, with the patient in either the upright or recumbent posture. In contrast, premonitory light-headedness, faintness, and "blacking out" usually precede simple emotional vasovagal syncope, which develops with the patient in the upright position and is relieved by the recumbent posture. If the heart of a patient with Möbitz type II 2:1 block is monitored during or shortly after the lapse of consciousness, ventricular standstill (or less commonly fibrillation) will be recorded during the syncopal period, often followed by complete block in the early recovery state, 2:1 block being restored after a variable interval. When a person with a slow heart rate or with an electrocardiogram showing second-degree block develops a characteristic syncopal attack, the diagnosis should be simple. However, in a number of patients, syncopal attacks may appear at relatively long intervals over a number of years, during which time the electrocardiogram between episodes remains normal and the PR interval stays well within the normal range. Ambulatory electrocardiographic monitoring or demonstration of latent conduction abnormalities with atrial pacing and His bundle recordings may be particularly useful in unmasking the diagnosis. Intravenous administration of atropine in such persons may reveal concealed block, since the AV conduction system may be unable to follow the accelerated sinus rate. Eventually, most people with type II block, whether overt or concealed, will develop complete block if they do not first succumb in a Stokes-Adams attack. When Möbitz type II block occurs in association with acute anterior myocardial infarction, its prognosis is extremely poor because its appearance generally reflects extensive necrosis involving the ventricular septum and free wall. Accordingly, it has been difficult to determine whether permanent pacing improves the mortality rate among patients who survive the acute episode. Nevertheless, a strong case can be made for permanent pacing for patients with bifascicular block, Möbitz type II block, or complete heart block appearing for the first time in association with acute myocardial infarction.

Complete, or third-degree, AV block (Fig. 237-2L) This advanced form of block is caused by any of the disorders responsible for type II second-degree block as well as by accidental surgical trauma to the AV node or His bundle. Occasionally, one encounters an otherwise normal person with congenital AV block, and rarely a patient with persistent complete block will be found at autopsy to display no demonstrable microscopic lesion in the conduction system. A transitory form, lasting a few seconds, may follow carotid sinus pressure, and it may also be a consequence of digitalis intoxication, disappearing a week or two after the drug is withdrawn. Most cases of chronic and persistent complete heart block are infra-AV nodal, i.e., due to block in the bundle of His or bilateral bundle branch block. When block occurs within the bundle of His, two depolarizations of the His bundle may be recognized on His bundle electrograms—one proximal to the block and following each nonconducted P wave, and the other distal to the block and temporally associated with each QRS complex. In the presence of complete heart block the ventricular rate is usually 45 beats per minute or less, although in congenital heart block, which is usually due to AV junctional block proximal to the His bundle, the rate may be as rapid as 60 beats per minute. In either case the rhythm is regular. Generally the rate increases only slightly or not at all after exercise, but some patients with congenital heart block exhibit acceleration of a junctional pacemaker and nearly normal heart rates with exercise. The lesion tends to occur proximal to the bifurcation of the bundle of His in patients with congenital heart block, while acquired third-degree AV block and Möbitz type II second-degree block are usually bilateral bundle branch or trifascicular blocks. When the subsidiary pacemaker is in the AV node or the bundle of His, as is usual in congenital heart block, the QRS complex is usually normal; when it is below the bifurcation of the bundle of His, i.e., within the Purkinje system, as is usual in acquired heart block, the QRS complex is prolonged, notched, and slurred. The intensity of the first heart sound varies from beat to beat, being sometimes almost inaudible and at other times so loud as to merit the term *bruit de canon;* faint atrial contractions can also often be heard, possibly because of diastolic mitral regurgitation caused by atrial relaxation with a momentary reduction of atrial pressure below the ventricular level.

Acute myocardial infarction often precipitates AV block (Chap. 245). Infarcts associated with ischemia in the distribution of the right coronary artery (e.g., inferior or posterior infarctions) commonly cause AV junctional block which is due to impaired conduction proximal to the His bundle bifurcation, is transient, and is usually first or second degree (Möbitz type I block). Even when third-degree block occurs in this setting, recovery of conduction may generally be anticipated. On the other hand, heart block associated with infarcts due to ischemia in the distribution of the left coronary artery is less common and more grave. It usually results from extensive damage of the His bundle and/or all three fascicles of the conduction system, is persistent, and presents as second-degree Möbitz type II or third-degree trifascicular block. The mortality rate associated with infarcts producing this type of block is high, even despite the indicated pacemaker therapy, because of the massive nature of the infarct responsible.

Because myocardial infarction is so common, it is by far the commonest cause of acute AV block. However, coronary artery disease is responsible for only a minority of cases of chronic and persistent complete heart block, which is usually due to primary or secondary degeneration or inflammation of the conduction system.

The prognosis of first- and second-degree Möbitz type I AV block is favorable. The outlook for high grades of block (second-degree Möbitz type II or complete AV block) is always uncertain, since the patient is constantly subject to the risk of Stokes-Adams attacks, any of which may be fatal. When such attacks occur frequently in patients with complete block and are uncontrolled, death usually occurs within a year. AV block occurring in the course of acute myocardial infarction is often transient (Chap. 244). Temporary transvenous pacemakers are useful when the block is progressive, when it leads to impaired cardiac performance with hemodynamic sequelae, or when it sets the stage for demonstrable increases in ectopic ventricular dysrhythmias. Patients who survive acute infarction with or without the aid of a transvenous pacemaker generally exhibit eventual restoration of sinus rhythm within several days. Since bifascicular block may progress to complete block, prophylactic insertion of a temporary transvenous pacemaker is often performed when the condition develops in association with acute myocardial infarction pending evolution or regression of block or the results of thorough subsequent electrophysiologic evaluation. Trifascicular block may require implantation of a permanent pacemaker, but most patients with infarction who develop this condition have sustained extensive infarction associated with profound hemodynamic impairment and high early mortality rate.

Treatment of heart block The important problem is the prevention of the Stokes-Adams attacks. Accordingly, in all patients with symptomatic or high-grade block, definitive therapy and the treatment of choice consist of implantation of a permanent pacemaker as described earlier in this chapter. Despite the occurrence of complications with this mode of therapy including infection, failure to pace due to electrode displacement or fracture, or perforation of the heart, therapy with permanent pacemakers has dramatically improved the outlook for patients with symptomatic AV block. The mortality rate in treated cohorts is in the range of 5 percent per year. It approximates the mortality rate in age- and sex-matched normal subjects except for death due to the higher prevalence of other disorders and not resulting from conduction system disease in the patient group.

In emergency situations, every effort should be made for prompt institution of pacemaker therapy without undue reliance on drugs. Atropine and isoproterenol or epinephrine are useful adjuncts to accelerate ventricular rate acutely and temporarily. However, since the latter two agents increase myocardial oxygen demand, they may increase ischemic injury or lead to prolonged anginal attacks, if used chronically. In life-threatening situations, external countershock may be applied for ventricular fibrillation, and life may be sustained by these measures and by closed-chest cardiac massage until intracardiac pacing by means of a catheter electrode has been achieved.

When AV block is not complete, digitalis therapy may either improve or worsen its degree. Hence the drug should be withheld unless congestive failure fails to respond to other measures and until a pacemaker has been implanted. Under no circumstances should quinidine, procainamide, disopyramide, or beta-adrenergic blockers be used in the presence of high-grade block unless the ventricular rhythm is first controlled by an artificial electrical pacemaker. However, these agents are useful in patients with complete heart block who manifest frequent ventricular premature contractions despite continued ventricular pacing.

Bundle branch block disorders (Fig. 237-2*P* and *Q*) These are examples of impaired conduction in a specific portion of the conducting system (Chap. 232). When the duration of the QRS complex exceeds 0.12 s and when the main deflection is positive in leads I and V_6 and negative in leads III and V_1, left bundle branch block is said to be present. Similar prolongation but with opposite directional deflections in the leads mentioned is characteristic of right bundle branch block. Lesser degrees of QRS lengthening are often designated as incomplete left or right bundle branch block. In some instances the ventricular complex may be markedly prolonged without these typical changes; such disturbances are usually considered to be *intraventricular blocks*.

The Wolff-Parkinson-White (WPW) syndrome (anomalous atrioventricular excitation) (Fig. 237-2*N*) This example of a group of *preexcitation syndromes* is a congenital or acquired disorder characterized by the presence of normal P waves, a PR interval of 0.11 s or less, increased QRS duration, a slur on the initial phase of the QRS complex (delta wave), and a pronounced tendency for the occurrence of atrial tachyarrhythmias, especially paroxysmal tachycardia, atrial flutter, and atrial fibrillation. The pathophysiologic common denominator of these disorders is premature activation of a portion of ventricular muscle in relation to atrial depolarization. Variations include the presence of some of but not all these electrocardiographic features, such as the *Lown-Ganong-Levine syndrome* (LGL syndrome), which is manifested by a short PR interval but no delta wave or QRS widening. Recent anatomic and electrophysiologic studies have led to a general concept embracing these disorders. The common denominator appears to be the presence of an anatomic and/or functional anomalous conduction pathway which bypasses the AV node (Fig. 237-3), often apparently because of persistent muscular bridges reflecting defects in embryologic partitioning of atria from ventricles. Conduction through the anomalous pathway may be manifest or occult. In the classic Wolff-Parkinson-White syndrome the sinus impulse is conducted concomitantly down the anomalous pathway and the normal pathway. Accordingly, the impulse fragments longitudinally. Ventricular excitation is a composite of early excitation (preexcitation) by the impulse traversing the anomalous pathway and hence not delayed in the AV node, and normal excitation by the impulse conducted normally through the AV node. Thus, "normal" beats are fusion beats

containing a delta (preexcitation) wave, accounting for QRS prolongation. The activation from the preexcitation impulse travels more slowly through ventricular myocardium than does the normal impulse through the specialized His-Purkinje system once it has traversed the AV node. Accordingly, a large portion of ventricular depolarization is due to normal conduction, and the preexcitation wave is extinguished by the activation front of the normally conducted impulse.

Accessory pathways of anomalous conduction (classically the bundle of Kent, bypass tracts of James, and fibers of Mahaim) underlie the genesis of the supraventricular tachyarrhythmias so common in patients with these disorders. An important feature is the disparity between the duration of the refractory period of the AV node and accessory pathway. Although conduction through the accessory pathway occurs more rapidly, generally its refractory period is longer than that in the AV node. The tachycardia, usually paroxysmal supraventricular tachycardia, is initiated by a premature supraventricular beat which finds the anomalous pathway refractory and the normal pathway excitable. Accordingly, impulse transmission proceeds antegrade through the normal pathway; the impulse fragments in the AV node; *antegrade* conduction proceeds within one fragment, leading to ventricular excitation; *retrograde* conduction of the other fragment proceeds through the anomalous pathway, which has become excitable by this time; and the tachyarrhythmia persists because when the impulse reaches the normal pathway again it can be retransmitted antegrade in a persistently reciprocating manner. Thus, during the tachycardia QRS complexes are normal and do not exhibit a delta wave. A fortuitously timed or induced premature beat will terminate the tachycardia by resetting the refractory period of one or both pathways so that the circus movement is interrupted. Termination may occur also by block in one or the other of the pathways, or in both of them, sufficient to interrupt the reciprocating impulse and allow reemergence of sinus pacemaker activity. When the refractory period of the accessory pathway is less than that of the AV node, premature atrial depolarizations may not initiate supraventricular tachycardia probably because of concealed conduction in the AV node, although premature ventricular depolarizations do initiate supraventricular tachycardia. Preexcitation manifested by atrial fibrillation with unusually rapid ventricular response is associated with accessory pathways with short refractory periods. Marked variation of QRS morphology occurs, reflecting changing contributions from accessory pathway and AV nodal conduction. The rate of the ventricular response is inversely related to the duration of the accessory pathway refractory period.

A similar mechanism probably underlies many so-called "ectopic" supraventricular tachyarrhythmias in patients without electrocardiographic evidence of preexcitation. In such cases the anomalous pathway may simply represent longitudinal functional stratification within the AV junction, allowing for fragmentation of impulse propagation because of disparity between recovery times of two or more longitudinal pathways. In many patients with preexcitation syndromes the electrocardiogram shifts between the abnormal preexcitation and the normal intraventricular conduction pattern. The normal pattern may reveal abnormalities masked by the preexcitation form.

Two classic Wolff-Parkinson-White patterns have been recognized. In group A the delta wave is directed anteriorly and QRS complexes are dominantly positive in the right precordial leads. In some instances deep Q waves are present in lead aVF. In group B the delta wave is directed to the left and posteriorly, resulting in dominantly negative right precordial QRS complexes. Therefore, in both types, the tracing may be mistaken for QRS abnormalities indicative of myocardial infarction. The shift to anomalous conduction can sometimes be induced by vagal stimulation, such as that produced by carotid sinus pressure or by digitalis given intravenously. The normal type of conduction may be elicited by vagal inhibition with atropine or exercise, and also by quinidine and procainamide. As noted earlier, during paroxysms of tachycardia, the widened ventricular complexes usually assume a normal configuration.

Intracardiac electrograms, programmed electrical stimulation of the heart, and epicardial mapping in those patients requiring surgery are essential for localization of the anatomic sites of accessory pathways. Recurrent paroxysmal supraventricular tachycardia, or atrial fibrillation refractory to medical management, may require surgical section of the accessory pathway, which also often normalizes the PR interval and QRS duration. Adequate electrophysiologic diagnostic studies are needed since (1) multiple accessory pathways may be present and identification of the one(s) responsible for the tachycardia is necessary, (2) tachycardia may be due to reentry through the AV node rather than through a demonstrable but clinically insignificant accessory pathway, and (3) the responsible accessory pathway may not correspond to the locus suggested by a delta wave on the electrocardiogram.

The preexcitation syndrome should be suspected in any person subject to paroxysms of tachycardia, particularly when they have occurred from youth. Although preexcitation has been associated with Ebstein's and other congenital cardiac abnormalities, mitral valve prolapse, hypertrophic cardiomyopathy, and hyperthyroidism, it is generally an isolated disorder. Any patient with a supraventricular tachyarrhythmia in which the ventricular rate exceeds 200 beats per minute is a likely candidate, because normal AV nodal delay of conduction usually precludes rates this rapid. Persistent tachycardia, particularly atrial fibrillation, often requires electrical cardioversion, the therapy of choice whenever hemodynamic embarrassment ensues. Alternatively, programmed atrial or ventricular pacing may be effective in terminating an individual attack, particularly when the site of stimulation can be selected on the basis of knowledge of the locus of the accessory pathway defined by electrophysiologic studies.

Pharmacologic therapy is designed to reduce the incidence of premature depolarizations potentially capable of initiating reentrant tachycardia, to diminish the disparity in length between effective refractory periods in the AV node and accessory pathways, or to prolong refractoriness in a portion of the tachycardia circuit so that propagation of the reentrant impulse is blocked. Digitalis may terminate a paroxysm of rapid heart action by increasing the AV nodal refractory period. However, with atrial fibrillation it may paradoxically increase the ventricular rate by facilitating conduction through the AV node–bypass pathway, and procainamide or quinidine is more effective. Administration of lidocaine intravenously occasionally terminates episodes of atrial flutter associated with preexcitation by prolonging conduction time in the bypass pathway.

Procainamide and quinidine diminish the frequency of attacks in some patients probably by diminishing the incidence of the precipitating premature beats. Propranolol generally slows conduction through the AV node rather than through the accessory pathway. In combination with quinidine, it may be effective not only in terminating an acute attack but also in reducing the frequency of recurrent attacks. Repetitive attacks may be disabling, and rarely sudden death occurs during an attack. If maintenance propranolol or other pharmacologic prophylaxis is ineffective, two procedures merit consideration: implantation of a transvenous atrial, coronary sinus, or ventricular pacemaker which can be activated to interrupt the tachycardia by initiating an appropriately timed beat. This procedure should not be performed without thorough electrophysiologic evaluation including His bundle electrocardiography, since atrial pacing may induce atrial fibrillation with potentially catastrophic results accompanying a very rapid ventricular response and since ventricular pacing may induce ventricular fibrillation. In cases refractory to pharmacologic therapy, with repetitive disabling attacks, relief may follow surgical interruption of the anomalous pathway defined by definitive electrophysiologic studies.

REFERENCES

BERNE RM (ed): Electrophysiology of the heart, in *Handbook of Physiology,* sec 2: *The Cardiovascular System,* vol 1: *The Heart.* Bethesda, American Physiological Society, 1979, pp 187-428

BIGGER JT: Arrhythmias: Mechanisms, diagnosis and treatment, in *Heart Disease,* E Braunwald (ed). Philadelphia, Saunders, 1980, chaps 19, 20

——— et al: Ventricular arrhythmias in ischemic heart disease: Mechanism, prevalence, significance, and management. Prog Cardiovasc Dis 19:255, 1977

CHARDACK WM: Cardiac pacemakers and heart block, in *Gibbon's Surgery of the Chest,* 3d ed, DC Sabiston, FC Spencer (eds). Philadelphia, Saunders, 1976, chap 50, p 1252

DURRER D, WELLENS HJJ: Medical and surgical treatment of the Wolff-Parkinson-White syndrome. Annu Rev Med 27, 1976

GETTES LS: Electrophysiologic basis of arrhythmias in acute myocardial ischemia, in *Modern Trends in Cardiology—3,* MF Oliver (ed). London, Butterworths, 1975, p 219

KENNEDY HL, CARALIS DG: Ambulatory electrocardiography: A clinical perspective. Ann Intern Med 87:729, 1977

KRIKLER DM, GOODWIN JF: *Cardiac Arrhythmias: The Modern Electrophysiological Approach.* Philadelphia, Saunders, 1975

LOWN B et al: Paroxysmal atrial tachycardia with block. Circulation 21:129, 1960

MUNDTH ED et al: Surgical treatment of ventricular irritability. J Thorac Cardiovasc Surg 66:943, 1973

NARULA OS: *His Bundle Electrocardiography and Clinical Electrophysiology.* Philadelphia, Davis, 1975

ROSEN KM: Cardiac electrophysiology symposium. Arch Intern Med 135:387, 1975

WELLENS HJJ, LIE HI: *The Conduction System of the Heart.* Philadelphia, Lea & Febiger, 1976

ZIPES DP et al: Role of the slow current in cardiac electrophysiology. Circulation 51:761, 1975

Medical treatment of heart disease

238
PHARMACOLOGIC TREATMENT OF CARDIOVASCULAR DISORDERS

EUGENE BRAUNWALD

The clinical pharmacology of positive inotropic agents (digitalis glycosides and sympathomimetic agents), antiarrhythmic drugs, and coronary vasodilator agents is presented in this chapter. Diuretics and vasodilators are discussed in Chap. 236, antihypertensive agents in Chap. 251, and adrenergic blocking agents in Chap. 72.

The *direct* cardiac action of drugs may be divided into four major areas: (1) an effect on contractility (inotropic effect), reflecting alterations in the myocardial force-velocity relation at any given initial muscle length (Chap. 235); (2) an effect on heart rate, expressed as an alteration in the rhythmicity, i.e., the frequency of discharge of normal pacemaker tissue, generally that in the sinoatrial node; (3) an effect on conductivity, i.e., on the velocity with which the depolarization wave travels through the myocardium and the atrioventricular conduction system; and (4) an effect on irritability, i.e., the tendency to develop ectopic pacemaker activity, which is dependent on the rate of diastolic depolarization and the threshold potential (Chap. 237). In addition to these direct effects, drugs may also affect any of or all these four properties *indirectly* by altering

(1) autonomic influences acting on the heart directly or reflexly, or (2) the relationship between myocardial oxygen supply (determined largely by coronary blood flow) and oxygen needs (Chap. 244).

DIGITALIS GLYCOSIDES

The basic molecular structure of the digitalis glycosides is a steroid nucleus to which an unsaturated lactone ring is attached at C-17 (Fig. 238-1*A*). These two elements together are called *aglycone* or *genin*, and it is this portion of the molecule which is responsible for the cardiotonic activity. The addition of a sugar to this basic structure enhances both the potency and duration of action of the glycoside, probably as a result of increasing solubility. The sugar residue may prevent alterations in the steric structure of the molecule, which would result in a loss of cardiotonic activity.

PHARMACOKINETICS Although, in the absence of severe malabsorption, digitalis is adequately absorbed from the intestinal tract even in the presence of vascular congestion secondary to heart failure, some glycosides, including ouabain, are poorly absorbed and, therefore, are effective only when administered parenterally; the intravenous route is preferable to the intramuscular, since absorption is erratic with the latter. When they are administered orally, absorption is close to complete within 2 h. The fraction of orally administered glycoside which

FIGURE 238-1

Chemical structure of various cardioactive drugs.

is absorbed varies. Approximately 40 percent of digitalis powder is absorbed, almost 100 percent of digitoxin, and 65 to 75 percent of digoxin. Considerable variability of bioavailability has been found in different commercial preparations of digoxin. Cholesterol-lowering resins, antidiarrheal agents containing pectin and kaolin, nonabsorbable antacids, and neomycin can reduce the absorption of digoxin and digitoxin. Varying degrees of protein-binding of glycosides occur in the bloodstream (for example, 97 percent for digitoxin and 25 percent for digoxin), and though these differences may account in part for the varying durations of the effect of different glycosides, they are not related to the speed of action of these drugs. The plasma contains only approximately 1 percent of the body stores of digoxin; digoxin is not effectively removed from the body by dialysis, exchange transfusions, or during cardiopulmonary bypass, presumably because of tissue binding. The major fraction of the glycosides is directly bound by various tissues including the heart, in which the concentration is approximately 30 times that in the plasma for digoxin and 7 times for digitoxin, which is less polar and more lipid-soluble than digoxin.

Digoxin, which has a half-life of 1.6 days, is filtered in the glomeruli, and 85 percent is excreted in the urine, most in unchanged form; only 10 to 15 percent of digoxin is eliminated in the stool through biliary excretion in the presence of normal renal function. The ratio of digoxin clearance to endogenous creatinine clearance is 0.8, and the percentage of the body's total stores of digoxin lost per day can be calculated as (14 ± 0.2) × creatinine clearance in milliliters per minute. In patients with normal renal function a plateau concentration in the blood and tissue is reached after 5 days of daily maintenance treatment without a loading dose (Fig. 70-2). Therefore, significant reductions of the glomerular filtration rate reduce the elimination of digoxin (but not of digitoxin) and, therefore, may prolong digoxin's effect, allowing it to accumulate to toxic levels. The administration of most diuretics does not alter the excretion of digoxin significantly, but spironolactone can inhibit tubular secretion of digoxin, resulting in significant accumulation of the drug. Serum levels and pharmacokinetics are essentially unchanged by massive weight loss. *Digitoxin,* with a half-life of approximately 5 days, is metabolized chiefly in the liver; only 15 percent is excreted in the urine unchanged and an equal fraction in the stool. Drugs such as phenobarbital and phenylbutazone that increase activity of hepatic microsomal enzymes accelerate the metabolism of digitoxin. To reach a steady state, digitoxin requires maintenance doses for 3 to 4 weeks. *Ouabain* is very rapid acting, exhibiting an onset of action 5 to 10 min and a peak effect 60 min following intravenous injection. It is poorly absorbed from the gastrointestinal tract and, therefore, is not suitable for oral use; it is excreted by the kidneys, has a half-life of 21 h, and is useful in emergencies.

MECHANISM OF ACTION The cardiac actions of all digitalis glycosides are alike. The clinical effects result from augmenting contractility and irritability and from slowing heart rate and atrioventricular conduction. In addition, the cardiac glycosides potentiate vagal influences on the heart.

The most important effect of digitalis on cardiac muscle is to shift its force-velocity relation upward (Chap. 235). This positive inotropic effect is exhibited in normal, nonfailing hypertrophied as well as in failing hearts. In the absence of heart failure, however, when cardiac output is not limited by cardiac contractility, the drug does not elevate the output. The finding that digitalis increases the contractility of the nonfailing heart has led to its use (1) in patients with heart disease but without heart failure prior to operation or other stressful situations such as serious infections, and (2) in the presence of a chronically increased load, such as hypertension without heart fail-

ure. However, definitive evidence of its efficacy in these circumstances has not been provided.

Excitation-contraction coupling is the membrane and intracellular process most likely involved in producing the positive inotropic effect of digitalis glycosides. These drugs inhibit transmembrane sodium and potassium movement by inhibition of the magnesium and ATP-dependent sodium- and potassium-activated transport enzyme complex. The latter, localized to the sarcolemma, and termed Na$^+$- and K$^+$-stimulated ATPase, appears to be the receptor for cardioactive glycosides. There is a correlation between inhibition of the enzyme and the inotropic potency of the glycoside. The resulting altered transmembrane distribution of sodium, i.e., the elevation of the intracellular concentration of this ion, according to one theory, then competes with calcium for efflux at internal membranes, so that less calcium is transported out of the cell and more is available to activate contractile sites. According to another concept, the increased intracellular sodium concentration enhances transmembrane exchange of sodium and calcium. Regardless of the precise mechanism involved, there is an increased myocardial uptake of calcium, which augments calcium released to the myofilaments during excitation and, therefore, invokes a positive inotropic response.

The action of glycosides on the inhibition of the sarcolemmal Na$^+$- and K$^+$-stimulated ATPase also produces alteration in the electrical properties of both the contractile cells and the specialized automatic cells. While low concentrations of glycosides produce little effect on the action potential, high concentrations result in a reduction in the resting potential (phase 4) with an augmented rate of diastolic depolarization (Chap. 237). The reduction in the resting potential brings the cell closer to the threshold for depolarization. These two effects lead to increased *rhythmicity* and ectopic impulse activity. With the lowering of the resting potential, the rate of rise of the action potential is reduced, resulting in a slowing of conduction velocity, which is conducive to the development of reentry. Thus, the known electrophysiologic effects of digitalis glycosides are capable of explaining both reentry and ectopic foci and the resultant arrhythmias associated with digitalis intoxication.

The glycosides also prolong the *functional refractory period* of the atrioventricular node, through a direct action, as well as an enhanced vagal effect. Digitalis also shortens the refractory period of the atrial and ventricular muscle. Small action potentials are propagated in a decremental fashion in the atrioventricular junction. Most do not reach the ventricles but leave some of the atrioventricular junctional cells in a refractory state. Together with the action of digitalis to augment vagal activity, this helps to explain the slowing of ventricular rate produced by digitalis glycosides in supraventricular tachycardias. In atrial fibrillation, the slowing of ventricular rate is explained by several factors, in addition to prolongation of the functional refractory period of the atrioventricular node, including increased fibrillation rate (shortened atrial refractory period) and increased concealed conduction with fewer impulses penetrating the atrioventricular junction owing to both direct and vagal effects of glycosides on junctional tissue.

Digitalis exerts a negative chronotropic action, which in part is a vagal effect and in part is due to a direct action on the sinus pacemaker. In heart failure, slowing of the sinus rate following the administration of digitalis results also from withdrawal of sympathetic activity secondary to general improvement in circulatory status due to the positive inotropic effect of the glycoside. In the nonfailing heart the slowing effect is negligible, and digitalis should not be used for the treatment of sinus tachycardia unless heart failure is present. The apparent suppression of pacemaker activity which may take place following high doses of digitalis is probably due not to arrest of the pacemaker but rather to a sinoatrial block related to a depression of conduction.

In addition, the digitalis glycosides also exert an action on the peripheral vasculature, causing venous and arterial constriction in normal individuals and reflex dilatation resulting from withdrawal of sympathetic constrictor activity in patients with congestive heart failure.

INDICATIONS The most important indication for the administration of digitalis is congestive heart failure (Chap. 236). By stimulating the contractile function of the heart, digitalis improves ventricular emptying; i.e., it augments the ejection fraction, increases cardiac output, promotes diuresis, and reduces the elevated diastolic pressure and volume and end-systolic volume of the failing ventricle with consequent reduction of symptoms resulting from pulmonary vascular congestion and elevated systemic venous pressure. It is most beneficial in patients in whom ventricular contractility is impaired secondary to chronic ischemic heart disease, or when hypertensive, valvular, or congenital heart disease imparts an excessive volume or pressure load. Digitalis is also indicated in both the prevention and the abolition of recurrent episodes of paroxysmal supraventricular tachycardia. It is helpful in slowing the rapid ventricular rate of patients with atrial flutter and fibrillation (Chap. 237). It is of relatively little value in most forms of cardiomyopathy, myocarditis, beriberi with heart failure, mitral stenosis, thyrotoxicosis and sinus rhythm, cor pulmonale when the lung disease is not being treated concurrently (Chap. 246), and chronic constrictive pericarditis (Chap. 249). Nonetheless, it is not contraindicated in these disorders and is frequently used since it may exert a beneficial effect, albeit not a striking one.

Digitalis is of little hemodynamic or clinical benefit in cardiogenic shock secondary to acute myocardial infarction, but is usually moderately effective in pulmonary edema and milder forms of heart failure secondary to myocardial infarction. Digitalis has variable effects on angina pectoris, sometimes reducing this symptom in the presence of cardiomegaly and heart failure but tending to increase it in their absence. In patients with second-degree atrioventricular block, digitalis may be harmful by inducing complete (third-degree) block, and in those with idiopathic hypertrophic subaortic stenosis (Chap. 247) by increasing obstruction to left ventricular outflow.

DIGITALIS INTOXICATION Although digitalis is one of the cornerstones of the treatment for heart failure, it is a two-edged sword, because intoxication due to digitalis excess is a common, serious, and potentially fatal complication of its use. The therapeutic-to-toxic ratios are identical for all cardiac glycosides. In most patients with heart failure the lethal dose of most glycosides is probably 5 to 10 times the minimal effective dose and only about twice the dose which leads to minor toxic manifestations. In addition, old age, acute myocardial infarction or ischemia, hypoxemia, magnesium depletion, renal insufficiency, hypercalcemia, carotid sinus massage, electrical cardioversion (Chap. 239), and hypothyroidism all may reduce the tolerance of the patient to the digitalis glycosides or provoke latent digitalis intoxication. The most common precipitating cause of digitalis intoxication, however, is depletion of potassium stores, which often occurs as a result of diuretic therapy and secondary hyperaldosteronism. Since it is not nec-

essary for a patient to receive a maximally tolerated dose of digitalis to derive a beneficial effect, even small doses provide some therapeutic action; this point should be considered if these drugs are to be used in patients prone to toxicity.

Anorexia, nausea, and vomiting, which are among the earliest signs of digitalis intoxication, are caused by direct stimulation of centers in the medulla and are not of gastrointestinal origin. The most frequent disturbance of cardiac rhythm caused by digitalis is premature ventricular beats, which may take the form of bigeminy because of increased myocardial irritability or facilitation of reentry. Atrioventricular block of varying degrees of severity may occur. Nonparoxysmal atrial tachycardia with variable atrioventricular block is quite characteristic of digitalis intoxication. Finally, sinus arrhythmia, sinoatrial block, sinus arrest, and atrioventricular junctional and multifocal ventricular tachycardia may also occur. These arrhythmias are due to action of the glycoside both on cardiac tissues and on the central nervous system. Chronic digitalis intoxication may be insidious in onset and characterized by exacerbations of heart failure, weight loss, cachexia, neuralgias, gynecomastia, yellow vision, and delirium. Digitalis-toxic cardiac arrhythmias precede extracardiac (gastrointestinal or central nervous system) toxicity in about one-half of cases.

Digitalis intoxication has been reported to occur in as many as 20 percent of hospitalized patients receiving a cardiac glycoside, which emphasizes the importance of the ability to diagnose this condition. The administration of quinidine to patients receiving digoxin raises the serum concentration of the latter and increases the incidence of digitalis intoxication. Therefore, serum digoxin concentrations and electrocardiograms should be followed carefully when quinidine is given to digitalized patients. The radioimmunoassays for digoxin and digitoxin make possible the correlation of serum glycoside levels with the presence of toxicity. In patients receiving standard maintenance doses of digoxin and digitoxin and in whom no sign of intoxication is present, serum concentrations approximate 1 to 1.5 and 20 to 25 ng/ml, respectively. When signs of intoxication are present, serum levels of more than 2 and 30 ng/ml, respectively, of these glycosides are often found. Since many factors other than the serum concentration determine digitalis intoxication, and since there is overlap in serum glycoside concentrations in patients with and without toxicity, it is clear that these levels cannot be used as a sole guide to digitalis dosage. However, when taken together with findings on the clinical examination and electrocardiogram, they add useful information to the clinical evaluations of digitalis intoxication. In addition they will indicate whether a patient for whom the history of digitalis intake is in doubt has, in fact, been receiving the drug.

Treatment of digitalis intoxication When tachyarrhythmias result from digitalis intoxication, withdrawal of the drug and treatment with potassium, phenytoin, propranolol, or lidocaine are indicated. Potassium should be administered cautiously and by the oral route whenever possible if hypokalemia is present, but small doses may also be helpful when serum potassium levels are normal; *potassium must not be employed in the presence of atrioventricular block or hyperkalemia,* when phenytoin is more appropriate. Propranolol should not be used to treat digitalis toxicity in the presence of severe heart failure or atrioventricular block; lidocaine is effective in the treatment of digitalis-induced ventricular tachyarrhythmias in the absence of preceding atrioventricular block. A cardiac pacemaker may be required in digitalis-induced atrioventricular block. Electrical conversion may not only be ineffective in treating these arrhythmias but may induce more serious arrhythmias (Chap. 239). However, it may be lifesaving in digitalis-induced ventricular fibrillation. Quinidine and procainamide are not useful in the treatment of digitalis intoxication. Fab fragments of purified, intact digitalis antibodies represent a potentially lifesaving approach to the treatment of severe intoxication.

CATECHOLAMINES AND SYMPATHOMIMETIC DRUGS (See also Chap. 72)

Norepinephrine, a catecholamine, is normally found in sympathetic nerve endings in the heart as well as in arterioles and venules. A large fraction of the endogenous stores of norepinephrine in the heart is synthesized within the cardiac sympathetic postganglionic nerve endings; the remainder is taken up from the circulation. Cardiac norepinephrine is protected from enzymatic degradation because it is stored in granules found in the postganglionic nerve endings. In the absence of endogenous catecholamines and in the presence of congestive heart failure, the heart's stores of norepinephrine are depleted (Chap. 236). However, sympathetic nerve stimulation is an important supporting mechanism for the heart in the presence of stress.

Catecholamines and other sympathomimetic drugs act upon the circulation of stimulating adrenergic receptors in the effector organs. Activation of alpha-adrenergic receptors results in vasoconstriction, leading to a pressor response. Stimulation of beta$_1$-adrenergic receptors results in stimulation of cardiac contractility, automaticity, conduction velocity, and irritability, while stimulation of beta$_2$ receptors results in relaxation of smooth muscle in the vascular bed and the tracheobronchial tree.

An intimate relation between changes in cyclic 3',5'-adenosine monophosphate (cyclic AMP) and contractility has been suggested but remains to be defined. It is clear that adenylate cyclase, a membrane-bound enzyme which catalyzes the production of cyclic AMP from adenosine triphosphate (ATP) in the presence of Ca^{2+}, is activated by sympathomimetic amines which attach to beta receptors on the cell membrane. Cyclic AMP, in turn, activates a class of enzymes in the cell known as *protein kinases* which phosphorylate a number of proteins in the cell and stimulate the transport of Ca^{2+} into the cell. Blockade of beta receptors interferes with both the inotropic response to the drug and the augmentation of cyclic AMP concentration in the heart.

The catecholamines are based on the β-phenylethylamine molecule, an aromatic nucleus consisting of a benzene ring and an aliphatic portion, ethylamine (Fig. 238-1*B*). In general, these compounds have a brief duration of action. When administered orally, they are rapidly inactivated in the intestinal wall and liver and are therefore ineffective. Epinephrine is rapidly absorbed after intramuscular injection. However, norepinephrine should be administered only intravenously, because it produces necrosis of tissue consequent to intense vasoconstriction when given intramuscularly or subcutaneously. Isoproterenol may be administered parenterally, as an aerosol, or sublingually.

Catecholamines may be inactivated by orthomethylation by the enzyme catechol orthomethyl transferase (COMT), or they may be deaminated by monoamine oxidase (MAO). The combined actions of MAO and COMT on epinephrine or norepinephrine lead to the production of vanillylmandelic acid (VMA), elevated urinary levels of which are useful in the diagnosis of pheochromocytoma (Chap. 337).

The specific effects of a catecholamine or a sympathomimetic amine depend on whether the drug is of the alpha-, beta$_1$-, or beta$_2$-adrenergic or mixed type, and whether its action is direct or due to release of stored catecholamines. Certain sympathomimetic drugs, similar in structure to the catecholamines but lacking the catechol nucleus, act by varying combinations of a direct action on the sympathetic receptor as well as by causing the release of stored catecholamines. Examples of this type are *metaraminol* (Aramine) and *mephentermine*

(Wyamine), which have both direct and catecholamine-releasing action. Tyramine, on the other hand, acts solely by releasing stored catecholamines. In addition, sympathomimetic agents may be used for the reflex effects which they frequently induce. *Methoxamine* (Vasoxyl) and *phenylephrine* (Neo-Synephrine), for instance, are essentially pure alpha-adrenergic stimulators and produce arteriolar constriction, thereby augmenting systemic vascular resistance. *Norepinephrine* (Levophed), on the other hand, exerts a predominant alpha-adrenergic action on the peripheral vascular bed but also stimulates beta receptors. Its effects include an increase in systolic and diastolic blood pressures, as well as an increase in total peripheral resistance with compensatory reflex slowing of the heart similar to that produced by methoxamine. Stroke volume is increased and cardiac output is essentially unchanged. Coronary blood flow is increased, but blood flow through kidney, brain, liver, and skeletal muscle is usually reduced. *Isoproterenol* (Isuprel) has pure beta-adrenergic activity. Its administration, therefore, leads to a reduction in peripheral vascular resistance with an increase in heart rate and contractility and, thus, an increase in cardiac output. Tachycardia and ventricular ectopic rhythms may also occur.

INDICATIONS Sympathomimetic amines are useful in the management of a variety of cardiovascular disorders. Isoproterenol is indicated in the treatment of a number of arrhythmias characterized by reduced automaticity and conductivity (Chap. 237). It may be administered as a continuous intravenous infusion (1 to 6 μg/min) or sublingually (10 to 20 mg every 2 to 4 h) in patients with sinus arrest, sinoatrial block, sinus bradycardia, various forms of atrioventricular conduction defects, and Stokes-Adams attacks. This amine is also indicated in a variety of low cardiac output states, including those following cardiac operations and those associated with septic and hemorrhagic shock, unless the peripheral vascular bed is already dilated; during isoproterenol infusion expansion of circulating volume is often necessary because the vasodilatation produced by the drug may greatly reduce central venous pressure and ventricular preload. Adverse effects include the development of sinus tachycardia and other tachyarrhythmias and increases in myocardial oxygen consumption due to enhanced myocardial contractility and heart rate; this may intensify myocardial ischemia if it is present.

Methoxamine and phenylephrine, which act almost exclusively by stimulating alpha receptors, are indicated in hypotensive states such as occur during spinal anesthesia secondary to loss of vasoconstrictor tone, when it is desired to augment peripheral resistance without increasing cardiac contractility or automaticity. These agents are not beneficial in shock due to myocardial infarction and other conditions in which depression of cardiac contractility plays an important role in the genesis of the hypotension, but are useful in patients with supraventricular tachycardia, when it is desired to induce hypertension and augment vagal tone while reducing adrenergic tone reflexly (Chap. 237).

Agents which stimulate both alpha and beta receptors, such as *norepinephrine, epinephrine,* and *metaraminol,* may be used to elevate arterial pressure when hypotension is secondary to both a depression of myocardial contractility and an inadequate vasoconstrictor response. However, in most hypotensive states peripheral vascular resistance is already increased, and the alpha-receptor stimulation provided by norepinephrine may actually be deleterious. However, in low doses [norepinephrine <0.03 (mg/kg)/min; epinephrine <0.01 (mg/kg)/min], these agents stimulate beta receptors almost exclu-

TABLE 238-1

Electrophysiologic and electrocardiographic effects and pharmacokinetics of antiarrhythmic drugs

| Drug | Automaticity | Conduction velocity | Effective refractory period | Action-potential duration | Interval | | | Gastrointestinal absorption, % | Half-life, h | Therapeutic plasma levels, μg/ml |
					PR	QRS	QT			
Quinidine	↓	↓	↑	↑	$= ↑$	↑	↑	> 95	6.5	2.5–8.0
Procainamide	↓	↓	↑	↑	$= ↑$	↑	↑	85	3.5	3–10
Disopyramide	↓	↓	↑	↑	$= ↑$	↑	↑	85	4.5	3–8
Lidocaine	↓	$= ↑$	↓	↓	$= ↓$	$=$	$= ↓$	< 30	0.5–2	1.5–6
Diphenylhydantoin	↓	$= ↑$	↓	↓	$= ↓$	$=$	↓	Slow	24–36	10–18
Propranolol	↓	↓	↑	↑	$= ↑$	$=$	↓	> 95	3–6	30–100

NOTE: ↑, *increased or prolonged;* ↓, *reduced or shortened;* =, *unchanged;* $= ↑$, *unchanged or prolonged;* $= ↓$, *unchanged or shortened.*

sively. In higher doses, both alpha and beta receptors are activated although norepinephrine is a predominant alpha-adrenergic agent while epinephrine is a dominant beta-stimulant.

Undesirable reactions to the catecholamines include headache, anxiety, severe hypertension, and cardiac arrhythmias. When norepinephrine extravasates from its site of intravenous administration, tissue necrosis and sloughing may occur. Infiltration of the area with an alpha-adrenergic blocking agent such as phentolamine (Regitine) may prevent necrosis by blocking vasoconstriction. Following prolonged administration of sympathomimetics for the support of arterial pressure, the dose may have to be tapered slowly and the blood volume expanded to prevent vascular collapse. The replacement of endogenous catecholamine stores with nonreleasable congeners such as metaraminol may explain in part the difficulties of weaning patients from these drugs.

Dopamine, the naturally occurring immediate precursor of norepinephrine, has a combination of actions which make it particularly useful in the treatment of a variety of hypotensive states and congestive heart failure. At very low doses, that is, 1 to 2 (μg/kg)/min, it dilates renal and mesenteric blood vessels through stimulation of specific dopaminergic receptors, thereby augmenting renal and mesenteric blood flow and sodium excretion. In the range of 2 to 10 (μg/kg)/min dopamine stimulates myocardial beta receptors but induces little tachycardia, while at higher doses it also stimulates alpha-adrenergic receptors and elevates arterial pressure.

Dobutamine is a synthetic catecholamine which acts primarily on beta$_1$-adrenergic receptors, and stimulates beta$_2$ and alpha receptors only slightly. Consequently, it exerts a potent inotropic action. It has only a modest cardioaccelerating effect and lowers peripheral vascular resistance, but since it raises cardiac output, it has little effect on systemic arterial pressure. Dobutamine, given in continuous infusions of 2.5 to 15 (μg/kg)/min, is useful in the treatment of acute heart failure without hypotension. Like other sympathomimetic amines it may be particularly valuable in the management of patients requiring relatively short-term inotropic support—up to 1 week—in conditions which are reversible, such as the cardiac depression which sometimes follows open-heart surgery, or in patients with acute heart failure who are being prepared for operation. Adverse effects include sinus tachycardia, tachyarrhythmias, and hypertension.

ANTIARRHYTHMIC AGENTS

QUINIDINE This drug, the D isomer of quinine (Fig. 238-1C), is one of some twenty alkaloids derived from the bark of the cinchona tree, found in certain regions of South America and the Far East.

The *electrophysiologic effects* of quinidine on ventricular and Purkinje fibers are shared by *procainamide* (Pronestyl), and the following summary applies equally to both drugs (Table 238-1). The durations both of the effective refractory period and of the action potential are prolonged, the former more than the latter. The slope of phase 4 of the action potential is also reduced, and it is this effect which is responsible for slowing the spontaneous frequency of discharge of ectopic pacemakers. The drug also has negative chronotropic effects, depressing the activity of both the sinoatrial node and ectopic pacemakers. However, this direct negative chronotropic effect of quinidine is often counteracted by its vagal blocking action, which may lead to no change, or an actual increase in heart rate, and reduce the refractory period of the atrioventricular junction. Quinidine slows conductivity in the atrioventricular junction; therefore, in the presence of depressed atrioventricular conduction, it must be used with great caution. However, its potent vagal blocking action may actually facilitate conduction through this system. Quinidine prolongs conduction in depressed portions of a reentrant pathway so that conduction is further delayed and block occurs, thereby terminating reentrant ventricular arrhythmias. Quinidine also increases the threshold of excitability, thereby making atrial, ventricular, and Purkinje tissue less irritable. Quinidine produces peripheral vasodilatation, which together with a decreased cardiac output may lead to hypotension.

There are various interpretations of the means by which quinidine is effective in converting atrial fibrillation to normal sinus rhythm. If atrial fibrillation results from the formation of rapid waves of depolarization in the atrium (Chap. 237), then by diminishing the rate of impulse of an ectopic pacemaker, quinidine may slow this rate below the frequency at which atrial fibrillation occurs. If, on the other hand, atrial fibrillation results from a circus movement of impulses around the atrium, the prolongation of the atrial refractory period by quinidine would interrupt the circus movement, even though the velocity of impulse transmission is also decreased.

Diminished intraventricular conduction velocity is reflected in an increase in the duration of the QRS complex, while the delayed repolarization is reflected in the prolongation of the QT interval of the electrocardiogram. The anticholinergic action of quinidine may produce sinus tachycardia. The drug may also lead to an increase in ventricular rate when it alone is used for the treatment of atrial flutter or fibrillation; the slowing of atrial rate produced by quinidine may reduce the repetitive concealed conduction of atrial impulses in the atrioven-

Protein binding, %	Percentage excreted unchanged	Adverse effects
80	20-50	Gastrointestinal symptoms, cinchonism, rashes, thrombocytopenia, hypotension, heart block, ventricular fibrillation
15	50-60	Lupus-like syndrome, gastrointestinal symptoms, hypotension, heart block
5-65	50	Cardiac decompensation, gastrointestinal symptoms, and anticholinergic effects
30	<10	Drowsiness, disorientation, agitation, convulsions, coma, paresthesias, myocardial depression
>50	<5	Ataxia, nystagmus, hypotension, bradycardia, skin rash
90	<2	Asthma, heart block, asystole, hypotension, heart failure, weakness, insomnia, lethargy

tricular junction, and the vagal blocking action may enhance atrioventricular conduction. As a consequence, a greater fraction of the impulses entering the atrioventricular junction may propagate to the ventricle. Therefore, digitalis should be administered in doses sufficient to increase the effective refractory period of the atrioventricular junction before treating either atrial flutter or fibrillation with quinidine.

Toxic doses induce premature ventricular beats, ventricular tachycardia and fibrillation, complete atrioventricular block, severe myocardial depression, and peripheral vasodilatation, which together with a decreased cardiac output may lead to serious hypotension.

Indications Although quinidine may be used to convert atrial fibrillation to sinus rhythm, electrical countershock is now employed more frequently because of its safety and effectiveness (Chap. 239). Quinidine is used most frequently for prevention of recurrent atrial fibrillation after sinus rhythm has been restored. It may also be used in atrial flutter after a trial of digitalis therapy has failed to convert this rhythm to normal sinus rhythm. In the treatment of atrial flutter, however, quinidine frequently leads to a progressive reduction in the degree of block from 4:1 or 2:1 to 1:1, and when this occurs the rapid ventricular response may be hazardous. Quinidine or procainamide is frequently used to prevent supraventricular and ventricular tachycardia and fibrillation in patients who have had episodes of these arrhythmias. However, if atrioventricular block is associated with ventricular tachycardia, quinidine is contraindicated, because suppression of the ventricular focus in the presence of complete heart block may lead to ventricular standstill or fibrillation. Quinidine and procainamide are also used in the treatment of ectopic premature supraventricular and ventricular beats, but are not indicated unless the frequency of these ectopic impulses seriously disturbs the patient or unless the onset of a more serious arrhythmia is feared, as in acute myocardial infarction (Chap. 245). When given orally, these drugs are useful in maintaining control of ventricular extrasystoles in patients with an acute myocardial infarction when a lidocaine infusion is terminated.

Pharmacokinetics These differ for quinidine and procainamide. Quinidine may be administered orally (generally as the sulfate) or intramuscularly as the gluconate. The drug is well absorbed following oral administration which produces maximum effects in 1 to 2 h. If the drug is given at intervals of 2 to 4 h, effects will be cumulative. Effects are negligible 8 h following administration. This point may be especially important in the prophylaxis of recurrent supraventricular arrhythmias. If

doses are spaced more than 6 h apart, less than therapeutic serum levels may occur between doses and prophylaxis may fail. More frequent rather than increased doses may avert this problem. Sustained-release preparations may also be used. Peak effects occur 30 to 90 min following intramuscular administration, but injection is painful and absorption erratic. Intravenous administration, however, does not produce instantaneous effects; therefore, when it is given by this route, the drug should be administered slowly and the dose should not be repeated before peak effect has been achieved. In heart failure, impaired elimination of the drug and/or a decreased volume of distribution may occur. Renal failure has little effect on quinidine's pharmacokinetics.

In therapeutic concentrations approximately 80 percent of quinidine is bound by plasma albumin. Blood concentrations may be measured easily; concentrations of the order of 2.5 μg/ml are necessary for therapeutic effects; approximately 10 μg/ml usually produces toxicity. Although metabolic degradation of quinidine, mostly to hydroxy derivatives which have minimal antiarrhythmic activity, occurs in most tissues, particularly in the liver, hepatic injury does not appear to influence the rate at which quinidine leaves the plasma. Both the metabolic end product (2-hydroxyquinidine) and the unchanged drug normally are rapidly excreted by the kidneys. Phenobarbital and phenytoin stimulate the hepatic metabolism of quinidine and can result in reductions in plasma levels and loss of antiarrhythmic effect.

Adverse reactions to quinidine include cinchonism, consisting of tinnitus, headache, nausea, and distorted vision. Diarrhea, anorexia, nausea, and vomiting are common side effects but may be controlled with the phenothiazines. Frequently, in order to convert atrial fibrillation to normal sinus rhythm, it may be necessary to accept moderate levels of toxicity, entailing nausea, vomiting, tinnitus, and minor widening of the QRS complex. Idiosyncratic reactions, thrombocytopenic purpura, and severe hypotension may occur. The myocardial depressant action of quinidine limits its usefulness in the presence of heart failure and hypotensive states. Its use is also contraindicated in patients with a history of thrombocytopenic purpura or in individuals with digitalis intoxication, particularly those who have an atrioventricular conduction disorder. Widening of the QRS complex to 0.12 or by 50 percent or greater of control values and reduction of arterial pressure by more than 20 mmHg are serious warning signs and necessitate discontinuation of the drug. The greatest hazard of quinidine is sudden death due to ventricular fibrillation. This may occur even in patients treated with moderate therapeutic doses.

PROCAINAMIDE In 1936 the discovery was made that procaine, applied directly to the heart, elevates the threshold of ventricular muscle to electrical stimulation. Its prominent central nervous system–stimulating effect and rapid enzymatic hydrolysis make it undesirable clinically. Procainamide (Pronestyl), which differs from procaine in that an amide structure (—CONH—) is present instead of an ester linkage (—COO—) (Fig. 238-1D), has negligible central nervous system effects and is protected from enzymatic hydrolysis by plasma esterases.

The electrophysiologic effects of procainamide on the heart are similar to those of quinidine (Table 238-1). Clinically, procainamide is generally used in the treatment or prevention of ventricular tachyarrhythmias, in which it appears to be slightly more effective than quinidine. Procainamide, especially when given by the intravenous route, may cause hypotension, and alpha-adrenergic stimulators should be available to counteract this effect.

Pharmacokinetics Procainamide may be administered by the oral, intramuscular, or intravenous routes. It is rapidly and almost completely absorbed from the gastrointestinal tract and has a peak effect in approximately 1 h. Oral absorption may be impaired in the early hours after an acute myocardial infarction. If given intravenously for rapid control of arrhythmia, it can be administered in doses of 100 mg at intervals of 5 min while blood pressure and ECG are continuously monitored, since arrhythmias and hypotension may occur. An intravenous infusion of 0.3 to 1.0 (mg/kg)/min is begun simultaneously. It is concentrated in most tissues to levels greater than in the plasma. Approximately 15 percent of procainamide is bound to plasma proteins. It is eliminated by both hepatic metabolism and renal excretion. Approximately 50 percent is excreted in the urine unchanged, and the remainder is acetylated to *N*-acetylprocainamide; this metabolite has some antiarrhythmic activity. The rate of acetylation of procainamide parallels that of isoniazide and hydralazine, varying widely among individuals and appearing to be genetically determined.

An initial loading dose of 1 g given intramuscularly will rapidly produce effective blood concentrations (3 to 10 μg/ml) which may be maintained with an average dose of 250 mg orally or intramuscularly every 3 h. Since the half-life is only 3 to 4 h, longer intervals between doses may cause undesirably great fluctuations in concentration. Renal excretion of procainamide is important, and renal insufficiency may predispose to toxicity. Low cardiac output prolongs the elimination of procainamide. Therefore, the dose should be reduced in patients with cardiac or renal failure.

Adverse effects These include nausea, vomiting, and diarrhea. Acute toxicity consists of cardiac depression, atrioventricular block, and death. During the chronic administration of procainamide periodic blood counts should be obtained, because this drug has caused fatal agranulocytosis. It is also frequently a cause of drug fever and drug eruptions, anorexia, nausea, and vomiting. The commonest problem encountered during chronic administration of procainamide is a lupus erythematosus-like syndrome. After several months of administration, arthralgias sometimes accompanied by fever and hepatomegaly are present in about one-third of patients; an even higher proportion have positive antinuclear antibody tests. Toxicity is more common in slow acetylators. Cross-sensitivity to procaine and other related drugs should also be anticipated. Procainamide is contraindicated in the presence of atrioventricular block and when there is a history of hypersensitivity to local anesthetics.

DISOPYRAMIDE (NORPACE) (Fig. 238-1*E*) This agent resembles quinidine and procainamide in that it reduces conduction velocity, prolongs the durations of the action potential and of the effective refractory period, and exerts vagolytic properties. In addition, it may also exert a potent local anesthetic effect and reduce the transcellular influx of calcium. Its therapeutic and toxic effects may be potentiated by a high plasma K concentration. It is well absorbed when given orally and cleared essentially equally by the liver and the kidney. The therapeutic plasma concentration is 2 to 4 μg/ml. The loading dose is 200 or 300 mg, and the maintenance dose 100 or 200 mg every 6 h. These doses should be reduced in the presence of renal or hepatic failure.

The principal use for oral disopyramide is the suppression of frequent ventricular extrasystoles, in patients with and without acute myocardial infarction. The incidence of adverse effects has been reported to be less than with quinidine, but they include aggravation of cardiac decompensation and atrioventricular block. Vomiting, diarrhea, and anticholinergic effects

including urinary retention, dry mouth, blurred vision, constipation, and aggravation of glaucoma have been reported. It appears to be an acceptable alternative to quinidine or procainamide, particularly in patients who cannot tolerate these medications.

LIDOCAINE Although lidocaine has some similarities to procainamide in its antiarrhythmic action, it is not similar to procaine and to the other local anesthetics in the aromatic portion of its structure (Fig. 238-1*F*). In addition, lidocaine lacks an ester linkage and may be given to persons sensitive to procaine. Unlike quinidine and procainamide, lidocaine does not prolong the effective refractory period of ventricular myocardium. It diminishes automaticity in the His-Purkinje system and raises the threshold of ventricular fibrillation. Lidocaine enhances conduction at the Purkinje fiber–myocardial junctions, an action that may diminish reentrant arrhythmias by causing their extinction (Chap. 237). Lidocaine is the drug of choice for ventricular arrhythmias complicating myocardial infarction (Chap. 245). Its use is indicated (1) if the number of unifocal premature contractions exceeds five per minute and in the presence of (2) multifocal premature contractions or early (R on T wave) premature contractions, (3) couplets, and (4) runs of ventricular tachycardia. Since the incidence of ventricular tachycardia and fibrillation is diminished when lidocaine is administered prophylactically to patients with acute myocardial infarction, some physicians use it in all patients with this condition (Chap. 245).

Pharmacokinetics These are described on pages 372 to 373 and in Fig. 70-1. The absorption, metabolism, and effectiveness of oral lidocaine are unpredictable. When administered intravenously, 70 percent of the lidocaine entering the liver is metabolized on a single pass. Less than 3 percent of an administered dose is excreted unchanged in the urine, and thus it acts almost instantaneously, but its action is quite transient. Because of these properties, it is particularly useful when there is expectation that the inciting cause of the arrhythmia will disappear. Lidocaine, therefore, is widely used during cardiac catheterization and during cardiac operations when the stimuli which produce arrhythmias are short-lived. However, arrhythmias abolished by single injections of lidocaine may reappear in 10 to 20 min.

In order to achieve adequate blood levels, which generally range from 1.5 to 6 μg/ml, administration should be initiated with a bolus intravenous injection of 1 mg per kilogram of body weight, with additional doses every 5 min until the arrhythmia is abolished or 5 mg/kg has been administered, followed by a continuous intravenous infusion of 20 to 40 (μg/kg)/min. It is also effective when injected intramuscularly (5 mg of 10% lidocaine per kilogram of body weight) into the deltoid muscle. This route is frequently used in patients with myocardial infarction while they are being transported to the hospital. The half-life of lidocaine is about 1 h, and its deactivation is dependent on hepatic metabolism. In the presence of congestive heart failure, liver disease, or shock, dosage should be reduced by as much as 50 percent to avoid toxic effects, which include myocardial depression, hypotension, and neurological abnormalities such as drowsiness, numbness, paresthesias, disorientation, respiratory depression, and convulsions. Two of the metabolites also exert convulsant properties. It is contraindicated in patients with sinoatrial block. Renal failure does not alter lidocaine's pharmacokinetics profoundly.

PHENYTOIN (DIPHENYLHYDANTOIN, DILANTIN) (Fig. 238-1*G*) In 1938, this agent was introduced in the treatment of epilepsy. During the following 20 years a number of studies in animals reported its effectiveness in experimentally produced cardiac arrhythmias, especially those induced by digitalis. Unlike quinidine, phenytoin does not reduce atrioventricular or intraventricular conduction velocity and does not prolong the ventricular refractory period. However, like quinidine, it reduces automaticity in Purkinje fibers and raises the atrial and ventricular fibrillation thresholds. Possibly a depressant action of phenytoin on sympathetic centers in the central nervous system may play a role in its antiarrhythmic properties.

Indications Phenytoin is particularly effective in supraventricular and ventricular arrhythmias, particularly those resulting from digitalis excess, because it does not interfere with atrioventricular conduction, as do several other antiarrhythmic agents. It may also be useful in the treatment and prevention of ventricular extrasystoles and tachycardia not caused by digitalis excess, as well as acute ventricular arrhythmias associated with anesthesia, cardioversion, cardiac catheterization, and cardiac surgery if the more standard agents such as quinidine, procainamide, and lidocaine are ineffective. Less success has been reported with phenytoin in the treatment of supraventricular tachyarrhythmias not secondary to digitalis excess or when administered prophylactically in attempts to reduce ventricular arrhythmias in patients with ischemic heart disease.

Pharmacokinetics Soon after intravenous administration, the drug is concentrated in liver, kidney, and salivary glands and to a lesser extent in brain, fat, and muscle. Plasma concentrations decrease rapidly, but the kinetics of disposition are nonlinear. The chief site of inactivation is the liver where it is parahydroxylated by microsomal enzymes and there is a substantial enterohepatic circulation of metabolites of the drug; urinary excretion of metabolites is also significant. There is considerable intersubject variability in metabolism, and other drugs may alter drug disposition further by inducing or inhibiting hepatic microsomal enzymes.

Phenytoin may be administered orally or intravenously. The drug is well absorbed, although slowly, when given orally. To reach antiarrhythmic plasma levels (10 to 18 $\mu g/ml$), an oral loading dose of 1000 mg is given the first day, 500 mg on each of the next 2 days, and 400 mg per day thereafter. Intravenous doses consist of 100 mg every 5 min until the arrhythmia is abolished or until adverse effects appear; the total dosage should not exceed 1000 mg. For emergency use, 50 to 100 mg is administered intravenously every 5 min until the arrhythmia is controlled, until 500 mg has been given, or until untoward effects appear. Lower maintenance doses are then required. Because of the complex pharmacokinetics serial determinations of plasma concentrations are often helpful.

Adverse effects These include transient hypotension and bradycardia; with long-term administration, ataxia, slurring of speech, nystagmus, lethargy, mild gastric upsets, and skin rashes occur in 2 to 5 percent of patients. Excessive intravenous doses may produce respiratory arrest, hypotension, asystole, ventricular fibrillation, and death. During chronic administration, hyperplasia of the gums develops in about 20 percent of patients. Hepatocellular injury, folate-responsive megaloblastic anemia, peripheral neuropathy, and pseudolymphoma are rare complications.

BRETYLIUM This drug is concentrated in postganglionic sympathetic neurons and first stimulates, then inhibits, the release of norepinephrine, thus blocking sympathetic nerve function. It has been reported to be useful for and approved for treatment of life-threatening ventricular tachycardia or fibrillation refractory to other therapy. Its half-life averages 10 h, and it is excreted unchanged in the urine. The dose (5 to 10 mg/kg every 6 h) can be administered intravenously or intramuscularly. The principal adverse effect is increased arrhythmia during norepinephrine release followed by hypotension.

BETA-ADRENERGIC RECEPTOR BLOCKING AGENTS

See Chap. 72.

NITRATES Glyceryl trinitrate (nitroglycerin) and amyl nitrite have been used for more than a century for their vasodilating properties. In recent years, however, numerous other nitrate compounds have been introduced which have a longer duration of action than nitroglycerin (Fig. 238-1*H*).

MECHANISM OF ACTION The vasodilators have only one specific therapeutic effect—to relax smooth muscle. The mechanism of this action is not known, and it cannot be blocked by any known inhibitors. For example, nitrite ion can relax smooth muscle even in the presence of the alpha-adrenergic-stimulating effects of norepinephrine. Administration of organic nitrates leads to generalized arterial and venous dilation, resulting in a fall in mean systemic arterial pressure and in peripheral pooling of blood. Pulse pressure, stroke volume, and central venous pressure decline, particularly when the patient is in the erect position. In the absence of heart failure hypotension evokes a compensatory tachycardia. Dilatation of blood vessels in the skin causes marked flushing of the head, neck, and chest, and severe pounding headache may occur because of dilatation of the meningeal vessels.

Though nitroglycerin increases coronary blood flow in normal individuals, there is considerable evidence that it does not always evoke this effect in the presence of diffuse, severe coronary artery disease. Therefore, it is difficult to relate the beneficial effects of this drug in angina pectoris to a direct increase in total coronary blood flow. Myocardial ischemia, however, relates not only to the amount of blood which reaches the coronary capillaries but also to the demands for oxygen (Chaps. 5 and 244). Since nitroglycerin regularly reduces arterial blood pressure, the work performance and the oxygen requirements of the heart are diminished. The venous dilatation produced by this drug leads to a reduction in heart size, which also tends to reduce myocardial oxygen consumption. Coronary blood flow, however, is not diminished, and therefore the major effect of nitroglycerin may be to improve the relationship between myocardial oxygen delivery and myocardial oxygen requirements. There is some evidence that nitroglycerin dilates coronary collateral vessels, increasing perfusion of ischemic areas. Finally, the reduction in left ventricular end-diastolic tension consequent to the venous dilatation induced by nitroglycerin reduces the compression of subendocardial coronary vessels and may thereby induce a more favorable distribution of myocardial perfusion to the subendocardium, which is the portion of the heart wall most subject to ischemia.

INDICATIONS The nitrates are primarily used for the treatment of angina pectoris; the chest pain is relieved within 2 to 4 min by sublingual nitroglycerin. Because the effects of this drug may persist for 30 min, it may also be used prophylactically to prevent angina pectoris when the patient predicts that it will occur. However, long-term prophylaxis with the longer-acting nitrates has been relatively unsuccessful except when used in conjunction with beta-adrenergic blocking agents.

PHARMACOKINETICS The *nitrite* ion is an active vasodilator in both inorganic and organic forms, but the *nitrate* ion is active only in organic form. The organic nitrates are absorbed most effectively from the sublingual or buccal mucosa. Many of the longer-acting nitrates, however, are also absorbed from

TABLE 238-2
Approximate dosage schedules for cardioactive drugs*

Drug	Initial or loading dose			Usual maintenance dosage
	Oral	Intramuscular	Intravenous	
Ouabain			0.5–1.0 mg in divided doses	
Digoxin	1.0–1.5 mg		0.5–1.0 mg in divided doses	0.125–0.50 mg PO daily
Digitoxin	1.0–1.5 mg			0.05–0.15 mg PO daily
Digitalis leaf	1.0–2.0 g			0.05–0.15 g PO daily
Disopyramide	200–300 mg			100–200 mg qid
Quinidine	200 mg every 4–6 h; increase dose by 200 mg until arrhythmia is controlled or dose of 600 mg every 4 h is reached		300–700 mg injected over 30 min	200–400 mg every 4 h
Procainamide	0.5–1.0 g	0.5–1.0 g	100 mg every 5 min up to 10 times	500 mg PO every 6 h
Lidocaine			75 mg (1 mg/kg)	20–40 (μg/kg)/min
Phenytoin	250 mg qid		100 mg every 5 min up to 5 times	100 mg PO every 6 h
Propranolol	10–80 mg PO qid or greater for angina 10–40 mg PO qid for arrhythmias		1.0 mg every 5 min up to 3 times for arrhythmias	Same as initial dose for angina
Bretylium		5–10 mg/kg	5–10 mg/kg	5–10 mg/kg IM every 6 h
Glyceryl trinitrate	0.3–0.6 mg sublingually			As needed
Isosorbide dinitrate				2.5–10 mg sublingually or 40 mg PO every 4 h

* *Dosage schedules represent broad ranges and must be modified for individual patients. Initial digitalis doses are total loading doses and should be given in fractional amounts.*

the gastrointestinal tract and may be administered orally. Despite this, oral administration may be of little value because of its almost complete degradation by the liver in some patients. Portions of absorbed nitrite ion may be converted to ammonia, and portions are excreted in the urine, but their metabolic fate is largely unknown.

The most useful of the longer-acting nitrates appears to be sublingual isosorbide dinitrate in doses of 2.5 to 10 mg. When given sublingually or transcutaneously by ointment (2 percent nitroglycerin) in adequate doses, nitrates regularly produce cutaneous flushing and headache; if the patient fails to be relieved of angina but also fails to show any side effects, it is possible that the dose of the drug is not adequate or that tolerance has developed.

ADVERSE EFFECTS These include headache, hypotension, dizziness, and syncope, as well as occasional drug eruptions. In addition, the nitrate ion readily oxidizes hemoglobin to methemoglobin, which may cause severe hypoxia if large enough doses are ingested.

DOSAGE SCHEDULES The approximate dosage schedules for cardioactive drugs are summarized in Table 238-2.

OTHER VASODILATORS

See Chap. 236.

REFERENCES

DANILO P JR et al: Effects of disopyramide on electrophysiologic properties of canine cardiac Purkinje fibers. J Pharmacol Exp Ther 201:701, 1977

FOWLER NO (ed): Digitalis intoxication and electrolyte imbalance, in *Cardiac Diagnosis and Treatment*, 2d ed. Hagerstown, Harper & Row, 1976, chap 49, p 1009

GOLDBERG LI: Newer catecholamines for treatment of heart failure and shock. Prog Cardiovasc Dis 19:327, 1977

GOODMAN LS, GILMAN A (eds): *The Pharmacological Basis of Therapeutics*, 5th ed. New York, Macmillan, 1975, pp 477, 653

HARRISON DC et al: Clinical pharmacology of antiarrhythmic drugs. Prog Cardiovasc Dis 20:217, 1977

HURST JW et al (eds): Pharmacology of cardiovascular drugs, in *The Heart*, 4th ed. New York, McGraw-Hill, 1978, chap 109, p 1942

JEWITT DE: Antiarrhythmic drugs and their mechanisms of actions, in *Modern Trends in Cardiology*, MF Oliver (ed). London, Butterworth, 1975, vol 3, p 333

SMITH TW, BRAUNWALD E: Management of heart failure, in *Heart Disease*, E Braunwald (ed), Philadelphia, Saunders, 1980, chap 16

SONNENBLICK EH et al: Dobutamine: A new synthetic cardioactive catecholamine. N Engl J Med, 1979 (in press)

TARAZI RC: Sympathomimetic agents in the treatment of shock. Ann Intern Med 81:364, 1974

WIT AL et al: Electrophysiology and pharmacology of cardiac arrhythmias. Am Heart J 88:380, 515, 664, 798, 1974; 89:115, 253, 391, 526, 665, 804, 1975; 90:117, 265, 397, 521, 665, 795, 1975

ZAINAL N et al: Oral disopyramide for the prevention of arrhythmias in patients with acute myocardial infarction admitted to open wards. Lancet 2:887, 1977

239
ELECTRICAL REVERSION OF CARDIAC ARRHYTHMIAS

BERNARD LOWN

Ectopic arrhythmias of the heart have generally been controlled by means of drugs. The use of antiarrhythmic drugs presents a number of problems. To reach an effective dose may require a time-consuming biologic titration involving frequent monitoring of the patient's condition. There is a high incidence of mild as well as serious toxic reactions. Furthermore, a number of rhythm disorders are refractory to drugs. A method is needed that is simple in application, restores sinus rhythm consistently, and is free from untoward side effects. These requirements are satisfied by the use of a specific type of electrical discharge across the intact chest.

THEORETICAL BASIS FOR THE USE OF ELECTRICAL DISCHARGE The use of electrical energy for terminating ectopic arrhythmias is based on three propositions:

1 Chronic ventricular and atrial arrhythmias are initiated by a multiplicity of interacting factors, some of which are transient. Once initiated, the abnormal mechanisms are self-sustaining, perhaps because of a continuing passage of recirculating wave fronts of excitation over fixed or variable pathways (circus movement).
2 When an ectopic disorder is momentarily extinguished, the sinus node, which has the highest rhythmicity in the heart, resumes as dominant pacemaker.
3 The heart can be depolarized across the intact chest by electrical discharge. When effective, such depolarization abolishes the ectopic mechanism and permits restoration of sinus rhythm.

If electrical discharge were safe, it would constitute an ideal form of antiarrhythmic therapy. Ventricular fibrillation has been terminated across the intact chest by 60-Hz alternating current (ac) shocks. When this type of electrical discharge is administered to normal animals, it may induce cardiac arrest or ventricular fibrillation. The danger of provoking such serious disruptions in cardiac mechanism has deterred adoption of alternating current for the treatment of arrhythmias.

CARDIOVERSION Capacitor discharge, or direct current (dc) shock, may also be employed to defibrillate the heart. A capacitor can be made to yield a great variety of waveforms, depending on the parameters of the discharge circuit. Incorporating an inductance in the circuit reduces the peak voltage released by a capacitor and lengthens the duration of discharge. A single monophasic pulse resulting from the use of an appropriate capacitor and inductor is more effective in depolarizing the heart, induces fewer arrhythmias and less tissue damage than alternating current, and, furthermore, does not provoke cardiac standstill. The one hazard remaining is the sporadic occurrence of ventricular fibrillation.

When the dc pulse is delivered systematically through the cardiac cycle, ventricular fibrillation occurs only when the discharge is triggered during the final one-third of systole. This vulnerable period appears to be an essential physiologic property of the mammalian heart. It generally has a duration of 30 ms and just precedes the apex of the T wave of the surface electrocardiogram. When a dc discharge is triggered outside this vulnerable period, ventricular fibrillation does not occur.

Thus by employing a capacitor discharge with a specific underdamped pulse and synchronizing the release of this pulse within a safe part of the cardiac cycle, that is, 30 ms after the beginning of the QRS complex, the twin dangers of electricity, namely, ventricular standstill and fibrillation, can be avoided. The use of synchronized capacitor shock has been designated *cardioversion* and is employed for terminating a diversity of ectopic arrhythmias.

TECHNIQUE OF CARDIOVERSION The technique employed is essentially the same irrespective of the type of arrhythmia. Cardioversion can be carried out as an outpatient procedure, although brief hospitalization is preferred. No special area is required. In the treatment of atrial fibrillation or atrial flutter, quinidine in a dose of 0.3 g every 6 h is initiated 24 to 48 h prior to the procedure. The objective is fourfold:

1 To build up an adequate level of drug in the body so that the arrhythmia will not recur soon after reversion
2 To determine whether quinidine is tolerated
3 To obtain a small dividend of reversion which occurs in about 10 percent of patients with chronic atrial fibrillation who are given this dose of quinidine
4 To decrease the occurrence of postcardioversion arrhythmias

Premedication is limited to a sedative drug given about an hour before the procedure. Amnesia is induced by means of small (10 to 15 mg) intravenous doses of diazepam.

The electrical discharge is applied by means of two insulated electrode paddles. These are covered with thick layers of conductive paste. One electrode is placed below the angle of the left scapula, the other is applied over the right parasternal area of the third intercostal space. The instrument is automatically synchronized to deliver the discharge during inscription of the QRS complex. The initial energy setting is 5 to 10 W·s, depending upon the severity of heart disease and uncertainty about the presence of overdigitalization. If reversion is not accomplished with these low-energy discharges, successive shocks are delivered without delay at increasing energies, proceeding to 25, 50, 100, 200, 300, up to 400 W·s. The patient's response consists of a single twitch of thoracic muscle, a slight jerk of the arms, and at times an audible sigh. Normal rhythm is restored instantly; at times a brief episode of nodal rhythm precedes establishment of sinus node dominance.

CLINICAL RESULTS Many thousands of patients have been treated with this method. The good results that have almost always occurred have confirmed theoretic expectations. Cardioversion has been found effective in many ectopic rhythm disorders, whether of ventricular, nodal, or atrial origin. The patient's underlying clinical condition is an important determinant of whether cardioversion will be successful. In those with

FIGURE 239-1
Ventricular tachycardia in a 42-year-old man with acute myocardial infarction. A single cardioversion discharge restores sinus rhythm.

FIGURE 239-2

Restoration of sinus rhythm in a patient with long-standing atrial fibrillation. The isoelectric interval of 1.56 s represents an artifact due to the massive electrical field across the chest. Note the marked slowing in ventricular rate.

acute pulmonary embolism or advanced pulmonary obstructive disease and accompanying severe hypoxia, the atrial arrhythmias are generally impervious to reversion, and if sinus rhythm is restored, it is but of transient duration. Similarly when the patient is actively thyrotoxic, has tight mitral stenosis, or is severely polycythemic, attention to the underlying illness should precede attempts to control the cardiac arrhythmia. However, when the ventricular rate exceeds 180 per minute and there is evident hemodynamic compromise, especially in the elderly or those with ischemic heart disease, cardioversion should not be delayed.

Ventricular tachycardia In the majority of instances, ventricular tachycardia arises in patients with serious organic heart disease; usually, it occurs in the wake of a myocardial infarction. The rapid heart action and aberrant activation of the myocardium seriously compromise cardiac function. This arrhythmia frequently constitutes a dire emergency. Antiarrhythmic drugs may reduce ventricular contractility and peripheral resistance, and thus further impair cardiac function. Cardioversion is devoid of these adverse actions. Restoration of sinus rhythm is immediate (Fig. 239-1). The median energy required for restoring sinus rhythm is 5 W·s, and 10 W·s will abolish ventricular tachycardia in the overwhelming majority. This method is nearly 100 percent effective and constitutes a treatment of choice for ventricular tachycardia when the disorder does not respond to a 50-mg bolus of lidocaine. In the case of the oft-recurring episodes of ventricular tachycardia which accompany acute myocardial infarction, the use of continuous intravenous infusion of lidocaine is the treatment of choice.

Atrial fibrillation This arrhythmia is the most common chronic disorder of the heartbeat. Even when quinidine is given to the point of toxicity, the rhythm of only 50 percent of patients can be restored to sinus rhythm. With cardioversion, atrial fibrillation can be terminated in more than 90 percent of patients. Failures are encountered mainly in patients with mitral valvular disease, with giant left atria, and with continuous arrhythmia for 2 years or longer. A typical example of cardioversion is illustrated in Fig. 239-2. At times, transitional mechanisms are encountered, consisting of nodal rhythm and ectopic atrial beats which generally last for 30 to 60 s, until the sinoatrial node "warms up." Slowing the ventricular rate is one immediate effect of restoration of sinus rhythm; not infrequently first-degree atrioventricular block is present. In patients with congestive heart failure, restoration of sinus rhythm results in an increase in the cardiac output. The patient generally feels improved and comments on the newly sensed "calm" in the chest. Compared with the use of quinidine, cardioversion is a more efficient and safer method. Nevertheless, quinidine continues as an invaluable antiarrhythmic drug for maintenance therapy. Without its use a majority of patients would experience recurrence of atrial fibrillation.

Atrial flutter and other arrhythmias Cardioversion has proved nearly 100 percent effective in chronic atrial flutter. Usually, a single low-energy discharge proves adequate. This method is also applicable to other atrial and atrioventricular nodal ectopic arrhythmias which have not responded to drug therapy.

Complications Immediate complications have been limited to the development of ventricular ectopic beats, ventricular tachycardia, and, rarely, even ventricular fibrillation. Such disorders can nearly always be avoided if the lowest effective amount of energy for reversion is employed, electrolyte deficits are corrected prior to the cardioversion, and treatment of overdigitalized patients is avoided. Furthermore, the electrical discharge should not be released in the presence of artifacts in the electrocardiogram. Such artifacts may trigger the discharge to occur during the vulnerable period, thereby precipitating ventricular fibrillation. It is probable that most, if not all, of the very rare fatalities which have been reported have been due either to neglect of these precautions or to the excessive and, at times, improper use of such drugs as digitalis and quinidine. Transthoracic electrical discharge causes release of skeletal muscle enzymes. When larger energies, in excess of 200 W·s are employed, cardiac injury may be induced, resulting in myocardial uptake of the radionuclide ^{99m}Tc stannous pyrophosphate.

In many patients electrical reversion is only temporarily successful and the arrhythmia soon recurs. It is therefore often necessary to continue the use of the drugs mentioned in Chap. 238. Moderate to large doses of quinidine, procainamide, or disopyramide may be needed. In refractory patients antithyroid substances such as propylthiouracil or radioiodine may at times be a useful supplement to the several antiarrhythmic drugs.

Summary Cardioversion is a simple and direct method for terminating various ectopic cardiac arrhythmias by depolarizing the heart transthoracically by means of a synchronized dc discharge. It is based on physiologic principles and is the most effective and safest means yet devised for restoring a sinus mechanism.

REFERENCES

DORNEY ER: The use of cardioversion and pacemakers in the management of arrhythmias, in *The Heart*, 4th ed, JW Hurst et al (ed). New York, McGraw-Hill, 1978

HORN RH, LOWN B: Cardioversion 1975: Foremost therapy for tachyarrhythmias. Geriatrics 30:75, 1975

RESNEKOV L: Present status of electroversion in management of cardiac dysrhythmias. Circulation 47:1356, 1973

——, MCDONALD L: Electroconversion of lone atrial fibrillation and flutter including haemodynamic studies at rest and on exercise. Br Heart J 33:339, 1971

Specific cardiac diseases

240
CONGENITAL HEART DISEASE

WILLIAM F. FRIEDMAN
EUGENE BRAUNWALD

GENERAL CONSIDERATIONS

INCIDENCE Approximately 9 births in 1000 are complicated by a cardiovascular malformation. If the problem is recognized early, these anomalies can now be diagnosed accurately, and most of these babies may be salvaged by aggressive medical and surgical management.

Children with congenital heart disease usually show an overall male preponderance. Moreover, specific defects may show a definite sex preponderance; patent ductus arteriosus and atrial septal defect are common in females, whereas valvular aortic stenosis, coarctation of the aorta, tetralogy of Fallot, and transposition of the great arteries are more common in males. Table 240-1 demonstrates the frequency of occurrence of specific cardiovascular malformations in clinical and pathologic studies.

ETIOLOGY Congenital cardiovascular malformations are generally the result of aberrant embryonic development of a normal structure or a failure of such a structure to progress beyond an early stage of embryonic development. Malformations appear to result from a complex interaction between multifactorial genetic and environmental systems that does not allow a single specification of etiology; only rarely may a causal factor be identified. Maternal rubella and chronic maternal alcohol abuse are environmental insults that are known to interfere with normal cardiogenesis in man. The *rubella syndrome* consists of cataracts, deafness, microcephaly, and, either singly or in combination, patent ductus arteriosus, pulmonary valvular and/or arterial stenosis, and ventricular septal defect (see Chap. 182). The *fetal alcohol syndrome* consists of microcephaly, micrognathia, microphthalmia, fetal growth retardation, developmental delay, and cardiac septal defects. Hypoxia, deficiency or excess of several vitamins, intake of several categories of drugs, and ionizing irradiation are teratogens that are capable of causing cardiac defects in experimental animals, but their precise relation to human malformations requires further definition.

A single gene mutation may be incriminated in the familial forms of atrial septal defect, mitral valve prolapse, ventricular septal defect, congenital heart block, situs inversus, the combination of supravalvular aortic stenosis and peripheral pulmonary arterial stenosis, idiopathic hypertrophic subaortic stenosis (Chap. 58), and the syndromes of Noonan, Holt-Oram, Ellis–van Creveld, and Kartagener. Table 240-2 provides a partial list of syndromes in which cardiovascular anomalies may be manifestations of the pleiotropic effects of single genes or examples of gross chromosomal defects. Despite the long list presented in Table 240-2, it must be appreciated that recognized chromosomal aberrations and mutations of single genes account for less than 10 percent of all cardiac malformations.

The finding that, with some exceptions, only one of a pair of monozygotic twins is affected by congenital heart disease indicates that the vast majority of cardiovascular malformations are not inherited in a simple manner. Family studies indicate a two- to fivefold increase in the incidence of congenital heart disease in the siblings of affected patients. The malformations are concordant or partially concordant in at least half of such cases. Nonetheless, the incidence of congenital heart disease in the siblings of an index patient is only 2 to 5 percent. With few exceptions, therefore, patients with isolated heart defects have a negative family history for malformations and a normal chromosome pattern, and it is rarely wise to discourage the parents of one affected child from having additional children. The low recurrence rate and the increasing possibilities for effective therapy for nearly all cardiac lesions usually justify a positive approach to family counseling. If, however, two or more members of a family are affected, the recurrence risk may be quite high, and a pedigree should be obtained prior to further counseling. If a dominant or recessive mendelian pattern is established, the mendelian laws apply, and the risk of recurrence in each pregnancy is equal.

PREVENTION The feasibility of preventive programs will depend upon what is learned in the future about the cause of the 90 percent or more of cardiovascular anomalies for which no cause is now known.

An effective rubella vaccine has been developed, and immunization of children with this vaccine may be anticipated to eradicate maternal rubella and its cardiac consequences. Strict testing in animals of new drugs that may be teratogenic when taken early in pregnancy may be expected to reduce the chances of another thalidomide tragedy. In this regard, no medications should be taken during pregnancy without prior consultation with a physician. Physicians dealing with pregnant women should be aware of known teratogens, as well as of drugs for which inadequate information exists relative to their teratogenic potential. Similarly, appropriate use of radiologic equipment and techniques for reducing gonadal and fetal radiation exposure may be expected to reduce the potential hazards of this likely cause of birth defects.

The presence of a cardiac malformation as one component of a multiple system involvement that may exist in Down's, Turner's, and the trisomy 13 to 15 (D_1) and 17 to 18 (E) syn-

TABLE 240-1
Frequency of occurrence of cardiac malformations at birth*

Disease	Percent
Ventricular septal defect	30.5
Atrial septal defect	9.8
Patent ductus arteriosus	9.7
Pulmonary stenosis	6.9
Coarctation of the aorta	6.8
Aortic stenosis	6.1
Tetralogy of Fallot	5.8
Complete transposition of the great arteries	4.2
Persistent truncus arteriosus	2.2
Tricuspid atresia	1.3
All others	16.5

* *2310 cases = 100 percent.*

TABLE 240-2
Syndromes with associated cardiovascular involvement

Syndrome	Major cardiovascular manifestations	Major noncardiac abnormalities
HERITABLE AND POSSIBLY HERITABLE		
Ellis–van Creveld	Single atrium or atrial septal defect	Chondrodystrophic dwarfism, nail dysplasia, polydactyly
TAR (thrombocytopenia-absent radius)	Atrial septal defect, tetralogy of Fallot	Radial aplasia or hypoplasia, thrombocytopenia
Holt-Oram	Atrial septal defect (other defects common)	Skeletal upper limb defect, hypoplasia of clavicles
Kartagener	Dextrocardia	Situs inversus, sinusitis, bronchiectasis
Laurence-Moon-Biedl-Bardot	Variable defects	Retinal pigmentation, obesity, polydactyly
Noonan	Pulmonary valve dysplasia	Webbed neck, pectus excavatum, cryptorchidism
Tuberous sclerosis	Rhabdomyoma, cardiomyopathy	Phacomatosis, bone lesions, hamartomatous skin lesions
Multiple lentigenes syndrome	Pulmonic stenosis	Basal-cell nevi, broad facies, rib anomalies
Rubenstein-Taybi	Patent ductus arteriosus (others)	Broad thumbs and toes, hypoplastic maxilla, slanted palpebral fissures
Familial deafness	Arrhythmias, sudden death	Sensorineural deafness
Friedreich's ataxia	Cardiomyopathy, conduction defects	Ataxia, speech defect, degeneration of spinal cord dorsal columns
Muscular dystrophy	Cardiomyopathy	Pseudohypertrophy of calf muscles, weakness of trunk and proximal limb muscles
Osler-Rendu-Weber	Arteriovenous fistulas (lung, liver, mucous membranes)	Multiple telangiectasia
CONNECTIVE TISSUE DISORDERS		
Cutis laxa	Peripheral pulmonic stenosis	Generalized disruption of elastic fibers, diminished skin resilience, hernias
Ehlers-Danlos	Arterial dilatation and rupture, mitral regurgitation	Hyperextensible joints, hyperelastic and friable skin
Marfan	Aortic dilatation, aortic and mitral incompetence	Gracile habitus, arachnodactyly with hyperextensibility, lens subluxation
Osteogenesis imperfecta	Aortic incompetence	Fragile bones, blue sclera
Pseudoxanthoma elasticum	Peripheral and coronary arterial disease	Degeneration of elastic fibers in skin, retinal angioid streaks
INBORN ERRORS OF METABOLISM		
Pompe's disease	Glycogen storage disease of heart	Acid maltase deficiency, muscular weakness
Homocystinuria	Aortic and pulmonary arterial dilatation, intravascular thrombosis	Cystathionine synthetase deficiency, lens subluxation, osteoporosis
Mucopolysaccharidosis:		
Hurler, Hunter	Multivalvular and coronary and great artery disease, cardiomyopathy	Hurler: Deficiency of α-L-iduronidase, corneal clouding, coarse features, growth and mental retardation Hunter: Deficiency of L-iduranosulfate sulfatase, coarse facies, clear cornea, growth and mental retardation
Morquio, Scheie, Morateaux-Lamy	Aortic incompetence	Morquio: Deficiency of N-acetylhexosamine sulfate sulfatase, cloudy cornea, normal intelligence, severe bony changes involving vertebrae and epiphyses Scheie: Deficiency of α-L-iduronidase, cloudy cornea, normal intelligence, peculiar facies Morateaux-Lamy: Deficiency of arylsulfatase B, cloudy cornea, osseous changes, normal intelligence
CHROMOSOMAL ABNORMALITIES		
Trisomy 21 (Down's syndrome)	Endocardial cushion defect, atrial or ventricular septal defect, tetralogy of Fallot	Hypotonia, hyperextensible joints, mongoloid facies, mental retardation
Trisomy 13 (D)	Ventricular septal defect, double-outlet right ventricle	Single midline intracerebral ventricle with midfacial defects, polydactyly, nail changes, mental retardation
Trisomy 18 (E)	Ventricular septal defect, patent ductus arteriosus, pulmonic stenosis	Clenched hand, short sternum, low-arch dermal-ridge pattern on fingertips, mental retardation
Cri-du-chat (short-arm deletion-5)	Ventricular septal defect	Cat cry, microcephaly, antimongoloid slant of palpebral fissures, mental retardation
XO (Turner)	Coarctation of aorta	Short female, broad chest, lymphedema, webbed neck
XXXY and XXXXX	Patent ductus arteriosus	XXXY: hypogenitalism, mental retardation, radial-ulnar synostosis XXXXX: small hands, incurving of fifth fingers, mental retardation

dromes may be anticipated in occasional pregnancies by the detection of abnormal chromosomes in fetal cells obtained from amniotic fluid. Similarly, identification in such cells of the enzyme disorders observed in Hurler's syndrome, homocystinuria, or type II glycogen storage disease may allow one to predict the ultimate presence of cardiac disease.

THE FETAL AND TRANSITIONAL CIRCULATIONS

The fetal circulation is a single circulation in which the pulmonary vasculature exists in parallel, not in series, with the systemic circulation. Prenatal survival is not endangered by extremely severe cardiac anomalies as long as one side of the heart can drive blood from the great veins to the aorta. Inferior vena caval blood is deflected across the foramen ovale into the left atrium. Most of the blood that reaches the right ventricle bypasses the high-resistance, unexpanded lungs and passes through the ductus arteriosus into the descending aorta. In fetal life, pulmonary arteries and arterioles are surrounded by a fluid medium, have relatively thick walls and small lumens, and resemble comparable arteries in the systemic circulation.

Although fetal somatic growth may be unimpaired, the hemodynamic effects in utero of some cardiac malformations may alter the development and structure of the fetal heart and circulation. Thus, premature closure in utero of the foramen ovale may result in hypoplasia of the left ventricle. Moreover, postnatally the caliber of the aortic isthmus may be reduced in the presence of lesions, such as aortic stenosis with ventricular septal defect, that divert a portion of left ventricular output away from the ascending aorta while increasing right ventricular output and ductus arteriosus flow in utero. Similarly, obstruction in utero to right ventricular outflow is associated with an increase in proximal aortic flow and diameter and almost never with aortic coarctation. In these and other examples it is important to recognize that malformations compatible with fetal survival may nonetheless result in abnormal development of the circulation in utero and also affect circulatory adjustments after birth.

Normally the fundamental change which occurs at birth is the division of this single circulation into two separate circulations operating in series. Inflation of the lungs at the first inspiration produces a marked reduction in pulmonary vascular resistance. Fetal pulmonary vessels, heretofore supported by fluid media, are suddenly suspended in air, reducing extravascular pressure. New vessels are opened, and already patent vessels enlarge. Pulmonary arteriolar vasodilatation results from the increase in oxygen tension to which these vessels are exposed. Pulmonary arterial pressure falls, and pulmonary blood flow increases greatly. The systemic vascular resistance rises when clamping the umbilical cord removes the low-resistance placental circulation. Increased pulmonary blood flow increases the return of blood to the left atrium and raises left atrial pressure, which in turn closes the foramen ovale. The shift in oxygen dependence from the placenta to the lungs produces a sudden increase in arterial blood oxygen tension, which, in concert with alterations in the local prostaglandin milieu, initiates constriction of the ductus arteriosus, and total anatomic closure follows within a few days.

PULMONARY HYPERTENSION Pulmonary hypertension frequently complicates congenital heart disease, and the status of the pulmonary vascular bed may be the principal determinant of the clinical picture, its rate of progression, and whether corrective surgical treatment is feasible. Elevation of pulmonary arterial pressure results from elevation of pulmonary blood flow and/or resistance, the latter often reflecting structural alterations in the pulmonary vascular bed. Normally, following the fall in the pulmonary arterial pressure, resistance, and vasomotor tone which occurs shortly after birth, there is a gradual postnatal reduction in the thickness of the media of the pulmonary arterioles and widening of the lumens. Hence, the pulmonary circulation of the normal adult has evolved from a high-pressure, high-resistance, highly reactive vascular bed with relatively small cross-sectional area, to a low-pressure, low-resistance, less reactive bed with a large cross-sectional area.

As in the other vascular beds, the pressure in the pulmonary artery is determined by the product of the volume of blood flow, per unit of time, and the resistance to that flow. Equalization of pressures in the systemic and pulmonary circulations may be expected if a large communication exists between the two great arteries or between the two ventricles in the absence of semilunar valve obstruction. Pulmonary vascular resistance is calculated as the transpulmonary pressure difference per unit of pulmonary blood flow (Chap. 234). When blood flow increases, existing patent vessels are distended and additional vessels are opened, so that calculated vascular resistance diminishes. Therefore, in a normal pulmonary vascular bed, pressure will rise substantially only if flow is very greatly increased. In the vast majority of patients with congenital heart disease and elevated pulmonary vascular resistance, the pulmonary arterioles are the principal locus of this abnormal resistance.

A delay in the normal involution of the pulmonary vascular bed often occurs postnatally in the presence of an intra- or extracardiac communication with a large left-to-right shunt. In patients having high pulmonary arterial pressure from birth, anatomic changes in the pulmonary vessels, in the form of medial thickening and intimal proliferation, usually progress so that in the older child or adult the vascular resistance may ultimately be fixed by obliterative changes in the pulmonary vascular bed. However, if pulmonary arterial hypertension is not present in infancy or childhood, it may never occur or may not develop until the third or fourth decade, or even later.

Because pulmonary vascular obstructive disease may be the factor limiting a decision concerning the advisability of operation, it is important to quantify and compare pulmonary to systemic flows and resistances in patients with severe pulmonary hypertension. Furthermore, the lability of the pulmonary vascular resistance should be evaluated; a marked reduction with the infusion of acetylcholine or tolazoline or the inhalation of oxygen suggests that resistance is not fixed and may fall after successful operation. Some defects between the left and right sides of the heart should be closed in order to eliminate a sizable left-to-right shunt, which, in turn, may result in a significant drop in pulmonary arterial pressure because of reduction of pulmonary blood flow. Conversely, little or no benefit and high mortality rates may be expected from the closure of defects that are associated with bidirectional or predominant right-to-left shunts in patients with high-resistance and obstructive pulmonary hypertension. The designation *Eisenmenger's reaction* is applied to this condition in patients who may have a large communication between the two circulations at the aortopulmonary, ventricular, or atrial levels. The actual mechanism for the persistence, delayed reduction, or late onset of elevated pulmonary vascular resistance is not known.

The clinical manifestations of the hyperkinetic form of pulmonary hypertension, i.e., that associated with a large left-to-right shunt, reflect the specific malformation responsible. When a significant right-to-left shunt exists, the patient is cyanotic, and polycythemia and clubbing of the digits may be noted (Chap. 28). A dominant *a* wave in the jugular venous pulse may be seen, reflecting vigorous right atrial contraction due to diminished compliance of the right ventricle; in some instances there are large systolic *c-v* waves, which suggest tricuspid regurgitation. A prominent right ventricular parasternal lift and palpable systolic expansion of the pulmonary artery are present. On auscultation, one often hears a soft pulmonary systolic ejection murmur following a loud ejection sound, marked accentuation of the pulmonic component of the second heart sound, and often, a fourth heart sound. The decrescendo diastolic murmur of pulmonary valvular regurgitation may be heard. The electrocardiogram shows right ventricular hypertrophy. Roentgenologic examination reveals enlargement of the right ventricle, a conspicuously enlarged pulmonary artery, prominent hilar pulmonary vascular markings, and attenuated peripheral vessels. The site of the underlying defect may be localized by means of cardiac catheterization and angiocardiography (Chap. 234). Pressures in the right side of the heart are essentially identical to systemic pressures in cyanotic patients if the shunt is at the ventricular or aortopulmonary levels, but they are usually lower than systemic pressure in patients with an interatrial shunt. No specific treatment has proved beneficial for obstructive pulmonary vascular disease.

CIRCULATORY SHUNTS

Although equal quantities of blood flow through the pulmonary and systemic circulations in normal subjects postnatally, systemic circulation has a flow resistance approximately six times that of the pulmonary circuit, which is reflected in the markedly higher arterial and ventricular systolic pressures in the systemic circulation; the lower compliance of the thicker left ventricle is reflected in higher ventricular end-diastolic and mean atrial pressures on the left side of the heart. Therefore, if an abnormal communication is present, blood will flow from the left to the right side of the heart. The size of the opening and the pressures on either side of it generally determine the direction and magnitude of the shunt flow. A right-to-left shunt usually requires either an obstructive lesion at some point in the right-sided circulation (i.e., tricuspid stenosis or atresia, pulmonary valvular or infundibular stenosis, elevated pulmonary vascular resistance), a mixing of systemic venous and arterialized blood (i.e., total anomalous pulmonary venous drainage, a single atrium or ventricle, or a persistent truncus arteriosus), or some form of obligatory recirculation of systemic venous blood (e.g., transposition of the great arteries). The location, direction, and magnitude of the right-to-left shunt may be determined during hemodynamic study by measuring the admixture of venous and arterial blood at various sites in the central circulation, by indicator-dilution curves, and by angiocardiography, as outlined in Chap. 234.

CLINICAL MANIFESTATIONS OF RIGHT-TO-LEFT SHUNTS
Cyanosis and polycythemia These signs are discussed in Chap. 28.

Clubbing A prominent accompaniment of arterial hypoxemia consists of a widening and thickening of the terminal phalanges of the fingers and toes, accompanied by convex nails. These digits have an increased number of capillaries with increased blood flow through extensive arteriovenous aneurysms, and an increase of connective tissue.

Hypoxic spells and squatting A sudden marked increase in cyanosis due to an abrupt reduction in pulmonary blood flow occurs in younger children with certain types of cyanotic heart disease, particularly tetralogy of Fallot. The spells may lead to convulsions and may even be fatal; they may be precipitated by fluctuations in intravascular volume or in arterial P_{CO_2} and pH, a sudden fall in systemic or increase in pulmonary vascular resistance, or an acute increase in the severity of right ventricular outflow tract obstruction, either by augmented contraction of the hypertrophied muscle in the right ventricular outflow tract or by a decrease in right ventricular cavity volume due to tachycardia. Treatment consists of oxygen administration, placing the child in the knee-chest position, and intravenous administration of fluids and of sodium bicarbonate to correct the accompanying acidosis. Additional medications that may prove of value include morphine, alpha-adrenergic receptor stimulants such as phenylephrine to raise peripheral resistance and to diminish right-to-left shunting, and beta-adrenergic blocking agents, which may increase ventricular volume by reducing heart rate and lessen infundibular obstruction by reducing contractility.

Patients with cyanotic heart disease, especially tetralogy of Fallot, typically assume a squatting posture after exertion to obtain relief from breathlessness. Squatting appears to hasten an increase in the arterial oxygen saturation by increasing systemic vascular resistance and thereby diminishing the right-to-left shunt and by trapping markedly unsaturated blood in the legs. Also, systemic venous return and therefore pulmonary blood flow may rise.

"Paradoxic" embolus and brain abscess In patients with cyanotic congenital heart disease, venous blood bypasses the normal filtering action of the lungs, and emboli arising in systemic veins may pass directly to the systemic circulation. Patients with severe cyanosis or polycythemia have often had previous occlusive microcirculatory damage to the central nervous system. These predisposing factors are primarily responsible for the relatively high incidence (2 to 4 percent) of brain abscess in such patients.

Impaired growth Physical underdevelopment and a delayed onset of adolescence are common features of many types of cyanotic and, to a lesser extent, acyanotic forms of congenital heart disease. Mental development is rarely affected. Various explanations for the mechanisms of growth interference have implicated malnutrition, tissue anoxia, diminished peripheral blood flow, hypermetabolic state, chronic cardiac decompensation, genetic and endocrine factors, and frequency of upper and lower respiratory infections.

SPECIFIC CARDIAC DEFECTS

Various classifications of congenital cardiovascular lesions have been proposed, depending on hemodynamic, anatomic, and radiographic factors. Although there is overlapping between groups, the following arrangement of the more common anomalies is used in this chapter:

1 Communications between the systemic and pulmonary circulation without cyanosis (left-to-right shunts)
2 Obstructing valvular and vascular lesions with or without associated right-to-left shunts
3 Abnormalities in the origins of the great arteries and veins; the transpositions
4 Malpositions of the heart

COMMUNICATIONS BETWEEN SYSTEMIC AND PULMONARY CIRCULATION WITHOUT CYANOSIS (LEFT-TO-RIGHT SHUNTS)
Atrial septal defect Atrial septal defect, the most commonly recognized congenital cardiac anomaly in adults,

occurs more frequently in females than in males. Defects of the *sinus venosus* type occur high in the atrial septum, near the entry of the superior vena cava, and are associated frequently with anomalous connection of pulmonary veins from the right lung to the junction of the superior vena cava and right atrium. Most often, an atrial defect involves the fossa ovalis, is midseptal in location, and is of the *ostium secundum* type. This type of defect should not be confused with a patent foramen ovale. Anatomic obliteration of the foramen ovale ordinarily follows its functional closure soon after birth, but residual "probe patency" is a common normal variation; atrial septal defect denotes a true deficiency of the atrial septum and implies functional as well as anatomic patency. *Ostium primum* anomalies are a form of endocardial cushion defect that lie immediately adjacent to the atrioventricular valves, either of which may be deformed and incompetent, or which may form together a common atrioventricular valve; this defect may also involve the basal portion of the interventricular septum. *Ostium primum defects* occur commonly in patients with *Down's syndrome* (mongolism), although the more complex endocardial cushion anomalies are more characteristic. *Lutembacher's syndrome* is the designation applied to the rare combination of atrial septal defect and mitral stenosis; this component of the malformation almost invariably is the result of acquired rheumatic valvulitis.

The magnitude of the left-to-right shunt through an atrial septal defect depends on the size of the defect, the relative compliance of the ventricles, and the relative resistances in the pulmonary and systemic circulations. The left-to-right shunt causes diastolic overloading of the right ventricle and increased pulmonary blood flow. The pulmonary vascular resistance is usually normal or low in the child and young adult with atrial septal defect, and the volume load is usually well tolerated even though pulmonary blood flow may be three to six times greater than systemic.

Patients with atrial septal defect are usually asymptomatic in early life although there may be some physical underdevelopment and respiratory infections; cardiorespiratory symptoms occur in many of the older patients. Beyond the fourth decade, a significant number of patients develop atrial arrhythmias, pulmonary arterial hypertension, bidirectional and then right-to-left shunting of blood, and cardiac failure. Patients exposed to the chronic environmental hypoxia of high altitude tend to develop pulmonary hypertension at younger ages. Historical features suggesting that the defect is of the endocardial cushion variety include the onset of disability, pulmonary hypertension, and heart failure in infancy or childhood.

Physical examination usually reveals a prominent right ventricular cardiac impulse and palpable pulmonary artery pulsation. The first heart sound is normal or split, with accentuation of the tricuspid valve closure sound. Increased flow across the pulmonic valve is responsible for a midsystolic pulmonary ejection murmur. The second sound is widely split and is relatively fixed in relation to respiration, because of reciprocal changes in the magnitude of the left-to-right shunt and of the systemic venous inflow into the right ventricle during respiration, so that filling of the right ventricle remains constant throughout the respiratory cycle. A middiastolic rumbling murmur at the fourth intercostal space and along the left sternal border reflects increased flow across the tricuspid valve. In patients with ostium primum defects, an apical thrill and holosystolic murmur indicate associated mitral or tricuspid incompetence or a ventricular septal defect.

The *physical findings* are altered when an increase in the pulmonary vascular resistance results in diminution of the left-to-right shunt. Both the pulmonary and tricuspid murmurs decrease in intensity, the pulmonic component of the second heart sound and a systolic ejection sound are accentuated, the

two components of the second heart sound may fuse, and a diastolic murmur of pulmonic incompetence appears. Cyanosis and clubbing accompany the development of a right-to-left shunt.

The *electrocardiagram* in patients with an ostium secundum defect usually shows right axis deviation, right ventricular hypertrophy, and a right intraventricular conduction defect. A coronary sinus pacemaker or first-degree heart block is occasionally noted in patients with defects of the sinus venosus type. In patients with an ostium primum defect, the right ventricular conduction defect is characteristically accompanied by left axis deviation and by superior orientation and counterclockwise rotation of the QRS loop in the frontal plane. Varying degrees of right ventricular and right atrial hypertrophy may be seen with each type of defect, depending on the height of the pulmonary artery pressure; prolongation of the PR interval is most common with defects of the ostium primum variety. Chest roentgenograms reveal enlargement of the right atrium and ventricle, dilatation of the pulmonary artery and its branches, and increased pulmonary vascular markings. Left atrial enlargement is extremely uncommon. Echocardiographic features include pulmonary arterial and right ventricular dilatation and anterior systolic (paradoxical) or "flat" interventricular septal motion if significant right ventricular volume overload is present. Prolapse of the posterior mitral leaflet has been recognized with increasing frequency in association with secundum defects. Abnormal "mitral" motion and septalatrioventricular valve relationships are typically observed in endocardial cushion anomalies.

The diagnosis may be confirmed readily at cardiac catheterization by passage of the catheter across the atrial defect. The site at which the catheter crosses, if high in the cardiac silhouette, may suggest a sinus venosus defect, or, if low, a primum defect. Serial determinations of the oxygen saturation, or indicator-dilution curve techniques, may be used to estimate the magnitude of the shunt. In young patients, pressures in the right side of the heart are often normal despite a large shunt; pulmonary arterial hypertension occurs with greater frequency in the older patients. If an endocardial cushion defect is present, a left ventricular angiogram will frequently demonstrate a "gooseneck" deformity of the left ventricular outflow tract caused by an abnormal anterior mitral valve leaflet; it may also show mitral regurgitation. When a high oxygen saturation is found in the superior vena cava, or when the catheter enters pulmonary veins directly from the right atrium, a sinus venosus defect is likely, and indicator-dilution curves and selective angiography will aid in identifying the number and location of the anomalous veins. *Partial anomalous pulmonary venous connection*, although generally associated with a sinus venosus defect, may occasionally accompany primum and secundum defects, or be unassociated with any defect of the interatrial septum.

Endocardial cushion anomalies more complex than the ostium primum defect are associated with high morbidity and mortality rates in infancy and childhood. Patients with atrial septal defect of the sinus venosus or secundum types rarely die before the fifth decade. During the fifth and sixth decades, the incidence of progressive symptoms, often leading to severe disability, increases substantially. Medical management should include prompt treatment of respiratory tract infections, antiarrhythmic medications for atrial fibrillation or supraventricular tachycardia, and the usual measures for heart failure (Chap. 236) if these complications occur. Although the risk of subacute bacterial endocarditis is low, antibiotics should be administered prophylactically prior to dental procedures (see Chap. 243).

Operative repair, ideally in patients between 3 and 6 years of age, should be advised for all patients with uncomplicated atrial septal defects in whom there is evidence of significant left-to-right shunting, i.e., with pulmonary-to-systemic flow ratios exceeding approximately 1.5:1.0. Excellent results may be anticipated, at low risk, even in patients beyond 40 years of age in the absence of pulmonary hypertension. The defect is closed by suture or with a patch of prosthetic material with the patient on cardiopulmonary bypass. Special attention must be given to the atrioventricular valves in patients with endocardial cushion defects; cleft, deformed, and incompetent valves may require repair or replacement to prevent significant regurgitation and failure in the postoperative period. The operative risk and the incidence of such complications as complete heart block and the persistence of significant mitral regurgitation are significantly higher in patients with endocardial cushion defects. Electrophysiologic mapping of the course of the conduction system during operation may substantially reduce the risk of postsurgical heart block. Operation should not be carried out in patients with small defects and trivial left-to-right shunts, or in those with severe pulmonary vascular disease without a significant left-to-right shunt.

Ventricular septal defect Isolated defects of the ventricular septum are among the commonest cardiac malformations, and they are encountered as one component of a combination of anomalies more often than any other. Most frequently, the opening is single and situated in the membranous portion of the septum. The functional disturbance caused by a ventricular septal defect is dependent primarily on its size and the status of the pulmonary vascular bed, rather than on the location of the defect. A substantial left-to-right ventricular pressure gradient occurs in the presence of a small defect (*maladie de Roger*), and a small shunt, limited by the size of the defect, occurs throughout systole. Larger defects offer less resistance to flow, while in the presence of very large defects both ventricles will function hemodynamically as a single pumping chamber with two outlets, equalizing the pressures in the systemic and pulmonary circulations. In such patients, the magnitude of the left-to-right shunt varies inversely with the ratio of pulmonary-to-systemic vascular resistance. In patients with large defects and large left-to-right shunts, the left ventricle is overloaded and may fail. Survival through infancy in many of these patients is predicated on delayed regression of the fetal pulmonary vascular pattern, the development of an elevated pulmonary vascular resistance, or the secondary development of infundibular hypertrophy and obstruction to right ventricular outflow. Irreversible obliterative changes in the pulmonary vessels with dominant right-to-left shunts and cyanosis become manifest in many patients with large defects after the second decade of life. Spontaneous closure of small and even large ventricular defects occurs in a significant number of patients, especially before the age of 3 years. In some others, the relative size of the interventricular communication may diminish as normal growth of the heart occurs with advancing age. Rarely, incompetence of the aortic valve resulting from insufficient cusp tissue or prolapse of a cusp through the interventricular defect complicates and dominates the clinical course of patients with ventricular septal defect.

The clinical picture varies greatly, depending on the patient's age, the size of the defect, and the level of the pulmonary vascular resistance. Patients with small defects are generally asymptomatic; moderate left-to-right shunts may be associated with effort intolerance and fatigue. Large defects are commonly accompanied by frequent pulmonary infections,

growth retardation, and cardiac failure in infancy, but survival past this period is often associated with an amelioration of symptoms until adulthood. In patients with severe pulmonary vascular obstruction, symptoms develop most often in adult life and consist of exertional dyspnea, chest pain, syncope, and hemoptysis. The right-to-left shunt leads to cyanosis, clubbing, and polycythemia.

Patients with moderate-sized defects exhibit cardiomegaly with a forceful left ventricular impulse and a prominent systolic thrill along the lower left sternal border. The second heart sound is normally or closely split, with moderate accentuation of the pulmonic component; a third heart sound and diastolic rumbling murmur, reflecting increased flow across the mitral valve during rapid ventricular filling, are often audible at the cardiac apex. The characteristic holosystolic murmur results from flow across the defect; it is best heard along the third and fourth interspaces to the left of the sternum, and is widely transmitted over the precordium. A basal midsystolic ejection murmur may also be heard, because of increased flow across the pulmonic valve. In patients with pulmonary vascular obstruction and small left-to-right shunts, both the systolic thrill and murmur decrease in intensity and duration and may disappear entirely, to be replaced by a marked right ventricular precordial lift, pulmonary ejection sound and soft systolic ejection murmur, a closely split second heart sound with accentuation of the pulmonic component, and the diastolic murmur of pulmonic incompetence.

The electrocardiographic pattern, the relative size and contour of the two ventricles roentgenographically, and the appearance of the lung fields serve as indicators of the underlying pathophysiologic condition. The electrocardiogram is generally normal in patients with small defects. Left or combined ventricular hypertrophy is seen with large left-to-right shunts; right ventricular hypertrophy occurs with pulmonary vascular obstruction. The roentgenograms may be normal in patients with small defects; large defects are characterized by an enlarged left atrium, biventricular hypertrophy, a prominent pulmonary artery segment, and increased pulmonary vascular markings. Relative diminution and attenuation of the peripheral pulmonary vasculature occur in patients with obstructive pulmonary vascular disease.

In approximately 90 percent of patients with this malformation, the defect occurs in the membranous septum. A shunt from the left ventricle to the right atrium may occur with a defect in the most superior portion of the ventricular septum, since the tricuspid valve is lower than the mitral valve. The clinical, electrocardiographic, and radiologic findings in these patients often do not differ appreciably from those with a simple ventricular septal defect, although right atrial enlargement and evidence of right ventricular volume overload may be present; the diagnosis can be established by left ventriculography. Prolapse of an aortic valve leaflet through a subpulmonary ventricular defect or the combination of subcristal ventricular septal defect and underdevelopment of an aortic valve commissure may produce aortic regurgitation that is frequently progressive and is the most significant hemodynamic lesion. In these patients complete operative repair may necessitate insertion of a prosthetic aortic valve.

The pathophysiology of a single or common ventricle resembles that of a large ventricular septal defect, although the two lesions are dissimilar embryologically. There is an obligatory admixture of systemic and pulmonary venous return in patients with a single ventricle, but there is occasionally little or no cyanosis if selective streaming and increased pulmonary blood flow occur. Severe pulmonary hypertension is invariably present unless pulmonic stenosis coexists. It is imperative to differentiate a large ventricular septal defect from a single ventricle by echocardiography and angiography, because attempts at corrective operation for single ventricles have met with little success.

The risk of bacterial endocarditis is higher in patients with small or moderate-sized defects than in those with large ones, but appropriate prophylaxis is essential in all. In the small infant with a large left-to-right shunt, congestive failure may be severe and intractable despite intensive medical management; this problem is managed best by primary closure of the defect. Operation is indicated in children and adults when there is a moderate or large left-to-right shunt with a pulmonary to systemic flow ratio which exceeds 1.5:1.0 or 2.0:1.0 regardless of the level of pulmonary artery pressure. Operation is contraindicated in patients with small defects and left-to-right shunts and in patients in whom the pulmonary vascular resistance is elevated to a level which eliminates the net left-to-right shunt and carries an increased risk whenever pulmonary resistance is significantly elevated.

Patent ductus arteriosus The ductus arteriosus is a vessel leading from the bifurcation of the pulmonary artery to the aorta just distal to the left subclavian artery. Normal closure of the ductus immediately after birth may be due to the sudden increase in arterial oxygen tension that accompanies ventilation and abrupt alterations in the disposition of vasoactive substances, particularly prostaglandins. Intimal proliferation and fibrosis proceed more gradually, so that total anatomic obliteration may not occur for several months after birth. Persistent patency of the ductus after birth is a relatively common anomaly, occurring more frequently in females, in the offspring of women whose pregnancies were complicated by first-trimester rubella, in premature infants, and in children born at high altitudes. A distinction should be made between patency of the ductus arteriosus in the preterm infant who lacks the normal mechanisms for postnatal ductal closure because of immaturity and the full-term newborn in whom patency of the ductus is a true congenital malformation related, most likely, to a primary anatomic defect of the elastic tissue within the wall of the vessel. Although the latter anomaly occurs most frequently in the isolated form, it may coexist with other malformations, particularly coarctation of the aorta, ventricular septal defect, pulmonic stenosis, and aortic stenosis. Patency of the ductus may provide the only route for maintaining pulmonary or systemic blood flow in the presence of such lesions as pulmonary atresia or aortic arch interruption.

The flow across the ductus is determined by the pressure and resistance relationships between the systemic and the pulmonary circulations, and by the cross-sectional area and length of the ductus itself. Most commonly, pulmonary pressures are normal, and a gradient and shunt from aorta to pulmonary artery persists throughout the cardiac cycle. Physical examination reveals a characteristic thrill and a continuous "machinery" murmur, with a late systolic accentuation at the upper left sternal border. The left atrium and ventricle enlarge to accommodate the increased pulmonary venous return, and flow murmurs across the mitral and aortic valves may be detected. With large or moderate-sized left-to-right shunts, the runoff of blood through the ductus causes a widened systemic pulse pressure and bounding peripheral pulses. The hemodynamic abnormality is reflected by left ventricular and, occasionally, left atrial hypertrophy on the electrocardiogram and by left atrial and ventricular enlargement, a prominent ascending aorta and pulmonary artery, and pulmonary vascular engorgement on the chest roentgenogram. Left atrial and ventricular size determined echocardiographically provide an estimate of the magnitude of left-to-right shunting.

The clinical recognition of patent ductus arteriosus may be difficult in infancy and in patients with pulmonary hypertension or heart failure. In these circumstances, the pressure gradient between the aorta and pulmonary artery is reduced or absent, as is the typical continuous murmur, and there may be only a systolic ejection murmur at the base, a diastolic blowing murmur of pulmonary regurgitation (Graham Steell), or no murmur audible at all. When severe pulmonary vascular disease results in reversal of flow through the ductus, unoxygenated blood is shunted to the descending aorta, and the toes, but not the fingers, become cyanotic and clubbed, a finding termed *differential cyanosis.*

Delayed spontaneous closure of the ductus arteriosus occurs in premature babies, even if heart failure was a problem in the neonatal period. The preterm infant lacks the normal mechanisms for postnatal ductal closure because of immaturity. This situation may be contrasted to the full-term infant in whom patency of the ductus arteriosus is a true congenital malformation related, most likely, to an elastic tissue defect within the wall of the vessel. Although a large ductus often results in cardiac failure and pulmonary edema in the premature infant, its occurrence in the full-term baby is often compatible with survival until adult life. The symptomatic preterm infant may be managed either by pharmacologic inhibition of prostaglandin synthesis with indomethacin to constrict and close the ductus or by surgical ligation. The leading causes of death in adults with patent ductus are cardiac failure and bacterial endocarditis. In older patients, severe pulmonary vascular obstruction may cause aneurysmal dilatation, calcification, and rupture of the ductus.

In the absence of severe pulmonary vascular disease with predominant right-to-left shunting of blood, the simple presence of a patent ductus is generally considered a sufficient indication for operation, at least in patients over 3 years of age. Ligation or division of the ductus is associated with a low risk (under 2 percent) when it is performed electively in an otherwise healthy person. The operative risk is reduced if cardiac failure can be treated successfully before operation. Operation should be deferred for several months in patients treated successfully for bacterial endarteritis, because the ductus may remain somewhat edematous and friable.

Aortopulmonary septal defect Aortopulmonary window, partial truncus arteriosis, and aortic septal defect are other designations applied to this relatively uncommon anomaly, which consists of a communication between the aorta and the pulmonary artery just above the semilunar valves. Such defects are usually large and are accompanied by varying degrees of obstructive pulmonary vascular disease and severe pulmonary arterial hypertension. The anomaly may be difficult to distinguish from patent ductus arteriosus with which it is often associated. Its presence should be suspected whenever a large shunt into the pulmonary artery is demonstrated at catheterization. Distinction from patent ductus and persistent truncus arteriosus is facilitated by catheter passage across the defect and selective angiocardiography, with the injection of contrast material into the left ventricle and/or the root of the aorta. Operative correction is usually indicated in patients with large left-to-right shunts; total cardiopulmonary bypass is required, and the defect is closed, generally with a prosthetic patch.

Aortic sinus aneurysm and fistula Congenital aneurysm of an aortic sinus of Valsalva, particularly the right coronary sinus, is an uncommon anomaly with a predilection for males; it consists of a separation, or lack of fusion, between the media of the aorta and the annulus fibrosus of the aortic valve. Progressive aneurysmal dilatation of the weakened area develops but may not be recognized until the third or fourth decade of life, when rupture into a cardiac chamber occurs. The receiving chamber of the aorticocardiac fistula is usually the right ventricle, but occasionally the fistula drains into the right atrium.

The unruptured aneurysm generally does not produce symptoms or a hemodynamic abnormality. Rupture is often of abrupt onset, causes chest pain, and creates continuous arteriovenous shunting and volume overloading of both right and left heart chambers, with resultant heart failure. Bacterial endocarditis may originate either on the edges of the aneurysm or on the jet lesions in the right side of the heart. This anomaly should be suspected in a patient with a history of recent onset of chest pain, symptoms of diminished cardiac reserve, bounding pulses, and a loud, superficial, continuous murmur accentuated in diastole when the fistula opens into the right ventricle, as well as a thrill along the right or left lower parasternal area. The diagnosis may be established definitively by retrograde thoracic aortography. Operation is indicated in patients with large left-to-right shunts.

Coronary arteriovenous fistula Coronary arteriovenous fistula is an unusual anomaly that most often consists of a communication between the right coronary artery and the right atrium or ventricle. The shunt is usually of small magnitude, and myocardial blood flow is not usually compromised. Potential complications include bacterial endocarditis, thrombus formation with occlusion or distal embolization, rupture of an aneurysmal fistula, and rarely, pulmonary hypertension and congestive failure. The finding of a loud, superficial, continuous murmur at the lower or midsternal border usually prompts a further evaluation of asymptomatic patients. Retrograde thoracic aortography or coronary arteriography permits identification of the size and anatomic features of the fistulous tract, which may be closed by suture obliteration.

Anomalous pulmonary origin of coronary artery In this rare malformation, the left coronary artery originates from the pulmonary artery. As the elevated pulmonary vascular resistance declines immediately after birth, perfusion of the left coronary artery from the pulmonary artery ceases and the direction of flow in the anomalous vessel reverses. Thus, blood flows from the aorta to the right coronary artery, then through collateral channels to the left coronary artery, and finally to the pulmonary artery. Total myocardial perfusion must pass through the right coronary artery and may be sufficient for normal activity if adequate collateral channels develop between the two coronary circulations. Myocardial infarction and fibrosis commonly develop during the first 6 months of life, leading to death within the first year. From 10 to 20 percent of patients survive to childhood or adolescence without surgical correction. Occasionally, in older children or adults one may find an example of mitral regurgitation which results from dysfunction of ischemic or infarcted papillary muscles. In some instances the coronary anomaly is unsuspected until a previously well adolescent or adult experiences angina, heart failure, or sudden death.

The diagnosis of anomalous origin of the coronary artery is supported by the electrocardiographic findings of an anterolateral myocardial infarction. Chest roentgenograms show moderate to severe enlargement of the left atrium and ventricle. Aortic root or coronary angiography demonstrates the retrograde drainage of the coronary vessel into the pulmonary artery and the presence of a single right coronary artery arising from the aorta.

Ideal operative management of these patients consists of anastomosis of the left coronary artery to the subclavian artery or to the aorta via a graft. The outcome of operation and ultimate prognosis are influenced significantly by the degree of myocardial damage suffered preoperatively.

Persistent truncus arteriosus Persistent truncus arteriosus is a rare but serious anomaly in which a single vessel forms the outlet of both ventricles and gives rise to the systemic, pulmonary, and coronary arteries. It is always accompanied by a ventricular septal defect. The designation "pseudotruncus arteriosus" refers to the condition in which a single vessel arises from the heart but is accompanied by a remnant of atretic pulmonary artery; pseudotruncus arteriosus does not differ from tetralogy of Fallot with pulmonary atresia (see below). In truncus arteriosus pulmonary flow is governed by the size of the pulmonary arteries and the pulmonary vascular resistance. Most often, mild cyanosis coexists with the cardiac findings of a large left-to-right shunt. The most frequent physical findings include cardiomegaly, a systolic ejection sound, a loud, single second heart sound, a harsh systolic murmur accompanied by a thrill, an early diastolic blowing murmur of truncal valve regurgitation, and a low-pitched middiastolic rumbling murmur. The diagnosis should be suspected at catheterization if the catheter fails to enter the central pulmonary arteries from the right ventricle despite evidence of increased pulmonary blood flow; aortography is the diagnostic procedure of choice.

The early fatal course and, in patients surviving infancy, the development of pulmonary vascular obstructive disease are responsible for the poor prognosis associated with persistent truncus arteriosus. Corrective operation employs a prosthetic tubular conduit incorporating a heterograft aortic valve to construct a pulmonary trunk. In infants palliative banding of one or both of the pulmonary arteries may be indicated when pulmonary flow is markedly excessive.

VALVULAR AND VASCULAR LESIONS WITH OR WITHOUT RIGHT-TO-LEFT SHUNT **Pulmonary stenosis with intact ventricular septum** Obstruction to right ventricular outflow is relatively common; it may be localized to the supravalvular, valvular, or subvalvular levels or occur at a combination of these sites. Multiple sites of narrowing of the peripheral pulmonary arteries are often a feature of rubella embryopathy and may be associated with both the familial and sporadic forms of supravalvular aortic stenosis. Valvular pulmonic stenosis is the most common form of isolated right ventricular obstruction.

The severity of the obstructing lesion, rather than the site of narrowing, is the most important determinant of the clinical course. In the presence of a normal cardiac output, a peak systolic transvalvular pressure gradient between 50 and 80 mmHg is considered to be moderate stenosis; levels below and above that range are classified as mild and severe, respectively. Patients with mild pulmonic stenosis are generally asymptomatic and demonstrate little or no progression in the severity of obstruction as they grow older. In patients with more significant stenosis, the severity of the obstruction may increase with time. Atresia of the pulmonary valve is commonly associated with a hypoplastic right ventricle and interatrial communications. Symptoms vary according to the degree of obstruction. Infants with pulmonary atresia often die from hypoxia. Fatigue, dyspnea, right ventricular failure, and syncope may limit the activity of older patients, in whom moderate or severe obstruction may prevent an augmentation of pulmonary blood flow with exercise.

In patients with severe obstruction, the systolic pressure in the right ventricle may exceed that in the left ventricle, since the ventricular septum is intact. Right ventricular ejection is prolonged in patients with moderate or severe stenosis, and the sound of pulmonary valve closure is delayed and soft. Right ventricular hypertrophy reduces the compliance of that chamber, and a forceful right atrial contraction is necessary to augment right ventricular filling. A fourth heart sound, prominent *a* waves in the jugular venous pulse, and occasionally, presystolic pulsations of the liver reflect the vigorous atrial contraction. The clinical diagnosis is further supported by the presence of a right parasternal lift and harsh systolic ejection murmur and thrill at the upper left sternal border, typically preceded by a systolic ejection sound if the obstruction is valvular. The systolic murmur becomes louder, and its crescendo occurs later in systole, with more severe degrees of valvular obstruction resulting in a greater prolongation of right ventricular systole. The holosystolic decrescendo murmur of tricuspid regurgitation may accompany severe pulmonic stenosis, especially in the presence of congestive heart failure. Cyanosis usually reflects venoarterial shunting through a patent foramen ovale or atrial septal defect. In patients with supravalvular or peripheral pulmonary arterial stenosis, the murmur is systolic or continuous and is best heard over the area of narrowing, with radiation to the peripheral lung fields.

The electrocardiogram may be helpful in assessing the degree of obstruction to right ventricular output. In mild cases, the electrocardiogram is often normal, whereas moderate and severe stenoses are associated with right axis deviation and right ventricular hypertrophy. A ventricular strain pattern, as well as high-amplitude P waves in leads II and V_1, indicating right atrial enlargement, is associated with severe stenosis. The chest roentgenogram in patients with mild or moderate pulmonic stenosis often shows a heart of normal size and normal vascularity of the lungs. In the presence of valvular stenosis, poststenotic dilatation of the main and left pulmonary arteries may be evident. In patients with severe obstruction and resultant right ventricular failure, right atrial and right ventricular enlargement are generally evident. The pulmonary vascularity may be reduced in patients with severe stenosis, right ventricular failure, and/or a venoarterial shunt at the atrial level.

Cardiac catheterization and angiocardiography with right ventricular injection are necessary to localize the site of obstruction and evaluate its severity and to document the coexistence of additional cardiac malformations. The treatment of moderate and severe degrees of pulmonary valvular and subvalvular stenosis is surgical. Direct surgical relief of the obstruction may usually be accomplished at a low risk. Multiple stenoses of the peripheral pulmonary arteries are usually inoperable, but narrowing of a single branch or at the bifurcation of the main pulmonary trunk may be corrected.

Tetralogy of Fallot The four components of this malformation are (1) ventricular septal defect, (2) obstruction to right ventricular outflow, (3) overriding of the aortic orifice above the ventricular defect, and (4) right ventricular hypertrophy. Systolic pressures are equal in the right ventricle and aorta as a consequence of the first two components. The overall incidence of tetralogy approaches 10 percent of all forms of congenital heart disease, and it is the most common anomaly responsible for cyanosis after the age of 1 year. The ventricular septal defect is usually large, approximating the aortic orifice in size, and located high in the septum beneath the crista supraventricularis and just below the aortic valve. The aortic root may be displaced anteriorly and straddle or override the septal defect. Infundibular stenosis occurs as the only major site of obstruction to right ventricular outflow in about one-half the patients and coexists with valvular obstruction in another 25 percent. Supravalvular and peripheral pulmonary arterial narrowing may be observed. When the main pulmonary artery, pulmonic valve, or right ventricular infundibulum is atretic, the condition may be called *pseudotruncus arteriosus* (see "Persistent Truncus Arteriosus" above). In such cases, the lungs are perfused through enlarged bronchial arteries and/or through the pulmonary arteries via a patent ductus arteriosus. A right-sided aortic knob, arch, and descending aorta occur in approximately 25 percent of patients with tetralogy of Fallot.

The relationship between the resistance to blood flow from the ventricles into the aorta and into the pulmonary vessels plays the major role in determining the hemodynamic and clinical picture. Therefore, it is the severity of obstruction to right ventricular outflow which is of fundamental significance. When right ventricular outflow obstruction is severe, the pulmonary blood flow is markedly reduced and a large volume of unsaturated systemic venous blood is shunted from right to left across the ventricular septal defect, severe cyanosis and polycythemia occur, and symptoms of systemic anoxia are prominent. The term *pink, or acyanotic, tetralogy of Fallot* is used often to describe an interventricular communication and a milder degree of obstruction to right ventricular outflow with no appreciable venoarterial shunting. In many patients the obstruction to right ventricular outflow is mild but progressive, so that early in life pulmonary exceeds systemic blood flow and the symptoms resemble those produced by a simple ventricular septal defect.

Most children with tetralogy of Fallot are cyanotic from birth or develop cyanosis before 1 year of age. Dyspnea with exertion, retarded growth and development, clubbing, and polycythemia are common. When resting after exertion, infants with tetralogy characteristically assume a squatting posture. Spells of severe anoxia and cyanosis (see "Hypoxic Spells" above) constitute a major threat to survival.

Physical examination reveals variable degrees of underdevelopment and cyanosis. Clubbing of the terminal digits may be prominent after the first year of life. A right ventricular impulse and systolic thrill may be palpable along the left sternal border; there is no generalized cardiomegaly. The second heart sound is single, and the pulmonic component is rarely audible. A systolic ejection murmur is produced by flow across the narrowed right ventricular outflow tract or pulmonic valve. The intensity and duration of the murmur vary inversely with the severity of obstruction, the opposite of the relation existing in patients with an intact ventricular septum and pulmonary stenosis. Polycythemia, decreased systemic vascular resistance, and increased obstruction to right ventricular outflow may all be responsible for a decrease in the intensity of the murmur. A continuous murmur over the paravertebral area may indicate collateral circulation to the lungs through bronchial arteries.

The electrocardiogram ordinarily shows right ventricular and, less often, right atrial hypertrophy. Radiologic examination characteristically reveals a normal-sized, boot-shaped heart (*coeur en sabot*) with prominence of the right ventricle and a concavity in the region of the pulmonary conus. The pulmonary vascular markings are typically diminished, and the aortic arch and knob may be on the right side. Echocardiography demonstrates discontinuity between the ventricular septum and anterior aortic wall, a thickened anterior wall of right ventricle, an enlarged, anteriorly displaced aorta, and small pulmonary artery. Selective angiocardiography with right ventricular injection is necessary to confirm the diagnosis and to evaluate the architecture of the right ventricular outflow tract, pulmonary valve and annulus, and caliber of the main branches of the pulmonary artery.

Among the factors that may complicate the management of patients with tetralogy are iron-deficiency anemia, infective endocarditis, paradoxic embolism, polycythemia, coagulation defects, and cerebral infarction of abscess. The paroxysmal cyanotic spells may respond quickly to oxygen, placing the child in the knee-chest position, and morphine. If the spell persists, metabolic acidosis will develop from prolonged anaerobic metabolism, and infusion of sodium bicarbonate may be necessary to interrupt the attack. Vasopressors, beta-adrenergic blockade, or general anesthesia may occasionally be necessary.

Total correction is ultimately advisable for almost all patients with tetralogy of Fallot. However, if cyanosis or symptoms are marked in an infant, the risk of primary repair may be high unless performed in a center prepared properly for intracardiac surgery, and a palliative operation designed to increase pulmonary blood flow may be recommended. These procedures include aortopulmonary or subclavian-pulmonary arterial anastomosis or transventricular infundibulectomy or valvulotomy. Total correction can then be carried out at a lower risk later in childhood or during adolescence.

Ebstein's anomaly In this rare anomaly there is abnormal morphogenesis of the tricuspid valve, with redundancy of tricuspid valve tissue, and the attachment of portions of the septal and posterior leaflets of the tricuspid valve is lower than normal; the leaflets originate from the right ventricular wall rather than from the atrioventricular ring. Hence, the portion of the right ventricle that lies between the atrioventricular ring and the origin of the valve is continuous with the right atrial chamber. The tricuspid valve is usually incompetent, the foramen ovale is patent, and the right ventricle exhibits varying degrees of hypoplasia. The clinical manifestations of Ebstein's anomaly are variable, depending on the severity of the anatomic changes in the tricuspid valve. Ultimately, however, progressive cyanosis resulting from the right-to-left shunt across the interatrial communication, symptoms resulting from right ventricular dysfunction, and/or paroxysmal arrhythmias develop.

A prominent systolic pulsation of the liver and a large *v* wave in the jugular venous pulse accompany the systolic thrill and murmur of tricuspid regurgitation. Wide splitting of the first and second heart sounds and prominent third and fourth heart sounds may produce a characteristically rhythmic auscultatory cadence. The electrocardiogram shows giant P waves, a prolonged PR interval, and complete or incomplete right bundle branch block. Roentgenography usually demonstrates an enlarged right atrium and a small right ventricle and pulmonary artery; reduced pulsations; the pulmonary vascularity may be reduced if a large right-to-left shunt is present. The principal echocardiographic findings include a large anterior tricuspid leaflet with delayed tricuspid valve closure with respect to mitral closure. At cardiac catheterization the intracavitary electrocardiogram recorded just proximal to the tricuspid valve shows a right ventricular type of complex, while the pressure recorded is that of the right atrium.

Most patients survive to the third decade at least. In some disabled patients moderate improvement has resulted from anastomosis of the superior vena cava to the right pulmonary artery to divert systemic venous return from the right atrium and to increase pulmonary blood flow. Patients beyond age 12 have occasionally benefited from prosthetic replacement of the tricuspid valve; at all ages, however, patients with Ebstein's anomaly are poor surgical risks.

Tricuspid atresia Atresia of the tricuspid valve, an interatrial communication, and, frequently, hypoplasia of the right ventricle and pulmonary artery, as well as transposition of the great arteries, exist in this malformation. Survival is dependent on a right-to-left shunt at the atrial level. Blood reaches the lungs through a patent ductus arteriosus, bronchial collateral vessels, or the right ventricle and pulmonary artery via a ventricular septal defect (if the great arteries are oriented normally). The clinical picture is usually dominated by symptoms resulting from greatly diminished pulmonary blood flow, with anoxic spells and severe cyanosis.

The electrocardiogram showing right atrial enlargement, left axis deviation, and left ventricular hypertrophy in a cyanotic child strongly suggests tricuspid atresia. Echocardiography reveals a small or absent right ventricle, large left ventricle, and absent tricuspid valve echoes. Many patients die in the first weeks or months of life. Balloon atrial septostomy and palliative operations consisting of increasing pulmonary blood flow, often by systemic arterial or venous–pulmonary artery anastomosis, are capable of producing clinical improvement in patients with diminished blood flow. Functional correction of the anomaly can be accomplished in selected patients with normal or low pulmonary arterial pressure by insertion of a prosthetic valve-containing conduit between the right atrium and pulmonary artery and closure of the interatrial communication.

Coarctation of the aorta Narrowing or constriction of the lumen of the aorta may occur anywhere along its length but is most commonly localized just distal to the origin of the left subclavian artery near the insertion of the ligamentum arteriosum. Coarctation is encountered in approximately 7 percent of patients with congenital heart disease and is twice as common in males as in females, although the lesion occurs frequently in patients with gonadal dysgenesis (Turner's syndrome, Chap. 342). Clinical manifestations depend on the site and extent of obstruction and the presence of associated cardiac anomalies, which occur in the majority of patients. These include most commonly bicuspid aortic valve, congenital aortic stenosis, patent ductus arteriosus, ventricular septal defect and mitral regurgitation. When diffuse narrowing of the aorta is located proximal to the ductus arteriosus, right ventricular hypertrophy develops in utero and pulmonary hypertension and congestive heart failure are common in early life. *Differential cyanosis* may result from preferential shunting of unsaturated pulmonary arterial blood through a patent ductus arteriosus to the lower part of the body.

More commonly, the coarctation is localized at or just distal to the attachment of the ductus or ligamentum arteriosus. The majority of children and young adults with isolated juxta- or postductal coarctation are asymptomatic. Headache, epistaxis, cold extremities, and claudication with exercise may be noted, although attention is usually directed to the cardiovascular system when a heart murmur or hypertension in the upper extremities is detected on routine physical examination. Mechanical factors, rather than those of renal origin, play the primary role in the production of hypertension.

Absence, marked diminution, or delayed pulsations in the femoral arteries and a low or unobtainable arterial pressure in the lower extremities with hypertension in the arms are the basic clues to the diagnosis. In adults, enlarged and pulsatile collateral vessels may be palpated in the intercostal spaces anteriorly, in the axillae, or posteriorly in the interscapular area. Also, the upper extremities and thorax may be preferentially more developed than the lower extremities. A midsystolic murmur over the anterior part of the chest, back, and spinous processes is most frequent, becoming continuous if the lumen is narrowed sufficiently to result in a high-velocity jet across the lesion throughout the cardiac cycle. Additional systolic and continuous murmurs over the lateral thoracic wall may reflect increased flow through dilated and tortuous collateral vessels. The *electrocardiogram* reveals left ventricular hypertrophy of varying degree, depending on the height of the arterial pressure proximal to the obstruction and the patient's age; predominant right or combined ventricular hypertrophy may be seen in infants and children, and usually implies a complicated lesion. *Roentgenograms* may show a dilated left subclavian artery high on the left mediastinal border and a dilated ascending aorta. Indentation of the aorta at the site of coarctation and pre- and poststenotic dilatation (the "3" sign) along the left paramediastinal shadow are almost pathognomonic. Notching of the ribs, an important radiographic sign, is due to erosion by dilated collateral vessels, increases with age, and usually becomes apparent between the sixth and twelfth years of life. Cardiac catheterization and aortography may be indicated to localize accurately the site of obstruction, determine the length of the coarctation, and identify associated malformations.

The *treatment* of uncomplicated coarctation of the aorta is surgical; resection and end-to-end anastomosis can be accomplished with excellent results in most patients, although it is occasionally necessary to use a tubular graft or patch in the repair if the narrowed segment is long. Paradoxic hypertension of short duration is often noted in the immediate postoperative period, and occasionally a necrotizing panarteritis of the small vessels of the gastrointestinal tract of uncertain cause complicates the course of recovery. In those who survive the first 2 years of life complications are uncommon before the second or third decade; operation on asymptomatic patients is advised ideally between the ages of 4 and 8. The chief hazards to patients with coarctation result from severe hypertension and include the development of cerebral aneurysms and hemorrhage, rupture of the aorta, left ventricular failure, and infective endocarditis. Systemic hypertension in the absence of residual coarctation has been observed in resting or exercise-stressed patients postoperatively and appears to be related to the duration of preoperative hypertension, as well as incomplete operative repair; lifelong observation is desirable because of the late onset of hypertension in some postoperative patients.

CONGENITAL AORTIC STENOSIS Malformations that cause obstruction to the ejection of blood from the left ventricle include congenital valvular aortic stenosis, the discrete form of congenital subaortic stenosis, congenital narrowing of the supravalvular ascending aorta, and idiopathic hypertrophic subaortic stenosis (Chap. 247).

Valvular aortic stenosis Valvular aortic stenosis occurs in approximately 4 percent of patients with congenital cardiovascular defects and occurs three to four times more often in males than in females. However, the congenital bicuspid aortic valve, which is not necessarily stenotic, may actually be the most common congenital malformation of the heart, although it may go undetected in early life. Because bicuspid valves may become stenotic with time or be the site of infective endocarditis, the lesion may become of clinical significance only in adult life, when it may be difficult to distinguish it anatomically from acquired rheumatic aortic stenosis. Commonly associated anomalies include patent ductus arteriosus and coarctation of the aorta.

The dynamics of blood flow associated with a congenitally deformed, rigid aortic valve commonly lead to thickening of the cusps and, in later life, to calcification. When the obstruction is hemodynamically significant, concentric hypertrophy of the left ventricular wall and dilatation of the ascending aorta occur.

The hemodynamic abnormalities produced by obstruction to left ventricular outflow are discussed in Chap. 242. A peak systolic pressure gradient exceeding 70 mmHg, in association with a normal cardiac output, or an effective aortic orifice less than 0.6 cm² per square meter of body surface, is considered to represent critical obstruction to left ventricular outflow. The resting cardiac output is generally within normal limits, but often fails to rise normally during muscular exercise.

Most children with congenital aortic stenosis are asymptomatic and grow and develop normally. Usually, a murmur is detected on a routine examination. At least moderately severe obstruction should be suspected if there is a definite history of fatigability and exertional dyspnea. In patients with severe obstruction, the inability of the left ventricle to increase its output and to maintain cerebral flow during exercise may result in

exertional syncope, while the disparity between the oxygen supply to the left ventricle and myocardial oxygen requirements may be responsible for anginal pain. The symptomatic patient with valvular aortic stenosis generally has critical stenosis, although a lack of symptoms does not preclude the presence of moderately severe obstruction. Sudden death is a distinct threat to patients with critical stenosis. Its precise cause is poorly understood, but ventricular arrhythmias, perhaps initiated by acute myocardial ischemia, may be responsible.

When obstruction is hemodynamically significant, a left ventricular lift is usually palpable and a precordial systolic thrill is felt over the base of the heart, with transmission to the jugular notch and along the carotid arteries. Presystolic expansion is often palpable. A systolic aortic ejection sound, signifying opening of the aortic valve, is typically present at the cardiac apex when the valve is mobile, particularly in patients with mild to moderate stenosis. Delayed closure of the stenotic aortic valve leads to a single or a closely split second heart sound, and paradoxic splitting may be present. A fourth heart sound is generally associated with severe obstruction. The systolic murmur starts after the completion of left ventricular isometric contraction, is rhomboid-shaped, loud, harsh, and best heard at the base of the heart. The murmur, like the thrill, radiates to the jugular notch and carotid vessels, as well as to the apex. In some patients, an early diastolic blowing murmur of aortic regurgitation is present, but unless the valve leaflets have been eroded by infective endocarditis, the regurgitation is usually not hemodynamically significant; occasionally, in patients with a congenital bicuspid valve, aortic regurgitation may be severe and the dominant lesion hemodynamically.

Electrocardiographically, left ventricular hypertrophy tends to vary with the severity of obstruction, although a *normal or near-normal electrocardiogram does not exclude severe aortic stenosis*. The left ventricular "strain pattern" generally indicates that severe aortic stenosis is present.

Roentgenographically, the overall heart size is most often normal or only slightly enlarged. Left atrial enlargement and concentric left ventricular hypertrophy accompany moderate or severe obstruction. Poststenotic dilatation of the ascending aorta is a common finding. Echocardiographic findings include multiple eccentric diastolic closure lines in the aortic lumen, thickening of the left ventricular posterior wall and septum, reduced separation of thickened aortic valve leaflets, and aortic dilatation. Cardiac catheterization is indicated when the clinical diagnosis of aortic stenosis has been established and when the history, clinical examination, roentgenogram, electrocardiogram, or echocardiogram suggests the possibility of severe obstruction. The site and severity of obstruction are established, and any associated malformations are identified. In patients with mild or moderate obstruction repeat left-sided heart catheterization should be carried out every 5 to 10 years because stenosis may progress.

The medical management of congenital valvular aortic stenosis includes prophylaxis against infective endocarditis and, in patients with diminished cardiac reserve, the administration of digitalis and diuretics and sodium restriction while awaiting operation. If severe aortic stenosis is present, avoidance of strenuous physical activity is advised even when the patient is asymptomatic, and participation in competitive sports should probably also be restricted in patients with milder degrees of obstruction. The decision concerning the advisability of operation depends on the severity of obstruction rather than on the symptoms described by the patient. Operation is carried out under direct vision with the aid of total cardiopulmonary bypass, and in children without valvular calcification the fused commissures are opened. Following commissurotomy the valves remain somewhat deformed. Further degenerative changes, including calcification, may lead to significant stenosis later. The treatment of congenital aortic stenosis in the adult is described in Chap. 242.

Subaortic stenosis The most common form of subaortic stenosis is the *idiopathic hypertrophic* variety, which occurs in a congenital form in about one-third of the patients and is discussed in Chap. 247. Both clinically and physiologically, however, it is the *discrete* form of subaortic stenosis which resembles valvular aortic stenosis. The lesion usually consists of a membranous diaphragm or fibrous ring encircling the left ventricular outflow tract just beneath the base of the aortic valve. It is less common than isolated valvular obstruction, but it also occurs more frequently in males than in females. There are no clinical criteria which can be relied upon to distinguish the two forms of obstruction, although a systolic ejection sound is rarely heard in patients with discrete subvalvular aortic stenosis and the diastolic murmur of aortic regurgitation is more common than in patients with valvular aortic stenosis. Valvular calcification is not observed roentgenographically in patients with subaortic stenosis. Echocardiography may demonstrate the subaortic obstruction, and usually reveals an abnormal pattern of motion of the aortic valve leaflets. Definitive differentiation between valvular and subvalvular obstruction is best accomplished at cardiac catheterization by recording pressure tracings as a cardiac catheter is withdrawn across the outflow tract and by left ventricular angiocardiography.

Because of the likelihood of progressive obstruction and aortic regurgitation, the presence of even mild or moderate subaortic stenosis warrants consideration of elective operation. Surgical correction consists of excising the membrane or fibrous ridge.

Occasionally, valvular and subvalvular aortic stenosis coexist in the same patient, producing a tunnel-like narrowing of the left ventricular outflow tract. Associated findings are often a small ascending aorta, hypoplasia of the aortic valve ring, and thickened valve leaflets. It may be recognized by angiography. Operative treatment frequently necessitates prosthetic replacement of the aortic valve, as well as enlarging the aortic annulus, proximal aorta, and left ventricular outflow tract, or the interposition of a valved conduit between the left ventricle apex and the ascending aorta.

Several anatomic lesions other than a membrane, ridge, or muscular band that may produce subaortic stenosis are listed in Table 240-3.

Supravalvular aortic stenosis Supravalvular aortic stenosis is a localized or diffuse narrowing of the ascending aorta, originating just above the level of the coronary arteries at the superior margin of the sinuses of Valsalva. In contrast to other forms of aortic stenosis, in the supravalvular variety the coronary arteries are subjected to the elevated pressures that exist

TABLE 240-3
Unusual causes of subaortic stenosis

  I Accessory tissue of the mitral valve
 II Prolapse of aneurysm of membranous septum into left ventricular outflow tract
III Restriction of movement of the anterior mitral valve leaflet
   A Anomalous basal attachment of anterior leaflet
   B Accessory chordae tendineae
   C Abnormal fusion of valvular tissue to the septal wall of the outflow tract
   D Convergence of all mitral chordae into one or two fused papillary muscles ("parachute" deformity)
 IV Deficiency of the ventricular septum (endocardial cushion defects)
  V Anomalous subaortic muscle bundle (corrected transposition)
 VI Type II glycogen storage disease

within the left ventricle, and are often dilated and tortuous. Adherence of the free edges of the aortic cusps to the sites of supravalvular stenosis may interfere with coronary arterial inflow.

The designation *supravalvular aortic stenosis syndrome* has been applied to the distinctive clinical picture produced by coexistence of the cardiovascular lesion and a metabolic disorder, idiopathic infantile hypercalcemia, that is probably related to deranged vitamin D metabolism. Other manifestations of this syndrome include mental retardation, a peculiar "elfin facies," craniosynostosis, strabismus, narrowing of peripheral systemic and pulmonary arteries, inguinal hernias, cryptorchidism in males, premature development of secondary sexual characteristics in females, and abnormalities of dental development. Supravalvular aortic stenosis and peripheral pulmonary arterial stenosis are also seen in familial and sporadic forms unassociated with the other features of the syndrome. Genetic studies suggest that when the anomaly is familial it is transmitted as an autosomal dominant trait with variable expression.

The physical findings resemble those in valvular aortic stenosis, except that the sound of aortic valve closure is accentuated, ejection sounds are infrequent, and transmission of the thrill and murmurs into the jugular notch and along the carotid vessels is more prominent; the systolic pressure in the right arm is characteristically higher than in the left. Poststenotic dilatation of the ascending aorta is rarely present.

The electrocardiogram reveals left ventricular hypertrophy. The diagnosis is confirmed by the demonstration at retrograde aortic catheterization of a pressure gradient just above the aortic valve, and a constriction at this level as revealed by aortography.

Surgical treatment consists of widening the lumen of the aorta by the insertion of a fabric prosthesis, and operative treatment is indicated if the obstruction is discrete and severe without generalized hypoplasia of the ascending aorta and arch.

Hypoplastic left-sided heart syndrome This designation is used to describe the condition of patients with an obstructive lesion on the left side of the heart associated with hypoplasia of the left ventricle and hypertrophy of the right ventricle. This syndrome, which is a significant cause of neonatal mortality, may be caused by atresia and/or hypoplasia of the aortic and mitral valves and of the aortic arch. The left atrium and ventricle often exhibit endocardial fibroelastosis. Echocardiographic findings may be diagnostic and include a diminutive aortic root and left ventricular cavity and absent or poor visualization of aortic and mitral valve echoes, which, when seen, are of diminished amplitude and mobility. Presently, the anatomic lesions are inoperable.

Malformations obstructing pulmonary venous flow A number of malformations at or upstream to the mitral valve may cause obstruction to flow of pulmonary venous blood into the left ventricle.

MITRAL STENOSIS Anatomic types of mitral stenosis include the "parachute" deformity of the valve, in which shortened chordae tendineae converge and insert into a single large papillary muscle, often associated with endocardial fibroelastosis of the left atrium and ventricle, and a supravalvular circumferential ridge of connective tissue arising at the base of the atrial aspect of the mitral leaflets; an anomalous arcade of obstructing papillary muscles; rudimentary valve commissures and thickened fibrotic leaflets.

COR TRIATRIATUM In this malformation an abnormal fibromuscular diaphragm divides the left atrium into a posterosuperior chamber, into which the pulmonary veins drain, and an anteroinferior chamber, which communicates with the mitral valve and atrial appendage. The diaphragm contains an opening, or occasionally several openings, the size of which determines the degree of obstruction to pulmonary venous return.

CONGENITAL PULMONARY VEIN STENOSIS This malformation may consist of a localized narrowing at or near the junctions of the pulmonary veins and the left atrium, or individual pulmonary veins may be hypoplastic for variable distances along their intra- or extrapulmonary portions.

The hemodynamic and clinical consequences of each of these lesions result from obstruction to pulmonary venous return. At cardiac catheterization cor triatriatum and pulmonary vein stenosis may be suspected if the pulmonary arterial wedge pressure is higher than a simultaneous left atrial pressure obtained by transseptal catheterization. A specific diagnosis of each of these anomalies may be established by visualizing the obstructing lesion angiographically. Although these malformations are rare, differential diagnosis is important, since cor triatriatum may be easily corrected at operation.

TRANSPOSITION COMPLEXES The term *transposition* identifies a complicated group of malformations that have in common abnormal relationships between the cardiac chambers and the great arteries.

Complete transposition of the great arteries The aorta arises from the right ventricle to the right of and anterior to the pulmonary artery, which emerges from the left ventricle. This results in two separate and parallel circulations, and some communication between the two circulations must exist after birth in order to sustain life. Almost all patients have an interatrial communication, two-thirds have a patent ductus arteriosus, and about one-third have an associated ventricular septal defect. Transposition occurs more frequently in the offspring of diabetic mothers and in more males than females. It is a leading cause of death due to congenital heart disease in the first 2 months of life and accounts for approximately 10 percent of all patients with cyanotic heart disease. Without treatment, about 70 percent of the patients with this malformation die by the age of 6 months. A few survive into childhood, and rarely a patient survives into young adult life. Those who live beyond infancy have, as a general rule, either an isolated large atrial septal defect or a single ventricle or ventricular septal defect and pulmonic stenosis.

The clinical course is determined by the degree of tissue hypoxia, the ability of each ventricle to sustain an increased workload in the presence of reduced coronary arterial oxygenation, the nature of the associated cardiovascular anomalies, and the anatomic and functional status of the pulmonary vascular bed. A bidirectional shunt is always present, because continuous unidirectional shunting would result in a progressive depletion of the circulating volume in either the pulmonary or the systemic vascular bed. The magnitude of both the arteriovenous and venoarterial shunts is modified by the number and size of intercirculatory communications that exist, the presence of associated obstructive intra- and extracardiac anomalies, and the relations between the pulmonary and systemic vascular resistances. Severe morphologic alterations develop in the pulmonary vascular bed by the age of 1 to 2 years in almost all patients with this anomaly with an associated large ventricular septal defect or large patent ductus arteriosus in the absence of obstruction to left ventricular outflow.

The usual clinical manifestations are dyspnea and cyanosis from birth, retardation of growth, and congestive heart failure. Murmurs are of little diagnostic significance and are absent or insignificant in approximately 30 percent of these infants.

The usual electrocardiographic findings include right axis

deviation, right atrial enlargement, and right ventricular hypertrophy, reflecting that the right ventricle is the systemic pumping chamber. Left ventricular hypertrophy is occasionally present in those patients with large ventricular septal defects and elevated pulmonary blood flow, or with obstruction to pulmonary blood flow. The roentgenographic findings are often highly suggestive of the diagnosis and consist of (1) progressive cardiac enlargement in early infancy, (2) characteristic oval or egg-shaped cardiac configuration in the anteroposterior view and a narrow vascular pedicle, and (3) increased pulmonary vascular markings. In the absence of dextrocardia, transverse cross-sectional echocardiography may strongly suggest the diagnosis by demonstrating that the anterior great artery (aorta) is to the right of the posterior great artery (pulmonary). Cardiac catheterization shows a lower oxygen saturation in the aorta than in the pulmonary artery. Angiocardiography is diagnostic and demonstrates that the anteriorly placed aorta arises from the right ventricle, and the posteriorly placed pulmonary artery in continuity with the mitral valve arises from the left ventricle.

Medical treatment includes use of oxygen, digitalis, diuretics, iron if an associated iron-deficiency anemia is present, and intravenous sodium bicarbonate for severe anoxemic metabolic acidosis. The creation or enlargement of an interatrial communication is the simplest procedure for providing increased intracardiac mixing of systemic and pulmonary venous blood; it may be achieved surgically or, preferably, by rupturing the valve of the foramen ovale with a balloon catheter during transseptal catheterization of the left side of the heart (Rashkind's procedure), balloon septostomy. Pulmonary artery banding should be considered as an adjunct in infants with ventricular septal defect, and high pulmonary arterial pressure. Systemic-pulmonary artery anastomosis may be indicated in the patient with severe obstruction to left ventricular outflow and diminished pulmonary blood flow. Intracardiac repair may be accomplished by rearranging the venous return so that the systemic venous blood is directed to the mitral valve and thence to the left ventricle and pulmonary artery, while the pulmonary venous blood is diverted through the tricuspid valve and right ventricle to the aorta (Mustard or Senning operation). The risk of this corrective operation is lowest in those patients with an intact ventricular septum and no obstruction to pulmonary flow. For those patients with a ventricular septal defect in whom it is necessary to bypass a severely obstructed left ventricular outflow tract, corrective operation employs an intracardiac ventricular baffle and extracardiac prosthetic conduit to replace the pulmonary artery (Rastelli's procedure).

Partial transposition This designation is usually applied to the anomaly referred to as *double-outlet right ventricle* or *origin of both great vessels from the right ventricle*. The aorta is transposed and arises entirely from the right ventricle, while the pulmonary artery takes its usual origin. A ventricular septal defect, which serves as the sole outlet of the left ventricle, is always present. The clinical and physiologic picture is determined by the size of the ventricular septal defect and the presence or absence of pulmonary stenosis. Because of the streaming of blood flow from the left ventricle across the outflow tract of the right ventricle to the aorta, these patients may resemble clinically those with isolated, large ventricular septal defects without cyanosis. However, when there is accompanying pulmonary stenosis, the clinical findings are similar to those of cyanotic tetralogy of Fallot. Diagnosis of these lesions is dependent on careful angiocardiographic analysis, and increased preoperative recognition of the partial transposition anomalies may be expected to result in improved operative results. In the *Taussig-Bing* form of partial transposition, the ventricular septal defect is related to a nonstenotic pulmonary orifice. This malformation resembles complete transposition with ventricular septal defect and pulmonary vascular obstruction clinically.

Corrected transposition The two fundamental anatomic derangements composing this malformation are transposition, or anteroposterior reversal of the ascending aorta and pulmonary trunk, and inversion, or right-left reversal of the ventricles. This arrangement of the great vessels and ventricles (in contrast to the uncorrected transposition) permits functional correction, so that systemic venous blood passes into the pulmonary trunk while arterialized pulmonary venous blood flows into the aorta. In corrected transposition, the systemic veins drain into the right atrium. Venous blood hence flows across an atrioventricular valve, which has the structure of a normal *mitral* valve, into the right-sided "venous ventricle." This chamber, however, has the morphologic characteristics of a normal left ventricle, i.e., its interior lining is finely trabeculated, it has no crista supraventricularis, and its atrioventricular valve is in continuity with a posteriorly placed semilunar valve. It ejects blood into the pulmonary trunk, which arises posterior to the ascending aorta. Oxygenated blood returns from the lungs to the left atrium, which is normal in position and structure, from which it flows into the left-sided "arterial ventricle" across an atrioventricular valve, which has the structure of a normal *tricuspid* valve. The interior lining of the arterial ventricle has the morphologic characteristics of a normal right ventricle, i.e., it has coarse trabeculations and a crista supraventricularis; the tricuspid atrioventricular valve is not in continuity with the anteriorly placed semilunar valve. The arterial ventricle ejects blood into the aorta, which arises anterior to the pulmonary trunk.

In complete, "uncorrected" transposition of the great arteries the maintenance of life is dependent on the presence of associated defects. In contrast, patients in whom corrected transposition exists as an isolated anomaly present no functional alterations and have no symptoms. Ebstein-type anomalies of the left-sided, tricuspid atrioventricular valve, ventricular septal defect, obstruction to outflow from the venous ventricle, and congenital heart block are those malformations most often associated with corrected transposition. Malposition of the heart may further complicate the altered anatomy.

In addition to the manifestations of the associated lesions, patients with corrected transposition frequently have an accentuated, single second heart sound in the second left intercostal space, representing closure of the aortic valve, which lies lateral and anterior to the pulmonic valve. An abnormal direction of initial (septal) ventricular depolarization is manifested electrocardiographically by a reversal of the precordial Q-wave pattern (Q waves are present in the right precordial leads and absent on the left). The His bundle is elongated because of the greater distance between the atrioventricular node and the base of the ventricular septum. This arrangement may be a causal factor in a variety of arrhythmias, and atrioventricular conduction disturbances are common. Roentgenographic examination characteristically reveals absence of the normal pulmonary artery segment and a smooth convexity of the left supracardiac border produced by the displaced ascending aorta. The displaced aorta may be visualized by radionuclide scintillation scans of the central circulation. The diagnosis of corrected transposition can usually be established by selective angiocardiography.

High operative morbidity and mortality rates have attended repair of the lesions associated with corrected transposition;

these rates are related to the elevated pulmonary vascular resistance which may exist in patients with associated ventricular septal defects, which are usually large, and to a high incidence of surgically induced heart block. The latter complication may be expected to diminish with the application of newly devised intraoperative techniques for electrophysiologic mapping of the course of the conduction system. In addition, the inversion of the coronary arterial system greatly limits and may preclude an incision into the venous ventricle, thereby interfering with exposure of interventricular septal defects in the usual manner.

Transposition of the pulmonary veins When all the pulmonary veins connect either to the right atrium directly or to the systemic veins or their tributaries, the condition is called total anomalous pulmonary venous connection (TAPVC). Because all venous blood returns to the right atrium, an interatrial communication is an integral part of this malformation. Additional major cardiac malformations occur in about one-third of these patients. TAPVC accounts for about 2 percent of the deaths from congenital heart disease in the first year of life. The anomalous connection is usually supradiaphragmatic and to the left brachiocephalic vein, right atrium, coronary sinus, or superior vena cava. The distal site of connection may be below the diaphragm, a condition which is hazardous because it is typically associated with marked obstruction to pulmonary venous return.

Most infants with the more usual, unobstructed form of supradiaphragmatic TAPVC fail to thrive, are subject to repeated respiratory infections, and have congestive heart failure by the age of 6 months. The physiologic consequences and, accordingly, the clinical picture depend on the size of the interatrial communication and on the magnitude of the pulmonary vascular resistance. When the interatrial communication is small, systemic blood flow is markedly limited, right atrial and systemic venous pressures are elevated, and hepatic enlargement and peripheral edema are present. On the other hand, the magnitude of the pulmonary blood flow and, therefore, the arterial oxygen saturation, which ranges from markedly reduced to normal values, is inversely related to the pulmonary vascular resistance. Therefore, cyanosis is not usually prominent in the absence of congestive failure unless the patient survives long enough to acquire secondary pulmonary vascular changes and a reduction in pulmonary blood flow.

A characteristic physical finding is the presence of multiple heart sounds, consisting of a first sound followed by an ejection click, a fixed, widely split second heart sound with an accentuated pulmonic component, and a third, and often a fourth, heart sound. The electrocardiogram shows right axis deviation, as well as right atrial and ventricular hypertrophy. Roentgenograms of the chest reveal increased pulmonary blood flow; the right atrium and ventricle are dilated and hypertrophied, and the pulmonary artery segment is enlarged. In addition, the specific site of anomalous connection may result in a characteristic appearance of the cardiac silhouette. Thus in patients with TAPVC to the left brachiocephalic vein, the superior vena cava on the right, left brachiocephalic vein superiorly, and left vertical vein on the left produce a cardiac shadow that resembles a "snowman" or figure-of-eight. The upper right cardiac border may be prominent when the anomalous connection is to the right superior vena cava. Echocardiography demonstrates marked enlargement of the right ventricle and a small left atrium. Selective pulmonary arteriography and indicator-dilution studies at cardiac catheterization are especially helpful in determining the drainage pathways of the pulmonary veins. Indicator injected into the right ventricle or pulmonary artery takes longer to reach the peripheral arterial sampling site than indicator injected into the venae cavae or right atrium. The contour of the dilution curves obtained from a peripheral artery after injection into both the right atrium and a pulmonary vein are identical and show a large right-to-left shunt while the left atrial curve is normal.

Balloon atrial septostomy may provide dramatic palliation for the infant in whom the small size of the interatrial communication limits the amount of blood reaching the left side of the heart and systemic circulation. Unless serious pulmonary vascular disease is present, results of operation for TAPVC in patients more than 1 year of age are good. The procedure consists of creating an anastomosis between the common pulmonary venous channel and left atrium and closing the atrial defect and the anomalous venous pathway.

Partial transposition of the pulmonary veins In this condition, one of the pulmonary veins (or more than one) is connected to the right atrium or to one or more of its tributaries. An atrial septal defect, particularly one of the sinus venosus type, usually accompanies partial transposition of the pulmonary veins, and the usual connection involves the veins of the right upper and middle lobes and the superior vena cava. In the absence of associated anomalies, the physiologic disturbance is determined by the number of anomalous veins and their site of connection, the presence and size of an atrial septal defect, the state of the pulmonary vascular bed, and associated anomalies. In the usual case of isolated partial transposition of the pulmonary veins, the hemodynamic state and physical findings are similar to those in atrial septal defect. Occasionally, drainage is into the inferior vena cava. This condition may be associated with pulmonary parenchymal abnormalities, hypoplasia of the right pulmonary artery and lung, and dextroposition of the heart. This complex has been designated the "scimitar syndrome," because of the characteristic roentgenographic finding of a crescent-like shadow in the right lower lung field which is produced by the anomalous venous channel.

MALPOSITIONS OF THE HEART Positional anomalies of the heart refer to conditions in which the cardiac apex is located in the right side of the chest (dextrocardia) or at the midline (mesocardia), or in which there is a normal location of the heart in the left side of the chest but abnormal position of the viscera (isolated levocardia). Knowledge of the position of the abdominal organs is important in diagnosing these malpositions. For example, a mirror-image dextrocardia is usually observed in a patient with complete situs inversus; this condition occurs more frequently in an otherwise normal person than in one with a malformed heart. In contrast, when dextrocardia occurs without situs inversus, associated cardiac malformations are the rule. When the heart occupies its normal position but situs inversus of the viscera is present, the heart is almost always seriously malformed. Moreover, when the visceral situs is indeterminate, there is a striking association of asplenia or polysplenia with complex, multiple cardiac anomalies, which usually include a combination of systemic and pulmonary venous abnormalities, defects in the atrial and ventricular septa, and endocardial cushion defects. In addition, pulmonary arterial obstruction and maldevelopment of the great arteries may occur with both asplenia and polysplenia but are more common in the former. Transposition of the great arteries occurs frequently in cardiac malposition, and double-outlet right ventricle is common in asplenia. It is important to recognize these complex syndromes in order to distinguish them from forms of cyanotic heart disease that may be amenable to corrective surgical therapy. The diagnosis is suggested by a symmetric liver shadow roentgenographically, and by the presence of Howell-Jolly and Heinz bodies in red blood cells demonstrated by blood smear, and confirmed by a negative or abnormal radioactive spleen scan.

Once the type of visceral situs is defined, it is necessary to describe the basic anatomic structure of the heart and its vascular connection. The atria exhibit a strong tendency to conform to the general orientation of the viscera so that the right, or venous, atrium lies on the same side of the body as the trilobed lung, liver, and inferior vena cava, while the morphologic left, or arterial, atrium tends to lie on the same side as the stomach, spleen, and bilobed lung. The visceral situs can usually be determined by the location of the stomach bubble and liver on a routine roentgenogram, and the inferior vena cava can be located by the position of the cardiac catheter or by means of a venous or radioisotope angiocardiogram. The location of the ventricles and the relationship between the great arteries may also be demonstrated angiocardiographically. The cardiac chambers should be diagnosed positionally (left- and right-sided), functionally (arterial and venous), and morphologically (in terms of their intrinsic anatomic characteristics). When the positional, functional and morphologic relationships are understood, the presence of associated anomalies is established and the principles of medical and surgical treatment can be applied to patients with cardiac malpositions just as they are in normally located hearts.

REFERENCES

General

ALPERT J, BRAUNWALD E: Congenital heart disease in the adult, in *Heart Disease*, E Braunwald (ed). Philadelphia, Saunders, 1980, chap 29

FRIEDMAN WF: Congenital heart disease in infancy and childhood, in ibid, chap 28

———— et al: *Neonatal Heart Disease.* New York, Grune & Stratton, 1973

GOOR DA, LILLEHEI CW: *Congenital Malformations of the Heart.* New York, Grune & Stratton, 1975

MOSS AJ et al: *Heart Disease in Infants, Children and Adolescents,* 2d ed. Baltimore, Williams & Wilkins, 1977

NORA JJ, NORA AH: *Genetics and Counseling in Cardiovascular Disease.* Springfield, Ill, Charles C Thomas, 1978

PERLOFF JK: *The Clinical Recognition of Congenital Heart Disease,* 2d ed. Philadelphia, Saunders, 1978

RUDOLPH AM: *Congenital Diseases of the Heart.* Chicago, Year Book, 1974

Anomalous pulmonary origin of coronary artery

GRACE RR et al: Aortic implantation of anomalous left coronary arising from the pulmonary artery. Am J Cardiol 39:608, 1977

Aortic sinus aneurysm and fistula

MYER J et al: Aneurysm and fistula of the sinus of Valsalva. Clinical considerations and surgical treatment of 45 patients. Ann Thorac Surg 19:170, 1975

Aortopulmonary septal defect

BLIEDEN LC, MOLAR JH: Aorticopulmonary septal defect. Br Heart J 36:630, 1974

Atrial septal defect

DAVE KF et al: Atrial septal defect in adults. Am J Cardiol 31:7, 1973

McCABE JC et al: Surgical treatment of endocardial cushion defect. Am J Cardiol 39:72, 1977

Coarctation of the aorta

SIMON AB, ZLOTTO AE: Coarctation of the aorta: Longitudinal assessment of operated patients. Circulation 50:456, 1974

Complete transposition of the great arteries

STARK J: Surgical treatment of patients with transposition of the great arteries. Johns Hopkins Med J 140:181, 1977

TRUSLER GA, MUSTER WT: Palliative and reparative procedures for transposition of the great arteries. Ann Thorac Surg 17:410, 1974

Congenital valvular aortic stenosis

FRIEDMAN WF: Congenital aortic valve disease: Natural history, indications and results of surgery, in *New Aspects in Congenital, Valvular, and Coronary Artery Disease,* D Morse (ed). Mt Kisco, NY, Futura, 1975, p 43

———— et al: Congenital aortic stenosis in adults. Cardiovasc Clin, vol 10, no 1, p 235

Coronary arteriovenous fistula

RUTTENHOUSE EA et al: Congenital coronary artery–cardiac chamber fistula. Review of operative management. Ann Thorac Surg 20:468, 1975

Corrected transposition

ALLWORK SP et al: Congenitally corrected transposition of the great arteries. Am J Cardiol 38:910, 1976

Cor triatriatum

THILENIUS OG et al: Subdivided left atrium: An expanded concept of cor triatriatum sinistrum. Am J Cardiol 37:743, 1976

Discrete subaortic stenosis

NEWFELD EA et al: Discrete subvalvular aortic stenosis in childhood. Am J Cardiol 38:53, 1976

Ebstein's anomaly

JUGDUTT BI et al: Surgical treatment of Ebstein's anomaly. J Thorac Cardiovasc Surg 73:114, 1977

Hypoplastic left-sided heart syndrome

MEYER RA, KAPLAN S: Echocardiography in the diagnosis of hypoplasia of the left and right ventricles in the neonate. Circulation 41:55, 1972

Malposition of the heart

STANGER P et al: Cardiac malpositions: An overview based on a study of 65 necropsy specimens. Circulation 56:159, 1977

Partial transposition

SONDHEIMER HM et al: Double outlet right ventricle: Clinical spectrum and prognosis. Am J Cardiol 39:709, 1977

STEWART S: Double outlet right ventricle. A collective review with a surgical viewpoint. J Thorac Cardiovasc Surg 71:355, 1976

Patent ductus arteriosus

FRIEDMAN WF: The patent ductus arteriosus in the newborn. Clin Perinatol 5:411, 1978

Pulmonary stenosis

MODY MR: The natural history of uncomplicated valvular pulmonary stenosis. Am Heart J 90:317, 1975

NEUGENT EW et al: Clinical course in pulmonary stenosis. Circulation 56:I-38, 1977

Supravalvular aortic stenosis

MARTIN EC, MOSELEY IF: Supravalvular aortic stenosis. Br Heart J 35:758, 1973

Tetralogy of Fallot

FINNIGAN P et al: Results of total correction of tetralogy of Fallot. Long-term hemodynamic evaluation at rest and during exercise. Br Heart J 38:934, 1976

PACIFICO AD et al: Surgical management of pulmonary stenosis in tetralogy of Fallot. J Thorac Cardiovasc Surg 74:382, 1977

Transposition of the pulmonary veins

DELISLE G et al: Total anomalous pulmonary venous connection: Report of 93 autopsy cases with emphasis on diagnostic and surgical considerations. Am Heart J 91:99, 1976

Tricuspid atresia

WILLIAMS WG et al: Tricuspid atresia: Results of treatment in 160 children. Am J Cardiol 38:235, 1976

Truncus arteriosus

MARCELETTI C et al: The natural history of truncus arteriosus. Circulation 54:108, 1976

Ventricular septal defect

WIEDMAN WH et al: Clinical course in ventricular septal defect. Natural history study. Circulation 56:I-56, 1977

241
RHEUMATIC FEVER

GENE H. STOLLERMAN

DEFINITION Rheumatic fever is an inflammatory disease which occurs as a delayed sequel to pharyngeal infection with group A streptococci. It involves principally the heart, joints, central nervous system, skin, and subcutaneous tissues. The usual manifestations in the acute form are migratory polyarthritis, fever, and carditis. Sydenham's chorea, subcutaneous nodules, and erythema marginatum may occur as other typical manifestations. No single symptom, sign, or laboratory test is pathognomonic of rheumatic fever, although several combinations of them are diagnostic. Although the name *acute rheumatic fever* emphasizes involvement of the joints, rheumatic fever owes its importance to the involvement of the heart, which can be fatal during the acute stage of the disease or can lead to rheumatic heart disease, a chronic condition due to scarring and deformity of the heart valves.

ETIOLOGY AND PATHOGENESIS The etiologic relationship of group A streptococci to rheumatic fever can be summarized briefly, as follows. (1) Numerous clinical and epidemiologic studies have shown a close association of group A streptococcal infections and rheumatic fever. (2) Antecedent streptococcal infection can almost always be demonstrated immunologically in the acute stage of rheumatic fever by increased titers of antibodies to streptococcal antigens. Moreover, in long-term prospective follow-up studies, rheumatic fever recurs only as a result of intercurrent streptococcal infections. (3) Both primary and secondary attacks of the disease can be prevented by prompt treatment or prevention of streptococcal infections with antimicrobial therapy. The pharyngeal route of infection is necessary to initiate the rheumatic process. Streptococcal skin infections do not do so. Furthermore, throat infections with some group A strains appear to produce rheumatic fever rarely or not at all.

The mechanism by which the group A streptococcus initiates the disease process remains unknown. A relatively small percentage of persons who suffer from streptococcal sore throats subsequently develops rheumatic fever. The organism is not demonstrable in the lesions when rheumatic fever appears several days or weeks after the acute streptococcal infection. No one product of the streptococcus has been incriminated as a cause of the lesions, either as a direct tissue toxin or as an antigen inducing hypersensitivity. Gamma globulin has been demonstrated by fluorescent antibody methods to be deposited in the sarcolemma of myocardial fibers of patients who have died of rheumatic carditis and in the biopsied auricular appendages of patients operated upon for mitral stenosis. Also streptococcal membrane antigens have been purified which cross-react immunologically with myocardial sarcolemma. Furthermore, patients with rheumatic carditis or chronic rheumatic heart disease often have circulating antibodies to heart tissue. This finding has led to the suggestion that the myocardial lesions of rheumatic fever are the result of some form of autoimmunity induced by streptococcal antigens. The validity of this concept has not been confirmed, however, since the immunologic phenomena might be secondary to cardiac tissue damage rather than a cause of it.

INCIDENCE AND EPIDEMIOLOGY Although rheumatic fever may occur at any age, it is extremely rare in infancy; it appears most commonly between the ages of 5 and 15 years, when streptococcal infection is most frequent and intense. Similarly, the geographic distribution, incidence, and severity of rheumatic fever are, in general, a reflection of the frequency and severity of streptococcal disease. The attack rate of rheumatic fever following exudative streptococcal pharyngitis in epidemics averages approximately 3 percent. When streptococcal pharyngitis is sporadic and mild or due to strains of lesser rheumatic potential, the attack rate of rheumatic fever may be very much lower. Two important variables of streptococcal infection which influence the attack rate of rheumatic fever have been emphasized: (1) the duration of throat carriage of group A streptococci during convalescence from the pharyngeal infection, and (2) the magnitude of the immune response to the antecedent streptococcal infection.

Environmental, bacterial, and host factors which appear to play a role in the development of rheumatic fever are important primarily as they are related to the incidence and severity of preceding streptococcal infection. Such factors as latitude, altitude, crowding, dampness, economic factors, and age all affect the incidence of rheumatic fever because they are related to the incidence of streptococcal infection in general.

The attack rate of rheumatic fever following streptococcal infections in patients who have had previous attacks of rheumatic fever is increased to as high as 5 to 50 percent and is also related to the virulence of the reactivating infection. Furthermore, the frequency of rheumatic recurrences following streptococcal infection is consistently greater in those with rheumatic heart disease than in those who escaped cardiac injury during prior attacks. The tendency to suffer recurrences of rheumatic fever following streptococcal infections declines with the passage of years since the preceding attack. It appears, therefore, that certain host variables, as well as probable qualitative and quantitative differences in the nature of the antecedent streptococcal infection, also influence the development of rheumatic fever. To what extent such variables are genetic or acquired has not been settled. It is common to obtain a family history of rheumatic fever as well as to encounter multiple cases among siblings of a single family. However, the concordance of rheumatic fever in identical twins is approximately 20 percent, which does not exceed that of poliomyelitis or tuberculosis, suggesting only a limited penetrance of genetic predisposition to rheumatic fever.

The mortality of acute rheumatic fever has been declining steadily for the past 30 years. It is still, however, a major cause of death and disability in children and adolescents. Rheumatic fever also remains a common cause of heart disease in patients below the age of 40, and is second only to hypertension and arteriosclerosis as a cause of heart disease in the older age groups. It is generally believed that the incidence of rheumatic fever, like that of streptococcal sore throat and scarlet fever, has been decreasing for several years in countries where housing and economic conditions have been improving steadily. The rate of decrease may have been accelerated by the wide use of antimicrobial therapy. The decrease also may be due to a change in the prevalence of rheumatogenic streptococcal strains. Rheumatic fever remains, however, a worldwide disease having its greatest incidence wherever poor economic conditions, overcrowding, and substandard housing are most common.

PATHOLOGY The lesions of rheumatic fever are disseminated widely throughout the body, with special predilection for connective tissues. Focal inflammatory lesions occur particularly around small blood vessels.

Cardiovascular lesions The heart is the site of the most characteristic and consequential involvement, and all its layers—endocardium, myocardium, and pericardium—may be involved. This generalized involvement gives rise to the term *rheumatic pancarditis.* The most characteristic and specific pattern of rheumatic inflammation is found in the *myocardial Aschoff body,* a submiliary granuloma. This lesion, when present in its classic form, is generally considered to be pathognomonic of rheumatic fever. In many areas the inflammatory lesion is accompanied by swelling and fragmentation of the collagen fibers and alteration in the staining properties of the ground substances of the connective tissues. This change is described as *fibrinoid degeneration of collagen,* but its chemical basis has not been established. Aschoff bodies with less exudative and more productive changes may persist for many years as the lingering traces of chronic rheumatic inflammation in patients with rheumatic heart disease, long after rheumatic fever has become clinically quiescent. The persistence of such lesions is most common in patients who develop severe mitral stenosis. Eventually the Aschoff body is converted into a spindle-shaped or triangular scar lying between the muscle bundles and surrounding blood vessels.

Rheumatic endocarditis produces the verrucous valvulitis of acute rheumatic fever which leads to the most serious permanent cardiac damage. It may heal with fibrous thickening and adhesion of the valve commissures and chordae tendineae, leading to variable degrees of valvular regurgitation and stenosis. Deformity resulting in functional impairment of the heart occurs most commonly in the mitral and aortic valves, less frequently in the tricuspid, and almost never in the pulmonic valves. *Rheumatic pericarditis* (Chap. 249) produces a serofibrinous effusion, with the deposit of shaggy elements of fibrin on the surface of the heart. The pericardium may become calcified, but pericardial constriction does not occur.

Extracardiac lesions Involvement of the *joints* is characterized by exudative rather than proliferative changes, and healing of these structures occurs without significant scarring or deformity. *Subcutaneous nodules,* seen during the acute phase of the disease, are composed of granulomas with localized areas of "fibrinoid" swelling of subcutaneous collagen bundles, and perivascular collections of large cells with pale nuclei and prominent nucleoli. Synovitis is usually mild and nonspecific. *Pulmonary* and *pleural* lesions are less definite and less characteristic. Fibrinous pleurisy and rheumatic pneumonitis may occur with exudative and proliferative lesions but without definite Aschoff bodies. Patients with active *chorea* rarely die. The pathologic findings which have been reported in the central nervous system are not consistent, and no characteristic lesion has been reported to explain this clinical manifestation. During active chorea the spinal fluid remains normal, being free of cells, with no increase in total protein and no change in the relative concentration of various proteins.

CLINICAL FEATURES The major clinical manifestations by which rheumatic fever can be recognized are polyarthritis, carditis, chorea, erythema marginatum, and subcutaneous nodules.

Arthritis The classic attack of rheumatic fever appears as an acute migratory polyarthritis accompanied by signs and symptoms of an acute febrile illness. The large joints of the extremities are most frequently affected, but no joint is impervious to the inflammatory process; one may find arthritis of the hands and feet but only rarely of the spine or of the sternoclavicular or temporomandibular joints. Joint effusions occur but are not persistent. As pain and swelling subside in one joint, others tend to become involved. Although such "migratory" involvement is characteristic, it is not invariable, and several large joints may be inflamed at one time. To be acceptable as a criterion for the diagnosis of rheumatic fever, the polyarthritis should involve two or more joints, should be associated with at least two minor manifestations such as fever and elevation of sedimentation rate, and should be associated with high titer of anti-streptolysin O or some other streptococcal antibody (Table 241-1).

Acute rheumatic carditis Acute rheumatic carditis first manifests itself by the appearance of the heart murmurs of either mitral or aortic regurgitation, the former most frequently. Signs and symptoms of pericarditis and of congestive heart failure may supervene in more severe cases. Death may result from heart failure during the acute stage of the disease, or permanent valvular damage may be sustained which results ultimately in serious disability. Carditis may vary from a fulminating, fatal course to a low-grade, inapparent inflammation. *It is well to bear in mind that the vast majority of patients with carditis do not have symptoms referable to the heart.* The latter occur only in more severe cases when heart failure or pericardial effusions produce characteristic symptoms. For this reason, unless extracardiac manifestations, such as polyarthritis and chorea, are present, patients whose rheumatic fever is manifested only by carditis are frequently not diagnosed and in later life may be discovered to have rheumatic heart disease without a definite history of rheumatic fever.

When carditis is manifest, there is usually tachycardia disproportionate to the degree of fever, gallop rhythms are often

TABLE 241-1
Jones criteria (revised)

Major manifestations	Minor manifestations
Carditis	Fever
Polyarthritis	Arthralgia
Chorea	Previous rheumatic fever or rheumatic heart disease
Erythema marginatum	Elevated ESR or positive CRP
Subcutaneous nodules	Prolonged PR interval

Plus supporting evidence of preceding streptococcal infection: history of recent scarlet fever; positive throat culture for group A streptococcus; increased ASO titer or other streptococcal antibodies.

SOURCE: *American Heart Association, 1965.*

heard, and the heart sounds may become fetal or "tic-tac" in quality. Occasionally, arrhythmias and/or a pericardial friction rub may be present. Prolongation of the conduction time may lead to dropped beats with varying degrees of heart block. Prolongation of the PR interval and other changes in the electrocardiogram are very common, but these findings, in the absence of clinical manifestations of carditis, have a benign prognosis. Therefore, changes in the electrocardiogram alone, unassociated with significant murmurs or cardiac enlargement, do not by themselves constitute an acceptable criterion for the diagnosis of rheumatic carditis. Pericarditis may cause precordial pain, and a friction rub may be audible.

A definite clinical diagnosis of carditis can be made if one or more of the following can be demonstrated: (1) the appearance of, or change in the character of, organic heart murmurs; (2) definite increase in heart size demonstrated by radiogram or fluoroscopy; (3) pericardial friction rub or effusion; or (4) signs of congestive heart failure. Rheumatic carditis is almost always associated with a significant murmur.

Subcutaneous nodules These are usually small, pea-sized, painless swellings over bony prominences and therefore frequently go unnoticed by the patient. The skin moves freely over them. Characteristic locations are the extensor tendons of the hands and feet, the elbows, margins of the patellae, the scalp, over the scapulae, and over the spinous processes of the vertebrae.

Chorea (Sydenham's chorea, chorea minor, Saint Vitus' dance) This is a disorder of the central nervous system characterized by sudden, aimless, irregular movements, often accompanied by muscle weakness and emotional instability. Chorea is a delayed manifestation of rheumatic fever, and other manifestations may or may not still be present at the time it appears. Polyarthritis, when part of the same attack, always subsides before chorea appears. Carditis is often discovered for the first time when the presenting feature of rheumatic fever is chorea. Chorea may appear after a long latent period (up to several months) from the antecedent streptococcal infection and at a time when all other manifestations of rheumatic fever have abated. When no previous rheumatic manifestations are noted, such cases are called *pure chorea.*

The clinical onset of chorea is often gradual. Patients may be unusually nervous and fidgety and may have difficulty in writing, drawing, and handiwork. They may stumble or fall, drop things, and grimace. As symptoms become more severe, spasmodic movements extend to all parts of the body, and muscular weakness may become so marked that patients cannot walk, talk, or sit up. Often the weakness is severe enough to simulate paralysis. The irregular, jerky, spasmodic movements may become so violent that cribs and beds must be padded to prevent injury. Symptoms are exaggerated by excitement, effort, or fatigue but subside during sleep. Emotional instability is almost invariable in patients with chorea, and it is thought by some that emotional trauma may precipitate the disorder. All degrees of speech disturbance are seen.

Erythema marginatum This evanescent pink rash is characteristic of rheumatic fever. The erythematous areas often have clear centers and round or serpiginous margins. They vary greatly in size and occur mainly on the trunk and proximal part of the extremities, never on the face. The erythema is transient, migratory, and may be brought out by the application of heat; it is nonpruritic, not indurated, and blanches on pressure.

Minor clinical criteria These are clinical features which occur frequently in rheumatic fever but are also common to many other diseases and are therefore of minor diagnostic value. They include fever, arthralgia, abdominal pain, tachycardia, and epistaxis.

LABORATORY FINDINGS   There is no specific laboratory test to indicate the presence of rheumatic fever. The appraisal of rheumatic activity by laboratory findings is, however, of value, since various tests may indicate *continued* rheumatic inflammation when clinical features are not apparent.

Streptococcal antibody tests to disclose preceding streptococcal infection   Streptococcal antibody titers differentiate preceding streptococcal from other acute respiratory infections and are increased following asymptomatic as well as symptomatic streptococcal infections. These antibody levels are increased in the early stages of acute rheumatic fever. They may be declining, or low, if the interval between the acute streptococcal infection and the detection of rheumatic fever has been longer than 2 months, a situation which occurs most often in patients whose presenting rheumatic manifestation is chorea. However, patients whose only major manifestation is rheumatic carditis also may have low antibody titers when first seen. Their rheumatic attack may have been in progress several months before becoming symptomatic and recognized. Except in these two instances, *one should be reluctant to make the diagnosis of acute rheumatic fever in the absence of serologic evidence of a recent streptococcal infection.* The anti-streptolysin O test (ASO) is the most widely used and best-standardized streptococcal antibody test. In general, single titers of at least 250 Todd units in adults and at least 333 units in children over 5 years of age are considered to be increased. Depending on the general prevalence of streptococcal infections, a varying percentage of the normal population may show titers of this magnitude.

About 20 percent of patients in the early stages of acute rheumatic fever, and most patients who present with chorea, have a low or borderline ASO titer. In these instances, it is advisable to obtain another streptococcal antibody test. Other streptococcal antibody tests that can be employed include the following: antihyaluronidase (AH), antideoxyribonucleotidase B (anti-DNase B), antinicotinamide-adenine dinucleotidase (anti-NADase), and anti-streptokinase (ASK). The anti-streptozyme test (ASTZ) is a hemagglutination reaction to a concentrate of extracellular streptococcal antigens absorbed to red blood cells. It is a very sensitive indicator of recent streptococcal infection; virtually all patients with acute rheumatic fever have titers greater than 200 units per milliliter. The real value of the ASTZ test is in *ruling out* rheumatic fever when the titer is low in patients with isolated polyarthritis. To date, the specific antigens involved in the ASTZ test remain unidentified and therefore the test has not yet been adequately standardized. A rise in titer of two dilution tubes or more can be demonstrated for at least one of the streptococcal antibodies in almost all recurrent as well as primary attacks of rheumatic fever (Table 241-2). Increased streptococcal antibodies, however, do not reflect rheumatic activity per se, and their rate of decline is independent of the course of the rheumatic attack.

Isolation of group A streptococci   Some patients continue to harbor group A streptococci at the onset of acute rheumatic fever, but these organisms are usually present in small numbers and may be difficult to isolate by a single throat culture. The administration of penicillin or other antibodies may also result in failure to isolate the infecting organism. In addition, a significant number of *normal* individuals, particularly children, may harbor group A streptococci in the upper respiratory tract. For these reasons, throat cultures are less satisfactory than antibody tests as supporting evidence of recent streptococcal infection.

Acute phase reactants   These tests offer objective but nonspecific confirmation of the presence of an inflammatory process. *The erythrocyte sedimentation rate* (ESR) and the test for *C-reactive protein* (CRP) in serum are used most commonly. Unless the patient has received corticosteroids or salicylates, these reactions are almost always abnormal in patients presenting with polyarthritis or acute carditis, whereas they are often normal in patients with chorea. Other laboratory findings which reflect inflammation include reactions such as leukocytosis, and increases in serum complement, mucoproteins, and α_2 and gamma globulins. Prolongation of the PR interval of the electrocardiogram, although neither specific for rheumatic fever nor diagnostic of serious cardiac involvement, is frequent in acute rheumatic fever (about 25 percent of all cases), and other nonspecific electrocardiographic changes are also common. Anemia, due to the suppression of erythropoiesis characteristic of chronic inflammatory diseases, is another feature of rheumatic activity.

COURSE AND PROGNOSIS   The course of rheumatic fever varies greatly and is impossible to predict at the onset of the disease. In general, however, approximately 75 percent of acute rheumatic attacks subside within 6 weeks, 90 percent within 12 weeks, and less than 5 percent persist more than 6 months. The latter usually consist of severe, intractable forms of rheumatic carditis or stubborn, prolonged attacks of Sydenham's chorea, both of which may persist for as long as several years. Once acute rheumatic fever has subsided and more than 2 months have elapsed after withdrawal of treatment with salicylates or adrenal corticosteroids, rheumatic fever does not recur in the absence of new streptococcal infections. Recurrences are most common within the first 5 years of the initial attack and tend to decline with increasing duration of freedom from rheumatic activity. The frequency of recurrences is dependent upon the frequency and severity of streptococcal infection, the presence or absence of rheumatic heart disease following an attack, and the duration of freedom from the last attack.

Approximately 70 percent of patients who develop carditis do so within the first week of the disease, 85 percent within the first 12 weeks of the disease, and almost all within 6 months from the onset of the acute attack. Thereafter, if significant murmurs have not appeared, the prognosis for a patient in whom recurrences are prevented is excellent.

Chronic rheumatic carditis and the course of rheumatic heart disease   The remarkable variability in the course of rheumatic carditis and rheumatic valvular disease stems from sev-

TABLE 241-2
Serologic results in patients with streptococcal disease

| Patient group (no.) | Percent of patients whose serums were "positive" | | | | |
	ASO	AH	Anti-DNase B	At least 1 of 3	ASTZ
Acute rheumatic fever (20)	90	65	85	95	100
Acute glomerulonephritis (22)	50	63	72	91	95
Convalescent pharyngitis (11)	81	54	54	91	91
Convalescent pyoderma (23)	35	35	91	96	91
Total (76)	61	54	79	93	95

SOURCE: *AL Bisno, I Ofek, Am J Dis Child 127:676, 1974.*

eral factors: (1) the variability in the duration and severity of the rheumatic inflammation; (2) the amount of scarring of the valves and myocardium following the abatement of the acute inflammation; (3) the location and severity of the hemodynamic lesion due to valvular insufficiency or stenosis; (4) the frequency of recurrent bouts of carditis; and (5) the progression of valvular calcification and sclerosis, which occurs as a secondary phenomenon in a deformed or injured valve without recurrent or persistent rheumatic inflammation (as seen in congenital valvular disease or following healed acute bacterial endocarditis). These factors, and possibly others not yet appreciated, produce striking variations in the clinical syndromes of rheumatic heart disease.

Chronic rheumatic myocarditis   In this syndrome, the presenting picture is one of chronic heart failure in a patient with a markedly dilated heart and with physical, roentgenographic, and electrocardiographic findings of mitral regurgitation. The differentiation of this syndrome from other forms of chronic myocarditis may be very difficult, if not impossible, when the associated extracardiac features of rheumatic fever (chorea, polyarthritis, and so forth) are not present. Although rheumatic fever does not produce *isolated* myocarditis, and is almost invariably a pancarditis, the pericardial inflammation may not be clearly evident, and the mitral valvulitis may not be distinguishable from mitral regurgitation due to dilation of the mitral ring. In such cases one must search diligently for an evanescent friction rub, evidence of pericardial effusion, appearance of a soft aortic regurgitation murmur, and extracardiac clues such as fever responding promptly to salicylates, arthralgias, transient subcutaneous nodules, evanescent erythema marginatum, and subtle signs of chorea.

The course of chronic rheumatic carditis may be intractable and end fatally after months or even several years. Often, however, the patient improves rather suddenly and even recovers cardiac reserve dramatically in association with the disappearance of systemic manifestations of the inflammatory process. The heart may remain large, may decrease somewhat in size, or in occasional instances may return to normal size with varying degrees of residual valvular deformity. Such a course signals the termination of the "toxic" phase of the rheumatic process, and thereafter the course of rheumatic heart disease depends on the variables in healing cited above.

DIFFERENTIAL DIAGNOSIS   Early cases of rheumatic fever may be confused with other diseases which begin with acute polyarthritis. It is wise to exclude *bacteremia* by blood cultures, particularly because such infections may be masked by penicillin given for presumed acute rheumatic fever. Polyarthritis due to *infective endocarditis* in a patient with preexisting rheumatic heart disease may be mistaken for a recurrence of acute rheumatic fever. If streptococcal antibodies are not increased, polyarthritis should be attributed to some cause other than rheumatic fever. Gonococcal polyarthritis may be distinguished from rheumatic fever by the dramatic response of the former to a therapeutic trial of penicillin. In rheumatoid arthritis, joint involvement will persist and characteristic joint deformities may appear. The latter are not seen in rheumatic fever. The rheumatoid factor so characteristic of rheumatoid arthritis is not present in rheumatic fever. Lupus erythematosus cells and antibodies against nuclear components are absent in rheumatic fever. Rheumatic pericarditis and myocarditis, associated with cardiac enlargement and heart failure, are both almost invariably associated with valvular lesions which produce significant murmurs.

Overdiagnosis of rheumatic fever should be avoided. Unless ill-defined febrile syndromes are clearly associated with a ma-

jor manifestation of rheumatic fever, the diagnosis of rheumatic fever should not be made. A common error is the premature, vigorous administration of corticosteroids or salicylates before the signs and symptoms of rheumatic fever are unmistakable. In the absence of a curative agent, one should not suppress the signs and symptoms of rheumatic fever until they are clearly expressed.

Particularly confusing in the differential diagnosis of rheumatic fever is the drug sensitivity with fever and polyarthritis which may occur after administration of penicillin for a previous pharyngitis. Urticaria or angioneurotic edema, if present, helps differentiate penicillin sensitivity in such cases. The abdominal pain of rheumatic fever may be mistaken for appendicitis, and the crisis of sickle-cell anemia may also be associated with joint pain, enlargement of the heart, and cardiac murmurs. The rapidity with which the arthritis symptoms of rheumatic fever are controlled with salicylates is characteristic of this disease. Dramatic response to salicylates does not in itself, however, establish a diagnosis of rheumatic fever.

In order to help clarify the diagnosis of rheumatic fever, the American Heart Association has accepted and modified criteria usually referred to as the *Jones criteria* (Table 241-1). They are not to be used as a substitute for good medical judgment but are recommended as a guide for careful study of questionable cases. The finding of two major criteria, or of one major and two minor criteria, indicates a high probability of the presence of rheumatic fever if supported by evidence of a preceding streptococcal infection. The absence of the latter should always make the diagnosis questionable, except in the situation in which rheumatic fever is first discovered after a long latent period from the antecedent infection (Sydenham's chorea or low-grade carditis). Because the prognosis may differ according to the major manifestations, for recording purposes the diagnosis of rheumatic fever should be followed by a list of the major manifestations present, e.g., rheumatic fever manifested by polyarthritis and carditis. An indication of the severity of carditis in terms of presence or absence of congestive heart failure and cardiomegaly is also advisable.

TREATMENT   There is no specific cure for rheumatic fever, and no known measures change the course of the attack. Good supportive therapy, however, can reduce the mortality and morbidity of the disease.

Chemotherapy   After rheumatic fever is first diagnosed, a course of penicillin should be given to eliminate group A streptococci. This is advisable even if bacteriologic examination yields throat cultures negative for streptococci, since the organisms may be present in areas inaccessible to swabs. It is preferable to administer penicillin parenterally. An effective course is a single injection of 1.2 million units of benzathine penicillin intramuscularly or 600,000 units of procaine penicillin intramuscularly daily for 10 days. Attempts to reduce ultimate heart damage by administering penicillin early in the acute rheumatic attack in larger doses have not been successful. After completion of the therapeutic course of penicillin, continuous protection from reinfection with streptococci should be provided by instituting one of the prophylactic regimens described below.

Suppressive therapy   For patients without carditis treatment with adrenal corticosteroids is unnecessary. Acute arthritis can be relieved with codeine or with salicylate, the latter being preferable to reduce fever and joint inflammation. When salicylate is used in the therapy of rheumatic fever, the dosage should be increased until the drug produces either a clinical effect or systemic toxicity characterized by tinnitus, headache, or hypernea. A starting daily dose of 15 to 20 mg/kg in children and 6 to 8 g in adults given in four or five divided doses is recommended. Of the various salicylate preparations ordinary aspirin is cheapest and most effective. Gastric intolerance can usually be diminished by administering aspirin after meals or by giving antacids 15 to 30 min after each dose of aspirin.

Many physicians prefer corticosteroids to salicylates for the treatment of carditis, despite the lack of a demonstrated advantage of these adrenal hormones in controlled clinical trials. Corticosteroids are more potent anti-inflammatory agents but are more likely to be followed by posttherapeutic "rebounds," and they have the additional disadvantage of more frequent side effects, particularly acne, hirsutism, and cushingoid changes in facies and habitus. For this reason it is preferable to begin treatment of patients who have carditis with salicylates; if these drugs fail to reduce fever and to ameliorate heart failure, therapy with corticosteroids may be initiated promptly. Prednisone is administered in doses of 60 to 120 mg or higher when necessary in four divided doses daily. After the inflammation has been brought under control by either salicylates or corticosteroids, treatment should be continued until the sedimentation rate approaches near-normal values and should be maintained for several weeks thereafter. To prevent poststeroid rebounds, an "overlap" course of salicylate therapy may be added when steroids are tapered off over a 2-week period. A useful method for tapering steroids is outlined in Chap. 336. Salicylates may then be continued for an additional 2 to 3 weeks. Rebounds of rheumatic activity are usually of short duration and, when mild, are best managed without resuming anti-inflammatory treatment, because a second or even a third rebound may occur when suppressive therapy is discontinued. About 5 percent of rheumatic attacks persist for 8 months or longer, either in the form of spontaneous acute recrudescences or as posttherapeutic rebounds. These "chronic" attacks are most likely to occur in patients with cardiac damage and with previous rheumatic episodes. Weekly tests for C-reactive protein in blood and for erythrocyte sedimentation rate are useful in following the healing process, particularly while treatment with corticosteroids or salicylates is gradually withdrawn.

Treatment of chorea The signs and symptoms of chorea usually do not respond well to treatment with antirheumatic agents. Because the patient with chorea is frequently emotionally unstable and because the manifestations of chorea may be exaggerated by emotional trauma, complete mental and physical rest is essential. Patients with chorea should be kept in a quiet room and cared for by sympathetic attendants. Corticosteroids or salicylates have little or no effect on chorea. Sedatives and tranquilizers, particularly diazepam and chlorpromazine, are useful. If the chorea is severe, large doses of phenobarbital rather than tranquilizers alone are usually necessary to control purposeless movements. Padded sideboards for the bed may be necessary to avoid injury to the patient. In the absence of other evidence of acute rheumatic disease, it is advisable to allow gradual resumption of physical activity when improvement is apparent rather than waiting for all choreiform movements to disappear, which may require many months.

Because of the great variability in the course of chorea, evaluating the effectiveness of various therapeutic measures is difficult. It is well to remember that chorea is a self-limited disease which is usually not followed by significant neurologic sequelae and that good results are almost invariably obtained by patient, attentive nursing care and by conservative medical management.

PREVENTION OF RECURRENCE The most efficient regimen for continuous prophylaxis against group A streptococci is a monthly intramuscular injection of 1.2 million units of benzathine penicillin. The disadvantages and discomfort of this regimen have to be weighed against the individual patient's susceptibility to recurrences. Those with rheumatic heart disease, recent rheumatic fever, and exposure to an environment in which the incidence of streptococcal infection is frequent deserve the most effective protection. As a second choice, prophylaxis may be administered orally with either 1 g sulfadiazine daily in a single dose or 200,000 units of penicillin given twice daily on an empty stomach. The duration of continuous prophylaxis cannot be fixed arbitrarily for all patients, although the safest generalization is that it be continued indefinitely. Certainly, those under the age of 18 years should receive a continuous prophylactic regimen. A minimum period of 5 years is recommended for patients who develop rheumatic fever without carditis over the age of 18 years. The decision to continue prophylaxis beyond this period should take into account a number of variables. Patients with rheumatic heart disease are more susceptible to reactivation of rheumatic fever if they contract a streptococcal infection. Moreover, patients who have had carditis in a previous attack are much more likely to suffer carditis again in a subsequent attack. Climate, age, occupation, household situation, cardiac status, and length of time since the previous attack are all significant variables which influence the risk of recurrence. The decline in recurrence rates with increasing age is due to (1) decreased rate of streptococcal infection and (2) decrease in the rate of rheumatic reactivation following streptococcal infection in older rheumatic subjects. Despite this decreased rate, however, the risk of rheumatic recurrence in adults remains relatively high when the streptococcal disease encountered is severe or epidemic.

PREVENTION OF INITIAL RHEUMATIC ATTACKS Early and adequate treatment of pharyngeal infection due to group A streptococci will prevent initial attacks of rheumatic fever. If clinical streptococcal disease were properly detected by throat cultures and adequately treated, the spread of infection in a given population would be prevented, the epidemiology of streptococcal disease would be modified markedly, and the incidence of rheumatic fever in the community would be diminished. In communities where group A streptococcal disease has been diagnosed early and treated well and where socioeconomic standards are high, the group A organisms cultured frequently from schoolchildren's throats may be of relatively low virulence and may cause rheumatic fever less frequently than do more virulent strains prevalent in many epidemics.

Streptococcal pharyngitis is adequately treated by a single intramuscular injection of 600,000 units of benzathine penicillin in children less than 10 years of age or 1.2 million units in older children and adults. Any alternate plan of parenteral therapy or combined parenteral and oral therapy should provide for treatment over a period of 10 days. If oral penicillin is employed, at least 800,000 units per day in four divided doses must be given for no less than 10 days to achieve results comparable with a single injection of benzathine penicillin. Erythromycin in daily doses of 1 g for 10 days may be substituted in penicillin-sensitive individuals. Tetracycline is not recommended because some strains of group A streptococci have acquired resistance to it. All group A streptococci have so far remained extremely sensitive to penicillin.

REFERENCES

AHA COMMITTEE ON RHEUMATIC FEVER AND BACTERIAL ENDOCARDITIS: Prevention of rheumatic fever. Circulation 55:1, 1977

AMERICAN HEART ASSOCIATION: Jones criteria (revised) for guidance in the diagnosis of rheumatic fever. Circulation 32:664, 1965

JOINT REPORT OF UK-US COOPERATIVE STUDY: The natural history of rheumatic fever and rheumatic heart disease. 10 year report of a cooperative clinical trial of ACTH, cortisone and aspirin. Circulation 32:457, 1965

READ S, ZABRISKIE JB (eds): *Streptococcal Disease and the Immune Response.* New York, Rockefeller Press, 1979

STOLLERMAN GH: *Rheumatic Fever and Streptococcal Infection.* New York, Grune & Stratton, 1975

————: Rheumatic fever, connective tissue disorders and heart disease, in *Heart Disease,* E Braunwald (ed). Philadelphia, Saunders, 1980, chap 47

WANNAMAKER LW, MATSEN JM (eds): *Streptococci and Streptococcal Diseases.* New York, Academic, 1972

242
VALVULAR HEART DISEASE

EUGENE BRAUNWALD

Specific valve abnormalities are discussed in this chapter. The role of physical examination in the evaluation of patients with these lesions is considered in Chap. 231; of echocardiography, phonocardiography, and other indirect graphic techniques in Chap. 233; and of cardiac catheterization and angiography in Chap. 234.

MITRAL STENOSIS

PATHOPHYSIOLOGY In normal adults the mitral valve orifice is 4 to 6 cm^2. In the presence of significant obstruction, i.e., when the orifice is less than one-half of normal, blood can flow from the left atrium to the left ventricle only if propelled by an abnormally elevated left atrioventricular pressure gradient; such a gradient is the hemodynamic hallmark of mitral stenosis. When the mitral valve opening is reduced to 1 cm^2, a left atrial pressure of approximately 25 mmHg is required to maintain a normal cardiac output. The elevated left atrial pressure in turn raises pulmonary venous and capillary pressures, resulting in exertional dyspnea. The first bouts of dyspnea are usually precipitated by an increased rate of blood flow across the mitral orifice, which results in further elevation of the left atrial pressure. In order to assess the severity of obstruction, it is essential to measure the transvalvular pressure gradient and flow rate. The latter is dependent not only on the cardiac output but on the heart rate as well. An increase in heart rate shortens diastole proportionately more than systole, and diminishes the time available for flow across the mitral valve. Therefore, at any given level of cardiac output tachycardia augments the transvalvular gradient and elevates left atrial pressure.

The left ventricular diastolic pressure is normal in pure mitral stenosis; coexisting mitral regurgitation, aortic valve disease, the residua of damage produced by rheumatic myocarditis, systemic hypertension, or ischemic heart disease may be responsible for elevations which reflect impaired left ventricular function and/or reduced left ventricular compliance. However, left ventricular dysfunction, as reflected in reduced ejection fraction and circumferential fiber shortening rate, occurs in about one-fifth of the patients. In pure mitral stenosis and sinus rhythm, the mean left atrial and pulmonary artery wedge pressures are usually elevated and the pressure pulse shows a prominent atrial contraction (*a* wave), and a gradual pressure decline after mitral valve opening (*y* descent). In patients with mild to moderate mitral stenosis without elevation of the pulmonary vascular resistance, the pulmonary arterial pressure may be normal at rest and may rise only with exercise. However, in severe mitral stenosis and whenever the pulmonary vascular resistance is significantly increased, the pulmonary arterial pressure is elevated even when the patient is at rest, and in extreme cases it may exceed the systemic arterial pressure. Further elevations of left atrial, pulmonary capillary, and pulmonary arterial pressures occur during exercise. When the pulmonary arterial systolic pressure exceeds 60 mmHg in patients with mitral stenosis, or for that matter with any valvular lesion, the mean right atrial and right ventricular end-diastolic pressures may also be elevated; the increased right ventricular afterload impedes the emptying of this chamber, and right ventricular end-diastolic pressure and volume (preload) rise as a compensatory mechanism.

Cardiac output varies considerably in patients with mitral stenosis. Thus, the hemodynamic response to a given degree of mitral obstruction may be characterized by a normal cardiac output and a high left atrioventricular pressure gradient or, at the opposite end of the hemodynamic spectrum, by a greatly reduced cardiac output and low transvalvular pressure gradient. In a small fraction of patients with moderately severe mitral stenosis, the cardiac output is normal at rest and rises normally during exertion; under these circumstances, the high atrioventricular pressure gradient elevates the left atrial and pulmonary capillary pressures, and this elevation is responsible for symptoms of pulmonary congestion. In the majority of patients with obstruction of equal severity the cardiac output is normal at rest but rises subnormally during exertion. In patients with severe stenosis, particularly those in whom the pulmonary vascular resistance is strikingly elevated, the cardiac output is subnormal at rest and may fail to rise or may even decline during activity. The depressed cardiac output in patients with mitral stenosis is related primarily to the obstruction of the mitral orifice but may also be due to the impairment of left ventricular function which can accompany it.

The clinical and hemodynamic features of mitral stenosis are dictated largely by the level of the pulmonary artery pressure. Pulmonary hypertension results from (1) the passive backward transmission of the elevated left atrial pressure, (2) arteriolar constriction, which presumably is triggered by left atrial and pulmonary venous hypertension (reactive pulmonary hypertension), and (3) organic obliterative changes in the pulmonary vascular bed. The elevation of pulmonary vascular resistance may be considered to be a complication of longstanding and severe mitral stenosis; in time, the resultant severe pulmonary hypertension results in tricuspid and pulmonary incompetence as well as right-sided heart failure. However, the changes in the pulmonary vascular bed may also be considered to exert a protective effect; the elevated precapillary resistance reduces the likelihood of symptoms of pulmonary congestion by tending to prevent blood from surging into the pulmonary capillary bed and damming up behind the stenotic mitral valve. However, this protection is at the expense of a decreased cardiac output.

ETIOLOGY AND PATHOLOGY Mitral stenosis is generally rheumatic in origin. A history of one or more attacks of acute rheumatic fever can be elicited from approximately two-thirds of adult patients with predominant or pure mitral stenosis. The valve leaflets are diffusely thickened by fibrous tissue and/or calcific deposits. The mitral commissures fuse, the chordae tendineae fuse and shorten, the valvular cusps become rigid, and these changes in turn lead to narrowing at the apex of the funnel-shaped valve. While the initial insult to the mitral valve is rheumatic, the later changes may be a nonspecific process resulting from trauma to the valve caused by altered flow patterns. Calcification of the stenotic mitral valve results in progressive immobility of the leaflets and narrowing of the orifice. Thrombus formation and arterial embolization may arise from the calcific valve itself. Pure or predominant mitral stenosis is a common valvular abnormality following rheumatic fever, occurring in approximately 40 percent of all patients with rheumatic heart disease. Two-thirds of all patients with mitral stenosis are females. Rarely, mitral stenosis is congenital in origin (Chap. 240), most commonly the so-called "parachute" mitral valve, in which all the chordae insert into a single left ventricular papillary muscle.

SYMPTOMS In temperate climates the latent period between the initial attack of carditis and the development of symptoms due to mitral stenosis is generally long, on the order of two decades; most patients begin to experience disability in the fourth decade. Once a patient with mitral stenosis becomes seriously symptomatic, continuous progression of the disease to death usually occurs in 2 to 5 years unless the stenosis is relieved by operation. In economically deprived areas, particularly in the Indian subcontinent, Central America, and the Middle East, mitral stenosis tends to progress more rapidly and frequently causes serious symptoms before the age of 20 years. On the other hand, slowly progressive mitral stenosis in the elderly is also being recognized with increasing frequency.

When valvular obstruction is trivial, the physical signs of mitral stenosis may be present in the absence of any symptoms. However, even in those patients whose mitral orifices are large enough to accommodate a normal blood flow with only mild elevations of left atrial pressure, extreme exertion, excitement, fever, severe anemia, paroxysmal tachycardia, sexual intercourse, pregnancy, and thyrotoxicosis may precipitate elevations of pulmonary capillary pressure and lead to dyspnea and cough. As stenosis progresses, the stresses that precipitate dyspnea become less severe, and the patient becomes limited in his daily activities. Redistribution of blood from the dependent portions of the body to the lungs, which occurs when the recumbent position is assumed, leads to orthopnea and paroxysmal nocturnal dyspnea. *Pulmonary edema* develops when there is a sudden increase in flow rate across a markedly narrowed mitral orifice (Chap. 27). When moderately severe mitral stenosis has existed for several years, *atrial arrhythmias*—premature contractions, paroxysmal tachycardia, flutter, and fibrillation—tend to occur with increasing frequency. The rapid ventricular rate associated with untreated or inadequately treated atrial fibrillation is frequently responsible for acute exacerbations of dyspnea. The development of permanent atrial fibrillation often marks a turning point in the patient's course and is generally associated with acceleration of the rate at which symptoms progress.

Hemoptysis (Chap. 26) results from rupture of pulmonary-bronchial venous connections. It tends to occur most frequently in patients who have elevated left atrial pressures without markedly elevated pulmonary vascular resistances. True hemoptysis must be distinguished from the bloody sputum that occurs with pulmonary edema, pulmonary infarction, and bronchitis, three conditions that occur with increased frequency in the presence of mitral stenosis. This complication is almost never fatal.

When the pulmonary vascular resistance rises or when tricuspid stenosis or regurgitation develops, symptoms secondary to pulmonary congestion may diminish, and the episodes of acute pulmonary edema and hemoptysis become reduced in frequency and severity. Elevation of pulmonary vascular resistance further increases right ventricular systolic pressure, ultimately leading to right ventricular failure, fatigue, weakness, abdominal discomfort due to hepatic congestion, and ankle edema (Chap. 236).

Recurrent pulmonary emboli with infarction (Chap. 266) are an important cause of morbidity and mortality late in the course of mitral stenosis, occurring most frequently in patients with right ventricular failure and markedly elevated pulmonary vascular resistance. *Pulmonary infections,* i.e., bronchitis, bronchopneumonia, and lobar pneumonia, commonly complicate untreated mitral stenosis. *Infective endocarditis* (Chap. 243) is rare in pure mitral stenosis but is not uncommon in patients with combined stenosis and regurgitation. *Chest pain* occurs in about 10 percent of patients with severe mitral stenosis; it may be due to pulmonary hypertension, myocardial ischemia secondary to coronary embolization or coronary atherosclerosis; most often the cause cannot be discovered despite careful investigation.

In addition to the aforementioned changes in the pulmonary vascular bed, extensive fibrosis of the alveolar walls and thickening of pulmonary capillary walls occur commonly in mitral stenosis. The vital capacity, total lung capacity, maximal breathing capacity, and oxygen uptake per unit of ventilation are reduced, and in patients with severe stenosis the latter fails to rise normally during exertion. There is uneven distribution of blood flow and ventilation, resulting in physiological dead space. As in other conditions in which left atrial pressure is elevated, pulmonary blood flow in the erect position is displaced from the basal to the superior segments of the lung (Chap. 255). The diffusing capacity may be reduced, particularly during exertion, as a result of structural changes in the diffusing surface and reduction of the pulmonary capillary blood volume. The reduction of pulmonary compliance that occurs generally correlates directly with the severity of the dyspnea and inversely with the left atrial pressure, and these changes are intensified during exercise. In some patients airway resistance is abnormally increased.

The changes in the lungs are due, in part, to increased transudation of fluid from the pulmonary capillaries into the interstitial and alveolar spaces as a consequence of the elevated pulmonary capillary pressure. A combination of the above-mentioned alterations in pulmonary function, particularly the diminution of pulmonary compliance, contributes to the increase of respiratory work and plays an important role in the genesis of dyspnea in mitral stenosis. However, the thickening of the alveolar and capillary walls tends to impede the transudation of fluid into the alveoli and the development of pulmonary edema at times when the pulmonary capillary pressure exceeds the plasma oncotic pressure. The increased capacity of the pulmonary lymphatic system to drain excess fluid also retards the development of pulmonary edema.

Thrombi may form in the left atria, particularly in the enlarged atrial appendages of patients with mitral stenosis. When they embolize, they do so to the systemic vessels, most commonly the brain, kidneys, spleen, and extremities. This complication occurs much more frequently in patients with atrial fibrillation or unstable rhythms, in older patients, and in those with a reduced cardiac output. However, it is not particularly more common in patients with extremely severe mitral valve obstruction than in those with only moderate degrees of obstruction; hence systemic embolization may be the presenting complaint in otherwise asymptomatic patients with mild mitral stenosis. At operation, thrombi are not found more frequently in the left atria of patients with past history of embolization than in those without this complication, indicating that it is usually the freshly formed clots that break off. Patients who have had one or more systemic emboli are more likely to have further embolic episodes than are patients with stenosis of comparable severity without previous embolization. Rarely, a large pedunculated thrombus or a free-floating clot may suddenly obstruct the stenotic mitral orifice. Such "ball valve" thrombi produce syncope, angina, and changing auscultatory signs with alterations in position, findings that resemble those produced by a left atrial myxoma (Chap. 248).

PHYSICAL FINDINGS (See also Chap. 231) Peripheral and facial *cyanosis* may occur in patients with extremely severe mitral stenosis. In advanced cases there is a malar flush and the facies appear pinched and blue. The jugular venous pulse reveals prominent *a* waves due to vigorous right atrial systole in patients with sinus rhythm who have associated tricuspid stenosis or severe pulmonary hypertension. When atrial fibrillation is present, the jugular pulse reveals only a single expansion during systole (*c-v* wave). The systemic arterial pressure is usually normal or slightly low. The heart generally presents a right ventricular tap along the left sternal border, signifying an enlarged right ventricle. The first heart sound may be palpable in patients with pliable valve leaflets. In patients with associated pulmonary hypertension, the impact of pulmonary valve closure can usually be felt in the second and third left intercostal spaces just to the left of the sternum; the left ventricle is not palpable in severe, pure mitral stenosis. A diastolic thrill may frequently be felt at the cardiac apex, particularly if the patient is turned into the left lateral recumbent position. The apex cardiogram (Chap. 233) reveals a slow rate of left ventricular filling during early diastole; when a rapid left ventricular filling phase is present, either mitral stenosis is very mild or there is associated mitral or aortic regurgitation.

On *auscultation*, the first heart sound is generally accentuated and snapping, and since the mitral valve does not close until the left ventricular pressure reaches the level of the elevated left atrial pressure, this sound is often slightly delayed, particularly in patients with severe stenosis. In patients with pulmonary hypertension, the pulmonary component of the second heart sound is often accentuated, and the two components of the second heart sound are closely split. A pulmonary systolic ejection click is heard commonly in patients with severe pulmonary hypertension and extensive dilatation of the pulmonary artery. The opening snap of the mitral valve is most readily audible in expiration at, or just medial to, the cardiac apex but may also be easily heard along the left sternal edge or at the base of the heart. This sound generally follows the sound of aortic valve closure by 0.06 to 0.12 s, that is, after the pulmonic valve closure sound. Since the opening snap of the mitral valve occurs at the instant at which the left ventricular pressure falls below the left atrial pressure, the time interval between aortic closure and the opening snap will tend to be short, that is, 0.06 to 0.07 s, in patients with severe obstruction and long, that is, 0.10 to 0.12 s, in patients with mild mitral stenosis. The intensities of the opening snap and the first heart sound correlate with the mobility of the anterior mitral leaflet.

The opening snap usually ushers in a low-pitched, rumbling, diastolic murmur, heard best at the apex with the patient in the left lateral recumbent position, and often accentuated by exercise carried out just before auscultation. In general, the duration of this murmur correlates with the severity of the stenosis. In patients with sinus rhythm the murmur often reappears or becomes reaccentuated during atrial systole, as atrial contraction reelevates the rate of blood flow across the narrowed orifice. Soft (grade I or II/VI) systolic murmurs are commonly heard at the apex or along the left sternal border in patients with mitral stenosis and do not necessarily signify the presence of mitral regurgitation. Hepatomegaly, ankle edema, ascites, and the physical finding of pleural effusion, particularly in the right pleural cavity, may occur in patients with mitral stenosis and right ventricular failure.

Associated lesions When severe pulmonary hypertension is present in a patient with mitral stenosis, a loud pansystolic murmur produced by functional tricuspid regurgitation may be audible along the left sternal border. This murmur is often accentuated by inspiration, diminishes during forced expiration or during performance of the Valsalva maneuver, may disappear as compensation is restored, and must not be confused with the apical pansystolic murmur of mitral regurgitation, since management is quite different if mitral regurgitation is present.

Once the diagnosis of mitral stenosis is established, the recognition of associated mitral regurgitation is of considerable clinical importance. A presystolic murmur and an accentuated first heart sound speak against the presence of serious associated mitral regurgitation; when the first heart sound and/or the opening snap are soft or absent in a patient with mitral valve disease, it is likely that significant mitral regurgitation and/or serious calcification of the deformed mitral valve leaflets are present. A third heart sound at the apex often signifies that the degree of associated mitral regurgitation is more than trivial. This sound is generally duller and lower pitched and follows the opening snap. Occasionally, in patients with pure mitral stenosis, physical signs may falsely suggest mitral regurgitation. Thus, in the presence of severe pulmonary hypertension and right ventricular failure, a third heart sound may originate from the right ventricle and be audible along the left sternal border. In such patients the enlarged right ventricle may rotate the heart in a clockwise direction and form the cardiac apex, giving the examiner the erroneous impression of left ventricular enlargement. Under these circumstances the rumbling diastolic murmur and the other auscultatory features of mitral stenosis become less prominent or may even disappear. When severe congestive heart failure exists in a patient with calcific mitral stenosis, none of the auscultatory findings typical of severe mitral stenosis may be detectable, but they may become apparent again as compensation is restored. Associated tricuspid stenosis also tends to obscure many of the physical signs of mitral stenosis.

The Graham Steell murmur of pulmonary regurgitation, a high-pitched, diastolic, decrescendo blowing murmur along the left sternal border, results from dilatation of the pulmonary valve ring and occurs in patients with mitral valve disease and serious pulmonary hypertension. This murmur may be indistinguishable from the more common murmur produced by mild aortic regurgitation except that it is rarely audible at the second right intercostal space, and may disappear following successful surgical treatment of the mitral stenosis.

Electrocardiogram The QRS complex may be normal, even in patients with critical mitral stenosis. However, with severe pulmonary hypertension, right axis deviation and right ventricular hypertrophy are usually found. When left ventricular hypertrophy is present in patients with mitral stenosis, it generally indicates that an additional lesion which places a burden on the left ventricle, such as mitral regurgitation, aortic valve disease, or hypertension, is present. In mitral stenosis and sinus rhythm the P wave usually suggests left atrial enlargement (Chap. 232). It may become tall and more peaked in lead II and upright in lead V_1 when severe pulmonary hypertension or tricuspid stenosis complicates mitral stenosis and right atrial enlargement occurs. When atrial fibrillation is present in patients with mitral valve disease, the base line shows coarser undulations than when this arrhythmia occurs as a consequence of coronary artery disease.

Echocardiogram (see also Chap. 233) The echocardiogram is the most sensitive and specific noninvasive method for diagnosing mitral stenosis. The M-mode tracing reveals that the anterior and posterior mitral leaflets do not separate widely in early diastole (i.e., less than 15 mm) and they maintain a fixed relation to each other throughout diastole. A reduction in the EF slope reflects failure of the anterior leaflet of the mitral valve to float back to midposition in middiastole, but this slope can not be utilized to estimate the severity of obstruction. In the presence of a mobile valve the EF slope is related to the severity of the obstruction. Calcification and thickening of the mitral valve are detected as multilayered echoes on the anterior leaflet of the mitral valve or a thickening of the echo pattern. Mitral orifice area is best determined with cross-sectional (two-dimensional) imaging systems. The left atrium is usually enlarged.

Roentgenographic features The earliest changes are straightening of the left border of the cardiac silhouette, prominence of the main pulmonary arteries, dilatation of the upper lobe pulmonary veins, and backward displacement of the esophagus by an enlarged left atrium. In patients with mild or moderate stenosis, the overall cardiac size is not grossly enlarged. In severe mitral stenosis, however, all chambers and vessels upstream to the narrowed valve are prominent, including the two atria, the pulmonary arteries and veins, right ventricle, and superior vena cava. Kerley B lines are fine, dense, opaque, horizontal lines which are most prominent in the lower and midlung fields and which result from distention of interlobular septa and lymphatics with edema. These lines usually signify a resting mean left atrial pressure of at least 20 mmHg. As the pulmonary arterial pressure rises, the smaller pulmonary arteries become attenuated, at first in the lower, then in the mid-, and finally in the upper lung fields. Deposits of hemosiderin occur in the lungs of patients who have had multiple hemoptyses; the hemosiderin-containing macrophages fill the air spaces, and if they become large enough and confluent result in a fine, diffuse nodulation most prominent in the lower lung fields. Ossified nodules are also more common in this region and are produced by true lamellar bone, which tends to develop in areas of interstitial pulmonary edema.

DIFFERENTIAL DIAGNOSIS Significant mitral regurgitation may be associated with a prominent diastolic murmur at the apex, but this murmur commences slightly later than in patients with stenosis, and there is often clear-cut evidence of left ventricular enlargement on physical examination, roentgenography, and electrocardiography. In addition, a pansystolic murmur of at least grade III/VI intensity as well as a third heart sound should arouse the suspicion of significant associated regurgitation. Similarly, the apical middiastolic murmur associated with aortic regurgitation (Austin Flint murmur) may be mistaken for mitral stenosis. However, in a patient with aortic regurgitation the absence of an opening snap or of presystolic accentuation if sinus rhythm is present points to the absence of mitral stenosis. Tricuspid stenosis, a valvular lesion that occurs very rarely in the absence of mitral stenosis, may mask many of the clinical features of mitral stenosis. The echocardiogram is particularly useful in detecting mitral stenosis in patients who have or are suspected of having other valve lesions.

Exertional dyspnea and recurrent pulmonary infections may be falsely ascribed to pulmonary emphysema in patients with both *chronic lung disease* and mitral stenosis. Careful auscultation, however, will generally reveal the characteristic opening snap and rumbling diastolic murmur. Similarly, the hemoptysis that occurs in many otherwise asymptomatic patients with mitral stenosis may be improperly attributed to bronchiectasis or tuberculosis. Actually, the latter condition is uncommon in patients with significant mitral obstruction.

Primary pulmonary hypertension (Chap. 265) results in a number of the clinical and laboratory features of mitral stenosis. It is seen most frequently in young women; however, the opening snap and diastolic rumbling murmur are absent, there is no left atrial enlargement on the electrocardiogram, roentgenogram, or echocardiogram, and the pulmonary artery wedge and left atrial pressures are normal.

Atrial septal defect (Chap. 240) may also be mistaken for mitral stenosis; in both conditions there is often clinical, electrocardiographic, and roentgenographic evidence of right ventricular enlargement and accentuation of the pulmonary vascularity. The widely split second heart sound of atrial septal defect may be confused with the mitral opening snap, and the diastolic flow murmur across the tricuspid valve considered to be the mitral diastolic murmur. However, the absence of left atrial enlargement on the roentgenogram, electrocardiogram, or echocardiogram, the absence of Kerley B lines, and demonstration of fixed splitting of the second heart sound all favor atrial septal defect over mitral stenosis.

Cor triatriatum is an unusual congenital malformation that consists of a fibrous ring within the left atrium (Chap. 240). It results in elevation of the pulmonary venous, capillary, and arterial pressures. This lesion can be recognized most readily by means of left atrial angiography.

A *left atrial myxoma* (Chap. 248) may obstruct left atrial emptying, resulting in dyspnea, a diastolic murmur, and hemodynamic changes that resemble those of mitral stenosis. However, patients with left atrial myxoma often demonstrate findings suggestive of a systemic disease, with weight loss, fever, anemia, systemic emboli and elevated erythrocyte sedimentation rate, and serum gamma-globulin concentration. Usually an opening snap is not audible, there is no clinical evidence of associated aortic valve disease, and the auscultatory findings frequently change with body position. The diagnosis can be established by demonstrating a characteristic echo-producing mass in the left atrium by echocardiography and a lobulated filling defect in the left atrium by angiocardiography.

Specialized techniques Left-side heart catheterization (Chap. 234) is extremely helpful in deciding whether valvulotomy is necessary in patients in whom it is difficult to estimate the severity of obstruction by clinical means alone. When combined with left ventricular angiocardiography, this procedure is particularly valuable in the detection and estimation of associated mitral regurgitation and of coexisting lesions such as aortic stenosis and regurgitation as well as left ventricular dysfunction. Left atrial thrombi and tumors may be detected or excluded by angiocardiography, particularly when the contrast medium is injected directly into the left atrium. Catheterization of the left side of the heart is also helpful in the detection of conditions that impair left ventricular function and would thereby contraindicate or reduce the effectiveness of mitral valvulotomy. Detailed physiological investigations are indicated for most patients who have undergone previous mitral valve operations and who have redeveloped serious symptoms; in such patients clinical assessment is particularly difficult, and the hemodynamic studies allow determination of the severity of the lesion, intelligent planning of the operative procedure when it is indicated, and a more informed estimate of the risk.

TREATMENT In the asymptomatic adolescent with mitral valve disease, penicillin prophylaxis of beta-hemolytic streptococcal infections (Chap. 241), prophylaxis for bacterial endocarditis (Chap. 243), and vocational counseling are particularly important; physically strenuous occupations should be avoided so that premature retirement will not be necessary should symptoms develop later. In symptomatic patients considerable improvement can be expected with restriction of sodium intake and maintenance doses of oral diuretics. Digitalis glycosides do not alter the hemodynamics and usually do not benefit patients with pure stenosis and sinus rhythm, but they are necessary for slowing the ventricular rate of patients with atrial fibrillation and for reducing the manifestations of right-sided heart failure in the advanced stages of the disease. Small doses of propranolol (10 to 20 mg qid) may be added when cardiac glycosides fail to control ventricular rate in patients with atrial fibrillation or flutter. Particular attention must be directed to detecting and treating anemia and infections. Hemoptysis is treated by measures designed to diminish pulmonary venous pressure, including bed rest, the sitting position, salt restriction, and diuresis. The administration of anticoagulants for at least 1 year is indicated in patients with mitral stenosis who have suffered systemic and/or pulmonary embolization and those with intermittent atrial fibrillation.

If atrial fibrillation is of relatively recent origin in a patient whose mitral stenosis is not severe enough to warrant surgical treatment, reversion to sinus rhythm, by means of either electrical countershock (Chap. 239) or quinidine (Chap. 238), is indicated. Usually this should be undertaken following 4 to 6 weeks of anticoagulant treatment. Conversion to sinus rhythm is rarely helpful in patients with severe mitral stenosis, particularly those in whom the left atrium is especially enlarged or in whom atrial fibrillation has been present for more than 1 year, since it is frequently impossible to maintain sinus rhythm, and reversion to atrial fibrillation is common.

Surgical treatment Unless there is a specific contraindication, operative treatment is indicated in the symptomatic patient with pure mitral stenosis whose effective orifice is less than approximately 1.5 cm². Operation not only usually results in striking symptomatic and hemodynamic improvement but also clearly prolongs survival. In uncomplicated cases, the surgical mortality rate should be less than 2 percent, and a comparison of the natural history of patients with serious symptoms treated by valvulotomy with those who did not receive the benefits of surgical therapy has shown considerable improvement following operation. However, there is no evidence that surgical treatment improves the prognosis of patients with slight or no functional impairment. Therefore, unless recurrent systemic embolization has occurred, valvulotomy is not indicated in patients who are entirely asymptomatic, regardless of hemodynamic findings. When there is little symptomatic improvement following valvulotomy, it is likely that the procedure was ineffective, that it induced mitral regurgitation, or that associated valvular or myocardial disease was present. The recurrence of symptoms several years after what appeared to be a satisfactory initial result is usually due to an inadequate valvulotomy, but progression of other valvular lesions, the development of myocardial disease, restenosis of the mitral valve, or some combination of these factors may also be responsible. In the pregnant patient with mitral stenosis operative treatment should be carried out if pulmonary congestion occurs despite medical treatment or when there is a history of pulmonary edema.

A closed operation (with "pump standby") is usually preferable for patients with pure mitral stenosis who have not been operated upon previously, in whom no valvular or perivalvular calcification is detected on fluoroscopic and/or echocardiographic examination, and in whom there is no suspicion of left atrial thrombosis. Many surgeons have found that transventricular instrumental dilatation of the mitral valve results in more effective relief of stenosis than transatrial finger fracture, and the importance of loosening any existing subvalvular fusion of papillary muscles and chordae tendineae must

be appreciated. In a number of patients with uncomplicated mitral stenosis, closed valvulotomy may be ineffective or may result in severe regurgitation. For these reasons, the ready availability of an extracorporeal system is prudent. Operative treatment of patients with extremely severe obstruction, significant associated mitral regurgitation, valvular calcification, left atrial thrombi, or a mitral valve distorted by previous operative manipulation is usually carried out under direct vision, with open-heart techniques. The valve may have to be replaced with a prosthesis or a heterograft in those patients who were severely symptomatic preoperatively and in whom the surgeon does not find it possible to improve valve function significantly. Since the operative mortality rate of replacement of the mitral valve is still approximately 5 to 10 percent in most hospitals, and since there is some uncertainty concerning the long-term fate of valve replacements, patients in whom preoperative evaluation suggests the possibility that replacement may be required should be operated on only if they are symptomatic on ordinary activity despite optimal medical therapy.

The results of valve replacement are dependent primarily on (1) the patient's myocardial function and level of pulmonary artery pressure at the time of operation, (2) the technical abilities of the operative team and the quality of the postoperative care, and (3) the durability and long-term functioning of the valve used for replacement. Increased operative mortality is associated with the degree of preoperative functional disability and pulmonary hypertension. In patients who have undergone valve replacement with a prosthesis, it is necessary to maintain the patient permanently on anticoagulants postoperatively. Late complications of replacement of any valve, which fortunately are declining in incidence, include paravalvular leakage, thromboemboli, bleeding due to anticoagulants, mechanical dysfunction of the prosthesis, and infective endocarditis. The primary advantage of tissue valves over prosthetics is the elimination of thromboembolic complications and the necessity for anticoagulants. One primary problem associated with their use is infective endocarditis, and late deterioration of the graft has been reported in a few instances.

The overall 5-year survival following mitral valve replacement approximates 70 percent. Long-term prognosis is worse in subgroups of older patients and those with marked disability and striking depression of the cardiac index preoperatively.

MITRAL REGURGITATION

PATHOPHYSIOLOGY The regurgitant mitral orifice may be considered to be in parallel with the aortic orifice, and therefore the resistance to left ventricular emptying is reduced in patients with mitral regurgitation. As a consequence, the left ventricle decompresses itself rapidly into the left atrium early during ejection, and with the marked reduction in left ventricular size there is a rapid decline in left ventricular tension. Therefore, a greater proportion of the contractile activity of the left ventricle is expended in shortening, and the cardiac output may be maintained at normal levels for many years even in patients with severe regurgitation. The initial compensation to mitral regurgitation consists of more complete systolic emptying of the left ventricle. However, a progressive increase in left ventricular end-diastolic volume occurs as the severity of the regurgitation increases and the function of the left ventricle deteriorates. The atrial contraction wave in the left atrial pressure pulse (a wave) is usually not as prominent as it is in mitral stenosis, but the v wave is often much taller, since it is inscribed during ventricular systole, when the left atrium fills from the pulmonary veins as well as from the left ventricle. During early diastole, as the distended left atrium suddenly empties, there is a particularly rapid y descent. The left ventricular end-diastolic pressure is either near the upper limits of normal or somewhat elevated. The effective cardiac output usually declines in seriously symptomatic patients. Although a left atrioventricular pressure gradient persisting throughout diastole signifies the presence of significant associated mitral stenosis, a brief, early diastolic gradient may occur in patients with pure regurgitation as a result of the torrential flow of blood across a normal-sized mitral orifice. In chronic mitral regurgitation, there is often an increase in left ventricular compliance, so that ventricular volume may be greatly increased with little elevation in end-diastolic pressure.

The diagnosis of mitral regurgitation can be established by means of left ventricular angiocardiography; the prompt appearance of contrast material indicator in the left atrium following its injection into the left ventricle signifies the presence of mitral regurgitation. The regurgitant volume can be measured by determining the difference between the total left ventricular stroke estimated angiocardiographically, while simultaneously measuring the effective forward stroke volume by Fick's method. The results of such studies suggest that the regurgitant volume may be of the same magnitude as the effective forward stroke volume or may even exceed it in patients with severe regurgitation. Qualitative, but clinically useful, estimates of the severity of regurgitation may be made by observation on cineangiograms of the degree of left atrial opacification following the injection of contrast material into the left ventricle.

Patients with severe mitral regurgitation may be divided into several subgroups, depending on the compliance, i.e., the pressure-volume relationship, of the left atrium and pulmonary venous bed, which appears to be capable of affecting the clinical and hemodynamic picture. Among patients with severe mitral regurgitation, three major conditions have been identified:

1 *Normal or reduced compliance.* In this group there is little enlargement of the left atrium, but marked elevation of the mean left atrial pressure, particularly of the *v* wave. In many patients in this group severe mitral regurgitation has developed suddenly, as in those in whom it follows rupture of chordae tendineae, infarction of one of the heads of a papillary muscle, or tear of a mitral leaflet. Marked elevation of pulmonary vascular resistance frequently occurs, presumably as a consequence of the left atrial hypertension, and therefore right-sided heart failure is a common clinical manifestation; sinus rhythm is usually present.

2 *Moderate increase in compliance.* By far the most common group consists of patients whose clinical and hemodynamic features are midway between those in the other two groups; i.e., they exhibit variable degrees of enlargement of the left atrium, associated with significant elevation of the left atrial pressure.

3 *Marked increase in compliance.* At the other end of the spectrum from group 1 are those patients with severe chronic mitral regurgitation, massive enlargement of the left atrium, and normal left atrial pressure. The pulmonary artery pressure and pulmonary vascular resistance are normal or only slightly elevated at rest. Clinically, these patients are usually disabled with fatigue and exhaustion, because of a low cardiac output, while symptoms resulting from pulmonary congestion are less prominent. In this group the mitral regurgitation is long-standing, and atrial fibrillation is almost invariably present. The association of a normal left atrial pressure with a markedly enlarged, thin-walled left atrium indicates that this chamber must be far more compliant than normal. Thus, long-standing mitral regurgitation may, in some instances, alter the physical properties of the left atrial wall and thereby displace the atrial pressure-volume curve, allowing a normal pressure to exist in a greatly enlarged left atrium.

ETIOLOGY In about half the patients mitral regurgitation is caused by chronic *rheumatic heart disease,* but in contrast to mitral stenosis, pure or predominantly rheumatic mitral regurgitation occurs more frequently in males. The rheumatic process produces rigidity, deformity, and retraction of the valve cusps, and commissural fusion, as well as shortening, contraction, and fusion of the chordae tendineae. Mitral regurgitation may also occur as a congenital anomaly (Chap. 240), most commonly as a consequence of (1) a defect of the endocardial cushions, (2) corrected transposition, (3) endocardial fibroelastosis, and (4) the "parachute" mitral valve. It may follow rupture or fibrosis of a papillary muscle or of one of its heads in ischemic heart disease. Myocardial infarction, fibrosis, or a ventricular aneurysm, at the base of the papillary muscle but not necessarily involving it, may lead to abnormal anchoring of the latter, also resulting in mitral regurgitation. The latter may also occur during transient periods of ischemia involving a papillary muscle or adjacent myocardium and may accompany bouts of angina pectoris. Mitral regurgitation may occur with marked left ventricular dilatation of any cause in which dilatation of the mitral annulus and lateral displacement of the papillary muscles interfere with coaptation of the valve leaflets. In idiopathic hypertrophic subaortic stenosis the anterior leaflet of the mitral valve is displaced anteriorly during systole, leading to regurgitation (Chap. 247). Systemic lupus erythematosus, rheumatoid arthritis, and ankylosing spondylitis are less common causes. Massive calcification of the mitral annulus of unknown cause, which occurs most commonly in elderly women, can also be responsible for significant mitral regurgitation. Mitral regurgitation may occur acutely in patients with infective endocarditis involving the valve or chordae tendineae, as a consequence of trauma or as a complication of cardiac surgery.

Abnormal elongation of chordae tendineae and/or redundant posterior cusps of the mitral valve with prolapse of the cusps into the left atrium, the so-called "floppy valve," leading to the syndrome of midsystolic click and midsystolic murmur, also referred to as the prolapsing mitral valve leaflet syndrome (see below), is another important cause of mitral regurgitation.

Regardless of etiology, significant mitral regurgitation tends to be gradually progressive since enlargement of the left atrium places tension on the posterior mitral leaflet, pulling it away from the mitral orifice, thereby aggravating the valvular dysfunction. Similarly, the dilatation of the left ventricle increases the regurgitation, which in turn further enlarges the left atrium and ventricle, resulting in a vicious cycle; hence the aphorism, "mitral regurgitation begets mitral regurgitation."

SYMPTOMS Only a fraction of patients with chronic mitral regurgitation ever experience any reduction of cardiac reserve, but in those who do become symptomatic, fatigue, exertional dyspnea, orthopnea, and nocturnal dyspnea are prominent complaints. Symptoms resulting from pulmonary congestion tend to be less episodic in nature than in mitral stenosis, since fluctuations of the mean pulmonary capillary pressure are less marked. Indeed, acute paroxysmal pulmonary edema is quite rare in patients with chronic mitral regurgitation. Similarly, hemoptysis and systemic embolism occur far less frequently in mitral regurgitation than in stenosis. On the other hand, fatigability, weakness, exhaustion, weight loss, and even cachexia are more prominent and occur most frequently in patients with marked reduction of cardiac output. Right-sided heart failure, characterized by painful hepatic congestion, ankle edema, distended neck veins, ascites, and evidence of tricuspid regurgitation, is observed commonly in patients with mitral regurgitation who have associated pulmonary vascular disease. In patients with acute severe mitral regurgitation, left ventricular failure with acute pulmonary edema and/or cardiovascular collapse is common. In contrast to patients with mitral stenosis, pure regurgitation rarely leads to hemoptysis, systemic emboli, or chest pain.

PHYSICAL FINDINGS Although the arterial pressure is usually normal, the arterial pulse is often characterized by a sharp upstroke. The jugular venous pulse shows abnormally prominent *a* waves in patients with sinus rhythm and marked pulmonary hypertension. A systolic thrill is usually palpable at the cardiac apex, the left ventricle is hyperdynamic with a brisk systolic impulse and a palpable rapid-filling wave, and the apex beat is often displaced laterally. When the left atrium is markedly enlarged, it may extend anteriorly, and its expansion may be palpable along the sternal border late during ventricular systole. The combination of the retraction of the left ventricle and expansion of the left atrium during systole may produce a characteristic rocking motion of the chest with each cardiac cycle. A right ventricular tap and the shock of pulmonary valve closure may be palpable in patients with marked pulmonary hypertension.

The first heart sound at the apex is generally absent, soft, or buried in the systolic heart murmur, and an accentuated mitral closure sound is useful in excluding severe regurgitation. A pulmonary ejection sound is often audible in patients with associated pulmonary hypertension. Splitting of the second heart sound is usually normal, but in patients with severe regurgitation, aortic valve closure may occur early, resulting in wide splitting of the second heart sound. An opening snap indicates associated mitral stenosis but does not exclude predominant regurgitation. A low-pitched third heart sound, occurring 0.12 to 0.17 s after the aortic valve closure sound, at the completion of the rapid-filling phase of the mitral valve, is believed to be caused by the sudden tensing of the papillary muscles, chordae tendineae, and valve leaflets and is an important auscultatory feature of severe mitral regurgitation. The absence of a third heart sound indicates that if mitral regurgitation exists, it may not be severe. The third heart sound may usher in a short, rumbling, diastolic murmur in the absence of mitral stenosis. A fourth heart sound is heard characteristically in patients with acute severe regurgitation in sinus rhythm. A presystolic murmur is not ordinarily heard in patients with pure regurgitation and sinus rhythm but is present when there is significant associated mitral stenosis.

A systolic murmur, grade III/VI in intensity or louder, is the most characteristic auscultatory finding in patients with severe mitral regurgitation. It is usually holosystolic (Chap. 231). Although the systolic murmur usually radiates into the axilla, in a minority of patients, particularly those with ruptured chordae tendineae or primary involvement of the posterior mitral leaflet, the regurgitant jet strikes the left atrial wall adjacent to the aortic root, and the systolic murmur is referred to the base of the heart and therefore may be confused with the murmur of aortic stenosis. In patients with ruptured chordae tendineae the systolic murmur may have a cooing or "sea gull" quality.

In patients with acute severe mitral regurgitation the systolic murmur may be decrescendo because the tall *v* wave in the left atrial pressure pulse results in a reduced late systolic left ventricular-atrial pressure gradient.

Electrocardiogram The electrocardiographic signs of ventricular hypertrophy are variable; in many patients there is no clear-cut electrocardiographic evidence of enlargement of either ventricle. In severe regurgitation the signs of left ventricu-

lar hypertrophy are often present, although in patients with pulmonary hypertension associated right ventricular hypertrophy is apparent. Electrocardiographic signs of pure right ventricular hypertrophy occur in patients with severe pulmonary hypertension, and, though unusual in patients with pure mitral regurgitation, they do not exclude this diagnosis. There is electrocardiographic evidence of left atrial enlargement in patients with sinus rhythm, but right atrial hypertrophy may be present when pulmonary hypertension is extreme. Prolonged, severe mitral regurgitation with marked left atrial enlargement is generally associated with atrial fibrillation.

Echocardiogram The left atrium is usually enlarged and/or exhibits increased pulsations. The left ventricle is hyperdynamic. With ruptured chordae tendineae there is coarse erratic motion of the mitral leaflets during diastole and multiple echoes in systole occurring over a wide portion of the flail leaflet. The echocardiogram in the syndrome of midsystolic click and midsystolic murmur is described below.

Roentgenographic features The left atrium and left ventricle are the dominant chambers; the latter may be enlarged to aneurysmal proportions and form the right border of the cardiac silhouette. Though both mitral stenosis and regurgitation tend to increase left atrial size, extreme left atrial enlargement usually signifies that regurgitation is the predominant lesion and has existed for many years. On fluoroscopic examination the left ventricle is hyperdynamic and the left atrium exhibits vigorous systolic expansions. Marked calcification of the mitral leaflets occurs commonly in patients with long-standing combined severe regurgitation and stenosis but is uncommon in patients with pure regurgitation. Cineangiography commonly reveals late systolic prolapse of a leaflet (usually the posterior) of the mitral valve into the left atrium in patients with the syndrome of mid-late systolic click and late systolic murmur. This abnormal movement of the mitral valve can also be detected by echocardiography.

TREATMENT The nonsurgical management of mitral regurgitation is directed toward restricting those physical activities which regularly produce extreme fatigue and dyspnea, reducing sodium intake, and enhancing sodium excretion with the appropriate use of diuretics (Chap. 236). Digitalis glycosides (Chap. 238) play a more important role in the treatment of mitral regurgitation than in treatment of mitral stenosis, since these drugs augment the output of the overburdened left ventricle even in the presence of sinus rhythm. The same considerations as in patients with mitral stenosis apply to the reversion of atrial fibrillation to sinus rhythm. In the late stages of the disease, anticoagulants and leg binders are used to diminish the likelihood of venous thrombi and pulmonary emboli. Effective surgical treatment of rheumatic mitral regurgitation generally requires valvular replacement with a suitable prosthesis or tissue valve. Though most patients who survive operation appear to be greatly improved, some degree of myocardial dysfunction may persist. The risks and complications attendant upon mitral valve replacement have been described (see "Surgical Treatment," above).

When surgical treatment is contemplated, detailed hemodynamic investigations and selective left ventricular angiocardiography are indicated. These studies are helpful in confirming the presence of severe regurgitation, and they aid in the identification of patients with primary myocardial disease and relatively mild, functional mitral regurgitation, who usually do not benefit from operation. Hemodynamic studies are also helpful in detecting and assessing the severity of associated valve lesions, which may have to be dealt with at the time of operation or which might limit the patient's ultimate improvement if they are left untreated.

In the selection of patients for surgical treatment, the chronic, often slowly progressive nature of the disease must be balanced against the immediate risks and long-term uncertainties attendant upon valve replacement. Patients with mitral regurgitation who are asymptomatic or who are limited only during severe exertion are not considered to be ideal candidates for surgical treatment, since they may live for many years with little deterioration. However, surgical treatment should be considered seriously in patients whose limitations do not allow them to work full time or carry out normal household activities despite optimal medical management. The risks of valve replacement rise sharply when the patient has developed congestive heart failure which is refractory to medical therapy, or associated severe tricuspid regurgitation. In addition, long-term survival of these patients is reduced (approximately 50 percent in 5 years). However, conservative management has little to offer these patients, so that operative treatment may be indicated even at these advanced stages of the disease, and occasionally the clinical and hemodynamic improvement following surgical treatment is dramatic. It is likely that the immediate results of surgical treatment will improve considerably and will lead to recommendations of operative treatment for selected patients with mitral regurgitation before they become severely disabled.

SYSTOLIC CLICK-MURMUR SYNDROME This is also variously termed the *prolapsing mitral valve leaflet syndrome, Barlow's syndrome, floppy-valve syndrome,* and *billowing mitral leaflet syndrome,* a common, but highly variable, clinical syndrome resulting from diverse pathogenic mechanisms of the mitral valve apparatus. Among these are excessive or redundant mitral leaflet tissue, which is commonly involved with myxomatous degeneration and greatly increased concentration of acid mucopolysaccharide. This is a frequent finding in patients who have the typical features of Marfan's syndrome or cystic medial necrosis (Chap. 252). In some patients myxomatous degeneration is confined to the mitral valve leaflets without other clinical or pathological manifestations of disease; the posterior leaflet is usually more affected than the anterior, and the mitral valve annulus is often greatly enlarged. In other patients, short, attenuated chordae tendineae as well as elongated redundant chordae have been identified. In still others, abnormalities of shortening and/or orientation of the papillary muscles, as well as localized or diffuse abnormalities of left ventricular contraction, appear to be responsible. There are probably several subsets of these patients, who differ in regard to the etiology and hemodynamic and clinical sequelae of abnormal mitral valve function. In the majority of patients, the etiology is unknown, but the condition may occur in acute rheumatic fever, chronic rheumatic heart disease, following mitral valvulotomy, in 20 percent of patients with atrial septal defect, and in ischemic heart disease. The resulting syndrome has protean manifestations.

This syndrome is a usually benign abnormality that may progress to a stage involving significant regurgitation and ventricular dilatation in some individuals. In these, prolapse of the valve leads to excessive stress on the papillary muscles, which in turn leads to dysfunction and ischemia of the papillary muscle and subjacent ventricular myocardium. The characteristic ventriculographic deformity (see below), the electrocardiogram showing changes of ischemia, and many of the recurrent arrhythmias appear to result from regional ventricular dysfunction related to abnormalities of the papillary muscles; these abnormalities do not appear to be manifestations of a diffuse cardiomyopathy, of some general disorder of the coronary circulation, or of myocardial metabolism.

The electrocardiogram most commonly shows biphasic or inverted T waves in leads II, III, and aVF. The echocardiogram characteristically shows an abrupt posterior displacement of the posterior or sometimes of both mitral valve leaflets in mid- to late systole immediately after the click and during the systolic murmur. Angiocardiography generally reveals prolapse of the posterior and sometimes of both mitral valve leaflets and, rarely, severe mitral regurgitation. Many patients have bulging of the posteroinferior wall of the left ventricle into the left ventricular cavity during systole and/or hypokinesis of the anterolateral left ventricular wall.

The syndrome is more common in females and occurs in a wide age range but most commonly between the ages of 14 and 30. Echocardiographic surveys have suggested that it may occur in as many as 10 percent of this group. There is an increased familial incidence suggesting an autosomal dominant form of inheritance. In many patients the echocardiographic abnormality is not accompanied by any other clinical manifestation of cardiac disease, and the significance of this finding is uncertain.

Most of the patients are asymptomatic, but arrhythmias, most commonly ventricular premature contractions and paroxysmal supraventricular and ventricular tachycardia, have been reported. In patients with supraventricular tachycardia a left-sided atrioventricular bypass tract can often be discerned. Patients with arrhythmias complain of palpitations, light-headedness, and syncope. Many patients have chest pain which is difficult to evaluate. It is often substernal, prolonged, and poorly related to exertion and rarely resembles typical angina pectoris.

The most common finding on physical examination is the mid- or late systolic click, which occurs 0.14 s or more after the first heart sound, and is thought to be generated by the sudden tensing of slack, elongated chordae tendineae or by the prolapsing mitral leaflet when it reaches its maximum posterior excursion; systolic clicks may be multiple and are often followed by a high-pitched late systolic crescendo-decrescendo murmur, occasionally "whooping" or "honking," heard best at the apex with the patient in the left lateral decubitus position. The click and murmur occur earlier with maneuvers such as standing, the Valsalva maneuver, or inhalation of amyl nitrite, all of which decrease left ventricular volume, exaggerating the propensity of mitral leaflet prolapse. Conversely, squatting or isometric exercise, which increases left ventricular end-diastolic volume, diminishes the propensity for the mitral valve leaflets to prolapse, and the click-murmur complex is delayed and may even disappear. Some patients have a midsystolic click without the murmur; others have the murmur without a click. Many patients with this syndrome but without overt features of Marfan's syndrome have certain bony abnormalities such as a high arched palate and deformities of the chest and thoracic spine.

The treatment of patients with mitral valve prolapse is directed toward the prevention of infective endocarditis and the relief of the atypical chest pain; propranolol has been found to be helpful in this regard, although its use is on an empiric basis. Antiarrhythmic agents are administered if frequent ventricular premature contractions are present at rest or during exercise, and propranolol has been advocated in patients with arrhythmias and prolongation of the QT interval. If mitral regurgitation is severe, mitral valve replacement is indicated.

AORTIC STENOSIS

Aortic stenosis occurs in about one-fourth of all patients with chronic valvular heart disease; approximately 80 percent of adult patients with symptomatic valvular aortic stenosis are male.

PATHOPHYSIOLOGY The primary hemodynamic abnormality in aortic stenosis is obstruction to left ventricular outflow which leads to a pressure gradient between the left ventricle and aorta during the systolic ejection period. When severe obstruction is suddenly produced experimentally, the left ventricle responds to this excessive afterload by dilatation and reduction of stroke volume. However, in clinical aortic stenosis, the obstruction may be present at birth or it increases gradually over the course of many years, and left ventricular output is maintained by the presence of left ventricular hypertrophy, which serves as a useful compensatory mechanism since it reduces toward normal the systolic stress developed by each segment of myocardium. A large pressure gradient across the aortic valve may exist for many years without a reduction of cardiac output, left ventricular dilatation, or the development of any symptoms. As aortic stenosis progresses in severity, the left ventricular systolic pressure continues to rise but rarely exceeds 300 mmHg.

A peak systolic pressure gradient exceeding 50 mmHg in the face of a normal cardiac output or an effective aortic orifice less than 0.7 cm² per square meter of body surface area, i.e., less than approximately one-third of the normal orifice, is generally considered to represent critical obstruction to left ventricular outflow. The left ventricular pressure pulse exhibits a rounded summit as the contraction of this chamber becomes progressively more isometric, and pulsus alternans in the left ventricle may occur in patients with severe stenosis. The elevated left ventricular end-diastolic pressure observed in many patients with severe aortic stenosis does not necessarily signify the presence of left ventricular failure or dilatation, but may instead reflect diminished compliance of the hypertrophied left ventricular wall.

A large *a* wave in the left atrial pressure pulse is usually present in patients with severe aortic stenosis, because of enhanced atrial contraction and diminished ventricular compliance. Atrial contraction tends to raise left ventricular end-diastolic pressure without producing a concomitant elevation of mean left atrial pressure. This "booster pump" function of the left atrium prevents the pulmonary venous and capillary pressures from rising to levels which would produce pulmonary congestion, while at the same time maintaining left ventricular end-diastolic pressure at the elevated level necessary for effective left ventricular contraction. Loss of appropriately timed, vigorous atrial contraction, as occurs in atrial fibrillation or atrioventricular dissociation, may result in a rapid aggravation of symptoms or cardiovascular collapse, even when the ventricular response is not particularly rapid.

The cardiac output and stroke volume at rest are within normal limits in the majority of patients with severe aortic stenosis. These variables may fail to rise normally during exercise. Late in the disease the cardiac output, stroke volume, and left ventricular-aortic pressure gradient decline, and the mean left atrial, pulmonary artery wedge, pulmonary arterial, and right ventricular pressures become elevated. At this stage, a prominent *a* wave in the right atrial pressure pulse is also commonly found, and hemodynamic evidence of mitral regurgitation, with a tall left atrial *v* wave and sharp *y* descent, may occur in association with marked left ventricular dilatation.

The hypertrophied left ventricular muscle mass elevates myocardial oxygen requirements. In addition, even in the absence of obstructive coronary artery disease, there may be interference with coronary blood flow, because the pressure compressing the coronary arteries exceeds the coronary perfusion pressure. Metabolic evidence of myocardial ischemia, i.e., lactate production, can be demonstrated in patients with aortic stenosis in both the presence and absence of coronary arterial

narrowing, when myocardial oxygen needs are stimulated by isoproterenol.

A significant fraction of patients with rheumatic aortic stenosis has associated mitral valve disease. Aortic stenosis intensifies the severity of mitral regurgitation by increasing the pressure driving blood from the left ventricle to the left atrium. The dilatation of the left ventricle which occurs late in the course in some patients with aortic stenosis further raises the mitral regurgitant flow.

Etiology Aortic stenosis may be congenital in origin, secondary to rheumatic inflammation of the aortic valve, or due to calcification of the aortic cusps of unknown cause. The *congenitally affected valve* may already be stenotic at birth and may gradually become calcified during the first three decades of life, becoming progressively more stenotic. The valve may also be congenitally bicuspid without serious narrowing of the aortic orifice during childhood; its abnormal architecture makes its leaflets susceptible to normal hemodynamic stresses, which ultimately lead to valvular calcification, increased rigidity, and narrowing of the aortic orifice.

Rheumatic endocarditis of the aortic leaflets produces commissural fusion, resulting, at first, in a bicuspid valve. This, in turn, also makes the leaflets more susceptible to trauma, and ultimately leads to calcification and further narrowing. By the time the obstruction to left ventricular outflow causes serious disability, the valve is usually a rigid calcified mass, and even careful examination may make it difficult or even impossible to determine whether the underlying process was rheumatic or congenital. Rheumatic aortic stenosis is almost always associated with rheumatic involvement of the mitral valve. A rheumatic etiology is also favored by a history of active rheumatic fever and by associated severe aortic regurgitation. *Idiopathic calcific aortic stenosis* occurs most often in the elderly and is occasionally associated with fibrosis and fusion of the valve cusps; the pathological process is considered to be a degenerative one—a "wear-and-tear" phenomenon. It may produce many of the characteristic physical signs of aortic stenosis. The valvular obstruction is usually relatively mild and of little if any hemodynamic significance; it may, however, on occasion, produce severe obstruction.

OTHER FORMS OF OBSTRUCTION TO LEFT VENTRICULAR OUTFLOW Besides valvular aortic stenosis, three other lesions may be responsible for obstruction to left ventricular outflow.

1 Idiopathic hypertrophic subaortic stenosis. This is the most important of these conditions numerically. It is characterized by marked hypertrophy of the left ventricle, involving in particular the interventricular septum of the left ventricular outflow tract, as described in Chap. 247.
2 Discrete congenital subvalvular aortic stenosis. This condition is produced by either a membranous diaphragm or a fibrous ridge just below the aortic valve (Chap. 240).
3 Supravalvular aortic stenosis. This uncommon congenital anomaly is produced by narrowing of the ascending aorta or by a fibrous diaphragm with a small opening just above the aortic valve (Chap. 240).

SYMPTOMS Aortic stenosis is rarely of hemodynamic or clinical importance until the valve orifice has narrowed to approximately one-third of normal. In contrast to mitral stenosis, which results in symptoms as soon as the obstruction becomes severe because the chamber just proximal to the narrowed valve, i.e., the left atrium, provides little compensation, severe aortic stenosis may exist for many years without producing any clinical disability because of the ability of the hypertrophied left ventricle to generate the elevated intraventricular pressures and the presence of the mitral valve upstream to the left ventricle.

Most patients with pure or predominant aortic stenosis have gradually increasing obstruction for years but do not become symptomatic until the fourth or fifth decade. Exertional dyspnea, angina pectoris, and syncope are the three cardinal symptoms. Often there is a history of insidious and subtle progression of fatigue and dyspnea associated with gradual curtailment of activities. Dyspnea results primarily from elevation of the pulmonary capillary pressures, which in turn results from elevations of left atrial and left ventricular end-diastolic pressures. Angina pectoris usually develops somewhat later and reflects an imbalance between the augmented myocardial oxygen requirements and oxygen availability; the former results from the increased myocardial mass and intraventricular pressure, while the latter may result from the coronary artery disease which is not uncommon in patients with aortic stenosis. Angina in severe aortic stenosis may occur without coronary narrowing, but the absence of angina usually signifies that severe coronary obstructive disease can be excluded. Exertional syncope may result from a decline in arterial pressure caused by vasodilatation in the exercising muscles and inadequate vasoconstriction in nonexercising muscles in the face of a fixed cardiac output, or from a sudden fall in cardiac output produced by an arrhythmia (Chap. 13). If prolonged, the syncopal episode may be accompanied by convulsions and loss of sphincteric control.

Since the cardiac output is usually well maintained at rest until the late stage of the disease, marked fatigability, weakness, peripheral cyanosis, and other clinical manifestations of a low cardiac output are usually not prominent until this stage is reached. Orthopnea, paroxysmal nocturnal dyspnea, and pulmonary edema, i.e., symptoms of left ventricular failure, also occur only in the advanced stages of the disease. Severe pulmonary hypertension leading to right ventricular failure and systemic venous hypertension, hepatomegaly, atrial fibrillation, and tricuspid regurgitation are usually preterminal findings.

When aortic stenosis and mitral stenosis coexist, the latter lesion masks many of the clinical findings of aortic stenosis. The reduction of cardiac output induced by mitral stenosis lowers the pressure gradient across the aortic valve, diminishes the frequency of anginal episodes, and retards the development of aortic calcification and severe left ventricular hypertrophy. On the other hand, symptoms considered more characteristic of mitral stenosis, such as pulmonary congestion and hemoptysis, occur more frequently in patients with combined stenotic lesions than in those with isolated aortic stenosis. Careful physical, electrocardiographic, and radiological examinations in patients with aortic and mitral stenosis generally reveal more evidence of left ventricular enlargement than in patients with pure mitral stenosis, and catheterization of the left side of the heart is helpful in defining the relative importance of each valvular abnormality.

PHYSICAL FINDINGS AND GRAPHIC TRACINGS The systemic arterial pressure is usually within normal limits. In the late stages, however, when stroke volume declines, the systolic pressure may fall and the pulse pressure narrows. Systemic hypertension is unusual in patients with marked aortic stenosis, and a basal systolic arterial pressure exceeding 200 mmHg practically excludes severe narrowing of this valve. The peripheral arterial pulse, as palpated in the carotid or brachial arteries, rises slowly, to a delayed sustained peak. Indirect recordings of the carotid pulse exhibit a gradually ascending limb, often with a prominent anacrotic notch or shoulder on the upstroke, as well as a delayed peak, with coarse systolic vibrations. The left ventricular ejection period is prolonged, even in heart failure; the preejection period is abbreviated, and the

ratio of these two, i.e., the preejection period/systolic ejection period, is characteristically reduced (Chap. 233). A palpable double systolic wave, the so-called "bisferiens pulse," excludes pure or predominant aortic stenosis and signifies dominant or pure aortic regurgitation or idiopathic hypertrophic subaortic stenosis (Chap. 247). In the late stages of the disease, when the pulse pressure is reduced, the pulse amplitude is so small that the anacrotic nature of the pulse and the delay in its upstroke may become more difficult to appreciate. The jugular venous pulse may be normal, although in many patients the *a* wave is accentuated. This results from the diminished distensibility of the right ventricular cavity caused by the bulging, hypertrophied, interventricular septum and/or the presence of pulmonary hypertension.

The apex beat is usually active and displaced inferiorly and laterally, reflecting the presence of left ventricular hypertrophy. A double apical impulse may be appreciated, particularly with the patient in the left lateral recumbent position; the first outward expansion occurs during atrial systole and reflects the important contribution made by atrial contraction to ventricular systole and is forceful and well sustained during ejection. The right ventricle is usually palpable only when pulmonary hypertension develops in the late stages of the disease. A systolic thrill is generally present at the base of the heart, in the jugular notch, and along the carotid arteries, but occasionally it is palpable only during expiration and with the patient leaning forward. In patients who do not have marked pulmonary emphysema, a thick chest wall, thoracic deformity, or heart failure, *the absence of a systolic thrill signifies that the aortic stenosis is relatively mild.*

The rhythm is generally regular; until very late in the course atrial fibrillation should call to mind the possibility of associated mitral valve disease. An early systolic ejection sound, actually the opening snap of the aortic valve, is frequently audible in children and adolescents with noncalcific valvular aortic stenosis. However, this sound usually disappears when the valve becomes calcified and rigid. The sound of aortic valve closure can also be identified most frequently in patients with aortic stenosis with pliable valves, and calcification tends to diminish the intensity of this sound. As aortic stenosis increases in severity, left ventricular systole may become prolonged so that the aortic valve closure sound no longer precedes the pulmonic valve closure sound, and the two components may become synchronous, or aortic valve closure may even follow pulmonic valve closure. This is called paradoxic splitting of the second heart sound (Chap. 231); in patients with aortic stenosis in the absence of a left intraventricular conduction defect this finding usually signifies severe obstruction to left ventricular outflow. Atrial (presystolic) gallop rhythm, audible at the apex in many patients with severe aortic stenosis, reflects the presence of left ventricular hypertrophy and an elevated left ventricular end-diastolic pressure; ventricular (protodiastolic) gallop rhythm in adults generally occurs when the left ventricle dilates and fails.

The systolic murmur in aortic stenosis is of the ejection type, i.e., it commences shortly after the first heart sound, increases in intensity to reach a peak toward the middle of the ejection period, and diminishes progressively thereafter to end just before aortic valve closure (Chaps. 231 and 233). The murmur is usually low-pitched, rough, and rasping in character and is loudest at the base of the heart, most commonly in the second intercostal space just to the right of the sternum. It is transmitted upward to the jugular notch and along the carotid arteries. In patients with mild degrees of obstruction or in those with severe stenosis in the late stage of the disease in whom the stroke volume is reduced, the murmur may be relatively soft and brief, and confined to midsystole. However, in almost all patients with significant obstruction, the murmur is at least grade III/VI. Occasionally, the murmur is transmitted downward and to the apex and may be confused with the systolic murmur of mitral regurgitation. However, this murmur is usually holosystolic, while that of aortic stenosis is diamond-shaped and of the ejection type (Chap. 231).

Electrocardiogram This reveals left ventricular hypertrophy in the majority of patients with severe aortic stenosis (Chap. 232). In advanced cases, ST-segment depression and T-wave inversion in standard leads I, aVL, and in the left precordial leads are evident. However, there is no close correlation between the electrocardiogram and the hemodynamic severity of obstruction, and the absence of electrocardiographic signs of left ventricular hypertrophy does not exclude severe obstruction. Left bundle branch block or the presence of intraventricular conduction defects with QRS prolongation suggests diffuse fibrotic involvement of the myocardium. The presence of left atrial enlargement should suggest the possibility of associated mitral valve disease.

Echocardiogram This reveals thickening of the left ventricular wall, and in patients with valvular calcification, multiple, bright, thick, echoes from within the aortic root, without the normal box-like separation of the aortic cusps during systole. While cusp calcification does not necessarily indicate significant valve stenosis, its absence can usually be used to exclude such a diagnosis. Eccentricity of the aortic valve cusps is characteristic of congenitally bicuspid valves (Chap. 233). Left ventricular dilatation and reduced systolic shortening reflecting impairment of left ventricular function can be recognized. Echocardiography is particularly useful for identifying valvular abnormalities such as mitral stenosis and aortic regurgitation which sometimes accompany aortic stenosis, and for differentiating valvular from idiopathic hypertrophic subaortic stenosis.

Roentgenographic features The chest roentgenogram may show no or little overall cardiac enlargement for many years, since the development of concentric left ventricular hypertrophy is the initial response to obstruction to left ventricular outflow. Considerable hypertrophy without dilatation may produce some rounding of the cardiac apex in the frontal projection and slight backward displacement in the lateral view; significant aortic stenosis is usually associated with poststenotic dilatation of the ascending aorta. Aortic calcification is usually readily apparent on fluoroscopic examination with an image intensifier or by echocardiography; indeed, *the absence of valvular calcification in an adult suggests that severe valvular aortic stenosis is not present.* In later stages of the disease as the left ventricle dilates, there is progressively more evidence of left ventricular enlargement, and there may also be roentgenologic signs of pulmonary congestion, as well as enlargement of the left atrium, pulmonary artery, right ventricle, and right atrium.

Catheterization and angiocardiography Catheterization of the left side of the heart should be carried out in the majority of patients suspected of having severe aortic stenosis, particularly before a final decision concerning operative treatment is made. The goals of catheterization of the left side of the heart are to document (1) the severity of the aortic obstruction, (2) the status of left ventricular function, and (3) the location of left ventricular outflow obstruction. These investigations are especially indicated in:

1 Young, asymptomatic patients with noncalcific aortic stenosis, in order to define the severity of their obstruction to left ventricular outflow, since operation may be indicated if severe aortic stenosis is present.
2 Patients in whom it is suspected that the obstruction to left ventricular outflow may not be at the aortic valve, but rather in the sub- or supravalvular regions.
3 Patients with clinical signs of aortic stenosis and symptoms of myocardial ischemia, in whom associated coronary artery disease is suspected. An effort should be made to determine whether aortic stenosis or coronary atherosclerosis is responsible for the symptoms in this group of patients, and coronary arteriography should be carried out in addition to catheterization of the left side of the heart.
4 Patients with multivalvular disease, in whom the role played by each valvular deformity must be defined before operative treatment is planned.

Angiocardiographic studies with left ventricular injection of contrast material are helpful in defining the size of the left ventricular cavity, the thickness of the wall, the site of obstruction, the degree of deformity and mobility of the aortic valve cusps, the diameter of the ascending aorta, and the presence and degree of accompanying mitral regurgitation. In patients with severe narrowing, a jet of contrast substance passing through the aortic orifice is readily visualized. When contrast substance is injected into the ascending aorta, the aortic valve cusps can also be outlined, and associated aortic regurgitation can be detected and its severity assessed.

NATURAL HISTORY The advanced age at death of patients with severe aortic stenosis is a consistent feature of this disease, and averages 63 years in men. In several studies, based on analysis of data obtained at postmortem examination, the average duration of various symptoms was as follows: angina pectoris, 3 years; syncope, 3 years; dyspnea, 2 years; and congestive heart failure, 1.5 to 2 years. Moreover, in more than 80 percent of these patients who died with aortic stenosis, symptoms had existed for less than 4 years. Congestive heart failure was considered to be the cause of death in one-half to two-thirds of patients.

Among adults dying with valvular aortic stenosis, sudden death, which presumably results from an arrhythmia, occurred in 10 to 20 percent, and at an average age of 60 years (Chap. 32). About one of every six patients dying suddenly has evidence of old or recent myocardial infarction at postmortem examination.

TREATMENT Strenuous physical activity should be avoided even in the asymptomatic stage in patients with *severe* aortic stenosis. Digitalis glycosides, sodium restriction, and diuretics are indicated in the treatment of congestive heart failure. While nitroglycerin is helpful in relieving angina pectoris, vasodilator therapy for heart failure should be avoided. The most critical decision in the management of aortic stenosis concerns the advisability of surgical treatment. The indications and results of operation, as well as the techniques, differ considerably, depending on the patient's age and the nature of the valvular deformity.

In children and adolescents with noncalcific aortic stenosis, considerable hemodynamic improvement can be anticipated from simple commissural incision under direct vision (Chap. 240). When carried out by an experienced surgical team, this procedure may be expected to enlarge the size of the valvular orifice significantly, without increasing the magnitude of aortic regurgitation, with a mortality rate of less than 3 percent. This operation is recommended not only for symptomatic patients but also for asymptomatic children and adolescents with hemodynamic evidence of severe obstruction to left ventricular outflow, with a peak systolic pressure gradient exceeding 50 mmHg when the cardiac output is normal, or a calculated effective orifice less than 0.7 cm² per square meter of body surface area. Though this procedure can be expected to result in complete or almost complete relief of obstruction in the majority of patients, the valve cannot be rendered entirely normal anatomically, and it may become deformed, calcified, and stenotic again, entailing the possibility of reoperation, and perhaps valve replacement at some later date.

In the majority of adults with calcific aortic stenosis, satisfactory valve function cannot be restored, even by deliberate sculpturing procedures carried out under direct vision, and replacement of the aortic valve is necessary. In most instances, it is prudent to postpone operation in patients with severe calcific aortic stenosis who are asymptomatic, since their future course is difficult to predict and they may continue to do well for many years. However, they should be followed carefully by clinical examination for the development of symptoms and by the various noninvasive tests for evidence of deteriorating left ventricular function. It is likely that as the results of surgical replacement of the aortic valve improve, many of these patients will become candidates for operation before their disease reaches the symptomatic stage. At this time replacement of the aortic valve should be undertaken in patients with symptoms believed to result primarily from aortic stenosis who also have hemodynamic evidence of severe obstruction.

It is clear that when symptoms of angina pectoris, syncope, or left ventricular decompensation develop in adults with valvular aortic stenosis, the outlook, despite medical treatment, is poor but can be improved significantly by replacement of the aortic valve with a prosthesis or tissue valve. Therefore, the risk entailed by operation in this group of patients is considerably lower than the risk involved by nonoperative treatment; moreover, the symptomatic improvement in many survivors of operation has been remarkable. However, the influence of aortic valve replacement on long-term survival and disability has not been established.

Operation should, if possible, be carried out before frank left ventricular failure supervenes; at this late stage, the operative risk is high (15 to 25 percent), and evidence of myocardial disease may persist even when the operation is technically successful. Furthermore, long-term postoperative survival correlates inversely with preoperative functional disability. Nonetheless, in view of the very poor prognosis of such patients when they are treated medically, there is usually little choice but to advise immediate surgical treatment. In patients in whom severe aortic stenosis and coronary artery disease coexist, relief of the aortic stenosis and revascularization of the myocardium by means of aortocoronary bypass grafting (Chap. 244) may result in striking clinical and hemodynamic improvement. Since many patients with calcific aortic stenosis are elderly, particular attention must be directed to the adequacy of hepatic, renal, and pulmonary function before valve replacement is recommended. At the present time aortic valve replacement in symptomatic patients with severe obstruction but without heart failure is associated with a higher immediate mortality rate than is aortic commissurotomy in childhood (5 to 12 percent in most centers), and the long-term results and complications associated with the use of the several available prostheses and heterografts show some variation. The mortality rate depends to a substantial extent on the patient's preoperative clinical and hemodynamic state. Accordingly, a more conservative approach to operative treatment is warranted in adults with calcific aortic stenosis than in children with noncalcific stenosis. The 8-year survival rate following aortic valve replacement is approximately 65 percent. Fortunately, there is evidence that regression of left ventricular hypertrophy may occur following relief of obstruction.

AORTIC REGURGITATION

PATHOPHYSIOLOGY The total stroke volume expelled by the left ventricle (i.e., the sum of the effective forward stroke volume and the volume of blood which regurgitates back into the left ventricle) is increased in aortic regurgitation. In contrast to mitral regurgitation, in which a fraction of the left ventricular stroke volume is delivered into the low-pressure left atrium, in aortic regurgitation the entire left ventricular stroke volume must be ejected into a high-pressure zone, the aorta. Although the low aortic diastolic pressure facilitates ventricular emptying during early systole, an increase of the left ventricular end-diastolic volume constitutes the major hemodynamic compensation to aortic regurgitation, and the total stroke volume is augmented. Measurements of aortic regurgitant flow by means of angiocardiographic techniques have revealed that in patients with free aortic regurgitation the volume of regurgitant flow may be of the same order of magnitude as the effective forward stroke volume. The dilatation of the left ventricle allows this chamber to expel a larger stroke volume without requiring any increase in the relative shortening of each myofibril. Therefore, severe aortic regurgitation may occur with a normal effective forward stroke volume and a normal ejection fraction [total (forward plus regurgitant) stroke volume/end-diastolic volume], together with an elevated left ventricular end-diastolic pressure and volume. On the other hand, through the operation of Laplace's law (which indicates that myocardial wall tension is the product of intracavitary pressure and left ventricular radius), left ventricular dilatation increases the left ventricular systolic tension required to develop any given level of systolic pressure. As left ventricular function deteriorates, the end-diastolic volume increases without further elevation of the aortic regurgitant volume; the ejection fraction and forward stroke volume decline. Deterioration of left ventricular function often precedes the development of symptoms. Considerable thickening of the left ventricular wall also occurs with chronic aortic regurgitation, and at autopsy the hearts of these patients may be among the largest encountered, occasionally exceeding 1000 g in weight.

The reduction of the aortic diastolic pressure in aortic regurgitation shortens the left ventricular isometric contraction period, which is helpful in prolonging the left ventricular ejection period. The reverse pressure gradient from aorta to left ventricle, which is responsible for the aortic regurgitant flow, falls progressively during diastole, accounting for the decrescendo nature of the diastolic murmur. Equilibration between aortic and left ventricular pressures may occur toward the end of diastole, particularly when the heart rate is slow, and the left ventricular end-diastolic pressure may be elevated, occasionally to extremely high levels (>40 mmHg). Rarely, the left ventricular pressure exceeds the left atrial pressure toward the end of diastole, and this reversed pressure gradient closes the mitral valve prematurely, or may cause diastolic mitral regurgitation.

In patients with free aortic regurgitation the effective forward cardiac output usually is normal or slightly reduced at rest, but often it fails to rise normally during exertion. In advanced stages there may be considerable elevation of the left atrial, pulmonary artery wedge, pulmonary arterial, and right ventricular pressures, and lowering of the cardiac output at rest. A qualitative index of the severity of aortic regurgitation may be obtained by determining the intensity of left ventricular opacification and the size of the left ventricle during thoracic cineaortography. In addition, this technique allows the detection of associated mitral regurgitation. However, quantitative angiographic techniques are required for accurate estimates of aortic regurgitant flow.

Myocardial ischemia occurs in patients with aortic regurgitation because both left ventricular dilatation and the elevated left ventricular systolic pressure tend to augment myocardial oxygen requirements. However, the major portion of coronary blood flow occurs during diastole, when arterial pressure is lower than normal; thus, coronary perfusion pressure is reduced. The result is a combination of increased oxygen supply and reduced demand.

ETIOLOGY Approximately three-fourths of all patients with pure or predominant regurgitation are males; however, females predominate among patients with aortic regurgitation who have associated mitral valve disease. In approximately 80 percent of patients with aortic regurgitation the disease is rheumatic in origin, resulting in a chronic form of the disorder with thickening, deformation, and shortening of the individual aortic valve cusps, changes which prevent their proper closure during diastole. A rheumatic etiology is less common in patients with isolated aortic regurgitation. Less commonly, infective endocarditis may attack a valve previously affected by rheumatic disease, a congenitally deformed valve, or rarely a normal aortic valve, and may result in the perforation or erosion of one or more of the leaflets, resulting in acute regurgitation. Patients with discrete membranous subaortic stenosis may develop thickening of the aortic valve leaflets, which in turn leads to mild or moderate degrees of aortic regurgitation and makes these valves particularly susceptible to endocarditis. Aortic regurgitation may also occur in patients with congenital bicuspid aortic valves. Prolapse of an aortic cusp, resulting in progressive chronic aortic regurgitation, occurs in approximately 15 percent of patients with ventricular septal defect (Chap. 240). Congenital fenestrations of the aortic valve occasionally produce mild or moderate degrees of aortic regurgitation. Traumatic rupture of the aortic valve is an uncommon cause of acute aortic regurgitation, but it represents the most frequent serious lesion observed in patients surviving nonpenetrating cardiac injuries. In patients with aortic regurgitation due to primary valvular disease, dilatation of the aortic annulus may occur secondarily and intensify the regurgitation.

Aortic regurgitation, both acute and chronic, may be due entirely to marked aortic dilatation, without primary involvement of the valve leaflets; widening of the aortic annulus and separation of the aortic leaflets are responsible for the aortic regurgitation. Syphilis and ankylosing rheumatoid spondylitis may be associated with cellular infiltration and scarring of the media of the thoracic aorta, leading to aortic dilatation, aneurysm formation, and severe regurgitation. In syphilis of the aorta (Chap. 250), the involvement of the intima may narrow the coronary ostia, which narrowing in turn may be responsible for coronary insufficiency. Cystic medial necrosis of the ascending aorta, which may or may not be associated with other manifestations of Marfan's syndrome (Chap. 250), idiopathic dilatation of the aorta, and severe hypertension may also widen the aortic annulus and lead to progressive aortic regurgitation. Occasionally, retrograde dissection of the aorta involving the aortic annulus produces aortic regurgitation.

The coexistence of hemodynamically significant aortic stenosis with aortic regurgitation usually excludes all the rarer forms of aortic regurgitation because it occurs almost entirely in patients whose aortic regurgitation is on a rheumatic or congenital basis.

SYMPTOMS A family history may frequently be elicited from patients with Marfan's syndrome, and a history of a heart murmur heard early in life may be obtained from patients with congenital aortic regurgitation. Patients with aortic regurgitation of obscure cause should also be questioned in detail about a positive serologic test for syphilis and about prior chest trauma; a history compatible with infective endocarditis may sometimes be elicited from patients with rheumatic or congenital involvement of the aortic valve, and the infection often precipitates or seriously aggravates preexisting symptoms. Ankylosing spondylitis is usually self-evident.

The interval between the first episode of acute rheumatic fever and the development of hemodynamically significant aortic regurgitation averages approximately 7 years, and this period is followed by an asymptomatic interval of approximately 10 to 20 years, during which the severity of the aortic regurgitation usually increases. Thus, severe aortic regurgitation may exist for many years without producing symptoms.

In chronic severe aortic regurgitation, the first complaint is often an uncomfortable awareness of the heartbeat, especially on lying down. Sinus tachycardia occurring during exertion or with emotion, or premature ventricular contractions, may produce particularly uncomfortable palpitations, as well as head pounding. These complaints may persist for many years before the development of exertional dyspnea, usually the first symptom of diminished cardiac reserve. This is followed by orthopnea, paroxysmal nocturnal dyspnea, and excessive diaphoresis. Symptoms of left ventricular failure are more common than symptoms of myocardial ischemia in patients with severe aortic regurgitation. Chest pain occurs frequently, even in younger patients, and invoking the presence of coronary artery disease is not necessary to explain this symptom in patients with aortic regurgitation. Chest pain may be due to myocardial ischemia, or it may originate from excessive cardiac pounding on the chest wall. Anginal pain may develop at rest as well as during exertion. Nocturnal angina may be a particularly troublesome symptom and is frequently accompanied by marked diaphoresis. The anginal episodes may be prolonged and often do not respond satisfactorily to sublingual nitroglycerin. Late in the course of the disease, evidence of systemic fluid accumulation, including congestive hepatomegaly, ankle edema, and ascites, may develop. Patients with severe aortic regurgitation tolerate high fevers, infections, or cardiac arrhythmias poorly, and may die in pulmonary edema as a result of one of these complications.

In patients with acute severe aortic regurgitation, as may occur in trauma or infective endocarditis, the left ventricle rapidly exhausts its ability to dilate, and left ventricular end-diastolic pressure rises rapidly with associated elevations of left atrial and pulmonary capillary pressures.

PHYSICAL FINDINGS The general examination should be directed toward the detection of causes predisposing to aortic regurgitation, such as Marfan's syndrome, rheumatoid spondylitis, syphilis, essential hypertension, and ventricular septal defect. Even prior to the examination of the heart of the patient with free aortic regurgitation, the jarring of the entire body and the bobbing motion of the head with each systole can be appreciated, and the abrupt distention and collapse of the larger arteries are easily visible. A rapidly rising "water-hammer" pulse, which collapses suddenly as arterial pressure falls rapidly during late systole and diastole (Corrigan's pulse), and capillary pulsations (Quincke's pulse), an alternate paling and flushing of the skin at the root of the nail while pressure is applied to the tip of the nail, are characteristic of free aortic regurgitation. A booming, "pistol-shot" sound can be heard over the femoral arteries, and a to-and-fro murmur (Duroziez's sign) is audible if the femoral artery is lightly compressed with a stethoscope.

The arterial pulse pressure is widened, with an elevation of the systolic pressure, sometimes to as high as 300 mmHg, and a depression of the diastolic arterial pressure. The measurement of arterial diastolic pressure with a sphygmomanometer may be complicated by the fact that systolic sounds are frequently heard with the cuff completely deflated. However, the level of cuff pressure at the time of muffling of the Korotkov sounds generally corresponds fairly closely to the true intraarterial diastolic pressure. The severity of aortic regurgitation does not always correlate directly with the arterial pulse pressure, and in many instances severe regurgitation exists in patients with arterial pressures in the range of 140/60. As the disease progresses, and the left ventricular end-diastolic pressure becomes markedly elevated, the arterial diastolic pressure may actually rise since the aortic diastolic pressure cannot fall below the left ventricular end-diastolic pressure.

The apex beat is displaced laterally and inferiorly. The left ventricle is hyperdynamic in patients with free regurgitation, and the systolic expansion and subsequent retraction of the apex are prominent and contrast sharply with the sustained systolic thrust characteristic of severe aortic stenosis. A diastolic thrill is often palpable along the left sternal border, and a prominent systolic thrill may be palpable in the jugular notch and transmitted upward along the carotid arteries. This thrill and the accompanying systolic murmur are due to the markedly increased blood flow across the aortic orifice, and do not necessarily signify the coexistence of aortic stenosis. Palpation, or indirect recording of the carotid arterial pulse, reveals it to be bisferiens, i.e., with two systolic waves separated by a trough, in many patients with pure aortic regurgitation, or with combined stenosis and regurgitation.

In patients with severe regurgitation the aortic valve closure sound is usually diminished or absent, and the indirectly recorded carotid arterial pulse does not usually show a clear-cut incisura. A third heart sound is common, and occasionally a fourth heart sound may also be heard. A loud systolic ejection sound is frequently audible; presumably it results from the sudden dilatation of the aorta by a greatly increased stroke volume.

The murmur of aortic regurgitation is typically a high-pitched, blowing, decrescendo diastolic murmur which is usually heard best in the third left intercostal space. In patients with mild regurgitation this murmur is brief and usually lasts less than one-third of diastole. However, as the severity increases, the murmur generally becomes louder and longer, and in patients with free aortic regurgitation it is usually holodiastolic. When the murmur is soft, it can be heard best with the diaphragm of the stethoscope and with the patient sitting up, leaning forward, and with the breath held in forced expiration. As it increases in intensity it tends to radiate widely, particularly down the lower sternal edge. In patients in whom the regurgitation is caused by primary valvular disease, the diastolic murmur is usually louder along the left than the right sternal border. However, when the decrescendo diastolic murmur is heard best along the right sternal border, it suggests that the aortic regurgitation is caused by dilatation or an aneurysm of the aortic root. "Cooing" or musical diastolic murmurs suggest eversion of an aortic cusp vibrating in the regurgitant stream.

On a purely statistic basis, a diastolic blowing murmur along the left sternal border is much more commonly caused by aortic than by pulmonic regurgitation. Unless it is trivial in magnitude, the aortic regurgitation can also be recognized by peripheral signs such as a widened pulse pressure or a collapsing pulse. On the other hand, the Graham Steell murmur of pulmonary regurgitation is usually accompanied by clinical evidence of severe pulmonary hypertension, including a loud and palpable pulmonary component of the second heart sound. In addition, the phonocardiogram reveals that the murmur of aortic regurgitation begins with the aortic second sound and therefore commences somewhat before the murmur of pulmonary regurgitation.

A systolic ejection murmur is generally heard best at the base of the heart and is transmitted to the jugular notch and along the carotid vessels. This murmur may be as loud as grade V or VI without indicating the presence of organic obstruction; it is often higher pitched, shorter, and less rasping in quality than the ejection systolic murmur heard in patients with predominant aortic stenosis.

The third murmur which is frequently heard in patients with aortic regurgitation is the Austin Flint murmur, a soft, low-pitched, rumbling middiastolic or presystolic bruit. It is probably produced by the displacement by the aortic regurgitation stream of the anterior leaflet of the mitral valve. However, this displacement of the mitral valve does not appear to be associated with hemodynamically significant obstruction to left ventricular filling; earlier onset and longer Austin Flint murmurs correlate with more severe aortic regurgitation. In patients with rheumatic aortic regurgitation it may be difficult to distinguish the Austin Flint murmur from the rumbling diastolic murmur of mitral stenosis. Both are loudest at the apex, but the murmur of mitral stenosis is usually accompanied by a loud first heart sound and immediately follows the opening snap of the mitral valve, while the Austin Flint murmur is often shorter in duration than the murmur of mitral stenosis, and in patients with sinus rhythm the latter more frequently is characterized by presystolic accentuation. The auscultatory features of aortic regurgitation are intensified by isometric exercise such as strenuous handgrip, which augments systemic resistance, and reduced by inhalation of amyl nitrite, which evokes the opposite effect. A blowing holosystolic murmur at the apex, which is transmitted to the axilla, may also be heard in patients with marked left ventricular dilatation and functional mitral regurgitation.

In *acute* severe aortic regurgitation, the elevation of left ventricular end-diastolic pressure may lead to early closure of the mitral valve, an associated middiastolic sound, a soft or absent S_1, a pulse pressure that is not particularly wide, and a soft, short diastolic murmur.

Electrocardiogram In patients with mild aortic regurgitation there may be no electrocardiographic abnormalities, but as the severity of aortic regurgitation increases, so do the electrocardiographic signs of left ventricular hypertrophy (Chap. 232). In addition to the abnormally tall R waves over the left precordium and deep S waves over the right precordium, patients with severe aortic regurgitation frequently exhibit ST-segment depressions and T-wave inversions in leads I, aVL, V_5, and V_6. Electrocardiographic signs of previous myocardial infarction generally indicate associated coronary artery disease. Left axis deviation and/or QRS prolongation denote diffuse myocardial disease, generally associated with patchy fibrosis; these signs are usually associated with a poor prognosis.

Echocardiogram This reveals increased systolic excursion of the posterior left ventricular wall; the velocity of wall motion is supernormal or normal until myocardial contractility declines. A rapid, high-frequency fluttering of the anterior leaflet of the mitral valve produced by the impact of the aortic regurgitant jet is a characteristic finding. The echocardiogram is also useful in detecting dilatation of the aortic root and of the left atrium in patients with aortic regurgitation.

Roentgenogram Moderate or severe degrees of regurgitation are always associated with varying degrees of left ventricular enlargement. The apex is displaced downward and to the left on the frontal projection, and frequently the cardiac shadow appears to extend below the left diaphragm. Left ventricular enlargement also occurs in the left anterior oblique and lateral projections, in which the left ventricle is displaced posteriorly and encroaches on the spine. In patients in whom primary valvular disease is responsible for the aortic regurgitation, the ascending aorta and aortic knob may be moderately dilated and may extend further to the right than the right atrial shadow in the frontal view. On fluoroscopic examination the aorta and left ventricle pulsate vigorously in opposite directions during systole. When aortic regurgitation is caused by primary disease of the aortic wall, aneurysmal dilatation of the aorta may be seen roentgenographically, and the aorta may fill the retrosternal space in the lateral view.

TREATMENT The left ventricular failure of chronic aortic regurgitation at first usually responds to treatment with digitalis glycosides, salt restriction, and diuretics. Digitalis may also be indicated in patients with severe regurgitation and dilated left ventricles without symptoms of frank left ventricular failure (Chap. 238). Cardiac arrhythmias and infections are poorly tolerated in patients with free aortic regurgitation, and must be treated promptly and vigorously. Although nitroglycerin and long-acting nitrites are not as helpful in relieving anginal pain as in patients with coronary artery disease or aortic stenosis, they are worth a trial. Patients with syphilitic aortitis should receive a full course of penicillin therapy (Chap. 146).

As in patients with other valvular lesions, the most critical decision in patients with aortic regurgitation concerns the advisability and proper timing of surgical treatment. Patients with chronic aortic regurgitation usually remain asymptomatic until after the development of myocardial dysfunction. Also, surgical treatment often does not restore normal left ventricular function. Therefore, careful clinical follow-up and repeated noninvasive testing, with judicious timing of catheterization of the left side of the heart when deterioration of cardiac function occurs, are desirable.

Replacement of the aortic valve with a suitable prosthesis or porcine heterograft is generally necessary in patients with rheumatic aortic regurgitation and in many patients with other forms of regurgitation. Rarely, when a leaflet has been perforated during an episode of infective endocarditis, or torn from its attachments to the aortic annulus, surgical repair may be possible. When aortic regurgitation is due to aneurysmal dilatation of the annulus and ascending aorta, rather than to primary valvular involvement, it may be possible to reduce the regurgitation by narrowing the annulus or by excising a portion of the aorta without operating on the aortic valve itself. More frequently, however, regurgitation can be eliminated only by replacing the aortic valve, excising the aneurysm responsible for the regurgitation, and replacing the latter with a graft. This formidable procedure entails a higher risk than aortic valve replacement alone.

As in patients with aortic stenosis, the operative risks of aortic valve replacement are largely dependent on the stage of the disease. Surgical treatment should be considered in patients who have free aortic regurgitation and who are symptomatic when engaged in ordinary activity in spite of medical therapy. Late mortality is also dependent on myocardial function at the time of operation; patients with marked cardiac enlargement and prolonged left ventricular dysfunction have a late mortality of approximately 5 percent per year. It is likely, however, that as in the case of aortic stenosis, further reductions of the operative mortality rate and increased confidence in the long-term effects of valvular prostheses and tissue valves will make it possible in the future to extend the recommendation for operative treatment to minimally symptomatic or even asymptomatic patients with severe regurgitation and cardiomegaly. In patients with acute, severe aortic regurgitation producing left ventricular failure, early surgical treatment is generally indicated and may be lifesaving. Long-term postoperative survival correlates inversely with the height and preoperative left ventricular end-diastolic pressure.

TRICUSPID STENOSIS

Tricuspid stenosis, a relatively uncommon valvular lesion, is generally rheumatic in origin and is much more common in women than in men. It does not usually occur as an isolated lesion or in patients with pure mitral regurgitation, but most commonly is observed in association with mitral stenosis, and sometimes with combined mitral and aortic stenosis. Hemodynamically significant tricuspid stenosis occurs in 5 to 10 percent of patients with severe mitral valve disease; rheumatic tricuspid stenosis is commonly associated with some degree of regurgitation. Carcinoid heart disease, fibroelastosis, and endomyocardial fibrosis are rare causes of tricuspid stenosis.

PATHOPHYSIOLOGY A diastolic pressure gradient between the right atrium and ventricle is the hemodynamic hallmark of tricuspid stenosis. This gradient can be recorded most accurately and conveniently with a double-lumen cardiac catheter, by placing the distal opening into the right ventricle and the proximal opening into the right atrium. It is augmented when the transvalvular blood flow increases during inspiration, and it is reduced when flow declines during expiration. A mean diastolic pressure gradient exceeding 5 mmHg is usually sufficient to elevate the mean right atrial pressure to levels which result in systemic venous congestion and, unless sodium intake has been restricted or diuretics have been given, is associated with ascites and edema. In patients with sinus rhythm, the right atrial *a* wave may be extremely tall and may even approach the level of the right ventricular systolic pressure. The resting cardiac output is usually quite reduced and fails to rise during exercise. The low cardiac output is responsible for the normal or only slightly elevated left atrial, pulmonary arterial, and right ventricular systolic pressures despite the presence of even moderately severe mitral stenosis.

SYMPTOMS Since mitral stenosis generally precedes the development of tricuspid stenosis, many patients initially have symptoms of pulmonary congestion. Amelioration of the symptoms of pulmonary congestion in a patient with mitral stenosis should raise the possibility that tricuspid stenosis may be developing. Characteristically, patients with hemodynamically significant tricuspid stenosis complain of relatively little dyspnea for the degree of hepatomegaly, ascites, and edema which they present. In some patients tricuspid stenosis may be suspected for the first time when symptoms of right ventricular failure persist after an adequate mitral valvulotomy. Weakness secondary to a low cardiac output and discomfort due to refractory edema, ascites, and marked hepatomegaly are common in patients with tricuspid stenosis and/or regurgitation.

PHYSICAL FINDINGS The diagnosis is often missed unless it is specifically considered and searched for. Severe tricuspid stenosis is associated with marked hepatic congestion, often resulting in cirrhosis, jaundice, serious malnutrition, severe edema, and ascites. Congestive hepatomegaly and, in advanced cases of tricuspid stenosis and/or regurgitation, splenomegaly are present. The jugular veins are distended, and in patients with sinus rhythm there may be giant *a* waves. The *v* waves are less conspicuous, and since tricuspid obstruction impedes right atrial emptying during diastole, there is a slow *y* descent. In patients with sinus rhythm there may be prominent presystolic pulsations of the enlarged liver as well.

The right ventricle and the shock of pulmonary valve closure are usually not easily palpable. Indeed, a giant *a* wave in the jugular venous pulse without palpatory evidence of pulmonary hypertension or right ventricular enlargement suggests the possibility of tricuspid stenosis. The pulmonic closure sound is not accentuated on auscultation, and occasionally an opening snap of the tricuspid valve may be heard or recorded phonocardiographically approximately 0.06 s after pulmonary valve closure. The diastolic rumbling murmur of tricuspid stenosis has many of the qualities of the mitral diastolic murmur, and since tricuspid stenosis almost always occurs in the presence of mitral stenosis, the less-common valvular lesion may be missed. However, the tricuspid murmur is generally most readily audible along the left lower sternal margin and over the xiphoid process and is most prominent during presystole in sinus rhythm. It is augmented during inspiration, when negative intrathoracic pressure increases the velocity of blood flow across the tricuspid orifice, and it is reduced during expiration and particularly during the Valsalva maneuver, when tricuspid blood flow is reduced. This finding (Carvallo's sign) is often most easily elicited when the patient is in the erect position. In patients with sinus rhythm the presystolic component is often loudest. The diastolic murmur is reduced in amplitude as the stethoscope is inched laterally, only to intensify or reappear as the mitral murmur at the apex. In patients with sinus rhythm the presystolic component is often louder at the tricuspid than at the mitral area; the tricuspid presystolic murmur commences before the mitral, and it often is of the crescendo-decrescendo type. As already indicated, severe tricuspid stenosis may obscure many of the physical signs of accompanying mitral stenosis.

Electrocardiogram and roentgenogram The features of right atrial enlargement (Chap. 232) include tall, peaked P waves in lead II, as well as prominent, upright P waves in lead V_1. The absence of electrocardiographic evidence of right ventricular hypertrophy in a patient with right-sided heart failure who is believed to have mitral stenosis should suggest the possibility of associated tricuspid valve disease. The chest roentgenograms in patients with combined tricuspid and mitral stenosis show particular prominence of the right atrium and superior vena cava without much enlargement of the pulmonary artery and with less evidence of pulmonary vascular congestion than occurs in patients with pure mitral valve disease.

TREATMENT Patients with tricuspid stenosis generally exhibit marked systemic venous congestion; intensive salt restriction, digitalization, and diuretic therapy are required during the preoperative period. Such a prolonged preparatory period may diminish hepatic congestion and thereby improve hepatic function sufficiently that the risks of operation are diminished. Surgical treatment of the tricuspid valve is not ordinarily indicated at the time of mitral valve surgery in patients with mild tricuspid stenosis. On the other hand, definitive surgical relief of the tricuspid stenosis should be carried out, preferably at the time of mitral valvulotomy, in patients with moderate or severe tricuspid stenosis who have mean diastolic pressure gradients exceeding 5 mmHg and tricuspid orifices less than 1.5 to 2.0 cm². Tricuspid stenosis is almost always accompanied by significant tricuspid regurgitation; simple finger-fracture valvulotomy often does not result in significant hemodynamic improvement, but may merely substitute severe regurgitation for stenosis. However, open operations utilizing cardiopulmonary bypass may permit substantial improvement of tricuspid valve function. If this cannot be accomplished, the tricuspid valve may have to be replaced with a prosthesis.

TRICUSPID REGURGITATION

Tricuspid regurgitation is usually functional and secondary to marked dilatation of the right ventricle and the tricuspid valve ring. Functional tricuspid regurgitation may complicate right ventricular failure of any cause, and is commonly seen in the late stages of heart failure due to rheumatic or congenital heart disease with severe pulmonary hypertension, i.e., with systolic pressures exceeding 60 mmHg, as well as ischemic heart disease, cardiomyopathy, and cor pulmonale. It is in part reversible if pulmonary hypertension is relieved. Rheumatic fever may also produce organic tricuspid regurgitation, which is associated with tricuspid stenosis in some instances. Less commonly, regurgitation results from congenitally deformed tricuspid valves, and it occurs with defects of the atrioventricular canal, as well as with Ebstein's malformation of the tricuspid valve (Chap. 240). Carcinoid heart disease, endomyocardial fibrosis, infective endocarditis, trauma, and infarction of right ventricular papillary muscles may also produce tricuspid regurgitation.

The clinical features of tricuspid regurgitation result primarily from systemic venous congestion and reduction of the cardiac output. With the onset of tricuspid regurgitation, as cardiac output declines, symptoms of pulmonary congestion diminish, but the clinical manifestations of right-sided heart failure become intensified. The neck veins are generally distended, with prominent *v* waves, and marked hepatomegaly, ascites, pleural effusions, edema, systolic pulsations of the liver, and positive hepatojugular reflux are common. A prominent right ventricular pulsation along the left parasternal region and a blowing holosystolic murmur along the lower left sternal margin which is generally intensified during inspiration and reduced during expiration or the Valsalva maneuver are characteristic findings; atrial fibrillation is usually present.

The electrocardiogram is usually characteristic of the lesion responsible for the enlargement of the right ventricle which leads to this form of valvular dysfunction. In the rare instances of isolated tricuspid regurgitation the electrocardiogram often shows incomplete right bundle branch block. Roentgenographic examination usually reveals enlargement of both the right ventricle and right atrium, and the latter chamber expands during systole. The cardiac output is usually markedly reduced, and the right atrial pressure pulse may exhibit no *x* descent during early systole, but a prominent *c-v* wave, with a rapid *y* descent. The mean right atrial and the right ventricular end-diastolic pressures are often elevated.

Isolated tricuspid regurgitation, without pulmonary hypertension, such as that occurring as a consequence of infective endocarditis or trauma, is usually well tolerated and does not require operation. Treatment of the underlying cause of heart failure usually reduces the severity of functional tricuspid regurgitation. In patients with mitral valve disease and tricuspid regurgitation due to pulmonary hypertension and massive right ventricular enlargement, effective surgical correction of the mitral valvular abnormality results in lowering of the pulmonary vascular pressures and gradual reduction or disappearance of the tricuspid regurgitation without direct treatment of the tricuspid valve. However, in patients with severe regurgitation secondary to deformity of the tricuspid valve due to rheumatic fever, particularly those without severe pulmonary hypertension, surgical treatment of the tricuspid regurgitation, consisting of either valve replacement or narrowing of the annulus, should be carried out.

PULMONIC VALVE DISEASE

The pulmonic valve is affected by rheumatic fever far less frequently than the other valves and is uncommonly the seat of infective endocarditis. The most common acquired abnormality affecting the pulmonic valve is regurgitation secondary to dilatation of the pulmonary valve ring as a consequence of severe pulmonary hypertension of any cause. This produces the Graham Steell murmur, a high-pitched, decrescendo, diastolic blowing murmur along the left sternal border, which is difficult to differentiate from the far more common murmur produced by aortic regurgitation. It is of little hemodynamic significance; indeed surgical removal or destruction of the pulmonic valve by infective endocarditis does not produce heart failure unless serious pulmonary hypertension is also present.

Congenital pulmonic stenosis is discussed in Chap. 240.

REFERENCES

BRAUNWALD E: Mitral regurgitation: Physiological, clinical and surgical considerations. N Engl J Med 281:425, 1969

————: Acquired valvular heart disease, in *Heart Disease,* E Braunwald (ed). Philadelphia, Saunders, 1980, chap 31

DEMARIA AN: Echocardiographic identification of the mitral valve prolapse syndrome. Am J Med 62:819, 1977

EL-SHERIF N: Rheumatic tricuspid stenosis: Hemodynamic correlations. Br Heart J 33:16, 1971

GOLDSCHLAGER N et al: The natural history of aortic regurgitation. Am J Med 54:577, 1973

HANNING CE, ROWE GC: Tricuspid insufficiency: A study of hemodynamics and pathogenesis. Circulation 45:793, 1972

JOHNSON AD et al: Medical and surgical management of patients with aortic valve disease. West J Med 126:460, 1977

MORGANROTH J et al: Acute severe aortic regurgitation. Ann Intern Med 87:223, 1977

O'ROURKE RA, CRAWFORD MH: The systolic click-murmur syndrome: Clinical recognition and management, in *Current Problems in Cardiology,* vol 1, no 1. Chicago, Yearbook, 1976

SONNENBLICK EH, LESCH M (eds): *Valvular Heart Disease.* New York, Grune & Stratton, 1974

Symposium on the Current Status of Valve Replacement. Am J Cardiol 35:221, 710, 1975

243
INFECTIVE ENDOCARDITIS

LAWRENCE L. PELLETIER, JR.
ROBERT G. PETERSDORF

DEFINITION Infective endocarditis is a microbial infection of the heart valves or of the endocardium in proximity to congenital or acquired cardiac defects. A similar clinical illness develops when there is infection of arteriovenous fistulas or aneurysms. The infection may develop abruptly or insidiously, may pursue a fulminant or prolonged course, and is fatal unless treated. The infection caused by indigenous microorganisms with low pathogenicity is ordinarily subacute, whereas infection by microorganisms with high pathogenicity is often acute. Fever, cardiac murmurs, splenomegaly, anemia, hematuria, mucocutaneous petechiae, and embolic manifestations are characteristic of the disease. Viridans streptococci are the commonest cause of bacterial endocarditis when superimposed upon congenital or rheumatic endocardial lesions and are usually associated with a subacute course.

ETIOLOGY AND EPIDEMIOLOGY Acute bacterial endocarditis is caused by relatively pathogenic microorganisms, exemplified by *Staphylococcus aureus,* pneumococcus, group A streptococcus, and less often gonococcus, *Histoplasma capsulatum, Brucella,* and *Listeria.* Endocarditis attributed to these organisms usually follows dissemination from an infected focus, which is often undetectable. Endocarditis caused by staphylococci, coliform bacilli, and *Candida* has been described frequently among intravenous drug users. Infection of the heart due to staphylococci, *Candida, Aspergillus,* or coliform bacilli and resembling endocarditis is a rare but serious complication of surgery in which sutures or prostheses have been placed in the heart or peripheral arteries. Primarily in alcoholics, endocarditis is sometimes observed in association with pneumococcal meningitis and bacteremia (Chap. 115). Staphylococcal endocarditis can result from bacteremia associated with septic thrombophlebitis due to infected intravenous catheters, hyperalimentation lines, or arteriovenous shunts; or a cutaneous, bone, or pulmonary infection. Group A streptococcal endocarditis is probably never a complication of streptococcal pharyngitis but may follow the bacteremia of streptococcal skin or puerperal infection. Polymicrobial infections may occur occasionally in parenteral drug addicts or after prosthetic valve surgery.

Subacute bacterial endocarditis usually develops in persons with rheumatic valvular or congenital cardiac lesions. It is most commonly caused by the viridans streptococci, which are part of the normal upper respiratory bacterial flora. *Streptococcus faecalis* (enterococcus), indigenous to the fecal and perineal flora, is an increasingly important cause of subacute bacterial endocarditis, particularly in elderly men with prostatism or women with genitourinary tract infections. *Staphylococcus aureus* may produce subacute as well as acute bacterial endocarditis. Suppuration, cellulitis, or other infected foci may precede subacute bacterial endocarditis but are recognized infrequently. Viridans streptococci are commonly found in the blood immediately after dental manipulation or extraction. Tonsillectomy and rigid bronchoscopy are also occasionally associated with transient bacteremia. Chewing of food or use of a water jet may result in bacteremia in patients with gingival disease or dental infection. Transient bacteremia of this sort is probably an important initiating factor in some cases of subacute bacterial endocarditis.

PATHOGENESIS Subacute bacterial endocarditis occurs most frequently in persons with preexisting heart disease. Infection most commonly involves the left side of the heart. The mitral, aortic, tricuspid, and pulmonary valves may be involved, in the order of frequency listed. Valves damaged by rheumatic fever are most commonly involved, but valves damaged by syphilis and arteriosclerosis are also susceptible to bacterial endocarditis. Enterococcal endocarditis in elderly men is associated with involvement of the aortic valve, and frequently results in marked valvular damage. Subacute bacterial endocarditis rarely involves interatrial septal defects. Prosthetic heart valves, mitral valve leaflet prolapse, or idiopathic hypertrophic subaortic stenosis may predispose to endocarditis. Infection in patients with interventricular septal defects often involves the endocardium opposite the septal defect in the direction of the shunt. Infection associated with patent ductus arteriosus develops on the pulmonary side of the ductus. Drug addicts frequently develop right-sided endocarditis involving the tricuspid valve. Valvular infection in association with rheumatic heart disease is usually on the valve edge along the line of closure.

Hemodynamic events are important in the pathogenesis of the disease. Alterations in blood flow can cause marked changes in vascular endothelium. It has been demonstrated experimentally that bacteria are deposited on the endothelium in areas of high flow with decreased lateral pressure. These factors are undoubtedly important in determining the situations and location where bacterial endocarditis develops. Infection in the heart is most often at a site of a structural change or abnormality. Thrombi that develop on endocardial irregularities have been implicated as foci for bacterial implantation, and it seems likely that a sterile vegetation consisting of platelets and fibrin is the nidus on which bacteria become implanted.

Serum antibodies in high titer against the infecting microorganisms are often found in patients with bacterial endocarditis and circulating antigen-antibody complexes are commonly found, associated with immune complex glomerulonephritis and possibly cutaneous vasculitis. The presence of opsonizing antibodies to bacteria may facilitate localization of organisms on the endocardium during transient bacteremias. However, the role of immunity in the development of bacterial endocarditis is not known.

Infective endocarditis leads to deposition of fibrin and platelets about the site of infection, producing a vegetation. Highly pathogenic microorganisms often cause rapid valvular destruction and ulceration. Less pathogenic microorganisms usually cause less valvular destruction or ulceration but can lead to development of large polypoid vegetations. The infection may extend from the valve to the surrounding mural endocardium or penetrate the valve ring to produce a mycotic aneurysm, myocardial abscess, or cardiac conduction defects. Involvement of chordae tendineae may lead to rupture and valvular insufficiency. Acute bacterial endocarditis, particularly when caused by *S. aureus,* often is associated with abscesses in the valve ring. Vascularization of involved valves may increase during endocarditis but rarely extends into the area of infection. Phagocytes are not prominent in the area of bacterial growth, which may explain why infection by microorganisms of low pathogenicity progresses uncontrolled without bactericidal antimicrobial therapy. The lack of vascularization of the granulation tissue in the vegetation also may account for ineffectiveness of host defenses and the requirement for intensive treatment.

The bacteremia of intravascular infections is ordinarily continuous. For this reason few blood cultures are required to demonstrate the microorganisms. The microorganisms are primarily cleared from the blood by the reticuloendothelial cells of the liver and spleen. There is no obvious reduction in the number of bacteria in the blood during circulation through the extremities. Arterial blood cultures, therefore, are no more likely to show bacteremia than are venous blood cultures.

Embolization is a characteristic feature of infective endocarditis. The friable fibrin vegetations may separate from the site of infection and be propelled as emboli into the systemic or pulmonary circulation, depending on whether the endocarditis involves the left or right side of the heart. Emboli vary in size and most often involve the brain, spleen, kidney, gastrointestinal tract, heart, or extremities. Emboli in fungal endocarditis tend to be large and occlude major vessels. Pulmonary infarction or abscess is common in right-sided endocarditis. Septic infarction is uncommon in subacute bacterial endocarditis caused by microorganisms of low pathogenicity, and suppurative complications are rarely seen at these sites when viridans streptococci are the offending agents. Osteomyelitis has been described, however, as an embolic complication of endocarditis due to viridans streptococci and enterococci. Septic infarction is common in acute bacterial endocarditis attributable to bacteria of high pathogenicity, as are metastatic abscesses. Involvement of major arteries by emboli produces mycotic aneurysms, which may rupture. Myocardial infarction may develop

after coronary embolization. In addition, focal myocarditis is common in subacute bacterial endocarditis and may be embolic.

The spleen is frequently enlarged, particularly in subacute cases. Three types of renal lesions may be produced. When large emboli find their way into the kidney, infarction may develop. Small emboli may produce a focal glomerulitis. In many instances, there is a diffuse glomerulonephritis that is indistinguishable from other types of immune complex glomerulonephritis. Petechial skin lesions, characterized histologically by acute vasculitis, are probably not embolic and may be immunologic in origin. Other skin lesions associated with pain, tenderness, and cellulitis, however, may be embolic.

MANIFESTATIONS Subacute bacterial endocarditis Patients ordinarily cannot date the onset of the infection. Symptoms begin insidiously, and gradually the illness becomes apparent. In some individuals, however, the onset of infection can be related to a recent dental extraction, urethral instrumentation, tonsillectomy, acute respiratory infection, or abortion.

Weakness, fatigability, weight loss, feverishness, night sweats, anorexia, and arthralgia are the usual symptoms of subacute bacterial endocarditis. Emboli may produce paralysis, chest pain due to myocardial or pulmonary infarction, acute vascular insufficiency with pain in the extremities, hematuria, acute abdominal pain, or sudden blindness. Painful fingers or toes and painful skin lessions may also be important symptoms. Chills are not common. Transient cerebral ischemic attacks, toxic encephalopathy, headache, brain abscess, subarachnoid hemorrhage from rupture of a mycotic aneurysm, or purulent meningitis may develop.

Physical examination may reveal a variety of findings, none of which alone is pathognomonic of subacute bacterial endocarditis. Physical examination may be normal early in the course of infection. The association of the different manifestations, however, usually provides a characteristic picture of the disease. The patient usually appears chronically ill and pale and has an elevated temperature. The fever is most often remittent, with afternoon or evening peaks. The pulse is usually rapid, and if cardiac failure complicates the infection, it may be greater than expected with the degree of fever.

Mucocutaneous lesions are common and vary in type. Petechiae are most frequent and may be found in the mucosa of the mouth, pharynx, or conjunctivas. These small, red, hemorrhagic-appearing lesions do not blanch on pressure and are not tender or painful. On the mucous membranes or conjunctivas these petechiae may have a pale center. Small, occasionally flame-shaped hemorrhages are found in the retina, and may also have pale centers (Roth's spots). Petechiae may be found anywhere on the skin but are most common over the upper part of the trunk anteriorly. They are frequently difficult to distinguish from angiomas, but they gradually become brownish and disappear. Frequently, petechiae continue to appear, even during convalescence. Linear hemorrhages (splinter hemorrhages) may be found under the nails, but these are difficult to differentiate from traumatic lesions, particularly in manual laborers. These mucocutaneous lesions are not specific for bacterial endocarditis but may be found in patients with other conditions such as profound anemia, leukemia, trichinosis, and sepsis without endocarditis.

The pulp of the fingers may show tender subcutaneous papules which are purplish or erythematous (Osler's nodes). Larger erythematous, painful, and tender nodules may develop on the palms of the hands or soles of the feet. These are probably embolic lesions. Emboli to larger peripheral arteries may result in gangrene of fingers, toes, or larger portions of the extremities.

Clubbing of the fingers is observed in long-standing or prolonged bacterial endocarditis. Mild jaundice is found occasionally.

Findings in the heart are usually those of underlying heart disease. Major changes in cardiac murmurs, primarily development of a new diastolic murmur, may be attributable to ulceration of a valve, dilatation of the heart or valve ring, rupture of chordae tendineae, or development of a very large vegetation. Minor changes in systolic bruits are usually of little significance. In rare instances, no cardiac murmurs are detected. In this situation, right-sided endocarditis or an infected mural thrombus, or pulmonary, or peripheral arteriovenous fistula should be suspected.

Splenomegaly is common in subacute bacterial endocarditis. Rarely is the spleen tender, but a friction rub may be heard over it when there is infarction. Hepatomegaly is not characteristic unless heart failure develops.

Arthralgia is relatively common, and arthritis resembling acute rheumatic fever may occur.

Embolic phenomena may precipitate awareness of the infection. Sudden development of hemiplegia, flank pain with hematuria, abdominal pain with melena, pleuritic pain and hemoptysis, left upper abdominal pain with splenic friction rub, blindness, or monoplegia in a patient with fever and cardiac murmurs makes bacterial endocarditis suspect. Pulmonary emboli in right-sided endocarditis may be confused with pneumonia.

Acute bacterial endocarditis Infectious endocarditis caused by highly pathogenic microorganisms usually begins abruptly. Suppurative infection commonly antedates the onset of endocarditis. For example, infection of the heart may develop as a complication of pneumococcal meningitis, septic thrombophlebitis, group A streptococcal cellulitis, or staphylococcal abscesses. The source of cardiovascular infection, therefore, is often evident.

Acute bacterial endocarditis often involves the normal heart, in contrast to the subacute infection, which almost invariably involves the abnormal heart. It is particularly common in intravenous drug users. The acute infection is fulminant and pursues a rapid course. Fever is often greater, may be intermittent, and in certain instances (as in gonococcal endocarditis) may be characterized by a double quotidian temperature curve. Chills are common. Petechiae may be numerous, and embolic phenomena are prominent. Osler's nodes and painful erythematous nodules of the palms and soles are uncommon. Hematuria is seen with embolic lesions of the kidney, and diffuse glomerulonephritis may occur. Destruction of the cardiac valves can be complicated by rupture of chordae tendineae or perforation of cusps, leading to rapidly progressing cardiac failure. Metastatic abscesses following septic emboli are frequent.

Prosthetic valve endocarditis Prosthetic valve infections develop in 1 to 2 percent of patients following prosthetic valve placement. About one-third of these infections develop *within 2 months of surgery* and are probably due to colonization of the prosthesis or suture sites during surgery. *Staphylococcus aureus, S. epidermidis,* coliform bacilli, *Candida* spp., *Aspergillus* spp., and diphtheroid organisms that cause early infections are often resistant to antimicrobial agents; such infections are associated with a high mortality rate due to septic shock, valve dehiscence, and myocardial invasion. Gram-negative bacteremia in the immediate postoperative period may originate from urinary tract, wound, pulmonary infections, or septic phlebitis and is often not associated with prosthetic valve infection.

Prosthetic valve infections that occur *more than 2 months after surgery* are frequently caused by viridans streptococci, enterococci, *S. aureus,* or *S. epidermidis.* These infections probably result from colonization of the prosthesis or its site of attachment during transient bacteremias. Patients with prosthetic valves should receive prophylactic antimicrobial agents when undergoing procedures known to produce bacteremia, and minor infections that might produce bacteremia should be treated promptly. Late onset infections caused by streptococci have a better prognosis than early infections and may be controlled with antibiotics alone.

Prosthetic valve infections often produce symptoms and signs indistinguishable from infections on natural valves, but there is a greater frequency of valve ring infection that may involve part or all of the circumference producing valve dehiscence or penetration into the myocardium or surrounding tissues. Myocardial abscess, conduction disturbances, sinus of Valsalva aneurysm, or fistulas into the right side of the heart or pericardium may result. Prolongation of the PR interval, a new left bundle branch block, or right bundle branch block with left anterior hemiblock should suggest involvement of the ventricular septum in aortic valve infections. Extension of infection from the mitral valve annulus may be associated with nonparoxysmal junctional tachycardia, or second- or third-degree heart block with a narrow QRS complex. Prosthetic valve stenosis due to vegetations narrowing the orifice or interfering with valve excursion may be detected by auscultation or phonocardiogram. A postoperative regurgitant murmur or abnormal position or movement of the valve on fluoroscopic examination or echocardiogram may indicate partial dehiscence of the prosthesis. Prosthetic valve infections complicated by valve stenosis, valve dehiscence with congestive heart failure, recurrent emboli, resistance to antimicrobial therapy, or evidence of myocardial invasion require early surgical intervention. Relapse following appropriate antimicrobial treatment or fungous infections also requires early surgical removal of the infected prosthesis.

LABORATORY FINDINGS Leukocytosis with neutrophilia is the rule but is by no means an invariable finding. Macrophages (histiocytes) may be found in the blood, particularly in the first drop obtained from the earlobe. Normocytic, normochromic anemia is almost always found in subacute bacterial endocarditis but may not be present early in acute bacterial endocarditis. The erythrocyte sedimentation rate is rapid. Serum immunoglobulins are increased but return to normal during convalescence. The anti-gamma globulin latex fixation test is commonly positive, and the Rose-Waaler test is negative. Mild bilirubinemia is detected occasionally. Proteinuria is common, and microscopic hematuria is frequently present. Serum total hemolytic complement and the third component of complement may be decreased.

An echocardiogram may identify high-risk patients with large vegetations or unsuspected preexisting valvular lesions, or it may provide an indication for early operation in patients with acute aortic insufficiency and severe volume overload of the left ventricle. The echocardiogram does not detect vegetations smaller than 2 mm, nor does it differentiate active from healed lesions.

Blood cultures are positive in the majority of cases. Three to five cultures of 10 ml of blood, taken at intervals determined by the patient's clinical status, are usually adequate to demonstrate the bacteremia, if it is demonstrable at all. Blood cultures may not become positive for several days, if at all, in patients who have received antibiotics prior to the time when cultures are obtained. Failure to demonstrate bacteremia or delayed growth in blood cultures also may be due to infection by unusual microorganisms such as *Histoplasma capsulatum, Brucella, Pasteurella, Hemophilus parainfluenzae,* or anaerobic streptococci that require special nutrient media or extended (up to 4 weeks) incubation. Thiol-requiring streptococcal variants may require pyridoxine- or cysteine-supplemented broth. Castañeda-type culture bottles are required for fungi and *Brucella. Aspergillus* endocarditis is seldom associated with positive blood cultures. *Coxiella burnetii* endocarditis and *Chlamydia psittaci* endocarditis are diagnosed by serologic tests, since blood cultures are always negative. Bone marrow cultures and serologic testing for *Candida, Histoplasma,* and *Brucella* may be helpful in culture-negative endocarditis. Endocarditis of the right side of the heart is as likely to produce bacteremia as is endocarditis involving the left side of the heart.

DIFFERENTIAL DIAGNOSIS When several of the manifestations of infective endocarditis occur together, the diganosis is not difficult. In particular, the presence of fever, petechiae, splenomegaly, microscopic hematuria, and anemia in a patient with cardiac murmurs is most suggestive of infection. When only a few manifestations are present, however, the diagnosis is not simple. Prolonged fever in a patient with rheumatic heart disease is particularly troublesome, but the diagnosis of bacterial endocarditis should be considered in every patient with fever and a heart murmur. The diagnosis becomes even more difficult when blood cultures show no growth.

Acute rheumatic fever with carditis is often difficult to distinguish from bacterial endocarditis, and in a few instances, active rheumatic fever has been found to coexist with the valvular infection. The diagnosis of rheumatic carditis hinges on a combination of clinical and laboratory criteria (Chap. 241).

Subacute bacterial endocarditis is a common cause of "fever of undetermined origin" (Chap. 10). It may be mistaken for a hidden neoplasm, systemic lupus erythematosus, periarteritis nodosa, poststreptococcal glomerulonephritis, and intracardiac tumors such as myxoma of the atrium. Dissecting aneurysms with acute aortic regurgitation also may mimic bacterial endocarditis. Drug fever may be erroneously diagnosed as bacterial endocarditis. Postoperative endocarditis should be suspected in patients who develop fever, anemia, and leukocytosis after cardiovascular surgery. In these postoperative patients, the various postthoracotomy and postcardiotomy syndromes must also be considered.

PROGNOSIS Recovery from untreated bacterial endocarditis is rare. With appropriate antibiotic therapy, however, over 70 percent of the patients with infection on endogenous valves and 50 percent with infection on prosthetic valves survive the infection. Intravenous drug users with right-sided staphylococcal endocarditis generally have a good prognosis. The infection has a poor prognosis under the following circumstances: (1) when congestive heart failure is present; (2) when bacteremia is not demonstrable; (3) when the organisms are resistant to multiple antimicrobials; (4) when therapy is delayed; or (5) when infection develops on a prosthetic valve. Prosthetic valve, gram-negative bacillus, fungous, and acute bacterial types of endocarditis are associated with the poorest prognosis.

The commonest cause of death in treated endocarditis is congestive heart failure, attributable either to valve destruction or to myocardial damage. Additionally, death may be precipitated by embolization to vital organs, by renal insufficiency, by rupture of a mycotic aneurysm, or by complications following cardiac surgery. Many patients recover completely without apparent worsening of the underlying cardiovascular disease. When recurrent endocarditis develops, it usually involves the same valve and is due to failure to kill microorganisms in an environment of suboptimal host resistance.

Further reduction in the mortality rate of infective endocarditis will depend primarily on the increased use of cardiac surgery in combination with antimicrobial therapy to eliminate refractory infections, and the early replacement of damaged valves in patients with congestive heart failure.

PROPHYLAXIS Patients with prosthetic heart valves and suspected congenital or acquired valvular heart disease should be given antibiotics immediately before any dental manipulation, periodontal surgery, obstetric delivery, urethral catheterization, and other forms of intubation. The rationale for this practice is that when these patients develop bacteremia, they are more likely to develop endocarditis. The best experimental evidence available holds that for prevention of endocarditis caused by viridans streptococci with penicillin, both a high concentration and relatively prolonged duration of action are necessary. It has been shown that penicillin and streptomycin act synergistically in killing viridans streptococci. These data suggest a regimen consisting of a single dose of 1.2 million units of aqueous procaine penicillin G plus 1.0 g streptomycin administered intramuscularly within 30 min of dental surgery, followed by penicillin V 0.5 g orally at 6-h intervals for four doses, is effective. A loading dose of 2 g penicillin V followed by 0.5 g of the drug at 6-h intervals for 24 h is probably equally effective. Patients who are allergic to penicillin should receive vancomycin, 1.0 g intravenously over 30 min, 1 h before the procedure or erythromycin, 1.0 g orally 1½ to 2 h before the procedure. Either antibiotic should be followed with erythromycin, 0.5 g orally every 6 h for four doses. The best regimen for preventing enterococcal endocarditis is ampicillin plus gentamicin. Ampicillin, 1 g, plus gentamicin, 1.5 mg/kg (not over 80 mg), should be given intramuscularly or intravenously 30 to 60 min before the procedure, and both agents should be repeated every 8 h for two doses. Penicillin-allergic patients should receive vancomycin, 1.0 g intravenously, and streptomycin, 1.0 g intramuscularly, 30 to 60 min before the procedure; administration of both agents is repeated 12 h later. Although not proved definitively, antistaphylococcal prophylaxis may be indicated during surgery associated with implantation of prosthetic heart valves, intracardiac materials, or vascular prostheses. Cephalothin or cefazolin, 1.0 g intravenously, every 4 to 6 h should be given 30 min prior to surgery and continued no longer than 72 h.

The prophylactic doses of penicillin used to prevent group A streptococcal infection and recurrent rheumatic fever will not prevent bacterial endocarditis, although the dose of penicillin G given for rheumatic fever prophylaxis does not predispose to bacterial endocarditis caused by penicillin-resistant microorganisms.

TREATMENT The best treatment of bacterial endocarditis is assured when treatment is begun early in the illness, when an effective *bactericidal* antimicrobial agent is selected, and when treatment is continued over a relatively long period of time.

Selection of the most effective antibiotic for treatment of bacterial endocarditis depends on the sensitivity of the infecting microorganism. When bacteremia is not demonstrated, selection of the therapeutic agent depends on predicting the most probable infecting bacteria and their probable antibiotic sensitivity.

Bacterial endocarditis in young persons with rheumatic or congenital disease is most often due to the viridans streptococci. These microorganisms are usually very sensitive to penicillin G. Administration of 2.4 to 6 million units of penicillin daily to these patients is usually effective in eliminating the infection when therapy is continued for 4 weeks. The penicillin should be given parenterally for 2 weeks but for the second 2 weeks may be given orally (penicillin V if adequate serum levels are assured by a peak serum bactericidal titer of more than 1:8 dilution). There is a synergistic effect of streptomycin with penicillin on viridans streptococci, and streptomycin in a dose of 0.5 g twice a day should be administered in addition to penicillin during the first 2 weeks of therapy.

Bacterial endocarditis in older men and women after abortion or endometritis is often due to enterococci (*S. faecalis, S. faecium, S. durans*). These microorganisms are relatively resistant to penicillin alone. Enterococci should be differentiated from group D nonenterococcal organisms (*S. bovis*) that are susceptible to penicillin alone. The combination of penicillin with gentamicin is synergistic against the enterococcus, and the administration of these two antibiotics together is the treatment of choice in the infection. Penicillin G should be given parenterally in a dose of 12 to 24 million units per day, together with gentamicin in a dose of 3 to 5 mg/kg per day divided into three doses. Ampicillin, in a dosage of 8 to 12 g per day, may be substituted for penicillin G. Treatment should be continued for a minimum of 4 weeks. Adjustment of the gentamicin dosage may be necessary in renal insufficiency or in the absence of therapeutic serum levels.

Penicillin G, 6 to 12 million units a day given parenterally, is satisfactory for treatment of pneumococcal and group A streptococcal endocarditis. Treatment should be continued for 4 weeks. Penicillinase-resistant penicillin analogues should be used in the initial treatment of staphylococcal endocarditis because of the high probability that the infection is due to a penicillin-resistant organism. Methicillin should be given intravenously in a dose of 12 g per day in divided doses at 4-h intervals in 50-ml volumes injected over 20 to 30 min. Oxacillin, nafcillin, cephalothin, cefazolin, or vancomycin may be administered in lieu of methicillin. The addition of gentamicin to a penicillinase-resistant penicillin or cephalosporin results in enhanced staphylococcal killing in vitro and may improve the clinical response in some patients. If the staphylococcus is found to be sensitive to penicillin G, this antibiotic should be given rather than methicillin, in a dose of 16 to 24 million units per day. Treatment should be continued for at least 4 weeks. In staphylococcal endocarditis in particular, attention must be given to possible metastatic abscesses requiring surgical drainage. Prosthetic valve infections should be treated 6 to 8 weeks.

In patients allergic to penicillin, the alternative drugs are cephalothin, cefazolin, and vancomycin. Vancomycin and streptomycin should be administered to penicillin-allergic patients with enterococcal endocarditis. If an allergic reaction to penicillin develops during the course of therapy, antihistamines or corticosteroids may be used to alleviate the manifestations of the reaction.

Usually fever begins to disappear within 3 to 7 days after the start of treatment of bacterial endocarditis. Embolic complications of the disease, heart failure, and infection with resistant microorganisms, however, may delay defervescence. Drug fever or phlebitis may occasionally supervene and complicate the febrile course. Cessation of all therapy for 72 h is not hazardous and may identify such a drug reaction readily. Sterile emboli or late valve rupture occurs occasionally up to 12 months after cessation of therapy.

Many patients with arteriovenous fistulas, valve ring abscess, recurrent embolization, endocarditis produced by resistant organisms, or infected cardiac prostheses require surgical intervention before the infection can be controlled. In addition, early valve replacement should be considered in patients who develop congestive heart failure associated with marked valvular damage (particularly aortic or mitral regurgitation) as a consequence of bacterial endocarditis. Valve replacement has been lifesaving and must be undertaken before intractable heart failure ensues.

Fungous endocarditis is usually fatal. However, a few survivors have been reported after surgical debridement and replacement of the infected valve combined with amphotericin B therapy.

When bacterial endocarditis recurs, it usually develops within 4 weeks after treatment is terminated. Reinstitution of antibiotic therapy is required, but the sensitivity of the microorganism to the antibiotic must be reevaluated. Relapse may indicate inadequate or inappropriate therapy, or the need for surgical intervention. Recrudescence of bacterial endocarditis more than 6 weeks after cessation of treatment usually connotes a new infection.

REFERENCES

DUMA RJ (ed): *Infections of Prosthetic Heart Valves and Vascular Grafts.* Baltimore, University Park Press, 1977

KAPLAN EL et al: Prevention of bacterial endocarditis. Circulation 56:139A, 1977

———, TARANTA AV (eds): *Infective Endocarditis: An American Heart Association Symposium*, Monograph 52. Dallas, American Heart Association, 1977

KARCHMER AW et al: Late prosthetic valve endocarditis. Am J Med 64:199, 1978

KAYE D (ed): *Infective Endocarditis.* Baltimore, University Park Press, 1976

KERR AJ JR: *Subacute Bacterial Endocarditis.* Springfield, Ill, Charles C Thomas, 1955

LERNER PI, WEINSTEIN L: Infective endocarditism in the antibiotic era. N Engl J Med 274:199, 1966

PELLETIER LL, PETERSDORF RG: Infective endocarditis: A review of 125 cases from the University of Washington hospitals, 1963-72. Medicine 56:287, 1977

PETERSDORF RG: Prophylaxis of bacterial endocarditis: Prudent caution or microbial overkill. Am J Med 65:220, 1978

ROY P et al: Spectrum of echocardiographic findings in bacterial endocarditis. Circulation 53:474, 1976

SIPES JN et al: Prophylaxis of infective endocarditis: A re-evaluation. Annu Rev Med 28:371, 1977

WILSON WR et al: Prosthetic valve endocarditis. Ann Intern Med 82:751, 1975

244
ISCHEMIC HEART DISEASE

EUGENE BRAUNWALD
PETER F. COHN
RICHARD S. ROSS

Ischemia refers to oxygen deprivation consequent to reduced perfusion. The term *ischemic heart disease* defines a disease spectrum of diverse etiology, with the common factor being an imbalance between myocardial oxygen supply and demand. This imbalance is usually related to either an absolute reduction in coronary blood flow or an inability to increase coronary blood flow relative to the needs of the heart, and is most often due to atherosclerotic obstruction of large coronary arteries. The myocardium can be rendered ischemic also by nonatheromatous coronary obstructive lesions, such as embolism, coronary ostial stenosis associated with luetic aortitis, coronary artery spasm, or very uncommonly an arteritis of the coronary vessels. Congenital abnormalities of the coronary circulation, especially anomalous origin of the left coronary artery from the pulmonary trunk, may cause myocardial ischemia in the infant or child and, rarely, in the adult. The imbalance between myocardial oxygen supply and demand may be less commonly due to an increase in myocardial oxygen demands exceeding the supply capabilities of a normal coronary circulation, as occurs in severe myocardial hypertrophy especially when aortic stenosis is present. Myocardial ischemia may occur when the oxygen-carrying capacity of the blood is reduced, as in anemia or the presence of carboxyhemoglobin, or as a consequence of an inadequate perfusion pressure due to hypotension of any cause.

The location of atherosclerotic lesions in the coronary circulation and the degree of luminal narrowing they cause serve to determine whether the lesions will bring about significant and clinically evident ischemia. Luminal narrowing is important because flow through a tubular conduit varies with the fourth power of the radius if other conditions are kept constant. Location is important because it relates to the mass of myocardium perfused by the vessel in question. Thus, occlusive disease of the proximal left anterior descending artery jeopardizes the septum and anterior left ventricular free wall, whereas a similar lesion in a distal branch of this vessel compromises the flow of a lesser mass of myocardium. The state of the collateral circulation also helps determine whether ischemic heart disease develops as a consequence of coronary atherosclerosis. Although all the factors responsible for collateral development and their influence on the course of the disease remain uncertain, it appears that the potential for the development of collaterals is present in many and possibly all hearts, but that these channels do not develop sufficiently to be visualized until the stimulus of ischemia is manifest.

Asymptomatic coronary arteriosclerosis develops at an unknown rate and is detected only when death occurs from another cause, such as trauma, or when the coronary vessels are visualized angiographically; the latter may be carried out when an exercise electrocardiogram or thallium 201 scan performed for screening purposes is positive. The disease begins early in life, as evidenced by the relatively frequent finding of significant obstructive lesions in the coronary arteries of young men killed in war. The symptomatic phase presents most commonly as angina pectoris, acute myocardial infarction (Chap. 245), or sudden death; the latter presumably is due to ventricular arrhythmia (Chap. 32). Alternatively, patients may present with a symptom complex that shares features of both acute myocardial infarction and angina and is termed *unstable angina* or the *intermediate syndrome* (Chap. 245). A less common presentation is with arrhythmias, generally ventricular electrical instability, of sufficient severity to cause symptoms in the absence of angina or infarction. Frequently, however, these arrhythmias do not result in symptoms, and the tentative diagnosis of ischemic heart disease is suggested only when arrhythmia is discovered on a routine physical examination or exercise testing. The recent enthusiasm for periodic physical examinations including rest and exercise electrocardiographic evaluation has defined a new presentation of coronary arteriosclerosis, i.e., the asymptomatic patient in whom coronary obstructive lesions are suspected on the basis of an abnormal electrocardiogram at rest or during the stress of an exercise test.

Once in the symptomatic phase, the patient may remain symptomatic with either a stable or progressive course, return to the asymptomatic stage, or die suddenly. The average mortality rate following entry into the symptomatic phase of ischemic heart disease is 4 percent per year irrespective of whether the initial event is the development of angina pectoris or a myocardial infarction from which the patient has recovered.

There are, however, subsets of this patient population with mortality rates that differ by a factor of 4. For example, patients with a normal electrocardiogram and arterial pressure have an expected mortality rate of only 2 percent per year, in contrast to those with hypertension and an abnormal electrocardiogram, for whom the expected annual mortality rate is 8 percent per year.

The two principal prognostic indicators are the *state of function of the left ventricle* and the *extent of coronary artery disease*. Patients with compromised ventricular function are at increased risk. Compromised function may be noted by symptoms of congestive heart failure, roentgenographic evidence of cardiac enlargement, and/or angiographic evidence of altered cardiac performance (reduced ejection fraction, elevated left ventricular end-diastolic volume, and, perhaps most importantly, elevated left ventricular end-systolic volume). The mortality rates in patients with normal left ventricular function and disease in all three or in two of the three major coronary arteries average 11 and 8 percent per year, respectively, as compared with 2 percent per year in patients with single-vessel involvement. In patients with obstruction in the left main coronary artery, mortality averages 15 percent. With any degree of coronary artery obstruction the mortality is correspondingly elevated in patients with impaired left ventricular function. Within each angiographic class, additional prognostic subsets have also been defined. For example, patients with obstructive lesions isolated to a single artery segregate into different mortality groups. Lesions isolated to the left anterior descending coronary artery appear to carry a greater risk than those to the right or left circumflex vessels. Data concerning mortality in patients with specific coronary arterial lesions have generally been obtained from patients with symptomatic disease. Prognosis of asymptomatic individuals with similar anatomic abnormalities is not well established. Ventricular ectopic activity is yet another index of increased risk (Chap. 32).

Although numerous variables which affect mortality in coronary artery disease have thus been identified, no matrix analysis incorporating all these factors into a coronary prognostic index is available. As such, it is best to conceptualize coronary atherosclerosis as a process that destroys myocardial tissue at an unpredictable rate, thus reducing cardiac reserve. The greater the degree of muscle cell death at any point in time, the less the cardiac reserve, the less the ability to tolerate additional myocardial damage, and therefore the higher the expected mortality rate. In this light, the various indexes of increased risk, such as an abnormal electrocardiogram and left ventricular failure, should be taken as evidence of advanced degrees of myocardial cell death. However, sudden death may occur in patients without much myocardial destruction, probably from an arrhythmia, generally in an individual with rather extensive coronary atherosclerosis (Chap. 32).

The pathogenesis of myocardial infarction remains a matter of debate. It is clear that the simplistic concept of thrombosis superimposed on an atheroma or of hemorrhage into an atheromatous lesion is not adequate and that different types of infarcts exist, each with a different pathogenesis. Severe atheromatous disease is usually present, but the role of thrombosis requires clarification. Further complicating any simplistic explanation of the pathogenesis of myocardial infarction are recent arteriographic studies documenting normal coronary anatomy in patients with evidence of remote acute myocardial infarction. Many investigators consider these to be examples of a recanalized embolus.

Variant (Prinzmetal's) angina (see "Angina Pectoris" below) has been demonstrated to result from spasm of a large coronary artery. Coronary artery spasm may also be an important contributing factor in some instances of typical angina pectoris and myocardial infarction.

PREVENTION

See Chap. 250.

PATHOPHYSIOLOGY

CORONARY CIRCULATION Under basal conditions, the heart extracts a high and relatively fixed percentage of the oxygen from coronary arterial blood. Since increased oxygen extraction is thus not possible, augmented myocardial oxygen demands must be met by increases in coronary blood flow. Blood flow in the coronary bed, as in other vascular beds, is related directly to coronary perfusion pressure and inversely to vascular resistance. Since arterial pressure does not increase sufficiently or at all during a stress, such as exercise, variation in the resistance vessels of the coronary bed is the mechanism by which coronary flow, and thus oxygen supply, are regulated. The immense dilatory reserve of the normal coronary circulation is proved by the observation that patients without coronary disease may tolerate prolonged periods of hypotension or severe anemia without sustaining ischemic myocardial damage.

Coronary vascular resistance is mediated at the level of the coronary arterioles, while the large coronary arteries located on the epicardium serve more of a conduit function. Pathological studies have defined the large conduit vessels as the major sites of atherosclerosis, and arteriographic studies have shown them to be the site of spasm in variant angina. In animal experiments it has been shown that when there is a significant narrowing of the lumen of the conduit vessel (i.e., greater than 80 percent) by the atherosclerotic process, flow through the vessel decreases in the basal state, and a pressure gradient across the obstruction develops. In response to the reduction in pressure distal to the obstruction, resistance vessels at this site dilate in order to maintain flow. In this manner, the dilatory reserve of the resistance coronary vessels is progressively diminished by the advancing atherosclerotic process. As stenotic lesions become critical, the resistance vessels become permanently dilated in order to maintain basal flow, thus explaining the inability of patients with ischemic heart disease to augment coronary flow appropriately in response to stress. The observation that myocardial infarction without coronary occlusion occurs most commonly in the presence of severe coronary artery disease is explained by the lack of dilatory reserve; i.e., if myocardial oxygen demands are augmented in excess of supply capability, infarction will occur in the absence of total obstruction once the discrepancy between oxygen supply and demand becomes too great for too long a period of time. In addition, the existence of pressure gradients across stenotic sections of coronary vessels explains the inability of patients with coronary artery disease to tolerate hypotension. In the presence of such obstruction, coronary flow declines as perfusion pressure drops, despite dilatation of the resistance vessels.

EFFECTS OF ISCHEMIA The state of inadequate myocardial oxygenation induced by the atherosclerotic process results in abnormalities of the biochemical, electrical, and mechanical function of the heart. One biochemical response to ischemia which is used to evaluate the adequacy of myocardial perfusion relates to the aerobic metabolism of the normal heart; i.e., in the nonischemic heart, glucose and glycogen are oxidized completely to CO_2 and H_2O, and intermediary metabolites of carbohydrate breakdown such as lactate neither accumulate in the myocardium nor appear in coronary sinus blood. Under conditions of impaired oxygenation, anaerobic patterns of metabolism are utilized and lactate is formed. Intracellular lactate accumulates and is eventually released into coronary sinus blood. Myocardial lactate production is thus an index of ischemia. Unfortunately, the use of coronary arteriovenous lactate analysis is of limited clinical value, since the blood sample obtained in the coronary sinus represents *mixed* coronary venous blood, and regional increases of lactate in coronary venous blood draining a small ischemic area may thus escape detection.

Ischemia alters the electrical properties of the heart, the most characteristic early changes in the electrocardiogram being those of the repolarization process, as evidenced by inversion of T waves and later by displacement of the ST segment (Chap. 232). ST-segment shifts are seen clinically during episodes of angina pectoris and also in the early stages of myocardial infarction. Another important consequence of myocardial ischemia is electrical instability, leading to ventricular tachycardia and ventricular fibrillation. Most patients who die suddenly from ischemic heart disease do so from a ventricular arrhythmia (Chap. 32).

The contractile function of ischemic myocardium is markedly impaired. Transient ischemia, as occurs with angina pectoris, induces a reversible depression of myocardial function. Prolonged ischemia and the resultant process of infarction create both necrosis and an area of ischemia in tissue adjacent to the necrotic core. The necrosis causes an irreversible loss of contractile function with eventual scar formation, while the impaired contractility of the ischemic zone remains potentially reversible. This ischemic zone may progress to necrosis or revert to a normal state, depending upon the interaction of numerous factors which are as yet only partially defined. The potential for worsening and/or improvement in the ischemic zone explains why abnormalities of contractile function noted in the early phase of acute infarction are not static and may either progress or resolve.

Coronary atherosclerosis is a regional process which causes nonuniform ischemia. This results in an asymmetric distribution of disordered contractility, which in turn alters the symmetry and synchrony of ventricular contraction and reduces the efficiency of myocardial pump function. When the ischemic process involves those segments of myocardium responsible for the normal function of the mitral valve, mitral regurgitation may also occur. The ischemic or infarcted portion of myocardium may bulge outward when the normal portion of the ventricle contracts, further reducing the effectiveness of ventricular systole.

ANGINA PECTORIS

Angina pectoris is a clinical syndrome resulting from transient myocardial ischemia. The various diseases that result in myocardial ischemia as well as the numerous pain syndromes that may be confused with angina are discussed in Chap. 5. Approximately four-fifths of all patients with angina pectoris are men, and an even larger fraction of those younger than 50 years of age are men. The typical patient is in his fifties or early sixties and seeks medical advice because of chest discomfort. The patient commonly declines to apply the word *pain* to his chest symptoms, may have difficulty describing the sensation, and will usually select words such as heaviness, pressure, smothering, tightness, choking, or squeezing. The typical discomfort is substernal in location, but other sites are also commonly involved (see below). The most important diagnostic feature of angina pectoris is its relation to exertion or emotion. The discomfort comes on during physical or emotional stress and is relieved by rest. Anger, fright, hurrying, or sexual activity may bring on the syndrome.

The threshold for the development of angina varies with the time of day more than from day to day. The typical patient may have to stop at exactly the same spot on his way to work each morning, yet by midday he may be able to cover many times that distance without discomfort. Symptoms which develop soon after arising are common, and the patient may not be able to shave without stopping; yet he may perform moderately heavy manual labor later in the day after he has "warmed up."

Manual chores which have been performed for many years may be well tolerated, whereas unfamiliar tasks requiring comparable effort may cause angina. This pattern is commonly observed in a laborer who is asymptomatic at work but notices chest discomfort with household or recreational activities. Relatively nonstressful activities which require the hands to be held at or above the level of the head (combing hair, shaving) frequently cause symptoms in patients who are asymptomatic while performing more strenuous chores which do not require elevation of the arms. This phenomenon is thought to be related to the increased total body oxygen requirements associated with continuous contraction of the antigravity muscles of the arms and shoulder girdles. The pain may occur during or after eating. Exposure to cold temperature or to wind may accentuate or precipitate the symptoms.

Variation in the location and character of the discomfort may occur, and so angina pectoris should not be ruled out just because the location of the pain is atypical, especially if there is a strong relation to exertion. Myocardial ischemia may be characterized by pain in the neck, jaw, throat, back, shoulder, abdomen, or arm, with no symptoms in the chest. Radiation to the arms, particularly the ulnar aspect of the left arm, is common in typical angina, and sometimes the only discomfort may be in the arms or wrists, where it is often described as numbness or heaviness. Sharp pains, especially those that are localized to the left submammary area and are of short duration, are rarely due to myocardial ischemia, but the words *knife-like* and *cutting* are occasionally utilized to describe angina.

The term *angina decubitus* has been applied to the variant of angina pectoris which develops while the patient is in the recumbent position. The patient may report that he is awakened at night by a sensation which is similar to his exertional pain. The syndrome of angina decubitus is similar to that of paroxysmal nocturnal dyspnea, and dyspnea actually often accompanies the chest discomfort. It is postulated, but not proved, that the pathophysiology is also similar and that angina decubitus is a form of left ventricular failure precipitated by the expansion of the intrathoracic blood volume which occurs with recumbency and which may increase myocardial oxygen requirements. Elevation of systemic arterial blood pressure has been demonstrated to precede attacks of pain in some instances and may be another precipitating factor. Dreaming has also been implicated in the pathogenesis of this relatively unusual variant of angina.

Variant angina, or *Prinzmetal's angina,* is characterized by the development of the anginal syndrome, usually at rest, and it may be accompanied by ventricular arrhythmias. Characteristically the electrocardiogram demonstrates ST-segment *elevations* during the episodes of pain, in contrast to the more characteristic ST-segment depression of the typical effort angina syndrome. Variant angina represents transmural ischemia, often due to spasm of one of the major coronary arteries. However, varying degrees of atherosclerotic obstruction in these patients have been described.

PHYSICAL EXAMINATION Although many patients are often overweight and of mesomorphic habitus, there are many exceptions to this traditionally accepted description. Evidence of atherosclerosis is often present in vessels other than the coronary arteries; the fundi may show an increased light reflex and arteriovenous nicking, the peripheral vessels may be thickened on palpation, and there may be bruits over the carotid arteries. Physical findings are often normal in the patient with angina pectoris between episodes, but transient abnormalities of contractile function induced by the ischemia associated with angina pectoris may result in transient auscultatory and palpatory evidence of ventricular dysfunction which helps to establish the diagnosis. These include third and fourth heart sounds and rarely paradoxical splitting of the second heart sound (Chap. 231). Frequently, an asymmetric contraction pattern, localized lack of contraction, or paradoxical contraction (akinesis or dyskinesis) may be palpated as a transient ectopic left ventricular impulse. The third and fourth sounds and aneurysmal lift are best appreciated with the patient in the left lateral decubitus position. Another manifestation of ischemia is dysfunction of the papillary muscles, which may be reflected in a systolic murmur of mitral regurgitation. The transient arterial hypertension induced by isometric handgrip may cause a previously undetectable murmur of mitral regurgitation associated with papillary muscle dysfunction to become detectable. While this maneuver is useful in the evaluation of patients with stable disease, it should not be utilized during the acute phase of acute myocardial infarction or during an episode of angina pectoris because of the severe degree of transient hypertension that typically occurs. In order to exclude left ventricular outflow tract obstruction as the etiology of the anginal syndrome, auscultatory evidence of aortic valve disease (Chap. 242) or idiopathic hypertrophic aortic stenosis (Chap. 247) should be sought.

Physical examination is also valuable in detecting evidence of a systemic disease, a metabolic state or risk factor which predisposes to coronary atherosclerosis. For example, systemic hypertension is a finding of great significance because it accelerates the atherosclerotic process and is amenable to treatment. Xanthelasma and xanthoma may indicate abnormalities of lipid metabolism which may be associated with an increased incidence of coronary atherosclerosis (Chaps. 100 and 250). Nicotine stains on the fingertips suggest prolonged, excessive smoking.

LABORATORY EXAMINATION The tentative diagnosis of ischemic heart disease may frequently be made by means of the history, but in the absence of a history of documented infarction, the definitive diagnosis requires laboratory confirmation. Laboratory evaluation of all patients with suspected or documented coronary disease should include an electrocardiogram and chest roentgenogram. When a diagnosis cannot be established with these techniques, the indicated procedure is electrocardiographic stress testing, which in certain instances is followed by coronary arteriography. A positive response to a therapeutic trial of nitroglycerin is also helpful in supporting the diagnosis of angina pectoris.

Electrocardiogram The electrocardiogram may establish the diagnosis of ischemic heart disease if characteristic changes are present. The absence of abnormalities, however, by no means excludes the diagnosis. The 12-lead electrocardiogram recorded at rest and in the absence of pain is normal in approximately one-half of patients with typical angina pectoris and arteriographically demonstrable coronary atherosclerosis. The most definite and diagnostic electrocardiographic changes are those of old myocardial infarction (Chap. 232). The characteristic Q-wave changes of a myocardial infarction, especially if they are of the anterior or anterolateral type with changes in leads 1, aVL, and the precordial leads, are almost specific for myocardial infarction. The common exception to this relates to the QS pattern in lead V_1 and poor precordial R-wave progression frequently noted in patients with hypertension or chronic obstructive pulmonary disease. Similarly, a Q wave in a single inferior lead is of little significance. The electrocardiographic diagnosis of acute myocardial infarction can be made with greater certainty when a previously normal electrocardiogram can be used as a reference. In some instances the vectorcardiogram may be helpful as well.

T-wave changes are more difficult to interpret as evidence of ischemic heart disease. Inverted T waves may appear as the only manifestation of ischemic heart disease, but they may also occur in other conditions which may be associated with chest pain, such as pericarditis, myocarditis, and abnormalities of vasoregulation.

Great diagnostic significance can be placed upon ST-segment and T-wave changes which occur during attacks of pain and disappear thereafter. The most characteristic change is displacement of the ST segment, with or without T-wave inversion, which is similar in every way to that induced during the course of an exercise test. Long-term monitoring with magnetic tape may be useful in documenting the association of ECG changes and chest pain. The ST segments are usually depressed but rarely may be strikingly elevated, as in the early stages of myocardial infarction, or in variant (Prinzmetal's) angina.

Chest roentgenogram The chest roentgenogram may aid in the diagnosis of ischemic heart disease when calcification in a coronary artery or a ventricular aneurysm is identified. Cardiac enlargement is a nonspecific finding, but in patients with ischemic heart disease it usually reflects the presence of a large quantity of infarcted myocardium.

Stress testing Two general classes of stress test have been defined for the evaluation of cardiac function. One, the measurement of cardiac output and intraventricular pressure, assesses the adequacy and/or reserve of myocardial pump function. Stress tests of this type are of little value in establishing the diagnosis of ischemic heart disease since the definition of impaired ventricular function does not establish the etiologic diagnosis of heart disease.

The second form measures the capability of the coronary circulation to augment coronary blood flow in response to increased myocardial oxygen demands. Although such evaluation may be occasionally obtained with catheterization techniques (coronary arteriovenous lactate analysis, atrial pacing), the application of invasive testing is obviously limited. The ideal test for application to a large number of patients would employ a form of stress that augments myocardial oxygen demands in a safe and reproducible fashion and in the presence of ischemic heart disease results in an easily observable and specific alteration of cardiovascular function. At the present time electrocardiographic stress testing is the best approximation of this ideal because electrocardiographic ST-segment displacement is a characteristic response to ischemia and occurs during and immediately following an exercise stress. Unfortunately, certain known factors (K^+, digitalis), and many as yet undefined factors, affect ST-segment morphology; therefore ST-segment depression is not specific for ischemia (i.e., false-positive responses may occur). Similarly, false-negative responses are known to occur and may be due to the complex geometry of the heart and the fact that certain areas of the heart are electrically silent. These limitations notwithstanding, the realization that ST-segment depression is the best readily available index of ischemia has prompted the development of standardized exercise tests which use ST-segment depression as the end point to define ischemia.

The ischemic ST-segment response is generally defined as a flat depression of the ST segment 0.1 mV below the base line, i.e., the PR segment, lasting more than 0.08 s (Fig. 244-1). The depression is of the "square-wave" or "plateau" type and is flat or slopes downward (unlike the ST-segment depression that slopes upward, which is referred to as a *junctional change* and does not constitute a positive test result unless the slope is shallow). T-wave abnormalities, ventricular arrhythmias, and conduction disturbances may develop with exercise but do not constitute certain evidence of myocardial ischemia. If 0.1 mV or more ST-segment depression is required before the test is considered to be positive, the percentage of false-positive results will be less than 10 percent, and only about 15 percent of patients with severe coronary atherosclerosis will have negative test results; these are usually patients with only single-vessel disease. If the threshold of positivity is set at 0.05 mV, there will be more false-positive tests and fewer false-negative ones.

FIGURE 244-1
Positive electrocardiographic exercise test. "Square-wave" ST-segment displacement in lead V_1 in postexercise record. Changes during exercise are probably abnormal also (slow upstroke).

CONTROL

EXERCISE 1½ min

POST EXERCISE 3 min

The duration of exercise, presence of anginal symptoms, heart rate, and blood pressure response are also important in evaluating the results of a stress electrocardiogram. Thus, false-positive results are *least* likely in those patients who demonstrate ST-segment depression *early* in the test, who experience typical angina during the test, or who have only minimal increases in heart rate and blood pressure (compared with the control values) when the ECG changes occur. It is also important to emphasize that, according to Bayes' theorem, the probability that coronary artery disease exists in the population under study must be considered along with the diagnostic features of the test in the interpretation of a positive or negative exercise test result. For example, on the basis of arteriographic studies, patients with typical angina, who have not had an exercise electrocardiogram, have a high (approximately 90 percent) probability of demonstrating coronary artery disease, patients with atypical angina have a 50 percent probability, patients with nonanginal chest pain about a 10 percent probability, and asymptomatic persons about a 5 percent probability. A positive exercise result indicates that the likelihood of coronary artery disease is 98 percent in patients with typical angina, 88 percent in patients with atypical pain, 44 percent in patients with nonanginal chest pain, and only 33 percent in asymptomatic persons.

Approximately 10 percent of patients with a positive test will have ST-segment changes only *during* exercise; hence, the sensitivity of the test is improved by monitoring during, in addition to immediately after, exercise. Exercise testing is safer with in-exercise monitoring because ST-segment changes or arrhythmias may develop before pain or other symptoms occur (or even in the absence of symptoms) and the stress can be discontinued before severe ischemia develops. Multiple leads should be recorded, and precordial leads should be included, because one-third of patients with a positive test will have changes only in one lead, which is most likely V_5 or V_6.

Three formats of stress testing are commonly used; tests with standardized external workloads, tests which are standardized by heart rate response, and tests designed to reach the maximal possible exercise load. The two-step system of exercise developed by Master is an example of the first variety. The second and third varieties employ a treadmill or bicycle and differ only with respect to the method of determining the end point of the exercise. In the *target heart rate* test, exercise is continued until the patient attains 80 to 90 percent of his predicted maximum heart rate, which can be obtained from available tables. In the *maximal exercise* test, exercise is progressively increased until maximal workload is attained. Both tests are discontinued at a lower level of work if the patient develops chest pain, signs of cerebral insufficiency, fall in blood pressure, or significant electrocardiographic changes. The percentage of positive tests in a population of patients with angina and arteriographically proved coronary atherosclerosis is greater with the graded exercise methods (85 to 90 percent) than with the tests standardized on the basis of external workload (double two-step test). A physician must be in attendance throughout the exercise test to observe the patient, to evaluate the in-exercise ECG and in-exercise blood pressure recordings, and to decide whether the testing should continue. The risk of an exercise test is small but real, being estimated at approximately one fatality and two nonfatal complications per 10,000 tests. The test is probably unusually hazardous and hence contraindicated in patients with unstable angina pectoris and patients who have suffered acute myocardial infarction during the preceding few weeks. Combining the exercise test with myocardial perfusion imaging (using thallium 201, for example) has been demonstrated to improve its diagnostic accuracy even further.

Other forms of stress testing have been developed for use in the recumbent subject during the course of cardiac catheterization and angiography. Under these circumstances the heart can be stressed by having the patient perform leg exercise with a bicycle device fixed to the catheterization table or having him do isometric handgrips by squeezing an ergometer. Probably the most widely used form of stress at catheterization is the pacing stress test, in which the heart rate is increased by electrical pacing with a pacing catheter in the right atrium. Pacing-induced tachycardia increases the myocardial oxygen demands and hence produces ischemia in the patient with limited ability to increase myocardial blood flow in proportion to oxygen demands. The rate is increased in stages from the basal level to 160 to 180 beats per minute, or until the patient develops chest pain or changes on the electrocardiogram consistent with ischemia. One of the advantages of this form of stress is that it can be conducted on a recumbent subject, and therefore hemodynamic measurements can be made during the test. The major disadvantage lies in the fact that pacing-induced tachycardia is not physiologically comparable with exercise in that the cardiac output does not increase, and hence the stroke volume declines as rate increases.

Other noninvasive procedures Two types of noninvasive *radionuclide studies* discussed in Chap. 233 are helpful in diagnosing ischemic heart disease. The first is myocardial perfusion imaging with thallium 201 in which areas of underperfused myocardium can be identified in the basal state or during stress. The second type of study, the gated radioisotopic angiogram, can provide a measure of ventricular volumes and ejection fraction at rest and during exercise and permits identification of disorders of global left ventricular function and of localized wall motion.

Echocardiography can also be used to evaluate regional left ventricular motion. Two-dimensional (cross-sectional) echocardiographic techniques allow much larger portions of the myocardium to be visualized than is possible with the M-mode technique.

Coronary arteriography (see also Chap. 234) Coronary arteriography is the only method which will provide unequivocal diagnostic information concerning the presence or absence of coronary atherosclerosis in living patients. It also permits estimation of the severity of obstructive lesions which may be present. Opinion is nearly unanimous that arteriography is indicated in the following specific situations: (1) Patients with either chronic, stable angina pectoris or one of the unstable angina syndromes (Chap. 245) who are refractory to medical treatment, and others who, on clinical grounds, are considered to be candidates for coronary bypass surgery, as discussed under "Operation" below. No uniform statement regarding the indications for arteriography in the evaluation and management of the patient with stable but unequivocal coronary disease can be made at present. The uses of arteriography in such patients vary among physicians and among institutions and are predicated upon the local definition of "intractable angina" and the prevailing attitude toward the indications for coronary bypass operations in such patients. (2) Patients with a variety of diagnostic problems in which the diagnosis of ischemic heart disease needs to be established or ruled out.

Six groups of patients exemplify the latter situation. (1) Patients with negative exercise tests and a disabling chest pain syndrome. Included in this group are patients with a chest pain syndrome that the physician believes is *probably* not angina but who need unequivocal evidence either for psychological reasons or for personal decisions relating to career planning, family planning, insurability, etc. (2) Patients with frequent hospital admissions with the diagnosis of possible myocardial infarction which has never been substantiated. (3) Commercial and military flight personnel or others with careers in which more than individual safety is concerned and in whom there is a reasonable doubt as to the status of the coronary circulation. (4) Patients with severe aortic valve disease and angina pectoris in whom this symptom could be secondary to the valvular lesions and/or to coronary arteriosclerosis. (5) Young patients (under age 45) with angina or documented myocardial infarction in whom none of the risk factors associated with premature coronary disease can be identified and who may not have extensive coronary atherosclerosis and, hence, a more favorable prognosis. (6) Patients with severe congestive heart failure suspected to be related to papillary muscle dysfunction, postmyocardial infarction, ventricular septal defect, or discrete aneurysm rather than global ventricular dysfunction.

The diversity of opinion concerning the role of arteriography in the evaluation of patients with suspected or documented coronary disease is due to a combination of factors: (1) the continuing controversy over the role of coronary artery bypass surgery in the management of patients with ischemic heart disease, (2) the invasive nature of the test and the attendant small but distinct morbidity and mortality, and (3) the fact that the quality of study and complication rate vary widely. In general, the performance record of laboratories doing less than 100 studies per year, for example, is not comparable with that of more active laboratories.

MANAGEMENT OF ANGINA PECTORIS   The term *management* is more appropriate than *treatment* with reference to angina pectoris because far more is required than the prescription of a drug or the recommendation of operation. The patient must be evaluated with particular reference to the interaction between his disease and life pattern. The physical and emotional stresses which precipitate pain and the pleasurable activities prohibited by angina must be identified. The management plan has six parts: (1) reassurance, (2) general measures directed toward preventing progression of ischemic heart disease, (3) definition of a protocol of activity designed to prevent and minimize the attacks of ischemia, (4) elimination of the possibility of coexistent disease capable of exacerbating angina, (5) institution of a program of drug therapy, and (6) definition of end points which will be indications for consideration of coronary bypass surgery.

Reassurance   The patient must be made to realize that long, useful life is possible even though he has angina pectoris. It is usually not advisable to quote statistics, but the recital of case histories of persons in public life may be of great value. A realistic explanation of the pathophysiology of the disease is worthwhile for the intelligent patient and can be used as a basis for the life plan which is to be described.

General measures   There is no definitive proof in humans that the lesions of coronary atherosclerosis can be made to regress, but extrapolation from animal experiments makes this appear likely. It is clear that certain factors accelerate the progression of these lesions. It seems reasonable, therefore, to make the reduction of these risk factors a keystone of treatment in all patients with coronary atherosclerosis. Ideal weight should be

attained and maintained, hypertension treated if present, and cigarette smoking forbidden. It has been demonstrated that the mortality rate of individuals who have discontinued cigarette smoking is the same as that for those who have never smoked. Thus, the facts do not support the excuse often offered by patients that it is too late to stop. Diabetes and the hyperlipidemias should be treated when they are present (Chap. 250). The patient should be encouraged to engage in steady dynamic exercise, such as walking; isometric exercise may actually be hazardous. The maintenance of good physical condition enables him to perform physical work more efficiently at a lower pulse rate and, therefore, reduces the frequency of anginal episodes. The patient in good physical condition also may have a better chance of surviving a myocardial infarction.

Activity   Specific therapy depends on the elimination of the discrepancy between the demand of the heart muscle for oxygen and the ability of the coronary circulation to meet this demand. Most patients can be made to understand this fundamental concept and utilize it in the rational programming of activity. The patient must be taught that many tasks which usually cause pain may be accomplished without symptoms if the speed with which the task is performed is lessened. He must appreciate the variation in tolerance with the time of day and reduce activity requirements in the morning and immediately after meals. It may be necessary to counsel a change in employment or residence to avoid physical stress, but with the exception of the manual laborer it is usually possible for the patient to continue to function merely by allowing more time for the completion of each task. Emotional tension is often neglected in the planning of a program for the patient with angina. In some patients, anger and frustration may be the most important precipitating factors in daily life. If these cannot be avoided, tranquilizing and sedative drugs should be prescribed. A treadmill exercise test to determine the approximate heart rate at which ischemic electrocardiographic changes or symptoms may occur may be of help in developing a specific exercise program. Electrocardiographic tape recording during daily activities may also be helpful in this regard. A conditioning program may reduce the heart rate and blood pressure produced by a specific degree of exertion, thereby lowering the oxygen requirements of the heart.

Exacerbating conditions   A number of illnesses, not primarily cardiac in nature, may either increase oxygen demand of, or decrease oxygen supply to, the myocardium. These conditions may exacerbate angina pectoris and must be considered. In the former category are hyperthyroidism (iatrogenic or spontaneous), hypertension, and anemia. Frequently, severe angina may be treated successfully by appropriate antihypertensive or antithyroid therapy. Decreased oxygen supply to the myocardium may be due to decreased oxygenation of the blood (intrinsic pulmonary disease, carboxyhemoglobin due to cigarette or cigar smoking) or decreased oxygen-carrying capacity (anemia).

Drug therapy   NITRATES   The mechanism of action of nitroglycerin, the most valuable drug in the treatment of angina pectoris, is discussed in Chap. 238. The activity of the agent depends upon its absorption, which is most rapid and complete through the mucous membranes. For this reason, nitroglycerin is administered sublingually, in tablets of 0.4 or 0.6 mg. Patients with angina should be instructed to take the medication to relieve an attack and also in anticipation of stress which is likely to induce angina. When the patient develops pain on exertion, he should cease activity and place a tablet under his tongue. The discomfort generally disappears more rapidly with nitroglycerin than would be expected if the drug were not administered. A flight of stairs, a walk up a hill, or sexual intercourse may produce pain consistently, but often the pain can be prevented by the anticipatory use of nitroglycerin.

The dose of nitroglycerin should be large enough to relieve pain but not large enough to produce a feeling of pulsating fullness in the head or a frank headache. The latter is the most common side effect of nitroglycerin and fortunately only rarely becomes disturbing at a dose required to relieve angina. Nitroglycerin deteriorates with exposure to air, moisture, and sunlight; therefore, if it produces neither relief of pain nor a headache, nor a slight sensation of burning at the sublingual site of absorption, the preparation may be inactive, and a fresh supply should be obtained. If the patient does not experience relief after the first dose of nitroglycerin, he may take a second, but should be instructed not to continue to take the medication if the first few doses prove unsuccessful. If pain continues despite nitroglycerin, the patient should consult his physician, who should then evaluate him for the possibility of an acute myocardial infarction, or, if the patient cannot do this, he should report promptly to a hospital emergency room for evaluation.

A diary or log of the time of occurrence of pains in relation to activity and other precipitating factors and nitroglycerin administration is often helpful to the physician attempting to tailor a management program for a new patient. A log may also be valuable in detecting a change in frequency and severity of pains which may herald an impending myocardial infarction (Chap. 245). The stable patient may keep the log only intermittently or discontinue it, especially if the recording of pains focuses attention on the disease and has undesirable psychologic consequences.

Unfortunately, none of the long-acting nitrates is as effective as nitroglycerin in the relief of angina pectoris. However, several of these preparations are useful in prolonging the time interval between attacks and, hence, in reducing the amount of nitroglycerin which has to be taken as therapy for acute attacks. Preparations which are chewed or taken sublingually and therefore depend upon absorption through the mucous membranes are more effective than those that are simply swallowed. If one preparation is ineffective, another should be tried, as many patients find one preparation more effective than others. There is marked variation among patients in the dose required to produce a result, especially in the preparations to be swallowed, just as there is variation in the dose of nitroglycerin required for relief of an acute attack. The dosage of the long-acting agent should be increased gradually until either a therapeutic or a toxic effect is encountered. It may be taken on a regular basis every few hours by patients with frequent anginal attacks, in addition to being taken in anticipation of events known to provoke angina. Nitroglycerin ointment applied to the chest can be utilized as a slow-release preparation which is especially useful in the treatment of angina decubitus. An application of ointment at bedtime may give the patient a night's sleep which had not been possible before.

CARDIAC GLYCOSIDES AND DIURETICS During an attack of angina pectoris, left ventricular function becomes impaired, and the left ventricular end-diastolic pressure rises, leading in turn to an elevation of pulmonary vascular pressures. Therefore, agents useful in the treatment of congestive heart failure (Chaps. 236 and 238) may also be valuable in the management of angina pectoris. The cardiac glycosides will be most effective in the patient with an enlarged heart. A decrease in heart size decreases wall tension and hence myocardial oxygen requirements. If the heart is of normal size, the cardiac glycosides may aggravate angina by increasing contractility and

hence the oxygen requirements. The addition of an oral diuretic will also prove useful in many patients. These measures are especially valuable in the prevention of attacks of nocturnal angina and of angina at rest, i.e., angina decubitus. When angina pectoris is refractory to the general measures outlined above, digitalis should be tried even though overt congestive failure may be absent.

BETA-ADRENERGIC BLOCKADE The beta-adrenergic blocking agents, such as propranolol, represent a useful addition to the pharmacological treatment of angina pectoris (Chap. 72). The effects of beta-adrenergic blockade are described best as being the opposite of those of isoproterenol, an agent which stimulates the cardiac beta receptors. Isoproterenol produces an increase in heart rate, myocardial contractility, cardiac output, and myocardial oxygen consumption, associated with a decrease in total peripheral resistance, while the beta-adrenergic blocking agents prevent these changes. The effects of these drugs are most apparent during exercise; there is only a small decrease in cardiac output and heart rate at rest, but beta blockade reduces these variables more strikingly during exercise. Propranolol is useful in angina pectoris because it reduces the workload associated with exercise, rather than because of any direct effect on the coronary arteries. Propranolol is usually administered in an initial dose of 40 mg per day in four divided doses and is increased as tolerated to doses of 160 to 320 mg per day. Some patients require much higher doses, as much as 1 g per day to obtain relief, however. If heart failure is present and/or there is cardiomegaly on radiographic examination, prior treatment with digitalis and a lower initial dose of propranolol are in order. Treatment is monitored by observation of the pulse rate and examination for signs of congestive failure: a resting pulse rate below 45 beats per minute and clinical evidence of impairment of left ventricular function are grounds for reduction of the dose or discontinuation of the drug. The goal of treatment with beta blockade is not only to decrease the resting heart rate but also to blunt the heart rate response to exercise.

Operation Numerous surgical procedures have been proposed for the treatment of ischemic heart disease, but the only procedure for which there is enthusiasm at present is the aortocoronary bypass graft. A section of vein, usually the saphenous, is used to form a connection between the aorta and the coronary artery distal to the obstructing lesion. Alternatively, the end of the mammary artery may be anastomosed to a coronary artery distal to the obstructing lesion. The operation is attractive because it represents a simple, direct mechanical attack on the obstructive lesions in the major coronary arteries.

Despite the controversy surrounding the indications for coronary bypass procedures and the problems enumerated above, certain areas of agreement can be identified: (1) The operation is relatively safe, with reported mortality rates as low as 1 percent in elective operations carried out by experienced surgical teams in patients with normal or near-normal left ventricular function. (2) Operative and postoperative mortality increases with left ventricular dysfunction and with surgical inexperience. (3) The graft procedure is surgically feasible, with patency rates of 70 to 80 percent reported at 2 to 3 years. Ultimate patency of the graft correlates with graft flow at the time of operation. The frequency of occlusion of grafts with flow rates exceeding 50 ml/min is very low. (4) Grafts that become occluded usually do so within 1 year. (5) When a bypass operation is performed on a partially occluded vessel, the probability of the partial obstruction in the native circulation progressing to completion is markedly increased. (6) Angina is unequivocally relieved in 85 percent of patients, although drug therapy may still be necessary in many. In most instances this relief can be attributed to increased blood flow to the ischemic myocardium, but this is not an adequate explanation in all patients. For example, relief of symptoms in the presence of occluded grafts could be due to infarction of the ischemic or angina-producing segment of the myocardium. The well-known placebo effect of operation is another possible mechanism for symptomatic improvement, but relief due to this mechanism would not be expected to be long-lasting. The fact that symptomatic relief is attributable to increased flow is also supported by the occasional fortuitous arteriographic demonstration that pain abruptly recurs when a graft becomes occluded, suggesting that the placebo effect is not entirely responsible for the relief of pain. (7) The inability to demonstrate ventriculographic or hemodynamic improvement of global ventricular function after bypass operation in some patients is not surprising when it is recognized that improvement could not be expected in those patients who have normal ventricular function prior to operation or in patients with ventricular function impaired by previous infarction and scar or aneurysm formation. (8) Perioperative and intraoperative myocardial infarction occurs in 8 to 15 percent of patients. In most instances these infarcts are small. (9) The mortality rate of patients with unoperated left main coronary artery lesions is exceedingly high, and the results of some studies suggest that this rate can be reduced by operative intervention. (10) The mortality of patients with unoperated single-vessel disease limited either to the circumflex or right coronary arteries is low and does not differ greatly from that of age-matched controls without any disease.

The objectives of surgical treatment include the relief of symptoms and improvement of exercise tolerance, improvement of ventricular function, prevention of myocardial infarction, and improvement of life expectancy. The impressive ability of the procedure to relieve pain in most patients has been discussed above. Available data have not shown unequivocally that the procedure is capable of improving ventricular function for the reasons discussed above. In general, dramatic clinical improvement in ventricular function should not be anticipated from bypass surgery unless the surgical procedure includes the correction of some mechanical deficit (i.e., repair of mitral regurgitation or closure of ventricular septal defect or resection of aneurysm).

Major controversy as to indications for bypass graft operations exists because of lack of knowledge of the effect of the operation on the natural history of the disease. The largest group of potential candidates for operation consists of patients with two- or three-vessel disease and some disorder of left ventricular function. The only certain effect of operation in this group is the relief of symptoms. However, recent data from some centers reporting on 3- to 7-year follow-up of surgically treated patients using the life table analysis technique *suggest, but do not prove,* that bypass graft surgery favorably affects the natural history of coronary artery disease when patients with similar degrees of angiographically proved disease who have been treated medically are used as controls. Whether the operation can forestall infarction or other complications of coronary artery disease is not known.

The considerable disagreement concerning the indications for, and/or results of, bypass surgery is attributable to a number of factors: (1) Although it is acknowledged that different subsets of patients with coronary artery disease exist, the morbidity and mortality of patients in each group have not been defined. Therefore, it is difficult to estimate the natural history of patients not treated by operation, and attempts to define a beneficial effect of operation are thereby compromised. (2) Most life table analyses of patients with ischemic heart disease utilize patients in whom the diagnosis was proved by coronary arteriography. As a rule, only symptomatic patients are subjected to arteriography. Thus, the use of life table analyses to document the history of untreated coronary disease may represent a biased approach since untreated, asymptomatic, or mildly symptomatic patients with comparable findings on coronary arteriography are excluded. (3) The indications for surgical treatment and the effectiveness of operation vary among institutions and surgeons, thus rendering interinstitutional comparisons of limited value.

In view of these considerations, the role of this operation in the treatment of ischemic heart disease cannot be defined precisely at this time, and it is, therefore, possible to list indications only in terms of current practice. Three factors are usually considered in arriving at a decision to advise coronary bypass operations: (1) symptomatic status and age of the patient, (2) coronary anatomy as demonstrated by coronary arteriography, and (3) ventricular function as determined by left ventricular angiography and hemodynamics. Most patients advised to undergo operation are symptomatic, although the severity of the symptoms in surgical candidates varies widely among institutions. The ideal candidate has severe (80 percent or greater) obstructive lesions in the proximal portions of at least two of the three major coronary arteries. In some centers, patients with lesions in a single vessel are also considered to be operative candidates. This seems justified if the left anterior descending rather than the right or circumflex coronary artery is the vessel involved. Patients with severe lesions in the left main coronary artery are at high risk and should have operative therapy if there are no contraindications. The best results are obtained in patients with normal ventricular function or at most a single area of impaired myocardial contractility.

Major controversy persists as to the indications for operation in the asymptomatic or mildly symptomatic patient with obstructive coronary artery disease. If the studies purporting to demonstrate a beneficial effect of the operation on the natural history of the disease can be confirmed, the indications will obviously be less stringent than if relief of symptoms is the only goal of the procedure. Patients who have definite symptomatology, but in whom significant relief with medical therapy is obtained, present a difficult problem. The definition of a level of symptomatology which indicates the need for operation must represent a joint decision between physician and patient. Older patients, i.e., those over 70 years, are generally treated medically unless the symptoms are truly disabling, whereas in a younger individual less disability is generally required before operation is advised. An important additional factor frequently not discussed relates to the technical skills of the surgical and diagnostic teams, and the quality of care in the early postoperative period. The variation in results of operative therapy from different institutions reflects this factor as well as differing selection criteria for operation. As a general rule, the poorest results are reported from institutions performing the least number of operations, and the advisability of having operation carried out by an experienced surgical team cannot be overemphasized. Operative mortality is also a function of case selection. If only patients with good ventricular function are selected, mortality may be less than 1 percent, but such a policy may exclude many patients who could benefit from the procedure.

MANAGEMENT OF THE PATIENT WITH ASYMPTOMATIC CORONARY ARTERIOSCLEROSIS

The widespread use of exercise testing during routine annual examinations has defined a heretofore unrecognized group of patients with asymptomatic coronary artery disease. Longitudinal studies of young military personnel have demonstrated an increased incidence of coronary events (sudden death, infarction, angina) in asymptomatic patients with positive exercise tests. In addition, patients who are asymptomatic after an infarct are nonetheless at greater risk for a second coronary event than the general population. Although medical therapy (elimination of smoking, antihypertensive medication, diet, etc.) aimed at preventing progression of the disease is indicated, recent surgical data suggesting that bypass surgery improves mortality in coronary patients have led some to advocate routine coronary arteriography to establish a diagnosis and subsequent bypass surgery if anatomically feasible despite the asymptomatic state. While such an approach cannot be condoned on the basis of available data, a number of factors should be considered when faced with this dilemma: (1) the degree of positivity of the exercise test and duration or stage of exercise at which it appears, (2) the ECG leads in which the test is positive (changes in the anterior precordial leads appear to indicate less favorable prognosis than changes in the inferior leads), (3) the age of the patient, and (4) the occupation of the patient. Whereas most would agree that the asymptomatic, young, commercial airline pilot with 4-mm ST-segment depression in leads V_1 to V_4 during mild exercise should have arteriograms and the asymptomatic sedentary 75-year-old retiree with 1-mm ST-segment depression in leads II and III during maximal exercise should not, there is no consensus about the appropriate procedure in less extreme situations.

REFERENCES

BRAUNWALD E (ed): Coronary artery disease, in *Heart Disease.* Philadelphia, Saunders, 1980, chaps 32–37

COHN PF (ed): *Diagnosis and Therapy of Coronary Artery Disease.* Boston, Little, Brown, 1979

CORYA BC: Echocardiography in ischemic heart disease. Am J Med 63:10, 1977

GROVES BM: Variant angina: An electrocardiographic and arteriographic spectrum produced by coronary artery spasm, in *Current Problems in Cardiology,* vol II, no 4. Chicago, Year Book, 1977

HILLIS LD, BRAUNWALD E: Myocardial ischemia. N Engl J Med 296:971, 1034, 1093, 1977

———, ———: Coronary artery spasm. N Engl J Med 299:695, 1978

JULIAN DG: Diagnosis and management of angina pectoris, in *Current Problems in Cardiology,* vol II, no 7. Chicago, Year Book, 1977

KOPPES G et al: Treadmill exercise testing, in *Current Problems in Cardiology,* vol VII, nos 8, 9. Chicago, Year Book, 1977

MCINTOSH HD, GARCIA JA: The first decade of aortocoronary bypass grafting, 1967–1977. A review. Circulation 57:405, 1978

PROUDFIT WL et al: Natural history of obstructive coronary artery disease: Ten-year study of 601 nonsurgical cases. Prog Cardiovasc Dis 21:53, 1978

REEVES TJ et al: Natural history of angina pectoris. Am J Cardiol 33:423, 1974

ROSS RS: Ischemic heart disease: An overview. Am J Cardiol 36:496, 1975

SHELDON WC et al: Surgical treatment of coronary artery disease: Pure graft operations with a study of 741 patients followed 3–7 years. Prog Cardiovasc Dis 18:237, 1975

VLODAVER A, EDWARDS JE: Pathology of coronary atherosclerosis. Prog Cardiovasc Dis 14:256, 1971

245

ACUTE MYOCARDIAL INFARCTION

EUGENE BRAUNWALD
JOSEPH S. ALPERT
RICHARD S. ROSS

CLINICAL PRESENTATION

Pain is the most frequent presenting complaint of the patient with myocardial infarction and in some instances may be severe enough to be described as the worst pain the patient has ever experienced (Chap. 5). It is a deep, visceral pain, and adjectives commonly used to describe it are "heavy," "squeezing," and "crushing." It is similar in character to the pain of angina pectoris but is usually more severe and lasts much longer. Typically the pain is gradual in onset, involves the central portion of the chest and epigastrium, and radiates to the arms in about 25 percent of cases. Less common sites of radiation are the abdomen, back, jaw, and neck. The pain of myocardial infarction does not radiate above the maxilla or below the umbilicus. The location of the pain beneath the xiphoid may be responsible for the mistaken diagnosis of acute indigestion. The pain is often accompanied by weakness, sweating, nausea, vomiting, giddiness, and marked anxiety. It may begin during a period of exertion but, in contrast to angina pectoris, may also begin with the patient at rest, and it does not usually subside with rest. Characteristically, the pain of myocardial infarction causes the patient to move about in an attempt to find a comfortable position. Again, this is in contrast to the pain of angina pectoris which causes the patient to remain relatively immobile for fear of making the pain reappear.

Although pain is the most common presenting complaint, it is by no means always present; a minimum of 15 to 20 percent of myocardial infarcts may be painless. The frequency of painless infarcts is probably higher than this estimate because patients without pain may not seek medical attention. The incidence of painless infarcts is greater in patients with diabetes and increases with age, and in the elderly the presenting complaint of a myocardial infarct may be the sudden onset of breathlessness, which may progress to pulmonary edema. Other less common presentations in the absence of pain include sudden loss of consciousness, a confusional state, a sensation of profound weakness, the appearance of an arrhythmia, or merely an unexplained drop in arterial blood pressure.

PHYSICAL FINDINGS

In many instances the dominant feature of the patient's presentation is his reaction to the chest pain. He is typically anxious and may be restless, attempting to relieve the pain by moving about in bed, squirming, stretching, belching, or even inducing vomiting. Pallor is common and is often associated with perspiration and coolness of the extremities. No alteration of pulse rate is specific for myocardial infarction, with bradycardia, normal sinus rhythm, and sinus tachycardia being observed both early and late in the course of the disease. This is not unexpected in view of the multiplicity of physiological derangements that may occur with infarction.

The precordium is usually quiet, and the apical impulse may be difficult to palpate. In about one-fourth of patients with anterior-wall infarction an abnormal systolic pulsation, distinguishable from the point of maximal impulse, develops in the periapical area within the first days of the illness and then may resolve. This represents a transient, palpable systolic bulging of the infarcted ventricle. This abnormality is best brought out with the patient in the left lateral decubitus position. Other physical signs of ventricular dysfunction that may be present include, in decreasing incidence, atrial (S_4) and ventricular filling (S_3) gallop sounds, decreased intensity of heart sounds, and paradoxical splitting of the second sound (Chap. 231). A transient apical systolic murmur, presumably due to mitral regurgitation secondary to papillary muscle dysfunction during acute infarction, may be midsystolic or late systolic in timing. A pericardial friction rub may be heard in many patients with transmural myocardial infarction at some time in their course if they are examined frequently enough. Temperature elevations in the range of 37 to 38°C, and occasionally as high as 39°C, may be observed during the first week following acute myocardial infarction; however, a temperature exceeding 38°C should prompt a search for other causes.

LABORATORY DIAGNOSIS

The laboratory tests of value in confirming the diagnosis of myocardial infarction may be divided into three groups: (1) nonspecific indexes of tissue necrosis and inflammation, (2) the electrocardiogram, and (3) serum enzyme changes.

The *nonspecific reaction* to myocardial injury is associated with polymorphonuclear leukocytosis, which appears within a few hours after the onset of pain, persists for 3 to 7 days, and often reaches levels of 12,000 to 15,000 leukocytes per cubic millimeter. The magnitude of the leukocytosis yields some information about the size of the infarct, the higher white blood cell counts being associated with larger infarcts. The erythrocyte sedimentation rate rises more slowly than the white blood cell count, peaking during the first week, and remaining elevated for several weeks.

FIGURE 245-1

The time course of serum enzyme concentration changes following a typical myocardial infarction. CPK, creatinine phosphokinase; LDH, lactic dehydrogenase; GOT, glutamic oxaloacetic transaminase.

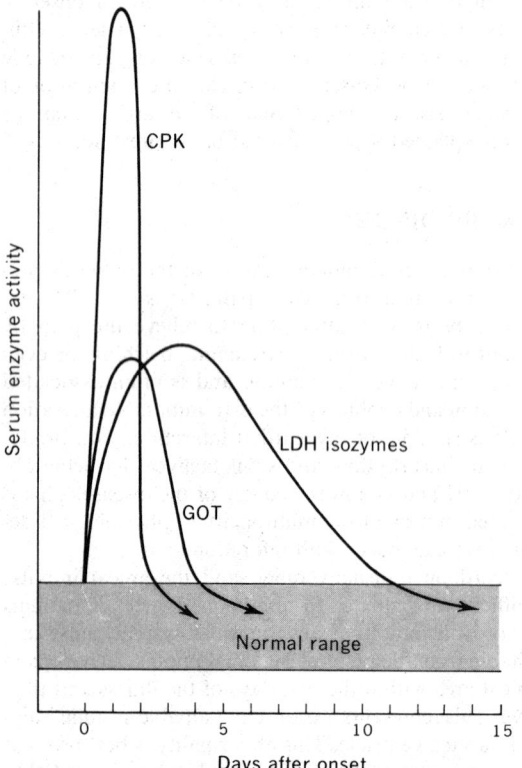

The *electrocardiographic manifestations* of transmural acute myocardial infarction are described in Chap. 232. The term *transmural* denotes an infarct which results in necrosis of the entire thickness of the wall of an area of myocardium. If the infarct does not involve the entire thickness of the myocardium, it is said to be *nontransmural* or *subendocardial*. In this situation, there are no Q waves, and the characteristic changes are limited to the ST segment and the T wave. The amplitude of the R waves in the precordial leads may also be decreased. The ST-segment and T-wave changes of nontransmural infarction are variable and nonspecific, and the diagnosis of infarction has to be supported by other clinical and laboratory information. Agreement between the electrocardiographic and pathological evidence of transmural or nontransmural infarction is far from perfect. For example, the electrocardiogram may exhibit only ST-segment and T-wave changes despite pathological demonstration of transmural infarction.

SERUM ENZYME STUDIES The discovery of increased concentration of serum glutamic oxaloacetic transaminase (SGOT) in patients with myocardial infarction ushered in an era of improved diagnostic accuracy. The release of other enzymes in large quantities into the blood from necrotic heart muscle following myocardial infarction was subsequently noted. The rate of liberation of specific enzymes differs following infarction, and the temporal pattern of enzyme release is of diagnostic importance. The time course of the serum concentration of the most commonly used enzymes is shown in Fig. 245-1. Levels of two of the enzymes, SGOT and creatinine phosphokinase (CPK), rise and fall rapidly, while that of lactic dehydrogenase (LDH) rises later and remains elevated longer. SGOT is most widely used, but has the disadvantage that it is also present in skeletal muscle, liver, and red blood cells and may be liberated from these extracardiac stores. CPK has an advantage over SGOT in that it is not present in significant concentrations in red blood cells, the kidney, liver, or lungs, but only in heart, skeletal muscle, and brain. Therefore, it is more specific and sensitive than SGOT. Since rises in serum concentration of CPK and SGOT are short-lived, they may be missed if initial blood samples are drawn more than 72 h after the infarct developed. In myocardial infarction, the level of LDH rises during the first day, peaks at 3 to 4 days, and returns to normal in 14 days.

Five common LDH isoenzymes may be separated by starch-gel electrophoresis. Tissues differ with respect to the specific isoenzyme patterns; the rapidly migrating isoenzyme which predominates in the heart is referred to as LDH_1, while the slowly migrating components predominate in liver and skeletal muscle. LDH_1 rises before total LDH in patients with myocardial infarction and may rise when there is no change in total LDH. Therefore, increased LDH_1 is a more sensitive indicator of myocardial infarction than total LDH. Its sensitivity exceeds 95 percent. CPK isoenzymes have also been demonstrated, and the isoenzyme designated MB is found almost exclusively in myocardium. As in LDH studies, the use of CPK isoenzyme determinations increases the accuracy of the enzymatic diagnosis of acute myocardial infarction. CPK isoenzymes are particularly useful when there has been skeletal muscle or brain damage since both tissues contain large amounts of the enzyme but none of the MB isoenzyme.

Of particular importance in the clinical situation is the fact that a two- to threefold elevation of CPK may follow an intramuscular injection. This may lead to the erroneous diagnosis of myocardial infarction in a patient who has been given an intramuscular injection of a narcotic for chest pain of noncardiac origin. Other potential sources of total CPK elevation worthy of note include (1) the myopathy associated with chronic alcoholism, (2) clofibrate therapy, (3) electrical cardioversion, (4) cardiac catheterization, (5) hypothyroidism, (6) stroke, and (7) surgery. Cardiac surgery and electrical cardioversion can also result in elevation of serum levels of MB isoenzyme. The use of CPK isoenzymes is particularly helpful when myocardial infarction is suspected in the presence of one of these disorders.

It has long been recognized that the amount of enzyme released correlates in some manner to the size of the infarct. Recent studies have demonstrated that the mass of heart muscle infarcted can be estimated from analysis of the concentration-time curve of the enzyme if the kinetics of the release, degradation, disposal, etc., of the enzyme are known. Although semiquantitative data as to the size of an infarct in terms of grams of infarcted tissue have been obtained by use of CPK, controversy as to the accuracy of this technique persists.

The best estimates of the accuracy of enzyme diagnosis are based on experience with SGOT. A characteristic rise occurs in more than 95 percent of patients with clinically proven myocardial infarction, and the SGOT level generally does not usually rise in unstable angina (page 1135), rheumatic carditis, or pericarditis. The rise in SGOT which follows pulmonary infarction occurs later and is of a lesser magnitude than that which follows myocardial infarction. The list of conditions other than myocardial infarction which may result in elevated SGOT includes (1) right ventricular failure with hepatic congestion, (2) the administration of salicylates, opiates, or coumarin-type anticoagulants, (3) primary muscle disease, including muscular dystrophy and surgical trauma, (4) cardiac operations, (5) acute pancreatitis, (6) extensive central nervous system damage, (7) toxemia of pregnancy, (8) hemolytic crisis, (9) crush injuries or burns, (10) infarction of kidney, spleen, or intestine, and (11) hypothyroidism.

Many patients with suspected infarction have base-line enzyme levels which are normal and increase threefold in a pattern consistent with infarction, although the absolute level of enzyme in the blood never exceeds the upper limits of normal. This situation is most commonly observed in patients with nontransmural infarction and, although not diagnostic, is highly suggestive of acute infarction. Isoenzyme studies are particularly helpful in this situation.

MANAGEMENT

By virtue of experience in the coronary care unit and the extensive research on acute myocardial infarction during the past decade, the management of this disorder has been substantially altered. Two general classes of complications have been defined: (1) electrical (arrhythmias) and (2) mechanical ("pump failure"). Ventricular fibrillation is the most common form of arrhythmic death in acute myocardial infarction. The observation that ventricular tachycardia or ventricular premature beats were almost uniformly present in all patients during the early phases of infarction and appeared to be harbingers of ventricular fibrillation led to the development of a therapeutic plan based upon the aggressive suppression of all ventricular ectopic activity. It was also realized that the potential for arrhythmic death was greatest during the early phase of infarction; that is, 65 percent of male subjects under 50 years of age who died of myocardial infarction did so within 1 h of the onset of symptoms, and 85 percent died within the first 24 h. Simultaneously, lidocaine (Chap. 238) was identified as an antiarrhythmic drug of unique effectiveness for the prophylactic treatment of ventricular ectopic activity in acute myocardial infarction. It became apparent that ventricular fibrillation could, in most instances, be prevented if the harbingers of this arrhythmia were aggressively treated, and the focus of coronary care changed from resuscitation to prevention. These developments led to the formulation of the therapeutic tenets which are now the hallmark of care for patients with acute

myocardial infarction. Reduction of in-hospital mortality for acute myocardial infarction from 30 to 15 percent is the result of institution of measures such as rapid transfer of patients with acute myocardial infarction to facilities with ECG monitoring capability staffed by personnel (not necessarily physicians) knowledgeable in the recognition and treatment of ventricular ectopic activity.

With sudden and unexpected in-hospital arrhythmic deaths essentially eliminated by the preventive approach to ventricular arrhythmias, attention has turned to the other major complication of acute myocardial infarction, i.e., pump failure. Although advances have been made in the treatment of pump failure, it remains the primary cause of in-hospital death from acute myocardial infarction. The degree of pump failure in acute myocardial infarction is a rough index of the extent of ischemic necrosis and thus the best predictive index of mortality. Hospital mortality can be related to the status of cardiac pump function on admission. A clinical classification originally proposed by Killip divides patients into four groups as follows: class I, no signs of pulmonary or venous congestion; class II, moderate heart failure as evidenced by rales at the lung bases, S_3 gallop, tachypnea, or signs of failure of the right side of the heart including venous and hepatic congestion; class III, severe heart failure, pulmonary edema; class IV, shock with systolic pressure less than 90 mmHg and evidence of peripheral constriction, diaphoresis, peripheral cyanosis, mental confusion, and decreased urine output. The expected hospital mortality rate of patients in these clinical classes has been established by a number of investigators as follows: class I, 0 to 5 percent; class II, 10 to 20 percent; class III, 35 to 45 percent; and class IV, 85 to 95 percent.

GENERAL CONSIDERATIONS The primary therapeutic objectives of management of the patient with myocardial infarction are to prevent death from arrhythmia and to minimize the mass of infarcted tissue.

Arrhythmias can usually be managed successfully if trained personnel and appropriate equipment are available when this complication develops. Since mortality from arrhythmia is greatest during the first few hours after infarction, it is obvious that the effectiveness of coronary care units relates directly to the speed with which patients come under medical observation. The biggest delay is not in transportation to the hospital but rather between the onset of pain and the patient's decision to call for help. One hopes that this delay can be reduced by education of the public concerning the significance of chest pain and the importance of seeking early medical attention.

Within the past decade, it has been demonstrated that the amount of myocardial tissue which becomes necrotic secondary to a vascular occlusion is determined by factors other than just the site of occlusion. Infarct size is now known to be variable with time and affected by therapeutic agents currently in use. The balance between myocardial oxygen supply and demand in areas rendered ischemic by an occlusion is the single most important factor determining the ultimate fate of these areas of jeopardized myocardium. While no routine therapeutic approach to reduce infarct size in all patients is currently available, the realization that infarct size may be increased by interventions which adversely alter the supply-demand balance has prompted the reevaluation of previously accepted therapeutic maneuvers in the management of patients with acute infarction.

A number of "common sense" rules in the management of acute myocardial infarction deserve particular emphasis. First and foremost, it is mandatory to maintain an optimal balance between myocardial oxygen supply and demand so that as much of the jeopardized zone of the myocardium surrounding the center of the infarct can be salvaged as possible. This can be accomplished by maintaining the patient at rest; analgesia when necessary, mild sedation, and a quiet atmosphere may reduce anxiety and thereby lower heart rate, a major determinant of myocardial oxygen consumption.

If the patient was receiving a beta-adrenergic blocking agent at the time the clinical manifestations of the infarct commenced, it is reasonable not to discontinue the drug unless a specific contraindication develops, such as left ventricular failure or a bradyarrhythmia. Marked sinus bradycardia (heart rate less than approximately 45 beats per minute) should be treated by leg elevation and atropine or by electrical pacing. However, the routine administration of atropine, with the resultant increase in heart rate, to patients without serious bradycardia seems unwise. All forms of tachyarrhythmias require prompt and direct treatment. Drugs that exert a positive inotropic effect, such as the digitalis glycosides and cardioactive sympathomimetics, should be administered only if there is evidence of ventricular failure—and should not be given prophylactically. Of the various sympathomimetic amines available, isoproterenol with its chronotropic and vasodilator effects is the least desirable. Dopamine and Dobutamine, which have less effect on heart rate and systemic vascular resistance, are more desirable when it is necessary to augment cardiac contractility. Obviously, diuretics are also indicated in the presence of heart failure and might, in fact, be used prior to and perhaps in place of cardiac stimulants unless the patient is already hypovolemic or unresponsive to their administration.

All patients should inhale oxygen-enriched air (see below). Particular attention must be paid to preserving arterial oxygenation in patients with hypoxemia, as occurs in those with chronic pulmonary disease, pneumonia, or left ventricular failure. Severe anemia, which can also extend the area of ischemic injury, should be corrected by the cautious administration of packed red blood cells, sometimes accompanied by a diuretic. Associated conditions, particularly infections and the accompanying tachycardia and elevated myocardial oxygen needs, require immediate attention. Systolic arterial pressure should not be allowed to deviate by more than 25 to 30 mmHg from the patient's usual level.

Coronary care units The development of coronary care units has resulted in improved care of patients with myocardial infarction, a reduction in mortality rates, and a major increase in knowledge about myocardial infarction. The coronary care unit is a specially designed *nursing unit*, the most important feature of which is a staff of highly trained nursing personnel with authority to take immediate action in emergency situations. The unit should be equipped with systems which permit continuous monitoring of the electrocardiogram of each patient. Defibrillators, respirators, and facilities for introducing pacing catheters and flow-directed balloon-tipped catheters should be available. However, equipment alone does not ensure an effective coronary care unit. Of prime importance is the organization of a highly trained team of nurses who can recognize arrhythmias, adjust the dosage of antiarrhythmic drugs, and perform cardiac resuscitation, including the application of electroshock when necessary. A physician should be available at all times, but many lives have been saved because nurses have treated ventricular tachycardia or fibrillation before the physician arrived.

The policies and procedures for admission to a coronary care unit should ensure that patients are admitted early in their illness when they may expect to derive maximum benefit from the care provided. The threshold for admission of patients with suspected infarction should be low, and this is best monitored in terms of the fraction of total admissions in whom myocardial infarction is eventually proved. If this fraction exceeds 50 percent, the admission policies may well be too restrictive, and not enough patients are being admitted for suspected myocardial infarction which did not develop. Mortality rates for myocardial infarction treated in coronary care units vary from 12 to 20 percent; this variation can be explained, in part, by variations in admission policies as regard age limitations, the type of population being served (tertiary care center versus community hospital), and other as yet unidentified factors.

TREATMENT OF THE PATIENT WITH AN UNCOMPLICATED INFARCT Analgesia Myocardial infarction usually announces itself with severe pain, and therefore one of the important initial therapeutic objectives is the relief of pain. Morphine, the agent traditionally used for this purpose, is still the most effective and remains the drug of choice. It may lower arterial pressure by reducing sympathetically mediated arteriolar and venous constriction. The resultant venous pooling may produce a reduction in cardiac output. This must be recognized but does not necessarily contraindicate its use. The skin may become cool and moist, and the patient may complain of nausea, but these events usually pass and are replaced by a feeling of well-being associated with the relief of pain. It is important to recognize this syndrome as one attributable to morphine, because the hypotension and signs of peripheral constriction may be incorrectly interpreted as manifestations of the shock syndrome and taken as grounds for the initiation of vasoconstrictor or other therapy which would be inappropriate. The hypotension associated with venous pooling usually responds promptly to elevation of the legs. Morphine also has a vagotonic effect and may cause bradycardia or advanced degrees of heart block, particularly in patients with diaphragmatic infarction. These side effects of morphine usually respond to atropine, and prophylactic atropine (0.4 mg intravenously) should be administered prior to the injection of morphine if bradycardia or any degree of heart block is present. Because of these potential side effects, it is advisable to select the minimal effective dose of morphine which relieves pain. This can be accomplished by the repetitive (every 5 min) intravenous injection of a small dose of drug (2 to 4 mg) rather than the administration of a larger quantity by either the intramuscular or subcutaneous route, from which sites absorption may be unpredictable in acute myocardial infarction. Demerol or Dilaudid may be effectively employed in place of morphine. Inhalation of 30 to 50 percent inspired nitrous oxide is effective in relieving both pain and anxiety associated with the discomfort of myocardial ischemia and/or necrosis. Nitrous oxide may be administered in addition to narcotic analgesics with little or no depression of left ventricular function.

Oxygen The routine use of oxygen is supported by the observation that the arterial P_{O_2} is reduced in many patients with myocardial infarction and that oxygen inhalation reduces infarct size in experimental animals. Inhalation of oxygen increases the P_{O_2} of the blood and hence increases the concentration gradient responsible for the diffusion of oxygen into the ischemic myocardium from adjacent, better-perfused areas. Although oxygen elevates peripheral resistance and lowers cardiac output slightly, and it is possible that these effects may be deleterious, the weight of evidence favors the administration of oxygen. The majority of patients should receive supplemental inspiratory oxygen. It should be administered by tent, face mask, or nasal prongs for the first 2 or 3 days after infarction.

Activity Factors which increase the work of the heart may increase the size of the myocardial infarct. Circumstances in which heart size, cardiac output, or myocardial contractility are increased should be avoided. It has been demonstrated that 6 to 8 weeks are required for the healing which takes place by the replacement of the infarcted myocardium by scar tissue. The purpose of reduced physical activity is to provide the most favorable possible circumstances for this healing.

All patients with myocardial infarction should be admitted to a coronary care unit and remain there for 3 or 4 days under constant observation by trained personnel utilizing continuous electrocardiographic monitoring. A catheter should be introduced into a peripheral vein, firmly fixed so that it is not easily dislodged, and kept open by the slow infusion of glucose solution. This is a route of administration for antiarrhythmic or other drugs which may be necessary. During the first 2 to 3 days in the absence of pump failure, the patient should be at bed rest most of the day, with one or two periods of 15 to 30 min in a bedside chair. The patient may use a bedside commode and should be bathed by a nurse. Patients may eat unassisted. The bed should be equipped with a footboard, and the patient should push his feet against the footboard firmly 10 times during each waking hour to prevent venous stasis and thromboembolism and to maintain muscle tone in the legs.

The usual patient whose course has been uncomplicated may be discharged from the coronary care unit on the third or fourth day. By this time, he or she should be spending 30 to 60 min in a chair twice a day. It is advisable at this stage to measure the patient's blood pressure when standing in order to be aware of postural hypotension, which may be a problem when ambulation is begun. Standing and gradual ambulation are usually begun somewhere between the fifth and eighth days postinfarction in patients with uncomplicated transmural and nontransmural myocardial infarction. Initial ambulation is to the bathroom if it is in the patient's room or nearby. Ambulation is progressively increased, eventually including walks about the hospital floor. The total duration of hospitalization in uncomplicated cases is usually 10 to 14 days, but many physicians still hospitalize patients with transmural infarction for 3 weeks, while others have reduced the period to as short as 1 week when the opportunities for home convalescence are ideal, without apparent ill effect. Patients in clinical class II or higher may require 3 or more weeks of hospitalization, depending upon the rapidity with which the congestive heart failure resolves and the home situation to which the patient is returning.

The remainder of the convalescent phase of myocardial infarction may be accomplished at home. Some physicians restrict the patient to one floor until he has completed 5 weeks of convalescence, and then allow only one trip upstairs a day. Other physicians allow patients to make one daily trip up and down a single flight of stairs beginning several days after discharge from the hospital. From 5 to 8 weeks, the patient should be encouraged to increase activity with walking about the house and outdoors in good weather. Patients should still spend 8 to 10 h in bed each night. Additional rest periods in the morning and afternoon may be advisable for selected patients.

From 8 weeks onward, the physician must regulate the patient's activity on the basis of his or her exercise tolerance. It is during this period of increasing activity that the patient may become aware of profound fatigue. Postural hypotension may still be a problem. Most patients will be able to return to work after 12 weeks. A definite trend toward earlier ambulation, hospital discharge, and resumption of full activity for patients recuperating from acute myocardial infarction has developed in recent years.

Diet During the first 5 days, a low-calorie diet divided into multiple small feedings is preferred. Cardiac output increases following ingestion of food, and therefore the quantity of feed-

ings should be kept small. If congestive heart failure is present, sodium intake should be modestly restricted. Since constipation commonly occurs during convalescence from myocardial infarction, it is reasonable to give average or even increased amounts of bulk in the diet. In addition, the ingestion of potassium-rich foods should be encouraged in patients receiving diuretics. During the second week, increasing amounts of food may be introduced into the diet. At this time, the importance of restriction of calories and saturated fat may be explained to the patient, and he or she can be started on an appropriate diet. Willingness to accept dietary restriction and to discontinue smoking is usually never greater than it is during this early period of convalescence.

Bowels Bed rest of 3 to 5 days and the effect of the narcotics utilized for the relief of pain often lead to constipation. Most patients are not comfortable using a bedpan. Attempts to use the bedpan frequently result in excessive straining at stool and/or isometric work as patients attempt to elevate themselves to accommodate the bedpan. This maneuver is highly undesirable because it serves as a vagal stimulant which may produce bradycardia and provoke arrhythmias. For these reasons, a bedside commode, a diet rich in bulk, and the routine use of a stool softener such as dioctyl sodium sulfosuccinate, 200 mg daily, is recommended. The patient should be reassured that it will not be deleterious to go without a bowel movement for several days. However, if the patient becomes distressed and uncomfortable, a laxative can be safely used. It is safe to perform a gentle rectal examination on patients with acute myocardial infarction.

Sedation Most patients require sedation during hospitalization in order to withstand the period of enforced inactivity with tranquillity. Chlordiazepoxide 10 mg, or diazepam 5 mg, given four times daily is usually effective. These drugs are preferable to phenobarbital in patients receiving warfarin-type anticoagulant drugs since the destruction of the latter is increased by phenobarbital (Chap. 70). Appropriate sleeping medication may be given at night to ensure adequate sleep. Chloral hydrate 0.5 to 1.0 g or flurazepam 15 to 30 mg is usually sufficient to induce sleep. Attention to this problem is especially important during the first few days in the coronary care unit, where the atmosphere of 24-h vigilance may interfere with the patient's sleep. Sedation is no substitute for a dark, quiet room.

Anticoagulants Few topics are more controversial than the use of anticoagulants in the routine treatment of acute myocardial infarction. The lack of any statistically clear-cut demonstration of a lower mortality rate in the first few weeks following myocardial infarction suggests that the benefit of anticoagulant therapy, if any, is small. The use of anticoagulant therapy to retard the process of coronary occlusion during the initial phases of myocardial infarction is not justified. However, there is agreement that anticoagulant therapy does reduce the incidence of both arterial and venous thromboembolic complications. Since the incidence of venous thromboembolic disease is known to be increased in patients with congestive heart failure, shock, and previous venous or thromboembolic disease, the routine, prophylactic use of anticoagulant drugs to prevent pulmonary embolism in the coronary care unit is recommended for those patients at high risk for this complication. Routine anticoagulation as prophylaxis against venous thromboembolism is not recommended in class I patients. Patients in classes III and IV are at greater risk for pulmonary embolism and should be routinely anticoagulated during the initial 10 to 14 days of hospitalization, or until ambulatory. This is best accomplished initially by the continuous intravenous administration of heparin with a constant infusion pump at a rate of 400 units per hour with frequent measurement of the clotting time or partial thromboplastin time to define the need for increasing or decreasing the infusion rate. Once the patient is out of the intensive care area, oral anticoagulants may be substituted for heparin. Controversy as to the need for anticoagulant therapy in class II patients persists. It would seem appropriate to anticoagulate these patients only if the signs of congestive heart failure persist for more than 3 or 4 days.

Small subcutaneous doses of heparin (5000 units every 8 to 12 h) have been advocated as a means of preventing deep venous thrombosis and subsequent pulmonary embolism in patients with myocardial infarction. Early ambulation schedules also reduce this complication, making "minidose" heparin, if employed, necessary for only 4 to 5 days.

The incidence of arterial embolism from clot originating in the ventricle at the site of infarct is small (i.e., less than 5 percent) but definite. Frequently, arterial embolism presents as a major complication, such as hemiparesis, when the cerebral circulation is involved, or hypertension if the renal circulation is compromised. The low incidence of this complication, contrasted with its severity, renders it impractical to establish firm guidelines for the use of anticoagulant drugs as prophylaxis against arterial embolism in acute myocardial infarction. The likelihood of intraventricular clot formation appears to increase with the extent of infarction and the resultant inflammation and endocardial stasis due to akinesis. Therefore, as is the case with venous thromboembolism, the indication for anticoagulation as prophylaxis against arterial embolism increases with the extent of infarction.

TREATMENT Arrhythmias (see also Chap. 237) The improved management of arrhythmias constitutes a most significant advance in the treatment of myocardial infarction. The prevention of serious and life-threatening arrhythmias depends on the early recognition and aggressive management of their precursors.

VENTRICULAR PREMATURE SYSTOLES These are the most frequent harbingers of more serious ventricular arrhythmias. Infrequent, sporadic ventricular premature systoles occur in almost all patients with infarction and do not require therapy, but prompt treatment is indicated if the premature systoles occur frequently or in certain patterns. Indications for suppression of ventricular ectopic beats are generally considered to be the following: (1) the presence of more than five isolated ectopic beats per minute, (2) the occurrence of consecutive or multifocal ventricular extrasystoles, and (3) the occurrence of ectopic ventricular beats early in diastole and hence superimposed on the T wave of the preceding beat (the so-called "R on T phenomenon"). Intravenous lidocaine has become the treatment of choice for ventricular premature beats and ventricular arrhythmias, because it acts rapidly and side effects disappear soon (15 to 20 min) after its administration is discontinued (Chap. 238). Lidocaine is given initially as a single intravenous injection of 50 to 100 mg to establish adequate blood levels quickly. This initial dose usually eliminates the ectopic activity and is followed by an intravenous infusion of 1 to 4 mg/min. Usually, ventricular premature beats spontaneously disappear after 72 to 96 h. If significant ventricular ectopic activity persists past this time, chronic antiarrhythmic therapy should be continued.

Procainamide and quinidine are most commonly used for the treatment of persistent ventricular ectopic activity, although propranolol (Chap. 72) is also effective occasionally. Disopyramide is also effective in abolishing ventricular ectopic activity in infarction patients. This agent should be used with great care in patients with manifest left ventricular failure as it has a significant negative inotropic action. If the usual doses of these drugs (Chap. 238), singly or in combination, are not effective, blood levels should be measured to ensure that adequate blood concentrations are being obtained. Frequent clinical and electrocardiographic assessment of the patient for signs of drug toxicity (Chap. 238) are mandatory when higher doses of these drugs are employed.

VENTRICULAR TACHYCARDIA AND VENTRICULAR FIBRILLATION Sustained ventricular tachycardia is treated first with lidocaine, and if it cannot be terminated by a 50- to 100-mg dose, electroconversion should be employed (Chap. 239). Electroshock is used immediately in patients with ventricular fibrillation, or when ventricular tachycardia causes hemodynamic deterioration. If fibrillation has persisted for more than a few seconds, the first shock may be unsuccessful, and in this situation it is advisable to administer closed-chest massage, mouth-to-mouth respiration, and intravenous sodium bicarbonate solution (40 to 90 meq) before attempting electroconversion again. Improvement of oxygenation and perfusion and correction of acidosis increase the likelihood of successful defibrillation (see also Chap. 32).

In consideration of the efficacy of therapy for ventricular fibrillation, it is useful to divide patients into groups based on the circumstances of origin of the arrhythmia. Long-term survival is good in patients with *primary* ventricular fibrillation, i.e., ventricular fibrillation resulting as a primary response to acute ischemia and not associated with predisposing factors such as congestive heart failure, shock, or ventricular aneurysm. In one series, 87 percent of patients with primary ventricular fibrillation left the hospital alive. This prognosis is in sharp contrast to that for patients who develop ventricular fibrillation *secondary* to severe pump failure. A far smaller percentage, 29 percent, of patients in this group was discharged from the hospital alive.

ACCELERATED IDIOVENTRICULAR RHYTHM Accelerated idioventricular rhythm (AIVR) has been found to occur in 25 percent of patients with myocardial infarction. It is especially frequent in diaphragmatic infarction, where it is usually associated with sinus bradycardia. The rate of AIVR is usually similar to that of the sinus rhythm which precedes and follows it, and this similarity of rate and the relatively minor hemodynamic effects make this rhythm impossible to detect other than by electrocardiographic monitoring. The QRS complexes are broad and identical in shape. The rhythm comes and goes spontaneously as fluctuation in sinus rate causes the atrial rate to fall below the accelerated escape level, usually 50 to 90 beats per minute. For the most part, this rhythm is benign and does not presage the development of classic ventricular tachycardia. However, a number of cases have been documented wherein AIVR was associated with more dangerous forms of ventricular ectopic activity or where AIVR degenerated into a potentially fatal ventricular arrhythmia. Since one cannot predict when this complication will occur, it may be best to treat AIVR whenever it is identified. This can be done by using a drug which decreases the ventricular escape rate (lidocaine) and/or one that increases the sinus rate (atropine).

SUPRAVENTRICULAR ARRHYTHMIAS The common arrhythmias in this group are junctional rhythm and tachycardia, atrial tachycardia, atrial flutter, and atrial fibrillation. These rhythm disturbances are often secondary to left ventricular failure. The administration of a short-acting glycoside, such as digoxin or ouabain, is the treatment of choice. If the abnormal rhythm persists for more than 2 h with a ventricular rate in excess of 120 beats per minute, treatment with electroshock should be considered. However, when tachycardia induces heart failure, shock, or ischemia (as manifested by pain or ECG changes), the situation should be considered an emergency and electroshock utilized immediately.

The frequency of junctional arrhythmias in acute myocardial infarction is low. These arrhythmias are of diverse etiology, are not indicative of any specific abnormality, and from a therapeutic viewpoint must be considered on an individual basis. Even in the presence of acute myocardial infarction, digitalis excess must be ruled out as a cause of junctional tachycardia. In some patients with severely compromised left ventricular function, the loss of appropriately timed atrial systole results in a marked decrease in cardiac output. Right atrial or coronary sinus pacing is indicated in such instances. The hemodynamic effects of these two modes of pacing are identical, but coronary sinus pacing offers the advantage of better catheter stability.

SINUS BRADYCARDIA The significance of bradycardia as a predisposing factor to ventricular fibrillation in acute myocardial infarction is controversial. While the incidence of ventricular tachycardia in patients with sustained bradycardia is twice that observed in patients with normal heart rates, sinus bradycardia has also been identified in hospitalized patients as an index of a favorable prognosis. Experience with mobile coronary care units indicates sinus bradycardia occurring within the first hour after infarction is more consistently associated with ventricular ectopic rhythms than that occurring later in the course of the illness. Since most ventricular tachycardia is presaged by ventricular premature beats, and these premature beats can often be abolished by increasing the sinus rate, treatment of sinus bradycardia is mandatory if significant ventricular ectopic activity is present or if hemodynamic compromise results from the slow heart rate. There is no agreement as to whether bradycardia should be treated in asymptomatic, normotensive, arrhythmia-free patients. Elevation of the legs and/or the foot of the bed is frequently helpful in the treatment of sinus bradycardia. Atropine is the most useful drug for increasing heart rate and should be given intravenously in doses of 0.4 to 0.6 mg. If the rate remains below 60 beats per minute, additional doses of 0.2 mg, up to a total of 2.0 mg, may be given in divided doses. Persistent bradycardia (< 40 beats per minute) despite atropine may be treated with electrical pacing.

CONDUCTION DISTURBANCES Malfunction of the conduction system in acute myocardial infarction is similar to that seen in other disease states in that block or failure to conduct may develop at three different levels in the conduction system: the atrioventricular (AV) node, the bundle of His, or the more peripheral portions of the conduction system (Chaps. 232 and 237). If the block occurs in the AV node, the escape rhythm originates in the AV junction and the QRS complexes are of normal duration; but when the block occurs distal to the AV node, the escape site is ventricular and the QRS configuration is abnormal and its duration is prolonged. Rosenbaum has directed attention to disturbances of conduction in the three peripheral branches of the conduction system as being of value in predicting the occurrence of AV nodal block (Chap. 232). When block occurs in any two of the three fascicles, bifascicular block is said to exist; trifascicular block, resulting in complete AV block, follows in approximately 35 percent of such patients. Patients with the combination of right bundle branch block and either left anterior or left posterior hemiblock have a particularly high risk of progression to complete heart block.

Conduction disturbances may occur in patients with anterior or inferior infarction. However, the mortality rate of patients with complete AV block in association with anterior infarction (80 to 90 percent) is almost three times that of patients who develop conduction disturbances with inferior infarction (30 percent), and the risk of subsequent death in those who survive to leave the hospital is also increased in the former group. This difference is related to the fact that heart block in inferior infarction is caused by AV nodal ischemia. The AV node is a discrete structure, and thus a small amount of necrosis, if strategically located, can result in AV nodal dysfunction. In anterior wall infarction, heart block is related to ischemic malfunction of the three fascicles of the conduction system and can thus result only from extensive myocardial necrosis.

Electrical pacing provides an effective means of increasing the heart rate of patients with bradycardia due to AV block, but it is not possible to be sure that such acceleration is always beneficial. For example, in patients with anterior wall infarction and complete heart block, the large size of the infarct is the major factor determining the outcome, and correction of the conduction deficit does not clearly improve the uniformly poor prognosis in this group. Pacing does appear to be beneficial, however, in patients with an inferior (diaphragmatic wall) infarct who have complete heart block associated with heart failure, hypotension, marked bradycardia, or significant ventricular ectopic activity.

Some cardiologists advocate the placement of a pacing catheter prophylactically in patients with conduction disturbances known to be precursors of complete heart block. Unanimity of opinion does not exist on this point. Pacing may diminish the risk of treating ventricular ectopic beats with antiarrhythmic agents such as procainamide or lidocaine in the presence of heart block or sinus bradycardia. Permanent pacing has been advocated for patients who develop persistent bifasicular and transient third-degree heart block during the acute phase of myocardial infarction. Retrospective studies in small numbers of such patients suggest that the incidence of sudden death is decreased in those in whom permanent pacing was instituted.

Congestive heart failure Some degree of transient congestive heart failure occurs in over half of the patients with myocardial infarction. The most common clinical signs are pulmonary rales and a protodiastolic gallop (S_3) rhythm. Pulmonary congestion is also frequently seen on chest roentgenogram. Elevation of left ventricular filling pressure and pulmonary artery pressure are the characteristic hemodynamic findings. The therapy of congestive failure in association with myocardial infarction is similar to that of congestive failure secondary to other forms of heart disease, with a few exceptions (Chap. 236). The major difference concerns the use of cardiac glycosides. The benefit following the administration of digitalis is less impressive in acute myocardial infarction. This is not surprising in that the agent would not be expected to improve the function of infarcted tissue, and the function of the noninfarcted tissue may be normal. On the other hand, diuretic agents are extremely effective in the treatment of congestive failure following myocardial infarction. A fall in left ventricular filling pressure and an improvement in orthopnea and dyspnea follow the intravenous administration of furosemide. This powerful drug should be used with caution, however, as it can result in a massive diuresis with associated decrease in plasma volume, cardiac output, systemic blood pressure, and hence coronary perfusion. The patient with pulmonary edema is treated in the manner described in Chap. 236. Recent studies with agents that reduce cardiac afterload, i.e., nitrates, alphablockers, hydralazine, prazosin, and sodium nitroprusside, indicate that the reduction in cardiac work which results from the lowered afterload may significantly improve left ventricular performance with a reduction of ventricular filling pressure and pulmonary congestion concomitant with an elevation of cardiac output.

Shock syndrome—power failure With the development of effective methods for treating arrhythmias, shock or "power failure" has become the most important fatal complication of myocardial infarction. It is useful to consider this syndrome as a severe form of left ventricular failure. Shock occurs in about 20 percent of patients with myocardial infarction and accounts for at least 70 percent of the in-hospital deaths, now that the mortality rate due to arrhythmias has been reduced. The mortality rate in myocardial infarction with shock (Killip class IV) ranges from 85 to 95 percent.

Hypotension alone is not a basis for the diagnosis of the shock syndrome, because many patients who make an uneventful recovery will have serious hypotension (systolic pressures < 80 mmHg) for several days. The shock syndrome is considered to be present when hypotension is accompanied by other clinical signs of circulatory inadequacy. The following criteria for the shock syndrome define a population of patients with a mortality rate of greater than 95 percent: (1) systolic arterial blood pressure less than 90 mmHg which has declined by at least 30 mmHg below the previous level, as recorded by direct intraarterial pressure measurements rather than sphygmomanometry; (2) clinical signs of peripheral circulatory insufficiency, e.g., cold, moist skin and cyanosis; (3) dulled sensorium; (4) oliguria with urine flow of less than 20 ml/h; and (5) failure of improvement following relief of pain and administration of oxygen. Specifically *excluded* are patients with hypotension secondary to vasovagal reaction, arrhythmia, drug reaction, or hypovolemia.

PATHOPHYSIOLOGY OF PUMP FAILURE   Marked reduction of the quantity of contracting myocardium is the cause of the

FIGURE 245-2
Diagram depicting the sequence of events in the vicious cycle in which coronary artery obstruction leads to cardiogenic shock and progressive circulatory deterioration.

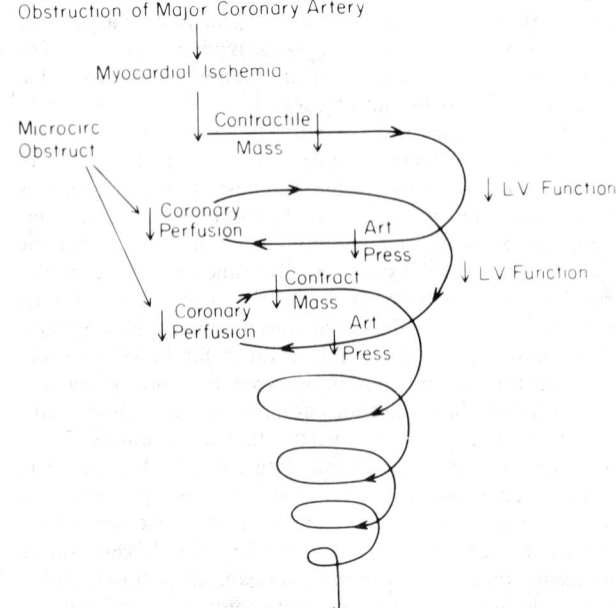

shock syndrome in myocardial infarction, although all organ systems are involved ultimately. The function of the heart is impaired by the initial insult; this results in a decrease in arterial pressure and hence in coronary blood flow because of its dependence on aortic perfusion pressure (Fig. 245-2). The reduction in coronary perfusion pressure and myocardial blood flow further impairs myocardial function and may increase the size of the myocardial infarction. Arrhythmias and metabolic acidosis also contribute to this deterioration because they are the result of inadequate perfusion, and both tend to perpetuate the precipitating conditions. It is this positive feedback loop (impaired cardiac function → arterial hypotension → reduced coronary blood flow → impaired cardiac function) which accounts for the high mortality rate associated with the shock syndrome.

Arterial blood pressure is a function of two factors—the cardiac output and total peripheral resistance—and a decrease in either without a compensatory rise in the other will result in a fall in arterial blood pressure. Cardiac output is lower in a population of patients with shock than in those who do not have the shock syndrome, but this is by no means the whole explanation. Many patients with myocardial infarction without shock have cardiac outputs in the same range as those in patients with shock, and therefore it is not possible to characterize these patients on the basis of reductions of cardiac output alone.

Total peripheral resistance, the other factor important in determining blood pressure, may be either normal or increased in myocardial infarction. Here again, a similar range of values for total peripheral resistance may be seen in patients in the absence of shock. Normally, a fall in cardiac output is accompanied by a compensatory rise in total peripheral resistance, but in patients with shock due to myocardial infarction, the appropriate response in peripheral resistance may fail to occur. In such patients, total peripheral resistance does not increase sufficiently to support blood pressure at the depressed level of cardiac output.

It is necessary to return to the heart itself as the site of the fundamental physiological alteration in the shock syndrome. It is axiomatic that if the diagnosis of myocardial infarction is correct, there will be a reduction in myocardial contractile function. Direct measurement of left ventricular filling pressure in the form of pulmonary capillary wedge pressure has demonstrated that left ventricular function may be impaired in the absence of the usual clinical manifestations of left-sided heart failure, such as pulmonary congestion.

A simple schematic diagram depicting the relationship between left ventricular work and filling pressure is seen in Fig. 245-3. The upper curve represents the familiar Frank-Starling relationship in the normal heart; the lower curve shows the relation which might be expected in the patient with shock secondary to myocardial infarction. It is obvious that at all levels of end-diastolic pressure, the left ventricular work of the patient with myocardial infarction is depressed. At point C, the end-diastolic pressure is elevated, but at point B, it may be normal despite the fact that myocardial work is well below that expected of the normal heart at this diastolic pressure, as indicated by point A.

Treatment of pump failure The gravity and complex physiology of this condition indicate that all patients with shock should, if possible, have continuous monitoring of arterial pressure and left ventricular filling pressure as reflected in the pulmonary capillary wedge pressure measured with a Swan-Ganz catheter, as well as frequent determinations of cardiac output. All patients with the shock syndrome should receive 100 percent oxygen continuously to help combat the hypoxemia which is universally present. The relief of pain is important, as some vasodepressor reflex activity may be a response to severe pain. However, narcotics should be used cautiously in view of their propensity to lower arterial pressure.

Treatment is directed at the interruption of the feedback loop (Fig. 245-2), whereby impaired myocardial function leads to a reduction in arterial pressure, decreased coronary blood flow, and further depression of left ventricular function. This objective is approached by attempting to maintain coronary perfusion by raising the arterial blood pressure with vasopressors or volume replacement to a level that ensures an optimum left ventricular filling pressure (approximately 18 to 20 mmHg).

Hypovolemia is an easily corrected condition which may contribute to the hypotension and vascular collapse associated with myocardial infarction in some patients. Fluid loss may be secondary to previous diuretic use, reduced intake during the early stages of the illness, and/or vomiting associated with pain or medications. In addition, a state of relative hypovolemia may exist; i.e., with the acute reduction in contractile function and ventricular compliance resulting from infarction, an increase in vascular volume is needed to maintain cardiac output. Owing to the acute nature of the process, there is insufficient time for compensatory fluid retention to accommodate this need, and relative hypovolemia in a normally hydrated patient results. Consequently, hypovolemia should be identified and corrected in patients with acute myocardial infarction and hypotension before embarking upon more vigorous forms of therapy. If left ventricular filling pressure is in the normal range, fluid should be administered until the left ventricular filling pressure increases to 18 to 20 mmHg. Central venous pressure measurements are inadequate in this situation, since left ventricular function is almost always affected much more adversely than is right ventricular function in acute myocardial infarction.

VASOPRESSORS   In the shock state, the coronary vascular bed distal to an obstructing lesion will be maximally dilated, and myocardial blood flow will be totally dependent on the perfusion pressure. Agents such as methoxamine, phenylephrine, and angiotensin, which are pure vasoconstrictors, have no place in the treatment of shock due to myocardial infarction, since failure of arterial constriction usually plays only a minor role.

Dopamine, a newly developed sympathomimetic drug, is useful in patients with the power failure syndrome (Chap. 238). This drug has both alpha- and beta-adrenergic effects, with the latter being predominant at lower doses. At low dosages, the drug has positive chronotropic and inotropic effects, and at high-dose ranges a vasoconstrictor effect as a result of the stimulation of alpha receptors is noted. It also has the unique effect of dilating the renal vascular bed. Experience with this drug in the treatment of pump failure syndromes has been favorable, although it is not clear that it reduces mortality in patients with cardiogenic shock. It appears that dopamine has little effect on myocardial oxygen consumption when employed at low dosages. Intravenous dopamine infusion is started at 2 to 5 (mg/kg)/min with increments in dosage every 2 to 5 min up to a maximum of 20 to 50 (mg/kg)/min. Systolic arterial blood pressure should be maintained at approximately 90 mmHg.

Norepinephrine should be administered intravenously through an indwelling catheter to avoid the risk of extravasation, which results in necrosis of subcutaneous tissue. It is desirable to determine the smallest effective dose of norepinephrine by starting with 4 mg dissolved in a liter of 5% glucose solution. The infusion rate is set to maintain a systolic pressure of around 90 mmHg, which should provide adequate perfusion of the heart, brain, and kidneys. To increase the pressure above this level imposes an unnecessary load on the heart and

may be undesirable. Should 4 μg/min (1 ml/min) prove inadequate to maintain systolic pressure near 90 mmHg, the concentration of the infused solution should be increased, but if pressure cannot be maintained with a dosage of 15 μg/min, it is unlikely that a further increase in dosage will be beneficial. The lack of response to norepinephrine probably indicates that the remaining functional myocardium is already maximally stimulated by endogenous catecholamines. Renal blood flow is decreased early in the development of circulatory failure, and therefore urine flow constitutes a sensitive indicator of the rate of renal perfusion, which may be considered adequate if a urine flow of 0.5 ml/min is maintained.

Every effort should be made to use the smallest effective dose of positive inotropic agent for the shortest possible time. Weaning the patient from pressors is often difficult and requires close observation and the exercise of considerable clinical judgment. The rate of administration must be reduced cautiously. The systolic arterial pressure may fall to 80 mmHg, but if there are no other clinical signs of circulatory insufficiency, i.e., cyanosis, clouded sensorium, or cold moist extremities, it is wise not to reinstitute therapy. Close observation often reveals that arterial pressure rises gradually with passage of time. If, on the other hand, the pressure falls further or clinical signs of circulatory inadequacy appear, therapy should be reinstituted. Pressor amines cause fluid to shift from the intravascular space to the extracellular fluid space, and their prolonged use may result in a depletion of intravascular volume in patients who do not lose weight and who may actually appear edematous. In such instances, blood pressure falls dramatically when pressor amine support is withdrawn. Hypovolemia which results from these internal fluid shifts must be treated in patients who cannot be weaned from pressor amines.

Isoproterenol is a synthetic sympathomimetic amine which has enjoyed unjustified popularity in the treatment of shock due to myocardial infarction. This agent increases myocardial contractility and heart rate and, unlike norepinephrine, produces peripheral vasodilatation. The increase in contractility results in an increase in myocardial oxygen consumption, which may extend the area of ischemic injury, and the increase

FIGURE 245-3

Schematic representation of the Frank-Starling relationship as applied to patients with the shock syndrome in myocardial infarction.

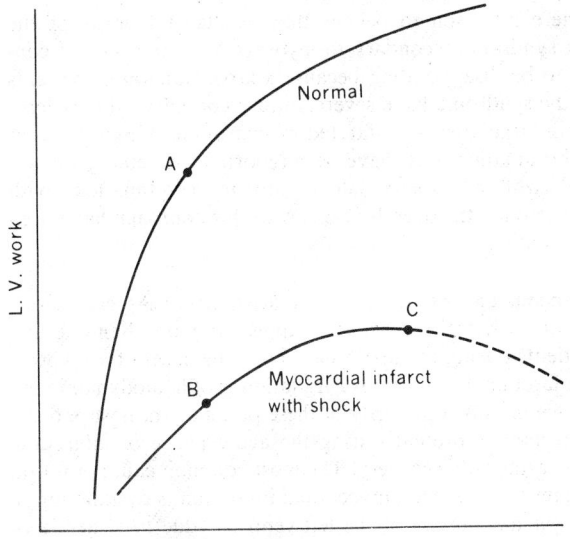

in wall tension produces a decrease in blood flow to the inner layers of the myocardium. It has also been demonstrated that isoproterenol results in metabolic deterioration, as evidenced by an increase in lactate production by the heart. For all these reasons, isoproterenol is of little if any value and may actually be detrimental in the treatment of shock due to myocardial infarction.

CARDIAC GLYCOSIDES Consideration of the central role of impaired myocardial function in the shock syndrome leads to the conclusion that cardiac glycosides should be administered to all patients with this condition. Controlled studies, however, have failed to demonstrate significant beneficial effects of glycoside therapy in the early phases (0 to 48 h) of acute myocardial infarction, and it is possible that digitalis increases myocardial irritability during this period. Hemodynamic improvement has been documented at later times, but this effect is marginal. Since cardiac glycosides cannot improve the function of necrotic myocardium and since pump failure is thought to be related to the total mass of infarcted tissue, digitalis therapy does not result in dramatic improvement in patients with acute myocardial infarction. Nonetheless, it is probably worthwhile to treat patients with signs and symptoms of left ventricular failure with digitalis. It has been demonstrated that when scrupulous attention is paid to the dosage, incidence of arrhythmias and cardiac rupture is no higher in patients with myocardial infarction treated with digitalis than in a control group, and therefore digitalis can be administered with relative safety.

NEWER FORMS OF THERAPY The basic defect in the shock syndrome is impaired myocardial function; therefore, many mechanical assist devices have been developed to supplement the pumping action of the heart. The largest body of clinical experience has been obtained with the intraaortic balloon system of diastolic pressure augmentation. A sausage-shaped balloon at the end of a catheter is introduced into the aorta via the femoral artery, and the balloon is inflated during early diastole, thereby enhancing both coronary blood flow and peripheral perfusion. The balloon collapses in early systole, thereby reducing the afterload against which left ventricular ejection takes place. Improvement in hemodynamic status has been observed with balloon pumping in a large number of patients, but long-term survival following this mode of therapy alone is still disappointing. The balloon system appears to be of greatest use for the support of patients during and after coronary arteriography and bypass surgery.

There is reason to believe that results of therapy of the shock syndrome secondary to myocardial infarction will continue to be disappointing because a large fraction of patients with the syndrome have severe, diffuse coronary atherosclerosis with large areas of infarcted myocardium. Although occasional dramatic results have been reported with emergency revascularization surgery alone, or in combination with infarctectomy, the overall results with this approach have been disappointing.

Other complications MITRAL REGURGITATION Apical systolic murmurs of mitral regurgitation appear in more than one-half of patients during the first 5 days after the onset of a myocardial infarction, but mitral regurgitation is of hemodynamic importance in only a minority of these patients. In most patients the murmur is present during the acute phase of infarction, disappearing with recovery. The most common cause of mitral regurgitation following myocardial infarction is dysfunction of the papillary muscles of the left ventricle, due to ischemia or infarction.

Other pathogenetic mechanisms may contribute to or be solely responsible for the development of mitral regurgitation after myocardial infarction. Mitral valve competence depends on the normal spatial relationships between the papillary muscles and the mitral valve; therefore, mitral regurgitation may be the result of alteration in the size or shape of the ventricle due to impaired contractility or to aneurysm formation. Either papillary muscle may rupture, the posterior one twice as frequently as the anterior. Left ventricular function is often compromised by the superimposition of mitral regurgitation, sometimes dramatically. The differential diagnosis includes perforation of the ventricular septum (see below), and the differentiation between mitral regurgitation is conveniently made at the bedside with a flow-directed balloon catheter; large *v* waves are recorded in the pulmonary capillary wedge position. Surgical replacement of the mitral valve may be followed by dramatic results in patients in whom acute heart failure results primarily from severe mitral regurgitation due to papillary muscle rupture or dysfunction and in whom myocardial function is relatively well maintained.

If aortic systolic pressure is lowered in patients with mitral regurgitation, a greater fraction of the left ventricular output will be ejected antegrade, thus lessening the regurgitant fraction. To this end, both intraaortic balloon counterpulsation, which lowers the aortic systolic pressure mechanically, and the infusion of sodium nitroprusside, 0.5 to 8.0 (μg/kg)/min, which reduces peripheral vascular resistance, have been used with success for the interim management of patients with mitral regurgitation in the setting of acute myocardial infarction; the results of definitive operative treatment are better if it can be postponed for 4 to 6 weeks after the infarct.

VENTRICULAR ASYNERGY—VENTRICULAR ANEURYSM The term *ventricular asynergy* describes a disorder of ventricular function which occurs in 25 to 35 percent of patients with ischemic heart disease. The term *ventricular aneurysm* is usually used to describe two forms of asynergy: (1) *dyskinesis* or local expansile paradoxical wall motion, and (2) *akinesis* or local absence of wall motion. Normally functioning myocardial fibers must shorten more if stroke volume and cardiac output are to be maintained, and if they are unable to do so, ventricular function is impaired.

The clinical manifestations of left ventricular aneurysm include congestive failure, arterial embolism, and ventricular arrhythmias. Apical aneurysms are the most common and the most easily detected by clinical examination. The physical finding of greatest value is a double, diffuse, or displaced apical impulse. The standard roentgenogram frequently reveals an abnormal bulge distorting the contour of the left side of the heart, but the roentgenogram may be entirely normal, especially with posterior aneurysms. The electrocardiographic finding of ST-segment elevation at rest is present in precordial leads in 25 percent of patients with either apical or anterior aneurysms. Ventricular aneurysms may cause persistent ventricular arrhythmias such as ventricular tachycardia.

THROMBOEMBOLISM Clinically apparent thromboembolism complicates myocardial infarction in approximately 10 percent of cases, but embolic lesions are found in 45 percent of patients in necropsy series, suggesting that thromboembolism is often unrecognized clinically. Thromboembolism is considered to be at least an important contributing cause of death in 25 percent of infarct patients. The left ventricle is the most common locus for mural thrombus, and the rarity of mural thrombi in the right ventricle is consistent with the belief that most pulmonary emboli arise in the leg veins. Thromboembolism most commonly occurs in association with large infarcts and in the presence of congestive failure. The high incidence of thromboembolism constitutes one of the best arguments for the use of anticoagulant therapy in patients with extensive infarction.

CARDIAC RUPTURE Myocardial rupture is a dramatic complication of myocardial infarction most likely to occur during the first week after the onset of symptoms; its frequency increases with the age of the patient. First infarction, female sex, and hypertension also seem to be associated with a higher incidence of cardiac rupture. The clinical presentation may often be that of a sudden disappearance of the pulse, blood pressure, and consciousness while the electrocardiogram continues to show sinus rhythm. The myocardium continues to contract, but forward flow is not maintained as blood escapes into the pericardium. Cardiac tamponade ensues (Chap. 249), and closed-chest massage is ineffective. Although almost universally fatal, there have been a few instances in which cardiac rupture has been recognized and successfully treated by operation.

SEPTAL PERFORATION The pathogenesis of perforation of the ventricular septum is similar to that of external rupture of the myocardium, but the therapeutic potential is greater. Patients with ventricular septal rupture present with congestive failure in association with the sudden appearance of a pansystolic murmur typical of a ventricular septal defect, often accompanied by a parasternal thrill. It is often impossible to differentiate this condition from rupture of a papillary muscle. The diagnosis can be established by the demonstration of a left-to-right shunt (i.e., an oxygen step-up at the level of the right ventricle) by limited cardiac catheterization performed at the bedside using a flow-directed balloon catheter. Rupture of the ventricular septum is amenable to immediate surgical treatment, albeit at a high mortality. If the clinical condition permits, however, surgical intervention should be postponed for 6 to 8 weeks, at which time the margins of the defect are composed of firm scar tissue, and surgical closure is easier and more likely to be successful. The physiology of acute mitral regurgitation and acute ventricular septal perforation are similar in that the level of aortic systolic pressure determines in part the regurgitant fraction, the difference being the chamber into which the regurgitant fraction is ejected. In septal perforation, a fraction of left ventricular output is ejected into the right ventricle; in a manner analogous to mitral regurgitation, lowering of aortic systolic pressure by mechanical (intraaortic balloon counterpulsation) or pharmacological (nitroglycerin or nitroprusside) means can decrease the hemodynamic compromise caused by perforation.

PERICARDITIS (see also Chap. 249) Pericardial friction rubs and/or pericardial pain are frequently encountered in patients with acute transmural myocardial infarction. This complication is easily managed with anti-inflammatory agents such as aspirin (650 mg qid) or indomethacin (25 mg tid). It is important to diagnose the chest pain of pericarditis accurately, since failure to appreciate it may lead to the erroneous diagnosis of recurrent ischemic pain and/or infarct extension with resultant inappropriate use of anticoagulants, nitrates, propranolol, or narcotics. No definite cause and effect relationship between anticoagulant administration and pericarditis or tamponade has been proved. Nonetheless, a sufficiently high probability of cause and effect exists to make the use of anticoagulants contraindicated in patients with pericarditis, as manifested by either pain or persistent rub. When pericarditis exists but there is a compelling indication for anticoagulant therapy such as arterial embolism, patients should be watched closely for signs of pericardial tamponade. If venous thromboembolism and recurrent pulmonary emboli are the indications for anticoagula-

tion in a patient with pericarditis, consideration should be given to a caval-interruption procedure, such as an inferior vena caval umbrella (Chap. 266).

POSTMYOCARDIAL INFARCTION SYNDROME—DRESSLER'S SYNDROME (see also Chap. 249) This syndrome, characterized by fever and pleuropericardial chest pain, was first described by Dressler and is thought to be due to an autoimmune pericarditis, pleuritis, and pneumonitis. It may begin from 1 to 6 weeks after myocardial infarction. The pain can often be distinguished from that of an extending infarction by its characteristic pericardial pattern: it is substernal, radiates to the neck and shoulders, is relieved by leaning forward, and exacerbated by deep breathing. The syndrome responds promptly to therapy with salicylates or indomethacin. On occasion, corticosteroids may be required to relieve discomfort of an unusual, refractory nature. Effusions associated with Dressler's syndrome may become hemorrhagic if anticoagulants are administered.

SHOULDER-HAND SYNDROME A few patients develop pain and stiffness of the left arm and shoulder following myocardial infarction. The syndrome is probably related to immobility during the early period of therapy and is less frequent in patients who have been mobilized at an early stage in convalescence.

UNSTABLE ANGINA OR INTERMEDIATE SYNDROME The manifestations of ischemic heart disease may be thought of as representing a spectrum ranging from angina pectoris at one end to acute myocardial infarction at the other. In angina pectoris, the myocardial blood supply is temporarily inadequate, but there is no death of tissue, whereas myocardial infarction is, by definition, characterized by death of myocardial tissue. Some patients develop manifestations which logically place them at an intermediate position between these two extremes, hence, the term *intermediate syndrome*. Included under this heading are syndromes known as acute coronary insufficiency, unstable angina, and preinfarctional angina. Unstable angina may be superimposed upon a background of stable exertional angina pectoris, or it may represent the first manifestation of symptomatic ischemic heart disease.

Unstable angina pectoris may be characterized by discrete episodes of severe ischemic chest discomfort which may come on at *rest*. On occasion, the discomfort begins during exertion and does not disappear with rest. The pain lasts 30 min or more and is of such severity that the diagnosis of myocardial infarction is considered. Although there may be electrocardiographic ST-segment and T-wave changes, myocardial infarction is ruled out by the absence of both evolutionary QRS changes in the electrocardiogram and diagnostic elevation of serum enzyme concentrations. Unstable angina may be superimposed upon chronic stable angina pectoris. The patient notes that his pain is precipitated by less severe exertion, comes more frequently, lasts longer, or has changed in pattern.

The specific implications of propensity to develop acute myocardial infarction are presently debatable, and the role of coronary artery bypass graft surgery in the treatment of these syndromes is thus particularly controversial. It appears that coronary bypass results in immediate relief of unstable angina pectoris in most patients, but long-term morbidity and mortality are similar to that seen in patients treated with aggressive medical regimens. Coronary arteriography in patients with unstable angina has revealed a spectrum of morphological abnormalities ranging from severe three-vessel involvement to normal coronary anatomy, indicating that the term *unstable* angina does not define a specific clinical entity but rather yet another pattern of presentation in the spectrum of coronary artery disease. Generalized statements as to either the prognosis of patients with unstable angina or the role of surgical therapy are thus not possible, and a graduated approach to therapy is indicated.

Most patients with unstable angina will stabilize with intensive medical therapy, i.e., hospitalization, bed rest, oxygen, sedation, and drug therapy with nitrates and beta-blocking agents. The adequate dose of beta-blocking agent varies from patient to patient, and increasing amounts of drug should be administered until the resting pulse rate is below 60 beats per minute. Patients with unstable angina pectoris should receive continuous electrocardiographic monitoring. Given the high success rate with medical therapy ($>$ 75 percent) and the slightly increased risk of coronary arteriography and coronary artery bypass graft surgery in patients with unstable angina, intensive medical therapy should be the initial approach in these patients. Should such therapy be successful, as defined by the disappearance of rest pain and/or the resumption of previous activity levels, the need for early coronary arteriography with a view toward emergency surgery is obviated. The question of coronary arteriography and coronary bypass graft surgery may then be considered on an elective basis as it would be in any patient with chronic stable coronary artery disease. On the other hand, if unstable angina persists despite intensive medical therapy, an advisable course is to carry out coronary arteriography and, if the anatomy is suitable, revascularization surgery. Often these procedures may be aided by stabilizing the patient with intraaortic balloon counterpulsation.

REFERENCES

ALPERT JS: *The Heart Attack Handbook: A Commonsense Guide to Treatment, Recovery, and Prevention.* Boston, Little, Brown, 1978

———, FRANCIS GS: *Manual of Coronary Care.* Boston, Little, Brown, 1977

BRAUNWALD E: *The Myocardium: Failure and Infarction.* New York, HP Publishing, 1974

———: Protection of the ischemic myocardium. Circulation, vol 53, suppl 1, 1976

———, MAROKO PR: Limitation of infarct size, in *Current Problems in Cardiology,* vol III, no 7, Chicago, Year Book, 1978

COHN JN, FRANCIOSA JA: Pathophysiology of shock in acute myocardial infarction, in *Progress in Cardiology,* PN Yu, JF Goodwin (eds). Philadelphia, Lea & Febiger, 1973, vol 2

FOWLER NO (ed): Treatment of acute myocardial infarction, in *Cardiac Diagnosis and Treatment,* 2d ed. New York, Harper & Row, 1976, chap 35, p 704

PANTRIDGE JF et al: *The Acute Coronary Attack.* New York, Grune & Stratton, 1975

RACKLEY CE et al: Modern approach to the patient with acute myocardial infarction, in *Current Problems in Cardiology,* vol I, no 10. Chicago, Year Book, 1977

246
COR PULMONALE

ALFRED P. FISHMAN

Cor pulmonale denotes enlargement of the right ventricle secondary to malfunctioning lungs. Often, but not invariably, hypertrophy and dilatation coexist; in chronic cor pulmonale, hypertrophy is more apt to predominate than in acute cor pul-

TABLE 246-1
Pulmonary disorders predisposing to chronic cor pulmonale

I Intrinsic disease of the lungs and airways
   A Chronic obstructive lung disease (COLD)
   B Diffuse pulmonary interstitial disease
   C Pulmonary vascular disease
II Malfunctioning chest bellows
   A Kyphoscoliosis
   B Neuromuscular incompetence
   C Marked obesity ("Pickwickian syndrome")
III Inadequate ventilatory drive from respiratory centers
   A Primary or idiopathic alveolar hypoventilation ("Ondine's curse")
   B Chronic mountain sickness

monale. Moreover, the abnormal performance of the lungs need not be due to intrinsic lung disease: in some instances, an abnormal chest bellows or a depressed ventilatory drive from the respiratory centers (Table 246-1) is the cause. Invariably, if the cause is in the lungs, the disease will be diffuse, bilateral, and extensive, in most cases affecting airways as well as parenchyma.

Pulmonary arterial hypertension invariably precedes cor pulmonale. Indeed, cor pulmonale is synonymous with pulmonary hypertensive heart disease. But before making the diagnosis of cor pulmonale, *disease of the left side of the heart* and *congenital heart disease* must be excluded. It is worth emphasizing that the term *cor pulmonale* does not automatically imply heart failure. However, it is understood that if the pulmonary hypertension that led to enlargement of the right ventricle is not relieved, cor pulmonale will become associated with right ventricular failure.

Hypertrophy and/or dilatation of the right ventricle are usually much more difficult to detect and to quantify, both clinically and at autopsy, than are left ventricular hypertrophy and dilatation. Consequently, in interpreting the size of the right ventricle it is helpful to understand the mechanisms that operated during life to impose an abnormal hemodynamic load upon it.

These caveats have several practical implications. By underscoring the critical role of abnormal pulmonary performance in the pathogenesis of cor pulmonale, the point is being emphasized that prognosis and treatment of cor pulmonale *depend more on the lungs and their response to treatment than on the heart.* Moreover, by stressing *enlargement* of the right ventricle as the hallmark of cor pulmonale they indicate that pulmonary hypertension may exist without straining the right ventricle to the stage of enlargement and that right ventricular failure is a complication, rather than an essential feature, of cor pulmonale.

TYPES OF COR PULMONALE By tradition, the designation "acute" is generally reserved for the dilatation of the right side of the heart which follows acute embolization of the lungs. The designation "chronic" is less specific. Usually chronicity is judged by the type and duration of the pulmonary disorder that led to the cardiac enlargement (Table 246-1). Just how long, and to what degree, the heart remains enlarged will depend on fluctuations in the level of pulmonary arterial pressure.

INCIDENCE Reliable estimates of the prevalence of chronic cor pulmonale are sparse. However, because obstructive disease of the airways is so prevalent and is so often the precursor of pulmonary hypertension, cor pulmonale is a common type of heart disease. Indeed, in parts of the world where cigarette smoking and air pollution have resulted in a high incidence of chronic bronchitis and emphysema (described in detail in Chap. 263), cor pulmonale may comprise up to one-quarter of all types of heart failure. By virtue of exposure rather than predisposition, men are more often affected than women. Chronic cor pulmonale is also a common sequel to cystic fibrosis of the pancreas. In contrast, it is an unusual complication of allergic asthma.

Most diffuse pulmonary diseases are either too limited in extent or too circumscribed in their effects on alveolar-capillary gas exchange to set in motion the train of events leading to cor pulmonale. Thus, the bulk of patients with silicosis, emphysema, or diffuse fibrosis suffer from breathlessness for years but fail to develop pulmonary hypertension or cardiomegaly.

PATHOGENESIS

Pulmonary hypertension is a prerequisite for cor pulmonale. Although a large cardiac output, tachycardia, an expanded blood volume, or myocardial damage from hypoxia and acidosis may contribute to the pulmonary hypertension, the crux in the pathogenetic sequence is an increase in pulmonary vascular resistance to blood flow through small muscular arteries and arterioles. The increase in vascular resistance may be anatomic or vasomotor in origin; often both mechanisms are involved (Table 246-2).

**ANATOMIC INCREASE IN PULMONARY VASCULAR RESIST-
ANCE** In the normal resting individual, the pulmonary circulation is a highly distensible, low-resistance circuit, accommodating the same blood flow as the systemic circulation at approximately one-fourth the mean blood pressure; during moderate exercise, tripling the blood flow elicits only slight increments in pulmonary arterial pressure. Even after pneumonectomy, the residual pulmonary vascular bed accepts considerable increments in pulmonary blood flow with only slight increase in pulmonary artery pressure as long as the lung is free of fibrosis, emphysema, or pulmonary vascular change. Similarly, disappearance of a large portion of the pulmonary capillary bed in emphysema generally fails to elicit pulmonary hypertension.

However, when pulmonary vascular reserve has been exhausted by progressive reduction in the extent and distensibility of the pulmonary vascular tree, even the increments in blood flow associated with daily living may suffice to elicit marked pulmonary hypertension. The essential component of this vulnerability is a decrease in the cross-sectional area of the pulmonary resistance vessels. The restricted vascular bed stems from widespread narrowing and obstruction of small pulmonary arteries and arterioles, usually accompanied by a decrease in the distensibility not only of the vessels but also of the adjacent lung.

**VASOMOTOR INCREASE IN PULMONARY VASCULAR RESIST-
ANCE (HYPOXIA AND ACIDOSIS)** The most potent stimulus for pulmonary vasoconstriction is alveolar hypoxia which acts directly on adjacent small pulmonary arteries and arterioles; systemic arterial hypoxemia supplements the local effects of alveolar hypoxia indirectly by way of the sympathetic nerves to the pulmonary circulation. Experiments in dogs indicate that severe acidosis (pH < 7.2) also elicits pulmonary vasoconstriction. In humans, acidosis acts synergistically with hypoxia, whereas alkalosis diminishes the pressor response to hypoxia. The biologic basis for this interplay remains unclear. In chronic hypoxia, the effects of these pulmonary hypertensive stimuli are often intensified by increased viscosity of the blood arising from secondary polycythemia.

HYPERCAPNIA In contrast to the effects of hypoxia and acidosis, the effects of CO_2 on the pulmonary circulation appear to be by way of the acidosis that it generates rather than by a direct action on pulmonary vessels. However, because heart failure in cor pulmonale is often associated with respiratory insufficiency, and because management of the respiratory insufficiency generally determines the prognosis, the noncardiac effects of hypercapnia merit consideration.

Hypercapnia affects mainly the central nervous system, producing cerebral vasodilatation, increased cerebrospinal fluid pressure, and neurologic derangements ranging from weakness, irritability, lassitude, and cloudy sensorium to somnolence, confusion, and coma. These derangements are most apt to occur if hypercapnia is acute in onset and severe, or if chronic hypercapnia is acutely aggravated. In contast, during chronic hypercapnia, the patient may be virtually free of central nervous system disturbances if respiratory acidosis is fully compensated. When severe hypoxemia and hypercapnia coexist, it may be impossible to distinguish between their neurologic effects because severe hypoxia causes anatomic damage to nervous tissues.

TABLE 246-2
Pathogenetic mechanisms in chronic pulmonary hypertension and cor pulmonale

Pathogenetic mechanism	Intermediaries	Examples
PRIMARY MECHANISMS		
Anatomic increase in pulmonary vascular resistance	Obliteration, obstruction, reduction, and stiffening of pulmonary vascular tree	*Vascular disease:* Primary pulmonary hypertension; recurrent pulmonary emboli *Extravascular disease:* Diffuse interstitial disease; fibrosing alveolitis; pneumoconiosis
Vasomotor increase in pulmonary vascular resistance	Pulmonary vasoconstriction by hypoxia and acidosis	*General alveolar hypoventilation with normal lungs:* *1* Disorders of chest bellows: neuromuscular; extreme obesity; kyphoscoliosis *2* Diminished ventilatory drive: primary alveolar hypoventilation; sleep; hypercapnia
Combined anatomic restriction and vasomotor	Combination of above	*Net alveolar hypoventilation with abnormal lungs:* Chronic obstructive lung disease: "blue bloater"; cystic fibrosis of pancreas
SECONDARY MECHANISMS		
Increase in cardiac output	Increase in metabolic rate; acute hypoxia	Daily activities; acute respiratory infection
Increase in blood viscosity	Secondary polycythemia	Chronic hypoxia
Tachycardia	Aggravation of hypoxia	Heart failure

Carbon dioxide retention, with elevated CO_2 tensions in the blood and tissues, is self-perpetuating. On the one hand, hypercapnia from any cause blunts the responsiveness of the respiratory center to the CO_2 stimulus; on the other, hypercapnia promotes retention of bicarbonate by the kidney. Not only the hypercapnia originating in disorders of the lungs or ventilation, but also the hypercapnia of metabolic alkalosis, such as that produced by powerful diuretics, causes ventilatory depression. This is why patients with chronic hypercapnia are particularly vulnerable to the effects of sedatives or oxygen breathing, both of which may cause calamitous increments in the degree of hypercapnia, sedatives by depressing further the respiratory centers in the brain, and oxygen by abolishing the hypoxic peripheral drive to ventilation. A large diuresis in which the loss of chloride is inordinate for the output of chloride maybe equally effective in depressing the ventilation. It is usually in the severely hypoxic, hypercapnic patient that right-sided heart failure occurs.

ALVEOLAR HYPOVENTILATION　A large disparity commonly exists between the degree of pulmonary hypertension recorded during life and the anatomic changes in the lungs and pulmonary vessels at autopsy. This discrepancy is particularly marked in patients with obstructive disease of the airways, in whom the anatomic changes in the gas-exchanging parts of the lungs consistently appear to be inadequate to explain either the blood-gas abnormalities or the pulmonary arterial pressor response. Similarly, the most extensive emphysema may be associated with normal levels of blood gases and normal pulmonary arterial pressures. Much of this discrepancy disappears when account is taken of alveolar hypoventilation, an important functional disorder which cannot be quantified at autopsy. Recognizing that alveolar hypoventilation is an essential component in the pathogenesis of cor pulmonale is critical for two reasons: (1) elimination of the initiating mechanism (e.g., acute respiratory infection) usually reverses the alveolar hypoventilation, and (2) unless alveolar ventilation is improved, other therapeutic measures are apt to be ineffective.

PULMONARY HYPERTENSION

Two distinct patterns characterize the natural history of cor pulmonale at sea level: (1) The pattern of *episodic* pulmonary hypertension, due to exacerbations of the underlying pulmonary disorder, is more common. Generally, each bout leaves its imprint and predisposes to continuing hypertension even though recovery from the early bouts frequently is associated with the return of pulmonary arterial pressures to normal. (2) The pattern of *progressive,* unremitting pulmonary hypertension and cor pulmonale leading inexorably to right-sided heart failure is generally a consequence either of progressive pulmonary vascular or interstitial disease or of unremitting hypoxia (as in continuing alveolar hypoventilation). Distinction between the two sequences tends to become blurred if intercurrent respiratory infections decrease the intervals between bouts of hypoxia and pulmonary hypertension. Also, each bout of pulmonary hypertension seems to predispose to a subsequent bout of cor pulmonale because of residual hypertrophy of the muscular pulmonary arteries or further curtailment of the extent and distensibility of the pulmonary vascular tree. Consequently, although relief of hypoxia may restore the pulmonary arterial pressure to normal or near-normal levels, with each attack the pulmonary vascular tree seems to lose some of its adaptability and the patient moves a little closer to the verge of persistent cor pulmonale.

FROM PULMONARY HYPERTENSION TO COR PULMONALE
In those who have clinical evidence of cor pulmonale, pulmonary hypertension is a regular occurrence. The evolution of the pulmonary hypertension depends on the underlying pulmonary disorder, but as a general rule, pulmonary hypertension appears in a predisposed individual either when blood flow is increased (exercise, fever) or during a bout of acute hypoxia (bronchopulmonary infection). In time, pulmonary hypertension is present even at rest. The highest pulmonary artery pressures occur in pulmonary vascular and interstitial disease; the levels of pulmonary hypertension are neither as high nor as fixed in chronic obstructive diseases of the airways, even during an acute exacerbation.

The pulmonary hypertension that comes on only during exercise or hypoxia is associated with normal end-diastolic pressure in the right ventricle. However, as pulmonary hypertension becomes persistent and severe, abnormally high filling (end-diastolic) pressure develops in the right ventricle as a result either of incomplete emptying of the ventricle as it dilates or of the decrease in ventricular compliance associated with hypertrophy; cardiac output is still normal at rest and increases normally during exercise (cor pulmonale without heart failure). Finally, the onset of right-sided heart failure is identified by abnormally high end-diastolic pressures in the right ventricle. At this stage, the cardiac output, which may still be normal at rest, fails to increase normally during exercise; the systemic veins are engorged, reflecting the inability of the right ventricle to empty normally.

THE LEFT VENTRICLE IN COR PULMONALE　Except for those few high-altitude dwellers who develop mountain sickness, the left ventricle does not share in the cardiomegaly of high altitude. Consequently, tolerable levels of hypoxia do not exert serious noxious effects on the myocardium; nor are they associated with an inordinate hemodynamic load on the left ventricle. Conversely, severe, intolerable levels of hypoxia and arterial hypoxemia at altitude may impair myocardial function of both ventricles as well as produce right ventricular overload. The left ventricle then enlarges and fails, primarily because of inadequate oxygen delivery to the myocardium.

At sea level, cor pulmonale is not associated with left ventricular enlargement as long as arterial hypoxemia is modest in degree, but in pulmonary disorders associated with severe hypoxemia, left ventricular enlargement and malfunction may occur. In the latter group, a complicated interplay seems to be involved in the pathogenesis of abnormal left ventricular performance: independent disease of the left ventricle, particularly arteriosclerotic heart disease, aggravated by the direct effects of inadequate oxygen delivery to the myocardium plus the noxious effect of severe hypoxemia and acidosis on the myocardium. In turn, the respiratory insufficiency which initiated the impaired myocardial performance by causing abnormal levels of arterial blood gases is intensified if left ventricular failure causes interstitial and alveolar pulmonary edema.

CLINICAL MANIFESTATIONS OF COR PULMONALE

The likelihood that a physician will recognize that a patient has cor pulmonale depends on his or her awareness that the underlying pulmonary disorder can culminate in pulmonary hypertension. The diagnosis is generally straightforward in obliterative diseases of the pulmonary circulation, e.g., multiple pulmonary emboli. It is much more elusive in obstructive disease of the airways because chronic bronchitis and bronchiolitis are not always self-evident, and clinical indexes of pulmonary hypertension are not always reliable. Therefore, the cor pulmonale that follows chronic bronchitis may be appreciated only retrospectively, i.e., after an episode of overt right ventricular failure. Detection may be particularly difficult if the systemic venous congestion and peripheral edema develop insidiously, over days to weeks, rather than suddenly in the course of an acute bronchopulmonary infection.

DIFFERENTIAL DIAGNOSIS Cor pulmonale is particularly important to recognize in the elderly patient who is old enough to have arteriosclerotic heart disease, has had cough and sputum for many years ("chronic bronchitis"), and clearly manifests right ventricular failure. Analyses of arterial blood gases are then most helpful in deciding whether the primary cardiac disorder is in the right or left ventricle, since appreciable arterial hypoxemia, hypercapnia, and acidosis are unusual in left-sided heart failure unless frank pulmonary edema is also present.

Support for the diagnosis of cor pulmonale may be adduced from roentgenographic and electrocardiographic evidence of right ventricular enlargement. Rarely is catheterization of the right side of the heart needed to settle the question, once suspicion of cor pulmonale is aroused. But, if necessary, cardiac catheterization will typically show pulmonary arterial hypertension, normal left atrial ("pulmonary wedge") pressures, and the classical hemodynamics of right ventricular failure.

The conventional signs of right ventricular enlargement include a cardiac thrust along the left sternal border, or immediately below the sternum, and a fourth heart sound arising in the hypertrophied ventricle. Concomitant pulmonary hypertension is suggested by a cardiac thrust in the second left interspace adjacent to the sternum, an unusually loud second component of the second heart sound in the same area, and occasionally the murmur of pulmonary valvular insufficiency. If the right ventricle fails, tricuspid insufficiency and a right ventricular gallop sound are often added. Hydrothorax is uncommon, even after the advent of overt right ventricular failure. Permanent arrhythmias, such as atrial flutter or fibrillation, are unusual, but transitory arrhythmias are common during severe hypoxia or when respiratory alkalosis has been induced by mechanical hyperventilation.

The diagnostic value of the *electrocardiogram* in cor pulmonale depends on the underlying pulmonary or ventilatory disorder (Table 246-3). It is most valuable in pulmonary vascular or interstitial disease, particularly if unassociated with obstructive disease of the airways, or in alveolar hypoventilation with normal lungs. Conversely, because of the hyperinflated lungs and the episodic nature of the pulmonary hypertension and right ventricular overload, patterns diagnostic of right ventricular hypertrophy are uncommon in cor pulmonale secondary to chronic bronchitis and emphysema. Consequently, even if right ventricular enlargement in the course of chronic bronchitis and emphysema is marked, as during a bout of acute upper respiratory infection, electrocardiographic evidence may be inconclusive because of rotation and displacement of the heart, widened distances between electrodes and the cardiac surface, and the predominance of dilatation over hypertrophy in the cardiac enlargement. Thus a reliable diagnosis of right ventricular enlargement can be expected in one-third of patients with chronic bronchitis and emphysema whose hearts show right ventricular hypertrophy at autopsy, whereas the diagnosis is easily and reliably made in the great majority of patients with cor pulmonale originating in pulmonary disorders other than chronic bronchitis and emphysema. With these qualifications in mind, the more reliable criteria for right ventricular hypertrophy in a patient who has chronic bronchitis and emphysema have proved to be an S_1Q_3 pattern; right axis deviation $\geq 110°$; an $S_1S_2S_3$ pattern; and an R/S ratio in $V_6 \leq$ 1.0. Combinations of these criteria enhance their diagnostic sensitivities.

Roentgenography has more diagnostic value in arousing suspicion of or confirming than in detecting enlargement of the right ventricle. Suspicion is aroused by evidences of an antecedent predisposing pulmonary disorder coupled with large central pulmonary arteries and a pruned peripheral arterial tree, i.e., evidence of pulmonary hypertension. Serial x-rays are generally more useful than a single examination for heart size, particularly in obstructive disease of the airways, where dramatic changes in heart size may occur between a bout of acute respiratory insufficiency and recovery.

Echocardiography has recently come into play as a tool for detecting pulmonary hypertension on the basis of movements of the pulmonary valve. The technique is not easy but is gaining in popularity. Unfortunately, present approaches in echocardiography do not provide reliable measurements of right ventricular dimensions.

CLINICAL FORMS OF COR PULMONALE AND THEIR TREATMENT

Regardless of the mechanism of initiation—anatomic, vasomotor, or both—chronic pulmonary hypertension tends to be self-perpetuating because of continuing narrowing and obliteration of the pulmonary vascular bed by muscular hypertrophy of small arteries and arterioles, arteriosclerosis, thrombosis, and devious malformations in the course of small arteries and arterioles (*glomus formations*).

ANATOMIC INCREASE IN PULMONARY VASCULAR RESISTANCE These abnormalities may be sorted into two general categories (Table 246-2): vascular disease and extravascular disease, as described below.

Vascular disease; occlusive disease of the small pulmonary arteries In these disorders, widespread occlusion of the small pulmonary vessels takes place over months to years. Most often, the cause is multiple pulmonary emboli (Chap. 266); less common are multiple thromboses such as those which complicate sickle-cell anemia. A rare cause is primary pulmonary hypertension (Chap. 265).

Tachypnea, persisting during sleep, is an outstanding feature of multiple pulmonary emboli. This increase in respiratory frequency is associated with alveolar hyperventilation as indicated by characteristically low values for alveolar and arterial P_{CO_2} and for serum bicarbonate. Incapacitating breathlessness occurs on mild exertion. Precordial or thoracic pain is not uncommon: occasionally the pain mimics angina; at other times

TABLE 246-3
ECG patterns in chronic cor pulmonale

I Chronic obstructive lung disease (suggestive, but not diagnostic, of right ventricular enlargement)*
  A "P pulmonale" (in leads II, III, aVF)
  B Right axis deviation $\geq 110°$
  C R/S ratio in $V_6 \leq 1$
  D rRS' in right chest leads
  E Right bundle branch block (partial or complete)
II Pulmonary vascular or interstitial disease; general alveolar hypoventilation (diagnostic of right ventricular enlargement)
  A Classic pattern in V_1 or V_3R (dominant R or R' with inverted T waves in right chest leads)
  B Often associated with "suggestive" criteria above

* Among the "suggestive" criteria, it is difficult to distinguish right ventricular enlargement (hypertrophy and dilatation) from changes in the anatomic and electrical positions of the heart produced by the hyperinflated lungs. Consequently, the "suggestive" criteria are more useful as confirmatory, than as diagnostic, evidence.

it is clearly pleuritic, intensifying during inspiration. Clinical criteria and roentgenographic and electrocardiographic characteristics are classical for right ventricular enlargement. Cyanosis, which is rarely impressive before heart failure, usually becomes striking after the right ventricle fails. Objective evidence for pulmonary emboli is conventionally sought by photoscanning and pulmonary angiography (Chaps. 256 and 266).

Of all patients who develop cor pulmonale, those with multiple pulmonary emboli have the highest pulmonary arterial pressures; these may equal or even exceed systemic arterial pressures. The cardiac output tends to be low. Mild arterial hypoxemia is the rule and seems to arise from shunting within the lungs. Whether the shunts represent blood flow through recanalized vessels (e.g., glomus formations) that are no longer in contact with alveoli, or too-rapid passage of the entire cardiac output through unoccluded and dilated portions of the pulmonary vascular tree, or blood flow through anatomic pulmonary arteriovenous channels that are ordinarily inoperative, is conjectural. During right-sided heart failure, these shunts cause profound arterial hypoxemia because the shunted (mixed venous) blood has an extremely low O_2 content.

Once pulmonary hypertension is fixed, treatment directed at the process in the lungs is rarely effective, since organization of emboli has led to irreversible occlusions of innumerable small arteries. Continuous administration of O_2-enriched mixtures is standard. Caution must be exercised to avoid oxygen toxicity by administering as little additional oxygen as possible. Unfortunately, compromises are often required, since arterial blood is not easily restored toward normal levels of oxygenation because of the magnitude of the venous shunts.

The grim outlook for treating the cor pulmonale of multiple pulmonary emboli, as well as the ever-present prospect of catastrophic pulmonary embolization, has emphasized the need for prophylactic measures in patients judged to be candidates for pulmonary emboli (Chap. 266). Heart failure is treated by the usual cardiotonic measures in conjunction with measures directed at improving arterial oxygenation. Rarely does it respond dramatically as long as the hemodynamic overload persists.

Diffuse interstitial fibrosis and granuloma Among the diverse entities included in this category are (1) sarcoidosis, berylliosis, and the "nonspecific" granulomatoses (Chap. 264); (2) scleroderma of the lung (Chap. 264), (3) the various interstitial or alveolar-septal fibroses such as "fibrosing alveolitis," radiation fibrosis, or pulmonary asbestosis, and the special progressive form of interstitial disease known as the Hamman-Rich syndrome (Chap. 264); (4) immunopathologic disease of the lungs, exemplified by "farmer's lung" (Chap. 258); and (5) diffuse carcinomatous infiltration of the lung, such as "alveolar-cell" or lymphangitic carcinoma (Chap. 268).

Clinically, the respiratory difficulty often begins with an acute respiratory illness that fails to resolve. Tachypnea persists. The roentgenogram shows the fine nodular or fibrotic lesions widely disseminated throughout both lung fields. In the resting subject, the arterial P_{O_2} is sustained at near-normal levels by chronic hyperventilation; during exercise, it drops precipitously. The arterial P_{CO_2} is normal or slightly low, reflecting the balance between the augmented ventilation, the oxygen consumption, which is often increased, and the partition of the augmented ventilation between the alveoli and the dead space.

As long as hypoxemia is mild, pulmonary hypertension is modest. But as the disease progresses and as hypoxemia increases—in part because of ventilation-perfusion abnormalities—the level of pulmonary hypertension also increases, and

cor pulmonale begins to evolve. Right ventricular failure generally occurs late in the course of the disease. At first, it responds well to oxygen mixtures and a cardiotonic program (Chap. 236). Oxygen therapy is quite useful since it affords relief of dyspnea and improves oxygenation without threat of carbon dioxide retention. However, oxygen dependence may become marked, and the hazards of oxygen toxicity increase pari passu with the increasing concentrations of inspired oxygen and the duration of exposure.

Relief of heart failure is usually transient unless the initiating mechanism is controlled. Rarely is the underlying lesion in the lung reversible, even though steroids occasionally have been associated with dramatic benefit, especially in some of the granulomatoses and "fibrosing alveolitis." More apt to be rewarding is the successful treatment of superimposed respiratory infection which has toppled a stable patient into heart failure.

VASOMOTOR INCREASE IN PULMONARY VASCULAR RESISTANCE For convenience, alveolar hypoventilation, a prime cause of elevated pulmonary vascular resistance, can be identified by a value for arterial P_{CO_2} greater than 45 mmHg; the disorder may be regarded as either "general" or "net."

Alveolar hypoventilation: general The critical importance of abnormal values for blood gases in the pathogenesis of cor pulmonale is illustrated by the syndrome of alveolar hypoventilation coexistent with normal lungs ("general alveolar hypoventilation"). In these patients, some abnormality, either in the regulation of ventilation or in the neuromuscular apparatus, rather than intrinsic pulmonary disease, is responsible for the hypoxia and hypercapnia. The syndrome may have diverse etiologies. The particular category of sleep-apnea syndromes is currently receiving considerable attention. These disorders and the pathways by which they lead to alveolar hypoventilation and cor pulmonale are considered in Chap. 270.

Alveolar hypoventilation: net The common denominator in this group of disorders is the imbalance between alveolar ventilation, blood flow, and diffusion, resulting in hypercapnia and hypoxemia. In contrast to *general* alveolar hypoventilation, in which the same abnormalities of arterial blood gas levels occur despite normal lungs, intrinsic lung disease is the basis for the abnormal values for blood gases in *net* alveolar hypoventilation.

The assortment of obstructive airways diseases predisposing to cor pulmonale has been pictured as a spectrum of bronchopulmonary disorders, ranging from pure obstruction of the airways at one end to pure emphysema at the other; between the two ends are the mixtures which are most prevalent (Chap. 263). Most likely to develop cor pulmonale is the patient with bronchitis and bronchiolitis, usually with some emphysema, in whom obstructive disease of the airways has so deranged the balance between alveolar ventilation, blood flow, and diffusion as to cause the characteristic syndrome of cyanosis (hypoxemia), somnolence (hypercapnia), and right ventricular failure; these are the "blue bloaters." In contrast, the "pink puffers," with comparable degrees of airways obstruction by conventional tests, do not develop hypoxia in the course of their breathless existence; only during an intercurrent respiratory infection, as hypoxia is superimposed, do they become candidates for cor pulmonale. Emphysema without bronchitis is rarely associated with cor pulmonale since alveolar ventilation and capillary blood flow seem to be commensurately curtailed, as after pulmonary resection, so that neither hypoxia nor pulmonary hypertension becomes appreciable.

Successful treatment of the "blue bloater" with cor pulmonale depends on relieving the bronchitis and bronchiolitis

(Chap. 272). Cardiotonic agents are useless unless oxygenation is improved. If the patient succeeds in maintaining good oxygenation, digitalis and diuretics can usually be discontinued. Relief of airways obstruction is more readily accomplished in some disorders than in others. For example, it is generally easier in chronic bronchitis than in cystic fibrosis of the pancreas, in which most of the airways remain plugged with abnormal thick, tenacious sputum despite heroic therapeutic efforts.

Cor pulmonale is uncommon in uncomplicated silicosis or tuberculosis. On the other hand, it is not uncommon when silicosis, anthrosilicosis, or long-standing fibrotic tuberculosis is complicated by extensive, conglomerate, massive fibrosis, distorted adjacent parenchyma, shrunken lobes, and bronchitis. The likelihood of cor pulmonale is increased further by chronic pleurisy, fibrothorax, or excisional surgery. In such cases, a combination of anatomic restriction of the vascular bed and disturbances in gas exchange is involved in the pathogenesis of the pulmonary hypertension. Indeed, the disturbances in gas exchange, often brought to clinical levels by an acute respiratory infection, are the most reversible element of this disorder.

Although it is convenient to separate "net" from "general" alveolar hypoventilation on pathogenetic grounds, the therapeutic principles are basically the same for both and are described in Chap. 272. The present section will deal only with the circulatory abnormalities.

Since the pulmonary hypertension in the most prevalent pulmonary disorders is rarely anatomically fixed but arises mainly from hypoxia and acidosis, relief of alveolar hypoventilation is usually remarkably successful in restoring the circulation to normal. Measures to improve alveolar ventilation vary considerably. In mild cases, simple measures, such as hydration, antibiotics, and bronchodilators, often suffice; in more severe degrees of hypoxemia and hypercapnia, in which heart failure is associated with respiratory insufficiency, mechanical aids to respiration are usually needed.

It has been noted above that treatment of right-sided heart failure is less important than restoring the blood gas values to tolerable levels. The usual therapeutic measures for heart failure (Chap. 236) apply: low salt regimen, digitalis, diuretics. However, measures to decrease the circulating blood volume (and hematocrit) are of greater importance. Several phlebotomies, each draining 300 to 400 ml, may be needed within a period of 2 to 3 weeks to bring hematocrit and blood volume back to normal; repeated phlebotomies at monthly or bimonthly intervals may have to be instituted to prevent return of the hypervolemia. Diuretics have to be given with more care than usual because the metabolic alkalosis, which may complicate the use of potent diuretics such as ethacrynic acid, aggravates ventilatory insufficiency by depressing the effectiveness of the CO_2 stimulus on the respiratory centers.

The effects of vigorous therapy, directed mainly to the pulmonary disorder, are often dramatic in improving the blood gas abnormalities and heart failure. Other manifestations usually clear more slowly. Indeed, several weeks to a month may elapse before the arterial blood gases, the hematocrit, cardiac output, and pulmonary arterial pressures return to optimal levels. But therapy throughout is guided by the fact that the final outcome in cor pulmonale usually depends on the ability to cope with the underlying pulmonary disorder rather than with the changes in the heart and circulation.

REFERENCES

BATTESTI JP et al: Chronic cor pulmonale in pulmonary sarcoidosis. Thorax 33:76, 1978

FISHMAN AP: Dynamics of the pulmonary circulation, in *Handbook of Physiology,* vol 2: *Circulation,* WF Hamilton, P Dow (eds). Washington, DC, American Physiological Society, 1963

————: Chronic cor pulmonale. State of the art. Am Rev Respir Dis 114:775, 1976

————: Hypoxia and its effects on the pulmonary circulation. Circ Res 38:221, 1976

————: *Pulmonary Diseases and Disorders.* New York, McGraw-Hill, 1980

FOWLER NO: Cor pulmonale caused by lung disease, in *Cardiac Diagnosis and Treatment,* 2d ed, NO Fowler (ed). New York, Harper & Row, 1976, chap 41, p 801

HEATH D, WILLIAMS DR: *Man at High Altitude.* Edinburgh, Churchill Livingstone, 1977

KOERNER SK, MALOVANY RJ: Acute respiratory insufficiency and cor pulmonale: Pathophysiology, clinical features and management. Am Heart J 88:115, 251, 1974

MURPHY ML, HUTCHESON F: The electrocardiographic diagnosis of right ventricular hypertrophy in chronic obstructive lung disease. Chest 65:622, 1974

STEELE P et al: Left ventricular ejection fraction in severe chronic obstructive airways disease. Am J Med 59:21, 1975

WAGENVOORT CA, WAGENVOORT N: *Pathology of Pulmonary Hypertension.* New York, Wiley, 1977

247
THE CARDIOMYOPATHIES AND MYOCARDITIDES

GERALD GLICK
EUGENE BRAUNWALD

CARDIOMYOPATHY

Until recent years, virtually all cases of symptomatic heart disease in adults were classified as ischemic, hypertensive, valvular, or congenital heart disease. When unequivocal evidence for one of these diagnoses was not present in an older patient, the diagnosis of ischemic heart disease was often made, even though a history of a myocardial infarction or angina pectoris could not be elicited. With the development of newer diagnostic techniques, particularly coronary arteriography, it has become clear that ischemic heart disease is not a diagnosis of exclusion, but must meet rigorous and specific criteria (Chap. 244). With this realization, various cardiomyopathies, previously considered uncommon, have emerged as important causes of morbidity and mortality.

The term *cardiomyopathy* is used here to indicate a disease entity in which the presenting signs and symptoms result entirely or predominantly from dysfunction of the myocardium. However, myocardial lesions produced by ischemic heart disease, hypertensive cardiovascular disease, cor pulmonale, valvular heart disease, and congenital heart disease are excluded, although these disease states may produce clinical and hemodynamic findings indistinguishable from the cardiomyopathies. These may be classified on a pathologic basis as resulting either from primary involvement of the myocardium or from secondary involvement as part of a generalized disease (Table 247-1). From a clinical point of view, however, it is more desirable to classify them on the basis of differences in their pathologic physiology and differences in clinical presentation (Table 247-2).

CONGESTIVE CARDIOMYOPATHY The hearts are always dilated and sometimes are also hypertrophied. Mural thrombi are frequently present in the left ventricle, left atrium, and right atrium. On histologic examination the major changes seen are fibrosis and myocardial degeneration and hypertrophy. Electron microscopy reveals disorganization, loss of contractile elements, and disorganization of the sarcoplasmic reticulum, both in idiopathic and alcoholic cardiomyopathies. Idiopathic cardiomyopathy most frequently occurs in middle-aged persons, who when first seen, have the signs and symptoms of congestive heart failure. The failure is both left- and right-sided and is manifested by dyspnea on exertion, fatigue, orthopnea, paraoxysmal nocturnal dyspnea, peripheral edema, and palpitations. Sometimes, the patient's initial clinical presentation is dominated by cardiac arrhythmias, rather than by congestive heart failure. In addition, pulmonary and systemic emboli are not uncommon.

Physical findings The pulse pressure is small, and in the presence of heart failure, the arterial diastolic pressure and the jugular venous pressure may be elevated. Cardiomegaly is usually present, and the apical impulse is hypodynamic. Protodiastolic and presystolic gallop sounds (Chap. 231) are present, and the tricuspid and mitral rings may be dilated, with consequent production of valvular regurgitation and the associated physical signs. However, diastolic murmurs and valvular calcification militate strongly against the diagnosis of cardiomyopathy and point toward a rheumatic origin. As the congestive failure improves with treatment, the abnormal physical findings, including the elevated arterial pressure, may return to normal.

Roentgenologic examination commonly reveals the heart to be grossly and diffusely enlarged; pericardial and pleural effusions may be present, and the lung fields may show evidence of venous hypertension and interstitial congestion. The most common abnormalities present in the *electrocardiogram* are left atrial enlargement, premature ventricular contractions, nonspecific ST-T wave changes, sinus tachycardia, and atrial fibrillation. Frequent premature ventricular contractions and paroxysmal ventricular tachycardia occurs not infrequently

TABLE 247-1
Pathologic classification of cardiomyopathies

I Primary myocardial involvement
  A Idiopathic
  B Familial
  C Alcoholic
  D Peripartum
  E Endocardial fibroelastosis
  F Endomyocardial fibrosis
  G Postcarditic
II Secondary myocardial involvement
  A Amyloidosis
  B Hemochromatosis
  C Sarcoidosis
  D Connective tissue disease
    1 Lupus erythematosus
    2 Polyarteritis
    3 Scleroderma
    4 Dermatomyositis
  E Neuromuscular disease
    1 Muscular dystrophy
    2 Myotonic dystrophy
    3 Friedreich's ataxia
    4 Refsum's disease
  F Neoplastic
  G Glycogen storage disease (Pompe's disease)
  H Lipidoses
    1 Hunter-Hurler syndrome
    2 Fabry's disease
    3 Sandhoff's disease

TABLE 247-2
Clinical classification of cardiomyopathies

1 Congestive: Characterized by cardiac dilatation, congestive heart failure, arrhythmias, emboli, and murmurs of mitral and tricuspid regurgitation
2 Restrictive: Characterized by restriction to ventricular filling
3 Hypertrophic: With or without obstruction to ventricular outflow

and without apparent cause. Left anterior fascicular block is common, and incomplete or complete left bundle branch block or, rarely, right bundle branch block may be present. Frequently, low voltage is noted, but left ventricular hypertrophy may be present. *Echocardiography* (Chap. 233) is helpful in excluding a pericardial effusion and revealing a dilated, poorly contracting left ventricle.

Hemodynamic study generally reveals a cardiac output which is moderately or severely reduced at rest and which does not increase normally with exertion. The end-diastolic pressures in both ventricles are usually elevated (the left more than the right), and consequently the mean atrial pressures are also elevated to abnormally high levels. Angiocardiography characteristically reveals left ventricular dilatation, a reduced ejection fraction, a variably thickened left ventricular wall, and, in some instances, mitral regurgitation. Localized or generalized hypokinesis and asynergy are often noted, particularly in advanced cases, and these findings are associated with a poor prognosis. Patients with ventricular dysfunction due to severe coronary artery disease, often associated with multiple myocardial infarctions, may present with identical findings.

Treatment In its early phases, the congestive heart failure associated with idiopathic cardiomyopathy responds to the usual therapeutic regimen of digitalis, salt restriction, and diuretics, but as the disease enters its more advanced stages it frequently becomes refractory to these standard therapeutic measures. Prolonged, strict bed rest for up to 1 year or more has been advocated for the optimal management of these patients, but the effectiveness of this form of therapy remains controversial and it is not feasible in most patients; one must usually rely, therefore, on the standard management for congestive heart failure supplemented by afterload reduction (Chap. 236). Excessive activity, however, is certainly contraindicated. The associated arrhythmias may also be extremely resistant to the usual antiarrhythmic drugs. Anticoagulants are indicated in patients with a history of embolization, atrial fibrillation, or a markedly reduced cardiac output. The usefulness of corticosteroid therapy has not been established.

Until recently, this form of cardiomyopathy, characterized by congestive heart failure, has usually been recognized only in its far-advanced stages; as a result, treatment has been difficult and the prognosis poor. As the diagnosis of this disease is established earlier, therapy may prove more effective and the prognosis may be improved; however, this point remains to be confirmed.

Familial cardiomyopathy In some families a genetic predisposition to cardiomyopathy exists. Aside from the familial occurrence, this type of cardiomyopathy resembles the idiopathic, nonfamilial form just described. Several different types of genetic abnormalities may manifest themselves as familial cardiomyopathy; they appear to be inherited as autosomal dominant traits with incomplete penetrance and variable expressivity.

Alcoholic cardiomyopathy Animal experiments, as well as studies in humans, have demonstrated that ethanol depresses ventricular performance, reduces myocardial uptake of free fatty acids but enhances uptake of triglycerides, and causes myocardial cell injury. Other experimental work has shown that acetaldehyde, a major product of ethanol biotransformation, interferes with normal cardiac protein synthesis. Moreover, alcoholic subjects develop higher acetaldehyde levels than nonalcoholic subjects receiving the same amount of ethanol. These experimental studies have their clinical expression in those patients who repeatedly develop congestive heart failure and/or cardiac arrhythmias after ingestion of large quantities of alcohol. Because successive insults to the myocardium may lead to increasing irreparable damage, these persons must be instructed to stop all alcoholic intake. Clinically, they resemble patients with idiopathic cardiomyopathy as described above, and should be treated similarly. When the myocardial damage has become widespread and severe, the prognosis is poor. In contrast, when the diagnosis is made early and appropriate measures are instituted, the prognosis improves considerably. Therefore, ingestion of alcohol must be interdicted as soon as possible in the course of the disease. Although thiamine deficiency may be present in many of these patients, alcoholic cardiomyopathy is associated with a low cardiac output and systemic vasoconstriction, in contrast to beriberi heart disease (Chap. 80), in which elevated cardiac output and diminished peripheral vascular resistance occur.

Peripartum cardiomyopathy When cardiac enlargement and congestive heart failure of unexplained causation develop for the first time in a patient during the last month of pregnancy or during the first 5 months after delivery, the diagnosis of peripartum cardiomyopathy should be considered. This temporal relation to delivery may not represent a direct consequence of pregnancy itself but may be conditioned by such factors as poor nutrition, familial or hereditary abnormalities, autoimmune mechanisms, unsuspected myocarditis, or some unknown cause. Nevertheless, a clinical picture quite characteristic of this entity has emerged. The patient is usually multiparous, black, and over the age of 30; has been undernourished; may have a history of hypertension; and may have had a pulmonary embolus. The symptoms and signs are similar to those in patients with idiopathic cardiomyopathy; a protodiastolic gallop, cardiomegaly, and frequent ventricular extrasystoles are common findings. The prognosis in these patients appears to be closely related to whether or not the heart size returns to normal after the first episode of congestive heart failure. If the peripartum heart returns to a normal size, subsequent pregnancies may sometimes be well tolerated; if the heart remains enlarged, however, further pregnancies frequently produce increasing myocardial damage, ultimately leading to refractory congestive heart failure and death. Therapy is the same as for patients with the idiopathic form of cardiomyopathy and includes bed rest, salt restriction, diuretics, anticoagulation, and antiarrhythmic medications. These patients apparently have an increased sensitivity to digitalis. Those who recover should be encouraged to improve their nutritional state and to avoid further pregnancies, especially if residual cardiomegaly exists.

Neuromuscular disease Cardiac involvement is common in many of the muscular dystrophies. In the *Duchenne type of progressive muscular dystrophy,* the myocardial involvement is most often detected electrocardiographically. The most characteristic abnormalities, which do not occur in other forms of muscular dystrophy, are an excessively tall R wave in lead V_1, with a ratio between the amplitude of the R wave and S wave in this lead which exceeds 1.0 but which is not caused by right ventricular hypertrophy, and deep Q waves in limb leads and lateral precordial leads. Rapidly progressive congestive heart failure leading to death may supervene after years of apparent circulatory stability during which the only detectable abnormalities are in the electrocardiogram. The carrier state in this

sex-linked recessive abnormality can sometimes be detected in women who manifest electrocardiographic changes similar to those recorded in affected male patients. *Myotonic dystrophy* is also marked by electrocardiographic abnormalities, viz., atrioventricular and intraventricular conduction disturbances, left anterior fascicular block, sinus bradycardia, and atrial fibrillation or atrial flutter with a relatively slow ventricular response. Sudden death may occur, but congestive heart failure is relatively uncommon. The heart is usually of normal size. In *limb girdle dystrophy,* cardiomyopathy manifested by congestive heart failure and arrhythmias may appear in middle life. In *fascioscapulohumeral dystrophy,* cardiac involvement is absent or exceedingly rare.

Refsum's disease, which results from an inability to metabolize phytanic acid (with consequent deposition of this material in various tissues), produces cardiac abnormalities, including intraventricular conduction defects, ST-T abnormalities, and complete heart block, and may result in sudden death.

RESTRICTIVE CARDIOMYOPATHY Certain of the cardiomyopathies are dominated by the features of restriction to ventricular filling, and the pathologic physiology and clinical presentation are similar even though the causes may be diverse. Thus, patients with restrictive cardiomyopathy resulting from primary amyloidosis, hemochromatosis, sarcoidosis, and Loeffler's fibroplastic endocarditis have similar cardiac findings. In many of these disease states, particularly those involving primarily the endocardium, the partial obliteration of the ventricular cavity by fibrous tissue and thrombus contributes to the abnormally elevated resistance to ventricular filling. As a result of persistently elevated venous pressure, these patients commonly have dependent edema, ascites, and an enlarged, tender liver. The jugular venous pressure is elevated and does not fall normally or may rise with inspiration (Kussmaul's sign). The heart is usually enlarged, the heart sounds are distant, and third and fourth sounds are common. Murmurs are not distinctive. The *electrocardiogram* shows low-voltage, nonspecific ST-T wave changes and various arrhythmias. The most important radiologic features are moderate cardiac enlargement and absence of pericardial calcification.

A given disease entity may present certain features of the congestive and restrictive cardiomyopathies simultaneously or sequentially, e.g., as the heart in the congestive form becomes progressively more fibrotic and therefore less distensible, or as the heart in idiopathic hypertrophic subaortic stenosis becomes excessively hypertrophied, it acquires some of the characteristics of the restrictive form of cardiomyopathy. Infiltrative diseases, such as amyloidosis, may present initially as either restrictive or congestive cardiomyopathies.

Echocardiography reveals a symmetrically thickened left ventricular wall and a normal ejection fraction in patients with restrictive cardiomyopathy. The velocity of mitral valve closure may be reduced and the left ventricular transverse dimension may be increased.

Cardiac catheterization shows a decreased cardiac output, elevation of right and left ventricular end-diastolic pressure, and a dip and plateau configuration of the diastolic portion of the ventricular pressure pulse. This form of cardiomyopathy may be indistinguishable from constrictive pericarditis (Chap. 249), both at the bedside and even with the benefit of cardiac catheterization. Certain clues in the differentiation, which are presented in Chap. 249, may be observed. However, thoracotomy and operative exploration may be necessary to make a definitive differentiation between a restrictive cardiomyopathy and chronic constrictive pericarditis. This distinction is of importance because the latter condition is potentially curable by operation.

Endocardial fibroelastosis This disease, also of unknown cause, is generally seen in infants and is a not uncommon cause of congestive heart failure in this age group. It occurs far less frequently in adults, and is characterized by a thickened endocardium that shows proliferation of elastic tissue. The process generally affects the left ventricle most extensively but may also involve the mitral and aortic valves. Mitral regurgitation is often present, and it may be difficult to determine to what extent the clinical picture results primarily from the endocardial or the valvular lesion. Involvement of the right side of the heart is less common. When first seen, the patient generally has congestive heart failure and shows stigmata of both the congestive and restrictive forms of cardiomyopathy. The electrocardiogram usually shows evidence of left ventricular hypertrophy, and the chest roentgenogram reveals left ventricular and atrial enlargement. Therapy is directed at the congestive failure but is generally unsatisfactory.

Endomyocardial fibrosis This is a progressive form of heart disease, seen in the tropics, especially in Africa, occurring most commonly in children and young adults; it resembles Loeffler's eosinophilic fibroplastic endocarditis and is characterized by fibrosis in the inflow tract and the apex of one or both of the ventricles. Fibrosis of the endocardium begins at the apex of either ventricle and extends toward the inflow tract to involve the tricuspid and mitral valves, and also toward the outflow portions of each ventricle. The apex of the ventricles may be obliterated by the buildup of fibrous tissue and thrombus. In addition, the disease process extends into the myocardium to produce muscle destruction, fibrosis, and occasionally calcification; tricuspid and/or mitral regurgitation are common.

The clinical picture depends upon which ventricle and atrioventricular valve show predominant involvement. The electrocardiogram generally shows low voltage, and roentgenologically the heart is usually enlarged, primarily as a consequence of atrial enlargement. The most prominent findings at cardiac catheterization are a decreased cardiac output, elevated central venous pressure, and the characteristics of *restrictive cardiomyopathy,* described above. Thus, endomyocardial fibrosis and endocardial fibroelastosis fall into the category of a cardiomyopathy that has features both of congestive and of restrictive disease.

Loeffler's endocarditis Also called *fibroplastic endocarditis,* this disease entity appears to be a subcategory of the hypereosinophilic syndrome, in which the heart is predominantly involved. Typically, the endocardium of either or both ventricles thickens markedly, with involvement of the underlying myocardium. Large mural thrombi may develop in either ventricle, thereby compromising the size of the ventricular cavity and serving as a source of pulmonary and systemic emboli. Hepatosplenomegaly and localized eosinophilic infiltration of other organs are usually present. It has been postulated that Loeffler's endocarditis is fundamentally the same disease as endomyocardial fibrosis, but represents its presentation in temperate climates. Steroids and immunosuppressive drugs have been used, but they have been generally of little value, with patients dying either rapidly or after a prolonged, debilitating illness. An operative procedure consisting of resection of the ventricular fibrosis including the atrioventricular valve, coupled with mitral or tricuspid valve replacement, has been advocated to treat this form of restrictive cardiomyopathy.

Differential diagnosis *Amyloidosis* may be diagnosed by biopsy of the rectal mucosa, tongue, gums, or liver. Amyloid deposits may involve the adventitia and media of the intramural coronary arteries, and in these patients angina pectoris and myocardial infarction may occur. Necropsy studies have demonstrated that the frequency of localized areas of amyloid deposition within the heart increases linearly with age. However, for amyloid to produce cardiac dysfunction, widespread and heavy deposits must be present which make the ventricle rubbery, firm, and noncompliant, but the cavity usually is not dilated. Digitalis frequently does not improve the congestive heart failure and may induce cardiac arrhythmias. The electrocardiogram is characterized by low-voltage complexes and arrhythmias. *Hemochromatosis* (Chap. 94) should be suspected if cardiomyopathy occurs in the setting of diabetes mellitus, hepatic cirrhosis, and increased skin pigmentation. Phlebotomy may lead to reversal of cardiomegaly and cardiac symptoms if begun early in the course of the disease. *Sarcoid* involvement of the heart (Chap. 216) is generally associated with other manifestations of generalized disease, such as uveitis, parotitis, hilar lymphadenopathy, pulmonary infiltrates, and cor pulmonale. Sarcoidosis may result in the involvement of any portion of the heart by noncaseating granulomas. Congestive heart failure with recurrent arrhythmias is the most common clinical feature, but rarely it may present as myocardial infarction, pericarditis, or valve involvement. Although the heart may be involved in *scleroderma,* the major symptoms result from esophageal, pulmonary, and cutaneous involvement.

Transvenous biopsy of the endomyocardium employing a catheter bioptome has been used increasingly to obtain specimens for histologic and electron-microscopic study. This technique is becoming important in the diagnosis of myocardial disease, particularly in the recognition of infiltrative diseases such as amyloidosis, hemochromatosis, and sarcoidosis.

HYPERTROPHIC CARDIOMYOPATHY Idiopathic hypertrophic subaortic stenosis (IHSS) This disease is also referred to as asymmetric septal hypertrophy (ASH), hypertrophic cardiomyopathy with or without obstruction, hypertrophic obstructive cardiomyopathy, muscular subaortic stenosis, and asymmetric ventricular hypertrophy. The various appellations all emphasize the characteristic abnormality, namely, marked hypertrophy of the left ventricle, most striking in the ventricular septum, without dilatation of the cavity. Deep clefts in the septum have been observed at necropsy in one-third of cases, associated in some instances with marked narrowing of small intramural coronary arteries in the region of hypertrophy. Histologic and electron-microscopic studies have shown profound abnormalities of the septum in all patients with the disease, irrespective of whether obstruction is present or not. Specifically, a marked disarray of myocardial architecture is observed, resulting from the presence of hypertrophied, bizarrely shaped, disorganized muscle cells. In patients *without* obstruction, similar changes are noted in the free ventricular wall, but, in contrast, in patients *with* obstruction, the myocardium forming the free wall is more normal. Obstruction to outflow occurs when the anterior mitral leaflet abuts on the hypertrophied septum during systole (Chap. 233).

In contrast to the obstruction to flow seen in patients with valvular aortic stenosis, in whom the size of the narrowed orifice is fixed, in patients with hypertrophic cardiomyopathy, the obstruction to outflow, when present, is dynamic and may change between examinations, from beat to beat, or even in the course of a single ejection period. The severity of obstruction is a function of the width of the outflow tract during systole, which in turn appears to be related to three major factors: (1) the left ventricular end-diastolic volume, (2) the myocardial contractile state, and (3) the pressure that distends the left ventricular outflow tract during systole. Muscular exercise, isoproterenol, and digitalis glycosides, all of which increase the force of myocardial contraction and decrease the size of the ventricle, intensify the obstruction. Similarly, when ventricular volume is decreased by the Valsalva maneuver, nitroglycerin, amyl nitrite, or tachycardia, the obstruction is also increased. Conversely, elevation of arterial pressure by phenylephrine, squatting, and isometric handgrip exercise, augmentation of venous return by raising the legs, and expansion of the blood volume all tend to increase the ventricular volume and to ameliorate the obstruction. Sometimes the hypertrophied septum bulges into the outflow tract of the right ventricle, thereby impeding the ejection of blood from this chamber as well.

Until recently, it was believed that most cases of hypertrophic cardiomyopathy were sporadic, rather than familial. However, with the advent of echocardiography and its ability to detect disproportional hypertrophy of the ventricular septum, it has become clear that almost 50 percent of first-degree relatives, i.e., parents, siblings, and children, have evidence of septal involvement, but frequently without obstruction or symptoms. Thus, in most instances, the disease is transmitted as an autosomal dominant trait with a high degree of penetrance.

CLINICAL FINDINGS The most common symptoms are dyspnea, angina, dizziness, syncope, and left ventricular failure. Physical examination usually reveals a prominent *a* wave in the jugular venous pulse, a double or triple apical impulse, a sharply rising peripheral pulse that is best appreciated in the carotid arteries, and a fourth heart sound. The second heart sound may be paradoxically split, and a third heart sound may be audible. A systolic ejection murmur is heard best along the left sternal border or at the apex, rather than at the aortic area or along the carotid arteries, as in patients with valvular aortic stenosis. Some degree of mitral regurgitation is present in the majority of patients, probably as a result of the displacement of the mitral valve by the grossly hypertrophied left ventricular myocardium. Indeed, IHSS must be distinguished both from isolated mitral regurgitation and from ventricular septal defect, conditions which it resembles superficially. The murmur, itself, probably results both from the obstruction to ventricular outflow and from the mitral regurgitation.

The *electrocardiogram* commonly shows left ventricular hypertrophy and widespread, abnormally deep, broad Q waves that suggest an old myocardial infarction but probably result from gross septal hypertrophy. Although *chest roentgenograms* reveal left ventricular hypertrophy, in contrast to valvular aortic stenosis, calcification of the aortic valve is not observed and poststenotic dilatation of the aorta is present only rarely. The indirectly recorded carotid arterial pressure pulse rises unusually rapidly and often displays a double peak during systole. *Echocardiography* usually, but not invariably, reveals disproportional hypertrophy of the ventricular septum compared with the posterior free wall, the former being at least 1.3 times as thick as the latter. Another typical feature includes abnormal motion of the anterior leaflet of the mitral valve, with reopening of the valve in midsystole and juxtaposition of the septum and anterior leaflet at the onset of obstruction—so-called "systolic anterior motion" (SAM) of the anterior mitral leaflet. The echocardiogram reveals that the septum is not hypercontractile, but rather shows a diminished amount of systolic thickening and a decreased extent of and velocity of contraction. This evidence of abnormal septal contraction reflects the abnormalities of myocardial cell structure. Systolic anterior motion, coupled with obstruction of the left ventricular outflow tract, but without disproportional septal hypertrophy, occurs in a small fraction of patients with IHSS.

Disproportional septal hypertrophy may be detected in patients with other forms of cardiac disease, including coronary artery disease, mitral valve prolapse, primary pulmonary hypertension, and various forms of congenital heart disease such as pulmonary stenosis and Eisenmenger's syndrome. In most of these patients it is clear that the septal hypertrophy does not represent IHSS because first-degree relatives do not display similar septal hypertrophy, systolic anterior motion of the mitral valve is not present, and, in those patients who have been studied at necropsy, myocardial cellular disarray is usually not present. Thus, most of these patients develop disproportionate septal hypertrophy as a hemodynamic consequence of their underlying heart disease. Because of the frequency of IHSS, however, some patients will inevitably have this disease along with other commonly occurring diseases, such as coronary artery disease.

When a pressure gradient is present, it is located between the body of the left ventricle and the area directly below the aortic valve. When a gradient is not present, it frequently can be induced by provocative maneuvers such as infusion of isoproterenol, inhalation of amyl nitrite, or the Valsalva maneuver. In some patients symptoms may be severe but obstruction to ventricular outflow may be minimal. In these patients the left ventricular end-diastolic pressure is generally elevated, and symptoms probably result from restriction to ventricular filling, a consequence of decreased ventricular compliance. Thus, IHSS may have features of a restrictive cardiomyopathy.

The natural history of IHSS is variable, with some patients improving, some deteriorating, and some remaining stable. Over a long period of time some of these patients lose their murmur as their condition deteriorates and the gradient decreases or disappears, quite likely because the failing heart becomes somewhat dilated and contracts less forcefully. Sudden death is now recognized as a frequent complication and accounts for approximately 30 percent of the deaths in IHSS. It does not seem related to the severity or type of previous symptoms or to the extent of obstruction. Apparently successful medical management or operative treatment does not obviate the possibility of sudden death. Subacute bacterial endocarditis may involve the aortic valve, the mitral valve, or both.

Cardiac glycosides or nitroglycerin are ordinarily not helpful, although once overt congestive failure has developed, digitalis may be tried cautiously. Beta-adrenergic receptor blocking agents reduce the frequency and severity of angina and syncope, but if symptoms remain intractable, surgical excision or incision of the hypertrophied portion of the outflow tract may be indicated. Frequently, as a result of operation the systolic anterior motion of the mitral valve is abolished or markedly decreased and both the obstruction to ventricular outflow and the mitral regurgitation are significantly improved. The size of the left atrium usually decreases postoperatively in patients under 40 years of age, although the size does not change postoperatively in older patients. Because atrial fibrillation develops only in patients with an enlarged left atrium, operation may reduce the risk of this arrhythmia in the young. Operative intervention, however, is not indicated in symptomatic patients without evidence of obstruction, or in asymptomatic patients with or without obstruction.

The heart is involved in about 50 percent of patients with *Friedreich's ataxia.* The picture is that of a hypertrophic cardiomyopathy associated with arrhythmias. The coronary arteries may either be normal or show extensive intimal proliferation leading to obstruction of both small and large arteries; atherosclerosis and thrombosis are generally not present. *Type*

II glycogen storage or Pompe's disease with cardiac involvement may also show features of obstruction to ventricular ejection. In addition, signs and symptoms of congestion and restriction may also be present.

Drugs Certain widely used drugs are capable of producing myocardial damage and the clinical picture of a rapidly progressive congestive cardiomyopathy. Other drugs may produce electrocardiographic abnormalities and cardiac arrhythmias. *Doxorubicin* (Adriamycin) and *daunorubicin* (Daunomycin) are anthracycline antibiotics that are powerful antineoplastic agents. When given in high doses (more than 550 mg/m² for doxorubicin), irreversible heart failure may develop. Factors that potentiate the cardiotoxicity of these agents are radiation to the heart and prior, concurrent, or subsequent treatment with dactinomycin, mithramycin, cyclophosphamide, or high-dose methotrexate. Electrocardiographic changes and arrhythmias may result from treatment with the *tricyclic antidepressants,* the *phenothiazines,* various *aerosol propellants,* and *emetine. Methysergide* is used primarily for the treatment of migraine headache. It may cause endocardial fibrosis, together with retroperitoneal and pleuropulmonary fibrosis. The cardiac lesions have been associated with the development of heart murmurs and valvular heart disease.

MYOCARDITIS

Generally, myocarditis is the result of an infectious process, but it may also be present in hypersensitivity states such as acute rheumatic fever (Chap. 241) or be caused by radiation therapy, chemical poisons, physical agents, or drugs. The myocarditides may be divided into the acute and chronic forms. In the United States, clinically significant acute myocarditis is caused most commonly by viruses. Thus far, the coxsackievirus A and B strains, the poliomyelitis, influenza, adeno, echo, rubeola, and rubella viruses have been the best-documented etiologic agents, but as viral studies become more widespread, other viruses probably will be implicated. Generally, when the heart is involved in these diseases, only transient ST-T wave abnormalities are noted and the myocardial involvement does not influence the course of the disease. However, sometimes myocarditis, which may develop either during or several weeks after the respiratory illness, may lead to acute heart failure which may be fatal, more frequently in infants than in adults, or it may lead to a variety of cardiac arrhythmias. Myocarditis is frequently associated with acute pericarditis, especially when it is caused by coxsackievirus B strains or echoviruses (Chap. 187).

Physical examination may show the first heart sound to be faint, a ventricular gallop (third heart) sound may be heard, and a soft apical systolic murmur is often present. A pericardial friction rub is usually heard in patients with associated pericarditis.

Measures to combat the congestive failure, such as use of digitalis, diuretics, and salt restriction, may be necessary. Patients with viral myocarditis are sometimes exceedingly sensitive to digitalis; therefore this drug should be given cautiously and a short-acting preparation should be used. The arrhythmias are occasionally extremely difficult to manage and may be refractory to the usual treatment with drugs such as quinidine, procainamide, diphenylhydantoin, lidocaine, or propranolol. When propranolol is used, care must be taken not to precipitate congestive heart failure. Deaths attributed to heart failure and arrhythmias have been reported, and it seems prudent to monitor patients with arrhythmias, especially during the acute illness. Prolonged bed rest may be helpful, but its efficacy remains to be established. Animal studies suggest that steroids and exercise may aggravate the myocardial involvement.

Though viral myocarditis is most often self-limited and without sequelae, active disease may recur, and it is likely that acute viral myocarditis occasionally progresses to a chronic form. Patients often give the history of a preceding upper respiratory febrile illness, and viral nasopharyngitis or tonsillitis may be evident clinically. The isolation of virus from the stool, pharyngeal washings, or other body fluids and changes in specific viral antibody titers are helpful clinically. It is possible that many of the instances of idiopathic congestive cardiomyopathy (page 1142) arise from mild or subclinical episodes of myocarditis.

ISOLATED MYOCARDITIS Also called *Fiedler's myocarditis,* this is a rare condition in which only the myocardium is involved and the cardiac involvement cannot be related to a previous or concurrent illness. The etiology of this disease is unknown, but a viral causation has been postulated. When first seen by the physician, the patient generally has fulminating congestive heart failure; corticosteroids are occasionally effective, but in general, therapy is unsatisfactory and a fatal outcome follows a brief illness.

Idiopathic giant-cell myocarditis is a newly recognized entity characterized by a short clinical course, with the frequent occurrence of sudden death, apparently as a result of an arrhythmia. Death may also result from severe congestive heart failure. Fever is usually present, and the electrocardiogram reveals evidence of widespread myocardial damage, together with bundle branch block and arrhythmias. At necropsy, the distinctive features include grossly visible serpiginous areas of myocardial necrosis in both ventricles and microscopically evident giant cells, apparently forming from degenerating muscle cells. It is possible that some of the reported cases of Fiedler's myocarditis may have been idiopathic giant-cell myocarditis. This condition has been reported alone and in association with other diseases, including thymoma, thyroiditis, thyrotoxicosis, sarcoidosis, lupus erythematosus, and tuberculosis.

Diphtheritic myocarditis is caused by an exotoxin produced by *Corynebacterium diphtheriae* (Chap. 133). Patients may die in acute congestive heart failure or as a result of complete heart block. Widespread immunization against diphtheria has virtually eliminated this disease.

TOXOPLASMOSIS (See also Chap. 203) Toxoplasmosis is a relatively common cause of acute myocarditis in the newborn. The parasite *Toxoplasma gondii* can pass in utero from the mother to the fetus, so that toxoplasmosis may occur in the fetus or in the newborn. Toxoplasma myocarditis may occur in several members of a family. In adults it occurs most often as an opportunistic infection in patients treated with corticosteroids, cytotoxic chemotherapy, or immunosuppressive agents. Myocarditis may be isolated or occur as a feature of miliary toxoplasmosis. This condition should be considered in the differential diagnosis of obscure acute myocarditis or cardiomyopathy. Markedly elevated or rising levels of complement in a complement fixation test or of antibody in the antibody dye test are valuable diagnostic aids. Therapy consists of administration of pyrimethamine and triple sulfonamides, as described in Chap. 203. *Aspergillus myocarditis* is another opportunistic infection that is being recognized more frequently.

CHAGAS' DISEASE (See also Chap. 202) Chagas' disease, caused by *Trypanosoma cruzi,* produces a form of myocarditis that occurs in well-defined acute and chronic forms. It is one of the most common causes of heart disease encountered in Central and South America, affecting more than 7 million people. Cardiac involvement is the most important clinical feature and accounts for 87 percent of the deaths attributable to this disease. The heart is enlarged, the sounds are distant, and a protodiastolic gallop sound may be present. The electrocardiogram may show first-degree atrioventricular dissociation and abnormal T waves. The acute myocarditis is usually self-limited, but some patients develop the chronic form, which may occur in patients without a history of an acute episode. The chronic form is characterized by dilation of the cardiac chambers, fibrosis and thinning of the ventricular wall, aneurysm formation in the areas of thinning, especially at the apex, and mural thrombi. At first, the electrocardiogram may show evidence of intraventricular block and occasional premature ventricular contractions. As the patient becomes symptomatic, signs and symptoms of congestive heart failure develop. Premature contractions become more frequent, and serious arrhythmias, such as ventricular tachycardia, may occur. The cause of death is either intractable congestive failure or an arrhythmia. Therapy is directed toward the treatment of the congestive heart failure and arrhythmias.

RADIATION MYOCARDITIS Patients who receive large doses of radiation therapy to the area of the heart (generally in excess of 4000 rads), most frequently for carcinoma of the lung or breast, lymphoma, or Hodgkin's disease, may develop acute pericarditis, chronic constrictive pericarditis, chronic myocarditis, and perhaps premature coronary artery disease. The myocardial fibrosis may be secondary to involvement of capillary endothelial cells which leads to obliteration of these vessels.

REFERENCES

ARNETT EN et al: Massive myocardial hemosiderosis. Am Heart J 90:777, 1975

BRAUNWALD E (ed): Cardiomyopathies and infiltrative diseases of the heart, in *Heart Disease*. Philadelphia, Saunders, 1980, chap 39

BRISTOW MR et al: Doxorubicin cardiomyopathy: Evaluation by phonocardiography, endomyocardial biopsy, and cardiac catheterization. Ann Intern Med 88:168, 1978

CHEW CY et al: Primary restrictive cardiomyopathy: Non-tropical endomyocardial fibrosis and hypereosinophilic heart disease. Br Heart J 39:413, 1977

COHEN J, SHAH PM (eds): Cardiac hypertrophy and cardiomyopathy. Circ Res, vol 35, suppl II, 1974

DAVIES MJ et al: Idiopathic giant cell myocarditis: A distinctive clinicopathological entity. Br Heart J 37:192, 1975

DEGLIN SM et al: Drug-induced cardiovascular diseases. Drugs 14:29, 1977

DEMAKIS JG et al: Natural course of peripartum cardiomyopathy. Circulation 44:1053, 1971

EPSTEIN SE et al: Asymmetric septal hypertrophy. Ann Intern Med 81:650, 1974

FAJARDO LF, STEWART JR: Pathogenesis of radiation-induced myocardial fibrosis. Lab Invest 29:244, 1973

FRANK S, BRAUNWALD E: Idiopathic hypertrophic subaortic stenosis: Clinical analysis of 126 patients with emphasis on the natural history. Circulation 37:759, 1968

HALL SW JR et al: Hypereosinophilic syndrome with biventricular involvement. Circulation 55:218, 1977

JAMES TN: Sarcoid heart disease. Circulation 56:320, 1977

LERNER AM et al: Enteroviruses and the heart. Mod Concepts Cardiovasc Dis 44:7, 1975

MARON BJ et al: Sudden death in patients with hypertrophic cardiomyopathy: Characterization of 26 patients without functional limitation. Am J Cardiol 41:803, 1978

MEHTA J et al: Electrocardiographic and vectorcardiographic abnormalities in Fabry's disease. Am Heart J 93:699, 1977

MINTZ GS et al: Systolic anterior motion of the mitral valve in the absence of asymmetric septal hypertrophy. Circulation 57:256, 1978

REGAN TJ et al: Role of ethanol in cardiac disease. Annu Rev Med 28:393, 1977

SANYAL SK et al: An ultrastructural basis for electrocardiographic alterations associated with Duchenne's progressive muscular dystrophy. Circulation 57:1122, 1978

SMITH ER et al: Hypertrophic cardiomyopathy: The heart disease of Freidreich's ataxia. Am Heart J 94:428, 1977

SOLLEY GO et al: Endomyocardiopathy with eosinophilia. Mayo Clin Proc 51:697, 1976

SWANTON RH et al: Systolic and diastolic ventricular function in cardiac amyloidosis. Am J Cardiol 39:658, 1977

248

CARDIAC TUMORS AND OTHER UNUSUAL FORMS OF HEART DISEASE

GERALD GLICK
EUGENE BRAUNWALD

TUMORS OF THE HEART

MYXOMA Cardiac myxomas, though rare causes of heart disease, are the commonest type of primary tumor of the heart seen in adults. Despite their rarity, myxomas are of clinical importance because they represent a potentially curable form of heart disease; therefore they always present a formidable diagnostic challenge to the clinician. They occur most frequently in the atria, the left atrium being involved three times as often as the right. Cardiac myxomas may be bilateral and familial. They are generally pedunculated, with the stem attached to the atrial septum in the region of the foramen ovale; they may be either firm and smooth or gelatinous and polypoid. When in the ventricles, myxomas are generally sessile. Microscopically, an abundant mucoid stroma and stellate-shaped cells with pleomorphic nuclei of varying degrees of differentiation are seen. The derivation of cardiac myxomas still remains unsettled, but the weight of evidence favors a neoplastic rather than a thrombotic origin. Metastases rarely, if ever, occur.

The clinical manifestations produced by cardiac myxomas may be divided into three separate groups: (1) symptoms resulting from impediment to blood flow through the heart as a result of mechanical obstruction produced by the tumor itself; (2) symptoms resulting from emboli released from the tumor into the pulmonary or systemic arterial beds; and (3) generalized constitutional abnormalities.

When the myxoma is located in the left atrium, the clinical findings suggest the diagnosis of mitral valve disease possibly complicated by bacterial endocarditis, or of a cardiomyopathy; it may mimic mitral stenosis because the pedunculated mass may fall into the mitral orifice, thereby obstructing blood flow into the left ventricle. Less commonly the clinical findings resemble those produced by combined mitral stenosis and regurgitation or pure mitral regurgitation. Presumably the tumor causes regurgitation by interfering with the function of the mitral valve leaflets. The left atrial pressure is elevated, and the increased pressure is transmitted through the pulmonary vascular bed, with consequent pulmonary congestion and pulmonary arterial hypertension. All the symptoms and some of the signs of mitral valve disease therefore may be produced (Chap.

242). In addition, episodes of syncope or sudden relief or exacerbation of symptoms with changes in posture may occur as the myxoma shifts its position in relation to the valve orifice.

The pertinent *physical findings* include splitting of the first heart sound, accentuation of the pulmonic component of the second heart sound, an early diastolic sound attributed to the hitting of the myxoma against the ventricular wall or to abrupt deceleration of the tumor (a tumor "plop"), and both apical pansystolic and middiastolic murmurs. The auscultatory findings may change with alterations in position. Systemic emboli, resulting from the breaking off of pieces of tumor tissue or from the formation of thrombi on the tumor, may involve any organ. In fact, when many organs are involved, attention may be diverted away from the heart. Intracardiac myxomas also produce constitutional symptoms such as weight loss, fever, weakness, arthralgias, myalgias, anemia, hyperglobulinemia, an elevated erythrocyte sedimentation rate, and abnormal liver function tests. These findings may also direct attention away from the heart. Coupled with the finding of changing heart murmurs, they may suggest the diagnosis of subacute bacterial endocarditis. Rarely, the tumor itself may become infected.

When the myxoma is located in the right atrium, it may produce the signs and symptoms of tricuspid stenosis. Embolization from these tumors produces pulmonary hypertension as a result of widespread obstruction of the pulmonary vascular bed. Constitutional symptoms are similar to those occurring with left atrial myxomas. Ventricular myxomas may obstruct ventricular outflow by involving the semilunar valves or subvalvular regions; they may also produce emboli.

The diagnosis of intracardiac myxoma can be made by echocardiography (Chap. 233) or selective angiocardiography, which may demonstrate a space-occupying lesion in one of the cardiac chambers. Early operative treatment is mandatory because of the high morbidity and mortality related, in particular, to embolization. Accordingly, echocardiography and, if the results are suggestive, angiocardiography should be carried out in patients with apparent valvular heart disease and unusual features or in those with obscure cardiac problems in whom the diagnosis is considered. Operative removal usually results in a complete cure, including relief of the constitutional symptoms. Because of potential recurrence, the endocardial attachment should be excised; follow-up echocardiography is desirable.

RHABDOMYOMA This is the most common form of primary cardiac tumor in young children. It is considered to be a hamartoma, i.e., it arises from normal embryonal elements found in the heart, and is therefore benign. It is frequently associated with tuberous sclerosis, a disease in which hamartomas of many organs occur. The left ventricle is the chamber most frequently involved, and multiple nodules are present in the ventricular septum and free wall. Another benign tumor is the *mesothelioma of the atrioventricular node* (conduction tumor). It produces heart block and may cause sudden death in infancy or adolescence.

SARCOMAS These comprise the malignant primary cardiac tumors. They occur most commonly in the right atrium; as a result they may occlude inflow into the atrium from either vena cava, and produce an inferior or superior vena caval syndrome. Right ventricular outflow may also be obstructed. Arrhythmias and intractable heart failure are common findings. Metastases to the vertebral column and to parenchymal organs are common. The tumors are named for the dominant cellular element involved, the most common being *fibrosarcomas, rhab-*

domyosarcomas (anaplastic malignant tumors which are composed of embryonal striated muscular elements), and *angiosarcomas.*

SECONDARY TUMOR INVOLVEMENT At autopsy the heart is involved in 25 percent of patients with Hodgkin's disease, 37 percent of patients with leukemia, and 60 percent of patients with malignant melanoma. In addition, metastases to the heart occur relatively often in individuals with bronchial carcinoma and carcinoma of the breast. More rarely, metastases may arise secondary to carcinoma of the pancreas, gastrointestinal tract, or kidney. The most common abnormalities produced by secondary involvement of the heart by tumor are the production of arrhythmias, including atrioventricular block, and bloody pericardial effusions. Atrial fibrillation is the commonest arrhythmia seen in these circumstances.

TUMORS OF THE PERICARDIUM See Chap. 249.

OTHER UNUSUAL FORMS OF HEART DISEASE

MALIGNANT CARCINOID In the usual form of carcinoid syndrome with gastrointestinal tumors and hepatic metastases (Chap. 91), the lesions in the heart are mainly on the right side and result in tricuspid regurgitation and pulmonic stenosis. The clinical manifestations consist of dilated neck veins with prominent *v* waves, hepatomegaly, ascites, and edema. Predominantly left-sided lesions of mitral stenosis have been reported in patients with bronchial carcinoid tumors and in patients with right-to-left shunts through a patent foramen ovale. It is probable that an as yet unidentified substance released by the tumor is responsible for the development of the valvular lesions, and that this substance is removed or detoxified in the pulmonary circulation.

OBESITY In extremely obese patients, the heart may be markedly enlarged, the left ventricle showing the greatest degree of hypertrophy. This form of heart disease must be distinguished from the Pickwickian syndrome (Chap. 270). The clinical course of obesity heart disease is marked by congestive heart failure, with both pulmonary and systemic venous congestion. Left ventricular end-diastolic pressure at rest is usually near the upper limits of normal, but it usually rises to abnormal levels during exercise. Since obesity without cardiac involvement may be responsible for dyspnea and ankle edema, evidence of superimposed congestive failure may be difficult to recognize; measurement of venous pressure and circulation time may be helpful. Also, a therapeutic trial of digitalis, salt restriction, diuretics, and weight loss may be indicated.

MYXEDEMA (See also Chap. 335) The heart appears often to be enlarged, and electrocardiographic abnormalities such as low voltage, prolonged PR interval, and T-wave alterations are common. Arrhythmias, such as paroxysmal atrial tachycardia and atrial fibrillation, and high-grade atrioventricular dissociation may occur. Disappearance of the electrocardiographic abnormalities and arrhythmias is usual after restoration of the euthyroid state. Echocardiographic studies have shown that in most cases the enlarged cardiac silhouette is due to a pericardial effusion and this effusion disappears with treatment. However, cardiomegaly will persist if it is the result of coronary artery disease or some other process. A large amount of fluid, of high protein content, may accumulate in the pericardial space but rarely produces tamponade. On histologic examination myxedema hearts reveal a variety of nonspecific degenerative changes. Lack of thyroid hormone per se depresses intrinsic myocardial contractility. Nevertheless, myxedema seldom, if ever, causes actual myocardial failure; when heart failure is present in patients with myxedema, it is likely that some other form of heart disease, such as ischemic heart disease, is associated with the myxedema or that myxedema is of long duration. Thyroid replacement therapy should be carried out with great caution, and the initial dose should be quite small because of the possibility of precipitating anginal attacks or cerebral dysfunction in patients whose arteries have been narrowed by atherosclerotic lesions and in whom, therefore, blood flow may be inadequate to meet the increased oxygen demands of the heart and brain produced by the hormone.

RHEUMATOID ARTHRITIS (See also Chap. 356) The heart may be involved in various ways in patients with rheumatoid arthritis. Granulomatous lesions resembling subcutaneous nodules in their histologic characteristics may affect all tissues of the heart. Involvement of the aortic and mitral valves may lead to severe valvular regurgitation. Other lesions that may occur include healed or active pericarditis, focal or diffuse myocarditis, valvular fibrosis, and healed or subacute arteritis. *Ankylosing spondylitis,* an entity probably distinct from rheumatoid arthritis, is associated in about 3 percent of cases with valvular regurgitation, most often of the aortic valve but occasionally of the mitral valve. Partial or complete atrioventricular block may also occur.

TRAUMATIC HEART DISEASE Cardiac damage may be due to both penetrating and nonpenetrating injuries. The most frequent cause of a nonpenetrating injury is impact of the chest against the steering wheel of an automobile. Serious injury of the heart may ensue even though no external sign of thoracic trauma is evident. Although the common type of injury is myocardial contusion, any structure of the heart may be affected by the trauma. If the valvular apparatus is ruptured, a loud heart murmur may appear, followed by the development of rapidly progressive heart failure. The most serious consequence of nonpenetrating injury is rupture either of the atria or of the ventricles, which is generally fatal; patients with ruptured ventricular or atrial septum may survive. Hemopericardium may also follow tear of a pericardial vessel or of a coronary artery. Myocardial contusion may cause arrhythmias, bundle branch block, or electrocardiographic abnormalities resembling those of infarction. Thus, it is important to bear trauma in mind as a cause of otherwise unexplained electrocardiographic changes. Similarly, myocardial contusion may produce positive radionuclide scans and regional impairment of ventricular function as occurs in patients with acute myocardial infarction. Pericardial effusion may occur weeks or even months after the accident, as a late manifestation of a nonpenetrating injury of the chest wall. In these cases, the pericardial effusion is a manifestation of the post-cardiac injury syndrome, which resembles the postpericardiotomy syndrome (Chap. 249).

Conservative medical treatment for acute myocardial failure resulting from rupture of a valve, most commonly the aortic, is rarely effective; operative correction is usually necessary. If the electrocardiographic abnormalities are those of myocardial infarction, it may be impossible to distinguish between myocardial contusion and infarction secondary to coronary artery injury; in either case, treatment is the same, namely, that indicated for myocardial infarction due to ischemic heart disease (Chap. 245). When pericardial hemorrhage leads to constrictive pericarditis, decortication is necessary.

Penetrating injuries of the heart produced by bullets or stab wounds usually result in immediate or very rapid death because of hemopericardium or massive hemorrhage. However, sometimes the patient survives the acute incident, and presents with a cardiac murmur and congestive heart failure. A left-to-right shunt due to traumatic ventricular septal defect, aorto-

pulmonary artery fistula, or coronary artery fistula may be suspected and confirmed by cardiac catheterization and angiocardiography. Operation is indicated if hemodynamically significant abnormalities are present or if a foreign body, e.g., a bullet, is lodged in the heart.

Immediate thoracotomy should be carried out if there is cardiac tamponade and/or shock, regardless of whether the trauma was penetrating or nonpenetrating. Pericardiocentesis may be helpful in patients with tamponade, but usually only as a holding maneuver.

REFERENCES

ALEXANDER JK, PETERSON KL: Cardiovascular effects of weight reduction. Circulation 45:310, 1972

COHN PF, BRAUNWALD E: Traumatic heart disease, in *Heart Disease,* E Braunwald (ed). Philadelphia, Saunders, 1980, chap 42

FELDMAN PS et al: An ultrastructural study of seven cardiac myxomas. Cancer 40:2216, 1977

FOWLER NO (ed): Uncommon varieties of heart disease, in *Cardiac Diagnosis and Treatment,* 2d ed. New York, Harper & Row, 1976, p 838

IVESON JMI et al: Aortic valve incompetence and replacement in rheumatoid arthritis. Ann Rheum Dis 34:312, 1975

JACKSON DH, MURPHY GW: Nonpenetrating cardiac trauma. Mod Concepts Cardiovasc Dis 45:123, 1976

KERBER RE, SHERMAN B: Echocardiographic evaluation of pericardial effusion in myxedema. Circulation 52:823, 1975

ROSS JS: Heart block, sudden death, and atrioventricular node mesothelioma. Am J Dis Child 131:1209, 1977

SELZER A et al: Protean clinical manifestations of primary tumors of the heart. Am J Med 52:9, 1972

STOLLERMAN E: Rheumatic fever, connective tissue disorders and heart disease, in *Heart Disease,* E Braunwald (ed). Philadelphia, Saunders, 1980, chap 47

WENGER NK: Cardiac tumors, in *The Heart,* 4th ed, JW Hurst et al (eds). New York, McGraw-Hill, 1978, pp 1668–1682

249
PERICARDIAL DISEASE

EUGENE BRAUNWALD

NORMAL FUNCTIONS OF THE PERICARDIUM The visceral pericardium is a serous membrane, separated by a small amount of fluid from a fibrous sac, the parietal pericardium. The pericardium prevents sudden dilatation of the cardiac chambers during exercise and hypervolemia, and facilitates atrial filling during ventricular systole, as the result of the development of a negative intrapericardial pressure during ejection. It holds the heart in a fixed anatomic position, minimizes friction between the heart and surrounding structures, prevents displacement of the heart and kinking of the great vessels, and probably retards the spread of infections from the lungs and pleural cavities to the heart. However, its total absence does not produce obvious clinical disease. In partial left pericardial defects the main pulmonary artery and left atrium bulge through the defect; rarely their herniation may cause sudden death.

It is useful to classify the types of pericarditis both clinically and etiologically (Table 249-1), as it is by far the most common pathological process involving the pericardium.

ACUTE PERICARDITIS

Pain, a pericardial friction rub, electrocardiographic changes, and pericardial effusion with cardiac tamponade and paradoxic pulse are cardinal manifestations of many forms of acute pericarditis and will be considered prior to a discussion of the most common varieties.

Pain is an important but not invariable symptom in various forms of acute pericarditis; it is usually present in the acute infectious types and in many of the forms presumed to be related to hypersensitivity or autoimmunity. Pain is often absent in a slowly developing tuberculous, postirradiation, or neoplastic pericarditis. The pain of pericarditis is often severe; its character and location have been described in Chap. 5. It is *usually* pleuritic, but occasionally the steady, constrictive pain, radiating into either arm or both arms and resembling that of myocardial ischemia, may overshadow the pleuritic pain, or it may occur along the arm at the onset of the illness, with the

TABLE 249-1
Classification of pericarditis

I Clinical classification
  A Acute pericarditis (<6 weeks)
    1 Fibrinous
    2 Effusive (or bloody)
  B Subacute pericarditis (6 weeks to 6 months)
    1 Constrictive
    2 Effusive-constrictive
  C Chronic pericarditis (>6 months)
    1 Constrictive
    2 Effusive
    3 Adhesive (nonconstrictive)
II Etiologic classification
  A Infectious pericarditis
    1 Viral
    2 Pyogenic
    3 Tuberculous
    4 Mycotic
    5 Other infections (syphilitic, parasitic)
  B Noninfectious pericarditis
    1 Acute myocardial infarction
    2 Uremia
    3 Neoplasia
      a Primary tumors (benign or malignant)
      b Tumors metastatic to pericardium
    4 Myxedema
    5 Cholesterol
    6 Chylopericardium
    7 Trauma
      a Penetrating chest wall
      b Nonpenetrating
    8 Aortic aneurysm (with leakage into pericardial sac)
    9 Postradiation
    10 Associated with atrial septal defect
    11 Associated with severe chronic anemia
    12 Infectious mononucleosis
    13 Familial Mediterranean fever
    14 Familial pericarditis
      a Mulibrey nanism*
    15 Sarcoidosis
    16 Acute idiopathic
  C Pericarditis presumably related to hypersensitivity or autoimmunity
    1 Rheumtic fever
    2 Collagen vascular disease
      a Systemic lupus erythematosus
      b Rheumatoid arthritis
      c Scleroderma
    3 Drug-induced
      a Procainamide
      b Hydralazine
      c Other
    4 Postcardiac injury
      a Postmyocardial infarction (Dressler's syndrome)
      b Postpericardiotomy

* *An autosomal recessive syndrome, characterized by growth failure, muscle hypotonia, hepatomegaly, ocular changes, enlarged cerebral ventricles, mental retardation, and chronic constrictive pericarditis.*

result that confusion with myocardial infarction is not infrequent. It may be in the epigastrium, referred to the left shoulder and relieved by leaning forward. This problem becomes even more perplexing when, with acute pericarditis, the serum transaminase level rises to about 80 units. However, the MB isoenzyme of creatine kinase does not rise in acute pericarditis. Suffice it to say that a pain felt either in the precordium or in one or both of the shoulders or trapezius ridges, aggravated by coughing, swallowing, inspiration, or rotation of the trunk, and relieved by sitting up and leaning forward should alert one to the possibility of an acute pericarditis.

The *pericardial friction rub* is the most important physical sign; it may have up to three components per cardiac cycle, as described in Chap. 231, and may sometimes be elicited only when firm pressure with the stethoscope is applied to the chest wall. It is heard most frequently during forced inspiration, with the patient leaning forward or on his or her hands and knees. The rub is likely to be inconstant and transitory, and a loud to-and-fro leathery sound may disappear within a few hours, possibly to reappear the following day.

The *electrocardiogram* in acute pericarditis without massive effusion usually displays elevation of the ST segments in two or three standard limb leads and V_2 to V_6, with reciprocal depressions only in aVR and V_1 and without significant changes in QRS complexes, except occasionally for some diminution in voltage. Several days later, the ST segments return to normal and the T waves then become inverted. In contrast, in acute myocardial infarction, reciprocal depression of ST segments is usually more prominent; QRS changes occur, particularly the development of Q waves; and T-wave inversions usually occur before the ST segments have become isoelectric. Sequential electrocardiograms are useful in distinguishing acute pericarditis from acute myocardial infarction and from early repolarization (see also Chap. 232). With large pericardial effusion, the QRS voltage is reduced. Atrial premature beats and atrial fibrillation are sometimes noted.

PERICARDIAL EFFUSION Usually associated with an enlargement of the cardiac silhouette, pericardial effusion is especially important when it develops within a relatively short time. Differentiation from heart enlargement may be difficult, but heart sounds tend to become faint; the friction rub may disappear or remain clearly audible, and the apex impulse may vanish, but sometimes it is felt well within the left border of cardiac dullness. The chest roentgenogram may show a "water bottle" configuration of the cardiac silhouette. Lucent pericardial fat lines may be seen deep within the cardiopericardial silhouette. Fluoroscopic examination may show the ventricular pulsations to be diminished. When the effusion is large, one often encounters an area of dullness and tubular breath sounds at the angle of the left scapula, probably caused by compression of the lung (Ewart's sign).

Diagnosis of pericardial effusion A number of laboratory techniques are available for establishing the diagnosis of pericardial effusion. Echocardiography (Chap. 233) has emerged as the most effective, since it is sensitive, simple, innocuous, noninvasive, and may be performed at the bedside. The presence of pericardial fluid is recorded as a relatively echo-free space between the posterior pericardium and the posterior left ventricular epicardium in patients with small effusions and such a space between the anterior right ventricle and the parietal pericardium just beneath the anterior chest wall with larger effusions (Fig. 249-1). In patients with large effusions the heart may swing freely within the pericardial sac; when severe, this motion may be associated with electrical alternans. The diagnosis of pericardial fluid or thickening may be confirmed by one of the following:

1 Cardiac catheterization. A catheter is introduced into the right atrium and rotated so that its tip makes contact with the lateral right atrial wall. In the presence of an effusion, or pericardial thickening, the tip of the catheter is seen to be separated from the radiolucent lungs by an opaque band.

2 Angiocardiography. Contrast medium is injected rapidly into the right atrium, and the lateral wall is outlined.

When examination of pericardial fluid is deemed essential, exploration of the pericardium may be required. To accomplish this, a needle should be attached to a properly grounded electrocardiographic lead, and intrapericardial pressure should be measured, utilizing the same apparatus employed for measuring cerebrospinal fluid pressure during lumbar puncture. When an effusion develops, the fluid nearly always has the physical characteristics of an exudate. Bloody fluid is commonly due to tuberculosis or tumor, but it may also be found in the effusion of rheumatic fever or in the post-cardiac injury syndrome (see below). Occasionally, bloody fluid may be found in the effusion of uremic pericarditis and in the hemopericardium following myocardial infarction, especially following the administration of anticoagulants.

CARDIAC TAMPONADE The accumulation of fluid in the pericardium in an amount sufficient to cause serious obstruction to the inflow of blood to the ventricles results in cardiac tamponade. The amount of fluid necessary to produce this critical state may be as small as 250 ml, when the fluid develops rapidly; or it may be over 1000 ml in slowly developing effusions when the pericardium has had the opportunity to stretch and adapt to the increasing volume of fluid. The volume of fluid required to produce tamponade varies directly with the thickness of the ventricular myocardium and inversely with the thickness of the parietal pericardium. Tamponade results most often from bleeding into the pericardial space following cardiac operations, trauma (including cardiac perforation during diagnostic procedures), tuberculosis, pyogenic infection, or tumor, but it may occur in acute viral or idiopathic pericarditis, the post-cardiac injury syndrome, postradiation pericarditis, and hemopericardium which may result when a patient with any form of acute pericarditis is treated with anticoagulants.

The clinical manifestations are due to the fall in cardiac output and to systemic venous congestion. However, the classic findings of arterial hypotension and of a small quiet heart with faint heart sounds usually are seen only with very rapidly developing, severe tamponade, as occurs with cardiac trauma.

More frequently, tamponade develops slowly and the clinical manifestations, resembling those of heart failure, include dyspnea, orthopnea, tachycardia, hepatic engorgement, and a positive hepatojugular reflux. A high index of suspicion is required, since, in many instances, no obvious cause for pericardial disease is apparent, and tamponade should be considered in any patient with hypotension and elevation of jugular venous pressure. A widening of the area of flatness to percussion across the anterior aspect of the chest wall, a paradoxical pulse (see below), clear lung fields, diminished pulsations of the cardiac silhouette on fluoroscopy, reduction in amplitude of the QRS complexes, and *electrical alternans* should raise the suspicion of cardiac tamponade. Since immediate treatment may be life-saving, prompt measures to establish the diagnosis (echocardiography, followed by cardiac catheterization and angiocardiography) should be undertaken.

Paradoxical pulse This important clue to the presence of cardiac tamponade consists of *a greater than normal (10 mmHg) inspiratory decrease in systolic arterial pressure.* When severe, it may be detected by palpating weakness or disappearance of the arterial pulse during inspiration, but usually sphygmomanometric measurement of systolic pressure during slow respiration is required (Fig. 249-2).

The mechanism of paradoxical pulse in cardiac tamponade is complex. Normally, the inspiratory decline in intrathoracic pressure enhances right ventricular filling by virtue of the increased pressure gradient between the extrathoracic veins and the chambers of the right side of the heart. Right ventricular output increases, but because of the time required for the transmission of this augmented output through the pulmonary vascular bed and left atrium, left ventricular output does not rise until the following expiration. Thus, normally there is a slight inspiratory diminution in systemic arterial pressure. This effect is enhanced by the relatively greater reduction of left ventricular stroke volume which occurs in cardiac tamponade, since the respiratory variation then involves a larger fraction of the total output. Also, respiratory distress increases the fluctuations in intrathoracic pressure, which, in addition to exaggerating the mechanism just described, are also transmitted directly to the intrathoracic aorta and hence to the peripheral arterial bed. In addition, the inspiratory increase in venous return distends the right atrium and right ventricle; since these chambers share a tight incompressible covering with the left side of the heart, the volume of the latter declines reciprocally and the fall of left ventricular stroke volume is greater than normal.

Paradoxical pulse is less common in constrictive pericarditis than in tamponade. Furthermore, it is important to bear in mind that paradoxical pulse is not pathognomonic of pericardial disease because it may be observed in various forms of restrictive cardiomyopathies (Chap. 247) and, indeed, in some cases of severe myocardial failure, hemorrhagic shock, chronic obstructive airways disease, and severe bronchial asthma.

TREATMENT All patients with acute pericarditis should be observed frequently and carefully for the possibility of a developing effusion or, if effusion is already present, for signs of tamponade. In the presence of an effusion, arterial and venous pressures and heart rate should be monitored continuously or carefully followed and serial echocardiograms and chest roentgenograms obtained. If manifestations of tamponade appear, pericardiocentesis must be carried out at once, since relief of the intrapericardial pressure may be lifesaving.

VIRAL OR IDIOPATHIC FORM OF ACUTE PERICARDITIS This disorder is an important clinical entity because of its frequency and because it may be confused with other more serious illnesses. In some cases an A or B coxsackievirus or the virus of influenza, echovirus type 8, mumps, herpes simplex, chickenpox, or adenovirus has been isolated from pericardial fluid and/or appropriate elevations in viral antibody titers have been noted; in other instances, acute pericarditis has occurred in association with illnesses of known viral origin and, presumably, was caused by the same agent. In others there is an antecedent infection of the respiratory tract, but in many patients such an association is not evident and viral isolation and serologic studies are negative. Frequently, a viral causation cannot be established nor can it be excluded; the term *acute idiopathic pericarditis* is then appropriate. However, regardless of the specific causative factor, the clinical manifestations are similar. This form of acute pericarditis occurs at all ages but is more frequent in young adults; it is often associated with pleural effusions and pneumonitis. The appearance of fever and precordial pain at about the same time, often 10 to 12 days after a viral illness, constitutes an important feature in the differentiation of acute pericarditis from myocardial infarction, in which pain precedes fever. The constitutional symptoms are usually mild to moderate, but occasionally the initial symptoms are stormy, the temperature rising to 40 to 40.6°C (104 to 105°F). The disease ordinarily runs its course in a few days to 2 weeks, but occasionally after the patient has apparently recovered he or she may have one or several recurrences, weeks or even months later. Tamponade is unusual, although accumulation of some pericardial fluid is common, and constrictive pericarditis develops rarely. A pericardial friction rub is often audible. The ST-T wave alterations in the electrocardiogram are usually transitory, but the abnormal T waves may persist for several years or indefinitely, constituting a subsequent source of confusion in persons without a clear history of pericarditis. Pleuritis and pneumonitis frequently accompany pericarditis.

There is no specific therapy, but anti-inflammatory treatment with aspirin, if necessary up to 900 mg qid, may be given. If this is ineffective, indomethacin or corticosteroids effectively suppress the clinical manifestations of the acute illness and may be useful in patients who do not respond to supportive nonspecific therapy after the purulent and tuberculous forms of pericarditis have been excluded. Recurrences occur in about one-fourth the patients, but the tendency to relapse decreases within 2 years after the initial episode. When recurrences persist beyond this period, pericardiectomy may be effective in terminating the illness.

POST-CARDIAC INJURY SYNDROME During the past few years, it has been recognized that a number of disorders, identical in their clinical manifestations, may appear under a variety of circumstances. They have one common feature: previous injury to the myocardium, with blood in the pericardial cavity. The syndrome has been observed when the injury has been induced in the course of a cardiac operation (postpericardiotomy syndrome or, as it was originally designated, postcommissurotomy syndrome). It may also follow myocardial infarction (Dressler's syndrome) or develop after trauma of the heart (e.g., stab wound, contusions following a nonpenetrating blow

FIGURE 249-2

Simultaneous recording of electrocardiogram (ECG), blood flow velocity in the superior vena cava (SVC), brachial arterial pressure (BA), and the pneumogram (Pneumo) in a patient with cardiac compression and para- *doxical pulse. A downward deflection of the pneumogram denotes significant inspiration, when SVC blood velocity rises and arterial pressure falls (paradoxical pulse). Arterial pressure is maintained during prolonged expiratory pause.*

to the chest, and following perforation of the heart with a pacemaker catheter).

The principal symptom is pain, which usually develops after an interval of 2 to 4 weeks following the cardiac injury but sometimes appears only after a lapse of months. Recurrences are common and may occur up to 2 years or more after the injury. Fever up to 38.9 to 40°C (102 to 104°F), pericarditis, pleuritis, and pneumonitis are the outstanding features, the bout of illness usually subsiding in 1 or 2 weeks. The pericarditis, which appears to be the most constant lesion, may be of the fibrinous variety, or it may be a pericardial effusion, which is often serosanguineous and sometimes causes tamponade. Concomitantly, arthralgias, leukocytosis, an increased sedimentation rate, and typical electrocardiographic changes may occur.

The mechanism whereby the clinical manifestations are induced is not certain, but there is a likelihood that they are the result of a hypersensitivity reaction in which the antigen originates from injured myocardial tissue and/or pericardium; the suggested designation of post-cardiac injury syndrome for this group of disorders implies that they may have a common pathogenetic mechanism. Circulating autoantibodies to myocardium occur frequently, but their precise role in this syndrome has not been defined.

The clinical picture mimics acute viral or acute idiopathic pericarditis. Moreover, it is possible that the recurrences that occur so frequently in the latter condition are not always caused by an exacerbation of the original (presumably viral) infection, but that the original injury may have initiated the sequence of events that culminates in the post-cardiac injury syndrome.

Often no treatment is necessary aside from analgesics for pain. The management of pericardial effusion and tamponade has already been discussed. When the illness is severe and is followed by a series of disabling recurrences, therapy with indomethacin or corticosteroids is usually effective.

Differential diagnosis   Differential diagnosis of *acute idiopathic pericarditis* is primarily one of exclusion, as there is no specific test for this disorder. Consequently all other disorders that may be associated with acute fibrinous pericarditis must be considered. When associated with *acute myocardial infarction,* acute fibrinous pericarditis may be confused with acute viral or idiopathic pericarditis; this complication of infarction, described on page 1135, must be differentiated by the occurrence of fever, pain, and a friction rub in the first 4 days following the development of the infarct. Electrocardiographic abnormalities (such as the appearance of Q waves and earlier T-wave changes in myocardial infarction), the extent of the elevations of myocardial enzymes, and the total clinical picture are helpful in the identification of the pericarditis of acute myocardial infarction. A common error is assuming that acute viral or idiopathic pericarditis represents acute myocardial infarction.

Acute pericarditis occurring as a component of the *post-cardiac injury* syndrome is most likely to be confused with acute idiopathic pericarditis when it follows myocardial infarction or a nonpenetrating bruise to the chest. Such pericarditis is differentiated from acute idiopathic pericarditis chiefly by timing. If it occurs within a few weeks of an infarction or a chest blow, concluding that the two are probably related is justified. If the infarct has been silent or the chest blow forgotten, the relationship to the pericarditis may not be recognized.

It is important to distinguish *pericarditis due to collagen disease* from acute idiopathic pericarditis. Most important in the differential diagnosis is the pericarditis due to systemic lupus erythematosus (Chap. 68). Sometimes it appears as an asymptomatic effusion; more often pain is present, and rarely tamponade develops. Very rarely, when pericarditis occurs in the absence of other evidence of the underlying disorder, differentiation from acute viral and idiopathic pericarditis or tuberculous pericarditis may be made on discovery of lupus erythematosus (LE) cells, a rise in antinuclear antibodies, or by the specific methods for diagnosing tuberculosis. Acute pericarditis is also an occasional complication of *rheumatoid arthritis, scleroderma,* and *periarteritis nodosa,* but again, other evidence of these diseases is usually obvious. Asymptomatic pericardial effusion is also frequent in these disorders. It is important to question every patient with acute pericarditis about the ingestion of *procainamide* and *hydralazine,* both of which can cause this syndrome.

The pericarditis of *acute rheumatic fever* is generally associated with evidence of severe pancarditis and with cardiac murmurs. *Pyogenic (purulent) pericarditis* is usually secondary to cardiothoracic operations, immunosuppressive therapy, rupture of the esophagus into the pericardial sac, and rupture of a ring abscess in a patient with infective endocarditis. It is now uncommonly due to pneumococcal pneumonia and pleuritis or staphylococcal septicemia. *Uremic pericarditis* is a common finding in patients with uremia. It may be fibrinous or associated with a serous or bloody effusion. A friction rub is common; pain and tamponade are unusual. Pericarditis due to *neoplastic diseases* results from mediastinal irradiation or extension of primary or metastatic tumors (most commonly carcinoma of the lung and breast, malignant melanoma, and lymphomas) to the pericardium or from invasion by a lymphomatous or leukemic process; pain, atrial arrhythmias, and tamponade are complications which occur occasionally. Unusual causes of acute pericarditis include syphilis, fungous infection (actinomycosis, histoplasmosis, coccidioidomycosis), and parasitic infestation (amebiasis, toxoplasmosis, echinococcosis, trichinosis).

TUBERCULOUS PERICARDIAL EFFUSION   Tuberculous involvement of the pericardium may present as an acute fibrinous pericarditis, but more frequently it presents as a chronic pericardial effusion. With the acute form, the history of precordial pain is inconstant and there may be no other evidence of tuberculosis (Chap. 143). The symptoms are those of a chronic, systemic illness in an individual with effusion. It is important to bear this condition in mind when a middle-aged or elderly person with fever has an apparent enlargement of the heart of undetermined origin, with or without congestive failure. Weight loss, fever, and fatigability are sometimes observed. Inasmuch as effective specific methods of therapy have now reduced strikingly the mortality rate from the previous figures of about 70 percent, overlooking a tuberculous pericardial effusion is a serious error. Consequently, no method of examination should be omitted to establish this diagnosis. Included are chest roentgenograms for pulmonary tuberculosis and a search for tuberculosis in other organs; tuberculin skin tests, repeated after several weeks; cultures and smears of gastric washings and of pleural and pericardial fluid. Finally, if the diagnosis is still obscure, a pericardial biopsy, preferably by a limited thoracotomy, should be performed after 1 or 2 weeks of preliminary antituberculous chemotherapy. If definitive evidence is then still lacking, but the specimen shows caseation necrosis, continuous antituberculous chemotherapy for at least 24 months is justified (Chap. 143). Pericardiectomy should be carried out in order to prevent the development of constriction if the biopsy specimen shows a thickened pericardium.

Differential diagnosis of chronic pericardial effusion   *Tuberculosis* is the most common cause of chronic pericardial effusion.

Myxedema may be responsible for a pericardial effusion that is sometimes massive. The other manifestations of myxedema should clarify the diagnosis, but unfortunately, even when they are present the diagnosis is frequently overlooked. It is important, therefore, to carry out appropriate tests for thyroid function (Chap. 335) in patients with an enlarged cardiac outline of undetermined origin.

Neoplasms, systemic lupus erythematosus, rheumatoid arthritis, mycotic infection, radiation therapy, pyogenic infections, severe chronic anemia, chylopericardium, and cholesterol deposits may also cause chronic pericardial effusion.

Aspiration and analysis of the pericardial fluid may often be helpful in diagnosis. In infections the organism can be identified by smear or on culture. Grossly sanguineous pericardial fluid results most commonly from a neoplasm, tuberculosis, or slow leakage from an aortic aneurysm.

CHRONIC CONSTRICTIVE PERICARDITIS

This disorder results when the healing of an acute fibrinous or serofibrinous pericarditis is followed by obliteration of the pericardial cavity, with the formation of granulation tissue which gradually contracts and forms a firm scar, encasing the heart and interfering with filling of the ventricles. In some reports, a high percentage of all cases has been of tuberculous origin. In other series, particularly those reported in the last decade, tuberculosis has been an infrequent cause. The condition also may follow purulent infection, trauma, radiation, histoplasmosis, neoplastic disease, and acute viral or idiopathic pericarditis, rheumatoid arthritis, lupus erythematosus, and chronic renal failure with uremia treated by chronic dialysis. In many patients the cause of the pericardial disease is undetermined. Rarely, routine fluoroscopic or radiographic examination may reveal calcification of the pericardium in a person who is free of all symptoms referable to the heart.

The basic physiological abnormality in symptomatic patients with chronic constrictive pericarditis, as in those with cardiac tamponade, is the inability of the ventricles to fill adequately during diastole because of the limitations imposed by the rigid, thickened pericardium or the tense pericardial fluid. Stroke volume is diminished, and the end-diastolic pressures in both ventricles, as well as the mean pressures in the atria, pulmonic veins, and systemic veins, are elevated to about the same levels. Despite these hemodynamic changes myocardial function may be normal; instead, the ventricles may be considered to be underloaded. In some instances fibrous obliteration of the pericardium is associated with myocardial fibrosis and impairment of left ventricular function. In constrictive pericarditis the central venous and right and left atrial pressure pulses display an M-shaped contour, with sharp *a* and *v* waves and *x* and *y* descents; the *y* descent is the most prominent deflection and is interrupted by a rapid rise in pressure during early diastole, when ventricular filling is impeded by the constricting pericardium. In cardiac tamponade the pressure contour differs in that the most prominent deflection is the *x* trough, while the *y* descent is usually absent. These characteristic changes are transmitted to the jugular veins, where they may be recorded or recognized by inspection. In constrictive pericarditis, but not in cardiac tamponade, both ventricular pressure pulses exhibit characteristic "square root" signs during diastole. These hemodynamic changes, although characteristic, are not pathognomonic of constrictive pericarditis but are also observed in cardiomyopathies characterized by restriction of ventricular filling, as discussed on page 1143.

CLINICAL FINDINGS IN PERICARDIAL CONSTRICTION

Weakness, fatigue, weight loss, and anorexia are common symptoms. The patients often appear to be chronically ill with decreased muscle mass, protuberant abdomen, and peripheral edema. Contrary to a widely held impression, dyspnea, though absent or minimal at rest, is often present on exertion, and orthopnea is commonly present in chronic constrictive pericarditis, although it is not severe. Attacks of acute left ventricular failure (acute pulmonary edema) practically never occur. The cervical veins are distended and remain so even after intensive diuretic treatment, and in about one-third of the cases a paradoxical pulse may be observed; this may be associated with increased inspiratory venous distention (Kussmaul's sign). Congestive hepatomegaly is pronounced and may impair hepatic function; ascites is common and is more prominent than dependent edema. In about half the patients, the heart is normal in size; if it is enlarged, the enlargement is rarely extreme. The apical pulse is reduced in intensity. The heart sounds may be distant, an early third heart sound, i.e., a pericardial knock, occurring 0.06 to 0.12 s after aortic valve closure, is often conspicuous, and murmurs are usually absent. The apex beat is poorly defined, and cardiac pulsations under fluoroscopic examination are diminished. Because of the high sustained venous pressure, congestive splenomegaly may be sufficiently pronounced to make the spleen palpable. In the absence of evidence of bacterial endocarditis or tricuspid valve disease, splenomegaly in a patient with congestive heart failure should arouse suspicion of constrictive pericarditis. Protein-losing gastroenteropathy due to impaired lymphatic drainage from the small intestine, and the nephrotic syndrome or sometimes only marked proteinuria or hypoalbuminemia, may complicate chronic constrictive pericarditis. The electrocardiogram frequently displays low voltage of the QRS complex and flattening or inversion of the T waves in most leads; P mitrale is frequently found in patients with sinus rhythm; atrial fibrillation is present in about one-third of these patients.

Systemic and/or pulmonary venous congestion is initially the result of impaired filling of the ventricles caused by the restrictive action of the inelastic pericardium. However, the fibrotic process may extend into the myocardium, and venous congestion may then be due to the combined effects of the myocardial and pericardial lesions. The interference with filling reduces the work of the heart and perhaps this leads to myocardial atrophy. The latter probably accounts for the delayed beneficial effects of operative treatment.

Inasmuch as the usual physical signs of cardiac disease (murmurs, cardiac enlargement) may be inconspicuous or entirely lacking, hepatic enlargement and dysfunction associated with intractable ascites may lead to a mistaken diagnosis of cirrhosis of the liver. This error should be avoided if the neck veins are inspected carefully in all patients with ascites and hepatomegaly. *Given a clinical picture resembling that of cirrhosis, but with the added feature of distended neck veins, careful search for calcification of the pericardium by chest roentgenograms should be carried out and may disclose a curable or remediable form of heart disease.* Calcification occurs in only about one-half of these patients and usually never in those that are not of long-standing. Therefore, surgical exploration of the pericardium is justifiable if the clinical picture and cardiac catheterization findings are suggestive even in the absence of pericardial calcification.

DIFFERENTIAL DIAGNOSIS Like cor pulmonable (Chap. 246), chronic constrictive pericarditis may be associated with severe systemic venous hypertension but with little or no pulmonary congestion; the heart may not appear to be enlarged, and a striking inspiratory fall in arterial pressure may be present. However, in contrast to constrictive pericarditis, in cor pulmonale there is also an inspiratory fall in venous pressure, and advanced parenchymal pulmonary disease is evident. *Tricuspid stenosis* may also simulate the picture of chronic constrictive pericarditis; congestive hepatomegaly and ascites may be equally prominent, and the manifestations of left-sided heart failure may be inconspicuous. However, in tricuspid stenosis, the characteristic murmur, the frequent presence of mitral stenosis, the absence of a paradoxic pulse, as well as the absence, in the jugular venous pulse, of the steep, deep *y* descent followed by a rapid ascent (manifested by the diastolic shock on palpation and its audible equivalent, the pericardial knock), should make the clinical differentiation possible.

It is of the greatest importance, though often difficult, to distinguish chronic constrictive pericarditis from various forms of heart disease which are characterized by a similar physiologic abnormality, i.e., restriction of ventricular filling, leading to a similar clinical picture. Described in Chap. 247, these include endomyocardial fibrosis, infiltrative cardiomyopathies such as amyloidosis, hemochromatosis, sarcoidosis, scleroderma and idiopathic myocardial hypertrophy, in which the marked thickening of the ventricular wall is responsible for the diminished compliance.

The features favoring the diagnosis of one of the above forms of cardiomyopathy are a well-defined apex beat, conspicuous enlargement of the heart, and pronounced orthopnea with attacks of acute left ventricular failure, left ventricular preponderance, bundle branch block, or significant Q waves in the electrocardiogram. At catheterization, patients with chronic constrictive pericarditis usually are found to have left atrial or pulmonary arterial wedge pressure equaling right atrial pressure, the latter often exceeding 15 mmHg following intensive medical treatment for heart failure; the pulmonary artery systolic pressure is often less than 50 mmHg, and the right ventricular end-diastolic pressure often reaches one-third of the systolic pressure; the cardiac output is slightly depressed. In contrast, in patients with cardiomyopathy, the left atrial usually exceeds the right atrial pressures by at least 10 mmHg, the mean right atrial pressure usually falls to below 15 mmHg following treatment, the pulmonary artery systolic pressure often exceeds 50 mmHg, and the right ventricular end-diastolic pressure is usually less than one-third the systolic pressure, while the cardiac output is markedly depressed. The volumes of the right and left ventricular cavities, as determined angiocardiographically (Chap. 234), are characteristically reduced or normal in constrictive pericarditis, and the ejection fractions are normal; the left ventricular end-diastolic volume may be normal in some cardiomyopathies but is frequently elevated in others, in whom the ejection fraction is reduced; the latter finding militates strongly against the diagnosis of constrictive pericarditis. The echocardiogram in chronic constrictive pericarditis characteristically shows pericardial thickening, i.e., a distinct echo posterior to the left ventricular wall and paradoxical septal motion. The left ventricular wall moves sharply outward in early diastole and then remains flat. The left ventricular cavity is small.

The lesson to be learned is that when a patient has progressive, disabling, and unresponsive congestive failure, and if he or she displays any of the phenomena of constrictive heart disease, the most careful and detailed clinical and laboratory studies must be carried out in order to detect or exclude constrictive pericarditis. In many instances cardiac catheterization, selective angiocardiography, and coronary arteriography may be required. However, when even these examinations do not yield a definitive diagnosis, the only decisive method of determining whether constrictive pericarditis is responsible for

the clinical manifestations of heart failure is by surgical exploration of the pericardium.

Occult constrictive disease Patients with this condition may have unexplained fatigue, dyspnea, and chest pain. No overt manifestations of pericardial disease are present, but following the rapid intravenous infusion of 1 liter of saline solution, atrial and ventricular pressure pulses and diastolic equilibration of intracardiac pressures, as in overt constrictive pericarditis, occur. Symptomatic improvement follows pericardiectomy.

TREATMENT Surgery is the only definitive treatment of constrictive pericarditis, but diuretic drugs and sodium restriction are useful during preoperative preparation for pericardial resection. Digitalis may be beneficial in the prevention of heart failure when resection of the thickened pericardium permits an increased inflow into the ventricles and hence an enhanced burden on an atrophic myocardium. The benefits derived from a complete cardiac decortication are often striking, and frequently the improvement, though slight at first, is progressive over a period of many months.

Many instances of constrictive pericarditis are of tuberculous origin. Antituberculous therapy during the phase of effusion may prevent the development of constriction, and such therapy should be carried out before and after operation, if a tuberculous origin is suspected or cannot be excluded in a patient with chronic constrictive pericarditis (Chap. 143).

SUBACUTE EFFUSIVE-CONSTRICTIVE PERICARDITIS This form of pericardial disease is characterized by tense effusion into a free pericardial space, as well as by constriction of the heart by the visceral pericardium, and thus it shares a number of features both with pericardial effusion producing cardiac compression and with pericardial constriction. It may be caused by tuberculosis, multiple attacks of acute idiopathic pericarditis, radiation, traumatic pericarditis, uremia, and scleroderma. The heart is generally enlarged, there are a paradoxical pulse and a prominent *x* descent in the atrial pressure pulse, and the atrial pressure may remain elevated even after pericardiocentesis. In many patients the condition progresses to the chronic constrictive form of the disease. Wide excision of both the visceral and parietal pericardium is usually effective.

OTHER DISORDERS OF THE PERICARDIUM

Pericardial cysts appear as rounded or lobulated deformities of the cardiac silhouette, most commonly at the right cardiophrenic angle. They do not cause symptoms, and their major clinical significance lies in the possibility of confusion with a tumor, ventricular aneurysm, or massive cardiomegaly. *Tumors* involving the pericardium are most commonly secondary to malignant neoplasms originating in or invading the mediastinum, including carcinoma of the bronchus and breast, lymphoma, and melanoma. The most common *primary* malignant tumor is the mesothelioma. The usual clinical picture of malignant pericardial tumor is an insidiously developing, often bloody, pericardial effusion. Surgical exploration is required to establish a definitive diagnosis and to carry out definitive or palliative treatment.

REFERENCES

BUSH CA et al: Occult pericardial disease. Circulation 56:924, 1977

EBERT PA: The pericardium, in *Gibbon's Surgery of the Chest,* 3d ed, DC Sabiston, FC Spencer (eds). Philadelphia, Saunders, 1976

FOWLER NO (ed): Pericardial disease, in *Cardiac Diagnosis and Treatment,* 2d ed. New York, Harper & Row, 1976, chap 44, p 858

HANCOCK EW: Subacute effusive-constrictive pericarditis. Circulation 43:183, 1971

HIRSCHMANN JV: Pericardial constriction. Am Heart J 96:110, 1978

IKRAM H et al: Clinical features of nontuberculous constrictive pericarditis. Thorax 29:204, 1974

LEWIS BS, GOTSMAN MS: Left ventricular function in systole and diastole in constrictive pericarditis. Am Heart J 86:23, 1973

MARTIN RG et al: Radiation-related pericarditis. Am J Cardiol 35:216, 1975

ROBERTS WC, SPRAY TL: Pericardial heart disease. Curr Probl Cardiol, vol 2, no 3, 1977

SPODICK DH (ed): *Pericardial Diseases (Cardiovascular Clinics).* Philadelphia, Davis, 1976, p 297

section 2 | **Disorders of the vascular system**

250

ATHEROSCLEROSIS AND OTHER FORMS OF ARTERIOSCLEROSIS

EDWIN L. BIERMAN

Arteriosclerosis, a generic term for thickening and hardening of the arterial wall, is responsible for the majority of deaths in the United States and most westernized societies. One type of arteriosclerosis is *atherosclerosis,* the disorder of the larger arteries that underlies most *coronary artery disease, aortic aneurysm,* and *arterial disease of the lower extremities* and also plays a major role in *cerebrovascular disease.* Atherosclerosis is by far the leading cause of death in the United States, both above and below age 65 (Table 250-1).

Other types of arteriosclerosis include focal calcific arteriosclerosis (*Mönckeberg's arteriosclerosis*) and *arteriolosclerosis.* The major arterial diseases other than arteriosclerosis include *congenital structural defects, inflammatory* or *granulomatous* diseases (e.g., syphilitic aortitis), and disorders affecting mainly the smaller vessels, such as *hypersensitivity* or autoimmune diseases.

TABLE 250-1
Deaths, by cause, in the United States, 1976

	No. of deaths, thousands			
	Below age 65		Age 65 and above	
Causes of death	Male	Female	Male	Female
All causes	427	237	625	620
All cardiovascular diseases	150	63	362	399
Ischemic heart disease	113	36	248	249
Cerebrovascular disease	16	14	65	94
Hypertensive disease*	2	2	5	8
All infectious disease	4	4	4	4
All cancer	81	71	124	101
Accidents	58	19	13	11

* *A substantial proportion of deaths of hypertensive persons occurs with ischemic heart disease or cerebrovascular disease; such deaths are classified in those categories.*
SOURCE: *Vital Statistics of the United States, 1976, vol II: Mortality. Division of Vital Statistics, National Center for Health Statistics.*

THE NORMAL ARTERY

STRUCTURE   The normal artery wall consists of three reasonably well-defined layers: the intima, the media, and the adventitia.

Intima   A single continuous layer of *endothelial cells* lines the lumen of all arteries. The intima is delimited on its outer aspect by a perforated tube of elastic tissue, the *internal elastic lamina.* This tube of elastic tissue is particularly prominent in the large elastic arteries and the medium-caliber muscular arteries, and it disappears in capillaries. The endothelial cells are attached to one another by a series of junctional complexes and are also attached, apparently somewhat tenuously, to an underlying meshwork of loose connective tissue, the *basal lamina.* These lining endothelial cells normally form a barrier that controls the entry of substances from the blood into the artery wall. Such substances usually enter the cells by specific transport systems. Normally, no other cell type is present in the intima of most arteries.

Media   The media consists of only one cell type, the *smooth-muscle cell,* arranged in either a single layer (as in small muscular arteries) or multiple lamellae (as in elastic arteries). These cells are surrounded by small amounts of collagen and elastic fibers, which they elaborate, and usually take the pattern of diagonal concentric spirals through the vessel wall. They are closely apposed to one another and may be attached by junctional complexes. The smooth-muscle cell appears to be the major connective tissue forming cell of the artery wall, producing collagen, elastic fibers, and proteoglycans (mucopolysaccharides). In that sense it is analogous to the fibroblast in skin, the osteoblast in bone, and the chondroblast in cartilage. The media is bounded on the luminal side by the internal elastic lamina and on the abluminal side by a less continuous sheet of elastic tissue, the *external elastic lamina.* In conducting or *elastic arteries,* like the aorta and the major pulmonary arteries, elastic lamellae are prominent. Such arteries expand and increase their elastic tension with the pulse of systole. In diastole, the elastic fibers recoil, helping to propel the blood distally and progressively dampening the pulsatile character of flow toward more terminal vessels. In distributing or *muscular arteries,* in which smooth-muscle cells predominate, peripheral flow is regulated, particularly in arterioles, by contraction (vasoconstriction) and relaxation (vasodilatation). Located about midway through the media of most arteries is a "nutritional water-shed." The outer portion is nourished from the small blood vessels (vasa vasorum) in the adventitia; the inner layers receive their nutrients from the lumen.

Adventitia The outermost layer of the artery is the adventitia, which is delimited on the luminal aspect by the external elastic lamina. This external coat consists of a loose interwoven admixture of thick bundles of collagen, elastic fibers of varying size, and a mixture of smooth-muscle cells and fibroblasts. This layer also contains the vasa vasorum and nerves.

METABOLISM AND FUNCTION The artery wall is a metabolically active organ that must meet a steady demand for energy production to maintain smooth-muscle tension and endothelial cell function, and to repair and replenish tissue constituents. Arteries are subjected to constant stresses and demands throughout life. They are conduits that must withstand the passage of a complex viscous suspension under high pressure. Their shape and internal diameter not only vary along the length of the vessel, but change cyclically with pulsatile flow. The mechanical forces on the arterial wall are complex, and considerable tensile stresses are imposed on it, mainly by hydraulic force. Shear or frictional stresses are especially prominent near the entrance regions of branches. The form and manner in which these forces are dissipated depend upon flow, the amount of elastic tension developed, and the tethering or external support provided by surrounding structures. Arteries are also permeable pipes, which constantly exchange fluid and solutes with the blood they carry.

Maintenance of the endothelial cell lining is critical. Endothelial cell turnover occurs at a slow rate but may be accelerated in focal areas by changing patterns of flow along the vessel wall. When intact, these cells selectively control the passage of circulating substances by active transport (endocytosis and exocytosis) through their cytoplasm and elaborate connecting tissue components to form their own substratum. In addition, intact endothelial cells function to prevent clotting partly by elaboration of a particular prostaglandin (prostacyclin or PGI_2) that inhibits platelet function, thereby enhancing unimpeded flow of blood. When the lining is damaged, platelets adhere to it, in part as the result of production of a different class of prostaglandins, the thromboxanes, and form a clot; endothelial cells function in the clotting process by elaboration of key substances, including factor VIII.

What is known about the metabolism of arteries in large part reflects the biochemistry of smooth-muscle cells. Recent studies of these cells in tissue culture under conditions in which they retain their differentiated phenotype have helped elucidate their metabolism and function. Arterial smooth-muscle cells form abundant collagen, elastic fibers, soluble and insoluble elastin, and glucosaminoglycans (mainly dermatan sulfate). Multiple anabolic and catabolic pathways are present. These cells metabolize glucose by both anaerobic and aerobic glycolysis. A variety of catabolic enzymes are present including fibrinolysins and lysosomal hydrolases. Because of the prominence of lipids in atherosclerotic lesions, much attention has been directed to lipid metabolism in arteries. Arterial wall cells can synthesize fatty acids, cholesterol, phospholipids, and triglycerides from endogenous substrates to satisfy their structural needs (membrane replenishment), but smooth-muscle cells appear preferentially to utilize lipids from plasma lipoproteins transported into the wall. Circulating lipoproteins traverse endothelial cells in pinocytotic vesicles. Smooth-muscle cells possess specific high-affinity surface receptors for certain apoproteins on the surface of lipid-rich lipoproteins, thus facilitating the entry of lipoproteins into the cell by adsorptive endocytosis. As has been shown for cultured skin fibroblasts, in

arterial smooth-muscle cells these vesicles fuse with lysosomes, resulting in catabolism of lipoprotein components (Chap. 100). Free cholesterol entering the cell in this manner inhibits endogenous cholesterol synthesis, facilitates its own esterification, and partially limits further entry of cholesterol by regulating the number of lipoprotein receptors.

Thus, many complex and interrelated metabolic processes are present in arterial wall cells. Although some of these may play a role in the production of arteriosclerosis, no one biochemical reaction can be singled out as culpable. Physiological factors, such as transfer processes across the endothelial lining, the flux of oxygen and substrates from both the luminal and adventitial sides of the wall, and the reverse flow of catabolic products, need to be considered as well. The ability of the arterial wall to maintain the integrity of its endothelium, prevent platelet aggregation, and ensure the nutrition of its middle portion may be the critical determinants of the arteriosclerotic process.

CHANGES WITH AGING The major change that occurs with normal aging in the arterial wall in humans is a slow, apparently continuous, symmetrical increase in the thickness of the intima. This intimal thickening results from a gradual accumulation of smooth-muscle cells (presumably resulting from migration of these cells from the media and their subsequent proliferation), surrounded by additional connective tissue. In the nondiseased artery wall, the lipid content, mainly cholesterol ester and phospholipid (particularly sphingomyelin), also progressively increases with age. Phospholipid synthesis rises with aging (perhaps in response to the need for more membrane formation for plasma membranes, vesicles, lysosomes, and other intracellular organelles) followed by a compensatory increase in activity of all phospholipases except sphingomyelinase. While most of the phospholipid in the normal artery wall appears to be derived from in situ synthesis, the cholesterol ester that accumulates with aging appears to be derived from plasma, since it contains principally linoleic acid, the major plasma cholesterol ester fatty acid. Furthermore, low-density lipoproteins (LDL) are immunologically detectable in the intima of normal arteries in direct relation to their concentration in plasma. It has been estimated that between the second and sixth decade, the normal intima accumulates approximately 10 mg cholesterol per gram of tissue. Thus, as the normal artery ages, smooth-muscle cells and connective tissue accumulate diffusely in the intima, leading to progressive thickening of this layer, coupled with progressive accumulation of sphingomyelin and cholesterol linoleate. This diffuse age-related intimal thickening is to be distinguished from focal discrete raised fibromuscular plaques, a characteristic feature of atherosclerosis.

Functionally, these changes with aging result in gradual increasing rigidity of vessels. The larger arteries may become dilated, elongated, and tortuous, and aneurysms may form in areas of an encroaching degenerating arteriosclerotic plaque. Such "wear-and-tear" changes are frequently proportional to the vessel diameter and correlated with branching, curvature, and anatomic points of attachment. The amount of external support also determines the ability of vessels, weakened by loss of elasticity, to withstand hydrostatic pressure. The unsupported cerebral arteries may be particularly vulnerable in this regard. Although senescence is accompanied by the intimal thickening that is a feature of localized atheromatosis, the changes of aging and arteriosclerosis appear to be separate and distinct processes.

NONATHEROMATOUS FORMS OF ARTERIOSCLEROSIS

Atherosclerosis involves primarily the intimal layer and occurs most commonly in the abdominal aorta and its large renal and lower extremity branches, the coronary arteries and the cerebral vasculature. It may accompany or accelerate the other major forms of arteriosclerosis, *focal calcification* and *arteriolosclerosis*.

FOCAL CALCIFICATION   Not to be confused with atherosclerosis is focal calcification of the media, particularly in the medium-sized muscular arteries. This type of arteriosclerosis is called *Mönckeberg's sclerosis* and is common in the lower extremities, upper extremities, and the arterial supply of the genital tract in both sexes. This disorder is rare in individuals below age 50 and affects both sexes indiscriminately. The process involves degeneration of smooth-muscle cells, followed by calcium deposition. The vessels become hard and tortuous, so that palpable vessels such as the radial artery can be felt as rigid tubes. The medial changes alone do not narrow the lumen, have little effect on the circulation, and have relatively little clinical significance. However, in the lower extremities, medial sclerosis is often associated with atherosclerosis, leading to arterial occlusion. These changes are common in the elderly, but in individuals with diabetes mellitus, focal calcification may be accelerated and severe.

ARTERIOLOSCLEROSIS   This disorder involves hyaline and degenerative changes affecting both the intima and media of small arteries and arterioles, particularly in the spleen, pancreas, adrenal, and kidney. In the kidney, but not necessarily elsewhere, arteriolosclerosis is almost invariably associated with hypertension. Lesser degrees of sustained hypertension characteristically cause *hyalinization* of renal arterioles; more severe or malignant hypertension produces a typical *fibrous and elastic hyperplasia,* and even necrosis, of the media and intima.

ATHEROSCLEROSIS (See Table 250-2)

HISTORY   Although a scourge of modern industrialized civilizations, atherosclerosis is an ancient disease that has been detected in Egyptian mummies and described in Greek writings. The term *atheroma* (from the Greek *athere,* "gruel") was re-

TABLE 250-2
Disorders associated with early arteriosclerosis

ATHEROSCLEROSIS

Diabetes mellitus
Hypertension
Familial hypercholesterolemia
Familial combined hyperlipidemia
Broad beta disease
Hypothyroidism
Werner's syndrome
Cholesterol ester storage disease

NONATHEROMATOUS ARTERIOSCLEROSIS

Diabetes mellitus
Chronic renal insufficiency
Chronic vitamin D intoxication
Pseudoxanthoma elasticum
Idiopathic arterial calcification in infancy
Werner's syndrome
Homocystinuria

vived by Albrecht von Haller of Bern (1755) to focus attention on the softening process which often accompanies the sclerosis and the aneurysms that had been emphasized earlier by da Vinci and then by Vesalius and other anatomists of the sixteenth and seventeenth centuries. For a time in the nineteenth century, it was believed that imbibition of substances from the blood (Virchow) or other events at the endothelial-blood interface might cause atheromas (Rokitansky); but by the time the term *atherosclerosis* was coined (Marchand, 1904), the dominant concept was that the lesions were intimal softenings secondary to an increase in subintimal connective tissue that in turn was due to irritative or mechanical forces. The present-day preoccupation with the etiologic importance of lipid infiltration began about 1910, with the demonstration of an increased amount of cholesterol in atheromas (Windhaus, Aschoff) and the experimental production of atherosclerosis by feeding cholesterol (Ignatowski, Anitschkow, and others). Many of the present assumptions about the causes of atherosclerosis are derived from epidemiologic observations based on the occurrence of the complications of the disease.

LESIONS   Morbid anatomy   Atherosclerosis is a patchy nodular type of arteriosclerosis. The lesions are commonly classified as *fatty streaks, fibrous plaques,* and *complicated lesions.* Fatty streaks may be the earliest lesions of atherosclerosis and are characterized by an accumulation of lipid-filled smooth-muscle cells (foam cells) and fibrous tissue in focal areas of the intima. They are stained distinctly by fat-soluble dyes, but may be visible without staining as yellowish or whitish patches on the intimal surface. The lipid is mainly cholesterol oleate, partly derived from synthesis in situ. The fatty streak is usually sessile and causes little obstruction and no symptoms. The lesion is universal, appearing in various segments of the arterial tree at different ages beginning in the aorta in infancy. In all children, regardless of race, sex, or environment, fatty streaks are present in the aorta by age 10 and increase to occupy as much as 30 to 50 percent of the aortic surface by age 25, but they do not appear to extend further with aging. Despite a presumed relation between fatty streaks and fibrous atherosclerotic plaques, aortic fatty streaks are not correlated with the location and extent of fibrous lesions. In the coronary arteries, the extent of fatty streaks may be a better indicator of the development of clinically significant raised lesions later in life. They are usually observed by age 15 and continue to involve more surface area with increasing age. Fatty streaks in the cerebral arteries are also present in all populations, develop during the third and fourth decade, and are more extensive in those populations having a higher incidence of cerebrovascular disease. It is generally believed that fatty streaks may be reversible, but the evidence is inconclusive.

Fibrous plaques, also called raised lesions or pearly plaques, are palpably elevated areas of intimal thickening and represent the most characteristic lesion of advancing atherosclerosis. They do not share with fatty streaks the ubiquitous distribution among populations. These plaques first appear in the abdominal aorta, coronary arteries, and carotid arteries in the third decade and increase progressively with age. They appear in men before women, in the aorta before the coronary arteries, and much later in the vertebral and intracranial cerebral arteries. Reasons for the difference in susceptibility of various segments of the arterial tree and the nonuniform distribution of lesions are not known. Typically, the fibrous plaque is firm, elevated, and dome-shaped, with an opaque glistening surface that bulges outward into the lumen. It consists of a central core of extracellular lipid and necrotic cell debris ("gruel") covered by a fibromuscular layer or cap containing large numbers of smooth-muscle cells and collagen. Thus the plaque is much thicker than normal intima. Although the lipid, like that of fatty streaks, is mainly cholesterol ester, linoleic rather than oleic is the principal esterified fatty acid. Thus plaque cholesterol ester composition differs from fatty streaks but resembles plasma lipoproteins.

The *complicated lesion* is a calcified fibrous plaque containing various degrees of necrosis, thrombosis, and ulceration. These are the lesions frequently associated with symptoms. With increasing necrosis and accumulation of gruel, the arterial wall progressively weakens, and rupture of the intima can occur, causing aneurysm and hemorrhage. Arterial emboli can form when fragments of plaque dislodge into the lumen. Stenosis and impaired organ function result from gradual occlusion as plaques thicken and thrombi form.

Localization Although the term "generalized atherosclerosis" is commonly used clinically, lesions are actually irregularly distributed; different vessels are involved at different ages and to varying degrees. The aorta, especially its abdominal portion, is involved earliest and most severely by atherosclerotic lesions, and it is the bellweather of lesions elsewhere. The *aorta* is usually most heavily involved in its abdominal portion, about the orifices of its branches, particularly at the level of the coronary and intercostal arteries, in the aortic arch, and frequently at its bifurcation into the iliac arteries. There is more atherosclerosis in the lower than in the upper limbs. In the legs, the incidence decreases peripherally, as the musculoelastic vessels give way to large muscular arteries and these become smaller vessels, such as the plantar or digital arteries. Plaques and thrombosis are particularly common in the *femoral* artery, in Hunter's canal, and in the *popliteal* artery just above the knee joint. The *anterior* and *posterior tibial* arteries are often occluded together, but in different sites—the posterior where it rounds the internal malleolus and the anterior where it is superficial and becomes the dorsalis pedis artery. The peroneal artery, which is well embedded in muscle, often escapes when other major vessels are occluded, and it may be the main blood supply to the extremity (*peroneal leg*). Atherosclerosis in abdominal branches, except for the renal and mesenteric arteries, causes less difficulty than in coronary and cerebral vessels.

In the *coronary arteries,* raised lesions are most prominent in the main stems, the highest incidence being a short distance beyond the ostia. Atherosclerosis is nearly always found in the epicardial (extramural) portions of the vessels, while the intramural coronary arteries are spared. Coronary atherosclerosis is often diffuse. The degree to which the lumen is narrowed varies, but once the process is present, all the intima of the extramural portions of the vessel is usually involved. A single tiny plaque occluding an otherwise normal coronary artery is rare. In the cervical and cerebral arteries the distribution of atherosclerosis is patchy, as it may be in other arteries. It first appears in the base of the brain in the carotid, basilar, and vertebral arteries. The proximal portion of the internal carotids in the neck is a site of special predilection. There is a concentration of lesions near bifurcations. Atherosclerosis in the *pulmonary artery* bears no relation to the severity of the disease in the aorta or other systemic arteries. There is some involvement in about half of adults over 50 years of age who have no reason to have pulmonary hypertension. Pulmonary hypertension per se, however, is associated with medial hypertrophy, intimal thickening, and great acceleration of atheroma formation.

THEORIES OF ATHEROGENESIS One generally accepted theory for the pathogenesis of atherosclerosis consistent with a variety of experimental evidence is the *reaction to injury* hypothesis. According to this idea the endothelial cells lining the intima are exposed to repeated or continuing insults to their integrity. The injury to the endothelium may be subtle or

gross, resulting in a loss of the ability of the cells to attach to one another and to the underlying connective tissue. The cells then become susceptible to the shearing stress of the blood flow and they may desquamate. Examples of types of "injury" to the endothelium include chemical injury, as in chronic hypercholesterolemia or homocystinemia, mechanical stress associated with hypertension, and immunologic injury, as may be seen after cardiac or renal transplantation. Loss of endothelial cells at susceptible sites in the arterial tree would lead to exposure of the subendothelial tissue to increased concentrations of plasma constituents, and a sequence of events including platelet adherence, platelet aggregation and formation of microthrombi, and release of platelet granular components, including a potent mitogenic factor. This platelet factor, in conjunction with other plasma constituents, including lipoproteins and hormones such as insulin, could stimulate both the migration of medial smooth-muscle cells into the intima and their proliferation at these sites of injury. These proliferating smooth-muscle cells would deposit a connective tissue matrix and accumulate lipid, a process that would be particularly enhanced with hyperlipidemia. Thus repeated or chronic injury could lead to a slowly progressing lesion involving a gradual increase in smooth-muscle cells, connective tissue, and lipid. Areas where the shearing stress on endothelial cells is increased, such as branch points or bifurcation of vessels, would be at greater risk. As the lesions progress and the intima becomes thicker, blood flow over the sites will be altered and potentially place the lining endothelial cells at even greater risk for further injury, leading to an inexorable cycle of events culminating in the complicated lesion. However, a single or a few injurious episodes may lead to a proliferative response that could regress, in contrast to continued or chronic injury. This reaction to injury hypothesis thus is consistent with the known intimal thickening observed during normal aging, would explain how many of the etiologic factors implicated in atherogenesis might enhance lesion formation, might explain how inhibitors of platelet aggregation could interfere with lesion formation, and fosters some optimism regarding the possibility of interrupting progression, or even producing regression of these lesions.

Other theories of atherogenesis are not mutually exclusive. The *monoclonal hypothesis* suggests, on the basis of single isoenzyme types found in lesions, that the intimal proliferative lesions result from the multiplication of single individual smooth-muscle cells, as do benign tumors. In this manner, factors that might stimulate smooth-muscle cell proliferation would act on single cells. Focal *clonal senescence* may explain how intrinsic aging processes contribute to atherosclerosis. According to this theory, the intimal smooth-muscle cells that proliferate to form an atheroma are normally under feedback control by diffusible agents (mitosis inhibitors) formed by the smooth-muscle cells in the contiguous media, and this feedback control system tends to fail with age as these controlling cells die and are not adequately replaced. This is consistent with the recent observation that cultured human arterial smooth-muscle cells, like fibroblasts, show a decline in their ability to replicate as a function of donor age. If this loss of replicative potential applies to a controlling population of smooth-muscle cells, then cells that are usually suppressed would be able to proliferate.

The *lysosomal theory* suggests that altered lysosomal function might contribute to atherogenesis. Since lysosomal enzymes can accomplish the generalized degradation of cellular components required for continuing renewal, this system has been implicated in cellular aging and the accumulation of lipofuscin or "age pigment." It has been suggested that increased deposition of lipids in arterial smooth-muscle cells may be related in part to a relative deficiency in the activity of lysosomal cholesterol ester hydrolase. This would result in increased accumulation of cholesterol esters within the cells, perhaps accentuated by lipid overloading of lysosomes, eventually leading to cell death and extracellular lipid deposition. Consonant with this idea, patients with the rare cholesterol ester storage disease, caused by a defect in lysosomal cholesterol ester hydrolase, have accelerated atherosclerosis.

RECOGNITION OF ATHEROSCLEROSIS There is no blood test for atherosclerosis, but recently several sophisticated noninvasive techniques have been developed for demonstrating its presence. Angiographic visualization of deformity in the lumen of a vessel remains the best presumptive test of silent atherosclerosis. Coronary angiography now permits visualization and assessment of arteries as small as 0.5 mm in diameter. Doppler probes for measuring velocity and amount of blood flow have been used noninvasively and adapted to determine vessel outlines. Ultrasonic techniques are not yet clinically useful for detection of plaques in the coronary arteries.

Functional tests based on pathophysiological or metabolic effects of a narrowed arterial lumen often give indirect clues. Assessment of electrocardiographic changes induced after standardized exercise is a relatively simple noninvasive aid to the diagnosis of coronary atherosclerosis with significant narrowing. Similarly, myocardial perfusion defects demonstrable with imaging techniques using radionuclides are usually attributable to atherosclerosis (Chap. 233). Digit plethysmography with exercise often unmasks significant atherosclerotic involvement of lower extremity arteries.

Radiographic demonstration of calcification in the location of arteries does not always indicate the presence of atherosclerosis. Although calcified coronary vessels usually indicate atherosclerosis, complete luminal obstruction may occur in the absence of any calcification. Calcification or beading of peripheral arteries is not correlated directly with atherosclerosis. Abnormalities in retinal arterioles evident upon funduscopic examination are not well correlated with atherosclerosis in arteries. Thus despite the availability of a variety of tests, detection of atherosclerosis usually awaits one of the clinical complications attending a critical decrease of blood flow in an involved vessel. Knowledge of the prevalence and incidence of arteriosclerosis and most of the inferences concerning its causes are derived from tabulations of the appearance of its complications.

Ischemic heart disease (IHD), synonymous with *coronary heart disease* or *arteriosclerotic heart disease* (Chap. 244), is the most useful indicator of atherosclerosis available today. Practically all patients with myocardial infarction, as defined by electrocardiographic and enzyme changes, have coronary atherosclerosis. Rare exceptions are due to congenital anomalies of the coronary vessels, emboli, or ostial occlusion due to other types of cardiac or vascular disease. Nontraumatic *sudden death* (Chap. 32) makes up a sizable portion of all deaths eventually certified as due to IHD. At autopsy, evidence of fresh myocardial infarction or of *coronary thrombosis* is usually absent. While ventricular fibrillation may have been due to sudden closure of a partially compromised vessel by a small thrombus or embolus, or to *spasm,* none of these need have preceded a fatal arrhythmia. The majority of victims of sudden death have had a previous diagnosis of IHD; the number who had diabetes or hypertension is also significant. In epidemiologic studies of IHD, *angina pectoris* and electrocardiographic

changes attributable to ischemia without infarction are considered "softer end points" and treated separately.

Cerebrovascular disease (stroke) is a less reliable criterion for the presence of atherosclerosis. It includes *cerebral hemorrhage* and *cerebral thrombosis* (Chap. 365). Cerebral thrombosis, including infarction or softening without evidence of embolus, is usually due to atherosclerosis. On the other hand, cerebral hemorrhage is most often the result of congenital aneurysms or of vascular defects peculiar to hypertension and diabetes. Dissections of the aorta (Chap. 252), *peripheral vascular disease* (Chap. 253), thrombosis of other major vessels, and ischemic renal disease (Chap. 282) likewise are not used to determine the prevalence of atherosclerosis in a population or as an index of atherosclerosis elsewhere. Therefore, from an epidemiologic standpoint, consideration of atherosclerosis focuses on IHD.

INCIDENCE AND PREVALENCE According to the National Health Examination Survey, about 5 million Americans have IHD. It is the leading cause of death in males after age 35 and in all persons after age 45. Premature deaths from IHD, arbitrarily defined as appearing before age 65, occur preponderantly in men, and a third of all deaths from IHD in males occur before age 65. In fact nearly all the excess premature mortality in American males is due to IHD. Between the ages of 35 and 55 the death rate is five times higher in white men than in white women in the United States (Table 250-3). The exceptions are women with hypertension, diabetes, hyperlipidemia, or premature (usually iatrogenic) menopause, who are at increased risk and often share the risk of the male. For both sexes, there is more than a fivefold increase in the average annual incidence of myocardial infarction between ages 40 and 60, according to the Framingham study. A distressing higher mortality rate in younger nonwhite women (Table 250-3) is probably due mainly to a greater incidence of hypertension in blacks. There is less difference between men and women in the prevalence of angina pectoris than in that of myocardial infarction; after age 65 more women than men have angina without a history of infarction.

Changing death rates Death rates in the United States from IHD rose appreciably between 1940 and 1960. Mortality peaked in 1963 and started to decline with the rate of decline accelerating in recent years for all ages, for both sexes, and for whites and nonwhites. This recent decline in mortality from coronary atherosclerosis (Table 250-4) is the first recorded in American history. In 1976 the reduction in IHD death rate averaged more than 20 percent for persons age 35 to 74. The trend remains unexplained, but there has been a concurrent

TABLE 250-3
Death rates in the United States from ischemic heart disease, 1976 (deaths per 100,000)

Sex	Age	White	Nonwhite
Male	25–34	6	13
	35–44	64	90
	45–54	276	326
	55–64	752	795
	65–74	1698	1488
	75–84	3869	2824
	85+	7954	4177
Female	25–34	1	5
	35–44	12	33
	45–54	59	148
	55–64	227	422
	65–74	731	983
	75–84	2485	2278
	85+	6596	3591

SOURCE: *National Center for Health Statistics, Division of Vital Statistics.*

TABLE 250-4
Age-adjusted death rates by cause in the United States, 1968 and 1976

	Rate per 100,000 population		
Cause of death	1968	1976	% change
All deaths	743.8	627.5	− 15.6
All cardiovascular diseases	361.8	284.4	− 21.4
Ischemic heart disease	241.6	191.6	− 20.7
Cerebrovascular disease	71.3	51.4	− 27.9
Rheumatic heart disease	7.2	4.7	− 34.7
Cancer	129.2	132.3	+ 2.4
Accidents and violence	76.5	67.2	− 12.2
All other diseases	176.3	143.6	− 18.5

SOURCE: *The National Center for Health Statistics, Division of Vital Statistics.*

change in living habits including reduced smoking among middle-aged males, decreased consumption of animal fats and cholesterol, better control of hypertension, and improved treatment of IHD.

There are many interesting differences in regional death rates from IHD within the population of the United States. The highest rates for both sexes combined are in the Middle Atlantic states. They exceed the lowest, found in the mountain states, by 25 percent. Even more striking differences may occur within one locality, such as Evans County, Georgia, where age-adjusted incidence of IHD in white males is more than three times that in black males, a discrepancy that appears best related to differences in amount of physical activity.

International comparisons In most industrialized countries, IHD is the major single cause of premature cardiovascular deaths. There are, however, marked differences in premature death rates among them. The seven having the highest rates in males between 45 and 54 years of age are, in descending order, Finland, the United States, Scotland, Northern Ireland, Australia, New Zealand, and Canada. Much lower age-adjusted death rates from IHD are found in most Western European countries, Latin America, and Japan. The rates in Japan are about one-fifth of those in the United States. Subsamples obtained in many countries convey the strong impression that upper socioeconomic classes that have adopted the culture of Western industrialized countries have far more IHD than lower socioeconomic classes. Among the most obvious cultural differences between these groups are total calories, fat content of the diet, and amount of physical work. Extensive epidemiologic studies have not revealed the reasons for differences between cultures that are superficially similar. Why, for example, do the Scots and North Americans have nearly twice the death rate from premature IHD as Swedes, a difference that can be extrapolated to excess of deaths before age 65 of about 60,000 males in the United States? Migrants to the United States tend to have a higher risk of death from premature IHD than age-matched relatives who remain at home. Although there are many instances in which different ethnic groups in the same locality have widely differing prevalences of IHD, the available data suggest that cultural factors are more important than genetic determination of IHD. Nevertheless, genetic heterogeneity undoubtedly underlies many of the striking differences in susceptibility seen among individuals sharing the same ethnic and cultural setting.

ETIOLOGY A number of conditions and habits present more frequently in individuals who develop atherosclerosis than in the general population; these factors have been termed *risk factors.* The majority of people below age 65 afflicted with atherosclerosis have one or more identifiable risk factors other than aging per se (Table 250-5). The risk factor concept implies that a person with at least one risk factor is more likely to

develop a clinical atherosclerotic event and to do so earlier than a person with no risk factors. The presence of multiple risk factors further accelerates atherosclerosis. They vary in terms of importance in the population of the United States. There is general agreement from an epidemiologic perspective that hypercholesterolemia, hypertension, and cigarette smoking may be the most potent factors involved in causation of atherosclerosis. Risk factors also vary in terms of their potential reversability with current techniques of preventive management.

Thus age, sex, and genetic factors are currently considered to be irreversible risk factors, whereas continually emerging evidence suggests that elimination of cigarette smoking and treatment of hypertension reverses the high risk for atherosclerosis attributable to those factors. Life insurance policyholder data suggest that reduction of obesity reduces total mortality, presumably by diminishing the sequelae of atherosclerosis. Potentially reversible factors currently under study include hyperglycemia and the various forms of hyperlipidemia.

These factors are not mutually exclusive since they clearly interact. For example, obesity appears to be causally associated with hypertension, hyperglycemia, hypercholesterolemia, and hypertriglyceridemia. Genetic factors may play a role by exerting direct effects on arterial wall cell structure and metabolism, or they may act indirectly via such factors as hypertension, hyperlipidemia, diabetes, and obesity. Aging appears to be one of the more complex factors associated with the development of atherosclerosis, since many of the risk factors in themselves are related to aging, e.g., elevated blood pressure, hyperglycemia, and hyperlipidemia. Thus in addition to the possible involvement of intrinsic aging in atherogenesis (perhaps through effects on arterial wall metabolism), a variety of associated metabolic factors are also age-dependent.

Hyperlipidemia Both *hypercholesterolemia* and *hypertriglyceridemia* appear to be important risk factors for atherosclerosis. While there is no absolute quantitative definition of hyperlipidemia, statistical definitions, based on the upper 5 or 10 percent of the distribution of plasma lipid levels within a population, are often used. Such definitions are likely to detect affected individuals from families with one of the familial hyperlipidemias or hyperlipidemia associated with other diseases or drugs, and also are useful for prediction of emergence of premature atherosclerosis and institution of preventive measures. However, these upper limits of "normality" are too high for defining those cholesterol and triglyceride levels that are

TABLE 250-5
Risk factors for atherosclerosis

I Not reversible
   A Aging
   B Male sex
   C Genetic traits—positive family history of premature atherosclerosis
II Reversible
   A Cigarette smoking
   B Hypertension
   C Obesity
III Potentially or partially reversible
   A Hyperlipidemia—hypercholesterolemia and/or hypertriglyceridemia
   B Hyperglycemia and diabetes mellitus
   C Low levels of high-density lipoproteins (HDL)
IV Other possible factors
   A Physical inactivity
   B Emotional stress and/or personality type

correlated with increasing risk of IHD in whole populations. Thus, correlations between the cholesterol concentrations in young men in North America and the incidence of premature IHD indicate that an increasing risk can be detected when the cholesterol level is higher than 220 mg per 100 ml, a value close to the mean for men from 40 to 49 years of age in this population. Extrapolation of similar data from other populations suggests that a cholesterol level at birth averages 60 mg per 100 ml. Within a month the average has risen to about 120 and by the first year to 175. A second rise begins in the third decade and continues to about age 50 in men and somewhat later in women.

A similar age-related increase in plasma triglyceride levels is also observed. The increases in cholesterol are associated mainly with a rise in *low-density lipoprotein* (LDL) concentrations, the increases in triglyceride with a rise in *very low density lipoproteins* (VLDL). Adiposity may play a key role in this age-associated rise in triglyceride and cholesterol levels since the increases in triglyceride, cholesterol, and body weight with age in whole populations occur concurrently. In primitive people who remain thin throughout adulthood, plasma lipids do not increase with age. Metabolic mechanisms have been postulated whereby obesity, which is associated with insulin resistance of peripheral tissues and compensatory hyperinsulinemia, promotes enhanced production of triglyceride- and cholesterol-rich lipoproteins by the liver. Current concepts of plasma lipoprotein transport suggest that accumulation of cholesterol in the circulation may in part be secondary to excessive production of triglyceride-rich lipoproteins.

Hyperlipidemia is associated unequivocally with increased incidence of premature IHD; however, its importance varies in relation to age. In the Framingham study, cholesterol levels in males below age 40 were closely related to the future development of IHD; this relation was much less pronounced in older individuals. For both sexes combined, the relative incidence of myocardial infarction in individuals between the ages of 30 and 49 with cholesterol levels greater than 260 mg per 100 ml was three to five times that for individuals with cholesterol levels less than 220. There appears to be a continuous gradient of risk as the cholesterol level ascends. These data are supported by comparisons of the prevalence of IHD and cholesterol (or LDL) in many other populations. The relationship of triglycerides and VLDL to IHD is confounded by a rise in cholesterol as VLDL increases. Nevertheless, in several population studies, increased triglycerides (or VLDL) are independently correlated with premature IHD.

Hypertriglyceridemia may be associated with premature atherosclerosis in some specific disorders; this association may not be apparent in studies of whole populations. Patients with high VLDL who come from families with familial combined

hyperlipidemia appear to be at the same increased risk as those affected members of these families with elevated LDL levels. In contrast, patients with comparably elevated VLDL levels who come from families with pure monogenic familial hypertriglyceridemia do not appear to have an increased risk. In addition, high VLDL may increase the risk for premature atherosclerosis when associated with other risk factors for coronary artery disease such as in diabetes, and in patients on chronic hemodialysis who smoke and are hypertensive. Individuals in whom remnant lipoproteins accumulate, with resulting elevations in both cholesterol and triglycerides (Chap. 100), also seem to be at risk for early development of atherosclerosis.

Some of these relationships were clarified in a comprehensive study in Seattle of the role of the genetics of hyperlipidemia in clinical atherosclerosis in which 500 consecutive survivors of myocardial infarction were tested. Hyperlipidemia was present in about one-third of the group. Approximately one-half of the males and two-thirds of the females below age 50 had either hypertriglyceridemia, hypercholesterolemia, or both. On the other hand, in individuals over age 70 the prevalence of atherosclerotic coronary disease was very high, yet virtually no males (and only about one-fourth of the females) had hyperlipidemia. Thus, in both sexes there appeared to be a progressive decline with age in the association of hyperlipidemia with myocardial infarction. More than half of the hyperlipidemic atherosclerotic survivors appeared to have simple monogenic familial disorders inherited as an autosomal dominant trait (*familial combined hyperlipidemia, familial hypertriglyceridemia,* and *familial hypercholesterolemia,* in descending order of frequency, Table 250-6). These simply inherited hyperlipidemias (particularly hypercholesterolemia) were more frequent in myocardial infarction survivors below age 60 than in those who were older. In contrast, nonmonogenic forms of hyperlipidemia occurred with equal frequency above and below age 60. Thus it appears that genes associated with the simply inherited hyperlipidemias accelerate changes seen with age, leading to atherosclerosis at an earlier age than usual. All studies indicate that hyperlipidemia is a more meaningful risk factor below age 50 and that it operates independently of, and in addition to, hypertension, diabetes, obesity, and other factors. For men and women over age 65, there is no evidence of a correlation between hyperlipidemia and atherosclerosis or its complications.

When the screening of individuals for hyperlipidemia occurs after a myocardial infarction, it is several decades too late. Screening at birth or in childhood for genetic hyperlipidemia is not practical or useful except in the instance of familial hypercholesterolemia, which may affect about 1 in 1000 children. This is detectable by LDL elevations in cord blood when one already knows that a parent is affected. Other genetic or nongenetic primary hyperlipidemia is often not apparent until the third decade. *Today, good health maintenance practice includes a test for detection of hyperlipidemia in all persons between 20 and 30 years of age. It is especially important in all young persons who have a family history of premature IHD.*

Hyperlipidemia is best detected by measurement of the concentration of cholesterol and triglycerides in serum or plasma in a sample obtained after an overnight fast. The measurements should be made by a reliable laboratory that follows a program of standardization. Routine use of lipoprotein electrophoresis provides little additional information, is nonspecific, and is not recommended for screening or for management. In adults less than 55 years of age, a cholesterol concentration (C) greater than 250 mg per 100 ml or a triglyceride concentration (TG) greater than 200 mg per 100 ml clearly indicates hyperlipidemia sufficient to require some attention by the physician to the items listed in Table 250-7. If hyperlipidemia is absent, the tests need not be repeated for

TABLE 250-6
Frequency of hyperlipidemia in survivors of myocardial infarction

Disorder	% of total myocardial infarction survivors		
	Under age 60	Over age 60	Ratio
I Monogenic hyperlipidemias	20.6	7.5	—
A Familial hypercholesterolemia	4.1	0.7	6:1
B Familial hypertriglyceridemia	5.2	2.7	2:1
C Familial combined hyperlipidemia	11.3	4.1	3:1
II Polygenic hypercholesterolemia	5.5	5.5	1:1
III Sporadic hypertriglyceridemia	5.8	6.9	1:1

SOURCE: *Goldstein et al.*

several years in an adult who maintains body weight and does not otherwise change in health or life-style. Vigor in pursuing the "causative factors" in Table 250-7 should increase in proportion to the degree of hyperlipidemia. If causes of *secondary hyperlipidemia* or offending drugs are absent, attention to the origin of *primary hyperlipidemia* turns mainly to diet and genetic causes. Severe hyperlipidemia (C > 350 mg per 100 ml or TG > 400 mg per 100 ml) usually reflects a genetic disorder; when xanthomas are present, it practically always does. Diagnosis always includes examination of first-degree relatives and proceeds according to information contained in Chap. 100.

Direct proof is still lacking that reduction of hyperlipidemia results in a decrease in progression of atherosclerosis in humans. It has been demonstrated directly in other primates, however, and several controlled trials of different diets which have been accompanied by fall in mean cholesterol levels in small test populations have shown a favorable effect on incidence of the overall complications of IHD. The weight of evidence strongly favors conservative measures to control hyperlipidemia in patients through middle age.

The first step in treatment of primary hyperlipidemia is attention to diet. All patients with mild to moderate hyperlipidemia should first be brought to normal weight if they exceed it, and then be maintained on a diet emphasizing decreases in intake of saturated fat and cholesterol. If hypertriglyceridemia is present, alcohol intake should be limited or eliminated. A single dietary approach to all forms of hyperlipidemia, including reduced intake of calories, cholesterol, and saturated fat, is appropriate for most patients. The degree of dietary restriction would be proportional to the degree and nature of the hyperlipidemia. The maximum effect of such a regimen will be observed within 2 months after body weight has stabilized. If at that time C is greater than 300 mg per 100 ml, a 2-month trial of a bile acid binding resin (cholestyramine or colestipol) should be considered. If TG is greater than 300 mg per 100 ml, clofibrate may be tried. These two drugs may be used simultaneously if both C and TG are high; their use remains empirical. Continued therapy with any hypolipidemic drug is dependent upon the demonstration that, when added to diet at stable weight, it is associated with at least a 15 percent further decrease in hyperlipidemia. Significant side effects dictate withdrawal of any hypolipidemic agent except under extraordinary circumstances.

High-density lipoproteins (HDL) On the basis of newer epidemiologic data, it has been recently reemphasized that HDL, which carries about 20 percent of the total plasma cholesterol, protects against the development of premature atherosclerosis, and therefore can be considered an "antirisk factor." HDL levels can be assessed simply by measurement of cholesterol in the supernatant fluid after the other lipoproteins in plasma have been precipitated. Thus individuals whose HDL cholesterol is elevated may be less likely to develop IHD; conversely low HDL cholesterol is associated with increased risk of IHD. In the Framingham study, low HDL cholesterol was a more potent lipid risk factor than was high cholesterol or LDL. At least five diverse population studies have confirmed a close correlation between IHD and low HDL, independent of other factors.

Consistent with differences in risk between the sexes, HDL cholesterol averages about 25 percent higher in women than in men. Estrogens tend to raise and androgens tend to lower HDL levels. In women, low HDL, particularly when associated with diabetes and obesity, markedly raises the risk of IHD. Octogenarians tend to have high HDL which may be partly familial. Of interest for preventive measures, cigarette smoking decreases and regular strenuous exercise increases HDL cholesterol. Regular exercise increases HDL even in individuals after myocardial infarction. A small daily intake of

alcohol has been associated with both reduced risk of IHD and high HDL levels. Mechanisms for these effects remain unknown.

HDL measurements are most helpful in individuals, especially women, with only a mild increase in plasma cholesterol and normal triglyceride levels to determine whether the increase is in HDL rather than in LDL for assessment of risk of IHD. Because of the close inverse relationship between plasma triglycerides (or VLDL) and HDL, measurement of HDL in hypertriglyceridemic persons, with or without hypercholesterolemia, gives little additional useful information.

Hypertension (Chap. 251) High blood pressure is an important risk factor for atherosclerosis, mainly IHD and cerebrovascular disease. The risk increases progressively with increasing blood pressure; in the Framingham study, IHD incidence in middle-aged men with blood pressures exceeding 160/95 was more than five times that in normotensive men (blood pressure 140/90 or less). Hypertensive men and women are both affected, with the diastolic pressure perhaps being more important. In industrialized populations, blood pressure appears to increase inexorably with age; however, the nature of this age relation varies among populations, since there are remote primitive populations that age without any changes in blood pressure levels. The age-associated blood pressure increase might be related to physical activity or dietary factors, particularly sodium and total caloric content. In contrast to the other age-related risk factors, hypertension appears to increase atherosclerosis throughout the age span. Thus, after the age of about 50, hypertension may be more potent than hypercholesterolemia as a risk factor.

Conversely, the risk for atherosclerosis appears diminished by therapeutic reduction of blood pressure. Recent intervention studies have shown convincingly that reduction of diastolic levels greater than 105 mmHg significantly reduces the incidence of strokes, IHD, and congestive heart failure in men. Even when patients with diastolic elevations between 90 and 105 mmHg are similarly maintained on adequate treatment, the incidence of some of these complications may be reduced. Special urgency for relief of hypertension obtains when hyperlipidemia or other risk factors are present.

Cigarette smoking Not only is cigarette smoking one of the more potent risk factors for atherosclerosis, it is also one of the factors that when reduced or eliminated clearly decreases the risk of developing atherosclerosis. Ample statistical evidence

TABLE 250-7
Factors to consider in patients with hyperlipidemia

I Disorders to which hyperlipidemia is secondary
   A Uncontrolled diabetes mellitus (insulin deficiency)
   B Hypothyroidism
   C Uremia
   D Nephrotic syndrome (hypoproteinemia)
   E Obstructive liver disease
   F Dysproteinemia (multiple myeloma, lupus erythematosus)
II Drugs producing hyperlipidemia
   A Oral contraceptives
   B Estrogens
   C Glucocorticoids
III Dietary factors
   A Caloric intake (recent weight gain)
   B Content of saturated fats and cholesterol
   C Alcohol intake
IV Genetic disorders (primary hyperlipidemias)
   A Family history of hyperlipidemia or xanthomas
   B History of pancreatitis or recurrent abdominal pain

supports a mean increase of about 70 percent in the death rate, and a three- to fivefold increase in risk of IHD, in men who smoke one pack of cigarettes per day compared with nonsmokers. In general, the increase in death rate is proportional to the amount smoked and decreases with age. Excess morbidity from myocardial infarction is also present in women smokers, but the relationship is somewhat less firm than in men. However, there is an impressive accentuation of IHD mortality in women taking oral contraceptives who in addition smoke cigarettes. In some atherosclerosis-prone populations, such as patients maintained on long-term hemodialysis, cigarette smoking interacts with other risk factors, resulting in a marked enhancement of atherosclerosis mortality. Such interaction is also likely, but not proved, for diabetic and hypertensive populations.

The association of smoking and increased IHD remains unexplained. Pipe and cigar smokers have a lesser increase in risk of IHD, presumably because less smoke is inhaled. Smokers dying of causes other than IHD have been found at autopsy to have more coronary atherosclerosis than nonsmokers. The major influence of smoking is upon the incidence of sudden death, however. Those who stop smoking show a prompt decline in risk and may reach the risk level of nonsmokers as early as after 1 year of abstention.

Hyperglycemia and diabetes mellitus (Chap. 338) Studies in a a variety of populations have shown an association of hyperglycemia with clinically evident atherosclerotic disease suggesting a role of hyperglycemia in atherogenesis. In known diabetics, both juvenile-onset and adult-onset types, there is at least a twofold increase in incidence of myocardial infarction compared with nondiabetics. This risk is markedly increased in younger diabetics, and diabetic women are even more prone to IHD than are diabetic men. There is an increased tendency toward cerebral thrombosis and infarction but not toward cerebral hemorrhage in diabetes. Gangrene of the lower extremities has been variously estimated to be from 8 to 150 times as frequent in diabetics as in nondiabetics. Diabetes is associated with an increase in atherosclerosis observed at autopsy in a variety of populations worldwide, whether the prevalence of atherosclerosis in a particular population is high or low. The approximately twofold increase in the frequency of hypertension among diabetics, particularly adult females, may accentuate the risk. This relationship is presumably associated with obesity.

The risk for atherosclerotic disease, however, does not appear to be grossly related to the degree of hyperglycemia. Results in the University Group Diabetes Program Study have suggested that reduction of blood glucose by insulin does not appear to influence mortality from established atherosclerosis during a 5-year period. Thus, although hyperglycemia and atherosclerosis are associated, since there is an increased prevalence of large vessel disease in known diabetics and, conversely, an increased prevalence of hyperglycemia in association with atherosclerotic disease, these associations remain unexplained and reversibility undocumented. The capillary microangiopathy, pathognomonic of diabetes and causing important dysfunction of the kidneys and retina, also has unknown clinical significance in relation to atherosclerotic disease in larger arteries.

Obesity In general, morbidity and mortality from IHD are higher in direct relation to the degree of overweight. Furthermore, from data obtained in the Framingham study, it appears that obesity may accelerate atherosclerosis since its effect is more apparent before age 50. Nevertheless, some of the major epidemiologic studies of coronary heart disease have not demonstrated an independent relationship between this condition and anything less than very severe obesity. However, obesity is a disorder closely associated with four other potent risk factors, i.e., hypertriglyceridemia, hypercholesterolemia, hyperglycemia, and hypertension. The relationship between obesity and atherosclerosis is thus multifaceted; and since in practice obesity does not occur "independently," it is of considerable importance as a risk factor.

Physical inactivity Study of the relationship of the prevalence of IHD to daily (occupational) physical activity is made difficult because so many variables are involved. Among prospective studies the Framingham data do indicate that the less sedentary an individual is, the less susceptible that individual is to sudden death. Physical work may be the major determinant of greatly differing incidences of IHD in Southern black and white males and in populations that move from rural areas to urbanized environments. How physical activity may operate to decrease death from IHD, or possibly atherogenesis, is not known. Beyond ameliorating hyperlipidemia by increasing caloric expenditure, no mechanism has been demonstrated. The meaning of the physical activity–induced increase in HDL, the antirisk factor for IHD, remains mysterious. Physical training has been shown to improve exercise performance in patients with IHD and angina pectoris. Regular physical activity is supported as a desirable element in a program of preventive health maintenance.

Stress and personality There is a valid clinical impression that psychic or emotional stress and anxiety are associated with precipitation of overt IHD and sudden death. Debate continues as to whether there may be distinct personality types prone to and relatively immune from premature IHD (the so-called "personality types A and B"), and whether the presumably more deleterious type is amenable to correction beyond elimination of cigarette smoking, adverse dietary patterns, and avoidance of stressful life situations. Many social and demographic analyses have so far failed to reach any agreement about the etiologic relationships of occupation and similar situational factors and the incidence of IHD.

Genetic factors Premature atherosclerosis often appears to be familial. In many instances this can be attributed to the inheritance of risk factors such as hypertension, diabetes mellitus, and hyperlipidemia. Occasionally, families with excessive premature vascular disease can be found in which none of the known risk factors appears to be operating. Genetic determinants of protective factors, such as HDL, need to be understood; undoubtedly other important determinants remain to be discovered. Nevertheless, family history is one of the more important factors to be weighed in assessment of risk in helping the physician to avoid missing treatable risk factors, and in institution of appropriate preventive measures.

ROLE OF DIET IN RISK FOR ATHEROSCLEROSIS The relationship of diet to IHD remains an area of intense interest and persistent controversy. In epidemiologic studies, no population habitually subsisting on a diet low in saturated fat and cholesterol has an appreciable amount of IHD. These populations also tend to have lower plasma lipid concentrations. There is a general upward shift of average cholesterol and triglyceride levels in highly developed countries, which is an effect of change in total culture and life-style as well as in diet. Dietary changes in migrant populations who move from more primitive to more industrialized societies commonly include increased intake of total calories, animal fats, cholesterol, and salt, leading to a diet-accentuated emergence of risk factors such as obesity, hyperlipidemia, and hypertension. There is no question that the plasma cholesterol (and LDL) level is sensitive to the amount of saturated fat and cholesterol in the diet. The "average" adult in the United States eats about 140 g fat per day and about 500 mg cholesterol. The mixture of fats ingested usually contains about three times as much saturated fatty acids (mainly palmitic and stearic) as polyunsaturated fatty acids (mainly linoleic and linolenic). If a healthy young adult switches from this diet to one containing the same amount of total fat in which the ratio of polyunsaturates to saturates is closer to unity and the cholesterol content is less than 300 mg per day, the cholesterol concentration will usually drop by 10 to 15 percent within 2 weeks, and remain depressed on continuation of the diet.

The average cholesterol level in most populations is most closely related to the amount of animal fats (meat, eggs, and milk products, major sources of long-chain saturated fatty acids and cholesterol) in the diet. Increased animal fat consumption also tends to be correlated with a greater proportion of dietary fats being saturated and with lesser intake of complex carbohydrates and vegetable fibers; these are dietary changes that may lead to a rise in plasma cholesterol levels. The average triglyceride level is more sensitive to total caloric balance and to alcohol intake. It is important to note that physical activity, emotional stress, smoking, and intake of coffee or tea have only weak or indirect influences on cholesterol and triglyceride concentrations.

In experimental animals added dietary cholesterol and fat are essential for the production of atherosclerosis. Typical American diets fed to subhuman primates produce aortic and coronary atherosclerosis which is reversible when a cholesterol-free diet is fed. Controlled metabolic studies in humans show a direct relation between dietary and plasma cholesterol below intakes of about 600 mg per day; no relation is observed at higher intakes when plasma cholesterol is already high. There appear to be marked genetic variations in the ability of dietary cholesterol to influence plasma cholesterol among individuals and among populations. The relation between dietary polyunsaturated/saturated fat ratio (P/S) and both cholesterol and triglyceride levels also has been amply established.

A definitive prospective study of the effect of diet on IHD in the general population has never been undertaken. Nevertheless, preliminary reports of newer studies of alterations of diet in high-risk populations, coupled with published findings of studies in selected populations, provide strong evidence of a reversible relation among diet, plasma lipids, and IHD. On this basis, although without definite proof of effectiveness, numerous authoritative nutrition councils have recommended prudent dietary modifications for the general population of Western countries to be instituted early in life and to include a caloric intake adjusted to achieve and maintain ideal body weight, a reduction in total fat calories to 30 to 35 percent of total calories achieved by a substantial reduction in dietary saturated fat to less than 10 percent of total calories, and a reduction in cholesterol intake to less than 300 mg per day. Although a causal relationship in humans between sodium intake and hypertension has not been firmly established, avoidance of excessive dietary sodium has also been recommended.

RISK FACTORS AND MECHANISMS OF ATHEROGENESIS

Adiposity produces insulin resistance in peripheral tissues (mainly muscle and adipose), which leads to compensatory hyperinsulinemia. The liver is not resistant to some effects of insulin, and enhanced production of triglyceride-rich lipoproteins results, leading to elevated plasma triglyceride and cholesterol levels. Thus it has been demonstrated that body weight is related not only to triglyceride levels but also to cholesterol levels. Concomitantly, obesity is associated with increased total body cholesterol synthesis. Obesity produces higher circulating levels of insulin, both in the basal state and after stimulation with glucose or other secretagogues. Since obesity is related to atherosclerosis—both directly and via hypertension, hypertriglyceridemia, hypercholesterolemia, and hyperglycemia—it is not surprising that many studies show a relationship between serum insulin levels, particularly after oral glucose intake, and atherosclerotic disease of the coronary and peripheral arteries. A few studies, however, suggest that this association between insulin and atherosclerosis occurs independently of obesity. It has been postulated that insulin may directly affect arterial wall metabolism, leading to increased endogenous lipid synthesis and thus predisposing to atherosclerosis. Insulin has been shown in physiological concentrations to stimulate proliferation of arterial smooth-muscle cells and enhance binding of LDL and VLDL to fibroblasts; it therefore may be one of the plasma factors gaining increased access to the intima and media after endothelial injury and thus may be an additional factor in atheroma formation.

Hypertension may enhance atherogenesis by directly producing injury via mechanical stress on endothelial cells at specific high-pressure sites in the arterial tree. This would allow the sequence of events in the chronic injury hypothesis of atherogenesis to take place. In addition, hypertension might allow more lipoproteins to be transported through intact endothelial lining cells by altering permeability. Hypertension markedly increases lysosomal enzyme activity, presumably owing to stimulation of the cellular disposal system by the internalization of increased amounts of plasma substances. This might lead to increased cell degeneration and release of the highly destructive enzymes (within the lysosomes) into the arterial wall. Experimental hypertension also increases the thickness of the intimal smooth-muscle layer in the arterial wall and increases connective tissue elements. It is still not known if continued high pressure within the artery produces changes in the ability of smooth-muscle cells or stem cells to proliferate.

Diabetes could provide a unique contribution to atherogenesis. Although the fundamental genetic abnormality in human diabetes mellitus remains unknown, it has been suggested that genetic diabetes in humans represents a primary cellular abnormality intrinsic to all cells, resulting in a decreased life span of individual cells, which in turn results in increased cell turnover in tissues. If arterial endothelial and smooth-muscle cells are intrinsically defective in diabetes, accelerated atherogenesis can be readily postulated on the basis of any one of the current theories of pathogenesis. Platelet dysfunction in diabetes might also play a role.

The role of glucose in atheroma formation, if any, is poorly understood. Hyperglycemia is known to affect aortic wall metabolism. Sorbitol, a product of the insulin-independent aldose reductase pathway of glucose metabolism (the polyol pathway) accumulates in the arterial wall in the presence of high glucose concentrations, resulting in osmotic effects including increased cell water content and decreased oxygenation. Increased glucose also appears to stimulate proliferation of cultured arterial smooth-muscle cells.

The development of atherosclerosis accelerates in approximate quantitative relation to the degree of *hyperlipidemia*. A long-established theory suggests that the higher the circulating levels of lipoprotein the more likely they are to gain entrance to the arterial wall. By an acceleration of the usual transendothelial transport, large concentrations of lipoproteins within the arterial wall could overwhelm the ability of smooth-muscle cells to metabolize them. Lipoproteins have been immunologically identified in atheroma, and in humans there is a close relationship between plasma cholesterol and arterial lipoprotein cholesterol concentration. It is possible that the lipid that accumulates in the arterial wall with increasing age results from infiltration of plasma lipoproteins. However, atheromatous lesions are associated with a marked increase in arterial wall lipids, which may result in part from additional "chemical" injury to the endothelium possibly produced by chronic hyperlipidemia, as was recently demonstrated in cholesterol-fed monkeys. A further mechanism for accelerated atherogenesis in hyperlipidemia is related to the demonstrated ability of LDL to stimulate proliferation of arterial smooth-muscle cells.

The effect of *chronic smoke inhalation* from cigarettes could result in repetitive injury to endothelial cells, thereby accelerating atherogenesis. Hypoxia stimulates proliferation of cultured human arterial smooth-muscle cells; thus, since cigarette smoking is associated with high levels of carboxyhemoglobin and low oxygen delivery to tissues, another mechanism for atherogenesis is suggested. Hypoxia could produce diminished lysosomal enzyme degradative ability, as evidenced by impaired degradation of LDL by smooth-muscle cells, causing LDL to accumulate in the cells. Consistent with this suggestion is the fact that aortic lesions that resemble atheroma have been produced in experimental animals by systemic hypoxia, and lipid accumulation in the arterial wall of cholesterol-fed rabbits and monkeys appears to be increased by hypoxia.

RISK FACTOR REVERSAL AND REGRESSION OF ATHEROSCLEROSIS

Although the emergence of clinical consequences of atherosclerosis can be lessened, no convincing instance of regression or interruption of progression of atherosclerosis, determined by direct or indirect examination of lesions, by removal or reversal of any single or group of risk factors has yet been proved in humans. Nevertheless, feasibility of such demonstrations is becoming established, and preliminary results are encouraging. Through mass-media educational efforts, whole communities can be influenced to reduce smoking, change diet, and lower blood pressure levels. Adult males in the United States have lowered cigarette consumption, although increases among teenage girls have kept total usage high. There has been a trend toward lower cholesterol and saturated fat consumption in the United States, coupled with increasing attention to reducing overweight and the use of exercise programs. Concomitantly, and perhaps causally, there has been the noted decline in IHD mortality. Treatment of hyperlipidemia in some instances has been shown to reduce atherosclerotic involvement of peripheral vessels by both invasive and noninvasive measurement. There is also some encouraging evidence in animals, most notably in primates, that relatively complicated plaques induced by hyperlipidemia will regress, and that further progression of atherosclerosis will cease when hyperlipidemia is removed. Therefore efforts to prevent atherogenesis, to interrupt progression, and perhaps to promote regression of existing lesions by risk factor reduction seem warranted.

PREVENTION

Although premature IHD is overall the most costly and common of the untimely complications of atherosclerosis, preoccupation with IHD must not blind one to the realization that angina pectoris and myocardial infarction are expressions of late-stage atherosclerotic lesions. Factors precipitating these clinical events may be independent of those leading to initiation of plaque formation or its progression to a complicated lesion. Steps taken to prevent recurrence of myocardial infarction or fatal arrhythmia, termed *secondary prevention,* will not necessarily be the same as those taken to delay or prevent formation of atherosclerosis (*primary prevention*). Since atherosclerotic plaques have been detected in the coronary arteries of American males as early as the second decade in autopsy studies of Korean and Vietnam war deaths, primary prevention of atherosclerosis must begin early in life, long before there is any suspicion of IHD.

Thus, *prevention of atherosclerosis, rather than treatment, is the goal* and one of the most important tasks facing those responsible for the health of the public and of individual persons. Although an effective program of prophylaxis has not been established, enough is known to guide in both identification of those with a higher risk and in development of conservative measures that probably will reduce that risk.

Prevention versus treatment The decline of American death rates from premature IHD today coincides with two trends in health practices. One is the increasing acceptance of the importance of detecting and attempting to correct some of the risk factors correlated with the complications of atherosclerosis. The other is a greater awareness of the dietary sources of cholesterol and saturated fats and a tendency of the public to restrict somewhat the intake of such foods. Whether these phenomena are causally related to the changes in death rate is not known. At least there is encouragement for maintenance of these health practices. Certainly it is desirable to continue finding and helping the members of the population most susceptible to early atherosclerosis. For the vast majority of these, the health maintenance responsibilities of the physician are confined largely to conservative treatment of hypertension and encouragement of good habits regarding diet, body weight, alcohol intake, smoking, and exercise. Drug treatment of hyperlipidemia should be limited to those individuals who do not respond adequately to dietary management. Although preliminary trials are encouraging, the long-term value of antiplatelet drugs in reducing either the mortality rate or incidence of myocardial infarction in individuals with IHD remains unproved, and trials are continuing. There is no agent proved to have any value in "treatment" of atherosclerosis unless it clearly reduces severe hyperlipidemia or obvious hypertension. In fact, there is no treatment of atherosclerosis, only of its complications. Prevention must be the paramount goal of both research and health care practice.

REFERENCES

BIERMAN EL, ROSS R: Aging and atherosclerosis, in *Atherosclerosis Reviews*, R Paoletti, AM Gotto Jr (eds). New York, Raven, 1977, pp 79–111

BRUNZELL JD et al: Pathophysiology of lipoprotein transport. Metabolism 27:1109, 1978

CAMERINI-DAVALOS RA et al (eds): *Atherogenesis.* New York, New York Academy of Sciences, 1976

DAWBER TR: Risk factors for atherosclerotic disease, in *Current Concepts.* The Upjohn Company, 1975

GLUECK CJ, CONNOR WE: Diet–coronary heart disease relationships reconnoitered. Am J Clin Nutr 31:727, 1978

GOLDSTEIN JL et al: Hyperlipidemia in coronary heart disease. J Clin Invest 52:1533, 1544, 1973

GORDON T et al: Diabetes, blood lipids, and the role of obesity in coronary heart disease risk for women. The Framingham study. Ann Intern Med 87:393, 1977

———— et al: High density lipoprotein as a protective factor against coronary heart disease. The Framingham study. Am J Med 62:707, 1977

INTER-SOCIETY COMMISSION FOR HEART DISEASE RESOURCES: Primary prevention of the atherosclerotic diseases. Circulation 42:A-55, 1970

KULLER LH: Epidemiology of cardiovascular diseases: Current perspectives. Am J Epidemiol 104:425, 1976

MCGILL HC JR (ed): The geographic pathology of atherosclerosis. Lab Invest 18:463, 1968

ROSS R, GLOMSET JA: The pathogenesis of atherosclerosis. N Engl J Med 295:369, 420, 1976

251

HYPERTENSIVE VASCULAR DISEASE

GORDON H. WILLIAMS
PAUL I. JAGGER
EUGENE BRAUNWALD

In 1971, the Hypertension Study Group reported "15–20% of adults in the United States have hypertension. . . . More than half of these have hypertensive heart disease . . . and the great majority are presently undetected, untreated, or inadequately treated." Thus, an elevated arterial pressure is probably the more important public health problem in developed countries—being common, asymptomatic, readily detectable, usually easily treatable, and often lethal if left untreated. As a result of extensive educational programs in the late 1960s and 1970s by both private and governmental agencies, the number of undiagnosed and/or untreated patients has been significantly reduced. This factor may be the most important one responsible for the decline in cardiovascular mortality which has taken place during the latter half of the 1970s (Chap. 250), although our understanding of the pathophysiology of an elevated arterial pressure has also increased. Unfortunately, in 90 to 95 percent of cases the etiology (and thus potentially the prevention or cure) is still unknown.

DEFINITION

One hundred years have past since Mahomed clearly distinguished hypertension from Bright's renal disease, yet defining who has hypertension and who should be treated remains controversial. Sir George Pickering has long argued "there is no dividing line" between normal and high blood pressure. "The relationship between arterial pressure and mortality is quantitative; the higher the pressure, the worse the prognosis." Thus, arbitrary levels have been established to define those who have an increased risk of developing a morbid cardiovascular event and/or will clearly benefit from medical therapy. These definitions should consider not only the level of diastolic pressure but also systolic pressure, age, sex, and race. For example, patients with a diastolic pressure greater than 105 mmHg will have a significant reduction in morbidity and mortality with adequate therapy. These, then, are patients who definitely have arterial pressure high enough to treat. Contrariwise, while the cardiovascular morbidity rate is twofold greater in untreated patients with diastolic pressures of 90 to 95 mmHg than in those with lower levels, the number of morbid events they have is not significantly reduced with adequate therapy even if it is continued for as long as 10 years. This statement does not imply that treatment is not helpful. It may mean simply that other risk factors for atherosclerotic complications, such as hyperlipoproteinemia and cigarette smoking, dilute the effect of the mild hypertension and that a very large population must be treated for a prolonged period of time before significance is achieved.

The level of systolic pressure is also important in assessing arterial pressure's influence on cardiovascular morbidity. Males with normal diastolic pressures ($<$ 82 mmHg) but elevated systolic pressures ($>$ 158 mmHg) have a 2½-fold increase in their cardiovascular mortality rates when compared with individuals with normal systolic pressures ($<$ 130 mmHg).

Other significant factors which modify blood pressure's influence on the frequency of morbid cardiovascular events are age, race, and sex with young black males being most adversely affected by hypertension.

Thus, even though in an adult hypertension is usually defined as a pressure greater than or equal to 160/95, a more appropriate definition may be:

Women at any age	$\geq$ 160/95
Men above age 45	$\geq$ 140/95
Men below age 45	$\geq$ 130/90

To date reduction of excess cardiovascular morbidity has been demonstrated clearly only in patients with diastolic pressures greater than 105 mmHg.

Individuals can be classified as being *normotensive* if arterial pressure is less than the levels noted above, as having *sustained* hypertension if the diastolic pressure always exceeds 105 mmHg, and *borderline* hypertension if the diastolic pressure is between 90 or 95 and 105 mmHg. Arterial pressure fluctuates in most persons, whether they are normotensive or hypertensive. Those who are classified as having *labile* hypertension are patients who sometimes but not always have arterial pressures within the hypertensive range.

Sustained hypertension can become accelerated or enter a malignant phase. Though a patient with *malignant hypertension* often has a blood pressure above 200/140, it is papilledema, usually accompanied by retinal hemorrhages and exudates, and not the absolute pressure level, that defines this condition. *Accelerated hypertension* signifies a significant recent increase over previous hypertensive levels associated with evidence of vascular damage on funduscopic examination but without papilledema.

Obviously these definitions are arbitrary. For example, if additional studies demonstrate that treating patients with initial diastolic pressures between 90 and 95 mmHg reduces their cardiovascular morbidity rate, then the definitions of sustained and borderline hypertension would be different.

FREQUENCY The prevalence of hypertension depends on both the racial composition of the studied population and the criteria used to define the condition. In a Caucasian suburban population as used in the Framingham study, nearly 20 percent would have blood pressures greater than 160/95 while 45 percent would have pressures greater than 140/90. An even higher prevalance has been documented in the nonwhite population.

ETIOLOGY

The cause of elevated arterial pressure is unknown in most cases. The prevalence of various forms of secondary hypertension depends on the nature of the population studied and how extensive the evaluation is. There are no available data to define the frequency of secondary hypertension in the general population, although in middle-aged males it has been reported to be 6 percent. On the other hand, in referral centers where patients undergo an extensive evaluation, it has been reported to be as high as 35 percent. The various forms of hypertension are outlined in Table 31-1, and their relative frequencies are given in Table 251-1.

ESSENTIAL HYPERTENSION Patients with arterial hypertension and no definable cause are said to have *primary, essential,* or *idiopathic hypertension.* By definition, the underlying mechanism(s) is unknown; however, the kidney probably plays a central role (see Chap. 31). Undoubtedly, this group represents a spectrum of diseases and includes as yet undefined forms of secondary hypertension. There are characteristics common to many patients in this group, however, including a positive family history for hypertension and evidence for increased vascular reactivity.

Heredity Genetic factors have long been assumed to be important in the genesis of hypertension. Data supporting this view can be found in animal studies as well as population studies in humans. One approach has been to assess the correlation of blood pressures within families (familial aggregation). From these studies the minimum size of the genetic factor can be expressed by a correlation coefficient of approximately 0.2. Most studies would also support the concept that the inheritance is probably multifactoral.

Environment A number of environmental factors have been specifically implicated in the development of hypertension including salt intake, obesity, occupation, family size, and crowding. These factors have all been assumed to be important in the increase in blood pressure with age in more affluent societies, in contrast to the decline in blood pressure with age in more primitive cultures. Indeed, even the familial aggregation of blood pressure has been suggested as being related to environmental rather than genetic factors. However, since adopted children do not demonstrate familial aggregation of blood pressure, this phenomenon is probably almost entirely the result of genetic factors.

Factors modifying the course of essential hypertension Age, race, sex, smoking, serum cholesterol, glucose intolerance, weight, and perhaps renin activity may all alter the prognosis of this disease. The younger the patient when hypertension is first noted, the greater the reduction in life expectancy if left untreated. In the United States, urban blacks have about twice the prevalence rate for hypertension as whites and more than four times the hypertension-induced morbidity rate. At all ages and in both white and nonwhite populations, females with hypertension fare better than males. Yet, females with hypertension run the same relative risk of a morbid cardiovascular event compared with their normotensive counterparts as males do. Accelerated atherosclerosis is an invariable companion of hypertension. Thus, it is not surprising that independent risk factors associated with the development of atherosclerosis, e.g., an elevated serum cholesterol, glucose intolerance, and/or cigarette smoking, significantly enhance the effect of hypertension on mortality rates regardless of age, sex, or race. There is no question that there is a positive correlation between obesity and arterial pressure. A gain in weight is associated with an increased frequency of hypertension in subjects with normal pressures, and weight loss in obese subjects with hypertension

TABLE 251-1
Prevalence of various forms of hypertension in the general population and in specialized referral clinics*

Diagnosis	General population, %	Specialty clinic, %
Essential hypertension	92–94	65–85
Renal hypertension:		
Parenchymal	2–3	4–5
Renovascular	1–2	4–16
Endocrine hypertension:		
Primary aldosteronism	0.3	0.5–12
Cushing's syndrome	<0.1	0.2
Pheochromocytoma	<0.1	0.2
Oral contraceptive-induced	2–4	1–2
Miscellaneous	0.2	1

* *Estimates based on a number of reports in the literature.*

TABLE 251-2
Factors indicating an adverse prognosis in hypertension

  I Black race
 II Youth
III Male
 IV Persistent diastolic pressure >115 mmHg
  V Smoking
 VI Diabetes mellitus
VII Hypercholesterolemia
VIII Obesity
 IX Evidence of end organ damage
    A Cardiac
       1 Cardiac enlargement
       2 ECG changes of ischemic or left ventricular strain
       3 Myocardial infarction
       4 Congestive heart failure
    B Eyes
       1 Retinal exudates and hemorrhages
       2 Papilledema
    C Renal: Impaired renal function
    D Nervous system: Cerebrovascular accident

increases their rate of remission. However, there are no convincing data that obesity adversely affects the hypertension-associated mortality rate. Plasma renin activity has also been reported by some to influence and correlate with the development of morbid cardiovascular events in patients with hypertension.

Natural history Because essential hypertension is a heterogenous disorder, variables in addition to the level of arterial pressure modify its course. Thus, the probability of developing a morbid cardiovascular event with a given arterial pressure may vary by as much as twentyfold depending on whether associated risk factors are present (Table 251-2). Although exceptions have been reported, most untreated adults with hypertension will have an increase in their arterial pressure with time. Furthermore, both from actuarial data and from experience in the era prior to effective therapy, it has been documented that untreated hypertension is associated with a shortening of life by 10 to 20 years, usually related to an acceleration of the atherosclerotic process, with the rate of acceleration in part related to the severity of the disease. Even individuals with relatively mild disease, i.e., without evidence of end organ damage, left untreated for 7 to 10 years have a high risk of developing significant complications. Nearly 30 percent will exhibit atherosclerotic complications, and more than 50 percent will have end organ damage related to the hypertension itself, e.g., cardiomegaly, congestive heart failure, retinopathy, a cerebrovascular accident, and/or renal insufficiency. Thus, even in its mild forms, hypertension is a progressively lethal disease, if left untreated.

SECONDARY HYPERTENSION As noted earlier, in only a small minority of patients with an elevated arterial pressure can a specific cause be identified. Yet, they should not be ignored for at least two reasons: (1) with correction of the cause their hypertension may be cured, and (2) the secondary forms may provide insight into the etiology of essential hypertension. Nearly all the secondary forms are related to an alteration in hormone secretion and/or renal function and are discussed in detail in other chapters.

Renal hypertension (see also Chap. 282) Hypertension produced by renal disease is the result of either (1) a derangement in the renal handling of sodium and fluids leading to volume expansion or (2) an alteration in renal secretion of vasoactive materials resulting in a systemic or local change in arteriolar tone. The main subdivisions of renal hypertension are renovascular hypertension, including preeclampsia and eclampsia, and renal parenchymal hypertension. A simple explanation for renal arterial hypertension is that decreased perfusion of renal tissue due to stenosis of a main or branch renal artery activates the renin-angiotensin system described in Chap. 336. The angiotensin elevates arterial pressure by direct vasoconstriction, by stimulation of aldosterone secretion with resultant sodium retention (Chap. 31), and/or by stimulating the adrenergic nervous system. In actual practice only about one-half of patients with renovascular hypertension have elevated absolute levels of renin activity in peripheral plasma, although when renin measurements are referenced against an index of sodium balance, a much higher fraction have inappropriately high values.

In recent years the use of the competitive angiotensin antagonist, saralasin (1-sar, 8-ala angiotensin II), has further clarified the role of angiotensin in the genesis of the hypertension in this disease. Nearly all patients with surgically correctable disease have exhibited a reduction of arterial pressure when given this agent in the sodium- or volume-depleted state.

Activation of the renin-angiotensin system also has been offered as an explanation for the hypertension in both acute and chronic renal parenchymal disease. In this formulation the only difference between renovascular and renal parenchymal hypertension is that the decreased perfusion of renal tissue in the latter case results from inflammatory and fibrotic changes involving multiple small intrarenal vessels. There are enough differences between the two conditions, however, to suggest that there are other mechanisms active in renal parenchymal disease: (1) peripheral plasma renin activity is elevated far less frequently in renal parenchymal than in renovascular hypertension; (2) cardiac output is said to be normal in the renal parenchymal type (unless uremia and anemia are present), but slightly elevated in renovascular hypertension; (3) circulatory responses to tilting and to the Valsalva maneuver are exaggerated in the latter condition; and (4) blood volume tends to be high in patients with severe renal parenchymal disease and low in patients with severe renovascular hypertension. Alternate explanations for the hypertension in renal parenchymal disease include the possibilities that the damaged kidneys (1) produce an unidentified vasopressor substance other than renin, (2) fail to produce a necessary humoral vasodilator substance (perhaps prostaglandin or bradykinin), (3) fail to inactivate circulating vasopressor substances, and/or (4) are ineffective in disposing of sodium, and the retained sodium is responsible for the hypertension (as outlined in Chap. 31). Though all these explanations, including participation of the renin-angiotensin system, probably have some validity, the hypothesis involving sodium retention is particularly attractive. It is supported by the observation that those patients with chronic pyelonephritis or polycystic renal disease who are salt wasters do not develop hypertension, and by the observation that removal of salt and water by dialysis or diuretics is effective in controlling arterial pressure in the majority of patients with uremia.

A recently described form of renal hypertension results from the excess secretion of renin by juxtaglomerular cell tumors or nephroblastomas. The initial presentation has been similar to that of hyperaldosteronism with hypertension, hypokalemia, and overproduction of aldosterone. However, in contrast to primary aldosteronism, peripheral renin activity is *elevated instead of subnormal*. This disease can be distinguished from other forms of secondary aldosteronism by the presence of normal renal function and with unilateral increases in renal vein renin concentration without a renal artery lesion.

Endocrine hypertension ADRENAL HYPERTENSION Hypertension is a feature of a variety of adrenal cortical abnormalities. In *primary aldosteronism* (Chap. 336) there is a clear relationship between the aldosterone-induced sodium retention and the hypertension. Normal individuals given aldosterone develop hypertension only if they also ingest sodium. Since aldosterone causes sodium retention by stimulating renal tubular

exchange of sodium for potassium, hypokalemia is a prominent feature in most patients with primary aldosteronism, and the measurement of serum potassium provides a simple screening test. The effect of sodium retention and volume expansion in chronically suppressing plasma renin activity is critically important for the definitive diagnosis. In most clinical situations plasma renin activity and plasma or urinary aldosterone levels parallel each other, but in patients with primary aldosteronism, aldosterone levels are high and relatively fixed because of autonomous aldosterone secretion, while plasma renin activity levels are suppressed and respond sluggishly to sodium depletion. Primary aldosteronism may be secondary either to a tumor or bilateral adrenal hyperplasia. It is important to distinguish between these two conditions preoperatively, as usually the hypertension in the latter is not modified by operation (Chap. 336).

The sodium-retaining effect of large amounts of glucocorticoids also offers an explanation for the hypertension in severe cases of *Cushing's syndrome* (Chap. 336). Moreover, increased production of mineralocorticoids also has been documented in some patients with Cushing's syndrome. However, the hypertension in many cases of Cushing's syndrome does not seem volume dependent, leading investigators to speculate that it may be secondary to glucocorticoid-induced production of renin substrate (angiotensin-mediated hypertension) or a steroid-induced change in vascular reactivity. In the forms of the adrenogenital syndrome due to C-11 or C-17 hydroxylase deficiency (Chap. 336) deoxycorticosterone accounts for the sodium retention and the resultant hypertension, which is accompanied by suppression of plasma renin activity.

In patients with *pheochromocytoma* increased secretion of epinephrine and norepinephrine by a tumor most often located in the adrenal medulla causes excessive stimulation of adrenergic receptors, which results in peripheral vasoconstriction and cardiac stimulation. This diagnosis is confirmed by demonstrating increased urinary excretion of epinephrine and norepinephrine or their metabolites (Chap. 337).

ACROMEGALY (see also Chap. 333) Hypertension, coronary atherosclerosis, and cardiac hypertrophy are frequent complications of this condition.

HYPERCALCEMIA (see also Chap. 349) The hypertension which occurs in up to one-third of patients with hyperparathyroidism ordinarily can be attributed to renal parenchymal damage due to nephrolithiasis and nephrocalcinosis. However, increased calcium levels can also have a direct vasoconstrictive effect. In some cases, the hypertension disappears when the hypercalcemia is corrected.

ORAL CONTRACEPTIVES The most common cause of endocrine hypertension is that resulting from the use of estrogen-containing oral contraceptives. Indeed, this may be the most common form of secondary hypertension. The mechanism producing the hypertension is likely to be secondary to activation of the renin-angiotensin-aldosterone system. Thus, both volume (aldosterone) and vasoconstrictor (angiotensin II) factors are important. The estrogen component of oral contraceptive agents stimulates the hepatic synthesis of renin substrate, which in turn favors the increased production of angiotensin II and secondary aldosteronism. Women taking oral contraceptives have increased plasma concentrations of angiotensin II and aldosterone with some increase in arterial pressure. However, only about 5 percent actually have an increase in arterial pressure to greater than 140/90. In about half, the hypertension will remit within 6 months of stopping the drug.

Why some women taking oral contraceptives develop hypertension and others do not is unclear but may be related to (1) increased vascular sensitivity to angiotensin II, (2) the presence of mild renal disease, (3) familial factors (over one-half have a positive family history for hypertension), (4) age (hypertension is significantly more prevalent in women over age 35), and/or (5) obesity. Indeed some investigators have suggested that the oral contraceptives are simply unmasking patients with essential hypertension.

Coarctation of the aorta (see also Chap. 240) The hypertension associated with coarctation may be caused by the constriction itself, or perhaps by the changes in the renal circulation which result in an unusual form of renal arterial hypertension. The diagnosis of coarctation is usually evident from physical examination and routine x-ray findings.

Low-renin essential hypertension Approximately 20 percent of patients who by all other criteria have essential hypertension have suppressed plasma renin activity. This occurs more frequently in black than in white patients. Though these patients are not hypokalemic, they have been reported to have expanded extracellular fluid volumes, and it is tempting to implicate sodium retention and renin suppression due to excessive production of an unidentified mineralocorticoid. Involvement of the adrenal cortex is suggested by the observation that large doses of spironolactone, the mineralocorticoid antagonist, and the inhibition of steroidogenesis by aminoglutethimide can result in sodium loss and lowering of blood pressure in these patients. A search for other mineralocorticoids occasionally reveals increased secretion of 18-hydroxy-11-deoxycorticosterone or 16-hydroxydehydroepiandrosterone in some patients. However, the frequency of these abnormalities is no greater than in patients with normal renin hypertension. Recent studies have suggested that many of these patients have an increased sensitivity to angiotensin II which may be the underlying mechanism. Since this altered sensitivity has been reported even in patients with normal renin hypertension, it is likely that patients with low-renin hypertension are not a distinct subset but rather form part of a continuum of patients with essential hypertension.

APPROACH TO THE PATIENT WITH HYPERTENSION

In evaluating patients with hypertension, the initial history, physical examination, and laboratory tests should be directed at (1) uncovering correctable secondary forms of hypertension (Table 31-1), (2) establishing a pretreatment base line, (3) assessing factors which may influence the type of therapy or which may be adversely modified by therapy, and (4) determining whether other risk factors for the development of arteriosclerotic cardiovascular disease are present (Chap. 250).

SYMPTOMS AND SIGNS The majority of patients with hypertension have no symptoms referable to their blood pressure elevation and will be identified only in the course of a physical examination. When symptoms do bring the patient to the physician, they fall into three categories. They are related to (1) the elevated pressure itself, (2) the hypertensive vascular disease, and (3) the underlying disease in the case of secondary hypertension. Though popularly considered a symptom of elevated pressure, headache is characteristic only of severe hyper-

tension; most commonly it is localized to the occipital region, is present when the patient awakens in the morning, and subsides spontaneously after several hours. Other possibly related complaints include dizziness, palpitations, and easy fatigability. Complaints referable to vascular disease include epistaxis, hematuria, blurring of vision owing to retinal changes, episodes of weakness or dizziness due to transient cerebral ischemia, angina pectoris, and dyspnea due to cardiac failure. Pain due to dissection of the aorta or to a leaking aneurysm is an occasional presenting symptom.

Examples of symptoms related to the underlying disease in secondary hypertension are polyuria, polydipsia, and muscle weakness secondary to hypokalemia in patients with primary aldosteronism, or weight gain and emotional lability in patients with Cushing's syndrome. The patient with a pheochromocytoma may present with episodic headaches, palpitations, diaphoresis, and postural dizziness.

CLINICAL EVALUATION History A strong family history of hypertension, along with the reported finding of intermittent pressure elevation in the past, favors the diagnosis of essential hypertension. Secondary hypertension often develops before the age of 35 or after the age of 55 years. The history of use of adrenal steroids or estrogens is of obvious significance. A history of repeated urinary tract infections or proteinuria suggests renal parenchymal disease; nocturia and polydipsia suggest renal or endocrine disease, while trauma to either flank or an episode of acute flank pain may be a clue to the presence of renal injury. A history of weight gain is compatible with Cushing's syndrome, while weight loss suggests pheochromocytoma. A number of aspects of the history aid in determining whether vascular disease has progressed to dangerous stages. These include chest pain due to myocardial ischemia and symptoms of cerebrovascular insufficiency, of congestive heart failure, and/or of peripheral vascular insufficiency. Other risk factors that could be elicited include cigarette smoking, diabetes mellitus, lipid disorders, and a family history of early deaths due to cardiovascular disease.

Physical examination The physical examination starts with the patient's general appearance. Are the round face and trunkal obesity of Cushing's syndrome present? Is muscular development in the upper extremities out of proportion to that in the lower extremities, suggesting coarctation of the aorta? The next step is to compare the blood pressures and pulses in both upper extremities. Also, measurements in the supine position should be compared with measurements taken during standing. A rise in diastolic pressure when the patient goes from the supine to the standing position is most compatible with essential hypertension; a fall, in the absence of antihypertensive medications, suggests other forms of secondary hypertension. Detailed examination of the ocular fundi is mandatory, since funduscopic findings provide one of the best indications of the duration of hypertension and of prognosis. The Keith-Wagener-Barker classification of funduscopic changes (Table 251-3) is useful; the specific changes should be recorded and a grade assigned. Palpation and auscultation of the carotid arteries for evidence of stenosis or occlusion are important; narrowing of a carotid artery may be a manifestation of hypertensive vascular disease, and it may also be a clue to the presence of a renal arterial lesion, since these two lesions may occur together. In examination of the heart and lungs, one should search for evidence of left ventricular hypertrophy and cardiac decompensation. Is there a left ventricular lift? Are third and fourth heart sounds present? Are there pulmonary rales? Chest examination also includes a search for extracardiac murmurs and palpable collateral vessels that may result from coarctation of the aorta. The most important part of the abdominal examination is aus-

TABLE 251-3
Classification of hypertensive and arteriolosclerotic retinopathy

| | Hypertension | | | | | Arteriolosclerosis | |
| | Arterioles | | | | | | |
Degree	General narrowing AV ratio*	Focal spasm†	Hemor-rhages	Exudates	Papilledema	Arteriolar light reflex	AV crossing‡ defects
Normal	3:4	1:1	0	0	0	Fine yellow line, red blood column	0
Grade I	1:2	1:1	0	0	0	Broadened yellow line, red blood column	Mild depression of vein
Grade II	1:3	2:3	0	0	0	Broad yellow line, "copper wire," blood column not visible	Depression or humping of vein
Grade III	1:4	1:3	+	+	0	Broad white line, "silver wire," blood column not visible	Right-angle deviation, tapering, and disappearance of vein under arteriole Distal dilatation of vein
Grade IV	Fine, fibrous cords	Obliteration of distal flow	+	+	+	Fibrous cords, blood column not visible	Same as grade III

* This is the ratio of arteriolar to venous diameters.
† This is the ratio of diameters of region of spasm to proximal arteriole.
‡ Arteriolar length and tortuosity increase with severity.

cultation for bruits originating in stenotic renal arteries. Bruits due to renal arterial narrowing nearly always have a diastolic component or may be continuous and are best heard just to the right or left of the midline above the umbilicus, or in the flanks; they are present in many patients with renal artery stenosis due to fibrous dysplasia and in 40 to 50 percent of those with functionally significant stenosis due to arteriosclerosis. The abdomen also should be palpated for abdominal aneurysm and for the enlarged kidneys of polycystic renal disease. The femoral pulses must be carefully felt, and, if they are decreased and/or delayed, blood pressure in the lower extremities must be measured. Even if the femoral pulse is normal to palpation, arterial pressure in the lower extremities should be recorded at least once in patients in whom hypertension is discovered before the age of 30 years. Finally examination of the extremities for edema and a search for evidence of a previous cerebrovascular accident and/or other intracranial pathology should be performed.

Laboratory investigation Controversy exists as to what laboratory studies should be performed in patients presenting with hypertension. In general, the disagreement resides in how extensively to evaluate the patient for secondary forms of hypertension. In the following discussion laboratory studies are divided into those which should be performed in all patients with sustained hypertension (basic group) and those which should be added if (1) from the initial evaluation a secondary form of hypertension is suggested and/or (2) arterial pressure is not controlled after first-step therapy (Table 251-4).

BASIC STUDIES Renal status is evaluated by assessing the presence of protein, blood, and glucose in the urine and measuring serum creatinine and/or blood urea nitrogen (BUN). Microscopic examination of the urine is also helpful. A serum potassium level is needed both as a screen for mineralocorticoid-induced hypertension and as a base line prior to initiating diuretic therapy.

Other blood chemistries may also be useful particularly since they can often be ordered as a battery of automated tests at minimal cost to the patient. For example, a blood glucose is helpful both because diabetes mellitus may be associated with accelerated arteriosclerosis, resultant renal vascular disease, and diabetic nephropathy, and because primary aldosteronism, Cushing's syndrome, and pheochromocytoma all can be associated with hyperglycemia. Furthermore, since subsequent

antihypertensive therapy with diuretics can raise the blood sugar level, it is important to establish a base line. The possibility of hypercalcemia may also be investigated. Serum uric acid is useful because of the increased incidence of hyperuricemia in patients with renal and essential hypertension and because, as with blood sugar, the level subsequently may be raised by treatment with diuretics. Serum cholesterol and triglycerides may be measured to identify other factors which predispose to the development of arteriosclerosis. An electrocardiogram should be obtained in all cases as an assessment of cardiac status, particularly if left ventricular hypertrophy is present, and as a base line. The chest roentgenogram may also be helpful by providing the opportunity to identify aortic dilatation or elongation and the rib notching that occurs in coarctation of the aorta.

SECONDARY STUDIES (Table 251-4) Certain clues from the history, physical examination, and basic laboratory studies suggest an unusual cause for the hypertension and dictate the need for special studies. For example, the abrupt onset of severe hypertension and/or the onset of hypertension of any severity under the age of 25 or after the age of 50 years should lead to laboratory tests to exclude renovascular hypertension and pheochromocytoma (Table 251-4). A history of headaches, palpitations, anxiety attacks, unusual sweating, and weight loss should lead to tests to exclude pheochromocytoma

TABLE 251-4
Laboratory tests and special studies for evaluation of hypertension

I Basic studies
  A Always included
    1 Urine for protein, blood, and glucose
    2 Hematocrit
    3 Serum potassium
    4 Serum creatinine and/or blood urea nitrogen
    5 Electrocardiogram
  B Usually included, depending on cost and other factors
    1 Microscopic urinalysis
    2 White blood cell count
    3 Serum glucose, cholesterol, and triglycerides
    4 Serum calcium, phosphate, and uric acid
    5 Chest x-ray
II Special studies to screen for secondary hypertension
  A Renovascular: Rapid sequence IVP, radioisotope renogram, and/or saralasin test
  B Pheochromocytoma: 24-h urine for creatinine, metanephrines, and catecholamines
  C Cushing's syndrome: Overnight dexamethasone suppression test

(as well as hyperglycemia). The presence of an abdominal bruit should lead to workup for renovascular hypertension, and the finding of bilateral upper abdominal masses on physical examination, consistent with polycystic renal disease, should lead to the performance of an intravenous pyelogram (Chap. 283). An elevated creatinine or blood urea nitrogen, associated with proteinuria and hematuria, should initiate a detailed workup for renal insufficiency (Chap. 274). Special studies are also indicated if there is therapeutic failure on the first-step drug program. The specific diagnostic measures depend on the most likely causes of secondary hypertension.

Pheochromocytoma. The easiest and best screening procedure for pheochromocytoma is the measurement of catecholamines or their metabolites in a 24-h urine collected during the time the patient is hypertensive. This test may be indicated even in patients who do not have spells, as over half the patients with pheochromocytoma have fixed hypertension. Provocative tests are seldom if ever indicated (Chap. 337).

Cushing's syndrome. A 24-h urine test for 17-hydroxysteroids and/or 17-ketosteroids or a plasma cortisol level can be used to screen for the presence of this condition; however, the more definitive test involves the administration of 1 mg dexamethasone at bedtime, followed by measurement of plasma cortisol at 7 to 10 A.M. Suppression of the plasma cortisol level to below 5 μg per 100 ml effectively rules out Cushing's syndrome (Chap. 336).

Renovascular hypertension. The standard test for renal vascular hypertension has been the rapid-sequence intravenous pyelogram (IVP). Features suggestive of renal ischemia include (1) unilateral delayed appearance and excretion of contrast material, (2) a difference in kidney size greater than 1.5 cm, (3) irregular contour of the renal silhouette, suggesting partial infarction or atrophy, (4) indentations on the ureter or renal pelvis, possibly due to dilated ureteral arteries (collateral notching), and (5) hyperconcentration of contrast medium in the collecting system of the smaller kidney. When these criteria are used, the false-positive rate is 11 percent and the false-negative rate 12 percent. The isotope renogram, which measures differential uptake and excretion by the two kidneys of one of several isotope-labeled substances, can be used as a further screening procedure. Its sensitivity and reliability are probably somewhat less than the IVP. The most recent screening test is the blood pressure response to saralasin, an angiotensin II antagonist. In preliminary studies, the false-positive rate appears to be the same or lower than with an IVP with a comparable false-negative rate. Since it is considerably easier to administer and less expensive than an IVP, it may be the best screening test for renovascular hypertension. Split renal function tests and measurements of random peripheral plasma renin activity are less useful and have been almost entirely replaced by one or more of the other three screening tests.

The definitive test of surgically correctable renal disease is the combination of a renal angiogram and renal vein renin determinations. The renal arteriogram both establishes the presence of a renal arterial lesion and aids in determining whether the lesion is due to atherosclerosis or to one of the fibrous or fibromuscular dysplasias. It does not, however, prove that the lesion is responsible for the hypertension, nor does it permit prediction of the chances of surgical cure; it must be noted that (1) renal artery stenosis is a frequent finding by angiography and at postmortem in normotensive individual, and (2) essential hypertension is a common condition and may occur in combination with renal arterial stenosis which actually may not be responsible for the hypertension. Bilateral renal vein catheterization for measurement of plasma renin activity is, therefore, used to assess the functional significance of any lesion. When one kidney is ischemic and the other is normal, all the renin released comes from the involved kidney. In the most straightforward situation, the ischemic kidney has a significantly higher venous plasma renin activity than the normal kidney by a factor of 1.5 or more. Moreover, the renal venous blood draining the uninvolved kidney exhibits levels similar to those in the inferior vena cava below the entrance of the renal veins. Significant benefit from operative correction may be anticipated in at least 80 percent of patients with the findings described above. When obstructing lesions in the branches of the renal arteries are demonstrated by arteriography, an attempt to obtain blood samples from the main branches of the renal vein should be made in an effort to identify a localized intrarenal arterial lesion responsible for the hypertension.

Primary aldosteronism. The diagnosis of this cause of secondary hypertension is discussed in Chap. 336. These patients almost always exhibit hypokalemia. Diuretic therapy often complicates the picture when the hypokalemia is first observed and needs to be assessed. Given hypokalemia, the relation between plasma renin activity and the aldosterone level becomes the key to the diagnosis of primary aldosteronism. The aldosterone concentration or excretion is high and plasma renin activity is low in primary aldosteronism, and these levels are relatively unaffected by changes in sodium balance. A critical part of the evaluation after primary aldosteronism has been established is to determine whether unilateral or bilateral disease is present since surgical removal of the lesion usually reduces arterial pressure only in those with unilateral disease.

Plasma renin activity measurements. Some studies have suggested that most hypertensive patients should have a plasma renin level measured and indexed against a 24-h urine sodium excretion rate to assess whether high, low, or normal levels are present. This information, it is argued, may be important for both therapeutic and prognostic reasons. However, it is unclear, on the basis of presently available data and treatment programs, that these measurements are really useful except in patients with findings suggestive of renal vascular disease or mineralocorticoid excess in whom lateralizing renal vein renin levels or suppressed peripheral renin levels may be of diagnostic and/or therapeutic significance.

TREATMENT Virtually every patient with diastolic hypertension is a candidate for diagnostic studies and for subsequent treatment. This conclusion must be tempered with the acknowledgment that no data exist which show the benefits of reduction of mild pressure elevations (diastolic pressure of 90 to 104 mmHg). Furthermore, at any given level of blood pressure elevation, the risk of developing hypertensive vascular complications is greater in men than in women, and in younger persons than in older ones. It may be argued, then, that it is hard to justify producing the uncomfortable side effects of therapy in, for example, an asymptomatic woman over 70 years of age with a diastolic pressure of 90 mmHg. On the other hand, it is easy to justify side effects in a man of 30 with a diastolic pressure of 104 mmHg, because such a person may be expected to receive the greatest benefit from therapy. Fortunately, the choice of treatment is such that a satisfactory program to control arterial pressure with minimal side effects can be developed for most patients. A reasonable guideline would be that all patients with diastolic pressure repeatedly above 100 mmHg should be treated unless specific contraindications exist. In patients with diastolic pressures of 90 to 100 mmHg, other features, including sex, age, and presence of other known risk factors for development of vascular disease, such as hyperglycemia and hypercholesterolemia, should be considered before deciding to treat. There is controversy regarding the advisability of treating isolated systolic hypertension. Until the results of a well-controlled prospective study provide evidence to the contrary, treatment of isolated systolic hypertension is not recommended. Patients with labile hypertension, borderline hypertension, or isolated systolic hypertension who are not treated should have regular follow-up examinations at 6-month intervals, because of the frequent development of progressive and/or sustained hypertension.

The identification of an operable form of secondary hypertension does not automatically mean that surgical treatment is indicated. The decision depends upon the age and general health of the patient, the natural history of the lesion, and the response of the pressure to drug therapy. In patients with renovascular hypertension the feasibility of vascular repair versus nephrectomy and the degree of overall renal function impairment must be considered. Age and general health are important in patients with renovascular hypertension due to arteriosclerosis, because there is no evidence that repair of the stenosis increases life expectancy in the elderly patient with other evidence of vascular disease. Knowledge of the natural history of the disease is especially important when approaching the decision in the young patient with renal-artery stenosis due to fibrous dysplasia. If the arteriographic appearance suggests that the stenosis is due to intimal or subadventitial fibroplasia, the lesion may be expected to progress and operation is required. Medial fibroplasia, on the other hand, often remains stable, and operation may not be necessary if pressure can be controlled by drug therapy. The decision regarding operation should also be considered particularly carefully in patients with primary aldosteronism when bilateral adrenal venography does not demonstrate a tumor, because such patients may prove to have multinodular hyperplasia. This means that bilateral adrenalectomy would be required to eliminate the aldosterone excess, and, even then, hypertension usually persists. If hypokalemia can be controlled by spironolactone or other drug therapy, and arterial pressure lowered with antihypertensive agents, then it is reasonable to withhold operative treatment.

General measures (Table 251-5) Nondrug therapeutic intervention is probably indicated in all patients with borderline or sustained hypertension and probably most with labile hypertension. The general measures employed include (1) relief of stress, (2) diet, (3) regular exercise, and (4) control of other risk factors contributing to the development of arteriosclerosis. Relief of emotional and environmental stress is one of the reasons for the improvement in hypertension that occurs when the patient is hospitalized. Though it is usually impossible to extricate the hypertensive patient from all his internal and external stresses, he should be advised to avoid any unnecessary tensions. In rare instances, it may be appropriate to recommend a change of job or of life-style. Recently it has been suggested

that relaxation techniques may also lower arterial pressure. However, it is uncertain that these techniques alone have much long-term effect.

Dietary management has three aspects:

1 Because of the documented efficacy of sodium restriction and volume contraction in lowering blood pressure, patients previously were instructed to curtail sodium intake drastically. The advent of effective oral diuretics provided an additional method of decreasing body sodium stores and led some to suggest that sodium restriction was no longer necessary. However, a number of reports have documented that while mild sodium restriction has little, if any, direct action on blood pressure, it significantly potentiates the effectiveness of nearly all antihypertensive agents. Thus, the most practical approach now is to advise mild dietary sodium restriction (up to 5 g NaCl per day).
2 Caloric restriction should be urged for the patient who is overweight. Some obese patients will show a significant reduction in pressure simply as a consequence of weight loss.
3 A moderate restriction in intake of cholesterol and saturated fats is recommended on the suggestive evidence that such a diet may diminish the incidence of arteriosclerotic complications. Regular exercise is indicated within the limits of the patient's cardiovascular status. Not only is exercise helpful in controlling weight, but in addition there is evidence that physical conditioning itself may lower arterial pressure. Isotonic exercises (jogging, swimming) are better than isometric exercises (weight lifting) since, if anything, the latter raises arterial pressure. The dietary management outlined above is aimed at the control of other risk factors. Probably the most significant additional step that could be taken in this area would be to convince the smoker to give up cigarettes.

Drug therapy (Table 251-6) To make rational use of antihypertensive drugs, the sites and mechanisms of their action must be understood. In general, there are four classes of drugs: diuretics, antiadrenergic agents, vasodilators, and angiotensin blockers.

DIURETICS (see also Chap. 236) Drugs active on the renal tubules affect arterial pressure primarily by causing sodium diuresis and volume depletion. The thiazides are the most frequently used and most extensively investigated members of this group, and their early effect certainly is related to the diuresis. A reduction in peripheral vascular resistance also has been reported by some workers to be important in the long term. Thiazide diuretics form the cornerstone of most therapeutic programs designed to lower arterial pressure. Their most frequent side effects are hypokalemia due to renal potassium loss, hyperuricemia due to uric acid retention, and carbohydrate intolerance. The more potent diuretics, furosemide and ethacrynic acid, also have been shown to be antihypertensive but have been less extensively used for this purpose primarily because of their shorter duration of action. Spironolactone causes renal sodium loss by blocking the effect of endogenous mineralocorticoids, and therefore it may be more effective in patients whose mineralocorticoids are present in excess, e.g., primary or secondary aldosteronism. Although it does not compete directly with aldosterone, triamterene acts at the same site as spironolactone to impede sodium reabsorption and is effective in the same situations as spironolactone. Spironolactone or triamterene can also be given along with thiazide diuretics to minimize renal potassium loss.

A new class of diuretics, derivatives of acetic acid, which are uricosuric has recently been developed to reduce the hyper-

TABLE 251-5
Treatment of patients with hypertension

GENERAL MEASURES

1 Relief of stress (relaxation techniques)
2 Dietary control
   a Restrict sodium chloride to 4 to 6 g per day
   b Restrict calories
   c Restrict cholesterol and saturated fats
3 Regular isotonic exercise
4 Stop cigarette smoking

DRUG THERAPY

Step 1: Thiazide diuretic
Step 2: Add an antiadrenergic agent: propranolol, methyldopa, or reserpine
Step 3: Add a vasodilator: hydralazine
Step 4: Add guanethidine or substitute clonidine or prazosin for a step 2 drug

TABLE 251-6
Drugs used in treatment of hypertension—listed according to site of action

Site of action	Drug	Dosage	Indications	Contraindications	Frequent or peculiar side effects
DIURETICS					
Renal tubule	Thiazides	Depends on specific drug	Mild hypertension, as adjunct in treatment of moderate to severe hypertension	Diabetes mellitus, hyperuricemia, primary aldosteronism	Potassium depletion, hyperglycemia, hyperuricemia, dermatitis, purpura
	Hydrochlorothiazide	Oral: 25–50 mg qd or bid			
	Furosemide	Oral: 20–40 mg qd or bid	Mild hypertension, as adjunct in severe or malignant hypertension	Hyperuricemia, primary aldosteronism	Potassium depletion, hyperuricemia, nausea, vomiting, diarrhea
	Ethacrynic acid	Oral: 25–50 mg qd or bid	Mild hypertension, as adjunct in severe or malignant hypertension	Hyperuricemia, primary aldosteronism	Potassium depletion, hyperuricemia, diarrhea
	Spironolactone	Oral: 25–100 mg tid or qid	Hypertension due to hypermineralocorticoidism, adjunct to thiazide therapy	Renal failure	Hyperkalemia, diarrhea, gynecomastia, menstrual irregularities
	Triamterene	Oral: 100 mg qd up to tid	Hypertension due to hypermineralocorticoidism, adjunct to thiazide therapy	Renal failure	Hyperkalemia, nausea, vomiting, leg cramps
ANTIADRENERGIC AGENTS					
Central	Clonidine	Oral: 0.2–0.6 mg qid	Mild to moderate hypertension, renal disease with hypertension		Postural hypotension, drowsiness, dry mouth, rebound hypertension after abrupt withdrawal
	Methyldopa (also acts by blocking sympathetic nerves)	Oral: 250–750 mg tid or qid; IV: 500–1000 mg every 4–6 h (tolerance may develop)	Mild to moderate hypertension (oral), malignant hypertension (IV)	Pheochromocytoma, active hepatic disease (IV), during MAO inhibitor administration	Postural hypotension, sedation, fatigue, diarrhea, impaired ejaculation, fever, gynecomastia, lactation, positive Coombs tests (occasionally associated with hemolysis)
	Sedatives and tranquilizers		Tense or anxious patient with hypertension		Drowsiness, fatigue
	Phenobarbital	Oral: 15–30 mg tid or qid			
	Diazepam	Oral: 2–10 mg qid			
Autonomic ganglia	Trimethaphan	IV: 1–10 mg/min	Severe or malignant hypertension	Severe coronary artery disease, cerebrovascular insufficiency, diabetes mellitus (on hypoglycemic therapy), glaucoma, prostatism	Postural hypotension, visual symptoms, dry mouth, constipation, urinary retention, impotence
Nerve endings	Rauwolfia alkaloids		Mild to moderate hypertension in young patient	Pheochromocytoma, peptic ulcer, depression, during MAO inhibitor administration	Depression, nightmares, nasal congestion, dyspepsia, diarrhea, impotence
	Reserpine	Oral: 0.1–0.5 mg qd			
	Guanethidine	Oral: 10–300 mg qd	Moderate to severe hypertension	Pheochromocytoma, severe coronary artery disease, cerebrovascular insufficiency, during MAO inhibitor administration	Postural hypotension, bradycardia, dry mouth, diarrhea, impaired ejaculation, fluid retention
Alpha receptors	Phentolamine	IV: 1–5 mg	Suspected or proved pheochromocytoma	Severe coronary artery disease	Tachycardia, weakness, dizziness, flushing
	Phenoxybenzamine	Oral: 10–50 mg qd or bid (tolerance may develop)	Proved pheochromocytoma		Postural hypotension, tachycardia, miosis, nasal congestion, dry mouth
	Prazosin	Oral: 1–5 mg bid or tid	Mild to moderate hypertension		Sudden syncope, headache, sedation, dizziness, tachycardia
Beta receptors	Propranolol	Oral: 10–120 mg qid	Mild to moderate hypertension (especially with evidence for hyperdynamic circulation), adjunct to hydralazine therapy	Congestive heart failure, asthma, diabetes mellitus (on hypoglycemic therapy), during MAO inhibitor administration	Dizziness, depression, bronchospasm, nausea, vomiting, diarrhea, constipation, heart failure
	Metoprolol	Oral: 50–225 mg bid			

TABLE 251-6 (continued)
Drugs used in treatment of hypertension—listed according to site of action

Site of action	Drug	Dosage	Indications	Contraindications	Frequent or peculiar side effects
VASODILATORS					
Vascular smooth muscle	Hydralazine	Oral: 10–75 mg qid IV or IM: 10–50 mg every 6 h (tolerance may develop)	As adjunct in treatment of moderate to severe hypertension (oral), malignant hypertension (IV or IM), renal disease with hypertension	Lupus erythematosus, severe coronary artery disease	Headache, tachycardia, angina pectoris, anorexia, nausea, vomiting, diarrhea, lupus-like syndrome
	Diazoxide	IV: 300 mg rapidly	Severe or malignant hypertension	Diabetes mellitus, hyperuricemia, congestive heart failure	Hyperglycemia, hyperuricemia, sodium retention
	Nitroprusside	IV: 0.5–8 (μg/kg)/min	Malignant hypertension		Apprehension, weakness, diaphoresis, nausea, vomiting, muscle twitching

uricemia associated with thiazide diuretics. However, it is too early to determine their usefulness. Indeed, even after two decades of diuretic usage, it is still unknown whether the chemical changes induced by these agents are harmful.

ANTIADRENERGIC AGENTS These drugs act at one or more sites either centrally on the vasomotor center, in peripheral neurons modifying catecholamine release, or by blocking adrenergic receptor sites on target tissue. Drugs that appear to have predominant *central actions* are *clonidine* and *methyldopa*. These drugs and their metabolites are predominantly alpha-receptor agonists. Stimulation of alpha receptors in the vasomotor centers of the brain *reduces* sympathetic outflow, thereby reducing arterial pressure. Usually a fall in cardiac output and heart rate also occurs, more commonly with clonidine, but the baroreceptor reflex is intact. Thus, postural symptoms are absent. However, rebound hypertension may rarely occur when these drugs, particularly clonidine, are stopped. This is probably secondary to the increase in norepinephrine release which had been inhibited by these agents secondary to their agonist effect on presynaptic alpha receptors.

Another class of antiadrenergic agents is the *ganglionic blocking* drugs. These compounds block ganglionic transmission in the autonomic nervous system. They have little effect when the patient is supine, but they prevent reflex vasoconstriction in the upright position. Ganglionic blocking agents interfere with parasympathetic as well as sympathetic function, and this results in such side effects as impairment of visual accommodation, paralytic ileus, retention of urine, and failure of erection and ejaculation. Because of these problems, ganglionic blocking agents are now usually reserved for the rapid lowering of arterial pressure by parenteral administration in patients with severe hypertension.

Various drugs act at *postganglionic nerve endings*. The *rauwolfia alkaloids* are the oldest members of the group; their long-term effect results from their ability to inhibit the storage of norepinephrine within the vesicles in adrenergic nerve endings, thus leading to depletion of catecholamine stores. When given parenterally, they also have a direct effect on vascular smooth muscle. The rauwolfia alkaloids, like the other drugs of this class, exhibit the side effects that result from the unopposed activity of the parasympathetic nervous system, including nasal congestion, diarrhea, impairment of sexual function, and increased gastric secretion. Depression is the most serious side effect of the rauwolfia alkaloids; this is most likely to occur in elderly patients. The rauwolfia alkaloids are most helpful in treatment by the oral route of mild to moderate hypertension. *Guanethidine* blocks the release of norepinephrine from the sympathetic nerve endings. It has a greater postural effect than the other drugs that work at the nerve endings, and

orthostatic hypotension is a frequent side effect. However, centrally mediated side effects (sedation, depression) are infrequently observed since guanethidine has a low lipid solubility and, therefore, only poorly enters the central nervous system.

The last group of drugs affecting the adrenergic system are those which block the *peripheral adrenergic receptors,* either alpha or beta. *Phentolamine* and *phenoxybenzamine* block the action of circulating norepinephrine at *alpha*-adrenergic receptor sites. Since high circulating levels of norepinephrine are not present in most patients with hypertension, alpha blockade usually is not effective in lowering pressure. The exception is the patient with pheochromocytoma. While the above two compounds block both pre- and postsynaptic alpha receptors, *prazosin* selectively blocks only the *postsynaptic alpha* receptor. Thus, presynaptic alpha action remains, suppressing norepinephrine release and probably contributing to the greater efficacy of this drug. A variety of effective *beta-adrenergic receptor blocking agents* (Chap. 72) are available (only propranolol and metoprolol in the United States) which block sympathetic effects on the heart and should be most effective in reducing cardiac output and in lowering arterial pressure when there is increased cardiac sympathetic nerve activity. In addition, they block the sympathetic nerve-mediated release of renin from the renal juxtaglomerular cells, and this action may be an important component of their blood pressure–lowering action. Beta-adrenergic blockers are particularly useful when employed in conjunction with vascular smooth-muscle relaxants, which tend to evoke a reflex increase in myocardial contractility, and with diuretics, the administration of which often results in an elevation of circulating renin activity. In practice, beta blockers appear to be effective even when there is no evidence of increased sympathetic tone with about one-half or more of all patients showing a fall in pressure. Propranolol can precipitate congestive heart failure and asthma in susceptible individuals, and it must be used with caution in diabetics receiving hypoglycemic therapy, because it inhibits the usual sympathetic responses to hypoglycemia. Cardioselective beta-blocking agents (so-called "beta₁ blockers") have been developed (metoprolol, atenolol) which may be superior to nonselective beta blockers such as propranolol in patients with bronchospasm.

VASODILATORS *Hydralazine* is the most versatile of the drugs that cause direct relaxation of vascular smooth muscle; it is effective both orally and parenterally, acting mainly on arterial resistance, rather than on venous capacitance vessels, as evidenced by lack of postural changes. Unfortunately, the effect of hydralazine on peripheral resistance is partly negated by reflex increases in sympathetic discharges that raise heart rate and cardiac output. These limit the usefulness of hydralazine, especially in patients with severe coronary artery disease.

However, the efficacy of hydralazine can be increased if it is given in conjunction with propranolol or drugs such as methyldopa, clonidine, or reserpine, all of which block reflex sympathetic stimulation of the heart. A serious side effect of doses of hydralazine exceeding 300 mg per day has been the production of a lupus erythematosus-like syndrome.

Minoxidil is even more potent but unfortunately produces significant hirsutism and, therefore, is mainly limited to patients with severe hypertension and renal insufficiency.

An interesting drug in the same category as hydralazine but restricted in its application to acute situations is the thiazide derivative *diazoxide*. It is not a diuretic; in fact, it causes sodium retention. However, like the other thiazides, it reduces carbohydrate tolerance. It must be given rapidly intravenously to guarantee effect. It begins to act immediately to lower blood pressure, and its effects may last for several hours. *Nitroprusside* given intravenously also acts as a direct vasodilator, with onset and offset of actions that are almost immediate. These latter two drugs are useful only for the treatment of hypertensive emergencies (Table 251-8).

ANGIOTENSIN BLOCKERS   Drugs from several of the categories discussed above have been shown to possess an additional action resulting in inhibition of renin secretion. These include clonidine, reserpine, methyldopa, and propranolol, with clonidine and propranolol being the most effective. There is also a group of analogues of angiotensin II, e.g., saralasin, that act by antagonizing the effects of angiotensin II. A third group of drugs in this class are those which inhibit the enzyme converting angiotensin I into angiotensin II, e.g., captopril. Use of these converting-enzyme inhibitors is still in an investigational stage. However, these agents are promising because they not only inhibit the generation of a potent vasoconstrictor (angiotensin II) but also retard the degradation of a potent vasodilator (bradykinin).

Approach to drug therapy (Table 251-5)   The aim of drug therapy is to use the agents just described, alone or in combination, to return arterial pressure to normal levels with minimal side effects. When used in combination, drugs should be chosen for their different sites of action. Since many effective antihypertensive agents are available, a number of useful therapeutic regimens have been developed. The approach recommended is the step-care program suggested by the Joint National Committee on Detection, Evaluation and Treatment of High Blood Pressure. In general this approach can be used in most patients with hypertension. Those who have significant hypertension, however (average diastolic pressure of 130 mmHg or more), will require more intensive therapy with several drugs simultaneously. The following plan is suggested for patients without contraindications to specific agents, such as those listed in Table 251-6. The first drug employed is a thiazide diuretic. Even if not effective by itself, it potentiates the action of other hypotensive agents. It should be started at less than maximal doses and gradually increased at 2- to 4-week intervals until either arterial pressure is reduced to normal, maximum levels are reached, or side effects become significant. Reduction of serum potassium levels below 3.3 meq per liter or the simultaneous administration of cardiac glycosides will require potassium supplementation or the addition of a potassium-sparing diuretic (spironolactone or triamterene). Asymptomatic hyperuricemia (less than 10 mg per 100 ml) usually does not require treatment.

If arterial pressure is not controlled and other reasons for poor therapeutic response are not present (Table 251-7), then the addition of a second drug is appropriate. Prior to this step a search for possible secondary forms of hypertension should be made by performing the following studies (if not previously obtained): rapid-sequence IVP, isotope renogram and/or saralasin test; microscopic urinalysis and urine culture; serum calcium and phosphate; serum potassium; 24-h urine for creatinine, metanephrines, and catecholamines; and, if appropriate, overnight dexamethasone suppression test. If these studies are normal, then one of the antiadrenergic drugs, usually either a beta blocker or a centrally acting alpha agonist (methyldopa), should be added. Again therapy should begin with small doses, gradually increased until either the hypertension is controlled or a maximum dose is reached (Table 251-6).

If arterial pressure is still not controlled, then the addition of a vasodilator (hydralazine) is indicated. Adequate diuretic therapy and sodium restriction are again important, as is the simultaneous use of a sympathetic blocking drug. Vasodilators should be used cautiously in patients with coronary artery disease (angina) since they may increase cardiac rate. There are only a few patients in whom blood pressure cannot be adequately controlled with the above approach. In these, use of other drugs discussed in the previous section should be considered. Failure to obtain adequate pressure control may be due to insufficient volume depletion, and more vigorous dietary sodium restriction and diuretic administration may be helpful in resistant cases. In those few patients who are still resistant, a fourth step is necessary. This consists of giving a different antiadrenergic agent such as clonidine or prazosin, in place of the initial one, or substituting or adding guanethidine in increasing doses.

While the recommendations outlined above are satisfactory for the majority of patients, it is important to use a flexible approach since individual patients may respond differently to each combination of drugs. For those patients requiring multiple drugs, once the appropriate combination has been found, the use of a single pill with the appropriate combination of drugs may simplify the regimen and thereby increase compliance. Every effort should be made to reduce the number of times each day the patient must interrupt his schedule for the medication.

As noted earlier, in those patients who present with markedly elevated diastolic pressure—greater than 125 mmHg—an accelerated treatment program is needed including the initial use of maximum therapeutic doses of two or more drugs.

Reduction of arterial pressure in hypertensive patients with impaired renal function is often accompanied by an initial increase in serum creatinine. This change does not represent further structural renal damage and should not deter continuation of therapy, since achievement of blood pressure control may eventually reduce the value toward normal. Therapy in the azotemic patient should emphasize the use of those drugs that have the least propensity to lower renal blood flow, namely, hydralazine, clonidine, and methyldopa. However, the latter drug may accumulate in the presence of renal failure, and the dosage might have to be reduced.

TABLE 251-7
Reasons for poor therapeutic response in patients with hypertension

  I Inadequate patient compliance
  II Volume expansion
    A Excessive sodium intake
    B Secondary to nondiuretic antihypertensive agent
  III Inadequate doses
  IV Drug antagonism
    A Cold remedies
    B Sympathomimetics
    C Oral contraceptives (estrogens)
    D Adrenal steroids
  V Secondary forms of hypertension
    A Pheochromocytoma
    B Renal disease
  VI Inappropriate combination therapy

Probably fewer than one-fourth of hypertensive patients in the United States are being treated effectively. Only a small number of these failures is related to drug unresponsiveness. The majority is related to (1) failure to detect hypertension, (2) failure to institute effective treatment of the asymptomatic hypertensive subject, and (3) failure of the asymptomatic hypertensive subject to adhere to therapy. In order to improve this deficiency, patients must be educated to continue treatment once an effective regimen has been identified. Side effects and inconveniences of treatment must be minimized or counteracted in order to obtain the patient's continued cooperation.

MALIGNANT HYPERTENSION

In addition to marked blood pressure elevation in association with papilledema and retinal hemorrhages and exudates, the full-blown picture of malignant hypertension may include manifestations of hypertensive encephalopathy, such as severe headache, vomiting, visual disturbances (including transient blindness), transient paralyses, convulsions, stupor, and coma. These have been attributed to spasms of cerebral vessels and to cerebral edema. In some patients who have died, multiple small thrombi have been found in the cerebral vessels. Cardiac decompensation and rapidly declining renal function are other critical features of malignant hypertension. Oliguria may, in fact, be the presenting feature. The vascular lesion characteristic of malignant hypertension is fibrinoid necrosis of the walls of small arteries and arterioles, and this can be reversed by effective antihypertensive therapy.

The pathogenesis of malignant hypertension is unknown. However, at least two independent processes, dilatation of cerebral arteries and generalized arteriolar fibrinoid necrosis, contribute to the associated signs and symptoms. The cerebral arteries dilate because the normal autoregulation of cerebral blood flow decompensates secondary to the markedly elevated arterial pressure. As a result, cerebral blood flow is excessive, producing the encephalopathy associated with malignant hypertension. Many patients also show evidence of a microangiopathic hemolytic anemia, but this appears to be a secondary phenomenon, which could, however, contribute to the deterioration of renal function. Most patients also have elevated levels of peripheral plasma renin activity and increased aldosterone production, and these may be involved in causing vascular damage.

About 1 percent of hypertensive patients develop the malignant phase, which occurs in the course of both essential and secondary hypertension. Rarely it is the first recognized manifestation of the blood pressure problem. The average age at diagnosis is 40, and men are more often affected than women. Prior to the availability of effective therapy, life expectancy after diagnosis of malignant hypertension was less than 2 years, with most deaths being due to renal failure, cerebral hemorrhage, or congestive heart failure. With the advent of effective antihypertensive therapy, at least half of patients survive for more than 5 years.

Malignant hypertension is a medical emergency and requires immediate therapy. The initial aim of therapy should be to reduce diastolic pressure toward, but not below, 90 mmHg. The drugs available for treatment of malignant hypertension can be divided into two groups on the basis of time of onset of action (Table 251-8). Those in the first group act within a few minutes but are not satisfactory for long-term management. If the patient is having convulsions, if arterial pressure must be reduced rapidly, then one from the immediate-acting group should be used. *Diazoxide* is the easiest to administer, for no individual titration of dosage is required. A dose of 300 mg is given rapidly intravenously, and the antihypertensive effect is noted in 1 to 2 min. The same dose can be repeated when the pressure begins to rise, usually after several hours. In an occasional patient, pressure may drop below normal levels after diazoxide administration. Because of this, some physicians use a modified program, giving 150 mg rather than 300 mg initially, followed by a second 150-mg dose in 5 min if the blood pressure response has been minimal. It should not be used in patients who may have a dissecting aneurysm. The other two agents in this group require continuous infusion and close monitoring. *Nitroprusside* is given by continuous intravenous infusion at a dose of 0.5 to 8.0 (µg/kg)/min. It has the advantage over the ganglionic blockers of not being associated with the development of tachyphylaxis and can be utilized for days with few side effects. The dosage must be controlled with an infusion pump. *Trimethaphan,* a ganglionic blocker, is given at a rate of 1 to 15 mg/min. The patient should be in the sitting position, and the pressure should be monitored closely, preferably in an intensive care unit.

Patients given any of these agents should also receive other medications effective for long-term control. Those in the second group require 30 min or more to obtain full effect, but have the advantage of being satisfactory for subsequent oral administration and for long-term management of the patient's hypertension (Table 251-8). If such a delay in attainment of full effect is acceptable, intravenous *methyldopa* is an effective drug with which to begin therapy if symptoms of encephalopathy are absent. A dose of 500 mg in 100 to 200 ml 5% dextrose in water is given intravenously over 30 min; if the effect is inadequate in 2 to 4 h, a second dose of 500 to 1000 mg is given. Additional intravenous doses may then be given every 6 h until the pressure is stabilized. Intravenous *hydralazine* is effective in many patients within 10 min; an effective protocol involves giving 10-mg doses intravenously every 10 to 15 min until the desired effect has been obtained or until a total of 50

TABLE 251-8
Therapeutic agents used to treat malignant hypertension

| Drug | Route | Time course of action | | | Oral preparation available |
		Onset	Peak	Duration	
IMMEDIATE ONSET					
Diazoxide	IV bolus	1–3 min	2–4 min	4–12 h	No
Nitroprusside	Continuous IV	<1 min	1–2 min	2–5 min	No
Trimethaphan	Continuous IV	<1 min	1–2 min	2–5 min	No
DELAYED ONSET					
Hydralazine	IV, IM	10–20 min	20–40 min	2–6 h	Yes
Methyldopa	IV	1–3 h	3–5 h	2–12 h	Yes
Reserpine	IM	2–3 h	3–4 h	6–24 h	Yes

mg has been administered. The total required for response may then be repeated intramuscularly or intravenously every 6 h. Hydralazine should be used with caution in patients with significant coronary artery disease and should be avoided in patients evidencing myocardial ischemia or dissecting aneurysm. The converting-enzyme inhibitor, *captopril*, while promising in preliminary studies, is still under investigation.

The potent diuretics furosemide and ethacrynic acid are important adjuncts to the therapy just discussed. Given either orally or intravenously, they serve to maintain sodium diuresis in the face of a falling arterial pressure, and thus will speed recovery from encephalopathy and congestive heart failure as well as maintain sensitivity to the primary antihypertensive drug. Digitalis (Chap. 238) also is indicated if there is evidence of cardiac decompensation.

In patients with malignant hypertension in whom the existence of pheochromocytoma is suspected, urine should be collected for measurement of the products of catecholamine metabolism, and drugs which might release additional catecholamines, such as methyldopa, reserpine, and guanethidine, must be avoided. The parenteral drug of choice in these patients is phentolamine administered with care to avoid a precipitous reduction in arterial pressure.

There is hope even for patients who fail to respond sufficiently to any of the forms of therapy and who show progressive deterioration in renal function. In some, a period of peritoneal dialysis or hemodialysis to deplete extracellular fluid has resulted in better blood pressure control and eventual improvement in renal function. In other patients with refractory hypertension and renal failure who do not respond to volume depletion or hypotensive therapy, including Minoxidil, particularly those with marked elevation of plasma renin activity, bilateral nephrectomy has resulted in amelioration of hypertension; subsequently these patients have been maintained on chronic dialysis or have received renal homografts. However, bilateral nephrectomy should be avoided where possible since (1) the loss of renal erythropoietin will contribute to the associated anemia, (2) vitamin D metabolism may be adversely affected, and (3) all residual renal function will be lost.

REFERENCES

BERGLUND G et al: Prevalence of primary and secondary hypertension: Studies in a random population sample. Br Med J 2:554, 1976

BOOKSTEIN JJ et al: Radiologic aspects of renovascular hypertension. Part 2. The role of urography in unilateral renovascular disease. JAMA 220:1225, 1972

FISCH IR, FRANK J: Oral contraceptives and blood pressure. JAMA 237:2499, 1977

GAVRAS H et al: Antihypertensive effect of the oral angiotensin converting-enzyme inhibitor SQ 14225 in man. N Engl J Med 298:991, 1978

GIFFORD RW, TARAZI R: Resistant hypertension: Diagnosis and management. Ann Intern Med 88:661, 1978

HOLLENBERG NK et al: Renin, angiotensin and an angiotensin antagonist: Response to saralasin in essential and secondary hypertension. Medicine 58:115, 1979

HUNT JC: Management and treatment of essential hypertension, in *Hypertension: Physiopathology and Treatment,* J Genest et al (eds). New York, McGraw-Hill, 1977, pp 1068–1085

KAPLAN NM: *Clinical Hypertension,* 2d ed. Baltimore, Williams & Wilkins, 1978

LARAGH JH: Vasoconstriction-volume analysis for understanding and treating hypertension: The use of renin and aldosterone profiles. Am J Med 55:261, 1973

LEE C et al: Bilateral nephrectomy for hypertension in patients with chronic renal failure on a dialysis program. J Urol 119:20, 1978

MOSER M: Report of the Joint National Committee on Detection, Evaluation, and Treatment of High Blood Pressure. JAMA 237:255, 1977

PAGE LB et al: Drugs in the treatment of hypertension. Am Heart J 91:810, 1975; 92:252, 1976

SMITH WM: Treatment of mild hypertension. Results of a ten-year intervention trial. Circ Res 25(suppl 1):98, 1977

STRANDGAARD S: Autoregulation of cerebral blood flow in hypertensive patients. Circulation 53:720, 1976

STREETEN DHP et al: Use of an angiotensin II antagonist (saralasin) in the recognition of "angiotensinogenic" hypertension. N Engl J Med 55:402, 1973

VETERANS ADMINISTRATION COOPERATIVE STUDY GROUP ON ANTIHYPERTENSIVE AGENTS: Effects of treatment on morbidity in hypertension. II. Results in patients with diastolic blood pressure averaging 90 through 114 mmHg. JAMA 213:1143, 1970

252

DISEASES OF THE AORTA

JAMES E. DALEN

The aorta is subject to a variety of stresses. Its walls must withstand the shearing effect of each systolic thrust of blood. With its large diameter, the aorta is under greater tension than the rest of the arterial system because wall tension is a direct function of diameter and pressure. For this reason also, the effects of hypertension are especially deleterious. In addition, the aorta is subject to infection, trauma, necrosis of the media, and, most notably, arteriosclerosis, which has replaced syphilis as the most frequent disease affecting the aorta. Arising from these stresses are four major diseases of the aorta: aneurysm, dissection, arteriosclerotic occlusive disease, and aortitis. The number of deaths due to disease of the aorta is uncertain because other cardiovascular disease, ischemic heart disease, hypertensive disease, and cerebrovascular disease often coexist and take priority in the coding of death certificates.

ANEURYSMS A "true" aortic aneurysm is an abnormal widening that involves all three layers of its wall. The basic defect is destruction of elastic fibers in the media, which permits the remaining fibrous tissue to stretch and leads to an increase in diameter, which in turn raises wall tension. As this process leads to further enlargement, rupture becomes increasingly possible. "False" aneurysms, which are usually caused by trauma, are those disruptions of the inner and medial segments of the wall which permit expansion of the aorta so that the wall of the aneurysm consists of only adventitia and/or perivascular clot.

The commonest aneurysms are *fusiform*, in which a segment of the aorta becomes diffusely dilated, its total circumference being affected. In contrast, *saccular* aneurysms involve a portion of the circumference and consist of an outpouching with a mouth.

The commonest underlying cause of aneurysm is arteriosclerosis, but cystic medial necrosis, trauma, and syphilis and other infections must also be noted as causes.

Aneurysms of the abdominal aorta The pathogenesis and pathophysiology of aneurysms vary according to their site of origin. Three-fourths occur in the abdominal aorta, just below the renal arteries. Nearly all aneurysms in the abdominal aorta are caused by arteriosclerosis. The majority of victims are men older than age 60; more than half have associated hypertension.

The *diagnosis* is often made by physical examination, which reveals a pulsating mass in the midepigastrium. The diagnosis may first be suspected by x-ray of the abdomen, which demonstrates curvilinear calcification in the wall of the aneurysm. Most patients are asymptomatic when the diagnosis is first made. When symptoms do occur, they consist of abdominal or low back pain. Aortography may be used to delineate the size and extent of the aneurysm in uncertain cases. However, a preferable diagnostic technique is *ultrasound.* Continuous ultrasonic B scanning can visualize the abdominal aorta in longitudinal and transverse sections. This permits delineation of the size of the abdominal aorta and the thickness of its walls. It also allows detection of intraluminal clot. Its noninvasive nature permits serial estimation of the size of the aneurysm.

The *prognosis* depends upon the size of the aneurysm and, very importantly, the presence of other arteriosclerotic cardiovascular diseases. The diameter of the normal abdominal aorta is 2.5 cm. When the diameter of the aneurysm is greater than 6 cm, the probability of rupture in a 10-year period is 45 to 50 percent, whereas it is only 15 to 20 percent when the diameter is less than 6 cm.

Ischemic arteriosclerotic heart disease, which is present in about one-half of patients with abdominal aneurysm also has a profound impact on the prognosis. In one series of patients who had not had surgery, 5-year survival without clinically evident associated coronary disease was 50 percent. With ischemic heart disease, 5-year survival was only 20 percent. Follow-up of patients without surgery for abdominal aneurysms has shown that about one-third die of rupture of the aneurysm and one-third die of associated cardiovascular disease.

In properly selected patients operation prolongs life by preventing rupture. Symptomatic or expanding aneurysms should have prompt surgical correction. Similarly, large aneurysms (more than 6 cm in diameter) should almost always be repaired. The therapeutic decision for patients with asymptomatic aneurysms of moderate size (4 to 6 cm) is more difficult. Operative mortality with elective surgery, that is, before rupture, is about 5 percent. It is influenced by the size of the aneurysm but far more by the presence of associated cardiovascular disease, especially ischemic heart disease, in which case even successful surgery may not improve the prognosis. If there is no significant associated cardiovascular disease, small (4 to 6 cm) asymptomatic aneurysms should usually have surgical correction. With significant associated disease, it may be appropriate to follow the patient with serial ultrasound examinations. Surgery should be performed if symptoms occur, or if there is a significant increase in the size of the aneurysm.

Some patients with ruptured aneurysms survive long enough to become candidates for emergency surgical repair. They usually present, in shock, with severe pain in the abdomen, the lower back, or both. A tender pulsatile mass may be palpated. The salvage rate with emergency surgery in these circumstances is about 50 percent.

Aneurysms of the descending aorta　The second most frequent site of aortic aneurysms is in the descending aorta just distal to the origin of the left subclavian artery. These aneurysms are usually fusiform and due to arteriosclerosis. Most patients are asymptomatic when the diagnosis is first suspected by chest x-ray and then confirmed by fluoroscopy or aortography. Resection of thoracic aneurysms is more difficult than is resection of abdominal aneurysms. The risk of operation, about 20 percent, is in large part determined by associated cardiovascular or pulmonary disease. Operative therapy is indicated if the aneurysm is symptomatic or enlarging rapidly, unless associated cardiovascular disease presents a prohibitive risk.

Traumatic, false aneurysms of the descending aorta may occur in patients who survive rupture of the aorta. The most frequent cause is deceleration injuries suffered in automobile accidents. The diagnosis is suspected by noting mediastinal widening by chest x-ray. These patients are likely to be young and without associated cardiovascular disease. Surgical resection is nearly always indicated.

Less frequently, aneurysms of the descending aorta are saccular owing to *lues* or other *infection* (mycotic aneurysms). Saccular aneurysms are particularly likely to rupture, and they are less difficult to treat surgically than are fusiform aneurysms.

Aneurysms of the ascending aorta　The ascending aorta is the site of aneurysms of a wide variety of etiologies. In a prior era, nearly all were due to *syphilis.* They were readily recognized by x-ray by the presence of calcification in the wall of the ascending aorta. Luetic aneurysms can become huge, causing signs and symptoms by compression of adjacent structures. At the present time, the two commonest causes of aneurysms of the ascending aorta are *arteriosclerosis* and *cystic medial necrosis*; the latter may occur in association with Marfan's syndrome or as an apparent response to hypertension and/or aging of the aorta, or it may be of unknown etiology.

Aneurysms of the ascending aorta, particularly when they are due to cystic medial necrosis, may cause aortic regurgitation and lead to left ventricular failure. In this circumstance, resection of the aneurysm and replacement of the aortic valve is indicated.

The most common symptom of large aneurysms of the ascending aorta is chest pain, usually described as a deep, diffuse, aching sensation. The decision to resect an asymptomatic aneurysm to prevent rupture depends upon its size and the presence of associated cardiovascular disease. Echocardiography is useful in assessing and following the size of aneurysms in this area.

Aneurysms of the aortic arch　These aneurysms—the least frequent of all—are the most likely to cause symptoms because they compress adjacent structures, thus causing dysphagia, dry cough, hoarseness, dyspnea, or pain. Arch aneurysms may be fusiform due to arteriosclerosis, or saccular due to syphilis or other infection. Surgical correction of aneurysms of the aortic arch carries an operative risk as high as 40 to 50 percent.

Management of concurrent hypertension　Hypertension, which is present in more than half of patients with aortic aneurysms, needs optimal management. Persistent systolic hypertension abets further enlargement of aneurysms and may predispose to their rupture. In addition to standard antihypertension medications, propranolol is appropriate to help control hypertension and, in addition, decrease stress to the aortic wall by blunting myocardial contractility.

DISSECTION OF THE AORTA　This occurs when the intima is interrupted so that blood enters the wall of the aorta and separates its layers. Even though it is relatively uncommon, dissection is the most important acute disease involving the aorta and, without treatment, is almost always fatal. With prompt diagnosis and appropriate therapy, the majority of patients survive.

As with aneurysm of the aorta, the basic defect that permits dissection is disease of the media. The commonest disorder of the media that predisposes to dissection is *cystic medial necrosis,* which, in some instances, may be associated with Marfan's syndrome or, more commonly, to disorders that increase the hemodynamic stress on the aorta such as hypertension, pregnancy, coarctation, or bicuspid aortic valve. The second commonest cause of disease of the media predisposing to dissection is arteriosclerosis.

Nearly all aortic dissections begin at one of two sites: the ascending aorta (2 to 5 cm above the aortic valve) or the descending aorta, just distal to the origin of the left subclavian artery. The aorta is relatively fixed in each of these two positions, but is mobile on each side. Thus, at these two points, the hemodynamic stress of each systolic pressure wave is maximal, and the intima overlying diseased media may tear there, permitting blood to enter and separate the layers of the aorta.

The signs and symptoms and, importantly, the therapeutic implications are quite different when dissection involves the ascending as opposed to the descending aorta.

Dissection of the ascending aorta Dissection here may extend around the arch into the descending and abdominal aorta. This type of aortic dissection (type I by the DeBakey classification) is the most common and the most lethal. The majority of these patients have cystic medial necrosis and are men under age 60. About one-half have hypertension.

Dissection of the ascending aorta is heralded by the very abrupt onset of very severe chest pain (Chap. 5). Unlike the pain of myocardial infarction, the pain is maximal at the onset. The pain is most frequent in the anterior chest, but may radiate to, or even be limited to, the midscapular area of the back. The pain is nearly always initially attributed to acute myocardial infarction. There are several ways that the appropriate diagnosis may be made. Since dissection of the ascending aorta involves the great vessels in the majority of cases, a discrepancy between the carotid pulses, or a difference in the blood pressure in the two arms, should lead to a search for other evidence of aortic dissection. Dissection involving the carotids can cause a sudden neurologic deficit that may be intermittent. If the dissection compromises the right coronary artery, bradyrhythmias may occur, and occasionally there may be electrocardiographic signs of acute myocardial infarction. In approximately one-half of patients, the dissection causes acute aortic regurgitation. The presence of a new murmur of aortic regurgitation in the setting of apparent myocardial infarction should suggest the possibility of dissection of the ascending aorta. In the most severe cases, dissection causes hemopericardium. The appearance of a pericardial friction rub may be rapidly followed by pericardial tamponade.

In some patients, dissection of the ascending aorta may end before the origin of the left subclavian artery. This type of dissection (type II by the DeBakey classification) is seen most frequently in young patients with Marfan's syndrome. Aortic regurgitation is nearly always present.

Chest x-ray provides the most important clue to the presence of dissection of the ascending aorta. The most consistent finding is widening of the superior mediastinum. The ascending aorta may be enlarged out of proportion to the descending aorta. If dissection is suspected by physical examination or chest x-ray, preparations for aortography to confirm the diagnosis should be made at once. Unless hypotension is present, medical treatment, aimed at lowering blood pressure and depressing myocardial contractility, should be begun. This is most appropriately effected by beginning an infusion of trimethaphan (Arfonad), 1 to 2 mg/ml, or nitroprusside.

Aortography performed by the retrograde arterial technique will usually demonstrate a false lumen, and possibly an intimal flap separating the true and false lumina in the ascending aorta. If the blood in the false lumen has clotted, the principal finding will be an abnormal narrowing of the true lumen.

Once the diagnosis of dissection of the ascending aorta has been established by aortography, the majority of patients should have surgical correction, which consists of resection of the portion of the aorta containing the intimal tear and replacement with a prosthetic graft. Concomitant aortic valve replacement may be required if aortic regurgitation is present. Surgical correction can be performed at a risk of about 20 percent. Although medical treatment is vital to stabilize the patient prior to operation, it rarely is definitive in patients with dissection of the ascending aorta because the majority develop life-threatening complications, such as hemopericardium, hypotension, compromise of the carotid or coronary arteries, or aortic regurgitation. Without treatment, death is due to rupture, usually into the pericardium.

Dissection of the descending aorta Dissection of the descending aorta (type III by the DeBakey classification) is most likely to occur in elderly hypertensive patients. The underlying disease of the media may be arteriosclerosis or cystic medial necrosis. Dissection ordinarily begins just beyond the origin of the left subclavian artery and proceeds distally to the diaphragm or into the abdominal aorta. Dissection of the descending aorta usually does not proceed in retrograde fashion. Therefore, aortic regurgitation and hemopericardium do not occur. The carotid pulses and blood pressure in the arms are usually not altered. The primary symptom is the sudden onset of chest pain, often interscapular, often radiating to the anterior chest. The prime supporting evidence of dissection is to be found in the chest roentgenogram, which usually shows a widening of the superior mediastinum and may show the descending to be larger than the ascending aorta. If there is calcification in the aortic knob, its distance from the outer border of the aortic shadow may be increased.

The diagnosis of dissection of the descending aorta should be confirmed by aortography. As with dissection of the ascending aorta, hypotensive treatment should begin when the diagnosis is first suspected. A continuous intravenous drip of trimethaphan or nitroprusside at an infusion rate sufficient to keep systolic pressure at 100 to 120 mmHg, are the ideal first drugs. Propranolol or reserpine should also be begun.

Patients with dissection of the descending aorta usually do not have urgent indications for surgical correction. Medical treatment to lower systolic pressure, and to depress myocardial contractility so as to blunt the force of systole, may control the dissection. If medical treatment does not relieve the pain, or if there is evidence of progression of the dissection by x-ray or the appearance of a left pleural effusion (due to hemothorax), surgical resection should be performed. Surgical correction of dissection of the descending aorta poses a higher risk than dissection of the ascending aorta because the patients are older and are more likely to have associated cardiovascular disease. Elective surgical correction may be indicated after the dissection is controlled with medical therapy.

Prolonged, optimal control of hypertension is essential in patients with dissection of the ascending or descending aorta. In the absence of overt or latent congestive heart failure, it is advisable to include propranolol in the regimen to help prevent recurrent dissection.

ARTERIOSCLEROTIC OCCLUSIVE DISEASE The majority of adults in the United States have some degree of arteriosclerosis of the aorta. However, the disease remains silent unless it causes aneurysm or dissection, or unless it is sufficiently advanced to cause occlusive disease. The mildest form of arteriosclerosis of the aorta, longitudinal fatty streaks of the intima, may be seen in children (Chap. 250). Elevated intimal plaques begin to appear in adult life. Occlusive disease of the aorta may occur if these plaques are complicated by hemorrhage, ulceration, calcification, or overlying thrombus formation.

Arteriosclerotic occlusive disease is more frequent in the abdominal aorta, where it involves the terminal part of the aorta and extends for a variable distance into the iliac and femoral arteries. Arteriosclerosis of the aorta may be complicated by superimposed thrombosis. Thrombotic occlusion of the aorta is termed the Leriche syndrome. Depending upon the adequacy of collateral circulation, arteriosclerotic occlusive disease may cause ischemia of the lower extremities.

The classic symptom is claudication, which is present in the buttocks and thighs or in the calves. Impotence may also occur. The femoral pulses are absent or diminished in the majority of cases. Arteriography is needed to delineate the extent of the disease.

Surgical treatment consists of aortic-femoral bypass grafting. Endarterectomy is indicated when the disease is limited to the terminal aorta and proximal iliac arteries. The results of operation are usually excellent; symptoms are relieved or decreased in more than 90 percent of the patients in some series. Patency rates of 80 to 90 percent at 5 years have been reported. As with aneurysms, operative and late mortality is usually due to associated ischemic heart disease, which is present in up to one-half of the patients. The status of coronary and cerebrovascular circulations should be assessed prior to operation.

Symptomatic arteriosclerotic occlusive disease is rare in the ascending or descending thoracic aorta but may occur in the arch, where it becomes symptomatic by compromising the origin of one or more of the arch vessels. The carotid pulses, and/or pulses of the upper extremities, may be obliterated; thus, arteriosclerotic occlusive disease is one of the causes of the aortic arch syndrome. Other causes of this syndrome (also called "pulseless disease") include Takayasu's arteritis, syphilis, trauma, and neoplasm. Symptoms may include ischemia of the upper extremities or, more commonly, cerebrovascular ischemia, dependent upon the location of the disease. Surgical correction is usually feasible; however, its appropriateness depends upon the extent of the disease, and the status of the coronary and cerebral circulations.

AORTITIS Several different diseases may cause aortitis, i.e., an inflammatory process involving the wall of the aorta. The pathophysiology of aortitis depends on the severity of the process and upon its location. Aortitis becomes most evident when it involves the origins of the vessels of the aortic arch. Under these circumstances, it can, as noted above, cause the aortic arch syndrome.

The best understood cause of aortitis is *syphilis.* Only 10 percent of patients with luetic aortitis develop complications that permit its detection during life: saccular thoracic aneurysms, aortic valvulitis causing aortic regurgitation, and stenosis of the coronary ostia. Uncomplicated luetic aortitis is recognized at postmortem as a chronic panarteritis that causes patchy destruction of smooth muscle and elastic tissue of the media, endarteritis obliterans of the vasa vasorum, and intimal atherosclerosis. The process is most marked in the ascending aorta because of the predilection of treponemas for its rich lymphatic supply. The only clinical correlates of uncomplicated luetic aortitis are dilatation of the ascending aorta with or without calcification and a tambour-like aortic second sound.

TAKAYASU'S DISEASE Takayasu's disease is a nonspecific arteritis that has a particular predilection for the aortic arch of young females. Although it is suspected to be an autoimmune disease, its exact etiology is unknown. In the majority of cases, the disease begins in the second or third decade of life. In its initial stage, constitutional symptoms may occur. These may include fever, malaise, anorexia, weight loss, night sweats, and at times arthralgias.

These constitutional symptoms are then replaced by signs and symptoms secondary to involvement of the large arteries, particularly the aortic arch and its main branches. The patho-

logic lesion is a panarteritis that seems to begin with inflammation of the adventitia, with subsequent disruption and fibrotic changes in the media, and marked proliferation of the intima. Involvement of the arch vessels may be heralded by local pain and the presence of bruits. Progression of the aortitis causes stenosis at, or obliteration of, the origins of the arch vessels, thereby causing the aortic arch syndrome. Obstruction of the carotid arteries causes blurred vision, syncope, and dizziness secondary to cerebral ischemia. Involvement of the subclavian arteries causes paresthesias, intermittent claudication, and loss of pulses of the upper extremities. Hypertension occurs in the majority of cases owing to involvement of the renal arteries or to suprarenal obstruction of the aorta. The presence of hypertension, with absent pulses in the upper extremities, has caused this syndrome to be called *reversed coarctation.*

Reconstructive vascular surgery may relieve symptoms; however, the disease follows a relentless course so that death usually occurs within 5 years of diagnosis. Although some studies have shown that corticosteroid therapy may alleviate some of the constitutional symptoms of this disease, there is no evidence that treatment improves life expectancy.

REFERENCES

ANAGNOSTOPOULOS CE et al: *Acute Aortic Dissections.* Baltimore, University Park Press, 1975

APPELBAUM A et al: Ascending vs descending aortic dissections. Ann Surg 3:296, 1976

BAHNSON HT et al: The aorta, in *Gibbon's Surgery of the Chest,* 3d ed, DC Sabiston, FC Spencer (eds). Philadelphia, Saunders, 1976, p 878

BERNSTEIN EF et al: Growth rates of small abdominal aortic aneurysms. Surgery 80:765, 1976

DALEN JE et al: Dissection of the thoracic aorta: Medical or surgical therapy? Am J Cardiol 34:803, 1974

DEBAKEY ME et al: Aneurysms of the thoracic aorta. Mod Concepts Cardiovasc Dis 10:53, 1975

FOWLER NO (ed): Diseases of the aorta, including syphilitic heart disease, in *Cardiac Diagnosis and Treatment,* 2d ed. New York, Harper & Row, 1976, chap 51, p 1054

ISHIKAWA K: Natural history and classification of occlusive thrombo-aortopathy (Takayasu's disease). Circulation 57:27, 1978

LUPI-HERRERA E et al: Takayasu's arteritis: Clinical study of 107 cases. Am Heart J 93:94, 1977

MALONE JM et al: The natural history of bilateral aortofemoral bypass grafts for ischemia of the lower extremities. Arch Surg 110:1300, 1975

NANDA NC: Echocardiography of the aortic root. Am J Med 62:836, 1977

REUL GJ JR et al: Dissecting aneurysm of the descending aorta. Arch Surg 110:632, 1975

SZILAGYI DE et al: Contribution of abdominal aortic aneurysmectomy to prolongation of life. Ann Surg 164:678, 1966

THOMPSON JE et al: Surgical management of abdominal aortic aneurysms. Ann Surg 181:654, 1975

253
VASCULAR DISEASES OF THE EXTREMITIES

D. EUGENE STRANDNESS, JR.

In approaching the patient with a suspected peripheral vascular disorder, the physician must seek answers to the following questions: (1) Is the disease arterial, venous, or lymphatic in origin? (2) Is the process primary or secondary to some underlying disorder? (3) What segment(s) of the vascular system is involved? (4) How useful and specific are the symptoms and signs in establishing the diagnosis? (5) Under what circumstances are special tests necessary to make a correct diagnosis and to plan therapy? (6) What are the complications associated with the disorder? and (7) What is the prognosis with and without therapy? The following discussion will present the pertinent, available information that permits at least a partial answer to some of these questions.

ARTERIAL DISORDERS

ACUTE ARTERIAL OCCLUSION Sudden interruption of the blood supply to all or a portion of an extremity results in a spectrum of symptoms and signs which are dependent upon the location and extent of the occlusion and the immediately available collateral circulation. The major causes of acute arterial occlusion are *embolism, thrombosis,* and *injury.* In the upper extremity the heart is the source of the emboli in 95 percent of the patients with this problem. Less common causes include emboli from ulcerated plaques in the subclavian artery and aorta (especially aneurysms) as well as paradoxic emboli via an interatrial septal defect.

In the lower extremity somewhat over half of emboli will lodge in either the superficial femoral or the popliteal artery. The abdominal aorta is occluded in about one-sixth of cases, with the iliac arteries involved in approximately one-fifth. The remaining emboli will lodge in the three major vessels distal to the popliteal artery. The heart is the most common source of emboli to the leg arteries, but they may also originate from ulcerated plaques and aneurysms in the thoracic and abdominal aorta.

A variety of diseases involving the heart must be considered when a patient has acute arterial occlusion. Diseases of the aortic or mitral valve secondary to rheumatic endocarditis, particularly when associated with left atrial enlargement, atrial fibrillation, or atrial flutter, are common sources of emboli. Mural thrombi on the wall of the left ventricle which form secondary to a myocardial infarction may also be a source of the problem. A prosthetic aortic or mitral valve should also be considered a possible source of arterial emboli. Infective endocarditis must always be considered in patients with acute arterial occlusion. Emboli from ulcerated plaques or thrombi in peripheral aneurysms may cause ischemia of the foot and digits. These are small, usually lodging in small arteries of the distal limb. If they arise from the thoracic or abdominal aorta, bilateral involvement is the rule. If the involvement is unilateral, popliteal aneurysm must be considered as a potential source.

Arterial thrombosis occurs secondary to a number of causes, which include injury to the arterial wall, arteriosclerosis obliterans, collagen vascular disorders, myeloproliferative disorders, disseminated intravascular coagulation, and the dysproteinemias. Determining the exact cause of acute arterial thrombosis is not always easy.

Symptoms and signs Acute arterial occlusion produces an immediate fall in both the mean and pulse pressures in the distal arteries. Tissue P_{O_2} decreases markedly during the initial period after the insult. If collateral artery function is adequate to sustain viability, both the distal arterial pressure and tissue P_{O_2} gradually rise. The rapidity with which perfusion improves depends largely upon the resistance offered by the collateral arteries.

If acute arterial occlusion involves a critical segment of the arterial system where the collateral potential is poor, the clinical picture is dramatic. The initial complaint is pain in the most distal part of the limb; this is rapidly accompanied by pallor, coldness, and a sensation of numbness. Cutaneous sensation is usually lost within the first hour. After about 6 h ischemic muscular contracture develops. Subcutaneous hemorrhage, focal gangrene, and fixed staining of the skin also develop after about 6 h. Fixed staining of the skin is a certain index of loss of viability.

If limb viability is not in question, the major findings include loss of pulses distal to the site of occlusion, a decrease in skin temperature, and a systolic pressure in the distal portion of the limb which is lower than normal. When the arterial inflow is marginal, ischemic pain at rest involving the distal foot and toes may be present. The foot is nearly always cool, with very reduced capillary filling, particularly of the toes.

Though the diagnosis is rarely difficult when the extent of the ischemia is as outlined above, there are important variations in the clinical picture. If the immediately available collateral circulation is sufficient to maintain viability, the patient may complain only of a sensation of numbness, usually accompanied by a decrease in the temperature of the part. Under these circumstances, the circulation will nearly always improve, with these minor symptoms disappearing over the course of several hours.

Diagnosis The physical examination is helpful in establishing the most proximal level of the occlusion and the extent of the peripheral ischemia. The combination of pain, pallor, and paralysis clearly indicates that limb viability will be lost unless the proximal occlusion can be immediately corrected. If limb viability is not in question, the major physical findings include loss of pulses distal to the site of occlusion and a decrease in skin temperature. Light touch sensation is usually intact, even though the patient may complain of numbness. Detection of a bruit from the subclavian artery is common when an arterial plaque or aneurysm is the source of emboli to the hand.

When the leg is affected, it is important to determine whether a previous history of arterial insufficiency existed. If there is a history of intermittent claudication, it is likely that the basis for the acute changes is thrombosis on a preexisting plaque. With *cholesterol emboli* from the aorta, the clinical picture may be confusing. If the emboli arise from the thoracic aorta it is common for the patient to present with hematuria, abdominal pain, and ischemic pain at rest in both feet. When the emboli arise from the abdominal aorta (including aneurysms), ischemic pain at rest in the feet is often the only complaint. The ischemic pain is accompanied by prominent livedo reticularis of both feet, as well as petechiae. Peripheral pulses are nearly always present, since emboli rarely pass through collateral circuits in sufficient quantity to produce serious ischemia in the foot. Bruits must be looked for from the level of the abdominal aorta to the popliteal fossa. If amputation is required, cholesterol clefts may often be demonstrated in the material occluding the small arteries.

It cannot be emphasized too strongly that arteriography is rarely necessary to make the diagnosis of major artery occlusion and results in needless, dangerous delay when severe ischemia is present.

Treatment In any situation where the collateral circulation is clearly inadequate, immediate operation is required, if feasible. Time is of the essence, since tissue damage is progressive, often reaching an irreversible stage in about 6 h. If limb viability is not in question, the indications for operation are not as clear. In the arm, occlusions of the radial, ulnar, or brachial artery can often be treated nonoperatively with good results. However, patients with brachial artery occlusions may later complain of arm claudication, particularly if their occupation requires heavy physical labor. In the leg, acute occlusions distal to the popliteal artery rarely require operative intervention. If the obstruction is in or proximal to the popliteal artery, embolectomy should be carried out (with few exceptions), because of the high incidence of limb loss and subsequent disability if nonoperative treatment is employed.

Operative extraction of emboli can now be successfully managed with a balloon catheter. Since this can be accomplished under local anesthesia if necessary, regardless of the site of occlusion, the operation should rarely be withheld, even in the critically ill patient.

Anticoagulants (with heparin) for the short term and oral coumadin for the long term are used to treat the underlying cause of the emboli and prevent extension of the peripheral thromboembolism (Chap. 266). If a cardiac lesion is the source of the embolus, serious consideration must be given to operative correction of the underlying problem. If that is not feasible, the patient should be given anticoagulants for an indefinite period. Patients with suspected cholesterol emboli from aortic atherosclerosis are treated expectantly, with the prognosis depending entirely upon the extent of occlusion. In some cases, amputation is required to control ischemic pain at rest and tissue loss which may occur.

Immediately after acute arterial occlusion, the head of the bed is elevated so that the legs are in the dependent position. The patient must be kept warm, but heat should not be applied to the ischemic limb; vasodilator drugs have not been shown to be helpful.

ARTERIOSCLEROSIS OBLITERANS The primary lesion of arteriosclerosis is the intimal plaque, which progressively narrows and, in many instances, leads to complete occlusion of large and medium-sized arteries. In the abdomen the disease has its highest incidence in the aorta and common iliac arteries. The external iliac arteries are often spared. Distal to the inguinal ligament occlusions are most common in the adductor canal, with the popliteal artery itself down to the level of its three major branches having a much lower incidence of involvement. In the lower leg, the posterior tibial artery at the ankle and the anterior tibial at its origin are most commonly diseased. Arteriosclerosis obliterans is usually a segmental disease, with marked variation from patient to patient in its extent.

Clinical features Unless complicated by thrombosis, the symptoms and signs that develop secondary to arteriosclerosis obliterans rarely have an abrupt onset, since the process is a gradual, progressive one. The most common symptom occurs with exercise and is termed *intermittent claudication,* i.e., the pain that occurs in a muscle(s) with an inadequate blood supply that is stressed by exercise. The patient often describes the discomfort as a cramp which disappears within 1 or 2 min after stopping the exercise. Occasionally, profound weakness will be noted as exercise progresses. The walking distance required to produce the claudication is usually quite constant from day to day. The pain is more severe and the walking distance is always shortened when the patient walks upstairs and up a hill.

A point not often appreciated is that with arteriosclerosis obliterans claudication does not occur with occlusions in the anterior tibial, posterior tibial, or peroneal arteries. The location of the involved muscle group(s) is useful in predicting the most proximal level of occlusion. For example, calf and thigh claudication suggests that the primary involvement is proximal to the origin of the thigh muscles, i.e., the profunda femoris artery. The combination of hip, thigh, and buttock claudication with impotence in the male indicates terminal aortic occlusion, *the Leriche syndrome.*

The second important group of symptoms consists of those which occur at rest and are the result of either multiple levels of occlusion or involvement of a critical arterial segment where the major collaterals are also obstructed. Paresthesias and indeed numbness may occur but are less common than continuous pain in the toes or foot, which may be partially or completely relieved by dependency. Ulceration and gangrene of the toes and distal foot are a common occurrence when the disease reaches this advanced stage.

The patient with diabetes mellitus often presents variations in the clinical picture. Approximately 30 percent of patients with diabetes have a peripheral neuropathy which results in loss of deep pain sensation and sympathetic tone. When diabetics with a neuropathy develop ulcers with or without arterial occlusion, the lesions are typically painless. The combination of chronic arterial occlusion, peripheral neuropathy, and a nonhealing ulcer is a difficult therapeutic problem.

The physical examination is useful in substantiating the diagnosis and localizing the levels of disease. Patients with single occlusions in the aortoiliac or superficial femoral artery often have limbs which are normal in appearance. Patients with far-advanced disease secondary to multiple levels of disease often have ulcers, gangrene, loss of hair, trophic nail changes, and dependent rubor. Chronic arterial narrowing and occlusion lead to loss of pulses distal to the most proximal level of disease. The pulses should be examined in the groin in the popliteal fossa, and at the level of the ankle. If the involvement results in narrowing only, bruits are commonly heard which are transmitted for varying distances downstream from the stenosis. Auscultation should be performed from the level of the midabdomen to the popliteal artery; one should listen for the characteristic sound which is diagnostic of arterial narrowing.

Special diagnostic tests The magnitude of the physiologic derangement can be assessed simply by measuring the ankle systolic blood pressure at rest and following exercise to the point of claudication. Since arterial occlusion forces the blood to follow alternate pathways (collaterals) whose resistance to flow exceeds that of the normal vessel, an abnormal pressure gradient develops which lowers the pressure recorded at the ankle. The pressure may be measured by a variety of plethysmographs or the ultrasonic velocity detector. In general, if the systolic pressure at the ankle is greater than one-half that recorded from the arm, occlusion of one segment is most likely. Ankle pressures less than one-half of the arm systolic pressure are most often observed with multiple levels of disease.

When the patient with intermittent claudication exercises to the point of pain, the postexercise ankle blood pressure falls, often to unrecordable levels, requiring several minutes to return to the prewalking level. With exercise there is a marked fall in arterial resistance in the muscle. The amount of inflow available through the collateral arteries is inadequate, because of their high resistance to flow. As a consequence, distal arterial pressure falls and blood is shunted away from the foot. These changes explain the pallor in the foot which is so commonly observed during and immediately following exercise to the point of claudication. This test is most useful in following the progress of disease with and without therapy and is the most sensitive index of change available. Its great utility lies in the fact that each patient can serve as his or her own control.

Arteriography is essential prior to operation to localize precisely the disease and the extent of the involvement. However, it is rarely required to establish the diagnosis of arterial narrowing or occlusion secondary to arteriosclerosis obliterans.

Differential diagnosis It is rarely difficult to make the diagnosis of chronic arterial narrowing or occlusion if the clinical picture is combined with measurements of ankle blood pressure. There is a recently recognized entity, referred to as "pseudoclaudication," which may be secondary to neurospinal disease. The features of the symptom complex which are useful in distinguishing it from true intermittent claudication include the following: (1) the exercise-pain-rest cycle is not constant; (2) the symptoms may include numbness, tingling, weakness, incoordination, and clumsiness; (3) patients with pseudoclaudication may have to sit down or even lie down for relief; and (4) the time required for the pain to disappear often exceeds the few minutes observed in claudication due to arterial occlusion.

Therapy Patients with mild or moderate intermittent claudication may benefit from a rigorous, daily exercise training program. The essential features of this program include (1) repetitive daily walks to 75 percent of the claudication distance with interspersed periods of rest (1 to 2 min); (2) weekly retesting of maximum walking time with readjustment of walking distance; and (3) continuation of the exercise program—this is essential, since evidence suggests that cessation of the daily walking periods will result in loss of improvement. Vasodilator drugs have been advocated and used for the treatment of intermittent claudication, but evidence supporting their efficacy is lacking.

Weight reduction can be useful in patients with intermittent claudication by simply reducing the workload involved. It is also important that *smoking be stopped* entirely. All patients with arteriosclerosis should have their serum lipid levels determined, since they may be found to have a treatable disorder (Chap. 250). Direct arterial surgery may be effective in bypassing or removing areas of occlusion but should be reserved for those patients with disabling claudication.

Most patients with ischemic rest pain, ulcers, or gangrene present serious problems which can be helped only by direct arterial surgery. Lumbar sympathectomy may be useful but should be used *only* in patients with mild rest pain. If the rest pain is controlled by nonnarcotic analgesics and transient dependency, about 50 percent of these patients can obtain permanent pain relief by lumbar sympathectomy.

The majority of patients with arteriosclerosis obliterans will never require surgical therapy even though they do suffer some disability. The nondiabetic will have a limb loss rate of about 2 percent per year; this rate increases to 7 percent per year if the patient has diabetes mellitus. Meticulous foot care, which includes properly fitting shoes, and immediate attention to cuts and blisters are critical in proper management. This is particularly true in patients with diabetes and a peripheral neuropathy who are unable to appreciate deep pain.

THROMBOANGIITIS OBLITERANS (BUERGER'S DISEASE) In 1908 Buerger described a nonatheromatous lesion involving arteries, veins, and nerves occurring in young males and frequently leading to nonhealing ulcers and gangrene. Though there has been some controversy concerning the existence of this disease as a specific entity, sufficient evidence is available to recommend its continued recognition. The exact pathogenesis is obscure, but there appears to be a definite relationship with tobacco smoking or chewing.

The disease typically occurs in young males and has a characteristic location and set of clinical manifestations. Whereas arteriosclerosis obliterans is a segmental disease of large and medium-sized arteries, Buerger's disease starts in the smaller arteries of the hands and feet. There is usually an intense in-

flammatory component, which in later stages results in arterial and venous occlusion as well as fibrous encasement of the entire neurovascular bundle.

Clinical features The diagnosis of Buerger's disease should be suspected when male patients in the 20- to 40-year age range give the following history. A superficial, migratory nodular phlebitis may occur early in the disease. These nodules are well localized, associated with cutaneous erythema, and tender to touch. Cold sensitivity of the Raynaud's type occurs in about one-half the patients and is frequently confined to the hands. The fingers turn white when exposed to cold, then blue, and finally red—the so-called "triphasic" color response.

One of the most characteristic and typical symptoms of Buerger's disease is instep claudication. Exercise results in pain in the instep, promptly relieved by rest. Calf claudication may occur but is unusual, since the disease does not commonly progress proximally to involve and occlude either the popliteal or superficial femoral artery. When there is hand involvement, the occlusions may be bilateral, are often symmetric, and may lead to the development of hand claudication and fingertip ulcers which are exquisitely painful and difficult to heal.

The following findings during *physical examination* should lead one to suspect Buerger's disease: (1) intense rubor of the feet; (2) absent foot pulses in the presence of a normal femoral and popliteal pulse; and (3) reduction or absence of the radial and/or ulnar pulses.

Therapy There is only one effective treatment, and that is permanent, complete abstinence from tobacco. However, for some unknown reason, patients with Buerger's disease rarely discontinue smoking even though amputation is usually the inevitable consequence and the only method available of controlling the severe rest pain and ulceration which ultimately develop.

ARTERIOVENOUS FISTULAS **Acquired** Most acquired arteriovenous fistulas occur secondary to penetrating injuries; however, they may in certain circumstances occur secondary to blunt trauma. Malignancy, infection, and arterial aneurysms have also been responsible for the development of arteriovenous communications.

CLINICAL PICTURE Patients with penetrating injuries of an extremity should all be suspected of having an arteriovenous fistula. Initially there are no distinguishing symptoms which alert the physician to the presence of the fistula. The diagnosis is made by noting a continuous murmur and palpable thrill over the abnormal communication. Compression of the feeding artery will obliterate the murmur and thrill. With large fistulas compression of the feeding artery results in an abrupt slowing of the heart rate (Branham's sign). In rare instances distal arterial perfusion may be so severely impaired that gangrene develops.

With chronic fistulas the clinical manifestations may mimic those of venous disease, with varicose veins, stasis pigmentation, and cutaneous ulcers. Cardiac enlargement with or without failure may be seen in long-standing fistulas. Infection (bacterial endarteritis) may complicate large fistulas.

THERAPY The proper treatment of arteriovenous fistulas is division of the communication with maintenance of arterial continuity. Immediate operation may be indicated with large fistulas between such vessels as the abdominal aorta and inferior vena cava where cardiac failure may develop very quickly.

Congenital The development of anomalous communications between arteries and veins can pose both diagnostic and therapeutic difficulties. When there is an arrest in the development of the circulation during the stage of an undifferentiated capillary network, a *cavernous hemangioma* results. There is at this period an interlacing system of blood spaces which contain mixed blood, and it is impossible to distinguish the arterial and venous components.

When the development is arrested at the stage of differentiation, intercommunicating arteriovenous channels may persist. If the fistulas are large enough to be visualized arteriographically, the term used is congenital *macrofistulous arteriovenous* aneurysm. When the fistulas are too small to be visualized by arteriography, the term *microfistulous communication* should be used. This classification, based upon the size of the communications, is useful from a therapeutic standpoint.

CLINICAL MANIFESTATIONS   The clinical manifestations are extremely variable and largely depend upon the location and extent of the abnormal communications. The most common symptoms are (1) cosmetic changes due to the presence of the fistulas in the subcutaneous tissue and skin, (2) limb swelling and hypertrophy, (3) visible pulsations in some cases with macrofistulous communications, and (4) varicose veins in atypical locations. In long-standing cases stasis pigmentation and cutaneous ulcers may develop in response to the continued venous hypertension.

DIAGNOSIS   The presence of arteriovenous fistulas should be suspected when the following findings are presented: (1) unilateral leg or arm swelling, (2) cutaneous hemangioma of the "port-wine" variety, (3) varicose veins in atypical locations, and (4) an increase in temperature of the part. An important syndrome which may be confused with congenital arteriovenous fistulas is the *Klippel-Trénaunay* syndrome. The triad of this syndrome consists of varicose veins, "port-wine" hemangioma of the skin, and bone and soft-tissue hypertrophy. Arteriovenous fistulas are usually not demonstrable on arteriographic studies, but there is either agenesis or obstruction of the deep venous system.

THERAPY   The management of congenital arteriovenous fistulas depends entirely upon location, extent, and clinical manifestations. Treatment is largely conservative, with support stockings used to control the venous hypertension and valvular incompetence which often produce symptoms identical with those of the postphlebitic syndrome. If the fistulas are limited in extent, it may be possible to excise the lesions in their entirety, but this is usually not feasible.

THORACIC OUTLET SYNDROMES   The neurovascular bundle, by virtue of its course from the neck and thorax, is subject to compression by both muscular and skeletal structures. Traditionally, the bases for the symptoms and signs have been subdivided into the underlying anatomic defect(s), which include the scalenus anticus, cervical rib, costoclavicular, and the hyperabduction syndromes. From a diagnostic standpoint, obliteration of the radial pulse in a variety of arm positions has been considered the distinguishing feature of the underlying problem. This should no longer be considered the key diagnostic test since it frequently occurs in normal subjects. Further, the symptoms are generally due to compression of the brachial plexus and not the subclavian artery.

Those patients with the most prominent symptoms and signs will have cervical ribs with an associated fibrous band which attaches to the first rib producing compression of the neurovascular bundle. The key diagnostic features in these patients are (1) prompt appearance of paresthesias and numbness with the arm abducted to 90° and externally rotated, (2) appearance of a prominent bruit in the supraclavicular fossa, and (3) immediate disappearance of the symptoms when the arm is returned to the neutral position. There is little doubt that chronic arterial compression can lead to aneurysmal dilatation of the subclavian artery with occlusion and/or emboli, but this is rare.

In the absence of a *clear-cut* relationship between arm position and the symptoms, it is essential to rule out other causes for the clinical picture, which includes a cervical disk, degenerative joint disease, and the carpal tunnel syndrome. If cold sensitivity is also present, the vasospastic syndromes discussed in the next section must be ruled out. Removal of the first rib is performed too frequently and must be reserved for only those patients in whom the diagnosis is clear and other causes have been ruled out. The best results will be obtained in patients with cervical ribs in whom the relationship between arm position and neurovascular compression is easily demonstrated.

VASOSPASTIC DISORDERS   Those diseases which are properly classified as arteriospastic disorders include acrocyanosis, livedo reticularis, and cold sensitivity of the Raynaud type. The challenge in dealing with these entities is not in making the correct clinical diagnosis but rather in differentiating between the primary and secondary forms of the diseases. The primary forms are benign, rarely lead to digit ulcers, and never terminate fatally. The secondary causes of the arteriospastic disorders are frequently serious and may have a fatal outcome.

Cold sensitivity of the Raynaud type   In evaluating and determining whether a patient has a true sensitivity to cold or emotional stimuli it is necessary to establish whether or not the "triphasic" color response occurs, i.e., pallor, cyanosis, and rubor, in sequence. The most important element from a diagnostic standpoint is the pallor, during which the digits turn absolutely white.

Livedo reticularis   Livedo reticularis presents with a persistent cyanotic mottling of the skin which has a typical "fishnet" appearance. In contrast to Raynaud's disease, a phenomenon which is confined to the digits, livedo reticularis may involve all parts of the extremities and trunk. This cutaneous pattern is often accentuated by exposure to cold.

Acrocyanosis   The most uncommon of the vasospastic disorders is acrocyanosis, which is characterized by a persistent diffuse cyanosis of the fingers, hands, toes, and feet. This disease is benign and not associated with an underlying disorder. The involved parts are nearly always cold, with excessive perspiration being a common accompanying feature.

Diagnosis   *Raynaud's disease* is more common in women, often starting in the late teens, is usually bilateral and symmetric, and uncommonly leads to fingertip ulceration or gangrene. The hands are much more commonly involved than are the feet. The factors in the clinical presentation which should lead the clinician to suspect that the Raynaud's phenomenon is secondary to some underlying disorder include (1) abrupt onset with rapid progression to tissue necrosis; (2) late onset in life ($>$ 50 years), particularly in men; (3) unilateral involvement, especially when only one or two digits are affected; and (4) associated symptoms compatible with a systemic disease.

Sorting out the underlying causes is often difficult because of the wide variety of diseases which may have Raynaud's phenomenon as a part of their clinical picture. The following diseases must be kept in mind: (1) chronic arterial disease, most particularly thromboangiitis obliterans; (2) the collagen vascular disorders, with scleroderma being the most common;

(3) occupational and industrial exposure to vibrating instruments; (4) poisoning with lead and arsenic; (5) ingestion of drugs, namely, the ergotamine preparations, methysergide, and propranolol; (6) hematologic disorders, namely, cryoglobulins, cold agglutinins, and dysproteinemias; (7) bilateral thoracic outlet syndromes; (8) late sequelae of bilateral cold injury; (9) primary pulmonary hypertension; and (10) occult carcinoma.

The secondary causes of livedo reticularis include (1) collagen diseases, in particular periarteritis nodosa and disseminated lupus erythematosus; (2) hematologic disorders, i.e., hyperviscosity syndrome, macroglobulinemia, and cryoglobulinemia; (3) cholesterol emboli arising from ulcerated plaques in the thoracic and abdominal aorta; (4) Cushing's syndrome; (5) drug ingestion, i.e., adrenal corticosteroids; (6) prolonged dependency or immobilization; (7) late result of cold injury; and (8) prolonged exposure to or the local application of heat.

Therapy The primary forms of cold sensitivity, i.e., livedo reticularis and acrocyanosis, rarely require treatment other than assurance and instruction relative to the dangers of prolonged exposure to cold. Sympathectomy has been widely applied, with inconsistent results, in the treatment of Raynaud's disease. Lumbar sympathectomy, probably because of the higher incidence of permanent denervation, is more likely to give good results than cervicodorsal sympathectomy. Sympathectomy, particularly in the upper extremity, should be performed only when conservative measures fail to control the symptoms. Reserpine and methyldopa have been reported to reduce the frequency and severity of the attacks.

When there are secondary causes for the vasospastic disorders, treatment is directed at the cause of the problem. It is important to remember that drugs and sympathectomy are rarely effective with the secondary forms of the disease.

ERYTHROMELALGIA This rare disorder of unknown etiology expresses itself as burning, tingling, and often itching of the foot and lower leg which appears as the ambient temperature increases. There is usually a critical temperature for each patient above which the symptoms appear [usually in the range of 31.7 to 36.1°C (89 to 97°F)]. During the attack the patient's feet and lower legs become bright red. The patient quickly finds that the symptoms are related to temperature and will assiduously avoid those circumstances which bring out the symptoms. Characteristically, patients wear sandals, avoid stockings, sleep with their feet outside the bedcovers, and use fans to reduce the skin temperature.

The *diagnosis* is established by the history and the examination of the extremities during an attack. The pedal pulses are intact, and the skin is warm and bright red. The disease is usually primary but has, in rare instances, been associated with myeloproliferative disorders.

Therapy is usually unsuccessful, but some patients have reported relief with aspirin or methysergide maleate.

VENOUS DISORDERS

VARICOSE VEINS Varicose veins are dilated, tortuous superficial veins with incompetent valves. The greater and lesser saphenous systems are most commonly involved, but it is not unusual for secondary branches of the superficial system of veins also to become dilated. They most often appear after the age of 20, but in women often develop in relation to puberty, during pregnancy, and with commencement of the menopause. In men there is a fairly even distribution in the onset of symptoms by decades up to age 70.

The etiology remains largely obscure, but varicose veins are known to be aggravated by hormonal factors in the female, increased intraabdominal pressure, and in rare instances, arteriovenous fistulas. Hereditary factors are important but have been poorly studied.

Classification It is important to classify varicose veins as either primary or secondary. Primary varicose veins occur in the absence of deep venous disease and generally have a benign course. Varicosities which occur secondary to obstruction and valvular incompetence of the deep venous system are much more serious.

Clinical features Primary varicose veins are brought to the attention of the patient first by the cosmetic deformity and second by the symptoms which develop with prolonged standing. The patient complains of a feeling of heaviness in the leg, combined with fatigue, that gets progressively worse toward the end of the day. Elevation of the legs will result in rapid and impressive relief from the symptoms. When the varicose veins are secondary to deep venous obstruction, loss of valves, and incompetent perforating veins, the symptoms are more severe and accompanied by swelling (see "Postphlebitic Syndrome" below).

Diagnosis The diagnosis of primary varicose veins is made largely by inspection of the legs in the upright position. The varicosities appear as dilated, often tortuous channels which are most commonly observed in the greater and lesser saphenous systems. When isolated clusters are observed in atypical locations, the possibility of an underlying incompetent perforating vein or arteriovenous fistula should be considered. To assess whether or not incompetent perforating veins are contributing factors, the Trendelenburg test may be employed. With the legs elevated and the superficial veins empty, a tourniquet is applied about the thigh close to the groin. The patient then quickly stands, and the pattern of filling is noted. If the superficial veins do not fill in 30 s, it is unlikely that incompetent perforating veins are contributing to the etiology of the varicose veins.

Therapy The majority of patients with symptomatic primary varicose veins should be treated initially with compression stockings. If the deep veins and perforating channels are patent and competent, it is very unusual for primary varicose veins to lead to stasis pigmentation and ulceration. In those rare instances in which treatment with compression stockings is inadequate, high ligation and stripping of the long and/or short saphenous veins may be required.

ACUTE VENOUS OCCLUSION Obstruction of superficial or deep veins occurs in two settings. The first is associated with an intense inflammatory component as usually observed with involvement of superficial veins. More common and potentially lethal is thrombosis of the deep veins where inflammation as either the inciting event or a clinical manifestation is uncommon. Thus, it is appropriate to separate these two entities since the clinical course and treatment are different.

Superficial thrombophlebitis Except for so-called "chemical" phlebitis secondary to direct intimal injury, the etiology remains obscure, but the clinical presentation is dramatic. The involved vein is exquisitely tender with surrounding erythema and edema. A fever is often present. While concern has been expressed regarding propagation of the thrombus into the deep venous system with subsequent pulmonary embolization, this rarely occurs. Treatment is directed at local measures to reduce the inflammation—application of heat, elevation of legs, and administration of anti-inflammatory agents such as phenylbutazone. It is important to be certain that the presenting symptoms are not signs due to a bacterial cellulitis or lymphangitis. The Doppler velocity detector is useful in distinguishing the above, since thrombophlebitis is always associated with thrombosis of the involved segment.

Acute venous thrombosis The most common in-hospital vascular disorder is thrombosis of the minor and major deep veins of the leg. In the initial stages, the soleus plexus of veins and sinus of the venous valve are the sites most commonly involved. When the thrombi remain confined to these areas they are not detectable unless prospective screening with ^{125}I-labeled fibrinogen has been carried out.

ETIOLOGY There are definite known precipitating factors, which include trauma and bacterial infection, but these are not the most common causes. The much larger group of patients who develop this problem fall into one or more of the following categories: (1) prolonged bed rest associated with a medical or surgical illness; (2) malignancy, particularly of the pancreas, lung, or gastrointestinal system; (3) administration of estrogens including oral contraceptives; (4) disseminated intravascular coagulation; (5) the postpartum period; and (6) paralysis.

CLINICAL FEATURES The most important factor concerning the symptoms and signs that develop is that they are not specific and may result from a variety of other diseases. Although edema and local tenderness with associated pain have been considered the most important findings, they are not sufficient to warrant either making the diagnosis of venous thrombosis or instituting therapy. Pulmonary embolization (Chap. 266) may, in fact, be the first clue that deep venous thrombosis is present.

DIAGNOSIS The bedside diagnosis of deep venous thrombosis is so inaccurate that it *must* be established by some independent means. The ^{125}I-labeled fibrinogen test is used for prospective studies but has limited application since it must be given prior to the initiation of the thrombosis. The most useful available noninvasive tests include Doppler ultrasound and plethysmography. Properly used, these tests have a rate of false-positive and false-negative results in the range of 5 to 10 percent. These methods are insensitive to thrombi confined to the muscular veins but can be used for sequential study to detect propagation into the major deep veins. If a vascular laboratory is present which has experience with these noninvasive tests, therapy can be based upon the results. However, if the tests are unavailable or the findings equivocal, contrast venography should be performed. A promising new approach is to carry out radionuclide venography with simultaneous lung scanning. This diagnostic test provides two critically important bits of information: the status of the major deep veins and a base-line perfusion lung scan.

THERAPY The treatment is directed at control of the thrombotic process already initiated. There is agreement that intravenous heparin is the most effective therapy. Until recently, it was common to give heparin intermittently (every 4 to 6 h). At present, the preferred method is continuous administration, starting with a loading dose of 5000 to 10,000 units and varying the dosage depending upon the partial thromboplastin time, which should be kept between two and three times the control time. The two major advantages of this approach are a more uniform level of anticoagulation and a lower incidence of hemorrhagic complications.

The duration of heparin therapy depends upon the degree of involvement and whether pulmonary embolization has occurred. With the latter, treatment must be continued for 10 to

14 days and even longer if the patient remains at risk. Oral therapy with one of the coumarin preparations should be started while the patient is still on heparin, which is discontinued only when a satisfactory level of anticoagulation has been achieved. The maintenance level varies considerably between 2 to 15 mg daily but must be carefully controlled to keep the one-stage prothrombin time approximately two times the control time.

The duration of oral anticoagulation is dependent upon the severity of the problem. For isolated calf vein thrombosis, therapy of 4 to 6 weeks is sufficient. However, for femoropopliteal or iliofemoral thrombosis, with or without pulmonary embolism, anticoagulation should be continued for 3 to 6 months.

PROPHYLACTIC MEASURES There is conflicting evidence that low-dose heparin (5000 units subcutaneously 2 h prior to operation, then three times daily) is effective in reducing the incidence of deep venous thrombosis as well as the occurrence of fatal and nonfatal pulmonary embolism.[1]

Operative therapy is usually applied to patients who either have sustained pulmonary embolism that is not controlled by adequate doses of heparin or have sustained hemorrhagic complications. The more commonly used procedures include ligation or partial occlusion of the inferior vena cava by a plastic clip. Patients who are not candidates for the direct operative approach may benefit from the transvenous placement of an "umbrella" in the vena cava just below the renal veins.

POSTPHLEBITIC SYNDROME Patients who have single or multiple episodes of deep venous thrombosis will frequently have irreversible changes in the veins which lead to further morbidity. The acute venous thrombosis often leads to residual chronic occlusion and destruction of the venous valves.

The loss of the valvular mechanism in the deep venous system forces the blood to follow abnormal pathways, particularly during exercise. In the standing position or during walking the muscle pump pushes the blood proximally, distally, and out through the perforating veins into the superficial system. By increasing venous and capillary pressures, this sequence of events, over a period of many years, leads to edema, and to rupture of small superficial veins in the vicinity of the perforating veins. The subcutaneous hemorrhage leads to deposition of hemosiderin pigment (stasis pigmentation), subcutaneous fibrosis, cutaneous atrophy, and lymphatic obstruction. These chronic changes lead to the development of stasis ulcers, which are difficult to manage.

Clinical features and diagnosis The important features of this disorder consist of swelling which is always worse at the end of the day, pain, cutaneous pigmentation (usually in the region of the medial malleolus), and nonhealing ulcers which develop secondary to minor trauma. Repeated trauma, subcutaneous hemorrhage, and cellulitis can produce changes in the skin and subcutaneous tissues that are indistinguishable from those of the postphlebitic state. In questionable cases venography is useful in establishing the cause of the problem.

Therapy The most important factor in the treatment of the postphlebitic syndrome is to reduce the hydrostatic pressure and to prevent "high-pressure leaks" through the perforating veins when the patient is erect. This can best be accomplished

---

[1] *The reader is directed to the writings of Strandness (1979) and Wessler for evaluations of the opposing views on this issue.*

by a tailored pressure-gradient stocking, which must be worn at all times that the patient is ambulatory, and by elevating legs when possible.

When an ulcer is present, healing may be accomplished by bed rest and elevation of the legs with or without concomitant skin grafting. In selected cases, removal of the incompetent superficial veins with ligation of the perforating veins may be necessary. Support stockings must be worn regardless of the therapy directed at the ulcer, because the deep venous system remains incompetent and edema will continue to develop without adequate external support.

LYMPHATIC DISORDERS

LYMPHEDEMA Lymphedema, an abnormal accumulation of lymph in the extremities, occurs from multiple causes, which include (1) lymphedema from organisms such as *Wuchereria bancrofti*; (2) infectious lymphedema resulting in thrombosis of lymphatics; (3) congenital lymphedema with arrest in lymph growth, which is apparent at birth or shortly thereafter; (4) traumatic lymphedema secondary to direct injury, burns, operations, and radiation; (5) essential lymphedema—so-called "Milroy's disease" which appears at puberty and is most commonly observed in women; (6) allergic lymphedema occurring secondary to exposure to drugs and pollens; (7) post-thrombotic lymphedema, which represents combined venous and lymphatic obstruction; and (8) malignant lymphedema, which occurs secondary to either direct invasion or obstruction of the lymphatics by tumor cells.

Clinical features Painless swelling of the involved extremity is the earliest and most common symptom and sign with most types of lymphedema. The swelling usually starts in the foot and ankle and then progresses proximally. Initially the swelling tends to subside somewhat at night, but as the process progresses, the swelling becomes permanent secondary to fibrosis of both the skin and subcutaneous tissues. Skin color and texture are normal until the late stages, when the skin becomes thickened and brown and has multiple papillary projections—so-called "lymphostatic verrucosis."

Diagnosis The location and nature of the edema readily separate lymphedema from edema due to other causes. In the legs, the dorsa of the toes and foot are nearly always involved; this is uncommon in other causes of swelling. The edema is often brawny in character and pits only with difficulty. Though the other forms of edema often improve with bed rest, elevation, and diuretics, lymphedema, even in early stages, responds poorly to these measures. In later stages when fibrosis develops in the skin and subcutaneous tissues, these conservative mea-

sures are of little, if any, value. Lymphangiography in selected cases may be of value in localizing and elucidating the cause of the lymphedema.

Therapy Therapy is directed at minimizing the amount of edema and prevention of recurrent attacks of cellulitis when a problem. Pressure-gradient stockings and the use of intermittent-pressure devices at night are helpful in controlling the edema. Since recurrent attacks of cellulitis due to the beta-hemolytic streptococcus are not uncommon and always result in further lymphatic destruction, prophylactic penicillin should be used indefinitely. Excision of the edematous tissue is reserved for only the most advanced stage of the disease when there is marked, irreversible swelling and disfigurement.

ANTERIOR TIBIAL COMPARTMENT SYNDROMES

Acute swelling of the anterior tibial compartment may occur secondary to intensive exercise, increased capillary permeability (with ischemia), or hematoma in the enclosed space. When arterial revascularization has been successful for prolonged ischemia, muscular swelling resulting in an increase in compartment pressure may lead to nerve damage, and muscle necrosis. This is recognized by the severe pain in the compartment, swelling, and local tenderness. If the anterior compartment is involved, there is anesthesia of a triangular area on the dorsum of the foot at the base of the first and second toes. *Immediate* fasciotomy is indicated, since a delay of even a few hours may result in irreversible changes.

REFERENCES

Bernstein EF (ed): *Symposium on Non-Invasive Testing.* St Louis, Mosby, 1978

Freeman LM, Blaufox MD: Thrombosis detection. Semin Nucl Med 7:3, July 1977

Nicolaides AW (ed): *Thromboembolism.* Baltimore, University Park Press, 1975

Rutherford RF (ed): *Vascular Surgery.* Philadelphia, Saunders, 1977

Salzman EW et al: Management of heparin therapy: Controlled prospective trial. N Engl J Med 292:1046, 1975

Strandness DE Jr: The case against low-dose heparin, in *Current Controversies in Cardiovascular Disease,* E Rapaport (ed). Philadelphia, Saunders, 1979 (in press)

———, Sumner DS: *Hemodynamics for Surgeons.* New York, Grune & Stratton, 1975

———, ———: *Ultrasonic Techniques in Angiology.* Berne, Switzerland, Hane Huber, 1975

——— et al: Present status of acute venous thrombosis. Surg Gynecol Obstet 145:433, 1977

Wessler SW: The case for low-dose heparin, in *Current Controversies in Cardiovascular Disease,* E Rapaport (ed). Philadelphia, Saunders, 1979 (in press)

Diagnostic methods

254
APPROACH TO THE PATIENT WITH DISEASE OF THE RESPIRATORY SYSTEM

EUGENE BRAUNWALD

As in other branches of medicine, a careful and detailed history and physical examination are the cornerstones of an accurate diagnosis in patients with disorders of the respiratory system. In addition, the roentgenographic examination occupies a particularly important role in the evaluation of patients with lung disease. Since abnormalities of the respiratory system are frequently a manifestation of a systemic process, attention must be focused not only on the chest; a comprehensive evaluation of the patient's entire health status is essential. For example, the presence of a pulmonary lesion may be due to metastatic disease, and hemoptysis may be due to a disorder of hemostasis. Diffuse scleroderma may result in diffuse pulmonary infiltrative disease (Chaps. 264 and 362), and multiple pulmonary cavities may be a manifestation of Wegener's granulomatosis (Chap. 67). Carcinoma of the lung (Chap. 268) may be accompanied by prominent extrathoracic manifestations, which may overshadow the pulmonary lesion. These include myopathy, peripheral neuropathy, hypertrophic pulmonary osteoarthropathy, and a variety of endocrine and metabolic manifestations, including Cushing's syndrome, the carcinoid syndrome, a hyperparathyroid-like picture, inappropriate secretion of antidiuretic hormone, gonadotropin (Chap. 347), and increased frequency of pulmonary infections.

In eliciting the history of patients with pulmonary disease, it must be appreciated that an increasing fraction of the population is exposed to materials which are potentially toxic to the lung (Chap. 259). The history must therefore contain a detailed *occupational and personal history* with a description of exposure to hazards such as coal, silica, asbestos, beryllium, bagasse, iron oxide, tin oxide, cotton dust, titanium oxide, silver, nitrogen dioxide, animals, moldy hay, air conditioners, and furnace humidifiers. It is useful to construct a work history, which includes the patient's duties, duration of exposure, use of protective devices, and illness in fellow workers. The occupational history should include information on a job-by-job basis as well as the military service. Contact with both wild and domestic animals may result in pulmonary symptoms, such as bronchospasm in the subject allergic to a pet, or acute pneumonitis in patients with ornithosis (Chap. 175), tularemia (Chap. 128), or Q fever (Chap. 170). A history of tobacco consumption must also be sought and should be quantified. A record of the patient's *previous residence* is of considerable importance in the diagnosis of histoplasmosis, coccidioidomycosis, or tropical eosinophilia. For example, pulmonary mass lesions in patients in the Mediterranean Basin may be due to hydatid cysts, hemop-

tysis in patients from Central China may be caused by paragonimiasis (Chap. 212), and cor pulmonale in Egypt frequently results from schistosomiasis (Chap. 211).

The *family history* should consider pulmonary diseases which may be genetic, such as cystic disease of the lung, pulmonary emphysema due to α_1-antitrypsin deficiency, cystic fibrosis, asthma, hereditary telangiectasia, Kartagener's syndrome, and alveolar microlithiasis, as well as infections due to the tubercle bacilli, fungi, and schistosoma where exposure to involved family members is important.

Dyspnea is a cardinal manifestation of diseases involving the respiratory and cardiovascular systems (Chap. 27). A detailed physical examination of both organ systems is therefore mandatory in every patient with this symptom. Dyspnea secondary to cardiac disease is often recognized by the presence of other evidence of heart failure, such as cardiac enlargement, gallop rhythms, and cardiac murmurs. It may be difficult to differentiate paroxysmal nocturnal dyspnea due to pulmonary edema of cardiac origin from nocturnal attacks of bronchial asthma, but a detailed description of the circumstances in which this symptom occurs is most useful. Dyspnea is a common functional complaint, and an important clue in the identification of this form is the observation that shortness of breath often occurs at rest and is relieved during exertion; the opposite is the case in patients in whom this symptom is secondary to disease of the lungs or heart. Equally important in the differential diagnosis is a careful elucidation of the relationship of dyspnea to other symptoms such as cough or angina pectoris.

Patients with diseases involving the respiratory system may also present with *chest pain* which is frequently caused by inflammation of the pleura, occurring in pneumonia, pulmonary thromboembolism, tuberculosis, and malignancy (Chap. 5). Pleuritic pain is usually localized to one side of the chest and is related to movements of the thorax and to respiration. Lesions confined to the pulmonary parenchyma do not produce pain, while diseases involving the organs in the mediastinum (Chap. 269) may cause local discomfort with radiation characteristic of the specific organ. Pain may also originate in or be referred to the chest wall; it may be due to intercostal neuritis, as in herpes zoster, or to compression of the intercostal nerves as they leave the spinal cord. Such pain is often superficial in character and may be related to coughing and straining. Thoracic pain may also be due to myositis, costochondral disturbances, myocardial ischemia, pericarditis, esophageal disease, and aortic dissection and aneurysm (Chap. 5).

Cough and *expectoration* are also cardinal features of pulmonary disease (Chap. 26). Few patients can describe the severity of cough or quantity of expectoration reliably, and it is therefore desirable for the physician to inspect a 24-h collection of sputum. Cough is often precipitated by foreign materials irritating nerve endings in airways and is frequently caused by inflammation of the bronchi; the latter may be persistent (as in patients with a cigarette cough and chronic bronchitis) or acute (as in a variety of viral and bacterial infections). The time of occurrence of the cough and the character and quantity of expectorated material may point to the diagnosis. For example, bronchiectasis and lung abscess produce purulent sputum which may have an offensive odor or be streaked with blood (Chaps. 260 and 261). In pulmonary edema, the sputum is pink, frothy, and watery (Chap. 27). Mucoid (translucent, viscid, shiny, white or gray) or mucopurulent (mucoid with flecks of yellow or green pus) sputum is characteristic of acute and chronic bronchitis. Sputum is bloody or rusty in pneumonia; it is thick, gelatinous, and brick red, laced with pus, in *Klebsiella* pneumonia. Paroxysmal cough may also be the presenting feature in patients with bronchial asthma, in whom physical examination reveals wheezing respirations and squeaking musical sounds (Chap. 257), as well as in patients with left ventricular failure, in whom it generally occurs at night and in the recumbent position (Chap. 236). Pulmonary tuberculosis (Chap. 143), though less common than previously, remains a common cause of chronic cough, as does neoplasm of the lung (Chap. 268). A change in the character of a chronic cough, unaccompanied by an acute infection, should alert the physician to the need of carrying out a detailed examination.

In addition to a detailed examination of the thorax, a meticulous *general physical examination* is mandatory in patients with disorders of the respiratory system. Tell-tale stains on the finger point to heavy cigarette smoking; characteristic cutaneous lesions may point to the presence of sarcoidosis (Chap. 216), collagen vascular disease, Wegener's granulomatosis, and berylliosis, all of which may have prominent pulmonary manifestations. Clubbing of the fingers, or when advanced, osteoarthropathy (Chap. 363) may point to carcinoma (Chap. 268) or suppurative disease (Chap. 260) of the lung; chronic hypoxemia, as occurs in patients with chronic bronchitis (Chap. 263); pulmonary arteriovenous fistula; or congenital heart disease with right-to-left shunt (Chap. 240). However, clubbing and hypertrophic osteoarthropathy are also seen in some patients with biliary cirrhosis of the liver, regional enteritis and ulcerative colitis. A careful search for infection in the teeth, gums, tonsils, or sinuses is recommended in patients known to have or to be suspected of having bronchiectasis or lung abscess. Neurologic findings including headache, drowsiness, papilledema, and other evidence of increased intracranial pressure may occur in patients with pulmonary disease who have hypoxia and hypercapnia. Vascular collapse is a late complication of carbon dioxide intoxication and is characterized by hypotension, flushed skin, sweating, and tachycardia.

Hemoptysis is often a frightening symptom (Chap. 26). Faint streaking of the sputum with blood may be observed in acute infections of the respiratory tract. However, many patients with bloody sputum have serious disease, such as pulmonary thromboembolism, tuberculosis, mitral stenosis, neoplasm of the lung, or bronchiectasis. In all instances it is necessary to exclude sources of blood in the nasopharynx and bleeding of gastric or esophageal origin. The character of the bloody expectorate should be defined, since it may be helpful in identifying the underlying disease process. Sputum which is frankly bloody without mucus or pus may be due to pulmonary thromboembolism (Chap. 266). When pus is present, pneumonia, bronchiectasis, or lung abscess should be considered. Dilute, pink, frothy sputum should suggest acute pulmonary edema (Chap. 27).

The *roentgenographic examination* of the chest represents the cornerstone of the diagnostic workup of the patient with suspected pulmonary disease, and it is the integration of the information obtained from the clinical examination and the roentgenogram which often provides the key to diagnosis. Unfortunately, in recent years, physical examination of the chest has been deemphasized, largely because of the recognition of the enormous value of radiographic techniques. However, abnormalities such as small or moderate amounts of fluid in the alveoli or in the mediastinum, bronchospasm, and pleural effusions can often be detected more accurately by physical examination than by chest roentgenography. Chest roentgenograms obtained in the lateral decubitus position will frequently reveal small pleural effusions not evident in the upright position. It must also be appreciated that a number of other abnormalities may be associated with normal roentgenograms. These include solitary lesions less than 6 mm in diameter, acute pulmonary thromboembolism without infarction, early interstitial pneumonia, diffuse granulomatous disease such as miliary tuberculosis, interstitial disease such as scleroderma and systemic lupus erythematosus, bronchiectasis, acute chronic bronchitis, mild to moderate emphysema, endobronchial masses only partially obstructing the airways, and the majority of instances of hypoventilation due to disorders of the central nervous system or neuromuscular disease. On the other hand, gross abnormalities of thoracic structure; pulmonary, mediastinal, and pleural masses; parenchymal consolidation, cysts, cavities, and abnormalities of the pulmonary vascular bed are all detected more reliably by roentgenographic than by physical examination.

An abnormal chest roentgenogram may be the presenting feature in an otherwise symptomless patient. In such circumstances the physician must make every effort to obtain earlier films in order to determine whether the lesion is new or old. Laminagraphy, computerized tomography, angiocardiography, and pulmonary photoscanning are additional procedures which may be helpful in establishing a diagnosis in a patient with an abnormality on the plain chest roentgenogram.

A variety of other diagnostic procedures are helpful in the workup of the patient with known or suspected pulmonary disease. These are presented in Chap. 256 and include skin tests for tuberculosis, scratch or intradermal tests to detect atopic reactions; appropriate serum complement fixation tests; and examination and culture of the sputum, pleural fluid, and bronchial washings. Bronchoscopy, bronchial brushings, and bronchoscopic biopsy have been greatly facilitated by the development of the fiberoptic bronchoscope. Mediastinoscopy, scalene node and mediastinal node biopsy, and pleural and lung biopsy may also be instrumental in establishing a diagnosis in an otherwise asymptomatic patient. Particularly important points which must be investigated in the history of the asymptomatic patient with a lesion discovered on a routine chest roentgenogram include exposure to individuals with tuberculosis; previous tuberculin and fungous skin tests; residence in or visits to areas where fungal disease is endemic; a history of smoking and of exposure to dusts; and symptoms of systemic disease such as fever, sweat, fatigue, and weight loss.

In the approach to a patient with pulmonary disease, consideration must be given to the observation that substantial changes in the relative incidence of disease affecting the respiratory system have taken place in the United States during the past three decades. Chronic infectious disorders such as tuberculosis, lung abscess, and bronchiectasis have decreased. On the other hand, patients with chronic bronchitis and with emphysema now survive longer and form an increasing fraction of patients with chronic respiratory disease, as do patients with environmental lung disease. Modern intercontinental travel has increased the appearance in the lung of parasitic infestations in the Western world. Also, the reduction of immunologic competence which occurs in the treatment of patients with a variety of malignancies and following organ transplantation (Chap. 69) has led to an increasing incidence of opportunistic infections of the lungs with a variety of microorganisms rarely pathogenic in the past. Physiologic (lung function) studies (Chap. 255) are of limited value in establishing an etiologic diagnosis in the patient with pulmonary disease. They are, of course, critical in assessing the physiologic consequence of disorders of the respiratory system and chest wall, as well as following the effects of their progression or remission.

REFERENCE

BAUM GL (ed): *Textbook of Pulmonary Diseases*, 2d ed. Boston, Little, Brown, 1974

FISHMAN AP (ed): *Pulmonary Diseases and Disorders.* New York, McGraw-Hill, 1980

255
DISTURBANCES OF RESPIRATORY FUNCTION

JOHN B. WEST

The prime function of the lung is to exchange gas between the inspired air and the venous blood. A convenient starting point, therefore, for a discussion of disturbances of respiratory function is the alveolar membrane across which gas exchange occurs (Fig. 255-1). This blood-gas barrier is less than 1 μm thick and has a surface area of some 100 m². It is therefore ideally suited to its gas exchange function.

Air is pumped to one side of this membrane and blood to the other. The air flows through conducting tubes, the bronchi; these are not lined with blood capillaries, with the result that no gas exchange can occur within them. These conducting airways, therefore, comprise a *dead space.* Beyond these airways is the *alveolar gas,* which makes up most of the volume of the lung. This gas is in a constant state of agitation because of molecular diffusion, and thus all the alveolar gas has access to the capillary blood via the alveolar membrane.

On the other side of the membrane, blood is pumped from the right side of the heart to the pulmonary capillaries. These delicate vessels have diameters of only about 10 μm, so that the blood is spread out in a thin film, one or two red blood cells thick, around the air sacs.

It is worth emphasizing two features of the basic lung unit shown in Fig. 255-1: (1) its symmetry, i.e., air and blood are equally important in the central process of gas exchange (this simple fact is sometimes forgotten in clinical medicine, where the patient's difficulties in moving air in and out of the lung often dominate the picture); (2) the simplicity of the lung unit compared with, say, the nephron. The structure of the lung is simple because its main role is simple, i.e., bringing together air and blood so that gas exchange can occur by passive diffusion. By contrast, the kidney carries out many functions involving active transport, and its structure is correspondingly complicated.

VENTILATION

This is the process of moving inspired air into the alveolar gas compartment, where the gas exchange with the blood occurs. It is worth attaching some typical values for ventilation to the lung shown in Fig. 255-1. A normal breath is about 500 ml, so that with a breathing frequency of 15 per minute some 7 to 8 liters of air enters the lung each minute. However, because the volume of the conducting airways (dead space) is about 150 ml, only 350 of the 500 ml of air inhaled with each breath reaches the alveolar gas compartment. The rest remains behind in the airways and is subsequently exhaled. Thus, the volume of fresh gas entering the alveoli each minute is about

350 ml × 15, or some 5 liters. This is known as the *alveolar ventilation* and is of key importance to gas exchange. Of the 5 liters of air entering the alveoli, some 300 ml of oxygen moves across into the blood each minute to be replaced by about 250 ml of carbon dioxide. Thus less than 5 percent of the gas volume inhaled is exchanged with the gas in the blood.

The above figures apply to resting conditions. On exercise, the oxygen uptake may rise as high as 4 to 6 liters per minute and the minute volume of air inspired may increase twentyfold. This is accomplished by an increase in both tidal volume and the frequency of breathing.

It should be noted that inspired air passes only a limited distance down the airways by ordinary bulk flow. Before it gets to the alveoli, its forward velocity is reduced to something like a millimeter per second, because of the enormous combined cross-sectional area of the small airways. In addition, the volume of gas in the bronchioles is so large that the alveoli and their ducts have completed their expansion before the fresh inspired air reaches them. The last few millimeters of its travel are therefore accomplished by molecular diffusion within the small airways. This process is very rapid for gas molecules but exceedingly slow for dust particles if they are over 0.5 μm in diameter. For this reason most inhaled dusts and aerosols never reach the alveoli, and many are deposited in the region of the terminal bronchioles.

MEASUREMENT OF VENTILATION The total volume of air passing the lips is easily measured by connecting a large bag or spirometer to the patient via a mouthpiece and one-way valve. The resting and exercise ventilations are increased when disease impairs the efficiency of pulmonary gas exchange, but the measurement of ventilation by itself is not often useful because it is partly under voluntary control and is often changed by the stress of the measurement.

The maximum ventilation, or maximum breathing capacity, can be measured by asking the patient to breathe as fast and deep as possible for 15 s. This measurement gives information about the mechanical properties of the lungs, but it has been replaced by a less demanding measurement, the forced expiratory volume (see below).

FIGURE 255-1
The functional lung unit. The alveolar membrane across which gas exchange takes place has alveolar gas on one side and pulmonary capillary blood on the other.

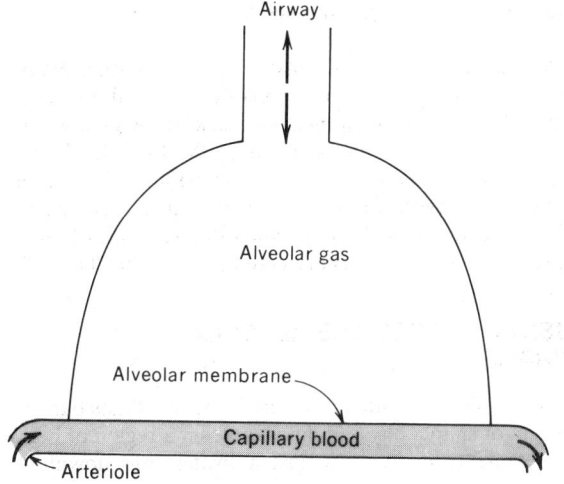

CONTROL OF VENTILATION The rhythmic act of breathing is initiated in the respiratory centers of the pons and medulla. The level of ventilation is closely controlled from minute to minute by the medullary chemoreceptors which respond to changes in the partial pressure of carbon dioxide (P_{CO_2}) in arterial blood. There is evidence that these chemoreceptors are exquisitely sensitive to a fall in pH of the cerebrospinal fluid near them, which occurs when carbon dioxide diffuses across the blood-brain barrier. This dissolved gas moves easily across the blood-brain barrier, whereas H^+ and HCO_3^- do not.

Arterial hypoxemia also increases the ventilation through its action on the peripheral chemoreceptors in the carotid bodies. This hypoxic stimulus is normally relatively weak and variable but may dominate during chronic hypoxia, for example, following ascent to high altitude. This is also often the situation in patients with chronic respiratory failure, with the result that the administration of oxygen may cause hypoventilation and severe carbon dioxide retention.

The pH of the arterial blood has an effect on ventilation which is independent of the P_{CO_2}. This is why ventilation may be increased during metabolic acidosis, thus reducing the arterial P_{CO_2}.

HYPOVENTILATION When inspired air reaches the alveoli, oxygen is removed from it and carbon dioxide is added. The concentrations, or partial pressures, of these two gases in the alveoli depend on a balance between two processes. On the one hand, the removal of oxygen from (or addition of carbon dioxide to) the alveolar gas is determined by the metabolic demands of the body. On the other hand, the addition of oxygen to (or removal of carbon dioxide from) the alveolar gas depends on the amount of alveolar ventilation. Thus, if the alveolar ventilation is low in relation to oxygen uptake and carbon dioxide output, the partial pressure of oxygen in alveolar gas and arterial blood falls, and the level of carbon dioxide rises. This is hypoventilation.

Hypoventilation is commonly caused by disease outside the respiratory system and often exists in the presence of normal lungs. Causes include depression of the respiratory center by drugs or anesthesia, damage to the medulla by disease, diseases affecting the nerve supply to the muscles of the thorax or the muscles themselves, injury to the chest wall, and obstruction to the airways. Because the lungs themselves are often normal, the prognosis may be excellent if the precipitating cause is removed. However, hypoventilation can be caused by primary disease of the lungs. Note that hypoventilation always causes both hypoxemia and hypercapnia, although the first can be abolished by adding oxygen to the inspired air. The carbon dioxide retention can be relieved only by increasing the ventilation, e.g., by using a ventilator. Disorders leading to hypoventilation are discussed in more detail in Chap. 270.

HYPERVENTILATION If the alveolar ventilation is abnormally high for the carbon dioxide production of the body, the arterial P_{CO_2} falls. This may occur in metabolic acidosis, e.g., uremia, in which the chemoreceptors respond to the low blood pH. Hysterical hyperventilation is also not uncommon. For more information on hyperventilation see Chap. 270. The sensation of respiratory distress, or *dyspnea,* which should be clearly distinguished from *hyperpnea,* is considered in detail in Chap. 27.

DIFFUSION ACROSS THE ALVEOLAR MEMBRANE

Oxygen and carbon dioxide move across the blood-gas barrier by a process of simple physical diffusion from a region of high partial pressure to one of low, just as water runs downhill.

Consider a red blood cell as it enters a pulmonary capillary. The P_{O_2} in mixed venous blood (in the pulmonary artery) is typically about 40 mmHg, and as the cell enters the capillary less than 1 μm away, the P_{O_2} in alveolar gas is approximately 100 mmHg. Oxygen therefore moves rapidly across the barrier into the cell to combine with hemoglobin, and the P_{O_2} rises. As a consequence, the oxygen pressure difference between the cell and the alveolar gas falls, and the rate of inflow of oxygen is reduced. However, under normal conditions, the diffusion properties of the alveolar membrane are so good and the rate of combination of oxygen with hemoglobin so rapid that before the cell has spent more than about a third of its time in the capillary, its P_{O_2} has virtually reached that of the alveolar gas. This transfer of oxygen is helped by the shape of the oxygen dissociation curve; the nearly flat upper part of the curve (see Fig. 53-1) ensures that the driving pressure difference is maintained until almost all the oxygen is moved across. Thus, under ordinary circumstances, there is no measurable difference between the P_{O_2} of alveolar gas and that of the blood at the end of the pulmonary capillary. Indeed, the normal lung has plenty of reserve diffusion in hand.

Two factors which stress the diffusion ability of the lung are exercise and alveolar hypoxia. During strenuous exercise, the time spent by the red blood cells in the capillaries is greatly reduced, perhaps to a third of that at rest, so that the time available for the diffusion process is curtailed. Even so, the P_{O_2} in the capillary blood almost reaches that of the alveolar gas, except possibly during the most exhausting work. Additional stress occurs if the lung inspires a low oxygen mixture, thus reducing the alveolar P_{O_2}. Because the pressure difference between the oxygen in the gas and that in the red blood cells as they enter the capillary is lowered, the rate of movement of oxygen across the membrane is slowed. There is evidence that heavy work when the inspired P_{O_2} is very low (e.g., at high altitude) causes lowering of the arterial P_{O_2} because of inadequate diffusion into the pulmonary capillary. It is generally argued that carbon dioxide transfer is never limited by diffusion across the alveolar membrane because of the much higher diffusion rate of this gas, but recent work suggests that this may not always be the case.

MEASUREMENT OF DIFFUSING CAPACITY This can be done using carbon monoxide. The subject inspires a low concentration (approximately 0.1 percent), and the rate of uptake of the gas by the blood is calculated from the difference between the inspired and expired concentrations. The measurement can be made during the course of a single 10-s breath-holding period, or over a minute or so of steady breathing. In both cases, the diffusing capacity is expressed as the milliliters per minute of carbon monoxide taken up by the lung per millimeter of mercury of partial pressure of carbon monoxide in the alveolar gas. Normal values are in the region of 20 (ml/min)/mmHg at rest, rising to 60 (ml/min)/mmHg or more on exercise.

The reason the uptake of carbon monoxide measures the diffusing capacity is the remarkable avidity of blood for this gas. This means that appreciable amounts of carbon monoxide can be combined with hemoglobin in the blood at an exceedingly low partial pressure. As a result, the rise in partial pressure of carbon monoxide in the red blood cells as they pass along the pulmonary capillaries is negligible, and the amount of the gas which is transferred into the blood is determined only by the diffusion properties of the alveolar membrane and the rate of combination of carbon monoxide with hemoglobin. The latter depends on the P_{O_2} in the alveoli; by measuring the carbon monoxide uptake at various inspired oxygen partial pressures, it is possible to determine separately the diffusing capacity of the alveolar membrane itself and the volume of blood in pulmonary capillaries.

The measurement of carbon monoxide uptake is a relatively simple procedure, and there is no problem in following changes of diffusing capacity in the normal lung under a variety of conditions. Unfortunately, however, it is very difficult to say how far the carbon monoxide uptake reflects the true diffusion characteristics of the alveolar membrane and the capillary blood in the presence of appreciable lung disease. The reason for this is that inequality of ventilation, diffusion characteristics, and blood volume reduce the carbon monoxide in an unpredictable way. For this reason, the test when used in the clinic is sometimes said to measure the *transfer factor* of the lung for carbon monoxide and should be looked upon as a general index of the efficiency of gas exchange in the lung rather than as a specific test of diffusion.

IMPAIRMENT OF DIFFUSION The diffusion properties of the alveolar membrane depend on its thickness and area. Thus, the diffusing capacity is reduced by diseases in which the thickness is increased, including diffuse interstitial fibrosis (Chap. 264), sarcoidosis (Chap. 216), asbestosis (Chap. 259), and alveolar cell carcinomatosis (Chap. 268). The diffusing capacity also falls when the area of the membrane is reduced. This occurs following pneumonectomy and in emphysema. In addition, as we saw above, the diffusing capacity falls when the capillary blood volume or the number of red blood cells in the capillaries is reduced. This is the case in anemia and in diseases such as pulmonary embolism.

The importance of diffusion impairment as a cause of hypoxemia has long been disputed. In those lung diseases such as diffuse interstitial fibrosis in which microscopically the alveolar wall is thickened, it is tempting to attribute any hypoxemia to defective diffusion. The term *alveolar-capillary block* was coined for this situation, and it is certainly an easy one to remember. However, recent work indicates that impaired diffusion is not the principal cause of the hypoxemia in these patients. It is probably impossible for normal ventilation and blood flow to occur in an alveolus which has a thickened wall, and several investigators have shown marked inequality of ventilation and blood flow in the lung in these conditions. Studies in which it is possible to assess the extent of ventilation-perfusion inequality in patients with interstitial lung disease using a multiple inert gas technique indicate that, at rest, all the hypoxemia can be attributed to uneven ventilation and blood flow. However, on exercise, a small component of the hypoxemia is apparently caused by diffusion impairment. Thus, most of the hypoxemia in patients with so-called "alveolar-capillary block" must be attributed to ventilation-perfusion inequality.

BLOOD FLOW

Mixed venous blood is pumped to the pulmonary capillaries directly from the right side of the heart so that the total *pulmonary blood flow* is equal to the cardiac output, say 5 or 6 liters per minute in a normal adult. We saw earlier that the volume of fresh inspired air entering the alveoli each minute, the *alveolar ventilation,* is some 5 liters. Thus, the overall ratio of ventilation to blood flow, or *ventilation/perfusion ratio,* is about 1.

Even though the volumes of fresh gas and blood reaching the alveoli each minute are about the same, the volumes involved in exchanging gas at any instant are very different. Thus, while the alveolar gas volume is 2 to 3 liters at the end of a normal expiration, the capillary blood volume is only some 70 ml. This is why the lung microscopist sees chiefly air.

The pressures in the pulmonary circulation have long been considered the domain of the cardiologist, but they have an important bearing on gas exchange in the lung. The normal pulmonary arterial pressure is only just sufficient to raise blood to the top of the upright lung; if the pressure is reduced, as in hemorrhagic shock, the upper part of the lung is unperfused and gas exchange is impaired. Alterations in the pulmonary venous pressure, too, affect the distribution of blood flow in the lung.

VENTILATION-PERFUSION RELATIONSHIPS

Up to this point, we have been assuming that all lung units behave identically. Thus, Fig. 255-1 has been taken to refer to an alveolus, a group of alveoli with their duct, a lobe, or even the whole lung. In fact, however, the lung is not homogeneous, and the differences in behavior between the millions of units are responsible for the great bulk of the hypoxemia and hypercarbia seen in clinical practice. We shall see that even in the normal lung, there are marked regional differences in blood flow and ventilation which affect gas exchange, while in diseased states, the inhomogeneity becomes so severe that respiratory failure may ultimately develop.

NORMAL DISTRIBUTION OF BLOOD FLOW It is possible to measure the regional distribution of blood flow and ventilation in the lung by using radioactive gases. In one technique, the inert gas xenon 133 is employed. To measure blood flow, the xenon is dissolved in saline and injected into a peripheral vein. On reaching the lung, it is evolved into alveolar gas because of its poor solubility; there it remains during breath holding, and its radiation can be detected by external counters. To measure ventilation, the patient inhales a single breath of the radioactive gas and again its regional distribution is measured. In both instances, a further measurement after a period of rebreathing of xenon allows a correction for lung volume to be made.

In the normal upright lung, blood flow per unit volume decreases rapidly from bottom to top, reaching very low values at the apex. This pattern is affected by change of posture and exercise. When the subject lies supine, the apical and basal blood flows become the same, but the posterior (dependent) part of the lung has a higher blood flow than the anterior region. In the lateral position, the dependent regions are best perfused. On exercise in the upright position, both apical and basal blood flows increase, so that the proportion of the total flow going to the apex rises.

The cause of this uneven distribution of blood flow lies in the hydrostatic pressure differences within the lung. The pulmonary circulation is unique in that air and blood are separated by a very delicate membrane over a vertical distance of some 30 cm, and consequently, the hydrostatic effect of this large column of blood determines the caliber of the small vessels. It has been shown that the distribution of blood flow depends on the relative magnitudes of the pulmonary arterial, venous, and alveolar pressures. In particular, if pulmonary arterial pressure falls (as in hemorrhage, shock, and anesthesia) or alveolar pressure is raised (as in positive-pressure ventilation), the distribution of blood flow becomes more uneven. The normal pattern is also commonly affected by both heart and lung disease.

NORMAL DISTRIBUTION OF VENTILATION Ventilation also increases down the upright lung, though the changes are less marked than for blood flow. This distribution of ventilation which is seen under normal resting conditions is altered at low lung volumes. It has been shown that when a normal subject exhales as far as possible (to residual volume) and then gradually inhales in small steps, initially very little air goes into the lower zones, but the upper zones are well ventilated. However, before this subject reaches a normal resting lung volume (functional residual capacity), this distribution is reversed and the lower zones are better ventilated than the upper. This pattern is then maintained right up to maximal volumes. The poor ventilation of the dependent regions of the lung at low lung volumes is seen in the erect, supine, and lateral situations, and it has important implications in clinical situations in which the lung volume is low, e.g., in obesity or following abdominal surgery. Since the dependent regions are the best perfused, the impairment of gas exchange may then be severe.

The cause of the normal uneven distribution of ventilation has to do with the way the lung is supported inside the chest. It is known that the expanding pressure on the lung is less in the dependent zones, presumably because these regions help to support the lung above them. Thus, the intrapleural pressure is less negative at the bottom of the lung than at the top. The reason for the greater ventilation of the dependent regions at normal volumes is twofold: (1) these alveoli have a smaller resting volume, and (2) their increase in volume is relatively large because, having a smaller volume, they are more distensible. By contrast, these dependent regions are poorly ventilated at low lung volumes because the expanding forces on them are then too weak to inflate them. Indeed, under these conditions, the airways to these alveoli may close and the alveoli become unventilated.

The volume at which the lower zone airways close (the *closing volume*) is considerably less than the functional residual capacity in normal young subjects. However, as the lung ages, and especially in the presence of chronic obstructive lung disease, the closing volume increases until it encroaches on the normal breathing range. Thus elderly normal subjects and patients with chronic bronchitis and emphysema frequently close their lower zone airways during resting breathing; this results in a poorly ventilated region which impairs gas exchange.

The closing volume can be measured by having the patient inhale a vital capacity breath of oxygen and then measuring the nitrogen concentration at the mouth during the subsequent full expiration. Because the apical regions of the lung are relatively poorly ventilated, the nitrogen there is less diluted by the breath of oxygen. During the subsequent expiration, an abrupt rise in nitrogen concentration measured at the mouth indicates preferential emptying of the apex and, therefore, signals closure of lower zone airways. There is some evidence that the measurement of closing volume is a sensitive test of early disease affecting the small airways. For example, cigarette smokers may have an increased closing volume when other tests of lung function are still normal.

VENTILATION/PERFUSION RATIO We have seen that while blood flow increases greatly down the upright lung, the change in ventilation is less. As a result, the ventilation/perfusion ratio varies from a high value at the top of the lung to a low value at the bottom. The ventilation/perfusion ratio is of key importance because it determines the gas exchange which occurs in any part of the lung.

Consider a lung unit as shown in Fig. 255-1. It can readily be seen that the partial pressure of oxygen in the alveolar gas (and therefore in the end-capillary blood) will be set by a balance between the rate of its removal by the blood flow, on the one hand, and the rate of its replenishment by the ventilation on the other. Thus, if the ventilation is gradually reduced but the blood flow is maintained, the oxygen partial pressure will gradually fall. The limit is reached when the unit is not ventilated and the P_{O_2} becomes that of venous blood. This is a ventilation/perfusion ratio of zero. By contrast, if perfusion is gradually reduced, the P_{O_2} will rise. The limit now occurs when the unit is unperfused and the P_{O_2} in the alveolus is the same as that of inspired air. This is a ventilation/perfusion ratio of infinity.

Thus, the crucial factor determining the oxygen partial pressure is the ventilation/perfusion ratio; this is also true for the partial pressure of carbon dioxide, and indeed of any other gas that might be present. It can be shown that regional differences of gas exchange occur in the normal upright lung as a consequence of the uneven ventilation/perfusion ratios.

OVERALL GAS EXCHANGE Though such regional differences in gas exchange are of interest, more important is the effect of uneven ventilation/perfusion ratios on overall gas exchange, i.e., the ability of the lung to take up oxygen and put out carbon dioxide. The reason gas transfer is impaired by uneven ventilation and blood flow is that those lung units which are overperfused in relation to their ventilation, and which therefore have a low P_{O_2}, contribute a disproportionate amount of the blood flow to the systemic arterial system. The net result is that the arterial P_{O_2} is depressed because it is loaded with less well oxygenated blood. In the same way, because these lung units have a relatively high P_{CO_2}, they tend to elevate the arterial P_{CO_2}. It is as if uneven ventilation/perfusion ratios set up a barrier between the gas and the blood, with the result that the arterial P_{O_2} is depressed and the P_{CO_2} is raised.

There is an additional reason why the arterial P_{O_2} is reduced by ventilation/perfusion ratio inequality. Though the oxygen content of blood draining from alveoli with a low ventilation/perfusion ratio is always abnormally low, alveoli with a high ventilation/perfusion ratio are not able to oxygenate their blood much more than normal alveoli. This is because the blood is normally almost fully saturated with oxygen owing to the shape of the oxygen dissociation curve. This additional reason does not apply to carbon dioxide.

In the normal lung, the effects of uneven ventilation/perfusion ratios on overall gas exchange are trivial; the arterial P_{O_2} is reduced by a few millimeters of mercury and the P_{CO_2} is raised by less than 1 mmHg, if all else remains the same. Both these liabilities can be met if the total ventilation of the lung and thus its overall ventilation/perfusion ratio are increased. Indeed, the level of overall ventilation is normally set by the medullary respiratory center via the arterial P_{CO_2}. Thus, if uneven ventilation/perfusion ratios elevate the arterial P_{CO_2}, this is brought back by the increased respiratory drive and the consequently higher overall ventilation.

In the diseased lung, the effects of ventilation/perfusion ratio inequality on gas transfer may be very severe because the degree of uneven ventilation and blood flow is far greater than in the normal lung. The arterial P_{O_2} may be depressed by 50 mmHg or more, and in practice no amount of increased ventilation can return it to its normal level. The P_{CO_2} however, is often maintained at the normal level by an increase in total ventilation. The reason an increase in ventilation to diseased lungs can reduce the arterial P_{CO_2} but not increase the P_{O_2} to normal levels lies in the different shapes of the two dissociation curves. If the ventilation is not increased, the P_{CO_2} remains elevated. Ventilation/perfusion ratio inequality is much the commonest cause of hypoxemia and hypercapnia in generalized lung disease.

MEASUREMENT OF VENTILATION/PERFUSION INEQUALITY Unfortunately, it is difficult to derive much information about the pattern of uneven ventilation and blood flow in the diseased lung. Because much of the inequality is at the microscopic level, radioactive gas detectors which "see" relatively large regions of lung give little indication of the extent of the unevenness. The best method as yet which is suitable for clinical practice is by the analysis of expired gas and arterial blood.

We have seen that the P_{O_2} of arterial blood is depressed in the presence of ventilation/perfusion ratio inequality because it is loaded with less well oxygenated blood from those alveoli which are overperfused in relation to their ventilation. By contrast, the expired alveolar gas receives a disproportionately high contribution from lung units which are overventilated in relation to their blood flow, where the P_{O_2} is high. An alveolar-arterial oxygen difference therefore develops, and the magnitude of this difference is a measure of the amount of ventilation/perfusion ratio inequality.

Though arterial blood can be collected by puncture, a representative sample of mixed alveolar gas is often impossible to obtain in the diseased lung because of its disturbed pattern of emptying. An alternative is to collect all the expired gas (including that from the dead space of the bronchi), using a valve box and a large bag or spirometer, and to calculate what is called the *ideal alveolar* P_{O_2}. This is the value which the alveolar gas would have in the absence of ventilation/perfusion ratio inequality. This calculation is made using the arterial P_{CO_2} and the alveolar gas equation.

The P_{O_2} difference between ideal alveolar gas and arterial blood chiefly reflects those alveoli with an abnormally *low* ventilation/perfusion ratio, i.e., the alveoli which are overperfused in relation to their ventilation. These alveoli cause the hypoxemia, and their presence has the same effect as the admixture of some venous blood with arterial blood. Indeed, it is possible to express their contribution *as if* a certain proportion of the venous blood bypassed the lung altogether and was then added to the arterial blood. This is called *venous admixture,* physiologic shunt, or wasted blood flow, and is calculated from the P_{O_2} difference between ideal alveolar gas and arterial blood. Normally, calculated venous admixture is only about 2 percent of the pulmonary blood flow, but it may rise to 30 percent or higher in the presence of severe ventilation/perfusion ratio inequality.

The alveoli with an abnormally *high* ventilation/perfusion ratio, i.e., those which are overventilated in relation to their perfusion, mainly affect carbon dioxide elimination. They behave as if a certain proportion of the inspired gas bypassed the alveoli altogether, i.e., as if the dead space were increased in size, thus resulting in wasted ventilation. Their contribution can be calculated from the P_{CO_2} of arterial blood and mixed expired gas, using Bohr's equation. This gives a value for the *physiologic dead space*, which includes not only the volume of the bronchi but also the so-called "alveolar dead space" attributable to the overventilated alveoli. Normally the physiologic dead space is less than 30 percent of the tidal volume at rest, but it may rise to 50 percent or more in the presence of severe disease. Both venous admixture and physiologic dead space are typically increased in chronic obstructive pulmonary disease (Chap. 263) and interstitial diseases of the lung (Chap. 264); in pulmonary thromboembolism (Chap. 266), an increase in dead space predominates.

Another method of measuring ventilation/perfusion inequality has recently been described. Rather than measuring the partial pressures of oxygen and carbon dioxide in arterial blood and expired gas, this method uses a continuous infusion of six foreign inert gases into the venous blood. After a steady state of gas exchange has been established, the consequent partial pressures in arterial blood and expired gas are then measured. From this information, it is possible to derive an almost continuous distribution of ventilation/perfusion ratios. Young normal subjects have very narrow distributions centered on the normal value of about 1. Patients with chronic obstructive lung disease and asthma, for example, often have bimodal distributions with substantial amounts of blood flow going to lung units with very low ventilation/perfusion ratios. As yet, this method is confined to the clinical research setting.

MEASUREMENT OF VENTILATION INEQUALITY Because the measurement of ventilation/perfusion ratio inequality is a relatively difficult procedure, the simpler measurement of uneven ventilation is often made. Although it would be theoretically possible for a patient to have ventilatory inequality but no mismatch of ventilation and blood flow, this is not seen in practice.

The simplest method of measuring uneven ventilation is the single-breath nitrogen wash-out test. For this, the patient takes a single inspiration of pure oxygen and then exhales fully. A rapid nitrogen meter at the lips measures expired nitrogen concentration, and expired volume is recorded simultaneously. After 750 ml has been expired (sufficient to clear the dead space), the rise in nitrogen concentration over the next 500 ml is measured. This is less than 1.5 percent in normal subjects. However, in patients with uneven ventilation, the nitrogen concentration rises more rapidly because the degree of dilution of the nitrogen by the inhaled oxygen varies throughout the lung, and also because the poorly ventilated regions (which receive little oxygen and therefore have the most nitrogen) always empty last. This is a simple, quick, and useful test, and it may also be used to give the closing volume (see earlier under "Normal Distribution of Ventilation").

Uneven ventilation can also be detected by a multibreath nitrogen wash-out test, but this is now seldom used.

VENTILATION/PERFUSION RATIO INEQUALITY IN DISEASE Virtually all generalized diseases of the lung, such as emphysema, chronic bronchitis, diffuse interstitial fibrosis, and the pneumoconioses, result in mismatch of ventilation and blood flow. As yet little is known about the pattern of unevenness in these conditions, though it is not difficult to imagine that an area of fibrosis or a bulla, for example, must interfere with both ventilation and blood flow.

There is evidence that in general, areas of the lung which are poorly ventilated are also poorly perfused. One reason for this is that local pathologic change tends to disturb both processes by its mechanical effects. However, there are other physiologic mechanisms which reduce the mismatch of ventilation and perfusion. One is the reduction in blood flow to a poorly ventilated, hypoxic region of the lung, which has now been demonstrated on many occasions. The precise mechanism is unknown, but it appears to be a local response to alveolar hypoxia, since it occurs in the isolated denervated lung. Another mechanism is the reduction of ventilation which has been shown to follow obstruction to a branch of the pulmonary artery. This is apparently due to an increase in resistance of the small airways caused by a fall in P_{CO_2} in the region. This mechanism is weak in human beings.

How far these two mechanisms operate in practice is unknown, but it has been shown that the administration of various bronchodilator and vasodilator drugs to patients with generalized lung disease can exaggerate their hypoxemia. For example, isoproterenol (by aerosol) and epinephrine and aminophylline (by injection) have been shown to reduce the arterial P_{O_2} of some patients with chronic obstructive lung disease and bronchial asthma. It is possible that one of the actions of these drugs is to interfere with these active mechanisms which reduce ventilation/perfusion ratio inequality.

MECHANICS OF BREATHING

This section deals with the forces involved in supporting and moving the lung and chest wall so that ventilation can be accomplished. The bellows function of the lung is one of the easiest to measure and also one of the most informative measurements in practice. Serious malfunction of the lung is almost always accompanied by a reduced ventilatory capacity.

LUNG AND CHEST WALL The lung is elastic and collapses if it is not held expanded. The pressure *inside* the lung (alveolar pressure) is the same as atmospheric pressure at the end of inspiration or expiration if the glottis is open. The pressure *outside* the lung (intrapleural pressure) is less than atmospheric pressure, or "negative." This pressure keeps the lung inflated and is developed by the chest wall, which is also elastic and tends to bow outward. If air is introduced into this space and a pneumothorax is produced, the lung collapses inward and the chest wall moves outward.

During quiet breathing, inspiration is produced chiefly by the action of the diaphragm assisted by the intercostal muscles, and expiration results from the passive elastic recoil of the lungs. During deep breathing, the accessory muscles such as the sternomastoids and scaleni are called upon, and patients with diseased lungs may use these even at rest. Under these conditions, expiration is often assisted by the abdominal muscles.

COMPLIANCE This is a term used to describe the elastic properties of the lung and chest wall. The normal lungs expand by about 200 ml when the expanding pressure (intrapleural pressure) changes by 1 cmH$_2$O. Thus the compliance (or distensibility) of the lungs is said to be 200 ml/cmH$_2$O. In fact, this figure only applies at normal resting lung volumes; at high lung volumes, the lungs are less easy to expand and their compliance falls. A more complete description of the elastic properties of the lungs, therefore, is the pressure-volume curve over the whole range of lung volumes; for this reason, this measurement is preferred in many pulmonary function laboratories. The compliance of the normal chest wall is about the same as that of the lungs, and the compliance of both lung and chest wall together is therefore about half this value, i.e., 100 ml/cmH$_2$O.

The compliance of lung depends very much on how much tissue is present. A single lobe, for example, will clearly not change its volume by as much as a whole lung for the same change in expanding pressure. Compliance is therefore sometimes corrected for lung volume and called *specific compliance*.

The normal elastic behavior of the lungs is only partly caused by the elastic tissue within it. An important component is the surface tension of the fluid lining the alveoli. The lungs may be regarded as composed of 300 million tiny bubbles which tend to collapse for the same reason that a soap bubble on the end of a bubble pipe does. The surface forces which tend to reduce the area of the surface thus tend to reduce the volume of the bubble. These surface forces therefore contribute to the elastic force of the lung. Fortunately some of the cells lining the alveoli produce a phospholipid which lowers the surface tension of the lining fluid to extremely low values. The substance is known as a *surfactant*. This lowering of the surface tension is of great physiologic importance, because it helps to maintain the stability of the alveoli and discourage atelectasis. About half the normal elastic recoil force of the lung is due to these surface forces.

The normal elastic behavior of the lung is disturbed by many diseases. Diffuse pulmonary fibrosis, pleural thickening, healed tuberculosis with scarring, and atelectasis all reduce the compliance of the lung. Heart disease, such as mitral stenosis and left ventricular failure, also commonly lowers compliance, although it is often difficult to be certain whether the volume of ventilating lung is reduced by edema in the airways, for

example, or whether the elastic behavior of the lung tissue itself is altered. An absence of surfactant is thought to be responsible for the alveolar collapse and the stiff lungs seen in hyaline membrane disease of the newborn. In emphysema and old age, the lungs become more compliant and have an abnormally large volume at normal expanding pressures.

AIRWAY RESISTANCE So far we have been looking at the static forces involved in maintaining the expansion of the lung. However, during ventilation, additional forces are required to move air along the airways, because of the resistance offered to flow. This is expressed as the pressure difference between the alveoli and the mouth per unit of airflow rate. The normal value is in the vicinity of 1 to 2 cmH$_2$O per liter per second of flow at normal flow rates. The resistance rises at higher flow rates.

Until recently it was thought that the chief site of resistance was the small airways. However, it is now known that most of the resistance lies in the medium-sized bronchi and that the bronchioles less than 2 mm in diameter contribute less than 20 percent of the total airway resistance. The reason for this is the prodigious number of small airways. As a consequence, substantial increases in resistance of these bronchioles will not be detected by the usual pulmonary function tests, and they are said to constitute a "silent zone." There is currently a good deal of interest in new tests designed to detect changes in the small airways. These include the measurement of closing volume referred to above, and the measurement of "frequency-dependent compliance," i.e., the apparent fall in lung compliance which occurs at high breathing rates. The clinical usefulness of these tests has not yet been established.

Various factors alter airway resistance. For example, the resistance is higher during expiration than inspiration, and it is greater at small lung volumes because the airways are then not held open so much. A single deep inspiration often reduces the resistance, but the inhalation of cigarette smoke or other irritants increases it, through reflex contraction of airway smooth muscle following stimulation of irritant receptors located in the airway wall.

A dramatic increase in airway resistance occurs during forced expiration. The cause of this is collapse of the airways, so-called "dynamic compression." The explanation is that the high intrapleural pressure is applied not only to the alveoli in an effort to empty them but also to the outside walls of the airways which lie within the chest. Consequently the airways are compressed, and as a result, the expiratory flow rate is independent of respiratory effort over a large range, since the greater the effort, the more the collapse. In normal subjects, this phenomenon takes place only during forced expirations, but it occurs much more readily in patients with chronic bronchitis and emphysema. This is because the airway walls are diseased and weakened, or because the airways lose their support by radial traction from the surrounding lung.

Diseases which increase airway resistance during normal breathing include bronchial asthma and chronic bronchitis. The resistance may rise to many times its normal value and even during clinical remissions of the disease can be shown to be abnormally high. Lung volume increases in these conditions, and this has two helpful consequences: the airways are pulled open more, thus limiting the increase in resistance, and the higher passive recoil pressure of the lung assists expiration.

WORK OF BREATHING To move the lungs and chest wall and force air along the airways, work is required and the respiratory muscles must consume oxygen. In normal subjects, the work of breathing is very small except during the large ventilation of heavy exercise. In patients with obstructive lung disease, however, the frictional resistance to airflow is high even at rest and the work of breathing is much increased, perhaps to five or ten times its normal value. Under these conditions, the oxygen cost of breathing may become an appreciable fraction of the total oxygen consumption.

Patients with a reduced compliance of the lungs or chest wall have a higher work of breathing, because the stiffer structures are more difficult to move. These patients tend to use rapid shallow breaths, which reduces their oxygen cost of ventilation. However, if breathing becomes too shallow, the volume of air merely moved in and out of the bronchial dead space becomes disproportionately high, and gas exchange is consequently impaired. A compromise is therefore reached.

MEASUREMENTS OF MECHANICS One of the most useful tests in the armamentarium of the pulmonary function laboratory is the analysis of a single forced expiration. The patient makes a full inspiration and then exhales as hard and as fast as possible into a lightweight spirometer. Typical records are shown in Fig. 255-2. It can be seen that for a normal subject the total volume exhaled is large. This is called the vital capacity or preferably, the *forced vital capacity* (FVC). (The word "forced" is added because the volume may be less than the vital capacity measured with a slow expiration.) Also, about 80 percent of this volume is exhaled in 1 s. This is called the *forced expiratory volume,* or FEV_1. In *obstructive lung disease,* e.g., emphysema, the forced vital capacity is reduced because the airways close and limit expiration before the patient has breathed out fully. In addition, the FEV_1 is grossly reduced as is the FEV/FVC percentage. This is because of the high airway resistance, which slows down the rate of expiration. In *restrictive lung disease,* e.g., ankylosing spondylitis, the FVC is low because of the limited expansion of the lung or chest wall. However, the FEV_1 is often not reduced proportionately, because airway resistance is normal. Thus the FEV/FVC percentage is normal or high.

Other indexes of ventilatory function can be derived from a forced expiration. One is the maximal midexpiratory flow rate (MMEFR) which is obtained by dividing the volume between 75 percent and 25 percent of the vital capacity by the corresponding elapsed time (Fig. 255-2). This correlates well with the FEV_1 but may be a more sensitive measure of airway obstruction in early chronic obstructive lung disease.

The FEV_1 is closely related to the maximum breathing capacity, and since it is a much simpler test to perform, it has replaced it in practice. Impaired lung function is almost always associated with a reduced FEV_1, and the test is therefore a valuable screening procedure. It is also useful in assessing the efficacy of bronchodilator therapy and in following the progress of patients with asthma or chronic obstructive lung disease.

Other lung volumes can also be measured at the same time. The *total lung capacity* is the total volume of gas in the lung at full inspiration. The *inspiratory capacity* is the maximum volume which can be inspired from the resting volume of the lungs, which is called the *functional residual capacity.* The maximum volume which can be expired from the resting level is the *expiratory reserve volume.* This leaves the *residual volume* still in the lungs, and this and the functional residual capacity can be measured only indirectly. One technique is to connect the patient to a spirometer circuit containing helium and measure the degree of dilution of this gas which occurs after several minutes of rebreathing. Another is to use a body plethysmograph (see below).

These volumes are often altered by disease. The functional residual capacity and residual volume are typically increased in diseases in which there is an increased airway resistance, for example, in emphysema, chronic bronchitis, and asthma. Indeed, at one time an elevated residual volume was regarded as an essential feature of emphysema, but less emphasis is placed on this test now. A reduced functional residual capacity and residual volume are often seen in patients with a reduced lung compliance, for example, in diffuse interstitial fibrosis. Here the lung is stiff and tends to recoil to a much smaller resting volume.

The measurement of compliance and airway resistance is more difficult. In order to determine lung compliance, i.e., volume change per unit of pressure change, the pressure expanding the lungs must be known. In practice this can be found by passing a small latex balloon connected to a manometer down into the esophagus. Esophageal pressure is then taken as a measure of intrapleural pressure. To measure airway resistance, i.e., the pressure drop along the airways per unit of airflow, alveolar pressure must be known. This can be found by seating the patient in a large airtight box, or plethysmograph. First, the patient is asked to try to breathe against a complete obstruction, and from the change in box pressure, lung volume can be calculated. Next, the patient is asked to pant, and again box pressure is recorded. Alveolar pressure can then be derived and airway resistance calculated. This equipment is available only in specialized centers.

Aging has an important influence on lung function. With increasing age there is a fall in vital capacity and forced expiratory volume and an increase in functional residual capacity, residual volume, and closing volume. Some inequality of ventilation and ventilation/perfusion ratios develops and the arterial P_{O_2} falls almost linearly with age. It is therefore impor-

FIGURE 255-2

Measurement of the forced expiratory volume, FEV_1, forced vital capacity, FVC, and maximum midexpiratory flow rate, MMFR. The patient makes a full inspiration and then exhales as hard and as fast as possible.

As the patient exhales the pen moves down. The FEV_1 is the volume exhaled in 1 s; the FVC is the total volume exhaled. The MMFR is the mean flow rate measured over the middle half of the FVC. Note the differences between the normal, obstructive, and restrictive patterns.

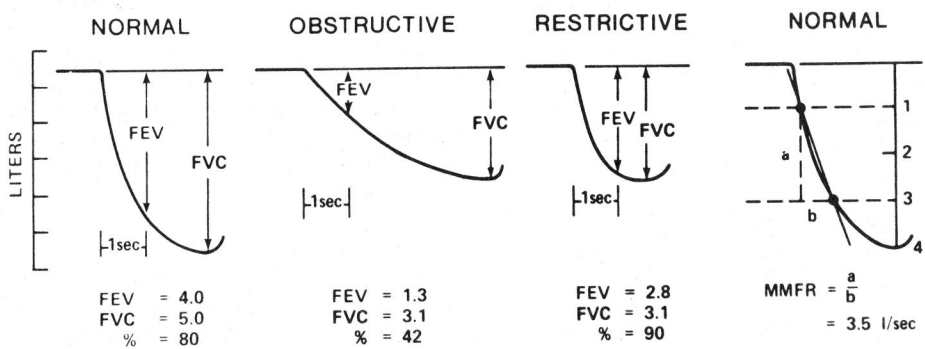

tant to take account of the age of the patient when interpreting many pulmonary function tests.

ACID-BASE DISTURBANCES If pulmonary gas exchange is impaired, the P_{CO_2} in the arterial blood may rise, thus tending to depress the pH and causing *respiratory acidosis*. The compensatory mechanisms which are then brought into play are discussed in Chap. 85.

MEASUREMENT OF BLOOD GASES Blood gas measurements play a vital role in the management of respiratory failure. Arterial blood can be obtained by direct puncture, and the oxygen and carbon dioxide partial pressures and the pH can be measured by electrodes. Oxygen saturation can be derived from the oxygen content of the blood using van Slyke's method before and after complete oxygenation, or the saturation can be calculated from an oxygen dissociation curve.

HYPOXEMIA

The four main causes of a low arterial P_{O_2} are (1) ventilation/perfusion ratio inequality, (2) right-to-left shunt, (3) hypoventilation, and (4) impaired diffusion. In addition, living at high altitude or deliberately inspiring a low oxygen mixture causes hypoxemia.

1 *Ventilation/perfusion ratio inequality* is the commonest cause and is responsible for almost all the hypoxemia seen in chronic lung disease. Specific tests of ventilation/perfusion inequality are not generally available, although the multiple inert gas infusion technique referred to earlier can be used in specialized centers. The demonstration of ventilatory inequality (see above) is a useful pointer. Mild degrees of ventilation/perfusion ratio inequality may be present without hypoxemia, and considerable inequality may exist without hypercapnia if overall ventilation is increased. However, carbon dioxide retention almost always develops eventually. The hypoxemia is eventually abolished by the administration of 100% oxygen. However, with severe equality, the arterial P_{O_2} may take so many minutes to rise to normal values because of very poorly ventilated areas that, in practice, the levels seen in normal subjects may not be attained. Exercise may or may not aggravate the hypoxemia and hypercapnia (see Table 255-1). The response of the arterial P_{O_2} to exercise depends to a large extent on the changes in total ventilation and blood flow.

2 *Shunted blood,* i.e., blood which has bypassed ventilated areas of the lung, causes hypoxemia. Patients with right-to-left shunts through congenital heart defects or a pulmonary arteriovenous fistula belong to this group. Patients with ven-

tilation/perfusion ratio inequality often have some parts of the lung completely unventilated, and the contribution of these regions is indistinguishable from that of a shunt. The hypoxemia due to shunt is not abolished (although it is reduced) by administering 100% oxygen, and this test will distinguish it from the other causes of hypoxemia. The level of the arterial P_{O_2} under these conditions allows the percentage of shunted blood to be measured. The arterial P_{O_2} rises to some extent because of the addition of dissolved oxygen to the pulmonary blood, and a measurement of arterial saturation may not permit detection of the hypoxemia. It is therefore important to measure P_{O_2}. The hypoxemia of shunt may be exaggerated by exercise. Hypercapnia does not occur unless the shunt is very gross, because the respiratory center increases the ventilation, thus holding the arterial P_{CO_2} down.

3 *Hypoventilation* always causes both hypoxemia and hypercapnia. Because of the shape of the oxygen dissociation curve, which means that a substantial fall in arterial P_{O_2} can occur with little reduction in oxygen saturation (see Fig. 53-4), considerable carbon dioxide retention may be present without recognizable cyanosis. If the patient is inhaling an enriched oxygen mixture, e.g., in the anesthetic recovery room, hypoxemia is not present but the hypercapnia may be severe.

4 *Impaired diffusion* rarely causes hypoxemia but not hypercapnia. The hypoxemia is accentuated by exercise but abolished if an enriched oxygen mixture is administered. As we have seen, diffusion impairment may occur in normal subjects during work at very high altitude, but its importance as a cause of hypoxemia in disease is minimal.

HYPERCAPNIA

The two chief causes of carbon dioxide retention are ventilation/perfusion ratio inequality and hypoventilation. Ventilation/perfusion ratio inequality is the commonest cause, although many patients have some degree of uneven ventilation and blood flow without hypercapnia. A combination of the two causes can occur.

Why does a patient with chronic lung disease develop hypercapnia? Progressive lung disease (perhaps aggravated by an acute infection) causes increasing mismatch of blood flow and ventilation and greater impairment of carbon dioxide transfer. For a time, the respiratory center is able to hold the arterial P_{CO_2} down to the normal level by increasing the ventilation, but the work of breathing is usually high because of airway obstruction, so that eventually a compromise is reached and the arterial and alveolar partial pressures are allowed to rise. This has the advantage that more carbon dioxide is put out for the same ventilation, so it may be looked upon as a compensatory mechanism albeit a hazardous one. As the ventilation/perfusion ratio inequality becomes worse, the tendency is for the arterial P_{CO_2} to rise further.

A particularly dangerous situation may arise if such a patient is given oxygen to breathe. The chief stimulus to ventilation in these patients is often hypoxemia, and when this is suddenly relieved, the ventilation may drop precipitously and the arterial P_{CO_2} climb rapidly. The carbon dioxide retention and acidosis may then cause clouding of consciousness, muscular twitching, and a raised intracranial pressure. Drugs which depress the respiratory center may produce a similar effect. Thus while oxygen administration is indicated in these patients because of their severe hypoxemia, it should be given with caution.

Another hazardous situation often arises when these patients are taken off oxygen because they are retaining too much carbon dioxide. Since the body stores of carbon dioxide are so large, many minutes elapse before the alveolar P_{CO_2} returns to

TABLE 255-1
Features helpful in distinguishing the various causes of hypoxemia and hypercapnia

	Hypoxemia	*Hypercapnia*	*Hypoxemia on exercise*	*Hypercapnia on exercise*	*Hypoxemia on 100% O$_2$*
Ventilation/perfusion ratio inequality	Yes	Yes or no	Yes	Yes or no	No
Shunt	Yes	No	Yes	Possible	Yes
Hypoventilation	Yes	Yes	Often severe	Often severe	No
Impaired diffusion	Yes (rarely)	No	Often severe	No	No

reasonable levels. During this recovery period, this high alveolar carbon dioxide dilutes the alveolar oxygen and may cause profound hypoxemia.

METABOLIC FUNCTIONS OF THE LUNG

In addition to its primary function of gas exchange, the lung has significant metabolic functions. One of the most important of these is the synthesis of phospholipids such as dipalmitoyl lecithin, a constituent of surfactant (see earlier under "Compliance"). In addition the lung modifies various substances circulating within the blood. For example, it converts the relatively inactive polypeptide, angiotensin I, into the potent vasoconstrictor, angiotensin II. Also the lung inactivates circulating serotonin, bradykinin, and some prostaglandins, while it takes up norepinephrine and histamine to some degree.

In disease, the lung has a remarkable potential for hormone production and secretion. For example, neoplasms such as bronchial carcinomas can produce a variety of polypeptide hormones.

REFERENCES

Cotes JF: *Lung Function,* 3d ed. Philadelphia, Lippincott, 1975
Murray JF: *The Normal Lung.* Philadelphia, Saunders, 1976
West JB: *Pulmonary Pathophysiology—the Essentials.* Baltimore, Williams & Wilkins, 1977

256
FIBEROPTIC BRONCHOSCOPY AND OTHER DIAGNOSTIC PROCEDURES

KENNETH M. MOSER

In seeking a definitive diagnosis in the patient with respiratory disease, a wide choice of diagnostic procedures is available. These procedures vary considerably, not only in diagnostic reliability and specificity, but also in terms of the discomfort and hazard to the patient. Hence, an orderly sequence of test selection is mandatory. This sequence should begin with procedures involving little risk and move on only if necessary to those which entail higher morbidity and mortality rates.

NONINVASIVE PROCEDURES

RADIOGRAPHIC PROCEDURES The *chest roentgenogram* serves two major roles in the search for a diagnosis in the patient with respiratory disease: *detector* and *guide.* Often, in its role as a detector, the routine chest roentgenogram initiates the diagnostic search by disclosing an abnormality in an asymptomatic individual. More commonly, it permits detection of pulmonary involvement in someone already ill. Rarely, detection may coincide with diagnosis; e.g., in spontaneous pneumothorax or when a radiopaque foreign body has been aspirated.

Far more frequently, however, the roentgenogram, having detected potential disease, provides a guide to the selection of subsequent diagnostic procedures. Many radiographic findings are quite characteristic of certain diseases. A number of radiographic patterns are sufficiently repetitive to warrant descriptive names, such as bilateral hilar adenopathy, solitary pulmonary nodule, diffuse interstitial infiltrate, alveolar filling pattern, multinodular lesion, and honeycomb lung. Thus, a particular radiographic finding, combined with other pertinent data, often permits establishment of a reasonable list of possi-

ble diagnoses. For example, the roentgenographic detection of bilateral hilar adenopathy in an asymptomatic, 26-year-old black male immediately places sarcoidosis at the top of the list. A chest roentgenogram disclosing upper lobe cavities in a febrile male whose brother recently was admitted to a tuberculosis sanitarium would make tuberculosis the most likely entity. Or a "diffuse interstitial" infiltrate—for which more than 100 causes exist—may yield a prompt diagnosis of varicella pneumonia when combined with the classical skin lesions.

In some instances, special radiographic techniques may provide valuable diagnostic insights.

Fluoroscopy allows visualization of the thoracic contents in a dynamic rather than static manner and also permits a wide range of special views. It also indicates whether a lesion is pulsatile, what its precise location in the thorax is, whether the hemidiaphragms move normally, i.e., whether they are fixed or move paradoxically, and how various zones of the lung behave during inspiration and expiration. Image intensification, permanent recording of fluoroscopy on videotape, and quantification of lung density from such recordings (videodensitometry) are extending the diagnostic capabilities of this simple procedure.

Tomography (laminagraphy, planigraphy) is a radiographic technique by which a sequence of roentgenograms, each representing a "slice of the lung" at a different depth, is obtained. Ordinarily, "cuts" are made at 0.5- to 1-cm distances through the area of interest. Tomograms can identify a number of features which were not appreciated on the "routine" roentgenogram, including the presence of calcium or cavity in a lesion; the presence of hilar adenopathy; abnormalities in configuration of the trachea and major bronchi; and the contours of masses in the mediastinal area.

Thoracic *computerized tomography (CT) scanning,* using the whole-body device, may provide useful information not available by other techniques for the definition of pleural lesions (e.g., differentiating fluid from tumor) and lesions in the mediastinum (nodes, tumors, vascular structures). The potential value of this procedure and its newer counterpart, the emission CT scanner, remains to be fully defined.

SKIN TESTS Having arrived at a tentative list of diagnostic possibilities based on the history, physical examination, and the radiographic appearance, the physician should move to other procedures. One of the simplest and most commonly overlooked is the application of *skin tests* with specific antigens. Antigens are now available to assist in the diagnosis of tuberculosis, histoplasmosis, coccidioidomycosis, blastomycosis, trichinosis, and toxoplasmosis. A negative battery of skin tests, particularly if it incorporates antigens such as mumps, streptokinase-streptodornase, *Trichophyton,* and *Monilia,* may provide a diagnostic clue by suggesting disorders associated with depressed cell-mediated immunity, such as Hodgkin's disease, sarcoidosis, disseminated tuberculosis, or coccidioidomycosis.

SEROLOGIC TESTS These tests also may be useful in the diagnosis of histoplasmosis, blastomycosis, coccidioidomycosis, toxoplasmosis, *Mycoplasma* pneumonia, Legionnaires' disease, and a variety of other infectious diseases involving the lungs. Often, more extensive diagnostic procedures can be avoided if appropriate serologic tests are obtained.

SPUTUM EXAMINATION Another rapid, innocuous diagnostic procedure is *sputum examination.* It is important that the specimen contain sputum, not saliva. The gross nature of the sputum—color, odor, and the presence of blood—may provide valuable clues. Carefully stained smears of the sputum should be examined next, for these will disclose the causative organism in many bacterial pneumonias, in tuberculosis, and in some fungous infections. Sputum eosinophilia can suggest the presence of reversible airway disease responsive to corticosteroids; hemosiderin-laden macrophages suggest the possibility of Goodpasture's syndrome. Often valuable time is lost because the sputum smear is not examined and results of culture are awaited instead.

Culture of expectorated sputum (spontaneous or induced) has fallen into disrepute because of uncertain yield and, particularly, because of frequent and unavoidable contamination by the oropharyngeal bacterial flora. Although such cultures are invaluable for identification of organisms responsible for tuberculous and fungous infections, their utility in detection of other bacterial agents responsible for pulmonary infection is often uncertain and can be misleading. Three procedures, described below, are now gaining wide acceptance because they limit oropharyngeal contamination and/or obtain representative samples of lung secretions from the area of lung involvement: (1) transtracheal aspiration, (2) catheter aspiration, and (3) percutaneous needle aspiration.

Exfoliative cytology of the sputum is helpful in the diagnosis of carcinoma of the lung. Proper handling of such specimens is essential. Sputum samples often can be obtained in a patient who is not coughing by having him inhale a heated mixture of a mildly irritative solution which induces cough.

PULMONARY FUNCTION TESTS These tests may serve as diagnostic guides. Certain "patterns" of derangement in spirometric tests, arterial blood gases, diffusing capacity, and other functional parameters are particularly suggestive of certain pulmonary diseases. For example, diffuse interstitial fibrotic diseases of the lungs produce a "restrictive" spirometric defect, reduced pulmonary compliance, and an alveolar-arterial pressure gradient which is widened at rest and widens further with exercise. Emphysema characteristically causes expiratory obstruction, lung hyperinflation, decreased static elastic recoil (increased compliance), and a reduced diffusing capacity (Chap. 255).

PULMONARY SCINTIPHOTOGRAPHY This technique can provide a visual image of the distribution of both blood flow and ventilation in the lungs, as well as quantitative data on such distribution. Scintiphotos ("scans") are obtained by a variety of "scanning" devices which record the pattern of pulmonary radioactivity after intravenous injection or inhalation of gamma-emitting radionuclides. Injection (perfusion) photoscans have proved especially valuable in detecting zones of absent or decreased blood flow compatible with embolism (Chap. 266). When ventilation scans, obtained with radioactive gases, are combined with perfusion studies, ventilation-perfusion patterns are provided which permit recognition of parenchymal lung diseases and vascular disorders, including embolism.

Another type of scan involves intravenous injection of radionuclides which have an affinity for intrathoracic inflammatory and neoplastic tissues. Concentration of gamma-emitting nuclides, defined by scanning, may permit detection of neoplastic or inflammatory disease in the lungs or mediastinal lymph nodes. Gallium 67 is the most useful of these radionuclides now available.

All the above procedures involve minimal risks and discomfort to the patient. These approaches should be exhausted before the techniques discussed below are considered, unless the condition of the patient demands immediate diagnosis.

INVASIVE PROCEDURES

BRONCHOSCOPY The introduction of the flexible, fiberoptic bronchoscope (FOB) has led to major advances in the diagnostic approach to pulmonary disease. The primary objectives of bronchoscopy include direct visualization of the tracheobronchial tree, including abnormalities such as tumors or granulomatous lesions; biopsy of suggestive or obvious endobronchial lesions; and brushing, washing, or biopsy of lung regions for cultural and cytologic examinations. But the *diagnostic reach of* and *accessibility to* bronchoscopy have been expanded by the FOB. This can be understood best by comparing the FOB with the "standard" rigid bronchoscope.

The rigid bronchoscope is a wide-bore metal tube which incorporates a lighted mirror-lens system. The FOB is composed of fiberoptic bundles which provide both illumination and visualization pathways. A small channel with a diameter of 1 to 3 mm traverses the FOB, through which instruments can be passed, fluids delivered, and suction applied. The rigid bronchoscope comes in various external diameters limited only by the feasibility of introducing the rigid device orally and through the larynx. Biopsy and other procedures are carried out through the rather capacious interior of the rigid tube. The FOB also is available in various external diameters, but all are substantially smaller than rigid bronchoscopes (since no "wall" exists in the FOB). The distal tip of FOB can be *flexed* easily to 90° and usually to 130° or more from the vertical.

Thus, the rigid bronchoscope permits visualization only of lobar bronchi and the orifices of some segmental bronchi. The flexible, smaller FOB extends the range of *view* to all segmental and subsegmental bronchi and the range for *biopsy and sampling* to the pulmonary parenchyma itself. A biopsy forceps, catheter, or brush passed through the FOB can be directed well beyond the tip of the bronchoscope itself, permitting *transbronchial lung biopsy, brushings,* or *aspiration of secretions* for cytologic examination from the most distal regions of the lung. Indeed, both forceps and brush can reach and perforate the pleura, leading to pneumothorax. Therefore, when the lesion being approached is distal, fluoroscopic guidance is essential. Not only does this permit placement of the FOB, forceps, catheter, or brush directly into the area of interest, but also it assures that the pleura will not be inadvertently reached and punctured. The FOB also allows *regional* lung lavage to obtain materials for cytologic examination and culture. The use of specially designed catheters (see below) placed through the FOB is quite useful in obtaining representative, noncontaminated secretions for culture, thus avoiding the problems mentioned previously with expectorated sputum.

Thus, the FOB has sharply increased the limited diagnostic reach previously available with rigid bronchoscopy. Equally important, the FOB has made bronchoscopy more available to the physician and more acceptable to the patient. The performance of rigid bronchoscopy requires the supine position for peroral insertion of the device; can be performed safely by a relatively few trained surgeons; and is often carried out under general anesthesia in an operating room. Therefore, it has been a procedure requiring significant preparation and hence delay. Fiberoptic bronchoscopy can be performed in the sitting or supine position, since the FOB is easily inserted transnasally; can be performed by a large number of trained pulmonary specialists as well as surgeons; usually requires only local anesthesia; and can be performed safely on the wards, in diagnostic rooms equipped with a "dentist-type" chair, and in intensive care units. The FOB can be used easily in intubated patients on ventilators with simple "side-arm" adaptors attached to the endotracheal tube. Therefore, when bronchoscopy is indicated, it is not surprising that fiberoptic bronchoscopy is now commonly the first choice. The roomier rigid bronchoscope is now usually reserved for situations in which the small biopsy-suction channel in the FOB may be inadequate (e.g., for removal of large foreign bodies). The FOB also has a widening range of therapeutic applications including aspiration of secretions in patients with airway obstruction or atelectasis due to retained secretions; obstruction of bleeding areas of the lung, with a wedged FOB itself or with a balloon catheter passed via the FOB, in patients who are poor surgical risks; removal of small foreign bodies; and placement of radionuclides in tumors.

The hazards of bronchoscopy are modest but should be recognized. In addition to the risk of general anesthesia which rigid bronchoscopy usually requires, they can include hypoxemia, laryngospasm, bronchospasm, pneumothorax, and, of course, bleeding following biopsy. Proper management before, during, and after bronchoscopy should prevent most of these complications. The primary contraindication to both rigid and fiberoptic bronchoscopy is the same: performance by inexperienced personnel. Lack of experience sharply reduces diagnostic and therapeutic yield while increasing risks.

BRONCHOGRAPHY In this method, radiopaque material is instilled into the tracheobronchial tree via a catheter or bronchoscope. Positioning of the patient and catheter permits the material to coat all portions of the tracheobronchial tree for a sufficient period so that their outline can be recorded on chest roentgenograms. Bronchography is required for the diagnosis of bronchiectasis, for the identification of obstruction in distal bronchi, and for the detection of other types of congenital and acquired forms of tracheobronchial distortion or malformation.

TRANSTRACHEAL, CATHETER, AND PERCUTANEOUS NEEDLE ASPIRATION OF THE LUNG All three of these procedures are used to obtain material for culture and microscopic examination. In the case of culture, all three techniques bypass the oropharyngeal flora, though transtracheal aspiration is the least certain in this regard.

Transtracheal aspiration involves needle puncture of the cricothyroid membrane, insertion of a plastic cannula and installation of a saline solution, followed by suctioning of a sample. The procedure cannot be performed in intubated patients; contamination rates are high in previously intubated patients or those who have aspirated oropharyngeal contents. Because the procedure entails risks, although these are minimized by meticulous technique and experience, clear indications for its use should exist. These include patients with apparent pulmonary infection who are unable to cough, in whom cough is nonproductive, or in whom there has been a lack of response to therapy based on smears or cultures from expectorated sputum.

In these same contexts, *catheters* specially designed with a distal plug to avoid oropharyngeal contamination can be used. These are manipulated (through an FOB or without it) into the trachea, the absorbable plug ejected, and the catheter wedged in the area of involvement. Aspirations, brushings, and washings are then obtained. Finally, an alternative procedure is direct percutaneous aspiration, which can be performed using a small (23 gauge), thin-walled, *noncutting* needle. The needle is introduced percutaneously into the lung area of interest and secretions are aspirated by syringe, with or without installation of 1 to 3 ml saline. Both the catheter and needle approaches are low-risk, high-yield, low-contamination procedures in experienced hands. Pneumothorax and bleeding are potential risks of the needle aspiration approach, and patients must be monitored for both.

THORACENTESIS AND PLEURAL BIOPSY Thoracentesis should be performed to obtain pleural fluid in all pleural effusions of uncertain etiology and may be indicated for relief of symptoms in some patients with effusion of known cause. In effusions of uncertain cause, closed (needle) pleural biopsy should be performed as part of the same procedure.

When pleural fluid is small in amount or when its presence or location is uncertain from routine or lateral decubitus roentgenograms, performance of the thoracentesis and biopsy under fluoroscopic or ultrasound guidance (or with CT scan views) enhances both yield and safety. Pleural fluid obtained should be examined for specific gravity, white blood cell count and differential, protein and glucose concentrations, LDH, pH, P_{CO_2} (sample collected anaerobically), and amylase. Gram stain, cultures, and exfoliative cytologic specimens should be obtained; and in some instances, rheumatoid factor and complement levels are measured. The gross appearance of the fluid, the quantity obtained, and the precise location of the thoracentesis should be recorded. A combination of a pleural fluid LDH above 200 IU, a pleural fluid/serum protein ratio greater than 0.5, and a pleural fluid/serum LDH ratio greater than 0.6 all indicate than an "exudative" rather than "transudative" process is present. A low pH (< 7.20) indicates that an empyema, probably requiring tube drainage, is present. Specific diagnostic findings in pleural fluid may include the opalescent, pearly fluid characteristic of chylothorax; positive smears or cultures for tuberculosis or other infections; a marked elevation of amylase indicative of effusion secondary to pancreatitis or a ruptured esophagus; and the very low glucose values often seen in effusions associated with rheumatoid arthritis.

As already noted, closed (needle) pleural biopsy should follow thoracentesis whenever the diagnosis is uncertain. It is important to leave some fluid in the pleural space as this makes biopsy easier and safer. Bleeding, pneumothorax, and bronchopleural fistula induced by cutting through the visceral pleura are all more likely in the absence of fluid, and a satisfactory biopsy specimen is less likely to be obtained. Several special needles are available for biopsy of the parietal pleura. All have a cutting edge and some device for retaining the biopsy. The needle is inserted into the pleural effusion, then withdrawn until it is seated on the parietal pleura, from which a biopsy is obtained with the cutting edge. Usually, three biopsies are taken from different sites at the same session. Care should be exercised to place the needle in a position least likely to impinge on the intercostal vessels. All diagnostic fluid should be removed before biopsy since postbiopsy bleeding may obscure the true character of the fluid.

In the absence of a pleural effusion, two other options exist for obtaining tissue from pleural based lesions: aspiration needle biopsy and open biopsy. The technique for aspiration biopsy is the same as that described above, although some physicians use "cutting" needles (see "Lung Biopsy," below). Open pleural biopsy involves a limited thoracotomy, requiring anesthesia. A small intercostal incision is made, and the parietal pleural is biopsied under direct visualization. The incision is then closed, often without an intercostal tube. "Open" biopsy has several advantages because a larger specimen is obtained and the pleura and underlying lung can be seen and palpated. When pleural involvement is "spotty," open biopsy increases the possibility of establishing a diagnosis.

PULMONARY AND BRONCHIAL ANGIOGRAPHY Just as bronchography outlines the tracheobronchial anatomy, pulmonary angiography permits visualization of the pulmonary vasculature. Radiopaque materials are injected rapidly by vein or via a catheter into the systemic veins, right chambers, or the pulmonary artery. The distribution of this material in the pulmonary vasculature is recorded on film (angiography), by a high-speed camera (cineangiography), or on videotape (Chap. 235). Angiography is frequently used to detect pulmonary emboli and a variety of congenital and acquired lesions of the pulmonary vessels. The procedure is not without risk, particularly in patients with pulmonary hypertension, and clear indication for it must exist as well as personnel experienced in its performance and interpretation.

Bronchial arteriography is now used in some centers to identify otherwise unidentified bleeding sites in the lungs. Transarterial placement of a catheter into the orifices or parent vessels of bronchial arteries can be accomplished by experienced operators. Radiopaque material is then injected so that these arteries can be visualized. If a bleeding site is identified, emboli can be injected via the catheter as a means for halting hemoptysis.

MEDIASTINOSCOPY AND MEDIASTINOTOMY Another favored site for biopsy is the lymph nodes in the mediastinum. Because they receive lymphatic drainage from the lungs, these nodes often disclose intrathoracic diseases such as carcinoma, granulomatous infections, and sarcoidosis. Biopsy of these nodes is accomplished during mediastinoscopy. This involves insertion of a lighted mirror-lens system, much like a bronchoscope, through an incision at the base of the neck anteriorly. The instrument is advanced under visual control into the mediastinum, where inspection and biopsy can be carried out. Because of its higher yield of diagnostic lymph nodes, mediastinoscopy has virtually replaced biopsy of the *scalene fat pad* for nodes of interest on the right side of the mediastinum. However, for anatomic reasons, mediastinoscopy on the left is less satisfactory and more hazardous. Nodes in this location are usually approached through a limited left anterior thoracotomy (mediastinotomy) or, occasionally, by scalene fat pad biopsy. Mediastinoscopy and mediastinotomy are low-risk, high-yield procedures. They are invaluable on the "staging" of patients with known or suspected pulmonary malignancy.

LUNG BIOPSY Finally, if the diagnosis still remains unclear, biopsy of the lung may be required. Again, "closed" and "open" approaches are available. Closed biopsies are of three types: transbronchial, aspiration, and "cutting needle." Transbronchial biopsy, carried out through the fiberoptic bronchoscope, is a highly useful procedure, particularly since larger forceps have been introduced and the taking of multiple biopsies during one procedure has become routine.

However, when lesions are small and/or anatomically located beyond the reach of the FOB, direct aspiration needle biopsy is often more rewarding. *Aspiration* biopsy, mentioned previously, provides cytologic material but does not actually obtain a specimen of lung whose architecture can be examined, a feature which may be necessary to establish a diagnosis. Various "cutting" needles are available which do provide a "core" of the involved lung. However, this approach has waned in popularity because of the high incidence of pneumothorax and bleeding, occasional deaths due to air embolism, and the small size of the biopsy specimen, which may limit diagnostic interpretation. Fluoroscopic guidance is essential in all these closed approaches, and they are contraindicated if pulmonary hypertension or a hemorrhagic diathesis is present.

Open lung biopsy, requiring thoracotomy, is the final diagnostic resort. It is, however, a relatively safe procedure even in patients with respiratory failure, hemorrhagic diathesis, or pulmonary hypertension if meticulous surgical and anesthetic techniques are observed. Direct visualization allows selection of an optimum biopsy site, and of course, a specimen of adequate size is obtained. In selecting among these closed and open options, consideration of local expertise in their performance is a key factor.

All specimens obtained by biopsy should be both cultured and processed for pathologic examination.

REFERENCES

ANDERSEN HA, FABER LP (eds): Diagnostic and therapeutic applications of the bronchoscope. Chest 73:685, 1978

BARTLETT JA: Diagnostic accuracy of transtracheal aspiration bacteriologic studies. Am Rev Respir Dis 115:778, 1977

BATES DV et al: *Respiratory Function in Disease.* Philadelphia, Saunders, 1971

BAUM GL: *Textbook of Pulmonary Diseases.* Boston, Little, Brown, 1974

BOOKSTEIN JJ et al: The role of bronchial arteriography and therapeutic embolization in hemoptysis. Chest 72:658, 1977

DAVIDSON M: Bacteriologic diagnosis of acute pneumonia: Comparison of sputum, transtracheal aspirate and lung aspirates. JAMA 235:158, 1976

FRASER RG, PARÉ JAP: *Diagnosis of Diseases of the Chest.* Philadelphia, Saunders, 1977

LIGHT RW, et al: Diagnostic significance of pleural fluid pH and P_{CO_2}. Chest 64:591, 1973

SACKNER MA: Bronchofiberoscopy: State of the art. Am Rev Respir Dis 111:62, 1975

Lung disease caused by immunologic and environmental injury

257
ASTHMA

E. R. McFADDEN, JR.
K. FRANK AUSTEN

DEFINITION Asthma is a disease of airways that is characterized by increased responsiveness of the tracheobronchial tree to a multiplicity of stimuli. Asthma is manifested physiologically by a widespread narrowing of the air passages which may be relieved spontaneously or as a result of therapy. Asthma is manifested clinically by paroxysms of dyspnea, cough, and wheezing. It is an episodic disease, acute exacerbations being interspersed with symptom-free periods. Typically, most attacks are short-lived, lasting minutes to hours, and after them the patient seems to recover completely clinically. However, there can be a phase in which the patient experiences some degree of airway obstruction daily. This phase can be mild, with or without superimposed severe episodes, or much more serious, with severe obstruction persisting for days or weeks, a condition known as *status asthmaticus.*

PREVALENCE AND ETIOLOGY The prevalence and incidence of asthma in various parts of the world is difficult to assess with certainty because of the lack of reliable population-based figures which have used uniform diagnostic criteria. However, data from a national health survey indicates that 3 percent of the population of the United States suffers from this disease. Similar figures have been reported from other countries, but for unknown reasons, asthma is uncommon in New Zealand highlanders, American Indians, Eskimos, and West Africans. Bronchial asthma occurs at all ages but predominantly in early life. About one-half of the cases develop before age 10 and another third occur before age 40. In childhood, there is a 2:1 male/female preponderance which equalizes by age 30.

From an etiologic standpoint, asthma is a heterogenous disease, and attempts to define it in etiologic or pathologic terms have proved difficult. It is useful for epidemiologic and clinical purposes to classify the forms of this disease by the principal stimuli that incite or are associated with acute episodes. However, it is important to emphasize that the common denominator underlying the asthmatic diathesis is a nonspecific hyperirritability of the tracheobronchial tree. Thus, the distinction between various types of asthma may often be artificial, and the response of a given subclassification may be initiated by more than one type of stimulus. With this reservation in mind, one can describe two broad groups: allergic and idiosyncratic.

Allergic asthma is often associated with a personal and/or family history of allergic diseases such as rhinitis, urticaria, and eczema; positive wheal-and-flare skin reactions to intradermal injection of extracts of airborne antigens; increased levels of IgE in the serum; and/or positive response to provocation tests involving the inhalation of specific antigen. Immunologic mechanisms appear to be causally related to the development of asthma in 25 to 35 percent of all cases, and contributory in perhaps another third. Allergic asthma is fre-

quently seasonal, and it is most often observed in children and young adults. A nonseasonal form may result from allergy to feathers, animal danders, molds, and other antigens present continuously in the environment.

A significant segment of the asthmatic population will present with negative family or personal histories of allergy, negative skin tests, and normal serum levels of IgE, and therefore cannot be classified on the basis of defined immunologic mechanisms. These we term *idiosyncratic.* Many of these will develop a typical symptom complex upon contracting an upper respiratory illness. The initial insult may be little more than a common cold, but after several days the patient begins to develop paroxysms of wheezing and dyspnea that can last for days to months. These individuals should not be confused with the so-called "infective asthmatics" or with persons in whom the symptoms of bronchospasm are superimposed upon chronic bronchitis (see Chap. 263).

Unfortunately, many patients will not clearly fit into either of the above categories but will fall into a mixed group with features of each. In general, those patients whose onset of disease is in early life will tend to have a strong allergic component to their illness while those who develop their asthma late tend to be nonallergic or to have mixed etiologies.

STIMULI THAT PROVOKE ASTHMA   Allergens Most of the allergens that provoke asthma are airborne, and in order to induce a state of sensitivity, they must be reasonably abundant for considerable periods of time. Once sensitization has occurred, however, the patient can then exhibit exquisite responsivity, so that minute amounts of the offending agent can produce significant exacerbations of the disease. The mechanism by which an inhaled antigen can provoke an acute episode of asthma in a susceptible individual is unknown, and several paradoxes remain to be solved. The first is that most aeroallergens are too large to stay suspended in the airstream when respired and are effectively removed by the filtering action of the nose and mouth. Second, even when directly applied to the nose or inhaled through the mouth, whole pollen grains fail to induce measurable airway obstruction in asthmatic subjects who respond vigorously to an aerosol of a solution of the same antigen. Third, because there are tight intercellular bridges in the lining epithelium of the airways, a dilemma exists about how the antigen can rapidly reach a submucosal mast cell to initiate an acute reaction. Along these same lines, it has also been difficult to explain the findings that substances such as charcoal dust, which are chemically and immunologically inert, can induce changes in airflow resistance in asthma.

Sufficient data that provide at least a partial insight into these problems have accumulated. It now seems likely that plant debris other than pollen may provide sufficiently small antigenic particles to allow penetration of the lung's defenses. Once this occurs, recent evidence demonstrates that there are two converging pathways in the initial reaction sequence, and that a stimulus may have a direct effect upon the smooth muscle of an airway while simultaneously activating subepithelial vagal receptors, thereby provoking reflex bronchoconstriction as well. Precise details on how these effects are elicited are lacking, but it is now known that mast cells are also located intramucosally in the airway lumen and not only submucosally as formerly thought. Thus, mast cell–antigen interaction can occur initially at the mucosal surface of the airway, and the chemical products of that interaction can facilitate penetration of additional antigen to the more numerous submucosal mast cells by opening the tight junctions. Evidence is also accumulating that the local release of the neurotransmitter of the parasympathetic nervous system can produce the same effect. In addition, it is possible that the inflammatory changes resulting from chronic antigen-induced release of chemical mediators lowers the response threshold of the airway irritant or rapidly adapting stretch receptors and so changes airway responsivity to a variety of stimuli.

Aspirin and related substances   In a group of patients ingestion of aspirin or other nonsteroidal anti-inflammatory agents such as indomethacin makes the asthma worse. These patients are usually adults with the triad of severe unremitting asthma, nasal polyposis, and sinusitis. However, aspirin sensitivity can be found in the absence of this triad and has also been reported in children. Other drug allergies are common in such patients, and, while they are sensitive to acetylsalicylic acid, they uniformly tolerate sodium salicylate. The reaction, which is sometimes alarming, usually occurs within 2 h of ingestion of as little as 300 mg aspirin. (In the laboratory 15 to 30 mg can induce the response.) In its most severe form, it is characterized by acute rhinitis, wheezing, skin flushing, pruritus, urticaria, hypotension, and syncope. An immunologic basis has not been demonstrated. Consequently, this reaction may be idiosyncratic, but the possibility of asthmatics coming into contact with substances related to aspirin in food additives (e.g., tartrazine yellow) and elsewhere in the environment is so great because of the widespread use of these compounds that this sensitivity may be the cause of the reaction rather than merely an exacerbating factor.

Environmental factors   An additional group of persons will become symptomatic when confronted with environmental conditions which promote the concentration of airborne pollutants and antigens. This type of asthma, the so-called "Tokyo-Yokohama" or "New Orleans asthma," tends to occur in individuals living in heavy industrial or dense urban areas during thermal inversions, or in other situations associated with stagnant air masses. Such atmospheric conditions generally make all types of asthma worse, but they also cause the de novo development of symptoms in some individuals who are not otherwise troubled. The reaction may be idiosyncratic, but it may also be toxic, resulting from exposure to chemicals like SO_2 that depress lung function in anyone if inhaled in sufficient concentration. Alternatively, inhalation of polluted air could alter the threshold of the irritant receptors in the airways of a latent asthmatic so as to create a response to other less noxious stimuli.

Occupational factors   A variety of compounds used in industry can cause asthma in susceptible individuals. Various names have been applied to this condition, such as meat wrappers' asthma, bakers' asthma, woodworkers' asthma, and they give some indication of the heterogeneity of the jobs in which reversible airway disease can be found. The underlying mechanisms appear to be three in number: (1) in some cases the offending agent results in the formation of a specific IgE, and the cause seems immunologic; (2) materials being employed, in other cases, cause a direct liberation of bronchoconstrictor

substances; and (3) work-related irritant substances, in still other cases, directly or reflexly stimulate the airways of either latent or frank asthmatics.

Infections   Respiratory infections are among the most common of the stimuli that evoke acute exacerbations of asthma. For many years, it was believed that bacterial infection was of prime importance, but well-controlled investigations have rather conclusively demonstrated that respiratory viruses are the major factors. In young children, the most important infectious agents are respiratory syncytial virus and parainfluenza virus. In older children and adults, rhinovirus and influenza virus predominate as pathogens. Most studies indicate that simple colonization of the tracheobronchial tree is insufficient to evoke acute episodes of bronchospasm and that attacks of asthma occur only when symptoms of an ongoing respiratory tract infection are, or have been, present. The mechanism by which viruses induce asthma is unknown, but the weight of current evidence suggests that the resulting inflammatory changes in the airway mucosa produce a reduction in the firing thresholds of the subepithelial receptors. Supporting evidence for this concept is derived from the fact that the airway responsiveness of normal nonasthmatic subjects to aerosols of histamine and methacholine are dramatically, but transiently, increased after a viral respiratory infection.

Exercise   Asthma can also be induced or made worse by physical exertion. Provocation of bronchospasm by exercise is probably operative to some extent in every asthmatic patient, and in some it may be the only trigger mechanism that will produce symptoms. In the latter circumstance, when such patients are followed for sufficient periods of time, one can often observe the development of recurring episodes of airway obstruction independent of exercise: thus, the onset of this problem can frequently serve as the first manifestation of the full-blown asthmatic syndrome. Exercise-induced asthma is particularly troublesome in children because of their usual high level of physical activity. There is a significant interaction between the climatic environment in which the exercise is performed and the magnitude of the postexertional obstruction. For example, the inhalation of cold air during physical exertion markedly enhances the response, while warm, humid air can blunt or abolish it. Consequently, activities such as ice hockey, skiing, or ice skating are more provocative than is swimming in an indoor heated pool. The mechanism by which exercise produces acute exacerbations of asthma has not been conclusively determined, but strong evidence is accumulating that indicates that it is related to the degree of cooling of intrathoracic airways that develops as heat and water are transferred to the inspired air to bring the latter to body conditions before it reaches the alveoli.

Emotional stress   Abundant objective data now exist that demonstrate that psychologic factors can interact with the asthmatic diathesis to worsen or ameliorate the disease process. The pathways and nature of the interactions are complex but probably operational to some extent in almost half of the patients studied. Changes in airway caliber seem to be mediated through modification of vagal efferent activity. The most frequently studied variable has been that of suggestion, and the weight of current evidence is that it can be quite an important influence in selected asthmatics. Recent investigations have shown that when responsive individuals are given the appropriate suggestion, they can actually decrease or increase the pharmacologic effects of adrenergic and cholinergic stimuli on their airways. The extent to which psychologic factors participate in the induction and/or continuation of any given acute exacerbation is unknown but probably varies from patient to patient and in the same patient from episode to episode.

PATHOLOGY In a patient who has died of acute asthma, the most striking feature of the lungs at necropsy is their gross overdistention and failure to collapse when the pleural cavities are opened. When the lungs are cut, numerous gelatinous plugs of exudate are found in the majority of the bronchial branches down to the terminal bronchiole. Histologic examination shows hypertrophy of the bronchial smooth muscle, mucosal edema, denudation of the surface epithelium, pronounced thickening of the basement membrane, and eosinophilic infiltrates in the bronchial wall. In asthmatic patients who die from trauma and causes other than asthma itself, mucous casts, basement membrane thickening, and eosinophilic infiltrates are frequently observed. In both situations there is an absence of any of the well-recognized forms of destructive emphysema.

IMMUNOPATHOLOGY The concurrence of allergic rhinitis and asthma in many patients with a familial background of such disorders, and the presence in the serum of passive transfer activity to the clinical allergen led Coca and Cooke in 1923 to introduce the term *atopy* for the propensity to develop an altered state of reactivity after "natural" exposure to specific allergens. As presently used, *atopic allergy* implies a familial tendency to manifest alone or in combination such conditions as asthma, rhinitis, urticaria, and eczematous (atopic) dermatitis; and the passive transfer factor is now known to be immunoglobulin E (IgE). The importance of specific IgE in atopic diseases is that this immunoglobulin fixes to tissue mast cells. When this occurs, these cells become the target of further antigen exposure and mast cell–derived mediators appear to be the effector principles of the subsequent symptom complex. Mast cells are located in respiratory tissues in both mucosal and deeper perivenular sites and can be triggered by either immune or nonimmune mechanisms. The end result is the generation and release of a diverse group of highly active pharmacologic materials which together possess all the necessary functions for a fully expressed but locally controlled biphasic inflammatory response. The early phase is edematous and acellular with an influx of plasma proteins, and the later response is characterized by the influx of specific phagocytic cells. The natural regulation of this process is multifactorial and includes the intensity and persistence of the event activating the mast cell, the intracellular controls regulating the generation and release of the mediators, feedback mechanisms by which released mediators modulate subsequent mast cell response, the reaction to mediator activity, and the rate at which the released mediators undergo biodegradation. Thus, because of their contents and strategic locations, tissue mast cells may well be immunologically specific gatekeepers at sites of potential host penetration. This view, however, does not exclude mechanisms for activation with function in the nonimmune host. Such a postulate also implies a potential for serving the host in either a beneficial or an adverse manner, depending upon the appropriateness of activation and capability for containment of the response.

Chemical mediators of immediate hypersensitivity Fragments of human lung or nasal polyps obtained from allergic individuals respond to challenge with specific antigens with the release of many of the chemical mediators listed in Table 257-1. Similar results are obtained when fragments from nonallergic persons are passively sensitized with IgE and then exposed to specific allergen. Those biologically active substances that are granule-associated are considered to be the primary mediators

of immediate hypersensitivity because of morphologic and chemical data indicating that the exocytosed granule is in contact with the extracellular environment. Once released, their putative activity may be expressed directly or may require further uncovering for full expression. In order to emphasize the striking differences in the immediate bioavailability of such mediators, they may be further divided into those which diffuse readily from the granule in physiologic buffer and those which are more tightly granule-associated and thus require a step beyond granule exocytosis for full expression of their possible functions. In reality, this distinction is composed of a spectrum: histamine, 5-hydroxytryptamine, the tetrapeptides of eosinophil chemotactic factor of anaphylaxis (ECF-A), and the oligopeptides with eosinophilotactic activity are readily diffusible from the discharged granule in physiologic ionic medium; acetyl-β-D-glucosaminidase exhibits partial releasibility from the discharged or isolated granule in physiologic solution and complete dissociation in 0.5 M NaCl; and macromolecular heparin and chymase are not released from the rat mast granule until it undergoes dissolution in 1.0 M salt. The relevance of the extracellular action and fate of the granule has been heightened by the recent demonstration of numerous metachromatic extracellular granules in human cutaneous tissues after experimental mast cell activation and their subsequent ingestion by infiltrating eosinophils after several hours. Those mediators which are not stored preformed in the mast cell and appear as a result of coupled activation-secretion of the granule are considered to be secondary. Thus, they can be by-products of that reaction, or of the perturbation of a second cell by the primary mediators, or both.

The functional characteristics of the primary and secondary chemical mediators tabulated in Table 257-1 are largely derived from in vitro actions. In vivo studies are limited. Histamine alters both large and small airways by direct and reflex cholinergic mechanisms in primates and other species, while slow-reacting substance of anaphylaxis (SRS-A), which has been adequately studied only in the guinea pig, acts directly on, and with a marked preference for, peripheral airways. Crude platelet activating factor(s) has been shown to have procoagulant activity in the rat and to be a permeability enhancing factor with platelet localizing activity in the rabbit skin. The synthetic tetrapeptides of human ECF-A cause the local accumulation of eosinophils after intracutaneous administration to humans or subhuman primates.

Role of the chemical mediators It has been known for about 20 years that the airways of individuals with asthma have an exquisite hyperreactivity to a wide variety of inhaled stimuli, including such chemical mediators as histamine, acetylcholine, and crude SRS-A. Furthermore, the response is augmented in the presence of beta-adrenergic blockers such as propranolol. Increased airway hyperreactivity has recently been demonstrated in a portion of clinically unaffected family members in large kindreds with asthmatic members, suggesting that overt clinical disease may require the presence of both airway hyperreactivity and a trigger such as episodic allergic mediator release. Whether persistent mediator release alone is sufficient to establish an acquired hyperreactivity is unknown. However, the capacity of mast cells to serve as a trigger is supported by their intraepithelial location and the arguments developed earlier in this chapter in the section on allergens.

Histamine has both direct effects and indirect cholinergic reflex effects on bronchomotor tone. It also increases the permeability of veins to proteins. Histamine-induced changes in

TABLE 257-1
Mediators of immediate hypersensitivity

Mediators	Structural characteristics	Assay(s)	Other functions	Inactivation
PRIMARY				
Histamine	β-Imidazolylethylamine (111 mol wt)	Contraction of guinea pig ileum; specific radio labeling by histamine N-methyltransferase	Increased vascular permeability; elevation of cyclic AMP; chemokinesis	Histaminase; histamine methyltransferase
Serotonin	5-Hydroxytryptamine (5-HT)	Biologic and enzymatic assays	Increases vascular permeability	5-HT deaminase
Eosinophilic chemotactic factor of anaphylaxis (ECF-A)	Hydrophobic acidic tetrapeptides (360-390 mol wt)	Chemotactic attraction of eosinophils and neutrophils	Eosinophil and neutrophil deactivation	Aminopeptidase carboxypeptidase
Intermediate-molecular weight ECF	1500-3000 mol wt	Chemotactic attraction of eosinophils and neutrophils	Eosinophil deactivation	
High-molecular-weight neutrophilic chemotactic factor (NCF)	$\geq$ 750,000 mol wt	Chemotactic attraction of neutrophils	Neutrophil deactivation	
Heparin	Macromolecular acidic proteoglycan ($\sim$ 750,000 mol wt)	Antithrombin III activation; metachromasia	Anticoagulant; anticomplementary activity	
Chymase	25,000 mol wt	Hydrolysis of BTEE	Proteolysis	
N-Acetyl-β-glucosaminidase	Protein (150,000 mol wt)	Hydrolysis of N-acetyl-β-glucosamine paranitrophenyl substrate		
Arylsulfatase A	115,000 mol wt	Hydrolysis of p-nitrocatechol sulfate	Inactivation of SRS-A	
SECONDARY				
Slow reacting substance of anaphylaxis (SRS-A)	Acidic hydrophilic sulfate ester (400 mol wt)	Contraction of antihistamine-treated guinea pig ileum	Contraction of human bronchiole; increased vascular permeability	Arylsulfatases A and B
Platelet activating factors (PAFs)	Lipid-like ($\sim$ 300-500 mol wt)	Release of [^{14}C]5-HT from platelets	Aggregation	Phospholipase D
Lipid chemotactic factor	Lipid-like products of arachidonate metabolism	Chemotactic attraction of neutrophils	Neutrophilic deactivation	
Lipid chemokinetic factor	Lipid-like products of arachidonate metabolism	Chemokinetic attraction of neutrophils		

bronchomotor tone and mucosal edema could contribute to lowering the threshold of the irritant receptors to nonspecific stimuli, but it seems unlikely that histamine alone is sufficient. In fact, histamine may decrease mediator release from primary and perhaps secondary target cells through a feedback mechanism involving the stimulation of membrane-associated histamine-2 receptor sites linked to adenylate cyclases.

SRS-A appears to be a potent constrictor of human bronchial smooth muscle in vitro, and the intravenous administration of SRS-A to unanesthetized guinea pigs results in decreases in pulmonary compliance with minimal decreases in conductance. The effects on compliance are not blocked by atropine, and exposure of atropinized isolated smooth muscle strips to SRS-A results in potentiation of the histamine responses.

The actions of both histamine and SRS-A on the smooth muscle of the target tissues in lung may result in the secondary elaboration of prostaglandins, which in turn may have profound effects on bronchomotor tone, the pulmonary vasculature, and the primary effector cells. The constrictor effects of $PGF_{2\alpha}$ could interact significantly with those of histamine and SRS-A and so amplify the response. Prostaglandins are highly active as potentiators of the vascular permeability changes induced by histamine and bradykinin. Low concentrations of PGE_1 and especially $PGF_{2\alpha}$ are capable of decreasing cellular levels of cyclic AMP and enhancing the antigen-induced re-

lease of chemical mediators, thereby augmenting the effects of the initial reaction. Thus, the primary and/or secondary mediators could alter tissue levels of cyclic nucleotides so as to facilitate further mediator release, mediator action on target tissue, or both, thereby making the irritant receptors more responsive.

In bringing about their pathobiologic effects, many of the primary and secondary mediators recruit the participation of non-IgE-sensitized effector cells. The tetrapeptides of ECF-A, the intermediate molecular weight of eosinophilotactic factors, histamine, and the lipid chemotactic and chemokinetic principles all contribute to the accumulation of eosinophils at sites of mast cell activation. The marked overall heterogeneity in terms of size, charge, and hydrophobicity of the chemotactic factors released after mast cell activation may create multiple gradients to which the eosinophil could respond; such gradients could contribute to net movement by utilizing different cell receptors or by presenting different concentrations along the path of movement. In the asthmatic lung, eosinophils are prominent in the bronchial walls and in the tenacious mucous plugs filling the bronchial lumens. Indeed, Charcot-Leyden crystals appear to be formed from crystalloids of the granules of degenerated eosinophils. Although the eosinophil could contribute to the inflammatory response, the bulk of current evidence favors a dampening effect: the eosinophil is rich in phospholipase D which inactivates platelet-activating factors

(PAFs), histaminase which destroys histamine, and arylsulfatase B which is capable of inactivating SRS-A. Since many of these chemotactic factors have a secondary specificity for neutrophilic polymorphonuclear leukocytes but not monocytes, their action as well as that of high-molecular-weight neutrophilic chemotactic factors could also account for the presence of neutrophils. Finally, PAFs may cause the release of platelet factors such as serotonin and factor III into the reaction site with both smooth muscle and procoagulant effects.

It is tempting to speculate that the purpose of mast cell activation in terms of a physiologic role in host defense is to recruit plasma proteins, including immunoglobulins and complement, and phagocytic tissue (eosinophils) and peripheral (neutrophils) blood cells to the reaction site. Once specific antibody and complement, followed in hours by polymorphonuclear leukocytes, have arrived at the reaction site, the essential ingredients of the *humoral* and *cellular phases* of local host defense would be in place. The phagocytic cells would then engage in phagocytosis, which would be facilitated by their interaction with the humoral factors such as specific antibody or C3b on the target particles. Tissue damage at the reaction site, possibly in part by lysosomal enzymes released during phagocytosis or in response to chemotactic stimuli, might require a controlled degradation of damaged structural elements before repair with fibroblast proliferation, capillary regeneration, and connective tissue formation can occur. The mast cell might facilitate such a process by contributing arylsulfatases, N-acetyl-β-glucosaminidase, chymase, and less well characterized enzymatic activities such as β-glucuronidase, acid phosphatase, and collagenase. The concept of a biphasic host inflammatory response based upon the nature of the mast cell-derived mediators is entirely consistent with the IgE-mediated cutaneous reaction in the human, which presents an immediate edematous acellular phase followed in hours by an indurated inflammatory lesion with a profound cellular infiltrate. It is of interest that there can also be a biphasic pulmonary response to antigen challenge with a time course that is the same as that observed after the intracutaneous administration of such materials. The initial reaction consists of bronchoconstriction which quickly subsides, followed thereafter by a more intense reaction characterized by fever, dyspnea, and the recurrence of airway obstruction 6 to 8 h later.

The immunopharmacologic data thus suggest that chronic allergic bronchial asthma may be regarded as the superimposition of acute and subacute inflammatory events upon a base line of airway hyperirritability. Circumvention of the endogenous regulatory mechanisms of mast cell activation would supply an obvious trigger in allergic asthma, but this cell may also be involved in the pathobiologic response to nonimmunologic stimuli. For instance, cromolyn sodium, a rather selective inhibitor of mast cell activation, has no action on the airways and yet has a prophylactic action in preventing exercise-induced abnormalities in pulmonary function in asthmatics with or without a demonstrable allergic diathesis.

PATHOPHYSIOLOGY AND CLINICAL CORRELATES The pathophysiologic hallmark of asthma is a reduction in airway diameter brought about by contraction of smooth muscle, edema of the bronchial wall, and thick tenacious secretions. Although the relative contributions of each component to the patient's ventilatory impairment is unknown, the net result is an increase in airway resistance, decreased forced expiratory volumes and flow rates, hyperinflation of the lungs and thorax, increased work of breathing, changes in elastic recoil, abnormal distribution of both ventilation and pulmonary blood flow, mismatched ratios, and altered arterial blood gases. Thus although asthma is considered to be primarily a disease of airways, virtually all aspects of pulmonary function are compro-

mised during an acute attack. In addition, in very symptomatic patients there frequently is electrocardiographic evidence of right ventricular hypertrophy. Pulmonary hypertension can be found, and the patient may develop a paradoxical pulse. This sign, and that of the use of the accessory muscles of respiration, have been found to be extremely valuable in indicating the severity of the obstruction. In the presence of either, pulmonary function tends to be significantly more impaired than in its absence.

The other signs and symptoms of asthma imperfectly reflect the physiologic alterations that are present, so much so that if one relies upon the loss of subjective complaints, or even the sign of wheezing, as being the end point at which therapy for an acute attack should be terminated, an enormous reservoir of residual disease is missed.

Hypoxemia is a universal finding during acute exacerbations, but frank ventilatory failure is relatively uncommon. Most asthmatics who present for treatment have hypocarbia and a respiratory alkalosis. Statistically, the finding of normal arterial carbon dioxide tension tends to be associated with quite severe levels of obstruction, and consequently when found in a symptomatic individual, should be viewed as impending respiratory failure and treated as such. Usually, there are no clinical counterparts to the derangements in blood gases. Cyanosis is a very late sign. Thus, a dangerous level of hypoxia can go undetected. Likewise the signs which are attributable to carbon dioxide retention such as sweating, tachycardia, and wide pulse pressure do not tend to be of great value in predicting the presence of hypercapnia in individual patients, for they are too frequently seen in anxious patients with more moderate disease to be of much use. Consequently, trying to judge the state of an acutely ill patient's ventilatory status on clinical grounds alone can be extremely hazardous, and should not be relied upon with any confidence. Arterial blood gas tensions, therefore, must be measured.

The symptoms of asthma consist of a triad of dyspnea, cough, and wheezing, the latter often being regarded as the sine qua non. In its most typical form asthma is an episodic disease, and all three symptoms coexist. Attacks often occur at night, for reasons which are not clear but may relate to circadian variation in airway receptor threshold. Attacks may also abruptly follow exposure to a specific allergen, physical exertion, a viral respiratory infection, or emotional excitement. At the onset the patient experiences a sense of constriction in the chest, often with a nonproductive cough. Respiration becomes audibly harsh, and wheezing in both phases of respiration becomes prominent. Patients frequently have tachypnea, and expiration becomes prolonged. The lungs rapidly become overinflated, and the anterior-posterior diameter of the thorax increases. If the attack is severe or prolonged, the accessory muscles become visibly active. Termination of the episode is frequently marked by a cough producing thick stringy mucus which often takes the form of casts of the distal airways (Curschmann's spirals), and when examined microscopically often shows eosinophils and Charcot-Leyden crystals. In extreme situations, wheezing may markedly lessen or even disappear completely, cough may become extremely ineffective, and the patient may begin a gasping type of respiratory pattern. These findings imply extensive mucous plugging and impending suffocation. Ventilatory assistance by mechanical means may be required. Atelectasis due to inspissated secretions may occasionally occur with asthmatic attacks, but spontaneous pneumothorax and/or mediastinal emphysema are rare.

Less typically, a patient with asthma may complain of intermittent episodes of nonproductive cough or dyspnea only on exertion. Unlike other asthmatics when examined during their symptomatic periods, these patients tend to have normal breath sounds but will wheeze after repeated forced exhalations and will show dynamic ventilatory impairments when tested in the laboratory.

The differentiation of asthma from other diseases associated with dyspnea and wheezing is usually not difficult, particularly if the patient is seen during an acute episode. The physical findings and symptoms listed above, and the history of periodic attacks, are quite characteristic. A personal or family history of allergic diseases such as eczema, rhinitis, or urticaria is valuable contributory evidence. *Upper airway obstruction by tumor* or *laryngeal edema* can occasionally be confused with asthma. Typically, such a patient will present with stridor, and the harsh respiratory sounds can be localized to the area of the trachea. Diffuse wheezing throughout both lung fields is usually absent. However, differentiation can sometimes be difficult, and indirect laryngoscopy or bronchoscopy may be required.

Persistent wheezing localized to one area of the chest in association with paroxysms of cough indicates *endobronchial disease* such as foreign-body aspiration, neoplasms, or bronchial stenosis.

The signs and symptoms of *acute left ventricular failure* can occasionally mimic asthma, but the findings of moist basilar rales, gallop rhythms, blood-tinged sputum, and other signs of heart failure (Chap. 236) allow the appropriate diagnosis to be reached.

Recurrent episodes of bronchospasm can occur with *carcinoid tumors* (Chap. 106), *recurrent pulmonary emboli* (Chap. 266), and *chronic bronchitis* (Chap. 263). In the latter there are no true symptom-free periods in that one can usually obtain a history of chronic cough and sputum production as a background upon which acute attacks of wheezing are superimposed. Recurrent emboli, particularly in young women on oral contraceptives, are occasionally very difficult to separate from asthma. Frequently, these patients will present with episodes of breathlessness, particularly on exertion, and they can sometimes wheeze. Pulmonary function studies may show evidence of peripheral airway obstruction (Chap. 255), and when these changes are present, lung scans may also be abnormal. The therapeutic response to bronchodilators, discontinuation of the contraceptives, and institution of anticoagulant therapy may be helpful, but pulmonary angiography may be necessary in order to establish the correct diagnosis.

Eosinophilic pneumonias (Chap. 258) are often associated with asthmatic symptoms as are various chemical pneumonias and exposures to insecticides and cholinergic drugs. Bronchospasm can occasionally be a manifestation of *polyarteritis*.

LABORATORY FINDINGS It is difficult to establish the diagnosis of asthma in the laboratory, for no single test is conclusive. Positive wheal-and-flare reactions to skin tests can be demonstrated to various allergens, but that finding does not necessarily correlate with the intrapulmonary events. Sputum and blood eosinophilia are also helpful but are not specific for asthma. Chest roentgenograms showing hyperinflation are nondiagnostic, as are tests of pulmonary function. The latter, however, are quite useful in that one can measure the degree of obstruction present, document its reversible nature, and, when combined with provocational challenges, demonstrate the airway hyperirritability so characteristic of this disease. Furthermore, the performance of forced vital capacity maneuvers is very helpful in the evaluation of acute asthmatic attacks. A reduction in the 1-s forced expiratory volume to less than 25 percent of that predicted or to less than 750 ml with little or no

response following the administration of a bronchodilator indicates that the patient should receive very careful surveillance in conjunction with intensive treatment.

THERAPY Elimination of the causative agent(s) from the environment of an allergic asthmatic is the most successful means available of treating this condition (for details on avoidance see Chap. 65). Desensitization or immunotherapy with extracts of the suspected allergens has enjoyed widespread favor, but controlled studies are limited and have not proved it to be highly effective.

Drug treatment The drugs used in the treatment of asthma may be conveniently broken down into five major categories: methylxanthines, beta-adrenergic agonists, glucocorticoids, chromones, and anticholinergics. This array attests to the fact that the perfect agent has yet to be developed, and because there are few controlled trials that have conclusively demonstrated the superiority of one regimen over the other, specific recommendations for therapy are difficult to make. Thus, the treatment for a given patient is often determined empirically and is based on the overall severity and chronicity of the illness, and the response to the chosen intervention. Since the degree of relief of airway obstruction is frequently incomplete with the use of a single agent, multiple drug regimens are commonplace.

METHYLXANTHINES Theophylline is the only agent of this class used for its bronchodilating activity, and it is a competitive inhibitor of phosphodiesterase, an enzyme that inactivates cyclic adenosine monophosphate (AMP). The action of this drug is thought to be mediated by an increase in intracellular cyclic AMP levels, although this is still debated. The therapeutic plasma concentrations of theophylline lie between 10 and 20 μg/ml, but the dosage required to achieve this plasma level varies widely from patient to patient due to differences in the disposition of the drug. Therefore, therapy must be individualized. Theophylline half-lives are prolonged in liver disease, in the elderly, and in the presence of a high carbohydrate diet. They can be appreciably shortened in cigarette smokers.

In contrast to the large number of oral compounds, aminophylline is the only preparation available for intravenous use. The current recommendations are 5.6 mg per kilogram of body weight as a loading dose followed by one of three maintenance schedules: 0.9 (mg/kg)/h in young patients; 0.68 (mg/kg)/h in those over 50 years of age; and 0.45 (mg/kg)/h in patients with liver disease or congestive heart failure. In patients who have taken the drug sporadically, half the loading is used, and it is best to eliminate it completely if the patient was on a seemingly adequate oral regimen.

ADRENERGIC STIMULANTS This class of compounds consists of catecholamines, resorcinols, saligenins, and ephedrine, which have their effects through stimulation of alpha-, beta$_1$-, and beta$_2$-adrenergic receptors (Chap. 72). Only the beta agonists are useful in the treatment of asthma. They produce their physiologic effects by activating adenyl cyclase and through that elevate cellular levels of cyclic AMP. The perfect bronchodilator of this class would be one with pure beta$_2$ activity. It would dilate airways, but would not have the undesirable effects of cardiac stimulation.

The catecholamines are norepinephrine, epinephrine, isoproterenol, and isoetharine. Since norepinephrine is predominantly an alpha agonist, it is not employed to treat asthma. The other drugs are useful bronchodilators, but they are short acting and not effective by oral administration. Epinephrine is about equal in its alpha and beta effects. The usual dose is 0.3 to 0.5 ml of a 1:100 solution administered subcutaneously. Isoproterenol is devoid of alpha activity and is the most potent agent of this group. It is usually administered in a 1:200 solution by inhalation, but it has also been used by the intravenous route in the management of status asthmaticus. In these circumstances, extremely careful monitoring of heart rate, rhythm, and blood pressure is an absolute requirement; and this therapy is not recommended save for very dire emergencies. Isoetharine is the most beta$_2$-selective compound of this class, but is a relatively weak bronchodilator. It is employed as an aerosol and supplied as a 1% solution. Ephedrine is not a catecholamine but its action in large part is mediated by enhancing the release of endogenous sympathomimetics. It therefore has both alpha and beta activity, and its usefulness is further limited by the possibility of self-blockade of its catecholamine-releasing effects.

Manipulation of the catecholamine molecule gives rise to the resorcinols and saligenins. These alterations confer more beta$_2$ selectivity and give these compounds longer duration of action and make them suitable for oral administration. Resorcinols in widespread clinical use include metaproterenol and terbutaline, while salbutamol, a saligenin, is a highly selective beta$_2$ agonist available in most countries other than the United States. Oral terbutaline and salbutamol appear equipotent and more effective than metaproterenol. Both have durations of action in excess of 6 h. A frequent side effect of these drugs is tremor. Aerosols of these three agents provide almost as much bronchodilation as does isoproterenol but with much less cardiac stimulation. However, it should be noted that when terbutaline is given parenterally, its beta$_2$ selectivity diminishes, and it can produce a beta$_1$ effect similar to that seen with epinephrine.

GLUCOCORTICOIDS Glucocorticoids have been used for over 25 years in the treatment of asthma, but controversy still surrounds such basic issues as their specific indication and dose. Although it is difficult to provide precise recommendations because objective data are lacking, there are several situations in the management of acute and chronic asthma in which all would agree that steroids should be employed. In acute illness, this is when severe airway obstruction is not resolving, or is even worsening despite intense optimal bronchodilator therapy, and in chronic disease, steroids are most helpful when there has been failure of a previously optimum regimen with frequent recurrences of symptoms of progressive severity.

Although many dosage schedules have been proposed, few objective data on pulmonary function are available to support them. Those that are indicate that plasma cortisol levels above 100 μg per 100 ml may be required to produce an effect. In acute situations, this can be achieved by the intravenous administration of 4 mg per kilogram of body weight of hydrocortisone as a loading dose, followed several hours later by an infusion regulated to deliver 3 mg/kg every 6 h. It should be emphasized that the effects of steroids in acute asthma are not immediate and may not be seen for 6 h or more after their initial administration. Consequently, it is mandatory to continue vigorous bronchodilator therapy during this interval. After 24 to 72 h, depending upon response, the patient can be switched to oral agents. A usual starting point is 60 mg prednisone as a single daily A.M. dose. The amount can then be reduced by 5 mg every third or fourth day. In situations in which it appears that continued steroid therapy will be needed, an alternate-day schedule should be instituted to minimize side effects. This is particularly important in children, since continuous corticosteroid administration interrupts growth. Long-acting preparations such as dexamethasone should not be used in this approach for they defeat the purpose of alternate-day schedules by causing prolonged suppression of the pituitary-adrenal axis.

Recently, inhaled steroids of high topical potency have been introduced. Of the compounds studied, beclomethasone appears to combine maximum antiasthmatic effect with a minimum of systemic absorption. The usual dose is two puffs (100 μg) four times daily, but double this amount has been used without hyperadrenal corticism or adrenal suppression. The major side effect is symptomatic oropharyngeal candidiasis.

CHROMONES Cromolyn sodium is not a bronchodilator, but has its effect by inhibiting degranulation of mast cells, thereby preventing the release of the chemical mediators of anaphylaxis. The drug does not inhibit the combination of antigen with antibody, nor does it affect the fixation of IgE to mast cells. Cromolyn has been shown to be of use in atopic and nonatopic asthmatics, and it blunts exercise-induced asthma in both children and adults. Numerous trials have shown that about 75 percent of patients derive worthwhile benefits from the drug in terms of reduction of medications and improvement in symptoms. Therapy is best initiated between attacks or in periods of relative remission. If no response is noted by 4 to 6 weeks, the drug can be discontinued.

ANTICHOLINERGICS Anticholinergic drugs, such as atropine, are known to produce bronchodilatation in patients with asthma, but their use has been limited by systemic side effects. Recently, newer nonabsorbable aerosol agents have undergone extensive trials and have been found to be both effective and remarkably free of untoward effects. These agents, when available, may be of particular benefit in patients with asthma and coexistent heart disease, in whom use of methylxanthines and beta stimulants may be dangerous.

MISCELLANEOUS Opiates, sedatives, and tranquilizers should be absolutely avoided in the acutely ill asthmatic because the risk of depressing alveolar ventilation is great and respiratory arrest has been reported to occur shortly after their use. Admittedly most individuals are anxious and frightened, but experience has shown that they can be calmed equally well by the physician's presence and reassurances. Beta-adrenergic blockers and parasympathetic agonists should be avoided, or used with great caution, for they can cause marked deterioration in lung function.

Expectorants and mucolytic agents have enjoyed great vogue in the past, but there is little evidence available to indicate that they add significantly to the treatment of the acute or chronic phases of this disease. Mucolytic agents such as acetylcysteine may actually produce bronchospasm when administered to susceptible asthmatics. This can be overcome by aerosolizing them in solution with a beta-adrenergic agent. The use of intravenous fluids in the treatment of acute asthma has also been advocated. There is little evidence to indicate that this adjunct hastens recovery, but it may prevent dehydration and through that forestall the inspissation of secretions, by replacing the larger insensible water losses that could occur with prolonged hyperventilation.

PROGNOSIS AND CLINICAL COURSE Death from asthma is uncommon. Mortality statistics for the United States for the year 1973 reveal 1912 deaths from asthma at all ages. In the age group 5 to 34 years, the ages in which few other diseases are likely to be confused with asthma, there were 250 deaths, yielding a death rate of approximately 0.3 per 100,000 persons.

The available information on the clinical course of asthma suggests that somewhere between 50 to 80 percent of all patients can expect to have a reasonably good prognosis, particularly those whose disease develops in childhood. The number of children still having asthma 7 to 10 years after the initial diagnosis varies from 26 to 78 percent with an average of 46 percent; however, the percentage who continue to have severe disease is relatively low (6 to 19 percent). The natural course of asthma in adult life has been little investigated. Some studies suggest that spontaneous remissions occur in approximately 20 percent of those who develop the disease as adults and 40 percent or so can be expected to improve with less frequent and severe attacks as they grow older.

REFERENCES

AUSTEN KF: Reaction mechanisms in the release of mediators of immediate hypersensitivity from human lung tissue. Fed Proc 33(11):2256, 1974

————: Biologic implications of the structural and functional characteristics of the chemical mediators of immediate hypersensitivity, in *The Harvey Lectures.* New York, Academic Press (in press)

FELDMAN NT, MCFADDEN ER: Asthma: Therapy old and new. Med Clin North Am 61:1239, 1977

MCFADDEN ER, FELDMAN NT: Asthma: Pathophysiology and clinical correlates. Med Clin North Am 61:1229, 1977

———— et al: Acute bronchial asthma: Relations between clinical and physiological manifestations. N Engl J Med 288:221, 1973

SEGAL MS, WEISS EB (eds): *Asthma: Mechanisms and Therapeutics.* Boston, Little, Brown, 1976

258
HYPERSENSITIVITY PNEUMONITIS

DANIEL J. STECHSCHULTE
K. FRANK AUSTEN

Hypersensitivity disease of the lung encompasses a number of related clinical entities of diverse etiology, with suspected related immunopathogenic inflammatory reactions. *Allergic alveolitis, extrinsic allergic pneumonia, allergic interstitial pneumonitis,* and *hypersensitivity pneumonitis* are all terms which refer to the same clinical entity and which reflect an immunologic reaction at several locations within the lung. The respiratory illnesses induced by a recognized exposure to the spores of thermophilic actinomycetes, particularly *Micropolyspora faeni* or *Thermoactinomyces vulgaris,* are termed *farmer's lung, mushroom picker's lung,* and *bagassosis,* depending on the occupation of the individual. Inhalations of the spores of *Aspergillus clavatus* or *Cryptostroma corticale* induce malt worker's disease and maple bark disease, respectively. Exposure to antigens derived from pituitary snuff, avian proteins, fish meal, and fur also produce descriptively named hypersensitivity diseases of the lung (Table 258-1). When colonization of the respiratory passages with the fungus *Aspergillus fumigatus* occurs in atopic or asthmatic individuals, a unique clinical syndrome termed *allergic bronchopulmonary aspergillosis* is observed. Adverse reactions to repeated administration of a variety of drugs, such as nitrofurantoin, hydrochlorothiazide, and sulfonamides, can also produce an inflammatory reaction in the lung with features common to the other hypersensitivity pneumonitides. Autoimmune reactions in the lung known to occur in systemic lupus erythematosus and Goodpasture's syndrome are considered elsewhere (Chaps. 67 and 68). Byssinosis (Chap. 259) is a respiratory disease caused by the inhalation of a number of chemically active compounds, but is not considered a hypersensitivity disease of the lung because there is no evidence to implicate an immunologically mediated inflammatory reaction. Similarly, the interpretation of adverse reactions to toluene diisocyanate is complicated by the marked chemical reactivity of this agent with proteins and cell surfaces, a reaction which would favor toxic effects irrespective of an immune response.

This chapter will consider selected hypersensitivity pneumonitides due to (1) inhalation of antigen, with farmer's lung discussed as the prototype of extrinsic allergic alveolitis, (2) fungal colonization of the large airways with subsequent antigen production as observed in allergic bronchopulmonary aspergillosis, and (3) administration of drugs such as nitrofurantoin which also serve as antigen for an immunologically related inflammatory reaction in the lung.

The disease process has an acute and a chronic form and their separate clinical presentations can be recognized. The acute form of the disease presents with chills, fever, malaise, dyspnea, and cough within 2 to 8 h after inhalation exposure to the appropriate antigen. This form of the disease must be differentiated from pulmonary edema, pulmonary embolism, pneumonia, and reactions due to inhalation of chemical irritants such as cotton fiber extracts (byssinosis), sulfur dioxide, ammonia, and thiocyanates. The chronic form of the disease is manifested by the insidious onset of fatigue, progressive dyspnea, and a nonproductive cough. The differential diagnosis at this stage includes entities such as pneumoconiosis, diffuse idiopathic interstitial fibrosis of the lung, tuberculosis and chronic fungal infection, sarcoidosis, and, rarely, idiopathic pulmonary hemosiderosis.

EOSINOPHILIC PULMONARY REACTIONS

Although the hypersensitivity pneumonitides, in particular allergic bronchopulmonary aspergillosis, may qualify as "eosinophilic pneumonia," it is preferable to utilize an etiologic term whenever possible. The eosinophilic leukocyte is a multifunctional cell capable of responding to a chemotactic gradient with subsequent localization and of modulating local inflammation by inactivating inflammatory mediators, phagocytizing immune complexes, and releasing lysosomal enzymes. Two of its major constituents, major basic protein and Charcot-Leyden crystals, are not functionally defined. The identification of

TABLE 258-1
Inhalant hypersensitivity pneumonitides

Clinical syndrome	Suspected source of antigen
Farmer's lung	*Micropolyspora faeni*
Bird-fancier's lung	Pigeon, budgerigar, hen, and turkey droppings
Humidifier and air-conditioning pneumonitis	Thermophilic actinomycetes
Maple bark disease	*Cryptostroma corticale*
Mushroom picker's lung	*Micropolyspora faeni*
Malt worker's lung	*Aspergillus clavatus*
Furrier's lung	Epithelial components
Bagassosis (sugarcane fiber)	*Thermoactinomyces vulgaris*
Pituitary snuff lung	Porcine and bovine proteins
Detergent worker's lung	*Bacillus subtilus* enzyme
Fish meal lung	Fish proteins
Suberosis (oak bark)	*Micropolyspora faeni*
Sequoiosis	*Graphium* and *Auerobasidium*
Wood pulp worker's disease	*Alternaria*
Cheese worker's lung	*Penicillium*
Wheat weevil disease	*Sitophilus granarius*
Wood dust pneumonitis	Oak and mahogany dust
Vineyard sprayer's lung	Copper
New Guinea lung	*Streptomyces olivaceus*
Coffee worker's lung	?

antibody-directed as well as nonantibody C3b-dependent eosinophil cytotoxicity for certain helminths demonstrates an important host-defense role for this cell. Although the bulk of the evidence indicates a regulatory and protective role for the eosinophil, an excessive accumulation of degranulating cells may well present a capacity for tissue destruction. *Primary eosinophilic reactions of the lung* or *eosinophilic pneumonia* are terms used to designate pulmonary infiltrations of unknown cause associated with blood eosinophilia (PIE syndrome) and also eosinophilic infiltrations of the lung with or without an associated increase in the eosinophil count in peripheral blood. A variety of hypersensitivity, infectious, toxic, autoimmune, granulomatous, and malignant inflammatory reactions in the lung produce an eosinophilia by either common or unique mechanisms and are labeled *secondary eosinophilic reactions of the lung*. Pulmonary eosinophilia was recognized many years ago and subdivided by clinical criteria to include the following categories:

1 *Loeffler's syndrome,* consisting of transient migratory pulmonary infiltrations associated with minimal, if any, respiratory or systemic symptoms.
2 *Prolonged pulmonary eosinophilia,* in which the symptoms are more marked and persist for longer than 1 month.
3 *Pulmonary eosinophilia with asthma* (Chap. 257), the primary manifestations being related to reversible airway disease.
4 *Eosinophilia associated with parasitic infestations,* including inflammatory reactions in the lung during the pulmonary migration phase of parasitic infections such as *Ascaris lumbricoides, Necator americanus, Ancylostoma braziliense, Trichinella spiralis,* and *Strongyloides stercoralis;* filariasis (tropical eosinophilia) such as infection with *Wuchereria bancrofti* or *malayi;* and mite infestation of the respiratory tract.
5 *Polyarteritis nodosa* (Chap. 67), characterized by pulmonary symptoms and eosinophilia when the lung is involved with this disease.

It is now apparent that this classification included both primary and arbitrarily some of the secondary eosinophilic reactions of the lung. It is anticipated that the list of recognized diseases causing secondary eosinophilic pulmonary reactions will expand as specific causes are identified and will then be divided as the mechanisms for inducing tissue and blood eosinophilia are elucidated.

The histologic picture of the eosinophilic pulmonary reactions is characterized by filling of alveoli with a mixture of large mononuclear cells and eosinophils, edema, and eosinophilic infiltration of the connective tissue as well as infiltration by varying numbers of small mononuclear cells and plasma cells. Fibrinous exudates are common, and granulomatous reactions occur with varying degrees of frequency and organization. Mucus plugging of bronchi and bronchioles with secondary atelectasis is observed. Cellular infiltration occurs about veins and venules, but necrotizing angiitis with fibrinoid necrosis is absent except for periarteritis with pulmonary involvement.

Therapy is ideally directed at the cause of the pulmonary eosinophilic reaction and emphasizes the need to identify the underlying disease process. Primary eosinophilic pulmonary reactions such as Loeffler's syndrome are frequently self-limited and require no therapy. However, the recognition that granulomatous reactions and organization of lung tissue are common features of this disease suggests that irreversible changes can occur. Thus, corticosteroids are indicated when symptoms are severe or prolonged, and the use of these drugs is associated with a dramatic recovery in a significant number of patients.

The eosinophilic pulmonary reactions are distinct from the hypereosinophilic syndrome, which is characterized by a persistent and marked eosinophilia of the blood associated with a diffuse eosinophilic infiltration of the cardiovascular, pulmonary, hematopoietic, and nervous systems as well as other organs. Progressive tissue destruction is observed in some patients with the latter syndrome, and neither corticosteroids nor cytotoxic drugs consistently control this process.

FARMER'S LUNG

A common inhalant hypersensitivity pneumonitis is termed farmer's lung disease. It is a specific respiratory illness which results from the inhalation of airborne material generated from moldy hay or similar vegetable matter. Harvested wet hay provides the environment for the rapid growth of fungi and bacteria. With fermentation and the production of heat, thermophilic actinomycetes predominate, and this hay, when dry, reportedly can contain more than 10^9 actinomycete spores per gram. Approximately 90 percent of patients with this disease have detectable serum antibody against moldy hay or *Micropolyspora faeni* or *Thermoactinomyces vulgaris* extracts, and the major antigen is derived from the spores of *M. faeni.* An aerosolized extract of *M. faeni* delivered to the bronchial tree reproduces the disease state in patients with farmer's lung without causing symptoms in normal individuals. Only a limited number of subjects exposed to the same environment develop the disease even though the antibody is demonstrated in a significant number of exposed individuals without the disease. Preliminary studies suggest an association between the presence of certain HLA antigens and hypersensitivity pneumonitides. Such a linkage dysequilibrium in the population would be compatible with a genetic predisposition to the development of the immune response related to the disease. An atopic history is rare in patients with farmer's lung disease. Acute and chronic disease states are thought to be due to the quantity of antigen inhaled and to the duration of exposure. There is no evidence that the spores which induce this type of hypersensitivity pneumonitis colonize and proliferate within the tracheobroncial tree.

PATHOLOGY The inflammatory reaction in hypersensitivity pneumonitis is the result of repeated antigenic challenge to the periphery of the lung, the resultant systemic and local immune response being implicated in the pathogenesis of this disease. Soluble molecules deposited in the respiratory tract readily appear in the circulation. Therefore, the inflammatory roles of both local and systemic antibody production and the compartmentalization of reactive lymphocytes must be considered in this disease.

The histopathology of farmer's lung varies depending on the duration of time between antigen exposure and examination of the tissue. Descriptions of the pathologic process present within weeks after the exposure to antigen, or the onset of clinical symptoms are limited in number. Diffuse miliary nodules with minimal distention of intervening parenchymal tissue and minimal hilar node enlargement are noted macroscopically. The nodules consist of proliferating alveolar epithelial cells with a prominent number of lymphocytes, some plasma cells, and a few neutrophils and eosinophils. An increased number of reticular and fine collagen fibers are present. Large mononuclear cells resembling histiocytes, multinuclear giant cells, and Langhans' giant cells are seen in some lesions. The nodules presumably vary depending on their state of evolution. Intact alveoli have thickened walls and a mononuclear cell infiltration. An acute vasculitis primarily affecting alveolar capillaries and some small arterioles with platelet and fibrin deposition and neutrophil infiltration of the walls is observed. A centrilobular broncheolitis occurs with neutrophil and mononuclear cell infiltration along with an occasional multinuclear giant cell. Thus, there is histologic evidence of alveolitis, an interstitial reaction, bronchiolitis, and vasculitis, and therefore the term *hypersensitivity pneumonitis* appropriately describes this syndrome. The localization of antigen, antibody, or complement protein in the acute stage of the disease has not been adequately studied.

Histologically, tissue obtained from patients who are in the stable phase or the resolving phase of their disease is characterized by a granulomatous bronchiolitis obliterans. Polymorphonuclear cellular infiltration is not evident, while various degrees of interstitial fibrosis are present. Immunofluorescent studies of biopsy material are limited even at this stage but demonstrate the presence of antigen in bronchiolar walls, immunoglobulin associated with lymphocytes and plasma cells distributed through the lung, and C3 associated with histiocytes. The failure to demonstrate immune reactants within vessel walls is consistent with the absence of vasculitis in the chronic form of this disease.

The presence of circulating antibody in most cases of farmer's lung disease and the onset of symptoms 4 to 6 h after exposure to antigen is strong circumstantial evidence implicating immune-complex deposition in this and related diseases. Although antiglobulin and antinuclear antibodies have been demonstrated in farmer's lung disease, it is unlikely that they play a direct role in the disease state. Because circulating antibodies predominantly of the IgG class, but including the IgM and the IgA classes, can be detected at similar levels in symptomatic and asymptomatic farmers and in pigeon breeders, the pathogenetic role of immune complexes in hypersensitivity pneumonitis is unclear. It can be argued that local antibody production or local changes in venular permeability mediated by an IgE response or some toxic materials associated with the antigen characterize the symptomatic group. Alternatively, cell-mediated immunity may contribute, since the pathology has a granulomatous element and in vitro tests of cell-mediated hypersensitivity are more likely to be positive in symptomatic than in asymptomatic persons with pigeon breeder's disease. Indeed in a recent study of pigeon breeder's disease, bronchioalveolar wash cells elaborated a lymphokine (migration inhibitory factor) in vitro in response to pigeon products at a time when the peripheral blood lymphocytes were not reactive. After aerosol challenge the bronchioalveolar wash cells were rendered selectively unresponsive to the pigeon products but not to other antigens, whereas the peripheral blood lymphocytes now responded to pigeon products with production of the lymphokine. It seems likely that both local humoral and cell-mediated hypersensitivity responses to inhaled antigens are responsible for the pathobiologic response of hypersensitivity pneumonitis.

CLINICAL FEATURES Inhalation of an undetermined amount of antigen over a period of 6 to 10 weeks results in primary sensitization of the exposed population. The development of the disease state after reexposure to antigen depends upon unknown factors that exist in a limited number of sensitized individuals who are generally not atopic persons. Two forms of the disease are recognized: The acute form develops 4 to 6 h after exposure to antigen and consists of malaise, chills, fever, nausea, cough, and dyspnea without wheezing. Symptoms subside spontaneously over a period of hours to days. Physical examination may reveal cyanosis, tachypnea, tachycardia, and fine crepitant basilar rales without wheezing. Leukocytosis with a left shift is usual, while eosinophilia is rare. Oxygen desatura-

tion may occur with a normal or reduced P_{CO_2}. An elevation of the serum immunoglobulin level is common with detectable low-titer antiglobulin and antinuclear antibody. Precipitating antibody against the appropriate antigen is present usually in high titer, but this reflects exposure with immunization rather than being specific for the disease state. The chest roentgenogram is not diagnostic but usually demonstrates multiple small nodular densities uniformly distributed with some sparing of the apexes and bases. Hilar adenopathy and pleural reaction with effusion are uncommon. Pulmonary function studies characteristically show a reduction in diffusing capacity and pulmonary compliance; ventilatory and total lung capacities are not consistently affected, but a decrease in the forced vital capacity (FVC) and the 1-s forced expiratory volume (FEV_1) with little change in the FEV_1/FVC ratio can occur. These characteristic changes in lung mechanics can be predictably recognized 4 to 6 h after antigen exposure. In patients with an atopic disposition, IgE and IgG antibodies are produced after antigen inhalation. Challenge of these patients results in a two-stage reaction: an immediate typical asthmatic reaction with a decrease in the FEV_1 and expiratory flow rates without a change in the diffusing capacity, and a 4- to 6-h reaction indistinguishable from that seen in the nonatopic patient.

The chronic form of the disease is the result of repeated acute episodes or presumably continual or repeated antigen exposure without the initiation or recognition of constitutional manifestations. The insidious onset of disabling, frequently irreversible respiratory symptoms due to pulmonary fibrosis is characteristic of this form of the disease. The immunoglobulin abnormalities are minimal, and precipitating antibody is present in approximately 50 percent of the patients at titers lower than those seen in the acute form. The chest film demonstrates progressive fibrotic changes with less nodular densities. A decrease in lung volume with shrinkage of the upper lobes may occur. Function studies show diminished flow rates, decreased diffusing capacity, or features consistent with a combination of airway obstruction and interstitial disease; reduction in O_2 saturation is variable.

Skin testing in patients with farmer's lung has been performed with partially characterized extracts of moldy hay or *M. faeni*. An Arthus-type reaction occurs 4 to 6 h after the injection of antigen. An immediate-type wheal-and-flare reaction would be expected only in an atopic individual with hypersensitivity pneumonitis, and has been difficult to evaluate because of the local irritative effect of the extracts. Delayed tuberculin-type reactions have not been reported.

THERAPY The most important aspect of treatment is the avoidance of reinhalation of antigen. Cromolyn sodium will inhibit the 4- to 6-h delayed onset reaction and merits consideration as a prophylactic agent in this disease as an adjunct to avoidance. The administration of high dosages of a corticosteroid is indicated in the acute form of the disease, especially when it is associated with hypoxia. Patients with the acute form of the disease experience recovery with proper therapy, whereas the chronic form of the disease with fibrotic noninflammatory changes of the lung is apparently not reversible with currently available therapy. A brief course of steroids may nonetheless be justifiable to establish whether any aspect of the apparent chronic form of the disease is reversible.

OTHER INHALANT HYPERSENSITIVITY PNEUMONITIDES

The list of inhalant hypersensitivity pneumonitides is continually being expanded. The clinical syndromes, including both acute and chronic forms, are very similar to those described for farmer's lung. The terms used to identify these clinical syndromes, in general, describe the environmental settings which are conducive to the development of the disease state. The growth of a particular fungus such as thermophilic actinomycetes in humidifiers or air conditioners can lead to the continual exposure of individuals in either the home or office to fungus spores. Trees, such as the maple and redwood, and plants, such as sugarcane, commonly provide a medium for sufficient fungous growth so that workers involved with processing the bark or bagasse, respectively, are candidates for developing hypersensitivity pneumonitis. However, for reasons which are not clear, only a limited number of individuals subjected to environmental exposure with organic materials such as fish proteins, epithelial components, or fungus spores develop the clinical syndrome. The minor variations reported in the specific entities are thought to be due to antigen deposition in different areas of the lung as determined by particle size and to the existence of enzymes and nonspecific inflammatory factors along with antigen in some inhalants. In all the syndromes there is evidence of circulating precipitating antibody against the suspected antigen. The evidence in pigeon-fancier's disease, associated with circulating antibody to pigeon antigen, that the development of the disease state is related to the existence of sensitized lymphocytes requires further analysis and extension to the other hypersensitivity pneumonitides.

ALLERGIC BRONCHOPULMONARY ASPERGILLOSIS

Allergic bronchopulmonary aspergillosis is a form of hypersensitivity pneumonitis due to the production and release of antigen from a fungus infection with *Aspergillus fumigatus,* uniquely localized in the tracheobronchial secretions. Other species of *Aspergillus,* such as *A. flavus, A. nidulans, A. terreus,* and *A. clavatus,* may infect humans, but *A. fumigatus* is the most common. Bronchial asthma is the underlying prerequisite condition. Viable fungus spores can be recovered from respiratory secretions for at least 1 month after a heavy exposure of a normal individual, and it is assumed that the quantity and quality of tracheobronchial secretions of the asthmatic patient somehow permit fungal growth; alternately, the defect may be in phagocytic or other clearance mechanisms. The spores of other fungi also are inhaled but apparently have growth characteristics not suited to this environment. It is estimated that approximately 15 percent of the asthmatic population in Great Britain has allergic bronchopulmonary aspergillosis. The exact incidence of this disease in the United States is not known, but it is reported to occur in less than 10 percent of the asthmatic patients. Allergic bronchopulmonary penicilliosis and allergic bronchopulmonary pseudomoniosis are uncommon entities clinically similar to allergic bronchopulmonary aspergillosis but are caused by *Penicillium rubrum* and *Pseudomonas aeruginosa* infections, respectively.

PATHOLOGY The histologic picture of lung tissue obtained from patients with allergic bronchopulmonary aspergillosis is rarely reported but appears to have features of both hypersensitivity pneumonitis and bronchial asthma. The segmented bronchi are filled with a thick, tenacious mucus containing fibrin, Curschmann's spirals, Charcot-Leyden crystals, inflammatory cells, and varying numbers of fungus hyphae. The bronchial mucosa is intact but edematous with a prominent infiltration of lymphocytes, plasma cells, and eosinophils. A decreasing inflammatory reaction extends to the small bronchioles. Atelectasis occurs with thickening of the alveolar walls and epithelization of the alveoli. Parenchymal granulomas are seen surrounded by a mixed inflammatory exudate in which plasma cells and eosinophils are prominent. Multinucleated

giant cells and vasculitis involving the pulmonary veins can also be part of this picture. Immunofluorescent techniques have demonstrated the presence of IgG, IgM, IgA, and C3 in cells believed to be eosinophils. The periphery of the granulomas stain for IgG, and there is evidence that pulmonary venules contain immunoglobulin, antigen, and complement. Sufficient information is not yet available to permit definite recognition of the immunopathogenic mechanisms, but multiple pathways involving IgE antibody sensitization, immune-complex deposition, and possibly activated lymphocytes must be considered.

CLINICAL FEATURES The clinical picture of asthma, eosinophilia, recurrent pulmonary infiltrations with systemic symptoms, and the presence of *A. fumigatus* in respiratory secretions leads to a diagnosis of allergic bronchopulmonary aspergillosis. It occurs at any age in both sexes. Skin testing with an extract of *A. fumigatus* elicits a dual response characterized by an immediate wheal-and-flare reaction followed 4 to 6 h later by an erythematous indurated reaction. Marked elevation of serum IgE is noted without a consistent change in the other immunoglobulin levels. Serum precipitins to *A. fumigatus antigen* are present in all patients but are not specific for the disease state. Roentgenograms of the chest demonstrate transient pulmonary infiltrates and a pattern consistent with mucoid impaction, atelectasis, and deflation, with a predilection for the upper lobes. Bronchography reveals a localized saccular dilatation occurring proximally in the bronchial branches, at the sites of previous segmental pulmonary infiltration. The peripheral bronchi fill normally.

TREATMENT The management of these patients rests primarily upon the use of corticosteroids to decrease the excessive mucus production and inflammation that exists in the chronic asthmatic. A variety of antifungal agents has been utilized, but their efficacy for clearing *Aspergillus* has not been documented, and the overall prognosis is difficult to assess because of the dual pathology of this disease.

DRUG-INDUCED HYPERSENSITIVITY LUNG DISEASE

The lung is a recognized site for adverse drug reactions. A number of drugs, particularly basic amines, accumulate in lung tissue and may achieve a lung tissue/blood ratio of 100:1 or more. This may be a factor in the increasing number of drugs such as nitrofurantoin, penicillin, hydrochlorothiazide, para-aminosalicylic acid, hydralazine, chlorpropamide, sulfadimethoxine, mecamylamine, mephenesin, aurothioglucose, methotrexate, D-penicillamine, pyrethrum, and sulfasalazine, which have been implicated in pulmonary syndromes described as acute alveolar, chronic interstitial, or pleuropulmonary reactions. The clinical evidence linking a drug to the disease process is usually the development of the pulmonary reaction while the drug is being administered, reversal of the reaction with discontinuation of the medication, and the induction of the signs and symptoms in an asymptomatic individual with readministration of the drug in question. The pathogenic mechanisms are not understood and little histologic information is available. However, in a number of instances the lymphocytes of an affected individual have undergone transformation or produced macrophage-inhibiting factor (MIF) after in vitro incubation with the drug.

NITROFURANTOIN-INDUCED LUNG DISEASE Among the drug-induced reactions nitrofurantoin is the best documented and is implicated in both acute and chronic pulmonary reactions that are clinically similar to the acute and chronic inhalant hypersensitivity pneumonitides. The preliminary evidence suggesting that the alveolar involvement as compared with the bronchiolar is relatively greater in situations of systemic exposure as compared with aerosolized exposure may merely reflect the mechanisms of antigen distribution.

Clinical features The acute form of this disease may occur within several hours to days after the administration of the drug. Symptoms include cough, fever, dyspnea, and malaise. Examination reveals bibasilar rales and occasionally a nonspecific rash. A leukocytosis with prominent eosinophilia is a common, but not consistent, finding. Antiglobulin and antinuclear antibodies have been observed. Chest roentgenograms are characterized by reticulonodular basilar densities with pleural fluid seen on occasion. The clinical syndrome subsides within a few days after discontinuation of the drug.

The chronic form of this disease has no distinctive features and occurs within months to years after the onset of drug therapy. Dyspnea is the usual complaint. Roentgenograms of the chest reveal a nonspecific pattern consistent with a diffuse bilateral interstitial infiltrate most prominent in the bases. Pleural effusion and eosinophilia are rare. Pulmonary function studies demonstrate a pattern of restrictive lung disease with impaired diffusing capacity. Transbronchoscopic biopsy material demonstrates a chronic interstitial pneumonitis with fibrosis. The reversibility of the disease is minimal if extensive fibrosis exists. Antibody specific for nitrofurantoin has not been demonstrated in either the acute or the chronic form of the disease; however, in vitro lymphocyte stimulation with mitogenesis and MIF production with this drug has been reported in both forms. As pathologic studies with immunofluorescence are lacking, the mechanism of tissue injury requires further definition.

Treatment The management of all drug-induced pulmonary reactions rests upon the discontinuation of the medication. The acute form of nitrofurantoin lung disease is self-limiting if the drug is discontinued. With severe reactions intravenous corticosteroids and general supportive measures are indicated. The chronic form of the disease with fibrosis and impaired diffusing capacity warrants a limited trial of corticosteroids because the degree of reversibility cannot be anticipated.

REFERENCES

CHAN-YEUNG M et al: Allergic bronchopulmonary aspergillosis: Clinical and pathological study of three cases. Chest 59:33, 1971

CHUSID MJ et al: The hypereosinophilic syndrome. Medicine 54:1, 1975

HOPKE EJ et al: Farmer's lung: A clinical, radiographic, functional and serological correlation of acute and chronic stages. Thorax 23:451, 1968

LIEBOW AA, CARRINGTON CB: The eosinophilic pneumonias. Medicine 48:251, 1969

PEARSALL HR et al: Nitrofurantoin lung sensitivity: Report of a case with prolonged nitrofurantoin lymphocyte sensitivity and interaction of nitrofurantoin-stimulated lymphocytes with alveolar cells. J Lab Clin Med 83:728, 1974

PEPYS J: Hypersensitivity diseases of the lung due to fungi and organic dusts, in *Monograph in Allergy,* vol 4. New York, Karger, 1969

REEDER WH, GOODRICH BE: Pulmonary infiltration with eosinophilia (PIE syndrome). Ann Intern Med 36:1217, 1952

ROBERTS RC, MOORE VL: Immunopathogenesis of hypersensitivity pneumonitis. Am Rev Resp Dis 116:1075, 1977

ROSENOW EC III: The spectrum of drug induced pulmonary disease. Ann Intern Med 77:977, 1972

SCHATZ M et al: Immunopathogenesis of hypersensitivity pneumonitis. J Allergy Clin Immunol 60:27, 1977

SCHLUETER DP: Response of the lung to inhaled antigens. Am J Med 57:476, 1974

SCHUYLER MR et al: Local pulmonary immunity in pigeon breeder's disease: A case study. Ann Intern Med 88:355, 1978

259
ENVIRONMENTAL LUNG DISEASE

AREND BOUHUYS
J. BERNARD L. GEE

The airways and lungs provide an 80-m² surface area for deposition, absorption, and biological action of many inhaled materials besides oxygen: allergens, virus, bacteria, smoke, toxic gases, and dusts. These inhalants interact with physiological mechanisms in the host tissue; they may also elicit unphysiological tissue responses. The clinical manifestations of these interactions—environmental lung disease—are often but the end stage of a protracted process, which begins with subtle physiological changes and advances to severe tissue damage, disability, and death.

Many lung diseases could be prevented if we breathed pure air at all times. Hence, control of the environment—outdoors, in work places, and in homes—is a straightforward way to prevent environmental lung disease. In terms of number of people affected, cigarette smoke is the most critical air pollutant (Chap. 219). However, exposures to industrial agents that cause lung disease are also widespread and cannot be controlled by the individual. For example, in a survey of some 800 establishments in the Chicago area, dust hazards were found in 20 percent of the plants visited. Since it is unlikely that environmental control alone can abolish all instances of environmental lung disease, it is important to identify host factors which increase or decrease risks. In the future, identification of host factors might, for example, assist in the selection of workers at minimum risk of developing disease despite some remaining industrial exposure. Before considering specific exposures, classified according to pathologic and physiologic criteria, some general principles of pulmonary transport require discussion.

TRANSPORT OF MATTER

VAPORS AND GASES A volatile substance can be absorbed from inspired air at a maximum rate equal to the product of its concentration and the alveolar ventilation. The quantity absorbed depends on its solubility in body tissues and fluids; the toxic effects depend, in addition, on its rates of excretion and metabolism. Effects of irritant gases on upper airways are common with highly soluble gases such as NH_3 and SO_2, which dissolve immediately in the mucus of the nose and throat, while only minimal amounts reach lower airways. Less soluble gases, such as Cl_2 and phosgene, are not as readily removed by the scrubbing action in the upper airways and can therefore elicit violent responses in the peripheral airways and pulmonary parenchyma.

AEROSOLS An aerosol is a suspension of liquid or solid particles in air. When inhaled, some particles are deposited in the airways and lungs, depending on their size, weight, shape, and especially their settling velocity. Large particles (> 10 μm in diameter) tend to impact or settle in the nose and upper airways, while very small particles (< 0.1 μm in diameter) may behave like very large molecules; if retained at all, they are deposited in small airways and alveoli. Particles of intermediate size tend to settle by gravity (sedimentation). Many aerosols of medical interest consist of particles in this intermediate size range (0.1 to 10 μm in diameter), for which it is difficult to define a precise pattern of deposition.

Most "natural" aerosols contain particles with a wide range of sizes; with liquid aerosols, a relatively small number of large particles contain more than 90 percent of the toxic or therapeutic substance. Thus, the effects depend primarily upon the site of deposition of the large particles, not on that of the much more numerous small particles, which account for only a small fraction of the total aerosol mass. For instance, bronchodilator aerosols with a few large droplets may deposit most of the drug in the upper airways, where they have no useful action, while systemic absorption from this site may cause undesirable side effects. Predominant deposition in smaller airways is obtained with aerosols of a more restricted size range, e.g., 0.5 to 5 μm in diameter. The deposition pattern of aerosols of solid particles (dusts) is more complex than that of liquid droplets, because it depends not only on their size but also on their shape and specific gravity; e.g., long, thin, straight fibers, such as asbestos, may penetrate to much smaller airways than round particles of equivalent mass.

ASPIRATION Solid food or fluids, including saliva, may be aspirated into the lungs in states of disturbed consciousness, in debilitating diseases, disorders of deglutition, obstructing lesions of the esophagus, after local anesthesia of the pharynx, and in drowning. Emulsions and oils may be aspirated even in the absence of overt disturbances of deglutition, particularly following their intranasal instillation, or in older persons who frequently ingest laxative mineral oils. Small amounts of such materials may coat the pharyngeal mucosa and may be aspirated without evoking a cough reflex.

MUCOCILIARY CLEARANCE Normally, small particles entering the bronchial tree are engulfed in a layer of mucus produced by bronchial glands and goblet cells. The respiratory cilia move this layer toward the pharynx, where it is swallowed. Since goblet cells are virtually absent from bronchioles, mucociliary clearance is probably only effective in airways larger than these. In smaller airways, phagocytes provide the most important clearance mechanism; these cells probably reach "the first rung of the mucociliary ladder" by their own motility.

The amount and regulation of normal mucus production are unknown; in experiments with animals, vagal stimulation increases mucus production in the tracheobronchial tree, while atropine decreases it. Mucus is not homogeneous and has elastic, plastic, and viscous properties. Two layers of mucus cover the airways—a watery layer, the sol phase, in which the cilia beat, and, superficial to that, a more viscous layer, the gel phase, which moves toward the pharynx. In addition to its important role in the removal of particulate matter from the lungs, mucus also has an antibacterial function, provided by secretory antibodies and lysozyme.

PHAGOCYTOSIS The two principal phagocytes in the lung are the leukocyte and the alveolar macrophage, both of which are mobilized in response to inhaled particles and vapors. Leukocytes respond vigorously to acute, high-intensity challenges and to the chemotaxis of inflammatory responses. Alveolar macrophages are mobilized in response to the more chronic application of less intense stimuli and to agents which evoke little acute inflammation, such as fibrogenic dusts and carbon, as well as in delayed hypersensitivity responses. Once ingested, particles are subjected to biochemical events within the cell. Lysosomal hydrolases may degrade inhaled organic materials and, together with the release of oxidizing free radicals, exert both a defensive antimicrobial action and a tissue-injuring effect, notably on endothelial cells. Other ingested materials injure the phagocytes and may kill them. Silica injures lysosomal membranes, and the release of lysosomal enzymes within the cell then initiates autodigestion. Yet other agents, including oxides of nitrogen and ozone, impair the ingestion of particles and modify the actions of lysosomal hydrolases. Alveolar macrophages obtained from the lungs of cigarette smokers show increases in glucose oxidation, in the activity of lysosomal hydrolases, and in the secretion of lysozyme, but the phagocytic competence of such cells does not seem to be impaired. Cell surface and membrane events may be of critical importance in determining particle ingestion. The lysosomal enzymes of the phagocytic cells usually exert important defensive actions, but the release of these enzymes, particularly the neutral proteinases (e.g., collagenase and elastase), may also lead to lung injury and inflammation.

Following ingestion of the particles, some phagocytes remain viable, migrate to lymphatics, and are trapped in regional lymph nodes, where they deposit the ingested material. Cells that die soon after particle ingestion, on the other hand, may either disintegrate locally or be removed via the mucociliary ladder.

GENERAL RESPONSES TO INHALED MATERIALS

PROTECTIVE REFLEXES Irritant gases cause subjective sensations such as unpleasant odor or throat irritation, which in turn elicit behavioral responses designed to avoid further exposure. In addition, reflex responses may lead to sneezing, glottal closure, apnea, or rapid shallow breathing, cough, and constriction of lower airways. Some of these responses can help to limit absorption or remove inhaled matter. The reflex responses also serve as warning signals to the patient to minimize exposure; noxious gases, such as phosgene, that do not elicit these reflexes can cause grave lung injury.

MUCUS PRODUCTION This is increased acutely by SO_2 and other irritant gases in high concentration, and chronically by cigarette smoke. An increase in mucus production occurs in the early years of smoking and results in hypertrophy of bronchial glands and an increase in goblet cells. Since mucus production often decreases when cigarette smoking is discontinued, it appears that the changes in the mucous glands are at least partially reversible.

PULMONARY EDEMA This is a prominent feature of the response to "deep-lung irritants" such as phosgene. The predominant symptom is dyspnea, followed by cyanosis and other signs of asphyxia (Chap. 27).

AIRWAY CONSTRICTION Airway caliber may decrease because of mucosal swelling, mucus accumulation, deposition of foreign matter, or contraction of smooth muscle. The latter occurs in many instances in response to allergens in asthma and to some toxic dusts. This response is mediated by locally released substances (Chap. 257). Reflex airway constriction can be induced by stimulation of the upper airway, larynx, or trachea with mechanical stimuli or irritant gases. This is usually a short-lived response.

EMPHYSEMA Epidemiologic data show an association of emphysema with cigarette smoking and certain occupational exposures. Loss of elastic recoil in the lung may occur in workers with enzyme detergents and textiles, suggesting structural damage of the kind found in emphysema (Chap. 263).

PARENCHYMAL RESPONSES The cellular reactions in environmental lung diseases include (1) acute necrotizing and inflammatory responses induced by chemicals; (2) edema and inflammatory responses with leukocyte mobilization induced by organic antigens (extrinsic allergic alveolitis, see Chap. 258); (3) formation of granulomas, as in beryllium exposure; (4) mobilization of macrophages after exposure to dusts; (5) pleomorphic cellular responses following exposure to asbestos and hard metals; and (6) fibrosis, a late reaction to many of the above.

Three forms of fibrosis occur: (1) diffuse interstitial, (2) focal or nodular, and (3) progressive massive fibrosis (PMF). These are progressively disabling conditions which restrict lung volumes and decrease gas transport and pulmonary compliance. Their early stages may include destruction of the alveolar basement membrane and release of lysosomal enzymes from macrophages. Injury to the alveolar basement membrane may be critical since this membrane serves a cytoarchitectural function providing a skeleton upon which other cells are organized. Much of the functional consequences of pulmonary fibrosis appear to depend on disorganized healing rather than a large net increase in collagen deposition. Indestructible particles, such as asbestos and silica, may recycle through macrophages and cause sustained low-grade inflammation. Collagen formation may depend on reactions to such inflammation or to products of autolyzed macrophages. These mechanisms do not explain the distribution of fibrous tissue, which, for example, is diffuse in asbestosis and nodular in silicosis. Instead, this distribution may result from different patterns of deposition, which in turn are a function of the size and shape of particles.

The fibrogenic properties of dusts vary. In some instances (e.g., siderosis) they depend on the varying silica contents of the inhaled material. The cause of PMF in patients with silicosis and coal worker's pneumoconiosis is unknown; it is manifested by confluent opacities on the chest roentgenogram of patients who usually have severe dyspnea, and it may progress to respiratory insufficiency. Tuberculous infection is not a prerequisite for its development. PMF lesions may develop cavities, perhaps from ischemic necrosis, and these lesions account for about 25 percent of all fatal cases of coal worker's pneumoconiosis.

COMBINED EXPOSURES Exposures to more than one agent are common and may result in independent or additive effects, or interactions between multiple agents may occur. The high risk of lung cancer in asbestos workers who smoke is one example of interaction. Since many workers exposed to occupational inhalants also smoke, assessing the relative risk of each agent requires that nonsmokers as well as smokers be studied.

Smoking and occupational exposure to irritant gases or dusts are common features of the history of patients with chronic bronchitis, emphysema, and other chronic obstructive lung diseases (Chap. 263). The terminal stages of these diseases include widespread obstruction of the small airways and ventilatory failure, but their early stages and natural history may differ considerably. For instance, patients with chronic airway obstruction may have cystic fibrosis, α_1-antitrypsin deficiency, or an occupational disease such as byssinosis. The majority of patients with chronic airway obstruction probably have some environmental injury (including cigarette smoking) to the lungs and airways.

HOST VARIABILITY Some individuals respond to environmental toxic agents that do not harm others. Such individual differences may result from atopy (Chap. 257), acquired sensitization, a normal distribution of sensitivities, or a bimodal distribution, with distinct groups of "reactors" and "nonreactors" in the population at risk. Among textile workers there are reactors who develop byssinosis and nonreactors who do not, a difference which is not acquired by sensitization. The autonomic innervation of airways may play a role in determining reactor status. Thus, a nonreactor to textile dust can temporarily be converted to a reactor by the blockade of beta-adrenergic receptors with propranolol (Chap. 72), while parasympathetic blockade with atropine renders a reactor temporarily insensitive. Propranolol also enhances the airway constrictor effect of cigarette smoke. Interaction between neural and humoral endogenous stimuli with environmental factors in airway smooth muscle may be an important determinant of individual sensitivity. Temporal variations in sensitivity include those induced by drugs (e.g., atropine, adrenergic agonists and antagonists, antihistamines), tachyphylaxis (temporary desensitization after exposure), the efficacy of the various protective mechanisms, and the state of the effector organ (e.g., normal versus constricted airways).

DIAGNOSTIC METHODS

HISTORY AND PHYSICAL EXAMINATION A detailed environmental and occupational history is usually the key to the diagnosis of environmental lung diseases (Chap. 254). It should include a complete, quantitative record of past and present smoking habits, residences since birth, and all jobs held since leaving school.

Respiratory symptoms may be effectively analyzed with a standard questionnaire. Inquiries must be made about exposures to irritant gases, fumes, dusts, and vapors at work or in hobbies. The nature of the work, characteristics of the workplace, and type of materials handled are more important than the title of the position. For example, an electrician may be exposed to silica in a foundry, to asbestos in construction work, or to cotton dust in a textile mill. A mesothelioma in an executive, diagnosed in 1980, may be due to exposure to asbestos during 2 years of work in a shipyard in World War II.

Exposures at home may include dust, smoke, paints, and solvents. Exposure to noxious agents occurs not only in modern industry but also in primitive societies. For example, the grinding of corn between siliceous stones indoors is a cause of silicosis in Africa, while the batting and hackling of flax or soft hemp fibers may cause disabling byssinosis.

IDENTIFICATION OF INHALED MATERIAL This may be less crucial for diagnosis than may appear at first sight. For instance, the presence of asbestos bodies in the sputum merely confirms that exposure has taken place, not that asbestos-induced disease is present. Similarly, the finding of free silica in tissue obtained by means of lung biopsy confirms that exposure has occurred but does not indicate the extent of the disease. Environmental monitoring of the workplace provides a simpler confirmation of exposure, without risk to the worker. Lung biopsy is rarely required to diagnose environmental lung disease, and in many instances the findings are nonspecific.

CHEST ROENTGENOGRAPHY Together with a history of exposure, the chest roentgenogram provides important information, in particular, in patients with silicosis and other mineral dust diseases. However, even with standardized methods of interpretation, observer error is large, especially when lesions are small, diffuse, and relatively translucent. Nevertheless, the chest x-ray offers a crude guide to dust exposure as long as one deals with a single type of dust. Thus, in large groups of coal miners, roentgenographic changes during life correlate with lung dust content at autopsy. But, similar amounts of different minerals may cause dissimilar x-ray shadows if their atomic weights differ. For example, heavy but innocuous tin oxide causes prominent x-ray changes but little tissue damage. In coal workers' pneumoconiosis, x-ray lesions may be minimal in spite of the presence of disabling chronic bronchitis, not visible on the roentgenogram. Thus, in many instances, the proper assessment of patients with environmental lung disease is functional, not radiological.

LUNG FUNCTION AND DISABILITY Sensitive tests are needed to detect early stages of lung disease; maximum expiratory flow-volume (MEFV) curves are useful for this purpose (Fig. 259-1). They offer several advantages: (1) VC (vital capacity) and FEV_1 (forced expiratory volume in 1 s) data are available (Chap. 255); (2) specific curve patterns are of diagnostic value; and (3) the portion of the MEFV curve which is independent of the patient's effort can be used to measure flow rates at small lung volumes. The latter are often reduced when other indexes of obstruction (e.g., FEV_1/VC) are still normal, e.g., in patients with asymptomatic asthma or in young cigarette smokers.

Restrictive lung function loss (Chaps. 255 and 264) occurs in environmental lung diseases with extensive fibrosis. The airways are not obstructed, and elastic recoil may be increased. Hence, expiratory flow rates are high, with an FEV_1/VC ratio approaching 1. The reduced VC and the high flow rates produce a typical MEFV curve pattern (Fig. 259-1A). In *obstructive lung function loss,* in which there is expiratory obstruction to airflow, forced expiratory flow rates are reduced, but VC may be normal. Flow reduction is usually most pronounced at low lung volumes, since the caliber of airways decreases with lung volume. This results in another typical configuration of the MEFV curve, with a curvature opposite in direction from that in restrictive function loss (Fig. 259-1A). The sensitivity of flow measurements on MEFV curves, at small volumes, is illustrated by an example taken from a study on teen-aged smokers (Fig. 259-1B). In that instance, maximum flows at 50 percent VC discriminated much better between smokers and nonsmokers than did the FEV_1. Among tests of gas exchange, the single-breath diffusing capacity for carbon monoxide (Chap. 255) is suitable for epidemiologic work on interstitial lung disease of occupational origin.

Airway obstruction and restrictive function loss are relatively simple to detect when overt clinical disease is present. In epidemiologic studies, however, it is important to detect lesser degrees of function loss related to environmental exposures. One may compare groups at risk with control groups; however, many variables (sex, race, age, height, weight, and smoking habits) must be taken into account in such comparisons. Hence, large numbers of persons with and without exposure need to be studied. Recent data on more than 3000 healthy black and white children and adults, nearly all lifetime nonsmokers, allow improved assessment of lung function in smokers and others at risk of environmental exposure (Fig. 259-1).

The clinician must often decide whether a certain degree of lung function loss provides a basis for disability. The Social Security Administration assumes total disability when the FEV_1 is less than 1.1 to 1.5 liters, depending on body height. Such patients are usually short of breath during minimal exertion. Persons whose jobs require physical exertion may be disabled, even though their FEV_1 is above these limits. Objective criteria for decreased work performance in lung disease are as yet unsatisfactory. Many persons with restrictive function loss or airways obstruction reach the limit of their exercise tolerance because of their limited ventilatory capacity. This can be

shown by comparing ventilation during exercise with maximum ventilatory performance (Fig. 259-2). In severe lung disease, an abnormally low arterial O_2 tension, if it occurs at rest or during light exercise, is an indicator of clinical disability.

ACUTE SPECIFIC EXPOSURES

CHEMICAL INFLAMMATION Many agents listed in Table 259-1 produce acute inflammation of mucous membranes (conjunctiva, nose, pharynx, larynx, and lower airways) and pulmonary edema. The more irritant chemicals (acid mists and ammonia) produce severe, immediate reactions, with intense

FIGURE 259-1

Maximum expiratory flow-volume (MEFV) curves. Ordinate shows flow in liters per second. Curves indicate maximum expiratory flow produced during forced expiration from total lung capacity. A. Abscissa shows lung volume in absolute values (thoracic gas volume). 1 = volume expired in 1 s (FEV_1). Solid line = normal. Long dashes = obstructive. Short dashes = restrictive. On the abscissa, total lung capacity is indicated by the dots at 5 and 8, residual volume by the circles at 1 and 2. The abscissa in B and C shows lung volume as percent of vital capacity (VC). X = maximum flow at 50 percent VC (MEF 50%). B. Solid line = nonsmoking teenager. Dashed line = smoking teenager. C. Textile worker before (solid line) and after (dashed line) 4 h of dust exposure. VC, FEV_1, MEF 50% depend in complex fashion on sex, race, age, body height, and body weight. Prediction equations and lower 95 percent confidence limits for healthy black and white men, women and children (age 7+; 2968 lifetime nonsmokers, 78 healthy smokers) are available (Schoenberg et al.).

A

B

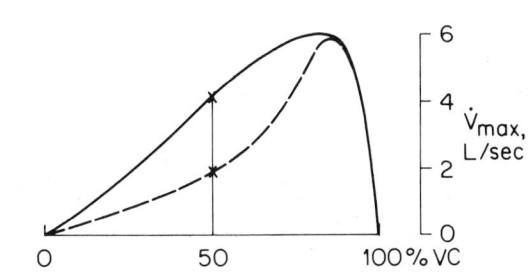

C

lacrimation, sore throat, and reflex cough. Other chemicals (oxides of nitrogen, chlorine, phosgene, and cadmium fumes) provoke less noxious effects immediately, and prolonged exposure may occur; since inflammation of lower airways and pulmonary edema may take several hours to develop, 24-h observation is indicated after exposure to these fumes. Clinical features following such exposure include cough, expectoration, chest tightness, cyanosis, and dyspnea, with rhonchi, diffuse rales, or both. Roentgenographic change may be minimal despite the presence of severe arterial desaturation; usually, however, pulmonary edema, an alveolar filling process, or an increase in interstitial markings is present on the roentgenogram. Arterial oxygen saturation is often low because of intrapulmonary shunting of blood. Treatment includes administration of oxygen to raise arterial P_{O_2} to between 50 and 60 mmHg; tracheostomy may be needed if laryngeal edema is present. Steroids may help to diminish the inflammatory response; the need for preventive use of antibiotics is arguable.

Similar but less acute responses occur in workers in polymerization processes such as the production of rubber and plastic, including polyurethanes. The specific chemicals involved have not been precisely identified, but diisocyanates, aromatic amines, and aldehydes may be involved. Continued exposure leads to chronic cough, mucus expectoration, and minor hemoptysis, sometimes with low-grade fever and malaise, initially worse at the beginning of the work week but more persistent later. FEV_1 and pulmonary diffusing capacity are reduced, and moderate arterial hypoxemia may be present;

TABLE 259-1
Acute chemical reactions

Agents	Industries
Ammonia	Chemical, refrigeration, coal distillation, fertilizers, explosives, tires
Nitrogen dioxide	Silage, metal etching, explosives, rocket fuels, welding
Acid fumes, HF, HCl, H_2SO_4, HNO_3	Chemical, steel, metal, bleaching, glass and metal etching, tires
Halides (Cl, Br, F)	Chemical, bleaching
Metal fumes, As_2O_3, Cd oxide, Hg, Ni, Zn, Mn, Cu, Co, Be, V, Al_2O_3	Metal industry, brass and zinc foundries, galvanizing, chrome plating, welding, metal grinding
Phosgene	Munitions, welding (chlorinated solvent)
Osmium tetroxide	Electron microscopy
Paraquat	Agriculture
Polymerizing chemicals, amine accelerator and hardeners, epoxy resins, isocyanates	Rubber, plastics, resins, electron microscopy, polyurethane foam rubber, tires
Plastics, polymers, Teflon, polyethylene	Machining and manufacture of plastics

partially reversible airway obstruction also occurs. The chest roentgenograms may show minor patchy and soft opacities. Most patients recover in a few weeks after termination of exposure, but residual disability and permanent lung damage may occur.

Exposure to oxides of nitrogen, as may occur in silo-filler's disease, may lead to progressive *bronchiolitis obliterans*, with disabling dyspnea due to closure and narrowing of peripheral airways and restrictive function loss. However, febrile reactions some weeks after silage exposure are probably cases of *farmer's lung* (Chap. 258), rather than of silo-filler's disease. Another hazard in agriculture is ingestion of paraquat, a herbicide which causes severe, often fatal, pulmonary edema and lung tissue damage. Like some other pollutants (e.g., ozone), it acts through formation of free radicals with oxidant action.

Metal fumes (Table 259-1) and products of combustion of polymers, notably Teflon, cause *metal fumes fever*, characterized by febrile reactions, shaking chills, diaphoresis, malaise, and leukocytosis. Pulmonary symptoms and signs may be sparse. Chest roentgenograms are usually normal, and the conditions appear to be benign, may pass for a viral syndrome, and usually last for 24 to 48 h. Some metals, in particular cadmium, cause severe chemical inflammation as well as fever. Acute *cadmium pneumonitis* is easily misdiagnosed as acute infection; since steroid therapy may be lifesaving in these cases, recognition of the exposure is imperative. A similar syndrome has been observed after severe acute exposures to *beryllium* and its salts.

Deaths in fires usually result from CO inhalation, thermal injury, or lack of oxygen. "Acute smoke inhalation" during fires may include effects of chemicals formed during combustion: ammonia, hydrochloric acid, sulfur dioxide, isocyanates (from plastics), hydrogen cyanide (paper, wool, silk, synthetics), or nitrogen dioxide. The latter, from burning nitrocellulose x-ray film, was largely responsible for 123 deaths in the 1929 Cleveland Clinic fire. The clinician must be alert for delayed pulmonary reactions (24 to 72 h) in fire victims; bronchiolitis obliterans with permanent loss of lung function occurs occasionally. Apart from a recurring risk of these acute episodes, fire fighters do not appear to sustain permanent lung injury from repeated lesser exposures to combustion products.

Allergic alveolitis (see also Chap. 258)   Many forms of allergic alveolitis need to be distinguished from the chemical pneumonias discussed above. The clinical picture does not always give

FIGURE 259-2

Expiratory flow volume curves. Dotted line = tidal expiration (V_T) at rest. Dashed line = V_T during moderate exercise. Solid line = V_T during heavy exercise. All expiratory flow volume loops are drawn within contours of MEFV curves in a healthy person (A) and in two patients with moderate (B) and severe (C) obstructive disease. Limits of expiratory performance are reached at rest in C, during moderate exercise in B, and during heavy work in A. Patient represented by C is dyspneic at rest, and the patient represented by B is dyspneic during moderate exercise.

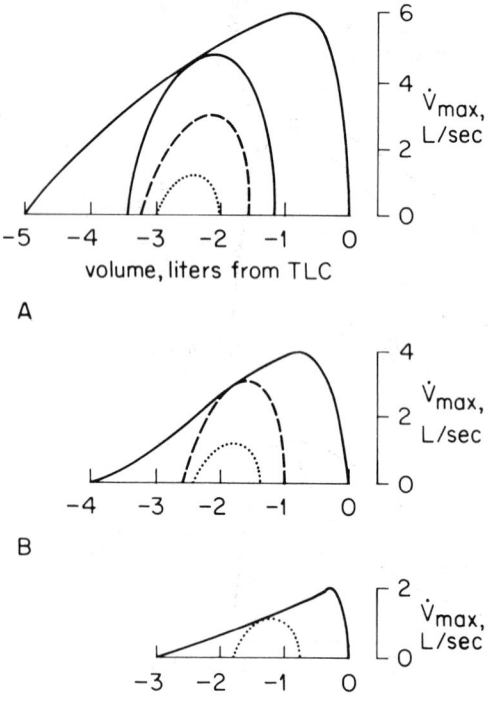

sufficient clues. Personal inspection of suspected workplaces by the physician may be needed to aid in diagnosis and also to prevent others from becoming ill from the same cause. In farmers, confusion can arise between farmer's lung and silo-filler's disease; methemoglobinemia points to the latter.

REVERSIBLE AIRWAY OBSTRUCTION Environmental exposures always need to be explored in patients with bronchial asthma (Chap. 257). Sensitization to organic materials occurs in many industries (Table 259-2), but not all these instances are related to IgE-mediated reaginic allergy. Other inhaled agents causing asthma act via direct release of histamine and other chemical mediators (Chap. 257), e.g., textile dusts, platinum salts. Airways obstruction may affect large as well as small bronchi and bronchioli. Small airway obstruction often predominates, but the site of obstruction cannot be determined with certainty from the results of lung function tests.

Byssinosis This disease occurs among cotton textile workers (carders and others) and among preparers of flax and soft hemp fibers. Its symptoms include chest tightness, cough, and wheezing, initially on first workdays after a temporary absence from work ("Monday dyspnea"). Chronic respiratory symptoms and permanent dyspnea follow in many cases after 10 to 20 years of exposure. The acute symptoms may occur in up to 70 to 80 percent of all workers exposed to dust in a cotton cardroom, and they are associated with decreases of FEV_1 and of flow rates on MEFV curves (Fig. 259-1*C*), and with impair-

ment of intrapulmonary mixing. Since isoproterenol reverses symptoms and function loss, the airway obstruction in byssinosis is probably caused by contraction of smooth muscle. It is of interest that textile dusts contain agents that release histamine from nonsensitized human lung in vitro; one of these is derived from the bracts of the cotton boll which contaminate raw cotton. Healthy, nonallergic laboratory subjects have chest tightness and airway obstruction after 10 to 20 min of inhalation of aerosols of tyrode extracts of cotton dust or bracts, the same effects as occur in textile workers after dust exposure. Thus, the acute stage of byssinosis can be adequately explained by chemical agents in textile dusts.

The chronic stage of byssinosis develops most frequently in workers who have suffered from the acute effects of the dust for years. Disabled persons with chronic byssinosis usually have severe airway obstruction and diminished elastic recoil. Varying degrees of chronic bronchitis and emphysema have been found at autopsy to provide a structural basis for these irreversible changes in lung function. Byssinosis was recognized as a compensable disease in Great Britain in 1940. A recent estimate is that about 30,000 textile workers in the United States are disabled because of byssinosis. The chronic disease progresses even after dust exposure ceases. The effects of smoking and of cotton dust exposure on lung function are additive.

TABLE 259-2
Chronic occupational lung diseases

Disease	Agent	Industries	Effects
MINERAL DUSTS			
Aluminum lung	Aluminum powder	Fireworks, explosives	Fibrosis
Antimony pneumo-coniosis	Antimony oxides	Mining, smelting	Dust deposits
Asbestosis	Asbestos: Chrysotile Amosite Crocidolite	Insulation, lagging, construction, ship-yards, brake linings, and textiles	Fibrosis, pleural plaques, lung cancer, mesothelioma
Baritosis	$BaSO_4$	Mining	Dust deposits
Bauxite lung (Shaver's disease, aluminosis)	Al_2O_3	Corundum smelting	Fibrosis, bullae, pneumothorax
Beryllium disease	Be compounds	Aircraft manufacturing, metallurgy, rocket fuels	Pneumonitis, granuloma, interstitial fibrosis
Coal worker's pneumoconiosis ("black lung")	Coal dust	Mining, coal trimming, graphite	Dust deposits, fibrosis, bronchitis, progressive massive fibrosis (PMF)
Hard-metal disease	Tungsten carbide with Co, Cr, Ni, Ti	Cutting tool industry	Interstitial fibrosis
Kaolinosis	Hydrated Al silicates	Porcelain	Dust deposits, fibrosis, PMF
Platinum asthma	Platinum salts	Electronics, chemical	Reversible airway obstruction
Siderosis	Iron oxide	Welding, iron ore mining, foundries	Dust deposits
Silicosis	Silica (SiO_2)	Mining (gold, tin, copper, graphite, coal), pottery, sand blasting, foundries, quarries and masonry (granite, slate, sandstone)	Dust deposits, fibrosis, PMF
Stannosis	Tin oxide	Smelting	Dust deposits
Talcosis	Hydrated Mg silicates	Rubber industry	Granulomas, interstitial fibrosis
ORGANIC DUSTS			
Asthma (see Chap. 257)	Castor bean Flour Tamarind seed Gum acacia Grain weevil Guinea pig hair Grass pollen	Castor oil manufacturing Bakeries Yarn finishing Printing industry Grain handlers Laboratory workers Gardeners, grounds keepers	Reversible airway obstruction
Allergic alveolitis (see Chap. 258)	Various fungi; vegetable dusts and animal matter		Acute and chronic interstitial pneumonitis, fibrosis
Byssinosis ("brown lung")	Cotton, flax, and hemp dust	Textiles	Airway obstruction, loss of elastic recoil

Diisocyanates These compounds, including toluene diisocyanate (TDI), which are used in the manufacture of polyurethane foam, can cause acute reversible airway obstruction, often more severe at the beginning of the work week. Responses vary from subclinical decreases in FEV_1 to overt wheezing and dyspnea. Chronic exposure may cause persistent reductions in FEV_1.

Enzyme detergents The "enzymes" in laundry detergents are concentrated autolysates from *Bacillus subtilis*. In workers exposed to dust of the concentrate, wheezing, chest tightness, dyspnea, and cough develop within a few hours after leaving work. Recent studies suggest that the risk has decreased by prevention of exposure in the industry.

CHRONIC SPECIFIC RESPONSES

The two main forms of chronic parenchymal response to mineral dusts are (1) diffuse interstitial responses, with pleomorphic cellular reactions and diffuse fibrosis, e.g., asbestosis; and (2) focal responses, which occur in silicosis and coal workers' pneumoconiosis. The former present functionally as purely restrictive disease; the latter may combine features of obstructive and restrictive disease.

DIFFUSE INTERSTITIAL RESPONSES These feature progressive dyspnea, dry cough, clubbing of the fingers, increased risk of spontaneous pneumothorax, and diffuse roentgenographic changes (Chap. 264).

Asbestos Asbestos includes several fibrous minerals, consisting of hydrated silicates. Asbestos fibers are resistant to heat and acid, and have high tensile strength and low electrical conductivity. These properties make asbestos a unique mineral with multiple uses. The same properties make asbestos fibers persist indefinitely in lung tissue, where they may cause *asbestosis, lung cancer, pleural plaques,* and *mesothelioma*. The risks vary with the type of asbestos: crocidolite (blue asbestos) is the most and chrysotile the least dangerous. The risks increase with the amounts inhaled. Some 40 percent of workers with heavy and prolonged exposures die of asbestos-related disease. Such exposures are becoming less common. But even brief (e.g., 1 to 2 years) exposures may lead to mesothelioma 20 to 40 years later; this tumor may also be traced to residence near asbestos factories. Autopsies have shown asbestos (or ferruginous) bodies in the lungs of city dwellers, similar to those in the sputum and lungs of asbestos workers. The origin of the inhaled asbestos is not clear, and there is no evidence for increased risk of asbestos-induced disease among urbanites in general. In addition, increased risk should not be confused with the proportion of those who become ill. A tenfold increased risk of a rare disease like mesothelioma still means that only few people with incidental asbestos exposure will develop mesothelioma. The widespread distribution of asbestos fibers and the associated risks have led to a search for safe asbestos substitutes. However, caution should be exercised with the use of any substitute material that is as persistent and indestructible as asbestos.

Asbestosis is an interstitial process which slowly develops into diffuse pulmonary fibrosis after a long latent period. There are instances of massive exposure with a rapid course, but the disease is usually recognized after 10 or more years of exposure and then continues to progress even after cessation of exposure. Its prevalence has been as high as 15 percent of those at risk in shipyard and insulation work. Early signs of asbestosis

include dyspnea, basal rales, and decreased vital capacity and CO diffusion capacity. Chronic bronchitis is not related to asbestos exposure.

Lung cancer (Chap. 268) among asbestos workers occurs nearly always in smokers; cigarette smoke and asbestos interact as etiologic agents. The most common abnormalities in asbestos workers are *pleural plaques,* symptomless calcified lesions which occur on the visceral pleura and in interlobar fissures, with frequent involvement of diaphragmatic and pericardial surfaces. *Mesotheliomas* of the pleura (Chap. 269) and the peritoneum are malignant tumors, often silent until local invasion has occurred. They are generally inoperable when diagnosed. Asbestos fibers, which are long and thin, probably cause pleural disease by inhalation and penetration of the pleura. The risk is greater with the straight fibers of amphibole asbestos (crocidolite, amosite) than with the curled chrysotile fibers, but both cause pleural disease when injected into the pleural cavity of animals.

Aluminum Exposure to metallic aluminum powder (fireworks, explosives) may cause fibrosis. A similar syndrome (bauxite lung, aluminosis, Shaver's disease) occurs in smelters of metallic corundum in the abrasives industry, in which Al_2O_3 is used. The usual course is a subacute interstitial pneumonitis with subsequent fibrosis; formation of bullae and spontaneous pneumothorax may occur.

Hard metal Machining, grinding, and polishing of hard metal (tungsten carbide with 3 to 25 percent cobalt and small amounts of other metals) may cause acute asthma or acute alveolitis, and also chronic interstitial pneumonitis and fibrosis. Cobalt is the most likely culprit.

Silicates Acute and chronic interstitial disease may occur after exposure to mica, kaolin, or talc dusts; the latter may contain free silica as well as asbestos fibers, which may account for its fibrogenic properties. Fatal cases of kaolin pneumoconiosis with massive fibrosis have been described. Talc has occasionally caused acute lethal disease in infants who were heavily exposed at home.

Beryllium Acute pneumonitis occurs after heavy exposures, but more commonly there is formation of focal, noncaseating granulomas which are difficult to distinguish from sarcoidosis (Chap. 216). There is, however, no lymph node or ocular involvement or hypercalcemia.

Mineral oil Aspiration of oils is rarely an occupational hazard. However, aspiration produces chronic low-grade inflammatory and granulomatous responses which sometimes evoke localized fibrotic reactions; symptoms are few and nonspecific. The chest roentgenogram may show patchy or nodular lesions, particularly at the lung bases. Occasionally, a larger or circumscribed lesion simulating a tumor, the so-called "paraffinoma," is produced. The diagnosis of lipoid pneumonitis is suggested by a long history of using oily nasal drops or mineral oil laxatives; it may be confirmed by demonstrating fat-filled macrophages in fresh sputum with Sudan III or IV. Smoking of tobacco "laced" with mineral oil ("black fat tobacco") can also cause lipid pneumonitis.

FOCAL RESPONSES Silicosis A major component of the earth's crust is free crystalline silica (SiO_2), which occurs in several crystal forms, such as quartz. Mines and other industries with exposure risks to silica dust are listed in Table 259-2. Acute forms of silicosis are now rare. Chronic silicosis, which still occurs in primitive as well as modern industries, usually has a latent period of 10 or more years, with gradual worsening of dyspnea on exertion, cough, expectoration, and eventual disability. Progressive massive fibrosis (see "Parenchymal Responses," above) is now the principal complication. In advanced cases patients may develop cor pulmonale, and there is an unexplained high incidence of scleroderma in silicosis. Tuberculosis is still a common complication, though less so than in the past, and adequate chemotherapy should be prolonged.

The radiologic patterns include diffuse nodular fibrosis, notably in the upper lobes, and "calcified rings" or "egg shells," which affect hilar and bronchopulmonary nodes. Lung-function changes are variable and do not correlate well with roentgenographic changes. There may be a combination of restrictive and obstructive lung disease, the former predominating in advanced cases. The early changes have been inadequately described, but it has been reported that reduction of arterial oxygen tension may occur during exercise at a time that lung volumes are near normal.

There is no specific therapy. In the early stages of the disease one must decide whether or not to advise the patient to stop work. Although there are no adequate data on postexposure progression, we believe that termination of exposure is advisable. Silicosis is still a significant hazard, especially when organized industrial medical surveillance is lacking.

Coal worker's pneumoconiosis (CWP) Lung disease among coal miners was recognized as a compensable occupational disease in Great Britain in 1929 and in some states in the United States in the 1960s. A "Black Lung" Act has provided compensation to all eligible coal miners in the United States since 1969. The prevalence of CWP varies with the type of coal mined, its silica content, and perhaps its content of aluminum and iron oxide. Silica increases the risk, while aluminum and iron oxide may render CWP more benign. Mechanization may increase dust production; construction of shafts and tunnels poses high risks. The prevalence of CWP is high; in one United States study which included retired miners, roentgenograms revealed pneumoconiosis in 46 percent.

Although inhaled dust contains carbon and varying amounts of silica, there is no longer any doubt that CWP can occur in the absence of silica exposure; typical lesions occur in lungs without silica deposits, and pure carbon dust (graphite) can cause CWP. The lesions include deposits of carbon dust along respiratory bronchioles, with development of a reticulin fiber network and bronchiolar widening due to loss of wall structure. Thus, early lesions in CWP include dilatation of respiratory bronchioles and centrilobular emphysema. At this stage ventilatory function may be normal, but gas distribution and ventilation-perfusion relations may already be disturbed. At a later stage, nodular lesions appear, with a radial type of fibrosis and a preponderance of reticulin rather than collagen fibers. Silicotic nodules may be found if there is concomitant SiO_2 exposure. *Caplan's syndrome* is an association between seropositive rheumatoid arthritis and CWP.

The correlation between x-ray lesions of CWP, on the one hand, and symptoms, disability, and lung function, on the other hand, is poor. Disabling function loss among coal workers is commonly due to chronic airway obstruction and bronchitis. Inhalation of gases and fumes at work, and also smoking, are probable causative factors, rather than inhalation of mineral dust. Nevertheless, dust exposure, too, must be minimized because the focal lesions of CWP may progress to disabling progressive massive fibrosis (see "Parenchymal Responses," above).

Other dust deposits Several mineral dusts are inhaled and deposited in the lungs and elicit only minimal tissue responses. These include iron oxide (siderosis), tin oxide (stannosis), and barium sulfate (baritosis). In mining iron oxide there may be associated SiO_2 exposure and thus silicosis.

CIGARETTE SMOKING The ill effects of smoking on the lungs (see Chap. 219) often compound the risk of occupational exposures. Smoking greatly enhances the risk of lung cancer in asbestos workers (see page 1220). In other instances, chronic airway obstruction may be attributed to smoking when it in fact results from an unrecognized exposure at work. Hence, smokers and nonsmokers should always be considered separately in studies of groups of workers at potential risk. Subtle inhalant risks may show only in nonsmokers; in smokers they may be overwhelmed by the effects of cigarette smoke. In other instances (e.g., byssinosis) cigarette smoking and dust exposure have additive effects on the development of chronic airway obstruction. As a result, the lungs of smoking textile workers age more rapidly than those of their nonsmoking colleagues. Disabled textile workers who smoke are on the average about 5 years younger than disabled workers who never smoked. Even though subtle effects of smoking occur at an early age (Fig. 259-1*B*), disabling obstructive lung function loss develops only in a minority of smokers but in many more if they are also exposed to textile dust. Why some smokers have chronic airway obstruction at an early age while others have only slight or no evidence of functional damage after 30 or more years of regular smoking is an unanswered question. Clearly, unraveling the relative contributions of smoking and occupational exposures to airway obstruction in smoking workers is only feasible in controlled studies of sufficiently large populations.

LUNG CANCER (See also Chap. 268) An increased risk of bronchogenic carcinoma occurs in workers exposed to asbestos, chromates, nickel, arsenic, radioactive dusts, and in those exposed to coke oven fumes. However, cigarette smoking remains the major causal factor in the development of lung cancer, in terms of the total number of persons affected.

AIR POLLUTION

In past decades, acute air pollution disasters occurring in Donora, Pennsylvania; in the Meuse Valley, Belgium; and in London have shown that stagnant air masses heavily contaminated with industrial and domestic air pollutants can cause large increases in morbidity and mortality from lung disease. Since the last of these tragic episodes (London, 1952), clean air regulations have improved air quality in the United States and in Western Europe. Recurrence of air pollution disasters now appears unlikely. However, complete control of toxic pollutant emissions has not been achieved, and probably never will be, in industrial societies. There remains widespread public concern about the harmful effects of current, relatively low, air pollutant concentrations. The two main types of polluted air masses are oxidant smog and reducing smog (SO_2 and particulates).

OXIDANT SMOG The "Los Angeles-type" smog arises by photochemical oxidation of automobile exhaust (NO, hydrocarbons) in atmospheric air. Oxidant smog is linked with sunlight and traffic patterns and shows striking diurnal variations, with peak levels occurring a few hours after the morning rush hour. Its main toxic components are ozone (O_3), nitrogen dioxide (NO_2), and peroxyacetyl nitrate. High concentrations of O_3 cause severe damage to lung tissue. Alveolar type I cells are destroyed and pulmonary edema may develop. Repair follows by proliferation of type II cells; this increases the thickness of the alveolar membrane and limits gas exchange. Nitrogen dioxide may cause bronchiolitis obliterans. Both NO_2 and O_3 impair defenses against bacteria and virus in animals, mainly through effects on alveolar macrophages. Other actions observed in animal experiments include accelerated aging of lung tissue, impairment of mucus lysozyme activity (O_3), and lipid peroxidation of unsaturated fatty acids (NO_2). Most of these actions occur at O_3 or NO_2 concentrations higher than those in polluted ambient air. Ozone concentrations similar to those in smog [0.37 part per million (ppm) or more] cause lung function changes (decreased maximum flow, increased airway resistance) in humans. These changes are enhanced by exercise, which increases the inhaled dose of O_3. Nitrogen dioxide (3 ppm or more) also increases airway resistance in man.

SULFUR OXIDES Sulfur dioxide is an irritant gas, soluble in water and hence largely absorbed in upper airways. In concentrations higher than those in urban air (1 to 5 ppm and more) it causes airway constriction. Sulfur dioxide may dissolve in airborne water droplets and form ionic SO_3 and sulfates. In animal experiments, ammonium sulfate is more of an irritant than SO_2, but this compound has little or no effect on humans (including asthmatic patients) in concentrations similar to those in severely polluted air. Sulfur dioxide concentrations in ambient air indicate the amount of air pollution produced by burning of fossil fuels in industry, homes, and power plants.

PARTICULATES Particles are responsible for lack of visibility, soiling, and similar undesirable effects of air pollution. Even chemically inert particles can affect the airways, although this requires very large amounts. The size and shape of particles and their chemical constituents are more important than their absolute quantities. Indoors, tobacco smoking is a prime source of particulate pollution. Outdoors, asbestos pollution near asbestos plants has been linked to mesothelioma (page 1220).

CARBON MONOXIDE (CO) Automobile exhaust, cigarette smoke, and fires are common sources of CO (see also Chap. 224). Increased but nonfatal concentrations of inspired CO, as in smoke-filled rooms, traffic tunnels, or parking garages, may lead to slight degrees of anoxia and subtle decrements in psychophysical performance. For nonsmokers, the resulting slight increase in CO hemoglobin is of little consequence. In smokers, CO hemoglobin induced by their own smoking is quantitatively much more important. Typical exposures to CO among traffic policemen and tunnel personnel are in the order of 30 to 100 ppm, several hours per day. The long-term effects, if any, of such low-level exposures are not well known.

LEAD (Pb) Because automobile exhaust often contains lead (see Chap. 225), widespread low-grade exposure to this heavy metal results. However, inhalation of lead from ambient air does not appear to be a significant health hazard.

EFFECTS OF AIR POLLUTION ON HUMAN HEALTH The principal concerns about air pollution relate to three disease categories: asthma, chronic bronchitis and airway obstruction, and lung cancer. There is no evidence that urban air pollution aggravates the incidence or severity of *asthma*. In fact, a history of asthma was found to be more common among rural residents in two parts of the United States than in urban residents of Connecticut, and a recent study in Los Angeles found no association between oxidant smog peaks and attacks of asthma. Other factors (allergens in particular) predominate in the pathogenesis of asthma. Earlier studies had suggested an

increased prevalence of *chronic bronchitis* among urban residents, and an increased prevalence of respiratory infections in children living in high-pollution areas in the United Kingdom. These studies concerned air pollution levels (SO_2 and particulates) much higher than those prevailing at present in the United States and Western Europe. Also, no convincing evidence of increased airway obstruction (as deduced from lung function tests) among urban residents has emerged. When race, sex, age, height, weight, and smoking habits are taken into account, sensitive tests of airway obstruction (MEF 50%; Fig. 259-1) show no differences between rural residents of Connecticut and South Carolina, on the one hand, and residents of a high-oxidant area in Los Angeles, on the other hand (nonsmoking men and women, age 45 to 64 years). The FEV_1 of rural, nonsmoking, black and white, adult males in 1972 to 1974 is similar to the FEV_1 of comparable men working outdoors in New York City in 1961 to 1962, at a time when SO_2 and particulate levels were much higher that at present. Urban and rural blacks in the United States and blacks living in a primitive African village have similar FVC and FEV_1 values when sex, age, height, and smoking are taken into account. Lastly, FVC, FEV_1 and MEF 50% are similar in rural U.S. children and in Czech children living in a town with high SO_2 and particulate levels (age 10 to 11 years). There is some evidence that urban adult nonsmokers in the United States have slightly more cough and phlegm than rural nonsmokers, but chronic bronchitis (usual cough and usual phlegm, more than 3 months per year, during at least 2 years) is equally uncommon among both these groups in Connecticut and among Los Angeles nonsmokers. Among smokers, any effect of urban residence is overwhelmed by that of smoking. Thus, residence in urban areas may be associated with a slight excess of respiratory symptoms, but there is no evidence that this leads to chronic bronchitis or airway obstruction. With respect to *lung cancer,* an excess incidence has been noted in urban residents in several countries. However, in several instances this can be explained by differences in cigarette smoking habits between urban and rural residents. Effects of outdoor air pollution, if any, on lung cancer incidence are minimal compared with those of smoking and occupational exposures.

For many people, even in urban areas, indoor air pollution by tobacco smoke (particulates, CO), gas stoves (NO_2), or cars in attached garages contributes more to their total pollutant load than exposure to ambient air outdoors. So far, however, no association between indoor pollution in homes, monitored with portable devices, and lung function or respiratory symptoms among the residents has been found. Among nonsmoking children and adults, lung function is similar whether they live in homes with smokers or with nonsmokers only.

The current concern about ill effects of relatively low air pollution levels in our cities thus appears to have little basis in fact. Aggravation of preexisting chronic lung disease by urban air pollution cannot be excluded, but there is little reason to think that it is an important factor. Improving the indoor environment of such patients by removing indoor pollutant sources and/or installing an air cleaner, may make more sense than a move to a rural area where other pathogenetic factors (e.g., pollens) may aggravate disease. Although urban air pollution may have been overestimated as a source of ill health, it should remain a matter of serious concern for reasons of hygiene, esthetics, ecology, and personal comfort.

PREVENTION AND CONTROL

The prime target for programs to prevent chronic respiratory disease and lung cancer should be cigarette smoking (see Chap. 219). Current programs to control outdoor sources of air pollution (car exhaust emissions, industrial effluents, domestic fuel use) are unlikely to have a significant impact on the prevalence or severity of respiratory diseases.

More benefit can be expected from attempts to control exposures in the occupational environment. Usually, one can determine who is at risk and what can be done to prevent exposures. Physicians can have a direct impact on such programs, since the absence of signs and symptoms of incipient or overt disease should be the final criterion for their success. Industrial exposures should first of all be limited by engineering methods: substitution of nonhazardous materials, prevention of accidents with irritants, enclosure of sources of pollutants, and suitable dust exhaust and collection systems. The effectiveness of such controls needs to be monitored by air sampling. Setting "safe" levels, termed "threshold limit values," for pollutants provides suitable goals for these control programs. Masks are needed during short hazardous exposures, or as emergency measures until engineering controls can be implemented.

For several substances (asbestos, cotton dust, and radioactive materials) no unequivocal "safe limits" can be set. As exposure decreases, the risk becomes less but does not disappear totally. In such instances, some persons may continue to experience ill effects on health from minimal exposures in workplaces protected with modern controls. Medical surveillance is required to detect and protect individuals at risk, in particular those who are highly sensitive. Medical surveillance includes preemployment and periodic medical examinations. Persons with preexisting lung disease should usually not be assigned to dusty work areas. Periodic examinations should include a full-sized chest roentgenogram and pulmonary function tests, including vital capacity and FEV_1, in all industries in which occupational lung diseases occur. Transfer to other work should be advised only after full consideration of medical as well as financial, social, and legal implications for the worker. For instance, the risk of progression of silicosis must be weighed against financial and social factors (decreased wage, loss of seniority) involved in a transfer. Such arbitrary judgments can largely be avoided if adequate environmental control is practiced in industry.

REFERENCES

BOGOVSKI P et al (eds): *Biological Effects of Asbestos,* IARC Scientific Publication no 8. Lyon, International Agency for Research on Cancer, 1973

BOUHUYS A: *The Physiology of Breathing.* New York, Grune & Stratton, 1977

——— et al: Epidemiology of chronic lung disease in a cotton mill community. Lung 154:167, 1977

——— et al: Do present levels of air pollution outdoors affect respiratory health? Nature 276:466, 1978

DOLL R: Strategy for detection of cancer hazards to man. Nature 265:589, 1977

MOHR U et al (eds): *Air Pollution and Cancer in Man,* IARC Scientific Publication no 16. Lyon, International Agency for Research on Cancer, 1977

NATIONAL RESEARCH COUNCIL, COMMITTEE ON MEDICAL AND BIOLOGIC EFFECTS OF ENVIRONMENTAL POLLUTANTS: *Medical and Biologic Effects of Environmental Pollutants: Nitrogen Oxides.* Washington, DC, National Academy of Sciences, 1977

NATIONAL RESEARCH COUNCIL, COMMITTEE ON MEDICAL AND BIOLOGIC EFFECTS OF ENVIRONMENTAL POLLUTANTS: *Ozone and Other Photochemical Oxidants.* Washington, DC, National Academy of Sciences, 1977

PARKER WR: *Occupational Lung Disorders.* London, Butterworth, 1974

SCHOENBERG JB et al: Growth air decay of pulmonary function in healthy blacks and whites. Respir Physiol 33:367, 1978

SPENCER H: *Pathology of the Lung,* 3d ed. Oxford, Pergamon, 1977, vols I, II

TERRIL JB et al: Toxic gases from fires. Science 200:1343, 1978

US DEPARTMENT OF HEALTH, EDUCATION, AND WELFARE, PUBLIC HEALTH SERVICE, NATIONAL INSTITUTE FOR OCCUPATIONAL SAFETY AND HEALTH: *Occupational Diseases: A Guide to Their Recognition,* NIOSH Publication no 77-81, June 1977

Pulmonary infections

260
PNEUMONIA AND LUNG ABSCESS

JAN V. HIRSCHMANN
JOHN F. MURRAY
ROBERT G. PETERSDORF

PNEUMONIA

DEFINITION Pneumonia is defined as inflammation in the lung parenchyma, the portion distal to the terminal bronchioles and comprising the respiratory bronchioles, alveolar ducts, alveolar sacs, and alveoli. While the inflammation may have many different causes and varying durations, the term *pneumonia* most commonly refers to acute infections.

PATHOGENESIS Organisms reach the lung to cause pneumonia by one of four routes: (1) inhalation of microbes present in the air, (2) aspiration of organisms from the naso- or oropharynx, the most common cause of bacterial pneumonia, (3) hematogenous spread from a distant focus of infection, or rarely, (4) direct spread from a contiguous site of infection.

Lung defense mechanisms Although inhalation of organisms and aspiration of oropharyngeal contents are probably common, even in healthy people, the airway distal to the larynx is normally sterile or possesses a sparse flora because of several protective mechanisms. The glottis reflexly closes when material is aspirated; whatever reaches the trachea and large bronchi usually evokes coughing, which expels the material from the tracheobronchial tree. The airway from the larynx to the terminal bronchioles is further protected by its lining of mucus-covered ciliated epithelium, which propels trapped inhaled matter from the smaller to the larger airways, where it can be eliminated by expectoration or swallowing.

The immunoglobulins constitute another defense mechanism. IgA, present in high concentrations in the upper respiratory tract, protects against viral infection. It is less abundant in the lower respiratory secretions, where it may help agglutinate bacteria, neutralize microbial toxins, and reduce bacterial attachment to mucosal surfaces. IgG in the serum and lower respiratory tract agglutinates and opsonizes bacteria; activates complement, promoting chemotaxis of granulocytes and macrophages; neutralizes bacterial toxins and viruses; and lyses gram-negative bacteria. Also present in the alveoli are alveolar macrophages, which ingest and kill organisms, and alveolar lining material, which may enhance phagocytic function. In addition, neutrophils, which ingest and kill organisms, and lymphocytes, providing humoral and cell-mediated immunity, are available from the bloodstream to help combat infection.

Predisposing conditions Pneumonia may occur in healthy people but is usually associated with conditions that impair one or more of the defense mechanisms listed above. Altered consciousness from alcoholism, cranial trauma, seizures, general anesthesia, drug overdose, cerebrovascular disease, or other causes, and old age depress the cough and glottic reflexes, allowing the aspiration of oropharyngeal contents. Pain from trauma or thoracic or upper abdominal surgery; weakness from malnutrition or neuromuscular disease; thoracic cage deformities such as serious kyphoscoliosis; or severe obstructive lung disease may prevent the full inspiration and brisk expiration necessary to generate an effective cough. An endotracheal tube or tracheostomy eliminates glottic closure and impedes effective coughing.

Mucociliary transport is impaired by alcohol, cigarette smoke, old age, and preceding viral respiratory infections, which may cause necrosis and desquamation of the tracheobronchial epithelium. Endobronchial obstruction from tumor, foreign body, or other causes compromises effective clearance mechanisms. Thick mucus from cystic fibrosis or chronic bronchitis makes the transport system less effective. Indeed, in chronic bronchitis, the tracheobronchial tree is typically colonized with an abundant flora, especially pneumococci and *Hemophilus influenzae.*

Lymphocyte disorders, including congenital and acquired immunodeficiencies, and granulocyte abnormalities may predispose to pneumonia (Chap. 107). Pulmonary infection may also occur when alveolar macrophage function is impaired by cigarette smoke, hypoxia, starvation, anemia, pulmonary edema, and viral respiratory infections.

Oropharyngeal flora Most pneumonias arise from the aspiration of oropharyngeal flora, normally a complex assortment of aerobic and anaerobic bacteria. Which of these organisms causes the pneumonia seems to depend upon the identity of the microbes present and the quantity of material aspirated. *Streptococcus pneumoniae, H. influenzae, Staphylococcus aureus,* and even *Neisseria meningitidis,* all potential pathogens, are often found in the oropharynx of healthy adults. Each of these organisms, as single agents, may cause pneumonia when aspirated into alveoli. Anaerobes, however, which outnumber aerobes severalfold in the oral cavity, are weak pathogens individually and usually cause infection by an interaction among several species. These organisms, therefore, are likely to cause pneumonia, usually as a polymicrobial infection, only when aspirated in relatively large quantities.

Coliforms, such as *Escherichia coli, Klebsiella,* and *Proteus,* are uncommon in the oropharynx of healthy adults. Several conditions, especially hospitalization, however, favor their growth. Serious underlying illness, confinement in an intensive care unit, the use of an endotracheal tube or tracheostomy, contaminated respiratory equipment, and antimicrobial ther-

apy, which frequently selects out organisms resistant to the agents used, especially encourage colonization with coliforms present in the hospital environment. Certain illnesses, such as acute granulocytic leukemia, alcoholism, and diabetes mellitus, are associated with an increased frequency of oropharyngeal colonization with aerobic gram-negative bacilli whether or not the patient is hospitalized.

CLINICAL MANIFESTATIONS The major symptoms of pneumonia, occurring in varying combinations, are cough, fever, chest pain, dyspnea, and the production of sputum, which may be mucoid, purulent, or even bloody. In some patients, especially the elderly or those with serious underlying disease, extrapulmonary features such as confusion or disorientation may predominate. Important in the history are inquiries about prodromal symptoms, the type of onset (abrupt or gradual), the presence of rigors and pleuritic chest pain, similar illness in family members or acquaintances, animal exposure, and recent travel.

Common physical findings are fever, tachycardia, and tachypnea. Severely hypoxemic patients may be cyanotic. On chest examination there may be decreased respiratory excursion on the affected side because of pleuritic pain and dullness to percussion from pneumonic consolidation or an accompanying pleural effusion. Among the earliest auscultatory findings is the presence of high-pitched, end-inspiratory crackles, originating from fluid-filled alveoli, that are often increased by, or heard only after, coughing. Secretions in the airways may cause lower-pitched, early or mid-inspiratory crackles. Consolidated lung surrounding a patent bronchus often gives rise to bronchial breath sounds, an accentuation of both the inspiratory and expiratory phases of breathing. In some patients, despite impressive roentgenographic abnormalities, physical examination of the chest is entirely normal. In patients whose pneumonia is secondary to hematogenous spread, the primary site of infection may be apparent. Alternatively, bacteremia arising from pneumonia may cause infection in distant sites, such as meningitis, septic arthritis, or pustular skin lesions.

The arterial blood gases commonly reveal hypoxemia and in the absence of other pulmonary disease, hypocarbia and respiratory alkalosis. These abnormalities result from ventilation-perfusion inequality, particularly the continued perfusion of the poorly ventilated areas affected by the pneumonia.

ROENTGENOGRAPHIC FINDINGS The microbial etiology of a pneumonia cannot be accurately predicted by its roentgenographic characteristics. Nevertheless, certain appearances are more typical of some organisms than others. Pneumonias tend to conform to one of three pathological and roentgenographic patterns (Fig. 260-1): (1) alveolar or air space pneumonia, (2) bronchopneumonia, or (3) interstitial pneumonia. In air space pneumonia the organism causes an inflammatory exudate that spreads from one alveolus to the next via the communicating channels, the pores of Kohn, and the canals of Lambert. Segmental boundaries are not preserved, and the bronchi, relatively uninvolved, remain patent. The roentgenographic result is nonsegmental consolidation with air bronchograms, the classic example being pneumococcal pneumonia. Some organisms produce bronchopneumonia, which consists of inflammation in the conducting airways, especially terminal and respiratory bronchioles, and the surrounding alveoli. Because interalveolar spread in the peripheral air spaces is minimal, the pneumonia tends to maintain a distribution corresponding to the involved pulmonary segment. Inflammation affects the bronchi themselves, sometimes causing atelectasis, and air bronchograms are absent. An example is staphylococcal pneumonia. *Mycoplasma pneumoniae* and viruses often cause an interstitial pneumonia, where inflammation is predominantly in the alveolar septa, producing a reticular radiographic appearance.

DIAGNOSTIC TECHNIQUES Among the most useful procedures to define a pneumonia's etiology is the microscopic examination of a Gram-stained sputum specimen. Although precise speciation of bacteria is impossible by Gram's stain alone, the appearance of organisms allows reasonable inferences about their identity. An acceptable sputum sample, one genuinely arising from the lower respiratory tract rather than the oropharynx, has more than 25 leukocytes per low-power field (100×). Squamous epithelial cells from the oropharynx are sparse, and alveolar macrophages are often present. Specimens that fail to meet these standards represent mostly saliva and are useless for further examination or culture. Acceptable specimens should be cultured on appropriate media.

Adequate staining of acceptable specimens is crucial for accurate interpretation. If cells, including the nuclei of leukocytes, are not gram-negative (red), the sample is underdecolorized. If gram-positive (blue) organisms are present near the gram-negative leukocytes, the stain is suitable. If the cells and all the organisms are gram-negative, the slide may be overdecolorized and may require restaining. The slide should be examined carefully for the predominant organism; bacteria overlying squamous epithelial cells should be disregarded.

Usually, sputum expectorated after a deep cough is acceptable for stain and culture by the criteria outlined above. When the specimen is unsatisfactory or the patient cannot produce one, suctioning with a catheter introduced through the nose into the posterior pharynx will often induce coughing and provide an adequate sample. Since sputum that is expectorated or obtained by nasotracheal suction is unavoidably contaminated by oropharyngeal flora, which normally contains anaerobic organisms, it is not appropriate for anaerobic cultures.

Another method of obtaining sputum is transtracheal aspiration with a polyethylene catheter inserted into the trachea through the cricothyroid membrane. This procedure is generally safe but should be accompanied by oxygen administration in those with hypoxemia and avoided in those with serious clotting disorders or platelet defects. This method avoids contamination with the abundant, complex mouth flora and yields a specimen suitable for anaerobic culture. An alternate way of obtaining lower respiratory secretions is transthoracic aspiration of the lung with a spinal needle attached to a syringe. The major complications are pneumothorax or pulmonary hemorrhage. Lower respiratory secretions may also be obtained by bronchoscopy. Because contamination with oropharyngeal flora is generally unavoidable, even with preceding endotracheal intubation, these specimens are approximately equivalent to good expectorated sputum samples.

Since bacteremia sometimes accompanies pneumonia, blood cultures taken from two separate venipuncture sites may grow the responsible organism. Similarly, the presence of a pleural effusion requires a thoracentesis, which may yield infected fluid. Skin lesions, joint effusions, and cerebrospinal fluid should be cultured if these areas appear infected.

Although viruses, *M. pneumoniae, Coxiella burnetti,* and *Francisella tularensis,* may grow from sputum specimens cultured on appropriate media, pneumonias due to these agents are usually diagnosed by serology. Since *Legionella pneumophila* rarely grows from sputum or pleural fluid, Legionnaires' disease also usually requires a serologic diagnosis. Acute and convalescent serum samples should be obtained when these agents are suspected.

DIFFERENTIAL DIAGNOSIS **Community-acquired pneumonias** Pneumococcal (Chap. 115) pneumonia, the most common bacterial pneumonia, in its classic form frequently follows an upper respiratory infection and begins abruptly with a single shaking chill, fever, pleuritic chest pain, and a cough productive of purulent, often bloody sputum. In some patients, especially the elderly and those with serious underlying disorders such as alcoholism or chronic obstructive lung disease, the illness is often considerably less dramatic, with the insidious onset of fever, cough, and dyspnea. Extrapulmonary features such as confusion or weakness may be more impressive than the respiratory complaints. The white blood cell count is usually elevated, with increased immature forms, but may be normal or low. The typical sputum Gram's stain shows numerous neutrophils and abundant, gram-positive lancet-shaped diplococci as the predominant organism. The chest roentgenogram characteristically demonstrates a unilateral, homogeneous, nonsegmental air space consolidation, usually abutting against a visceral pleural surface. Unilateral or bilateral multilobar involvement may occur, and in patients with emphysema the consolidation may have an inhomogeneous appearance of multiple "holes" from the radiolucent, uninvolved bullae. Cavitation rarely occurs, but pleural effusions, usually small but occasionally voluminous, are frequent.

Pneumonia from *S. pyogenes* (Chap. 117) is very uncommon. It may follow pharyngitis or a viral illness, especially influenza, or occasionally occurs as outbreaks in closed populations, such as military recruits. The onset is typically abrupt,

FIGURE 260-1

Roentgenographic appearances of pneumonia. A. Air space pneumonia. There is a dense, homogeneous, nonsegmental consolidation in the right lower lobe with a visible air bronchogram. B. Interstitial pneumonia. A *linear or reticular pattern involves the lower lung fields bilaterally, more on the right. C. Bronchopneumonia. A segmental infiltrate without a visible air bronchogram appears in the left lower lung field.*

A   B   C

with multiple rigors, fever, a productive cough, and pleuritic chest pain. Pharyngitis is often present. The white blood cell count is commonly elevated, and immature forms increased. The sputum Gram's stain shows multiple neutrophils and gram-positive cocci in chains. The chest roentgenogram usually reveals unilateral bronchopneumonia and large pleural effusions, which develop rapidly after the onset of illness. Cavitation is frequent.

Pneumonia from *S. aureus* (Chap. 116), also quite uncommon, tends to follow an influenza attack. The onset is generally abrupt and the course rapid, with fever, multiple rigors, purulent sputum production, and pleuritic chest pain. The white blood cell count is elevated, and immature forms are increased. The sputum smear shows numerous neutrophils and gram-positive cocci in clumps. The chest roentgenogram reveals bronchopneumonia, often bilateral, frequently with cavitation and pleural effusions.

Pneumonia due to *N. meningitidis* (Chap. 118) may occur in sporadic cases, following viral respiratory infections, or especially in military recruits. The onset may be abrupt, resembling pneumococcal pneumonia, or more gradual, with cough, fever, sore throat, and chest pain. Meningitis or cutaneous evidence of meningococcemia is uncommon, and blood cultures are typically sterile. Neutrophilic leukocytosis is usual. The sputum smear shows gram-negative diplococci that are often present within the cytoplasm of neutrophils. The chest film most commonly demonstrates patchy alveolar consolidation, predominantly in the lower lobes. Pleural effusions and pulmonary cavitation are rare.

Although *H. influenzae* (Chap. 125) pneumonia may occur in healthy young adults, the typical patient is over 50 years old and has chronic obstructive lung disease or alcoholism. The onset may be abrupt but is more frequently gradual. The major complaints are fever, productive cough, chills, dyspnea, and pleuritic chest pain. Neutrophilic leukocytosis is usual. The sputum smear shows abundant neutrophils and many pleomorphic gram-negative organisms that range from cocci to bacilli of various sizes and are often especially predominant in the cytoplasm of the white blood cells. The bacilli are slender, unlike the typical plump appearance of enteric organisms. The chest film usually discloses diffuse bronchopneumonia, often bilateral, although air space consolidation sometimes occurs. Pleural effusions developing rapidly in the course of disease are common, but lung abscess formation is rare.

Klebsiella pneumoniae (Chap. 120) pneumonia is very uncommon. It typically occurs in middle-aged or elderly patients with underlying chronic disease, especially alcoholism and diabetes mellitus. The illness begins abruptly with fever, rigors, productive cough, and dyspnea. Neutrophilic leukocytosis is usual. The sputum may be tenacious and bloody. Plump gram-negative bacilli of uniform size are visible on the sputum smear. The chest roentgenogram shows an air space pneumonia usually in one of the upper lobes and frequently complicated by abscess formation and a pleural effusion. The inflammatory exudate in the lung may be so voluminous that the interlobar fissure bulges, a characteristic, but not pathognomonic, appearance.

Pneumonia from *anaerobic organisms* (Chap. 142) usually occurs in patients with periodontal disease, which increases their number in the mouth, and in patients with a propensity to aspirate because of swallowing disorders, altered consciousness, or other causes. The onset may be abrupt but is usually gradual, with several days to weeks of fever, weight loss, and a productive cough. The sputum may be foul smelling, a feature diagnostic of anaerobic infection. The sputum smear typically shows many neutrophils, and several different organisms, usually both gram-positive and gram-negative, are profuse. Many anaerobic bacteria have a characteristic appearance. *Actinomyces,* eubacterium, and Bifidobacterium are filamentous, branching, thin gram-positive rods. Peptostreptococci are tiny gram-positive cocci in chains. *Fusobacterium* appears as a long, fusiform gram-negative rod with pointed ends, while *Bacteroides* are pleomorphic gram-negative bacilli that range from coccoid to long, filamentous structures. Understandably, aerobic cultures typically fail to grow a likely pathogen. Chest films demonstrate consolidation in the segments where gravitation favors the flow of aspirated material. These are the posterior segments of the upper lobes and the superior segments of the lower lobes, when aspiration has occurred in the supine position, and the basilar segments of the lower lobes for the upright position. Single or multiple areas of cavitation and pleural effusions are very common.

Pneumonia due to *L. pneumophila* (Legionnaires' disease, Chap. 138) may occur in outbreaks or sporadically. The first symptoms of myalgia and headache are followed by fever, chills, and a cough that is nonproductive or yields small amounts of mucoid sputum. Diarrhea, chest pain that is often pleuritic, and confusion or delirium are common. Sputum smears show few leukocytes and rare bacteria. The organism itself is not visible on Gram's stain. The chest film reveals air space consolidation that may develop into unilateral or bilateral, poorly marginated, rounded opacities. Pleural effusions, if present, are usually small, and cavitation does not occur.

Pneumonia due to *Francisella tularensis* (Chap. 128) follows tick bites or exposure to infected animals. A cutaneous ulcer and regional lymphadenopathy may be present but are absent in the typhoidal form. The illness typically begins abruptly with fever, chills, headache, and cough, which is usually nonproductive. The leukocyte count is usually normal but may be elevated. The sputum smear may show neutrophils, but the organism is rarely seen. The chest roentgenogram typically shows a bronchopneumonia, often with hilar adenopathy, a finding seldom seen in other bacterial pneumonias. Sometimes the pneumonia appears as a distinctive, oval, homogeneous consolidation. Pleural effusions are common, but cavitation is rare.

The most frequent cause of community-acquired, nonbacterial pneumonia is *M. pneumoniae* (Chap. 172). It occurs most commonly in children or young adults, but may develop in older persons, especially during outbreaks in a family group. It differs from the bacterial pneumonias described above in many respects. It has an insidious, rather than abrupt, onset and a cough that is nonproductive or yields only small amounts of mucoid sputum. Pleuritic chest pain, rigors, and hemoptysis are distinctly uncommon. The temperature is generally less than 38.9°C (102°F), and headache is a prominent symptom. As in other nonbacterial pneumonias, the sputum smear typically demonstrates mononuclear leukocytes or neutrophils but few organisms, since the agent is not visible on Gram's staining. The white blood cell count is usually normal or only mildly elevated, with a normal differential. The chest roentgenogram demonstrates segmental bronchopneumonia, or sometimes a predominant interstitial pattern, mostly affecting the lower lung fields. Bilateral involvement is common, but, unlike many bacterial pneumonias, substantial pleural effusions or cavitation are rare. The extent of radiographic involvement is often more impressive than the clinical examination would suggest.

Other community-acquired nonbacterial pneumonias are Q fever, psittacosis, and viral pneumonia. Q fever (Chap. 170) occurs from the inhalation of aerosolized particles containing *Coxiella burnetti,* the usual sources being placental tissues, amniotic fluid, milk, and feces of infected cattle, sheep, and goats. It is, thus, largely an occupational disease of those exposed to livestock. It begins abruptly with headache, fever, chills, and myalgias. Chest pain, often pleuritic, and a nonproductive cough follow. The white blood cell count is usually normal, and the chest film typically shows segmental consolidation that is predominantly in the lower lobes.

Psittacosis (Chap. 175), also an occupational disease, occurs in those exposed to infected birds. Fever, an excruciating headache, myalgias, and an unproductive cough are the predominant symptoms. Splenomegaly, rare in most pneumonias, is frequent. The white blood cell count is usually normal. The roentgenographic appearance varies from homogeneous to patchy consolidation, which may be segmental or lobar in distribution. Sometimes the chest film shows nodular or miliary opacities.

Viral pneumonias are quite uncommon in civilian adults who are not immunosuppressed, and this diagnosis should be made only with strong clinical or epidemiologic evidence, supported by viral cultures and serologic studies. The overwhelming majority of pneumonias in adults are due to the agents discussed above, not viruses. The most frequent viral pneumonia is *influenza* (Chap. 179), which tends to occur in patients with underlying cardiac or pulmonary disease. It begins as typical influenza, with fever, myalgias, and headache. Twelve to thirty-six hours later dyspnea and cyanosis may develop rapidly and often proceed to a fatal outcome. The chest roentgenogram shows diffuse, patchy, unilateral or bilateral air space pneumonia. Even with these typical clinical features, a bacterial superinfection, especially with pneumococci or *S. aureus,* may be responsible for the pneumonia, instead of the virus itself.

Varicella (Chap. 185) can cause pneumonia in adults and typically begins 2 to 3 days after the vesicular eruption appears. Fever, cough, dyspnea, hemoptysis, and pleuritic chest pain are the major symptoms. The chest film demonstrates patchy, diffuse, generally discrete air space consolidations that are almost nodular.

Measles (Chap. 181) pneumonia in adults generally occurs in military recruits and may begin just before, with, or after the skin rash. The chest film shows a diffuse bilateral reticular pattern.

Adenovirus (Chap. 178) pneumonia also occurs predominantly in military recruits. Fever, cough, rhinitis, and pharyngitis are the major features. The chest film shows patchy consolidation, generally in the lower lung fields.

Hospital-acquired pneumonia Because of changes in oropharyngeal flora with hospitalization, hospital-acquired pneumonias, unlike community-acquired ones, are likely to be due to a wide variety of aerobic gram-negative bacilli with varying antimicrobial susceptibilities and, less frequently, *S. aureus.* Only rarely is it possible to distinguish among pneumonias caused by different species of gram-negative rods on the basis of the clinical or roentgenographic features. Adequate sputum Gram's stains and cultures, therefore, are especially important in defining the etiologic agent and suggesting the appropriate antibiotic therapy.

Hospitalized patients with endotracheal tubes or tracheostomies receiving mechanical ventilation are an important group in whom the diagnosis of pneumonia is particularly difficult to make. Shortly after intubation, the tracheobronchial tree becomes colonized with organisms, and a purulent tracheobronchitis commonly ensues. Even though there is purulent sputum with plentiful organisms, this tracheobronchitis requires no antimicrobial therapy, which only encourages the growth of drug-resistant organisms, unless pneumonia is present. The diagnosis of pneumonia requires evidence of parenchymal lung involvement and in this setting depends upon the presence of purulent tracheobronchial secretions *plus* fever, leukocytosis, and a new or progressive pulmonary infiltrate on chest films.

TREATMENT Community-acquired pneumonia Patients whose history or physical examination suggests the likelihood of pneumonia should have a chest roentgenogram to confirm the diagnosis and delineate the pattern and extent of pulmonary involvement. Most patients with mild to moderate disease on clinical and radiologic assessment can be treated as outpatients. In them, a white blood cell count may be useful in the differential diagnosis, but routine blood cultures and arterial blood gases are unnecessary. The clinical and radiographic features and the sputum Gram stain should dictate the choice of antimicrobial therapy. If sputum is unobtainable or unhelpful and the other information inconclusive, erythromycin is a good choice. It is effective against pneumococci and *M. pneumoniae,* the two most frequent causes of community-acquired pneumonia, but also should be satisfactory to treat Legionnaires' disease, *H. influenzae* pneumonia, and most anaerobic pneumonias. Auxiliary measures should include adequate hydration, analgesics to relieve chest pain, if present, and cough suppressants for those with the harassing, unproductive cough characteristic of *M. pneumoniae.* In patients with good clinical improvement, a repeat chest film after 4 to 6 weeks is appropriate to document radiographic resolution.

Indications for hospitalization include severe dyspnea or hypoxemia; evidence of empyema or extrapulmonary foci of infections, such as meningitis; shock; serious underlying disease, especially cardiac or pulmonary; severe systemic manifestations such as delirium; or social circumstances making treatment at home unfeasible. These patients should have two blood cultures obtained from separate venipuncture sites; a complete blood count, including white blood cell differential; and arterial blood gas measurements if there is marked tachypnea, severe dyspnea, altered mental status potentially attributable to hypoxemia, cyanosis, or serious underlying cardiopulmonary disease. The clinical and radiographic features and, especially, the sputum Gram's stain should indicate the proper antibiotic choice. Since the most common community-acquired pneumonia requiring hospitalization is pneumococcal, the appropriate agent usually is penicillin. If the sputum smear is unsatisfactory or unobtainable by expectoration or nasotracheal suctioning, transtracheal aspiration may be indicated, particularly if the patient has an underlying illness like alcoholism that makes gram-negative pneumonia more likely.

Auxiliary measures include adequate hydration, the administration of humidified oxygen, relief of chest pain by adequate analgesics, and the encouragement of coughing to expectorate sputum. Intermittent positive pressure breathing (IPPB), however, is not helpful, and postural drainage should generally be reserved for those with bronchiectasis or lung abscess. Mechanical ventilation is required when the diffuseness of the pneumonia or the severity of underlying cardiopulmonary disease prevents adequate oxygenation with spontaneous respiration and supplemental oxygen by mask or nasal prongs.

Hospital-acquired pneumonia Since the range of organisms causing hospital-acquired pneumonias is so wide and their antimicrobial susceptibilities so variable, precise bacteriologic diagnosis is crucial. Patients with hospital-acquired pneumonias should have blood cultures, and vigorous attempts must be made to obtain sputum by expectoration, nasotracheal suctioning, or, if these are unsuccessful, transtracheal aspiration. When gram-negative rods are the predominant organism on Gram's stain, an aminoglycoside effective against *Pseudomonas aeruginosa,* like gentamicin or carbenicillin, should be given. If gram-positive cocci resembling *S. aureus* are present, a penicillinase-resistant penicillin is appropriate. If a mixture of these organisms is present or no sputum is obtainable, a combination of an aminoglycoside plus a penicillinase-resistant penicillin or a cephalosporin is a good choice. The regimen should be altered later according to the identity and susceptibility of the organisms isolated. If the sputum smear reveals organisms characteristic of pneumococci, anaerobes, or *H. influenzae*, which sometimes cause nosocomial pneumonias, the appropriate therapy for these organisms recommended in Chap. 111 should be given.

Pneumonia in compromised hosts (see also Chap. 107) Compromised hosts with pneumonia require special consideration. Patients who are severely neutropenic from acute leukemia or from cytotoxic agents generally develop pneumonia from aerobic gram-negative bacilli. Unless the Gram's stains strongly indicate otherwise, these patients should receive an aminoglycoside effective against *P. aeruginosa* and either carbenicillin or ticarcillin until the culture results return.

In severely immunosuppressed patients without neutropenia, the possible causes of fever and a new pulmonary infiltrate are legion. They fall into four categories: (1) the disease itself, such as Hodgkin's disease of the lung; (2) the effects of treatment, such as radiation pneumonitis or pulmonary toxicity from agents like methotrexate; (3) infections; and (4) miscellaneous disorders such as pulmonary emboli and intrapulmonary hemorrhage. Possible infectious causes include not only bacteria but also fungi, like *Candida* or *Aspergillus*; viruses, especially cytomegalovirus; and protozoa, particularly *Pneumocystis carinii* (Chap. 204). In these patients unless the initial evaluation, including sputum smears and blood cultures, strongly indicates a specific diagnosis, lung tissue, obtained by bronchoscopic biopsy, transthoracic needle biopsy, or, preferably, open-lung biopsy is necessary for definitive diagnosis. Empiric treatment with an assortment of antimicrobial agents in the absence of a specific diagnosis is usually unwise.

LUNG ABSCESS

DEFINITION A lung abscess is a necrotic area of lung parenchyma containing purulent material. An etiologic classification appears in Table 260-1.

PATHOGENESIS The pathogenesis of lung abscesses is nearly identical to that of pneumonia as discussed earlier in this chapter. Most arise from the aspiration of naso- or oropharyngeal contents. The development of a lung abscess, instead of just pneumonia, depends upon the infecting organism's ability to

TABLE 260-1
Classification of lung abscesses according to cause

I Necrotizing infections
  A Pyogenic bacteria (*S. aureus, Klebsiella,* group A streptococcus, *Bacteroides, Fusobacterium,* anaerobic and microaerophilic cocci and streptococci, other anaerobes, *Nocardia*)
  B Mycobacteria (Mycobacterium tuberculosis, M. kansasii, M. intracellularis)
  C Fungi (*Histoplasma, Coccidioides*)
  D Parasites (amoebas, lung flukes)
II Cavitary infarction
  A Bland embolism
  B Septic embolism (various anerobes, *Staphylococcus, Candida*)
  C Vasculitis (Wegener's granulomatosis, periarteritis)
III Cavitary malignancy
  A Primary bronchogenic carcinoma
  B Metastatic malignancies (very uncommon)
IV Other
  A Infected cysts
  B Necrotic conglomerate lesions (silicosis, coal miner's pneumoconiosis)

cause necrosis of lung tissue. Pneumococci, *H. influenzae, M. pneumoniae,* and viruses rarely cause necrosis, but it is common in pulmonary infections due to *K. pneumoniae* and other enteric gram-negative bacilli, *S. aureus,* and *S. pyogenes.* Anaerobic organisms are the most frequent cause of pyogenic lung abscesses and tend to occur when large quantities of oropharyngeal material are aspirated because of disordered consciousness or impaired swallowing.

Less frequently, abscesses arise from hematogenous spread of organisms to the lung. This may occur during bacteremia originating from a distant site of infection or as a result of septic emboli either from right-sided endocarditis or from septic thrombophlebitis associated with infections in the extremities or the abdominal cavity.

Patients with tuberculosis (Chap. 143), pulmonary fungal infections (Chaps. 150 to 161), and pleuropulmonary amebiasis (Chap. 199) may develop one or more areas of lung necrosis. Although usually labeled "cavities," these lesions are really abscesses. While the clinical course typically distinguishes these conditions from pyogenic lung abscess, there may be many similarities that cause confusion in the differential diagnosis.

CLINICAL MANIFESTATIONS Anaerobic lung abscess The clinical features of pulmonary infections due to staphylococci, streptococci, and aerobic gram-negative bacilli are discussed earlier in this chapter and in the chapters dealing with the specific organisms. These are usually acute, rapidly progressive infections.

While the spectrum of illness in anaerobic lung abscess may vary from a mild productive cough to acute disease with severe systemic manifestations, the onset is usually insidious, with the disease gradually worsening over several weeks. The most common feature is a cough productive of moderate to large amounts of purulent sputum that is often fetid and bloody. Fever, pleuritic or dull chest pain, dyspnea, weakness, anorexia, and weight loss, which can be considerable, are common. A condition predisposing to aspiration, such as alcoholism or epilepsy, is usually present.

Most patients are febrile. Oral examination usually discloses poor dentition, with caries, gingivitis, and periodontal infection, conditions which increase the number of anaerobes in the oral cavity. The chest examination may be normal or may include signs of consolidation, rales, and, occasionally, amphoric or cavernous breath sounds over the involved area. Patients with an associated empyema may have dullness to percussion and decreased breath sounds. Clubbing, although uncommon, may occur. Neutrophilic leukocytosis with an increase in immature forms is usual, and, if the infection has persisted for several weeks, anemia and hypoalbuminemia may be present. The medical history, physical findings, and routine laboratory results are often nonspecific; foul-smelling sputum present in about half the patients, however, clearly indicates an anaerobic pulmonary infection. Definitive diagnosis rests on the demonstration of an abscess cavity on chest films and the identification of the causative organisms on culture.

The chest roentgenogram reveals an area of consolidation containing a radiolucency. Not all radiolucent areas are abscess, however, and either a wall or a border completely surrounding the lucent area or a fluid level within it should be present to diagnose an abscess cavity. Even these criteria are not definitive, since infected bullae or cysts or an empyema with a bronchopleural fistula may have an identical appearance. The location of the abscess cavities is in those segments that are most dependent at the time of aspiration: the posterior segment of the upper or superior segment of the lower lobes, especially on the right, when the patient is supine or the basilar segments of the lower lobes when upright.

Examination of the sputum by both microscopy and culture is essential to establish the correct diagnosis. In staphylococcal and aerobic gram-negative bacillary infections, the single causative organism clearly predominates on smear and culture. Gram's stain of sputum from an anaerobic abscess reveals abundant neutrophils and numerous organisms, including gram-positive cocci and rods and gram-negative rods of varying size and configuration. Since expectorated sputum is unavoidably contaminated by the normal anaerobic oral flora, anaerobic sputum cultures are appropriate only for specimens obtained by transtracheal or transthoracic aspiration. Secretions aspirated through the fiberoptic bronchoscope are unsuitable because the instrument is contaminated as it passes through the naso- or oropharynx, even with preceding endotracheal intubation. Appropriately collected and cultured sputum specimens usually grow two or more anaerobic organisms, most commonly *Peptococcus, Peptostreptococcus, Fusobacterium nucleatumi,* and *Bacteroides melaninogenicus.* In about 60 percent of cases the infecting flora is exclusively anaerobic; in 40 percent both aerobes and anaerobes are present. The most common aerobic isolates are *S. aureus* and enteric gram-negative bacilli.

Associated pleural effusions should be aspirated and cultured aerobically and anaerobically. Blood cultures are usually sterile.

Septic pulmonary emboli In patients with septic pulmonary emboli, the site of origin is usually tricuspid valve endocarditis, particularly in heroin addicts, or septic thrombophlebitis, which may occur in the arm veins of patients with infected intravenous catheter sites, infected injection sites from intravenous drug abuse, or infected arteriovenous shunts used in hemodialysis. Other areas of septic thrombophlebitis include pelvic veins with postpartum or postoperative pelvic infections, peritonsillar and internal jugular veins with pharyngeal infections, and veins adjacent to undrained suppuration, such as soft tissue infections or osteomyelitis. Rigors, high fever, dyspnea, cough, tachycardia, and tachypnea are the major clinical manifestations in these acutely ill patients. Neutrophilic leukocytosis is usual. The chest film typically discloses multiple, bilateral, round, or wedge-shaped opacities. These frequently and rapidly excavate to form thin-walled cavities, often without fluid levels. Blood cultures are usually positive. Patients may not produce sputum, but if they do, it usually reveals the responsible organism, most commonly *S. aureus,* on Gram's stain and culture.

TREATMENT The history, physical examination, chest roentgenograms, and most importantly, Gram's and acid-fast sputum stains usually indicate whether an abscess is caused by aerobic organisms, anaerobes, or tubercle bacilli. Abscesses caused by aerobic organisms or tubercle bacilli should be treated according to the recommendations outlined in the chapters dealing with them.

Where septic pulmonary emboli from septic thrombophlebitis are suspected, it is important not only to institute appropriate antimicrobial therapy but also to identify the source. Removal of catheters, incision and drainage of systemic abscesses or infected veins, or ligation of the inferior vena cava may be necessary to prevent further embolization.

When the clinical findings and the sputum Gram's stain suggest an anaerobic abscess, penicillin is the drug of choice. It is usually given intravenously in doses of 5 to 10 million units daily until clinical improvement (return of appetite, defervescence) occurs. Oral penicillin in doses of about 500 mg four times daily is then given for the duration of therapy. Some clinicians use oral medication from the start. Penicillin is effective in virtually all cases, even when *B. fragilis,* which is resistant in vitro to penicillin, is isolated as part of the anaerobic flora. It is also effective when there is a mixture of aerobic and anaerobic organisms. Alternative agents for penicillin-allergic patients or the rare case that fails to respond to penicillin are clindamycin and chloramphenicol. Because of relapses with shorter courses, antibiotics are usually given for at least 6 weeks. The optimal duration of therapy is unknown, but some clinicians continue treatment until the chest roentgenogram is clear or shows a stable residual lesion.

Ancillary measures include postural drainage and chest physiotherapy to help drain the abscess cavity. The role of bronchoscopy is unsettled. Some physicians believe that every patient with a lung abscess deserves bronchoscopy; others reserve its use for patients who fail to respond as anticipated to antibiotic therapy, who have evidence of an obstructing tumor or foreign body, or who have poorly communicating cavities that fail to drain adequately.

Except for the tube thoracostomy drainage of an associated empyema, surgery for lung abscess is rarely necessary. Incomplete roentgenographic resolution is not a sufficient reason for resectional surgery since delayed closure is common. Resection is indicated for massive hemoptysis, malignancy, or associated symptomatic bronchiectasis. Rarely, tube thoracostomy or some other form of surgical drainage may be necessary to manage uncontrolled sepsis arising from a poorly draining abscess.

REFERENCES

Pneumonia

BARTLETT JG, FINEGOLD SM: Anaerobic infections of the lung and pleural space. Am Rev Respir Dis 110:56, 1974
FRASER RG, PARE JAP: *Diagnosis of Diseases of the Chest.* Philadelphia, Saunders, 1978, vol II, chap 6
GREEN GM et al: Defense mechanisms of the respiratory membrane. Ann Rev Respir Dis 115:479, 1977
KNIGHT V: *Viral and Mycoplasmal Infections of the Respiratory Tract.* Philadelphia, Lea & Febiger, 1973, chaps 5, 6, 14
PIERCE AK, SANFORD JP: Aerobic gram-negative bacillary pneumonias. Am Rev Respir Dis 110:647, 1974

Lung abscess

BARNETT TB, HERRING CL: Lung abscess: Initial and late results of medical therapy. Arch Intern Med 127:217, 1971
BARTLETT JG et al: Bacteriology and treatment of primary lung abscess. Am Rev Respir Dis 109:510, 1974
———, FINEGOLD SM: Anaerobic infections of the lung and pleural space. Am Rev Respir Dis 110:56, 1974

261
BRONCHIECTASIS AND BRONCHOLITHIASIS

JOHN F. MURRAY

These disorders both involve branches of the tracheobronchial system, have numerous, rather than single, underlying causes, and occasionally coexist. However, the pathogenesis, clinical manifestations, treatment, and prognosis of the two conditions are remarkably different.

BRONCHIECTASIS

DEFINITION Bronchiectasis can be defined as a permanent abnormal dilatation of one or more large (greater than 2 mm in diameter) bronchi due to destruction of the elastic and muscular components of the bronchial wall. This definition is not completely satisfactory because bronchi are also abnormally dilated in chronic bronchitis. Thus chronic bronchitis merges into bronchiectasis, and the distinction between them depends upon the *degree* of dilatation. The semantic problem is complicated further by the fact that the two conditions frequently coexist.

Classification is therefore difficult and is not useful in indicating the clinical severity of the disease; however, certain descriptive terms are commonly used to describe the appearance of bronchi displayed by bronchography. *Saccular (cystic) bronchiectasis* occurs mainly in the proximal large bronchi; affected airways show marked dilatation ending in large sacs at about the fourth bronchial division. *Cylindrical (fusiform) bronchiectasis* involves airways from the sixth to the tenth generation; the bronchographic appearance shows mild to moderate uneven widening, without a great increase in diameter, of bronchi that often look beaded and end squarely and abruptly. *Varicose bronchiectasis* is intermediate between saccular and cylindrical changes and is used to describe bronchi that resemble varicose veins. Saccular, varicose, and cylindrical bronchiectasis represent stages in a continuum of involvement, and all three may be present in the same patient.

Although "true" bronchiectasis is not reversible, the concept of reversibility is an important one, because abnormalities displayed by bronchography in some patients with reversible lung diseases (atelectasis, tracheobronchitis) may simulate bronchiectasis. Atelectasis causes shortening and tortuosity of airways in the involved region, producing an accordion-like appearance on bronchography. Similarly, ulcerations of the bronchial mucosa, which are common in viral infections of the lower respiratory tract, appear as an irregular pattern on bronchography. Both conditions resemble cylindrical bronchiectasis. Reexpansion of the collapsed lung and/or regeneration of the epithelium results in reversibility of the "pseudobronchiectasis." Thus bronchography, if indicated, should be delayed for several months after an episode of tracheobronchitis, pneumonia, or atelectasis.

PATHOGENESIS Since bronchiectasis is defined by the presence of morphologic changes in the caliber of large bronchi, its pathogenesis depends on antecedent factors that either cause or lead to necrosis of the bronchial wall and supporting tissues. The origin of the destructive process is nearly always a bacterial infection, but other factors—hereditary, congenital, or mechanical—may also be present that predispose to the development of the infection. The infection may be a primary event, such as suppurative necrotizing pneumonia, or it may be secondary to local or systemic abnormalities that impair defense mechanisms (i.e., cellular, humoral, and clearance) and promote bacterial growth. Now, because the use of vaccines and antibiotic drugs has resulted in a marked decline in the incidence of severe necrotizing pneumonias and their bronchiectatic complications, this sequence is infrequently encountered; however, bronchiectasis as a complication of underlying systemic disorders appears to be increasing.

Hereditary and congenital factors Several hereditary and congenital disorders have been identified in which there is a high incidence of secondary bronchiectasis. *Congenital bronchiectasis* occurs at the site of a pre- or postnatal development defect of the bronchial system. The formation of cysts, cul-de-sacs, or bronchomalacia leads to pooling of secretions and bacterial infection. The generalized disorder of exocrine gland secretions in patients with *cystic fibrosis,* discussed in Chap. 262, affects the physical properties of tracheobronchial mucus and/or the adequacy of mucociliary clearance; this causes retention of secretions, with partial or complete plugging of airways, that provides a nidus for implantation and growth of bacteria. Most deaths (95 percent) of patients with cystic fibrosis who survive beyond 1 year of age are now caused by the consequences of chronic bronchopulmonary suppuration. The diffuse bronchiectasis rarely encountered with patients with *atopic bronchial asthma,* in whom there is often a strong familial association (Chap. 257), presumably is related to diffuse obstruction, as described below.

A variety of hereditary *immune-deficiency diseases,* secondary to either cellular or humoral defects, is associated with a high incidence of bacterial infections. Involvement of the sinuses and airways is particularly common, and the tendency for infections to recur in the lower airways often leads to bronchiectasis in patients with impaired immunologic mechanisms.

A newly designated group of genetically determined disorders called the *immotile cilia syndrome,* which includes *Kartagener's syndrome* (bronchiectasis, dextrocardia, and sinusitis) is characterized by ultrastructural changes causing immotility of cilia in the respiratory tract epithelium, sperm, and other cells. These abnormalities lead to recurrent sinopulmonary infections, infertility, and presumably disturbances during embryogenesis. The high incidence of unexplained bronchiectasis in Eskimo families and in the Maoris of New Zealand may also be hereditary in origin.

Obstruction Postobstructive bronchiectasis was much commoner in preantibiotic years than it is today. The availability of antimicrobial therapy and corrective surgical procedures accounts for the decreased incidence in this form of the disease. It is now recognized that obstruction per se does *not cause* bronchiectasis but *favors its development* by impairing clearance mechanisms, which enhances bacterial infection. Any process that leads to bronchial obstruction, therefore, may be associated with bronchiectasis distal to the site of involvement. Since the disorders causing obstruction are usually confined to one part of the bronchial system, postobstructive bronchiectasis is of the localized rather than the diffuse variety found in most forms of congenital-hereditary bronchiectasis. An exception is the bronchiectasis associated with diffuse obstruction of airways in patients with chronic bronchitis, atopic asthma, and cystic fibrosis. Patients with atopic asthma are liable to have secondary infections with *Aspergillus,* which produces the syndrome of bronchopulmonary aspergillosis characterized by proximal airway bronchiectasis, eosinophilia, and recurrent bouts of mucous plugging (Chap. 257).

Endobronchial tumors or foreign bodies, compression of airways from enlarged hilar lymph nodes or tumor masses, and bronchostenosis from endobronchial inflammatory disease (especially tuberculosis) all cause bronchial obstruction and may favor the development of postobstructive bronchiectasis.

Necrotizing inflammation Virtually all forms of bronchiectasis are associated with bacterial infections. Other causative factors may be present, such as hereditary disorders and bronchial obstruction, that predispose the patient to secondary bacterial involvement, but bronchiectasis can occur as the result of necrotizing infections in a previously healthy individual. This presumably is the mechanism underlying the bronchiectasis that follows tuberculosis and the staphylococcal or other suppurative pneumonias that occasionally complicate measles, pertussis, adenovirus infections, and influenza.

In rare instances, bronchiectasis may follow the introduction of corrosive chemical substances, commonly hydrocarbons, into the tracheobronchial tree. Similarly, the repeated aspiration of gastric fluid into the lungs may cause bronchiectasis. Since ulceration from chemical causes is invariably associated with secondary bacterial infection, it is difficult to dissociate the contributions of these two factors.

CLINICAL MANIFESTATIONS The signs and symptoms of bronchiectasis depend on the extent, severity, location, and presence of complications of the disease, but the hallmarks of the disease are chronic cough with sputum production, hemoptysis, and recurrent pneumonia. Even these vary greatly in frequency and severity and may be absent if the disease is mild or involves only the upper lobes of the lung.

The most frequent symptom is a *chronic cough* that produces sputum. The amount of sputum varies considerably but may be voluminous and is apt to be purulent during bouts of intercurrent infections. Streaks of blood in the sputum are common, and frank hemoptysis of large amounts of blood may develop if necrosis of the mucosa is severe. Exacerbation of chronic bronchial infection is frequent and may progress to pneumonia, occasionally with lung abscess or empyema formation. Associated systemic features of bronchiectasis are fever, weight loss, anemia, and weakness; these usually indicate the presence of active sepsis from severe disease or untreated intercurrent bacterial infection.

In what was once the typical patient with bronchiectasis, symptoms develop during infancy or early childhood; the onset is usually acute and follows suppurative pneumonia or pulmonary infection complicating measles or pertussis. However, because of the success of antimicrobials and vaccines in treating or preventing these disorders, acute onset of bronchiectasis at an early age is becoming infrequent, except in those areas of the United States and other countries where, owing to isolation or poverty, good medical care is not available.

Although chronic childhood bronchiectasis is decreasing, another group of patients with a different form of the disease appears to be increasing: these patients have recurrent lower respiratory tract infections that initially respond to treatment, with symptom-free intervals between episodes. The infections usually begin during childhood or young adulthood. As the number of recurrent bouts increases, the time between them tends to shorten and the response to treatment becomes less complete. Finally, chronic symptoms of cough and sputum develop. Patients in this category are likely to have cystic fibrosis, immune-deficiency diseases, or atopic asthma.

Sinusitis is a common accompaniment of diffuse bronchiectasis and may be an expression of the vulnerability of the entire respiratory tract in these patients. Development of digital clubbing, metastatic abscesses (often brain), and amyloidosis were common complications in the past but are less frequent now. If the disease is widespread, it may resemble other forms of chronic obstructive lung disease, with generalized wheezing and ultimate progression to cor pulmonale; this constellation is particularly apt to occur in patients with underlying systemic abnormalities that lead to diffuse pulmonary involvement.

DIAGNOSIS Bronchiectasis is defined as a morphologic disorder; hence its diagnosis depends on demonstrating the abnormal anatomy of the bronchial system. Ordinarily this is accomplished by roentgenographic techniques, usually *bronchography*. The diagnosis should be *suspected* in any patient with chronic productive cough, especially if the sputum intermittently becomes more purulent and streaked with blood. Physical examination seldom reveals the severity and extent of distribution of the disease. Inspiratory rales are often the only evidence of pulmonary involvement. Occasionally, advanced cases of saccular bronchiectasis can be diagnosed by routine (plain) chest roentgenography; in such cases multiple 1- to 2-cm cystic lesions or fluid levels in poorly delineated sacs can be

seen. More often, however, plain chest roentgenograms show only streaky infiltrations and loss of volume in involved areas; at times the chest x-rays may appear completely normal.

Bronchography (Chap. 256) should not be performed routinely in all patients with suggestive symptoms, but is indicated primarily in the evaluation of patients for possible operation, those with recurrent, localized pneumonias or severe hemoptysis. Since the information from bronchography contributes little to the management of patients in whom surgery is contraindicated, such as those with minimal disability, with generalized involvement, or with obstructive airways disease, the procedure should be avoided in these patients because of its hazards. When bronchography is indicated, it should not be performed in patients during exacerbations of their cough and sputum production, but only after the manifestations have been thoroughly treated (see next section) and the volume of secretions is minimal. Postural drainage and vigorous tracheobronchial toilet help to prepare patients with copious secretions for bronchography. It is safer and advisable to study one lung at a time, owing to alterations in pulmonary function and to occasional inflammatory reactions induced by the procedure. Filling must be adequate and all segments must be visualized if the study is to be considered satisfactory for diagnostic purposes.

Bronchoscopy does not establish the diagnosis of bronchiectasis but may be useful in identifying the source of secretions in patients with cough and sputum and in determining the site of bleeding in patients with hemoptysis.

All patients with multiple episodes of sinopulmonary infections should have an immunologic survey to detect immune-deficiency diseases. Similarly, patients with suspected cystic fibrosis should have measurements of the concentrations of sodium and chloride in two or more samples of sweat (Chap. 262). Electron photomicrographic studies of sperm or mucosal biopsies from the respiratory tract reveal characteristic abnormalities in patients with the immotile cilia syndrome. Patients with asthma and suspected bronchiectasis from bronchopulmonary aspergillosis should have sputum cultures for *Aspergillus* and serologic studies for aspergillin precipitins.

The sputum volume, color, cellular content, and bacterial inhabitants are useful guides to the presence of active infection. During exacerbations of the disease, the sputum increases in volume, becomes more purulent, and contains large numbers of polymorphonuclear leukocytes and bacteria that can be identified by Gram's stain. Culture of the sputum often reveals normal nasopharyngeal flora and, less commonly, *Diplococcus pneumoniae* or *Hemophilus influenzae*. Fetid sputum signifies the presence of anaerobic microorganisms. Sputum from patients receiving prolonged or frequent treatment with broad-spectrum antibiotic drugs may grow *Staphylococcus* species or *Pseudomonas aeruginosa;* this finding is especially common in patients with cystic fibrosis.

The blood count is apt to be within the normal range but may reveal anemia, reflecting chronic infection, or leukocytosis, signifying active suppuration. The urinalysis is normal except in the rare instances of *amyloidosis,* when proteinuria occurs. The electrocardiogram is normal until the late stages, when *cor pulmonale* may supervene. Owing to the wide variations in the extent and severity of the disease, only broad generalizations about pulmonary function abnormalities are possible, although a correlation exists between the overall impairment of lung function and the number of involved segments. Vital capacity and expiratory flow rates tend to be reduced but may be within normal limits if the disease is mild. In the late stages of diffuse bronchiectasis, functional abnormalities similar to those of emphysema are found, except that the total lung capacity is usually reduced. A mild to moderate reduction in arterial oxygen tension (P_{O_2}) reflects regional abnormalities in the distribution of ventilation with respect to perfusion. Mismatching of ventilation and perfusion is the physiologic hallmark of bronchiectasis and can now be examined in regions of the lung by the use of radioactive gases, e.g., ^{133}Xe (Chap. 255). Pulmonary function studies are helpful in defining the extent and severity of abnormalities, in assessing the effects of therapy, and in evaluating patients for surgery.

TREATMENT Since bacterial infections are associated with most forms of bronchiectasis initially and are responsible for its exacerbation, antibiotics are the major weapons for its prevention and treatment. The choice of antimicrobial agents should be guided by the results of sputum culture; however, as indicated, these may reveal "normal flora" and no conspicuous pathogen. The drug of choice for patients with this finding is ampicillin; patients allergic to the penicillins usually respond to one of the tetracyclines. When pneumococci are present, it is best to avoid the tetracycline drugs, as some pneumococcal strains are resistant to these agents. Antibiotics should be given until sputum production becomes minimal and purulence disappears; this desirable therapeutic result is usually achieved swiftly (5 to 7 days) if antibiotics are started early in the course of an exacerbation—as soon as the patient's cough increases and becomes productive of sputum in greater quantity and purulence than customary—but much longer periods are required if the infection is well established. Antibiotics should be administered either orally or by injection, *not* by nebulization (owing to failure of delivery, inactivation of the antibiotic, and risk of sensitization).

Adjuvant medical measures are of great benefit in diminishing the consequences of bronchiectasis. Postural drainage and physical therapy facilitate removal of secretions. The treatment regimen depends on the location of the disease segments and is best administered under the supervision of a skilled respiratory physical therapist. Bronchodilators, expectorants, and humidifiers are of questionable value in many patients but are useful in those with bronchospasm or thick tenacious sputum. The need for expectorants can be reduced if the patient maintains a good fluid intake and stays well hydrated. Fiberoptic bronchoscopy is useful in identifying sites of endobronchial disease (Chap. 256) and sources of secretions and hemoptysis and permits removal of secretions by aspiration under direct vision. Repeated bronchoscopies are helpful in the management of the unusual patient with problems of sputum retention. Similarly, bronchial lavage has been tried as a "last resort" in patients with large volumes of inspissated secretions. Oxygen should be given to patients with hypoxia during acute exacerbations; it can be administered outside the hospital to patients who are severely and chronically hypoxic. Inflammation from any cause will aggravate the effects of chronic bronchiectasis; therefore, smoking should be prohibited, exposure to air which is excessively polluted should be avoided, and influenza and pneumococcal vaccines should be administered yearly.

Resectional surgery, once the mainstay of treatment, is used far less often now than previously for two reasons: (1) medical management is very effective in controlling bronchiectasis and preventing disability from it; (2) many patients with bronchiectasis have a generalized disorder that makes their entire tracheobronchial system vulnerable; although their bronchiectasis may appear well localized when evaluated initially, new

sites of involvement may appear later. Operation should be considered in patients with localized (i.e., resectable) lesions who do not respond to medical management or who are sufficiently disabled by complications so that either their livelihood or their emotional life is impaired. Bouts of hemoptysis, especially if massive, and recurrent localized pneumonias are the usual complications that require hospitalization, cause repeated disability, and indicate the need for surgery.

PREVENTION The best approach to bronchiectasis is prevention. Patients with heritable diseases that predispose to bronchiectasis and their families should obtain genetic counseling to minimize the incidence of these disorders. Prompt diagnosis and effective antimicrobial treatment of bacterial infections of the lower respiratory tract constitute the best way of avoiding their potential chronic sequelae. The eradication of measles and pertussis by vaccines should eliminate these diseases as harbingers of bronchiectasis.

Prompt removal of foreign bodies, tumors, and other causes of bronchial obstruction should diminish postobstructive bronchiectasis.

BRONCHOLITHIASIS

Broncholiths, or bronchial stones, occur when calcified particles in a lymph node or the lung parenchyma erode into a contiguous bronchus. Broncholithiasis, therefore, is a secondary complication of an antecedent disease that has resulted in residual intrathoracic calcifications. Numerous disorders leave calcified deposits that can be detected by chest roentgenography, but clinically significant broncholithiasis is rare. It is usually a late complication of one of the three common granulomatous infections: tuberculosis, histoplasmosis, and coccidioidomycosis. Of these, histoplasmosis has the greatest tendency to heal with multiple residual calcifications, and coccidioidomycosis has the least; hence broncholithiasis in the United States, especially in the Central and Eastern regions, is most likely to be related to previous infection with *Histoplasma capsulatum*.

The clinical consequences of broncholithiasis are related to the movement of stones through the airway wall and their release into the lumen. The process of erosion is often accompanied by paroxysms of cough, intermittent hemoptysis, and bronchopulmonary infection. The overlying inflammatory reaction impairs bronchial clearance and narrows the lumen; these conditions may lead to distal bronchiectasis or, if the obstruction is complete, atelectasis. The hallmark of broncholithiasis is the coughing and expectoration of chalky sediment, sandy (gritty) particles, or stones. Such episodes are usually single but may be multiple.

Broncholithiasis should be suspected in any patient with recurrent cough and hemoptysis whose chest roentgenograms show multiple calcifications in the lung and/or mediastinal lymph nodes. The diagnosis can be established by recovering stones in the sputum, by visualizing broncholiths penetrating the bronchial wall at the time of bronchoscopy, or by establishing that calcified particles have disappeared on serial chest x-ray films. Tomography may be helpful in determining with greater precision than routine roentgenograms the presence and location of calcifications in and around bronchi.

Treatment depends on the magnitude of the symptoms. The disorder is self-limiting once the stone has eroded into the lumen and is coughed up; however, ulceration of the particle may be slow and attended by significant symptoms. Antimicrobial agents are useful in the treatment of associated bacterial infection. Bronchoscopy should be performed and the stone removed if possible. At times, thoracotomy and lung resection are necessary, usually for obstructive complications or massive hemoptysis.

REFERENCES

Bronchiectasis

BASS H et al: Regional structure and function in bronchiectasis: A correlative study using bronchography and [133]Xe. Am Rev Respir Dis 97:598, 1968

CROFTON J: Diagnosis and treatment of bronchiectasis: I. Diagnosis. II. Treatment and prevention. Br Med J 1:721, 783, 1966

ELIASSON R et al: The immotile-cilia syndrome: A congenital ciliary abnormality as an etiologic factor in chronic airway infections and male sterility. N Engl J Med 297:1, 1977

FIELD CE: Bronchiectasis: Third report on a follow-up study of medical and surgical cases from childhood. Arch Dis Child 44:551, 1969

SHWACHMAN H et al: Cystic fibrosis: A new outlook. 70 patients above 25 years of age. Medicine 56:129, 1977

Broncholithiasis

ARRIGONI MG et al: Broncholithiasis. J Thorac Cardiovasc Surg 62:231, 1971

WEED LA, ANDERSEN HA: Etiology of broncholithiasis. Dis Chest 37:270, 1960

262
CYSTIC FIBROSIS

HARRY L. SHWACHMAN

DEFINITION Cystic fibrosis (CF) is an autosomal recessive disease characterized by abnormally thick secretions from mucous glands, pancreatic insufficiency in approximately 80 percent of patients and a three- to fivefold increase in the concentration of sodium and chloride in sweat. The main clinical features are related to the dysfunction of the pancreas and to a chronic, diffuse, obstructive pulmonary process. Although the disease is commonly diagnosed and treated by the pediatrician, an increasing number of patients survive to or are diagnosed for the first time in adulthood.

ETIOLOGY AND EPIDEMIOLOGY The disease occurs predominantly in Caucasians with a frequency of 1 in 1600 births. The gene frequency in the Caucasian population is 1 in 20. It is only one-tenth as common in Negroes. Although both sexes are equally affected, males survive longer than females. In the past cystic fibrosis was considered a fatal disease of infancy and childhood. As a result of early diagnosis and the detection of mild cases combined with improved methods of treatment, the life expectancy has increased from approximately 2 years in 1948 to 19 years at present.

There is no reliable test to detect the heterozygote, although many studies offer the promise that this might be accomplished in the near future. The etiology of this disease remains obscure and there is a considerable body of conflicting reports in the literature. Many investigators believe that there is a "CF factor," in the form of an abnormal α_2 macroglobulin complex, in serum which characterizes the disease. The absence of an isoenzyme of arginine esterase has been detected. The transport of electrolytes is abnormal, and the defect in the sweat glands is due to a substance that inhibits sodium transport within the lumen of the duct. The chemical composition of the mucus secreted by the various glands may reveal minor differences

from the normal in that the ratio of fucose to sialic acid differs. One group of investigators suspects this to be a disorder of lysosomes, in spite of the fact that there is no appreciable accumulation of a metabolite within the cell. Studies utilizing cultured skin fibroblasts have yielded a great deal of information about differences in the biological behavior when compared with control cultures.

CLINICAL MANIFESTATIONS Cystic fibrosis has diverse clinical manifestations (Table 262-1). The initial manifestation occurs in the newborn in the form of meconium ileus, which occurs in approximately 10 percent of all cases of cystic fibrosis. When the intestinal obstruction is uncomplicated, the sticky meconium can be displaced by Gastrografin enemas. In the presence of complications such as volvulus, secondary atresia, or perforation, surgical correction is necessary. With rare exceptions survivors develop the typical clinical manifestations of the disease as they grow. The meconium in cystic fibrosis contains a high content of albumin and an increase in activity of lactase. These characteristics are used as signals in screening for cystic fibrosis in the neonate.

The early clinical findings include a rapid respiratory rate and a cough which often becomes persistent. At times the

TABLE 262-1
Principal clinical manifestations of cystic fibrosis

I Viscid secretions→small duct obstruction
  A Respiratory
    1 Sinusitis, nasal polyposis
    2 Atelectasis
    3 Emphysema
    4 Bronchitis, bronchopneumonia, bronchiectasis, lung abscess, aspergillosis
    5 Respiratory failure
    6 Cor pulmonale
II Intestinal
  A Meconium ileus
    1 Volvulus
    2 Peritonitis
    3 Ileal atresia
    4 Obstruction
  B Pancreas
    1 Nutritional failure due to pancreatic insufficiency
    2 Steatorrhea and creatorrhea
    3 Diabetes mellitus
    4 Vitamin deficiencies
    5 Loss of bile salts
III Hepatobiliary
  A Mucous hypersecretion
  B Atrophic gallbladder
  C Focal biliary cirrhosis
  D Laennec's cirrhosis
  E Hepar lobatum
  F Portal hypertension
  G Esophageal varices
  H Hypersplenism
IV Reproductive system
  A Males: sterility; absent vas deferens, epididymis, and seminal vesicles
  B Females: decreased fertility
V Skeletal
  A Retardation of bone age
  B Demineralization
VI Other
  A Salt depletion
  B Heat stroke
  C Salivary gland hypertrophy
  D Retinal hemorrhage
  E Hypertrophy of apocrine glands

SOURCE: *After H Shwachman, RJ Grand, in Gastrointestinal Disease, M Sleisenger, J Fordtran (eds), Philadelphia, Saunders, 1978.*

cough is paroxysmal and resembles pertussis. Failure to gain weight and the passage of large, frequent bowel movements accompanied by an excessive appetite are characteristic features in early life. Many gastrointestinal complications, including rectal prolapse, steatorrhea and creatorrhea, pot belly, hypoproteinemia, anemia and hypoprothrombinemia, growth retardation, and other features secondary to malabsorption can be avoided by prompt therapy.

Although the lungs are normal at birth, the pulmonary lesion may be progressive. The earliest defect is the elaboration of a thick mucus which results in either complete or partial obstruction of the bronchioles. Infection supervenes, but fever is rarely present. Patchy atelectasis, irregular aeration, and air trapping are seen on the chest x-ray. The infection persists and the initial flora, which usually includes *Staphylococcus aureus* is later replaced by gram-negative bacteria. *Pseudomonas aeruginosa* becomes the predominant inhabitant, and the smooth strain may soon be accompanied or replaced by a mucoid strain. Thus, *P. aeruginosa* and staphylococci, usually coagulase positive, are the predominant microorganisms isolated from the lungs post mortem. Other pathogens such as *Escherichia coli, Proteus,* and *Aspergillus* may also occur. The mucoid strain of *P. aeruginosa* is rarely encountered in other disease states.

The pulmonary complications include pneumonia, bronchiectasis, atelectasis, abscesses of varying sizes, empyema, pneumothorax, and hemoptysis. The immune response appears intact and bacteremia is rare, even in the presence of extensive pulmonary infection.

With longer survival of patients with cystic fibrosis new complications have been observed, and the clinical challenges of dealing with these patients consists in recognizing and treating these complications. Either a viral or a bacterial infection, or some environmental condition, sets off the process which leads to the pulmonary manifestations. There may be no increase in susceptibility to infection, but once the infection becomes established, it is apt to become more severe and prolonged. Death in cystic fibrosis is primarily due to the extensive pulmonary infection which leads to respiratory failure. *Cor pulmonale* is a common late complication. Pulmonary function tests combined with a clinical evaluation and chest roentgenograms provide an indication of the severity of the disease.

The *liver* reveals changes in approximately 10 percent of cases. It seldom accounts for jaundice in the neonatal period. The earliest change is a focal biliary cirrhosis; bile plugging and proliferation of the bile ductules are pathognomonic. The lesion may progress to a multilobular cirrhosis. Portal hypertension occurs in approximately 3 percent of patients, and this may be followed by hypersplenism. Most of these patients have pancreatic insufficiency. Portal hypertension has not been seen in the 20 percent of the CF population with persistent pancreatic function. Rarely, patients may present with portal hypertension as the initial complaint.

The *male genital tract* is of special importance in CF since the great majority of adult males (approximately 97 percent) are sterile, owing to structural defects in the Wolffian duct derivatives, the vas deferens, the seminal vesicles, and the epididymis. However, sexual function and secondary sex characteristics are normal. The female may be unable to become pregnant because of the increased viscosity of cervical mucus or the presence of a mucus cervical plug. The fertility rate is approximately one-fifth that of healthy women of the same age group. However, births to well over 120 women with CF have been recorded. The chances of having a baby with CF is 1 in 40 and three such cases have been recorded. The vast majority of babies have had normal sweat tests and are healthy; they are obligate heterozygotes.

A small group of patients have an incomplete expression of the disease. The major features are the typical pulmonary lesion, normal or borderline sweat electrolytes, sterility in the adult male, and minimal or no pancreatic disease.

DIAGNOSIS Clinical suspicion must be high to suggest this disease. A positive family history is helpful, but the most accurate diagnostic test for CF is the sweat test, which should be performed in a laboratory known for its accuracy. The level of sweat electrolytes does not reflect the severity of the disease. A variety of sweat tests is available but unfortunately many results are not reliable because of inaccuracy, lack of experience, or unstandardized procedures and equipment. The recommended procedure is the quantitative pilocarpine iontophoresis method, in which sweat from the forearm (stimulated by pilocarpine iontophoresis) is absorbed onto a weighed gauze pad, eluted, and the Na and Cl concentrations determined. This procedure requires approximately 40 min. The least amount of sweat for analysis should be 50 mg. Patients with CF should yield values of at least 65 meq per liter for both Na and Cl. In the presence of elevated sweat electrolytes in a patient who is symptomless and has a clear chest x-ray, the diagnosis of CF cannot be made. A positive sweat test does not establish a diagnosis, but will confirm the diagnosis in a patient with some of the clinical features of the disease.

The sweat test must be standardized, since one can achieve high electrolyte values by a variety of stimuli including exercise or exposure to heat or any method that produces a rapid sweat rate. Although the values for healthy adults are greater than those for healthy children, the quantitative pilocarpine procedure will identify the adult with CF. A number of procedures has been used, including the chloride ion electrode and conductivity methods. In expert hands these methods are valid and reproducible, but in the hands of the average technician, erratic results are very common. In view of the profound medical and personal implications of the diagnosis of CF, it should be made only with a great deal of circumspection, and a second sweat test is recommended for confirmation.

THERAPY Since the disease varies greatly from mild to severe, treatment must be individualized. The management of pancreatic insufficiency includes the use of a potent pancreatic preparation with each meal, such as pancreatin (Viokase) or pancrelipase (Cotazym), the reduction of fat in the diet, the liberal use of multivitamins, and a high caloric intake (Chap. 309). The use of added salt should be considered in hot weather, with fever, or whenever sweating is excessive. This will prevent heat exhaustion and salt depletion. In those patients with adequate pancreatic function no dietary restriction is necessary.

The management of the pulmonary disease includes postural drainage, an exercise program, and the use of antibiotics either singly or in combination to combat the pulmonary infection. Aerosols are also advocated in patients with early bronchiectasis; these include *N*-acetylcysteine (Mucomyst), neomycin or colistin, and isoproterenol (Isuprel). Bronchodilators may be used if there is evidence of bronchospasm.

Attention must be paid to the social, emotional, and financial aspects; and assistance through various agencies may be necessary. The cooperation of social workers, nutritionists, physical therapists, and nurses is important in the continuing care of these patients. Constant encouragement and education are essential.

REFERENCES

DI SANT'AGNESE PA, DAVIS PB: Research in cystic fibrosis. N Engl J Med 295:481, 534, 597, 1976

MANGOS JA: Cystic fibrosis, in *Physiology of Membrane Disorders,* IL Andreoti et al (eds), chap 46

MARK EJ, SHWACHMAN H: Progressive respiratory failure in a 46-year-old man with a positive sweat test. N Engl J Med 296:1519, 1977

NADLER HL et al: Cystic fibrosis, in *The Metabolic Basis of Inherited Disease,* 4th ed, JB Stanbury et al (eds). New York, McGraw-Hill 1978, p 1683

SHWACHMAN H et al: Mucoviscidosis, in *Advances in Pediatrics,* 7th ed, SV Levine (ed). Chicago, Year Book, 1955, p 249

——— et al: Cystic fibrosis: A new outlook. 70 patients above 25 years of age. Medicine 56:129, 1977

WOOD RE et al: Cystic fibrosis. Am Rev Respir Dis 113:833, 1976

Diffuse lung disease

263
CHRONIC BRONCHITIS, EMPHYSEMA, AND CHRONIC AIRWAYS OBSTRUCTION

ROLAND H. INGRAM, JR.

Chronic bronchitis and emphysema are two distinct processes, often present in combination in patients with chronic airways obstruction. The diagnosis of chronic bronchitis is made by history, chronic airways obstruction is assessed physiologically, and emphysema can be diagnosed with certainty only by histologic examination of sections of whole lung fixed at inflation. Although the relationships between clinical characteristics, physiologic derangements, and morphologic changes have been diligently studied for many years, reasonably certain and uniform clinical criteria are still not available. Definitions and classifications have evolved, but these are not universally accepted. Nonetheless, the following definitions along with brief qualifications and descriptions are currently used by most persons involved in the diagnosis, treatment, and epidemiology of the chronic obstructive airways syndromes.

DEFINITIONS *Chronic bronchitis* is a condition associated with excessive tracheobronchial mucus production sufficient to cause cough with expectoration for at least 3 months of the year for more than 2 consecutive years. Several subclassifications have been proposed. *Simple chronic bronchitis* describes a condition characterized by mucoid sputum production. *Chronic mucopurulent bronchitis* is characterized by persistent or recurrent purulence of sputum in the absence of localized suppurative diseases such as bronchiectasis. Since there may or may not be obstruction as assessed by the use of the forced expiratory vital capacity maneuver, *chronic bronchitis with obstruction* deserves a separate classification. There is a further subset of patients with chronic bronchitis and obstruction who experience severe dyspnea and wheezing in association with inhaled irritants or during acute respiratory infections. Such patients are said to have *chronic infective asthma* or *chronic asthmatic bronchitis.* Confusion is possible between patients with this condition and those with asthma (Chap. 257) who may also have *chronic airways obstruction.* The patient with chronic asthmatic bronchitis has a long history of cough and sputum production with a later onset of wheezing, whereas the asthmatic with chronic obstruction gives a long history of wheezing with later onset of chronic productive cough.

Emphysema is defined as distention of the air spaces distal to the terminal bronchiole with destruction of alveolar septa. *Chronic obstructive lung disease* is defined as a condition in which there is chronic obstruction to airflow due to chronic bronchitis and/or emphysema. Although the degree of obstruction may be less when the patient is free from respiratory infection and may improve somewhat with bronchodilator drugs, some obstruction is always present.

PREVALENCE Since chronic bronchitis, with or without obstruction by usual functional criteria, can be diagnosed by history as derived from standard questionnaires, it is not surprising that there are good prevalence data only for chronic bronchitis. Approximately 20 percent of adult males have the condition, yet only a minority is clinically disabled. According to all surveys females are less often affected than males. Although cigarette smoking is the single most important etiologic factor, occupational and environmental exposures are now receiving more attention.

Since no criteria have been agreed upon for making the diagnosis of emphysema during life, the incidence data are derived solely from postmortem surveys. It is rare to find adult lungs completely free of emphysema. There is a distinct increase in the extent of emphysema in the fifth decade with further increases through the seventh decade and little increase after that. Approximately two-thirds of adult males and one-fourth females (most without recognized dysfunction) will have well-defined emphysema, which is often limited in extent. Therefore, the majority of those with emphysema will not have had disability or even symptoms associated with it. The situation is analogous to atherosclerosis in that the morphologic changes are far more frequent than the clinical manifestations attributable to the changes.

PATHOLOGY *Chronic bronchitis* is associated with hyperplasia and hypertrophy of the mucus-producing glands found in the submucosa of large cartilaginous airways. Quantitation of this anatomic change, known as the Reid index, is based upon the ratio of the thickness of the submucosal glands to that of the bronchial wall. In persons without a history of chronic bronchitis the mean ratio is 0.44 with a standard deviation ±0.09, whereas those with such a history have a mean ratio of 0.52 ± 0.08. Although a low index is *rarely* associated with symptoms and a high index is commonly associated with symptoms during life, there is a great deal of overlap. Therefore many persons will have morphologic changes in large airways without having had chronic bronchitis.

Perhaps more important than the abnormalities in large airways are the changes often found in the small noncartilaginous airways. Goblet-cell hyperplasia, mucosal and submucosal inflammatory cells, and edema, peribronchial fibrosis, intraluminal mucus plugs, and increased smooth muscle are characteristic findings in small airways. The frequency of these latter findings in relation to premortem clinical and functional status has not been determined. However, in lungs from patients with chronic obstructive lung disease which have been studied at postmortem, the major site of airflow obstruction has been shown to be in the small airways.

Emphysema is classified according to the pattern of involvement of the gas-exchanging units (acini) of the lung distal to the terminal bronchiole. Although several morphologic patterns have been described, the two most important in the context of this discussion are those involving the respiratory bronchioles and alveolar ducts in the center of the acinus (centroacinar emphysema) and those involving the entire acinus (panacinar emphysema). Quite often both morphologic patterns are present in a single lung of a patient dying from chronic obstructive lung disease, although one type may predominate over the other.

With centroacinar emphysema the distention and destruction are mainly limited to the respiratory bronchiole and alveolar ducts, with relatively less change peripherally in the acinus. Because of the large functional reserve in the lung, many units must be involved in order for overall dysfunction to be detectable. The centrally destroyed regions of the acinus have a high ventilation/perfusion ratio because the capillaries are missing yet ventilation continues. This results in increased wasted ventilation (Vd/Vt), while the peripheral portions of the acinus have crowded and small alveoli with intact, perfused capillaries giving a low ventilation/perfusion ratio. This results in wasted blood flow to give a high alveolar-arterial P_{O_2} difference ($PA_{O_2} - Pa_{O_2}$) (Chap. 255). Mild degrees of centroacinar emphysema, often limited to the lung apices, are extremely common in lungs from persons above age 50 and are practically considered a normal finding.

Panacinar emphysema involves both the central and peripheral portions of the acinus which results, if the process is extensive, in a reduction of the alveolar-capillary gas exchange surface and loss of elastic recoil properties. When emphysema is severe, it may be difficult to distinguish between the two types which most often coexist in the same lung.

CONTRIBUTORY FACTORS **Smoking** Cigarette smoking is the most commonly identified correlate with both chronic bronchitis during life and extent of emphysema at postmortem. Experimental studies have shown that prolonged cigarette smoking impairs ciliary movement, inhibits function of alveolar macrophages, and leads to hypertrophy and hyperplasia of mucus-secreting glands; massive exposure in dogs can produce emphysematous changes. Inhaled cigarette smoke can produce an acute increase in airways resistance due to vagally mediated smooth-muscle constriction, presumably by way of stimulating submucosal irritant receptors. The relationship of such recurrent episodes of acute bronchial constriction to the development and progression of chronic airways obstruction is uncertain.

Evidence is accumulating that even young asymptomatic smokers often have considerable obstruction in small airways without there being either an increase of airway resistance or a diminution in the forced expiratory volume in 1 s. Since small airways, because of their large total cross-sectional areas, con-tribute very little to overall airflow resistance, more sensitive tests must be used to detect mild degrees of small-airways obstruction. Some tests, such as a decrease in compliance and resistance at rapid breathing rates, are based upon nonuniform behavior of the lung which is apparent only at increased frequencies. Obstruction of small airways also results in airways closure at higher lung volumes than in persons of the same age with unobstructed airways (Chap. 255). The measurements of closing volume and frequency dependence of resistance and compliance require special equipment not often available to clinicians. However, the simple spirogram is useful since flow rates at or below the midvital capacity range are often diminished in persons with mild small-airways obstruction. It has been shown that obstruction of small airways is the earliest demonstrable mechanical defect in young cigarette smokers and that the obstruction may disappear after cessation of smoking. It is possible, but has not been established with certainty, that those with small-airways obstruction are at greater risk of developing disabling chronic airways obstruction at some future time.

Not only is cigarette smoking the most common single factor leading to chronic airways obstruction, it also interacts with virtually every other contributory factor to be discussed below.

Air pollution The incidence and mortality rates of both chronic bronchitis and emphysema may be higher in heavily industrialized urban areas. Exacerbations of bronchitis are clearly related to periods of heavy pollution with SO_2 and particulate matter (Chap. 259).

Occupation Chronic bronchitis is more prevalent in workers who engage in occupations exposing them to either inorganic or organic dusts or to noxious gases. Epidemiologic surveys have succeeded in demonstrating an accelerated decline in lung function in many such workers—e.g., workers in plastics plants exposed to toluene diisocyanate and carding room workers in cotton mills (Chap. 259)—suggesting that their occupational exposure contributes to their future disability.

Infection Morbidity, mortality, and frequency of acute respiratory illnesses are higher in patients with chronic bronchitis. Existing evidence relates these illnesses to infection with viruses, mycoplasmas, and bacteria. It is intuitively appealing to assign some role to respiratory infections in the pathogenesis and progression of chronic obstructive lung disease, and although this question is under study, there has been no conclusion to date. Recent epidemiologic studies, however, implicate acute respiratory illness as one of the major factors associated with the etiology as well as the progression of chronic airways obstruction. It has been shown that cigarette smokers may either transitorily develop or worsen small airways obstruction in association with even mild viral respiratory infections. There is also some evidence that severe viral pneumonia early in life may lead to chronic obstruction, predominantly in small airways.

Familial and genetic factors Familial aggregation of chronic bronchitis has been well demonstrated in the past. Recent surveys have shown that children of smoking parents may experience more frequent and severe respiratory illnesses and have a higher prevalence of chronic respiratory symptoms. In addition, nonsmokers who remain in the presence of cigarette smokers have increased blood levels of carbon monoxide which indicates that they are significantly exposed to smoke. Thus a part of the familial aggregation may be related to home air pollution generated by smoking family members. However, some studies of monozygotic twins have suggested some genetic predisposition to the development of chronic bronchitis independent of personal or familial smoking habits. The exact genetic mode of transmission, if it exists at all, is uncertain.

The protease inhibitor α_1-antitrypsin is an acute-phase reactant, and normally the serum levels rise in association with many inflammatory reactions and with estrogen administration. Either deficient or absent serum levels of α_1-antitrypsin are found in some patients with the early onset of emphysema. By use of the techniques of acid starch gel and immunoelectrophoresis, genetic typing of the protease inhibitor (Pi) types has been possible. Most of the normal population have two M genes, designated as Pi type MM, and have α_1-antitrypsin levels in excess of 250 mg per 100 ml serum. Several genes are associated with alterations in levels of serum α_1-antitrypsin, but the commonest ones associated with emphysema are the Z and S genes. Individuals who are homozygous ZZ or SS have serum levels less than 50 mg per 100 ml and develop severe panacinar emphysema in the third and fourth decades of life. The panacinar process predominates at the lung bases. Progressive dyspnea with minimal cough characterizes the clinical presentation, although chronic bronchitis is prominent in smokers. The MZ and MS heterozygotes have intermediate levels of serum α_1-antitrypsin (i.e., between 50 and 250 mg per 100 ml); hence the genetic expression is that of an autosomal codominant allele. It is a matter of some controversy whether the heterozygous state is associated with lung function abnormalities. Published studies are in direct conflict on this point, and further data are needed to be certain. The matter is of some importance, since the heterozygous state is common, with incidence estimates varying between 5 and 14 percent of the general population.

The precise way in which antitrypsin deficiency produces emphysema is unclear. In addition to inhibition of trypsin, α_1-antitrypsin is an effective inhibitor of elastase and collagenase, as well as several other enzymes. There is experimental evidence that the structural integrity of lung elastin and collagen depends upon this antienzyme which protects the lung from proteases released from leukocytes. It is tempting to speculate that recurrent inflammatory reactions related to infection and pollutants play some role in pathogenesis by calling forth leukocytes whose released proteases are uninhibited and are free to cause the damage.

PATHOPHYSIOLOGY On the basis of the use of flow rates from forced expiratory vital capacity maneuvers and more sophisticated measures of airways resistance and elastic recoil properties of the lung, it has become clear that both chronic bronchitis and emphysema can exist without evidence of obstruction. However, by the time a patient begins to experience dyspnea as a result of these processes, obstruction is always demonstrable. Since chronic bronchitis and emphysema are usually combined, it might appear fruitless to determine the role of each in producing an individual patient's disability. However, one process may predominate over the other, and to the extent that inflammatory airways disease, secretions, and bronchospasm are present, there are therapeutic possibilities with some hope for improvement. Therefore it is of value to understand the mechanisms of airways obstruction in order to guide therapy and anticipate results.

Both chronic bronchitis and emphysema result in airways narrowing. In addition to the primary airways processes of chronic bronchitis, loss of elastic recoil of the lung in emphysema accounts for a decrease in airways caliber through loss of radial traction on airways. Narrowing of airways is often associated with both an increase in airways resistance and a diminution in maximal expiratory flow rates.

There are occasions in which a normal or only slightly elevated airways resistance is accompanied by low maximal expiratory flow rates. Under such circumstances an increase in the dynamic collapsibility of intrathoracic airways during forced exhalation is a possible explanation. Also in this context, the elastic recoil pressure of the lung must be considered in a slightly different way. In addition to providing radial support to airways during quiet breathing, the elastic recoil properties of the lung serve as a major determinant of maximal expiratory flow rates. The static recoil pressure of the lung is the difference between alveolar and intrapleural pressure. During forced exhalations, when alveolar and intrapleural pressures are high, there are points in the airway at which bronchial pressure equals pleural pressure. Flow does not increase with higher pleural pressure after these points become fixed so that the effective driving pressure between alveoli and such points is the elastic recoil pressure of the lung. Hence maximal expiratory flow rates represent a complex and dynamic interplay between airways caliber, elastic recoil pressures, and collapsibility of airways. As a direct consequence of the altered pressure-airflow relationships, the work of breathing is increased in bronchitis and emphysema. Since flow-resistive work is flow rate-dependent, there is a disproportionate increase in the work of breathing with increased ventilation.

The designated subdivisions of the lung volume outlined in Chap. 255 are abnormal to varying degrees in both bronchitis and emphysema. The residual volume (RV) and functional residual capacity (FRC) are almost always higher than normal. Since the normal FRC is the volume at which the inward recoil of the lung is balanced by the outward recoil of the chest wall, loss of elastic recoil of the lung would clearly result in a higher static FRC. In addition, prolongation of expiration in association with obstruction would lead to a dynamic increase in FRC if inspiration is initiated before the respiratory system reaches its static balance point. Elevations of total lung capacity (TLC) are frequent. The exact cause is uncertain, but increases in TLC are often found in association with decreases in the elastic recoil of the lung. The vital capacity is frequently decreased, yet significant airways obstruction can be present with a normal to near-normal vital capacity.

The consequences of the airways and parenchymal processes are far more extensive than just the mechanical alterations discussed above. Maldistribution of inspired gas and blood flow is always present to some extent. When the mismatching is severe, impairment of gas exchange is reflected in abnormalities of arterial blood gases. There are regions of the lung with ventilation in excess of perfusion which increase the wasted ventilation ratio (that is, Vd/Vt; Chap. 255). At a normal resting CO_2 production, the net effective alveolar ventilation, as reflected by the arterial P_{CO_2}, may be excessive, normal, or insufficient depending upon the relationship of the overall minute volume to the wasted ventilation ratio. The net contribution of regions with perfusion in excess of ventilation can be assessed by either estimating or measuring the alveolar-arterial P_{O_2} difference (that is, $P_{A_{O_2}} - Pa_{O_2}$; Chap. 255). Whatever the clinical syndrome associated with chronic bronchitis and emphysema, there are to some degree increases in both wasted ventilation and wasted blood flow.

The clinical manifestations depend, in large part, upon the ventilatory response to the disordered lung function. Some patients, at the cost of extremely high effort of breathing and chronic dyspnea, will maintain a strikingly increased minute volume, which results both in a normal to low arterial P_{CO_2}, despite the high Vd/Vt, and a relatively high arterial P_{O_2}, despite the high difference, $P_{A_{O_2}} - Pa_{O_2}$. Other patients with only modest increases in effort of breathing and less dyspnea will maintain a normal to only moderately elevated minute volume at the cost of accepting a high arterial P_{CO_2} and a severely depressed arterial P_{O_2}.

Factors which account for clear differences in ventilatory responses between patients have been studied and debated for years. The bulk of available evidence suggests that those patients who maintain relatively normal or low arterial P_{CO_2} levels are those with an increased ventilatory drive and those who chronically maintain high arterial P_{CO_2} and lower P_{O_2} levels have a diminished ventilatory drive. It is not at all certain whether individual differences are accounted for by variations in peripheral or central chemoreceptor sensitivity or through other afferent pathways. Perhaps of more immediate value is the fact that patients with predominant emphysema are either normally or excessively responsive both to hypercapnia and to exercise, whereas those with predominant bronchitis are less responsive to both, despite similar degrees of airways obstruction by spirometry.

The pulmonary circulation malfunctions not only in terms of regional distribution of blood flow but in terms of abnormal overall pressure-flow relationships. There is often mild to severe pulmonary hypertension at rest with further increases disproportionate to cardiac output elevations during exercise. A reduction in the total cross-sectional area of the pulmonary vascular bed can be attributed to anatomic changes and constriction of vascular smooth muscle in pulmonary arteries and arterioles as well as destruction of alveolar septa with loss of capillaries. Rarely does loss of capillaries alone lead to severe pulmonary hypertension with cor pulmonale, except as a terminal event. Of more importance and interest is the constriction of pulmonary vessels in response to alveolar hypoxia. The constriction is reversible upon increase in alveolar P_{O_2} with therapy. There is a synergism between hypoxia and acidosis which assumes importance during episodes of acute or chronic respiratory insufficiency. Chronic hypoxia leads not only to pulmonary vascular constriction but also to secondary erythrocytosis. The latter, although not proved to be a significant contributor to pulmonary hypertension, could add an unfavorable rheologic load. As discussed in Chap. 246, the chronic afterload on the right ventricle leads to hypertrophy and, in association with disordered blood gases, ultimately to failure.

CLINICAL-FUNCTIONAL CORRELATIONS Dyspnea and impairment of physical work capacity are characteristic only of severe to moderately severe airways obstruction. There is considerable variation among patients, and those with predominant emphysema have greater dyspnea and restriction of physical activity with lesser degrees of obstruction than those in whom chronic bronchitis predominates. The majority of patients have functionally mixed disease, will usually experience exertional dyspnea when the forced expiratory volume in 1 s (FEV_1) falls below 50 percent of that predicted, and will have dyspnea at rest when the FEV_1 is less than 25 percent of that predicted. In addition to dyspnea at rest, carbon dioxide retention and cor pulmonale frequently occur when the FEV_1 falls to 25 percent of that predicted. However, those with predominant bronchitis often have carbon dioxide retention and cor pulmonale with FEV_1 values above 25 percent of normal, in contrast to patients with predominant emphysema whose FEV_1 usually falls well below that level before the onset of carbon dioxide retention and cor pulmonale. With a respiratory infection, small changes in the degree of obstruction can make a large difference in symptoms and gas exchange. Thus small therapeutic gains have rewarding results.

In general, the more severe the obstruction, the poorer the prognosis. Despite the general relationship, 20 to 30 percent of patients with severe obstruction and carbon dioxide retention will survive beyond 5 years.

CLINICAL SYNDROMES It is clear that the clinical presentation can vary in severity from simple chronic bronchitis without disability to the severely disabled state with chronic respiratory failure. From a practical standpoint, it is well to consider that any symptom or any measurable abnormality may foreshadow the development of severe disabling disease; hence cessation of smoking and avoidance of environmental irritants and toxins are to be advised. However, the advice to modify behavior and life patterns is rarely taken, and most physicians are called upon to categorize and treat patients with fully developed, chronic airways obstruction. Thus the approach taken here is to describe two polar opposite types of fully developed, chronic obstructive pulmonary disease with the realization that the majority of patients will have some features of both types. The salient features of each type are outlined in Table 263-1.

Predominant emphysema These patients often give a long history of exertional dyspnea with minimal cough which is productive of only small amounts of mucoid sputum. Mucopurulent exacerbations in association with infections are not frequent. The body build is asthenic with evidence of weight loss. The patient appears distressed with obvious use of accessory muscles of respiration which serve to lift the sternum in an anterosuperior direction with each inspiration. There is tachypnea with a relatively prolonged expiration through pursed lips, or expiration is begun with a grunting sound. While sitting, these patients often lean forward, extending the arms to brace themselves. The neck veins may be distended during ex-

TABLE 263-1
Chronic obstructive lung disease: salient features of the two types

	Predominant emphysema	*Predominant bronchitis*
Age at time of diagnosis	60±	50±
Dyspnea	Severe	Mild
Cough	After dyspnea starts	Before dyspnea starts
Sputum	Scanty, mucoid	Copious, purulent
Bronchial infections	Less frequent	More frequent
Respiratory insufficiency episodes	Often terminal	Repeated
Chest film	"Hyperinflation" ± bullous changes, small heart	Increased bronchovascular markings at bases, large heart
Chronic Pa_{CO_2}, mmHg	35–40	50–60
Chronic Pa_{O_2}, mmHg	65–75	45–60
Hematocrit, %	35–45	50–55
Pulmonary hypertension:		
Rest	None to mild	Moderate to severe
Exercise	Moderate	Worsens
Cor pulmonale	Rare, except terminally	Common
Elastic recoil	Severely decreased	Normal
Resistance	Normal to slight increase	High
Diffusing capacity	Decreased	Normal to slight decrease

piration, yet they collapse briskly with inspiration. The lower intercostal spaces retract with each inspiration, and by palpation the lower lateral chest wall can be felt to move inward. The percussion note is hyperresonant, and by auscultation the breath sounds are diminished, with faint, high-pitched rhonchi heard toward the end of expiration. The cardiac impulse, if at all visible, is seen only in the xiphoid and subxiphoid regions, and cardiac dullness is either absent or severely reduced. By palpation there is frequently a sustained forward and downward right ventricular impulse in the subxiphoid region, and a presystolic gallop accentuated during inspiration is commonly heard.

The arterial P_{O_2} is often in the mid 70s (mmHg), and the P_{CO_2} is low to normal. Because of the maintained increase in minute volume and the maintenance of arterial P_{O_2} sufficient to nearly saturate hemoglobin, these patients have been referred to as "pink puffers."

The TLC and RV are invariably increased, the vital capacity is low, and the maximal expiratory flow rates are diminished. The elastic recoil properties of the lung are severely impaired, and in direct proportion to this impairment, the capacity of the lung to transfer carbon monoxide is lowered.

On radiographic examination the diaphragms are low and flattened, the bronchovascular shadows do not extend to the periphery of the lung, and the cardiac silhouette is lengthened and narrowed. These findings in association with a large retrosternal translucency on lateral chest radiographs are interpreted as hyperinflation which correlates well with increases in TLC and loss of elastic recoil. Peripheral attenuation of bronchovascular markings and increased retrosternal lucency correlate best with subsequent postmortem demonstration of extensive and severe emphysema which is predominantly of the panacinar type.

It is fortunate that the patient with predominant emphysema is less prone to mucopurulent relapses than is the patient with predominant bronchitis, since such relapses frequently lead to severe respiratory failure and death. That is to say, right-sided heart failure and hypercapnic respiratory failure are often terminal events in those patients with predominant emphysema. In the absence of such relapses, the clinical course is characterized by severe and progressive dyspnea for which little can be done. The physician's role is to seek out and treat any factor that is possibly reversible and strive to avoid pollutants and infections.

Predominant bronchitis The patient with predominant bronchitis usually has an impressive history of cough and sputum production for many years with an immodest history of cigarette smoking. Initially the cough is present only in the winter months, and the patient is apt to seek medical attention, if at all, only during the more severe of the frequent mucopurulent relapses. Over the years the cough progresses from hibernal to perennial, and mucopurulent relapses increase in frequency, duration, and severity. After beginning to experience exertional dyspnea, the patient often seeks medical help and will be found to have a severe degree of obstruction. Occasionally such a patient will seek out a physician only after the onset of peripheral edema secondary to overt right ventricular failure. More rarely the initial medical contact is made by family members who present the physician with a deeply cyanotic, edematous, and stuporous patient with acute respiratory insufficiency.

The patient with predominant bronchitis is often overweight and cyanotic. There is usually no apparent distress at rest, the respiratory rate is normal or only slightly increased, and there is no apparent usage of accessory muscles. The chest percussion note is normally resonant, and by auscultation, one can usually hear coarse rhonchi and wheezes which change in location and intensity after a deep and productive cough.

There may be a sustained heave along the lower left sternal border which indicates right ventricular hypertrophy. In the presence of right ventricular failure there are often an early diastolic gallop and occasionally a holosystolic murmur, both of which are accentuated by inspiration. The latter finding is indicative of functional tricuspid regurgitation which is frequently accompanied by neck vein distention characterized by large v waves and brisk y descents. With right ventricular failure the cyanosis deepens and peripheral edema becomes prominent. Clubbing of the digits is unusual.

With or without right ventricular failure, the minute volume is either normal or only slightly increased. Failure to increase minute volume in the face of significant proportions of wasted ventilation and blood flow results in severely deranged arterial blood gases, with arterial P_{CO_2} values which are chronically increased to the range of the high 40s to low 50s (mmHg). The lowered P_{O_2} produces desaturation of hemoglobin, serves to stimulate erythropoiesis, and results in hypoxic pulmonary vasoconstriction. Desaturation and erythrocytosis combine to produce the cyanosis, and hypoxic pulmonary vasoconstriction accentuates the right-sided heart failure. Because of cyanosis and edema secondary to heart failure, such patients have been referred to as "blue bloaters."

The TLC is often normal, and there is a moderate elevation of RV. The vital capacity is mildly diminished, and maximal expiratory flow rates are invariably low. The elastic recoil properties of the lung are normal or only slightly impaired, and the capacity of the lung to transfer carbon monoxide is either normal or minimally decreased.

On radiographic examination the diaphragms are well rounded, the bronchovascular markings are increased in the lower lung fields, and the cardiac silhouette is somewhat enlarged. In association with right ventricular failure the cardiac silhouette enlarges further, pulmonary arteries become more prominent, and an antigravity distribution of perfusion is apparent.

Despite well-planned management (see below) the patient with predominant bronchitis may experience many episodes of respiratory failure from which recovery is frequent with proper therapy (see Chap. 272). The ability to recover from such repeated episodes in those patients is in striking contrast to the frequently fatal outcome of such events in those with predominant emphysema. Ultimately, the lungs at postmortem will be found to have severe bronchitic changes in both large and small airways and only moderate emphysema, predominantly of the centroacinar variety.

PRINCIPLES OF MANAGEMENT Intelligent management must be based upon as complete knowledge as possible of the degree of obstruction, the extent of disability, and the relative reversibility of the patient's illness. To the extent that obstructive processes in the airways are contributory, there is a chance for treatment to be effective. Since emphysema is an irreversible process, prevention of progression and avoidance of acute insults constitute the only approach. History, physical examination, and chest radiographs should be supplemented by tests of lung function performed during a symptomatically stable period. Ideally, complete spirometry, plethysmographic lung volumes, airways resistance, transfer of carbon monoxide, arterial blood gases, and lung elastic recoil properties should be measured. Spirometry, lung volumes, and resistance should be remeasured after the administration of bronchodilators in order to assess the degree of acutely reversible airways obstruction. Failure to see an acute change with bronchodilator drugs does not rule out the possibility of improvement with more prolonged administration of these agents. In instances in which the degree of exertional dyspnea appears to be disproportionately greater than the degree of obstruction, measurements of blood gases, minute volume, CO_2 production, and O_2 consumption during exercise are indicated in order to determine whether impaired lung function is sufficient to account for the symptoms. After the initial assessment the physician has some idea of the relative emphasis to be placed upon patient education, preventive measures, and direct therapeutic interventions in management of the patient and the illness.

Cessation of smoking is the only certain means of influencing the progression of the chronic obstructive airways syndromes, and such behavior modification is most effective at early stages of the disease processes. In the instances in which occupational or environmental exposures are thought to play a significant role, change of occupation or relocation of dwelling is advisable. The validity of such advice should be carefully considered since the impact on both the patient and the family is likely to be great. A simpler environmental change is that of eliminating aerosol sprays such as deodorants, hair sprays, and insecticides from the household. Hair sprays have been shown to produce acute airways responses even in normal subjects. Other preventive measures include yearly vaccination against the common or expected influenza virus strains.

Infections cannot be totally avoided, and the patient should be made aware that increasing purulence, viscosity, or volume of secretions signals the onset of an infection which should be treated early. The commonest pathogenic bacteria found are *Hemophilus influenzae* and *Streptococcus pneumoniae*. Either tetracycline or ampicillin should be given for a 7- to 10-day course. It is practical to have the patient keep a 7- to 10-day supply of antibiotics at home and to begin treatment at the onset of symptoms. In Great Britain it is common practice to give continuous antibiotic therapy during winter months in order to prevent mucopurulent relapses. Although there is evidence that both viruses and mycoplasmas are frequent causes of mucopurulent relapses, clinical studies have shown that the standard antibiotic regimens decrease the duration and severity of infective episodes unrelated to culturable bacterial pathogens. Microscopic examination and culture of sputum are indicated if there are chills, fever, or chest pain or if purulence fails to respond to usually administered antibiotics.

It has been shown repeatedly that exercise programs, although not accompanied by measurable improvement in lung function, result in increased exercise tolerance and an improved sense of well-being. The improvement is usually task-specific, so that most physicians advise walking in preference to the use of special apparatus, such as stationary bicycles or wall gyms.

Bronchodilator drugs are often quite helpful in alleviating symptoms, especially in those patients who respond to them acutely in the laboratory. These drugs form three categories: the methylxanthines, sympathomimetics with strong beta-adrenergic-stimulating properties, and anticholinergics. Theophylline, the most commonly used methylxanthine, can be given orally, rectally, or parenterally; in addition to bronchodilatation, it stimulates respiration and has cardiotonic and diuretic properties. The most commonly used beta-adrenergic agent, isoproterenol, is given mainly as an aerosol. More selective beta$_2$-stimulating drugs have recently been developed, and these can be given both orally and by aerosol with fewer cardiac side effects. Anticholinergic agents such as atropine have been avoided in the past because of their tendency to desiccate secretions, but such drugs are effective bronchodilators; new

analogues with less effect on secretions are now being developed and tested and may be found useful in the future.

Bronchopulmonary drainage must be maintained in patients with hypersecretion. If the coughing mechanism is either ineffective or if paroxysms of coughing are exhausting, postural drainage is often a useful adjunct. Although liquefaction of secretions by means of orally administered expectorants or aerosol delivery of mucolytic agents is an appealing idea, it has never been shown by properly designed trials to be more effective than simple maintenance of total body hydration.

Intermittent positive pressure breathing (IPPB) devices have long been advocated for home management. The various rationales include diminution in the work of breathing, promotion of bronchopulmonary drainage, and more efficient delivery of bronchodilator drugs. The first of the rationales has been shown to have no basis in fact and the goals of the last two have been shown to be as well accomplished by postural drainage and use of less elaborate aerosol generators. Hence the use of intermittent positive pressure breathing for home management cannot be justified.

When hypoxemia is persistent and severe, portable oxygen therapy is often considered. There are suggestive data indicating that supplemental oxygen improves exercise tolerance and alleviates pulmonary hypertension. However, the data are not conclusive concerning prolongation of life. In view of the expense of such therapy and the dangers of uncontrolled oxygen delivery, it should be given only when it can be carefully monitored and objectively assessed.

Secondary erythrocytosis with the hematocrit in excess of 50 percent is most easily viewed as a mechanism allowing greater oxygen delivery to compensate for the chronically lowered arterial P_{O_2}. Since erythrocytosis results in elevation of blood viscosity at all shear rates, the proposal has been made that pulmonary vascular hypertension is aggravated by its presence. However, no study has demonstrated an objective improvement following phlebotomy. Nonetheless, some patients who complain of headaches and a sense of head fullness show a favorable subjective response to periodic phlebotomy when the hematocrit is in excess of 55 percent.

Chronic cor pulmonale and acute respiratory failure are common complications often present in combination. These two processes are discussed in Chaps. 246 and 272, respectively.

FACTORS PRECIPITATING ACUTE RESPIRATORY FAILURE
Infection of the tracheobronchial tree is the most common cause of acute respiratory failure in chronic obstructive lung disease. Increasing airways obstruction with airways inflammation and secretion, especially in association with a blunted ventilatory drive, leads to worsening hypoxemia and increasing CO_2 retention. Some patients apparently depend upon hypoxemia as a major stimulus to breathing; and uncontrolled oxygen therapy, by removing the hypoxic drive, can result in further elevations of P_{CO_2} with coma and apnea. Thus, during episodes of increasing hypoxemia, oxygen should be administered in low concentrations, and the resulting arterial blood gas values must be carefully monitored. The physician must be alert to the possible need for endotracheal intubation and mechanical ventilatory assistance if hypercapnic stupor and coma occur with oxygen therapy. Agitation, insomnia, and increasing dyspnea with impending respiratory failure are occasionally treated, mistakenly, with either sedatives or narcotics, and these, too, may precipitate frank respiratory failure. In fact such depressant drugs which impair ventilatory drive should be avoided at all times in patients with severe chronic obstructive lung disease. Major episodes of air pollution can also lead to respiratory failure, and the physicians responsible for pa-

tients with severe bronchitis and emphysema should be alert to these environmental events.

In the setting of impending respiratory failure, pneumonia, thromboembolism, left ventricular failure, and pneumothorax occasionally occur and are extremely difficult to detect unless considered and specifically sought. Such processes may actually precipitate respiratory failure rather than accompany it. As a minimum, chest radiographs, electrocardiograms, and sputum examinations should be obtained in addition to arterial blood gas measurements in all patients with respiratory failure. The incidence of peptic ulcer is increased in these patients. This complication may first become manifest as hypotension secondary to gastrointestinal hemorrhage during the course of respiratory failure, and awareness of the possibility increases the likelihood of detection and prompt treatment.

PROGNOSIS　On the average, data collected on large populations demonstrate a slow and relentless diminution in ventilatory function in patients with chronic airways obstruction. Although slow, the decrement in function with time far exceeds the rate of change seen with normal aging. In general, the likelihood of episodes of acute respiratory failure increases when the FEV_1 falls below 25 percent of predicted normal values. Although the in-hospital mortality rate averages 30 percent for a single episode and the 5-year survival rate after the initial episode of respiratory failure averages only 15 to 20 percent, the clinical syndrome is extremely important in determining both the short- and long-range prognosis. As noted above, those patients with predominant emphysema have a poorer prognosis after the onset of respiratory failure than do those with predominant bronchitis.

BULLOUS EMPHYSEMA　Confluent air spaces with diameters in excess of 1 cm are occasionally congenital but most often are found in association with generalized emphysema or progressive fibrotic processes. Gradual increases in size of such air spaces (or bullae) result from traction applied by regions with better elastic recoil properties, and such regions lose volume as the bullae become enlarged. If disability is severe, if the bulla is extremely large, and if either lobar gas sampling or ventilation and perfusion scans demonstrate that sufficient function remains in the nonbullous regions, surgical excision of the bulla may lead to functional improvement. Usually, however, improvement is relatively transitory because other emphysematous regions gradually enlarge into bullae after surgery.

VARIANTS OF EMPHYSEMA　In addition to the centroacinar and panacinar forms of emphysema described above, other structural patterns have been described but are functionally less important. Often there is overdistention and alveolar septal destruction in lung regions surrounding scar tissue (paracicatricial or scar emphysema) or along the borders of the acinus (paraseptal emphysema). The latter form, when it occurs at the visceral pleural surface, may predispose to episodes of spontaneous pneumothorax (Chap. 269). Infants rarely develop a check valve mechanism in a lobar bronchus which leads to rapid and life-threatening overdistention (congenital lober emphysema). Unilateral emphysema may be an incidental radiographic finding (Macleod's or Swyer-James's syndromes). Since, in this condition, the airways are normal in number and structure but the alveoli are reduced in number, this form of unilateral emphysema has been attributed to disease occurring before the age of 8 years when alveoli are normally increasing in number. Overdistention and alveolar septal destruction are not present, and so this condition does not fit the definition of true emphysema. Most often the pulmonary artery on the affected side is hypoplastic. Although usually an incidental finding, the affected lung may become repeatedly infected so that surgical excision may be indicated.

REFERENCES

Cosio M et al: The relations between structural changes in small airways and pulmonary function tests. N Engl J Med 298:1277, 1978

Diener CF, Burrows B: Further observation on the course and prognosis of chronic obstructive lung disease. Am Rev Respir Dis 111:719, 1975

Fraser RG: The radiologist and obstructive airway disease. Am J Roentgenol Radium Ther Nucl Med 120:737, 1974

Hugh-Jones P, Waimster W: The etiology and management of disabling emphysema: State of the art. Am Rev Respir Dis 117:343, 1978

Macklem PT: The pathophysiology of chronic bronchitis and emphysema. Med Clin Am 57:669, 1973

Thurlbeck WM: *Chronic Airflow Obstruction in Lung Disease.* Philadelphia, Saunders, 1976

———, Simon G: Radiographic appearance of the chest in emphysema. Am J Roentgenol 130:429, 1978

264
DIFFUSE INFILTRATIVE DISEASES OF THE LUNG

JOHN F. MURRAY

Infiltration means the diffusion into, or accumulation in, a tissue of substances not normal to it. Infiltrates of the lung are usually either cellular (e.g., inflammatory or neoplastic infiltration) or noncellular (e.g., infiltration by edema fluid, collagen, or other substances). Numerous clinicopathologic entities, therefore, are associated with diffuse infiltration of the lung. Although these disorders differ considerably in their pathogenesis—which is obscure in many instances—they share the common features of widespread structural involvement and characteristic alterations in pulmonary function. Because of these similarities, they are often accompanied by identical signs, symptoms, and roentgenographic changes.

The lung, like other organs, has a limited capacity to react to injury; accordingly, the interstitial pneumonias, the most common cause of diffuse pulmonary infiltration, are regarded as a spectrum of pathologic changes that represent a common response to diverse stimuli. In contrast to the acute polymorphonuclear *intra*alveolar exudative process that characterizes most bacterial pneumonias, the reaction in the infiltrative diseases is primarily *inter*alveolar. In the latter the acute cellular infiltrate is usually composed of round cells (histiocytes, lymphocytes, and plasma cells) and is accompanied by interstitial edema and a proteinaceous exudate, containing some cells or cellular debris, that accumulates in alveolar spaces and bronchioles; organization of this material leads to hyaline membrane formation. In many patients with extensive damage to the alveolar-capillary membrane, the acute exudative response to injury appears to be completely reversible and normal lung architecture is restored. In other patients, for unknown reasons, the repair process is characterized by abundant hyperplasia and/or metaplasia of bronchial and alveolar epithelium. The process of reepithelialization and scarring progressively incorporates the intraalveolar inflammatory exudate (fibrosing alveolitis) and widens the interalveolar septum; this eventually causes extensive fibrosis with gross lung destruction and "honeycombing." When the changes become advanced ("end-stage lung"), any specific histologic or identifying hallmarks that were present are usually lost. Although the cellular popu-

TABLE 264-1
Causes of diffuse infiltrative diseases of the lungs

I Infections*
  A Viruses: influenza, cytomegalovirus, measles, varicella zoster
  B Bacteria: miliary tuberculosis, staphylococcal infection, streptococcal infection, *Klebsiella* infection, mycoplasma infection, brucellosis, salmonellosis, shigellosis, tularemia, glanders, pneumonic plague, pertussis, psittacosis (ornithosis), lymphopathia venereum, Q fever, Rocky Mountain spotted fever, nocardiosis
  C Fungi: histoplasmosis, coccidioidomycosis, blastomycosis, cryptococcosis, candidiasis, aspergillosis, geotrichosis, sporotrichosis
  D Parasites: schistosomiasis, *Pneumocystis carinii* infection, filariasis, toxoplasmosis, paragonimiasis, ascariasis, trichinosis, hookworm infestation, strongyloides, visceral larva migrans, amebiasis, echinococcosis
II Occupational causes
  A Mineral dusts: silicosis; asbestosis; berylliosis; coal miner's pneumoconiosis; Shaver's disease (bauxite); diatomaceous earth disease; talc pneumoconiosis; siderosis (arc welder's disease); pneumoconiosis from barium, silver, tin, vanadium, manganese
  B Chemical fumes: nitrogen dioxide (silo-filler's disease), chlorine, ammonia, sulfur dioxide, phosgenes, acetylene, kerosene, carbon tetrachloride, bromine, hydrogen fluoride, hydrochloric acid, nitric acid, picric acid
III Neoplastic causes: bronchioloalveolar carcinoma, hematogenous metastases, lymphangitic carcinomatosis, leukemia, lymphoma, polycythemia vera
IV Congenital or familial causes: cystic fibrosis, Niemann-Pick disease, Gaucher's disease, neurofibromatosis, tuberous sclerosis, familial dysautonomia (Riley-Day syndrome), pulmonary alveolar microlithiasis, familial idiopathic pulmonary fibrosis (congenital cystic disease with pulmonary fibrosis and familial fibrocystic pulmonary dysplasia)
V Metabolic causes: uremic pneumonitis, hypercalcemia, paraquat poisoning
VI Physical agents: postirradiation fibrosis, thermal injury, oxygen toxicity, blast injury
VII Circulatory causes
  A Thromboembolic: multiple pulmonary emboli, fat embolism, lymphangiography, sickle-cell anemia, foreign-body vasculitis (drug addicts, schistosomiasis)
  B Hemodynamic: pulmonary edema, chronic passive congestion with fibrosis (possibly with hemosiderosis and/or bone deposition)
VIII Immunologic causes
  A Hypersensitivity pneumonia
    1 Inhaled antigens: farmer's lung, bagassosis, bird fancier's disease, maple bark disease, sequoiosis, mushroom grower's disease, malt worker's lung, pneumonitis from pituitary snuff, exposure to *Bacillus subtilis* enzymes (detergent manufacturing), or smallpox vaccine
    2 Drug reactions: sensitivity to hydralazine, busulfan, nitrofurantoin, hexamethonium, mecamylamine, methysergid(e), and bleomycin
  B Collagen diseases: scleroderma, rheumatoid arthritis, lupus erythematosus, periarteritis nodosa, Wegener's granulomatosis, dermatomyositis, Sjögren's syndrome
  C Goodpasture's syndrome
IX Unknown origin
  A Sarcoidosis
  B Histiocytosis X: Letterer-Siwe disease, Hand-Schüller-Christian disease, eosinophilic granuloma
  C Idiopathic hemosiderosis
  D Pulmonary alveolar proteinosis
  E Diffuse idiopathic pulmonary fibrosis (synonyms: organizing interstitial pneumonia, usual interstitial pneumonia, chronic interstitial pneumonitis, idiopathic interstitial pulmonary fibrosis, acute diffuse interstitial fibrosis of the lungs, diffuse fibrosing alveolitis, chronic diffuse sclerosing alveolitis, chronic Hamman-Rich syndrome, bronchiolar emphysema, and muscular cirrhosis of the lung)

* *Infections are not a common cause of diffuse infiltrative disease of the lungs. More commonly they cause focal processes.*

lation causing the infiltrate differs considerably depending on whether infiltration is initiated by infectious agents, mineral dusts, immunologic phenomena, or other causes, the resulting functional alterations and clinical consequences are remarkably similar.

It follows from these considerations that the number of diffuse infiltrative diseases of the lung is large. Table 264-1 lists the most important causes but is by no means inclusive.

PATHOGENESIS Infections Several members of each of the major classes of infectious agents are known to cause diffuse infiltration of the lung parenchyma. Viruses that affect the lower respiratory tract cause an acute interstitial inflammatory infiltration of lymphocytes, histiocytes, and plasma cells that may be accompanied by occasional hyaline membranes. Although most viral interstitial pneumonias resolve without significant residual lesions, experimental and clinical evidence has linked viruses with chronic, progressive diffuse interstitial disease. Necrotizing pyogenic bacterial infections that may heal with permanent scarring are usually focal rather than diffuse because they are acquired by aspiration through the tracheobronchial tree. In contrast, hematogenous infections, such as miliary tuberculosis, disseminated mycoses, and the migration of certain parasites, typically cause widespread pulmonary involvement. However, infections are not a common cause of *diffuse* infiltration of the lung, but they are important to recognize because most of them are treatable.

Neoplastic disease Widespread pulmonary neoplasms (Chap. 268) are an important cause of diffuse pulmonary infiltrations and may occur in three different locations: (1) the surface epithelium, (2) the blood vessels and lymph channels and their surrounding spaces, and (3) the interstitial tissues. Bronchioloalveolar carcinoma is a primary lung cancer that may cause either focal tumor deposits or extensive epithelial infiltration (pulmonary adenomatosis). Some varieties grow slowly and are not invasive; others spread rapidly and are highly malignant. The lung parenchyma may become diffusely infiltrated by hematogenous or lymphatic metastases from a primary tumor anywhere in the body. Similarly, widespread interstitial pulmonary involvement may occur during the course of any of the lymphomas (Hodgkin's disease, lymphosarcoma, reticulum cell sarcoma), in mycosis fungoides, and in Kaposi's sarcoma.

Infiltration of the lung with leukemic cells can be identified microscopically in a high proportion of patients with leukemia, but the involvement, in most cases, is not associated either with radiographically recognizable lesions or with clinically significant symptoms. Acute and chronic lymphatic leukemias are much more likely than myelogenous leukemias to cause pulmonary infiltrations. Fever and detectable pulmonary infiltrations in a patient with leukemia usually indicate the presence of an infection, often by an "opportunistic" organism, and these conditions should not be regarded as leukemic until a thorough search has been made for potential pathogens. Untreated polycythemia vera is often associated with congestion of the pulmonary circulation and occasionally has been reported to cause interstitial pulmonary fibrosis.

Congenital or familial diseases Several unrelated congenital or familial diseases are associated with diffuse pulmonary infiltration; most are systemic disorders, and the pulmonary component may be overshadowed by involvement of other organs that are more important and frequent sources of morbidity and mortality. *Familial dysautonomia* may be associated with pulmonary scarring secondary to pneumonitis resulting from frequent aspiration caused by autonomic nervous system dysfunction. Diffuse pulmonary fibrosis has been found in 10 to 20 percent of patients with *tuberous sclerosis* or *neurofibromatosis* (von Recklinghausen's disease). In *Niemann-Pick disease* and

Gaucher's disease (usually in infantile form), chest roentgenograms may reveal fine reticulonodular shadows that reflect the presence of diffuse infiltration by histiocytes containing the abnormal lipids that characterize the diseases. Diffuse parenchymal scarring occurs in *cystic fibrosis* secondary to widespread bronchiectasis and recurrent pyogenic infections.

Pulmonary microlithiasis is a sporadic or familial disease in which there are innumerable intraalveolar calcified particles. The disorder presumably begins at an early age and is often recognized accidentally by chest roentgenography in an asymptomatic patient. There are no identifiable alterations in calcium and phosphorus metabolism, but local physicochemical abnormalities in lung tissue may account for the deposition of calcium salts. *Familial idiopathic pulmonary fibrosis* is identical to organizing interstitial pneumonia (described in more detail later) but has, in addition, a definite familial incidence and a tendency to afflict younger persons. The pathogenesis in both sporadic and familial cases remains obscure.

Metabolic disorders Two relatively common clinical disorders, uremia and hypercalcemia, are associated with diffuse pulmonary infiltration. The pathologic findings in *uremic pneumonitis* consist of a fibrinous exudate in the alveoli (most marked in the hilar regions of the lung), often organized into dense hyaline membranes, and an interstitial pneumonia with varying degrees of organization. Similar changes have been observed in chronic left ventricular failure in the absence of uremia; a controversy exists about whether the lung lesions are caused by uremia, since congestive heart failure often accompanies uremia, or are related to the associated heart disease. Available data indicate that in patients with uremia, a dialyzable substance may accumulate that affects capillary permeability generally and contributes to the development of lung lesions.

Hypercalcemia from virtually any cause, e.g., hyperparathyroidism, extensive bone malignancy, and hypervitaminosis D, may be associated with multiple deposits of calcium salts in the lungs. The lung, like the gastric mucosa and renal tubules, is a preferred site of involvement, presumably owing to local changes in pH which favor calcification. Although metastatic calcification of the lung parenchyma may be extensive when examined microscopically, it is often undetectable by chest roentgenography and seldom produces symptoms.

Accidental or deliberate ingestion of the herbicide *paraquat* produces injury in several organs, including the lung. If the patient survives the acute episode, chronic lung disease may result, consisting of diffuse inflammatory thickening of the interalveolar septa and interstitial fibrosis. The mechanism of tissue injury is not clear but may involve induction of metabolic abnormalities in type II alveolar epithelial cells.

Physical agents *Radiation pneumonitis* results from the cytotoxic effects of irradiation of the lung. The areas of involvement are usually sharply confined to the target sites, but if either the area irradiated or the secondary scatter is extensive, much of the lung parenchyma may be involved. The pathologic process consists of varying degrees of capillary congestion, interstitial edema, cellular infiltration, lymphangiectasis, and hyaline membrane formation. In the chronic phase, dense interstitial fibrosis develops, and blood vessels become narrowed or obliterated. Virtually every patient who acquires radiation pneumonitis also develops radiation fibrosis; however, fibrosis may occur in the absence of a clinically significant acute phase, presumably through the organization of a subacute and more indolent reaction. Use of certain drugs may potentiate the effects of irradiation, but this does not completely account for the wide variation in the response of patients to a given dose suggesting that "host factors" may also

be important. *Thermal and blast injuries* initiate a similar series of pathogenetic events: diffuse parenchymal injury, followed by organization and repair. There is also abundant experimental and clinical evidence that *oxygen,* given in high concentrations for several days, also injures the lung; moreover, its acute effects and subsequent evolution are similar to those of irradiation but proceed more rapidly. Exposure to high concentrations of oxygen (60 to 100 percent) damages pulmonary capillary endothelium and initiates an acute infiltrative-edematous phase, often with hyaline membrane formation, followed by a proliferative phase leading to fibrosis and collagen deposition.

Circulatory disorders Numerous thromboembolic conditions and a variety of hemodynamic complications of disorders of the left side of the heart and the pulmonary venous system may cause obliteration of, or leakage from, small pulmonary blood vessels. Diffuse pulmonary infiltrations ensue if *thromboemboli* elicit a perivascular inflammatory response or if abnormal hydrostatic forces cause chronic accumulation of fluid in the interstitium; when excessive fluid is retained in the lung parenchyma for prolonged periods, as in *mitral stenosis* and *chronic left ventricular failure,* hemosiderin is deposited, and possibly it or other factors cause slowly progressive interstitial fibrosis. At times, focal organization may progress to bone deposition.

Immunologic disorders The disorders in this category are presumed to originate through aberrant immunologic mechanisms; this assumption remains unproved because antigen, antibody, and (at times) complement have not been consistently demonstrated at the sites of the pulmonary lesions and in other involved organs. Three major subgroups can be differentiated on the basis of their clinical manifestations and immunologic characteristics:

HYPERSENSITIVITY PNEUMONIA (see also Chap. 258) A good example of how numerous apparently varied disorders express themselves through a common pathogenetic mechanism can be found in hypersensitivity pneumonia (also called extrinsic allergic alveolitis and allergic interstitial pneumonitis). The factors that determine the pathogenesis of pulmonary infiltration following inhalation of dust include the immunologic reactivity of the host, the nature and size of the inhaled organic dust and the degree and duration of exposure. The onset may be acute if exposure is great or if the patient is exquisitely sensitive to the antigen; conversely, the onset may be insidious in weakly sensitized subjects or when exposure is mild.

Hypersensitivity to a suspected (specific) antigen can be established by demonstrating precipitating antibodies in the patient's serum, and by the presence of a positive intermediate skin reaction (Arthus type) 4 to 8 h after intradermal testing. Finding precipitating antibodies alone is not diagnostic because they are often found in exposed persons without lung disease. Evidence for an etiologic role for the antigen is obtained by reproducing an acute attack, with attendant pulmonary function abnormalities, following inhalation of an aerosol containing the antigen. Evidence such as the presence of granulomas and sensitized T lymphocytes implicates type IV cell-mediated immune responses, in addition to type III immune-complex phenomena, in the pathogenesis of hypersensitivity pneumonitis.

The pathogenesis of pulmonary lesions following the long-term ingestion of certain drugs is unclear. The acute interstitial pulmonary inflammatory reaction they provoke is similar to that found following the inhalation of sensitizing antigens, but direct evidence of an allergic mechanism is lacking and their classification is inferential. Specific examples of immunologic disorders involving the lung are detailed in Chap. 258.

"COLLAGEN DISEASES" Diseases in this group share such common features as multisystem involvement, considerable overlap in organ dysfunction (e.g., arthritis, nephritis), and the presence of excessive quantities of immunoglobulins and circulating non-organ-specific "autoantibodies." Although antigen-antibody complexes have been implicated in the pathogenesis of the nephritis of lupus erythematosus, there is no direct evidence that they cause the associated pulmonary infiltrates, nor have immune complexes been identified in the other "collagen diseases." Pathologically, the prototype lesion is vascular, and pulmonary vasculitis is found in periarteritis nodosa (and related disorders like Churg-Strauss allergic granulomatosis) and Wegener's granulomatosis. Vasculitis may also be present in scleroderma, rheumatoid arthritis, lupus erythematosus, dermatomyositis, and Sjögren's syndrome, but a more common pulmonary lesion is diffuse interstitial fibrosis. The pathogenesis of organizing interstitial pneumonias is unknown but may pertain to the unique vulnerability of the lung. The lung receives more blood flow, and hence more circulating antigens, antibodies, or immune complexes, than other organs and offers a much greater surface area than the skin for contact with environmental antigens. Procainamide-induced lupus erythematosus, for example, is associated with a higher incidence of pulmonary infiltration than the naturally occurring disease.

GOODPASTURE'S SYNDROME This syndrome is differentiated from the collagen diseases on the basis of clinical and experimental evidence that is mediated by a cytotoxic tissue-specific antibody rather than by immune complexes. There appear to be antigenic similarities between alveolar and glomerular basement membranes, and antibodies to them have been identified in the serum and on the basement membranes of the respective organs. However, it is not known how the presence of the specific antibodies induces injury after combination with tissue antigens or why the disorder afflicts chiefly men 16 to 25 years of age.

Occupational causes A wide variety of mineral dusts and chemical fumes may be inhaled (Chap. 259). Whether or not disease is produced depends on a number of factors, including the duration of exposure and concentration of the agent, its chemical properties (e.g., whether or not it is inert, fibrogenic, granuloma-inducing), and the susceptibility (including immunologic responsiveness) of the host. The long-standing notion that a "host factor" exists has received support from the presence of rheumatoid factor and antinuclear factor in the serum of many patients with various pneumoconioses, particularly of a severe or accelerated variety.

Diffuse parenchymal infiltration results from the tissue injury produced by the toxic substances and the cellular response they provoke and from the subsequent organization and evolution of the reaction. Once exposure ceases, the process may remain stable, as in early ("simple") silicosis, or it may progress slowly and become clinically apparent only many years later, as in asbestosis. The growth and conglomeration of the early small infiltrates in patients with coal miner's pneumoconiosis or silicosis into progressive massive fibrosis may occur spontaneously, but often signifies the presence of either rheumatoid disease (Caplan's syndrome or rheumatoid pneumoconiosis), or coexisting infection with *Mycobacterium tuberculosis* or other mycobacteria.

Unknown origin Although the basic pathogenesis of many of the diseases just discussed (e.g., drug reactions, congenital disorders, immunologic diseases) is not known, they can be classified according to major subject headings that allow inferences to be made concerning their etiology. There remain several important diffuse infiltrative diseases of the lung that cannot be conveniently grouped and so are listed separately under disorders of unknown origin.

SARCOIDOSIS Sarcoidosis (Chap. 216) is a multisystem disease with characteristic, but *not* pathognomonic, noncaseating granulomas commonly involving the lungs, lymph nodes, and liver. Interalveolar and interstitial granulomas may be undetectable roentgenographically but can be recognized by sensitive tests of pulmonary function. The natural history of sarcoidosis is variable and capricious. Spontaneously, the pulmonary lesions may either resolve completely or organize by extensive scarring and disruption of alveoli (honeycombing) with devastating loss of pulmonary function.

HISTIOCYTOSIS X Histiocytosis X (Chap. 322) is a generic term that includes *Letterer-Siwe disease, Hand-Schüller-Christian disease, eosinophilic granuloma*, and their variants. The disorder is characterized by proliferation of, and infiltration by, histiocytes into various tissues. The stimulus for the histiocytic proliferation is unknown, and inflammatory, immunologic, and neoplastic causes have been considered. Tissue eosinophilia may occur, and the presence of foam cells, collagenization, and fibrosis indicates older organizing lesions. The major variations of histiocytosis X depend on the age of the patient, the extent of involvement, and the duration of the disease. The pulmonary complications vary, therefore, in a manner analogous to the progression in sarcoidosis, from acute cellular infiltration to chronic extensive scarring of the lung parenchyma.

IDIOPATHIC PULMONARY HEMOSIDEROSIS This uncommon disease affects infants and children and is extremely rare in persons more than 20 years of age; its chief manifestations are diffuse pulmonary infiltration, anemia, and hemoptysis. Bleeding into the lung interstitium accounts for the anemia and, when brisk, for the hemoptysis. Hemosiderin-filled macrophages, the clinical hallmark of the disease, can be found in the sputum during exacerbations and are abundant in the lung at all times. The presence of blood or blood products appears to initiate a fibrogenic response that leads to an increase in reticulum, collagen, and, ultimately, fibrous tissue. The prognosis is poor, and death usually occurs during an acute episode of bleeding; however, if the patient survives for several years, extensive interstitial fibrosis may result. Theories about etiology have included immunologic mechanisms, vascular defects, and abnormal iron storage, but none is proved.

PULMONARY ALVEOLAR PROTEINOSIS In 1958 Rosen, Castleman, and Liebow described 27 cases of a new entity they called pulmonary alveolar proteinosis. The disorder is characterized by diffuse pulmonary infiltrations, which, in contrast to the disorders described earlier, are confined to alveolar spaces; alveoli in involved areas are filled with a dense granular material that stains vividly with the periodic acid-Schiff technique. The material has been identified as a lipoprotein with many chemical similarities to pulmonary surfactant, but with different physical properties. Although hyperplasia of alveolar epithelium is usually present, inflammation and fibrous thickening of the interalveolar septa are conspicuously absent, and, in the absence of infection, fibrous tissue organization to the stage of honeycombing has been reported only once. In contrast to the relatively uniform roentgenographic and pathologic appearance of the lungs in pulmonary alveolar proteinosis, the clinical manifestations are extremely varied; they range from asymptomatic involvement to total disability or death from hypoxia, cor pulmonale, or secondary infection (often with "opportunistic" microorganisms, notably *Nocardia*). The etiology is unknown, and the natural history is poorly defined and appears to be variable: both spontaneous resolution and worsening have been reported.

DIFFUSE IDIOPATHIC INTERSTITIAL FIBROSIS   The lack of specificity of the pulmonary pathologic reaction in the large number of diffuse pulmonary infiltrative disorders is best illustrated by the many known causes of or associations with diffuse interstitial fibrosis. *Identical* pathologic findings have been documented in cases caused by infections, occupational exposure, hypersensitivity reactions, a variety of familial disorders, irradiation or oxygen inhalation, prolonged circulatory failure, "collagen disease," and desquamative interstitial pneumonia. The term *"usual* organizing interstitial pneumonia" (UIP) has been recommended for all these disorders, because it correctly describes the similar pulmonary pathology in all of them, but, being descriptive, it ignores what is known about etiology and pathogenesis. In most large series of cases of UIP, the etiology or pathogenesis can be identified in about half, and the remaining half are labeled "idiopathic." The patients in whom a specific diagnosis cannot be made have been described by a variety of terms, but the most common one used in the United States is diffuse idiopathic interstitial fibrosis. The confusion about nomenclature is reflected in the number of synonyms listed in Table 264-1 that are mainly descriptive, each having some advantages and some disadvantages over the others. The term *Hamman-Rich disease* should be reserved for patients with acute rapidly progressive diffuse interstitial pneumonitis with fibrosis; this variant is much less common than chronic idiopathic pulmonary fibrosis.

Until recently, *desquamative interstitial pneumonia* (DIP) was considered sufficiently distinct to warrant classification as a separate entity. In patients with DIP, there is striking hyperplasia of the type II alveolar epithelial cells and filling of alveolar spaces with macrophages; in addition, there is an impressive interstitial cellular infiltration and an interstitial fibrotic reaction of varying severity. Evidence of progression from DIP to UIP on serial biopsies has led to the belief that the DIP is probably a stage in the development of the more commonly observed UIP.

CLINICAL MANIFESTATIONS   The symptoms, signs, and results of laboratory tests obviously vary, depending on the extent of the pulmonary process and its rate of progress. Moreover, if diffuse pulmonary infiltration is but one component of a systemic disorder (e.g., in collagen diseases), the clinical manifestations may pertain to other organ system disease. In addition, pulmonary involvement is substantially augmented by the presence of secondary complications—infection, cor pulmonale, and pneumothorax.

The predominant complaint caused by pulmonary infiltration is dyspnea, which is usually insidious in development, related primarily to exercise at its onset, and progressive. Weakness and fatigue often occur and are difficult to dissociate from breathlessness. Cough is present much less commonly than in other pulmonary diseases, and, if productive, especially if associated with fever, signifies the coexistence of bronchopulmonary infection. A variety of uncharacteristic and variable pleuritic and substernal chest pains may develop during the evolution of the disorder. Findings on physical examination may be unremarkable, especially in the early stages. The most characteristic findings are increased transmission of breath sounds and showers of superficial crackling rales at the lung bases. Clubbing of the digits and cyanosis indicate more severe involvement; signs of cor pulmonale (loud pulmonary second sound, parasternal heave, venous distention, hepatomegaly,

and peripheral edema) imply advanced lung dysfunction with hypoxia and obliteration of the pulmonary vascular bed.

Chest roentgenograms characteristically reveal diffuse reticular or reticulonodular densities that are most marked in the lung bases. At times roentgenograms may not show any abnormalities, even in the presence of significant symptoms and pulmonary function abnormalities, or the lungs may have a homogeneous "ground-glass" haziness. With progression of the process, the linear densities become coarser; small cystic lesions appear (honeycombing); marked loss of lung volume occurs (shown primarily by elevation of the diaphragm); and central pulmonary arterial dilatation and right ventricular enlargement may become apparent. Pleural involvement (thickening, effusions, plaques, and calcification) is uncommon except in asbestosis and collagen diseases.

Routine laboratory studies are not very helpful. Anemia may be present in chronic infection, hemosiderosis, or collagen diseases. Polycythemia may be present if hypoxia has been severe and prolonged. Pulmonary function studies, however, provide valuable documentation of the severity of impairment that is useful in deciding whether lung disease is present in symptomatic patients with normal chest roentgenograms, whether treatment is indicated, and in defining prognosis; they are also useful in following the course of the disease and objectively determining its response to treatment. However, pulmonary function studies do *not* delineate etiology or pathogenesis, because, as might be anticipated from the similar pathologic involvement of the lungs in the various disorders, the functional impairment is also similar.

The earliest easily measured physiologic abnormality is a reduction in the diffusing capacity, which reflects mainly a loss of pulmonary capillaries or, less likely, an increase in the diffusion pathway from the alveolar spaces to the interior of the red blood cells, or both. Another basic functional disturbance in the lungs of patients with diffuse interstitial infiltrative disorders is a decrease in pulmonary compliance (i.e., the lungs become stiffer); this explains why these diseases are the classic cause of a restrictive ventilatory defect, manifested by a loss of both vital capacity and residual volume, the former proportionately more than the latter.

Gas exchange abnormalities consist of a decrease in resting arterial oxygen tension or, more precisely, an increase in the alveolar-arterial oxygen tension difference. Unwarranted emphasis has been placed on the contribution of impaired diffusion of oxygen (the so-called "alveolar-capillary block syndrome") to the alveolar-arterial oxygen tension difference, which is now recognized as being caused by mismatching of the distribution of inspired air and blood flow (ventilation-perfusion imbalance) (Chap. 255). However, the abnormality of diffusion is responsible for the characteristic finding of a worsening of arterial oxygen tension in these patients during exercise.

A corollary finding is alveolar hyperventilation (presumably owing to stimuli from hypoxia and intrapulmonary reflexes) that occurs despite an increased physiologic dead space. Arterial carbon dioxide tension is thereby reduced while the disease process progresses through most of its course; carbon dioxide tension becomes normal and finally elevated only in the terminal stages of the illness.

DIAGNOSIS   Careful historical examination is essential to the diagnosis of occupational lung diseases and hypersensitivity pneumonias. Chills, fever, weight loss, fatigue, and other nonspecific symptoms suggest that either an infectious process or a systemic disorder underlies the diffuse pulmonary infiltration.

Physical examination is not likely to contribute to the differential diagnosis of those disorders confined to the lungs but may reveal important evidence of multisystem involvement in infectious, neoplastic, familial, metabolic, immunologic, and circulatory diseases as well as in sarcoidosis and histiocytosis X.

The results of routine blood counts, urinalysis, and blood chemistries are not likely to reveal important abnormalities or provide clues to the etiology of the underlying pulmonary disorder. Infections may be identified by appropriate cultural or serologic studies; hypersensitivity and immunologic diseases may be established by finding circulating antibodies or immune complexes; and neoplasms may be diagnosed by cytologic examination of the sputum. However, specific diagnosis of most diffuse infiltrative diseases, if it can be made at all, requires examination of tissue.

Biopsy is often the only method of documenting the type and cause of pulmonary disorder. The source of biopsy material is determined by the likelihood of obtaining diagnostic tissue and by the risks inherent in the procedure. Skin, lymph nodes, and liver are useful biopsy sites in disseminated infections, neoplasms, and at times sarcoidosis. But finding noncaseating granulomas is by no means pathognomonic of sarcoidosis, and a biopsy from within the thorax is more likely than one from a more peripheral organ to discriminate among the multiple causes of granulomas. If cervical or supraclavicular lymph nodes are palpable, they should be examined histologically and culturally. If nodes are not palpable, but paratracheal or mediastinal nodes are evident roentgenographically, mediastinoscopy is indicated. At times, anterior mediastinotomy provides a useful approach to hilar nodes.

The majority of diffuse pulmonary infiltrative diseases are not associated with significant lymphadenopathy; if a diagnosis cannot be documented by other means, lung biopsy is indicated. Three types of lung biopsy are available: percutaneous, transbronchial, and open. Transbronchial biopsy is gradually replacing percutaneous biopsy and has proved useful in patients with diffuse infiltrative disease of the lung. However, the amount of tissue sampled is small, which limits diagnostic investigation. For this reason, open lung biopsy is recommended because it allows removal of a suitable piece of selected lung tissue that can be cultured and examined histologically by light and electron microscopy; in addition, a portion can be frozen for special studies at a later date (virus cultures, chemical or spectroscopic analysis). Transbronchial biopsy is the procedure of choice in the seriously ill patient in whom diagnostic information is imperative and the risks of thoracotomy are grave.

Recently, it has been shown that the uptake of radioactive gallium by the lungs, assessed by external counters, correlates with the cellularity found on lung biopsy. Similarly, the cellular and immunoglobulin composition of fluid lavaged from the lung during fiberoptic bronchoscopy has been correlated with the cellularity of the infiltrative process. At present, the results of these procedures do not appear to have diagnostic specificity but may indicate responsiveness to anti-inflammatory drugs and provide a means of assessing the influence of therapy.

TREATMENT The majority of diffuse pulmonary infiltrations do not respond well to therapy, but some are eminently treatable, and the value of making an etiologic diagnosis lies in determining which of the many available therapeutic agents should be used. Specific chemotherapy is available for most infectious agents. Removal from exposure diminishes the risk of occupational pulmonary diseases and may allow clearing of hypersensitivity pneumonias. Lung lavage is indicated in severely disabled patients with pulmonary alveolar proteinosis. Plasmapheresis to remove circulating antibasement membrane

antibodies has proved effective in controlling Goodpasture's syndrome.

Corticosteroids are useful in the treatment of many of the causes of organizing interstitial pneumonia, especially when administered early. They are helpful in patients with hypersensitivity pneumonias, chemical injuries of the lungs, sarcoidosis, histiocytosis X, and desquamative interstitial pneumonia; their role in idiopathic hemosiderosis and acute idiopathic interstitial pneumonia (Hamman-Rich disease) is questionable. They are seldom of benefit in the treatment of collagen diseases, diseases due to occupational dusts, and chronic diffuse interstitial fibrosis of known or idiopathic origin.

When corticosteroids are used, they should be given in sufficient doses to ensure that a response will occur if one can be elicited. Patients with disorders that usually improve (sarcoidosis, etc.), customarily improve when given prednisone, 40 to 60 mg per day (or its equivalent); the dosage is reduced 5 to 10 mg per day each week until maintenance levels are reached—usually 5 to 15 mg per day or 10 to 30 mg every other day. The patient's response must be followed objectively by serial chest roentgenograms and, more importantly, by appropriate tests of pulmonary function (arterial blood gases, lung volumes, diffusing capacity), since subjective responses to corticosteroids are notoriously unreliable. Measurements of gas exchange during exercise, such as the change in arterial P_{O_2} or alveolar-arterial P_{O_2} difference divided by the change in O_2 consumption, are reported to be the most sensitive tests of responsiveness to treatment. Patients with infiltrative disorders in which improvement is less predictable (organizing interstitial pneumonia, collagen diseases) should be started on even higher doses (60 to 100 mg prednisone per day) in an attempt to achieve a response; if pulmonary function studies document that no improvement has occurred, the drug should be rapidly discontinued.

Immunosuppressive therapy has produced striking long-term remissions of severe forms of Wegener's granulomatosis, usually a progressive and fatal disease. Rheumatoid arthritis and lupus erythematosus nephritis have responded to cytotoxic drugs in short-term controlled trials, but whether the fibrotic pulmonary infiltrations associated with these diseases will resolve remains to be determined. Thus far, the results from uncontrolled trials are not encouraging. Drugs that inhibit fibrogenesis are being tried in controlled studies, but none is available for routine use.

PROGNOSIS It follows from the information presented in previous sections that the course and prognosis of diffuse infiltrative diseases of the lung are extremely variable. The outlook is determined by the natural history of the underlying cause of the disorder, how far advanced it is when diagnosed, its response to therapy, and the presence of complications. The prognosis is favorable in those diseases with reversible component, either spontaneous or induced by easily tolerated therapy (infections, chemical injuries, hypersensitivity pneumonias, and sarcoidosis). The prognosis is poor in most collagen diseases, progressive occupational dust diseases, chronic diffuse idiopathic interstitial fibrosis, and in any condition that has advanced to severe lung fibrosis and honeycombing; these disorders·are associated with slow but relentless lung destruction, with progressive hypoxia, and finally with death from cor pulmonale or secondary bronchopulmonary infection.

REFERENCES

CARRINGTON CB et al: Natural history and treated course of usual and desquamative interstitial pneumonia. N Engl J Med 298:801, 1978

CRYSTAL RG et al: Idiopathic pulmonary fibrosis: Clinical, histologic, radiographic, physiologic, scintigraphic, cytologic, and biochemical aspects. Ann Intern Med 85:769, 1976

DREISIN RB et al: Circulating immune complexes in the idiopathic interstitial pneumonias. N Engl J Med 298:353, 1978

EPLER GR et al: Normal chest roentgenograms in chronic diffuse infiltrative lung disease. N Engl J Med 298:934, 1978

KAO D et al: Advances in the treatment of pulmonary alveolar proteinosis. Am Rev Respir Dis 111:361, 1975

LEWIS JG: Eosinophilic granuloma and its variants with special reference to lung involvement. Q J Med 33:337, 1964

LIVINGSTON JL et al: Diffuse interstitial pulmonary fibrosis: A clinical, radiological, and pathological study based on 45 patients. Q J Med 33:71, 1964

MATTHAY RA et al: Pulmonary manifestations of systemic lupus erythematosus: Review of twelve cases of acute lupus pneumonitis. Medicine 54:397, 1975

MCCOMBS RP: Diseases due to immunologic reactions in the lungs. N Engl J Med 286:1186, 1245, 1972

SCADDING JG: Diffuse pulmonary alveolar fibrosis. Thorax 29:271, 1974

Vascular diseases of the lung

265
PRIMARY PULMONARY HYPERTENSION

JOHN ROSS, JR.

Primary (or idiopathic) pulmonary hypertension is an uncommon disease, the diagnosis of which can be established only after a thorough search for the usual causes of pulmonary hypertension. The patient with primary pulmonary hypertension typically is a young female between the ages of 20 and 40, although older and younger patients of either sex have been described. The clinical and laboratory features of severe pulmonary hypertension are present, but there is no evidence of parenchymal pulmonary disease or of primary heart disease, nor is there evidence for the occurrence of pulmonary emboli. Anatomic verification often has been necessary to distinguish clearly the primary form of pulmonary hypertension from that due to multiple pulmonary emboli, although angiography and radioisotope scanning methods have facilitated this differentiation considerably.

PATHOLOGY The findings on pathologic examination of patients with primary pulmonary hypertension usually are confined to the right side of the heart and lungs. The right atrium often is enlarged and the right ventricle is hypertrophied. Frequently, the large pulmonary arteries exhibit atherosclerotic plaques. The disease process involves the small pulmonary arteries (between 40 and 300 μm in diameter), which exhibit muscular hypertrophy and intimal hyperplasia, sometimes with fibrosis. On occasion, a necrotizing arteritis may be encountered. Other histologic studies have shown a reduced number of small arteries, as well as fewer capillaries in the alveolar wall. Electron-microscopic studies have documented an increase in thickness of the endothelial cells and basement membranes of alveolar capillaries, and some capillaries are blocked by the abnormal epithelial cells. Medial hypertrophy of muscular pulmonary arteries may be the first response to prolonged pulmonary vasoconstriction, but in later stages of the disease concentric laminar intimal fibrosis and plexiform lesions appearing as cellular, intraluminal tufts (so-called "plexogenic pulmonary arteriopathy") may develop. Patients with recurrent pulmonary thromboembolism may clinically resemble patients with primary pulmonary hypertension, but his-

tologic sections of the lung exhibit various degrees of organization of pulmonary thromboemboli; some may be recanalized, there may be fibrous septa and eccentric fibrosis in the vessels; secondary medial hypertrophy of muscular arteries may be marked, but plexiform lesions are not present. In infants and young children with pulmonary venoocclusive disease the clinical picture may suggest primary pulmonary hypertension, and the pulmonary wedge pressure may be normal. Organized thrombotic disease is found in the venules and small veins, together with proximal hypertrophy of the muscular venous wall and secondary medial hypertrophy in the pulmonary arterioles.

Rarely, disease of the systemic arterial vascular bed resembling that found in the pulmonary blood vessels has been described. The syncope and sudden death which may occur in this disease have been attributed to involvement of the coronary arterial branch supplying the sinoatrial node in some patients.

ETIOLOGY The cause of primary pulmonary hypertension is unknown, but a number of possible etiologic factors have been suggested. A few patients with primary pulmonary hypertension have been reported in whom minimal changes were found in the pulmonary vessels on pathologic examination, and this observation has raised the possibility that a neurohumoral vasoconstrictor mechanism is involved. Support for this view has been provided by the observation that the pulmonary vascular resistance can be acutely reduced in some patients with this disease by the intrapulmonary injection of vasodilators, or by breathing oxygen. A febrile illness may precede the onset of the disease by a variable period and has been implicated in the etiology. The occurrence of the disease in young females has prompted the suggestion that unrecognized thromboemboli or amniotic fluid emboli during pregnancy may play a role. In other patients, it seems quite possible that the disease may represent an end stage of earlier, unrecognized emboli originating from the legs or pelvic veins. An apparent association between an increased occurrence of primary pulmonary hypertension and use of the anoretic agent aminorex fumarate (Menocil), an agent having structural similarity to ephedrine, was observed in Europe between 1967 and 1970. The alkaloids in many species of crotalaria plants used in herbal brews may cause pulmonary hypertension in humans, as demonstrated experimentally in rats. The use of oral contraceptives may bear a relation to the occurrence of pulmonary hypertension, particularly in patients with predisposing factors such as systemic lupus erythematosus or a family history of primary pulmonary hypertension.

Raynaud's phenomenon precedes the onset of primary pulmonary hypertensive disease by a number of years in an appreciable number of patients. This association and the occurrence of Raynaud's disease in scleroderma, disseminated lupus erythematosus, rheumatoid arthritis, and dermatomyositis have led to the speculation that primary pulmonary hypertension may represent a form of collagen vascular disease. Moreover, primary pulmonary hypertension and collagen vascular disease, including lupus erythematosus, have been reported to occur simultaneously in a number of patients. It also has been suggested that the disease may be congenital and present from birth; however, the closely packed, parallel elastic fibers in the main pulmonary arteries in patients having Eisenmenger's syndrome from birth, described by some investigators, usually have not been observed in patients with primary pulmonary hypertension. Finally, primary pulmonary hypertension has been reported in a number of families; sometimes more than two members and up to three generations have been affected. A fibrinolytic defect was reported in one family study.

PATHOPHYSIOLOGY Some studies have suggested that the response of the pulmonary vascular bed is labile early in the course of this disease, as evidenced by a response to vasodilating agents and oxygen. It also has been proposed that the disease tends to progress. Thus, serial cardiac catheterizations have shown a tendency for the pulmonary vascular resistance to increase and to become fixed. With the development of severe pulmonary vascular disease, abnormal elevation of the pulmonary arterial pressure occurs, often to a striking degree, and the pulmonary arterial pressure may be equal to that in the systemic arterial bed. The pulmonary arterial wedge pressure is normal in patients with primary pulmonary hypertension, the cardiac output is normal or reduced, and no intracardiac shunts are detected. In many patients the mean right atrial pressure is elevated, and the a wave in the right atrium may be markedly elevated, an indication of the forceful atrial contraction necessary to fill the hypertrophied right ventricle. With the long-standing overload on the right side of the heart, right ventricular failure finally develops. In some patients, peripheral cyanosis\occurs secondary to reduced cardiac output, and occasionally central cyanosis becomes evident at the end stage of the disease because of right to left shunting through a patent foramen ovale. Mild systemic arterial desaturation is quite common, even in the absence of heart failure, and may be due to shunting within the lungs. Pulmonary function in patients with primary pulmonary hypertension generally is normal, although hyperventilation often is present, resulting in hypocapnia and a decreased serum bicarbonate concentration. A low carbon monoxide-diffusing capacity has been described in some patients.

CLINICAL PICTURE The patient, usually a young female, gives a history of relatively recent onset of symptoms. Ordinarily, the natural course of the disease encompasses less than 5 years, but occasionally survival for 25 years or more has been reported. Not uncommonly, patients with primary pulmonary hypertension are classified as neurotic early in the course of their disease because of the hyperventilation, chest discomfort, and the relative paucity of objective findings. Precordial pain on exertion occurs in from 25 to 50 percent of patients, and occasionally severe chest pain has been associated with a dissection of the main pulmonary artery. Other common symptoms are weakness, fatigue, exertional dyspnea, and effort syncope. Hoarseness may be noted because of compression of the left recurrent laryngeal nerve by the enlarged pulmonary artery. Unexplained sudden death occurs relatively often. Sudden death also has occurred during cardiac catheterization or surgical procedures and after the administration of barbiturates or anesthetic agents. The terminal course usually is characterized by right-sided heart failure. Very rarely, spontaneous regression of the disease has been reported.

On physical examination, the jugular venous pulse usually shows a prominent a wave, there is a right ventricular heave, and an impulse may be felt over the region of the main pulmonary artery. An ejection click may be audible at the pulmonic area, the second heart sound is narrowly split, and the pulmonic closure sound is markedly accentuated and may be palpable. Often, an atrial gallop sound is heard at the lower left sternal border, and in some patients there is an ejection murmur at the pulmonic area, or the early diastolic murmur of pulmonic regurgitation. The chest roentgenogram may show cardiac enlargement with right ventricular and right atrial prominence, and there is marked dilation of the pulmonary artery segment. Peripherally, the pulmonary arteries taper sharply, and the lung fields may appear oligemic. The electrocardiogram almost always shows some evidence of right ventricular enlargement, with right axis deviation, right ventricular hypertrophy in the precordial leads, and sometimes inverted T waves over the right precordium. Right atrial enlargement also may be evident on the electrocardiogram.

DIFFERENTIAL DIAGNOSIS It is imperative that the diagnosis of primary pulmonary hypertension not be made until potentially treatable causes of elevated pulmonary arterial pressure have been excluded. The presence of pulmonary hypertension and cor pulmonale caused by chronic pulmonary disease can be established readily by finding abnormalities in pulmonary function. Cardiac catheterization studies are necessary to search for a primary cardiac defect, and angiography or radioactive lung-scanning studies also may be indicated to detect pulmonary emboli (Chap. 266). In performing pulmonary arteriography, injection of small amounts of contrast medium is advisable since sudden death has occasionally occurred. Patients having chronic emboli to the lungs are difficult to distinguish from those with primary pulmonary hypertension, but the distinction is important because anticoagulants, inferior vena caval or common femoral vein interruption, and pulmonary embolectomy sometimes have been effective in patients with embolic disease. The lung scan and pulmonary arteriogram are typically normal in primary pulmonary hypertension, but with thromboembolic pulmonary hypertension perfusion defects on lung scan or pulmonary arterial occlusions and filling defects on angiography often are visible. With pulmonary embolism, serial chest x-rays may show evidence of pulmonary infarction. Open lung biopsy has been used occasionally to differentiate primary pulmonary hypertension from the thromboembolic variety. Sometimes a site of origin for emboli cannot be identified in the leg veins, and other possible sources should be considered, such as right atrial thrombus, or ovarian and pelvic vein thromboses.

Several congenital cardiac conditions must be considered and excluded by appropriate cardiac catheterization studies. Valvular pulmonic stenosis usually can be distinguished from pulmonary hypertension by identification of the delayed, soft pulmonic closure sound, but peripheral stenoses of the pulmonary arteries may be associated with an increased second heart sound. A left-to-right shunt at the pulmonary arterial, ventricular, or atrial levels should be sought. The wide, fixed splitting of the second heart sound should be helpful in identifying patients with atrial septal defect. Eisenmenger's syndrome in a patient with ventricular septal defect or patent ductus arteriosus (Chap. 240) may be confused with primary pulmonary hypertension, but usually in Eisenmenger's syndrome cyanosis, polycythemia, and clubbing are present, and at cardiac catheterization a large right-to-left shunt at the ventricular or pulmonary arterial level can be demonstrated.

The murmurs of tricuspid or pulmonic regurgitation and the atrial gallop sounds heard in patients with primary pulmonary hypertension may be mistaken for the murmurs of rheumatic mitral and aortic valve disease, or vice versa. Before making the diagnosis of primary pulmonary hypertension, the presence of left atrial hypertension due to undetected mitral stenosis, or to a more unusual lesion such as left atrial myxoma or cor triatriatum, should be specifically sought and excluded. This can be done by obtaining pulmonary arterial wedge pressure tracings or by catheterization of the left side of the heart, with angiography if necessary.

THERAPY Presently, no definitive treatment is available for patients with primary pulmonary hypertension, and therapy during their progressive downhill course therefore must be palliative. The use of anticoagulants is of doubtful value, provided chronic pulmonary embolic phenomena can be excluded. Right-sided heart failure should be treated with a cardiotonic and diuretic regimen (Chap. 236). Since there is no hypercapnia in these patients, the hypoxia which may accompany heart failure can be treated safely with oxygen therapy.

Pharmacologic approaches to therapy have proved disappointing, and though transient reductions in pulmonary vascular resistance may be observed with intrapulmonary arterial injection of acetylcholine or tolazoline, the chronic oral use of these agents usually has not been effective. Administration of isoproterenol also may lower the pulmonary vascular resistance, and favorable effects on syncope and dyspnea were reported in a young patient treated for 3 years with sublingual isoproterenol.

REFERENCES

ALPERT JS, BRAUNWALD E: Primary pulmonary hypertension, in *Heart Disease,* E Braunwald (ed). Philadelphia, Saunders, 1980, chap 44

BOURDILLON PDV, OAKELY CM: Regression of primary pulmonary hypertension. Br Heart J 38:264, 1976

EDWARDS WD, EDWARDS JE: Clinical primary pulmonary hypertension. Three pathologic types. Circulation 56:884, 1977

FOLLATH F et al: Drug-induced pulmonary hypertension? Br Med J 1:265, 1971

FOWLER NO: Cor pulmonale: Pulmonary embolism and idiopathic pulmonary hypertension, in *Cardiac Diagnosis and Treatment,* 2d ed, NO Fowler (ed). New York, Harper & Row, 1976, p 816

HARRIS P, HEATH D: Unexplained pulmonary hypertension, in *The Human Pulmonary Circulation.* Edinburgh, Churchill, Livingstone, 1977, pp 418–440

HATANO S, STRASSER T (eds): Primary pulmonary hypertension: Report on a WHO meeting. Geneva, World Health Organization, 1975

WAGENVOORT CA, WAGENVOORT N: *Pathology of Pulmonary Hypertension.* New York, Wiley, 1977, p 345

266
PULMONARY THROMBOEMBOLISM

KENNETH M. MOSER

Pulmonary thromboembolism (PTE) is a leading cause of morbidity and mortality, and can appear in many clinical contexts. Epidemiologic surveys indicate that PTE is responsible for more than 50,000 deaths in the United States annually. However, available data suggest that less than 10 percent of all pulmonary emboli result in death. Thus, the incidence of fatal plus nonfatal emboli in this nation probably exceeds 500,000

annually. This overall incidence seems verified by autopsy statistics. Evidence of recent or old embolism is detected in 25 to 30 percent of routine autopsies; with special techniques, this figure exceeds 60 percent. Even these data underestimate incidence, since many emboli resolve without trace and are not found at postmortem examination. The high incidence of PTE at autopsy contrasts sharply with the incidence of antemortem diagnosis. Available information suggests that an antemortem diagnosis has been made in only 10 to 30 percent of all cases in which old or recent embolism is demonstrated at autopsy.

The three factors involved in thrombogenesis are stasis, abnormalities in the vessel wall, and alterations in the blood coagulation system. Coagulation alterations have been studied extensively, but as yet there is no reliable test for a state of "hypercoagulability" in a given patient. Conditions which are associated with a high risk of venous thromboembolism include the postoperative period; pregnancy, particularly the postpartum period; in the opinion of many, the use of anovulatory drugs; congestive heart failure; chronic pulmonary disease; fractures or other injuries of the lower extremities; chronic deep venous insufficiency of the legs; prolonged bed rest; and carcinoma.

Although there is increasing awareness of the conditions which predispose to PTE, detection of embolism in the majority of patients remains poor. One reason is inadequate understanding of the natural history of pulmonary embolism.

NATURAL HISTORY OF EMBOLISM

THE ACUTE EVENTS The immediate result of thromboembolism is complete or partial obstruction of the pulmonary arterial blood flow to the distal lung. This obstruction leads to a series of pathophysiologic events which can be categorized as the "respiratory" and "hemodynamic" consequences of PTE.

Respiratory consequences Embolic obstruction produces a zone of the lung which is ventilated but not perfused—an intrapulmonary "dead space" (Chap. 255). Because it cannot participate in the process of gas exchange, ventilation of this nonperfused area is "wasted," in the functional sense. A potential consequence of embolic obstruction is constriction of the air spaces and airways in the affected lung zone. In animal experiments in which each lung is ventilated separately, this "pneumoconstriction" appears to be due to the marked bronchoalveolar hypocapnia that results from cessation of pulmonary capillary blood flow because it is abolished by inhalation of carbon dioxide–enriched air. This probably occurs very rarely in patients who inhale dead space air (rich in carbon dioxide) into embolized lung zones.

Another disturbance caused by embolic obstruction—loss of alveolar surfactant—does not occur immediately. This surface-active lipoprotein is required to maintain alveolar stability. In its absence, alveolar collapse occurs. Cessation of pulmonary capillary blood flow leads to reduction in surfactant within 2 or 3 h, which becomes severe at 12 to 15 h. Frank atelectasis—the morphologic expression of alveolar instability—can be detected at 24 to 48 h after interruption of blood flow.

Arterial hypoxemia is a common, though by no means universal, consequence of embolism. The mechanisms responsible for hypoxemia are still debated. It appears that, acutely, hypoxemia is a consequence of ventilation/perfusion disturbances and/or cardiac failure with a lowered mixed venous P_{O_2} (widened arteriovenous P_{O_2} difference). Both of these abnormalities require rather massive occlusion to develop, and hypoxemia is characteristically most frequent and marked in massive embolism. Other mechanisms for hypoxemia which may be present at the outset or develop subsequently include perfusion of lung zones in which congestive atelectasis occurs as a result of surfactant loss; perfusion of zones partially collapsed by pleural fluid; and obligatory perfusion of lung zones which are poorly ventilated due to preexisting airways or parenchymal disease.

Hemodynamic consequences The primary hemodynamic consequence of thromboembolic obstruction is a reduction in the available cross-sectional area of the pulmonary arterial bed. This loss of vascular capacity increases the resistance to pulmonary blood flow; this resistance, if marked, leads to pulmonary hypertension and acute failure of the right ventricle. Tachycardia and often a decline in cardiac output also occur.

The factors which determine the severity of these hemodynamic changes have been a subject of continued debate. There is agreement that the *extent of embolic obstruction* is a key factor. However, the reserve capacity of the pulmonary arteriocapillary bed is so extensive that more than 50 percent of the vascular area must be obstructed before significant elevation in pulmonary arterial pressure results. Because pulmonary hypertension occurs in some patients with occlusion of lesser extent, investigators have searched for reflex or humoral vasoconstrictor mechanisms associated with embolism. Despite long and careful search for such mechanisms, their extent and frequency in human PTE remains unknown. Hence, some workers maintain that the degree of embolic obstruction itself is the only determinant of hemodynamic impairment. They suggest that instances of apparent disparity between the extent of embolism and clinical response reflect only clinical underestimation of the magnitude of the embolism. Other investigators, however, have presented compelling evidence to support the occurrence of vasoconstriction with embolism. Some have demonstrated that constriction is associated with obstruction of the smaller, but not the larger, pulmonary arterial vessels. Another thesis holds that serotonin, a known pulmonary vasoconstrictive-bronchoconstrictive substance, is released from platelets, coating fresh emboli as they lodge in the pulmonary tree. This thesis introduces the attractive concept that an embolus should be regarded as a packet with pharmacologic, as well as obstructive, potential. A consensus view, then, suggests that, while the extent of embolism is a key factor, humoral and/or reflex influences probably are operative in certain patients and compromise the pulmonary circulation to a greater extent than might be expected on an anatomic basis alone.

The cardiopulmonary status of the patient prior to embolism is also critical in determining the clinical severity of embolism. A small embolus may have limited impact upon an otherwise healthy individual but may have serious consequences in someone with advanced cardiac or pulmonary disease.

Both experimental and clinical studies have established that infarction—death of lung tissue—rarely accompanies embolic occlusion. It is likely that less than 10 percent of emboli in humans lead to infarction. That infarction rarely follows embolism should occasion little surprise. The lung has three avenues for obtaining its oxygen requirements: the pulmonary arterial circulation; the bronchial arterial circulation; and the airways. Thus, infarction occurs infrequently, and its appearance usually is associated with compromise of bronchial arterial flow and/or airways to the involved area. Such compromise is promoted by the existence of other cardiac or pulmonary diseases, such as left ventricular failure, mitral stenosis, and chronic obstructive lung disease. Thus, infarction may occur in 30 percent or more of such patients, while it is

quite rare in individuals who are free of cardiopulmonary disease.

BEYOND THE ACUTE STATE The vast majority of pulmonary emboli resolve, and resolve rather quickly. Resolution of fresh emboli begins within the first few days and is well advanced in 10 to 14 days. Two powerful mechanisms promote restoration of vascular patency: the fibrinolytic system and the process of organization. The fibrinolytic system seems specifically designed to dissolve fibrin thrombi wherever they occur in the body and is responsible for the rapid phase of thromboembolic resolution. Organization is a slower process, requiring some days. As it proceeds, the thrombus is gradually transformed into a small scar attached to the vascular wall.

The availability of these two efficient mechanisms raises the question as to why not all emboli resolve. There may be some impairment of the intrinsic fibrinolytic system. The emboli may have been well organized prior to their lodgment in the lung so that they are subject to neither fibrinolytic attack nor further organization. Alternatively, some emboli may be recurrent, so that their failure to resolve is more apparent than real.

Another important element of the natural history of thromboembolism is the development of bronchial arterial collateral circulation. If pulmonary arterial obstruction persists, bronchial arterial flow increases substantially over a period of several weeks, restoring flow to the capillary bed. With the return of flow, surfactant production is restored, so that alveolar stability is regained and congestive atelectasis resolves.

Finally, it should be recognized that most emboli are not totally occlusive. Some distal pulmonary arterial flow often persists and modifies the cardiopulmonary events described above.

DIAGNOSTIC FEATURES

Sudden onset of unexplained dyspnea should suggest the diagnosis of embolism. This symptom, related to the sudden addition of alveolar "dead space," is usually the only one which occurs. *Pleuritic chest pain and hemoptysis are present only when infarction has occurred* and, because bland embolism rarely leads to infarction, are usually absent. With extensive embolism, severe substernal oppressive discomfort may be present. Patients also may present with syncope, suggesting a neurologic disorder. The most reliable symptom, however, is breathlessness. Severe, persistent dyspnea is an ominous sign, for it usually indicates extensive embolic occlusion.

PHYSICAL EXAMINATION Findings on physical examination, like the history, may be deceptively normal. Examination of the lungs may disclose a few atelectatic rales; localized wheezes rarely are heard. A pleural friction rub or evidence of pleural effusion will not be present unless infarction has occurred.

On cardiac examination, the single consistent finding is tachycardia. Only in the rare cases of massive embolism will such signs as a right ventricular gallop, a palpable "lift" over the right ventricle, a loud pulmonary closure sound, or prominent *a* waves in the jugular venous pulse be found. A scratchy systolic ejection-type murmur may be heard in the pulmonic area. Also, a systolic or continuous murmur accentuated by inspiration may be audible over the lung fields. These murmurs appear to be generated by turbulence of flow in vessels partially obstructed by emboli since they disappear after resection or resolution of emboli. They should be carefully sought in any patient suspected of having PTE. Wide, often fixed, splitting of the second heart sound may be present. This indicates extensive embolic obstruction and implies both severe pulmonary hypertension and right ventricular failure. As embolic resolution occurs, this finding disappears. Absence of an accentuated pulmonic closure sound is not a reliable guide to the severity of PTE, since, when embolism is sufficiently massive to reduce cardiac output, pulmonary closure may be normal or diminished.

The detection of *deep venous thrombosis* qualifies as an excellent clue to the diagnosis of embolism, but its absence should by no means rule out the diagnosis. Even when sought with diligence, *clinical* evidence of thrombophlebitis is found in less than half of patients with PTE, even though thrombi *can* be detected by laboratory methods (e.g., radiolabeled fibrinogen). *Fever* in patients with pulmonary embolism is uncommon without complicating infection or infarction. With infarction, fever of 37.8 to 38.3°C [100 to 101°F (oral)] is the rule; but temperature elevations to 38.4°C (103°F) or above may occur, making difficult the differentiation between pulmonary infarction and infection.

On clinical grounds alone, then, a firm diagnosis of embolism cannot be made; the clinical *suspicion* of embolism requires confirmation by laboratory studies.

LABORATORY STUDIES   Routine laboratory studies contribute little toward the diagnosis. Leukocytosis and elevation of the sedimentation rate are rarely present in the absence of infarction. A diagnostic "triad" of elevation of serum lactic dehydrogenase (LDH) and bilirubin levels with a normal serum glutamic oxalacetic transaminase (SGOT) level has been proposed but is of limited value. Other blood tests, such as assay for specific fibrinopeptides or fibrin degradation products, have not been shown to be diagnostically reliable or specific.

Aside from tachycardia, the *electrocardiogram* is normal in most patients. With extensive embolization, there may be evidence of acute pulmonary hypertension, rightward shift of the QRS axis, a tall, peaked P wave, and ST-T changes indicative of right ventricular "strain" and "ischemia." These changes are often transient, lasting minutes to hours, but when persistent, suggest severe pulmonary vascular obstruction.

The *chest roentgenogram* may show a parenchymal infiltrate and evidence of a pleural effusion if *infarction* has occurred. Characteristically, the infiltrates caused by infarction abut against the pleura. However, their shape varies, and they do not usually appear until 12 to 36 h after the infarction has occurred. The effusion, which often precedes the infiltrate, is characteristically small. Thoracentesis usually, but by no means invariably, yields hemorrhagic fluid, with the characteristics of an exudate.

The radiographic findings with embolism alone are more subtle. *Differences in diameter between vessels which should be of equivalent size* should raise the suspicion of embolism. For example, embolic obstruction of the right main pulmonary artery can lead to dilation of the left main pulmonary artery because that vessel must accept the entire pulmonary flow. There may be abrupt *"cutoff"* of a vessel; i.e., as the vessel is traced distally, it suddenly disappears. Clot has the same radiodensity as blood, accounting for the proximal shadow; the absence of flow beyond the clot explains the sudden radiographic "disappearance" of the vessel.

Organization of a clot within a pulmonary artery may lead to retraction of the vessel's walls and a so-called "rattail configuration," in which the vessel is relatively normal proximally and suddenly tapers to a sharp point. Finally, there may be *abnormal radiolucency* in some lung zones due to absent or decreased flow. Such abnormally lucent areas, indicative of proximal arterial obstruction, are best appreciated by examining comparable areas in the two lung fields.

Even in embolization without infarction, the roentgenogram may show small infiltrates, which appear in about 24 h and

reflect atelectasis secondary to surfactant depletion. They are not associated with effusion, may fail to touch a pleural surface, and disappear without the linear scarring characteristic of infarction. It should be emphasized that a *normal chest roentgenogram does not exclude the diagnosis of PTE.* Indeed, a *normal* chest roentgenogram is the *most common* finding in embolic disease.

Fluoroscopy   Although clot and blood have the same radiodensity, a vessel containing clot will exhibit reduced or absent pulsations. Fluoroscopic discovery of a nonpulsatile vessel is a good clue to PTE.

Analysis of arterial blood gases   This may be of value, since massive embolism is commonly associated with arterial hypoxemia, hypocapnia, and respiratory alkalosis. In addition, the difference between alveolar P_{CO_2} and arterial P_{CO_2} ($P_{A_{CO_2}} - Pa_{CO_2}$) may be widened owing to the increase in alveolar dead space (Chap. 255); but a normal P_{O_2} does not exclude the diagnosis.

The laboratory tests discussed thus far are often negative in PTE and are relatively nonspecific. Therefore, it is usually necessary to proceed to two more definitive techniques: pulmonary perfusion and ventilation radiophotoscans and the pulmonary angiogram.

Pulmonary perfusion and ventilation scintiphotography   Perfusion scintiphotographs (photoscans) are obtained by intravenous injection of gamma-emitting radionuclides. The most commonly used materials are microspheres or macroaggregates of albumin (MAA), labeled with a gamma-emitting isotope such as technetium 99m. The radioactive particles, 50 to 100 μm in diameter, are trapped in the pulmonary capillary bed because the pulmonary capillaries approximate 10 μm in diameter. Alternatively, xenon 133 gas, dissolved in saline solution, may be used, but patients must hold their breath. The distribution of labeled particles entrapped in capillaries, or of xenon 133 evolved from them, accurately depicts the distribution of pulmonary blood flow.

After injection, a gamma-detecting device records the pattern of radioactivity within the lungs. This radioactive image can be recorded on radiographic film, on special photographic film, as a television image, or on video tape. Normal scans exhibit homogeneous distribution of radioactivity, smooth margins, and a configuration which corresponds to the normal anatomy of the lungs. Any deviation from these characteristics requires explanation because it represents an abnormality in blood flow distribution.

The perfusion lung photoscan is quite valuable in the diagnosis of embolism. A properly performed perfusion scan which is *normal* essentially excludes the diagnosis of clinically significant pulmonary embolism. On the other hand, a scan demonstrating zones of absent or sharply decreased radioactivity in the patient whose other findings are compatible with PTE provide substantial diagnostic support. Scanning is simple, safe, and rapid. It can be repeated to define the resolution, or recurrence, of obstructive vascular phenomena. Like any laboratory test, however, the photoscan must be applied and interpreted with care. It is important, for example, to obtain multiple scan views because lesions not apparent in one view may be easily detected in another. Furthermore, the lung photoscan demonstrates only abnormalities of the *distribution of blood flow.* It does not provide anatomic information. Many disorders other than PTE are associated with abnormalities in the distribution of pulmonary blood flow. Any disease process, such as pneumonia, atelectasis, or pneumothorax, which reduces the ventilation of a lung zone will decrease its perfusion. Parenchymal diseases, such as emphysema, sarcoidosis, bronchogenic carcinoma, and tuberculosis, can all produce scan defects. Therefore a perfusion defect lacks specificity. Specificity is enhanced by also assessing the distribution of *ventilation* in the region(s) of abnormal blood flow. This is accomplished by performing a ventilation scan. This is achieved by having the patients breathe a radioactive gas such as xenon 133 or xenon 127. If vascular obstruction (e.g., embolism) is present, scans will demonstrate normal wash-in and, more important, normal wash-out of radioactivity from the embolized lung zones. However, if parenchymal disease is responsible for the perfusion abnormality, wash-in and/or wash-out will be abnormal. Thus, "mismatch" of perfusion and ventilation is characteristic of vascular obstruction; "match" is indicative of parenchymal disease.

Pulmonary angiography   This is the only means for providing anatomic information about the pulmonary vasculature. Injection of radiopaque material, preferably through a cardiac catheter advanced into the pulmonary artery, provides a visual image of the pulmonary vessels. Cardiac catheterization and angiography require specialized personnel and a reasonable period for preparation and performance, and they entail more risk than the procedures discussed above. However, the procedure has the advantage of providing valuable hemodynamic data which may be necessary for therapeutic decisions. Interpretive limitations of angiography are of three types: (1) *Injection artifacts* may occur which suggest absence of flow to a vessel. Injection should be repeated whenever the question of such artifacts exists. (2) The inability to evaluate the patency of small vessels is another limitation. Emboli in vessels below the resolving capability of the method cannot be detected with certainty although magnification techniques can extend resolving capability. (3) Interpretive errors may also be a consequence of *not looking for the proper type of defect.* Classically, the angiogram shows an *abrupt "cutoff"* of a vessel at the point of embolic impaction. However, complete embolic obstruction is uncommon. Therefore, *filling defects* are the most frequent finding; i.e., the embolus creates a "negative" shadow as the radiopaque material flows around it. Also, a *decrease in filling* of a lung zone suggests embolic obstruction. The major contraindication to angiography is the absence of personnel who are experienced in both performing the procedure and interpreting the results. Serious diagnostic errors are commonplace if optimal techniques are not used or the complexities of interpretation are not appreciated.

How far one should proceed down the diagnostic pathway outlined above depends on many factors, the major ones being the severity of the patient's symptoms and the hazards of contemplated therapy. Both condition the need for precise diagnosis. If misdiagnosis in either direction carries high risk, precision is mandatory. If this is not provided by photoscanning, then there should be no hesitancy in proceeding to angiography. However, if local expertise is lacking in either scanning or angiography, that procedure which is most reliable should be performed—or the patient should be transferred to a facility where such procedures are known to be reliable.

TREATMENT

Initial intravenous administration of heparin is the therapy of choice for PTE. With a strong *suspicion* of embolism based on clinical and routine laboratory tests, such therapy should be instituted immediately, without awaiting diagnostic confirmation, unless the initial dose of heparin places the patient at clear risk (i.e., in patients with recent or active bleeding or a known hemostatic defect). Except in such patients, heparin therapy should not await diagnostic confirmation; one can always stop therapy if such confirmation is not forthcoming.

The goals of therapy of PTE are several: (1) immediate inhibition of thrombus growth in the lung and elsewhere, (2) promotion of thrombus resolution, and (3) prevention of embolic recurrence. Heparin achieves the first goal; it encourages the second by allowing fibrinolytic dissolution to be achieved unopposed by thrombus growth; and it assists in, although it does not assure, prevention of recurrence by accomplishing the first two goals. In addition, heparin inhibits platelet aggregation (and therefore serotonin release) at the embolic site, and its anticoagulant action is promptly reversible.

There is consensus that therapy should be initiated with an intravenous bolus of 15,000 to 20,000 units of heparin. However, there is substantial controversy regarding the safest, most efficacious regimen beyond that point. The two most popular regimens, begun 2 to 4 h after the initial bolus, are a continuous intravenous infusion at approximately 1000 units per hour or 5000 to 7500 units given intravenously every 4 h. If intravenous therapy cannot be maintained reliably, heparin should be given subcutaneously in doses of 7500 units every 6 h or 10,000 units every 8 h. Intramuscular injection should be avoided because hematomas result. The need for clotting times (CT) or partial thromboplastin times (PTT) and their utility in guiding therapy are debated. If done improperly or poorly timed, these tests are worthless and may be misleading. If used appropriately, the usual objective is to keep CT or PTT, measured *just prior to the next intermittent dose,* two times the base-line CT or PTT or, with continuous infusion, at 1.5 to 2.5 times normal. However, existing data do not establish that use of such coagulation tests ensures either safer or more effective heparin therapy than does the use of the empiric doses noted above. Heparin therapy should be maintained until the patient's cardiopulmonary status has stabilized and any evidence of venous thrombosis has resolved. Because thrombi become firmly attached to vessel wall and are well along the road toward organization within 5 to 7 days, bed rest should be maintained for at least that period. If possible, ambulation is begun while the patient is on heparin therapy, with elastic supports applied to the legs. If symptoms do not recur, the heparin may be tapered over the next 36 to 48 h and then discontinued.

Prothrombinopenic drugs are not suitable for initial therapy in embolism. Their only role is in maintaining anticoagulant protection for prolonged periods. The decision for "long-term" protection depends upon the presence of risk factors which might predispose to recurrence of venous thrombosis and embolism, such as congestive heart failure, chronic venous insufficiency of the lower extremities, or the need for prolonged bed rest. In the absence of such indications, heparin alone suffices. If prothrombinopenic drugs are to be used, the patient should be "in range" as defined by a prothrombin time 1.5 to 2.5 times the control time for 3 to 5 days before heparin is discontinued. An alternative to prothrombinopenic agents, now under exploration, is the use of self-injected subcutaneous "mini-dose" heparin (see below).

Thrombolytic (fibrinolytic) agents such as streptokinase and urokinase can hasten the resolution of emboli. Despite extensive study, it has not been established that these agents reduce the morbidity or mortality rate in patients with embolism. Both drugs are associated with hemorrhagic risk. If they do have a place in the therapy of PTE, it is in the treatment of patients with massive embolism in whom surgical intervention would otherwise be contemplated.

Surgical therapy should be reserved for those patients in whom heparin therapy is deemed inadequate or impractical. Anticoagulant therapy may be contraindicated by the presence of a bleeding diathesis, or the patient may be in such critical condition that it is felt unwise to await a response to medical therapy. In such instances *venous interruption* and *pulmonary embolectomy* must be considered.

The objective of venous interruption is to prevent immediate recurrence of embolism. Ligation of the superficial femoral vein offers no protection against embolization from the deep femoral venous system, and ligation of the common femoral vein is unacceptable because of severe obstruction to venous drainage. Furthermore, these procedures must be bilateral to grant protection from a suspected embolic focus in the legs. For these reasons, interruption of the inferior vena cava has replaced more distal ligation procedures. A number of surgical procedures have been applied to the inferior vena cava; simple ligation; plication, in which fine channels are preserved; and the application of totally or partially occlusive "clips." Nonsurgical interruption also can be accomplished by introducing "umbrella" or balloon devices, attached to catheters, into the inferior vena cava via neck or upper-extremity veins. Each procedure has advantages and disadvantages. For example, total interruption leads to variable degrees of edema of the legs; successful plication does not prevent small emboli from reaching the lungs; devices introduced into the cava may migrate upward or be badly placed. Unfortunately, no form of inferior vena caval interruption precludes embolic recurrence. There are several reasons for this; sizable collateral channels develop weeks to months after interruption of the cava, through which embolization may recur; thromboembolism may originate at the site of caval manipulation; caval blockade does not prevent embolization from foci within the right cardiac chambers. Therefore, because most pulmonary emboli do resolve, caval interruption should be regarded as a *lifesaving procedure* to be restricted to patients who could not tolerate an *immediate* embolic recurrence. To elect this procedure, definite evidence of cardiopulmonary compromise by embolism is required, and there should be reasonable assurance that the embolic source is in the caval drainage area.

Caval interruption is not a formidable surgical procedure but may be associated with substantial morbidity. It should be used therefore only when required, and with recognition that it does not necessarily provide long-term protection. There is one instance, however, in which prompt caval ligation is the therapy of choice: septic thrombophlebitis of pelvic origin with multiple septic pulmonary emboli. If these patients do not respond promptly to a heparin-antibiotic regimen, they may die unless caval (and left ovarian vein) ligation is carried out promptly.

The decision to carry out emergency *pulmonary embolectomy* has many features in common with the decision to interrupt the inferior vena cava. In addition, since embolectomy is a major, complex operation which has been associated with a 50 percent mortality rate, the decision to carry out this procedure is a difficult one. However, there is agreement that two criteria should be met before embolectomy is performed: (1) there must be evidence of severe hemodynamic compromise due to embolism which is not responsive to supportive measures, particularly sustained systemic hypotension, and (2) the personnel and equipment required for embolectomy must be available.

These criteria require angiographic confirmation of the extent and location of the embolus except under the most unusual circumstances when a scan might suffice. Hemodynamic measurements are extremely helpful. Facilities for cardiopulmonary bypass should be available. Unless these requirements are met, the opportunity for error is great and the chance of a successful outcome is limited—indeed, it is less than with medical therapy. Therefore, emergency pulmonary embolectomy is rarely indicated.

SPECIAL CONSIDERATIONS Total resolution of emboli does not always occur. If residual vascular obstruction is substantial, the patient may present, months or years after the actual embolic events, with dyspnea and pulmonary hypertension of uncertain cause. Multiple undetected recurrent small emboli may produce the same picture. The latter condition may be misdiagnosed as "chronic lung disease" or "primary" pulmonary hypertension (Chap. 265).

Such patients should be studied by appropriate techniques, since larger emboli are potentially resectable, even after having been present for months to years. These conditions are potentially curable forms of otherwise fatal pulmonary hypertensive disease.

Embolism should also be suspected in other clinical contexts: as a precipitating cause for cardiac arrhythmia; as a reason for sudden or progressive worsening of congestive heart failure (Chap. 236); as an explanation for sudden deterioration in the patient with chronic obstructive pulmonary disease; and as a possible alternative to the diagnosis of "psychic" hyperventilation.

PROGNOSIS IN PULMONARY EMBOLISM The prognosis of the patient with pulmonary embolism *in whom therapy is promptly instituted* is excellent. As stated at the outset of this chapter, less than one embolic event in ten is lethal. The majority of these deaths occur suddenly and can be avoided only by prophylaxis (see below). The remainder appear to be due to embolic extension or recurrence, which therapy can moderate. Thus, of patients who survive long enough to reach medical attention and receive heparin, the outlook is quite good. Morbidity following embolism is uncommon since embolic resolution is the rule and few patients develop the pulmonary hypertensive problem noted above.

Limited reliable data are available regarding recurrence rates in the months and years after a single embolic event (with or without prolonged postembolic anticoagulant therapy). In the absence of risk factors, recurrence appears to be uncommon, but more precise data are needed.

PROPHYLAXIS The ultimate goal in the management of pulmonary embolism is its prevention. Two related approaches to this goal exist: (1) improved methods for early detection of deep venous thrombosis (DVT) and (2) application of prophylactic therapy to individuals at "high risk" of having DVT.

Three noninvasive methods now promise improved early detection and follow-up of DVT: impedance plethysmography; the ultrasonic (Doppler) flow technique; and the radiolabeled fibrinogen method. Each of these simple approaches correlates well with the definitive (but invasive) standard test for diagnosis of DVT—i.e., *ascending contrast phlebography*—but each also has significant limitations which must be recognized. Available reports indicate that the combination of impedance phlebography and radiofibrinogen leg scanning is equal in sensitivity and reliability to contrast venography.

Application of these noninvasive approaches to the early diagnosis and follow-up of patients at high risk for DVT already has led to a significant change in approach to the prophylaxis of DVT (and therefore of PTE), namely, the use of small doses of subcutaneous heparin ("mini-dose heparin"). Multiple studies, chiefly using radioactive fibrinogen, have shown the high incidence of DVT in certain groups: patients over the age of 40 years with fractures of lower extremities for whom a period of 10 days or more of immobilization is anticipated; patients with severe congestive heart failure; patients with myocardial infarction; patients undergoing major abdominal, thoracic, or gynecologic surgery. Furthermore, in the last group of patients these studies have shown a significant decrease in the incidence of DVT, PTE, and lethal PTE when "mini-doses" of heparin are given before, during, and after surgery; i.e., 5000 units every 12 h subcutaneously, beginning before surgery (or on admission to the hospital) and continued until the patient is ambulatory. A consensus would agree that this prophylactic approach, which leaves CT and PTT virtually unaffected and is associated with limited hemorrhagic hazard, also should be applied to all medical patients at high risk of DVT and PTE. In the case of acute myocardial infarction, high risk would be imposed by the development of congestive failure, the presence of severe obesity, chronic venous insufficiency, or a prior history of DVT or PTE. In other medical patients, clear definition of risk factors that warrant mini-doses of heparin has not been achieved. Better definition of "risk" and of alternatives to mini-doses of heparin (e.g., dextran, antiplatelet agents such as aspirin and sulfinpyrazone) is required. In the interim, the decision to apply such prophylaxis must be made by assessing the risk and benefit in the specific patient.

NONTHROMBOTIC EMBOLISM

Because the lung vasculature serves as a filter of the venous circulation, it is the recipient of diverse materials which can gain entry into venous blood, including bone marrow, foreign bodies, parasites, and tumor cells. The most frequently encountered form of nonthrombotic embolism is *fat embolism.* This dramatic and controversial entity follows the introduction of neutral fat into the venous circulation, most commonly after bone trauma or fracture (marrow fat), but occasionally after trauma to adipose tissue or liver infiltrated by fat. The clinical sequence is characteristic. After a latent period of 12 to 36 h or more, during which the patient is asymptomatic, sudden cardiopulmonary and neurologic deterioration appears. Mental aberrations, delirium, and coma develop. Dyspnea, tachypnea, and tachycardia occur, and the chest roentgenographic and

physiologic components of the "adult respiratory distress syndrome" appear (see Chap. 271). Anemia and thrombocytopenia are common, as are petechiae on the upper thorax and arms. The pathogenesis of the syndrome is not clear, but it seems likely that two events occur: release of free fatty acids (by action of lipases on the neutral fat) which induces a toxic vasculitis, followed by platelet-fibrin thrombosis; and actual obstruction of small pulmonary arteries by macroaggregates of fat. Several forms of therapy have been proposed (corticosteroids, heparin, ethanol), but treatment remains supportive and mortality rate high.

Another dramatic form of nonthrombotic embolism is *amniotic fluid embolism.* This occurs during both spontaneous delivery and cesarean section. Sudden and massive obstruction of the pulmonary microvasculature occurs, leading to shock and, often, death. With survival of the initial phase of the disease, the picture of disseminated intravascular coagulation appears. The syndrome is due to the entrance of a significant quantity of amniotic fluid into the venous circulation. This fluid is a potent thromboplastic agent which induces thrombosis in the pulmonary vasculature and elsewhere. The fluid also contains particulates which lodge in the lung. Treatment consists of supportive measures.

REFERENCES

BIVINS BA et al: Fat embolism revisited. South Med J 69:899, 1976
Current problems in pulmonary embolism. Prog Cardiovasc Dis 17:161, 239, 329, 1974–1975
MOSER KM: Pulmonary embolism: State of the art. Am Rev Respir Dis 115:829, 1977
———, STEIN MS (eds): *Advances in Cardiopulmonary Diseases—Pulmonary Thromboembolism.* Chicago, Year Book, 1973
PARASKOS JA et al: Late prognosis of acute pulmonary embolism. N Engl J Med 289:55, 1973
Prevention of fatal post-operative pulmonary embolism by low doses of heparin: An international multicenter trial. Lancet 2:45, 1975
Prophylactic Therapy of Deep Vein Thrombosis and Pulmonary Embolism, US Department of Health, Education and Welfare Publication (NIH) 76–866, 1977

Other abnormalities of the respiratory tract

267
DISEASES OF THE UPPER RESPIRATORY TRACT

LOUIS WEINSTEIN

Disorders of the upper respiratory tract (nose, nasopharynx, paranasal sinuses, and larynx) are among the commonest forms of human illness. In most instances, they result in discomfort which is more annoying and distracting than disabling, and while they may interfere with the individual's function sufficiently to prevent participation in normal activities, they are not life-threatening nor do they usually lead to serious chronic disability. Less commonly, more serious disorders may present with symptoms referable to the upper respiratory tract.

NOSE

ANOSMIA Total loss of olfactory sense is most common as a transient manifestation of acute infections of the upper respiratory tract. It may be present with chronic nasal obstruction due to edema of the mucosa or marked swelling of the turbinates and with congenital defects, ozena, tumors (see below), trauma involving the olfactory nerves, and nasal polyps.

RHINOPHYMA This is a progressive, deforming, nodular enlargement of the alae nasi due to hypertrophy of sebaceous follicles in association with chronic, severe acne rosacea. There is no specific treatment. Plastic surgery may produce a dramatic degree of improvement.

RHINITIS AND NASAL OBSTRUCTION Intermittent or persistent nasal discharge may be caused by a variety of disorders, including hay fever, vasomotor rhinitis and complicating nasal polyposis, acute coryza, and other forms of viral rhinitis, the upper respiratory manifestations of measles, syphilis (the "snuffles" of the congenital disease), and nasal diphtheria, intranasal foreign bodies, and chronic use of vasoconstrictor drugs.

Acute and self-limited nasal obstruction is usually associated with acute upper respiratory tract infections, most commonly viral. Hypertrophy and inflammation of the turbinates leading to nasal obstruction, with or without persistent nasal discharge, may be caused by allergic reactions. A common reason for difficulty in breathing through the nose is a deviated septum. Menstruation is associated, in some instances, with bogginess of the turbinates to a degree sufficient to produce retardation of airflow through the nose; pregnancy may produce the same phenomenon.

RHINORRHEA Although unilateral nasal discharge may be caused by intranasal foreign bodies, when it is intermittent or persistent, the possibility that it is due to *cerebrospinal fluid (CSF) rhinorrhea* must be considered. This condition may be diagnosed by injecting a marker such as a dye (fluorescein) or a radioactive tracer into the CSF and following its appearance in nasal secretions. A positive reaction for glucose indicates that the nasal discharge is cerebrospinal fluid.

OZENA This is a severe chronic rhinitis of unknown cause, characterized by thick, greenish discharge, mucosal crusts, atrophy of the turbinates, and an offensive odor. Patients eventually become anosmic. Even when the nasal passages are widened and resistance to airflow is decreased, obstruction is a constant complaint. Cultures grow gram-negative bacilli (*Klebsiella, Pseudomonas,* etc.). Treatment, aimed at reducing the odor, includes use of local or systemic antibiotics and large doses of vasodilators (Priscoline, nicotinic acid). Local cleansing by means of repeated saline irrigation is extremely important to eliminate foul-smelling crusts.

PERFORATION OF THE NASAL SEPTUM A variety of conditions may cause perforation of the nasal septum, including chronic nose "picking," prolonged use of potent vasoconstrictors, chronic sniffing of cocaine, cautery of the nasal septum for repeated episodes of epistaxis, tumors of the nose invading the septum, nasal septal surgery, rheumatoid arthritis, syphilis, the espundia type of American leishmaniasis, South American blastomycosis, midline granuloma, Wegener's granulomatosis, and phycomycosis.

EPISTAXIS Probably the commonest cause is nose picking, leading to tearing of the rich network of veins in the anterior nares (Kiesselbach's plexus). Among the infections in which acute nosebleed may develop are typhoid fever, unilateral nasal diphtheria, pertussis, and malaria. Minor epistaxis may also appear in the course of viral infections of the upper respiratory tract. Other causes of intermittent or repeated episodes of epistaxis are atheromas of the nasal vessels, hypertension, vicarious menstruation, bleeding diatheses including thrombocytopenia of different etiologies and deficiencies of clotting factors, polycythemia vera, rhinoliths, acute sinusitis especially involving the ethmoid sinus, tumors of the nose and paranasal sinuses, and nasal angiomas. Episodes of bleeding or the severity of attacks are frequently increased in patients receiving aspirin. Vitamin C and prothrombin deficiency are *not* associated with isolated epistaxis, although this may occur with bleeding from other sites. In hereditary hemorrhagic telangiectasia (Osler-Rendu-Weber syndrome) the only site of bleeding may be the nose; a family history of repeated hemorrhages from this and other sites should suggest this diagnosis.

NASAL FURUNCULOSIS Furuncles involving the internal or external surfaces of the nose pose potential threats to life because of the possibility of spread to the cavernous sinus via the draining veins. When seen in their early stage, they respond rapidly to antimicrobial therapy which should be directed primarily against *Staphylococcus aureus* and given in large doses (Chap. 116). Oral treatment may be adequate in the early stages of the disease, but parenteral therapy is necessary when the constitutional reaction is severe and there is marked edema of the intra- or extranasal tissues. *Under no circumstances should these lesions be squeezed* because of the danger of spread of organisms to intracranial venous sinuses. Also, incision for drainage should not be carried out unless pain becomes severe or the lesion has become large.

NASAL TUMORS Basal cell carcinoma of the skin covering the nose is the commonest malignant tumor of this organ. Rodent ulcer resulting from local spread of a basal cell lesion may involve not only the skin over the external nasal surface and adjacent areas of the face, but may also invade intranasally and produce marked destruction of the internal structures.

PHARYNX

ACUTE PHARYNGITIS The outstanding symptom of acute pharyngitis, regardless of cause, is a sore throat. About two-thirds of all acute illnesses in families are viral infections of the upper respiratory tract, with varying degrees of pharyngeal discomfort present. The acute pharyngitides can be classified into three groups: (1) treatable infections, (2) untreatable infections, and (3) noninfectious disorders (Table 267-1).

Physical examination of the pharyngeal mucosa may reveal changes varying in intensity from mild redness and congestion of blood vessels (many viral infections) to intense red-purple color, patchy yellow exudate, hypertrophy of all the lymphoid tissue, and marked vascular injection (e.g., severe disease due to group A *Streptococcus pyogenes*). Symptoms may be variable and may range from a complaint of "scratchy throat" to pain so severe that swallowing of saliva is difficult. The presence of exudate does not establish a specific etiology and may be noted in infections due to *S. pyogenes, Hemophilus influenzae, H. parainfluenzae* (children), *Corynebacterium diphtheriae, Streptococcus pneumoniae* (rare) as well as in some viral diseases, such as those caused by adenovirus. Ulcerations involving the posterior pharyngeal wall and/or tonsils are characteristically present in fusobacterial infections (Plaut-Vincent's angina), pharyngeal tularemia, syphilis (primary chancre), tuberculosis, following local trauma to the pharynx, and in immunosuppressed and agranulocytic patients in whom invasion by fusobacteria or other members of the indigenous pharyngeal microflora takes place. The presence of limited or extensive pseudomembrane does not always indicate a specific microbial cause. While most characteristic of faucial diphtheria, such lesions may be present in infectious mononucleosis, agranulocytosis, staphylococcal pharyngitis, and diffuse injury to the pharyngeal mucosa following direct trauma or chemical or thermal burns.

The tonsils are often involved in the course of viral and bacterial pharyngitis; they may be markedly reddened and swollen and contain exudate in the crypts.

The etiologic diagnosis of acute pharyngitis is difficult to establish on the basis of visual examination of the throat. However, in some instances in which characteristic findings are present, such as the typical pseudomembrane and suggestive odor of diphtheria, severe group A streptococcal infection, the ulceration and anaerobic odor of fusobacterial disease, or the white irregular patches overlying shallow ulcers produced by *Candida,* a specific cause may be suspected.

Cultures of the pharyngeal mucosa, tonsils, or exudate will usually reveal the bacteria responsible for the disease and determine the choice of antimicrobial agent. It should be stressed, however, that these are not always rewarding. For example, only 70 percent of single throat cultures yield group A *S. pyogenes,* even when pharyngitis due to this organism is severe. Patients suspected of having streptococcal pharyngitis but whose throat cultures fail to yield the organism should be treated if this kind of disease is known to be present in the community in which they live at the time they present. The sore throat of subacute thyroiditis may be relieved occasionally by the administration of thyroid hormone or prednisone. None of the viral pharyngitides is treatable.

Gonococcal pharyngitis is almost always the result of orogenital contact. The incidence of the disease in heterosexual men varies from 0.2 to 1.4 percent. It ranges from 5 to 25 percent in homosexual males; 20 percent of those with genital infection have simultaneous involvement of the throat. From 5 to 18 percent of women with other manifestations of gonorrhea have pharyngitis; in 1 to 3 percent this is the only disease. While mild to severe sore throat is present in about 30 percent of patients, the majority are asymptomatic. Because the clinical features of gonococcal pharyngitis may mimic disease produced by other organisms, the diagnosis is based on isolation

TABLE 267-1
Etiology of pharyngitis

I Infections
  A Treatable
     1 Group A *Streptococcus pyogenes*
     2 *Hemophilus influenzae*
     3 *H. parainfluenzae*
     4 *Neisseria gonorrhoeae*
     5 *N. meningitidis*
     6 *Corynebacterium diphtheriae*
     7 *Spirochaeta pallida*
     8 *Fusobacterium*
     9 *F. tularensis*
     10 *Candida*
     11 *Cryptococcus*
     12 *Histoplasma*
     13 *Mycoplasma pneumoniae* (?)
     14 *Streptococcus pneumoniae* (?)
     15 *Staphylococcus aureus* or gram-negative bacilli are rare and are usually found in neutropenic patients or those treated with antibiotics
  B Untreatable
     1 Primary
        a Influenza virus
        b Rhinovirus
        c Coxsackievirus A
        d Epstein-Barr virus
        e Echovirus
        f Herpes simplex
        g Reovirus
     2 Manifestation of systemic disease
        a Poliomyelitis
        b Measles
        c Chickenpox
        d Smallpox
        e Viral hepatitis
        f Rubella
        g Pertussis
II Noninfectious
  A Trauma by heat, sharp objects, etc.
  B Inhalation of irritants
  C Dehydration—mouth breathing
  D Glossopharyngeal neuralgia
  E Subacute thyroiditis (tends to be prolonged or frequently recurrent, often associated with low-grade fever)
  F Psychogenic (see comment above)
  G Monomyelocytic leukemia
  H Immunosuppressed state

and identification of *Neisseria gonorrhoeae.* This is accomplished by culturing pharyngeal secretions on Thayer-Martin medium immediately after they are obtained; incubation in an atmosphere of 5% CO_2 is required. The isolated organism must be confirmed as the gonococcus by its biological properties because of the presence of other *Neisseria* in the pharynges of most normal individuals.

PERITONSILLAR CELLULITIS AND ABSCESS (QUINSY) This condition is most often a complication of acute pharyngitis. The organisms commonly involved are group A *S. pyogenes* and *S. aureus.* The first sign of this disease is marked enlargement of the tonsils, which are surrounded by red, edematous pillars. The tonsillar and peritonsillar hypertrophy may progress to a degree threatening occlusion of the upper airway. High-grade fever and leukocytosis are present, and severe rigors may occur. In its early stages, the process is a cellulitis, but, in the absence of therapy, abscess develops as infection progresses and involves one or both tonsils; at this time, soft grayish white exudate may cover the tonsillar surfaces. The diagnosis is made purely on the basis of the physical findings. If detected early when only peritonsillar cellulitis is present, administration of a properly selected antimicrobial agent may clear the infection and abort the development of abscess. Antimicrobial therapy alone is inadequate after abscess has developed. The optimal treatment at this stage is incision and drainage of the involved tonsil(s).

PARAPHARYNGEAL SPACE ABSCESS This syndrome is always a complication of acute pharyngitis. Primary or secondary bacterial invasion of one of the tonsils results in the development of an intratonsillar abscess accompanied by considerable edema and inflammatory reaction in the parapharyngeal space. The lesion is usually unilateral; there is frequently very little pharyngeal discomfort, but there is marked tenderness at the angle of the jaw on the same side as the tonsillar abscess. The remainder of the throat frequently has a benign appearance. There is usually considerable fever and leukocytosis. If unrecognized and not treated early in its course, the infection spreads through the tonsillar veins to the jugular vein, where it produces thrombophlebitis. Septic emboli from this source may be widely disseminated and cause widespread metastatic thrombosis and infection, a highly fatal syndrome termed *postanginal sepsis.* Early recognition and institution of therapy before spread to the jugular vein results in rapid clearing of the infection.

RETROPHARYNGEAL ABSCESS Infection of the retropharyngeal lymph nodes occurs most often as a complication of acute bacterial pharyngitis in children 3 years of age or younger; these nodes disappear rapidly after this age. Adults usually acquire the disease as a result of injury to the posterior pharyngeal wall by a sharp object, as a complication of neglected acute infections of the middle ear, during the course of tuberculosis, or secondary to suppurative parotitis. A universal symptom is the sensation of a "lump in the throat that cannot be swallowed." Dyspnea that is present in the sitting position and absent when patients lie on their back and pain on swallowing are common. The voice has a characteristic quality that has been likened to the cry of a duck (*cri du canard*). Coughing, snoring, choking, and stertorous breathing are often present. As the abscess enlarges, progressive airway obstruction develops, marked edema and redness of the entire posterior pharynx and cervical lymphadenopathy are common, and there is usually high fever. When recognized early, most retropharyngeal abscesses respond promptly to antimicrobial therapy. Because most of the organisms involved are gram-positive cocci, parenteral administration of a penicillinase-resistant penicillin or a cephalosporin compound is usually effective; in young children, therapy must include agents effective against *H. influenzae.* If the abscess comes to attention late in its course, or if obstruction of the airway is progressing rapidly, the lesion must be drained surgically and chemotherapy must be given before, during, and after the procedure. Tracheostomy may be necessary in far-advanced cases.

TUMORS OF THE TONSILS Carcinoma of the tonsil is the second commonest tumor of the upper airway (osteoma being the commonest; see below). Other neoplastic tonsillar lesions include lymphoma and Hodgkin's disease. Persistence of pain in one enlarged firm tonsil, in the absence of an infectious process, is an indication for biopsy. The presence of fever does not rule out a neoplastic lesion, because considerable elevation of the temperature may be present when lymphoma is the cause.

LINGUAL TONSILS These are situated on the posterior borders of the tongue and extend from the circumvallate papillae to the epiglottis. Infection produces lingual pain that may be severe and markedly increased by movement of the tongue. Sore throat is often absent or mild; when the responsible organism is *S. pyogenes,* fever is present. Examination of the posterior tongue reveals swelling and redness of the lymphoid masses; yellow exudate is present in the crypts when group A streptococci are the cause of the disease. The pharynx may appear normal or only slightly reddened.

SINUSES

ACUTE SINUSITIS The organisms most often responsible for acute sinusitis are *S. pneumoniae,* group A *S. pyogenes, S. aureus,* and *H. influenzae.* Other bacteria may be involved in patients receiving immunosuppressive therapy, in those who have received antibiotics, or in whom penetrating trauma, local tumors, or vasculitis is a predisposing factor. The etiology of chronic sinusitis may be the same as that of the acute form, but more than one pathogen may be present. In many instances, however, cultures yield only members of the indigenous microflora of the upper respiratory tract.

The commonest predisposing factor of acute purulent sinusitis is viral infection of the upper respiratory tract, which may lead to obstruction of drainage of the paranasal sinuses and the development of localized pain, tenderness, and low-grade fever. These manifestations usually clear as the viral disease subsides. In a number of instances, however, invasion by pyogenic bacteria supervenes and is responsible for the development of purulent sinusitis. Obstruction of meatal drainage of any type or direct introduction of bacteria into the sinuses may lead to the development of acute infection of the paranasal sinuses. Abscesses of the roots of the upper bicuspid or molar teeth that rupture into the maxillary sinuses, swimming and diving, and direct local injury may be inciting mechanisms. Fractures of the bones encompassing the sinuses, especially the frontals and ethmoids, may be followed by infection. Wegener's granulomatosis and tumors of the meatuses of the turbinates may produce the clinical picture of acute or chronic sinusitis. In some of these patients, bacterial infection is superimposed, and these patients are studied only after infection develops, the underlying lesion often being overlooked. This underscores the fact that recurrent or prolonged episodes of sinusitis that are refractory to antimicrobial therapy, or that relapse soon after treatment is discontinued, must be investigated thoroughly for the presence of a noninfectious obstructing lesion.

The diagnosis of acute purulent sinusitis is usually made when constitutional manifestations are present, such as fever, chills, pain and tenderness of the involved sinuses, nasal obstruction, and recurrent headaches that change in intensity with position and disappear shortly after getting out of bed.

Isolation of a pathogenic organism from the nasal secretions or from material draining into the meatuses of the nasal turbinates may help to solidify the diagnosis. When there is marked swelling of the turbinates, they can be shrunk by the local application of cocaine or other potent vasoconstrictors. This exposes the meatuses and permits the collection of exudate draining directly from the involved sinus. Transillumination of the sinuses is also helpful, while radiologic study is of value in identifying the specific sinus involved.

Frontal sinusitis is characterized by pain over the forehead approximately in the area of the underlying sinus. Although the overlying site is usually normal, it may be swollen and reddened over an area outlining the sinuses. Pressure applied over the sinuses and on the lateral edge of the orbital ridges produces pain. Examination of the nasal turbinates shows purulent exudate in the middle meatus if drainage is not prevented by swelling of these structures. Pain, swelling, and tenderness in the anterior portions of the maxillae are the outstanding features of *maxillary sinusitis.* When the infection is severe, pain may be referred to the upper teeth which may become loosened, and hemorrhage may be present in the surrounding tissues. Pus is visible in the middle meatus of the turbinates. The symptoms and signs of *ethmoid sinusitis* are pain in the upper lateral areas of the nose, frontal headache, and redness of the skin and tenderness to pressure over the upper lateral areas of the nasal bones adjacent to the inner canthi of the eyes. Pus is visible in the middle meatus when the anterior cells of the sinus are involved, and in the superior meatus if the posterior cells are infected; in most instances, both areas of the sinus are involved and exudate is present in both meatuses. The manifestations of infection of the *sphenoid sinus* are tenderness and pain over the vertex of the skull, the mastoid bones (in the presence of normal tympanic membranes), and the occipital portion of the head. Rarely, streaks of redness may be detectable over both zygomas as a result of irritation of a branch of the trigeminal nerve that lies in close proximity to the sinus.

Osteomyelitis of the frontal bone is a rare complication of frontal sinusitis. This is characterized by fever, chills, leukocytosis, frontal headache, and the presence of cool, pale edema over the forehead (Pott's puffy tumor). Despite absence of signs of inflammation in the overlying skin, aspiration of the subgaleal area frequently yields purulent exudate. Involvement of the bone in which the ethmoid sinus lies may be manifest by unilateral or bilateral exophthalmos when one or both sinuses are involved. This is usually due to a sterile or pyogenic orbital cellulitis secondary to a "sympathetic" inflammation or perforation of the lamina papyracea, the lateral wall of the sinus, and the medial wall of the orbit. Complications of venous return from the orbits may supervene because of intracranial spread of infection from the sinuses through the diploic veins. Among these are meningitis, infection, and thrombosis of the superficial cerebral veins or cavernous and sagittal venous sinuses, cranial nerve palsies, and extradural abscess.

Bacterial meningitis is also a rare complication of purulent sinusitis, usually involving the frontal sinuses, and associated with cranial osteomyelitis and subdural and brain abscess. Sudden onset of convulsions, hemiplegia, and aphasia in a patient with acute frontal sinusitis should suggest the possibility of subdural abscess with thrombophlebitis of the sagittal sinus or superficial cerebral veins. Infections of the ethmoid sinus may be complicated by paralysis of the third cranial nerve due to invasion of the dural sinuses, or profuse epistaxis as a result of thrombosis of the ethmoidal veins that drain into the cavernous sinus, which may become thrombosed. Chronic or recurrent purulent sinusitis may eventually be responsible for the development of bronchiectasis. An unusual form of chronic sinusitis in association with bronchiectasis and situs inversus is *Kartagener's syndrome.* Patients with these disorders have been noted to have delayed mucociliary transport in the lower airways—the immotile ciliary syndrome; this is accompanied in men by lack of motility of sperm, the numbers of which are normal.

TABLE 267-2
Differential diagnosis of hoarseness and other manifestations of laryngeal dysfunction

I Intralaryngeal disease
  A Infectious
    1 Common cold
    2 Viral laryngitis
    3 Hemophilus influenzae
    4 Membranous laryngitis *(Streptococcus pyogenes, Pseudomonas, Fusobacterium)*
    5 Diphtheria (laryngeal membrane)
    6 Herpes simplex
    7 Actinomycosis
    8 Candidiasis
    9 Blastomycosis
    10 Tuberculosis (ulcers)
    11 Syphilis (secondary stage, chondritis, gumma)
  B Noninfectious
    1 Trauma (edema or hematoma)
    2 Vocal cord nodules (singer's nodes)
    3 Papillomas of vocal cords
    4 Pachyderma of vocal cords
    5 Inhalation of smoke, fire, irritating gases, tobacco smoke
    6 Leukoplakia of vocal cords
    7 Rheumatoid arthritis (involvement of cricoarytenoid joint)
    8 Chronic alcoholism
    9 Benign tumors
    10 Cancer
    11 Foreign bodies
II Extralaryngeal disease
  A Lesions in neck [produce hoarseness because of (1) pressure on larynx that interferes with movement of vocal cords, (2) edema secondary to decreased venous and lymphatic drainage, and (3) impingement on laryngeal nerves with paresis or paralysis of cords]
    1 Hemorrhages and/or edema due to trauma, severe traction of neck, thyroidectomy, tracheostomy, and biopsy of scalene node
    2 Tumors of hypopharynx
    3 Tumors of carotid body
    4 Thrombophlebitis of jugular bulb
  B Local and systemic disorders outside neck (produce hoarseness by pressure on laryngeal nerves anywhere along the course outside the neck, or paresis or paralysis of the vocal cords as a manifestation of generalized neurologic dysfunction)
    1 Local lesions
      a Bacterial meningitis
      b Meningovascular syphilis
      c Infectious mononucleosis (enlarged mediastinal nodes)
      d Angioneurotic edema
      e Mitral stenosis (enlarged pulmonary artery)
      f Aneurysms of arch of aorta, carotid or innominate arteries
      g Ligation of patent ductus arteriosus
      h Tumors of mediastinal structures
      i Tumors of parotid gland
      j Relapsing polychondritis
      k Neoplastic disease of meninges
      l Fracture of base of skull
      m Cancer or nodules of thyroid
      n Goiter
    2 Systemic disorders
      a Diphtheria (peripheral neuritis)
      b Poliomyelitis (bulbar)
      c Infectious mononucleosis (nervous system involvement)
      d Herpes zoster
      e Mucoviscidosis
      f Myxedema
      g Acromegaly
      h Wegener's granulomatosis
      i Lupus erythematosus
      j Diabetic neuropathy
      k Poisoning by lead, mercury, arsenic, botulinus toxin

CHRONIC SINUSITIS It is difficult to establish the diagnosis of chronic sinusitis in the absence of documented recurrences of acute purulent infection. Many patients complaining of headaches, often frontal in nature, and troubled by obstruction of the nasal airway, may have some degree of tenderness over any of the paranasal sinuses. X-ray examinations of the sinuses often reveal thickening of the mucous membranes. Cultures of the nose or nasal discharge frequently yield no pathogenic organisms. In many instances, an allergic background is present in individuals with this syndrome; in these cases, relief of symptoms is often produced by the judicious use of nasal vasoconstrictors, and treatment is directed to the specific allergy. Occasionally, chronic sinusitis is due to persistent infection, as demonstrated by repeated isolation of a pathogenic organism. However, there is considerable experience to suggest that the manifestations presented by many patients are not related to chronic infection, but are due to other factors such as irritating dusts or gases or excessive exposure to tobacco smoke.

Effective management of acute sinusitis rests on demonstration of a specific pathogenic organism in the secretion present in the nose or drained from the sinuses, testing of the organism for sensitivity to a variety of antimicrobial agents, and administration of the most active agent in adequate dose. The antibiotics most effective for the bacteria most frequently involved in this disease are discussed in Chap. 111. Vasoconstrictors are of help in producing transient relief of symptoms, but must not be used excessively. Surgical drainage may be indicated when infection becomes prolonged or local or intracranial complications develop.

TUMORS OF THE SINUSES The commonest benign tumor of the paranasal sinuses is osteoma. Fifty percent of cases involve the frontal, 40 percent the ethmoid, and 10 percent the maxillary and sphenoid sinuses. The malignant tumors include carcinoma of the maxilla, sarcoma, Burkitt's lymphoma, myeloma, and adenocarcinoma. Melanoma of the nasal cavity may extend into the paranasal sinuses. Other malignant diseases originating in the sinuses may invade the nasal cavity and, because they produce obstruction, lead to consideration of the nose as the primary site of the lesion. A neoplastic lesion should be ruled out in patients who experience repeated episodes of acute sinusitis or who have chronic symptoms, particularly repeated epistaxis in the absence of an identifiable pathogenic organism.

LARYNX

SYMPTOMS AND SIGNS OF LARYNGEAL DISEASE There are three main causes of laryngeal disease: (1) intralaryngeal lesions, (2) extralaryngeal processes that produce other manifestations by direct pressure on either the larynx or the nerves that supply the vocal cords, and (3) disorders in which either local or diffuse disease of the nervous system leads to dysfunction of the vocal cords. A differential diagnosis of the various disorders of the larynx is presented in Table 267-2.

Hoarseness is the commonest symptom of disorders of the larynx, regardless of etiology. The common denominator of the numerous causes of this symptom is interference with normal phonatory function of the larynx. Both inflammatory and noninflammatory diseases of this organ as well as functional disturbances (hysterical aphonia) may be causative factors. Although hoarseness is usually of short duration with acute self-limited processes such as infections, it may persist for long periods.

Cough is common with any type of laryngeal disease. *Pain* occurs occasionally, while *stridor* and *dyspnea* are uncommon manifestations of laryngeal involvement. However, when present, the latter are ominous because they indicate the development of airway obstruction which may rapidly become complete. Obstruction to breathing is not only associated with intralaryngeal lesions or those which exert pressure directly on this organ, but may occur as a result of neurologic disorders in which paralysis of both vocal cords develops.

The exact cause of laryngeal obstruction can be detected only by direct or indirect examination of the larynx. *This is usually necessary when manifestations have persisted for longer than 2 or 3 weeks.* However, if serious obstruction of the airway develops rapidly in acute disorders of the larynx, laryngoscopic examination should be carried out promptly and tracheostomy performed if necessary.

The three disorders of the larynx described below require specific and early diagnosis because of their life-threatening potential.

ACUTE EPIGLOTTITIS Acute infections of the epiglottis are most commonly caused by *H. influenzae* in children; this organism, as well as the pneumococcus and group A streptococci, may be responsible for the disease in all age groups. The onset of symptoms is often very rapid and is characterized by varying degrees of fever, severe sore throat, pooling of pharyngeal secretions, drooling, and dysphagia. Stridor is rapidly followed by increasing difficulty in breathing as airway obstruction develops. If untreated, there is increasing use of the accessory muscles of respiration followed by cyanosis, prostration, and finally shock.

Examination of the hypopharynx reveals a markedly swollen, cherry red epiglottis, which may be necrotic when *S. pyogenes* is involved. Treatment must be undertaken early, preferably before there is evidence of severe respiratory distress. In such instances, the administration of ampicillin or any other antimicrobial agent effective against the organisms most often involved, together with inhalation of moist air and oxygen, will often prevent progression of the disease. When it is clear that the airway is seriously threatened, tracheostomy, in addition to chemotherapy, is urgently indicated.

FOREIGN BODY Inhalation of a foreign body rapidly produces symptoms. *Pain* is "sticking" in quality and localized to the larynx. *Laryngeal spasm* is usually present. *Dyspnea* may develop as a result of edema and lead to a degree of obstruction sufficient to compromise the airway. There is often a *change in the quality of the voice;* complete *aphonia* may occur. If the inhaled object is sharp, as a chicken bone, there is rapid development of local swelling and progressive obstruction to breathing. Perforation of the larynx may occur and lead to infection that extends from the local site to other areas in the neck and mediastinum. If the inhaled object is lying loosely in the larynx, three diagnostic signs are helpful. These are the *wheeze, palpatory thud* (palpating fingers detect a thud over the larynx during respirations), and *auscultatory slap* (a slapping noise is heard over the larynx as its walls are hit by the foreign body when it moves while breathing). Suspicion of a foreign body makes mirror or laryngoscopic examination an emergency procedure.

CANCER OF THE LARYNX This lesion develops at an average age of 60 years and is 10 times more common in men than in women. Cancers of the larynx are of two types: *intrinsic,* arising on the vocal cords (70 percent of the cases), and *extrinsic,* extending beyond the vocal cords. Although hoarseness develops early in the course of intrinsic lesions, it is frequently late in onset with extrinsic ones. The treatment of choice for this disease is surgery.

Small lesions of the middle third of the cord often respond to radiation alone. Total or partial laryngectomy is required in the majority of cases. When the cancer involves the epiglottis and/or the false cords, partial supraglottic laryngectomy is the preferred operative procedure because it does not result in loss of normal speech and has a high chance of cure. In some instances, preoperative irradiation of the larynx and surrounding lymph nodes may help in the eradication of the tumor. About 90 percent of cancers of the larynx are cured if detected and treated early.

REFERENCES

DeWeese DD, Saunders WH: *Textbook of Otolaryngology,* 4th ed. St Louis, Mosby, 1973

Eliasson R et al: The immotile-cilia syndrome. A congenital ciliary abnormality as an etiologic factor in chronic airway infections and male sterility. N Engl J Med 297:1, 1977

Scott-Brown WG: *Diseases of the Ear, Nose and Throat,* vol 3: *The Nose,* 3d ed, V Ballantine, J Groves (eds). Philadelphia, Lippincott, 1971

———: *Diseases of the Ear, Nose and Throat,* vol 4: *The Throat,* 3d ed, V Ballantine, J Groves (eds). Philadelphia, Lippincott, 1971

Wiesner PJ: Gonococcal pharyngeal infection. Obstet Gynecol 18:121, 1975

268
NEOPLASMS OF THE LUNG

GENNARO M. TISI

At the turn of the century Adler, in his classic monograph, was able to collect only 374 cases of cancer of the lung from the world's literature. During the past 60 years, there has been a slow but steady increase in the incidence of cancer of the lung. Currently, lung cancer is the most common form of malignancy in the male, reaching a peak between the fifth and seventh decades and accounting for one in four male cancer deaths. The sex incidence is at least 5:1, male to female, but with the current changes in the pattern of cigarette smoking in the female this difference in incidence may narrow in the future. The alarming increase in the incidence of lung cancer in both smoking men and women may be referred to as the "lung cancer epidemic."

EPIDEMIOLOGY Extensive statistical analysis has confirmed the relationship between lung cancer and heavy cigarette smoking. Cigarette smoke is a heterogeneous mixture of gases, uncondensed vapors, and liquid particulate matter. Although many carcinogenic polycyclic hydrocarbons have been isolated from cigarette smoke, 3,4-benzpyrine has the highest carcinogenic rating. It has been demonstrated that the more cigarettes a person smokes, the greater is the risk of developing cancer of the lung. Hammond and Horn report the death rate in cancer of the lung per hundred thousand is 3.4 in the male nonsmoker, 59.3 for 10 to 20 cigarettes daily, and 217.3 for 40 or more cigarettes daily. A person who stops smoking is less likely to develop lung cancer than one who continues to smoke. Although smoking has attracted the principal interest in the epidemiology of lung cancer, other factors also have been implicated. Considerable attention has been directed to the potential role of air pollution, exposure to ionizing radiation, and numerous occupational hazards, including exposure to chromates, metallic iron and iron oxides, arsenic, nickel, beryllium, and asbestos. The chances of an individual's developing cancer of the lung as a consequence of exposure to an industrial carcinogen are increased if that person is also a cigarette smoker (e.g., an asbestos worker or a uranium miner). In many tissues, chronic inflammatory changes are known to precede cancer. In the lung, fibrosis may follow focal destructive and proliferative lesions. Numerous studies report an increased incidence of peripheral adenocarcinomas in such areas of chronic scarring (so-called "scar-carcinoma"). This incidence is particularly high in patients with scleroderma and chronic interstitial fibrosis of the usual type.

Recent work has established an interesting link between naturally occurring carcinogens and membrane-bound enzymes. The majority of the chemical carcinogens must be metabolically converted in the target tissue into a carcinogenic form. In keeping with this concept the polycyclic aromatic hydrocarbons contained in cigarette smoke are metabolized by certain mixed-function oxidases to reactive intermediates, which in turn can elicit cell transformation, cytotoxicity, and mutagenicity. Aryl hydrocarbon hydroxylase (one of the mixed-function oxidases) is such an inducible, membrane-bound enzyme. Studies on the lymphocytes of patients with bronchogenic carcinoma indicate that susceptibility to bronchogenic carcinoma is associated with higher levels of this enzyme than normal.

PATHOLOGY Primary cancer of the lung can be classified, in terms of its anatomic location, into *central* or *peripheral* categories. Central lesions involve the tracheobronchial tree from the primary to the distal bronchi, while peripheral lesions involve the distal bronchi and bronchioles. The relative frequency of cancer of the lung, when divided into these broad anatomic categories, is approximately equal. This simple classification helps in understanding many of the vagaries of the clinical presentation, the pattern of growth, the avenues of metastasis, and the preferential diagnostic approach.

There is not universal agreement on the histologic classification of primary pulmonary carcinoma. The classification offered here has been selected because it stresses the correlation between a histologic pattern and particular mode of clinical-pathologic behavior. Four basic histologic patterns of primary lung cancer and their approximate relative incidences are recognized: (1) *squamous cell* carcinoma (epidermoid carcinoma), 60 percent; (2) *adenocarcinoma,* 15 percent; (3) *undifferentiated* or anaplastic carcinoma including the round-cell, large-cell, and oat-cell types, 20 percent; and (4) *bronchioloalveolar* cell carcinoma (alveolar cell carcinoma), 2 percent. In some instances it is difficult to discern a uniform histologic pattern, and this leads to the diagnosis of mixed patterns.

With reference to this histologic classification, the following observations should be considered:

1 *Squamous cell* or *epidermoid carcinoma* is virtually always associated with cigarette smoking, usually occurs in central locations on the chest roentgenogram, produces earlier symptoms because of the potential for bronchial obstruction, spreads generally by continuity, and may undergo cavitation.
2 *Adenocarcinoma* has been associated with focal lung scars and chronic interstitial fibrosis, occurs primarily in peripheral locations on the chest roentgenogram, may spread by all routes but particularly by the bloodstream, and often remains clinically silent until distant hematogenous metastases occur.
3 *Undifferentiated carcinoma* is found in a relatively younger age group than the other types, occurs predominantly in the male (as does squamous cell carcinoma), occurs with equal frequency in central and peripheral areas, and metastasizes early.

4 *Bronchioloalveolar cell carcinoma* classically presents with a diffuse or multinodular type of lesion, significant bronchorrhea, progressive dyspnea, and increasing hypoxemia usually associated with hyperventilation. This combination of hypoxemia and hypocapnia is typical of diffuse interstitial processes.

Considerable controversy centers on whether alveolar cell carcinoma has a multicentric or unicentric origin. The principal evidence favors a unicentric origin, providing philosophically a bright approach to therapy.

Primary carcinoma of the lung may spread by any of four routes: (1) direct local extension, (2) hematogenous dissemination, (3) lymphatic spread and, uncommonly, (4) transbronchial spread. The preferential sites of extrapulmonary metastasis include the prescalene lymph nodes, liver, brain, adrenal glands, and bones.

CLINICAL PRESENTATION   Primary tumors   The clinical presentation of carcinoma of the lung depends upon many variables, including cell type; site of origin; the concept of biologic predetermination of cancer behavior; and immunologic mechanisms, at present poorly understood. The resulting symptom complexes should be viewed as constituting two modes of presentation: early and late.

The *early* mode of presentation has special clinical significance because a reasonable expectation of cure can be anticipated. In this stage of the disease, a patient may present with symptoms attributable to an intrabronchial lesion, such as a mild cough or a change in the pattern of a chronic cigarette cough. Symptoms secondary to local bronchial obstruction and/or surrounding inflammation including fever, chills, sputum production, a localized wheeze, or hemoptysis, may also be present. The last of these is alarming but a presenting symptom in only 7 to 10 percent of patients. In many instances a patient may be entirely asymptomatic, the sole reason for referral to medical attention being an abnormal chest roentgenogram. Unfortunately, in the early cases, the physical examination may be entirely negative. A localized wheeze over a segmental bronchus brought out by a forced expiratory or panting maneuver may be an early sign. As the lesion progresses, the classical physical signs due to obstruction may develop, including those of atelectasis, pneumonitis, abscess formation, and loss of lung volume.

The *late* mode of presentation indicates that a lesion has extended beyond the stage of resectional or curative surgery. In this stage of the disease, depending upon the degree or direction of spread, a patient may present with one or a combination of the following: (1) nonspecific systemic symptoms, (2) signs and symptoms of intrathoracic spread, (3) signs and symptoms of extrathoracic extension, and (4) classical systemic syndromes.

A patient with advanced disease may present with *nonspecific systemic* symptoms such as weight loss, anorexia, nausea and vomiting, and weakness. The longer the duration of such symptoms, the more likely it is that the lesion is nonresectable.

When the patient is first seen, evidence for *intrathoracic spread* already may be present. Evidence for such spread includes hoarseness due to involvement of the recurrent laryngeal nerve; pleuritis, with or without effusion, due to pleural extension; a unilaterally paralyzed diaphragm with paradoxical motion, due to involvement of the phrenic nerve; dysphagia due to esophageal involvement; Horner's syndrome due to involvement of the cervical thoracic sympathetic nerves; and superior vena caval obstruction due to entrapment of the superior vena cava.

Symptoms of *extrathoracic spread* or distant metastasis may also be present. The symptoms in any given patient depend upon the sites of metastasis. Commonly involved are one or more of the following: prescalene lymph nodes, brain, liver, adrenal glands, and bone.

The fourth symptom complex includes numerous *systemic syndromes.* These syndromes are of diagnostic value in that, in some instances, they may antedate the roentgenographic appearance of a pulmonary lesion. The list of syndromes associated with cancer of the lung (particularly the oat-cell variety) continues to grow. This intriguing array of classical systemic syndromes can be divided into five categories:

1 Metabolic, including hypercalcemia, the syndrome of inappropriate ADH secretion, Cushing's syndrome, gynecomastia, and carcinoid syndrome (the latter is usually associated with bronchial adenoma).
2 Neuromuscular, including peripheral neuropathy, corticocerebellar degeneration, and nonspecific myopathy.
3 Dermatologic abnormalities, including acanthosis nigricans and dermatomyositis.
4 Vascular abnormalities, including thrombocytopenic purpura, leukemoid reaction, myelophthisic anemia, and nonbacterial thrombotic endocarditis.
5 Connective tissue abnormalities, including hypertrophic pulmonary osteoarthropathy (HPO), clubbing, and nonspecific arthralgias.

The terms clubbing and HPO are not synonymous. Clubbing is often seen in the absence of HPO, while virtually all patients with HPO have clubbing. The clinical significance of these two signs is that they should lead to a search for malignancy, especially intrathoracic. Malignant lung tumors, usually squamous cell carcinomas, account for over 90 percent of the cases of HPO.

Two modes of presentation deserve separate mention: the patient with a bronchial adenoma and the patient with a Pancoast tumor.

Bronchial adenomas (carcinoid bronchial adenoma) comprise 3 to 10 percent of all surgically excised pulmonary neoplasms. They are primarily central in location, with approximately 90 percent visible at bronchoscopy. The characteristics of central location, slow growth, and marked vascularity account for the common types of clinical presentation: (1) recurrent hemoptysis, (2) localized wheezing, (3) infection distal to bronchial obstruction, and (4) history often antedating diagnosis by 5 or more years. Due to the vascularity of this tumor, biopsy at the time of bronchoscopy has been reported, rarely, to produce hemoptysis, which if massive can even result in asphyxiation. Distant blood-borne metastases are rare. Bronchial adenoma, like oat-cell carcinoma, has been associated with multiple endocrinopathies.

Tumors arising in the apex of the lung have been referred to as *Pancoast* or superior sulcus tumors; with few exceptions they are squamous cell carcinomas. Since there are many crossing shadows at the apex of the lung, apical lesions may escape detection. If there is any question as to the normality of this region, apical lordotic views or midchest tomograms should be obtained. Tumors in the apex have a propensity for early invasion of surrounding structures, including bone, pleura, chest wall, the tracheal plexus, and the cervical sympathetic plexus. Extension to these neural structures can result in *Horner's syndrome* (enophthalmos, ptosis, miosis, and anhidrosis on the side of the lesion) and intractable pain out of proportion to the size of the apical lesion. The extent of the local involvement will determine whether such tumors are resectable. Patients whose tumors are nonresectable are candidates for palliative irradiation. In some series preoperative external irradiation has resulted in higher resectability percentages, with 5-year survivorship statistics surprisingly approaching 20 to 25 percent.

Solitary pulmonary nodules A common and difficult problem in diagnosis and treatment is presented by the patient, usually asymptomatic, with a solitary pulmonary nodule on a chest roentgenogram. To qualify for the designation of a solitary pulmonary nodule, the mass must have minimal satellite lesions and must have normal aerated lung around it; it is usually in the middle or lateral one-third of the lung fields. Its shape may be round or oval; lobulations, if present, must be minimal. Its margins are circumscribed and its contour is smooth, and there must be minimal, if any, associated atelectasis, pneumonitis, or regional adenopathy. The prevalence of solitary pulmonary nodules is increased in those geographic areas where common fungal diseases may produce granulomatous nodules in the course of their healing (e.g., coccidioidomycosis in the Southwestern United States, histoplasmosis in the Midwestern United States). The sequence of diagnostic evaluation of an asymptomatic patient with a solitary pulmonary nodule can be divided into three phases: (1) noninvasive approaches, (2) invasive techniques, and (3) exploratory thoracotomy. How far an individual patient progresses in this sequence is a function of the following:

Noninvasive evaluation begins with consideration of the age of the patient and the pattern of calcification of the mass. Statistics indicate that below age 30, such lesions are infrequently malignant (less than 2 percent). Thereafter, the incidence of malignancy is a direct function of age (i.e., the older the patient the higher the incidence of malignancy: ages 35 to 44, 15 percent; 45 to 49, 26 percent; 50 to 59, 41 percent; 60 to 69, 50 percent; 70 to 79, 70 percent; 80 and older, almost 100 percent). The major percentage of the benign lesions is accounted for by granulomas, with hamartomas accounting for an additional minor subgroup. The *pattern of calcification* within a lesion is also of diagnostic significance. The presence of a calcific flex or of peripheral calcification does not exclude the presence of a malignant lesion. However, dense generalized calcification as seen in a Gohn tubercle, laminated calcification as seen in granuloma, and "popcorn" type of calcification as seen in hamartomas are generally associated with benign lesions. Tomograms of the chest may be required to determine whether calcium is present and its specific pattern. Each patient should be carefully interrogated as to the availability of old chest roentgenograms. If any chest x-rays were taken within the recent or distant past, further evaluation should be halted until these films are obtained and carefully reviewed. The concept of *doubling time* is of particular importance in reviewing such old films. The time required for an increase in the diameter of a lesion which results in a doubling of the volume of that lesion is referred to as the doubling time. Most carcinomas have a doubling time between 5 weeks and 18 months. Lesions with shorter doubling times are often inflammatory, while those with longer times are infrequently malignant, and those which show no change in size for 18 months (stable lesions) are almost never malignant. Current evidence indicates that the faster the rate of growth of a tumor, the worse the prognosis, including a shortened 5-year survival rate following resectional surgery. Composite analyses of these three features of age, calcific pattern, and doubling time will determine whether the lesion can be diagnosed as benign, or whether further evaluation is necessary to establish a cause.

The invasive evaluation of such mass lesions includes percutaneous transthoracic aspiration needle biopsy and those techniques which can be performed at the time of fiberoptic bronchoscopy, including biopsy, localized washings, and peripheral brushings under fluoroscopic control (see "Diagnostic

Evaluation," further on). The diagnostic yield of such techniques is a direct expression of the experience of the bronchoscopist.

If evaluation up to this point has either established the diagnosis of a malignant lesion or not excluded this possibility, then exploratory thoracotomy should be recommended. This recommendation will depend upon the characterization of the patient as an operative candidate (see "Treatment," further on). In general, since the incidence of mediastinal metastasis is low for such lesions (usually less than 10 to 20 percent), exploratory thoracotomy is usually not preceded by separate staging mediastinoscopy. Approximately 90 to 95 percent of all malignant solitary pulmonary nodules are primary lung tumors. The 5-year survival rate in a patient presenting with an asymptomatic, malignant solitary pulmonary nodule has been reported to be as high as 50 percent. Since the mortality and morbidity rates of exploratory thoracotomy are low (significantly less than 1 percent mortality), risk-salvage statistics have been used to support a surgical approach for all middle-aged patients with undiagnosed, uncalcified solitary pulmonary nodules of uncertain duration.

Metastatic tumors The pulmonary capillaries, with a mean cross-sectional diameter of 12 μm, are ideally suited to the entrapment of tumor emboli. This feature and the rich lymphatic supply of the lung account, in large part, for the high incidence of metastatic (secondary) carcinoma in the lung. The great majority of pulmonary metastatic lesions are adenocarcinomas from the gastrointestinal tract, genitourinary tract, and glandular tissues. Metastases to the lung are usually spherical in shape, variable in size, multiple, and bilateral. These roentgenographic features combined with symptoms suggesting an extrapulmonary source help in the differential diagnosis of primary from metastatic carcinoma.

Early diagnosis and improved therapy have produced an increase in the number of long-term survivors of nonpulmonary primary malignancies. If such a surviving patient presents with a new pulmonary lesion during long-term follow-up care, what are the etiologic possibilities? The problem of distinguishing among late metastasis to the lung, a new primary in the lung, or a benign pulmonary lesion has been reviewed by Adkins. The majority of such patients will present with ancillary evidence of metastatic spread from the original primary tumor. The pattern of spread will depend upon the sites of predilection of the original primary. However, if the patient is asymptomatic and if diagnostic evaluation fails to provide evidence for other distant metastases, a substantial percentage of such lesions will prove to be either a new primary or a benign lesion.

DIAGNOSTIC EVALUATION There are three principal aims in the diagnostic evaluation of a patient with carcinoma of the lung: (1) identification of the lesion as a carcinoma; (2) determination whether the pulmonary lesion has extended (a) beyond the pulmonary parenchyma and (b) beyond the thoracic cavity; and (3) preoperative cardiopulmonary evaluation to determine whether the patient with an operable lesion will be able to tolerate the degree of resection anticipated.

In most instances, the initial diagnostic approach is *roentgenographic*. Many times the x-ray may display the only abnormality in an asymptomatic patient. In all cases, inquiries about past roentgenograms should be made, and every attempt should be made to obtain these films promptly. The initial x-ray lesion may be of any size, shape, or location. Early roentgenographic signs include a large central hilar mass, the solitary pulmonary nodule, areas of localized overinflation due to intrabronchial obstruction, atelectasis with unilateral loss of volume, and the appearance of localized inflammatory changes. All patients over the age of 40 with pneumonia should be followed with serial chest films to the point of complete resolution. Such an approach may lead to the diagnosis of a slowly resolving pneumonia and be the first indication of carcinoma of the lung. Roentgenographic signs of intrathoracic spread include pleural thickening and/or effusion (providing an inflammatory basis is excluded), elevation of a diaphragm, rib erosion, hilar metastasis, and lymphatic obstruction with Kerly B lines. Multiple roentgenographic views, including lateral and oblique projections, and tomography may be invaluable in defining the features described above, particularly the presence of calcification within solitary pulmonary nodules. Above all else, roentgen evaluation should establish that a potential mass lesion is in the chest and not on the chest wall or due to an artifact. Common chest wall lesions include warts, hemangiomas, neurofibromas, and nipple shadows, while artifacts include shadows produced by hair braids and defects due to film processing.

The nonradiographic evaluation of lung cancer includes the triad of fiberoptic bronchoscopy, mediastinoscopy, and sputum cytology. Experience with *fiberoptic bronchoscopy* has established that the tracheobronchial tree is now much more accessible to diagnosis than previously. In contrast to the rigid scope, fiberoptic bronchoscopy allows examination of the upper lobe bronchi, the superior segments of the lower lobes, and the more distal segmental and subsegmental bronchi. This is particularly critical in view of the upper lobe prevalence of carcinoma of the lung. The technique provides for biopsy, regional lung washings, and cytologic brushing of both central and peripheral lesions. The yield of these manipulations depends directly upon the experience of the bronchoscopist. When dealing with peripheral lesions, the diagnostic yield is significantly improved by performing bronchoscopy and peripheral brushing under fluoroscopic control. *Mediastinoscopy* has virtually replaced scalene node biopsy in most centers. This procedure is not only a routine method of establishing a tissue diagnosis but a primary method of staging a patient with lung cancer. The mediastinal lymph node chain on the right is highly accessible to mediastinoscopy, while the aorta limits accessibility on the left side and results in the substitution of anterior thoracotomy for this procedure. The performance of mediastinoscopy as part of routine preoperative assessment has led to improved selection of patients for operation and a resultant higher resectability rate. Positive mediastinal nodes generally identify a patient as having a nonresectable lesion and result in sparing such a patient unrewarding thoracic exploration. Contraindications to thoracotomy based on mediastinoscopy or anterior thoracotomy include (1) bilateral nodal metastasis, (2) contralateral nodal metastasis, (3) tumor invasion of the mediastinum, and (4) fixed nodes with fixation of the carina. The presence of positive lobar nodes which can be included in the block of a surgical resection does not constitute a contraindication to surgery. *Sputum cytology* is the least invasive technique for arriving at a potential diagnosis of malignancy. It has the highest rate of positivity when the lesion (1) is located in the upper lobes, (2) communicates with a bronchus, (3) has a central location, and (4) has a significant mass.

The highest yield in cytodiagnosis is obtained from bronchoscopy specimens, postbronchoscopy specimens, and induced sputums. If ordinary sputum samples are to be employed, an early morning deep cough specimen is preferred. The combination of the triad of bronchoscopy, mediastinoscopy, and sputum cytology should provide a positive diagnosis in over 80 percent of all patients with central epidermoid carcinoma.

If a pleural effusion is observed as an isolated presentation or related to a parenchymal lesion, *thoracentesis* and *needle biopsy* of the *pleura* should be performed. The fluid should be sent for cytologic analysis. The character of the pleural fluid in malignancy is usually exudative (specific gravity greater than 1.015 and protein greater than 3.5 g per 100 ml) with an increased red blood cell count (greater than 10,000 red blood cells per milliliter).

When the initial clinical presentation, physical examination, or initial laboratory examination suggests one of the classical patterns of metastatic spread to liver, brain, or bone, further evaluation should include, in the instance of suspected brain metastasis, skull films, echoencephalogram, brain scan, and lumbar puncture; in the instance of suspected liver metastasis, liver function tests and liver scan and biopsy; and in the instance of bone metastasis a radioisotopic bone scanning. The bone scan has replaced the skeletal x-ray survey in the evaluation of skeletal metastasis. However, when a localized skeletal metastasis is suspected clinically, x-rays of the area in question should be obtained. If such films are consistent with metastatic disease and the site is accessible, local biopsy should provide a tissue diagnosis. In patients with central hilar and mediastinal mass lesions in whom a diagnosis of oat-cell carcinoma is being considered, a bone marrow biopsy should be performed; such a biopsy has been reported to be positive in 30 to 50 percent of patients with oat-cell carcinoma. Such data stress the early, widespread metastasis and the nonsurgical nature of this cell type.

The efficacy of percutaneous transthoracic aspiration needle biopsy of the lung in establishing a diagnosis of pulmonary carcinoma has been stressed by many centers. In experienced hands this procedure (Chap. 256) provides a high diagnostic yield, particularly for peripheral roentgenographic lesions. The benefits of this procedure include saving the patient an exploratory thoracotomy in the diagnosis of benign disease and providing a preoperative diagnosis of lung cancer in a patient whose lesion is resectable; the gain in making the latter diagnosis preoperatively is that anesthesia time during thoracotomy is reduced by the time required to obtain a frozen section.

In patients with carcinoma of the lung, *pulmonary scintiphotoscans* with radioisotope-labeled macroaggregated albumin may provide nonspecific information on the status of arteriocapillary pulmonary perfusion. The combination of ventilation and perfusion scintiphotoscans should allow differentiation of primary perfusion defects from those which are secondary to decreased or absent ventilation (Chap. 256). It is hoped that pulmonary scintiphotoscans and pulmonary angiograms in selected patients may provide potentially valuable and reliable information on resectability and operability.

Although a patient may have a pulmonary lesion which by all criteria is operable, with potential for a curative resection, a decisive problem remains. Will the patient's cardiopulmonary reserve be sufficient to tolerate the degree of pulmonary resection anticipated? If there are no clinical signs of cardiopulmonary disability, simple determination of static lung volumes, dynamic flow rates, and resting arterial blood gas tensions and pH is sufficient, but if results of these studies are abnormal, further evaluation is indicated. The patient with obvious pulmonary disability presents a more complex physiologic problem. In this group of patients the determination of the type and degree of disability is essential. The more extensive the patient's clinical disability, the more extensive and sophisticated should be the preoperative evaluation.

Indications of nonoperability include laboratory evidence of (1) a *severe* restrictive and/or obstructive defect (determined by static lung volumes, dynamic flow rates, and measurement of pulmonary compliance and pulmonary resistance by body plethysmography (Chap. 255); (2) a *markedly reduced* functional pulmonary arteriocapillary bed (determined by a decreased diffusion capacity for carbon monoxide, an increase in

calculated wasted ventilation, i.e., ventilation of nonperfused areas, and resting hypoxemia with a widening of the alveolar-arterial oxygen gradient under conditions of exercise); (3) *grossly abnormal* ventilation-perfusion relationships [determined by pulmonary scintiphotoscans with radioisotope-labeled macroaggregated albumin, xenon (^{133}Xe) ventilation-perfusion scans, and pulmonary angiography]; (4) *marked alveolar hypoventilation* (determined by a level of alveolar ventilation inadequate to maintain a normal arterial carbon dioxide tension); and (5) *serious* pulmonary hypertension and cor pulmonale (determined by right-sided heart catheterization with measurement of cardiac output, pulmonary artery pressure, and total pulmonary vascular resistance).

Staging of lung cancer The numerous patterns of clinical presentation, the potential variations in diagnostic approach, and the impact and extent of disease on therapeutic options and prognosis make a system for the clinical staging of lung cancer essential. Staging of a lesion may be according to the characteristics of the local tumor (T), its regional and hilar-mediastinal nodal metastasis (N), and its distant hematogenous metastasis (M) (see Table 268-1).

Once an intrathoracic lesion is defined as a malignant lesion of the non-oat-cell type or a primary tumor whose cell type cannot be determined, then staging of the tumor should proceed. This can be viewed in terms of matching available diagnostic techniques to the TNM classification: (1) to define the T characteristics routine chest roentgenogram and fiberoptic bronchoscopy are required; (2) to define the N characteristics some combination of routine chest roentgenography, midchest tomography, gallium imaging of the lung and mediastinum, and mediastinoscopy are required; (3) to define the M characteristics the triad of history, physical examination, and an admission chemistry panel including liver function tests is recommended. Available data indicate that unless an abnormality is identified by one of the above, routine screening by means of liver, brain, and bone scans is not productive.

TABLE 268-1
TNM classification

PRIMARY TUMOR (T)

T_1	Lesion less than 3 cm in greatest diameter without bronchoscopic invasion proximal to a lobar bronchus
T_2	Greater than 3 cm in diameter, or tumor of any size, which, with its associated atelectasis or obstructive pneumonitis, extends to hilum; lesion must be further than 2 cm from the carina and there must be no intrathoracic spread
T_3	Lesion of any size with intrathoracic spread

REGIONAL LYMPH NODES (N)

N_0	Negative hilar or mediastinal nodes
N_1	Positive ipsilateral hilar nodes
N_2	Positive mediastinal nodes

DISTANT METASTASIS (M)

M_0	No distant metastasis
M_1	Systemic metastasis

STAGE GROUPING

Stage 1	T_1, N_0, M_0 lesion
	T_1, N_1, M_0 lesion
	T_2, N_0, M_0 lesion
Stage 2	T_2, N_1, M_0 lesion
Stage 3	T_3 with any N or M
	N_2 with any T or M
	M_1 with any T or N

TREATMENT Surgery If a patient has had adequate diagnostic evaluation, the therapeutic approach will follow naturally. The currently preferred therapeutic approach is surgical resection of the primary pulmonary carcinoma. In most instances, in an attempt to conserve pulmonary function, lobectomy rather than pneumonectomy is the operation of choice, provided the lesion can be excised completely by lobectomy.

An operative candidate is an individual who has no demonstrable evidence of intra- or extrathoracic spread of the malignancy and whose cardiopulmonary status does not preclude resectional surgery. Accepted contraindications to thoracotomy and pulmonary resection for primary carcinoma include (1) evidence of metastatic lymph node involvement; (2) superior vena caval obstruction; (3) recurrent laryngeal or phrenic nerve paralysis; (4) pleural thickening and/or effusion, with histologic evidence of carcinomatous involvement of the pleura, and/or the presence of malignant cells in the pleural fluid; (5) distant metastasis to liver, brain, adrenal glands, or bones; (6) multicentric or multilobar distribution of the lesion; and finally (7) a *serious* cardiopulmonary functional defect.

The *classical systemic syndromes* with which a patient may present do not by themselves constitute contraindications to resection. On the contrary, since they may contribute significantly to the patient's discomfort and demise, resection of the pulmonary parenchymal lesion may offer significant palliation. As a rule, many of these syndromes abate with resection and recur with metastasis.

Chemotherapy The response of lung cancer to current chemotherapeutic protocols is a direct function of cell type. To date, the impact of current protocols on survivorship in both squamous carcinoma and adenocarcinoma has been discouraging. However, several studies now demonstrate that multiple drug chemotherapy (protocols usually including some combination of cyclophosphamide, methotrexate, methyl-CCNU, and vincristine) has increased survivorship in oat-cell carcinoma. Such protocols involve sequential therapy with highly reactive and cell cycle–nonspecific agents (e.g., alkylating agents) followed by cell cycle–specific anticancer agents (e.g., antimetabolites). This approach is based on the concept that reduction in the viable tumor cell population is followed by an increase in growth and increased sensitivity to antimetabolite drugs.

Radiotherapy Radiation therapy alone does not alter the 5-year survival seen in the natural history of squamous cell and adenocarcinomas. However, radiotherapy does have a vital role in the *palliative* treatment of patients with disabling manifestations of bone pain, superior vena caval obstruction, and the consequences of endobronchial obstruction including bleeding, atelectasis, distal pneumonia, and abscess formation. The approach to patients with oat-cell carcinoma differs in that this tumor is exquisitely radiosensitive. Several protocols employing radiation to the tumor site, prophylactic brain irradiation, and multiple drug chemotherapeutic programs are currently under study in patients with this tumor type. Initial data indicate that such protocols significantly prolong survivorship.

Immunotherapy The newest avenue which has opened for the treatment of lung cancer is immunotherapy. This modality holds considerable promise as an adjuvant form of therapy in that (1) it is a systemic form of therapy, (2) it may operate by zero-order kinetics by affecting every cell at risk at the same time, and (3) it has exquisite specificity for tumor cells as opposed to normal cells. Multiple clinical studies have been instituted using BCG (bacillus Calmette-Guérin) and *Corynebacte-*

rium parvum in this country and Levamisol in Europe. Current clinical trials are based on the findings that (1) nonspecific immune stimulation can kill tumor cells, (2) alterations of surface antigens of tumor cells may increase their immunogenicity, (3) the immune response is not able to deal with large tumor burdens, and (4) common tumor antigens may promote tumor immunity. To date this work is in its preliminary stages. Currently, only patients participating in study protocols should be treated with adjuvant immunotherapy so that basic data on tumor immunology can be collected in addition to data on survivorship. In this regard, it is interesting that unresectability, poor prognosis, and multiple metastases have been correlated with skin test anergy to standard antigens and inability to produce sensitization to 2,4-dinitrochlorobenzene.

PROGNOSIS Data on the interrelationships between cell type and stage and 5-year prognosis have been provided by the American Joint Commission for Cancer Staging and End Results Reporting. The important characteristics of these data can be summarized as follows:

1 *Squamous cell carcinoma.* The highest 5-year survival for any cell type is for stage 1 squamous cell carcinoma (40 to 50 percent). Prognosis is directly related to stage: for stages 1 and 3 the curves asymptote at 2 years, and 8 to 10 percent of patients with stage 3 disease survive 5 years.
2 *Adenocarcinoma.* For stage 1 disease, the 5-year survivorship is somewhat lower than that for stage 1 squamous cell carcinoma (approximately 35 to 40 percent). Once again prognosis is directly related to stage: for stages 1 and 2 the curves asymptote at 2 years, and 2 to 4 percent of patients with stage 3 disease survive 5 years.
3 *Oat-cell carcinoma.* The survivorship data for oat-cell carcinoma are usually poor and unaffected by stage.

Many clinical messages may be drawn from these data:

1 Early detection of localized disease is associated with significant survivorship for squamous cell and adenocarcinomas.
2 Although it is usual to speak of 5-year cures, the tendency of the curves for squamous cell carcinoma and adenocarcinoma to asymptote after 2 years indicates that particular attention should be focused on the detection of tumor spread during the first 2 years following diagnosis.
3 The natural history for untreated squamous cell carcinoma and adenocarcinoma are indicated by stage 3 disease. These data are essential in evaluating the response of these cell types to current and future protocols of chemotherapy, radiotherapy, immunotherapy, and combination therapy.
4 Despite surgical removal of all clinically recognized disease, more than 50 percent of patients with stage 2 squamous cell carcinoma die within 5 years, indicating that systemic micrometastases must be present at the time of surgical resection. Such a conclusion leads inescapably to the need for the development of adjuvant therapy in addition to surgery. However, in keeping with the adage that the best therapy is prevention, cessation of smoking offers the best current means of halting the epidemic of lung cancer.

REFERENCES

ADKINS PC: Thoracotomy on the patient with previous malignancy. Metastasis or new primary. J Thorac Cardiovasc Surg 56:351, 1968

ALAZRAKI NP et al: Reliability of gallium scan and chest radiography compared to mediastinoscopy for evaluating mediastinal spread in cancer. Am Rev Respir Dis 117:415, 1978

THE AMERICAN JOINT COMMITTEE FOR CANCER STAGING AND END RESULTS REPORTING: Clinical staging system for carcinoma of the lung. Cancer 24:87, 1974

BERGH NP et al: Bronchogenic carcinoma. Follow-up study of a surgically treated series with special reference to the prognostic significance of lymph node metastasis. Acta Chir Scand Suppl 347:1, 1965

RAMSDELL JW et al: Multiorgan scans for staging lung cancer. J Thorac Cardiovasc Surg 73:653, 1977

SAGEL SS et al: Percutaneous transthoracic aspiration needle biopsy. Ann Thorac Surg 26:399, 1978

269
DISEASES OF THE PLEURA, MEDIASTINUM, AND DIAPHRAGM

NICHOLAS A. SAUNDERS
ROLAND H. INGRAM, JR.

THE PLEURA

The visceral and parietal pleurae form a continuous membrane that encloses a potential space which normally contains only a small amount of liquid. This liquid is dynamic, and, as with all movements of liquid between the vascular and extravascular compartments, the principles of the Starling equation (Chap. 27) apply. Under normal circumstances, the liquid is filtered out of the parietal pleura which is supplied by systemic capillaries at a mean pressure of 30 cmH$_2$O and is taken up at the visceral pleura supplied by the pulmonary circulation that has a mean capillary pressure of 11 cmH$_2$O. Abnormal accumulations of liquid, designated as pleural effusions, occur with changes in hydrostatic and oncotic forces (transudation) or with alterations in membrane permeability (exudation) such as occurs with inflammation or neoplastic involvement.

The parietal pleura is supplied by segmental nerves and when inflamed gives rise to pain which is referred to superficial regions supplied by the intercostal nerves and the thoracic segments. This pain is sharp and superficial, and is aggravated during inspiration (Chap. 5). Since the location of the pain is determined by the distribution of the somatic afferents, pain may be referred to the shoulder if the diaphragmatic pleura (C3 to C5) is involved or to the upper abdomen if the lower thoracic intercostals are affected. The visceral pleura is supplied by visceral afferents that do not produce sharp and localizable pain.

The patient with pleuritic chest pain frequently has shallow, rapid breathing, and there may be lesser excursion of the affected hemithorax than the unaffected side (splinting). Inflammation of the pleural surfaces may also cause a pleural friction rub which may be localized or may be best heard at the lower thorax posteriorly, the region where there is greatest respiratory excursion. A pleural friction rub has a harsh, scratchy quality and is heard throughout the respiratory cycle; it is maximal toward the end of inspiration and early in expiration.

PLEURITIS Inflammation of the pleura can occur with or without apparent underlying pulmonary disease and has many causes, including pneumonia, tuberculosis, pulmonary infarction, and neoplasm. Pleural pain in the *absence of physical and roentgenographic findings* suggests the diagnosis of epidemic pleurodynia (Bornholm's disease, Chap. 187), other viral infections of the pleura, or connective tissue disorders such as systemic lupus erythematosus. The *presence of parenchymal disease on the chest roentgenogram* in a patient with pleuritic chest pain and fever suggests an infectious process such as acute bacterial pneumonia (Chap. 260). Pulmonary infarction secondary to pulmonary embolism (Chap. 266) may also cause inflammation of the pleural surface. Under these circum-

stances, hemoptysis is a common presenting feature. The finding of a *pleural effusion in the absence of parenchymal disease* suggests tuberculosis, subdiaphragmatic abscess, mesothelioma, or primary bacterial infection of the pleural space.

Treatment of pleuritis is directed toward the underlying disease and relief of pain. Analgesics frequently suppress pain, but generally they do not completely eradicate the pain associated with deep breaths and coughing. If pain prevents the patient from coughing up secretions, regional anesthesia by blockade of the appropriate intercostal nerves with a medium-duration local anesthetic is helpful. Occasionally, acute pleuritis leads to chronic adhesive pleuritis as a sequela of tuberculosis, empyema, or hemothorax. Adhesive pleuritis is characterized by marked thickening of the pleura, which may interfere with pulmonary function. Under these circumstances, the thickened pleura encases the lung and "traps" it, so that the lung behaves as if it were small and stiff, despite having intrinsically normal mechanical properties. If symptoms such as dyspnea are severe, surgical removal of the thickened pleura (decortication) may be indicated.

PLEURAL EFFUSION Pleural effusions may or may not be associated with disease of the pleura. In general, effusions due to pleural disease more nearly resemble plasma (exudates), while those occurring with a normal pleura are ultrafiltrates of the plasma (transudates). Effusions in association with pleuritis are due to increased permeability of the parietal pleura secondary to inflammatory or neoplastic involvement. A good example of pleural effusion with a normal pleura is that associated with congestive heart failure. Both increased fluid formation from the parietal pleura due to systemic capillary hypertension and decreased reabsorption from the visceral pleura secondary to elevations in pulmonary capillary pressure account for the abnormal collection of pleural liquid in this condition. Hypoalbuminemia, as occurs in nephrosis or cirrhosis, also leads to increased formation and decreased resorption of pleural liquid on the basis of decreased intravascular oncotic pressures. An additional mechanism, lymphatic obstruction, also leads to effusions in the absence of pleural disease. In this case the sharp distinction between exudates and transudates may become fuzzy. Since the lymphatic channels provide the only route for reabsorption of protein from the pleural space, protein concentrations in the effusion are often high, even though the pleura is not abnormally permeable.

The extent to which a pleural effusion compromises lung volume will depend in part on the relative stiffness of the lung and chest wall. At lung volumes in the normal breathing range, the chest wall tends to recoil outward while the lung tends to recoil inward. Thus, a pleural effusion of 1 liter would not be expected on a purely mechanical basis to reduce lung volumes by an identical amount, since part of the volume is taken up by outward movement of the chest wall. Ventilation is reduced in the lung underlying the effusion due to damping of pleural pressure swings by the liquid, and by some degree of atelectasis.

Many pleural effusions are asymptomatic, but patients may complain of shortness of breath, pleuritic chest pain, or a dull sensation in the chest. The physical signs include deviation of the trachea away from the affected side, dullness to percussion, and diminished breath sounds over the affected side. Egophony may be heard at the upper border of the effusion.

The most common appearance of a pleural effusion on chest roentgenogram is obliteration of the sharp angle between the diaphragm and rib cage (costophrenic angle) with an upward concavity of the liquid level. Occasionally, effusions lie underneath the lung (*subpulmonic effusion*) and give the appearance of an elevated hemidiaphragm. A chest roentgenogram in the lateral decubitus position (affected side down) will show the pleural fluid layering out along the lateral chest wall, provided the fluid is not loculated. A clue to the presence of a subpulmonic effusion in the left hemithorax from the chest roentgenograph taken in the upright posture is a wide density between the gastric air bubble and the apparent upper border of the diaphragm. Pleural effusions may be missed on anteroposterior roentgenograms taken in the supine posture since the liquid layers out posteriorly. In this case it produces a generally hazy shadow that is difficult to detect when unilateral and impossible to detect when bilateral. Occasionally, effusions may form between lobes of the lungs and produce a rounded opacity on the chest roentgenogram that resembles a solitary nodule. Since these often disappear with resolution of the effusion, they are referred to as *phantom tumors*.

Aspiration of the pleural effusion under local anesthesia should always be performed if the etiology of the effusion is in doubt, or if the effusion is causing dyspnea. If the diagnosis of neoplasm or tuberculosis is seriously considered, closed pleural biopsy with an Abrams or Cope needle should be performed at the time of the initial thoracentesis.

Pleural fluid that is bloodstained is suggestive of neoplasm or pulmonary infarction; however, blood may also be present in effusions due to infection, congestive heart failure, and trauma. The differentiation of pleural effusions into *transudates* and *exudates* is of considerable diagnostic importance. Many different tests on the pleural liquid have been advocated (Table 269-1); however no single test is diagnostic. Effusions which have a high protein content, high pleural liquid-to-serum LDH activity ratios, and many white blood cells are indic-

*Draw blood sample simultaneously to compare with pleural fluid values

FIGURE 269-1

Approach to the diagnosis of pleural effusions.

ative of exudates. However, transudates secondary to congestive heart failure may have high protein contents after the volume of the effusion decreases with diuresis; any effusion that contains cellular debris may have a high pleural liquid-to-serum LDH ratio; and there is no absolute leukocyte count that clearly differentiates transudates from exudates. Clearly the diagnosis depends on interpretation of the test results in the context of the patient's illness. In addition to chemical tests, exudative pleural liquid should receive complete cytologic and microbiologic examinations. Figure 269-1 presents an approach to the evaluation of pleural effusions. Despite an orderly and complete approach, no cause will be found for the pleural effusion in up to 25 percent of patients.

Postprimary tuberculous effusions present as isolated pleural effusions in the absence of radiologically demonstrable parenchymal disease and occur within months of primary subclinical infection. The patient may be asymptomatic or, more commonly, presents with fever, malaise, and weight loss. Occasionally, high fever and pleuritic chest pain are present. More than 90 percent of patients have a positive tuberculin skin test. Thoracentesis reveals an exudative effusion, with predominant lymphocytosis. Acid-fast bacilli are rarely seen on direct smear, and cultures are positive in fewer than 20 percent of pleural effusions due to tuberculosis. The diagnostic yield is higher with closed pleural biopsy, which will reveal noncaseating granulomas and/or positive culture material in more than 50 percent of the cases.

Neoplastic pleural effusions are common. *Bronchogenic carcinoma* is the commonest malignancy causing pleural effusions and may do so by direct extension to the pleural surface, obstruction to lymphatic drainage (secondary to mediastinal spread), or by pleural inflammation secondary to pneumonia behind an obstructed bronchus. Patients usually present with symptoms referable to the primary lesion (Chap. 268), but may present with dyspnea or pleuritic chest pain. The effusion is invariably an exudate with or without blood. Pleural liquid cytology and pleural biopsy will confirm the diagnosis in up to 60 percent of cases. *Metastatic carcinoma,* most commonly from the breast, may also cause pleural effusions and is a more frequent cause of bilateral pleural effusions than bronchogenic carcinoma. *Lymphoma* may directly involve the pleura or may obstruct lymphatic drainage leading to a pleural effusion. Malignant effusions reaccumulate rapidly after aspiration, and repeated aspirations are not warranted. Instillation of sclerosing compounds such as tetracycline or cytotoxic agents may suc-

TABLE 269-1
Constituents of pleural effusions

	Transudate	Exudate
ROUTINE TESTS		
Protein	<3.0 g/100 ml	>3.0 g/100 ml
Lactic dehydrogenase	Low	High
Pleural fluid/serum LDH ratio	<0.6	>0.6
SPECIAL TESTS		
RBC	<10,000/mm³	Indeterminant >100,000/mm³ suggests neoplasm, infarction, trauma
WBC	<1000/mm³	Usually >1000/mm³
Differential WBC	Usually >50% lymphocytes or mononuclear cells	>50% lymphocytes (tuberculosis, neoplasm) >50% polymorphonuclear (acute inflammation)
pH	>7.3	<7.3 (inflammatory)
Glucose	Same as blood (±)	Low (infection) Extremely low (rheumatoid arthritis, occasionally neoplasm)
Amylase		>500 units/ml (pancreatitis; occasionally neoplasm, infection)
Specific proteins		Low C3, C4 components of complement (SLE, rheumatoid arthritis) Rheumatoid factor Antinuclear factor

ceed in producing adhesions between parietal and visceral pleural surfaces and decrease the rate of liquid accumulation.

Rheumatoid arthritis (Chap. 356) may cause pleural effusions with or without nodular changes in the pulmonary parenchyma or on the pleural surface. Patients are most often males, and subcutaneous nodules are usually associated with the arthritis. The pleural liquid is characteristically turbid and greenish yellow and has a very low glucose concentration (less than 20 mg per 100 ml) due to impaired glucose transport into the pleural liquid. These effusions are usually asymptomatic and do not require specific therapy.

Symptoms and signs referable to the chest very frequently accompany *subphrenic (subdiaphragmatic) abscess.* Fever, pleuritic chest pain, and an exudative pleural effusion are common. The chest roentgenogram usually reveals elevation of the hemidiaphragm, a small pleural effusion, and basal atelectasis, but is rarely diagnostic. Thoracentesis usually reveals sterile liquid, but an empyema due to direct extension of the infection may be present. It should be emphasized that pleural effusions following abdominal surgery are very common and should not be taken as a sign of a subdiaphragmatic abscess in the absence of other clinical features.

In *pancreatitis,* a left-sided pleural effusion may be present in up to 15 percent of patients with acute pancreatitis or pancreatic pseudocysts. Effusions are typically exudative and have a high amylase concentration. A high pleural fluid amylase concentration has occasionally been reported in neoplasm and infection, and may also be found in cases of esophageal rupture where the amylase is of salivary origin. No specific therapy of pleural effusion secondary to pancreatitis is indicated.

Pleural effusion and ascites in association with nonmetastatic pelvic tumors in women has been designated as *Meigs's syndrome.* The pleural effusion is most commonly right sided, may be an exudate or transudate, and is thought to develop from movement of ascitic liquid across the diaphragm. Both the ascites and pleural liquid dramatically resolve following removal of the pelvic tumor.

Eosinophilic pleural effusion is defined as the finding of eosinophils in excess of 10 percent in the pleural liquid; this attention-getting yet nonspecific finding may be present in effusions due to acute bacterial pneumonia, viral pleuritis, pancreatitis, neoplasm, and trauma.

Patients have been described with the triad of *yellow nails, lymphedema of the extremities, and pleural effusions.* The effusions have a high protein concentration, and are thought to be due to impaired lymphatic drainage of the pleural space rather than to pleural disease.

CHYLOTHORAX Leakage of thoracic duct lymph into the pleural space may be due to trauma to the thoracic duct or obstruction of the duct by a malignant process (lymphoma, mediastinal spread of bronchogenic carcinoma) or mediastinal fibrosis. A rare disorder, *lymphangiomyomatosis,* is frequently accompanied by chylothorax. Physical findings and the chest roentgenogram in patients with chylothorax are usually nonspecific, although mediastinal widening may be present in patients with lymphoma or bronchogenic carcinoma. Thoracentesis reveals a milky white liquid which is characteristically an exudate. Fat globules may be seen microscopically on staining with Sudan III dye. Total fat content ranges from 1 to 4 g per 100 ml. In cases of traumatic rupture of the thoracic duct, conservative management by repeated aspiration or thoracostomy-tube drainage and by cessation of oral feedings is tried initially. If this fails, lymphangiography followed by surgical ligation of the thoracic duct may be indicated. A chylothorax secondary to malignancy should not be repeatedly aspirated, since it reaccumulates rapidly.

Pseudochylous effusions do not contain fat globules but have a cloudy, milky appearance due to high concentrations of cho-

lesterol in the pleural liquid. Cholesterol crystals may give a metallic sheen to the pleural liquid. This condition most frequently occurs in long-standing pleural effusions, and the most frequent underlying diagnoses are tuberculosis and rheumatoid lung disease.

HEMOTHORAX Hemothorax due to frank bleeding into the pleural space most commonly follows blunt or penetrating trauma to the chest. A small amount of bleeding may complicate a spontaneous pneumothorax, producing a hemopneumothorax. Patients with hematologic disorders or who are taking anticoagulants may bleed into the pleural space following procedures such as closed pleural biopsy; therefore, a pleural biopsy should never be performed without first assuring that the patient's coagulation status is adequate. Treatment of hemothorax is directed toward adequate drainage of the pleural space. Bleeding originating from the lung is usually self-limiting, but bleeding from the chest wall is often progressive. Continued bleeding, inadequate drainage, or shock unresponsive to blood replacement require thoracotomy. Inadequate drainage of a hemothorax may lead to an intense, fibrous reaction (fibrothorax) where the thickened pleura encases the lung (trapped lung); early decortication is indicated.

EMPYEMA The presence of infected liquid or frank pus in the pleural space is termed an empyema. In the majority of cases it is the result of spread of infection from a contiguous structure and may complicate the course of bacterial pneumonia, subdiaphragmatic abscess, lung abscess, or esophageal perforation. Up to 20 percent of empyemas follow thoracic surgery or instrumentation of the pleural space (thoracentesis, inadvertent entry of the pleural space during puncture of the subclavian vein). Direct infection of the pleural space without involvement of the underlying lung by hematogenous spread of organisms from a distant site accounts for the remaining cases and is more common in children than adults. Bacteria implicated in the etiology of empyema include *Staphylococcus aureus* (most common in all ages), *Pseudomonas aeruginosa, Klebsiella pneumoniae, Escherichia coli, Pneumococcus* spp., and anaerobic bacteria.

Chest pain, fever and night sweats, cough, and weight loss are common complaints. These symptoms may be mild if an empyema develops during the course of antibiotic treatment for bacterial pneumonia; hence the empyema may go unrecognized. Signs of a pleural effusion will be present, and the chest roentgenogram will reveal pleural liquid and usually underlying parenchymal disease. Thoracentesis may reveal thick, purulent liquid, but in the early stages of the disease, thin, serous liquid with a high leukocyte count (>5000 per cubic millimeter; polymorphonuclear cells predominate), high protein content (>3 g per 100 ml), and low glucose concentration (<20 mg per 100 ml) may be obtained. Gram's stain usually reveals the causative organism.

Treatment is directed at providing adequate drainage of the pleural space in addition to appropriate antimicrobial therapy. If the pleural liquid is thin, drainage may occasionally be achieved by repeated thoracenteses. Most commonly, closed thoracostomy-tube drainage will be required; multiple thoracostomy tubes may be needed if the empyema is loculated and not free-flowing. If closed drainage of the pleural space does not result in the disappearance of fever and general improvement of the patient within 4 to 5 days, a limited thoracotomy is indicated, at which time resection of a small portion of the overlying rib and manual breakdown of pleural adhesions is performed. If this approach fails, or if treatment has been delayed, decortication with removal of the thick, fibrous tissue covering the lung (pleural peel) may be necessary to obtain lung expansion and obliteration of the empyema cavity. Rarely, an unrecognized empyema may rupture through the chest wall and spontaneously drain onto the body surface (*empyema necessitans*).

The mortality of empyema is high among patients who are elderly, who have serious underlying disease, or in whom treatment is delayed.

PNEUMOTHORAX A pneumothorax is a collection of gas in the pleural space that results in complete or partial collapse of the lung. Normally, the pressure in the pleural space at the end of a quiet breath is subatmospheric due to a balance between the tendency of the lung to recoil inward and the tendency of the chest wall to recoil outward (Chap. 255). The lung may therefore be thought to be held in an expanded position by the surrounding negative pleural pressure much as a balloon would be held inflated when surrounded by a vacuum. When air enters the pleural space, pleural pressure in the affected hemithorax tends toward atmospheric pressure; the less negative the pleural pressure, the greater the degree of lung collapse. The mediastinum shifts toward the unaffected side as a result of the normal elastic recoil of the unaffected lung. If pressure inside the pneumothorax becomes above atmospheric, as may occur with a one-way leak into the pleural space ("ball-valve" leak) or when a pneumothorax occurs as a complication of positive pressure ventilation, a *tension pneumothorax* is present. Under these circumstances the affected lung is compressed, the mediastinum is further shifted toward the unaffected side, and cardiac output may be severely compromised due to the positive intrathoracic pressure decreasing venous return to the heart. Tension pneumothorax is a medical emergency.

A pneumothorax may occur spontaneously or may be secondary to underlying lung disease, chest trauma, mechanical ventilation, or perforated esophagus.

SPONTANEOUS PNEUMOTHORAX Spontaneous pneumothorax most commonly occurs in previously healthy adults between 20 and 40 years of age. In such patients there is a strong tendency toward recurrence of the pneumothorax. Air leaks into the pleural space due to rupture of small blebs on the surface of the visceral pleura; the etiology of these blebs is unclear. They tend to be at the apex of the lung, perhaps due to the more negative pleural pressure around the lung apex. Some patients have been found to have small pleural nodules consisting of histiocytes, giant cells, and other inflammatory cells (*reactive eosinophilic pleuritis*). These lesions should be differentiated from pulmonary eosinophilic granuloma.

Pleuritic chest pain and dyspnea are the commonest complaints in patients with pneumothorax. Physical examination reveals tachypnea, asymmetrical expansion of the chest on the affected side (due to outward recoil of the chest wall as the lung collapses), mediastinal shift with deviation of the trachea and apex beat away from the pneumothorax, and hyperresonance to percussion and diminished breath sounds over the affected side. The chest roentgenogram reveals a visible visceral pleural edge with no lung markings between this edge and the chest wall. Chest roentgenograms should be taken in the upright position before a pneumothorax can be excluded, since in the supine posture upward movement of air with approximation of visceral and parietal pleurae laterally may obscure its presence. Small pneumothoraxes may be more easily seen if the chest roentgenogram is taken at the end of a maximal expiration. If pneumothorax is associated with tearing of

adhesions in the pleural space, *hemopneumothorax* may develop, with a gas-liquid level visible in the pleural space.

Treatment depends on the size of the pneumothorax. A small pneumothorax needs only close observation, since the air leak has usually sealed by the time the patient presents. The air in the pleural space will be reabsorbed spontaneously, since the sum of the partial pressures of the gases in the pleural space (i.e., air = 760 mmHg at sea level) is greater than the sum of the partial pressures of gases in the end-capillary blood due to the low end-capillary P_{O_2}. Larger pneumothoraxes should be aspirated or treated with closed thoracostomy-tube drainage. Failure of the lung to reexpand, despite application of suction to the chest tube, indicates that the lung is "trapped," that a major bronchus is occluded, or that there is a large continuing air leak through a major communication between the pleural space and lung (*bronchopleural fistula*). A bronchopleural fistula rarely occurs spontaneously unless there is underlying lung disease such as rupture of a lung abscess into the pleural space or necrotizing pneumonia, but may occur following lung resection or chest trauma or during mechanical ventilation (barotrauma). Spontaneous *tension* pneumothorax is unusual, but if present, it should be treated by immediate aspiration through a wide bore needle placed in the pleural space at the level of the second intercostal space anteriorly at the midclavicular line. If there is circulatory collapse and severe dyspnea, tension pneumothorax should be suspected and treated without waiting for roentgenographic confirmation.

Approximately 50 percent of patients with spontaneous pneumothorax have a recurrence, and the incidence of further recurrence is even higher following the second episode. Repeated spontaneous pneumothorax should be treated surgically by application of irritants to the pleural surfaces so that they adhere to each other (*pleurodesis*) or by performing a *parietal pleurectomy*. Because of the tendency of pneumothorax to recur, if both sides are ever involved, even at different times, surgical intervention is indicated.

Patients with pneumothorax should not be moved in unpressurized aircraft because the decrease in atmospheric pressure may result in enlargement of the pneumothorax to an extent that it may seriously compromise ventilatory and cardiac function. Similarly, patients with a history of spontaneous pneumothorax should not pilot aircraft or undertake scuba diving. Should a pneumothorax occur underwater, enlargement of the pneumothorax on ascent may be catastrophic.

Pneumothorax may occur spontaneously in patients with a wide variety of lung diseases, such as asthma, emphysema, lung abscess, neoplasm, eosinophilic granuloma, and the adult respiratory distress syndrome. In the presence of underlying lung disease closed thoracotomy-tube drainage will almost always be needed. *Catamenial pneumothorax* is a rare disorder characterized by spontaneous pneumothorax at the time of the menstrual period. The right side is more frequently, but not invariably, affected. The pathogenesis of this disorder is not understood but may be related to intrathoracic endometriosis. Hormonal therapy with suppression of ovulation is usually successful.

PLEURAL TUMORS Two types of *mesothelioma*, a rare tumor of the visceral and parietal pleura, are recognized. The *localized form* is a solitary growth on the pleural surface that only occasionally causes a pleural effusion and may be cured by surgical resection. Patients are often asymptomatic or may complain of chest pain and cough. The *diffuse mesothelioma* is a highly malignant tumor that is usually associated with a serous or blood-stained pleural effusion. There is no effective therapy for this tumor. Clubbing of the digits and hypertrophic pulmonary osteoarthropathy are associated with pleural-based tumors. The diagnosis of mesothelioma may be obtained from cytologic examination of the pleural liquid or closed pleural biopsy, but difficulty may be encountered distinguishing this tumor histologically from adenocarcinoma. There is an increased incidence of pleural and peritoneal mesotheliomas among persons exposed to asbestos; a higher incidence is found among those engaged in the processing and use of asbestos products than those in the mining industry. The interval between exposure and tumor development often exceeds 20 years; continuous exposure to asbestos is not necessary. In addition to primary tumors, the pleura is a common site for *metastases* from neoplasms of the bronchus, breast, ovary, and gastrointestinal tract.

MEDIASTINUM

The mediastinum occupies the central portion of the chest and is anatomically defined by the thoracic inlet above, the diaphragm below, the mediastinal pleura laterally, the paravertebral gutter and ribs posteriorly, and the sternum anteriorly. The mediastinum is divided into four compartments for descriptive purposes (Fig. 269-2). The *superior mediastinum* is bounded above by the plane of the first rib and below by an imaginary line drawn anteroposteriorly from the sternal angle to the lower edge of the fourth thoracic vertebra. It contains the trachea, upper esophagus, thymus gland, thoracic duct, great veins, arch of the aorta and its branches, and the phrenic, vagus, and left recurrent laryngeal nerves. Below the superior mediastinum lie three further compartments. The *anterior mediastinum* contains fibroareolar tissue and lymph nodes, but no major structures. The *middle mediastinum* contains the heart, ascending aorta, great veins, pulmonary artery, and phrenic nerves. The *posterior mediastinum* contains the esophagus, thoracic duct, descending aorta, sympathetic chain, and intercostal and vagal nerves.

TUMORS AND CYSTS The commonest mediastinal masses in adults are metastatic carcinomas (most commonly bronchogenic carcinoma) and lymphomas. Neurogenic tumors, teratodermoids, thymomas, and bronchogenic cysts account for approximately two-thirds of the remaining mediastinal masses.

One-third of patients are asymptomatic, with the mediastinal mass detected on a routine chest roentgenogram. In the remainder, chest pain, cough, dyspnea, and symptoms due to compression or invasion of structures in the mediastinum may be present (e.g., dysphagia, hoarseness due to recurrent laryngeal nerve involvement, superior vena caval obstruction). Symptoms are more common with malignant tumors.

Investigation of a mediastinal mass begins with posteroanterior and lateral chest roentgenograms to which are added oblique views, a contrast study of the esophagus, and tomogra-

phy, if needed, to more clearly define the anatomic location and borders of the mass. The anatomic site of the lesion is of diagnostic importance, and may determine the next step in the diagnostic workup (Fig. 269-2). Computerized tomography of the chest with injection of contrast material into a peripheral vein, or angiography of the pulmonary circulation or aorta may be needed to distinguish vascular from nonvascular lesions, a differentiation of particular importance if biopsy of the mass is considered. Mediastinoscopy and biopsy are useful in the diagnosis of mediastinal masses if metastatic carcinoma, lymphoma, or sarcoidosis are considered likely. Lymph nodes behind the trachea and below the aortic arch on the left side are not accessible for biopsy using this approach. Scalene lymph node biopsy in the absence of palpable nodes may provide the diagnosis if lymphoma or metastatic carcinoma is suspected. Bronchoscopy is unlikely to be helpful in the diagnostic workup unless there are symptoms suggestive of an endobronchial lesion (e.g., hemoptysis) or unless there is evidence of lobar collapse, consolidation, or a mass lesion in the lung parenchyma on chest roentgenograph. Special tests such as radionuclide scanning with ^{131}I to detect an active retrosternal goiter may also be helpful.

Neurogenic tumors are the most common primary mediastinal neoplasms and are found almost exclusively in the posterior mediastinum near the paravertebral gutter. The majority of these neoplasms are benign; neurofibromas, schwannomas, and ganglioneuromas are the commonest tumors seen. Vague chest pain and cough may be present but "root" pain is an infrequent complaint. *Neurofibromas* may occur singly or in association with von Recklinghausen's disease (Chap. 374). *Ganglioneuromas* arise from the sympathetic chain and, together with *neuroblastomas*, may secrete hormones which lead to diarrhea, flushing, and hypertension. Vanillylmandelic acid (VMA) may be found in the urine. Mediastinal *neuroblastoma* usually occurs in children, is particularly responsive to irradiation, and has a better prognosis than neuroblastomas of the abdomen or retroperitoneal space. *Pheochromocytoma* is a rare mediastinal tumor which may secrete catecholamines and present the same clinical picture as the more common (but still rare) abdominal form (Chap. 337). The treatment of all neurogenic tumors of the mediastinum is surgical, with postoperative irradiation for patients with neuroblastomas.

Teratodermoids most commonly arise in the anterior mediastinum. Dermoid tumors consist only of ectodermal structures and may be cystic or solid. However, the majority of these tumors also contain elements derived from endoderm (bron-

FIGURE 269-2
Common sites for mediastinal masses.

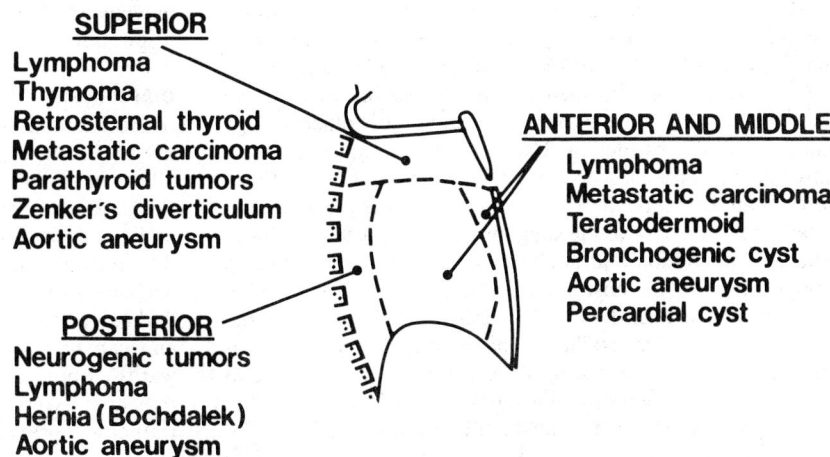

SUPERIOR
Lymphoma
Thymoma
Retrosternal thyroid
Metastatic carcinoma
Parathyroid tumors
Zenker's diverticulum
Aortic aneurysm

ANTERIOR AND MIDDLE
Lymphoma
Metastatic carcinoma
Teratodermoid
Bronchogenic cyst
Aortic aneurysm
Percardial cyst

POSTERIOR
Neurogenic tumors
Lymphoma
Hernia (Bochdalek)
Aortic aneurysm

chial or intestinal epithelium) and mesoderm (smooth muscle, bone) and are more correctly termed teratodermoid tumors. Most tumors are detected in early adult life and approximately 10 to 20 percent undergo malignant changes. Teratodermoids frequently contain linear calcification of the lining of a cyst, and bone and teeth may be evident on chest roentgenogram. Teratodermoids are treated by surgical excision.

Thymomas account for 10 percent of primary mediastinal neoplasms and are found in the superior and anterior mediastinum. Approximately one-fourth are malignant, but they rarely metastasize. Myasthenia gravis (Chap. 381) occurs in about 50 percent of patients with thymoma; however, the majority of patients with myasthenia gravis do not have a thymic tumor. Agammaglobulinemia, pure red blood cell aplasia, and Cushing's syndrome have been reported to be associated with thymoma. Because of compression of the trachea by the tumor, patients may complain of dyspnea in the supine posture. Symptoms may also arise from local invasion or compression of other surrounding structures. Treatment is by surgical excision; malignant thymomas are usually radiation-sensitive.

Benign cysts most commonly arise in the anterior and middle mediastinum. Most do not produce symptoms and are detected only on routine chest roentgenography. *Bronchogenic cysts* most commonly develop in the paratracheal area or near the carina. The cysts are lined with ciliated respiratory epithelium and contain smooth muscle and cartilage in their walls. They are liquid-filled and therefore have a uniform density on chest roentgenogram, where they appear as rounded or tear-shaped opacities. Usually the cyst has no demonstrable communication with the tracheobronchial tree; however, they may become infected. *Enteric cysts* occur along the esophagus and are lined by gastric or intestinal epithelium. As with bronchogenic cysts, infection and abscess formation may occur. If the cyst contains acid-secreting cells, ulcer formation, perforation, and hemorrhage may occur. The *pericardial cyst* is a developmental anomaly and is attached to the pericardium but only rarely communicates with the pericardial cavity.

SUPERIOR VENA CAVAL SYNDROME Obstruction of the superior vena cava (SVC) secondary to compression or infiltration by superior mediastinal tumors results in a characteristic constellation of physical findings with dilatation of collateral veins of the upper thorax and neck, plethora and edema of the face and neck, conjunctival edema, and headache. Visual disturbances and alterations in the state of consciousness may occur. Compression of the adjacent esophagus and trachea may cause dysphagia, wheeze, and shortness of breath.

Obstruction of the SVC is almost invariably due to malignant disease, approximately 75 percent of the cases being due to *bronchogenic carcinoma. Lymphoma* accounts for almost all the remaining cases. Right-sided tumors much more frequently produce the syndrome as would be expected on an anatomic basis. Rarely, this syndrome occurs with *fibrosing mediastinitis* that is either idiopathic or secondary to histoplasmosis or occurs in association with methylsergide ingestion. *Retrosternal thyroid* and *aortic aneurysms* are among the other benign causes of SVC obstruction. Using invasive diagnostic procedures such as bronchoscopy, esophagoscopy, and mediastinoscopy in an attempt to obtain a tissue diagnosis is contraindicated due to the risk of bleeding during the procedure. Unless clinical examination and noninvasive investigations suggest a benign cause for the obstruction, or unless there is tissue elsewhere to biopsy (e.g., lymphadenopathy, skin lesions), the patient should receive irradiation or chemotherapy before attempts are made to obtain a tissue diagnosis. Corticosteroids are sometimes given during the initial stages of management in an effort to decrease edema at the site of obstruction.

PNEUMOMEDIASTINUM (MEDIASTINAL EMPHYSEMA) Air within the planes of the mediastinum may appear spontaneously or may be secondary to chest trauma, perforation of the trachea, bronchus, or esophagus, spread of air from the fascial planes of the neck or pharynx, or from dissection of air from the retroperitoneal space. When pneumomediastinum occurs with no apparent cause it is referred to as a *spontaneous pneumomediastinum.* In contrast to spontaneous pneumothorax, there is no tendency for recurrence. Air is thought to dissect from alveoli to the interstitial space and into the vascular adventitia to the hilum. From there it moves into the mediastinum, neck, or retroperitoneal space. Predisposing factors include raised intrathoracic pressure, as with coughing, vomiting, and Valsalva maneuvers. Rapid decompression such as occurs with sudden ascent during diving has also been implicated. Pneumomediastinum may also occur spontaneously during an attack of asthma. The patient with pneumomediastinum may be asymptomatic but usually complains of retrosternal pain and dyspnea; less commonly there is sore throat due to dissection of air into the retropharyngeal space. Examination may reveal subcutaneous crepitus in the upper body, and a crunching sound synchronous with the heart beat may be heard over the precordium (Hamman's sign). Fever and mild leukocytosis are common with uncomplicated pneumomediastinum. Occasionally, cardiac function is compromised with physical signs of cardiac tamponade (Chap. 249). A lateral chest roentgenogram should always be obtained if pneumomediastinum is suspected since abnormalities may be seen only on this view. Air is seen outlining the pulmonary artery trunk and root of aorta and may be seen tracking into the neck.

Pneumomediastinum secondary to *esophageal perforation* may follow endoscopy or may occur with vomiting (Boerhaave's syndrome). Esophageal perforation is a surgical emergency and should be suspected if there is increasing pain aggravated by swallowing or fever and when signs of increasing mediastinal width and left pleural effusion occur on chest roentgenogram. Acute and fulminant mediastinitis is a frequent sequela and should be treated with immediate surgical drainage, closure of the perforation site, and broad-spectrum antibiotic therapy.

THE DIAPHRAGM

The diaphragm is the major muscle of inspiration and is derived embryonically from the septum transversum and the pleuroperitoneal membranes. Its motor nerve supply is from the phrenic nerves (C3 to C5); the afferent supply is derived both from the phrenic and lower intercostal nerves. When the diaphragm contracts, intrathoracic pressure is lowered and intraabdominal pressure is increased. Thus, the diaphragm acts as if it were "pulling" on the lung (by lowering intrathoracic pressure) and "pushing" on the rib cage (by raising abdominal pressure), resulting in an increase in lung volume and outward movement of both rib cage and abdomen as it descends on inspiration.

DIAPHRAGMATIC PARALYSIS *Unilateral diaphragmatic paralysis* is usually the result of injury to a phrenic nerve secondary to trauma or tumor in the mediastinum. The lesion is usually asymptomatic but the patient may complain of dyspnea in the supine posture when the diaphragm, weakened by unilateral paralysis, must work against the added load of the abdominal contents. Unilateral paralysis results in only a small decrease in vital capacity. The diagnosis is suggested by the finding of an elevated hemidiaphragm on chest roentgenogram and can be confirmed by fluoroscopy. Paradoxical (i.e., upward) motion of the affected hemidiaphragm occurs when the patient is asked to sniff, a maneuver that suddenly lowers intrathoracic pressure.

Bilateral diaphragmatic paralysis is less common than unilateral paralysis, but it has far greater consequences on respiration. Bilateral paralysis may be due to high cervical cord injury, motor neuron disease, poliomyelitis, polyneuropathies, or bilateral involvement of the phrenic nerve by mediastinal lesions. The patient usually has severe shortness of breath, particularly in the supine position, and often hypercapnic respiratory failure is present. In most patients with bilateral diaphragmatic paralysis, there is paradoxical (i.e., inward) motion of the abdomen on inspiration, a finding easily observed at the bedside, particularly with the patient supine. This is due to passive ascent of the diaphragm as intrathoracic pressure is lowered by the intercostal and accessory muscles. In a few patients paradoxical abdominal motion may not be obvious with the patient erect due to use of the abdominal muscles during expiration. Here, abdominal motion will appear normal as contraction of the abdominal muscles causes inward abdominal motion on expiration and relaxation results in outward abdominal motion on inspiration. Under these circumstances the diaphragm may appear to move normally at fluoroscopy, and the diagnosis of diaphragmatic paralysis will be missed.

The vital capacity which is reduced in the upright posture is even more severely reduced when the patient is supine because the paralyzed diaphragm is sucked upward during a maximal inspiration with displacement of abdominal contents into the thorax. The diagnosis of bilateral diaphragmatic paralysis is established by assessment of transdiaphragmatic pressure obtained by comparison of simultaneous measurements of esophageal and gastric pressures. Treatment of this disorder may be conservative, using a rocking bed at night; in patients with intact phrenic nerves, electrical pacing of those nerves has been successful.

ELEVATION OF THE HEMIDIAPHRAGM ON CHEST ROENTGENOGRAPH The physician is often confronted with a chest roentgenogram that shows elevation of one hemidiaphragm. Normally, the right side of the diaphragm is approximately 4 cm higher than the left due to displacement by the liver. *Apparent elevation* of one hemidiaphragm is due to a subpulmonic pleural effusion, and a lateral decubitus chest roentgenogram will establish this diagnosis. *True elevation* of one hemidiaphragm is most commonly due to upward displacement secondary to intraabdominal masses or ascites, or it may be due to loss of lung volume on the affected side secondary to pulmonary collapse or fibrosis. *Eventration of the diaphragm* is a rare congenital disorder more common on the left side. The anterior two-thirds of the diaphragm is replaced by a thin membrane, resulting in upward movement of abdominal contents into the thoracic cage. Patients are usually asymptomatic, and the diagnosis is made following a routine chest roentgenogram. No treatment is necessary. Rarely, eventration of the diaphragm may seriously compromise ventilatory function in the newborn. Plication of the hemidiaphragm is then performed. Eventration must be distinguished from *diaphragmatic hernias* through which abdominal contents are displaced into the chest. The most common location is at the esophageal hiatus with displacement of part of the stomach into the posterior mediastinum (Chap. 289).

MISCELLANEOUS DISEASES OF THE DIAPHRAGM Neoplasms of the diaphragm are rare; they include lipomas, fibromas, neurofibromas, and cysts. These benign tumors are approximately 1 to 1½ times more frequent than the malignant fibrosarcoma. The diaphragm may be involved by direct extension of primary lung or abdominal tumors and may be the site of metastases from distant tumors.

REFERENCES

BENJAMIN SP et al: Primary tumors of the mediastinum. Chest 62:297, 1972

BLACK LF: The pleural space and pleural fluid. Mayo Clin Proc 47:493, 1972

GAENSLER EA, KAPLAN AI: Asbestos pleural effusions. Ann Intern Med 74:178, 1971

LIGHT RW et al: Pleural effusions: The diagnostic separation of transudates and exudates. Ann Intern Med 77:507, 1972

MUNSELL WP: Pneumomediastinum. JAMA 202:689, 1967

NEWSOM DAVIS J et al: Diaphragm function and alveolar hypoventilation. Q J Med 177:87, 1976

POKORNY WI, SHERMAN JO: Mediastinal masses in infants and children. J Thorac Cardiovasc Surg 86:869, 1974

ROGERS PM et al: Catamenial pneumothorax. Am J Obstet Gynecol 118:572, 1974

SABISTON DC JR, OLDHAM HN JR: The mediastinum, in *Gibbon's Surgery of the Chest*, 3d ed, DC Sabiston Jr, FC Spencer (eds). Philadelphia, Saunders, 1976, p 406

270
DISORDERS OF REGULATION OF RESPIRATION

JOHN B. WEST

The principles governing pulmonary ventilation and its regulation are discussed in Chap. 255. The fine control of ventilation is normally carried out by the central chemoreceptors near the ventral surface of the medulla which respond to changes in pH of the cerebrospinal fluid near them. For example, a fall in pH caused by diffusion of carbon dioxide across the blood-brain barrier increases respiratory drive, thus holding the arterial P_{CO_2}[1] within close limits (Fig. 270-1). The extreme sensitivity of this feedback control is seen when a normal subject inhales air containing carbon dioxide. Typically the ventilation may double for a rise in P_{CO_2} of only 2 to 3 mmHg.

Arterial hypoxemia constitutes a coarse control through its action on the peripheral chemoreceptors in the carotid bodies. Although this control is minor under normal conditions, it becomes very important during chronic hypoxia, as in people living at high altitude, or in patients with chronic lung disease. Under these conditions the increased ventilation lowers the P_{CO_2} of the arterial blood and cerebrospinal fluid, but the pH of the cerebrospinal fluid is reset to its normal level of about 7.32 by outward movement of bicarbonate.

Additional control is afforded by changes in pH of the arterial blood irrespective of its P_{CO_2}. This relatively weak regulation apparently occurs through stimulation of the peripheral chemoreceptors, and although it is seldom seen under normal conditions, it may dominate in the control of ventilation in metabolic acidosis.

Disorders of the regulation of respiration include hypoventilation, hyperventilation, and abnormal patterns of breathing. A cardinal feature of hypoventilation is carbon dioxide retention (Table 270-1), and indeed these terms are often used virtually interchangeably. This can be misleading, but following common usage, the various types of carbon dioxide retention are grouped here under the heading of hypoventilation.

---

[1] *Unless otherwise stated, the partial pressures refer to arterial blood.*

FIGURE 270-1

Scheme to illustrate the various causes of carbon dioxide retention. These include (1) disorders of the respiratory center or (2) of the supplying nerves or (3) of muscles of ventilation or (4) some mechanical problem in lung or chest wall, including obstruction to the upper airways. All these conditions result in hypoventilation. However, chronic obstruction pulmonary disease (5) in effect diverts blood from the ventilated regions, so that carbon dioxide retention occurs in spite of a normal (or high) ventilation. In addition, the ventilatory response is inappropriate for the level of carbon dioxide in these patients because of the increased work of breathing and sometimes also because of a reduced sensitivity of the respiratory center.

HYPOVENTILATION

CARBON DIOXIDE RETENTION CAUSED BY PURE HYPOVENTILATION (NORMAL LUNGS) In this group of diseases, the amount of air going into the lungs each minute is reduced. Strictly it is the volume of air entering the alveoli, or *alveolar ventilation,* which is crucial (Chap. 255). However, in practice,

TABLE 270-1
Causes of carbon dioxide retention

I Pure hypoventilation (normal lungs)
  A Respiratory center depression—morphine derivatives, barbiturates, some general anesthetics
  B Diseases of the brainstem—encephalitis, hemorrhage, trauma, neoplasm (rare)
  C Abnormalities of spinal cord conducting pathways—high cervical dislocation
  D Anterior horn cell disease—poliomyelitis
  E Diseases of nerves to respiratory muscles—Guillain-Barré syndrome, diphtheria
  F Diseases of the myoneural junction—myasthenia gravis, anticholinesterase poisoning
  G Diseases of the respiratory muscles—progressive muscular dystrophy
  H Thoracic cage abnormalities—crushed chest, kyphoscoliosis (lungs may be abnormal)
  I Upper airway obstruction—thymoma, aortic aneurysm
  J Hypoventilation associated with extreme obesity (Pickwickian syndrome)
  K Idiopathic hypoventilation
  L Other causes—metabolic alkalosis
II CO₂ retention associated with chronic lung disease

the volume of the conducting airways remains fairly constant so that, if the amount of air passing the lips is abnormally low, hypoventilation is said to be present.

The alveolar ventilation and alveolar P_{CO_2} are related by the following equation:

$$\text{Alveolar } P_{CO_2} = \frac{CO_2 \text{ output}}{\text{alveolar ventilation}}$$

In normal lungs, the P_{CO_2} of arterial blood is virtually the same as that in alveolar gas, and the carbon dioxide output at rest remains fairly constant. Thus the expression implies that if the alveolar ventilation is halved, the arterial P_{CO_2} is doubled.

The level of alveolar ventilation also influences the P_{CO_2}. As the ventilation falls and the P_{CO_2} rises, the P_{O_2} falls. An important practical point is that, if the P_{CO_2} is considerably increased by pure hypoventilation, say to 70 mmHg, the P_{O_2} may still be well above the level at which cyanosis can be detected clinically. Thus a patient may have serious carbon dioxide retention and yet appear a "healthy" pink color. Note also that if a patient is given an oxygen-enriched mixture to breathe, the hypoxemia will be abolished, but the hypercapnia remains (Chap. 272).

Conditions affecting the respiratory center During normal *sleep,* the P_{CO_2} rises by 3 or 4 mmHg. Patients with idiopathic hypoventilation or with the "Pickwickian syndrome" (see below) are particularly likely to develop depressed breathing when they are asleep. One of the commonest causes of hypoventilation is depression of the respiratory center by *drugs.* These include many anesthetics, the barbiturates, and morphine and its derivatives. Respiratory center depression is often seen in the recovery room, before the effects of anesthetic and preoperative sedatives have worn off, and also in the emergency room in patients who have taken an overdose of barbiturate (Chap. 228). In these circumstances, the arterial P_{CO_2} should be measured, and assisted ventilation following endotracheal intubation or tracheostomy may be lifesaving. Depression of the respiratory center is often accompanied by impairment of the cough reflex and difficulties with swallowing, so that aspiration of fluid into the lungs may occur and lead to pneumonia. An additional advantage of intubation is that it allows the airways to be sucked free of secretions and inhaled material (Chap. 272).

Brainstem abnormalities Conditions which may cause hypoventilation include inflammation, hemorrhage, trauma, and rarely neoplasms. Encephalitis and acute bulbar poliomyelitis (in the absence of involvement of the respiratory muscles) may cause slowing and shallowness of respiration. Irregularities of rhythm and periods of apnea may develop. The first signs of these abnormalities often appear during sleep. The ventilatory response to inhaled CO₂ mixtures is depressed. These patients can return their blood gases to normal by voluntarily increasing their ventilation, and indeed they can sometimes be managed by being reminded to breathe when periods of apnea develop. However, they may die because of apnea during sleep. Respiratory depression may be associated with loss of the cough and swallowing reflexes and consequent accumulation of secretions.

Neuromuscular disorders Neuromuscular disorders affecting the spinal conducting pathways, the anterior horn cells, the nerves to the respiratory muscles, and the respiratory muscles themselves are important causes of hypoventilation (Table 270-1). Examples include compression of the cervical cord, poliomyelitis, the Guillain-Barré syndrome, and myasthenia gravis. The most important muscle of respiration is the diaphragm, and patients with progressive disease often do not complain of dyspnea until the diaphragm is involved. By then their ventilatory reserve is severely compromised, and they must be carefully observed. The converse also occurs. Patients with neurologic disease such as amyotrophic lateral sclerosis may complain of dyspnea as their initial symptom at a time when their neurologic findings may be extremely subtle. The progress of the disease can be monitored by measuring the vital capacity and the arterial blood gases. Again, the treatment of hypoventilation in these conditions is assisted ventilation either by oropharyngeal intubation in acute states, or with a tracheostomy for long-term management (Chap. 272). Patients with chronic paresis of their respiratory muscles are likely to develop chest infections because of their difficulty in getting rid of secretions.

Thoracic cage abnormalities CRUSHED CHEST An increasingly common cause of hypoventilation is trauma to the thoracic cage resulting from automobile accidents. Frequently this is caused by impact of the steering wheel with the sternum, or the chest is crushed when a wheel of a car runs over it. Usually there are multiple injuries. There may be dissociation of movement of the chest wall, so that one region is sucked in while the remainder of the chest wall moves out during inspiration ("flail chest"). Prompt intubation and assisted ventilation is often required, and careful monitoring of the arterial blood gases is mandatory.

SCOLIOSIS Bony deformity of the chest can lead to respiratory failure with a raised arterial P_{CO_2}. Scoliosis refers to lateral curvature of the spine, and kyphosis to posterior curvature. The effects of scoliosis on cardiopulmonary function are the more serious, especially if the angulation is situated high in the vertebral column. Scoliosis is frequently associated with rotation of the spine and backward protuberance of the ribs, giving the appearance of an added kyphosis. In fact, the term kyphoscoliosis is often used for this condition, although true kyphoscoliosis is rare. Some 80 percent of cases of scoliosis are idiopathic in origin. The rest are caused by neuromuscular disorders such as poliomyelitis or are congenital in origin.

The initial complaint is dyspnea on exertion. Later hypoxemia develops; eventually carbon dioxide retention and signs of failure of the right side of the heart may supervene. Sometimes bronchitis may complicate the picture, especially in smokers. The chief cause of the CO_2 retention is the deformity of the respiratory muscles and a great increase in the work of breathing. The compliance of the chest wall is reduced (it is stiffer), especially in older patients, and this results in rapid shallow breathing, so that an increasingly large fraction of the tidal volume is wasted in the dead space of the bronchi. The hypoventilation causes not only hypercapnia but also hypoxemia. Pulmonary vasoconstriction results, pulmonary artery pressure rises, and the work of the right side of the heart is also raised by the polycythemia which develops (Chap. 246).

It should be noted, however, that these patients also have abnormal lungs. These tend to be remarkably small, and the restricted pulmonary vascular bed probably also plays a role in the development of pulmonary hypertension. Areas of atelectasis are common, presumably because the volume of the thoracic cage is greatly reduced. Uneven ventilation of the lungs has been demonstrated in many cases, so that ventilation-perfusion inequality contributes to the hypoxemia.

Pulmonary function tests show a reduction in all lung volumes; indeed the total lung capacity may be reduced to half the predicted normal value. Some of the inequality of ventilation can be explained by airway closure in dependent regions of the lung as a result of the gross reduction of lung volume. Airway resistance in relation to lung volume is approximately

normal, but the maximum breathing capacity is reduced because of the restricted vital capacity. The diffusing capacity of the lung for carbon monoxide is not markedly abnormal when related to lung volume. In advanced disease, a reduced ventilatory response to inhaled carbon dioxide can be demonstrated. This is probably related to the large increase in work of breathing caused by the deformity of the chest wall. Not only is the chest wall stiff, but the respiratory muscles operate inefficiently.

Little specific therapy is available. Just as the cause of most cases of the disease is unknown, so are the factors determining its progression poorly understood. Some help can be obtained from orthopedic braces such as the Milwaukee brace, in the early stages of the disease. Corrective surgery such as the Harrington procedure during adolescence improves the appearance and may relieve back pain. However, the long-term effects on cardiopulmonary function are unknown. Any pulmonary infection should be promptly and vigorously treated with appropriate antibiotics. If hypoxia is severe and O_2 therapy is required (Chap. 272), the patient should be carefully watched for evidence of increasing hypoventilation. Cor pulmonale and right-sided heart failure should be treated with diuretics, digitalis, and perhaps phlebotomy if the polycythemia is severe.

OTHER CONDITIONS Also associated with an abnormal chest wall are ankylosing spondylitis and pectus excavatum. In *ankylosing spondylitis* there is immobility of the vertebral joints and fixation of the ribs, so that movement of the chest wall may be grossly reduced. There is a reduction of vital capacity and total lung capacity, but good movement of the diaphragm is preserved so that the ventilatory capacity is unimpaired. Some fall in the compliance of the chest wall has been reported and also some uneven ventilation, the latter possibly caused by the reduced lung volume. In general, however, the lungs are virtually normal and do not show the pathologic changes seen in kyphoscoliosis. Hypoventilation is not a feature, and secondary heart failure does not occur.

Pectus excavatum is a congenital abnormality in which the lower part of the sternum is depressed toward the spine. In spite of the bizarre appearance of the chest, little interference with pulmonary function is the rule. There may be a slight reduction in vital capacity, total lung capacity, and maximum breathing capacity, but gas exchange is virtually normal, and hypoventilation does not occur. Surgical correction for cosmetic reasons may be considered.

Obstruction to the upper airways Tracheal stenosis can be caused by neoplasms such as thymoma in structures adjacent to the trachea, by scarring following injury, by aortic aneurysm, or by a congenital abnormality. Tumors originating in the upper airways and foreign bodies may also be responsible for airways obstruction. Hypoventilation with CO_2 retention may occur, and this may be of long standing. It is possible to distinguish tracheal obstruction from the airway obstruction of chronic obstructive lung disease by the stridor and by the flow patterns of maximal inspiration and expiration. In addition, pulmonary function tests show no inequality of ventilation. Intermittent upper airway obstruction may occur in obese people during sleep (see "Sleep Apnea" below).

Hypoventilation associated with extreme obesity ("Pickwickian syndrome") Some extremely obese patients hypoventilate, and the association of obesity, somnolence, polycythemia, and excessive appetite has been dubbed the *Pickwickian syndrome*, after the fat boy, Joe, in Charles Dickens' *Pickwick Papers.* Apart from the obesity, the clinical features are similar to those in patients with idiopathic hypoventilation (see below); in the fully developed form they include marked obesity (body weight typically over 300 lb), somnolence, twitching, cyanosis, periodic respiration, secondary polycythemia, right ventricular hypertrophy, and right-sided heart failure.

The obesity may have been present for years, but in some cases a recent rapid gain in weight has been described. The somnolence may be a striking feature, the patient sometimes dozing off halfway through a sentence. The cyanosis and periodic breathing are particularly marked during sleep. Sleep apnea may occur (see below) and in some patients this is caused by upper airway obstruction as a result of collapse of the pharyngeal walls. Ankle edema is a common symptom, and an enlarged liver and engorged neck veins are seen.

Blood gas measurements show an elevated P_{CO_2} and depressed P_{O_2}; the former may be as high as 70 mmHg. Lung function tests show a reduction in lung volumes, particularly in the expiratory reserve volume (the volume which can be forcibly exhaled from normal end-expiration). The vital capacity is also reduced, as is the compliance of the chest cage. The abdominal pressure is raised, especially when the patient is supine, thus forcing the diaphragm into the chest. There are no indications of airway obstruction and little inequality of ventilation, but the energy cost of moving the chest wall is abnormally high. The ventilatory response to inhaled CO_2 is therefore generally greatly decreased. In these respects the syndrome is similar to kyphoscoliosis. However, in addition, some patients have a diminished sensitivity of the respiratory center to CO_2. The reduction of lung volume causes airway closure in the dependent regions of the lung, and this contributes to the hypoxemia. There is an increase in the resting oxygen consumption of these patients which aggravates the effects of their impaired ventilation.

A striking feature of this syndrome is the dramatic improvement that takes place in all symptoms when the patient loses weight. Objective indices of improvement include a fall in arterial P_{CO_2}, rise in P_{O_2}, increases in vital capacity, total lung capacity, and total ventilation, and an enhanced ventilatory response to inhaled CO_2. In addition, signs of heart failure often disappear. Even a loss of 30 to 40 lb is often sufficient to bring about a remarkable improvement in well-being. Treatment by caloric restriction is indicated. In addition, recent work shows that some patients respond well to progesterone. If upper airway obstruction causes sleep apnea, tracheostomy is often very beneficial.

It is important to note that not all extremely obese patients develop hypoventilation. Some investigators have suggested that the Pickwickian individual is simply a patient with idiopathic hypoventilation who happens to be obese. The term "Pickwickian syndrome" is often used rather loosely. It should be reserved for very obese patients who have an increased P_{CO_2} without evidence of lung disease. The cause of the hypoventilation is not clear but presumably is related to the high energy cost of moving the chest wall. In addition the reduction in lung volumes caused by elevation of the diaphragm causes shallow inefficient breathing. However the association of marked somnolence and voracious appetite suggests that, in some patients at least, there is an abnormality in the central nervous system.

Idiopathic hypoventilation Idiopathic, or primary, hypoventilation is a rare disease of unknown cause occurring in patients whose lungs and chest wall are normal. A colorful name sometimes given to this condition is Ondine's curse after the fairy whose human lover lost the ability to breathe automatically and had to will himself to do so. Most of the reported patients have been between 20 and 60 years of age, and there has been a preponderance of males. Typical symptoms include lack of energy, somnolence, headache, and some breathlessness on exertion. Cyanosis, especially when the patient is asleep, is a common observation, this being caused by a combination of the hypoxemia and polycythemia. Periodic breathing is often noted at night. Occasionally unusual sensitivity to sedatives or hypnotic drugs given preoperatively has been a feature. In some cases, an acute respiratory infection has prompted awareness of the condition. Several patients have had a past history of encephalitis, neurosyphilis, or schizophrenia. Signs of heart failure including engorged neck veins, enlarged heart, palpable liver, and peripheral edema have been described in severe cases.

The P_{CO_2} is elevated, generally in the range of 55 to 80 mmHg, and the P_{O_2} is depressed; these can rapidly be restored to near normal by asking the patient to increase ventilation voluntarily. Indeed some observers have found considerable variability in the P_{CO_2}, because, when the patients are tested and become aware of their breathing, they tend to breathe more. For this reason the finding of a raised plasma bicarbonate may be a useful diagnostic pointer. The hematocrit is typically between 50 and 70 percent. The ventilatory response to inhaled CO_2 is greatly impaired, though the work of breathing is not increased. Tests of pulmonary function are generally normal with no indication of airway obstruction. The pulmonary arterial pressure is typically increased because of the alveolar hypoxia.

No specific pathologic changes have been found in the central nervous system of these patients. Congestive heart failure and respiratory infections should be treated vigorously.

Metabolic alkalosis A few patients with metabolic alkalosis hypoventilate, although this causes no symptoms and is difficult to detect clinically. The commonest causes include severe vomiting, and potassium and chloride loss such as that caused by diuretics or steroid therapy. The arterial pH is always raised, indicating only partial respiratory compensation, and many patients do not hypoventilate at all.

Sleep apnea Recently a number of patients have been described in whom breathing periodically stops during sleep as a result of upper airway obstruction. Initially this was noted in extremely obese patients (see above), but it is now recognized that the condition is not confined to these. Airway obstruction can be caused by backward movement of the tongue, collapse of the pharyngeal walls, or greatly enlarged tonsils or adenoids. Loud snoring is a feature, and the patient may wake violently after an apneic episode. There is often chronic sleep deprivation, and the patient may exhibit daytime somnolence, chronic fatigue, morning headaches, and often personality disturbances such as paranoia, hostility, and agitated depression. Long-term tracheostomy has been used successfully, and weight loss is valuable if the patient is obese.

CARBON DIOXIDE RETENTION ASSOCIATED WITH CHRONIC LUNG DISEASE The commonest clinical situation in which CO_2 retention is seen is chronic lung disease. Patients with this condition are often said to be "hypoventilating," but the cause of their hypercapnia is clearly very different from that in patients with normal lungs whom we have considered so far. Historically it is easy to see how the term hypoventilation came to be applied so indiscriminately. When in the late 1950s it became possible to measure the P_{CO_2} of arterial blood in the clinical setting, CO_2 retention was found to be a common and serious complication of chronic lung disease which could always be abolished by artificially increasing the ventilation. Thus it was natural to say that these patients had a reduced ventilation, and this term had the advantage of keeping an important therapeutic option in the forefront.

It is important to understand the factors leading to CO_2 retention in these patients if their disease is to be managed most effectively. Figure 270-1 shows a scheme of the factors determining CO_2 elimination in patients with lung disease. CO_2 is produced in the tissues at a rate which depends on the level of metabolic activity; at rest there is little variation. It is transported to the lungs in the venous blood and pumped out by the ventilation. The speed of the pump is normally set by the level of the P_{CO_2} via the medullary chemoreceptors. In the presence of lung disease, the efficiency of the pump is impaired. Thus, for the same level of ventilation, less CO_2 is eliminated. This is principally because ventilation and blood flow are unevenly matched within the lung (see Chap. 255). In any event the result is that for a normal level of ventilation, inadequate amounts of CO_2 are excreted, and CO_2 retention occurs.

When the increased arterial P_{CO_2} causes a fall in the cerebrospinal fluid pH which is sensed by the medullary chemoreceptors, the ventilation is increased. This usually returns the P_{CO_2} to normal, because fortunately even lungs with grossly mismatched ventilation and blood flow can greatly increase their elimination of CO_2 when their ventilation is raised. (Contrast this with the behavior of O_2, where uneven ventilation and blood flow invariably result in low P_{O_2}; this follows from the shape of the O_2 dissociation curve as discussed in Chap. 255.) Thus a common end result is a normal P_{CO_2}, but at the expense of increased ventilation. However, in the presence of severe disease, the ventilation may not be increased enough to restore the P_{CO_2} to normal, and CO_2 retention therefore occurs.

The ventilatory response to CO_2 in these patients can be reduced for two reasons. One is an increased work of breathing. It has been shown that if normal subjects breathe through a resistance, their ventilatory response to inhaled CO_2 is depressed. Indeed, the relationship between increase in ventilation and inspired CO_2 concentration may become indistinguishable from that observed in patients with chronic airway obstruction. In most cases of chronic obstructive lung disease, the resistance to airflow is high so that the increase in ventilation for a given rise in arterial P_{CO_2} is depressed. Such patients may have a normal neural output of the respiratory center in response to an increased P_{CO_2} but nevertheless the ventilatory response is impaired.

However, some patients also have a reduced neural output of the respiratory center in response to an increased arterial P_{CO_2}. This can be established by specialized tests such as measurement of the mechanical work performed during inspiration or the inspiratory pressure developed during a brief period of airway occlusion. The reason for the diminished sensitivity of the respiratory center in these patients is not understood though in some cases it may be congenital. There is evidence that the sensitivity of the respiratory center to CO_2 (and hypoxia) varies considerably among normal subjects. It may be that those patients who have good respiratory center sensitivity are more distressed by dyspnea, while those who respond weakly may succumb to CO_2 retention and respiratory failure.

When CO_2 retention becomes established, the respiratory center becomes reset at a higher arterial P_{CO_2}. This can be explained by an increase in bicarbonate concentration in the cerebrospinal fluid because of transport of bicarbonate across the blood-gas barrier. As a result the pH of the cerebrospinal fluid is returned to near its normal value of 7.32 in spite of its increased P_{CO_2}. Since this pH apparently chiefly determines the response of the medullary chemoreceptors, respiratory drive may then not be much increased despite the raised P_{CO_2}.

Further CO_2 retention occurs in some patients with chronic lung disease, especially following the administration of oxygen.

These patients have chronic hypercapnia and hypoxemia but a near normal pH in their arterial blood (compensated respiratory acidosis) and in their cerebrospinal fluid. Their main stimulus to ventilation may be the arterial hypoxemia via the peripheral chemoreceptors, so that, when this is relieved, ventilation almost ceases. The ensuing rise in P_{CO_2} may further depress ventilation because of the narcotic effect of high levels of carbon dioxide. This extremely dangerous situation should be avoided by giving carefully controlled O_2 concentrations, for example, 24 to 28 percent, assiduously watching the patient, and measuring the arterial P_{CO_2} from time to time. CO_2 retention in chronic obstructive lung disease is considered in Chap. 263, and the treatment of acute and chronic respiratory failure in Chap. 272.

HYPERVENTILATION

Hyperventilation is most commonly caused by lesions of the central nervous system, metabolic acidosis, and anxiety states. In addition, hyperventilation may be seen in salicylate poisoning, acute or chronic hypoxia (as at high altitude), severe hypoglycemia, and hepatic coma. A patient with severe cerebral hemorrhage causing coma may exhibit deep, regular respirations of a mechanical nature. This causes a reduced P_{CO_2} in the arterial blood, which initially shows a high pH and a normal base excess. Irregularities of breathing such as Cheyne-Stokes respiration may also occur. In metabolic acidosis caused, for example, by uncontrolled diabetes mellitus or by chronic renal insufficiency, deep regular respiration known as *Kussmaul breathing* is frequently seen. Active rather than passive expiratory movements are a feature of this pattern. Here the low P_{CO_2} is accompanied by reduction in base excess and a low pH (see Chap. 85).

In the hyperventilation of anxiety states, the patient may be very apprehensive and complain of shortness of breath, difficulty in taking a deep breath, a feeling of chest tightness, or a sense of suffocation. The patient is often a nervous, anxious woman who has other functional disturbances due to tension. There are often accompanying symptoms such as numbness in the limbs, palpitations, and epigastric discomfort. The fall in P_{CO_2} and the consequent alkalosis may be severe and cause tetany with carpopedal spasm. The reduced plasma bicarbonate level and relatively normal arterial pH (compensated respiratory alkalosis) distinguish chronic hyperventilation from the acute hyperventilation with fall in P_{CO_2} which frequently accompanies an arterial puncture. The patient may complain of fainting spells and blurring of vision; these are probably related to the reduction in cerebral blood flow caused by low P_{CO_2}. The finding of slow waves of high voltage in the EEG suggests that these changes may be the result of hypoxia. The changes can be reversed by hyperbaric oxygenation. The serum calcium level remains normal. It is likely that some of the cardiovascular symptoms are related to the release of epinephrine.

These patients are usually not aware of the overbreathing, although they may admit to periods of sighing. It is often possible to reproduce many of the symptoms of an attack by encouraging them to overbreathe spontaneously. It is also useful to demonstrate to these patients that they can hold a breath for a considerable period even during an attack. An attack can sometimes be terminated by having the patient breathe in and out of a plastic bag, or inhale a 5% CO_2 mixture. However, attention to the underlying anxiety state is indicated.

ABNORMAL PATTERNS OF VENTILATION

CHEYNE-STOKES BREATHING This is a form of periodic breathing characterized by alternating periods of apnea and hyperpnea. The patient often lies motionless for 15 to 20 s and then begins to breathe shallowly at first, then with increasing amplitude, and finally shallowly again. The respirations during this period of breathing are regular in time.

The cause of this disturbance presumably lies in some delay in the control process which results in "hunting" for the equilibrium condition. Periodic breathing can be produced in experimental animals by lengthening the distance over which blood travels from the thorax to the brain. As a result, the response of the medullary chemoreceptors lags behind the blood gas changes produced by the lungs, and a cyclical chain of events is created. Conditions in which Cheyne-Stokes breathing is seen include congestive heart failure when the circulation time is prolonged (Chap. 236), brain damage caused by trauma or cerebral hemorrhage, and chronic hypoxia. It occurs in normal subjects living at high altitude, especially during sleep.

BIOT'S BREATHING This is another form of periodic breathing in which periods of apnea are punctuated by a few deep breaths which may be irregular and which do not have the waxing and waning pattern of Cheyne-Stokes respiration. It is most frequently associated with brain damage.

REFERENCES

BURWELL CS et al: Extreme obesity associated with alveolar hypoventilation—a Pickwickian syndrome. Am J Med 21:811, 1956

FISHMAN AP: The syndrome of chronic alveolar hypoventilation. Bull Physio-Pathol Respir 8:971, 1972 (contains some 25 papers from a symposium on hypoventilation)

GUILLEMINAULT C et al: The sleep apnea syndromes. Annu Rev Med 27:465, 1976

SACKNER MA et al: Periodic sleep apnea: Chronic sleep deprivation related to intermittent airway obstruction and central nervous system disturbance. Chest 67:164, 1975

WEST JB: Causes of carbon dioxide retention in lung disease. N Engl J Med 284:1232, 1971

271

ADULT RESPIRATORY DISTRESS SYNDROME

ROLAND H. INGRAM, JR.

Adult respiratory distress syndrome is a descriptive term that has been applied to many acute, diffuse infiltrative lung lesions of diverse etiologies when they are accompanied by severe arterial hypoxemia. The term was chosen because of several clinical and pathologic similarities between such acute illnesses in adults and the neonatal respiratory distress syndrome. However, in the neonatal form, immaturity of alveolar surfactant production and a highly compliant chest wall are primarily involved in the pathophysiology, whereas in the adult, alveolar surfactant changes are secondary to the primary process, and the chest wall is not compliant. Despite the large number of causes (Table 271-1), the clinical characteristics, respiratory pathophysiologic derangement, and current techniques for management of these acute abnormalities are remarkably simi-

TABLE 271-1
Conditions which may lead to the adult respiratory distress syndrome

1 Diffuse pulmonary infections (e.g., viral, bacterial, fungal, pneumocystis)
2 Aspiration (e.g., gastric contents with Mendelson's syndrome, water with near-drowning)
3 Inhalation of toxins and irritants (e.g., chlorine gas, NO_2, smoke, ozone, high concentrations of oxygen)
4 Narcotic overdose pulmonary edema (e.g., heroin, methadone, morphine, dextropropoxyphene)
5 Nonnarcotic drug effects (e.g., nitrofurantoin)
6 Immunologic response to host antigens (e.g., Goodpasture's syndrome, systemic lupus erythematosus)
7 Effects of nonthoracic trauma with hypotension ("shock lung")
8 In association with systemic reactions to processes initiated outside the lung (e.g., gram-negative septicemia, hemorrhagic pancreatitis, amniotic fluid embolism, fat embolism)
9 Postcardiopulmonary bypass ("pump lung," "postperfusion lung")

lar. It has been argued that the "lumping" of such processes of different etiologies obscures the unique features of each in terms of pathogenesis, prevention, and specificity of treatment. It is clear that the conditions listed do not always lead to respiratory failure and that specific treatment of the underlying processes will often be different. Therefore, the reader is urged to refer to the appropriate sections of this text for the unique characteristics of each condition and to recognize that only the common features at the onset of respiratory failure will be focused upon in this chapter. It should be further emphasized that many of the listed conditions are often present in combination and may come into play at different times in the clinical course of the adult respiratory distress syndrome.

PATHOPHYSIOLOGY Regardless of the initiating process, the adult respiratory distress syndrome is invariably associated with increased liquid in the lungs. Thus it is a form of pulmonary edema, yet it is distinct from cardiogenic pulmonary edema because pulmonary capillary hydrostatic pressures are not elevated (Chap. 27). Initially there is injury to the alveolar-capillary membrane that results in leakage of liquid, macromolecules, and cellular components from the blood vessels into the interstitial space and, with increasing severity, into the alveoli. Alveolar collapse occurs secondary to the effect of the alveolar liquid, especially its fibrinogen, that interferes with normal surfactant activity and because of possible impairment of further surfactant production by injury to the granular pneumocytes. Though radiographically diffuse, the regional dysfunction is nonhomogeneous; it leads to severe ventilation-perfusion imbalance and the shunting of blood through regions in which alveoli are collapsed or filled with liquid. The lungs become less compliant—i.e., stiffen on the bases of interstitial edema, alveolar collapse, and increase in surface forces. Because of the decreased compliance, large inspiratory pressures must be generated by the respiratory muscles so that the work of breathing is elevated. Both hypoxemia and the stimulation of receptors in the stiff lung parenchyma cause an increase in respiratory frequency, decrease in tidal volume, and deterioration in gas exchange.

PATHOLOGY In the absence of demonstrable specific pathogens, the pathology is remarkably similar among the various conditions leading to the adult respiratory distress syndrome, since the lung has a limited number of ways in which it reacts to an almost limitless number of injuries. Grossly, the lungs are heavy, edematous, and almost airless with regions of hemorrhage, atelectasis, and consolidation. By light microscopy there is edema and cellular infiltration of interalveolar septa and interstitial spaces surrounding airways and blood vessels, atelectasis and hyaline membranes in many regions, engorgement of vessels with red blood cells, and aggregates of platelets along with interstitial and alveolar hemorrhage. In addition, both hyperplasia and dysplasia of the granular pneumocytes are often present.

If the illness has been prolonged beyond 10 days, there is often a surprising amount of fibrosis in addition to the acute changes. In instances of recovery and subsequent death from another cause, significant interstitial fibrosis and emphysematous changes may be found in the lung. A significant number of patients, however, will recover completely and have normal pulmonary function with no respiratory symptoms. Hence aggressive clinical management is both indicated and often rewarding.

CLINICAL CHARACTERISTICS At the time of initial injury and for several hours thereafter the patient may be free of respiratory symptoms or signs. The earliest sign often is an increase in respiratory frequency followed shortly by dyspnea. Arterial blood gas measurement in the earlier period will disclose a depressed P_{O_2} despite a decreased P_{CO_2} so that the alveolar-arterial difference for oxygen (Chap. 255) is increased. At this early stage, administration of oxygen by mask or nasal prongs results in a significant increase in the arterial P_{O_2}. The brisk rise in P_{O_2} indicates that ventilation-perfusion mismatching and, possibly, diffusion impairment account for the widened alveolar-arterial P_{O_2} difference ($P_{A_{O_2}} - Pa_{O_2}$) initially. Physical examination may be unremarkable, although a few fine inspiratory rales may be audible. Radiographically the lung fields may be clear or demonstrate only minimal and scattered interstitial infiltrates. With progression, the patient becomes cyanotic and increasingly dyspneic and tachypneic. Rales are more prominent and are easily heard throughout both lung fields along with regions of tubular breath sounds; the chest radiograph demonstrates diffuse, extensive bilateral interstitial and alveolar infiltrates (Fig. 271-1). At this point hypoxemia cannot be corrected by the simple expedient of in-

FIGURE 271-1

A standard posteroanterior chest radiograph from a patient with the adult respiratory distress syndrome secondary to a severe viral pneumonitis. Such a diffuse radiographic change is typical of all conditions listed in Table 271-1 when they are severe enough to cause acute hypoxemic respiratory failure. A similar radiographic picture is also seen in pulmonary edema due to left ventricular failure (Chap. 27). Often in such acutely ill patients, the radiograph must be taken with a portable unit and the film exposed from the anterior direction. Both the anteroposterior exposure and the failure to take a deep inspiration result in an apparent enlargement of the cardiac silhouette which further obscures the reliable detection of left ventricular failure.

creasing the oxygen concentration of the inspired gas, and mechanical ventilatory assistance or control must be started (Chap. 272). Right-to-left shunting of blood through collapsed or filled alveoli becomes the major mechanism for arterial hypoxemia at this more advanced stage. In contrast to ventilation-perfusion mismatching and diffusion impairment, with right-to-left shunts, $P_{A_{O_2}} - Pa_{O_2}$ remains high with breathing of pure oxygen. Positive end-expiratory pressure (PEEP) serves to increase lung volume, which in turn opens collapsed alveoli and decreases shunting. With further progression, and if mechanical ventilator and PEEP therapy are delayed, the combination of increasing tachypnea and decreasing tidal volumes results in alveolar hypoventilation, a rising P_{CO_2}, and worsening hypoxemia; these represent a near-terminal constellation of findings.

COMPLICATIONS Increasing severity of the clinical illness and continued radiographic progression in association with the primary process often obscure complications that arise during the course of acute hypoxemic respiratory failure. The development of left ventricular failure is a good example of a common, easily missed complication. With deterioration, left ventricular failure should be suspected; it is helpful to insert a balloon-tipped (Swan-Ganz) catheter which can be used to monitor pulmonary arterial pressure continuously and pulmonary artery wedge (pulmonary capillary) pressure and oxygen of mixed venous blood intermittently. There are two special precautions that must be taken with regard to interpretation of vascular pressures within the thorax when PEEP is being used. First, if pleural pressure is greater than atmospheric, as is often the case with PEEP, the true effective pressure (i.e., intravascular minus pleural) may be overestimated. Second, in the capillary "wedge" position, if the capillaries are closed by the high alveolar pressure with PEEP, the pressure registered will be higher than the true wedge or left atrial pressure. Either misinterpretation could lead to errors in both assessment and management. With a diffuse radiographic pattern, a secondary bacterial infection is easily overlooked, so frequent sputum smears and cultures should be obtained, especially when there is fever. With many conditions—e.g., gram-negative septicemia, acute hemorrhagic pancreatitis, and "shock lung"—there may be associated disseminated intravascular coagulation, which leads to gastrointestinal and intrapulmonary hemorrhage. Frequent monitoring of platelet count, fibrinogen level, and partial thromboplastin and prothrombin times is helpful in the early detection of this complication and in guiding treatment (see Chap. 318). Finally, in the course of treating the illness with mechanical ventilators and high inflation pressures (see Chap. 272), pneumothorax or pneumomediastinum may develop and may be impossible to detect except radiologically. Any deterioration should lead the physician to suspect the complication, repeat the chest radiograph, and institute immediate treatment should pneumothorax be present. If deterioration is sudden, tension pneumothorax should be suspected; if physical signs are present, a pleural catheter should be inserted immediately without radiographic confirmation. It is important to realize that high oxygen concentrations (>0.60) for prolonged periods can produce both the lesions and the clinical picture of the adult respiratory distress syndrome. Therefore, as discussed under clinical management (Chap. 272), the *minimal* oxygen concentration associated with acceptable arterial oxygenation should always be used.

PROGNOSIS Given the diversity of the etiologies and the frequency of associated diseases, it is difficult, if not impossible, to give meaningful prognostic figures for the adult respiratory distress syndrome. If all recently published series are taken together, the mortality rate runs between 50 and 60 percent. This represents an improved survival rate over the virtual 100 percent mortality rate of a few years ago and is a result of the application of modern treatment techniques discussed in Chap. 272. If the syndrome is due to drug overdose, the mortality rate is low; if associated with shock, the chances of a fatal outcome are much greater. Other etiologies and associated diseases are between these two extremes. The following factors appear to be associated with a poor outcome: an increase in $PA_{O_2} - Pa_{O_2}$, requiring increasing inspired O_2 concentrations and PEEP; decreasing compliance, requiring greater inflation pressures; either low or falling colloid osmotic pressures; and the onset of systemic arterial hypotension not responding to intravascular volume replacement.

CLINICAL MANAGEMENT   See Chap. 272.

REFERENCES

HOPEWELL PC, MURRAY JF: The adult respiratory distress syndrome. Annu Rev Med 27:343, 1976

PETTY TL, ASHBAUGH DG: The adult respiratory distress syndrome. Chest 60:233, 1971

SIMPSON DL et al: Long term follow-up and bronchial reactivity testing in survivors of the adult respiratory distress syndrome. Am Rev Respir Dis 117:449, 1978

WEIL MH et al: Relationship between colloid osmotic pressure and pulmonary artery wedge pressure in patients with acute cardiorespiratory failure. Am J Med 64:643, 1978

272
MANAGEMENT OF ACUTE RESPIRATORY FAILURE

KENNETH M. MOSER

The management of acute respiratory failure is simple in terms of the concepts which guide therapy but complex with respect to the specific means applied. Furthermore, the fundamental concepts of therapy are well established, while the specifics are continuously evolving. This chapter focuses upon the principles of the management of acute respiratory failure, a condition which is said to exist when, as a consequence of acutely impaired respiratory function, arterial hypoxemia and/or hypercapnia are present; at sea level and with the patient at rest, an arterial $P_{O_2} < 60$ mmHg and a $P_{CO_2} > 45$ mmHg are useful guidelines in establishing the diagnosis. Clearly, substantial mechanical, biochemical, hemodynamic, and structural abnormalities may long antedate significant impairment of pulmonary gas exchange. Furthermore, a substantial number of patients with severe, chronic lung disease have long-term respiratory failure with arterial P_{O_2} and P_{CO_2} values in the stipulated "failure category"; in them, *acute* respiratory failure is signaled by a worsening of their preexisting hypercapnia and/or hypoxemia.

Therefore, acute respiratory failure is a laboratory diagnosis, defined in terms of failure to maintain adequate gas exchange. Its detection requires (1) arterial puncture, a simple, safe procedure which should be familiar to any physician responsible for the diagnosis and treatment of patients with acute respiratory failure; and (2) determination of the P_{O_2},[1] P_{CO_2}, and pH. The development of instrumentation which can analyze the P_{O_2}, P_{CO_2}, and pH precisely and within minutes has helped to shape the modern management of acute respiratory failure.

In clinical practice, two forms of acute respiratory failure are encountered: the hypercapnic type, in which the P_{CO_2} is elevated and the P_{O_2} is lowered, and the nonhypercapnic type, in which hypoxemia is present despite a P_{CO_2} that is normal or even depressed. These two forms differ with respect to pathogenesis, clinical presentation, pathophysiology, and therapy.

HYPERCAPNIC RESPIRATORY FAILURE   Patients with acute hypercapnic respiratory failure are categorized into two major groups: those with essentially normal lungs and those with intrinsic lung disease. Carbon dioxide retention in the first group is due to an absolute reduction in alveolar ventilation because of abnormalities in respiratory control, in the neuromuscular events required to maintain ventilation, or in the behavior of the chest wall (Chap. 270). Acute respiratory failure is often overlooked in these patients, who do not have pulmonary disease. The second type of patient with acute hypercapnic respiratory failure has intrinsic lung disease—most often emphysema, bronchitis, and/or asthma (Chap. 263). In these patients, alterations in the mechanical and gas exchange characteristics of the lungs lead to inadequate CO_2 elimination (alveolar hypoventilation), even though minute ventilation may be normal to increased (Chap. 270). Occasionally, mixed forms occur. A common example is the patient with chronic obstructive lung disease who receives sedatives or narcotics because of anxiety or because of a misdiagnosis of left ventricular failure. Such therapy, by depressing ventilation, may make the patient appear to be more comfortable. However, since a high level of ventilation is required to maintain adequate elimination of CO_2, the decreased ventilation may lead to acute respiratory failure and, often, to hypercapnic coma.

Consequences of hypercapnia   Regardless of the events responsible for hypercapnia, all forms are complicated by hypoxemia, by respiratory acidosis if hypercapnia develops acutely, by an increase in pulmonary arteriolar resistance, and by dilatation of the cerebral vessels; such dilatation leads to the increase in intracranial pressure which is sometimes seen in acute respiratory failure, including the development of papilledema, and perhaps the asterixis, seen in some patients. This increase in intracranial pressure, combined with the direct effects of hypercapnia and hypoxemia on cerebral function, also explains the disorientation, personality changes, and coma that may appear in the course of respiratory insufficiency. Hypoxemia is an inevitable consequence of hypercapnia because as alveolar P_{CO_2} rises, the alveolar P_{O_2} must fall. However, if hypercapnia *alone* is responsible for hypoxemia, the alveolar-arterial P_{O_2} difference ($PA_{O_2} - Pa_{O_2}$) is not widened. If this difference *is* widened, hypoxemia is more severe than can be accounted for by hypercapnia alone and must be due to the presence of low V/Q zones and/or right-to-left shunt.

NORMOCAPNIC RESPIRATORY FAILURE   In this form of acute respiratory insufficiency, the central problem is failure of the lungs to deliver sufficient O_2 to the pulmonary capillary blood, resulting in arterial hypoxemia. Carbon dioxide elimination is normal or even increased in these patients, so that the P_{CO_2} is normal or reduced. This form of respiratory failure occurs in a variety of circumstances, including a group of disorders which may be grouped under the label "adult respiratory distress syndrome" (Chap. 271).

---

[1] *Unless otherwise stated in this chapter, P_{O_2} and P_{CO_2} refer to the partial pressures of these gases in arterial blood.*

Diffuse pulmonary infiltrates seen on the chest roentgenogram are characteristic as this form of respiratory failure develops. The hypoxemia is due to severe ventilation-perfusion imbalance as manifested by an increase in $P_{A_{O_2}} - P_{a_{O_2}}$ (Chap. 255). In multiple zones of the lung there is diminished to absent ventilation, while perfusion continues. Where alveoli are filled with exudate, a true intrapulmonary shunt exists. Reduced lung compliance is due to the extensive accumulation of fluid, first in lung interstitial spaces and later within alveoli. Some degree of pulmonary hypertension is usually present because of arteriolar constriction from focal alveolar hypoxia and arteriolar compression by fluid in the perivascular space. Ventilation is markedly increased because of the hypoxemia and the stimuli arising from the stiff pulmonary parenchyma.

MANAGEMENT OF THE PATIENT WITH ACUTE RESPIRATORY FAILURE

The most dangerous feature of respiratory failure, the abnormality which threatens the patient's life, is the impairment of gas exchange. Therefore, the first goal of therapy is to assure that hypoxemia, hypercapnia, and acidosis do not reach hazardous levels, which are defined rather arbitrarily, since coexisting conditions modify such definitions. For example, a degree of hypoxemia which may be tolerated by a young adult with barbiturate overdosage may be dangerous in an elderly person who has recently sustained a myocardial infarction. However, there is reasonable agreement that P_{O_2} levels below 40 mmHg are poorly tolerated by adults. Such levels are commonly associated with cardiac arrhythmias, impaired cardiac and cerebral function, and functional or anatomic damage to other organs, such as the liver and kidney. The danger level of pH is more difficult to establish, but strenuous efforts should be made to avoid or correct values below 7.2. Patients have survived brief episodes of pH 6.9 and below, but the mortality rate increases with each decrement below 7.2. The deleterious effects of severe acidosis potentiate the actions of hypoxemia and include the induction of pulmonary hypertension, depression of myocardial contractility, and compromise of cellular function throughout the body. There is no generally accepted "danger" level of P_{CO_2}, because the injurious effects of P_{CO_2} relate importantly to the degree of associated acidosis. Thus, chronic hypercapnia of 60 mmHg with a nearly normal pH is not dangerous, while a sudden rise to 60 mmHg sharply elevates hydrogen ion concentration and has much greater functional impact. However, when the P_{CO_2} exceeds 70 mmHg, even when this level has been reached slowly, many patients become confused or comatose.

MAINTENANCE OF ADEQUATE OXYGENATION The principle guiding oxygenation is to use the simplest method and the lowest inspired P_{O_2} which will achieve the desired result. Reference to the oxyhemoglobin dissociation curve (Chap. 53) provides general guidance in defining the latter. At a P_{O_2} of approximately 50 to 60 mmHg, the curve reaches its flat portion. Above this level, substantial increments in P_{O_2} lead to only modest increments in hemoglobin saturation and total O_2 content of the arterial blood. Therefore, a reasonable objective of O_2 therapy is to achieve a P_{O_2} of 50 to 60 mmHg. It is not necessary to attempt to achieve a normal or even supernormal P_{O_2} because there is little gain in O_2 content of the blood, as noted above. Also, any increase in arterial P_{O_2} carries significant risk of causing respiratory depression in the patient with chronic hypercapnia and direct lung injury as a consequence of the high inspiratory oxygen concentrations.

The hazard of respiratory depression with O_2 is confined to patients with the hypercapnic form of respiratory failure in whom the normal stimuli to ventilation are compromised. The major central drives to respiration are reviewed in Chap. 270.

Acute CO_2 retention provides potent drives to respiration through a decline in the pH of cerebrospinal fluid, a fall in arterial pH, and a decrease in the P_{O_2}. However, with chronic hypercapnia, cerebrospinal fluid pH readjusts to normal within 24 h and arterial pH returns toward normal within 3 to 5 days by rises in cerebrospinal fluid and blood bicarbonate levels respectively. Thus, after several days, hypercapnia itself no longer provides a major stimulus to ventilation. Only hypoxemia and cortical factors remain. If the patient is sedated or obtunded, little cortical "drive" is provided to respiration. Therefore, hypoxemia is the major residual drive to respiration. When oxygen is given, this drive is blunted, the patient ventilates less, and the P_{CO_2} climbs. Hypercapnic coma and death may ensue.

It is critical, then, to avoid both sedatives and excessive O_2 delivery in patients with chronic hypercapnia. Such patients *need* O_2 and, while fears of respiratory depression should not prevent adequate relief of hypoxemia, use of O_2 should be judicious, with frequent monitoring of P_{O_2} and P_{CO_2}, i.e., the administration of a concentration of O_2 in the inspired gas ($F_{I_{O_2}}$) which restores the P_{O_2} to acceptable levels of 50 to 60 mmHg, without raising P_{CO_2} or lowering pH significantly.

The second toxic risk of a high $F_{I_{O_2}}$ is direct injury to the lung. The mechanisms underlying this injury are debated, but its nature and gravity are well established. High concentrations of inspired O_2 injure some component(s) of the alveolar-capillary membrane, presumably the endothelium of the pulmonary capillary, and/or the type I alveolar cell, with consequent increase in permeability and the leak of blood components into the interstitial and alveolar spaces. Some alveoli are flooded with proteinaceous fluid and red blood cells; in others, hyaline membranes form. In their advanced form, the lesions induced are lethal, because of progressive hypoxemia. In its end stage the lung damage by O_2 resembles that of the infant dying with hyaline membrane disease or the adult dying with devastating viral pneumonia or "shock lung."

The risks of O_2 toxicity are related to at least two factors; the $F_{I_{O_2}}$ and the duration of O_2 administration. For example, hyperbaric O_2 at several atmospheres of pressure can induce the lesion of O_2 toxicity within hours. As the $F_{I_{O_2}}$ is lowered, the period of safe exposure lengthens. Thus an $F_{I_{O_2}}$ of 1.0, i.e., 100% O_2 at ambient partial pressure, may take several days to produce lung injury. Whether an inspired $F_{I_{O_2}}$ below 0.50 is safe when given for many days is debatable. All available data indicate that the best rule is to use the lowest $F_{I_{O_2}}$ possible to maintain adequate oxygenation and for the shortest time necessary.

Means for delivering O_2 These are multiple; soft nasal prongs through which O_2 is delivered at the required flow rate are used most commonly. The net $F_{I_{O_2}}$ entering the trachea will be determined by the minute ventilation of the patient, and the flow rate of O_2. The best procedure is to start at very low rates (0.5 to 1.0 liter per minute) and measure the response of the P_{O_2}, P_{CO_2}, and pH, gradually increasing the flow rate until the desired response has been achieved. Such "titration" by monitoring the arterial blood gases provides a safe way to guide O_2 administration.

An alternative method of O_2 delivery involves the use of masks which have been designed to deliver known, fixed concentrations of O_2. Such masks achieve a fixed concentration (regardless of the oxygen flow rate to the mask) by the *Venturi* principle. These "Venturi" masks can be obtained in related concentration ($F_{I_{O_2}} = 0.24$, 0.28, etc.). They are "high-flow" masks, fitting lightly over nose and mouth, thus providing the patient with a microenvironment of fixed $F_{I_{O_2}}$. The major advantage of masks over nasal prongs is that, regardless of the total ventilation, $F_{I_{O_2}}$ remains constant. With prongs delivering a fixed flow, $F_{I_{O_2}}$ varies inversely with total ventilation. The disadvantage of masks is that the dyspneic patient often cannot tolerate a device over the nose and mouth.

These simple means of O_2 delivery suffice in the great majority of patients with hypoxemia. However, in some patients with hypercapnic respiratory failure, masks and prongs may be unable to achieve adequate P_{O_2} without inducing marked hypercapnia, and in some patients with hypoxemic respiratory failure, it may not be possible to achieve the desired P_{O_2}. The next step is to provide the patient with a mechanical device, i.e., a ventilator, to assist respiration, and simultaneously to raise P_{O_2} and lower P_{CO_2}. This is a major decision, since it requires tracheal intubation and attachment of the patient to a mechanical device. Thus, these patients are placed in a "closed system" over which they can exert only limited control, and they become heavily dependent, or if obtunded, totally dependent, on those attending them. Furthermore, intubation and ventilation expose the patient to the additional risks described below. Therefore, it is a decision which should not be undertaken until it is clear that simpler measures will not suffice.

If assisted ventilation is required, basically two kinds of ventilator are available: the pressure-cycled and volume-cycled devices. The inspiratory phase of a pressure-cycled ventilator can be initiated by the negative-pressure inspiratory effort of the patient or by an automatic timer. Inspiration is terminated when the pressure in the device reaches a preset value of positive pressure. Thus, the volume delivered is determined by the inspiratory flow rate and the time required to reach the preset pressure limit. In a volume-cycled device, the operator sets the desired volume and either the inspiratory time or the inspiratory flow rate. The machine generates whatever pressure is required to achieve the volume selected.

Each type of ventilator has its advantages and disadvantages. The major limitation of pressure-cycled devices is their inability to attain the high inspiratory pressure which may be required in patients with very high airway resistance (e.g., severe asthma) or very low lung compliance (e.g., adult respiratory distress syndrome). Pressure-cycled ventilators in such patients may not maintain adequate gas exchange and, in some cases, may compromise gas exchange by repetitively ending inspiration *prematurely* as the preset maximum pressure is achieved after small inspiratory volumes are delivered. The major hazard of volume-cycled respirators is the very high pressures which they can achieve, with potential deleterious effects on venous return and cardiac output and an increased risk of pneumothorax. Patients with normocapnic respiratory failure usually have poorly compliant lungs and require a volume ventilator. Most patients with hypercapnic respiratory failure, who have normal or highly compliant lungs, can be managed with pressure-cycled devices which are less costly.

In *hypercapnic respiratory failure,* ventilatory assistance provides several potential gains: (1) concern about respiratory depression of ventilatory drive due to increased $F_{I_{O_2}}$ is reduced, since the respirator will continue to ventilate the patient even if respiratory drive ceases, as long as the device is set to cycle automatically; (2) ventilation can be augmented at will, thus decreasing the P_{CO_2} and leading to a rise in P_{O_2} (often allowing the use of an $F_{I_{O_2}}$ approaching room air); (3) the patient's own ventilatory effort may be reduced, making the patient more comfortable and decreasing both O_2 needs and CO_2 production.

In *normocapnic respiratory failure,* the ventilator is used to achieve improvement of oxygenation, by assuring adequate lung inflation and restoring a better match between ventilation and perfusion. Even areas of the lung with marked disturbances in airway resistance and compliance can be ventilated. An additional dividend is that O_2 requirements may diminish as the respirator assumes a portion of the patient's ventilatory workload.

In some patients assisted ventilation does not suffice. They "fight" the respirator and are unable to cycle with it effectively; their ventilation must therefore be controlled. This usually can be accomplished by sedation and setting the respirator to cycle automatically. If sedation does not achieve this goal, the patient can be paralyzed with curare-like drugs.

The condition of almost all patients with hypercapnic respiratory failure can be managed by the maneuvers described above. However, some patients with severe normocapnic failure remain dangerously hypoxemic—even with controlled volume ventilation at 100% O_2. Clearly, in this situation, there is the risk of inducing O_2 toxicity in an effort to maintain the patient's life. Two additional maneuvers may be considered at this point. One is the use of positive end-expiratory pressure (5 to 15 cmH$_2$O), or maintenance of a continuous positive airway pressure. Positive end-expiratory pressure (PEEP) increases arterial P_{O_2} in many such patients and allows a reduction in $F_{I_{O_2}}$. However, it may also decrease venous return and cardiac output. If the increase of continuous or end-expiratory pressure required to elevate P_{O_2} is large, it may be necessary to measure cardiac output to determine whether oxygen delivery has actually been increased, since the arterial P_{O_2} alone may be misleading—if it rises at the expense of a sharp decline in cardiac output and mixed venous P_{O_2}.

The second and final resort in severely hypoxemic patients is the application of cardiopulmonary bypass. Membrane oxygenators capable of maintaining adequate gas exchange for many days are now available. They appear capable of sustaining patients who cannot be saved with respirators or who are placed at hazard by the need for prolonged administration of 100% O_2 at high pressures via respirators. To date, application of these devices has not reduced the mortality rate in selected patients with severe hypoxemia.

How rapidly these escalating maneuvers to assure adequate oxygenation must be employed depends on the clinical situation. Patients who have severe hypoventilatory respiratory failure because they have inadvertently received excess sedation or O_2 may require immediate intubation and ventilation, as do many patients with a fulminant form of the acute respiratory distress syndrome. Guided by the condition of the arterial blood gases, the physician can make these decisions rapidly and evaluate the patient's response.

TREATMENT OF THE PRIMARY PROBLEM Once the life-threatening derangements of gas exchange have been controlled, attention can be focused on the treatment of the problem which induced respiratory failure. In patients with absolute hypoventilation, the primary problem usually can be identified rapidly and appropriate treatment initiated. In patients with drug overdosage, treatment with dialysis or other methods to enhance drug excretion should be considered. Similar specific measures are available for patients with myasthenia gravis (Chap. 381) or myxedema (Chap. 335). In other patients, such as those with Guillain-Barré syndrome (Chap. 377), long-term ventilatory support is required until the process runs its course.

In patients with relative hypoventilation due to obstructive lung disease, therapy is directed toward removing the problems which caused acute deterioration in the effectiveness of gas exchange. The most frequent problems are accumulation of secretions, bronchospasm, and infection. Treatment of these abnormalities will improve the mechanical dysfunction of the lungs, restore ventilation-perfusion relationships toward normal, and thereby reduce the disturbances in gas exchange.

If bronchospasm is present, therapy usually begins with administration of xanthine drugs such as aminophylline, parenterally, by mouth, or rectally; or with administration of beta-adrenergic stimulating drugs (e.g., isoproterenol) by aerosol. The usual adult dose of intravenous aminophylline is 250 to 500 mg dissolved in 10 to 20 ml diluent and delivered as an initial loading dose (4 to 6 mg/kg in 15 to 30 min) followed by continuous infusion [0.5 to 1.0 (mg/kg)/h], with the objective a blood level of 10 to 20 mg/ml. Rectal and oral doses are comparable. Isoproterenol is usually delivered by nebulizer as a 1:200 solution for 5 to 10 deep inhalations; it may be repeated hourly if necessary. The new, "more pure" $beta_2$-adrenergic agents (metaproterenol, terbutaline) are generally being substituted for isoproterenol, as they become available in solutions for aerosol use, because of their less marked hemodynamic effects. If severe bronchospasm persists, adrenocortical steroids should be administered promptly by mouth or parenterally. A starting dose of 100 to 200 mg hydrocortisone is appropriate and may be repeated at hourly intervals until bronchospasm is controlled, at which point both dose size and frequency are reduced. Again, only blood gas analysis can determine how rapidly therapy should be escalated and tapered.

The attack upon secretions is two-pronged and should include measures to liquefy and to remove them. Liquefaction is best achieved by adequately hydrating the patient. Drugs which may assist in liquefaction of sputum include inorganic iodide preparations (10 drops saturated solution of potassium iodide in a glass of liquid every 6 h or equivalent intravenous potassium iodide), glyceryl guaiacolate (15 to 30 ml by mouth every 4 to 5 h), and acetylcysteine (5 ml of a 10% solution delivered by aerosol every 2 to 6 h). However, the value of these agents is marginal; by far the most effective technique for liquefying sputum is fluid administration, and adequate hydration is the keystone to sputum mobilization. If adequate hydration cannot be accomplished by mouth, oral delivery can be supplemented intravenously or by aerosol delivery of water. Furthermore, all inspired gases (oxygen or compressed air delivered from wall sources or via ventilators) should be well humidified to avoid dehydration and the accompanying thickening of nasotracheobronchial secretions.

Secretions are best removed by encouraging the patient to cough. The likelihood that coughing will be productive is greatly enhanced if a skilled respiratory or physical therapist is available to encourage the patient, assure that proper postural drainage positions are used, and supplement the patient's efforts with percussion and vibration. When spontaneous cough is either depressed or inadequate, nasotracheal or transtracheal insertion of a catheter will assist in inducing cough and removing secretions. Transtracheal catheters, which must be kept scrupulously clean, can also be used for instillation of water and other agents and for obtaining reliable sputum for culture. Finally, bronchoscopy, which is no longer a formidable procedure since introduction of the flexible fiberoptic bronchoscope, can be performed even in patients receiving continuous ventilator support. This procedure has special value in assessing the extent and distribution of secretions and in assuring that they have been removed.

Respiratory infection   This is both a frequent cause and a common complication of respiratory failure in patients with obstructive lung disease. Indeed, it is so common that therapy is usually initiated with broad-spectrum antibiotics (ampicillin, tetracycline) on the presumption that infection is present. The antibiotic regimen is altered, if necessary, on the basis of the results of sputum smear and appropriately obtained cultures. Finally, there should be a thorough search for other factors which may have induced respiratory failure, particularly left ventricular failure and pulmonary embolism.

In the normocapnic type of acute respiratory failure, treatment of the primary problem is usually not feasible, since injury to the alveolar-capillary membrane is involved and no effective method is available for restoring its integrity. Therefore, treatment usually consists of maintenance of adequate gas exchange while awaiting resolution of the initial injury. If the latter has been caused by an infectious agent, identification and appropriate treatment are important. Occasionally, open or closed lung biopsy may be required for the rapid identification or exclusion of infectious agents, particularly in the case of viral and *Pneumocystis carinii* infections, although specimens obtained by fiberoptic bronchoscopy should be examined first.

Corticosteroids often are useful in those forms of normocapnic respiratory failure which are mediated through the immune system or are responses to injurious inhalants (e.g., irritant gases, chemical substances, or thermal injuries). High doses of these agents should be used in an effort to halt inflammation and restore the integrity of cell membranes (e.g., 100 to 200 mg hydrocortisone or its equivalent every 2 to 4 h). If a response is to occur, it should be apparent within a few days and the dose of corticosteroids should then be tapered. The value of corticosteroids remains controversial in many of the forms of normocapnic respiratory failure, such as aspiration pneumonia and fat embolism. Nevertheless, their use is warranted when the lung injury is severe. It is also essential that the presence of left ventricular failure, masquerading as or complicating the adult respiratory distress syndrome, be ruled out.

Tracheostomy   There are three major indications for tracheostomy in patients with acute respiratory failure: (1) to bypass upper airway obstruction (e.g., croup, allergic edema); (2) to provide a port for long-term ventilator attachment; (3) to facilitate removal of secretions. These indications are relative, since an endotracheal or nasotracheal tube can be used for attaching ventilators and other means for removal of secretions are available. However, when copious secretions are a major problem, tracheostomy often is of great value in reversing respiratory failure. Tracheostomy is preferable to an endo- or nasotracheal tube in patients who require ventilatory assistance for more than a few days, particularly alert patients.

THE RESPIRATORY INTENSIVE CARE UNIT   The patient with acute respiratory insufficiency requires expert care in terms of both monitoring and therapy. These special requirements are intensified if the patient requires ventilatory support. Such requirements are best satisfied in a unit specifically devoted to the care of such patients, i.e., a respiratory intensive care unit. The central elements of such a unit include (1) a staff of physicians and nurses highly trained in the diagnosis and therapy of respiratory failure, supported by respiratory and chest physical therapists; (2) immediate and continuous availability of special equipment for ventilation, resuscitation, aspiration, and of monitoring equipment, including instruments for arterial blood gas analysis; and (3) a geographic area designed for these purposes. Such a pooling of personnel and resources available 24 h a day, 7 days a week, is an expensive undertaking, but this cost appears to be justified by the more favorable results of therapy. Though not every hospital needs to develop a respiratory intensive care unit, one such unit should be available within a reasonable transport time for patients in any given geographic region. Indeed, many respiratory intensive care units now offer transport teams which move patients to the unit from their homes or from other medical facilities.

Complications of respiratory intensive care   Certain complications occur frequently in patients being treated for acute respiratory failure; when sudden deterioration of the patient with acute respiratory failure occurs, the reasons will usually be among those listed below:

1   *Cardiac arrhythmias* of all types are very common. Potential causes of arrhythmias in respiratory failure are multiple: hypoxemia, wide swings in pH, electrolyte disturbances, and the action or interaction of pharmacologic agents such as aminophylline and beta-adrenergic agents employed in the treatment of acute respiratory failure. Digitalis toxicity, for example, is potentiated by hypoxemia, and the arrhythmic potential of isoproterenol is well recognized. For these reasons, continuous monitoring of the cardiac rhythm is essential.
2   *Gastrointestinal hemorrhage* is also frequently seen in these patients. In part, this reflects the high incidence of peptic ulcer in patients with obstructive lung disease, but it also is related to other factors such as stress, the possible effects of severe blood gas derangements and of alterations in cardiac output upon the gastrointestinal circulation, and the use of adrenocortical steroids, aminophylline, aspirin, and other drugs. Bleeding occurs almost exclusively from the stomach and duodenum and may be both massive and sudden.
3   *Pulmonary infection* already has been mentioned. Scrupulous cleansing of respiratory equipment is essential, lest these devices populate the patient's lungs with pathogenic bacteria. All personnel caring for such patients must observe strict aseptic techniques in all manipulations of the patient (e.g., nasotracheal suction, cleaning tracheostomy tubes).
4   *Pneumothorax* occurs with more than chance frequency in patients with acute respiratory failure, especially in those requiring ventilator support. Volume ventilators and end-expiratory positive pressure in particular predispose to this complication, although the likelihood of such barotrauma cannot be related specifically to the pressures used. Sudden respirator malfunction or respiratory distress should promote a prompt search for a pneumothorax, since its persistence may be lethal and its correction can be accomplished simply and rapidly.
5   *Bronchial obstruction by endotracheal or tracheostomy tubes* often occurs. These tubes, when too long or poorly anchored, slide into one main bronchus, usually the right one because of its less angulated origin from the trachea. The tube then blocks ventilation of the other main bronchus, and atelectasis may ensue. Such an event usually causes abrupt deterioration in the patient with respiratory failure. It is detected readily by physical examination, which reveals the absence of breath sounds over the occluded lung. The tube should immediately be pulled back slowly if this complication is suspected.

Other common complications during acute respiratory failure include (1) acute right ventricular failure due to pulmonary hypertension and hypoxia (Chap. 246); (2) left ventricular failure, detectable by means of right-sided heart catheterization carried out at the bedside with flow-guided catheters; (3) pulmonary interstitial and alveolar edema from overhydration and increased pulmonary capillary permeability; (4) pulmonary oxygen toxicity, reviewed previously; (5) convulsions due to hypoxia or to sudden induction of respiratory alkalosis with ventilators; and (6) tracheal injury due to excessive pressure in the occluding cuffs of endotracheal-tracheostomy tubes or pressure exerted by the tubes themselves.

Those caring for patients with acute respiratory failure must be alert to all these complications. Their prevention—or prompt detection and reversal—often spell the difference between survival and death. The ability of all personnel in the respiratory intensive care unit to deal with these problems is another factor which enhances the likelihood of survival of the patient in the respiratory intensive care unit environment.

VENTILATOR MANAGEMENT AND WEANING   Modern ventilators allow a high degree of flexibility in determining the type of ventilatory pattern, as well as the volume of ventilation, delivered to a specific patient. Most such devices now incorporate controls and/or monitors for rate, depth, inspiratory flow rate, peak inspiratory pressure, inspiratory "hold," air temperature and humidity, $F_{I_{O_2}}$, and the application of positive end-expiratory pressure (PEEP) and intermittent mandatory ventilation (IMV). Such flexibility is of value not only during early management but also in that critical period when the patient is being withdrawn from ventilatory support ("weaning"). The ease and speed with which weaning can be accomplished depends upon the extent to which the three variables *inducing* acute respiratory failure have resolved, namely, the pulmonary disease causing abnormalities in gas exchange, aberrations in respiratory control, and dysfunction of the neuromuscular apparatus. The first can be monitored easily; the latter two cannot presently be assessed in clinical situations. However, new methods for assessing them are being developed (e.g., measurement of early inspiratory pressures, transdiaphragmatic pressures). Until such measurements are available, weaning "trials" guided by gas exchange data are utilized. IMV has aided this semiempiric approach significantly by allowing the patient to participate in the weaning process. With skillful use of IMV, gradual and safe withdrawal from mechanical ventilatory support now presents problems only in the exceptional case (e.g., patients with serious neuromuscular or pulmonary parenchymal deficits).

MANAGEMENT OF CHRONIC RESPIRATORY FAILURE   See Chap. 263.

REFERENCES

CLARK JM, LAMBERTSON CJ: Pulmonary oxygen toxicity: A review. Pharmacol Rev 23:37, 1971

Conference on the Scientific Basis of Respiratory Therapy. Am Rev Respir Dis 110(suppl):1, 1974

DOWNS JB et al: Intermittent mandatory ventilation. Arch Surg 109:519, 1974

INTER-SOCIETY COMMISSION FOR HEART DISEASE RESOURCES, STUDY GROUP ON PULMONARY HEART DISEASE: Resources for the optimal care of acute respiratory failure. Circulation 43:A185, 1971

MILIC-EMILI J et al: Workshop on assessment of respiratory control in humans. Am Rev Respir Dis 115:177, 363, 365, 1977

ROGERS RM (ed): Symposium on Cardiopulmonary Intensive Care. Chest 62(suppl):1S, 1972

SAHN SA et al: Weaning from mechanical ventilation. JAMA 235:2208, 1976

SUTER PM et al: Optimum end-expiratory airway pressure in patients with acute pulmonary failure. N Engl J Med 292:284, 1975

UNGER K et al: Evaluation of left ventricular performance in acutely ill patients with chronic obstructive lung disease. Chest 68:135, 1975

ZWILLICH GW et al: Complications of assisted ventilation. A prospective study of 354 consecutive episodes. Am J Med 57:161, 1974

273
APPROACH TO THE PATIENT WITH DISEASES OF THE KIDNEYS AND URINARY TRACT

FREDRIC L. COE
BARRY M. BRENNER

Diseases affecting the kidneys or the lower urinary tract can often be detected, even in asymptomatic patients, from clues derived from routine clinical and laboratory examination. Physicians have long appreciated that specific lesions of the urinary tract frequently give rise to a consistent array of clinical signs, symptoms, and laboratory findings which, when taken together, constitute syndromes that effectively narrow the range of causal entities to be considered in the search for an exact diagnosis. Ten such nephrological syndromes have been recognized and are listed in Table 273-1. Although the findings derived from routine evaluation are often sufficient to suggest the presence of one of these syndromes, they are rarely adequate for precise diagnosis. Instead, additional biochemical, serologic, radiological, and/or urologic evaluation is usually required, as is sequential clinical observation. Occasionally, even these approaches prove inadequate, and precise diagnosis must await the results of renal biopsy or exploratory laparotomy. Nevertheless, these syndromes serve as useful frameworks upon which an orderly system of diagnostic nephrology can be based. The purpose of this chapter is to present the general features of these syndromes and the clinical and laboratory data base required for their recognition. Succeeding chapters in this section will then be concerned with detailed descriptions of the various disease entities known to cause the syndromes.

THE MAJOR SYNDROMES IN NEPHROLOGY Acute or rapidly progressive renal failure This syndrome exists in patients in whom glomerular filtration rate (GFR) falls drastically over a period of days (acute) to several weeks (rapidly progressive). Severe oligoanuria and progressive azotemia often accompany the decline in GFR, adding further to the notion of acuteness, since life could not have been sustained for very long with such inadequate renal function. Acute tubular necrosis, considered in detail in Chap. 275, whether due to sepsis, exposure to a known nephrotoxin, or to any of a number of other causes, is usually responsible for acute renal failure. Extracapillary proliferative (crescentic) glomerulonephritis,[1] due to glomerular immunological injury or to vasculitis, leads to deterioration of renal function in a period of weeks to a few months and is, therefore, also an important cause of this syndrome (Chap. 278).

A number of clinical and laboratory abnormalities can be recognized in patients with the syndrome of acute or rapidly progressive renal failure (Table 273-1). Proof for the existence of the syndrome, however, requires documentation of severe oliguria or anuria and a rapid decline in GFR. If these findings are not present, the other clinical and laboratory abnormalities listed in Table 273-1 can be regarded only as clues consistent with, but not proof of, the existence of this syndrome. Ultimately the syndrome of acute or rapidly progressive renal failure can be established only by serial observations, and especially serial determinations of urine flow rate and blood urea nitrogen (BUN) or serum creatinine levels. The causes of this important syndrome and the steps required to invoke or exclude them in a given patient are considered principally in Chap. 275, while other potentially important causes of acute or rapidly progressive renal failure including rapidly progressive glomerulonephritis (Chap. 278), acute interstitial edema (Chap. 281), major renal vascular accidents (Chap. 282), and urinary tract obstruction (Chap. 285) are discussed elsewhere in this section.

Chronic renal failure Chronic renal failure is a syndrome which results from progressive and irreversible destruction of nephrons, regardless of cause (Chap. 276). This syndrome may be considered to exist when GFR is found to be reduced and is known to have been reduced for at least 3 to 6 months (Table 273-1). Often, in fact, a gradual decline in GFR can be documented over a period of years. Proof of chronicity is also provided by the demonstration by abdominal scout film, ultrasonography, intravenous pyelography, or tomography of bilateral reduction of kidney size. Other findings consistent with long-standing renal failure, such as renal osteodystrophy or signs and symptoms of uremia, also help to establish this syndrome (Table 273-1). Several laboratory abnormalities are often regarded as reliable indicators of chronicity of renal disease, such as anemia, hyperphosphatemia, or hypocalcemia, but these are not specific and may be misleading (Chap. 274). In contrast, the finding of broad casts in the urinary sediment (Chap. 42) is quite specific for chronic renal failure, the wide diameters of these casts reflecting the compensatory dilatation and hypertrophy of surviving nephrons. Proteinuria is a frequent but nonspecific finding, as is hematuria. Chronic obstructive uropathy, polycystic and medullary cystic diseases, analgesic nephropathy, and the inactive end stage of any chronic tubulointerstitial nephropathy are excellent examples of conditions in which the urine often contains little or no protein, cells, or casts even though nephron destruction has progressed to the stage of chronic renal failure.

When acute renal failure occurs and there is also clear evidence of chronic renal failure, the acute component must be evaluated as if chronic renal failure were not present, largely because the acute component is potentially reversible. In most instances, depletion of extracellular fluid volume accounts for the acute deterioration of renal function, but other factors such as urinary tract obstruction, drug-induced nephrotoxicity, or exacerbation of the underlying renal disease may also be responsible (Chap. 276).

---

[1] *The term* rapidly progressive glomerulonephritis *is often used to denote renal failure associated with extensive extracapillary proliferation in glomeruli, which leads to crescent formation.*

TABLE 273-1
Initial clinical and laboratory data base for defining major syndromes in nephrology

Syndromes	Important clues to diagnosis	Findings which are common but not of diagnostic value	Location of discussion of diseases causing syndrome
Acute or rapidly progressive renal failure	Anuria Oliguria Documented recent decline in GFR	Hypertension Hematuria Proteinuria Pyuria Casts Edema	Chaps. 275, 278, 281, 282, 285
Chronic renal failure	Azotemia for > 3 months Prolonged symptoms or signs of uremia Symptoms or signs of renal osteodystrophy Kidneys reduced in size bilaterally Broad casts in urinary sediment	Hematuria Proteinuria Casts Oliguria Polyuria, nocturia Edema Hypertension Electrolyte disorders	Chaps. 274, 276
Acute nephritis	Hematuria RBC casts Azotemia Oliguria Edema Hypertension	Proteinuria Pyuria	Chaps. 277 to 279
Nephrotic syndrome	Proteinuria > 3.5 g per 1.73 m² per 24 h Hypoalbuminemia Hyperlipidemia Lipiduria	Casts	Chaps. 278, 279
Asymptomatic urinary abnormalities	Hematuria Proteinuria (below nephrotic range) Sterile pyuria Casts		Chap. 278
Urinary tract infection	Bacteriuria > 10⁵ colonies per milliliter Other infectious agent documented in urine Pyuria, leukocyte casts Frequency, urgency Bladder tenderness Flank tenderness	Hematuria Mild azotemia Mild proteinuria Fever	Chap. 280
Renal tubule defects	Electrolyte disorders Polyuria, nocturia Symptoms or signs of renal osteodystrophy Large kidneys Renal transport defects	Hematuria "Tubular" proteinuria Enuresis	Chaps. 281, 283
Hypertension	Systolic/diastolic hypertension	Proteinuria Casts Azotemia	Chaps. 31, 251, 282
Nephrolithiasis	Previous history of stone passage or removal Previous history of stone seen by x-ray Renal colic	Hematuria Pyuria Frequency, urgency	Chap. 284
Urinary tract obstruction	Azotemia Oliguria, anuria Polyuria, nocturia Urinary retention Slowing of urinary stream Large prostate Large kidneys Flank tenderness	Hematuria Pyuria Enuresis, dysuria	Chap. 285

Acute nephritis A number of diseases involve the glomeruli and, to a generally lesser extent, the tubules in an acute but *transient* inflammatory process, manifested clinically by acute reduction in GFR, rapidly progressive azotemia, oliguria, and salt and water retention. The resulting expansion of the extracellular volume, if marked, leads to hypertension, pulmonary vascular congestion, and facial and peripheral edema (Chap. 278). Damage of the glomerular wall is usually severe enough in almost all causes of this syndrome to permit red blood cells and plasma proteins to gain access to the urinary space (Chap. 42). Gross or microscopic hematuria, red blood cell casts, and proteinuria, therefore, occur with great regularity; their absence should alert the physician to other diagnostic possibilities. In the acute nephritic syndrome these various clinical and laboratory abnormalities (Table 273-1) exhibit a remarkable tendency to wax and wane in synchrony over a period of from several days to a few weeks.

Acute poststreptococcal glomerulonephritis due to infection with group A streptococci is the prototype of the syndrome of acute nephritis (Chap. 278). Immune complexes become deposited in the subepithelial region of the glomerular capillary wall, between the basement membrane and the visceral epithelial cells that separate the membrane from the urinary space. The process is usually self-limited, with renal function returning to normal within weeks to months in the vast majority of affected patients. Acute nephritis can occur during the course of a wide variety of other bacterial and viral infections (Chap. 278), with deposition of immune complexes again believed to be responsible for the usually transient renal damage that occurs. Immune complexes are also believed to be critical to the pathogenesis of lupus nephritis, membranoproliferative glomerulonephritis, and Henoch-Schönlein purpura (Chaps. 277 to 279).

It is important to recognize that all the forms of acute glomerulonephritis and vasculitis that cause acute or rapidly progressive renal failure may mimic the syndrome of acute nephritis at their onset, largely because hematuria, proteinuria, and fluid retention occur commonly during all forms of acute renal failure. But in many of these disorders, the features of renal failure do not wane. This distinction highlights the transient character of the acute nephritic syndrome, because progression to chronic renal failure is uncommon. Acute tubulointerstitial nephritis (Chap. 281), mixed IgG/IgM cryoglobulinemia (Chap. 279), and membranoproliferative glomerulonephritis (Chap. 278) are exceptions to this general principle, however, and often cause chronic renal failure.

Patients with the acute nephritic syndrome usually have a proliferative form of glomerulonephritis, and the prognosis and treatment are influenced strongly by the precise histological and ultrastructural pattern, as well as the types of immune complexes and immunoglobulins deposited in the renal tissues. Renal biopsy is, therefore, a cornerstone in the evaluation of most patients with this syndrome.

Nephrotic syndrome This syndrome is generally held to be present when a patient demonstrates massive proteinuria (usually defined as more than 3.5 g protein per 1.73 m² per 24 h and consisting mainly of albumin), reduced serum albumin concentration, edema, and hyperlipidemia (Table 273-1). Massive proteinuria alone has come to define the syndrome since this finding connotes serious renal disease whether or not the protein losses lead to hypoalbuminemia, lipid disturbances, or edema (Chap. 42). Provided the proteins appearing in the urine are not abnormal paraproteins readily excreted by the normal kidney (e.g., light chains in multiple myeloma), massive proteinuria must be evaluated carefully and completely, irrespective of the physiologic consequences of protein loss.

Common causes of the nephrotic syndrome include lipoid nephrosis, idiopathic membranous nephropathy, focal sclerosing glomerulonephropathy, and diabetic glomerulosclerosis (Chaps. 278 and 279). These diseases typically cause less inflammation than is seen in diseases associated with the acute nephritic syndrome; therefore, the urine contains fewer cellular elements. Acute changes in GFR and urine volume are also uncommon. Hematuria may be a frequent manifestation of some forms of nephrotic syndrome, however, especially chronic membranoproliferative glomerulonephritis (Chap. 278). The presence of many cellular or granular casts should suggest lupus nephritis (Chap. 279) or one of the several known causes of acute nephritis associated with massive proteinuria (Chap. 278).

Asymptomatic urinary abnormalities As indicated in Table 273-1, mild degrees of microscopic hematuria, pyuria, casts, or less than 3.5 g protein per 1.73 m² per 24 h may be present in the urine of a patient lacking concurrent evidence of other nephrological syndromes. By exclusion, these patients are best considered to belong to the syndrome of asymptomatic urinary abnormalities. Isolated hematuria or proteinuria, or unexplained pyuria, are the most frequent abnormalities that occur in this syndrome.

Isolated hematuria, without proteinuria or casts, may be the sole clue to the presence of neoplasm, stone, or infection (e.g., tuberculosis) in any part of the urinary tract (Chaps. 42, 280, 284, and 286). Isolated hematuria may also arise from renal papillae in analgesic and sickle-cell nephropathies (Chaps. 281

and 282). Persistent isolated hematuria often requires intravenous pyelography, cystoscopy, and, occasionally, renal arteriography, to identify the source of bleeding. *Nephronal hematuria,* with red blood cell or pigmented granular casts (Chap. 42), again without proteinuria, occurs mainly in benign recurrent hematuria and Berger's disease (Chap. 278). *Nephronal hematuria and proteinuria* occur together in many specific renal diseases that may eventually lead to chronic renal failure (Chap. 276). In general, the combination of nephronal hematuria and proteinuria suggests a worse prognosis than either one alone.

Isolated proteinuria, without red blood cells or other formed elements in the urinary sediment, is characteristic of many renal diseases which manifest little or no inflammatory reaction within the glomeruli (e.g., diabetes mellitus, amyloidosis). Less than nephrotic-range proteinuria is common in mild forms of all the diseases that can cause overt nephrotic syndrome (Chaps. 278 and 279). "Tubular" proteinuria (Chap. 42) is the rule in cystinosis, heavy metal intoxication from cadmium, lead, or mercury, and in the peculiar Balkan nephropathy localized to only a small region along the Danube River (Chap. 281).

Pyuria may also be a sole urinary abnormality and frequently reflects infection of inflammation of the lower urinary tract, rather than intrinsic parenchymal renal disease. Nevertheless, prominent pyuria can occur in any inflammatory disease of the kidneys, especially tubulointerstitial nephritis, lupus nephritis, pyelonephritis, and renal transplant rejection, but usually in association with mild proteinuria or hematuria. The finding of leukocyte casts (Chap. 42) establishes the kidney as the site of the inflammatory reaction.

Urinary tract infection This syndrome is defined by the demonstration in urine of pathogenic organisms, either bacteria, tubercle bacilli, or fungi (Chap. 280). When urine specimens are obtained for culture, the condition under which the urine is collected must minimize contamination from external genitourinary surfaces. Women should void into a wide-mouthed sterile container after preliminary cleansing of the vulva with a moist, sterile gauze pledget. In men, midstream collection is usually adequate. Bacterial colony counts of 10⁵ organisms per milliliter or greater in urine generally indicate urinary tract colonization and infection. Levels between 10⁴ and 10⁵ colonies per milliliter are usually viewed as suspicious and require reculture. When the urinary tract is anatomically normal, *Escherichia coli* is the usual bacterial pathogen. After prolonged antibiotic treatment of persistent infections, particularly when urinary drainage is impaired or stones are present, *Klebsiella, Enterobacter,* and *Proteus* species predominate.

As discussed in Chap. 280, the presence of a positive urine culture need not imply that an organism is producing tissue inflammation or injury. In some patients, tissue effects may be trivial; in others, injury may be occurring even though symptoms or urinary abnormalities are not present at the time of evaluation. When bacteriuria is associated with tissue inflammation or injury, clinical manifestations usually depend upon the site(s) involved. Dysuria, frequency, urgency and suprapubic tenderness are common symptoms of bladder and urethral inflammation (Chap. 44 and Table 273-1). Prostatitis also leads to frequency, dysuria, and urgency, and the prostate may be boggy and tender on rectal examination. Flank pain, chills, fever, nausea and vomiting, hypotension from sepsis, and leukocyte casts all suggest true renal parenchymal infection, i.e., pyelonephritis (Chap. 280).

Whether or not remediable causes are found, predisposing factors and visible sequelae of urinary tract infection must be sought because they alter prognosis and, therefore, the approach to treatment. The approaches involved and the basis for decision making in this common clinical syndrome are discussed in Chap. 280.

Renal tubule defects This syndrome encompasses a large number of acquired and hereditary disorders, all of which tend to affect tubules more than glomeruli. Hereditary anatomic defects, including such entities as polycystic renal disease, medullary cystic disease, and medullary sponge kidney, are readily detected by intravenous pyelography, which is usually performed because of hematuria, bacteriuria, flank pain, or unexplained azotemia (Chap. 283).

Defects in tubule transport functions, on the other hand, tend not to be associated with prominent renal anatomic defects and arise either as inherited traits (Chap. 283) or during the course of acquired renal disease (Chap. 281). In general, these functional defects impair secretion and/or reabsorption of electrolytes and organic solutes, or limit urinary concentrating and diluting ability (Table 273-1). Typical manifestations of such functional disturbances include polyuria and nocturia (Chap. 43), metabolic acidosis (Chap. 84), and various disorders of fluid and electrolyte balance (Chap. 83). Such defects are defined by direct physiological measurements; their elucidation requires a sound understanding of normal renal physiology.

Hypertension The syndrome of hypertension is considered to exist when the average of a series of reliable blood pressure measurements exceeds 145 mmHg systolic or 95 mmHg diastolic (Table 273-1). The pathogenetic mechanisms, clinical and laboratory manifestations, and therapeutic approaches are discussed in detail elsewhere (Chaps. 23 and 251). In addition, a number of renal complications of hypertension are reviewed in Chap. 282, as is the entity of renal artery stenosis, an infrequent but potentially curable cause of hypertension.

Nephrolithiasis This syndrome is established with certainty when a stone is passed, visualized by x-ray, or removed at surgery or cystoscopy (Table 273-1 and Chap. 284). Less certain, but highly suggestive, evidence of nephrolithiasis exists in the patient with renal colic, painful hematuria or unexplained pyuria, dysuria, and urinary frequency (Chap. 44). Colic varies in its symptomatology but usually begins suddenly in one flank, radiates downward toward the groin, and is excruciatingly painful.

Most renal stones are composed of calcium, uric acid, cystine, or struvite (magnesium ammonium phosphate). All are radiopaque except for those composed solely of uric acid and are, therefore, visible by routine abdominal radiography. Uric acid stones appear as radiolucent filling defects and can be mistaken for tumor or blood clot. The causes of stones are diverse; the approach to their detection, treatment, and prevention is discussed in Chap. 284.

Urinary tract obstruction Documentation of the various structural or functional causes of urinary tract obstruction usually requires radiological or surgical visualization. The manifestations of obstruction, which initiate the search for its causes, are numerous (Table 273-1) and are reviewed in Chap. 285. Anuria in an adult is almost always due to obstruction of bladder outflow. Less commonly, blockage of upper urinary drainage from both kidneys, or from a solitary functioning kidney, accounts for total or near-total cessation of urine flow. A large bladder after voiding is a sign of outflow obstruction, usually due to urethral stricture, tumor, stone, neurogenic causes, or prostatic hypertrophy. Nocturia, frequency and overflow incontinence, and slowing or hesitancy of micturition are also suggestive of outflow obstruction (Chaps. 43 and 44). Upper tract obstruction often produces few clinical manifestations. When it is incomplete or unilateral urine volume may be normal, or even elevated because of a loss of renal concentrating ability (Chap. 43). Urinary stasis secondary to obstruction commonly predisposes to recurrent urinary tract infection.

MISCELLANEOUS DISORDERS In addition to the 10 major syndromes of nephrology that serve as the basis for organization of subsequent chapters in this section, tumors of the urinary tract (Chap. 286) and a variety of vascular disorders that affect the kidneys (Chap. 282) are also considered in this section. The entities considered in these two chapters are heterogeneous, in both their pathogenesis and clinical expression and, therefore, do not lend themselves readily to the syndromic approach.

REFERENCES

BLACK DAK: Diagnosis and renal disease, in *Renal Disease*, DAK Black (ed). New York, Oxford, 1972

CAMERON JS: The natural history of glomerulonephritis, in ibid, p 295

COE FL: The clinical and laboratory assessment of the patient with renal disease, in *The Kidney*, 2d ed, BM Brenner, FC Rector Jr (eds). Philadelphia, Saunders, 1980

274
DISTURBANCES OF RENAL FUNCTION

BARRY M. BRENNER
THOMAS H. HOSTETTER

Near constancy of the composition of the internal environment, including the volume and compartmental distribution of the body fluids, is a condition essential to human survival. With unrelenting acquisition of food and fluids, which vary from day to day in amount as well as composition, preservation of the internal environment requires the continuous excretion of the by-products of these substances, and in amounts that balance precisely the quantities acquired by ingestion and metabolic transformation. Although losses from skin, lungs, and intestine normally contribute to this excretory capacity, by far the greatest responsibility for solute and water excretion is borne by the kidneys.

The kidneys operate primarily to maintain the integrity of the *extracellular* environment. The continuous exchange of water and solutes that takes place across all cell membranes during life, however, permits the kidneys to contribute significantly to the regulation of the volume, composition, and tonicity of the *intracellular* fluids as well. To accomplish these tasks, the human kidney has evolved a number of physiological mechanisms that enable the individual to excrete any excesses of water and nonmetabolized solute contained in the diet, as well as the nonvolatile and end products of nitrogen metabolism, such as urea and creatinine. By contrast, when faced with deficits of water and/or any of the other major constituents of the body fluids, renal excretion of these substances can be curtailed, reducing the likelihood of severe volume or solute depletion. The purpose of this chapter is to review the major functions of the normal kidney and to examine the way these functions are affected by disorders that impair the operations of this organ in humans.

MECHANISMS OF RENAL EXCRETORY FUNCTION WITH NORMAL AND REDUCED NEPHRON MASS

The volume of urine excreted per day (about 1.5 liters, or roughly 1 ml/min) is the small residuum of two very large, and in many ways opposing, processes—namely, *ultrafiltration* of 180 liters or more fluid per day (approximately 125 ml/min) across glomerular capillaries on the one hand and, on the other, *reclamation* (or *reabsorption*) of more than 99 percent of this ultrafiltrate by transport processes operating in the renal tubules. The enormity of the initial step in this process in humans is underscored by the fact that, in humans under resting conditions, about 20 percent of the cardiac output passes through the kidneys, which together comprise less than 1 percent of body weight. Hence, per unit weight of tissue, the rate of blood flow to the kidneys is much greater than that to other solid organs generally considered to be well-perfused, including the heart, brain, and liver.

GLOMERULAR ULTRAFILTRATION Urine formation begins with the elaboration of a protein-free ultrafiltrate of plasma across the walls of the glomerular capillaries. The rate of ultrafiltration (glomerular filtration rate, GFR) is determined by three factors: (1) the balance of pressures acting across the capillary wall (the glomerular capillary hydrostatic and Bowman's space oncotic pressures tend to favor filtration, while glomerular capillary oncotic and Bowman's space hydrostatic pressures tend to retard it), (2) the rate at which plasma flows through the glomeruli, and (3) the permeability and the total surface area of the filtering capillaries. A decrease in GFR can be expected when (1) glomerular hydrostatic pressure is reduced (as in hypotensive shock), (2) tubule (hence, Bowman's space) hydrostatic pressure is increased (ureteral or bladder neck obstruction), (3) plasma oncotic pressure rises to unusually high levels (hemoconcentration due to dehydration; multiple myeloma or other dysproteinemias), (4) renal (hence, glomerular) blood and plasma flow are decreased (circulatory collapse, profound heart failure), and (5) permeability and/or total filtering surface area is reduced (acute or chronic glomerulonephritis).

Despite the extraordinarily high rate of water movement across the glomerular capillary wall, all but the smallest of the circulating plasma proteins are excluded from passage through this barrier. Molecules the size of inulin (approximately 5200 molecular weight), or smaller, normally appear in glomerular urine in the same concentrations as in plasma water, whereas the transport of substances of increasingly greater size diminishes progressively, normally approaching very low values as the size of serum albumin is approached. The *glomerular capillary basement membrane* and the *slit-like diaphragms* that connect adjacent epithelial cell foot processes on the urinary aspect of the glomerular capillary wall are believed to serve as major barriers to protein filtration. In addition to these mechanical gates, *electrostatic factors* also serve to retard the filtration of plasma proteins, especially albumin. The albumin molecule behaves as a polyanion in physiological solution, and is therefore retarded by the highly anionic glycoproteins contained in the various component layers of the glomerular wall. With disruption of these mechanical and electrostatic barriers, as seen in many forms of glomerular injury (see Chaps. 277 to 279), abnormally large quantities of plasma proteins gain access to the urine.

BIOLOGICAL CONSEQUENCES OF SUSTAINED REDUCTIONS IN GFR Measurement of total GFR of both kidneys provides a sensitive and commonly employed index of overall renal excretory function. When renal excretory function is impaired, either acutely or chronically, one or more of the determinants of GFR in affected nephrons is altered unfavorably so that total GFR declines. The magnitude of the decline is determined by the sum of the impairments of function of individual glomeruli. Initially, the effect of such impairments in single-nephron GFR (SNGFR), no matter how small, is to reduce the total rate of excretion of water and those solutes normally contained in the glomerular ultrafiltrate. In the steady state, these reduced rates of filtration, when accompanied by comparably reduced rates of excretion, lead to *retention* and *accumulation* of the unexcreted substances in the body fluids. Further reduction in GFR augments the degree to which these substances are retained.

Figure 274-1 depicts the major patterns of response to these impairments in filtration. The degree of reduction in total GFR is plotted on the abscissa, expressed as a percentage of normal (100 percent). For the various solutes normally contained in glomerular filtrate, three general types of response are common, depicted by curves A, B, and C. Curve A describes the pattern seen with substances, such as creatinine and urea, which normally depend largely on glomerular filtration for their excretion into the urine; i.e., secretion fails to influence urinary excretion appreciably. Therefore, as GFR falls, plasma levels of creatinine, urea, and other substances normally excreted largely by filtration rise progressively, albeit in the nonlinear manner illustrated.

The clinical course of chronic renal failure (CRF) usually also conforms to the pattern described by *curve A*. Patients with CRF usually pass from a long asymptomatic period of "compensation" to a more accelerated and clinically symptomatic terminal phase. In other words, chronic forms of renal

FIGURE 274-1

Representative patterns of adaptation for different types of solutes in body fluids in chronic renal failure. (After NS Bricker et al, in Brenner and Rector.)

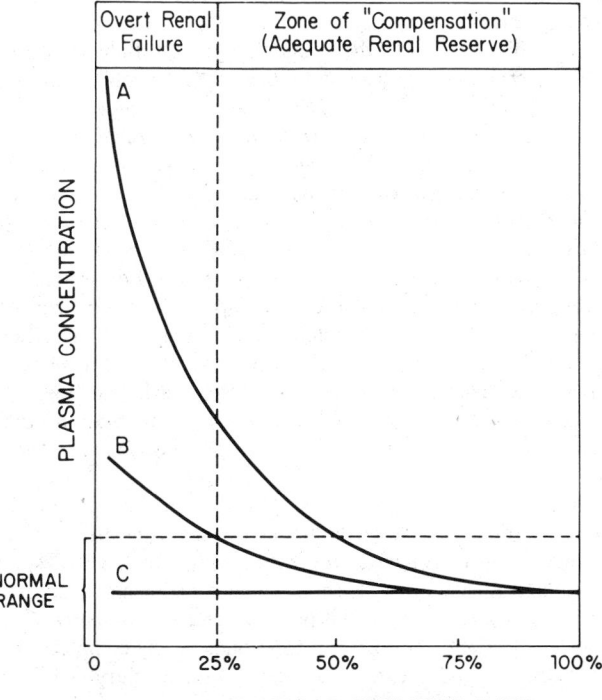

TOTAL GLOMERULAR FILTRATION RATE
(PERCENT OF NORMAL)

injury which lead to slow but inexorable destruction of nephron mass usually lead to progressive but modest elevations in creatinine and urea levels in plasma, but not to levels beyond the range of normal, despite loss of as much as 50 percent of total GFR. With further loss of nephron mass, and further reduction in GFR, however (even though the rate of nephron destruction may not be accelerated), the limits of renal reserve are exceeded, and continued accumulation of *curve A type solutes* leads to plasma concentrations clearly beyond the range of normal (Fig. 274-1). Because these retained solutes are believed to exert "toxic" effects on virtually all organ systems, manifestations of CRF now become overt. As a result, for patients with reduced renal mass, even small additional decrements in total GFR may spell the difference between "compensation" and overt uremia.

Despite this tendency for *curve A type solutes* to accumulate with progressive renal failure, external balance for these solutes can still be achieved. In the case of creatinine, for example, assuming a constant rate of creatinine production, a 50 percent reduction in GFR results in an approximate doubling of the plasma creatinine concentration. The latter restores the filtered load of creatinine (that is, GFR × plasma creatinine concentration) to the preillness level, and urinary excretion rate again becomes equivalent to the rate of creatinine production. Unfortunately, since no mechanism exists for augmenting creatinine excretion beyond this level, elimination of retained creatinine is not possible, and plasma concentration remains twice normal. With progressive reduction in GFR, plasma creatinine levels rise further, due both to the most recent loss of function and to the retention associated with earlier nephron destruction (Fig. 274-1). *In practice, so long as the net rates of acquisition and production remain reasonably constant, the inverse relationship between plasma concentrations of solutes such as creatinine and urea and GFR is sufficiently reliable and predictable to allow plasma levels of such solutes to serve as useful clinical indexes of GFR.*

In contrast to solutes of the *curve A type*, plasma levels of substances such as phosphate, urate, and potassium (K^+) and hydrogen (H^+) ions usually fail to rise above the normal range until GFR falls to a small percentage of normal. With progressive renal failure this pattern of response, depicted by *curve B* in Fig. 274-1, reflects the participation of tubule transport mechanisms that contribute to the excretion of these substances. In other words, *as GFR declines, the tubules facilitate the excretion of progressively greater fractions of the filtered load of these solutes, either by enhancing their net secretion or by diminishing their net reabsorption.* Plasma levels of *curve B type solutes,* therefore, rise much less than do those of *curve A* because, with progressive reduction in GFR, *excretion rate per nephron* and, therefore, *fractional excretion* both increase. Eventually, however, enhanced fractional excretion can no longer offset the inevitable retention of these solutes caused by diminished GFR, and plasma levels rise above the normal range (Fig. 274-1). For urate, phosphate, and K^+ at least, increased fractional excretion usually serves to maintain normal plasma levels until GFR falls to less than one-fourth of normal.

Finally, for certain solutes, such as sodium chloride (NaCl), concentrations in plasma remain virtually constant, and at normal levels, throughout the entire course of CRF, despite continued ingestion of these substances in normal amounts. Such solutes conform to the pattern described by *curve C* in Fig. 274-1. The extent of compensation is nearly complete and represents a fundamental adaptation to renal injury. To illustrate the magnitude of the adaptation involved, it is useful to compare the pattern of Na^+ excretion in an individual with

normal renal excretory function (GFR of 125 ml/min) with that in an individual with advanced renal insufficiency (GFR of 2 ml/min). Both subjects are allowed to ingest a diet containing 7 g salt per day (120 meq Na^+). With a normal serum Na^+ concentration of 140 meq per liter, external Na^+ balance is achieved in the normal individual by excreting approximately 0.5 percent of the filtered load of Na^+. By contrast, for external balance to be maintained in the patient with CRF, fractional excretion of Na^+ must rise to 30 percent. *In other words, external balance for Na^+ demands that the same quantity of Na^+ (120 meq) be excreted into the urine each day in the subject with CRF as in the normal subject.* Given the drastic reduction in GFR faced by the patient with CRF, external balance can be achieved only by a progressive transformation of the Na^+ reabsorptive processes in surviving tubules, so that a progressively larger fraction of the filtered load of Na^+ escapes reabsorption and appears in final urine. In short, *the rate of excretion of Na^+ per surviving nephron increases in inverse proportion to the composite GFR of surviving nephrons.*

MECHANISMS OF TUBULE TRANSPORT WITH NORMAL AND REDUCED NEPHRON MASS Loss of renal function with nearly all forms of progressive renal disease is usually attended by a progressive distortion of renal morphology and architecture. Despite this structural disarray, glomerular and tubular functions often remain as closely integrated (i.e., *glomerulotubular balance*) in the diseased kidney as they do in the normal organ, at least until the final stages of CRF. A fundamental feature of this *intact nephron hypothesis* is that following loss of nephron mass, residual renal function derives primarily from the operation of surviving healthy nephrons, while the diseased nephrons are believed to cease functioning. Despite progressive nephron destruction, there is considerable evidence to suggest that many of the mechanisms that contribute to the maintenance of solute and water balance differ only quantitatively, and not qualitatively, from those believed to govern fluid and solute homeostasis under normal physiological conditions. The most important of these are considered below.

Tubule transport of sodium chloride and water in health Most of the filtered water and Na^+ salts are reabsorbed by the tubules, leaving small and variable amounts, equivalent on a day-to-day basis to the quantities ingested, to reach the final urine. About two-thirds of the glomerular ultrafiltrate is reabsorbed in the *proximal tubule* without changing the osmolality or Na^+ concentration of the unreabsorbed fraction (Fig. 274-2). In other words, fluid reabsorption in the proximal tubule is *isosmotic*. Reabsorption of Na^+ across the proximal tubule cell involves a two-step process. Since the Na^+ concentration in the cell is lower, and the voltage more negative, than in either the tubule lumen or peritubular fluid, the movement of Na^+ from lumen to cell proceeds down electrochemical gradients and is therefore a passive process. Efflux of Na^+ from tubule cell to peritubular interstitial fluid is believed to be due to an active, energy-dependent process, although the mechanism involved is not well understood. According to current concepts, salts of Na^+ enter proximal tubule cells through the luminal brush border membrane and then are transported from the cells into *lateral intercellular channels*. As a result, salt concentration (and osmolality) within the channels exceeds that in adjacent tubule cells or surrounding interstitium, causing movement of water from tubule lumen and cell interior into the channels by osmosis. As a consequence, the hydrostatic pressure within the channels rises, driving fluid into the surrounding peritubular interstitium.

The rate of reabsorption of fluid from proximal convoluted tubules and peritubular interstitium is sensitive to the effects of *physical factors*, i.e., the hydrostatic and colloid osmotic (or oncotic) pressures acting across the walls of the peritubular

PROXIMAL CONVOLUTED TUBULE

DISTAL CONVOLUTED TUBULE

FIGURE 274-2

Transport functions of the various anatomic segments of the mammalian nephron. Fluid reabsorption across the proximal tubule is isosmotic and accounts for approximately two-thirds of the reabsorption of filtered Na^+ and H_2O. The major portions of the filtered HCO_3^-, amino acids, and glucose are reabsorbed in the early proximal convoluted tubule. Reabsorption of glucose and amino acids is coupled to Na^+ transport and thereby generates a negative potential difference within the tubule lumen. At the same time, $NaHCO_3^-$ is reabsorbed by a nonelectrogenic mechanism, most likely via H^+ secretion. The active transport of these solutes results in transepithelial concentration and effective osmotic pressure gradients promoting H_2O flow across the proximal tubule, into the peritubular capillaries. The rise in tubule fluid Cl^- concentration is a necessary reciprocal consequence of the decreased luminal HCO_3^- concentration. The resultant high concentration of Cl^- becomes an important force for the outward passive transport of Cl^- down its concentration gradient, resulting in a lumen positive potential difference in the late proximal convoluted tubule. The pars recta of the proximal tubule is capable of active electrogenic transport of Na^+ independent of organic solute transport. Under normal conditions, approximately one-third of the glomerular filtrate enters the descending limb of Henle's loop. Because the thin descending limb is incapable of active outward NaCl transport and is characterized by low permeability to Na^+ but high H_2O permeability, H_2O is abstracted passively as the fluid approaches the bend of Henle's loop.

Hypertonic fluid with a greater NaCl concentration but lower urea concentration than the surrounding medullary interstitium thus enters the thin ascending limb of Henle. This segment differs from the descending limb in that it is largely impermeable to H_2O and urea but highly permeable to NaCl. These characteristics allow for passive diffusion of NaCl out of the ascending limb. Active electrogenic Cl^- transport across the water-impermeable thick ascending limb of Henle, with Na^+ following passively, allows for separation of solute and water. In consequence tubule fluid becomes dilute, and the medullary interstitium hypertonic. Irrespective of the final osmolality of the urine, the fluid that enters the distal convoluted tubule is always hypoosmotic. This segment exhibits active Na^+ reabsorption. All but the terminal portion of the distal convoluted tubule is water impermeable, even in the presence of ADH. Aldosterone exerts its effect in this segment by enhancing Na^+ reabsorption, which is variably coupled to K^+ and H^+ secretion. The cortical and papillary portions of the collecting duct are sites where ADH exerts its principal effect. The permeability of these segments to H_2O in the absence of ADH is very low but can be greatly enhanced in the presence of ADH. These segments are also characterized by active Na^+ reabsorption, which appears to depend on the presence of mineralocorticoid. In the absence of ADH, the collecting tubule is water impermeable so that hypotonic tubule fluid courses through it. However, in the presence of ADH, water is avidly reabsorbed here, resulting in hypertonic final urine.

capillaries. Because the plasma proteins in glomerular capillaries are concentrated by ultrafiltration, there is a marked rise in the oncotic pressure as plasma flows along the glomerular capillary network. This step-up in plasma oncotic pressure is transmitted largely unchanged to the peritubular capillaries, via the efferent arterioles. These resistance vessels cause a substantial drop in hydrostatic pressure, however, so that when the plasma reaches the peritubular capillaries, oncotic pressure greatly exceeds hydrostatic pressure. These *Starling forces* are

therefore oriented in an *uptake mode*, in contrast to the *filtration mode* at the glomerulus, where hydrostatic pressure exceeds oncotic. The extent to which oncotic pressure exceeds hydrostatic pressure in the peritubular capillary network is thought to modulate the overall rate of reabsorption of fluid by the proximal tubules. Therefore, when peritubular oncotic pressure falls, or hydrostatic pressure rises, uptake of fluid by these capillaries is reduced. As a result, fluid is retained in the interstitial space, altering the hydrostatic pressure in the space, and ultimately retarding the egress of fluid from the lateral intercellular channels. Without an adequate route of drainage, fluid in the channels leaks back into the tubule lumen and diminishes *net fluid reabsorption* by this tubule segment. The opposite occurs in states in which peritubular oncotic pressure increases (increased filtration fraction), or hydrostatic pressure decreases (enhanced efferent arteriolar tone). Under these circumstances, peritubular capillary uptake of reabsorbate is augmented, leading ultimately to *enhanced net fluid reabsorption* by the proximal tubule.

In contrast to the proximal tubule, active outward transport of NaCl from tubule lumen to peritubular blood has not been established for the *thin limbs of Henle's loop*. In the next segment of the nephron, the *medullary thick ascending limb of Henle,* the concentration of NaCl is reduced below the level that prevails at the beginning of this segment. Here the means for lowering the salt concentration involves the *active transport of Cl⁻*, with Na⁺ following passively to preserve electroneutrality. Since the ascending limb of Henle is always impermeable to water, net NaCl reabsorption not only generates hypotonic tubule fluid, but also gives rise to the high NaCl concentration of the outer medullary interstitium (Fig. 274-2).

The fluid leaving the thick ascending limb of Henle is normally low in NaCl concentration, a condition largely independent of the organism's diet or state of hydration. In the *distal convoluted tubule,* water reabsorption is variable, depending on the state of hydration or, more specifically, on the presence or absence of the *antidiuretic hormone (ADH)* in plasma. In the absence of ADH, this and more distal nephron segments are impermeable to water, so that the hypotonic fluid entering this segment is excreted as *dilute urine.* Indeed, continued salt reabsorption along the distal convoluted tubule results in further dilution of the urine. In the presence of ADH, the permeability of the late portion of this segment to water increases, and as a result, the osmolality of the late distal tubule fluid rises to a value close to that of plasma. NaCl continues to be reabsorbed from the tubule lumen, against moderately steep chemical and electrical gradients. The reabsorptive process for NaCl at this site is enhanced by *aldosterone.*

The *cortical collecting tubule* possesses an extremely low permeability to water in the absence of ADH, whereas this permeability increases greatly in the presence of the hormone. The sensitivity of this segment to ADH appears to be more pronounced than is that of the distal convoluted tubule. As with the distal convoluted tubule, the cortical collecting tubule is capable of further net reabsorption of NaCl.

The terminal segment of the distal nephron is the highly branched *papillary collecting duct.* Continued electrolyte transport in this segment results in the large ion concentration differences that normally exist between urine and plasma. As in the cortical collecting tubule, Na⁺ transport appears to be active since reabsorption proceeds against sizable electrochemical gradients. The rate of Na⁺ transport in this segment depends on the diet and on the load of Na⁺ delivered from more proximal segments, and is affected by aldosterone. The permeability of this segment to water also increases markedly in the presence of ADH.

Effects of reduced nephron mass on sodium chloride transport in surviving nephrons   With progressive destruction of nephrons, *maintenance of external balance for NaCl requires that fractional salt excretion increases as GFR decreases.* Very likely several mechanisms contribute to this adaptive increase in fractional salt excretion. With losses of functioning nephron units, peritubular capillary hydrostatic and oncotic pressures are probably altered in directions that serve to suppress proximal tubule reabsorption of NaCl and water. For example, a rise in peritubular capillary hydrostatic pressure, which tends to inhibit net proximal fluid reabsorption, might be anticipated with arterial hypertension, a common feature of renal insufficiency. Similarly, peritubular oncotic pressure might be expected to decline with renal injury, owing both to reductions in filtration fraction and to hypoalbuminemia. While such alterations in peritubular factors clearly account for diminution in proximal fluid reabsorption in response to falling levels of GFR in animals, such alterations have not been established with certainty in humans. Aldosterone, normally an important determinant of Na⁺ reabsorption in distal portions of the nephron, is probably not a major factor responsible for reducing fractional Na⁺ reabsorption, since aldosterone levels in plasma are rarely reduced in CRF. Furthermore, external Na⁺ balance has been shown to be preserved in bilaterally adrenalectomized uremic dogs maintained on fixed doses of mineralocorticoid hormones. Yet another factor that has received attention in contributing to the suppression of fractional NaCl reabsorption in CRF relates to the retention of solutes as GFR declines. In addition to urea and creatinine, a host of *organic acids* (including *hippurates*) also accumulate. These substances are normally excreted by both filtration and tubule secretion; the latter process involves a carrier-mediated organic acid transport system in proximal tubule epithelia. When GFR is reduced and plasma levels of these organic acids increase, sufficient fluid may accompany the secretion of these organic anions into the proximal tubule lumen (by osmosis) to diminish net fluid reabsorption, and even favor net fluid secretion. Evidence in support of this intriguing mechanism derives from studies in which uremic serums were capable of inducing net fluid secretion in isolated proximal tubules of rabbits studied in vitro.

It has also been suggested that NaCl transport across the mammalian renal tubule may be governed, at least in part, by a *natriuretic hormone*. In support of this possibility, serums and urine from patients and dogs with uremia have been reported to contain factors capable of inhibiting NaCl transport across frog skin, toad bladder, and rat renal tubule. However, accumulation of natriuretic factors in uremia may not be without cost; the "trade-off" for maintenance of external Na⁺ balance is the possibility of abnormalities occurring in Na⁺ transport across cell membranes, which often occurs in advanced renal insufficiency. This possibility is discussed in greater detail in Chap. 276.

The obligatorily high rate of solute excretion per surviving nephron (so-called "osmotic diuresis" due to urea and other retained solutes) may also contribute to enhancing fractional NaCl excretion, much as occurs in normal subjects following administration of nonreabsorbable solutes such as mannitol. Finally, certain forms of CRF tend to be associated with unusually pronounced salt losses in urine. These *salt-wasting nephropathies* include chronic pyelonephritis and other tubulointerstitial diseases (see Chap. 281) as well as polycystic and medullary cystic diseases. These disorders have in common greater destruction of medullary and interstitial, than cortical and glomerular, portions of the renal parenchyma. Preferential impairment of tubule reabsorptive function, rather than a primary reduction in GFR, may, therefore, underlie the salt-losing tendency in these disorders. A number of clinical derangements associated with the altered renal handling of NaCl in CRF (including hypo- and hypervolemia, hypertension, etc.) are considered in Chap. 276.

Effects of reduced nephron mass on water reabsorption in surviving nephrons   As with NaCl, there is a progressive increase in the fractional excretion of water with advancing renal insufficiency, so that even the patient with a total GFR of 5 ml/min or less can usually maintain external water balance. The adaptations in the handling of water by the tubules of the diseased kidney are of importance in the pathogenesis of the urinary concentrating defect and, hence, of the polyuria and nocturia seen commonly in CRF (see Chap. 43). To appreciate the mechanisms involved, the responses of a normal and a uremic subject in maintaining external water balance need to be compared. Assuming that both subjects ingest the same diet and also the same amount of fluid, total solute and volume excretion in each subject should be identical as well. If the *obligatory solute load* to be excreted in each is assumed to be 600 mosmol per day, and urine osmolality is 300 mosmol/kg, a urine volume of 2 liters per day will be required to excrete the total solute load in each subject. If GFR in normal and uremic subjects is 180 and 4 liters per day, respectively, urinary volume excretion of 2 liters per day represents excretion of slightly more than 1 percent of the filtered water in the normal individual, compared with a much larger value, 50 percent, in the uremic subject. Since the range of urine osmolalities that the diseased kidney can achieve (250 to 350 mosmol/kg) is much narrower than in the normal (40 to 1200 mosmol/kg), the individual with normal function is able to excrete the obligatory daily solute load of 600 mosmol in as little as 500 ml urine per day or as much as 15 liters per day, compared with the much narrower range in the patient with renal insufficiency, from about 1.7 to 2.4 liters per day.

In CRF, the limited ability to concentrate the urine usually correlates closely with other measures of impaired renal function. Isosthenuria is, therefore, a nearly universal finding when GFR falls below 25 ml/min. At this level of GFR and below, urine osmolality becomes insensitive even to supramaximal doses of ADH, suggesting that the concentrating defect is related not only to loss of diseased nephrons but also to impaired concentrating ability in surviving nephrons. As has been discussed, with diminution in functioning nephron mass, there is a concurrent increase in fractional excretion of a number of solutes. As a consequence, solute diuresis per nephron obligates a nearly isosmotic amount of water and prevents the elaboration of hypertonic urine, even in the presence of adequate amounts of ADH. Disease-induced abnormalities of the architecture of the renal medulla (loops of Henle, vasa rectae), aberrations in renal medullary blood flow, and defective transport of NaCl in the ascending limb of Henle undoubtedly also contribute to this defect in urine concentration. Finally, there is suggestive evidence that uremia per se may impair the responsiveness of terminal nephron segments to ADH.

Since patients with renal insufficiency are usually unable to excrete concentrated urine, they must have access to adequate amounts of water in order to ensure the excretion of total daily solute loads. For this reason, restriction of fluid intake may prove extremely hazardous in patients with CRF. Likewise, impairment of diluting capacity may prevent many patients from excreting large amounts of ingested fluids. The consequences of the abnormal water excretion patterns in CRF, including the tendencies to development of hypo- and hypernatremia, are considered in Chaps. 84 and 276.

Tubule transport of phosphate with normal and reduced nephron mass Under normal physiological conditions, about 80 to 90 percent of the filtered load of phosphate is reabsorbed, mainly in the proximal tubule. *Parathyroid hormone (PTH)* augments phosphate excretion by inhibiting this proximal reabsorptive process (Chap. 349). Hence, with enhanced PTH secretion, reabsorption of phosphate can fall markedly, to as little as 15 percent of the amount filtered. By modifying phosphate reabsorption, PTH plays a key role in phosphate homeostasis. In normal humans, when dietary phosphate intake increases, a *transient* rise in plasma phosphate concentration is usually observed. This results in a similarly transient reduction in the plasma ionized calcium concentration (due largely to calcium-phosphate deposition in bone), which, in turn, stimulates PTH

secretion. By enhancing fractional phosphate excretion, PTH restores external phosphate balance and normophosphatemia. This then enables plasma ionized calcium levels to return to normal, thereby removing the stimulus to PTH release, and restoring all elements of the phosphate control system to the original steady state.

With advancing renal disease, and constant dietary intake of phosphate, external phosphate balance is achieved by progressive reduction in fractional phosphate reabsorption. Enhanced PTH secretion is an important determinant of this phosphaturic response to reduced nephron mass. Figure 274-3 provides a schematic summary of the mechanisms believed to be involved. As shown, with each succeeding decrement in GFR, the total amount of phosphate filtered by surviving glomeruli is reduced, leading to transient retention of phosphate and, therefore, a rise (albeit small) in the phosphate concentration in extracellular fluid, including plasma. This rise in plasma phosphate concentration leads to a reciprocal small decline in plasma ionized calcium concentration and a corresponding increase in PTH secretion. Although the phosphaturic response of surviving tubules to this elevation in circulating PTH is thought to restore plasma phosphate and, therefore, calcium levels to normal (at least in the "compensated" stage of CRF described by the relatively flat portion of curve B in Fig. 274-1), the biological cost of this return to normophosphatemia and normocalcemia is a *persistent elevation in the plasma PTH level*. As shown in Fig. 274-3, with successive decrements in GFR, each stage in this overall process is repeated, but at an ever-increasing cost, namely, *progressive elevation in the circulating level of PTH*. At least two additional processes are thought to contribute to elevated PTH levels in renal failure. One relates to the skeletal resistance to the calcemic effect of PTH seen in uremia. This resistance necessitates a greater than normal level of circulating PTH to effect an increment in serum calcium concentration. The other derives from evidence indicating that reductions in renal mass impair the ability of the kidneys to degrade circulating PTH. The fact that phosphate conforms more to a curve B than curve C type solute in Fig. 274-1 indicates that these forms of adaptation are limited; ultimately phosphate retention occurs when GFR falls below about 25 ml/min.

FIGURE 274-3

The "Bricker" model for return to external phosphate balance in chronic renal failure. (From NS Bricker et al, in Brenner and Rector.)

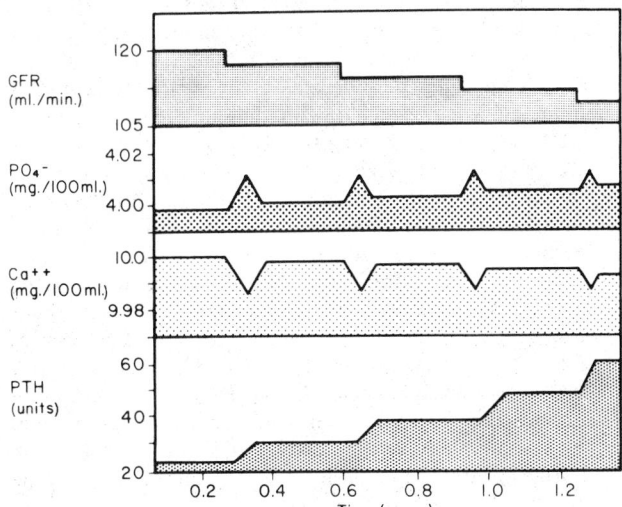

Since PTH exerts major biological effects on bone, as well as renal tubules, the external balance of phosphate in CRF is achieved at the expense of elevated PTH levels, which, in turn, account for many of the bone changes of renal osteodystrophy (i.e., *secondary hyperparathyroidism,* Fig. 276-1). In support of this ingenious *trade-off hypothesis,* studies in animals with CRF suggest that when dietary phosphate intake is reduced in proportion to the reduction in GFR, external balance of phosphate no longer requires augmentation of fractional phosphate excretion in surviving nephrons. Accordingly, circulating PTH levels no longer rise, and the typical bone changes of secondary hyperparathyroidism are diminished, if not prevented.

Destruction of renal mass also impairs phosphate, calcium, and skeletal metabolism by mechanisms largely independent of impaired excretory function. The kidneys are normally the major site of *metabolic conversion of vitamin D to its active metabolites.* Whereas the tendency to secondary hyperparathyroidism begins, at least theoretically, when a single nephron unit is destroyed, impaired vitamin D biotransformation is not usually apparent until GFR falls to below 25 percent of normal. As discussed in detail in Chap. 351, precursors of the active form of vitamin D, synthesized in skin or acquired from foods, undergo initial hydroxylation in the liver to form 25-hydroxyvitamin D_3 [25-(OH)D_3]. The kidney is the site of a second important hydroxylation step, to form 1,25-dihydroxyvitamin D_3 [1,25-(OH)$_2D_3$]. This activated form of vitamin D operates to enhance intestinal calcium and phosphate absorption, as well as to promote resorption of these ions from bone. In addition, 1,25-(OH)$_2D_3$ probably opposes the phosphaturic action of PTH at the level of the renal tubule, by augmenting, rather than diminishing, phosphate reabsorption. With advancing renal disease, reduction in renal mass causes vitamin D hydroxylation to be impaired; phosphate retention has also been shown to suppress this important hydroxylation reaction. Reduction in circulating 1,25-(OH)$_2D_3$ levels, by suppressing calcium absorption from gut, contributes further to the development of the hypocalcemia and PTH excess of CRF, the conditions of which are considered in Chap. 276.

Hydrogen and bicarbonate transport with normal and reduced nephron mass   As discussed in Chap. 85, the pH of extracellular fluid in humans is normally maintained within a narrow range, 7.36 to 7.44, despite day-to-day variations in the quantity of acids entering the body fluids from dietary and metabolic sources (approximately 1 meq H$^+$/kg per day). These acids consume buffer, of which bicarbonate (HCO$_3^-$) is the most important. Such buffering minimizes the changes in pH that would otherwise occur. The HCO$_3^-$ buffer system would be of little long-term benefit were it not for homeostatic mechanisms, however, since with unrelenting acquisition of nonvolatile acids from dietary and metabolic sources, buffering capacity would ultimately be exhausted, eventually culminating in fatal acidosis. The kidneys normally function to prevent this possibility by *regenerating* HCO$_3^-$ and, thereby, maintaining the concentration of HCO$_3^-$ in the plasma. In addition to generating HCO$_3^-$, the kidneys also *reclaim* essentially all the HCO$_3^-$ present in the glomerular ultrafiltrate. This reabsorptive process takes place in the proximal tubule and is virtually complete below a critical serum HCO$_3^-$ concentration—the threshold concentration—which in humans is normally about 26 meq per liter, identical to the concentration of HCO$_3^-$ in plasma. As a consequence, urinary wastage of HCO$_3^-$ is prevented. Alternatively, when plasma HCO$_3^-$ concentration rises above this threshold level, reabsorption of HCO$_3^-$ becomes less complete, and the excess HCO$_3^-$ escapes into the final urine, returning the plasma HCO$_3^-$ concentration to the threshold level. Despite reabsorption of all the filtered HCO$_3^-$, metabolic acidosis would still ensue if HCO$_3^-$ consumed in buffering nonvolatile strong acids were not constantly regenerated.

The *reabsorption* of filtered HCO$_3^-$ and the *regeneration* of new HCO$_3^-$ occur by a single mechanism. In proximal tubule cells, H$^+$, formed by the splitting of water into H$^+$ and OH$^-$, is secreted into the tubule lumen, very likely in exchange for Na$^+$. The OH$^-$ ion, under the influence of *carbonic anhydrase,* combines with CO$_2$ to form HCO$_3^-$, which diffuses across the peritubular cell membrane to enter the extracellular HCO$_3^-$ pool. The H$^+$ secreted into the tubule lumen combines with a filtered HCO$_3^-$, forming H$_2$CO$_3$. Dehydration of the latter in the proximal tubule lumen leads to the formation of CO$_2$ which also diffuses from lumen to peritubular blood. As a result, *a filtered HCO$_3^-$ ion is reclaimed.* Secreted H$^+$ ions are also free to combine with non-HCO$_3^-$ buffers (e.g., phosphate or ammonia) in the tubule fluid and to be excreted in these forms in the final urine. HCO$_3^-$, the other original product of the breakdown of H$_2$CO$_3$, formed within the tubule cell, enters the peritubular blood, and *a HCO$_3^-$ ion is regenerated.*

Hydrogen ions in the urine are bound primarily to filtered buffers (e.g., phosphate) in an amount (the so-called "titratable acid") equivalent to the amount of alkali required to titrate the pH of the urine to the pH of blood. It is usually not possible, however, to excrete all the daily acid load as titratable acid alone. To serve as additional buffer, the cells of the renal tubules generate ammonia (NH$_3$), largely from the hydrolysis of glutamine. NH$_3$ diffuses from these cells into the tubule lumen where it combines with H$^+$ to form NH$_4^+$. As noted above, each mole of NH$_4^+$ excreted into the urine is associated with the regeneration of one mole of HCO$_3^-$. *Ammoniagenesis,* a process which occurs within proximal tubule cells, is responsive to the acid-base needs of the individual. When faced with an acute acid burden and an increased need for HCO$_3^-$ regeneration, the rate of renal ammonia synthesis increases sharply.

The quantity of hydrogen ions excreted as titratable acid and NH$_4^+$ is equal to the quantity of HCO$_3^-$ regenerated in tubule cells and added to the plasma. Under steady-state conditions, the quantity of net acid excreted into the urine (the sum of titratable acid and NH$_4^+$ minus HCO$_3^-$) must equal the quantity of acid gained by the extracellular fluid from all sources. Metabolic acidosis and alkalosis result when this delicate balance is perturbed, the former the result of *insufficient* net acid excretion, the latter due to *excessive* acid excretion.

Progressive loss of renal function usually causes little or no change in arterial pH, plasma bicarbonate concentration, or arterial carbon dioxide tension (P_{CO_2}) until GFR falls below 50 percent of normal. Thereafter, all three quantities tend to decline as *metabolic acidosis* ensues. In general, the metabolic acidosis of CRF is not due to overproduction of endogenous acids, but is largely a reflection of the reduction in renal mass, which limits the amount of NH$_3$ (and therefore HCO$_3^-$) that can be generated. Although surviving nephrons are probably capable of generating supernormal quantities of NH$_3$ *per nephron,* the diminished nephron population causes overall NH$_3$ production to be reduced to an extent inadequate to permit sufficient buffering of H$^+$ in urine. Though patients with CRF may acidify the urine normally (i.e., urine pH as low as 4.5), the defect in NH$_3$ production limits total daily acid excretion to 30 to 40 meq, or half to two-thirds the quantity of nonvolatile acid formed in the same time period. Metabolic acidosis is the inevitable consequence of this positive balance for H$^+$, which in most patients with stable CRF is relatively mild and nonprogressive (arterial pH of approximately 7.33 to 7.37).

Given this substantial daily accumulation of H$^+$, and the typically stable and nonprogressive nature of the resulting acidosis, including the observed relative constancy of the plasma

HCO$_3^-$ concentration (albeit at reduced levels of 14 to 20 meq per liter), it follows that some large tissue source of buffering must account for the stability of the acidosis in CRF. Bone is the most likely candidate, particularly in view of its large reservoir of alkaline salts (calcium phosphate and calcium carbonate). Dissolution of this buffer source probably contributes to the osteodystrophy of CRF (see Fig. 276-1).

Although the acidosis of CRF is a consequence of the reduction in total renal mass and is therefore tubular in origin, it nevertheless depends to a large extent on the level of GFR. When GFR is reduced to only a moderate extent (i.e., to about 50 percent of normal), retention of anions, principally sulfates and phosphate, is not pronounced, so that as the plasma HCO$_3^-$ level falls owing to tubular dysfunction, retention of Cl$^-$ by the kidneys leads to the development of *hyperchloremic acidosis*. At this stage, therefore, *the anion gap is normal*. With further reduction in GFR and more pronounced azotemia, however, retention of phosphates, sulfates, and other *unmeasured* anions is the rule, and plasma Cl$^-$ concentration falls to normal levels despite the reduction in plasma HCO$_3^-$ concentration. *A moderate to large anion gap therefore develops.*

Tubule potassium transport with normal and reduced nephron mass As with H$^+$, the concentration of K$^+$ in extracellular fluid is normally maintained within a relatively narrow range, 4 to 5 meq per liter. Ninety-five percent or more of total body K$^+$ is in the intracellular fluid compartment, where the intracellular concentration is approximately 160 meq per liter. Normal individuals maintain external K$^+$ balance by excreting into the urine an amount of K$^+$ per day equivalent to the amount ingested, minus the relatively small amounts lost in stool and sweat. K$^+$ is freely filtered at the glomerulus, although the amount excreted usually represents no more than about 20 percent of the quantity filtered. The great bulk of the filtered K$^+$ is *reabsorbed* in the early portions of the nephron, about two-thirds in the proximal tubule, and an additional 20 to 25 percent in the loop of Henle. A K$^+$ *secretory process* operates in the distal tubule and terminal nephron segments. This process is largely dependent on exchange of K$^+$ for Na$^+$, the reabsorbed Na$^+$ creating an electrical gradient across the tubule wall, lumen negative. K$^+$ therefore diffuses from the cell interior into the lumens of distal tubules and collecting ducts, down this electrical gradient.

The ability to maintain external K$^+$ balance and normal plasma K$^+$ concentration as well, until relatively late in the course of CRF, is a consequence primarily of a progressive increase in fractional excretion of K$^+$. Greatly enhanced rates of K$^+$ secretion in distal portions of surviving tubules appear to underlie this adaptation. The augmented secretion rate of aldosterone is believed to contribute to enhanced tubule secretion of K$^+$, as does the osmotic diuresis and enhanced luminal electronegativity created by retention of highly nonpermeating anions such as phosphate and sulfate. Aldosterone also stimulates net entry of K$^+$ into the lumen of the colon, a mechanism known to be enhanced in CRF. More detailed discussions of the abnormalities in K$^+$ homeostasis in acute and chronic forms of renal failure are given in Chaps. 275 and 276.

REFERENCES

BRENNER BM, RECTOR FC JR (eds): *The Kidney*, 2d ed. Philadelphia, Saunders, 1980

BRICKER NS: On the pathogenesis of the uremic state: An exposition of the "trade-off" hypothesis. N Engl J Med 286:1093, 1972

MAXWELL MH, KLEEMAN CR: *Clinical Disorders of Fluid and Electrolyte Metabolism*, 3d ed. New York, McGraw-Hill, 1978

ROSE BD: *Clinical Physiology of Acid-Base and Electrolyte Disorders*. New York, McGraw-Hill, 1977

275

ACUTE RENAL FAILURE

ROBERT J. ANDERSON
ROBERT W. SCHRIER

INTRODUCTION Acute renal failure is broadly defined as a rapid deterioration in renal function sufficient to result in accumulation of nitrogenous wastes in the body. The causes of such deterioration may have a prerenal, postrenal, or renal parenchymal origin (Table 275-1) and therefore include renal hypoperfusion, obstructive uropathy, and intrinsic renal diseases such as acute glomerulonephritis. This chapter deals with acute reversible renal failure (see Table 275-1), a condition commonly termed *acute tubular necrosis* even though the histological findings of tubular necrosis are not consistently present.

ETIOLOGY Sixty percent of all cases of acute reversible renal failure are related to surgery or trauma, 40 percent occur in a medical setting, and 1 to 2 percent are related to pregnancy. The most common cause is renal ischemia. Clinical conditions associated with renal ischemia include rapid hemorrhage, profound volume depletion, intraoperative hypotension, cardiogenic shock, and operative procedures associated with interruption of renal circulation. Duration of renal hypoperfusion is important. If it is brief, correction of defects in intravascular

TABLE 275-1
Major causes of acute deterioration in renal function

Diseases	Examples
PRERENAL FAILURE	
Hypovolemia	Skin, gastrointestinal, or renal volume loss; hemorrhage; sequestration of extracellular fluid (burns, pancreatitis, peritonitis)
Cardiovascular failure	Impaired cardiac output (infarction, tamponade); vascular pooling (anaphylaxis, sepsis, drugs)
POSTRENAL FAILURE	
Obstruction	Urethral obstruction; bladder, pelvic, prostatic, or retroperitoneal neoplasms; prostatism; surgical accidents; medications; calculi
Bladder rupture	Trauma
ACUTE REVERSIBLE RENAL FAILURE (ACUTE TUBULAR NECROSIS)	
Postischemic	All conditions listed above for prerenal failure
Pigment-induced	Hemolysis (transfusion reaction, malaria); rhabdomyolysis (trauma, muscle disease, coma, heat stroke, severe exercise, potassium or phosphate depletion)
Toxin-induced	Antibiotics; contrast material; anesthetic agents, heavy metals; organic solvents
Pregnancy-related	Septic abortion; uterine hemorrhage; eclampsia
OTHER RENAL DISEASES	
Vascular disease	Vasculitis; malignant hypertension; thrombotic thrombocytopenic purpura; scleroderma; arterial or venous occlusion
Acute glomerulonephritis	Poststreptococcal; bacterial endocarditis; systemic lupus erythematosus
Interstitial disease	Drugs; idiopathic
Intratubular precipitation	Multiple myeloma; uric acid; oxalate; methotrexate; sulfonamides
Miscellaneous	Hypercalcemia; diffuse pyelonephritis

volume or cardiac output can restore renal function. With longer duration of renal hypoperfusion, acute tubular necrosis may supervene.

Nephrotoxic agents are a frequent cause of acute renal failure. In the past, heavy metals, organic solvents, and glycols were common inducers of acute renal failure. Although these toxins are less frequently encountered currently, their occasional occurrence serves to illustrate the importance of seeking a history of occupational and environmental toxin exposure in each patient with acute renal failure. More recent studies suggest that aminoglycoside antibiotics are now the leading nephrotoxic cause of acute renal failure. The acute renal failure associated with these drugs is enhanced by depletion of intravascular volume, advancing age, the presence of underlying renal disease, and the concomitant use of other nephrotoxic agents or potent diuretics. Some anesthetic agents (methoxyflurane and enflurane) and radiographic contrast agents also may induce renal failure. Contrast agent–induced nephrotoxicity is especially common in dehydrated patients with underlying diabetic nephropathy.

Release of large amounts of myoglobin into the circulation is recognized with increasing frequency as a cause of acute renal failure. Rhabdomyolysis is often due to extensive trauma and crush injuries. However, nontraumatic rhabdomyolysis associated with increased muscle oxygen consumption (heat stroke, severe exercise, and seizures), decreased muscle energy production (hypokalemia, hypophosphatemia, and genetic enzymatic deficiencies), muscle ischemia (arterial insufficiency, drug overdosage with resultant coma and muscle compression), infections (influenza), and direct toxins (alcohol) also can produce rhabdomyolysis resulting in acute renal failure. Careful questioning of patients with acute renal failure for muscular symptoms as well as examination for tender, swollen muscles is important, although many of these patients may have muscle necrosis without muscle symptoms. The exact mechanism whereby myoglobinuria results in acute renal failure is uncertain. There is substantial evidence that myoglobin is not directly nephrotoxic. However, direct nephrotoxicity of other muscle breakdown products, as well as tubular obstruction due to myoglobin precipitation and cast formation, has been proposed. Most patients with rhabdomyolysis-associated acute renal failure also have concomitant depletion of intravascular volume and renal hypoperfusion.

Intravascular hemolysis may also cause acute renal failure. Although pure hemoglobin per se is not a potent nephrotoxin, toxic substances from red blood cell stroma and concomitant renal hypoperfusion may act synergistically to induce renal failure. In spite of intensive investigation, experienced clinicians are often unable to establish a definite etiology for some cases of acute renal failure. In other cases, multiple etiologies are likely, as in patients with shock who are volume depleted, have received transfusions, are septic, and have received antibiotics.

PATHOPHYSIOLOGY A unifying pathogenic schema of acute renal failure must account for several observed clinical phenomena: the severe reduction in glomerular filtration as measured clinically by creatinine clearance, the moderate reduction in renal blood flow which remains in a range compatible with life-sustaining glomerular filtration rate, the variability of renal histological alterations, the variability in urine flow rate ranging from extreme oliguria to polyuria, the ability of both ischemic and toxic insults to result in a clinically identical syndrome of acute renal failure, and the potential for complete reversibility of the renal functional and histological abnormalities.

Current pathogenic theories developed largely in animal models can be divided into those suggesting either a tubular or a vascular basis for acute renal failure. One tubular theory suggests that casts and debris obstruct tubular lumina with resultant increases in intratubular pressure sufficient to decrease net glomerular filtration pressure. Alternatively, it has been suggested that severe constriction of the afferent arteriole provides a vascular basis for a marked reduction in glomerular filtration pressure. The mechanisms of this afferent arteriolar constriction may be related to renal nerve stimulation or to the effect of humoral substances such as angiotensin II or catecholamines. Both supporting and contradicting evidence can be found for each of these theories. While a precise pathogenic schema of acute renal failure is not presently available, it is likely that both tubular and vascular events are of pathogenic importance. Additional studies are needed to define the relative importance of each factor and to differentiate between mechanisms that initiate and maintain acute renal failure.

PATHOLOGY The histopathologic alterations observed in kidneys of patients with acute renal failure are variable. Frequently, no abnormalities are observed. Varying degrees of tubular necrosis with disrupted, necrotic, or regenerating tubular epithelium, intratubular casts, interstitial edema, and interstitial cellular infiltration can be seen. Both tubular collapse and dilated tubules can be observed. Unless either disseminated intravascular coagulation or severe, prolonged ischemic insults are present, intrarenal blood vessels and glomeruli are normal by light and electron microscopy. Microdissection studies demonstrate two general types of renal lesion. Following direct nephrotoxic injury, a uniform, diffuse necrosis of proximal tubular cells, especially of proximal convoluted tubules, with intact tubular basement membrane, is observed. In contrast, following renal ischemia, mild, patchy necrosis occurs throughout the nephron which tends to be most marked in distal tubular segments at the corticomedullary junction. Disruption of tubular basement membrane is also observed. A striking lack of correlation between renal histopathologic changes and renal function parameters is often noted in acute renal failure. Renal biopsies performed after recovery from acute renal failure either demonstrate minor abnormalities or are normal.

DIFFERENTIAL DIAGNOSIS (Table 275-1) The diagnosis of acute renal failure is a diagnosis of exclusion since prerenal (renal hypoperfusion), postrenal (obstruction of urine flow), and other intrarenal disorders (glomerulonephritis, renal interstitial and vascular diseases, and intrarenal crystal precipitation) may all lead to an identical clinical syndrome of deteriorating renal function. In contrast to acute renal failure, however, prerenal, postrenal, and other intrarenal disorders are often specifically treatable.

Impaired renal perfusion from extrarenal cause may result in sufficient reduction in glomerular filtration so that the daily endogenous load of nitrogenous wastes cannot be excreted. The azotemia can be reversed if the cause of the renal ischemia is corrected. This may require expansion of extracellular fluid volume, improvement in cardiac output, or restoration of normal renal perfusion pressure. A careful history with regard to volume loss or sequestration and symptoms of impaired cardiac output is necessary in patients with declining renal function. In addition, physical examination with specific attention to orthostatic hypotension and tachycardia, decreased jugular venous pressure, cardiac dysfunction, and skin turgor should be an initial undertaking in any patient with renal deterioration.

Obstruction to urine flow at any level of the urinary tract must be considered in every patient with renal failure. At the bladder, urinary retention secondary to anatomic (prostatic disease) or functional (organic or drug-induced neuropathy) bladder neck obstruction is a relatively common cause of renal failure and can be evaluated by suprapubic palpation and percussion as well as a single bladder catheterization to measure postvoiding residual volume. Obstruction of the upper urinary tract is a less common cause of renal failure since it requires simultaneous obstruction of both ureters or unilateral ureteric obstruction with absence of, or severe disease in, the contralateral kidney. Causes of bilateral urinary tract obstruction include retroperitoneal fibrosis and space-occupying processes such as tumor or abscess, surgical accident, and bilateral intraureteric occlusion (stones, papillary tissue, blood clots, or pus). A careful rectal and pelvic examination is essential in evaluation. A plain film of the abdomen may help detect retroperitoneal disease or radiopaque calculi. If obstruction of the upper urinary tract cannot be excluded by infusion pyelography, ultrasound, or computerized tomography (CT scanning), investigation of the patency of the ureter(s) by retrograde pyelography may be required. Knowledge of normal renal function prior to the renal failure allows examination for patency of only one ureter since bilateral urinary tract obstruction would be necessary to cause azotemia. On the other hand, unilateral ureteric obstruction occurring on the background of chronic renal failure may be sufficient to precipitate symptoms of uremia. In this setting, documentation of patency of both ureters is necessary to exclude a contributing role for urinary tract obstruction in causing the decline in renal function.

Intrarenal parenchymal or vascular diseases which are listed in Table 275-1 can also cause an acute decline in renal function. Although these disorders are less frequent than acute tubular necrosis, they are often amenable to specific therapy and should be considered in each case of deterioration in renal function.

The initial presentation of the patient with end-stage renal failure may be confused with acute renal failure when there is no information about renal function prior to presentation. Under these circumstances, the presence of uremic osteodystrophy, uremic neuropathy, small kidney size on abdominal films, and unexplained anemia suggest chronic renal failure. Some end-stage renal diseases such as amyloidosis, diabetic glomerulosclerosis, scleroderma, and rapidly progressive glomerulonephritis may have normal-sized kidneys, necessitating time for continued observation and, in some circumstances, renal biopsy to distinguish between potentially reversible forms of acute renal failure and end-stage chronic renal failure.

Observation of the pattern of urine flow may provide a diagnostic clue as to the cause of declining renal function. Complete anuria (no urine by catheterization) virtually never occurs in acute tubular necrosis. Potential causes of total anuria include complete bilateral ureteric obstruction, diffuse cortical necrosis, rapidly progressive glomerulonephritis, and bilateral renal artery occlusion. Wide fluctuations in daily urine output suggest intermittent obstructive uropathy. Polyuria ($>$ 3 liters per day) can be a hallmark of partial urinary tract obstruction. This occurs secondary to the accompanying defect in renal concentrating ability. Although oliguria ($<$ 400 ml per day) has been considered to be a cardinal feature of acute renal failure, a substantial portion of patients have urine volumes of greater than 1 liter per day (nonoliguric acute renal failure).

Examination of the urinary sediment is of great value in the differential diagnosis of acute renal failure. Sediment containing few formed elements or only hyalin casts strongly suggests prerenal azotemia or obstructive uropathy. With acute tubular necrosis, brownish pigmented cellular casts and many renal tubular epithelial cells are observed in over 75 percent of patients. Red blood cell casts suggest the presence of glomerular or vascular inflammatory diseases of the kidney and rarely, if ever, occur with acute tubular necrosis. The presence of large numbers of polymorphonuclear leukocytes singly or in clumps suggests acute diffuse pyelonephritis or papillary necrosis. Eosinophilic casts on Wright's stain of urine sediment supports a diagnosis of acute allergic interstitial nephritis. The combination of brownish pigmented granular casts and positive occult blood tests on urine in the absence of hematuria indicates either hemoglobinuria or myoglobinuria. In acute renal failure, the finding in fresh, warm urine of large numbers of uric acid crystals may suggest a diagnosis of acute uric acid nephropathy, while the finding of large numbers of oxalic acid or hippuric acid crystals suggests ethylene glycol toxicity. The presence of large numbers of broad casts (greater than two to three white blood cells in diameter) suggests chronic renal disease.

Chemical analysis of urine composition is also helpful in differentiating acute tubular necrosis from prerenal azotemia and is depicted in Table 42-1. It is important to recall that other disorders associated with abrupt deterioration in renal function and intact renal tubular integrity such as glomerulonephritis and early (few hours) obstructive uropathy have urine chemical values similar to those encountered in prerenal azotemia. Prior administration of diuretic agents as well as osmotic diuresis due to glycosuria may interfere with avid renal tubular reabsorption of sodium and water and thus alter urinary chemical indexes. Acute uric acid nephropathy may be differentiated from other causes of acute renal failure by a urinary uric acid to creatinine concentration ratio of greater than 1.

CLINICAL COURSE The clinical course of acute renal failure can be divided into an initiating phase, a maintenance phase, and a recovery phase. The initiating phase is the period of time between the precipitating event and the appearance of renal failure no longer reversible by manipulation of extrarenal factors. Recognition of the initiating phase of acute renal failure is extremely important since early correction of the underlying cause of renal failure may prevent the development of the maintenance phase. However, the initiating phase of acute renal failure may come to the attention of the clinician only in retrospect because it lacks characteristic signs and symptoms.

Oliguria has been considered the cardinal feature of the initiating and maintenance phases of acute renal failure. However, recent studies suggest that 25 to 50 percent of all patients with acute renal failure are nonoliguric ($>$ 800 ml per day). Although progressive renal failure without oliguria can result from any type of renal insult, including both ischemic and toxic insults, this form of renal failure appears to be particularly frequent following nephrotoxic (e.g., aminoglycoside) drug administration. Progressive azotemia occurs in nonoliguric patients owing to the marked impairment in glomerular filtration rate and renal concentrating capacity. For example, maximal concentrating ability of the nonoliguric patient averages only 350 mosmol/kg water. Therefore, with a urine output of 1000 ml per day, 350 mosmol solute can be excreted daily. In acute renal failure, daily solute loads may be increased from normal values of 600 mosmol to values to as high as a 1000 mosmol. Thus, a positive solute (predominately urea and creatinine) balance and azotemia would occur despite a daily urine output of 1 liter.

Oliguria characterizes the maintenance phase of acute renal failure in more than 50 percent of cases. When oliguria occurs, it starts shortly following the inciting event and lasts an average of 10 to 14 days. However, the oliguric phase may be as short as a few hours or as long as 6 to 8 weeks. Prolonged oliguria is common in the elderly patient with underlying vascular disease. If oliguria persists for longer than 4 weeks, the diagnosis of acute tubular necrosis should be reconsidered, and entities such as diffuse cortical necrosis, rapidly progressive glomerulonephritis, renal artery occlusion, and renal vasculitis should be evaluated. Anuria is not characteristic of acute tubular necrosis. However, a few days of severe oliguria with urine volume less than 100 ml per day may be encountered with acute tubular necrosis.

Urinary elimination of nitrogenous wastes, water, electrolytes, and acid is impaired in the initiating and maintenance phases of acute renal failure. The magnitude of resultant abnormalities in blood chemistry depends on whether the patient is oliguric or nonoliguric and on the catabolic state of the patient. Nonoliguric patients have higher levels of glomerular filtration than do oliguric patients and thus excrete more water and electrolytes in their urine. Hence, abnormalities in blood chemistry are generally milder in nonoliguric than oliguric patients with acute renal failure.

In the afebrile, noncatabolic, oliguric patient with acute renal failure, the daily increments in blood urea nitrogen (BUN) and serum creatinine average 10 to 20 and 0.5 to 1.0 mg per 100 ml, respectively. In catabolic patients with fever, sepsis, or extensive trauma, daily increments in BUN and serum creatinine may be as high as 40 to 100 and 2 to 5 mg per 100 ml, respectively. In patients with acute renal failure due to rhabdomyolysis, the daily increment in serum creatinine may be disproportionately high compared with the BUN. This is due to release of creatine from muscle which is converted by nonenzymatic hydrolysis to creatinine.

Salt and water overload with resultant hyponatremia, edema, and pulmonary congestion are ever-present dangers in patients with acute renal failure, particularly in oliguric patients. Hyponatremia results from excessive water intake and edema from excessive sodium and water intake. Rarely, the nonoliguric patient with a relatively high rate of urine flow and high concentration of urine sodium will develop intravascular volume depletion which may retard recovery of renal function.

Hyperkalemia due to decreased renal elimination of potassium occurring with continued tissue potassium release is a frequent accompaniment of acute renal failure. The usual rate of increase in serum potassium in the noncatabolic, oliguric patient is 0.3 to 0.5 meq per day. Higher rates of rise in serum potassium concentration should suggest the possibility of an endogenous (tissue destruction) or exogenous (medication, diet, blood transfusion) potassium load or of cellular shift of potassium due to acidemia. Generally, hyperkalemia is asymptomatic until serum potassium increases to values greater than 6.0 to 6.5 meq per liter. Above that level, electrocardiographic abnormalities (bradycardia, recent appearance of left axis deviation, peaked T waves, prolonged QRS complexes, prolonged PR interval, and decreased amplitude of the P waves) and ultimately cardiac arrest can occur. Hyperkalemia can also result in muscle weakness and flaccid quadriparesis.

Hyperphosphatemia, hypocalcemia, and mild *hypermagnesemia* are usually present in acute renal failure. Hyperphosphatemia results from decreased renal phosphorus elimination in the face of continued release of phosphorus from tissues. The serum phosphorus is usually in the range of 6 to 8 mg per 100 ml, but much higher values may be encountered in the traumatized, catabolic patient as well as in one with rhabdomyolysis. Hypocalcemia in the range of 6 to 9 mg per 100 ml often develops during acute renal failure. The reason for this decrease in serum calcium concentration is not clear. Increases in serum magnesium to levels of 2 to 3 mg per 100 ml are often observed in acute renal failure. The serum magnesium elevation is mild unless magnesium-containing compounds such as antacids are ingested.

Metabolic acidosis is a regular accompaniment of acute renal failure. The daily production of approximately 1 meq per kilogram of body weight of nonvolatile acid from endogenous metabolic sources can no longer be eliminated by the damaged kidney. A resultant retention of organic acids occurs which is sufficient to produce a daily decrease of 1 to 2 meq in plasma bicarbonate and metabolic acidosis with an anion gap occurs.

Hyperuricemia in the range of 9 to 12 mg per 100 ml due to decreased renal uric acid excretion is usually present in acute renal failure. In catabolic patients with extensive tissue damage, much higher values of serum uric acid may be observed. Elevation of serum amylase due to impaired renal amylase excretion may be observed in the absence of clinical evidence of pancreatitis. The elevations of amylase are mild and less than twice the upper limit of normal.

Abnormalities in the hematologic examination are usually present in acute renal failure. A normocytic normochromic anemia develops shortly following the onset of significant azotemia, and the hematocrit usually stabilizes between values of 20 to 30 percent. This anemia is due to impaired erythropoiesis as well as to a mild and variable degree of extracorpuscular hemolysis. Additional factors that often contribute to anemia include hemodilution, gastrointestinal blood loss, and suppressed erythropoiesis due to infections or drug administration. White blood cell production is not severely disturbed in acute renal failure. However, since acute renal failure usually occurs in the setting of stress and tissue damage, mild leukocytosis is usually present. Leukocytosis persisting after the initial week of acute renal failure should suggest the possibility of infection. Mild degrees of thrombocytopenia due to reduction of bone marrow platelet production may be observed early in the course of acute renal failure. Qualitative defects in platelet function occur and, in association with additional poorly defined coagulation disturbances, contribute to the bleeding tendency of acute renal failure. Acute renal failure may be a complication of several primary hematologic or vascular disorders that have major hematologic manifestations such as disseminated intravascular coagulation, thrombotic thrombocytopenic purpura, hemolytic uremic syndrome, and systemic lupus erythematosus.

Cardiovascular complications of acute renal failure involve circulatory congestion, hypertension, arrhythmias, and pericarditis. Circulatory congestion is usually due to excessive sodium and water administration. Mild hypertension is seen in 15 to 25 percent of cases and usually appears in the second week of oliguria. This hypertension is usually a manifestation of extracellular fluid volume overload. Supraventricular arrythmias may complicate 20 to 30 percent of cases of acute renal failure. Known causes for these arrythmias include congestive heart failure, electrolyte abnormalities, digitalis intoxication, pericarditis, and anemia. Pericarditis currently occurs infrequently, probably because of the early institution of dialytic therapy.

Neurological abnormalities are common in acute renal failure. In undialyzed patients, lethargy, somnolence, confusion, disorientation, asterixis, agitation, myoclonic muscle twitching, and generalized seizures may be observed. These neurological abnormalities are most often encountered in the elderly patient and generally respond well to dialytic therapy. In addition to renal failure per se, drug administration, electrolyte abnormalities, and primary neurological disease should be considered as potential causes of neurological disturbances in the patient with acute renal failure.

Gastrointestinal complications of acute renal failure are common and include anorexia, nausea, vomiting, ileus, and poorly defined abdominal pains. The combination of stress of acute illness and hemostatic abnormalities can lead to gastrointestinal hemorrhage in 10 to 30 percent of patients. Fortunately, the gastrointestinal hemorrhage is usually mild in nature and easily controlled with conservative therapy.

Infections complicate 30 to 70 percent of all cases of acute renal failure and are a leading cause of morbidity and mortality. The sites of infection include the respiratory tract, operative sites, and urinary tract. Resultant septicemia is frequent, and both gram-positive and gram-negative organisms are encountered. Although the exact factors responsible for the high rate of infection remain to be determined, disruption of normal anatomic barriers with intravenous infusions and indwelling catheters may play a role.

The recovery phase of acute renal failure commences when the glomerular filtration rate increases so that the BUN and serum creatinine concentrations no longer continue to increase. In oliguric acute renal failure, the recovery phase is heralded by a progressive increase in urine volume. Generally, in the first days the urine volume may double daily, and in some cases a daily urine volume of greater than 2 liters may be observed for a few days. In nonoliguric patients, a marked diuretic phase is usually not observed. The duration of BUN and serum creatinine concentrations greater than 50 and 5 mg per 100 ml, respectively, averages 15 to 25 days in oliguric patients and 5 to 10 days in nonoliguric patients. The major complications of acute renal failure such as infections, gastrointestinal hemorrhage, fluid and electrolyte disturbances, and cardiovascular dysfunction may persist or first appear during the recovery phase of acute renal failure. In addition, persistent abnormalities in glomerular and tubular function can lead to over- or underhydration or electrolyte disturbances unless continued careful daily weight, intake and output, biochemical, and clinical monitoring are undertaken during the recovery phase of acute renal failure. In particular, hypercalcemia has been observed to occur during the diuretic phase of acute renal failure, especially in patients with rhabdomyolysis. The cause of this complication remains obscure.

Although the major improvement in renal function occurs within the first 1 to 2 weeks of the recovery phase, renal function continues to improve for up to 12 months following acute renal failure. Sensitive tests of glomerular and tubular function suggest that mild defects in renal function persist indefinitely following acute tubular necrosis. However, the vast majority of patients achieve clinically normal renal function, and there is no evidence of later progression of renal dysfunction or of complications such as hypertension.

The mortality rates in large series of patients with acute renal failure vary from 30 to 60 percent. The mortality rates are highest in postoperative or traumatized patients (50 to 70 percent), intermediate in patients with acute renal failure encountered in a medical setting (30 to 50 percent), and lowest in acute renal failure observed in an obstetrical setting (10 to 20 percent). Advanced age, the presence of serious underlying illness, and the development of multiple medical complications during the course of acute renal failure are associated with higher mortality rates. Nonoliguric acute renal failure is associated with a lower mortality rate than oliguric acute renal failure. Infections, complications resulting from fluid and electrolyte disturbances, gastrointestinal hemorrhage, and progression of the primary underlying disease are the major causes of mortality in acute renal failure.

MANAGEMENT The first principle of therapy in acute renal failure is to exclude causes of deterioration in renal function which are potentially remedial. A search for prerenal factors, obstructive uropathy, glomerulonephritis, renal vascular and interstitial disease, and intrarenal crystal precipitation should be performed. Once the diagnosis of acute tubular necrosis is made by exclusion, little specific therapy is available. Dialysis for the removal of nephrotoxins such as carbon tetrachloride and ethylene glycol may be indicated. Even in the presence of acute tubular necrosis, any prerenal factors should be corrected both to improve the circulation and avoid delay in the onset of the renal recovery. In the oliguric patient in whom prerenal factors have been corrected, it has become common clinical practice to administer either a potent loop diuretic or mannitol in an attempt to enhance urine flow. The rationale for such therapy is based on the thought that there is an early phase of renal failure during which the correction of prerenal factors and establishment of urine flow can lead to a nonoliguric state. Prospective studies have demonstrated lower morbidity and mortality in nonoliguric as compared with oliguric acute renal failure. However, a prospective study of the utility of potent diuretics in early acute renal failure is needed.

Conservative therapy is capable of controlling many of the manifestations of acute renal failure. After any defects in intravascular volume have been corrected, fluid intake should equal measured output plus estimated insensible losses. Sodium and potassium administration should not exceed measured losses. Daily monitoring of fluid balance and body weight allow assessment of the patient's volume status. A weight loss of 0.2 to 0.5 kg per day occurs in the well-managed patient with acute renal failure. Greater weight loss suggests hypercatabolism or volume depletion, and lesser weight loss suggests excessive salt and water administration. The serum sodium concentration provides a guideline for water administration. A decrease in serum sodium concentration indicates that excess water is present, while an abnormally high serum sodium concentration indicates a deficiency of water.

In an effort to minimize catabolism, intake should include at least 100 g carbohydrate per day. Recently some studies suggest that central intravenous administration of a mixture of amino acids and hypertonic glucose improves morbidity and mortality in patients with acute renal failure following surgical procedures or trauma. Since parenteral hyperalimentation may be associated with significant complications, confirmatory studies, as well as studies on noncatabolic patients with acute renal failure in a medical setting, are needed. Alternative means of alimentation in acute renal failure include peripheral intravenous alimentation utilizing lipid and glucose solutions and the utilization of a small nasogastric feeding tube. In the past, anabolic androgens have been utilized in the hope of decreasing protein catabolism and diminishing the rate of rise of blood urea nitrogen. Such therapy is not generally utilized at present. Additional means of minimizing catabolism include early removal or debridement of necrotic tissue, control of pyrexia, and early, specific antimicrobial therapy.

The mild metabolic acidosis associated with acute renal failure is generally not treated unless serum bicarbonate falls to below 10 meq per liter. Rapid correction of acidemia by acute alkali administration may decrease ionized calcium concentrations and precipitate tetany. Hypocalcemia rarely requires specific therapy. Hyperphosphatemia should be controlled with 30 to 60 ml aluminum hydroxide administered orally four to six times per day, since a high calcium-phosphorus product ($>$ 70) may cause soft-tissue calcification. For the occasional patient with profound hyperphosphatemia, early dialysis therapy and intravenous alimentation may help control elevated serum phosphate concentration. Unless acute uric acid nephropathy is a diagnostic consideration, the secondary hyperuricemia of acute renal failure is usually not treated with allopurinol. Because of the low glomerular filtration rate, the filtered load of uric acid, and thus intratubular deposition, are low. Also, for unknown reasons, clinical gout rarely complicates acute renal failure despite hyperuricemia. Careful observation of the hematocrit and stool for occult fluid is important in the early detection of gastrointestinal blood loss. If a decrease in hematocrit out of proportion of renal failure occurs, alternative causes of anemia should be sought.

Congestive heart failure and hypertension indicate the presence of volume overload and should be treated accordingly, recognizing, of course, that many drugs such as digoxin are excreted largely by the kidneys. Hypertension occasionally may persist, however, in the absence of volume overload, and factors such as hyperreninemia may contribute to this hypertension. Selective histamine-2 receptor blockade (cimetidine) therapy has been of benefit in preventing gastrointestinal bleeding in some seriously ill patients but has not yet been studied in acute renal failure. Avoidance and early detection of infection require minimization of interruption of normal anatomic barriers, including avoidance of long-term catheterization of urinary bladder, provision of mouth and skin care, promotion of early mobilization, utilization of aseptic techniques for intravenous and tracheostomy sites, and close clinical and temperature monitoring. Fever and suspected infection should be promptly evaluated with careful inspection of lung, wound, urinary tract, and intravenous sites. Since the metabolism and elimination of many drugs are impaired in acute renal failure, careful adjustment of drug doses is required.

Hyperkalemia is an ever-present threat in acute renal failure. Mild elevations of serum potassium (< 6.0 meq per liter) can best be treated by withdrawal of all sources of potassium and by continued close laboratory observation. If serum potassium increases to values greater than 6.5 meq per liter and particularly if any electrocardiographic changes appear, active therapy should be instituted. Therapy of such hyperkalemia can be divided into emergent and nonemergent forms. Emergent therapy includes intravenous administration of calcium (5 to 10 ml of 10% calcium chloride solution intravenously over 2 min with electrocardiographic monitoring) and of bicarbonate (44 meq intravenously over 5 min), insulin and glucose (200 to 300 ml of 20% glucose with 20 to 30 units regular insulin given intravenously over 30 min). Nonemergent therapy includes administration of potassium-binding ion exchange resins such as sodium polystyrene sulfonate (Kayexalate). This can be administered orally every 3 to 4 h in 25 to 50-g doses with 100 ml 20% sorbitol (to avoid constipation). Alternatively, in the patient who cannot take oral medications, 50 g Kayexalate and 50 g sorbitol in 200 ml water can be given as a retention enema at 1- to 2-h intervals. With refractory hyperkalemia, hemodialysis may be necessary.

Some patients with acute renal failure, particularly those that are nonoliguric and noncatabolic, can be successfully managed with minimal or no dialytic therapy. There has been an increasing tendency to use dialysis therapy early in acute renal failure in an attempt to minimize the development of complications. Early use of dialysis frequently simplifies management, allowing more liberal fluid and potassium intake and improvement of the general well-being of the patient. Absolute indications for dialysis include symptomatic uremia (usually manifest by central nervous system and/or gastrointestinal symptomatology), development of resistant hyperkalemia, severe acidemia or fluid overload not responsive to medical therapy, and pericarditis. In addition, many centers attempt to keep predialysis levels of BUN and serum creatinine less than 100 and 8 mg per 100 ml, respectively. Doing so may require infrequent dialysis in the noncatabolic, nonoliguric patient or daily dialysis in the catabolic, traumatized patient. Peritoneal dialysis is an acceptable means of dialysis even in the postoperative patient. However, because of the relative lack of efficiency of peritoneal dialysis, its use is often contraindicated in the catabolic patient, and it is most useful when the need for infrequent dialysis is anticipated.

PREVENTION Because of the high mortality and morbidity rates of acute renal failure, prophylactic therapy deserves special mention. A major reduction in deaths secondary to acute renal failure occurred from the Korean War (1 in 200 casualties) to the Vietnamese conflict (1 in 1900 casualties). This reduction in the incidence of acute renal failure paralleled earlier evacuation from the field and early expansion of intravascular volume. Thus, identification of patients at high risk for the development of acute renal failure is important. Such high-risk patients include those with multiple trauma, burns, rhabdomyolysis, and intravascular hemolysis, those receiving potential nephrotoxins, and those undergoing operative procedures necessitating interruption of renal blood flow. In these patients, particular attention should be given to maintaining optimal intravascular volume, cardiac output, and urine flow rates. Care in the use of potential nephrotoxic drugs combined with frequent monitoring of renal failure, early therapy of cardiogenic shock, sepsis, and eclampsia of pregnancy may also reduce the occurrence of acute renal failure.

ACUTE RENAL FAILURE IN PREGNANCY When acute renal failure occurs during pregnancy, it is usually in the earliest or latest stages. During the first trimester of pregnancy, acute renal failure usually occurs in the setting of nontherapeutic, nonsterile abortion. In these cases, volume depletion, sepsis, and nephrotoxins contribute to renal failure. This form of renal failure has markedly declined with the current widespread availability of sterile abortion.

Acute renal failure can also occur because of either excessive postpartum hemorrhage or preeclampsia in the latter stages of pregnancy. The majority of patients with this type of acute renal failure totally recover renal function. A small number of pregnant patients with acute renal failure have not recovered renal function, and histological evidence of diffuse cortical necrosis is present. This entity usually complicates severe hemorrhage of abruptio placentae and is associated with clinical and laboratory evidence of intravascular coagulation.

A rare form of acute renal failure occurring 1 to 12 weeks following uncomplicated pregnancy has been described in a few cases (postpartum glomerulosclerosis). This form of renal failure is usually characterized by irreversible, rapidly progressive renal failure, although milder cases have been described. All these patients have an associated microangiopathic hemolytic anemia. The renal histopathologic changes are indistinguishable from malignant hypertension or scleroderma. The pathophysiology of this disorder has not been defined. No therapeutic modality is consistently successful, although heparin therapy is widely advocated.

HEPATORENAL SYNDROME The hepatorenal syndrome is a serious complication of advanced liver disease in which renal failure occurs in the absence of clinical, laboratory, or anatomic evidence of other causes of renal dysfunction. The renal failure is usually associated with oliguria, an unremarkable urinary sediment, and low urinary sodium concentrations (< 10 meq per liter). Generally, the renal failure occurs in the setting of advanced hepatic cirrhosis complicated by jaundice, ascites, and hepatic encephalopathy. Occasionally, this syndrome may complicate fulminant hepatitis. The mechanism of the renal failure is not known. The lack of consistent histopathologic alterations in kidneys of patients with this syndrome and the restoration of normal renal function when kidneys from donors with hepatorenal syndrome are transplanted into recipients without liver disease suggest a functional renal hemodynamic defect.

Treatment of the hepatorenal syndrome is usually unsuccessful. Care should be taken in the cirrhotic patient not to induce major changes in intravascular volume by large paracentesis or aggressive diuresis, maneuvers which may precipitate hepatorenal syndrome. Since this syndrome mimics prerenal azotemia, a cautious trial of expansion of intravascular volume is warranted. In a few cases, recovery has followed either portacaval shunting or insertion of an abdominal-venous (Leveen) shunt. These treatment modalities have not been subjected to controlled trials. Improvement in hepatic function often results in parallel improvement in renal function. Every effort should be made to ensure that more specifically treatable causes of concomitant liver and renal dysfunction such as infections (leptospirosis, hepatitis with immune complex disease), toxins (aminoglycosides, carbon tetrachloride), and circulatory disorders (severe heart failure, shock) are not present. It should also be recalled that jaundiced patients with liver disease are also susceptible to acute tubular necrosis.

REFERENCES

ANDERSON RJ et al: Nonoliguric acute renal failure. N Engl J Med 296:1134, 1977

LEVINSKY NG, ALEXANDER EA: Acute renal failure, in *The Kidney,* BM Brenner, FC Rector Jr (eds). Philadelphia, Saunders, 1976, p 806

SCHRIER RW, CONGER JD: Acute renal failure: Pathogenesis, diagnosis and management, in *Renal and Electrolyte Disorders,* RW Schrier (ed). Boston, Little, Brown, 1976, p 2891

STEIN JH et al: Current concepts on the pathophysiology of acute renal failure. Am J Physiol 234:F171, 1978

276
CHRONIC RENAL FAILURE

BARRY M. BRENNER
J. MICHAEL LAZARUS

In contrast to the remarkable capacity of the kidney to regain function following the various forms of acute renal injury discussed in the preceding chapter, renal injury of a more sustained nature is often not reversible but leads instead to progressive destruction of nephron mass. Glomerulonephritis, tubulointerstitial diseases, diabetic nephropathy, and nephrosclerosis are among the most common causes of chronic renal failure. These and other progressive forms of renal disease are considered in detail in the remaining chapters of this section. Irrespective of cause, the eventual impact of severe reduction in nephron mass is an alteration in function of virtually every organ system in the body. *Uremia* is the term generally applied to the clinical syndrome observed in patients suffering from profound loss of renal function. Although the cause(s) of the syndrome remain unknown, the term uremia was adopted originally because of the presumption that the abnormalities seen in patients with chronic renal failure (CRF) resulted from *retention* in the blood of urea and the other end products of metabolism normally excreted into the urine. It is clear that the uremic state represents more than failure of renal excretory function alone, because a host of metabolic and endocrine functions normally subserved by the intact kidney are also impaired in CRF. Furthermore, the inexorably progressive course to renal failure is often accompanied by severe malnutrition, impaired metabolism of carbohydrates, fats, and proteins, and defective utilization of energy. Because CRF involves more than just retention of normal urinary constituents in blood, the term *uremia* in current usage is devoid of any pathophysiologic connotation, but is employed instead to refer, in a general sense, to the constellation of signs and symptoms associated with CRF, regardless of etiology.

The presentation and severity of signs and symptoms of uremia often vary greatly from patient to patient, depending, at least in part, on the magnitude of the reduction in functioning renal mass as well as the rapidity with which renal function is lost. As discussed in Chap. 274, in the relatively early stage of CRF [i.e., when total glomerular filtration rate (GFR) is reduced but not to levels below about 35 to 50 percent of normal], overall renal function is sufficient to maintain the patient symptom-free, although renal reserve may be diminished. At this stage of renal impairment base-line excretory, biosynthetic, and other regulatory functions of the kidney are generally well maintained. At a somewhat later stage in the course of CRF (GFR about 20 to 35 percent of normal), *azotemia* occurs, and initial manifestations of renal insufficiency usually appear, with *hypertension* and *anemia* being the most common early abnormalities. Other derangements include *carbohydrate intolerance, hyperuricemia, hypertriglyceridemia,* and impaired ability to elaborate concentrated urine, the latter leading to *polyuria* and *nocturia* (see Chap. 43). Although patients are relatively asymptomatic at this stage, renal reserve is diminished sufficiently that any sudden stress, such as intercurrent infection, urinary tract obstruction, dehydration, or administration of a nephrotoxic drug, may compromise renal function still further, often leading to signs and symptoms of overt uremia. Return to a more stable base line can frequently be achieved in such patients by prompt correction of the underlying acute disturbance. With further loss of nephron mass (GFR below 20 to 25 percent of normal), the patient develops *overt renal failure,* which, in addition to increased severity of the anemia and hypertension, is characterized by *metabolic acidosis, fluid overload,* and various disturbances of the *gastrointestinal, cardiovascular,* and *nervous systems.* At this stage there is still sufficient capacity to excrete potassium so that clinically significant hyperkalemia is not a problem. Uremia may be viewed as the final stage in this inexorable process, when many of or all the untoward manifestations of CRF become evident clinically. In this chapter the causes and clinical characteristics of the disturbances of the various organ systems seen in patients with CRF will be considered.

PATHOPHYSIOLOGY AND BIOCHEMISTRY OF UREMIA

ROLE OF RETAINED TOXIC METABOLITES The finding that serums from patients with uremia exert toxic effects in a variety of biological test systems has motivated a diligent search to identify the responsible toxin(s). The most likely candidates thought to qualify as toxins in uremia are the *by-products of protein and amino acid metabolism.* Unlike fats and carbohydrates, which are eventually metabolized to carbon dioxide and water, substances which are easily excreted even in uremic subjects via lungs and skin, the products of protein and amino acid metabolism depend largely on the kidneys for excretion. A vast number of such products have been identified, with urea being quantitatively the most important. *Urea* represents some 80 percent or more of the total nitrogen excreted into the urine in patients with CRF maintained on diets containing 40 or more g protein per day. The *guanidino compounds* are the next most abundant of the nitrogenous end products of protein metabolism and include substances such as guanidine, methyl- and dimethylguanidine, creatinine, creatine, and guanidinosuccinic acid. As with urea, guanidines are derived, at least in part, from urea cycle amino acids. Other metabolic products of amino acid and protein catabolism that have been implicated as possible uremic toxins include *urates and other end products of nucleic acid metabolism, aliphatic amines,* a variety of *peptides,* and, finally, several *derivatives of the aromatic amino acids tryptophan, tyrosine, and phenylalanine.* The role of these substances in the pathogenesis of the clinical and biochemical abnormalities seen in CRF is unclear. It is generally believed that uremic symptoms correlate only in a rough and inconsistent way with concentrations of urea in blood. Nevertheless, although urea is probably not a major cause of overt uremic toxicity, it may account for some of the less serious clinical abnormalities, including anorexia, malaise, vomiting, and headache. On the other hand, elevated levels of plasma *guanidinosuccinic acid,* by interfering with activation of platelet factor III by adenosine diphosphate (ADP), have been shown to contribute to the impaired platelet function seen in CRF. *Creatinine,* generally regarded as a nontoxic substance, may cause adverse effects in uremic subjects following conversion to more toxic metabolites such as sarcosine and methylguanidine. Whether these substances, as well as *creatine,* a metabolic precursor of creatinine, and the other compounds cited above, are of clinical importance in the pathogenesis of uremic toxicity remains to be established.

Nitrogenous compounds of larger molecular weight are also retained in CRF. A toxic role for these substances has been suggested, on the impression that patients treated with intermittent peritoneal dialysis are less troubled with neuropathy than patients maintained on chronic hemodialysis, despite higher levels of urea and creatinine in blood. Since the clearance of small molecules depends mainly upon blood and dialysate flow rates, which are higher with hemodialysis, whereas clearance of larger molecules depends more on membrane surface area and time, which are greater with peritoneal dialysis, this form of therapy may be a more effective means of removing these substances of larger molecular weight. Using a variety of chemical separation procedures, several groups of workers have obtained evidence in support of this "middle-molecule hypothesis" by observing differences in composition between normal and uremic plasmas, with prominent abnormal "uremic peaks" in the molecular weight range of about 300 to 3500. Evidence from amino acid analysis suggests that these substances of larger molecular weight are polypeptides. Despite the foregoing, proof that efficient removal of middle molecules is associated with objective evidence of clinical well-being, and improvement in neuropathy in particular, remains to be provided. On the other hand, when there is insufficient removal of substances of smaller molecular weight (e.g., urea), symptoms of uremia are frequently aggravated.

Not all these middle-sized molecules accumulate in uremic plasma because of decreased renal excretion alone. The kidney normally *catabolizes* a number of circulating plasma proteins and polypeptides; with reduced renal mass, this capacity may be impaired greatly. Furthermore, plasma levels of many polypeptide hormones [including parathyroid hormone (PTH), insulin, glucagon, growth hormone, luteinizing hormone, and prolactin] rise with advancing renal failure, often markedly so, not only because of impaired renal catabolism but also because of enhanced endocrine secretion. The consequences of high circulating levels of many of these hormones in CRF are considered below and in Chap. 274.

EFFECTS OF UREMIA ON CELLULAR FUNCTIONS

Alterations in the composition of intracellular and extracellular fluids in CRF have long been recognized. Such abnormalities are believed to be a consequence, at least in part, of *defective ion transport* across cell membranes generally, with

retained uremic toxins possibly mediating these alterations in transmembrane ion transport. Integrity of cellular volume and composition depends to a large extent on the active outward transport of Na^+ from cell interior to exterior, the resulting intracellular fluid being relatively low in Na^+ and high in K^+, whereas the reverse is true for extracellular fluid. Active Na^+ transport is a metabolically costly process, accounting for a major fraction of basal energy utilization and oxygen consumption. The consequences of this efflux of Na^+ from cells are many and include, most notably, (1) the generation of a resting electrical potential difference across the cell membrane (with this transcellular voltage oriented so that cell interior is electronegative to cell exterior), and (2) a mechanism for enhancing the influx of K^+ into cells.

In experimental animals, partial inhibition of this active efflux mechanism for Na^+ across cell membranes leads to alterations in body composition and cell functions similar to those demonstrable in erythrocytes, leukocytes, skeletal muscle, and other tissues obtained from uremic subjects. These include increased and decreased intracellular concentrations of Na^+ and K^+, respectively, and reduction in magnitude of the transcellular voltage. These alterations have been shown to be largely reversed by efficient hemodialysis and, for erythrocytes at least, to be recreated when cells from normal subjects are incubated in uremic serums. Other derangements in cellular function have also been implicated as causes for altered body composition in uremia. For example, Na^+- and K^+-stimulated ATPase activity has been shown to be decreased in erythrocytes and brain tissue derived from uremic patients and animals, respectively. Whether the "uremic toxins" which account for these derangements in cellular function represent abnormally retained products of metabolism which fail to be excreted, or normal substances present in increased quantities in response to reduced renal mass, remains unknown. *Parathyroid and natriuretic hormones,* examples of this category of substances, are discussed in this context in Chap. 274.

EFFECTS OF UREMIA ON WHOLE-BODY COMPOSITION

What is the impact of these disturbances in active transcellular Na^+ transport on the uremic organism as a whole? From the pathophysiologic considerations already discussed, CRF is likely to lead to abnormally high intracellular Na^+ concentrations, and hence to osmotically induced overhydration of cells generally, whereas these same cells are thought to be relatively deficient in K^+. With the inevitable onset of malaise, anorexia, nausea, vomiting, and diarrhea, patients with CRF may eventually develop classic protein-calorie malnutrition and negative nitrogen balance, often with profound losses of lean body mass and fat deposits. Owing to the concomitant tendency for salt and water retention, these losses often go unnoticed until the late stages of CRF. Whereas a large fraction of the increase in total body water in uremia is the result of expansion of intracellular volume, extracellular volume expansion also is observed commonly. With initiation of intermittent hemodialysis or renal transplantation, there is often an immediate and substantial loss of body weight, due primarily to correction of this overhydration. With successful transplantation, the initial diuresis is followed by a period of impressive weight gain, due to restoration of lean body mass and fat deposits to preillness levels. For patients on chronic dialysis, the anabolic response is less dramatic, even when therapy is regarded as optimal, involving mainly reaccumulation of fat deposits. The failure to restore lean body mass to normal with chronic dialysis may reflect insufficient intake of protein, which, in adequately dialyzed patients, should be maintained at levels of 0.8 to 1.4 g/kg per day.

The occurrence of deficits in intracellular K^+ concentration in CRF has already been mentioned and may result from inadequate intake (poor diet or overzealous K^+ restriction by the physician), excessive losses (vomiting, diarrhea, diuretics), reduction of Na^+- and K^+-stimulated ATPase, or a combination of these. In addition to promoting losses of K^+ into urine (which may be substantial if urine volume remains relatively normal in uremic subjects), the high levels of plasma aldosterone often seen in CRF may also augment net secretion of K^+ into the colon, thereby contributing to marked K^+ losses in stool or diarrheal fluids. Despite deficits in intracellular K^+ concentration, serum K^+ is usually normal or high in CRF, owing most often to metabolic acidosis, which induces an efflux of K^+ from cells. Additionally, uremic patients are relatively resistant to the action of insulin (see below), a hormone which normally enhances K^+ uptake by skeletal muscle.

EFFECTS OF UREMIA ON METABOLISM

HYPOTHERMIA In experimental animals injections of urine, urea, or other retained toxic metabolites can induce hypothermia, and basal heat production diminishes soon after nephrectomy. Since active Na^+ transport across cell membranes accounts for a major proportion of basal energy production, it is generally believed that the inverse relationship between body temperature and degree of azotemia is due, in part, to inhibition of the sodium pump by some retained toxin(s). Dialysis usually returns body temperature to normal.

CARBOHYDRATE METABOLISM The ability to metabolize an exogenous glucose load is impaired in most patients with CRF. The defect largely involves a slowing of the rate at which blood glucose concentration declines to the normal range after administration of a glucose load. Fasting blood sugar levels are usually normal or only slightly elevated; severe hyperglycemia and/or ketosis is uncommon. Consequently, the *glucose intolerance of CRF* usually does not require specific therapy (hence the term *azotemic pseudodiabetes*). Because insulin depends to a large extent on the kidney for its removal from plasma and eventual degradation, circulating insulin levels tend to be increased in uremia. Whereas insulin levels in plasma are only slightly to moderately increased in most fasting uremic subjects, levels considerably in excess of normal are usually found in response to a glucose load. The response to intravenous insulin in patients with CRF is also abnormal, and the rate of utilization of glucose by peripheral tissues often is diminished substantially. The glucose intolerance of uremia is thought to result largely from this peripheral resistance to the action of insulin.

In normal subjects, deficits of K^+ induced by administration of cation exchange resins or thiazide diuretics may result in glucose intolerance. The possibility exists, therefore, that in uremia the intracellular deficits of K^+ (described above) may also contribute to carbohydrate intolerance. It is likely that metabolic acidosis also contributes to impaired carbohydrate metabolism in uremia since this acid-base disturbance has been shown to depress glycolysis, impair glucose utilization, and interfere with the peripheral action of insulin. A role for *glucagon* in the abnormal carbohydrate metabolism of uremia has also been suggested, on the observation that plasma glucagon levels are usually increased in CRF and the fact that glucagon plays a major role in hepatic glycogenolysis. In part, hyperglucagonemia may be a consequence of reduced renal mass since this hormone, as does insulin, depends on the kidneys for its clearance and catabolism. Finally, the possible contributions of other hormones in the pathogenesis of this glucose intolerance, including catecholamines, growth hormone, and prolactin, as well as the myriad of potentially toxic metabolites retained in CRF, remain to be determined.

NITROGEN AND LIPID METABOLISM Given that the capacity to eliminate the nitrogenous end products of protein catabolism is reduced drastically, CRF may be regarded as a state of *protein intolerance.* As discussed above, retention of these end products of nitrogen metabolism is thought to represent a dominant cause of the signs and symptoms of uremic toxicity.

Hypertriglyceridemia and decreased high-density lipoprotein cholesterol are common in uremia, whereas cholesterol levels in plasma are usually normal. Whether uremia accelerates triglyceride production by the liver and intestine is unknown. The well-known lipogenic effect of hyperinsulinism may contribute to increased triglyceride synthesis. The rate of removal of triglycerides from the circulation, which depends in large part on the enzyme *lipoprotein lipase,* has been shown to be depressed in uremia, an effect not corrected appreciably by hemodialysis. The high incidence of premature atherosclerosis seen in patients on chronic dialysis (see "Cardiovascular and Pulmonary Abnormalities" below) may be related, at least in part, to these abnormalities in lipid metabolism.

CLINICAL SPECTRUM OF ABNORMALITIES IN UREMIA

As noted earlier, CRF leads ultimately to disturbances in function of every organ system in the body. With the advent and increasingly greater application of chronic dialysis in the past two decades, the incidence and severity of these disturbances have been modified enormously, so that virtually everywhere that modern medicine is practiced, the overt and florid manifestations of uremia have largely disappeared. Unfortunately, however, even optimal dialysis therapy is not a panacea for the patient with CRF, because, as indicated in Table 276-1, some disturbances resulting from impaired renal function fail to respond fully, while others may even progress despite dialysis treatment. Furthermore, as with many modern and complex therapeutic modalities, intermittent dialysis may be responsible for the appearance of unique abnormalities not seen prior to initiation of therapy; these abnormalities should be viewed as complications of dialysis.

FLUID, ELECTROLYTE, AND ACID-BASE DISORDERS (See also Chaps. 84 and 85) **Sodium and volume homeostasis** In most patients with stable CRF, modest increases in total body Na^+ and water content can be documented, although objective signs of extracellular fluid (ECF) volume expansion may not be apparent clinically. With ingestion of excessive amounts of salt and water, however, control of excess volume becomes an important clinical and therapeutic consideration. In general, excessive *salt* ingestion contributes to, or aggravates, congestive heart failure, hypertension, ascites, and edema formation. On the other hand, hyponatremia and weight gain are the typical consequences of excessive ingestion of *water,* abnormalities which in most patients are relatively mild and asymptomatic. In the majority of patients, daily intake of fluid equal in volume to urine volume per day plus about 500 ml usually will maintain the serum Na^+ concentration at normal levels. Hypernatremia is encountered relatively infrequently in CRF, although its occurrence has been noted during peritoneal dialysis when high glucose concentrations are added to the dialysate. In dialysis patients with evidence of extracellular volume expansion, management should include ultrafiltration and restriction of salt and water intake between dialyses. In the patient with CRF not maintained on dialysis, diuretics and modest restriction of salt and water intake are the mainstays of therapy.

TABLE 276-1
Clinical spectrum of abnormalities in uremia*

FLUID AND ELECTROLYTE DISTURBANCES
___

Volume expansion and contraction (I)
Hypernatremia and hyponatremia (I)
Hyperkalemia and hypokalemia (I)
Metabolic acidosis (I)
Hyperphosphatemia and hypophosphatemia (I)
Hypocalcemia (I)

ENDOCRINE-METABOLIC DISTURBANCES
___

Renal osteodystrophy (I or P)
Secondary hyperparathyroidism (I or P)
Carbohydrate intolerance (I)
Hyperuricemia (I or P)
Hypothermia (I)
Hypertriglyceridemia (P)
Protein-calorie malnutrition (I or P)
Impaired growth and development (P)
Infertility and sexual dysfunction (P)
Amenorrhea (P)

NEUROMUSCULAR DISTURBANCES
___

Fatigue (I)
Sleep disorders (P)
Headache (I or P)
Impaired mentation (I)
Lethargy (I)
Asterixis (I)
Muscular irritability (I)
Peripheral neuropathy (I or P)
Restless legs syndrome (I or P)
Paralysis (I or P)
Myoclonus (I)
Seizures (I or P)
Coma (I)
Muscle cramps (D)
Dialysis disequilibrium syndrome (D)
Dialysis dementia (D)

CARDIOVASCULAR AND PULMONARY DISTURBANCES
___

Arterial hypertension (I or P)
Congestive heart failure (I)
Pericarditis (I)
Cardiomyopathy (I or P)
Uremic lung (I)
Accelerated atherosclerosis (P or D)

DERMATOLOGIC DISTURBANCES
___

Pallor (I or P)
Hyperpigmentation (I or P)
Pruritus (P)
Ecchymoses (I or P)
Uremic frost (I)

GASTROINTESTINAL DISTURBANCES
___

Anorexia (I)
Nausea and vomiting (I)
Uremic fetor (I)
Gastroenteritis (I)
Peptic ulcer (I or P)
GI bleeding (I, P, or D)
Hepatitis (D)
Refractory ascites (D)

HEMATOLOGIC AND IMMUNOLOGIC DISTURBANCES
___

Normocytic, normochromic anemia (P)
Lymphocytopenia (P)
Bleeding diathesis (I)
Increased susceptibility to infection (I or P)
Splenomegaly and hypersplenism (P)
Leukopenia (D)
Hypocomplementemia (D)

* *Virtually all the abnormalities contained in this table are completely reversed by successful renal transplantation. The response of these abnormalities to intermittent hemo- or peritoneal dialysis therapy is more variable. I denotes an abnormality which usually improves with an optimal program of intermittent dialysis and related therapy. P denotes an abnormality which tends to persist, or even progress, despite an optimal dialysis program. D denotes an abnormality which develops only after initiation of dialysis therapy.*

Patients with CRF have grossly impaired renal mechanisms for conserving Na^+ and water (discussed in detail in Chap. 274). When confronted with an *extrarenal* cause for increased fluid loss (e.g., vomiting, diarrhea, fever), these patients are prone to develop ECF volume depletion, with signs and symptoms of dry mouth and other mucous membranes, dizziness, syncope, tachycardia, decreased filling of jugular veins, orthostatic hypotension, and even vascular collapse. Depletion of extracellular fluid volume typically results in deterioration of residual renal function and, in the previously stable and asymptomatic patient with mild CRF, signs and symptoms of overt uremia. Cautious fluid repletion usually restores extracellular and intravascular volumes to normal and often, but not always, returns renal function to previously stable levels.

Potassium homeostasis Derangements in K^+ balance (see also Chaps. 84 and 274) are occasionally documented by laboratory analysis in patients with CRF, but are rarely responsible for clinical symptoms unless GFR is below 5 ml/min or an endogenous (hemolysis trauma, infection) or exogenous (stored blood, K^+-containing medications) K^+ load is administered. Despite progression of renal failure, most patients maintain normal serum K^+ concentrations until the final stages of uremia. As discussed in Chap. 274, this ability to sustain K^+ balance with advancing renal failure is due to adaptations in the renal distal tubules and colon, sites where aldosterone and other factors serve to enhance K^+ secretion. Not surprisingly, oliguria, or disruption of key adaptive mechanisms, can lead to *hyperkalemia* and its potentially ominous effects on cardiac function. Antikaliuretic drugs, such as spironolactone or triamterene, should be used with extreme caution in CRF. Hyperkalemia in CRF may also be induced by abrupt lowering of arterial blood pH, since acidosis is associated with efflux of K^+ from intracellular to extracellular fluids. A clinically useful index of the magnitude of this hydrogen-potassium exchange is that for every 0.1 unit change in blood pH, there will be a reciprocal change in serum K^+ concentration of approximately 0.6 meq per liter. Correction of acidosis-induced hyperkalemia with sodium bicarbonate is the treatment of choice. Intravenous insulin and dextrose are useful in lowering serum potassium acutely, while the ion exchange resin Kayexalate is useful in longer-term control of hyperkalemia. Patients in whom hyperkalemia persists in the absence of excessive K^+ intake, oliguria, or acute acidosis should be evaluated for the possibility of *hyporeninemic hypoaldosteronism*. Patients with this syndrome have reduced circulating levels of renin and aldosterone in the plasma and often also have diabetes mellitus.

Hypokalemia due to diminished ability of the kidneys to conserve K^+ is uncommon in most forms of CRF. When hypokalemia occurs in these patients, poor dietary K^+ intake, usually in association with excessive diuretic therapy or gastrointestinal losses, is likely to be the underlying cause. When hypokalemia occurs as a result of primary K^+ wasting in urine, it may represent a solitary renal reabsorptive defect or, more commonly, be associated with other solute transport abnormalities, as in Fanconi's syndrome, renal tubular acidosis, or other forms of hereditary or acquired tubulointerstitial diseases (see Chaps. 281 and 283). A detailed discussion of the clinical consequences and management of hypokalemia and hyperkalemia is given in Chap. 84.

Metabolic acidosis With advancing renal failure, total daily acid excretion falls below the level needed to maintain external balance of hydrogen ions. Metabolic acidosis is the inevitable result, and the mechanisms involved are considered in Chap. 274. In most patients with stable renal insufficiency, administration of 20 to 30 meq sodium bicarbonate or sodium citrate per day will usually correct the acidosis. In response to a sudden acid challenge (whether from an endogenous or exogenous source), however, patients with CRF are particularly susceptible to profound acidosis, which requires more substantial quantities of alkali for correction. Administration of sodium must be carried out with careful attention to the patient's volume status.

Phosphate, calcium, and bone   As discussed in detail in Chap. 274, serum phosphate concentration begins to rise when GFR falls below about 25 percent of normal. Calcium deposition in bone is critically dependent upon the availability of phosphate; retention of phosphate in plasma, therefore, facilitates calcium entry into bone and thereby contributes to the *hypocalcemia* and *elevations in plasma PTH* levels seen in CRF. Hypocalcemia in CRF also results from the impaired ability of the diseased kidney to synthesize *1,25-dihydroxyvitamin D$_3$* [1,25-(OH)$_2$D$_3$], the active metabolite of vitamin D (Fig. 276-1). Reabsorption of calcium in the gut is impaired when circulating levels of this active metabolite are low. Finally, in patients with advanced CRF, the ability of PTH to mobilize calcium salts from bone may be altered. Despite these various causes of hypocalcemia, symptoms such as tetany are rare unless patients are treated with large amounts of alkali.

Overproduction of parathyroid hormone, disordered vitamin D metabolism, chronic metabolic acidosis, and excessive fecal losses of calcium all contribute to the occurrence of bone diseases in uremia (Fig. 276-1). *Renal* and *uremic osteodystrophy* are broad and imprecise terms that encompass a number of distinct skeletal abnormalities, including osteomalacia, osteitis fibrosa, osteosclerosis, and, in children especially, impaired bone growth. Although clinical symptoms of bone disease are uncommon, occurring in less than 10 percent of patients with advanced renal failure, radiological and histological abnormalities are observed in about 35 and 90 percent, respectively. Renal osteodystrophy is seen more often in growing children than in adults, and especially in patients with congenital renal anomalies associated with very slowly progressive renal insufficiency. On radiological examination, three types of lesions can be identified: (1) changes analogous to those described in children with nutritional rickets, namely, widened osteoid seams at the growth margin of bones (so-called "renal rickets"); (2) the bone changes of *secondary hyperparathyroidism* (*osteitis fibrosa*), characterized by osteoclastic bone resorption and mani-

fested by subperiosteal erosions, especially of the phalanges, long bones, and distal ends of the clavicles; and (3) *osteosclerosis*, often best noted by enhanced bone density in the upper and lower margins of vertebrae, producing the so-called "rugger jersey spine." Since patients with osteosclerosis are usually in negative calcium balance, sclerosis is due mainly to bone remodelling and redistribution. With very rapid mobilization of skeletal calcium, as occurs in dialysis when the bath is low in calcium, or following prolonged bed rest, osteosclerosis is usually replaced by loss of bone density and osteoporosis.

With renal osteodystrophy there is a tendency to *spontaneous fractures,* which are often slow to heal. The ribs are most commonly involved. Painful joints may occur in association with renal osteodystrophy due to calcium deposition in bursas and other periarticular structures. When bone pain is severe, a proximal *myopathy* may coexist, giving rise to gait abnormalities and even leading to cessation of ambulation. The incidence of *aseptic necrosis of the hip* is increased in renal transplant recipients, probably related to such factors as chronic corticosteroid therapy, secondary hyperparathyroidism, and altered vitamin D metabolism. In CRF there is often a tendency to *extraosseous,* or *metastatic, calcification,* especially when the calcium-phosphate product exceeds 60. Medium-sized blood vessels, subcutaneous, articular, and periarticular tissues, myocardium, eyes, and lungs are common sites of metastatic calcification.

Management of patients with renal osteodystrophy includes reduction in dietary phosphate available for absorption through the use of aluminum hydroxide binding agents. When such treatment is instituted early in CRF, signs and symptoms of renal osteodystrophy and parathyroid gland hypertrophy may largely be prevented. Daily vitamin D supplementation, in the form of 1,25-dihydroxycholecalciferol or dihydrotachysterol, is also of value, particularly to improve osteomalacia, osteitis fibrosa, and myopathy. Supplementation of dietary calcium intake (to 1 to 1.5 g per day) as well as judicious increases in calcium ion concentration in the dialysate is also useful for treating or preventing hypocalcemia, but should not be insti-

FIGURE 276-1
Pathogenesis of bone diseases in chronic renal failure.

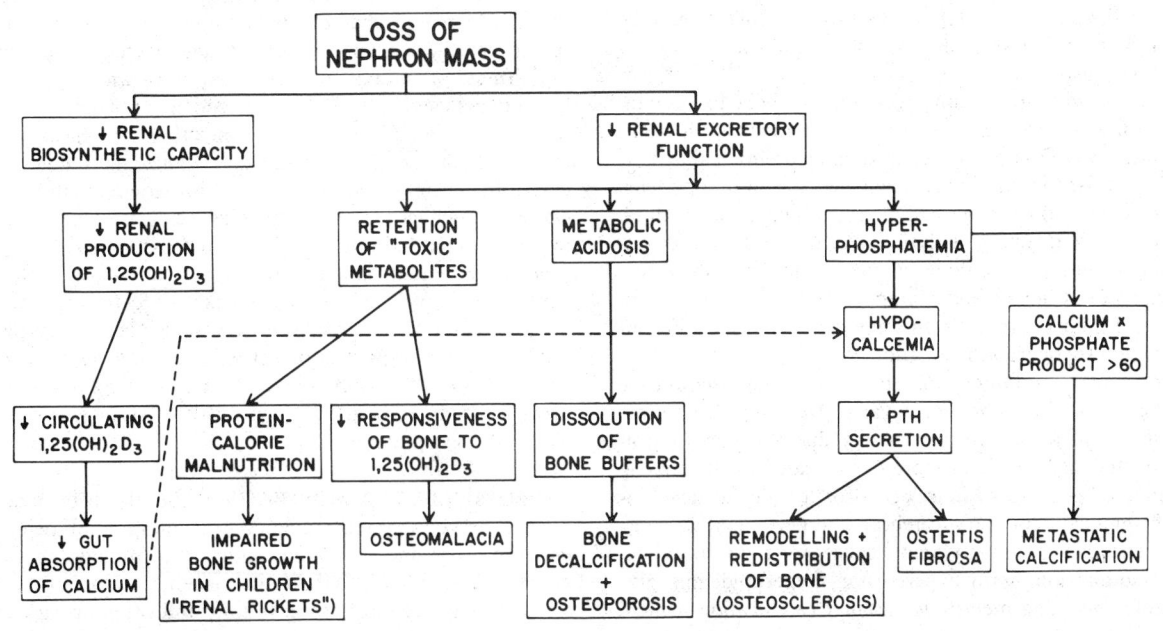

tuted until hyperphosphatemia is corrected. Close monitoring of serum calcium and phosphate concentrations is required to avoid serious hypercalcemia and metastatic calcification.

Other solutes Other inorganic solute derangements in CRF include *hyperuricemia* and *hypermagnesemia.* Uric acid retention is a common feature of CRF but rarely leads to symptomatic gout. Hypophosphatemia is usually a consequence of overzealous oral administration of phosphate-binding gels. Because serum magnesium levels tend to rise in CRF, magnesium-containing antacids and cathartics should be avoided.

CARDIOVASCULAR AND PULMONARY ABNORMALITIES
Fluid retention in uremic patients often results in congestive heart failure and/or pulmonary edema. A unique form of pulmonary congestion and edema may be seen in uremia even in the absence of volume overload and is typically associated with normal or mildly elevated intracardiac and pulmonary wedge pressures. This entity, referred to as *uremic lung,* is characterized radiologically by perihilar vascular congestion (the peripheral lung regions appear uninvolved), giving rise to the impression of a "butterfly wing" distribution. Uremic lung, as well as cardiopulmonary abnormalities associated with circulatory overload, usually respond promptly and dramatically to vigorous dialysis.

Arterial hypertension is the most commonly observed complication of end-stage renal disease. When it is not present, the patient is either receiving antihypertensive therapy or is volume-depleted, the latter condition usually due to excessive gastrointestinal fluid losses, overzealous or surreptitious diuretic therapy, or salt-wasting forms of renal disease (e.g., polycystic or medullary cystic disease or chronic pyelonephritis). Since fluid overload is the major cause of hypertension in uremic subjects, the normotensive state can usually be restored by dialysis. Nevertheless, some patients remain hypertensive, despite rigorous salt and water restriction and ultrafiltration, because of hyperreninemia. In the majority of these cases, antihypertensive drug therapy is effective. A small minority of these patients develop *accelerated or malignant hypertension,* manifested by markedly elevated systolic and diastolic pressures, severe hyperreninemia, encephalopathy, seizures, retinal changes, and papilledema. Use of more potent drugs such as minoxidil and nitroprusside may prove useful; however, when malignant hypertension fails to respond to maximum antihypertensive therapy and rigorous dialysis, patients should be considered for bilateral nephrectomy to which they may respond dramatically.

As is likely with uremic lung, retained metabolic toxins contribute to the occurrence of *pericarditis* in patients with CRF. The clinical presentation of pericarditis in uremic subjects is generally similar to that of other etiologies, except that pericardiocentesis for effusions usually yields hemorrhagic fluid. Treatment with intensive dialysis is recommended, and systemic anticoagulation should be avoided to minimize the possible occurrence of hemorrhagic tamponade. Oral indomethacin may be useful for pericarditis. In some patients, pericardiocentesis with intrapericardial instillation of air or steroids is effective for pericardial tamponade. Pericardiectomy should be considered only after more conservative treatment has failed.

Clinical experience with chronically dialyzed patients followed for the past decade or more has revealed the disturbing occurrence of *accelerated atherosclerosis,* leading to development of significant coronary, cerebral, and peripheral vascular disease. There are seemingly ample causes for these complications, including long-term hypertension, hyperlipidemia, glucose intolerance, and metastatic vascular calcification, which,

by interfering with the atrioventricular conduction system of the heart, have been known to cause cardiac arrhythmias and sudden death.

HEMATOLOGIC ABNORMALITIES *Normochromic, normocytic anemia* occurs regularly in CRF and contributes to fatigability and listlessness in these patients. Erythropoiesis is depressed in CRF, due both to the effects of retained toxins on bone marrow and to diminished biosynthesis of erythropoietin by the diseased kidney. *Hemolysis* also occurs and involves an extracorpuscular defect since survival of erythrocytes from normal subjects is reduced when these cells are transfused into uremic patients, and erythrocytes from patients with CRF have relatively normal survival times when transfused into normal individuals. Gastrointestinal and chronic dialyzer *blood loss* contributes to anemia, as does *hypersplenism* in the occasional patient. Blood loss is exaggerated in hemodialysis patients because of the need for heparin (during dialysis) and oral anticoagulants (between dialyses) to minimize clotting of vascular access devices. Transfusions may contribute to suppression of erythropoiesis in CRF and, due to increased risk of hepatitis, should be avoided unless anemia aggravates other underlying disorders (for example, coronary or cerebrovascular disease). Androgen therapy has been shown to improve erythropoiesis in some dialysis patients not previously subjected to nephrectomy. Parenteral or oral iron therapy and vitamin supplementation are also indicated in most patients, the former to correct deficits due to chronic blood loss and the latter, especially folic and ascorbic acids and the soluble B vitamins, to offset chronic losses of these substances through dialyzer membranes.

Abnormal hemostasis is another common hematologic derangement in CRF, characterized by a tendency to abnormal bleeding and bruising. Bleeding into gastrointestinal tract, pericardial sac, and intracranial vault, in the form of subdural hematoma or intracerebral hemorrhage, is of greatest concern. Prolongation of bleeding time, decreased platelet factor III activity, abnormal platelet aggregation and adhesiveness, and impaired prothrombin consumption contribute to the clotting defects in uremia. The abnormality in factor III correlates with increased plasma levels of guanidinosuccinic acid and can largely be corrected by dialysis.

A wide variety of changes in leukocyte formation and function also occur in uremia leading to *enhanced susceptibility to infection.* Lymphocytopenia and atrophy of lymphoid structures occur in CRF, whereas neutrophil production is relatively unimpaired. Nevertheless, there is evidence to suggest that all leukocyte cell types are affected adversely by uremic serum. Decreased chemotaxis is among the best documented of the defects occurring in uremic leukocytes, with resulting impairment of acute inflammatory response and decreased delayed hypersensitivity. There is a tendency for uremic patients to have less fever in response to infection. For these reasons, infections may be more difficult to recognize in uremia. Leukocyte function may also be impaired in patients with CRF because of such coexisting factors as acidosis, hyperglycemia, protein-calorie malnutrition, serum and tissue hyperosmolarity (due to azotemia), and reduced serum immunoglobulin and complement levels. Mucosal barriers to infection may also be defective, and, in dialysis patients, vascular access devices also serve as common portals of entry for pathogens, particularly staphylococci. Anti-inflammatory steroids and immunosuppressive drugs add further to the risk of serious infection in many of these patients.

NEUROMUSCULAR ABNORMALITIES Subtle disturbances of central nervous system function, including mild behavioral changes, drowsiness, and insomnia, are among the earliest symptoms of uremia. Inability to concentrate, loss of memory, and errors in judgment soon follow, and often are associated with signs of neuromuscular irritability, including hiccups, cramps, and fasciculations and twitching of large muscle groups. Asterixis, myoclonus, and chorea are common in terminal uremia, as are stupor, seizures, and coma. Many of these neuromuscular complications of severe uremia resolve with dialysis, although nonspecific EEG abnormalities may persist.

Peripheral neuropathy is a relatively common complication of advanced CRF. Initially, sensory nerve involvement exceeds motor, lower extremities are involved more than the upper, and the distal portions of the extremities more than proximal. The "restless legs syndrome," characterized by ill-defined sensations of discomfort in the feet and lower legs and frequent leg movement, is a disturbing complication in some uremic patients. If dialysis is not instituted soon after onset of sensory abnormalities, motor involvement follows, often leading to loss of deep tendon reflexes, weakness, peroneal nerve palsy (foot drop), and, eventually, flaccid quadriplegia. Accordingly, early evidence of peripheral neuropathy is generally taken as a firm indication to initiate dialysis or transplantation.

Two types of neurological disturbances appear to be unique to patients on chronic dialysis. One is the syndrome of *dialysis dementia,* seen in patients who have been on dialysis for a number of years. This syndrome is characterized by speech dyspraxia, myoclonus, dementia, and eventually seizures and death. The possibility of aluminum intoxication has been suggested, with aluminum hydroxide (phosphate-binding) gels as the likely source. The other disturbance occurs during the first few dialyses, in association with rapid reduction of blood urea levels. Nausea, vomiting, drowsiness, headache, and even grand mal seizures have been attributed to the more rapid (dialysis-induced) reduction in osmolality of extracellular than intracellular fluids within the cranium, leading to cerebral edema and raised intracranial pressure—hence the term *dialysis dysequilibrium syndrome.*

GASTROINTESTINAL ABNORMALITIES Anorexia, hiccups, nausea, and vomiting are common and early manifestations of uremia and contribute to the protein-calorie malnutrition of this disorder. *Uremic fetor,* a uriniferous odor to the breath, derives from the breakdown of urea in saliva to ammonia and is often associated with unpleasant taste sensation. Mucosal ulcerations leading to blood loss can occur at any level of the gastrointestinal tract in later stages of CRF—so-called "uremic gastroenteritis." Peptic ulcer disease is particularly common, occurring in as many as one-fourth of uremic subjects. Whether this high incidence is related to increased gastric acidity, hypersecretion of gastrin, or secondary hyperparathyroidism is unknown. Most of the gastrointestinal symptoms, except those related to peptic ulcer disease, usually improve with dialysis.

Viral hepatitis (see also Chaps. 108 and 302), though not a complication of uremia per se, is a common problem encountered in chronic dialysis patients because of frequent blood transfusions. A recent national cooperative study in the United States has reported detecting hepatitis B type antigen in almost 17 percent of chronic dialysis patients and in 2.5 percent of dialysis support personnel. This prevalence is higher than in the general population and indicates transmission of infection between patients and support staff. Type B, as well as type A, viral hepatitis in dialysis patients tends to be milder, indeed, often subclinical, in comparison with nonuremic victims. Jaundice and hyperbilirubinemia are uncommon; the abnormalities consist of mild hepatomegaly, modest elevations in SGOT, SGPT, and alkaline phosphatase, and moderate Bromsulphthalein retention. Type B antigen is usually present and may persist long after other features of the illness have resolved. In addition to serum hepatitis, hemodialysis patients are also susceptible to other infectious forms of hepatitis, particularly that caused by cytomegalovirus (Chap. 194). Hepatitis associated with hypersensitivity or toxic reactions to commonly employed drugs and solvents may also occur.

ENDOCRINE-METABOLIC DISTURBANCES The common disturbances in parathyroid function, glucose, and insulin metabolism, as well as the lipid, protein-calorie, and other nutritional abnormalities of uremia have already been considered. In general, pituitary, thyroid, and adrenal gland functions are relatively normal, often despite measurable abnormalities in circulating thyroxine, growth hormone, aldosterone, and cortisol levels. In women, amenorrhea and inability to carry pregnancies to term are early manifestations of uremia. While menses frequently reappear after chronic dialysis is initiated, successful pregnancies remain rare. In men with CRF, including those on chronic dialysis, impotence, oligospermia, and germinal cell dysplasia are common, as are reduced plasma testosterone levels. As with growth, sexual maturation is often impaired in adolescent children, even among those on chronic dialysis.

DERMATOLOGIC ABNORMALITIES The skin shows many abnormalities. This is not surprising in view of anemia (pallor), defective hemostasis (ecchymoses and hematomas), calcium deposition and secondary hyperparathyroidism (pruritus, excoriations), dehydration (poor skin turgor, dry mucous membranes), and the general cutaneous consequences of protein-calorie malnutrition. A sallow, yellow cast may reflect the combined influences of anemia and retention of a variety of pigmented metabolites, or *urochromes.* In advanced uremia urea concentrations in sweat may reach sufficiently high levels that, after evaporation, a fine white powder can be found on the skin surface—so-called "uremic (urea) frost." Although many of these cutaneous abnormalities improve with dialysis, *uremic pruritus* may persist and is usually resistant to most systemic and topical therapies. Regular bathing and lubrication of the skin with bland ointments are helpful in preventing superficial infection and excessive dryness.

MANAGEMENT OF CHRONIC RENAL FAILURE

Despite the tendency to inexorable progression, every effort should be made to detect and correct any of the numerous potentially reversible acute complications that may arise in patients with CRF. Included among these are active infection, uncontrolled hypertension, congestive heart failure, volume depletion, urinary tract obstruction and/or stone formation, hypercalcemia, hyperuricemia, and injudicious use of nephrotoxic drugs.

CONSERVATIVE MANAGEMENT Involved in conservative management is the use of measures other than dialysis or transplantation to reverse, or at least slow, the progression of renal insufficiency. Specific measures such as antibiotics, antihypertensive and cardiac drugs, phosphate-binding gels, immunosuppressive agents, and glucocorticoids are considered elsewhere in this section, as are drugs to control fluid and electrolyte imbalances and anemia. This discussion will deal with *dietary therapy,* and in particular *protein restriction,* in an effort to control the rate of production and accumulation of nitrogenous end products of metabolism.

Protein restriction to about 40 g per day, together with supplements of carbohydrates and vitamins, has been employed for decades as a means for maintaining nitrogen balance in patients with other than severe uremia, while at the same time reducing slightly the level of blood urea nitrogen and the rate of accumulation of metabolic toxins. The major benefit derived from this effort has been to lessen the symptoms of nausea and vomiting. Nitrogen balance can also be achieved with substantially lower daily intakes of protein (20 g per day), at least in some patients, provided that the proportion of essential amino acids in the protein employed is high (e.g., eggs and milk). Substitution of nitrogen-free α-keto analogues of essential amino acids has been shown in experimental studies to reduce nitrogen-intake requirements, decrease synthesis of urea, and, in some patients, postpone the need for dialysis. While these conservative approaches are likely to prove useful in nonoliguric patients with GFR above 3 to 5 percent of normal, many experts believe that protein restriction may add to the debility of patients with CRF and, therefore, recommend initiation of dialysis and/or transplantation with continued adequate protein intake.

DIALYSIS AND TRANSPLANTATION When CRF progresses to the stage at which oliguria, hyperkalemia, advanced neuropathy, intractable hypertension, congestive heart failure, and pericarditis appear, conservative measures usually no longer suffice, and, if life is to continue, dialysis and/or transplantation is required.

It is important to emphasize, however, that such therapies should not be withheld until more conservative measures fail. Instead, dialysis or transplantation is indicated when conservative approaches no longer sustain a *reasonable quality of life* and no longer avoid psychological discouragement or physical debility, as may occur with severe peripheral neuropathy or renal osteodystrophy. The choice between intermittent chronic dialysis and transplantation is usually a matter of personal preference, based on consideration of relative risks, rather than clear-cut medical judgment. Generally, transplantation is the preferred treatment in relatively young and healthy patients, when a living related donor is available (ideally an identical twin or HLA-identical sibling), when the uremic patient is a preadolescent child, or when dialysis proves to be a serious hardship for medical or personal reasons. Chronic hemodialysis and/or peritoneal dialysis is a generally preferred therapy in elderly patients and those with malignancies or certain systemic diseases in whom immunosuppression and chronic corticosteroid therapy may pose additional serious risks. It is generally agreed that, if successful, transplantation offers the greatest likelihood of total rehabilitation and recovery for the patient with CRF, since virtually all the complications and untoward metabolic consequences of uremia tend to be reversed completely. Rehabilitation tends not to be as dramatic or complete with chronic dialysis, even when therapy is considered optimal. Moreover, dialysis, at best, is a costly, demanding, and time-consuming therapy, itself chronic and unrelenting in nature.

Intermittent hemodialysis therapy At the present time, some 26,000 patients are maintained on intermittent hemodialysis therapy in the United States. The majority are dialyzed for 3 to 5 h three times per week. Although the design of the various artificial kidneys varies considerably, most employ cellophane-type membranes which permit exchange of small molecules and water between blood and dialysate, with differences in transmembrane hydrostatic and osmotic pressure accounting for the movement of exchangeable substances. This extracorporeal molecular exchange process requires repeated access to the circulation. For this purpose, surgically created subcutaneous arteriovenous fistulas (accessible by needle puncture) have

generally replaced external shunts, largely because of fewer complications, such as infections and clotting. Heparin is employed during the dialysis procedure to prevent clotting of the extracorporeal circulation. In the United States, most patients are now dialyzed in out-patient centers or at home, in contrast to a decade ago when nearly all treatment was limited to hospital-based programs. Home dialysis is generally regarded as preferable, since patient independence is fostered, treatment schedules can be tailored to the individual, and expense is reduced. These advantages are not without cost, however, because the demands on the helpers, usually family members, are high. Medical suitability and patient and family preference for this form of therapy are important considerations.

Complications related to dialysis per se, in addition to those already discussed, derive largely from the sustained need for access to the circulation and include infection, bleeding, and thrombosis of fistulas and shunts. Technical problems related to errors in preparation of dialysate, air embolus, and inadvertent hypovolemic shock (usually due to excessive ultrafiltration) may also occur.

Most centers report that a small percentage of chronically dialyzed patients are in excellent health, free of hypertension, anemia, renal osteodystrophy, or other complications. A similar small percentage of patients benefit little, if at all, from dialysis and remain debilitated and incapacitated. The remainder of the population on chronic dialysis improves in general health and well-being substantially, and 60 to 70 percent are effectively rehabilitated. Nevertheless, they may continue to have some manifestations of CRF, including hypertension, intermittent volume overload, osteodystrophy, and/or peripheral neuropathy, infertility, sexual dysfunction, and a host of psychological abnormalities not unlike those seen in other chronic illnesses.

The mortality of chronic dialysis has been reduced to about 10 percent per year, even with broadened criteria for acceptance of patients. Cardiovascular complications (myocardial infarction and cerebrovascular disease) account for about 50 percent of deaths, with sepsis accounting for another 25 percent. Progression of extrarenal diseases, voluntary withdrawal from a dialysis program, and complications of therapy account for remaining deaths.

Intermittent peritoneal dialysis Technical advances in recent years have resulted in the development of effective and reliable peritoneal access devices and automated, closed delivery and drainage systems which make repeated peritoneal dialysis possible for an increasing number of patients. Since exchange rates for dialyzable solutes are generally slower than with hemodialysis, peritoneal dialysis requires considerably more therapeutic time, about 36 to 42 h per week (conveniently planned as three dialyses a week, each for 12 to 14 h, usually at night). Chronic ambulatory peritoneal dialysis is a new technique utilizing long dwell times; in early trials it appears to offer another suitable form of therapy. Recurrent peritonitis is no longer a common problem due to improved techniques, and protein losses (via the peritoneal fluid) can be countered by increased protein intake. For patients with inadequate vascular access, severe cardiovascular instability, or lack of an available home dialysis helper, peritoneal dialysis has proved increasingly effective and enjoys growing acceptance and popularity.

DRUG THERAPY IN CHRONIC RENAL FAILURE The broad expression of clinical signs and symptoms in CRF often results in the treatment of such patients with a multiplicity of drugs. Unfortunately, these patients are more susceptible to the risk of untoward drug reactions, for reasons that are readily understandable. Drugs normally eliminated largely or entirely by renal excretory mechanisms require reduction in dosage and frequency of administration in order to avoid excessive levels in blood and tissues. Decreased protein binding and reduced volumes of distribution of numerous drugs also contribute to excessive blood and tissue levels in CRF. In addition, patients with CRF exhibit increased sensitivity to many drugs, even when blood levels are within the desired range. For more detailed discussion of this important aspect of patient management in CRF, the reader is referred to Chaps. 70 and 111 and Table 111-1.

REFERENCES

ANDERSON RJ et al: *Clinical Use of Drugs in Renal Failure.* Springfield, Ill, Charles C Thomas, 1976

DEFRONZO RA et al: Carbohydrate metabolism in uremia: A review. Medicine 52:469, 1973

DELUCA HF: The kidney as an endocrine organ involved in the function of vitamin D. Am J Med 58:39, 1975

ESCHBACH JW et al: Iron balance in hemodialysis patients. Ann Intern Med 87:710, 1977

FELDMAN HA, SINGER I: Endocrinology and metabolism in uremia and dialysis: A clinical review. Medicine 54:345, 1974

GIORDANO C (ed): Uremia. Kidney Int 7(suppl 3):S267, 1975

GOTCH F, KRUEGER K (eds): Adequacy of dialysis. Kidney Int 7(suppl 2):S1, 1975

HAMPERS C et al: *Long Term Hemodialysis,* 2d ed. New York, Grune & Stratton, 1973

KOPPLE JD, SWENDSEID ME: Protein and amino acid metabolism in uremic patients undergoing maintenance hemodialysis. Kidney Int 7(suppl 2):S64, 1975

LAZARUS JM, KJELLSTRAND C: Medical aspects of dialysis, in *The Kidney,* 2d ed, BM Brenner, FC Rector Jr (eds). Philadelphia, Saunders, 1980, chap 48

—— et al: Hypertension in chronic renal failure. Treatment with hemodialysis and nephrectomy. Arch Intern Med 133:1059, 1974

LOWRIE EG et al: Survival of patients undergoing chronic hemodialysis and renal transplantation. N Engl J Med 288:863, 1973

NOLPH KD: Short dialysis, middle molecules and uremia. Ann Intern Med 86:93, 1977

SCRIBNER BH, BABB AL: Evidence for toxins of "middle" molecular weights. Kidney Int 7(suppl 2):349, 1975

SHERRARD DJ et al: Advances in peritoneal dialysis. Kidney Int 7(suppl 3):422, 1975

277
IMMUNOPATHOGENETIC MECHANISMS OF RENAL INJURY

RICHARD J. GLASSOCK
BARRY M. BRENNER

Recognition of the important role played by aberrant immunologic processes in many forms of renal injury, especially those involving the glomerular circulation, constitutes one of the most significant conceptual advances made in the understanding of renal diseases during the last quarter century. Although the fine details of these abnormal processes have been elucidated for many disease entities, large gaps in knowledge still exist concerning both the initiating events and the etiological factors involved in renal disease.

In its broadest conceptual framework the immunopathogenesis of renal injury can be simplified to a few fundamental mechanisms. One involves the reaction of a circulating antibody with its respective renal antigen in situ. The antigen may be either an intrinsic constituent of the kidney or one which has been bound to the tissue by some special biochemical or immunological reaction. Antigens in basement membranes of glomerular capillaries or renal tubules and antibodies to these basement membranes are prime components of this mechanism, often referred to as *anti-basement membrane antibody disease.* These mechanisms should be considered in relation to the other immunopathologic mechanisms which can cause tissue damage and which are described in Chap. 62.

Another pathogenetic category, by far the most prevalent in human renal disease, involves the localization of circulating macromolecular aggregates composed of antigens and antibodies (i.e., circulating immune complexes) within renal structures, principally glomeruli. This mechanism is referred to as *immune-complex-mediated disease.* The immune complexes need not bear any special immunochemical relationships to renal structures; thus the kidney can be viewed as a passive participant or an innocent party, damaged by processes originating elsewhere. The source of the antigen may be either *endogenous* (*autologous*) or *exogenous* (*environmental*). Further, exogenous antigens may be biologically inert or derived from an organism capable of self-replication (e.g., bacteria, viruses, etc.). Under special circumstances environmental agents may also combine with autologous substances to result in new antigenic compounds (hapten-protein conjugates), which may act in concert with antibodies to form immune complexes. In contrast to the above mechanisms, *cell-mediated* immune processes are far less well established as possible mechanisms in glomerular and vascular diseases of the kidney. Finally, certain human glomerular diseases are prominently associated with abnormal activation of the *alternative pathway of the complement cascade.*

ANTI-BASEMENT MEMBRANE ANTIBODY MEDIATED RENAL INJURY This form of renal injury is relatively rare in man, accounting for less than 5 percent of all immunologically mediated glomerulonephritides. The experimental prototype of this mechanism is nephrotoxic serum nephritis (NSN). Here an antibody to glomerular basement membrane (GBM) of one species (e.g., rat) is raised in another species (e.g., rabbit) and is administered intravenously to the species originally providing the immunogen (e.g., rat). The *heterologous* antibody binds rapidly to its respective antigen in the GBM. In this instance the antigen is a glycoprotein and is uniformly distributed along the glomerular capillary wall as repeating subunits. Therefore, the deposited immunoglobulin (Ig) will assume a linear pattern by immunofluorescence microscopy (Fig. 277-1*A*). If sufficient heterologous antibody has been administered and bound, various mediator factors are induced. These include the complement and coagulation cascades, vasoactive peptides and amines, and polymorphonuclear leukocytes and macrophages (monocytes). These mediators act to disturb the functional and anatomical integrity of the glomerular capillary wall, leading to proteinuria. Proliferation of cellular elements within the glomerulus, by causing capillary luminal obstruction and hemodynamic alterations, results in a reduction in the glomerular filtration rate. Local enzyme release from storage sites in infiltrating cells may lead to fragmentation of the GBM and leakage of macromolecules, such as fibrinogen, as well as migration of cellular elements, such as macrophages and erythrocytes, into Bowman's space. In the presence of severe glomerular capillary wall damage there may be associated extracapillary

FIGURE 277-1

A. Immunofluorescence photomicrograph of a portion of a glomerulus from a patient with antiglomerular basement membrane antibody-mediated glomerular injury. Note the linear deposits (fluorescein-labeled antihuman IgG). B. Immunofluorescence photomicrograph of a portion of a glomerulus from a patient with immune-complex-mediated glomerular injury. Note the irregular, granular deposits (fluorescein-labeled antihuman IgG). C. Electron micrograph of a portion of a glomerular capillary from a patient with immune-complex-mediated glomerular injury. Note the electron-dense deposits (D).

proliferation (crescents). Under many circumstances such extracapillary proliferation is dependent upon the polymerization of fibrin within Bowman's space. Although the activation of the complement cascade facilitates injury by virtue of chemotactic and cytolytic effects, glomerular injury may occur independent of complement activation. For example, by virtue of surface receptors for an altered Fc portion of Ig, cells such as polymorphonuclear leukocytes and macrophages are attracted to sites of antibody deposition. This *heterologous phase* of NSN would be self-limited were it not for the fact that the deposited Ig is foreign to the host and therefore quite distinct from the original GBM antigen reacting with the heterologous antibody. As a consequence, a host-directed response to the deposited foreign Ig perpetuates the glomerular injury and leads to chronic disease. This is referred to as the *autologous phase* of NSN. Remarkably little "foreign" antigen is required to initiate this phase, so little in fact that amounts, classes, or subunits of heterologous antibody to GBM incapable of initiating injury in their own right can induce an autologous phase if the host response is magnified by preimmunization to foreign Ig.

Glomerular injury of the type seen in the laboratory model of NSN rarely occurs in humans. However, in the early days of renal transplantation some preparations of heterologous antilymphocyte serum used to suppress allograft rejection were contaminated with antibodies to human GBM antigens, and NSN was inadvertently produced in transplant recipients in the treatment of rejection with these preparations. Some drugs are capable of binding to renal structures (e.g., penicillins) and may act as "planted" antigens in a fashion similar to the foreign Ig in NSN. Circulating antibody to renal structures likewise may result if transplanted kidneys possess antigens not shared by the recipient. Binding of these antibodies to relevant antigens in the donor kidney can be viewed in the same conceptual framework as NSN. Finally, antibody directed to antigens *not uniformly* represented along basement membrane structures may give rise to rather discontinuous deposits of Ig by immunofluorescence microscopy and may resemble the in situ formation or deposition of immune complexes (see below).

The formation of antibodies to autologous renal structures may also be induced by intentional immunization of animals with renal antigens (e.g., GBM or tubule basement membranes, TBM), usually in conjunction with adjuvants. Under most circumstances the antigen consists of semipurified extracts of homologous or heterologous GBM or TBM. These antigens possess some degree of cross reactivity with autologous antigens. It is also theoretically possible that altered autologous antigens, released into the circulation consequent to tissue injury, might induce antibody production to normal autologous antigens. The active induction of antitissue autoantibody disease by immunization with organ extracts and adjuvants is a well-studied phenomenon. Such immunization results in the termination of natural tolerance to autologous tissue antigens. The precise mechanism by which this is brought about is unknown, but may involve the calling forth of T-helper cells to interact with dormant B cells already genetically programmed to synthesize antibody to self-constituents. The expansion of autoreactive clones of B cells leads to production of circulating antibody. Other mechanisms may also be involved, including modulation of the activity of T-suppressor cells. In any case, the primary distinction between *active* and *passive* models of antitissue antibody diseases involves the source of antibody. Since in the former the antibody is endogenous and not immunogenetic in the ordinary sense, an autologous phase does not occur, unless, of course, anti-idiotype or antiantibody production develops. By and large, progressive injury in the active models is dependent upon a continuing source of antibody. Mediation of injury presumably occurs by pathways similar to those operating in the heterologous phase of NSN.

Certain diseases occurring in man virtually duplicate the events which transpire in the model of actively induced antitissue antibody-mediated renal disease. The best studied is the clinicopathologic entity known as *Goodpasture's syndrome,* or lung purpura with nephritis (see also Chap. 279). This syndrome is generally believed to be mediated by antibody to GBM; however, the etiologic factors are largely unknown. It has been suggested that exposure to viral infection may release altered autologous antigens capable of abrogating natural tolerance. Goodpasture's syndrome fulfills the criteria of an anti-basement membrane antibody-induced disease, namely,

1 Circulating antibody to normal human GBM is present. This antibody also reacts to a limited extent with primate GBM and to basement membrane antigens of alveoli and renal tubules.
2 "Linear" deposits of IgG, and rarely IgA, are found deposited in diseased tissue.
3 Eluates of diseased tissue contain antibody to normal GBM.
4 Circulating or eluted antibody is capable of inducing glomerular disease in subhuman primates.
5 Renal transplant recipients may acquire the disease if transplantation is performed when the disease is active.

The pulmonary manifestations set Goodpasture's syndrome apart from the experimental models of anti-basement membrane antibody disease in which such manifestations usually do not occur, despite the fact that there is extensive cross reaction between GBM and alveolar capillary basement membrane. Linear Ig deposits are found along the alveolar basement membrane, serum and eluates of lung tissue will react in vivo with normal lung and kidney basement membranes, and serum and eluates of kidney react in vitro with normal lung alveolar basement membrane. The precise mechanisms responsible for pulmonary hemorrhage in anti-basement membrane antibody-induced disease are not well understood. The level of circulating anti-basement membrane antibody does not relate well to the severity of pulmonary hemorrhage. Although GBM antigens are the principal targets of the immune response in this disease, TBM antigens may also be the site of deposition of antibody. "Linear" deposits of Ig along TBM, circulating anti-TBM antibody, and eluates containing anti-TBM antibody are characteristically present. The development of an anti-TBM antibody response exclusively has been recorded occasionally in human diseases: most notably in occasional cases of acute methicillin-induced hypersensitivity interstitial nephritis, in rare cases of poststreptococcal glomerulonephritis, in chronic idiopathic interstitial nephritis, and in renal allograft rejection.

IMMUNE-COMPLEX-MEDIATED RENAL INJURY The deposition in the kidney of immune complexes formed in the circulation account for over 75 percent of all diseases of the kidney for which there is clear evidence of participation of some immunologic process. At the experimental level a multitude of models have been studied, each illustrating important points regarding the details of the pathogenetic processes involved. As mentioned previously, immune-complex-mediated renal diseases involve either replicating or nonreplicating exogenous or endogenous antigens. The best studied of these models, illustrative of the exogenous, nonreplicating category, has been that of *acute and chronic serum sickness.* These models are developed by single or multiple injections, respectively, of soluble immunogenetic foreign serum protein. Figure 277-2 depicts the sequence of events which occurs following the intravenous in-

jection of a single dose of such foreign serum proteins. Initially the protein equilibrates with the intra- and extravascular fluids and undergoes slow metabolic degradation. Subsequently, as a clone of specifically activated B cells begins to secrete antibody into the extracellular fluid, the rate of elimination of the antigen from the circulation will accelerate (i.e., immune elimination) and circulating immune complexes will be formed. At first these immune complexes will be generated in a large excess of antigen and therefore will be relatively small and highly soluble. Few of these complexes possess properties which favor tissue localization and little disease results. With clonal expansion, antibody secretion accelerates still further, so that the ratio of antibody to antigen will approach equivalence and favor the formation of soluble aggregates of increasing size and complexity. A small portion of these will then localize within the glomerular mesangium; in the walls of peripheral capillaries; and in joints, heart valves, choroid plexus, splenic sinusoids, and larger blood vessels, particularly at sites of turbulent flow. The localization of these complexes depends in part on changes in capillary permeability brought about by the release of vasoactive amines, such as histamine, from cellular storage sites. In experimental animals, platelets, basophils, and IgE antibody interact to bring about this release of permeability factors. Once deposited, these complexes possess unique properties which evoke an inflammatory response at the site of deposition. This appears to be especially true of complexes localized within the microvasculature outside the kidney. If the antibody is capable of fixing C1q, the classical complement cascade will be activated; complement components will then be consumed in the process. The antigen itself may also be involved in complement activation. Polysaccharide antigens

FIGURE 277-2

Circulating antigen, antibody, antigen-antibody complexes, and hemolytic complement activity following intravenous injection of soluble serum protein (e.g., bovine serum albumin). Ordinate (log scale) refers to percent of injected antigen remaining in circulation; amount of free antibody as micrograms of antigen bound per milliliter of serum; antigen-antibody complexes as percent injected antigen in immune complexes; complement as percent of normal serum. [After FJ Dixon, in Immunological Diseases, 2d ed, M Samter (ed), Boston, Little, Brown, 1971.]

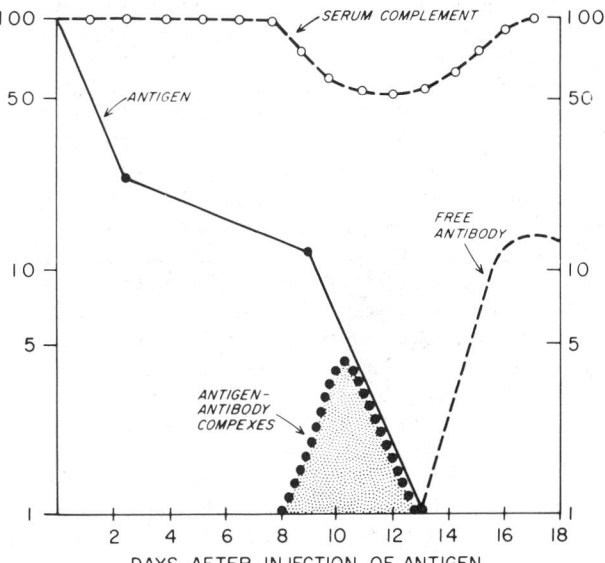

may be independently capable of initiating complement activation via the alternative pathway.

Ultimately the supply of antigen is exhausted. However, antibody synthesis proceeds unabated, leading eventually to a state of antibody excess, which, in the case of multivalent antigens such as soluble serum proteins, favors extensive polymerization of the immune complex, the formation of a lattice network, and a great increase in the size of the immune complex. These immune complexes formed in antibody excess are then treated as particulate material by the reticuloendothelial system and removed rapidly. Once all the antigen is eliminated only free antibody can be detected in the circulation. The immune complexes deposited in the kidney during the immune elimination phase will be metabolized and degraded and the inflammatory process will eventually subside spontaneously.

On the other hand, if the antigen is administered repeatedly (thus resembling the situation which prevails when antigens are released from endogenous sites or from replicating organisms), then the opportunity exists for the development of a continuing or fluctuating level of soluble circulating immune complexes of varying molecular composition and phlogistic activity. In this circumstance, modifying the function of the reticuloendothelial system, the release of factors which alter glomerular capillary permeability, the rate of antigen egress into the vascular fluids, or the rate of antibody formation all would be expected to have far-reaching consequences on the amount of immune complexes localizing within renal structures.

Although this formulation presupposes that immune complexes form within the circulation and then are deposited in vascular structures, it is also possible for immune complexes to be formed in the extravascular (interstitial) compartment by virtue of diffusion into this fluid compartment of cell-derived antigens and circulating antibody. Such a phenomenon may explain the deposition of immune complexes in the interstitial areas of the kidney, with relative sparing of the glomerular circulation. Regardless of the nature of the antibody or antigen or the particular circumstances surrounding the immunologic events, a valuable clue to the presence of immune-complex deposition is the morphologic pattern found when tissues are examined by immunofluorescence or electron microscopic techniques. Granular, discontinuous, and irregular deposits of Ig, often in conjunction with complement components, are found by immunofluorescence (Fig. 277-1B), whereas electron-dense deposits are seen by electron microscopy (Fig. 277-1C). Sometimes these deposits acquire a definite substructure, but for the most part they are rather homogeneous. The deposits may develop in several locations within the glomerulus: beneath the epithelial cells (subepithelial), within the basement membrane (intramembranous), beneath the endothelium (subendothelial), and within the mesangial matrix. Immune complexes may also localize in the peritubular capillary network. The precise reason for localization at these differing sites is not well understood but may involve factors such as size or charge of the complexes, receptors for the Fc or complement components within glomerular structures, or local hemodynamic events. The deposits appear to increase in size by aggregation, and there is some evidence that glomerular cells may participate in their removal. The persistence of deposits is related to the rate of formation balanced by the activity of removal systems. Finally, an antibody reacting with an intrinsic basement membrane antigen which is irregularly distributed along the GBM could also give rise to the appearance of "granular" deposits of Ig by immunofluorescence. Thus, although granular immunofluorescence for Ig and electron-dense deposits are generally regarded as being reliable signposts of circulating immune-complex deposition, other pathogenetic mechanisms may be responsible for this pattern. Once deposited in glomeruli, circulating immune complexes evoke local inflammatory and functional changes, which at least for the glomerular circulation may be relatively independent of complement or polymorphonuclear leukocytes. Furthermore, the morphologic lesions which result from immune-complex deposition may vary considerably, from diffuse proliferative to nonproliferative membranous or sclerosing lesions. Coagulation, platelet agglutination, activation of the complement cascade, and release of vasoactive amines may participate in determining the pattern of morphologic response.

The *exogenous* antigens involved in circulating immune-complex-mediated disease are derived chiefly from infectious agents such as bacteria, viruses, or parasites. Replication of the organism provides a continuing source of antigen. The best studied examples of these in humans are *infective endocarditis*, *leprosy*, *syphilis*, *hepatitis B*, and *malaria*. The *endogenous* antigens involved in human disease vary considerably and include *DNA*, *thyroglobulin*, *autologous immunoglobulins*, *erthrocyte stroma*, *renal tubular antigens*, and *tumor-specific* or *tumor-associated* antigens.

COMPLEMENT-ASSOCIATED GLOMERULAR INJURY Although there is little evidence that complement activation, independent of antitissue antibody or circulating immune complexes, can bring about glomerular injury, there are certain associations between complement and renal disease in man. The clinicopathologic entity known as *idiopathic membranoproliferative glomerulonephritis* (see also Chap. 278) may be associated with patterns of serum complement component deposition within glomeruli suggestive of involvement of the alternative pathway of complement activation, perhaps independent of immune-complex deposition. These patterns are not, however, necessarily unique to this group of disorders since they may also be observed in a wide variety of postinfectious glomerulonephritides and in certain collagen vascular diseases.

As discussed in greater detail in Chap. 62, the alternative pathway mechanism of complement activation depends upon the interaction of aggregated or immune-complex IgA, polysaccharides, or lipopolysaccharides with a serum-initiating factor of unknown biochemical composition. Subsequently, an enzyme capable of cleaving native C3 is generated from the interaction of factors B, D, native C3, and Mg^{2+}. The C3 convertase thus assembled is composed of a fragment of C3 (C3b) and an altered form of factor B (Bb) and known as C3bBb. This alternative pathway convertase is analogous to the C3 convertase generated in the classical pathway of complement activation (also known as C4b2a). The alternative pathway C3 convertase is stabilized by binding to properdin and degraded by several inactivators (C3b inactivator, β1H). Alternative pathway C3 convertase cleaves C3 into C3a (anaphylatoxin I) and C3b, which is further cleaved by C3 inactivator into C3c and C3d, biologically inactive fragments. The C3b formed in this manner can also autocatalytically form additional alternative pathway C3 convertase in the presence of factors B, D, and Mg^{2+}. The hallmarks of activation of the alternative pathway are depressed serum levels of native C3, circulating fragments of C3 (C3c, C3d), low levels of factor B, and circulating fragments of B (Bb), all occurring in the absence of perturbations in the early classical components C1q, C4, and C2. The terminal complement components C5 through C9 may also be activated and even result in lysis of cells in the absence of antibody. Depression of the synthesis of C3 may also contribute to diminished serum levels, since circulating fragments of C3 may reduce cellular production.

In *idiopathic membranoproliferative glomerulonephritis,* particularly the subset known as "dense deposit disease," serum C3 levels are depressed; C4, C1, and C2 levels tend to be normal; and C3 may be deposited in glomeruli without Ig (see also Chap. 278). In addition, an oligoclonal autoantibody (an immunoconglutinin) to $\overline{C3bBb}$ is frequently found in the circulation. This autoantibody reacts with a conformational neoantigen of the $\overline{C3bBb}$ complex and acts to stabilize this enzyme from the influence of C3b inactivator and $\beta1H$ in a fashion similar to properdin. As a result serums containing this autoantibody are capable of inducing C3 cleavage in vitro by permitting the assembly of a stable fluid phase C3 convertase. This antibody is also known as C3 nephritic factor (C3NeF), and was first described in the serums of patients with glomerulonephritis and persistent depression of C3 levels.

The relationship between these aberrations in the complement pathway and glomerular injury is uncertain. No experimental models of persistent activation of the alternative pathway have been associated with glomerulonephritis. Glomerulonephritis may be a closely associated but pathogenetically unrelated phenomenon, perhaps genetically determined. On the other hand, some have suggested that persistent hypocomplementemia may interfere with the normal removal processes for environmental antigens such as viruses. Such a defect might favor the persistence of these antigens in the circulation and enhance the likelihood of formation of circulating immune complexes.

CELL-MEDIATED IMMUNITY IN GLOMERULAR AND TUBULO-INTERSTITIAL DISEASES The roles of specifically sensitized cells acting independently of antibody (i.e., T-killer cells) and antibody-dependent lymphoid cell-mediated (ADCC) or "armed" macrophages in the pathogenesis of glomerular and tubulointerstitial diseases have been difficult to establish firmly except in one clear-cut example. The rejection of renal allografts in nonsensitized recipients is clearly a cell-mediated process. This subject is dealt with in greater detail in Chap. 69.

It is true that by utilizing a variety of in vitro techniques cell-mediated hypersensitivity to both environmental and endogenous antigens may be demonstrable in several diseases of the kidney, including glomerulonephritis. The precise role such "sensitized" cells play in the actual tissue injury is unclear, especially in human glomerular disease. No doubt the burgeoning knowledge in the field of cell-cell interactions will eventually clarify these uncertainties. It is very likely that some diseases which do not fit into an antibody or immune-complex–mediated category will find an explanation in reactions of the cell-mediated variety. One likely candidate for this category is so-called "minimal change disease," one of the morphological subsets of idiopathic nephrotic syndrome. Furthermore, because of the prominence of lymphoid cell infiltration, various forms of chronic tubulointerstitial nephritis have also been suggested as examples of cell-mediated reactions (see Chap. 281).

REFERENCES

McCluskey RT, Klaasen J: Immunologically mediated glomerular, tubular and interstitial renal disease. N Engl J Med 290:564, 1973

Peters DK: The immunological basis of glomerulonephritis. Proc R Soc Med 67:557, 1974

Wilson CB, Dixon FJ: The renal response to immunological injury, in *The Kidney,* 2d ed, BM Brenner, FC Rector Jr (eds). Philadelphia, Saunders, 1980

Wilson CB et al (eds): Immunologic mechanisms of renal disease, in *Contemporary Issues in Nephrology,* vol 3. New York, Churchill Livingstone, 1979

278

THE MAJOR GLOMERULOPATHIES

RICHARD J. GLASSOCK
BARRY M. BRENNER

Disease-induced alterations of the structural and functional integrity of the glomerular capillary circulation are often associated with the findings, either singly or in combination, of hematuria, proteinuria, reduced glomerular filtration rate (GFR), and hypertension. Five major glomerulopathic syndromes are recognized: *acute glomerulonephritis, rapidly progressive glomerulonephritis, chronic glomerulonephritis,* the *nephrotic syndrome,* and *asymptomatic urinary abnormalities.* This chapter deals with each of these syndromes in some detail, describing diseases in which the kidney is either the sole or predominant organ involved (i.e., the primary glomerulopathies) or is involved as a complication of infection or drug exposure. Glomerular injury associated with multisystem disorders or heredofamilial conditions is discussed in Chap. 279.

ACUTE GLOMERULONEPHRITIS (AGN)

The causes of AGN are given in Table 278-1. The "acute nephritic syndrome" consists of the abrupt onset of *hematuria* and *proteinuria,* accompanied by evidence of *azotemia* (i.e., reduced GFR) and renal *salt and water retention.* If GFR is reduced markedly, oligoanuria may be present (see also Chaps. 43, 275). Salt and water retention leads to circulatory congestion, hypertension, and edema. Fluid retention appears to be due both to diminished GFR and to exaggerated salt and water reabsorption, particularly in distal nephron segments.

The edema of acute glomerulonephritis tends to appear initially in areas of low tissue pressure, such as the *periorbital* areas, but may subsequently progress to involve dependent portions of the body and lead to *ascites* and/or *pleural effusions. Circulatory congestion* is manifested by an increase in systemic and pulmonary vascular pressures, normal or increased cardiac output, and a shortened circulation time. In the absence of underlying valvular, myocardial, or coronary artery disease or severe diastolic hypertension there is little likelihood that true left ventricular congestive heart failure will develop. If left atrial filling pressure rises above the opposing plasma oncotic pressure, however, pulmonary edema may ensue. *Arterial diastolic hypertension* is the consequence of several factors, including extracellular fluid volume expansion, enhanced cardiac output, and modest increases in peripheral vascular resistance. Plasma renin activity, aldosterone, and the

TABLE 278-1
Causes of acute glomerulonephritis

I Infectious diseases
  A Poststreptococcal glomerulonephritis
  B Nonpoststreptococcal glomerulonephritis
    1 Bacterial: Infective endocarditis, "shunt nephritis," sepsis, pneumococcal pneumonia, typhoid fever, secondary syphilis, meningococcemia
    2 Viral: Hepatitis B, infectious mononucleosis, mumps, measles, varicella, vaccinia, echovirus, and coxsackievirus
    3 Parasitic: Malaria, toxoplasmosis
II Multisystem diseases: Systemic lupus erythematosus, vasculitis, Schönlein-Henoch purpura, Goodpasture's syndrome
III Primary glomerular diseases: Membranoproliferative glomerulonephritis, Berger's disease, "pure" mesangial proliferative glomerulonephritis
IV Miscellaneous: Guillain-Barré syndrome, irradiation of Wilms's tumor, self-administered diphtheria-pertussis-tetanus vaccine, serum sickness

sympathetic nervous system are relatively suppressed. Hypertension may at times be accompanied by encephalopathy, particularly in young children.

The extent and severity of urinary abnormalities in AGN vary considerably. Gross (macroscopic) *hematuria* is the most common, and is often described by the patient as smoky, coffee, or cola colored urine. Lesser degrees of hematuria may go unrecognized by the patient or parent; for this reason, the features of fluid retention and hypertension may be ascribed erroneously to other illnesses if a careful examination of the urine sediment is omitted from the initial laboratory evaluation. Hematuria is often, but not invariably, accompanied by the excretion of *red cell casts.* Leukocyturia and leukocyte casts may also occur, indicating the presence of inflammation in the glomerulus. The degree of *proteinuria* varies according to the nature and severity of the underlying glomerular lesions. Rarely, protein excretion rates may fall within the normal range, but generally are between 0.2 and 3 g per day. If proteinuria is marked and sustained, features of the nephrotic syndrome may appear (see below).

The short-term evolution of acute nephritis generally depends upon the nature of the underlying glomerular lesion; however, within a week or so of onset most patients with postinfectious AGN will begin to experience spontaneous resolution of fluid retention and hypertension. Urinary abnormalities often take longer to resolve. A few patients with the acute nephritic syndrome will go on in the ensuing weeks or months to develop a rapidly progressive form of renal failure (i.e., rapidly progressive glomerulonephritis, discussed below). The long-term outlook for patients with AGN, in the context of treatment of specific lesions, is considered below.

ACUTE POSTSTREPTOCOCCAL GLOMERULONEPHRITIS (PSGN) Clinical features and diagnosis This disorder can be viewed as the archetype of AGN. PSGN follows in the wake of *pharyngeal or cutaneous infection* with one of a limited number of strains of *group A beta-hemolytic streptococci.* These potentially "nephritogenic" streptococci may be identified by serotyping of a cell wall antigen (M protein). Among outbreaks of infection with proved "nephritogenic" strains of streptococci the PSGN attack rate is relatively uniform, averaging about 10 percent, but because of variation in the nephritogenicity among group A streptococci, attack rates among outbreaks of infection may vary considerably. Immunity to M protein is type specific, long lasting, and protective. Repeated episodes of PSGN are therefore unusual. Outbreaks of pharyngeal infection–associated PSGN are commonest in children aged 6 to 10. AGN following cutaneous streptococcal infection is more commonly associated with factors such as poor personal hygiene, overcrowding, and concomitant cutaneous disease, such as scabies infestation. Seasonal and geographic variations in prevalence of AGN are more marked for pharyngeal than for cutaneous disease.

An important feature of PSGN is the existence of a *latent period* between the earliest manifestations of infection and the onset of recognizable signs and symptoms of nephritis. The latent period is more apparent following pharyngeal infections, where it usually is 6 to 10 days in duration. Cutaneous infections are associated with longer latent periods, averaging about 2 weeks. Definitive signs of glomerular inflammation occurring at the same time as, or shortly after, infection usually indicate an *exacerbation* of a preexisting chronic glomerular disease (see below).

The diagnosis of PSGN rests upon the demonstration of at least two of the following features: (1) The presence of a group A beta-hemolytic streptococcus of a potentially nephritogenic M-protein type in a throat or skin lesion. (2) The demonstra-

tion of an immune response to one or more of the streptococcal *exoenzymes,* including anti-streptolysin O (ASO), antistreptokinase (ASK), anti-deoxyribonuclease B (ADNAase B), anti-nicotinyl adenine dinucleotidase (ANADase), or antihyaluronidase (AH). ASO responses are typically brisk in pharyngeal infections, but often absent in cutaneous infection; whereas AH, ADNAase, and ANADase responses occur after the latter. Testing for multiple antibody responses and serial determinations are necessary to achieve a diagnostic accuracy of 90 percent. Early antimicrobial therapy may prevent the antibody response to exoenzymes and render throat cultures negative, but may not interfere with the development of AGN; this makes accurate serologic diagnosis difficult or impossible. (3) The demonstration of a transient decline in the serum concentration of C3 component of complement, with a return to normal within 8 weeks after the first signs of renal disease. Other complement components (i.e., C1q and C4) are frequently less depressed. In addition to these laboratory features it is desirable to document a latent period appropriate to the nature of the infection. Furthermore, the patient should not have any known preexisting renal disease.

Other laboratory features commonly observed in PSGN include transient cryoimmunoglobulinemia, positive tests for circulating immune complexes, and circulating high-molecular-weight fibrinogen complexes. The erythrocyte sedimentation rate is usually elevated, while C-reactive protein and rheumatoid factor are generally normal or absent. Mild anemia and hypoalbuminemia, both largely dilutional in origin, may be present. Severe hypoalbuminemia may be encountered if heavy proteinuria is present and prolonged. Excretion rates of urinary protein in excess of 3.5 g per day occur in less than 20 percent of hospitalized patients. Proteinuria is usually of a nonselective character and frequently contains high concentrations of fibrin-degradation products (FDP) and C3 protein, particularly during the diuretic phase. Hyponatremia, hyperkalemia, and metabolic acidosis may be seen in azotemic or oliguric patients, especially those having free access to water or potassium. Urinary sodium concentration is usually low, reflecting avid salt reabsorption in the distal nephron. Abdominal films reveal normal or enlarged kidneys. The chest x-ray may be normal or reveal a slightly enlarged heart, often accompanied by signs of pulmonary congestion. The electrocardiogram may reveal nonspecific T-wave abnormalities. Rheumatic fever rarely coexists with acute PSGN.

The differential diagnosis of PSGN includes other infectious or primary renal diseases which may produce an identical acute nephritic syndrome (Table 278-1). Finally, multisystem diseases such as SLE, Schönlein-Henoch purpura, and vasculitis may present initially as acute nephritis (Chap. 279). Predominantly nonglomerular diseases, including thrombotic thrombocytopenic purpura, hemolytic-uremic syndrome, and acute hypersensitivity interstitial nephritis may also present the features of the acute nephritic syndrome (Chaps. 281 and 282).

Pathology and pathogenesis Renal biopsies performed early in the course of PSGN reveal *diffuse, endocapillary proliferative glomerulonephritis.* Infiltration of glomeruli with polymorphonuclear leukocytes and monocytes is also common. The glomerular capillary walls are usually thin and delicate and free of necrosis. Occasional discrete proteinaceous deposits projecting from the outer aspects of the capillary wall toward the urinary space (humps) may be recognized by light microscopy and coincide with the electron-dense deposits seen by electron microscopy. Segmental extracapillary proliferation (crescents) may involve a few glomeruli, but diffuse crescent formation is uncommon except among a subset of patients presenting with severe and rapidly progressive acute renal failure (see section below on rapidly progressive glomerulonephritis). Extraglomerular vessels and tubulointerstitial areas are usually normal. Red blood cells are frequently seen in the lumens of distal tubules, where they form red blood cell casts.

By immunofluorescence microscopy, granular deposits of IgG are seen in peripheral capillary loops and mesangium, nearly always accompanied by C3 and properdin, but less commonly by C1q and C4 (Chap. 277). These deposits may also be recognized by electron microscopy and probably represent immune complexes, although the precise nature of the antigen-antibody systems involved remains unknown. Most likely the antigen is derived from the streptococcal organism itself, but this has been difficult to verify. The profile of altered serum complement components described above, and the prominent C3 and properdin deposition in glomeruli, are suggestive of involvement of the alternative pathway of complement activation (Chap. 277).

Course and treatment   The ultimate *prognosis* for PSGN appears to differ between sporadic and epidemic forms and between adults and children. *Epidemic* forms of the disease in *children* have a uniformly favorable short- and long-term prognosis. Few patients die of complications of renal failure (many fewer than 1 percent), and nearly all experience a spontaneous resolution of abnormal clinical signs within a week after the onset of illness. Abnormalities in the urinary sediment subside slowly in the ensuing months; in a few cases, several years elapse before the urinary sediment becomes consistently normal. Among children with PSGN during epidemics of streptococcal infection, and in whom some form of preexisting chronic glomerular disease was absent, long-term follow-up has revealed little or no evidence of progression to chronic renal disease. A very small percentage may develop extensive crescentic glomerulonephritis with its relentlessly progressive course. The site of the streptococcal infection, the type of M protein, the severity in abnormalities of complement components or urinary sediment, or the extent of the rise in antibody response to exoenzymes have little or no bearing on the ultimate prognosis of PSGN. Prolonged and persistent heavy proteinuria and/or abnormal GFR imply a more unfavorable outcome. *Sporadic* cases of PSGN among *children* may have more serious long-term consequences, although this remains controversial. After the subsidence of the acute disease, some children subsequently develop slowly progressive glomerular capillary obliteration (global glomerulosclerosis), reduced GFR, and hypertension; after several decades, end-stage renal failure from chronic glomerulonephritis may result. The persistence of abnormal proteinuria is the rule in such cases.

The prognosis for *adults* with PSGN seems to be less favorable than for children. The reason for this apparent age difference is poorly understood. Although the overall prognosis for PSGN in *epidemics* seems good, *sporadic* PSGN in adults appears to be associated with lasting and/or progressive deterioration in renal function in approximately one-third to one-half of all cases. This may take the form of persistent proteinuria and/or hematuria, or of slowly progressive glomerulosclerosis and renal failure, often accompanied by hypertension. This evolution seems more likely to occur when the initial disease has been unusually severe. Whether milder forms of sporadic PSGN can lead to chronic disease is an important but unresolved issue (see "Chronic Glomerulonephritis," below).

The *treatment* of acute PSGN is supportive. It seems reasonable to recommend bed rest until the signs of glomerular inflammation and circulatory congestion (primarily hypertension) subside, but prolonged forced periods of inactivity are of no demonstrable benefit in the healing process. Fluid retention, circulatory congestion, and edema may be treated with sodium and fluid restriction, or loop diuretics. Diuresis alone will often ameliorate mild to moderate hypertension. If severe hypertension is present, vasodilator drugs such as nitroprus-

side, hydralazine, or diazoxide may be useful. Encephalopathy and pulmonary congestion will generally improve with lowering of blood pressure and the relief of circulatory overload. Digitalis preparations should be avoided except in instances of well-documented organic heart disease with congestive failure. Treatment with ion exchange resins and/or dialysis may be required for cases of severe oliguria, fluid overload, and hyperkalemia. Mild protein restriction is desirable for azotemic patients. A 7- to 10-day course of antimicrobials (e.g., penicillin or erythromycin) should be given if streptococcal infection is documented. Long-term chemoprophylaxis is not indicated. Steroids and cytotoxic drugs have not been shown to be of value.

NONSTREPTOCOCCAL ACUTE GLOMERULONEPHRITIS
Clinical features and diagnosis   A variety of infectious illnesses other than those caused by group A beta-hemolytic streptococci may also be associated with AGN (Table 278-1). These include *bacteremic states* and various *viral* and *parasitic* diseases. Ordinarily these diseases can be diagnosed by the presence of typical extrarenal clinical features or by bacteriologic or serologic findings. A substantial body of evidence indicates that circulating immune complexes play an important role in the pathogenesis of AGN in these diseases. Bacteremic states are frequently associated with persistent depression of serum concentrations of complement components C1q, C4, and C3, elevated levels of rheumatoid factor, circulating cryoimmunoglobulins, and strongly positive tests for circulating immune complexes. Control of infection usually results in the resolution of the signs of glomerular inflammation, although, in occasional instances, rapidly progressive or chronic glomerulonephritis may ensue.

RAPIDLY PROGRESSIVE GLOMERULONEPHRITIS (RPGN)

A minority of patients with AGN develop azotemia, which is *transient,* usually in association with a short period of oliguria. A diuresis usually follows within days or a few weeks and GFR returns to normal. On the other hand, some cases of AGN are characterized by a *rapidly progressive* form of renal failure, which often develops abruptly and displays little tendency for spontaneous or complete recovery. The clinical term *rapidly progressive glomerulonephritis (RPGN)* is often applied to this group to connote the development of renal failure in a period of weeks to months, rather than years or decades, as is typical of chronic glomerulonephritis (see below). Usually, but not invariably, extensive *extracapillary (crescentic) glomerulonephritis* is found as the pathologic lesion underlying the syndrome of RPGN and the two terms are often used interchangeably.

RPGN can arise in three clinical settings (Table 278-2): (1) as a renal complication of an acute or subacute infectious disease, (2) as a renal complication in many multisystem diseases, and (3) as a primary or idiopathic glomerular disease. The first category is discussed in Chap. 277, the second in Chap. 279, and the third will be considered here.

IDIOPATHIC RAPIDLY PROGRESSIVE GLOMERULONEPHRITIS
Clinical features and diagnosis   This disorder affects individuals in a broad age distribution and has a predilection for males. Wide geographic differences in the prevalence of the disease have been noted, and outbreaks ("miniepidemics") may occur. Some patients have had recent heavy exposure to volatile hydrocarbons, but there is little evidence to support a

TABLE 278-2
Causes of rapidly progressive glomerulonephritis

I Infectious diseases
   A Poststreptococcal glomerulonephritis
   B Infective endocarditis
   C Occult visceral sepsis
II Multisystem diseases
   A Systemic lupus erythematosus
   B Schönlein-Henoch purpura
   C Vasculitis (including Wegener's granulomatosis)
   D Goodpasture's syndrome
   E Essential cryoimmunoglobulinemia
   F Malignancy (rare)
III Primary glomerular diseases
   A Idiopathic crescentic glomerulonephritis
   B Membranoproliferative glomerulonephritis
   C Berger's disease (rare)
   D Membranous glomerulopathy complicated by anti-glomerular basement membrane antibody formation (rare)

cause-and-effect relationship. While a flu-like or viral prodrome may occur, frank arthritis, sinusitis, otitis, skin rash, neuritis, or encephalopathy are uncommon and are more in keeping with a multisystems disease. Symptoms of weakness, nausea, and vomiting (indicative of azotemia) usually dominate the clinical picture. Oliguria, abdominal or flank pain, and hemoptysis may also be present (see "Goodpasture's Syndrome," Chap. 279). The blood pressure is usually normal or only modestly elevated. Urinalysis typically reveals hematuria and red cell casts, but exceptional cases with relatively benign urine sediments have been observed. Proteinuria is always present and may occasionally be massive. Other biochemical features of the nephrotic syndrome are uncommon, probably because of the concomitant reduction in GFR. Proteinuria is typically nonselective, and high concentrations of FDP are found in urine. Azotemia develops early and tends to progress at a rapid rate. Other clinical and laboratory features relate to the underlying pathology and pathogenesis.

Pathology and pathogenesis It is clear that idiopathic RPGN is far from a homogeneous disease. By light microscopy the characteristic abnormality found in the kidneys is *extensive extracapillary proliferation,* i.e., *crescents.* The extent and degree of glomerular involvement varies considerably; however, among patients with rapid deterioration of renal function it is usual for more than 70 percent of glomeruli to be involved with circumferential crescents. Endocapillary proliferation may also be seen, but if very prominent, suggests the presence of antigen-antibody complexes. Fibrin-related antigens are nearly always demonstrable within the crescents by special stains or by immunofluorescence. Interestingly, antihemophilic globulin has not been found in a similar distribution, suggesting that fibrin polymerization occurs by non-thrombin-dependent mechanisms. Gaps or focal discontinuities in the glomerular basement membrane (GBM) are observed in association with crescents.

Variations in the underlying pathogenetic mechanisms responsible for RPGN are revealed by immunofluorescence studies of renal biopsies (Chap. 277). In approximately one-third of cases, *linear deposits* of IgG, often accompanied by C3, indicate involvement of *anti-GBM antibodies.* Circulating anti-GBM antibodies are found in this group by indirect immunofluorescence, hemagglutination, or radioimmunoassay techniques. Patients falling into this pathogenetic subgroup tend to have normal serum complement levels and a marked tendency to develop hemoptysis (see also "Goodpasture's Syndrome," Chap. 279). About one-third of cases will have findings indicative of *immune-complex–mediated disease,* namely, *granular deposits* of immunoglobulin by immunofluorescence microscopy and electron-dense deposits by electron microscopy. This mechanism of RPGN tends to occur in older individuals, to produce more constitutional symptoms, and to result in more

disturbances of the complement pathways than does anti-GBM antibody mediated disease. Hemoptysis may also occur, but circulating anti-GBM antibodies are absent. The remainder of cases of RPGN reveal scanty or no immunoglobulins or complement by immunofluorescence; their pathogenesis is unknown. This group also tends to include older individuals, in whom serum complement concentrations are normal and anti-GBM antibodies are absent. Occasionally, mild hemoptysis may occur.

It is obvious from the foregoing discussion that lung hemorrhage may be observed in a variety of circumstances associated with RPGN. This subject is covered in greater detail in the section on Goodpasture's syndrome in Chap. 279. As noted in Table 278-2, other idiopathic (primary) renal diseases may, from time to time, be accompanied by a prominent tendency for crescent formation and a rapidly progressive course.

Course and treatment In general, the prognosis for preservation of renal function in RPGN is poor. Patients with crescent formation in 70 percent or more of glomeruli, oliguria or severe reduction in GFR (less than 5 ml/min) at the time of presentation, or an anti-GBM antibody mediated process have the worst prognosis. Although advances in treatment are changing the outlook for patients with RPGN, at least one-half to two-thirds of patients currently require maintenance hemodialysis within 6 months of discovery of the illness. Exceptional patients with crescentic glomerulonephritis will have a more protracted illness. Spontaneous resolution is very uncommon, except among patients with infection as the basis for formation of antigen-antibody complexes, where removal of antigen can take place.

The treatment of RPGN is currently undergoing reevaluation. *Corticosteroids,* in the form of "pulses" of parenteral methylprednisolone in high doses, or continuous oral prednisone daily, often combined with *cytotoxic agents* (azathioprine or cyclophosphamide), have yielded varying degrees of success. Since no controlled studies have been conducted, however, it is difficult to verify the exact value of these approaches. The addition of *anticoagulants* (heparin or coumadin) and antithrombotic agents (cyproheptadine, dipyridamole, sulfinpyrazone) seems rational on the basis of evidence suggesting involvement of the coagulation process in the genesis of crescent formation. However, objective evidence of benefit from such therapies in animals afflicted with experimentally induced crescentic glomerulonephritis has been inconsistent, in part because of variations in the severity of the disease models, the timing of treatment, and the nature of the anticoagulant or antithrombotic agent used. *Ancrod,* a fibrinogenolytic agent not yet released in the United States, may yet prove to be the most effective agent. Very recently, intensive plasma exchange (2 to 4 liters of plasma daily or three times weekly), combined with steroids and cytotoxic agents, has been employed in patients with RPGN with very encouraging preliminary results. Beneficial effects appear to be greatest when such combined therapy is instituted early in the course of disease, before glomerular abnormalities are advanced. Despite aggressive therapy, patients with oliguria continue to do poorly. Clearly, treatment must be individualized, and because regular dialysis therapy and/or transplantation are available to virtually all patients with RPGN, one should probably err on the side of a conservative approach, unless compelling evidence in support of potential reversibility is present.

RPGN may recur in the renal transplant. It is difficult to be certain of the precise risk in individual cases. At present it seems prudent to recommend that, after initiating dialysis, a period of 3 to 6 months be allowed to elapse before undertaking renal transplantation in patients who have circulating anti-

THE NEPHROTIC SYNDROME (NS)

In its overt form, NS is characterized by *albuminuria, hypoalbuminemia, hyperlipidemia,* and *edema*. These abnormalities are direct or indirect consequences of excessive glomerular leakage of plasma proteins into the urine (see also Chap. 42). *Heavy proteinuria* is the hallmark of the nephrotic state. Arbitrarily, protein excretion rates in excess of 3.5 g per 1.73 m² per day are considered to be in the nephrotic range, primarily because proteinuria of this magnitude is seldom observed in tubulointerstitial and vascular diseases of the kidney. Sustained heavy proteinuria is often, but not invariably, accompanied by *hypoalbuminemia*. Excessive urinary losses, increased renal catabolism, and inadequate hepatic synthesis of albumin all contribute to this depression of plasma albumin. The resulting decrease in plasma oncotic pressure leads to a disturbance in the Starling forces acting across peripheral capillaries. Intravascular fluid migrates into the interstitial tissue (i.e., *edema*), particularly in areas of low tissue pressure. These disturbances initiate a series of homeostatic adjustments designed to correct the resulting deficit in effective plasma volume. These include activation of the renin-angiotensin-aldosterone system, enhanced antidiuretic hormone secretion, stimulation of the sympathetic nervous system, and perhaps a reduction in the secretion of a postulated "natriuretic hormone." These and other poorly understood adjustments lead to renal sodium and water retention, primarily because of avid reabsorption in distal nephron segments, resulting in unrelenting edema. The severity of edema correlates with the level of serum albumin and with the extent of urinary protein losses. The extent and severity of edema is significantly conditioned by the presence of other factors such as heart disease or peripheral vascular disease.

The diminished plasma oncotic pressure also appears to stimulate hepatic lipoprotein synthesis, and *hyperlipidemia* is a frequent accompaniment of the nephrotic state. Low-density lipoproteins and cholesterol are elevated most frequently, but as the plasma oncotic pressure falls to very low levels, very low density lipoproteins and tryglycerides also increase. Excessive urinary losses of plasma protein factors regulating lipoprotein synthesis or disposal may also contribute to the hyperlipidemic state. These lipid abnormalities may contribute to the accelerated atherosclerosis which occurs in patients with NS. Lipid bodies (fatty casts, oval fat bodies) commonly appear in the urine.

Urine losses of plasma proteins other than albumin are also of importance in NS. Loss of thyroxine-binding globulin may produce abnormalities in thyroid function tests, including a low T4 and an enhanced resin T3 uptake. Loss of cholecalciferol-binding protein may lead to a vitamin D deficiency state, secondary hyperparathyroidism, and bone disease, and also may contribute to the hypocalcemia and hypocalciuria seen commonly in NS. Enhanced urinary excretion of transferrin may produce an iron-resistant microcytic hypochromic anemia. Zinc and copper deficiency may result from urinary losses of metal binding proteins. Loss of antithrombin III (heparin cofactor) in the urine may be associated with increased coagulability, which may or may not be balanced by losses of procoagulant factors in the urine. If it is not, it may produce a hypercoagulable state, and the increased tendency to thrombosis may lead to renal vein thrombosis.

Some patients with NS develop severe IgG deficiency, in part due to urinary losses and hypercatabolism. Low-molecular-weight complement components may also be lost in the urine and contribute to defects in the opsonization of bacteria. Various drug-binding proteins (chiefly albumin) may be decreased, altering the pharmacokinetic and toxicity properties of many drugs. Cellulose acetate electrophoresis of serum reveals, in addition to diminished albumin levels, increases of alpha and beta globulins.

COMPLICATIONS AND MANAGEMENT OF THE NEPHROTIC SYNDROME *Edema* should be managed cautiously and conservatively. Overly vigorous diuresis with potent loop diuretics (furosemide or ethacrynic acid) may result in a further lowering of effective plasma volume, and GFR, and lead to postural hypotension. Severe extracellular volume depletion may predispose to the development of acute renal failure. The temptation to administer concentrated salt-poor albumin should be resisted, as nearly all the administered protein will be excreted in 24 to 48 h, so that any beneficial effect on plasma oncotic pressure will be transient. However, such treatment may be necessary in severely hypoalbuminemic patients suffering from profound postural symptoms or very refractory anasarca.

The treatment of *hyperlipidemia* is difficult at best and its influence on morbidity and mortality uncertain. Most agents effective in reducing cholesterol and/or triglyceride levels are either too toxic (e.g., clofibrate) or poorly tolerated (e.g., cholestyramine) for chronic use. The value of newer agents in the management of hyperlipidemia in NS is not well established.

The *thromboembolic complications* of NS are reasonably common and have a broad range of clinical manifestations, including spontaneous peripheral venous and/or arterial thromboses, as well as pulmonary arterial and renal venous occlusions. *Renal vein thrombosis,* either unilateral or bilateral, is a particularly distressing complication of NS. In the past, this was regarded as a cause rather than a consequence of NS, a conclusion no longer held to be true. Certain glomerular lesions are more likely than others to be associated with renal vein thrombosis. These include membranous nephropathy, membranoproliferative glomerulonephritis, and amyloidosis. Features which are suggestive of renal vein thrombosis include unilateral or bilateral flank or loin pain, gross hematuria, widely fluctuating GFR and urinary protein excretion rates, asymmetry of renal size and/or function, scalloping of the ureters (due to collateral circulation) and evidence of pulmonary emboli and/or infarction (Chap. 282). Renal vein thrombosis is best documented by selective renal venous angiography. The presence of a documented thromboembolic complication of NS is usually regarded as a clear indication for long-term oral anticoagulation. The effectiveness of heparin may be impaired by concomitant antithrombin III deficiency, a plasma factor required for the full expression of the heparin-induced antithrombin effect.

To offset protein malnutrition, a diet rich in protein of high biological value should be provided unless marked azotemia is present. Correction of transport protein deficiencies is not feasible. Supplemental vitamin D might be desirable if overt deficiency is present, but this has not been evaluated clinically. In rare circumstances, profound protein malnutrition or other complications of massive proteinuria may justify bilateral nephrectomy.

A classification of the causes of NS is provided in Table 278-3. The multisystemic, heredofamilial, neoplastic, and metabolic causes are discussed in Chap. 279. The primary (idiopathic) glomerular diseases associated with NS, as well as the diseases secondary to infectious or drug etiologies are considered below.

TABLE 278-3
Causes of the nephrotic syndrome

I Primary glomerular diseases
  A Minimal change disease
  B Focal and segmental glomerulosclerosis and hyalinosis
  C Membranous glomerulopathy
  D Proliferative glomerulonephritis
    1 Membranoproliferative glomerulonephritis
    2 Crescentic glomerulonephritis
    3 "Pure" mesangial proliferative glomerulonephritis
    4 Focal and segmental proliferative glomerulonephritis
II Secondary to other diseases
  A Infections: Poststreptococcal glomerulonephritis, endocarditis, "shunt nephritis," secondary syphilis, leprosy, hepatitis B, infectious mononucleosis, malaria, schistosomiasis, filariasis
  B Drugs: Organic gold; inorganic, organic, and elemental mercury; penicillamine; "street" heroin; probenicid; tridione; mesantoin; perchlorate; antivenom; antitoxins; contrast media
  C Neoplasia: Hodgkin's disease, lymphomas, leukemia, carcinomata, melanoma, Wilms's tumor
  D Multisystem: Systemic lupus erythematosus, Schönlein-Henoch purpura, vasculitis, Goodpasture's syndrome, dermatomyositis, dermatitis herpetiformis, amyloidosis, sarcoidosis, Sjögren's syndrome
  E Heredofamilial: Diabetes mellitus, Alport's syndrome, sickle-cell disease, Fabry's disease, nail-patella syndrome, lipodystrophy, congenital nephrotic syndrome
  F Miscellaneous: Preeclamptic toxemia, thyroiditis, myxedema, malignant obesity, renovascular hypertension, chronic interstitial nephritis with vesicoureteric reflux, chronic allograft rejection, bee stings

IDIOPATHIC NEPHROTIC SYNDROME This diagnosis is arrived at by exclusion of known causes of NS, such as infections, drug exposure, multisystem disease, or hereditary disorders. The idiopathic forms of NS are further classified according to the morphologic features found on renal biopsy. Performance of a renal biopsy, at least among adults, is required for the accurate diagnosis of idiopathic NS and for the formulation of a rational plan of treatment. Children need not always be subjected to renal biopsy since careful clinical study can often lead to accurate diagnosis.

Minimal change disease This is often referred to as *lipoid nephrosis, nil lesion,* or *foot process disease.* In this form of idiopathic NS, although little or no alterations of the glomerular capillaries are demonstrable by light microscopy (hence the designation "minimal change"), *diffuse epithelial foot process effacement*[1] is evident by electron microscopy. Immunofluorescence microscopy reveals absent or irregular and nonspecific deposits of immunoglobulin and complement components. Nil lesion is the most frequently encountered form of idiopathic NS in children, accounting for more than 70 to 80 percent of cases diagnosed before the age of 8. This lesion is not rare in adults, either, representing 10 to 20 percent of cases of idiopathic NS in patients over the age of 16. There is a slight predilection for males. Typically patients present with overt NS, normal blood pressure, normal or slightly reduced GFR, and a "benign" urinary sediment. Varying degrees of microscopic hematuria are found in up to 20 percent of cases. Urinary protein is typically highly selective in children, but is variable in adults. Fibrin split products and C3 are absent in the urine. Serum levels of complement components are normal, except for a slight reduction in C1q. IgG concentrations are often quite depressed during relapse, whereas IgM levels are modestly increased, both during remission and relapse. Some cases may have associated atopy, a history of recent immunization, or upper respiratory infection. The histocompatibility antigen HLA-B12 is more prevalent when minimal change dis-

ease is associated with atopy, indicating a possible genetically based predisposition to this disease. Thromboembolic manifestations occur, but renal vein thrombosis is uncommon.

Spontaneous remissions and relapses of heavy proteinuria may occur, usually for reasons which are unexplained. Interestingly, an identical lesion is often encountered in patients with Hodgkin's disease, in whom NS develops, suggesting a role for lymphocytes in its pathogenesis. Except for patients who develop focal and segmental sclerosing lesions (see below), a progressive decline in GFR does not occur. Acute renal failure is rare. In the preantibiotic era infection with encapsulated organisms (e.g., pneumococci) was a leading cause of death, but now the mortality rate is exceedingly low and most deaths are associated with complications of treatment rather than the disease itself.

Since the etiology and pathogenesis are unknown, treatment is empirical and symptomatic. A large body of evidence indicates that corticosteroids markedly enhance the natural tendency for this disease to undergo spontaneous remission. Daily or alternate-day oral steroid therapy seem to be equally effective, the latter associated with fewer steroid-related complications. Prednisone, in a dose of 2 mg per kilogram of body weight given every other day as a single morning dose, or 1 mg/kg daily for 8 weeks or less, is usually effective in inducing remission. The vast majority of patients who respond do so within the first 4 weeks of treatment, but occasionally a favorable response requires more prolonged therapy. The absence of a response within 8 weeks is usually indicative of an error in diagnosis and should provoke a review of the renal biopsy. In many patients who respond, withdrawal of steroid treatment is often accompanied by relapse; this usually occurs within the first year after cessation of treatment. A steroid-dependent patient or one with multiple relapses may be benefited by a brief course of cyclophosphamide (1 to 2 mg/kg per day) or chlorambucil (0.1 to 0.2 mg/kg per day) for 8 to 12 weeks. When given with steroids to patients to induce remissions, either of these agents reduces the likelihood of a subsequent relapse. However, these agents have serious adverse effects on bone marrow, and in the case of cyclophosphamide, the gonads and urinary bladder. They may also be oncogenic. Azathioprine has been demonstrated to be ineffective in inducing prolonged remissions. The use of cytotoxic agents should be reserved for patients who develop serious or life-threatening complications of multiple courses of steroid therapy. The long-term prognosis of patients with the minimal change lesion is excellent; a 10-year survival in excess of 90 percent can be expected, but a few develop renal failure usually as a consequence of the lesion described in the next section.

Focal and segmental glomerulosclerosis (focal sclerosis) This lesion is characterized by sclerosis and hyalinization of some, but not all, glomeruli (hence the term *focal*). Among affected glomeruli, only a portion of the glomerular tuft is abnormal (hence, segmental). There is a predilection for these lesions initially to affect the *juxtamedullary glomeruli* and to be associated with progressive tubulointerstitial damage. By immunofluorescence, granular and nodular deposits of IgM and C3 are found in the segmental sclerosing lesion. By electron microscopy, focal basement membrane collapse and denudation of epithelial surface are noted. Affected glomeruli reveal diffuse epithelial foot process effacement. This lesion accounts for 5 to 10 percent and 10 to 20 percent of cases of idiopathic NS seen among children and adults, respectively. Males tend to be affected slightly more often than females. Many investigators believe that focal sclerosis represents a stage in the evolution of a subgroup of patients with minimal change disease. In more than two-thirds of cases of focal sclerosis overt NS will be

---

[1] The term "fusion" is often used to describe these changes in foot processes, although true fusion of cell membranes does not occur.

present at the time of diagnosis; in the remainder only isolated proteinuria in the nonnephrotic range is present. Hypertension, reduced GFR, abnormal tubular function, and abnormal urinary sediment occur commonly. It is important to emphasize that focal sclerosis may have clinical features indistinguishable from either minimal change disease or membranous glomerulopathy (see below). Proteinuria is nearly always nonselective or becomes so on follow-up. FDP and C3 may be present in the urine. Serum levels of C3 are normal and IgG levels are reduced, but not as severely as in minimal change disease. Similar lesions may be seen in association with "street" heroin abuse, vesicoureteric reflux, and renal allograft rejection. Abnormalities in the prevalence of HLA antigens have not been described. Renal vein thrombosis is uncommon.

There is little tendency for spontaneous remission, except among children. A progressive decline in GFR is the rule, albeit at variable rates. A subset of patients with focal sclerosis, who have extremely heavy proteinuria (i.e., greater than 15 to 20 g per day) and profound hypoalbuminemia, progress quite rapidly to end-stage renal failure, occasionally in a period of only a few months. Rarely, acute renal failure without recovery occurs. The etiology and pathogenesis of focal sclerosis are unknown. Immune-complex–mediated disease has been postulated, primarily on the basis of immunofluorescence findings, and circulating immune complexes have been found in a small minority of cases. There is no convincing evidence that any form of treatment is effective in forestalling the ultimate development of end-stage renal failure among patients with documented focal sclerosis. Some patients may experience a reduction in daily protein excretion with steroid therapy. Partial remissions of proteinuria, i.e., reductions to less than 2 g per day, seem to be associated with an improved long-term prognosis. At least 50 percent of patients develop end-stage renal failure or die of intercurrent illnesses within 10 years of diagnosis. The prognosis is much poorer for those patients with persistent NS or in whom azotemia or hypertension are evident at time of diagnosis. This lesion has, at times, been found to recur in renal allografts, occasionally within a few hours of transplantation, suggesting the possibility of a circulating glomerular permeability "toxin" in its pathogenesis.

Membranous glomerulopathy This lesion is characterized by the presence of irregular, discontinuous proteinaceous deposits along the outer (or subepithelial) aspect of the glomerular capillary wall. These deposits contain IgG and appear dense by electron microscopy. Unlike focal sclerosis, *all glomeruli are involved uniformly.* At an early stage all glomeruli may appear normal by light microscopy, but as the disease progresses, immune deposits coalesce, causing the capillary wall to thicken. Eventually, increased amounts of basement membrane material project outward between deposits toward the urinary space, giving the appearance of "spikes." There is little proliferation of capillary endothelial or mesangial cells, although mesangial sclerosis may occur in advanced cases. Tubulointerstitial atrophy and vascular lesions are other late manifestations.

This disorder accounts for 30 to 50 percent of cases of idiopathic NS in adults but is quite rare in children. In over 80 percent of cases overt NS is present. In the remainder only isolated proteinuria is found. Males tend to be affected more often than females. Blood pressure, GFR, and urinary sediment tend to be normal early in the course, making it extremely difficult to distinguish membranous glomerulopathy from minimal change disease on clinical grounds alone. Urinary protein selectivity is quite variable. Serum complement components are normal, but IgG levels are usually modestly depressed. Membranous glomerulopathy may develop in association with systemic lupus erythematosus (Chap. 279), certain

chronic infections (e.g., malaria, hepatitis B), solid tumors (e.g., melanoma and cancer of the lung and colon), or after exposure to heavy metals (gold, mercury) or drugs (penicillamine). A careful search for these causes is warranted in every case of idiopathic NS due to membranous glomerulopathy. There appears to be a high frequency of renal vein thrombosis in affected patients (see above).

Spontaneous complete remissions of NS are quite common in children with membranous nephropathy but take place in only 20 percent of adults. Steroid treatment does not greatly influence the development of lasting complete remissions, but may induce a reduction of proteinuria to nonnephrotic levels. A beneficial effect of steroids is still a source of controversy, since spontaneous partial remissions also occur, although somewhat less frequently than in steroid-treated patients. There is presently no agreement about optimal dosage and duration of therapy; however, alternative-day steroid therapy seems to be the safest approach. Cytotoxic agents appear to be of no benefit.

Slowly progressive renal functional impairment occurs almost exclusively among those patients with persistent proteinuria in the nephrotic range. Partial or complete spontaneous or treatment-associated remissions provide nearly complete protection from renal failure. Complete or partial remissions occur at variable times after the discovery of the disease, but renal failure is unlikely to develop in the first few years. Within 10 years of the time of the diagnosis, however, about 50 percent of patients will die of intercurrent illness or develop end-stage renal failure. The vast majority of survivors will have had complete or partial remission of proteinuria. Rare cases have occurred in renal transplants. A few patients are known to have developed superimposed anti-GBM antibody mediated disease and RPGN.

Membranoproliferative glomerulonephritis This group of disorders is characterized by proliferation of mesangial cells, often with segmental or diffuse interposition of these cells or their cytoplasm into peripheral capillary loops. There is evidence of increased synthesis of mesangial matrix as well. The glomerular capillary wall is irregularly thickened, by virtue of the mesangial extensions and the attendant synthesis of basement membrane–like material. This group of disorders is also known as *mesangiocapillary* or *lobular glomerulonephritis.* Several immunofluorescence and electron microscopic patterns are present and are believed to reflect heterogeneous mechanisms of pathogenesis. In the ultrastructural *type I* lesion, subendothelial electron-dense deposits are present. C3 is deposited in a granular pattern indicative of immune-complex pathogenesis, but IgG and the early components of complement are present inconsistently. In the ultrastructural *type II* lesion the lamina densa of the GBM is transformed into an extremely electron-dense character, giving rise to the term *dense deposit disease.* Basement membranes in Bowman's capsules and in tubules are similarly affected. C3 is found irregularly in the GBM and in granules or rings in the mesangium. Small amounts of Ig (typically IgM) are present, but the early acting complement components are absent from the deposits. Properdin deposition is variable. Additional ultrastructural variants, based upon location of deposit and basement membrane changes, have also been described.

Membranoproliferative glomerulonephritis, types I and II, are found in 5 to 10 percent of cases of idiopathic NS in children, particularly between the ages of 8 to 16 years, and somewhat less commonly in adults. Type I accounts for at least two-thirds of cases. Sexes are affected equally. In 50 to 75 percent of patients, a full-blown NS is present, often with features of AGN. In the remainder, proteinuria is in the nonnephrotic range and is nearly always accompanied by microscopic hematuria. Blood pressure and GFR are frequently abnormal, and the urinary sediment is typically active. Functional abnormalities of the renal tubules are common. Urinary protein selectivity is usually poor; FDP and C3 are found in the urine. Serum C3 levels are reduced in 70 to 80 percent of cases of type I and in over 90 percent of type II disease. The early acting complement components C1q, C4, and C2 are often normal, however, especially in type II disease. This pattern may be indicative of activation of the alternate complement pathway (see Chap. 277). C3 nephritic factor (C3NeF) is often found in the serums of patients with type II, especially if the C3 level is quite low. Circulating immune complexes are found in type I. Lesions similar to type I membranoproliferative glomerulonephritis may also be found in SLE, hemolytic-uremic syndrome, transplant rejection, chronic hepatitis B antigenemia, and "shunt" nephritis. Renal vein thrombosis may occur. Type II nephritis may be associated with partial lipodystrophy.

Spontaneous remissions are uncommon. There is little evidence favoring a beneficial effect of any form of therapy, but long-term, alternate-day steroid therapy (0.3 to 0.5 mg/kg every other day) may delay the progression of the disease. Treatment regimens which combine steroids, cytotoxic agents, and anticoagulants are not of proven value. The course is usually relentlessly progressive, and more than 50 to 60 percent of patients die or develop end-stage renal failure within 10 years of the diagnosis. The prognosis for type II lesions seems somewhat worse than for type I. Type II disease almost invariably recurs in the transplanted kidney but does not always result in the premature loss of the allograft.

Other forms of idiopathic nephrotic syndrome In a small percentage of adults and children with idiopathic NS (i.e., 5 to 10 percent) other lesions are encountered on renal biopsy. These include *"pure" mesangial proliferative glomerulonephritis, crescentic glomerulonephritis,* and *segmental proliferative glomerulonephritis.* The pathogenetic mechanisms responsible for these lesions vary. For example, some of the cases of focal and segmental, or pure mesangial, glomerulonephritis may have extensive mesangial IgA deposits and fit into the category of Berger's disease (see below). Others may exhibit diffuse IgM deposits. Serum C3 levels are usually normal. The clinical characteristics, natural history, and response to treatment of these lesions are not well defined. Hematuria is common and may be recurrent. Proteinuria tends to be nonselective. Spontaneous remissions of NS are known, mostly among patients with "pure" mesangial proliferation. Since no controlled studies have been conducted, it is not possible to evaluate the effectiveness of treatment. Crescentic glomerulonephritis is likely to have a poor prognosis, whereas mesangial and focal and segmental proliferative glomerulonephritis have a more favorable long-term outlook.

NEPHROTIC SYNDROME CAUSED BY INFECTIOUS AGENTS, DRUGS, OR CHEMICALS Table 278-3 lists the common infectious and drug-related etiologies of NS. In many instances, NS will abate following cure of the infection or withdrawal of the offending medication. In patients receiving organic gold therapy for rheumatoid arthritis, or in those exposed to inorganic, organic, or elemental mercury or to penicillamine therapy, membranous glomerulopathy is usually the lesion responsible for NS. NS is known to follow immunization and antiserum treatment of tetanus or snakebite and to occur in situations associated with atopy.

ASYMPTOMATIC URINARY ABNORMALITIES

This group of patients is identified principally by the findings of *proteinuria in the nonnephrotic range and/or hematuria,* unaccompanied by edema, reduced GFR, or hypertension. Abnormalities are often discovered incidentally and may be persistent or recurrent. This syndrome may, of course, be but a phase in the natural history of other glomerulopathic syndromes, especially NS or chronic glomerulonephritis. Common glomerular disorders which present as asymptomatic proteinuria and/or hematuria at some point in their natural history are listed in Table 278-4. The heredofamilial and multisystem diseases are discussed in Chap. 279.

IDIOPATHIC RENAL HEMATURIA (See also Chap. 42) **Berger's disease (IgA nephropathy)** This disorder was first described by Berger and Hinglais in 1968 and is characterized by recurrent episodes of gross or microscopic hematuria. The diagnosis depends on the finding of prominent IgA deposits in the mesangium by immunofluorescence microscopy. Berger's disease is the most common cause of recurrent hematuria of glomerular origin. It most commonly affects young adults, mostly males. Typically, episodes of macroscopic hematuria are associated with minor flu-like illnesses or vigorous exercise. Patients frequently complain of vague constitutional symptoms, but skin rash, arthritis, or abdominal pain are absent. Urine protein excretion rates are usually less than 3.5 g per day; not uncommonly protein excretion is normal or only mildly increased. The nephrotic syndrome develops occasionally. Blood pressure, GFR, and serum albumin are normal, at least early in the disease. Serum IgA levels are increased in about 50 percent of cases, while serum complement component levels remain normal. Biopsy of the skin of the volar surface of the forearm will often reveal dermal capillary deposits of IgA, C3, and fibrin, but not early acting complement components or IgA secretory fragments. Similar skin biopsy findings may be encountered in Schönlein-Henoch purpura (Chap. 279). Indeed, Berger's disease may be a forme fruste of Schönlein-Henoch purpura.

Renal biopsy reveals a spectrum of changes by light microscopy, but focal and segmental proliferative glomerulonephritis is found most often. In some cases glomerular morphology may be normal by light microscopy; rarely, crescents may be found. The distinguishing feature is the finding by immunofluorescence microscopy of *diffuse mesangial deposition of IgA,*

TABLE 278-4
Glomerular causes of asymptomatic urinary abnormalities

I Hematuria with or without proteinuria
  A Primary glomerular diseases
    1 Berger's disease (IgA nephropathy)
    2 Membranoproliferative glomerulonephritis
    3 Other primary glomerular hematurias accompanied by "pure" mesangial proliferation, focal and segmental proliferative glomerulonephritis, or other lesions
  B Associated with multisystems or heredofamilial diseases
    1 Alport's syndrome and other "benign" familial hematurias
    2 Fabry's disease
    3 Sickle-cell disease
  C Associated with infections
    1 Resolving poststreptococcal glomerulonephritis
    2 Other postinfectious glomerulonephritides
II Isolated nonnephrotic proteinuria
  A Primary glomerular diseases
    1 "Orthostatic" proteinuria
    2 Focal and segmental glomerulosclerosis
    3 Membranous glomerulopathy
  B Associated with multisystems or heredofamilial diseases
    1 Diabetes mellitus
    2 Amyloidosis
    3 Nail-patella syndrome

often accompanied by lesser amounts of IgG and nearly always by C3 and properdin, but not by C1q or C4. Fibrin reactive antigens are also commonly demonstrable in the mesangium or in association with crescents if the latter are present.

The prognosis is variable, but, in general, the disease tends to progress slowly. It has been estimated that approximately 50 percent of patients can be expected to develop end-stage renal failure within 25 years of the time of diagnosis. Azotemia, hypertension, or proteinuria in the nephrotic range at the time of diagnosis are associated with a poor prognosis. At present, there is no evidence to suggest that any form of therapy greatly influences the natural history. Some have suggested that intermittent steroid therapy may reduce the frequency of episodes of gross hematuria.

Other primary renal hematurias Some cases of recurrent hematuria do not reveal the typical immunofluorescence findings seen in Berger's disease. This group of patients is poorly defined, and in them the etiology and pathogenesis is varied. Some may represent resolving episodes of acute glomerulonephritis or early examples of membranoproliferative or hereditary glomerulonephritis (Alport's syndrome, see Chap. 279). The morphologic lesions most commonly encountered are focal and segmental or diffuse mesangial proliferative glomerulonephritis, although mild and nonspecific glomerular changes may also be observed. Immunofluorescence studies reveal varying degrees of immunoglobulin deposition (principally IgM) in the mesangium. Some cases show linear deposits of IgG, suggesting a possible anti-GBM antibody pathogenesis. Electron microscopy may reveal dense deposits in the mesangium. Overall, this group of patients is believed to have an excellent prognosis, with spontaneous permanent remissions of recurrent hematuria. Progressive renal insufficiency is unusual. Because of the benign prognosis no treatment is indicated.

ISOLATED NONNEPHROTIC PROTEINURIA OF GLOMERULAR ORIGIN (See also Chap. 42) The discovery of mild to moderate degrees of proteinuria (i.e., greater than 150 mg but less than 3.5 g per day), unaccompanied by abnormalities in the urinary sediment or evidence of hypertension or reduced renal function, is a common problem in internal medicine. Such patients may display other features of heredofamilial or multisystem diseases, including diabetes mellitus, amyloidosis, rheumatoid arthritis, or cancer. Among cases of isolated proteinuria consequent to primary glomerular disease the abnormality may either be persistent or evanescent. Proteinuria may occur primarily in the upright posture (*orthostatic proteinuria*) or be present both in recumbent and erect positions. Persistent nonnephrotic proteinuria, demonstrable in both orthostatic and recumbent positions, generally indicates the presence of some significant and readily demonstrable glomerular pathology. Some of the lesions which might be encountered have been discussed in the context of idiopathic NS. Other patients may prove to have a clinically unsuspected disease such as amyloidosis or diabetes mellitus. In the remainder, the lesions are usually trivial and nonspecific and their long-term significance is quite uncertain. In the case of primary glomerular diseases, so long as urinary protein excretion remains modest, the prognosis is excellent and deterioration of renal function is uncommon. On the other hand, orthostatic proteinuria is more often than not associated with mild and entirely nonspecific glomerular alterations which have little tendency for progression. Furthermore, orthostatic proteinuria commonly disappears during prolonged follow-up. Renal biopsy is commonly undertaken in patients with persistent and isolated proteinuria, largely as a means of accurately estimating long-term prognosis. This does not result in useful information.

CHRONIC GLOMERULONEPHRITIS (CGN)

The syndrome of CGN is characterized chiefly by *persistent urinary abnormalities* (e.g., proteinuria and/or hematuria) and by *slowly progressive impairment of renal function,* eventuating in hypertension, contracted granular kidneys, and end-stage renal failure. With the possible exception of the minimal change lesion associated with idiopathic nephrotic syndrome (see above) all the disorders described in this chapter and in Chap. 279 can lead eventually to CGN. The pathophysiology of the syndrome of CGN as it appears in the context of renal failure is described in Chaps. 274 and 276.

The glomerular structural alterations that underlie this syndrome may be categorized as *proliferative* (including endo- and/or extracapillary proliferative glomerulonephritis and focal and segmental proliferative glomerulonephritis), *sclerosing* (including focal and diffuse glomerular sclerosis), and *membranous*. Such lesions are found in the vast majority of patients with CGN. In the small remainder, the underlying lesions are not readily categorized morphologically. These are often referred to as *chronic "nonspecific" glomerulonephritis.*

The clinical characteristics of the specific lesions are described in other sections of this chapter. The etiologic and pathogenetic origins of chronic nonspecific glomerulonephritis are unknown but are undoubtedly heterogeneous. Complicating vascular disease contributes to the glomerular obliteration seen in this group of disorders. It is quite reasonable to suspect that some of the patients categorized as having chronic nonspecific glomerulonephritis may have had an earlier unrecognized or undiagnosed episode of acute PSGN. However, such patients usually fail to recall a specific episode of acute nephritis.

The detection of CGN usually occurs in one of several ways: (1) by the incidental finding of abnormal urine, impaired renal function, or hypertension during multiphasic screening of asymptomatic individuals or during evaluation of such individuals for an unrelated illness; (2) as the result of the insidious onset of progressive symptoms or signs of advanced renal disease, especially anemia and hypertension; or (3) after an exacerbation of glomerulonephritis, usually during the course of a nonspecific viral or bacterial illness. In advanced stages of the syndrome, the clinical separation of CGN from other causes of renal failure may be difficult; however, the presence of symmetrically contracted kidneys, moderate to heavy proteinuria, abnormal urinary sediment (especially red blood cell casts), and x-ray evidence of normal pyelocalyceal systems are all suggestive of CGN.

The evolution of CGN varies considerably, depending upon the nature of the underlying disease and the presence or absence of complications, especially hypertension. Ten, fifteen, twenty, or more years may elapse from the first discovery of an abnormal urine sediment until the development of end-stage renal failure. Renal biopsy is necessary to define the precise nature of the underlying glomerular lesion. The principal advantage of a morphologic evaluation among patients presenting with the syndrome of CGN is to determine prognosis rather than therapy.

Treatment of patients with CGN is supportive and symptomatic. Despite many years of controlled and uncontrolled trials, unequivocal evidence of a favorable effect of treatment with steroids, cytotoxic agents, nonsteroidal anti-inflammatory agents, and anticoagulants has yet to be provided. The management of specific lesions is discussed in greater detail in the relevant sections of this chapter. Hypertension and symptomatic urinary tract infections should be treated vigorously, taking care to avoid nephrotoxic agents. Diuretics should generally be employed only as adjuncts to antihypertensive management or to deal with debilitating degrees of edema. Fluid and sodium should be provided according to the dictates of blood pressure control. Rigorous salt restriction is usually unnecessary and may be hazardous. In the absence of congestive heart failure or marked hypoalbuminemia, severe edema rarely occurs in CGN until the terminal phases of the illness. Potassium restriction is usually unnecessary.

REFERENCES

GLASSOCK RJ: Clinical aspects of acute, rapidly progressive and chronic glomerulonephritis, in *Diseases of the Kidney,* 3d ed, LE Earley, C Gottschalk (eds). Boston, Little, Brown, 1979

———— et al: The glomerulopathies: The major clinical syndromes, in *The Kidney,* 2d ed, BM Brenner, FC Rector Jr (eds). Philadelphia, Saunders, 1980

HAYSLETT JP et al: Clinicopathologic correlations in the nephrotic syndrome due to primary renal disease. Medicine 52:93, 1973

HEPTINSTALL RH (ed): *Pathology of the Kidney,* 2d ed. Boston, Little, Brown, 1974

ROW PG et al: Membranous nephropathy: Long-term followup and association with neoplasia. Q J Med 44:207, 1975

279

GLOMERULOPATHIES ASSOCIATED WITH MULTISYSTEM AND HEREDOFAMILIAL DISEASES

RICHARD J. GLASSOCK
BARRY M. BRENNER

Glomerular injury may be a prominent feature of diseases which affect multiple organs and systems. By and large the etiologies of these diseases are unknown, but aberrant immunologic processes, neoplasia, metabolic disturbances, and genetically based biochemical abnormalities are believed to be dominant factors in their pathogenesis.

MULTISYSTEM DISEASES

SYSTEMIC LUPUS ERYTHEMATOSUS (See also Chap. 68) Systemic lupus erythematosus (SLE) is the archetype of an immune-complex-mediated disease (see Chap. 277) and is representative of the group of multisystem diseases in which renal involvement is extremely common. The etiology of SLE is unknown; however, a growing body of evidence suggests that viral infection, genetic factors, and abnormal immune responsiveness interact to produce the disease. The prevalence of clinically evident renal involvement in SLE has been variously reported, ranging from as low as 35 percent to more than 90 percent. Clinical manifestations of renal disease range from mild abnormalities of the urinary sediment (predominantly hematuria) to massive proteinuria, and from chronic indolent glomerulonephritis to a fulminant inflammatory process leading to progressive renal failure.

Morphological evidence of renal involvement may exist with or without clinical manifestations. If immunofluorescence and electron microscopic studies of renal tissue are performed, abnormalities are present in virtually every patient with SLE. The diagnosis and extrarenal manifestations of SLE are more fully described in Chap. 68. This section will deal with the clinical features of the various forms of renal involvement of SLE. Although extrarenal features often dominate the clinical picture, SLE may present initially solely with renal manifestations. The glomerular morphological lesions observed in SLE form a spectrum which may be divided, somewhat arbitrarily, into several categories based upon correlative light and electron microscopic and immunofluorescence studies of renal biopsies.

Mesangial lupus glomerulonephritis This pattern is characterized by mild to moderate diffuse mesangial cell proliferation and/or mesangial sclerosis. Immunofluorescence studies reveal immunoglobulins (IgG, IgM, and IgA) and complement components (C1q, C4, C3) deposited in a granular pattern exclusively in the mesangium. Electron-dense deposits are also confined to the mesangium by electron microscopy. This morphological appearance may be found in the absence of clinical evidence of renal disease or may be associated with only minor abnormalities in the urinary sediment and modest proteinuria. Glomerular filtration rate (GFR) is almost always normal. Hypertension may or may not be present. It is thought that mesangial lupus glomerulonephritis may be the initial stage of renal involvement in SLE, from which all other patterns evolve. Associated serologic abnormalities depend upon the degree of extrarenal activity. These include positive antinuclear antibodies (ANA), increased levels of antibody to denatured, single-stranded (ssDNA) or native, double-stranded (dsDNA), depressed serum levels of C3, C4, and C1q, and detectable levels of circulating immune complexes (CIC) (Table 279-1).

Focal lupus glomerulonephritis This pattern is characterized by focal and segmental cellular proliferation, often associated with necrosis, superimposed on diffuse mesangial hypercellularity. Granular deposits of immunoglobulins and complement components are more extensive than in the mesangial form and involve both the mesangium and occasional glomerular capillary loops. By electron microscopy subendothelial dense deposits are found in the mesangium and in a few peripheral capillary loops. Clinical and laboratory evidence of renal injury is observed more commonly than in mesangial lupus glomerulonephritis. Nephrotic syndrome may occur in 10 to 20 percent of patients, but in general GFR is well preserved. This lesion may persist, resolve, or progress to diffuse proliferative lupus glomerulonephritis. Serologic features of active disease are often present in untreated patients. A recent study suggests that patients in this category who have necrosis have the same prognosis as those with diffuse glomerulonephritis.

Diffuse proliferative lupus glomerulonephritis This pattern is characterized by diffuse mesangial and endothelial cell proliferation which may include extensive peripheral capillary wall interposition of mesangial cells (i.e., membranoproliferative glomerulonephritis; see Chap. 278). In addition focal cellular necrosis, hematoxylinophilic bodies, fibrinoid necrosis, and "wire loops" (capillaries whose basement membranes are thickened markedly owing to subendothelial deposits) may be present. Extensive extracapillary proliferative (crescentic) glomerulonephritis, vasculitis, and interstitial nephritis may also be found occasionally. Granular deposits of immunoglobulins and complement components are extensive and involve the mesangium and nearly every capillary loop. Electron microscopy reveals extensive subendothelial and mesangial electron-dense deposits as well as occasional intramembranous or subepithelial deposits. Most patients will have an active urinary sediment, heavy proteinuria, and progressive impairment of renal function; occasionally, however, clinical evidence of renal involvement is lacking. In the untreated patient evidence of serologic activity is usually present, including positive ANA,

TABLE 279-1

Serologic findings in multisystem and heredofamilial diseases

Disease	C3	Ig	FANA	Anti-dsDNA	Anti-GBM	Cryo-Ig	CIC
Systemic lupus erythematosus	+ to +++	↑ IgG	+++	+++	−	++	+++
Goodpasture's syndrome	−	−	−	−	+++	−	±
Henoch-Schönlein purpura	−	↑ IgA	−	−	−	±	+
Polyarteritis	+	↑ IgG	+	±	−	++	+++
Wegener's granulomatosis	±	↑ IgA, IgE	−	−	−	±	++
Cryoimmunoglobulinemia	++	±	−	−	−	+++	++
Multiple myeloma	−	↓↑IgG, IgA, IgD, IgE	−	−	−	+	±
Waldenström's macroglobulinemia	−	↑ IgM	−	−	−	−	−
Amyloidosis	−	± Ig	−	−	−	−	−
Alport's syndrome	−	−	−	−	−	−	−
Fabry's disease	−	−	−	−	−	−	−
Sickle-cell disease	−	−	−	−	−	−	±
Diabetic nephropathy	−	−	−	−	−	−	±

NOTE: C3 = C3 component of complement, B_1C/B_1A; Ig = immunoglobulin levels; FANA = fluorescent antinuclear antibody assay; anti-dsDNA = antibody to double-stranded (native) DNA; anti-GBM = antibody to glomerular basement membrane antigens; cryo-Ig = cryoimmunoglobulin; CIC = circulating immune complexes; − = normal; + = occasionally slightly abnormal; ++ = often abnormal; +++ = severely abnormal.

markedly depressed serum C3 and C4 concentrations, high levels of precipitating and nonprecipitating complement-fixing antibody to dsDNA, cryoimmunoglobulinemia, and circulating immune complexes (CIC). This lesion usually is associated with an ominous prognosis, although vigorous treatment may greatly modify the course (see below).

Membranous lupus glomerulopathy This pattern is nearly identical to that described for idiopathic membranous glomerulopathy (Chap. 278), except that mesangial deposits and mesangial proliferation are seen more frequently. There is thickening of the glomerular capillary wall due to the presence of immunoglobulin and complement-containing electron-dense deposits in the subepithelial space, often associated with a spike-like basement membrane reaction. Nearly all patients manifest heavy proteinuria and the nephrotic syndrome. Although GFR may be normal initially, most patients ultimately develop progressive renal failure. A proliferative lesion may occasionally evolve in these patients, and the prognosis then assumes that of the diffuse proliferative form of glomerulonephritis. Serologic features of SLE may or may not be present at the time of diagnosis of this nephropathy. Antibody to dsDNA tends to be nonprecipitating; for this reason, some patients with membranous lupus glomerulopathy may be erroneously categorized as having idiopathic membranous glomerulopathy (see Chap. 278). Careful serial serologic investigations, measurement of the level of antibody to dsDNA, circulating immune complexes, and biopsies of skin for dermal-epidermal deposits of Ig ("lupus band test") may prove helpful for diagnosis in such cases.

Sclerosing or end-stage lupus glomerulonephritis This pattern is characterized by obliterative and sclerosing lesions of portions of the glomeruli, and probably represents a late stage of proliferative lesions. Immunofluorescence studies may be only weakly positive for immunoglobulins; subendothelial deposits are seen infrequently. Hypertension and impaired renal function are common. Serologic parameters of activity of SLE may or may not be present.

Prognosis and treatment The prognosis and treatment of SLE with renal involvement depends to a large extent upon the nature of the underlying renal lesion. Patients with milder forms of renal disease (e.g., mesangial or focal lupus glomerulonephritis) tend to do well if treatment is primarily directed to control of the extrarenal manifestations of the disease. Corticosteroids in modest doses, salicylates, or antimalarials are usually sufficient. Potent nonsteroidal, anti-inflammatory agents may cause functional depression of GFR and should be used with caution in patients with known renal involvement. Serologic parameters, including anti-dsDNA and complement components (C3, C4), should be followed serially. Fluorescent antinuclear antibody tests have little value in prognosis or in following the effectiveness of treatment in patients with SLE. A return to normal values for antibody to dsDNA and/or complement components is a favorable sign; however, persistently abnormal serologic features do not necessarily indicate worsening or progressive renal involvement, especially in patients with active extrarenal manifestations. For patients with mild lesions which have not evolved into diffuse proliferative lupus glomerulonephritis, overall survival is excellent, and 85 percent or more of patients with mesangial or focal lupus glomerulonephritis can be expected to survive at least 10 years. Patients with membranous lupus glomerulopathy who receive treatment directed primarily at the extrarenal features also have favorable long-term prognosis. On the other hand, patients with diffuse proliferative lupus glomerulonephritis do less well and, therefore, warrant a more aggressive approach toward ameliorating the renal disease. Unfortunately, it has been difficult to prove unequivocally that aggressive forms of treatment, such as high doses of oral or parenteral steroids or combinations of steroids and cytotoxic drugs (immunosuppressive therapy), are truly beneficial in the management of these patients. It has been suggested that high doses of steroids, either given as "pulses" of parenteral methylprednisolone (5 to 15 mg/kg for 3 to 15 doses) or oral prednisone (1 to 2 mg/kg per day) for weeks or months, are required to suppress clinical manifestations of glomerular disease (restore GFR, improve urine sediment, and reduce proteinuria). Unfortunately, some patients will continue to manifest active and progressive renal disease despite such aggressive steroid therapy. A large body of experience, mostly uncontrolled, has suggested that the addition of a cytotoxic agent (i.e., azathioprine, cyclophosphamide, or chlorambucil) will exert a "steroid-sparing" effect and act to bring the disease under better control. This suggestion has been difficult to confirm in controlled studies. Cytotoxic agents have serious side effects (e.g., enhanced susceptibility to infections, bladder irritation, damaging effects on the gonads, and possible oncogenic potential). These very real hazards notwithstanding, selected patients with diffuse proliferative glomerulonephritis treated with a combination of steroids and cytotoxic drugs seem to have done better than would be expected. A trial of such therapy seems indicated providing no contraindications exist, fully informed consent is obtained, and there is sufficient histopathologic evidence to support the notion that the renal lesions are, in fact, potentially reversible. Little is to be gained by using a combined steroid-cytotoxic approach in patients with advanced renal failure due to progressive glomerular capillary obliteration and sclerosis. These patients are best referred for dialysis and/or transplantation. The role of intensive plasma exchange accompanied by immunosuppressive therapy for fulminating disease has not yet been established, but early experience appears extremely promising. In some centers an aggressive steroid-cytotoxic drug approach has been associated with an approximate 85 percent 5-year survival in diffuse proliferative lupus glomerulonephritis. Serologic studies, especially serial measurements of antibody to dsDNA, complement components, and circulating immune complexes, are useful parameters to follow in patients under therapy. Normalization of these parameters usually indicates satisfactory control of disease and provides reassurance that drug dosage can be safely diminished. These measurements also need to be monitored in order to guide resumption of more aggressive therapy.

Overall, long-term prognosis for patients with SLE and renal involvement has improved steadily over the past decade. Whether improvements in methods of diagnosis, serologic monitoring, or treatment are responsible is unknown. Progression to end-stage renal disease is now relatively uncommon even for patients with diffuse proliferative glomerulonephritis. Cerebral involvement and infectious complications now loom as major causes of morbidity and mortality in SLE. Patients with SLE seem to do well on regular chronic dialysis; moreover, as uremia develops, some patients have noted remissions of extrarenal activity. In transplanted patients, recurrence of SLE in the renal allograft has been quite uncommon. These observations indicate that patients with SLE and nephritis are satisfactory candidates for both dialysis and transplantation.

GOODPASTURE'S SYNDROME This disorder consists of a triad of findings: *pulmonary hemorrhage, glomerulonephritis,* and *antibody to basement membrane antigens.* Its etiology is unknown. Goodpasture's syndrome typically affects young males but may appear at any age. Pulmonary hemorrhage may be extremely mild and easily overlooked, or severe and life-threatening. The initial manifestations of pulmonary involvement are cough, mild shortness of breath, and hemoptysis. Hilar pulmonary infiltrates may be seen by chest x-ray, and hypoxia is frequent. With marked intraalveolar hemorrhage pulmonary carbon monoxide uptake is increased, and the pulmonary clearance of radioactive carbon monoxide is depressed. Pulmonary iron sequestration may be documented by scanning of the lungs with ^{59}Fe. Hemosiderin-laden macrophages may be seen in the sputum, but this is a nonspecific finding. Iron-deficiency anemia may result if pulmonary bleeding is prolonged and severe. A history of recent inhalation of volatile hydrocarbons or viral influenza may be obtained. Fever, arthralgias, and other systemic symptoms are generally mild or absent at the time of presentation. Pulmonary hemorrhage may also be associated with renal failure in SLE, polyarteritis, Wegener's granulomatosis, cryoimmunoglobulinemia,

Henoch-Schönlein purpura, pulmonary embolism consequent to renal vein thrombosis, Legionnaires' disease, and as a feature of congestive heart failure occurring in patients with end-stage renal disease. These disorders can ordinarily be differentiated from Goodpasture's syndrome by their extrarenal clinical features and by typical serologic findings (Table 279-1).

The appearance of glomeruli in Goodpasture's syndrome ranges from normal or nearly normal to focal proliferative and necrotizing glomerulonephritis; most often there is extensive extracapillary proliferation (crescents). Rapidly progressive renal failure is the most common clinical feature of the syndrome, although patients may initially present only with microscopic abnormalities in the urinary sediment and normal renal function. Immunofluorescence studies of renal biopsy material reveal the typical *linear deposits* of anti-basement membrane antibody, often but not necessarily always accompanied by C3 deposition. Anti-basement membrane antibodies can be eluted from such tissue by appropriate in vitro techniques. Electron-microscopic studies do not reveal electron-dense deposits.

Circulating antibody to basement membrane (glomerular, alveolar, and tubular) antigens are found in over 90 percent of cases if serums are examined early in the course of the disease by such sensitive assays as immunofluorescence or radioimmunoassay (Table 279-1). The level of circulating antibody does not correlate well with the severity of the renal or pulmonary manifestations. Measurements of circulating antibody are principally of diagnostic value and have no established prognostic significance. Serum complement components are nearly always normal; CIC and cryoimmunoglobulin are absent.

The course of the disorder is quite variable. Patients surviving an initial bout of severe hemoptysis may undergo long-term remissions of pulmonary disease or may have repeated bouts of pulmonary hemorrhage. Mild forms of glomerular injury may not progress, and the principal clinical problems may be related to recurrent hemoptysis. The diagnosis in such patients may be confused clinically with idiopathic pulmonary hemosiderosis. More commonly the renal disease is progressive, sometimes fulminant, leading to oliguric renal failure in a matter of a few weeks or months (i.e., rapidly progressive glomerulonephritis).

The treatment of Goodpasture's syndrome is undergoing a rapid and dramatic change. Life-threatening degrees of pulmonary hemorrhage may respond temporarily to high doses of parenteral methylprednisolone (7 to 15 mg/kg) given over short periods. The effectiveness of such steroid therapy in reversing extensive crescentic glomerular lesions is not well established. Anticoagulants are contraindicated in the face of active pulmonary hemorrhage. Intensive plasma exchange (2 to 4 liters of plasma per day), employed in combination with cytotoxic drugs and modest doses of steroids, has been associated with dramatic remissions of pulmonary hemorrhage and improvement of the glomerular lesions. This is particularly true if treatment is initiated early in patients with relatively acute disease in whom oliguria has not yet developed. The duration and frequency of plasma exchanges need to be individualized, depending upon the clinical response of the patient and results of monitoring levels of circulating antibody to glomerular basement membrane antigens. Renal biopsy is helpful in guiding the management, but even in the presence of very extensive crescent formation satisfactory responses have been obtained. If irreversible glomerular obliteration, extensive interstitial fibrosis, and tubular atrophy are found, especially in the oliguric patient with long-standing disease, intensive plasma exchange offers little hope for improving the renal lesion. Such patients are best referred for regular hemodialysis and/or transplantation. Although recurrences may occasionally develop after renal transplantation, Goodpasture's syndrome is not a contraindication to transplantation so long as transplantation is delayed until circulating anti-basement membrane antibody has fallen to undetectable levels.

HENOCH-SCHÖNLEIN PURPURA (See also Chap. 317) This disorder is characterized by the development of non-thrombocytopenic purpura, arthralgias, abdominal pain, and glomerulonephritis. Typically, children and adolescents are affected, but the disorder may appear at any age. Purpura is due to cutaneous vasculitis and chiefly involves the buttocks and lower extremities. Cutaneous involvement may occur in bouts, often associated with other systemic features. Arthralgias and abdominal pain may vary in severity, and occasionally the latter may be associated with gastrointestinal bleeding and/or perforation. Renal involvement is very common and is manifested chiefly by hematuria and proteinuria. In some instances renal involvement is severe, leading to rapidly progressive glomerulonephritis or nephrotic syndrome. The onset of the disease may resemble acute postinfectious glomerulonephritis. Serum complement component levels are usually normal. Serum IgA levels are increased in about half the patients (Table 279-1). Renal biopsy reveals a spectrum of abnormalities depending upon the severity of clinical renal disease. Mild diffuse mesangial cell proliferation and/or focal and segmental proliferative glomerulonephritis is noted most commonly when bouts of macroscopic hematuria accompanied by modest proteinuria are found clinically. More severe and diffuse proliferative glomerulonephritis, sometimes accompanied by extracapillary proliferation (crescents), is seen among patients with heavy proteinuria and/or rapidly diminishing GFR. Characteristically immunofluorescence studies reveal mesangial and peripheral capillary granular deposits of IgA, IgG, C3, properdin, and fibrinogen but not C1q, C4, IgA secretory piece, or IgM. Similar immunofluorescence findings are noted in the dermal capillaries of biopsies of involved and uninvolved skin. Electron microscopy reveals electron-dense deposits principally confined to the mesangium. These findings suggest that Henoch-Schönlein purpura is due to circulating IgA-containing immune complexes. Circulating cryoimmunoglobulins and immune complexes have been noted in some instances; however, the nature of the antigen, and the antibody reactivity of the IgA, are unknown. Although food allergies and upper respiratory infections may be present, there is no clear-cut etiologic relationship. *Berger's disease* (IgA nephropathy, Chap. 278) may represent a form of Henoch-Schönlein purpura.

The diagnosis of Henoch-Schönlein purpura is ordinarily not difficult when the typical clinical features mentioned above are present. The differential diagnosis includes SLE, polyarteritis, infective endocarditis, postinfectious glomerulonephritis, and essential cryoimmunoglobulinemia.

The course is benign in the majority of cases; however, in some patients progressive renal failure may occur. Renal biopsy is a useful prognostic tool. Patients with persisting urinary abnormalities may experience deterioration of renal function several years after diagnosis. Treatment is symptomatic and there is no convincing evidence that steroid or immunosuppressive therapy is beneficial for the renal lesion, although these treatments may ameliorate some of the extrarenal features. Patients with rapidly progressive (crescentic) glomerulonephritis may be benefited by intensive plasma exchange or immunosuppressive drugs combined with anticoagulant and antithrombotic agents (see Chap. 278).

DISSEMINATED VASCULITIS (POLYARTERITIS) (See also Chap. 67) Glomerular involvement is common in the heterogeneous group of disorders which result from widespread inflammatory lesions of blood vessels. Several clinical and pathological variations are recognized, including microscopic polyarteritis (hypersensitivity angiitis), macroscopic polyarteri-

tis (periarteritis nodosa), Wegener's granulomatosis, allergic granulomatous arteritis, rheumatoid vasculitis, temporal arteritis, and Takayasu's syndrome. Henoch-Schönlein syndrome and SLE can also be considered as examples of vasculitis.

Renal involvement in *macroscopic polyarteritis* consists principally of inflammatory lesions of the relatively large blood vessels. Lesions of various ages are found. Fibrotic vascular occlusion, intrarenal aneurysms, and segmental renal infarctions may be noted. Hypertension tends to be severe and may be associated with a microangiopathic hemolytic anemia. Glomerular lesions of ischemia or necrosis may be seen. The disorder tends to affect older males, and there may be a history of drug abuse (amphetamines) or concomitant chronic hepatitis B infection. Fever, neuritis, cutaneous ulcers, purpura, abdominal pain, central nervous system disturbances, and coronary artery disease may also be found. Complement component levels are variable, but tests for CIC are often positive (Table 279-1). Renal failure is usually slowly progressive in nature and late in onset. The pathogenesis is presumed to be related to vascular deposits of circulating immune complexes; in some instances these complexes are composed of hepatitis B surface antigens, antibody, and complement.

Microscopic polyarteritis (hypersensitivity angiitis) tends to involve smaller vessels of the kidney and other organs. Pulmonary involvement is particularly common so that this disease superficially resembles the anti-basement membrane antibody-mediated diseases (Goodpasture's syndrome). Eosinophilia is found commonly in patients with pulmonary involvement. Renal disease is often rapidly progressive and is associated with segmental or diffuse glomerular capillary necrosis and extensive crescent formation. Deposits of IgG or IgM may be seen in affected glomeruli, but, in general, such deposits are scanty and evanescent.

Some patients with macroscopic or microscopic forms of polyarteritis may have long-standing underlying rheumatoid arthritis. For reasons that are only poorly understood, the disseminated vasculitis accompanying rheumatoid arthritis seldom affects the kidney. Renal involvement in Takayasu's syndrome and in temporal arteritis is likewise unusual.

The overall prognosis for microscopic and macroscopic forms of polyarteritis is poor with or without renal involvement. High doses of corticosteroids, combined with cytotoxic agents, are claimed to exert a beneficial effect. Patients with rapidly progressive glomerulonephritis may benefit from aggressive therapy including plasma exchange if such treatment is instituted early.

Wegener's granulomatosis (see also Chap. 67) is a special variety of disseminated vasculitis characterized by its predilection to affect the upper and lower respiratory tract and the kidneys. Hemoptysis may be present; thus, these cases may be confused with Goodpasture's syndrome. Serum levels of IgA and IgE may be increased, and complement component levels are usually normal (Table 279-1). Pathologically, a granulomatous necrotizing vasculitis is seen in kidneys, lungs, and other organs. Immunofluorescence studies reveal scattered granular deposits of immunoglobulin and complement, suggesting an immune-complex-mediated pathogenesis. The antigen and antibody systems are unknown. The prognosis of untreated patients with Wegener's granulomatosis is very poor. The use of steroids and cytotoxic drugs, particularly cyclophosphamide, has radically altered the course of this disease. Long-term survival and prolonged disease-free intervals have been produced by aggressive treatment with cyclophosphamide. Response of the pulmonary lesion is especially dramatic.

Allergic granulomatous arteritis (Churg and Strauss syndrome) is a rare form of vasculitis in which severe asthma, fever, and eosinophilia are associated with necrotizing granulomas and extensive tissue infiltration with eosinophils. Necrotizing glomerulonephritis may be found. Steroids seem to be effective in the treatment of this disorder.

DYSPROTEINEMIAS AND PARAPROTEINEMIAS Essential (mixed) cryoimmunoglobulinemia This disorder is associated with high serum levels of circulating cold precipitable immunoglobulins (cryoimmunoglobulins), usually consisting of IgG and IgM; the latter possess rheumatoid factor activity. Purpura, necrotizing skin lesions in cold-exposed areas, arthralgias, fever, and hepatosplenomegaly are found frequently. Hepatitis B infection and other occult fungal, bacterial, or viral infections may be the cause of this syndrome. Cryoimmunoglobulins are also found in the circulation in many diseases, particularly chronic infections, and probably represent circulating immune complexes with unusual physical properties. Glomerular disease is common, resulting from the precipitation of the cryoimmunoglobulin in the glomerular capillaries. Acute renal failure, rapidly progressive (crescentic) glomerulonephritis, or the nephrotic syndrome may result. Serum complement components are depressed, and CIC are present (Table 279-1). Pathologically, a diffuse proliferative glomerulonephritis may be seen, with immunofluorescence findings consistent with the deposition of the circulating cryoimmunoglobulin. Eradication of the underlying infection, if possible, is of great value in treatment. Intensive plasma exchange, accompanied by steroids and cytotoxic agents, has been used with some success in severe cases.

Monoclonal gammopathies *Multiple myeloma* (Chap. 63) may be associated with at least three types of glomerular injury. Amyloidosis (Chap. 64) (see below) occurs in 10 to 15 percent of patients with proved multiple myeloma. Lesions resembling nodular diabetic glomerular sclerosis are seen occasionally. Monoclonal cryoimmunoglobulins occasionally may be deposited in glomeruli. Proteinuria and the nephrotic syndrome are common clinical features of glomerular injury in multiple myeloma. *Waldenström's macroglobulinemia* may be associated with acute renal failure when the homogeneous IgM paraprotein precipitates in glomerular capillaries as "thrombi." Intensive plasma exchange, accompanied by therapy with alkylating agents, may be beneficial. Hyperviscosity may occasionally result in functional alterations in GFR. Renal amyloidosis occurs uncommonly. *Benign monoclonal gammopathies* are seldom associated with glomerular complications, except for mild asymptomatic proteinuria and, rarely, nephrotic syndrome.

Amyloidosis (see also Chap. 64) This disorder may occur in the absence of systemic disease (primary amyloidosis), may be secondary to chronic inflammatory processes (e.g., rheumatoid arthritis, osteomyelitis, paraplegia), multiple myeloma, other neoplastic diseases, or may occur in a heredofamilial form (e.g., familial Mediterranean fever). All forms may affect the glomeruli.

Primary amyloidosis commonly affects the kidneys. It usually occurs in older age groups. Proteinuria, often of nephrotic proportions, is the most common clinical manifestation of renal involvement. The urine sediment tends to be benign. The degree of proteinuria is not necessarily related to the extent of glomerular deposition of amyloid. Enlarged kidneys may be noted in patients with well-preserved renal function, but this is a nonspecific finding. The blood pressure is normal unless advanced uremia is present. Pathologically, the classic features include hypocellular glomeruli infiltrated with amorphous deposits which are positive with Congo red stains and reveal apple-green birefringence under polarized light. The typical fibrillar nature of the amyloid deposits can be demonstrated by electron microscopy. The fibrils in primary amyloidosis are related immunologically to the IgG light chain. A similar immunochemical relationship is noted in multiple myeloma. Immunofluorescence studies reveal amorphous deposits of immunoglobulin and complement in glomeruli. Renal vein thrombosis may complicate the course of amyloidosis. The diagnosis of amyloidosis is usually made by tissue biopsy. Rectal biopsy is a reasonably safe procedure and has a low prevalence of false-negative results. Patients with primary amyloidosis may have increased plasmacytosis in bone marrow aspirates and may reveal paraprotein abnormalities by serum and urinary protein electrophoresis.

Renal amyloidosis is a progressive disease for which there is no established form of treatment. Remissions may occur in secondary amyloidosis if the cause can be found and eliminated. Remissions in primary amyloidosis have been exceedingly rare; however, a few reports describe remissions following the use of cytotoxic agents. Overall the 5-year survival for patients with primary amyloidosis is less than 20 percent. Azotemia, persistent nephrotic syndrome, and clinically evident myocardial involvement confer an even more ominous prognosis.

Neoplastic disease Glomerular alterations may develop in close association with a variety of neoplastic diseases. *Carcinomas,* especially adenocarcinoma of lung, colon, stomach, and breast, may be accompanied by glomerular lesions resembling idiopathic membranous glomerulopathy, although, on occasion, crescentic or focal and segmental proliferative glomerulonephritis or amyloidosis may be seen. Nephrotic syndrome is the most common clinical renal manifestation. Approximately 6 to 10 percent of patients with idiopathic nephrotic syndrome associated with membranous glomerulopathy harbor an underlying malignancy. Successful treatment of the tumor, especially by surgical means, may lead to a remission of the clinical findings. Presumably the glomerular lesions arise because of the deposition of circulating immune complexes, which are composed of tumor antigen and antitumor antibody.

Lymphomas and leukemias may also give rise to glomerular abnormalities. Hodgkin's disease is most commonly associated with the findings of idiopathic nephrotic syndrome (minimal change disease). Other glomerular lesions including membranous glomerulopathy and focal proliferative and sclerosing glomerulonephritis may also be seen. The mechanism of the association of Hodgkin's disease with minimal change disease is unknown, but an underlying T-cell abnormality has been suggested. The nephrotic syndrome is the chief clinical manifestation of glomerular involvement in Hodgkin's disease. Proteinuria may wax and wane with fluctuations in the clinical activity of the Hodgkin's disease. Remissions may be produced by local x-ray irradiation of involved lymph nodes or by systemic chemotherapy.

MISCELLANEOUS MULTISYSTEM DISEASES OCCASIONALLY AFFECTING GLOMERULI Mixed connective tissue disease (MCTD) This disorder consists of a mixture of clinical, serologic, and pathological features of SLE, scleroderma, and dermatomyositis. Raynaud's phenomena, myositis, altered esophageal motility, normal serum complement components, and high titers of antibody to a ribonuclease-sensitive saline extractable nuclear antigen (ENA) are found. A "speckled" pattern is seen in fluorescent antinuclear antibody assay (FANA) tests, low titers of antibody to ds and ssDNA may be found, and LE cell preparations are usually negative. Renal disease is uncommon and, if present, is usually mild. Clinical manifestations include hematuria and proteinuria and occasionally nephrotic syndrome. Pathologically, membranous glomerulopathy or membranoproliferative glomerulonephritis is seen. The prognosis is generally favorable, and treatment is directed at extrarenal manifestations.

Rheumatoid arthritis Several forms of glomerular injury may occur in rheumatoid arthritis (Chap. 356). Secondary amyloidosis occurs in 5 to 10 percent of patients with long-standing arthritis. Nephrotic syndrome is a complication of both gold therapy and penicillamine (see Chap. 278). In addition, the kidney may share in the vasculitis seen occasionally in patients with severe rheumatoid arthritis. Finally, patients with rheumatoid arthritis may develop a mild proliferative glomerulitis or diffuse membranous glomerulopathy which resembles lesions seen in SLE. Proteinuria, sometimes with nephrotic syndrome, is the principal clinical feature of these lesions.

Other disorders *Acute rheumatic fever* (Chap. 241) may be associated with a mild proliferative glomerulonephritis of little clinical significance. *Sjögren's syndrome* (Chap. 356) may be associated with nephrotic syndrome due to membranous or membranoproliferative glomerulonephritis (type I). More frequently, interstitial nephritis is seen. *Sarcoidosis* is rarely complicated by membranous nephropathy. *Partial or total lipodystrophy* may be associated with membranoproliferative glomerulonephritis (type II, dense deposit disease) (see Chap. 278). Complement abnormalities are found, consisting of depressed C3 levels, normal C1q and C4 levels, and circulating C3 lytic factors (i.e., C3 nephritic factor).

Chronic liver disease may be complicated by glomerular disease. The nephrotic syndrome may appear in the course of *chronic active hepatitis* associated with persistent hepatitis B surface antigenemia. Glomerular lesions include membranous glomerulopathy or membranoproliferative (type I) glomerulonephritis. Immunofluorescence studies in such patients reveal granular deposits of immunoglobulins, complement components, and hepatitis B surface antigen, indicating an immune complex disease. Serum C3 levels are often reduced, and tests for CIC and cryoimmunoglobulins are frequently positive. Occasionally patients will have little clinical evidence of liver disease, yet develop distinct glomerular lesions secondary to chronic hepatitis B infection. *Acute viral hepatitis* may be associated with transient hematuria or proteinuria and resemble other postinfectious glomerulonephritides (see Chap. 278). Severe *chronic liver disease* (cirrhosis) may be associated with diffuse glomerulosclerosis. Few clinical manifestations of glomerular disease are found. Prominent mesangial IgA deposits, of unknown pathogenetic significance, have been noted in patients with alcoholic (Laennec's) cirrhosis.

HEREDOFAMILIAL DISEASES

DIABETIC NEPHROPATHY (See also Chap. 338) Diabetes mellitus affects the structure and function of the kidney in many ways. *Diabetic nephropathy* is a generic term which encompasses all the lesions occurring in the kidneys of patients with diabetes mellitus. These lesions include *glomerulosclerosis* (diffuse or nodular), *arterionephrosclerosis, chronic interstitial nephritis, papillary necrosis,* and various tubular lesions. Diabetic nephropathy is associated with a variety of clinical syndromes, including mild asymptomatic proteinuria, nephrotic syndrome, progressive renal failure (acute, rapidly progressive, or chronic), and hypertension. Glomerular lesions are particularly common and account for the majority of abnormal clinical findings referable to the kidney. *Diffuse diabetic glomerulosclerosis* (diffuse intercapillary glomerulosclerosis) is the most common lesion and can be identified in the vast majority of

diabetic patients regardless of the presence or absence of abnormal clinical findings referable to the kidney. This lesion consists of a mild diffuse increase in mesangial matrix accompanied by an increased width of the glomerular basement membrane. Various exudative lesions, such as capsular drops and fibrin caps, may also be present. Hyaline arteriosclerosis, particularly of the efferent arteriole, is also found commonly. Taken together, these lesions strongly suggest the diagnosis of diabetes mellitus, but individually they are not specific. *Nodular glomerulosclerosis* (Kimmelstiel-Wilson lesion), on the other hand, is reasonably specific for juvenile onset or islet-cell antibody-positive diabetes mellitus. This lesion consists of PAS-positive, laminated, intercapillary nodules developing on a background of a diffuse increase in mesangial matrix. At the periphery of the nodules open glomerular capillary loops are found. The nodules are relatively acellular, in contrast to the cellular lesions sometimes seen in membranoproliferative glomerulonephritis (often referred to as *lobular glomerulonephritis*). A variable percentage of glomeruli may be affected.

The pathogenesis of diffuse or nodular diabetic glomerulosclerosis is poorly understood. Evidence supporting a role for both the abnormal diabetic milieu (e.g., insulinopenia, hyperglycemia, hyperglycosuria) and genetic factors is reviewed in Chap. 338.

The principal clinical manifestation of diabetic glomerular disease is proteinuria. Initially proteinuria is mild and asymptomatic. Overt carbohydrate intolerance nearly always precedes the development of proteinuria by one or more decades; however, in exceptional cases proteinuria either develops in concert with overt hyperglycemia or even may precede the clinical appearance of diabetes mellitus. GFR is normal or even increased in early diabetic glomerulopathy. The diastolic blood pressure is normal initially. The urine sediment is typically benign, although pyuria may be present if urinary tract infection coexists. An active urinary sediment suggests the chance occurrence of another form of glomerulopathy. Diabetic retinopathy strongly indicates the presence of underlying glomerulopathy, but exceptions have been recorded. With the passage of time, the quantity of protein excreted increases, often with the development of overt nephrotic syndrome. Hypertension appears and progressively worsens but seldom is of malignant proportions. Typically, plasma renin activity is normal or decreased. Acquired hyporeninemic hypoaldosteronism, with persistent hyperkalemia and mild hyperchloremic metabolic acidosis, is not uncommon. From the time of appearance of proteinuria, progressive loss of GFR and end-stage renal failure can be expected to occur within 5 to 7 years. For reasons that are unknown, the rate of loss of GFR in diabetic nephropathy exceeds that of many of the common primary glomerulopathies, including membranoproliferative glomerulonephritis, membranous glomerulopathy, and focal glomerular sclerosis.

Until the cause (or causes) of diabetic mellitus is (are) found, prevention of the glomerulopathy will not be feasible. If the abnormal diabetic milieu is responsible for the vascular complications (including glomerular disease), as some have suggested, then very precise regulation of blood sugar (e.g., meticulous attention to diet, exercise, insulin dosage, servo-feedback devices for insulin administration) may be effective in reducing the prevalence of diabetic nephropathy. Once developed to a clinically recognizable stage, no form of treatment has unequivocally altered the natural history of diabetic nephropathy. Pancreatic allotransplantation may be the best ultimate hope. Patients with end-stage renal failure due to diabetic nephropathy are poor candidates for long-term dialysis, primarily because of concomitant multiple organ dysfunction secondary to widespread arteriovascular disease. Mortality rates among diabetics on chronic dialysis are three to five times higher than among similarly treated nondiabetics of comparable age. Renal transplantation has been successfully undertaken in the younger diabetic, especially if a living related donor is available. The success rate is somewhat less than in the nondiabetic population, but transplantation is a viable alternative to dialysis in selected patients. Recurrence of typical diabetic glomerular lesions has been documented in renal allografts, but thus far, with short-term follow up, progressive loss of GFR secondary to recurrent disease has not been noted.

ALPORT'S SYNDROME This disorder consists of sensorineural deafness associated with hereditary nephritis. Renal disease manifests itself at an early age, principally as recurrent hematuria. Males are more frequently and severely affected than females. Slowly progressive renal insufficiency, terminating in end-stage renal disease in the second to third decade, is common among males. There is no clear-cut relationship between the onset or severity of the hearing abnormality and the clinical extent of renal disease. Other associated abnormalities include spherophakia, lenticonus, thrombocytopathia, hyperprolinemia, and cerebral dysfunction. Complement component levels are normal. Family studies have indicated an autosomal dominant or X-linked mode of inheritance, with variable penetrance and expressivity. Renal failure seems to be preferentially associated with the X chromosome. The pathogenesis of this disorder is unknown but may be due to defective synthesis of glycopeptide (noncollagenous) components of glomerular and tubular basement membranes.

The pathological features by light microscopy are nonspecific, and a diagnosis cannot be established by optical microscopy alone. Both glomerular and interstitial lesions are present. Focal and diffuse glomerular proliferation, with segmental sclerosis, is common. Interstitial foam cells are nonspecific findings. Electron microscopy reveals thinning, splitting, and delamination of both glomerular and tubular basement membranes, thought by some to be specific for Alport's syndrome. Immunofluorescence studies fail to reveal deposits of immunoglobulins or complement components. The autoantibody to basement membrane antigens found in patients with Goodpasture's syndrome does not react with the glomeruli of patients with Alport's syndrome. Treatment is supportive; steroids and cytotoxic agents are ineffective. The disease is not known to recur following transplantation.

FABRY'S DISEASE (See also Chap. 101) This disorder, angiokeratoma corporus diffusum, is an X-linked inborn error of glycosphingolipid metabolism which leads to the accumulation of neutral glycosphingolipids in many tissues including the kidney. A specific deficiency of alpha-galactosidase, ceramide trihexosidase A has been described. Clinical manifestations include punctate, purple-colored macules in mucous membranes and skin, particularly over the lower body and scrotum, acroparesthesias, corneal dystrophy, and premature coronary artery disease. Rarely, affected females may develop renal disease without the usual cutaneous features. Renal manifestations include hematuria and modest proteinuria, often associated with slowly progressive renal failure. Light-microscopic findings include foamy alterations of the epithelial cells of the glomerulus. Staining of these cells with Sudan black reveals them to contain lipid. Electron microscopy reveals these same cells to contain intracellular rounded laminated bodies ("myelin figures"). The disorder is untreatable unless replacement

of the deficient enzyme can be assured. Some investigators have claimed that successful renal transplantation corrects the enzyme deficiency. Perhaps transplantation of other tissues (e.g., bone marrow) may ultimately become the treatment of choice.

NAIL-PATELLA SYNDROME This disorder is an autosomal dominant disease, linked to the ABO blood groups and characterized by dystrophic nails, absence of one or both patellae, iliac horns, and renal disease. The renal manifestations include isolated proteinuria and hematuria, and occasionally the nephrotic syndrome. Progressive renal failure is relatively uncommon. Glomerular lesions by light microscopy are nonspecific, but electron microscopy reveals a characteristic moth-eaten appearance of the glomerular basement membrane associated with intramembranous collagen fibrils. The prognosis is generally favorable. No treatment is known to be effective.

CONGENITAL NEPHROTIC SYNDROME This disorder is an autosomal recessive trait characterized by the development of nephrotic syndrome at the time of or shortly after birth. It occurs with highest frequency in families of Finnish extraction. Affected individuals have very large placentas, low birth weight, anasarca, polycythemia, and an initially normal GFR. α-Fetoprotein levels are increased in amniotic fluid and maternal serum. Proteinuria is usually heavy and very nonselective. Nephrotic syndrome appearing several months after birth is usually due to other causes, especially minimal change disease or focal glomerular sclerosis (Chap. 278). Congenital syphilis or congenital toxoplasmosis may produce a similar syndrome and must be excluded. Pathologically, microcystic transformation of the cortical nephrons, due to proximal tubular dilatation, is found. Glomerular changes are nonspecific. Extensive effacement of the foot processes and sclerosis of the glomerular tufts are seen by electron microscopy. Immunofluorescence findings are either negative or nonspecific. The course is progressive, and few patients survive the first year of life. Death is usually due to inanition, infection, or renal failure. All forms of treatment have been ineffective. A few patients may survive long enough to be considered for renal transplantation.

SICKLE-CELL DISEASE (See also Chaps. 282 and 315) This disorder is an autosomal dominant trait characterized by the development of an abnormal hemoglobin (hemoglobin S). Glomerular lesions occur infrequently in homozygous sickle-cell disease. The medulla seems to be preferentially affected, leading to impaired concentrating ability and acid excretion and, occasionally, papillary necrosis. Some patients develop mainly glomerular lesions, often accompanied by proteinuria and a nephrotic syndrome. These glomerular lesions conform to either membranous or membranoproliferative glomerulonephritis. Immunofluorescence findings are usually positive, with both immunoglobulin and complement components deposited in a granular pattern suggesting immune-complex-mediated disease. In a few instances, renal tubuloepithelial antigens have been localized in these deposits, suggesting that ischemic damage of the kidney may release autologous renal antigens to provoke the immune-complex disease. The course in patients with sickle-cell disease complicated by glomerulopathy is often relentlessly progressive, leading ultimately to the development of end-stage renal disease. No form of treatment is known to be effective. Transplantation has been successful occasionally.

REFERENCES

BALDWIN DS et al: Lupus nephritis. Clinical course as related to morphologic forms and their transitions. Am J Med 62:12, 1977

CRAWFURD MD, TOGHILL PT: Alport's syndrome of hereditary nephritis with deafness. Q J Med 37:563, 1968

GLASSOCK RJ, COHEN AJ: Glomerulopathies in multisystem disease, in *The Kidney*, 2d ed, BM Brenner, FC Rector Jr (eds). Philadelphia, Saunders, 1980

SUKI WN, EKNOYAN G (eds): *The Kidney in Systemic Disease*, New York, Wiley, 1976

280

URINARY TRACT INFECTION, PYELONEPHRITIS, AND RELATED CONDITIONS

WALTER STAMM
MARVIN TURCK

DEFINITIONS Urinary tract infection exists when a significant number of microorganisms are detected in the urine. In most instances, more than 10^5 organisms per milliliter grown from a properly collected midstream "clean catch" urine or from a catheter specimen indicates infection. A smaller number of bacteria (10^3 to 10^5 per milliliter) may also indicate infection, especially from urine obtained by suprapubic aspiration or "in and out" catheterization, or from a patient with an indwelling catheter. Without associated cystitis, acute infections of the urethra and prostate do not usually result in significant bacteriuria and hence are not generally classified as acute urinary tract infections. Significant bacteriuria may also be absent in some circumstances when true urinary tract infection exists. These circumstances include recent antibiotic therapy, early hematogenous pyelonephritis, total urinary obstruction or urine of high osmolarity, high urea concentration, or low pH.

Considerable confusion has arisen about the clinical and pathologic terms used to describe urinary tract infections. Acute infections can be subdivided into two general anatomic categories: lower tract infection (urethritis, cystitis, and prostatitis) and upper tract infection (acute pyelonephritis). The latter term should be reserved for acute bacterial infections that involve the renal interstitium; it should not be used to refer to lower urinary tract infections. Cystitis and acute pyelonephritis may occur together or independently. Either infection may be asymptomatic or present as the clinical syndromes outlined below. Symptoms of dysuria, urgency, and frequency unaccompanied by significant bacteriuria have been termed the urethral syndrome. Chronic pyelonephritis refers to chronic interstitial nephritis believed to result from bacterial infection of the kidney (Chap. 281). Many noninfectious diseases also cause an interstitial nephritis indistinguishable pathologically from chronic pyelonephritis.

ACUTE INFECTIONS OF THE URINARY TRACT: CYSTITIS, ACUTE PYELONEPHRITIS, URETHRAL SYNDROME

EPIDEMIOLOGY Acute urinary tract infections are very common, involving at least 15 percent of all females at some time during their lives. Some studies show that 20 percent of adult women, regardless of age, experience dysuria each year. However, only 50 percent, mostly younger women, seek medical attention. Males rarely develop symptomatic urinary tract infections until after age 45 unless urologic abnormalities are present.

Many urinary tract infections remain asymptomatic. Approximately 1 percent of male infants and fewer female infants acquire asymptomatic bacteriuria. After infancy, asymptomatic bacteriuria occurs in fewer than 1 percent of males until age 45 to 50; in older males, up to 5 percent have bacteriuria. During childhood, 1 to 2 percent of females have asymptomatic bacteriuria. This increases to 2 to 5 percent during the childbearing years, 2 to 10 percent during pregnancy, and 5 to 15 percent in older women.

ETIOLOGY Many different microorganisms can infect the urinary tract, but by far the most common agents are the gram-negative bacilli. *Escherichia coli* causes approximately 90 percent of acute infections in patients without urologic abnormalities or calculi. Other gram-negative rods, including *Proteus, Klebsiella, Enterobacter, Serratia,* and *Pseudomonas* account for a smaller proportion of uncomplicated infections. These organisms assume increasing importance in recurrent infections and infections associated with urologic manipulation, calculi, or obstruction. They play a major role in nosocomial, catheter-associated infections (see below). *Proteus* species, by virtue of urease production, and *Klebsiella* species, through production of extracellular slime and polysaccharides, predispose to stone formation and are isolated more frequently from patients with calculi.

Gram-positive cocci play a lesser role in urinary tract infections. Enterococci and *Staphylococcus aureus* most often cause infections in patients with renal stones or previous instrumentation. Isolation of *S. aureus* should arouse suspicion of bacteremic infection of the kidney. *Staphylococcus saprophyticus,* a novobiocin-resistant, urease-positive, coagulase-negative staphylococcus, has been recognized as an important cause of acute symptomatic urinary tract infections in young females.

About one-third of women with dysuria and frequency have either a nonsignificant number of bacteria in urine cultures or completely sterile cultures, and have been defined as having the "urethral syndrome." While it seems likely that the majority of these women have an infection, the responsible etiologic agent(s) have not been defined.

Viruses can produce pyelonephritis in animals and may increase the kidney's susceptibility to infection with coliform bacteria. In humans, viruses are most commonly recovered from the urine without evidence of acute urinary disease, although some adenoviruses have been implicated as a cause of hemorrhagic cystitis. Similarly, candida and other fungi may colonize the urine of catheterized patients or diabetics, but they rarely cause acute symptomatic infection.

PATHOGENESIS AND SOURCES OF INFECTION The distal urethra is normally colonized with diphtheroids, streptococcal species, and staphylococcal species but not with the enteric gram-negative bacilli that commonly cause urinary tract infections. In females prone to development of cystitis, however, enteric gram-negative organisms residing in the bowel colonize the introitus, the periurethral skin, and the distal urethra prior to and during episodes of bacteriuria. Factors predisposing to periurethral colonization with coliforms remain poorly understood but may involve absence of local antibody and/or enhanced attachment of organisms to the epithelial cells of infection-prone women. A small number of periurethral bacteria probably gain entry to the bladder frequently, perhaps facilitated in some women by trauma during intercourse. Whether infection ensues then depends upon a number of factors, including the pathogenicity of the strain, the inoculum size, and local and systemic host defense mechanisms.

Under normal circumstances, a large number of bacteria placed in the bladder are rapidly cleared in humans or experimental animals. This results partly from the flushing and dilutional effects of voiding, but also from direct antibacterial properties of urine. Due mostly to high urea concentration and high osmolarity, the bladder urine of many normal persons inhibits or kills bacteria. Prostatic secretions possess antibacterial properties as well. Polymorphonuclear leukocytes in the bladder wall also appear to play a role in clearing bacteriuria. The role of locally produced antibody remains unclear.

The urinary tract should be viewed as a single anatomic unit connected by a continuous column of urine that extends from the urethra to the kidney. In the vast majority of infections, bacteria gain access to the bladder via the urethra. Ascent of bacteria from the bladder may then follow and is probably the usual pathway for most renal parenchymal infections. However, at least 50 percent of patients with bacteriuria do not have evidence of pyelonephritis.

Hematogenous pyelonephritis occurs most often in debilitated patients who either have chronic illnesses or who are receiving immunosuppressive therapy. Staphylococcal pyelonephritis may follow bacteremia from distant foci of infection in the bone, skin, endothelium, or elsewhere.

CONDITIONS AFFECTING PATHOGENESIS Sex The female urethra appears particularly prone to colonization with colonic gram-negative bacilli, owing to its proximity to the anus, its short length (about 4 cm), and its termination beneath the labia. Urethral trauma, as occurs during sexual intercourse, may cause introduction of bacteria into the bladder. The precise role of intercourse in the pathogenesis of urinary infections remains unclear, however. In males, prostatitis or urethral obstruction due to prostatic hypertrophy are important factors predisposing to bacteriuria.

Pregnancy Depending on socioeconomic status, urinary infections are detected in 2 to 8 percent of pregnant women. In particular, symptomatic infections occur more commonly during pregnancy; fully 20 to 40 percent of pregnant women with asymptomatic bacteriuria subsequently develop pyelonephritis. Bladder catheterization during or after delivery causes additional infections. Cystitis and pyelonephritis are no more common in women with toxemia of pregnancy than in other pregnant women. Increased prematurity and newborn mortality may result from urinary infections during pregnancy.

Obstructive uropathy Any impediment to the free flow of urine—tumor, stricture, stone, or prostatic hypertrophy—results in hydronephrosis and greatly increased frequency of urinary tract infection. Infection superimposed on urinary tract obstruction may lead to rapid destruction of renal tissue. It is of utmost importance, therefore, when infection is present to repair obstructive lesions. On the other hand, with minor degrees of obstruction that are not progressive or associated with infection, great caution must be exercised in attempting surgical correction. The introduction of infection in such patients may be more damaging than uncorrected minor obstructions which do not significantly impair renal function.

Neurogenic bladder dysfunction Interference with the nerve supply to the bladder, as in spinal cord injury, tabes dorsalis, multiple sclerosis, diabetes, or other diseases, may be associated with urinary tract infection. The infection may be initiated by the use of catheters for bladder drainage and is favored by the prolonged standing of urine in the bladder. An additional factor often present in these patients is bone demineralization due to immobilization, which causes hypercalciuria, calculus formation, and obstructive uropathy.

Vesicoureteral reflux This condition is defined as reflux of urine from the bladder cavity up into the ureters and sometimes into the renal pelvis. It occurs during voiding or with elevation of pressure in the bladder. In practice, vesicoureteral reflux exists when retrograde movement of radiopaque or radioactive material can be demonstrated. However, since a fluid connection between the bladder and kidney always exists in the patent urinary system, in infections some retrograde movement of bacteria probably occurs normally but is not detected by radiologic techniques. An anatomically impaired ureterovesical junction facilitates reflux of bacteria.

Vesicoureteral reflux is common in children with anatomic abnormalities of the urinary tract and in children with anatomically normal but infected urinary tracts. In the latter group, reflux disappears with advancing age and probably results from rather than causes urinary infection. Follow-up of children with urinary tract infection who were found to have reflux establishes that renal damage correlates with massive reflux, not with infection.

The routine search for reflux would be aided by development of noninvasive tests applicable to young children, where the need is greatest. In the meantime, it appears reasonable to search for massive reflux in anyone with unexplained failure of renal growth or renal scarring, because urinary tract infection per se is an insufficient explanation for these abnormalities. On the other hand, it is doubtful that all children with recurrent urinary tract infections but normal tracts on pyelography should be subjected to voiding cystoureterography merely to detect the rare patient with massive reflux that did not reveal itself on the intravenous pyelogram.

Renal disease and hypertension Experimental and clinical evidence indicate that various renal diseases may increase the kidney's susceptibility to infection. These include diabetic nephropathy, gout, nephrocalcinosis, sickle cell disease, hypercalcemia, and hypokalemia. In surveys of nonhospital populations, mean blood pressure levels are likely to be slightly higher in women with urinary infections than in those without infections. However, whether hypertension or urinary infection is primary remains unclear. Because persons with abnormal urinalyses or hypertension often undergo urinary tract instrumentation, thereby providing access of bacteria to the urinary tract, it is possible that repeated catheterizations rather than underlying renal disease predisposes these patients to infection.

Diabetes mellitus Despite reports that chronic pyelonephritis at autopsy is very common in diabetics, clinical surveys of hospital and nonhospital populations have failed to document any convincing difference in the prevalence of urinary tract infections in diabetic and nondiabetic persons of the same age. This suggests either that diabetics with urinary infections are more likely to develop pyelonephritis or that in the presence of severe vascular and glomerular lesions in diabetic kidneys, morphologic changes result which are similar to those of bacterial infection. The problem requires further study. Irritation of the vulva in women with heavy uncontrolled glucosuria probably increases the rate of false positive voided cultures and may predispose to bladder infection. When diabetic neuropathy has interfered with normal bladder function, persistent infections of the urine are frequent.

Urinary tract infections in diabetics may produce difficulties in the regulation of carbohydrate metabolism and may precipitate diabetic acidosis. The risk of additional renal disease caused by infection in persons already subject to severe vascular and glomerular disease must, of course, be avoided whenever possible. Diabetics are also likely to develop necrotizing papillitis, a fulminating form of renal disease usually associated with infection (see below).

EXPERIMENTAL EVIDENCE Urinary tract infections can be produced in experimental animals by inoculation of bacteria into the renal pelvis or into the bladder urine. Certain organisms such as *Pseudomonas,* enterococci, staphylococci, and *Candida* are capable of causing infection in the normal kidney when they are injected by the intravenous route. Coliform organisms will generally not do this unless intrarenal hydronephrosis or acute obstruction of the ureter is present. Renal damage resulting from a viral or staphylococcal infection can also render the kidney susceptible to infection by coliforms injected intravenously.

The frequent association of urinary tract infection with an obstructive lesion has led to the widespread view that stasis of urinary flow is a prime factor in the development of infection. Since urine readily supports growth of bacteria, prolonged opportunity for multiplication during slow passage along the urinary tract would provide a heavier inoculum to which the kidneys and urinary tissues are exposed. The effect of increased hydrostatic pressure may be an additional factor to explain the association between obstruction and urinary infection. The relative importance of stasis and increased pressure cannot be readily assessed since slowing of urine flow inevitably accompanies obstruction and dilatation of the passages above the obstruction. However, even when profuse diuresis occurs in a patient with a partially obstructed urinary tract, this seldom if ever cures the infection, whereas relief of the obstruction, with or without diuresis, may be followed by subsidence of infection. Even without curing the urinary infection, relief of obstruction materially reduces the risk of renal damage.

Interaction between the tissues and the urine itself is important in the pathogenesis of urinary tract infection, and infection beginning in one can spread to the other. In the urine, phagocytosis is probably less effective than in tissues, and elimination of bacteria may call for more than simply bacteriostasis. This line of reasoning would suggest that optimal drug treatment should include the use of an agent or combination of agents capable of killing the infecting bacteria both in tissues and in the urine. However, there is no clinical or experimental proof to support this contention.

Clinical and experimental evidence has shown that the papillae and medulla of the kidney are particularly susceptible to bacterial infection. Bacterial multiplication in animals with pyelonephritis begins in the medulla, and in this normally hypertonic environment at least some host defense mechanisms such as leukocyte migration, phagocytosis, and complement activity are likely to be impaired. In addition, cell wall defective bacteria can survive in the hypertonic environment of the renal medulla, whereas they are lysed in tissues isotonic to plasma. In patients without urinary obstruction, decreasing the osmolarity of the papillae by drinking large quantities of water would be expected to increase resistance to infection. However, experiments testing the effect of water diuresis on urinary infections vary in outcome, depending on animal species, test organism, means by which bacteria gain access to the urinary tract, and presence of underlying renal disease. In humans, water diuresis may temporarily lower the concentration of bacteria in the urine, but the long-term consequences of water diuresis on the natural history of urinary infections or on the outcome of antibiotic treatment are unknown.

Infections involving the upper urinary tract usually cause a significant rise in serum antibodies directed against the O antigen of the infecting strain. They also produce a temporary defect in renal concentrating ability in many patients, and may be associated with formation of leukocyte casts. Lower tract infections rarely result in increased antibody titers, concentrating defects, or white cell casts. Unfortunately, these methods of distinguishing renal parenchymal infection from cystitis are neither reliable nor convenient enough for routine clinical use. More sensitive tests for distinguishing pyelonephritis from cystitis (bilateral ureteral catheterization and the bladder washout technique originated by Fairley) are inherently invasive and too complex for clinical practice. The development of a simpler and clinically applicable test to separate upper and lower tract infections based upon antibody coating of bacteria in the urine appears to be an important advance. In this test, bacteria from patients with pyelonephritis demonstrate antibody coating on their surface when they have been exposed to a fluorescein-labeled antihuman globulin and are viewed under a fluorescence microscope. No surface antibodies can be visualized on bacteria from patients with cystitis. This antibody response consists mainly of IgG and can be reproduced in an experimental pyelonephritis model in animals. In males, prostatitis may also give rise to antibody-coated bacteriuria.

CLINICAL PRESENTATION Clinical signs and symptoms cannot be relied upon to diagnose urinary tract infection correctly or to localize the site of infection. Approximately one-half of patients with significant bacteriuria (including some with upper tract infection) have no symptoms at all. Of those with significant bacteriuria and symptoms, about one-half have cystitis and one-half have pyelonephritis. Clinical symptoms and signs, though often suggestive, cannot reliably distinguish between upper and lower tract infection. Furthermore, among women presenting with dysuria and frequency, only 60 to 70 percent have significant bacteriuria. The remaining patients (with what is termed *urethral syndrome* or *symptomatic abacteriuria*) cannot be differentiated from those with significant bacteriuria except by urine culture.

Enumeration of the number of bacteria in the urine is therefore an extremely important diagnostic procedure. In symptomatic infections of the urinary tract, bacteria are virtually always easily demonstrable in the urine in large numbers. The absence of easily demonstrable bacteria in uncentrifuged bladder urine indicates that urinary infection does not explain the patient's symptoms. Quantitative estimation of the number of bacteria in the urine, as a rule, makes it possible to distinguish contaminants from true bacteriuria.

A quantitative estimate can be made by means of Gram's stain or microscopic examination of uncentrifuged, freshly voided urine. If bacteria can be found by this method, it may be assumed that the number present approximates 100,000 per milliliter. Since bacteria multiply in urine, they usually achieve concentrations in excess of 100,000 viable units per milliliter in infected patients. In culturing voided urine specimens, contamination often occurs. It is essential, therefore, to examine two or three urine specimens bacteriologically before instituting treatment in patients with few or no symptoms. In patients who are sufficiently ill to require prompt antibiotic therapy, a single quantitative estimate of the number of bacteria in the urine combined with symptoms typical of infection is sufficient to make the diagnosis of urinary infection. If fewer than 10,000 viable bacterial units per milliliter are cultured from a voided urine specimen, they are likely to be of no significance. If 10,000 to 100,000 are present, no positive conclusion can be drawn. Since the large number of bacteria in the bladder urine is due in part to bacterial multiplication during residence in the bladder cavity, samples of urine from the ureters or renal pelvis might contain fewer than 10^5 bacteria per milliliter and yet indicate infection. If the urine contains antibacterial substances or if the pH is 5.0 or lower, inhibition of bacterial multiplication will also result in a lower number of bacteria in the presence of infection. For this reason, antiseptic solutions should not be used in washing the periurethral area prior to collection of the urine specimen.

Cystitis Many physicians refer to significant bacteriuria associated with dysuria, frequency, urgency, and suprapubic pain as cystitis. In actuality, both urethritis and cystitis are usually present. The urine often becomes grossly cloudy, malodorous, and, in some cases, bloody. Pyuria without leukocyte casts, and bacteria should be present on examination of the unspun urine. Physical examination generally reveals only a reddened, tender urethra or suprapubic tenderness. If a purulent urethral discharge or a vaginal discharge is present, especially with fewer than 10^5 bacteria per milliliter on culture, other causes of urethritis, vaginitis, and cervicitis such as gonorrhea, *Trichomonas, Candida,* and herpesvirus hominis should be ruled out. Prominent systemic manifestations like fever over 101°F, nausea, vomiting, and costovertebral angle tenderness usually indicate concomitant renal infection. However, the absence of these findings does not insure that infection is limited to the bladder and urethra.

Acute pyelonephritis Symptoms generally develop rapidly over a few hours or a day and include fever which is often 103°F or greater, shaking chills, nausea, vomiting, and diarrhea. Symptoms of cystitis may or may not be present. Besides fever, tachycardia, and generalized muscle tenderness, physical examination reveals marked tenderness on deep pressure in one or both costovertebral areas or on deep abdominal palpation. In some patients, signs and symptoms of gram-negative sepsis predominate. Most patients have significant leukocytosis, pyuria with leukocyte casts in the urine, and bacteria on a Gram's stain of unspun urine. Hematuria may be present during the acute phase of the disease, but if it persists after acute manifestations of infection have subsided, a stone, tumor, or tuberculosis should be considered.

Except in individuals with papillary necrosis or urinary obstruction, the manifestations of acute pyelonephritis usually subside within a few days, even without specific antibacterial therapy. However, despite the absence of symptoms, bacteriuria or pyuria may persist. With severe pyelonephritis, fever subsides more slowly and may not disappear for several days, even after appropriate antibiotic treatment has been instituted.

Urethral syndrome Approximately 30 to 40 percent of women with dysuria and frequency have cultures that show either no growth or nonsignificant growth. Clinical signs and symptoms cannot distinguish women with significant bacteriuria from those without it; in particular, fever and costovertebral angle tenderness may be seen in the urethral syndrome. Pyuria, absence of leukocyte casts or hematuria, and a negative Gram's stain characterize the microscopic examination of the urine. Symptoms generally subside without therapy within 5 to 7 days or may remit with pyridium.

Catheter-associated urinary tract infections Significant bacteriuria frequently occurs in hospitalized patients with indwelling urethral catheters. *Proteus, Pseudomonas, Klebsiella,* and *Serratia,* in addition to *E. coli,* usually cause these infections. Many infecting strains show marked antimicrobial resistance compared with organisms that cause community-acquired urinary infections.

Infection occurs when bacteria reach the bladder by migrating through the column of urine in the catheter lumen or up the mucous sheath outside the catheter. Hospital-acquired pathogens reach the patient's catheter or urine-collecting system on the hands of hospital personnel, in contaminated solutions or irrigants, and via contaminated instruments or disinfectants. In addition, the patient's own bowel flora often migrate to the perineal skin and periurethral area and reach the bladder via the conduit provided by the catheter.

Most catheter-associated infections appear to be benign. They cause minimal symptoms, no fever or pyuria, and often resolve after withdrawal of the catheter. The frequency of upper tract infection associated with catheter-induced bacteriuria remains unknown. Gram-negative bacteremia, which follows 1 to 2 percent of cases of catheter-associated bacteriuria, is the most significantly recognized complication of catheter-induced urinary infections.

These infections can be partially prevented in patients catheterized less than 2 weeks by use of a sterile closed collecting system, attention to aseptic technique during insertion and care of the catheter, and by measures to minimize cross infection. Despite these precautions, the majority of patients catheterized longer than 2 weeks develop bacteriuria. The optimal treatment for such patients has not been established. Removal of the catheter and a short course of antibiotics to which the organism is susceptible is probably the best course of action and nearly always eradicates the bacteriuria. If the catheter cannot be removed, antibiotic therapy usually proves to be unsuccessful and may result in infection with a more resistant strain. In this situation, the bacteriuria should be ignored unless the patient develops symptoms or is at high risk of developing bacteremia. In these cases, systemic antibiotics or urinary bladder antiseptics may reduce the degree of bacteriuria and the likelihood of bacteremia.

TREATMENT Several therapeutic principles should underlie treatment of urinary tract infections:

1 Quantitative urine cultures must be obtained to document infections reliably and to differentiate the urethral syndrome from bacterial cystitis or pyelonephritis.
2 Antimicrobial sensitivity testing should be used to direct therapy in patients with recurrent infections.
3 Factors predisposing to infection, such as obstruction, neurogenic bladder, calculi, etc., should be identified and corrected if possible.
4 Relief of clinical symptoms does not indicate bacteriologic cure, and follow-up cultures after therapy must be obtained.
5 After completion of therapy and follow-up cultures, each treatment episode should be classified as failure (bacteriuria not eradicated during therapy or upon the immediate posttreatment culture) or a cure (elimination of bacteriuria). Recurrent infections should be classified as relapses or reinfections. Relapses are defined as recurrent infection with the same strain occurring less than 14 days (usually less than 5 days) after cessation of therapy. Reinfection indicates a new infection with a different strain, usually occurring weeks or months after administration of antibiotics is discontinued.
6 In general, uncomplicated infections confined to the lower urinary tract respond to low doses and short courses of therapy, while upper tract infections require longer periods of treatment. Relapses usually indicate an upper tract focus of infection while reinfection more often indicates lower tract infection.
7 Community-acquired infections, especially initial infections, are nearly always due to antibiotic-sensitive strains.
8 Patients with repeated infections, instrumentation, or recent hospitalization should be suspected of harboring resistant strains.

Until recently, most antibiotic trials did not distinguish lower urinary tract infections from upper tract infections in assessing therapeutic outcome. In such trials, many antibiotics (ampicillin, sulfonamides, tetracyclines, penicillin, cephalosporins, nitrofurantoin, aminoglycosides, and others) achieved cure rates of approximately 80 percent. However, data utilizing the antibody-coated bacteria method suggest that the location of a urinary tract infection greatly influences success or failure of a therapeutic agent. Bladder bacteriuria can usually be eliminated with nearly any regimen to which the infecting strain is sensitive, and as little as a single dose of 3.0 g ampicillin or 500 mg intramuscular kanamycin will eliminate bladder bacteriuria in most patients. A 7-day course of therapy with oral drugs appears more than adequate. With upper tract infections, however, single-dose therapy fails in the majority of cases and even a 7-day course will be unsuccessful in some patients. Longer periods of treatment (2 to 6 weeks) aimed at eradicating a persistent focus of infection may be necessary in cases of relapse. If available, the antibody-coated bacteria test can be used to distinguish upper and lower tract infections and guide therapy in patients with recurrent infections. In most hospitals, this test has not become available and empiric therapy should be based upon the clinical situation.

For patients with their first episode of *acute uncomplicated cystitis,* a 7-day course of a sulfonamide, ampicillin, nitrofurantoin, nalidixic acid, or tetracycline will be highly effective. More than 90 percent of these infections are due to *E. coli,* and most strains are sensitive to many antibiotics. Single-dose therapy with ampicillin, kanamycin, and trimethoprim-sulfamethoxazole has also been effective. In the absence of calculi or urologic abnormality, recurrent episodes of cystitis can be treated similarly, except that increased antibiotic resistance and infection with strains other than *E. coli* should be anticipated, and antimicrobial sensitivities must be obtained to guide therapy.

Acute pyelonephritis without accompanying clinical evidence of calculi or urologic disease is due to *E. coli* in most cases. A 7-to-10-day course of ampicillin or cephalosporin usually provides adequate therapy. Some of these patients relapse following therapy and should be investigated to determine whether unrecognized calculi or urologic disease are present. If not, treatment should be extended to 2 to 6 weeks to eliminate a presumed upper tract focus causing recurrent bacteriuria.

When suspected *gram-negative sepsis* complicates acute pyelonephritis, hospitalization, prompt parenteral therapy with an aminoglycoside, and ancillary measures to treat sepsis should be provided (Chap. 109). When the antibiotic sensitivities of the infecting strain are available, therapy can be changed to a less toxic agent. Similar therapy should be used for infected patients with calculi or urologic abnormalities who have suspected sepsis.

Optimal treatment regimens for patients with *catheter-associated urinary tract infections* have not been well established. These infections often remit spontaneously or with short-term antibiotic therapy if the catheter can be removed. If the catheter cannot be removed, systemic antibiotics or urinary antiseptics may reduce bacteriuria, but do not usually eliminate it. Asymptomatic bacteriuria in catheterized patients can probably be left untreated in most patients who are not immunosuppressed or who are not at high risk for sepsis because of old age, severe underlying disease, diabetes, or pregnancy.

PROGNOSIS In patients with uncomplicated cystitis or pyelonephritis, treatment ordinarily results in complete resolution of symptoms. In fact, symptoms usually remit even without specific therapy. Lower tract infections in adult women are of concern mainly because they cause discomfort, minor morbidity, and time lost from work. Cystitis may also result in

upper tract infection or in bacteremia (especially during instrumentation), but there is little evidence to suggest that renal impairment follows. When repeated episodes of cystitis occur, they are nearly always reinfections, not relapses.

Uncomplicated acute pyelonephritis in adults rarely progresses to functional impairment and chronic renal disease. Repeated upper tract infections often indicate relapse rather than reinfection, and a vigorous search for renal calculi or an underlying urologic abnormality should be undertaken. If neither is found, 6 weeks of chemotherapy may be useful in eradicating an unresolved focus of infection.

Repeated symptomatic urinary tract infections in children, and in adults with obstructive uropathy, neurogenic bladder, structural renal disease, or diabetes more often progress to chronic renal disease. Asymptomatic bacteriuria in these groups, as well as in adults without urologic disease or obstruction, predisposes to increased episodes of symptomatic infection but does not result in renal impairment in most instances.

PREVENTION Patients with frequent symptomatic infections may benefit from long-term low-dose antibiotics directed at preventing recurrences. A single dose of trimethoprim-sulfamethoxazole (80 mg trimethoprim and 400 mg sulfamethoxazole daily) or nitrofurantoin (50 mg daily) have been particularly effective. Suppressive therapy should be initiated only after bacteriuria has been eradicated with a full-dose treatment regimen. Women having more than two infections every 6 months should be considered for preventive antibiotics. Low-dose antibiotics (nitrofurantoin 50 to 100 mg) after sexual intercourse may also be of benefit in preventing episodes of symptomatic infections. Other situations in which prophylaxis appears to have some merit include men with chronic prostatitis; patients undergoing prostatectomy, both during the operation and postoperative periods; and pregnant women with asymptomatic bacteriuria.

CHRONIC PYELONEPHRITIS

Chronic interstitial nephritis thought to result from bacterial infection of the kidney has been termed *chronic pyelonephritis.* It may occur in patients with predisposing urologic abnormalities (obstruction, vesicoureteral reflux, or neurogenic bladder) or in patients with apparently normal urinary tracts. Unlike acute urinary tract infections, for which simple diagnostic criteria and characteristic clinical syndromes exist, no pathognomonic clinical, laboratory, or pathologic criteria can be used to identify cases of chronic pyelonephritis, and few reliable data on the incidence or prevalence of this condition have been collected. Many patients with renal lesions that fulfill the pathologic criteria for chronic pyelonephritis at autopsy have sterile urine cultures and were not known to have had clinical episodes of bacterial urinary tract infection or urinary obstruction during life. Such cases suggest that other forms of renal injury result in morphologic changes indistinguishable from those produced by bacterial infection. Conversely, relatively few individuals with acute urinary infection develop chronic infection or progressive renal impairment. Most often, this occurs in patients with anatomic obstruction, neurogenic bladder, or vesicoureteral reflux.

Patients with many episodes of urinary tract infection; impaired renal function; pyuria with white cell casts; bacteriuria; an intravenous pyelogram showing an irregularly outlined renal pelvis with calicectasis and cortical scars; and typical pathologic changes can be diagnosed as having chronic pyelonephritis. In less typical patients, the relationship of infection to renal damage is uncertain and the diagnosis often remains unclear.

PATHOLOGY Characteristically, the kidneys are asymmetric in size, scarred, and irregularly pitted on the surface. Pathologic changes usually begin in the interstitial tissue of the medulla and papillae, with connective tissue, lymphocytes, and plasma cells completely replacing interstitium and tubules. Foci of active interstitial inflammation may be seen throughout the medulla, and leukocyte casts are found in some tubules. Other tubules contain large amounts of eosinophilic material and colloid casts, and may be dilated. Early in the disease, most glomeruli appear relatively normal. A proliferative endarteritis may be present. With progression, involvement of glomeruli and vessels becomes more pronounced and uniform, eventually resulting in an "end-stage" kidney.

None of the foregoing changes is pathognomonic for chronic pyelonephritis. Similar morphologic features may result from the nephropathy of chronic hypokalemia, nephrocalcinosis, chronic analgesic abuse, primary vascular disease of the kidneys, obstruction, diabetes mellitus, and Balkan nephropathy (Chap. 281).

CLINICAL FEATURES Early signs and symptoms are minimal and nonspecific and often include hypertension. During this stage, the disease may be detected when hypertension, an elevated BUN, or abnormal urinalysis are noted. Patients usually seek medical attention only after renal failure appears. Clinical manifestations at this stage often include fatigue, lassitude, nausea, easy bruising, anorexia, weight loss, polyuria, and nocturia.

In general, glomerular filtration and renal blood flow decline together as pyelonephritis progresses, giving rise to the laboratory features characteristic of uremia (Chap. 276). Reduced maximum concentrating ability, impaired sodium conservation, and hyperchloremic acidosis due to reduced renal excretion of acid and reabsorption of bicarbonate are often more prominent in chronic pyelonephritis than in glomerular diseases. Proteinuria infrequently exceeds 2 g daily.

The appearance of white blood cell casts in the urine suggest the diagnosis of chronic pyelonephritis. However, bacteria, leukocytes, and leukocyte casts may appear only intermittently and often are not present during the chronic stage of the disease. Intravenous pyelography is often normal early in the course of the disease but subsequently shows bilateral small kidneys with irregular outlines, calyceal blunting or dilatation, and cortical scarring. Renal biopsy may be normal owing to the focal nature of the disease early in its course.

PROGNOSIS The course of chronic pyelonephritis may be prolonged and compatible with a comfortable life even after considerable impairment of renal function. Associated hypertension generally worsens the prognosis. In perhaps no other renal disease can fluctuations in renal function be so marked or frequent. During acute infections or episodes of dehydration, renal decompensation may progress to the stage of advanced uremia; yet the patient may recover and regain adequate renal function for years. Correction of obstructing lesions may prevent progression of the disease.

TREATMENT Surgically approachable obstructive lesions should be promptly corrected. Antibiotic therapy for proved infections should be given and should be based on antimicro-

bial sensitivity tests. Hypertension should be controlled to reduce renal vascular complications. The treatment of chronic renal failure is discussed in Chap. 276.

PAPILLARY NECROSIS

The renal papilla is of major importance in the pathogenesis of chronic interstitial nephritis and, when complicated by bacterial infection, pyelonephritis. The peculiar susceptibility of the renal papilla to bacterial infection has been discussed earlier in this chapter (see "Experimental evidence"). It has become evident that a variety of underlying conditions cause primary renal papillary damage, resulting eventually in the renal lesions of chronic interstitial nephritis. When urinary infection does not supervene, the resulting renal disease may progress slowly and silently to the point of renal insufficiency. The pathology of this renal injury may be indistinguishable from that of pyelonephritis. In addition to common diseases such as gout and diabetes mellitus, which cause renal papillary damage, many medications, which achieve enormous concentrations in the urine traversing the renal papilla, may be toxic for that zone of the kidney. The best known of these are phenacetin-containing analgesic mixtures. This problem is much more common than generally recognized, and diagnosis requires careful attention to historical information obtained from the patient.

It is not known how many other substances may be important in the pathogenesis of primary renal papillary disease. However, in view of the benignity of urinary infection in persons without underlying renal papillary damage, it is reasonable to assume the presence of primary underlying renal papillary damage in any patient with urinary infection who shows the development or progression of renal damage.

When severe infection of the renal pyramids is present in association with vascular diseases of the kidney or with urinary tract obstruction, renal papillary necrosis is likely to result. Patients with diabetes, sickle cell disease, chronic alcoholism, and vascular disease seem peculiarly susceptible to this complication. Hematuria, pain in the flank or abdomen, and chills and fever are the most common presenting symptoms. Acute renal failure with oliguria or anuria sometimes occurs. Rarely, sloughing of a pyramid may take place without symptoms in a patient with chronic urinary infection, and the diagnosis is made when the necrotic tissue is passed in the urine or identified as a "ring shadow" on pyelography. If renal function deteriorates suddenly in a diabetic or a patient with chronic obstruction, the diagnosis of renal papillary necrosis should be entertained, even in the absence of fever or pain. Although renal papillary necrosis is often bilateral, when it is unilateral, nephrectomy may be lifesaving in the management of overwhelming infection.

RENAL AND PERINEPHRIC ABSCESS

See Chap. 110.

PROSTATITIS

The term *prostatitis* designates various inflammatory conditions affecting the prostate, including acute and chronic infections with specific bacteria and, more commonly, instances in which signs and symptoms of prostatic inflammation are present but no specific organisms can be detected (prostatosis). Patients in this category usually have low back pain and perineal or testicular discomfort; less often, mild dysuria may be present. Microscopic pyuria or hematuria without any other evidence of genitourinary disease may be the only manifestation of prostatic disease. Such patients may respond to prostatic massage and warm sitz baths. Antibiotic therapy produces variable results. In some cases infection may be secondary to *Chlamydia* or t-strain mycoplasma, which have been incriminated in the pathogenesis of urethritis (Chap. 174). In these cases, treatment with tetracycline or doxycyline for 2 to 6 weeks may be successful.

ACUTE BACTERIAL PROSTATITIS   This disease generally affects young male adults when it occurs spontaneously, but it may be associated with an indwelling urethral catheter. It is characterized by fever, chills, dysuria, and a tense or boggy, extremely tender, prostate. Palpation of the prostate is the key to diagnosis. Although prostatic massage usually produces purulent secretions with a large number of bacteria on culture, bacteremia may result from manipulation of the inflamed gland. For this reason, and because the etiologic agent can usually be identified on urine culture, massage should be avoided unless antibiotic treatment has been instituted. The infection is generally due to one of the common gram-negative urinary tract pathogens or *Staphylococcus aureus*. Despite the fact that the antibiotics used to treat this entity penetrate poorly into prostatic secretions, the response to antibiotics is usually prompt, perhaps because the drugs penetrate more readily into the acutely inflamed prostate. The long-term prognosis is good, although in some instances acute infection may result in abscess formation, epididymoorchitis, seminal vesiculitis, septicemia, and residual chronic bacterial prostatitis. Since the advent of antibiotics, the frequency of acute bacterial prostatitis has diminished markedly. Many so-called cases of "acute prostatitis" are probably posterior urethritis.

CHRONIC BACTERIAL PROSTATITIS   This entity is less well defined and difficult to diagnose. It is a major cause of recurrent bacteriuria in males. Symptoms are usually absent, the prostate feels normal on palpation, and although many white blood cells may be seen in the urinary sediment, results of conventional bacteriologic studies are negative. A small number of bacteria may be cultured from the expressed prostatic secretion or postmassage urine. The presence of these bacteria can be determined only by careful quantitative bacteriologic techniques when the bladder urine is sterile. The method used by Stamey and colleagues should be employed. The usual symptoms of frequency and dysuria occur when infection spreads to the bladder urine. Antibiotics are of limited value in eradicating the focus of chronic infection in the prostate, but they usually do relieve the symptoms of the acute exacerbations promptly. The relative ineffectiveness of antimicrobials in part results from the poor penetration of most antibiotics into the prostate because the low pH which prevails in this organ precludes solubility of most drugs. The macrolide group of drugs (erythromycin, oleandomycin) do enter the prostatic secretions, but these agents are generally ineffective against gram-negative organisms. Sulfonamide-trimethroprim has been employed with considerable success in some of these infections. Patients with frequent episodes of acute cystitis should be treated with prolonged courses of antimicrobials with a view toward suppressing symptoms and keeping the bladder urine sterile. Total prostatectomy produces cure of chronic prostatitis but is associated with considerable morbidity. Transurethral prostatectomy is safer but cures only one-third of patients.

Urinary infections are much less common in men than in women, perhaps because of the antibacterial properties of prostatic fluid. The pattern of recurrent bladder infection in the male with chronic bacterial prostatitis is clinically not very different from that seen in the recurrent cystourethritis of the female. It has been suggested that this pattern of infection in women is due to chronic bacterial infection of the paraurethral glands and ducts, which are, in fact, vestigial remnants of the prostate.

REFERENCES

BRUMFITT W, ASSCHER AW: *Urinary Tract Infection.* New York, Oxford University Press, 1973

GALLAGHER DJ et al: Acute infections of the urinary tract and the urethral syndrome in general practice. Br Med J 1:622, 1965

JONES SR et al: Localization of urinary tract infection by detection of antibody-coated bacteria in urine sediment. N Engl J Med 290:591, 1975

KUNIN CM: *Detection, Prevention and Management of Urinary Tract Infections.* Philadelphia, Lea & Febiger, 1976

MOND NC et al: Presentation, diagnosis and treatment of urinary tract infections in general practice. Lancet 1:514, 1965

SANFORD JP: Urinary tract symptoms and infection. Annu Rev Med 26:485, 1975

STAMEY TA: *Urinary Infections.* Baltimore, Williams & Wilkins, 1972

———, SEXTON CC: The role of vaginal colonization with enterobacteriacae in recurrent urinary infections. J Urol 113:214, 1975

Symposium on Urinary Infections. Kidney Int, vol 4, suppl, 1975

281
TUBULOINTERSTITIAL DISEASES OF THE KIDNEY

BARRY M. BRENNER
THOMAS H. HOSTETTER
H. DAVID HUMES

A large and etiologically diverse group of bilateral renal diseases can be distinguished from those considered in Chaps. 278 and 279 because the histological and functional abnormalities involve the tubules and interstitium to a greater degree than the glomeruli and renal vasculature (see Table 281-1). Morphologically, acute forms of these tubulointerstitial disorders are characterized predominantly by interstitial edema, often associated with cortical and medullary infiltration by polymorphonuclear leukocytes and patchy areas of tubule cell necrosis. In more chronic forms, interstitial fibrosis predominates, inflammatory cells are typically mononuclear, and abnormalities of the tubules tend to be more widespread, as evidenced by atrophy, luminal dilatation, and thickening of tubule basement membranes. In the past, the diagnosis of chronic pyelonephritis was almost universally applied when these chronic tubulointerstitial abnormalities were found. It is now apparent that only a small proportion of these lesions results from infection. Nonbacterial factors, including exogenous toxins and metabolic and immunologic derangements, constitute the major pathogenetic mechanisms thought to be involved. Irrespective of etiology, the extent of tubular dysfunction often correlates closely with the extent of structural distortion of the tubules and interstitium. Defects in tubule function are usually expressed clinically as manifestations of impaired concentrating ability (polyuria, nocturia), diminished ammoniagenesis and net acid excretion (metabolic acidosis), and diminished reabsorption of filtered solutes, particularly amino acids, urate, phosphate, sodium, chloride, and potassium (salt wasting and Fanconi's syndrome). In any given patient, regardless of cause, these tubule abnormalities may be either latent or overt and may occur as isolated defects or in various combinations. However, although the major structural defects originate in the tubules and interstitium, progressive reduction in GFR is a common functional accompaniment of most, if not all, forms of tubulointerstitial damage, reflecting secondary injury to glomeruli and other elements of the renal microcirculation.

TOXINS

A number of factors make the renal tubules and interstitium particularly prone to toxic injury. Although the kidneys constitute less than 1 percent of total body mass, they receive approximately 20 percent of the cardiac output, and 90 percent or more of this very large renal blood flow is distributed to the renal cortex. Exposure of tubules and interstitium of the renal cortex to circulating toxins is, therefore, quantitatively greater than is that of most other tissues. Transport processes operating in renal tubules contribute further to the intrarenal accumulation of toxins, thereby enhancing local concentrations of noxious agents. Furthermore, the urinary concentrating mechanism can establish high levels of toxins within medullary and papillary portions of the kidney, predisposing these regions to chemical injury. Finally, the relatively acid pH of the fluid within most nephron segments may affect the ionization characteristics of potentially toxic compounds and thereby influence local concentration and solubility. Although these normal physiological processes render the kidney particularly vulnerable to toxic injury, the role of nephrotoxins in the causation of renal damage often goes unrecognized, largely because the manifestations of such injury are usually nonspecific in nature and insidious in onset. Diagnosis largely depends upon obtaining a history of exposure to a certain toxin, a difficult matter since exposure may be occult. Particular attention should, therefore, be paid to the patient's occupational history, as well as to an assessment of exposure, current as well as remote, to pharmaceutical agents, especially antibiotics and analgesics. The clinical recognition of a potential association between a patient's renal disease and exposure to a nephrotoxin is of crucial importance because, unlike many other forms of renal disease, progression of the functional and morphological abnormalities associated with toxin-induced nephropathies may be prevented, and even reversed, simply by eliminating additional exposure.

EXOGENOUS TOXINS **Analgesic nephropathy** Over the past three decades, numerous studies have established that individuals who ingest large quantities of analgesic drugs are particularly prone to develop tubulointerstitial damage and papillary necrosis. Indeed, in Australia, Switzerland, and Sweden, analgesic abuse ranks as one of the most common causes of chronic renal failure, and it is now recognized as an important cause of renal insufficiency in the United States as well. Studies in animals have demonstrated that *phenacetin* and *aspirin* can induce papillary necrosis when either of these drugs is given in quantities far in excess of usual therapeutic doses. However, these chemicals are far more likely to cause renal damage, and clinically apparent renal disease, when ingested in combination. Epidemiologic studies leave no doubt that the chronic ingestion of mixtures of these analgesics produces permanent and irreversible renal injury in humans.

Morphologically, analgesic nephropathy is characterized by papillary necrosis and tubulointerstitial inflammation. At an early stage prior to overt papillary necrosis, damage to the vascular supply of the inner medulla (vasa rectae) leads to a local interstitial inflammatory reaction and, eventually, to papillary ischemia, fibrosis, necrosis, and calcification. Destruction of papillae usually precedes extension of the tubulointerstitial abnormalities to the renal cortex and, therefore, occurs before renal size and GFR are reduced significantly. It is important to recognize that although papillary necrosis is a common finding in patients with the nephropathy of analgesic abuse, necrosis of papillae may also be seen in patients with chronic pyelonephritis, diabetes mellitus, sickle-cell disease, and obstructive uropathy. The susceptibility of the renal papilla to damage by analgesic compounds which contain phenacetin is believed to be related to the establishment of a renal corticomedullary gradient for the phenacetin metabolite, *acetaminophen,* resulting in papillary tip concentrations which are more than tenfold higher than those present in renal cortex. Hydration serves to dissipate this gradient and may explain the protective effect of this maneuver in preventing phenacetin-induced papillary necrosis in animals. The aspirin in these analgesic compounds is also believed to contribute to renal injury, by uncoupling oxidative phosphorylation in renal mitochondria and by inhibiting the synthesis of renal prostaglandins, which are potent endogenous renal vasodilator hormones. Both effects of aspirin favor hypoxia in renal tissues and, therefore, enhance the susceptibility of the inner medulla to nephrotoxic injury.

Clinically, analgesic nephropathy occurs some three to five times more commonly in women than men. A direct relationship exists between the total amount of analgesic compounds ingested and the degree of renal impairment. An intake of 1.0 g phenacetin per day for 1 to 3 years, or total ingestion of 2 kg phenacetin in combination with other analgesics, appears to represent minimum requirements for the development of analgesic nephropathy. In such patients, renal function usually declines gradually, in association with chronic necrosis of papillae and diffuse tubulointerstitial damage to the renal cortex. Occasionally, papillary necrosis may be associated with gross hematuria, and even renal colic, due to obstruction of a ureter by a fragment of necrotic tissue. More than half of patients with analgesic nephropathy have pyuria, which, if persistently associated with sterile urine, provides an important clue to the diagnosis. Nonetheless, active pyelonephritis may coexist in patients with analgesic nephropathy. Proteinuria, if present, is typically mild (less than 1 g per 24 h). Patients with analgesic nephropathy are usually unable to generate maximally concentrated urine, reflecting the underlying medullary and papillary damage. An acquired form of distal renal tubular acidosis has been described and may contribute to the development of *nephrocalcinosis*. The occurrence of anemia out of proportion to the degree of azotemia may also provide a useful clue to the diagnosis of analgesic nephropathy. Occult gastrointestinal bleeding (usually secondary to analgesic-induced gastritis) and, in an occasional patient, hemolysis (particularly in those with glucose 6-phosphate dehydrogenase deficiency) are believed to contribute to the severity of the anemia. Vague abdominal complaints, as well as nonspecific headaches and arthralgias, are common in these patients. Moderate hypertension is also a common finding. It progresses to a malignant phase in only a small minority of patients. When analgesic nephropathy has progressed to the stage of moderate to severe renal insufficiency, the kidneys usually appear bilaterally shrunken on intravenous pyelography, and the calyces are deformed. A "ring sign" on the pyelogram, representing radiolucency of the area at the base of a papilla, is pathognomonic of papillary necrosis, but it is present in only a few of these patients.

Every effort must be made to convince the patient who ingests excessive quantities of analgesics to discontinue this hazardous practice. When renal damage is at an early stage, cessation of drug abuse will usually arrest the progression of the nephrotoxic process; not infrequently, overall renal function will improve with time. With continued abuse of these drugs, however, progressive renal damage leads invariably to chronic renal failure.

Lead nephropathy (see also Chap. 225) Children and adults suffering from lead intoxication often develop a chronic form of tubulointerstitial renal disease. In children, lead poisoning usually results from ingestion of lead-based paints (pica). The oxide of lead liberated from paint, or present in the vapor arising from the welding of metals covered with lead-based paint, may be inhaled in substantial quantities, thereby constituting an industrial form of exposure in adults. Alcohol, illegally distilled in an apparatus constructed from automobile radiators (so-called "moonshine"), is yet another source of lead poisoning. Tubule transport processes enhance the accumulation of lead within renal cells, particularly of the proximal convoluted tubule, leading to cell degeneration, mitochondrial swelling, and eosinophilic intranuclear inclusion bodies rich in lead. In addition to tubule degeneration and atrophy, lead nephropathy is associated with ischemic changes in the glomeruli, fibrosis of the adventitia of small renal arterioles, and focal areas of cortical scarring. Eventually, the kidneys become grossly atrophic. In addition to progressive azotemia, abnormalities of tubule function may occur, particularly *renal glycosuria* and *aminoaciduria*. Urinary excretion of lead, bile pigments, and porphyrin precursors, particularly δ-aminolevulinic acid, coproporphyrin, and urobilinogen, is increased. Patients with chronic lead nephropathy are characteristically *hyperuricemic*, a consequence of enhanced reabsorption of filtered urate. Acute gouty arthritis (so-called "saturnine gout") occurs in about 50 percent of patients with lead nephropathy, in striking contrast to other forms of chronic renal failure in which gout is rare. Hypertension is also a frequent complication of this disorder. Therefore, in any patient with slowly progressive renal failure, atrophic kidneys, gout, and hypertension, the diagnosis of lead intoxication should be seriously considered. In addition to these manifestations, patients with chronic lead poisoning often complain of frequent episodes of abdominal colic and have evidence of anemia, peripheral neuropathy, and encephalopathy. The diagnosis is suspected by finding elevated serum levels of lead and can be confirmed by documenting an increment of more than 0.6 mg per day in the urinary excretion of lead following a standardized infusion of calcium ethylenediaminetetraacetic acid (EDTA). Treatment includes removing the patient from the source of exposure and augmenting lead excretion with a chelating agent such as disodium calcium EDTA.

Miscellaneous nephrotoxins Many agents which commonly lead to acute renal failure are also capable of producing tubulointerstitial injury (see Chap. 275). These include antibiotics (e.g., aminoglycosides, amphotericin B), radiographic contrast agents, various hydrocarbons (e.g., carbon tetrachloride), and heavy metals (e.g., mercury, cadmium, and bismuth).

METABOLIC TOXINS Acute uric acid nephropathy Disorders characterized by acute overproduction of uric acid and extreme hyperuricemia often lead to a rapidly progressive form of renal insufficiency, so-called "acute uric acid nephropathy." This tubulointerstitial disease is usually seen in patients given cytotoxic drugs for the treatment of lymphoproliferative or myeloproliferative disorders, but may also occur in these patients even before such treatment is begun. The pathological changes associated with acute uric acid nephropathy are largely the result of deposition of uric acid crystals in the kidneys and their collecting systems leading to partial or complete obstruction of collecting ducts, renal pelvis, or ureter. Since obstruction is often bilateral, patients typically show the clinical course of acute renal failure, characterized by oliguria and rapidly rising serum creatinine concentration. In the early phase of this disorder, uric acid crystals can often be found in urine, usually in association with microscopic or gross hematuria. Peak serum uric acid levels vary but are almost always above 20 mg per 100 ml and may even exceed 60 mg per 100 ml.

Prevention of hyperuricemia in patients at risk, by treatment with allopurinol in doses of 200 to 800 mg per day prior to cytotoxic therapy, greatly reduces the danger of acute uric acid nephropathy. Once hyperuricemia develops, however, efforts should be directed to preventing deposition of uric acid within the urinary tract. Increasing urine volume with potent diuretics (furosemide or mannitol) effectively lowers intratubular uric acid concentrations, and alkalinization of the urine to pH 7 or greater with sodium bicarbonate and/or a carbonic anhydrase inhibitor (acetazolamide) enhances uric acid solubility. If these efforts, together with allopurinol therapy, are ineffective in preventing acute renal failure, dialysis should be instituted to lower the serum uric acid concentration as well as to treat the acute manifestations of uremia. The combination of conservative therapy and hemodialysis allows most patients with acute uric acid nephropathy to survive this form of acute renal failure and ultimately recover renal function essentially completely.

Gouty nephropathy Patients with less severe but more prolonged forms of hyperuricemia are predisposed to a more chronic tubulointerstitial disorder, often referred to as *gouty nephropathy*. The severity of renal involvement in this disorder correlates well with the duration and magnitude of the elevation of the serum uric acid concentration. Histologically, the distinctive feature of gouty nephropathy is the presence of crystalline deposits of uric acid and monosodium urate salts in kidney parenchyma. These deposits are believed to represent the primary pathogenetic process in gouty nephropathy, with intraluminal crystallization of uric acid taking place in distal tubules and collecting ducts where urine pH is generally quite low and where uric acid concentrations are considerably in excess of levels in plasma. These deposits not only cause intrarenal obstruction, but also incite an inflammatory response, leading to lymphocytic infiltration, foreign-body giant-cell reaction, and eventual fibrosis, especially of medullary and papillary regions of the kidney. Bacteriuria and pyelonephritis occur in about one-fourth of cases, presumably as complications of intrarenal urinary stasis. Since patients with gout frequently suffer from hypertension and hyperlipidemia, degenerative changes of the renal arterioles may constitute a striking feature of the histological abnormality, often out of proportion to other morphological defects. Clinically, gouty nephropathy is an insidious cause of renal insufficiency. Early in its course, GFR may be near normal, often despite focal morphological changes in medullary and cortical interstitium, proteinuria, and diminished urinary concentrating ability. If hyperuricemia is permitted to persist, the interstitial fibrosis may result in frank renal failure. Treatment for progressive gouty nephropathy must, therefore, be directed at returning serum uric acid concentrations to normal with allopurinol. However, the value of prophylactic treatment of asymptomatic persons with chronic hyperuricemia has not been clearly demonstrated.

Hypercalcemic nephropathy   Chronic hypercalcemia, as occurs in primary hyperparathyroidism, sarcoidosis, multiple myeloma, vitamin D intoxication, or metastatic bone disease, is a well known cause of tubulointerstitial damage and progressive renal insufficiency. Pathologically, the earliest renal lesion induced by hypercalcemia is a focal degenerative change in renal epithelia, primarily in collecting ducts, distal convoluted tubules, and loops of Henle. Tubule cell necrosis leads to nephron obstruction and stasis of intrarenal urine, favoring local precipitation of calcium salts and infection. Dilatation and atrophy of tubules eventually occur, as does interstitial fibrosis, mononuclear leukocyte infiltration, and interstitial calcium deposition (nephrocalcinosis). Calcium deposition may also occur in glomeruli and the walls of renal arterioles. Clinically, the most striking defect is an inability to concentrate the urine maximally, resulting in polyuria and nocturia. Defective transport of chloride in the ascending limb of Henle's loop is believed to be responsible, at least in part, for this concentrating defect. Additionally, reduced collecting duct responsiveness to ADH may contribute to this abnormality. Reductions in GFR and renal blood flow also occur, both in states of acute severe hypercalcemia as well as with prolonged hypercalcemia of lesser severity. Distal renal tubular acidosis and sodium and potassium wasting have also been described in these chronic states. Eventually, uncontrolled hypercalcemia leads to severe tubulointerstitial damage and overt renal failure. Urinalysis is rarely a clue to the presence of hypercalcemic renal failure, but abdominal x-rays may demonstrate nephrocalcinosis as well as nephrolithiasis, the latter due to the hypercalcinuria which often accompanies hypercalcemia. Treatment for hypercalcemic nephropathy consists of reducing the serum calcium concentration toward normal and correcting the primary abnormality of calcium metabolism. The management of hypercalcemia is discussed in Chap. 350. Prognosis for recovery of renal function depends upon the severity of the renal lesion at the time hypercalcemia is corrected. Renal dysfunction of recent onset secondary to acute hypercalcemia may be completely reversible. Gradual, progressive renal insufficiency related to chronic hypercalcemia, however, may not improve with correction of the calcium disorder. Nonetheless, every effort should be made to return serum calcium concentration to normal in order to minimize further loss of renal function.

Hypokalemic nephropathy   Disturbances of renal structure and function are observed commonly in patients with moderate to severe potassium depletion of at least several weeks' duration. Histologically, renal epithelial cells are often seen to contain numerous vacuoles, most marked in proximal, and to a lesser extent, distal convoluted tubules. These findings usually disappear with potassium repletion. Glomeruli and blood vessels are usually uninvolved. Whether prolonged or recurrent potassium deficiency results in irreversible tubulointerstitial fibrosis, scarring, and atrophy is still a controversial issue. Loss of urinary concentrating ability is the most commonly encountered functional defect. Experimental studies in animals have shown that this urinary concentrating abnormality is preceded by a period of primary polydipsia. The reduced concentrating capacity which eventually develops is due, at least in part, to defective operation of the countercurrent multiplier system. Elevated rates of intrarenal prostaglandin synthesis may also contribute to this concentrating defect, since prostaglandins are known to antagonize the hydroosmotic action of antidiuretic hormone on collecting-duct epithelium. Symptoms of nocturia, polyuria, and polydipsia are frequently encountered in patients with chronic potassium depletion, although, occasionally, patients with severe hypokalemia have no complaints referable to the urinary tract. It has been suggested that patients with hypokalemic nephropathy have an enhanced susceptibility to pyelonephritis, but this issue remains unresolved. The polydipsia is probably due to both the impaired renal concentrating ability and a primary disorder of the thirst mechanism, which is believed to be a common feature of most chronic potassium depletion states. Urinalysis often reveals no abnormalities except for mild proteinuria. Serum creatinine and urea nitrogen concentrations usually remain within normal limits. Treatment should be directed at repleting body potassium stores and correcting the primary process responsible for potassium loss. With correction of body potassium stores, functional and histological abnormalities of the kidneys usually disappear, although maximum urinary concentrating ability may not return to normal for several months.

Miscellaneous metabolic toxins   Urinary oxalate, derived from the metabolism of glycine and, to a variable extent, from ingested oxalate, may deposit as insoluble intratubular calcium oxalate crystals and result in chronic tubulointerstitial damage in patients with hereditary or acquired forms of *hyperoxaluria*. *Cystinosis* and *Fabry's disease* are other hereditary depositional disorders affecting the renal tubules and interstitium. The reader is referred to Chaps. 279, 283, and 284 for more detailed discussions of these and other uncommon metabolic causes of tubulointerstitial injury.

NEOPLASIA

In addition to being the site of origin of several benign and malignant neoplasms (see Chap. 286), the kidneys are frequently affected by neoplasms arising outside the urinary tract. Except for the glomerulopathies associated with lymphomas and several solid tumors (see Chap. 278), the renal manifestations of primary extrarenal neoplastic processes are confined mainly to the interstitium and tubules. Although metastatic renal involvement by solid tumors is unusual, the kidneys are often invaded by neoplastic cells in various lymphomas and leukemias and in multiple myeloma. In postmortem studies of patients with *lymphoma*, renal involvement is found in approximately one-half of cases. The involvement may be focal, in the form of multiple discrete nodules, or diffuse, with lymphomatous infiltration throughout the renal parenchyma. Diffuse infiltration is seen most commonly in lymphomas other than

Hodgkin's disease. There may be flank pain related to massive renal infiltration, and x-rays may show enlargement of one or both kidneys. Renal insufficiency occurs in a distinct minority of cases, and overt uremia is rare. Treatment of the primary disease may improve renal function in these cases.

The kidneys are also commonly involved in various forms of *leukemia*. At postmortem examination, bilateral renal involvement can be demonstrated in approximately 50 percent of cases. As with lymphoma, uremia is rarely, if ever, a consequence of leukemic infiltration of the kidneys. The kidneys can also be involved in leukemias because of the associated high incidence of hyperuricemia, hypercalcemia, and lysozymuria. The myelogenous leukemias, particularly of the monocytic type, may be complicated by tubule defects involving potassium, magnesium, and calcium conservation.

In contrast, infiltration of the kidneys with *myeloma* cells is infrequent. When it occurs, the process is usually focal, so that renal insufficiency from this cause is also uncommon. The more usual lesion is *"myeloma kidney,"* which is characterized histologically by atrophic tubules, many with eosinophilic intraluminal casts, and numerous multinucleated giant cells within tubule walls as well as in the interstitium. The frequent occurrence of myeloma kidney in patients with Bence-Jones proteinuria has suggested a causal relation. Bence-Jones proteins are thought to cause myeloma kidney through direct toxicity to renal tubule cells. In addition, Bence-Jones proteins may precipitate within the distal nephron where the high concentrations of these proteins and the acid composition of the tubule fluid favor intraluminal cast formation and intrarenal obstruction. Indeed, positive immunofluorescence staining for light chains can often be demonstrated in casts found in myeloma kidneys. Occasionally, acute renal failure occurs after intravenous pyelography in patients with multiple myeloma and is believed to result from the further precipitation of Bence-Jones proteins induced by dehydration prior to radiographic study. Routine dehydration of the patient with myeloma in preparation for intravenous pyelography should, therefore, be avoided. Multiple myeloma may also affect the kidneys indirectly. Hypercalcemia or hyperuricemia may occur and lead to the nephropathies described above. Proximal tubule disorders are also seen occasionally in patients with myeloma, including type 2 proximal renal tubular acidosis and the Fanconi syndrome. Additionally, intrarenal deposits of *amyloid* (see below) may contribute to impaired excretory function in patients with multiple myeloma.

IMMUNE DISORDERS

HYPERSENSITIVITY NEPHROPATHY   An acute diffuse tubulointerstitial reaction may result from hypersensitivity to a number of drugs. First reported after the use of sulfonamides, acute tubulointerstitial damage is now seen most often with the antibiotic *methicillin,* although other drugs, including *ampicillin, penicillin, cephalothin, phenindione, thiazides,* and *furosemide,* have also been implicated. Grossly, the kidneys are usually enlarged. Histologically, the glomeruli appear normal. The principal pathological abnormalities are in the interstitium of the kidney, which reveals pronounced edema and infiltration with polymorphonuclear leukocytes, lymphocytes, plasma cells, and, in some cases, large numbers of eosinophils. If the process is severe, tubule cell necrosis and regeneration may also be apparent. Immunofluorescence studies in a number of cases either have been unrevealing or have demonstrated a linear pattern of immunoglobin and complement deposition along tubule basement membranes. In a few cases of methicillin-induced acute tubulointerstitial disease, circulating anti-tubule basement membrane antibodies have also been found, suggesting that autoantibody formation may have been in-

duced by the penicilloyl hapten of methicillin (by conjugation of hapten with tubule basement membrane proteins, thereby altering the native antigenicity of the basement membrane). Evidence for an immunologic basis for these various drug-related nephropathies also derives from the facts that the onset of nephropathy does not appear to be dose-related, often follows a second exposure to the drug presumed to be responsible for the renal injury, and often is associated with increased levels of serum IgE. In the case of methicillin, the patients usually develop evidence of renal injury after about 2 weeks of drug administration. Hematuria, fever, skin rash, and eosinophilia are prominent. Many patients develop azotemia which typically resolves after withdrawal of the offending drug. Proteinuria and pyuria often accompany the hematuria, and occasionally eosinophils are found in the urine sediment. The clinical picture may be confused with acute glomerulonephritis, but when acute azotemia and hematuria are accompanied by eosinophilia, skin rash, and a history of drug exposure, a hypersensitivity reaction leading to acute tubulointerstitial nephritis should be regarded as the leading diagnostic possibility. Discontinuation of the drug usually results in complete reversal of the renal injury; rarely, renal damage may be irreversible. Corticosteroids have been used, but their value in this disorder has not been established with certainty.

SJÖGREN'S SYNDROME   Keratoconjunctivitis sicca (see Chap. 356), or Sjögren's syndrome, is an immunologic disorder characterized by dryness of mucous membranes and mononuclear cell infiltration of salivary and lacrimal glands; it is often seen in patients with rheumatoid arthritis. When the kidneys are involved in Sjögren's syndrome, the predominant histological findings are those of chronic tubulointerstitial disease. Interstitial infiltrates are composed primarily of lymphocytes, causing the histology of the renal parenchyma in these patients to resemble that of the salivary and lacrimal glands. Renal functional defects associated with this disorder include diminished urinary concentrating ability and distal renal tubular acidosis. Urinalysis may show pyuria (predominantly lymphocyturia) and mild proteinuria.

AMYLOIDOSIS (See also Chap. 64)   Renal deposition of amyloid occurs in approximately 80 percent of cases of amyloidosis secondary to chronic suppuration, as compared with 30 percent of patients with primary amyloidosis. Glomerular pathology usually predominates and leads to heavy proteinuria and azotemia. However, tubule function may also be deranged, giving rise to a nephrogenic form of diabetes insipidus and to distal renal tubular acidosis. In several cases these functional abnormalities have been correlated with peritubular deposition of amyloid, particularly in areas surrounding vasa rectae, loops of Henle, and collecting ducts. Bilateral enlargement of the kidneys, especially in a patient with massive proteinuria and evidence for tubule dysfunction, should raise the possibility of amyloid renal disease. Characteristic amyloid fibrils have been identified by electron microscopy in the urinary sediment of patients with renal amyloid deposits, but these fibrils may also be found in proteinuric states other than amyloidosis.

TUBULOINTERSTITIAL ABNORMALITIES ASSOCIATED WITH GLOMERULONEPHRITIS   A number of primary glomerulopathies may also be associated with damage to tubules and interstitium. Pathogenetically, the extraglomerular component in these renal disorders often involves the same mechanisms that are responsible for the more pronounced glomerular injury.

For example, in more than half of patients with the nephropathy associated with systemic lupus erythematosus, deposits of immune complexes can be identified in tubule basement membranes, usually accompanied by an interstitial mononuclear inflammatory reaction. Similarly, in many patients with glomerulonephritis associated with antiglomerular basement membrane antibody, the same antibody can be shown to be reactive against tubule basement membranes as well.

MISCELLANEOUS DISORDERS

RADIATION NEPHRITIS Clinical renal dysfunction can be expected to occur if 2300 R or more of x-ray irradiation is administered to both kidneys during a period of 5 weeks or less. Histological examination of the affected kidneys reveals hyalinized glomeruli, atrophic tubules, extensive interstitial fibrosis, and hyalinization of the media of renal arterioles. Radiation-induced renal ischemia is believed to be the main pathogenetic factor responsible for the widespread tubulointerstitial damage, which may not become evident clinically for weeks to months after completion of irradiation. The clinical presentation of acute radiation nephritis includes rapidly progressive azotemia, moderate to malignant hypertension, anemia, and proteinuria, which may reach the nephrotic range. More than 50 percent of these cases progress to chronic renal failure. A more insidious form of radiation nephritis may also occur; it is characterized by slower development of azotemia, anemia, and nephrotic syndrome. Malignant hypertension has also been known to follow unilateral renal irradiation and to resolve with ipsilateral nephrectomy. Radiation nephritis in recent years has all but vanished because of heightened awareness of its pathogenesis by radiotherapists.

BALKAN NEPHROPATHY Balkan nephropathy is an acquired, endemic disorder restricted to the small geographic region where Yugoslavia, Romania, and Bulgaria meet to form the Danubian basin. The renal lesions seen in affected patients from this region progress from focal tubular atrophy, interstitial edema, and mononuclear cell infiltration to diffuse interstitial fibrosis, leading eventually to bilaterally shrunken, atrophic kidneys. Epidemiologic studies point to an environmental toxin as the cause, but the offending agent has not yet been identified. Defects in urinary concentrating ability, low-molecular-weight ("tubular") proteinuria, and renal tubular acidosis are common. In most cases, the disease is progressive, leading eventually to chronic renal failure. A high incidence of papillary transitional carcinoma of the renal pelvis and upper ureter appears to be a late complication in patients with this endemic nephropathy.

REFERENCES

COTRAN RS: Tubulo-interstitial diseases, in *The Kidney*, 2d ed, BM Brenner, FC Rector Jr (eds). Philadelphia, Saunders, 1980, chap 28

DITLOVE J et al: Methicillin nephritis. Medicine 56:483, 1977

HALL PW, DAMMIN GJ: Balkan nephropathy. Nephron 22:281, 1978

KINCAID-SMITH P (ed): Symposium on analgesic nephropathy. Kidney Int 13:1, 1978

PORTER GA, BENNETT WM: Toxic nephropathies, in *The Kidney*, 2d ed, BM Brenner, FC Rector Jr (eds). Philadelphia, Saunders, 1980, chap 39

WILSON CB, DIXON FJ: The renal response to immunologic injury, in *The Kidney*, 2d ed, BM Brenner, FC Rector Jr (eds). Philadelphia, Saunders, 1980, chap 25

282

VASCULAR INJURY TO THE KIDNEY

NORMAN K. HOLLENBERG

Processes ranging from renal artery stenosis and occlusion to arteriolar nephrosclerosis, polyarteritis nodosa, the hemolytic uremic syndromes, scleroderma, and preeclampsia share a sufficient number of clinical features, morphologic characteristics, and pathogenetic consequences to justify their consideration in this chapter. The clinical, functional, and morphological expressions of interrupting the renal blood supply are dependent on several factors including the degree of obstruction to flow, the rate at which the occlusion occurs, the level of vessel or vessels involved, and the total mass of ischemic parenchyma. Because the intrarenal arterial tree is made up of end arteries, sudden occlusion results in infarction with clinical manifestations that vary with the level at which the occlusion occurs. More gradual partial occlusion, on the other hand, results in ischemic atrophy and a different functional and clinical picture.

Renal blood flow, averaging 4.0 (ml/g)/min, exceeds by three- to fivefold the flow in such metabolically active organs as the heart, liver, and brain. Renal blood flow is adjusted not to satisfy metabolic need, but rather to provide the plasma flow and pressure to the glomerular capillary bed in order to sustain an appropriate level of glomerular filtration. Renal perfusion is also an important determinant of sodium handling by the kidney. For these reasons, a reduction in renal blood flow too small to result in cell death has important consequences including a reduction in filtration rate, increased sodium reabsorption, increased renin release, and hypertension, which to a varying extent are features common to the syndromes resulting from abnormalities in the renal circulation.

ACUTE ARTERIAL OCCLUSION Acute, complete occlusion of the main renal artery or a major intrarenal arterial branch may follow secondary to blunt trauma to the abdomen or back or to renal arterial embolism occurring in patients with a number of conditions, most commonly mitral stenosis and atrial fibrillation, infective endocarditis, mural thrombi overlying myocardial infarcts, or ulcerating atherosclerotic disease of the aorta. The kidneys receive about one-fifth of the cardiac output, making embolic occlusion of the small intrarenal arteries common. Acute occlusion results in coagulation necrosis in the region supplied by the obstructed artery, the size of the wedge-shaped infarct varying with the level of the occlusion.

The clinical features also depend on the size of the infarct. Small infarcts, involving a portion of the renal cortex, are often clinically silent. Larger infarcts may induce a sudden, sharp unremitting pain in the flank or upper abdomen associated with fever, leukocytosis, and gross or microscopic hematuria. The impact on renal function also varies. Even total occlusion of one main renal artery may leave the blood urea nitrogen (BUN) and serum creatinine in the normal range in the presence of a healthy contralateral kidney which can undergo hypertrophy. When the patient has only a solitary functioning kidney, arterial occlusion enters the differential diagnosis of acute oliguric renal failure. Although total destruction of the kidney will generally occur within hours of occlusion, at least a dozen case reports of restoration of renal function after days to weeks of total occlusion have appeared, generally in a setting in which prior partial occlusion has led to a rich collateral arterial blood supply sufficient to provide nutrition for the renal parenchyma, although inadequate to maintain renal function. Angiography is necessary to establish the diagnosis. Evidence of collateral filling of the intrarenal arterial tree suggests that operation may restore renal function.

RENAL ARTERY STENOSIS (See also Chap. 251) Partial occlusion of the renal artery or its major branches by atherosclerotic narrowing or by fibromuscular dysplasia is responsible for about 1 to 2 percent of cases of hypertension; its importance lies in the fact that it represents the most common curable form of hypertension. *Renal arterial atherosclerosis,* as with atherosclerosis elsewhere, is more frequent in males, and its incidence increases with advancing age, previous hypertension, or diabetes mellitus. The *fibromuscular dysplasias* of the renal artery are a heterogeneous group of lesions in which fibrous or fibromuscular thickening may involve the intima, the media, or the subadventitial region. The process is frequently bilateral and may extend into the intrarenal tree. The fibrous renal artery dysplasias are ten times more common in females than males, appear most often in the third and fourth decades, and, presumably because the individuals are younger, are associated with a lower surgical morbidity and a higher cure rate than are atherosclerotic renal arterial lesions.

The clinical features which may be helpful in detecting renal artery stenosis include a history of the onset of hypertension at an age which is unusual for essential hypertension, i.e., under 30 or over 50 years of age, or of a poor response to medical therapy. Physical examination may reveal a bruit in the flank or upper abdominal region. Routine laboratory evaluation often reveals evidence of secondary hyperaldosteronism including hypokalemia, metabolic alkalosis, and an alkaline urine. As in primary aldosteronism, hypokalemia may be masked by a restricted sodium intake.

The intravenous pyelogram (IVP) and the radionuclide Hippuran renogram are the most widely used screening tests for renovascular hypertension. Characteristics in the pyelogram suggesting renal artery stenosis include a reduction in renal size of at least 1.5 cm compared with the opposite kidney, a delay in the appearance of contrast in the involved kidney when films are obtained at 1, 2, and 3 min after injection of the contrast agent, hyperconcentration of contrast on the involved side in the late films, and filling defects in the renal pelvis and ureter reflecting the local effects of dilated collateral arteries. In the Cooperative Study on Renovascular Hypertension, the characteristic triad of the late appearance of contrast medium in a small kidney, which showed late hyperconcentration of contrast in the renal pelvis, was never seen in patients with essential hypertension. Unfortunately, only 22 percent of patients with renovascular hypertension had this triad, and so it was relatively insensitive. The presence of any single abnormality was found in 78 percent of patients with renovascular hypertension, but with a sharp reduction in specificity since 11 percent of patients with essential hypertension had at least one of these manifestations, most commonly a significant difference in renal size. The characteristics of a radiohippuran renogram which suggest renal artery stenosis include a delay in the rate of rise of the tracer in the kidney, a delay in the time to reach the peak, and a reduced rate of disappearance from the kidney. The renogram identified 75 percent of patients with renovascular hypertension, with a false-positive rate of 24 percent. Because both the IVP and the renogram compare the two kidneys, they are less often positive when stenosis is bilateral.

Because of the high incidence of hypertension and the low yield of renovascular hypertension when a detailed evaluation is undertaken, the clinical indications for laboratory investigations in search of renovascular hypertension are gradually undergoing modification. No more than 1 to 2 percent of patients with hypertension have a curable renal arterial lesion. The evaluation is costly, amounting to approximately $700 in 1980. Finally, operation, especially in patients with atherosclerosis, carries considerable risk. For these reasons a detailed evaluation for renal artery stenosis is currently recommended only in circumstances when the yield is likely to be high, including patients in whom the onset of hypertension has occurred be-

fore the age of 30 years, in the presence of a bruit, or when hypertension is severe and responds poorly to medical therapy.

Identification of renal artery stenosis can be accomplished only by arteriography. Because all arterial lesions are not hemodynamically significant, ancillary tests are used to assess the hemodynamic significance of the stenosis. The most widely used test involves the measurement of renin activity in blood samples obtained from both renal veins and either the lower inferior vena cava or the aorta. A positive test, strongly suggestive of curable renovascular hypertension, reveals a plasma renin activity from the involved renal veins which exceeds the contralateral renal vein concentration by at least 50 percent, and evidence of suppression of renin-release from the intact contralateral kidney, i.e., identical renin activity in the arterial and contralateral renal venous plasma. With these criteria the false-positive rate is only 7 percent, but there is a quantitatively important false-negative rate. There is considerable current interest in the potential utility of angiotensin antagonists in identifying curable, renin-mediated renovascular hypertension. Preliminary data obtained suggest that a 10-mmHg fall in diastolic pressure following the injection of saralasin (1-Sar, 8-Ala angiotensin II) will identify 86 percent of curable patients, with a false-positive rate of 8.5 percent, which compares favorably with the available alternatives. Bilateral ureteral catheterization to obtain urine samples for measurement of osmolality and creatinine and sodium concentrations in urine from each kidney (the Howard, Stamey, and Rapaport tests) is no longer widely employed. At present we employ renal arteriography and renal vein renin determinations as the standard approach in patients in whom the history, physical examination, and preliminary laboratory evaluation make renovascular hypertension likely.

The Cooperative Study on Renovascular Disease has provided a clear picture of the current results of operation. When renal artery stenosis was due to fibromuscular disease, the cure rate exceeded 90 percent with a mortality of no more than 3 percent—probably reflecting the youth of the population which was largely free of additional systemic disease. In patients with atherosclerotic disease, on the other hand, the mortality was 9 percent and the failure rate exceeded 25 percent. For these reasons evaluation for renal artery surgery in older patients who are likely to have atherosclerotic disease is restricted in many centers to patients in whom medical management fails.

ARTERIOLAR NEPHROSCLEROSIS Small-vessel changes in the kidney are so intimately associated with hypertension, on the one hand, and with the normal aging process, on the other, that it is difficult to define the boundary between normal and disease and to discuss the vascular lesion without discussing hypertension. At least some degree of small-vessel lesion is found in about 70 percent of random necropsy examinations of normotensive individuals who die after the age of 60 years. The frequency and severity of the arteriolar and small-artery lesions are increased in younger age groups in association with predisposing factors, which include hypertension and diabetes. Large and medium-sized arteries at the interlobar and arcuate levels show intimal thickening of variable degree. Typically more widespread and more severe abnormalities are seen in the small arteries and arterioles where, in addition, there is an eosinophilic hyalin thickening which results in a variable degree of vascular narrowing. As a consequence there is patchy ischemic atrophy. The severity of the ischemic atrophy and glomerular sclerosis, in general, parallels that of the vascular change.

The vascular changes described above presumably account for most of the loss of renal function which accompanies normal aging. The modest reductions in renal plasma flow and glomerular filtration rate are of little clinical importance, except for the loss of an element of functional reserve, making older individuals more prone to develop azotemia when faced with volume depletion or surgical stress. The increased incidence of drug-induced complications in the elderly presumably reflects the important role played by glomerular filtration in the excretion of drugs and metabolites. Some examples are the propensity of the elderly to develop eighth nerve toxicity with streptomycin and to be particularly sensitive to digoxin. Other features of arteriolar nephrosclerosis include a moderate loss of concentrating power and often mild proteinuria. Occasionally more profound renal functional abnormalities occur, but marked renal insufficiency is uncommon.

On the other hand, "accelerated nephrosclerosis" associated with malignant hypertension is a dramatic complication of all forms of hypertension in which an abrupt change in course, renal insufficiency, and a uremic death were common before effective therapy became available (Chap. 251). The onset of the malignant phase is characterized by a sharp increase in blood pressure, with diastolic pressures typically exceeding 130 mmHg. In essential hypertension, the malignant phase is usually preceded by a benign period of variable duration, but occasionally occurs de novo. This process also occurs as a complication of all forms of secondary hypertension including glomerulonephritis, pyelonephritis, vasculitis, renal artery stenosis, scleroderma, polycystic kidney disease, Cushing's syndrome, pheochromocytoma, and hypertension associated with use of oral contraceptives. Until recently it was suggested that accelerated nephrosclerosis does not complicate the course of primary aldosteronism, but several well-documented cases now exist. In pheochromocytoma accelerated hypertension is typically associated with preserved renal function.

The morphological hallmarks of the renal lesion include petechial hemorrhages of the cortical surface, responsible for the characteristic "flea-bitten" appearance; fibrinoid necrosis of afferent arterioles; a hyperplastic endarteritis of the interlobular and arcuate arteries, and severe ischemic atrophy or infarction distal to the abnormal vessels. Immunofluorescent and electromicroscopic studies have shown that the amorphous material in the arteriolar wall consists of fibrin. Several lines of investigation suggest that the severe hypertension, per se, is responsible for the vascular necrosis, probably due to endothelial injury and leakage of fibrin and other plasma constituents into the arteriolar wall.

The clinical features include severe hypertension, neuroretinopathy with blurring of vision, retinal hemorrhages, exudates, and papilledema. Hypertensive encephalopathy is evidenced by severe headache, changes in the sensorium, and seizures. Congestive heart failure and rapidly progressive uremia are common. The renal manifestations include gross or microscopic hematuria, marked proteinuria, and a rapid rise in BUN and creatinine. As in renal artery stenosis, evidence of secondary aldosteronism is common with hypokalemia and a metabolic alkalosis, until the metabolic acidosis of renal failure supervenes.

Prior to the availability of effective therapy for the hypertension, the mortality in patients with this syndrome approximated 50 percent in 3 months and 90 percent within 1 year. In the past two decades, the availability of effective antihypertensive therapy (Chap. 251) has greatly improved the prognosis of accelerated nephrosclerosis. In the early 1950s a BUN which exceeded 30 mg per 100 ml at the time the diagnosis was made guaranteed a rapid demise. Today a patient with a BUN which exceeds this level by three or fourfold may have a stable course with effective therapy.

SCLERODERMA (PROGRESSIVE SYSTEMIC SCLEROSIS) (See also Chap. 362) The renal aspects of scleroderma are considered in some detail here because renal involvement is second only to that of heart and lungs as a cause of death, and the characteristic morphological lesions and clinical course closely resemble those associated with accelerated nephrosclerosis.

As in accelerated nephrosclerosis, the morphological features include kidneys which are generally normal or only slightly reduced in size even in patients who have died with renal failure. Petechial hemorrhages and wedge-shaped cortical infarcts are common. The most striking and distinctive abnormality is seen at the level of the intralobular arteries which are markedly narrowed or occluded as a result of fibrinoid change and deposition of fibrin and acid mucopolysaccarides. The afferent arterioles in some patients also show fibrinoid necrosis and occasional occlusion by fibrin thrombi. Distal to the occlusion ischemic atrophy and infarction are evident. It has been suggested, in part because of the similarity to the changes in accelerated nephrosclerosis, that the renal vascular lesions are secondary to the hypertension, but such vascular changes have been well documented at necropsy in patients with scleroderma who have never been hypertensive.

Renal involvement is rarely the presenting feature. In one study renal involvement was found at presentation in only 3 percent of patients with scleroderma. However, in a 20-year longitudinal survey, 47 percent of patients ultimately developed a clinically important renal lesion. There is uniform agreement that renal failure contributes to or is primarily responsible for 40 to 50 percent of all deaths attributable to scleroderma. The presence of renal involvement is associated with a poor prognosis in patients with this condition; most patients with clinically evident renal disease die in less than 1 year and often within 3 months. Indeed, in the aforementioned longitudinal study only 10 percent of patients without renal involvement died, whereas 60 percent of patients with proteinuria, azotemia, or hypertension succumbed.

The clinical expression of renal involvement in scleroderma which is most widely recognized is characterized by an abrupt onset and an explosive course; accelerated hypertension is followed by oliguria and a uremic death within months. Presentation of scleroderma with this syndrome is uncommon; clinical evidence of major renal involvement is typically noted 3 to 5 years after the onset of manifestations in the skin and other systems. Occasionally, however, renal disease antedates obvious skin involvement.

A second, less distinct clinical expression of renal involvement is also being recognized. Isolated proteinuria unaccompanied by either hypertension or azotemia adversely affects prognosis but less strikingly than does the syndrome of malignant hypertension. Mild hypertension, without proteinuria or azotemia, occurs with greater frequency in scleroderma than would be anticipated from known prevalence rates of essential hypertension. Mild hypertension without proteinuria or azotemia occurs later than the malignant form and has a much less grave prognosis.

No specific therapy exists for scleroderma. Preliminary evidence suggests that the hypertension is renin-mediated and that antihypertensive drugs acting on this system might be most effective. When hypertension is refractory to antihypertensive medication and hemodialysis, bilateral nephrectomy has been effective. Occasionally, renal transplantation has been carried out; in one patient there was nothing to suggest recurrence of scleroderma in the transplanted kidney 4 years after transplantation. In another person, however, lesions indistinguishable from scleroderma recurred in the allograft within 6 weeks, despite immunosuppressive therapy. Insufficient information is available to suggest that renal transplantation should be denied to patients with scleroderma.

SICKLE-CELL NEPHROPATHY (See also Chap. 315) Sickle-cell disease, sickle-cell trait, sickle thalassemia, and other combinations of hemoglobin S with abnormal hemoglobins often have clinically important disorders of renal structure and function. The most dramatic of the renal manifestations of sickle hemoglobinopathy is gross painless hematuria. A history of mild trauma to the renal area may be obtained. The source of bleeding has been identified as arising from miliary gross and microscopic infarcts in the papillae, renal pelvis, and renal cortex. For unknown reasons the bleeding occurs from the left side in 80 percent of cases and, despite the systemic nature of the primary process, is bilateral in only 11 percent. Abnormalities in the IVP, most commonly a pelvic filling defect, are frequent and have led to unnecessary surgical intervention. Despite the failure of conservative therapy such as bed rest to influence the bleeding, most cases remit spontaneously. Because causes other than sickle-cell anemia may be responsible for hematuria in these patients, a complete urologic assessment is generally performed (Chap. 42). When filling defects are found, serial studies are recommended; surgical exploration should be considered only if they persist. Operation may also be required in rare instances of life-threatening hemorrhage.

Failure of urinary concentration is the most consistent feature of sickle-cell nephropathy. In very young children with sickle-cell anemia the concentrating defect can be reversed by multiple transfusions, but the capacity for improvement is lost with age, becoming negligible in patients after 15 years of age. In older adults the maximum concentration of the urine rarely exceeds 400 mosmol per liter. The failure of urinary concentration is typically attributed to a disorder of perfusion of the renal medulla. This, in turn, may be due to the sickling process per se or to an abnormality of the microvasculature. Because both hypoxia and an increased osmolality precipitate the sickling phenomenon and because sickle cells increase blood viscosity significantly, this condition may impede the normal circulation through the vasa rectae which normally have a very high resistance to flow. In addition, microangiographic studies on kidneys from cadavers have revealed obliteration and distortion of the remaining vasa recta.

Appreciable proteinuria is common in sickle-cell disease and occurred in 31 percent of patients in one series. On occasion proteinuria is sufficiently severe that the nephrotic syndrome develops.

With increasing age, the growing number and size of cortical infarcts results in a progressive reduction in glomerular filtration rate and renal plasma flow, which are typically higher than normal in the young patients with sickle-cell disease. Deterioration of renal function caused by sickle-cell anemia to the point at which dialysis becomes necessary has not been described. However, it has been shown that patients with sickle-cell disease can be maintained on chronic hemodialysis without encountering undue complications.

HEMOLYTIC-UREMIC SYNDROME (See also Chap. 314) The coincidence of acute renal failure, hemolytic anemia, and thrombocytopenia has emerged as a clearly defined, relatively common entity in which infants or children develop acute anemia, signs of renal and central nervous system injury, and gastrointestinal bleeding after a prodrome of digestive, respiratory, and systemic symptoms. The hallmarks of the syndrome are hemolysis due to red blood cell fragmentation, a reduction in platelet count, and biochemical and pathological evidence of intravascular coagulation. The differential diagnosis includes thrombotic thrombocytopenic purpura, renal cortical necrosis as part of the Shwartzman reaction in gram-negative sepsis, severe vasculitis, and "necrotizing glomerulonephritis." The differentiation among these entities may be extremely difficult, even at necropsy.

Initially only severe, generally fatal cases were recognized, but with increasing familiarity patients with mild or moderate lesions have been identified. The immediate prognosis is related to the degree of renal failure and the severity of involvement of the central nervous system. If the patient survives, the hematologic abnormality is short-lived and does not recur. In some patients the extent of renal destruction precludes prolonged survival without the help of dialysis. In a few others severe neurological sequelae have been permanently disabling. In many patients the renal lesions heal completely, but on occasion slowly progressive renal failure occurs after the initial insult.

Although primarily a disease of children, familiarity with the process has led to its increasing recognition in adults. In adults the prodrome, which resembles a nondescript viral illness, is less striking, but associations have been found with pregnancy and the postpartum period, use of oral contraceptive agents, and infection, including typhoid fever, gram-negative bacteremia, mumps, and infectious mononucleosis. The clinical manifestations are similar to those in children, and the prognosis appears to be poorer.

Because chemical evidence of coagulation disturbances and fibrin deposition in small arteries and arterioles is common and because the syndrome is accompanied by a microangiopathic hemolytic anemia, there is widespread belief that disseminated intravascular coagulation plays a major role in the pathogenesis. The commonly observed coagulation disturbances include thrombocytopenia, a prolonged prothrombin time, and accumulation of fibrin degradation products in the serum. For unknown reasons the kidney is the most extensively involved organ in the hemolytic-uremic syndrome. Because in adults pregnancy and oral contraceptive agents appear to predispose to cortical necrosis and pregnancy also predisposes to the Shwartzman reaction induced by endotoxin in animals, it has been suggested that the Shwartzman reaction and the hemolytic-uremic syndrome share a common mechanism. The morphological lesions are also strikingly similar; immunofluorescent studies have revealed intense staining with antibody to fibrin in both conditions.

The treatment is largely supportive. There is major controversy as to whether heparin therapy modifies the natural history. Controlled studies have been disappointing, but in individual patients heparin therapy has been temporally associated with improvement in renal function. Other forms of therapy including steroids, immunosuppressive agents, antimetabolities, exchange transfusions, and dextran have met with equivocal results.

RENAL VEIN THROMBOSIS Thrombosis of one or both of the renal veins is an uncommon cause of the nephrotic syndrome. Occlusion of both renal veins usually, but not necessarily, implies thrombosis of the inferior vena cava as well. Renal vein thrombosis is most commonly associated with membranous glomerulonephritis. It is not clear whether the glomerulonephritis predisposes to renal vein thrombosis or vice versa, but the weight of evidence favors the former possibility (page 1315). Other causes of renal vein thrombosis include local trauma, invasion of the renal vein by hypernephroma, and severe dehydration, especially in children.

Clinical features and morphological change depend on the availability of an adequate collateral venous drainage. Sudden complete thrombosis of a renal vein, without adequate collateral drainage, causes severe lumbar pain, hematuria, and loss of function of the involved kidney. The kidney is enlarged and suffers hemorrhagic infarction. When the process is bilateral or involves a solitary kidney this sequence leads to oliguria and renal failure. If the occlusion is more gradual, especially if adequate collateral venous channels develop, renal function is preserved, and massive proteinuria results in the nephrotic syndrome. Hypertension is uncommon, and the urinary sediment may be entirely normal or contain only a few red blood cells.

The diagnosis is suggested by a history of trauma, pain, or a predisposing factor such as prolonged travel in a cramped position. A history of pulmonary embolism should also lead to suspicion of this diagnosis. Physical examination may reveal a venous collateral map on the anterior abdominal wall if the inferior vena cava is involved. The intravenous pyelogram may show filling defects in the renal pelvis and ureter reflecting collateral draining veins. The diagnosis is established by inferior vena caval and selective renal venography.

Surgical removal of a clot from the renal venous system has been successful in a small number of patients, especially in children in whom the onset is often in association with dehydration and occurs acutely. In most circumstances, however, medical management with anticoagulants has been used. Recanalization of the renal veins has led to amelioration of the nephrotic syndrome in occasional patients. Typically, however, anticoagulants are employed to prevent pulmonary embolism and extension of the thrombus into the open collateral veins.

PREECLAMPSIA AND ECLAMPSIA: TOXEMIAS OF PREGNANCY Toxemia of pregnancy is characterized by the appearance, during gestation or within 7 days of delivery, of a constellation of abnormalities which includes hypertension, edema, and proteinuria (preeclampsia). When hypertension is more severe, convulsions and coma may occur (eclampsia). Preeclampsia usually begins after the thirty-second week of pregnancy but may begin earlier, particularly in women with preexisting renal disease or hypertension. Preeclampsia in the first trimester occurs in hydatidiform mole. Toxemia has a bimodal frequency with peak incidence in the young primipara and in multiparous women over 35 years of age. In the United States toxemia occurs in approximately 7 percent of pregnancies. Perhaps as a reflection of an increased prevalence in the economically underprivileged, the incidence reaches 30 percent in Puerto Rico. Most series include many patients in whom preexisting renal disease or hypertension either begins during or is exacerbated by pregnancy, but there is clearly, in addition, a specific process affecting the kidney and the vascular system which in most patients improve dramatically when, or soon after, pregnancy is terminated.

The morphological features in the kidney include reversible generalized swelling of the glomerular tufts and apparent thickening of the glomerular basement membrane due to an increase of the cytoplasm of the endothelial cells with narrowing of the capillary lumina, a finding termed *glomerular endotheliosis,* and sub- or interendothelial fibrinoid deposition. In patients who die of acute toxemia of pregnancy, necrosis of renal tubules and of liver cells is frequent in addition, along with evidence of disseminated intravascular coagulation and petechial hemorrhage in the brain.

The pathogenesis of the process is not clearly understood, but it appears to be focused on the renin-angiotensin-aldosterone axis and its interaction with sodium balance. Sodium retention and an increase in blood volume are normal concomitants of pregnancy. Considerable evidence suggests that plasma volume is *lower* in the toxemic than normal pregnancy, and from this observation debate about the role of too little or too much sodium intake has emerged. Whether the reduced plasma volume is a cause or consequence of the process is unclear. The evidence suggests that uteroplacental ischemia occurs with toxemia. The uterus, like the kidney, synthesizes both vasoconstrictors (renin) and vasodilators (prostaglandins of the E series). One current hypothesis is that the release of small amounts of renin from the uterus in a setting of well-documented increased sensitivity to angiotensin is responsible for the severe hypertension.

The onset is typically insidious but may also be abrupt. Because arterial blood pressure normally falls during pregnancy, pressures which exceed 125/75 should be considered abnormal, especially if they are rising. In association, headache, visual disturbances, epigastric distress, and apprehension are frequent symptoms. Edema usually appears coincident with hypertension; it is typically generalized, being particularly evident in the face and hands. Proteinuria generally follows the onset of the syndrome within several days but occasionally precedes the hypertension and edema. Examination of the optic fundi reveals segmental arteriolar narrowing and a glistening retinal sheen indicative of edema. Hemorrhages and exudates occur late and only in severe cases.

Examination of the urine reveals from a trace to 10 g protein per 24 h, as well as granular and hyalin casts, but red blood cells and cellular casts are infrequent. Because of the physiological increase of glomerular filtration rate and reduction in serum urea and creatinine concentration which occurs in a normal pregnancy, a blood urea nitrogen of 20 mg per 100 ml is usually indicative of a sharp diminution in filtration rate. A more striking increase in blood uric acid is common, reflecting a reduction in urate clearance.

Treatment varies with the severity of the process. In patients with mild hypertension and minimal proteinuria, antihypertensive agents are routinely used: whether restriction of sodium intake, which is required to control edema, may be a precipitating factor in preeclampsia is the subject of debate. If the process is more severe, patients are admitted to the hospital for bed rest and closer control of sodium intake and blood pressure. Involvement of the central nervous system with convulsions and marked hypertension are unequivocal indications for termination of pregnancy, which is usually followed by prompt improvement of the mother. Emptying of the uterus is the most effective treatment. Proteinuria and hypertension usually disappear within 1 or 2 weeks but on occasion may persist for as long as 6 months. A substantial fraction of patients with preeclampsia are left with a process which is indistinguishable from essential hypertension. Whether such patients were candidates for development of essential hypertension which became apparent during, or was precipitated by, pregnancy is not yet clear.

POLYARTERITIS NODOSA (See also Chap. 67) The genre *necrotizing vasculitis* includes polyarteritis nodosa, hypersensitivity angiitis (also known as the microscopic form of polyarteritis), and allergic granulomatous angiitis. Because renal involvement occurs in at least 80 percent of patients with polyarteritis nodosa and contributes to death in a substantial number, they are considered here. Other vasculitides such as rheumatic arteritis and temporal arteritis rarely involve the kidney. Various attempts at classification reflect a sorting of clinical syndromes, primarily by site and size of vessel involved, major presenting symptoms, and clinical course. They are not based on an understanding of the etiology or pathogenesis, and no classification is totally satisfactory. Moreover, attempts at classification have been made primarily by information based on necropsy, and distinctions among polyarteritis nodosa, hypersensitivity angiitis, and granulomatous angiitis are indistinct in many patients because of overlap of these syndromes.

Polyarteritis nodosa is a recurrent or progressive, necrotizing inflammatory disease of the medium and small-sized muscular arteries. Involvement of multiple viscera is typical, resulting in a variety of clinical manifestations which commonly include fever, myalgia, arthritis, weight loss, gastrointestinal, cardiac, and neurological signs and symptoms. The disease, three times more frequent in males than in females, may occur at any age.

The kidney is the most common organ involved, with estimates ranging upwards of 70 percent, and renal failure is one of the major causes of death. Hypertension occurs in about 50 percent of patients and is usually a late manifestation, probably reflecting renal ischemia which develops during the healing phase. The hypertension often terminates in a malignant phase with hypertensive encephalopathy or heart failure. Renal involvement may be manifested by proteinuria, microscopic or gross hematuria, urinary casts, azotemia, and edema.

In polyarteritis nodosa, the lesions involve only the medium and small muscular arteries, especially at sites of branching. There is disagreement concerning the involvement of capillaries and veins. Classically there are subendothelial and medial edema and fibrinoid necrosis; infiltration of all vessel coats with an inflammatory exudate including polymorphonuclear leukocytes, eosinophils, lymphocytes, and plasma cells; destruction of the media and internal elastica; proliferation of fibroblasts which generally starts in the adventitia and progresses during a stage of granulation through the vessel wall with healing, and a reduction in the acute inflammatory process; and healed lesions in which the vessel wall is replaced by fibrous tissue and the lumen is generally narrowed or occluded. Glomerular lesions consisting of focal or diffuse proliferative changes or ischemic necrosis are common. Any or all of these stages may be present at any given time in the kidney. Renal insufficiency and hypertension characteristically develop during the healing stages. Because larger vessels are involved, a renal biopsy of the cortex may miss the characteristic lesion.

The pathogenetic factors responsible for polyarteritis are becoming clearer. Multiple lines of evidence have implicated an immunologic mechanism, and since 1970 a number of studies have implicated hepatitis B as the responsible antigen in as many as 30 percent of patients with necrotizing vasculitis and the polyarteritis nodosa syndrome. A vasculitis indistinguishable from periarteritis nodosa is also being recognized in an increasing number of young drug abusers. Because of the multiplicity of the chemical agents injected, and the high probability of contamination, the exact etiologic agent has not been unequivocally defined, but methamphetamine appears to be a common denominator.

Hypersensitivity angiitis differs from classic polyarteritis nodosa. It is often a fulminating illness characterized by an acute necrotizing inflammatory process involving small arteries, arterioles, capillaries, and venules; the involvement in all vessels appears to be at the same stage. Clinically, the process may be characterized by its fulminating course, the typical absence of hypertension, and eosinophilia. Proteinuria and hematuria, however, are present in virtually every patient.

Allergic granulomatous angiitis is also a diffuse systemic vascular disease, but, in addition, there are widespread extravascular granulomatous, necrotizing lesions. Azotemia occurs in some cases but with less frequency than in hypersensitivity angiitis or classic polyarteritis. In addition there may be focal glomerular lesions and fibrosis.

Therapy of the vasculitides is discussed in Chap. 67. General supportive measures include control of hypertension, which is required in most patients with renal involvement. Corticosteroids are widely employed and with immunosuppressive agents are the only presently available therapy of any

potential value. In patients with renal involvement steroids may have an initial adverse effect on the clinical course because vascular healing is frequently associated with obliteration of arteries, resulting in focal renal infarction, increasing hypertension, and azotemia.

REFERENCES

ALFREY AC: The renal response to vascular injury, in *The Kidney*, 2d ed, BM Brenner, FC Rector Jr (eds). Philadelphia, Saunders, 1980, chap 30

ALLEYNE GAQ et al: The kidney in sickle cell anemia. Kidney Int 7:371, 1975

CITRON BP et al: Necrotizing angiitis associated with drug abuse. N Engl J Med 283:1003, 1970

FERRIS TF: Toxemia and hypertension, in *Medical Complications during Pregnancy*, GN Burrow, TF Ferris (eds). Philadelphia, Saunders, 1975

GIANANTONIO CA et al: The hemolytic-uremic syndrome. Nephron 11:174, 1973

LLACH F et al: Renal vein thrombosis and nephrotic syndrome. Ann Intern Med 83:8, 1975

MAXWELL MH: Cooperative study of renovascular hypertension: Current status. Kidney Int 8:S153, 1975

OLIVER JA, CANNON PJ: The kidney in scleroderma. Nephron 18:141, 1977

ROSEMANN E et al: Renal vein thrombosis in the adult: A clinical and pathological study based on renal biopsies. Medicine 47:219, 1968

SERGENT JS et al: Vasculitis with hepatitis B antigenemia: Long-term observations in nine patients. Medicine 55:1, 1976

283
HEREDITARY TUBULAR DISORDERS

SATISH KATHPALIA
FREDRIC L. COE

POLYCYSTIC RENAL DISEASE IN ADULTS

ETIOLOGY AND PATHOLOGY This disease is found in 1 in 500 autopsies and 1 in 3000 hospital admissions and accounts for approximately 5 percent of all instances of end-stage renal failure. Inheritance is autosomal dominant, and penetrance is nearly 100 percent in carriers who survive until the eighth decade. The cortex and medulla of both kidneys are usually filled with thin-walled, spherical cysts, ranging from millimeters to several centimeters in diameter, that enlarge the organs and interfere with their functioning, presumably by compressing the nephrons and causing localized intrarenal obstruction. The cysts, which are lined by a low cuboidal epithelium, contain straw-colored fluid that becomes hemorrhagic with trauma or infection. The intervening renal parenchyma may be normal or show changes of nephrosclerosis or interstitial nephritis.

CLINICAL FEATURES Flank pain, which is the most common symptom, as well as gross and microscopic hematuria, occurring especially after trauma, and nocturia, due to severe impairment of osmotic concentrating ability, usually begin in the third or fourth decades. Ten percent of patients pass renal calculi whose composition and pathogenesis have not been well studied. Stones and blood clots both cause renal colic. Usually the kidneys are palpable and asymmetrical and have a knobby surface. Hypertension develops in 75 percent of patients, and progression to chronic renal failure usually occurs.

Proteinuria is the most common laboratory abnormality, but it rarely exceeds 2 g per day. Urinary infection ultimately occurs in most patients, especially as a consequence of instrumentation and renal calculi, while erythrocytosis may occur because of high circulating erythropoietin levels; in other patients anemia may result from the hematuria.

Acute renal failure can result from infection, ureteral obstruction due to clots or stone, or sudden angulation of a ureter by a nearby cyst. Azotemia progresses slowly in the absence of these complications. Patients with end-stage chronic renal failure tend to have higher hematocrits than their counterparts with other renal diseases. Fluid overload is infrequent because of a tendency for renal salt wasting.

Hepatic cysts are present in about 30 percent of patients with polycystic kidneys. Hepatic function is usually normal, and the liver cysts usually are asymptomatic but can cause epigastric discomfort or biliary colic, or can become infected. Cysts also may occur in the spleen, pancreas, lungs, ovaries, testes, epididymis, thyroid, uterus, broad ligament, and bladder. Subarachnoid hemorrhage from an intracranial aneurysm is the cause of death in about 9 percent of patients.

DIAGNOSIS Palpable kidneys, hypertension, or asymptomatic urinary abnormalities are often the only manifestations. Excretory or retrograde urography typically shows large kidneys with elongated pelvises and flat calyces that are indented by cysts. Ultrasonography and radioisotopic renal scanning can both demonstrate the cysts quite well. Gray scale sonography may be an alternative to intravenous pyelography for screening individuals with an affected parent, especially when genetic counseling is desired.

TREATMENT Superimposed renal damage such as that produced by analgesics, obstruction, urinary infection, nephrotoxic antibiotics, and hypertension must be guarded against. Dehydration and inadequate intake of sodium chloride (less than 100 mM per day) should be avoided. The management of chronic renal failure is simplified because fluid overload is not a usual problem and the hypertension is usually amenable to treatment, but the cysts can cause special problems, such as pain, bleeding, infection, or ureteral obstruction. Puncture of cysts, and in some instances even nephrectomy, may be necessary for treatment.

POLYCYSTIC RENAL DISEASE IN INFANTS AND CHILDREN

The *infantile form* manifests itself at birth by diffusely enlarged kidneys, renal failure, and maldevelopment of intrahepatic bile ducts. The *childhood form* consists of medullary ductal ectasia which is usually asymptomatic, in association with congenital hepatic fibrosis and portal hypertension. Inheritance of both the infantile and childhood forms is autosomal recessive. Renal failure develops frequently in both forms, but death usually results as a consequence of hepatic disease in the childhood form.

MORPHOLOGY In the infantile form, the distal tubules and collecting ducts are dilated into elongated cysts that are arranged in a radial fashion, particularly in the cortex, and make the kidneys very large and spongy. In the childhood form, cysts are fewer in number, cortical collecting ducts are less involved, and the kidneys are not as large. Small intrahepatic bile ducts are irregularly dilated, and large interconnecting spaces, lined by hyperplastic epithelium, fill the portal areas.

There is portal fibrosis rather than dilatation and proliferation of small bile ducts, and portal hypertension is the rule by late childhood.

DIAGNOSIS AND TREATMENT Infantile polycystic kidneys may be large enough to cause dystocia. At birth they do not function, and oliguric renal failure, respiratory distress, hypertension, and congestive heart failure appear. Intravenous pyelography may reveal a mottled nephrogram with variable retention of contrast material in cysts that correspond to dilated cortical and medullary collecting ducts. On retrograde urography the calyces are blunted, and abnormal pyelotubular reflux may be seen. In the childhood type the intravenous pyelogram may suggest medullary sponge kidney, because medullary tubular ectasia is prominent. Renal failure is an inconstant feature, though chronic infection is common.

MEDULLARY SPONGE KIDNEY

PATHOLOGY In this condition the ducts of Bellini, i.e., the terminal collecting ducts that reach to the ends of the papillae and drain the final urine into the renal pelvis, are dilated to cystic proportions and frequently contain small calcium oxalate calculi. The kidneys are involved asymmetrically, and the more abnormal kidney is usually the larger of the two. One or more medullary cysts are found near the tip of each involved papilla, and calculi form in the terminal collecting ducts in, or proximal to, the cysts (Fig. 283-1). Parenchymal alterations are secondary to intrarenal obstruction. The cysts are lined by cuboidal and, sometimes, by pseudostratified and stratified squamous epithelium.

CLINICAL DIAGNOSIS AND TREATMENT Medullary sponge kidney has been found in 1 of 200 unselected intravenous pyelograms. Although most cases are sporadic, familial instances with autosomal dominant inheritance have been described. The disease has a bimodal pattern of appearance, the first in adolescence and the second during the third and fourth decades. Calculi, infection, and hematuria occur in 60, 35, and 30 percent of patients, respectively. Papillary nephrocalcinosis due to clusters of stones in cysts is a common feature. Hypercalciuria occurs in nearly half of stone-forming patients but is equally frequent in other forms of calcium stone disease (Chap. 284). Hypertension is no more common than in the general population. Renal failure is rare, unless nephrolithiasis and/or renal infections are unusually severe.

The diagnosis of medullary sponge kidney is made by intravenous urography. The magnitude of pyelotubular backflow may vary from a simple papillary blush to frank tubular ectasia at the tips of the papillae. Small pyramidal cysts and nephrocalcinosis are frequent, and papillary concretions are obscured by the urographic contrast medium. Ectatic collecting ducts are usually difficult to fill during retrograde pyelography, and so the contrast material remains separate from papillary concretions in the cysts.

Asymptomatic patients require no treatment except advice to avoid dehydration and thereby reduce the risk of stone formation. The metabolic etiology of stones should be sought and treated conventionally, while infection and urological consequences of stones should be treated as described in Chap. 284. Medullary sponge kidneys are abnormally vulnerable to infection, and urological instrumentation should, therefore, be minimized.

MEDULLARY CYSTIC DISEASE (NEPHRONOPHTHISIS COMPLEX)

ETIOLOGY This is a mixture of hereditary medullary cystic diseases that have similar morphology but differing patterns of

A

B

FIGURE 283-1

A. Radiographic appearance of medullary sponge kidney. Abdominal flat plate reveals multiple bilateral calcifications. B. Radiographic contrast material accumulates in the dilated and cystic terminal collecting ducts and obscures the calcifications.

inheritance. The recessive form is associated with renal failure before 20 years of age (early-onset type), whereas the dominant form causes renal failure only after the second decade (adult-onset type). Both sexes are affected. When renal disease is associated with retinal degenerative changes (renal retinal dysplasia), inheritance is always recessive, but renal failure occurs during adult life.

PATHOLOGY In either form, most of the cysts are in the medulla and the corticomedullary region and have been localized by microdissection to collecting ducts and distal convoluted tubules. Cysts have a low, frequently atrophic, epithelium and range from microscopic dimensions to several millimeters in size. The kidneys usually are asymmetrically scarred and shrunken. Both tubular atrophy and periglomerular fibrosis are present, but the former is more severe than the latter. In advanced cases, glomeruli become sclerotic and hyalinized, cortical fibrosis and cellular interstitial infiltration appear, and the histology becomes difficult to differentiate from that of chronic interstitial nephritis.

DIAGNOSIS AND TREATMENT Concentrating ability, acid excretion, and sodium conservation are defective as might be expected from a lesion that damages late segments of the nephron. The disease is marked by polyuria, progressive renal failure, stunted growth, severe anemia, hyperchloremic metabolic acidosis, and poor sodium conservation. In adults, the inability to conserve sodium may cause a salt-wasting syndrome that resembles Addison's disease but that is unresponsive to mineralocorticoids. Hypertension usually is a terminal event. The urinalysis is normal at first, but mild proteinuria may develop. On intravenous pyelography, the kidneys are small, scarred, and without calcification. The calyces are distorted by numerous cysts in the corticomedullary area.

In the presence of acidosis, high sodium and water intake and alkali replacement are needed. Treatment of infections, anemia, hypertension, and other aspects of end-stage renal failure are as discussed in Chap. 276. Genetic counseling may be helpful in family planning and in selection of a related donor for renal transplantation.

FUNCTIONAL TUBULAR DISORDERS

BARTTER'S SYNDROME In 1962, Bartter described a syndrome consisting of hypokalemia due to renal potassium wasting, elevated plasma renin activity and aldosterone secretion, normotension, hyporesponsiveness of blood pressure to infused angiotensin II, and hyperplasia of the granular cells of the juxtaglomerular apparatus. Weakness, or periodic paralysis,

and polyuria occur because of chronic potassium depletion. Hyperplasia of renal medullary interstitial cells, which produce prostaglandins (PG) E and F, has been described in some patients, along with very elevated PGE_2 production. Inheritance is autosomal recessive, and manifestations commonly begin in childhood.

Pathogenesis While the pathogenetic sequence has not been proved with certainty, depressed reabsorption of sodium chloride in the proximal tubule or thick ascending limb of the loop of Henle is thought to be the basic underlying defect in this syndrome. The exact basis for the tubular reabsorptive defect is uncertain, but it may be part of a widespread inherited disorder. Sodium transport by skeletal muscles and erythrocytes may be defective, and, in the relatives of some patients, erythrocyte sodium transport has also been demonstrated to be abnormal. Excessive sodium chloride and water losses in the urine cause depletion of extracellular fluid volume, which in turn stimulates hyperplasia of the granular cells of the juxtaglomerular apparatus and increases renin production. The resulting increase in angiotensin II production stimulates aldosterone secretion. The renal tubular defect permits continued delivery of sodium to the sodium-potassium exchange sites in the distal nephron, which are stimulated by a supernormal concentration of serum aldosterone, and renal wasting of potassium ensues. Blood pressure remains normal because the pressor effects of angiotensin II are offset by depletion of extracellular volume. Infusion of angiotensin II produces less than the usual rise in arterial pressure because angiotensin II levels are already elevated.

Excessive production of PGE_2 may result from hypokalemia or elevated concentration of angiotensin II, both known stimulators of PGE_2 synthesis, and may therefore be a secondary consequence of the syndrome. In some cases blockade of PGE_2 production with indomethacin lowered renin levels and restored vascular response to angiotensin II infusion, but did not reduce potassium wasting. This observation supports the notion that overproduction of PGE_2 may be a secondary phenomenon.

Treatment The dietary intake of sodium chloride and potassium should be liberal; often potassium supplements are required despite a high dietary intake. Pharmacological blockade of aldosterone effects on distal tubules with spironolactone can prevent potassium wasting, though sodium intake must be increased. Inhibition of prostaglandin synthesis with indomethacin has met with varying success, as indicated above. Beta-adrenergic blockade has also been used, with some success, to lower renin production.

LIDDLE'S SYNDROME (PSEUDOHYPERALDOSTERONISM)

This rare inherited disorder is characterized by hypertension, hypokalemic alkalosis, and negligible aldosterone secretion. It appears to be due to an unusual tendency of distal tubules or collecting ducts to conserve sodium and excrete potassium despite the virtual absence of aldosterone. No other biochemical abnormalities have been described. These patients respond to 100 mg per day of triamterene (Chap. 236), a diuretic agent that blocks sodium and potassium exchange in the distal tubule.

FAMILIAL NEPHROGENIC DIABETES (DI)

In this disease the distal tubules and collecting ducts are unresponsive to vasopressin because of a sex-linked recessive disease, with variable penetrance in heterozygous females. Affected individuals excrete large volumes of very hypotonic urine even when plasma osmolality and vasopressin concentration are both high. Polyuria, polydipsia, and hypertonic dehydration following restriction of fluid intake all result from renal tubular insensitivity to antidiuretic hormone (ADH). Unresponsiveness to vasopressin may be due to reduced production of cyclic adenosine 5'-monophosphate (cyclic AMP) in the epithelium of the collecting ducts, to the inability of cyclic AMP to increase the permeability of collecting duct luminal cell membranes to water, or to a combination of the two. Other hereditary tubular defects such as juvenile nephronophthisis, medullary cystic and polycystic diseases, as well as cystinosis and congenital or acquired chronic urinary tract obstruction can cause vasopressin-resistant (nephrogenic) DI, but in these syndromes the characteristic findings of the underlying disorder are obvious.

Affected infants easily become dehydrated, hypernatremic, and hyperthermic, and damage of the central nervous system and resultant mental retardation may result. In the absence of dehydration, overall renal function is normal. On intravenous pyelography the renal pelvis, ureters, and bladder are dilated, as in any form of DI, because of massive diuresis.

Oral hydration usually is adequate treatment except during early infancy, when hypotonic parenteral fluids may be required. Vasopressin and its synthetic analogues are ineffective, but diuretic agents such as chlorothiazide reduce polyuria. This drug inhibits NaCl reabsorption in the thick ascending limb of the loop of Henle, thereby reducing production of free water. In addition, chlorothiazide produces a diuresis that causes contraction of extracellular fluid volume which, in turn, stimulates reabsorption of NaCl and water in the proximal tubule and limits their delivery to the thick ascending limb.

RENAL TUBULAR ACIDOSIS (RTA)

In this group of disorders renal excretion of acid is reduced out of proportion to any reduction of glomerular filtration rate that may be present. Metabolic acidosis results, but in contrast to renal failure the anions that accompany surplus hydrogen ions in the blood, such as sulfate and phosphate, are excreted normally and are unavailable to balance any fall in serum bicarbonate that occurs. Therefore, the kidneys reabsorb chloride in unusually large amounts, and serum chloride rises to preserve electroneutrality in the extracellular fluid. The result is *hyperchloremic acidosis,* and the unmeasured anion gap is normal. There is general agreement that four types of RTA exist. Types 1 and 2 are often hereditary. Type 3 is a rare mixture of types 1 and 2. Type 4 is acquired and is associated with either hyporeninemic hypoaldosteronism or tubular hyporesponsiveness to circulating mineralocorticoid hormones.

TYPE 1 (DISTAL) RTA Sporadic cases occur, but autosomal dominant inheritance is usually present. The kidney does not lower urine pH normally, either because the collecting ducts permit excessive back-diffusion of hydrogen ions from lumen to blood or fail to transport hydrogen ions against a steep pH gradient. Since titration of urine buffers and diffusion trapping of NH_4^+ in the tubules both depend upon a low intraluminal pH, excretion of acid is deficient. Urinary osmotic concentration and potassium conservation also tend to be impaired.

Chronic acidosis lowers tubule reabsorption of calcium, causing renal hypercalciuria and mild secondary hyperparathyroidism. The hypercalciuria, alkaline urine, and low levels of urine citrate—which normally complexes about 40 percent of urine calcium and is deficient during systemic acidosis—cause calcium phosphate stones and papillary nephrocalcinosis. Growth is stunted in children because of rickets; this growth defect responds dramatically to amelioration of the acidosis with sodium bicarbonate or other alkali. In the adult bone disease takes the form of osteomalacia. In both children and adults, bone disease results, at least in part from acidosis-induced loss of bone mineral as well as from inadequate production of 1,25-dihydroxyvitamin D_3 [1,25-$(OH)_2D_3$]. Since the kidney does not conserve potassium or concentrate the urine normally, polyuria and hypokalemia occur. Given the stress of an intercurrent illness, acidosis and hypokalemia can become life-threatening.

The diagnosis is suggested by osteomalacia or rickets, hyperchloremic acidosis associated with alkaline urine, and calcium phosphate stones or nephrocalcinosis. To prove that the urine pH cannot be lowered normally, the oral ammonium chloride (NH_4Cl) loading test should be carried out: 0.1 g (1.9 mmol) NH_4Cl per kilogram is administered, and the course of blood and urine pH are followed. Although systemic acidosis worsens, urine pH does not fall below 5.5. Urinary infection must not be present during this test because bacteria may possess urease which hydrolyzes urea to ammonia and produces a very alkaline urine. When hyperchloremic acidosis is severe and the urine is grossly alkaline, the test is unnecessary.

It can be difficult to distinguish primary RTA from RTA secondary to stone disease, infection, or other forms of renal disease. Several useful clues are that urine calcium excretion is normal or elevated in hereditary type 1 RTA but usually is below normal, i.e., less than 100 mg per day, in acquired forms and that hypokalemia occurs in hereditary but not commonly in acquired RTA. A clinically confusing situation may occur when type 1 RTA results from nephrocalcinosis due to hereditary idiopathic hypercalciuria. In this circumstance, stones usually are composed of calcium oxalate, and hypokalemia is absent. Other hereditary diseases that cause RTA, medullary sponge kidney, galactosemia, Ehler-Danlos syndrome, Fabry's disease, and hereditary elliptocytosis, can be excluded by clinical findings. The relatives of patients with type 1 RTA should be screened because they may have this treatable cause of renal damage.

Treatment Sodium bicarbonate tablets (10 grains = 7.2 meq base) and Shohl's solution (1 meq base per milliliter, as Na and K citrate) are both convenient for treatment; the dose should be 0.5 to 2.0 meq/kg in four or five divided doses daily. The total dose of alkali should be raised until acidosis and hypercalciuria are both eliminated, and the patients should then be followed by measurements of serum chloride and CO_2 content and of urine calcium excretion approximately twice yearly. Potassium supplementation usually is not required. Requirements for alkali usually increase during intercurrent illnesses.

TYPE 2 (PROXIMAL) RTA Proximal RTA usually occurs as part of a generalized disorder of proximal tubule function, but this section refers to the rare isolated form which can occur as an autosomal dominant, autosomal recessive, or sex-linked recessive trait and is usually recognized in childhood. Bicarbonate reabsorption in the proximal tubule is defective, and renal bicarbonate wasting occurs at a normal concentration of plasma bicarbonate. As plasma bicarbonate falls, the filtered load drops to a level that the defective tubule can reabsorb. Then the urine is free of bicarbonate and has a low pH. Potassium wasting and hypokalemia occur, especially when supplementary alkali is given, because bicarbonate is excreted in the urine partly as the potassium salt. There is moderate hypercalciuria, and stone formation is rare. During the NH_4Cl loading test, urine pH falls below 5.5.

Treatment is often not required. When it is, because of severe acidosis, bicarbonate must be given in large amounts daily, often above 4 meq/kg, and even up to 10 meq/kg per day, because bicarbonate is rapidly excreted in the urine. Another approach is to use thiazides and a low-salt diet which induce mild volume depletion and enhance proximal bicarbonate reabsorption, thereby reducing the required dose. Potassium supplements are needed during treatment because excessive sodium bicarbonate reaches the distal nephron where much of the sodium is exchanged for potassium, which is then lost in the urine.

VITAMIN D DISORDERS

FAMILIAL X-LINKED HYPOPHOSPHATEMIC VITAMIN D-REFRACTORY RICKETS (See also Chap. 352) Reduced tubular reabsorption of phosphate by the proximal tubule and hypophosphatemia occur in this sex-linked dominant disease, which can also be termed *renal phosphate leak*. Although they may be asymptomatic, patients usually are short and their bones rachitic; their legs are particularly short and deformed, and they develop osteomalacia in adult life. Bone age and dentition are retarded, and the teeth are poorly developed. The skull becomes deformed, and the maxillofacial region may develop abnormally. Overgrowth of bone at sites of muscular attachment can limit movement or compress nerves. Bony abnormalities are less common in females. Serum alkaline phosphatase levels are elevated, serum parathyroid levels are normal or high, while serum calcium concentration is usually normal, and urinary calcium excretion rate is normal or low.

The hypophosphatemia arises in part from decreased tubular reabsorption of phosphate and increased fractional excretion of phosphate. Intestinal absorption of calcium and phosphate may be decreased in untreated patients but increased during treatment with vitamin D. Although glycinuria and mild glucosuria have been reported, most patients exhibit only a defect in excretion of phosphate. Absence of hyperchloremic acidosis and a normal serum calcium concentration help to exclude RTA, malabsorption syndrome, and nutritional rickets.

Treatment requires oral neutral phosphate, 1 to 4 g daily, in divided doses, and 10,000 to 50,000 units of vitamin D; one must watch for hypercalcemia. Bony deformities require orthopedic management, but corrective surgery, except for genu valgum, should be postponed until active growth is completed.

VITAMIN D-DEPENDENT RICKETS Also known as hereditary pseudovitamin D deficiency rickets, this disease is inherited as an autosomal recessive trait, and there is a high incidence of parental consanguinity. Defective production of $1,25\text{-}(OH)_2D_3$, perhaps because of a genetic defect in 25-hydroxycalciferol 1α-hydroxylase, has been proposed as the basis for the disease. But the dose of $1,25\text{-}(OH)_2D_3$ or 1α-hydroxyvitamin D_3 [1α-$(OH)D_3$] required to heal rickets is higher than that for vitamin D–deficiency rickets, suggesting an attenuated response to, or excessive degradation of, $1,25\text{-}(OH)_2D_3$.

Rickets usually appears before 2 years of age. Serum calcium is low, parathyroid hormone concentration and alkaline phosphatase are high, and plasma phosphorus is variable. Urinary calcium is decreased, fecal calcium is increased, and tubular phosphate reabsorption is reduced. Serum levels of $1,25\text{-}(OH)_2D_3$ are undetectable. Aminoaciduria and hyperchloremic acidosis can occur, but urinary cyclic AMP increases normally in response to PTH infusion.

The 1α-hydroxylated metabolites of vitamin D bypass the enzyme defect and produce a dramatic healing of rickets. Vitamin D_2, 10,000 to 40,000 units per day, is also effective, but oral calcium, 0.5 to 2.0 g per day, is needed as well. The need for vitamin D persists throughout life. $1,25\text{-}(OH)_2D_3$, an ideal replacement therapy, will provide safer therapy when it becomes available.

RENAL GLUCOSURIA

See Chap. 90.

ISOLATED HYPOURICEMIA (See also Chap. 90)

This disorder is familial, but its pattern of inheritance is not known. Hypouricemia can occur in the Fanconi syndrome, Hartnup's disease, and Wilson's disease, but may also appear as an isolated trait. Uric acid clearance is high, and urine oxypurine levels are normal, excluding hereditary xanthinuria. Patients are asymptomatic except for occasional uric acid nephrolithiasis. No specific treatment is needed except the avoidance of dehydration. Coexistent hypercalciuria and decreased bone density have been described in a few patients, who may have a related disease with recessive inheritance.

SELECTIVE DISORDERS OF AMINO ACID TRANSPORT

CYSTINURIA (See also Chaps. 90 and 284) Renal and intestinal transport of cystine and the other dibasic amino acids, lysine, arginine, and ornithine, are defective, and excessive amounts are lost in the urine. Clinical disease is due solely to the insolubility of cystine, which forms stones. Patients are short, probably because of a linked inherited tendency rather than amino acid losses. Cystinuria is transmitted as an autosomal recessive trait whose prevalence in newborns is 1 in 7000.

Pathogenesis The weight of available evidence indicates that cystinuria occurs because of defective transport of amino acids by the brush borders of renal tubule and intestinal epithelial cells. Cystine, lysine, arginine, and ornithine appear to share a common renal transport pathway, because infusion of lysine decreases tubular reabsorption of the other three. But cystine also seems to be transported by a separate transport mechanism, because cystinuria and dibasic aminoaciduria can each occur independently. The inheritance of the brush border transport defects is complex. The intestinal defects are not similar in all patients who are homozygous for cystinuria, and the extent of aminoaciduria in those relatives of cystinuric pa-

TABLE 283-1
Classification of cystinuria into three subtypes*

	Type I	Type II	Type III
Intestinal transport:			
Cystine	0	↓↓	N − ↓
Lysine	0	0	↓
Arginine	0	−	−
Urine excretion in heterozygotes:			
Cystine	N	↑	↑
Lysine	N	↑	↑

NOTE: ↑, *increased;* ↓, *reduced;* ↓↓, *very reduced;* 0, *absent transport;* N, *normal urinary excretion rates;* −, *not known.*

tients who are heterozygous carriers of the defect, for example, their siblings, varies from family to family. Thus far three types of inheritance have been described (Table 283-1).

Diagnosis and treatment Cystine stones are formed only by patients with cystinuria, but 10 percent of stones formed by cystinuric patients do not contain cystine; therefore, every stone former should be screened for the disease. The sediment from a first morning urine specimen in many patients with homozygous cystinuria reveals typical flat hexagonal platelike cystine crystals. Cystinuria can also be detected using the sodium nitroprusside test on a urine sample. The test gives a positive response to 75 to 125 mg cystine per liter of urine, a concentration lower than that found in the urine of patients with homozygous cystinuria but well above the levels encountered in normal urine. Because the test is sensitive, it will be positive in many individuals who are heterozygous for cystinuria, most of whom do not form cystine stones (Table 283-1). A positive nitroprusside test or the finding of cystine crystals in the urine sediment should be evaluated by measurement of daily cystine excretion. Normal adults excrete 40 to 60 mg per gram of creatinine; heterozygotes usually excrete less than 300 mg/g; and patients with homozygous cystinuria almost always excrete above 250 mg/g.

Treatment consists of a high fluid intake, even at night. Daily urine volume should exceed 3 liters (Chap. 284). Raising urine pH with alkali is helpful, provided the resulting daily urine pH exceeds 7.0. Because drug side effects are frequent, D-penicillamine, which forms the soluble mixed disulfide cysteine-penicillamine, should be used only when fluid loading and alkali therapy have been ineffective. *N*-Acetyl-D-penicillamine has a similar mode of action and may have fewer side effects, but is not available for routine use. Mercaptopropionyl-glycine has been used to dissolve renal calculi by perfusion of the renal pelvis and has been given by mouth to prevent stones, but also is experimental. Low methionine diets have not proved to be practical for clinical use.

HARTNUP'S DISEASE (See also Chap. 90) In this rare autosomal recessive disorder, renal and intestinal transport of monoamino-monocarboxylic amino acids are defective. An erythematous, scaly, pellagra-like rash appears after exposure to sunlight, and episodic cerebellar ataxia, emotional instability, delirium, and aminoaciduria all occur. The prevalence is 1 in 15,000 newborns and is higher in the offspring of consanguineous marriages.

Dietary monoamino-monocarboxylic amino acids remain in the intestinal lumen where they undergo bacterial degradation. At the same time, they are lost in the urine. Inadequate tryptophan availability limits nicotinamide synthesis and leads to pellagra. The products of tryptophan degradation appear to cause central nervous system symptoms. Decreased absorption

and urine loss of the other monoamino-monocarboxylic amino acids can cause generalized malnutrition.

The diagnosis is based upon demonstration of massive urine losses of alanine, serine, threonine, asparagine, glutamine, valine, leucine, isoleucine, phenylalanine, tyrosine, tryptophan, histidine, glycine, and citrulline. Hypouricemia may also occur. Renal function is otherwise normal. Most patients respond to treatment with oral nicotinamide, 40 to 200 mg per day, and a high-protein diet to compensate for amino acid malabsorption and loss. The ultimate prognosis is good, and the disease often improves with adulthood.

FAMILIAL IMINOGLYCINURIA (See also Chap. 90) This autosomal recessive trait is characterized by excessive urinary excretion of proline, hydroxyproline, and glycine despite normal plasma levels of these amino acids, probably because of deletion or alteration of a membrane transport protein of the renal tubule cells. The patients are well. Iminoglycinuria can occur in normal newborn infants for up to 3 months.

FANCONI SYNDROME

Fanconi syndrome is a constellation of transport defects in the proximal tubule involving amino acids, monosaccharides, sodium, potassium, calcium, phosphate, bicarbonate, uric acid, and proteins. Generalized aminoaciduria, glucosuria, salt wasting, hypercalciuria, hypophosphatemia, proximal renal tubular acidosis, hypouricemia, and tubular proteinuria (Chap. 42) all may result. Fanconi syndrome can be acquired or arise from systemic inherited diseases such as cystinosis, tyrosinemia, galactosemia, fructose intolerance, glycogen storage disease (type 1), Wilson's disease, familial nephrosis, and hereditary amyloidosis. Lowe's (or oculocerebrorenal) syndrome is an X-linked recessive form of the Fanconi syndrome associated with ocular and cerebral abnormalities.

An autosomal recessive disease, *adult Fanconi syndrome*, occurs in the absence of any systemic disorder. The term *adult* is misleading since cases are recognized in childhood, but no abnormalities are apparent at birth. Dwarfism and hypophosphatemic rickets occur along with the laboratory abnormalities of Fanconi syndrome. Renal failure is rare, and the prognosis is usually good when the systemic effects of Fanconi syndrome are treated. Typically, there is a "swan neck" deformity of the initial portion of the proximal tubule which, in all probability, is the anatomic basis of this tubular disorder. There is cellular atrophy in the deformed tubular segment. The consequences of each of the transport defects that involve water, sodium, potassium, acid, and phosphate excretion often require treatment. Water, sodium, and potassium intake must be liberal, and phosphate supplements may be needed. Metabolic acidosis may be corrected by the administration of alkali. Vitamin D may be needed to help promote bone healing. Glucosuria, uricosuria, and tubular proteinuria do not require treatment.

REFERENCES

ANDREOLI TE, SCHAFER JA: Nephrogenic diabetes insipidus, in *The Metabolic Basis of Inherited Disease,* 4th ed, JB Stanbury et al (eds). New York, McGraw-Hill, 1978, p 1634

BARTTER FC et al: Bartter's syndrome. Adv Nephrol 7:191, 1977

BERNES LG et al: Familial proximal renal tubular acidosis. Am J Med 52:244, 1977

BERNSTEIN J, KISSANE JM: Hereditary disorders of the kidney, part 1: Parenchymal defects and malformations. Perspect Ped Pathol 1:117, 1973

DANOVITCH GM: Clinical features and pathophysiology of polycystic disease in man, in *Cystic Diseases of the Kidney,* KD Gardner (ed). New York, Wiley, 1976, p 123

Ekstrom T et al: *Medullary Sponge Kidney.* Stockholm, Almqvist and Wiksell, 1959

Feest TG, Wrong OM: Inherited defects in distal tubular acidification. Ann Intern Med 82:584, 1975

Gardner KD: Juvenile nephronophthisis and renal medullary cystic disease, in *Cystic Diseases of the Kidney,* KD Gardner (ed). New York, Wiley, 1976, p 125

Jepson JB: Hartnup disease, in *The Metabolic Basis of Inherited Disease,* 4th ed, JB Stanbury et al (eds). New York, McGraw-Hill, 1978, p 1563

Liddle GW et al: A familial renal disorder simulating primary aldosteronism but with negligible aldosterone secretion. Trans Ann Am Phys 76:199, 1963

Newcombe DS: Isolated deficiency in renal tubular reabsorption of urate, in *Inherited Biochemical Disorders and Uric Acid Metabolism.* Baltimore, University Park Press, 1975, p 232

Perkoff GT: The hereditary renal diseases. N Engl J Med 277:79, 129, 1967

Rasmussen H, Anast C: Familial hypophosphatemic (vitamin D resistant) rickets and vitamin D dependent rickets, in *The Metabolic Basis of Inherited Disease,* 4th ed, JB Stanbury et al (eds). New York, McGraw-Hill, 1978, p 1537

Rector FC Jr: Renal acidification, in *The Kidney,* 2d ed, BM Brenner, FC Rector (eds). Philadelphia, Saunders, 1980, chap 10

Scriver CR: Familial iminoglycinuria, in *The Metabolic Basis of Inherited Disease,* 4th ed, JB Stanbury et al (eds). New York, McGraw-Hill, 1978, p 1593

——— et al: Genetic aspects of renal tubular transport: Diversity and topology of carriers. Kid Int 9:149, 1976

Segal S: Disorders of renal amino acid transport. N Engl J Med 294:1044, 1976

Thier SO, Segal S: Cystinuria, in *The Metabolic Basis of Inherited Disease,* 4th ed, JB Stanbury et al (eds). New York, McGraw-Hill, 1978, p 1578

Walton J: Familial hypophosphatemic rickets. Clin Pediatr 15:1007, 1976

284

NEPHROLITHIASIS

FREDRIC L. COE
MURRAY J. FAVUS

TYPES OF STONES

Calcium salts, uric acid, cystine, and struvite ($MgNH_4PO_4$) are the basis of virtually all kidney stones formed by patients residing in the Western Hemisphere. Calcium oxalate and calcium phosphate stones comprise 75 to 85 percent of the total (Table 284-1) and may be admixed in the same stone. Calcium phosphates in stones are usually hydroxyapatite [$Ca_5(PO_4)_3OH$] or, less commonly, brushite ($CaHPO_4$).

Calcium stones are formed mainly by men; the average age of onset is the third decade. Most persons who form a single calcium stone will eventually form another, and the intervals between successive stones shorten or remain constant, suggesting that stone-forming activity usually does not wane with time. The average rate of new stone formation in patients who have previously formed a stone is about one stone every 2 or 3 years. Calcium stone disease is strongly familial.

In the urine, calcium oxalate monohydrate crystals (whewellite) usually grow as biconcave ovals that resemble red blood cells in shape and size, but also occur in a larger, "dumbbell" form. In polarized light the crystals appear bright against a dark background, a property known as *birefringence*. Calcium oxalate dihydrate crystals (weddellite) are bipyramidal and only weakly birefringent. Apatite crystals do not exhibit birefringence and appear amorphous, because the actual crystals

are too small to be resolved by light microscopy. Brushite produces elongated lathlike (narrow, long, rectangular) crystals.

Uric acid stones are radiolucent, account for 5 to 8 percent of all stones (Table 284-1), and are also formed mainly by men. Half of patients who form uric acid stones have gout; whether or not gout is present, uric acid lithiasis is familial. In urine, uric acid crystals become red-orange colored because they adsorb the pigment uricine. Anhydrous uric acid produces very small crystals that appear amorphous by light microscopy. They are indistinguishable from apatite crystals, except for their birefringence. Uric acid dihydrate tends to form teardrop-shaped crystals as well as flat, square plates; both are strongly birefringent. Uric acid gravel appears like red dust, and the stones are also orange or red on some occasions. *Cystine stones* are very uncommon (less than 1 percent of all stones), are lemon yellow, and sparkle; they are radiopaque because they contain sulfur. Cystine crystals appear in the urine as flat, hexagonal plates.

Struvite stones are common (Table 284-1) and potentially dangerous. These stones, formed mainly by women, result from urinary tract infection with bacteria that posses urease, usually *Proteus* species. The stones can grow to a large size and fill the renal pelvis and calyces to produce a "staghorn" appearance. They are radiopaque and have a variable internal density. In urine, struvite crystals are rectangular prisms that have been likened to coffin lids.

MANIFESTATIONS OF STONES

As stones grow upon the surfaces of the renal papillae or within the urinary collecting system, they need not produce symptoms. Accordingly, asymptomatic stones are often discovered during the course of abdominal radiographic studies undertaken for unrelated reasons. Sometimes stones cause only gross or microscopic hematuria. In fact, stones rank, along with benign and malignant neoplasms, renal cysts, and genitourinary tuberculosis, as among the most common causes of isolated hematuria. Much of the time, however, stones break loose and enter the ureter, or occlude the ureteropelvic junction, causing pain and obstruction.

STONE PASSAGE A stone can traverse the ureter without symptoms, but most of the time passage produces pain and bleeding. The pain begins gradually, usually in the flank, but increases over the next 20 to 60 min to become very severe, and narcotic drugs are often needed for its control. The pain may remain in the flank or spread downward and anteriorly toward the loins, the testicles, or vulva. Pain that migrates downward always indicates that the stone has passed to the lower third of the ureter, but if the pain does not migrate, the position of the stone cannot be predicted. A stone in the portion of the ureter within the bladder wall causes frequency, urgency, and dysuria that may be confused with urinary tract infection. Hematuria is the rule with passage of a stone.

OTHER SYNDROMES Staghorn calculi Struvite, cystine, and uric acid stones often grow too large to enter the ureter. They gradually fill the renal pelvis and may extend outward through the infundibula to the calyxes themselves.

Nephrocalcinosis Calcium stones grow on the renal papillae. Most break loose and cause colic, but sometimes they remain in place so that multiple papillary calcifications are found by x-ray, a condition termed *nephrocalcinosis.* Papillary nephro-

TABLE 284-1
Major cause of renal stones

Stone type and causes	Percent of all stones*	Percent occurrence of specific causes*	Ratio of men to women	Etiology	Diagnosis	Treatment
Calcium stones:	75–85		2:1 to 3:1			
Idiopathic hypercalcinuria		50–55	2:1	Hereditary (?)	Normocalcemia, unexplained hypercalciuria†	Thiazide diuretic agents
Hyperuricosuria		20	4:1	Diet	Urine uric acid > 750 mg per 24 h (women), > 800 mg per 24 h (men)	Allopurinol or diet
Primary hyperparathyroidism		5	3:10	Neoplasia	Unexplained hypercalcemia	Surgery
Distal renal tubular acidosis		~1–2	1:1	Hereditary	Hyperchloremic acidosis, minimum urine pH > 5.5	Alkali replacement
Intestinal hyperoxaluria		~1–2	1:1	Bowel surgery	Urine oxalate > 50 mg per 24 h	Cholestyramine or oral calcium loading
Hereditary hyperoxaluria		Rare	1:1	Hereditary	Urine oxalate and glycolic or L-glyceric acid increased	Fluids and pyridoxine
Idiopathic stone disease		20	2:1	Unknown	None of the above present	Oral phosphate, fluids
Uric acid stones:	5–8					
Gout		~50	3:1 to 4:1	Hereditary	Clinical diagnosis	Alkali to raise urine pH
Idiopathic		~50	1:1	Hereditary (?)	Uric acid stones, no gout	Allopurinol if daily urine uric acid above 1000 mg
Dehydration		?	1:1	Intestinal, habit	History, intestinal fluid loss	Alkali, fluids, reversal of cause
Lesch-Nyhan syndrome		Rare	Men	Hereditary	Reduced hypoxanthine guanine phosphoribosyltransferase level	Allopurinol
Malignant tumors		Rare	1:1	Neoplasia	Clinical diagnosis	Allopurinol
Cystine stones	1		1:1	Hereditary	Stone type; elevated cystine excretion	Massive fluids, alkali, D-penicillamine if needed
Struvite stones	10–15		2:10	Infection	Stone type	Antimicrobial agents and judicious surgery

* *Values are percent of patients who form a particular type of stone and who display each specific cause of stones.*
† *Urine calcium above 300 mg per 24 h (men), 250 mg per 24 h (women), or 4 mg/kg per 24 h either sex. Hyperthyroidism, Cushing syndrome, sarcoidosis, malignant tumors, immobilization, vitamin D intoxication, rapidly progressive bone disease, and Paget's disease all cause hypercalciuria and must be excluded in diagnosis of idiopathic hypercalciuria.*

calcinosis is very common in hereditary distal renal tubular acidosis and in other states characterized by severe hypercalciuria. In medullary sponge kidney disease (page 1344) calcification may occur in dilated distal collecting ducts.

Sludge There can be enough uric acid or cystine in the urine to plug both ureters with precipitate. Calcium oxalate crystals do not do this because usually less than 100 mg oxalate is excreted daily in the urine in even severe hyperoxaluric states, compared with 1000 mg uric acid in patients with ordinary hyperuricosuria and 200 to 400 mg cystine in patients with homozygous cystinuria. Calcium phosphate crystals can render the urine milky but do not plug the urinary tract.

INFECTION Although urinary tract infection is not a direct consequence of stone disease, it is a frequent complication that arises from instrumentation and surgery of the urinary tract, which are frequently required in the treatment of stone disease. Stone disease and urinary infection can enhance the seriousness of one another and interfere with treatment. Obstruction of an infected kidney by a stone may lead to sepsis and extensive damage of renal tissue, since it converts the urinary tract proximal to the obstruction into a closed, or partially closed, space that can become an abscess. On the other hand, some forms of infection, those due to bacteria that possess the enzyme urease, can produce stones composed of struvite.

ACTIVITY OF STONE DISEASE *Active disease* means that new stones are forming or that preformed stones are growing. Sequential radiographs of the renal areas are needed to document the growth or appearance of new stones and to assure that stones which pass are actually newly formed, not preexistent ones.

PATHOGENESIS OF STONES

Urinary stones usually arise because of the breakdown of a delicate balance. On the one hand the kidneys must conserve water, but they must also excrete materials that have a low solubility. These two opposing requirements must be balanced against one another during adaptation to a particular combination of diet, climate, and activity. The problem is mitigated to some extent by the fact that urine contains some substances that inhibit crystallization of calcium salts and others that bind calcium in soluble complexes. But these protective mechanisms are less than perfect. When the urine becomes saturated with insoluble materials, because their excretion rates are excessive, and/or because water conservation is extreme, crystals form and may grow and aggregate with one another to form a stone.

SUPERSATURATION Consider a solution that is in equilibrium with crystals of calcium oxalate. The product of the chemical activities of the calcium and oxalate ions in the solution is termed the *equilibrium solubility product,* because it is the activity product that is unique to the equilibrium condition. If the crystals are removed, and if either calcium or oxalate is added to the solution, the activity product will rise, but the solution will remain clear; no new crystals form. Such a solution is considered to be *metastably supersaturated.* If new calcium oxalate seed crystals are now added, they will grow in size. Ultimately, the activity product will reach a critical value at which a solid phase begins to develop spontaneously. This value is called the *upper limit of metastability,* or the *formation product.* Stone growth in the urinary tract requires a urine that, on the average, is above the equilibrium solubility product. Persistence of a stone requires an average saturation at least equal to the solubility product. In general there is agreement that excessive supersaturation is a factor common to the formation of most stones.

Calcium, oxalate, and phosphate form many stable soluble complexes among themselves and with other substances in urine, such as calcium citrate. As a result, their free ion activities are considerably below their chemical concentrations and can be measured only by indirect techniques. Urine saturation can be increased by a deficiency of inhibitors of crystal growth (see below), by dehydration, or by overexcretion of calcium, oxalate, or phosphate. Saturation of the urine with cystine or uric acid also rises when overexcretion or low urine volume is present. Urine pH can also be an important factor; phosphate and uric acid are weak acids that dissociate readily over the physiological range of urine pH. Alkaline urine contains more urate and dissociated phosphate, favoring deposits of sodium hydrogen urate, octocalcium phosphate, and apatite. Below a urine pH of 5.5, uric acid crystals (pK 5.47) predominate, whereas phosphate crystals are rare. The solubility of calcium oxalate, on the other hand, is not influenced by changes in urine pH. Measurements of saturation in a 24-h urine sample are averages that probably underestimate the risk of precipitation. Transient dehydration or postprandial bursts of overexcretion may cause values that are considerably above the average.

NUCLEATION **Homogeneous nucleation** When urine is supersaturated with respect to calcium oxalate, clusters of ions form at random as saturation rises. Most of them disperse when their mass is small because the internal forces between ions that tend to hold the clusters together are too weak to overcome the random tendency of ions to move away. Clusters of over 100 ions can remain stable because attractive forces balance surface losses. Once they are stable, nuclei can grow at a saturation far below that needed for their creation. The formation product marks the point at which stable nuclei become frequent enough to create a permanent solid phase.

Heterogeneous nucleation If a supersaturated urine is seeded with preformed nuclei of a crystal that is similar in structure to calcium oxalate, calcium and oxalate ions in solution will precipitate on the crystal's surface as they would upon a seed crystal of calcium oxalate itself. The organized growth of one crystal on the surface of another is called *epitaxial growth,* and the seeding of a supersaturated solution by foreign nuclei is called *heterogeneous nucleation.* Sodium hydrogen urate, uric acid, and hydroxyapatite crystals can serve as heterogeneous nuclei for calcium oxalate. Brushite can be transformed to hydroxy apatite and cause heterogeneous nucleation of sodium hydrogen urate; as a consequence, calcium oxalate stones can form even if urine calcium oxalate saturation never exceeds the metastable limit.

INHIBITORS OF CRYSTAL GROWTH AND AGGREGATION Stable nuclei must grow and aggregate to produce a stone of clinical significance. Urine contains potent inhibitors of both of these processes for calcium oxalate and calcium phosphate, but not for uric acid, cystine, or struvite crystals. Inorganic pyrophosphate is a potent inhibitor which appears to affect calcium phosphate more than calcium oxalate crystals. Other urine inhibitors that appear to be glycoproteins strongly inhibit the growth of calcium oxalate crystals. Slowing of crystal growth must raise the apparent upper limit of metastability, because the critical growth of ion clusters into stable nuclei is hindered. As a consequence of the presence of these inhibitors, crystal growth in urine is very slow compared with simple salt solutions, and the upper limit of metastability is higher.

EVALUATION AND TREATMENT OF PATIENTS WITH NEPHROLITHIASIS

A majority of patients with nephrolithiasis harbor remediable metabolic disorders that cause stones and can be detected by chemical analysis of the serum and urine. A practical outpatient evaluation consists of three 24-h urine collections, each with a corresponding blood sample. Serum and urine calcium, uric acid and creatinine, urine oxalate and serum electrolyte measurements should be made. Whenever possible, the composition of kidney stones should be determined because treatment depends on stone type (Table 284-1). No matter what disorders are found, every patient should be counseled to avoid dehydration and to drink six to eight glasses of water daily. Since treatment is prolonged, the use of medications must be justified by the activity and severity of stone disease and the desire the patient may have for protection against new stones.

The management of stones that are already present in the kidneys or urinary tract requires a combined medical and surgical approach. The specific treatment for any individual patient depends upon the details of the location of the stone, the extent of obstruction, the function of the affected and unaffected kidneys, the presence or absence of urinary tract infection, the progress of stone passage, and the overall clinical state of the patient, as it affects the risk of operation or anesthesia. For this reason, treatment must be individualized. Nevertheless, a few broad rules do apply. In general, when severe obstruction, infection, intractable pain, or serious bleeding occur, removal of a stone by operation upon the kidney, renal pelvis, or ureter, or by passing a flexible basket retrograde up the ureter from the bladder during the course of cystoscopy is usually attempted. This dictum applies whether the stone is small and in the ureter or is a large staghorn calculus that fills the renal pelvis.

CALCIUM STONES **Idiopathic hypercalciuria** (see also Chap. 350) This condition appears to be hereditary, and its diagnosis is straightforward (Table 284-1). In some patients, primary intestinal hyperabsorption of calcium causes transient postprandial hypercalcemia that suppresses secretion of parathyroid hormone. The renal tubules are deprived of their most potent normal stimulus to reabsorb calcium at the same time that the filtered load of calcium is increased. In other patients, reabsorption of calcium by the renal tubules appears to be defective, and secondary hyperparathyroidism is evoked by urinary losses of calcium. Renal activation of 1,25-dihydroxy-vitamin D is increased, producing intestinal hyperabsorption of calcium. Hypercalciuria contributes to stone formation by raising urine saturation with respect to calcium oxalate and calcium phosphate.

Thiazide diuretics lower urine calcium in both types of hypercalciuria and are very effective in preventing the formation of stones. The drug effect requires slight contraction of the extracellular fluid volume, and massive use of NaCl will reduce its therapeutic effect.

Primary hyperparathyroidism (see also Chap. 350) The diagnosis of this condition, which is more common in women than men, is aided by the finding of unexplained phosphate stones and is established by documenting hypercalcemia that cannot be otherwise explained accompanied by inappropriately elevated serum concentrations of parathyroid hormone. Hypercalciuria, which is usually present, raises the urine saturation of calcium phosphate and/or calcium oxalate (Table 284-1). It is important to establish the diagnosis since parathyroidectomy is effective treatment and should be carried out before renal damage has occurred.

Distal renal tubular acidosis (see also Chap. 283) The defect in this condition seems to reside in the distal nephron, which cannot establish a normal pH gradient between urine and blood, leading to hyperchloremic acidosis. The minimum urine pH in response to an oral challenge with NH_4Cl, 1.9 mmol/kg, is above 5.5. Hypercalciuria, an alkaline urine, and a low urine citrate concentration cause supersaturation with respect to calcium phosphate. Calcium phosphate stones are formed, nephrocalcinosis is common, and osteomalacia or rickets may occur. Renal damage is frequent, and a gradual fall in glomerular filtration rate usually occurs. Treatment with supplemental alkali reverses hypercalciuria and limits the production of new stones. The usual dose of sodium bicarbonate is 0.5 to 2.0 meq/kg, in four to six divided doses. An alternative is Schohl's solution, which contains citrate and citric acid.

Hyperuricosuria About 20 percent of calcium oxalate stone formers are hyperuricosuric, primarily because of an excessive intake of purine from meat, fish, and poultry. The mechanism of stone formation probably is heterogeneous nucleation of calcium oxalate by crystals of sodium hydrogen urate or uric acid that lodge in the terminal ends of the collecting ducts and produce an anchored site on which calcium oxalate can deposit. A change in diet is ideal treatment but difficult for many patients to achieve. The alternative is allopurinol, usually 100 mg bid. Some patients eventually alter their diets so that allopurinol can be withdrawn.

Hyperoxaluria Overabsorption of dietary oxalate and consequent oxaluria, i.e., so-called "intestinal oxaluria," has been ascribed to fat malabsorption (Chap. 292). The latter can be caused by a variety of conditions, including bacterial overgrowth syndromes, chronic disease of the pancreas and biliary tract, jejunoileal bypass in treatment of obesity, or ileal resection greater than 22 cm for inflammatory bowel disease. With fat malabsorption, calcium in the bowel lumen is bound by fatty acids instead of precipitating with oxalate, which is left free for absorption. Dietary excess of oxalate, ascorbic acid loading, and hereditary hyperoxaluric states due to overproduction of oxalate are much less common causes of hyperoxaluria. Hyperoxaluria from any cause can produce tubulointerstitial nephropathy (Chap. 281) and lead to stone formation.

Cholestyramine, a resin that can bind oxalate, at a dose of 8 to 16 g per day, correction of fat malabsorption, and a low-fat diet are effective treatments for oxaluria secondary to intestinal absorption. Calcium lactate, 8 to 14 g per day, which acts by precipitating oxalate in the gut lumen is an alternative form of therapy. There is no effective treatment for hereditary hyperoxaluria, a disorder characterized by an enzymatic defect involving the metabolism of the precursor of oxalate and transmitted as an autosomal recessive. A high fluid intake, phosphate, and pyridoxine (200 mg per day) are recommended, but irreversible renal failure secondary to recurrent stone formation usually occurs before the age of 20 years.

Idiopathic calcium lithiasis At least 20 percent of patients have no obvious cause for stones (Table 284-1). The best treatment for them appears to be a high fluid intake, so that the urine specific gravity remains below approximately 1.005 throughout the day and night. Oral phosphate at a dose of 2 g phosphorus daily may lower urine calcium and increases urine pyrophosphate excretion, and thereby may bring about a reduction in the rate of recurrence of stones. Orthophosphate causes mild nausea and diarrhea initially, but tolerance may improve with continued intake. Thiazide treatment to reduce calcium excretion and allopurinol to diminish uric acid output may also be helpful. There are no adequate studies to support the use of supplemental magnesium, pyridoxine, or methylene blue, commonly mentioned remedies.

URIC ACID STONES These stones form because the urine becomes supersaturated with undissociated uric acid. In gout, idiopathic uric acid lithiasis, and dehydration, the average pH is abnormally low, usually below 5.4, and often below 5.0. Undissociated uric acid (pK 5.47), which is very insoluble and cannot be dissolved in urine in concentrations exceeding 200 to 300 mg per liter, predominates. Hyperuricosuria, when present, worsens supersaturation; but urine of low pH can be excessively supersaturated with undissociated uric acid, even though the daily excretion rate is normal. Myeloproliferative syndromes, chemotherapeutic treatment of malignant tumors, and the Lesch-Nyhan syndrome cause such massive production of uric acid and consequent hyperuricosuria that stones and urine sludge occur even at a normal urine pH. The renal collecting tubules can be plugged by uric acid with consequent acute renal failure.

The two goals of treatment are to raise urine pH and to lower urine uric acid excretion, when it is very high, i.e., above 1000 mg per day. Supplemental alkali, 1 to 3 meq/kg per day, should be given in three or four evenly spaced divided doses, one of which should be reserved for bedtime. If the overnight urine pH is below 5.5, the evening dose of bicarbonate may be raised, or 250 mg acetazolamide added at bedtime. With massive overexcretion of uric acid, high doses of allopurinol, exceeding 300 mg daily, may be needed. Treatment with allopurinol should be instituted before chemotherapy of highly cellular tumors, since massive hyperuricosuria can be expected. Alkali treatment must be avoided if hypercalciuria is also present.

CYSTINE STONES (See also Chap. 283) Like uric acid, cystine is more soluble in alkaline urine. However, improvement in solubility begins only above pH 7, and alkali confers only limited benefits. The major treatment is sufficient water to create 3 to 4 liters urine per day, and deliberate nocturia is an unavoidable part of treatment. If fluids and alkali are insufficient, D-penicillamine may be added. The side effects of this drug, i.e., anosmia and loss of taste, usually respond to replacement of zinc. Development of the nephrotic syndrome is a common serious side effect of D-penicillamine that contraindicates further use of the drug.

STRUVITE STONES These stones are always a result of urinary infection with bacteria, usually *Proteus* species, which possess urease, an enzyme that degrades urea to NH_3 and CO_2.

The NH_3 hydrolyzes to NH_4^+ and raises pH, usually to 8 or 9. The CO_2 hydrates to H_2CO_3 and then dissociates to CO_3^{2-} which precipitates with calcium as $CaCO_3$. The NH_4^+ precipitates PO_4^{2-} and Mg^{2+} to form the triple salt $MgNH_4PO_4$. The result is a stone of calcium carbonate admixed with struvite. It is impossible to form struvite in urine without infection, because NH_4^+ concentration is very low in urine that is alkaline in response to physiological stimuli. Chronic proteus infection can occur because of impaired urinary drainage, infection of retained stones of any type, urologic instrumentation or surgery, and especially chronic antibiotic treatment, which can favor the emergence of *Proteus* as the predominant urinary tract flora.

Treatment Mandelamine, which lowers urine pH and liberates formaldehyde, is used for chronic suppression of infection when a stone is present. More extreme lowering of urine pH with chronic administration of NH_4Cl may retard stone growth but may also raise urine calcium level and promote the formation of calcium oxalate stones. Antimicrobial treatment is best reserved for dealing with acute exacerbation of infection and for maintenance of a sterile urine after surgery, in the hope of preventing recurrence or minimizing stone growth. Surgery should be reserved for severe obstruction, intractable pain, bleeding, or serious manifestations of urinary infection. Since stones can regrow from any infected fragment which is left behind, recurrences following operation are quite common.

REFERENCES

COE FL: Nephrolithiasis: Pathogenesis and treatment. Chicago, Year Book, 1978
———, FAVUS MJ: Disorders of stone formation, in *The Kidney,* 2d ed, BM Brenner, FC Rector Jr, (eds). Philadelphia, Saunders, 1980, chap 37
FLEISCH H et al (eds): *Urolithiasis Research.* New York, Plenum, 1976
PAK CYC (ed): Urolithiasis. Kidney Int 13:341, 1978

285
URINARY TRACT OBSTRUCTION

BARRY M. BRENNER
H. DAVID HUMES

Obstruction to the flow of urine, with attendant stasis and elevation in urinary tract pressure, impairs renal and urinary conduit functions and represents a common cause of acute and chronic renal failure. With early relief of obstruction, these defects in function usually disappear completely. However, chronic obstruction may produce profound and permanent loss of renal mass (renal atrophy) and excretory capability, as well as enhanced susceptibility to local infection and stone formation. Early and accurate diagnosis and prompt and appropriate therapy are, therefore, essential to minimize the otherwise devastating effects of obstruction on urinary tract structure and function.

ETIOLOGY Obstruction to urine flow can result from *intrinsic* or *extrinsic mechanical blockade* as well as from *functional defects* not associated with fixed occlusion of the urinary drainage system. Lesions causing mechanical obstruction can occur at any level of the urinary tract, from the renal calyxes to the external urethral meatus. Normal points of narrowing, such as the ureteropelvic and ureterovesical junctions, bladder neck, and urethral meatus, are common sites of obstruction. When blockage is above the level of the bladder, unilateral dilatation

of the ureter (*hydroureter*) and renal pyelocalyceal system (*hydronephrosis*) occur; when the lesion is at or below the level of the bladder, bilateral involvement is the rule.

Common forms of mechanical obstruction are listed in Table 285-1. In childhood, *congenital malformations,* including marked narrowing of the ureteropelvic junction, anomalous (retrocaval) location of the ureter, and posterior urethral valves predominate. The latter defect is the most common cause of bilateral hydronephrosis in the male child. Children may also have bladder dysfunction secondary to congenital urethral stricture, urethral meatal stenosis, or bladder neck obstruction. In adults, urinary tract obstruction is due mainly to *acquired defects.* Pelvic tumors, calculi, and urethral stricture predominate. Ligation of, or injury to, the ureter during pelvic or colonic surgery can lead to hydronephrosis which, if unilateral, may remain relatively silent and undetected. Obstructive uropathy may also result from extrinsic neoplastic (carcinoma of cervix or colon, retroperitoneal lymphoma) or inflammatory disorders. One such inflammatory disorder is retroperitoneal fibrosis, a process of unknown cause seen most commonly in middle-aged males, which occasionally leads to bilateral ureteral obstruction. Occurring in some patients taking methysergide for relief of migraine, retroperitoneal fibrosis must be distinguished from other retroperitoneal causes of ureteral obstruction, particularly lymphomas and pelvic neoplasms.

Functional impairment of urine flow usually results from disorders which involve both the ureter and bladder. Common functional lesions include neurogenic bladder, often with adynamic ureter, and vesicoureteral reflux. Reflux of urine from

TABLE 285-1
Common mechanical causes of urinary tract obstruction

Ureter*	Bladder outlet†	Urethra†
CONGENITAL		
Ureteropelvic junction narrowing or obstruction	Bladder neck obstruction	Posterior urethral valves
Ureterovesical junction narrowing or obstruction	Ureterocele	Anterior urethral valves
Ureterocele		Stricture
Retrocaval ureter		Meatal stenosis
		Phimosis
ACQUIRED INTRINSIC DEFECTS		
Calculi	Benign prostatic hypertrophy	Stricture
Inflammation	Cancer of prostate	Tumor
Trauma	Cancer of bladder	Calculi
Sloughed papillae	Calculi	Trauma
Tumor	Diabetic neuropathy	Phimosis
Blood clots	Spinal cord disease	
Uric acid crystals		
ACQUIRED EXTRINSIC DEFECTS		
Pregnant uterus	Carcinoma of cervix, colon	Trauma
Retroperitoneal fibrosis	Trauma	
Aortic aneurysm		
Uterine leiomyomata		
Carcinoma of uterus, prostate, bladder, colon, rectum		
Retroperitoneal lymphoma		
Accidental surgical ligation		

* *Lesions are typically associated with unilateral obstruction.*
† *Lesions are typically associated with bilateral obstruction.*

bladder to ureter(s) is more common in children than adults and may result in severe unilateral or bilateral hydroureter and hydronephrosis. Abnormal insertion of the ureter into the bladder is the most common cause of vesicoureteral reflux in children. Reflux occurring in the absence of urinary tract infection or bladder neck obstruction usually does not lead to renal parenchymal damage and often resolves spontaneously as the child matures. Surgical reinsertion of the ureter into the bladder is indicated if reflux is severe and unlikely to improve spontaneously, if renal function deteriorates, or if urinary tract infections recur despite chronic antimicrobial therapy.

CLINICAL FEATURES Pain is the symptom which most commonly provokes the need for medical attention. The pain of urinary tract obstruction is due to distention of the collecting system or renal capsule. The severity of the pain is influenced more by the rate at which distention develops than the degree of distention. Acute supravesical obstruction, as from a stone lodged in a ureter (Chap. 284), is associated with excruciatingly severe pain, usually called *renal colic*. This pain is relatively steady and continuous, with little fluctuation in intensity, and often radiates to the lower abdomen, testes, or labia. The patient with renal colic is usually restless and unable to remain still. By contrast, more insidious causes of obstruction, such as chronic narrowing of the ureteropelvic junction, may produce little or no pain, yet result in total destruction of the affected kidney. Flank pain which comes on only with micturition is pathognomonic of vesicoureteral reflux.

Symptoms of *polyuria* and *nocturia* commonly accompany chronic partial urinary tract obstruction and result from impaired renal concentrating ability. This defect usually does not improve with administration of exogenous vasopressin and is therefore a form of acquired nephrogenic diabetes insipidus. Disturbances in sodium chloride transport in the ascending limb of Henle and, in azotemic patients, the osmotic (urea) diuresis per nephron lead to decreased medullary hypertonicity and, hence, a concentrating defect. Partial obstruction, therefore, may be associated with increased rather than decreased urine output. Indeed, wide fluctuations in urinary output in a patient with azotemia should always raise the possibility of intermittent or partial urinary tract obstruction. If fluid intake becomes inadequate in these patients, severe dehydration and hypernatremia may develop. On the other hand, complete and bilateral obstruction, or complete unilateral obstruction in a patient with only one previously functioning kidney, results in *total anuria*. Hesitancy and straining to initiate the urinary stream, postvoid dribbling, urinary frequency, and (overflow) incontinence are complaints common to patients with obstruction at or below the level of the bladder (see Chap. 44).

In addition to loss of urinary concentrating ability and azotemia, partial bilateral urinary tract obstruction often results in other derangements of renal function, including *acquired distal renal tubular acidosis* and *renal salt wasting*. These defects in tubule function are often accompanied by histological evidence of widespread renal tubulointerstitial damage. Morphological abnormalities appear early in the course of obstruction; initially the interstitium becomes edematous and infiltrated with mononuclear inflammatory cells. With continued obstruction, the interstitium becomes fibrotic; scarring and atrophy of the papilla and medulla occur and precede these processes in the cortex.

The possibility of urinary tract obstruction must always be considered in patients with urinary tract infections or urolithiasis. Urinary stasis encourages the growth of organisms as well as the formation of crystals, especially magnesium ammonium

phosphate (struvite). Systemic manifestations of urinary tract obstruction include *hypertension* and *polycythemia*. Hypertension is seen frequently in acute and subacute forms of unilateral obstruction and is usually a consequence of increased release of renin by the involved kidney. Chronic unilateral or bilateral hydronephrosis, in the absence of extracellular volume expansion or other forms of renal disease, rarely results in significant hypertension. Polycythemia, an infrequent complication of obstructive uropathy, is probably secondary to increased erythropoietin production by the obstructed kidney.

DIAGNOSIS A history of difficulty in voiding, pain, infection, or changes in urinary volume is common. Evidence for distention of the kidney or urinary bladder often can be obtained by palpation and percussion of the abdomen. A careful rectal examination may reveal enlargement or nodularity of the prostate, abnormal rectal sphincter tone, or a rectal or pelvic mass. The penis should be inspected for evidence of meatal stenosis or phimosis. In the female, vaginal, uterine, and rectal lesions responsible for urinary tract obstruction are usually revealed by inspection and palpation.

Urinalysis and examination of the urine sediment may reveal hematuria, pyuria, and bacteriuria. Often, however, the urine sediment is devoid of abnormal elements, even when obstruction leads to marked azotemia and extensive structural damage. An abdominal scout film should be obtained to evaluate the possibility of nephrocalcinosis or a radiopaque stone at any level of the urinary collecting system. Once urinary tract obstruction is suspected, definitive diagnosis invariably requires intravenous pyelography. If the patient is not azotemic, a standard dose of contrast medium usually provides adequate information. With renal insufficiency, however, high-dose (drip-infusion) pyelography with nephrotomography is usually required for adequate visualization. In the presence of obstruction, the appearance time of the nephrogram is often delayed but eventually becomes more dense than normal because of slow tubular fluid flow rate which results in enhanced water reabsorption by the nephrons and greater concentration of contrast medium within tubules. The kidney involved by an acute obstructive process is usually slightly enlarged, and there is dilatation of the calyxes, renal pelvis, and ureter above the obstruction. The ureter, however, is not tortuous, as is the case when the obstruction is chronic. In comparison with the nephrogram, the pyelogram may be extremely faint, especially if the dilated renal pelvis is voluminous, causing dilution of the contrast medium. The radiographic study should be continued until the site of obstruction is determined or the contrast medium is excreted. Delayed films taken as long as 48 h after contrast administration may be necessary to determine the exact site of obstruction.

Patients with intermittent ureteropelvic obstruction (whether functional or mechanical) should have radiological evaluation while they are in pain, since a normal pyelogram is commonly seen during asymptomatic periods. Hydration or mannitol infusion often helps to provoke a symptomatic attack. Patients with obstruction at or below the level of the bladder exhibit thickening, trabeculation, and diverticula of the bladder wall. Postvoiding films reveal residual urine. Voiding cystourethrography is of great value in the diagnosis of vesicoureteral reflux and bladder neck and urethral obstructions. If these radiographic studies fail to provide adequate information for diagnosis, endoscopic visualization by the urologist often permits precise identification of lesions involving the urethra, prostate, bladder, and ureteral orifices; insertion of retrograde ureteral catheters enables evaluation of ureters and renal collecting systems (retrograde pyelography) but is associated with risk of infection. Renal imaging with radionuclides, and ultrasonography, is also proving increasingly useful and reliable in the diagnosis of urinary tract obstruction. Finally, the diagnosis of functional obstruction may be facilitated by cineradiographic studies of ureteral peristalsis and bladder emptying.

TREATMENT AND PROGNOSIS An individual with any form of urinary tract obstruction complicated by infection requires relief of obstruction as soon as possible to prevent development of generalized sepsis and progressive renal damage. On a temporary basis, depending on the site of obstruction, drainage is often satisfactorily achieved by nephrostomy, ureterostomy, or ureteral, urethral, or suprapubic catheterization. When infection is not present, immediate surgery often is not required, even in the presence of complete obstruction and anuria (because of the availability of dialysis), at least until acid-base, fluid and electrolyte, and cardiovascular status have returned to normal. Nevertheless, the site of obstruction should be ascertained as soon as feasible, in part because of the possibility that sepsis may occur and necessitate prompt urologic intervention. Elective relief of obstruction is usually recommended in patients with urinary retention, recurrent urinary tract infections, persistent pain, or progressive loss of renal function. Infrequently, mechanical obstruction can be alleviated by nonsurgical means, as with radiation therapy for retroperitoneal lymphoma. Likewise, functional obstruction secondary to neurogenic bladder may be decreased with the combination of frequent voiding and cholinergic drugs. The approach to obstruction secondary to renal stones is discussed in Chap. 284.

With relief of obstruction, the *prognosis* regarding return of renal function depends largely upon whether irreversible renal damage has occurred. When obstruction is not relieved, the patient's course will depend mainly on whether the obstruction is complete or incomplete, bilateral or unilateral, and whether urinary tract infection is also present. Complete obstruction with infection can lead to total destruction of the kidney within days. Experimental studies in dogs suggest that relief of complete obstruction of 1 and 2 weeks' duration restores glomerular filtration rate to 60 and 30 percent of normal, respectively; after 8 weeks, recovery does not occur. If an obstructed kidney has no possibility of regaining function, surgical intervention is rarely indicated.

POSTOBSTRUCTIVE DIURESIS Relief of bilateral, but not unilateral, complete urinary tract obstruction commonly leads to a postobstructive diuresis, characterized by polyuria, which may be massive. The urine is usually hypotonic and may contain a large amount of sodium chloride. The natriuresis is due, at least in part, to the excretion of retained urea, which acts as a poorly reabsorbable solute and diminishes salt and water reabsorption in the tubules (osmotic diuresis). The increase in intratubular pressure very likely also contributes to the impairment in net sodium chloride reabsorption, especially in the terminal nephron segments. It has been suggested that natriuretic factors (other than urea) also accumulate during uremia induced by obstruction and serve to depress tubule salt and water reabsorption when urine flow is reestablished. In the vast majority of patients this diuresis is physiological, resulting in the *appropriate* excretion of the excesses of salt and water retained during the period of obstruction. When extracellular volume and composition return to normal, the diuresis usually abates spontaneously. Therefore, replacement of urinary losses should serve only to prevent hypovolemia, hypotension, or disturbances in serum electrolyte concentrations. Occasionally, iatrogenic expansion of extracellular volume, secondary to administration of excessive quantities of intravenous fluids, is responsible for, or sustains, the diuresis observed in the postobstructive period. Replacement of no more than two-thirds of urinary volume losses per day is usually effective in avoiding

this complication. In a rare patient, however, relief of obstruction may be followed by urinary salt and water losses severe enough to provoke profound dehydration and vascular collapse. In these patients, an intrinsic defect in tubule reabsorptive function is probably responsible for the marked diuresis. Appropriate therapy in such patients includes intravenous administration of large quantities of salt-containing solutions to replace sodium and volume deficits.

REFERENCES

GUGGENHEIM SJ, SCHRIER RW: Obstructive nephropathy: Pathophysiology and management, in *Renal and Electrolyte Disorders*, RW Schrier (ed). Boston, Little, Brown, 1976

HARRIS RH, YARGER WE: The pathogenesis of post-obstructive diuresis. J Clin Invest 56:880, 1975

WILSON DR: Renal function during and following obstruction. Annu Rev Med, 28:329, 1977

WRIGHT FS, HOWARDS SS: Obstructive injury, in *The Kidney*, 2d ed, BM Brenner, FC Rector Jr (eds). Philadelphia, Saunders, 1980, chap 38

286
TUMORS OF THE URINARY TRACT

BARRY M. BRENNER
H. DAVID HUMES

TUMORS OF THE KIDNEY

BENIGN RENAL TUMORS Several benign tumors are known to arise in renal parenchyma. They usually remain small in size and are recognized as incidental findings at autopsy or nephrectomy, the latter performed for other reasons. *Adenomas* are the most common benign renal tumors, occurring as small (5- to 10-mm) nodules in from 10 to 20 percent of all kidneys examined grossly. With other less frequently encountered benign lesions, including hamartomas (angiomyolipomas) and hemangiopericytomas, adenomas may be responsible for recurrent painless hematuria. Since adenomas are believed to undergo malignant transformation and are histologically indistinguishable from some renal-cell carcinomas, nephrectomy is appropriate when they are detected clinically. *Hamartomas* are observed commonly in patients with tuberous sclerosis but also occur in individuals without this ectodermal defect. Hamartomas may be unilateral or bilateral, contain vascular, fat, and smooth-muscle components, and rarely, if ever, undergo malignant change. By angiography, these highly vascular lesions often reveal multiple small arterial aneurysms. *Hemangiopericytomas* are uncommon benign renal tumors arising from capillary pericytes in the region of the juxtaglomerular apparatus. They have been associated with increased renin production and hypertension, both of which usually disappear with resection of the tumor.

MALIGNANT RENAL TUMORS **Renal-cell carcinoma (hypernephroma, adenocarcinoma of kidney)** This is the most common renal neoplasm, occurring almost exclusively in adults over age 20. The yellow color of this fleshy tumor initially led to the erroneous impression that is arises from "adrenal rests"—hence the term *hypernephroma*. Instead, renal-cell carcinoma is of tubular epithelial origin, with tumor cells often arranged in a tubular or cord-like distribution.

CLINICAL FEATURES Renal-cell carcinoma has been called the "internist's tumor" because the lesion is often diagnosed, even in the absence of metastases, from *systemic* rather than urologic manifestations. The triad of *gross hematuria, flank pain,* and a *palpable abdominal mass,* although considered as classic evidence for the clinical diagnosis of renal-cell carcinoma, is encountered relatively infrequently, appearing in less than 10 percent of cases. Clinically, the most common presenting abnormality is *hematuria,* which occurs in about 60 percent of cases. Unfortunately, although microscopic hematuria is a consistent abnormality of the urinary sediment examination, bleeding is not usually evident grossly, so that the tumor often grows to large size before symptoms appear. These include pain and a sensation of fullness in the flank. By this time, the tumor has often invaded the renal capsule and local renal veins which provide the main route to distant metastases, especially to lungs, brain, and bone. Local spread to liver and perirenal lymph nodes is also common.

Systemic symptoms of *fatigability, weight loss,* and *cachexia* are found in about half the patients with renal-cell carcinoma. *Intermittent fever,* unassociated with evidence of infection, occurs occasionally and may be the only sign of this renal neoplasm. *Anemia* is common and is a presenting sign in approximately 50 percent of cases. *Erythrocytosis,* on the other hand, seen in about 5 percent of patients, is almost certainly due to erythropoietin production by tumor cells. *Eosinophilia, leukemoid reactions, thrombocytosis,* and *increased erythrocyte sedimentation rate* are other hematologic abnormalities associated with this tumor. Renal-cell carcinomas are capable of producing a number of hormones or hormone-like substances, including *parathyroid hormone* and *prostaglandins* (which, in turn, may lead to hypercalcemia), *prolactin* (galactorrhea), *renin* (hypertension), *gonadotropins* (feminization or masculinization), and *glucocorticoids* (Cushing's syndrome). In very vascular tumors, *intrarenal arteriovenous fistulas* may predispose to high-output congestive heart failure. Tumor invasion of the renal vein and inferior vena cava may result in symptomatic left *varicocele* and *dependent edema,* respectively. Alternatively, hepatic vein occlusion by tumor, with or without vena caval obstruction, may lead to *hepatosplenomegaly* and *ascites* formation. Reversible disturbances in liver function are sometimes found in affected patients, even in the absence of liver metastases. These include Bromsulphalein retention, elevated alkaline phosphatase, hypoalbuminemia, and prolongation of the prothrombin time. Finally, nearly two-thirds of patients with von Hippel-Lindau disease, characterized by hereditary vascular malformations of the retina and cerebellum, develop renal-cell carcinomas, which are often multiple and bilateral.

DIAGNOSIS Although intrarenal calcifications and/or alterations in renal contours seen on the abdominal scout film may suggest the presence of a renal-cell carcinoma, excretion urography (with nephrotomography) is the primary examination by which most renal masses are detected and initially evaluated. Renal ultrasonography and needle aspiration of cystic lesions, with evaluation of fluid for cytology and fat content, are additional diagnostic tools to distinguish simple cysts from tumor. Selective renal arteriography reveals abnormal tumor vessels (neovascularization) in approximately 95 percent of patients with renal-cell carcinoma. Renal arteriographic abnormalities associated with this neoplasm include hypervascularity, arteriovenous communications (pooling of contrast media in venous sinusoids within the tumor mass), and evidence of tumor invasion of the major renal veins and inferior vena cava. Whereas nontumor vasculature undergoes brisk vasoconstriction in response to local renal arterial infusion of epinephrine, the abnormal tumor vessels fail to constrict and, therefore, persist as a "tumor blush" when epinephrine is infused. Examination of urinary cytology, although useful in the diagnosis of neoplasms of the renal pelvis, ureter, and bladder, has not been helpful in renal cell carcinoma. Once the diagnosis of renal-cell carcinoma is established, chest x-ray and scans of bone, liver, and brain should be obtained to evaluate the possibility of metastatic involvement.

PROGNOSIS AND TREATMENT The prognosis in patients with renal-cell carcinoma is largely dependent upon the extent of tumor involvement at the time of diagnosis. The current overall 5-year survival rate is about 45 percent. If distant metastases are not evident, this survival rate increases to nearly 65 percent. The conventional approach to treatment in patients without evidence of metastases is *radical nephrectomy.* An aggressive approach has also been endorsed by some surgeons for patients having evidence of a solitary metastasis. Although scattered reports in the literature suggest the possibility of spontaneous regression of various metastatic foci following surgical removal of the primary lesion, it is generally believed that nephrectomy in patients with disseminated disease should be employed mainly to relieve symptoms resulting from the primary tumor, such as severe pain or bleeding. The response of metastatic renal-cell carcinoma to treatment with chemotherapy, hormonal agents, or radiotherapy has generally been unsatisfactory.

Nephroblastoma (Wilms's tumor) Nephroblastoma is the second most common malignant tumor of the kidney and is the most common malignancy of the urinary tract in children. Peak incidence occurs between the ages of 2 and 4 years, with 90 percent of cases recognized under the age of 8. Fewer than 150 cases have been reported in adults. This tumor arises from mesonephric mesoderm (embryonic nephrogenic tissue) and contains a multitude of cell types, including epithelia, muscle, bone, and cartilage. The tumor often reaches very large size, may be bilateral, and presents as a palpable mass in 50 percent or more of cases. Hematuria, pain, fever, and hypertension are other common abnormalities noted at time of diagnosis. All these manifestations of nephroblastoma respond favorably to nephrectomy. Although once considered an incurable tumor, aggressive programs of pre- and postoperative irradiation and postoperative chemotherapy with actinomycin D (often in combination with vincristine) have improved the prognosis markedly, and the 5-year survival now exceeds 75 percent.

TUMORS OF THE URINARY COLLECTING SYSTEM

Tumors of the renal pelvis, ureter, and urinary bladder, derived from transitional epithelia, account for 10 to 15 percent of all primary malignancies in adults. These *urothelial* carcinomas are multicentric in nature and often occur (and recur) at multiple sites in the lower urinary tract in an affected patient. The wall of the urinary bladder is the most commonly involved site of involvement. Epidemiologic studies have confirmed a markedly increased incidence of bladder cancer in workers exposed to various aromatic amines employed in the dyeing, chemical, and rubber industries. It has been suggested that exposure to synthetic sweeteners, food colors, tobacco, and coffee may account for a large proportion of other cases.

Hematuria is the sole presenting complaint in nearly all cases, irrespective of the exact level of urinary tract involvement. When the tumor arises in the renal pelvis or upper ureter, gross hematuria may be associated with signs and symptoms of *ureteral colic,* due to obstruction by blood clots. Intravenous and/or retrograde pyelography, cystoscopy with biopsy, and urine cytology are the main approaches to establishing the site, nature, and extent of involvement of tumors of the collecting system. Endoscopic brush biopsy is used for upper tract lesions. Urothelial tumors tend to spread by local invasion. Prognosis is, therefore, dependent upon extent of invasion and degree of anaplasia at time of diagnosis, with patients with bladder carcinoma having less than a 30 percent chance for 5-year survival when tumor extends beyond the bladder wall. The prognosis is considerably better when the tumor is confined to the bladder and is treated with cystectomy, usually in combination with local radiotherapy. Nephroureterectomy is the treatment of choice for urothelial tumors of the renal pelvis or ureter.

Squamous-cell carcinoma is a less frequent neoplasm of the renal pelvis than is the papillary, transitional-cell variety and has an extremely poor prognosis. Squamous-cell tumors have been shown to occur more commonly in patients with recurrent nephrolithiasis and upper urinary tract infections. A high incidence of bladder cancer of the squamous type has been found in patients with chronic parasitic infestation due to *Schistosoma haematobium.*

Benign hypertrophy and adenocarcinoma of the prostate, extremely common disorders in men beyond age 50, are considered in Chap. 341.

REFERENCES

CAMPBELL MF, HARRISON JH (eds): *Urology,* 4th ed. Philadelphia, Saunders, 1978

CRONIN RE et al: Renal cell carcinoma: Unusual systemic manifestations. Medicine 55:291, 1976

RICHIE JP, SKINNER DG: Renal neoplasia, in *The Kidney,* 2d ed, BM Brenner, FC Rector Jr (eds). Philadelphia, Saunders, 1980, chap 40

section 5 | Disorders of the alimentary tract

287
APPROACH TO THE PATIENT WITH GASTROINTESTINAL DISEASE

KURT J. ISSELBACHER
ROGER J. MAY

GENERAL CONSIDERATIONS Gastrointestinal symptoms occur not only with primary gastrointestinal tract disease but frequently as manifestations of other systemic diseases. Thus anorexia, nausea, and vomiting may be seen in congestive failure and uremia, and diarrhea or constipation may be seen as a consequence of metabolic derangements such as electrolyte changes or alterations in thyroid function. With today's technical advances one finds too often that the physician is willing to diagnose (or misdiagnose) gastrointestinal disease simply by relying on routine x-ray studies of the upper and lower parts of the gastrointestinal tract. Such an overwhelming dependence on technical procedures often leads to great pitfalls. In order to define the most probable and profitable area to study, the proper approach requires careful attention to the history and physical examination before ordering the appropriate diagnostic tests.

IMPORTANCE OF THE HISTORY To evaluate gastrointestinal symptoms, a careful history is crucial. Pain or indigestion is the most common intestinal complaint. Correlation between pain and gastrointestinal function must of necessity be chronologic. There should be a meticulous inquiry as to the frequency and specificity of the complaint. The questioning should include the location of the pain and whether it is circumscribed or diffuse. It is important to determine what factors aggravate or relieve the discomfort. *Does eating produce the symptom?* If so, determine whether the discomfort occurs *while eating* (as in esophageal disorders and abdominal angina), shortly *after the meal* (as often occurs in biliary tract disease), or *30 to 90 min later* (as typically seen with peptic ulcer). *Does eating relieve*

the symptom, and if so, for how long? Temporary relief of epigastric pain is characteristic of gastritis and peptic ulceration. Many patients have tried or taken antacids by the time they come to the physician, and a history indicating relief of epigastric pain by antacids is suggestive of peptic disease of the upper part of the intestine. *What is the relation of pain to bowel movements?* The patient with ulcerative colitis often obtains temporary relief from lower abdominal cramps by defecation.

Attention should be paid to *anorexia* and weight *loss;* their combined occurrence should make one suspicious of an underlying malignancy. If weight loss is accompanied by an increased appetite, one must consider the diagnosis of malabsorption or maldigestion as well as a hypermetabolic state, such as thyrotoxicosis. If *diarrhea* is present, one should determine the average number of the stools and their consistency. To some patients, diarrhea means an increased number of stools, even though they are relatively normal in consistency; to others, diarrhea means watery stools. In a patient with diarrhea one should ask about stool *odor* (malodorous stools being typical of pancreatic insufficiency and sprue), change in stool *color* (light-colored stools are seen with steatorrhea or cholestasis), and whether blood or mucus has been noted. (Blood is characteristic of ulcerative colitis but is hardly ever noted in functional bowel disease.)

Finally, careful attention must be given to a "drug history." We are living in a "medicated society." Unless asked, patients may forget to mention that they take aspirin almost daily for headache, and this may indeed account for occult blood in stool. Many patients take daily laxatives, which may explain chronic diarrhea and colonic changes on x-ray.

PHYSICAL EXAMINATION AND ENDOSCOPY A vague history of abdominal distress may be brought into focus by a thorough physical examination. Upper abdominal distress together with tenderness in the right upper quadrant suggests that cholecystitis or hepatitis may be present. The history of intermittent abdominal pain together with a palpable mass or tender loop of bowel in the right lower quadrant should make one suspicious of regional enteritis. All too often, however, in gastrointestinal diseases the routine physical examination is negative, and other techniques for examining the intestine are needed. Among the techniques which should almost be routine as an extension of the physical examination is *sigmoidoscopy*. This technique is important in the diagnosis of colonic cancer because (1) approximately 50 percent of large-intestine malignancies are within the reach of the sigmoidoscope; and (2) small rectosigmoid tumors may be missed on examination after a barium enema because of the tortuosity and redundancy of the intestine in this area. Sigmoidoscopy also permits inspection of the mucosa for edema, erythema, friability, or ulceration. In a patient with diarrhea due to nonspecific causes, the mucosa may be normal; with dysentery due to agents such as *Shigella,* the mucosa may become friable, edematous, and hyperemic; if the latter findings are combined with extensive ulcerations, ulcerative or amebic colitis may be present.

With the advent of *fiberoptic instruments,* it has become much easier and less hazardous to perform endoscopic procedures. Gastroscopy is valuable in helping to determine whether a gastric ulcer is benign or malignant. Endoscopy has become an increasingly routine technique in the approach to selected patients with upper gastrointestinal bleeding. Colonoscopy with fiberoptic equipment permits direct examination of mucosa beyond the customary 25 cm of the rigid sigmoidoscope. (For details see Chap. 288.)

RADIOLOGIC EXAMINATION Perhaps in no other organ system is the use of x-ray examination as important to diagnosis as in disorders of the intestinal tract. In fact, with few exceptions, investigation of the patient with gastrointestinal symptoms is not complete without appropriate x-ray examination. However, all too often x-ray examination is ordered by the physician without attention to a number of important factors.

Initial considerations by the internist To obtain the best and most effective use of gastrointestinal x-rays, the physician must decide (1) which *organ system* is most likely to be involved, (2) in what *sequence* to perform the x-rays, and (3) whether there are any *contraindications* to the proposed radiologic study.

After ordering an upper gastrointestinal series and finding the results negative, the physician may decide to order a barium enema only to learn that it must be delayed because of the presence of barium from the prior study. Therefore, if a thorough study of the intestinal tract is contemplated, the sequence should be (1) oral cholecystogram, (2) barium enema, and (3) upper gastrointestinal series. Preparation or prior cleansing of the intestinal tract is important for a proper barium enema examination, but the physician must keep in mind that with obstructing lesions of the colon or small intestine or in the presence of active ulcerative colitis, the use of strong cathartics may be hazardous and even life-threatening. *No x-ray preparation should be considered routine.* In fact, the barium examination itself may aggravate an acute ulcerative colitis or precipitate colonic perforation or the onset of toxic megacolon. Similarly, if partial obstruction of the intestine is detected by plain x-ray of the abdomen, the physician must be wary of introducing barium from above for fear of producing further or complete intestinal obstruction.

Consultation with the radiologist One cannot overemphasize the importance of providing the radiologist with as much information as possible about the nature of the disease process under investigation. Though this can be done in writing (on the x-ray requisition), it is often preferable to do it verbally. In fact, in difficult cases it is advantageous for the physician to join the radiologist during the study. In addition, the radiologist may suggest, for example, that instead of barium an iodinated ra-

diopaque dye may be preferable; that the study should be supplemented with angiography, especially in the patient with gastrointestinal bleeding or portal hypertension; or that the examination be repeated with more adequate preparation of the patient.

Interpretation All too often the busy physician allows a negative x-ray report to be the decisive factor in the diagnosis. If the patient has had weight loss and a change in bowel habits and the physician suspects a colonic neoplasm, inspection of the x-rays (personally or preferably with the radiologist) may in fact reveal that the patient had too much retained fecal material in his colon or that the area of concern was never well visualized. Similarly, if the patient has typical ulcer symptoms or a classic history of biliary colic, the physician should not discard the diagnosis merely because of a negative x-ray report.

On the other hand the physician must be able to determine whether the abnormal finding is causally related to the symptoms. This is especially true in older patients where the presence of a hiatus hernia, gallstones, or diverticulosis is not unusual and hence may be coincidental.

DIAGNOSTIC APPROACHES Problems of swallowing The approach should be as follows:

1 Careful visual and *neurologic examination* of the pharynx, with tests for myasthenia gravis if indicated.
2 *Routine esophageal x-rays* in the upright and lateral or Trendelenburg position. The horizontal views are essential for demonstration of the swallowing mechanism, unaided by gravity, and of the esophagogastric junction. For details of the pharyngoesophageal area cineradiography is necessary because of the rapidity with which the contrast media passes through. Hiatus hernia is extremely common (in 15 to 35 percent of persons over 50) and often asymptomatic unless reflux of gastric contents can be demonstrated to occur repeatedly.
3 *Esophagoscopy* is desirable to describe lesions suggested by x-ray, or if the lesion is unsuspected, to obtain biopsies from masses or abnormal mucosa, and to obtain washings for exfoliative cytologic study. The diagnosis of peptic esophagitis is best made endoscopically. Esophageal varices can be identified by this approach when they are too small to be seen radiologically, although the latter technique will pick up 70 percent of large varices.
4 *Manometric studies* of the upper esophagus, particularly in conjunction with cineradiography, at present offer the best differential between disorders primary in the central nervous system, primary pharyngeal muscular disease, and cricopharyngeal dystonia. Manometry of the lower esophagus is useful in the diagnosis of diffuse esophageal spasm, achalasia, and infiltrative diseases which can alter esophageal motility.

Peptic or digestive disorders The approaches to these disorders include:

1 *Insertion of a nasogastric tube.* This is used to establish whether significant gastric retention (more than 75 ml of gastric contents in the fasting state) exists, and whether there is acid, bile, blood, or other material in these contents. If pyloric obstruction or gastric atony is present, the tube is used to maintain suction while the patient's electrolyte and fluid balance is restored to normal; the stomach is kept as clean as possible so that reliable radiologic investigation may be carried out.
2 *Radiologic examination* of stomach, duodenum, and the upper part of the jejunum is the most important single procedure in this area. The single examination of the stomach carries an overall accuracy of about 80 percent if the lumen is carefully cleaned out beforehand; duodenal lesions are

most precisely identified (90 percent). However, gastritis and superficial ulcers of the duodenum may be missed with routine barium studies. The hypotonic duodenogram is an important technique for the demonstration of intra- or extraduodenal lesions. This is accomplished by giving an anticholinergic agent or glucagon intravenously to produce atony of the duodenum and allow better definition of mucosal detail by the barium.

3 When lesions are noted radiographically in the stomach, *upper intestinal endoscopy* may be very helpful in identifying the diffuseness of the mucosal response in gastritis or, together with biopsy and brushings for cytology, in differentiating between peptic and neoplastic ulcerating lesions. Gastroscopy may permit the diagnosis of superficial erosive gastritis and the Mallory-Weiss syndrome as a cause of bleeding when the x-ray examination is negative. It may identify a specific bleeding site in clinical situations where several potential bleeding sites could exist, such as in the patient with portal hypertension. Gastroscopy is also particularly helpful in inspecting the postoperative stomach, especially when stomal ulceration is expected. It is useful in detecting bile reflux. The first and second portions of the duodenum can also be examined with the fiberoptic gastroscope, and important information about ulcers and other lesions can be obtained by this procedure.

4 *Gastric acid secretory studies* are useful in the diagnosis of the Zollinger-Ellison syndrome and suspected carcinoma or atrophic gastritis, and for determination of completeness of vagotomy. They should not be obtained for the routine diagnosis of uncomplicated duodenal ulcer. There is no convincing evidence that acid studies are useful in determining the type of surgery for duodenal ulcer.

The only reliable technique for measuring rates of gastric acid production employs an indwelling tube and requires careful attention to details of tube placement, handling of samples, and analysis. Presently this method is used in one of two ways: (1) *Basal secretion* is that obtained in the morning after an overnight fast in an unstimulated stomach; it measures vagal plus hormonal factors acting on the gastric mucosa. After discarding the first aspirate, four samples are taken over a period of an hour, while the patient expectorates any saliva. The absence of hydrochloric acid in any of the four samples is considered incompatible with the presence of an active duodenal ulcer. (2) *Maximum acid output* is assessed by collecting samples every 15 min for an hour in a patient who has previously received parenteral histamine equal to 0.04 mg histamine acid phosphate per kilogram of body weight; if the safer analogue, betazole, is used, 2 mg per kilogram of body weight is administered. One may also give pentagastrin (6 μg/kg) intramuscularly. With these drugs one attempts to obtain maximal stimulation of parietal cells. The maximum output is proportional to the total "parietal cell mass." Achlorhydria is defined as the failure of the stomach so stimulated to produce a juice with a pH less than 6. The normal basal fasting secretion is 30 to 70 ml/h, with acid production being 1 to 5 meq/h. Average maximal acid output is 20 meq/h with the upper limit of normal approximately 40 meq/h. In the Zollinger-Ellison syndrome basal acid secretion is usually greater than 10 meq/h and exceeds 60 percent of the maximal acid output. Increased serum gastrin level may confirm the diagnosis.

Obstructive and vascular disorders of the small intestine When intestinal problems present as obstructive syndromes, the plain x-ray of the abdomen is the most important diagnostic adjunct to careful physical examination. Patterns of dilatation of individual loops of intestine may be characteristic, as in volvulus or acute pancreatitis; erect and decubitus views will often show fluid levels in the affected segments. Air under the diaphragm is diagnostic of a perforated viscus; air in the portal vein usually results from intestinal necrosis secondary to mesenteric vascular occlusion. The diagnostic accuracy of the plain x-ray in all types of intestinal obstruction is about 75 percent. Celiac artery angiography is of particular value in the diagnosis of mesenteric vascular disease.

Inflammatory and neoplastic diseases of small and large intestine Patients with these conditions are usually identified by history, physical examination, and careful examination of the stools for exudate and blood. Sigmoidoscopy is valuable in identifying mucosal and neoplastic lesions of the lower 25 cm of the colon. The mucosal surface of the entire colon and terminal ileum can be examined directly and biopsied through the fiberoptic colonoscope. This technique is valuable in differentiating between inflammatory and neoplastic stricture, or in evaluating polypoid lesions beyond the reach of the sigmoidoscope. The radiologic examination of the small intestine is highly reliable in identifying the prestenotic and stenotic lesions of Crohn's disease. In the colon a single examination in a well-prepared patient has a diagnostic accuracy of 80 to 85 percent; the addition of air-contrast technique brings the accuracy up over 90 percent, but none of these figures is meaningful if the patient is poorly prepared for the examination. In the demonstration of small polyps the degree of accuracy is understandably not so high, but for polyps larger than 1 cm, which are of greater clinical importance, it is satisfactory. The cecal area is the hardest to examine adequately because of its anatomy; flat plaquelike lesions on the posterior wall are particularly hard to demonstrate. The rectal area is usually better visualized proctoscopically than it is radiologically. The immunologic assay for the carcinoembryonic antigen has not proved to be specific for colonic cancer; nevertheless, it does contribute to the evaluation of the extent of tumor and to the detection of residual or recurrent disease in postoperative patients.

Peroral biopsy of the small intestine and forceps biopsy of the rectosigmoid are of considerable importance in revealing mucosal disease. Rectal biopsy is an excellent means of demonstrating amyloidosis, schistosomiasis, and amebiasis. Submucosal disease is not seen in these superficial biopsies. Hirschsprung's disease is histologically diagnosed by a deep surgical biopsy of the lower part of the rectum.

Malabsorption syndromes Malabsorption may be suspected on the basis of history and physical examination and is confirmed by examination of the stools. Radiologic examination is of general help in ruling out local lesions and suggesting motor and secretory dysfunction, but it is rarely diagnostic unless an abnormal small-bowel mucosa or fistulas between intestine and stomach are demonstrated.

The tests useful in the diagnosis of malabsorption are discussed in Chap. 291. A simple screening test for excessive fat in the stools can be accomplished by the microscopic examination of a stool specimen stained with Sudan. Chemical analysis of 3-day stool collection for fat, with the patient on a standard diet, is used to establish the diagnosis of malabsorption. The D-xylose absorption test is about 90 percent accurate in separating mucosal disease from pancreatic insufficiency. Peroral biopsy of the small intestine is of value in the diagnosis of celiac disease, and may show the less common infiltrations of the mucosa by amyloid or bacterial mucoproteins (Whipple's disease). Leakage of protein into the intestinal lumen may cause hypoproteinemia and can be demonstrated by the recovery in stools of intravenously administered markers such as albumin labeled with iodine or chromium isotopes.

Pancreas The pancreas is difficult to study directly because of its anatomic location and relative inaccessibility. Calcification of the pancreas on a plain abdominal film is highly suggestive of chronic pancreatitis and may be associated with fat malabsorption. Pancreatic exocrine insufficiency can be documented by intubation of the duodenum and collection of pancreatic juice after stimulation with secretin or a test meal. The pancreatic duct can be cannulated via the fiberoptic duodenoscope; pancreatic juice can then be collected for cytology, or the duct visualized by the injection of a radiopaque dye. This latter is helpful in the diagnosis of pancreatic tumors and cysts. Angiography, abdominal ultrasound, and computerized tomography may also be useful in the diagnosis of pancreatic disease. See Chaps. 308 and 309.

288
GASTROINTESTINAL ENDOSCOPY

FRED E. SILVERSTEIN
CYRUS E. RUBIN

Fiberendoscopes have revolutionized the examination of the gastrointestinal tract. Because of the flexibility of the fiberoptic bundles and because of controllability of the instrument tip, the operator can steer the instrument around multiple bends under visual control. A side channel permits passage of a variety of endoscopic tools such as biopsy forceps, foreign-body forceps, cytology brushes, wash tubes, and electrocautery snares. The viewing window and the light at the instrument's distal end can be washed free of obscuring material. Fluid can be aspirated from hollow organs, and air can be insufflated as needed to improve visualization.

The usefulness of fiberendoscopy in diagnosing gastrointestinal disease is well established. Shallow lesions such as erosions or healing ulcers may be missed by routine x-ray but not by endoscopy. The brilliant success of polypectomy via the colonoscope has led to the development of other endoscopic methods of treatment which may replace some invasive surgical techniques; the most significant advances in the future will probably be in this area.

Although esophagogastroduodenoscopy (EGD) is not a procedure for the occasional operator, it should be available in every general hospital. It is a relatively easy procedure to perform technically, but training and continued experience are necessary for optimal diagnostic accuracy. Complications are most frequent when the operator is inexperienced. Before the procedure the competent endoscopist always takes a history and examines the patient. Prior evaluation of cardiac status and clotting mechanisms is also essential.

The more complex procedures such as colonoscopy and endoscopic retrograde cholangiopancreatography (ERCP) require special dexterity, a substantial investment of time for learning, and constant practice to maintain adequate skill; they are probably best accomplished by subspecialists. Colonoscopy, one hopes, will be simplified so that it can be as widely available as esophagogastroduodenoscopy.

UPPER GASTROINTESTINAL ENDOSCOPY Forward-viewing, oblique, and side-viewing instruments may be used for EGD. After a careful explanation of the procedure to the patient, pharyngeal topical anesthesia with viscous lidocaine is followed by intravenous diazepam to the point of somnolence. The tip of the endoscope is placed at the upper cricopharyn-

geal sphincter of the esophagus and the patient is encouraged to swallow while gentle pressure is exerted. Small amounts of air are passed through the endoscope to visualize the esophageal lumen. The endoscope is then passed under direct vision into the stomach. The gastric body and antrum are carefully examined. The instrument tip is retroflexed to view the gastric cardia and the whole lesser curvature. The pylorus is traversed, and the first and second portions of the duodenum are visualized. The whole examination is repeated as the instrument is withdrawn. Visualized lesions can be recorded on still photographs, movies, or television tape. Biopsies and brush cytological examinations can be obtained from suspicious areas.

EGD is a relatively safe procedure in experienced hands. A nationwide survey revealed a morbidity of 0.13 percent and a mortality of 0.004 percent. The main causes of mortality were cardiopulmonary complications and perforations by the instrument. Upper endoscopy is usually substituted for x-ray in the urgent diagnosis of gastrointestinal illness in women who might be pregnant.

Peptic regurgitant esophagitis Esophagitis is one of the commonest benign diseases of the upper gastrointestinal tract. Esophageal pain may be confused with cardiac disease, or esophagitis may present as painless blood loss. Because esophagitis usually involves only the superficial mucosa, it cannot be diagnosed by x-ray. At endoscopy, the diffuse bleeding of erosive esophagitis is clearly visible. Not every patient with heartburn requires esophagoscopy, but the procedure is indicated if x-ray shows a stricture or an ulcer, or if antireflux surgery is contemplated.

The squamous mucosa of the esophagus is far more vulnerable to peptic digestion than the columnar epithelium of the stomach. Thus, bleeding esophagitis is located on the squamous side of the esophagogastric junction and is most severe in the distal esophagus where the squamous mucosa is most exposed to regurgitated acid and pepsin from the stomach. Discrete peptic ulceration of the esophagus is uncommon.

A short area of esophagitis or a stricture can be seen at levels as high as the arch of the aorta. This is explained by progressive replacement of distal eroded squamous mucosa with metaplastic gastric epithelium which is more resistant to peptic digestion (Barrett's epithelium). This finding can be documented by biopsy. Such epithelium is more prone to malignant transformation and, therefore, may merit regular surveillance with esophagoscopy and/or exfoliative cytology.

Esophagitis may progress to scarring and stricture formation. The endoscopic appearance of a benign stricture is characteristic but not diagnostic because a malignancy can be missed and should be ruled out before medical treatment is undertaken with dilation and antacids; therefore, the whole length of the stricture should be sampled to rule out cancer, if necessary, after dilatation (biopsy and cytology).

Dilations of difficult strictures are best initiated by passing a flexible-tipped guide wire via the side channel of the endoscope through the stricture under direct vision. The endoscope can then be withdrawn over the wire which serves as a guide for passage of progressively larger metal olives through the stricture under fluoroscopic control.

Peptic ulcer It is now generally agreed that esophagogastroduodenoscopy is more accurate than upper gastrointestinal x-ray in detecting ulcers. It has been suggested that x-ray be abandoned entirely in favor of endoscopy for detecting ulcers. This makes sense when seeking the source of acute upper gastrointestinal bleeding if urgent surgical intervention is being considered; in such situations, obscuring barium would make endoscopy impossible. However, in the workup of the patient with less pressing ulcer complaints, an upper gastrointestinal x-ray is more cost-effective. As more radiologists routinely use air contrast to obtain better mucosal detail, diagnostic sensitivity for superficial lesions will increase. The greater expense and discomfort of endoscopy are justified if the x-ray is equivocal, if the ulcer is possibly malignant, if the x-ray is negative but the clinical picture is suggestive of peptic ulceration, or if the patient is about to be operated for ulcer and there is a need to be sure that an ulcer is present and that other lesions have not been missed. Patients with duodenal ulcers by x-ray or with classic ulcer deformities of the duodenal bulb do not require endoscopy for diagnosis if the presenting symptoms are characteristic and if the symptomatic response to strict antacid or cimetidine treatment is good.

There are some situations in which x-ray reveals ulcers missed by endoscopy, e.g., ulcers in hourglass constrictions of the stomach or in small duodenal bulbs incompletely visualized by currently available instruments. Fiberendoscopy is especially useful in visualizing postbulbar ulcers, giant duodenal ulcers, and stomal ulceration after partial gastrectomy, all of which can be missed by x-ray. In most circumstances, patients with duodenal ulcers do not need to be reendoscoped to see if the ulcer has healed.

In the enthusiasm for fiberendoscopy one must not forget that visual interpretation of gross pathology is subjective—one observer's ulcer is another's erosion. An erosion is confined to the mucosa and heals without a trace, whereas an ulcer is deeper and usually implies a chronic recurrent disease. Endoscopically, erosions are superficial, small, and multiple; ulcers are deeper and larger and tend to be solitary. In the future it is likely that lesions seen endoscopically will be photographically documented just as currently all lesions seen fluoroscopically are demonstrated in spot films.

Cancer The endoscopic appearance of upper gastrointestinal cancer may seem obvious, especially if there is a mass growing into the lumen. On the other hand, malignant ulcers, infiltrative carcinomas, or small early carcinomas are frequently impossible to diagnose by their gross appearance. The biopsies obtained with currently available forceps are very small, and deeper lesions can be missed. Only one of multiple biopsies may reveal the cancer. A larger particle of tissue may be removed from a suspicious area with an electrocautery snare, and this may facilitate diagnosis. Experience and skill in choosing the biopsy site improve the accuracy. An exfoliative or cytological examination of the lavage or brush specimen adds to the diagnostic accuracy in all areas of the upper gastrointestinal tract (see Chap. 291).

It may be impossible to differentiate severe esophagitis from infiltrative cancer by the gross appearance at esophagoscopy. Biopsies from patients with cancer may show only the associated inflammation. Thus, all such lesions should have careful cytological examination, either by lavage or by brushing. Because chronic inflammation may predispose to esophageal cancer, patients with lye stricture, peptic regurgitant esophagitis, or the stasis esophagitis of achalasia merit esophagoscopy and cytological examination when they are first seen and whenever their symptom patterns change.

Radiological demonstration of healing of a benign-appearing gastric ulcer is very reassuring but not infallible in excluding cancer. Diagnostic accuracy in differentiating benign from malignant gastric ulcer by exfoliative cytological lavage, endoscopic biopsy, or brush cytology depends very much upon the combined skills of endoscopists, cytologists, and pathologists. Among North American communities accuracy in diagnosing cancer may vary from 50 to 90 percent. Physicians must individually decide which patients should be examined by methods that have proved accurate in their own community, and which patients should be referred to centers with greater resources. The effort expended in diagnosing gastric cancer tends to be proportional to the frequency of the disease in a community. What is done in Japan may not be justified in the United States (see Chap. 291).

Primary gastric lymphoma is a diagnosis well worth making because the 5-year survival is far higher than for adenocarcinoma. It can mimic benign gastric ulcer or adenocarcinoma by gastroscopy or x-ray. It can be diagnosed by biopsy or cytology, although the accuracy is not as high as in adenocarcinoma.

If a polypoid lesion of the stomach is covered by mucosa that appears normal by gastroscopy, the likelihood of malignancy is very small. Most such lesions are intramural, extramucosal benign tumors such as leiomyomas or pancreatic rests. Polyps covered by abnormal-appearing mucosa can be benign or malignant. Random biopsy can miss carcinoma within a polyp. If technically feasible, polyps should, therefore, be removed in their entirety by snare cautery for histological examination. If over 2 cm in diameter, they are more likely to contain cancer (see Chap. 291).

Ampullary carcinoma may be diagnosed by biopsy and brush cytology during duodenoscopy. Other primary duodenal malignancies are very rare. Extensions from pancreatic or biliary tract cancer are difficult to diagnose because the tumor may not have extended into the mucosa and may therefore not be accessible for biopsy or cytological examination. In these secondary tumors, diagnosis must depend upon some combination of echography, hypotonic duodenography, selective pancreatic angiography, and endoscopic retrograde cholangiopancreatography, with cytological examination of ductal contents.

Upper gastrointestinal bleeding (see also Chap. 38) Endoscopy within the first 12 to 24 h of an upper gastrointestinal hemorrhage can be very helpful in planning rational therapy by visualizing the bleeding source. Shallow lesions not visible by x-ray may be seen (esophagitis, Mallory-Weiss tear, erosive gastritis, shallow stress ulcer, and telangiectasia). Lesions which are visible by x-ray may not be the source of bleeding. Only endoscopy can determine the actual bleeding site which may affect treatment. For example, visualization of a spurting artery which is flooding the stomach indicates massive ongoing bleeding requiring prompt operative intervention.

A conservative estimate of the diagnostic accuracy of emergency endoscopy in upper gastrointestinal bleeding is 80 to 85 percent, which is far superior to emergency x-ray examination. Endoscopic diagnoses of bleeding erosive gastritis may be made too frequently when blood from another unsuspected source spreads over the gastric mucosa or when trauma from overly vigorous antecedent lavage creates ecchymoses. To avoid overdiagnosis of erosive gastritis, portions of the gastric wall should be washed free of blood to determine the true appearance of the underlying gastric mucosa.

Every patient having endoscopy for upper gastrointestinal bleeding merits a complete endoscopic examination of the esophagus, stomach, and duodenum. Finding a potential bleeding lesion is not proof that this is the source of hemorrhage unless active bleeding is seen. Approximately one-half of patients with esophageal varices can be shown endoscopically to be bleeding from another source such as erosive gastritis, duodenal ulcer, or gastric ulcer. Occasionally it is not possible to diagnose the exact lesion which is bleeding, but localizing the area of bleeding can be very helpful; for example, bright red arterial blood may be seen pouring from the duodenum when the esophagus and stomach are relatively free of blood.

There are three controversial areas. First, *do all bleeders need endoscopy?* We feel that endoscopy is indicated in all patients who may require surgery because of continual bleeding or rebleeding. Although 85 percent of upper gastrointestinal bleeders stop spontaneously, it is impossible to predict which ones will; therefore, we endoscope most bleeders. Second, *how early should endoscopy be performed in the acutely bleeding patient?* Most studies suggest that the diagnostic accuracy of esophagogastroduodenoscopy remains high for the first 12 to 24 h after the bleeding episode. All would agree that it is desirable to delay endoscopy until vital signs have been stabilized after adequate blood replacement. Upper endoscopy is best performed during waking hours at a time during the first day of bleeding when the patient's vital signs are stable and when the full endoscopic team is available. Emergency endoscopy at night should be reserved for those patients with continued massive bleeding or rebleeding requiring an immediate decision regarding surgery or other treatment. If the patient is exsanguinating, endoscopy can follow induction of anesthesia just preceding surgery. Finally, *does endoscopy affect the clinical outcome?* Current studies suggest that it does not. This may be more a reflection on the inadequacies of medical therapy and the dangers of nonelective surgical treatment of bleeding patients who are severely ill than on the usefulness of more accurate endoscopic detection of the bleeding source. If endoscopic methods of stopping bleeding prove to be safe in controlled trials, more accurate endoscopic diagnosis may indeed affect outcome favorably.

Emergency endoscopy is not for the inexperienced. It requires considerable technical skill and interpretative experience and the best available instruments.

Other indications Most patients with *dysphagia* merit esophagoscopy because the cause is frequently organic and may be missed by x-ray. On the other hand, dysphagia caused by esophageal spasm or dysrhythmia is best diagnosed by manometry or cineradiography. *Painful swallowing* (odynophagia), especially in immunosuppressed or diabetic patients, may merit esophagoscopy because biopsy and scrapings of the involved esophageal wall may reveal monilial, herpetic, or cytomegalic virus infections. Soon after ingestion of a corrosive agent, limited and gentle esophagoscopy is useful in evaluating the severity of injury. Many impacted foreign bodies can be removed from the esophagus or stomach with a snare or forceps; sharp foreign bodies are usually best removed by pulling them into the lumen of a rigid tubular esophagoscope. Careful esophagoscopy after removal of a foreign body is important to determine whether there is an underlying lesion which caused the impaction (e.g., cancer, benign stricture, peptic esophagitis).

In the postoperative stomach, gastroscopy is especially useful in detecting carcinoma, recurrent ulceration, retrograde intussusception, and stomal stricture. Several European studies indicate a definite threat of carcinoma developing in the gastric stump 10 to 20 years after a Billroth II gastrectomy. The diagnosis of such postoperative carcinomas may require many biopsies of seemingly normal mucosa near the anastomosis. Prospective data on the natural history of this condition in the United States are badly needed because, if the European studies are confirmed, such patients should be endoscoped and biopsied on a regular basis.

When the duodenal bulb shows reddening or nodularity, many endoscopists diagnose "duodenitis." There is little evidence to suggest that this picture is of significance. On the other hand, diffuse and bleeding erosions of the duodenal bulb merit a diagnosis of "erosive duodenitis" because they may be a significant source of bleeding, especially after ingestion of gastric irritants such as aspirin; such erosions may also be a precursor of frank ulcerations. A nodular or narrow duodenum

will occasionally yield granulomas on biopsy, indicative of Crohn's disease.

ENDOSCOPIC RETROGRADE CHOLANGIOPANCREATOGRAPHY (ERCP) This endoscopic technique involves placing a side-viewing instrument in the descending duodenum. The papilla of Vater is cannulated, contrast medium is injected, and the pancreatic ducts and hepatobiliary tree are visualized radiologically. Skilled operators can visualize 90 to 95 percent of pancreatic ducts and 80 to 85 percent of biliary ducts.

ERCP is performed on an x-ray table. The oropharynx is anesthetized with topical lidocaine, and the patient is sedated with intravenous diazepam. Atropine and glucagon are given intravenously to induce duodenal hypotonia. The pancreatic duct is usually visualized first and gently filled throughout its entire length with 2 to 5 ml contrast material (Fig. 288-1*A*). Injection is continued until the first side branches are seen or until the patient complains of pain. Overfilling is avoided. By insertion of the cannula at a more acute cephalad angle, the common bile duct and the whole biliary tract including the gallbladder are visualized (Fig. 288-1*B*).

At present not all indications for ERCP are clearly established. Those for the hepatobiliary tree are clearer than those for the pancreatic duct. Because ERCP is not without risk, it is justified only to seek an operable lesion or to prevent an unnecessary operation. Asymptomatic amylase elevations occur in 30 to 40 percent of patients after the procedure and are rarely of clinical significance. Pancreatitis occurs in only 1 percent of patients but is usually benign and self-limited. In a nationwide survey of complications, morbidity was 3 percent and mortality 0.2 percent. It is significant that the complication rate was highest for the inexperienced operator (7 percent). The morbidity and mortality rates are substantially lower from large centers with great experience. The main serious complication is retained, nonsterile contrast material proximal to an obstructed duct causing cholangitis or pancreatic sepsis. All patients with obstructed ducts and retained dye should be covered immediately with antibiotics and drained surgically within 36 h. No patient should have ERCP unless advance arrangements for possible operation have been made with the patient and a surgical consultant.

Retrograde cholangiography This procedure is especially useful in patients with persistent jaundice whose cause cannot be established by conventional diagnostic methods. The important differential diagnosis is between "surgical" and "medical" jaundice. When the cause of jaundice is unclear, approximately 15 percent of patients thought to have "medical" jaundice prove to have extrahepatic biliary obstruction requiring surgery, and, conversely, the same percentage of patients thought to have "surgical" jaundice prove to have an open ductal system by ERCP and can be spared unnecessary surgery.

Remediable causes of obstructive jaundice which can be diagnosed by retrograde cholangiography include common duct stones (Fig. 288-1*C*), gallbladder stones, benign strictures, and, occasionally, resectable ductal carcinomas. In jaundiced patients with suspected primary liver disease such as sclerosing cholangitis or primary biliary cirrhosis, ERCP can relieve the worry that an operable obstruction is being missed.

In addition to ERCP, there are three other methods of visualizing the biliary tree in the jaundiced patient. Which test to use first depends on the clinical situation, the availability of equipment, and the experience of the specialists using the techniques. The first method is *percutaneous transhepatic cholangiography (PTC)* in which contrast material is injected from the exterior via a "skinny" needle into the intrahepatic bile ducts under fluoroscopic control; success in visualizing the ducts is

FIGURE 288-1

A. A tapering pancreatic duct (arrow) of normal diameter is seen and may be compared with the endoscope (E) 1 cm in diameter. B. Normal cholangiogram. The diameter of the common duct (CD) is normal. The intrahepatic ducts branch normally, and the gallbladder (GB) can be seen. The *endoscope (E) is seen in the duodenum. C. Three stones (arrows) are visible in an obstructed, dilated common duct (CD). The intrahepatic ducts (IHD) are also grossly dilated. Regurgitated contrast material is seen in the duodenum (DUO). D. The sharp cutoff (arrow) of the pancreatic duct (P) is caused by a carcinoma of the body of the pancreas.*

90 to 100 percent if they are dilated, but only approximately 66 percent if they are not dilated. PTC is generally safe, but complications do occur (sepsis, bleeding, bile leak, etc.); precise morbidity and mortality figures are not yet established. The two other methods, which are noninvasive, use *ultrasound* (echo) and *computerized tomography* (CT scan); these techniques employ sound waves or x-rays to visualize organs and any stones, cysts, or solid masses within them. They can also be used to determine whether the biliary ducts or gallbladder are enlarged.

The relative usefulness of these four tests is not established. Many physicians first try the noninvasive echo or CT scan to see whether the biliary ducts are dilated and to seek a clear cause of the patient's jaundice (stones, pancreatic mass, etc.). Direct visualization is undertaken if the diagnosis is not established, PTC first if the hepatic ducts are dilated, and ERCP if not. In the event of a technical failure or incomplete information resulting from either ERCP or PTC, one of the other techniques is tried. This approach detects most lesions requiring surgical intervention.

ERCP or PTC can also be useful in patients with biliary pain, cholangitis, or impaired liver function after previous biliary surgery. Remediable postoperative lesions such as strictures can be discovered, and their precise anatomy outlined so that reoperation is less difficult.

Retrograde pancreatography Patients with recurrent or chronic pancreatitis may merit retrograde pancreatography to seek a lesion which can be approached surgically, such as cyst, localized pancreatitis in the tail, or ductal pathology amenable to drainage which may be found in nearly 50 percent of these patients. Finding concomitant unsuspected stones in the gallbladder or common duct may direct surgical intervention toward the underlying problem.

Patients with symptoms, signs, or laboratory findings suggesting pancreatic carcinoma may have pancreatograms suggesting malignancy with a narrowed, encased, or sharply "cutoff" pancreatic duct (Fig. 288-1D). Differentiation of such pancreatic ductal findings from benign inflammatory disease can be difficult. Cytologic examination of pancreatic duct contents obtained during ERCP may prove helpful. Unfortunately, most patients with symptomatic pancreatic cancer diagnosed by ERCP are inoperable.

Patients presenting with painless steatorrhea of pancreatic origin may be shown to have a ductal pattern suggesting chronic pancreatitis or pancreatic carcinoma. Some of these carcinomas may be resectable, although it is as yet unknown whether this represents palliation or the more remote possibility of cure.

Pancreatography has not been useful in the study of obscure upper abdominal pain. Pancreatic cysts can be better diagnosed by noninvasive techniques such as echography, and pancreatography should be reserved for those cases where the diagnosis is unclear or when the surgeon desires precise outlining of the anatomy prior to surgery. Pancreatography alone does not seem promising as a method of screening for early pancreatic carcinoma, although cytological examination of ductal fluid may prove useful.

Therapeutic ERCP Successful endoscopic papillotomy of the sphincter of Vater with extraction of retained stones has now been reported by several groups. An electrosurgical wire attached to the ERCP catheter can be used to cut the sphincter of Vater. Certainly this approach will be used increasingly in patients who are poor operative risks. Manometry of the sphincter presents certain technical difficulties, but it may yet prove invaluable in the diagnosis of periampullary stenosis.

Other diagnostic techniques Critical comparative studies are needed of the various approaches to biliary tree disorders and to pancreatic diseases (ERCP, PTC, angiography, CT scanning, and ultrasound).

COLONOSCOPY The interior of the entire length of the colon from anus to cecum can be visualized by the experienced colonoscopist. This method may prove to be the most significant diagnostic and therapeutic application of fiberoptic endoscopy because it can diagnose potentially curable colonic cancers missed by other techniques.

Approximately one-half of colonoscopies are performed because of an abnormal barium enema showing a polyp or a narrowing or filling defect suggesting carcinoma. Approximately one-quarter of colonoscopies are done because of chronic occult gastrointestinal bleeding. The ability to examine the whole colon is proving valuable in the management of some patients with inflammatory bowel disease.

Patients are prepared for colonoscopy with a liquid diet for 2 days, magnesium citrate laxation the evening before examination, and tap water enemas the morning of the procedure. Immediately before the procedure the patients are lightly sedated with intravenous diazepam and meperidine. Intravenous anticholinergics and glucagon are used when needed to relax local spasm. Vasovagal bradycardial reactions can be reversed quickly by intravenous anticholinergics.

The main complications of colonoscopy are hemorrhage and perforation (morbidity is 0.5 to 1.3 percent, mortality is 0.02 percent). The complication rate for polypectomy is 1 to 2 percent. Most complications occur during the first 40 procedures by a new colonoscopist. Diverticular or ischemic disease and prior irradiation make the procedure more difficult and hazardous.

Polyps A polyp seen on barium enema merits colonoscopy for several reasons: it may be an artifact or a cancer, and a second polyp or cancer may have been missed. The polyp can usually be excised with a lower morbidity and mortality than with surgery. The best way to rule out cancer within a polyp is to remove it completely for histological examination. The most common colonic polyps are hyperplastic histologically, and they do not develop cancer; colonic polyps which show benign neoplasia histologically may become malignant (adenomatous and villous polyps). The risk of neoplastic polyps being cancerous increases with their size. Those over 1 cm in diameter have at least a 10 percent chance of being malignant. Pedunculated polyps with cancer confined to the mucosa and with an uninvolved stalk can be cured by removal with an electrocautery snare during colonoscopy. Thus, most colonoscopists will remove all polyps more than 0.5 cm in diameter. It is more difficult to know what to do with polyps smaller than 0.5 cm in diameter because some are adenomatous, although most are hyperplastic. A coagulating biopsy technique can be used to both biopsy and destroy even the smallest adenomatous polyp in the hope that the subsequent risk of developing colonic can-

cer will be reduced. The wisdom of this course of action is suggested by a sigmoidoscopic study in which the removal of all polyps reduced the expected incidence and invasiveness of subsequently developing cancers. Most agree that the patient with adenomatous polyps is more likely to develop another polyp or cancer and therefore merits some regular screening program.

Cancer screening by x-ray All filling defects on barium enema merit evaluation by colonoscopy. If the lesion is a pedunculated polyp, it can be removed for histological examination; if its appearance suggests a cancer it can be biopsied and brushed for histological and cytological confirmation. When a carcinoma is found, the remainder of the colon should be screened for additional polyps and synchronous carcinoma. This avoids multiple colotomies to search for a second lesion and reduces surgical morbidity. Approximately 10 percent of lesions diagnosed as carcinoma by x-ray are not present on colonoscopy or are found to be caused by other diseases.

Narrowing by x-ray An etiologic diagnosis of segmental narrowing may be difficult by x-ray. Colonoscopy often determines the cause of segmental narrowing and differentiates adenocarcinoma from inflammation secondary to ischemia, irradiation, diverticular disease, or Crohn's colitis. Even the most classic "apple-core" lesion by x-ray may be covered by normal mucosa at colonoscopy, suggesting an extrinsic inflammatory lesion. Narrowed segments present on x-ray are not visualized (in 10 to 30 percent of patients) during colonoscopy because they are probably areas of temporary spasm. Such findings avoid unnecessary operations.

Chronic bleeding (x-ray and sigmoidoscopy negative) This condition leads to approximately 25 percent of colonoscopies. The cause of bleeding is found in approximately 40 percent of such patients. The common bleeding sources are adenomatous polyp (15 percent), adenocarcinoma (15 percent), and Crohn's disease (7 percent). Many of these carcinomas are resectable, and this group may benefit most from colonoscopy. If no bleeding source is found, a search may be appropriate for an upper gastrointestinal source with an upper gastrointestinal x-ray and/or upper endoscopy. Narrowing or masses on x-ray can be studied colonoscopically to see if they are due to inflammation, malignancy, or an artifact. Colonoscopy may be indicated in patients with ulcerative colitis of more than 10 years' duration because of the increased risk of carcinoma; it is hoped that repeated colonoscopies will serve to detect these malignancies earlier than x-ray and while the lesions are still curable. The prognostic value of "precancer" or "dysplastic" changes revealed by multiple colonic biopsies in patients with long-standing ulcerative colitis remains to be established.

Other indications The short fiberoptic colonoscope may replace the rigid 25-cm sigmoidoscope for routine screening because it can be passed to 40 to 60 cm with minimal preparation. There is less discomfort and a higher diagnostic yield. However, the question remains whether flexible sigmoidoscopy will pick up significant lesions missed by screening stools for occult blood. At this time, rigid sigmoidoscopy remains an important method of evaluating colorectal symptoms. After segmental colonic resection for carcinoma, colonoscopy may detect early mucosal recurrence and differentiate it from benign anastomotic strictures or bleeding suture granulomas. Colonoscopy is occasionally used during laparotomy to assist the surgeon in ruling out other lesions. The colonoscope can be advanced to the cecum rapidly with the surgeon's assistance, and additional polyps removed without colotomy. We believe that the best diagnostic approach to acute bleeding is selective angiography; this may be useful not only for finding lesions such as angiodysplasia and bleeding diverticulas but also for permitting treatment with vasoconstrictors. Visualizing a bleeding site by colonoscopy may be difficult when there is massive bleeding.

Colonoscopy detects some carriers of the dominant familial polyposis gene before diagnosis by barium enema and sigmoidoscopy. Such information is useful for genetic counseling of patients regarding their decision to have children. Carcinoma is a great threat only in those familial syndromes which produce many adenomatous polyps (familial polyposis and Gardner's syndrome); in these conditions, polypectomy is useful for diagnosis, but colectomy is the only treatment which prevents development of carcinoma. Peutz-Jeghers syndrome and generalized juvenile polyposis produce mostly hamartomatous polyps and, therefore, have a very much lower incidence of gastrointestinal carcinoma; the cancers that develop in these patients may be related to occasional polyps undergoing adenomatous change.

Malignant tumors develop in 2 to 3 percent of patients with Peutz-Jeghers syndrome, and they are mostly located in the stomach and duodenum. Thus these patients may merit regular upper endoscopy and prophylactic polypectomy.

CONSCIOUS LAPAROSCOPY The potentialities for laparoscopy in conscious patients have not been as fully appreciated in North America as they have been in other countries where it has been used widely for over 20 years. This procedure has an extremely low mortality and morbidity in experienced hands. The instrument used for laparoscopy is a stiff tube with a lens system that provides a superb view. Under local anesthesia pneumoperitoneum is gradually induced with air or nitrous oxide. To avoid intraabdominal trauma, the extent of the gas cavity must be determined by probing with a spinal needle before the sharp trocar is carefully pushed through the abdominal wall into this cavity. The sharp obturator is removed and the laparoscope introduced through the airtight trocar to visualize the peritoneal cavity.

Much of the exterior of the liver, gallbladder, spleen, peritoneum, diaphragm, and pelvic organs can be clearly visualized. Portions of the colon and small bowel can also be seen, depending upon the location and size of the greater omentum. Lesions can be biopsied under direct vision, and any resultant bleeding controlled by electrocoagulation. Furthermore, in centers with extensive experience contrast material can be injected into the liver to visualize vascular, lymphatic, and biliary systems.

Laparoscopy should be considered an indispensable diagnostic tool. It permits one to make a difficult diagnosis without resorting to laparotomy by biopsying localized hepatic disease under direct vision, and can often help differentiate "medical" from "surgical" jaundice. It may also enable staging of malignant disease without laparotomy.

REFERENCES

BECK K et al: *Color Atlas of Laparoscopy.* New York, FK Schattauer Verlag, 1970

BLOOM BS et al: Fiberoptics: Morbidity and cost. N Engl J Med 288:368, 1973

COTTON PB, BEALES JSM: Endoscopic pancreatography in management of relapsing acute pancreatitis. Br Med J 1:608, 1974

DEYHLE P: Coloscopy in the management of bowel disease. Hosp Pract 9:121, 1974

EASTWOOD GL: Does early endoscopy benefit the patient with active upper gastrointestinal bleeding? Gastroenterology 72:737, 1977

KATON RM, SMITH FW: Panendoscopy in the early diagnosis of acute upper gastrointestinal bleeding. Gastroenterology 65:728, 1973

KOCH H: Operative endoscopy. Gastrointest Endosc 24:65, 1977

OVERHOLT BF: Colonoscopy: A review. Gastroenterology 68:1308, 1975

TEAGUE RH et al: Colonoscopy for investigation of unexplained rectal bleeding. Lancet 1:1350, 1978

VENNES JA et al: Endoscopic cholangiography for biliary system diagnosis. Ann Intern Med 80:61, 1974

WAYE JD: The current status of flexible fiberoptic endoscopy. Mt Sinai J Med NY 42:1, 1975

289
DISEASES OF THE ESOPHAGUS

THOMAS R. HENDRIX

Although the exact correlation of anatomic, radiologic, and functional features of the esophagus and the cardioesophageal junction in particular continues to be debated, it is useful to consider disorders of the esophagus in functional terms. In normal swallowing the activities of the striated muscle of the pharynx and upper esophagus and the smooth muscle of the lower esophagus are so closely integrated that they function as a single tissue. The esophagus proper is separated from adjacent segments of the alimentary tract by two sphincters. (A sphincter is a segment that has a resting tone greater than the adjacent segments and that relaxes in response to the appropriate stimulus—swallowing in the case of the esophagus.) The upper esophageal sphincter (cricopharyngeus) separates the pharynx from the esophagus and prevents air from filling the esophagus during inspiration. The lower esophageal sphincter is the primary barrier to reflux of gastric juice into the esophagus. It relaxes during swallowing, regurgitation, belching, and vomiting. The pressure in the lower esophageal sphincter is not static; rather it is responsive to need. Its pressure increases in response to increased intraabdominal pressure and is modified by changes in hormone levels associated with the ingestion of a meal. (A protein meal increases and a fatty meal decreases sphincter pressure.)

Other structures illustrated diagrammatically in Fig. 289-1 have been assigned varying roles in preventing reflux. These include the infradiaphragmatic segment of the lower esophageal sphincter, the possible flap valve mechanism provided by the angle of His, and the diaphragm itself. The first phase of swallowing, the movement of the bolus from the mouth to the pharynx, is voluntary, but subsequent events are involuntary. As the upper sphincter relaxes, the bolus is propelled into the esophagus. The lower esophageal sphincter relaxes prior to the arrival of the bolus in the lower esophagus. Finally, the esophagus is swept clean by a peristaltic wave proceeding from the pharynx to the lower esophageal sphincter.

SYMPTOMATOLOGY

DYSPHAGIA (See Chap. 34) Difficulty in swallowing can be produced by the derangement or incoordination of any part of the swallowing act as well as by the narrowing of the lumen by a tumor or an inflammatory stricture. Dysphagia of oropharyngeal origin is characterized by failure to move a bolus out of the mouth, regurgitation into the nose, or aspiration into the trachea. Esophageal dysphagia is characterized by the complaint that food is sticking somewhere behind the sternum. Dysphagia occurs only with swallowing and must be differentiated from globus hystericus, a persistent sensation of a lump or tightness in the throat.

Dysphagia is usually localized to the level of the lower sternum corresponding to the most frequent site of esophageal disease. In other instances dysphagia is localized higher in the chest or at the base of the neck, either because the responsible lesion is situated higher in the esophagus or because in some patients sensations from the distal esophagus are referred to the level of the sternal notch.

Dysphagia may be painless, but more often it is distressing and sometimes causes pain of alarming proportions. It commonly appears gradually or in intermittent attacks, although on occasion the onset is abrupt and reaches maximum intensity rapidly. Certain foods, notably beef and soft breads, are often the first offenders, probably because these elastic solids are wedged by peristalsis into the segment narrowed by esophageal disease. The impacted bolus may be forced through the narrowed area by drinking liquids, or forceful retching may be required to dislodge the food, and on occasion it must be removed through use of the esophagoscope.

PAIN Heartburn, or pyrosis, is the most common type of esophageal pain. It is a burning, tight, or searing sensation which appears intermittently beneath the lower sternum and spreads upward in a wavelike fashion to the throat or even into the angles of the jaw. It is often associated with increased salivation. Heartburn is most likely to occur 10 to 60 min after eating, especially after overindulging, and is accentuated by bending over or lying down. Heartburn is the consequence of reflux of irritant material into the esophagus.

Esophageal pain frequently accompanies dysphagia and may be severe if the bolus is unable to pass the constricted segment. In addition, esophageal pain may occur in the absence of dysphagia or obvious heartburn. At times its onset is so abrupt and severe that myocardial infarction is the initial diagnosis. Esophageal pain may mimic ischemic heart pain

even to the radiation of pain down the ulnar aspect of the arms. Referral of esophageal pain to the epigastrium is common, and referral to the back is encountered on occasion.

BELCHING A belch is caused by the forceful regurgitation of air from the stomach or esophagus. Although belching is an esophageal phenomenon, it is not a common manifestation of esophageal disease. More often it is a functional disorder or is indicative of peptic, cardiac, or biliary tract disease.

REGURGITATION Regurgitation, as contrasted to vomiting, is the effortless appearance of esophageal or gastric contents in the mouth. Its appearance may be the consequence of an incompetent lower esophageal sphincter or obstruction of the esophagus.

GASTROESOPHAGEAL REFLUX AND ESOPHAGITIS

Reflux of small amounts of gastric juice into the lower part of the esophagus is a common event. Its frequency is increased by overindulgence. Whether reflux occurs and whether it produces symptoms are determined by three factors: (1) the competency of the lower esophageal sphincter, the primary barrier to reflux, (2) the irritant nature of the refluxed material, and (3) the sensitivity of the esophageal mucosa to the refluxed material. Although the symptoms of reflux were attributed in the past to inflammation of the esophagus, i.e., esophagitis, it is clear that esophagitis is a complication of severe reflux rather than the cause of the symptoms associated with reflux. On the other hand, the competency of the lower esophageal sphincter correlates well with the presence or absence of reflux. Refluxed acid gastric juice is the most common cause of reflux symptoms, but there is increasing evidence that refluxed bile acids also play an important role. Bile acids may enter the stomach and then the esophagus because of an incompetent pyloric sphincter or alterations produced by gastric surgery.

Symptoms Heartburn, the typical symptom of reflux, is characterized by burning epigastric or retrosternal pain which spreads upward. Typically, heartburn appears after meals, especially large meals, and is aggravated by bending over, lying down, or straining. It is relieved by standing up or drinking something, especially antacids. In severe episodes, the pain may radiate to the base of the neck, the angles of the jaw, or down one or both arms, simulating angina pectoris. Although heartburn is often a trivial complaint without serious consequences, it must be differentiated from other causes of chest pain and may be the manifestation of esophagitis. In some cases, when the patient is asleep, there is a reflux of material into the hypopharynx and this material is aspirated. The patient awakens coughing and strangling on the refluxed material. If this process is severe or recurrent, pneumonitis or pulmonary fibrosis may ensue.

Diagnosis To establish that a patient's chest pain is caused by reflux, it must be shown that reflux occurs and that the esophagus is sensitive to the refluxed fluid. The most sensitive test of reflux is to measure intraesophageal pH after instilling a volume (300 ml) of 0.1 N HCl into the stomach. If the sphincter is competent, intraesophageal pH will remain above 5 or 6. In patients with reflux the pH falls intermittently to 1.5 or 2, and in those with free reflux the pH never rises above intragastric levels as the pH electrode is withdrawn from the stomach into the esophagus. A more physiologic test is to record intraesophageal pH over a 12-h period, noting the frequency and duration of low pH. Radiographic studies can demonstrate reflux in no more than 40 percent of symptomatic patients. Recently, gastroesophageal Scintiscan has been advocated as a simple

FIGURE 289-1

Diagrammatic representation of the structure and relations of the lower esophagus. A. Normal esophagus. B. Rolling hernia. C. Sliding hernia. In the sliding hernia the distinction between the lower esophageal sphincter and the herniated cardia is lost, and the angle of His has become obtuse. L.E.S. = lower esophageal sphincter, P.E.L. = phrenoesophageal ligament. The location of the gastroesophageal junction is a matter of opinion. It may be defined as located at the level where the tube of the esophagus widens into the sac of the stomach, but sometimes the transition from one shape to the other is gradual rather than abrupt. Alternatively, the junction is placed at the serrated line where squamous esophageal and glandular gastric mucosa meet, but this epithelial boundary is located somewhat above the level of the angle of His and thus does not coincide with a division of stomach and esophagus based on gross shape and muscular function.

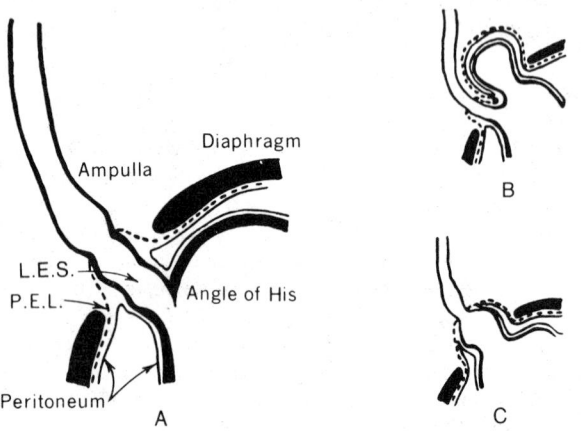

technique for detection of gastroesophageal reflux. After the ingestion of ^{99m}Tc in water, gamma camera images of the precordium are taken to detect esophageal reflux while abdominal pressures are increased stepwise to 35 mmHg. The advantage of the gastroesophageal Scintiscan technique in the detection of reflux is its simplicity without the necessity of intubation; its disadvantages are the use of costly equipment and radioisotopes to answer a relatively straightforward clinical question. To determine if reflux causes the patient's symptom, reflux may be mimicked by perfusing the esophagus alternately with saline solution and 0.1 N HC1 at 120 drops per minute. In patients with symptoms due to reflux, pain is produced by acid perfusion but not with saline, whereas the asymptomatic individual or a patient with chest pain of different origin is unable to distinguish between saline and acid perfusion.

Treatment Medical management aims to protect the esophagus by decreasing reflux of gastric juice and by decreasing the irritant effect of the refluxed juice. The first aim may be achieved by decreasing the volume of gastric contents available for reflux, by positioning the patient so that gravity acts to impede reflux, and by improving the function of the lower esophageal sphincter. In practical terms, the patient is advised to take small meals and not to eat in the 2 to 3 h before retiring. Patients should avoid those foods which they may have found to be associated with dyspepsia and heartburn. Four- to six-inch blocks elevating the head of the bed lessen nocturnal gastroesophageal regurgitation.

Although anticholinergic drugs decrease the volume of gastric secretion, they are not indicated in the treatment of reflux symptoms because in effective doses they also decrease the volume of alkaline saliva, decrease the tone of the lower esophageal sphincter, and decrease the frequency of secondary peristalsis, which functions to return refluxed gastric juice to the stomach. To aid in decreasing the irritant effect of refluxed gastric juice, a liquid, viscous antacid preparation, such as aluminum-magnesium hydroxide gel, should be taken 1 and 3 h after meals and at bedtime. Alternatively, taking two antacid tablets after meals and at bedtime also decreases the irritant quality of reflux. After 2 weeks the frequency usually can be decreased because the esophageal mucosa has become less sensitive to the refluxed material. If symptoms are severe or unresponsive to antacids, bethanechol (Urecholine), 25 mg before meals and at bedtime, should be added. Bethanechol decreases esophageal reflux by increasing lower esophageal sphincter tone. In addition, the efficacy of bethanechol may be due in part to increased gastric emptying, which limits the reflux of bile acids from the duodenum.

Finally, in stocky or obese patients, weight loss helps.

CHRONIC REFLUX ESOPHAGITIS Reflux esophagitis is inflammation of the esophageal mucosa caused by reflux of acid gastric or alkaline intestinal juice. One-fourth of patients with symptoms severe enough to be thought indicative of reflux esophagitis have nearly normal esophageal biopsies; less than 20 percent have acute inflammatory changes. On the other hand, esophagitis is the precursor of the complications of reflux, namely, bleeding, stricture, and change in esophageal epithelium from squamous to columnar. Bleeding is usually slow and chronic. Acute massive bleeding occasionally occurs with esophagitis but is usually due to an associated peptic ulcer of the esophagus. Both severe esophagitis and peptic ulcer of the esophagus lead to peptic strictures. Barrett's esophagus or an esophagus lined by columnar epithelium is also a complication of severe esophagitis. As the squamous epithelium is destroyed, it is replaced by columnar epithelium usually similar to adjacent gastric mucosa of the cardia. This epithelium, as the gastric epithelium, may in turn show metaplastic changes which are believed to be premalignant. The squamocolumnar junc-

tion is particularly prone to develop peptic ulcers which may bleed or lead to stricture. A benign midesophageal stricture is almost always due to Barrett's esophagus if ingestion of corrosives has been ruled out.

Symptoms The symptoms of esophagitis are symptoms of reflux. In some patients heartburn worsens, cold and hot foods and slightly acid foods are increasingly painful to swallow, and eventually dysphagia appears. Dysphagia is most frequently due to acid-induced esophageal spasm. In some patients, not necessarily those with the most impressive reflux symptoms, an inflammatory stricture develops, causing progressive dysphagia. With advancing disease, malnutrition is inevitable, and occasionally slow blood loss occurs.

Diagnosis The diagnosis of esophagitis may be suspected on clinical, radiographic, and esophagoscopic findings but is established by demonstrating inflammatory changes in an esophageal biopsy. Esophagitis is not necessarily a primary process but may be the manifestation of a variety of diseases such as peptic ulcer, cancer, and scleroderma.

Treatment The treatment of esophagitis is the treatment of reflux, but the end point in addition to relief of symptoms is healing of the inflammatory process so that strictures do not develop. If healing does not occur, cimetidine, an H$_2$ antagonist which blocks gastric acid secretion, should be tried before turning to surgical therapy (300 mg before meals and at bedtime).[1] If esophagitis is not healed or reflux-induced symptoms are not controlled within 3 months of medical therapy, surgery should be considered. The fundoplication operations of Belsey, Hill, or Nissen have given the best results. If a severe stricture has developed, it may be necessary to resect the involved segment and interpose a segment of colon.

HIATAL HERNIA Hiatal hernia is defined as a herniation of a portion of the stomach into the chest through the esophageal hiatus of the diaphragm. Hernias are classified as rolling, or paraesophageal, and sliding, or direct. In the first, the gastric cardia rolls through the hiatus beside a gastroesophageal junction that is normally situated with respect to the diaphragmatic hiatus (Fig. 289-1*B*). In the second, the sliding, or direct, hernia, both the stomach and the gastroesophageal junction slip up into the chest, thereby placing the gastroesophageal junction above the diaphragmatic hiatus (Fig. 289-1*C*). Many hernias are mixed and present features of both types.

Sliding hernia is three to ten times as common as the rolling and mixed hernias combined. Rolling hernias are primarily a disorder of women, being ten times as frequent in women as in men.

Symptoms Most hiatal hernias are symptomatic, although a variety of diverse symptoms resembling coronary insufficiency, cholelithiasis, peptic ulcer, and functional digestive disorders have been attributed to hiatal hernia. Such an association, however, does not establish a cause and effect relationship.

Symptoms due to the herniated pouch of the stomach are almost exclusively limited to the rolling or mixed type of hernia. On rare occasions a patient with a rolling hernia comes to the physician with acute prostration due to strangulation of the hernia. Although chronic and acute bleeding commonly are attributed to hernias, bleeding most often originates in muco-

---

[1] *This drug has not been approved for this purpose in the United States by the Food and Drug Administration at the time of publication.*

sal erosions, peptic ulcers, and esophagitis, all of which may be associated with diaphragmatic hernia.

Diagnosis The diagnosis of diaphragmatic hernia is often suspected on the basis of reflux symptoms. The definitive diagnosis, however, must rest on radiographic evidence. The clinically important question is not whether a hiatal hernia is present but whether the patient has gastroesophageal reflux and whether the reflux has led to esophagitis or stricture. Most hiatal hernias are asymptomatic and clinically of no importance.

Treatment The aim of treatment is to decrease gastroesophageal reflux. Operative repair of rolling hernias is indicated if they cause esophageal obstruction, respiratory symptoms, perforation, strangulation, repeated or chronic bleeding, or severe distress not remedied by intensive medical measures.

ACUTE ESOPHAGITIS Mild acute esophagitis, with substernal pain aggravated by swallowing, may complicate infections of the upper part of the respiratory tract. Severe esophageal inflammation with variable necrosis may occur in moribund states, in diseases of the central nervous system, after extensive burns or trauma, and after operations, especially if vomiting is pronounced or gastric intubation prolonged. Acute esophagitis due to *Candida* and a variety of viruses such as herpes simplex and cytomegalovirus are increasingly common with the widespread use of immunosuppressive drugs, broad-spectrum antibiotics, and corticosteroids. Acute esophagitis is a particularly troublesome complication, frequently encountered in oncology patients under treatment with a variety of chemotherapeutic agents. Although moniliasis often can be controlled with oral nystatin, the appearance of acute esophagitis often necessitates cessation of chemotherapy.

The ingestion of alkaline corrosive agents produces a form of acute esophagitis which, if not immediately fatal, may terminate in extensive esophageal stenosis. Immediate treatment consists of administration of parenteral analgesics for pain and avoidance of oral intake for 3 to 7 days. The use of adrenocorticosteroids to contain the tissue reaction responsible for the stricture, intubation to maintain an esophageal lumen, and antibiotics to prevent mediastinitis are controversial.

DIFFUSE ESOPHAGEAL SPASM

Diffuse esophageal spasm is not a specific disease but a common disorder of esophageal motility which is caused by several unrelated conditions. It may be a manifestation of aging (presbyesophagus), ganglion degeneration (as seen in early stages of achalasia), mucosal irritation (most commonly encountered in gastroesophageal reflux and esophageal moniliasis), obstruction at the cardia, neuromuscular disorders such as diabetic neuropathy and amyotrophic lateral sclerosis, or if none of these features is present, it may be labeled idiopathic. Diffuse spasm in severe form produces retrosternal pain, dysphagia, or both. Many patients may, however, have radiographic or manometric evidence of the disorder without symptoms. In patients with this disorder, peristalsis is initiated normally by swallowing, but as the wave approaches the distal third of the esophagus, the progressive contraction is supplanted by "spastic" or simultaneous contractions. One-third of symptomatic patients have elevated resting pressure and incomplete relaxation of the lower esophageal sphincter with swallowing, dysfunction similar to that of achalasia.

Symptoms Dysphagia or substernal distress occurs episodically. Symptoms frequently, although not necessarily, are trig-

gered by ingestion of elastic boluses (such as meat) or cold or carbonated beverages, and by eating when tense or upset. On occasion a bolus becomes so firmly lodged in the "spastic" segment that relief is achieved only by retching and regurgitating the offending bolus. Following such an episode the patient usually can return to the table and finish the meal without incident. Weight loss and aspiration pneumonia are rarely features of diffuse spasm. Substernal pain of esophageal origin may be acute and severe, and may be confused with angina pectoris, especially if symptoms are not associated with eating.

Diagnosis The diagnosis is suggested by the history of intermittent dysphagia and chest pain. X-ray findings (with barium swallow) confirm the existence of disordered esophageal motility. The mildest abnormality is tertiary or segmental contractions without a peristaltic wave in the distal esophagus. The contour of the lower esophagus may take a variety of bizarre shapes described as curling, pseudodiverticulosis, corkscrew, or rosary-bead esophagus. Symptoms, however, do not clearly correlate with the extent of the abnormality seen on barium swallow. Indeed, only a minority of patients with this disturbed motor pattern have significant symptoms. The motility abnormalities of diffuse esophageal spasm may be recorded by esophageal manometry.

Treatment The first step in the treatment of diffuse spasm is to assure the patient that it is a benign condition. The second step is to minimize the contribution of gastroesophageal reflux by prescribing antacids and small meals and elevation of the head of the bed as already described under "Gastroesophageal Reflux and Esophagitis."

An occasional patient obtains gratifying control of symptoms with the use of sublingual nitroglycerin at mealtime. Anticholinergic drugs, however, have not provided symptomatic relief. In patients with sphincter abnormality and severe, poorly controlled symptoms forceful distention of the lower esophagus and sphincter by a pneumostatic dilator may be employed. As a last resort, a longitudinal myotomy of the entire distal esophagus has been successful in providing relief. This is, however, an extensive operation for a benign disorder and is very rarely required.

ACHALASIA

The terms *achalasia* and *cardiospasm* are used interchangeably for a disease usually presenting as slowly progressive dysphagia. Neither describes the nature of the disease completely. Actually, achalasia is a motor disorder involving the entire distal two-thirds of the esophagus. The pressure within the lower esophageal sphincter is greater than normal, relaxation of the sphincter in response to a swallow is incomplete, and the sphincter is supersensitive to gastrin. In addition, there is no peristaltic response to swallowing in the esophagus. For this reason, the name *aperistalsis* is used in Brazil. Finally, the massive dilatation seen in some patients has, in turn, given rise to the name *megaesophagus*.

The motor disorder of achalasia appears to reflect impaired cholinergic innervation of the esophagus. Although the greatest attention has been given to the damage and loss of postganglionic parasympathetic neurons of the myenteric plexuses, pathologic lesions have also been described in the brainstem and extrinsic vagal fibers. Pharmacologic studies have shown that the administration of a cholinergic agent produces violent, segmental contractions of the affected esophagus. This response, when interpreted in the light of Cannon's finding that denervated structures respond maximally to neurohumoral stimulation, provides additional evidence that in achalasia the cholinergic innervation of the esophagus is deficient. Recently, the response of the lower esophageal sphincter to gastrin, which is mediated through the postganglionic parasympathetic fibers, has been shown to be hyperactive in achalasia. Since the normal neuromuscular interactions and the pathology of achalasia are incompletely understood, it is not possible to define the mechanisms responsible for the loss of peristalsis and normal sphincter function in achalasia. In Brazil, the remarkable prevalence of achalasia in areas where Chagas' disease is prevalent has fostered the conviction that the intrinsic esophageal denervation is a late result of esophageal infestation by *Trypanosoma cruzi*. This agent cannot be implicated in achalasia in the United States.

Symptoms Achalasia affects patients of all ages and both sexes. Its course is usually chronic, with dysphagia gradually worsening over months to years, leading to progressive weight loss. In some patients, the process is painless; in others spasms of substernal pain may follow eating. Occasionally the initial episode of dysphagia appears with dramatic suddenness, either after bolting food or after an emotional upset. In either case, however, the condition has probably been present in latent form before the acute episode. As the disease progresses, extreme and tortuous dilatation of the esophagus may develop. When the patient lies down, the copious amount of food residue and saliva contained in the spacious esophageal sac may flow into the pharynx and mouth. If the regurgitated material is aspirated, recurrent aspiration pneumonia is a potential serious complication. Although stagnation of food in the esophagus may be striking, esophagitis rarely if ever occurs in untreated achalasia.

Diagnosis Diagnosis is usually made without difficulty on the basis of the history and the characteristic radiologic findings of abnormal esophageal motor function with smooth, beaklike narrowing of the distal esophageal segment. In untreated achalasia an air-fluid level is always maintained in the esophagus. An occasional case presents as diffuse esophageal spasm and evolves into typical achalasia only after many years of symptoms. In some cases, cancer originating in the gastric cardia and infiltrating the esophagus may present a somewhat similar x-ray appearance. This possibility is best excluded by esophagoscopic examination of the distal esophagus and cardia. These problems in differential diagnosis would be less frequent if it is remembered that the radiologic abnormalities of achalasia consist of deranged peristalsis as well as narrowing in the area of the sphincter.

Treatment Symptomatic medical treatment consisting of sedatives, semisoft foods, nitrites, and anticholinergic drugs is not effective. The best available therapy is forceful dilation of the unrelaxing sphincter with the specific purpose of tearing some of the muscle fibers in this area. Passing graduated mercury-tipped bougies does not accomplish this purpose and therefore relieves dysphagia only briefly. It is necessary to use bags that can be inflated under pressure or a mechanical (Starck) dilator. In experienced hands, these instruments, when positioned under fluoroscopic control, rarely cause esophageal rupture, and dysphagia is relieved successfully for years, or even permanently, in over 75 percent of patients. Forceful dilation does not restore normal esophageal motility, but it impairs the contractile power of the sphincter and thus permits the esophagus to empty by means of gravity and transmitted oropharyngeal pressures. Improved esophageal emptying, in turn, prevents further distention of the lumen and aspiration of esophageal contents.

When the esophagus is extremely dilated and sufficiently tortuous to warrant the adjective *sigmoid,* mechanical dilation of the narrowed area is often not feasible and surgical myotomy becomes necessary. Unfortunately any procedure that removes the sphincter between the dilated esophagus and the

stomach permits, when the patient lies, reflux of gastric contents into an already damaged esophagus which cannot muster the peristaltic force necessary to return the gastric contents to the stomach. As a consequence severe esophagitis, which is often more distressing than the achalasia and may also be a major source of blood loss, occurs. If technically feasible, the surgical procedure favored at present is the Heller myotomy, which is based on the same principle as forceful dilation: the contractile power of the sphincter is reduced by placing a longitudinal cut through the muscle, but not the mucosa, of the narrowed segment. However, myotomy is not invariably successful in alleviating dysphagia or preventing reflux esophagitis. In advanced cases, with unsuccessful previous operative procedures, colonic interposition may have to be used to replace the hopelessly malfunctioning gastroesophageal segment.

CANCER

Symptoms The importance of dysphagia as a symptom and the urgent necessity of determining its cause are no better exemplified than by the patient with esophageal cancer. No cancer, with the possible exception of carcinoma of the pancreas, has a worse prognosis. Difficulty in swallowing solids is the patient's first and usually only complaint as the tumor encroaches upon the lumen. Although initially intermittent, the dysphagia is inexorably progressive over a course of rarely more than 6 months. Pain under the sternum, the back, or in the neck is common and may merely be caused by associated spasm or esophagitis, but it usually indicates spread of the tumor through the wall of the esophagus. In some cases an early symptom not to be ignored is substernal burning on swallowing hot liquids. Slow oozing of blood is a frequent complication, but brisk bleeding is rare. When esophageal stenosis is severe, regurgitation of esophageal contents, which are sometimes blood-flecked, is common.

Approximately 25 percent of squamous esophageal cancers are in the upper third, 50 percent in the middle, and 25 percent in the lower third of the organ. Lesions in the upper two-thirds are derived from squamous esophageal mucosa. In the distal esophagus over half the cases prove to be adenocarcinomas, indicating that many cancers in this area are gastric in origin. Origin in the stomach is, in fact, often evident at operation in cases which radiologically appear to be purely esophageal.

Course Physical examination is usually negative, and even those patients with advanced disease may present no more than the signs of malnutrition. Although metastases to lymph nodes occur in three-fourths of the cases, only 5 percent have palpable nodes in the supraclavicular or other accessible areas. Because the liver and lung each are involved eventually in 20 to 25 percent of the cases, hepatomegaly or pulmonary lesions may be evident. Other organs subject to metastatic foci are bone, kidneys, and adrenal glands. Sometimes direct invasion of adjoining structures leads to dramatic complications: (1) mediastinitis with subcutaneous emphysema in the neck, (2) tracheoesophageal or bronchoesophageal fistula with an apoplectic cough induced by swallowing liquids, or (3) aortic perforation with precipitous exsanguination.

Diagnosis Esophageal cancer occurs in the usual cancer age groups, and predominantly in males in a ratio of 4:1. In the United States and Europe it accounts for only 7 percent of all cancers in males, whereas in some parts of Asia it is one of the most common cancers. In the United States there is a strong correlation between heavy use of alcohol and cigarettes and esophageal cancer. In addition, the incidence of esophageal cancer appears increased in patients with severe corrosive burns of the esophagus and Barrett's esophagus. Less well substantiated is the reported association with achalasia. X-ray often reveals the irregular and sometimes surprisingly long luminal defect caused by esophageal cancer, but supplemental diagnostic information must usually be sought by esophagoscopy, biopsy, and brushings of the lesion for cytological examination. The initial examination is not invariably adequate in differentiating cancer from inflammatory stricture. In these cases, repeat esophagoscopy with biopsy and brushings as well as cytologic examination of material obtained by esophageal lavage is indicated.

Treatment Lesions that appear to be resectable are usually treated surgically. Calculated on the basis of all esophageal cancer patients who enter a hospital, the 5-year cure rate is still no higher than 7 percent. In some selected series, 5-year cure rates of 15 percent have been reported in patients with cancer of the lower third of the esophagus who have no gross evidence of extension at operation. Somewhat better results have been obtained by combining resection with preoperative irradiation. Successful resection of middle and upper-third lesions is more difficult or impossible, and such lesions are usually treated with radiotherapy. Since esophageal cancer is so rarely curable, the clinical question usually is what will provide the simplest, most effective palliation. In many patients dysphagia can be minimized by regular bougienage or placement of a silastic tube through the neoplastic stricture. The misery of starvation and repeated aspiration thus is avoided.

OTHER ESOPHAGEAL DISORDERS

DIVERTICULA Diverticula are found in the esophagus in about 5 percent of older patients who are given a swallow of barium. Most of these pouches occur in the midesophagus and distal esophagus, but they are usually small (1 to 4 cm in diameter) and do not cause symptoms. Extremely rarely an esophageal diverticulum is subject to ulceration or becomes large enough to cause dysphagia. A diverticulum of great clinical importance, however, is Zenker's diverticulum, a pouch which actually arises in the posterior aspect of the hypopharynx above the upper esophageal sphincter but which extends downward between the spine and the esophagus. Patients with this condition—elderly men for the most part—suffer dysphagia because swallowed material tends to fill the diverticular sac, which then compresses the esophagus. Regurgitation of stagnant food and nocturnal fits of coughing may complicate the picture. The diagnosis can usually be made by x-ray provided the pharynx is adequately studied as the patient swallows barium. Surgical treatment is necessary to relieve the symptoms of Zenker's diverticulum. Myotomy of the upper sphincter has improved the results of surgical treatment.

LOWER ESOPHAGEAL RING This is the name given to a thin, symmetric, diaphragm-like structure located 1 to 4 cm above the diaphragmatic hiatus. Ten to twenty percent of adults have asymptomatic rings, but if the residual lumen is less than 12 mm in diameter, the ring may cause a highly characteristic syndrome consisting of intermittent attacks of dysphagia, recurring over years, unassociated with any other esophageal abnormality and precipitated only when the patient swallows meat or other elastic chunks without proper chewing. Treatment usually consists of avoiding hasty swallowing. Dilation is inconstantly successful. In a few, unusually severe cases, surgical treatment with cutting or fracture of the diaphragm is indicated.

SCLERODERMA (PROGRESSIVE SYSTEMIC SCLEROSIS)
Scleroderma is associated with loss of esophageal peristalsis and sphincter tone in more than 80 percent of the cases. Although gastroesophageal reflux and esophagitis are common, heartburn is not a prominent feature, and dysphagia, which is much less striking than that encountered with achalasia, does not become prominent until esophagitis has led to stricture of the esophagus. Chronic blood loss may be an important complication. Esophageal aperistalsis is not limited to scleroderma but may be seen occasionally in other disorders, particularly those associated with Raynaud's phenomenon. Since all defenses against gastroesophageal reflux are compromised in patients with scleroderma and other symptoms appear later, they should all be treated with antireflux measures.

DERMATOMYOSITIS Oropharyngeal dysphagia (see Chap. 34) complicates the course of patients with dermatomyositis because of involvement of the striated muscle of the pharynx. Difficulty in propelling the bolus from the mouth into the esophagus, regurgitation into the nose, and aspiration are the consequences of pharyngeal muscle weakness. Aperistalsis of the esophagus is seen occasionally in patients with polymyositis. It is sometimes difficult to categorize these patients, because they may have features of both scleroderma and dermatomyositis.

PEPTIC ULCER A solitary peptic ulcer is occasionally found in the distal esophagus. This lesion differs from peptic esophagitis in that the ulcer is sharply localized, penetrates deeply, and may perforate or cause massive bleeding. The solitary peptic ulcer in the distal esophagus resembles a benign gastric ulcer in many respects. Most frequently they occur at the junction between squamous and columnar epithelium. Healing frequently leads to stricture.

PERFORATION AND RUPTURE Perforation of the esophagus may complicate esophagitis, peptic ulcer, or neoplasm. Rupture may be induced by external trauma or, more commonly, during instrumentation of the esophagus. Sometimes it develops spontaneously in a previously healthy organ. The consequences are a syndrome comprising (1) severe pain, usually substernal but occasionally epigastric or precordial, intensified by swallowing; (2) free air in the mediastinum, producing a mediastinal crunch and subcutaneous emphysema palpable within 1 to 12 h; (3) digestion of mediastinal pleura by pressure and gastric juice with resultant hydropneumothorax or hemopneumothorax and respiratory embarrassment; (4) shock; and (5) secondary infection.

Spontaneous rupture is a specific entity that develops suddenly during vomiting or coughing, or occasionally merely after injudicious gluttony. The tear, 1 to 8 cm in length, almost invariably is in the posterolateral portion of the esophagus immediately proximal to the diaphragmatic hiatus. The diagnosis should be suspected in patients who suddenly have pain while vomiting or coughing; it is established by x-ray (air in the mediastinum or neck or demonstration of laceration by having the patient swallow radiopaque material). Mediastinal emphysema is usually a late finding so the diagnosis should not be delayed because of its absence. Spontaneous rupture of the esophagus is often mistakenly diagnosed as myocardial infarction, pancreatitis, or ruptured abdominal viscus. Confusion is avoided if it is remembered that vomiting precedes pain in rupture of the esophagus, whereas vomiting, if it occurs, follows pain in those disease states most commonly mistaken for rupture of the esophagus.

Perforation of the esophagus is fatal if not treated vigorously. In early cases, constant esophageal suction and parenteral administration of antibiotics, which are active against both enteric gram-negative organisms and enterococci, should be given. Surgical drainage and repair of the laceration are indicated as soon as possible.

A disorder closely allied to spontaneous esophageal rupture is vertical laceration of the gastroesophageal junction producing severe and occasionally exsanguinating hemorrhage. This so-called "Mallory-Weiss syndrome" usually develops when vomiting follows an alcoholic bout.

KELLY-PATTERSON (PLUMMER-VINSON) SYNDROME This syndrome, also known as *sideropenic dysphagia,* is a cause of dysphagia in women with hypochromic anemia. A crescentic fold indenting the anterior aspect of the cricopharyngeal area and mucosal atrophy and inflammation of the hypopharynx are features of this disorder. A good diet and iron are usually therapeutically effective. This lesion predisposes to pharyngeal carcinoma.

FOREIGN BODIES Foreign bodies may cause dysphagia, pain, or perforation of the esophagus. Rigid bodies usually are arrested above the aortic arch, and elastic material usually is held up in the distal esophagus. Not infrequently a structural abnormality or disease of the esophagus is responsible for stopping the foreign body.

VARICES Esophageal varices are discussed in Chaps. 38 and 304. They do not cause dysphagia or other esophageal symptoms. Radiologically, however, they may be confused with cancer or esophagitis.

BENIGN INTRAMURAL TUMORS OF THE ESOPHAGUS Tumors such as cysts (usually of respiratory tract origin), leiomyoma, fibroma, and neurofibroma may cause intermittent dysphagia and sharply defined radiologic defects with smooth margins. Some benign tumors, especially adenomas, may produce intraluminal polyps.

The esophagus may be affected by leukoplakia, acanthosis nigricans, sarcoma, Hodgkin's disease, and leukemia.

EXTRINSIC DISEASE Diseases of the aorta, heart, respiratory tract, or mediastinal lymph nodes often displace the esophagus and may appear to narrow the lumen. Aneurysms of the aortic arch and an aberrant right subclavian artery may compress the esophageal lumen; however, dysphagia is rarely produced by extrinsic esophageal masses. Invasion of the esophagus by bronchogenic carcinoma occurs rarely.

REFERENCES

ATKINSON M: Disorders of oesophageal motility. Clin Gastroenterol 5:1, 1976

BEHAR J et al: Medical and surgical management of reflux esophagitis. N Engl J Med 293:263, 1975

———— et al: Evaluation of esophageal tests in the diagnosis of reflux esophagitis. Gastroenterology 71:9, 1976

BENNETT JR, HENDRIX TR: Diffuse esophageal spasm: A disorder with more than one cause. Gastroenterology 59:273, 1970

BRAND DL et al: Esophageal manometrics in patients with angina-like chest pain. Am J Dig Dis 22:300, 1977

COHEN S, HARRIS LD: Does hiatus hernia affect competence of the gastroesophageal sphincter? N Engl J Med 284:1053, 1971

DIMARINO AJ, COHN S: Characteristics of lower esophageal sphincter function in symptomatic diffuse esophageal spasm. Gastroenterology 66:1, 1974

HEIT HA et al: Palliative dilation for dysphagia in esophageal carcinoma. Ann Int Med 89:629, 1978

POPE CE II: Pathophysiology and diagnosis of reflux esophagitis. Gastroenterology 70:445, 1976

Symposium on Esophageal Motility. Arch Intern Med 136:511, 1976

VANTRAPPEN G et al: Achalasia, diffuse esophageal spasm and related motility disorders. Gastroenterology 76:450, 1979

290
PEPTIC ULCER

JAMES E. McGUIGAN

Peptic ulcer is a term used to refer to a group of ulcerative disorders of the upper gastrointestinal tract, which appear to have in common the participation of acid-pepsin in their pathogenesis. The major forms are chronic duodenal and gastric ulcer. The Zollinger-Ellison syndrome (gastrinoma) may also be considered a form of peptic ulcer.

Although our present knowledge of the etiology of peptic ulcer is incomplete, studies in humans and in experimental animals indicate that acid-pepsin is crucial for development of peptic ulcer. The presence or absence of peptic ulcer is determined by the delicate interplay between gastric acid secretion and mucosal resistance. Why do not all humans develop peptic ulcer? The normal capacity of gastric and proximal duodenal mucosa to resist the corrosive effects of acid-pepsin is extraordinary and unique. This resistance is not shared by other tissues—hence the susceptibility of the esophageal mucosa when exposed to refluxed gastric juice and the almost inevitable ulceration of the small intestine at the site of surgical attachment to actively secreting gastric mucosa.

Much has been learned concerning the mechanisms regulating gastric secretion and the factors which appear important in development of peptic ulcer. Consideration of gastric physiology provides an understanding of some elements responsible for the development of peptic ulcers and also a rational basis for its treatment.

GASTRIC PHYSIOLOGY RELATED TO PEPTIC ULCER

The gastric mucosa possesses an extraordinary capacity to secrete acid. Parietal (oxyntic) cells secrete hydrochloric acid by a process involving oxidative phosphorylation. Parietal cells, located in mucosal glands in the body and fundus of the stomach, can secrete hydrogen ions at a concentration 3 million times that found in blood. The estimated concentration of HCl secreted directly by parietal cells is approximately 160 mM. Each secreted hydrogen ion (H^+) is accompanied by a chloride ion (Cl^-). With increased gastric hydrogen ion secretion, there is a reciprocal decrease in sodium ion secretion. For each hydrogen ion (H^+) secreted into the gastric lumen one bicarbonate ion (HCO_3^-) is returned via the gastric venous circulation, accounting for the *alkaline tide,* which directly reflects the magnitude of gastric H^+ secretion. Bicarbonate is released from carbonic acid; the latter is generated from carbon dioxide by carbonic anhydrase of the parietal cell. The two-component hypothesis for secretion of gastric juice proposes that parietal cells secrete pure HCl, which is mixed (in various proportions) with nonparietal cell alkaline secretions, similar in ionic composition to extracellular fluid.

Both *neural* and *hormonal* factors participate in regulation of gastric acid secretion. Acid secretion is stimulated by gastrin and by cholinergic postganglionic vagal fibers via muscarinic receptors on parietal cells. Gastrin, the most potent known stimulant of gastric acid secretion, consists of a family of polypeptides, present in cells of the antral pyloric glands. The major form of tissue gastrin is heptadecapeptide gastrin (G-17) containing 17 amino acid residues. Gastrin II is a form in which the tyrosyl residue is sulfated at position 12, and gastrin I is the nonsulfated form. Approximately two-thirds of circulating gastrin consists of a larger molecular species of gastrin, namely, "big gastrin" or G-34, which contains 34 amino acids, the final 17 of which are identical to heptadecapeptide gastrins. G-17 has a shorter half-life than G-34. Although most circulating gastrin is G-34, the major hormonal stimulus to gastric acid secretion after feeding is due to G-17. On a molar basis circulating G-17 is approximately six times as potent as G-34 in stimulating gastric acid secretion.

More than 90 percent of antral mucosal gastrin is in the form of G-17. Gastrin is also present in duodenal mucosa, the highest concentration being in the most proximal duodenum (at 10 percent of the antral concentration).

The effects of gastrin and the vagus on gastric acid secretion are intimately related. Vagal action enhances gastric acid secretion by (1) directly stimulating parietal cells, (2) stimulating release of gastrin into the circulation, and (3) lowering the parietal cell threshold to circulating gastrin concentrations. While the roles of gastrin and acetylcholine (the vagal effector) in parietal cell acid secretion have been well established, controversy remains regarding the exact role of histamine in this process. Histamine is present in large concentrations in mast cells in the parietal cell–containing regions of the gastric mucosa. Views on the importance of histamine differ enormously. Some have suggested that histamine is the "final common pathway" for cholinergic and gastrin stimulation of parietal cell acid secretion; others have been skeptical about any role of histamine in this process.

The role of histamine on acid secretion has been renewed by the discovery of H$_2$-receptor antagonists which inhibit the action of histamine on H$_2$ receptors (located on gastric parietal, cardiac atrial, and uterine smooth-muscle cells). These drugs exert negligible effect on H$_1$ receptors, which are readily inhibited by conventional antihistamines. H$_2$-receptor antagonists (e.g., cimetidine) inhibit basal acid secretion and secretory responses to feeding, gastrin, histamine, and vagal stimulation. Most of the available data support the concept that (1) histamine plays a role in stimulating acid secretion, (2) it acts in concert with gastrin and cholinergic activity, but (3) it is probably not the final common effector molecule in the stimulation of parietal cell secretion.

Food ingestion is the major physiological stimulus of gastric acid secretion. Traditionally, gastric acid secretion has been divided into three phases—cephalic, gastric, and intestinal. This classification is of some value in examining the multiple factors which regulate gastric acid secretion. The cephalic phase represents the secretory response to the sight, smell, taste, and anticipation of food. The gastric phase is induced by the presence of food in the stomach. The intestinal phase is due to the entry or presence of food within the lumen of the small intestine. Although these three phases provide a convenience for consideration of the diverse contributions to gastric acid secretion, each phase is complex and probably not due to a single stimulatory control mechanism.

The cephalic phase is mediated by the vagus which in turn leads to acid secretion by stimulation of parietal cells directly and by an increased release of gastrin. The gastric phase involves stimulation of chemical and mechanical receptors in the gastric wall luminal contents. Mechanical distention of the stomach stimulates gastric acid secretion but not gastrin release; this mechanical effect is inhibited by atropine and appears to be mediated by vagal reflexes. Food in the stomach promotes acid secretion by increasing gastrin release, principally due to the protein content of the meal; oral glucose and fat cause slight increases in serum gastrin but do not stimulate gastric acid secretion. Food in the proximal small intestine stimulates the intestinal phase of gastric acid secretion. A peptone meal introduced into the small intestine stimulates gastric acid secretion but not gastrin release. It has been proposed that

food in the small intestine induces release of an intestinal hormone, presumably a polypeptide, which stimulates gastric acid secretion. This substance is believed to be distinct from gastrin and, unlike gastrin, appears to be degraded substantially during its portal transit through the liver.

Ingestion of coffee (either caffeine-containing or caffeine-free) stimulates gastric acid secretion; the mechanism has not been defined but appears not to involve increased gastrin release. In humans ethanol ingestion does not stimulate gastrin release or acid secretion; in fact, at concentrations sufficient to interrupt the gastric mucosal barrier (i.e., greater than 14 percent), ethanol reduces gastric acid output. Intravenous calcium stimulates acid secretion and produces minimal increases in serum gastrin levels. Oral calcium can stimulate gastric acid secretion directly, i.e., without an increase in serum calcium or gastrin concentrations. Except in patients with gastrinoma, hypercalcemia is usually not associated with acid hypersecretion or increases in serum gastrin.

Inhibition of acid secretion can be produced by several mechanisms. Acid secretion may be inhibited by acid in the stomach or duodenum, by hyperglycemia, or by hypertonic fluids or fat in the duodenum. Reduction of the intragastric pH to 3.0 produces a partial inhibition of gastrin release; further reduction to pH 1.5 or below blocks the release of gastrin to almost all stimuli. Acid in the duodenum inhibits gastric acid secretion by stimulation of secretin release. Secretin is a linear polypeptide which contains 27 amino acids and bears structural similarities to glucagon. Secretin is contained in the cytoplasm of cells (S cells) in the mucosa of the small intestine. Fat in the duodenum appears to inhibit acid secretion by the intestinal release of gastric inhibitory peptide (GIP) or cholecystokinin (CCK). GIP directly inhibits gastric acid secretion, whereas CCK (a polypeptide containing 33 amino acids and having some structural similarities to gastrin) is a weak gastrin agonist and it inhibits gastrin-mediated acid secretion. The mechanisms by which hyperglycemia or intraduodenal hyperosmolality inhibits gastric acid secretion are not known. A large number of peptides have been identified in the mucosa of the gastrointestinal tract which have the capacity to inhibit gastric acid secretion. These peptides include somatostatin, glucagon, vasoactive intestinal peptide (VIP) and urogastrone. The latter appears to be structurally and functionally identical to epidermal growth factor. The extent to which these peptides contribute to the overall regulation of acid secretion is not clear.

The proteolytic effects of pepsin and the corrosive effects of acid appear to be integral components in the tissue injury which leads to peptic ulceration. Acid autocatalytically cleaves inactive pepsinogen molecules to active pepsins and also provides the pH required for pepsin activity. Pepsin activity is almost completely abolished above pH 3.0, and these enzymes are inactivated irreversibly at neutral or alkaline pH. There are a variety of pepsinogens and pepsins in gastric juice. Pepsinogens (and their corresponding active pepsins) have been classified by immunochemical techniques as either PG I (pepsinogens 1 through 5) or PG II (pepsinogens 6 and 7). Pepsinogen I is present in chief and mucous cells in the body and fundus of the stomach. Pepsinogen II is located in cells of the pyloric glands, Brunner's glands of the duodenum, mucous cells of the gastric cardiac glands, and the same cells in which PG I is found. Both PG I and PG II are found in plasma, while only PG I can be detected in urine. A high degree of correlation exists between serum concentrations of PG I and maximal gastric acid secretion. In general, agents which stimulate gastric acid secretion also stimulate pepsinogen secretion. Cholinergic action is particularly potent in promoting pepsinogen secretion. Secretin, although it inhibits gastric acid secretion, serves as a stimulus to pepsinogen secretion.

Parietal cells also secrete *intrinsic factor.* Thus agents which stimulate gastric acid secretion also lead to secretion of intrinsic factor.

Gastric *mucus,* secreted by gastric mucous cells, is a gelatinous material which coats the mucosal surface. Mucus secretion is enhanced by mechanical or chemical irritation and by cholinergic stimulation. Gastric mucus contains mucopolysaccharides and glycoproteins, including blood group substances. Approximately three-fourths of the population secrete gastric juice containing AB(H) substances and are referred to as *secretors.* Although the physiological role of gastric mucus is not well understood, there is doubt that mucus contributes significantly to neutralization of stimulated gastric acid secretions.

The precise mechanism by which the normal stomach and duodenum resist the corrosive effects of acid-pepsin has not been defined. The importance of gastric mucus to mucosal resistance is controversial, and there appears to be no convincing evidence that gastric mucus contributes significantly to mucosal resistance to acid-pepsin. The *gastric mucosal barrier,* however, may participate in mucosal resistance to acid-peptic ulceration. Normally the gastric luminal epithelial cell surfaces and intercellular tight junctions provide an almost completely impermeable barrier to back-diffusion of hydrogen ions from the lumen. This barrier may be interrupted by various agents including bile acids, salicylates, alcohol, and weak organic acids and thus permit back-diffusion of hydrogen ions from the lumen to intercellular sites. Such back-diffusion may result in cellular injury, release of histamine from mast cells, further stimulation of acid secretion, damage to small blood vessels, mucosal hemorrhage, and superficial ulceration. Interruption of the gastric mucosal barrier may be responsible (at least in part) for the hemorrhagic erosive gastritis associated with salicylate and ethanol ingestion, and may also contribute to other forms of gastric mucosal injury.

The relationship between the gastric mucosal barrier and mucosal resistance to chronic peptic ulcer has not been completely elucidated. Other mucosal factors, some of which are genetic, apparently contribute to the ability of the gastric mucosa to resist or permit the development of peptic ulceration.

MEASUREMENT OF GASTRIC ACID SECRETION

Since hydrochloric acid secretion by the stomach appears to be an important factor in the production of peptic ulcer disease, measurement of basal and stimulated acid secretion by the stomach may be of value in the assessment of peptic ulcer patients. In general, basal and stimulated acid outputs in females are approximately two-thirds to three-fourths those found in males. The range for normal-value subjects is extremely broad and overlaps substantially with that found in patients with duodenal ulcer, gastric ulcer, and even the Zollinger-Ellison syndrome. Mean basal acid output (BAO) in normal males without known ulcer disease is about 1.5 to 2.0 meq/h. In individual ulcer patients mean basal acid output averages from 4 to 6 meq/h, again with a wide degree of variation. Patients with gastric ulcer tend to have gastric acid secretory rates which are normal or even slightly below those of normal subjects.

Measurement of gastric acid output is not helpful in either diagnosing peptic ulcer or excluding it. Thus measuring gastric acid secretion is clearly not necessary in all patients with duodenal ulcer disease. However, detection of gastric acid hypersecretion is of value in patients in whom the Zollinger-Ellison syndrome is suspected. Measurement of gastric acid output is useful to detect achlorhydria as found in patients with pernicious anemia. Since patients with benign gastric ulcer virtually always secrete some acid, pentagastrin-fast achlorhydria in a patient with a gastric ulcer almost always indicates malignancy. Measurement of gastric acid secretion is indicated in the assessment of patients in whom recurrence of ulcer is suspected after surgery for peptic ulcer.

In order to measure gastric acid output, a radiopaque gastric tube is passed so that its tip is located in the most dependent portion of the stomach. With the patient in a reclining or semirecumbent position on the left side, the position of the tube is verified by fluoroscopy. Gastric contents are aspirated and discarded. Basal gastric acid secretions are then collected in four consecutive 15-min intervals to determine the 1-h basal acid output. Secretion volume and acid concentration (titrated with 0.1 N sodium hydroxide to pH 7.0) are measured, and acid output is expressed as milliequivalents per hour.

A variety of substances have been used to produce maximal acid output (MAO) by the stomach. These have included histamine, betazole (Histalog)—a structural analog of histamine, and pentagastrin (Peptavalon). *Histamine,* the first standard stimulant to be used for gastric acid secretory testing, requires the simultaneous administration of an antihistaminic agent to inhibit untoward systemic side effects. *Betazole* possesses less of the undesired side effects of histamine and does not require the concomitant administration of an antihistamine. *Pentagastrin* (*N-tert*-butyloxycarbonyl-β-Ala-Trp-Met-Asp-Phe-NH$_2$) contains the carboxyl-terminal tetrapeptide amide portion of the gastrin molecule and is currently the preferred agent to induce maximal acid secretion. Gastric juice is again collected for four consecutive 15-min periods after the subcutaneous injection of pentagastrin (6 μg/kg). The MAO is determined by the milliequivalent of acid aspirated 1 h after pentagastrin administration. Peak acid output (PAO) is calculated by combining the two highest consecutive 15-min acid outputs and multiplying by 2.

DUODENAL ULCER

GENERAL CONSIDERATIONS Duodenal ulcer is a chronic and recurrent disease. The ulcer is usually deep and sharply demarcated. It tends to penetrate through the submucosa and often into the muscularis propria. The ulcer floor contains no intact epithelium and usually consists of a zone of eosinophilic necrosis resting on a base of granulation tissue surrounded by variable amounts of fibrosis. The ulcer bed may be clear or contain either blood or a proteinaceous exudate with entrapped erythrocytes and acute and chronic inflammatory cells. More than 95 percent of duodenal ulcers occur in the first portion of the duodenum, and approximately 90 percent of these are located within 3 cm of the junction of the pyloric and duodenal mucosa. Duodenal ulcers are usually round or oval but may be irregular or elliptic. They are usually less than 1 cm in diameter. Rarely, duodenal ulcers may be extremely large (3 to 6 cm diameter) and may be mistaken radiographically for the entire duodenal bulb. These giant ulcers are usually identified only endoscopically or at surgery or postmortem examination.

The absolute prevalence of duodenal ulcer in the population is not known. Estimates have ranged from 6 to 15 percent. This variation may be related to the populations examined, differences in study design and diagnostic methods (e.g., endoscopy vs. radiological examination), and perhaps to actual changes in frequency of duodenal ulcer disease. The best current estimates suggest that approximately 10 percent of the population has a clinical evidence of duodenal ulcer at some time in their lifetimes. Duodenal ulcer is approximately twice as common in males as in females and is four times as frequent as clinically recognized gastric ulcer. Some studies suggest that the frequency of duodenal ulcer has been decreasing in the United States and England during the past 25 years. If these observations are valid, there is no current explanation for this reduction.

Although much is now known concerning factors which contribute to development of duodenal ulcer, we do not completely understand its pathogenesis. Acid secretion by the stomach is required for production of a duodenal ulcer, but the factors which render the acid-secreting subject susceptible to duodenal ulceration are not completely understood. As a group, the ulcer patients secrete more acid than normal; however, from one-half to two-thirds of duodenal ulcer patients have gastric acid secretory rates (both BAO and MAO) within normal range. A duodenal ulcer tends to develop when there is an unfavorable balance between acid-pepsin secretion and mucosal resistance. In duodenal ulcer disease, the evidence favors the etiologic importance of absolute or relative gastric acid hypersecretion. In patients with gastric ulcer defective mucosal resistance appears to be the dominant major permissive factor.

Fasting *serum gastrin* levels are normal in duodenal ulcer patients. However, in response to a protein-containing meal, more gastrin is released into the circulation in duodenal ulcer patients than in normal subjects. Duodenal ulcer patients also have a greater response to gastrin than normal persons. Thus pentagastrin produces a greater acid secretory response for a given dose, and smaller doses of pentagastrin are required to achieve the same fraction of the maximal acid secretory response in duodenal ulcer patients compared with normal subjects. In addition, in duodenal ulcer patients intragastric acid appears to have less of an effect in inhibiting gastrin release. Therefore, although fasting serum gastrin levels are normal in duodenal ulcer patients, gastrin may still play an important role in the acid hypersecretion which is often observed in duodenal ulcer disease.

Genetic factors appear to be important. Duodenal ulcers are approximately three times as common in first-degree relatives of duodenal ulcer patients when compared with the population at large. Patients with duodenal ulcers have an increased frequency of blood group O and of the nonsecretory status [those who do not secrete AB(H) antigens in their gastric juice], but these associations are weak. An increased incidence of HLA-B5 antigen in white male subjects with duodenal ulcer has also been shown. Previously no strong genetic marker for the disease was identified, but recently elevated serum pepsinogen I (PG I) levels have been found to be inherited as an autosomal dominant trait. It thus appears that an elevated PG I level may prove to be a subclinical marker of the duodenal ulcer diathesis in families with this autosomal dominant form of peptic ulcer disease.

Cigarette smoking has been associated with increased duodenal ulcer frequency, decreased responses to therapy, and an increased mortality (from duodenal ulcer). The incidence of duodenal ulcer is also increased in patients with chronic renal failure, alcoholic cirrhosis, and chronic obstructive pulmonary disease.

The importance of psychological factors in the pathogenesis of duodenal ulcer is controversial. Contrary to earlier views, there is no single characteristic duodenal ulcer personality. There are no identifiable differences in frequency of duodenal ulcer among different socioeconomic classes or occupational groups. Chronic anxiety and psychologic stress may, however, be factors in exacerbation of ulcer activity.

CLINICAL FEATURES Epigastric pain is by far the most frequent symptom of duodenal ulcer. The pain is often described as burning or gnawing. Just as frequently, however, the pain may be ill-defined, boring, or aching, or perceived as abdominal pressure or fullness, or as a sensation of hunger. In approximately 10 percent of patients the pain is located to the right of the midepigastrium. The pain characteristically occurs from 90 min to 3 h after eating. It frequently awakens the patient at night. Pain on awakening before breakfast is sufficiently rare in patients with duodenal ulcer disease as to challenge the diagnosis. The pain is usually relieved within a few minutes by food or antacids. The severity of symptoms varies substantially from patient to patient, and symptoms tend to be recurrent and episodic. Episodes of pain may persist for periods of several days to weeks or months. Periods of remission may last from weeks to years, and are almost always longer than the episodes of pain. In some patients the disease is more aggressive, with frequent persistent symptoms and development of complications. Pain relief (whether with antacids or food) is believed to result from acid neutralization. Ingestion of food leads to a transient partial neutralization of gastric acid, which is followed by gastrin release and resultant stimulation of acid secretion. With subsequent gastric emptying and increasing gastric acid secretion, a sufficiently low pH is achieved that pain results. Acid-induced pain in patients with duodenal ulcer is believed due to (1) acid stimulation of chemical receptors and/or (2) alterations in gastric motility.

Changes in the character of the pain often indicate the presence of complications. For example, ulcer pain which becomes constant, is no longer relieved by food or antacids, or radiates to the back or upper quadrant may herald *penetration* of the ulcer (often into the pancreas). Ulcer pain which is accentuated rather than relieved by food, or is accompanied by vomiting, often indicates *gastric outlet obstruction*. Abrupt, severe, or generalized abdominal pain is characteristic of free *perforation* into the peritoneal cavity. Weight loss, in the absence of some degree of gastric outlet obstruction, is unusual. Acute gastrointestinal bleeding may occur which may present with vomiting of blood or coffee-grounds material, or with melena, and the passage of black tarry stools or even frank red blood if the bleeding is massive.

It is important to note that *many patients with active disease have no ulcer symptoms*. This leads to a significant, although not quantifiable, underestimation of duodenal ulcer frequency and recurrence in the population. Recent studies, especially those using duodenoscopy, indicate that there is poor correlation between resolution of symptoms and ulcer healing. Since many duodenal ulcer patients are asymptomatic, the absence of a history of ulcer symptoms does not exclude duodenal ulcer as a potential cause for spontaneous gastrointestinal hemorrhage or abrupt ulcer perforation.

On *physical examination* epigastric tenderness is the most frequent abnormal finding. The area of tenderness is usually in the midline, often midway between the umbilicus and the xiphoid process. In 20 to 30 percent of patients the tender area is to the right of the midline. Acute free perforation of the ulcer into the peritoneal cavity often produces a rigid, board-like abdomen, usually with generalized rebound tenderness. In patients with gastric outlet obstruction caused by a duodenal or pyloric channel ulcer one may find a "succussion splash," due to both fluid and air in the distended stomach. Tachycardia or hypotension, in some instances demonstrable only by orthostatic maneuvers, may reflect acute hemorrhage from duodenal ulcer. Cutaneous and mucosal pallor may be seen when there is anemia from chronic blood loss.

Only about five percent of duodenal ulcers are located distal to the duodenal bulb, and these are usually in the immediate postbulbar portion of the first part of the duodenum. Most postbulbar ulcers in this area are of the common duodenal ulcer variety. However, postbulbar ulceration, when located at or beyond the second portion of the duodenum, suggests the Zollinger-Ellison syndrome. Postbulbar ulcer pain may be in the right upper quadrant or radiate through to the back. Obstruction and hemorrhage are more frequent with postbulbar ulcers than with those in the duodenal bulb.

The pyloric channel, which is 1 to 2 cm in length, is the narrowest portion of the gastric outlet. Ulcers in this location may produce symptoms similar to those of a duodenal ulcer; however, these symptoms tend to be less responsive to food and antacids. With pyloric channel ulcers food may accentuate rather than relieve abdominal discomfort or even result in vomiting because of the frequent occurrence of outlet obstruction. In general, surgery is required more frequently with channel ulcers than with those in the duodenal bulb.

DIAGNOSIS Epigastric pain readily relieved by food or antacids strongly suggests duodenal ulcer. It must be reemphasized, however, that many patients with ulcer-like symptoms may have no evidence of an ulcer even after careful radiographic and endoscopic examination. Barium examination of the upper gastrointestinal tract is of value in identifying duodenal ulcer. The proportion of ulcers which are identified radiographically depends on the skill, persistence, enthusiasm, and diagnostic criteria of the radiologist. Using conventional barium contrast techniques, 70 to 80 percent of duodenal ulcers demonstrated by endoscopy can be identified by x-ray examination. With newer radiographic techniques, including double-contrast examinations, it is possible to detect approximately 90 percent of duodenal ulcers. On x-ray the typical duodenal ulcer is usually perceived as a discrete crater in the proximal portion of the duodenal bulb. Marked deformity of the duodenal bulb, common in patients with chronic recurrent duodenal ulcer, may make radiographic identification of the ulcer difficult or impossible (Figs. 290-1 and 290-2).

Use of fiberoptic endoscopic instruments for examination of the upper gastrointestinal tract has facilitated accurate diagnosis of duodenal ulcer disease. Duodenoscopy is not required for diagnosis of duodenal ulcer when it has been established by barium radiographic examination. Endoscopy may be of great value, however, (1) in detecting suspected duodenal ulcer in the absence of radiographically demonstrable ulcer and in pa-

FIGURE 290-1

Deformed duodenal bulb with ulcer crater.

FIGURE 290-2

Distortion of the duodenal bulb with "cloverleaf" deformity.

tients with radiographic deformity and uncertainty regarding activity of the disease, (2) in identifying ulcers too small or too superficial to be recognized by x-ray, and (3) in identifying an ulcer as the source and site of active gastrointestinal hemorrhage. Duodenoscopy also permits direct visualization and photographic documentation of the character of the ulcer, its size, shape, and location, and it may provide a reference basis for the assessment of subsequent healing. Endoscopic studies have shown that 85 percent of duodenal ulcers are less than 1 cm in diameter with approximately 70 percent having a diameter between 0.5 and 1 cm.

Measurement of gastric acid secretion is not necessary in most patients with clinical features of a typical duodenal ulcer. Determination of serum gastrin is recommended in those patients in whom surgery is planned or gastrinoma is suspected.

MEDICAL TREATMENT Major objectives of therapy are relief of pain and ulcer healing. Prevention of ulcer recurrence and complications are additional objectives. The literature describing duodenal ulcer treatment is voluminous.

In the past enthusiasm has been expressed for virtually every mode of treatment which has ever been tried for this disease. In many instances positive results have been due to spontaneous healing. Specific agents currently available and recommended for use in the treatment of duodenal ulcer are described and considered below.

Antacids Administration of antacids has been the major accepted form of treatment for duodenal ulcer. However, only recently have data been obtained which establish the effectiveness of antacids in duodenal ulcer healing. The ideal antacid should be potent in neutralizing acid, inexpensive, not adsorbed from the gastrointestinal tract, and contain negligible amounts of sodium. It should be sufficiently palatable to be readily tolerated and should be free from side effects. Although the ideal antacid is yet to be developed, a number of preparations are available which can be used in treatment of patients with duodenal ulcer. Individual antacids differ substantially in their capacities to neutralize acid, their sodium contents, their absorption properties, and their potential adverse effects (see Table 290-1).

Calcium carbonate is a potent and inexpensive antacid. In neutralizing acid, it is converted to calcium chloride in the stomach. Approximately 10 percent of calcium ingested as calcium carbonate is absorbed from the small intestine. Unfortunately, calcium carbonate administration may be associated with the milk-alkali syndrome, producing elevations of serum calcium, phosphate, blood urea nitrogen, creatinine, and bicarbonate. These patients may develop renal calcinosis and progressive renal insufficiency. Calcium carbonate is unique among the antacids in that its ingestion is followed by stimulation of gastric acid secretion (a genuine "acid rebound" phenomenon). This is due primarily to the direct action of calcium in stimulating parietal cell acid secretion and, to a lesser extent, to calcium-mediated stimulation of gastrin release. Because of its potential adverse effects, calcium carbonate is not recommended for use as an antacid for treatment of patients with peptic ulcer.

Sodium bicarbonate is a potent, rapidly acting, inexpensive antacid. However, because of its tendency to induce systemic alkalosis and its high sodium content, it should not be used as an antacid in treatment of peptic ulcer.

TABLE 290-1
Relative potency of liquid antacid preparations

Antacid	Contents	meq/30 ml*
Delcid	Al and Mg hydroxides	256
Mylanta II	Mg and Al hydroxides, simethicone	124
Titralac	Glycine, Ca carbonate	118
Camalox	Al and Mg hydroxides, Ca carbonate	108
Basaljel	Al carbonate	100
Aludrox	Al hydroxide gel, Mg hydroxide	84
Maalox	Mg and Al hydroxide	78
Cremalin	Hexitol-stabilized Al hydroxide gel, magnesium hydroxide	78
Di-Gel	Al and Mg hydroxides, simethicone	76
Mylanta	Mg and Al hydroxides, simethicone	72
Silain-Gel	Mg and Al hydroxides, simethicone	70
Marblen	Mg and Ca carbonates, Al hydroxide, Mg phosphate, Mg trisilicate	70
WinGel	Al and Mg hydroxides, hexitol stabilized	70
Gelusil M	Mg trisilicate, Al hydroxide, Mg hydroxide	66
Riopan	Mg and Al hydroxides	66
Amphojel	Al hydroxide gel	58
A-M-T	Mg trisilicate, Al hydroxide gel	54
Kolantyl Gel	Bentyl, Al hydroxide, Mg hydroxide, methylcellulose	52
Trisogel	Mg trisilicate, Al hydroxide gel	52
Malcogel	Mg trisilicate, Al hydroxide gel	48
Gelusil	Mg trisilicate, Al hydroxide gel	40
Robalate	Dihydroxyaluminum aminoacetate	34
Phosphaljel	Al phosphate gel	12

* *Indicates the capacity, expressed in milliequivalents, to raise the pH of 0.1 N HCl and maintain it at pH 3.0 for 2 h.*
SOURCE: *After Fordtran et al.*

The most widely used antacid preparations are mixtures of *aluminum hydroxide* and *magnesium hydroxide,* in some instances with additional agents. Aluminum hydroxide neutralizes hydrochloric acid with the production of aluminum chloride and water. Use of aluminum hydroxide tends to produce constipation. Aluminum binds phosphate within the gut lumen, thereby facilitating its excretion. As a consequence, prolonged and regular use of aluminum hydroxide may induce systemic phosphate depletion with resultant weakness, malaise, and anorexia.

Magnesium hydroxide is a potent antacid which neutralizes hydrochloric acid to produce magnesium chloride and water. Magnesium hydroxide may produce loosening of the stools. This laxative effect and the constipating effects of aluminum hydroxide can be overcome by using these agents in combination, or by alternating their use. Antacid combinations vary enormously in their capacities to neutralize hydrochloric acid. Table 290-1 provides examples of some available liquid antacid preparations and their neutralizing capacities, as defined by their ability to increase and maintain the pH of 0.1 N hydrochloric acid at 3.0 for 2 h. Magnesium trisilicate, which is frequently included in various antacid mixtures, is a slow-acting or weak antacid. In contrast to liquid formulations, tablet preparations of magnesium hydroxide and/or aluminum hydroxide possess little acid-neutralizing capacity and are not recommended in the treatment of duodenal ulcer.

Acceptance of the crucial role of acid in the pathogenesis of duodenal ulcer provides a rational basis for the use of antacids in treatment of patients with duodenal ulcer. However, there are some controlled studies on the effects of antacids on duodenal ulcer healing, in which vigorous antacid therapy has been compared with placebo, and ulcer response has been verified by endoscopy. In one study, 4 weeks of treatment with a potent magnesium and aluminum hydroxide antacid mixture increased duodenal ulcer healing. Ulcer healing occurred in 45 percent of patients receiving placebo and in 78 percent of those treated with the antacid (144 meq given 1 and 3 h after meals and at bedtime).

H₂-receptor antagonists It has been known for decades that conventional antihistamines, which readily block the actions of histamine on smooth muscle of the gut or bronchi, do not inhibit histamine-stimulated gastric acid secretion by the stomach. The parietal cell receptor for histamine has been termed the H_2 receptor and that blocked by classic antihistamines, the H_1 receptor. The H_2-receptor antagonist, *cimetidine,* is now used widely in the treatment of duodenal ulcer. Cimetidine is related structurally to histamine (Fig. 290-3), sharing the same imidazole ring but bearing an extended side chain which contains a cyanoguanidine group. Cimetidine at a dose of 300 mg inhibits basal acid secretion by more than 80 percent and meal-stimulated acid secretion by approximately 70 percent. It strikingly reduces acid secretory responses to histamine, caffeine, insulin, and gastrin. Cimetidine has been shown to be more effective than placebo in promoting endoscopically verified duodenal ulcer healing. Its effectiveness in promoting duodenal ulcer healing appears to be comparable with that of vigorous antacid therapy. The recommended oral dose of cimetidine for treatment of patients with duodenal ulcer is 300 mg four times daily, with meals and at bedtime. Treatment of active duodenal ulcer with cimetidine is continued for periods from 4 to 8 weeks. In spite of the large numbers of patients treated with cimetidine, few serious adverse effects have been experienced. Cimetidine administration has been associated with slight and reversible increases in serum transaminase and creatinine levels. Instances of diarrhea, malaise, and mental confusion have also been described. Tender gynecomastia has been observed in a small number of patients treated with large

$CH_2CH_2NH_2$

HISTAMINE

CH_3 $CH_2SCH_2CH_2NHCNHCH_3$
$\quad\quad\quad\quad\quad\quad\quad N-C\equiv N$

CIMETIDINE

FIGURE 290-3

Chemical structures of histamine and the H₂-receptor antagonist cimetidine. Note the common imidazole ring and the cyanoguanidine group in the cimetidine side chain.

doses for prolonged periods of time (e.g., for the Zollinger-Ellison syndrome). Increased serum prolactin levels can also result.

Anticholinergic agents Anticholinergic drugs act by inhibiting the effects of acetylcholine on muscarinic receptors. These agents decrease gastric acid secretion, but not as effectively as H₂-receptor antagonists. Anticholinergics reduce basal gastric acid secretion by approximately 50 percent, histamine- or gastrin-stimulated acid secretion by 40 percent, and postprandial acid secretion by 30 percent. They also delay gastric emptying. Most studies have *not* shown that anticholinergic agents hasten healing or improve symptoms of duodenal ulcer; therefore, they are not recommended as primary therapy for duodenal ulcer. However, anticholinergic agents may be useful when combined with antacids or cimetidine. Side effects of anticholinergic agents include dryness of mouth, blurring of vision, and urinary retention. They should not be used in patients with glaucoma, impaired gastric emptying, or history or symptoms of urinary retention. Because of their capacity to relax the lower esophageal sphincter and decrease gastric emptying, it is unwise to use anticholinergic agents in patients with gastroesophageal reflux.

Diet Many different dietary programs have been recommended and used for treatment of patients with duodenal ulcer. There is no evidence that bland diets reduce gastric acid secretion, promote healing, or relieve symptoms in patients with duodenal ulcer. Similarly soft diets or diets free of spices or fruit juices have not proved of benefit. Traditionally, milk and cream have been prescribed. These diets may contribute to development of the milk-alkali syndrome and may be associated with increased atherogenesis. They may promote gastric acid secretion by direct calcium effects and by gastrin release stimulated by milk protein and calcium.

What dietary measures, if any, should be recommended in the treatment of duodenal ulcer? Clearly, strict diet control is not necessary. Milk should not be used as a component of treatment of patients with duodenal ulcer. If patients experience symptoms after ingestion of certain foods, these should be avoided. A regular diet can be combined with antacids as described below. It has been common practice to restrict caffeine-containing beverages in patients with duodenal ulcer. Al-

though ethanol does not stimulate gastric secretion in humans, it is often omitted from the diet of patients with duodenal ulcer.

General therapeutic considerations How does one integrate available information concerning treatment of duodenal ulcer to construct a reasonable therapeutic formulation? Clinical studies indicate the effectiveness of *antacids* and of the H₂-receptor antagonists such as *cimetidine* in the promotion of duodenal ulcer healing. On the basis of present knowledge, there appear to be two primary approaches to the medical treatment for duodenal ulcer—namely, either the neutralization of gastric acid by the frequent use of potent antacids or the inhibition of acid secretion by H₂-receptor antagonists.

Antacid treatment of duodenal ulcer should consist of frequent doses of a potent liquid antacid. However, the minimal or optimal doses of antacids required for duodenal ulcer healing are not precisely known. In one effective program, it is recommended that the antacid (100 to 140 meq of neutralizing activity; for most antacids this equals 30 to 60 ml) be given 1 and 3 h after each meal and at bedtime. Such a regimen should be continued for approximately six weeks. Symptom recurrence may be treated by shorter periods of therapy, at similar dose levels. When cimetidine is used, a 300-mg tablet is recommended with each meal and at bedtime for 6 to 8 weeks. When anticholinergics are used in conjunction with antacids or cimetidine, they are administered either once a day at bedtime or four times a day (i.e., before meals and at bedtime).

It is useful clinically to separate the approach to gastric and duodenal ulcers because the implications of the two disorders are very different, although the ulcers are similar pathologically.

GASTRIC ULCER

INCIDENCE AND ANATOMIC LOCATION The peak incidence for gastric ulcer is in the sixth decade, approximately 10 years later than for duodenal ulcer. Gastric ulcers, just as duodenal ulcers, are more common in males. They are also histologically similar to duodenal ulcers. Gastric ulcers are characteristically deep, extending beyond the mucosa of the stomach. Almost all benign gastric ulcers are located in the *antrum,* in a zone immediately distal to the junction of the antral mucosa with the acid-secreting mucosa of the body of the stomach. The location of this junction is variable, especially on the lesser gastric curvature. In general, the antrum extends approximately two-thirds of the way up the lesser curvature and one-third of the way up the greater curvature of the stomach. Benign gastric ulcers are almost always accompanied by gastritis and by variable amounts of mucosal atrophy of antrum and, in some instances, of the entire stomach. Gastritis may be absent with aspirin-associated gastric ulcers; the latter are usually located in the antrum, but are not confined to the junction of the antral and parietal-cell mucosa.

ETIOLOGY AND PATHOGENESIS Acid-pepsin appears to be important in the pathogenesis of gastric ulcer. In contrast to duodenal ulcer, however, gastric ulcer patients generally have acid secretory rates which are normal or even reduced when compared with nonulcer subjects. Although many patients with gastric ulcer have reduced rates of acid secretion, *true achlorhydria* in response to stimulation *almost never occurs* in patients with benign gastric ulcer. Ten to twenty percent of patients with gastric ulcer also have duodenal ulcer disease. In many instances the duodenal ulcer precedes development of the gastric ulcer. Patients with both duodenal and gastric ulcers tend to have acid secretory patterns which parallel those of duodenal ulcer. Patients with pyloric channel ulcers have acid secretory rates that are also usually similar to those associated with duodenal ulcers.

Various factors have been considered as being involved in the pathogenesis of gastric ulcer. Most evidence supports the importance of primary defects in gastric mucosal resistance and/or direct gastric mucosal injury as the most important elements. Serum gastrin levels are increased in some gastric ulcer patients, but these increases are limited to those with acid hyposecretion. It has been suggested that gastric regurgitation of duodenal contents, especially those containing bile, may induce gastric mucosal injury and subsequent gastric ulceration. Gastric ulcer patients have been shown to have increased duodenal-gastric reflux of bile and greater concentrations of bile in the stomach when compared with nonulcer subjects and with duodenal ulcer patients. It has been proposed that bile acids injure the gastric mucosa by interruption of the gastric mucosal barrier with resultant back-diffusion of secreted hydrogen ions. Although the factors producing duodenal-gastric reflux in gastric ulcer patients have not been clearly established, a defect in pyloric sphincter function has been proposed. In normal individuals cholecystokinin and secretin appear to increase pyloric sphincter tone and competence, but in gastric ulcer patients these hormones fail to increase pyloric sphincter tone. Bile acid perfusion of the antrum or intact stomach has been shown to stimulate release of gastrin into the circulation. Gastrin antagonizes the effects of cholecystokinin

FIGURE 290-4

Benign lesser curvature gastric ulcer. Note ulceration beyond the projected margins of the stomach and the collar of edema.

on the pyloric sphincter and decreases pyloric sphincter pressure. Thus, it is possible, although not proved, that gastrin may contribute to defective pyloric sphincter function.

CLINICAL FEATURES As with duodenal ulcer, epigastric pain is the most common symptom in patients with gastric ulcer. However, the symptoms are much less typical and unpredictable than in patients with duodenal ulcer. While the pain may be similar to that noted with duodenal ulcers, some gastric ulcer patients experience no relief of pain with eating, and pain may actually be precipitated or accentuated by food. Relief of symptoms with antacids is also less consistent with gastric than with duodenal ulcers. Gastric ulcers tend to heal but then recur. Recognizable episodes of recurrent gastric ulcer activity are usually less frequent than with duodenal ulcer. The precise incidence of gastric ulcer is not known, since many gastric ulcer patients are asymptomatic. While nausea and vomiting almost always indicate gastric outlet obstruction in duodenal ulcer patients, these symptoms may occur in patients with gastric ulcer in the absence of mechanical obstruction. Weight loss occurs in approximately 40 percent of patients due to anorexia or to food aversion from discomfort produced by eating.

Gastric outlet obstruction may develop with ulcers in the pyloric channel or most distal antrum. Hemorrhage is a common complication, occurring in approximately 25 percent. Gastric ulcer perforation is less frequent than hemorrhage. Mortality with perforation of gastric ulcers is approximately three times that which occurs with duodenal ulcers. This increased mortality appears related to the increased age of gastric ulcer patients. The greater mortality may also be due to uncertainty and delay in diagnosis, as well as to greater soilage of the peritoneum with gastric ulcer perforation.

DIAGNOSIS The history may be of value in suspecting gastric ulcer, but it is not as characteristic as in duodenal ulcer. The two major methods for diagnosis are barium examination of the upper gastrointestinal tract and endoscopy. Gastric ulcer can usually be identified by barium examination with an accuracy that approaches 90 percent. Superficial ulcerations and erosions, however, may escape radiographic identification. Approximately 4 percent of gastric ulcers which appear benign radiographically prove to be malignant (by endoscopic biopsy or at surgery). Benign gastric ulcers occur more commonly on the lesser than on the greater curvature (Fig. 290-4). Radiation of gastric mucosal folds from the margin of the ulcer crater suggests a benign lesion. Large gastric ulcers, i.e., those greater than 3 cm in diameter, are more often malignant than smaller ones. An ulcer within a mass, as defined radiographically, also suggests malignancy.

Endoscopic visualization of the ulcer allows one to define its size, location, and, by biopsy, general morphological characteristics. At gastroscopy at least six biopsies should be obtained from the inner margin of the ulcer. If accurate cytology is available, brushings of the ulcer should be performed prior to biopsy. By application of combined radiographic, endoscopic, and histological techniques, distinguishing malignant from benign gastric ulcer should be possible with at least 99 percent confidence.

Gastric ulcer in association with achlorhydria almost always indicates that one is dealing with a gastric carcinoma. However, most patients with gastric carcinoma (about two-thirds to three-fourths) are capable of secreting some gastric acid, although usually less than normal.

MEDICAL TREATMENT At present, antacid administration is the most widely accepted primary treatment for peptic ulcer. The ideal dose and frequency for antacid therapy for gastric ulcer healing are not known. However, since acid hypersecretion is not characteristic of the disease, smaller doses of antacid may possibly be required than for treatment of duodenal ulcer. It is suggested that 15 to 30 ml of a potent liquid antacid be taken 1 and 3 h after meals and at bedtime. Anticholinergic agents have been recommended by some physicians. However, because of substantial side effects of anticholinergic drugs, their tendency to reduce gastric emptying, the fact that gastric ulcer patients are often older and, therefore, more susceptible to the complications of these agents, and the lack of evidence for their benefit, the use of anticholinergic drugs in gastric ulcer treatment does not appear justified. Some studies suggest that hospitalization is of benefit in gastric ulcer healing.

Experience with the use of H$_2$-receptor antagonists in the treatment of patients with gastric ulcer is limited. Early results suggest that cimetidine may be of value when administered in a dose of 300 mg four times per day, with meals and at bedtime. With further study, cimetidine may prove to be an alternative to antacid administration as primary therapy for benign gastric ulcer.

Since salicylate ingestion has been associated with development of gastric ulcers (often in atypical locations), it is strongly recommended that patients with gastric ulcer not ingest salicylates. Alcohol, because of its injurious effects on the gastric mucosa, should be avoided. Milk and cream, as well as bland or homogenized diets, have not been shown to be of value in treatment. In general, it is probably sufficient to recommend that patients take a diet of their own choice. Since caffeine-containing liquids stimulate gastric acid secretion, it may be of benefit to omit these beverages.

Carbenoxolone has been used in many countries (other than the United States) in the treatment of patients with gastric ulcer. This drug is a hydrolytic product of glycyrrhizinic acid (derived from licorice) and has been shown to improve symptoms and increase the rate of gastric ulcer healing. Carbenoxolone is not an antacid, nor does it decrease gastric acid secretion. It increases the life span of gastric mucosal epithelial cells and increases the secretion and viscosity of gastric mucus. Carbenoxolone possesses aldosterone-like effects, and thus sodium and water retention tend to occur. It is possible to inhibit the aldosterone-like effects of carbenoxolone by use of aldosterone antagonists; however, the latter also abolish the beneficial effects of carbenoxolone in gastric ulcer healing. Carbenoxolone has not been approved for general use in the United States.

One must be alert to the occasional "healing" of an ulcerating gastric carcinoma, especially with cimetidine treatment. The failure of a gastric ulcer to decrease satisfactorily in size and to heal with antacid treatment should suggest a gastric malignancy. Benign gastric ulcers should heal completely after 3 months of vigorous antacid therapy. Upper gastrointestinal barium examination or gastroscopy should be performed after 4 weeks of antacid therapy, at which time definite healing should be demonstrable in benign gastric ulcers—the diameter of most ulcers should be reduced by more than 50 percent. If at 4 weeks the ulcer is not reduced in size, malignancy must be considered and looked for by appropriate biopsies of the ulcer. If the ulcer has not healed completely at 4 weeks, x-ray and endoscopic examination should be repeated in another month, at which time most benign gastric ulcers should have healed. In general, large gastric ulcers heal more slowly than smaller ones.

COMPLICATIONS AND SURGERY FOR PEPTIC ULCER

Surgery is reserved for patients with complications of both duodenal and gastric ulcer. These include hemorrhage, obstruction, perforation, and refractoriness to medical therapy.

Hemorrhage occurs in approximately 15 to 20 percent of patients with duodenal ulcer; there may be a recurrence of bleeding in about 40 percent. In most patients hemorrhage from peptic ulcer responds satisfactorily to medical management—including gastric suction and antacid administration (see Chap. 38).

Free *perforation* into the peritoneal cavity occurs in approximately 6 percent of patients with duodenal ulcer. Five to ten percent of these patients will have had no prior recognizable ulcer symptoms. Simultaneous hemorrhage occurs in about 10 percent of patients with duodenal ulcer perforation; the mortality in this group is greatly increased. Duodenal ulcers, especially those located posteriorly, may penetrate into adjacent structures, most often the pancreas—frequently resulting in increased levels of serum amylase. Duodenal ulcers less commonly may penetrate into the liver, biliary tract, or colon.

Gastric outlet obstruction occurs in 2 to 4 percent of patients admitted to hospital with duodenal or pyloric channel ulcers. Symptoms include abdominal bloating, nausea, vomiting, and weight loss. These patients usually have had ulcer symptoms for many years and often obstructive symptoms for several months.

Failure to respond satisfactorily to medical treatment generally requires consideration of surgery. The true incidence of lack of ulcer healing with vigorous medical programs is not known; it is clear, however, that most patients with peptic ulcer can be treated successfully without surgery.

Decisions regarding surgery for patients with complication of peptic ulcer must be individualized. Risks of surgery must be balanced with risks of the disease. The patient's discomfort, costs of medical care and hospitalization, and time lost from work must be weighed in relation to the morbidity and possible mortality associated with surgery and anesthesia, risks of recurrent ulcer, and long-term postoperative sequelae. The skill and experience of the surgeon must be weighed as a major factor in considering operation.

SURGERY FOR DUODENAL ULCER No single surgical procedure has been accepted universally as the most satisfactory duodenal ulcer operation. At present the most commonly performed surgical procedures are vagotomy with antrectomy and vagotomy with pyloroplasty. With standard vagotomy and antrectomy, the vagal trunks are transected, the antrum is removed, and gastrointestinal continuity is reestablished by anastomosis of the remaining stomach with the proximal duodenum (Billroth I anastomosis) or with a loop of the jejunum (Billroth II anastomosis). Vagotomy and antrectomy is an effective procedure with a low recurrence rate (approximately one percent). Morbidity and mortality with vagotomy and antrectomy are variable, depend upon patient selection and the skill of the surgeon, but are probably slightly greater than with vagotomy and pyloroplasty.

When vagotomy and pyloroplasty are selected, the pyloroplasty is performed to facilitate gastric drainage after truncal or selective vagotomy. Vagotomy is performed to inhibit vagal stimulation of gastric acid secretion. It does not inhibit gastrin release; in fact, release of gastrin is enhanced after vagal interruption. Three types of vagotomy are now used in the surgical treatment of duodenal ulcer, namely, *truncal vagotomy, selective vagotomy,* and *parietal cell vagotomy* (also referred to as *superselective* or *proximal gastric vagotomy*). Pyloroplasty with truncal vagotomy, which is still the most commonly performed method for vagal transection in the United States, is associated with approximately one percent mortality. Ulcer recurrence during the 5 years after surgery is about 5 to 8 percent. With selective vagotomy only the branches of the vagus which supply the stomach are transected, preserving the vagal innervation of the other abdominal viscera. Selective vagotomy has been found by some surgeons to result in a more complete vagotomy, less ulcer recurrence, and fewer postvagotomy complications than truncal vagotomy. Parietal cell vagotomy is the most recently introduced form of vagotomy. This procedure spares the branches of the vagus which innervate the antrum, and a drainage procedure is unnecessary. Both immediate and late postoperative complications are less common with parietal cell vagotomy than with truncal vagotomy, but reduction in acid secretion with parietal cell vagotomy is generally comparable with that produced with truncal and selective vagotomy. Mortality with parietal cell vagotomy is less than 1 percent. Although most studies suggest that recurrence is comparable with other forms of vagotomy with pyloroplasty, some studies have shown disturbingly high rates of ulcer recurrence. Thus, while the long-term incidence of ulcer recurrence after parietal cell vagotomy remains to be established, it would appear that this procedure is an effective and safe surgical therapy for duodenal ulcer.

SURGERY FOR GASTRIC ULCER Surgical treatment is required for gastric ulcer patients who do not respond satisfactorily to medical therapy or who develop complications similar to those described for duodenal ulcer. With the accuracy of careful radiographic examination, endoscopy, biopsy of the ulcer margins, and exfoliative cytology, it should rarely be necessary to operate because of a remaining uncertainty regarding the malignant or benign nature of the ulcer. The recommended surgical procedure for the treatment of gastric ulcer is antrectomy with gastroduodenal (Billroth I) anastomosis. It is not necessary to perform a vagotomy when antrectomy is performed for gastric ulcer.

CONSEQUENCES AND SYNDROMES AFTER PEPTIC ULCER SURGERY

Modern surgery for peptic ulcer is effective in both the treatment of ulcer complications and the prevention of ulcer recurrence. However, numerous postoperative sequelae and syndromes may occur.

TABLE 290-2
Provocative gastrin tests*

Disorder	Gastrin response (change from basal level)		
	After secretin injection	After calcium infusion	After test meal
Zollinger-Ellison (gastrinoma)	Increase (usually greater than 400 pg/ml)	Increase (usually more than 50% or more than 500 pg/ml)	Little or no increase (increase less than 50%)
Common duodenal ulcer	Decrease or no change	Small increase (usually less than 50%; always less than 500 pg/ml)	Moderate increase (often slightly more than normal, but less than in gastrin cell hyperplasia)
Antral gastrin cell hyperplasia	Decrease	May or may not increase greater than 50%	Striking increase (greater than 50%)

* Responses and results are based on currently available data and are subject to change as further information becomes available.

RECURRENT ULCERATION Recurrent ulceration occurs in approximately 5 percent of patients after surgery for peptic ulcer. Approximately 95 percent of the recurrences follow surgery for duodenal ulcer disease. The risk of development of recurrent ulcer is 3 to 10 percent after surgery for duodenal ulcer and approximately 2 percent after gastric ulcer surgery. Recurrence is more common after vagotomy and pyloroplasty than after vagotomy and antrectomy. When ulcers occur after partial gastric resection, the site is usually at or immediately distal to the anastomosis. Abdominal pain is the most common symptom in patients with a stomal (or marginal) ulcer. The pain is usually epigastric but is often not characteristic of common duodenal ulcer. It is usually, but not always, relieved by meals or antacids and tends to be more persistent and progressive than that observed with duodenal ulcer. Hemorrhage or anemia due to blood loss, nausea and vomiting from obstruction, weight loss, or symptoms from perforation may occur. The development of a stomal ulcer after duodenal ulcer surgery almost always indicates that an incomplete vagotomy was performed. Inadequate gastric resection, when performed without vagotomy, is also associated with stomal ulceration. Additional causes for the development of a recurrent ulcer include an excessively long jejunal afferent loop, an inadvertently performed gastroileal or gastrocolic anastomosis, or poor gastric drainage. Less commonly, a marginal ulcer may be caused by gastrinoma or the retained-antrum syndrome. If patients with gastrinomas are treated by gastroenterostomy, even with a complete vagotomy, stomal ulceration is almost inevitable.

Radiographic examination with barium is of limited diagnostic value and identifies only from 50 to 65 percent of stomal ulcerations. Surgical deformity at the anastomotic site may often mimic stomal ulcer in its absence, or conceal it when present. When suspected, endoscopic examination is required to identify stomal ulceration. Medical treatment is almost always unsatisfactory in patients with stomal ulcer, while surgery is usually necessary and successful. In patients with recurrent ulcer provocative tests should be performed with infusions of calcium or secretin and measurements of serum gastrin to identify or exclude gastrinoma (see below).

RECURRENT ULCER DUE TO RETAINED ANTRUM Recurrent ulcers have been described in a small number of patients after antrectomy with gastrojejunostomy (Billroth II anastomosis) in which the antral resection is not complete. In these patients the distal antrum, inadvertently not resected, remains in continuity with the duodenum after surgery. These patients usually develop or continue to have gastric acid hypersection due to gastrin release by the residual antral mucosa which is no longer in contact with gastric acid, the normal inhibitor of gastrin release. In these patients fasting serum gastrin may be normal to moderately increased. Patients with retained antrum can be distinguished from those with gastrinoma by intravenous injection of secretin with measurements of serum gastrin. Gastrinoma patients exhibit paradoxical increases in serum gastrin, whereas in those with retained antrum serum gastrin levels decrease after secretin administration (see Table 290-2). These patients can be treated successfully by surgical removal of the remaining antrum.

AFFERENT LOOP SYNDROMES Patients with partial gastric resection with gastrojejunostomy (Billroth II anastomosis) may experience abdominal bloating and pain 20 min to 1 h after eating, frequently followed by nausea and vomiting. The vomitus often contains large amounts of bile. Characteristically, the bloating and abdominal discomfort are relieved by vomiting. This syndrome is believed to be caused by distention of an incompletely draining afferent intestinal loop by pancreatic and biliary secretions which are stimulated by eating. Serum amylase levels may be mildly or moderately increased. Because of partial obstruction it is often difficult to demonstrate the afferent loop by barium meal examination. Treatment is surgical correction of the incomplete afferent loop obstruction, and, in some instances, revision to a gastroduodenal anastomosis.

A second form of afferent loop dysfunction is that due to stasis with bacterial overgrowth within the afferent loop. These patients may exhibit the same characteristics as are found with other forms of small intestinal bacterial overgrowth or blind-loop syndromes (see Chap. 292). These include malabsorption, especially of fat and vitamin B_{12}. Correction of the afferent loop bacterial overgrowth syndrome can be accomplished by surgical revision of the afferent loop.

BILE REFLUX GASTRITIS After peptic ulcer surgery a small proportion of patients experience early satiety, abdominal discomfort, and vomiting, which is believed due to reflux of duodenal contents into the stomach. Endoscopic examination usually reveals regurgitated bile in the stomach and diffuse gastritis, often involving the entire gastric remnant. Various terms assigned to this entity include *alkaline reflux gastritis, bile reflux gastritis,* and *bilious vomiting.* The mechanisms accounting for these symptoms have not been defined. Although the term *bile reflux gastritis* has been used, there is no certainty that regurgitated bile is responsible for the syndrome. Administration of cholestyramine, intended to bind bile acids and facilitate their excretion, has not been of benefit in this disorder. Some surgeons have reported successful treatment of bile reflux gastritis by diversion of duodenal contents from proximity to the stomach with a Roux-en-Y anastomosis.

DUMPING SYNDROME Following peptic ulcer surgery some patients experience an assortment of vasomotor symptoms after eating. These include palpitation, tachycardia, lightheadedness, diaphoresis, and, less frequently, postural hypotension. Abdominal discomfort and vomiting may also occur. The vasomotor symptoms, referred to as the *early dumping syndrome,* are usually experienced within 30 min after eating and are believed to result from rapid emptying of hyperosmolar gastric contents into the proximal small intestine. This leads to a shift of fluid into the gut lumen and produces intestinal distention and contraction of plasma volume. Additional proposed mechanisms for these symptoms include stimulation of autonomic reflexes secondary to small intestinal distention and/or release of hormones from the gut in response to rapid entry of gastric contents into the duodenum or jejunum. Hormone candidates have included serotonin, vasoactive intestinal peptide (VIP), and gastric inhibitory peptide (GIP).

The *late dumping syndrome* refers to a symptom complex comprising dizziness, lightheadedness, palpitation, diaphoresis, confusion, and, in rare instances, syncope, occurring 90 min to 3 h after eating. The symptoms can often be precipitated by meals rich in simple carbohydrates, especially sucrose. The syndrome appears to result from hypoglycemia due to insulin release stimulated by abrupt increases in blood glucose secondary to rapid emptying of sugar-containing meals into the proximal small intestine.

Both forms of the dumping syndrome are treated by dietary measures. These include limitation of simple sugar-containing liquids and solids (sweets), elimination of liquids at mealtime, and frequent small meals.

POSTVAGOTOMY DIARRHEA A significant number of patients experience diarrhea after peptic ulcer surgery, especially when there has been a vagotomy. Diarrhea usually occurs within 2 h of eating. Although the mechanism is not clear, interruption of vagal fibers to the abdominal viscera appears to play an important role in the production of the diarrhea. Selective and proximal vagotomy are associated with less diarrhea than truncal vagotomy. Rapid emptying of gastric contents into the small intestine, resulting in increased fluid volume within the intestinal lumen, due to the osmotic action of the meal, may also contribute to the diarrhea.

HEMATOLOGIC COMPLICATIONS Intrinsic factor secreted by gastric parietal cells is necessary for active absorption of vitamin B_{12} by the distal ileum. Patients who have had a total gastrectomy will invariably develop malabsorption of vitamin B_{12} and should receive monthly intramuscular injections of vitamin B_{12} (50 to 100 μg indefinitely). Inasmuch as the stomach secretes intrinsic factor 100-fold in excess of need, peptic ulcer patients treated with partial gastric resection seldom develop severe vitamin B_{12} deficiency. However, they may develop decreased serum levels due to reduced absorption of food-bound vitamin B_{12}; these patients will have a normal absorption of free vitamin B_{12}, as used in the Schilling test. The precise mechanism for the malabsorption of food-bound vitamin B_{12} is not known. It may be due in part to rapid emptying of gastric contents, with reduced efficiency of intrinsic factor binding of B_{12}. Anemia after peptic ulcer surgery may also result from deficiency in iron or folate. A combined deficiency of vitamin B_{12}, iron, and folate is common in patients with anemia following partial or subtotal gastric resection. Iron deficiency is the most common single hematologic defect after peptic ulcer surgery resulting from either blood loss (e.g., with persistent or recurrent ulcer) or iron malabsorption. Patients with gastric resection malabsorb dietary iron but have normal absorption of iron salts. Folate deficiency may result from either reduced dietary intake or impaired absorption. Except for the anemia associated with early recurrent ulcer disease, the development of anemia after peptic ulcer surgery is gradual, usually occurring several years postoperatively.

The nature of the anemia after ulcer surgery should be clarified by observation of the red blood cell morphology and by measurements of serum iron, folate, and vitamin B_{12}. Iron or folate deficiency may be treated by oral replacement. Vitamin B_{12} deficiency should be treated with monthly intramuscular injections of the vitamin.

OSTEOMALACIA AND OSTEOPOROSIS Osteoporosis and osteomalacia may develop after partial or complete gastrectomy but rarely occur after vagotomy and pyloroplasty. These bone changes are believed to result from malabsorption of calcium and vitamin D. Patients may develop bone pain and have pathological fractures. Reduced bone density requires years to develop and can be identified by x-ray. Patients with osteomalacia will have reduced levels of serum calcium and increased levels of alkaline phosphatase. These patients should be treated by supplemental oral vitamin D and calcium.

GENERAL MALABSORPTION (See Chap. 292) Mild, chemically demonstrable steatorrhea is common in patients after ulcer surgery. However, the major cause of weight loss after peptic ulcer surgery is reduced food intake. On a 100-g fat diet, loss of stool fat seldom exceeds 15 g per day. In general, weight loss and malabsorption are greater in patients with gastric resection, with or without vagotomy, than in those with vagotomy and pyloroplasty. The causes of maldigestion and malabsorption after peptic ulcer surgery include rapid gastric emptying, reduced dispersion of food in the stomach, reduced bile concentrations in the gut lumen, increased rate of transit of the meal through the small intestine, and reduced or delayed pancreatic secretory responses to feeding. Steatorrhea, weight loss, and vitamin B_{12} malabsorption may also develop as a result of bacterial overgrowth, especially in patients with afferent loop bacterial stasis.

CARCINOMA AFTER PARTIAL GASTRECTOMY Several studies have documented an increased incidence of adenocarcinoma of the stomach following partial gastric resection. This usually develops 10 or more years after ulcer surgery. The possibility of carcinoma of the stomach should be considered when abdominal symptoms, which may be similar to those due to the original ulcer, appear many years after apparently successful surgery.

ZOLLINGER-ELLISON SYNDROME (GASTRINOMA)

In 1955 Zollinger and Ellison described the syndrome which bears their name, i.e., ulcer disease of the upper gastrointestinal tract, marked increase of gastric acid secretion, and non-beta islet-cell tumors of the pancreas.

ETIOLOGY AND PATHOGENESIS Zollinger and Ellison initially suggested that the disease resulted from liberation of a secretagogue from the islet-cell tumors which accounted for the often enormously increased rates of gastric acid secretion. In 1960 extracts of Zollinger-Ellison tumors were shown to stimulate gastric acid secretion. Subsequently, it was shown that these pancreatic tumors contained gastrin and that large amounts of this hormone were released into the circulation, producing the pathophysiologic characteristics of the syndrome. These gastrin-containing tumors are, therefore, now referred to as *gastrinomas*. Gastrin has been demonstrated in these tumors by chemical isolation of polypeptides with an amino acid composition and peptide mapping patterns identical to those of human gastrin. In addition, large amounts of gastrin have been demonstrated in gastrinomas and in the serums of patients with the Zollinger-Ellison syndrome by radioimmunoassay.

Approximately 90 percent of gastrinomas are found within the pancreas, 5 percent in the proximal duodenum, and the remainder in other sites including the hilum of the spleen and the stomach. In rare instances, the Zollinger-Ellison syndrome has resulted from ectopic gastrin-containing tumors, e.g., parathyroid and ovarian adenomas. A small number of gastrin-containing islet-cell tumors have been described which contained multiple hormones, for example, adrenocorticotropic hormone, glucagon, insulin, and vasoactive intestinal peptide. Pancreatic gastrinomas may be single or multiple and may vary in size from 2 mm to more than 20 cm in diameter. In from one-half to two-thirds of patients multiple gastrinomas are found within the pancreas. Pancreatic gastrinomas are most common in the body or tail. Approximately two-thirds of gastrinomas are histologically or biologically malignant. Gastrinomas have light-microscopic similarities to carcinoid tumors and, particularly when arising from the mucosa of the small intestine or stomach, may be mistaken for carcinoid tumors. From one-half to two-thirds of patients with gastrinomas have metastases, most commonly to regional lymph nodes and liver, but also may involve peritoneal surfaces, spleen, bone, skin, or mediastinum. However when death occurs, it is usually not due to the malignant invasion of the tumor but rather due to the excess gastrin-producing marked acid secretion and fulminant ulcer disease.

In most gastrinomas approximately 90 to 95 percent of gastrin is in the form of heptadecapeptide gastrin (G-17 or little gastrin), with most of the remainder being big gastrin (G-34).

In contrast, approximately two-thirds of circulating gastrin in gastrinoma patients is G-34; most of the remainder of circulating gastrin is G-17. However, small amounts of even larger forms of gastrin and smaller gastrin fragments can be detected in the serum. The parietal cell mass is substantially expanded secondary to the trophic effects of gastrin on parietal cells. The parietal cell mass in gastrinoma patients is estimated to be three to six times normal.

In some instances the gastrinoma is a component of the multiple endocrine adenomatosis type (MEA-1) syndrome, an autosomal dominant disorder with a high degree of penetrance and great variability in expressivity. Patients with MEA-1 may have hyperplasia, adenomas, or carcinoma. The involved organs are the parathyroid glands, pancreatic islets and pituitary, in that order of frequency. Hyperparathyroidism is present in 87 percent of patients with the MEA-1 syndrome, and gastrinoma is present in approximately half of these patients (see Chap. 348).

While the true incidence of gastrinomas is not known, estimates are that they account for 0.1 to 1 percent of peptic ulcers. They may occur at any age, but initial manifestations are most common between ages 20 and 50.

CLINICAL FEATURES From 90 to 95 percent of patients with gastrinomas develop ulceration of the gastrointestinal tract at some point during the course of their disease. Profound gastric hypersecretion is found in most, but not all, patients. Symptoms are often similar to those seen in patients with typical peptic ulcer disease. However, the ulcer symptoms may be more fulminant, progressive, and persistent, and usually respond poorly to medical and surgical peptic ulcer treatment programs. The anatomic site of the ulcers in patients with gastrinoma is similar, but not identical, to that of patients with common types of peptic ulcer. Seventy-five percent of gastrinoma patients have ulcers in the first portion of the duodenum or in the stomach. The ulcers are usually single but may be multiple. When multiple ulcers occur, they are frequently located not only in the first portion of the duodenum, but also in the remainder of the duodenum or even the jejunum. In one large series, 14 percent of the ulcers were found in the duodenum beyond its first portion and 11 percent in the jejunum. Prompt recurrence of ulcer, often with hemorrhage or perforation, after usual peptic ulcer surgery (in which the Zollinger-Ellison syndrome had not been recognized) is characteristic of gastrinoma.

Diarrhea occurs in about 40 percent of patients, although about 7 percent of patients may have diarrhea in the absence of ulcer disease. The diarrhea is due to the outpouring of large amounts of hydrochloric acid into the proximal duodenum and can be reduced or eliminated by aspiration of gastric juice. The excessive acid reduces the pH within the lumen of the proximal and distal jejunum to as low as 1 and 3.6, respectively. Inflammatory changes may develop in the mucosa of the small intestine presumably secondary to the injurious effect of the increased amounts of acid and pepsin. Steatorrhea may also occur owing to inactivation of pancreatic lipase by the increased acid in the proximal small intestine and decrease in luminal bile salts. The decrease in bile salts may occur owing to precipitation of the major bile acids at the low pH. This leads to impaired micelle formation which, in turn, reduces the intestinal absorption of fatty acids and monoglycerides (see Chap. 292). Vitamin B_{12} malabsorption, not correctable by addition of intrinsic factor, can be detected in some patients with gastrinoma. Although the secretion of intrinsic factor appears normal, the reduced pH within the gut interferes with intrinsic factor mediation of vitamin B_{12} absorption. This can be corrected by neutralizing the pH within the gut lumen. The mechanism by which low pH in the gut interferes with intrinsic factor action is not known.

Diarrhea in patients with gastrinoma is invariably accompanied by gastric acid *hypersecretion*. This must be distinguished from the severe diarrhea seen with nonbeta islet-cell tumors of the pancreas, which is usually associated with *hyposecretion* of gastric acid or even achlorhydria [pancreatic cholera or WDHA (watery diarrhea, hypokalemia, and achlorhydria) syndrome]. The pancreatic cholera syndrome appears due to tumor release of VIP (see Chaps. 309 and 348).

DIAGNOSIS The presence of a gastrinoma should be suspected in patients with a compatible clinical history, especially in those with evidence of marked acid hypersecretion. Two-thirds of gastrinoma patients have basal gastric acid outputs (BAO) which exceed 10 meq/h. However, as stated earlier, there is substantial overlap in the rates of gastric acid secretion in patients with gastrinoma, duodenal ulcer, and in normal subjects. Gastrinoma patients often have basal acid output rates greater than 60 percent of those induced by maximal stimulation (MAO). In most normal subjects and duodenal ulcer patients basal acid secretory rates are substantially less than 60 percent of maximal secretion. Because of frequent patient variations, the use of the BAO/MAO ratio is of limited value in identifying gastrinoma patients.

Some radiographic features may suggest and support the diagnosis of Zollinger-Ellison syndrome. Prominence of mucosal folds may be demonstrated in the stomach, throughout the duodenum, and, in some instances, in the jejunum. The lumen of the stomach and small intestine may often contain large amounts of fluid. Radiographic features of most ulcers in these patients, except when they are multiple or distal in location, do not assist in distinguishing them from common peptic ulcer. Arteriography is of limited value in identifying patients with gastrinoma; abnormalities are noted in from 20 to 40 percent of patients.

The diagnosis of the Zollinger-Ellison syndrome depends upon the demonstration of *increased serum gastrin levels* by radioimmunoassay. Fasting serum gastrin levels in normal subjects and patients with typical duodenal ulcer average approximately 60 pg/ml and usually do not exceed 160 pg/ml. Patients with gastrinoma almost always have fasting serum gastrin levels which are greater than 200 pg/ml and have been reported as high as 450,000 pg/ml.

Several provocative tests are of value in identifying gastrinoma patients. These tests are of greatest assistance in identifying patients with gastrinoma who do not exhibit striking hypergastrinemia, i.e., fasting serum gastrin greater than 1000 pg/ml. These tests involve the measurement of serum gastrin levels in response to calcium infusion, secretin injection, or a standard test meal (see Table 290-2).

In the *calcium infusion test* a constant 3-h intravenous infusion of calcium gluconate is given (5 mg calcium per kilogram per hour). Serums for gastrin measurements are obtained before and at 30-min intervals for 4 h after initiation of infusion. In gastrinoma patients serum gastrin concentrations usually increase above the basal serum gastrin by at least 50 percent or by 500 pg/ml. In the *secretin injection test*, secretin (GIH secretin, 2 units per kilogram) is given over 30 to 60 s intravenously. (Boots secretin is approximately one-sixth as potent as GIH secretin supplied by the Karolinska Institute, Stockholm.) Gastrin is measured in serum samples obtained before injection of secretin and at 5-min intervals thereafter for 30 min. In normal individuals and duodenal ulcer patients secretin produces either no change or small reductions in serum gastrin levels. By contrast, in gastrinoma patients intravenous secretin induces paradoxical increases in serum gastrin. The gastrin levels increase promptly, usually at 5 min and by at least 50 percent, or by at least 400 pg/ml. The third provocative test involves the *feeding of a standard meal;* gastrin is measured in serums obtained before the meal and at 15-min intervals for 90 min. In gastrinoma patients peak serum gastrin levels are usually less than 50 percent greater than fasting serum gastrin concentrations (see Table 290-2).

The precise frequency with which gastrinoma patients conform to the criteria suggested for these provocative tests is not known. However, with what information is now available, the following conclusions appear warranted. *The secretin infusion test appears to be the provocative test of greatest value in identifying gastrinoma patients.* Positive serum gastrin responses to intravenous secretin are detected in more than 90 percent of patients with gastrinoma. Such paradoxical increases in serum gastrin following secretin injection have not been found in other patients. Enhanced release of gastrin in response to calcium infusion is found in more than 80 percent of gastrinoma patients; however, this exaggerated response to infusion has been observed in some nongastrinoma patients with hypergastrinemia (e.g., achlorhydria with or without pernicious anemia). In gastrinoma patients enhanced gastrin release with calcium infusion is rarely, if ever, observed in the absence of paradoxical gastrin release in response to secretin.

In an extremely small proportion of patients with duodenal ulcer (less than 1 percent) gastric acid hypersecretion may be accompanied by increased serum gastrin levels, which appear to result from hyperplasia of antral gastrin cells (G cells). These patients can be distinguished from those with gastrinoma by the secretin and meal stimulation tests. In patients with antral gastrin cell hyperplasia, intravenous secretin reduces serum gastrin, but the test meal leads to striking increases in serum gastrin levels, exceeding the fasting serum gastrin concentrations by more than 50 percent.

TREATMENT Ulceration of the upper gastrointestinal tract in patients with gastrinoma is usually resistant to conventional forms of medical and surgical treatment for common peptic ulcer. Antacid treatment may yield transient symptomatic relief but seldom induces ulcer healing or sustained relief of symptoms. Partial gastric resection or vagotomy with pyloroplasty is almost invariably followed by prompt and often fulminant ulcer recurrence. Many patients with gastrinoma have had multiple surgical procedures, particularly when the diagnosis was not established initially. Mortality is lowest when gastrectomy has been performed as the initial surgical procedure. Total gastrectomy is the surgical procedure of choice; subtotal gastric resections should not be performed. It would be desirable if one could remove the tumor at the time of surgery, but unfortunately the gastrinomas are usually multiple or are associated with nonresectable metastases at the time of laparotomy. Approximately 50 percent of duodenal gastrinomas are solitary and without metastases. Therefore, in some patients resection of the duodenal tumor may be indicated, with recognition that occult metastases may later become evident.

The H_2-receptor antagonist, cimetidine, has been used successfully in the medical treatment of patients with gastrinoma. Its use has been associated with improvement in clinical symptoms, ulcer healing, and decreases in gastric acid output. Many, but not all, of these patients have responded sufficiently well so as to not require surgery. Cimetidine doses are often 1.5 to 2 times those used in the treatment of common duodenal ulcer, in order to adequately suppress gastric acid secretion. Cimetidine treatment is of great value in those patients who are not good surgical candidates, as well as in preoperative management prior to total gastrectomy. At present, insufficient data are available to assess the role of H_2-receptor antagonists in the long-term treatment of gastrinoma patients.

STRESS ULCERS AND EROSIONS

A variety of acute ulcerative lesions of the gastrointestinal tract are distinct clinically from chronic peptic ulcer. Among these are the acute upper gastrointestinal erosions and ulcerations which are often observed in patients with shock, burns, sepsis, and severe trauma. These are often referred to as *stress erosions* and *ulcers*. These lesions, which are frequently multiple, are most common in the acid-secreting portion of the stomach, but may also occur in the antrum and duodenum. Acute stress erosions and ulcerations are usually superficial, with necrosis limited to the mucosa. These erosions and superficial ulcers occur in about 90 percent of patients with massive injuries and burns.

The most common clinical finding in patients with acute erosions or ulcerations is painless gastrointestinal hemorrhage. Blood loss may be minimal or substantial. Erosions usually occur approximately 24 h after trauma. Small amounts of blood loss may be detected in the first 24 to 48 h after trauma. However, massive hemorrhage usually occurs more than 2 or 3 days after the acute insult. The diagnosis is best established by upper gastrointestinal endoscopy. The ulcerative lesions are frequently too superficial to be recognized by barium examination of the upper gastrointestinal tract. The lesions should be suspected when there is evidence of upper gastrointestinal bleeding in patients with severe injuries, burns, infections, and shock.

Gastric acid appears to be involved in the production of these acute stress erosions and ulcers, although there is usually no evidence of acid hypersecretion. The lesions cannot be produced in experimental animals in the absence of acid.

Many theories have been proposed to explain stress-associated acute mucosal ulceration, but the mechanism for the mucosal injury is still not clear. The two major mechanisms which have been proposed are mucosal ischemia and enhanced back-diffusion of hydrogen ions. Studies have shown that the gastric mucosal barrier is intact after severe burns and injuries. A number of studies support the concept that mucosal ischemia may be most important in the production of stress ulceration.

The treatment of acute stress ulcerations and erosions is principally preventive. In high-risk patients the frequency of stress ulcerations can be diminished by the vigorous use of antacids to neutralize gastric contents. While anticholinergics are of no value, there is preliminary evidence that inhibition of acid secretion by cimetidine may be effective in both prevention and treatment. Intravenous vasopressin infusion or its selective intraarterial infusion into the left gastric artery has been found to decrease hemorrhage in patients with stress erosions. When medical therapy fails to arrest bleeding, surgical approaches have varied from total gastrectomy to pyloroplasty and vagotomy. In general, medical treatment should be instituted initially, and if surgery is required, vagotomy and pyloroplasty should be performed. Only if these measures are unsuccessful should gastrectomy be considered.

The term *Cushing's ulcer* has been applied to acute ulceration of the upper gastrointestinal tract associated with intracranial injury or increases in intracranial pressure, e.g., with brain tumors. These ulcers may involve the stomach, proximal duodenum, or esophagus, and frequently lead to hemorrhage or perforation. They do not differ histologically from acute stress ulcerations. Unlike stress ulceration, however, Cushing's ulcer is usually accompanied by increases in gastric acid secretion; hypergastrinemia has also been observed in some of these patients. Treatment includes correction of increased intracranial pressure, when possible, and the usual measures for treatment of acute erosions and ulcerations.

DRUG-ASSOCIATED ULCER AND EROSIONS

Gastric and duodenal ulcers have been described following administration of many drugs. Salicylate ingestion has been shown to be associated with an increased incidence of gastric ulcer, and these drugs are a frequent cause of hemorrhagic gastric erosions. There is no evidence of an increased frequency of duodenal ulcer among patients treated with salicylates. The mechanism by which salicylates induce, or are associated with, gastric ulcer has not been established. It has been suggested that salicylates contribute to development of gastric ulcer by mucosal injury induced by interruption of the gastric mucosal barrier. This is the mechanism by which salicylates produce erosive gastritis. Patients with gastric ulcer should avoid salicylates, and many physicians also withhold recommending salicylates in patients with duodenal ulcer.

Administration of corticosteroids has been reported to be associated with development of ulcer disease of the upper gastrointestinal tract. Although for the most part this proposal has been widely accepted, there are no firm data conclusively establishing the association between corticosteroids and gastric or duodenal ulcers. Most control studies have failed to demonstrate an increased incidence of ulcers in patients treated with corticosteroids for a variety of disorders. Some studies have suggested an increased incidence of ulcer disease in patients with rheumatoid arthritis, and this may account for an apparent increase in ulcer frequency when these patients receive corticosteroids. Thus, data do not establish with certainty a direct association between treatment with corticosteroids and an increased incidence of duodenal or gastric ulcer.

Other drugs which have been reported to be associated with ulceration of the upper gastrointestinal tract include indomethacin, phenylbutazone, and reserpine. It is uncertain whether these drugs are responsible for the associated ulcer disease and, if so, by what mechanism the ulceration is produced. Because of the potential suspected ulcerogenicity of corticosteroids, indomethacin, phenylbutazone, and reserpine, most physicians limit their use, when possible, in patients with known peptic ulcer disease. In addition to salicylates and indomethacin, acute gastric erosions have been reported after ingestion of other anti-inflammatory agents used in the treatment of arthritis, including ibuprofen and naproxen. When possible, their use should also be limited in patients with ulcer disease.

REFERENCES

BARDHAN KD et al: Double blind comparison of cimetidine and placebo in the maintenance and healing of chronic duodenal ulceration. Gut 20:158, 1979

FORDTRAN JS et al: In vivo and in vitro evaluation of liquid antacids. N Engl J Med 288:923, 1973

ISENBERG JI et al: Increased sensitivity to stimulation of acid secretion by pentagastrin in duodenal ulcer. J Clin Invest 55:330, 1975

LAMERS CBH, VAN TONGEREN JHM: Comparative study of the value of calcium, secretin, and meal stimulated increase in serum gastrin to the diagnosis of the Zollinger-Ellison syndrome. Gut 18:128, 1977

MACDONALD WC: Correlation of mucosal histology and aspirin intake in chronic gastric ulcer. Gastroenterology 65:381, 1973

MCCARTHY DM: Report on the United States experience with cimetidine in Zollinger-Ellison syndrome and other hypersecretory states. Gastroenterology 74:453, 1978

MCGUIGAN JE, TRUDEAU WL: Differences in rates of gastrin release in normal persons and patients with duodenal ulcer. N Engl J Med 288:64, 1973

MENDELOFF AI: What has been happening to duodenal ulcer? Gastroenterology 67:1020, 1974

PETERSON WL et al: Healing of duodenal ulcer with an antacid regime. N Engl J Med 297:341, 1977

ROTTER JI et al: Duodenal ulcer disease associated with elevated serum pepsinogen I. An inherited autosomal disorder. N Engl J Med 300:63, 1979

SAWYERS JL et al: Proximal gastric vagotomy compared with vagotomy and antrectomy and selective gastric vagotomy pyloroplasty. Ann Surg 196:510, 1977

SKILLMAN JJ, SILEN W: Stress ulceration in the acutely ill. Annu Rev Med 27:9, 1976

STABILE BE, PASSARO E JR: Progress in gastroenterology. Recurrent peptic ulcer. Gastroenterology 70:124, 1976

WALSH JH, GROSSMAN MI: Gastrin. N Engl J Med 292:1324, 1975

WINSHIP DH: Cimetidine in the treatment of duodenal ulcer. Review and commentary. Gastroenterology 74:402, 1978

291
CANCER, BENIGN TUMORS, GASTRITIS, AND OTHER GASTRIC DISEASES

WALTER C. MacDONALD
CYRUS E. RUBIN

CANCER

CARCINOMA Throughout the world gastric cancer is one of the most common lethal malignancies. Although its frequency is decreasing in the United States, it still causes about 15,000 deaths each year. Because early symptoms are often minimal or nonexistent in the potentially curable phase, patients usually seek medical advice too late. Thus, less than 10 percent of patients survive 5 years, despite improved diagnostic and surgical techniques.

Epidemiology Whereas gastric cancer is very common in Japan, Chile, and parts of Eastern Europe, it is uncommon in the United States, Mexico, and Malaysia. Over the past 40 years in the United States there has been a remarkable but unexplained fall in the annual mortality from 30 to 8 per 100,000. A lesser decline is apparent in Western Europe. Japanese migrating to the United States continue to have a high incidence, but their children have a much lower incidence, suggesting the importance of environmental factors in pathogenesis. Throughout the world, men are affected about twice as often as women. The mean age usually quoted is 55 years, but the patients are even older in some North American series. Only 5 percent of patients are less than 40 years of age.

Etiology The cause of gastric cancer is unknown, but diet has been implicated. Gastric cancer can be readily induced in some animals by the oral administration of N-methyl-N^1-nitrosoguanidine. It has been suggested that gastric cancer may be related to the formation of N-nitroso compounds by the conversion of food nitrates to nitrites, which then interact in the stomach with secondary or tertiary amines. Interestingly, this reaction is inhibited by ascorbic acid.

Predisposing factors Gastric cancer is two to four times more common in relatives of patients with the disease than in a control population. The concordance rate is greater for identical than dizygotic twins. The disease is marginally more common in persons with blood group A. These data suggest a small genetic element in pathogenesis.

Atrophic gastric mucosa, especially when associated with intestinal metaplasia, probably increases the risk of gastric cancer. Such mucosal changes are invariably seen in Addisonian pernicious anemia, and 6 percent of these patients develop stomach cancer. Comparison of Japanese and American autopsy results shows that the high-risk Japanese have more extensive atrophic gastritis and intestinal metaplasia than the low-risk Americans. Serial biopsy studies also suggest that persons with atrophic gastritis are more likely to develop gastric cancer than those with normal mucosa. It must, however, be recognized that atrophic gastritis is common in normal older people without cancer, and that some patients with gastric cancer have no gastritis in the uninvolved portions of the stomach.

Adenomatous gastric polyps more than 2 cm in diameter frequently contain adenocarcinoma. It is not known whether these uncommon larger polyps contain cancer from the onset or whether they were originally benign. Certainly most gastric cancers do not begin as polyps. Patients with benign epithelial gastric polyps are predisposed to cancer elsewhere in the stomach, and this is possibly related to the atrophic gastritis which is regularly seen surrounding such polyps.

Benign gastric ulcer without operation has not been shown to be a precursor of gastric cancer. Ten to twenty years after a Billroth II partial gastrectomy for peptic ulcer there is an increased risk of gastric cancer.

Pathology Gastric cancers are almost always adenocarcinomas. Gross and microscopic classification of these carcinomas is frequently impossible because many are of mixed pattern. In general, there are five macroscopic types: polypoid, ulcerative, combined ulcerative and infiltrative, diffuse infiltrative (linitis plastica), and superficial spreading. Microscopic classification is particularly difficult, but three cell types are discernible: intestinal, gastric (pylorocardiac), and diffuse (mucous cell). When classifiable, the gross and microscopic categorizations have limited prognostic value. Polypoid, ulcerative, and superficial spreading cancers are often less malignant than the infiltrative types. Microscopically, the intestinal cell type has a slightly better prognosis than the diffuse mucous cell variety. However, the most important morphologic factors in prognosis are the depth of invasion and the presence or absence of metastases. Stromal reaction with lymphocytes, plasma cells, and young fibroblasts is indicative of host resistance and improves the prognosis.

Cancer originates with equal frequency in the antrum and body of the stomach and involves the lesser curvature more often than the greater. Ten to twenty percent occur at the cardia. The cancer spreads by direct extension along the gastric wall and through it to the perigastric tissues. Sometimes direct extension involves the pancreas, colon, or liver. Proximal gastric tumors often invade the esophagus, but distal ones less commonly cross the pylorus into the duodenum. Lymph node metastases to the perigastric nodes are usually present; nodes in the preaortic area, porta hepatis, and hilum of the spleen are often involved as well. Spread via the thoracic duct can involve the left supraclavicular (Virchow's) lymph nodes. Peritoneal metastases are evident in about 20 percent of patients at laparoscopy or operation. Intraabdominal metastases may be confined to the ovary or prerectal pouch. Blood-borne metastases to the liver are apparent in about 30 percent of patients at operation; less often, the lungs, brain, or other organs are involved.

Clinical features The history is of little help in distinguishing benign from malignant gastric ulcer because many of the varied symptoms may be seen in both diseases. Approximately 25 percent of patients with cancer have classic ulcer symptoms.

The most common presenting complaint, however, is upper abdominal discomfort of insidious onset. This is often mild but varies greatly in severity from a vague, postprandial fullness to a severe, steady pain. Anorexia, often with slight nausea, is very common but is not the usual presenting complaint. Weight loss is observed in about 50 percent of patients. Nausea and vomiting are particularly prominent with tumors of the pylorus, but can occur with advanced disease elsewhere in the stomach. Dysphagia is the major symptom of cardia tumors. Weakness, hematemesis, melena, and alteration in bowel habits are other presenting complaints. Some patients suffer from the symptoms of anemia, or their anemia may be discovered on routine examination. Occasionally, an ulcerating carcinoma perforates, and rarely a gastrocolic fistula develops.

The initial symptoms may be related to metastases. These include abdominal distention by malignant ascites; jaundice from biliary tract obstruction by nodes at the porta hepatis or by intrahepatic metastases; pain from bone involvement; neurologic symptoms secondary to brain metastases; and shortness of breath from lung spread. Mechanical bowel obstruction can be secondary to peritoneal metastases, and pelvic symptoms can result from ovarian spread.

The duration of symptoms before patients see a physician is remarkably variable but averages 6 months. Symptoms of several years' duration are not uncommon. Some patients with long-standing functional gastrointestinal complaints may notice a change in their pain pattern. In North America, less than 10 percent of patients with symptoms have disease confined to the mucosa or submucosa. Screening studies in Japan confirm that most patients with early curable gastric cancer are asymptomatic.

An epigastric mass is palpable in only a minority of patients; it is a poor prognostic sign but does not exclude the possibility of cure. Abdominal tenderness is found in about one-third of patients. Pallor or cachexia may be observed, and occasionally a gastric succussion splash is demonstrable. Physical signs suggesting metastases should be carefully sought because distant metastases that are proved by biopsy exclude curative surgery. These include hepatomegaly, jaundice, enlargement of left supraclavicular or pectoral nodes, a shelf-like mass in the prerectal pouch above the prostate or cervix (Blumer's shelf), an ovarian mass on vaginal or abdominal examination (Krukenberg's tumor), ascites, an umbilical mass, and skin nodules. A low-grade fever may occur with advanced disease, particularly with liver metastases. Rarely gastric cancer is associated with dermatomyositis, acanthosis nigricans, neuromyopathy, or hypoglycemia.

Laboratory findings Iron-deficiency anemia because of occult bleeding is found in about two-thirds of patients. Occasionally the cancer is associated with pernicious anemia. Rarely a pancytopenia is caused by bone marrow replacement. A "leukemoid" reaction and disseminated intravascular coagulation are other rare findings. Occult blood is demonstrable in the stools in about 80 percent of patients if repeated tests are done. Elevation of 5'-nucleotidase suggests the presence of liver metastases, and liver scan can confirm it. The serum albumin may be low because of protein leakage from the involved gastric mucosa. Measurement of gastric secretion is considered less helpful than in the past. Achlorhydria after stimulation with pentagastrin usually excludes a benign peptic ulcer, but the test is of limited value because most patients with a malignant ulcer secrete some acid. A rise in the carcinoembryonic antigen (CEA) after treatment suggests recurrence of carcinoma, but the test is of little initial diagnostic value.

Diagnosis In North America x-ray of the stomach is the initial method used for detecting gastric carcinoma. In more than 90 percent of symptomatic patients, x-ray detects a gastric abnormality. However, experienced radiologists fail to differentiate benign from malignant gastric lesions in approximately 25 percent of cases. Thus, gastroscopy with biopsy and brush or exfoliative cytology must be used to confirm or exclude a diagnosis of cancer (see Chap. 288). It is as important to the patient to exclude gastric cancer as it is to diagnose it because unnecessary emotional trauma and surgical morbidity or mortality can be avoided by definitive diagnosis of benign disease.

The diagnostic accuracy of x-ray is greatest when it is used wisely. Equivocal examinations should always be repeated. The use of double contrast techniques helps to detect small lesions by improving mucosal detail. The stomach should be distended at some time during every x-ray examination because decreased distensibility may be the only indication of a diffuse infiltrative carcinoma. Although gastric ulcers can be detected fairly easily, it may be impossible to distinguish benign from malignant ulcers radiologically. Differential x-ray diagnosis is also difficult when the antrum is narrowed or when mucosal folds are enlarged. Cancer of the proximal stomach invading the neural plexuses of the esophagus may mimic achalasia by x-ray. In cancer of the cardia the x-ray appearance may be considered normal or may be confused with benign mucosal distortion secondary to a hiatus hernia. It is impossible to differentiate adenocarcinoma from lymphoma radiologically. Cancer of the pancreas or colon invading the stomach may be confused with primary gastric neoplasm.

Fiberoptic gastroscopy with biopsy and brush cytology is especially useful for confirming the diagnosis of cancer suspected by x-ray, differentiating cancer from lymphoma, clarifying equivocal radiologic findings, and checking suspicious clinical findings despite negative x-rays. At least six biopsies should be taken from suitable areas of a suspected neoplasm; if the tissue is serially sectioned and thoroughly examined by an expert, accuracy in the diagnosis of cancer approaching 90 percent can be achieved. The addition of brush cytology raises the accuracy in detecting cancer even higher but slightly raises the risk of a false diagnosis of cancer. Diffuse infiltrative tumors and recurrent cancers can be impossible to diagnose even by these methods because malignant cells may not be present in the biopsied mucosal layer. Expertly performed exfoliative cytology by "blind" gastric lavage yields cancer cells in over 85 percent of patients with a false-positive rate of less than 1 percent. The procedure is particularly useful in elderly or poor-risk patients and in those in whom endoscopy is unsuccessful or equivocal. If all techniques are used, gastric cancer is seldom missed, but occasionally laparoscopy or laparotomy is required for diagnosis.

The x-ray demonstration of a benign-appearing gastric ulcer presents special problems. Some physicians feel that gastroscopy is not mandatory if the x-ray features are typically benign, if healing at 6 weeks is complete by x-ray, and if a follow-up x-ray examination several months later is negative. Other physicians, however, feel that gastroscopic biopsy and brush cytology are required for all patients with a gastric ulcer in order to exclude carcinoma or lymphoma. The marked drop in the incidence of malignant gastric ulcers in North America has raised the question whether it is cost-effective to endoscope all patients with gastric ulcer rather than to perform endoscopy only in those with a suspicious x-ray or clinical course.

Using x-ray and intragastric photography for mass screening, the Japanese have detected many early curable cancers of the stomach. In North America, such screening methods are probably not cost-effective because the disease is relatively uncommon. However, special attention must be paid to patients over 40 years of age who are predisposed to gastric cancer because of pernicious anemia, the presence or history of an adenomatous gastric polyp, a family history of gastric cancer, Billroth II gastrectomy 10 to 20 years previously, or birth in countries where gastric cancer is common. In addition, one must be certain that all gastric ulcers treated medically are indeed benign.

Treatment Surgical removal of the tumor offers the only chance for cure. A careful evaluation for evidence of distant metastases will avoid unnecessary surgery. Physical examination is supplemented by chest x-ray, liver function tests, liver scan, and, in selected cases, abdominal ultrasound (echo) or computerized tomography (CT scan). Suspected areas of metastasis should be sampled, for example, lymph nodes or liver and pleural or peritoneal effusions. If metastases are suspected but unproved, laparoscopy under local anesthesia with direct biopsy of suspected areas of metastasis is particularly helpful in assessing operability. Cancer of the distal and midstomach is usually treated by subtotal gastrectomy; removal of the regional lymph nodes requires resection of the greater and lesser omentum and sometimes the spleen. Tumors of the proximal stomach are treated by distal esophagectomy and proximal gastrectomy. Total gastrectomy is indicated only occasionally. If obstruction is present or if bleeding is a problem, palliative resection may be worthwhile even though the disease is found to be incurable at operation. The operative mortality rate for gastric cancer is still higher than 10 percent in many hospitals.

It is often difficult to assess the reported results of surgical treatment. Careful and standardized descriptions by surgeon and pathologist would facilitate comparison of different series. These should include depth of tumor penetration, extent of lymph node involvement, and presence of distant metastases. More than 80 percent of cancers confined to the mucosa or submucosa are curable, compared with 10 to 20 percent when the tumor extends through the serosa. Up to 50 percent survive 5 years after curative resection if the lymph nodes are not involved. Tumor diameter of less than 2 cm and a long history of symptoms are good prognostic signs. However, in North America fewer than 10 percent survive 5 years after diagnosis. Rarely, patients live for 5 years without treatment or for many years after a palliative resection.

Chemotherapy with 5-fluorouracil (5-FU) causes some tumor regression in about 10 percent of patients. Combination chemotherapy (e.g., 5-FU plus methyl-CCNU and adriamycin) appears to induce a response in a somewhat higher percentage of patients (see Chap. 324). The effectiveness of adjuvant or palliative radiotherapy, or of adjuvant chemotherapy, remains to be demonstrated. Other palliative measures include replacement of iron and vitamin B_{12}, dilatation of obstructing cardia tumors with or without placement of plastic tubular stents, treatment of postgastrectomy problems, and the judicious use of analgesics and antiemetics.

LYMPHOMA Primary gastric lymphomas account for about 5 percent of gastric malignancies and about 60 percent of gastric sarcomas. Most are histiocytic lymphomas (reticulum-cell sarcomas) or lymphocytic lymphomas; Hodgkin's disease is relatively uncommon, and plasmacytoma is rare. Some gastric lymphomas present a varied histologic picture that defies classification. Gastric involvement secondary to disseminated lymphoma is more common than the primary form. In one large series, one-third of histiocytic lymphomas and one-sixth of lymphosarcomas eventually spread to the stomach. The sexes are affected equally, and the mean age is about 55 years.

The symptoms are indistinguishable from those of gastric ulcer or cancer. Hematemesis (20 percent) and perforation (10 percent) occur more often than with carcinoma. An abdominal mass is palpable in approximately one-third of patients. Ap-

proximately half of patients have iron-deficiency anemia, usually with occult blood demonstrable in the stools.

X-ray studies usually show an abnormality which can seldom be distinguished from adenocarcinoma. Large rigid folds, multiple ulcers, or duodenal involvement suggest the possibility of lymphoma. The x-ray appearance may also be confused with that of Ménétrier's disease or benign peptic ulcer. The tumor is usually obvious at gastroscopy, but its gross appearance is seldom diagnostic. A preoperative diagnosis can often be made by the combination of endoscopic biopsy and cytologic examination, but even these methods may fail. Pseudolymphoma cannot be distinguished from true lymphoma prior to surgical excision.

Primary gastric lymphoma should be treated by a combination of surgical excision and radiation therapy. Usually surgery precedes radiotherapy, but it may be advantageous to shrink large tumors with radiation before attempting to excise them. Thirty to fifty percent of patients so treated survive 5 years. Survival is particularly good if the tumor does not penetrate the serosa or involve the perigastric nodes. A careful search for evidence of disseminated disease should be made before operation. Laparoscopy is especially useful for such staging. Some patients with nonresectable tumors have survived 5 years after treatment with radiotherapy alone. Disseminated lymphoma with gastric involvement is treated by chemotherapy and radiotherapy as discussed in Chap. 324.

LEIOMYOSARCOMA These tumors account for 1 to 3 percent of gastric malignancies. The mean age of the persons affected is about 60 years, and the sexes are affected equally. The tumors are usually large, spherical, and in the upper half of the stomach; they tend to ulcerate and become necrotic in their center. The tumor may spread to the peritoneum or liver but rarely to lymph nodes. Most patients complain of pain. The majority are anemic, and massive bleeding occurs in about one-third. A mass is palpable in more than 50 percent. X-ray studies show a large, smooth tumor, often with central ulceration and sometimes with a sinus tract to the center of the neoplasm. It is impossible to differentiate leiomyosarcoma by x-ray from benign leiomyomas except that they tend to be larger. Endoscopic biopsy rarely provides a correct preoperative diagnosis, but brush cytology of the ulceration may. Treatment is by wide surgical excision if feasible; about 40 percent of patients are cured. Expert chemotherapists have used adriamycin in combination with various other agents to successfully palliate some patients with advanced disease. Radiotherapy is ineffective.

Carcinoid tumors and other malignancies Gastric carcinoids are uncommon. They are often symptomless but can cause bleeding or epigastric pain. The roentgenographic appearance is that of a smooth, rounded, sessile filling defect sometimes with ulceration. About 20 percent are malignant, but only a small minority cause the malignant carcinoid syndrome. Small carcinoids can be excised locally; those larger than 2 cm and those that are malignant require partial gastrectomy. The malignant carcinoid syndrome and its treatment are described in Chap. 91.

Rare primary gastric malignancies include carcinosarcoma, hemangiopericytoma, neurogenic sarcoma, fibrosarcoma, and liposarcoma. Approximately 10 percent of leiomyoblastomas are malignant. Metastases to the stomach most often originate from generalized lymphoma, lung cancer, breast cancer, or malignant melanoma.

BENIGN TUMORS

EPITHELIAL POLYPS After cancer, benign epithelial polyps are the most common tumors of the stomach (5 to 10 percent). There is considerable confusion regarding the nomenclature of these epithelial polyps. What is important to remember is that 80 to 90 percent of them are not neoplastic, and probably never become malignant. The most common nonneoplastic polyp is *hyperplastic*, i.e., is composed almost completely of normal surface mucous cells and at times of mucus-secreting pyloric glands. Greater than 90 percent of such polyps are less than 1.5 cm in diameter and do not enlarge with the passage of time. They may be single or multiple or pedunculated or sessile and can occur in any part of the stomach. They are covered with normal-appearing mucosa and frequently have a superficial ulceration on their tip. The mucosa surrounding them often shows chronic gastritis or atrophy. Although hyperplastic polyps almost never become malignant, carcinoma in other parts of the same stomach is more frequent.

Ten to twenty percent of benign epithelial polyps are composed of neoplastic epithelium and are called *adenomas*. They are usually larger than 2 cm in diameter and do enlarge with the passage of time. As many as 40 percent of all adenomatous gastric polyps are already malignant when first diagnosed and the rest may become malignant. They can be pedunculated or sessile and are solitary in two-thirds of cases. They are covered with abnormal reddened velvety mucosa which may be lobulated or mammillated. Most are located in the antrum. The mucosa surrounding them is usually atrophic, and carcinoma elsewhere in the stomach is common (30 percent or more in various series).

Both hyperplastic and adenomatous polyps occur more frequently in patients over 50 years of age, and 80 percent or more of these patients are achlorhydric. From 6 to 20 percent of patients with pernicious anemia have epithelial polyps. Occult bleeding is the most important clinical manifestation and at times is associated with vague epigastric stress. Rarely, vomiting results from prolapse of a large, pedunculated antral polyp into the duodenum. Radiologically, the polyps appear as smooth, rounded, or lobulated filling defects, with or without a stalk. Although those greater than 2 cm in diameter are more likely to be adenomas or polypoid carcinomas, exceptions are not uncommon.

Hyperplastic polyps may have a different gross appearance from adenomas at endoscopy, but one cannot differentiate between the two with certainty even after sampling them by forceps biopsy. To determine the histologic nature of a polyp and to exclude malignancy, the whole lesion is best examined. Most pedunculated or small sessile polyps can be removed with an electrocautery snare during gastroscopy by an experienced endoscopist. It may be dangerous to attempt endoscopic removal of larger sessile polyps or those with a broad pedicle. Such lesions can be biopsied endoscopically by removing a sizable superficial portion of the polyp with a coagulating cautery snare, or the diagnosis can be established by surgical excision. Once the histological diagnosis of adenoma has been made, excision is the appropriate treatment. Because of the high risk of cancer in the surrounding mucosa, such patients must be followed regularly with endoscopic and cytologic examinations. Partial or even total gastrectomy may eventually be needed.

Rare hamartomatous gastric polyps are made up of the various benign epithelial cells normally present in the gastric mucosa. They are usually part of two familial polyposis syndromes: Peutz-Jeghers and juvenile polyposis. Twenty-five percent of Peutz-Jeghers cases involve the stomach or duodenum and 2 to 3 percent develop gastric or duodenal carcinoma. Malignant change in gastric juvenile polyposis is either very rare or absent. Cronkhite-Canada syndrome is a rare cause of benign gastric retention polyps composed of dilated cystic glands with markedly edematous stroma.

Diffuse gastric polyposis is a rare and poorly defined condition in which the gastric mucosa is covered with numerous sessile or pedunculated epithelial polyps. This condition must not be confused with a variant of chronic gastritis in which the mucosa has a diffusely polypoid appearance; this entity is diagnosed by biopsy. Multiple gastric polyps are usually proved to be hyperplastic by snare excision. Such patients should be followed by regular endoscopic and cytologic examinations because of the higher frequency of cancer in the surrounding mucosa. Multiple gastric adenomas are very rare. They may be seen in familial polyposis or Gardner's syndrome. Because of the high risk of cancer they may require partial or even total gastrectomy.

LEIOMYOMAS AND RARE BENIGN TUMORS Most leiomyomas are tiny and of no clinical significance. Larger ones, usually 3 cm or more in diameter, may cause massive or occult bleeding or epigastric pain. The x-ray appearance is that of a smooth, rounded, sessile filling defect, often with a central ulcer. The gastroscopic appearance is highly suggestive but not diagnostic. Mucosal biopsies are too superficial for diagnosis, but brush cytology of the ulcerated area may help rule out leiomyosarcoma. Small symptomatic lesions may be treated by local surgical excision, and larger ones by partial gastrectomy. Other rare benign gastric tumors include lipomas, schwannomas, leiomyoblastomas, hemangiomas, lymphangiomas, and fibromas.

PSEUDOTUMORS A number of gastric conditions other than peptic ulcer simulate neoplasms by x-ray. These include hypertrophic pyloric stenosis; antral gastritis; inflammatory polyps; Ménétrier's disease and other gastric hyperplasias; pseudolymphoma; heterotopic pancreas; gastric eosinophilic granuloma; Crohn's disease; gastric varices; hematoma, deformity after fundoplication (Nissen repair); extrinsic pressure by the liver, pancreas, or spleen; and bezoars or retained food. Often endoscopic evaluation and consideration of the total clinical picture solve these problems, but in rare cases surgical exploration is necessary to exclude malignancy.

GASTRITIS

ACUTE EROSIVE GASTRITIS Erosive gastritis (also known as hemorrhagic gastritis or multiple gastric erosions) is an important cause of upper gastrointestinal bleeding. By endoscopy, multiple bleeding erosions are distributed diffusely throughout the gastric mucosa or are localized to the fundus, body, or antrum. The mucosa may appear reddened and friable, or it may appear normal.

Histologically, the mucosal destruction by erosions does not extend below the muscularis mucosae; characteristically, the mucosal lesions heal completely. At any one time, different erosions can be observed in various stages of evolution and regression. Between erosions there may be areas of surface epithelium depleted of mucus and focal or diffuse extravasation of blood into the lamina propria. Erosions may develop in any type of gastritis or in normal mucosa. When erosions enlarge and extend below the muscularis mucosae into the submucosa, they form acute ulcers.

Erosive gastritis can occur for no apparent reason. Many cases, however, are associated with aspirin ingestion. The low pK_a of aspirin facilitates its gastric absorption in the acid milieu of the gastric lumen because it is un-ionized and liposoluble at a low pH and is therefore absorbed readily by passive nonionic diffusion. At the neutral intracellular pH of the gastric surface epithelium aspirin becomes an ionized acid which can destroy the cells and provide an entry point for acid-peptic digestion. When aspirin is given with sodium bicarbonate, it may not be injurious because it cannot be absorbed by the gastric mucosa in its ionized form. Acute alcoholism and ingestion of certain anti-inflammatory prostaglandin inhibitors such as phenylbutazone or indomethacin may also be associated with erosive gastritis.

Severe stress secondary to burns, sepsis, trauma, surgery, shock, or respiratory, renal, or liver failure often causes gastric erosions or acute ulcers. Their pathogenesis is poorly understood and probably varies with different predisposing conditions. There are data suggesting that alterations in mucosal blood flow lead to areas of microinfarction with further evolution of the lesion dependent upon acid-peptic digestion. Erosive gastritis is a less frequent problem now that hyperalimentation and a strict antacid regimen are regularly used in severely stressed patients.

Patients present with hematemesis and/or melena. Many have no other symptoms, but some notice mild epigastric discomfort or nausea. The diagnosis is best made by gastroscopy on the same day as the bleeding episode, because otherwise the lesions may have healed and disappeared. Standard x-ray examination is of no help because the lesions are too superficial to change the barium silhouette. They may, however, be demonstrated by double-contrast studies. Many clinical diagnoses of erosive gastritis are made in patients with upper gastrointestinal bleeding and negative x-rays. Unfortunately, such presumptive diagnoses can be wrong. Erosive gastritis is best diagnosed by early gastroscopy.

The usual measures for restoring circulating blood volume should be undertaken promptly (Chap. 42). Not uncommonly, the bleeding has stopped by the time a tube is passed. If not, lavage of the stomach with iced isotonic saline through a large-diameter Ewald tube is traditional, but its efficacy is unproved in this spontaneously remitting illness. In any event, such lavage may facilitate diagnostic gastroscopy by washing out the stomach. Gravity drainage, *not suction,* should be used for emptying the iced saline from the stomach, lest suction artifacts be produced which are indistinguishable from acute erosions endoscopically.

If bleeding stops, a regimen of hourly antacids or cimetidine is instituted. If bleeding continues, or if rebleeding fails to respond to iced saline lavage, an attempt at control by selective infusion of Pitressin into the left gastric artery may stop the bleeding. In the rare case in which bleeding continues and is life-threatening, the erosions have usually progressed to deeper acute ulcers and emergency operation is necessary. Antrectomy with vagotomy appears to be the most effective surgical treatment but is not always successful. Very rarely persistent severe bleeding requires total gastrectomy.

CHRONIC GASTRITIS This is a histologic diagnosis and not a clinically recognizable entity because it has never been proved to be a direct cause of symptoms. The diagnosis can be made with certainty only by biopsy. There are two main types: fundal gland gastritis and "antral" or pyloric gland gastritis. In many persons, however, both gastric areas are involved, often in a patchy manner.

Chronic fundal gland gastritis This condition diffusely affects the mucosa of the body and fundus but may spare the antrum. There are three pathologic types: superficial gastritis, atrophic gastritis, and gastric atrophy. In superficial gastritis, acute and chronic inflammation and epithelial abnormalities are confined to the superficial nonglandular mucosa. In atrophic gastritis, there is partial loss of fundal glands and an increased number of lymphocytes and plasma cells within the lamina propria. To

varying degrees the chief and parietal cells of the fundal glands are replaced by intestinal or mucous cells. In gastric atrophy, the fundal glands have mostly disappeared and are almost completely replaced by mucous or intestinal cells; there is usually no histologic evidence of inflammation. Severe fundal gland atrophy is invariably present in Addisonian pernicious anemia. The relationship, if any, between the three types of chronic gastritis is uncertain, although some biopsy studies suggest that the superficial type sometimes progresses to atrophic gastritis and atrophy.

Chronic fundal gland gastritis is a very common histologic finding in the general population, particularly in older age groups. The atrophic type is especially common in patients with thyroid disease or idiopathic iron-deficiency anemia and in relatives of patients with pernicious anemia. Chronic fundal gland gastritis does not have a characteristic gross appearance by barium x-ray or gastroscopy unless there is severe mucosal atrophy; then, the fold pattern may be flattened in the fundus and body by x-ray, and pallor, absent folds, and submucosal vessels may be seen by gastroscopy.

Patients with superficial fundal gland gastritis usually have normal or slightly reduced acid secretion. Those with atrophic fundal gastritis are hypochlorhydric, and those with fundal atrophy are achlorhydric. In pernicious anemia the parietal cells which secrete intrinsic factor are virtually absent, and as a result food vitamin B_{12} is not absorbed. Serum gastrin levels are high in patients with pernicious anemia and in some patients with severe atrophic fundal gastritis because the uninvolved antrum secretes gastrin continuously in the absence of acid to inhibit it. Antibodies to parietal cells are present in the serum of about 60 percent of persons with atrophic gastritis and 80 to 90 percent of those with pernicious anemia. Antibodies to intrinsic factor are present in the serum or gastric juice of most patients with pernicious anemia but are not found in patients with superficial or atrophic gastritis. The relationship between these immunologic phenomena and the gastric mucosal atrophy of pernicious anemia is uncertain.

Ordinarily, chronic superficial or atrophic fundal gastritis requires no treatment. After adequate investigation has excluded other disease, those patients who have abdominal distress should be reassured. It is essential to rule out vitamin B_{12} malabsorption in persons who are found to be achlorhydric. If pernicious anemia is proved, it is treated as discussed in Chap. 311. The iron-deficiency anemia which may be associated with atrophic gastritis responds to medicinal iron.

Although severe atrophic gastritis and especially gastric fundal atrophy predispose to gastric cancer, diagnostic screening of patients so affected has not been productive. It is prudent nonetheless to investigate thoroughly unexplained abdominal symptoms in such patients.

Chronic antral gastritis So-called "antral" or pyloric gland gastritis is common in asymptomatic persons. With age, this type of gastritis probably tends to extend proximally into the fundal gland area. Patients with peptic ulcer almost invariably have an associated pyloric gland gastritis except for some patients with aspirin-related ulcers. If the peptic ulcer is located in the upper stomach, pyloric gland gastritis may extend far proximally. Gastric cancer is often associated with pyloric gland gastritis involving the antrum, as well as pyloric gland metaplasia and inflammation of much of the fundal gland area. Acid secretion may be normal or low, depending upon the extent of fundal gland involvement. In contrast to chronic fundal gastritis, serum gastrin levels tend to be low, and parietal cell antibodies are not found in the serum. It has been postulated that regurgitation of duodenal contents, particularly bile salts, into the stomach causes pyloric gland gastritis.

In most cases, pyloric gland gastritis does not cause symptoms and does not require treatment. Occasionally, it is associated with narrowing of the antrum on x-ray examination suggestive of malignancy; often such patients complain of ulcer-like pain and may indeed prove to have ulcers subsequently. At gastroscopy, normal antral motility suggests pliability, and malignancy can usually be excluded. The symptoms often respond to antacids.

GASTRIC HYPERPLASIA ("HYPERTROPHIC" GASTRITIS) Hypertrophic gastritis is a histologic misnomer. The individual mucosal epithelial cells are not enlarged (hypertrophic), but there are more of them (hyperplasia), and thus the mucosa is thickened. There are three benign causes for gastric mucosal hyperplasia: Ménétrier's disease, hypersecretory gastropathy, and Zollinger-Ellison syndrome (gastrinoma; see Chap. 290). Most hyperplastic mucosal conditions produce enlarged gastric folds which are often indistinguishable by x-ray or endoscopy from infiltrative cancer, lymphoma, or a functional abnormality.

Ménétrier's disease This is an uncommon type of gastric mucosal hyperplasia of unknown cause. It is characterized grossly by tortuous enlargement of the gastric mucosal folds resembling cerebral convolutions, and histologically by a thickened mucosa with hyperplasia of mucous cells and loss of most parietal and chief cells. The gastric pits are markedly elongated and tortuous and often exhibit cystic dilatation; these cysts may penetrate through the muscularis mucosae into the submucosa. The lamina propria often contains increased numbers of lymphocytes. Intestinal metaplasia may be present. The mucosal involvement may be localized or diffuse, and tends to be most prominent on the greater curvature.

Epigastric pain is the most common complaint. Anorexia, nausea, vomiting, weight loss, or diarrhea are other symptoms. Bleeding is not uncommon because of superficial erosions. Some patients develop a gastric ulcer. Carcinoma may develop rarely. Loss of protein through the mucosa often causes hypoalbuminemia, and sometimes edema. The gastric juice contains little or no hydrochloric acid and often excessive mucus. X-ray studies show very large folds and sometimes hypomotility. Ménétrier's disease is difficult to differentiate radiologically from the heavy folds of cancer, lymphoma, Zollinger-Ellison syndrome, or a variant seen in normal persons. The diagnosis can usually be made from clinical, radiologic, and laboratory data supplemented by gastroscopy with biopsy and cytology. Occasionally, laparotomy with full-thickness biopsy of the stomach is necessary to establish the diagnosis and to exclude malignancy.

There is no specific treatment, but frequent small meals may give some symptomatic relief. Those with gastric ulcers should receive antacids or cimetidine. A high-protein diet should be given to patients with hypoalbuminemia, but intravenous human albumin may be necessary for those with severe edema. Treatment with anticholinergic drugs may reduce protein loss. Partial gastrectomy may be helpful for intractable symptoms if the disease is sufficiently well localized. Rarely, total gastrectomy may be necessary. This gesture of desperation should be deferred as long as possible because of reports of spontaneous improvement or complete reversal of chronic disease.

Hypersecretory gastropathy This is a far more common cause of gastric mucosal hyperplasia than Ménétrier's disease or gastrinoma. There is some question whether it is really a separate

entity. The majority of these patients probably represent the upper end of the spectrum of increased fundal gland mass seen in patients with duodenal ulcer. Patients with this syndrome differ from those with classic Ménétrier's disease because they secrete gastric acid normally or excessively, but not at the high rate seen in gastrinoma; furthermore, their blood gastrin levels are normal. Grossly, the gastric mucosa is indistinguishable from that found in Ménétrier's disease, but histologically it is composed of lengthened fundal glands composed of increased numbers of parietal and chief cells. Ulcer symptoms may improve after antacids or cimetidine, but some patients may require surgery. Substantial loss of protein through the mucosa occurs only rarely; when present, it may be difficult to control unless the disease remits spontaneously.

Gastrinoma (Zollinger-Ellison syndrome) This is a fundal gland hyperplasia caused by excessive gastrin secretion by a gastrinoma, usually located in the pancreas. The pathogenesis, clinical features, and treatment are described in the previous chapter on peptic ulcer.

POSTGASTRECTOMY GASTRITIS After partial gastrectomy, gastritis often develops in the gastric remnant, especially if the stomach has been connected to the jejunum as in a Billroth II operation. Inflammation is usually accompanied by loss of parietal and chief cells, resulting in hypochlorhydria or achlorhydria, which protect against recurrent ulceration. Occasionally, secretion of intrinsic factor is insufficient for adequate vitamin B_{12} absorption. The pathogenesis of the gastritis is not well understood, but it is probably caused by reflux of bile and pancreatic juice through the large stoma and by loss of the trophic effect of gastrin secondary to antrectomy.

Usually, the histologic evidence of gastritis is not associated with symptoms. Occasionally, severe inflammation, especially near the stoma, is associated with epigastric pain, which may be aggravated by eating. Bilious vomiting and symptoms of regurgitant esophagitis may also be present. Similar symptoms occasionally occur after vagotomy and pyloroplasty, even though gastritis is usually less severe. Gastroscopy often shows a red, edematous mucosa, a finding which appears to correlate better with symptoms than does histologic evidence of gastritis. Precise data regarding the diagnosis of symptomatic postgastrectomy gastritis remain scarce.

Asymptomatic patients require no treatment but should be observed for evidence of iron or vitamin B_{12} deficiency. Some symptomatic patients respond to six small meals daily and, strangely enough, to the frequent use of antacids. The head of the bed should be raised if there is any suggestion of esophageal reflux. Attempts to bind the presumably irritating bile salts with cholestyramine have been disappointing. Surgical diversion of bile from the stoma by a Roux-en-Y loop may relieve severe symptoms unresponsive to medical management, but it is impossible to predict which patients will respond favorably to surgical treatment.

Alarming reports of frequent precancerous dysplasia and carcinoma within the residual gastric mucosa 10 to 20 years after Billroth II gastrectomy raise the question of the desirability of endoscopy with biopsy and cytology at regular intervals in all such patients.

CORROSIVE GASTRITIS The accidental or suicidal ingestion of strong alkali, such as lye, or of acids, such as hydrochloric or carbolic, can cause necrosis of the gastric wall, particularly in the prepyloric region. Alkali usually injures the esophagus more severely than the stomach, whereas the reverse tends to occur with acid. The degree of gastric injury varies with the quantity and concentration of irritant ingested and the amount of food present in the stomach. Patients complain of burning of the mouth, throat, and retrosternal area. With gastric injury, there is severe epigastric pain, often with vomiting. Perforation, peritonitis, or massive hemorrhage may occur shortly after corrosive ingestion, or may be delayed. Later, scarring may cause esophageal or pyloric stenosis.

If the patient is seen shortly after ingesting a corrosive, the stomach should be gently emptied via a small, soft rubber tube. Orange juice or dilute vinegar can be given for alkali and antacids for acid. Intravenous therapy, sedation, analgesia, supportive measures, and careful observation are instituted. Corticosteroids may be helpful if edema threatens the airway, and antibiotics may help treat aspiration pneumonia. If perforation or peritonitis is suspected, laparotomy should be performed, and a partial gastrectomy done if full-thickness injury to the wall is found. Surgical treatment may be necessary also for acute massive bleeding or for late obstruction caused by scarring.

PHLEGMONOUS GASTRITIS This rare condition should be considered when a patient presents with acute upper abdominal pain, signs of peritonitis, fever, purulent ascitic fluid, nausea or vomiting, and a normal serum amylase. It is a bacterial infection of the gastric wall, most often caused by streptococci, although staphylococci, pneumococci, *Escherichia coli,* or gas-forming bacteria can be responsible. Alcoholism, upper-respiratory or other infection, peptic ulcer, and gastric surgery are predisposing conditions. Vigorous antibiotic therapy including penicillin should be followed immediately by laparotomy which is both diagnostic and therapeutic. Depending upon the operative findings, drainage or partial gastrectomy should be performed. Without surgery the mortality is 100 percent: with surgery it is approximately 20 percent.

OTHER GASTRIC DISEASES

ACUTE GASTRIC DILATATION This is an uncommon but serious condition. The use of nasogastric suction has greatly reduced its frequency in the postoperative period. Gastric dilatation may also occur after trauma, the use of body casts, pneumonia, diabetic acidosis, or large doses of anticholinergic drugs. It is a rare complication of many diseases and also may occur for no apparent reason. The patient complains of anorexia and epigastric fullness and often vomits small amounts of fluid. Increasing abdominal distention with tympany, especially in the left hypochondrium, and a succussion splash are demonstrable. Untreated, large volumes of fluid are sequestered in a gastric "third space" with resultant saline and potassium depletion. The patient becomes restless and listless; hypovolemia, tachycardia, reduced urine output, and, finally, shock develop. Aspiration pneumonia may occur. A plain x-ray film of the abdomen shows massive gastric distention with an air-fluid level. Continuous nasogastric suction and restoration of fluid and electrolyte balance result in rapid improvement.

ADULT HYPERTROPHIC PYLORIC STENOSIS In this uncommon condition, the pyloric muscle is enlarged because of hypertrophy and possibly hyperplasia of the fibers of the circular layer. Many cases are associated with a peptic ulcer near the pylorus. In others, the pyloric muscle hypertrophy has been attributed to associated antral gastritis or neoplasm. A minority of cases without other gastric disease may be due to unrecognized infantile hypertrophic pyloric stenosis. Most often symptoms of pyloric obstruction such as nausea, vomiting, and gastric retention develop in mid-adult life, although occasionally mild symptoms are lifelong. An epigastric mass is not palpable in adults as it is in infants. Barium x-ray studies show a long, narrowed pyloric canal, often with triangular outpouchings within the canal. Gastroscopy shows a narrowed pylorus that is fixed in the open position. Although the diagnosis often appears highly likely from the above studies, an infiltrating

cancer often cannot be excluded without operation. A limited gastric resection is said to give better symptomatic relief than a pyloromyotomy, and in addition provides an exact histologic diagnosis. The frequently associated juxtapyloric ulcers merit vagotomy.

MALLORY-WEISS SYNDROME A longitudinal laceration in the cardioesophageal region is the cause of about 5 percent of massive episodes of upper gastrointestinal bleeding. About 60 percent of tears are located just below the gastroesophageal junction; the remainder involve the cardioesophageal junction and least frequently the esophagus alone. The tear is often related to retching, although other causes of increased abdominal pressure have been implicated. These include severe coughing, straining, convulsions, trauma, and childbirth. Often the patients are alcoholic. Many have a hiatus hernia. A history of vomiting normal gastric contents followed by hematemesis or melena suggests the diagnosis. Not uncommonly, however, the history is not helpful. The diagnosis is best made by endoscopy. If endoscopic visualization is inadequate, then the site of bleeding can often be determined by arteriography. Barium x-ray examination is almost always negative. The initial treatment is supportive and expectant. If bleeding stops, it rarely recurs. If bleeding continues, selective arteriography with infusion of pitressin can be tried. In a minority of cases, persistent bleeding requires that the laceration be sutured via a gastrotomy. Treatment of perforation complicating an esophageal tear is discussed in Chap. 289.

BEZOARS AND FOREIGN BODIES Conglomerates of food and mucus or phytobezoars composed of vegetable matter sometimes form in the gastric remnant after partial gastrectomy, especially if a vagotomy was also performed. They occur less often after vagotomy and pyloroplasty. Autonomic neuropathy associated with diabetes mellitus is another predisposing condition. Patients complain of anorexia, epigastric fullness, nausea, or vomiting. The diagnosis is often apparent from the barium x-ray examination, but endoscopy may be needed to distinguish the food mass from a neoplasm. The food conglomerate or bezoar can often be removed by vigorous and repeated gastric lavage. Fragmenting the lesion at gastroscopy may facilitate removal by lavage. Some phytobezoars can be partially digested with cellulase and then broken up successfully by lavage. Occasionally surgical removal is necessary. If the mass passes into the small bowel, it can cause obstruction requiring surgery. Treatment with metoclopromide may be tried to prevent recurrence.

Bezoars in the intact stomach are rare. Phytobezoars are most common, a well-known type being the persimmon ball. Trichobezoars are composed of hair. Concretions of inorganic substances such as shellac, asphalt, or calcium carbonate are occasionally seen. Bezoars of the intact stomach often require surgical removal, although nonoperative methods may be successful for phytobezoars. Persimmon balls have responded to treatment with papain and sodium bicarbonate.

Small foreign bodies such as coins, marbles, or even closed safety pins usually pass through the stomach and bowel without difficulty. Elongated, sharp objects such as needles, toothpicks, or open safety pins may hold up at some point and cause obstruction, ulceration, bleeding, abscess, or peritonitis. Occasionally, large objects such as forks or knives are swallowed by emotionally disturbed persons. Patients who have swallowed dangerous objects should be promptly referred to an experienced endoscopist who may elect endoscopic removal, observation, or surgical treatment, depending on the circumstances.

GASTRIC DIVERTICULA These uncommon lesions usually occur just below the cardia on the posterior wall near the lesser curvature. Almost all are asymptomatic and require no treatment. Pain, bleeding, or perforation is a very rare complication. Surgery should not be undertaken except for severe intractable symptoms that cannot be attributed to another cause. The x-ray appearance is usually diagnostic, but occasionally gastroscopy is needed to distinguish the lesion from a peptic ulcer.

GASTRIC VOLVULUS OR TORSION Rarely the stomach can twist about its longitudinal axis, thus turning itself upside down and obstructing the lower esophagus. The volvulus may be acute or more often chronic. It tends to be associated with a paraesophageal hernia or eventration of the diaphragm. The stomach can also twist about the vertical axis of the gastrohepatic omentum to produce a torsion rather than a true volvulus. Acute volvulus is associated with severe upper abdominal pain and retching which produces saliva rather than gastric or duodenal contents. Passage of a nasogastric tube beyond the cardia is usually impossible. Plain x-ray films of the abdomen show distention of the stomach; the finding of two separate fluid levels is diagnostic. Acute volvulus may be of short duration and subside spontaneously or may be associated with strangulation and require emergency surgical treatment. Those with chronic volvulus may be asymptomatic or have intermittent pain, often associated with eating. Severe symptoms may require surgical correction of the volvulus, including repair of an associated paraesophageal hernia, if present.

RARE GASTRIC DISEASES Pseudolymphoma This benign lymphoid hyperplasia may involve the stomach. Grossly the lesion is usually single and ulcerated. Some lesions are nodular; others may present as enlarged folds. Multiple lesions are not found. There is a marked lymphocytic infiltration of the gastric wall. The lesion is distinguished from true lymphoma by the maturity of the germinal centers and by the presence of inflammatory cells other than lymphocytes. The x-ray and endoscopic findings usually suggest malignancy or peptic ulcer. Partial gastrectomy is usually required for diagnosis.

Eosinophilic gastroenteritis The antrum may be involved in this condition which is usually associated with marked peripheral eosinophilic leukocytosis. The diagnosis can be made by mucosal biopsy, and chronic treatment with small doses of corticosteroids is usually effective.

Eosinophilic granuloma is usually a circumscribed lesion of the antrum and is not associated with peripheral eosinophilic leukocytosis. It does not respond to corticosteroid treatment and may require excision because of pyloric obstruction or other symptoms.

Tuberculosis and tertiary syphilis rarely affect the stomach. The diagnosis can sometimes be made from the clinical picture and endoscopic biopsy, but more often operation is needed to exclude malignancy. Appropriate antibiotic therapy is effective. Other rare gastric infections include herpes simplex, candidiasis, and histoplasmosis.

REFERENCES

Bockus HL (ed): *Gastroenterology*, vol 1, 3d ed. Philadelphia, Saunders, 1974

Buell P, Dunn JE: Cancer mortality among the Japanese issei and nisei of California. Cancer 18:656, 1965

Clémençon G et al: Das Karzinom des operierten Magens. Dtsch Med Wochenschr 101:1, 1976

Dupont JB et al: Adenocarcinoma of the stomach: Review of 1497 cases. Cancer 41:941, 1978

Imai T et al: Chronic gastritis in Japanese with reference to high incidence of gastric carcinoma. J Natl Cancer Inst 47:179, 1971

Ming S: Tumors of the esophagus and stomach, in *Atlas of Tumor Pathology*, 2d ser. Washington, DC, Armed Forces Institute of Pathology, 1971, fasc 7

Moertel CG: Chemotherapy of gastrointestinal cancer. N Engl J Med 299:1049, 1978

Morson BC, Dawson, IMP: *Gastrointestinal Pathology*. Oxford, Blackwell, 1971

Vandelli C et al: Autoantibodies to gastrin-producing cells in antral (type B) chronic gastritis. N Engl J Med 300:1406, 1979

292
DISORDERS OF ABSORPTION

NORTON J. GREENBERGER
KURT J. ISSELBACHER

MECHANISMS OF ABSORPTION

Diseases of the small intestine are frequently accompanied by alterations in intestinal function, and clinically this impaired function is seen as the malabsorption syndrome. In order to obtain a better appreciation of the derangements which occur in the many disorders of intestinal function, the processes of normal absorption will first be reviewed.

It is important to distinguish between digestion and absorption, since an increased loss of nutrients in the stool may be a reflection of a derangement of either process. Digestion involves the breakdown or hydrolysis of nutrients to smaller molecules in order to prepare the ingested substances for absorption, or transport across the intestinal cell. It will be recalled that most of the digestive process is initiated in the stomach by acid and pepsin and is continued in the upper small intestine primarily by the action of pancreatic enzymes such as lipase, amylase, and trypsin. As a result of these digestive actions carbohydrates are broken down to monosaccharides and disaccharides, proteins to peptides and amino acids, and fats to monoglycerides and fatty acids. In the adult it is in this form that nutrients are, to a large extent, transported across the epithelial surface of the intestinal cell.

ANATOMIC AND PHYSIOLOGIC FACTORS The intestine has an enormous surface area. This can be attributed in large part to its length, which in the adult is more than 12 ft, and to the foldings of the surface plicae. At the light microscopic level, the villi of the small intestine provide additional surface area, which is further augmented by the presence of microvilli (approximately 2×10^8 per square centimeter) on the outer, or brush border, region of epithelial cells. Thus the total absorptive area of the small intestine is enormous.

Motility (contractility) of the bowel is an important process which permits nutrients to remain in intimate contact with the intestinal cells and possibly influences the continued movement of the nutrients *into* and along the absorbing channels, such as the lymphatics. Two types of motility aid in this process: the gross motility of the intestine itself and the motility of individual villi. Entrance of the nutrients into the general circulation is achieved via the capillaries into the portal system or via the lacteals into the intestinal lymphatics.

TYPES OF ABSORPTION Four mechanisms have been considered to be important in the transport of substances across the intestinal cell membrane, namely, active transport, passive diffusion, facilitated diffusion, and pinocytosis (Table 292-1).

Active transport involves the transport of a substance across the cell against an electric or chemical gradient; this process requires energy, is carrier-mediated, and is subject to competitive inhibition. *Passive diffusion* is the opposite of this process; energy is not required, transport is with (rather than against) the electric or chemical gradient, the process is not carrier-mediated, and it does not show properties of competitive inhibition. Thus active transport may be viewed as "uphill" transport, whereas passive diffusion is equivalent to "downhill" transport. *Facilitated diffusion* is similar to passive diffusion except that such a process shows evidence of being carrier-mediated and frequently subject to competitive inhibition.

Pinocytosis, or endocytosis, is a process akin to phagocytosis. By this mechanism nutrients (soluble or particulate) upon entering the cell are surrounded by the components of the outer plasma cell membrane. In the intestinal tract pinocytosis occurs in the neonatal period and, contrary to earlier belief, also occurs to a limited extent in the adult organism. While quantitatively limited, it appears to account, for example, for uptake of antigens.

SITES OF ABSORPTION While many substances are absorbed throughout the length of the small intestine, certain nutrients tend to be absorbed more in one region than in other regions. The proximal intestine is a major area for the absorption of iron, calcium, water-soluble vitamins, and fat (monoglycerides and fatty acids). Sugars are absorbed in the proximal and also midintestine. While the amino acids appear to be absorbed primarily in the middle of the small intestine or jejunum, some absorption also occurs in the upper and lower areas. The distal small intestine appears to be the *major* absorptive area for bile salts and vitamin B_{12}. As is emphasized below, this factor is of clinical significance in circumstances where there has been removal or disease of the ileum.

The colon is important for the absorption of water and electrolytes, a process which occurs predominantly in the cecum. Although the rectum is not a usual site for absorption of ingested foodstuffs, drugs introduced by rectum may be absorbed there. Thus drugs introduced by this route, such as salicylates or steroids, may be absorbed systemically.

ABSORPTION OF SPECIFIC NUTRIENTS Carbohydrate absorption Much of the carbohydrate we ingest is in the form of starch, a complex polysaccharide consisting of many hexose units (attached either in a 1,4 or 1,6 linkage). By the action of salivary and pancreatic amylase, starch is hydrolyzed to oligosaccharides and then to dissacharides (mostly maltose). While monosaccharides such as glucose are readily absorbed, disaccharides are not. Disaccharides are split enzymatically into their component sugars by disaccharidases (or oligosaccharidases) located on or within the microvilli of intestinal epithelial cells. The two types of disaccharidases are β-galactosidases (lactase) and α-glucosidases (sucrase, maltase). By the action of these enzymes, lactose is split into glucose and galactose, sucrose into glucose and fructose, and maltose into two molecules of glucose. The resultant monosaccharides are then transported through the cell into the portal circulation. Most disaccharides are hydrolyzed so rapidly by brush border enzymes that the capacity of the transport mechanism is exceeded and some monosaccharides diffuse back into the intestinal lumen. Lactose, however, is hydrolyzed at a slower rate, and thus lactose hydrolysis is the rate-limiting step in lactose absorption.

Sugars such as glucose and galactose are absorbed by an active transport mechanism. The transport rate of sugars can be related to the substrate concentration by the expression K_t, where K_t stands for the monosaccharide substrate concentration that produces half the maximal transport rate. Published K_t values for glucose transport have varied widely, partly because of failure to consider the unstirred water layer, which constitutes a diffusion barrier for solutes.

The exact mechanism for the active transport of sugars such as glucose and galactose has not been elucidated. However, *sodium* ions appear necessary for the *entry* of the sugar into the cell, and *energy* is required for the *accumulation* of the sugars within the cell. Glucose and galactose presumably are transported by a hexose "carrier," but the nature of this carrier remains to be determined. Glucose-galactose malabsorption, a congenital defect in sugar transport, is characterized by severe fermentative diarrhea and increased intestinal secretion of water and electrolytes. The basic defect in this disorder is believed to be a reduced number of functioning sugar carriers at the microvillus membrane, resulting in decreased uptake of glucose and galactose.

Protein and amino acid absorption Dietary proteins are initially subject to degradation in the stomach by pepsin. However, complete hydrolysis is largely achieved by the action of the pancreatic enzymes trypsin, chymotrypsin, and carboxypeptidase. By these enzymatic processes oligopeptides, dipeptides, and amino acids are formed. Just as there are disaccharidases in mucosal cells to digest disaccharides, there are also oligopeptidases to split small peptides. Dipeptidases are located in the cytoplasm as well as on the microvilli. Dipeptides are absorbed more rapidly than amino acids, and presumably their uptake involves a separate mechanism. As indicated above, contrary to earlier beliefs proteins can also be absorbed by the adult intestine. Although quantitatively limited, protein absorption probably is immunologically significant.

Most naturally occurring amino acids are L-amino acids, and these are subject to a number of different transport processes. *Neutral* amino acids seem to share a common carrier mechanism; thus amino acids such as tryptophan and alanine show competitive inhibition. Among the *dibasic* amino acids which appear to have a distinct transport mechanism are arginine, ornithine, and lysine. The neutral amino acid cystine shares this mechanism. There is also a separate transport system for *glycine* and the *imino acids* proline and hydroxyproline. There is also a transport system for *dicarboxylic* acids such as glutamic and aspartic acids. Therefore, in genetic disorders, such as cystinuria, one will find impaired absorption not only of cystine but also of arginine, ornithine, and lysine. Similarly in Hartnup disease, a defect in the transport of neutral amino acids (especially of tryptophan, phenylalanine, histidine) is found. In these genetic disorders uptake and absorption of dipeptides is normal.

The actual mechanism of the absorption of amino acids by the intestine has not been elucidated. As in the case of carbohydrates, sodium ions appear to be required for the entry of

TABLE 292-1
Mechanisms of transport across the intestinal cell

Types of transport	Properties			
	Energy-dependent	Carrier-mediated	Competitive inhibition	Electric or chemical gradient
Active	+	+	+	+
Diffusion:				
Passive	0	0	0	0
Facilitated	0	+	+ /0	0
Pinocytosis	?	0	0	0

these acids and the energy needed for their concentration within the cell. Some amino acids have affinity for more than one mechanism. For example, glycine may be transported by both the neutral and imino acid transport systems.

Fat absorption (Fig. 292-1) Most of the ingested dietary fats are in the form of long-chain triglycerides. These triglycerides contain both saturated fatty acids (such as palmitic and stearic) and unsaturated fatty acids (such as oleic and linoleic). The particle size of the fat is decreased largely by the churning action of the stomach. The entry of fat into the duodenum plus the presence of acid causes release of secretin and pancreozymin-cholecystokinin, which in turn leads to a stimulation of the flow of bile and pancreatic juice.

ROLE OF PANCREATIC LIPASE The hydrolysis of triglycerides by pancreatic lipase is a complex process involving lipase, colipase, and bile salts. Pancreatic lipase is an enzyme that binds to the oil-water interface of an emulsified triglyceride substrate. The detergent properties of bile salts permit pancreatic lipase to gain access to water-insoluble lipids. One of the important functions of bile salts is to clear the oil-water interface of dietary fat from proteins of exogenous and endogenous origin, thus making it available for pancreatic lipolysis. Colipase, a protein present in pancreatic juice, is also essential for the action of lipase; its function is to anchor the lipase close to the surface of the triglyceride droplet. All three components, i.e., pancreatic lipase, colipase, and bile salts form a *ternary complex,* which generates lipolytic products that diffuse away from the complex and are absorbed. With colipase present, lipase remains at the interface and forms 2-monoglycerides and fatty acids, which are the major end products of triglyceride hydrolysis. Less than 5 percent of ingested fat remains in the form of diglycerides and triglycerides. Without colipase, bile acids would actually wash pancreatic lipase away from the interface and its hydrolytic rate would be reduced.

ROLE OF BILE SALTS (Fig. 292-2) Bile salts play an important role in the digestion and absorption of fat. They are synthesized in the liver (approximately 200 to 600 mg daily) from cholesterol and excreted in the bile in the form of their glycine or taurine conjugates. In humans the principal bile acids excreted are conjugates of cholic and chenodeoxycholic acid.

Bile salts are good detergents, because they have both polar (hydrophilic) and nonpolar (hydrophobic) groups. During digestion the concentration of conjugated bile salts in the lumen is in the range of 5 to 15 μmol/ml, and at these concentrations the bile salts aggregate to form *micelles.* Fatty acids and monoglycerides enter these micelles, forming mixed micelles. An emulsion of triglyceride is turbid; mixed micelles containing bile salts, fatty acids, and monoglycerides are clear solutions. The formation of *mixed micelles* and hence the solubilization of fatty acids and monoglycerides are much more effectively achieved with *conjugated bile salts* at the pH which normally exists in the intestinal lumen (Fig. 292-2).

There are additional properties of bile salts important in fat absorption and digestion. Bile salts shift the pH optimum of pancreatic lipase from 8.5 to 6.5. This is important because the pH in the upper small intestine is normally 6 to 6.5. Most conjugated bile salts are absorbed in the ileum and after entering the portal vein are subject to an enterohepatic circulation. By this process about 90 percent of the conjugated bile salts reaching the ileum are reabsorbed. As a consequence only about 200 to 600 mg bile salts is excreted in the feces per day, while, as part of the enterohepatic circulation, as much as 20 to 30 g bile salts recirculates daily between the liver and intestine. When the enterohepatic circulation is intact, the size of the bile salt pool is largely determined by the frequency of the enterohepatic circulation, i.e., the number of cycles per day (see also Chap. 307). If the ileum is diseased or removed, absorption of bile salts is impaired, and a significant fecal loss of bile salts will occur. As a consequence of this bile salt depletion, the concentration of bile salts in the intestinal lumen will also decrease, leading to further impairment of fat absorption. A similar result will occur if bile salt reabsorption is prevented by chelating agents, such as cholestyramine (see "Regional Enteritis," below).

INTRAMUCOSAL ASPECTS OF FAT ABSORPTION (Fig. 292-1) After the hydrolysis of fatty acids to monoglycerides and their interaction with bile salts to form mixed micelles, the lipids pass through an "unstirred" water layer covering the cell surface. The mixed micelles apparently do not enter the cell, but instead the component fatty acids and monoglycerides are released from the micellar phase and then enter the cell by diffusion. Upon entry fatty acids may interact with specific binding proteins. The subsequent fate of the intracellular lipid is strongly influenced by the fatty acid chain length. Fatty acids and monoglycerides derived from long-chain triglycerides (i.e., containing C-16 to C-18 fatty acids) are promptly *reesterified to triglycerides* by enzymes of the endoplasmic reticulum. These

FIGURE 292-1
Scheme of intestinal digestion, absorption, esterification, and transport of dietary triglycerides. TG, triglycerides; FA, fatty acids; MG, monoglyceride; BS, bile salts.

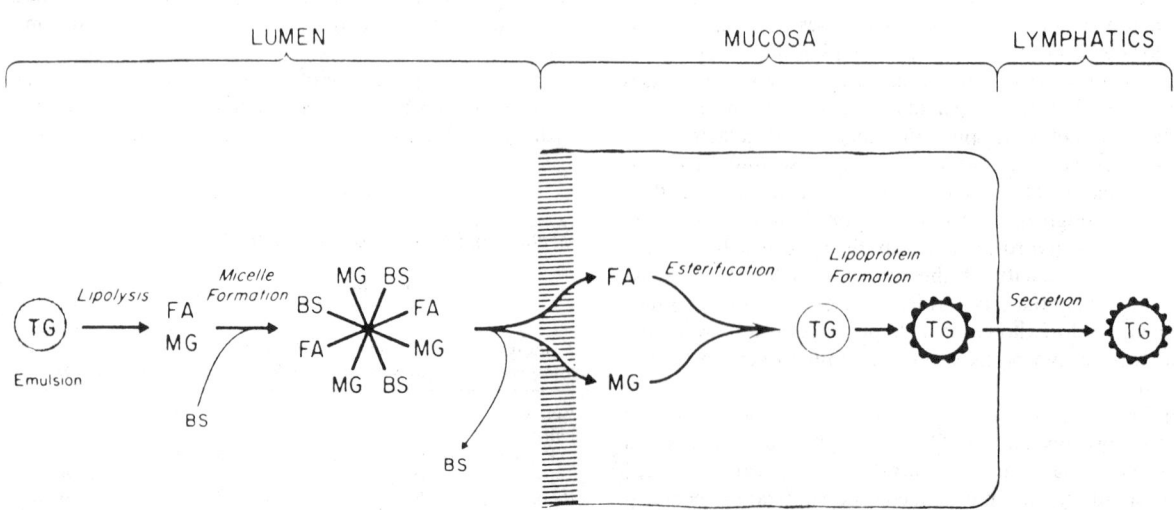

triglycerides then interact with specific apolipoproteins plus cholesterol and phospholipid to form chylomicrons and very low density lipoproteins. These initially accumulate in the Golgi region of the cell and then are secreted into the lacteals and the intestinal lymph. There are thus four major steps in the absorption of long-chain fatty acids and monoglycerides: (1) mucosal uptake and interaction with binding proteins, (2) reesterification to triglycerides, (3) lipoprotein formation, and (4) secretion into lymph.

By contrast, fatty acids derived from medium-chain triglycerides (i.e., containing C-8 and C-12 fatty acids) are *not reesterified* to any significant extent within the cell and are not incorporated into lipoproteins. Instead, they rapidly enter the portal venous system, where they are transported as fatty acids bound to albumin. The major aspects of fat absorption are summarized in Fig. 292-1.

Absorption of cholesterol and fat-soluble vitamins (A, D, E, K) In addition to contributing significantly to the total body synthesis of cholesterol, the intestine also plays an active role in the absorption of cholesterol and its esters. Within the lumen, cholesterol esters from the bile and diet are hydrolyzed by a pancreatic esterase. There is also a separate cholesterol esterase in the intestinal microvilli, which completes this hydrolysis. As a result only free cholesterol appears to enter the intestinal cell. However, just as in the case of long-chain fatty acids, much of the cholesterol is reesterified and is then secreted primarily into lymph.

The absorption mechanisms of the fat-soluble vitamins A, D, E, and K are not well understood. The intestine is able to convert β-carotene into vitamin A. The vitamin A thus formed or absorbed from the lumen is esterified in the mucosa primarily with palmitic acid, transported in the chylomicrons of the lymph, and stored as retinyl palmitate in the liver. The other lipid-soluble vitamins also appear in lymph chylomicrons, but esterification with fatty acids does not appear to be necessary for their transport.

Water and sodium absorption In spite of extensive investigations the main mechanisms of water and electrolyte transport are not well understood. Individual intestinal mucosa cells are joined near their apex by a "tight junction," and ions and water traverse this pathway during absorption and secretion. It is believed that the tight junction pathway contains aqueous-filled channels or pores. Such intercellular spaces are closed in the resting state and dilated during absorption. Considerable evidence has accumulated indicating that pumps and carriers are involved in intestinal water and solute transport. For example, the basolateral membrane is believed to contain a Na^+ pump which actively transports Na^+ out of the mucosal cell and into the intercellular space. After Na^+ and Cl^- are transported across the brush border membrane into the cell, Na^+ is pumped across the basolateral membrane and Cl^- either follows passively or is also pumped into the intercellular space. Since Na^+,K^+-ATPase is present in the basolateral but not in the brush border membrane, it could be the biochemical mediator of this pump. Bulk water movement obviously influences the movement of Na^+, K^+, and Cl^-. This "solvent drag" effect is explained by two mechanisms: (1) solutes may be caught in a moving stream of water and transported across a membrane, and (2) water movement results in increased concentration of solute on the side of the membrane from which water was transported which causes solute to diffuse through the direction of flow. Diarrhea can be simply defined as impaired net absorption of water and electrolytes by the small intestine or colon. Some mechanisms producing diarrhea are listed in Table 292-2.

Calcium absorption Calcium is actively transported by the small intestine, and this process is intimately linked to the action of vitamin D metabolites. Vitamin D_3 or cholecalciferol is hydroxylated to 25-hydroxycholecalciferol in the liver; the 25-hydroxycholecalciferol is further metabolized in the kidney to 1,25-dihydroxycholecalciferol, which represents the biologically active form of cholecalciferol in the intestine. The impaired absorption of calcium found in renal rickets, uremia, and anephric individuals may be due to decreased synthesis of vitamin D metabolites.

FIGURE 292-2

Scheme of hepatic and intestinal metabolism of bile salts and the enterohepatic circulation (from ileum to liver). Note that bacteria lead to the formation of secondary bile acids; of the latter, only deoxycholic acid is absorbed to any appreciable extent.

Iron absorption The formation of soluble iron complexes is important for maintaining intraluminal iron in an absorbable form. Gastric acid facilitates the chelation of inorganic iron with substances such as ascorbic acid, sugars, amino acids, and bile; these macromolecular complexes then remain soluble in the more alkaline duodenum and jejunum. A regulatory mechanism for the absorption of inorganic iron appears to exist within the small-intestinal mucosal cells. Iron is actively transported by the small intestine, and the duodenum is the principal site of iron absorption. The absorption of elemental iron in man and animals involves at least two distinct steps: (1) mucosal uptake of iron from the lumen and (2) mucosal transfer of iron to the plasma. Much of the iron entering the mucosal cell is not transferred to the plasma but remains trapped within the cell and is excreted into the lumen when the cell is shed. Iron lost by this mechanism seems to vary inversely with body iron stores. However, this mucosal regulatory mechanism can be overcome when pharmacologic doses of iron are ingested. Hemoglobin iron is also absorbed by human subjects, depending upon body requirements for iron; the heme is split from globin in the lumen and absorbed as an intact metalloporphyrin. The absorption of inorganic iron is increased by ascorbic acid. Similarly, the presence of anemia, liver injury, pregnancy, idiopathic hemochromatosis, or a portacaval shunt may result in increased iron absorption. Conversely, the prior ingestion of large doses of iron and the presence in the lumen of phosphates, carbonates, and phytates may lead to decreased absorption of inorganic iron. Impaired absorption of iron is frequent in disorders (such as nontropical sprue) which involve the duodenal mucosa.

Water-soluble vitamins *Vitamin B₁₂ absorption* is discussed in Chap. 311. In the case of *folic acid absorption*, it should be emphasized that folates exist in food conjugated with glutamyl peptides. These *polyglutamates* must be deconjugated (by folic deconjugase) to monoglutamates for absorption to occur. Certain drugs (such as oral contraceptives, sulfasalazine, trimethoprim, and pyrimethamine) inhibit the absorption of dietary folate and hence can cause folate deficiency. Sulfasalazine, for example, competitively inhibits three enzymes important in the intestinal metabolism of folate, i.e., dehydrofolate reductase, methylene tetrahydrofolate reductase, and serine transhydroxymethylase. Thiamine and riboflavin appear to be absorbed by passive diffusion.

TESTS USEFUL IN THE DIAGNOSIS OF MALABSORPTION

Most of the tests useful in the diagnosis of malabsorption indicate the presence of abnormal absorptive or digestive function, and only a few tests may suggest a specific diagnosis. Accordingly, it is frequently necessary to employ a combination of tests to establish a diagnosis. To illustrate the use of various tests, the characteristic findings in nontropical sprue, an example of a primary malabsorptive disorder, and pancreatic insufficiency, an example of impaired digestion, are compared in Table 292-3.

Stool fat The qualitative examination of the stool for undigested muscle fibers, neutral fat, and split fat is a simple and reliable screening test for steatorrhea. The finding of an increased number of muscle fibers indicates impaired intraluminal digestion. Properly performed, the qualitative microscopic examination of a stool specimen with the Sudan III stain is of value and correlates well with the quantitative determination of fecal fat by the Van de Kamer method. The latter remains the most reliable measurement of steatorrhea. A normal fecal fat excretion is less than 6 g for 24 h, or less than 6 percent of ingested fat.

In preliminary reports, it has been suggested that oral [¹⁴C]triolein can be used as an effective test for fat absorption. During the digestive process the triolein is hydrolyzed, and the labeled glycerol is absorbed and metabolized by the liver. The ¹⁴CO₂ produced is exhaled and can then be measured hourly (for 6 h) in the expired air. Normally more than 3.5 percent of the administered label (5 μCi) appears in the breath per hour.

Xylose absorption In the most commonly employed form of the xylose absorption test, the patient ingests 25 g D-xylose. A 5-h urine xylose excretion of 4.5 g or greater is considered normal. There is some decreased renal excretion with age, and over age sixty-five 3.5 g is the normal value. Falsely low values may be obtained in patients with ascites, intestinal bacterial overgrowth, or renal insufficiency, after administration of certain drugs (e.g., acetylsalicylic acid, indomethacin), and most commonly if the urine collection is incomplete. To obviate difficulties in interpreting the test, it is advisable to determine the blood xylose level 2 h after ingestion of xylose. A blood xylose level of 30 mg per 100 ml or greater indicates normal absorption of D-xylose. An abnormal D-xylose absorption test is found most frequently in disorders affecting the mucosa of the proximal small intestine, such as nontropical and tropical sprue.

Gastrointestinal x-ray studies All patients with malabsorption should have radiographic examinations of the small intestine and, in many cases, of the esophagus, stomach, and colon as well. Occasionally, the latter two examinations may provide

TABLE 292-2
Some mechanisms in the production of diarrhea

I Secretory diarrhea
  A Secretory agents associated with adenylate cyclase system
    1 Enterotoxin producing bacteria *(Vibrio cholera, Escherichia coli)*
    2 Methylxanthines (caffeine, theophylline)
    3 Prostaglandins
    4 Vasoactive intestinal peptide (VIP)
    5 Dihydroxy bile acids (affect colon primarily; effects seen after ileal resection)
  B Secretory agents not associated with adenylate-cyclate system
    1 Glucagon, secretin, cholecystokin-pancreozymin, serotonin, calcitonin, gastrin inhibitory polypeptide (GIP)
    2 Some laxatives* (ricinoleic acid, bisacodyl; phenolphthalein, dioctyl sodium sulfosuccinate)
    3 Bacterial enterotoxins *(Shigella, Staphylococcus aureus, Clostridium perfringens)*
  C Mucosal injury, altered cell permeability
    1 *Salmonella, Shigella,* invasive *E. coli,* gastroenteritis viruses
    2 Celiac sprue
    3 Inflammatory bowel disease (ulcerative colitis, regional enteritis)
  D Neoplasms with or without hormone production
    1 Gastrinoma (gastrin)
    2 Carcinoid syndrome (serotonin, prostaglandins)
    3 Medullary carcinoma thyroid (calcitonin, prostaglandins)
    4 Pancreatic cholera syndrome (? VIP)
    5 Villous adenoma
II Osmotic diarrhea
  A Impaired carbohydrate absorption
    1 Disaccharidase deficiency (lactose or sucrose-isomaltose intolerance)
    2 Glucose-galactose malabsorption
  B Laxative-ingestion or abuse
    1 Nonabsorbable osmotically active agents (lactulose, sorbitol, mannitol)
    2 Saline purgatives (magnesium phosphate, magnesium hydroxide-containing antacids)
  C Postsurgical
    1 Vagotomy and pyloroplasty*
    2 Gastrojejunostomy* (Billroth I and II)
III Motility disorders
  A Laxative abuse*
  B Irritable bowel syndrome
  C Diverticular disease of the colon
  D Diabetic diarrhea with visceral neuropathy

* *Multiple mechanisms involved in production of diarrhea.*

TABLE 292-3
Tests useful in the diagnosis of malabsorptive disorders

Test	Normal values	Malabsorption (nontropical sprue)	Maldigestion (pancreatic insufficiency)	Comment
		Typical findings in:		
Quantitative determination of stool fat	<6 g/24 h; >95% coefficient of fat absorption	>6 g/24 h	>6 g/24 h	Best test for establishing presence of steatorrhea
D-Xylose absorption (25-g oral dose)	5-h urinary excretion >4.5 g; peak blood level >30 mg/100 ml	↓	Normal	A good screening test for carbohydrate absorption
Small-intestinal x-rays		Malabsorption pattern	Normal or minimal malabsorption pattern; occasionally pancreatic calcification	Moulage sign and other abnormalities may be present in several disorders (see text)
Small-intestinal mucosal biopsy		Abnormal	Normal	A specific diagnosis can be established in a small number of disorders (see text)
Schilling test for vitamin B$_{12}$ absorption	>8% urinary excretion in 48 h	Frequently ↓	Frequently ↓	Useful in determining whether vitamin B$_{12}$ malabsorption is due to gastric or small-intestinal disorders
Secretin test	Volume >1.8 (ml/kg)/h Bicarbonate concentration >80 meq/liter	Normal	Abnormal	See discussion of pancreatic insufficiency in Chaps. 308 and 309
Serum calcium	9–11 mg/100 ml	Frequently ↓	Usually normal	
Serum albumin	3.5–5.5 g/100 ml	Frequently ↓	Usually normal	Decreased levels of both serum albumin and globulins should raise the question of protein-losing enteropathy
Serum cholesterol	150–250 mg/100 ml	↓	Frequently ↓	Usually decreased in disorders associated with significant steatorrhea
Serum iron	80–150 μg/100 ml	Frequently ↓	Normal	Low values may reflect decreased body iron stores
Serum carotenes	>100 IU/100 ml	↓	Usually ↓	Fairly satisfactory screening tests for malabsorption
Serum vitamin A	>100 IU/100 ml	↓		
Prothrombin time	70–100%; 12–15 s	Frequently ↓	Frequently ↓	
Urine 5-hydroxyindoleacetic acid (5-HIAA)	2–9 mg/24 h	↑	Normal	Slightly increased level (12–16 mg/24 h) characteristically found in nontropical sprue
Breath H$_2$ (after 50 g lactose)	Minimal breath H$_2$	May be ↑	Normal	Secondary to lactase deficiency (see text)
Duodenal fluid analysis:				
Conjugated bile salts	> 2 mmol/ml	Normal	Normal	May be decreased with bacterial overgrowth, ileal resection, or ileal inflammatory disease
Unconjugated bile salts	Not present	Normal	Normal	Increased with bacterial overgrowth
Micellar lipid	>50% ingested lipid in micellar phase	Normal or decreased	Decreased	Decreased with a deficiency of conjugated bile salts or pancreatic lipase
Bacteria (culture)	<10^3 organisms/ml	Normal	Normal	>10^5 organisms/ml indicate bacterial overgrowth
Glycocholic acid metabolism (oral glycine-1-[^{14}C]glycocholate)	<1% of dose excreted as $^{14}CO_2$ in 4 h	Normal	Normal	Increased $^{14}CO_2$ excretion with bacterial overgrowth or bile acid malabsorption (due to ileal resection or inflammatory disease)
	<4% of dose excreted in stools			Increased fecal excretion of ^{14}C in bile acid malabsorption
[^{14}C]Triolein absorption (breath test)	>3.5% of dose as breath $^{14}CO_2$ per hour	Decreased	Decreased	Correlates well with chemical stool fat; recently introduced test

important clues to the presence of such disorders as gastroileostomy, scleroderma, Zollinger-Ellison syndrome, ulcerative colitis, and intestinal fistulas. The typical small-bowel radiographic abnormalities in patients with a malabsorption syndrome are a breaking up of the barium column with segmentation, clumping, and coarsening of the mucosal folds. Segmentation or clumping of the barium in a small-bowel loop is often termed a *moulage sign*. Less frequently there is dilatation of the proximal small bowel and loss of a normal mucosal pattern. Collectively, these changes have been referred to as a *malabsorption pattern*. These findings are nonspecific and may be found in several of the disorders listed in Table 292-4. Some representative examples of abnormal small-bowel radiographs are shown in Fig. 292-3.

A

B

C

FIGURE 292-3

A. X-ray of a normal small intestine showing good mucosal pattern. B. Intestinal x-ray of a patient with nontropical sprue. Note dilatation of small bowel, lack of mucosal markings, and segmentation and clumping of barium. C. Intestinal x-ray of patient with obstructed lymphatics due to Köhlmeier-Degos disease. Note "accordion-pleated" pattern at lower edge of film.

Small-intestinal biopsy The most commonly used instruments for obtaining peroral biopsy specimens from the small intestine include the Rubin and Shiner tubes and the Crosby, Carey, and Ross-Moore capsules. Examination of small-bowel biopsy specimens has proved to be of considerable value in the differential diagnosis of malabsorptive disorders. Table 292-4 lists disorders associated with abnormalities in intestinal biopsies, and Fig. 292-4 depicts some illustrative lesions.

Schilling test for vitamin B$_{12}$ absorption The Schilling test is valuable in the differential diagnosis of malabsorption and is frequently carried out in three stages: (1) without intrinsic factor, (2) with intrinsic factor, and (3) after a course of treatment with antibiotics. Since vitamin B$_{12}$ is absorbed primarily in the distal ileum, an abnormal Schilling test may indicate a pathologic condition of the distal small bowel. In disorders affecting the terminal ileum such as regional enteritis and lymphomas, the first-stage Schilling test is frequently abnormal. The ileal receptor site appears to be damaged in these disorders, and the impaired absorption of B$_{12}$ is not corrected by the addition of intrinsic factor or the use of antibiotics. The Schilling test may also be useful in establishing a diagnosis of abnormal bacterial overgrowth of the small bowel which may be present in disorders such as blind-loop syndrome, scleroderma, and multiple small-bowel diverticula (Table 292-3). In the blind-loop syndrome, for example, the bacteria can actually take up vitamin B$_{12}$ with resultant impaired absorption of B$_{12}$. Under these conditions the first-stage Schilling test is frequently abnormal. After appropriate antibiotic treatment the Schilling test usually returns to normal. Vitamin B$_{12}$ absorption is frequently abnormal in patients with exocrine pancreatic insufficiency (see Chap. 309).

Secretin test The secretin test, secretin pancreozymin test, and intraduodenal perfusion with essential amino acids, which may be useful in establishing a diagnosis of pancreatic insufficiency, are discussed in detail in Chap. 308.

Serum calcium, albumin, cholesterol, magnesium, and iron Abnormal serum calcium, albumin, cholesterol, magnesium, and iron values may be found in several malabsorptive disorders. The primary value of such tests is to suggest that abnormal intestinal absorptive function may be present. These tests

TABLE 292-4
Disorders associated with abnormalities in small-bowel biopsy specimens

I Disorders in which biopsy is of diagnostic value
  A Celiac sprue: Shortened or absent villi; hypertrophied crypts; damaged surface epithelium; mononuclear infiltrate
  B Whipple's disease: Lamina propria infiltrated with macrophages containing PAS-positive glycoproteins
  C Abetalipoproteinemia: Villus structure normal; epithelial cells vacuolated due to excess fat
  D Agammaglobulinemia: Flattened or absent villi; increased lymphocyte infiltration; absence of plasma cells
II Disorders in which biopsy may be of diagnostic value
  A Intestinal lymphoma: Infiltration of lamina propria and submucosa with malignant cells
  B Intestinal lymphangiectasia: Dilated lacteals and lymphatics in lamina propria; clubbed villi
  C Eosinophilic enteritis: Diffuse or patchy eosinophilic infiltration in lamina propria and mucosa
  D Amyloidosis: Presence of amyloid confirmed by special stains
  E Regional enteritis: Noncaseating granulomas
  F Parasitic infestations: Parasitic invasion of mucosa; adherence of trophozoites to mucosal surface
  G Systemic mastocytosis: Mast cell infiltration of lamina propria
III Disorders in which biopsy may be abnormal but not diagnostic
  A Tropical sprue: Lesion similar to celiac sprue with shortened or absent villi; lymphocyte infiltration
  B Folate deficiency: Shortened villi; megalocytosis; decreased mitoses in crypts
  C Vitamin B_{12} deficiency: Similar to folate deficiency
  D Acute radiation enteritis: Similar to folate deficiency
  E Systemic scleroderma: Fibrosis around Brunner's glands
  F Bacterial overgrowth syndromes: Patchy damage to villi and increased lymphocyte infiltration

are usually of limited value in the *differential diagnosis* of malabsorption, but if abnormal, may be helpful in supporting this diagnosis.

Serum carotenes, vitamin A, and prothrombin time Absorption of the fat-soluble vitamins A, D, K, and E is frequently impaired in patients with steatorrhea. Measurements of serum carotene and vitamin A levels are useful as screening tests for malabsorption. However, other tests not only are more sensitive but often give more specific information than the serum carotene and vitamin A levels. The blood prothrombin time is an important test, since patients with malabsorption may present with abnormal bleeding due to vitamin K deficiency. If the decreased prothrombin activity is due to malabsorption, it should be readily correctable with parenteral vitamin K.

Breath tests The bile acid breath test utilizing [^{14}C]cholylglycine is a reasonably reliable screening test for bacterial overgrowth syndromes. Approximately two-thirds of patients with a positive small-bowel culture will have an abnormal bile acid breath test. However, in patients with suspected malabsorption of bile acids the test is rather insensitive without the additional determination of fecal bile acid excretion. The excretion of breath hydrogen after ingestion of lactose is a sensitive, specific, and noninvasive test for detecting lactase deficiency. Lactulose and [^{14}C]xylose breath tests for bacterial overgrowth have also been found helpful.

PATHOPHYSIOLOGIC BASIS FOR SYMPTOMS AND SIGNS IN MALABSORPTIVE DISORDERS The common symptoms and signs found in malabsorptive disorders are listed in Table 292-5. The most frequent symptoms are those of malnutrition, weight loss, and diarrhea. However, in each of the clinical settings listed in Table 292-5, it is important to consider the cause of the malabsorption.

DISORDERS ASSOCIATED WITH MALABSORPTION

INADEQUATE DIGESTION   Liver and biliary tract disease It is not generally appreciated that patients with acute or chronic liver disease may develop malabsorption due to impaired intraluminal digestion. Steatorrhea has been described in acute viral hepatitis, chronic extrahepatic biliary tract obstruction, primary biliary cirrhosis, and postnecrotic and nutritional cirrhosis. Absorption of D-xylose and vitamin B_{12} are usually normal, and small-intestinal mucosal biopsy specimens are generally unremarkable. The steatorrhea associated with liver and biliary tract disease is thought to be due to impaired hepatic synthesis or excretion of conjugated bile salts, resulting in impaired formation of micellar lipid. In addition to steatorrhea, patients with liver disease may have impaired absorption of vitamin D and calcium, resulting in severe metabolic bone disease. This is particularly common in patients with primary biliary cirrhosis. Skeletal roentgenograms may show increased porosity of bone, cortical thinning, vertebral compression, and spontaneous pathologic fractures. Patients with alcohol-induced liver disease may also have exocrine pancreatic insufficiency. Accordingly, pancreatic function should be evaluated in patients with liver disease and malabsorption.

Postgastrectomy malabsorption The presence of a malabsorption syndrome has been documented frequently in patients after subtotal gastrectomy. Steatorrhea is more common with a Billroth II than a Billroth I type of anastomosis. Usually the fat loss is minimal, ranging from 7 to 10 g per 24 h. Patients with gross steatorrhea usually have impaired intraluminal fat digestion due to several factors: (1) With a Billroth II anastomosis the duodenum is bypassed, and there is a decreased entry of stomach contents into the proximal duodenum (i.e., afferent loop). This leads to a decreased stimulus for the release of *secretin* and *pancreozymin* from the duodenum and may result in a depressed pancreatic enzyme response. (2) There may

TABLE 292-5
Pathophysiologic basis for symptoms and signs in malabsorptive disorders

Symptom or sign	Pathophysiology
Generalized malnutrition and weight loss	Malabsorption of fat, carbohydrate, and protein → loss of calories
Diarrhea	Impaired absorption or increased intestinal secretion of water and electrolytes; unabsorbed dihydroxy bile acids and fatty acids → lowered absorption of water and electrolytes; excess load of fluid and electrolytes presented to the colon may exceed its absorptive capacity
Nocturia	Delayed absorption of water; hypokalemia
Anemia	Impaired absorption of iron, vitamin B_{12}, and folic acid
Glossitis, cheilosis	Deficiency of iron, vitamin B_{12}, folate, and other vitamins
Peripheral neuritis	Deficiency of vitamin B_{12}
Edema	Impaired absorption of amino acids → protein depletion → hypoproteinemia
Amenorrhea, ↓ libido	Protein depletion and "caloric starvation" → secondary hypopituitarism
Bone pain	Protein depletion → impaired bone formation →osteoporosis; Calcium malabsorption → demineralization of bone → osteomalacia
Tetany, paresthesias	Calcium malabsorption → hypocalcemia; magnesium malabsorption → hypomagnesemia
Hemorrhagic phenomena	Vitamin K malabsorption → hypoprothrombinemia
Weakness	Anemia; electrolyte depletion (hypokalemia)
Eczema	Cause uncertain
Night blindness	Impaired absorption of vitamin A

FIGURE 292-4
Typical peroral intestinal biopsies.

A. Jejunal mucosa of patient with nontropical sprue. Note virtual absence of villi, elongated crypts (some are cut in cross section), mononuclear infiltrate, cuboidal instead of columnar epithelium on top of villi (300×).

B. Biopsy from the same patient as in (A), after 9 months on a gluten-free diet. Note the reappearance of villi with normal-appearing columnar cells, and reduction in infiltrate and crypt height (300×).

C. Biopsy from patient with agammaglobulinemia. The features bear a striking resemblance to those of nontropical sprue. There is a marked mononuclear infiltration, some of it in aggregates (200×).

be *inadequate mixing* of the pancreatic enzymes and bile salts secreted into the proximal duodenum with the gastric contents entering the jejunum. (3) There may be *stasis* of intestinal contents in the afferent loop, resulting in abnormal bacterial proliferation in the proximal small bowel. This in turn may lead to abnormalities in bile salt metabolism (see "Pathophysiology," below). (4) The presence of maldigestion may lead to *protein depletion,* which in turn may produce further impairment in pancreatic function. (5) The *loss of the reservoir function of the stomach* may result in decreased intestinal transit time. Perhaps the most important factor is rapid gastric emptying, which results in low luminal concentrations of digestive secretions for the first 60 to 80 min after a meal. Such a disorder has been described in patients with subtotal gastrectomy and duodenostomy (Billroth I), gastrojejunostomy (Billroth II), and truncal vagotomy and pyloroplasty (V&P). That gastric emptying rates are somewhat slower in patients with V&P may account for the overall less severe nutritional deficiencies in such patients. In some patients treatment with pancreatic enzymes may lead to significant improvement. Specimens of duodenal or jejunal fluid should be obtained for culture of both aerobic and anaerobic organisms and appropriate antibiotic therapy instituted if there is evidence of abnormal bacterial overgrowth (colony count of greater than 10^5 per milliliter of jejunal fluid). Because the duodenum is the principal site of absorption of iron and calcium, in patients with a Billroth II anastomosis impaired absorption of calcium and iron may also develop.

INADEQUATE ABSORPTIVE SURFACE (SHORT BOWEL SYNDROME) Extensive intestinal resection often results in the short bowel syndrome. The most common disorders resulting in short bowel syndrome are (1) massive intestinal resection following a vascular insult to the small intestine, (2) regional enteritis with multiple bowel resections, and (3) jejunoileal bypass for morbid obesity. In general, the absorption of nutrients will be influenced by the extent and site of small bowel resected, the presence of the ileocecal valve, and adaptation of the remaining small bowel. Resection of 40 to 50 percent of the small bowel is usually well tolerated, provided the proximal duodenum, the distal half of the ileum, and the ileocecal valve are spared. By contrast, resection of the ileum and the ileocecal valve alone may induce severe diarrhea and malabsorption, even though less than 30 percent of the small intestine is resected.

Several measures are important in the management of short bowel syndrome: (1) The diet should contain at least 2500 cal and consist primarily of carbohydrate and protein with fat restricted to less than 40 g per day. A fat-restricted diet is effective in reducing diarrhea, presumably because there is decreased production of hydroxy fatty acids from long-chain fats. Such hydroxy fatty acids, in essence, are cathartics and increase net secretion of water and electrolytes by the colon as well as the small bowel. (2) It is often necessary to provide vitamin and mineral supplements, which usually include K^+, Cl^-, Mg^{2+}, Ca^{2+}, trace metals (Zn, Cd, Mn), iron, folate, vitamin B_{12}, other vitamins (A, D, E, K, B_1, B_2, B_6, biotin), and

D. Close-up of villi of patient with protein-losing enteropathy. Tips of villi are broadened and dilated. Lymphatic spaces are present (arrows) (450×).

E. Intestinal biopsy from patient with abetalipoproteinemia. The villus tips have a "lacy" appearance (arrow) due to retained fat (300×). (This is more apparent at the higher magnification shown in F.)

F. High-power micrograph of villus from patient with abetalipoproteinemia. The vacuoles are filled with lipid (750×). Insert shows dark-staining (osmium) lipid droplets in mucosal cells (osmium counterstained with Giemsa; 800×).

essential fatty acids. (3) Specific drugs (for example, belladonna alkaloids, diphenoxylate, loperamide, and codeine), which decrease intestinal motility and prolong mucosal contact time, are helpful in controlling diarrhea. These agents also decrease ileostomy outputs. (4) A bile salt–sequestering agent such as cholestyramine blunts the effects of bile salts, which stimulate net secretion of water and electrolytes by the colon. (5) Patients with short bowel syndrome may have gastric acid hypersecretion, which results in dilution of pancreatic secretions as well as inactivation of pancreatic enzymes. Under these conditions, the histamine H_2-receptor antagonist, cimetidine, is useful because it will suppress gastric acid secretion and decrease the volume of fluid entering the proximal small bowel, thus leading to an increased concentration of pancreatic enzymes. In addition, supplemental pancreatic enzyme therapy may be required. (6) A bypassed colon can be used to receive infusions of fluid and electrolytes since a portion of the colon can still absorb 1000 to 1500 ml fluid per day. Finally, (7) total parenteral nutrition is frequently required during the first 6 months after massive intestinal resection until some degree of adaptation has occurred. Such patients may also require long-term parenteral hyperalimentation with a silicone rubber catheter in the superior vena cava.

For a discussion of regional enteritis see Chap. 293.

MALABSORPTION DUE TO BACTERIAL OVERGROWTH OF THE SMALL BOWEL The proximal small intestine is often bacteriologically sterile. When bacteria are isolated from the upper small bowel, they are frequently contaminants transported from the mouth and upper respiratory tract, and the colony count rarely exceeds 10^4 per milliliter of jejunal fluid. The major mechanism limiting the growth of bacteria in the small intestine is normal peristalsis. Any disorder leading to impaired intestinal motility may result in abnormal stasis of intestinal contents with ineffective mechanical cleansing of bacteria. This in turn may lead to abnormal bacterial proliferation and malabsorption. Several malabsorptive disorders have been associated with bacterial overgrowth of the small bowel, and these are listed in Table 292-6.

Pathophysiology Bacterial overgrowth may result in changes in bile salt metabolism, and these are believed directly and indirectly to account for the steatorrhea. First, bacteria (especially anaerobic gram-positive bacteria) may lead to the intraluminal deconjugation of bile salts with a consequent production of free bile acids. In contrast to conjugated bile salts, unconjugated bile salts may be absorbed in the proximal small bowel by nonionic diffusion, resulting in decreased intraluminal concentrations of bile salts in the jejunum. Second, the decreased bile salt concentrations, the increase of unconjugated bile salts, and the decrease of the conjugated salts all serve to contribute to impaired intraluminal micelle formation and hence fat malabsorption. In addition to abnormalities in bile salt metabolism, intestinal mucosal lesions have been demonstrated in patients with intestinal stasis. Such lesions are often patchy in distribution, and the histologic appearance ranges in severity from minimal changes in villus architecture to severe lesions with virtual absence of villi. The etiology of these lesions is unclear; possible causes include damage caused by bacterial invasion, bacterial toxins, or metabolic products such as unconjugated bile salts. The impaired absorption of vitamin B_{12} is not related to the disturbed bile salt metabolism but appears to be due to uptake of vitamin B_{12} by microorganisms.

Many of the above abnormalities in bile salt metabolism may be reversed by appropriate antibiotic therapy. When such treatment is instituted, unconjugated bile salts in the jejunal fluid decrease, an increase in the micellar lipid phase will oc-

TABLE 292-6
Classification of the malabsorption syndromes

I Inadequate digestion
  A Postgastrectomy steatorrhea*
  B Deficiency or inactivation of pancreatic lipase
    1 Exocrine pancreatic insufficiency
      a Chronic pancreatitis
      b Pancreatic carcinoma
      c Cystic fibrosis
      d Pancreatic resection
    2 Ulcerogenic tumor of the pancreas (Zollinger-Ellison syndrome, gastrinoma)*
II Reduced intestinal bile salt concentration (with impaired micelle formation)
  A Liver disease
    1 Parenchymal liver disease
    2 Cholestasis (intrahepatic or extrahepatic)
  B Abnormal bacterial proliferation in the small bowel
    1 Afferent loop stasis
    2 Strictures
    3 Fistulas
    4 Blind loops
    5 Multiple diverticula of the small bowel
    6 Hypomotility states (diabetes, scleroderma, intestinal pseudoobstruction)
  C Interrupted enterohepatic circulation of bile salts
    1 Ileal resection
    2 Ileal inflammatory disease (regional ileitis)
  D Drugs (by sequestration or precipitation of bile salts)
    1 Neomycin
    2 Calcium carbonate
    3 Cholestyramine
III Inadequate absorptive surface
  A Intestinal resection or bypass
    1 Mesenteric vascular disease with massive intestinal resection
    2 Regional enteritis with multiple bowel resections
    3 Jejunoileal bypass
  B Gastroileostomy (inadvertent)
IV Lymphatic obstruction
  A Intestinal lymphangiectasia
  B Whipple's disease*
  C Lymphoma
V Cardiovascular disorders
  A Constrictive pericarditis
  B Congestive heart failure
  C Mesenteric vascular insufficiency
  D Vasculitis
VI Primary mucosal absorptive defects
  A Inflammatory or infiltrative disorders
    1 Regional enteritis*
    2 Amyloidosis
    3 Scleroderma*
    4 Lymphoma*
    5 Radiation enteritis
    6 Eosinophilic enteritis
    7 Tropical sprue
    8 Infectious enteritis (e.g., salmonellosis)
    9 Collagenous sprue
    10 Nonspecific ulcerative jejunitis
    11 Mastocytosis
    12 Dermatologic disorders (e.g., dermatitis herpetiformis)
  B Biochemical or genetic abnormalities
    1 Nontropical sprue (gluten-induced enteropathy); celiac sprue
    2 Disaccharidase deficiency
    3 Hypogammaglobulinemia
    4 Abetalipoproteinemia
    5 Hartnup disease
    6 Cystinuria
    7 Monosaccharide malabsorption
VII Endocrine and metabolic disorders
  A Diabetes mellitus*
  B Hypoparathyroidism
  C Adrenal insufficiency
  D Hyperthyroidism
  E Ulcerogenic tumor of the pancreas (Zollinger-Ellison syndrome, gastrinoma)*
  F Carcinoid syndrome

* Malabsorption caused by multiple defects.

cur, and steatorrhea diminishes or disappears. In addition, significant improvement in the absorption of vitamin B_{12} will occur with broad-spectrum antibiotics such as tetracycline.

Clinical manifestations Breath tests, i.e., ^{14}C-labeled bile acid, [^{14}C]xylose, and lactulose, are useful screening tests for malabsorption syndrome due to abnormal bacterial overgrowth of the small intestine. A definitive diagnosis is established by demonstrating larger numbers of microorganisms (greater than 10^5 per milliliter) in cultures of duodenal or jejunal fluid. Other clinical features include the following: (1) steatorrhea of a moderate degree, usually in the range of 15 to 30 g fecal fat per 24 h; (2) macrocytic anemia with a megaloblastic bone marrow; (3) impaired absorption of vitamin B_{12} which is not corrected by intrinsic factor; and (4) correction of steatorrhea and impaired vitamin B_{12} absorption by antibiotic therapy. Absorption of D-xylose, peroral small-intestinal biopsy specimens, and other tests of absorptive function (Table 292-3) may be normal in these patients.

Tropical sprue Tropical sprue is a malabsorptive disorder of unknown cause affecting residents or visitors to tropical regions. Both epidemic and endemic forms of the disease have been recognized. The etiology of the disorder has not been elucidated, but it might well result from one or more of the following: (1) a nutritional deficiency, (2) a transmissible infectious microorganism, and (3) a toxin elaborated by a microorganism or contained in the diet. It is of interest that coliform organisms, shown to produce an enterotoxin causing fluid secretion, have been isolated from the jejunum of tropical sprue patients but not from other patients with bacterial overgrowth of the proximal small bowel. Anorexia, diarrhea, weight loss, symptoms of anemia, sequelae of nutritional deficiency (Table 292-5), and abdominal distention are common findings. Patients are frequently deficient in iron as well as vitamin B_{12} and folate. Laboratory studies usually reveal anemia (megaloblastic in 60 percent of cases) and impaired absorption of fat, xylose, and vitamin B_{12}. Malabsorption of at least two nutrients is considered essential for the diagnosis. Jejunal biopsy classically reveals shortened and thickened villi, increased crypt depth, and increased infiltration of mononuclear cells in the lamina propria and epithelium (Table 292-4). However, these biopsy findings are not specific, and in addition, interpretation is difficult because "control" biopsies from asymptomatic residents in the same tropical region are often considered abnormal when compared with normal biopsies from patients in temperate zones. Such histological findings have been termed *tropical jejunitis*. Treatment with vitamin B_{12}, folate, and antibiotics have all been effective in inducing a remission. A short course, i.e., 2 to 4 weeks, of therapy with a sulfonamide or tetracycline is usually given. Occasional patients require more prolonged antibiotic therapy.

Scleroderma Although there are numerous reports of small-intestinal involvement in scleroderma, frank malabsorption has been reported infrequently. It has been suggested that malabsorption may be due to several factors: (1) lymphatic obstruction; (2) reduced arterial blood supply to the gut; (3) impaired intestinal motility leading to relative stasis of intestinal contents and hence bacterial overgrowth; and (4) involvement of the intestinal wall by the disease. At present there is little evidence to support the first two postulated mechanisms. In some cases abnormal bacterial proliferation in the upper small bowel has been documented, and in these patients antibiotic therapy has resulted in decrease in steatorrhea, gain in weight, and increased absorption of vitamin B_{12}. In the intestinal wall there may also be extensive deposition of collagen, especially in the muscular mucosa, submucosa, and muscularis externa, with significant muscle atrophy. Electron microscopic studies have revealed a paucity of nexuses (cell junctions) between adjacent muscle cells in the small intestine of these patients. Studies of duodenal myoelectric activity in scleroderma revealed normal slow-wave frequency and propagation velocity but decreased excitability of the bowel to mechanical stimuli such as distention and humoral stimuli such as pentagastrin and secretin. This motor dysfunction may be important. Since nexuses are involved in the propagation of electric impulses, the loss of contact between muscle cells may result in impairment of muscular contraction. This may be an important factor in the dilatation, atony, and stasis of intestinal contents in scleroderma.

DISORDERS ASSOCIATED WITH LYMPHATIC OBSTRUCTION
Whipple's disease This is a rare disorder characterized clinically by arthralgia, abdominal pain, diarrhea, progressive weight loss, and impaired intestinal absorption. Wasting, low-grade fever, increased skin pigmentation, and peripheral lymphadenopathy are frequently present. Laboratory examination usually reveals the presence of steatorrhea, impaired xylose absorption, abnormal small-bowel x-rays, hypoalbuminemia, and anemia. Hypoalbuminemia is due to excessive loss of serum albumin into the gastrointestinal tract as well as impaired synthesis of albumin. Serum calcium, cholesterol, and iron levels are usually low and often inversely correlated with the degree of malabsorption.

The diagnosis is established by demonstrating the presence in the mucosa of macrophages containing large cytoplasmic granules which give a brilliant magenta stain with periodic acid-Schiff reagent (PAS). Such macrophages may also be seen in other tissues such as lymph nodes, spleen, or liver. The finding of PAS-positive macrophages in the lamina propria is not specific for Whipple's disease, but virtual replacement of most cellular elements in the lamina propria by these macrophages has been seen only in this disorder. In addition to the PAS-positive macrophages, jejunal biopsies frequently show dilated lymphatics and some degree of blunting of the intestinal mucosal villi.

Electron microscopic studies have revealed the presence of rod-shaped structures (or bacilliform bodies) 0.3 by 1.5 to 2.5 μm within and adjacent to the macrophages in the lamina propria as well as within epithelial cells, and polymorphonuclear leukocytes. The ultrastructural features of these bacilliform bodies suggest that they are microorganisms. It is of particular interest that after treatment with antibiotics the bacilliform bodies decrease or disappear together with a decrease in the number of PAS-positive macrophages. In addition, the reappearance of the bacteria often heralds the onset of a clinical relapse after antibiotics have been withdrawn.

Whipple's disease at one time was thought to be invariably fatal. However, it is now clear that therapy with antibiotics, with or without corticosteroids, will usually induce a clinical remission. In a few cases there has been complete reversal of the histologic abnormalities in the jejunal mucosa, and some of these cases have been followed for 10 years. It is recommended that patients with Whipple's disease be treated with antibiotics such as tetracycline for at least 1 year and then followed closely with serial small-bowel biopsies. The most important parameter for following the disease and predicting its course is the presence or absence of bacilli in sections of small-bowel biopsies.

Intestinal lymphoma Steatorrhea is a manifestation of *primary* intestinal lymphoma. The disease occurs predominantly in men, and the mean age of onset of symptoms is about 50 years. The diagnosis should be suspected in patients with malabsorption with the following findings: (1) a malabsorption syndrome in which clinical and biopsy features resemble those of non-

tropical sprue but in which there is an incomplete response to a gluten-free diet, (2) the presence of *abdominal pain* and *fever*, and (3) signs of symptoms of intestinal obstruction. The usual stigmata of generalized lymphoma are frequently absent. Hepatomegaly, splenomegaly, palpable abdominal masses, and peripheral adenopathy are usually not found. Lymphangiography may reveal abnormal intraabdominal nodes. The diagnosis can be established by laparotomy and often may be made by thorough examination of multiple mucosal biopsy specimens obtained perorally. There may be a total absence of villi or lesser degrees of blunting and shortening of the villi. In contrast to nontropical sprue, the lamina propria is usually massively infiltrated with lymphoid cells. Malignancy may be diagnosed by demonstrating lymphoid cells with the cytologic features of malignancy, the presence of reticulum cells outside germinal centers, and infiltration and destruction of crypts by pleomorphic lymphoid cells. Some patients elaborate or secrete a fragment of the heavy chain of IgA immunoglobulins (*alpha chain disease*). The latter is probably a variant of intestinal lymphoma.

The mechanism of malabsorption in intestinal lymphoma may be related to several factors: (1) diffuse involvement of the small-intestinal mucosa; (2) involvement of the bowel wall with lymphatic obstruction; and (3) localized stenosis with stasis of intestinal contents and bacterial overgrowth. It should be emphasized that it is often difficult, by clinical and morphologic features alone, to distinguish nontropical sprue from intestinal lymphoma. Indeed, there is evidence to suggest that lymphoma may develop as a late complication of nontropical sprue.

The course of intestinal lymphoma has ranged from 4 months to 4 years from the onset of symptoms. Perforation, bleeding, and intestinal obstruction are common terminal complications. There is insufficient evidence to determine whether radiation therapy, chemotherapy, or localized surgical resection modify the natural course of the disease.

CARDIOVASCULAR DISORDERS Steatorrhea has been described in patients with chronic congestive heart failure, superior mesenteric artery insufficiency, and constrictive pericarditis. Abnormal dilated mucosal lymphatics and excessive enteric loss of protein have been demonstrated in patients with constrictive pericarditis. The mechanism of steatorrhea in patients with chronic heart failure remains uncertain. It might be due to congestion and edema of the mucosa, mucosal hypoxia, or abnormalities in pancreatic function. Although pronounced steatorrhea is uncommon in congestive heart failure, these patients are frequently anorectic, and a low fat intake could mask a latent steatorrhea. Steatorrhea is quite infrequent in patients with vasculitis and is thought to be due to segmental infarction of the small bowel in addition to intestinal ischemia.

DEFECTS IN MUCOSAL FUNCTION

INFLAMMATORY OR INFILTRATIVE DISORDERS Regional enteritis The clinical features of regional enteritis are described in Chap. 293. Malabsorption in regional enteritis may result from several factors; these are listed in Table 292-7. Active ileal disease and/or ileal resection resulting in an interrupted enterohepatic circulation of and deficiency of conjugated bile salts appears to be the major factor responsible for steatorrhea as well as impaired absorption of vitamin B_{12}. Small-bowel absorptive function has been correlated with the extent of ileal disease or resection. When the length of ileal dysfunction exceeds 90 to 100 cm, virtually all patients will have steatorrhea and vitamin B_{12} malabsorption. After intestinal resection, the functional capacity of the remaining small bowel will depend on the site and extent of resection as well as the presence of residual inflammatory disease. Massive intestinal resection usually results in impaired absorption of all food constituents. When the malabsorption is due to strictures and blind loops as a result of previous surgical therapy, antibiotic therapy may be helpful, but surgical removal of these areas is usually necessary for long-term improvement. With diffuse inflammatory disease a florid malabsorption syndrome may occur with steatorrhea, hypocalcemia, impaired vitamin B_{12} absorption; and hypoalbuminemia due to increased enteric protein loss. Treatment with sulfasalazine and corticosteroid drugs may be beneficial (see Chap. 293).

After *ileal resection,* patients frequently have bothersome diarrhea. This appears to be due to *interruption of the enterohepatic circulation* whereby increased amounts of bile salts reach the colon, where they interfere with water and electrolyte absorption and thus have a cathartic effect. The *bile salt–induced diarrhea* after ileal resection may respond to treatment with cholestyramine, an exchange resin which binds bile salts and causes them to lose their biochemical effect on the bowel. Patients with ileal resection of less than 100 cm and fecal fat excretion less than 20 g per day show the best symptomatic response to cholestyramine.

Amyloidosis This disorder is discussed in detail in Chap. 64.

Radiation injury to the small bowel Extensive morphologic damage of the small-intestinal mucosa often follows normal or excessive abdominal irradiation. These changes include a decrease in crypt mitoses, marked shortening of the villi, megalocytosis of epithelial cells, and inflammatory cell infiltration of the lamina propria. This may be associated with transient diarrhea and impaired intestinal absorption. However, restoration of normal intestinal architecture is usually complete within 2 weeks after cessation of therapy. Persistent diarrhea and malabsorption may develop shortly after x-ray therapy, or there may be a latent period of several years before the onset of diarrhea. Steatorrhea, ranging from 10 to 40 g per day, has been frequently observed, but impaired absorption of calcium, iron, D-xylose, or vitamin B_{12} is less common. In some patients intestinal strictures may develop following irradiation, and thus stasis of intestinal contents and abnormal bacterial proliferation may occur. In others, intestinal lymphangiectasia, presumably due to lymphatic obstruction, has been documented. Diarrhea and malabsorption may be refractory to all methods of management. Treatment with antibiotics, pancreatic enzymes, gluten-free diet, adrenal corticosteroids, anticholinergic drugs, and opiates has met with but limited success.

Eosinophilic enteritis Eosinophilic gastroenteritis is an uncommon disorder of the stomach, small bowel, and colon of unknown etiology characterized by peripheral blood eosinophilia and eosinophilic infiltration of the gut wall but without evidence of vasculitis. The clinical manifestations, usually recurrent, are protean and relate to the site of gastrointestinal tract involvement. Three main patterns have been identified: (1) Predominant mucosal disease manifested by iron deficiency anemia, hypoalbuminemia due to protein-losing enteropathy, and mild steatorrhea. Patients in this group often present with a malabsorption syndrome and a history of intolerance to specific foods. (2) Predominant muscle layer disease characterized by marked thickening and rigidity of the stomach and proximal small bowel with obstructive symptoms and radiologic features of pyloric narrowing and obstruction. The obstructive form of eosinophilic gastroenteritis accounts for half of the reported cases since 1970. Accordingly, eosinophilic enteritis should be considered in the differential diagnosis of gastric outlet obstruction, diffuse small-bowel disease, and ileocolitis. Indeed, eosinophilic enteritis often mimics regional enteritis. (3) Predominant subserosal disease in which the cardinal manifestation is ascites with marked eosinophilia in the ascitic fluid. Although the above classification based on tissue layer of major involvement is useful in understanding the principal manifestations, it should be emphasized that multiple clinical forms, e.g., ascites (serosal involvement) and obstruction (muscular involvement), also occur.

Previous reports have emphasized food allergy and mucosal features of this disease. However, food sensitivity is related to symptoms in less than 20 percent of patients. In such patients fasting serum IgE levels are often elevated, and challenge with offending foods frequently evokes symptoms of abdominal pain and diarrhea in addition to a marked increase in serum IgE levels. In most patients with eosinophilic enteritis, however, immunological studies including serum immunoglobulins, serum complement, lymphocyte quantitation, and lymphocyte response to nonspecific nitrogens reveal no abnormalities. Thus, both IgE-mediated and IgE-dependent mechanisms may be operative in different patients with eosinophilic gastroenteritis. Several nonreaginic factors influence peripheral blood and tissue eosinophilia. It seems clear that evidence of allergy or food sensitivity is often absent and is not required for the diagnosis of eosinophilic enteritis. In addition, even in patients with food allergies, elimination diets are frequently ineffective and such patients may require prolonged corticosteroid therapy to remain well. Surgical treatment for relief of obstructive symptoms and corticosteroids are the mainstays of therapy.

Dermatitis and malabsorption A malabsorption syndrome, usually mild, has been reported in patients with a variety of dermatological disorders, including psoriasis, eczematoid dermatitis, and dermatitis herpetiformis. Proximal intestinal mucosal abnormalities are almost invariably found in patients with dermatitis herpetiformis. In one study 21 of 22 patients had lesions ranging in severity from a completely "flat" to an almost normal intestinal mucosa. The mucosal lesions were often patchy in distribution. Clinical and laboratory evidence of significant malabsorption was infrequent, possibly due to the limited length of small intestine involved in this skin disorder. In some patients with dermatitis herpetiformis, blunted and flattened intestinal mucosal lesions, and steatorrhea, there may be a striking improvement in villous architecture and regression of steatorrhea after withdrawal of gluten from the diet. Further, in patients with dermatitis herpetiformis and a morphologically normal small-intestinal mucosa, administra-

TABLE 292-7
Mechanisms of malabsorption in regional enteritis

I Deficiency of conjugated bile salts producing impaired micelle formation
   A Interruption of enterohepatic circulation of bile salts by ileal disease or resection
   B Deconjugation of bile salts due to bacterial overgrowth
      1 Strictures
      2 Fistulas
II Active inflammatory bowel disease decreasing mucosal cell function
III Sequelae of intestinal resection
   A Inadequate absorptive surface
   B Rapid intestinal transit
IV Sequelae of protein depletion producing impaired exocrine pancreatic function
V Miscellaneous
   A Fistulas (→ decreased absorptive surface)
   B Acquired lactase deficiency
   C Increased lumenal concentrations of dihydroxy bile salts, fatty acids, or hydroxy fatty acids

tion of a high-gluten diet may result in blunted and flattened mucosal lesions indistinguishable from those of celiac sprue. These observations raise the interesting question as to whether certain patients with dermatitis herpetiformis and a malabsorption syndrome have latent nontropical sprue.

BIOCHEMICAL OR GENETIC ABNORMALITIES Nontropical sprue DEFINITION Nontropical sprue is a disorder characterized by malabsorption, abnormal small-bowel structure, and intolerance to gluten, a protein found in wheat and wheat products. It has been appropriately referred to as *gluten-induced enteropathy.* Celiac disease in children and nontropical sprue of the adult are probably one and the same disorder with the same pathogenesis.

There are insufficient data to provide an accurate estimation of the incidence of nontropical sprue in any population. This is largely because the severity of the disease varies greatly and individuals may have typical mucosal change and yet have no overt symptoms. Seventy percent of the cases in most reported series are women. The incidence in siblings appears to be many times higher than that in the general population, and it has been suggested that sprue may be inherited through a dominant gene of incomplete penetrance. Celiac sprue patients have an increased frequency of serum histocompatibility antigens, particularly of the HLA-B8 type. The HLA-B8 phenotype has been found in 85 to 90 percent of sprue patients as compared with 20 to 25 percent in normal subjects. The HLA-B8 antigen may be linked to immune response genes which may determine the immunologic recognition of certain substances. It has been suggested that such genetic factors may predispose to immunologic tolerance of dietary proteins such as the peptides in gluten or to the production of pathogenic antigluten antibodies which could result in binding of gluten to epithelial cells with subsequent tissue damage.

PATHOPHYSIOLOGY Gluten and the related substance gliadin are high-molecular-weight proteins found especially in wheat. These proteins are unique in that glutamine accounts for about 40 percent of the component amino acids. These proteins as well as the larger peptide hydrolysis products (containing glutamine) are toxic when administered to patients with sprue in remission. The exact mechanism for this effect is not clear, but two theories have been proposed, namely, a "toxic" and an immunologic theory. One possible mechanism is that patients with sprue lack a specific mucosal peptidase, such that gluten or its larger glutamine-containing peptides are not effectively hydrolyzed to smaller peptides (i.e., dipeptides or amino acids). As a consequence "toxic" peptides might accumulate in the mucosa. It has been demonstrated that patients with sprue in remission will develop steatorrhea and typical mucosal changes when they are given gluten. Similar results will occur with the administration of peptide hydrolyzates containing at least eight amino acids with a terminal glutamine residue. It has been shown that when gluten is instilled into the *ileum* of sprue patients, histologic changes begin to occur within hours, but not in the upper jejunum, suggesting that the effect is immediate and local rather than systemic. After noxious gluten fractions damage surface absorptive cells, the damaged cells are sloughed rapidly from the mucosal surface into the gut lumen. To compensate for this, cell proliferation increases, crypts hypertrophy, and cell migration is accelerated to replace the damaged and sloughed epithelial cells. This more rapid than normal epithelial cell renewal can be reversed by a gluten-free diet. The intestinal mucosa of patients with sprue shows many enzyme alterations including decreased levels of disaccharidases, alkaline phosphatase, and peptide hydrolases as well as impaired ability to digest gluten peptides. However, these abnormalities usually revert toward normal after successful treatment with a gluten-free diet. There is additional evi-

dence supporting the concept of toxicity of gluten and gluten breakdown products in sprue. First, gliadin is toxic to sprue mucosa maintained in organ culture, causing ultrastructural changes and depression of disaccharidase activity. Second, sprue mucosa hydrolyzes a specific fraction of a gliadin digest (i.e., fraction 9) in a defective manner, and fraction 9 is selectively toxic to sprue mucosa. Third, specific fractions of gluten fed to sprue patients cause transient alterations in mucosal histology and depression of disaccharidase activity, but full recovery is observed in 72 h. The rapid onset of these changes and prompt recovery are consistent with a direct toxic effect. Despite intensive study, however, no persistent, specific, or selective peptidase deficiency has been demonstrated.

It has also been suggested that gluten or gluten metabolites may initiate an *immunologic reaction* in the intestinal mucosa. The presence of a mononuclear inflammatory cell infiltrate in the lamina propria of the mucosa, the beneficial response to corticosteroid drugs, the finding of abnormal antibodies to gliadin in the serum of sprue patients, the synthesis of increased amounts of antigliadin antibody by sprue mucosa maintained in organ culture, and the elaboration of lymphokines such as migration inhibitory factor (MIF) by sprue mucosa incubated with gliadin have all been cited as evidence in support of this hypothesis. However, the evidence indicating that an abnormal (immune) mechanism is important in initiating or perpetuating this disease process remains to be determined.

Jejunal biopsy specimens from patients with nontropical sprue usually show a characteristic lesion. There is blunting and flattening of the mucosal surface, with villi either absent or broad and short. The crypts are elongated, and there is generally a dense infiltration of inflammatory cells in the lamina propria. The surface epithelium is altered with a sparse brush border, cuboidal rather than the normal columnar cells, and infiltration of inflammatory cells in the epithelial layer. These changes are usually most severe in the proximal small bowel, presumably because this area of the bowel is exposed to the highest gluten concentration. The typical morphologic changes illustrated in Fig. 292-4 are characteristic of nontropical sprue but are not specific. Similar changes have been described in other conditions, including lymphoma, tropical sprue, and hypogammaglobulinemia associated with malabsorption. Many biochemical abnormalities have been demonstrated in mucosal biopsy specimens from nontropical sprue patients. Impaired esterification of fatty acids to triglycerides, decreased uptake of amino acids, and decreased activity of intestinal disaccharidases (especially lactase) have been well documented. The latter observation may account for the high incidence of milk intolerance in untreated sprue patients or those in relapse. However, the greater abundance of undifferentiated crypt cells may be important, since crypt cells normally have a decreased capacity for nutrient uptake than villus cells.

Since the mucosa is damaged and altered in patients with nontropical sprue, there may be *decreased release of pancreatic tropic hormones* (secretin and cholecystokinin-pancreozymin). This results in decreased stimulation of the pancreas with lower than normal intraluminal levels of pancreatic enzymes in response to a meal. In addition, the gallbladder appears to be resistant to the action of cholecystokinin, resulting in absent or minimal contractions of the gallbladder, in turn leading to sequestration of bile salts in an inert gallbladder. These two defects may result in impaired intraluminal digestion of fat and protein which will be superimposed on the defect in intestinal transport caused by a damaged mucosa.

Diarrhea is common in sprue patients and is due to a number of factors, including *impaired absorption* of salt and water by duodenum and jejunum, net *secretion* of water and electrolytes by an abnormally permeable jejunal mucosa, and net colonic secretion of water and electrolytes induced by unabsorbed fatty acids and hydroxy fatty acids. However, the distal small intestine in sprue has the ability to adapt to the damage and loss of absorptive capacity in the proximal small intestine. Indeed, increased ileal absorption of sodium, chloride, and water has been demonstrated in sprue patients.

CLINICAL FEATURES Most patients with nontropical sprue will have a typical malabsorption syndrome characterized by weight loss, abdominal distention and bloating, diarrhea, steatorrhea, and abnormal tests of absorptive function. The characteristic alterations in tests of intestinal absorption are outlined in Table 292-3. It should be emphasized, however, that some sprue patients may present with isolated abnormalities which initially do not suggest the diagnosis of nontropical sprue. Thus, a patient may be admitted for investigation of iron deficiency anemia without apparent blood loss or of abnormal bleeding due to hypoprothrombinemia, but not have diarrhea or overt steatorrhea. Likewise, sprue patients may present with puzzling metabolic bone disease without diarrhea or steatorrhea. Such patients usually complain of bone pain and tenderness and frequently are found to have extensive demineralization of bone, compression deformities, kyphoscoliosis, and Milkman's fractures. Emotional disturbances are common in these patients, and many individuals with a diagnosis of weight loss initially considered related to severe anxiety and depression are subsequently found to have nontropical sprue. In each of the above clinical settings, the diagnosis of sprue should be considered in the differential diagnosis.

Since there is no specific diagnostic test, three criteria should be met in order to establish a definite diagnosis of nontropical sprue: (1) evidence of malabsorption, (2) an abnormal small-bowel (jejunal) biopsy showing blunting and flattening of the villi along with changes in the surface epithelium, and (3) clinical, biochemical, and histologic improvement after institution of a gluten-free diet. In equivocal cases, the patient can be challenged with 30 to 50 g gluten orally, and if this promptly results in increased diarrhea and steatorrhea, the diagnosis of gluten-induced enteropathy is established. It should be emphasized that tests of intestinal absorption may reveal abnormalities which range from very minimal alterations to severe changes. Abnormalities in absorption tests have been shown to correlate reasonably well with the length of small-bowel involvement and to a lesser extent with the severity of the proximal lesion. A possible variant of celiac sprue is *collagenous* sprue. In this disorder small-bowel biopsy specimens characteristically reveal a blunted and flattened mucosa and large masses of eosinophilic hyalin material in the lamina propria. In one study of 349 jejunal biopsy specimens from 145 patients with celiac sprue, 45 (31 percent) showed basement membrane thickening often associated with collagen deposition, but dense collagen deposition was found in only 11 patients. Interestingly, fatal, unremitting malabsorption developed in four of the latter patients. These observations suggest that collagenous membrane thickening is a fairly frequent finding in jejunal biopsies from patients with sprue but that dense collagen deposits are an unusual feature and may indicate a poor prognosis.

TREATMENT Despite the uncertainties concerned with the diagnosis of nontropical sprue, approximately 80 percent of the patients improve after institution of a *gluten-free diet.* Symptomatic improvement usually occurs within a few weeks, but improvement in tests of absorptive function and small-bowel histologic characteristics may not occur for months. It has been repeatedly demonstrated that strict adherence to a gluten-free diet more consistently results in improvement than suboptimal gluten restriction. Nevertheless, even with strict diet adherence some cases show little improvement in intestinal histologic features. Patients with nontropical sprue treated with corticosteroids but continuing a normal gluten-containing diet have shown symptomatic improvement as well as improvement in intestinal histology and tests of intestinal absorptive function. The mechanism by which corticosteroids protect the mucosa from the effects of gluten is not clear.

If a patient with nontropical sprue does not respond to a gluten-free diet, other possibilities or complicative factors must be considered: (1) the diagnosis is incorrect; (2) the patient is not adhering strictly to the diet; (3) there may be another concurrent disease, such as pancreatic insufficiency; (4) the patient may have ulceration of the jejunum or ileum; (5) lactase deficiency may be present with resultant milk intolerance; (6) the patient may have collagenous sprue; or (7) he or she may have developed intestinal lymphoma, a disease which appears to occur more frequently in sprue than in the general population. Finally, it should be emphasized that a small number of patients show a markedly delayed response to a gluten-free diet, with significant improvement occurring only after 24 to 36 months of therapy.

Disaccharidase deficiency syndromes As indicated above, the hydrolysis of disaccharides occurs on or within the brush border (microvilli) of intestinal epithelial cells by specific disaccharidases located there. As would be anticipated, both primary (genetic or familial) and secondary (acquired) deficiencies of these disaccharidases have been observed.

LACTASE DEFICIENCY IN THE ADULT Instances of isolated deficiency of mucosal lactase occur which are associated with symptoms of lactose intolerance. Since lactose is the principal carbohydrate of milk, such individuals show milk intolerance with symptoms of abdominal cramps, bloating or distention, and diarrhea. Similar symptoms will occur following the ingestion of lactose. The symptoms are due to the fact that lactose when not hydrolyzed is not absorbed and its osmotic effect in the lumen leads to shifts of fluid into the intestinal tract. The pH of the stool will also decrease because of the production of lactic acid and short-chain fatty acids from the fermentation of lactose by colonic bacteria. Although primary intestinal lactase deficiency seems to be hereditary, lactose or milk intolerance may not become clinically evident until puberty or late adolescence. There are significant racial differences in the incidence of this entity. It would appear that about 5 to 15 percent of the adult white population shows intestinal lactase deficiency, but in American Negroes, Bantus, and Orientals, the incidence has been reported as high as 80 to 90 percent.

The diagnosis may be suspected by obtaining a history of gastrointestinal symptoms following milk ingestion. It should be emphasized that the ingestion of only moderate amounts of lactose, e.g., 5 to 12 g or the amount contained in 100 to 240 ml milk, often results in symptoms. Bloating, cramps, and flatulence, but not diarrhea, are usually produced with ingestion of small to moderate amounts of lactose. The vast majority of lactose-intolerant patients are aware that they are milk-intolerant and avoid milk. That these symptoms are not due to allergic reactions to the proteins in milk (i.e., milk allergy or hypersensitivity) can be demonstrated by performing a lactose tolerance test. This test consists of administering an oral dose of lactose (usually from 0.75 to 1.5 g per kilogram of body weight) and obtaining serial blood samples for measurements of blood glucose. In a positive test, intestinal symptoms occur, and the blood glucose increases less than 20 mg per 100 ml above the fasting level. However, false-positive and -negative tests occur in 20 percent of normal subjects because the test is influenced by gastric emptying and glucose metabolism. Measurement of breath hydrogen after ingestion of 50 g lactose is a more sensitive and specific test. The rationale for this test is that unabsorbed lactose is converted to hydrogen by colonic bacteria and breath hydrogen excretion subsequently rises. The test is noninvasive and is not influenced by gastric emptying or metabolic factors.

Acquired lactase deficiency is often seen in association with a variety of gastrointestinal diseases, in many of which there is histologic evidence of mucosal damage. The disorders in which lactose intolerance and lactase deficiency may occur include nontropical and tropical sprue, regional enteritis, bacterial infections of the intestinal tract, giardiasis, abetalipoproteinemia, cystic fibrosis, and ulcerative colitis.

DEFICIENCY OF OTHER DISACCHARIDASES Damage to the intestinal mucosa may produce decreased levels of other disaccharidases such as sucrase-isomaltase, but usually these are not as depressed as lactase, and symptoms of specific intolerance, such as sucrose intolerance, are uncommon. There are instances of primary and apparently hereditary sucrose intolerance, but these always occur in association with sucrase-isomaltase deficiency.

Hypogammaglobulinemia There are several reports documenting the association of malabsorption in hypogammaglobulinemia or agammaglobulinemia. The hypogammaglobulinemia may be of the congenital or the acquired type, with the onset either in childhood or adulthood. When malabsorption has been noted, it has included impaired absorption of fat, D-xylose, and vitamin B_{12}. Peroral intestinal biopsy may reveal changes comparable to those seen in nontropical sprue, but often one finds a more striking mononuclear infiltrate giving a nodular appearance to the mucosa both microscopically and macroscopically. Diarrhea and steatorrhea may precede or follow the development of hypogammaglobulinemia, and these may worsen during infections and subside after the infection is controlled with antibiotics. Intestinal infestation with *Giardia lamblia* is common in hypogammaglobulinemic patients. Meticulous collection and culture of intestinal fluids has revealed excessive numbers of anaerobic bacteria in the small bowel of some patients with hypogammaglobulinemia. However, the relationship between such overgrowth with anaerobes and diarrhea and steatorrhea remains to be clarified. Arthritis, resembling rheumatoid arthritis, and thymoma have also been described in patients with this syndrome. In some patients improvement in diarrhea and malabsorption may occur spontaneously, whereas in others improvement may follow treatment with a gluten-free diet, corticosteroids, antibiotics, injections of γ globulin, and cholestyramine. These forms of therapy have not been uniformly successful. Although transient improvement is common, complete cessation of symptoms is distinctly unusual.

The relationship between hypogammaglobulinemia and malabsorption remains obscure. There is no evidence to date indicating that excessive enteric loss of γ globulin or alteration of the intestinal microflora occurs, but abnormalities in IgA metabolism may be important in this syndrome. This immunoglobulin is the predominant one in the intestinal mucosa and is found in many exocrine secretions, including tears, saliva, gastric juice, and intestinal juice. A few patients have been described with malabsorption and selective deficiency of IgA.

Abetalipoproteinemia See Chap. 100.

Hartnup disease, cystinuria See Chap. 90.

ENDOCRINE AND METABOLIC DISORDERS **Diabetes mellitus** The occurrence of diarrhea and steatorrhea in patients with diabetes mellitus has been well documented. When steatorrhea

accompanies diabetes, it may be due to the presence of (1) exocrine pancreatic insufficiency, (2) coexistent nontropical sprue, (3) abnormal bacterial proliferation in the proximal small bowel, or (4) severe and uncontrolled diabetes per se (e.g., so-called "diabetic diarrhea"). Patients falling into the first three categories will usually respond in a satisfactory manner to treatment with pancreatic extracts, a gluten-free diet, and antibiotics, respectively. The pathogenesis of diarrhea and steatorrhea in patients in the fourth category remains poorly understood, and the response to various forms of therapy has been quite variable. It has been demonstrated that patients with "diabetic diarrhea" and steatorrhea may have involvement of the autonomic nervous system with degenerative changes in the sympathetic and parasympathetic nerves and ganglia. In some patients bacterial overgrowth in the stomach and proximal small bowel may occur and contribute to the diarrhea and steatorrhea.

The clinical features in patients with diarrhea and steatorrhea due to diabetes per se seem to be fairly uniform. Diabetes usually develops at a young age and is often severe and difficult to control. There is a distinct predominance of males. Several signs of autonomic neuropathy are usually present, including postural hypotension, anhydrosis, impotence, and bladder irregularities. Peripheral vascular disease and peripheral neuropathy are also common. Gastrointestinal x-rays may show delayed gastric emptying and disordered transit through the small bowel. Peroral small-bowel biopsy specimens are normal. Tests of intestinal absorptive function are normal except for steatorrhea and azotorrhea. There has been no consistent response to therapy with pancreatic extracts, gluten-free diet, or corticosteroids. When bacterial overgrowth is present, broad-spectrum antibiotics may be helpful.

Hypoparathyroidism Steatorrhea has been documented in several patients with idiopathic hypoparathyroidism. In addition to hypocalcemia, impaired absorption of D-xylose and vitamin B_{12}, decreased serum iron values, and abnormal small-intestinal roentgenograms have been demonstrated in some cases. In such patients the serum phosphorus level is elevated (due to the hypoparathyroidism) rather than low (as in primary malabsorption). The cause of malabsorption in this disorder is unclear. With regard to steatorrhea, however, preliminary studies suggest that luminal calcium modifies esterification and transport of absorbed fatty acids.

Adrenal insufficiency Although there are few studies on fat excretion in adrenal insufficiency in man, malabsorption, especially of fat, appears to occur more frequently than has been generally appreciated. Patients with adrenal insufficiency have been found to have steatorrhea which was corrected by therapy with adrenal corticosteroids.

Hyperthyroidism There are few detailed studies on intestinal absorptive function in patients with hyperthyroidism. Mild to moderate steatorrhea and hypoalbuminemia have been reported, but absorption of D-xylose and vitamin B_{12} is frequently normal. Steatorrhea usually remits after successful treatment of hyperthyroidism. Experimental studies suggest that steatorrhea in hyperthyroidism is not due to any defect of pancreatic, biliary, or small-intestinal mucosal function, but is a result of hyperphagia with ingestion of unusually large amounts of fat occurring in association with rapid gastric emptying and intestinal transit.

Ulcerogenic tumor of the pancreas (Zollinger-Ellison syndrome) The clinical features of ulcerogenic tumor of the pancreas are described in Chap. 290. Malabsorption is frequently found in this disease. The acidification and dilution of intestinal contents caused by gastric acid hypersecretion leads to major disturbances in fat digestion and absorption. Impaired formation of micellar lipid due to inactivation of pancreatic lipase is probably the major factor in the production of steatorrhea. Other factors contributing to fat malabsorption in this disorder include (1) precipitation of glycine conjugated bile salts due to low intraluminal pH, (2) alteration of the intestinal mucosa with ulceration and metaplasia, and (3) impaired fatty acid esterification and chylomicron formation.

Carcinoid syndrome (see Chap. 91)   Although diarrhea is common in the carcinoid syndrome, malabsorption with significant steatorrhea is unusual. In many of the cases of carcinoid syndrome with steatorrhea there has been a prior intestinal resection (usually ileal), and in these cases the resection is the important factor in the causation of steatorrhea. However, direct involvement of the bowel wall and mesentery by the carcinoid tumor have been well documented. That abnormalities in serotonin metabolism may also be important is suggested from the decrease in the steatorrhea observed in some of these patients when treated with the antiserotonin drug methysergide. Although side effects may occur, for control of diarrhea and steatorrhea, patients may be given a trial of 8 to 12 mg methysergide per day.

DRUG-INDUCED ABSORPTIVE DEFECTS   See Table 292-8.

PROTEIN-LOSING ENTEROPATHY   The gastrointestinal tract has been shown to play a significant role in the metabolism and physiologic degradation of plasma proteins. The exact magnitude of the normal gastrointestinal protein loss in man has remained unclear, but studies with ^{125}I-labeled and ^{51}Cr-labeled albumin have suggested that between 10 and 20 percent of the normal turnover of albumin may be accounted for by enteric protein loss. However, under certain pathologic conditions, excessive gastrointestinal protein loss may develop. An extensive number of disorders have been found to be associated with intestinal protein loss. Some of these are listed in Table 292-9.

Pathophysiology   Several mechanisms have been proposed for the passage of plasma proteins across the gastrointestinal mucosa, both normally and in certain disease states. First, plasma proteins may pass into the gastrointestinal tract through an inflamed or ulcerated mucosa and account for the protein loss occasionally seen in regional enteritis and ulcerative colitis. Second, plasma protein loss may occur as a result of disordered mucosal cell structure. For example, patients with nontropical sprue have abnormal villous structure and surface epithelium, and these changes could facilitate the diffusion of plasma protein between the cells. Third, in the presence of increased lymphatic pressure, there may be increased passage of plasma proteins into the lumen via the intercellular spaces of the mucosal epithelium. This might be expected to occur in disorders in which there is granulomatous or neoplastic involvement of lymphatics. Fourth, dilated lymph vessels in the mucosa may rupture through the surface epithelium, discharging their contents into the intestinal lumen. This is thought to be important in the pathogenesis of steatorrhea and hypoproteinemia in patients with idiopathic intestinal lymphangiectasia (see "Intestinal Lymphangiectasia," below).

Several techniques have been developed for the detection and quantitation of gastrointestinal protein loss. Most of these involve the use of intravenously administered radioactive-labeled macromolecules such as ^{125}I-labeled serum albumin, ^{51}CrCl$_3$, ^{51}Cr-labeled albumin, and [^{67}Cu]ceruloplasmin. ^{51}Cr-labeled albumin and ^{51}CrCl$_3$ (both of which rapidly become attached to circulating transferrin) are the compounds used most frequently. After the intravenous administration of 25 to 30 μCi of the labeled compound to normal subjects, between 0.1 and 0.7 percent of the administered radioactivity is recovered in the stool over a 4-day period. Patients with excessive enteric protein loss may excrete from 2 to 40 percent of the injected radioactive label. False-positive results may be obtained if the stool specimen is contaminated with urine.

Using intravenously administered radioiodinated albumin, the decline in radioactivity in the serum and whole body can be followed, and the rate of albumin synthesis and degradation determined. Such studies carried out in patients with protein-losing enteropathies have demonstrated a reduced circulating (intravascular) and total body pool of albumin, a normal or increased rate of albumin synthesis, markedly shortened albumin survival, and increased fecal protein loss. Whereas normal subjects catabolize 5 to 10 percent of their intravascular albumin pool each day (the fractional catabolic rate), patients with excessive enteric protein loss may have fractional catabolic rates of 50 to 60 percent.

Studies utilizing radioiodinated immunoglobulins have

TABLE 292-9
Disorders associated with protein-losing enteropathy

I Stomach
   A Gastric carcinoma
   B Giant hypertrophy of the gastric mucosa
   C Atrophic gastritis
   D Postgastrectomy syndrome
II Small intestine
   A Nontropic sprue
   B Tropical sprue
   C Regional enteritis
   D Whipple's disease
   E Lymphoma
   F Intestinal lymphangiectasia
   G Intestinal tuberculosis
   H Acute infectious enteritis
   I Scleroderma
   J Jejunal diverticulosis
   K Allergic gastroenteropathy
III Colon
   A Colonic neoplasm
   B Ulcerative colitis
   C Granulomatous colitis
   D Megacolon
IV Cardiac
   A Congestive heart failure
   B Constrictive pericarditis
   C Interatrial septal defect
   D Primary cardiomyopathy
V Miscellaneous
   A Esophageal carcinoma
   B Gastrocolic fistula
   C Agammaglobulinemia
   D Nephrosis

TABLE 292-8
Some drug-induced absorptive defects

Drug	Absorptive defect
Antacids	Phosphorus
Anticonvulsants	Folates
Biguanides (DBI)	Glucose, amino acids, vitamin B$_{12}$
Cholestyramine	Warfarin, thyroid hormone, cardiac glycosides, phenylbutazone
Colchicine	Xylose, vitamin B$_{12}$, cholesterol
Ethanol	Xylose, vitamin B$_{12}$, folate, glucose, amino acids
Methotrexate	Xylose, folic acid
Neomycin	Fatty acids, xylose, vitamin B$_{12}$
p-Aminosalicylic acid (PAS)	Cholesterol, vitamin B$_{12}$
Sulfasalazine	Folate
Tetracycline	Ferrous ions

SOURCE: *Longstreth and Newcomer.*

demonstrated a decreased intravascular globulin pool and increased fractional catabolic rate. However, the synthesis of IgG is usually normal, suggesting that a decreased level of IgG and increased enteric protein loss is not a potent stimulus for IgG synthesis. The increase in fractional catabolic rate is comparable for albumin, IgG, and IgM immunoglobulins, further suggesting that there is bulk loss of plasma proteins into the intestinal tract and not a selective loss of certain proteins. The finding of decreased globulins often is an ancillary aid in excluding renal, cardiac, and hepatic cases of hypoalbuminemia.

Abnormalities in albumin and globulin metabolism in patients with a protein-losing enteropathy may be reversed or diminished within a few months after the institution of appropriate therapy. It is obviously important that a specific etiologic diagnosis should be established in all patients with treatable disorders, who may be expected to have a remission induced by the appropriate therapy for the underlying disease. The intestinal protein loss in patients with nontropical sprue, Whipple's disease, constrictive pericarditis, regional enteritis, ulcerative colitis, and Ménétrier's disease has been ameliorated by therapy appropriate for the underlying disorder.

Intestinal lymphangiectasia PATHOPHYSIOLOGY The disorder intestinal lymphangiectasia is characterized by increased enteric loss of protein, hypoproteinemia, edema, lymphocytopenia, malabsorption, and abnormal dilated lymphatic channels in the small intestine. The high incidence of chylous effusions and abnormal peripheral, retroperitoneal, and thoracic lymphatics indicates that intestinal lymphangiectasia is part of a generalized congenital disorder of the lymphatic system. It has been suggested that the hypoplastic visceral lymphatic channels result in obstruction to lymph flow, with the subsequent development of increased intestinal lymphatic pressure. This in turn may lead to dilated lymphatic vessels throughout the small-bowel wall and mesentery. Hypoproteinemia and steatorrhea are thought to be due to rupture of the dilated lymphatic vessels with discharge of lymph into the bowel lumen. In adults approximately 1500 ml lymph, containing 70 g fat and 50 g albumin, passes through the thoracic duct each day. The leakage of a small amount of this lymph might be expected to result in considerable loss of protein and fat into the intestinal lumen. In addition, absorption of dietary long-chain triglycerides stimulates lymph flow, and this may increase further the retrograde leakage of intestinal lymph into the lumen. Three lines of evidence support the concept of intestinal leakage of lymph in intestinal lymphangiectasia: (1) chylous fluid has been recovered from the duodenum in these patients; (2) retrograde passage of contrast material from retroperitoneal lymphatics into the duodenum and jejunum has been documented; and (3) significant steatorrhea may persist in patients after institution of a completely fat-free diet, suggesting an increased enteric loss of endogenous fat present in lymph.

CLINICAL FEATURES The disease affects primarily children and young adults. All patients have edema, which may be asymmetrical because of hypoplastic peripheral lymphatics. Chylous effusions and diarrhea are common symptoms. The primary laboratory finding is hypoproteinemia with decreased serum levels of albumin, immunoglobulins IgG, IgA, and IgM, transferrin, and ceruloplasmin. Despite moderate to severe hypogammaglobulinemia there does not appear to be an increased incidence of pyogenic bacterial infections. In addition, circulating antibody response to challenge with *Brucella* and typhoid antigens is normal. Steatorrhea is usually mild, although in some instances fat loss may be as much as 40 g per day. Some patients have hypocalcemia and impaired absorption of vitamin B_{12}. Lymphocytopenia (due to the loss of lymphocytes in lymph) is common, with lymphocyte counts ranging from 400 to 1000 per milliliter (normal: 1500 to 4000 per

milliliter. This is associated with abnormal delayed hypersensitivity, as evidenced by prolonged homograft survival and impaired cutaneous responsiveness to antigens such as mumps and monilia.

Small-bowel roentgenograms are frequently abnormal, showing changes of mucosal edema and a malabsorption pattern. Lymphangiograms may demonstrate hypoplastic peripheral and visceral lymphatics with the absence of groups of retroperitoneal lymph nodes. Specimens of jejunal mucosa characteristically reveal dilated and telangiectatic lymphatic vessels in the lamina propria and submucosa. The villi may be club-shaped because of distortion from grossly dilated lymphatics (Fig. 292-4). Such changes in the intestinal mucosa may be reversed after appropriate therapy. The diagnosis of intestinal lymphangiectasia is therefore established by (1) small-intestinal biopsy and (2) demonstration of increased enteric protein loss using radioactive macromolecules.

TREATMENT A low-fat diet, by decreasing lymph flow, usually results in significant improvement with decreased fecal fat excretion, decreased enteric protein loss, increased serum calcium and albumin levels, and an increased half-life of injected ^{131}I-labeled albumin. Similar results may be obtained by the substitution of medium-chain triglycerides (MCT) for dietary long-chain triglycerides, since MCT are transported as medium-chain fatty acids by the portal vein rather than via the lymph.

REFERENCES

AMENT ME et al: Pathogenesis of steatorrhea in 3 cases of small intestinal stasis syndrome. Gastroenterology 63:728, 1972

——— et al: Structure and function of the gastrointestinal tract in primary immunodeficiency syndromes. Medicine 52:227, 1973

BAYLESS TM et al: Lactose and milk intolerance: Clinical implications. N Engl J Med 292:1156, 1975

BOND JH, LEVITT MD: Use of breath hydrogen (H_2) in the study of carbohydrate absorption. Am J Dig Dis 22:379, 1977

CALDWELL JH et al: Eosinophilic gastroenteritis with obstruction. Immunological studies of seven patients. Gastroenterology 74:825, 1978

CHUNG YC et al: Protein digestion and absorption in human small intestine. Gastroenterology 76:1415, 1979

FALCHUK ZM et al: In vitro model of gluten sensitive enteropathy: Effect of gliadin on intestinal epithelial cells of patients with gluten-sensitive enteropathy in organ culture. J Clin Invest 53:487, 1974

GRAY GM: Carbohydrate digestion and absorption: Role of the small intestine. N Engl J Med 292:1225, 1975

HOFMANN AF, POLEY JR: Role of bile acid malabsorption in pathogenesis of diarrhea and steatorrhea in patients with ileal resection. Gastroenterology 62:918, 1972

LONGSTRETH GF, NEWCOMER AD: Drug-induced malabsorption. Mayo Clin Proc 50:284, 1975

MACGREGOR I et al: Gastric emptying of liquid meals and pancreatic and biliary secretion after subtotal gastrectomy or truncal vagotomy and pyloroplasty in man. Gastroenterology 72:195, 1977

MATTHEWS, DM, ADIBI SA: Peptide absorption. Gastroenterology 71:151, 1976

NEWCOMER AD et al: Triolein breath test. A sensitive and specific test for fat malabsorption. Gastroenterology 76:6, 1979

PENA AS et al: Genetic basis of gluten-sensitive enteropathy. Gastroenterology 75:233, 1978

ROMMEL K et al: *Lipid Absorption: Biochemical and Clinical Aspects.* Lancaster, England, MTP Press, 1976

TRIER JS et al: Celiac sprue and refractory sprue. Gastroenterology 75:307, 1978

293

DISEASES OF THE SMALL INTESTINE

ROBERT M. GLICKMAN
KURT J. ISSELBACHER

SYMPTOMS OF SMALL-BOWEL DISEASE

The major symptoms of small-bowel disease are those due to *motility disturbances,* abdominal *pain,* gastrointestinal *bleeding,* and *malabsorption.* An alteration in the normal propulsive activity of the small intestine is a common manifestation of a variety of diseases. The presentation may be one of decreased motility such as ileus or intestinal obstruction (Chap. 295) due to any process which directly infiltrates or obstructs the lumen of the bowel. An impairment of the blood supply to the intestine or involvement of the serosal surface by a contiguous inflammation (i.e., peritonitis) is usually associated with the development of ileus. A variety of nonintestinal but metabolic disturbances (e.g., uremia, hypokalemia, hypercalcemia) can alter small-bowel propulsive activity and thus secondarily produce a paralytic type of ileus. Diarrhea frequently accompanies small-bowel disease (see Chap. 37) resulting from direct involvement of the mucosa by inflammatory or infiltrative lesions (sprue, regional enteritis). The associated malabsorption of fat and bile salts are important factors in the pathogenesis of diarrhea in these conditions (Chaps. 37 and 292).

Abdominal pain due to small-intestinal disease is usually periumbilical or supraumbilical and often poorly localized. With obstruction, pain is classically described as intermittent or colicky. As the intestine becomes progressively dilated with loss of muscular tone, the colicky nature of the pain may become less apparent. Acute inflammation of the small intestine which involves the visceral or parietal peritoneum is associated with steady, aching pain, usually located directly over the inflamed area, and often is accompanied by guarding and rebound tenderness. *Gastrointestinal bleeding* due to small-bowel disease may be detected as occult bleeding or, less commonly, brisk hemorrhage. In general, brisk bleeding from a source beyond the ligament of Treitz is not acted on by gastric acid and appears as a dark maroon color in contrast to the black, tarry melena which often results from gastric or duodenal bleeding. Obviously, the appearance of blood in the stool depends not only on site of bleeding but also on the briskness of the hemorrhage and the rapidity of transit; thus localization of the bleeding site by stool appearance alone may be misleading. An important clue to the presence of small-bowel diseases is the demonstration of some abnormality in intestinal absorption. With extensive mucosal damage or lymphatic obstruction, the presenting symptoms may relate to any of the features of a malabsorption syndrome or protein-losing enteropathy (Chap. 292) and should direct attention to the small intestine.

USEFUL DIAGNOSTIC PROCEDURES

Careful *examination* of the abdomen may disclose a mass or fistula associated with inflammatory or neoplastic disease, localized tenderness, or abdominal distention resulting from ileus or intestinal obstruction. The physical examination and findings in the patient with acute abdominal pain are discussed in Chap. 6.

Thorough examination may also reveal extraintestinal findings associated with small-intestinal diseases. Thus buccal pigmentation or telangiectasia may indicate coexistent small-bowel polyposis or telangiectasia and may clarify episodes of abdominal pain or chronic bleeding. Similarly, evidence of iritis, arthritis, or erythema nodosum may suggest the presence of inflammatory bowel disease.

Laboratory features of anemia, leukocytosis, or specific evidence of malabsorption, which may accompany many diseases of the small bowel, usually reflect the underlying pathologic process and are rarely diagnostic. The considerable length of the small intestine (some 12 to 22 ft in the adult) makes *radiologic studies* of the small bowel of prime importance and usually forms the basis for the diagnosis of small-bowel diseases. *Small-bowel x-rays* are not usually part of a routine upper gastrointestinal series and must be specifically requested. In view of the length of the small bowel and wide variations in transit time, it is essential to provide the radiologist with as much information as possible, since the precise nature of the problem may determine various technical aspects of the examination. It is only through sequential examination of the barium column as it progresses through the small bowel that localized abnormalities such as tumors, fistulas, areas of ischemia, or inflammatory bowel disease may be apparent. Visualization of the terminal ileum is often possible on *barium enema* when barium refluxes through the ileocecal valve and is of major value in the diagnosis of regional ileitis. *Mesenteric angiography* often is of help in the diagnosis of vascular insufficiency of the small bowel, localization of bleeding to a small bowel source, and in the demonstration of vascular malformations and small tumors.

Gastrointestinal endoscopy permits direct visualization and biopsy of most duodenal lesions; biopsy of the more distal bowel can be carried out using peroral biopsy instruments (see Chap. 292). Intestinal biopsy is of great value in the diagnosis of generalized inflammatory or infiltrative diseases such as sprue, amyloidosis, or generalized lymphoma.

DIVERTICULOSIS

Diverticula may occur in any portion of the small intestine; however, with the exception of Meckel's diverticulum, the most common locations are in the duodenum and jejunum. Histologically, congenital diverticula are herniations of the entire thickness of the intestinal wall, while the more common acquired diverticula consist only of herniated mucosa and serosa. The incidence of diverticula rises with age, presumably representing acquired weakness of the bowel wall, usually at the points where the nutrient arteries penetrate the serosal and muscular layers.

Most often diverticula are asymptomatic and discovered incidentally on upper gastrointestinal x-rays. On occasion, however, they may cause symptoms either because of their anatomic proximity to other structures or rarely from inflammation or bleeding.

Duodenal diverticula usually are single and found most commonly on the medial surface of the second portion of the duodenum. Rarely, they may become inflamed and present as acute diverticulitis with abdominal pain, fever, gastrointestinal bleeding, or, rarely, perforation. Adjacent structures, such as the bile or pancreatic ducts, may become involved, and cases of common-duct obstruction and pancreatitis have been reported. Jejunal diverticula, while less common, may also be the site of acute inflammation, bleeding, or perforation with resulting abscess or peritonitis.

Multiple jejunal diverticula may be associated with a malabsorption syndrome related to bacterial overgrowth within the diverticula, similar to other situations where intestinal stasis (i.e., blind loops) permits bacterial proliferation. The consequences of bacterial proliferation with resultant mucosal damage, deconjugation of bile salts, and vitamin B_{12} malabsorption are discussed in Chap. 292.

Meckel's diverticulum represents a persistence of the omphalomesenteric duct and is the most frequent congenital anomaly of the digestive tract, occurring in approximately 2 percent of autopsied adults. It arises from the antimesenteric border of the ileum, usually within 100 cm of the ileocecal valve. The diverticulum is usually wide-mouthed, approximately 2 in long, and usually ends blindly. All layers of the digestive tract are present. The diverticulum may be lined with normal ileal mucosa (approximately 50 percent) or contain gastric, duodenal, ectopic pancreatic, or colonic mucosa. While usually asymptomatic, massive gastrointestinal bleeding and inflammation are two prominent complications of a Meckel's diverticulum. In children, gastrointestinal bleeding is the striking clinical feature and accounts for half of all lower gastrointestinal bleeding in this age group. Numerous cases have also been reported in young adults. Usually, the onset of bleeding is painless and the stool may appear maroon, suggesting a bleeding site beyond the stomach. The source of bleeding is almost invariably an ileal ulceration, usually of peptic origin. The gastric mucosa in a Meckel's diverticulum has been shown to secrete acid peptic juice, which leads to ulceration of adjacent ileal epithelium. Conventional gastrointestinal x-rays usually do not demonstrate the diverticulum; however on occasion it may fill with barium. Mesenteric angiography during active bleeding may demonstrate an ileal source for the bleeding. Technetium scans are valuable in the diagnosis of Meckel's diverticulum (Fig. 293-1), the isotope being taken up and concentrated within the secretory epithelium lining the diverticulum.

Meckel's diverticulum should be considered in the differential diagnosis of painless gastrointestinal bleeding, especially when conventional x-rays are negative. Technetium scanning or mesenteric angiography may yield the correct diagnosis. The treatment is entirely surgical. In the young adult, the clinical presentation may change, with inflammatory features becoming more prominent. A picture indistinguishable from acute appendicitis may result, and failure to find an inflamed

FIGURE 293-1

Meckel's diverticulum (technetium abdominal scan). After the intravenous administration of ^{99m}Tc, the abdominal scan shows the isotope concentrated in the gastric mucosa (s), the urinary bladder (b), and in an ectopic area (m) surgically proved to be Meckel's diverticulum. (Courtesy of S Treves.)

appendix should prompt the surgeon to search for a Meckel's diverticulum.

REGIONAL ENTERITIS (CROHN'S DISEASE)

DEFINITION Regional enteritis is a chronic inflammatory disorder of unknown etiology, often with granulomatous reaction, which may involve any portion of the gastrointestinal tract. The original description of the disease by Crohn, Ginzberg, and Oppenheimer in 1932 localized the disease to segments of ileum. However, it is now known that the same process may involve the esophagus, stomach, and duodenum, as well as the jejunum and ileum. In addition, a similar inflammatory picture may occur in the colon, either alone or with accompanying small-intestinal involvement. In most instances, this granulomatous colitis can be distinguished clinically and pathologically from ulcerative colitis (see Chap. 294) and is also referred to as Crohn's disease of the colon. Clinically, regional enteritis is characterized by recurrent inflammatory involvement of intestinal segments with diverse clinical manifestations and often resulting in a chronic, unpredictable course.

EPIDEMIOLOGY Regional enteritis is worldwide in distribution and occurs in all races. While the disease has been reported to be less common in nonwhites, it is difficult to determine the influence of varying awareness and detection facilities on such statistics. In the United States the annual incidence is about 2 to 3 per 100,000, and this incidence seems to be on the increase. Both sexes are equally affected. While peak occurrence of the disease is between the ages of 15 and 35, it has been reported in every decade of life. Patients often are of Jewish origin; surveys in the United States indicated that the disease is two to three times more common in Jews than non-Jews. A familial occurrence of the disease has been noted in most large series, with estimates that 2 to 5 percent of persons with regional enteritis or ulcerative colitis will have one or more relatives affected. The disease has also been described in monozygotic twins. In spite of this apparent familial clustering, no simple pattern of mendelian inheritance is apparent, and it remains to be determined whether a single gene is involved or whether a possible hereditary basis involves many genes plus a strong environmental component (see below).

ETIOLOGY AND PATHOGENESIS While the cause of regional enteritis is unknown, certain features of the disease have suggested several areas of possible etiologic importance. These include familial, or genetic, infectious, and immunologic factors.

The observations that regional enteritis is more common in whites, occurs with an increased incidence in Jews, and exhibits familial clustering have suggested that there may be a *genetic predisposition* to the development of the disease. This has prompted a search for genetic markers which might be of value in identifying susceptible individuals. One approach has been to survey the major histocompatibility antigens in patients with regional enteritis. While none of the antigens surveyed appears to be specific for patients with regional enteritis, 75 percent of patients who exhibit associated ankylosing spondylitis are positive for HLA-B27, a histocompatibility antigen present in approximately 8 percent of normal individuals. A similarly high incidence of HLA-B27 has been found in idiopathic ankylosing spondylitis unassociated with inflammatory bowel disease. Therefore, while not specific for regional enteritis, the association of ankylosing spondylitis with inflammatory bowel disease in those patients who are HLA-B27–positive may indicate a possible underlying genetic susceptibility.

The chronic inflammatory nature of regional enteritis coupled with a granulomatous reaction has prompted a continuing search for a possible *infectious basis* for the disease. In spite of numerous attempts to find known bacterial, fungal, or viral agents, no etiologic agent has thus far been isolated. Studies have been carried out to determine whether a transmissible agent is present in intestinal and lymphatic tissue of patients with regional enteritis by injecting extracts of these tissues (obtained at surgery) into laboratory animals. A granulomatous inflammatory reaction has been produced in the footpads of mice after such injections, but the specificity of such a response remains to be determined. A more extensive granulomatous response, with many of the pathologic features of regional enteritis, has been described following the serosal injection of tissue extracts into the ileum of rabbits. While it remains to be demonstrated that such responses can be serially transmitted, these observations have raised the possibility that a transmissible agent may be involved in the etiology of the disease. While there are increasing reports concerning the isolation of a variety of agents (viruses, L forms of bacteria) from Crohn's disease tissues, the specificity of these isolates remains to be determined. In one instance, however, a specific infectious agent has been associated with an infectious form of ileitis. *Yersinia enterocolitis* infection has been shown to result in a syndrome of acute ileitis, which in many respects resembles regional enteritis (see below). While *Yersinia* infection cannot be implicated in most cases of regional enteritis, it has heightened interest in the search for an infectious etiology of this disease.

The theory than an *immune mechanism* may be involved is based on the concept that the extracolonic manifestations of the disease (e.g., arthritis, pericholangitis) may represent autoimmune phenomena and that agents such as corticosteroids and azathioprine, which are often helpful in treatment of the disease, may exert their effects via immunosuppressive mechanisms. Patients with inflammatory bowel disease may have humoral antibodies to colon cells and to bacterial antigens such as *Escherichia coli* 0 to 14. However, there is no clear evidence that these antibody changes are of primary pathogenic significance, and they may simply be the response to secondary intestinal epithelial damage.

Abnormalities of cell-mediated immunity have also been described in patients with regional enteritis. These include decreased skin test responsiveness to tuberculin and dinitrochlorobenzene, diminished responsiveness of lymphocytes to various mitogens, as well as a decrease in the number of T (thymus-derived) cells in the peripheral blood. In addition, lymphocyte-mediated cytotoxicity for colonic epithelial cells have been demonstrated, utilizing lymphocytes from both patients with ulcerative colitis and those with regional enteritis. In addition, experimental colitis has been produced in laboratory animals by prior sensitization with dinitrochlorobenzene, suggesting a T cell–dependent mechanism of tissue injury. Despite these provocative observations, it remains to be demonstrated that alterations in cellular immunity are of primary importance in the pathogenesis of regional enteritis.

PATHOLOGY A thorough familiarity with the pathologic changes seen in regional enteritis will greatly aid the clinician in understanding the diverse radiologic and clinical manifestations of this disease. The disease is characterized by chronic inflammation extending through *all layers of the intestinal wall* and involving the mesentery as well as regional lymph nodes.

The earliest pathologic changes in regional enteritis are poorly defined since surgery is usually not electively undertaken early in the course of the disease. However, in a small group of patients, the initial presentation is associated with the acute onset of right lower quadrant pain suggestive of acute appendicitis. At laparotomy, rather than finding acute appendicitis, the surgeon may find the terminal ileum to be hyperemic and boggy, with the mesentery and mesenteric lymph nodes swollen and reddened. At this early stage, the bowel wall, although edematous, is usually pliable. While some patients with this initial presentation will subsequently develop typical regional enteritis, a significant number will recover completely. This acute form of ileitis will undoubtedly be shown to have diverse etiologies. Indeed, a small number of patients with this presentation have been shown to be infected with *Y. enterocolitis,* an organism apparently capable of producing self-limited acute inflammatory ileitis.

As the disease progresses, the gross appearance assumes a characteristic picture. The bowel appears greatly thickened and leathery with the lumen narrowed (Fig. 293-2). This characteristic stenosis, most often present in the terminal ileum, can occur in any portion of the intestine and may be associated with varying degrees of intestinal obstruction (Fig. 293-3). The mesentery appears greatly thickened, fatty, and often extends over the serosal surface of the bowel in characteristic finger-like projections. The appearance of the mucosa is variable, depending on the severity and stage of the disease, but may appear relatively normal. In more advanced cases, the mucosa appears nodular with a "cobblestoned" look. This is the result of submucosal thickening and mucosal ulceration, often linear

FIGURE 293-2
Regional enteritis. Resected specimen of terminal ileum demonstrates thickened bowel wall and chronically inflamed mucosa. Note the relatively sharp demarcation of the diseased segment with grossly normal mucosa on the left.

FIGURE 293-3

Regional enteritis. Radiograph showing extensive involvement and narrowing of distal ileum.

in the long axis of the bowel at the base of mucosal folds. These ulcerations may penetrate into the submucosa and muscularis and coalesce to form intramural channels.

Microscopically, an inflammatory response largely consisting of lymphocytes and plasma cells involves all layers of the bowel wall. In approximately 50 percent of cases there are well-defined, noncaseating granulomas, containing multinucleated giant cells. While usually present in the submucosa, they may be found in any portion of the intestinal wall as well as in

the mesentery, regional lymph nodes, and liver. While granulomas are most helpful in distinguishing regional enteritis from other forms of inflammatory bowel disease, it is the chronic inflammation involving all layers of the intestinal wall which is most characteristic.

The transmural inflammatory process, involving serosa and mesentery, also accounts for other characteristic features of this disease, namely, fistula and abscess formation. As a result of serosal inflammation, adjacent loops of small intestine may become adherent and matted together by a fibrous peritoneal reaction. Clinically this may lead to and account for fullness or a palpable mass, most often in the right lower quadrant. Chronic inflammation between adjacent loops of bowel may lead to fistula formation and to communications between adherent loops of intestine (Fig. 293-4). Thus fistula formation may occur between segments of small intestine, colon, or other adjacent organs such as the bladder or vagina. Fistulous tracts may also lead to the skin or end blindly within the peritoneum or retroperitoneum, surrounded by adherent loops of bowel and inflammatory tissue. The latter are essentially abscess cavities communicating with the lumen of the bowel. They may pursue an indolent course or present abruptly with systemic evidence of severe sepsis (see below).

The disease process is often discontinuous in that severely involved segments of bowel are separated from each other with intervening segments of apparently normal bowel producing so-called "skip areas." The terminal ileum is the most common location of the disease, but in 10 to 15 percent of patients there may be diffuse and extensive ulceration of jejunum and ileum. This *diffuse ileojejunitis* is most often seen in children and adolescents and represents a particularly severe form of the disease.

Crohn's disease of the colon (Chap. 294) is indistinguishable pathologically from regional enteritis; in fact, small-bowel and colonic disease frequently coexist. Approximately 10 percent

FIGURE 293-4

Regional enteritis. X-ray showing fistulas between loops of bowel. Insert is a compression film of this area; note fistulas between adjacent loops of bowel.

of patients with granulomatous inflammatory bowel disease have colonic disease alone, and about 30 percent of cases have coexistent small-bowel and colonic involvement. For this reason, rectal biopsy may be of value in determining the nature of inflammatory bowel disease involving the small bowel and colon.

CLINICAL FEATURES The diverse pathologic features and variable intestinal involvement of the disease account for the multitude of clinical presentations which the clinician may encounter. The clinical features are a direct reflection of the location of the inflammatory lesion, its extent and acuteness, and its relationship to contiguous structures. Typically, the disease has its onset in a young adult with a history of fatigue, variable weight loss, right lower quadrant discomfort or pain, and diarrhea. Low-grade fever, anorexia, nausea, and vomiting may also be present. The abdominal pain may be steady and localized to the right lower quadrant or may assume a colicky or crampy pattern, reflecting variable degrees of intestinal stenosis. The diarrhea is often moderate, usually without gross blood; in the absence of rectal involvement, tenesmus is absent. Physical examination at this time often reveals right lower quadrant tenderness with an associated fullness or mass reflecting adherent loops of bowel. At this time the patient may have mild anemia, mild to moderate leukocytosis, and an elevated sedimentation rate.

Since *acute ileitis* may have an abrupt onset with fever, leukocytosis, and right lower quadrant pain, the clinical picture may be indistinguishable from acute appendicitis. The diagnosis can be made only at laparotomy when the characteristic beefy-red terminal ileum, boggy mesenteric fat, and succulent mesenteric lymph nodes indicate that appendicitis alone could not produce this picture.

While the symptoms of diarrhea and abdominal pain will usually alert the clinician to the possibility of regional enteritis, other symptoms may dominate the clinical presentation. In children and the aged, *fever of undetermined origin* and unexplained *weight loss* may be prominent and initially make one suspect underlying malignancy. In some patients the first manifestations of the disease may be *intestinal obstruction;* in others the disease may present with *fistula formation* in the form of perianal sepsis or urinary tract infection resulting from an enterovesical fistula. Similarly, right *ureteral obstruction* and *hydronephrosis* may occur due to external compression of the ureter by a right lower quadrant inflammatory mass. On occasion, often in the setting of extensive small-bowel involvement, features of malabsorption may be prominent. These may include (1) secondary disaccharidase deficiency, (2) protein-losing enteropathy, (3) malabsorption of sugars, amino acids, and fats, (4) bacterial overgrowth, and (5) bile salt deficiency resulting from impaired ileal reabsorption of bile salts. These features, along with anorexia and the catabolic effects of the chronic inflammatory process, may combine to produce striking degrees of weight loss.

The complications of the disease can be divided into (1) local complications, resulting from intestinal inflammation and involvement of adjacent structures, and (2) extraintestinal manifestations.

Intestinal obstruction is a frequent complication occurring in 20 to 30 percent of patients during the course of the disease. In the initial stages, the obstruction usually is due to the acute inflammation and edema of the involved intestinal segment. However as the disease progresses and fibrosis develops, obstruction may be due to fixed narrowing of the bowel.

Fistula formation is a frequent complication of chronic regional enteritis. Fistulas may occur between contiguous segments of intestine; they may also burrow into the retroperito-

neal spaces and present as cutaneous fistulas or indolent abscesses. In a significant number of patients, the first indication of the disease may be the presence of persistent rectal fissures, a perirectal abscess, or a rectal fistula. Although uncommon, pneumaturia should raise the suspicion of enterovesical fistula and is often associated with a persistent urinary tract infection.

Since regional enteritis is a transmural disease with the bowel wall greatly thickened, free intestinal *perforation* is uncommon. In a small number of cases, however, it may be the presenting feature, and the disease is first discovered at the time of laparotomy for a perforated viscus. While occult blood in the stool can be detected in many patients, gross lower-intestinal bleeding is uncommon. The passage per rectum of bright-red blood should alert one to the possible coexistence of rectal involvement (i.e., ileocolitis).

The *extracolonic manifestations* of regional enteritis are similar to those seen in ulcerative colitis (Chap. 294) but occur less frequently. They include erythema nodosum, iritis, clubbing, pericholangitis, and arthritis, or frequently, ankylosing spondylitis. As discussed above, a high percentage of patients with ankylosing spondylitis are HLA-B27–positive. The joint manifestations may antedate the development of clinical bowel disease and often do not correlate with the activity of the associated bowel disease.

There are increasing reports of *small-bowel malignancy* developing in the setting of long-standing regional enteritis. However, while the risk of developing malignancy is statistically increased, the complication is uncommon when compared with the frequency of malignancy in ulcerative colitis (Chap. 294). As in other chronic inflammatory diseases, patients with long-standing regional enteritis may develop *amyloidosis,* which may involve the liver, spleen, intestine, and kidneys. The development of hepatosplenomegaly or significant proteinuria should suggest this complication. The presence of extensive ileal disease, resulting in bile salt malabsorption, is associated with a decreased bile salt pool and an increased lithogenesis of bile (see Chap. 307). These changes probably account for an increased incidence of *cholelithiasis,* and it is estimated that up to 30 percent of patients with extensive ileal disease will develop gallstones. Also, in the setting of ileal disease, there is increased intestinal absorption of dietary oxalate with resultant hyperoxaluria and the development of *urinary oxalate stones.*

Sigmoidoscopy should be performed in all cases of regional enteritis to evaluate possible colonic involvement, which occurs in approximately 30 percent of cases. The features of granulomatous colitis are discussed in Chap. 294.

DIAGNOSIS Regional enteritis should be suspected in the patient with intermittent diarrhea and abdominal pain, especially if there is also evidence of fever, weight loss, persistent perianal sepsis, or any of the extraintestinal manifestations of the disease. It should also be considered in the differential diagnosis of all types of malabsorption syndrome, intermittent intestinal obstruction, fever of unexplained origin, amyloidosis, and polyarthritis.

The *laboratory features* of regional enteritis are largely nonspecific and either reflect the inflammatory process or are secondary to intestinal malabsorption. Mild degrees of leukocytosis and an elevated erythrocyte sedimentation rate are common. Patients usually have a variable degree of anemia, which may result from occult blood loss or the effect of chronic inflammation on the bone marrow. Folate or vitamin B_{12} malabsorption may also contribute to the anemia. Serum vitamin B_{12} levels may be low. While the Schilling test may be abnormal in patients with extensive ileal disease, frank macrocytic anemia due to vitamin B_{12} malabsorption alone is unusual, attesting to the marked efficiency of ileal absorption of the vitamin. When there is significant diarrhea, electrolyte abnormalities (hypokalemia, hypomagnesemia) may be prominent. Hypocalcemia may reflect extensive mucosal involvement and malabsorption of vitamin D. Hypoalbuminemia may result from amino acid malabsorption as well as from protein-losing enteropathy. In the setting of bile salt depletion and mucosal damage, variable degrees of steatorrhea may be found. Mild abnormalities of liver function (especially an increased serum alkaline phosphatase) may reflect the development of a fatty liver in the malnourished patient or a coexisting pericholangitis. Significant jaundice is unusual.

Radiologic examination of the bowel provides the most definitive aid in establishing the diagnosis of regional enteritis. Careful x-ray examination of the small bowel may demonstrate loss of mucosal detail and rigidity of involved segments resulting from submucosal edema or stenosis. The submucosal inflammation may lead to the characteristic radiologic cobble-stoned appearance of the mucosa. With more advanced disease, fibrosis and strictures may develop (Fig. 293-2) and fistulous tracts may be seen, especially in the ileocecal area. Involvement of the stomach and duodenum usually appears radiologically as stiffening and infiltration of the mucosa, and can mimic an infiltrative tumor. If such an appearance is due to regional enteritis, there is almost always coexistent involvement of either the jejunum or ileum. A barium enema should be performed, since colonic involvement coexists in about one-third of patients with regional enteritis. The radiologic appearance of granulomatous colitis is discussed in Chap. 294 and shares many of the radiologic features of regional enteritis.

While in most patients with the typical clinical features and characteristic x-ray findings the diagnosis is clear; on occasion histologic confirmation of the granulomatous inflammation is desirable. Since ileal biopsy by noninvasive techniques is usually not feasible, and since coexisting colonic involvement occurs in a significant number of cases, rectal biopsy may be of value. Direct biopsy of perianal inflammatory lesions as well as areas of rectal disease seen at sigmoidoscopy will often show features compatible with granulomatous inflammation. While not as well established, rectal biopsy of seemingly "uninvolved" areas noted at sigmoidoscopy may also show microscopic evidence of granulomatous inflammation. When gastric or duodenal involvement is suspected, biopsy of involved areas via the endoscope is often of value.

DIFFERENTIAL DIAGNOSIS The differential diagnosis of regional enteritis may be difficult before characteristic clinical and radiologic features are apparent. Many such patients, early in their diseases, are thought to have functional diarrhea. The presence of constitutional symptoms such as fatigue, fever, and weight loss, coupled with laboratory features of anemia, elevated erythrocyte sedimentation rate, or occult blood in the stool should alert the clinician to the possibility of inflammatory bowel disease. Similarly, the finding of leukocytes in a stained stool specimen points to an inflammatory basis for the diarrhea. In all cases, stool cultures and parasitologic examination of the stool are required to rule out enteric bacterial pathogens or amebiasis. With diffuse involvement of the jejunum and ileum, regional enteritis must be distinguished from *nongranulomatous ulcerative jejunoileitis.* Abdominal pain and diarrhea are prominent features of this disorder, and weight loss, malabsorption, and hypoproteinemia tend to be more prominent than in regional enteritis. Small-bowel biopsy shows a more diffuse lesion with flattened villi (similar to celiac sprue), infiltration of the lamina propria, and mucosal ulcerations. Abdominal *lymphoma* may likewise present with clinical and radiologic features difficult to distinguish from regional enteritis. Hepatosplenomegaly and peripheral adenopathy, when present, are helpful clues; however, not uncommonly the

disease may appear confined to the intestine. In such cases, laparotomy is usually required to make the definitive histologic diagnosis.

The advanced presentation of regional enteritis with areas of stenosis and draining fistulas may also be seen with chronic *fungal infection* of the bowel, particularly with actinomycosis, aspergillosis, and blastomycosis. These infections often are seen in debilitated patients with impaired host defenses. Fungal skin tests and examination of fistula drainage and biopsy material for characteristic granules and fungi are helpful in making the diagnosis.

Intestinal *tuberculosis* characteristically produces stenotic lesions, usually in the terminal ileum, also often involving the contiguous cecum and ascending colon. Unlike regional enteritis, "skip areas" are unusual. Histologically, the granulomatous inflammation seen with *Mycobacterium tuberculosis* may be indistinguishable from regional enteritis; acid-fast stains and cultures are required. Fortunately in Western countries primary intestinal tuberculosis is now rare; when intestinal involvement does occur, it invariably is associated with pulmonary tuberculosis.

PROGNOSIS *Acute regional enteritis,* often discovered at surgery for suspected appendicitis, has an excellent prognosis. More than two-thirds of such patients show no subsequent evidence of regional enteritis after resolution of the initial attack. As discussed above, despite the resemblance at surgery to regional enteritis, this form of acute ileitis may well be due to diverse etiologies. Prevailing surgical opinion favors a conservative approach in this situation, and in most instances operative resection is not indicated.

By contrast, *chronic regional enteritis* (i.e., typical Crohn's disease) has a variable natural history, and in general the course is chronic and intermittent; in most cases one or more complications will occur, such as intestinal obstruction or fistula formation. In some patients, the disease process pursues a surprisingly benign course and eventually appears to "burn out." In others, the extent of the disease and its complications dominate the clinical picture, requiring multiple hospitalizations and aggressive therapy. The case fatality rate for all patients with regional enteritis, regardless of therapy, probably ranges from 5 to 10 percent, with most deaths occurring from peritonitis and sepsis.

Faced with a chronic disease of unknown etiology and variable natural history, the relationship between physician and patient is among the most difficult and assumes particular importance. The elements of trust and mutual understanding, essential in the therapy of any chronic disease, are of particular importance in the long-term management of patients with regional enteritis. Often these patients are intelligent young adults and are frequently resentful of a disease affecting them during the most productive period of their lives. Through compassionate understanding, and often time-consuming discussions between doctor and patient, many patients are able to lead reasonably stable and productive lives. While there is no evidence that a psychiatric disorder underlies or determines the onset or progression of the disease, careful attention to personality and emotional factors should form part of the continuing therapy for this disorder. In most instances, emotional support during discouraging periods can be provided by the physician and informed family members. In certain instances, however, formal psychiatric assistance will be required.

TREATMENT The therapy of regional enteritis must be individualized since the manifestations of the disease are so protean. Maintaining adequate nutrition and avoiding excess fatigue during periods of disease activity are supportive measures indicated in all patients. During an acute exacerbation of the disease, the patient should be placed at bed rest. Diarrhea and crampy abdominal pain may be relieved by the use of codeine, diphenoxylate, loperamide, paregoric, or deodorized tincture of opium. These agents should be used with discretion and are contraindicated if significant intestinal obstruction is present. In patients with evidence of small-bowel obstruction or ileus, continuous nasogastric suction and supplemental intravenous fluids for several days may allow subsidence of acute edema and swelling. Electrolyte deficiencies resulting from diarrhea or vomiting should be corrected. In many patients, especially early in the disease, definite improvement will occur with supportive therapy alone. Many authorities will often add salicylazosulfapyridine (sulfasalazine, Azulfidine) in a dose of 2 to 6 g daily upon resumption of oral food intake. A recent U.S. national cooperative study on the treatment of Crohn's disease determined that salicylazosulfapyridine is effective in the treatment of mild to moderate disease. Although the drug does not appear to be as effective in suppressing recurrent disease as in ulcerative colitis, many authorities will continue the drug as maintenance therapy (2 to 3 g daily) with the hope of suppressing recurrent activity of the disease.

In some patients, however, clinical improvement fails to occur with supportive therapy alone, and there is evidence of persistent partial intestinal obstruction or active disease. If pain or high fever dominate the clinical picture, perforation with abscess formation should be suspected. In the absence of these complications, the persistence of active disease usually requires treatment with *corticosteroids*. Such therapy, especially early in the course of the disease, is often effective, presumably by reducing the inflammatory process and decreasing the edema. There is no evidence that any particular corticosteroid preparation is more effective than another when comparably administered and used in equivalent dosage. The choice is one of individual preference; however, oral *prednisone* (45 to 60 mg daily) is often employed initially. Alternatively, intravenous *ACTH* may be given (40 to 60 units) over an 8-h drip infusion. In the severely ill patient, parenteral administration of corticosteroids is preferable to avoid the uncertainty of adequate oral absorption. Usually after 7 to 10 days of such therapy, improvement occurs, and prednisone can be administered. It is desirable gradually to decrease the dose of corticosteroids over a period of several months until reaching the minimal dose required to suppress the clinical signs of inflammation. However, there is no evidence that chronic steroid administration favorably influences the long-term outlook of the disease or that recurrences can in fact be prevented by this form of therapy alone. These drugs, therefore, should be used to suppress active inflammatory disease and not with the hope of maintaining the patient in remission.

While corticosteroids are generally effective early in the course of the disease, they are less effective in resolving obstruction due to fixed small-bowel narrowing and fibrosis. In addition, their use is contraindicated in the presence of intraabdominal sepsis resulting from fistula or abscess formation. The presence of fistulas alone is not a contraindication to the use of corticosteroids; however, constant attention is required to detect evidence of sepsis, which can be masked by these agents.

When corticosteroids fail or when the dosage required to reduce inflammation is too high, *azathioprine* may be added to the regimen at a dose of 1.5 to 2.0 mg/kg. Results of this therapy are unpredictable, but dramatic improvement has resulted in a small percentage of patients so treated. As with other diseases which are treated with corticosteroids, the addition of azathioprine often results in a "steroid sparing" effect, permitting a reduction in corticosteroid dosage when this is desirable. As with corticosteroids, the presence of sepsis is contraindication to the use of this agent.

Refinements in the technique of *parenteral alimentation* have made it possible to provide a patient's total daily caloric intake intravenously for a period of weeks or even months. In part, parenteral alimentation has been employed with increasing frequency in the severely ill patient as a means of placing the gastrointestinal tract "at rest." While there is no evidence that this form of therapy exerts a primary effect on the disease process, this approach permits one to provide adequate nutrition in the debilitated patient with regional enteritis. Similarly, the use of oral *elemental diets* may be of value in selected patients.

Surgery is generally reserved for the complications of regional enteritis rather than as a primary form of therapy. Experience in most major hospital centers has shown that there is at least 50 percent recurrence rate following surgical extirpation of the diseased bowel segment. Yet surgery has a definite place in the management of the disease, and approximately 70 percent of patients with chronic regional enteritis will require at least one operation during the course of their disease. Although each case and situation must be individualized, in general, surgical therapy may be required for persistent or fixed bowel narrowing or obstruction, symptomatic fistula formation to the bladder, vagina, or skin, persistent anal fistulas or abscesses, and for intraabdominal abscesses or free perforation. The role of surgery in the management of Crohn's disease of the colon is discussed in Chap. 294. The therapy of regional enteritis in children often presents special problems since normal growth and development may be retarded in the presence of active disease. While each patient must be managed individually, the goals of treatment have been to attain clinical remission of disease and to promote growth while permitting the children to function as normally as possible. When the disease is confined to the small bowel, control of disease is often achieved by medical therapy. The use of alternate-day corticosteroids may be of benefit in this circumstance. In other patients intensive nutritional therapy or the judicious use of surgery may be indicated.

Once the acute manifestations of the disease have subsided, an important therapeutic aspect involves the maintenance of adequate nutrition. In patients with extensive small-bowel involvement or in those patients with a short bowel resulting from extensive bowel resection, supplementation of electrolytes, minerals, and vitamins will be required. Extensive ileal disease or resection often results in diarrhea induced by bile salts and in malabsorption; in such patients cholestyramine may be needed to control the diarrhea, and medium-chain triglycerides may be added to reduce fat malabsorption. In patients with stenotic segments of intestine, a low-residue (low-fiber) diet should be recommended. If there is an associated lactase deficiency, a lactose-free diet should be instituted. Except for these specific dietary measures, other forms of dietary restrictions have not been shown to have any beneficial effect on the primary disease process, and patients should be encouraged to eat a nutritious, appealing diet of their own choosing. It is through the meticulous long-term attention to the nutritional aspects of the disease and supportive therapy during periods of exacerbation and remission that the physician can be of the greatest service to patients with regional enteritis.

VASCULAR DISORDERS OF THE SMALL INTESTINE

The splanchnic circulation derives its arterial blood supply from the celiac axis and the superior and inferior mesenteric arteries. The small intestine is supplied by the celiac and superior mesenteric arteries; the colon is supplied by branches of the superior and inferior mesenteric. A rich network of anastomotic vessels and the possible development of collateral circulation determine the clinical picture of acute or chronic intestinal arterial insufficiency.

Acute ischemia or infarction of the small intestine may result from embolic occlusion, mesenteric arterial thrombosis (most commonly due to advanced arteriosclerotic disease), or nonthrombotic intestinal infarction (often associated with poor tissue perfusion). Abdominal pain is the presenting symptom. Early in the course the pain may be crampy and periumbilical in location, and bowel sounds may be hyperactive. If unrecognized, ischemia will progress to infarction with the development of ileus, loss of bowel sounds, development of generalized peritonitis, sepsis, hemoconcentration, and shock. Vascular insufficiency and ischemia should be suspected in the patient who has the acute onset of abdominal pain in association with (1) atrial fibrillation, often in the setting of rheumatic or arteriosclerotic heart disease; (2) extensive atherosclerosis; (3) poor tissue perfusion, especially associated with severe congestive failure, shock, or hypoxemia; and (4) prior symptoms of abdominal angina (see below). Early diagnosis is of paramount importance but may be difficult since no single test is diagnostic. Plain and erect films of the abdomen most often show evidence of ileus; thickening of the bowel wall due to mucosal edema or hemorrhage is helpful when present. Upper gastrointestinal x-rays can be of benefit to help exclude other disorders.

The role of mesenteric angiography is controversial. In cases of suspected embolization, occlusion of the superior mesenteric artery and the lack of significant collateral circulation help to establish the diagnosis. However, when there is poor tissue perfusion and nonthrombotic intestinal infarction, angiography is of less value. Since a significant proportion of older individuals may have no abdominal symptoms and yet have variable narrowing of abdominal vessels, it is often difficult to correlate angiographic findings with clinical findings. The diagnosis most often depends on a high index of suspicion in a patient with abdominal pain and on one or more of the predisposing factors mentioned above. The decision to operate for impending intestinal infarction is often difficult since many such patients are poor surgical risks and the mortality of a major operative procedure must be balanced against the extremely high mortality of the disease process itself.

Chronic arterial insufficiency may precede acute vascular insufficiency and may present abdominal angina. As in angina pectoris, vascular insufficiency occurs under conditions where there is a need for increased splanchnic blood flow. Typically intermittent dull or cramping midabdominal pain occurs 15 to 30 min after a meal and may last for several hours postprandially. Significant weight loss is primarily due to a decreased food intake; however, chronic intestinal ischemia may produce mucosal damage and malabsorption, which in turn aggravate the weight loss. Since abdominal angina may progress to bowel infarction, serious consideration should be given to performing arteriographic studies to confirm the diagnosis in those patients who are candidates for abdominal vascular surgery. The only definitive treatment is surgical removal of the obstruction or the construction of bypass arterial grafts to the ischemic bowel.

A variety of systemic conditions are associated with *vasculitis* of large and small arteries supplying the intestine. Most often, these disorders can be recognized by the associated extraintestinal manifestations as in polyarteritis nodosa, lupus erythematosus, dermatomyositis, Henoch-Schönlein purpura (allergic vasculitis), and rheumatoid vasculitis. When larger arteries are involved, as in polyarteritis nodosa, the picture of acute intestinal infarction is similar to embolic or atherosclerotic vascular occlusion. Often the involvement of smaller

vessels leads to areas of intramural hemorrhage and edema leading to abdominal pain, variable degrees of intestinal obstruction, and bleeding. Plain abdominal x-rays may show "thumbprinting" and "spiculation" due to localized edema, hemorrhage, and ulceration. In many instances, treatment of the underlying disorder may lead to regression of symptoms. If signs of an acute abdomen develop, surgical exploration is usually indicated.

Intramural small-intestinal hemorrhage may occur with vasculitis, trauma, or impaired coagulation, especially in patients receiving anticoagulants. The clinical and radiologic features are similar to those seen with vasculitis and local mucosal hemorrhage.

PRIMARY NONSPECIFIC ULCERATION OF THE SMALL INTESTINE

Although the existence of rare solitary and unexplained ulcers of the small intestine has been recognized for many years, a recent sharp increase in their incidence has suggested vascular factors producing ischemic necrosis of the mucosa in one or more areas of the small bowel. Most of these ulcers occur in patients receiving enteric-coated drugs known to be irritating to the mucosa; the most commonly implicated agent is potassium chloride, given to patients on chronic diuretic therapy. The symptoms are those of abdominal pain and obstruction, rarely with peritonitis and perforation. The treatment is discontinuance of the medication and surgical excision of the ulcerated or stenotic intestinal segment.

TUMORS OF THE SMALL INTESTINE

Small-bowel tumors are relatively rare and compose only 3 to 6 percent of gastrointestinal neoplasms. While uncommon, these tumors present great difficulty in diagnosis. Abdominal symptoms are usually vague and poorly defined, and conventional x-ray studies of the upper and lower intestinal tract are usually normal. Small-bowel tumors should be considered and careful radiologic studies of the entire small intestine carried out under the following situations: (1) recurrent, unexplained episodes of crampy abdominal pain; (2) intermittent bouts of intestinal obstruction, especially in the absence of inflammatory bowel disease or prior abdominal surgery; (3) intussusception in the adult; and (4) evidence of chronic intestinal bleeding in the face of negative conventional x-rays.

BENIGN TUMORS In general, the specific nature of small-bowel tumors is difficult to identify on clinical and radiologic grounds alone. The symptomatology is not distinctive, with pain, obstruction, and hemorrhage being the most frequent symptoms. These tumors are often discovered in the fifth and sixth decades of life, and their frequency is greater in the distal rather than the proximal small intestine. The most common small-bowel tumors are adenomas, lyomyomas, lipomas, and angiomas.

Adenomas These tumors include those of the islet cells and Brunner's glands as well as polypoid adenomas. *Islet-cell adenomas* are occasionally located outside the pancreas, and the associated syndromes are discussed in Chap. 340. *Brunner's gland adenomas* are not truly neoplastic but represent a hypertrophy or hyperplasia of submucosal duodenal glands. Occasionally x-rays of the duodenal bulb may show prominence of these structures. Most often this is an incidental finding on x-ray and not associated with any clinical disorder.

Polypoid adenomas Approximately 25 percent of benign small-bowel tumors are polypoid adenomas. They may present as single polypoid lesions or less commonly as papillary villous adenomas. As in the colon (see Chap. 294), the sessile or papillary form of the tumor is sometimes associated with coexistent carcinoma. Multiple polypoid tumors may occur throughout the small bowel in the Peutz-Jehgers syndrome (Chap. 51) and are usually hamartomas. The malignant potential of these lesions is low.

Lyomyomas These arise from smooth-muscle components of the intestine and are usually intramural lesions effacing the overlying mucosa. A central ulceration may be present and is responsible for gastrointestinal hemorrhage of varying severity.

Lipomas These tumors occur with greatest frequency in the distal ileum and at the ileocecal valve. Their radiolucent appearance on x-ray is characteristic. They are usually intramural and asymptomatic but may on occasion be associated with bleeding.

Angiomas While uncommon these are important small-bowel tumors since a high percentage of patients with these lesions will have evidence of intestinal bleeding. They may take the form of telangiectasia or hemangiomas. Multiple intestinal telangiectasia occurs in a nonhereditary form confined to the gastrointestinal tract or as a part of the hereditary Osler-Weber-Rendu syndrome. The latter syndrome is described in Chap. 317. Vascular tumors may also take the form of isolated hemangiomas, most commonly in the jejunum. Bleeding is common, and angiography is the procedure of choice in evaluating these lesions.

MALIGNANT TUMORS While not too common, small-bowel malignancies occur in patients with long-standing regional enteritis and celiac sprue with greater frequency than in the general population. In contrast to benign tumors, malignant tumors of the small bowel are frequently associated with fever, weight loss, anorexia, bleeding, and an abdominal mass on physical examination. If ampullary carcinomas are excluded (discussed in Chap. 309), the most frequent small-bowel malignancies are adenocarcinomas, lymphomas, leiomyosarcomas, and carcinoid tumors.

Adenocarcinomas These occur with highest frequency in the duodenum. Like adenocarcinomas elsewhere, they tend to ulcerate and cause hemorrhage or obstruction. Radiologically, they may resemble chronic duodenal ulcer disease. Diagnosis may also be difficult if the patient has long-standing regional enteritis. The diagnosis is best made by endoscopy of the duodenum and biopsy under direct vision.

Leiomyosarcomas Large, bulky tumors, leiomyosarcomas often are greater than 5 cm in diameter and may be palpable on abdominal examination. Bleeding, obstruction, or perforation are the most common manifestations.

Lymphomas All histologic types of lymphomas may involve the small bowel either primarily or secondarily. In both instances, lymphosarcomas and reticulum-cell sarcomas are more common than Hodgkin's disease. Involvement is more common in the jejunum and ileum than in the duodenum. Grossly, lymphomas may infiltrate the bowel wall or present as a large polypoid mass, often with central ulceration. Involvement of the adjacent mesentery and lymph nodes is common. Occasionally the small intestine may be diffusely involved, leading to malabsorption. This type of involvement, which for unknown reasons is more common in the Middle East, may be difficult to differentiate from celiac disease, since in the latter there is an increased incidence of lymphoma. An uncommon variant of Mediterranean lymphoma is *alpha-chain disease* found primarily in young people of Mediterranean origin. It leads to severe diarrhea, malabsorption, and often hypoproteinemia. The intestine is infiltrated with plasma cells, and fragments of the IgA heavy chains are found in blood and urine.

In most instances laparotomy is required for the diagnosis of primary intestinal lymphomas. Infiltrating lymphomas of the distal bowel must be distinguished from benign infiltrating lesions such as regional enteritis. Stenosis of bowel segments, involvement of both large and small bowel, and the extracolonic manifestations of inflammatory bowel disease suggest regional enteritis. Peroral intestinal biopsy and lymphangiography are useful in the diagnosis of diffuse intestinal lymphoma. Treatment of localized lymphoma is surgical resection, and the prognosis is good if the disease has not spread. Chemotherapy and radiotherapy are employed in the management of more extensive disease, but the results have been uniformly poor.

Carcinoid tumors Among the most common epithelial tumors of the small intestine are carcinoid tumors. They arise from argentaffin cells of the crypts of Lieberkühn and are most commonly found from the midduodenum to the transverse colon, areas embryologically derived from the midgut. The appendix is the most common location for gastrointestinal carcinoids, and often the tumors are found incidentally at the time of appendectomy. Most intestinal carcinoids are asymptomatic and of low malignant potential, but invasion and metastases may occur and lead to the *carcinoid syndrome* (see Chap. 91).

REFERENCES

Regional enteritis (Crohn's disease)

COOK WT, SWAN CHJ: Diffuse jejuno-ileitis of Crohn's disease. Q J Med 43:583, 1974

DONALDSON RM JR: Crohn's disease of the small bowel, in *Gastrointestinal Diseases,* 2d ed, MH Sleisenger, JS Fordtran (eds). Philadelphia, Saunders, 1978, chap 66

FIASSE R et al: Circulating immune complexes and disease activity in Crohn's disease. Gut 19:611, 1978

GREENSTEIN AJ et al: Reoperation and recurrence in Crohn's colitis and ileocolitis. N Engl J Med 293:658, 1975

GRYBOSKI JB, SPIRO HM: Prognosis in children with Crohn's disease. Gastroenterology 74:807, 1978

KAUFMAN S et al: A prospective study of the course of Crohn's disease. Dig Dis Sci 24:269, 1979

KLEIN M et al: Treatment of Crohn's disease with azathioprine: A controlled evaluation. Gastroenterology 66:916, 1974

SMITH RC et al: Low dose steroids and clinical relapse in Crohn's disease: a controlled trial. Gut 19:606, 1978

VANTRAPPEN G et al: Yersinia enteritis and enterocolitis: Gastroenterological aspects. Gastroenterology 72:220, 1977

Vascular disorders of the small intestine

CINETTA JM, KOLODNY M: Mesenteric venous thrombosis associated with oral contraceptives. Gastroenterology 58:713, 1970

JONA J et al: Recurrent primary mesenteric venous thrombosis. JAMA 227:1033, 1974

OTTINGER LW: The surgical management of acute occlusion of the superior mesenteric artery. Ann Surg 188:721, 1978

WILLIAMS LF JR: Vascular insufficiency of the intestine. Gastroenterology 61:757, 1971

Tumors of the small intestine

FREUND H et al: Primary neoplasms of the small bowel. Am J Surg 135:757, 1978

Nagvi MS et al: Lymphoma of the gastrointestinal tract: Prognostic guides based on 162 cases. Ann Surg 170:221, 1969

Novis BH et al: Abdominal lymphoma presenting with malabsorption. Q J Med 40:521, 1971

Seligman M, Rambaud JC: IgA abnormalities in abdominal lymphoma (α-chain disease). Isr J Med Sci 5:151, 1969

Steinberg LS, Shieber LS: Villous adenomas of the small intestine. Surgery 71:423, 1971

294
DISEASES OF THE COLON AND RECTUM

J. THOMAS LaMONT
KURT J. ISSELBACHER

SYMPTOMS OF COLONIC AND RECTAL DISEASE

The major symptoms of colonic disease are *alteration in bowel habit, rectal bleeding,* and *pain.* Alteration in bowel habit implies a change from previous patterns of defecation; hence a detailed history is important. Normal individuals have one to three movements of well-formed stools each day. *Diarrhea* means the passage of watery or loose stools usually with increased frequency, while *constipation* implies infrequent passage of hard, dry stools; *obstipation* is the absence of spontaneous bowel movements. A persistent change in bowel habit, particularly in older individuals with no previous irregularity, is usually an important early symptom of organic disease of the colon and should never be labeled *functional* unless a thorough diagnostic evaluation is negative. The appearance of the stool may also provide important diagnostic clues. Blood coating the exterior of a formed stool implies a lesion in the anal canal or rectum, while blood admixed with the feces indicates a bleeding source higher in the colon. Brisk hemorrhage from the colon or distal small intestine results in passage of fresh blood, called *hematochezia.* This may appear as fresh blood and clots if the lesion is in the left colon, or darker maroon-colored blood if the bleeding source is in the right colon. However, very brisk upper intestinal bleeding may result in hematochezia because the blood stimulates intestinal motility and is rapidly eliminated. Obviously, the appearance of blood in the stool depends largely on two factors, the site of the lesion and the rate of blood loss.

Pain resulting from colonic disease is usually localized to either of the lower abdominal quadrants, as opposed to pain of small-intestinal origin which is localized to the periumbilical area or higher. Rectal pain is often felt deep in the pelvis, while pain in the anal canal is accurately localized to the perineum. The mechanisms of colonic pain are similar to those in other intestinal viscera (see Chap. 6). Distention from gas or fluid causes crampy or colicky pain from stretching of the muscle layers and resulting contraction or spasm. Pain of this type is often relieved by passage of flatus or stool. Pain may also result if the colonic wall is inflamed or infiltrated by tumor. Acute colonic inflammation which involves the visceral or parietal peritoneum produces sharply localized pain, which may be accompanied by abdominal guarding and rebound tenderness. An important symptom of rectal disease is *tenesmus.* The patient complains of a painful urge to defecate and a sensation of incomplete emptying after defecation. This symptom can be caused by retention of stool in the rectum, by tumors of the rectum which simulate retained stools, or by colonic inflammation.

DIAGNOSTIC PROCEDURES

PHYSICAL EXAMINATION The abdomen should be carefully examined for the presence of colonic distention, an important sign of obstruction. The cecum, owing to its greater capacity and distensibility, may be greatly dilated in the presence of distal colonic obstruction from tumor or stricture. In nonobese individuals the stool-filled sigmoid colon may be palpable in the left lower quadrant, and tenderness may be elicited in colitis or diverticulitis. Perhaps the most important part of the physical examination in the diagnosis of colonic diseases is the *digital rectal examination.* This procedure should never be omitted for reasons of modesty or fear of embarrassment because it is essential in the diagnosis of perianal, sphincteric, and ampullary lesions; prostatic and uterine abnormalities; and even small rectal masses. A metastatic tumor may be felt in the perirectal tissues as a shelf-like deformity, especially anteriorly above the prostate. The fecal material on the glove should be immediately tested chemically for occult blood. Approximately one-half of all rectal carcinomas lie within the reach of the index finger, and omission of the rectal examination may delay diagnosis and worsen the prognosis.

SIGMOIDOSCOPY Contrary to the general impression, the technique of sigmoidoscopy is not difficult to master, and with practice the discomfort to the patient is minimal. The physician should learn to evaluate mucosal friability (one of the earliest signs of proctitis and colitis) and to recognize abnormal vascular patterns, edema, ulcerations, and polyps. Ninety percent of tumors of the rectum and rectosigmoid can be directly visualized with this instrument. Approximately half of all tumors of the large intestine lie within the terminal 25 cm of the colon and within the reach of the sigmoidoscope. It is important to remember that the distal 20 to 25 cm of the colon is difficult to examine by barium enema. A rectal carcinoma can be missed on routine barium enema yet easily visualized and biopsied through the sigmoidoscope. Furthermore, the earliest changes of ulcerative colitis may not be demonstrated radiographically but may be obvious through the sigmoidoscope. Rectal biopsy is easily and painlessly accomplished through the instrument and is associated with minimal morbidity except in the presence of bleeding disorders.

STOOL EXAMINATION Abnormal stools constitute important objective evidence of colonic disease. Stools should be examined by the physician as soon as possible after defecation for the presence of visible blood on the surface or within the specimen. A small sample should be tested for occult blood. Microscopic examination of fresh stool is important in the diagnosis of parasitic diseases, particularly in amoebic colitis when motile trophozoites can be seen in fresh, warm stool suspensions. Stool suspensions can also be stained with a drop of methylene blue for polymorphonuclear leukocytes, which indicate the presence of an acute inflammatory exudate characteristic of ulcerative colitis, amoebic colitis, and bacillary dysentery. Fixed and stained slides of stool may also reveal amoebas and other parasites. Stool culture is essential for the diagnosis of bacillary dysentery.

BARIUM ENEMA This is an extremely accurate diagnostic tool for the identification of structural abnormalities of the colon. A careful study in a well-prepared patient can demonstrate mucosal lesions as small as 0.5 cm. For high-quality resolution of subtle lesions such as small polyps or early changes of ulcerative colitis, an air-contrast barium enema is useful. In this study the mucosa is outlined by a thin coat of barium, after which air is injected to enhance contrast and outline small lesions. The combined use of the digital examination, proctosigmoidoscopy, and barium enema will identify 95 percent of significant colonic lesions. Negative results of these procedures constitute strong evidence that a functional disorder may be present.

COLONOSCOPY See Chap. 288.

DISORDERS OF COLONIC MOTILITY

MEGACOLON Megacolon, or giant colon, is characterized by massive distention of the colon usually accompanied by severe constipation or obstipation. This condition can be either congenital or acquired and is seen in all age groups. Acute toxic megacolon is a severe complication of chronic ulcerative colitis (see below).

Aganglionic megacolon (Hirschsprung's disease) This is a congenital disorder which becomes manifest in early infancy, occurring more frequently in males, and is often familial. These infants have massive abdominal distention, absent bowel movements, and impaired nutrition due to chronic obstruction of the colon. In some individuals with less severe symptoms the disease may not be diagnosed until adolescence or early adulthood. The inability to defecate is caused by the congenital absence in a small segment of the distal colon of ganglion cells in the submucosal (Meissner's) or myenteric (Auerbach's) plexuses. This aganglionic segment is unable to relax to permit passage of stool, and thus the normal colon proximal to it becomes greatly dilated. On rectal examination the ampulla is empty of feces and the anal sphincter is normal. Barium enema reveals a narrowed segment in the rectosigmoid area, with massive dilatation above (Fig. 294-1). Diagnosis is made by deep surgical biopsy under anesthesia and demonstration of absent ganglion cells in the diseased segment. In most patients the aganglionic segment is in the rectosigmoid colon; in rare instances the lesion may involve more proximal bowel or even the entire colon. The treatment is usually surgical, although milder cases may be treated by enemas to empty the colon. The most effective operation is a pull-through procedure in which normally innervated colon is anastomosed to the distal rectum just above the internal sphincter, thus bypassing the contracted aganglionic segment.

Chronic idiopathic megacolon This condition, also called *psychogenic megacolon,* has its onset later in childhood, usually at the time toilet training begins. It is characterized by severe chronic constipation and distention, and in contrast to Hirschsprung's disease, digital examination reveals the rectal ampulla to be invariably distended with feces. Barium enema shows the entire colon to be distended from the anal sphincter cephalad; no narrowed segment is seen, and rectal biopsy discloses the normal complement of ganglion cells in Auerbach's plexus. Treatment is based on education in normal bowel habits, but a long course of enemas or large doses of mineral oil may be required until the patient acquires more normal bowel movements.

Acquired megacolon In Central and South America infection with *Trypanosoma cruzi* (Chagas' disease) can result in destruction of ganglion cells of the colon, producing a clinical picture similar to congenital megacolon, except that the onset is in adult life rather than childhood. A number of other diseases are associated with megacolon in adults. Patients with schizophrenia or depression, particularly institutionalized patients, may have obstipation and massive colonic dilatation. Severe neurologic disorders including cerebral atrophy, spinal cord injury, and parkinsonism may also cause megacolon. Myxedema, infiltrative diseases such as amyloidosis, and scleroderma can also reduce colonic motility and produce marked colonic distention. Narcotic drugs, particularly morphine and codeine, can cause severe constipation, especially when administered to bedridden patients. Digital rectal examination reveals a rectum distended with feces, as opposed to the empty rectum in aganglionic megacolon. Treatment is aimed at the underlying disease and includes the careful use of enemas and cathartics.

COLONIC DIVERTICULA Diverticula of the colon are herniations or saclike protrusions of the mucosa through the muscularis. These outpouchings are composed of mucosa and serosa and follow the course of a nutrient artery within the muscularis of the bowel wall. Diverticula occur most commonly in the sigmoid colon and decrease in frequency in the proximal colon. They increase with age, and the incidence ranges between 20 and 50 percent in Western populations over age 50. The exact mechanism for their formation is unknown but may be related to an increase in intraluminal pressure. Since thickening of the muscle coat of the colon is often present, it has been suggested that herniations of mucosa are caused by the increased force produced by colonic muscle contractions. The rarity of colonic diverticula in underdeveloped nations in contrast to their frequent occurrence in Western countries has stimulated a number of epidemiologic studies. Some have suggested that diverticula result from the highly refined Western diet, which is deficient in dietary fiber or roughage. It is pro-

FIGURE 294-1
Aganglionic megacolon with narrowed rectal segment (arrows).

posed that such diets result in decreased fecal bulk, narrowing of the colon, and an increase in intraluminal pressure in order to move the smaller fecal mass. The role of dietary fiber in the etiology and treatment of diverticular disease remains to be determined.

Colonic diverticula are usually an incidental finding on a barium enema performed for other reasons and in most patients cause no symptoms. The major complications are inflammation, both acute and chronic, and hemorrhage. Since diverticulosis is quite common in older patients, one must avoid the temptation of attributing symptoms to the diverticula unless other conditions, especially colonic neoplasm, have been excluded.

Diverticulitis Inflammation can occur in or around the diverticular sac. The cause of diverticulitis is probably mechanical, related to retention in the diverticula of undigested food residues and bacteria, which may form a hard mass called a *fecalith*. This compromises the blood supply to the thin-walled sac (made up solely of mucosa and serosa) and renders it susceptible to invasion by colonic bacteria. The inflammatory process may vary from a small intramural or pericolic abscess to generalized peritonitis. Some attacks are accompanied by minimal symptoms and seem to heal spontaneously. Studies of resected specimens indicate that most perforations of the diverticular sac are small and result in inflammation of the sac itself and the corresponding serosal surface. Diverticulitis occurs more often in men than women, and three times as often in the left than in the right colon. This suggests that diverticulitis may be related to the higher intraluminal pressures and the more solid fecal material in the sigmoid and descending colon.

Acute diverticulitis is a disease of variable severity characterized by lower abdominal pain and tenderness. The clinical features are lower abdominal pain, made worse by defecation, and signs of peritoneal irritation—muscle spasm, guarding, rebound tenderness, fever, and leukocytosis. Rectal examination may reveal a tender mass if the area of inflammation is close to the rectum. Although constipation may not have been noted prior to the onset of the illness, the inflammation around the colon often results in some degree of constipation. Rectal bleeding, usually microscopic, is noted in 25 percent of cases; it is rarely massive. Complications include free perforation, which results in acute peritonitis, sepsis, and shock, particularly in the elderly. The perforation may be walled off by adherent omentum or neighboring structures such as bladder or small bowel. Abscess formation or fistulas may then occur as the inflammatory mass burrows into other organs. Severe pericolitis may cause a dense, fibrous reaction or stricture around the bowel which can be associated with colonic obstruction. Repeated attacks may result in fistulas between the diverticulum and neighboring organs, especially the bladder and vagina.

Differential diagnosis in the less acute situation is principally that of a neoplasm in the area of the diverticulosis. Sigmoidoscopy may show an acutely inflamed mucosa over an apparent extrinsic mass; passing the instrument through the contracted lumen is usually impossible. During the acute phase of diverticulitis, barium enema may be hazardous, since contrast material under pressure may lead to rupture of an inflamed diverticulum and convert a walled-off inflammatory lesion to a free perforation. The examination is usually safe after adequate treatment and healing of the diverticulitis. The radiologic findings on barium enema suggestive of diverticulitis are leakage of barium from a diverticular sac, stricture formation, and the presence of a pericolic inflammatory mass. Radiologic findings on barium enema may be diagnostic (see Fig. 294-2), but often the distortion caused by inflammation prevents a clear distinction between cancer and diverticulitis. Such a distinction may be difficult, even at the time of laparotomy.

Treatment in the mild case without signs of perforation consists of bed rest, stool softeners, a liquid diet, and a wide-spectrum antibiotic such as tetracycline or ampicillin. Hospitalized patients with acute peritoneal signs, suspected abscess, or perforation require intravenous antibiotics directed against

FIGURE 294-2
A. Diverticulosis with marked spasm of sigmoid colon. B. Diverticulosis with fistula to urinary bladder which is filled with barium.

A

B

gram-negative anaerobic bacteria. Surgical intervention is frequently necessary to drain abscesses or to resect an obstructing inflammatory mass. The usual procedure is a diverting colostomy with resection of the involved colon; reanastomosis is then performed at a second operation. Fistulas are particularly difficult to manage surgically, and there is considerable difference of opinion as to the proper surgical approach. There is general agreement that, if after careful medical management, repeated attacks of diverticulitis occur in the same area of the left colon, surgical resection of the involved segments is indicated.

Painful diverticular disease without diverticulitis Some patients with diverticulosis develop recurrent left lower quadrant colicky pain without clinical or pathologic evidence of acute diverticulitis. They often have bouts of alternating constipation and diarrhea, and the pain may be relieved by defecation or passage of flatus. These features suggest the coexistence of the irritable bowel syndrome (see below). Examination during a bout of pain reveals tenderness of the sigmoid colon, but signs of peritoneal inflammation such as rebound tenderness, muscle guarding, fever, and leukocytosis are absent. Barium enema shows typical diverticula without evidence of inflammation and stricture, plus a "sawtooth" irregularity of the lumen reflecting associated muscle spasm. In some patients the pain is severe enough to warrant observation in hospital and restriction of food since feeding aggravates the pain by causing colonic contraction. Anticholinergics, which reduce sigmoid contractions, and mild sedation are usually all that is required. The patient should be started on a high-residue diet or given a bulk laxative such as hemicellulose, unprocessed bran, or psyllium extract. Surgical excision is usually not indicated unless acute diverticulitis or its complications occur.

Hemorrhage from diverticula This rare complication of diverticulosis occurs in elderly patients, usually in the absence of signs or symptoms of diverticulitis. The pathogenesis is presumably erosion of a vessel by a fecalith within the diverticular sac. The degree of bleeding is often mild, although in some patients massive life-threatening hemorrhage occurs. In the majority of cases of mild or moderate hemorrhage the bleeding stops spontaneously with bed rest and blood transfusion. In patients with severe hemorrhage mesenteric angiography can be both diagnostic in localizing the bleeding site and therapeutic since vasoconstrictive drugs infused intraarterially can effectively control hemorrhage. Angiographic techniques can be extremely helpful in directing the surgeon to the area of bleeding if surgery is required for continued or recurrent bleeding. In several series the location of bleeding diverticula demonstrated at angiography has been more commonly in the right colon, particularly the ascending colon, in contrast to the sigmoid colon, where diverticula are more numerous.

FUNCTIONAL DISTURBANCES

IRRITABLE BOWEL SYNDROME The irritable bowel syndrome is the most common gastrointestinal disease in clinical practice, and although not a life-threatening illness, causes great distress to those afflicted and a feeling of helplessness and frustration for the physician attempting to treat it. The patient with irritable bowel syndrome may present with one of *three clinical variants*. Patients with so-called "spastic colitis" complain primarily of chronic abdominal pain and constipation. A second group have chronic intermittent watery diarrhea, often without pain. Some patients have both features and complain of alternating constipation and diarrhea.

The basic pathophysiologic abnormality in the irritable bowel syndrome is an alteration in intestinal motility. Patients with the spastic colon variant (pain and constipation) have *increased* resting colonic motility; in contrast those presenting primarily with diarrhea have *decreased* resting colonic motility. Both groups have an increase in colonic motility after injection of cholinergic drugs, the intestinal hormone cholecystokinin or during psychologic stress. It has been suggested that cholecystokinin may be a normal stimulus of intestinal motility, and that the spastic colon may result from an exaggerated response to the normal increased blood level of this hormone after eating.

It has also been shown that patients with the irritable bowel syndrome exhibit an abnormal basic electrical rhythm in the colon characterized by an increase in 3 cycle per minute slow-wave activity. It is not clear, however, whether these abnormalities of smooth-muscle contraction are primary or secondary to some other underlying abnormality of intestinal neuromuscular function.

Many investigators have also described evidence of significant psychological disturbances in the majority of patients with irritable bowel syndrome. Depression, hysteria, and obsessive-compulsive traits are common, and psychologic stress frequently triggers an exacerbation of symptoms. It should be noted however, that in normal individuals colonic motility is altered by stress. For example, increased intracolonic pressure has been observed in normal volunteers during a stressful interview. This suggests that psychologic stress may be a nonspecific trigger of symptoms in the irritable bowel syndrome, as has been observed in many other illnesses of diverse etiology.

Clinical features The irritable bowel syndrome is a disease of young or middle-aged adults, with a female/male ratio of 2:1. The predominant feature is a history of chronic constipation, diarrhea, or both. The typical patient describes watery diarrhea occurring *intermittently* for months or years. The diarrhea is usually worse in the morning upon arising or after breakfast. After the passage of three or four loose stools with excessive mucus the patient may be well for the rest of the day. Diarrhea throughout the day or nocturnal diarrhea is unusual. The diarrhea may last weeks or months, then disappear spontaneously for variable periods of time. Some patients may describe "pencil-like" pasty stools rather than diarrhea. Another typical presentation is that of chronic abdominal pain with constipation, or with alternating constipation and diarrhea. These patients describe intermittent crampy lower abdominal pain, often over the sigmoid colon, which is usually relieved by passage of flatus or stool. A variety of other complaints, such as heartburn, excessive bloating, back pain, weakness, faintness, and palpitations, are frequent in patients with irritable bowel syndrome.

Physical examination reveals these patients to be anxious but otherwise normal. During intense pain, the abdomen may be distended, but no visible peristalsis is noted; the abdominal musculature is relaxed, and a tender sigmoid full of feces may be palpated in the left lower quadrant. Characteristically, the rectal ampulla is empty of feces. Sigmoidoscopic examination is usually normal or at most shows a prominent vascular pattern. There may be difficulty in negotiating the rectosigmoid curve at 13 to 15 cm from the anus because of spasm. Large amounts of clear mucus are frequently encountered during the examination.

The *diagnosis* of the irritable colon syndrome is suggested by the long duration of symptoms without obvious signs of physical deterioration, the intermittent character of the disability, and the relation of symptoms to environmental or emotional stress. Nevertheless, each patient presenting such symptoms deserves not only a careful history but also a complete physical examination including sigmoidoscopy, stool examination (for occult blood, parasites, and pathogenic bacteria), and a barium enema. The radiographic study serves to rule out other lesions since there are no findings diagnostic for this syndrome, although spasticity of the sigmoid, accentuated haustra, and tubular descending colon may be observed when the patient is symptomatic. Lactase deficiency may masquerade as irritable colon syndrome and should be excluded by a trial of milk restriction or the more definitive lactose tolerance test (see Chap. 292). Thyrotoxicosis may be confused with this syndrome but is ruled out by careful physical examination and appropriate laboratory studies.

Treatment of the irritable colon syndrome requires both skill and patience. It is important that the patient be reassured that this condition normally does not lead to the development of inflammatory bowel disease (i.e., ulcerative colitis) or colonic malignancy. It is also important for both the patient and the physician to realize that the condition is chronic and probably cannot be cured. Treatment is aimed at encouraging the patient to adapt to the symptoms and minimize their impact on his or her life-style. The physician should not imply that the symptoms are entirely or largely emotional or psychological in origin, since this is usually rejected by the patient. It is appropriate, however, to emphasize the relationship between psychologic stress and the onset of severity of symptoms, since this may allow the patient to better deal with the disease. After the diagnosis is established, repeated x-rays and endoscopies are not necessary; general physical examinations, hemograms, and stool examinations, however, should be carried out at regular intervals.

Treatment is also aimed at altering the abnormal colonic motility in this disease. Patients with constipation may respond to increase in dietary bulk in the form of unprocessed bran or other nonabsorbed bulk laxatives. Mild sedation with phenobarbital or tranquilizers may be indicated, and anticholinergic drugs are useful in some patients. Troublesome diarrhea may respond to diphenoxylate (Lomotil) or paregoric. Unfortunately, there is no specific drug or dietary regimen which affords good relief in all patients, and thus in many instances a number of therapeutic maneuvers need to be tried.

CHRONIC CONSTIPATION   In Chap. 37 the mechanism of defecation is discussed. Disorders involving the sensory or motor components of this mechanism may arise from destruction of the nerves subserving these functions, from invasion or inflammation of the rectosigmoid itself, or from central nervous system lesions. If the afferent stimulus from the rectum does not reach the brain, or if, upon reaching it, there is no efferent response, defecation does not occur. If defecation is initiated but muscular contraction is lessened or lost, the act is not carried to completion. Most cases of chronic constipation arise from habitual neglect of afferent impulses, failure to initiate defecation, and accumulation of large, dry fecal masses in the rectum. This voluntary suppression of the call to stool may arise during the period of toilet training in childhood, or later in life because of a sense of social impropriety, unaccustomed surroundings, uncomfortable toilet facilities, or illnesses which require confinement to bed. As constant distention of the rectum with feces becomes chronic, the patient grows less aware of rectal fullness. Bowel movements become progressively more difficult, and painful hemorrhoids or anal fissures reinforce suppression of the urge to defecate. To avoid these problems, the patient begins the chronic use of laxatives or enemas, without which defecation becomes impossible.

Treatment   The physician should make every attempt to educate the patient about the chain of events which has led to chronic constipation. Attempts should be made to alter patterns of many years' duration, and the patient must recognize the importance of responding to, rather than suppressing, the urge to defecate. It is helpful to initiate a routine whereby defecation is attempted at a given time each day. In most individuals the call to stool occurs in the morning after breakfast. Physical exercise such as a brisk walk just before attempts at defecation may be helpful. Patients are instructed to increase dietary bulk with foods rich in fiber, such as green vegetables and unprocessed cereal grains, or by the regular use of bulk laxatives, such as hemicellulose, psyllium extract, and powdered unprocessed bran. The success of such a regimen depends to some extent on the duration of symptoms. Elderly patients with long-standing constipation and reliance on enemas or laxatives are more resistant to these measures than younger patients whose bowel patterns are less established. Poor muscle tone, reduced physical activity, and increased incidence of contributory conditions make the problem more difficult in the older age group. Bedridden elderly patients may develop severe constipation and even fecal impaction unless preventive measures are taken. This applies not only to patients with previous constipation but also to those with regular bowel movements prior to their confining illness. Regular administration of stool softeners, bulk laxatives, or mild cathartics is necessary until full ambulation and a normal diet is regained. The onset of fecal impaction in bedridden patients is heralded by a feeling of rectal distention, urgency of defecation, or tenesmus. Occasionally the fecal impaction will result in low-grade chronic obstruction and dilatation and increased fluid content proximal to the impaction; "paradoxical diarrhea" may thus occur as fluid moves past the obstructing fecal mass. This situation will be aggravated if antidiarrheal drugs are given because the underlying constipation will be worsened. The appropriate maneuver is to manually disimpact the rectum, or to administer gentle enemas if the impaction is beyond the reach of the finger.

ACUTE INFLAMMATION OF THE COLON

Acute inflammation of the colon can be caused by a number of infectious agents including viruses, bacteria, or parasites. The clinical manifestations of such infections include fever, crampy lower abdominal pain, and diarrhea, which may be bloody (see Chap. 37). Shigellosis (i.e., infection with *Shigella* organisms) is the most common form of bacterial dysentery. In severe cases gross blood may be present in the stool, and the clinical and sigmoidoscopic picture can mimic acute ulcerative colitis. Definitive diagnosis is established by culture of the organism. Certain pathogenic strains of *Escherichia coli* can invade the colonic epithelium and cause a picture similar to shigellosis. *Salmonella* infections may involve the colon and produce an illness with blood and pus in the stools. Microscopic examination of the stool for leukocytes is a useful technique for differentiating between bacterial dysentery and diarrhea induced by a virus or toxin (e.g., staphylococcal, cholera, or *E. coli* toxin). A fresh stool suspension is mixed with a few drops of methylene blue, which stains the nuclei dark blue, facilitating identification of polymorphonuclear leukocytes. Acute inflammatory cells are seen in *Shigella* or *Salmonella* infections, acute amoebic colitis, or idiopathic ulcerative colitis; they are absent in viral gastroenteritis or enterotoxin-induced diarrheas. Acute amoebic colitis is accompanied by a wide range of symptoms, from mild diarrhea to severe fulminant colitis with megacolon. The diagnosis can be made by demonstrating motile trophozoites of *Entamoeba histolytica* in a freshly passed stool or from swabbings of the mucosa taken during sigmoidoscopy. The colonic appearance is variable, but spotty ulcerations in areas of normal-looking mucosa are quite typical. Trophozoites may occasionally be seen on rectal biopsy. (For further descriptions of the above entities see Chaps. 120, 123, 124, 187, and 199.)

Antibiotic-associated colitis is an important consideration in the differential diagnosis of acute inflammation of the colon. A number of antibiotics, including lincomycin, clindamycin, ampicillin, and tetracycline, have been associated with a spectrum of symptoms, from mild diarrhea to severe fulminant pseudomembranous colitis. *Pseudomembranous colitis* is characterized by diarrhea, crampy abdominal pain, and fever. In most cases of clindamycin-associated pseudomembranous colitis the onset of diarrhea occurs within 4 to 14 days of starting the drug and is more frequent after oral than parenteral use. The rectal mucosa is edematous and hyperemic and is studded with plaque-like pseudomembranes composed of mucus, inflammatory cells, and sloughed epithelial cells. It has been shown that there is an overgrowth of *Clostridium difficile* in the stools of patients with pseudomembranous colitis associated with clindamycin, ampicillin, and various combinations of these and other antibiotics. The clostridia release a *toxin* which causes necrosis of the colonic epithelium and which can be detected in the stools of these patients. Management of antibiotic-associated colitis includes immediate cessation of the offending antibiotics and intravenous replacement of fluid and electrolyte losses. Oral vancomycin (250 mg four times daily) may hasten recovery by eliminating *C. difficile* from the colon. An occasional patient with megacolon or perforation will require emergency colectomy. The majority of patients recover spontaneously in 7 to 10 days.

CHRONIC INFLAMMATORY DISEASES OF THE COLON

Chronic inflammatory bowel disease may be divided into two major entities, chronic nonspecific ulcerative colitis and Crohn's disease of the colon (granulomatous colitis). Although these two disorders share many clinical, pathologic, and epidemiologic features, there are sufficient differences to allow their separation as distinct clinical entities (Table 294-1). However, in approximately 10 to 20 percent of cases the degree of overlap is such that a definite distinction between the two disorders may not be possible. The etiology of both types of chronic inflammatory bowel disease is unknown; hence, the current classification will undoubtedly undergo progressive revision as our knowledge of these entities increases. It is quite possible that ulcerative colitis and Crohn's disease of the colon are variations in the host response to the same etiologic agent.

Detailed epidemiologic studies of the populations in which these two major entities are found have not shown major differences. They are extremely rare in Africa, India, and the Orient. Both are more common in whites than in nonwhites, in urban than in rural settings, in Jews than in non-Jews, and both seem to be increasing in incidence. The best figures available for the Western world suggest that ulcerative colitis, including proctitis, occurs at an annual incidence rate just under 10 per 100,000 white adults at risk, and that Crohn's disease of the colon occurs at a rate of about 2 to 3 per 100,000. Crohn's disease of the small intestine (exclusive of the colon) has an incidence of about 2 per 100,000. In Europe the figures may be slightly lower, and for many areas of the United States no reliable data are available. Both diseases may occur in the same family, but with no regular interrelations. Generally in the same sibship only one disease is found, but parents or children may have the other disease. Multiple cases in families have been found in 10 to 20 percent of all families at risk.

CHRONIC NONSPECIFIC ULCERATIVE COLITIS Pathology

This disorder is characterized by an inflammatory reaction of the mucosa of the colon, including the rectum. The primary response always involves the mucosal epithelial cell, both at the luminal surface and along the crypts. This inflammatory response may be mild or intense, but early in the course of disease one sees neutrophils and eosinophils throughout the lamina propria, often actually invading damaged epithelial cells. As the process becomes more chronic, plasma cells and lymphocytes fill the lamina propria, the crypt goblet cells are replaced with non-mucus-producing cells, the crypts become irregular and may drop out entirely, and mild submucosal fibrosis is noted. Throughout the mucosa one sees intense hyperemia with very little variation in the entire area of involvement; the epithelium loses its integrity, and many small to moderate ulcerations can be identified. The muscular layer and the serosa of the colon do not participate in these responses except in toxic megacolon or in long-standing disease with foreshortening of the colon. In biopsy specimens a purulent exudate mixed with blood can be noted on the luminal surface; small abscesses around and inside the crypts (crypt abscesses) are common but not pathognomonic. The features are those of an acute or subacute mucosal inflammation which is strikingly uniform throughout the involved area of the rectum and colon; however, within a few centimeters of the proximal margin of involvement one finds an abrupt change toward normal.

In the century since the disease was first described, no agreement has been reached on its pathogenesis. According to Morson, in early active colitis there appears to be a vascular response, perhaps consistent with a state of tissue hypersensitivity. It is then converted into the characteristic inflammatory picture as a result of secondary infection by colonic bacteria. Immune responses to bacterial or dietary antigens or altered host proteins may add to the chronic inflammatory response.

The repeated bouts of inflammation produce a number of characteristic pathologic features. The bowel tends to become shorter, largely because of a peculiar retraction of longitudinal muscles rather than fibrosis. The rectum is nearly always markedly contracted, but often looks endoscopically less involved grossly than the colon more proximal to it. The colonic serosa is usually moist, shiny, and hyperemic, but not thickened or adherent to other intraabdominal structures. The submucosa is thin, and the mucosa markedly hyperemic and usually hemorrhagic. With continuing inflammation and loss of

TABLE 294-1
Chronic inflammatory bowel disease

Features	Ulcerative colitis	Crohn's disease of colon
Clinical:		
Rectal bleeding	Common, continuous	Infrequent
Fistula formation	Rare	Common
Perianal, perirectal abscess	Occasional	Common
Toxic megacolon	Occasional	Rare
Sigmoidoscopic:		
Rectal involvement	95%	50%
Friability	Frequent	Uncommon
Radiologic:		
Type of involvement	Continuous	Discontinuous
Right colon involvement	Occasional	Frequent
Terminal ileum, if involved	Widened, patulous	Narrow, stiff
Small bowel	Normal	Often involved
Pathologic:		
Depth of involvement	Mucosa and submucosa	Transmural
Granulomas	Rare	Common
Fissures, fistulas	Rare	Common
Mesenteric fat and lymph nodes	Not involved	Edematous and hyperplastic
Occurrence of malignancy	Occasional	Rare

crypts, the mucosa may be thinned to the point of denudation. Hyperplastic overgrowth of regenerating mucosa produces the characteristic inflammatory polyps or *pseudopolyps* (Fig. 294-4). A pseudopolyp is an island of inflamed mucosa surrounded by areas of denuded mucosa; hence the pseudopolyp appears as a raised area projecting into the lumen. In the severe acute form of colitis known as *toxic megacolon,* large areas of mucosa may become necrotic, leaving exposed the muscular coats which are friable and thinned out. Neural elements in the remaining wall may be severely damaged, and the entire wall is easily torn at surgery or subject to spontaneous perforation. When such severe damage to the muscular elements is present, the colon, particularly the transverse colon, is often grossly dilated and may be filled with blood and purulent exudate.

Etiology The etiology of ulcerative colitis is still unknown. Suggestions include genetic factors, transmissible agents (such as viruses or other microorganisms), reactions to allergens (such as milk proteins and bacterial polysaccharides), autoimmune phenomena, or a combination of these mechanisms. Some evidence for each of these possibilities has come from clinical studies (e.g., familial incidence) and animal experiments (e.g., suggestion of filterable agents in patients' colonic tissue and nodes able to produce lesions similar to colitis in animals). Some features of the disease, e.g., hemorrhagic necrosis of mucosa and vasculitis in the submucosa, have been experimentally produced by modifications of the Arthus or Shwartzman phenomena. In the dog a severe acute colitis with histiocytic proliferation has been observed as a naturally occurring disease. In none of these conditions or models has the full range of the pathologic or clinical features of the human disorder been seen.

The role of immune mechanisms in chronic ulcerative colitis has received much attention. The disease may be associated with erythema nodosum, arthritis, uveitis, and autoimmune hemolytic anemia, conditions suspected of having an immune basis. Furthermore, the serum of some patients with ulcerative colitis contains an antibody to colon epithelial cells. This antibody probably results from tissue injury and has been found in patients with a number of unrelated gastrointestinal diseases. Lymphocytotoxic antibodies occur in the serum in about 40 percent of patients. Several studies have suggested that abnormalities of cell-mediated immunity may be important in both chronic ulcerative colitis and Crohn's disease of the colon. Peripheral lymphocytes from patients with both diseases are cytotoxic to colon epithelial cells grown in tissue culture. Lymphocytes from patients with either disorder also release a substance which inhibits macrophage migration. Some patients with chronic inflammatory bowel disease are anergic to a number of antigenic stimuli, and the proportion of circulating thymus-derived lymphocytes (T cells) is diminished in some patients with Crohn's disease. Immunoglobulin levels in serum and colonic secretions are normal, but the proportion of circulating lymphocytes bearing surface immunoglobulin is significantly increased in both ulcerative colitis and Crohn's disease. Similar findings have been demonstrated in other chronic inflammatory diseases, suggesting that alterations in lymphocyte number and function are nonspecific responses to various pathogenic stimuli. Thus, the role of immune mechanisms in initiating or perpetuating the inflammatory response in the colon is unknown.

Psychologic features of patients with ulcerative colitis have also been stressed. There have been many suggestions of a relation between the onset of the disorder and major psychologic stress such as loss of a family member. Emphasis has been placed on the juvenile appearance of such patients, as well as their frequent feelings of helplessness or hopelessness in meeting routine life stresses. They often display an underlying hostility and have poorly developed interpersonal relation-

ships. On the other hand, about half the patients with ulcerative colitis appear to be normal in their psychologic behavior; these subjects have a resilient personal and work history; are successful in their educational pursuits, trade, or profession; and have maintained strong interpersonal relations.

A small number of patients have been studied prior to and subsequent to total colectomy; of these, about half have shown dramatic improvement of their depressive and despondent reactions, whereas underlying personality disorders persist in the remainder. The disease itself, with its relapses and remissions and its cost in time, money, and damaged career hopes, is usually associated with some degree of depression and anxiety in all patients. These reactions are important factors in modifying the course of the disease and the response to therapy. There is little doubt that in a significant proportion of patients with ulcerative colitis deep-seated personality disorders exist. However, it is not at all clear whether or how such psychopathology is related to the colonic inflammatory process.

Clinical features The major symptoms of chronic ulcerative colitis are *bloody diarrhea, abdominal pain, fever,* and *weight loss.* The extent of bleeding and diarrhea is quite variable, ranging from several semiformed stools per day to frequent passage, up to 20 times daily, of liquid stools with blood and pus. It should be emphasized that in a small percentage of patients, specific symptoms referable to the colon may be minimal or absent and only such nonspecific complaints as fatigue, malaise, or failure to thrive (in children) can be elicited. Rarely, a patient with ulcerative colitis may present with constipation, particularly those with predominantly rectal disease. In most patients, very little will be found on routine physical examination, except that the abdomen may be distended. In some patients one finds signs of extracolonic manifestations such as ocular inflammation, arthritis, or jaundice.

Laboratory findings in ulcerative colitis are quite nonspecific. Anemia due to a combination of iron deficiency and chronic inflammation is common. Leukocytosis with a shift to the left is frequent, especially during acute febrile exacerbations. Hypoalbuminemia, electrolyte disturbances, a mild increase in serum alkaline phosphatase, and elevations of the sedimentation rate are often found.

The *clinical course of chronic ulcerative colitis is highly variable* and relates in part to the extent of involvement and the intensity of the inflammatory process. Most patients give a history of intermittent symptoms interspersed with periods of normal or near-normal health. In others the disease is chronic and unremitting with continuous diarrhea, anemia, and nonspecific symptoms. Still others have an acute initial attack followed by apparent good health for periods ranging up to 10 or 15 years. In the majority of patients the symptoms are mild with fewer than four or five bowel movements per day and minimal blood loss, fever, or pain. Others have moderate or severe symptoms with disabling diarrhea, blood loss, abdominal pain, fever, and extracolonic complications. Fulminant disease occurs in 15 percent or less of patients. These patients are usually hospitalized with severe hemorrhagic diarrhea, fevers, abdominal pain and tenderness, dehydration, and electrolyte disturbances. A subset of this group will develop toxic megacolon (see below), which is associated with a significant mortality during the acute attack.

The extent of colonic involvement in ulcerative colitis is also quite variable. In two-thirds of patients the left half of the colon is involved; in many of these the rectum is initially involved, and the disease spreads proximally to involve the sigmoid and descending colon. The remainder of patients exhibit pancolitis, with the disease process involving the entire colon up to the ileocecal valve. In some of these the process will involve a small segment of the terminal ileum (so-called "backwash" ileitis). Except for the latter finding, *ulcerative colitis does not involve the small intestine,* a distinguishing feature from Crohn's disease which may involve both large and small intestine.

Diagnosis The diagnosis of chronic ulcerative colitis should be entertained in patients presenting with bloody diarrhea, the most common symptom of this disease. The atypical presentations of the disease are more confusing and often misdiagnosed. As mentioned above, constipation occurs in some patients, particularly with rectal or left colon involvement. Others present with a fever of unknown etiology but no bowel complaints, or with extracolonic manifestations such as arthritis or liver disease which may antedate or overshadow the bowel involvement. The most important diagnostic studies are sigmoidoscopy and barium enema.

The typical *sigmoidoscopic appearance* in ulcerative colitis consists of loss of the normal mucosal detail, increase in mucosal friability, and the presence of a thick inflammatory exudate composed of pus, mucus, and blood. Normally the rectal mucosa appears wet and shiny, and through it the finely branched submucosal vessels are visible. Bleeding is absent except when the tip of the instrument traumatizes the epithelial surface. In ulcerative colitis this fine mucosal detail is lost because of submucosal edema and inflammatory cell infiltration, and the blood vessels may be invisible. Heaped-up areas of inflammation cause the appearance of granularity, and the mucosa may appear redder than normal because of hyperemia. The *most characteristic finding is increased mucosal friability,* which is demonstrated by wiping the mucosa with a cotton-tipped swab and noting the appearance of minute bleeding points. Pseudopolyps and strictures are occasionally observed. Frank ulcerations are uncommon in the rectosigmoid area, as compared with their frequent occurrence more proximally in surgical specimens. Confirmation of the inflammatory process is obtained by rectal biopsy of the involved area. In ulcerative colitis, the sigmoidoscopic examination may be extremely painful and thus threatening for the patient. This is due in part to the

physician's desire to pass the instrument to its full length (25 cm) in order to establish the upper extent of disease. In patients with acute severe disease or painful perirectal complications (e.g., hemorrhoids or fissures), it is more prudent to examine only the distal 8 to 10 cm, postponing the complete examination until the disease is quiescent. Some patients are so traumatized by sigmoidoscopy that they become very reluctant to allow repeat examinations.

The *barium enema* is most helpful in assessing extent of disease and the presence of complications such as stricture, pseudopolyposis, or carcinoma (Figs. 294-3 and 294-4). It must be stressed, however, that patients with severe acute colitis may not tolerate a barium enema, and, in some, toxic megacolon has resulted from a barium study or the vigorous cleansing measures that proceed it. In many instances it is wisest to postpone the barium enema until the acute attack has subsided and the patient's general condition has improved. The physician should carefully review the standard preparation for barium enema and modify it to suit the individual patient's clinical condition.

The abnormalities on barium enema reflect the extent and duration of the inflammatory process. Early in the course of the disease or in disease localized to the rectum, the barium enema may be entirely normal. The earliest abnormality is a finely serrated or spiculated appearance of the mucosal surface caused by penetration of the barium into shallow ulcerations. As the disease progresses, these erosions become deeper and burrow laterally, producing a "collar button" ulcer. With chronic disease the bowel becomes a rigid, foreshortened tube which lacks the usual haustral markings (Fig. 294-5*A*). Other findings include appearance of pseudopolyps, strictures, or mass lesions indicative of a carcinoma.

Colonoscopy is useful in the diagnostic evaluation of certain patients with ulcerative colitis. In very early colitis, colonoscopy is the best method for evaluating extent of disease, since it is much more sensitive than the barium enema in detecting minimal mucosal abnormalities. Colonoscopic biopsies may also be useful in differentiating benign from malignant stric-

FIGURE 294-4

Pseudopolyposis of the entire colon secondary to chronic ulcerative colitis of 12 years' duration.

FIGURE 294-3

Adenomatous polyp of sigmoid colon on a long stalk.

tures and in the evaluation of polypoid lesions in patients with colitis. Colonoscopy is not routinely required in all patients with colitis, since the diagnosis can usually be established by barium enema and sigmoidoscopy.

Differential diagnosis In distinguishing ulcerative colitis from other disorders, one must consider primarily the clinical symptoms together with the sigmoidoscopic and radiologic features. When the primary complaint is rectal bleeding, *hemorrhoids* are commonly found, but should never be considered the sole cause of rectal bleeding until sigmoidoscopy and barium enema have ruled out other lesions. The next most important cause of rectal bleeding is *carcinoma* of the colon; here the combination of sigmoidoscopy and barium enema will serve to differentiate most cases. However, it must be remembered that ulcerative colitis and carcinoma may coexist. *Crohn's disease of the colon* may present with rectal bleeding; the differential diagnostic features are found in Table 294-1. *Amoebiasis* may present as rectal bleeding, and such bleeding is commonly found even when other features are more prominent. Sigmoidoscopic demonstration of discrete ulcers, microscopic studies of the fecal swabbings showing motile trophozoites, and the presence of trophozoites in rectal biopsies are the most important differential findings. *Radiation proctitis* shows localized telangiectasia, submucosal atrophy, and friability in the mid-rectum; such a patient has a history of prior pelvic irradiation. Large rectal ulcers, aphthous oral ulcers, uveitis, and urethritis occur in *Behçet's syndrome,* a type of vasculitis.

When diarrhea is the presenting symptom, the most important entities to be differentiated are the specific intestinal infections. Acute *bacillary dysentery,* especially shigellosis, produces hemorrhagic and purulent involvement of mucosa, which may be sigmoidoscopically indistinguishable from ulcerative colitis. The diagnosis therefore must be made by stool culture and serologic studies since mucosal biopsy is not diagnostic. *Tuberculosis* of the intestine characteristically involves the terminal ileum and adjacent cecum; advanced pulmonary lesions are usually present. The lesion in tuberculosis is usually a hyperplastic process, so that x-ray findings tend to resemble Crohn's disease or carcinoma of the ileocecal area rather than ulcerative colitis. *Celiac sprue* or *Whipple's disease* can on occasion be initially confused with ulcerative colitis, but the absence of colonic pathology and positive findings on upper gastrointestinal barium studies and small-bowel biopsy serve to separate these entities.

Abdominal pain in association with rectal bleeding and sudden disturbance of bowel habits may be due to *ischemic colitis,* usually seen in older patients with generalized vascular disease. The sigmoidoscopic examination is usually normal, unless the ischemic area involves the rectum. If the affected area is visible, one may observe edema, hyperemia, bleeding, and occasionally ulceration, which can be confused with ulcerative colitis. The radiologic features of ischemic colitis have been well described and usually permit one to make the diagnosis.

Disturbance in bowel function, particularly constipation with rectal urgency (i.e., tenesmus with inability to expel stool), but with passage of mucus, blood, or pus, is a feature of *ulcerative proctitis.* This diagnosis is totally dependent on proper interpretation of sigmoidoscopic findings since x-ray studies are usually negative. Stinging rectal pain with creamy pus in the rectum suggests *gonorrheal proctitis.* In such patients, the discharge should be cultured for gonococci, and a history of anal intercourse should be sought. The *irritable bow-*

FIGURE 294-5

Inflammatory disease of colon. A. Chronic ulcerative colitis with loss of haustral marking in left colon, pseudopolyps in right and transverse colon. B. Crohn's disease with skip areas in descending colon and cecum.

A

B

el syndrome (see above) usually first manifests itself in persons of the same age and sex as those at greatest risk of developing ulcerative colitis, but they do not have abnormal sigmoidoscopic findings, fever, leukocytosis, or blood and pus in the stools, and the barium enema is normal. Patients with *chronic laxative abuse* may give a history of diarrhea which may be associated with hypokalemia and evidence of right-sided colonic dysfunction—very voluminous watery stools, but without the sigmoidoscopic features of inflammation. The radiologic picture is quite characteristic, showing slowly changing muscular contractions, dilated ascending colon, and loss of haustrations of the left colon. The history of chronic laxative ingestion, although often concealed, will confirm this diagnosis.

Complications of ulcerative colitis The complications of this disease may be either local or systemic (see Table 294-2). Since the bowel wall is thinned by the disease process, perforation may develop. Acute perforation occurs most often with the first severe attack and is more likely to occur with extensive colonic involvement. Perforation may involve any site, but the sigmoid colon is most often involved. The features are those of peritonitis, with evidence of systemic toxicity; diagnosis is confirmed by the radiological demonstration of free air under the diaphragm. Conservative management of such patients carries a high mortality; in general, perforation is an indication for immediate colectomy.

Toxic megacolon can occur in amoebic or granulomatous colitis, but is most often seen in severe or fulminant ulcerative colitis. The patient typically has high fever, tachycardia, electrolyte imbalance, hypoalbuminemia, and pronounced diarrhea. Sometimes acute dilatation occurs suddenly in a patient with pancolitis in remission, with the onset of distention, abdominal pain, cessation of stools, and anorexia. Events which often precede this complication are excessive use of antidiarrheal drugs (such as diphenoxylate, codeine, or paregoric) or vigorous use of cathartics and enemas in preparation for barium studies. This process probably goes unrecognized in many patients with chronic colitis and may be spontaneously reversible. Toxic megacolon can be described as a paralysis of the motor function of the transverse colon, with rapid dilatation of that segment of the bowel, best diagnosed by the plain film of the abdomen. The diameter of the colon exceeds 6 cm, and the wall may be noted to contain gas. Often the borders on the luminal side are shaggy, and islands of necrotic mucosa can be seen to alternate with preserved mucosa. The predilection of the dilatation for the transverse colon probably results from the fact that in the supine position air collects in the transverse colon because it is higher than the rest of the large bowel. Toxic megacolon, occurring usually in patients with severe pancolitis, is associated with a mortality of up to 30 percent. Death results from localized perforation and septic shock.

TABLE 294-2
Systemic complications of inflammatory bowel disease

I Nutritional and metabolic changes
   A Loss of muscle mass
   B Electrolyte losses (K^+, Ca^{2+}, Mg^{2+})
   C Hypoalbuminemia
   D Iron-deficiency anemia
   E Vitamin deficiencies
   F Growth retardation in children
II Arthritis
III Liver disease
IV Skin disorders
V Uveitis
VI Stomatitis
VII Venous thrombosis and thromboembolism
VIII Renal stones

Anorectal complications such as fissures, fistulas, and abscesses may be the presenting symptoms, particularly in granulomatous ileocolitis. Many of the anal complaints are secondary to the diarrhea itself. The discomfort and anxiety produced by anorectal complications are often of more concern than the other symptoms of colitis; the discomfort may discourage attempts by the physician to examine the patient with the sigmoidoscope or to carry out necessary diagnostic studies. Local anesthetics may be helpful under such circumstances; short-acting general anesthesia is warranted if it is impossible otherwise to carry out such studies because of pain. The management of such complications consists of the local measures, as noted below, and treatment of the colitis itself. In some patients the entire function of the anorectal segment is lost; this is an indication for colectomy and ileostomy. Rectovaginal fistula results from breakdown or perforation of the wall between the rectum and vagina. This complication may allow the passage of stool or flatus from the vagina if the opening is large enough. In other patients, the fistula will be quite small and demonstrable only with a probe.

The development of *colonic strictures* may be caused by muscular hypertrophy, fibrosis, or malignancy. Inflammation and hypertrophy of the muscularis may cause narrowing which varies over the course of time. Hence, "strictures" of this sort may be reversible. True fibrosis is unusual in ulcerative colitis but when present may mimic a constricting carcinoma. For this reason, when a narrowed segment or stricture is found, it is important to exclude the presence of carcinoma; if the narrowed area can be seen and reached directly, biopsy and brush cytology may be diagnostic. The radiologic differentiation of benign from malignant stricture is not simple; colonoscopic examination may be helpful.

Inflammatory polyps, or *pseudopolyps,* may appear within a few months of a first attack of severe colitis; more commonly, however, they are noted within the first or second year after the onset of the colitis. They are a response to mucosal ulceration and thus define to some extent the severity of the mucosal damage. They are not of themselves precancerous, but they occur in the patients with severe disease who are more likely to develop colon cancer. They produce no symptoms and require no specific treatment. When present, they may make it difficult for the endoscopist to detect early carcinoma developing in mucosa adjacent to the polypoid changes.

Carcinoma of the colon is a serious complication of ulcerative colitis, although the overall incidence is difficult to define unless one subgroups the colitic population. Patients with localized ulcerative proctitis are not subject to increased risk of carcinoma of either rectum or colon. If colitis begins before age 15, the risk of colon cancer reaches 20 percent in those who have the disease for 20 years. This risk continues and increases with age. Factors increasing the risk are (1) duration of active disease greater than 10 years, (2) pancolitis, and (3) family history of colonic cancer. In general, patients with ulcerative colitis (other than proctitis) have an incidence of colonic cancer which is at least 10 times greater than that of a matched control population.

Carcinoma of the colon in patients with colitis tends to be difficult to diagnose for many reasons. Symptoms are often those of colitis. The tumors often arise multicentrically and are poorly defined radiologically because of spreading, indurated margins which blend into the abnormal colitic mucosa. In some patients the cancer is already metastatic when discovered, making surgical cure impossible. Since the diagnosis is so difficult, other means of diagnosing carcinoma have been proposed. Morson and Pang believe that a generalized precancerous stage (dysplasia) can be identified in rectal or rectosigmoid biopsies of patients who either have or will soon develop cancer of the colon. In their view, suspicious microscopic changes consist of epithelial tubules penetrating the muscularis and atypical epithelial cells with stratification of enlarged nuclei and increased mitotic activity. Detection of these changes requires examination of multiple biopsies by a skilled pathologist with a special interest in this field. Because of these factors, this approach has been utilized in only a few centers. Until better methods are available, one must depend upon radiologic criteria, change in clinical status, and frequent sigmoidoscopy or colonoscopy (with biopsies) to aid in the detection of malignancy.

Systemic complications (see Table 294-3) *Nutritional* and *metabolic complications* result from deficient colonic intake as well as from increased nutritional requirements and losses. Most patients with moderately severe ulcerative colitis have some anorexia; severely ill patients have in addition nausea and often vomiting. Weight loss and loss of muscle mass are to be expected under such circumstances. The negative nitrogen balance seen in all febrile inflammatory states is enhanced by increased corticosteroid production and increased levels of circulating catecholamines; these serve to mobilize fat from adipose tissue and stimulate gluconeogenesis. Muscle breakdown releases potassium from cells, and potassium deficits resulting from this mechanism as well as chronic diarrhea are common in these ill patients. Many such patients are initially unable to take oral feedings and are given parenteral fluids which are usually deficient in calcium and magnesium. Magnesium deficiency is an important complication and may account for some of the irritability seen in severely ill patients. The large surface area of mucosal ulceration also permits losses of albumin, red blood cells, and potassium in the stools. Anemia may be due to iron deficiency or secondary to chronic inflammation. Occasional patients develop an autoimmune hemolytic anemia. Drug-induced hemolytic anemia may develop in patients with deficiency of erythrocyte glucose 6-phosphate dehydrogenase who receive sulfasalazine or other drugs. Defects in blood coagulation may also occur; most often this is manifest as increased coagulability, with the production of thromboembolic phenomena. In both ulcerative colitis and Crohn's disease there may be an increase in the number of circulating platelets when the disease is active.

Liver disease is another major systemic complication. The incidence of liver biopsy abnormalities in patients with colitis range from 50 to 90 percent; however, the incidence of significant clinical liver disease is approximately 1 to 3 percent. *Fatty infiltration* is a common histologic abnormality, especially in autopsy material, and is related to poor nutrition and chronic inflammation. *Pericholangitis* is characterized pathologically by inflammation of the portal tract, bile duct proliferation, and fibrosis around the bile ductules. These changes may be related to portal bacteremia which occurs intermittently in some patients with colitis. Patients with pericholangitis may have only mildly abnormal liver function tests, particularly mild increases in serum alkaline phosphatase. Others present with jaundice plus elevation of alkaline phosphatase and the clinical features of cholestasis. *Sclerosing cholangitis* is a chronic low-grade inflammation of the extrahepatic biliary tree which results in thickening of the bile ducts and gradual obliteration of the lumen. These patients present with obstructive jaundice and ascending cholangitis, which progresses to secondary biliary cirrhosis if untreated. *Cholangiocarcinoma* is apparently increased in patients with chronic ulcerative colitis, perhaps as a result of chronic cholangitis. The tumor may arise in the distal common bile duct or more proximally at the bifurcation of the hepatic ducts. Finally, *chronic active hepatitis* and subsequent postnecrotic cirrhosis may complicate colitis. Colectomy may dramatically arrest the progress of pericholangitis or sclerosing cholangitis in some patients; however, this benefit must be weighed against the increased surgical morbidity and mortality in colitis patients with concomitant liver disease.

A variety of *skin and eye lesions* may occur in up to 5 percent of patients. Erythema nodosum appears most often in young women with colitis. Pyoderma gangrenosum is a suppurative ulcerating lesion found on the legs and ankles, usually in patients with very active colitis. These lesions often improve as the colitis is brought under control, either by medical or surgical treatment. However, some patients have persistent pyoderma in the face of inactive colitis, even after removal of the colon. Uveitis has been reported in 3 to 10 percent of patients. Although the uveitis may respond well to local or systemic corticosteroid therapy, dramatic disappearance of the lesion may be noted when colectomy is done for other indications.

Joint manifestations are quite common in patients with inflammatory bowel disease. In most cases patients have *arthralgias* or aching in various joints or periarticular tissues rather than true arthritis. Acute *arthritis,* as evidenced by joint swelling, tenderness, and limitation of motion, occurs in 5 percent of patients. The arthritis is often migratory, affecting several larger joints, particularly knees and ankles, although one joint may be primarily involved. The aspirated joint fluid will reveal an acute inflammatory exudate; negative culture of the joint fluid and negative serologic tests for rheumatoid factor, antinuclear antibody, and LE factor help to differentiate it from other arthritides. The bouts of arthritis correlate fairly well with the activity of the colitis and with other extracolonic manifestations such as uveitis or skin disease. Permanent deformity is rare, and in most cases the arthritis lasts less than 1 year. Sometimes the joint symptoms may precede the onset of colitis by weeks or months. The arthritis generally disappears after total colectomy.

Ankylosing spondylitis is 20 times more frequent in patients with inflammatory bowel disease than in the general population. This complication is characterized by inflammation of the sacroiliac joint and spondylitis of the lumbar spine, which may eventually progress upward and cause fusion of the entire vertebral column. Ankylosing spondylitis in patients with inflammatory bowel disease is similar to the syndrome in patients without bowel disease, except that there is a greater preponderance of females affected which reduces the male/female ratio from approximately 20:1 to 4:1. The spondylitis may precede the colitis by several years or more, is usually not well correlated with the activity of the disease, and often persists after total colectomy. Patients with inflammatory bowel disease and ankylosing spondylitis have an increased likelihood of bearing the HLA-B27 histocompatibility antigen, but the significance of this association is unclear.

Treatment MEDICAL MANAGEMENT Except for those patients with mild disease, or disease limited to the rectum, the acute attack of ulcerative colitis is best treated in the hospital setting rather than on an outpatient basis. The disease can be explosive, and it is often difficult to anticipate its course from the initial presentation. The aims of therapy are to control the inflammation and replace nutritional losses, both of which are necessary before the patient can resume normal activity. Many patients respond best to bed rest, no food other than clear liquids, and intravenous feedings to replace fluid and electrolyte losses. Severe anemia requires blood transfusion, as these patients do not respond to iron therapy or other hematinics during the stage of acute inflammation. The use of opiates or diphenoxylate (Lomotil) in moderately or severely ill patients is fraught with danger since they may precipitate toxic megacolon. They are indicated only in patients whose acute disease is controlled or in whom frequent diarrheal stools are troublesome.

The technique of *intravenous alimentation* has been successfully employed in a number of patients with severe colitis, although it is not without risk. By stopping all oral feedings, the intestinal tract is put to rest and the stool volume decreases. The patient can be supplied with all the nutrients, vitamins, and minerals required for healing of the ulcerative process and restoration of weight. This approach is useful in restoring positive nutritional balance in severely ill patients, particularly in those who are awaiting surgery. In some patients intravenous alimentation and complete bowel rest have allowed more effective control of the disease and prevented surgical intervention. Low-residue or elemental diets provide good nutrition with low fecal volume, thus allowing the bowel to "rest." Restriction of milk products in the diet may reduce the frequency of diarrhea inasmuch as some patients with colitis have coexistent lactose intolerance.

Antibiotics are not indicated in acute ulcerative colitis unless a focus of bacterial infection such as a perirectal abscess can be demonstrated. The *anti-inflammatory drugs* which are the most useful in treating the disease process are (1) *adrenal corticosteroids* given either as prednisone, prednisolone, or hydrocortisone or *ACTH* (which stimulates the endogenous production of adrenal corticosteroids), and (2) *sulfasalazine* (Azulfidine). The rationale for the use of corticosteroids is their known anti-inflammatory response, although immune suppression may also be an additional factor in their usefulness. Sulfasalazine is composed of an antibiotic (sulfapyridine) linked to a salicylate (5-aminosalicylic acid). This compound is not absorbed in the stomach or upper small intestine and passes into the distal small intestine and colon, where it is split by bacteria. Sulfapyridine is absorbed and excreted in the urine; the salicylate moiety remains in the colon and is excreted in the stool. The effectiveness of sulfasalazine in ulcerative colitis is attributed to the anti-inflammatory action of the salicylate moiety rather than to the antimicrobial activity of the sulfapyridine. The major goal of sulfasalazine therapy is to prevent recurrences of colitis; it is usually not effective in the control of acute, severe colitis.

For the acutely ill patient the administration of corticosteroids or ACTH is the initial treatment of choice. Some clinicians prefer ACTH to prednisone or other corticosteroids, although the rationale for this preference has never been established by controlled clinical trials. The usual practice is to give 40 to 80 units per day of ACTH in a slow intravenous drip, reducing this as the symptoms improve and substituting oral corticosteroids after 7 to 10 days. If treatment is begun with oral steroids, usually 40 to 60 mg prednisone per day is given initially, with the dose tapered gradually as improvement occurs. The goal of corticosteroid therapy is to reduce the inflammatory process as reflected by reduction in diarrhea, abdominal pain, and fever and improvement in appetite. In the majority of patients this is noted within 7 to 10 days of starting therapy.

After initial improvement has occurred, oral feedings may be resumed and the dosage of prednisone reduced. Sulfasalazine is started at a dosage of 500 mg twice daily, then increased after several days to 500 mg four times daily. A dosage of 4 to 6 g daily is usually not exceeded. Prednisone can then usually be tapered to 10 mg per day over the next 2 to 6 months. Ideally, the patient should be maintained on sulfasalazine in the hope of preventing relapse as corticosteroids are withdrawn altogether to avoid the serious side effects of their long-term usage. Some patients have persistent symptoms which worsen as attempts are made to reduce the dosage of prednisone, and these individuals are usually maintained on prednisone at 10 to 15 mg daily. Patients who require higher doses of prednisone to suppress continuous activity may develop severe side effects such as osteoporosis, hypertension, diabetes, and increased susceptibility to infection (see Chap. 336). Alternate-day corticosteroid therapy may be useful in minimizing certain side effects, but this schedule is often therapeutically ineffective.

Immunosuppressive therapy with azathioprine has been used on the assumption that cellular immune mechanisms are important in the pathogenesis of ulcerative colitis. Some studies suggest that azathioprine may be useful after remission has been produced with corticosteroids. Most clinicians feel that the drug should be tried only in those patients who do not tolerate, or have had complications from, corticosteroids or sulfasalazine. The usual procedure is to administer azathioprine at a dose of 1.5 to 2 mg/kg while gradually tapering corticosteroids. In many instances, the adult patient will be on a maintenance dose of 10 mg prednisone and 100 mg azathioprine. The white blood cell count is measured at frequent intervals, and patients carefully observed for signs of infection.

Toxic megacolon is a major complication of ulcerative colitis which requires careful management by both internist and surgeon. Opinion is divided as to the most effective therapeutic approach; some advocate emergency colectomy as soon as possible in all patients, while others recommend continued medical therapy with colectomy performed only if perforation occurs or seems imminent. Each case must be judged individually on the basis of frequent bedside evaluations and plain abdominal x-rays. Some patients will improve on the measures outlined above, and surgery can be carried out electively or postponed. The patient who fails to improve or continues to deteriorate will require prompt colectomy.

In patients with *ulcerative proctitis* or *mild ulcerative colitis*, a less vigorous approach may be taken. These patients do not require hospitalization and may respond initially to sulfasalazine. The usual dosage is 0.5 to 1 g four times daily with meals. If tenesmus continues, improvement may be obtained with the intrarectal instillation of steroids, of which there are many available preparations. In general, 20 mg prednisone (or 100 mg hydrocortisone) in 60 to 100 ml saline administered rectally at bedtime may provide beneficial effects without producing appreciable steroid side effects. Disposable retention enema units or foams containing hydrocortisone are a practical approach to the problem. If large doses of rectal steroids are needed to control symptoms, it is preferable to use oral prednisone at doses of about 20 mg per day. Such patients may do well on alternate-day prednisone, at levels of 20 to 40 mg per day.

PSYCHOTHERAPY   Most psychiatrists agree that the acutely ill patient is approachable only with the most superficial forms of supportive psychotherapy. This is best supplied by the physician managing the case, who must establish a strong physician-patient relationship. The physician should search the patient's history and behavior for indications of inner resources and motivations which can be converted to therapeutic use. Attempts to manipulate the immediate home and work environment of the patient are necessary, but may require professional psychiatric assistance. This is particularly true in children and pregnant women. Ulcerative colitis beginning during pregnancy is occasionally very severe and creates profound psychologic disturbances. The attending physician should create an attitude of optimism, warm concern, and orderly management; frequent visits and examinations are the cornerstone of good medical management.

In the chronically ill patient, in particular, children or adolescents, psychiatric help is often crucial in assessing and strengthening adaptive response and in preparing patients for colectomy. When ulcerative colitis occurs in elderly patients, it is often in a setting of despondency which may require emergency psychiatric care. Suicide accounts for a small but appreciable number of deaths from this disease.

SURGICAL THERAPY Perhaps the most urgent indication for colectomy is toxic megacolon. Another group of patients with severe, acute colitis, but without the full-blown picture of toxic megacolon, may also require surgery, but under less urgent conditions. These patients fail to improve in 2 or 3 weeks of intensive medical management and continue to have severe diarrhea, rectal bleeding, pain, fever, and weight loss. The decision for surgery versus continued medical therapy is a difficult one and requires expert clinical judgment. Other indications for colectomy include severe life-threatening hemorrhage, stricture or suspected malignancy, and chronic debilitating disease poorly controlled by medical management.

Prophylactic colectomy to prevent colon cancer still remains a controversial issue. The decision is especially difficult in patients with long-standing quiescent disease who are leading a normal life but are at high risk for developing colon cancer. Total colectomy is associated with a significant mortality rate (2 to 5 percent), the chance of producing impotence in males, and the burden of a permanent ileostomy. Given the present diagnostic limitations, many recommend alternating barium enema examinations (one year) and colonoscopy (next year) to detect early cancer. Colonoscopy, with multiple biopsies of areas without active inflammation, may allow for the selection of patients who are at high risk for the development of colon cancer.

Many patients are extremely reluctant to undergo colectomy and require much support prior to operation. In most large cities there are ileostomy groups who visit patients about to undergo surgery. The patient is usually visited by an individual of his own age and sex who is symptom-free and leading a normal life with a permanent ileostomy. It is also advisable to educate the patient about the function and care of the ileostomy prior to surgery, and in this situation a former patient volunteer or a nurse familiar with stoma care can be most effective.

Prognosis The prognosis of ulcerative colitis has been favorably influenced by the introduction of corticosteroids and sulfasalazine, as well as improvement in supportive techniques such as intravenous alimentation. The probability of inducing remission in hospitalized patients with ulcerative colitis is very high. In a large series in England the incidence of remission from an acute attack was 86 percent; colectomy was necessary in 0.8 percent, and death was recorded in 4.5 percent. As one might expect, the mortality rate was much higher in patients with severe disease involving the entire colon, particularly in those over age 60. In general the short-term outlook, except for toxic megacolon, is excellent.

The long-term prognosis of chronic ulcerative colitis and the effects of therapy are more difficult to assess, because of the extreme variability of the disease process. Patients with mild disease limited to the left colon or rectum have the best prognosis and rarely require hospitalization. With moderate activity and more extensive colonic involvement the course is punctuated by more frequent relapses and complications, and the time spent in hospital or out of work increases. About 75 percent of patients will experience recurrences, and with each acute relapse both morbidity and mortality are increased. The 5-year mortality in patients with severe or moderately severe first attacks ranges between 5 and 15 percent. Approximately 20 to 25 percent of patients with ulcerative colitis will require colectomy during the course of the disease. Colectomy is curative for chronic ulcerative colitis, except for the rare patient in whom extracolonic complications persist.

Colitis and pregnancy The presence of ulcerative colitis probably reduces fertility in both men and women because of the debilitating nature of the disease, malnutrition, and depression. However, the disease itself is not a contraindication to pregnancy or an indication for therapeutic abortion unless the life of the mother is threatened. Furthermore, the pregnancy itself is not adversely affected by the existence of colitis; of women with preexisting colitis who become pregnant, 85 percent will deliver normal babies. However, it appears from several studies that colitis developing during pregnancy is more severe. Preexisting colitis is occasionally worsened during pregnancy, but the relapse rate in one series was not greater than in patients of childbearing age who were not pregnant. Corticosteroid treatment is possibly hazardous to the fetus, particularly in the first trimester, and for this reason it is prudent to treat with sulfasalazine, which has not been associated with fetal damage. The delivery itself is conducted in the usual fashion unless severe perirectal complications preclude vaginal delivery.

Ulcerative proctitis This is a mild form of ulcerative colitis which involves only the rectum (distal 12 to 14 cm of colon). The presenting symptoms are rectal bleeding which may be associated with constipation rather than diarrhea, suggesting a hemorrhoid or fissure. The diagnosis depends on sigmoidoscopy which reveals friability, increased mucus, and an inflammatory exudate; the barium enema is usually normal except in long-standing disease when pronounced narrowing of the rectum and obliteration of the normal folds may be seen. The incidence of complications, both local and systemic, is reduced. Of particular importance is the very low incidence of carcinoma compared with patients with diffuse colonic involvement. Sulfasalazine or steroid enemas are usually effective treatment, and intensive in-patient treatment is not required.

CROHN'S DISEASE OF THE COLON (GRANULOMATOUS COLITIS) In the last decade numerous studies have confirmed the existence of a chronic inflammatory colitis with features similar to Crohn's disease of the small intestine and distinct from chronic ulcerative colitis. This entity is called *Crohn's disease of the colon or granulomatous colitis.* (The latter term is less accurate since not all cases have granulomas.) Although the pathologic and clinical features overlap with those of ulcerative colitis, there are sufficient differences to allow Crohn's disease of the colon to be defined as a separate entity (see Table 294-1). However, a significant number of patients cannot be categorized as having either Crohn's disease or ulcerative colitis because features of both entities coexist.

Pathology The major findings are similar to those seen in the intestine in regional enteritis (see Chap. 293). The presence of sinus tracts and granulomas in the colon help to distinguish it from ulcerative colitis. This is a transmural disease, affecting all layers of the colon, the mucosa least severely. The bowel becomes thickened and attached to adjacent tissues or viscera, leading ultimately to enteroenteric fistulas. Perianal fistulas and abscesses are common, and fistulas to the bladder and vagina also occur. The principal feature of the inflammation is its patchy distribution. The rectum is often spared; in fact, isolated rectal disease, so commonly observed in ulcerative colitis, is not a feature of Crohn's colitis. The disease may involve only the right colon, segments of the transverse or descending colon, or the entire colon including the rectum. However, the involvement is not of the continuous and symmetric character of ulcerative colitis. Inflammation limited only to the colon occurs in about 10 percent of all cases of Crohn's disease; the colon and small bowel are both involved in about 30 percent of cases. It is estimated that Crohn's disease of the colon comprises up to 50 percent of all cases of chronic inflammatory bowel disease admitted to hospital.

Epidemiology and etiology The features are generally those of ulcerative colitis. The sex ratio is more nearly equal compared with ulcerative colitis. The disorder probably begins somewhat earlier in life; approximately 20 to 30 percent of cases occur before the age of 20. However, it is not uncommon to find the first evidence of the disease over the age of 50. Epidemiologic studies suffer from the insidious onset of this disorder, associated lesions such as diverticulosis, and inadequacy of initial studies because the early complaints are often vague. Extensive Crohn's disease has been found at autopsy in patients with no prior history of gastrointestinal symptoms. At present the etiologic considerations are similar to those of Crohn's disease of the small bowel (Chap. 293).

Clinical features Fever, abdominal pain, diarrhea often without urgency, and generalized fatigability are the principal complaints. The presence of severe *anorectal complications* such as fistula and abscess formation are important and often the initial clinical clues. The radiographic features of this disease include cobblestoning, skip areas (Fig. 294-5*B*), internal fistulas, and asymmetric involvement of the bowel wall. These findings are often localized to the proximal colon and terminal ileum. The main complications include arthritis, uveitis, aphthous ulcerations of the oral or genital mucosa, hepatic functional derangements (including pericholangitis), and fistulous involvement of the anal and pudendal areas. As with the small-intestinal form, colonic Crohn's disease is a recurrent, often low-grade inflammatory process which varies in severity from mild diarrhea to toxic megacolon indistinguishable from that seen in ulcerative colitis. Colonic malignancy is significantly more common in these patients than in the general population, but the incidence is not as great as in ulcerative colitis.

Differential diagnosis The principal features of ulcerative colitis versus Crohn's colitis are outlined in Table 294-1. The other diseases from which the disease must be distinguished are tuberculosis, lymphoma, ischemic colitis, diverticulitis, and colon cancer.

Treatment The approaches to medical management are similar to those used for ulcerative colitis, but sulfasalazine and corticosteroids are not as effective in Crohn's disease. Results are usually satisfactory with respect to control of fever, diarrhea, and systemic manifestations. Temporary remissions as well as recurrences are common. The disease tends to be less explosive than ulcerative colitis; free perforations or general peritonitis are not frequent. Of importance is the fact that the disease tends to progress despite apparent clinical well-being. Azathioprine has been tried in several studies but is not more effective than either prednisone or sulfasalazine. Some patients do quite well on low doses of sulfasalazine after a remission has been induced by prednisone.

Another problem in management relates to the results of surgery. Whereas total proctocolectomy in ulcerative colitis may be regarded as curative, this is not necessarily the case in Crohn's colitis, particularly when there is small-bowel involvement. Patients with isolated colonic involvement or small-bowel involvement of only the terminal ileum may do quite well after colectomy and ileostomy. It is commonly observed that 50 percent of these patients will require stoma revisions, but in general the prognosis is somewhat better than in patients with progressive regional enteritis of the small bowel. Most surgeons are somewhat more reluctant to perform colectomy and ileostomy in Crohn's colitis than in ulcerative colitis, particularly when diseased small bowel is left behind. Since the disease may involve only the terminal ileum and right colon, some patients undergo primary resection and reanastomosis of ileum to transverse colon. Despite the fact that medical and surgical therapy of Crohn's colitis is less effective than for ulcerative colitis, the majority of patients are able to function reasonably well with this disease.

ISCHEMIC COLITIS

Ischemia of the colon most often affects the elderly population because of the greater frequency of vascular disease in that group. Although some cases of large-bowel infarction are caused by embolus or thrombosis of the mesenteric artery, the majority of cases do not have a demonstrable arterial occlusion. In these patients, ischemia is probably secondary to spasm of mucosal vessels or shunting of blood flow away from the end arterioles. The exact pathogenesis of nonocclusive ischemic colitis is not clear.

Ischemic colitis can present as acute fulminant colitis, subacute colitis, or postischemic stricture. In *acute fulminant colitis* there is severe lower abdominal pain and massive rectal bleeding, often accompanied by shock. Since perforation of the colon is common, barium enema should not be performed. Arteriography may reveal an obstruction of the inferior mesenteric artery or severe spasm of mucosal vessels. Irreversible necrosis and gangrene of the colon are frequently found; hence, surgical resection is usually required.

Subacute ischemic colitis is the commonest clinical variant of ischemic colonic disease. These patients have lesser degrees of pain and bleeding, often occurring over several days or weeks. The left colon may be involved, but the rectum is usually spared, a distinguishing feature from acute ulcerative colitis. Arteriography may reveal tapering or spasm of the colonic vessels, but occlusion is not observed. Barium enema shows irregularity and cobblestoning of the mucosa caused by submucosal hemorrhage and edema, often referred to as *thumbprinting* by the radiologist. Occasionally *stricture formation* may follow a bout of ischemic colitis or may present de novo without a history of antecedent pain or bloody diarrhea. Most cases of nonocclusive ischemic colitis resolve in 2 to 4 weeks and do not recur. Surgery is not required except for obstruction secondary to postischemic stricture.

TUMORS OF THE LARGE INTESTINE

Neoplasms of the colon, either benign or malignant, are very commonly encountered in clinical practice. The clinician must be alert to the possibility that a variety of colonic symptoms, but particularly blood in the stools, can indicate the presence of a polyp or carcinoma. It is also of importance to recognize the settings in which colonic malignancy is more prevalent, and to strive for earlier diagnosis in order to increase the 5-year survival rate.

POLYPS OF THE COLON A polyp is a structure arising from a mucosal surface and projecting into the lumen. This definition includes benign lesions, while the designation *polypoid carcinoma* refers to a malignant lesion whose gross appearance resembles a polyp. The most common polyp is the *adenomatous polyp,* which may be solitary or multiple, sessile (flat, not on a stalk), or pedunculated (on a stalk as in Fig. 294-3). In adults single adenomatous polyps are believed to occur in 2 to 15 percent of the population. Polyps are not to be confused with small hyperplastic mucosal tags which are very common and of no clinical or pathologic significance. Adenomatous polyps are more common in the rectum and sigmoid colon (80 percent) compared with the rest of the colon (20 percent). Clinically, adenomatous polyps are usually silent. When they produce symptoms, these usually consist of recurrent episodes of bleeding or intermittent obstruction if the polyp is large and capable of leading to intussusception. The clinical significance of adenomatous polyps relates to the possibility that they may represent a premalignant lesion. Some experts argue that there is no relationship between adenomatous polyps and malignancy, while others believe that progression to malignancy will occur in a high percentage of benign polyps unless they are removed. The argument is difficult to resolve because the natural history of adenomatous polyps has not been studied in detail. The contention that polyps are premalignant is based on the observations that (1) foci of atypia or carcinoma in situ are occasionally found in polyps, (2) the incidences of polyps and carcinoma of the colon follow a similar age and anatomic distribution, and (3) patients with multiple congenital polyposis of the colon have a marked increase in incidence of colon cancer. The opposing viewpoint is based on the facts that (1) areas of malignancy are rarely found in adenomatous polyps, (2) true progression from adenomatous polyp to carcinoma has rarely been demonstrated, and (3) carcinoma of the colon would be much more frequent if even a small percentage of adenomas underwent malignant change. The truth probably lies somewhere between the two opposite views; a small but significant percentage of polyps may have malignant foci or undergo malignant change, and for this reason a polypoid lesion in the colon must be viewed with concern.

Treatment of polyps in adults is influenced by the debate as to their possible malignant transformation. Polyps in the sigmoid colon or rectum should be removed via the sigmoidoscope whenever possible. Polyps higher in the colon which are less than 1 cm in length are rarely malignant. However, recent experience with colonoscopic polypectomy has shown that even small polyps or polyps on stalks may be malignant. For this reason many authorities recommend removal of polyps via the colonoscope unless there is some contraindication to the procedure. This spares the patient a laparotomy and may occasionally detect a tumor in what otherwise would have been considered a benign polyp. In 40 to 50 percent of patients who have had polyps removed new polyps will develop in the subsequent decade. Therefore, it is recommended that follow-up barium enemas or colonoscopies should be performed periodically (perhaps every 2 to 3 years) to detect new polyps.

Villous adenoma is a polypoid lesion of the colon with a definite malignant potential. The majority of these occur in the rectum or sigmoid and usually are larger than adenomatous polyps. They are soft, frond-like masses which are quite friable and bleed easily. The histologic pattern is one of atypical cells which resemble surface epithelial cells; evidence of malignant degeneration is present in 40 to 60 percent. Rarely these tumors will cause protracted watery diarrhea with excessive potassium loss leading to profound hypokalemia and dehydra-

tion. Most villous adenomas call attention to their presence by bleeding or passage of mucus per rectum. Proper treatment involves surgical resection with follow-up sigmoidoscopies and barium enema examinations because recurrence can be expected in a small but significant percentage.

Familial colonic polyposis is a rare genetic (autosomal dominant) disorder characterized by the appearance of numerous (often 1000 or more) adenomatous polyps involving the entire colon. Occasional cases appear to have no family history and presumably result from a spontaneous mutation. The polyps are not present at birth but appear in childhood and adolescence, giving rise to diarrhea or rectal bleeding. Once this disease is diagnosed, it is imperative that the entire family be examined by sigmoidoscopy and barium enema. The probability of cancer of the colon occurring in affected individuals is nearly 100 percent by age 40. Hence prophylactic colectomy is indicated, usually after the patient has attained full adult growth. Most surgeons prefer total colectomy and ileostomy, while others leave the rectum, which allows the patient to have normal bowel movements. These patients require careful follow-up sigmoidoscopy and removal of all polyps in the rectal stump. However, the rate of carcinoma in the rectal stump is so high that total colectomy should probably be considered the treatment of choice.

Gardner's syndrome refers to the coexistence of multiple colonic adenomatous polyps and various benign tumors elsewhere, such as lipomas, fibromas, sebaceous cysts, and osteomas, particularly of the jaw and skull bones. The colonic polyps develop at a later age than in multiple colonic polyposis, but the malignant potential is the same and thus colectomy is also recommended. Some patients with Gardner's syndrome have gastric and duodenal polyps, and malignancies of the duodenum have been reported in some of these individuals.

An entity easily confused with multiple colonic polyposis is *juvenile polyposis,* in which inflammatory polyps occur in the colon or in both large and small bowel. Histologically these polyps are composed of columnar epithelium and mucus cysts; inflammatory cells are often present and account for the designation "inflammatory polyp." Juvenile polyposis coli also occurs in kindreds and causes rectal bleeding or features of growth retardation, making differentiation from multiple adenomatous polyps difficult. However, the risk of malignancy is not increased, and hence colectomy is not recommended. The Peutz-Jeghers syndrome is characterized by multiple hamartomatous polyps of the entire gastrointestinal tract, associated with melanotic spots on the skin, lips, and buccal mucosa. Although the polyps in this syndrome are most prevalent in the small intestine, colonic polyps also occur. Several cases of malignant degeneration of duodenal polyps have been reported. Clinical features alone do not allow accurate differentiation of the various hereditary polyp syndromes (Table 294-3). For this

TABLE 294-3
Hereditable gastrointestinal polyp syndromes

Syndrome	Distribution of polyps	Histologic type	Malignant degeneration	Associated lesions
Familial colonic polyposis	Large intestine	Adenoma	100%	None
Gardner's syndrome	Large intestine	Adenoma	100%	Osteomas, fibromas, lipomas, epidermoid cysts
Peutz-Jeghers syndrome	Small and large intestine	Hamartoma	Rare	Mucocutaneous pigmentation
Juvenile polyposis	Small and large intestine	Inflammatory polyp	Absent	None

reason, careful histologic examination of polyps from several areas should always be obtained prior to colectomy in patients with suspected polyposis coli.

CANCER OF THE COLON Cancer of the large bowel accounts for about 20 percent of all deaths due to malignant disease in the United States. The colon is the second most common site for carcinoma in both males and females. Unfortunately, the death rate for this disease has not changed for the past 40 years and will undoubtedly remain the same until methods for earlier detection and improved treatment are available.

Etiology The cause of colon cancer is unknown. The greater incidence in Western society suggests that dietary factors may be involved, but the association may be circumstantial rather than causal. As mentioned above, while there is a possibility that adenomatous polyps may become malignant, villous adenomas are definitely associated with cancer. It appears that a colon bearing a polyp may develop a cancer elsewhere. Congenital multiple polyposis of the colon has an astonishingly high malignant potential; ulcerative colitis also seems to potentiate or stimulate the development of carcinoma in the diseased bowel. Other lesions of the large intestine seem to bear no causal relation to cancer. As with other malignant diseases, familial aggregates of the disease are well documented.

Pathology Colon carcinomas affect women more often than men; rectal carcinomas are seen more commonly in men. They have been recorded at all ages, but the peak incidence is in the fifth, sixth, and seventh decades. The cecum and ascending colon are involved in 15 percent of all carcinomas of the large bowel; the transverse colon in 10 percent; and the descending colon, rectosigmoid, and rectum in 75 percent. Approximately half of all cancers of the large intestine are within reach of the sigmoidoscope. In most series multiple primary colonic cancers are found in about 3 percent of patients operated on or autopsied for the disease.

Adenocarcinoma is the commonest type of colon cancer. The degree of differentiation varies widely but is not well correlated with degree of invasiveness or rapidity of growth. Classifications of the tumors according to their microscopic appearance—papillary, medullary, scirrhous, or colloid—are not of great assistance to the physician. Scirrhous carcinomas tend to constrict the lumen of the bowel and produce obstructive syndromes, especially in the sigmoid area. Colloid tumors, most common in the right colon, can grow to enormous bulky mucinous masses, often forming mucous fistulas to the overlying skin. The common medullary tumor grows as a solid mass, the bulk of which may produce intermittent obstructive symptoms. Papillary tumors of the distal colon usually bleed early. All tumors tend to invade regional lymph nodes and spread through the lymphatics and portal vein to the liver; direct spread into the paravertebral venous plexus is occasionally seen.

Clinical features Symptoms of colon carcinoma are usually vague and nonspecific at the outset. Weight loss and malaise are common and often disregarded by the patient. It is convenient to divide cancers of the colon into those affecting the right and left sides. Cancers of the cecum and ascending colon are usually flat or polypoid and often "silent" clinically because they do not obstruct the lumen or cause visible melena. Cancer of the rectosigmoid may obstruct the lumen or bleed and hence cause the patient to seek medical advice. The following symptoms are important clues to the presence of colonic carcinoma.

1 *Changes in bowel habits* are most frequent when carcinoma affects the left colon. These changes are often minimal but progressive and include diarrhea, constipation, and a sensation of incomplete rectal emptying (tenesmus).
2 *Rectal bleeding* occurs in left-sided lesions in about 70 percent of cases and is usually noticed by the patient. When the lesion is in the ascending colon or cecum, fewer than 25 percent of patients notice any blood in the stools, no doubt because the blood is thoroughly admixed with the fecal slurry in the right colon. Rectal bleeding should never be attributed to hemorrhoids or rectal fissures, especially in older individuals, unless a malignancy has been ruled out by barium enema and proctosigmoidoscopy.
3 *Pain* in the lower part of the abdomen is occasionally a symptom of lesions of the cecum or ascending colon. Pain in left colonic lesions may be related to varying degrees of bowel obstruction above a constricting carcinoma. Occasionally a sigmoid carcinoma may present as an acute bowel obstruction or acute perforation with peritonitis.
4 Symptoms of *anemia* are frequent in right-sided colonic cancer. Cardiac failure or angina pectoris may be the presenting symptoms.
5 *Anorexia, weight loss,* and *malaise* may occur at any time.

Diagnosis Carcinoma of the colon is one of the most common malignancies, and the physician must be alert to symptoms such as weight loss, blood in the stool, or change in bowel habit. The potentially serious nature of these symptoms must be recognized and not attributed to hemorrhoids or other minor conditions until carcinoma has been definitely excluded. It must be stressed that cancer of the large bowel is curable if discovered early in the course and that delay in diagnosis is the most significant factor in poor prognosis.

The most efficient and economical screening procedure for colon cancer involves testing the stool for occult blood (guaiac test). Most colonic malignancies bleed slowly into the lumen even before they reach sufficient size to cause symptoms. Thus the presence of occult blood in the stool should alert the physician to the possibility of colon cancer, particularly in individuals above the age of 40. As usually performed, the guaiac test suffers from variable sensitivity due to instability of the dye. Commercially prepared cards impregnated with the dye (Hemoccult test) are available in which the dye appears to be stable and the number of false-positive tests are reduced. False-positive tests can also be diminished if patients do not eat meat for several days prior to the test. A screening protocol for colon cancer has been devised which involves Hemoccult testing of six stool samples while the patient is on a meat-free diet. This simple screening technique appears to increase the detection of presymptomatic colon cancers amenable to surgical cure.

The *digital rectal examination* is the most important aspect of the physical examination, since approximately half of rectal cancers are within reach of the finger. Physical findings such as ascites, jaundice, or palpable abdominal masses indicate metastatic disease. Iron-deficiency anemia is present in over half of patients with right-sided lesions. Patients with left-sided lesions may also be anemic but less frequently and to a much less severe degree, since their blood loss is more easily appreciated by the appearance of the stools. In the presence of liver metastases the serum alkaline phosphatase and 5′-nucleotidase retention are elevated. The carcinoembryonic antigen (CEA) is not specific for colon cancer, and a normal level does not exclude the diagnosis. It is useful, however, in following patients after surgery, since return to normal of previously elevated CEA levels indicates successful removal of tumor, while persistently elevated or increasing CEA levels postoperatively suggest residual tumor or metastatic spread.

FIGURE 294-6
Filling defect in the cecum produced by a carcinoma.

Complications Since it is characteristic for tumors to invade, many tumors of the colon are first diagnosed because of a complication of the original lesion. The tumor may perforate the bowel wall, giving rise to acute peritonitis; may perforate slowly and wall itself off, giving rise to a local inflammatory mass and localized peritonitis; or may invade blood vessels to produce an episode of brisk rectal bleeding. More often, the tumor partially obstructs the bowel lumen for a long period of time, during which the colon proximal to the tumor dilates slowly without dramatic change in symptoms until frank obstruction occurs. This happens most often when the tumor is in the sigmoid, where the stool is driest. Tumors also weaken the colonic wall in such a way that an intussusception may occur, the tumor leading the intussusception. Similarly, fixation of the bowel wall by a tumor may produce a volvulus, which is most frequently seen in the sigmoid colon. Very large and slowly growing tumors may produce symptoms by pressure on neighboring organs such as uterus, bladder, or ureters. Inguinal hernias may become apparent as the first sign of such increased pressure. Fistulas between the colon and pelvic organs should lead to a thorough search for an underlying neoplastic infiltration. Abscesses inside the peritoneal cavity and cellulitis of the abdominal wall secondary to tumor infiltration are occasionally seen.

Treatment The current approach to treatment of colon cancer is primarily surgical. Some surgeons prefer preoperative radiation therapy to prevent metastases, but it has not been convincingly demonstrated that this improves survival. Surgeons generally prefer abdominoperineal resection and colostomy for tumors located below the peritoneal reflection; above this area there is considerably more freedom of choice, depending primarily on the size and extent of the lesion. Even patients with

Any patient suspected of having a colonic carcinoma should undergo sigmoidoscopy. This procedure is particularly useful in the diagnosis of low-lying rectal cancers which can be missed on barium enema. Sigmoidoscopy also allows for the diagnosis of other bleeding lesions in the rectum or sigmoid colon, particularly hemorrhoids, polyps, and proctitis.

A careful barium enema in a well-prepared colon is the next diagnostic maneuver. Important aspects of this examination are the following: (1) Tumors may project into the bowel, giving rise to a filling defect in the barium column (Fig. 294-6). (2) They may partially or completely encircle the bowel, producing a narrowing of the barium column proximal to which the bowel is often dilated (Fig. 294-7). (3) They may, by contiguous infiltration, distort the position of the colon, so that the barium is not free to follow gravity during the radiologist's examination of the patient. (4) After the barium has been expelled, films of the mucosal relief may show defects due to tumor which has not penetrated the muscular coat. (5) Some tumors give rise to no specific defects but interfere with peristalsis, so that irritability, fluid retention, and spasticity may be noted. It is worth emphasizing that the accuracy of barium enema in the diagnosis of low-lying rectal cancer is not high. It is imperative, therefore, that a careful sigmoidoscopic examination precede the barium enema. Colonoscopy and biopsy are useful in the diagnosis of suspicious lesions seen on barium enema which are above the reach of the sigmoidoscope.

Differential diagnosis of colon cancer include almost all the entities which affect that organ because changes in bowel habit and bleeding are common symptoms. Thus colitis, diverticular disease, polyps, and ischemic disease can be easily confused with colon carcinoma. Even more important is the fact that these diseases can coexist with or lead to malignancy. Filling defects of the cecum can occur in amoebic colitis, owing to the presence of a large inflammatory mass (amoeboma). This is rare except in patients with long-standing chronic amoebiasis. Tuberculosis, endometriosis, lymphogranuloma venereum, carcinoid tumors, and lymphoma may all masquerade as colon carcinoma. Metastatic cancer from other organs can occasionally involve the colon extrinsically and produce symptoms. Thus metastases to the perirectal area can produce diarrhea or obstructive symptoms. Such tumors produce extrinsic compression of the lumen and may be palpated through the rectum as a shelf (Blumer's shelf) or mass.

FIGURE 294-7
Obstructing carcinoma of the sigmoid.

obvious metastases usually benefit from a limited palliative resection, since this will relieve or prevent painful obstruction and hemorrhage. The overall operative mortality for colectomy is about 5 percent, except for emergency resections for perforation or obstruction. The operative mortality is somewhat higher for lesions in the left colon and for tumors which have perforated. Discussion of the complications of surgical therapy and the management of colostomies can be found in surgical texts.

The overall 5-year survival rate for all patients undergoing resection for colonic malignancy is approximately 50 percent. The 5-year survival rate after resection for patients free of local or distant spread is 75 to 80 percent. When nodal metastases are found at the time of resection, only 25 percent of these patients will be alive at 5 years. Palliative surgical attempts should not be discouraged because the symptomatic relief they produce may allow the patient to live in comfort for the remaining months of life. Chemotherapy with 5-fluorouracil or other agents is used in patients with metastases to the liver, but temporary improvement is obtained only in 25 percent or less of cases, and overall survival is not significantly affected. (For further details regarding chemotherapy, see Chap. 325.)

ANORECTAL PROBLEMS

HEMORRHOIDS The internal hemorrhoidal plexus of veins is located in the submucosal space above the valves of Morgagni. The anal canal separates it from the external hemorrhoidal venous plexus, but the two spaces communicate under the anal canal, the submucosa of which is attached to underlying tissue to form the interhemorrhoidal depression. Whenever the internal hemorrhoidal plexus is enlarged, there is associated increase in supporting tissue mass, and the resultant venous swelling is called an *internal hemorrhoid*. When veins in the external hemorrhoidal plexus become enlarged or thrombosed, the resultant bluish mass is called an *external hemorrhoid*.

Both types of hemorrhoids are very common and are associated with increased hydrostatic pressure in the portal venous system, such as during pregnancy, straining at stool, or with cirrhosis. When internal hemorrhoids enlarge, pain is not a usual feature until the situation is complicated by thrombosis, infection, or erosion of the overlying mucosal surface. Most persons complain of bright red blood on the toilet tissue or coating the stool, with a feeling of vague anal discomfort. The discomfort is increased when the hemorroid enlarges or prolapses through the anus; prolapse is often accompanied by edema and sphincteric spasm. Prolapse, if not treated, usually becomes chronic as the muscularis stays stretched, and the patient complains of constant soiling of underclothing with very little pain. Prolapsed hemorrhoids may become infected or thrombosed; the overlying mucous membrane may bleed profusely as the result of the trauma of defecation.

External hemorrhoids, because they lie under the skin, are quite often painful, particularly if there is a sudden increase in their mass. These episodes result in a tender blue swelling at the anal verge due to thrombosis of a vein in the external plexus and need not be associated with enlargement of the internal veins. Since the thrombus usually lies at the level of the sphincteric muscles, anal spasm often occurs.

The diagnosis of internal and external hemorrhoids is made by inspection, digital examination, and direct vision through the anoscope and proctoscope. Since such lesions are very common, they must not be regarded as the cause of rectal bleeding or chronic hypochromic anemia until a thorough investigation has been made of the more proximal gastrointestinal tract. Acute blood loss can occasionally be attributed to internal hemorrhoids. Chronic anemia in the presence of large but not definitely bleeding hemorrhoids should provoke a search for a polyp, cancer, or ulcer.

Most hemorrhoids respond to conservative therapy such as sitz baths or other forms of moist heat, suppositories, stool softeners, and bed rest. Internal hemorrhoids which remain permanently prolapsed are best treated surgically; milder degrees of prolapse or enlargement with pruritus ani or intermittent bleeding can be successfully handled by the injection of sclerosing solutions. External hemorrhoids which become acutely thrombosed are treated by incision, extraction of the clot, and compression of the incised area following clot removal. No surgical procedure should be carried out in the presence of acute inflammation of the anus, ulcerative proctitis, or ulcerative colitis. Both proctoscopy and barium enema should always be performed before a patient is subjected to hemorrhoidectomy.

ANAL INFLAMMATION Perianal inflammatory lesions may be primary or may be associated with inflammatory bowel disease or diverticular disease as mentioned above. Anal *fissures* are superficial erosions of the anal canal which usually heal rapidly with conservative therapy. Anal *ulcers* are more chronic and deep and give symptoms largely as the result of painful spasm of the external anal sphincter during and after defecation. Bleeding may occur with either fissure or ulcer; healing of the ulcer often is associated with a hypertrophied anal papilla and some degrees of anal contracture. *Fistula in ano,* a tract leading from the rectal lumen to the perianal skin, usually results from local crypt abscesses; fewer than 5 percent of such lesions found in medical practice in the United States are due to tuberculosis or cancer. The fistula is a chronically inflamed canal made up of fibrous tissue surrounding granulation tissue, the lumen of which may be difficult to demonstrate. Perirectal *abscesses* often represent the tracking down into the anal area of purulent material escaping from the rectosigmoid; diverticulitis, Crohn's disease, or colitis may be the underlying cause. Previous anal or rectal surgical therapy may be causal. Fistulas between the rectum and vagina and between the rectum and bladder represent serious complications of granulomatous, septic, or malignant disorders and require the patient to be hospitalized for definitive diagnostic and therapeutic procedures.

REFERENCES

BULL DM et al: Crohn's disease of the colon. Gastroenterology 76:607, 1979

BUNTAIN WL et al: Collective review: Premalignancy of polyps of the colon. Surg Gynecol Obstet 134:499, 1972

BURKITT DP: Epidemiology of cancer of the colon and rectum. Cancer 28:3, 1971

BUSSEY HJ et al: Genetics of gastrointestinal polyposis. Gastroenterology 74:1325, 1978

DOBBINS WO: Current status of the precancer lesion in ulcerative colitis. Gastroenterology 73:1431, 1977

DROSSMAN DA et al: The irritable bowel syndrome. Gastroenterology 73:811, 1977

FLEISCHNER F: Diverticular disease of the colon. Gastroenterology 60:316, 1971

GOLDMAN P, PEPPERCORN MA: Sulfasalazine. N Engl J Med 293:20, 1975

MOERTEL CG: Chemotherapy of gastrointestinal cancer. N Engl J Med 299:1049, 1978

RITCHIE JK et al: Clinical outcome of the first ten years of ulcerative colitis and proctitis. Lancet 1:1140, 1978

STEINBERG DM et al: Sequelae of colectomy and ileostomy: Comparison between Crohn's colitis and ulcerative colitis. Gastroenterology 68:33, 1975

WILLIAMS LF: Vascular insufficiency of the intestines. Gastroenterology 61:757, 1971

WINAWER SJ et al: Screening for colon cancer. Gastroenterology 70:783, 1976

WOLFE WI, SHINYA H: Polypectomy via the fiberoptic colonoscope. N Engl J Med 288:329, 1973

YARDLEY YH et al: Cancer in ulcerative colitis. Gastroenterology 76:221, 1979

295
ACUTE INTESTINAL OBSTRUCTION

WILLIAM SILEN

ETIOLOGY AND CLASSIFICATION Intestinal obstruction may be *mechanical* or *nonmechanical* (resulting from neuromuscular disturbances which produce either *adynamic* or *dynamic ileus*). The causes of mechanical obstruction of the lumen are conveniently divided into (1) lesions *extrinsic* to the intestine, e.g., adhesive bands, internal and external hernias; (2) lesions *intrinsic* to the wall of the intestine, e.g., diverticulitis, carcinoma, regional enteritis; and (3) obturation of the lumen, e.g., gallstone obstruction, intussusception. From the clinical standpoint, however, it is most useful to consider whether the obstructive mechanism involves the small or large intestine, because the causes, symptoms, and treatment are different (see below). Adhesions and external hernias are the most common causes of obstruction of the small intestine, constituting 70 to 75 percent of cases of this type. Adhesions, however, almost never produce obstruction of the colon, while carcinoma, sigmoid diverticulitis, and volvulus, in that order, are the most common etiologies and together account for about 90 percent of the cases.

Adynamic ileus is probably the most common overall cause of obstruction. Recent studies indicate that the development of this condition is mediated via the hormonal component of the sympathoadrenal system. Adynamic ileus will occur after any peritoneal insult, and its severity and duration will be dependent to some degree on the type of peritoneal injury. Hydrochloric acid, colonic contents, and pancreatic enzymes are among the most irritating substances, whereas blood and urine are less so. Adynamic ileus occurs to some degree after any abdominal operation, and its severity varies directly with the amount of intestinal handling and the length of the operation; it usually lasts 2 to 3 days after most operative procedures. Retroperitoneal hematomas, particularly associated with vertebral fracture, commonly cause severe adynamic ileus and the latter may occur with other retroperitoneal conditions such as ureteral calculus or severe pyelonephritis. Thoracic diseases including lower-lobe pneumonia, fractured ribs, and myocardial infarction frequently produce adynamic ileus, as do electrolyte disturbances, particularly potassium depletion. Finally intestinal ischemia, whether the result of vascular occlusion or intestinal distention itself, may perpetuate an adynamic ileus. Spastic or dynamic ileus is very uncommon and results from extreme and prolonged contraction of the intestine. It has been observed in heavy metal poisoning, uremia, porphyria, and extensive intestinal ulcerations.

PATHOPHYSIOLOGY Distention of the intestine is caused by the accumulation of gas and fluid proximal to and within the obstructed segment. Seventy to eighty percent of intestinal gas consists of swallowed air, and because this is composed mainly of nitrogen, which is poorly absorbed from the intestinal lumen, removal of air by continuous gastric suction is an important adjunct in the treatment of intestinal distention. The accumulation of fluid proximal to the obstructing mechanism results not only from ingested fluid, swallowed saliva, gastric juice, and biliary and pancreatic secretions but also from interference with normal sodium and water transport. During the first 12 to 24 h of obstruction there is a marked depression of flux from lumen to blood of sodium and consequently water in the distended proximal intestine. After 24 h, there is also movement of sodium and water into the lumen, contributing further to the distention and fluid losses. Intraluminal pressure rises from a normal of 2 to 4 cmH$_2$O to 8 to 10 cmH$_2$O. During peristalsis, when simple obstruction or a "closed loop" is present, pressures reach 30 to 60 cmH$_2$O. Closed-loop obstruction of the small intestine results when the lumen is occluded at two points by a single mechanism such as a hernial ring or adhesive band, thus producing a closed loop whose blood supply is often obstructed at the same time. Strangulation of the loop itself is thus common in association with marked distention proximal to the involved loop. A form of closed-loop obstruction is encountered when complete obstruction of the colon exists in the presence of a competent ileocecal valve (85 percent of individuals). Although the blood supply of the colon is not entrapped within the obstructing mechanism, distention of the cecum is extreme because of its greater diameter (LaPlace's law), and impairment of the intramural blood supply is considerable with consequent gangrene of the cecal wall, usually anteriorly. Necrosis of the small intestine may occur by the same mechanism of interference with intramural blood flow when distention is extreme, but this sequence is uncommon in the small intestine. Once impairment of blood supply occurs, bacterial invasion supervenes and subsequent peritonitis develops. The systemic effects of extreme distention include elevation of the diaphragms with restricted ventilation and subsequent atelectasis. Venous return via the inferior vena cava may also be impaired.

The loss of fluids and electrolytes may be extreme, and unless replacement is prompt, leads to hemoconcentration, hypovolemia, renal insufficiency, shock, and death. Vomiting, accumulation of fluids within the lumen by the mechanisms described above, and the sequestration of fluid into the edematous intestinal wall and peritoneal cavity as a result of impairment of venous return from the intestine all contribute to massive loss of fluid and electrolytes. As soon as significant impedance to venous return is present, the intestine becomes severely congested, and blood begins to seep into the intestinal lumen. Blood loss may reach significant levels when long segments of intestine are involved.

SYMPTOMS *Mechanical small-intestinal obstruction* is characterized by cramping midabdominal pain which tends to be more severe the higher the obstruction. The pain occurs in paroxysms, and the patient is relatively comfortable in the intervals between the pains. Audible borborygmi are often noted by the patient simultaneously with the paroxysms of pain. The pain may become less severe as distention progresses, probably because motility is impaired in the edematous intestine. When strangulation is present, the pain is usually more localized and may be steady and severe without a colicky component, a fact which often causes delay in diagnosis of obstruction. Vomiting is almost unavoidable, and it is earlier and more profuse the higher the obstruction. The vomitus initially contains bile and mucus and remains as such if the obstruction is high in the intestine. With low ileal obstruction, the vomitus becomes feculent, i.e., orange-brown in color with a foul odor, which results from the overgrowth of bacteria proximal to the obstruction. Singultus is common. Obstipation and failure to pass gas by rectum are invariably present when the obstruction is complete, although some stool and gas may be passed spontaneously or after an enema shortly after onset of the complete obstruction. Diarrhea is occasionally observed in partial obstruction. Blood in the stool is rare, even in the completely obstructed patient but does occur in cases of intussusception. Other than some minor but inconsistent differences in pain patterns noted above, the symptoms of strangulating obstructions cannot be distinguished from those of nonstrangulating obstructions.

Mechanical colonic obstruction produces colicky abdominal pain similar in quality to that of small-intestinal obstruction but of much lower intensity. Complaints of pain are occasionally absent in stoic elderly patients. Vomiting occurs late, if at all, particularly if the ileocecal valve is competent. Paradoxically, feculent vomitus is very rare. A history of recent alterations in bowel habits and blood in the stool is common because carcinoma and diverticulitis are the most frequent causes. Constipation becomes progressive, and obstipation with failure to pass gas ensues. Acute symptoms may develop over a period of a week.

In *adynamic ileus,* colicky pain is absent, and only discomfort from distention is evident. Vomiting may be frequent but is rarely profuse. It usually consists of gastric contents and bile and is almost never feculent. Complete obstipation may or may not occur. Singultus is very common.

PHYSICAL FINDINGS *Abdominal distention* is the hallmark of all forms of intestinal obstruction. It is least marked in cases of obstruction high in the small intestine and most marked in colonic obstruction. Early in the course of the disease, especially in closed-loop strangulating small-bowel obstruction, distention may be barely perceptible or absent. Tenderness and rigidity are usually minimal; the temperature is rarely above 100°F in nonstrangulating obstruction of the small and large intestine. Contrary to popular belief the same is true of strangulating obstruction until very late in the course of the disease, a fact which has often resulted in unfortunate delay in treatment. Signs and symptoms of shock also occur *very late* in strangulating obstruction. The appearance of shock, tenderness, rigidity, and fever often means that there has been contamination of the peritoneum with infected intestinal content. The presence of a palpable abdominal mass usually signifies a closed-loop strangulating small-bowel obstruction because the tense fluid-filled loop is the palpable lesion. Auscultation may reveal loud high-pitched borborygmi coincident with the colicky pain, but this classic finding is often not present late in strangulating or nonstrangulating obstruction. A quiet abdomen does not eliminate the possibility of obstruction, nor does it necessarily establish the diagnosis of adynamic ileus.

LABORATORY AND X-RAY FINDINGS Leukocytosis, with shift to the left, usually occurs when strangulation is present, but a normal white blood cell count does not exclude strangulation. Elevation of the serum amylase is encountered occasionally in all forms of intestinal obstruction, especially the strangulating variety.

The x-ray is extremely valuable but under certain circumstances may also be misleading. In nonstrangulating complete small-bowel obstruction, x-rays are almost completely reliable. Distention of fluid- and gas-filled loops of small intestine usually arranged in a "stepladder" pattern with air-fluid levels and an absence or paucity of colonic gas are pathognomonic (Fig. 295-1). These findings, however, are absent in slightly over half the cases of strangulating small-bowel obstruction, especially early in the disease. A general haze due to peritoneal fluid and

FIGURE 295-1

Acute mechanical obstruction of small intestine (upright film). Note air-fluid levels, marked distention of bowel loops, and absence of colonic gas.

sometimes a "coffee-bean" shaped mass are seen in strangulating obstruction. Occasionally the films are normal, but when symptoms are consistent with obstruction of the small intestine, a normal film should suggest strangulation. Roentgenographic differentiation of partial mechanical small-bowel obstruction from adynamic ileus may be impossible since gas is present in both small and large intestine; however, colonic distention is usually more prominent in adynamic ileus. A radiopaque dye given by mouth is useful in making this distinction.

Colonic obstruction with a competent ileocecal valve is easily recognized because distention with gas is mainly confined to the colon. Barium enema is usually advisable to determine the nature of the lesion except when concomitant perforation is suspected, a rare occurrence. When the ileocecal valve is incompetent, the films resemble those of partial small-bowel obstruction or adynamic ileus, and barium enema is necessary to establish the correct diagnosis. Barium given by mouth is perfectly safe when obstruction is in the small intestine since the barium sulfate does not become inspissated in this location. *Barium should never be given by mouth to a patient with possible colonic obstruction* until that possibility has been excluded by barium enema.

MESENTERIC VASCULAR OCCLUSION This term refers to a form of intestinal obstruction in which there is no mechanical occlusion of the intestine but ischemia is the basic feature. About 75 percent of cases result from occlusion of the superior mesenteric artery due to emboli or atherosclerotic narrowing. An additional 15 percent of cases are due to nonocclusive ischemia, a condition which usually occurs in elderly patients with congestive heart failure taking digitalis glycosides. The latter drugs have been shown to decrease splanchnic blood flow. The remainder are cases of pure venous mesenteric occlusion due to thrombi. Any patient with severe heart disease, particularly in the presence of auricular fibrillation, who complains of abdominal pain should be considered to have intestinal ischemia until proved otherwise. Over 70 percent of cases have a 2- to 3-

day history of low-grade colicky abdominal pain, often with diarrhea containing microscopic blood; this is followed by catastrophic shock, severe abdominal tenderness, rigidity, leukocytosis, and fever. Only in venous infarction, the rarest form of mesenteric vascular occlusion, are these findings encountered early. X-ray examination shows a nonspecific adynamic ileus, but selective angiography is usually diagnostic. Occasionally, barium enema is useful if the lesion is confined to the colon and shows characteristic "thumb printing," representing edematous and hemorrhagic mucosal folds most often in the region of the splenic flexure (see also Chap. 293).

PROGNOSIS AND TREATMENT   Small-intestinal obstruction
The overall mortality for obstruction of the small intestine is about 10 percent, even under the most optimal conditions. While the mortality for nonstrangulating obstruction is as low as 5 to 8 percent, that for strangulating obstruction has been reported to be between 20 and 75 percent. Well over half of the deaths from small-bowel obstruction occur in those with strangulation; however, the latter constitute only one-fourth to one-third of the cases. Careful studies indicate that the clinical, laboratory, and x-ray findings are not reliable in distinguishing strangulating from nonstrangulating obstruction when obstruction is complete. Complete obstruction is suggested when there has been a total cessation in the passage of gas or stool per rectum and when gas is absent in the distal intestine by x-ray. Since strangulating small-bowel obstruction is always complete, operation should always be undertaken in such patients after suitable preparation. Prior to operation, fluid and electrolyte balance should be restored, and decompression instituted by means of a nasogastric tube. Six to eight hours of preparation may be necessary. During this period broad-spectrum antibiotics are indicated if strangulation is felt to be likely, but operation should not be delayed unless there is unequivocal clinical and roentgenographic evidence of resolution of the obstruction during the period of preparation. Attempts to pass a long tube into the small intestine usually fail while putting the patient through uncomfortable unproductive manipulations which delay appropriate fluid replacement and decompression. *There are probably few if any indications for the use of a long intestinal tube.* Procrastination of operation because of improvement in well-being of the patient during resuscitation and gastric decompression usually leads to unnecessary and hazardous delay in proper treatment. Purely nonoperative therapy is safe only in the presence of incomplete obstruction and is best utilized in patients with (1) repeated episodes of partial obstruction, (2) recent postoperative partial obstruction, and (3) partial obstruction following a recent episode of diffuse peritonitis.

Colonic obstruction   The mortality rate for colonic obstruction is about 20 percent. As in small-bowel obstruction, nonoperative treatment is contraindicated unless the obstruction is incomplete. Occasionally, but not always, when the obstruction is incomplete, nonoperative therapy may result in sufficient decompression that a definitive operative procedure can be undertaken at a later date. This can usually be accomplished by discontinuation of all oral intake and perhaps by nasogastric suction, although attempts to decompress a *completely* obstructed colon by intubation are almost invariably futile. A long intestinal tube will not decompress an obstructed colon with a competent ileocecal valve. When obstruction is complete, early operation is mandatory, especially when the ileocecal valve is competent; cecal gangrene is likely if the cecal diameter exceeds 10 cm on plain abdominal film. For obstruction on the left side of the colon, the most common site, preliminary operative decompression by cecostomy or transverse colostomy followed by definitive resection of the primary lesion is the treatment of choice. For a lesion of the right or

transverse colon, primary resection and anastomosis can safely be performed because distention of the ileum with consequent discrepancy in size and hazard in suture are not present.

Adynamic ileus   This type of ileus usually responds to nonoperative continuous decompression and adequate treatment of the primary disease. The prognosis is usually good. Rarely, adynamic colonic distention may become so great that cecostomy is required if cecal gangrene is feared. Spastic ileus usually responds to treatment of the primary disease.

Mesenteric vascular occlusion   The mortality for mesenteric vascular occlusion usually is greater than 80 percent. For occlusive mesenteric ischemia, early operation is mandatory. Vascular reconstruction with resection of nonviable intestine is the procedure of choice unless intestinal gangrene is irreversible, in which case resection alone is indicated. If diffuse nonocclusive ischemia can be diagnosed by selective angiography, treatment involves adequate volume replacement and 24-h perfusion of the superior mesenteric artery with vasodilating agents, followed by operation to resect intestine of questionable viability. Although some instances of survival have been reported in this condition, these are rare.

REFERENCES

BECKER WF: Acute adhesive ileus: A study of 412 cases with particular reference to the abuse of tube decompression in treatment. Surg Gynecol Obstet 95:472, 1952

BROOKS DH, CARY LC: Base deficit in superior mesenteric artery occlusion: Aid to early diagnosis. Ann Surg 177:352, 1973

COHN I, ATIK M: Strangulation obstruction: Closed loop studies. Ann Surg 153:94, 1961

COPE Z: *The Early Diagnosis of the Acute Abdomen,* 14th ed. London, Oxford University Press, 1972

DUBOIS A et al: Postoperative ileus: Physiopathology, etiology and treatment. Ann Surg 178:781, 1973

FAULK DL et al: Chronic intestinal pseudoobstruction. Gastroenterology 74:922, 1978

MARSTON A et al: Ischaemic colitis. Gut 7:1, 1966

SHIELDS R: The absorption and secretion of fluid and electrolytes by the obstructed bowel. Br J Surg 52:774, 1965

SILEN W et al: Strangulation obstruction of the small intestine. Arch Surg 85:121, 1962

296
ACUTE APPENDICITIS

WILLIAM SILEN

INCIDENCE AND EPIDEMIOLOGY   The maximum incidence of acute appendicitis occurs in the second and third decades of life. While the disease may be encountered at any time of life, it is relatively rare at the extremes of age. Males and females are equally affected except between puberty and age 25, when males predominate in a 3:2 ratio. Perforation is relatively much more common in infancy and in the aged, during which periods mortality rates are highest. The mortality rate has decreased steadily in Europe and the United States from 8.1 per 100,000 of the population in 1941 to less than 1 per 100,000 in 1970. The absolute incidence of the disease also decreased by about 40 percent between 1940 and 1960 but since then has remained unchanged. Although various factors such as changing dietary habits, altered intestinal flora, and better nutrition and intake of vitamins have been suggested to explain the reduced incidence, the exact reasons have not been elucidated. Of interest is that the overall incidence of appendicitis is much lower in underdeveloped countries, especially parts of Africa, and in lower socioeconomic groups.

PATHOGENESIS The primary pathogenetic hallmark has always been thought to be luminal obstruction. While obstruction can be identified by careful examination in 30 to 40 percent of cases, recent studies have shown that ulceration of the mucosa is the initial event in the majority. The causation of the ulceration is unknown, although a viral etiology has been postulated. Whether the inflammatory reaction attendant with ulceration is sufficient to obstruct the tiny appendiceal lumen even transiently is also not clear. Obstruction, when present, is most commonly caused by a fecalith which results from accumulation and inspissation of fecal matter around vegetable fibers. Enlarged lymphoid follicles associated with viral infections (e.g., measles), inspissated barium, worms (e.g., pinworms, *Ascaris,* and *Taenia*), and tumors (e.g., carcinoid or carcinoma) may also obstruct the lumen. Secretion of mucus distends the organ, which has a capacity of only 0.1 to 0.2 ml, and luminal pressures rise as high as 60 cmH$_2$O. Luminal bacteria multiply and invade the appendiceal wall as venous engorgement and subsequent arterial compromise result from the high intraluminal pressures. Finally, gangrene and perforation occur. If the process evolves slowly, adjacent organs such as the terminal ileum, cecum, and omentum may wall off the appendiceal area so that a localized abscess will develop, whereas rapid progression of vascular impairment may cause perforation with free access to the peritoneal cavity. Subsequent rupture of primary appendiceal abscesses may produce fistulas between the appendix and bladder, small intestine, sigmoid, or cecum. Occasionally, acute appendicitis may be the first manifestation of Crohn's disease. While chronic infection of the appendix with tuberculosis, amebiasis, and actinomycosis may occur, a useful clinical aphorism states that *chronic appendiceal inflammation is not usually the cause of prolonged abdominal pain of weeks or months duration.* In contrast, it is clear that recurrent acute appendicitis does occur, often with complete resolution of inflammation and symptoms between attacks. Recurrent acute appendicitis may become more frequent as antibiotics are dispensed more freely.

CLINICAL MANIFESTATION The history and sequence of symptoms are among the most important diagnostic features of appendicitis. The initial symptom is almost invariably *abdominal pain* of the visceral type, resulting from appendiceal contractions or distention of the lumen. It is usually poorly localized in the periumbilical or epigastric regions. There is often an accompanying urge to defecate or pass flatus, neither of which relieves the distress. This visceral pain is mild, often cramping, and rarely catastrophic in nature, usually lasting 4 to 6 h, but may not be noted by stoic individuals or by some patients during sleep. As inflammation spreads to the parietal peritoneal surfaces, the pain becomes somatic, steady, and more severe, aggravated by motion or cough and usually located in the *right lower quadrant. Anorexia* is so frequent that the presence of hunger should arouse serious suspicion of the diagnosis of acute appendicitis. *Nausea* and *vomiting* occur in 50 to 60 percent of cases, but vomiting is rarely profuse and protracted. The development of nausea and vomiting before the onset of pain is extremely rare. Change in bowel habit is of little diagnostic value since any or no alteration may be observed, although the presence of diarrhea caused by an in-

flamed appendix in juxtaposition to the sigmoid may cause serious diagnostic difficulties. Urinary frequency and dysuria occur if the appendix lies adjacent to the bladder. The typical sequence of symptoms (poorly localized periumbilical pain followed by nausea and vomiting with subsequent shift of pain to the right lower quadrant) occurs in only 50 to 60 percent of patients, and some variations are considered below.

Physical findings vary with time after onset of the illness and according to the location of the appendix, which may be situated deep in the pelvic cul-de-sac, in the right lower quadrant in any relation to the peritoneum, cecum, and small intestine, in the right upper quadrant, or even in the left lower quadrant. *The diagnosis cannot be established unless tenderness can be elicited.* While tenderness is sometimes absent in the early visceral stage of the disease, it ultimately always develops and is found in any location corresponding to the position of the appendix. Abdominal tenderness may be completely absent if a retrocecal or pelvic appendix is present, in which case the sole physical finding may be tenderness in the flank or on rectal or pelvic examination. Percussion, rebound tenderness, and referred rebound tenderness are often, but not invariably, present; they are most likely to be absent early in the illness. Flexion of the right hip and guarded movement by the patient are due to parietal peritoneal involvement. Hyperesthesia of the skin of the right lower quadrant and a positive psoas or obturator sign are often late findings and are rarely of diagnostic value. When the inflamed appendix is in close proximity to the anterior parietal peritoneum, muscular rigidity is present, yet is often minimal early. The temperature is usually normal or slightly elevated (99 to 100.5°F), but a temperature above 101°F should always suggest the presence of perforation. Tachycardia is commensurate with the elevation of the temperature. Rigidity and tenderness become more marked as the disease progresses to perforation and localized or diffuse peritonitis. Distention is rare unless severe diffuse peritonitis has developed. The alleged disappearance of pain and tenderness just prior to perforation is extremely unusual. A mass may develop if localized perforation has occurred but usually will not be detectable before 3 days after onset of the disease. Earlier presence of a mass suggests carcinoma of the cecum or Crohn's disease. Perforation is rare before 24 h after onset of symptoms but may be as high as 80 percent after 48 h.

Laboratory examination does not establish the diagnosis since the latter is based primarily on clinical grounds. Although moderate leukocytosis of 10,000 to 18,000 cells per cubic millimeter is frequent (with a concomitant shift to immature cells), the absence of leukocytosis does not eliminate the possibility of acute appendicitis. Leukocytosis of greater than 20,000 cells per cubic millimeter should alert the clinician to the probability of perforation. Anemia and blood in the stool suggest a primary diagnosis of carcinoma of the cecum, especially in elderly individuals. The urine may contain a few white or red blood cells without bacteria if the appendix lies close to the right ureter or bladder.

Urinalysis is most useful, however, in excluding genitourinary conditions which may mimic acute appendicitis. X-rays are rarely of value except when an opaque fecalith (5 percent of patients) is observed in the right lower quadrant (especially in children) together with other clinical findings consistent with appendicitis. Consequently there is no routine need to obtain films of the abdomen unless there is a possibility of other conditions such as intestinal obstruction or ureteral calculus.

While the typical historical sequence and physical findings are present in 50 to 60 percent of cases, it is obvious that a wide variety of atypical patterns of disease are encountered, especially at the age extremes and during pregnancy. The 70 to 80 percent incidence of perforation and generalized peritonitis in infants under 2 years of age is dramatic testimony to the importance of the history in the early detection of the disease. Any infant or child with diarrhea, vomiting, and abdominal pain is highly suspect. Fever is much more common in this age group, and abdominal distention is often the only physical finding. In the elderly, pain and tenderness are often obtunded, and thus the diagnosis is frequently delayed. A 30 percent incidence of perforation in patients over 70 attests to the importance of this delay. Elderly patients often present themselves initially with a painless mass (a primary appendiceal abscess), or sometimes appear with adhesive intestinal obstruction 5 or 6 days after a previously undetected perforated appendix. Appendicitis occurs about once in every 1000 pregnancies and is the most common extrauterine condition requiring abdominal operation. The diagnosis may be missed or delayed because of the frequent occurrence of mild abdominal discomfort and nausea and vomiting during pregnancy. During the last trimester when the mortality rate from appendicitis is highest, uterine displacement of the appendix to the right upper quadrant and laterally leads to confusion in diagnosis.

DIFFERENTIAL DIAGNOSIS A listing of the differential diagnoses of acute appendicitis would produce an encyclopedic compendium of all conditions which cause abdominal pain since appendicitis may simulate any of these diseases. Diagnostic accuracy is about 75 to 80 percent for experienced clinicians and must be based solely on the clinical criteria outlined above. It is probably better to err slightly in the direction of overdiagnosis since delay is associated with perforation and increased morbidity and mortality. In unperforated appendicitis the mortality rate is 0.1 percent, little more than that associated with general anesthesia; for perforated appendicitis there is an overall mortality of 3 percent, a figure which increases to 15 percent in the elderly. Four to six hours of observation in doubtful cases is always more beneficial than harmful, however. The most common conditions discovered at operation when acute appendicitis is erroneously diagnosed are, in rough order of frequency, mesenteric lymphadenitis, no organic disease, acute pelvic inflammatory disease, ruptured graafian follicle or corpus luteum cyst, and acute gastroenteritis. In addition, acute cholecystitis, perforated ulcer, acute pancreatitis, acute diverticulitis, strangulating intestinal obstruction, ureteral calculus, and pyelonephritis frequently present diagnostic difficulties.

It is useful to consider separately some of the more common and difficult diagnostic possibilities, especially in the female. Differentiation of *pelvic inflammatory disease* from acute appendicitis may be virtually impossible. Gram-negative intracellular diplococci on cervical smear are not pathognomonic unless *Neisseria gonorrhea* can be cultured. Pain on movement of the cervix is not specific and may occur in appendicitis if perforation has occurred or if the appendix lies adjacent to the uterus or adnexa. *Rupture of a graafian follicle* (mittelschmerz) occurs at midcycle with spill of blood and fluid to produce pain and tenderness more diffuse and usually of a less severe degree than in appendicitis. Fever and leukocytosis are usually absent. *Rupture of a corpus luteum cyst* is identical clinically to rupture of a graafian follicle but develops about the time of menstruation. The presence of an adnexal mass and evidence of blood loss help differentiate *ruptured tubal pregnancy*. *Twisted ovarian cyst* and *endometriosis* occasionally are difficult to distinguish from appendicitis.

Acute mesenteric lymphadenitis is the appellation usually given when enlarged, slightly reddened lymph nodes at the root of the mesentery and a normal appendix are encountered at operation. Whether this is a single, discrete entity is unclear since the causative factor is not known. The diagnosis is essentially impossible clinically, although retrospectively there often

appears to have been more diffuse pain and tenderness, perhaps associated with lymphocytosis. Children seem to be affected more frequently than adults. Operation should be undertaken unless there is rapid resolution of all symptoms and findings. *Acute gastroenteritis* usually causes profuse watery diarrhea, often with nausea and vomiting but without localized findings. Between cramps, the abdomen is completely relaxed. In salmonella gastroenteritis the abdominal findings are similar, although the pain may be more severe and more localized, and fever and chills are common. The occurrence of similar symptoms among other members of the family may be helpful. When the diagnosis of acute pelvic appendicitis with perforation has been missed, gastroenteritis is the most common previous working diagnosis. Persistent abdominal or rectal tenderness should eliminate the diagnosis of gastroenteritis. *Regional enteritis* (Crohn's disease) is usually associated with a more prolonged history, often with previous exacerbations regarded by the patient or physician as episodes of gastroenteritis unless the diagnosis has been established previously. *Meckel's diverticulitis* usually cannot be distinguished from acute appendicitis but is very rare.

TREATMENT Cathartics and frequent enemas should be avoided if appendicitis is under consideration, and antibiotics should not be administered when the diagnosis is in question, as they will only mask the presence or development of perforation. The treatment is early operation and appendectomy as soon as the patient can be prepared. Preparation rarely takes more than 1 to 2 h in early appendicitis but may require 6 to 8 h in cases of severe sepsis and dehydration associated with late perforation. The *only* circumstance in which operation is *not* indicated is the presence of a palpable mass 3 to 5 days after the onset of symptoms. Should operation be undertaken at that time, a phlegmon rather than a definitive abscess will be found, and complications from dissection of such a phlegmon are frequent. Such patients treated with broad-spectrum antibiotics, parenteral fluids, and rest usually show resolution of the mass and symptoms within 1 week. *Interval appendectomy* can and should be done safely 3 months later. Should the mass enlarge or the patient become more toxic, drainage of the abscess is necessary. The complications of subphrenic, pelvic, or other intraabdominal abscesses usually follow perforation with generalized peritonitis, and can be avoided by early diagnosis of the disease.

REFERENCES

BOLTON JP: Assessment of the value of the white cell count in management of suspected acute appendicitis. Br J Surg 62:906, 1975

CANTRELL JR, STAFFORD ES: The diminishing mortality from appendicitis. Ann Surg 141:749, 1955

FITZ RH: Perforating inflammation of the vermiform appendix: With special reference to its early diagnosis and treatment. Trans Assoc Am Physicians 1:107, 1886

HYMAN P, WESTRING DW: Leukocytosis in acute appendicitis: Observed racial differences. JAMA 229:1630, 1974

SAKOVER RP, DEL FAVA RL: Frequency of visualization of normal appendix with barium enema examination. Am J Roentgenol Radium Ther Nucl Med 121:312, 1974

SISSON RG et al: Superficial mucosal ulceration and pathogenesis of acute appendicitis. Am J Surg 122:378, 1971

THOMAS DR: Conservative management of appendix mass. Surgery 73:677, 1973

THORBJARNARSON B: Acute appendicitis in patients over the age of 60. Surg Gynecol Obstet 125:1277, 1967

297

DISEASES OF THE PERITONEUM AND MESENTERY

KURT J. ISSELBACHER
J. THOMAS LaMONT

ACUTE PERITONITIS Peritonitis is a localized or generalized inflammatory process of the peritoneum that may appear in both acute and chronic forms. In the acute form the motor activity of the intestine is decreased, and the intestinal lumen becomes distended with gas and fluid. Fluid accumulates as a result of failure to reabsorb the 7 or 8 liters normally secreted daily into the lumen and absorbed from the distal small bowel and colon. There is also accumulation of fluid in the peritoneal cavity as well as decreased oral intake. These combined losses can lead to rapid depletion of the plasma volume with impaired cardiac and renal function.

Etiology Peritonitis may be due to entry of bacteria into the peritoneal cavity from a perforation in the gastrointestinal tract or from an external penetrating wound. It may be secondary to severe chemical reactions from the release of pancreatic enzymes, the digestive juices of the upper gastrointestinal tract, or bile as a result of injury or perforation of the intestine or biliary tract.

The most common causes of bacterial peritonitis are appendicitis, perforations associated with diverticulitis, peptic ulcer, gangrenous gallbladder, and gangrenous obstruction of the small bowel from adhesive bands, incarcerated hernia, or volvulus. Any lesion leading to the escape of intestinal bacteria may be a source, including a perforating carcinoma, foreign body, and ulcerative colitis. The peritoneal cavity is remarkably resistant to contamination, and unless continuing contamination occurs, the disease process becomes localized. Patients with alcoholic cirrhosis and ascites have an increased susceptibility to spontaneous bacterial peritonitis, usually from enteric pathogens. This complication occurs in the absence of recognizable perforation of a viscus, and may be due to leakage of bacteria through the intestinal wall.

Clinical features These usually consist of increasing abdominal pain, distention, nausea and vomiting, inability to pass feces or flatus, fever, hypotension, tachycardia, thirst, and oliguria. On physical examination the patient appears acutely ill, febrile, and has a variable degree of abdominal distention. The abdomen is usually acutely tender and tympanitic, often with rebound tenderness. The location of the pain and tenderness depends on the underlying cause and whether the inflammation is localized or generalized. In *localized* peritonitis, as seen in uncomplicated appendicitis or diverticulitis, the physical findings are limited to the area of inflammation. With widespread peritoneal inflammation there is *generalized* peritonitis with diffuse abdominal tenderness and rebound.

Peristalsis may be present initially but usually disappears as the illness progresses. Hypotension is common, as is leukocytosis, which often is greater than 20,000 cells per cubic millimeter. X-ray examination of the abdomen shows dilatation of the large and small bowel with edema of the small-bowel wall as evidenced by the distance between adjacent loops of gas-filled small intestine. Diagnostic paracentesis is valuable in determining the nature of the exudate as well as whether bacteria can be demonstrated or cultured. Lead colic, gastric crises of syphilis, and acute porphyria may cause severe abdominal symptoms that resemble the picture of acute peritonitis.

GONOCOCCAL PERITONITIS This usually involves an extension of gonococcal infection from a primary focus in the female reproductive tract. The signs of inflammation usually are limited to the pelvis, but there may be findings of a mild generalized peritonitis. Occasionally the patient has right upper quadrant pain and tenderness caused by gonococcal perihepatitis involving the liver capsule and adjacent peritoneum (Fitz-Hugh–Curtis syndrome; see also Chap. 119).

STARCH PERITONITIS An acute granulomatous peritonitis can develop in some patients as a foreign-body reaction to cornstarch used to powder surgical gloves. The clinical picture is that of acute abdominal pain and fever 10 to 30 days after an abdominal operation. The diagnosis can be made by paracentesis and demonstration of starch granules in monocytes. However, most patients are reexplored because of the fear of abscess or bacterial peritonitis, with the finding of foreign-body granuloma studding the peritoneum.

PSEUDOMYXOMA PERITONEI This is a rare condition resulting from rupture of a mucocele of the appendix or of a mucinous ovarian cyst. The abdomen becomes filled with masses of jelly-like material. Occasionally, with removal of the mucocele or the ovarian cyst and most of the myxomatous material, a cure may ensue. In other cases, however, the mucoid material recurs, leading to progressive wasting and eventual death. Colloid carcinoma arising from the stomach or colon with peritoneal implants may resemble pseudomyxoma at laparotomy. The course of this type of highly malignant tumor is one of rapid cachexia and early death. The diagnosis can usually be made by the appearance of many highly malignant cells in the peritoneal implants.

CANCER OF THE PERITONEUM Aside from mesothelioma, which in most patients is caused by previous exposure to asbestos, cancer of the peritoneum is usually secondary to a neoplasm within the abdomen, most commonly of the stomach and ovary. Invariably this type of metastatic malignancy is associated with progressive ascites with a high specific gravity and high protein content, often with large numbers of red blood cells or even gross blood. The diagnosis is established by demonstrating malignant cells in the fluid. The clinical progress of this malignant spread can sometimes be arrested by installations of radioactive gold, nitrogen mustard, or chloroquine.

FAMILIAL MEDITERRANEAN FEVER See Chap. 217.

PNEUMATOSIS CYSTOIDES INTESTINALIS This is a condition in which multiple gas-filled blebs or cysts accumulate in the intestinal wall beneath the serosal surface of the bowel. The exact source of the gas has not been explained satisfactorily. In some instances, this disease is associated with specific ulceration of the intestinal mucosa, in particular peptic ulcer with outlet obstruction. Cysts in the wall of the small bowel are seen as an occasional complication of mesenteric vascular occlusion. In the large bowel, these cysts are usually benign, may be seen with a variety of other disorders, and usually disappear in time.

There are no specific physical findings secondary to the pneumatosis, and the diagnosis is made either by x-ray or at laparotomy. Occasionally the subserosal cysts may rupture, resulting in pneumoperitoneum.

CHYLOUS ASCITES This term refers to the accumulation of chyle (intestinal lymph) in the peritoneal cavity. The condition is sometimes associated with chylothorax. The fluid in the peritoneal cavity appears milky or creamy because of the presence of chylomicrons. This fat may be demonstrated microscopically by staining with Sudan III and may be removed by acidification of the fluid followed by extraction with ether. The chyle (lipid) will then go into the ether phase. Many conditions may be associated with the cloudy or milky-appearing peritoneal fluid, so-called "pseudochylous ascites." The milky or turbid appearance is usually due to the presence of protein and desquamated cells. The turbidity of this fluid will not be removed with the ether but will clear with addition of alkali.

The causes of chylous ascites include (1) penetrating or nonpenetrating trauma that damages the main duct in the lymphatic system within the abdomen, (2) intestinal obstruction if it is associated with rupture of a major lymphatic channel, (3) congenital lymphangiectasia, (4) malignant disease or tuberculous infection that obstructs the intestinal lymphatics, (5) filariasis, or (6) cirrhosis.

The sudden accumulation of chyle in the peritoneal cavity often results in abdominal pain, signs of peritoneal irritation, and leukocytosis. These symptoms gradually subside, leaving the patient with a distended but nontender, fluid-filled abdomen. Lymphangiography is of value in determining the location of the leak or site of obstruction to the lymphatic channels. The course depends upon the underlying etiologic factors.

MESENTERIC LIPODYSTROPHY This is a rare disorder usually affecting middle-aged women and characterized pathologically by infiltration of the mesentery with lipid-laden macrophages and fibrous tissue. These patients present with ill-defined abdominal pain and occasionally an abdominal mass. The diagnosis is made at laparotomy by demonstration of thick fibrofatty masses at the root of the mesentery with retraction and distortion of the bowel loops.

REFERENCES

Conn HO, Fessel JM: Spontaneous bacterial peritonitis in cirrhosis. Medicine 50:161, 1971

Kipfer RE et al: Mesenteric lipodystrophy. Ann Intern Med 80:582, 1974

Rhoads JE et al: *Surgery: Principles and Practice.* Philadelphia, Lippincott, 1970

Warshaw AL: Diagnosis of starch peritonitis by paracentesis. Lancet 2:1054, 1972

section 6 | Disorders of the hepatobiliary system

298
APPROACH TO THE PATIENT WITH LIVER DISEASE

KURT J. ISSELBACHER

GENERAL CONSIDERATIONS While disease of the liver or biliary tract may be directly responsible for the symptoms that bring the patient to the physician, examination for nonhepatic complaints may occasionally provide the clues to otherwise asymptomatic or occult hepatobiliary disease. Liver function studies and other diagnostic procedures such as biopsy (as discussed in Chap. 300) are crucial, but much valuable information as to the possible nature and extent of liver disease can be obtained by a carefully elicited history and thorough physical examination.

Importance of clinical history Since laboratory tests often do not establish the specific cause of liver disease, the history is of the greatest significance. *Family history* is important with respect to jaundice, anemia, splenectomy, or cholecystectomy; a positive history may be helpful in diagnosing hemolytic anemia, congenital or familial hyperbilirubinemia, or gallstones. In Wilson's disease (hepatolenticular degeneration), there may be a family history of tremor or neurologic abnormalities. *Occupation* should be reviewed in detail, and *environmental factors* need to be examined. Note should be made of any contact with rats or other animals possibly carrying Weil's disease and of exposure to toxins such as carbon tetrachloride, beryllium, or vinyl chloride. The patient should be asked about travel to other countries, especially to areas where hepatitis may be endemic. Careful questioning regarding alcohol intake is important in most cases. Since the alcoholic often denies or understates the amounts consumed, it is desirable to check the validity of the history with close friends or relatives of the patient.

Contact with jaundiced patients should be noted, especially in hospitals, schools, or the military where viral hepatitis is frequent. If the patient has had any *injections* in the previous 6 months, hepatitis B infection may be the underlying disease. Injections include blood tests, blood or plasma transfusions, tattooing, and dental treatment. The patient should be asked about narcotics, hallucinogens, or stimulant *drugs* taken parenterally, as well as about agents taken orally, such as chlorpromazine or contraceptive drugs known to affect liver function.

A previous history of indigestion, fat intolerance, and right upper quadrant pain suggests cholelithiasis or choledocholithiasis. Jaundice following shortly after operation on the biliary tract suggests residual stone, that which occurs within 6 months suggests hepatitis B (or non-A, non-B hepatitis), and that occurring after 1 or more years may be due to stricture of the common bile duct. Postoperative jaundice may be due to the anesthetic, especially multiple uses of halothane, or to the impaired hepatic excretory function resulting from relative hypoxemia of liver cells during the operative or postoperative period.

The *onset of the illness* should be noted. The relatively abrupt onset of nausea, anorexia, and aversion to smoking followed by progressive jaundice suggests infection with hepatitis A virus. A gradual development of jaundice associated with pruritus suggests cholestasis. Jaundice associated with fever and chills makes cholangitis and extrahepatic biliary obstruction likely possibilities.

The patient with hepatitis generally feels ill, and dark urine and light stools occur before the appearance of scleral or skin icterus. In cholestatic hepatitis, the patient may feel relatively well and complain only of symptoms due to the obstruction, such as pruritus.

Physical examination Pallor indicative of anemia may be a reflection of hemolysis, cirrhosis, or neoplasm. Significant cachexia, especially of the extremities, may be associated with cancer or active cirrhosis. Jaundice is looked for in the sclera as well as the skin. In the alcoholic, one should look for stigmas of cirrhosis such as parotid gland enlargement, Dupuytren's contracture, gynecomastia, testicular atrophy, and diminished axillary or pubic hair.

The *skin examination* may reveal ecchymoses due to prothrombin deficiency, or purpura due to thrombocytopenia. *Palmar erythema* or *spider angiomas* may reflect acute or chronic liver disease. Spider angiomas are usually found above the umbilicus and especially on the face, neck, shoulders, forearms, and dorsum of the hands. The presence of a few spider angiomas is not abnormal in women, especially during pregnancy. However, their appearance in men is always abnormal and should be carefully searched for. In chronic cholestasis, *scratch marks, finger clubbing,* and *xanthoma* of the eyelids and extensor surfaces of the tendons of the wrists and ankles may be found. A *slate color* to the skin due to increased melanin should suggest the presence of hemochromatosis.

Evaluation of the *mental state* and *neurologic function* is important. Slight deterioration of the intellect and minimal personality changes may suggest hepatocellular disease or the presence of portal-systemic venous shunts, but care must be taken to exclude other causes such as primary or metastatic brain tumors. The presence of flapping tremor of the hands (asterixis) may be found in association with portal-systemic encephalopathy or impending hepatic coma.

Abdominal examination may reveal ascites, which, together with dilated periumbilical veins, suggests cirrhosis and extensive portal collateral circulation. A very large nodular and rock-hard liver suggests the presence of hepatoma or hepatic metastases. Careful percussion is necessary to evaluate the size of a nonpalpable liver. A small liver may indicate cirrhosis (especially postnecrotic); a small liver which diminishes in size suggests severe hepatitis or massive hepatic necrosis. In the alcoholic, fatty infiltration and cirrhosis often produce a uniform enlargement of the liver. The liver edge is tender in hepatitis, in congestive heart failure, and occasionally in malignant disease and with alcoholism (especially "alcoholic hepatitis").

A palpable and sometimes visibly enlarged gallbladder (Courvoisier's sign) suggests extrahepatic biliary obstruction often due to pancreatic cancer. A tender gallbladder and positive Murphy's sign suggests cholelithiasis or choledocholithiasis. A palpable spleen may indicate hepatitis; significant splenomegaly may be a reflection of portal hypertension.

Abdominal auscultation may reveal the presence of a venous hum over dilated collateral veins radiating from the umbilicus, the so-called "caput medusae." In advanced cirrhosis this venous hum is virtually diagnostic of significant portal hypertension. A bruit may sometimes be heard over large regenerating nodules in cirrhosis, and occasionally over hepatomas and metastatic nodules in the liver. The presence of a friction rub strongly suggests neoplastic disease or a hepatic abscess. A friction rub may occasionally be heard over hepatomas and metastatic liver nodules.

Diagnostic procedures These are reviewed in Chap. 300. For the proper evaluation of liver and biliary tract diseases chemical and biochemical tests of blood, urine, and stool are essential, and liver biopsy is often needed to help determine the nature of the liver disease. In addition, laparoscopy and special radiologic techniques such as cholangiography, angiography, or scintiscans of the liver may be employed. In a significant number of cases it may be impossible to distinguish between intrahepatic and extrahepatic disease. These patients should undergo cholangiography, either percutaneous or via the fiber-optic endoscope. If the situation is still in doubt, an exploratory laparotomy, including liver biopsy and operative cholangiography, should be performed.

CLASSIFICATION OF LIVER DISEASE The classification of the various types of liver disease has been difficult because in many instances the etiology and pathogenetic mechanism are obscure. As a consequence, one finds an abundance of labels and names applied to hepatic disorders. Some individuals use the term *hepatitis* to imply viral infection, others simply to connote evidence of hepatic inflammation. One finds ambiguity in the use of the words *acute, subacute,* and *chronic. Chronicity* should refer to continuing or recurrent disease (i.e., duration). *Activity* should refer to evidence of the presence of perpetuation of liver cell injury; this is most readily identified on biopsy by the degree of hepatocellular necrosis and by serum transaminase elevations.

Because of the difficulties involved in defining the etiology of many types of liver disease, in most instances the process is best defined and described by an examination of the morphologic character of the lesion. Therefore, a *morphologic classification* of liver disease, as outlined in Table 298-1, appears at present more practical than one based on etiology.

TABLE 298-1
Classification of liver disease

I Parenchymal
  A Hepatitis (viral, drug-induced, toxic)
    1 Acute
    2 Chronic (persistent or active)
  B Cirrhosis
    1 Alcoholic (portal, nutritional, Laennec's cirrhosis)
    2 Postnecrotic
    3 Biliary
    4 Hemochromatosis
    5 Rare types (e.g., Wilson's disease, galactosemia, cystic fibrosis of pancreas, α_1-antitrypsin deficiency)
  C Infiltrations
    1 Glycogen
    2 Fat (neutral fat, cholesterol, gangliosides, cerebrosides)
    3 Amyloid
    4 Lymphoma, leukemia
    5 Granuloma (e.g., sarcoidosis, tuberculosis, idiopathic)
  D Space-occupying lesions
    1 Hepatoma, metastatic tumor
    2 Abscess (pyogenic, amoebic)
    3 Cysts (polycystic disease, *Echinococcus*)
    4 Gummas
  E Functional disorders associated with jaundice
    1 Gilbert's syndrome
    2 Crigler-Najjar syndrome
    3 Dubin-Johnson and Rotor syndromes
    4 Cholestasis of pregnancy and benign recurrent cholestasis
II Hepatobiliary
  A Extrahepatic biliary obstruction (by stone, stricture, or tumor)
  B Cholangitis
III Vascular
  A Chronic passive congestion and cardiac cirrhosis
  B Hepatic vein thrombosis (Budd-Chiari syndrome)
  C Portal vein thrombosis
  D Pylephlebitis
  E Arteriovenous malformations

REFERENCES

SCHIFF L: *Diseases of the Liver,* 4th ed. Philadelphia, Lippincott, 1975
SHERLOCK S: *Diseases of the Liver and Biliary System,* 5th ed. Philadelphia, Davis, 1975

DERANGEMENTS OF HEPATIC METABOLISM

DAVID A. SHAFRITZ
SING HEIM YAP
KURT J. ISSELBACHER

The liver serves a variety of important functions related to macromolecular synthesis, energy generation and storage, catabolism, and disposal of toxic substances and waste products of intermediary metabolism. The hepatic parenchyma is comprised of three major cell types—the hepatocyte, biliary epithelial cell, and Kupffer cell—but the hepatocyte comprises approximately 80 percent of total liver mass. From analysis of specific liver functions and their derangements, certain general principles can be established: (1) Since the liver plays a major role in generalized metabolic events, acute or chronic liver dysfunction often leads to biochemical abnormalities. (2) The liver has considerable reserve capacity, so that minor or moderate dysfunction may not be reflected by changes in certain metabolic parameters (i.e., "liver function" tests based on biosynthesis or metabolic activity are of limited value). (3) Some functions of the liver are more sensitive to injury than others, so that liver injury may or may not be demonstrable by certain tests. (4) Since the liver performs many varied functions, *no one single test effectively measures total liver function.* Therefore, an understanding of the many known biochemical and metabolic functions of this organ is required to appreciate the wide variety of responses which may occur in acute or chronic liver failure.

The biochemical functions in which the liver plays a major role include (1) the metabolism of amino acids, ammonia, protein, carbohydrates, and lipids; (2) biochemical oxidations; and (3) metabolism and detoxification of drugs, vitamins, and hormones. These general topics are discussed below. The metabolism of bilirubin, porphyrins, and bile salts are described elsewhere (see Chaps. 96, 292, 301, and 307).

AMINO ACID METABOLISM Through a variety of anabolic and catabolic processes, the liver is the major site of amino acid interconversion. Amino acids utilized for hepatic protein synthesis are derived from dietary protein, metabolic turnover of endogenous protein (primarily from muscle), and direct synthesis in the liver. The bulk of amino acids entering the liver via the portal vein are catabolized to urea (except for the branched-chain amino acids leucine, isoleucine, and valine). A lesser amount is released into the general circulation as free amino acids, and a small portion is utilized for synthesis of liver intracellular proteins, plasma proteins, and special compounds such as glutathione, glutamine, taurine, carnosine, and creatine. Catabolism or degradation of amino acids in the liver involves two major reactions: *transamination* and *oxidative deamination.*

Transamination, the process by which the amino group of an amino acid is transferred to a keto acid, is catalyzed by a specific group of enzymes, *aminotransferases.* These enzymes are found in very high amount in liver but are also present in other tissues, such as kidney, muscle, heart, lung, and brain. Glutamic-oxaloacetic acid transaminase (asparatate aminotransferase) and glutamic-pyruvic acid transaminase (alanine aminotransferase) have been studied most extensively, and increased levels are found in the serum in various types of liver injury. As a result of transamination reactions, amino acids can enter the citric acid cycle to function in the intermediary metabolism of carbohydrates and lipids (see Chap. 86). At the same time, depending on the level of specific substrates, aminotransferases can catalyze the reverse reaction, namely, the synthesis of amino acids from certain keto acids. Therefore, transamination is a bidirectional process. Most of the nonessential amino acids are synthesized in the liver by transamination. *Oxidative deamination,* which results in conversion of an amino acid to a keto acid (and ammonia), is catalyzed by L-amino acid oxidases, with two exceptions: glycine oxidation is catalyzed by glycine oxidase, and glutamic acid oxidation is catalyzed by glutamic dehydrogenase. When the liver is severely damaged (e.g., in massive hepatic necrosis), utilization of amino acids is impaired, free amino acids in the bloodstream increase, and an "overflow" type of amino aciduria may occur.

AMMONIA METABOLISM Ammonia, a toxic product of nitrogen metabolism, is converted rapidly and almost exclusively in the liver into the nontoxic end product, urea. The intermediate steps in the urea (Krebs-Henseleit) cycle are shown in Fig. 299-1. This process involves four specific amino acids: ornithine, citrulline, arginine, and aspartic acid. Because the conversion of arginine to ornithine and urea by the enzyme arginase is irreversible, this pathway is unidirectional. In severe liver injury, urea synthesis is often depressed. This may result in significant reduction in blood urea nitrogen (BUN), an ominous sign of liver failure. A similar phenomenon may be observed in the later stages of chronic liver disease, such as in patients with alcoholic cirrhosis.

Approximately 25 percent of blood urea is excreted into the intestine, where NH_3 is produced. However, the major source of intestinal NH_3 is from bacterial deamination of undigested dietary protein, unabsorbed amino acids, and sloughed mucosal cells. NH_3 formed in the intestine enters the portal vein and is detoxified rapidly in the liver by conversion to urea. Under conditions of protein "overload," as in gastrointestinal bleeding, production of intestinal NH_3 and other nitrogenous substances is increased. When the liver is incapable of metabolizing the NH_3 and the other nitrogenous substances it receives, hepatic encephlopathy may ensue. In severe liver failure, either acute or chronic, this may occur, even in face of reduced protein intake (see Chap. 304).

Five principal mechanisms leading to an increased blood NH_3 level in chronic liver disease are illustrated in Fig. 299-2: (1) If there is *excessive nitrogenous material* in the intestine (from bleeding or dietary protein), excessive amounts of NH_3

FIGURE 299-1

The chemical steps of the urea (Krebs-Henseleit) cycle.

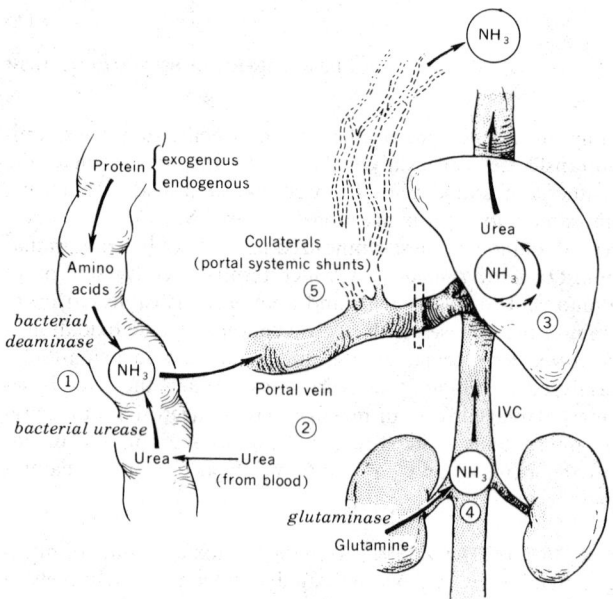

FIGURE 299-2

Major factors (steps 1 to 4) influencing the level of blood ammonia. In cirrhosis with portal hypertension, venous collaterals allow ammonia to bypass the liver (5), allowing for the entry of ammonia into the systemic circulation (portal-systemic shunting).

will be formed by bacterial deamination of amino acids. (2) If urine output falls (as in the hepatorenal syndrome), blood urea nitrogen rises, leading to increased diffusion of urea into the intestine, where bacterial urease converts it to ammonia. (3) If hepatic function is significantly depressed, *decreased urea synthesis* may occur with reduced removal of NH_3. (4) If metabolic alkalosis and hypokalemia accompany hepatic decompensation, there may be decreased H^+ ions. Thus, the NH_3 produced from glutamine by the action of renal glutaminase is shunted into the renal vein, leading to increased peripheral blood NH_3 levels. (5) If portal hypertension accompanies cirrhosis, venous anastomoses develop between the portal vein and systemic venous channels, and these *portal-systemic shunts* allow NH_3 to escape hepatic detoxification, leading to elevated blood NH_3 levels.

Two additional factors are probably important in determining whether a given NH_3 level in the blood will be injurious to the tissues. First, NH_3 is removed from the blood by a variety of tissues, including brain, lungs, and muscle, and the degree of utilization is affected by the presence of arteriovenous (AV) shunts, which often occur in chronic liver disease. Second, the more alkaline the blood pH, the more toxic a given level of NH_3 is likely to be. At 37°C the pK of NH_3 is 8.9, that is, close enough to the pH of blood so that small changes of blood pH might affect the NH_4^+/NH_3 ratio. Because un-ionized NH_3 crosses membranes more readily than ionized NH_4^+ ions, alkalosis favors the entry of ammonia into the brain by shifting the equilibrium of the following reaction to the right:

$$NH_4^+ + OH \rightleftharpoons NH_3 + HOH$$

Alkalosis then not only increases the peripheral blood levels of NH_3 by renal mechanisms but also increases tissue levels by its effect on the diffusion of NH_3 ions.

PROTEIN SYNTHESIS AND METABOLISM
The liver synthesizes all the proteins required for general cellular function, as well as certain proteins for specialized functions. Many plasma proteins are synthesized in the liver, and of these, *albumin* is synthesized in the greatest amount. The major functions of albumin in the serum are regulation of oncotic pressure and binding and transport of certain hormones, fatty acids, bilirubin, trace metals, and toxic products. The body contains about 5 g albumin per kilogram of body weight, and approximately 40 percent of this protein is found in the circulation. Albumin is synthesized exclusively in the liver, and in the normal adult, daily production is approximately 120 to 220 mg per kilogram of body weight. The normal half-life of serum albumin is 17 to 20 days. Under conditions of reduced albumin half-life from excessive losses from the body, as, for example, in massive proteinuria or protein-losing gastroenteropathy, synthesis can be increased two- to threefold. As shown in Fig. 299-3, secretory proteins such as albumin are synthesized by membrane-bound polyribosomes in the hepatocyte. Protein synthesis begins by the association of messenger RNA (in the form of messenger ribonucleoprotein particles, mRNPs) with free ribosomal subunits in the cytosol. From experimental studies in rats, it has been shown that albumin is synthesized as a precursor molecule, preproalbumin, containing 24 extra amino acids with a net hydrophobic charge in the *N*-terminal precursor segment. The hydrophobic nascent chain of polyribosomes synthesizing albumin directs these polyribosomes to associate with membranes to form the rough endoplasmic reticulum (RER). The "pre" portion of preproalbumin is cleaved within the RER even before protein synthesis is completed; subsequently the "pro" segment is removed within the lumen of the ER to form the final product, albumin. In contrast, proteins that are synthesized primarily for intracellular use, such as ferritin, remain on free polyribosomes in the cytosol and do not undergo these precursor-processing events.

Once albumin synthesis and processing is completed, it is transported through the vesicles of the ER to the hepatocyte surface and is secreted into the hepatic sinusoid by mechanisms that are still unclear. With liver injury, changes in albumin synthesis may occur at the level of messenger RNA tran-

FIGURE 299-3

Schematic diagram illustrating major steps in synthesis, processing, and secretion of albumin by the liver. Ribosomal subunits and mRNA (in the form of mRNPs) form polysome complexes to initiate protein synthesis. Polyribosomes synthesizing albumin associate with membranes to form membrane-bound polysomes (i.e., the rough endoplasmic reticulum). Synthesis of an albumin precursor molecule "preproalbumin" occurs, followed by stepwise proteolytic cleavage to albumin and secretion from the cell.

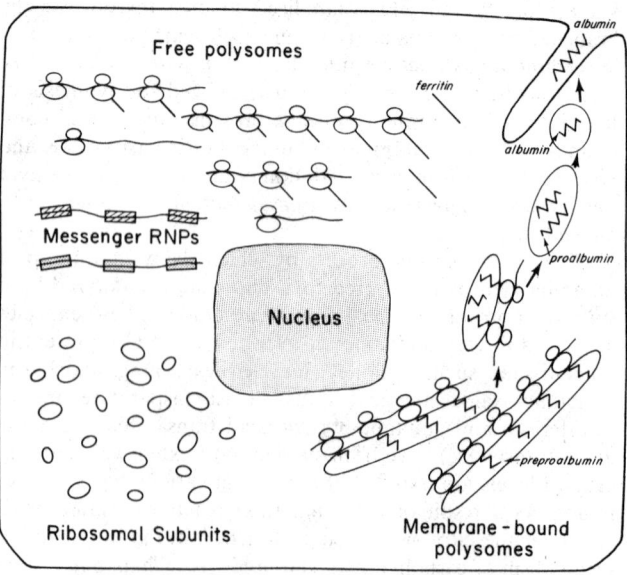

scription or at subsequent steps in translation. Abnormalities in the intracellular transport or secretion of albumin may also occur, and oncotic pressure has been implicated in the feedback regulation of albumin synthesis. Reduced serum albumin levels are found in most cases of advanced and diffuse hepatocellular disease.

Clinically decreased albumin synthesis can also result from an inadequate amino acid supply, as in starvation, protein-calorie malnutrition, or malabsorption syndromes. Hypothyroidism and chronic renal failure in experimental animals have also been reported to decrease albumin synthesis. Several patients have been found with congenital analbuminemia, a rare, probably inherited disorder associated with lack of albumin synthesis. Aside from pretibial edema, this syndrome has not been associated with major physiologic abnormalities. Variations in the amino acid structure of albumin have also been described, suggesting specific mutations or polymorphism in the albumin gene.

Far less is known about albumin catabolism than about synthesis. The major site of albumin degradation has not been established; clearly it is not the liver. In disease states, albumin may be lost in excessive amounts in urine, feces, extravascular fluid (ascites or exudates), and acute burn areas, leading to severe hypoalbuminemia. Intravenous replacement therapy is generally helpful only when losses are acute. With the possible exceptions of hemoconcentration from dehydration and overvigorous albumin infusion, hyperalbuminemia does not occur. Experimental evidence suggests that an increased rate of albumin catabolism provides a powerful means for correcting albumin excess.

Other proteins produced by the liver include many of the blood-clotting factors: fibrinogen (factor I), prothrombin (factor II), and factors V, VII, IX, and X. Factors II, VII, IX, and X are vitamin K–responsive and thus are dependent upon normal intestinal fat absorption. It is now established that vitamin K activates an enzyme system in liver endoplasmic reticulum, catalyzing γ-carboxylation of selected glutamyl residues in a prothrombin precursor. γ-Carboxylation enhances Ca^{2+} and phospholipid binding capacity of prothrombin and permits its rapid conversion to thrombin in the presence of factors V and X. In complete biliary obstruction with vitamin K malabsorption or in patients treated with "coumarin-like" anticoagulants (competitive antagonists for the phospholipid binding site), the prothrombin times become prolonged. This effect can be corrected by parenteral administration of vitamin K. With active hepatocellular disease, deficiencies in factors II, V, VII, and X may occur. All these clotting factors have a biological half-life shorter than that of albumin, varying from 4 h (factor VII: proconvertin) to 3 to 5 days (factor II: prothrombin). Therefore, when fresh blood is administered, levels of these factors will be elevated only transiently. Under normal circumstances, prothrombin is catabolized directly without formation of thrombin. For some proteins, e.g., fibrinogen, the fractional degradation rate is relatively constant, irrespective of plasma concentration. Since pathological conditions with reduced breakdown of fibrinogen are very rare, increased plasma levels of this protein (fibrinogen) usually reflect enhanced synthesis. Such conditions include posttraumatic states such as burns, surgical procedures, bacterial infections, and myocardial infarction, as well as cancer, rheumatoid arthritis, and pregnancy. Nutritional deficiency does not prevent the development of hyperfibrinogenemia. In several patients congenital hypo- or afibrinogenemia has been observed. Except in advanced cirrhosis, acquired conditions with reduced fibrinogen synthesis have not been described. In addition to fibrinogen, the liver demonstrates increased synthesis of other proteins in response to tissue damage. All these proteins are referred to as acute phase reactants. The best-known examples are orosomucoid, the C-reactive proteins, haptoglobin, ceruloplasmin, and

transferrin. Much of the serum α and β globulins are also synthesized in the liver, but most γ globulins are produced by plasma cells.

ENZYMES USED IN CLINICAL TESTS In connection with the many biochemical reactions performed by the liver, this organ contains thousands of protein catalysts or enzymes. Although some of these enzymes are unique to the liver, many are also found in nonhepatic tissues. Hence, measurements of serum enzyme activities to assess deranged liver function must be interpreted in combination with other pertinent clinical and laboratory data. When increased serum levels of enzymes such as the aminotransferases (transaminases) are found, several points must be kept in mind: (1) loss of enzymes from liver cells occurs with necrosis and also with changes in cell permeability produced by ischemia or hypoxia; (2) only minimal cell changes may be needed to cause a rise in serum enzyme levels and there is no direct quantitative correlation between the amount of liver cell injury and the height of serum enzyme levels, although in general, higher levels are found with more severe injury; (3) if measurement of serum enzymes is delayed after acute insult or injury, the initial increase may be missed, and normal or low-serum enzyme levels may be found subsequently as a consequence of a decreased functioning liver cell mass; and (4) some enzymes (e.g., aminotransferases) are elevated by injury or ischemia of nonhepatic tissues, particularly muscle, heart, and kidney. These and other enzymes (e.g., lactic dehydrogenase) often represent a series of different proteins in different tissues catalyzing the same reaction (isoenzymes). The specific tissue of origin can often be established by analysis of isoenzyme patterns. Alkaline phosphatase is present in bone, intestine, kidney, and placenta as well as in the liver. A variety of techniques are available to distinguish various alkaline phosphatase isoenzymes. Electrophoresis may be used to separate some of these isoenzymes; heat treatment tends to inactivate bone alkaline phosphatase; L-phenylalanine selectively inhibits the intestinal enzyme. Another useful approach to determine whether an elevated alkaline phosphatase level reflects hepatic disease is to measure a related enzyme, 5'-nucleotidase, which is elaborated by hepatic canalicular microvilli but is not found in bone.

In the hepatocyte, alanine aminotransferase (GPT) is present free in the cytosol, whereas aspartate aminotransferase (GOT) is demonstrable in both mitochondria and the cytosol. The activity of aspartate aminotransferase in liver is higher than that of alanine aminotransferase, but 40 to 60 percent of aspartate aminotransferase is located in the mitochondria. Aspartate aminotransferase activity in human serum (SGOT) is derived largely from the cytosolic enzyme of myocardium and hepatic parenchyma, but the mitochondrial enzyme is also invariably present in the serum. In healthy individuals, the ratio of SGOT to SGPT (serum activities) is usually less than 2:1. In acute liver injury, e.g., acute viral hepatitis, loss of mainly cytosolic enzymes occurs, producing a greater rise in SGPT and an SGOT/SGPT ratio which is often less than 1. In alcoholic-induced liver injury (e.g., alcoholic hepatitis) the SGOT/SGPT ratio may be increased up to 2 or more. This may be due to loss of aspartate aminotransferase from damaged liver mitochrondia and from other injured tissues, such as muscle.

CARBOHYDRATE METABOLISM The liver plays a vital role in glucose homeostasis. Unless given intravenous glucose supplements, patients with acute massive liver injury (viral or toxic hepatitis) die quickly from hypoglycemia. The liver maintains the level of blood glucose by (1) uptake and storage of glucose in the form of glycogen (*glycogenesis*), (2) conversion of stored glycogen into glucose upon specific need (*glycogenolysis*), and (3) formation of glucose from noncarbohydrate sources (*gluconeogenesis*). Several hormones, including insulin, glucagon, growth hormone, and certain catechol amines, are involved in this process. Following ingestion of glucose in a normal fasted individual, blood glucose starts to rise and insulin release is stimulated. This facilitates glucose uptake into cells. Fifty-five to 60 percent of an oral glucose load is taken up by the liver and is utilized for glycogen synthesis, triglyceride formation, and to a small extent, for glycolysis. Twenty-five percent escapes the liver and is used for needs of the brain and noninsulin-dependent tissues (glycogen sparing). In fasting, the liver contributes to glucose homeostasis by glycogenolysis and gluconeogenesis in response to hypoinsulinemia and hyperglucagonemia. Glycogen in the liver accounts for 5 to 7 percent of the normal tissue weight. Because the capacity of the liver to store glycogen is limited (~70 g) and glucose consumption (particularly in the brain) continues at a constant rate (~150 g per day), hepatic glycogen stores are depleted after 1 day of fasting. To compensate for this relative lack of available glycogen in fasting, hepatic gluconeogenesis is stimulated. In liver disease, both the ability to synthesize and store glycogen and the balance between hepatic glucose production and glucose utilization may be affected. This often leads either to hypoglycemia or to glucose intolerance, depending on specific circumstances. However, there is no correlation between abnormalities of carbohydrate metabolism and other liver function tests.

Hypoglycemia in severe liver damage may be due to (1) decreased hepatic glycogen stores, diminished glucagon responsiveness, and failure of glycogen repletion following a high carbohydrate intake, as in fulminant hepatitis or end-stage cirrhosis; (2) increased glucose utilization, as in hyperinsulinemic hypoglycemia in patients with fulminant viral hepatitis or postpartum toxic hepatitis; (3) decreased delivery of substrates for gluconeogenesis from diminished hepatic blood flow, as in severe passive congestion of the liver (chronic congestive heart disease); (4) toxic inhibition of gluconeogenesis from acute alcohol ingestion, especially when hepatic glycogen stores are

depleted by fasting; or (5) increased "insulin-like" activity in the serum in some patients with hepatocellular carcinoma.

Hyperglycemia and glucose intolerance occurs in relatively high frequency in patients with cirrhosis. This condition is often associated with normal or increased plasma insulin. These findings suggest that insulin resistance rather than insulin deficiency is responsible for glucose intolerance in liver disease. Glucagon, which is also metabolized by the liver, is increased in the plasma in patients with portal systemic shunting. In addition, the cirrhotic liver may have a reduced capacity to metabolize a large glucose load. Therefore, a variety of factors contribute to hyperglycemia in chronic liver disease. The high level of insulin in patients with cirrhosis may account for the rarity of diabetic angiopathy. Diabetes mellitus is also a frequent finding in patients with hemochromatosis. In such cases, carbohydrate intolerance is generally more severe than in alcoholic cirrhosis and the insulin response to glucose is reduced. Galactose is metabolized primarily by the liver, and impaired galactose tolerance occurs in liver disease. Increased serum lactic acid levels may occur with diffuse liver disease, because lactate uptake by the liver is also decreased under these circumstances. The liver is active in the synthesis of lipids, especially triglycerides. While some remain in the liver, most triglycerides are excreted into the bloodstream in the form of lipoproteins. The major steps in hepatic fatty acid and triglyceride metabolism are shown in Fig. 299-4.

Under normal conditions, most of the *fatty acids* taken up by the liver and *esterified to triglyceride* are derived from adipose tissue or the diet. Some fatty acids (especially saturated ones) are synthesized in the liver from acetate. The fatty acids may then be converted enzymatically to triglyceride, esterified with cholesterol, incorporated into phospholipids, or oxidized to CO_2 or ketone bodies. Most of the triglyceride is produced for export and in order to be secreted must be converted to *lipoproteins* by combining with relatively specific apoprotein moieties. Thus, protein synthesis is important for the release and secretion of triglyceride from the liver.

Studies on the production of a fatty liver have shown that singly or in combinations one or more of these steps depicted numerically in Fig. 299-4 may lead to excessive hepatic triglyceride accumulation and hence a fatty liver. *Increased influx* of fatty acids (1), such as may occur with drugs (e.g., ethanol or corticosteroids) producing lipid mobilization from adipose tissue or in diabetic ketosis, may lead to a fatty liver. Similarly *increased levels of fatty acids in the liver,* either from enhanced fatty acid synthesis (2) or from decreased oxidation (3), may lead to increased triglyceride formation. In some instances (e.g., ethanol excess) there may also be *increases* in the carbohydrate backbone, α-glycerophosphate, involved in fatty acid esterification to triglyceride (4). Since release of triglyceride involves the formation of lipoproteins, lipid accumulation may occur because of *decreased apoprotein synthesis* (5). In the case of fatty livers produced by toxins such as carbon tetrachloride, phosphorus, and ethionine, and by antibiotics like tetracycline, the major mechanism for lipid accumulation appears to be impaired apoprotein synthesis. Finally, there may be impaired lipoprotein synthesis (i.e., coupling of lipid with *apoprotein*) (6), or impaired lipoprotein secretion from the liver (7). Alcohol is perhaps the most common agent leading to a fatty liver, but the mechanism whereby alcohol leads to increased liver triglyceride is not clear. Alcohol administration, depending on dose or duration, may affect any of the seven steps shown in Fig. 299-4, and the primary factor for the production of the alcohol-induced fatty liver still remains to be determined.

Cholesterol and *bile acid synthesis* is carried out primarily by the liver. In the plasma cholesterol exists either *free* or combined with fatty acids in the form of *cholesterol esters;* both are found primarily in association with β-lipoproteins. The plasma and liver also contain cholesterol acyl transferase, an enzyme

FIGURE 299-4

Factors in the uptake and esterification of fatty acids to triglyceride by the liver including the formation and release of triglyceride as lipoprotein. The numbers refer to steps, which, if altered, may result in increased liver triglyceride (i.e., fatty liver).

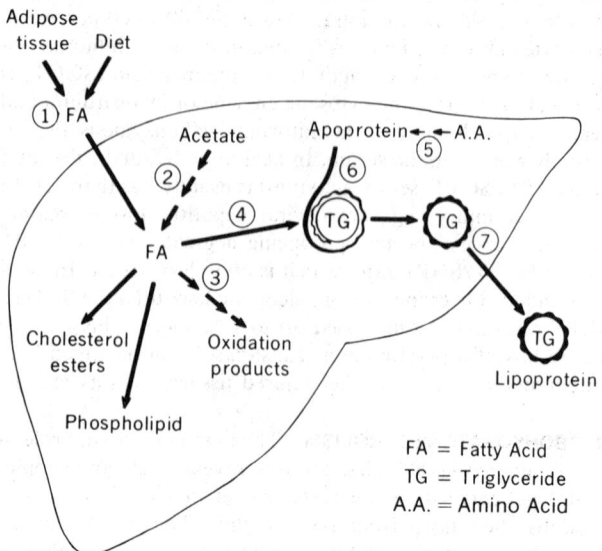

FA = Fatty Acid
TG = Triglyceride
A.A. = Amino Acid

involved in the conversion of free cholesterol to its esterified form. Free cholesterol exchanges readily between tissues, and thus changes in plasma cholesterol levels reflect changes in total body cholesterol. However, decreases in plasma cholesterol esters may reflect hepatic damage.

Severe liver injury often leads to a decrease in total serum cholesterol levels, including both free and esterified fractions. This may be due to decreased cholesterol and cholesterol ester synthesis, decreased apolipoprotein synthesis, or both. In cholestasis (intra- or extrahepatic) *total serum cholesterol often increases* strikingly. On the other hand, the serum cholesterol ester level increases to a much lesser extent, with the result that there is a *decrease* in the *ester fraction* (i.e., ester/total). An abnormal serum lipoprotein (lipoprotein X) which contains apolipoprotein C, and large quantities of both phospholipid and unesterified cholesterol has also been found in severe liver disease. The cholesterol elevation in cholestasis may be related in part to increased production of this abnormal lipoprotein.

BIOCHEMICAL OXIDATIONS (ENERGY PRODUCTION) The major source of energy in all animal cells is *aerobic respiration,* a process which occurs in the mitochondria (see Chap. 86). *Aerobic respiration* involves a series of reactions (the tricarboxylic acid cycle and the electron transport chain) to oxidize carbon-hydrogen bonds (fuel) to CO_2 and H_2O. During this process, energy is transferred to ATP and reduced pyridine and flavin nucleotides (NADH, NADPH, $FADH_2$, etc.), which are then used for various types of biochemical work. In energy production, the liver is unique, because it is rich in both mitochondria and enzymes which feed large quantities of substrates (carbohydrates, protein, and fat) into the tricarboxylic acid cycle (see Fig. 86-2).

In liver disease, numerous defects in hepatic metabolism of carbohydrate, protein, and fat have been described (see preceding sections). Such abnormalities would be expected to impair oxidative processes and energy production, but specific documentation for derangements in mitochondrial function has been difficult to obtain. In two specific instances, Reye's syndrome (see Chap. 306) and hypoglycin A toxicity (Jamaica vomiting sickness), the combined findings of hypoglycemia, metabolic acidosis, coma, and death suggest mitochondrial dysfunction. Electron microscopic evidence for abnormalities in mitochondrial structure (mitochondrial swelling and distortion of cristae) has been described in these syndromes, but similar changes are also found in other types of acute cellular injury.

DETOXIFICATION MECHANISMS The liver plays a key role in the detoxification of many substances, both endogenous (e.g., hormones) and exogenous (e.g., drugs or ingested substances). This is accomplished by numerous mechanisms, such as oxidation reduction, hydroxylation, sulfoxidation, deamination, dealkylation, and/or methylation, which reduce pharmacological activity of these compounds. These reactions involve several enzymatic systems, including the mixed function oxidases, cytochromes b_5 and P_{450} (microsomal), and glutathione S-aryltransferases (cytoplasmic). In addition, conjugation reactions with glucuronic acids, sulfate, taurine, and glycine produce water-soluble derivatives from less soluble substrates, so that these substances can be excreted in bile and urine. In other cases, certain drugs must be metabolized in the liver to form biochemically active intermediates. For example, in addition to its storage function, the liver converts dietary vitamin D to a metabolically more active 25-hydroxyl derivative. More recently, it has been discovered that in certain types of drug toxicity, hepatic metabolism actually generates the toxic intermediate (e.g., isonicotinic hydrazide and acetaminophen toxicity). Activation of certain carcinogens also occurs by formation of highly reactive epoxide intermediates in the liver.

Some hormones (e.g., insulin and glucagon) are inactivated in the liver by proteolysis or deamination. Thyroxine and triiodothyronine are metabolized in the liver by reactions involving deiodination as well as proteolysis. Steroid hormones, such as corticosteroids and aldosterone, are first inactivated by reduction of the Δ^4 double bond and the 3-keto group to their tetrahydro derivates, followed by conjugation mostly with glucuronic acid. Other alterations of cortisol, catalyzed by hepatic enzymes, include hydroxylations at C-2 and C-6, reduction of the carbonyl group at C-20, and reversible oxidation of the hydroxyl group at C-11 to produce cortisone. Testosterone is metabolized to the isomeric 17-ketosteroids, androsterone and etiocholanolone, and excreted mostly as sulfate conjugates in the urine. Estrogens, such as estradiol, may be converted to estriol and estrone and then conjugated with glucuronic acid or sulfate. Abnormalities in estrogen metabolism have often been considered the cause of spider angiomas, gynecomastia, loss of axillary or pubic hair, and testicular atrophy.

Estrogens also act directly on the liver by impairing hepatic secretory activity. Estradiol and related estrogens, such as those present in contraceptive pills, interfere with sodium sulfobromophthalein (Bromsulphalein, BSP) and bile salt excretion and may also elevate plasma alkaline phosphatase levels (see Chap. 300). Related steroids such as etiocholanolone and pregnanediol have also been shown to stimulate δ-aminolevulinic acid (ALA) synthetase activity leading to porphyrinuria. Since these steroids exert these effects only in their free (i.e., nonglucuronide) form, the increased hepatic levels of δ-aminolevulinic acid synthetase in patients with Laennec's cirrhosis may be due to the effect of gonadal steroids.

The ability of the liver to metabolize and detoxify drugs is an important consideration when treating patients with liver disease. Some drugs, such as phenobarbital and ethanol, can stimulate the smooth endoplasmic reticulum, thereby increasing activity of detoxifying enzymes. Thus, the efficacy of certain drugs may be reduced when taken in combination with other agents. In contrast, impaired drug metabolism often occurs in acute or chronic liver disease, and this may lead to a decreased dosage requirement or a reduction in the range between therapeutic and toxic levels. For example, morphine derivatives and all barbiturates, except barbital, are metabolized primarily in the liver, as are many other sedatives (chlordiazepoxide, paraldehyde, etc). Agitation, confusion, and irrational behavior are conditions for which such drugs are often prescribed but may also be early signs of impending hepatic coma. Therefore, the use of sedatives, tranquilizers, and depressant drugs in patients with hepatic insufficiency, either acute or chronic, should be viewed with extreme caution.

REFERENCES

ALBERTI KGMM: Some metabolic aspects of liver disease, in *Topics in Gastroenterology,* vol 2, SC Truelove, J Trowell (eds). London, Blackwell, 1975, p 341

COODLEY EI: Enzyme diagnosis in hepatic disease. Am J Gastroenterol 56:413, 1971

FISHMAN WH: Perspectives on alkaline phosphatase isoenzymes. Am J Med 56:617, 1974

LEHNINGER AL: The molecular basis of cell structure and function, in *Biochemistry,* 2d ed. New York, Worth, 1975

POPPER H, SCHAFFNER F: *Progress in Liver Diseases,* vol V. New York, Grune & Stratton, 1976

ROTHSCHILD MA et al: Albumin synthesis. N Engl J Med 286:748, 1972

SCHENKER S et al: Hepatic encephalopathy: Current status. Gastroenterology 66:121, 1974

SCHIFF L: *Diseases of the Liver,* 4th ed. Philadelphia, Lippincott, 1975

SHAFRITZ DA, ISSELBACHER KJ: Current concepts of hepatic protein synthesis, in *The Liver and Its Diseases,* F Schaffner et al (eds). New York, Intercontinental Medical Book Corp, 1974, pp 43–53

TRIGER DR: Hyperglobulinemia in liver disease, in *Topics in Gastroenterology,* vol 2, SC Truelove, J Trowell (eds). London, Blackwell, 1975, p 329

300 DIAGNOSTIC PROCEDURES IN LIVER DISEASE

KURT J. ISSELBACHER
J. THOMAS LaMONT

Prompt recognition of liver disease and determination of its nature and extent require an understanding of the physiologic bases of a wide variety of techniques that assess liver function. Since no "battery" of tests is universally applicable, those most appropriate to a given clinical problem must be selected, their potential value and risk considered, and the results interpreted in relation to the clinical findings.

LIVER FUNCTION TESTS

Many liver function tests are based on a wide variety of biochemical reactions, such that the clinician can select combinations of tests that often measure different aspects of hepatic function. Many tests, however, are still empiric and semiquantitative, and no single test is universally helpful in diagnosis. Some methods are too sensitive and lack diagnostic specificity, others are affected by nonhepatic factors, and many simply do not measure any true physiologic function of the liver.

The physician concerned with clinical liver disease should be guided by several practical principles: (1) the tests selected should assess different parameters of liver function; (2) liver function tests should be used *serially* in order to evaluate the evolution or course of the disease; and (3) all such tests should be interpreted within the total clinical context with the recognition that any laboratory test may be fallible. The discussion that follows deals with representative and commonly used tests and should be read in conjunction with Chaps. 39 and 299.

SERUM BILIRUBIN (See also Chaps. 39 and 301) Spectrophotometric determinations of serum bilirubin in the clinical laboratory measure two pigment fractions: (1) the water-soluble conjugated fraction that gives a *direct reaction* with the diazo reagent and consists largely of bilirubin diglucuronide, and (2) the lipid-soluble *indirect-reaction* fraction that represents primarily unconjugated bilirubin. The serum of normal adults contains less than 0.25 mg direct-reacting bilirubin per 100 ml and 1 mg or less of total bilirubin per 100 ml. As noted in Chap. 39, in classifying the type of jaundice it is initially helpful to measure both the direct and total serum bilirubin in order to determine whether the patient has predominantly unconjugated or conjugated hyperbilirubinemia.

URINE BILIRUBIN Bilirubinuria causes the urine to become smoky or tea-colored; this appearance is also caused by hemoglobin or myoglobin in the urine, which can be differentiated by appropriate tests. Clinically significant concentrations of urine bilirubin are measured by the foam test, Harrison spot test, or the Ictotest tablet method. Bilirubinuria occurs only when there is an increase in the serum direct or conjugated bilirubin. This is an important point in the diagnosis of conditions characterized by unconjugated hyperbilirubinemia in which bilirubinuria is not noted. Bilirubinuria occurs with even minimal degrees of jaundice, and in fact may be detected before the patient becomes jaundiced.

URINE UROBILINOGEN Although of limited usefulness as a test of liver function, semiquantitative measurements of urobilinogen can be made on a freshly collected 2-h urine specimen by the Watson method (normal values 0.2 to 1.2 units). In complete bile duct obstruction there is no excretion of bilirubin into the gut; hence, there is no conversion of bilirubin to urobilinogen by intestinal bacteria. This results in disappearance of urobilinogen from the urine. However, urinary urobilinogen varies with many other factors, and its measurement is of limited clinical usefulness.

BROMSULPHALEIN (BSP) EXCRETION BSP is a dye which is taken up by the hepatocytes and secreted into the bile. In all types of liver disease, the ability of the liver to concentrate and secrete this dye is impaired, and hence a decrease in BSP clearance can be used as an indication of liver damage. The BSP test is simple, quantitative, and sensitive but nonspecific, and it is this latter factor which limits its usefulness. The test is performed by injecting intravenously 5 mg BSP per kilogram of body weight and obtaining a sample of venous blood from another venous site after 45 min. The result is expressed as the percentage of injected dye remaining, which in normal persons is less than 5 percent. The test is not widely used because of its lack of specificity and occasional severe side effects, including anaphylactic reactions. Abnormal values are found in all types of liver disease, as well as in heart failure, shock, fever, or ascites.

SERUM ENZYME ASSAYS Measurements of many serum enzymes have been used to quantify liver damage or to distinguish between hepatocellular (i.e., functional) and mechanical cholestasis. No specific or truly diagnostic test has been devised to solve either problem, but the enzymatic liver function tests described below have proved helpful in the clinical study of many hepatobiliary diseases.

Alkaline phosphatase Serum contains alkaline phosphatase, an enzyme which hydrolyzes synthetic phosphate esters at pH 9. As indicated in Chap. 299, this enzyme is produced by many tissues, especially bone, intestine, liver, and placenta, and is excreted in bile. Most of the enzyme present in normal serum is derived from bone. In hepatobiliary disease, there is an increased release of the hepatic enzyme into the bloodstream, apparently owing to increased enzyme synthesis. In the absence of bone disease and pregnancy, an elevated serum alkaline phosphatase level generally reflects impaired hepatic excretory function.

Several methods of comparable accuracy and sensitivity are available to measure alkaline phosphatase activity. The most widely used are the Bodansky (normal: 1.5 to 4.5 units) and the King-Armstrong methods (normal: 4 to 13 units). Growing children and women in late pregnancy have serum levels that may be twice normal.

Slight to moderate increases in alkaline phosphatase (6 to 10 Bodansky units) occur in many patients with parenchymal liver disorders such as hepatitis and cirrhosis, and transient increases may occur in all types of liver disease. The most striking increases occur with extrahepatic biliary obstruction or in intrahepatic cholestasis, such as drug cholestasis or primary biliary cirrhosis. The alkaline phosphatase is almost always elevated in metastatic liver disease, and in many cases is the only abnormality on routine liver function tests. As already noted, the enzyme may be elevated in incomplete biliary obstruction or obstruction of one hepatic duct, namely, under conditions when the serum bilirubin is normal or only slightly elevated. Since bone is a source of the enzyme, extensive Paget's disease, bony metastases, and other diseases associated with increased osteoblastic activity may produce high levels of alkaline phosphatase in the absence of liver disease.

5'-Nucleotidase This enzyme is another phosphatase which originates largely in the liver and is used clinically to determine whether an elevation of the alkaline phosphatase is caused by liver or bone disease. In hepatic disease both 5'-nucleotidase and alkaline phosphatase are elevated, while in primary bone disease the alkaline phosphatase is elevated but the 5'-nucleotidase is usually normal. However, there are exceptions to this observation, and other liver function tests are usually required to establish the presence or absence of liver disease.

Transaminases (aminotransferases) Assays of many serum enzymes have been proposed as measures of hepatocellular damage. Of these, the serum glutamic-oxaloacetic (SGOT) and glutamic-pyruvic (SGPT) transaminases (aminotransferases) have proved to be the most practical. GOT occurs in all body tissues, especially in heart, liver, and skeletal muscle. GPT is present primarily in the liver and to a lesser extent in kidney and skeletal muscle. Although many studies have shown that the height and duration of serum enzyme elevations parallel the extent of liver cell damage (i.e., necrosis or altered cell permeability), precise quantitative correlations cannot be made in most clinical conditions (Chap. 299). Normal serum contains less than 40 Karmen units of GOT and less than 40 Karmen units of GPT.

In the absence of acute necrosis or ischemia of other organs such as the myocardium, high SGOT and SGPT levels suggest liver cell damage. With extensive acute hepatic necrosis, as in severe viral hepatitis, serum enzyme levels of 1000 to 3000 units may be found. Less severe necrosis produces transient levels of 500 to 1000 units. Mild chronic or focal liver diseases (e.g., subclinical or anicteric viral hepatitis, Laennec's cirrhosis, granulomatous infiltrations, and tumor invasion) may be associated with transaminase levels of 50 to 200 units. With intrahepatic or extrahepatic cholestasis (in the absence of hepatic cell necrosis) SGOT and SGPT levels usually are not significantly elevated and rarely exceed 300 units.

Serial determinations of SGOT and SGPT are helpful in following the course of a patient with liver disease, especially with acute or chronic hepatitis. Caution is needed in the interpretation of abnormal levels. Serum transaminases may actually *decrease* in some patients with fulminant hepatitis, because of the previous excessive release of enzymes from the liver. Laennec's cirrhosis and postnecrotic cirrhosis may be associated with only slightly elevated or even normal transaminase levels.

Lactic dehydrogenase (LDH) Measurement of total serum LDH is usually not helpful diagnostically because it is present in all organs and released into the serum from a variety of tissue injuries. Fractionation of LDH into its five tissue-specific isoenzymes may give useful information about the site of origin of the LDH elevation. Moderate elevations of LDH levels are common in acute viral hepatitis and in cirrhosis; biliary tract disease may produce slight elevations. High serum levels may be found in metastatic carcinoma of the liver.

Other enzymes A very sensitive enzyme for the detection of minimal hepatocellular damage is γ-glutamyl transpeptidase (GGT). This enzyme is found in high concentration in kidney and liver, and is elevated in the serum of almost all patients with hepatobiliary disorders. An elevated level can be demonstrated in the serum of heavy drinkers before other liver function tests are abnormal; thus GGT is a sensitive test for alcoholic liver disease. Ornithine carbamyl transferase (OCT) is a urea cycle enzyme present only in liver and intestinal tissue. Elevation of this enzyme occurs primarily in liver disease; however, it is not specific for any particular type of liver disease, and its diagnostic usefulness is therefore limited.

SERUM PROTEINS Albumin, prothrombin, fibrinogen, and several other serum proteins are synthesized exclusively by liver cells, and extensive liver damage may lead to decreased blood levels of these proteins. The level of serum immunoglobulins, produced by lymphocytes and plasma cells, varies widely in hepatobiliary disease and reflects inflammatory or immune responses rather than liver cell dysfunction. Thus, analyses of the various serum proteins may provide helpful insights into the nature and extent of liver disease. However, as noted in Chap. 299, many nonhepatic factors also affect the metabolism of these proteins.

Albumin and globulins Total concentrations of serum albumin (normally 3.5 to 5 g per 100 ml) and globulin (normally 2 to 3.5 g per 100 ml) may be determined chemically. The level of each should be evaluated separately, because the *albumin/globulin (A/G) ratio* has no physiologic significance. Concentrations of α_1, α_2, β, and γ globulins are usually measured by electrophoretic methods.

Hypoalbuminemia may occur in subacute and massive hepatic necrosis, chronic active hepatitis, cirrhosis, and other disorders with significant destruction or replacement of liver cells. The serum albumin level also serves as a useful guide to prognosis and therapy in these diseases. *Hyperglobulinemia* suggests the presence of chronic inflammatory disorders such as cirrhosis and chronic active hepatitis. Neoplastic and inflammatory diseases of the liver may produce increased levels of α_2 globulins, and some patients with bile duct obstruction have high β-globulin levels.

Immunoglobulins Nonspecific immunoglobulin abnormalities occur in a variety of acute and chronic liver diseases. The major immunoglobulin fractions may be increased slightly in the course of acute viral hepatitis. Increased concentrations of IgA and IgG are common in Laennec's cirrhosis, striking elevations of IgG levels are characteristic of chronic active hepatitis, and high levels of IgM may be seen in primary biliary cirrhosis. None of these changes, however, is specific or diagnostic.

Clotting factors The serum activities of several clotting factors are useful indicators of hepatic synthetic function and are important in patients with liver disease who are bleeding or about to undergo surgery. The *one-stage prothrombin time,* which reflects the activities of prothrombin, fibrinogen, and factors V, VII, and X, is dependent upon both hepatic synthesis of these factors and intestinal uptake of vitamin K. Prolongation of the prothrombin time may occur in severe hepatocellular necrosis as in hepatitis or cirrhosis. In acute viral hepatitis an abnormality of this test may indicate the presence of severe fulminant necrosis. Obstruction of the bile duct or prolonged intrahepatic cholestasis may cause vitamin K deficiency because of impaired lipid absorption. Parenteral injection of vitamin K (10 mg per day) will cause normalization of the prothrombin time in 48 h unless there is coexistent hepatocellular necrosis and impaired synthesis of clotting proteins. The *partial thromboplastin time,* which reflects the activities of fibrinogen, prothrombin, and factors V, X, VIII, IX, XI, and XII, may also be prolonged in patients with liver disease. It is necessary to assess the clotting mechanism in all patients with liver disease before any surgical procedure including liver biopsy. This can be accomplished by measuring the prothrombin time, partial thromboplastin time, platelet count, and bleeding time (see Chaps. 54 and 318).

SERUM AMMONIA Ammonia is elevated in the blood of some patients with liver disease, either acute or chronic. In acute fulminant hepatitis a markedly elevated serum ammonia reflects severe hepatocellular necrosis and the consequent inability of the liver to convert ammonia to urea. Cirrhotic patients, in particular those who have undergone a portacaval shunt, may also have varying degrees of hyperammonemia and hepatic encephalopathy. In these patients the ammonia produced by colonic bacteria and carried in portal venous blood is shunted around the liver and enters the systemic circulation. There is only a rough correlation between the serum ammonia levels and the degree of hepatic encephalopathy. Some patients will function normally with a twofold elevation, while others will be stuporous at the same level. Serum ammonia levels may also increase before the onset of coma and return to normal some 48 to 72 h before improvement of the neurologic status. This lag between the elevation of ammonia levels and onset of encephalopathy may indicate the relatively slow transport of ammonia into the central nervous system. However, metabolites other than ammonia also appear to be important in the pathogenesis of hepatic encephalopathy, and this may help to explain the observed lack of correlation between ammonia levels and hepatic coma.

BLOOD LIPIDS Measurements of serum total cholesterol (normal: 130 to 230 mg per 100 ml) and cholesterol esters (normal: 50 to 70 percent of total cholesterol) are frequently made in patients with liver disease. Acute or chronic diffuse liver disease often results in decreased total values and a decrease in the ester fraction; cholestasis, whether functional or mechanical, characteristically produces moderate to extreme elevations of the total cholesterol level but with a decrease in the percent esterified. In cholestasis one also finds variable elevations of serum triglycerides and of an abnormal lipoprotein (lipoprotein X).

IMMUNOLOGIC TESTS Immunologic derangements occur in a variety of liver diseases. Antimitochondrial antibodies are frequently found in primary biliary cirrhosis (85 percent of cases), although they may also be positive in some patients with chronic active hepatitis and drug hepatitis. In chronic active hepatitis the LE cell test may be positive, and antinuclear as well as antismooth muscle antibodies may be present in the blood. Immunologic methods are the key to the detection of the hepatitis B surface antigen (HBsAg) in long-incubation or serum hepatitis and are discussed in detail in Chap. 302. Alpha fetoprotein is of value in the diagnosis of hepatoma. Measurements of α_1-antitrypsin should be performed in infants with cirrhosis or hepatitis since they may have a hereditary deficiency of this enzyme.

RADIOLOGIC PROCEDURES

ABDOMINAL ROENTGENOGRAM Films of the upper abdomen and lower thorax rarely provide accurate estimates of liver size and shape, but gross hepatomegaly and hepatic masses that elevate or distort the diaphragm may be detected. However, the abdominal film is more accurate in determining the presence of splenomegaly and is often helpful in detecting minimal degrees of splenic enlargement. Plain films of the abdomen may reveal calcific densities in the gallbladder, biliary tree, pancreas, or liver (as echinococcal cysts, hemangioma, or, rarely, a metastatic tumor mass).

BARIUM STUDIES OF THE GASTROINTESTINAL TRACT An upper gastrointestinal series should be performed in suspected cases of portal hypertension, because esophagogastric varices can be demonstrated with about 70 to 90 percent accuracy when they are present. Enlargement of the left lobe of the liver (as with tumor, abscess, or cirrhosis) may displace the barium-filled stomach laterally and anteriorly. Tumors of the head of the pancreas often produce displacement or irregularity of the second portion of the duodenum. The radiologist can increase the diagnostic accuracy of a search for lesions involving the head of the pancreas or papilla of Vater by performing a hypotonic duodenogram. This involves injection of an anticholinergic drug or glucagon to inhibit motility; it often permits a better view of the mucosa and provides data concerning the distensibility of the duodenum.

CHOLECYSTOGRAPHY AND CHOLANGIOGRAPHY The *oral cholecystogram* provides limited information in most patients with overt hepatobiliary disease, because parenchymal dysfunction and impaired bile excretion lead to decreased excretion of the contrast material and hence nonvisualization of the gallbladder. An *intravenous cholangiogram* may permit demonstration of the intrahepatic and extrahepatic bile ducts and the localization of obstructing lesions of the major ducts. Even faint visualization of a normal-sized biliary tree may be helpful in the differential diagnosis of obstructive jaundice. However, as with the oral cholecystography, liver dysfunction and moderate cholestasis may prevent adequate secretion of dye to permit visualization on x-ray. In general, intravenous cholangiography will not be successful if the serum bilirubin is greater than 3 mg per 100 ml.

Percutaneous transhepatic cholangiography with a very thin needle is sometimes used to distinguish between mechanical biliary obstruction and intrahepatic cholestasis. This approach is used when decreased liver function precludes the use of intravenous cholangiography. With experience and proper precautions, dilated major ducts proximal to an obstructing lesion can be cannulated and visualized in up to 90 percent of cases; the normal or small ducts associated with intrahepatic cholestasis are more difficult to demonstrate, but with modern techniques, they can be demonstrated in up to 75 percent of cases.

Endoscopic retrograde cholangiopancreatography (ERCP) with the fiberoptic duodenoscope is another method of demonstrating the bile ducts radiographically in jaundiced patients. The papilla of Vater is cannulated under direct vision, and contrast material is injected into the biliary and pancreatic ducts. ERCP is particularly useful in jaundiced patients with suspected lesions of the head of the pancreas or ampulla of Vater, since in addition to contrast studies one may also obtain washings or brushings for cytology, or biopsies of intraduodenal mass lesions. ERCP does not rely upon dilatation of the bile ducts for success, and since the liver itself is not punctured, there is no risk of bile peritonitis in patients with high-grade biliary obstruction. However, acute pancreatitis may result from injection of contrast material into the pancreatic duct.

ANGIOGRAPHY An increasingly useful and effective approach for visualizing the hepatic and portal circulation involves *selective angiography* of the celiac, superior mesenteric, and hepatic arteries. In most centers it has replaced splenoportography since by injection of these arteries one can visualize both the arterial (hepatic) and venous (hepatic and portal) systems. Selective arteriography is quite safe. It is useful (1) in demonstrating the hepatic arterial circulation which will be deranged in cirrhosis and in the diagnosis of primary and secondary liver tumor masses, and (2) in visualizing the portal circulation for evidence of a collateral circulation, venous obstruction, anomalous vessels, etc. In major medical centers, this angiographic method is increasingly used as a diagnostic tool for the study of chronic liver disease and portal hypertension.

RADIOISOTOPE LIVER SCANS (SCINTISCANS) Hepatic scintiscans are performed with gamma-emitting isotopes that are extracted selectively by the liver, followed by external radiation scanning of the upper abdomen. There are basically three types of liver scans: the colloidal scan which depends on uptake of labeled colloid by Kupffer cells, the rose bengal scan in which the dye is taken up and excreted by hepatocytes, and the gallium scan in which the radionuclide ^{67}Ga is concentrated in neoplastic and inflammatory cells to a greater degree than in hepatocytes. Hence, a hepatoma or liver abscess will produce an area of reduced uptake or "hole" using a colloid or rose bengal scan, but there will be an area of increased uptake or "hot spot" with a gallium scan. The colloidal scan with ^{198}Au colloidal gold or ^{99m}Tc sulfur colloid is most commonly used. This technique can demonstrate filling defects greater than 2 to 3 cm in diameter; hence, in metastatic liver disease with smaller diffuse deposits, the scan will be falsely negative. False-positive scans are frequently observed in cirrhosis, because the distorted lobular architecture will result in irregular uptake and sometimes produce filling defects. The gallium scan may be helpful in diagnosing neoplastic infiltration in the patient with cirrhosis since the tumor will show increased uptake, while fibrous bands will show decreased uptake. The rose bengal scan has been used as a method of differentiating intrahepatic cholestasis from extrahepatic obstruction. With complete biliary obstruction there is failure of the isotope to enter the duodenum, while in intrahepatic cholestasis some isotope will be seen in the lumen of the small bowel. However, a clearcut distinction of these entities with the rose bengal scan is unusual, and the procedure has limited clinical usefulness.

ULTRASONOGRAPHY (See also Chaps. 307 to 309) Diagnostic ultrasound is approximately as accurate as oral cholecystography in detecting gallstones and has the added advantage of being independent of liver function. It can therefore be used to detect gallstones in the gallbladder or biliary tree in patients with jaundice. Ultrasound is also very useful in detecting mass lesions such as tumors, cysts, or liver abscess. Lesions as small as 1 to 2 cm can be visualized with this technique. Ultrasound of the upper abdomen is also quite useful in evaluating the possible causes of extrahepatic biliary obstruction. Abdominal computerized tomography (CT) scanning and ultrasound are approximately equal in their diagnostic sensitivity in evaluating patients with suspected mass lesions, gallstones, or obstructive jaundice. In general, ultrasound is the procedure of choice since it is less expensive than CT scanning and does not expose the patient to radiation.

COMPUTERIZED TOMOGRAPHY (CT SCAN) The CT scan of the abdomen provides a visual image of the abdominal viscera without injection of contrast material. This technique is particularly useful in the diagnosis of mass lesions in the liver or pancreas, where it has an accuracy and sensitivity comparable to that obtained with ultrasound. The test is particularly useful in differentiating intrahepatic fluid collections such as cysts, abscesses, and hematomas, since the density of the fluid can be determined with relative accuracy. Dilatation of the gallbladder, extrahepatic bile ducts or portal vein can be diagnosed on the CT scan. The major advantage of CT scanning is the ability to obtain an excellent image of solid intraabdominal organs

such as pancreas, liver, and spleen with modest doses of radiation, thus avoiding more invasive techniques such as angiography, cholangiography, or ERCP.

OTHER DIAGNOSTIC PROCEDURES

PORTAL AND HEPATIC VEIN MANOMETRY Measurement of the splenic pulp pressure (a reliable reflection of the actual portal venous pressure) by *percutaneous portal manometry* and estimation of the wedged hepatic venous pressure (WHVP, an approximation of the postsinusoidal intrahepatic venous pressure) by *hepatic vein catheterization* are useful in the study of patients with known or presumed portal hypertension. While determination of the WHVP is not a routine procedure, the demonstration of a normal or slightly elevated WHVP in a patient with proved portal hypertension serves to localize the obstruction to the extrahepatic portion of the portal vein, the portal inflow system (as in schistosomiasis), or the presinusoidal vessels (as in some cases of fatty liver or portal fibrosis). Splenic pulp pressure greater than 25 to 30 cm saline solution indicates significant portal hypertension.

PERCUTANEOUS NEEDLE BIOPSY OF THE LIVER Percutaneous needle biopsy is a safe, simple, and valuable method of diagnosing liver disease. Although the needle biopsy sample is small, *diffuse parenchymal disorders* such as cirrhosis, hepatitis, and drug reactions may be diagnosed with remarkable accuracy. In *disseminated focal diseases* (such as granulomas or tumor infiltrates) serial sections may demonstrate the lesion.

The biopsy is performed under local anesthesia, usually with the Menghini (aspiration) or Vim-Silverman (cutting) needle, by means of either the transpleural or subcostal approach. If the operator is skillful and the patient is carefully selected, morbidity should be low and limited to occasional postbiopsy pain or vasovagal reactions. The mortality of liver biopsy as reported in several large series is approximately 1 death in 5000 biopsies when the Menghini technique is used.

Some of the major indications for needle biopsy are (1) unexplained hepatomegaly or hepatosplenomegaly, (2) cholestasis of uncertain cause, (3) persistently abnormal liver function tests, (4) suspected systemic or infiltrative diseases such as sarcoidosis or miliary tuberculosis, and (5) suspected primary or metastatic liver tumor.

Needle biopsy should not be performed if (1) the patient is not able to cooperate; (2) clinical or laboratory evidence indicates impaired hemostasis (for example, the one-stage prothrombin time is prolonged by 3 s or more over control), thrombocytopenia (less than 80,000 to 100,000 platelets per cubic millimeter) or purpura is present, or the partial thromboplastin time or bleeding time is prolonged; (3) there is infection of the right pleural space or septic cholangitis; (4) profound anemia or tense ascites is present; or (5) compatible blood is not available for transfusion in case of hemorrhage. Amyloidosis and carcinoma of the liver may increase the hazard of postbiopsy hemorrhage. Although biopsy in mechanical biliary obstruction may lead occasionally to the escape of bile and localized bile peritonitis, this complication is uncommon.

PERITONEOSCOPY With this technique the serosal lining, liver, gallbladder, spleen, and other abdominal organs can be visualized with minimum discomfort and hazard. Diagnosis may be made by inspection or directed needle biopsy. Peritoneoscopy is useful in the study of patients with suspected intraabdominal malignancy since it may obviate the need for exploratory laparotomy to establish a diagnosis.

LAPAROTOMY When the most thorough clinical, laboratory, and biopsy studies fail to define the precise nature of hepatobiliary disease, exploratory laparotomy may be necessary. However, it must be reemphasized that when there is evidence of significant hepatocellular necrosis (e.g., markedly elevated SGOT levels), laparotomy will often be accompanied by an increased morbidity and mortality owing to postoperative liver decompensation. When laparotomy is performed, the medicosurgical team should be prepared to obtain full benefit from this direct approach, using biopsy, culture, cholangiography, and angiography as required.

REFERENCES

BAGGENSTOSS AH: Morphologic and etiologic diagnosis from hepatic biopsies without clinical data. Medicine 45:435, 1966

BLACK M: Diagnostic methods in liver disease. Med Clin North Am 59:1015, 1975

BRENSILVER HL, KAPLAN MM: Significance of elevated liver alkaline phosphatase in serum. Gastroenterology 68:1556, 1975

COTTON PB et al: Cannulation of papilla of Vater via fiberduodenoscope. Lancet 1:53, 1972

LOMAS F et al: Increased specificity of liver scanning with the use of ^{67}gallium citrate. N Engl J Med 286:1323, 1972

PEREIRAS R et al: Percutaneous transhepatic cholangiography with the "skinny" needle. Ann Intern Med 86:562, 1977

VALLON AG et al: Grey-scale ultrasonography in cholestatic jaundice. Gut 20:54, 1979

WITTENBERG J, FERRUCCI J: Computed body tomography. Gastroenterology 74:287, 1978

301
DISTURBANCES OF BILIRUBIN METABOLISM

KURT J. ISSELBACHER

The normal metabolism of bilirubin and the approach to the patient with jaundice have been presented in Chap. 39. With a consideration of these pathways, the disorders of bilirubin metabolism can be divided into four major categories, namely, those due to (1) increased pigment production, (2) reduced hepatic uptake of bilirubin, (3) impaired hepatic conjugation, and (4) decreased excretion of the conjugated pigment from the liver into bile. The first three of these disorders are associated with predominantly unconjugated hyperbilirubinemia (i.e., more than 80 percent of serum bilirubin is unconjugated, or indirect-reacting). The fourth group, defective excretion, is associated with predominantly conjugated hyperbilirubinemia (i.e., more than 50 percent of serum bilirubin is conjugated, or direct-reacting) and with bilirubinuria.

DISORDERS CAUSING PREDOMINANTLY UNCONJUGATED HYPERBILIRUBINEMIA

The plasma concentration of unconjugated bilirubin is determined by (1) the rate at which newly synthesized bilirubin enters the plasma (bilirubin turnover) and (2) the rate of irreversible removal of bilirubin by the liver (hepatic bilirubin clearance). The latter can result from derangements of hepatic bilirubin uptake, conjugation, or both. Measurements of these variables, although not routinely available, permit a classifica-

tion of patients into those with *increased bilirubin turnover* (e.g., hemolysis), those with *decreased bilirubin clearance* (e.g., Gilbert's syndrome), and those in whom both mechanisms operate.

OVERPRODUCTION OF BILIRUBIN (INCREASED TURNOVER)

Increased destruction of circulating erythrocytes (intravascular and extravascular hemolysis) In disorders associated with hemolysis, most commonly the hemolytic anemias, the rate of bilirubin production is increased and may even exceed the amount that can be removed by a normal liver. The resulting jaundice is primarily an unconjugated hyperbilirubinemia. There is often also a small but definite increase in the serum conjugated bilirubin, when the amount of bilirubin glucuronide formed exceeds the amount that the liver can excrete (see Chap. 39). If there is significant anemia or if other adverse factors are present (e.g., fever, sepsis, hypoxemia, or vascular collapse), the ability of the liver to handle the pigment load will be compromised, and the degree of jaundice will be greater.

The clinical and diagnostic features of the various hemolytic anemias are described in Chap. 314. The presence of reticulocytosis, shortened red blood cell survival, and increased fecal urobilinogen, in the absence of clinical and laboratory evidence of liver disease, strongly suggest hemolysis and overproduction of bilirubin as the cause of the jaundice. It is obvious, however, that in some cases (e.g., cirrhosis, tumors, and sepsis), hemolysis *plus* deranged liver function may be present. In most cases of uncomplicated hemolytic states, the mean serum bilirubin level will be in the range of 3 to 5 mg per 100 ml; rarely, levels up to 10 mg may be seen.

Jaundice due to increased pigment production may also be seen as a consequence of *tissue infarction* (e.g., pulmonary infarcts) and large *collections of blood in tissues* (e.g., leakage from blood vessels after catheterization studies, rupture of an aortic aneurysm). If hypotension and hypoxemia also supervene, jaundice is usually more pronounced, and the resulting impairment of liver function may also lead to a significant increase in the serum conjugated bilirubin level (see "Postoperative Jaundice" below).

Except in early infancy, elevations of serum unconjugated bilirubin levels are not generally harmful per se, and the prognosis is that of the hemolytic process itself. However, in the neonatal state and infancy, unconjugated bilirubin levels above 20 mg per 100 ml may lead to *kernicterus* due to bilirubin deposition in the lipid-rich basal ganglia (see Chap. 371). Chronic overproduction of bilirubin may result in the formation of gallstones composed predominantly of bilirubin ("pigment stones"). In this situation, all the potential complications of calculus disease of the biliary tract (Chap. 307) may be superimposed on the chronic hemolytic state which produced it.

Increased production of bilirubin from sources other than circulating erythrocytes As indicated in Chap. 39, about 15 to 20 percent of the circulating bilirubin is normally derived from sources other than the destruction of circulating red blood cells. This represents the so-called "early-labeled fraction"; it includes the synthesis of bilirubin from nonhemoglobin heme in the liver and from hemoglobin heme in the marrow.

In some conditions, jaundice results from an increased destruction of red blood cells or their precursors in the marrow—a process referred to as *ineffective erythropoiesis* (see Chaps. 39 and 53). In patients with thalassemia, pernicious anemia, and congenital erythropoietic porphyria, such an increased rate of formation of the early-labeled bilirubin fraction has been demonstrated. It is possible that some cases of unexplained unconjugated hyperbilirubinemia may be caused by an increased hepatic production of bilirubin from nonhemoglobin heme, but this phenomenon has not yet been demonstrated clinically.

IMPAIRED HEPATIC UPTAKE OF BILIRUBIN Drugs While numerous drugs may theoretically interfere with uptake of bilirubin by the liver, only a few agents have been definitely shown to influence this process. Flavaspidic acid, used in the treatment of tapeworm infestation, may cause unconjugated hyperbilirubinemia, as well as impairment of Bromsulphalein (BSP) clearance, during its administration. The jaundice readily subsides following treatment. Flavaspidic acid competes with bilirubin for intrahepatic binding proteins (ligandins), leading thereby to unconjugated hyperbilirubinemia. The jaundice which may occur with novobiocin is also apparently due to an interference in bilirubin uptake.

Gilbert's syndrome Some cases of this syndrome of chronic unconjugated hyperbilirubinemia may be due to a defect in hepatic uptake (as reflected by alteration in BSP kinetics). In most cases, however, a deficiency of bilirubin glucuronyl transferase can be demonstrated. Hence this syndrome is best considered as a defect in bilirubin conjugation. (For discussion, see below.)

IMPAIRED BILIRUBIN CONJUGATION (DECREASED ACTIVITY OF BILIRUBIN GLUCURONYL TRANSFERASE) Neonatal jaundice (physiological jaundice of the newborn) Almost every infant exhibits some transient unconjugated hyperbilirubinemia between the second and fifth days of life. While during gestation the placenta serves to clear bilirubin from the fetus, after birth infants must detoxify the pigments themselves. However, at this stage the hepatic enzyme system is still "immature" and inadequate for the task. As a result, unconjugated bilirubinemia develops, usually not exceeding 5 mg per 100 ml serum. The activity of glucuronyl transferase increases within several days to 2 weeks after birth, and concomitantly the serum bilirubin returns to normal. In the premature infant the glucuronyl transferase activity is less, and the neonatal jaundice may be more pronounced. The "maturation" of the fetal and neonatal liver may be enhanced by treatment of the pregnant mother or the newborn infant with phenobarbital or related drugs. This results in a clear-cut reduction of the degree and duration of unconjugated hyperbilirubinemia in the newborn. In infants with a superimposed hemolytic process (e.g., erythroblastosis), the excessive pigment load leads to more pronounced jaundice, and bilirubin levels may exceed 20 mg per 100 ml serum. It should be emphasized that neonatal jaundice is not present at the time of delivery; if jaundice is present at birth, other causes must be considered.

Two soluble, low-molecular-weight cytoplasmic liver cell proteins (ligandins Y and Z) have been described. These appear to be involved in the normal binding of bilirubin and drugs by the liver (Chap. 39). In experimental animals the Y protein which appears to bind bilirubin is low in the neonatal state and increases with age. It has been proposed that deficiency of this protein may contribute to neonatal jaundice.

An additional facet of the "immature" liver is a concomitant defect in the excretion of *conjugated* bilirubin. Rarely this defect persists beyond the time needed for the development of adequate glucuronide conjugation and may explain the occasional presence of conjugated hyperbilirubinemia in infants with erythroblastosis (*inspissated-bile syndrome*).

When in the neonatal state unconjugated bilirubin levels approach 20 mg per 100 ml, the infants may develop and die of *kernicterus*. This condition results from unconjugated bilirubin deposition in the lipid-rich basal ganglia. In the past treatment consisted of exchange transfusions. Albumin infusions may

also be given to increase binding of bilirubin in the circulation and diminish its entry into the brain. The current approach is *phototherapy;* intense illumination of these patients with strong white or blue light leads to photooxidation of bilirubin to water-soluble derivatives that are rapidly excreted in the bile and urine without the need of conjugation.

Hereditary glucuronyl transferase deficiency There are currently three syndromes that fall into this category. As indicated in Table 301-1, they reflect progressive decreases in the activity of glucuronyl transferase and thus may be part of a spectrum, i.e., from minimal deficiency to complete absence of bilirubin glucuronyl transferase.

GILBERT'S SYNDROME Since the original report by Gilbert in 1907, there has been an increased recognition of this benign but chronic disorder characterized by mild, persistent, unconjugated hyperbilirubinemia. The patient usually does not manifest this disorder until after the second decade and is often unaware of the jaundice until it is detected by physical examination or routine laboratory testing. The total serum bilirubin level usually ranges and fluctuates from 1.2 to 3 mg per 100 ml, and rarely exceeds 5 mg per 100 ml. Less than 20 percent of the total serum bilirubin is conjugated. Typically the jaundice fluctuates and is exacerbated following prolonged fasting (see below), surgery, fever or infection, and excessive exertion or alcohol ingestion. Liver function tests are normal, and liver histology shows no specific changes.

With the exception of hemolytic anemias, this disorder is probably the most common cause of mild unconjugated hyperbilirubinemia. Detailed studies show these patients to have a partial deficiency of bilirubin glucuronyl transferase. Some patients also manifest decreased bilirubin uptake and increased hemolysis. Decreased glucuronyl transferase alone or together with a decrease in bilirubin uptake appears to account for the observed *decrease in hepatic bilirubin clearance.*

Previously Gilbert's syndrome was traditionally defined as mild, chronic, unconjugated hyperbilirubinemia occurring in the absence of hemolysis. However, with the use of radiobilirubin kinetics and erythrocyte half-life studies, two forms of Gilbert's syndrome have been described. One group includes pa-

TABLE 301-1
Hereditary unconjugated hyperbilirubinemias with deficiency of glucuronyl transferase

Features	Mild (Gilbert's syndrome)	Moderate (Crigler-Najjar syndrome type II)	Severe (Crigler-Najjar syndrome type I)
Inheritance	Unclear*	Dominant†	Recessive
Serum bilirubin, mg per 100 ml	1–6	6–20	20–45
Kernicterus	No	Rare	Yes
Conjugated bilirubin in bile	Yes (↑ monoconjugates)	Yes (↑↑ monoconjugates)	No
Response to phenobarbital	Yes	Yes	No
Bilirubin conjugation	↓‡	↓↓	Absent

* *Many cases are without familial incidence.*
† *Variable expressivity.*
‡ *Other defects such as occult hemolysis and ↓ bilirubin uptake may coexist.*

tients with decreased bilirubin clearance and *no hemolysis*. A second group includes those who also have *evidence of hemolysis* (often occult) and hence increased bilirubin turnover. It would appear that the simultaneous presence of both derangements is a chance occurrence of two not uncommon disorders occurring in the same patient and does not imply a causal relationship. A feature of Gilbert's syndrome which can be useful diagnostically is the increase in serum bilirubin following prolonged fasting or calorie deprivation. Thus, patients with this disorder, when placed on 300 cal per day for 2 days, will increase their serum bilirubin by 1.5 mg per 100 ml or more, with the major increase being in the unconjugated fraction. It appears that a decrease in glucuronyl transferase activity is needed in order to obtain this effect. Patients with hemolysis do not show an increase in serum bilirubin with fasting. As a reflection of the mild decrease in glucuronyl transferase (1) their bilirubin levels will decrease when the enzyme activity is enhanced following phenobarbital administration, and (2) their bile shows a modest increase in monoconjugates of bilirubin (see Table 301-1).

In general, the diagnosis of this benign but not uncommon disorder is made by exclusion. The diagnosis is suspected in a patient with low-grade unconjugated hyperbilirubinemia when there are (1) no systemic symptoms, (2) *no overt* or clinically recognizable hemolysis, (3) normal tests of routine liver function, and (4) a liver biopsy (although usually not necessary) that is normal.

CRIGLER-NAJJAR SYNDROME (TYPES I AND II)   This disorder is known to exist in two forms. Type I is the clinically *severe* form (originally described by Crigler and Najjar) and is due to *absence of glucuronyl transferase*. Type II has more *moderate* clinical findings due to *partial deficiency of glucuronyl transferase*. The major differences between the two variants are summarized in Table 301-1.

Type I (Crigler-Najjar) is a rare disorder. Infants develop high unconjugated bilirubin levels in the serum (20 to 45 mg per 100 ml). Absence of the enzyme can be demonstrated in the liver. Routine liver function tests are normal, as is the liver histology. Because of the absence of glucuronyl transferase no conjugated bilirubin is formed by the liver; hence no bilirubin is secreted by the liver, and the bile is colorless.

Phototherapy may temporarily and transiently reduce the unconjugated bilirubin level. Phenobarbital has no effect since the enzyme defect is complete and no drug "induction" is therefore possible. Affected infants usually die within the first year of life, although some patients have survived to the second and third decade of life. Death is usually from kernicterus.

A strain of rats (Gunn rat) with the type I defect exists and is widely used as an animal model of the Crigler-Najjar syndrome.

Type II patients have a partial deficiency of glucuronyl transferase, and their disorder is less severe. Serum unconjugated bilirubin levels are lower (6 to 20 mg per 100 ml), jaundice may not appear until adolescence, and neurological complications are uncommon. The bile contains variable amounts of conjugated bilirubin with a significant increase in monoconjugates. Phenobarbital is effective in lowering the serum bilirubin level in type II patients. However, the disorder is relatively benign in those patients whose bilirubin is less than 18 to 20 mg per 100 ml.

Acquired deficiency of glucuronyl transferase   As with any enzyme, glucuronyl transferase is susceptible to inhibition by a variety of agents, and because of the decreased activity of the enzyme in the neonatal state, such inhibition may be more evident at that time. Neonatal jaundice may be aggravated or

prolonged in infants treated with *drugs* such as chloramphenicol or novobiocin, or with *vitamin K*. In some breast-fed infants jaundice has been ascribed to the presence in *breast milk* of pregnane-3β,20α-diol, a good inhibitor of glucuronyl transferase. When the infant is removed from the breast, the "breast-milk jaundice" subsides.

Hypothyroidism delays the normal "maturation" of glucuronyl transferase. In cretins, neonatal jaundice may be prolonged for weeks or months. In fact, the presence of prolonged unconjugated hyperbilirubinemia after birth may be a clue to an underlying hypothyroidism.

In the infant, as well as in the adult, *liver cell damage* leads to impairment in glucuronide conjugation as a result of decreased transferase activity. However, since excretion is probably the rate-limiting step in bilirubin metabolism and since this step is always interfered with to a greater extent than conjugation in parenchymal liver disease, the pigment which accumulates in the blood is predominantly conjugated bilirubin.

DISORDERS CAUSING PREDOMINANTLY CONJUGATED HYPERBILIRUBINEMIA

In jaundice due to primary liver disease, the plasma usually exhibits elevated levels of both conjugated and unconjugated bilirubin, and *urine contains bilirubin*. The relative proportions of the two pigments are highly variable. In many familial hepatic abnormalities (described below) and in some forms of drug-induced liver injury, the jaundice is almost entirely due to conjugated hyperbilirubinemia, 60 to 80 percent of the serum bilirubin giving a direct van den Bergh reaction. Such a pigment pattern is also seen with extrahepatic biliary obstruction.

In jaundice associated with diffuse liver cell damage, as in hepatitis and cirrhosis, the conjugated bilirubin levels may be somewhat less than in the above cholestatic syndromes, with the direct-reacting values ranging from 50 to 70 percent of the total serum bilirubin. However, the pattern is quite variable, and in all the above hepatic disorders, once the serum bilirubin components have been measured, repeated fractionation during the course of the disease is of little diagnostic or prognostic value. One cannot differentiate intrahepatic and extrahepatic causes of jaundice from either the levels or proportions of the two pigment types (i.e., unconjugated and conjugated bilirubin) in plasma. Thus the main purpose of the initial fractionation of the plasma bilirubin is to distinguish hepatic parenchymal and biliary obstructive disease from the disorders associated with predominantly unconjugated hyperbilirubinemia.

FAMILIAL DEFECTS IN HEPATIC EXCRETORY FUNCTION Dubin-Johnson syndrome   This disorder, also called *chronic idiopathic jaundice*, is a benign, autosomally inherited hyperbilirubinemia characterized by the presence of a dark pigment in the centrilobular region of the liver cells. Functionally there exists a *defect in biliary excretion* of bilirubin, cholephilic dyes, and porphyrins. The hyperbilirubinemia, which may begin at any age, is predominantly of the conjugated type, with total serum levels usually ranging from 3 to 10 mg per 100 ml. The patient may be asymptomatic or have vague constitutional or gastrointestinal symptoms. Not infrequently the liver is slightly enlarged; in about one-fourth of the cases there is mild hepatic tenderness. Oral and intravenous cholangiography fails to visualize the biliary tract. There is typically and characteristically a late rise in the plasma BSP elimination curve at *90 min*. This is caused by the reflux from the liver of the conjugated dye and reflects the defect in the hepatic excretory transport maximum (T_m). It is noteworthy that there is no secondary rise in plasma when dyes which are not conjugated by the liver are given, such as indocyanine green. In the liver the striking feature is the presence of a brown or black pigment in the hepatocytes. Earlier findings suggested that this unique pigment was melanin; however, electron spin resonance studies have not confirmed this. In fact, in some patients who also developed hepatitis, the pigment disappears from the liver and is excreted in the urine.

These patients also show an abnormality in coproporphyrin excretion. Normal urine contains mostly coproporphyrin III and small amounts of coproporphyrin I; Dubin-Johnson patients show a reversal of this pattern, i.e., a predominant excretion of coproporphyrin I. Heterozygotes show an intermediate excretory pattern.

There is impaired excretion of many metabolites, including conjugated bilirubin, BSP, and iodinated dyes. Excretion of bile acids, however, is normal. Oral contraceptive agents may accentuate hyperbilirubinemia or may produce jaundice for the first time. Features of cholestasis such as pruritus or steatorrhea are usually lacking, but serum alkaline phosphatase levels are *not* elevated. Impairment in the excretion of epinephrine metabolites may account for the accumulation of the melanin pigments. The overall prognosis of the disorder is excellent.

Rotor syndrome is similar in many respects to the Dubin-Johnson syndrome. However, *there is no pigment in the liver cells,* the gallbladder is usually visualized on cholecystography, and there is an increase in the total urinary coproporphyrins, but not an increased percentage excretion of coproporphyrin I. The BSP excretion pattern does *not* show a secondary rise at 90 min. The impairment in excretion which is typical of Dubin-Johnson syndrome is not present; instead in most cases of the Rotor syndrome there is impairment of *hepatic storage capacity (S)*. This rare syndrome is inherited as an autosomal recessive trait and is genetically distinct from Dubin-Johnson syndrome.

Benign familial recurrent cholestasis This is a relatively rare syndrome characterized by recurrent attacks of pruritus and jaundice. During an attack the serum alkaline phosphatase and bile acid levels are markedly elevated, and liver biopsy shows the morphological features of cholestasis. However, at laparotomy, biliary obstruction is not found, and operative cholangiography reveals a patent and apparently normal biliary tree. Remissions are the rule, and at such times hepatic function tests and liver morphological features are usually normal. The cause of the disorder is unknown; cirrhosis does not develop, and the disorder is benign. A congenital origin has been postulated on the basis of the early age of onset and familial incidence.

Recurrent jaundice of pregnancy This form of jaundice is also known as *intrahepatic cholestasis of pregnancy.* During a normal pregnancy some changes in liver function occur, especially during the last trimester. Usually these consist of slight increases in BSP retention and of serum alkaline phosphatase. This mild increase in alkaline phosphatase during pregnancy is normally of placental rather than hepatic origin. Bilirubin increases never exceed 2 mg per 100 ml serum and usually are hardly detectable.

In a small number of pregnant women an intrahepatic cholestasis may appear. This usually occurs in the third trimester but may develop any time after the seventh week of gestation. The clinical features consist primarily of pruritus and jaundice. Serum bilirubin levels are usually less than 6 mg and rarely higher than 8 mg per 100 ml. The serum alkaline phosphatase and cholesterol levels are elevated significantly, while other liver function tests are only mildly deranged. Histologically the liver shows varying degrees of cholestasis but only a few parenchymal cell changes. The clinical and laboratory abnormalities subside promptly after delivery and are usually completely normal within 7 to 14 days.

This condition has been seen more frequently in Scandinavia and Europe than in the United States. Since steroid hormones and specifically estrogens can induce changes in hepatic excretory function in normal individuals (see Chap. 299), these patients probably have an increased susceptibility or sensitivity to the hepatic effects of estrogenic and progestational hormones. The intrahepatic cholestasis is usually termed *recurrent*, since the syndrome often (but not always) reappears in subsequent pregnancies. The process is benign and self-limited, and treatment is usually not needed, but cholestyramine administration will diminish the pruritus. This disorder must be distinguished from the many other causes of jaundice not unique to pregnancy, such as viral hepatitis. It must also be distinguished from the idiopathic *acute fatty liver of pregnancy* and the *tetracycline-induced* fatty liver. The latter two conditions are rare, occur in the last trimester, and have a high fatality rate: however, in these disorders there is evidence of diffuse parenchymal damage and not just cholestasis.

ACQUIRED DEFECTS OF HEPATIC EXCRETORY FUNCTION
Drug-induced cholestasis A condition entirely analogous to the intrahepatic cholestasis of pregnancy may occur in some women following the use of oral contraceptive agents. A significant number of individuals using these drugs show mild increases in BSP retention, and even more have decreased BSP excretory capacity as measured by infusion tests. In some, mild cholestatic jaundice may occur, liver function returns to normal when the drugs are withdrawn, and chronic liver disease does not appear to result. It is relevant that one-third of the reported patients with jaundice due to oral contraceptives also have a history of recurrent intrahepatic cholestasis of pregnancy.

The nature of these changes produced by the natural and synthetic female sex hormones is very similar to those resulting from the administration of certain testosterone analogues, especially those with α substitutions at the 17 position of the steroid nucleus. These agents (such as methyltestosterone and norethandrolone) commonly cause BSP retention and less commonly cause jaundice or significant changes in other liver functions. However, unlike the female hormones, these agents have been implicated as a cause of chronic liver disease, especially biliary cirrhosis.

Because of these phenomena, synthetic steroid sex hormones should not be used in patients with liver disease. Conversely, in individuals using these agents the appearance of jaundice or elevations in serum aminotransferase (transaminase) levels or alkaline phosphatase contraindicates their further use. However, mild to moderate increases in BSP retention alone are probably not of clinical significance, although liver function tests should be carried out periodically.

As is discussed in detail in Chap. 302, there are many drugs which may produce not simply cholestasis but liver injury resembling acute hepatitis or cholestatic hepatitis. In contrast to the jaundice produced by the steroid hormones, the clinical features are those of fever, rash, arthralgia, and eosinophilia, with the liver showing a pronounced inflammatory reaction. These features suggest that such reactions are *allergic* or *toxic* in nature and therefore differ from the effects caused by the steroid hormones, which probably represent an exaggerated response by the liver to the normal action of these hormones.

Postoperative jaundice The occurrence of postoperative jaundice is a problem of increasing importance. It is perhaps seen more frequently now than in earlier years, because patients are able to undergo major surgical procedures (i.e., cardiac sur-

TABLE 301-2
Conditions causing or contributing to postoperative jaundice

I Increased pigment load
  A Hemolytic anemia
  B Transfusions (especially of stored blood)
  C Resorption of hematomas, blood in extravascular spaces
II Impaired hepatocellular function
  A Hepatitis-like picture
    1 Halothane anesthesia
    2 Drugs
    3 Shock
    4 Infection with hepatitis viruses
  B Cholestatic picture
    1 Hypotension, hypoxemia
    2 Drugs
    3 Sepsis
III Extrahepatic obstruction
  A Bile duct injury
  B Choledocholithiasis

gery, repair of ruptured aneurysms) and survive. In approaching this problem the possible pathogenic mechanisms listed in Table 301-2 need to be considered. The patient may have *pigment overload*, especially from blood transfusions (due to hemolysis of stored blood), from resorption of blood in extravascular spaces, and less commonly from hemolytic anemia. *Hepatocellular damage* and decreased liver cell function may occur due to concurrent use of hepatotoxic drugs (Chap. 302)

or anesthetics such as halothane. Hepatocellular necrosis may follow profound shock; with lesser degrees of hypotension or hypoxemia, morphological damage may be slight, but significant impairment of function may occur. Hence, prior shock or hypotension plus pigment overload may produce significant jaundice. Extensive sepsis can also produce jaundice, often of a cholestatic type. Concurrent renal impairment due to hypotension and hypoxemia may enhance the degree of jaundice because the renal excretion of conjugated bilirubin is decreased. *Extrahepatic obstruction* due to surgical damage or stones needs to be considered, but may be difficult to exclude.

A form of jaundice referred to as *benign postoperative intrahepatic cholestasis* may be seen. In the typical case the patient has had major and prolonged surgery for a catastrophic event such as a ruptured aortic aneurysm complicated by hypotension and hypoxemia, extensive blood loss into tissues, and massive blood replacement. Jaundice may be noted on the second or third postoperative day, and the serum bilirubin, predominantly conjugated, may reach 20 to 40 mg per 100 ml by the eighth to tenth day. Serum alkaline phosphatase levels may be elevated three- to tenfold. Typically the SGOT is only mildly elevated. The liver morphology is striking in that necrosis is not seen but only cholestasis and erythrophagocytosis.

The cause of this type of postoperative cholestatic jaundice is uncertain. However, in all likelihood it reflects (1) increased

TABLE 301-3
Laboratory features in icteric states

Bilirubin disorder	Serum bilirubin		Urine bilirubin	Comments
	Unconjugated	Conjugated		
I Overproduction				
A Hemolysis (intra- and extravascular)	↑	N	0	↑ Bilirubin turnover
B Ineffective erythropoiesis	↑	N	0	Splenomegaly; normal RBC survival; normoblasts in marrow
II Defective hepatic uptake	↑	N	0	Normal liver biopsy; direct/total serum bilirubin <20%
A Some drugs (e.g., flavaspidic acid, novobiocin)				
B Gilbert's syndrome (some cases)				
III Defective conjugation	↑	Low	0	
A Neonatal jaundice				↓ Glucuronyl transferase; ? ↓ ligandins
B Gilbert's syndrome				↓ Glucuronyl transferase; some may have ↑ hemolysis and ↓ bilirubin uptake; bile contains ↑ monoconjugates
C Conjugated nonhemolytic jaundice (types I and II)				Type I = absence of transferase Type II = deficiency of transferase; bile contains ↑↑ monoconjugates
IV Defective excretion				
A Intrahepatic obstruction				
1 Familial syndromes				
a Dubin-Johnson	↑	↑↑	+	Abnormal BSP curve, hepatic lipochrome pigment; ↑ urinary coproporphyrin type I
b Rotor				No liver pigment; ↑ total urinary coproporphyrin
2 Drugs (e.g., chloramphenicol, methyltestosterone)	↑	↑↑	+	↑ Alkaline phosphatase but other function tests usually normal
3 Benign recurrent cholestasis	↑	↑↑	+	↑ Alkaline phosphatase
4 Recurrent jaundice of pregnancy (third trimester)	↑	↑↑	+	↑ Alkaline phosphatase; may be reproduced in afflicted subjects by estrogens or progesterone
B Extrahepatic obstruction (tumors, stone, stricture of bile duct)				↑↑ Alkaline phosphatase (often > fourfold)
1 Partial	↑	↑↑	+	
2 Complete	↑	↑↑	+	
V Hepatocellular disease*				
A Hepatitis	↑	↑↑	+	Direct/total serum bilirubin >50-70%; liver biopsy important for diagnosis
B Cirrhosis: Same as hepatitis	↑	↑↑		

* *Note that in hepatocellular disease there is generally an interference in all pathways of bilirubin metabolism (i.e., impaired uptake, conjugation, and excretion).*

pigment load, (2) decreased liver function due to hypoxemia and hypotension, and (3) decreased renal bilirubin excretion due to varying degrees of tubular necrosis as a result of shock. This diagnostic possibility must be considered in the postoperative patient with marked cholestatic jaundice. The course of the jaundice is self-limited and will subside if the other systemic complications do not predominate and lead to death.

Hepatitis and cirrhosis   These disorders, discussed in detail in Chaps. 302 to 304, constitute the *most common disorders associated with jaundice.* As has been stated previously, when the liver cell is damaged, as in viral hepatitis, there is often impairment in all three major hepatic phases of bilirubin metabolism, namely, uptake, conjugation, and excretion. Since the excretory step is the one which is rate-limiting and most readily affected by injury, significant amounts of conjugated bilirubin reenter the systemic circulation. There are also usually lesser increases in the serum unconjugated bilirubin. The latter is probably a reflection of the impaired uptake and conjugation, and is due in part to the shortened life span of red blood cells often found in liver disease. In most patients with hepatitis and cirrhosis, the total serum bilirubin levels tend not to exceed 50 mg per 100 ml, but on rare occasions levels of up to 90 or 95 mg per 100 ml have been described. (For a summary of laboratory features in icteric states, see Table 301-3.)

EXTRAHEPATIC BILIARY OBSTRUCTION   Anatomic or mechanical obstruction of the bile ducts is most commonly due to stones, tumors, or strictures. The clinical picture is quite similar to that of intrahepatic cholestasis with pronounced elevation of the alkaline phosphatase level. Usually, but not always, fever, pain, and chills may be present. While the amount of direct-reacting (conjugated) bilirubin predominates in the serum, the amount of the total serum bilirubin which is direct-reacting is variable (60 to 80 percent) and of no real diagnostic or prognostic significance. In contrast to hepatitis and cirrhosis, the serum bilirubin level often tends to plateau and rarely exceeds levels of 35 mg per 100 ml. The reason for this plateau is not clear but may be related to renal excretion of conjugated bilirubin or alternative pathways of bilirubin catabolism in obstructive jaundice.

REFERENCES

Benign familial recurrent cholestasis

DePagter AGF et al: Familial benign intrahepatic cholestasis. Gastroenterology 71:202, 1976

Endo T et al: Bile acid metabolism in benign recurrent intrahepatic cholestasis. Gastroenterology 76:1002, 1979

Dubin-Johnson and Rotor syndromes

Berk PD et al: Inborn errors of bilirubin metabolism. Med Clin North Am 59:803, 1975

Swartz HM et al: On the nature and excretion of the hepatic pigment in the Dubin-Johnson syndrome. Gastroenterology 76:958, 1979

Wolkoff AW et al: Rotor's syndrome: A distinct inheritable pathophysiologic entity. Am J Med 60:173, 1976

Glucuronyl transferase deficiency states

Berk PD et al: Unconjugated hyperbilirubinemia: Physiologic evaluation and approaches to therapy. Ann Intern Med 82:552, 1975

Berthelot P, Dhumeaus D: New insights into the classification and mechanisms of hereditary, chronic, non-hemolytic hyperbilirubinemia. Gut 19:474, 1978

Felsher BF, Carpio NM: Caloric intake and unconjugated hyperbilirubinemia. Gastroenterology 69:42, 1975

Fevery J et al: Unconjugated bilirubin and an increased proportion of bilirubin monoconjugates in the bile of patients with Gilbert's syndrome and Crigler-Najjar disease. J Clin Invest 60:970, 1977

Hunter JO et al: Inheritance of type 2 Crigler-Najjar hyperbilirubinaemia. Gut 14:46, 1973

Postoperative jaundice

Koff RS: Postoperative jaundice. Med Clin North Am 59:823, 1975

LaMont JT, Isselbacher KJ: Postoperative jaundice. N Engl J Med 288:305, 1973

302
ACUTE HEPATITIS

JULES L. DIENSTAG
JACK R. WANDS
RAYMOND S. KOFF

ACUTE VIRAL HEPATITIS

Acute viral hepatitis is a systemic infection affecting the liver predominantly. Classically two types of viruses (A and B) had been implicated as the etiologic agents in this systemic infection; however, recently others (non-A, non-B) have been described. Viruses A and B can now be distinguished by their antigenic properties but are known to produce clinically similar diseases in humans. Synonyms used to describe hepatitis A include infectious hepatitis, short-incubation hepatitis, and MS-1 hepatitis. Hepatitis B has also been referred to as serum hepatitis, long-incubation hepatitis, MS-2 hepatitis, or hepatitis B surface antigen (HBsAg)-positive hepatitis.

ANTIGENIC PROPERTIES OF HEPATITIS VIRUSES   Hepatitis A   Hepatitis A virus (HAV) is a nonenveloped 27-nm (Fig. 302-1), heat-, acid-, and ether-resistant RNA virus with biophysical characteristics of the enterovirus subgroup of picornaviruses. Inactivation of viral activity can be achieved by boiling for 1 min, by contact with formaldehyde and chlorine, or by ultraviolet irradiation. All strains of this virus identified to date are immunologically indistinguishable and belong to one serotype. The virus is present in the liver, bile, stools, and blood during the late incubation period and acute preicteric phase of illness, but viral shedding in feces and viremia diminish rapidly once jaundice becomes apparent.

Hepatitis B   This viral infection is unique in that concentrations of viral antigen in the blood may reach 50 mg per 100 ml. Electron microscopic studies of serum have demonstrated the morphologic appearance of the various particles related to hepatitis B infection (see Fig. 302-1). Three types of particles have been observed (Table 302-1). The most numerous are the 22-nm particles which appear as spherical or long filamentous forms; these are antigenically identical with the outer surface or coat of the hepatitis B virus and are thought to represent excess viral coat protein. Less frequently seen in serum are large 42-nm spherical Dane particles, which are believed to represent the intact hepatitis B virus (HBV). These large particles characteristically have an outer coat and an inner icosahedral core measuring 27 nm in diameter. Previous studies have shown that antiserum obtained from hemophiliacs, who were presumably repeatedly exposed to hepatitis viruses through multiple blood transfusions, would form a precipitin line by

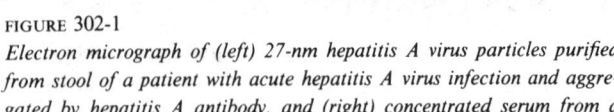

FIGURE 302-1

Electron micrograph of (left) 27-nm hepatitis A virus particles purified from stool of a patient with acute hepatitis A virus infection and aggregated by hepatitis A antibody, and (right) concentrated serum from a *patient with acute hepatitis B infection demonstrating the 42-nm virion, tubular forms, and spherical 22-nm particles of hepatitis B surface antigen (132,000×).*

diffusion in agar gel with an antigen present in hepatitis serum. This antigen was originally called the Australia antigen or hepatitis-associated antigen and subsequently referred to as the hepatitis B surface antigen (HBsAg). These observations provided the first serologic test to distinguish hepatitis B from non-B hepatitis. Isolation from serum of the various virus-associated particles related to hepatitis B infection and detection of antibodies to the antigens associated with these particles have permitted a more complete understanding of the antigenic composition of the hepatitis B virus (see Table 302-1). The long, tubular and small, spherical particles (22 nm) possess HBsAg, which is also present on the surface of the 42-nm Dane particle. HBsAg can be measured in clinical laboratories and is specific for hepatitis B infection. "Spurs" of immunoprecipitate are produced by certain combinations of HBsAg and antibody reactants in double immunodiffusion studies. Analysis of these reactions has led to the recognition of a number of different antigenic determinants. There is a common group-reactive antigen, *a*, shared by all HBsAg-positive serums. In addition, HBsAg may contain several type-specific antigens—namely, *d* or *y*, *w* or *r*, as well as others. These HBsAg *subtypes* provide additional epidemiologic markers in evaluating the transmission of hepatitis B infection in that subtypes "breed true." For example, studies of hepatitis outbreaks among patients and staff in hemodialysis units have shown that index cases and their contacts have identical HBsAg subtypes. Clinical course and outcome, however, are independent of subtype.

The intact 42-nm virion can be disrupted by mild detergents and the 27-nm core particle isolated. Naked core particles do not circulate in serum. The antigen is referred to as the hepatitis B core antigen (HBcAg), and the corresponding antibody is anti-HBc. HBcAg does not cross-react with HBsAg. Within the core particle is a predominantly double-stranded DNA which is associated with a DNA polymerase; the latter presumably directs replication or repair of viral DNA. Thus, the *hepatitis B virus can be classified as a DNA virus.*

A number of laboratory techniques are employed for the measurement of HBsAg in serum. The least sensitive is Ouchterlony gel diffusion. Counterimmunoelectrophoresis (CIEP) is approximately ten times more sensitive. *Radioimmunoassay* is the most sensitive and preferred technique for the measurement of HBsAg in serum. It is approximately 1000 times more sensitive than gel diffusion.

A third antigen associated with hepatitis B is *hepatitis B e antigen (HBeAg)*. HBeAg is a soluble, nonparticulate antigen, which is found only in HBsAg-positive serum and which is immunologically and biochemically distinct from HBsAg, HBcAg, and DNA polymerase. This antigen has not been completely characterized. Originally HBeAg and its antibody (anti-HBe) were detected by a relatively insensitive gel immunodiffusion technique, but more sensitive methods are now being evaluated. HBsAg-positive serum containing HBeAg is more likely to be highly infectious and to be associated with the presence of Dane particles and DNA polymerase than HBeAg-negative or anti-HBe-positive serum. For example, asymptomatic HBsAg carrier mothers who are HBeAg-positive almost invariably transmit hepatitis B infection to their offspring. Every individual with acute hepatitis B infection develops HBeAg transiently, early in the course of illness, but persistent HBeAg positivity correlates with ongoing viral replication and may be associated with chronic hepatitis.

Non-A, non-B hepatitis Sensitive serologic tests for identifying both types A and B hepatitis have led to the identification of hepatitis cases with incubation periods and modes of transmission consistent with an infectious disease but without serologic evidence of hepatitis A or B infection. Identified initially among recipients of transfused blood, these cases of so-called "non-A, non-B" hepatitis have not been associated serologically with Epstein-Barr virus or cytomegalovirus or with other viruses known to involve the liver. One or more of these non-A, non-B viruses exist and have been implicated in a variety of epidemiologic forms of hepatitis transmission (see below). Al-

TABLE 302-1
Nomenclature and features of hepatitis antigens and antibodies

Hepatitis type*	Particle diameter,nm	Description	Antigen (abbreviation)	Corresponding antibody (abbreviation)	Remarks
A	27	Icosahedral virus particle	Hepatitis A virus (HAV)	Hepatitis A antibody (anti-HAV)	RNA-type virus; present in stool and serum early in course of hepatitis A
B	42	Intact virus (surface and core); spherical (Dane particle)	Hepatitis B surface antigen (HBsAg) Hepatitis B core antigen (HBcAg)	Hepatitis B surface antibody (anti-HBs) Hepatitis B core antibody (anti-HBc)	DNA-type virus; found in serum
	27	Core of Dane particle; icosahedral	HBcAg	Anti-HBc	Core contains DNA and DNA polymerase; present in hepatocyte nuclei but not in serum Anti-HBc detected in serum during and after acute infection with virus
	22	Appear as spherical and filamentous forms; both have same antigenic properties as surface of Dane particle; represent excess viral coat material	HBsAg	Anti-HBs	HBsAg detectable in > 80% of patients with acute hepatitis B; found in serum, body fluids, and hepatocyte cytoplasm Anti-HBs appears following B infection; probably protective antibody
		Antigen subtypes: Group reactive	/a	Anti-/a	Antigen common to all HBsAg particles
		Type specific	/d or y; w or r	Anti-; d or y; w or r	Useful in epidemiologic investigation
	Nonparticulate	Soluble protein	HBeAg	Anti-HBe	HBeAg found in HBsAg-positive serum only, correlates with infectivity and presence of intact virus particles

* Non-A, non-B hepatitis is a transmissible hepatitis agent(s), but no immunologic marker or virus particle has yet been satisfactorily demonstrated.

though the virus(es) or virus antigens have not been identified definitively, chimpanzees are a susceptible host and may prove useful in the isolation, characterization, and serological identification of these agents.

HUMORAL RESPONSE TO HEPATITIS VIRUS INFECTION
There is a nonspecific increase in serum immunoglobulins during acute viral hepatitis. Serum IgG and IgM are elevated in about one-third of patients during the acute phase of infection, but serum IgM elevation is seen more characteristically during acute type A hepatitis. During the acute phase of viral hepatitis, antibodies to smooth muscle and other cell constituents may be present, and low titers of rheumatoid factor, antinuclear antibody, and heterophile antibody can also be found occasionally. These antibodies are nonspecific and can also be associated with other viral and systemic diseases.

Antibodies of hepatitis A Anti-HAV can be detected during acute illness when serum transaminase activity is elevated and fecal HAV shedding is still occurring. This early antibody response is predominantly of the IgM class and persists from several weeks to months. During convalescence, however, anti-HAV of the IgG class becomes the predominant antibody. Therefore, a diagnosis can be made during acute illness by demonstrating high-titer anti-HAV of the IgM class. Alternatively, diagnosis can be based on an increase in anti-HAV titers between acute and convalescent serum samples. Following acute illness, anti-HAV remains detectable indefinitely, and patients with serum anti-HAV are immune to reinfection. In-

deed, the anti-HAV present in immune serum globulin preparations accounts for the protection it affords against hepatitis A infection.

In the general population, anti-HAV increases in prevalence as a function of increasing age and of decreasing socioeconomic status. Serologic evidence of prior hepatitis A infection occurs in about 40 percent of urban populations, fewer than 5 percent of whom recall having had a symptomatic case of hepatitis. In older age groups (>50 years) evidence of previous hepatitis A infection approaches 80 percent, regardless of socioeconomic class. In developing countries, exposure, infection, and subsequent immunity is almost universal in childhood.

Antibodies to hepatitis B Specific antibody to HBsAg in serum (anti-HBs) has been demonstrated by radioimmunoassay in both the general population and patients convalescing from acute hepatitis B. Both IgM and IgG anti-HBs response have been demonstrated in prospectively studied adult patients. The appearance of IgM anti-HBs after primary exposure is transient, whereas IgG anti-HBs persists for years after infection. In volunteer blood donors, the prevalence of anti-HBs ranges from 5 to 10 percent, but the prevalence is higher in lower socioeconomic strata, older age groups, and persons frequently exposed to blood products.

A primary immune response with the production of anti-HBs occurs after acute infection or immunization. A subsequent and more pronounced rise in anti-HBs titers suggests an anamnestic response. Such a presumed anamnestic anti-HBs response has been observed in patients and medical personnel with preexisting anti-HBs following their reexposure to HBsAg, either through blood transfusions or hospital contacts. These individuals do not develop biochemical or clinical evidence of acute hepatitis B following this exposure, suggesting that *anti-HBs protects against reinfection with the hepatitis B virus.*

There is significant variability in the time of appearance of anti-HBs following exposure to HBsAg or acute hepatitis B infection. In some patients, anti-HBs is detectable 2 weeks to 2 months after HBsAg disappears from the serum; however in many instances anti-HBs is not detectable until 4 to 6 months after the disappearance of HBsAg. Measurement of serum anti-HBs titers is clinically and epidemiologically useful in documenting previous clinical or subclinical hepatitis B infection and may aid in documenting reexposure to HBsAg. Anti-HBs is rarely detectable in chronic carriers of HBsAg.

Antibody to the core antigen (anti-HBc) appears in the serum in high titer approximately 2 to 10 weeks after the appearance of HBsAg; it precedes detectable levels of anti-HBs by weeks to months (Fig. 302-2). During the "gap" between disappearance of HBsAg and the emergence of anti-HBs, anti-HBc may be the only serologic marker of recent HBV infection. This interval may be brief, as with acute infection, or may last many months following resolution of chronic infection. In the absence of HBsAg and anti-HBs, anti-HBc in high titer reflects ongoing viral replication; such anti-HBc–positive blood has been implicated in the development of transfusion-associated type B hepatitis in a small number of recipients. Following recovery, however, the anti-HBc titer is generally low, and anti-HBs is present as well. Immune individuals who are reexposed to hepatitis B develop a secondary anamnestic anti-HBs response, but anti-HBc titer does not change.

Antibodies to non-A, non-B agents Serologic tests to identify antigens and antibodies associated with non-A, non-B virus have not been developed. Details of the humoral immune response remain to be described.

FIGURE 302-2

Scheme showing typical time relationship of clinical and laboratory features and appearance of hepatitis B antigen and antibodies. Anti-HBc is measurable in the serum during active infection and gradually declines in titer during recovery. Anti-HBs has a variable appearance but in almost all patients is found after recovery from acute hepatitis B.

IMMUNOPATHOGENIC MECHANISM IN ACUTE VIRAL HEPATITIS While data on the immunopathogenesis of hepatitis A are very limited, there is increasing evidence that the clinical manifestations of acute hepatitis B are determined by the immunologic responses of the host. Immune-complex–mediated tissue damage plays a major pathogenetic role in the extrahepatic manifestations of acute hepatitis B. The occasional prodomal "serum sickness-like" syndrome observed in acute hepatitis B appears to be related to the presence of circulating immune complexes leading to activation of the complement system. The clinical consequences of this activation are rash, angioedema, and arthritis. In these patients during the early prodrome of hepatitis B, HBsAg in high titer in association with small amounts of anti-HBs lead to the formation of soluble, circulating immune complexes (in antigen excess). Complement components in the serum are depressed during the arthritic phase of the illness and are also detectable in the circulating immune complexes. In addition to complement components, these complexes contain the intact virus, tubules, and 22-nm spheres (HBsAg), anti-HBs, IgG, IgM, and IgA. These immune complexes disappear after recovery from the serum sickness-like syndrome.

In patients who become chronic carriers of HBsAg following acute hepatitis, other types of immune-complex diseases may be seen. *Glomerulonephritis* with the nephrotic syndrome is occasionally observed: HBsAg, immunoglobulins, and C3 deposition has been found on the glomerular basement membrane. Twenty to thirty percent of patients with *polyarteritis nodosa* have HBsAg in the serum, and in these patients the affected small and medium-sized arteries have been shown to contain HBsAg, immunoglobulins, and complement components.

Cellular immunity (delayed hyerpsensitivity) may be important in the host's response to hepatitis B infection. Patients with depressed T lymphocyte function have a high frequency of chronic infection with the hepatitis B virus. Lymphocytes appear to mediate liver injury as reflected by the ability of circulating lymphocytes from patients with acute hepatitis B to produce liver cell damage in vitro. Other evidence suggests that alterations in the host's cellular immune response may be important in the development of the chronic HBsAg carrier state and progression from acute hepatitis B to chronic active hepatitis.

PATHOLOGY The typical morphologic lesions of hepatitis A and B and non-A and non-B are often similar and consist of panlobular infiltration with mononuclear cells, hepatic cell necrosis, hyperplasia of Kupffer cells, and variable degrees of cholestasis. Hepatic cell regeneration is present, as evidenced by numerous mitotic figures, multinucleated cells, and "rosette" or "pseudoacinar" formation. The mononuclear infiltration consists primarily of small lymphocytes, although plasma cells and eosinophils are occasionally seen. Liver cell damage consists of hepatic cell degeneration and necrosis, cell dropout, ballooning of cells, and acidophilic degeneration of hepatocytes (so-called "Councilman bodies"). Large hepatocytes with a ground-glass appearance of the cytoplasm may be seen in chronic but not acute hepatitis B; these cells have been shown to contain HBsAg. In uncomplicated viral hepatitis the reticulin framework is preserved.

A more severe histologic lesion, *bridging hepatic necrosis,* also termed *subacute* or *confluent necrosis,* is occasionally observed in some patients with acute hepatitis. "Bridging" between lobules results from large areas of hepatic cell dropout, with collapse of the reticulin framework. Characteristically, the "bridge" consists of condensed reticulum, inflammatory debris, and degenerating liver cells that span adjacent portal areas, portal to central veins, or central vein to central vein. This lesion may have prognostic significance since substantially many affected individuals may either have a subacute course terminating in death within several weeks to months or develop chronic active hepatitis and postnecrotic cirrhosis. The incidence of bridging in uncomplicated acute hepatitis is probably on the order of 1 to 5 percent; however, in hospitalized patients with severe hepatitis B the incidence may be higher. When confluent necrosis is more severe and spans several lobules, the lesion is called *multilobular hepatic necrosis*. This lesion appears to be associated with a poor prognosis. In *massive hepatic necrosis* (fulminant hepatitis, acute yellow atrophy), the striking feature at postmortem examination is the finding of a small, shrunken, and soft liver. Histologic examination reveals massive necrosis and dropout of liver cells of most lobules with extensive collapse and condensation of the reticulin framework.

Immunofluorescence antibody studies have shown HBsAg in the cytoplasm of infected liver cells. In contrast, HBcAg predominates in the nucleus but occasionally is also seen in the cytoplasm. Electron microscopic studies of liver biopsy material have demonstrated the presence of HBsAg particles in the cytoplasm and HBcAg particles in the nucleus of liver cells during hepatitis B infection. These morphologic observations suggest that DNA is synthesized and packaged within core particles in the nucleus, while the surface coat is assembled in the cytoplasm, resulting in the formation of the intact hepatitis B virus.

EPIDEMIOLOGY Traditionally, viral hepatitis had been classified into two epidemiologically distinct types: infectious hepatitis (hepatitis A) and serum hepatitis (hepatitis B). These distinctions were based on earlier observations that hepatitis A had a shorter incubation period (15 to 45 days), high contagion rate, and usually a fecal-oral route of transmission; while hepatitis B had a longer incubation period (30 to 180 days), was less contagious, and was thought to be transmitted only by the parenteral route. It is now recognized that *a clear distinction between hepatitis A and B cannot be made solely by clinical or epidemiologic features* (Table 302-2), that modes of transmission overlap, and moreover, that other hepatitis viruses exist besides hepatitis A and B. The most accurate means to distinguish the various types of viral hepatitis involves specific serologic testing.

Hepatitis A is transmitted almost exclusively by the fecal-oral route. Spread of this virus is enhanced by poor personal hygiene and overcrowding, and large outbreaks as well as sporadic cases have been traced to contaminated food, water,

milk, and shellfish. Intrafamily and intrainstitutional spread are also common. There appears to be a predilection for hepatitis A to occur in late fall and early winter. In temperate zones, epidemic waves had been recorded every 5 to 20 years as new segments of nonimmune population appeared; however, in developed countries, the incidence of type A hepatitis has been declining, presumably as a function of improved sanitation, and these cyclic patterns are no longer being observed. No chronic HAV carrier state has been identified after acute type A hepatitis infection; perpetuation of the virus in nature depends presumably on nonepidemic, inapparent subclinical infection. In contrast, the major route of hepatitis B transmission is percutaneous; however, in many patients with acute hepatitis B, there is no history of known parenteral exposure, raising the possibility of obscure routes of transmission for hepatitis B infection. Indeed, inadvertent parenteral, oral, and as yet other unidentified routes of transmission may be responsible for many cases. HBsAg has been identified in seminal fluid, saliva, breast milk, tears, synovial fluid, intestinal fluid, gastric juice, and rarely in urine and feces; but, except for saliva and seminal fluid, the infective nature of these body fluids is not yet clearly established. Maternal hepatitis B does not appear to be directly transmitted transplacentally to the fetus in utero. However HBsAg has been found in the serum of infants whose mothers had hepatitis B, especially mothers with hepatitis during the last trimester of pregnancy, suggesting that the most likely route of transmission was either a break in the maternal-fetal circulation during the last trimester or at the time of delivery, or close contact between mother and child during the postpartum period. High attack rates of hepatitis B in spouses and sexual partners of affected patients, in family members of chronic HBsAg carriers, among male homosexuals, and in institutions also support the belief that transmission can occur via nonpercutaneous or covert percutaneous routes. The over 120 million chronic HBsAg carriers in the world constitute the main reservoir of hepatitis B in man. Serum HBsAg is infrequent (0.1 to 0.5 percent) in normal populations in the United States and Western Europe; however, a prevalence of up to 5 to 15 percent has been found in some tropical countries, and as high as 30 percent in patients with Down's syndrome, lepromatous leprosy, leukemia, Hodgkin's disease,

TABLE 302-2
Comparisons of type A, type B, and non-A, non-B hepatitis

Feature	Hepatitis A (infectious hepatitis, MS-1, short-incubation hepatitis)	Hepatitis B (serum hepatitis, MS-2, long-incubation hepatitis)	Non-A, non-B hepatitis
Incubation	15–45 days (mean 30)	45–160 days (mean 60–90)	15–160 (mean 50)
Onset	Acute	Often insidious	Insidious
Seasonal incidence	Fall, winter	Year round	Year round
Age preference	Children, young adults	Any age	Any age but more common in adults
Transmission route:			
Fecal-oral	+++	+/−	Unknown
Other nonpercutaneous*	+/−	++	++
Percutaneous	+/−	+++	+++
Severity	Mild	Often severe	Moderate
Prognosis	Generally good	Worse with age, debility	Moderate
Progression to chronicity	None	Occasional	Occasional
Immune serum globulin (ISG) prophylaxis	Good	Partial	?
Hepatitis B immune globulin (very high titer anti-HBs) prophylaxis	(Not applicable)	Good after needle stick	(Not applicable)
Carrier state	Rare, if ever	0.1–1.0%	Exists but prevalence unknown

* *For example, sexual or maternal-fetal contact.*

polyarteritis nodosa, in patients with chronic renal disease on hemodialysis, and in needle-using drug addicts.

Routine screening of blood donors for HBsAg and the elimination of commercial blood sources has markedly decreased the incidence of hepatitis B after transfusion, but *posttransfusion hepatitis* still remains a significant medical problem. The incidence of posttransfusion hepatitis has been reported to be from 0.3 to 9 cases per 1000 transfused units, or between 0.5 and 13 cases per 100 patients transfused. The risk of anicteric hepatitis following transfusion is much greater than that of clinical hepatitis with jaundice. The risk of viral hepatitis after transfusion of blood derivatives is dependent on the methods by which these products are processed. The *greatest risk* follows the use of multiple pooled donor products such as concentrates of factors II, VII, VIII, IX, and X. Hepatitis has developed in 20 to 30 percent of individuals receiving these pooled products for the first time. Blood products associated with an *average risk* include whole blood, packed red blood cells, single donor platelets, and plasma. Products involving *no risk* include human albumin and immune and hyperimmune serum globulin because of prior treatment of these substances by heating to 60°C and cold ethanol extraction. It has been suggested that frozen glycerol-treated red blood cells may carry a reduced risk of hepatitis, but this has not been confirmed. Elimination of HBsAg-negative blood that is positive for anti-HBc may prevent the few residual cases of transfusion-associated type B hepatitis, but this would lead to the loss of many noninfectious units and compromise the available blood supply. More of a problem than the relatively rare posttransfusion type B hepatitis is the occurrence of non-A, non-B posttransfusion hepatitis, which accounts for approximately 90 percent of cases following transfusion of voluntarily donated blood prescreened for HBsAg. The fact that it is transmitted by transfused blood from asymptomatic donors (Table 302-2) and that it can be transmitted to chimpanzees by blood from patients with chronic hepatitis suggests that there is a chronic carrier state for non-A, non-B hepatitis. Moreover, in addition to being transmitted by transfusion, non-A, non-B hepatitis cases have been observed in other settings of percutaneous and nonpercutaneous exposure (e.g., intrafamily contact, intravenous drug abuse, occupational contact, nosocomial infection, hemodialysis units, renal transplantation, and intrainstitutional contact). Non-A, non-B hepatitis accounts for approximately 20 percent of sporadic cases presenting for medical evaluation. Occurrence of multiple bouts of non-A, non-B hepatitis among drug abusers and of cases with either short or long incubation periods suggests that there may be more than one non-A, non-B hepatitis agent.

CLINICAL AND LABORATORY FEATURES Symptoms and signs
The *prodromal symptoms* of acute viral hepatitis are variable and systemic. Constitutional symptoms of anorexia, nausea and vomiting, fatigue, malaise, arthralgias, myalgias, headache, photophobia, pharyngitis, cough, and coryza may precede the onset of jaundice by 1 to 2 weeks. The nausea, vomiting, and anorexia are frequently associated with alterations in olfaction and taste. A low-grade fever between 100 and 102°F is more often present in hepatitis A than in B, except when hepatitis B is heralded by a "serum sickness-like" syndrome; rarely a fever of 103 to 104°F may accompany the constitutional symptoms. Dark urine and clay-colored stools may be noticed by the patient from 1 to 5 days prior to the onset of clinical jaundice.

With the onset of *clinical jaundice* the constitutional prodromal symptoms usually diminish, but in some patients mild weight loss (2.5 to 5 kg) is common and may continue during the entire icteric phase. The liver becomes enlarged and tender and may be associated with right upper quadrant pain and discomfort. Infrequently, patients present with a cholestatic picture, suggesting extrahepatic biliary obstruction. Splenomegaly and cervical adenopathy are present in 10 to 20 percent of patients with acute hepatitis. Rarely, a few spider angiomas appear during the icteric phase and disappear during convalescence. During the *recovery phase,* constitutional symptoms disappear, but usually some liver enlargement and abnormalities in hepatic function are still evident. The duration of the posticteric phase is variable, ranging from 2 to 12 weeks, and usually is more prolonged in acute hepatitis B and in non-A, non-B hepatitis. Complete clinical and biochemical recovery is to be expected 3 to 4 months after the onset of jaundice in three-quarters of uncomplicated cases. In the remainder biochemical recovery may be delayed.

Laboratory features   The serum transaminases (aminotransferases; SGOT and SGPT) show a variable increase during the prodromal phase of acute viral hepatitis and precede the rise in bilirubin level (see Fig. 302-2). The actual level of these enzymes, however, does not correlate well with the degree of liver cell damage. Peak levels vary from 400 to 4000 IU or more; these levels are usually reached at the time the patient is clinically icteric and progressively diminish during the recovery phase of acute hepatitis. The diagnosis of *anicteric* hepatitis is difficult and requires a high index of suspicion; it is often based solely on transaminase elevations, although mild increases in conjugated bilirubin may also be found.

Jaundice is usually visible in the sclera or skin when the serum bilirubin value exceeds 2.5 mg per 100 ml. When jaundice appears, the serum bilirubin typically rises to levels ranging from 5 to 20 mg per 100 ml. The serum bilirubin may continue to rise despite falling serum transaminase levels. In most instances the total bilirubin is equally divided between the conjugated and unconjugated fractions. The absolute level of the serum bilirubin appears to have some prognostic significance; *levels above 20 mg per 100 ml extending and persisting late into the course of viral hepatitis may indicate more severe disease.* In certain patients with underlying hemolytic anemia, however, such as glucose 6-phosphate dehydrogenase deficiency and sickle-cell anemia, high serum bilirubin is common, due to superimposed hemolysis. In such patients bilirubin levels greater than 30 mg per 100 ml have been observed and do not necessarily indicate a worse prognosis.

Neutropenia and lymphopenia are transient and are followed by a relative lymphocytosis. Atypical lymphocytes (varying between 2 and 20 percent) are common during the acute phase. These atypical lymphocytes are indistinguishable from those seen with infectious mononucleosis. It is important to measure the *prothrombin time* (PT) in patients with acute viral hepatitis, for a prolonged value may signify extensive hepatocellular necrosis and indicate a worse prognosis. Occasionally a prolonged PT may occur with only mild increases of the serum bilirubin and transaminase levels. A blood sugar determination is often helpful in patients with symptoms of *hypoglycemia.* Prolonged nausea and vomiting, inadequate carbohydrate intake, and poor hepatic glycogen reserve may contribute to very rare episodes of hypoglycemia in the patient with uncomplicated viral hepatitis. Serum alkaline phosphatase may be normal or only mildly elevated to levels of 80 to 240 IU. A diffuse but mild elevation of the gamma globulin fraction is common. In some patients mild and transient steatorrhea has been noted as well as slight microscopic hematuria and minimal proteinuria.

The presence of *circulating* HBsAg is the only test readily available in most clinical laboratories to distinguish between type B and non-B hepatitis. Sequential measurement of HBsAg during the course of hepatitis B has shown that the appearance of HBsAg precedes the rise in SGOT and clinical symptoms (Fig. 302-2). HBsAg may remain detectable during the entire icteric phase of acute hepatitis B. However, occasionally it may have reached low or undetectable levels when the patient is first seen. HBsAg usually is undetectable by serologic measurements 1 to 2 months following the onset of jaundice in most patients. Tests for anti-HBc and anti-HBs during acute illness and convalescence may help to establish the diagnosis of hepatitis B, especially in the approximately 10 to 25 percent of cases who never develop detectable HBsAg.

The titer of HBsAg bears little relationship to the severity of clinical disease. Indeed, there is an inverse correlation between the serum concentration of HBsAg and the degree of liver cell damage. Titers are *highest* in immunosuppressed patients and in normal carriers, lower in chronic liver disease (but higher in chronic persistent than in chronic active hepatitis), and *very low* in acute fulminant hepatitis. These observations suggest that in hepatitis B the degree of liver cell damage and the clinical course are probably related to variations in the patient's immune response to hepatitis B virus rather than to the amount of circulating HBsAg.

Tests for fecal or serum hepatitis A virus are not routinely available. Therefore, in most cases, a diagnosis of type A hepatitis is based on negative serologic testing for hepatitis B markers, the presence of high or rising titers of anti-HAV, especially of the IgM class, and a classical epidemiologic setting.

PROGNOSIS Virtually all previously healthy patients with hepatitis A recover completely from their illness with no clinical sequelae. Similarly in acute hepatitis B, the majority of patients have a favorable course and recover completely. There are, however, certain clinical and laboratory features which suggest a more complicated and protracted course. Patients with advanced age and serious underlying medical disorders, such as congestive heart failure, severe anemia, diabetes mellitus, and malignancy, may have a prolonged course and are more likely to develop severe hepatitis. Initial presenting features such as ascites, peripheral edema, and symptoms of hepatic encephalopathy suggest a poorer prognosis. In addition, a prolonged prothrombin time, low serum albumin, hypoglycemia, and serum bilirubin values greater than 20 mg per 100 ml suggest severe hepatocellular disease. Patients with these clinical and laboratory features deserve prompt hospital admission. The case fatality rate in hepatitis A and B is very low (<0.1 percent), but the case fatality rate in hepatitis A and B is significantly increased by age and underlying debilitating disorders. Non-A, non-B hepatitis is less severe in the acute phase than type B hepatitis and is more commonly anicteric, but the case fatality rate is not known.

COMPLICATIONS AND SEQUELAE During the prodromal phase of acute hepatitis B some patients may develop a "serum sickness-like" syndrome characterized by arthralgia or arthritis, rash, angioedema, and rarely hematuria and proteinuria. This syndrome occurs prior to the onset of clinical jaundice, and these patients are often erroneously diagnosed as having rheumatoid arthritis or other collagen vascular diseases such as systemic lupus erythematosus. This syndrome occurs in about 5 to 10 percent of hepatitis B patients. The diagnosis can be established by measuring the serum transaminase values, which are almost invariably elevated, and serum HBsAg.

The most feared complication of viral hepatitis is *fulminant hepatitis* (massive hepatic necrosis). This is primarily seen in hepatitis B and fortunately is rare. Patients usually present with signs and symptoms of encephalopathy and, in fact, many progress to deep coma. The liver is usually small, and the prothrombin time excessively prolonged. The combination of a rapidly shrinking liver size, rapidly rising bilirubin levels, and significant prolongation of the prothrombin time, together with clinical signs of confusion, disorientation, somnolence, ascites,

and edema indicates that the patient has hepatic failure with encephalopathy. Cerebral edema is common; evidence of brainstem compression as well as gastrointestinal bleeding, sepsis, respiratory failure, cardiovascular collapse, and renal failure are terminal events. The mortality is exceedingly high (greater than 80 percent in patients with deep coma), but patients who survive may have a complete biochemical and histologic recovery.

After acute type B hepatitis, approximately 10 percent of patients remain HBsAg-positive for more than 6 months. Most of these individuals clear the antigen from their circulation during the next several years, but a small percentage remain chronic HBsAg carriers. In their serum, anti-HBc is present in high titer, but anti-HBs is rarely detected. These carriers may (1) be asymptomatic, (2) have low-grade chronic persistent hepatitis, or (3) have chronic active hepatitis.

Chronic active hepatitis is a major late complication of acute hepatitis B occurring in approximately 3 to 5 percent of cases (see Chap. 303). This complication rarely, if ever, occurs after hepatitis A but may occur after non-A, non-B hepatitis. Certain clinical and laboratory features suggest progression of acute hepatitis to chronic active hepatitis: (1) lack of complete resolution of clinical symptoms of anorexia, weight loss, and fatigue and the persistence of hepatomegaly; (2) the presence of "bridging" or multilobular hepatic necrosis on liver biopsy during protracted, severe acute viral hepatitis; (3) failure of the serum transaminase, bilirubin, and alkaline phosphatase levels to return to normal within 6 to 12 months following the acute illness; and (4) the *continued presence of HBsAg* 6 months or more after acute hepatitis, suggesting chronic viral infection of the liver. Recent studies have shown that HBsAg-positive patients whose serum remains persistently positive for HBeAg are more likely to develop chronic active hepatitis than patients without persistent HBe antigenemia.

Rare complications of viral hepatitis include pancreatitis, myocarditis, atypical pneumonia, aplastic anemia, transverse myelitis, and peripheral neuropathy. Lifelong carriers of HBsAg appear to have an enhanced risk of developing hepatocellular carcinoma (see Chap. 305). In children, hepatitis B may rarely present with anicteric hepatitis, a nonpruritic papular rash of the face, buttocks, and limbs, and lymphadenopathy (papular acrodermatitis of childhood or Gianotti-Crosti syndrome).

DIFFERENTIAL DIAGNOSIS Viral diseases such as infectious mononucleosis; those due to cytomegalovirus, herpes simplex, and coxsackievirus; and toxoplasmosis may share certain clinical features with viral hepatitis and cause elevation in the serum transaminase and less commonly the serum bilirubin levels. Serologic tests such as the differential heterophile, Epstein-Barr virus antibody, and complement fixation tests for these agents may be helpful in the differential diagnosis if the HBsAg determination is negative. A complete drug history is particularly important since many drugs can produce either a picture of acute hepatitis or cholestasis (see below). Equally important is a past history of unexplained "repeated episodes" of acute hepatitis. This should alert the physician to the possibility that the underlying disorder is chronic active hepatitis. Alcoholic hepatitis must also be considered, but usually the serum transaminases are not as markedly elevated, other stigmata of alcoholism may be present, and the finding on liver biopsy of fatty infiltration, a neutrophilic inflammatory reaction, and "alcoholic hyalin" would be consistent with alcohol-induced rather than viral liver injury. Because acute hepatitis may present with right upper quadrant abdominal pain, nausea and vomiting, fever and icterus, it is often confused with acute cholecystitis, common duct stone, or ascending cholangitis. Patients with acute viral hepatitis tolerate surgery poorly; therefore it is important to exclude this diagnosis, and a percutaneous liver biopsy may be necessary prior to laparotomy. Viral hepatitis in the elderly is often misdiagnosed as obstructive jaundice due to common duct stone or carcinoma of the pancreas. Because acute hepatitis in the elderly may be quite severe and the operative mortality high, a thorough evaluation including laboratory tests (among them SGOT, HBsAg, and prothrombin time), radiographic studies of the biliary tree, and even liver biopsy may be necessary to exclude primary parenchymal liver disease.

MANAGEMENT AND PREVENTION   **Treatment of acute attack**
There is no specific treatment for *typical acute viral hepatitis.* Hospitalization may be required for correct diagnosis, for clinically severe illness, and for the elderly patient because of the high mortality. Forced and prolonged bed rest is not essential for full recovery, but many patients will feel better with restricted physical activity. A high-calorie diet is desirable, and because many patients may experience nausea late in the day, the major caloric intake is best tolerated in the morning. Intravenous feeding is necessary in the acute stage if the patient has persistent vomiting and cannot maintain oral intake. Drugs capable of producing adverse reactions such as cholestasis or those metabolized by the liver should be avoided. If significant pruritus is present, the use of a bile-salt-sequestering resin, such as cholestyramine, will usually alleviate this symptom. Corticosteroid therapy has no value in uncomplicated typical acute viral hepatitis.

Isolation of the patient with acute hepatitis to a single room and bathroom is probably unnecessary; however, both patient and hospital staff must be reminded of proper prophylactic techniques, such as washing hands after examining the patient, careful handling of body fluids and excreta, and the wearing of gloves when drawing blood, particularly from patients with hepatitis B.

Patients may be discharged from the hospital when there is substantial symptomatic improvement, a significant downward trend in the serum transaminase and bilirubin values, and normal prothrombin time. Mild transaminase elevations should not be considered contraindications to the gradual resumption of normal activity.

For patients with acute *severe clinical hepatitis,* or "bridging necrosis," corticosteroid therapy has often been used. However, the effectiveness of steroids in reversing this form of severe hepatitis has not been established, and steroid therapy may, in fact, be hazardous to some patients.

In *fulminant hepatitis,* the goal of therapy is to support the patient by maintenance of fluid balance and an open airway, support of circulation, control of bleeding, correction of hypoglycemia, and treatment of other complications of the comatose state in anticipation of liver regeneration and repair. Protein intake should be restricted and oral neomycin or lactulose administered. Although massive doses of corticosteroids have been administered, the value of this modality has never been proved. Likewise, exchange transfusion, plasmapheresis, human cross-circulation, porcine liver cross-perfusion, and hemoperfusion have not been proved to enhance survival.

Hazards to medical and paramedical personnel   Sporadic outbreaks of acute viral hepatitis, primarily type B, have been reported in blood bank employees, laboratory technicians, nurses, physicians, and dentists. Exposure to hepatitis viruses may result from contact with blood or other body fluids by pipeting, starting and maintaining intravenous cannulas, drawing blood, changing surgical dressings, emptying bedpans, caring for catheters, handling surgical instruments and pathologic specimens, and other patient care procedures. Defective gloves are common after long surgical procedures, and point source epidemics of acute hepatitis B have been reported among surgeons. Similarly, outbreaks of acute hepatitis have occurred in physicians and nurses working in hemodialysis and oncology units and in clinical laboratory employees; prevalence of exposure to hepatitis B in such health care settings is related directly to the extent of contact with blood rather than patients per se.

Asymptomatic HBsAg-positive carriers represent the greatest risk to health personnel because there are no readily identifiable clinical features, such as jaundice, that allow recognition and subsequent precautionary measures. Patients with a past history of hepatitis or multiple transfusions and those with parenteral drug abuse, chronic liver disease, chronic renal failure, leukemia, Hodgkin's disease, polyarteritis nodosa, Down's syndrome, and leprosy should have routine HBsAg determinations performed because of the high frequency of the HBsAg carrier state in these groups. If positive, they should be treated as potentially infectious, and appropriate precautions should be employed during operative or other acute care procedures. In dialysis units introduction of gloves and gowns, patient and staff education, routine periodic screening for HBsAg and transaminase elevations, and segregation of HBsAg-positive from susceptible patients have greatly reduced the incidence of hepatitis in both patients and medical personnel.

Prophylaxis   All preparations of immune serum globulin (ISG) contain anti-HAV, although the titers may vary. When administered before exposure or during the early incubation period, ISG is effective in preventing clinically apparent type A hepatitis. In some cases, ISG does not abort infection but, by ameliorating it, renders it inapparent. As a result long-lasting "passive-active" immunity occurs. For intimate contacts (household, institutional) of hepatitis A patients, administration of 0.02 ml/kg is recommended. It is not necessary for casual contacts (office, factory, school, hospital) nor for elderly individuals who are almost invariably immune. By the time common-source outbreaks of type A hepatitis are recognized, it is usually too late during the incubation period for ISG to be effective; however, prophylaxis may prevent illness in secondary cases. For travelers to tropical and developing countries, ISG prophylaxis is recommended. When such travel lasts less than 3 months, 0.02 ml/kg is given; for longer travel, a dose of 0.05 ml/kg every 4 to 6 months is recommended.

For passive immunoprophylaxis against hepatitis B, both standard ISG (with very modest levels of anti-HBs) and a high anti-HBs titer hepatitis B immune globulin (HBIG) have been evaluated. Currently HBIG is recommended only for postexposure prophylaxis of persons who have sustained an accidental needle stick with or who have ingested HBsAg-positive material. A dose of 0.05 to 0.07 ml/kg is given as soon after exposure as possible (or if HBIG is unavailable, 0.1 ml/kg ISG). This dose should be repeated 1 month later. The efficacy of HBIG vs. ISG in other postexposure settings (e.g., spouse of a patient with *acute* type B hepatitis, newborn of a HBsAg-positive mother) has not been clearly established; therefore, in these situations either preparation may be given. For preexposure prophylaxis against hepatitis B in endemic settings (e.g., travel to endemic areas, hemodialysis patients and staff), ISG is as effective as HBIG in preventing acute infection. In these settings, however, environmental and hygienic measures may be sufficient to abort hepatitis B virus transmission. When this is not the case, however, ISG should be given at a dose of 0.05 to 0.07 ml/kg at 4-month intervals. Anti-HBs–positive persons require no immunoprophylaxis. Active immunization against HBV will probably be available to high-risk populations in the near future. Tests are being conducted on a vaccine prepared from purified noninfectious 22-nm spherical forms of HBsAg derived from the plasma of chronic carriers.

For non-A, non-B hepatitis the effectiveness of ISG prophylaxis has not been demonstrated consistently. The only effective measures thus far which have reduced posttransfusion hepatitis are elimination of commercially obtained blood and screening for HBsAg.

COMMON PROBLEMS IN CLINICAL PRACTICE Expert opinion is divided regarding the *indications for liver biopsy* in the hospitalized patient with acute viral hepatitis. However, most agree that a liver biopsy is indicated when there is (1) a question about the diagnosis or (2) clinical evidence suggesting chronic active hepatitis. Liver biopsy should be performed only by physicians thoroughly familiar with this procedure in order to ensure adequate tissue for pathologic examination and to minimize the risk to the patient.

Serum HBsAg may persist for variable periods of time or indefinitely following hepatitis B infection. For example, immunosuppressed transplant recipients and patients with myeloproliferative and lymphoproliferative disorders are particularly susceptible to the acquisition of HBsAg from repeated blood transfusions; 10 to 30 percent of these patients become chronic carriers of HBsAg but may have little, if any, clinical evidence of liver disease. In contrast, the occasional persistence of HBsAg following acute icteric or anicteric hepatitis in normal individuals may be associated with the development of chronic liver disease. Therefore, it is particularly important to document the disappearance of serum HBsAg following apparent clinical recovery from acute hepatitis B. If HBsAg is detectable 6 to 12 months after acute hepatitis B, and serum transaminases remain elevated, a liver biopsy should be performed to exclude the development of chronic active hepatitis and differentiate this disorder from chronic persistent hepatitis (see Chap. 303).

Routine screening of blood donors by blood banks has identified numerous carriers of HBsAg who are often then referred to a physician for evaluation. Typically, such individuals are asymptomatic and have no signs of liver disease on physical examination. Liver function studies are either normal or show only mild abnormalities. Follow-up examinations will establish whether the patient is in the early prodrome of anicteric or icteric acute hepatitis B. However, if there is evidence on clinical examination of chronic liver disease and abnormal liver function tests, a diagnostic liver biopsy should be performed. If the patient is entirely asymptomatic with a normal examination and liver function tests are normal on several separate determinations, then the patient is a chronic carrier of HBsAg, and liver biopsy is probably not indicated since progression to chronic liver disease is very unusual. Asymptomatic patients with mild elevations in the serum transaminase or alkaline phosphatase, bilirubin, and gamma globulin determinations should have a liver biopsy to exclude chronic active hepatitis.

TOXIC AND DRUG-INDUCED HEPATITIS

Liver injury may follow the inhalation, ingestion, or parenteral administration of a number of chemical agents. These include industrial toxins (e.g., carbon tetrachloride, trichloroethylene, yellow phosphorus), the toxic cyclic peptides of certain species of *Amanita* and *Galerina* (mushroom poisoning), and, more commonly, pharmacologic agents used in medical therapy. It is essential that any patient presenting with jaundice or impaired liver function be questioned carefully about exposure to chemicals used in work or at home and drugs taken by prescription or bought "over the counter." In general, two major types of chemical hepatotoxicity have been recognized: (1) direct toxic and (2) idiosyncratic.

As shown in Table 302-3, toxic hepatitis is one which occurs with predictable regularity in individuals exposed to the offending agent and is dose-dependent. The latent period between exposure and liver injury is usually short (often several hours), although clinical manifestations may be delayed for 24 to 48 h. Agents producing toxic hepatitis are generally systemic poisons or are converted in the liver to toxic metabolites. The direct hepatotoxins result in morphologic abnormalities which are reasonably characteristic and reproducible for each toxin. For example, carbon tetrachloride and trichloroethylene characteristically produce a centrilobular zonal necrosis, whereas yellow phosphorus poisoning typically results in periportal injury. *Amanita phalloides* toxin usually produces massive hepatic necrosis. Tetracycline, when administered in intravenous doses greater than 1.5 g daily, leads to microvesicular fat deposits in the liver. Liver injury is often only one facet of the toxicity produced by the direct hepatotoxins, and it may go unrecognized until jaundice appears.

In idiosyncratic drug reactions the occurrence of hepatitis is usually infrequent and unpredictable, the response is not dose-dependent and may occur at any time during or shortly after exposure to the drug. Idiosyncratic reactions may be due to unique host susceptibility (metabolic reactivity) to specific agents or may be immunologically mediated. Immunologic evidence of classic hypersensitivity mechanisms (i.e., the demonstration of specific circulating or tissue-fixing antibodies) is not available. Similarly, a role for lymphocyte-mediated immune mechanisms in drug-induced hepatitis has been postulated but not proved. However, extrahepatic manifestations of hypersensitivity are common in some drug reactions and include arthralgias, rashes, fever, leukocytosis, and eosinophilia. Idiosyncratic reactions lead to a morphologic pattern that is more variable than those produced by direct toxins; a single agent is often capable of causing a variety of lesions, although certain patterns tend to predominate. Depending on the agent involved, idiosyncratic hepatitis may result in a clinical and morphologic picture indistinguishable from viral hepatitis (e.g.,

TABLE 302-3
Some features of toxic and drug-induced hepatic injury

| Features | Direct toxic effect | | Idiosyncratic | | | Other |
	(Carbon tetrachloride, e.g.)	(Acetaminophen, e.g.)	(Halothane, e.g.)	(Isoniazid, e.g.)	(Chlorpromazine, e.g.)	(Oral contraceptive agents, e.g.)
Predictable and dose-related toxicity	+	+	0	0	0	+
Latent period	Short	Short	Variable	Variable	Variable	Variable
Arthralgia, fever, rash, eosinophilia	0	0	+	0	+	0
Liver morphology	Necrosis, fatty infiltration	Centrilobular necrosis	Similar to viral hepatitis	Similar to viral hepatitis	Cholestasis with portal inflammation	Cholestasis without portal inflammation

halothane) or may clinically simulate extrahepatic bile duct obstruction with morphologic evidence of cholestasis and minimal hepatocellular damage (e.g., chlorpromazine). Morphologic alterations may also include submassive hepatic necrosis (e.g., α-methyldopa), or, infrequently, hepatic granulomas (e.g., sulfonamides).

Not all adverse hepatic drug reactions can be described as either toxic or idiosyncratic in type. For example, oral contraceptives, which combine estrogenic and progestational compounds, may result in impairment of hepatic function and occasionally in jaundice. However they do not produce necrosis or fatty change (in lower species), manifestations of hypersensitivity are generally absent, but genetic susceptibility to the development of oral contraceptive–induced cholestasis is well documented.

Because viral hepatitis is often a presumptive diagnosis and many adverse drug reactions produce a clinicopathologic picture resembling it, evidence of a causal relationship between the use of a drug and subsequent liver injury may be most difficult. The relation is most convincing for the direct hepatotoxins for which the frequency of hepatic impairment is usually high and the latent period between the start of therapy and impaired function is short. Idiosyncratic reactions may be reproduced, in some instances, when rechallenge, after an asymptomatic period, results in a recurrence of signs, symptoms, and morphologic and biochemical abnormalities. Rechallenge is often ethically unfeasible, and documentation of adverse hepatic reactions must often await the collection of other clinical cases.

Treatment of toxic and drug-induced hepatic disease is largely supportive as in acute viral hepatitis. Withdrawal of the suspected agent is indicated at the first sign of an adverse reaction. In the case of the direct toxins, liver involvement should not divert attention from renal or other organ involvement which may also threaten survival.

In Table 302-4, several classes of chemical agents are listed together with examples of the pattern of liver injury produced by them. It should be noted that certain drugs appear to be responsible for the development of chronic as well as acute hepatic injury. For example, oxyphenisatin, α-methyldopa, and isoniazid have been associated with chronic active hepatitis, and halothane and methotrexate have been implicated in

TABLE 302-4
Principal alterations of hepatic morphology produced by some commonly used drugs and chemicals

Principal morphologic change	*Class of agent*	*Example*
Cholestasis	Anabolic steroid	Methyl testosterone*
	Antithyroid	Methimazole
	Chemotherapeutic	Erythromycin estolate
	Oral contraceptive	Norethynodrel with mestranol
	Oral hypoglycemic	Chlorpropamide
	Tranquilizer	Chlorpromazine*
Fatty liver	Chemotherapeutic	Tetracycline
Hepatitis	Anesthetic	Halothane†
	Anticonvulsant	Diphenylhydantoin
	Antihypertensive	α-Methyldopa†
	Chemotherapeutic	Isoniazid†
	Diuretic	Chlorothiazide
	Laxative	Oxyphenisatin†
Toxic (necrosis)	Hydrocarbon	Carbon tetrachloride
	Metal	Yellow phosphorus
	Mushroom	*Amanita phalloides*
	Analgesic	Acetaminophen

* *Rarely associated with primary biliary cirrhosis.*
† *Occasionally associated with chronic active hepatitis or submassive hepatic necrosis and cirrhosis.*

the development of cirrhosis. A syndrome resembling primary biliary cirrhosis has been described following treatment with chlorpromazine, methyl testosterone, tolbutamide, and other drugs. Portal hypertension in the absence of cirrhosis may result from alterations in hepatic architecture produced by vitamin A or arsenic intoxication, industrial exposure to vinyl chloride, or administration of Thorotrast (thorium dioxide). The latter three agents have also been associated with angiosarcoma of the liver. Oral contraceptives have been implicated in the development of hepatic adenoma and, rarely, hepatic cell carcinoma and occlusion of the hepatic vein. Another unusual lesion, peliosis hepatis (blood cysts of the liver), has been observed in some patients treated with anabolic steroids. The existence of these hepatic disorders expands the spectrum of liver injury induced by chemical agents and emphasizes the need for a thorough drug history in all patients with liver dysfunction.

The following are the patterns of adverse hepatic reactions for some prototypic agents.

CARBON TETRACHLORIDE HEPATOTOXICITY (DIRECT TOXIN)
Poisoning may result from inhalation and accidental or purposeful ingestion, or possibly from skin absorption. Initial clinical manifestations include headache, dizziness, drowsiness, nausea, vomiting, and vasomotor collapse. Liver injury may be evident 1 to 4 days following intoxication, with jaundice and hepatomegaly, and serum transaminase levels may be markedly elevated. The striking pathologic features are centrilobular hepatic necrosis and diffuse fatty infiltration. Renal injury may be evident concomitantly or shortly thereafter, with azotemia, albuminuria, and oliguria progressing to anuria. Fatalities during the first week are usually due to liver injury, while deaths later in the course are usually the result of renal damage. When recovery occurs, it is complete by 4 to 6 weeks. Residual liver or renal disease has not been clearly demonstrated following a single acute exposure.

ACETAMINOPHEN HEPATOTOXICITY (DIRECT TOXIN) Acetaminophen (Tylenol), an analgesic and antipyretic that is available without a prescription, has caused severe centrilobular hepatic necrosis when ingested in large amounts in suicide attempts or accidently by children. A single dose of 10 to 15 g, occasionally less, may produce clinical evidence of liver injury. Fatal fulminant disease is usually associated with ingestion of 25 g or more, although not invariably. Blood levels of acetaminophen correlate with the severity of hepatic injury (levels above 300 μg/ml at 4 h after ingestion are predictive of the development of severe damage). Nausea, vomiting, diarrhea, abdominal pain, and shock are early manifestations occurring 4 to 12 h after ingestion. Twenty-four to forty-eight hours later, when these features are abating, hepatic injury becomes apparent. Maximal abnormalities and hepatic failure may not be evident until 4 to 6 days after ingestion. Renal failure and myocardial injury may be present.

Acetaminophen hepatotoxicity is mediated by a toxic reactive metabolite formed from the parent compound by the cytochrome P_{450} mixed-function oxidase system of the hepatocyte. This metabolite is detoxified by binding to glutathione. When excessive amounts of the metabolite are formed, glutathione levels in liver fall, and the metabolite is covalently bound to nucleophilic hepatocyte macromolecules. The latter process is believed to lead to hepatocyte necrosis; the precise sequence and mechanism are unknown. Hepatic injury may be potentiated by prior administration of alcohol or other drugs which stimulate the mixed-function oxidase system, or alternately by conditions, such as starvation, which reduce hepatic glutathione levels.

Treatment of acetaminophen overdosage includes gastric lavage, supportive measures, and oral administration of activated charcoal or cholestyramine to prevent absorption of residual drug. In patients with high acetaminophen blood levels, measured 4 to 10 h after ingestion, the administration of sulfhydryl compounds (e.g., cysteamine, cysteine, or *N*-acetylcysteine) within 12 h of ingestion appears to reduce the severity of hepatic necrosis. These agents act either by repleting hepatic glutathione, binding the reactive metabolite, or inhibiting its production. Late administration of sulfhydryl compounds is of uncertain value.

Although survivors of acute acetaminophen overdose usually have no evidence of hepatic sequelae, in a few patients prolonged or repeated administration of acetaminophen in therapeutic doses has led to the development of chronic active hepatitis and cirrhosis.

HALOTHANE HEPATOTOXICITY (IDIOSYNCRATIC REACTION)
Halothane, a nonexplosive fluorinated hydrocarbon anesthetic agent, structurally similar to chloroform, has been reported to result in severe hepatic necrosis in a small number of individuals, many of whom have previously been exposed to this agent. The failure to produce similar hepatic lesions in animals, the rarity of the hepatic impairment in humans, and the delayed appearance of hepatic injury suggest that halothane is not a direct hepatotoxin but may be a sensitizing agent. Fever, moderate leukocytosis, and eosinophilia may occur in the first week following halothane administration. Jaundice usually is noted 7 to 10 days after exposure but may occur earlier in previously exposed patients. Nausea and vomiting may precede the onset of jaundice. Hepatomegaly is often mild, but liver tenderness is common. The serum transaminases are elevated. The pathologic changes at autopsy are indistinguishable from massive hepatic necrosis due to viral hepatitis. The case fatality rate of halothane hepatitis is not known but may vary from 20 to 40 percent in cases with severe liver involvement. In rare instances cirrhosis has been observed following repeated bouts of halothane hepatitis. It is strongly suggested that patients in whom unexplained spiking fever, especially delayed fever, or jaundice develops after halothane anesthesia not receive this agent again. Because cross-reactions between halothane and methoxyflurane have been reported, the latter agent should probably not be used after halothane reactions.

ISONIAZID HEPATOTOXICITY (TOXIC AND IDIOSYNCRATIC REACTION)
Approximately 10 percent of patients treated with the antituberculosis agent isoniazid will develop elevated serum transaminase levels during the first few weeks of therapy; this appears to represent a toxic reaction to a metabolite of the drug. Whether or not isoniazid is continued, these values (usually < 200 units) return to normal in a few weeks. About 1 percent of treated patients develop an illness indistinguishable from viral hepatitis; approximately half of these occur within the first 2 months of treatment, while in the remainder clinical disease may be delayed for many months. Liver biopsy reveals morphologic changes similar to viral hepatitis or bridging hepatic necrosis. The disease may be severe, with a case fatality rate of 10 percent. Important liver injury appears to be age-related; the highest frequency is in patients over age 50, the lowest under the age 20. Fever, rash, eosinophilia, and other manifestations of drug allergy are distinctly unusual. A correlation of liver injury with rapid acetylation of isoniazid has been suggested. A picture resembling chronic active hepatitis has been observed in a few patients.

CHLORPROMAZINE HEPATOTOXICITY (CHOLESTATIC IDIOSYNCRATIC REACTION)
About 1 percent of patients receiving chlorpromazine develop intrahepatic cholestasis with jaundice after 1 to 4 weeks of treatment. In rare instances, jaundice has been reported after a single exposure. Anicteric reactions are frequent. The onset may be abrupt with fever, rash, ar-

thralgias, lymphadenopathy, nausea, vomiting, and epigastric or right upper quadrant pain. Pruritus may precede the appearance of jaundice, dark urine, and light stools. Eosinophilia with or without mild leukocytosis may be present, and conjugated hyperbilirubinemia, moderately elevated serum alkaline phosphatase, and mildly elevated serum transaminase levels (100 to 200 units) are noted. Liver biopsy reveals cholestasis, bile plugs in dilated bile canaliculi, and a dense portal infiltrate of polymorphonuclear, eosinophilic, and mononuclear leukocytes. Occasionally, scattered foci of hepatic parenchymal necrosis may be evident. Jaundice and pruritus usually subside within 4 to 8 weeks following cessation of therapy, without sequelae, and fatalities are rare. Cholestyramine may be of value in relieving severe pruritus. In a small number of patients, jaundice is prolonged for several months to years; rarely, a disorder resembling primary biliary cirrhosis may develop.

ORAL CONTRACEPTIVE HEPATOTOXICITY (CHOLESTATIC REACTION)
The administration of oral contraceptive combinations of estrogenic and progestational steroids results in significant BSP retention in a high proportion of patients, and, to a far lesser extent, elevation of serum alkaline phosphatase. Weeks to months after taking these agents, intrahepatic cholestasis with pruritus and jaundice is noted in a small number of patients. Especially susceptible seem to be patients with recurrent idiopathic jaundice of pregnancy, severe pruritus of pregnancy, or a family history of these disorders. Laboratory studies, with the exception of liver function tests, are normal, and extrahepatic manifestations of hypersensitivity are absent. Liver biopsy reveals cholestasis with bile plugs in dilated canaliculi and striking bilirubin staining of liver cells. In contrast to chlorpromazine-induced cholestasis, portal inflammation is absent. The lesion is reversible on withdrawal of the agent, and sequelae have not been reported. The two steroid components appear to act synergistically on hepatic function, although the estrogen may be primarily responsible. Oral contraceptives are contraindicated in patients with a history of recurrent jaundice of pregnancy. As indicated above, neoplasms of the liver and hepatic vein occlusion have also been associated with oral contraceptive therapy.

REFERENCES

DIENSTAG JL et al: Hepatitis A virus infection: New insights from seroepidemiologic studies. J Infect Dis 137:328, 1978

FEINSTONE SM, PURCELL RH: Non-A, non-B hepatitis. Annu Rev Med 29:359, 1978

GREGORY PB et al: Steroid therapy in severe viral hepatitis: A double blind, randomized trial of methyl-prednisolone versus placebo. N Engl J Med 294:681, 1976

KRUGMAN S et al: Viral hepatitis, type B: Studies on natural history and prevention re-examined. N Engl J Med 300:101, 1979

POPPER H: Clinical pathological correlation in viral hepatitis: The effect of the virus on the liver. Am J Pathol 81:609, 1975

Proceedings of a symposium on viral hepatitis. Am J Med Sci 270:1, 1975

VYAS GN et al (eds): *Viral Hepatitis.* Philadelphia, Franklin Institute Press, 1978

WANDS JR et al: Hepatitis-B in an oncology unit. N Engl J Med 291:1371, 1974

——— et al: Pathogenesis of arthritis associated with hepatitis-B surface antigen-positive hepatitis: Complement activation and characterization of circulating immune complexes. J Clin Invest 55:930, 1975

Toxic and drug-induced hepatitis

BLACK M et al: Isoniazid-associated hepatitis in 114 patients. Gastroenterology 69:389, 1975

ISHAK KG, IREY NS: Hepatic injury associated with the phenothiazines: Clinicopathologic and follow-up study of 36 patients. Arch Pathol 93:283, 1972

MITCHELL JR, JOLLOW DJ: Metabolic activation of drugs to toxic substances. Gastroenterology 68:392, 1975

ZIMMERMAN HJ: *Hepatotoxicity.* New York, Appleton-Century-Crofts, 1978

303
CHRONIC ACTIVE HEPATITIS

JACK R. WANDS
RAYMOND S. KOFF
KURT J. ISSELBACHER

DEFINITION Chronic active hepatitis is a disorder characterized by continuing hepatic necrosis, active inflammation, and fibrosis which may lead to or be accompanied by cirrhosis. While signs and symptoms of chronic liver disease are typical, manifestations of systemic involvement are common, and extrahepatic features and seroimmunologic abnormalities may dominate the clinical presentation. The prominence of these manifestations has led to the use of a variety of terms to describe this disorder. These terms include autoimmune hepatitis, lupoid hepatitis, acute juvenile cirrhosis, plasma cell hepatitis, subacute hepatitis, and chronic active liver disease. Chronic active hepatitis seems to be the most appropriate designation for this clinicopathologic entity, regardless of the etiology and the clinical variations.

PATHOLOGY Although chronic active hepatitis may be suspected from the clinical history and the physical findings, *liver biopsy is necessary to establish the diagnosis.* The cardinal histopathologic features observed in the liver include (1) a dense mononuclear and plasma cell infiltration of the portal zones which greatly expands these areas with extension of the inflammatory infiltrate into the liver lobule; (2) destruction of the hepatocytes at the periphery of the lobule (so-called "piecemeal necrosis") with erosion of the limiting plate; (3) connective tissue septa extending from the portal zones into the lobule, isolating parenchymal cells into clusters and enveloping bile ducts; and (4) evidence of hepatic regeneration with "rosette" formation, thickened liver-cell plates, and regenerative "pseudolobules." This process may be patchy, and individual liver lobules may remain uninvolved. Councilman-like bodies may be seen in the periportal areas representing necrosis of single liver cells. Early in the course of chronic active hepatitis the lesion of bridging hepatic necrosis may be seen in some patients. This lesion or its more extensive variant, multilobular bridging hepatic necrosis, suggests the presence of severe disease.

There is substantial morphologic evidence that in some instances chronic active hepatitis will progress to or is accompanied by the development of cirrhosis. On liver biopsy, cirrhosis can be demonstrated in 30 to 50 percent of patients, even early in the course of the disease, and at autopsy postnecrotic cirrhosis may be found. It is also possible that many cases of so-called "cryptogenic cirrhosis" are the result of chronic active

hepatitis after inflammation and necrosis have subsided. In other patients fibrosis is not progressive and morphologic evidence of cirrhosis cannot be found.

Chronic persistent hepatitis is often confused with chronic active hepatitis. While the clinical features of chronic persistent and chronic active hepatitis may be somewhat similar, the important distinction between these two entities is that chronic persistent hepatitis rarely if ever progresses to cirrhosis or produces portal hypertension or parenchymal liver failure. The diagnosis can be established with certainty only by liver biopsy. In typical chronic persistent hepatitis there is infiltration of the portal areas with mononuclear cells, but there is no erosion of the limiting plate (piecemeal necrosis) or extension of the inflammation into the liver lobule. A "cobblestone" arrangement of liver cells, indicative of hepatic regenerative activity, is a common feature. Minimal fibrosis may be observed, but cirrhosis is characteristically absent. The morphologic features of chronic active hepatitis and chronic persistent hepatitis are compared in Table 303-1.

ETIOLOGY Multiple etiologic agents may initiate chronic active hepatitis. Probably the most important and common triggering factors are infection with hepatitis B virus or the non-A, non-B hepatitis viruses. In about one-third of patients the disease begins abruptly following an illness typical of acute viral hepatitis. Persistence of the hepatitis B surface antigen (HBsAg) in the serum is found in 20 to 30 percent of patients with chronic active hepatitis, suggesting that persistent hepatitis B virus infection may be related to the development of chronic active hepatitis. Similarly persistent non-A, non-B hepatitis virus infections may be responsible for cases of chronic active hepatitis following transfusion-associated hepatitis. Furthermore, the transition of hepatitis B–induced bridging hepatic necrosis (see Chap. 301) to chronic active hepatitis has been observed and infection by non-A, non-B agents may be involved in the pathogenesis of some cases of chronic active hepatitis observed in immunosuppressed renal transplant recipients. Drugs are also involved in the pathogenesis. Features typical of chronic active hepatitis have been found in some patients in association with the ingestion of laxative preparations containing oxyphenisatin. In these patients challenge with oxyphenisatin has led to increased activity of the disease, while discontinuance has resulted in clinical, biochemical, and histologic improvement. α-Methyldopa, isoniazid, and other drugs have also been incriminated as etiologic agents in a few patients with chronic active hepatitis. Thus, chemical as well as viral agents may play a role in the production of chronic

TABLE 303-1
Distinguishing features of chronic active and chronic persistent hepatitis

Features	Chronic active hepatitis	Chronic persistent hepatitis
Clinical:		
Onset like acute viral hepatitis	30%	70%
Recurrent acute episodes	Common	Infrequent
Extrahepatic involvement (e.g., arthralgias, pleuritis, colitis)	Common	Rare
Prognosis	Variable	Good
Liver histology:		
Piecemeal necrosis	Characteristic	Inconstant
Site of inflammation	Portal extending into lobule	Portal
Lobular architecture	Distorted	Preserved
Fibrosis	Common	Slight
Progression to cirrhosis	Common	Rare

active hepatitis. The existence of other triggering factors seems likely, but their nature and mechanisms of action remain to be determined.

IMMUNOPATHOGENESIS There is increasing evidence that the progressive parenchymal-cell destruction in patients with chronic active hepatitis involves an interaction with the immune system which may be conditioned or controlled by genetic factors. Evidence to support this concept includes the following facts: (1) In the liver the histopathologic lesions are composed predominantly of *small lymphocytes* and plasma cells in association with progressive liver-cell destruction and replacement by fibrous tissue. (2) A variety of circulating "autoantibodies" are frequently detected, such as antismooth muscle, antimitochondrial, and antithyroid antibodies (see Table 303-2). (3) The persistence of HBsAg in the serum and the hepatitis B core antigen (HBcAg) in the liver cell following an attack of acute hepatitis B is frequently associated with the development of chronic active or chronic persistent hepatitis. (4) Other "autoimmune" diseases such as thyroiditis, ulcerative colitis, Coombs-positive hemolytic anemia, proliferative glomerulonephritis, and Sjögren's syndrome may be associated with chronic active hepatitis or are observed in relatives of affected patients. (5) Histocompatibility antigen HLA-B1 or -B8 are more prevalent than expected in patients with chronic active hepatitis without HBsAg. (6) Finally, the use of corticosteroids, believed to be effective in a variety of immunologic and autoimmune disorders, is often beneficial in the treatment of severe chronic active hepatitis.

There is increasing evidence that cellular immune reactions may be important in the pathogenesis of chronic active hepatitis. It has been suggested that lymphocytes become sensitized to altered or new antigens present on the surface membranes of hepatocytes. This hypothesis is supported in part by studies demonstrating that circulating lymphocytes may have the capability of causing liver cell damage in vitro.

Humoral immune mechanisms may be responsible for some of the clinical manifestations of chronic active hepatitis. Thus, extrahepatic features such as arthralgias, arthritis, rash, and glomerulonephritis appear to be mediated by the deposition of circulating immune complexes. Furthermore, complement activation, as demonstrated by low serum complement levels, and the presence of complement components in immune complexes suggest that circulating immune complexes may be involved in mediating extrahepatic inflammation and tissue damage.

CLINICAL FEATURES The clinical spectrum of chronic active hepatitis extends from asymptomatic illness at one end to fatal hepatic failure at the other. It affects all age groups but the idiopathic disorder is more common in young women and adolescents. In approximately two-thirds of patients the disease has an *insidious onset* over a period of several weeks to months. In a number of individuals the disease is discovered inciden-

TABLE 303-2
Serological abnormalities in chronic active hepatitis

Serological tests or reactions	Frequency, %
Increased serum IgG, IgM, IgA	50–70
Smooth-muscle antibodies	40–80
Antinuclear antibodies	20–50
Antimitochondrial antibodies	10–20
Lupus erythematosus (LE) cells	10–20
Rheumatoid factor	10–20
Heterophile reaction	5–10
Antigastric, antithyroid, antiadrenal antibodies	<5
False-positive syphilis test	<5

tally, and the duration of the illness is uncertain. In the remainder an abrupt onset similar to acute viral hepatitis is seen, but features of chronic active hepatitis usually develop during the ensuing 12 to 24 months. The clinical and laboratory features suggesting progression from acute hepatitis to chronic active hepatitis are discussed in Chap. 302. *Fatigue* is a common symptom. Persistent or recurrent *jaundice* is noted in about 80 percent of typical cases. Intermittent deepening of jaundice and recurrent symptoms of *malaise, anorexia,* and *low-grade fever,* suggestive of a superimposed acute hepatitis, are common throughout the course of the illness. In some patients complications of cirrhosis may first bring the patient to medical attention. In others the extrahepatic features dominate the clinical picture, and liver disease is entirely unsuspected. Extrahepatic presenting features may include amenorrhea, bloody diarrhea (due to associated ulcerative colitis), abdominal pain, arthralgia or arthritis, macular or papular eruptions, acne, erythema nodosum, pleurisy, pericarditis, anemia, azotemia, and sicca syndrome (of keratoconjunctivitis and xerostomia). These extrahepatic features and abnormal serologic reactions tend to be more frequent in women than men and in patients without serologic evidence of preceding hepatitis B.

The *course* of chronic active hepatitis is variable, and the disease may persist for long periods without clinically overt liver disease. This appears to be particularly true of chronic active hepatitis associated with hepatitis B. The condition may occasionally remit into a clinically inactive phase, although continuing hepatocellular necrosis or progression to cirrhosis may also occur. The histologic lesion may reverse itself completely before the development of cirrhosis in some HBsAg-positive patients after their antigenemia has spontaneously cleared. If untreated, the case fatality rate may be high (50 to 75 percent) during the first few years of illness, especially in patients with clinically severe disease and histologically confirmed chronic active hepatitis with cirrhosis and in those with bridging or multilobular hepatic necrosis, when death occurs as a result of liver failure and hepatic coma. Later death is often due to a complication of cirrhosis—variceal hemorrhage or intercurrent infection. Primary hepatocellular carcinoma is an uncommon complication of chronic active hepatitis, particularly in HBsAg-positive individuals and when the disease has progressed to postnecrotic cirrhosis. In a small number of patients clinical and histologic features of primary biliary cirrhosis may be noted during the course of typical chronic active hepatitis which emphasizes the clinical similarity between these two liver disorders, particularly in the early phase of illness. In most instances, however, a clinical and histologic distinction between these conditions can eventually be made.

LABORATORY FINDINGS Liver function tests are invariably abnormal but may not correlate with the clinical severity or histopathologic findings in the individual case. In fact, some patients have normal serum bilirubin, alkaline phosphatase, and globulin determinations with only minimal transaminase (aminotransferase) elevations or HBsAg positivity and yet have a liver biopsy consistent with severe chronic active hepatitis. In typical cases the serum bilirubin is moderately elevated (3 to 10 mg per 100 ml). Serum aspartate aminotransferase (SGOT) levels are increased and fluctuate in the range of 100 to 1000 units in most cases, although values as high as 4000 units have been reported.

The hepatitis B surface antigen may be found in 20 to 30 percent of patients with chronic active hepatitis and more commonly in men than women. Hypergammaglobulinemia (>

2.5 g per 100 ml) is common, particularly in patients with extensive plasma-cell infiltration of the liver. Mild hypoalbuminemia occurs in patients with active disease or in those with advanced cirrhosis. Serum alkaline phosphatase levels may be moderately elevated or near normal. The prothrombin time is often prolonged, particularly late in the disease or during active phases.

A variety of abnormal serologic reactions and circulating "autoantibodies" are found in chronic active hepatitis. Some of these serologic reactions are nonspecific and may be seen in other viral diseases. Circulating autoantibodies against DNA, IgG, smooth muscle, and mitochondria support the concept that chronic active hepatitis is indeed a systemic disease. Table 303-2 depicts some of the abnormal serologic reactions observed in chronic active hepatitis.

DIFFERENTIAL DIAGNOSIS Early in the course of chronic active hepatitis the disease may resemble typical *acute viral hepatitis*. However, the persistence of symptoms, including biochemical abnormalities such as elevated serum transaminase and bilirubin levels or circulating HBsAg over the ensuing months indicates that a chronic liver disorder is present. The major entity which is often confused with chronic active hepatitis is *chronic persistent hepatitis*. As indicated in Table 303-1, in chronic persistent hepatitis the onset of the illness frequently resembles acute hepatitis. The transaminase enzymes are usually elevated to a mild degree in chronic persistent hepatitis, and HBsAg may be present in serum. Fatigue, anorexia, malaise, right upper quadrant discomfort, and hepatomegaly may be associated with either chronic persistent or chronic active hepatitis. Thus, a definitive diagnosis can be established by liver biopsy since a *differentiation between chronic active and chronic persistent hepatitis cannot be made by clinical and biochemical criteria*. This distinction is important because chronic persistent hepatitis is not a progressive disorder, rarely if ever results in cirrhosis, and requires no therapy.

The presence of extrahepatic manifestations in chronic active hepatitis such as pleuritis, arthritis, and arthralgias may cause confusion with *connective tissue disorders* such as rheumatoid arthritis and systemic lupus erythematosus. The existence of clinical and biochemical features suggestive of progressive liver disease clearly distinguishes chronic active hepatitis from these disorders. In adolescence, *Wilson's disease* may present with features of chronic active hepatitis before the neurologic manifestations become apparent; serum ceruloplasmin, serum and urinary copper determination, and measurement of the liver copper levels will establish the diagnosis. Late in the course of chronic active hepatitis some patients may present with *postnecrotic cirrhosis* without evidence of active hepatitis. This lesion, termed cryptogenic cirrhosis, may also represent an end stage of other destructive liver diseases (e.g., primary biliary cirrhosis). *Primary biliary cirrhosis,* as previously mentioned, may share histologic similarities with chronic active hepatitis particularly early in the disease. However, in primary biliary cirrhosis the prominence of pruritus plus markedly elevated serum alkaline phosphatase and cholesterol levels, the presence of high titers of antimitochondrial antibodies (in contrast to the low levels seen in chronic active hepatitis), and the pattern of histologic progression will usually permit differentiation from chronic active hepatitis.

MANAGEMENT During episodes of active disease the patient should be managed as in acute viral hepatitis with general supportive care. Hospitalization may be required to define the severity and extent of disease, to verify the presence of extrahepatic involvement, and to confirm the diagnosis by percutaneous liver biopsy. Restriction of activity is indicated during active phases, but prolonged bed rest following remission is unnecessary. Corticosteroid therapy is the treatment of choice in symptomatic HBsAg-negative chronic active hepatitis and bridging or multilobular hepatic necrosis. Corticosteroids have been shown to be effective in prolonging survival of these patients during the first few years of illness when the mortality rate is high. A therapeutic response characterized by a complete clinical, biochemical, and histologic remission is to be expected in 60 to 80 percent of patients. Prednisone or prednisolone therapy should be initiated at a dose of 40 to 60 mg daily. This dose can usually be gradually tapered within 2 to 3 months to 15 to 20 mg daily. The beneficial effects of corticosteroid treatment on the course and prognosis of patients with mild or asymptomatic chronic active hepatitis (in the absence of cirrhosis or multilobular necrosis) remain to be determined.

The effect of corticosteroids on the natural course of HBsAg-positive chronic active hepatitis is less clear. It is difficult to justify treatment of *asymptomatic* HBsAg carriers who have evidence only of chronic active hepatitis on liver biopsy. In such patients, the disease may be mild and corticosteroid therapy is often associated with little improvement in aminotransferase (transaminase) values and liver histology. Similarly, in *symptomatic* HBsAg-positive patients with chronic active hepatitis the value of corticosteroids has not been shown with certainty. Close follow-up examinations and a repeat liver biopsy 6 months to 1 year following the initial evaluation is often helpful to establish the natural course of the disease and to determine whether fibrosis or cirrhosis has developed. If the disease has progressed, a trial of corticosteroids may be warranted. However, if objective improvement in the clinical and biochemical features of the disease is not apparent after several months of therapy, corticosteroids should be discontinued.

When corticosteroids are used, improvement of fatigue and anorexia is noted within days to several weeks. Biochemical improvement is to be expected over several weeks to months, with a fall in serum bilirubin and globulin levels and a rise in serum albumin. The serum transaminase level usually drops promptly, but the absolute value of the transaminase *alone* does not appear to be a useful marker of recovery in the individual patient. Histologic improvement, characterized by a decrease in mononuclear infiltration and subsequent improvement in the extent of hepatocellular necrosis, may be delayed for 6 to 24 months. After a favorable clinical and biochemical response, repeat liver biopsy may show features consistent with chronic persistent hepatitis.

Reduction of the suppressive corticosteroid doses should be performed cautiously, particularly at lower prednisone levels, since even small decrements in therapy may be associated with clinical worsening, and increasing dosage may be needed for control of spontaneous exacerbation. Unless major complications require discontinuation of corticosteroids, they should be prescribed for at least 12 months or longer, even after clinical and biochemical recovery, in order to prevent a high relapse rate.

Other therapeutic approaches have been used in the treatment of chronic active hepatitis, particularly in the elderly and in patients with major side effects from corticosteroids. An initial prednisone dosage of 30 mg, tapered down to 10 to 20 mg in combination with 50 to 75 mg azathioprine has been demonstrated to be effective; this treatment avoids the adverse effects of high dosage of corticosteroids. However, *azathioprine alone is not effective* in the treatment of chronic active hepatitis. Alternate-day prednisone therapy diminishes steroid side effects but usually does not provide adequate therapy.

REFERENCES

BOYER JL: Chronic hepatitis—a perspective on classification and determinants of prognosis. Gastroenterology 70:1161, 1976

GOLDING PL et al: Multisystem involvement in chronic liver disease. Studies on the incidence and pathogenesis. Am J Med 55:772, 1973

SCHALM SW et al: Contrasting features and responses to treatment of severe chronic active liver disease with and without hepatitis Bs antigen. Gut 17:781, 1976

WANDS JR et al: Arthritis associated with chronic active hepatitis: Complement activation and characterization of circulating immune complex. Gastroenterology 69:1286, 1975

WRIGHT EC et al: Treatment of chronic active hepatitis: An analysis of three controlled trials. Gastroenterology 73:1422, 1977

304
CIRRHOSIS

J. THOMAS LaMONT
RAYMOND S. KOFF
KURT J. ISSELBACHER

DEFINITION Morphologic Cirrhosis is a generic term that includes all forms of chronic diffuse liver disease characterized by extensive loss of liver cells and collapse and fibrosis of the supporting reticulin network, with distortion of the vascular bed and nodular regeneration of the remaining liver cell masses which are surrounded by fibrous tissue. The sine qua non of cirrhosis is extensive disorganization of the hepatic lobular architecture. The basic precursor of this lesion is believed to be diffuse liver cell death; however, evidence of necrosis may no longer be apparent when liver tissue is examined. The network of scars, the regenerating cell masses, and the changes in hepatic circulation develop secondarily. Less constant pathologic features of most types of cirrhosis include intralobular or portal inflammation, focal or widespread cholestasis, and proliferation of bile ductules.

Clinical and functional The morphologic elements of cirrhosis often have dramatic clinical counterparts. Progressive reduction of liver cell mass may produce jaundice, ascites and edema, central nervous system dysfunction, and cachexia—the syndrome of hepatic insufficiency. The advancing fibrosis leads to distortion of the intrahepatic vasculature, which in turn contributes to the development of portal venous hypertension with resultant esophageal and gastric varices and splenomegaly. Nodular regeneration often leads to distortion of liver shape and compression of intrahepatic venous and lymphatic radicles, which also contribute to portal hypertension and ascites. No clinical, etiologic, or morphologic classification of cirrhosis is satisfactory at present. Clinical signs and symptoms may not reflect accurately the extent and precise nature of the cirrhotic process or its stage of evolution or activity. In addition, pathologic patterns may represent nonspecific hepatic responses to many different forms of liver cell injury, while a variety of morphological patterns may be produced by a specific etiology in a single patient. However, in spite of these limitations, it is possible to categorize most cases of cirrhosis clinically, adding qualifying morphologic or etiologic terms when possible. Most types of cirrhosis can be classified as follows: (1) alcoholic, (2) postnecrotic, (3) biliary (either primary or secondary), (4) hemochromatosis, (5) cardiac or congestive, or (6) rare forms and cirrhosis of uncertain etiology.

ALCOHOLIC LIVER DISEASE AND CIRRHOSIS

DEFINITION Alcoholic liver disease is the term used to describe the spectrum of liver injury associated with acute and chronic alcoholism. Three components are recognized: (1) alcoholic fatty liver, (2) alcoholic hepatitis, and (3) alcoholic cirrhosis. These entities may exist independently, or coexist in the same liver. Furthermore, while fatty liver is a regular feature of both acute and chronic alcoholism, available evidence suggests that by itself fatty liver does not lead to the development of cirrhosis. On the other hand alcoholic hepatitis in some cases appears to be the precursor of alcoholic cirrhosis, although progression to cirrhosis is not invariable. Since alcohol may stimulate fibrogenesis and collagen synthesis in the liver, it is possible that cirrhosis may occur, at least in some instances, without preceding alcoholic hepatitis.

Alcoholic cirrhosis, the most common variety encountered in North America and many parts of Western Europe and South America, is characterized by diffuse fine scarring, a fairly uniform loss of liver cells, and small (often less than lobule-sized) islands of preserved or regenerating parenchyma. The terms *Laennec's, micronodular, portal,* and *fatty cirrhosis* have also been used to describe this type of chronic liver disease. While the eponym has some historical value, each of the other terms has misleading implications: etiologic factors other than alcohol may lead to micronodular cirrhosis and in late stages of alcoholic disease macronodular lesions may predominate; the fibrosis and scarring may not be centered about the portal triads; and cirrhosis may develop in the absence of important fatty infiltration of liver cells.

ETIOLOGY Experimental studies of both normal and alcoholic subjects have shown that ethanol (in moderate to large doses) produces liver dysfunction and fatty infiltration (Chap. 299) despite the ingestion of a well-balanced diet. This pattern of liver injury (*alcoholic fatty liver*) is completely reversible on cessation of alcoholism. If alcoholism continues, fatty liver persists. Most alcoholics with fatty liver do not develop alcoholic hepatitis or cirrhosis. However, some individuals develop an inflammatory reaction with polymorphonuclear infiltration and liver cell necrosis in addition to fatty changes. This lesion of *alcoholic hepatitis* may be the forerunner of cirrhosis, because healing with fibrosis distorts the normal lobular architecture. Many epidemiologic studies have implicated chronic alcoholism as the major cause of alcoholic cirrhosis: Between 10 and 20 percent of chronic alcoholic patients in the United States have clinical or morphologic evidence of cirrhosis. The quantity and duration of drinking necessary to cause cirrhosis is unknown, but average social usage is not sufficient to cause permanent liver damage. The typical alcoholic with cirrhosis has consumed a pint or more of whisky, several quarts of wine, or an equivalent amount of beer per day for at least 10 years. The amount of ethanol, rather than the type of alcoholic beverage, is the determinant factor.

Most chronic alcoholics consume protein- and vitamin-poor diets and may develop other clinical syndromes clearly related to faulty nutrition (exemplified by folate deficiency or Korsakoff-Wernicke's disease); treatment of cirrhotic patients with protein-rich diets often produces clinical and morphologic improvement. For these and other reasons, including the observation of a hepatic lesion closely resembling alcoholic injury in patients undergoing intestinal bypass operations for the control of obesity, absolute or relative *malnutrition* is regarded as a contributing factor to the evolution of cirrhosis. Although malnutrition per se does not lead to cirrhosis, a reasonable concept, based on much circumstantial evidence, is that a combination of *chronic alcohol ingestion plus impaired nutrition* leads to alcoholic hepatitis and cirrhosis.

Intercurrent bacterial *infections* are common in cirrhotic patients and seem, on occasion, to accelerate the course of the disease. There are, however, no firm data to implicate overt or latent infection in the pathogenesis of alcoholic cirrhosis. Icteric or anicteric bridging hepatic necrosis, presumably of viral origin, may occasionally lead to the development of a finely nodular cirrhosis resembling alcoholic cirrhosis in its general morphologic character, perhaps explaining the frequent reports of portal cirrhosis in nonalcoholic patients in England. Serial biopsies in these cases do not show many of the characteristic histologic features of progressive alcoholic cirrhosis (see below), and such cases may represent variants of postnecrotic cirrhosis.

Although rates of ethanol metabolism are under genetic control, no *metabolic defect* has been identified in cirrhotic patients or their families to suggest a unique "susceptibility" to ethanol or its toxic effects. Nonetheless, it is clear that individual tolerance to ethanol and its capacity to induce cirrhosis varies widely and that a true biologic predisposition to ethanol-induced liver diseases may exist.

PATHOLOGY AND PATHOGENESIS **Alcoholic fatty liver** The liver is enlarged, yellow, greasy, and firm. The parenchymal cells are usually diffusely abnormal, and many are distended by cytoplasmic fat vacuoles. When large, these triglyceride-containing vacuoles may push the hepatocyte nucleus to the periphery of the cell and flatten it against the cell membrane. Alcohol-induced hepatic triglyceride accumulation results from a number of alterations in fat metabolism; however, decreased mitochondrial fatty acid oxidation may play a key role. Triglyceride disappears with therapy and abstinence and recurs promptly after resumption of alcohol ingestion.

Alcoholic hepatitis Morphologic features include hepatic cell degeneration and necrosis, often with ballooned cells, accompanied by an infiltrate consisting of polymorphonuclear leukocytes and lymphocytes. The polymorphonuclears may encircle damaged hepatocytes which contain intracytoplasmic *Mallory bodies* or *alcoholic hyaline.* These irregular, dendritic, or bead-like clumps of perinuclear, deeply eosinophilic material have a fibrillar or tubular appearance on electron microscopy. They may represent aggregates of intracellular (actin) filaments. In some patients Mallory bodies and hepatic cell necrosis are prominent in the centrilobular region, producing the lesion of *sclerosing hyaline necrosis.* In patients with cirrhosis and recurrent or continuing alcoholic hepatitis the Mallory bodies tend to be found in liver cells at the periphery of nodules. Mallory bodies are highly suggestive but *not specific* for alcoholic hepatitis since morphologically similar material has been seen in occasional patients with Wilson's disease, primary biliary cirrhosis, hepatocellular carcinoma, and following intestinal bypass surgery. They are commonly found in Indian juvenile cirrhosis.

Immunological mechanisms may have a role in the pathogenesis of alcoholic hepatitis. Thymus-derived (T) lymphocytes are sequestered in the liver and may be reduced in the peripheral blood. Sensitization of T lymphocytes and a humoral response to alcoholic hyaline antigens have been described. The precise responsible mechanism remains to be determined.

Both alcoholic hepatitis and cirrhosis have been reported to occur in baboons given large amounts of alcohol for prolonged periods, but this model has not yet been confirmed.

Alcoholic cirrhosis As alcoholism continues and the liver disease advances, hepatocytes are destroyed, fibroblasts are found at the sites of injury, and collagen formation is stimulated. *Web-like septa of connective tissue appear in periportal and pericentral zones.* These fibrous septa become denser and more confluent, connecting portal triads and central veins. The fine connective tissue network contains small vessels, lymphatics, and other remnants of portal triads and surrounds small masses of liver cells. These lobular remnants undergo regeneration and form nodules. Inflammation is usually minimal and transient, but may be a prominent morphologic feature during acute exacerbations of alcoholic hepatitis. As the liver cell mass diminishes, the liver shrinks in size, acquires a finely nodular (hobnail) appearance, and becomes hard.

Alcoholic cirrhosis is basically a progressive disease, but appropriate therapy and strict avoidance of alcohol may arrest the disease at most stages and permit repair and functional improvement. Continued loss of liver cells by focal necrosis due to alcoholic hepatitis or continued stimulation of collagen formation results in progressive stromal collapse, fibrosis, and vascular distortion. Although regeneration occurs within the small remnants of parenchyma, cell loss eventually exceeds replacement, the liver cell mass dwindles, and a phase of irreversible, or end-stage, cirrhosis is reached.

CLINICAL FEATURES **Signs and symptoms** Clinical manifestations of alcoholic *fatty liver* are usually minimal or entirely absent, and the disorder may not be recognized unless another illness (e.g., alcoholic pancreatitis) brings the patient to medical attention. Hepatomegaly may be the only finding which signals the presence of alcoholic fatty liver. Jaundice, ascites, and edema are usually absent unless more serious liver injury is present.

The clinical spectrum of *alcoholic hepatitis* is extremely broad, varying from patients who are completely asymptomatic to those with severe hepatic insufficiency which may be fatal. Initial episodes are more likely to be clinically silent than recurrent or continuing bouts of alcoholic hepatitis in which clinical manifestations may be striking. Clinical features resemble those of viral or toxic liver injury. Anorexia, nausea and vomiting, malaise, weight loss, abdominal distress, and jaundice are common presenting complaints. Fever may be seen in about 50 percent of patients. Hepatomegaly is the most common physical finding. Liver tenderness may be present. Arterial "spider" angiomata, jaundice, ascites, and edema are common, and the spleen is enlarged in about a third of cases.

In many patients alcoholic hepatitis is superimposed upon or presents concurrently with alcoholic cirrhosis, but it is the former which is responsible for clinical manifestations. Jaundice and other signs of hepatic dysfunction may subside with therapy, but continued alcoholic excess and poor dietary habits lead to further episodes of hepatic decompensation. Acute acceleration of alcoholic liver damage may follow protracted drinking bouts. Fever, nausea and vomiting, deepening jaundice, hepatic encephalopathy, and ascites may occur rapidly in association with widespread liver cell loss and inflammation. Although some patients die during the acute exacerbations, most recover after several weeks or months. A few patients experience one or more transient episodes of cholestatic jaundice during the course of alcoholic liver disease. Clinical and laboratory studies may suggest the presence of mechanical biliary obstruction, but liver biopsy and the response to conservative therapy usually support the diagnosis of intrahepatic cholestasis.

Alcoholic cirrhosis also may be clinically silent, and about 10 percent of cases are discovered incidentally at laparotomy or autopsy. Men are affected more frequently than women, but this sex difference has decreased steadily in recent years as drinking habits have changed in many Western countries. Although the average age of onset of symptoms is about 50 years, cirrhosis may be found in alcoholic patients in the third or fourth decade of life.

Typically, after 10 or more years of alcohol excess, progressive liver dysfunction, fluid retention, and portal hypertension may become evident. After a period of weeks or months, the patient notes gradually increasing weakness and fatigability, anorexia, slight weight loss, jaundice, intermittent ankle edema, and increasing abdominal girth due to ascites. A firm and enlarged liver may be the only sign of disease, but additional typical findings include muscle wasting, jaundice, spider angiomas, gynecomastia and testicular atrophy (in men), menstrual irregularity or amenorrhea (in women), palmar erythema, splenomegaly, and ascites. Loss of body hair, parotid gland enlargement, purpura, clubbing of the fingers, and diffuse hyperpigmentation of the skin are common but less specific clinical signs. Dupuytren's contractures are not infrequent in alcoholics but are not specifically related to cirrhosis. Low-grade fever without shaking chills is frequent.

Over a period of 3 to 5 years, the cirrhotic patient becomes emaciated, weak, and chronically jaundiced; and ascites and signs of portal hypertension become increasingly prominent. Most patients with advanced cirrhosis die in hepatic coma, often precipitated by hemorrhage from esophageal varices or intercurrent infection. Acute and chronic pancreatitis and peptic ulceration occur with greater frequency in cirrhotic patients than in normal subjects. Gram-negative bacteremia, acute bacterial peritonitis, and hepatocellular carcinoma are uncommon complications.

Laboratory findings Laboratory studies are often unremarkable in alcoholic fatty liver except for minimal SGOT (aspartate aminotransferase) elevations. In more severe alcoholic liver disease laboratory abnormalities are characteristic. Anemia is often present. The etiology is almost always complex, and acute and chronic gastrointestinal blood loss, folic acid deficiency, hypersplenism, and a direct toxic effect of alcohol on the bone marrow are contributing causes. Hemolytic anemia accompanied by hypercholesterolemia and unusual spur-like projections of the erythrocyte membrane (acanthocytosis) have been described in some alcoholics with cirrhosis. Leukopenia and thrombocytopenia may result from hypersplenism or be a direct effect of alcohol on the bone marrow. Many patients have marked leukocytosis and a leukemoid reaction may be seen in a few. Liver function tests reveal hyperbilirubinemia and variable elevations of serum alkaline phosphatase. The SGOT is usually less than 250 units, although the SGPT (alanine aminotransferase) is usually lower and may be nearly normal. (A ratio of SGOT/SGPT greater than 2 is found more frequently in patients with alcoholic hepatitis than with viral hepatitis.) In patients with the lesion of sclerosing hyaline necrosis, SGOT levels may be considerably higher and may exceed 500 units. The serum albumin is usually depressed, while globulins are increased. Quantitative immunoglobulin determinations reveal elevations of all classes, especially IgG. In severe cases clotting factor deficiencies are common, as manifested by prolongation of the prothrombin and partial thromboplastin times. Elevated blood ammonia levels reflect a combination of impaired liver function and shunting of portal blood around the liver into the systemic circulation.

A diabetic type of glucose tolerance may occur in cirrhosis and appears to be a reflection of endogenous insulin resistance; however, clinical diabetes is uncommon. Respiratory alkalosis is frequently present, and reflects a tendency to hyperpnea seen in these patients. Hypomagnesemia is also common, and results from dietary deficiency and increased urinary losses. Dilutional hyponatremia and hypokalemia from excessive urinary loss are frequent in patients with ascites and edema, and reflect secondary hyperaldosteronism.

DIAGNOSIS Alcoholic fatty liver should be suspected in alcoholic patients with hepatomegaly. Alcoholic hepatitis should be considered in an alcoholic with recent heavy drinking who presents with an enlarged tender liver, jaundice, fever, and ascites. This variant of alcoholic liver disease can be fatal; and variceal bleeding, infection, and hepatic encephalopathy are

common. Although corticosteroids and propylthiouracil may cause a decrease in serum transaminase and bilirubin, their role in altering the prognosis of alcoholic hepatitis remains to be determined.

Alcoholic cirrhosis should be strongly suspected in patients with a history of prolonged or excessive alcohol intake, hepatomegaly and other signs of chronic liver disease, plus laboratory evidence of hepatic dysfunction. If there are no contraindications, most patients should have a percutaneous needle biopsy of the liver to confirm the diagnosis as well as to determine the stage and activity of the disease process. When the course of an otherwise stable cirrhotic patient changes without obvious explanation, complicating conditions such as occult bleeding, infection, hepatocellular carcinoma, and portal vein thrombosis should be sought.

PROGNOSIS Both retrospective and prospective studies of the natural history of severe alcoholic liver disease show that early, vigorous, and meticulous medical care will prolong life, decrease morbidity, and delay or prevent the appearance of certain complications. Patients with cirrhosis who abstain from alcohol and consume nutritious diets have a 5-year survival rate of about 60 percent, whereas those who continue to drink have a 40 percent 5-year survival rate. Mortality rates are higher in patients with complications, such as variceal bleeding or ascites, in whom abstinence may not improve survival rates. Massive variceal hemorrhage is a major direct or contributing cause of death in many patients. Although surgical shunts are effective in reducing portal hypertension, the overall prognosis remains poor in patients with advanced, irreversible liver disease.

TREATMENT Alcoholic hepatitis and cirrhosis are serious illnesses that require prolonged medical supervision and management. In most instances it is desirable to hospitalize the patient for initial study and assessment of the response to therapy as well as for dietary and medical instruction.

In the absence of signs of impending hepatic coma, a *diet* containing at least 1 g protein per kilogram of body weight and 2000 to 3000 cal per day should be prescribed. Because the patient with alcoholic hepatitis is often anorectic or nauseated, these dietary aims may be achieved by offering the patient three or four small meals with supplemental feedings of eggnog or ice cream. Vitamin supplements, in the form of multivitamin capsules, may be given, but there is no rationale for the clinical use of lipotropic agents. In the presence of Wernicke-Korsakoff disease (see Chap. 371) the patient should receive large parenteral doses of thiamine. The patient should understand clearly that neither nutritious diet nor added vitamins will protect the liver against the effects of further alcohol ingestion. *Therefore, alcohol should be absolutely forbidden.*

Ascites and edema may disappear with bed rest alone. More persistent fluid retention should be treated with *salt restriction,* utilizing diets that contain 1 to 2 g sodium chloride per day. Water restriction, limiting fluid intake to volumes that equal the measured fluid loss of the prior day, may be necessary if hyponatremia is present. In patients with active disease (i.e., jaundice, or signs of hepatic insufficiency) diuretics should be used with great caution in order to prevent electrolyte depletion, hypovolemia, and hepatic encephalopathy (see "Ascites" later in this chapter).

Confusion, drowsiness, or other signs of impending *hepatic coma* should be treated by prompt decrease in protein intake to levels of 20 to 30 g daily of less. A careful search for intercurrent bacterial infection and for gastrointestinal hemorrhage should be made, including the aspiration of gastric contents, and appropriate therapy to control infection or bleeding should be instituted. Possible offending drugs, especially diuretics and sedatives, should be omitted and any electrolyte imbalance corrected promptly (see "Hepatic Encephalopathy," below). Despite randomized studies from several studies the role of corticosteroids in acute alcoholic hepatitis remains controversial. In several studies a beneficial response was observed with prednisone or prednisolone 40 mg per day, while other investigators have been unable to confirm this. Preliminary studies suggest that propylthiouracil may be helpful.

Anemia should be characterized and corrected by appropriate means. Folic acid deficiency is particularly common in alcoholics and requires replacement therapy. *Fever,* especially when low-grade and unaccompanied by chills or other signs of infection, may be a manifestation of alcoholic hepatitis. However, the presence of hectic or persistent fever or shaking chills requires a vigorous search for septic processes, especially urinary tract infection, pneumonia, gram-negative bacteremia, or peritonitis.

POSTNECROTIC CIRRHOSIS

DEFINITION This form of chronic liver disease, the most common type of cirrhosis on a worldwide basis, is characterized morphologically by (1) confluent, often extensive loss of liver cells, (2) stromal collapse and fibrosis that produce broad bands of connective tissue containing the remains of many triads, and (3) irregular, large nodules, varying in size from microscopic to grossly visible, of intake or regenerating parenchyma. This pattern, which may vary considerably in extent and severity, results from an overall but unequal injury to the liver. As with other forms of cirrhosis, the appearance of advanced postnecrotic disease offers little insight into the original or potentiating causes of the liver cell damage.

The terms *toxic cirrhosis, coarsely nodular cirrhosis, posthepatic cirrhosis, cryptogenic cirrhosis,* and *multilobular cirrhosis,* are synonymous with postnecrotic cirrhosis.

ETIOLOGY The cause of postnecrotic cirrhosis is still unknown, but epidemiologic and serologic evidence suggests that viral hepatitis is an antecedent factor in many instances. In the United States, about 25 percent of patients with postnecrotic cirrhosis have a history compatible with recent or remote attacks of acute viral hepatitis. Furthermore, the progression of bridging hepatic necrosis through chronic active hepatitis (see Chap. 303) to postnecrotic cirrhosis is well documented. Approximately 5 to 20 percent of patients with established postnecrotic disease have positive serologic tests for HBsAg. A few patients with postnecrotic cirrhosis associated with hepatitis B have negative blood tests but have hepatitis B antigens present in liver tissue. Non-A, non-B viral hepatitis may be responsible for some cases, but hepatitis A is not an established cause.

A small percentage of cases stem from documented *intoxications* with industrial *chemicals* (e.g., phosphorus), poisons (e.g., *Amanita phalloides* toxins), or drugs (oxyphenisatin, α-methyldopa). Finally, certain *infections* (e.g., brucellosis), *parasitic infections* (clonorchiasis), *metabolic disorders* (hepatolenticular degeneration), and *advanced alcoholic liver disease* may produce confluent cell loss and result in postnecrotic cirrhosis.

PATHOLOGY AND PATHOGENESIS Typically, the postnecrotic liver is small, grossly distorted in shape, and composed of nodules of liver cells separated by dense, wide, sunken scars. Microscopically, the established lesion includes (1) large islands of parenchymal cells with rounded (inactive) or ragged (active) margins; (2) interdigitating broad to thin fibrous septa containing distorted vessels, lymphatics, and bile ducts derived from many portal areas; and (3) prominent mononuclear inflammatory infiltrates, often in the form of follicles or clusters. In some sections of liver, lobular architecture appears nearly normal, but central veins are absent or markedly displaced.

Current evidence suggests that infectious, toxic, metabolic, or nutritional factors initiate the postnecrotic process. The destruction appears to progress as the result of similar repeated or persistent insults or possibly on the basis of "autoimmune" liver cell injury.

CLINICAL FEATURES Postnecrotic cirrhosis affects women at least as often as men and should be suspected in nonalcoholic patients with evidence of chronic liver disease, especially in those in the younger age group. Like those with alcoholic cirrhosis, a few patients with postnecrotic disease may have little clinical evidence of advanced cirrhosis, the diagnosis being made at operation or postmortem examination or by a needle biopsy performed to investigate asymptomatic hepatosplenomegaly. About 25 percent of patients present with signs and symptoms suggesting active hepatitis, but often with atypical features such as prolonged illness, intense and protracted jaundice, ascites, or manifestations of portal hypertension. Splenomegaly may be the only sign of postnecrotic cirrhosis, and hypersplenism may be prominent. Some patients have bouts of upper abdominal pain, the sudden onset of unexplained ascites, episodes of hepatic encephalopathy, or massive variceal hemorrhage as the major or initial clinical feature. The signs and symptoms of postnecrotic cirrhosis resemble those of alcoholic cirrhosis and reflect the loss of liver cell reserve, advancing portal hypertension, and disorders of salt and water metabolism. In general, however, patients with postnecrotic cirrhosis show less wasting and more persistent jaundice early in their clinical illness than do patients with alcoholic cirrhosis.

The results of hematologic and liver function tests resemble those of alcoholic cirrhosis, but protracted and pronounced hyperbilirubinemia, persistent moderate elevations of serum transaminases (aminotransferases), and hypergammaglobulinemia (3 to 4 g per 100 ml serum) are often present.

DIAGNOSIS AND PROGNOSIS Postnecrotic cirrhosis should be suspected in young persons and nonalcoholic adults with signs and symptoms of cirrhosis or portal hypertension. Most laboratory and radiologic studies are nondiagnostic, and needle or operative liver biopsies are the definitive diagnostic procedures, but nonuniformity of the pathologic process may result in confusing sampling errors. About 75 percent of cases tend to progress despite supportive therapy and after 1 to 5 years terminate in death from exsanguinating variceal hemorrhage, hepatic coma, or superimposed hepatocellular carcinoma.

TREATMENT Because the primary cause of this disease is rarely detectable or treatable, long-term care must include appropriate test, control of ascites (see below), avoidance of drugs or excessive protein intake that may induce hepatic coma (see below), prompt treatment of infections, and surgical treatment of portal hypertension (see below) if variceal hemorrhage occurs. Patients with coexistent or antecedent chronic active hepatitis and cirrhosis may respond to therapy as described in Chap. 303.

BILIARY CIRRHOSIS

DEFINITION *Biliary cirrhosis* refers to a disorder characterized by clinical and chemical signs of chronic impairment of bile excretion and morphologic evidence of progressive liver destruction centered about the intrahepatic bile ducts. Major clinical concomitants of impaired bile excretion (cholestasis) include protracted itching, progressive and prolonged jaundice, steatorrhea, the development of cutaneous xanthelasmas and xanthomas, hepatomegaly, and marked elevations of serum alkaline phosphatase, cholesterol, and other lipid fractions. Morphologically, most forms of biliary cirrhosis evolve from chronic inflammatory lesions of the interlobular ducts, bile ductules, and periportal liver cells. True cirrhosis represents a late and often nonspecific phase.

Biliary cirrhosis can be *primary,* in which case the process is related to chronic inflammation and fibrosis of the intrahepatic bile ductules, or *secondary* to obstruction of the common bile duct or its large branches.

ETIOLOGY The cause of *primary biliary cirrhosis* is still unknown. The observation that 90 percent of cases occur in middle-aged women strongly suggests an endocrine contribution. The occasional onset of primary biliary cirrhosis following a bout of atypical (so-called "cholestatic") hepatitis has led to speculation that viral destruction of liver and duct cells initiates the disease process. Supporting serological data are lacking, however. Although no drug has produced a picture typical of progressive biliary cirrhosis, the occasional appearance of many elements of the syndrome in patients treated with phenothiazine suggests that drug hypersensitivity may be one etiologic factor. Hepatic copper levels are elevated, but this appears to be a nonspecific, secondary phenomenon resulting from impaired hepatic excretion of copper into bile due to chronic cholestasis. The occasional association of this form of cirrhosis with calcinosis, Raynaud's phenomenon, sclerodactyly, and telangiectasia (so-called "CRST syndrome") suggests that in some cases abnormalities of connective tissue may be related to primary biliary cirrhosis.

The "Sicca complex" of dry eyes and dry mouth, autoimmune thyroiditis, and renal tubular acidosis also may be present and indicate that primary biliary cirrhosis may be a systemic disorder.

Primary biliary cirrhosis is associated with a number of specific and nonspecific immunologic abnormalities:

1 A circulating mitochondrial antibody (IgG) is present in the serum of more than 95 percent of patients with primary biliary cirrhosis and only rarely in other forms of liver disease.
2 Elevated serum levels of IgM are seen in about 80 percent of patients with primary biliary cirrhosis, and cryoproteins, composed of IgM or IgM and IgG, are present in 90 to 95 percent. These cryoproteins consist of complement-fixing immune complexes which appear to activate the alternate complement pathway.
3 Circulating antibodies that react with bile canaliculi and the cytoplasm of bile ductular cells have been demonstrated in primary biliary cirrhosis. However, similar antibodies occur in many patients with acute hepatitis.
4 Impaired lymphocyte transformation has been documented in some patients, suggesting derangement of cell-mediated immune responses.

These observations suggest strongly that disordered immune responses play a major role in the initiation or progression of the chronic hepatic lesion of biliary cirrhosis, but the exact mechanisms involved are unclear.

Most instances of *secondary biliary cirrhosis* result from partial or total obstruction of the common bile duct or its major branches for more than a year. In adults, chronic bile duct obstruction by postoperative strictures or by gallstones, usually with superimposed infectious cholangitis, is the most common cause of this type of biliary cirrhosis. Tumors of the pancreas, biliary tree, or gallbladder that produce obstruction of the common bile duct occasionally induce cirrhosis but only rarely permit survival to this stage. A few patients with the peculiar pericholangitis of ulcerative colitis or with idiopathic scleros-

ing cholangitis develop secondary biliary cirrhosis. Congenital atresia of the intra- or extrahepatic bile duct system, a relatively common anomaly, induces rapidly advancing periportal fibrosis in infants; most cases are inoperable and eventually fatal. In neither acquired nor congenital biliary obstruction is the exact pathogenesis of the cirrhotic process understood. Simple effects of pressure, local toxicity of bile constituents, or secondary infection do not alone appear to explain the morphologic events satisfactorily.

PATHOLOGY AND PATHOGENESIS The earliest recognizable lesion of *primary biliary cirrhosis* might be termed "chronic nonsuppurative destructive cholangitis," a diffuse necrotizing and inflammatory process centered about the portal triads. This is characterized by destruction of medium and small bile duct cells, infiltration with acute and chronic inflammatory cells, local fibroblastic reaction, and variable bile stasis. At times, periductal granuloma and lymph follicles may be seen. Mallory (hyaline) bodies may be present in periportal hepatocytes. Progression of this process over a period of months to years (usually 3 to 5 years) leads to loss of liver cells, the formation of pseudolobules, expansion of periportal fibrosis into a network of connective tissue scars, with apparent loss of interlobular ducts and the development of cirrhosis with a micronodular configuration. However, end-stage primary biliary cirrhosis may be indistinguishable from postnecrotic cirrhosis in its gross and microscopic appearance.

Unrelieved obstruction of the extrahepatic bile ducts leads to (1) centrilobular bile stasis, cell degeneration, and focal areas of necrosis; (2) proliferation and dilatation of the portal ducts and ductules; (3) sterile or infected cholangitis with accumulation of polymorphonuclear infiltrates around bile ducts; and (4) progressive expansion of portal tracts by edema and fibrosis. Extravasation of bile from ruptured canaliculi, ductules, or ducts leads to the formation of "bile lakes" surrounded by cholesterol-rich pseudoxanthomatous cells. These changes are followed by a finely nodular cirrhosis with isolated islands of hepatocytes surrounded by dense fibrous septa. The duration of biliary obstruction necessary to cause cirrhosis is at least 1 year, and relief of the blockage is frequently accompanied by biochemical and morphological improvement. In both primary and secondary biliary cirrhosis, the liver is initially enlarged and greenish-yellow in appearance, but evolves to a smaller, firmer, more coarsely nodular organ as the disease progresses.

CLINICAL FEATURES **Signs and symptoms** Although not diagnostic, the early clinical course of *primary biliary cirrhosis* is quite characteristic. Typically, the patient is a middle-aged woman who develops persistent generalized itching (the earliest symptom in about 50 percent of cases), followed by dark urine, pale stools, and jaundice, with some darkening (melanosis) of the exposed areas of the skin. In contrast to many other forms of cirrhosis, there are few early signs of liver cell failure and hepatic fibrosis, and most of the features reflect impaired bile excretion. Steatorrhea with associated malabsorption of lipid-soluble vitamins often produce purpura, diarrhea, and osteomalacia; the last may be manifested by backache and bone pain. Protracted elevation of serum lipids, especially cholesterol, leads to the deposit of yellowish plaques or nodules in the subcutaneous tissues in the form of periorbital xanthelasmas and xanthomas over joints, in skin folds, and at sites of trauma. Over a period of months to years, the itching, jaundice, and hyperpigmentation slowly increase. At that time the pruritus and skin lipid deposits may decrease, ascites and edema usually appear, and signs of liver cell failure and portal hypertension supervene. Most symptomatic patients die within 5 to 10 years from the first signs of the illness. However, asymptomatic patients discovered primarily on the basis of finding an elevated serum alkaline phosphatase have a much better prognosis, and may remain asymptomatic for 10 years or more. Death usually is due to hepatic insufficiency and is often precipitated by variceal bleeding, intercurrent infection, or surgical procedures.

Physical examination may be entirely normal in the early phase of the disease, when pruritus is the sole complaint. Later there may be jaundice of varying intensity, hyperpigmentation of the exposed skin areas, xanthelasmas and xanthomas, moderate to striking hepatomegaly, splenomegaly, and clubbing of the fingers. Fever and chills are rare and usually indicate mechanical biliary obstruction or other associated diseases. Muscle wasting, spider angiomas, palmar erythema, ascites and edema, and the bony tenderness of osteomalacia appear in advanced stages of the disease.

Secondary biliary cirrhosis is difficult to differentiate from primary biliary cirrhosis on the basis of clinical features alone. Secondary biliary cirrhosis should be strongly considered in patients with a history of previous biliary tract surgery or gallstones, bouts of ascending cholangitis, and right upper quadrant pain.

Laboratory findings Biliary cirrhosis is frequently diagnosed at a presymptomatic stage because of the widespread use of blood chemistry screening tests. The earliest laboratory abnormality is a two- to fivefold elevation of the serum alkaline phosphatase, accompanied by normal or slightly increased bilirubin and transaminases. As the disease evolves, the bilirubin becomes progressively elevated and in the final stages may reach 30 mg per 100 ml or more. Transaminase (aminotransferase) values rarely exceed 150 to 200 units. Marked elevation of IgM is frequent in primary biliary cirrhosis; elevation of IgG also occurs. Hyperlipidemia is common, the most striking elevation being in unesterified cholesterol. An abnormal, unique lipoprotein (lipoprotein X) found in the plasma of patients with cholestasis is also present in this disorder. Serum bile salts (especially trihydroxy) are increased, but neither serum nor skin levels can be correlated with the intensity of itching. Hypoprothrombinemia and mild to moderate steatorrhea result from a deficiency of bile salts in the gut and impaired absorption of the fat-soluble vitamins and dietary lipids. The mitochondrial antibody test is positive in most cases of primary but usually not in secondary biliary cirrhosis. Patients with primary biliary cirrhosis have elevated liver copper levels; however, the relation of these derangements in copper metabolism to the pathogenesis of this disease is not clear.

DIAGNOSIS Biliary cirrhosis should be considered in any patient with signs, symptoms, and laboratory evidence of protracted obstruction to bile flow. Liver biopsy may be diagnostic of primary biliary cirrhosis. A positive mitochondrial antibody test suggests the presence of primary biliary cirrhosis. However, since false-positive results occur, this test should not be used by itself to make the diagnosis but rather be combined with liver biopsy, cholangiography, or laparotomy. The major diagnostic challenge, regardless of the duration of symptoms, is to exclude remediable causes of mechanical bile duct obstruction before permanent liver damage has occurred. This can usually be accomplished by either a transhepatic cholangiogram or by ERCP. If these attempts are unsuccessful or if the situation is confusing, an exploratory laparotomy with an operative cholangiogram may be required.

TREATMENT Complete correction of any mechanical obstruction to bile flow is the most important step in the prevention and therapy of *secondary biliary cirrhosis*. There is no known medical therapy which alters the slowly progressive course of primary biliary cirrhosis. Therapeutic efforts are therefore directed at the many bothersome symptoms or complications of the disease as they develop. Itching may be helped by antihistamines or topical lotions containing menthol. Systemic corticosteroids and various synthetic androgen compounds may decrease itching but are accompanied by serious side effects (especially exacerbation of osteopenia) and do not alter the course of the disease. The bile salt–sequestering resin *cholestyramine,* in doses of 8 to 12 g per day, usually relieves itching. Penicillamine, the copper-chelating agent, appears to enhance copper excretion in patients with primary biliary cirrhosis but its effect on the overall course of the disease is unclear. Steatorrhea can be treated by reduction in dietary long-chain triglycerides and substitution of medium-chain triglycerides which do not require bile salts for absorption. The *fat-soluble vitamins* D, A, and K should be given by parenteral injection at regular intervals to help prevent or correct osteomalacia and hypoprothrombinemia. Salt restriction and judicious use of oral diuretic agents usually prevent disabling ascites and edema (see "Ascites" later in this chapter). The occurrence of esophagogastric variceal hemorrhage may require surgery.

HEMOCHROMATOSIS

See Chap. 94.

CARDIAC CIRRHOSIS

DEFINITION *Cardiac cirrhosis* is a relatively rare complication of severe right-sided congestive heart failure of long-standing duration in patients with cor pulmonale, tricuspid insufficiency, or constrictive pericarditis. Cardiac cirrhosis must be distinguished from *acute passive congestion* of the liver which occurs in the setting of acute heart failure, and is reversible upon correction or improvement of the heart disease.

PATHOLOGY Acute heart failure of any cause may produce acute passive congestion of the liver. This results from elevation of right ventricular pressure which is transmitted to the liver via the inferior vena cava and hepatic veins. The acutely congested liver is tensely swollen and the hepatic sinusoids are dilated and engorged with blood. In the presence of superimposed hypotension or hypoxemia there may be centrilobular necrosis of hepatocytes. These morphologic changes are transient, and full recovery occurs if the heart disease can be corrected. Severe and prolonged heart failure causes fibrosis around the central veins, which extends outward as stellate scars, ultimately producing nodular regeneration and cirrhosis.

CLINICAL FEATURES In acute passive congestion the liver is enlarged and tender, and the patient may complain of severe right upper quadrant pain due to stretching of Glisson's capsule. Abnormalities of liver function are quite variable, ranging from mild elevations of bilirubin and transaminases to a syndrome resembling acute viral hepatitis with a bilirubin of 10 mg or greater and transaminases greater than 1000 units per 100 ml serum. Serum albumin is usually normal or only slightly decreased. Prothrombin concentration may be strikingly reduced in the presence of centrilobular necrosis. In long-standing right-sided heart failure the liver is enlarged, firm, and usually nontender. Splenomegaly may result from simple passive congestion and does not necessarily indicate cirrhosis. In cases of tricuspid insufficiency the liver may be pulsatile, but this finding disappears as cirrhosis develops. Cardiac cirrhosis is infrequently diagnosed antemortem because the signs and symptoms of heart failure greatly overshadow the liver disease. Bleeding from esophageal varices is rarely observed.

DIAGNOSIS The findings of a firm, enlarged liver with mild abnormalities of liver function tests, ascites, and peripheral edema in a patient with valvular heart disease, constrictive pericarditis, or cor pulmonale of long duration (greater than 10 years) should suggest the diagnosis of cardiac cirrhosis. Heart failure and hepatomegaly are quite common in hemochromatosis and amyloidosis, but these entities can be easily differentiated by appropriate blood tests and liver biopsy.

Budd-Chiari syndrome or occlusion of the hepatic veins is easily confused with congestive hepatomegaly, particularly the acute variety. In this condition the liver is grossly enlarged and tender, and severe intractable ascites is present. However, signs and symptoms of heart failure are notably absent. The clinical course may be indolent if the obstruction is gradual, or may be rapidly downhill in acute obstruction. The usual cause is thrombosis of the hepatic veins, often in the setting of polycythemia rubra vera or hypernephroma invading the inferior vena cava; occasionally congenital fibrous webs occlude the main hepatic veins. Hepatic venography or liver biopsy showing centrilobular congestion and necrosis and sinusoidal dilatation in the absence of right-sided heart failure establishes the diagnosis.

TREATMENT Prevention or treatment of cardiac cirrhosis depends on proper diagnosis and therapy of the underlying cardiovascular disorder. If constrictive pericarditis is present and pericardectomy is possible, liver function may improve within 6 to 12 months and fibrous bands will become narrower and avascular.

FORMS OF CIRRHOSIS OF UNKNOWN ETIOLOGY

Clinical, etiologic, and morphologic classifications of cirrhosis do not encompass all cases. Classification criteria and the study of patients with cirrhosis vary widely throughout the world, but *unexpected and unexplained cirrhosis accounts for about 10 percent of chronic liver disease* seen at autopsy. Equally important, many patients with cirrhosis are "classified" improperly during life, and small and unrepresentative biopsy specimens from patients with a poor history often account for the errors in diagnosis.

Cirrhosis may be found in association with the following diseases:

1 *Metabolic disorders:* galactosemia, hereditary fructose intolerance, glycogen storage diseases, hereditary tyrosinemia, α_1-antitrypsin deficiency, and the Fanconi syndrome
2 *Infectious diseases:* brucellosis, schistosomiasis, neonatal cytomegalovirus, and toxoplasma infections
3 *Infiltrative diseases:* sarcoidosis
4 *Gastrointestinal disorders:* chronic inflammatory bowel disease and cystic fibrosis of the pancreas
5 *Chemical intoxications:* pyrrolidizine alkaloids (venoocclusive disease) and arsenic

NONCIRRHOTIC FIBROSIS OF THE LIVER

Several diseases, either congenital or acquired, may be associated with localized or generalized hepatic fibrosis. The clinical manifestations in such cases may suggest on occasion the diagnosis of true cirrhosis, but the absence of clinical and functional evidence of hepatocellular damage, the lack of nodular

regenerative activity, and the localized nature of the scarring usually serve to distinguish these conditions from true cirrhosis.

IDIOPATHIC PORTAL HYPERTENSION (NONCIRRHOTIC PORTAL FIBROSIS) Not infrequently patients with portal hypertension and splenomegaly have no clinical or morphologic evidence of cirrhosis. Instead of cirrhosis, careful inspection of the liver often shows some fibrosis in the portal areas and variable thickening of the walls of the portal vein branches in the liver. There appear to be three variants of the process. Some patients have only *intrahepatic phlebosclerosis* and *fibrosis,* others have in addition segmental thickening or *sclerosis of the portal and splenic veins,* and a third group may show actual *thrombosis* of these vessels. Such cases have been reported from many parts of the world, some of them under the term "Banti's syndrome."

SCHISTOSOMIASIS (See also Chap. 211) The ova of *Schistosoma mansoni* elicit granulomatous and fibrotic reactions along the portal tracts, the result of a delayed hypersensitivity reaction modulated by an antigen-antibody immune-complex reaction. The characteristic hepatic lesion of schistosomiasis is, therefore, noncirrhotic portal ("pipestem") fibrosis, which produces progressive occlusion of the portal venules with resultant presinusoidal portal hypertension. In advanced cases sinusoidal portal hypertension may be seen. True cirrhosis may be present in some cases, but nutritional deficiencies and other factors, e.g., hepatitis B infection, contribute to this process. Clinically, the signs of portal hypertension predominate and variceal hemorrhage is the usual presentation. The liver and spleen are moderately enlarged. Hepatocellular function is usually normal, but jaundice and serum alkaline phosphatase elevations may be noted.

CONGENITAL HEPATIC FIBROSIS This rare variant of polycystic disease of the liver is probably transmitted as an autosomal recessive trait and may be associated with cystic renal disease. Typically, the patient is young, has no history or signs of hepatocellular disease, and presents with unexplained hepatosplenomegaly, hemorrhage from esophagogastric varices due to presinusoidal portal hypertension, or renal failure. Surgical correction of the portal hypertension may permit long-term survival in patients without renal involvement because progressive liver failure is rare. The biopsy findings are distinctive; normal masses of liver parenchyma are separated by mature fibrous bands containing networks of bile ducts; large cysts (typical of polycystic disease) are not found. The cellular damage, inflammation, and nodular regeneration of cirrhosis are notably absent.

MAJOR SEQUELAE OF CIRRHOSIS

Patients with any form of cirrhosis, with its progressive loss of liver cell function and advancing distortion of intrahepatic vasculature, are threatened by three major complications: *portal hypertension* and its associated complications of variceal hemorrhage and splenomegaly, disabling *fluid retention* in the form of ascites and edema, and *hepatic encephalopathy (hepatic coma).* One-third of deaths in patients with alcoholic cirrhosis are related to variceal hemorrhage; ascites occurs in 60 to 85 percent of cases of advanced cirrhosis; and about 50 percent of patients with cirrhosis die in hepatic coma. Other complications include portal vein thrombosis and hepatocellular carcinoma (especially in postnecrotic cirrhosis and hemochromatosis).

PORTAL HYPERTENSION   Definition   The normal adult liver is perfused by about 1500 ml blood per minute. Approximately two-thirds of hepatic blood flow and one-half of the oxygen supply is provided by the portal vein; the remainder is derived from the hepatic artery. Normally the pressure in the portal vein is quite low (10 and 15 cm saline), since the vascular resistance in the hepatic sinusoids is also low. The nodular regeneration and distortion of the lobular architecture of the cirrhotic liver produce an increase in vascular resistance in the portal venous bed, and a rise in portal venous pressure (portal hypertension) owing to the impairment of blood flow. Portal hypertension is defined as a portal pressure of over 30 cm saline when measured at surgery, or a wedged hepatic vein pressure greater than 4 mmHg above the inferior vena cava pressure.

Pathogenesis   Portal hypertension usually results from obstruction to portal blood flow. Anatomically this obstruction can occur at three levels: (1) hepatic veins (Budd-Chiari syndrome), (2) intrahepatic (cirrhosis, metastatic tumors), (3) portal vein (thrombosis, tumor involvement). Portal hypertension can also result from increased portal blood flow in the absence of obstruction, as in myeloid metaplasia with massive splenomegaly.

The commonest cause of portal hypertension in the United States is *cirrhosis,* which produces impedance of blood flow through the liver by fibrosis, thrombosis, and nodular regeneration. About 30 to 60 percent of patients with cirrhosis have an important degree of portal hypertension. The second most common cause of portal hypertension is *mechanical obstruction* of the extrahepatic portal vein, usually the result of thrombosis or tumor invasion. *Occlusion of the major hepatic veins* (Budd-Chiari syndrome) or their small intrahepatic branches (as in venoocclusive disease) may lead to portal hypertension. About 5 percent of patients with cirrhosis and portal hypertension have associated *portal vein thrombosis.* As mentioned above, a small but significant number of patients with sustained portal hypertension have no evidence of cirrhosis but show variable degrees of fibrosis and sclerosis of the intrahepatic portal veins (noncirrhotic portal fibrosis).

Clinical features   Many patients with portal hypertension of intra- or extrahepatic origin have symptoms or signs related only to the primary disease, and portal hypertension is tolerated without incident for years. Four major clinical consequences of portal hypertension may, however, lead to its recognition: (1) the development of extensive *portal-systemic venous collaterals,* with gastrointestinal hemorrhage; (2) the appearance of *congestive splenomegaly* with hypersplenism; (3) the onset of episodic stupor or *hepatic (portal-systemic) encephalopathy;* and (4) the development of *ascites.*

The development of collateral channels between the portal and systemic venous beds is the most characteristic consequence of portal hypertension. Major sites of collateral flow involve dilated veins around the rectum (hemorrhoids), cardioesophageal junction (esophagogastric varices), and retroperitoneal space and the falciform ligament of the liver (periumbilical or abdominal wall collaterals). Although hemorrhoids bleed frequently and varices of the bowel rupture occasionally, massive hemorrhage from thin-walled varices in the upper stomach and lower esophagus is the major complication of

portal hypertension. Variceal bleeding occurs without obvious precipitating cause and presents usually as painless massive hematemesis or melena. Abdominal wall collaterals are helpful clinical signs of portal hypertension and appear as slightly tortuous epigastic vessels (caput medusae) that radiate from the umbilicus toward the xiphoid and rib margins. Vascular bruits may be heard over the upper abdomen. *Splenomegaly,* the result of passive congestion, fibrosis, and siderosis, is present in most patients with significant and long-standing portal hypertension. The absence of splenomegaly does not rule out portal hypertension, because splenic size correlates poorly with the level of portal pressure. As noted in Chap. 320, splenic enlargement may be accompanied by abnormal sequestration and destruction of the circulating blood cells (hypersplenism). Patients with portal hypertension and with extensive portal-systemic venous shunting may experience bouts of *hepatic (portal-systemic) encephalopathy or hepatic coma.* These episodes are often precipitated by gastrointestinal hemorrhage and a moderate to high protein diet. Ascites is not a feature of portal vein obstruction or other forms of presinusoidal portal hypertension but is a common occurrence in portal hypertension associated with cirrhosis or hepatic venous blockade.

Diagnosis   The diagnosis of portal hypertension is usually based on indirect evidence such as the presence of esophageal varices, abdominal collateral veins, or hypersplenism or ascites in a patient with cirrhosis. Esophageal varices are visualized in the majority of cases by a careful *barium swallow* or *fiberoptic endoscopy.* The finding on a liver scan of significant uptake of radioactivity in the spleen and bone marrow suggest shunting of blood away from the liver and is suggestive of cirrhosis. Direct measurement of portal venous pressure by transhepatic catheterization is technically difficult and is not usually performed except during surgery. In certain patients with suspected portal vein thrombosis or previous portacaval shunt surgery it is useful to obtain measurement of portal pressure and visualization of the portal system prior to operation. Splenoportography, which requires percutaneous needle puncture of the spleen, is not widely used because it is technically difficult and hazardous. Mesenteric and hepatic angiography are frequently obtained prior to shunt surgery to visualize the hepatic arterial bed as well as the portal system during the venous runoff phase. This allows the surgeon to plan the operative approach, and also provides valuable information regarding the presence of unsuspected lesions such as hepatocellular carcinoma or Budd-Chiari lesions. In addition, measurement of wedged hepatic vein pressure (WHVP) can be obtained by wedging the catheter into the hepatic parenchyma. Elevation of WHVP occurs in portal hypertension due to cirrhosis, while WHVP is normal in portal vein thrombosis.

Treatment   GENERAL   Vigorous treatment of patients with alcoholic hepatitis superimposed on alcoholic cirrhosis, chronic active hepatitis, and other liver diseases may lead to a fall in portal pressure and to the disappearance of varices. As a rule, however, portal hypertension caused by established cirrhosis or portal vein occlusion is not reversible, and variceal hemorrhage remains a grave threat. No precise prognosis can be made in individual cases, but more than 30 percent of patients with cirrhosis and varices experience a major hemorrhage within 5 years and have an overall mortality of 60 to 80 percent. In contrast, patients with normal liver function and variceal hemorrhage secondary to portal vein block tolerate episodes of hemorrhage relatively well. Despite technical improvements in surgical methods of portal vein or variceal decompression, shunts should be reserved for patients who bleed from varices.

ACUTE VARICEAL HEMORRHAGE   Prompt and effective care of the patient with massive hematemesis or melena from a ruptured varix requires coordinated medical-surgical efforts. The basic elements of management include the following:

Quantitative replacement of blood loss is essential to prevent further deterioration of liver function. It is often advisable to use fresh blood if massive replacement therapy is required. *Demonstration of esophageal varices, location of the actual bleeding site,* and *exclusion of other causes of gastrointestinal hemorrhage* by endoscopy or radiography are critical. It should not be assumed that cirrhotics with proved or probable varices are bleeding from the varices, because at least one-third have other potential bleeding sites in the upper gastrointestinal tract.

Temporary control of variceal bleeding may be achieved by vasopressin infusions, balloon tamponade, or left gastric vein occlusion. Continuous infusion of 0.4 unit of vasopressin per minute through a peripheral vein may lead to a temporary decrease or cessation in variceal hemorrhage by lowering splanchnic blood flow and portal pressure. Vasopressin dosage is then tapered and discontinued 48 h after bleeding has stopped. Transient decreases in cardiac output, cardiac arrhythmias, and water retention may make the use of vasopressin hazardous to patients with ischemic heart disease. Mesenteric angiography is useful in both diagnosis and treatment of variceal bleeding. The injection of contrast material into the mesenteric, celiac, or gastric arteries is used to localize the site of hemorrhage. Temporary control of bleeding can be achieved in a high percentage of patients by infusion of vasopressin directly into the splanchnic bed via the superior mesenteric artery. This method has no clear advantage over peripheral vein infusion. The Sengstaken-Blakemore tube or a modified single-balloon tube may be inserted into the stomach, inflated, and attached to traction to provide local compression of the submucosal veins. Although often effective in producing temporary control of massive hemorrhage, this device is difficult to place accurately and is uncomfortable for the patient; and its use is often complicated by rebleeding, esophageal erosions, airway obstruction, or aspiration. The use of balloon tamponade or vasopressin infusion should be regarded as temporary therapy with a significant incidence of relapse. If both methods fail to control bleeding, transhepatic catheterization and occlusion of the left gastric vein may result in the cessation of variceal hemorrhage. This method requires further clinical evaluation for both efficacy and safety. Active steps must be taken to prevent or treat impending hepatic coma (see "Hepatic Encephalopathy" later in this chapter).

Evaluation of liver function and *assessment of operative risk* are important but difficult. No single clinical test of liver function can predict accurately the immediate postoperative morbidity and mortality. In general, however, patients with compensated or stable cirrhosis have a much more favorable outlook than those with deepening jaundice, ascites, or signs of encephalopathy. Careful medical management for 2 or 3 weeks may permit considerable recovery of liver function in patients with active alcoholic cirrhosis.

Emergency surgical shunting procedures to arrest bleeding may be performed within a few days. The mortality is 25 to 50 percent in the typical patient, but the operation does prevent exsanguination, usually prevents future variceal bleeding, and may permit considerable recovery of liver function.

In many patients, *elective shunt surgery* may be advisable. The results of large clinical series indicate that effective portacaval shunt surgery does not improve longevity but does prevent recurrent variceal hemorrhage. The type of surgical shunt procedure (e.g., portacaval, splenorenal) often depends on the experience and judgment of the surgeon. Portal decompression does not usually correct the pancytopenia of hypersplenism. In infants and in other patients with extensive portal vein disease,

effective portal-systemic shunts may be constructed, using other branches of the portal vein and the trunk of the inferior vena cava. Late complications in patients with functioning portacaval shunts include hepatic coma (15 to 20 percent), peptic ulceration (10 to 15 percent), slight unconjugated hyperbilirubinemia, and, rarely, accumulation of iron within the cirrhotic liver. A *selective,* distal splenorenal shunt with portalazygous ligation appears to decompress varices without dramatically altering portal pressure and may be relatively free of the complication of disabling encephalopathy.

ASCITES   See also Chap. 40.

Definition   Ascites, the accumulation of excessive volumes of fluid within the peritoneal cavity, is a frequent manifestation of cirrhosis and other types of diffuse parenchymal liver disease. The development of ascites is often accompanied by hemodilution, edema, and decreased urine volume. These and other clinical findings reflect the complex abnormalities of electrolyte, water, and protein metabolism that may complicate severe liver disease and other disturbances of the hepatic circulation.

Pathogenesis   Ascites is usually demonstrable clinically when 500 ml or more of fluid has accumulated in the peritoneal cavity. It results from disturbances of both local and systemic mechanisms that regulate the passage of fluid and solutes across vascular and serosal membranes. The *local or intraabdominal factors* favoring ascites formation in cirrhosis include the following:

1 Portal hypertension. The role of portal hypertension in the formation of ascites is not clearly understood. Patients with portal hypertension due to extrahepatic portal vein block do not generally have ascites. On the other hand reduction in portal vein pressure by a side-to-side portacaval anastomosis often results in improvement in ascites. It is likely that portal hypertension combined with other factors contributes to the formation and persistence of ascites in the cirrhotic patient.
2 Increased flow of hepatic lymph. Weeping of lymph from the surface of the cirrhotic liver can be observed at surgery. This presumably results from distortion and blockage of the hepatic sinusoids and lymphatics resulting in extravasation of protein-rich lymph into the peritoneal cavity. This mechanism may be quite important in the formation of ascites in the Budd-Chiari syndrome, in which the ascitic fluid has a high protein level.

The most important systemic factors include the following:

1 Decreased plasma colloid oncotic pressure. The serum albumin is low in cirrhotic patients because of a combination of expansion of the plasma volume, causing dilution of serum proteins, impaired hepatic synthesis, and loss of albumin from the vascular space into the peritoneal cavity. Up to one-fourth of total body albumin may be present in the ascitic fluid. Hypoalbuminemia is associated with reduction of the plasma oncotic pressure and loss of water into the extravascular space.
2 Hyperaldosteronism. Secondary hyperaldosteronism is common in the cirrhotic patient with ascites and leads to excessive reabsorption of sodium in the distal tubule. Hyperaldosteronism results from increased aldosterone secretion by the adrenal gland, presumably due to a reduction in renal blood flow and impaired hepatic metabolism and excretion of aldosterone.

3 Impaired water excretion. Patients with ascites have impaired renal excretion of a water load, which is due to reduced renal vascular flow and in some patients to excessive serum levels of antidiuretic hormone.

Treatment In some patients with reversible liver disease, particularly acute alcoholic hepatitis or chronic active hepatitis, improvement in liver function may be accompanied by spontaneous diuresis. However, in patients with stable cirrhosis there may be little or no improvement in liver function after a period of observation, and therapy directed against the ascites is indicated. It should be remembered that ascites develops quite slowly, and *must be removed slowly* in order to avoid acute changes in plasma volume, which can be disastrous. The goal of therapy should be the loss of not more than 1.0 kg per day if both ascites and peripheral edema are present, or no more than 0.5 kg per day in patients with ascites only. Fluid loss during treatment can be monitored by accurate daily weights.

Bed rest and strict fluid and sodium restriction are the first measures to be tried in the cirrhotic patient with ascites. Sodium intake should be restricted to 30 meq per day and fluid intake may be limited to 1500 ml per day if hyponatremia is marked. Unfortunately this degree of sodium restriction is not well tolerated by patients, and caloric intake may decline. It is therefore important to supply adequate low-sodium snacks or supplements to insure an adequate intake of calories and protein essential for healing of the damaged liver. If after 1 week there has been no change in weight, spironolactone 25 mg four times daily is added. If this dose is inadequate, spironolactone is increased in stepwise increments every 4 days until a maximum dose 100 mg four times daily is reached. If the ascites is still refractory, one may cautiously try furosemide 40 to 80 mg per day. Aggressive diuretic therapy may be complicated by depletion of plasma volume and reduction of renal function, which in turn may precipitate the hepatorenal syndrome (see below). Brisk diuresis may also cause hypokalemic alkalosis, which in turn enhances hepatic encephalopathy. Therefore frequent assessment of fluid and electrolyte status is mandatory, and restoration of plasma volume with infusions of albumin may be required if significant intravascular volume depletion occurs.

The conservative management of ascites is successful in the majority of cirrhotics, especially if sodium and water intake are strictly limited, usually in a hospital setting. In general, diuresis is more likely to occur in those patients in whom improvement in liver function occurs. A minority of patients with advanced cirrhosis fail to respond, despite intensive medical therapy. In some of these patients with intractable ascites a side-to-side portacaval shunt may result in improvement in ascites, presumably due to reduction of portal pressure. However, these patients are extremely poor surgical risks, and operative mortality and morbidity are high. Surgical implantation of a plastic shunt between the peritoneal cavity and the superior vena cava has also been used successfully to reduce intractable ascites. This type of peritoneovenous shunt (LeVeen) has a pressure-sensitive, one-way valve which allows ascites fluid to flow from the abdominal cavity to the superior vena cava. Although this technique may be useful in obtaining short-term control of ascites, it is accompanied by significant complications, including infection and disseminated intravascular coagulation; its overall efficacy remains to be determined.

Therapeutic *paracentesis* may be required in patients with respiratory embarrassment due to massive ascites. Up to 3 liters of fluid may be removed over a 4-h period using a plastic indwelling catheter or small-bore needle. Since the ascites usually reaccumulates within several days, it may be necessary to repeat the procedure until a diuresis can be initiated. Repeated therapeutic paracenteses should not be performed in patients with cirrhosis, since this may be complicated by infection of the ascites, chronic ascites leak, hemorrhage, and volume and protein depletion.

Hepatorenal syndrome is a serious complication of cirrhosis, characterized by advancing azotemia, oliguria, and intractable ascites. This may follow a bout of severe gastrointestinal bleeding, sepsis, and too rapid attempts at diuresis or paracentesis; or it may occur without a recognized precipitant. The urine output falls to 200 to 400 ml per day, with gradual elevation of the serum creatinine and marked sodium retention. Death may occur from uremia, gastrointestinal bleeding, or hepatic coma. The exact cause of renal failure in cirrhosis is unknown, but altered renal hemodynamics appears to be responsible for this functional disorder. Contributing factors include decrease in renal cortical perfusion, marked hyperaldosteronism, decreased effective circulating plasma volume, and increased intraabdominal pressure from tense ascites. The kidneys are structurally intact; urinalysis, pyelography, and renal biopsy are usually normal. Treatment is usually unsuccessful, although some patients with hypotension and decreased plasma volume may respond to infusions of salt-poor albumin with increasing urine output and gradual loss of ascites. Salt and water restriction and diuretic therapy are also usually employed, but recovery seems to be most closely correlated with improvement in liver function. In a few patients, recovery has followed a portacaval shunt or liver transplantation; however, most patients are extremely poor candidates for major surgery because of their severe liver disease and precarious general condition. It has been suggested but not proved that peritoneovenous shunt may reverse renal failure in some patients.

SPONTANEOUS BACTERIAL PERITONITIS   Patients with cirrhosis, particularly alcoholic cirrhosis and ascites, may develop acute bacterial peritonitis without an obvious precipitating event. The classic presentation is the abrupt onset of fever, chills, generalized abdominal pain, and rebound tenderness accompanied by cloudy ascitic fluid with a high white cell count and bacteria. However, a more common presentation is that of fever of unknown origin with mild abdominal pain which may be attributed to other causes. The diagnosis of spontaneous bacterial peritonitis is based upon careful examination of the ascites fluid. The presence of a white cell count greater than 300 cells per cubic millimeter, with more than 75 percent polymorphonuclear leukocytes, should suggest the diagnosis; this should be confirmed by demonstrating bacteria by Gram's stain and by culture. Enteric gram-negative bacilli are found in the majority of cases; pneumococci and other gram-positive organisms are occasionally found. The mechanism by which bacteria infect the ascites fluid is not known. Hematogenous spread during spontaneous bacteremia or leakage of bacteria from the intestinal tract are possible sources of infection. In the majority of cases a focus of infection is not present elsewhere in the body and the route of contamination remains unknown.

Bacterial peritonitis is a serious complication of cirrhosis, with a significant morbidity and mortality; not uncommonly the infection results in hepatic encephalopathy and worsening of liver function. The patient with suspected bacterial peritonitis should be treated initially with broad-spectrum antibiotics effective against gram-negative and gram-positive organisms. More specific antibiotics may be selected after the results of culture and sensitivity tests are available.

HEPATIC ENCEPHALOPATHY Definition Hepatic (portalsystemic) encephalopathy is a complex organic brain syndrome characterized by disturbances in consciousness, fluctuating neurologic signs, asterixis or "flapping tremor," and distinctive electroencephalographic changes. This metabolic disorder of the nervous system may appear in the course of acute or chronic hepatocellular disease or as a complication of portal-systemic venous shunting. It may be *acute* and self-limiting or *chronic* and progressive.

Diagnosis The recognition of hepatic encephalopathy or coma depends on four major elements: (1) The patient should have evidence of advanced hepatocellular disease, extensive portal-systemic collateral shunts, or both. The liver disease may be acute and massive, as in toxic or fulminant viral hepatitis; or chronic and advanced, as in cirrhosis. The portal-systemic venous shunts, which must permit a significant portion of the portal blood to bypass the liver, may be either *spontaneous* (e.g., naturally developing collaterals) or *surgical* (e.g., large portacaval anastomoses). Most of the patients who develop hepatic encephalopathy have, in fact, elements of both liver disease and portal-systemic shunting. (2) Disturbances of awareness and mentation are characteristic, and forgetfulness and confusion progress to stupor and finally to deep coma. (3) Mental changes are accompanied by shifting combinations of neurologic signs, which include rigidity, hyperreflexia, extensor plantar signs, and, rarely, seizures. A peculiar "flapping tremor" (asterixis), which is a nonrhythmic asymmetric lapse in voluntary sustained posture of extremities, head, and trunk, is often seen in precoma and in advancing hepatic encephalopathy but cannot be elicited in the presence of coma. This neurologic picture is nonspecific and is encountered also in patients with uremia, ventilatory failure, and other forms of metabolic brain disease. (4) Most patients with the clinical features of hepatic coma have characteristic symmetrical, high-voltage, slow-wave (2 to 5 per second) patterns on the electroencephalogram. *Fetor hepaticus*, a unique musty odor of the breath and urine, may be noted in patients with hepatic coma and also in those with extensive collateral circulation. Several clinical variants of the "classic" syndrome of hepatic encephalopathy have been recognized. *Chronic progressive hepatocerebral degeneration*, which may develop in patients with stable liver disease or with portacaval anastomoses, is characterized by a slow decline in intellectual function, psychiatric symptoms, cerebellar ataxia, tremor, and choreoathetosis. Isolated signs of *myelopathy*, including spasticity and hyperreflexia of the legs, may antedate the other elements of hepatic coma by several months. Both of these conditions must be distinguished from other nonhepatic causes of deranged nervous system function, as well as from Wilson's disease.

A number of conditions can mimic the clinical features of hepatic encephalopathy, particularly in the alcoholic patient with cirrhosis. Acute alcoholic intoxication, delirium tremens, Wernicke's encephalopathy, and Korsakoff's psychosis are accompanied by confusion and tremor and thus are easily confused with hepatic encephalopathy. *Subdural hematoma* is common in the alcoholic and may present with stupor or coma unaccompanied by localizing neurologic signs. *Meningitis* may produce alteration of consciousness without the usual clinical features. For example, lack of a febrile response to acute infection is quite common in the cirrhotic and may lead to delayed diagnosis. *Drug overdose*, particularly with sedatives, tranquilizers, or narcotics, may result from altered hepatic excretion of these agents, and can produce confusion or stupor. *Hypoglycemia* caused by poor nutrition, inadequate glycogen stores in the liver, and alcohol-induced impairment of gluconeogenesis occasionally occurs in the cirrhotic and may be accompanied by alteration of mental function. The diagnosis of hepatic encephalopathy is usually one of exclusion. A careful neurologic examination and judicious use of lumbar puncture, brain scan, skull films, and computerized tomography (CT scan) are generally required to eliminate intracranial hemorrhage or infection, while hypoglycemia, drug overdose, or alcohol intoxication are diagnosed by appropriate blood measurements.

Pathogenesis No single biochemical or physiologic defect has been shown to be the actual cause of hepatic encephalopathy or coma. Most studies have shown that hepatic coma and its associated disorders of cerebral function result from (1) the shunting of portal blood directly into the systemic circulation, so that the blood largely bypasses the liver, and (2) severe hepatocellular damage and dysfunction. Both circumstances have a common result: various toxic substances absorbed from the intestine are not metabolized by the liver, thus allowing them to accumulate within the brain. Ammonia is one such compound, and many patients with hepatic encephalopathy have elevated systemic arterial and venous blood levels of ammonia. Hyperammonemia is most often found in patients with portal-systemic venous shunting and in hepatic cell failure.

Undoubtedly, "toxic" substances other than ammonia are involved in the genesis of hepatic encephalopathy. The administration of methionine to patients with portal-systemic shunts has been shown to precipitate stupor or encephalopathy in the absence of hyperammonemia. Other putative factors include short-chain fatty acids, false neurotransmitter substances, and alterations in plasma levels of aromatic and branched-chain amino acids. The liver also is believed to produce substances that are essential for normal brain metabolism, and in liver failure these may be reduced. Decreased cerebral oxygen uptake and impaired intermediary metabolism of glucose in the brain are common but nonspecific features of hepatic encephalopathy.

Most patients with chronic forms of hepatic encephalopathy have distinctive enlargement and proliferation of protoplasmic astrocytes in many areas of the brain, and a few develop band-like cerebral cortical necrosis. These findings suggest that the syndrome may progress from a functional to a structural or irreversible phase.

PRECIPITATING FACTORS In the patient with stable inactive cirrhosis, hepatic encephalopathy often follows a precipitating event. Perhaps the most common predisposing factor is *gastrointestinal bleeding*, which causes an increase in the production of ammonia and other nitrogenous substances in the colon. *Increased dietary protein* may also result in a similar increase in nitrogenous substances by colonic bacteria. *Electrolyte disturbances*, particularly hypokalemic alkalosis secondary to excessive diuresis or vomiting, may precipitate hepatic encephalopathy. In systemic alkalosis there is an increase in the relative concentration of uncharged ammonia (NH_3) and a decrease in ammonium ions (NH_4^+). The uncharged ammonia can more readily cross the blood-brain barrier and accumulate in the central nervous system. Hypokalemia also increases renal ammonia production, some of which enters the systemic circulation by the renal vein. Acute *infections* often trigger hepatic encephalopathy, although the mechanisms involved are not clear. The features of encephalopathy may overshadow the signs of infection and delay diagnosis and treatment. Therefore all patients in hepatic coma should be carefully evaluated for precipitating conditions, such as pneumonia, peritonitis, urinary tract infections, or pancreatitis. *Deterioration of liver function* from any cause will usually precipitate hepatic encephalopathy in the stable cirrhotic. Acute viral hepatitis, alcoholic hepatitis, or extrahepatic obstruction are all accompanied by worsening liver function and impairment of the liver's metabolic capacity. Liver function may also worsen after surgery, or in the presence of other diseases such as heart failure or infection.

Treatment Early recognition and prompt treatment of hepatic encephalopathy are essential, because patients in profound coma respond poorly to all forms of therapy and are vulnerable to the added hazards of coma itself. Alterations in personality, mood disturbances, slight confusion, deterioration in self-care and handwriting, unusual somnolence, and asterixis should be noted. It may be desirable to grade or classify the stages of hepatic encephalopathy, since this is often helpful in charting the course of the illness and gauging the effects of therapy. One useful classification is based on the severity of mental and neurological signs, and ranges from grade I (slight apathy or euphoria with or without objective neurologic signs) to grade V (true coma).

The patient with severe hepatic encephalopathy requires careful attention to the usual supportive measures for the comatose patient, including a nasogastric tube and urinary catheter. Careful monitoring of fluid intake and output is essential. The deeply comatose patient with an absent gag reflex should undergo endotracheal intubation to avoid aspiration pneumonia and insure adequate delivery of oxygen.

Specific treatment of hepatic encephalopathy is aimed at (1) decreasing ammonia production in the colon and (2) elimination or treatment of precipitating factors. In the presence of acute gastrointestinal bleeding the blood in the bowel lumen should be promptly evacuated with enemas and laxatives in order to reduce the nitrogen load. Ammonia production can also be decreased by oral administration of neomycin, a nonabsorbable antibiotic, at a dosage of 1 g every 6 h. Ammonia absorption can be decreased with oral administration or enemas of lactulose, a nonabsorbable disaccharide. The sugar enters the colon where it is metabolized by colonic bacteria to organic acids, which lower the pH in the colon. The excess hydrogen ions convert ammonia (NH_3) to ammonium (NH_4^+), which, because of its positive charge, is not readily absorbed and bacteria assimilation of NH_3 appears to be increased. Lactulose usually produces a reduction in serum ammonia and improvement in encephalopathy within 24 to 48 h. Lactulose is administered in a loading dose of 50 ml syrup (65 g per 100 ml) every 2 h until diarrhea occurs; thereafter the dose is adjusted so that the patient has two to four loose stools per day.

Elimination or treatment of precipitating factors is of prime importance in the treatment of hepatic encephalopathy. Bleeding from the upper gastrointestinal tract must be promptly controlled to prevent worsening encephalopathy. This is usually difficult in the typical cirrhotic with bleeding varices or hemorrhagic gastritis who represents a poor surgical risk. Temporary elimination of all dietary protein is required until the patient improves to the point at which protein can be tolerated. Fluid and electrolyte abnormalities, particularly hypokalemic alkalosis, should be corrected promptly. Sedatives, analgesics, and tranquilizers should be discontinued, and antibiotics administered as indicated to patients with evidence of infection. Heroic measures such as extracorporeal charcoal column perfusion or exchange transfusion have not been convincingly shown to benefit the acutely encephalopathic patient.

Chronic hepatic encephalopathy is best treated with modest protein restriction (30 or 40 g per day) accompanied by small doses of either neomycin or lactulose. Treatment is adjusted to obtain a reasonable functional level of the patient with the least amount of protein restriction and neomycin or lactulose. Since most of the ammonia in serum is produced in and absorbed from the colon, colectomy or isolation of the colon from the fecal stream has been used successfully in some patients with disabling chronic encephalopathy unresponsive to

medical management. This approach is not widely used, however, because of the high operative morbidity and mortality and the low success rate.

REFERENCES

Alcoholic and postnecrotic cirrhosis

ANTHONY PP et al: The morphology of cirrhosis: Definition, nomenclature and classification. Bull WHO 55(4):521, 1977

CHOPRA IJ et al: Estrogen-androgen imbalance in hepatic cirrhosis. Ann Intern Med 79:198, 1973

MADDREY WC et al: Corticosteroid therapy of alcoholic hepatitis. Gastroenterology 75:193, 1978

ORREGO H et al: Effect of short-term therapy with propylthiouracil in patients with alcoholic liver disease. Gastroenterology 76:388, 1979

Biliary and other types of cirrhosis

GALBRAITH RM: High prevalence of seroimmunologic abnormalities in relatives of patients with active chronic hepatitis or primary biliary cirrhosis. N Engl J Med 290:64, 1974

JONES EA (moderator): Primary biliary cirrhosis and the complement system. Ann Intern Med 90:72, 1979

SHERLOCK S, SCHEUER PJ: The presentation and diagnosis of 100 patients with primary biliary cirrhosis. N Engl J Med 289:689, 1973

WANDS JR et al: Circulating immune complexes and complement activation in primary biliary cirrhosis. N Engl J Med 298:233, 1978

Hepatic encephalopathy

ATTERBURY CE et al: Neomycin-sorbitol and lactulose in the treatment of acute portal-systemic encephalopathy. Am J Digest Dis 23:398, 1978

CASCINO A et al: Plasma amino acid imbalance in patients with liver disease. Am J Digest Dis 23:591, 1978

CONN HO et al: Comparison of lactulose and neomycin in the treatment of chronic portal-systemic encephalopathy: A double-blind controlled trial. Gastroenterology 72:573, 1977

HOYUMPA AM JR et al: Hepatic encephalopathy. Gastroenterology 76:184, 1979

RIKKERS L et al: Subclinical hepatic encephelopathy: Detection prevalence and relation to nitrogen metabolism. Gastroenterology 75:462, 1978

Portal hypertension and ascites

EPSTEIN M: Deranged sodium homeostasis in cirrhosis. Gastroenterology 76:607, 1979

GABUZDA GH: Cirrhotic ascites: An etiologic approach to management. Hosp Practice 7:67, 1973

MALT RA: Portasystemic venous shunts. N Engl J Med 295:24, 1976

SHERLOCK S: Portal circulation and portal hypertension. Gut 19:70, 1978

305
TUMORS OF THE LIVER

ELLIOT ALPERT
KURT J. ISSELBACHER

PRIMARY CARCINOMA Carcinomas arising within the liver may be of liver cell (*hepatocellular*), bile duct cell (*cholangiocellular*), or mixed origin. Hepatocellular carcinoma (primary liver cell carcinoma) accounts for 80 to 90 percent of liver carcinomas. There is, however, little practical purpose in distinguishing between the two types, since both may be found in different parts of the same tumor and the clinical courses are similar.

Incidence and epidemiology Primary liver cancers account for only 1 to 2 percent of malignant tumors found at autopsy in

North and South America and Europe. However, in parts of Africa and Asia they may account for up to 20 to 30 percent of all types of malignancy. Liver cell carcinoma occurs two to four times more frequently in men than in women. The peak incidence occurs in the fifth and sixth decades of life in the United States, but one to two decades earlier in areas with a high prevalence of liver carcinoma. Cirrhosis, usually macronodular or postnecrotic, is found in 60 to 75 percent of autopsied patients with primary liver cell carcinoma in all parts of the world.

There is wide variation in the incidence of hepatocellular carcinoma in different parts of the world, and a number of etiologic factors may be important.

1 Chronic liver disease of any etiology also appears to predispose to the development of carcinoma. A variety of metabolic, alcoholic, viral, or idiopathic chronic liver diseases can lead to liver cell carcinoma. *Hemochromatosis* has the highest risk of malignant degeneration, presumably owing to the long duration of the chronic liver inflammation. The etiology of liver cell carcinoma in about a third of patients with no underlying liver disease is less clear.

2 Viral hepatitis is endemic in many areas of Africa and Asia. The prevalence of hepatitis B antigenemia in the normal population is 1 to 10 percent in some parts of Africa. In these areas, most patients with hepatocellular carcinoma superimposed on chronic liver disease will have serologic evidence of hepatitis B infection. Therefore, hepatitis B virus infection is probably a significant cause of chronic liver disease and subsequent liver carcinoma in these parts of the world.

3 Mycotoxins, metabolites of saprophytic fungi, including certain known hepatic carcinogens (e.g., aflatoxins), are continuously ingested in foodstuffs in small amounts and are found in high concentrations in foods in parts of Africa and Asia, where liver cell carcinoma is found more frequently. Ingested mycotoxins and viral inflammation may possibly act synergistically to increase the risk of malignant hepatocellular transformation.

4 The male predominance in liver cancer and the effect of sex hormones on experimental carcinogenesis suggest that *hormonal factors* may be important. Significantly, hepatocellular carcinoma has been reported in some patients on long-term androgenic therapy.

Clinical features Hepatic cancers may escape clinical recognition during life because they often occur in patients with underlying cirrhosis, and the symptoms and signs may initially suggest a progression of the underlying liver disease. *Hepatomegaly,* with *pain* or *tenderness,* usually moderate in degree and localized to the upper abdomen or the right upper quadrant, is a major complaint in more than half the cases. Other clinical features which should alert the clinician to the diagnosis include a *mass* in the liver, particularly if tender; the presence of a *friction rub* or *bruit* over the liver; and *blood-tinged ascites* (hemoperitoneum) which occurs in about 20 percent of cases. On rare occasions one may find metabolic disturbances such as polycythemia, hypoglycemia, acquired porphyria, hypercalcemia, and dysglobulinemia. Jaundice is characteristic of cholangiocarcinoma but is relatively uncommon in hepatocellular carcinoma in the absence of active liver disease.

Anemia, leukocytosis, and elevated alkaline phosphatase levels are common laboratory findings. In a patient with cirrhosis, a disproportionately high serum alkaline phosphatase in relation to other abnormal liver function tests is often a clue to an infiltrating or partially obstructing liver carcinoma.

Diagnosis The clinical features outlined above should suggest the possibility of primary liver carcinoma. Liver scintiscans may indicate the presence of one or more hepatic masses but frequently cannot distinguish between regenerating nodules in a cirrhotic liver and primary or metastatic liver tumors. Gallium 67 scans showing hepatocellular uptake in the abnormal area may be more helpful than ^{99m}Tc scans. Celiac axis *angiography* may reveal distortion or obstructions of vessels or "tumor blushes" characteristic of neovascularization, and usually can define the extent of the tumor. Angiography cannot, however, distinguish between types of tumor and may not be able to differentiate benign from malignant solitary tumors.

A unique fetal α_1 globulin, *α-fetoprotein* (AFP), is found in the serum of a high percentage of patients with hepatocellular carcinoma (as well as in embryonal teratoblastoma of the gonads). α-Fetoprotein serum concentrations, between 500 ng/ml and 5 mg/ml, occur in 75 to 95 percent of hepatocellular carcinoma patients in Africa and in up to 70 percent of patients in the United States. The serum AFP may be slightly elevated in about 5 to 10 percent of patients with hepatic metastases from gastrointestinal tumors, and in some patients with acute or chronic viral hepatitis, but only rarely to levels over 1000 ng/ml in these conditions. Minimally elevated levels of AFP may persist in some patients with chronic hepatitis. AFP is also elevated up to 500 ng/ml in maternal serums during pregnancy. Higher levels can occur in maternal serums with fetal distress or death. The detection and persistence of *high levels* of serum AFP in an adult (over 500 or 1000 ng/ml) in the absence of an obvious gastrointestinal tract tumor strongly suggest the presence of primary liver carcinoma. Ectopic hormones, such as chorionic gonadotropin are rarely found. Several variant isoenzymes (including aldolase, alkaline phosphatase, and 5'-nucleotide phosphodiesterase) have been reported in some liver cancer patients and also may be helpful diagnostically when present.

Percutaneous *liver biopsy* can be diagnostic, especially if the biopsy is taken in the area of a palpable nodule. False negatives may occur in as many as one-fourth of patients if the biopsy is performed in a routine, blind manner with the intercostal approach. Since cytologic examination of ascitic fluid is usually negative for tumor cells, *peritoneoscopy* or *laparotomy* with open liver biopsy is often required for diagnosis. This direct approach has the additional advantage of identifying the occasional patient with localized resectable tumor who may be suitable for partial hepatectomy.

Course and management The course of the disease is fatal and usually rapid. Most patients die within 6 months from gastrointestinal hemorrhage, progressive cachexia, or hepatic failure.

If the patient is young, in good general health, and has no obvious extrahepatic involvement, solitary hepatic lesions may be excised, or *partial hepatectomy* carried out, but the 5-year survival rate is low. Persistently high or rising levels of AFP after excision of the tumor are indicative of residual or recurrent tumor. Hepatocellular carcinoma may respond for brief periods to systemic or intraarterial chemotherapy. Further trials of combined drug therapy are in progress. Liver transplantation has been attempted in the treatment of hepatic cancer, but recurrence of tumor and frequent appearance of metastases after transplantation have limited the usefulness of this procedure. It is possible that, in the future, aggressive surgery or transplantation may prove to be of value in the treatment of small, localized tumors if diagnosed early.

OTHER BENIGN AND MALIGNANT TUMORS These tumors are very rare. Hepatoblastomas are histologically distinct primary malignant tumors of the liver occurring only in infancy and early childhood. Since they are usually solitary masses, they are more usually resectable than hepatocellular carcinoma. *Hemangiomas,* the most common of the benign tumors, are usually single and small, but may present as a large hepatic nodule. Percutaneous needle liver biopsy is contraindicated if the diagnosis is suspected because of the danger of hemorrhage. Scintillation scanning using radioactive ^{99m}Tc or ^{67}Ga will show a defect in the liver. In contrast, a labeled albumin scan may result in the accumulation of the isotope in the vascular tumors. The diagnosis can frequently be made by angiography. Surgical excision is usually not indicated unless the tumors are large and symptomatic or a malignant lesion cannot be excluded. *Hemangioendotheliomas* or *angiosarcomas* are rare malignant vascular tumors. They have occurred in some patients in association with chronic *vinyl chloride* exposure. These tumors have also begun to occur 15 to 20 years after the administration of Thorotrast, a radioactive contrast agent widely used for diagnostic purposes between 1930 and the mid-1950s.

Benign hepatic adenomas and focal nodular hyperplasia, although quite rare, have been reported with increasing frequency, particularly in women taking oral contraceptives. Other rare tumors include benign cholangiomas, rhabdomyomas, and rhabdomyosarcomas. These tumors usually present as a palpable mass in the liver or with intraabdominal hemorrhage. They can be visualized and their extent defined by angiography. Surgical exploration and open biopsy are usually required for definitive diagnosis and to determine resectability.

METASTATIC TUMORS Metastatic malignant tumors of the liver are common in clinical practice, ranking second only to cirrhosis as a cause of fatal liver disease. In the United States the incidence of clinically significant metastatic carcinoma is at least 20 times greater than that of primary carcinoma. Hepatic metastases have been reported at autopsies in 30 to 50 percent of patients dying from malignant disease.

Pathogenesis The liver is uniquely vulnerable to invasion by tumor cells: its size, high rate of blood flow, and double perfusion by hepatic artery and portal vein combine to make it the most common site of metastases except for the lymph nodes. In addition, local tissue factors appear to support the growth of metastatic implants. Virtually all types of neoplasms except those primary in the brain may metastasize to the liver. The most common primary tumors are those of the gastrointestinal tract, lung, and breast, and melanomas. Less common are metastases from tumors of the thyroid, prostate, and skin.

Clinical features Most patients with metastatic malignancy of the liver present with (1) symptoms referable only to the primary tumor, with asymptomatic hepatic involvement discovered in the course of clinical evaluation; (2) nonspecific symptoms of weakness, weight loss, fever, sweating, and loss of appetite; or, rarely, (3) features indicating active hepatic disease, especially abdominal pain, hepatomegaly, ascites, or jaundice.

Patients with widespread metastatic liver involvement usually have suggestive clinical signs of cancer and hepatic enlargement; some have localized induration or tenderness of the liver; signs of portal hypertension may be present; or a friction rub may be found, usually over tender areas of the liver.

Abnormal liver function tests are frequent but often mild and nonspecific. They reflect the effects of fever and wasting, as well as the infiltrating neoplastic process itself. An increase in serum alkaline phosphatase is the most common and frequently the only abnormality noted. Hypoalbuminemia, anemia, and occasional mild elevation of transaminase levels may also be found with more widespread disease.

Diagnosis Evidence of metastatic invasion of the liver should be sought actively in any patient with a primary malignancy, especially of the lung, gastrointestinal tract, or breast, before therapy is undertaken. Serial studies of liver function and hepatic scintiscans may provide a presumptive diagnosis. Needle biopsy of the liver is usually indicated, affording positive diagnoses in 60 to 80 percent of cases with established metastases. Serial sectioning of specimens, two or three repeat biopsies, or cytologic examination of biopsy smears may increase the diagnostic yield by 10 to 15 percent. Liver biopsy may, on occasion, be the first and only preoperative proof of widespread malignancy when the primary tumor is occult.

Treatment Most metastatic carcinomas respond poorly to all forms of treatment, which is usually only palliative. Surgical removal of a large metastasis is rarely feasible. Systemic chemotherapy with 5-fluorouracil or methotrexate is believed to slow tumor growth and reduce symptoms in some patients but probably does not significantly alter the prognosis. It remains to be determined whether newer drugs or combination chemotherapy will prove to be more effective.

REFERENCES

ALPERT E: Alpha-fetoprotein: Developmental biology and clinical significance, in *Progress in Liver Disease*, vol 5, H Popper, F Schaffner (eds). New York, Grune & Stratton, 1975

————: Primary hepatic tumor. Gastroenterology 74:759, 1978

BERMAN C: *Primary Carcinoma of the Liver: A Study in Incidence, Clinical Manifestations, Pathology and Etiology.* London, Lewis, 1951

FENSTER LF, KLATSKIN G: Manifestations of metastatic tumors of the liver. Am J Med 31:238, 1961

KLATSKIN G: Hepatic tumors: Possible relationship to use of oral contraceptives. Gastroenterology 73:386, 1977

MARGOLIS S, HOWEY C: Systemic manifestations of hepatoma. Medicine 51:381, 1972

OKUDA K: Clinical aspects of hepatocellular carcinoma: Analysis of 134 cases, in *Hepatocellular Carcinoma,* K Okuda, RL Peters (eds). New York, Wiley, 1976

OMATA M et al: Hepatocellular carcinoma in the USA: Etiologic considerations. Localization of hepatitis B antigens. Gastroenterology 76:279, 1979

SELIKOFF IJ, HAMMOND EC (eds): Toxicity of vinyl chloride–polyvinyl chloride. Ann NY Acad Sci 246:1975

WOGAN G: Aflatoxin in carcinogenesis and its implications in man, in *Hepatocellular Carcinoma,* K Okuda, RL Peters (eds). New York, Wiley, 1976

306

INFILTRATIVE AND METABOLIC DISEASES AFFECTING THE LIVER

KURT J. ISSELBACHER
J. THOMAS LaMONT

Many disseminated, systemic, or metabolic diseases involve the liver in a diffuse manner by the infiltration of abnormal cells or the accumulation of chemical substances or metabolites. Although infiltrative diseases may vary widely in their etiology and extrahepatic manifestations, the findings in the liver may be quite similar. Generalized enlargement and firmness of the liver, gradual and nonspecific deterioration of liver function, and, less often, signs of portal hypertension or ascites are typical features of this group of diseases. Differential diagnosis by clinical means may be difficult on occasion, but the diffusely infiltrated liver provides an excellent source of tissue for diagnostic purposes.

The infiltrative process may involve one or more of the structural components of the liver: the hepatocytes, the Kupffer cells and other elements of the reticuloendothelial system, the interstitial tissue, or the blood vessels.

LIPID INFILTRATIONS

FATTY LIVER Slight to moderate enlargement of the liver due to diffuse infiltration of liver cells by neutral fat (triglyceride) is a common clinical and pathologic finding. Although minimal fatty changes are often transient and have no clinical significance, persistent or extensive fatty infiltration may produce dysfunction and symptoms that require careful evaluation.

Etiology The major causes of fatty liver encountered in clinical practice depend on the age, geographic location, and metabolic-nutritional status of the patient population. *Chronic alcoholism* is the most common cause of fatty liver in this country and in other countries with a high alcohol intake. The severity of fatty involvement is roughly proportional to the duration and degree of alcoholic excess. *Protein malnutrition,* especially in infancy and early childhood, accounts for most cases of severe fatty liver in the tropical zones of Africa, South America, and Asia. The hepatic changes may be associated with other clinical and pathologic features of kwashiorkor. Patients with adult-onset *diabetes mellitus,* especially those who are overweight and are poorly controlled, often have fatty livers. *Obesity* is commonly associated with fatty infiltration of the liver, which recedes as weight reduction occurs. However, *jejunoileal bypass* for surgical treatment of morbid obesity is sometimes associated with severe fatty liver and hepatic failure which may be fatal. In patients with Cushing's syndrome and in those receiving large doses of corticosteroids, fatty infiltration of the liver may occur. In many *chronic illnesses,* especially those complicated by impaired nutrition of malabsorption, increased fat is found in liver cells. For example, patients with ulcerative colitis, chronic pancreatitis, or protracted heart failure frequently have moderately fatty livers at the time of death. Patients maintained on prolonged *intravenous hyperalimentation* may also develop a fatty liver.

Acute fatty liver is caused by a number of hepatotoxins and is frequently accompanied by signs and symptoms of liver failure. Carbon tetrachloride intoxication, DDT poisoning, and ingestion of substances containing yellow phosphorus result in severe fatty liver. Acute and prolonged alcohol ingestion may also be considered in this category and may be associated with a rapidly enlarging and fat-laden liver. Minor degrees of fatty infiltration are seen following acute alcoholic intoxication, but this is rarely of clinical significance. Two types of acute fatty liver deserve special comment: *Acute fatty liver of pregnancy,* a rare but often fatal condition seen during the third trimester of pregnancy, is characterized by nausea, vomiting, abdominal pain, renal failure, and coma. *Massive tetracycline therapy,* in amounts of 3 to 12 g administered intravenously is a rare cause of acute fatty liver and fatal hepatic coma, especially during pregnancy.

Pathogenesis The hepatic lipid deposits, which consist largely of triglycerides and lesser amounts of phospholipid and cholesterol, appear as vacuoles of varying size within the cytoplasm of liver cells. In extreme cases, every liver cell is involved, and lipids comprise up to 30 to 40 percent of the total liver weight.

The biochemical mechanisms leading to hepatic triglyceride accumulation are described in Chap. 299. Fatty infiltration has been produced in experimental animals by a variety of toxic agents and drugs, such as alcohol, carbon tetrachloride, and orotic acid. Dietary deficiencies, such as choline deficiency, readily lead to increased fat in the liver in the rat. However, with few exceptions these experimental studies cannot be used directly to explain the pathogenesis of fatty liver in clinical disease. Moderate doses of ethanol may produce both acute and chronic fatty changes in human subjects, probably by its direct effects on hepatic triglyceride and fatty acid metabolism (Chap. 299). Protein deficiency seems to account for the fatty liver of kwashiorkor, and impaired protein synthesis for the fat accumulation following tetracycline and carbon tetrachloride administration. In diabetes mellitus and in starvation, increased mobilization of fatty acids from adipose tissue may be involved.

Clinical features The signs and symptoms of fatty liver are related to the degree of fat infiltration, the time course of its accumulation, and the underlying cause. The obese or diabetic patient with chronic fatty liver is usually asymptomatic and has only mild tenderness over the enlarged liver. The liver function tests are normal or show mild elevations of alkaline phosphatase, transaminases, or aminotransferases. In contrast, alcoholic patients with acute fatty liver following a bout of heavy drinking may have right upper quadrant pain and tenderness with laboratory evidence of cholestasis. The clinical presentation of acute fatty liver of pregnancy or fatty liver from hepatotoxins is that of fulminant hepatic failure of any cause, with evidence of hepatic encephalopathy, marked elevations of prothrombin time and transaminases, and variable degrees of jaundice.

Diagnosis The findings of a firm, nontender, and generally enlarged liver with minimal hepatic dysfunction in a patient with chronic alcoholism, malnutrition, poorly controlled diabetes mellitus, or obesity should suggest a fatty liver. Needle biopsy of the liver will demonstrate the increased fatty content and possibly the underlying primary disorder. In acute fatty liver of pregnancy, especially when associated with tetracycline therapy, and in most cases of Reye's syndrome (see below), fat accumulates in small vacuoles rather than in large cytoplasmic droplets.

Treatment Attention to nutritional factors, removal of alcohol or offending toxins, and correction of any associated metabolic disorders usually result in recovery. There is no clinical rationale for the use of lipotropic agents such as choline. When indicated, attention should be directed to abstinence from alcohol, careful control of diabetes, weight loss, or correction of intestinal absorptive defects. In the alcoholic fatty liver there is gradual disappearance of fat from the liver after 4 to 8 weeks of adequate diet and abstinence from alcohol.

REYE'S SYNDROME (FATTY LIVER WITH ENCEPHALOPATHY)
This acute illness has been described in children up to 15 years of age. It is characterized by vomiting, progressive central nervous system damage, signs of hepatic injury, hypoglycemia, and morphologically by extensive fatty vacuolization of the liver and renal tubules. The cause is unknown, although viral and toxic agents have been implicated. Cases have been reported from several countries; infants and children of either sex are affected and familial occurrences have been described. In fatal cases, the liver is enlarged and yellow, with striking diffuse fatty microvacuolization of cells. Peripheral zonal hepatic necrosis has also been present in some cases. Fatty changes of the renal tubular cells, cerebral edema, and neuronal degeneration of the brain are the major extrahepatic changes.

The onset often follows an upper respiratory tract infection in a previously healthy child. Within 1 to 3 days persistent vomiting occurs together with stupor, which usually progresses rapidly to generalized convulsions and coma. The liver is enlarged, but *jaundice is characteristically absent or minimal.* Marked increases in serum transaminases and prothrombin time, hypoglycemia, metabolic acidosis, and elevated serum ammonia levels are the major laboratory findings. The mortality rate in Reye's syndrome is approximately 50 percent. Therapy consists of infusions of glucose and fresh frozen plasma, as well as intravenous mannitol, to reduce the cerebral edema. Chronic liver disease has not been reported in survivors.

Since the disease appears typically to follow apparent upper respiratory tract infections, chickenpox, or influenza, virologic studies have been carried out. Isolations from stool and tissues have included coxsackievirus, influenza viruses, echovirus 11, and adenovirus type 3. The role of these viral agents in the pathogenesis of the disease is still unclear. Electron-microscopic studies show structural alterations of the mitochondria of liver, brain, and muscle. Hyperammonemia in Reye's syndrome results in part from a transient dysfunction of several hepatic mitochondrial enzymes which convert ammonia to urea. These findings suggest that the hepatic and neurologic manifestations of Reye's syndrome may result from virally induced damage to the mitochondria of the liver and brain.

NIEMANN-PICK DISEASE (See Chap. 322)   This rare heritable disorder, found mainly in Jewish infants, is characterized by the accumulation of sphingomyelin and cholesterol in reticuloendothelial cells of the liver, spleen, bone marrow, and brain. Hepatomegaly and splenomegaly are present, but jaundice and other evidence of hepatic dysfunction are rare. The liver shows clusters of lipid-filled, foamy Kupffer cells. Diagnosis is made by lipid analysis of the tissue.

GAUCHER'S DISEASE (See Chap. 322)   Accumulations of large reticuloendothelial cells containing glucocerebrosides (Gaucher's cells) in the liver and spleen account for the characteristic moderate to massive hepatosplenomegaly. Rarely, ascites or portal hypertension is produced by compression of the intrahepatic vasculature. The diagnosis may be made readily by liver biopsy and demonstration of the Gaucher's cells.

WOLMAN'S AND CHOLESTEROL ESTER STORAGE DISEASES
Wolman's disease is a rare and fatal familial lipidosis of infancy producing hepatosplenomegaly and stippled calcification of the adrenal glands. Liver biopsy shows clusters of foam cells (reticuloendothelial cells filled with cholesterol ester and triglycerides), hepatocytes containing fat, and patchy fibrosis. A related but less severe genetic disorder is cholesterol ester storage disease. In this condition there is hypercholesterolemia and accumulation of both cholesterol esters and triglycerides in hepatic lysosomes. Both these storage disorders are associated with hepatic deficiencies of cholesterol ester hydrolase and triglyceride lipase.

Other rare lipid disorders associated with hepatomegaly and increased fat in the liver include abetalipoproteinemia (Chap. 100), Tangier disease (Chap. 100), Fabry's disease (Chap. 100), and type I and V hyperlipoproteinemia (Chap. 100).

HEPATIC GLYCOGEN ACCUMULATION

DIABETIC GLYCOGENOSIS   Hepatic enlargement caused by distention of liver cells with glycogen is present in some poorly controlled and often juvenile diabetic patients. Ketoacidosis

and vigorous insulin therapy may further enhance hepatic enlargement and glycogen deposition. In the absence of cirrhosis, the hepatomegaly usually decreases with careful control of the diabetes.

GLYCOGEN STORAGE DISEASE (See Chap. 97)   The normal liver contains 1 to 5 percent glycogen (by weight). In types I, II, and VI hereditary glycogen storage disease, increased amounts of glycogen (and fat) are found. Types III and IV are associated with derangements of glycogen structure, and cirrhosis may be present. Enzymatic and chemical analysis of liver tissue is usually needed for diagnosis.

GALACTOSEMIA (See also Chap. 98)

Hepatic changes are common in patients with unrecognized or untreated galactosemia. In early weeks of life fatty infiltration and cholestasis may be noted in acutely ill infants. If the disease goes unrecognized for months or years, cirrhosis may develop.

OTHER INFILTRATIVE DISEASES

HURLER'S SYNDROME (See Chap. 103)   This is an uncommon hereditary disease that is characterized by the widespread tissue deposition of mucopolysaccharide (chondroitin sulfate B and heparin sulfate) in many tissues. The liver is frequently enlarged and firm. Microscopically, Kupffer cells and other macrophages are enlarged and filled with metachromatic granular material. Cirrhosis may be a late complication.

α_1-ANTITRYPSIN DEFICIENCY   Patients with homozygous deficiency of serum α_1-antitrypsin (α_1-AT) are prone to develop emphysema in adult life. Hepatocytes of some patients with this deficiency contain periodic acid Schiff (PAS)-positive globules which have been shown to be α_1-AT. Approximately 10 percent of children with homozygous deficiency (ZZ phenotype) of α_1-AT will develop significant liver disease including neonatal hepatitis and progressive cirrhosis. It has been suggested that 15 to 20 percent of all chronic liver disease in infancy may be attributed to α_1-AT deficiency. Some adults have PAS-positive globules and portal fibrosis or cirrhosis. The occurrence of liver disease in these patients is not dependent upon the development of lung disease.

RETICULOENDOTHELIAL DISORDERS (See also Chaps. 322 and 327)

Moderate to massive hepatomegaly and splenomegaly occur frequently in the various types of leukemia and lymphoma. Jaundice, when present, is usually slight and results from hemolysis. Deep and protracted jaundice is distinctly rare and is caused by obstruction of the intrahepatic or extrahepatic bile ducts by tumor. Liver biopsy specimens reveal portal and sinusoidal infiltrates in most cases of leukemia, but the cellular pattern may be mixed and nonspecific. Liver biopsy may provide a tissue diagnosis in patients with lymphoma or Hodgkin's disease; however, if the biopsy needle misses the tumor nodules, the cellular infiltrates may show a nondiagnostic pattern.

Myeloid metaplasia and other myeloproliferative disorders associated with extramedullary hematopoiesis produce hepatomegaly which may reach huge proportions, especially following splenectomy. Bromosulphalein (BSP) retention and alkaline phosphatase elevations are often found. Ascites and portal hypertension, apparently caused by diffuse involvement of portal venules and lymphatics, are rare complications.

GRANULOMATOUS INFILTRATIONS

Systemic granulomatous diseases, including sarcoidosis, miliary tuberculosis, histoplasmosis, brucellosis, schistosomiasis, berylliosis, and drug reactions, produce focal infiltrative hepatic lesions with great regularity. In addition, isolated granulomas of no diagnostic importance may be found occasionally in patients with various forms of cirrhosis and hepatitis. The liver infiltrated by granulomas may be slightly enlarged and firm, but hepatic dysfunction is usually limited to BSP retention and increased serum alkaline phosphatase levels. In a few patients with sarcoidosis or brucellosis portal hypertension may develop, and extensive postnecrotic scarring or postnecrotic cirrhosis may follow healing of the granulomatous lesions.

Needle biopsy of the liver reveals granulomas and often provides the first definite evidence of a systemic or disseminated granulomatous disease. In patients with sarcoidosis who have neither clinical nor laboratory evidence of hepatic involvement, needle biopsy is positive in about 80 percent of cases. In cases of suspected miliary tuberculosis a portion of the biopsy should be cultured and stained for mycobacteria. The organism can be detected in the majority of cases, particularly when caseating granuloma are present. Serial sections of the biopsy specimen should be examined if granulomas are not apparent. Individual granulomas are rarely specific in their microscopic appearance, and final diagnosis usually requires other clinical, laboratory, or histologic data.

AMYLOIDOSIS (See also Chap. 64)

Systemic amyloidosis, whether primary and idiopathic, familial, or secondary to chronic inflammatory or neoplastic diseases, often involves the liver. Grossly, the liver infiltrated with amyloid is enlarged and pale and rubbery in consistency. Microscopically, the birefringent amyloid deposits appear as homogeneous waxy material within the space of Disse, often being concentrated in the periportal areas with atrophy of adjacent liver cell plates. Selective involvement of the walls of blood vessels, especially of the hepatic arterioles, may be a striking feature of primary amyloidosis. With this possible exception, however, the hepatic lesions are the same in all forms of amyloidosis and are present in 60 to 90 percent of cases.

An enlarged and firm liver is found in about 60 percent of patients, and ascites occurs in advanced stages of the disease in about 20 percent. Jaundice, portal hypertension, and other signs of chronic liver disease are usually absent. Liver function changes, although frequent, correlate poorly with the extent of liver infiltration. Hypoalbuminemia, BSP retention, and elevated serum alkaline phosphatase levels are common. The diagnosis is established by biopsy of rectum, skin, liver, or other involved organs.

REFERENCES

ALPERS DH, ISSELBACHER KJ: Fatty liver: Clinical and biochemical aspects, in *Diseases of the Liver*, 4th ed, L Schiff (ed). Philadelphia, Lippincott, 1974

GUCKIAN JC, PARRY JE: Granulomatous hepatitis. Ann Intern Med 65:1081, 1966

ISHAK KG et al: Cirrhosis of the liver associated with α_1-antitrypsin deficiency. Arch Pathol 94:445, 1972

MADDREY WC et al: Sarcoidosis and chronic hepatic disease: A clinical and pathologic study of 20 patients. Medicine 49:375, 1970

PARTIN JC: Reye's syndrome (encephalopathy and fatty liver). Gastroenterology 69:511, 1975

SVEGER T: Liver disease in α_1-antitrypsin deficiency. N Engl J Med 294:1316, 1976

307

DISEASES OF THE GALLBLADDER AND BILE DUCTS

LESLIE J. SCHOENFIELD

PHYSIOLOGY AND CHEMISTRY

BILE SECRETION AND COMPOSITION Bile formation begins at the level of the microvillus membrane of the bile canaliculus. The canaliculus is the most proximal portion of the biliary system and is formed from the cell membranes of two opposing hepatic cells. Bile flow is determined by three mechanisms (two canalicular and one ductular), each contributing approximately one-third to the daily bile volume of about 500 to 1200 ml. The *canalicular* mechanisms involve (1) active transport of the conjugated bile acids and (2) bile acid–independent active transport of sodium. *Ductular* transport depends on active secretion of sodium and bicarbonate; it responds to secretin, is mediated by cyclic adenosine monophosphate (AMP), and maintains bile isosmotic with plasma. The hepatic secretion of water, therefore, is primarily passive in response to osmotic gradients produced by solute transport. Some ductular reabsorption of water and solute also occurs.

Bile acids returning to the liver via the enterohepatic circulation account for 95 percent of bile acids secreted by the liver; the remainder represents new bile acid synthesis by the liver. An increase in the rate of bile secretion is associated with an increase in cholesterol secretion; the secretion of lecithin similarly is dependent primarily on the secretion of bile acids. There is no secretion of phospholipids and cholesterol in the absence of bile acid secretion. It is noteworthy, however, that at low rates of bile acid secretion relatively more cholesterol than lecithin is secreted. Thus, when bile acid secretion rates are less than 10 (μmol/kg)/h, bile becomes saturated with cholesterol; this occurs normally during fasting. The average daily output of bile acids is 27 mmol, of lecithin 14 mmol, and of cholesterol 3 mmol.

BILE ACIDS **Enterophepatic circulation** Under normal conditions, most of the conjugated bile acids entering the intestinal lumen are reabsorbed by an *active transport* mechanism in the terminal 100 cm ileum (see Chap. 292). A second, quantitatively less significant absorptive mechanism is *nonionic diffusion* or passive transport which occurs in the jejunum and colon. Nonionic diffusion is dependent on the variable ability of each bile acid to remain undissociated at the pH of the jejunal contents; this property is a function of the dissociation constant of the individual bile acids. Thus, unconjugated bile acids, deoxycholic acid, and the glycine conjugates of chenodeoxycholic acid will be in an un-ionized form and be reabsorbed by this mechanism. The reabsorbed bile acids enter the portal venous system (tightly bound to protein) and are largely taken up by the liver to be reconjugated and secreted into the bile (enterohepatic circulation). The bile acid pool, normally about 2 to 4 g, circulates 5 to 10 times daily. The daily fecal loss of bile acids is 0.3 to 0.6 g, an amount equal to the daily hepatic synthesis. Bile acids returning to the liver suppress hepatic synthesis by inhibiting the rate-limiting microsomal enzyme, cholesterol 7α-hydroxylase. When bile acid reabsorption is decreased, there is a compensatory increase in hepatic synthesis. However, when there is severe bile acid loss, the maximum hepatic synthesis rate of 5 g per day may be insufficient to restore biliary and intestinal bile acid concentrations to normal.

Primary and secondary bile acids (see also Chap. 292) The primary bile acids, cholic and chenodeoxycholic acids, are synthesized from cholesterol and conjugated with glycine or taurine in the liver. The secondary bile acids, deoxycholic and lithocholic acids, are formed in the colon by bacterial 7α-dehydroxylation of cholic and chenodeoxycholic acids. Deoxycholic acid is absorbed readily from the colon, returns to the liver, and is conjugated with glycine and taurine. Lithocholic acid is absorbed less efficiently; the small amount which reaches the liver is conjugated, sulfated, and secreted into the bile. The bile acid content of normal human bile is shown in Table 307-1. The ratio of glycine to taurine conjugates is about 3:1.

Functions Bile acids provide the main excretory route for biliary cholesterol and are necessary for efficient intestinal absorption of lipids (see Chap. 292). They also serve as major regulators of hepatic bile flow and lipid secretion as well as of intestinal electrolyte and water transport. Bile acids are water-soluble, amphiphilic, detergent-like molecules which in aqueous solutions and above a critical concentration (about 2 mM) form aggregates called *micelles*. The addition of lecithin to bile acid micelles enhances the ability of the micelles to incorporate cholesterol. The amount of cholesterol that can be solubilized in these mixed micelles is limited and depends on the total lipid concentration and the relative molar percentages of bile acids and lecithin (Fig. 307-1). The degree of saturation with cholesterol also can be expressed numerically as a lithogenic (saturation) index. Bile which is saturated has an index of 1, supersaturated bile has an index greater than 1, and unsaturated bile has an index of less than 1.

GALLBLADDER FUNCTION **Absorption and concentration** (see Table 307-2) The gallbladder concentrates bile by selective absorption of electrolytes and water at a rate of approximately 20 percent of its volume per hour. This process results in an increase of solids in bile from about 3 to 16 percent of bile weight (see Table 307-2). Gallbladder absorption involves energy-dependent, carrier-mediated, electrically neutral transport of NaCl, NaHCO₃, and water in isotonic proportions. The normal gallbladder is impermeable to conjugated bile acids, bilirubin, or iodinated contrast agents such as iopanoic acid (Telepaque). If, however, these compounds are rendered lipid-soluble by bacterial deconjugation, or if the gallbladder mucosa is damaged, they may be absorbed.

Storage and evacuation Bile is stored in the gallbladder and is discharged into the intestinal lumen following the ingestion of a meal. Between meals the pressure in the common bile duct averages 12 cmH₂O. This is less than the resistance of the sphincter of Oddi but exceeds the resting pressure in the gallbladder. Under these conditions bile enters and fills the gallbladder. After an overnight fast the gallbladder volume is

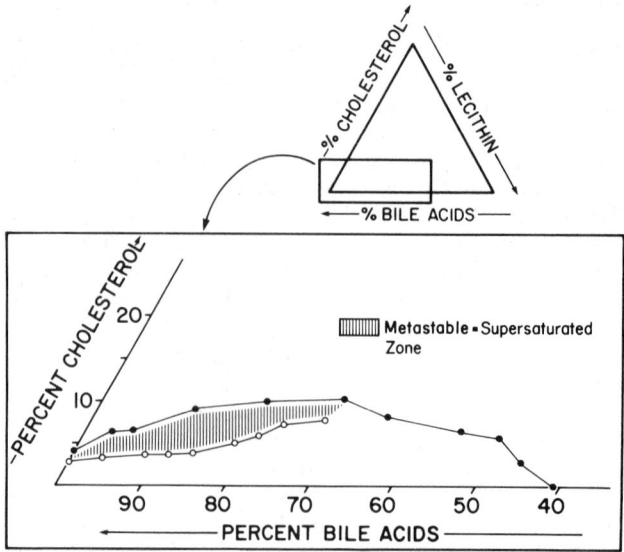

FIGURE 307-1

The relative concentrations of bile acid, cholesterol, and phospholipid are expressed on triangular coordinates as mole percentages totaling 100 percent. Points below the equilibrium solubility limit represent bile that is not saturated with cholesterol. Supersaturated bile is metastable when precipitation of cholesterol is slow (metastable zone) and labile when it is rapid (above the metastable-labile limit). With sufficient time supersaturated bile reverts to the equilibrium solubility limit, and the excess micellar cholesterol is transformed to a crystalline or liquid crystalline phase. (After Carey and Small.)

about 50 ml, sufficient to sequester the entire bile acid pool. During digestion, cholecystokinin-pancreozymin (CCK-PZ) is released (see Chap. 292), which causes increased hepatic secretion of bile, contraction of the gallbladder (increasing its pressure to about 26 cmH₂O), and decreased resistance of the sphincter of Oddi. Under these conditions bile enters the duodenum. The action of cholecystokinin on gallbladder muscle is mediated by the cyclic nucleotides, cyclic AMP and cyclic guanosine monophosphate (GMP).

GALLSTONES

FREQUENCY AND TYPES An estimated 20 million Americans have gallstones, and 1 million develop them each year. In autopsy studies in the United States, gallstones have been found in 20 percent of women and 8 percent of men. The prevalence, however, varies considerably among racial and national groups. For example, about 70 percent of American Indian women over age 30 have gallstones. In the United States, cholesterol stones account for 80 percent and pigment stones for 20 percent of gallstones. Although some cholesterol gallstones are virtually pure, most are mixed, containing more than 70 percent cholesterol monohydrate plus calcium salts, bile acids, bile pigments, fatty acids, protein, and phospholipids. Pigment stones are primarily calcium bilirubinate and contain less than 10 percent cholesterol.

PATHOGENESIS The solubility of cholesterol in bile depends on the relative molar concentrations of cholesterol, bile acids, and lecithin (Fig. 307-1). Saturated bile is secreted by the liver. Although not sufficient as a sole abnormality, cholesterol-saturated bile is a prerequisite for cholesterol gallstone formation. In some gallstone patients (but not all), the bile acid pool is reduced to about one-half of normal. This defect has been postulated to be secondary to decreased hepatic synthesis. In fact, patients with cholesterol gallstones have reduced activity

TABLE 307-1
Bile acids in normal human bile

	Percent (as Na⁺ and K⁺ salts)
Primary acids:	
Cholic	36
Chenodeoxycholic	36
Secondary acids:	
Deoxycholic	23
Sulfated lithocholic	4
Lithocholic	1
Ursodeoxycholic	0–5

TABLE 307-2
Chemical composition of normal gallbladder bile

	Percent (by weight)	Total lipids, mol %
Water	82	
Bile salts	12	72
Phospholipids (>95% lecithin)	4	24
Cholesterol (nonesterified)	0.7	4
Others (conjugated bilirubin, proteins, electrolytes, etc.)	>1	

of hepatic cholesterol 7α-hydroxylase, the rate-limiting enzyme for bile acid synthesis. The most important cause of saturated bile, however, appears to be *increased biliary secretion of cholesterol,* possibly due to increased activity of hepatic hydroxymethylglutaryl coenzyme A (HMG CoA) reductase, the rate-limiting enzyme of cholesterol synthesis. Substances such as mucoproteins probably trap microcrystals of cholesterol. Scanning electron micrographs have shown that during gallstone growth, laminated cholesterol crystals aggregate radially, concentrically, or randomly. After cholecystectomy and in some cases of nonvisualization of the gallbladder on cholecystogram, bile may again become unsaturated, possibly because of increased enterohepatic cycling and augmented secretion of bile acids.

In regard to pigment gallstone formation, hemolysis may be a contributory factor because it leads to increased biliary secretion of conjugated bilirubin. The enzyme β-glucuronidase, perhaps of bacterial origin, is thought to deconjugate bilirubin diglucuronide to free bilirubin. This insoluble pigment then combines with calcium to form calcium bilirubinate. Stagnation of bile may often abet the process. In Oriental subjects, gallstone formation has been associated with the presence of bacterial infection of bile; under these conditions, bacterial β-glucuronidase may be involved in the hydrolysis of conjugated bilirubin. In the United States, where biliary infections are less frequent than in the Orient, pigment stones are also less frequent.

PREDISPOSING FACTORS (See Table 307-3) The incidence of cholesterol gallstones is almost three times greater among women than men and increases with age. Obesity and possibly multiparity appear to be predisposing factors. Clofibrate, oral contraceptives, and estrogens increase biliary cholesterol secretion and appear to double the incidence of gallstones. Forty percent of patients with chronic ileal disease and extensive ileal resection develop gallstones, probably secondary to depletion of the bile acid pool. A marked increase in gallstone formation has been reported after truncal vagotomy and in patients with diabetes mellitus, possibly because of delayed emptying of the gallbladder and resultant stagnation of bile. Pigment gallstones occur in association with chronic hemolytic disorders, alcoholic liver disease, biliary infection, and with obstruction or anomalies of the biliary tree.

NATURAL COURSE Stones in the gallbladder usually cause symptoms only when they migrate to obstruct either the cystic duct or the common bile duct. Symptoms of biliary colic or acute cholecystitis are prominent manifestations of cystic duct obstruction and are eventually experienced by about one-half of patients with gallstones. Common duct stones may occur in up to 10 to 15 percent of patients with gallstones, and the incidence of choledocholithiasis increases with the duration of the stone-predisposing disease process. Development of biliary colic, cholangitis, obstructive jaundice, or pancreatitis occurs

subsequently in about 75 percent of patients with duct stones. In one study of patients with mild or moderate symptoms (not requiring cholecystectomy) for 1 year after their initial diagnosis of cholecystolithiasis, 35 percent developed severe symptoms (e.g., acute cholecystitis) requiring cholecystectomy over the subsequent decade of study.

RADIOLOGICAL DIAGNOSTIC PROCEDURES   Plain abdominal radiograph Approximately 20 percent of gallstones contain enough calcium for visualization on the plain film of the abdomen. Characteristic diagnostic features may also be seen with emphysematous cholecystitis (air in the gallbladder wall or lumen), porcelain gallbladder, milk of calcium bile, and gallstone ileus.

Oral cholecystography The patient is instructed to ingest tablets of iopanoic acid (Telepaque) the evening prior to study and to refrain from eating or drinking until the examination is finished. The contrast agent is absorbed from the intestine, conjugated with glucuronide in the liver, secreted in bile, and eventually concentrated in the gallbladder. Films are obtained about 12 h after the drug is ingested. Agents such as calcium ipodate (Oragrafin) designed for more rapid contrast visualization are also available. If the gallbladder is opacified, radiolucent stones may be seen in the lumen. Upright or lateral decubitus spot films are taken to detect stones which often aggregate in the dependent portion of the gallbladder. A fatty meal may be given during cholecystography to stimulate gallbladder contraction and evacuation; this can enhance detection of small stones and aid in the diagnosis of the hyperplastic cholecystoses. Oral cholecystography provides a correct diagnosis in 95 percent of patients, and less than 2 percent of gallbladders which are normal by cholecystogram contain previously undetected stones.

Nonvisualization of a diseased gallbladder most commonly occurs in the presence of cystic duct obstruction or because the contrast material is absorbed across the inflamed gallbladder mucosa. Approximately 60 percent of poorly visualized gallbladders and 30 percent of gallbladders nonvisualizing after a single dose will opacify following a second dose of a contrast agent. Extrabiliary factors responsible for nonvisualization include failure to ingest the contrast material, gastric retention, vomiting, diarrhea, and diminished intestinal absorption. In addition, the gallbladder will not usually visualize if the serum

TABLE 307-3
Predisposing (risk) factors for gallstones

I Cholesterol stones
  A Demography: Northern Europe; North and South America more than the Orient; American Indians; probable familial predisposition
  B Obesity, high-calorie diet
  C Clofibrate therapy
  D Malabsorption of bile acids (e.g., ileal disease or resection)
  E Cystic fibrosis
  F Female sex hormones: Women more than men, after puberty; oral contraceptives and other estrogens
  G Age, especially among males
  H Probable factors: Pregnancy, diabetes mellitus, dietary polyunsaturated fats
II Pigment stones
  A Demography: Oriental more than Occidental
  B Chronic hemolysis
  C Alcoholic liver disease
  D Biliary infection
  E Age

SOURCE: *After Bennion and Grundy.*

bilirubin level is 3 mg per 100 ml or more, or if there is impaired hepatic secretion due to liver disease or extrahepatic biliary obstruction. When extrabiliary and other hepatobiliary causes are excluded, nonvisualization after ingestion of Telepaque for two consecutive days provides evidence for underlying gallbladder disease. Failure of the gallbladder to contract or poor visualization has no specific diagnostic value.

Echography (see Fig. 307-2A) Reflected ultrasound provides images based on the differences in acoustic impedance among solid tissues of differing density, fluid, and air. Echography has an overall accuracy of 96 percent in the diagnosis of cholelithiasis. This rapid, reliable noninvasive technique is useful in patients allergic to contrast media, in those with jaundice, or in those with nonvisualization on oral cholecystography due to extrabiliary factors. It is also useful in pregnant patients and adolescents in whom excessive exposure to ionizing radiation is undesirable. Echography may occasionally detect small calculi not visible on an oral cholecystogram. Its accuracy in detection of common-duct stones remains to be substantiated.

Intravenous cholangiography (IVC) Oral cholecystography identifies duct or ductal stones in only about 15 percent of patients who have them. For improved visualization of the bile ducts, sodium iodipamide (Cholografin) may be administered intravenously. The clinical indications for intravenous cholangiography include upper abdominal pain after cholecystectomy, oral cholecystographic nonvisualization due to extrabiliary factors, and undiagnosed acute upper abdominal pain. The larger biliary channels opacify within 10 to 30 min, reaching maximal concentrations at 30 to 40 min (provided liver function is normal). Visualization rarely occurs when the serum bilirubin is greater than 3 mg per 100 ml. With an unimpeded flow of contrast material into the duodenum, the radiodensity should decrease within 60 min of injection. Partial obstruction of the common duct prevents normal emptying and prolongs maximum ductal opacification up to 2 h. If the gallbladder

fails to opacify by 2 h, follow-up radiographs should be made at 4 and 24 h. Fluoroscopy and tomography may aid radiographic visualization of the ducts and gallbladder. The normal common duct diameter ranges from 4 to 12 mm on intravenous cholangiograms. A common bile duct known to be previously enlarged rarely demonstrates a complete return to normal size; thus, knowledge of ductal size at surgery or prior examinations may be helpful in interpreting the finding of a dilated common duct. Adverse reactions with Cholografin injection occasionally occur; these include vasomotor reactions (nausea, vomiting, hypotension), urticaria, and (rarely) anaphylaxis.

Transhepatic cholangiography A long (6 to 9 in), thin (22 to 25 gauge), flexible Chiba needle is inserted through the eighth or ninth intercostal space in the midaxillary line into the liver under fluoroscopic guidance. During withdrawal of the needle, radiopaque dye is injected to locate an intrahepatic bile duct radicle; with cannulization of the radicle, dye is then injected to define the biliary anatomy. Through an indwelling catheter a dilated biliary tree can be decompressed either by draining either percutaneously or into the duodenum if the catheter can be advanced past the point of obstruction into the distal common bile duct or ampulla. Prophylactic ampicillin usually is administered 24 h before and up to 72 h after the procedure. Percutaneous transhepatic cholangiography is a technique of considerable use in (1) clarifying the diagnosis of cholestatic jaundice, (2) evaluating postcholecystectomy abdominal pain, and (3) visualizing the proximal biliary tree when a distal obstruction precludes retrograde opacification. The major contraindications are the presence of cholangitis and an uncorrectable coagulopathy. A successful examination is possible in nearly every patient with a dilated biliary tree and in about 70 percent of those patients with a normal biliary system. If after numerous (up to six) hepatic punctures a dilated duct is not entered, the jaundice is assumed to be of hepatocellular origin (such an assumption will be correct in 90 percent of cases). Bleeding, septicemia, or bile peritonitis occur in about 3 percent of patients undergoing this procedure.

FIGURE 307-2

Diagnosis of biliary tract disease. A. Grey-scale echogram: A gallstone (upper arrow) is seen within the gallbladder lucency; the stone attenuates the echoes and causes a lucent shadowing (lower arrow). B. Endoscopic retrograde cholangiogram: A common-duct stone (arrowhead) is apparent. (From Schoenfield.)

A

B

Endoscopic retrograde cholangiopancreatography (ERCP) (see Fig. 307-2*B*) A flexible, fiberoptic, side-viewing duodenoscope is introduced into the second portion of the duodenum, and, after identification of the structure, the ampulla of Vater is catheterized. Contrast medium is administered through the catheter in the ampulla of Vater into the biliary and pancreatic ducts and the anatomy defined. Experienced endoscopists obtain cholangiograms in 80 percent and pancreatograms in 95 percent of patients. The major indications are for (1) the differential diagnosis of jaundice, (2) the evaluation of postcholecystectomy abdominal pain, and (3) suspected cancer of the pancreas or ampulla. ERCP is successful in providing a correct diagnosis of gallbladder or common-duct calculi more often than intravenous cholangiography. The upper normal diameter of the common duct is 9 mm on retrograde cholangiograms. The principal contraindications to retrograde studies include the presence of acute pancreatitis and recent (within 6 weeks) myocardial infarction. Pancreatitis occurs in approximately 1 percent of patients successfully cannulated. Antibiotics may be administered to obviate cholangitis when biliary obstruction is expected or encountered during retrograde study of the bile ducts.

Manometry Operative manometry provides data on pressures within the ducts and gallbladder, and may supplement fluoroscopic observation of motility and cholangiographic visualization of anatomy. Manometry performed during retrograde cholangiopancreatography in unanesthetized patients is also being evaluated. The clinical significance of intraoperative manometry, however, remains to be determined.

BILIARY COLIC AND ACUTE CHOLECYSTITIS (CYSTIC DUCT OBSTRUCTION) Pathophysiology and clinical manifestations
BILIARY COLIC Sudden obstruction of the cystic duct by a calculus produces increased intraluminal pressure that cannot be relieved by stimulated biliary contractions. The resulting visceral pain is termed *biliary colic*. Sudden obstruction of the common duct by a calculus also produces increased intraductal pressure, distention, and biliary colic. The discrete attacks of colic occur at unpredictable intervals over periods of days to months and at any time of day or night. No evidence exists to support the idea that ingestion of a fatty meal specifically precipitates biliary colic. "Colic" is something of a misnomer because the pain does not customarily wax and wane. It is more often perceived as a steady, severe aching or pressure in the epigastrium or right upper quadrant which frequently radiates to the interscapular area, right scapula, or shoulder. The pain characteristically begins suddenly, persists for 1 to 3 h (range 15 min to 6 h), subsides rapidly or gradually, and may leave a residual aching discomfort 24 h afterward. The pain is not intensified by moving about; most patients are restless and pace the floor in an attempt to find a position which affords relief. Nausea (frequently) and vomiting (occasionally) accompany biliary colic and probably represent associated reflex phenomena.

ACUTE CHOLECYSTITIS The primary event in more than 90 percent of patients with gallstones who present with symptoms of biliary disease is obstruction of the cystic duct by a calculus. If cystic duct obstruction is not subsequently relieved (presumably by the stone falling back into the gallbladder or passing into the common bile duct), acute cholecystitis ensues. The presence of persistent obstruction triggers inflammation which is thought to be caused mechanically (increased intraluminal pressure and ischemia) and/or chemically (phospholipase activation releasing lysolecithin). Bacterial infection may supervene, and enteric microorganisms have been cultured from the bile of 75 percent of patients with cystic duct obstruction.

In contrast to biliary colic, the upper abdominal pain of acute cholecystitis is generalized and worsened by jarring or respiration. The patient prefers to remain motionless. Nausea is common, but jaundice is unusual. The gallbladder is generally enlarged and is palpable in about half the cases, but palpation may be difficult because of local guarding. Deep inspiration during palpation of the right upper quadrant produces increased tenderness and inspiratory arrest (Murphy's sign). Fever is usually low grade (average 38°C); shaking chills do not characteristically occur. A leucocyte count of 10,000 to 15,000 per cubic millimeter with a shift to the left is usual. About 75 percent of patients have spontaneous remission of symptoms within 48 to 72 h. In follow-up studies, cholecystitis has been shown to recur in 25 percent of patients in 1 year and in 60 percent within 6 years. The remaining 25 percent of patients presenting with acute cholecystitis show no remission of symptomatology, and the inflammatory process progresses. Empyema, necrosis, or perforation of the gallbladder may occur unless effective treatment is initiated.

DIAGNOSIS In acute cholecystitis the typical findings are pronounced right upper quadrant tenderness, fever, and leukocytosis. Liver function tests may remain normal if the process results from cystic duct obstruction, but in large series of patients with acute cholecystitis, 45 percent have increased levels of serum bilirubin (less than 5 mg per 100 ml), 25 percent have elevated levels of serum alkaline phosphatase (usually less than twice normal), and 40 percent have increases in serum transaminases (usually less than 5 times normal but sometimes higher). These abnormalities usually resolve within 1 week of resolution of symptoms. During an attack, the diagnosis of acute cholecystitis is supported by identifying stones on echography (ultrasound). The gallbladder will often not visualize on oral or intravenous cholecystography for a period of 4 to 6 weeks after an acute attack. In a patient with a normal oral cholecystogram and a clinical history suggestive of biliary colic or cholecystitis, the clinician may resort to techniques such as echography, intravenous cholangiography, and transhepatic or retrograde cholangiography to aid in making the diagnosis.

The symptoms of biliary colic and acute cholecystitis are mimicked most often by myocardial infarction, angina pectoris, peptic ulcer, esophageal disease, pancreatitis, or intestinal obstruction, and less often by appendicitis, lesions in the right colon, congestive heart failure, pleurodynia, pulmonary embolism, pyelonephritis, renal colic, herpes zoster, radiculitis, or gonococcal perihepatitis (see Chap. 119).

Treatment MEDICAL Patients with acute cholecystitis usually require hospitalization. The major goal of medical treatment should be to attain a more optimal condition of the patient prior to cholecystectomy. Temperature, pulse, white blood cell count, and abdominal pain, tenderness, and mass are serially monitored to assess the clinical course. Elimination of oral intake and institution of nasogastric suction remove stimuli to cholecystokinin release and may help to improve ileus. For relief of biliary tract pain, the use of meperidine may be preferable to other analgesics because it produces less of an increase in biliary pressure. Intravenous fluids are administered to prevent and correct dehydration, volume depletion, and electrolyte abnormalities. Empiric antibiotic administration is advisable in severe acute cholecystitis, especially in elderly or diabetic patients, to treat potential biliary tract infection and reduce postoperative septic complications. Ampicillin or a cephalosporin usually provides adequate coverage. Initiation of combination therapy with ampicillin plus gentamicin or tobramycin is preferable in patients with more severe disease.

SURGICAL Cholecystectomy is indicated for almost all patients with recurrent biliary colic or with acute cholecystitis, unless other diseases impose too great an operative risk. Cholecystectomy is usually advocated as an elective procedure during the acute stage of cholecystitis. In general surgery it should be performed within the first 72 h if the diagnosis is clear. Intraoperative cholangiography is performed routinely during cholecystectomy because radiographic demonstration of the presence or absence of stones in the common bile duct decreases the need for subsequent exploratory choledochotomy by nearly 50 percent, doubles the proportion of positive common-duct explorations, does not itself increase the morbidity or mortality of the surgical procedure (in contrast to the increased risk imposed by "blind" common-duct explorations), and reduces the incidence of subsequent morbidity from retained duct stones. Emergency operation is necessary in about 10 percent of patients because of an uncertain diagnosis, emphysematous cholecystitis, or signs of progressive peritonitis. The operative mortality for *elective* cholecystectomy is about 0.5 percent and for *emergency* cholecystectomy 3 percent; most postoperative deaths occur in elderly patients with cardiac or respiratory disease. Some surgeons recommend cholecystostomy and decompression of the biliary tree as the initial procedure of choice in the high-risk patient with cholecystitis who may be unable to tolerate early cholecystectomy.

COMPLICATIONS OF CHOLECYSTITIS Empyema, hydrops
The term *empyema of the gallbladder* indicates the presence of an intraluminal gallbladder abscess usually associated with severe right upper quadrant pain, prostration, and elevations of fever and white blood cell count. It results from persistent, complete obstruction of the cystic duct and progression of unresolved acute cholecystitis. The medical treatment is much the same as for severe acute cholecystitis and is aimed at preparing the patient for operative intervention. Prompt cholecystectomy is usually required.

Hydrops is also caused by prolonged, complete cystic duct obstruction. However, in this instance the gallbladder tends to be distended by clear mucus (so-called "white bile") resulting in the formation of a mucocele. The hydropic gallbladder may cause chronic right upper quadrant abdominal discomfort or may be asymptomatic. The examiner may find a visible, palpable, and nontender mass in the right upper quadrant. Cholecystectomy is usually indicated since empyema, gangrene, or perforation may supervene.

Perforation, fistulas, gallstone ileus Perforation of the gallbladder usually occurs in patients with acute necrotizing cholecystitis or empyema; it leads to a localized abscess or fistulization into an adjacent organ more often than to free rupture. Clinical suspicion of localized or free perforation warrants prompt cholecystectomy and abscess draining. Biliary fistulas are found, often incidentally, in 5 percent of patients undergoing gallbladder operations. Fistulas to the duodenum (accounting for 70 percent), colon, or stomach are more common than fistulization to the abdominal wall. Most cases of fistulous tract formation are asymptomatic. In gallstone ileus, the stone usually migrates through a cholecystoduodenal fistula and passes caudad with small-bowel contents to obstruct the intestine at the ileocecal valve. It is responsible for 2 percent of all mechanical small-bowel obstructions and occurs almost exclusively in the elderly. A history suggesting biliary tract disease is obtained in only one-half of the patients. The diagnosis can sometimes be made from the characteristic findings on a plain film (e.g., small-intestinal obstruction and gas in the biliary tree together with a calcified ectopic gallstone). Enterolithotomy, excision of the fistula, cholangiography, and cholecyst-

ectomy may sometimes be performed in one stage. If the patient is very ill or represents a poor operative risk, however, only the obstruction should be treated at the initial operation.

Limy bile, porcelain gallbladder Limy (milk of calcium) bile is formed by precipitation of calcium salts in the lumen of a hydropic gallbladder. The calcium is secreted by the gallbladder itself and causes a viscous opacification of the bile visible on a plain abdominal film. The clinical implications, course, and treatment are the same as for patients with calculous cholecystitis or hydrops of the gallbladder.

In the porcelain gallbladder, calcium deposition within the wall of the gallbladder produces interrupted mural calcification which is usually apparent on a plain film of the abdomen. Although the porcelain gallbladder rarely causes symptoms, up to 25 to 50 percent of patients with this finding subsequently develop biliary cancer. Prophylactic cholecystectomy, therefore, is indicated when a radiographic diagnosis of porcelain gallbladder has been made.

ASYMPTOMATIC CHRONIC CALCULOUS CHOLECYSTITIS
Chronic cholecystitis is invariably present in patients with gallstones, including those who have been clinically asymptomatic. Microorganisms may be cultured from bile of only one-third of these patients. Eventually, with or without recurrent bouts of acute cholecystitis, the gallbladder becomes fibrotic, thickened, and shrunken, and may adhere to the omentum or surrounding organs.

Diagnosis There are no symptoms, signs, or biochemical abnormalities in the serum which can be used to define uncomplicated chronic calculous cholecystitis. Pyrosis, eructation, and vague epigastric discomfort, often attributed to fatty-food intolerance, are not unique symptoms of gallstone disease and are present with equal frequency in patients with and without gallstones. The diagnosis may be clinically suggested by a previous history of biliary colic, acute cholecystitis, or cholangitis and may be radiographically revealed by the incidental discovery of gallstones on a plain film of the abdomen or by oral cholecystography in patients with unrelated gastrointestinal symptoms. Gallstones are occasionally discovered by palpation during laparotomy performed for other reasons in patients without biliary-related symptoms.

Treatment Management of the patient with asymptomatic calculous disease of the gallbladder remains an area of controversy. In asymptomatic patients under age 50, cholecystectomy is usually recommended. In asymptomatic patients over age 50, medical observation is often advised since (1) the disease remains asymptomatic in fully one-half of these patients when followed for 20 years, (2) 75 percent of patients who do develop symptoms will experience biliary colic, and cholecystectomy can usually be performed electively at that time, and (3) the 30-year mortality for gallstone disease has been estimated to be only about 1 percent, a figure closely approximating the overall mortality rate for cholecystectomy. On the other hand, some 20 percent of patients previously asymptomatic will develop acute cholecystitis or severe symptoms. In the latter group, the operative mortality risk increases (1) in those with age-related diseases of other organ systems, (2) in patients with prolonged calculous disease and the long-term complications of cholelithiasis, and (3) with the necessity for emergency as opposed to elective surgery. The actual mortality in a series of nearly 5000 operations performed for gallstone disease was 0.4 percent in patients under the age of 60 and 4.2 percent for those over 60. These data, coupled with studies showing an increased frequency of complications in patients over age 60 having "silent stones," have led to numerous articles and editorials in the surgical and medical literature advocating "prophylactic" cholecystectomy in young and elderly patients with asymptomatic gallstones (provided major contraindications to surgery are absent). The small potential risk (about 1 to 2 percent) of the subsequent development of cancer of the gallbladder in gallstone patients is not cited as an indication for prophylactic cholecystectomy since projected numbers of operative versus cancer deaths are comparable. It seems reasonable to suggest that cholecystectomy be performed (1) in all patients with symptomatic gallstones, (2) in asymptomatic patients under age 50, and (3) in those patients with "silent stones" over age 50 to 60 whose medical condition or economic and social activities warrant prophylactic surgery as opposed to prolonged medical follow-up.

Cholecystectomy is hazardous in patients with active angina pectoris and is relatively contraindicated within 3 to 6 months of acute myocardial infarction because of the high perioperative mortality. Marked obesity and severe hepatic cirrhosis are relative contraindications. The association of diabetes mellitus with cholelithiasis, even if asymptomatic, may represent an indication for prophylactic cholecystectomy because diabetes predisposes the patient to the septic complications of gallstone disease. Prophylactic cholecystectomy may also be advisable in asymptomatic gallstone patients with nonvisualization of the gallbladder on double-dose cholecystogram, since these patients appear to be more apt to subsequently develop symptomatic biliary disease than those patients whose gallstones are visualized on oral cholecystography.

MEDICAL DISSOLUTION OF GALLSTONES Chenodeoxycholic acid (CDC, chenic acid) has been used experimentally to dissolve cholesterol gallstones. Treatment with this bile acid accomplishes stone dissolution successfully in about 60 percent of patients treated with oral CDC in doses of 10 to 15 mg/kg per day for 6 to 24 months. After initial dissolution of stones and withdrawal of CDC therapy, recurrence of cholecystolithiasis is likely. Thus far, gallstone recurrence has been observed in 25 percent of CDC-treated patients followed for periods of 1 to 4 years. The relative indications for CDC treatment versus cholecystectomy or simply clinical observation have yet to be established. Elderly patients with mild or asymptomatic disease, and patients who are at high risk for surgical intervention, may eventually be appropriate for CDC. It is estimated that half of the patients with gallstones should meet criteria for CDC treatment. Unresponsiveness may be attributable to an inadequate dose of CDC, the presence of calcified or pigment gallstones, or poor gallbladder function as assessed by the oral cholecystogram. It is believed that CDC dissolves gallstones because it decreases the cholesterol saturation of bile by decreasing hepatic synthesis of cholesterol (secondary to a decrease in HMG CoA reductase activity) and by decreasing biliary secretion of cholesterol.

Hepatic injury in certain animals treated with CDC has been described and appears to be a result of a lower capacity than that demonstrable in humans to detoxify CDC-derived lithocholic acid by sulfation. Hepatotoxicity has not occurred in humans, but about 20 percent of CDC-treated patients have unexplained, transient, mild (two- to threefold) elevations of the serum transaminases during the period of treatment. Diarrhea (probably due to bile acid stimulation of intestinal mucosal cyclic AMP) is the most frequent side effect but is dose-dependent and often disappears with continued administration. Serum lipid abnormalities have not been encountered. The long-term safety of the therapeutic administration of this bile acid remains to be proved by showing that CDC does not cause chronic liver disease, bowel cancer, or atherosclerosis. *Ursodeoxycholic acid* has also been shown to dissolve cholesterol gallstones. This 7β epimer of CDC may have an advantage over CDC in that effective doses (5 to 10 mg/kg per day)

do not appear to produce diarrhea or derangements of liver function.

ACALCULOUS CHOLECYSTITIS Cholecystitis without demonstrable gallstones occurs in only 5 percent of patients presenting with acute cholecystitis. Acalculous cholecystitis is most frequently encountered in diabetes with emphysematous cholecystitis, in patients with vasculitis (especially periarteritis nodosa) or biliary anomalies, and in children with leptospirosis or streptococcal disease. In addition, it may be precipitated by burns, trauma, operation, or acute severe illness. The manifestations are not distinctive from calculous cholecystitis, although in general the presenting symptoms are more severe and the subsequent complications more frequent. Most patients require cholecystectomy. In some instances symptomatic acalculous inflammation of the gallbladder may occur with typhoid fever, tuberculosis, syphilis, actinomycosis, and in cases of certain parasitic infections (e.g., *Ascaris lumbricoides, Opisthorchis felineus* or *viverrini*, and *Fasciola hepatica*).

POSTCHOLECYSTECTOMY COMPLICATIONS Cholecystectomy predictably may relieve the specific biliary symptoms that precipitated surgery but may not affect complaints of nonspecific pyrosis, eructation, or vague epigastric discomfort in patients with cholelithiasis. Postoperative symptoms are often found to be caused by esophageal reflux, peptic ulcer, or irritable bowel, which preoperatively were unrecognized as responsible for the complaints. Absence of the gallbladder does not impair intestinal digestion, absorption, or motility. A cystic duct or gallbladder remnant is asymptomatic unless it contains a stone. Spasm of the sphincter of Oddi (biliary dyskinesia) has been proposed as a mechanism for postcholecystectomy pain but requires documentation as a valid entity. Fibrotic stenosis of the papilla of Vater may produce symptomatic choledochal distention and dilatation. This diagnosis is supported by consistent findings with cholangiography and manometry, but the therapeutic value of sphincteroplasty in relief of the symptom complex remains to be determined.

Duct stricture In about 1 in 500 cholecystectomies, injury to the common duct results in the development of a stricture. The initial clinical clue to the presence of stricture postoperatively is often the documentation of excessive leakage of bile along the drains or through the T-tube tract. Jaundice or cholangitis (signaling the onset of stricture) may, however, occur months or years later and may frequently be intermittent. The diagnosis of common-duct stricture is made by cholangiography. A Roux-en-Y jejunal reconstruction using the involved proximal segment of the common duct is the treatment of choice. Some distal common-duct strictures may be treated by performing a choledochoduodenostomy.

Retained stones Duct stones are left behind in about 1 percent of cholecystectomies and in 5 to 10 percent of common-duct explorations. As a rule, retained stones eventually will cause obstruction, although sometimes such obstruction will be evident years following cholecystectomy. Calculi rarely form de novo within the ducts after cholecystectomy, and when they do occur are usually secondary to ductal obstruction. The diagnosis of retained stones may be made by cholangiography, ultrasound, or computerized tomography (CT scan). Bile acids or monooctanoin (an experimental medium-chain glyceride) have been infused postoperatively through the T tube in attempts to dissolve and flush retained duct stones. It is important to note, however, that these infusions may cause cholangitis, probably as a result of increased intraductal pressure with the infusate. In many patients, retained duct stones may be extracted with a basket catheter inserted into the common duct through the T-tube tract up to 6 weeks after the operation. Oral administration of chenodeoxycholic acid is being evaluated for potential use in dissolution of retained duct stones. Reoperation may be required in some patients, although endoscopic papillotomy and stone removal may be considered as an alternative to surgery, especially in high-risk patients.

CHOLEDOCHOLITHIASIS Pathophysiology and clinical features Gallstones may pass from the gallbladder into the common bile duct where they may give rise to biliary obstruction. While the majority of stones originate in the gallbladder, they may on rare occasions also form in the intrahepatic or common bile ducts. The stones may remain free in the duct, obstruct partially or completely, or obstruct intermittently like a ball valve. Choledocholithiasis may present without symptoms, or with biliary colic, cholangitis, or pancreatitis. *Biliary colic* due to choledocholithiasis is caused by increasing biliary pressure due to sudden interference in bile flow. *Acute cholangitis* is an inflammation of the bile ducts caused by sudden, complete, or partial common-duct obstruction. The clinical manifestations are *spiking fever* and shaking chills, often associated with biliary *colic* and *jaundice* (Charcot's triad). The bile in 75 percent of patients contains culturable bacteria. The organisms are thought to ascend from the intestine to the ducts from which they may disseminate into the bloodstream. Nonsuppurative cholangitis usually subsides in 1 to 3 days. Less often, the common duct becomes completely obstructed, producing *acute suppurative cholangitis*. In the latter case, purulent material accumulates under increasing pressure in the ducts and may lead to septicemia, shock, or miliary hepatic abscesses. Acute suppurative cholangitis is a surgical emergency; without surgery for relief of obstruction and drainage of infected bile, the mortality approaches 100 percent.

Jaundice The time interval between common-duct obstruction and the onset of jaundice depends on the distensibility of the gallbladder and bile ducts, the rate of bile flow, and the absorptive capacity of the gallbladder. When a normal biliary system is obstructed, these "accommodating" factors initially stabilize intraductal pressure. Eventually the rate of hepatic bile secretion exceeds the rate of gallbladder absorption, the biliary tract distends maximally, and intraductal pressure rises. When the pressure exceeds about 25 cmH$_2$O, hepatic bile flow is suppressed and conjugated bilirubin regurgitates via lymphatics into the blood. With a normal gallbladder, jaundice may not occur for several days, but with an absent or diseased gallbladder (the rule rather than the exception in common-duct obstruction), jaundice usually occurs within 24 h.

Prolonged common-duct obstruction Continued or intermittent common-duct obstruction may lead to secondary biliary cirrhosis (see Chap. 304). Pruritus is a common sequel to the development of biliary cirrhosis and probably results from excessive accumulation of bile acids which stimulate sensory nerve endings in the skin. Since bile acids are necessary for the absorption of lipids, their absence from the intestine in cases of complete biliary obstruction produces steatorrhea and loss of fat-soluble vitamins, A, D, E, and K. Vitamin K deficiency develops rapidly (within 1 to 3 weeks) and depresses the synthesis of prothrombin and coagulation factors VII, IX, and X, leading, therefore, to coagulopathy and the development of bleeding tendencies. The loss of vitamins A, D, and E is of consequence only when obstruction is more prolonged. Pan-

creatitis may accompany or complicate common-duct obstruction perhaps because the stone interferes with the outflow of pancreatic secretions (see Chap. 309). The serum bilirubin is elevated in most patients with common-duct obstruction, usually is less than 12 mg per 100 ml, and returns to normal within 2 weeks if the obstruction resolves. The serum alkaline phosphatase is usually increased, the increase may precede the jaundice, and the elevation remains abnormal longer than the serum bilirubin following relief of obstruction. About 75 percent of patients with common-duct obstruction have an increase in serum transaminases (aminotransferases), usually by two- to fivefold but occasionally by as much as ten- to twentyfold. With resolution of the obstruction, elevated transaminase levels rapidly return toward normal.

Choledocholithiasis may be difficult to distinguish from obstructive tumors of the biliary tract or pancreas, bile duct stricture, acute pancreatitis, sclerosing cholangitis, choledochal cyst, or parasitic infestation. Malignant biliary obstruction rarely causes biliary colic or cholangitis. Neoplastic processes, by virtue of their relatively slow progression to complete obstruction, are usually associated with a constant or progressive pain or *painless jaundice,* anemia, weight loss, and a clinically dilated, nontender gallbladder. The latter is the basis for *Courvoisier's law,* i.e., the presence of an enlarged palpable gallbladder in a jaundiced patient suggests that the obstruction is secondary to an underlying malignancy. In contrast, fully 80 percent of gallbladders associated with choledochal stones are fibrotic and unable to enlarge or dilate in response to complete obstruction of the biliary tree.

The approach to the diagnosis of partial or complete obstruction of the biliary tree may vary depending on the availability of and experience with a variety of radiographic techniques at a given medical institution. When dilated bile ducts have been demonstrated by echography or with CT scanning, radio-contrast demonstration of the site or nature of the obstruction may be attempted by transhepatic cholangiography or by ERCP. If the serum bilirubin is less than 3 mg per 100 ml, intravenous cholangiography (IVC) will successfully demonstrate common-duct stones in 60 percent of patients who have them and may indirectly reveal the presence of underlying choledocholithiasis in an additional 20 percent by demonstration of delayed emptying or common-duct dilatation. If the biliary tree is not well visualized on IVC, if further definition of the obstructive process is necessary, or if the serum bilirubin is greater than 3 mg per 100 ml, then retrograde or transhepatic cholangiography may be utilized. In experienced hands, the transhepatic study is a rapid, low-risk procedure and offers the potential for good visualization of the biliary tree proximal to a site of obstruction as well as the opportunity for percutaneous decompression and drainage of the bile ducts in cases of complete biliary obstruction. ERCP is technically more difficult but has the added advantage of pancreatography in cases where pancreatic pathology is suspected and may offer the potential for endoscopic papillotomy and stone removal in cases of choledocholithiasis.

Treatment Medical treatment for cholangitis does not differ from that of severe acute cholecystitis and is a prelude to surgery unless strong clinical factors mitigate against exploration. In suppurative cholangitis treatment of septic shock and emergency operative decompression of the common duct are required. Associated pancreatitis, unless it is mild, may mandate temporary deferral of surgical exploration because of an increased operative morbidity and mortality. The preoperative indications for common-duct exploration include the presence of ductal stones demonstrated by contrast radiography and the clinical findings of jaundice or cholangitis, each of which is associated with a high probability of finding duct stones at exploration. Fiberoptic choledochoscopy during the operation further improves the detection of common-duct stones. Cholecystectomy and choledocholithotomy with T-tube drainage are the treatment of choice for choledocholithiasis. A T tube is inserted through the choledochotomy and allowed to drain percutaneously in order to decompress the biliary tree and to permit performance of T-tube cholangiography postoperatively. The T tube is usually removed on about the tenth postoperative day if recovery is uneventful.

CONGENITAL DISORDERS

Most congenital disorders of the bile ducts and gallbladder (including its congenital absence) are asymptomatic. These minor congenital anomalies may, however, cause biliary stasis and thus predispose to the development of jaundice or of pigment gallstones. Choledochal cysts may be developmental as well as congenital and usually involve the common duct. They occasionally produce their initial manifestations in adults, presenting with jaundice, cholangitis, and a right upper quadrant mass. The incidence of bile duct cancer is increased in patients with choledochal cysts. The diagnosis is made by cholangiography, and the treatment is usually cyst excision followed by Roux-en-Y jejunal anastomosis to the hepatic duct.

The fibropolycystic diseases of the biliary tree comprise a spectrum of rare disorders of recessive inheritance which often present their initial symptoms in young adults. Intrahepatic ductal ectasia (Caroli's disease) is characterized by findings of intrahepatic calculi and cholangitis. Congenital hepatic fibrosis is associated with development of portal hypertension. These manifestations may overlap, and they may be associated with concomitant formation of choledochal and renal cysts.

HEMOBILIA

The most common cause of hemobilia is hepatic trauma (blunt, biopsy, or operative) which results in formation of an intrahepatic hematoma, a false aneurysm, or an arteriobiliary fistula. Less common causative factors are mycotic or atheromatous aneurysms, gallstones, hepatoma, angioma, cholangiocarcinoma, and parasitic infestation of the biliary tree. The principal manifestation is usually onset of biliary colic, often in association with a palpable and distended gallbladder, obstructive jaundice, and upper gastrointestinal bleeding. The finding of blood clot casts of the bile ducts in gastroduodenal contents or the direct duodenoscopic observation of bleeding from the papilla of Vater establishes the diagnosis. Selective angiography can identify the precise bleeding site. Treatment consists of excision or ligation of an aneurysm, hepatic resection or arterial ligation for intrahepatic causes, and occasionally nonoperative management for small, peripheral, self-limited, or transient lesions.

EXTRINSIC BILE DUCT COMPRESSION

Expanding carcinoma of the head of the pancreas (see Chap. 309) is the most common cause of extrinsic bile duct compression. Chronic pancreatitis occasionally produces a smooth, fibrotic compression of the common duct. Enlarged lymph nodes in the porta hepatis (involved with lymphoma or metastatic cancer) may produce common bile duct compression. Duodenal disorders (villous adenomas, diverticula, or peptic ulceration), hepatic artery aneurysms, or enlarging renal masses may on rare occasions produce biliary compression and bile stasis. The clinical and biochemical manifestations do not differ from those of intrinsic obstruction. The specific diagnosis and treatment depends on radiographic delineation of the site of compression and subsequent identification of the primary disease.

HYPERPLASTIC CHOLECYSTOSES

The hyperplastic cholecystoses are degenerative, usually noninflammatory lesions characterized by proliferation of normal tissue components without malignant potential. Adenomyomatosis (proliferation of glands and muscle), cholesterolosis (deposition of esterified cholesterol in the lamina propria), and their localized forms (biliary adenomyomata and cholesterol polyps, respectively) are the most common of these entities. Manifestations of the hyperplastic cholecystoses are seen in about 5 percent of cholecystograms; half of affected patients are shown to have associated cholelithiasis. Symptoms of biliary colic and acute cholecystitis are usually attributable to coexistent calculi. Cholecystography often demonstrates a hyperconcentrated gallbladder and Rokitansky-Aschoff sinuses (evagination of surface mucosa into or through the muscle layer). Cholesterol polyps are seen as small, fixed, unevenly distributed filling defects, while adenomyomas present a dimpled filling defect or discrete compartmentalization of contrast at the fundus. Cholecystectomy is indicated where there is associated cholelithiasis.

CANCER OF THE GALLBLADDER

Cancer of the gallbladder is found mostly in women over age 65. Carcinoma of the gallbladder has been reported in 0.43 percent of routine antopsies and in 1 percent of patients with gallstones. Cholelithiasis is present as an associated finding in about 80 percent of patients with gallbladder adenocarcinoma. An upper abdominal mass and unremitting right upper quadrant pain, jaundice, and weight loss are the common presentations. Patients with these symptoms usually die within a year of presentation and diagnosis from biliary tract obstruction and liver failure. The cancerous gallbladder rarely visualizes on oral cholecystography. Radiographic contrast studies may demonstrate an obstructing lesion, but the diagnosis is more often made at laparotomy. In situ cancer may be cured by cholecystectomy, but invasive cancer is usually not operable. Results of trials attempting to treat carcinoma of the gallbladder with radiation or chemotherapy have not been encouraging.

CANCER OF THE EXTRAHEPATIC BILE DUCTS

Extrahepatic bile duct cancer is more prevalent in men than women and is most commonly found in the seventh decade. In patients with chronic ulcerative colitis, *Clonorchis sinensis* infestation, or choledochal cyst, cholangiocarcinoma occurs with increased frequency and at an earlier age. These biliary neoplasms are usually diffuse, infiltrating, fibrosing adenocarcinomas. The most frequent presenting symptoms are unremitting jaundice, pruritus, and weight loss. Upper abdominal pain occurs in 50 percent of patients, but biliary colic and cholangitis are uncommon. Jaundice is usually absent with cancer involving only one hepatic duct; it may be chronic and low grade (bilirubin less than 8 mg per 100 ml) with a Klatskin tumor (cancer at the junction of the hepatic ducts). The gallbladder may become palpably distended if obstruction occurs below the confluence of the cystic and common hepatic ducts. The serum alkaline phosphatase is almost always elevated (usually two- to tenfold), but the serum transaminase elevation is often modest (less than threefold). A prolonged prothrombin time is usually corrected by parenteral vitamin K unless protracted obstruction has produced secondary liver damage. The diagnosis is established by transhepatic or retrograde cholangiography. Cholestyramine, an anion exchange resin that binds bile acids, may be effective in relief of pruritus when duct obstruction is incomplete. Most cholangiocarcinomas are not surgically resectable. Excision of the carcinoma or surgical bypass with biliary-enteric anastomosis or silastic catheter drainage usually yields poor results. Occasionally, palliative hepaticoenterostomy may prove valuable.

CANCER OF THE PAPILLA OF VATER

After carcinoma of the gallbladder, cancer of the papilla of Vater is the most common malignant neoplasm of the biliary tract. Papillary carcinoma usually grows slowly and frequently causes obstructive jaundice before it has spread widely. Gross bleeding and ulcerative sloughing of the tumor are uncommon. Since the differential diagnosis at presentation usually includes cancer of the pancreas, sclerosing cholangitis, and biliary cirrhosis, an ERCP study is preferable to transhepatic cholangiography because it permits visualization of the pancreatic and small bile ducts and often provides a direct look at the lesion itself, allowing endoscopic biopsy. Cancer of the papilla has the best prognosis among biliary tract cancers; the 5-year survival after a radical pancreaticoduodenectomy (Whipple procedure) is as high as 40 percent.

SCLEROSING CHOLANGITIS

Primary sclerosing cholangitis is a rare, idiopathic, chronic inflammatory condition resulting in focal or diffuse fibrosis of the bile ducts. The lesion is most prevalent in men over age 40. It often appears as an isolated entity, without disease in other organ systems, but may be associated with ulcerative colitis (in 30 percent) or multifocal fibrosclerosis (retroperitoneal, mediastinal, or periureteral fibrosis, Riedel's struma, and pseudotumor of the orbit). Sclerosing cholangitis may also be *secondary* to common-duct stones or cancer, operative trauma, or contiguous inflammation. Involvement of the bile ducts in both forms of sclerosing cholangitis may be segmental or diffuse and extrahepatic or intrahepatic. The ducts are thickened and have narrow, beaded lumens. Affected patients usually present clinically with chronic or intermittent jaundice, pruritus, right upper quadrant abdominal pain, and cholangitis. Ultimately, secondary biliary cirrhosis, portal hypertension with bleeding varices, and liver failure may develop. The mean patient survival after diagnosis is 10 years. A diagnosis of sclerosing cholangitis is usually suggested by retrograde cholangiography and is established by operative cholangiography and biopsy. Excluding the possibility of biliary malignancy may prove difficult unless the intrahepatic ducts are clearly shown to be involved. Prolonged T-tube or internal drainage of the biliary tree may alleviate symptoms of obstruction, cholestyramine may relieve pruritus, and antibiotics may control cholangitis, but none of these interventions has been shown to alter progression of the disease. Corticosteroid therapy may be initiated if the duct lumens become virtually obliterated or if jaundice recurs after removal of the T tube. The results of most steroid trials have not shown much therapeutic efficacy in this disease. In patients with chronic ulcerative colitis, colectomy does not influence the course of sclerosing cholangitis. Progression of ductal sclerosis may occasionally stabilize after surgery (or for no apparent external reason).

REFERENCES

BENNION LJ, GRUNDY SM: Risk factors for the development of cholelithiasis in man. N Engl J Med 299:1161, 1221, 1978

BERK RN, CLEMETT AR: *Radiology of the Gallbladder and Biliary System.* Philadelphia, Saunders, 1977

CAREY MC, SMALL DM: The physical chemistry of cholesterol solubility in bile. Relationship to gallstone formation and dissolution in man. J Clin Invest 61:998, 1978

GOODHART GL et al: Pigment vs. cholesterol cholelithiasis. Bacteriology of gallbladder stone, bile and tissue correlated with biliary lipid analysis. Am J Dig Dis 23:877, 1978

LONGMIRE WP: When is cholangitis sclerosing? Am J Surg 135:312, 1978

SCHOENFIELD LJ: *Diseases of the Gallbladder and Biliary System.* New York, Wiley, 1977

THISTLE JL et al: Chenotherapy for gallstone dissolution. JAMA 239:1041, 1138, 1978

VALLON AG et al: Grey-scale ultrasonography in cholestatic jaundice. Gut 20:54, 1979

section 7 | Disorders of the pancreas

308
APPROACH TO THE PATIENT WITH PANCREATIC DISEASE

NORTON J. GREENBERGER
PHILLIP P. TOSKES

GENERAL CONSIDERATIONS

Inflammatory disease of the pancreas may be acute, relapsing, or chronic. Although good data exist concerning the frequency of acute pancreatitis (about 5000 new cases per year in the United States with a mortality rate of about 10 percent), the number of patients who suffer with relapsing pancreatitis or chronic pancreatitis is largely undefined. The relative inaccessibility of the pancreas to direct examination and the nonspecificity of the abdominal pain associated with pancreatitis make the diagnosis of pancreatitis difficult and usually dependent on elevation of blood amylase levels. Many patients with relapsing pancreatitis and the majority of patients with chronic pancreatitis do not have elevated blood amylase levels. Some patients with chronic pancreatitis develop signs and symptoms of pancreatic exocrine insufficiency, and thus objective evidence for pancreatic disease can be demonstrated. However, greater than 90 percent of the pancreas must be damaged before maldigestion of fat and protein is manifested. Obviously there is a very large reservoir of pancreatic exocrine function, and the signs and symptoms usually associated with exocrine insufficiency are late manifestations, depending on virtually complete destruction of the gland. Even the secretin stimulation test, which is the most sensitive method of assessing pancreatic exocrine function, is probably abnormal only when greater than 75 percent of exocrine function has been lost. Thus, the number of patients who have subclinical exocrine dysfunction (i.e., less than 90 percent loss of function) is unknown.

The clinical manifestations of acute and chronic pancreatitis and pancreatic insufficiency are protean. Thus, patients may present with hyperlipidemia, vitamin B$_{12}$ malabsorption, hypercalcemia, hypocalcemia, hyperglycemia, ascites, pleural effusions, and chronic abdominal pain with normal amylase levels. Indeed, if the clinician considers pancreatitis as a possible diagnosis only when presented with a patient having classic symptoms (i.e., severe constant epigastric pain that radiates through to the back along with an elevated blood amylase level), only a minority of the patients with pancreatitis will be correctly diagnosed.

As emphasized in Chap. 309, the etiologies as well as the clinical manifestations are quite varied. Although it is well appreciated that *pancreatitis* is frequently secondary to alcohol abuse and biliary tract disease, pancreatitis is also caused by drugs, trauma, and viral infections, and is associated with metabolic and connective tissue disorders. In addition, in 10 to 20 percent of patients with chronic pancreatitis, the etiology is obscure.

The incidence of *pancreatic cancer* in the United States has increased threefold since 1930. Associations have been made with cigarette smoking, exposure to some industrial carcinogens, and diabetes. The outlook for early diagnosis and effective treatment remains dismal.

Cystic fibrosis is usually considered a disease of childhood. However, an appreciable number of children with this disease reach adulthood because of more effective therapy for pulmonary complications. Eighty-five percent of patients with cystic fibrosis have pancreatic exocrine insufficiency; in some, pancreatic impairment may represent the primary clinical defect. This disease, in which the metabolic defect has not yet been clearly defined, affects many organ systems in addition to the gastrointestinal tract.

TESTS USEFUL IN THE DIAGNOSIS OF PANCREATIC DISEASE

Several tests have proved of value in the evaluation of pancreatic exocrine function. Examples of specific tests and usefulness in the diagnosis of acute and chronic pancreatitis are summarized in Table 308-1.

PANCREATIC ENZYMES IN BODY FLUIDS The serum amylase is widely used as a screening test for acute pancreatitis in the patient with acute abdominal or back pain. A value greater than 150 Somogyi units per 100 ml should raise the question of acute pancreatitis; levels greater than 300 units make the diagnosis more likely. In acute pancreatitis the serum amylase is usually elevated within 24 h and remains so for 1 to 3 days. Levels return to normal within 3 to 5 days unless there is extensive pancreatic necrosis, incomplete ductal obstruction, or pseudocyst formation. Approximately 75 percent of patients with acute pancreatitis will have an elevated serum amylase. Normal values, however, may occur if (1) there is a delay (2 to 5 days) in obtaining blood samples, (2) the underlying disorder is relapsing chronic pancreatitis rather than acute pancreatitis, and (3) hypertriglyceridemia is present. Patients with hypertri-

glyceridemia and proved pancreatitis have been found to have spuriously low levels of amylase activity presumably because of a circulating amylase inhibitor; serial dilutions of plasma will correct this abnormality and permit identification of hyperamylasemia.

The serum amylase is often elevated in other conditions (Table 308-2), in part because the enzyme is found in many organs in addition to the pancreas (salivary glands, liver, small intestine, kidney, fallopian tube) and can be produced by various tumors (carcinoma of the lung, esophagus, and ovary).

Urine amylase is increased in acute pancreatitis and may be elevated for 7 to 10 days after serum values have returned to normal. The finding that the renal clearance of amylase is higher than that of creatinine in acute pancreatitis has led to the suggestion that the amylase/creatinine clearance ratio (C_{am}/C_{cr}) may be a more specific test for the diagnosis of acute pancreatitis. It also may serve to identify patients with pancreatitis who do not have hyperamylasemia. The ratio is calculated by the formula:

$$\frac{C_{am}}{C_{cr}} = \frac{\text{urine amylase}}{\text{serum amylase}} \times \frac{\text{serum creatinine}}{\text{urine creatinine}} \times 100$$

The normal range of C_{am}/C_{cr} is 1 to 5 percent. In acute pancreatitis, the ratio usually exceeds 5 percent and may range up to 14 percent. The mechanism of increased renal amylase clearance in acute pancreatitis is not clear, but preliminary studies suggest that there is a reversible renal tubular defect which results in decreased amylase reabsorption.

The specificity of the C_{am}/C_{cr} ratio has, however, been questioned because of the observation that the ratio is increased in a number of disorders, e.g., diabetic ketoacidosis, burns, pancreatic neoplasms, renal failure, chronic hemodialysis, and fulminant alcoholic liver disease. Thus, (1) while the ratio is usually elevated in patients who have severe, obvious acute pancreatitis and an elevated serum amylase, there is incomplete information concerning this ratio in mild cases of pancreatitis, in acute pancreatitis with normal serum amylase levels, or in chronic pancreatitis. (2) This ratio probably will be elevated in any condition associated with defective tubular reabsorption of protein. (3) More accurate assessment of the diagnostic value of the ratio will be difficult because of lack of a reliable means of determining the presence of pancreatitis.

Elevation of ascitic fluid amylase occurs in acute pancreatitis as well as (1) in pancreatogenous ascites due to disruption of the main pancreatic duct of a leaking pseudocyst and (2) in other abdominal disorders which simulate pancreatitis (e.g., intestinal obstruction, intestinal infarction, and perforated peptic ulcer). Elevation of pleural fluid amylase occurs in acute pancreatitis, chronic pancreatitis, carcinoma of the lung, and esophageal perforation.

In the past, serum lipase levels were not frequently performed because of methodological problems. However, newer methods are now available. In a representative study, lipase levels were elevated in 63 percent of patients with acute pancreatitis, amylase levels in 70 percent, and both enzymes in 83 percent. Increased lipase levels have also been found in ascitic fluid in patients with acute pancreatitis.

STUDIES PERTAINING TO PANCREATIC STRUCTURE **Radiologic tests** Plain films of the abdomen provide useful information in 30 to 50 percent of patients with acute pancreatitis.

TABLE 308-1
Tests useful in the diagnosis of acute and chronic pancreatitis

Test	Principle	Comment
I Pancreatic enzymes in body fluids		
A Amylase		
1 Serum	Pancreatic inflammation leads to increased enzyme levels	Simple; reliable; false negatives and positives
2 Urine	Renal clearance of amylase is increased in acute pancreatitis	May be abnormal when serum levels normal; false negatives and positives
3 Amylase/creatinine clearance ratio (C_{am}/C_{cr})	Renal clearance of amylase greater than clearance of creatinine	Sensitivity and specificity not fully defined (see text)
4 Ascitic fluid	Disruption of gland or main pancreatic duct leads to increased amylase	Can establish diagnosis of pancreatitis; false positives with intestinal obstruction and perforated ulcer
5 Pleural fluid	Exudative pleural effusion with pancreatitis	False positives with carcinoma of the lung and esophageal perforation
B Serum lipase	Pancreatic inflammation leads to increased enzyme levels	New methods of determination greatly simplified; positive in 60–70% of cases
II Studies pertaining to pancreatic structure		
A Radiological and radionuclide tests		
1 Plan film of the abdomen	Abnormal in acute and chronic pancreatitis	Simple; normal in more than 50% of both acute and chronic pancreatitis
2 Upper gastrointestinal x-rays	Displacement of stomach or widening of duodenal loop suggests a pancreatic mass (inflammatory, neoplastic, cystic)	Simple; frequently normal
3 Hypotonic duodenography or air contrast	Inhibition of duodenal peristaltic activity enhances visualization of duodenal mucosal changes by barium studies	Can detect pancreatic inflammation and neoplasms; anticholinergic side effects
4 Ultrasonography	Echographic appearances can provide information on edema, inflammation, calcification, pseudocysts, and mass lesions	Simple, noninvasive; sequential studies quite feasible; procedure of choice for diagnosis of pseudocyst
5 Computerized tomography (CT scan)	Permits detailed visualization of pancreas and surrounding structures	Useful in the diagnosis of pancreatic calcification, dilated pancreatic ducts, and pancreatic tumors; may not be able to distinguish between inflammatory and neoplastic mass lesions; high cost
6 Selective angiography	Can identify pancreatic neoplasms (1) by sheathing of celiac or superior mesenteric branches by tumor or (2) by tumor straining; displacement of vessels by tumor	High cost; false negatives
B Endoscopic retrograde cholangio-pancreatography (ERCP)	Cannulation of pancreatic and common bile duct permits visualization of pancreatic-biliary ductal system	Provides diagnostic data in 60–85% of cases; differentiation of chronic pancreatitis from pancreatic carcinoma may be difficult
C Pancreatic biopsy with ultrasound guidance	Percutaneous biopsy with skinny needle and localization of lesion by sonography	High diagnostic yield; laparotomy avoided; requires special technical skills
III Tests of exocrine pancreatic function		
A Direct stimulation of the pancreas with analysis of duodenal contents		
1 Secretin-pancreozymin (CCK-PZ) test	Secretin leads to increased output of pancreatic juice and HCO_3^-; CCK-PZ leads to increased output of pancreatic enzymes; pancreatic secretory response related to functional mass of pancreatic tissue	Sensitive enough to detect occult disease; duodenal intubation; fluoroscopy; poorly defined normal enzyme response; overlap in chronic pancreatitis; large secretory reserve capacity of the pancreas
B Indirect stimulation of pancreas with measurement of pancreatic enzymes		
1 Lundh test meal	Test meal (fat, carbohydrate, and protein) causes increased release of CCK-PZ, which causes increased enzyme output; trypsin concentration measured	Useful in patients with pancreatic exocrine insufficiency; false negatives with delayed gastric emptying; false positives in patients with primary mucosal disease of the gut and choledocholithiasis; does not measure secretory capacity
2 Benzoyl-tyrosyl-*p*-aminobenzoic (Bz-Ty-PABA, tripeptide hydrolysis) test	Synthetic peptide (Bz-Ty-PABA) specifically cleaved by chymotrypsin liberating PABA which is absorbed and excreted in the urine	Simple and reliable test of pancreatic exocrine function; sensitivity and specificity not yet fully defined
C Measurement of intraluminal digestion products		
1 Microscopic examination of stool for undigested meat fibers and fat	Lack of proteolytic enzymes causes decreased digestion of meat fibers	Simple, reliable; not sensitive enough to detect milder cases of pancreatic insufficiency
2 Quantitative stool fat determination	Lack of lipolytic enzymes brings about impaired fat digestion	Reliable, reference standard for defining severity of malabsorption; does not distinguish between maldigestion and malabsorption
3 Fecal nitrogen	Lack of proteolytic enzymes leads to impaired protein digestion, causing increase in stool nitrogen	Does not distinguish between maldigestion and malabsorption
D Measurement of pancreatic enzymes in feces		
1 Chymotrypsin	Pancreatic output of proteolytic enzymes	May be useful in evaluating cystic fibrosis patients; tedious; 10% false positives and false negatives

TABLE 308-2
Causes of hyperamylasemia and hyperamylasuria

I Pancreatic disease
  A Pancreatitis
    1 Acute
    2 Chronic: Ductal obstruction
    3 Complications of pancreatitis
      a Pancreatic pseudocyst
      b Pancreatogenous ascites
      c Pancreatic abscess
  B Pancreatic trauma
  C Pancreatic carcinoma
II Nonpancreatic disorders
  A Renal insufficiency
  B Salivary gland lesions
    1 Mumps
    2 Calculus
    3 Irradiation sialadenitis
    4 Maxillofacial surgery
  C "Tumor" hyperamylasemia
    1 Carcinoma of the lung
    2 Carcinoma of the esophagus
    3 Ovarian carcinoma
  D Macroamylasemia
  E Burns
  F Diabetic ketoacidosis
  G Pregnancy
  H Renal transplantation
  I Cerebral trauma
  J Drugs: Morphine
III Other abdominal disorders
  A Biliary tract disease: Cholecystitis, choledocholithiasis
  B Intraabdominal disease
    1 Perforated or penetrating peptic ulcer
    2 Intestinal obstruction or infarction
    3 Ruptured ectopic pregnancy
    4 Peritonitis
    5 Aortic aneurysm
    6 Chronic liver disease
    7 Postoperative hyperamylasemia

SOURCE: *After WB Salt II, S Schenker, Medicine 55:269, 1976.*

The most frequent abnormalities include (1) a localized ileus usually involving the jejunum ("sentinel loop"); (2) a generalized ileus with air-fluid levels; (3) the "colon cutoff sign," which results from isolated distention of the transverse colon; (4) duodenal distention with air-fluid levels; and (5) a mass, which is frequently a pseudocyst. In chronic pancreatitis, an important radiographic finding is pancreatic calcification, which characteristically is localized adjacent to and superimposed on the second lumbar vertebra (Fig. 309-1).

Upper gastrointestinal x-rays may reveal displacement of the stomach by the retroperitoneal mass (Fig. 309-2A) or widening and effacement of the duodenal C loop which also suggests the presence of a pancreatic mass that could be an inflammatory, cystic, or neoplastic process. The use of hypotonic duodenography or good-quality air-contrast studies increases the diagnostic yield of upper gastrointestinal x-rays in patients with carcinoma of the head of the pancreas.

Ultrasonography (echography) can provide important information in patients with acute pancreatitis, chronic pancreatitis, pancreatic calcification, pseudocyst, and pancreatic carcinoma. Echographic appearances can indicate the presence of edema, inflammation, and calcification (not obvious on plain films of the abdomen) as well as pseudocysts and mass lesions (see Figs. 309-1 to 309-3). In acute pancreatitis the pancreas is characteristically enlarged. In pancreatic pseudocyst the usual appearance is that of an echo-free, smooth, round fluid collection. Pancreatic carcinoma distorts the usual landmarks, and mass lesions greater than 3.0 cm are usually detected as localized echo-free solid lesions. *Ultrasound should be the initial investigation for most patients with suspected pancreatic disease.* However, obesity, excess small- and large-bowel gas, and re-

cently performed barium contrast examinations can interfere with ultrasound studies.

Computerized tomography (CT scan) is useful in the detection of pancreatic tumors, fluid-containing lesions such as pseudocysts and abscesses, and calcium deposits. Most lesions are characterized by (1) enlargement of the pancreatic outline, (2) distortion of the pancreatic contour, or (3) fluid-containing lesions that have different attenuation coefficients than normal pancreas. However, it is occasionally difficult to distinguish between inflammatory and neoplastic lesions. Oral water-soluble contrast agents may be used to opacify the stomach and duodenum during CT scans; this permits more precise delineation of various organs as well as mass lesions.

Selective catheterization of the celiac and superior mesenteric arteries combined with superselective catheterization of others such as the hepatic, splenic, and gastroduodenal arteries permits visualization of the pancreas and detection of pancreatic neoplasms and pseudocysts. Pancreatic neoplasms can be identified by the sheathing of blood vessels by a mass lesion (Fig. 309-3). Hormone-producing pancreatic tumors are especially likely to exhibit increased vascularity and tumor staining. Angiographic abnormalities are noted in many patients with pancreatic carcinoma but are uncommon in patients without pancreatic disease. Angiography complements ultrasonography and endoscopic retrograde cholangiopancreatography (ERCP) in the study of a patient with a suspected pancreatic lesion and is often carried out if ERCP is either unsuccessful or nondiagnostic.

Endoscopic retrograde cholangiopancreatography ERCP may provide useful information on the status of the pancreatic ductal system and thus aid in the differential diagnosis of pancreatic disease (Figs. 309-2 and 309-3). Pancreatic carcinoma is characterized by stenosis or obstruction of either the pancreatic duct or common bile duct; both ductal systems are often abnormal. In chronic pancreatitis ERCP abnormalities include (1) luminal narrowing, (2) irregularities in the ductal system with stenosis, dilatation, sacculation, and ectasia, and (3) blockage of the pancreatic duct by calcium deposits. Differentiation from carcinoma may be difficult because of similar overlapping features, i.e., ductal stenosis and irregularity. Elevated serum amylase levels following ERCP have been reported in 25 to 75 percent of patients, but clinical pancreatitis is uncommon. In a series of 300 patients pancreatitis occurred in only five patients following ERCP.

Pancreatic biopsy with radiologic guidance Percutaneous aspiration biopsy of the pancreas under ultrasound or CT guidance can provide a definitive diagnosis of pancreatic neoplasms.

TESTS OF EXOCRINE PANCREATIC FUNCTION
(See Table 308-1)

Pancreatic function tests can be divided into the following categories:

1 Direct stimulation of the pancreas by intravenous infusion of secretin or secretin plus cholecystokinin (CCK) followed by collection and measurement of duodenal contents.
2 Indirect stimulation of the pancreas utilizing nutrients or amino acids, fatty acids, and synthetic peptides followed by assay of proteolytic, lipolytic, and amylolytic enzymes.
3 Study of *intraluminal digestion products* such as undigested meat fibers, stool fat, and fecal nitrogen.

4 *Measurement of fecal pancreatic enzymes* such as chymotrypsin.

The secretin test, used to detect diffuse pancreatic disease, is based on the physiological principle that the pancreatic secretory response is directly related to the functional mass of pancreatic tissue. In the standard assay, secretin is given intravenously in a dose of 1 clinical unit (CU) per kilogram, either as a bolus or continuous infusion. Obviously, results will vary with the secretin preparation used, dose, mode of administration, and completeness of collection of duodenal contents. Normal values for the standard secretin test are (1) volume output > 2.0 ml/kg in 80 min, (2) bicarbonate (HCO_3^-) concentration > 80 meq per liter, and (3) HCO_3^- output > 10 meq in 30 min. The most reproducible measurement having the highest level of discrimination between normal subjects and patients with chronic pancreatitis appears to be the maximal bicarbonate concentration.

The *combined secretin-CCK test* permits measurement of pancreatic amylase, lipase, trypsin, and chymotrypsin. Although there is overlap in the distribution of enzyme output in normal subjects and patients with pancreatitis, markedly decreased enzyme outputs suggest advanced damage and destruction of acinar cells. With frank exocrine pancreatic insufficiency there is usually an overall reduction in both HCO_3^- concentration and output of several enzymes. However, with lesser degrees of pancreatic damage there may be a dissociation between HCO_3^- concentration and enzyme output. There may also be a dissociation between the results of the secretin test and other tests of absorptive function. For example, patients with chronic pancreatitis often have abnormally low outputs of HCO_3^- after secretin but normal fecal fat excretion. Thus, the secretin test measures the secretory capacity of ductular epithelium, while fecal fat excretion indirectly reflects intraluminal lipolytic activity. Steatorrhea does not occur until intraluminal levels of lipase are markedly reduced, underscoring the fact that only small amounts of enzymes are necessary for intraluminal digestive activities. An abnormal secretin test should suggest only that chronic pancreatic damage is present; it will not consistently distinguish between chronic pancreatitis and pancreatic carcinoma.

Another test of exocrine pancreatic function, which indirectly reflects intraluminal chymotrypsin activity, has recently been evaluated in patients with pancreatic disease. This test (the *tripeptide hydrolysis test*) utilizes a synthetic peptide, N-benzoyl-L-tyrosyl-p-aminobenzoic acid (Bz-Ty-PABA), that is specifically cleaved by chymotrypsin to Bz-Ty and PABA. Normally, after oral administration, the peptide reaches the small intestine where it is hydrolyzed by chymotrypsin with the liberation of PABA which is rapidly absorbed and excreted in the urine. Results in over 200 patients with chronic pancreatitis and other disorders indicate that PABA excretion is significantly lower in chronic pancreatitis compared with controls. The overall sensitivity and specificity of the test remains to be determined.

Measurement of *intraluminal digestion products,* i.e., undigested muscle fibers, stool fat, and fecal nitrogen, is discussed in Chap. 292. Measurement of chymotrypsin in stool reflects pancreatic output of this proteolytic enzyme. Decreased chymotrypsin activity in stool has been reported in patients with chronic pancreatitis and cystic fibrosis. However, normal values may occur in patients with pancreatic insufficiency, and false-positive results have been reported in up to 10 percent of normal individuals.

Tests useful in the diagnosis of exocrine pancreatic insufficiency and the differential diagnosis of malabsorption are also discussed in Chaps. 292 and 309.

309

DISEASES OF THE PANCREAS

NORTON J. GREENBERGER
PHILLIP P. TOSKES
KURT J. ISSELBACHER

BIOCHEMISTRY AND PHYSIOLOGY OF PANCREATIC EXOCRINE SECRETION

GENERAL CONSIDERATIONS The pancreas secretes 1500 to 3000 ml isosmotic alkaline (pH > 8.0) fluid per day containing about 12 g digestive enzymes. The pancreatic secretions provide the enzymes needed to effect the major digestive activity of the gastrointestinal tract and to provide an optimum pH for the function of these enzymes.

REGULATION OF PANCREATIC SECRETION **Hormonal and neural mechanisms** The exocrine pancreas is under both hormonal and neural control, with hormonal control being of primary importance. Gastric *acid* is the stimulus for the release of secretin, a peptide with 27 amino acids. Sensitive radioimmunoassay studies for secretin suggest that the pH threshold for the release of secretin from the duodenum and jejunum is 4.5. Secretin stimulates the secretion of pancreatic juice rich in *water and electrolytes.* Release of cholecystokinin-pancreozymin (CCK-PZ) from duodenum and jejunum is largely produced by long-chain fatty acids, certain essential amino acids (tryptophan, phenylalanine, valine, methionine), and acid itself. CCK-PZ (a peptide with 33 amino acids) evokes an *enzyme-rich secretion from the pancreas.* Gastrin, although it shares an identical terminal tetrapeptide with CCK-PZ, is a weak stimulus for pancreatic enzyme output. The *parasympathetic nervous system* (via the vagus) exerts some control over pancreatic secretion. Part of this is mediated by the release of gastrin, and part is secondary to a direct effect of acetylcholine on the pancreatic acinar cell. In addition, vagal stimulation effects release of vasoactive intestinal peptide (VIP), a secretin agonist. Vagal control of pancreatic secretion seems to be most important following a truncal vagotomy, but even in such patients severe maldigestion does not ensue. Bile salts also stimulate pancreatic secretion, thereby integrating the functions of the biliary tract, pancreas, and small intestine.

Pancreatic secretion at the cellular level Studies with isolated pancreatic acinar cells indicate that secretin and VIP interact with receptors on the acinar cell, leading to the release of cyclic adenosine monophosphate (AMP). CCK-PZ and acetylcholine react with other receptors to cause the release of membrane-bound calcium, which in turn leads to the release of cyclic guanosine monophosphate (GMP). Cyclic AMP and GMP are believed to act as "second messengers" in stimulating pancreatic secretion.

WATER AND ELECTROLYTE SECRETION Although sodium, potassium, chloride, calcium, zinc, phosphate, and sulfate are found within pancreatic secretion, *bicarbonate is the ion of primary physiological importance.* In the acini and in the ducts, secretin causes the cells to add water and bicarbonate to the fluid. In the ducts an exchange occurs between bicarbonate and chloride. There is a good correlation between the maximal bicarbonate output after stimulation with secretin and the pancreatic mass. The bicarbonate output of 120 to 300 meq per day neutralizes gastric acid production and creates the appropriate pH for the activity of the pancreatic enzymes.

ENZYME SECRETION The pancreas secretes amylolytic, lipolytic, and proteolytic enzymes. Amylolytic enzymes such as amylase hydrolyze starch to oligosaccharides and to the disaccharide maltose. The *lipolytic enzymes* include lipase, phospholipase A, and cholesterol esterase. Bile salts *inhibit* lipase, but colipase, another constituent of pancreatic secretion, binds to lipase and prevents this inhibition. Bile salts *activate* phospholipase A and cholesterol esterase. *Proteolytic enzymes* include *endopeptidases* (trypsin, chymotrypsin), which act on the internal peptide bonds of proteins and polypeptides; *exopeptidases* (carboxypeptidases, aminopeptidases), which act on the free carboxyl terminal end and free amino terminal end of peptides, respectively; and elastase. The proteolytic enzymes are secreted as inactive precursors (zymogens). Ribonucleases (deoxyribonucleases, ribonuclease) are also secreted. *Enterokinase,* an enzyme found within the duodenal mucosa, cleaves the lysine-isoleucine bond of trypsinogen to form trypsin. Trypsin then activates the other proteolytic zymogens in a cascade phenomenon. All pancreatic enzymes have pH optima in the alkaline range.

AUTOPROTECTION OF THE PANCREAS   Autodigestion of the pancreas is prevented by the packaging of proteases in precursor form and by the synthesis of protease inhibitors. These protease inhibitors are found within the acinar cell, the pancreatic secretions, and the α_1 and α_2 globulin fractions of plasma.

EXOCRINE-ENDOCRINE RELATIONSHIPS   Pancreatic glucagon (29 amino acid residues), has a high degree of structural similarity to secretin. It decreases volume and enzyme secretion by the pancreas but not bicarbonate secretion. Glucose, in large concentrations, may also inhibit pancreatic exocrine secretion. The choleretic and insulinotropic effects of secretin are shared by glucagon.

ACUTE PANCREATITIS

GENERAL CONSIDERATIONS   Pancreatic inflammatory disease may be classified as follows: (1) acute pancreatitis, (2) relapsing acute pancreatitis, (3) relapsing chronic pancreatitis, and (4) chronic pancreatitis. This classification is based primarily on clinical criteria with the obvious difference between the acute and chronic varieties; restoration of normal function occurs in the former and permanent residual damage occurs in the latter. The pathologic spectrum of acute pancreatitis varies from *edematous pancreatitis,* which is usually a mild and self-limited disorder, to *necrotizing pancreatitis,* in which the degree of pancreatic necrosis correlates with the severity of the attack and its systemic manifestations. *Hemorrhagic pancreatitis* is less meaningful because variable amounts of interstitial hemorrhage can be found in pancreatitis as well as in other disorders such as pancreatic trauma, pancreatic carcinoma, and severe congestive heart failure.

The incidence of pancreatitis varies in different countries and depends upon etiological factors, e.g., alcohol, gallstones, metabolic factors, and drugs (Table 309-1). In the United States, for example, acute pancreatitis is related to alcohol ingestion more commonly than to gallstones; in England the opposite obtains. Epidemiologic data based on autopsy data indicate that in the United States the overall prevalence of acute pancreatitis is approximately 0.5 percent. An upward trend has been noted in the crude death rate in recent years from 1.0 per 100,000 in 1955 to 1.3 in 1965.

ETIOLOGY AND PATHOGENESIS   There are many causative factors in the pathogenesis of acute pancreatitis (Table 309-1), but the mechanisms by which these conditions trigger pancreatic inflammation have not been identified. Alcoholic patients with pancreatitis may represent a special subset, since most alcoholics do not develop pancreatitis. The list of identifiable

causes is growing, and it is likely that pancreatitis related to viral infections and drugs is more common than heretofore recognized.

Autodigestion is one pathogenetic theory which proposes that proteolytic enzymes (e.g., trypsinogen, chymotrypsinogen, proelastase, and phospholipase A) are activated within the pancreas rather than in the intestinal lumen. A variety of factors (such as endotoxins, exotoxins, viral infections, ischemia, anoxia, and direct trauma) are believed to activate these proenzymes. Activated proteolytic enzymes, especially trypsin, not only digest pancreatic and peripancreatic tissues but also can activate other enzymes such as elastase and phospholipase. The active enzymes then digest cellular membranes and cause proteolysis, edema, interstitial hemorrhage, vascular damage, coagulation necrosis, fat necrosis, and parenchymal cell necrosis. Cellular injury and death result in the liberation of activated enzymes. In addition, activation and release of bradykinin peptides and vasoactive substances (e.g., histamine) is believed to produce vasodilatation, increased vascular perme-

TABLE 309-1
Causes of acute pancreatitis

 I Alcohol ingestion (acute and chronic alcoholism)
 II Biliary tract disease (gallstones)
 III Postoperative (abdominal, nonabdominal)
 IV Post-endoscopic retrograde cholangiopancreatography (ERCP)
 V Trauma (especially blunt abdominal type)
 VI Metabolic
  A Hyperlipidemia
  B Hyperparathyroidism
  C Renal failure
  D After renal transplantation*
  E Acute fatty liver of pregnancy†
 VII Hereditary pancreatitis
 VIII Infections
  A Mumps
  B Viral hepatitis
  C Other viral infections (coxsackievirus, echovirus)
  D Ascariasis
  E Mycoplasma
 IX Drug-associated
  A Diuretics and antihypertensive drugs
   1 Thiazides
   2 Furosemide
   3 Ethacrynic acid
   4 Clonidine‡
  B Anti-inflammatory and immunosuppressive agents
   1 Azathioprine
   2 6-Mercaptopurine
   3 Sulfasalazine
   4 Corticosteroids
   5 L-Asparaginase
   6 Acetaminophen‡
  C Antimicrobials
   1 Isoniazid‡
   2 Tetracycline
   3 Rifampin‡
  D Miscellaneous
   1 Oral contraceptives
   2 Phenformin
   3 Propoxyphene‡
 X Connective tissue disorders with vasculitis
  A Systemic lupus erythematosus
  B Necrotizing angiitis
  C Thrombotic thrombocytopenic purpura
 XI Penetrating duodenal ulcer
 XII Obstruction of the ampulla of Vater
  A Regional enteritis
  B Duodenal diverticulum
XIII Other

* *Pancreatitis occurs in 3 percent of renal transplant patients and is due to many factors including surgery, hypercalcemia, drugs (corticosteroids, azathioprine, L-asparaginase, diuretics), and viral infections.*
† *Pancreatitis also occurs in otherwise uncomplicated pregnancy and is most often associated with cholelithiasis.*
‡ *Isolated case reports only.*

ability, and edema. There is thus a cascade of events culminating in the development of acute necrotizing pancreatitis.

The autodigestion theory has largely eclipsed two older theories. The "common channel" theory holds that such an anatomic arrangement facilitates reflux of bile into the pancreatic duct, and this results in activation of pancreatic enzymes. (Actually, a common channel with free communication between the common bile duct and main pancreatic duct is infrequently encountered.) The second theory is that obstruction and hypersecretion are pivotal in the development of pancreatitis. Obstruction of the main pancreatic duct, however, produces pancreatic edema but not pancreatitis.

CLINICAL FEATURES *Abdominal pain* is the major symptom of acute pancreatitis. Pain may vary from a mild and tolerable discomfort to severe, constant, and incapacitating distress. Characteristically, the pain which is steady and boring in character, is located in the epigastrium and periumbilical region and often radiates to the back as well as to the chest, flanks, and lower abdomen. The pain is frequently more intense when the patient is supine, and patients often obtain relief by sitting with the trunk flexed and knees drawn up. Nausea, vomiting, and abdominal distention due to gastric and intestinal hypomotility and chemical peritonitis are also frequent complaints.

Physical examination frequently reveals a distressed and anxious patient. Low-grade fever, tachycardia, and hypotension are fairly common. Shock is not unusual and may result from (1) hypovolemia secondary to exudation of blood and plasma proteins into the retroperitoneal space, i.e., a "retroperitoneal burn"; (2) increased formation and release of kinin peptides which cause vasodilatation and increased vascular permeability; (3) systemic effects of proteolytic and lipolytic enzymes released into the circulation; and (4) impairment of myocardial contractility by kinins and other poorly characterized peptides. Jaundice occurs infrequently; when present it usually is due to edema of the head of the pancreas with compression of the intrapancreatic portion of the common bile duct. Erythematous skin nodules due to subcutaneous fat necrosis may occur. In 10 to 20 percent of patients there are pulmonary findings, including basilar rales, atelectasis, and pleural effusion, the latter most frequently left-sided. Abdominal tenderness and muscle rigidity are present to a variable degree but compared with the intense pain, these signs may be unimpressive. Bowel sounds are usually diminished or absent. A pancreatic pseudocyst may be palpable in the upper abdomen. A faint blue discoloration around the umbilicus (Cullen's sign) may occur as the result of hemoperitoneum and a blue-red-purple or green-brown discoloration of the flanks (Turner's sign) reflects tissue catabolism of hemoglobin. The latter two findings, which are uncommon, indicate the presence of a severe necrotizing pancreatitis.

LABORATORY DATA The diagnosis of acute pancreatitis is usually established by the presence of an increased serum amylase exceeding 200 Somogyi units. However, there appears to be no definite correlation between the severity of pancreatitis and the degree of serum amylase elevation. After 48 to 72 h, even with continuing evidence of pancreatitis, amylase values tend to return to normal. It will be recalled that amylase elevations in serum and urine occur in many conditions other than pancreatitis (Table 308-2). The C_{am}/C_{cr} ratio is usually elevated in patients with severe obvious pancreatitis. Serum lipase activity increases in parallel with amylase activity, and measurement of both enzymes increases the diagnostic yield. Markedly increased levels of peritoneal or pleural fluid amylase (>5000 units per 100 ml) are also helpful, if present, in establishing the diagnosis.

Leukocytosis (15,000 to 20,000 leukocytes per cubic millimeter) occurs frequently. More severe cases may show hemoconcentration with hematocrit values exceeding 50 percent because of loss of plasma into the retroperitoneal space and peritoneal cavity. *Hyperglycemia* is common and is due to multiple factors that include decreased insulin release, increased glucagon release, and increased output of adrenal glucocorticoids and catecholamines. *Hypocalcemia* occurs in approximately 25 percent of cases and its pathogenesis is incompletely understood. It is apparently due to an impaired parathyroid gland response to a decrease in ionized calcium. Intraperitoneal saponification of calcium by fatty acids in areas of fat necrosis occurs as well as increased plasma levels of glucagon and calcitonin, but it is felt that these abnormalities do not account for the hypocalcemia. *Hyperbilirubinemia* (serum bilirubin > 4.0 mg per 100 ml) occurs in approximately 10 percent of patients. However, jaundice is transient and serum bilirubin levels return to normal in 4 to 7 days. Serum alkaline phosphatase and aspartate aminotransferase (SGOT) levels are also transiently elevated and parallel serum bilirubin values. Serum albumin is decreased to ≤ 3.0 g per 100 ml in about 10 percent of cases and is associated with more severe pancreatitis and an increased mortality rate (Table 309-2). Methemalbumin, a circulating heme metabolite attached to albumin, has been considered as a useful index of severe necrotizing pancreatitis. Its usefulness, however, has been limited by its nonspecificity for pancreatitis (it occurs, for example, in abdominal trauma, bone fractures, soft-tissue trauma, and retroperitoneal hematoma) and its absence in the majority of cases of severe necrotizing pancreatitis. *Hypertriglyceridemia* occurs in 15 to 20 percent of cases, and serum amylase levels in such patients are often spuriously normal (see Chap. 308). Most patients with hypertriglyceridemia and pancreatitis, when subsequently examined, show evidence of an underlying derangement in lipid metabolism which probably antedated the pancreatitis. Approximately 25 percent of patients have *hypoxemia* (arterial $P_{O_2} \leq$ 60 mmHg), which may herald the onset of adult respiratory distress syndrome. Finally, the electrocardiogram is occasionally abnormal in acute pancreatitis with ST-segment and T-wave abnormalities simulating myocardial ischemia.

Radiologic studies useful in the diagnosis of acute pancreatitis are listed in Table 308-1 and discussed in Chap. 308. Although one or more of the abnormalities are found in over 50 percent of patients, the findings are inconstant and nonspecific. Conventional x-rays have been superseded, to some extent, by *ultrasonography;* their chief value in acute pancreatitis is to help exclude other diagnoses, especially a perforated viscus. Intravenous cholangiography has been used to visualize the gallbladder and common duct and to exclude choledocholithi-

TABLE 309-2
Factors adversely influencing survival in acute pancreatitis*

I Risk factors identifiable upon admission to hospital
 A Increasing age
 B Hypotension
 C Tachycardia
 D Abnormal pulmonary findings
 E Abdominal mass
 F Fever
 G Leukocytosis
 H Hyperglycemia
 I First attack of pancreatitis
II Risk factors identifiable during initial 48 h of hospitalization
 A Fall in hematocrit > 10 percent with hydration and/or hematocrit < 30 percent
 B Necessity for massive fluid and colloid replacement
 C Hypocalcemia
 D Hypoxemia with or without adult respiratory distress syndrome
 E Hypoalbuminemia
 F Azotemia

* *Increased mortality with three or more risk factors.*

asis. However, it is often not helpful during the acute illness. While earlier studies suggested that oral cholecystography performed shortly after an attack of pancreatitis failed to opacify the gallbladder in more than half of patients, more recent studies indicate that in nonjaundiced, alcoholic patients with acute pancreatitis not caused by gallstones, oral cholecystography *after resumption of a solid diet* and *before hospital discharge* is successful in opacifying the gallbladder in 90 percent of patients.

DIAGNOSIS Any severe acute pain in the abdomen or back should suggest acute pancreatitis. The diagnosis is usually entertained when a patient with a possible predisposition to pancreatitis presents with severe and constant abdominal pain, nausea, emesis, fever, tachycardia, and abnormal findings on abdominal examination. Laboratory studies frequently reveal leukocytosis, abnormal x-rays of the abdomen and chest, hypocalcemia, and hyperglycemia. The diagnosis is usually confirmed by finding an elevated serum amylase or elevated amylase/creatinine clearance ratio. Obviously, not all the above features have to be present for the diagnosis to be established.

The *differential diagnosis* should include consideration of the following disorders: (1) perforated viscus, especially peptic ulcer; (2) acute cholecystitis and biliary colic; (3) acute intestinal obstruction; (4) mesenteric vascular occlusion; (5) renal colic; (6) myocardial infarction; (7) dissecting aortic aneurysm; (8) connective tissue disorders with vasculitis; (9) pneumonia; and (10) diabetic ketoacidosis. A penetrating duodenal ulcer can usually be identified by upper gastrointestinal x-rays and/or endoscopy. A perforated duodenal ulcer is readily diagnosed by the presence of free intraperitoneal air. It may be difficult to differentiate acute cholecystitis from acute pancreatitis since an elevated serum amylase may be found in both disorders. Pain of biliary tract origin is more right-sided and gradual in onset, and ileus is usually absent. Intestinal obstruction due to mechanical factors can be differentiated from pancreatitis by the history of colicky pain, findings on abdominal examination, and x-rays of the abdomen showing characteristic changes of mechanical obstruction. Acute mesenteric vascular occlusion is usually evident in elderly debilitated patients with brisk leukocytosis, abdominal distention, and bloody diarrhea, in whom paracentesis shows sanguinous fluid and arteriography shows vascular occlusion. Serum as well as peritoneal fluid amylase levels are increased, however, in patients with intestinal infarction. Systemic lupus erythematous and polyarteritis nodosa may be confused with pancreatitis, especially since pancreatitis may develop as a complication of those diseases. Diabetic ketoacidosis is often accompanied by abdominal pain, elevated serum amylase levels, and an abnormal amylase/creatinine clearance ratio, thus closely mimicking acute pancreatitis. The serum lipase is not elevated in diabetic ketoacidosis.

COURSE OF THE DISEASE AND COMPLICATIONS There is an increased mortality rate with three or more risk factors identifiable either at the time of admission to hospital or during the initial 48 h of hospitalization (see Table 309-2). It is important to identify the patient with acute pancreatitis with an increased risk of dying. In one large series such a subgroup was characterized by at least three of the following features: (1) respiratory failure requiring intubation, (2) shock, (3) massive colloid replacement, and (4) serum calcium < 8.0 mg per 100 ml. The survival rate was only 29 percent in the patients treated with medical measures but increased to 64 percent with operative treatment. The high mortality of such severely ill patients, despite maximal medical treatment, suggests that alternative therapeutic approaches such as peritoneal lavage or early surgical intervention merit broader consideration.

COMPLICATIONS The local and systemic complications of acute pancreatitis are listed in Table 309-3. Patients frequently develop an inflammatory mass in the first 2 to 3 weeks after pancreatitis. These may be phlegmons, abscesses, or pseudocysts (see below).

Systemic complications include pulmonary, cardiovascular, hematologic, renal, metabolic, and central nervous system abnormalities. Metabolic complications include hyperglycemia, hypocalcemia, and hypertriglyceridemia. Pancreatitis, hypertriglyceridemia, and alcoholism constitute a triad in which cause and effect remain incompletely understood. However, several reasonable conclusions can be drawn. First, hypertriglyceridemia can precede and apparently cause the development of pancreatitis. Second, the vast majority (> 80 percent) of patients with acute pancreatitis do not have hypertriglyceridemia. Third, almost all patients with pancreatitis and hypertriglyceridemia are *either* alcoholics who have been drinking shortly before the onset of pancreatitis *or* patients with preex-

TABLE 309-3
Complications of acute pancreatitis

I Local
  A Pancreatic phlegmon
  B Pancreatic abscess
  C Pancreatic pseudocyst
    1 Pain
    2 Rupture
    3 Hemorrhage
    4 Infection
  D Pancreatic ascites
    1 Disruption of main pancreatic duct
    2 Leaking pseudocyst
  E Involvement of contiguous organs by necrotizing pancreatitis
    1 Massive intraperitoneal hemorrhage
    2 Thrombosis of blood vessels
    3 Bowel infarction
  F Obstructive jaundice
II Systemic
  A Pulmonary
    1 Pleural effusion
    2 Atelectasis
    3 Mediastinal abscess
    4 Pneumonitis
    5 Adult respiratory distress syndrome
  B Cardiovascular
    1 Hypotension
      a Hypovolemia
      b Hypoalbuminemia
    2 Sudden death
    3 Nonspecific ST-T changes in electrocardiogram simulating myocardial infarction
    4 Pericardial effusion
  C Hematologic
    1 Disseminated intravascular coagulation (DIC)
  D Gastrointestinal hemorrhage *
    1 Peptic ulcer disease
    2 Erosive gastritis
    3 Hemorrhagic pancreatic necrosis with erosion into major blood vessels
    4 Portal vein thrombosis, variceal hemorrhage
  E Renal
    1 Oliguria
    2 Azotemia
    3 Renal artery and/or renal vein thrombosis
  F Metabolic
    1 Hyperglycemia
    2 Hypertriglyceridemia
    3 Hypocalcemia
  G Central nervous system
    1 Psychosis
    2 Fat emboli
  H Fat necrosis
    1 Subcutaneous tissues (erythematous nodules)
    2 Bone
    3 Miscellaneous (mediastinum, pleura, nervous system)

* All are aggravated by coagulation abnormalities (DIC).

istent hypertriglyceridemia. Finally, many of the patients with this triad have persistent hypertriglyceridemia after recovery from pancreatitis and abstention from alcohol.

TREATMENT In most patients (approximately 85 to 90 percent) with acute pancreatitis, the disease is self-limited and subsides spontaneously, usually within 2 to 5 days after treatment is instituted. Medical therapy is aimed at reducing pancreatic secretion and, in essence, "putting the pancreas at rest." Conventional measures include (1) analgesics for pain, (2) intravenous fluids and colloids to maintain normal intravascular volume, (3) no oral alimentation, and (4) nasogastric suction to decrease gastrin release from the stomach and prevent gastric contents from entering the duodenum. Recent controlled trials, however, have shown that nasogastric suction offers no clear-cut advantages in the treatment of mild to moderately severe acute alcohol-associated pancreatitis. Its use, therefore, must be considered elective rather than mandatory.

Anticholinergic drugs have previously been considered standard therapy in patients with acute pancreatitis, the rationale being to blunt stimulation of the pancreas. However, there are no controlled trials, demonstrating that anticholinergic drugs are superior to placebo. Moreover, anticholinergics may make it difficult to determine whether tachycardia, bowel hypomotility, need for additional fluid replacement, and signs of toxicity are due to the drugs or to a worsening of the pancreatitis. Accordingly, their use is not recommended. Although antibiotics have been used in the treatment of acute pancreatitis, two recent randomized prospective trials have shown no benefit from the use of antibiotics in acute pancreatitis of mild to moderate severity. However, because secondary infection of necrotic pancreatic tissue (phlegmon, abscess, pseudocyst) or obstructed biliary passages (ascending cholangitis, complicating choledocholithiasis) contributes to much of the late mortality, appropriate *antibiotic therapy of established infection* is obviously quite important. Previous reports suggested that glucagon was useful in acute pancreatitis, but controlled trials have not provided convincing evidence of effectiveness. Similarly, aprotinin (Trasylol) has not proved effective.

The patient with mild to moderate pancreatitis usually requires treatment with intravenous fluids, fasting, and possibly nasogastric suction for 2 to 4 days. A clear liquid diet is frequently started on the fifth day and a regular diet by the seventh day. The patient with unremitting *fulminant pancreatitis* usually requires inordinate amounts of fluid and close attention to complications such as cardiovascular collapse and respiratory insufficiency. Removal of toxic pancreatic exudate from the peritoneal cavity appears to alter the course of this lethal situation. This can be accomplished by either *peritoneal lavage* via a percutaneous dialysis catheter or *laparotomy* with wide sump drainage. If peritoneal lavage does not halt the patient's deterioration, laparotomy should be considered. The use of parenteral nutrition makes it possible to give nutritional support to patients with severe, acute, or protracted pancreatitis who are unable to eat normally.

PANCREATIC PHLEGMON, ABSCESS, AND PSEUDOCYST

The *phlegmon* is a solid mass of swollen, inflamed pancreas often containing patchy areas of necrosis; it may be present for 1 to 2 weeks. This prolonged inflammatory process should not be confused with a pseudocyst, a differentiation which is usually accomplished by sonography. Occasionally, extensive areas of pancreatic necrosis develop in phlegmons and require incision and drainage. Phlegmons may also be secondarily infected, resulting in abscess formation. The latter occurs in 5 to 10 percent of patients with acute pancreatitis and may arise from infection of necrotic tissue by colonic flora. Severe pancreatitis with the presence of three or more risk factors, postoperative pancreatitis, early oral feeding, and early laparotomy predispose to the development of pancreatic abscess. Pancreatic abscess may also develop because of communication of a pseudocyst with the colon, after inadequate surgical drainage of a pseudocyst, or after needling of a pseudocyst. The characteristic signs of abscess are fever, leukocytosis, ileus, and rapid deterioration in a patient initially recovering from pancreatitis. However, the only manifestations may be persistent fever and signs of continuing pancreatic inflammation. Laparotomy with radical sump drainage is mandatory because the mortality for undrained pancreatic abscess approaches 100 percent. Multiple abscesses are common and reoperation is frequently required.

Pseudocysts of the pancreas are collections of tissue, fluid, debris, pancreatic enzymes, and blood, which develop over a period of 1 to 4 weeks after the onset of acute pancreatitis. In contrast to true cysts, pseudocysts do not have epithelial lining and the walls consist of necrotic tissue, granulation tissue, and fibrous tissue. Disruption of the pancreatic ductal system is common. However, the subsequent course of this disruption varies widely, namely, from spontaneous healing to continuous leakage of pancreatic juice causing tense ascites. Pseudocysts are preceded by pancreatitis in 90 percent of cases and by trauma in 10 percent. Approximately 85 percent are located in the body or tail of the pancreas and 15 percent in the head. Some patients have two or more pseudocysts. Abdominal pain, with or without radiation to the back, is the usual presenting complaint. Usually a palpable, tender mass is found in the middle or left upper abdomen. The serum amylase is elevated in 75 percent of cases and may fluctuate markedly.

Pseudocysts displace some portion of the gastrointestinal tract on x-ray examination in 75 percent of cases (Fig. 309-1). Sonography, however, has proved to be reliable in detecting pseudocysts and should be the initial diagnostic procedure in a patient suspected of having a pseudocyst (Fig. 309-1). Sonography also permits differentiation between an edematous and an inflamed pancreas (pancreatic phlegmon), which can give rise to a palpable mass and an actual pseudocyst. Furthermore, serial ultrasound studies will indicate whether a pseudocyst has resolved. Computerized tomography (CT scanning) complements the use of ultrasound in the diagnosis of pancreatic pseudocyst (Fig. 309-2), especially when it is infected.

The management of pseudocysts is compromised by incomplete knowledge of the natural history of this disorder. Thus, in some patients there may be spontaneous resolution of pseudocysts, however, the frequency of this is not clear. In others, serious complications may occur such as (1) pain caused by expansion of the lesion and pressure on other viscera, (2) rupture, (3) hemorrhage, and (4) abscess. Rupture of a pancreatic pseudocyst is a particularly serious complication. Shock almost always supervenes and mortality rates range from 14 percent if the rupture is not associated with hemorrhage to over 60 percent if hemorrhage has occurred. Rupture and hemorrhage are the prime causes of mortality in pancreatic pseudocyst. A triad of findings, e.g., increase in size of the mass, localized bruit over the mass, and a sudden decrease in hemoglobin and hematocrit levels without obvious signs of external blood loss should alert one to the diagnosis of hemorrhage from a pseudocyst. Thus, in pseudocyst patients who are stable and uncomplicated, and in whom serial ultrasound studies show a decreasing pseudocyst, conservative therapy is indicated. Conversely, patients with a pseudocyst which is expanding and which is complicated by rupture, hemorrhage, and abscess should be operated on. Surgical therapy consists of external or internal drainage of the cyst. Prolonged observation of a nonresolving pancreatic pseudocyst exposes the patient to increased risks which exceed those of elective surgery.

A

B

C

FIGURE 309-1

Pseudocyst of the pancreas. A. Upper gastrointestinal x-ray showing displacement of stomach by pseudocyst. B. Sonogram showing pseudocyst (Ps), K = kidney, a = aorta, L = liver. C. CT scan showing pseudocyst compressing left kidney.

of the leak. If ascites continues to recur after 2 to 3 weeks of medical management, the patient should be operated on following pancreatography to define the anatomy of the abnormal duct.

CHRONIC PANCREATITIS AND PANCREATIC EXOCRINE INSUFFICIENCY

GENERAL AND ETIOLOGICAL CONSIDERATIONS Chronic inflammatory disease of the pancreas may take the form of relapsing chronic pancreatitis or chronic pancreatitis. In relapsing chronic pancreatitis there are episodes of acute inflammation superimposed upon a previously injured pancreas. The causes of relapsing chronic pancreatitis are similar to those of acute pancreatitis (Table 309-2), except that there is an appreciable incidence of cases of undetermined origin. In addition, the pancreatitis associated with gallstones is predominantly acute or relapsing acute in nature. A cholecystectomy is almost always performed in patients after the first or second attack of gallstone-associated pancreatitis. Patients with chronic pancreatitis may present with persistent abdominal pain, with or without steatorrhea, and some may present with steatorrhea and no pain.

Patients with chronic pancreatitis who develop extensive destruction of the pancreas (i.e., less than 10 percent of exocrine function remaining) will demonstrate steatorrhea and azotorrhea. In the adult in the United States, alcoholism is the most common cause of clinically apparent pancreatic exocrine insufficiency, while cystic fibrosis is the most frequent cause in children. In other parts of the world, severe protein calorie malnutrition is a common etiology. Table 309-4 lists other causes of pancreatic exocrine insufficiency, but they are relatively uncommon.

PATHOPHYSIOLOGY Unfortunately, the events that initiate an inflammatory process within the pancreas are still not well understood, and the many hypotheses will not be reviewed. In the case of alcohol-induced pancreatitis, however, it has been suggested that the primary defect may be the precipitation of protein (inspissated enzymes) within the ducts. The resulting ductal obstruction can lead to duct dilatation, diffuse atrophy

PANCREATIC ASCITES AND PANCREATIC PLEURAL EFFUSIONS Pancreatic ascites is usually due to disruption of the main pancreatic duct, often associated with an internal fistula between the duct and the peritoneal cavity (see also Chap. 40). The diagnosis of pancreatic ascites is suggested in a patient with an elevated serum amylase who also has increased levels of albumin (> 3.0 g per 100 ml) and amylase in the ascitic fluid. In addition, endoscopic retrograde cholangiopancreatography (ERCP) will often demonstrate passage of contrast material from a major pancreatic duct or a pseudocyst into the peritoneal cavity. As many as 15 percent of patients with pseudocysts have concurrent pancreatic ascites. The differential diagnosis should include intraperitoneal carcinomatosis, tuberculous peritonitis, constrictive pericarditis, and Budd-Chiari syndrome.

If the pancreatic duct disruption is posterior, an internal fistula may develop between the pancreatic duct and pleural space producing a pleural effusion, which is usually left-sided and often massive.

Treatment usually involves placing the patient on nasogastric solution and parenteral alimentation to decrease pancreatic secretion. In addition, paracentesis is performed to keep the peritoneal cavity free of fluid and hopefully effect sealing

A

B

C

D

FIGURE 309-2
Carcinoma of the pancreas. A. Sonogram showing pancreatic carcinoma (P), dilated intrahepatic bile ducts (d), dilated portal vein (pv), and inferior vena cava (IVC). B. CT scan showing pancreatic carcinoma (arrow).

C. ERCP showing abrupt cut off of the duct of Wirsung (arrow). D. Arteriogram showing sheathing of splenic artery by tumor encasement (arrow).

TABLE 309-4
Causes of pancreatic exocrine insufficiency

  I Alcohol, chronic alcoholism
 II Cystic fibrosis
III Severe protein calorie malnutrition with hypoalbuminemia
 IV Pancreatic and duodenal neoplasms
  V Pancreatic resection
 VI Gastric surgery
   A Subtotal gastrectomy with Billroth II anastomosis
   B Subtotal gastrectomy with Billroth I anastomosis
   C Truncal vagotomy and pyloroplasty
VII Gastrinoma (Zollinger-Ellison syndrome)
VIII Hereditary pancreatitis
 IX Traumatic pancreatitis
  X Idiopathic pancreatitis
 XI Hemochromatosis
XII Shwachman's syndrome (pancreatic insufficiency and bone marrow dysfunction)
XIII Trypsinogen deficiency
XIV Enterokinase deficiency
 XV Isolated deficiencies of amylase, lipase, or proteases
XVI α_1-Antitrypsin deficiency

of the acinar cells, fibrosis, and eventual calcification of some of the protein plugs. While patients with alcohol-induced pancreatitis generally consume large amounts of alcohol, some consume very little (i.e., 50 g or less per day). Thus, prolonged consumption of "socially acceptable" amounts of alcohol is compatible with the development of pancreatitis. In addition, the finding of extensive pancreatic fibrosis in patients who have expired during their first attack of clinical acute alcohol-induced pancreatitis supports the concept that such patients may already have chronic pancreatitis.

CLINICAL FEATURES Patients with relapsing chronic pancreatitis may present with symptoms identical with those found in acute pancreatitis, but their pain may be continuous or intermittent, or pain may be absent. The pathogenesis of this pain is poorly understood. Although the classic description is that of epigastric pain radiating through the back, the pain pattern is often atypical. The pain may be maximal in the right

FIGURE 309-3

Radiological abnormalities in chronic pancreatitis. A. Pancreatic calcification (arrows) and stenosis (tapering) of the intrapancreatic portion of the common bile duct demonstrated by percutaneous transhepatic cholangiography. B. Pancreatic calcification (Ca) demonstrated by sonography.

gb = gallbladder; K = kidney; a = aorta. C. Pancreatic calcification (vertical arrows) and dilated pancreatic duct (horizontal arrow) demonstrated by CT scan. D. Abnormal ERCP in chronic pancreatitis showing ductular ectasia (short arrows) and pseudocyst (long arrows).

or left upper quadrants in the back or diffuse throughout the upper abdomen; it may even be referred to the anterior chest or flank. Characteristically, the pain is persistent, deep-seated, and unresponsive to antacids. It often is increased by alcohol and ingestion of heavy meals (especially foods rich in fat). Often the pain is so severe as to require the frequent use of narcotics.

Weight loss, abnormal stools, and other signs of symptoms suggestive of malabsorption (Table 292-5) are common in chronic pancreatitis. However, clinically apparent deficiencies of fat-soluble vitamins are surprisingly rare. The physical findings in these patients are usually not impressive such that there is a disparity between the severity of the abdominal pain and the paucity of physical signs (save some abdominal tenderness and mild temperature elevation).

DIAGNOSTIC EVALUATION (See Chap. 308) In contrast to patients with relapsing acute pancreatitis, the serum amylase

and lipase levels are usually not elevated. Slight elevation of the serum bilirubin and alkaline phosphatase may indicate cholestasis secondary to chronic inflammation around the common bile duct (Fig. 309-3). Most patients demonstrate impaired glucose tolerance and may have an elevated fasting blood glucose level.

The classic triad of pancreatic calcification, steatorrhea, and diabetes mellitus usually establishes the diagnosis of chronic pancreatitis and exocrine pancreatic insufficiency but is found in less than one-third of chronic pancreatitis patients. Accordingly, it is often necessary to perform the *secretin stimulation test*, which usually becomes abnormal when 75 percent or more of pancreatic exocrine function has been lost. Approximately 40 percent of patients with chronic pancreatitis have *vitamin B$_{12}$ malabsorption* which is corrected by the administration of oral pancreatic enzymes. There is usually a marked excretion of fecal fat (see Chap. 292), which can be reduced with the administration of oral pancreatic extract. The *tripeptide* function test (Chap. 308) and D-xylose urinary excretion test are useful in patients with "pancreatic steatorrhea," since the tripeptide test will be abnormal and the D-xylose excretion usually normal.

The radiographic hallmark of chronic pancreatitis is the presence of scattered calcification throughout the pancreas (Fig. 309-3). Pancreatic calcification indicates that significant damage has occurred and obviates the need for the secretin test. Alcohol by far is the most common cause of pancreatic calcification but may also be seen in severe protein calorie malnutrition, hyperparathyroidism, hereditary pancreatitis, posttraumatic pancreatitis, and islet-cell tumors.

Special techniques such as sonography, CT scanning, and ERCP have added new dimensions to the diagnosis of pancreatic disease. In addition to excluding pseudocysts and pancreatic cancer, sonography may show calcification or dilated ducts associated with chronic pancreatitis (Fig. 309-3). Similar benefits can be derived from CT scans, but the availability and lower cost make sonography preferable at present. ERCP is the only nonoperative technique which provides a direct view of the pancreatic duct. In chronic pancreatitis, ERCP is most useful in the patient with nonalcohol-induced pancreatitis who presents with chronic abdominal pain. ERCP is performed in these patients with the hope of finding a surgically correctable stricture in the pancreatic duct.

COMPLICATIONS OF CHRONIC PANCREATITIS The complications of chronic pancreatitis are protean. *Vitamin B_{12} malabsorption* occurs in 40 percent of patients with alcohol-induced chronic pancreatitis and virtually all with cystic fibrosis. The vitamin B_{12} malabsorption is consistently corrected by the administration of pancreatic enzymes (containing proteases). The vitamin B_{12} malabsorption may be due to excessive binding of vitamin B_{12} by nonintrinsic factor B_{12}–binding proteins. The latter are ordinarily destroyed by pancreatic proteases, but with pancreatic insufficiency the nonspecific binding proteins escape degradation and compete with intrinsic factor for vitamin B_{12} binding. Although the majority of patients show *impaired glucose tolerance,* the development of diabetic ketoacidosis and coma are uncommon. Similarly, end organ damage (retinopathy, neuropathy, nephropathy) is also uncommon, and the appearance of these complications should raise the question of concomitant genetic diabetes mellitus. High amylase containing *effusions* occur within the pleura, pericardium, or peritoneum. *Gastrointestinal bleeding* may occur from ruptured varices secondary to splenic vein thrombosis due to inflammation of the tail of the pancreas. Mild *icterus* may occur, owing to either edema of the head of the pancreas compressing the common bile duct or chronic cholestasis secondary to chronic inflammatory reaction around the intrapancreatic portion of the common bile duct (Fig. 309-3). This chronic obstruction may lead to cholangitis and ultimately biliary cirrhosis. *Subcutaneous fat necrosis* may appear as tender red nodules on the lower extremities. *Bone pain* may be secondary to intramedullary fat necrosis. Inflammation of the large and small joints of the upper and lower extremities may occur. The incidence of pancreatic carcinoma is probably increased. Perhaps the most common and troublesome complication is addiction to narcotics.

TREATMENT AND APPROACH TO MANAGEMENT Therapy for patients with chronic pancreatitis is directed to two major problems, namely, pain and malabsorption. Patients with relapsing chronic pancreatitis are essentially treated like those with acute pancreatitis (see above). Patients with severe and persistent pain should avoid alcohol completely and avoid large meals rich in fat. Since the pain is often severe enough to require frequent use of narcotics (and hence addiction), a number of surgical procedures have been developed for pain relief. ERCP allows the surgeon to plan the operative approach. If there is a stricture of the pancreatic duct, then a *local resection* may ameliorate the pain. Unfortunately isolated localized strictures are not common and in most patients with alcohol-induced disease, the pancreas is diffusely involved and surgically correctible localized ductal disease is rare. When there is primary ductal obstruction, side-to-side pancreaticojejunostomy may provide effective pain palliation. In the majority of these patients, however, pain relief can only be achieved by resecting 50 to 95 percent of the gland. Although pain relief is achieved in three-quarters of these patients, they tend to develop pancreatic endocrine and exocrine insufficiency. It is important to screen the patients carefully, for such radical surgery is contraindicated in those who are severely depressed or suicidal or continue to drink. Procedures such as sphincteroplasty, splanchnicectomy and celiac ganglionectomy, and nerve blocks usually bring only temporary relief and are not recommended.

Large doses of pancreatic extract (see below) seem to ameliorate and even abort the pain in some patients with chronic pancreatitis. These clinical observations seem to fit in with data in experimental animals, in which the administration of large doses of oral trypsin decreases pancreatic secretion, perhaps by binding to the surface of the small intestinal cell and inhibiting the release of CCK-PZ. It seems reasonable to approach the patient with severe persistent or continuous abdominal pain thought to be secondary to chronic pancreatitis in the following manner. After other causes of abdominal pain (peptic ulcer, gallstones, etc.) have been appropriately excluded, a pancreatic *sonogram* should be done. If no mass is found, a *secretin test* may be performed, since with chronic pancreatitis and pain this test will be abnormal. If the secretin test is abnormal (i.e., decreased bicarbonate concentration or volume output) a 3- to 4-week *trial of pancreatic extract* is appropriate. If no relief is obtained, and especially if the volume secreted during the secretin test is very low, *ERCP* should be performed. If a localized ductal obstruction is found, surgery should be considered. If no surgically remedial lesion is found and severe pain continues despite abstinence from alcohol, subtotal pancreatic resection may be necessary.

The treatment of malabsorption rests upon the use of pancreatic enzyme replacement therapy. Although diarrhea and steatorrhea are usually improved, the results are frequently less than satisfactory. The major problem is delivery of enough active enzyme into the duodenum. Steatorrhea can be abolished if 10 percent of the normal amount of lipase could be delivered into the duodenum at the proper time. This concentration of lipase cannot be achieved with the presently available preparations of pancreatic enzymes, even if the latter are given in large doses. These poor results may be due to inactivation of lipase by gastric acid, food emptying from the stomach more rapidly than the exogenously administered pancreatic enzymes, and variation in the enzyme activity of various batches of commercially available pancreatic extracts. The use of the H_2-receptor antagonist cimetidine has proved to be a useful adjunct in patients failing to respond to pancreatic extract alone.

For the usual patient four to eight tablets or capsules of a potent enzyme preparation should be administered with meals. If this program fails, then the enzymes may be given more frequently (in the same total dose but every 2 h while awake) or together with cimetidine. Although theoretically antacids could buffer the gastric acid, cimetidine appears to be superior, perhaps because it also decreases the volume of gastric secretions, thus resulting in greater intraduodenal concentrations of enzymes.

Patients with severe exocrine pancreatic insufficiency secondary to alcohol who continue to drink have a high mortality (in one series 50 percent were dead when followed for 5 to 12 years) and significant morbidity (weight loss, lassitude, vitamin deficiency, and narcotic addiction). Those with pain usually do not have steatorrhea and are approached as described above. If steatorrhea develops, the pain usually abates. If abstinence is pursued and vigorous replacement therapy is utilized for the maldigestion-malabsorption, the patients do reasonably well.

HEREDITARY PANCREATITIS Hereditary pancreatitis is a rare disease similar to chronic relapsing pancreatitis except for an early age of onset and evidence of hereditary factors (involving an autosomal dominant gene with incomplete penetrance). These patients have recurring attacks of severe abdominal pain which may last from a few days to a few weeks. The serum amylase and lipase levels may be elevated during acute attacks. Patients frequently develop pancreatic calcification, diabetes mellitus, and steatorrhea, and in addition, they have an increased incidence of pancreatic carcinoma. Abdominal complaints in relatives of patients with hereditary pancreatitis should raise the question of pancreatic disease.

CYSTIC FIBROSIS

GENERAL CONSIDERATIONS Cystic fibrosis is the most common hereditary lethal disease in Caucasian children. It is transmitted as an autosomal recessive trait, with a prevalence of 1 per 1500 to 2500 births and with approximately 1 in 20 Caucasians being heterozygous for the condition. Patients with cystic fibrosis have a dysfunction of the mucus-producing exocrine glands in the bronchi, pancreas, liver, and intestine. However, the basic metabolic defect is unknown. This disease is no longer one of childhood and adolescence. With improvement in the therapy of patients with cystic fibrosis, an increasing number of patients are reaching adulthood. Twenty years ago the mean survival was only 1 year; presently, the mean survival is 16 years.

CLINICAL FEATURES Although the triad of recurrent pulmonary infections, maldigestion-malabsorption, and an abnormal sweat test are characteristic, patients are frequently seen without these classical manifestations. Approximately 85 percent of patients with cystic fibrosis have impairment of pancreatic exocrine function. Steatorrhea is often marked and accompanied by deficiencies of fat-soluble vitamins (e.g., low prothrombin levels). A small number of patients may have recurrent pancreatitis with abdominal pain and elevated amylase levels. Biliary cirrhosis develops in 5 to 10 percent. Approximately 15 percent of patients may develop intestinal obstruction at birth because of the thick, tenacious intestinal secretions. Similarly, children or adults may develop small- or large-bowel obstruction, ileocolic intussusception, cecal or sigmoid volvulus, rectal impaction, and rectal prolapse. Vitamin B_{12} and bile acid malabsorption are common but correctable by oral pancreatic extract. Vitamin B_{12} deficiency is rare, perhaps due to the almost universal administration of pancreatic extract to these patients beginning at an early age. The incidence of gallstones is increased.

DIAGNOSIS A properly performed and interpreted sweat test (quantitative pilocarpine iontophoresis) is essential for the diagnosis of cystic fibrosis. In almost all patients the sweat chloride is greater than 60 meq per liter. Secretin or CCK-PZ tests will usually demonstrate severe impairment of bicarbonate output and pancreatic enzymes, respectively. The tripeptide hydrolysis test (Chap. 308) is usually abnormal. Suction biopsy of the rectum will often show dilated crypts containing excessive amounts of mucus, but the specificity of these findings has been questioned.

THERAPY Treatment includes antibiotics for recurrent pulmonary infections, inhalation and physical therapy, pancreatic extracts, and vitamin supplementation, as well as psychological and emotional support. Although complete correction of fat malabsorption is usually not achieved, satisfactory weight gain is often attained. Elevated blood and urine uric acid levels may occur in children taking excessive doses of pancreatic extract, but this is reversible with reduction in dosage.

CANCER OF THE PANCREAS

GENERAL CONSIDERATIONS Carcinoma of the pancreas is now the fourth commonest cancer causing death in the United States; only cancer of the lung, colon, and breast occur more frequently. It accounts for 10 percent of all tumors of digestive organs and over 20,000 deaths per year. The incidence has increased 300 percent since 1930 to approximately 11 per 100,000 population. The disease is more common in males than females (1.5:1), and the peak incidence between the ages of 60 to 70. Although the etiologic factors in most cases are not known, incidence of carcinoma of the pancreas is 2.0 to 2.5 times greater in *smokers* than in nonsmokers, and about 2 times greater in patients with *diabetes mellitus*. Patients with *calcific pancreatitis* also have an increased incidence of pancreatic carcinoma. The tumors are usually adenocarcinomas arising from ductal epithelium. The head of the pancreas is involved in about 65 percent, the body and tail in 30 percent, and the tail alone in 5 percent. At the time of diagnosis the tumor is confined to the pancreas in only 15 percent of patients; 25 percent demonstrate local invasion or regional lymph node spread, and the remaining 60 percent exhibit distinct metastases.

CLINICAL FEATURES Weight loss, abdominal pain, anorexia, and jaundice are the classic symptoms. Nausea, weakness and fatigue, vomiting, diarrhea, dyspepsia, and back pain are also fairly common. The weight loss in carcinoma is extensive (average total loss about 25 lb) and is not fully explained by anorexia and maldigestion. The weight loss in patients with lesions in the body and tail, in whom malabsorption should be minimal, is often as pronounced as when the carcinoma is in the head of the pancreas.

Pain occurs at some time in the course of the disease in 75 to 90 percent of patients. With tumors of the head of the pancreas, the pain is likely to be in the epigastrium and right upper quadrant; with lesions in the body of the pancreas, pain often localizes in the midline, whereas with lesions in the tail, pain may be referred to the left upper quadrant. Abdominal pain may be vague or be a steady dull, aching, or boring pain often radiating through to the back. Severe and unrelenting pain suggests extension into the retroperitoneal area with invasion of the neural plexus around the celiac axis ganglion.

Jaundice occurs some time in the course of the disease in 80 to 90 percent of patients with carcinoma of the head, and in 10 to 40 percent in patients with tumors of the body and tail. When it occurs it is progressive and accompanied by pruritus. Both constipation and diarrhea have been cited as the predominant alteration of bowel habits. Emotional disturbances frequently occur in cancer of the pancreas and may take the form of insomnia, restlessness, rage, anxiety, depression, suicidal tendencies, and a sense of impending doom.

Physical examination frequently reveals evidence of weight loss, jaundice, and enlarged liver and abdominal tenderness. Although the gallbladder is usually enlarged, it is palpable in only 15 to 40 percent of cases (Courvoisier's sign). The finding of an enlarged gallbladder in a jaundiced patient without biliary colic should suggest malignant obstruction of the extrahepatic biliary tree. Splenomegaly may result from compression, invasion, and thrombosis of the portal venous system, especially the splenic vein. Erosion of the duodenal mucosa may cause occult or frank gastrointestinal bleeding. In carcinoma of the body and tail, an abdominal mass can be felt in 40 to 50 percent of patients; hepatomegaly is less common than in tumors of the head of the pancreas, and obvious hepatic enlargement should suggest hepatic metastasis. An important physical finding is an abdominal bruit which is usually heard in the periumbilical area and left upper quadrant, and this is due to invasion and/or compression of the splenic artery by tumor. Thrombophlebitis occurs in approximately 10 percent of patients and is more common with the tumors of the body or tail of the pancreas. In acinar-cell carcinomas, which are uncommon, tender subcutaneous nodules due to subcutaneous fat necrosis and polyarthralgia occur.

The diagnosis of pancreatic carcinoma should be suspected in patients past the age of 50 who present with any of the following findings: weight loss of uncertain cause, back pain, unexplained abdominal pain, and jaundice with obstructive features. Carcinoma of the hepatic duct bifurcation, of the ampulla of Vater, and of the duodenum also need to be considered in the differential diagnosis, but these all occur quite infrequently.

LABORATORY FINDINGS Laboratory data are only occasionally helpful in suggesting the diagnosis of pancreatic carcinoma. The serum amylase and lipase values are abnormal in only 10 percent of cases. About 20 percent of patients have fasting hyperglycemia or glycosuria, although the glucose tolerance test is abnormal in 50 percent. Anemia, which occurs in one-third of patients, and occult blood in the stool, which occurs in one-half of patients, are usually due to erosion of the duodenal mucosa by tumor. Although the stools may have a greasy or pultaceous consistency, frank steatorrhea occurs in only about 10 percent of patients. Carcinoma of the head of the pancreas with bile duct obstruction is accompanied by hyperbilirubinemia and clay-colored stools. By contrast, the blood, urine, and feces in patients with carcinoma of the body

and tail of the pancreas are often normal. The serum alkaline phosphatase is usually elevated in patients with jaundice (and may antedate the hyperbilirubinemia). It is elevated in about 35 percent of cases without jaundice.

DIAGNOSTIC PROCEDURES (See Table 309-5) Although standard gastrointestinal x-rays may suggest the presence of carcinoma of the head of the pancreas, the tumor is usually of considerable size before it distorts the duodenal mucosa and the configuration of the duodenal loop. Thus, only 50 percent of patients with carcinoma of the head of the pancreas have an abnormal examination. The frequency of abnormal exams is even lower with lesions in the body and tail of the pancreas.

Ultrasound is valuable in the diagnosis of pancreatic carcinoma, especially as an initial screening procedure; abnormalities are found in 70 to 90 percent of patients with pancreatic carcinoma. Sonography is most likely to be positive if the tumor is over 2 cm in diameter and lies in the head or body of the pancreas; lesions in the body and tail of the pancreas are more difficult to recognize.

If available, tests of exocrine pancreatic function with duodenal intubation and aspiration of duodenal contents after intravenous injection of secretin or secretin plus cholecystokinin are useful. Such tests are abnormal in approximately 80 percent of cases. Two types of abnormal responses are observed. First, the volumes of aspirated duodenal contents is markedly reduced, while the concentration of bicarbonate and enzymes remain normal or minimally altered. Second, there may be marked pancreatic achylia with sharply decreased volume output and concentration of bicarbonate and enzymes—a pattern indistinguishable from the secretory response of patients with chronic pancreatitis. Thus, pancreatic function tests do not permit discrimination between chronic pancreatic carcinoma and chronic pancreatitis.

Cytologic examination of pancreatic fluid and pancreatic secretory studies obtained after secretin-cholecystokinin stimulation should theoretically be useful but practically has been found not to be reliable enough to diagnose pancreatic cancer.

CT scanning is frequently abnormal in pancreatic carcinoma; in most series of proved cases, CT scans detected the lesion in over 80 percent. False-positive results have been reported in about 5 to 10 percent of cases where no tumor was found at laparotomy. Such false-positive results will perhaps be less in the future. CT scanning has slight advantages over ultrasound, such as better definition of the body and tail of the pancreas as well as contiguous organs, but the cost is considerably greater. Selective and superselective angiography is of definite value in the diagnosis of pancreatic carcinoma. Advantages of angiography include (1) detection of carcinoma in the body and tail of the pancreas by observing vessel sheathing (Fig. 309-2), vessel displacement, and vascular occlusion; (2) detection of metastatic spread to the liver; and (3) assessment

TABLE 309-5
Diagnostic procedures for pancreatic carcinoma*

Location of carcinoma	Sonography	Exocrine pancreatic function tests	Cytologic examination duodenal fluid	Computerized tomography (CT scan)	Endoscopic retrograde cholangiopancreatography (ERCP)	Percutaneous transhepatic cholangiogram (PTC)	Selective arteriography	Percutaneous pancreatic biopsy with radiologic guidance	Upper gastrointestinal x-rays
Head	+ +	+ +	+	+ + +	+ + +	+ + +	+ + +	+ + + +	+
Body	+ +	+ +	+	+ + +	+ + +	+	+ + +	+ + + +	+
Tail	+ +	+ +	+	+ + +	+ + +	0	+ + +	+ + + +	+

* If the ultrasound examination shows a pancreatic mass with dilated intrahepatic ducts, a PTC is the logical next step. If the patient has a mass on ultrasound examination but without dilated ducts, ERCP should be done. If clinical suspicion is high or exocrine pancreatic function tests are abnormal, ERCP should be considered. If ERCP is unsuccessful, selective arteriography is recommended. If arteriography shows encasement of vessels or hepatic metastases, percutaneous pancreatic biopsy should be considered as an alternative to laparotomy.

NOTE: + = helpful occasionally (<50 percent cases); + + = useful, especially as initial screening procedure; + + + = frequently (> 50 percent cases) abnormal; + + + + = often diagnostic.

of the degree of involvement of huge pancreatic vessels which may be an important consideration preoperatively. When the arteriogram is positive, about 85 percent of patients can be expected to have pancreatic cancer; however, false negatives occur in about 15 percent of patients.

ERCP may be diagnostic in 75 to 85 percent of cases. The characteristic findings are stenosis or obstruction of either the pancreatic or the common bile duct; both duct systems are abnormal in over half the cases. The differentiation, however, between carcinoma and chronic pancreatitis by ERCP can be quite difficult if both diseases are present. False-negative results with ERCP are quite low (less than 5 percent). Finally, *percutaneous aspiration biopsy of the pancreas* under ultrasonic guidance is a new procedure which can provide a definitive diagnosis and may obviate surgical exploration.

Patients with carcinoma of the pancreas are frequently investigated for several months before a diagnosis is established. Even laparotomy may not provide a definitive diagnosis because chronic pancreatitis may produce a hard mass in the head of the pancreas indistinguishable from carcinoma by palpation. Furthermore, biopsy of such a mass may not show neoplastic tissue and reveal only evidence of pancreatitis because the carcinoma is often surrounded by edematous, inflamed, and fibrotic tissue, e.g., changes of chronic pancreatitis.

TREATMENT AND COURSE When the diagnosis is confirmed at laparotomy, the tumor is usually inoperable. The resectability rate in most series is only about 15 to 20 percent. If the tumor is localized and has not spread to portal lymph nodes, and is not fixed to other structures (e.g., portal vein, superior mesenteric vein, and common bile duct), the lesion should be considered resectable. Resection under these circumstances offers an opportunity for palliation, although survival does not appear to be prolonged. Importantly, the mortality rate with a Whipple procedure (pancreatoduodenal resection) is about 20 percent in most series. The median survival is 6 months from the time of diagnosis. Approximately 10 percent of patients survive 1 year, and in most reported series, the 5-year survival rate is a dismal 1 to 2 percent.

PANCREATIC ENDOCRINE TUMORS

Pancreatic endocrine tumors are summarized in Table 309-6 and discussed in Chap. 340.

OTHER CONDITIONS

ANNULAR PANCREAS When there is a failure in communication of the ventral and dorsal anlage of the pancreas, a ring of pancreatic tissue encircles the duodenum. Such an annular pancreas may cause intestinal obstruction in the neonate or the adult. Symptoms of postprandial fullness, epigastric pain, nausea, and vomiting may be present for years before the diagnosis is entertained. The radiographic findings are symmetric dilatation of the proximal duodenum with bulging of the recesses on either side of the annular band, effacement of the duodenal mucosa without destruction of the mucosa, accentuation of the findings in the right anterior oblique position, and the lack of change on repeated examinations. The differential diagnosis should include duodenal webs, tumors of the pancreas or duodenum, postbulbar peptic ulcer regional enteritis, and adhesions. Patients with annular pancreas have an increased incidence of pancreatitis and peptic ulcer. The treatment is surgical even though the condition has been present for years because of the potential complications. Retrocolic duodeno-jejunostomy is the procedure of choice, although some surgeons advocate Billroth II gastrectomy, gastroenterostomy, and vagotomy.

TABLE 309-6
Pancreatic endocrine tumors

Syndrome	Hormone(s) produced	Primary hormone effects	Pathologic features	Clinical features
Zollinger-Ellison	Gastrin	Gastric acid hypersecretion with basal acid outputs usually >15 meq/h	Non-beta-cell islet tumors; 10% aberrant (duodenal); 60% malignant	Severe peptic ulcer disease often refractory to therapy; ectopic ulcers; diarrhea; multiple endocrine adenomas (parathyroid, pituitary, adrenal, thyroid)
Insulinoma	Insulin	Hypoglycemia with inappropriately increased serum insulin levels	Beta-cell islet tumors; 80-90% benign	Hypoglycemic symptoms
Glucagonoma	Glucagon	Hyperglucagonemia →glucose intolerance	Alpha-cell islet tumors; 60% malignant	Slow growing pancreatic tumor; hyperglycemia; bullous and eczematoid dermatitis; weight loss; anemia
Somatostatinoma	Somatostatin	Somatostatin inhibition of insulin, gastrin and pancreatic enzyme secretion	Delta-cell islet tumor	Pancreatic tumor; diarrhea; anemia
Pancreatic cholera	Vasoactive intestinal peptide (VIP) ? Gastrin ? Glucagon ? Gastric inhibitory polypeptide	Hormones cause altered salt and water transport by gut	? Delta-cell tumor; > 50% malignant	Pancreatic tumor with severe watery diarrhea flushing; weight loss, hypercalcemia; hypochlorhydria; inordinate fecal water and electrolyte losses
Carcinoid	Serotonin Prostaglandins	Altered gut motility; diarrhea	Non-beta-cell islet tumors	Carcinoid syndrome with flushing; wheezing; diarrhea; alcohol intolerance; hepatomegaly

PANCREAS DIVISUM This condition is receiving increased attention because of the performance of ERCP. In pancreas divisum, the duct of Wirsung is no more than 2 cm in length, while the duct of Santorini becomes the major ductal system and maintains its communication with the duodenum through the minor papilla. Approximately 2 to 3 percent of the population may have this anatomic anomaly. Pancreas divisum is suspected when a patient who is having ERCP performed complains of abdominal pain with the injection of small amounts of contrast material due to overdistention of the small duct of Wirsung. When such pain occurs, no further contrast material should be given and a film of the pancreas should be taken. Failure to opacify the main pancreatic duct suggests pancreas divisum.

REFERENCES

ARVANITAKIS C et al: Diagnostic tests of exocrine pancreatic function and disease. Gastroenterology 74:932, 1978

CREUTZFELDT W, SCHMIDT H: Aetiology and pathogenesis of pancreatitis (current concepts). Scand J Gastroenterol Suppl 6:47, 1970

DIMAGNO EP et al: Relations between pancreatic enzyme outputs and malabsorption in severe pancreatic insufficiency. N Engl J Med 288:813, 1973

———— et al: A prospective comparison of current diagnostic tests for pancreatic cancer. N Engl J Med 297:737, 1977

LEVITT MD et al: Is the C_{am}/C_{cr} ratio of value for the diagnosis of pancreatitis? Gastroenterology 75:118, 1978

MORGAN RGH, WORMSLEY KG: Progress report. Cancer of the pancreas. Gut 18:550, 1977

RUSSELL JGB et al: Ultrasonic scanning in pancreatic disease. Gut 19:1027, 1978

SARLES H: Chronic calcifying pancreatitis—chronic alcoholic pancreatitis. Gastroenterology 66:604, 1974

SCHWACHMAN H et al: Cystic fibrosis: A new outlook: 70 patients above 25 years of age. Medicine 56:129, 1977

SINGH M, WEBSTER PD: Neurohormonal control of pancreatic secretion. A review. Gastroenterology 74:193, 1978

WARSHAW A: Acute pancreatitis. Viewpoints Dig Dis, vol 9, no 5, November 1977

WINSHIP D et al: Pancreatitis: Pancreatic pseudocysts and their complications. Gastroenterology 73:593, 1977

section 8 | Disorders of the hematopoietic system

Red blood cell disorders

310

IRON-DEFICIENCY ANEMIA AND THE SIDEROBLASTIC ANEMIAS

G. RICHARD LEE
MAXWELL M. WINTROBE
H. FRANKLIN BUNN

IRON-DEFICIENCY ANEMIA

INCIDENCE Iron deficiency is, by far, the most common cause of anemia worldwide. In the United States, about 20 percent of adult women, 50 percent of pregnant women, and 3 percent of adult males are iron-deficient. Furthermore, iron deficiency is found in about 30 percent of preschool children with a peak incidence at 12 to 24 months of age. In Asia, the Middle East, and some parts of Africa and Central and South America, this anemia is not only very prevalent but may be very severe, particularly where hookworm is endemic.

IRON METABOLISM Iron is normally obtained by digestion of food. The newborn infant starts with a supply derived from its mother, but as growth occurs, dietary sources are necessary to meet the demands of the ever-expanding red blood cell mass. In the female, with the onset of menarche, additional iron is needed to compensate for the loss of blood. Later, the demands of pregnancy exceed the saving due to amenorrhea.

The distribution of iron in normal individuals is shown in Table 310-1. The body of a normal adult man contains approximately 50 mg iron per kilogram of body weight; that of a woman contains 35 mg/kg. About two-thirds of this amount is found in hemoglobin, and only about 3 mg circulates in the plasma as transferrin, a β_1 globulin. A very small proportion of the total body iron is present in myoglobin and the heme enzymes (150 mg). The remainder (about 1000 mg in men, 100 to 400 mg in women) represents a reserve which can be called upon for hemoglobin production and is stored in the liver, spleen, and bone marrow as ferritin and hemosiderin.

The average adult diet in the United States provides about 6 mg iron per 1000 kcal, or about 10 to 20 mg per day. However, only 5 to 10 percent of this amount is absorbed. When there is increased need for iron, absorption may be more efficient (10 to 20 percent). Iron derived from hemoglobin and other heme proteins of animal origin is absorbed as the intact heme molecule. Most other forms of iron must be converted to ferrous iron in the stomach and duodenum in order to be absorbed. Absorption is most efficient in the duodenum and upper part of the small intestine. Iron is transported through the

TABLE 310-1
Distribution of iron in normal individuals

Protein	Total iron in compound, mg	Function
Hemoglobin	2500	O_2 transport, blood
Myoglobin	140	O_2 transport, muscle
Ferritin and hemosiderin	1000 (males), 100–400 (females)	Storage
Transferrin	3	Transport
Enzymes	~ 1	O_2 utilization, etc.

mucosal cell, but the exact mechanism is still uncertain. The absorbed iron is then bound by plasma transferrin and transported to the bone marrow for hemoglobin synthesis. The normal plasma iron level is 60 to 190 μg per 100 ml, but it is more useful to think of the serum iron in terms of percentage saturation of transferrin, normally 20 to 45 percent. Iron turnover is rapid, so that 25 to 40 mg iron is transported in the plasma per day. The great bulk of this transport is to marrow erythroblasts. Since the total red blood cell mass contains approximately 2500 mg iron and the red blood cell life span is 120 days, about 20 mg iron is delivered each day to the erythron.

Conservation is the characteristic feature of iron metabolism. The iron derived from the breakdown of hemoglobin joins the body pool and is used again and again. Loss of iron from the body is minimal: probably about 1 mg per day in men and an average of 2 mg per day in menstruating women. Most of this amount is contained in cells desquamated from the intestinal mucosa or the skin. In women, menstrual iron loss is highly variable but, undoubtedly, is the greatest normal cause of iron loss. A normal woman loses an average of 17 mg iron during a normal period. The net loss of iron during a normal pregnancy is about 700 mg, i.e., an average of about 2.5 mg per day. These factors contribute to the lower iron stores in women of the childbearing age group.

It follows that, in a temperate climate, the requirement for iron in a normal man or postmenopausal woman is 0.5 to 1 mg per day. For menstruating women, it is 1.5 mg per day. During pregnancy, at least 2.5 mg per day is required. The iron requirement for growth during infancy and childhood varies with the growth rate at different periods. During the first year of life, the need may be as high as 1 mg per day, but averages 0.6 mg; during childhood, the average is about 1.0 to 1.5 mg per day.

CAUSES OF IRON DEFICIENCY From this review of the iron economy of the body, it follows that children, female adolescents, and women in their reproductive years are most in danger of developing iron deficiency. However, any circumstance which leads to increased demand on the iron stores of the body can result in iron deficiency. The possible factors leading to iron deficiency are (1) insufficient iron in the diet, (2) impaired absorption, (3) increased requirements, and (4) loss of blood. In many instances, more than one of these factors is responsible for the resulting deficiency.

Except in infants and in rapidly growing children, chronic loss of blood by hemorrhage is by far the most common cause of iron deficiency. Excessive menstruation and occult bleeding from the gastrointestinal tract (peptic ulcer, neoplasm, hookworm infection, esophageal varices, hemorrhoids, salicylate ingestion with associated gastritis) are the most common types of bleeding which may result in iron deficiency. A woman may lose as much as 200 ml blood during each menstrual period and not be aware that the loss is excessive. In the adult male and the postmenopausal female, the discovery of iron-deficiency anemia should cause a diligent search for a source of bleeding, and this is most likely to be found in the gastrointestinal tract. Chronic gastrointestinal blood loss may be due to a generalized bleeding diathesis rather than to a single anatomic lesion. Patients with hereditary telangiectasia often develop iron-deficiency anemia. Chronic and acute gastrointestinal blood loss is more commonly observed with thrombocytopenia or qualitative platelet abnormalities, such as von Willebrand's disease, than with deficiencies of soluble coagulation factors.

On the other hand, decreased assimilation of iron, whether from dietary deficiency of iron, impaired absorption, or both, is rarely an important cause of iron deficiency unless the iron stores are already poor, demands for iron (as by rapid growth or frequent pregnancies) are great, or blood loss has occurred. Since milk is a relatively poor source of iron, infants fed only

milk are particularly prone to develop iron deficiency. Similarly, diets high in cereal content and low in animal protein are relatively poor sources of iron. Furthermore, the nature of the diet itself, other than its iron content, influences the absorption of iron. Thus, both phosphates in the diet and phytates in cereals form a complex with iron and reduce its absorption. Ascorbic acid favors iron absorption, probably by promoting the reduction of ferric iron in food to the ferrous form. Some protection against dietary iron deficiency is being provided in the United States and elsewhere by fortification of flour, bread, and infant cereals with iron, but the influence of long-established cultural practices, food faddism, and generally poor dietary habits is hard to overcome.

The gastric hydrochloric acid favors ionization and thus absorption, yet many persons are found in whom achlorhydria has existed for years without iron deficiency developing. Nevertheless, iron deficiency frequently develops after total or partial gastrectomy in the absence of evidence of bleeding. In such patients increased motility or bypass of the actively absorbing segments of the duodenum may also reduce iron absorption. Likewise, chronic small bowel diarrhea prevents efficient absorption, and, in steatorrhea, iron absorption has been shown to be impaired. Not only is the absorption of dietary iron inefficient in these situations, but increased absorption in response to need, which occurs normally, does not take place.

Nevertheless, since the normal loss of iron from the body is relatively small, none of these circumstances of impaired iron assimilation is likely to be an important cause of iron deficiency unless blood loss or increased needs have developed. The high requirements for iron in infants, children, adolescents, and premenopausal women have been outlined above.

The syndrome of chlorosis, the "green sickness" of the last century and before, may have been no more than iron deficiency in adolescent girls in whom dietary iron was insufficient to meet the needs for growth and menstruation. Likewise, the chronic hypochromic anemia of women 30 to 45 years of age represents the ultimate combined effect of chronic loss of blood, frequent pregnancies, and poor diet in persons whose iron deficiency may have had its beginning in adolescence. It is of interest that, in many of these patients, certain constitutional features similar to those encountered in pernicious anemia have been observed, such as early graying of the hair and achlorhydria.

CLINICAL MANIFESTATIONS Most individuals with iron deficiency are asymptomatic. Patients develop symptoms in proportion to the degree of anemia. With more severe anemia, depending on the constitution of the patient and the cause of the deficiency, the accompanying clinical manifestations are those common to all chronic anemias, such as increasing fatigability, headache, tachycardia, exertional dyspnea, ankle edema, and pallor. It is evident that such symptoms are also sometimes found in the absence of anemia. Attempts to relate some of these manifestations to deficiencies of cellular iron metalloenzymes have not been successful. Pica (perverted appetite) may be a striking manifestation. Affected individuals may crave earth or clay (geophagia), starch (amylophagia), or ice (pagophagia).

Abnormalities in epithelial tissues, including sore or atrophic tongue, sore mouth, angular stomatitis, thinning or spooning of the nails (koilonychia), or dysphagia, may occur in an occasional patient who is iron-deficient. The Plummer-Vinson syndrome (sideropenic dysphagia) is characterized by the feeling of food sticking in the throat; a stricture in the postcricoid region of the laryngopharynx may be found, or the opening may be partially closed by a thin, mucous membrane web which can be demonstrated roentgenographically and is easily ruptured by the passage of an endoscope.

Menstrual disturbances are common—menorrhagia, irregularity of flow, or even amenorrhea. When present, menorrhagia may aggravate the iron-deficiency state. As in other causes of severe anemia, retinal hemorrhages and exudates may be found in cases of advanced iron deficiency (hemoglobin less than 5 g per 100 ml).

In the fully developed state, the clinical picture is striking; a tired, lifeless appearance, pallor, inelastic and often dry and wrinkled skin, sometimes with a brownish hue; dry and often scanty hair and pearly white scleras are found. In many cases, some degree of papillary atrophy of the tongue, slight cardiac enlargement, functional systolic murmurs, and a slightly enlarged liver are discernible. When the deficiency is severe, the nails may be flattened, longitudinally ridged, or even concave (koilonychia), and may break easily. Findings on neurologic examination are nearly always normal.

LABORATORY FINDINGS Most patients with iron deficiency have minimal anemia or none at all. As shown in Table 310-2, in mild iron deficiency red blood cells are usually normocytic or slightly microcytic. Hypochromia does not develop unless the deficiency is more advanced. When significant anemia is present, a blood smear will reveal small, pale red blood corpuscles poorly filled with hemoglobin (see Plate 9-7). In severe cases, these may be mere rings. Tiny microcytes, "target-like" cells, elliptical cells, and bizarre poikilocytes are also found as well as a certain portion of normally filled corpuscles. The red corpuscle count may be normal or nearly so or even greater than normal, while the hemoglobin and hematocrit are greatly reduced. The anemia is hypochromic and microcytic. The percentage of reticulocytes is usually normal but may increase temporarily following an acute episode of blood loss. The leukocyte count is normal or slightly reduced, and the platelet count is variable. The bone marrow reveals moderate erythroid hyperplasia. Many of the late normoblasts appear to have scanty cytoplasm.

The functioning of the gastric mucosa is often affected in iron deficiency. The augmented histamine test has shown true achlorhydria in 16 percent of patients. Superficial gastritis or moderate atrophy has been demonstrated by gastric mucosal biopsy in many instances. In this setting, iron absorption may be impaired, resulting in a vicious cycle. Iron therapy may be associated with return of free hydrochloric acid secretion, especially in younger persons, but in many patients, neither the secretory nor the morphologic changes in the stomach are relieved.

DIAGNOSIS Several stages of iron deficiency can be encountered clinically and are summarized in Table 310-2. Before significant anemia will occur, the iron stores must be depleted.

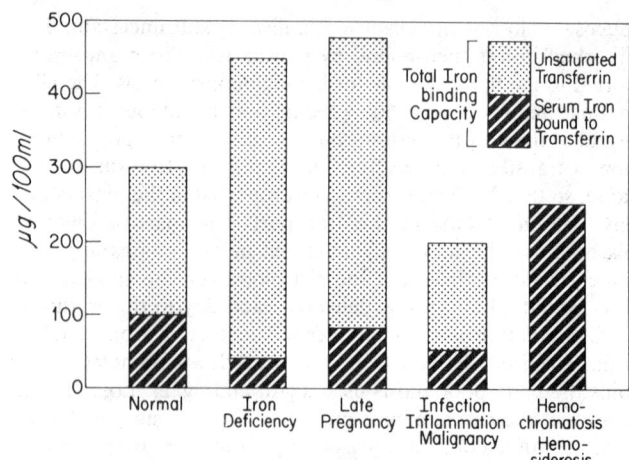

FIGURE 310-1
Serum iron and iron-binding capacity in various disorders.

It is useful to measure the serum iron and the iron-binding protein. The serum iron is reduced both in iron deficiency and in association with chronic disorders (Chap. 313); however, in the latter the iron-binding capacity characteristically falls below normal, while in the former it is usually increased (greater than 400 to 450 μg per 100 ml; see Fig. 310-1).

An additional useful procedure is the examination of the bone marrow after staining for iron. In iron-deficient subjects, no stainable iron will be visible, whereas marrow iron is normal or increased in the anemia of chronic disorders. Absence of detectable iron stores in the marrow occurs early in the development of iron deficiency. Measurement of serum ferritin will also provide a reliable estimate of iron stores and may obviate the necessity of doing a bone marrow examination. In patients with iron-deficiency anemia, serum ferritin levels are about one-tenth of normal, and the free erythrocyte porphyrin is elevated. If these tests are not available, a therapeutic trial of iron may aid in establishing the diagnosis. The clearest results from therapeutic trials are obtained when the anemia is severe and when there are no complicating illnesses to prevent an adequate response. If such a trial is undertaken, it is helpful if serial observations of the reticulocyte count are made during the first 10 days of therapy. A significant reticulocytosis occurring 7 to 10 days after commencement of iron administration indicates a response. During a therapeutic trial period of 3 to 4 weeks, a positive response is reflected in an increase in hemoglobin of about 0.2 g per 100 ml per day.

Examination of the stool for occult blood is an essential part of the workup of any patient with anemia, particularly one who appears to be iron-deficient. The most commonly used chemical test, the stool guaiac, can detect as little as 10 ml of fecal blood loss per day. Since gastrointestinal blood loss may be intermittent, it is advisable to check several specimens at periodic intervals.

TABLE 310-2
Stages in the development of iron deficiency

	Normal	Mild	Moderate	Severe
Hemoglobin:	15 g/100 ml	13 g/100 ml	10 g/100 ml	5 g/100 ml
MCV	N	↓	↓	↓↓
MCHC	N	N	↓	↓↓
Marrow Fe stores	Present	Absent	Absent	Absent
Serum Fe/TIBC, μg/100 ml	100/300	~ 75/300	~ 50/450	~ 25/600
Fe enzymes	N	N	N	↓

NOTE: *MCV, mean corpuscular volume; MCHC, mean corpuscular hemoglobin concentration; TIBC, total iron-binding capacity; N, normal.*

Iron deficiency is not the only cause of hypochromic microcytic anemia, even though it is the most common one. Other microcytic hypochromic anemias are discussed in the next section.

Mild iron-deficiency anemia may readily be confused with β-thalassemia and α-thalassemia traits. The peripheral blood smears and red blood cell indexes are quite similar in these disorders. Measurement of serum iron and iron-binding capacity and hemoglobin A_2 are useful in distinguishing between them. Hemoglobin A_2 is elevated in the β-thalassemia trait and is decreased in iron deficiency. However, hemoglobin A_2 is normal in the α-thalassemia trait (Chap. 315).

TREATMENT True iron deficiency can be relieved by the administration of iron, but this alone does not constitute adequate therapy; it is imperative to seek and, if possible, to correct the cause. Here the onus rests heavily with the physician, since effective iron therapy alone will correct the anemia temporarily but the opportunity to cure a malignant neoplasm (e.g., carcinoma of the cecum) or some other treatable condition may be lost if the cause is not discovered.

Regarding the type of iron preparation to be prescribed, nothing better has been devised for the correction of iron deficiency than ferrous sulfate. The addition of other minerals such as cobalt or copper, combination with vitamins, and the introduction of devices to improve absorption have accomplished nothing other than to increase the cost of therapy to the patient. Ferrous sulfate (300 mg hydrated ferrous sulfate or 200 mg of the anhydrous salt), three or four tablets per day, is recommended. With this dose, about one-quarter of patients complain of gastrointestinal side effects such as nausea, abdominal cramps, and diarrhea. However, about 13 percent of patients receiving a placebo also note such symptoms. The dose should be increased gradually (one tablet the first day, two the second, etc.) because tolerance for iron is thereby built up, and fewer gastrointestinal side effects develop. It is easier to take iron when the stomach contains food, but if it can be tolerated when the stomach contains little food, absorption is better. About 15 percent of orally administered iron is absorbed during the first 3 weeks of therapy. Thereafter, absorption decreases, averaging about 5 percent. Treatment for at least 6 months is needed in most cases if the body stores are to be replenished.

It is rare that parenteral therapy is required. When iron is absorbed poorly, as in some cases of steatorrhea or when a condition such as regional ileitis, ulcerative colitis, iliostomy, or colostomy prevents its use, iron dextran may be given intramuscularly. The first dose should be limited to 50 mg because reactions occur which are sometimes severe. By repeated injections, a total of 1.5 to 2.0 g may be given in this way. Although more likely to produce an adverse reaction, intravenous administration also is possible in patients who cannot tolerate intramuscular injections. The iron dextran solution can be given by direct infusion, or it can be diluted in about 200 ml sterile saline and administered by intravenous drip. One or two drops should be given intravenously and then, if no untoward symptoms develop in the next 5 min, 500 mg is infused slowly. The total amount of parenteral iron that should be given is based on the calculated deficit in red blood cell mass, plus an additional 1000 mg to replenish iron stores.

Transfusion of blood is rarely needed.

OTHER HYPOCHROMIC MICROCYTIC ANEMIAS

Although iron deficiency is, by far, the most common cause of hypochromic, microcytic anemia, other causes should be considered. Thalassemia (Chap. 315) results in hypochromia and microcytosis with little or no anemia in the heterozygous or

"minor" form and causes severe hypochromic, microcytic anemia with features of hemolysis in the homozygous or "major" form.

The anemia of chronic disorders (Chap. 313) usually is normocytic and normochromic. Occasionally, when the condition is long-standing, modest hypochromia and even microcytosis are observed. An incorrect diagnosis of iron deficiency may be made, not only because of the morphologic changes but because the serum iron concentration may be reduced. In contrast to iron deficiency, however, the iron-binding capacity is normal or reduced (Fig. 310-1), and iron is found in appropriately stained bone marrow specimens.

SIDEROBLASTIC ANEMIAS These anemias (Table 310-3) are a group of heterogeneous disorders in which a population of circulating hypochromic, microcytic erythrocytes is found in the blood, and "ringed" sideroblasts are present in the bone marrow. Sideroblasts are red blood cell precursors containing nonheme iron granules that stain with Prussian blue. In normal subjects, one to three small, blue granules may be seen in 30 to 50 percent of normoblasts. In patients with sideroblastic anemias, both the size and number of these iron-containing granules are increased, and the granules tend to form a ring around the nucleus. By electron microscopy, these "ringed" sideroblasts are characterized by extensive mitochondrial iron deposits. In contrast, visible nonheme iron in normal erythroblasts is found in the cytoplasm in the form of ferritin. As Fig. 53-3 shows, several of the enzymatic steps in heme synthesis take place in mitochondria, including the initial condensation of succinyl CoA and glycine to form δ-aminolevulinic acid (ALA). Mitochondrial function may be impaired by the presence of iron overload. In general, sideroblastic anemias are characterized by a defect in the synthesis of heme and, therefore, hemoglobin. As a result, red blood cells are often hypochromic and microcytic. Characteristically, a hypochromic population of cells is seen side by side with relatively normal cells ("partial hypochromia").

Sideroblastic anemias may be accompanied by increased total body iron. This is manifested by increased serum iron concentration with complete or nearly complete saturation of the iron-binding protein and by markedly increased mononuclear-phagocyte iron stores and deposition of iron in parenchymal organs. Iron deposition may be severe enough to cause hyperpigmentation of the skin and impaired function of the liver, pancreas, and heart. Hepatosplenomegaly may be found on examination. The leukocyte and platelet counts are usually normal, but may be reduced.

Kinetic studies usually reveal *ineffective erythropoiesis* with

TABLE 310-3
The sideroblastic anemias

I Hereditary or congenital sideroblastic anemias (usually pyridoxine-responsive)
  A X-linked
  B Autosomal recessive
II Acquired sideroblastic anemias
  A Idiopathic refractory sideroblastic anemia
  B Complicating other diseases
    1 Neoplastic (e.g., myeloma, lymphoma)
    2 Inflammatory (e.g., rheumatoid arthritis)
    3 Hematologic disorders (e.g., myelofibrosis, hemolytic anemia)
    4 Metabolic (e.g., myxedema, uremia)
  C Associated with drugs or toxins
    1 Ethanol
    2 Lead
    3 Antituberculosis agents (isoniazid, cycloserine)
    4 Chloramphenicol
    5 Antineoplastic agents

increased plasma iron turnover but impaired incorporation of iron into red blood cells. Red blood cell survival is normal or only slightly reduced and there is erythroblastic hyperplasia in the marrow, but the reticulocyte count is normal. There may be modest "indirect" hyperbilirubinemia and increased fecal urobilinogen excretion.

Sideroblastic anemias may be divided into two categories, hereditary (or congenital) and acquired (Table 310-3). Most patients with hereditary sideroblastic anemia respond to pyridoxine (vitamin B_6) therapy with reticulocytosis and an increase in blood hemoglobin concentration. It is unlikely that correction of a pyridoxine-deficient state accounts for the improvement since (1) the amount of pyridoxine required greatly exceeds the estimated daily nutritional requirement; (2) the response is usually incomplete—the anemia is not completely relieved, and morphologic abnormalities in the erythrocytes persist; (3) prompt relapse occurs when therapy is discontinued; and (4) no neurologic signs of vitamin B_6 deficiency are found. The mechanism underlying the response of some patients to pyridoxine is not well understood. Pharmacologic doses of pyridoxine may overcome a block in ALA synthesis, a mitochondrial reaction which requires pyridoxal phosphate as a cofactor (Chap. 53).

Most of the patients with hereditary or congenital sideroblastic anemia are males. An X-linked hereditary pattern has been demonstrated in several families. In one family, the affected patients were females, in whom there was a striking difference in the appearance of the normal and abnormal red blood cell populations, possibly on the basis of X-chromosome inactivation. In some of the reported patients, the free erythrocyte protoporphyrin content was reduced prior to institution of pyridoxine therapy and became normal or increased with treatment.

A congenital form of sideroblastic anemia which does not respond to pyridoxine also appears to be inherited as an X-linked trait. In patients with this disorder, the free erythrocyte coproporphyrin is markedly increased, and the free erythrocyte protoporphyrin is reduced. This finding suggests a deficiency in the enzyme coproporphyrinogen oxidase (Chap. 53).

Idiopathic refractory sideroblastic anemia usually is found in middle-aged or elderly subjects. In this condition, the proportion of hypochromic erythrocytes is usually small, as a rule, so that the mean corpuscular hemoglobin concentration (MCHC) is not abnormal; however, a careful examination of the blood smear will detect the abnormal erythrocytes (partial hypochromia). In some of these cells, basophilic stippling is present. The pathogenesis is not known. In a few of these patients, the anemia is partially relieved by the administration of pyridoxine, but in the great majority this does not occur. Occasional patients have responded to the parenteral administration of pyridoxal phosphate, the coenzyme form of vitamin B_6. Among those who fail to respond, some have such severe anemia that periodic transfusions are necessary. High-dose androgen therapy is sometimes useful in the latter group. The prognosis generally is fairly good; median survival is about 10 years. However, about 10 percent of the patients develop acute myeloblastic leukemia.

Secondary sideroblastic anemia has been observed in association with certain underlying illnesses. These include malignancies, such as Hodgkin's disease, multiple myeloma, and carcinoma of the prostate, and chronic inflammatory diseases, e.g., rheumatoid arthritis. Certain drugs (isoniazid, cycloserine, pyrazinamide, chloramphenicol) have been reported to induce sideroblastic anemia, apparently by interfering with vitamin B_6 metabolism. The drug-induced syndromes may be corrected by administering pyridoxine or by withdrawing the offending agent.

Sideroblastic anemia occurs in about 30 percent of alcoholics who are ill enough to require hospitalization. In addition to the usual findings of sideroblastic anemia, vacuolization of erythrocyte precursors is prominent. These morphologic abnormalities generally disappear shortly after cessation of alcohol ingestion.

Lead inhibits several of the enzymes of heme synthesis, and lead poisoning may occasionally be accompanied by sideroblastic anemia.

TREATMENT Management of patients with sideroblastic anemia requires that all possible offending drugs be withdrawn and underlying diseases searched for and treated. If these steps are ineffective, the patients should be given pyridoxine in a dose of 50 to 200 mg per day for about 2 months. If no response occurs, further pyridoxine therapy is of no value. Some patients who do not respond to pyridoxine will improve when given androgens in a regimen similar to that used in aplastic anemia (Chap. 312). Since the ultimate prognosis often is related to the degree of iron loading, it follows that iron-containing medications are contraindicated and blood transfusions should be kept to a minimum. It is rarely necessary to maintain the hematocrit at a level greater than 25. Selected patients may benefit from long-term therapy with an iron chelating agent.

REFERENCES

BOTHWELL TH, FINCH CA: *Iron Metabolism.* Boston, Little, Brown, 1962

BOTTOMLEY S: Porphyrin and iron metabolism in sideroblastic anemia. Semin Hematol 14:169, 1977

CARTWRIGHT GE, DEISS A: Sideroblasts, siderocyte and sideroblastic anemia. N Engl J Med 292:185, 1975

CROSBY WH: Current concepts in nutrition: Who needs iron? N Engl J Med 297:543, 1977

DAGG JS, GOLDBERG A: Detection and treatment of iron deficiency. Clin Hematol 2:365, 1973

JACOBS A, WORWOOD M: The biochemistry of ferritin and its clinical implications. Progr Hematol 9:1, 1975

KUSHNER J, CARTWRIGHT GE: The sideroblastic anemias. Adv Intern Med 1976

LEE GR et al: Hereditary X-linked sideroblastic anemia. Blood 32:59, 1968

WINTROBE MM et al: Anemias characterized by impaired iron metabolism, in *Clinical Hematology*, 7th ed. Philadelphia, Lea & Febiger, 1974, sec 3

311
MEGALOBLASTIC ANEMIAS

BERNARD M. BABIOR
H. FRANKLIN BUNN

The megaloblastic anemias are important examples of disordered erythroid maturation with distinctive blood and bone marrow morphology. The biochemical and physiological bases of the megaloblastic anemias are relatively well understood, thanks to a highly productive series of biochemical and clinical investigations over the past 40 years. These disorders are characterized by impairment of deoxyribonucleic acid (DNA) synthesis. Cells primarily affected include those having a relatively rapid turnover such as hematopoietic precursors in the bone marrow and the mucosal epithelium of the gastrointestinal tract. Although cell division is sluggish, cytoplasmic development progresses normally. Thus, megaloblastic cells tend to be large, with an increased ratio of ribonucleic acid (RNA) to

TABLE 311-1
Classification of the megaloblastic anemias

I Vitamin B_{12} deficiency
  A Inadequate intake: Vegetarians (rare)
  B Malabsorption
    1 Inadequate production of intrinsic factor (IF)
      a Pernicious anemia
      b Gastrectomy
      c Congenital absence of IF; congenital production of func-
        tionally abnormal IF (rare)
    2 Disorders of terminal ileum
      a Tropical sprue
      b Nontropical sprue
      c Regional enteritis
      d Intestinal resection
      e Neoplasms and granulomatous disorders (rare)
      f Selective vitamin B_{12} malabsorption (Imerslund's syn-
        drome) (rare)
    3 Competition for vitamin B_{12}
      a Fish tapeworm
      b Bacteria: Blind loop syndrome
    4 Drugs: *p*-Aminosalicylic acid, colchicine, neomycin
  C Transcobalamin II deficiency (rare)
II Folic acid deficiency
  A Inadequate intake: Unbalanced diet, excessive cooking (com-
    mon in alcoholics, teen-agers, some infants)
  B Malabsorption
    1 Tropical sprue
    2 Nontropical sprue
    3 Drugs: Phenytoin, barbiturates, (?) ethanol
  C Increased requirements
    1 Pregnancy
    2 Infancy
    3 Malignancy
    4 Increased hematopoiesis (chronic hemolytic anemias)
  D Impaired metabolism
    1 Inhibitors of dihydrofolate reductase: Methotrexate, pyri-
      methamine, triamterine, pentamidine, etc.
    2 Alcohol
    3 Rare enzyme deficiencies: Formiminotransferase, dihydro-
      folate reductase, etc.
III Other causes
  A Drugs which impair DNA metabolism
    1 Purine antagonists: 6-Mercaptopurine, azathioprine, etc.
    2 Pyrimidine antagonists: 5-Fluorouracil, cytosine arabinoside,
      etc.
    3 Others: Procarbazine, hydroxyurea
  B Metabolic disorders (rare)
    1 Hereditary orotic aciduria
    2 Others
  C Megalobastic anemia of unknown etiology
    1 Refractory megalobastic anemia
    2 Di Guglielmo's syndrome*

* *Atypical, dysplastic changes in erythroid and myeloid disorders.*

DNA. The red blood cells that emerge from the bone marrow are macrocytic. The asynchrony between nuclear and cytoplasmic development is one of the prime morphological abnormalities seen in bone marrow cells (see below). Megaloblastic cells tend to be destroyed in the marrow in excessive numbers, an abnormality termed *ineffective erythropoiesis*. In a severely megaloblastic patient, as many as 90 percent of the red blood cell precursors may be destroyed before they are released into the bloodstream, compared with 10 to 15 percent in the normal subject. Megaloblastic leukocytes and megakaryocytes are also thought to be unusually susceptible to intramedullary destruction.

Most megaloblastic anemias are due to a deficiency of vitamin B_{12} and/or folic acid. The various clinical entities associated with megaloblastic anemia are listed in Table 311-1. This classification is easier to comprehend if the physiological and biochemical principles discussed below are kept in mind.

PHYSIOLOGICAL CONSIDERATIONS

VITAMIN B_{12} This vitamin is a complex organometallic compound in which a cobalt atom is situated within a corrin ring, a structure similar but not identical to the porphyrin from which heme is formed (Fig. 53-1). As with heme, both δ-

aminolevulinic acid and porphobilinogen are precursors in the biosynthesis of vitamin B_{12}. However, unlike heme, vitamin B_{12} cannot be synthesized in the human body and must be supplied in the diet; it is synthesized by a variety of microorganisms including some normally present in intestinal flora, but not by plants. Accordingly, the chief dietary source of vitamin B_{12} is animal products: meat and dairy foods. The minimum daily requirement for vitamin B_{12} is about 2.5 μg.

During gastric digestion, vitamin B_{12} in food is released and forms a stable complex with gastric R binder, one of a group of closely related glycoproteins of unknown function which are found in secretions (e.g., saliva, milk, gastric juice, bile), granulocytes, and plasma. On entering the duodenum, the vitamin B_{12}–R binder complex is digested, releasing the vitamin B_{12}, which then binds to intrinsic factor (IF). This glycoprotein of molecular weight 50,000 is produced by the parietal cells of the stomach. The secretion of intrinsic factor generally parallels that of hydrochloric acid. The vitamin B_{12}–intrinsic factor complex is resistant to proteolytic digestion and travels to the distal ileum, where specific receptors on the mucosal brush border bind the vitamin B_{12}–intrinsic factor complex, thereby enabling the vitamin to be absorbed. Thus, intrinsic factor serves as a cell-directed carrier protein. Vitamin B_{12} is transferred from the ileal receptor across the mucosa to the capillary circulation where it binds initially to a transport protein, transcobalamin II (TC II). The vitamin B_{12}-TC II complex is rapidly taken up by the liver, the bone marrow, and other proliferating cells. Normally, about 2 mg vitamin B_{12} is stored in the liver, and another 2 mg is stored elsewhere in the body. In view of the minimum daily requirement, about 3 to 6 years would be required for a deficiency state to develop if absorption of vitamin B_{12} were to cease abruptly in an individual with normal stores.

Although TC II is the acceptor for newly absorbed vitamin B_{12}, most circulating vitamin B_{12} is bound to transcobalamin I (TC I), a glycoprotein closely related to gastric R binder. TC I appears to be derived in part from leukocytes. The paradox that most circulating vitamin B_{12} is bound to TC I rather than TC II, even though TC II receives all the vitamin B_{12} which is absorbed by the intestine, is explained by the fact that vitamin B_{12} bound to TC II is rapidly cleared from the blood ($T_{1/2}$ about 1 h), while clearance of vitamin B_{12} bound to TC I requires many days. The function of TC I is unknown.

FOLIC ACID Folic acid is the common name for pteroylmonoglutamic acid. The *prime function* of this vitamin is to transfer one-carbon moieties such as methyl and formyl groups to various organic compounds, as in the donation of a one-carbon moiety in the formation of thymidine from deoxyuridine. Folic acid is required at two steps in the biosynthesis of purines. Furthermore, as shown in the reaction in Fig. 311-1, folic acid derivatives provide methyl groups required for the conversion of homocysteine to methionine and for the conversion of uridylate to thymidylate. It is apparent that folic acid plays a pivotal role in the biosynthesis of DNA.

Folic acid is synthesized by many different plants and bacteria. Fruits and vegetables constitute the primary dietary source of the vitamin. Some forms of dietary folic acid are labile and may be destroyed by cooking. The minimum daily requirement is normally about 50 μg but may be increased severalfold during periods of enhanced metabolic demand such as pregnancy.

The assimilation of adequate amounts of folic acid is dependent on the nature of the diet and its means of preparation. Folates in various foodstuffs are largely conjugated to polyglu-

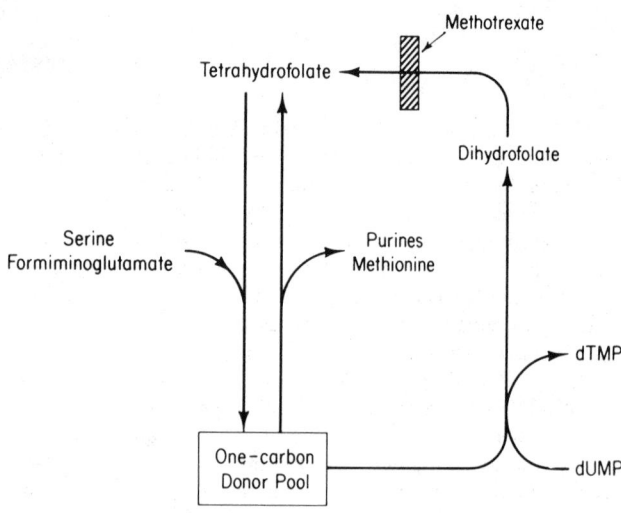

FIGURE 311-1

Scheme of folate metabolism.

tamic acid. This highly polar side chain impairs the intestinal absorption of the vitamin. However, conjugases (γ-glutamyl carboxypeptidases) in the lumen of the gut convert polyglutamates to mono- and diglutamates, which are readily absorbed in the proximal jejunum.

There are specific binding proteins in plasma for folates, but as yet their physiological significance is unclear. Plasma folate is primarily in the form of N^5-methyltetrahydrofolate, a monoglutamate. N^5-Methyltetrahydrofolate is transported into cells by a carrier which is specific for the tetrahydro forms of the vitamin. Once in the cell, the folate is reconverted to the polyglutamate form, after removal of the N^5-methyl group in a vitamin B_{12}–requiring reaction (see below). The polyglutamate form may be useful for retention of folate by the cell.

Normal individuals have about 5 to 20 mg folic acid in various body stores, half in the liver. In light of the minimum daily requirement, it is not surprising that a deficiency will occur within months if dietary intake or intestinal absorption is curtailed.

BIOCHEMICAL CONSIDERATIONS

FOLATE In the form of its tetrahydro derivative, folate functions as a participant in one-carbon transfer reactions (see scheme in Fig. 311-1). The source of the one-carbon fragments is usually serine, which reacts with tetrahydrofolate to produce glycine and $N^{5,10}$-methylenetetrahydrofolate. An alternative source is formiminoglutamic acid, an intermediate in histidine catabolism, which gives up its formimino group to tetrahydrofolate to yield N^5-formiminotetrahydrofolate and glutamic acid. These derivatives provide entry into an interconvertible donor pool consisting of tetrahydrofolate derivatives carrying one-carbon fragments at various levels of oxidation. The constituents of this pool can donate their one-carbon fragments to appropriate acceptor compounds to form metabolic intermediates which are ultimately converted to building blocks used in the synthesis of biological macromolecules. The most important such building blocks are (1) purines, in which the C-2 and C-8 atoms are introduced in folate-dependent reactions; (2) deoxythymidylate monophosphate (dTMP), synthesized from $N^{5,10}$-methylenetetrahydrofolate and deoxyuridylate monophosphate (dUMP); and (3) methionine, formed by the transfer of a methyl group from N^5-methyltetrahydrofolate to homocysteine. Vitamin B_{12} is also required for the formation of methionine from homocysteine (see below).

In all but one of the one-carbon transfer reactions, tetrahydrofolate is produced. It can immediately accept a one-carbon fragment and reenter the donor pool. The single exception is the thymidylate synthetase reaction (dUMP → dTMP), in which dihydrofolate is the product. This must be reduced to tetrahydrofolate by the enzyme dihydrofolate reductase before it can reenter the donor pool. A number of drugs are able to inhibit dihydrofolate reductase, thereby diverting folate from the donor pool and producing what amounts to a state of folate deficiency in the face of normal tissue folate concentrations.

VITAMIN B_{12} In humans there are two metabolically active forms of vitamin B_{12}, identified by the alkyl group attached to the sixth coordination position of the cobalt atom: adenosylcobalamin and methylcobalamin. The vitamin preparation which is used therapeutically is cyanocobalamin. The cyanide ligand is avidly taken up by cobalamin and is acquired during purification. Cyanocobalamin, however, has no known physiological role and must be converted to a biologically active form before it can be used by tissues.[1]

Adenosylcobalamin is required for the conversion of methylmalonyl coenzyme A (CoA) to succinyl coenzyme A. Lack of this cofactor leads to large increases in the tissue levels of methylmalonyl CoA and its precursor, propionyl CoA. As a consequence, nonphysiological fatty acids containing an odd number of carbon atoms are synthesized and incorporated into neuronal lipids. This biochemical abnormality may underlie the neurological complications of vitamin B_{12} deficiency (see below).

Methylcobalamin is an essential cofactor in the conversion of homocysteine to methionine (Fig. 311-2). When this reaction is deficient, folate metabolism is deranged, and it is this derangement which is thought to underlie the defect in DNA synthesis and the megaloblastic maturation pattern in patients who are deficient in vitamin B_{12} (see Fig. 311-2). What appears to happen in vitamin B_{12} deficiency is that the unconjugated N^5-methyltetrahydrofolate newly taken from the bloodstream cannot be converted to other forms of tetrahydrofolate by methyl transfer. This is the so-called "folate trap" hypothesis. Since N^5-methyltetrahydrofolate is a poor substrate for the conjugating enzyme (this has been shown in rats but has not yet been demonstrated in humans), it largely remains in the unconjugated form and slowly leaks from the cell. Tissue folate deficiency therefore develops, and this results in megaloblastic hematopoiesis. This hypothesis explains the fact that tissue folate stores in vitamin B_{12} deficiency are substantially reduced, with a disproportionate reduction in conjugated as compared with unconjugated folates, despite normal or supranormal se-

---

[1] *Strictly speaking, vitamin B_{12} refers only to cyanocobalamin. However, in this chapter, the term* vitamin B_{12} *will refer to both cyanocobalamin and biologically active cobalamins.*

FIGURE 311-2

Diagram showing the interrelationship between vitamin B_{12} (methylcobalamin) and folate metabolism within the cell.

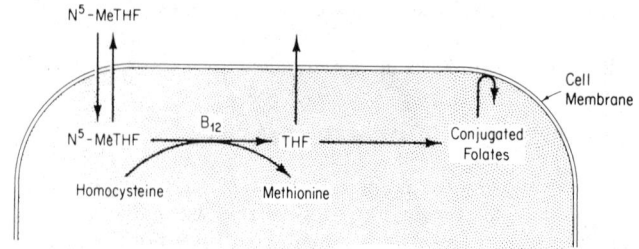

rum folate levels. It also explains why large doses of folate can produce a partial hematologic remission in patients with vitamin B_{12} deficiency.

CLINICAL DISORDERS

CLASSIFICATION OF MEGALOBLASTIC ANEMIAS The etiology of megaloblastic anemia varies in different parts of the world. In temperate zones, alcoholism and pernicious anemia are the common causes of megaloblastic anemias. In certain areas close to the equator, tropical sprue is endemic and an important cause. In Finland, megaloblastic anemia is sometimes secondary to infestation by the fish tapeworm *Diphyllobothrium latum.*

The dietary intake of vitamin B_{12} is more than adequate for the body's requirements. The only exceptions are rare individuals who subsist on a purely vegetable diet and their breast-fed infants. Thus, deficiency of vitamin B_{12} is almost always due to malabsorption. As explained in the section above, the absorption of vitamin B_{12} depends upon a specific binding protein produced in the stomach and uptake by a specific receptor in the mucosa of the distal ileum. Accordingly, several steps in this process can go awry and lead to malabsorption. These are listed in Table 311-1. In contrast, the dietary intake of folic acid is marginal in many parts of the world. Furthermore, since the body's stores of folate are relatively low, folic acid deficiency can arise rather suddenly during periods of decreased dietary intake or increased metabolic demand. Finally, folic acid deficiency may be due to malabsorption. Often two or more of these factors are at play in a given patient.

Combined deficiencies of vitamin B_{12} and folic acid are not uncommon. Patients with tropical sprue are often deficient in both vitamins. The biochemical lesion that results in megaloblastic maturation of bone marrow cells also causes structural and functional abnormalities of the rapidly proliferating epithelial cells of the intestinal mucosa. Thus, severe deficiency of one vitamin can lead to malabsorption of the other. Furthermore, as discussed above, a deficiency of vitamin B_{12} causes a secondary reduction in cellular folic acid. The secondary loss of intracellular folic acid is thought to be the basis for the impairment of DNA synthesis in marrow cells deficient in vitamin B_{12} and its partial correction by folate.

Finally, megaloblastic anemias may occasionally be induced by factors unrelated to a vitamin deficiency. Most such cases are caused by one or more of the many drugs which produce megaloblastic anemia as a side effect. Less common causes include certain acquired defects of hematopoietic stem cells. Rarest of all are certain congenital enzyme deficiencies in which megaloblastic anemia is characteristically encountered.

VITAMIN B_{12} DEFICIENCY There are many conditions in which vitamin B_{12} deficiency may develop. Although each has its own characteristic manifestations, certain clinical features are common to all. These clinical features involve the blood, the gastrointestinal tract, and the nervous system.

The hematologic manifestations are almost entirely the result of the anemia which characterizes vitamin B_{12} deficiency, although very rarely purpura may appear, due to thrombocytopenia. Symptoms may include weakness, lightheadedness, vertigo, and tinnitus, as well as palpitations, angina, and the symptoms of congestive failure. On physical examination, the patient with florid vitamin B_{12} deficiency is pale, with slightly icteric skin and eyes. The pulse is rapid, and the heart may be enlarged; auscultation will reveal a systolic flow murmur. The spleen and liver may be somewhat enlarged. There may be a slight fever.

The gastrointestinal manifestations reflect the effect of vitamin B_{12} deficiency on the rapidly turning over gastrointestinal epithelium. The patient sometimes complains of a sore tongue, which on inspection will be smooth and beefy red. Anorexia with moderate weight loss will also be evident, possibly accompanied by diarrhea and other gastrointestinal symptoms. These latter manifestations may be in part caused by megaloblastosis of the small intestinal epithelium, which results in malabsorption.

The neurological manifestations are the most worrisome of all, because they may not remit completely on treatment. They begin pathologically with demyelination, followed by axonal degeneration and eventual neuronal death; the final stage, of course, is irreversible. The typical site of involvement is the spinal cord, where the posterior and lateral columns undergo demyelination. However, peripheral nerves are also affected, as is the cerebrum itself. Signs and symptoms include numbness and paresthesias in the extremities (the earliest neurological manifestations), weakness, ataxia, and poor finger coordination. There may be sphincter disturbances. Reflexes may be diminished or increased. The Romberg and Babinski signs may be positive, and position sense will be diminished. Disturbances of mentation will vary from mild irritability and forgetfulness to severe dementia or frank psychosis. It should be emphasized that occasionally *neurological disease may occur in a patient with a normal hematocrit.*

In the usual patient, in whom hematologic problems predominate, the blood and bone marrow show characteristic megaloblastic changes which are described under "Diagnosis" below. The anemia may be very severe—hematocrits of 15 to 20 are not infrequent—but is surprisingly well tolerated by the patient because it develops so slowly.

Pernicious anemia The most common cause of vitamin B_{12} deficiency in temperate climates is pernicious anemia, in which intrinsic factor secretion ceases owing to atrophy of the gastric mucosa. It is most frequently seen in individuals of Northern European descent and is much less common in Southern Europeans, blacks, and Orientals. Men and women are equally affected. It is a disease of the elderly, the average patient presenting near age 60; it is rare under 30, although typical pernicious anemia can be seen in children under 10 (juvenile pernicious anemia). An inherited condition in which an abnormal intrinsic factor is secreted by a histologically normal stomach will cause vitamin B_{12} deficiency which appears in infancy or early childhood.

On the basis of incomplete evidence, pernicious anemia is currently thought to be caused by an autoimmune reaction against gastric parietal cells. There is considerable evidence for immunologic abnormalities in pernicious anemia. The incidence of pernicious anemia is substantially increased in patients with other diseases thought to be of immunologic origin, including Graves' disease, myxedema, thyroiditis, idiopathic adrenocortical insufficiency, vitiligo, and hypoparathyroidism. Patients with pernicious anemia also have abnormal circulating antibodies related to their disease: antiparietal cell antibody is present in 90 percent of patients with pernicious anemia, and anti-intrinsic factor is found in 60 percent of these patients. Antiparietal cell antibody is also found in 50 percent of patients with gastric atrophy without pernicious anemia as well as in 10 to 15 percent of an unselected patient population, but anti-intrinsic factor antibody is usually absent from these patients. Relatives of patients with pernicious anemia show an increased incidence of the disease, and even clinically unaffected relatives may have anti-intrinsic factor antibody in their serum. A final point supporting an immunologic basis for pernicious anemia is the fact that corticosteroids have been reported to reverse the disease both pathologically and clinically.

The destruction of parietal cells in pernicious anemia is thought to be mediated by the cellular immune system. Humoral factors such as anti-intrinsic factor antibody probably have little role in the pathogenesis of the disease, a view supported by the observation that pernicious anemia is usually common in patients with agammaglobulinemia.

Pathologically, the most characteristic finding in pernicious anemia is gastric atrophy which involves only the acid- and pepsin-secreting portion of the stomach; the antrum is spared. Other pathological changes, which are secondary to the deficiency of vitamin B_{12}, include megaloblastoid alterations in the gastric and intestinal epithelium and the neurological changes described above. The abnormalities in the gastric epithelium are evident as cellular atypia in gastric cytology specimens, a finding which must be carefully distinguished from the cytological abnormalities seen in gastric malignancy.

The *clinical manifestations* are primarily those of vitamin B_{12} deficiency, as described above. The disease is of insidious onset and progresses slowly. An additional physical finding is the tendency of patients with pernicious anemia to be fair-haired or prematurely gray. Laboratory examination will reveal histamine-fast achlorhydria as well as the hematologic and other laboratory abnormalities discussed below in "Diagnosis."

Through appropriate replacement therapy, patients with pernicious anemia should experience complete and lifelong correction of all abnormalities which are due to vitamin B_{12} deficiency, except to the extent that irreversible changes in the nervous system may have occurred prior to treatment. These patients, however, are unusually subject to certain gastric problems, including gastric polyps and cancer of the stomach. In view of the latter complication, patients should be followed with frequent stool guaiac examinations together with further diagnostic studies when indicated.

Postgastrectomy Following total gastrectomy or extensive damage to gastric mucosa as, for example, by ingestion of corrosive agents, megaloblastic anemia may develop because the source of intrinsic factor has been removed. In such patients the absorption of orally administered vitamin B_{12} is impaired. Megaloblastic anemia may also follow partial gastrectomy, but the incidence is lower than after total gastrectomy, in which vitamin B_{12} malabsorption occurs in 100 percent of patients. The cause of vitamin B_{12} deficiency after partial gastrectomy may be intestinal overgrowth of bacteria, but it does not always respond to antibiotics.

Intestinal organisms The macrocytic anemia seen in association with intestinal strictures, diverticula, anastomoses, and "blind loops" may be attributed to colonization of the small intestine by large masses of bacteria which divert vitamin B_{12} from the host. Steatorrhea may also be seen under these circumstances, because bile salt metabolism is disturbed when the intestine is heavily colonized with bacteria. Hematologic responses have been observed after administration of oral antibiotics such as tetracycline and ampicillin.

Megaloblastic anemia is seen, in Finland especially, in persons harboring the tapeworm *D. latum.* The anemia has been attributed to competition by the worm for vitamin B_{12}. Destruction of the worm eliminates the problem.

Ileal abnormalities Vitamin B_{12} deficiency is commonly found in tropical sprue, while it is an unusual complication of non-tropical sprue (gluten-sensitive enteropathy; see Chap. 292).

Virtually any disorder which compromises the absorptive capacity of the distal ileum can result in vitamin B_{12} deficiency. Specific entities include regional enteritis, Whipple's disease, and tuberculosis. Segmental involvement of the distal ileum by disease can cause megaloblastic anemia without any other manifestations of intestinal malabsorption such as steatorrhea. Vitamin B_{12} malabsorption is also seen after ileal resection. Finally, there is a rare congenital disorder, described by Imerslund, in which a selective defect in vitamin B_{12} absorption is accompanied by proteinuria.

FOLIC ACID DEFICIENCY Patients with folic acid deficiency are more apt to be malnourished than those with vitamin B_{12} deficiency. Accordingly, they are likely to appear wasted rather than flabby. The gastrointestinal manifestations are similar to but may be more widespread and more severe than those of pernicious anemia. Diarrhea is often present, and cheilosis and glossitis are also encountered. However, neurological abnormalities like those seen in pernicious anemia do not occur.

The hematologic manifestations of folic acid deficiency are the same as those of vitamin B_{12} deficiency. Folic acid deficiency can generally be attributed to one or more of the following factors: increased demand for folate, inadequate intake, and malabsorption.

Increased demand Tissues with a relatively high rate of cell division such as the bone marrow or gut mucosa have a large requirement for folate. Therefore, patients with chronic hemolytic anemias or other causes of very active erythropoiesis may become deficient if their high folate requirement is not met by dietary intake. Likewise, a pregnant woman may become deficient in folic acid because of the high demand of the developing fetus. Folate deficiency may also occur during the growth spurts of infancy and adolescence.

Inadequate intake of folic acid is commonly encountered among a number of groups. Alcoholics frequently become folate-deficient because their main source of caloric intake is in the form of alcoholic beverages. Distilled spirits are virtually devoid of folic acid, while beer and wine do not contain enough of the vitamin to satisfy the daily requirement. In addition, alcohol may interfere with folate metabolism. Narcotic addicts are also prone to become folate-deficient because of malnutrition. In general, indigent and elderly individuals who subsist primarily on canned foods or "tea and toast" and teenagers whose diet consists of soft drinks and potato chips are likely to develop folate deficiency.

Malabsorption syndromes Folic acid deficiency is a common accompaniment of tropical sprue. Both the gastrointestinal symptoms and malabsorption are improved by the administration of either folic acid or antibiotics by mouth. Patients with nontropical sprue (gluten-sensitive enteropathy) may also develop significant folic acid deficiency which parallels other parameters of malabsorption. Similarly, alcohol-related folate deficiency may be due in part to malabsorption. In addition, other primary small-bowel disorders are sometimes associated with vitamin deficiency. These entities are all discussed in Chap. 292.

DRUGS Next to deficiency of folate or vitamin B_{12}, the most common cause of megaloblastic anemia is drug ingestion. Drugs which cause megaloblastic anemia do so by interfering with DNA synthesis, either directly or by antagonizing the action of folate. They can be classified as follows:

1 *Direct inhibitors of DNA synthesis.* All the drugs in this category are used in the treatment of malignancy. Their efficacy depends on their ability to disrupt DNA synthesis. They

include alkylating agents (nitrogen mustard, cyclophospha-mide, etc.), purine and pyrimidine analogues (5-fluorouracil, cytosine arabinoside, 6-thioguanine, 6-mercaptopurine, etc.), and other drugs which interfere with DNA synthesis by a variety of mechanisms (adriamycin, bleomycin, hydroxy-urea).

2 *Folate antagonists.* The most toxic of these is methotrexate, an exceedingly powerful inhibitor of dihydrofolate reductase which is used in the treatment of certain malignancies. Much less toxic, but still capable of inducing a megaloblastic anemia, are several weak dihydrofolate reductase inhibitors which are used to treat a variety of nonmalignant condi-tions. These include pentamidine, trimethoptrine, triam-terine, and pyrimethamine.

3 *Others.* A number of drugs antagonize folate by mechanisms which are poorly understood but are thought to involve an effect on absorption of the vitamin by the intestine. In this category are certain anticonvulsants [phenytoin (Dilantin), primidone (Mysoline)], phenobarbital (Luminal), neomycin, *p*-aminosalicylic acid, colchicine, estrogens, and ethanol. Megaloblastic anemia induced by these agents is mild.

OTHER Hereditary Megaloblastic anemia may be seen in several hereditary disorders. It is a regular feature of orotic aciduria, a defect in pyrimidine metabolism which is also char-acterized by retarded growth and development as well as the excretion of large amounts of orotic acid, and which is due to a deficiency of orotidylic decarboxylase and phosphorylase. Megaloblastic anemia has been reported in a single case of the Lesch-Nyhan syndrome, a condition resulting from a defi-ciency of hypoxanthine-guanine phosphoribosyltransferase whose clinical manifestations include gout, mental retardation, and self-mutilation. Congenital folate malabsorption also causes megaloblastic anemia, accompanied by ataxia and men-tal retardation. Megaloblastic anemia has been reported to ac-company the congenital deficiency of other folate-metabolizing enzymes including formiminotransferase, dihydrofolate reduc-tase, and N^5-methyltetrahydrofolate reductase. These deficien-cies are less well documented than is congenital folate malab-sorption. Megaloblastic changes as well as multinuclearity of red blood cell precursors are seen in the marrow of certain patients with congenital dyserythropoietic anemia, a group of inherited disorders characterized by mild to moderate anemia presenting at any age and pursuing a benign course.

Transcobalamin II deficiency, as well as the congenital ab-normalities in vitamin B_{12} absorption described previously, causes pronounced deficiencies in vitamin B_{12} in infancy or early childhood, with all the accompanying manifestations. Megaloblastic anemia is not seen in hereditary transcobalamin I deficiency, nor, surprisingly, is it a prominent feature of the methylmalonic acidurias, a group of conditions in which vita-min B_{12} metabolism is severely deranged.

Acquired idiopathic anemia Some patients with acquired sid-eroblastic anemia show megaloblastic changes in the marrow. In addition, megaloblastic erythropoiesis is characteristic of some patients with refractory anemia unresponsive to vitamin B_{12}, folate, and pyridoxine (Chap. 310). In both of these condi-tions, the megaloblastic changes are restricted to the red blood cell series; large granulocyte precursors and giant metamyelo-cytes are not seen (see below). Both are said to be associated with an increased incidence of acute leukemia.

Megaloblastic changes are seen in erythremic myelosis and other forms of acute nonlymphocytic leukemia where red blood cell precursors are prominently involved. Here, the mar-row is characterized by bizarre erythroid maturation, with multinuclearity and multipolar mitotic figures in the red blood cell precursors. Erythremic myelosis is discussed further in Chap. 325.

DIAGNOSIS The finding of significant macrocytosis [mean corpuscular volume (MCV) > 96 fl] suggests the presence of a megaloblastic anemia. Other causes of macrocytosis include hemolysis, liver disease, hypothyroidism, and aplastic anemia. If the macrocytosis is marked (MCV > 110 fl), the patient is much more likely to have a megaloblastic anemia. The reticu-locyte count is low, and the leukocyte and platelet count may also be decreased, particularly in severely anemic patients. The blood smear (Plate 9-6) demonstrates marked anisocytosis and poikilocytosis, together with the macroovalocyte, a large, oval, fully hemoglobinized erythrocyte which is the typical cell of megaloblastic anemias. There is some basophilic stippling, and an occasional nucleated red blood cell may be seen. In the white blood cell series, the neutrophils show hypersegmenta-tion of the nucleus. This is such a typical finding that a single cell with a nucleus of six lobes or more should raise the imme-diate suspicion of a megaloblastic anemia. A rare myelocyte may also be seen. Bizarre, misshapen platelets are also ob-served. The bone marrow examination is very helpful in the diagnosis of megaloblastic anemia. As shown in Plate 9-6, the marrow is hypercellular with a decreased myeloid/erythroid ratio and abundant stainable iron. Red blood cell precursors are abnormally large and have nuclei that appear much less mature than would be expected from the development of the cytoplasm (nuclear-cytoplasmic asynchrony). The nuclear chromatin is more dispersed that it should be and conse-quently stains less intensely than normal. To the extent that it is aggregated, it condenses in a peculiar fenestrated pattern which is very characteristic of megaloblastic erythropoiesis. Abnormal mitoses may be seen. Granulocyte precursors are also affected, many being larger than normal, including giant bands and metamyelocytes. Megakaryocytes are decreased and show abnormal morphology.

Megaloblastic anemias are characterized by ineffective erythropoiesis (Chap. 53). Enhanced intramedullary destruc-tion of erythroblasts results in an increase in unconjugated bili-rubin and lactic acid dehydrogenase (isoenzyme 1) in plasma. Abnormalities in iron kinetics also attest to the presence of ineffective erythropoiesis with increased iron turnover but low incorporation of labeled iron into circulating red blood cells.

In evaluating a patient with megaloblastic anemia, it is im-portant to determine whether there is a deficiency of vitamin B_{12} or of folate. In many hospitals, specific assays for serum vitamin B_{12} and folate are available. Radioisotopic dilution techniques are easier to perform than microbiologic assays. However, the radioisotopic measurement of serum vitamin B_{12} sometimes gives falsely high values, a problem not encoun-tered with the microbiologic assay. The normal range of vita-min B_{12} in serum is 200 to 900 pg/ml; values less than 100 pg/ml indicate clinically significant deficiency.

The normal serum concentration of folic acid ranges from 6 to 20 ng/ml; values of 4 ng/ml or less are generally considered to be diagnostic of folate deficiency. However, it must be re-membered that the organisms used for the microbiological as-say of folic acid are affected by many antibiotics. Thus, a se-rum sample from a patient who is on antibiotics may rarely give a falsely low reading. Unlike serum vitamin B_{12}, serum folate levels may reflect recent alterations in dietary intake. Measurement of red blood cell folate occasionally provides useful information since it is less subject to short-term fluctu-ations in folate intake and, consequently, a better index of tissue folate stores.

Once vitamin B_{12} deficiency has been established, its patho-genesis can be delineated by means of a Schilling test. A pa-tient is given radioactive vitamin B_{12} by mouth followed shortly thereafter by an intramuscular injection of unlabeled vitamin B_{12}. The proportion of the administered radioactivity excreted in the urine during the next 24 h provides an accurate measure of absorption of vitamin B_{12}, assuming that a complete urine sample has been collected. Since vitamin B_{12} deficiency is almost always due to malabsorption (Table 311-1), this first stage of the Schilling test should be abnormal. The patient is then given labeled vitamin B_{12} bound to intrinsic factor. Absorption of the vitamin will now approach normal if the patient has pernicious anemia or some other type of intrinsic factor deficiency. If vitamin B_{12} absorption is still decreased, the patient may have bacterial overgrowth (blind loop syndrome), ileal disease, or even an ileal absorptive defect secondary to vitamin B_{12} deficiency. The former type of vitamin B_{12} malabsorption can usually be corrected by the administration of antibiotics. The Schilling test can provide equally reliable information after the patient has had adequate therapy with parenteral vitamin B_{12}.

Patients with pernicious anemia have atrophic gastritis with histamine-fast achlorhydria and hypergastrinemia. As discussed in "Pernicious Anemia" above, these individuals have a very high incidence of antiparietal cell antibody and a somewhat lesser incidence of anti-intrinsic factor antibody.

TREATMENT

VITAMIN B_{12} DEFICIENCY Apart from specific therapy related to the underlying disorder (e.g., antibiotics for intestinal overgrowth with bacteria), the mainstay of treatment for B_{12} deficiency is replacement therapy. Since the defect is one of absorption, replacement should be administered parenterally, specifically in the form of intramuscular cyanocobalamin. (If intramuscular administration is contraindicated or refused, vitamin B_{12} deficiency can be managed by oral replacement therapy, but at doses of 300 to 1000 μg daily, it is an exceedingly expensive mode of treatment which requires very close medical supervision to avoid relapse.) Treatment should be started with 100 μg vitamin B_{12} per day for a week. The frequency of administration of the vitamin may then be decreased, the goal being to give a total of 2000 μg during the first 6 weeks. The patient may then be placed on 100 μg cyanocobalamin intramuscularly every month, a regimen that must be maintained for the rest of the patient's life. If necessary, larger doses may be given at less frequent intervals (e.g., 1 mg every 2 to 4 months), but the risk of relapse is substantially greater than if the vitamin is given monthly.

FIGURE 311-3

Hematologic response of a patient with pernicious anemia to an intramuscular injection of 100 μg vitamin B_{12} on day 0. (From A Erslev, TG Gabuzda, Pathophysiology of Blood, Philadelphia, Saunders, 1975.)

The response to treatment is gratifying. Shortly after treatment is begun, and several days before a hematologic response is evident in the peripheral blood, the patient will experience an increase in strength and an improved sense of well-being. Marrow morphology begins to revert toward normal within a few hours after treatment is initiated. Reticulocytosis begins 4 to 5 days after therapy is started and peaks at about day 7 (Fig. 311-3), with subsequent remission of the anemia over the next several weeks. If a reticulocytosis does not occur, or if it is less brisk than expected from the level of the hematocrit, a search should be made for other factors contributing to the anemia (e.g., infection, coexisting folate deficiency, or hypothyroidism). The sudden development of hypokalemia and salt retention may occur early in the course of therapy; usually these are of no consequence, but occasionally they may represent clinical problems.

In most cases, replacement therapy is all that is needed for the treatment of vitamin B_{12} deficiency. Occasionally, however, a patient with a severe anemia will have such a precarious cardiovascular status that emergency transfusion is necessary. This must be done with great care, since it is very easy to precipitate florid congestive failure in such patients by fluid overload. Blood must be administered slowly in the form of packed cells, with very close observation, giving as an initial dose no more than 100 ml. This small volume will frequently be enough to ameliorate the cardiovascular problems sufficiently that further therapy can be restricted to vitamin B_{12} replacement. If necessary, blood may be administered by exchanging patient blood (mostly plasma) for packed cells.

With lifelong treatment, patients should experience no further manifestations of B_{12} deficiency. As previously stated, neurological symptoms may not be fully corrected even by optimal therapy. The potential for late development of gastric carcinoma in pernicious anemia necessitates careful follow-up of the patient.

FOLATE DEFICIENCY Like vitamin B_{12} deficiency, folate deficiency is treated by replacement therapy. The usual dose of folate is 1 mg per day, by mouth, but higher doses (up to 5 mg per day) may be required for folate deficiency due to malabsorption. Parenteral folate is rarely necessary. The hematologic response is similar to that seen after replacement therapy for vitamin B_{12} deficiency—that is, a brisk reticulocytosis after about 4 days, followed by correction of the anemia over the next 1 to 2 months. The duration of therapy depends on the basis of the deficiency state. Patients with a continuously increased requirement (such as patients with hemolytic anemia) or those with malabsorption or chronic malnutrition should continue to receive oral folic acid indefinitely. In addition, the patient should be encouraged to maintain an optimal diet containing adequate amounts of folate.

It is important to note that folate, particularly in large doses, can correct the megaloblastic anemia of vitamin B_{12} deficiency without altering the neurological abnormalities. Some think that the neurological abnormalities are aggravated by folate therapy. Vitamin B_{12} deficiency can thus be masked in patients who for one reason or another are taking large doses of folate. For this reason, a hematologic response to folate must never be used to rule out vitamin B_{12} deficiency in a given patient; vitamin B_{12} deficiency can be excluded only by appropriate laboratory evaluation.

OTHER CAUSES OF MEGALOBLASTIC ANEMIA Megaloblastic anemia due to drugs can be treated, if necessary, by reducing the dose of the drug or eliminating it altogether. The effects of folate antagonists which inhibit dihydrofolate reductase can be counteracted by folinic acid (citrovorum factor) in a dose of 100 to 200 mg per day. Since folinic acid is a derivative of tetrahydrofolate, it circumvents the block in folate metabolism imposed by dihydrofolate reductase inhibitors, replenishing the tissues with a form of folate which can directly enter the one-carbon donor pool.

Certain of the congenital megaloblastic anemia–producing enzyme deficiencies can be treated by appropriate specific therapeutic regimens. The anemia of orotic aciduria is corrected by uridine, and the anemia in one case of Lesch-Nyhan syndrome responded to adenine. Both congenital folate malabsorption and homocystinuria have been treated successfully with oral folate, the former with very large doses (40 mg per day). Transcobalamin II deficiency can be treated with cyanocobalamin, but the vitamin has to be administered parenterally in very large large doses so that it can enter cells by mass action without the aid of TC II.

For the megaloblastic forms of sideroblastic anemia, pyridoxine in pharmacologic doses (as high as 300 mg per day) should be tried. A few patients will respond to this therapy. Simple supportive measures are all that appear to be in order for treatment of refractory megaloblastic anemia. Erythemic myelosis and di Guglielmo's disease are sometimes treated like other types of acute nonlymphocytic leukemia (see Chap. 325).

REFERENCES

ALLEN RH: Human vitamin B$_{12}$ transport proteins. Prog Hematol 9:57, 1975

BABIOR BM (ed): *Cobalamin. Biochemistry and Pathophysiology.* New York, Interscience-Wiley, 1975

BECK WS: Erythrocyte disorders—anemias related to disturbance of DNA synthesis (megaloblastic anemias), in *Hematology,* WJ Williams et al (eds). New York, McGraw-Hill, 1974

CHANARIN I: Investigation and management of megaloblastic anemia. Clin Haematol 5:747, 1976

EICHNER ER, HILLMAN RS: The evolution of anemia in alcoholic patients. Am J Med 50:218, 1971

ERBE R: Inborn errors of folate metabolism. N Engl J Med 293:753, 807, 1975

KASS L: *Major Problems in Internal Medicine,* vol 7: *Pernicious Anemia.* Philadelphia, Saunders, 1976

LAWSON DH et al: Early mortality in the megaloblastic anemias. Q J Med 41:1, 1972

ROSENBERG IH: Folate absorption and malabsorption. N Engl J Med 293:1303, 1975

STEBBINS R et al: Drug induced megaloblastic anemias. Semin Hematol 10:235, 1975

312
BONE MARROW FAILURE: APLASTIC ANEMIA AND OTHER DISORDERS OF THE BONE MARROW

JOEL M. RAPPEPORT
H. FRANKLIN BUNN

An important group of anemias is caused by disorders of the bone marrow which impair the formation of erythropoietic precursors. The term *aplastic anemia* should be restricted to conditions in which an acellular or markedly hypocellular bone marrow results in pancytopenia (anemia, neutropenia, and thrombocytopenia). Rare patients develop selective aplasia of only erythroid cells (*pure red blood cell aplasia*). Alternatively, in *myelophthisic anemia,* erythropoiesis is suppressed because the marrow is infiltrated with tumor or granulomata. This type of anemia is often accompanied by characteristic abnormalities in the peripheral blood smear (leukoerythroblas-

tic picture). Aplasia and myelophthisis cause a severe and progressive anemia that is normochromic and normocytic. The pathophysiology, differential diagnosis, and treatment of these entities are discussed in this chapter.

APLASTIC ANEMIA

In 1888, Paul Ehrlich described a patient with severe anemia accompanied by fever, neutropenia, and bleeding. Postmortem examination revealed a yellow, hypocellular bone marrow. The term *aplastic anemia* was applied to all patients with refractory and progressive pancytopenia until the advent of bone marrow examination for diagnostic purposes. Since then it has become apparent that a variety of pathological processes can lead to pancytopenia (see Table 312-1). By convention, the term *aplastic anemia* should be reserved for patients who have a fatty or "empty" bone marrow due to severe hypoplasia of the erythroid, myeloid, and thrombopoietic cell lines. In occasional patients, pancytopenia may be associated with a normocellular or even hypercellular marrow. The term *refractory anemia* is more appropriate for such cases.

ETIOLOGY Aplastic anemia is thought to be due to injury or destruction of a common pluripotential stem cell, affecting all subsequent cell populations. The diverse factors associated with the development of aplastic anemia are listed in Table 312-2. In approximately half of the cases of aplastic anemia in the United States, no etiologic agent is identifiable, although this figure may vary with the vigor with which an agent is sought. In other areas of the world where a larger percentage of the population may be exposed to toxins such as insecticides and benzenes in uncontrolled dose, the percentage of idiopathic cases is probably less. Both clinical observations and in vitro studies have suggested that in a small minority of patients aplasia is mediated by immunologic factors. After having received immunosuppressive therapy with or without allogeneic bone marrow, a few patients have had spontaneous recovery of their own marrow. Most patients, however, have failed to respond to this therapy. Bone marrow specimens from occasional patients with aplastic anemia have inhibited the growth of normal marrow in tissue culture. These observations must be viewed cautiously because most patients had multiple transfusions, and the in vitro tests could have reflected a transfusion-induced sensitization against either human lymphocyte antigens (HLA) or minor histocompatibility antigens.

Congenital Constitutional aplastic anemia (Fanconi's anemia) is a relatively uncommon disease appearing in childhood, although occasionally the diagnosis is made in young adults. It may be associated with multiple congenital anomalies such as

TABLE 312-1
Causes of pancytopenia

I Aplastic anemia
II Pancytopenia with normal or increased bone marrow cellularity
  A Idiopathic refractory anemia
  B Hypersplenism (Chap. 322)
  C Vitamin B$_{12}$ or folate deficiency (Chap. 311)
  D Paroxysmal nocturnal hemoglobinuria (Chap. 314) (variable cellularity)
III Bone marrow replacement
  A Hematologic malignancies
  B Nonhematologic metastatic tumor
  C Storage-cell disorders (Chap. 322)
  D Osteopetrosis (Chap. 354)
  E Myelofibrosis (Chap. 321)

hypoplasia of the kidney, hyposplenism, and bony abnormalities, particularly hypoplastic (or absent) thumbs or radii. There is often a family history, and chromosomal abnormalities have been frequently observed. If the patient survives the complications of aplasia, there is a high risk of the development of leukemia.

Drugs and toxins Multiple and seemingly unrelated drugs and chemical agents have been incriminated as etiologic agents in aplastic anemia. The association has a varying spectrum from predictable dose-related aplasia with antineoplastic agents to idiosyncratic reactions unrelated to dose.

The agents which in an adequate dose will predictably produce bone marrow depression are the antineoplastic and immunosuppressive drugs along with ionizing radiation. The degree of aplasia is dose-related but may vary from individual to individual. These drugs include folic acid antagonists, alkylating agents, the anthracyclines, nitrosoureas, purine and pyrimidine analogues, and the vinca alkaloids. The effects of combination chemotherapy are both additive and cumulative. Withdrawal of the drug usually permits recovery of the marrow elements, although irreversible aplasia is occasionally noted. Marrow aplasia may also be induced by therapeutic x-rays or, less commonly, by acute exposure from a laboratory or industrial accident. The severity of aplasia is dependent upon the dose and rate of the exposure to the bone marrow.

Benzene derivatives have been associated with multiple hematologic abnormalities including aplastic anemia. These volatile solvents are heavily utilized both commercially and domestically. Safety regulations in the United States control the industrial use of benzene derivatives but not the use in the home of benzene-containing products such as paint removers, kerosene, and degreasers. Benzene-induced marrow aplasia is usually reversible, although mild abnormalities such as macrocytosis may persist. Other hematologic abnormalities may either precede or follow the aplasia or occur independently; they include hemolytic anemia, refractory anemia with hypercellular marrow, myeloid metaplasia, and leukemia. The mechanism by which benzene induces aplasia or other hematologic disorders is not known.

Chloramphenicol, a commonly used broad-spectrum antibiotic, is associated with two forms of bone marrow toxicity.

TABLE 312-2
Causes of aplastic anemia

  I Idiopathic
 II Constitutional (Fanconi's anemia)
III Chemical and physical agents
    A Dose-related
      1 Chloramphenicol
      2 Benzene
      3 Ionizing irradiation
      4 Alkylating agents
      5 Antimetabolites (folic acid antagonists, purine and pyrimidine analogues)
      6 Mitotic inhibitors
      7 Anthracyclines
      8 Inorganic arsenicals
    B Idiosyncratic
      1 Chloramphenicol
      2 Phenylbutazone
      3 Sulfa drugs
      4 Methylphenylethylhydantoin
      5 Gold compounds
      6 Organic arsenicals
      7 Insecticides
 IV Hepatitis
  V Immunologically mediated aplasia
 VI Pregnancy
VII Paroxysmal nocturnal hemoglobinuria
VIII Miscellaneous: Systemic lupus erythematosus, pancreatitis, miliary tuberculosis, Simmonds' disease, viral infections

The more common effect upon the bone marrow is a reversible dose-related suppression of erythroid and, on occasion, granulocytic and megakaryocytic precursors. This condition is characterized by a transient anemia, associated with a drop in reticulocytes and elevation of serum iron. Occasionally neutropenia and thrombocytopenia are seen. The bone marrow is normocellular with vacuolization of the cytoplasm of early erythroid and occasionally granulocytic precursors. This bone marrow suppression is related to the dose and duration of administration of chloramphenicol. Patients with liver disease are more susceptible. The marrow morphology reverts to normal after cessation of the drug. In this setting chloramphenicol inhibits mitochondrial protein synthesis. Similar morphological and ferrokinetic changes are seen in some patients who have ingested large amounts of alcohol.

The second and more serious form of bone marrow failure associated with chloramphenicol is an "idiosyncratic" reaction perhaps occurring in genetically predisposed individuals. This nitrobenzene compound has been the single most commonly incriminated drug in cases of aplastic anemia. These patients develop severe pancytopenia and often irreversible marrow aplasia, resulting in death. This syndrome occurs in approximately 1 in 30,000 patients at risk. The development of aplastic anemia seems to be unrelated to the total dosage of drug administered. Less is known about the mechanism involved in this form of chloramphenicol toxicity. Chloramphenicol-induced marrow aplasia cannot be anticipated or prevented by hematologic monitoring since it may appear long after cessation of the drug. There is incomplete evidence that when chloramphenicol is administered intravenously, the chance of developing aplastic anemia is markedly decreased. Unfortunately many cases of fatal aplastic anemia have occurred in patients who received chloramphenicol for trivial or dubious reasons. Chloramphenicol is a useful antibiotic for specific infections in hospitalized patients but should not be used when there are reasonable alternatives (Chap. 111).

Other unrelated chemicals and drugs may be responsible for the development of aplastic anemia. These agents can be placed into two classes: those in which a number of associations have been reported and, therefore, a definite toxic potential has been established, and those in which only a single or few reported cases exist and, therefore, only a possible toxic potential exists at present. The establishment of these relationships is often further confused by the fact that many of the patients have taken multiple drugs. Those agents in which a definite potential toxicity exists are shown in Table 312-2. In addition, other drugs have been incriminated in occasional patients with aplastic anemia, but etiologic relationships have not yet been clearly established.

Infectious hepatitis A number of cases of aplastic anemia have been reported following infectious hepatitis. The antecedent hepatitis is not distinguished by its severity, and the aplastic anemia appears as the hepatitis resolves. Aplasia has followed both A and B types of hepatitis. Unfortunately, the aplasia tends to be severe with a frequently fatal outcome. The most likely explanation of this relationship is a direct toxic effect of the virus upon both liver and bone marrow. Other viruses have been implicated in aplastic anemia. Many cases of so-called "idiopathic aplastic anemia" are preceded by a benign-appearing viral respiratory illness. Aplastic anemia associated with viral infections including infectious hepatitis may be the result of virus-induced autoimmune disease. However, this presumed mechanism would apply to a small minority of patients with "idiopathic" aplastic anemia.

Aplastic anemia has also been reported in association with a number of other illnesses (Table 312-2). Aplastic anemia that develops during pregnancy may remit following delivery of the fetus.

CLINICAL MANIFESTATIONS The onset of aplastic anemia is usually insidious. Initial presenting symptoms include mild progressive weakness and fatigue attributable to the anemia, and ecchymoses, petechiae, or hemorrhage from the nose, gums, vagina, or gastrointestinal tract due to the thrombocytopenia. The bleeding is usually mild, but occasionally bleeding into the retina or central nervous system may be the initial mode of presentation. Although the patient may be severely neutropenic, it is less common for the initial presentation to be a bacterial infection.

Physical examination generally reveals pallor. The skin and mucous membranes may also demonstrate petechiae or ecchymoses. The conjunctivas and fundi may also be involved. Like other conditions in which there is severe thrombocytopenia, the areas most commonly involved with petechiae are those in which there is an increased capillary pressure or areas subject to trauma. Lymphadenopathy and hepatosplenomegaly are absent. Fever may be present, but despite the presence of an infection, the usual signs of inflammation may be absent because of the neutropenia.

The *course* of the disease is often determined by the severity of the aplastic anemia. Furthermore, disease which is initially mild can progress. Conversely, partial recovery of one or more cell lines may develop. It is of great importance to obtain an accurate assessment of the degree of aplasia. Severe aplasia is defined as marked pancytopenia with at least two of the following criteria: granulocytes fewer than 500 per cubic millimeter, platelets fewer than 20,000 per cubic millimeter, anemia with corrected reticulocyte count less than 1 percent. The bone marrow is markedly hypoplastic and depleted of hematopoietic cells. Patients with severe disease have a high risk of dying from bleeding and/or infections in a matter of months, while patients with a milder form of the disease may live for years. The clinical course of the disease is affected primarily by the nature and location of bleeding and infections. Although infections may not dominate the clinical picture initially, they assume great importance with the passage of time. Because of the need for multiple red blood cell and platelet transfusions, over a period of time one may encounter the sequelae of hemosiderosis and/or hepatitis. Other clinical manifestations may be due to side effects from the administration of corticosteroids and androgens. Even those patients who recover may have mild thrombocytopenia for many years. The course of the disease and the chances of recovery seem to relate to the severity of disease rather than the etiology, although some agents such as chloramphenicol and infectious hepatitis seem to be associated with poor prognosis.

LABORATORY DIAGNOSIS The diagnosis of aplastic anemia and the assessment of its relative severity depend upon a thorough laboratory evaluation. The peripheral blood usually manifests pancytopenia. The white blood cell count may be low normal but is composed predominantly of normal lymphocytes. The red blood cells are normochromic, normocytic, or mildly macrocytic, and the reticulocyte index is very low or zero. The degree of depression of any cell line may be variable. Not infrequently the initial absolute granulocyte count may be low normal but becomes progressively depressed. Since the incidence of serious bleeding and/or infection correlates with the degree of thrombocytopenia or neutropenia, these values must be determined initially and followed periodically. A bone marrow aspirate may yield a "dry tap," but a bone marrow biopsy will reveal a severely hypocellular or aplastic marrow with a variable degree of replacement with fat. There is usually a severe depression or total absence of megakaryocytes, a marked depression of all myeloid cells, and a marked but relatively less severe depression of the erythroid precursors. The other scattered cells present include normal lymphocytes, histiocytes, reticulum cells, mast cells, and plasma cells. There is a lack of infiltration by fibrosis, leukemia, or tumor. Occasionally, small nests of normal marrow cells may be seen and are always a cause of debate as to whether they may represent a recovering state. The significance of these nests is usually resolved by the subsequent course. For obtaining a truly representative sampling of the marrow, multiple bone marrow biopsies may be necessary.

The serum iron concentration is elevated, and the iron-binding capacity is normal. Serum folate and vitamin B_{12} levels are normal, and there is no evidence of increased red blood cell destruction. As predicted from the nature of this disease, plasma iron clearance is prolonged, and incorporation of iron into red blood cells is markedly decreased. The absolute level of fetal hemoglobin, which was at one time thought to be of prognostic value, may be low, normal, or increased.

DIFFERENTIAL DIAGNOSIS The diagnosis of aplastic anemia implies the exclusion of the other causes of pancytopenia that are listed in Table 312-1. Splenomegaly and/or lymphadenopathy dictate strongly against aplastic anemia. Malignant and nonmalignant invasion of the bone marrow must be excluded. Either preleukemia or an early leukemia may present as a pancytopenia and calls for careful bone marrow examination. Similarly, ineffective cell production due to myelofibrosis and myeloid metaplasia can be identified by microscopic examination of the bone marrow. Paroxysmal nocturnal hemoglobinuria and systemic lupus erythematosus should be excluded by appropriate tests. Nutritional deficiency can be excluded by serum assays and morphological changes. Pancytopenia rarely may be secondary to various infections.

Before aplastic anemia can be classified as idiopathic, a careful history must exclude exposure to all known and suspected agents. In our complex society, all patients are exposed to potentially toxic agents in their environment. Nevertheless this difficulty should not discourage a careful and extensive search for an etiology.

TREATMENT The management of aplastic anemia has become one of the most challenging aspects of modern medicine, requiring a diligent multidisciplinary team of physicians and advanced forms of support. The aim of therapy is to provide support in expectation of spontaneous recovery. Patients with severe aplasia should receive a bone marrow transplantation, if a suitable donor is available. The efficacy of this treatment has been most clearly demonstrated in younger patients.

Supportive care Regardless of the therapy chosen, the mainstay of treatment is good supportive care. The first and most immediate step is the removal of any suspected etiologic agent. If the disease is mild at presentation, no further supportive care need be instituted, unless there is a subsequent further deterioration. If a severe neutropenia exists (polymorphonuclear leukocytes < 500 per cubic millimeter), the patient should be shielded from potential infections. This includes protection against environmentally acquired infections and prophylaxis against endogenous infections from nasopharynx, mouth, and gastrointestinal tract. The latter demands a dental evaluation with the institution of good mouth and dental care. In addition, food having a low content of bacteria and a bowel preparation composed of nonabsorbable antibiotics may be instituted, particularly in the setting of a sterile environment. Prophylactic systemic antibiotics should not be utilized. Intramuscular injections should be minimized and, if necessary, should be administered with care. Established infections should be treated vigorously with specific antibiotics, and fever of undetermined etiology may, after appropriate evaluation, call for broad-spectrum antibiotic coverage until a specific diagnosis is established.

Transfusions should be used judiciously. Only component therapy should be administered. Red blood cells should be administered to maintain the well-being of the patient rather than to establish a certain hemoglobin level. Maintaining a lower than normal hemoglobin to promote the secretion of endogenous erythropoietin has not been demonstrated to increase the rate of recovery. Transfusions pose significant risks such as hepatitis, hemosiderosis, and sensitization to both red blood cell antigens and transplantation antigens. Platelet transfusions should be administered in the face of serious hemorrhage, particularly central nervous system, mucous membrane, and gastrointestinal bleeding. The use of prophylactic platelet transfusions varies from center to center. Some groups administer platelet transfusions only when serious bleeding exists, while other groups employ prophylactic transfusions when the platelet count is lower than 20,000 per cubic millimeter. Responses to platelet transfusions may be blunted by the presence of infection. Over a period of time many patients will develop HLA antibodies and resistance to subsequent transfusions. Sensitization may be decreased by the utilization of single-donor platelet concentrates, and when sensitization develops, HLA-compatible donors should be sought. Should a bone marrow transplant be considered, family members should be avoided as a source of HLA-compatible donors, since the patient may develop antibodies to minor transplantation antigens. The use of prophylactic leukocyte transfusions is controversial. Donor white blood cells are difficult to obtain in adequate yields and survive only a few hours in the circulation. However, white blood cell infusions are of value in septic patients with severe neutropenia.

Marrow-stimulating agents A variety of agents have been utilized in an attempt to stimulate regeneration of the marrow. These include phytohemagglutinin, cobalt, vitamin B_{12}, and irradiation. None of these has been of value. Since 1961, various claims have been made about the efficacy of androgens as a hematopoietic stimulant in aplastic anemia. Occasional patients do seem to respond to androgens, and in fact a few have appeared to be androgen-dependent. The overall efficacy of these agents in aplastic anemia is uncertain. A randomized study has demonstrated no statistical advantage of androgen therapy in severe aplastic anemia. In mild cases in which hematopoietic elements still exist, and where there is a good chance of surviving 3 to 6 months, patients should be treated with androgens as the initial mode of therapy. Currently studies have been undertaken to systematically evaluate various androgen preparations. There is some evidence that individual patients may respond to one form of androgen but not to others. The most widely used drugs at present are oxymetholone, fluoxymesterone, and nandrolone decanoate. Side effects include hepatic dysfunction in 17α-alkylated androgens and masculinization and fluid retention in most of the drugs in this class.

Adrenal corticosteroids have also been advocated as myelostimulants, but there is no evidence for their efficacy. Corticosteroids may also lessen capillary fragility and prolong the survival of transfused red blood cells and platelets. If utilized, adrenal corticosteroids should be administered in low dosages since large doses probably have a deleterious effect, promoting gastrointestinal bleeding and increasing the chances of opportunistic infections.

In general, splenectomy has no role in the management of aplastic anemia.

Bone marrow transplantation In the mid-1950s, E. D. Thomas and his associates began investigating bone marrow transplantation as a possible therapeutic modality in aplastic anemia. Although nearly all early efforts were doomed to failure, recent advances in transplantation immunology and means of support have made bone marrow transplantation a therapeutic alternative in severe aplastic anemia. If aplastic anemia is a consequence of damage to the pluripotential stem cell, marrow transplantation is a reasonable therapeutic approach. On the other hand, if the disease results from damage to the microenvironment of the bone marrow, the procedure has far less rationale. The fact that patients with aplastic anemia have had successful marrow grafts provides strong support for the former mechanism. In patients with severe aplastic anemia, marrow transplantation offers the best chance for survival.

As mentioned above, the primary treatment of aplastic anemia consists mainly of supportive measures. Unfortunately, problems of life-threatening infection, severe hemorrhage, and presensitization to a potential donor are commonly encountered during the application of such conservative therapy. For this reason it is very important initially to classify the disease as mild, moderate, or severe and monitor the patient closely for any change in status. In cases of severe aplasia, histocompatibility testing should be done immediately on the patient and his or her siblings.

The HLA transplantation antigens include those of the A, B, and C histocompatibility loci and the D antigens detected by the mixed lymphocyte culture (MLC) reaction (see Chap. 61). Identity at the HLA-A, HLA-B, and HLA-D loci seems to be a minimal requirement for successful engraftment, although a few exceptions have been noted. While the chance of finding such a donor from the random population is extremely remote, there is a 25 percent chance that any given sibling will match completely at these loci. Despite such identity, other unnamed minor transplantation antigens may preclude a successful "take." For this reason the recipient must have his or her intact immune system completely suppressed. This may be accomplished by administering lethal doses of total body irradiation or extremely high doses of cyclophosphamide. Occasionally, antilymphocyte serum is also given. The side effects from such therapy may be extreme even if caution is used. Preparatory immunosuppression is not necessary if the recipient and donor are monozygotic twins, in whom one would expect identity even at minor loci. ABO identity is not required, in contrast to renal transplantation.

After preparation, the bone marrow is aspirated from the donor and administered intravenously to the recipient. During the next 2 to 3 weeks the emergence of donor cells in the circulation of the recipient indicates that engraftment has been successful (see Fig. 312-1). During this period and until adequate counts are established, the recipient must be protected from bacterial and fungal infection by isolation and sterilization of the gastrointestinal tract, and from bleeding by platelet transfusions. If an infection develops, granulocyte transfusions should be given.

Eighty percent of immunosuppressed HLA-identical, MLC-nonreactive sibling transplants (allogeneic) will have engraftment without rejection, and in one series all five monozygotic twins (syngeneic) had successful engraftment. All the monozygotic twins are doing well without immunosuppression 2 to 12 years later.

The 20 percent who fail to have successful engraftment usually have been presensitized to antigens distinct from the major histocompatibility region. Such sensitization probably arises through prior pregnancies or transfusion therapy. The likelihood of presensitization is increased if a family member is used for transfusion therapy, but exposure to these antigens may also occur through random donors. It is possible to detect such

FIGURE 312-1

Clinical course of a patient with aplastic anemia following successful bone marrow transplantation. Arrows indicate transfusion of platelets and leukocytes. (From B Camitta et al, Blood 43:473, 1974.)

sensitization and to overcome it by more intensive immunosuppressive therapy.

A major stumbling block in allogenic marrow transplantation, and the major factor differentiating this procedure from any other organ transplantation, is the development of graft-versus-host (GVH) disease. GVH disease is thought to result from the recognition by the newly engrafted immunologically competent cells of transplant antigens in the host, which are lacking in the graft. Alternatively the disorder may result from an imbalance of the newly engrafted immune system. Clinically, this disorder develops in approximately 70 percent of bone marrow transplant recipients. About half of these patients die from GVH or GVH-related infections. This problem may be acute or chronic and affects primarily the skin, liver, and gastrointestinal tract. It is thought that spontaneous cessation may occur either by the development of tolerance (suppressor T cells) or by the formation of blocking antibody. After the transplantation, methotrexate is utilized to ameliorate the course of acute GVH disease. Established acute GVH disease can be successfully treated with antilymphocyte serum in about one-third of cases. Chronic GVH disease has not yet been significantly modified by chemotherapy. GVH disease clinically resembles certain collagen vascular disorders, and, therefore, therapeutic advances in GVH may have a wider application.

An additional problem following transplantation is the susceptibility to opportunistic infections such as fungal and viral agents. Infection is an important cause of death, even in patients who have had successful engraftment.

Despite the complex problems outlined above, the chance of long-term survival at present in an experienced program is approximately 50 percent, a significant improvement over the 10 percent survival of severe aplastic anemia. Currently, the procedure is available only to the 40 percent of the population who have a suitable donor. The patient's physician must evaluate the therapeutic alternatives available at the time of diagnosis and determine the course of therapy in a manner that does not jeopardize the patient's chances for a successful transplant. This means maintaining the patient as free as possible of major infections and hemorrhage and yet keeping the patient from becoming sensitized to potential donor transplant antigens.

Bone marrow transplants have also been used with a lesser degree of success in acute leukemia. The same basic principles apply as in aplastic anemia, but an added problem is the recurrence of the underlying disorder. A third disease treated with bone marrow transplantation is severe combined immune deficiency; however, this situation differs from either aplasia or leukemia in two respects. Since the host has no immune defenses, no immunosuppression is necessary. Only small infusions of marrow are required to reconstitute the immune system. Successful engraftment has also been achieved in both the Wiskott-Aldrich syndrome and various genetic granulocyte disorders.

PURE RED CELL APLASIA

Pure red blood cell aplasia involves a selective failure in the production of erythroid elements in the bone marrow. Granulopoiesis and megakaryocytopoiesis remain normal. Patients have a normochromic normocytic anemia with normal granulocyte count and platelet count. Severe reticulocytopenia exists, and the bone marrow is characterized by a virtual absence of any erythroid precursors in the face of otherwise normal cellular elements. An increase in lymphocytes may be seen in the marrow. Red blood cell aplasia is distinct from both aplastic anemia which represents a pluripotential stem-cell failure and the relative failure of erythroid production associated with chronic inflammatory diseases.

CONSTITUTIONAL RED CELL APLASIA A rare chronic constitutional red blood cell aplasia known as Blackfan-Diamond syndrome may appear in infants from the time of birth to the age of 2 years. Twenty-five percent of patients have minor congenital anomalies. The disorder is of unknown etiology.

ACQUIRED RED CELL APLASIA A rare but fascinating syndrome is the acquired idiopathic form of pure red blood cell aplasia seen predominantly in middle-aged adults. About one-third of patients have thymomas, which are usually encapsulated spindle-cell tumors, although occasional malignant thymomas have been noted. Five percent of all patients with thymomas have pure red blood cell aplasia. The association between thymoma and myasthenia gravis is somewhat stronger. The thymoma may be of long standing prior to the development of the anemia. In those patients studied to date, both with and without thymomas, an inhibitor of hematopoiesis in bone marrow cell cultures has been commonly noted prior to therapy with disappearance in the remission state. This inhibitor has been shown to be a complement-fixing IgG immunoglobulin which has selective cytotoxicity to marrow erythroblasts. A much smaller group of patients have been noted to have an inhibitor against erythropoietin.

Treatment Since these patients have virtually no endogenous red blood cell production, they are totally dependent on red blood cell transfusion. If thymic enlargement is noted, a thymectomy may induce a remission in approximately 50 percent of patients. If the thymus is normal, thymectomy is of no benefit. The best therapy for patients without thymoma or those with an unsuccessful thymectomy seems to be a combination of corticosteroids and an immunosuppressive agent such as cyclophosphamide. The results to date demonstrate both prolonged clinical remission and disappearance of the inhibitor in many patients. Relapses may occur, and a significant mortality still exists with this disorder, generally from the chronic complications of blood transfusion therapy.

DRUG-INDUCED RED CELL APLASIA Drug-associated red blood cell aplasia has been rarely noted in all age groups. The drugs that have been incriminated are chloramphenicol, phenytoin, isoniazid, and tolbutamide. Except for chloramphenicol, this drug-related toxicity is less common than other hematologic effects associated with drugs. Unlike drug-induced aplastic anemia, the drug-related red blood cell aplasias are usually reversible with discontinuance of the offending agent.

MYELOPHTHISIC ANEMIA

Infiltration of the bone marrow with tumor or granulomas can result in the development of a severe anemia. Tumor may be derived from cell lines indigenous to the bone marrow such as leukemia, lymphoma, or myeloma, or the marrow may be invaded by metastatic deposits of solid tumor, usually carcinoma. Among the solid tumors most frequently associated with myelophthisic anemia are carcinoma of the breast, prostate, lung, and thyroid. Granulomatous involvement of the bone marrow is usually due to advanced tuberculosis. Primary lipid storage disorders such as Gaucher's disease and Niemann-Pick disease occasionally produce a myelophthisic anemia, and the rare disorder osteopetrosis, or marble bone disease, may also give a similar hematologic picture. In contrast, the development of fibrosis in the bone marrow is encountered relatively frequently, usually in association with myeloid metaplasia. This entity is discussed in Chap. 321.

The mechanism underlying the anemia in myelophthisis is not well understood. The invasion of the bone marrow by tumor or granulomas impairs both erythropoiesis and thrombopoiesis. In contrast, neutrophil production is generally normal or increased. It is unlikely that the anemia and thrombocytopenia are due merely to "crowding" of the bone marrow space by extrinsic cells. Myelophthisis also causes a distortion of the microcirculation of the marrow, with premature release of normoblasts and immature myeloid cells.

Myelophthisis usually results in a severe normochromic normocytic anemia. A variety of misshapen erythrocytes are noted, particularly teardrop cells and fragmented cells with some basophilic stippling. In addition, normoblasts are usually seen in the peripheral blood. The reticulocyte percentage is often slightly increased (4 to 7 percent). However, when corrected for the anemia and the premature release from the bone marrow, the absolute reticulocyte count is actually reduced

and reflects a decrease in red blood cell production. While thrombocytopenia is usually present, the white blood cell count is often elevated, with a marked shift to the left in the differential count. The combination of immature myeloid cells and normoblasts in the peripheral blood constitutes the "leukoerythroblastic" morphology so characteristic of myelophthisic anemia. Striking abnormalities are usually seen on examination of the bone marrow. Often an aspirate yields a "dry tap," due to the infiltration of the marrow with abnormal tissue. Marrow biopsy is more likely to be diagnostic, revealing leukemia, lymphoma, or foci of metastatic tumors or granulomas. However, marrow involvement is often segmental, so that the primary pathological process may be missed on a single biopsy.

The diagnosis of myelophthisic anemia is often straightforward if the characteristic peripheral blood picture is encountered in a patient with known cancer or tuberculosis. However, a wide variety of hematologic findings may be seen in tuberculosis. Occasionally, the diagnosis of disseminated tuberculosis is established on the basis of a bone marrow biopsy. If the patient has a markedly enlarged spleen in combination with the peripheral blood findings described above, he or she is likely to have myelofibrosis (see Chap. 321).

The treatment of myelophthisic anemia consists of attempts to reverse the primary pathological process. Disseminated tumors of the breast or prostate may respond remarkably well to appropriate hormonal therapy. It is particularly important to search for the presence of tuberculosis since this disease is readily treatable. More often, however, the disease is not amenable to therapy, and supportive measures, such as blood transfusions, must be employed.

REFERENCES

Ellman L: Bone marrow biopsy in the evaluation of lymphoma, carcinoma and granulomatous disease. Am J Med 60:1, 1976

Krantz SB: Pure red-cell aplasia. N Engl J Med 291:345, 1974

Thomas ED (ed): Aplastic anemia. Clin Hematol 7:429, 1978

——— et al: Bone marrow transplantation. N Engl J Med 292:832, 895, 1975

Williams DM et al: Drug induced aplastic anemia. Semin Hematol 10:195, 1973

313
ANEMIA ASSOCIATED WITH CHRONIC SYSTEMIC DISORDERS

H. FRANKLIN BUNN

Among the most commonly encountered anemias are those associated with a variety of chronic underlying diseases. These anemias will be corrected only if the primary condition can be reversed. As shown in Table 313-1, these anemias can be sub-

TABLE 313-1
Anemias secondary to chronic systemic diseases

I Anemia of chronic inflammation
   A Infection
   B Connective tissue disorders, etc.
   C Malignancy
II Anemia of uremia
III Anemia due to endocrine failure
IV Anemia of liver disease

divided into several groups. In contrast to the other anemias listed here, those associated with chronic inflammation are characterized by an abnormality in iron metabolism.

ANEMIA OF CHRONIC INFLAMMATION

CLINICAL DESCRIPTION Patients who have a chronic systemic inflammatory disorder persisting more than a month usually develop an anemia which is of mild or moderate severity. The extent of the anemia is roughly proportional to the duration and severity of the inflammatory process. These disorders include chronic infections such as subacute infective endocarditis, osteomyelitis, lung abscess, tuberculosis, and pyelonephritis. Among noninfectious causes of anemia of chronic inflammation, the most common is rheumatoid arthritis. Other noninfectious inflammatory disorders often associated with chronic anemia include systemic lupus erythematosis, vasculitides (such as temporal arteritis), sarcoidosis, and regional enteritis.

This kind of anemia is also commonly encountered in neoplastic disorders, including Hodgkin's disease and a variety of solid tumors such as carcinoma of the lung and breast. Other factors may contribute to the development of more severe anemia in cancer patients. In those with gastrointestinal cancer, blood loss can be the predominant factor. Chronic gastrointestinal bleeding will lead to iron deficiency. Furthermore, cancer patients may develop progressive anemia if the bone marrow is invaded with tumor cells. Myelophthisic anemia is discussed in detail in Chap. 312. Rarely, patients with disseminated malignancy develop severe microangiopathic hemolytic anemia (Chap. 314). Finally, suppression of hematopoiesis by chemotherapeutic agents or radiation therapy may aggravate anemia.

HEMATOLOGIC DESCRIPTION Hemoglobin values generally range between 9 and 11 g per 100 ml. A hemoglobin level less than 8 g per 100 ml indicates the presence of one or more of the contributing factors mentioned above. Although this group of anemias is generally classified as normocytic-normochromic, red blood cells often contain a subnormal amount of hemoglobin and may even be microcytic. It is not uncommon for the mean corpuscular volume to be as low as 70 fl. The mean corpuscular hemoglobin concentration is usually below 32 g per 100 ml. Examination of the bone marrow reveals normal erythroid maturation. However, the red blood cell precursors have less stainable iron than normal (i.e., fewer sideroblasts), while the macrophages in the marrow usually contain increased amounts of iron. Myeloid hyperplasia and an increase in plasma cells may be seen in certain chronic infections.

The reticulocyte count is usually normal ($<$ 3 percent). Careful measurement of red blood cell survival generally reveals moderately shortened erythrocyte life span. Cross-transfusion studies point to an extracorpuscular mechanism, perhaps hyperplasia of the mononuclear-phagocyte system. There is seldom any other evidence of significant hemolysis. However, in certain chronic infections such as subacute infective endocarditis and miliary tuberculosis, splenomegaly can contribute to further shortening of the red blood cell life span, thereby increasing the severity of the anemia. In this setting spherocytes may be seen on the blood smear.

Serum iron is characteristically subnormal in this group of anemias, and, in contrast to iron deficiency, the total transferrin level is also reduced but to a lesser extent (see Fig. 310-1). Hence the fractional saturation of transferrin is slightly lower than normal. The serum iron falls within days following the onset of the inflammation, whereas several weeks elapse before the transferrin level falls. Serum ferritin is increased in patients with inflammatory disorders. Certain other plasma proteins are characteristically elevated in chronic inflammation. These "phase reactants" include gamma globulin, the third component of complement, haptoglobin, α_1-antitrypsin, orosomucoid, and fibrinogen. The latter is usually not measured since protein electrophoresis is routinely done on serum rather than plasma. Elevation of these proteins is responsible for the increased rate of red blood cell sedimentation which is so commonly observed.

It is often difficult to detect iron deficiency in a patient with chronic inflammation. The serum iron is low, and red blood cell protoporphyrin is increased in both conditions. When iron deficiency is superimposed on a chronic inflammatory state, the serum ferritin falls and transferrin level rises, usually to within normal limits. Under such circumstances, detection of storage iron in the bone marrow is unpredictable. This problem is commonly encountered in patients with rheumatoid arthritis who may have developed iron deficiency owing to gastrointestinal blood loss. Because of this diagnostic uncertainty, it is often prudent to give such a patient a trial of iron and ascertain whether the hemoglobin level increases. However, it is important to avoid prolonged administration of iron unless a true deficiency state persists.

PATHOGENESIS The anemia of chronic inflammation is primarily due to defective red blood cell production and failure to compensate for the slightly decreased red blood cell life span. The subnormal amounts of iron in erythroblasts, in spite of an abundance of storage iron, suggests a defect in the transfer of iron to the developing erythroid cells. The cells that are formed are somewhat "iron deficient," and therefore tend to be small and pale. As in true iron deficiency, increased red blood cell protoporphyrin reflects the reduced availability of iron for heme synthesis. This defect can be quantitated by iron kinetic studies. If radioactive iron bound to transferrin is administered, there is normal uptake into the marrow and incorporation into circulating red cells. In contrast, if hemoglobin labeled with radioactive iron is injected, the incorporation of label into circulating red cells is only half normal. The hyperplastic mononuclear phagocyte system which is responsible for decreased survival of circulating red cells probably traps the hemoglobin iron and prevents its transfer to the bone marrow. For unexplained reasons, erythropoietin levels tend to be lower than expected for the degree of anemia. However, erythropoietin levels are not as low as in the anemia of renal failure (see below) and may not play a significant role in the pathogenesis of the anemia.

MANAGEMENT The anemia of chronic inflammation is not responsive to hematinic agents such as iron, folic acid, or vitamin B_{12}. Since the anemia is seldom severe, blood transfusion is rarely indicated. Efforts should be directed toward correcting the underlying disorder. In addition, if the anemia is more severe than expected, it is essential to search for other factors such as blood loss or drug-induced myelosuppression that could contribute to the reduction of red blood cell mass.

ANEMIA OF UREMIA

Anemia almost always accompanies the uremic syndrome. Although the hemoglobin level is highly variable among uremic patients, the severity of the anemia is roughly proportional to the degree of azotemia. The etiology of the renal failure usually has little bearing on the extent of anemia. However, for any level of serum creatinine patients with polycystic disease tend to be less anemic than those with other types of renal disease. In contrast to anemias associated with other chronic disorders discussed in this chapter, the anemia of uremia can be very severe, with hemoglobin levels as low as 4 g per 100 ml. However, patients often tolerate such marked anemia remarkably well. This is largely due to compensatory adjustments such as redistribution of blood flow and a decrease in the oxygen affinity of the blood (see Chap. 53).

The anemia of uremia is normochromic and normocytic. Red blood cell morphology is usually normal. Examination of the bone marrow seldom reveals any abnormalities. In about one-third of patients, so-called "burr" cells are seen in the peripheral blood smear. These red blood cells have a characteristic evenly scalloped border (see Plate 9-10). Neither the degree of anemia nor the red blood cell life span is influenced by the presence of burr cells. In most patients the reticulocyte count is normal and the red blood cell survival is only modestly decreased. Thus the low red blood cell mass is due to decreased red blood cell production. The primary basis for this defect is that the diseased kidneys are unable to secrete adequate amounts of erythropoietin. Plasma erythropoietin levels are lower than those of nonuremic patients with a comparable degree of uremia. Erythropoiesis is further impaired but not abolished in patients who have undergone bilateral nephrectomy. In addition, red blood cell production may be suppressed by the accumulation of substances that are normally cleared by the kidneys. Iron kinetic measurements reveal impaired incorporation of iron into circulating red blood cells. Thus, it is likely that the anemia is due in part to ineffective erythropoiesis (see Chap. 53). Improvement in the rate of utilization of iron by the bone marrow has been noted following hemodialysis.

A small minority of uremic patients, particularly those with advanced disease, have brisk hemolysis. Red blood cell survival studies indicate that the hemolysis is due to extracorpuscular factors. Both metabolic and mechanical factors contribute to the hemolysis. Some patients may acquire a defect in the hexose monophosphate shunt which renders the red blood cell vulnerable to the formation of Heinz bodies (see Chap. 314). The hemolysis can be aggravated by oxidant drugs or oxidant compounds such as chloramine in the dialysis bath. If the renal failure is due to thrombotic thrombocytopenic purpura or hemolytic-uremic syndrome, patients will have a severe form of microangiopathic hemolytic anemia, with characteristic abnormalities of red blood cell morphology (see Chap. 314).

Treatment of the anemia of uremia should focus on an attempt to reverse the renal failure. The anemia may be modestly improved following hemodialysis. A prompt and dramatic correction of the anemia follows successful renal transplantation. Occasionally, polycythemia may be encountered following the renal engraftment, and may be a harbinger of impending rejection. In those patients who are not candidates for renal transplantation the administration of androgens has proved effective in stimulating erythropoiesis, particularly in patients who have not undergone bilateral nephrectomy.

It is important to be aware of other factors that may aggravate the anemia of renal disease. Uremic patients have a propensity to hemorrhage, owing to a qualitative defect in platelet function. Thus, gastrointestinal blood loss is commonly encountered. Furthermore a small but significant amount of blood loss occurs during hemodialysis. For these reasons some uremic patients become iron deficient. Folic acid deficiency may also occur, owing to the poor nutrition of many patients or to the loss of this dialysable vitamin during dialysis.

ANEMIA SECONDARY TO ENDOCRINE FAILURE

A number of hormones, including thyroxine, glucocorticoids, testosterone, and growth hormone are known to affect proliferation of human erythroid cells in vitro. Therefore it is not surprising that a mild to moderate normochromic-normocytic anemia generally accompanies a number of endocrine deficiency states, including hypothyroidism, Addison's disease, hypogonadism, and panhypopituitarism. It is possible that the anemias associated with hypothyroidism and hypopituitarism are related to the decreased need for oxygen transport, since oxygen consumption is reduced when thyroid hormone or growth hormone is lacking.

The anemia of myxedema is usually normocytic. Red blood cell life span is normal and erythropoiesis is effective. A minority of patients have macrocytic red blood cells which can usually be attributed to either folic acid or B_{12} deficiency. Patients with myxedema have an increased incidence of pernicious anemia. Hypothyroid patients, particularly females with menorrhagia, often develop iron deficiency and a microcytic anemia. Because the plasma volume may be reduced along with the red blood cell mass, the anemia of hypothyroidism may be masked. Since the signs and symptoms of myxedema are sometimes elusive, this diagnosis should be considered in the evaluation of any patient with unexplained anemia.

The anemia of Addison's disease is also marked by a decrease in plasma volume. Untreated patients have an average hemoglobin level of about 13 g per 100 ml. Upon hormone replacement, the plasma volume is rapidly reconstituted and the hemoglobin level falls to 80 percent of its pretreatment value. With time, the red blood cell mass is restored toward normal.

Testosterone has a physiologic influence on red blood cell mass. During passage through adolescence the mean hemoglobin level of males increases from 13 to 15 g per 100 ml. Eunuchoid males generally have a mild decrease in hemoglobin, averaging 13 g per 100 ml. Pituitary dysfunction or ablation is associated with a mild normochromic normocytic anemia as well as occasional leukopenia.

The anemias secondary to endocrine failure are all readily corrected when adequate hormone replacement is given.

ANEMIA OF LIVER DISEASE

Anemia of varying severity is commonly encountered in patients with alcoholic liver disease. Many factors can contribute to the development of anemia. Alcohol is a direct suppressor of erythropoiesis. In alcoholics who have continued to drink up to the time of clinical evaluation, the bone marrow often reveals vacuoles in the cytoplasm of red and white blood cell precursors. In addition, ringed sideroblasts may be observed, particularly in patients who are malnourished. In alcoholics there often is suboptimal intake of dietary folic acid and impairment of folate utilization. Furthermore, alcoholics commonly develop significant hemorrhage from gastritis, esophageal varices, or duodenal ulcer, which contributes to the anemia. The risk of gastrointestinal blood loss is further increased by the presence of thrombocytopenia or deficiencies in soluble clotting factors. Although alcoholics usually have increased iron stores, they may become iron-deficient after prolonged gastrointestinal bleeding.

Even in the absence of such complications, patients with chronic liver disease usually have a mild to moderate anemia which is normocytic or slightly macrocytic. The bone marrow fails to compensate for a moderate shortening of red blood cell life span. Rarely patients with cirrhosis develop a severe hemolytic anemia accompanied by the appearance of rigid red blood cells with irregular borders called acanthocytes or "spur" cells (see Plate 9-12). More commonly morphology is normal, except for the presence of target cells and occasionally stomatocytes, which have increased deposits of cholesterol and phospholipid, resulting in an increase in the surface area of the red blood cell membrane. The anemia persists as long as hepatic function is defective, but it may be corrected if normal hepatic function can be restored.

REFERENCES

BUCHWALD D: Effect of nandrolone decanoate on the anemia of chronic hemo-dialysis patients. Nephron 18:232, 1977

BUDMAN DR, STEINBERG AD: Hematologic aspects of systemic lupus erythematosus. Ann Intern Med 86:220, 1977

CARTWRIGHT GE, LEE GR: The anemia of chronic disorders. Br J Haematol 21:147, 1971

DOUGLAS SW, ADAMSON JW: The anemia of chronic disorders: Studies of marrow regulation and iron metabolism. Blood 45:55, 1975

FRIED W: Erythropoietin and the kidney. Nephron 15:327, 1975

MOWAT AG: Hematologic abnormalities in rheumatoid arthritis. Semin Arthritis Rheum 1:195, 1972

NAETS JP: Hematologic disorders in renal failure. Nephron 14:181, 1975

STRAUSS DJ: Hematologic aspects of alcoholism. Semin Hematol 19:183, 1973

YAWATA Y, JACOB HS: Abnormal red cell metabolism in patients with chronic uremia: Nature of the defect and its persistence despite adequate hemodialysis. Blood 45:231, 1975

ZUCKER S et al: Bone marrow erythropoiesis in the anemia of infection, inflammation and malignancy. J Clin Invest 53:1132, 1974

314
HEMOLYTIC ANEMIAS

RICHARD A. COOPER
H. FRANKLIN BUNN

PATHOGENESIS OF RED CELL DESTRUCTION

Red blood cells undergo premature destruction by two general mechanisms. First, red blood cells lyse in the circulation with the release of their contents directly into the peripheral blood (intravascular lysis). Second, and more commonly, red blood cells are taken up by macrophages in the spleen and liver (mononuclear-phagocyte system) where they are destroyed and digested (extravascular lysis).

Intravascular lysis occurs when red blood cells in small blood vessels are exposed to excessive external trauma, as in march hemoglobinuria, or when they are exposed to the high shear stress of turbulent blood flow, as through a defective cardiac valve prosthesis. Similarly, it occurs when red blood cells stream through fibrin deposited in arterioles in disorders such as thrombotic thrombocytopenic purpura, the hemolytic uremic syndrome, and disseminated intravascular coagulation. Complement lysis is another mechanism whereby red blood cells are disrupted in the circulation; however, this phenomenon is unusual in humans. It occurs during some hemolytic transfusion reactions, and it is the major mode of red blood cell destruction in paroxysmal nocturnal hemoglobinuria and in paroxysmal cold hemoglobinuria. More commonly, the complement sequence is not completed; rather, it stops after the third component of complement has become fixed to the red blood cell membrane. Certain toxins of exogenous origin also may lyse human red blood cells. These include the venom of the cobra snake, the poison of the brown recluse spider, and the toxin of *Clostridium welchii*. Most other forms of red blood cell injury are not sufficiently severe to cause intravascular lysis. Rather, recognition, trapping, and destruction of the abnormal red blood cells occur primarily in the spleen and liver.

The spleen is capable of trapping and destroying red blood cells which have subtle abnormalities. The liver lacks the spleen's fine discrimination and is unable to recognize these cells. However, because the blood flow to the liver is about 7 times that to the spleen, the liver has a greater capacity for clearing red blood cells that have gross abnormalities. Phagocytosis of red blood cells induces a proliferative response in the spleen, and to a lesser extent in the liver, leading to hyperplasia, increased blood flow, and functional overactivity, thereby further augmenting the clearance of the abnormal red blood cells which instigated this process. When this proliferative response is stimulated by other factors, such as systemic inflammatory disease, or when the circulation of red blood cells through the spleen is retarded owing to anatomic factors, such as in cirrhosis, the spleen damages and then destroys otherwise normal red blood cells.

The mononuclear-phagocyte system clears red blood cells from the circulation under two general conditions: First, when the surface of the red blood cell possesses chemical properties for which macrophages present in the mononuclear-phagocyte system have specific receptors; and second, when the red blood cell possesses physical characteristics that limit its ability to traverse the fine filtering system of the spleen. It is the ability of macrophages to recognize IgG on the surface of the red blood cell that accounts for the spherocytosis and hemolysis which occur in immunohemolytic anemias. Similarly, the mononuclear-phagocyte system's ability to recognize C3 on the red blood cell surface accounts for the destruction of red cells in the cold hemagglutin disorders, and it plays a synergistic role in those hemolytic processes due to IgG where C3 is also fixed.

Extreme deformations of shape are required for red blood cells to traverse orifices of diameter smaller than their own, as they must in the spleen. Their discoid shape favors deformability, providing a surface area that is 60 to 70 percent in excess of the minimum necessary to encompass the contents of red blood cells, thus permitting a portion of the cell surface to accommodate changes in cell shape. The red blood cell membrane can be readily bent; however, it offers a high resistance to stretch. The limits of deformability, therefore, depend on the surface area-to-volume ratio of the red blood cell. Osmotic fragility is a useful test of this ratio. The deformability of hereditary spherocytes and hereditary elliptocytes is decreased because their surface area is decreased, and these cells are selectively sequestered in the spleen. When pooled in the spleen pulp, red blood cells undergo a process known as "conditioning" wherein the spleen itself causes red blood cells to lose surface area. This also occurs when normal red blood cells become pooled in a hyperplastic or congested spleen, when they stagnate in the spleen owing to an abnormality of red blood cell structure, or when they are trapped in the spleen because of the presence of IgG on their surface. The result in each case is a further reduction in the red blood cell's surface area and in its ability to pass the spleen filter again, leading ultimately to irreversible trapping and destruction in the spleen.

A modification of the structural properties of the red blood cell membrane may also impair the cell's ability to flow through the spleen. The fluid properties of the membrane depend on a fixed relationship between the amounts of cholesterol and phospholipid present in the membrane. When, as in spur-cell anemia, the amount of cholesterol becomes excessive relative to the amount of phospholipid, the fluidity of the membrane decreases, resulting in splenic pooling, conditioning, and destruction of spur cells in the spleen. The elastic properties of the red blood cell membrane depend on the structure of proteins within the membrane and on the interaction of these proteins with ATP and calcium. Red blood cells undergo a disk-to-sphere transformation when they become ATP-depleted, as occurs when a glycolytic enzyme is deficient. This phenomenon also may play a role in the destruction of red blood cells in other disorders, such as hereditary spherocytosis. A change in the physical properties of the red blood cell membrane which occurs during the process of sickling in sickle-cell anemia appears to account for the rigidity of permanently sickled cells in this disorder.

The flow properties of the red blood cell are strongly influenced by the nature of the red blood cell's contents. A striking increase in intracellular viscosity accompanies sickling in sickle-cell anemia. A rise in internal viscosity also appears to play a role in the destruction of red blood cells in hemoglobin C disease (see below). Finally, the passage of red blood cells through the spleen filter is impeded by the presence of inclusion bodies within the red blood cell that consist of precipitated hemoglobin. Examples of this are the α-chain inclusions in β thalassemia, the unstable β tetramers in α thalassemia, and the hemoglobin which is precipitated as Heinz bodies in patients with unstable hemoglobins and during oxidant hemolysis in patients deficient in the enzyme glucose 6-phosphate dehydrogenase (G6PD); all are discussed later in this chapter.

RED CELL MORPHOLOGY AS A CLUE TO HEMOLYSIS

Most hemolytic disorders are associated with a change in the morphologic appearance of red blood cells. Some of these are depicted in Plate 9. Spherocytes are the most common morphologic abnormality in hemolytic diseases, and small numbers occur in many disorders. They are most striking in patients with hereditary spherocytosis and in patients with warm antibody-induced immunohemolytic disease (Plates 9-13 and 9-14). Some patients with oxidant hemolysis have increased numbers of spherocytes, and spherocytes are the hallmark of splenic conditioning. Fragmented red blood cells raise the possibility of valve hemolysis, or one of the microangiopathic hemolytic anemias such as thrombotic thrombocytopenic purpura (Plate 9-15), hemolytic uremic syndrome, or disseminated intravascular coagulation. Target-shaped red blood cells which are well filled with hemoglobin occur in the absence of demonstrable disease in patients with hemoglobin C trait. They are prevalent in sickle-cell anemia, where they were first described, and they are found in patients with the underhydrated form of the hereditary stomatocytosis syndrome. The most common cause of target cells is liver disease of many etiologies. A distinctive type of target cell, with a crystalloid appearance, occurs in patients homozygous for hemoglobin C. Target cells which are deficient in hemoglobin (hypochromic) are the hallmark of the thalassemia syndromes.

Spiculated red blood cells often cause confusion because of the frequency with which they are induced as an artifact during the preparation of a blood smear. Under these conditions, they are particularly frequent at the edges of the smear. When surrounded by otherwise normal-appearing red blood cells, spiculated red blood cells can be a clue to diagnosis. They occur, usually in small numbers, in conjunction with uremia, and they are seen in small numbers following splenectomy even in the absence of an underlying red blood cell disorder. Bizarrely spiculated red blood cells (acanthocytes) occur in the rare condition abetalipoproteinemia (Chap. 100) and in anorexia nervosa; however, in each of these instances minimal hemolysis is present. As discussed below, acanthocytes are a striking feature of spur-cell anemia (Plate 9-12).

Permanently sickled, crescent-shaped red blood cells (Plate 9-16) are the hallmark of sickle-cell anemia (discussed below). Modifications of their structure to a boat-shape is a clue to the double heterozygous state of hemoglobin SC disease (see below). The presence of both crescent-shaped cells and hypochromic target cells on the same smear is suggestive of the doubly heterozygous state, sickle-cell–thalassemia disease.

While in no case can the peripheral blood smear be totally diagnostic, in many it is a low-cost, important clue to the diagnosis.

EXTRINSIC CAUSES OF HEMOLYSIS

SPLENOMEGALY The spleen is particularly efficient in trapping and destroying red blood cells which have minimal defects, often so mild as to be undetectable by in vitro techniques. This unique ability of the spleen to filter mildly damaged red blood cells results from its unusual vascular anatomy. Almost all the blood circulating through the spleen flows directly from arterioles in the white pulp to sinuses in the spleen's red pulp, and then on into the venous system. In contrast, a small portion of splenic blood flow (normally 1 to 2 percent) leaves the arterioles of the white pulp to enter a nonendothelialized portion of the spleen. In this sense, it is extravascular, although the entire spleen may be considered as a specialized part of the vascular system. This blood passes into the "marginal zone" of the lymphatic white pulp. Although the reticuloendothelial cells which occupy this zone are not phagocytic, they serve as a mechanical filter hindering the progress of damaged red blood cells. As red blood cells leave this zone and enter the red pulp, they flow into narrow cords which end blindly but which communicate with sinuses through small openings between the lining cells of the sinuses. These openings, averaging 3 μm in diameter, test the ability of red blood cells to undergo a deformation of shape. Red blood cells which do not pass the stringent test imposed upon them by the spleen filter are engulfed by phagocytic cells and destroyed.

The normal spleen poses no threat to normal red blood cells. However, splenomegaly exaggerates the adverse conditions to which red blood cells are exposed. Splenic enlargement may be considered in three broad categories. In the first are infiltrative disease (such as myeloproliferative disorders, Chaps. 320, 325, and 326), lymphomas (Chap. 327), and storage diseases (such as Gaucher's disease, Chap. 322). In the second are systemic inflammatory diseases leading to splenic hypertrophy. In the third are diseases in which the red blood cell's passage through the spleen is retarded by congestive splenomegaly. The second and third categories are considered in detail in Chap. 322, "Disorders of the Spleen and Reticuloendothelial System." These latter two categories are associated with an increased hemolytic rate. Hemolysis may occur whenever the spleen is enlarged. Its occurrence is least predictable in infiltrative diseases of the spleen where substantial splenomegaly may exist with no apparent hemolysis. Inflammatory and congestive splenomegaly are commonly associated with mild to moderate shortening of red blood cell survival.

RED CELL ANTIBODIES Immune hemolysis in the adult may be induced by three general types of antibodies:

1 Alloantibodies acquired by blood transfusions or pregnancies and directed against transfused red blood cells.
2 Antibodies reactive at body temperature and directed against the patient's own red blood cells. These may be formed in the absence of other disease manifestations or in association with certain drugs or with another disease, commonly one related to the immune system.
3 Antibodies reactive in the cold and directed against the patient's own red blood cells and which, like warm antibodies, may be formed in association with diseases of the immune system (Table 314-1).

Coombs' antiglobulin test is the major tool for diagnosing these disorders. This test relies on the ability of antibodies prepared in rabbits, goats, or other animals and directed against specific human serum proteins to agglutinate red blood cells if these human serum proteins are present on the red blood cell surface. The serum proteins of particular interest are IgG and C3. The ability of anti-IgG or anti-C3 antiserums to agglutinate the patient's red blood cells is referred to as the *direct Coombs test*. At times it is advantageous to know whether there is antibody in the serum of patients which is reactive against other human red blood cells. This is important in cross matching prior to blood transfusion (Chap. 319), and it is of prognostic significance in patients with warm-antibody hemolytic anemia. To determine this, an *indirect Coombs test* is performed by incubating ABO- and Rh-compatible red blood cells with the patient's serum and subsequently performing a direct Coombs test on these incubated red cells.

Alloantibodies Problems arising from the transfusion of incompatible red blood cells are discussed in Chap. 319.

"Warm" antibodies Antibodies which react at body temperature are usually of the IgG class, although occasionally they are of the IgA class. They induce a pattern of hemolysis which affects both the patient's own cells and normal transfused cells. This acquired syndrome is frequently designated *autoimmune hemolytic anemia*. In recent years, as a number of drugs which induce this clinical syndrome have become recognized, attention has focused on the exogenous factors which may underlie the formation of these red blood cell antibodies, and the expression *immunohemolytic anemia* is preferred.

CLINICAL MANIFESTATIONS Warm-antibody immunohemolytic anemia occurs at all ages but is most common in adults, women more frequently than men, and individuals in the fourth, fifth, and sixth decades more frequently than younger adults. In approximately one-fourth of patients this disorder occurs as a complication of an underlying disease affecting the immune system. The most common are chronic lymphocytic leukemia, non-Hodgkin's lymphoma, and systemic lupus erythematosus (SLE). This syndrome occasionally is seen in patients with advanced, active Hodgkin's disease. Case reports link it to a variety of nonlymphoid neoplasms.

The presentation and course of immunohemolytic anemia is quite variable. In its mildest form, the only manifestation is a positive Coombs test. In this instance, insufficient antibody is present on the red blood cell surface to permit the reticuloendothelial system to recognize the cell as abnormal. This is particularly common in SLE. A large fraction of patients with immunohemolytic anemia have a chronic mild anemia and splenomegaly. The direct Coombs test is positive for IgG but not for C3, and the indirect Coombs test is negative. In other cases this disorder may be more severe, with hemoglobin levels less than 7.0 g per 100 ml and reticulocyte counts of 30 percent and higher. Spherocytosis is usually marked. Coombs' test is

positive for IgG and frequently for C3 as well. This latter finding relates to the large number of antibody molecules per red blood cell providing the opportunity for two molecules to be close enough together on the cell surface to fix complement. The large quantity of antibody is also demonstrable by the indirect Coombs test, which demonstrates antibody not only on the patient's red blood cells but also in the patient's serum. Thrombocytopenia may also be present, and the coexistence of immune destruction of red blood cells and platelets is referred to as *Evans' syndrome*. Possibly because they all reflect the presence of a large amount of antibody, a positive Coombs test for C3, a positive indirect Coombs test, and thrombocytopenia are all poor prognostic signs. In its most severe form, immunohemolytic anemia presents with fulminant, overwhelming hemolysis associated with hemoglobinemia, hemoglobinuria, and shock, a syndrome which may be fatal.

Associated findings include hyperbilirubinemia, decreased haptoglobin levels, and occasionally hepatomegaly. Fever and abdominal pain occur in some patients. Venous thrombosis occurs commonly, the most frequent site being the deep veins of the legs, but thrombosis of mesenteric and portal veins has also been reported. Arterial thromboses occur as well.

PATHOGENESIS Little is known about the origin of red blood cell antibodies in the immunohemolytic anemias. Much more information exists concerning the mechanism of destruction of red blood cells coated with IgG antibodies. Although spherocytosis is often a prominent feature of hemolysis in vivo, the simple exposure of normal red blood cells to IgG antibodies does not lead to spherocytosis in vitro. However, human red blood cells coated with IgG antibodies are bound to the surface of monocytes or splenic macrophages and undergo a spherical transformation. The ability to cause this red blood cell–leukocyte interaction is greatest with IgG of subclasses 1 and 3 (the most common subclasses). It is not shared by IgM or IgA. However, C3 on the red blood cell surface also promotes this cell-cell interaction, but binding may be more transient because of the ability of the plasma C3 inactivator to release bound cells. Indeed, IgG and C3 behave in a synergistic fashion in this regard, accounting for the more severe hemolytic disease in patients in whom both IgG and C3 are present on the red blood cell surface. The slow flow compartment of the spleen is particularly efficient in trapping red blood cells which are coated with IgG antibodies, and the spleen is the major site of red blood cell destruction in this disorder.

THERAPY AND PROGNOSIS In the initial evaluation of the patient, it is important to rule out drugs which are known to cause immunohemolytic anemia. This topic is discussed below.

TABLE 314-1
Hemolysis due to antibodies

I Warm-antibody immunohemolytic anemia
  A Idiopathic
  B Lymphomas: Chronic lymphocytic leukemia, non-Hodgkin's lymphomas, Hodgkin's disease (infrequent)
  C Systemic lupus erythematosus
  D Tumors (rare)
  E Drugs
    1 α-Methyldopa type
    2 Penicillin type (hapten)
    3 Quinidine type (innocent bystander)
II Cold-antibody immunohemolytic anemia
  A Cold agglutinin disease
    1 Acute: Mycoplasma infection, infectious mononucleosis
    2 Chronic: Idiopathic, lymphoma
  B Paroxysmal cold hemoglobinuria

Patients having a mild degree of hemolysis usually do not require therapy. In those with clinically significant hemolysis, initial therapy consists of corticosteroids (e.g., prednisone, 1.0 mg/kg per day). A fall in reticulocytes and rise in hemoglobin are frequently noted within 3 or 4 days and occur in most patients within 1 week. Prednisone is continued until the hemoglobin level has risen to normal values, and thereafter it is tapered slowly over the course of several months. More than 75 percent of patients will achieve a significant and sustained improvement; however, in half of these patients the disease will relapse either during the period of steroid tapering or following the cessation of steroid therapy. Steroids appear to have two modes of action. An immediate effect is seen due to a steroid-induced inhibition of the monocytes' recognition of IgG-coated red blood cells. A second effect is the steroid-induced inhibition of antibody synthesis.

Patients with severe anemia may require blood transfusions. Because the antibody in this disease is a "panagglutinin," reacting with all normal donor cells, cross matching may be impossible. It is a practice of most hematologists to select donor cells which are ABO-compatible and appear to give the least amount of agglutination when Coombs' test is performed subsequent to incubation with the patient's serum. These red blood cells are administered slowly with attention paid to the possibility of an immediate-type transfusion reaction.

Splenectomy is the second line of therapy in this disorder. It is recommended for patients who cannot tolerate steroid therapy, in whom steroid therapy has been insufficient to control the disease process, or in whom a normal hematologic status can be maintained only with excessive doses of steroids. When red blood cells are labeled with chromium, their site of destruction can be determined. In 75 percent of patients, the spleen is the dominant site, whereas the liver predominates in the remaining patients. While it was hoped that this test would serve as a useful method of selecting those patients who would respond to splenectomy, this has not been the general experience. Rather, a favorable response to splenectomy is obtained in approximately two-thirds of patients in whom a splenic pattern of localization is found and in approximately one-third of patients in whom it is not found. Therefore, splenectomy must be undertaken on clinical grounds alone. Unlike hereditary spherocytosis, where splenectomy carries a very low morbidity and mortality, it poses a greater risk to patients with immunohemolytic anemia, particularly those with an underlying disease of the lymphoid system.

In recent years, patients who have been refractory to steroid therapy and to splenectomy have been treated with immunosuppressive drugs. The greatest experience is with azathioprine (Imuran) and cyclophosphamide (Cytoxan). A variable success rate has been reported with each.

In the majority of patients, this disease is controlled by steroid therapy alone, by splenectomy, or by a combination. In most of the remaining patients, a partial degree of control is achieved. Fatalities occur among three categories of patients: first, those with overwhelming hemolysis and in whom death is directly attributable to anemia; second, those with major thrombotic or infectious complications following splenectomy; third, those whose host defenses are impaired by corticosteroids, splenectomy, and/or immunosuppressives. In patients in whom immunohemolysis develops as a complication of an underlying disorder, the prognosis is dominated by that of the primary disease.

Immunohemolytic anemia secondary to drugs Drugs which have been directly related to immunohemolytic anemia are of three kinds, as distinguished by their three mechanisms of action: (1) Drugs, such as α-methyldopa (Chap. 251), which induce a disorder identical almost in every respect to the warm-antibody immunohemolytic anemia described above. (2) Drugs of the penicillin type which can become associated with the red blood cell surface and induce the formation of an antibody directed against the red blood cell–drug complex. (3) Drugs, such as quinidine, that form a complex with plasma proteins to which an antibody forms; this drug–plasma protein–antibody complex settles out on red blood cells or platelets to involve them in a destructive process on an "innocent bystander" basis.

α-METHYLDOPA-TYPE ANTIBODIES A positive direct Coombs test is observed in up to 10 percent of patients receiving α-methyldopa therapy in a dose of 2.0 g daily. A small minority of these patients develop spherocytosis and hemolysis, often of severe degree. Two distinctive features are that the indirect Coombs test is positive in almost all patients with hemolysis and that there are no reports of patients who also have C3 on their red blood cell surface. Hemolysis decreases over the course of several weeks after cessation of drug therapy, although the direct Coombs test may remain positive for more than 1 year.

PENICILLIN (HAPTEN)-INDUCED IMMUNOHEMOLYSIS An antibody directed against "penicillinized" red blood cells induces spherocytosis and hemolysis in patients receiving large, intravenous doses of penicillin and penicillin-type antibiotics (e.g., 15 to 20 million units of penicillin per day, or 12 to 15 g oxacillin per day). Hemolysis usually begins 7 to 14 days after the start of penicillin therapy and is associated with spherocytosis and hyperbilirubinemia. The patient's red blood cells are Coombs-positive for IgG during the period of penicillin therapy. An indirect Coombs test can be demonstrated with the patient's serum using normal red blood cells "penicillinized" in vitro. Hemolysis ceases abruptly when penicillin therapy is stopped, although the serum antibody can be demonstrated for many weeks.

INNOCENT BYSTANDER IMMUNOHEMOLYSIS Innocent bystander antibodies may be of either the IgG or IgM class, and the antigen-antibody complexes which adhere to the red blood cell surface are capable of fixing complement. The drug-antibody complex dissociates from the red blood cell, leaving only C3 to be detected by Coombs' test. The pattern of hemolysis may be primarily extravascular red blood cell destruction, or it may be intravascular hemolysis due to complement lysis with hemoglobinemia, hemoglobinuria, and acute renal failure. This is an uncommon form of hemolysis despite the fact that the drugs associated with it are in very common usage. They include quinine and quinidine, isoniazid, sulfonamides, plenacetin, stibophen, p-aminosalicylic acid, dipyrone, and various insecticides.

Immune hemolysis due to cold-reactive antibodies Antibodies which are reactive in the cold induce hemolysis under two general conditions. First, in cold agglutinin disease IgM antibodies, usually reactive with the I antigen, occur spontaneously, in the course of a lymphoproliferative disease or as a complication of infectious mononucleosis or mycoplasma pneumonia. Second, in paroxysmal cold hemoglobinuria, antibodies of the IgG class (Donath-Landsteiner) occur spontaneously or as a complication of syphilis or of certain viral diseases.

COLD AGGLUTININ DISEASE *Clinical manifestations.* Agglutination of red blood cells by IgM cold agglutinins is most profound at very low temperatures, and disagglutination occurs quickly upon warming. In most patients agglutination ceases at 32°C. The fixation of complement is a warm-reactive process. Therefore, patients may have very high titers of cold agglutinins as measured at low temperatures, but these antibodies may be inefficient in fixing complement to the cell surface and totally unable to induce agglutination at temperatures achieved in the bloodstream. Most cold agglutinins cause little or no shortening of red blood cell survival.

In mycoplasma pneumonia, cold agglutinins are very common, whereas only the occasional patient will have sufficient hemolysis to develop an acutely falling hematocrit associated with reticulocytosis. Spherocytes may be seen occasionally, but the red blood cell morphology is usually normal. The antibody is directed against the I antigen, and the entire process is self-limited.

The cold agglutinin in infectious mononucleosis is most frequently directed against the i antigen, an antigen accessible on the surface of fetal red blood cells but not adult red blood cells. Therefore, this cold agglutinin is of serologic interest, but rarely induces hemolysis in humans. Antibody directed against the I antigen and complex antibodies involving both antigens have also been reported, with hemolysis.

A chronic form of cold-induced hemolysis occurs in patients spontaneously or in association with lymphoid neoplasms, most commonly affecting individuals in their seventh or eighth decades. The clinical manifestations relate to hemolysis and less commonly to agglutination of red blood cells in capillaries in those portions of the body exposed to low temperature, causing acrocyanosis. Gangrene is uncommon. Hemoglobin levels are usually above 10 g per 100 ml and rarely below 7 g. Reticulocytes are fewer in number than might be anticipated, presumably because of the selective destruction of young cells (including reticulocytes) in this disorder.

In most patients with cold agglutinin disease, the antibody titer is very high (e.g., 1:10,000) at 4°C and very low (e.g., 1:16) at 37°C. In some patients the antibody shows a flatter thermal spectrum with a moderately high titer at 4°C (e.g., 1:320) and a readily demonstrable titer at 37°C (e.g., 1:64). Hemolysis tends to be more severe in this latter group. The Coombs' test demonstrates the presence of C3 on the red blood cell surface, but IgM is usually not found, and IgG is not present.

Pathogenesis. The etiology of the antibody is unknown. It appears to exert its hemolytic effect not through agglutination per se but rather by the fixation of C3 to the red blood cell surface. The liver is particularly efficient at detecting red blood cells coated with C3 in the form of C3b and clearing them from the circulation. A plasma enzyme, C3 inactivator, is capable of cleaving C3b into a small fragment (C3c) which leaves the cell surface and reenters the plasma, and C3d, which adheres to the red blood cell surface where it is recognized as C3 in Coombs' test but not as C3 by the mononuclear phagocyte system. The presence of C3d on the red blood cell surface decreases the ability of IgM anti-I to begin anew the complement sequence and thereby reestablish C3b on the red cell surface. Because of this, red blood cells that have survived in the circulation for a period of time have become "protected," while the younger red blood cells are in greater jeopardy.

Therapy. The cutaneous manifestations of this disorder are best treated by maintaining the patient in a warm environment. Because transfusion of normal blood presents to the patient a large number of red blood cells which have not previously been exposed to the cold agglutinin and are therefore not "protected," transfusion may be associated with an acceleration of the hemolytic process. Splenectomy is usually not of value in this disorder. Corticosteroids are of limited value, although patients with the panthermal variety of cold agglutinin disease may respond favorably to this therapy. Chlorambucil and cyclophosphamide are the most commonly employed agents in those patients in whom therapy is indicated. Al-

though some patients have experienced a dramatic improvement, the effectiveness of this therapy is marginal in most patients.

Cold agglutinin disease tends to be chronic and unremitting. The overall prognosis is dominated by the underlying lymphoproliferative disease, if present. In those patients in whom cold agglutinin disease appears to arise spontaneously, lymphoproliferative disease may become apparent after several years.

PAROXYSMAL COLD HEMOGLOBINURIA (PCH)   Now a rare disorder, PCH was more frequent at a time when tertiary syphilis was more prevalent. It results from the formation of the Donath-Landsteiner antibody, an IgG antibody directed against the P-antigen of the red blood cell surface. Attacks are precipitated by exposure to cold and are associated with hemoglobinemia and hemoglobinuria, chills and fever, back, leg, and abdominal pain, headache, and malaise. Recovery from the acute episode is prompt, and between episodes patients are asymptomatic. When this syndrome accompanies acute viral infections (e.g., measles and mumps), it is self-limited. When secondary to syphilis, it responds favorably to specific therapy for this disorder. No specific therapy exists for idiopathic cases. Despite the severity of individual episodes, the natural history of this disease extends over many years.

TRAUMA IN THE CIRCULATION   Red blood cells are exposed to trauma which disrupts their integrity under three general conditions: (1) when they flow through small vessels over the surface of bony prominences and are subject to impact trauma in the course of various physical activities; (2) when they flow across a pressure gradient created by an abnormal heart valve or valve prosthesis and undergo a shear stress which disrupts them; (3) when the deposition of fibrin in the microvasculature exposes them to a physical impediment that fragments them (Table 314-2).

External impact   Hemoglobinemia and hemoglobinuria have been observed in individuals who have undergone a prolonged

TABLE 314-2
Disturbances of the formed elements of blood secondary to intravascular trauma

Etiology	Fragments	Hemolysis	Thrombocytopenia
Impact: march hemoglobinuria, karate, playing bongo drums, etc.	0	+	0
Cardiac (turbulence):			
Aortic valve prosthesis	+ + +	+ + + +	0
Ostium primum repair	+ + + +	+ + + +	0
Mitral valve prosthesis	+ +	+ +	0
Calcific aortic stenoses	+	±	0
Vessel disease: Malignant hypertension Eclampsia Renal graft rejection Hemangiomas Immune disease (scleroderma)	+ + +	+	+
Thrombotic thrombocytopenic purpura	+ + + +	+ + + +	+ + + +
Hemolytic uremic syndrome	+ + + +	+ + + +	+ + +
Disseminated intravascular coagulation	+ +	±	+ + + +

march or a prolonged jog, most typically on a hard surface and while wearing thin-soled shoes. The role of direct external trauma in this process has been demonstrated by the fact that hemolysis can be prevented by the insertion of a soft inner sole in the runner's shoes. Similar types of hemolysis have been described following karate and the playing of bongo drums. No abnormality of red blood cell morphology has been demonstrated, even during the acute episode, and no underlying red blood cell abnormality has been uncovered. A large percentage of individuals will develop hemoglobinemia and hemoglobinuria when exposed to the conditions described above. Myoglobinuria commonly accompanies this process, a manifestation of muscle damage also occurring during some of these activities. There are no known instances of renal impairment, and no specific therapy is required.

Cardiac hemolysis   Hemolysis associated with fragmented red blood cells (Plate 9-15) occurs in approximately 10 percent of patients with artificial aortic valve prostheses, and this incidence is somewhat greater with valves having stellite rather than silastic occluders, greater with small valves as compared with larger valves, and greater when valves are cloth-covered. Traumatic hemolysis is much less common in recipients of porcine valves. Severe hemolysis occurs after repair of ostium primum or endocardial cushion defects with a prosthetic patch. Mitral valve prostheses have also been associated with hemolysis, but since the pressure gradient across these is lower than across aortic protheses, the incidence is lower. A moderately shortened red blood cell survival (chromium half-survivals of 15 to 20 days) with little or no anemia occurs in some patients with severe calcific aortic stenosis. Indeed, almost any intracardiac lesion which alters hemodynamics may lead to some shortening of red blood cell survival. In addition, traumatic hemolysis has been observed in patients who have undergone aortofemoral bypass.

CLINICAL MANIFESTATIONS   In severe cases hemoglobin levels fall to 5.0 to 7.0 g per 100 ml with reticulocytosis, fragmented red blood cells in the peripheral blood, depressed haptoglobin, elevated serum lactic dehydrogenase, and hemoglobinemia and hemoglobinuria. Iron loss (as hemoglobin or hemosiderin) in the urine may lead to iron deficiency. Coombs' test may become positive.

PATHOGENESIS   A number of factors combine to cause the fragmentation and destruction of red blood cells in this disorder. Direct mechanical trauma of red blood cells at the time of seating of the occluder of the prosthetic valve, the deposition of fibrin across disrupted attachment points, but probably most important, the shear stress resulting from turbulent blood flow may all result in the fragmentation of red blood cells. The last explains the higher incidence of hemolysis in patients who have a paravalvular leak and therefore greater velocity of blood flow across the aortic orifice during systole.

THERAPY AND PROGNOSIS   Iron deficiency should be corrected by the administration of oral iron, and the elevated hemoglobin which results may permit a decrease in the cardiac output and a slowing of the hemolytic rate. Corticosteroid therapy has been successful in partially alleviating the hemolysis in some patients. A limitation in physical activity usually lessens the hemolytic rate. When these measures fail, any paravalvular leak must be repaired or the prosthetic valve removed and replaced by a tissue valve.

Deposition of fibrin in the microvasculature   Fibrin becomes deposited in the microvasculature where it traps platelets and fragments red blood cells, under three general conditions: (1) abnormalities of the vessel wall in recognized disorders, such as malignant hypertension, eclampsia, rejection of a renal allograft, disseminated cancer, and hemangiomas; (2) two potentially fatal syndromes of unknown etiology, thrombotic thrombocytopenic purpura and the hemolytic uremic syndrome; and (3) disseminated intravascular coagulation.

ABNORMALITIES OF THE VESSEL WALL IN RECOGNIZED DISORDERS   The degree of hemolysis induced by this family of disorders is usually quite mild, although the number of fragments in the peripheral blood may be striking. In occasional patients, thrombocytopenia may be severe. In each case, therapy is best directed at the primary disease. Thus, reversal of renal graft rejection, treatment of malignant hypertension and eclampsia, control of cancer, etc., lead to a cessation of the hemolytic process. The relative importance of the primary vascular abnormality and of the deposition of fibrin in causing hemolysis is unclear.

THROMBOTIC THROMBOCYTOPENIC PURPURA (TTP)   This disease of unknown etiology affects individuals of all ages but primarily young adults, more often women.

   Clinical manifestations. Hemolysis is a striking feature of this disease. Anemia occurs in association with fragmented red blood cells, nucleated red cells in the peripheral blood, an elevated reticulocyte count, and thrombocytopenia of varying degree. Platelet counts range from 5000 to 100,000 per cubic millimeter. Jaundice is common, and petechiae may be present, although usually to a less striking degree than in idiopathic thrombocytopenic purpura (ITP). Tests of coagulation, such as the prothrombin time, partial thromboplastin time, fibrinogen concentration, and the level of fibrinogen split products, are usually entirely normal. If the coagulation tests indicate disseminated intravascular coagulation, the diagnosis of TTP is doubtful. Erythroid hyperplasia and an increased number of megakaryocytes are present in the bone marrow. The life span of platelets is decreased to hours, and no site of organ localization of destroyed platelets is observed. A positive lupus erythematosus cell test or antinuclear antibody is obtained in approximately 20 percent of patients. Some patients experience significant bleeding of uterine, gastrointestinal, or other origin, but severe bleeding is not common. Fever is present in almost all patients, and many experience nonspecific constitutional symptoms such as nausea, abdominal pain, and arthralgias. The spleen and liver may be palpable.

   The course of TTP spans days to weeks in most patients, but occasionally continues for months. As the disease progresses, the brain and kidneys become progressively involved, and their dysfunction is the ultimate cause of death in the majority of patients. Proteinuria and a moderate elevation of blood urea nitrogen may be present on initial presentation, and there is a continued rise in blood urea nitrogen and a fall in urine output as the disease progresses. Neurologic symptoms evolve in more than 90 percent of patients whose disease terminates in death. Initially, there may be changes in mental status such as confusion, delirium, or altered states of consciousness. Focal findings include seizures, hemiparesis, aphasia, and visual field defects. These neurologic symptoms may fluctuate and terminate in coma. Involvement of myocardial blood vessels may be a cause of sudden death in some patients.

   Pathogenesis. The etiology of TTP is unknown. Arterioles are filled with hyalin material, presumably fibrin and platelets, and similar material may be seen beneath the endothelium of otherwise uninvolved vessels. Immunofluorescence studies have shown the presence of immunoglobulin and complement in arterioles. Microaneurysms of arterioles are often present. Controversy exists concerning the specificity of these changes, some authorities noting them in the hemolytic uremic syndrome and in disseminated intravascular coagulation. An association with systemic lupus erythematosus (SLE), scleroderma, and Sjögren's syndrome suggests an immunologic etiology.

Diagnosis. The combination of hemolytic anemia with fragmented and nucleated red blood cells, thrombocytopenia, fever, neurologic disorders, and renal dysfunction is virtually pathognomonic for TTP. The diagnosis is further supported by the finding of normal coagulation tests, although occasional patients have an isolated abnormality of coagulation. In about 50 percent of cases, a biopsy of skin and muscle, gingiva, lymph node, or bone marrow will reveal pathologic abnormalities described above. It is advantageous to establish the diagnosis prior to the onset of renal or neurologic disease. When these two complications are absent, the major differential is idiopathic thrombocytopenic purpura, and TTP should be considered in every patient in whom the diagnosis of ITP or Evans' syndrome (ITP plus immunohemolytic anemia) is made. Because the clinical course can fluctuate widely, therapy is difficult to evaluate. The finding of fragmented red blood cells in the peripheral blood is particularly helpful in this regard.

Therapy and prognosis. Until recently, this disease was almost universally fatal. A large number of therapeutic modalities have been attempted with variable success. These include corticosteroids, exchange transfusion, splenectomy, heparin, and antiplatelet drugs. Patients are initially treated with high doses of corticosteroids (100 to 1000 mg prednisone per day). However, additional therapy is indicated once the diagnosis has been established. The most consistent improvement has been noted with exchange transfusion. It is unclear whether plasmapheresis is as effective as exchange transfusion. In some patients the response may depend upon the infusion of plasma. Splenectomy may also be effective, but this procedure poses additional risk in these critically ill patients. The additional benefit of antiplatelet drugs (Dipyridamole, sulfinpyrazone, dextran, aspirin) is unclear, but they are commonly used together with the therapeutic measures described above. Aspirin may increase the risk of bleeding and should be employed with caution. A few patients have improved after heparin infusion. Because of the ever-present risk of sudden death, therapy should be instituted promptly. Even deep coma is not a contraindication to therapy since full neurologic recovery is the rule in patients responding to therapy. If treatment is instituted early in the disease, remission occurs in at least one-third and possibly as many as two-thirds of patients. Relapses have been noted but are usually responsive to therapeutic intervention.

HEMOLYTIC UREMIC SYNDROME The hemolytic uremic syndrome is a disorder usually encountered in young children with laboratory features similar to those of TTP. Often the patient has a prodrome of a viral-like illness. Less commonly, the disorder appears to be familial. Patients present with acute hemolytic anemia, thrombocytopenic purpura, and acute oliguric renal failure. Most patients have either hemoglobinuria or anuria. Unlike TTP, neurologic manifestations are uncommon. The peripheral blood findings, coagulation tests, and pathologic changes on biopsy specimens are usually indistinguishable from those of TTP. Patients are treated with dialysis and transfusions. The efficacy of corticosteroids, dextran, and heparin is uncertain. The mortality in children ranges from 5 to 20 percent, but is considerably higher in adults.

DISSEMINATED INTRAVASCULAR COAGULATION (DIC) Red blood cell fragmentation in the microvasculature (microangiopathic hemolytic anemia) is a common accompaniment of DIC (Chap. 318). The degree of hemolysis is much less in DIC than in either TTP or the hemolytic uremic syndrome, and anemia with reticulocytosis and nucleated red blood cells is distinctly

rare. Indeed, fragmented red blood cells are seen in only 30 to 40 percent of patients with DIC.

DIRECT TOXIC EFFECTS A variety of infections may be associated with severe hemolysis. The causative agents in bartonellosis and malaria directly parasitize red blood cells. These two disorders are discussed in detail in Chaps. 136 and 200. Babesiosis also may cause a mild to moderate hemolytic anemia by direct parisitation of red blood cells.

Other infectious organisms exert their damaging effect on red blood cells indirectly. The most striking is that resulting from septicemia with *Clostridium welchii* (Chap. 141). The phospholipase produced by this organism is capable of cleaving the phosphoryl bond of lecithin thereby lysing human red blood cells. A mild, transient hemolysis frequently accompanies bacteremia with diverse organisms such as pneumococci, staphylococci, and *Escherichia coli*.

Hemolysis may result from the direct action of snake and spider venoms on the red blood cell. Although cobra venom is directly lytic in vitro, the clinical disease induced by the bite of the cobra is one of moderate hemolysis associated with spherocytosis. Spider bites are known to induce acute intravascular hemolysis associated with spherocytosis. It is thought that the brown recluse spider which inhabits the central and southern portions of the United States and portions of South America is responsible. The hemolytic disease continues for several days up to 1 week.

Copper has a direct hemolytic effect on red blood cells. Hemolysis has been observed following exposure of individuals to copper salts (such as during hemodialysis). In addition, the transient episodes of hemolysis observed in patients with Wilson's disease are probably due to copper toxicity.

The red blood cell membrane is unstable at temperatures above 49°C. When studied in vitro, the red blood cell undergoes a process of budding, cleavage, and resealing above this temperature. The same process is observed in individuals who have suffered extensive burns. Hemoglobinemia and hemoglobinuria may accompany this process, and spherocytosis is common.

MEMBRANE ABNORMALITIES

ACQUIRED DISORDERS OF THE MEMBRANE Spur-cell anemia Hemolytic anemia with bizarre-shaped red blood cells occurs in some patients with severe hepatocellular disease. Most patients with spur-cell anemia have advanced Laennec's cirrhosis, and this hemolytic disorder is observed in approximately 5 percent of patients with other manifestations of severe cirrhosis, such as ascites, jaundice, and hepatic encephalopathy. Spur-cell anemia has also been reported in neonatal hepatitis.

CLINICAL MANIFESTATIONS Anemia is moderate to severe, with hematocrit levels ranging from 16 to 30 percent. Thus, the anemia is more severe than is observed in otherwise uncomplicated cirrhosis, in which hematocrit levels are rarely below 28 percent, unless there is accompanying folic acid deficiency, blood loss, iron deficiency, etc. Splenomegaly is a constant feature, and the spleen is generally more prominent than in patients who have cirrhosis but who do not have spur-cell anemia. Jaundice is also a constant feature, and hepatic encephalopathy is common. Other tests of liver function are similar to values obtained in most patients with severe cirrhosis, although there is a tendency to longer prothrombin times. Chromium half-survival times of red blood cells are decreased to as short as 6 days (normal being 26 to 32 days), and red cell destruction is localized to the spleen. Normal transfused red blood cells have a survival similar to that of the patient's own red blood cells. Red blood cells are irregularly shaped with multiple spicules, and a small number of bizarre-shaped fragments are commonly seen on peripheral blood smears (see Fig. 53-7). Red blood cell osmotic fragility is within normal limits; however, both a "tail" of cells with increased fragility and a shoulder of osmotically resistant cells are commonly observed. Reticulocytes range from 5 to 15 percent.

PATHOGENESIS The surface membrane of spur cells contains 50 to 70 percent excess cholesterol, but its total phospholipid content is normal. In this way, spur cells are distinct from the more usual target red blood cells in liver disease, which possess an excess of both cholesterol and phospholipid. Cholesterol out of proportion of phospholipid decreases the fluidity of the spur-cell membrane, and therefore cell deformability. Normal red blood cells acquire the spur abnormality when incubated in serum from affected patients. This results from the presence in serum of an abnormal low-density lipoprotein with an increased mole ratio of free (unesterified) cholesterol to phospholipid. Thus, red blood cells in spur-cell anemia may be considered to be "innocent bystanders." These rigid, cholesterol-laden red blood cells are detected by the filtering system of the spleen, aided by congestive splenomegaly in cirrhosis. In contrast to circulating spur cells, normal red blood cells which have acquired cholesterol in vitro have an increased surface area and a decreased osmotic fragility, and they have a regular pattern of spicule deformity. This is also true in vivo for normal red blood cells during their initial 24 h in the circulation. However, during continued circulation in vivo in the presence of the spleen, cholesterol-rich spur cells lose surface area and transform to the irregular pattern of spiculation associated with acanthocytes (see "Red Blood Cell Morphology" above). This process of membrane "conditioning" by the spleen continues, and the cell is destroyed in the spleen.

DIAGNOSIS Increasing anemia in a patient with chronic cirrhosis most commonly results from blood loss, folic acid deficiency, or iron deficiency. The hemolytic rate may increase transiently during periods of acute fatty liver. The combination of an elevated reticulocyte count and elevated bilirubin in the presence of the characteristic morphologic abnormality on peripheral blood smear is diagnostic. Red blood cells of similar morphologic appearance are seen in patients with abetalipoproteinemia. However, these individuals have a minimal amount of hemolysis.

Spur cells and acanthocytes must be distinguished from regularly scalloped, crenated red blood cells (echinocytes). These are a frequent artifact on blood smears, and they are present in small numbers of patients with uremia ("burr cells"). Small, dense crenated spheres (spheroechinocytes) are seen in small numbers of patients with congenital nonspherocytic hemolytic anemia due to enzyme deficiencies in the Embden-Meyerhof pathway.

TREATMENT Since normal red blood cells acquire the spur abnormality when transfused into patients with this form of anemia, transfusion therapy is of limited benefit. Attempts to influence red blood cell cholesterol by the use of various lipid-lowering agents have thus far been unsuccessful. Splenectomy has been reported to prevent both the conditioning of red blood cells in the spleen and their premature destruction. However, splenectomy carries a high risk in patients with severe liver disease complicated by portal hypertension and co-

agulation defects, and it must be reserved for selected patients in whom hemolysis is a major clinical problem and who appear to be relatively good surgical risks.

PROGNOSIS In most patients spur-cell anemia occurs during the late stages of cirrhosis, and more than 90 percent of patients succumb to their underlying liver disease within 1 year of the diagnosis of spur-cell anemia.

Paroxysmal nocturnal hemoglobinuria (PNH) This condition is distinctive among hemolytic disorders in humans because it is an acquired, intracorpuscular defect. It occurs primarily in young adults, but it has also been reported in other age groups.

CLINICAL MANIFESTATIONS Anemia is of exceedingly variable degree with hematocrit values of 20 percent and lower in occasional patients and normal values in others. Mild granulocytopenia and thrombocytopenia are commonly present. Although hemoglobinuria is the classic feature of this disease, gross hemoglobinuria is present only intermittently in most patients, and in some gross hemoglobinuria never occurs. Hemosiderinuria is usually present. Other features of diagnostic significance are a low leukocyte alkaline phosphatase and a low red blood cell acetylcholinesterase. This disorder masquerades, often for several years, as a refractory anemia or as hypoplastic anemia with hyperplastic bone marrow. Red blood cells are normochromic and normocytic unless iron deficiency has occurred from the chronic loss of iron in the urine. The diagnosis is established by a positive acid hemolysis test or sucrose lysis test. Venous thromboses are a common complication of this disorder, and they have been reported in peripheral veins as well as in mesenteric, hepatic, portal, and cerebral veins. Thromboses are a common cause of death in patients severely affected with PNH. A second complication, possibly related to thromboses in small veins, is the occurrence of back and abdominal pain similar in character to that which occurs in sickle-cell anemia. Headache has also been reported. Since the widespread use of the sucrose lysis test, many patients have been discovered with mild, chronic disease.

PATHOGENESIS The underlying abnormality which affects red blood cells, granulocytes, and platelets in PNH is an inordinate sensitivity to complement. This may be demonstrated in vitro using a complement-fixing antibody. PNH red blood cells fix more Cl than normal red cells per unit of antibody present, and this Cl promotes more C3 fixation per molecule of Cl than is seen with normal red cells. However, antibody is not necessary for the lysis of red blood cells in PNH. Rather, C3 is readily fixed to the red blood cell surface by means of the alternate (properdin) pathway. Careful analytic procedures have demonstrated two and in some cases three separate populations of red blood cells with varying sensitivities to complement in patients with PNH. The clinical manifestations relate directly to the proportion of the red blood cells produced that are most sensitive to complement. Although platelets share with red blood cells this sensitivity to complement, platelet survival is normal in PNH. However, a functional modification of platelets induced by complement may underlie the thrombotic complications of this disease.

Since it affects granulocytes, platelets, and red blood cells but not lymphocytes, this defect is thought to occur because of an acquired change in the stem cell which generates these cells. In this respect it is similar to both acute myelogenous leukemia and the myeloproliferative syndromes, disorders which appear to affect the stem cells responsible for platelet, granulocyte, and red blood cell production. Both acute myelogenous leukemia and PNH may be secondary manifestations of a primary bone marrow injury that is manifested initially as aplastic anemia. Moreover, a number of patients with PNH have subsequently developed acute myelogenous leukemia. The red blood cell abnormality characteristic of PNH (complement sensitivity) occurs to a mild degree in some patients with aplastic anemia and in some with myelofibrosis, further linking this series of bone marrow disorders. Thus, although the precise mechanism has not been identified, it appears likely that PNH results from a mutation in the marrow stem-cell pool. The exact phenotypic representation of this presumed mutation is not known. Because the treatment of normal red blood cells with high concentrations of sulfhydryl reactive compounds (such as cysteine and glutathione) causes a PNH-like abnormality, the basic defect may involve membrane proteins with functionally important sulfhydryl groups.

DIAGNOSIS   As indicated above, PNH is commonly undiagnosed for a period of months to years. The classic manifestation of gross hemoglobinuria may be present only intermittently, and an awareness of its presence may be obtained only by repeated questioning of the patient. In some patients, a chronic hemolytic process occurs without gross hemoglobinuria. Therefore, diagnoses such as refractory anemia, hemolytic anemia of unknown etiology, and pancytopenia are common in patients subsequently diagnosed as having PNH. A decreased leukocyte alkaline phosphatase is a clue to the diagnosis, and the presence of hemosiderin in the urine sediment is strongly suggestive. Hemosiderinuria may occur with intravascular hemolysis of any etiology. However, only a few disorders in humans result in intravascular hemolysis. These are PNH, paroxysmal cold hemoglobinuria, hemolytic transfusion reaction, traumatic hemolysis, and hemolysis due to lysins (snake venom, *C. welchii* bacteremia) or to extensive acute burns. The acid hemolysis test is also positive in the rare congenital disorder, hereditary erythrocytic multinuclearity with positive acidified-serum test (HEMPAS). In this latter disorder, complement sensitivity results from an inordinate fixation of C4 molecules per molecule of C1. Since this sensitivity exists in the classic (antibody-mediated) pathway but not in the alternate (properdin) pathway, spontaneous fixation of complement with lysis in vivo is not a feature of the HEMPAS disorder.

It should be noted that chromium survival studies often produce information which is confusing in PNH. This results from the bi- or trimodal population of red blood cells. The cells most sensitive to complement have a very short survival, and they account for a minority of circulating red blood cells, whereas the cells less sensitive to complement have a more normal survival and account for the majority of circulating cells. Thus, the chromium survival is longer than might be anticipated from other measures of hemoglobin turnover.

TREATMENT   Transfusion therapy is useful in PNH not only for raising the hemoglobin level but also for suppressing the marrow production of red blood cells during episodes of sustained hemoglobinuria or of sustained painful crisis. The transfusion of blood prior to surgery may reduce the incidence of postoperative thrombotic complications. For reasons that are still unclear, whole blood transfusions frequently cause an exacerbation of the hemolytic process. This can be prevented by using washed red blood cells rather than whole blood.

Therapy with androgens frequently results in a rise of hemoglobin level. Either testosterone cyclopentylpropionate, 1 g per week parenterally, or fluoxymesterone, 20 to 30 mg per day, can be used. Adrenocorticoids are generally without benefit, although occasional patients may experience an amelioration of their disease with modest daily doses (e.g., 10 to 20 mg prednisone per day).

Because of iron loss in the urine, iron deficiency is common. An exacerbation of hemolysis often follows the administration of iron because of the formation of a large number of young red blood cells, many of which are sensitive to complement.

This may be minimized by suppressing the bone marrow with transfusions.

Splenectomy has been undertaken in some patients with the hope of decreasing the hemolytic rate and the transfusion requirement. However, because of the limited therapeutic benefit and the high risk attendant upon surgery in patients with PNH, splenectomy cannot be recommended.

Anticoagulation with coumarin-type drugs may have some benefit in preventing thromboses, particularly in the postsurgical patient. On the other hand, therapy with heparin has been noted to cause an increased amount of hemolysis in some patients with PNH, and caution must be exercised when using this drug.

PROGNOSIS   Most patients with classic PNH have a life expectancy of less than 10 years, although some survive for much longer. A recent series of 17 patients surviving more than 20 years was compiled by questioning hematologists nationally. In more than one-third of these patients, there had been an amelioration of disease symptoms, and in two patients PNH was totally quiescent. The major morbidity relates to venous thromboses. Despite the overwhelming degree of iron deposition in the kidney, death from renal failure is rare. The prognosis is uncertain in patients in whom the manifestations of PNH are more subtle and in whom the diagnosis was made because of the widespread use of the sucrose lysis test. Some patients may lead a normal life.

CONGENITAL ABNORMALITIES OF THE RED CELL MEMBRANE   Hereditary spherocytosis   This is a disease of autosomal dominant inheritance in which intrinsically abnormal red blood cells are destroyed in the presence of an otherwise normal spleen. Its incidence is approximately 1:4500. In 20 percent of patients no family history can be obtained, and the genetic mutation appears to have arisen de novo. It is sometimes clinically apparent in early infancy, but often escapes detection until adult life.

CLINICAL MANIFESTATIONS   The major clinical features of hereditary spherocytosis are anemia, splenomegaly, and jaundice. The prominence of the latter finding accounts for its prior designation "congenital hemolytic jaundice" and is due to an increased concentration of unconjugated (indirect-reacting) bilirubin in plasma. Jaundice may be intermittent and tends to be less pronounced in early childhood. Because of the increased bile pigment metabolism, gallstones of pigment type are common, even in childhood. Compensatory normoblastic hyperplasia of the bone marrow occurs with the extension of red marrow into the midshafts of long bones and occasionally with extramedullary erythropoiesis, at times leading to the formation of paravertebral masses visible on chest x-ray. Because the bone marrow's capacity to increase erythropoiesis by six- to tenfold exceeds the usual rate of hemolysis in this disease, anemia is usually mild or moderate and is absent in an otherwise healthy individual. Compensation may be temporarily interrupted by episodes of erythroid hypoplasia precipitated by infections, often of a minor nature. Splenomegaly is a constant feature of hereditary spherocytosis. The hemolytic rate may increase transiently during systemic infections which induce further splenic enlargement. Chronic leg ulcers, similar to those observed in sickle-cell anemia, occasionally occur.

The characteristic erythrocyte abnormality is the spherocyte (Plate 9-13). Its mean corpuscular volume (MCV) is usually normal or slightly decreased, and its mean corpuscular hemoglobin concentration (MCHC) is increased to 35 to 38 g per 100 ml. Spheroidicity may be quantitatively assessed in terms of osmotic fragility (Fig. 314-1). Because spherocytes have a decreased surface area per unit volume, they lyse more readily when exposed to solutions of low salt concentration. On microscopic examination spherocytes are usually detected even when present in very small numbers (see Plate 9-13). However, they will ordinarily not influence the osmotic fragility test unless they constitute more than 1 or 2 percent of the total cell population. A prominent increase in the osmotic fragility of red blood cells following sterile incubation of whole blood for 24 h at 37°C is also characteristic of hereditary spherocytosis. The autohemolysis test is an extension of this latter procedure and measures the amount of spontaneous hemolysis occurring after 48 h of sterile incubation. In hereditary spherocytosis about 10 to 50 percent of the red blood cells are lysed (versus less than 4 percent of normal red blood cells). Autohemolysis of these red blood cells is largely prevented by the addition of glucose prior to incubation.

PATHOGENESIS Although the exact defect in hereditary spherocytosis is unknown, it is clear that it resides in the membrane and imparts a number of unusual characteristics to it. First, the surface area of these erythrocytes is decreased, in part because of a reduced quantity of membrane lipid. However, the decrease in surface area is out of proportion to the reduction in the amount of lipid, suggesting that an abnormality of lipid-protein association may be of fundamental importance. Second, the red blood cell membrane shows increased permeability to sodium. Compensation is achieved by an increased rate of glucose metabolism to generate an increased amount of ATP with which the red blood cell extrudes this excess sodium. Thus, these red blood cells must remain metabolically active in order to maintain their integrity. Third, the red blood cell membrane is more rigid than normal, suggesting that membrane proteins may have an abnormal interaction with ATP

FIGURE 314-1
Osmotic fragility of red blood cells in hereditary spherocytosis. When the spleen is present, a small subpopulation of cells which are "conditioned" in the spleen form the fragile "tail" of the osmotic fragility curve. After splenectomy a single population exists which is more osmotically fragile than normal.

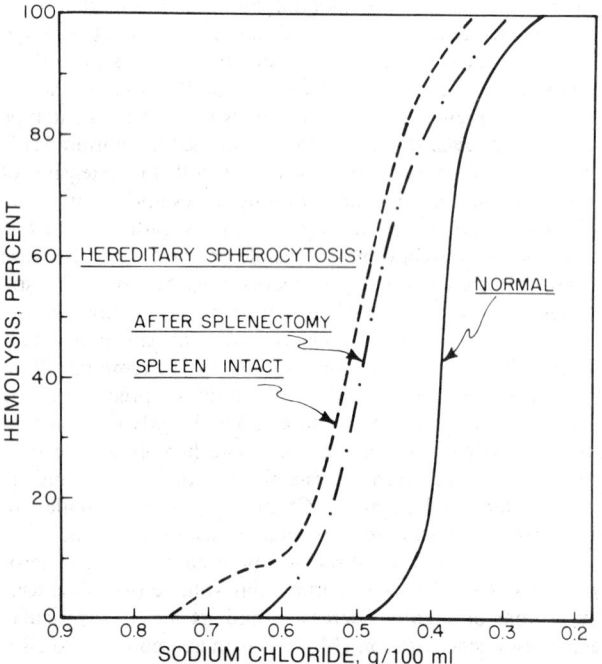

and calcium. Although it is assumed that these abnormalities relate to a basic structural defect in a membrane protein, none has yet been documented.

Spheroidal contour and rigid structure of the red blood cells impede their passage through the spleen. There, the red blood cells are exposed to an environment in which their increased metabolic rate cannot be sustained. The first injury imposed upon them by the spleen is a further loss of surface membrane "conditioning," which produces a subpopulation of hyperspheroidal red blood cells in the peripheral blood. These are subsequently destroyed in the spleen. The intracorpuscular nature of the red blood cell defect in hereditary spherocytosis is demonstrated by a diminished life span of the patient's red cells in normal subjects when the spleen is present and a normal survival of normal cells transfused into patients with hereditary spherocytosis.

DIAGNOSIS Hereditary spherocytosis must be distinguished from the spherocytic hemolytic anemias associated with red blood cell antibodies. The family history is helpful, when present, but in 20 percent of patients with the disease, a family history is lacking. The diagnosis of immune spherocytosis is usually readily made by use of Coombs' test. Autohemolysis is increased in immune spherocytosis, but it is not corrected by glucose. Spherocytes, often in considerable numbers, are seen in association with hemolysis induced by splenomegaly in patients with cirrhosis or chronic infections, and a few spherocytes are seen in the course of a wide variety of hemolytic processes, particularly glucose 6-phosphate dehydrogenase deficiency.

TREATMENT AND PROGNOSIS Splenectomy reliably corrects the anemia, although the red blood cell defect persists. The operative risk is low. The spleen is darkly congested with blood and usually weighs between 500 and 2000 g. Much of this weight is accounted for by red blood cells which are pooled there. Histologically the spleen pulp cords are congested with red blood cells while the sinuses are often dilated and empty. Red blood cell survival after splenectomy is normal or nearly so. Rare relapses have been reported and are probably attributable to postoperative growth of splenic autotransplants or to hyperplasia of secondary spleens which were overlooked at operation. Because of the potential for gallstones and for episodes of bone marrow hypoplasia or hemolytic crises, splenectomy should be performed in most individuals with hereditary spherocytosis, even those with mild anemia. Splenectomy in children should be postponed until the age of four years, if possible, although it may be performed at any age. Beyond age three, severe infections following splenectomy in hereditary spherocytosis are rare. Because of the increased requirement for folic acid in patients with hemolysis, a deficiency of this vitamin may exist, and therapy with folic acid may result in an increased hemoglobin level.

Hereditary elliptocytosis Red blood cells of oval or elliptic shape are normally found in birds, reptiles, camels, and llamas; however, they occur in appreciable numbers in humans only in *hereditary elliptocytosis*, a disorder which is transmitted as an autosomal dominant and affects 1 per 4000 to 5000 of the population, a frequency similar to that of hereditary spherocytosis. It is also referred to as *hereditary ovalocytosis*.

The great majority of patients manifest only mild hemolysis, with hemoglobin levels above 12 g per 100 ml, reticulocytes less than 4 percent, depressed haptoglobin levels, and red blood cell survivals within or just under the normal range. In 10 to 15 percent of patients the rate of hemolysis is substantially increased with chromium half-survival times of red blood cells as short as 5 days and reticulocytes ranging to 20 percent. Hemoglobin levels rarely fall below 9 to 10 g per 100 ml. Red blood cell destruction occurs predominantly in the spleen, which is enlarged in patients with overt hemolysis, and hemolysis is corrected by splenectomy.

In both the anemic and nonanemic varieties of this disorder the red blood cells are normochromic and normocytic. At least 25 percent and, more commonly, greater than 75 percent of red blood cells are elliptic, with an axial ratio (width/length) of less than 0.78. Patients with hemolysis frequently have microovalocytes, bizarre-shaped red blood cells, and red cell fragments, and these increase in number following splenectomy. The degree of hemolysis does not correlate with the percentage of elliptocytes. Osmotic fragility is usually normal but may be increased in patients with overt hemolysis. The pathogenesis of the red blood cell defect is thought to be similar to that of hereditary spherocytosis.

Hereditary stomatocytosis Stomatocytes are red blood cells having a slit-like central zone of pallor on dried smears. The syndrome of hereditary hemolytic anemia and stomatocytic red blood cells is inherited as an autosomal dominant. It may represent a number of discrete entities. Two major red blood cell defects have been delineated in this syndrome. First, red blood cells have an increased surface area associated with an increase in membrane lipid content. Second, the red blood cells have an increased permeability to sodium and potassium, which is compensated for by an increased active transport of these cations. In some patients, the red blood cell is swollen with an excess of ions and water and a decreased mean corpuscular hemoglobin concentration (overhydrated stomatocytes); in other patients the red cell is shrunken with a decreased ion and water content and an increased mean corpuscular hemoglobin concentration (dehydrated stomatocytes). Those patients in whom the red blood cells are overhydrated have true stomatocytes on dried smears. Dehydrated stomatocytes assume the morphology of target cells on dried smears. In both instances, red blood cells are cup- or bowl-shaped when examined in wet preparation. Osmotic fragility is increased in overhydrated stomatocytes and decreased in underhydrated stomatocytes. Autohemolysis is increased and is corrected by glucose.

Most patients have splenomegaly and mild anemia. Splenectomy decreases but does not totally correct the hemolytic process. Its indications are similar to those for hereditary spherocytosis.

DISORDERS OF THE INTERIOR OF THE RED CELL

RED CELL ENZYME DEFECTS During its maturation, the red blood cell loses its nucleus, ribosomes, and mitochondria and thus its capability for protein synthesis and oxidative phosphorylation. The mature circulating red blood cell has a relatively simple pattern of intermediary metabolism (Fig. 314-2) in keeping with its modest metabolic obligations. As discussed in Chap. 53, some ATP must be generated from the Embden-Meyerhof pathway to drive the cation pump which maintains the ionic milieu within the red blood cell. Smaller amounts of energy are needed for the preservation of hemoglobin iron in the ferrous (Fe^{2+}) state, and perhaps for the renewal of the lipids in the red blood cell membrane. About 10 percent of the glucose consumed by the red blood cell is metabolized via the hexose-monophosphate shunt (Fig. 314-2). This pathway protects both hemoglobin and the membrane from exogenous oxidants including certain drugs.

Studies of red blood cell enzyme defects have provided valuable information on the metabolic control of normal erythrocytes. Figure 314-2 shows a large number of recognized specific enzyme deficiency states affecting the glycolytic pathway, the hexose-monophosphate shunt, and a number of other

reactions involved in nucleotide synthesis and regulation. Many of these enzyme abnormalities appear to be restricted to red blood cells. In some cases, other isoenzymes may function adequately in nonerythroid cells. In addition, the long life span of the red blood cell and its inability to synthesize proteins poses a challenge to the stability of its enzymes. A mutation resulting in decreased stability will be expressed more readily in the red blood cell compared with other tissues.

Defects in the Embden-Meyerhof pathway Deficiencies of most of the enzymes of the Embden-Meyerhof (or glycolytic) pathway have been reported. Many of these have been encountered only in isolated families. In general, all these enzymopathies have similar pathophysiologic and clinical features. Patients present with a congenital nonspherocytic hemolytic anemia of variable severity. As a rule, the red blood cells are relatively deficient in ATP, considering their young age. As a result, there is an increased leak of potassium ion from inside these cells. Abnormalities in red blood cell morphology (see below) also indicate that the red cell membrane is secondarily affected by the enzyme defect. These red blood cells are apt to be rigid and thus more readily sequestered by the mononuclear-phagocyte system.

Some of these glycolytic enzyme deficiencies such as pyruvate kinase (PK) deficiency and hexokinase deficiency appear to be restricted to the red blood cell. There is no apparent metabolic abnormality in leukocytes or other cells that have been studied. In other disorders, the enzyme deficiency is more widespread. Glucose phosphate isomerase deficiency and phosphoglycerate kinase deficiency also involve leukocytes, although affected individuals have no apparent abnormalities of white blood cell function. Individuals with deficiency of triose phosphate isomerase have decreased levels of enzyme in leukocytes, muscle cells, and central nervous system fluid. Furthermore, they have a progressive neurologic disorder. Some patients with phosphofructokinase deficiency have a myopathy.

Among the reported defects of glycolytic enzymes, about 95 percent are due to PK deficiency and about 4 percent are due to glucose phosphate isomerase deficiency. The remainder shown in Fig. 314-2 are extremely rare. Most have been encountered in isolated families. There is considerable heterogeneity in the clinical manifestation and laboratory findings among reported cases of PK deficiency. This is probably due to the fact that a number of different PK variants have been reported. The high degree of polymorphism found in G6PD deficiency (see below) probably also applies to the other less common glycolytic enzyme defects. Therefore, the clinical manifestations of these disorders are somewhat variable.

GENETICS Most of the glycolytic enzyme defects are inherited in an autosomal recessive pattern. Thus, the parents of affected patients are heterozygotes. Since the gene frequency for this group of enzymopathies is low, it is not surprising that homozygotes are often the offspring of a consanguineous mating. Heterozygotes generally possess half-normal levels of enzyme activity which are more than adequate for normal metabolic function. Thus, these individuals are entirely asymptomatic. The only exception among the glycolytic enzymopathies is phosphoglycerate kinase deficiency which is inherited as a sex-linked disorder. Affected males have a severe hemolytic anemia while female carriers may have a mild hemolytic process.

CLINICAL MANIFESTATIONS Patients with severe hemolysis usually present during early childhood with anemia, icterus,

FIGURE 314-2

Metabolic pathways in the red blood cell. The glycolytic pathway is outlined vertically from glucose to lactate. The pentose phosphate pathway is shown on the right. Known enzyme deficiency states are shown. Bold solid lines denote common states, light solid lines less common ones, and dotted lines rare ones. (From WN Valentine, Semin Hematol 8:309, 1971.)

ever, in the hypoxic environment of the spleen, aerobic metabolism is curtailed and the ATP-depleted cells are destroyed in situ. It is of interest that following splenectomy patients with PK deficiency often have a marked increase in circulating reticulocytes. Patients with deficiency of glucose phosphate isomerase may also be improved by splenectomy. There is not sufficient information to indicate whether this operation would help individuals with other glycolytic enzymopathies.

Defects in the hexose-monophosphate shunt The normal red blood cell is well endowed to protect itself against oxidant stress. Upon exposure to an offending drug or toxin, the amount of glucose that is metabolized via the hexose-monophosphate shunt is increased severalfold. In this way reduced glutathione is regenerated, protecting the sulfhydryl groups of hemoglobin and perhaps the red blood cell membrane from oxidation. Individuals with an inherited defect in the hexose-monophosphate shunt are unable to maintain an adequate level of reduced glutathione in their red blood cells. As a result, hemoglobin sulfhydryl groups become oxidized, and the hemoglobin tends to precipitate within the red blood cell forming Heinz bodies.

Among the congenital shunt defects, by far the most common is *G6PD deficiency*. It affects millions of people throughout the world. Like the glycolytic enzymopathies, there is considerable genetic polymorphism among affected individuals. Indeed, over 100 variants of G6PD have been described. In contrast to the hemoglobin variants (Chap. 315) differences in primary structure among the G6PD variants have not yet been established but are presumed to exist on the basis of differences in electrophoretic mobility, enzyme kinetics, pH optimum, and heat stability. Like the hemoglobin variants, many of these G6PD mutants were discovered by chance and are not associated with any significant functional abnormalities. The normal or "wild" form of G6PD is designated by type B. About 20 percent of blacks have a G6PD (designated A+) which differs electrophoretically but is functionally normal. Among the clinically significant G6PD variants, the most common is the so-called A− type encountered primarily in blacks who originated from central Africa. The A− G6PD has the same electrophoretic mobility as the A+ type, but it is unstable and has abnormal kinetic properties. Like the HbS gene, the A− type of G6PD may confer protection against malaria. This variant is found in about 15 percent of black males in the United States. A second relatively common G6PD variant has been discovered in peoples of the Eastern Mediterranean area, particularly Sephardic Jews.

The G6PD gene is located on the X chromosome. Thus the deficiency state is a sex-linked trait. Affected males (hemizygotes) inherit the abnormal gene from their mothers who are usually carriers (heterozygotes). Because of inactivation of one of the two X chromosomes (Lyon hypothesis, see Chap. 58), the heterozygote has two populations of red blood cells: nor-

and splenomegaly. Other stigmata of chronic hemolysis are occasionally seen. Occasionally, siblings are similarly affected.

LABORATORY FINDINGS Patients have a normocytic (or slightly macrocytic) normochromic anemia with reticulocytosis. In those with PK deficiency, bizarre erythrocytes are noted on the peripheral smear with large numbers of spiculated red blood cells. Spherocytes are usually infrequent or absent. Hence, the term *congenital nonspherocytic hemolytic anemia* has been applied to these disorders. Unlike hereditary spherocytosis, the osmotic fragility of freshly drawn blood is usually normal. Incubation brings out an osmotically fragile population of red blood cells. When a blood specimen is incubated under sterile conditions for 48 h, an abnormal amount of "autohemolysis" is noted. In contrast to hereditary spherocytosis, the degree of autohemolysis in these disorders is not corrected by the addition of glucose.

The diagnosis of this group of anemias depends upon specific enzymatic assays. An abnormality in enzyme kinetics may be demonstrated. In addition, differences in electrophoretic mobility, pH optimum, or heat stability may be noted. This information is useful in documenting polymorphism among enzyme variants.

TREATMENT Most patients do not require therapy. Those with severe hemolysis should be given a daily supplement of folic acid (1 mg per day). Blood transfusions may be necessary during a hypoplastic crisis. Patients with PK deficiency may be benefited by splenectomy. Because of their enzymatic defect, the younger cells (reticulocytes) depend on mitochondrial respiration rather than glycolysis for maintenance of ATP. How-

TABLE 314-3

1545

CHAPTER 314
HEMOLYTIC ANEMIAS

Drugs causing hemolysis in subjects deficient in G6PD

Antimalarials: Primaquine, pamaquine, chloroquine, dapsone
Sulfonamides: Sulfanilamide, sulfasoxazole, etc.
Nitrofurans
Analgesics: Phenacetin, acetanilid
Miscellaneous: Vitamin K (water-soluble form), probenecid, methylene blue, *p*-aminosalicylic acid, nalidixic acid, quinine,* quinidine,* chloramphenicol*

* *Not known to cause hemolysis in blacks with A − type G6PD.*

mal and deficient in G6PD. Most female carriers are asymptomatic. Those who happen to have a high proportion of deficient cells resemble the male hemizygotes.

G6PD activity normally declines about 50 percent during the 120-day life span of the red blood cell. This decay is moderately accelerated in A − red blood cells and markedly so in red blood cells containing the Mediterranean variant. Individuals with the A − variant may have a slightly shortened red blood cell survival, but they are not anemic. Clinical problems arise only when the affected individual is subjected to some type of environmental stress. Most often, hemolytic episodes are triggered by viral and bacterial infections. The mechanism for this is unknown. Drugs or toxins which pose an oxidant threat to the red blood cell also cause hemolysis in individuals deficient in G6PD (see Table 314-3). Of these, sulfa drugs, antimalarials, and nitrofurantoins are most commonly incriminated. Although aspirin is frequently mentioned as a likely offender, it appears to have no deleterious effect in A − individuals. Occasionally, accidental ingestion of toxic compounds such as naphthalene (found in moth balls) can cause severe hemolysis. Finally, metabolic acidosis can precipitate an episode of hemolysis in subjects deficient in G6PD.

CLINICAL AND LABORATORY FEATURES   The patient may experience an acute hemolytic crisis within hours of exposure to the oxidant stress. In severe cases, hemoglobinuria and peripheral vascular collapse can develop. Since only the older population of red blood cells is rapidly destroyed, the hemolytic crisis is usually self-limited, even if the exposure to the oxidant continues. During the period of acute hemolysis, a rapid drop in hematocrit is accompanied by a rise in plasma hemoglobin and unconjugated bilirubin and a decrease in plasma haptoglobin. The peripheral smear is often unimpressive, but on occasion spherocytes and fragmented red blood cells may be seen. The demonstration of Heinz bodies requires the use of a supravital stain such as crystal violet. However, Heinz bodies are usually not seen after the first day or so, since these inclusions are readily removed by the spleen.

Individuals with the *Mediterranean type G6PD* have a more unstable enzyme and, therefore, a much lower overall enzyme activity than blacks with the A − variant. As a result, they have more severe clinical manifestations. Some have a chronic hemolytic anemia, even in the absence of any exposure to oxidants. A minority of patients is exquisitely sensitive to fava beans and will develop a fulminant hemolytic crisis following exposure. Sensitivity to *Vicia fava* is a poorly understood phenomenon that appears to be determined by a separate gene. Favism is not encountered in blacks with the A − variant. Individuals with the Mediterranean variant sometimes have a temporary episode of hemolysis during the newborn period.

The *diagnosis* of G6PD deficiency should be considered in any individual, particularly a black male, who experiences an acute hemolytic episode. The patient should be thoroughly questioned about possible exposure to oxidant agents. A number of screening tests are available to establish the diagnosis. However, since the deficiency occurs primarily in older red blood cells, a false-negative test may be seen during a hemolytic episode when there is a high proportion of young red

blood cells. It may be necessary to repeat these diagnostic tests after the patient has recovered. Unusual features in the case should prompt further investigation including a more complete and specific characterization of the enzyme.

TREATMENT   Since hemolysis in patients deficient in A − G6PD is usually self-limited, no specific treatment is necessary. Splenectomy does not appear to be of benefit to Mediterranean patients with chronic hemolysis. Blood transfusions are rarely indicated. If a patient develops a severe hemolytic episode with hemoglobinuria, maintaining adequate urine output is important.

Attention should be directed toward the *prevention* of hemolytic episodes. Infections ought to be treated promptly. Subjects deficient in G6PD should be warned about risks posed by oxidant drugs and fava beans. Any black patient about to be given an oxidant drug should be screened for G6PD deficiency.

Other defects of the hexose-monophosphate shunt   A few kindreds have been found to have congenital deficiency in red blood cell glutathione due to a defect in one of the two enzymes responsible for the synthesis of this tripeptide. Affected individuals have a hemolytic anemia with Heinz bodies that is aggravated by oxidant drugs. Deficiency of glutathione reductase has been reported, but its relationship to clinically significant hemolysis is not well established. Sometimes the deficiency state can be corrected by the administration of riboflavin (5 mg per day). There are also isolated reports of deficiencies of glutathione peroxidase and 6-phosphogluconate dehydrogenase, but, again, their association with hemolysis is uncertain.

HEMOGLOBINOPATHIES   The sickling disorders constitute an important form of congenital hemolytic anemia. Less commonly, hemolysis may be due to the inheritance of an unstable hemoglobin variant. These disorders of hemoglobin are discussed in Chap. 315.

REFERENCES

AMOROSI EL, ULTMANN JE: Thrombotic thrombocytopenic purpura: Report of 16 cases and review of the literature. Medicine 45:139, 1966

BRAIN MC: Microangiopathic haemolytic anemia. Br J Haematol 23 (suppl):25, 1972

BUNN HF et al: *Human Hemoglobins.* Philadelphia, Saunders, 1977

CHAPLIN H: Clinical usefulness of specific antiglobulin reagents in autoimmune hemolytic anemias. Prog Hematol 8:25, 1973

COOPER RA: Abnormalities of cell-membrane fluidity in the pathogenesis of disease. N Engl J Med 297:371, 1977

———, JANDL JL: Hereditary spherocytosis, in *The Metabolic Basis of Inherited Disease,* 4th ed, JB Stanbury et al (eds). New York, McGraw-Hill, 1976

——— et al: Role of the spleen in membrane conditioning and hemolysis of spur cells in liver disease. N Engl J Med 290:1279, 1974

FRANK MM et al: Pathophysiology of immune hemolytic anemias. Ann Intern Med 87:210, 1977

GOLDENFARB PB, FINCH SC: Thrombotic thrombocytopenic purpura: A ten year survey. JAMA 226:644, 1973

HINZ CF: Acid hemolysis revisited. Semin Hematol 13:201, 1976

LOHRMAN HP: Microangiopathic hemolytic anemia in metastatic carcinoma. Ann Intern Med 79:386, 1973

MAGALHAES RL et al: Microangiopathic hemolytic anemia in renal allotransplantation. Am J Med 58:862, 1975

MARSH GW, LEWIS SM: Cardiac hemolytic anemia. Semin Hematol 6:133, 1969

PETZ LD, FUDENBERG HN: Immunologic mechanisms in drug induced cytopenias. Prog Hematol 9:185, 1975

PIROFSKY B: Clinical aspects of autoimmune hemolytic anemia. Semin Hematol 13:251, 1976

PRUZANSKI W, SHUMAK KH: Biologic activity of cold-reacting autoantibodies. N Engl J Med 297:538, 583, 1977

VALENTINE WN: Red cell enzyme deficiencies as a cause of hemolytic disorders. Annu Rev Med 23:93, 1972

WILEY JS et al: Characteristics of the membrane defect in the hereditary stomatocytosis syndrome. Blood 46:337, 1975

315
DISORDERS OF HEMOGLOBIN STRUCTURE, FUNCTION, AND SYNTHESIS

H. FRANKLIN BUNN

In 1910, Herrick described a medical student from Jamaica who had a hemolytic anemia in conjunction with elongated "sickled" red blood cells on blood smear. Subsequently, it was shown that all the red blood cells of such patients assume a classic holly leaf or sickle shape following deoxygenation of the blood. In 1949, Itano and Pauling showed that sickle-cell anemia was associated with an electrophoretically abnormal hemoglobin. Eight years later, Ingram demonstrated that this hemoglobin (designated HbS) differed from normal HbA by the substitution of valine for glutamic acid at the sixth position of the β chain. Since then, over 300 structurally different human hemoglobin variants have been discovered in widely scattered parts of the world. Generally, a new hemoglobin is named after the place where it is first encountered. No more than a third of these mutant hemoglobins are associated with significant clinical manifestations. The remainder have been discovered by serendipity or as a result of large population surveys. All told, the hemoglobinopathies have taught us many valuable lessons in such diverse areas as the mechanisms underlying red blood cell destruction, the pathophysiology of oxygen transport, the stereochemistry of hemoglobin function, and the genetic bases of protein synthesis.

This chapter focuses on the clinically significant variants. In addition, disorders of the biosynthesis of globin (the thalassemias) and methemoglobinemia are discussed.

GENETIC CONSIDERATIONS The synthesis of each of the subunits of hemoglobin (α, β, γ, δ, ϵ, ζ) is governed by separate genes. The ϵ and ζ subunits are found only in embryonic hemoglobin. Each individual inherits two β-chain genes (one from each parent), probably four α-chain genes, and at least four γ-chain genes. The γ-, δ-, and β-chain genes are thought to occupy adjacent loci on the same chromosome. The inheritance of abnormal hemoglobins follows classic mendelian genetics. If two parents are heterozygous for a hemoglobin variant such as HbS, statistically one-quarter of the offspring will be SS homozygotes, another quarter will be normal (AA genotype), and half will have sickle trait (AS). The commonly encountered hemoglobinopathies such as S, C, and E are β-chain variants. Occasionally, an individual inherits two different β-chain variants, one from each parent. Hemoglobin SC disease is an example of such a double heterozygous state. The gene for β thalassemia is very closely linked to the β-chain structural gene. Therefore, the two genes can be considered allelic. Accordingly, an individual can inherit from one parent (and pass on to a child) either β thalassemia or a β-chain variant, but not both. Among the hemoglobinopathies associated with sickling (described below), only the homozygous state (Hb SS) or double heterozygous state (SThal or SC) has important clinical manifestations. In contrast, the unstable variants and those having abnormal oxygen-binding properties are encountered only in heterozygotes. In many cases, the homozygous state would be incompatible with life.

About 90 percent of these abnormal hemoglobins are single amino acid substitutions, due to a single base substitution in the corresponding triplet codon. The structural information accumulated on human mutant hemoglobins has provided ample verification of the fidelity of the genetic code. Other genetic mechanisms must be invoked to explain the structure of a few interesting hemoglobin variants. The Lepore hemoglobins have arisen because of nonhomologous crossover between the adjacent δ- and β-chain genes, giving rise to a fusion subunit in which the *N*-terminal end has the amino acid sequence of the δ chain and the *C*-terminal end has the sequence of the β chain. Some of the unstable hemoglobins have deletions of one or more residues in sequence within a subunit. Finally there are a few variants which have elongated subunits. These have arisen either because of a base substitution in the termination codon or because of a frame shift which puts the termination codon out of phase.

CLINICAL CLASSIFICATION The clinically significant hemoglobin variants are classified in Table 315-1. By far the most important and prevalent type of hemoglobinopathy is due to the presence of sickle hemoglobin, either in the homozygous state or in conjunction with another type of hemoglobin abnormality. The inheritance of an unstable hemoglobin variant may give rise to congenital hemolytic anemia associated with the presence of inclusions of precipitated hemoglobin within the red blood cells (Heinz bodies). Finally, hemoglobin variants may have abnormal functional or spectral properties, giving rise to such diverse clinical manifestations as familial erythrocytosis or familial cyanosis.

SICKLE SYNDROMES

SICKLE-CELL TRAIT About 8 percent of black Americans are heterozygous for HbS. The gene frequency is highest in central Africa, particularly in regions where malaria is endemic. In some parts of Nigeria, over 30 percent of the population has sickle trait. The gene has persisted because heterozygotes gain a slight protection against falciparum malaria. This is a well-accepted form of balanced polymorphism.

The diagnosis of sickle trait or any of the other sickle syndromes depends upon the demonstration of sickling under reduced oxygen tension. In the widely used sickle preparation, sickled cells can be visualized microscopically after the addition of an oxygen-consuming reagent such as metabisulfite. Many clinical laboratories prefer a solubility test which depends on the fact that deoxyhemoglobin S has a low solubility at high ionic strength. Hemoglobin S also has an increased rate of surface denaturation and will form a precipitate when a dilute solution is shaken vigorously. All these tests are reasonably specific for HbS although some of the unstable variants

TABLE 315-1
Clinically important hemoglobin variants

I Sickle syndromes
  A Sickle-cell trait (AS)
  B Sickle-cell anemia (SS)
  C Double heterozygous states: Sickle-β-thalassemia, sickle-C disease (SC), sickle-D disease (SD)
II Unstable hemoglobin variants (congenital Heinz body hemolytic anemia)
III Variants with high oxygen affinity: Hb Chesapeake, Hb Yakima, Hb Kempsey, Hb Mälmo, etc.
IV M hemoglobins (see Table 315-3)

may give false-positive solubility and mechanical precipitation tests. Therefore, if one of these screening tests is positive, hemoglobin electrophoresis should be performed. Individuals with sickle trait usually have about 35 percent HbS and 60 percent HbA.

Hemoglobin S heterozygotes have minimal clinical problems. Their overall life expectancy and frequency of hospitalization are no different from those of a comparable group of individuals with hemoglobin A. AS red blood cells require a much lower oxygen tension for sickling than SS red cells. Accordingly, individuals with sickle trait may develop sickle-cell crises only if they become severely hypoxic. They may occasionally sustain a splenic infarct. The renal medulla is particularly susceptible to sickling. Many AS individuals have impaired ability to form concentrated urine, and a few have recurrent episodes of painless hematuria as a result of medullary infarction. Infarction due to sickling has been encountered in other organs in sickle trait but is extremely rare. For these reasons, AS individuals should not be placed in any high-risk group for employment or insurance considerations.

SICKLE-CELL ANEMIA Sickle-cell anemia is the most prevalent form of congenital hemolytic anemia. About 0.15 percent of black children in the United States have the disease. The incidence is lower among adults because patients with sickle-cell anemia have a decreased life expectancy. The protean clinical manifestations of this disorder can all be attributed to a specific molecular lesion: the substitution of valine for glutamic acid at the sixth residue of the β chain.

Molecular pathogenesis Upon deoxygenation, a red blood cell containing HbS changes from a biconcave disk to an elongated crescent-shaped or "sickle"-shaped cell (see Plate 9-16). Electron micrographs, shown in Fig. 315-1, reveal the presence of fibers having a diameter of about 18 nm. It is likely that each sickle fiber consists of a helical polymer with four strands in an inner core and 10 strands in an outer core. The orientation of the individual HbS molecules in the fiber is not known. It is likely that both hydrophobic and electrostatic bonds are involved in the stabilization of the helical polymers. In addition, there are probably interactions between neighboring fibers. Sickling, both within the intact red blood cell and in free solution, is greatly affected by the presence of non-S hemoglobin. HbC participates more readily than HbA in copolymerization with HbS, while HbF appears to inhibit sickling. These experimental results fit well with the well-known differences in clinical severity of the various sickle syndromes: SS, SC, and sickle trait (AS).

Cellular pathogenesis As discussed in Chap. 53, the ability of red blood cells to traverse the microcirculation depends in large part on their pliability. As a red blood cell sickles, it becomes rigid, and, as a result, may obstruct capillary blood flow. The deoxygenation of blood from patients with sickle-cell disease is associated with a marked increase in viscosity. It is likely that obstruction to flow leads to local tissue hypoxia. As a result, further deoxygenation takes place, leading to further sickling. This vicious cycle may result in the amplification of microscopic obstruction into a larger area of infarction. The oxygen-dependent sickle cycle is ordinarily reversible. However, the membrane of SS red blood cells may become sufficiently damaged so that the cells lose potassium and water, leading to the formation of irreversibly sickled forms. In these cells, the characteristic sickle shape persists even after they are exposed to ambient oxygen tension at room temperature and can readily be seen on examination of Wright-stained blood films (see Plate 9-16). The percentage of irreversibly sickled cells varies from 2 to 30 percent in homozygous sicklers and is not correlated with clinical severity. Hemoglobin F is distrib-

uted unevenly among red blood cells of SS patients, and composes between 2 and 20 percent of the total hemoglobin. (The remainder is almost entirely HbS.) Since HbF inhibits the polymerization of HbS, those cells that are relatively rich in HbF are protected from sickling, whereas those cells that have relatively small amounts of HbF are likely to become irreversibly sickled. It is not surprising that these rigid cells are readily culled from the circulation and destroyed. The continuous formation and destruction of irreversibly sickled cells probably contributes significantly to the severe hemolytic anemia shared by all patients with sickle-cell anemia. Furthermore, these rigid cells may initiate small-vessel occlusions.

Factors which lower the oxygen affinity of red blood cells will enhance the formation of deoxyhemoglobin and, therefore, promote sickling. Thus, at a reduced oxygen tension, elevation of both intracellular 2,3-DPG and H^+ concentration (acidosis) will result in increased numbers of sickled cells. In addition, sickling is highly dependent on hemoglobin concentration. Any pathophysiologic process which tends to pull water out of sickle red blood cells will greatly increase their chance of sickling. Thus, the hypertonic environment of the renal medulla can cause local sickling and the formation of papillary infarcts, even in individuals with sickle trait.

Clinical manifestations Patients with homozygous sickle-cell anemia have a variety of clinical problems broadly outlined in Table 315-2. Signs and symptoms usually do not appear until after the sixth month of life, at which time most of the HbF has been replaced by HbS. Among the *constitutional* manifes-

FIGURE 315-1

Electron micrograph of deoxygenated SS hemoglobin. A. Transverse section showing bundles of fibers, each about 18 nm in diameter. B. Longitudinal section cut parallel to the long axis of sickling. (From JT Finch et al, Proc Natl Acad Sci USA 70:718, 1973.)

tations of sickle-cell anemia are impairment of growth and development and a general failure to thrive. In addition, these patients have an increased tendency to develop serious infections, particularly due to pneumococcus. There are several reasons for increased susceptibility to infection. Sicklers have marked impairment of splenic function, preventing effective clearance of circulating bacteria. With the passage of time, the organ develops recurrent infarcts and eventually becomes a nubbin of fibrous tissue. In addition, sicklers appear to have a defect in the alternative pathway for complement activation, preventing effective clearance of certain bacteria. As shown in Table 315-2, infections may trigger the development of painful crises and can cause a transient suppression of red blood cell production, resulting in worsening of anemia.

ANEMIA SS homozygotes invariably have a severe hemolytic anemia with hematocrit values which usually range between 18 and 30 percent. The destruction of red blood cells is independent of cell age. The mean red blood cell survival is about 10 to 15 days. Those cells having relatively low levels of Hb F have a shorter life span, in part due to a greater chance of becoming irreversibly sickled. As a result of accelerated red blood cell breakdown, patients with sickle-cell disease have characteristic clinical and laboratory findings discussed in Chap. 53. Even though hemolysis is primarily extravascular, plasma haptoglobin is generally low or absent, and plasma hemoglobin levels are moderately elevated.

The anemia becomes increasingly severe if erythropoiesis is suppressed. There are two main causes of "aplastic crises"—infection and folic acid deficiency. As discussed in Chap. 313, infection brings about a transient reduction in red blood cell production. In patients with severe ongoing hemolysis, this may result in a rapid drop in hematocrit.

VASOOCCLUSIVE PHENOMENA The morbidity and mortality of sickle-cell disease are due primarily to recurrent vasoocclusive phenomena. As shown in Table 315-2, these can be divided into two groups. Throughout their lives, sicklers are plagued by recurrent *painful crises*. These episodes may appear with explosive suddenness and attack various parts of the body, particularly the abdomen, chest, and the joints. About a third of painful crises are preceded by a viral or bacterial infection. The frequency of painful crises is highly variable. A given patient may have months or even years without a crisis and then have a cluster of frequent severe attacks. In some individuals, crises occur more frequently in cold weather, perhaps precipitated by reflex vasospasm. In others, crises come more often in warm weather, during times when patients are likely to become dehydrated. It is often difficult to distinguish between painful sickle crisis and some other type of acute process such as biliary colic, appendicitis, or a perforated viscus. Many patients have undergone surgical exploration under the impression that they had acute surgical abdomens. Patients having abdominal sickle crises usually have normal bowel sounds and

no rebound tenderness. If the abdominal pain is due to sickling, the surgeon generally finds no gross evidence of infarction or ischemia.

SS homozygotes frequently develop attacks of acute pleuritic chest pain with fever. Although the initial chest x-ray is often unremarkable, an infiltrate may evolve. The important differential is between pneumonitis and pulmonary infarction. Culture and Gram's stain of the sputum will be helpful in establishing the presence of pneumonia. In these patients, pulmonary infarctions are more likely due to thrombosis in situ than to emboli. Occasionally, pulmonary infarcts become secondarily infected.

When a sickle crisis is localized in the extremities, it may mimic osteomyelitis or an acute arthritis such as gout or rheumatoid arthritis. Patients commonly develop acute synovitis with joint effusion. Examination of the joint fluid is helpful in this differential diagnosis. If the effusion is due to sickling, the fluid will be clear and yellow, with a low white blood cell count (100 to 1000 mononuclear cells per cubic millimeter) and an absence of crystals or bacteria. Synovial biopsy may show sickled red blood cells in the lumen of small vessels.

Sickle crises may occasionally involve the central nervous system. Patients can present with a seizure, stroke, or coma. Although such crises are frequently reversible, they may be fatal.

CHRONIC ORGAN DAMAGE By the time that patients reach adulthood, there is often objective evidence of anatomic or functional damage to various tissues, due to the cumulative effect of recurrent vasoocclusive episodes. Almost any organ may be involved, but most commonly the lungs, kidneys, liver, skeleton, and skin.

Cardiopulmonary. Impairment of pulmonary function is a common complication of sickle-cell disease. Resting arterial P_{O_2} is usually reduced in part because of intrapulmonary arterial-venous shunting. Since SS red blood cells have decreased oxygen affinity, arterial blood will be significantly undersaturated, leading to an increased tendency for red cells to sickle when they reach the peripheral circulation. SS homozygotes frequently develop congestive heart failure. The chronic severe anemia and hypoxemia impose a sustained burden on the heart. Most patients have a systolic ejection murmur as a result of their hyperdynamic circulation. Even though more oxygen is extracted by the myocardium than any other tissue, SS patients rarely develop myocardial infarction.

Hepatobiliary. Like other patients with congenital hemolytic anemia, those with sickle-cell anemia have icterus and an increased tendency to form gallstones. It is often difficult to distinguish between the abdominal pain of acute cholecystitis and that due to a sickle crisis. Jaundice deepens markedly if a patient develops choledocholithiasis, and bilirubin levels as high as 50 mg per 100 ml have been reported. As a rule, cholecystectomy is not recommended unless gallstones cause symptoms. In addition, patients with sickle-cell anemia may develop hepatic infarcts which occasionally become infected, resulting in abscess formation. If a significant portion of hepatic parenchyma becomes infarcted, fibrosis and deterioration of liver function may result, with deepening of jaundice.

Genitourinary. The hypertonic and acidic environment of the renal medulla promotes sickling, resulting in microinfarcts. Virtually all patients have isosthenuria. The inability of the patient with sickle-cell anemia to form concentrated urine increases his risk of becoming significantly dehydrated. In addition, like those with sickle trait or SC disease, SS homozygotes may develop significant and prolonged painless hematuria as a result of papillary infarcts. Hematuria may be so extensive that iron deficiency develops. ε-Aminocaproic acid has proved to be effective in severe cases but must be used with caution since it may prevent the lysis of clots in the renal pelvis.

TABLE 315-2
Clinical manifestations of sickle-cell anemia

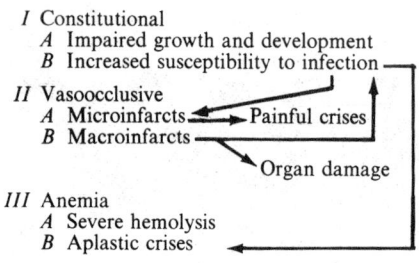

I Constitutional
  A Impaired growth and development
  B Increased susceptibility to infection

II Vasoocclusive
  A Microinfarcts
  B Macroinfarcts
    Painful crises
    Organ damage

III Anemia
  A Severe hemolysis
  B Aplastic crises

A small number of patients develop frank renal failure, sometimes following the nephrotic syndrome. The pathogenesis of the glomerular lesions is not well understood. Mild nitrogen retention is commonly encountered, accompanied by moderate hyperuricemia. However, patients rarely develop uric acid nephropathy or gout. Male patients with sickle-cell anemia occasionally develop priapism (spontaneous and painful engorgement of the penis). This distressing complication occurs with about equal frequency in prepubertal and postpubertal patients, although the latter are more difficult to treat and may develop impotence following the acute episode. Patients should be treated conservatively with sedation, analgesia, and intravenous fluids. The administration of packed red blood cells may also be effective. Surgical intervention is rarely indicated.

Skeletal. Like other patients with congenital hemolytic anemia, patients with sickle-cell anemia demonstrate radiologic abnormalities due to the expansion of red marrow. However, the development of bony infarcts results in more characteristic x-ray abnormalities. The biconcave or "fishmouth" vertebrae are pathognomonic of sickle-cell disease. Skeletal infarction generally leads to increased bony trabeculation and sclerosis. Aseptic necrosis of the head of the femur is particularly common in patients with sickle-cell disease and can lead to considerable disability. Like infarcts in other organs, bony infarctions are more likely to become infected. In patients who develop osteomyelitis, salmonella is a frequent pathogen.

Ocular. A variety of ocular abnormalities are encountered in patients with SS and SC disease. These include retinal infarcts, peripheral vessel disease, arteriovenous anomalies, vitreous hemorrhage, retinitis proliferans, and retinal detachment. In addition, when viewed with a strong magnifying lens, angulated and "corkscrew" vessels can be seen in the bulbar conjunctiva. The major ocular complications are more commonly encountered in SC patients than in SS patients. The early diagnosis of retinal lesions in SC and SS disease is important since retinal detachment may be prevented by appropriate therapy.

Skin. Chronic skin ulcers often occur in the distal lower extremities. The lesions appear to be commoner in patients with more severe anemia. Ankle ulcers have also been encountered in rare patients with other types of congenital hemolytic anemia. This complication is more commonly seen in tropical areas. Ankle ulcers generally respond to conservative management, such as elevation of the leg, maintenance of strict cleanliness, and application of a mild chemical debriding agent such as Dakin's solution. The weekly application of Unna boots has been effective. In patients with refractory ulcers, a hypertransfusion regimen is probably indicated. Skin grafting should be undertaken only after all other measures have failed.

Neurologic. A variety of neurologic manifestations may be encountered in sickle-cell anemia, primarily due to cerebral thromboses. A patient has about a 25 percent chance of developing some type of neurologic complication during his lifetime. Hemiplegia is encountered more frequently than coma, convulsions, or visual disturbances. Patients generally make a full recovery, particularly from their first cerebral vascular accident. Preliminary studies in children indicate that a hypertransfusion program is beneficial to those who have sustained a major neurologic complication.

Diagnosis The diagnosis of sickle-cell anemia should be considered in any black patient with a hemolytic anemia. The history of painful crises, arthropathy, ankle ulcers, etc., can be very helpful. If a patient has a relatively mild form of the disease, the diagnosis may not have been made during childhood. A number of laboratory tests are useful in distinguishing sickle-cell anemia from other hemoglobinopathies. Examination of the peripheral blood smear reveals normochromic normocytic red blood cells, many of which appear as targets. The

presence of irreversibly sickled forms is very helpful (see Plate 9-16). In addition, the presence of Howell-Jolly bodies, siderocytes, and occasional normoblasts suggests the absence of effective splenic function. A positive test for sickling, such as the metabisulfite preparation or the solubility test, indicates the presence of HbS but does not distinguish between SS, AS, and double heterozygotes (SThal, SC). Hemoglobin electrophoresis is necessary to establish the diagnosis. Patients with homozygous sickle-cell anemia have about 2 to 20 percent HbF and 2 to 4 percent HbA_2. The remainder is HbS. No HbA is detected unless the patient has been transfused within the past 4 months. Patients with sickle thalassemia will have hypochromic microcytic red blood cells, fewer irreversibly sickled forms, and a variable proportion of HbA (0 to 30 percent). SC diseases can be readily diagnosed by hemoglobin electrophoresis. In hemoglobin SD disease, the two hemoglobin variants comigrate during conventional electrophoresis at pH 8.6 but are usually separable upon agar gel electrophoresis at pH 6.0 to 6.5.

Treatment The understanding of the molecular pathogenesis of sickling has not yet led to an effective form of therapy. A large array of antisickling regimens has been proposed with varying rationale, but thus far none has stood the test of time. Currently accepted management of sickle-cell anemia is primarily supportive and conservative. Since patients with sickle-cell anemia are at increased risk of developing infections, many of which trigger painful and aplastic crises, it is very important to detect infection early and give appropriate antibiotics promptly. Malaria prophylaxis should be administered in endemic areas. The development of pneumococcal sepsis in children may be prevented by the administration of the polyvalent vaccine.

The anemia of sickle-cell disease increases markedly if the patient becomes deficient in folic acid. Since these patients have a continuous increased requirement for folic acid, it is reasonable to maintain them on a daily oral supplement. Testosterone has been demonstrated to increase the red blood cell mass in patients with sickle-cell anemia. However, the potential risk of hepatotoxicity, and of priapism in males, limits its utility.

Painful crises should be treated promptly with adequate analgesia and hydration. Some patients feel that their crises can be aborted if treated early. Therefore, it is reasonable to give patients a supply of analgesics such as codeine or meperidine which can be taken at home. However, these patients are at high risk of becoming addicted to opiates.

Blood transfusions play a limited role in the management of sickle-cell anemia. Between crises, patients tolerate anemia quite well and do not derive much subjective benefit from transfusions. However, partial replacement of the patients' red blood cells by transfused red cells (hypertransfusion) may be an effective way of preventing vasoocclusive crises. In order to lower the viscosity of the patient's blood significantly, it is necessary that over 50 percent of the patient's red blood cells be of donor origin. Hypertransfusion is often a reasonable approach to getting a patient through a limited period of risk such as pregnancy or surgery. However, the problems of isoimmunization, iron overload, and hepatitis dictate against its widespread use.

Prevention Genetic counseling can play an important role in the prevention of sickle-cell anemia. If both marital partners are AS heterozygotes, they may elect not to have children, knowing that there is a 25 percent chance that their offspring will be homozygous. The antenatal diagnosis of sickle-cell anemia can now be made in the second trimester of pregnancy by the testing of a very small sample of fetal blood obtained from the placenta. If it is established that the fetus is a SS homozygote, the parents may decide to interrupt the pregnancy.

Prognosis The clinical course of patients with sickle-cell anemia is highly variable. Many assessments of prognosis that have appeared in the literature have been unduly pessimistic. During the past 30 years there has been considerable improvement in the care of patients with sickle-cell anemia. In the United States, an increasing number of patients are surviving into adulthood and even bearing offspring. There has also been a decline in the mortality of SS mothers during pregnancy and childbirth. However, in underdeveloped nations, the mortality in sickle-cell anemia remains very high.

No single clinical or laboratory finding is a consistent predictor of prognosis in sickle-cell disease. Although those patients who have relatively high amounts of HbF tend to have milder clinical manifestations, this relationship is of no prognostic value in any given patient. Considerable variation in the severity of sickle-cell disease has been reported among different ethnic and geographical groups. A group of Shi Arabs from Saudi Arabia has been found to have a very benign form of sickle-cell anemia with very high levels of HbF (15 to 30 percent). A mild type of sickle-cell anemia has also been seen among the Veddoids of India.

SICKLE-β-THALASSEMIA This disease is highly variable in its clinical severity and complications. It is commonly encountered in people from the Mediterranean countries as well as those from central Africa. Sickle-β-thalassemia tends to be milder in blacks, just as homozygous β thalassemia is much less severe in blacks than in the Mediterranean populations. Patients have a congenital hemolytic anemia of variable severity, accompanied by splenomegaly in about 70 percent of the cases. They may have all the various types of vasoocclusive phenomena described above for homozygous sickle-cell anemia. However, painful crises are generally much less frequent and less severe.

Examination of the blood film reveals hypochromic microcytic red blood cells, with polychromatophilia, target cells, stippling, and rare fixed sickle forms. The electrophoretic pattern shows from 60 to 90 percent HbS and 10 to 30 percent HbF. Hemoglobin A will be about 10 to 30 percent if the β-thalassemia gene is capable of producing some β^A chains (β^+ thalassemia, see below). In patients who have sickle-β^0-thalassemia, no HbA will be present, and therefore the disorder may be difficult to distinguish from homozygous sickle-cell anemia. Hemoglobin A_2 is moderately elevated in sickle-β-thalassemia, but it is difficult to measure this minor component accurately in the presence of HbS. Most patients with sickle-β-thalassemia do not require close medical attention or specific therapy. Occasional patients may derive benefit from splenectomy if the spleen is sequestering a significant amount of red blood cells.

SICKLE-C DISEASE Although the gene frequency for HbC ($\alpha_2\beta_2^{6Glu\rightarrow Lys}$) is only one-fourth that for HbS, the prevalence of SC disease among adults is almost as high as SS disease since the former group of patients has a nearly normal life expectancy. These individuals have a mild to moderate hemolytic anemia, usually accompanied by splenomegaly. On peripheral blood smears, target cells and occasional plump sickled forms are seen. Patients with SC disease may occasionally have painful crises or organ infarcts. They are at particular risk of developing ocular complications described above, including proliferative retinopathy and retinal detachment. In addition,

patients with SC disease are at relatively high risk of developing hematuria from renal medullary infarcts and avascular necrosis of the femoral heads. Pregnant women with SC disease have a high rate of complications during pregnancy. Individuals with an electrophoretic pattern suggestive of Hb SC disease but with more severe clinical manifestations are likely to be double heterozygotes for HbS and HbO Arab ($\alpha_2\beta_2^{121Glu\rightarrow Lys}$).

SICKLE-D DISEASE A number of hemoglobins comigrate with HbS on routine electrophoresis. The most commonly encountered variant is HbD Los Angeles ($\alpha_2\beta_2^{121Glu\rightarrow Gln}$). Hemoglobins S and D can be separated by special electrophoretic methods. The diagnosis of Hb SD disease is suggested by the demonstration of a positive sickle-cell preparation in one of the patient's two parents. SD double heterozygotes have moderately severe anemia.

HOMOZYGOUS HbC DISEASE This disease is a mild congenital hemolytic anemia accompanied by splenomegaly. Hemoglobin C has a tendency to form intracellular crystals, particularly if red blood cells are suspended in a hypertonic medium. The blood film reveals striking target cells. Red blood cell osmotic fragility is decreased. Patients rarely develop significant complications. No specific therapy is indicated.

UNSTABLE HEMOGLOBIN VARIANTS

In the early 1950s a group of patients in England were found to have congenital nonspherocytic hemolytic anemia associated with inclusions of precipitated hemoglobin (Heinz bodies) within red blood cells. The presence of an abnormal hemoglobin was suspected by the fact that a precipitate was formed when the patients' hemolysates were gently heated. Currently, over 60 different unstable hemoglobin variants have been identified. The great majority are single amino acid substitutions in the β chain. A few are due to deletion of one or more amino acids within the β chain. Patients present with a hemolytic anemia of variable degree. Severe cases are usually detected in late infancy or early childhood and have jaundice, splenomegaly, and dark-colored urine. An autosomal dominant mode of inheritance can usually be established, although about a fifth of the cases appear to be spontaneous mutants.

Pathogenesis These hemoglobin variants have structural alterations at sites in the molecule that drastically affect its stability and solubility. Many involve an amino acid substitution in the portion of the subunit where heme is inserted. In such instances, the heme may be displaced from the heme pocket. As a result, the solubility of the subunit is decreased, and the abnormal hemoglobin forms an intracellular precipitate (Heinz body). Red blood cells which contain this type of inclusion are recognized by the mononuclear-phagocyte system and are either cleansed of their intracellular debris (pitting) or destroyed. The displaced heme moiety is aberrantly catabolized, forming dipyrroles, such as mesobilifuscin, instead of bilirubin. Pigmenturia is probably due to the excretion of these dipyrroles. The degree of instability of these hemoglobin variants and, therefore, the extent of hemolysis vary considerably. In some, such as Hb Zürich, an additional oxidant stress, such as the ingestion of certain drugs, is required for significant hemolysis. In contrast, patients with Hb Hammersmith have continuous and marked red blood cell breakdown. The degree of anemia is influenced not only by the severity of the hemolysis but also by the ability of the blood to unload oxygen. Thus, patients having unstable variants with high oxygen affinity, such as Hb Köln, may have a near-normal hemoglobin level, i.e., compensated hemolysis. In contrast, the hemoglobin level is apt to be much lower in patients having variants with decreased oxygen affinity such as Hb Hammersmith.

Diagnosis The red blood cell morphology is somewhat variable. Often, patients with a functioning spleen have normal-looking red blood cells. Slight hypochromia and basophilic stippling are not uncommon. The blood may have to be incubated in order to bring out Heinz bodies. In some cases, red blood cells appear as if a bite had been taken from a margin. It is tempting to speculate that at this site a Heinz body had been pitted. Following splenectomy, red blood cells appear much more abnormal. Heinz bodies are larger and more numerous. The extent of clinical symptomatology varies markedly with the degree of anemia.

The diagnosis of a congenital Heinz body hemolytic anemia is established by the following laboratory tests and results:

1 *Hemoglobin electrophoresis* will often reveal an abnormal component, usually composing less than 30 percent of the total.
2 *Heinz bodies* can be demonstrated by incubating a freshly drawn sample of blood with a supravital strain.
3 A significant *precipitate* is formed when the hemolysate is incubated at 50°C, or in the presence of 17% isopropanol.
4 The unstable hemoglobins often have an abnormal *oxygen dissociation curve.*

If these tests are negative in a patient with congenital nonspherocytic hemolytic anemia, a defect of one of the red blood cell glycolytic enzymes is likely.

Treatment The treatment of congenital Heinz body hemolytic anemia is primarily supportive. Anemia is rarely severe enough to warrant blood transfusion. Oxidant drugs should be avoided. Like others with chronic hemolysis, these patients have an increased requirement for folic acid. Those with severe hemolysis should benefit from prophylactic folate therapy. The red blood cell mass may fall during a period of bone marrow suppression, such as that resulting from folate deficiency or acute infection. Although patients with severe hemolysis may benefit from splenectomy, this operation is not curative. Because of the risk of bacterial sepsis in infants and young children who have been splenectomized, this treatment should be postponed until the child is over 4 years old. The diagnostic tests cited above become more abnormal following splenectomy. For this reason, in some cases the diagnosis may not be definitely established until after the operation.

STABLE VARIANTS HAVING ABNORMAL O$_2$ AFFINITY

In 1966 it was discovered that certain members of a large family had erythrocytosis in association with an electrophoretically abnormal hemoglobin, Hb Chesapeake, which was found to have a very high affinity for oxygen. Since then, more than 20 other stable hemoglobin variants have been encountered which also have a significant increase in oxygen affinity. Their structural alterations tend to be at sites which influence hemoglobin's functional behavior. As a result of the hemoglobin's increased oxygen affinity, oxygen unloading to tissues is decreased, and there is an erythropoietin-mediated stimulus to erythropoiesis. Accordingly, these individuals have secondary erythrocytosis. This disorder is manifested in the heterozygous state and follows an autosomal codominant pattern of inheritance. Hematocrit levels are rarely high enough to cause a significant increase in blood viscosity. Thus, affected individuals are generally asymptomatic and lack any pertinent physical findings other than a ruddy complexion. The diagnosis should be suspected in all patients with unexplained erythrocytosis, particularly when other family members are similarly affected, and can be established by the demonstration of increased oxygen affinity of the whole blood. About two-thirds

TABLE 315-3
Differential diagnosis of cyanosis

I Decreased oxygenation of hemoglobin (↑ deoxyhemoglobin)
  A Reduced arterial oxygen tension (common)
    1 Pulmonary disease
    2 Cardiac right-to-left shunt
  B Hemoglobin variant having decreased oxygen affinity (rare): Hb Kansas, Hb Beth Israel
II Methemoglobinemia
  A Hereditary
    1 M hemoglobins:
      a HbM Boston (α_2 $^{58His \to Tyr}\beta_2$)
      b HbM Iwate ($\alpha_2^{87His \to Tyr}\beta_2$)
      c HbM Saskatoon ($\alpha_2\beta_2^{63His \to Tyr}$)
      d HbM Hyde Park ($\alpha_2\beta_2^{92His \to Tyr}$)
      e HbM Milwaukee ($\alpha_2\beta_2^{67Val \to Glu}$)
    2 Methemoglobin reductase deficiency
  B Acquired
    1 Nitrites and nitrates: Sodium nitrite, amyl nitrite, nitroglycerin, nitroprusside, silver nitrate
    2 Aniline dyes
    3 Acetanilid and phenacetin
    4 Sulfonamides
    5 Other: Lidocaine, chlorate, phenazopyridine

of the high affinity variants can be readily separated from HbA by electrophoresis. No treatment is indicated. The patient should be reassured that the disorder is benign.

Hemoglobin variants having a marked decrease in oxygen affinity cause one form of familial cyanosis (Table 315-3). Except for this cosmetic problem, individuals with Hb Kansas or Hb Beth Israel have no other clinical manifestations. Because of the abnormality of hemoglobin function, arterial blood is partially unsaturated despite normal oxygen tension. Blood values are otherwise normal.

METHEMOGLOBINEMIA

Oxygen transport depends on the maintenance of intracellular hemoglobin in the reduced (Fe^{2+}) state. When hemoglobin is oxidized to methemoglobin, the heme iron becomes Fe^{3+} and is incapable of binding oxygen. Normal red cells contain less than 1 percent methemoglobin. A small amount of hemoglobin autooxidizes as red cells circulate. This process probably occurs by the dissociation of the superoxide anion from oxyhemoglobin:

$$Hb^{2+}O_2 \to Hb^{3+} + O_2^-$$

Normally, the methemoglobin that is formed is reduced enzymatically by the following reaction:

$$Hb^{3+} + NADH \xrightarrow[\text{(Diaphorase I)}]{\text{Methemoglobin reductase}} Hb^{2+} + NAD$$

Hereditary methemoglobinemia is due either to the presence of one of the M hemoglobins or to the deficiency of the enzyme methemoglobin reductase (Table 315-3). These inherited disorders are clinically mild, while the induction of methemoglobinemia by drugs or toxins can be life threatening.

If methemoglobin exceeds 1.5 g per 100 ml (10 percent of the total hemoglobin), affected individuals will have clinically obvious cyanosis. The color of the skin is indistinguishable from the much commoner cyanosis due to the impairment of oxygen saturation that may occur in pulmonary and cardiac disorders (Table 315-3). With higher amounts of methemoglobin, patients become symptomatic. At a methemoglobin level of about 35 percent, the affected individual experiences headache, weakness, and breathlessness. Levels in excess of 70 percent are probably incompatible with life.

The toxicity of methemoglobinemia can be readily explained in terms of the current understanding of hemoglobin function. The fact that a certain proportion of the heme moieties is no longer able to bind oxygen is not a serious physiological handicap per se. A proportion of 30 percent methemoglobin is much more deleterious than a 30 percent decrement in red cell mass, because the oxidized hemes have a profound effect on the remaining functional hemes in the hemoglobin tetramer. The conformation of methemoglobin (like that of carboxyhemoglobin) is very similar to that of oxyhemoglobin. Thus, a partially oxidized hemoglobin tetramer has the same tertiary and quaternary structure as a molecule which is comparably oxygenated. In each case, the affinity of the remaining hemes for oxygen is increased. For this reason, methemoglobinemia (as well as carbon monoxide) causes a "shift to the left" of the oxyhemoglobin dissociation curve and, consequently, impaired unloading of oxygen to tissues.

M HEMOGLOBINS Five hemoglobin variants listed in Table 315-3 have abnormal absorbance spectra, owing to the oxidation of the heme iron in the affected subunit. They involve amino acid substitutions of residues responsible for the binding of the heme iron to the globin. These so-called "M hemoglobins" result in a rare form of congenital and familial cyanosis. Individuals with the α-chain variants HbM Boston and HbM Iwate are cyanotic at birth, while cyanosis does not appear in those with the β-chain variants (HbM Saskatoon, HbM Hyde Park, and HbM Milwaukee) until about 4 to 6 months of age, when fetal hemoglobin has been replaced by adult hemoglobin. As with the unstable and high-affinity variants, an autosomal codominant inheritance pattern is found. Except for cyanosis, patients are asymptomatic.

METHEMOGLOBIN REDUCTASE (NADH-DIAPHORASE) DEFICIENCY This condition is inherited in an autosomal recessive pattern. The enzyme is thought to be a flavoprotein having properties similar to those of liver microsomal cytochrome b_5 reductase. The erythrocyte and hepatic enzymes have long segments of identical primary structure.

Individuals with diaphorase I deficiency have lifelong cyanosis of variable degree but usually have no associated symptoms or other physical findings. Some may have mild polycythemia. Others have been noted to be mentally retarded. Untreated individuals usually have 15 to 30 percent methemoglobin. Methemoglobin levels are higher in the older population of red cells because the activity of the abnormal enzyme declines markedly with red cell age. There appears to be considerable polymorphism in the variant enzymes from different families, as shown by differences in their electrophoretic mobility and kinetic parameters. In these ways, diaphorase I deficiency resembles glucose 6-phosphate dehydrogenase deficiency.

ACQUIRED METHEMOGLOBINEMIA This disorder is generally due to exposure to certain drugs or toxins. (Compounds which can cause clinically significant methemoglobinemia are listed in Table 315-3.) Some agents such as nitrite and chlorate oxidize the heme iron directly. Others such as sulfa drugs and aniline must undergo biochemical transformation before they cause methemoglobinemia. Few if any drugs currently in use cause significant methemoglobinemia, unless the individual is unusually susceptible. As might be expected, individuals heterozygous for methemoglobin reductase deficiency are much more likely than normal individuals to develop clinically apparent methemoglobinemia after exposure to an oxidant stress. The extent of methemoglobinemia depends not only on the dose of the toxic agent but also on the susceptibility of the exposed individual.

DIAGNOSIS Methemoglobinemia should be considered in any cyanotic patient with no evidence of heart or lung disease. If the cyanosis is due to decreased oxygen saturation, a blood specimen will change from a purple to a red color upon mixing with air. In contrast, a blood specimen from a methemoglobinemic individual remains a chocolate brown color irrespective of exposure to air. Methemoglobinemia can be documented by spectroscopic examination of the hemolysate. Individuals with hereditary methemoglobinemia will have lower levels than patients symptomatic from acquired methemoglobinemia. Occasional patients may have an additional hemoglobin derivative of unknown structure called sulfhemoglobin, which is also induced by oxidant-type drugs or toxins. Sulfhemoglobinemia tends to cause cyanosis even more readily than methemoglobinemia. Unlike methemoglobin, the absorbance of sulfhemoglobin at 620 to 630 nm is not decreased by the addition of cyanide. The M hemoglobins have characteristic spectral abnormalities which differ from normal hemoglobin (HbA), which is partially oxidized. Furthermore, these hemoglobin variants can be detected by hemoglobin electrophoresis.

TREATMENT In individuals with methemoglobin reductase deficiency, the oral administration of methylene blue (100 to 300 mg per day) or ascorbic acid (300 to 500 mg per day) will result in a marked reduction in the level of methemoglobin. The purpose of treatment is primarily cosmetic. Severe toxic methemoglobinemia is treated by the intravenous administration of methylene blue (2 mg/kg, repeat if needed). Usually, within an hour, the methemoglobin level is reduced by at least 50 percent. Treatment is neither necessary nor possible in individuals having HbM.

THALASSEMIAS

The thalassemias are a group of congenital disorders in which there is a defect in the synthesis of one (or more) of the subunits of hemoglobin. As a result of decreased production of hemoglobin, the red blood cells are hypochromic and microcytic (Table 53-1). The thalassemias which are due to decreased production of β chains are found primarily in peoples from the Mediterranean basin. The gene frequency for β-thalassemia trait is approximately 10 percent in southern Italy and certain Mediterranean islands. β thalassemia is also encountered quite commonly in central Africa, Asia, the South Pacific, and certain parts of India. In contrast, α thalassemia is found primarily among southern Orientals and in a milder form among blacks. From both a genetic and clinical viewpoint, the thalassemias are a heterogeneous group of disorders varying widely in prevalence, severity, and pathogenesis. A classification of the commonly encountered thalassemias is shown in Table 315-4.

GENETICS The inheritance pattern of β thalassemia is autosomal codominant, analogous to that for β-chain structural variants. As described in detail below, the heterozygous state has minimal clinical manifestations. Statistically, one-quarter of the offspring of two parents with β-thalassemia trait will have the homozygous state: β thalassemia major or Cooley's anemia. An individual may inherit the β-thalassemia gene from one parent and a β-chain structural variant from the other. Sickle-β-thalassemia (discussed above) is a commonly encountered example of such a double heterozygous state.

The genetic basis of the α thalassemias is less well understood. There is considerable evidence that normal individuals have four α-chain genes, two from each parent. If so, then four types of α thalassemia shown in Table 315-4 can be attributed to gene dosage with the silent carrier having only one α-thalas-

TABLE 315-4
Classification of the thalassemias

Diagnosis	Globin chain synthesis in reticulocytes β/α*	RBC morphology	Hb electrophoresis	Clinical severity
β thalassemia:				
Heterozygous	0.5	↓ MCV,† stippling	↑ A₂ (± ↑ HbF)	0 to +
Homozygous	0–0.3	↓ MCV, hypochromic Nucleated RBC, targets bizarre shapes	↑↑ HbF	4+ (major) 2–3+ (intermedia)
α thalassemia:	α/β*			
Silent carrier	0.9	Normal	Normal	0
α-thalassemia trait	0.7	↓ MCV	Normal	0
HbH disease	0.3	↓ MCV Heinz bodies	↑HbH (β₄) (10–15%)	2+
Hydrops fetalis	0	↑↑ Nucleated RBC	↑↑ Hb Barts (γ₄)	4+

* *Normal = 1.*
† *MCV = mean corpuscular volume.*

semia gene and three normal genes, and the stillborn baby having four abnormal (or absent) genes. However, the genetics of some of the α thalassemias (i.e., in blacks) may be even more complex than what is summarized here.

MOLECULAR PATHOGENESIS In contrast to the *qualitative* hemoglobin abnormalities listed in Table 315-1, the thalassemias are *quantitative* abnormalities of subunit synthesis. Thus, the β chains of patients with β thalassemia major have normal structure but are produced in reduced and sometimes in undetectable amounts. The impairment in globin chain synthesis can be demonstrated in vitro by incubating reticulocytes with labeled amino acids and determining the incorporation of radioactivity into globin subunits. As shown in Table 315-4, in β thalassemia major, the incorporation of label into β chains is markedly reduced or absent ($\beta/\alpha = 0$ to 0.3). In β thalassemia minor, the β/α synthesis ratio is ∼ 0.5. Similar results are obtained when the incubations are performed in a cell-free system. As shown in Table 315-4, β/α synthesis ratios are increased in the α thalassemias. Direct measurements utilizing RNA-DNA hybridization have revealed a quantitative decrease in β-mRNA in some cases of β thalassemia and of α-mRNA in the α thalassemias. In some of the β thalassemias, there appears to be a defect in transcription of β-globin-DNA into mRNA. Thus, β thalassemia may be due to an abnormality of an operator gene for the β chain. In contrast, α thalassemia usually involves an actual deletion of the DNA which codes for the α chain.

CELLULAR PATHOGENESIS As a result of imbalance in globin chain synthesis, the thalassemias have varying degrees of ineffective erythropoiesis and hemolysis. In β thalassemia major there is a marked relative excess of α-chain production. Free α chains have decreased solubility and will form insoluble aggregates or inclusions within red blood cell precursors in the bone marrow. Like congenital Heinz body hemolytic anemia due to unstable hemoglobin variants, the inclusion bodies in thalassemia bring about abnormalities in membrane permeability as well as entrapment and destruction of red blood cells by the macrophages in the mononuclear-phagocyte system. As a result, β thalassemia is characterized by both intramedullary erythroid destruction and also a marked shortening of the life span of circulating red blood cells that emerge from the bone marrow. Thus, these patients have the characteristic parameters of both ineffective erythropoiesis (increased plasma iron turnover, decreased incorporation of ^{59}Fe into red blood cells) and peripheral hemolysis. Because these red blood cells are under double jeopardy, there is an enormous compensatory stimulus to erythropoiesis, resulting both in expansion of the red marrow and in extramedullary hematopoiesis in the liver

and spleen. Chain imbalance in β thalassemia is attenuated to a variable degree by the "compensatory" synthesis of γ chains which are able to combine with excess free α chains and form a stable tetramer (HbF). Patients with Cooley's anemia who have a relatively high rate of γ-chain production have a less severe clinical course. Individuals with β thalassemia minor have absent or very mild ineffective erythropoiesis and hemolysis, detectable in some patients by a slight elevation in fecal urobilinogen and a modest shortening of the red blood cell life span.

In the α thalassemias a relative excess production of non-α chains can be detected, leading to the formation of Hb Barts (γ₄) in the newborn and young infant and HbH (β₄) in children and adults. In contrast to the α-chain inclusions found in β thalassemia, the Heinz bodies due to HbH are more stable and develop in mature circulating red blood cells. As a result, HbH disease is primarily a hemolytic disorder without a significant amount of ineffective erythropoiesis.

CLINICAL FEATURES AND LABORATORY FINDINGS β **thalassemia minor** This common entity is rarely associated with significant clinical manifestations. The diagnosis is generally made in patients being evaluated for mild anemia or in follow-up of abnormalities found on routine blood studies. Probably most individuals with β-thalassemia trait go without diagnosis. About one-fifth of affected individuals have splenomegaly. Icterus is occasionally noted, particularly in those individuals who also have Gilbert's disease, another common and benign congenital disorder (Chap. 301).

In otherwise healthy individuals with β-thalassemia trait, the mean hemoglobin level is about 15 percent lower than in normal persons of the same age and sex; the red blood cell count is usually elevated, and the cells are microcytic. Indeed, at any level of hematocrit, patients with β thalassemia minor will have more marked microcytosis than those with iron deficiency. In addition to microcytosis and mild hypochromia, examination of the blood film reveals occasional target cells, cigar-shaped cells, and a moderate amount of basophilic stippling; the reticulocyte count is normal. Special isotope techniques are required to demonstrate a slightly reduced red blood cell life span. The red blood cells have decreased osmotic fragility. Serum iron is normal unless the patient also happens to be iron-deficient. Hemoglobin electrophoresis is very useful in establishing the diagnosis of β thalassemia minor. Most affected individuals will have a twofold increase in HbA₂ (5 percent versus normal of 2.5 percent). In contrast, HbA₂ is subnormal in iron deficiency and sideroblastic anemias. Patients with β-thalassemia trait who become iron-deficient usually have a "normal" level of HbA₂ which increases to above normal after correction of the deficiency. Almost half of individuals with β thalassemia minor also have moderate elevation of HbF (2 to 5 percent). In rare instances, the thalassemic state also affects the adjacent δ-chain gene: $\delta\beta$ or F thalassemia. If so, HbA_2 levels will be normal, but HbF is increased (5 to 15 percent).

No treatment is indicated for individuals with β-thalassemia trait. They should be reassured that they do not have a serious hematologic problem. The genetic implications of thalassemia should be explained, particularly to those of childbearing age. Many individuals have been given long-term iron treatment on the mistaken impression that they had iron-deficiency anemia. These patients may gradually develop clinically significant siderosis. Establishing the diagnosis of β thalassemia minor should prevent such inappropriate therapy.

β thalassemia major Cooley's anemia is probably the most severe form of congenital hemolytic anemia. Clinical manifestations generally appear after the first four to six months of life when the switch from γ-chain to β-chain production usually occurs. Patients develop a severe anemia with a hematocrit of less than 20 unless they are supported by transfusions. Accordingly, patients have all the signs and symptoms associated with severe anemia. In addition, they have findings related to severe intramedullary and peripheral hemolysis and to iron overload. Patients with β thalassemia major often have marked wasting and appear malnourished. Children have slow rates of growth and development. In adolescents, the onset and development of secondary sex characteristics are delayed. Patients have a peculiar skin color due to a combination of icterus and increased melanin deposition. They usually have skeletal abnormalities, secondary to expansion of the erythroid marrow. Enlargement of the malar bones may give the characteristic "chipmunk" facies or cause malocclusion of the jaw. Patients invariably have cardiomegaly which may be accompanied by signs of congestive heart failure. Marked hepatomegaly and splenomegaly are always found in these patients.

The *diagnosis* of β thalassemia major should be entertained in any patient with a severe hemolytic anemia and hypochromic microcytic red blood cells. Examination of the peripheral blood smear reveals marked variations in the size and shape of red blood cells, including many target cells as well as teardrop and cigar-shaped cells. Normoblasts are usually seen, particularly if the patient has undergone splenectomy. Hemoglobin electrophoresis shows the presence of large amounts of HbF and variable amounts of HbA. In patients who are homozygous for β^0 thalassemia, no HbA can be detected. Hemoglobin A_2 is usually increased about twofold, although it can be normal in β thalassemia major.

Patients with β thalassemia major have a short life expectancy. It is unusual for a patient with the most severe form of the disease to survive into adulthood. Most patients have such severe anemia that they are dependent upon transfusions. The chronic administration of large amounts of blood along with an inappropriate increase in iron absorption from the gastrointestinal tract inevitably leads to clinically significant hemosiderosis. As a result of iron overload, these patients develop abnormalities in hepatic, pancreatic, and cardiac function. The combination of chronic hypoxia and myocardial siderosis leads to cardiac arrhythmias, congestive failure, and ultimately death.

Homozygotes who survive into adulthood are likely to have a milder form of the disease, designated as *β thalassemia intermedia*. There are several genetic subtypes which are associated with less severe clinical manifestations: (1) β thalassemia with unusually high levels of HbF synthesis, (2) $\beta\delta$ thalassemia in which there is suppression of δ-chain as well as β-chain synthesis, and (3) the presence of heterozygous α thalassemia in combination with homozygous β thalassemia, leading to more balanced subunit synthesis. A milder clinical course is also seen in individuals who are doubly heterozygous for β thalassemia and hereditary persistence of HbF. These patients usually have moderately severe anemia, but do not require transfusions.

Treatment of β thalassemia major is primarily supportive. The obvious benefits of transfusion therapy are partially offset by the risk of iron overload, hepatitis, and isoimmunization. Despite these problems, children with Cooley's anemia fare better if their hemoglobin is maintained at greater than 9 g per 100 ml. In view of the increased demands of the hyperplastic marrow, it is reasonable to maintain these patients on a daily supplement of folic acid. Since splenic sequestration contributes to shortened red blood cell survival, many patients derive some benefit from splenectomy. The prevention and treatment of iron overload is a continuing concern in these patients. It has recently been demonstrated that the combination of continuous subcutaneous injection of desferrioxamine and oral ascorbic acid permits the mobilization and excretion of significant amounts of iron. However, the long-term efficacy of this therapy has not yet been established.

Considerations of genetic counseling and antenatal diagnosis are as relevant in the *prevention* of β thalassemia major as they are for sickle-cell anemia (see above).

REFERENCES

BUNN HF et al: *Human Hemoglobins.* Philadelphia, Saunders, 1977

CASTLE WB: From man to molecule and back to mankind. Semin Hematol 13:159, 1976

DEAN J, SCHECHTER AN: Sickle cell anemia: Molecular and cellular bases of therapeutic approaches. N Engl J Med 299:752, 804, 863, 1978

EATON WA et al: Delay time of gelation: A possible determinant of severity of sickle cell disease. Blood 47:621, 1976

KAN YW: Prenatal diagnosis of hemoglobin disorders. Prog Hematol 10:91, 1977

KIESE M: *Methemoglobinemia: A Comprehensive Treatise.* West Palm Beach, CRC Press, 1977

LESSIN LS, JENSEN WN: Sickle cell symposium. Arch Intern Med 133:529, 1974

NIENHUIS AW, BENZ EJ: Regulation of hemoglobin synthesis during the development of the red cell. N Engl J Med 197:1318, 1430, 1977

ORKIN S, NATHAN DG: Thalassemia: Genetics and molecular pathogenesis. N Engl J Med 295:710, 1976

POWARS DR: Natural history of sickle cell disease: The first ten years. Semin Hematol 12:267, 1975

WEATHERALL DJ, CLEGG JB: *The Thalassemia Syndromes.* Oxford, Blackwell, 1972

WOOD WG et al: Developmental biology of human hemoglobins. Prog Hematol 10:43, 1977

Clotting disorders

316
PLATELET DISORDERS

HYMIE L. NOSSEL

Platelet disorders may be due to altered number of function of the platelets. Disorders of platelet number include thrombocytopenia and thrombocythemia (thrombocytosis). The most common serious bleeding disorder involving platelets is thrombocytopenia.

THROMBOCYTOPENIA

CLINICAL CONSIDERATIONS The normal platelet count ranges from 150,000 to 400,000 per cubic millimeter. A platelet count of less than 100,000 per cubic millimeter is generally considered to constitute thrombocytopenia. There is an approximate relationship between the platelet count and severity of bleeding. A sudden drop in the platelet count, fever, and anemia aggravate the hemostatic defect of thrombocytopenia. With platelet counts above 40,000 per cubic millimeter, bleeding may occur after injury or surgery, but spontaneous bleeding is uncommon. Spontaneous bleeding is common with platelet counts between 10,000 and 20,000 per cubic millimeter; with counts below 10,000 per cubic millimeter, it is usual and often severe.

Spontaneous bleeding into the skin manifests as petechiae, purpuric spots, or confluent ecchymoses. In the mouth, blood-filled bullae are almost pathognomonic for thrombocytopenia. Bleeding may occur from any mucosal surface, including the nose and uterus and the gastrointestinal, urinary, or respiratory tracts. The most serious site for spontaneous bleeding is the central nervous system, where it may be fatal. Bleeding due to trauma in a thrombocytopenic patient presents a number of features distinct from bleeding in a patient with a coagulation factor disorder: (1) it occurs immediately after the trauma; (2) in mild cases it may cease in response to local pressure; and (3) it usually stops within 48 h and does not readily recur.

MECHANISMS A low platelet count may result from one or a combination of mechanisms. These include abnormal platelet production, disordered platelet distribution, and increased rate of destruction (Table 316-1).

Defective production of platelets may result from decreased production or from defective maturation. When platelet production is significantly diminished, the number of megakaryocytes visible in a bone marrow aspirate is usually significantly decreased.

Reduced production may result from (1) the administration of drugs such as the cytotoxic agents used in cancer chemotherapy (this is the commonest cause of thrombocytopenia in a large medical center), gold, sulfonamides, and ethanol and irradiation of the bone marrow; (2) generalized decrease in production of all marrow cells (aplastic anemia); (3) marrow replacement or infiltration, including marrow fibrosis (myelophthisis), leukemia, and metastatic carcinoma; and (4) congenital deficiency of a thrombopoietic factor.

Defective maturation is associated with vitamin B_{12} or folate deficiency, the myeloproliferative disorders, paroxysmal nocturnal hemoglobinuria, and two hereditary disorders, the Wiskott-Aldrich syndrome and the May-Hegglin anomaly. In these disorders the bone marrow shows a normal or increased number of megakaryocytes, but thrombopoiesis is ineffective in a manner analogous to ineffective erythropoiesis.

Disordered distribution of platelets may be the cause of thrombocytopenia. In normal individuals about 30 percent of the circulating platelets are present in the spleen, whereas with massive splenomegaly up to 80 percent of the total number of circulating platelets may be in the spleen, resulting in thrombocytopenia in the peripheral blood. Thrombocytopenia may occur in any patient with a significantly enlarged spleen. However, the thrombocytopenia is rarely severe enough to produce hemorrhagic disease, and splenectomy will restore the platelet count to normal levels, but is not usually required.

Accelerated destruction of platelets is a frequent cause of thrombocytopenia. The survival time of platelets is markedly decreased from the normal of 10 days to less than 1 day. The commonest causes of accelerated platelet destruction are antibody-mediated platelet injury, increased platelet utilization in disseminated intravascular coagulation, and massive blood transfusion.

Antibody-mediated thrombocytopenia may be due to (1) *autoantibodies* in idiopathic thrombocytopenic purpura, systemic lupus erythematosus, chronic lymphocytic leukemia, and in association with autoimmune hemolytic anemia; (2) alloantibodies associated with pregnancy or transfusion; (3) antibodies associated with the administration of certain drugs such as quinidine, quinine, and sulfonamides.

TABLE 316-1
Causes of thrombocytopenia

I Production defect
  A Reduced thrombopoiesis (reduced megakaryocytes)
    1 Marrow injury: Drugs, chemicals, radiation, infection
    2 Marrow failure: Acquired, congenital (Fanconi's syndrome, amegakaryocytic)
    3 Marrow invasion: Carcinoma, leukemia, lymphoma, fibrosis
    4 Lack of marrow stimulus: Thrombopoietin deficiency
  B Defective maturation (normal or increased megakaryocytes)
    1 Vitamin B_{12} deficiency, folic acid deficiency
    2 Hereditary: Wiskott-Aldrich syndrome, May-Hegglin anomaly
II Sequestration (disordered distribution)
  A Splenomegaly
  B Hypothermic anesthesia
III Accelerated destruction
  A Antibodies
    1 Autoantibodies
      a ITP, systemic lupus erythematosus, hemolytic anemias, lymphoreticular disorders
      b Drugs
    2 Alloantibodies
      a Fetal-maternal incompatibility
      b Following transfusions
  B Nonimmunologic
    1 Injury due to:
      a Infection
      b Prosthetic heart valves
    2 Consumption
      a Thrombin in disseminated intravascular coagulation
      b Thrombotic thrombocytopenic purpura
    3 Loss by hemorrhage and massive transfusion

IDIOPATHIC THROMBOCYTOPENIC PURPURA (ITP) Clinical features This disorder may be considered the prototype thrombocytopenic state. The chief sign is purpura over the limbs, upper chest, and neck. Mucosal bleeding may occur. There is no adenopathy. The spleen is not palpable in 90 percent of patients and when palpable does not usually extend more than 1 cm below the left costal margin. Fever and malaise are uncommon.

The course of the disorder may be acute or chronic. The acute form of the disease occurs most commonly in children between the ages of 2 and 6 years, but is seen in adults as well. Bleeding starts suddenly, usually being most severe at the onset. The risk of cerebral hemorrhage is greatest at this time. Bleeding usually ceases within a few days, although some patients may display a bleeding tendency for several months. When bleeding persists for 6 months or more, the disease is considered to be chronic. The chronic recurrent form occurs most often in women between 20 and 40 years of age. The onset is usually more gradual and intermittent than in the acute form. Characteristically, transient remissions occur and may last weeks, months, or years.

Idiopathic thrombocytopenic purpura may present with bleeding localized to one site only, e.g., menorrhagia, hematuria, or epistaxis. In such patients idiopathic thrombocytopenic purpura should be suspected, and the platelet count should be measured.

Laboratory tests A low platelet count is present in the peripheral blood, and the platelets are normal morphologically, although occasionally large and atypical forms may be present. The bleeding time is prolonged, usually in proportion to the degree of thrombocytopenia. The whole-blood clotting time test is normal, but clot retraction is poor or absent when the platelet count is below 40,000 per cubic millimeter. Anemia is present only to the extent of blood loss; the erythrocyte sedimentation rate is usually normal. Bone marrow examination reveals megakaryocytes in normal or increased numbers with normal morphology. Platelet antibodies can be demonstrated in vitro (see below), but these tests are difficult to perform and are not yet part of routine laboratory studies.

Differential diagnosis A significant degree of splenomegaly, fever, disproportionate anemia, or a high sedimentation rate suggests another diagnosis. Bone marrow examination is essential in order to exclude other marrow diseases; the histology of the spleen should be examined for the same reason if the spleen is removed for therapeutic reasons. It is important to exclude other diagnoses, in particular drug-induced thrombocytopenia on a sensitization basis because the clinical and hematologic pictures of idiopathic and drug-induced hypersensitivity thrombocytopenic purpura are indistinguishable. A careful history is the only clue to the possibility of drug-induced thrombocytopenia. Systemic lupus erythematosus and other diseases associated with platelet antibodies should be considered, and appropriate serologic tests for lupus erythematosus should be carried out. When thrombocytopenia results from platelet sequestration in a large spleen, anemia and leukopenia are usually associated. In leukemia, disproportionate anemia is frequent and the marrow is diagnostic. In aplastic anemia, pancytopenia is characteristic, and bone marrow biopsy should reveal hypocellularity. In patients with bone marrow infiltration, large platelets or megakaryocyte fragments may be present, the patient is usually anemic, normoblasts and myelocytes are found in the peripheral blood, and the marrow is diagnostic.

Pathogenesis Platelet antibodies are present in the plasma of most patients with ITP. For this reason the term *autoimmune thrombocytopenia* has been proposed. Transfusion of plasma from patients with this disease causes transient thrombocytopenia and clinical purpura in the recipient. It is also known that transient thrombocytopenia may occur in infants born to mothers with ITP, suggesting transplacental passage of the antiplatelet factor.

In vitro demonstration of platelet antibodies in ITP has been difficult because the antibodies do not fix complement. Agglutination techniques have been unreliable because of the tendency of platelets to adhere. Antibodies have been demonstrated by measuring platelet factor 3 after exposure to IgG fractions from serum, release of platelet serotonin or lymphocyte stimulation by platelet-serum fraction complexes. Convincing evidence has been obtained of increased IgG bound to the platelets of patients with ITP. Patients who respond to corticosteroid therapy have less platelet-bound IgG. With response to therapy the amount of bound IgG decreases.

The antibody has been shown to be an IgG which sensitizes platelets for sequestration. Antibody synthesis has been shown to occur in the spleen.

Treatment of acute ITP More than 80 percent of patients with acute ITP will recover in time regardless of therapy; hence conservative management is favored. Treatment should take into account the following possibilities.

1 Corticosteroids do not appear to shorten the duration of thrombocytopenia, but prednisone, 1 mg per kilogram of body weight per day in children or 40 to 60 mg per day in adults, is advisable during the first 2 to 4 weeks because of a possible beneficial effect on capillary integrity.
2 Platelet transfusions may be of transient benefit in treating severe hemorrhage.
3 About 20 percent of children with ITP fail to recover in 6 months, and their course is similar to that of adults with chronic ITP. Of these 20 percent, about one-third have no or mild symptoms and do not require therapy. Purpura in the remainder can generally be controlled with prednisone. Splenectomy is generally advised if large doses of steroids are required beyond 3 to 6 months, although alternate-day steroid therapy may permit normal growth and minimize other undesirable side effects.
4 Splenectomy carried out on such patients is beneficial in 85 percent of cases.
5 Immunosuppressive therapy may be considered if splenectomy fails.

Treatment of chronic ITP The most important modes of treatment are the following.

1 Adrenocortical steroids produce a beneficial effect by improving the life span of antibody-coated platelets, by suppressing the phagocytic activity of the reticuloendothelial system and of the spleen in particular. Recent studies suggest that antibody synthesis is inhibited as well. A dose of 0.5 mg prednisone per kilogram per day will elevate the platelet count in mild cases; 1 mg/kg may be needed for cases of intermediate severity; 2 mg/kg or more per day may be necessary if the platelet count is less than 10,000 per cubic millimeter. The platelet count usually rises after several days, and by 14 days the majority of patients will show an elevation of platelet level. If improvement does not occur within 2 to 3 weeks or can be maintained only with massive doses of steroids, the spleen should be removed. In the patients who respond to steroids, dosage should be gradually reduced over a several-week period until the platelet count is about 60,000 per cubic millimeter. Splenectomy is favored in

patients who fail to recover spontaneously within 3 to 6 months, who require more than 5 to 10 mg prednisone per day, and who are suitable operative risks.

2 Splenectomy removes the major site of platelet destruction and also a significant source of platelet antibody synthesis. Prior to surgery the prednisone dosage should be increased to raise the platelet count. Platelet transfusion may be used in the presence of severe thrombocytopenia but is usually not required in the less severe cases. Eighty percent of patients improve after splenectomy, and the platelet count is restored to normal levels permanently in two-thirds of patients. The count may rise within 24 h or within a week of surgery. There is no certain method of predicting a successful response to splenectomy. Following splenectomy, steroids should be withdrawn gradually over a 3-week period. If steroids are still required to prevent purpura or severe thrombocytopenia, immunosuppression should be considered.

3 Patients in whom splenectomy has failed may show an immunosuppressive response to vincristine, cyclophosphamide, or azathioprine. An initial response rate of 50 to 70 percent to each of these drugs has been reported but is often not sustained. The clinical response with each of the three drugs has been approximately the same, but vincristine might be considered as the initial agent because of its marrow sparing effect.

4 Platelet transfusion is often effective in treating life-threatening hemorrhage but should not be used prophylactically because of the short platelet life span and because of alloantibody formation.

OTHER AUTOANTIBODY THROMBOCYTOPENIAS Thrombocytopenia occurs in about 10 percent of patients with systemic lupus erythematosus. The thrombocytopenia usually results from platelet autoantibodies, and hemolysis due to red blood cell autoantibodies is often present as well. The treatment and the results of treatment are the same as in ITP. Autoimmune thrombocytopenic purpura may also occur in association with a Coombs-positive hemolytic anemia (Evans syndrome) and in association with chronic lymphocytic leukemia.

Thrombocytopenia due to drugs and chemicals (see Table 316-2) In every adult patient with thrombocytopenia a drug etiology should be considered. Thrombocytopenia may be part of the marrow depression which occurs with the cytotoxic agents used in the therapy of leukemia, lymphoma, and carcinoma. Generalized marrow depression and consequent pancytopenia may also occur with other drugs such as gold or the sulfonamides. Selective thrombocytopenia may result from a specific effect on the megakaryocytes or as part of a hypersensitivity reaction in the peripheral blood. In the latter case the drug is thought to act as a hapten and bind to a plasma protein to form the primary antigen. Antibodies stimulated by the primary antigen bind the drug, and thrombocytopenia occurs when antigen-antibody complexes form which have a high affinity for the platelet membrane. The drugs most commonly associated with hypersensitivity reactions are quinidine, quinine, and sulfonamides.

The clinical manifestation of drug-induced thrombocytopenia is bleeding. In hypersensitivity reactions bleeding usually occurs within hours or days of initial drug administration, although it may occur after weeks or months of ingestion of the drug. Thrombocytopenia often develops abruptly. Bleeding is often severe and sudden in onset and may be associated with fever and systemic symptoms when toxic suppression of the marrow is involved. Thrombocytopenia usually develops gradually.

TABLE 316-2
Drugs implicated in thrombocytopenia

I Suppression of platelet production
  A Myelosuppressive drugs
    1 Severe: Cytosine arabinoside, daunorubicin
    2 Moderate: Cyclophosphamide, busulfan, methotrexate, 6-mercaptopurine
    3 Mild: Vinca alkaloids
  B Thiazide diuretics
  C Ethanol
  D Estrogens
II Immunologic platelet destruction
  A Clinical suspicion plus convincing experimental evidence
    1 Antibiotics: Sulfathiazole, novobiocin, p-aminosalicylate
    2 Cinchona alkaloids: Quinidine, quinine
    3 Foods: Beans
    4 Sedatives, hypnotics, anticonvulsants: Sedormid, carbamazepine, Centalun
    5 Arsenical drugs used to treat syphilis
    6 Digitoxin
    7 Methyldopa
    8 Stibophen
  B Clinical suspicion (major drugs implicated)
    1 Aspirin
    2 Chlorpropamide
    3 Chloroquine
    4 Chlorothiazide and hydrochlorothiazide
    5 Gold salts
    6 Insecticides
    7 Sulfadiazine, sulfisoxazole, sulfamerazine, sulfamethazine, sulfamethoxypyridazine, sulfamethoxazole, sulfatolamide

The bone marrow may show increased numbers of megakaryocytes when peripheral blood destruction of platelets is the mechanism of thrombocytopenia (hypersensitivity reactions), or a reduced number of megakaryocytes and other marrow elements in marrow depression. Evidence of drug hypersensitivity may be demonstrable in vitro. The drug may inhibit clot retraction when added to the patient's blood, but this is an insensitive test. Complement fixation is a far more sensitive test for drug hypersensitivity.

Patients with hypersensitivity thrombocytopenia generally recover briskly in response to withdrawal of the offending drug. Adrenocorticosteroids should be given for control of bleeding, and platelet transfusion is indicated if the bleeding is potentially fatal. Splenectomy is *not* indicated. Patients should be given a card to carry with them, indicating the drug sensitivity. When thrombocytopenia is part of aplastic anemia, the prognosis is that of the cause of the underlying anemia.

Thrombocytopenic purpura due to alloantibodies Alloantibodies may occur following immunization of the mother against fetal platelets with subsequent transplacental transfer of the antibody. The infant may manifest purpura at birth; if it is severe, steroids, exchange transfusion, and transfusion with maternal platelets may be tried.

A complement-fixing platelet alloantibody may develop in the blood of a patient following blood transfusion. This disorder results from sensitization of the patient to an antigen in the transfused platelets. The antigen Pl^{A1} occurs in 98 percent of the population and is absent from the platelets of a recipient who develops the disorder. Thrombocytopenic purpura may develop suddenly about 1 week after the transfusion and may persist for 6 weeks. The mechanism of the thrombocytopenia is not clear. There is some evidence that antibody provoked by Pl^{A1} antigen reacts with the antigen to form soluble immune complexes with a special affinity for the patient's own Pl^{A1}-negative platelets. The mechanism of this special affinity is unclear. If the thrombocytopenia is severe (below 10,000 per cubic millimeter), large doses of steroids and exchange transfusion should be used.

NONIMMUNOLOGIC THROMBOCYTOPENIC PURPURA Nonimmunologic causes of purpura include several forms of platelet injury and consumption.

Platelet injury INFECTION Thrombocytopenia occurring in acute infection may be due to marrow suppression, injury to the platelets caused directly by the organism or by exotoxins released by staphylococci or streptococci or endotoxins from gram-negative organisms. Disseminated intravascular coagulation may occur and contribute to the thrombocytopenia.

PROSTHETIC HEART VALVES Thrombocytopenia may occur with or without a hemolytic anemia with fragmented red blood cells in patients with malfunctioning prosthetic heart valves. It has been suggested that extreme turbulence is responsible for the hemolysis.

Platelet consumption DISSEMINATED INTRAVASCULAR COAGULATION In this condition thrombin aggregates platelets and reduces the circulating platelet count. Patients with diffuse intravascular clotting occasionally have fragmented red blood cells.

THROMBOTIC THROMBOCYTOPENIC PURPURA (TTP) This is a fulminating, generally lethal disorder characterized by a Coombs-negative hemolytic anemia with severely fragmented red blood cells (microangiopathic hemolytic anemia), thrombocytopenic purpura, fever, renal failure, and fluctuating, often bizarre, neurologic manifestations. Most patients die within a few weeks of the onset of the disease. The anemia is usually severe, the packed cell volume often being below 20 percent with a marked reticulocytosis. An essential diagnostic requirement is the presence of severely fragmented red blood cells in the peripheral blood smear. The diagnosis can be confirmed by the presence of hyalin thrombi in the lumina of arterioles and capillaries in the absence of vessel wall damage or inflammation. Lymph node, marrow, or gingival biopsy specimens may give a positive diagnosis in a significant number of patients. Fibrin has been demonstrated in the thrombotic lesions by immunofluorescence. The deposits are composed of platelets and fibrin. Blood coagulation tests generally show normal values with elevated fibrinogen levels in the early stages of the disease. Hypofibrinogenemia and elevated fibrinogen degradation product levels occur occasionally. Platelet survival is markedly decreased, and fibrinogen survival is only moderately reduced. Electron microscopy has revealed subendothelial accumulations of platelets and fibrin in patent capillaries. The cause of TTP is unknown. The available evidence does not support disseminated intravascular coagulation as having a primary pathogenic role. Platelet consumption is important, but it is not known whether the platelets or the vessel wall are primarily involved. The red blood cell fragmentation and hemolysis may result from contact with fibrin deposited in vessels. Some cases have occurred in association with systemic lupus erythematosus, rheumatoid arthritis, polyarteritis, or Sjögrens syndrome.

Acute TTP constitutes a medical emergency. Therapy unfortunately is empiric and quite unpredictable in its effects. Large doses of prednisone with splenectomy have been associated with remission in a number of cases. Remissions have been reported following plasmapheresis with or without plasma transfusion. However, the best method of therapy still remains to be determined. When the patient is improving, or in mild cases, recovery may be accelerated by the use of aspirin and dipyridamole which inhibit platelet aggregation. Heparin therapy is generally ineffective.

HEMOLYTIC-UREMIC SYNDROME This syndrome is a disease of infancy (6 to 12 months) or early childhood (until age 6) characterized by the acute onset of fever, renal failure, microangiopathic hemolytic anemia, and thrombocytopenia. Hypertension is often present. A minor febrile illness with diarrhea or respiratory symptoms may precede the illness, and it has been postulated that virus-related immune complexes play a primary role in the pathogenesis of the syndrome. Laboratory studies reveal markedly decreased platelet survival but only moderately decreased fibrinogen survival. An occasional patient may show evidence of disseminated intravascular coagulation. Biopsy reveals hyalin occlusions in the afferent arterioles and glomerular capillaries of the kidneys, but other organs are usually not affected. With regard to therapy, corticosteroids and heparin have equivocal effects. Dialysis and the judicious use of red blood cell transfusions are helpful and with their aid the mortality rate in the acute stage may be as low as 5 percent. Half of the survivors develop chronic renal disease.

OTHER CAUSES Thrombocytopenia and hemolysis with fragmented red blood cells may also occur with neoplasms, with widespread metastatic tumors. They may also occur as a complication of pregnancy or the puerperium when toxemia is present. The pathogenetic mechanism is not established.

PLATELET TRANSFUSIONS

Platelet transfusions are useful in preventing or stopping bleeding due to thrombocytopenia. Ideally the platelets should be transfused within 6 h of collection since they lose function after that time but are helpful if used within 24 h. Generally, in adults, transfusions involving platelets derived from 8 to 15 units of blood are used and elevate the platelet count temporarily above 30,000 per cubic millimeter.

Repeated platelet transfusion results in alloimmunization and failure of response to further infusion. Following alloimmunization a satisfactory response to HLA-compatible platelets generally occurs and may persist indefinitely. Platelet transfusions are indicated in the therapy of life-threatening or serious hemorrhage and to tide a patient over an acute period of severe thrombocytopenia of less than 10,000 per cubic millimeter. Conditions in which platelet transfusions may be used, on the basis of these principles, include:

1 Acute leukemia
2 Aplastic anemia with serious hemorrhage
3 Acute thrombocytopenia manifesting serious bleeding
4 Exsanguinating blood loss requiring massive blood transfusion
5 Uremia with bleeding while awaiting dialysis

THROMBOCYTOSIS AND THROMBOCYTHEMIA *Thrombocytosis* is a term used to describe a temporary elevation of platelet count above 400,000 per cubic millimeter which may occur after severe hemorrhage, surgery, or splenectomy and in iron deficiency. Thrombocytosis may also occur in chronic inflammatory disorders and following recovery from acute infection. Malignant diseases such as carcinoma and Hodgkin's disease may also be associated with thrombocytosis.

The term *thrombocythemia* refers to a sustained elevation of platelet count, usually above 800,000 per cubic millimeter. In this condition, which is generally considered to be a myeloproliferative disorder, the spleen is almost always palpably enlarged. Thrombocythemia may occur as part of polycythemia vera, chronic myelogenous leukemia, or myelosclerosis, or it may occur alone, in which case it is termed essential (hemorrhagic) thrombocythemia. Patients with essential thrombocythemia frequently manifest spontaneous bleeding as well as venous and arterial thromboses. Platelet function studies such as aggregation and platelet factor 3 activity are often abnormal. The treatment of primary thrombocythemia involves therapy to decrease the autonomous growth of megakaryocytes and thus the excessive platelet production. Phosphorus 32 or busulfan is used for this purpose. Heparin therapy is required if thrombosis develops; aspirin and dipyridamole may prove useful in preventing thrombosis. The prognosis of primary thrombocythemia is that of the basic myeloproliferative disorder.

FUNCTIONAL DISORDERS OF PLATELETS The finding of a prolonged bleeding time in association with a normal platelet count suggests a disorder of platelet function. These disorders can be classified according to mechanism.

Defective adhesion A *defect in adhesion* appears to be the functional disturbance present in von Willebrand's disease, in which the primary defect is in a plasma protein. Platelet aggregation is normal with ADP, epinephrine, thrombin, and collagen, but is defective in response to ristocetin. Similar findings due to a primary platelet disorder occur in the Bernard-Soulier (giant-platelet) syndrome in which a platelet membrane glycoprotein abnormality has been reported. Platelet adhesion is also defective in complete afibrinogenemia.

Defective primary aggregation A defect in the primary aggregation response is characteristic of a congenital disorder termed *thrombasthenia*. This disorder is associated with a severe hemorrhagic diathesis with a markedly prolonged bleeding time, absent clot retraction, and absent platelet aggregation in response to ADP or collagen. A defect in a membrane glycopeptide has been identified in the platelets of some patients with this disorder.

Defective platelet release reaction There are two distinct types of functional defect associated with defective ADP release. In one type, termed *storage pool disease*, the storage pool of ADP is defective, and the disorder occurs congenitally with or without albinism. In another type of congenital disorder the storage pool of ADP is normal, but the release reaction is defective. A patient with a congenitally defective release reaction associated with cyclo-oxygenase deficiency has been reported. In other patients the mechanism of defective release has not yet been established. Drugs may impair platelet function by inhibiting the release reaction. Aspirin inhibits release by acetylating cyclo-oxygenase, thereby blocking the production of thromboxane A_2, which mediates the release reaction. The aspirin effect persists for the life span of the platelet. Drugs which inhibit platelet release include phenylbutazone, indomethacin, and many others with an anti-inflammatory action. Analgesic drugs without effect on platelets include codeine, acetaminophen (Tylenol), and propoxyphene (Darvon). The plasma expander dextran may also inhibit platelet function and prolong the bleeding time. The drugs which inhibit platelet function do not produce a bleeding diathesis by themselves but may aggravate an underlying disorder of hemostasis. They lengthen the bleeding time of normal individuals, which generally still remains within the normal range. The secondary wave of platelet aggregation in response to ADP and epinephrine is defective, platelet factor 3 activity is reduced, and clot retraction is normal.

Platelets from patients with a myeloproliferative syndrome and from patients with cirrhosis have functional defects which have not been completely characterized. A defect of platelet function occurs in *uremia* and may be associated with generalized bleeding from mucosal surfaces such as the nose, gastrointestinal tract, or renal tract, as well as cutaneous bleeding. This defect in platelet function is reversed by dialysis. Some patients with *dysproteinemia* may have defective platelet function. In

patients with macroglobulinemia or myeloma, the abnormal globulin is thought to coat the platelet and interfere with its proper function.

REFERENCES

ASTER RH: Thrombocytopenia due to enhanced platelet destruction, in *Hematology*, 2d ed, WJ Williams et al (eds). New York, McGraw-Hill, 1977, chap 145

——, KEENE WR: Sites of platelet destruction in idiopathic thrombocytopenic purpura. Br J Haematol 16:61, 1969

DIXON R et al: Quantitative determination of antibody in idiopathic thrombocytopenic purpura. N Engl J Med 292:230, 1975

HARDISTY RM: Disorders of platelet function. Br Med Bull 33:207, 1977

MONCADA S, VANE JR: Arachidonic acid metabolites and the interactions between platelets and blood vessel walls. N Engl J Med 300:1142, 1979

MUSTARD JF, PACKHAM MA: Clinical pharmacology of platelets. Blood 50:555, 1977

317
BLEEDING DISORDERS DUE TO VESSEL WALL ABNORMALITIES

HYMIE L. NOSSEL

INTRODUCTION Vascular defects (nonthrombocytopenic purpuras) are common, but they usually do not cause serious bleeding problems. Bleeding mainly occurs from mucous membranes or into the skin, starts immediately following injury, ceases in less than 24 to 48 h, and rarely recurs. The mechanism of bleeding is thought to be damage to capillary endothelium. The platelet count is usually normal, but tests of platelet function may be normal or abnormal. In those cases where a platelet function defect is demonstrable, the actual role of the vascular defect in the pathogenesis of the bleeding syndrome is uncertain, and there is no current method of diagnosing the vascular defect under such circumstances. In many cases, the diagnosis of a vascular defect underlying the bleeding syndrome is by exclusion. The platelet count and bleeding time are usually normal. A number of disease syndromes may be accompanied by bleeding thought to be due to vascular defects.

INFECTIONS Many severe infections may be associated with bleeding manifestations, especially meningococcemia, septicemia, typhoid fever, subacute bacterial endocarditis, and sometimes childhood viral infections such as measles. Disorders of platelet function, thrombocytopenia, and coagulation (defibrination) may play a role as well as vascular defects.

DRUGS In addition to purpura, urticarial or maculopapular rashes may be present. Drugs which may be associated with purpura include penicillin and the sulfonamides.

SCURVY The pathogenetic mechanism in scurvy is defective intercellular substance of capillary walls. There is a failure in collagen formation associated with defective hydroxyproline synthesis. Ascorbic acid is essential for synthesis of hydroxyproline. In addition, a defect of platelet function has been described in scurvy. Bleeding may occur in the skin, where it is often perifollicular, in the muscles, particularly the calf muscles, in the gastrointestinal tract, or into the urine. Clinical signs which suggest scurvy are swelling of the gums and hyperkeratosis of the skin. If the diagnosis is suspected, it can be confirmed by demonstrating a low ascorbic acid content in the white blood cells. Treatment is administration of vitamin C.

CUSHING'S SYNDROME The basic pathologic defect in this disorder, characterized by excessive cortisol production, is thought to be the protein-wasting effect of the increased blood steroid level with loss of perivascular supporting tissue.

HENOCH-SCHÖNLEIN SYNDROME Also known as allergic purpura or hypersensitivity angiitis, this relatively uncommon disorder is thought to be a hypersensitivity reaction related to acute nephritis and rheumatic fever and is most common between the ages of 2 and 20. Pathologically, an acute inflammatory reaction of the capillaries and mesangial tissues of the small arterioles is found associated with increased vascular permeability, exudation, and hemorrhage into the tissues. IgA and alternate pathway complement components have been identified in the capillaries of patients with the disease. Food, drugs, and bacteria have been implicated in hypersensitivity angiitis without definitive evidence for any of these. The syndrome is most common in children and is often preceded by streptococcal sore throat 1 to 3 weeks before the onset of hemorrhagic manifestations. The clinical pattern includes:

1 *Purpuric rash,* with either small or large spots. Initially they may be urticarial, and they often have a characteristic distribution on the extensor surfaces of the arms, legs, and buttocks. The character and distribution of the rash may be the only clue to the diagnosis of the disorder. Tests of platelet function and coagulation are normal.
2 *Abdominal manifestations,* among them colicky pain due to extravasation of fluid and blood into the intestinal wall.
3 *Polyarthralgia and polyarthritis*—tenderness and swelling are mainly periarticular.
4 *Hematuria,* often with albuminuria, casts, and the clinical spectrum of acute diffuse glomerulonephritis, with edema and hypertension. The majority of cases recover completely, but an occasional patient may die in acute renal failure and 5 to 10 percent develop chronic nephritis. Tests of platelet function and coagulation are normal. Corticosteroids do not appear to affect the course of the disease but may control edema and joint and abdominal pain.

SENILE PURPURA This condition occurs most commonly in thin, elderly people and usually affects the extensor surfaces of the arms. Irregular dark purple areas with clear-cut margins are present on the arms, and the skin is freely mobile over the deeper tissues. The disorder is thought to be due to atrophy of collagen so that the skin is poorly anchored to deeper tissues and movements easily rupture vessels.

HEREDITARY HEMORRHAGIC TELANGIECTASIA This syndrome is transmitted as a simple dominant trait affecting both sexes equally. The telangiectases are due to multiple dilatations of capillaries and arterioles, which are lined by a thin layer of endothelial cells. The bleeding tendency is thought to be due to mechanical fragility of the dilated vessel. Clinically, the telangiectases may be on any part of the skin as well as the mucosae of the nose and mouth, gastrointestinal tract, or renal tract. Bleeding may occur from any one of these sites in a recurrent fashion. Telangiectases present on the skin blanch on pressure, since the blood is not extravascular but within the capillary dilatation. The diagnosis is made from the clinical triad of telangiectasia, hemorrhage, and familial pattern.

DYSPROTEINEMIA Vascular purpura may occur in macroglobulinemia, multiple myeloma, and cryoglobulinemia. Pathogenic mechanisms may involve damage by the proteins to the vessel walls and capillary anoxia associated with hyperviscosity. Platelet and coagulation function may be disturbed. A malignant type of maculopapular purpura may occur in association with mixed cryoglobulinemia. The vascular lesions are due to immune-complex damage to the vessel walls. Mixed cryoglobulinemia (often a complex of IgG and anti-IgG) may be associated with a variety of disorders including infection and autoimmune disorders. Mixed cryoglobulinemia and purpura may be associated with arthralgia, weakness, and nephritis without an identifiable primary disorder. Plasmapheresis with removal of cryoglobulin will have short-term benefit. Long-term management is that of the underlying disease. In the condition termed *benign hyperglobulinemic purpura,* purpuric spots are found characteristically on the anterior aspects of the lower limbs, in association with an elevated gamma globulin level in the serum.

REFERENCES

Capra DJ et al: Hyperglobulinemic purpura. Studies on the unusual anti-globulins characteristic of the sera of these patients. Medicine 50:125, 1971

Cream JJ et al: Schönlein-Henoch purpura in the adult. Q J Med 39:461, 1970

Gottlieb AJ: in *Hematology,* 2d ed, WJ Williams et al (eds). New York, McGraw-Hill, 1977, chaps 151, 153, 154

Wintrobe MM: *Clinical Hematology,* 7th ed. Philadelphia, Lea & Febiger, 1974

318

DISORDERS OF BLOOD COAGULATION FACTORS

HYMIE L. NOSSEL

CONGENITAL DISORDERS

Congenital disorders of coagulation characteristically involve a single coagulation protein, and transmission of the defect is genetically determined. A severe functional defect may be transmitted either as an autosomal recessive or dominant trait or as an X-linked recessive characteristically manifest in male hemizygotes and in the rare female homozygotes. In many instances a coagulation protein is present in the blood in normal concentrations as measured immunologically but is functionally defective. Since the plasma concentrations of most of the coagulation proteins are very low, evidence for the presence of a normal amount of the protein principally depends on measurement of a normal amount of antigenic activity. The coagulation proteins may then be measured as clot-promoting activity and as antigenic activity. In normal individuals these two activities correlate, whereas in some patients with coagulation factor disorders, clot-promoting activity may be sharply reduced and antigenic activity may be normal, reflecting an abnormal molecule. In other patients both coagulant and antigenic activity may be similarly reduced, possibly owing to the presence of fewer molecules of the factor.

HEMOPHILIA Hemophilia is a bleeding disorder due to inherited deficiency in the procoagulant activity of factor VIII, the antihemophilic factor. It is the most common of the congenital coagulation factor disorders, occurring in 1 in 10,000 of the population. The gene is transmitted in a sex-linked recessive pattern. Female heterozygotes (carriers) transmit the disorder to one-half of their sons and the gene to one-half of their daughters. Female carriers rarely manifest any bleeding tendency. The measured level of factor VIII coagulant activity cannot absolutely establish whether the sister of a hemophilic male is a carrier (heterozygote) or is normal. When both factor VIII coagulant activity and antigenic activity are measured, 30 percent of carriers can be detected at the 99 percent level of confidence and 50 percent at the 95 percent confidence level. Males with the disorder (hemizygotes) transmit the gene to all their daughters, who rarely have a bleeding tendency; their sons are all normal. In 30 percent of cases, no family history can be elicited.

Molecular defect Material has been isolated from human or bovine plasma which has the following characteristics. It has a molecular weight of 1.1×10^6 daltons and, following reduction of disulfide bonds, is split into subunits of 1 to 2×10^5 daltons. Preparations isolated by different workers have a similar amino acid composition and all of them contain carbohydrate. This material has been termed factor VIII and has two distinct functional activities. It corrects the coagulation defect of hemophilic plasma and also a functional defect in von Willebrand's disease plasma. The von Willebrand's disease defect involves the failure to promote platelet aggregation by ristocetin and platelet reaction with subendothelial tissues. The two functional activities may be dissociated by gel filtration at high salt (NaCl or $CaCl_2$) concentration. Almost all the protein is associated with the von Willebrand factor activity, hence antibodies to the material detect the von Willebrand factor moiety and very little protein is associated with the activity which corrects the coagulation defect of hemopholic plasma. The exact relationship between these two activities is not established. Further understanding will require isolation in sufficient quantity and characterization of the clot-promoting activity. Currently these activities are referred to as factor VIII_{AHF} (procoagulant activity), factor VIII_{VWF} (von Willebrand factor), and factor VIII_{AGN} (antigenic activity allied not to the procoagulant activity but to the von Willebrand factor). Since the molecular nature of the procoagulant activity is not known, the site of synthesis and plasma concentration are also unknown. However, functional procoagulant activity is readily measured and much is known about conditions which elevate or lower it.

Clinical features BLEEDING IN GENERAL It will be recalled (Chap. 54) that platelet plug formation is the first line of defense against bleeding, followed by coagulation. Since platelet plug formation is normal in hemophilia, the onset of bleeding is characteristically delayed for several hours or days after injury. Bleeding may, however, persist for several days or weeks since coagulation is important in maintenance of the occlusive plug. The clinical manifestations of hemophilia vary greatly depending on the level of factor VIII coagulant activity (Table 318-1). In milder cases, spontaneous bleeding does not occur, but exsanguinating hemorrhage may follow injury or surgery. In severe cases spontaneous recurrent bleeding episodes are characteristic and may be associated with chronic joint deformity. Large hematomas may be associated with fever, anemia, and hyperbilirubinemia.

BLEEDING IN SPECIFIC LOCATIONS As one would anticipate from the defect in the maintenance stage of hemostasis, bruises, ecchymoses, and deep subcutaneous and intramuscular hematomas occur frequently, whereas petechiae and purpura do not occur. Recurrent hemarthroses are a characteristic feature and often result in permanent joint damage with destruction of the edges of the bones forming the joints, osteophyte formation with limitation of joint movement, and even-

tual fibrous or bony ankylosis. Bleeding following dental extractions is often a problem. Bleeding also often occurs from mucosal surfaces such as the frenum of the tongue and the urogenital and gastrointestinal tracts. Gastrointestinal hemorrhage is frequently associated with a local lesion. Any organ in the body may be the site of bleeding. Hemorrhage is potentially lethal, owing to local pressure effects when it is intracranial, lingual, laryngeal, retropharyngeal, pericardial, or pleural in location.

Diagnosis Hemophilia should be suspected from the sex of the patient, a familial pattern if present, the age of onset, and the type of bleeding. A family tree should be drawn while taking the history. Laboratory tests establish the diagnosis. Tests of platelet function, bleeding time, and platelet count are normal. Tests of coagulation show a prolonged whole-blood clotting time in severe hemophilia; in mild hemophilia the clotting time may be normal. The prothrombin time is normal, and the partial thromboplastin time is prolonged. Low factor VIII procoagulant activity is diagnostic. Factor VIII antigenic activity is usually normal.

Treatment Following diagnosis, patients or their parents should be instructed in detail about the care, prognosis, and hereditary nature of the disorder. Children should be reared in as normal a way as is compatible with physical safety since emotional crippling can be as serious as that resulting from hemorrhage. As they grow older, patients should be encouraged to participate in sports such as swimming or golf and to avoid those involving body contact. A vocation should be sought which is not inherently dangerous. The aim should be to encourage patients to become self-supporting adults capable of looking after themselves and living a full life.

The basis for therapy of bleeding episodes is transfusion of material containing factor VIII procoagulant activity which temporarily corrects the specific defect. Whole blood is not used for this purpose, and its use is restricted to restoration of blood volume following severe loss. Plasma with a high factor VIII content may be used, but factor VIII concentrates are the preferred method of treatment since the content of antihemophilic factor is known and the load on the blood volume is less. Following infusion, about 90 percent of the infused activity may be found in the patient's plasma. Hence, if the amount of factor VIII infused and the patient's plasma volume are both

TABLE 318-1
Relationship of factor VIII blood levels to severity of bleeding

Factor VIII coagulant activity, % normal	*Type of bleeding*
50–100	None
25–50	Bleeding may be excessive after major trauma
5–25	Severe bleeding after surgical operations and some bleeding after minor trauma; no spontaneous bleeding
1–5	Severe bleeding after minor injury; occasional spontaneous hemorrhages
0	Severe hemophilia with spontaneous bleeding into muscles and joints

known, it is possible to predict the rise in factor VIII level resulting from the infusion. Following transfusion, factor VIII activity disappears rapidly, about half remaining after 12 h, so that repeated infusion is required till the bleeding stops. In the event of major injury or surgery, factor VIII levels should be elevated to above 50 percent of the normal level and maintained above 30 percent at all times until the wound has healed completely. The amount of factor VIII required may be calculated as follows: 1 unit of factor VIII (the average activity in 1 ml normal plasma) per kilogram of body weight elevates the factor VIII level about 1.8 percent of the normal. Following an initial dose of 50 units per kilogram, about 30 units per kilogram should be given every 8 h for the first 2 days. Infusions every 12 h of a suitably adjusted dose may then be given if clinical progress is satisfactory and factor VIII levels are in the desired range. For dental extraction an initial elevation of the factor VIII level to 75 percent of the normal level should be accompanied by the administration of ε-aminocaproic acid (EACA) (24 g per day in a 70-kg adult, orally for 7 days). The EACA greatly reduces the infusion requirement, probably by inhibiting salivary plasmin which otherwise dissolves clots as they form. A second similar dose of factor VIII should be given on the fourth or fifth day following the procedure. Sockets of extracted teeth should not be sutured since if hemostasis is not effective, blood accumulating under the sutures may track into the soft tissues of the neck or lingual area.

Transfusion of factor VIII is also useful in aborting bleeding into joints if given in the early stages. The factor VIII level in the patient should be elevated to 30 to 50 percent of normal. Acutely swollen joints should be immobilized, and local chilling in the early stages may be beneficial. Aspiration may be helpful but should be performed only after adequate infusion therapy. After bleeding has stopped, active motion without weight bearing is important to prevent chronic limitation of movement. Careful use of physiotherapy and splints may be helpful in preventing and correcting deformities and useful in avoiding later reparative surgery. Development and maintenance of strength of the muscles surrounding the joints should be an important aim of management so that the muscles will be able to assist the joints in weight bearing. Infusion therapy at home permits the early therapy of bleeding episodes which are thereby often aborted with a marked reduction in morbidity, absenteeism from work, time in hospital, and attendance of the outpatient clinic. These factors result in a high degree of patient satisfaction with home infusion therapy. It is important that regular contact between patient and physician be maintained.

For minor bleeding occurring from an accessible site, local measures such as application of thrombin, cold, and gentle pressure may be helpful. Hemophiliacs should not be given intramuscular injections, and following venipuncture, local pressure should be maintained until bleeding has stopped (usually within 5 min). Immunization against tetanus is important because patients with hemophilia may be prone to infection with this organism. Immunizations should be given while the patient is receiving factor VIII replacement therapy. Regular prophylactic care of the teeth should be provided. It is wise to avoid aspirin which increases the hazard of bleeding by impairing platelet function. Acetaminophen and propoxyphene are analgesics which do not impair hemostasis. It has been found that infusion of a synthetic analogue of the antidiuretic hormone [1-deamino-8-D-arginine vasopressin (DDAVP)] will transiently elevate the factor VIII level threefold in normal individuals and in hemophiliacs with measurable activity but not when the factor VIII level is below 1 percent. It has been suggested that DDAVP infusion may be useful to treat or pre-

vent bleeding in hemophiliacs with factor VIII levels of about 10 percent or higher. The place of such therapy remains to be determined.

About 5 percent of hemophiliacs develop antibodies to factor VIII (circulating anticoagulants) which vitiate the beneficial effect of infusion. Such patients should not undergo surgery, and infusion therapy should be avoided as far as possible to avoid unnecessarily raising the antibody titer.

Course and prognosis Patients with milder forms of hemophilia usually live a virtually normal life but may have severe hemorrhage after dental extraction, injury, or surgery. Patients with severe disease may require frequent admission to the hospital and may develop crippling joint deformities. Home transfusion therapy permits early treatment of the bleeding and significantly reduces morbidity. The patient or his family can be trained to give infusions at home and thereby avert many visits to the hospital emergency room. Regular contact with an experienced physician should be maintained so that when hospital therapy is required, it is not delayed unnecessarily. Many patients with severe disease may live productive lives, whereas others are chronic invalids. Although life expectancy has been greatly prolonged by replacement therapy, death as a complication of hemorrhage still occurs quite frequently.

VON WILLEBRAND'S DISEASE Von Willebrand's disease is a hereditary hemorrhagic disorder transmitted as an autosomal dominant trait and characterized by a prolonged bleeding time associated with reduced factor VIII coagulant activity, generally to less than 50 percent of the normal level.

Pathogenesis The pathogenesis of the prolonged bleeding time appears to involve a defect in platelet adhesion to the subendothelial collagen of the capillary wall. The von Willebrand protein is not required for normal adhesion of platelets to collagen under the flow conditions used for in vitro tests of this function. Under in vivo flow conditions, the von Willebrand protein is necessary for normal platelet adhesion. Since platelet adherence to the subendothelial tissues is abnormal, hemostatic plug formation is delayed, and the bleeding time is prolonged. The von Willebrand factor is required for normal platelet aggregation induced by ristocetin and in platelet-rich plasma from a patient with von Willebrand's disease ristocetin does not induce platelet aggregation. The protein which mediates platelet adhesion to subendothelial tissues under in vivo flow conditions and platelet aggregation with ristocetin in vitro is the large-molecular-weight component of the "factor VIII complex," discussed above. As noted above, this protein is the principal antigen in the factor VIII complex. Hence, *factor VIII (von Willebrand Factor) antigen is reduced or absent in the plasma of patients with von Willebrand's disease.* Immunofluorescence techniques demonstrate close association of von Willebrand antigen with endothelial cells lining blood vessels throughout the body. There is evidence that the antigen is synthesized in endothelial cells. In addition to the platelet adherence defect, in von Willebrand's disease factor VIII procoagulant activity is reduced approximately to the same degree as the von Willebrand antigen. The reason for the reduction in factor VIII coagulant activity is unknown, but in most patients with von Willebrand's disease infusion of plasma from a hemophilia patient lacking antihemophilic factor is accompanied by a slow and major increase in factor VIII procoagulant activity.

Clinical features In most cases, the hemorrhagic diathesis is mild; the symptoms include epistaxis, easy bruising in response to trauma, and troublesome bleeding for a few days after minor lacerations or dental extractions. If the coagulation defect is unusually severe, prolonged bleeding and hemarthroses may occur.

Diagnosis The diagnosis is based on the laboratory findings of a prolonged bleeding time, low factor VIII procoagulant activity, and defective in vitro platelet aggregation in response to ristocetin. Unlike hemophilia, there is an approximately parallel reduction in factor VIII antigenic and coagulant activities. In addition, abnormal platelet function may be demonstrated by decreased platelet trapping when whole blood is passed through a column of glass beads. Other tests of platelet function, including clot retraction and platelet aggregation in response to adenosine diphosphate, collagen, thrombin, and norepinephrine, are normal.

Treatment Local measures, as in hemophilia, are used in mild bleeding in von Willebrand's disease. Transfusion of normal plasma has a sustained effect on the factor VIII level in most patients, unlike the brief elevation in hemophilia (see Chap. 54). A cryoprecipitate rich in factor VIII prepared from normal plasma may be used in the therapy of von Willebrand's disease and produces both a prolonged increase in factor VIII activity and improvement in hemostasis. The hemostatic effectiveness of more purified factor VIII preparations is uncertain since it is not established that normal hemostasis is directly related to the level of factor VIII coagulant activity—the prolonged bleeding time should also be corrected. Infusion of DDAVP elevates the von Willebrand protein level in plasma transiently. The therapeutic benefit of this phenomenon remains to be determined.

CONGENITAL DEFICIENCY OF OTHER COAGULATION FACTORS Congenital deficiencies of each of the other coagulation factors occur, and may be associated with a hemorrhagic tendency except for factor XII deficiency. Laboratory diagnosis is made in a manner similar to that described for hemophilia; the results of different laboratory tests are summarized in Table 54-4. The principles of therapy are similar to those described for hemophilia. Replacement transfusion therapy is modified from that described for hemophilia according to the availability of concentrates and the recovery and in vivo survival times of the deficient factor (Table 54-3).

Factor IX deficiency Factor IX deficiency [also termed plasma thromboplastin component (PTC) or Christmas factor deficiency] occurs about one-sixth as frequently as factor VIII deficiency. The clinical manifestations and inheritance are exactly as in hemophilia, but a different protein is defective and a different concentrate is used in therapy. There is evidence that many patients with factor IX deficiency actually synthesize a factor IX-like protein with antigenic activity but with defective coagulant activity.

Concentrates containing factor IX are used in the treatment of the congenital deficiency. These concentrates (prothrombin complex concentrates) generally contain prothrombin and factors VII, IX, and X. Many of the concentrates contain some activated factors as well; when they are infused very rapidly, intravascular coagulation may result. The indications for use of the concentrates should be severe bleeding in the presence of established deficiency of one or more of the four factors listed above. The infusion should be given slowly over a period of at least 1 h. In addition, certain manufacturers recommend adding small amounts of heparin to the preparation.

Factor XI deficiency Clinically, deficiency of factor XI [which is also termed plasma thromboplastin antecedent (PTA)] resembles mild to moderate hemophilia. It is even less common than factor IX deficiency, occurs most often in people of Jewish origin, and is transmitted as an autosomal dominant characteristic. About one-third of affected individuals appear to

have no excessive bleeding at all. In individuals who do bleed excessively, the disorder is readily treated with infusions of fresh frozen plasma.

Factor XII deficiency Deficiency of this factor (also known as Hageman factor) is usually asymptomatic, and therapy is not required. The whole-blood clotting time and partial thromboplastin time tests are grossly prolonged. The explanation for the lack of hemorrhagic diathesis is unknown.

Factor XIII deficiency Deficiency of factor XIII appears to be inherited in two patterns—as an autosomal recessive trait in some families, confined to males in others. Clinically, a moderately severe bleeding tendency occurs. Fibrin clots formed in this disorder are not cross-linked and are very susceptible to dissolution by plasmin or by mechanical stress. Excessive bleeding from the umbilicus and production of keloid scar tissue, often on the forehead, following bleeding from injury is suggestive of the disorder. Recurrent abortion in early pregnancy is characteristic. The screening test for factor XIII deficiency is based on solubility of the non-cross-linked clot in 5 M urea or 1% monochloroacetic acid. There are other causes of abnormal clot solubility, and the diagnosis should be confirmed by a quantitative assay of factor XIII activity. All other coagulation tests are normal in this disorder. Transfusion with plasma temporarily restores normal hemostasis, the $T_{1/2}$ of the infused activity being 4 to 7 days.

Fibrinogen deficiency is generally transmitted as an autosomal recessive trait and may manifest as a complete or partial absence of fibrinogen from the blood plasma. Clinically, the disease resembles moderate or mild hemophilia, but hemarthroses do not occur. When there is complete absence of fibrinogen, the whole-blood clotting time, the one-stage prothrombin time, and thrombin clotting time all are grossly prolonged. Control of bleeding is achieved by transfusion of fibrinogen contained in freshly frozen plasma. With fibrinogen levels above 50 mg per 100 ml, the screening coagulation tests may show only minor abnormality, and a quantitative measure of the fibrinogen level is required to indicate the presence of a deficiency.

Congenital fibrinogen abnormality may also be due to the hereditary synthesis of structurally and functionally abnormal fibrinogen molecules, a situation analogous to some of the hemoglobinopathies. In fibrinogen Detroit the amino acid serine is substituted for arginine at position 19 on the Aα-polypeptide chain; the propositus with this defect presented with a severe bleeding tendency. More than 50 additional patients with molecular abnormalities of fibrinogen have been identified, although the biochemical defect has not been established in each case. Some of these patients display a severe hemorrhagic syndrome, whereas others are asymptomatic. The laboratory finding most useful in identifying these abnormalities is a prolonged thrombin clotting time.

ACQUIRED COAGULATION DISORDERS

These disorders occur much more often than do the congenital disorders and constitute the bulk of coagulation disorders encountered.

VITAMIN K DEFICIENCY Vitamin K is a fat-soluble vitamin essential for the synthesis of normal prothrombin and factors VII, IX, and X molecules, which are referred to as the K-dependent coagulation factors. Normal prothrombin has 10 γ-carboxyglutamic acid residues grouped near the NH$_2$-terminal

FIGURE 318-1

Precursor

Glutamyl residues

$$\alpha\ CH_2$$
$$\beta\ CH_2$$
$$\gamma\ COOH$$

$\xrightarrow[\text{"Carboxylase"}]{HCO_3^-}$

γ-Carboxyglutamyl residues

$$\alpha\ CH_2$$
$$\beta\ CH_2$$
$$\gamma\ CH$$
$$HOOC \qquad COOH$$

Vitamin K-dependent carboxylase. Vitamin K is a required cofactor in the reaction that converts glutamyl residues in microsomal precursors of prothrombin to γ-carboxyglutamyl residues in prothrombin.

end of the molecule which bind calcium and via calcium serve to bind phospholipid and factor X_a. Prothrombin synthesized in the absence of vitamin K has glutamic acid in place of the γ-carboxyglutamic acid, since vitamin K is required for postribosomal γ-carboxylation of glutamic acid (see Fig. 318-1). When glutamic acid replaces γ-carboxyglutamic acid, there is defective binding of calcium, phospholipid, and factor X_a to prothrombin. This impaired binding is responsible for the defective biological function of vitamin K–deficient prothrombin. Similar abnormalities are responsible for the defective activity of factors VII, IX, and X.

The natural sources of vitamin K are food and the intestinal bacterial flora. The principal food sources are green leafy vegetables. There are relatively small body stores of vitamin K, and if intake of the vitamin is stopped, deficiency may develop within 1 to 3 weeks. The diagnosis of vitamin K deficiency is confirmed if a prolonged prothrombin time test is corrected in 12 to 24 h by the parenteral administration of vitamin K.

Etiology In most patients, multiple factors are involved. Vitamin K deficiency may occur from impaired absorption due to lack of bile salts as in obstructive jaundice or biliary fistula. Intestinal malabsorption syndromes can also produce vitamin K deficiency. Oral administration of antibiotics which leads to decreased gut flora in association with total or partial parenteral alimentation, may lead to vitamin K deficiency.

Clinical features Bleeding associated with deficiency of the vitamin K–dependent factors is similar to that occurring with other coagulation defects. It may be severe or even fatal.

Treatment Proper therapy must involve correction of the underlying cause. Vitamin K administration will immediately correct the defect; it can be administered either as the naturally occurring oil-soluble vitamin K_1 (oral and intravenous forms are available) or as the synthetic vitamin K. Vitamin K_1 is the most potent and rapidly acting form, measurably correcting clotting tests within 6 to 12 h of intravenous administration; it should be used for treatment of hemorrhagic disease in the newborn or for any vitamin K deficiency if bleeding is active. Oral and parenteral preparations of synthetic vitamin K are also available and may be used for treatment in the absence of bleeding and for maintenance vitamin K replacement. Intravenous injection of vitamin K_1 has been associated with anaphylactic reactions and should be avoided. Synthetic preparations should not be used in the neonate since they may cause hemolysis and kernicterus in infants with glucose 6-phosphate dehydrogenase deficiency and in premature infants. Response to therapy should always be confirmed by repeating the prothrombin time 24 h after administration of vitamin K. Failure to correct the prothrombin time signifies failure to absorb the vitamin K or the presence of liver disease. If more urgent correction of the hemostatic defect is required than can be provided by administration of vitamin K, plasma or a concentrate of the vitamin K-dependent factors (prothrombin complex) should be infused.

ANTICOAGULANT DRUGS The commonly used anticoagulant drugs include the coumarin derivatives and heparin. The *coumarins* act by antagonizing the action of vitamin K and lead to the same clotting abnormalities as vitamin K deficiency (Fig. 318-2). Coumarin therapy prolongs the prothrombin and partial thromboplastin time tests and reduces the levels of prothrombin and factors VII, IX, and X. Abnormal bleeding is the chief complication of overdosage, which may be due to error, accident, or attempted suicide. The drugs usually implicated are dicoumarol (half-life 24 h) and warfarin (half-life 40 h). Treatment consists of administration of vitamin K and infusion of plasma or a prothrombin complex concentrate if bleeding is severe.

The best known action of *heparin* is the inactivation of thrombin, which prevents it from acting on fibrinogen. Blood contains a naturally occurring inhibitor of thrombin, termed *antithrombin III,* which combines with the thrombin molecule on a 1:1 basis and inactivates it. Heparin binds to the lysine residues on the antithrombin III molecule, thereby markedly accelerating the stoichiometric reaction between thrombin and antithrombin III in the inactivation of thrombin. Heparin also acts earlier in the coagulation sequence by accelerating the combination of antithrombin III with factors IX_a, X_a, XI_a, and XII_a. Some of the activated factors, notably factor X_a, are inactivated by much lower concentrations of heparin than are required to inactivate thrombin. This may be the reason that low-dose heparin, although without influence on the clotting time, nevertheless reduces the incidence of postoperative venous thrombosis and pulmonary embolism. All coagulation tests are affected by heparin, including the one-stage prothrombin time. The most sensitive tests usually used to monitor the pharmacologic effect of heparin are the whole-blood clotting time, the partial thromboplastin time, and the thrombin time. An average dose of heparin is cleared from the blood in about 6 h by excretion in the urine and inactivation by a liver heparinase.

The treatment of bleeding associated with an excessive blood level of heparin is relatively simple. Heparin is a strongly negatively charged molecule and is rapidly neutral-

FIGURE 318-2

Vitamin K is converted to vitamin K epoxide by a microsomal epoxidase in the liver, and vitamin K epoxide is converted back to vitamin K by a microsomal reductase. Warfarin blocks the action of the reductase, resulting in accumulation of vitamin K epoxide. The exact way in which this effect of warfarin antagonizes the action of vitamin K in carboxylation of coagulation proteins is not established.

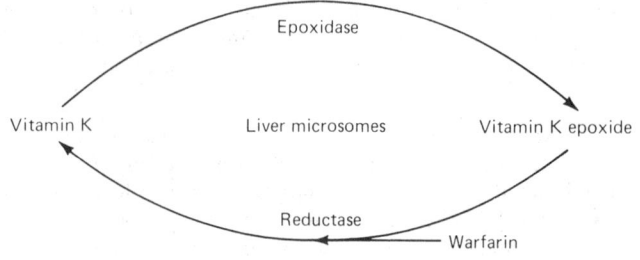

ized, milligram for milligram, by intravenous protamine sulfate which is strongly positively charged. The amount of protamine required to neutralize the circulating heparin can be determined in vitro by a protamine titration test.

LIVER DISEASE Liver disease is one of the commonest causes of impaired coagulation. The principal functional changes appear to be decreased hepatic protein synthesis and increased plasma proteolytic activity, perhaps due to a decrease in the liver's capacity to remove proteases from the circulation. Increased fibrinolytic activity is often found in patients with cirrhosis and liver failure. There is evidence that intravascular coagulation may also occur in liver failure. The net effect of these derangements is to reduce the levels of all coagulation factors except for factor VIII, the level of which is often significantly increased. Hemostasis is frequently further impaired by thrombocytopenia and platelet dysfunction.

In severe liver disease, a common pattern of hemostatic abnormalities includes a low plasma fibrinogen level, a prolonged prothrombin time, and a normal or increased partial thromboplastin time. The normal partial thromboplastin time may be the result of an elevated factor VIII level which can compensate for low levels of the other factors. The reason for the increased factor VIII concentration is not known. A low level of factor VII which does not affect the partial thromboplastin time may also contribute to a disproportionately prolonged prothrombin time. The thrombin clotting time is moderately prolonged in some patients with liver disease. The sialic acid content of the fibrinogen of these patients is increased and may be responsible for the prolonged thrombin clotting time. Heparin infusions may transiently elevate the fibrinogen level, suggesting that hypofibrinogenemia may in part be due to catabolism from thrombin-mediated proteolysis, but the low fibrinogen level is often not restored to normal. The effect of heparin on clinical hemostasis is variable; it is apt to be associated with increased bleeding due to the anticoagulant effect of heparin. Fibrinolytic inhibitors appear to have at best a transient beneficial effect. In the management of frank bleeding, infusion of plasma may be preferable to infusion of coagulation factor concentrates. Some concentrates contain active coagulation enzymes which, being poorly cleared by the failing liver, can aggravate intravascular clotting and compound the problem. If there is an associated vitamin K deficiency it should be treated. In general, bleeding due to liver failure responds poorly to therapy unless improvement in liver-cell function occurs.

FIBRINOGEN DEFICIENCY

The normal plasma concentration of fibrinogen is 200 to 400 mg per 100 ml. Elevated levels occur during pregnancy, during acute febrile reactions, and in many chronic diseases.

Acquired deficiency of fibrinogen may be due to impaired synthesis and/or accelerated destruction of the protein. Impaired synthesis occurs in hepatitis, hepatic necrosis, and following administration of L-asparaginase for the treatment of leukemia. Accelerated destruction usually results from increased blood proteolytic activity. The commonest causes of increased proteolytic activity are discussed in the following section.

DISSEMINATED INTRAVASCULAR COAGULATION

Abbreviated DIC, this condition constitutes a series of syndromes recognized with increasing frequency over the last several years. The pathogenesis, diagnosis, and management of the disorder are complex. It is inferred that thrombin action on

fibrinogen is the basis of the disorder, but the evidence for this inference is not very definite, as will be apparent from the discussion.

BIOCHEMISTRY AND PHYSIOLOGY The principal target protein in disseminated intravascular coagulation is fibrinogen. The principal enzymes which attack fibrinogen are thrombin and plasmin. The biochemistry of the actions of these enzymes is discussed in Chap. 54. Besides acting on fibrinogen, thrombin also digests factors V and VIII and aggregates platelets. The products of plasmin digestion are termed fibrinogen/fibrin degradation products. Tests for increased serum concentrations of the degradation products are important in the diagnosis of disseminated intravascular coagulation. The degradation products also have significant physiologic effects. They inhibit the clotting of normal blood by acting as anticoagulants. They delay the polymerization of fibrin and thus prolong the thrombin clotting time. The fibrinogen/fibrin degradation products may also interpose between fibrin polymers as they are forming, producing a weak, disordered fibrin clot. Platelet aggregation by ADP is also inhibited. It is thought that the α_2 globulin inhibitor of plasma reacts with plasmin and prevents significant plasmin degradation of fibrinogen. When a fibrin thrombus forms, plasmin is thought to be absorbed to the fibrin strands. Thus freed from the inhibitors, it is able to digest the fibrin. Plasmin also digests factors V and VIII.

The normal concentration of fibrinogen reflects a balance between synthesis and catabolism. Synthesis is in the liver and normally can be increased up to tenfold. The $T_{1/2}$ of fibrinogen in normal individuals is 100 h. The pathways of catabolism are not known nor is the extent to which enzyme action contributes normally. Thrombin action is believed to contribute less than 2 percent to normal fibrinogen catabolism. Coagulated fibrin is removed immediately from the circulating blood, and soluble fibrin and fibrinogen degradation products are removed more rapidly than is fibrinogen. Hence fibrinogen catabolism can be greatly accelerated by excessive enzyme action. If the synthetic reserve capacity is reduced as in liver failure, a lesser increase in catabolic rate would produce hypofibrinogenemia. Excessive proteolysis may reduce the fibrinogen concentration from an elevated level to the normal range or from the normal range to hypofibrinogenemic levels.

EXPERIMENTAL INTRAVASCULAR COAGULATION Intravascular coagulation can be induced experimentally. Rapid injection of thrombin into a large vein causes local thrombosis. Slower infusion of thrombin results in hypofibrinogenemia and usually no thrombi except sometimes in small vessels in the kidneys and adrenals. The reticuloendothelial system, particularly in the liver, removes fibrin and activated coagulation factors from the circulation, and suppression of reticuloendothelial activity enhances susceptibility to disseminated intravascular coagulation. Inhibition of fibrinolysis promotes the occurrence of organ thrombosis. In experimental intravascular coagulation, thrombin action results in reduced levels of fibrinogen, factors V and VIII, and in thrombocytopenia. Hemolysis and fragmented red blood cells may occur owing to red blood cell disruption by contact with fibrin strands, and shock and hemorrhage may be evident. Prior administration of heparin will prevent the coagulation changes, thrombocytopenia, red cell hemolysis, and reduce the severity of shock.

LABORATORY DIAGNOSIS The cardinal laboratory sign of disseminated intravascular coagulation is a quantitative and/or qualitative change in the plasma fibrinogen. The fibrinogen concentration is classically low but may be in the normal range, representing a reduction from a previously elevated level or may actually be elevated if the rate of synthesis exceeds the catabolic rate, even though the latter is elevated. An index of alteration in the fibrinogen molecule is the presence in the blood of increased concentrations of fibrinogen degradation products. There are two main types of degradation product—those reflecting plasmin action and those indicating thrombin action. The tests used as a reflection of plasmin action are the thrombin clotting time test, which is not specific for the products of plasmin action, and tests for fibrinogen derivatives in serum. Theoretically, when fibrinogen is clotted with thrombin, only fibrinopeptides A and B remain in the serum. In practice, serum derived from the clotting of normal blood contains very low concentrations of larger fibrinogen derivatives. These derivatives may be detected by immunologic techniques such as hemagglutination inhibition, immunodiffusion, or immunoelectrophoresis, or by their ability to clump certain strains of staphylococci. It is generally inferred that fibrinogen derivatives measured by these tests are derived principally by plasmin proteolysis of fibrin in most clinical circumstances. However, there is no direct evidence for this inference, and there is uncertainty about the contribution of plasmin proteolysis of fibrinogen to fibrinogen degradation product levels.

Tests which specifically reflect thrombin action in vivo are still at the research stage and include (1) the measurement of free fibrinopeptide A and (2) evidence for the presence of fibrin monomer in solution. Abnormalities in other laboratory tests may be useful as ancillary evidence of disseminated intravascular coagulation. Classically, factor V and VIII activity is reduced and thrombocytopenia is present. The coagulation factor abnormalities often result in a prolonged prothrombin and partial thromboplastin time. However, factor V and VIII levels may be normal or even grossly increased. The abnormalities in the coagulation factors presumably represent the effect of thrombin which initially increases the activity of factors V and VIII and subsequently inactivates these factors.

CLINICAL SYNDROMES Disorders with hypofibrinogenemia and intravascular coagulation are outlined in Table 318-2.

DIC with hypofibrinogenemia LOCALIZED In certain clinical syndromes, the stimulus to intravascular coagulation appears to be localized, yet the hematologic changes are manifest throughout the circulating blood. Such conditions include the Kasabach-Merritt syndrome, some cases of dissecting aneurysm of the aorta, and occasional cases of massive venous thrombosis or pulmonary embolism. In the Kasabach-Merritt syndrome, a congenital hemangioma is associated with throm-

TABLE 318-2
Disorders with hypofibrinogenemia and intravascular coagulation

I Local stimulus to clotting
  A Vascular: Giant hemangioma, aortic aneurysm, massive thrombosis, or pulmonary embolism
  B Tissue damage: Burns, retained dead fetus, premature placental separation, amniotic fluid embolism
II Generalized stimulus to clotting
  A Exogenous agents: Snake venoms
  B Shock: Hypovolemic, cardiogenic
  C Infections: Gram-negative and gram-positive septicemia, viremia, miliary tuberculosis, Rocky Mountain spotted fever, subacute bacterial endocarditis, malaria
  D Immunologic: Anaphylaxis
  E Neoplasms: Carcinoma of the prostate, pancreas, lung; leukemia, lymphoma
III Defective regulation (liver failure): Impaired clearance of activated factors and defective fibrinogen synthesis

bocytopenia, hypofibrinogenemia, and elevated levels of fibrinopeptide A and fibrinogen degradation products. The survival time of radiolabeled fibrinogen in the circulating blood is shortened, and can be prolonged by heparin infusion. The radiolabeled fibrinogen accumulates in the hemangioma. All the hematologic changes revert to normal following extirpation of the hemangioma. This type of case offers a clear demonstration that the stimulus to intravascular coagulation is local. It is not known whether the increased proteolytic activity becomes disseminated through the blood, and this question is also unanswered for the other diseases listed in this section.

Localized tissue damage appears to provide the stimulus for intravascular coagulation in burn injuries, retained dead fetus, premature placental separation, and amniotic fluid embolism.

GENERALIZED In other disease states it seems possible that the stimulus to intravascular coagulation may be generalized. It should be recognized that further work may well result in transfer of diseases from the generalized category to the localized, and vice versa. The disorders in this category with the clearest pathogenesis result from the action of coagulant enzymes present in snake venoms. The proteolytic enzyme may be introduced into the bloodstream by the fangs of the snake or as therapy by the physician. Preparations used therapeutically include Ancrod, derived from the venom of the Malayan pit viper, and reptilase, derived from *Bothrops atrox*. These preparations act specifically on fibrinogen but not on platelets or factors V and VIII, and hence do not alter their levels.

Shock of whatever cause (hypovolemic, cardiogenic) is frequently accompanied by disseminated intravascular coagulation, which rapidly ceases when the shock is reversed. The pathogenesis is unknown but may be related to tissue or vessel wall damage.

Sepsis is one of the commonest of the disorders associated with disseminated intravascular coagulation. Classically, the sepsis is due to gram-negative organisms such as in meningococcemia, but the syndrome may be encountered with infection with gram-positive organisms, viruses, plasmodia, and even in infectious mononucleosis. In animal experimental work, it has been found that endotoxin-induced intravascular coagulation is prevented by prior production of granulocytopenia with nitrogen mustard. Intravascular coagulation can be produced by infusion of extracts of leukocytes from endotoxin-treated animals. On the basis of these findings, it is thought that leukocytes may participate in intravascular coagulation accompanying certain cases with sepsis. Acute hemolysis associated with incompatible blood transfusion reaction or with near-drowning may be associated with disseminated intravascular coagulation, to which procoagulant materials released from the red blood cells contribute. Anaphylactic shock is frequently accompanied by intravascular coagulation. Disseminated intravascular coagulation may occur in association with malignant neoplasia. Carcinoma of the prostate is the most well-recognized of these, but the disorder is also encountered with many other neoplasms, including pancreatic and pulmonary neoplasms, acute leukemia, and lymphoma.

Clinical features present in patients with disseminated intravascular coagulation include the features of the primary condition, which frequently includes shock. Bleeding may be from a single site but is particularly suggestive of disseminated intravascular coagulation when it occurs from multiple bleeding sites, from venipuncture wounds, and from skin suture sites. Purpura and ecchymoses may be present. When the disorder is present chronically, as for example in the Kasabach-Merritt syndrome, the patient experiences no shock or bleeding but will bleed excessively following injury and from venipuncture wounds.

The primary *treatment* of intravascular coagulation is that of the underlying disease. The Kasabach-Merritt syndrome is cured by removal of the hemangioma. Intravascular coagulation associated with placental separation or with fetal death should be treated by removal of the uterine contents. When shock is the precipitating factor, every effort should be made to reverse it as rapidly as possible. Intravascular coagulation associated with metastatic prostatic carcinoma will often diminish very rapidly after the start of estrogen therapy, depending on the responsiveness of the tumor. A second line of therapy involves replacement of blood components. Without question, blood loss should be replaced. If fibrinogen is replaced without effectively controlling clotting, it will merely provide more substrate for the enzymes. Since it is difficult to be certain that clotting is controlled and because of the likelihood of hepatitis virus contamination, fibrinogen is best withheld. If the basic condition has been reversed or if heparin is being given, coagulation factor deficiencies should be replaced with plasma, and significant thrombocytopenia treated with platelet transfusion. When the primary disease cannot be treated effectively, heparin will inhibit intravascular clotting and elevate clotting factor levels, but the platelet count almost invariably remains low. Bleeding is frequently enhanced by heparin alone, and platelets and plasma should also be given. Approximately 100 units heparin per kilogram of body weight may be given to initiate therapy followed by 10 to 15 units per kilogram per hour by constant intravenous infusion. The best index of hemostatic effectiveness is cessation or reduction of bleeding. The most rapid and specific indication that coagulation has been interrupted is provided by a drop in fibrinopeptide A concentration to the normal level within 15 min of starting heparin. Of the available laboratory tests, elevation in fibrinogen level and reduction in degradation product level provide evidence that intravascular proteolysis has been interrupted. Larger doses of heparin than usual may be needed in some patients, and smaller than usual doses should be used in the presence of severe thrombocytopenia. When there is a large open wound, as after surgery, the risk of local bleeding limits the usefulness of heparin therapy. Heparin therapy is most useful when gross thrombosis or purpura fulminans is present.

Purpura fulminans is an acute disorder which occurs most often in children following a bacterial or viral infection. Following a latent period after the infection, swollen purple purpuric lesions, possibly with a necrotic center, occur on the limbs, back, buttocks, or face. The laboratory signs of disseminated intravascular coagulation are present; histologically, widespread thrombosis of capillaries and venules with a surrounding perivascular inflammatory reaction is found. Heparin can stop the progress of the disease, and vigorous therapy is recommended for about a week, to be succeeded by warfarin for several weeks.

Intravascular coagulation with normal or elevated fibrinogen concentrations In a large number of diseases, laboratory changes have been described comprising elevated levels of fibrinogen degradation products, plasma coagulation on addition of protamine or ethanol, and variations in the platelet count, partial thromboplastin time, prothrombin time, and thrombin clotting time. It is contended that these changes reflect increased intravascular coagulation and that although insufficient to produce hypofibrinogenemia, the clotting may be sufficient to produce ischemic tissue damage. A listing of such disorders is given in Table 318-3. It is not clear that the laboratory changes do signify the presence of disseminated intravascular coagulation. It is also not clear to what extent intravascular coagulation, if present, contributes to the pathogenesis of the disorders. With these uncertainties, the role of anticoagulant therapy in these conditions remains to be determined. As in the hypofibrinogenemic syndromes, heparin therapy is most clearly indicated when thrombosis is present.

TABLE 318-3
Disorders with normal or elevated fibrinogen levels associated with intravascular coagulation

I Local vascular alterations: Glomerulonephritis, nephrotic syndrome with proliferative glomerulonephritis, polyarteritis nodosum, thrombotic thrombocytopenic purpura, hemolytic-uremic syndrome, organ transplant rejection
II Generalized derangements
  A Hemolysis: Paroxysmal nocturnal hemoglobinuria, hemolytic-uremic syndrome
  B Immunologic: Systemic lupus erythematosus
  C Infections: Bacterial, viral, rickettsial, fungal, malaria, bubonic plague, subacute bacterial endocarditis
  D Neoplasms: Gastric, pulmonary, breast, renal

FIBRINOLYTIC STATES

In certain conditions it is thought that plasmin may be formed in the circulating blood separately from thrombin formation. The only definite condition in this category is produced by the therapeutic infusion of streptokinase or urokinase. In such circumstances, the concentration of fibrinogen and factors V and VIII in the circulating blood may drop, and increased fibrinogen degradation products may be present in the serum, whereas the platelet count may remain in the normal range.

It is uncertain whether a similar state may arise in patients not receiving thrombolytic therapy. Patients have been encountered in which a similar set of laboratory findings has occurred in association with rapid lysis of whole-blood clots formed in vitro and with rapid euglobulin lysis times. These circumstances have been accompanied by generalized oozing of blood. None of these patients has been studied in sufficient detail to know whether intravascular coagulation, i.e., excessive thrombin action, was an accompaniment.

There is evidence that localized plasmin action promotes bleeding following prostatectomy and dental extraction. Systemic administration of an inhibitor of plasmin formation, epsilon-aminocaproic acid, diminishes postprostatectomy hemorrhage and markedly reduces the requirement for replacement therapy in hemophiliacs undergoing dental extraction. One should be cautious about using EACA in patients diagnosed as having primary fibrinolysis until there is evidence concerning the degree of thrombin action in these patients. There is clinical and pathologic evidence that the drug will promote thrombosis in a potentially disastrous fashion if given alone when intravascular coagulation is present.

The extent to which plasmin digests fibrinogen in clinical disorders is not clear, but there is evidence that plasmin digests a formed fibrin clot much more effectively than fibrinogen in plasma.

CIRCULATING ANTICOAGULANTS

Most naturally occurring circulating anticoagulants are actually antibodies to specific clotting factors. Patients have been described with antibodies to fibrinogen, factors V, VIII, IX, X, XI, and XIII. Antibodies may arise in patients with congenitally deficient factor activity or in patients with a previously normal coagulation system. In the latter case, the antibody may be an isolated finding or may be only part of a complex autoimmune syndrome such as systemic lupus erythematosus.

The clinical findings in patients with *antibody-type circulating anticoagulants* are similar to those in patients with congenital deficiency of the designated factor. The principal difference is that replacement therapy is ineffective in the presence of such anticoagulants. Steroid treatment is generally also ineffective unless the primary disease (e.g., systemic lupus erythematosus) is responsive to steroids. The disorder may persist indefinitely or may remit spontaneously and unpredictably.

Laboratory studies reveal all the features of deficiency of the specific factor. For example, if the antibody is to factor VIII, there is a long partial thromboplastin time, low factor VIII level, and normal prothrombin time. Furthermore, the patient's plasma induces factor VIII deficiency in normal plasma when the two are mixed. The patient's plasma will also inactivate purified factor VIII in a time-dependent reaction. Antibodies to factor VIII are the commonest antibodies encountered; they occur in about 5 to 10 percent of hemophiliacs, transiently and occasionally in postpartum women, in association with penicillin allergy, systemic lupus erythematosus, and rheumatoid arthritis, and at times without apparent cause. Despite lack of laboratory evidence of an increase in specific factor level, infusion of the appropriate concentrate may be lifesaving. There appears to be a difference in the response to immunosuppressive (azathioprine) therapy in patients with antibodies to factor VIII, depending on whether the patient was previously normal or had hemophilia. Antibodies in previously normal individuals have in some instances disappeared as a response to azathioprine therapy, whereas in hemophilia, such therapy has been uniformly ineffective. Because of the likelihood of an anamnestic rise in antibody titer, therapy should be vigorous and prompt. Once hemostasis has been achieved, the rise in inhibitor level will not be deleterious. If hemostasis has not been secured, the high titer of antibody will render further therapy useless. A novel approach to treatment of bleeding in patients with factor VIII inhibitors is the infusion of certain "activated" commercial vitamin K–dependent factor concentrates. Hemostasis has been achieved in a number of instances. The beneficial effect is thought to depend on a poorly defined activated coagulant moiety which bypasses the factor VIII–dependent steps and produces a mild state of intravascular coagulation. A number of reports of thromboembolism, and even of death, in patients receiving these concentrates mandate great caution in their use. Patients with impaired liver function may be especially prone to thrombosis following infusion of these concentrates. Nevertheless, their use may be considered when no alternative therapy is feasible.

In addition to the antibody directed against a specific coagulation factor, patients with *systemic lupus erythematosus* may develop antibodies directed against prothrombin activator, or a component of the prothrombin activator complex. The prothrombin activator complex is composed of factor X_a, factor V, and calcium ions bound to the lipoprotein surface of the platelet membrane. In a number of instances, the antibody in systemic lupus appears to be directed against the lipid component. Clinically, there is usually no excessive bleeding other than bruising. Bleeding in these patients depends on the presence of associated thrombocytopenia. Thrombophlebitis has been reported in some patients. Laboratory features of the disorder include a prolonged whole-blood clotting time, prothrombin time, and partial thromboplastin time. When individual coagulation factors are assayed, the patient's prothrombin level may be low. Other factor assays are normal. A mixture of patient's and normal plasma has a long prothrombin and partial thromboplastin time immediately following mixing. This condition usually responds rapidly to steroid therapy, often with return to normal of the coagulation findings within a week, but the coagulation findings themselves are not an indication for steroid therapy, which should be used as indicated for the underlying disease.

REFERENCES

Biggs R (ed): *Human Blood Coagulation, Hemostasis and Thrombosis*, 2d ed. Oxford, Blackwell, 1976

———— (ed): *The Treatment of Haemophilia A and B and von Willebrand's Disease*. Oxford, Blackwell, 1978

Feinstein DI, Rapaport SI: Acquired inhibitors of blood coagulation, in *Progress in Hemostasis and Thrombosis*, vol 1, TH Spaet (ed). New York, Grune & Stratton, 1972

Hardisty RM, Ingram GIC: *Bleeding Disorders, Investigation and Management*. Philadelphia, Davis, 1965

Lorand L: Haemorrhagic disorders of fibrin-stabilization, in *Haemostasis*, D Ogston, B Bennett (eds). New York, Wiley, 1977

Minna JD et al: *Disseminated Intravascular Coagulation in Man*. Springfield, Ill, Charles C Thomas, 1974

Ratnoff OD (ed): *Treatment of Hemorrhagic Disorders*. New York, Harper & Row, 1968

Rosenberg RD, Damus PS: Actions and interactions of antithrombin and heparin. N Engl J Med 292:146, 1975

Suttie JW, Jackson CM: Prothrombin structure, activation and biosynthesis. Physiol Rev 57:1, 1977

Williams WJ et al (eds): *Hematology*, 2d ed. New York, McGraw-Hill, 1977, chaps 128–162

Other hematologic disorders

319
BLOOD GROUPS AND BLOOD TRANSFUSION

ELOISE R. GIBLETT

BLOOD GROUP ANTIGENS AND ANTIBODIES

INTRODUCTION Human red blood cell membranes contain over 300 different antigenic determinants, the molecular structure of which is dictated by genes at an unknown number of chromosomal loci. The term *blood group* is applied to any well-defined system of red blood cell antigens controlled by a locus having a variable number of allelic genes, such as *A*, *B*, and *O* in the ABO system. Twenty-one blood group systems are currently recognized. The term *blood type* refers to the antigen phenotype, which is the serologic expression of the inherited blood group genes.

Most of the blood group antigens are very difficult to characterize chemically, because the only source is the highly complex red blood cell membrane. However, a few of the antigens on red blood cells are also present as soluble substances in body fluids, facilitating their purification and analysis.

Alloantibodies specific for the blood group antigens may occur "naturally" (i.e., in the absence of known stimulus by foreign red blood cells) or in response to transfusion or pregnancy. Naturally occurring antibodies tend to be IgM molecules, and many of them (notably excepting anti-A and anti-B) react poorly at body temperature but readily agglutinate red blood cells at 5 to 20°C. Antibodies formed in response to exposure to another person's red blood cells or soluble blood group substances may initially belong to the IgM class but usually change to the IgG class within a few weeks or months. In general, these "immune" antibodies react best at body temperature, and special laboratory procedures are required for their detection.

BLOOD GROUP SYSTEMS   ABO system: genes and antigens

There are four major allelic genes in this system: *A¹, A², B,* and *O.* The locus for these alleles is on the long arm of chromosome 9. The actual products of the first three genes are glycosyltransferases which select specific sugars, *N*-acetyl-D-galactosamine (GalNAc) by the *A¹* and *A²* transferases and D-galactose (Gal) by the *B* transferase, attaching them by alpha-linkage to short (oligo) saccharide chains. These chains comprise the carbohydrate moiety of glycolipid and glycoprotein molecules on the red blood cells or in other tissues and fluids. Although the *A¹* and *A²* transferases perform the same function, they have different rate constants, so people who inherit an *A¹* gene have more A-reactive sites than those with an *A²* gene. The *O* gene product is a protein which cross-reacts immunologically with the *A* and *B* transferase molecules but has no detectable enzyme activity; thus it is functionally "silent."

Nearly all individuals produce "naturally occurring" antibodies against the A or B antigens not present on their own red blood cells, as shown in Table 319-1. This fact is used as the basis for confirming the red blood cell type. Most of the major phenotypes represent more than one genotype. Thus, in the absence of family studies, it is possible to infer the genotype from only three phenotypes: A₁B, A₂B, and O. In routine practice, the ABO type is determined by testing the red blood cells with anti-A and anti-B and by testing the serum against A, B, and O red blood cells. Under special circumstances, a further distinction between A and AB types is made by using anti-A₁, an antiserum prepared by absorbing anti-A typing serum with A₂ red blood cells. The remaining unabsorbed antibodies have A₁ specificity, reacting with A₁ and A₁B, but not with A₂ and A₂B cells. (Alternatively, anti-A₁ is prepared as a lectin from

extracts of certain seeds.) The frequencies of the various phenotypes in two American blood donor populations are also given in Table 319-1.

Red blood cells of types O and A₂ have large amounts of another antigen, called H, which is the immediate precursor to A and B. H specificity depends on the presence of a fucose (Fuc) residue attached to the oligosaccharides by a transferase that is the product of a very common gene called *H.* (The H and ABO loci are not genetically linked.) In very rare individuals who fail to inherit an *H* gene from either parent (i.e., they are homozygous for its allele, *h*), the *H* transferase is not made, and the H-determining fucose is not attached. This prevents the addition of specific sugars by the *A* and *B* transferases. As a result, even if an *A* or *B* gene has been inherited, the red blood cells are not agglutinated by anti-A, anti-B, or anti-H, while the serum contains all three antibodies. When a patient requiring transfusion has this so-called O_h (or Bombay) phenotype, special arrangements are necessary to obtain blood of the same rare type from a source such as the Red Cross.

About 80 percent of people are either homozygous or heterozygous for the "secretor," or *Se,* gene, which has no effect on the formation of antigens intrinsic to red blood cells but which activates the *H* gene to produce its fucosyltransferase in secretory tissues. Homozygotes for the apparently inactive allele *se* are called *nonsecretors* because their secretory cells do not produce the *H* transferase, so their body fluids lack H, A, and B antigen activities.

Antibodies in ABO system

Red blood cells of newborn infants have decreased numbers of H, A, and B reactive sites, and their plasma normally contains very little anti-A or anti-B. The latter finding is due to the fact that fetal immunoglobulin production is minimal, while most of the anti-A and anti-B produced in the mother are IgM molecules which cannot cross the placenta. However, in some type O adults, the anti-A, anti-B, and anti-AB (a cross-reacting antibody sometimes called anti-C) are of the IgG class and are strong hemolysins. Thus, ABO hemolytic disease of the newborn usually occurs in A (or B) infants of O mothers. Similarly, hemolytic transfusion reactions tend to be most severe in type O patients who receive ABO-incompatible blood.

TABLE 319-1
Blood types of the ABO system (including Hh)

Genotype*	Phenotype	Antigens on red blood cells†	Antibodies in serum‡	Phenotype frequencies in Americans, %	
				Western European descent	African descent
A^1A^1 A^1A^2 A^1O	A₁	A₁, (H)	Anti-B (anti-H)	35	23
A^2A^2 A^2O	A₂	A₂, H	Anti-B (anti-A₁)	10	6
BB BO	B	B, (H)	Anti-A, A₁	8	17
A^1B	A₁B	A, A₁, B	(Anti-H)	3	3
A^2B	A₂B	A, B, H	(Anti-A₁)	1	1
OO	O	H	Anti-A, A₁ Anti-B	43	50
hh	O_h	None	Anti-A, A₁ Anti-B Anti-H	Very rare	Very rare

* *In all types except the last, the H allele is present as HH or Hh.*
† *(H) indicates occasional presence of weakly reacting H antigen.*
‡ *Antibodies in parentheses are, if present, weak cold agglutinins.*
SOURCE: *Race and Sanger.*

It is not acceptable medical practice to transfuse A, B, or AB blood to patients whose red blood cells lack the corresponding antigens, since their plasma contains incompatible antibodies. However, it is acceptable to give A or B blood (preferably as packed red blood cells) to AB recipients, or to give O packed red blood cells (*not* whole blood, except in severe emergencies) to patients of type A, B, or AB when the transfusion requirement exceeds the supply of type-specific blood. Although antibodies with A_1 specificity frequently occur in the plasma of A_2 and A_2B subjects, they are almost always weak cold agglutinins. Thus, if anti-A_1 has been identified in a transfusion patient, it can be ignored unless it reacts in vitro with A_1 red blood cells at 37°C.

Lewis system Antigens in the Lewis system are not produced by red blood cells but rather are taken up as glycosphingolipid molecules from the surrounding plasma. About 80 percent of Western Europeans are either homozygous or heterozygous for the *Le* gene. The other 20 percent are homozygous for its presumably inactive allele, *le*. There are two well-defined Lewis antigenic determinants, Le^a and Le^b, both of which are structurally related to the H, A, and B antigens (Table 319-2). The *Le* gene product, like the *H* gene product, is a fucosyltransferase, but it attaches fucose to a different sugar (*N*-acetyl-D-glucosamine instead of D-galactose) in the oligosaccharide chains. The Le^a determinant is a monofucosyl structure which lacks the fucose attached by the *H* transferase. The Le^b determinant has two fucose residues placed there by the *H* and *Le* transferases, in that order.

As shown in Table 319-3, individuals who lack an *Se* gene (i.e., nonsecretors of H, A, and B) cannot produce molecules with the difucosyl structure. If they have an *Le* gene, their secretions and plasma contain a large amount of Le^a, but no Le^b, and their blood cells have the phenotype $Le(a+b-)$. However, secretors of H(A,B) who have an *Le* gene produce only a small amount of Le^a and a much larger amount of Le^b antigen. Their red blood cells are usually $Le(a-b+)$, although they may be $Le(a+b+)$, reacting with both anti-Le^a and anti-Le^b. The red blood cells of *le* homozygotes are $Le(a-b-)$, even if they inherit both *H* and *Se* genes, since they lack the necessary *Le* transferase to form either Le^a or Le^b determinants.

TABLE 319-2
Structure of oligosaccharides with H, A, B, and Lewis specificities

Antigen specificity	Structure*
H	β-Gal-β-GlcNAc-β-Gal-R† ↑ α-Fuc
A_1 or A_2	α-GalNAc-β-Gal-β-GlcNAc-β-Gal-R ↑ α-Fuc
B	α-Gal-β-Gal-β-GlcNAc-β-Gal-R ↑ α-Fuc

Le^a	β-Gal-β-GlcNAc-β-Gal-R
	      ↑
	      α-Fuc

Le^b	β-Gal-β-GlcNAc-β-Gal-R ↑ ↑ α-Fuc α-Fuc

* *See text for explanation of abbreviations. Specific bonds between sugars are omitted.*
† *R is the rest of the molecule, consisting of more monosaccharides, usually attached to peptide or lipid carriers.*
SOURCE: *Watkins.*

TABLE 319-3
Associations of various genes with H, A, B, and Lewis antigen activities

Genes present	Antigens on red blood cells		Antigens in plasma and secretions			
	H, AB	Le^a	Le^b	H,* AB	Le^a	Le^b
H, AB, Se, Le	+++		++	+++	+	++
H, AB, sese, Le	+++	+++			+++	
H, AB, Se, lele	+++			+++		
H, Ab, sese, lele	+++					
hh, AB, Se or sese, Le	†	+++			+++	
hh, AB, Se or sese, lele						

* *H antigen activity is demonstrable in secreted glycoproteins but not in the plasma glycosphingolipids.*
† *Individuals who lack the H gene belong to the very rare O_h phenotype.*
SOURCE: *Watkins.*

Anti-Le^a and anti-Le^b are fairly common naturally occurring antibodies, produced mainly by subjects of phenotype O, $Le(a-b-)$. Nearly all examples of these antibodies are of the IgM class, so they rarely, if ever, can cross the placenta during pregnancy. Were they to do so, destruction of the infant's red blood cells would be highly unlikely, since the Lewis glycosphingolipids are very poorly developed during fetal life.

Lewis antibodies (particularly anti-Le^a) are complement-binders, and thus anti-Le^a is occasionally the cause of a transfusion reaction with intravascular hemolysis. However, the plasma of $Le(a+)$ donors usually contains enough soluble Le^a antigen to neutralize the patient's anti-Le^a before it can attack the vulnerable red blood cells. Nevertheless, patients whose plasma contains anti-Le^a, which strongly hemolyzes $Le(a+)$ red blood cells or agglutinates them at temperatures above 30°C, should be given blood from either $Le(a-b+)$ or $Le(a-b-)$ donors. Anti-Le^b is virtually never a transfusion hazard.

P system Several structurally related antigens are considered together under the heading of a single system called P. As in the ABO and Lewis systems, the gene products are glycosyltransferases, attaching either D-galactose, *N*-acetyl-D-galactosamine, or *N*-acetyl-D-glucosamine to glycosphingolipids on the red blood cell membrane. P_1 and P_2, the major antigenic determinants, were previously thought to represent the expression of two allelic genes at the same locus, analogous to A^1 and A^2 in the ABO system. However, it is clear that these two antigens represent quite different sugar sequences, and the current genetic interpretation will require radical revision as soon as all biochemical analyses are completed.

Table 319-4 shows the five interrelated phenotypes in this "system," with their corresponding antigens and antibodies. P_1 is the most common phenotype in most populations, while P_1-negative individuals nearly always have the P_2 type. P_1^k, P_2^k, and p phenotypes are extremely rare, but they are clinically important, being associated with the presence of naturally occurring antibodies with strong hemolytic activity. On the other hand, anti-P_1, which frequently occurs in people of type P_2, is virtually never capable of causing red blood cell destruction—the exceptions being those rare examples which react strongly with P_1 red blood cells in vitro at 37°C. In patients with paroxysmal cold hemoglobinuria, the so-called Donath-Landsteiner autoantibodies frequently react with globoside, a very common red blood cell glycosphingolipid with P specificity.

I system The I and i antigenic determinants are structurally heterogeneous. Their inheritance is not well defined, but they are known to be biochemically related to the H, A, B, Le, and

TABLE 319-4
Characteristics of the P phenotypes

Phenotype	Approximate frequency	Antigens on red blood cells	Antibodies in plasma
P_1	75%	P_1,* P	None
P_2	25%	P*	Anti-P_1 (often)
P_1^k	Very rare	P_1, P^k	Anti-P
P_2^k	Very rare	P^k	Anti-P
p	Very rare	None	Anti-P_1PP^k

* P^k is also present on these cells but is not ordinarily detected by routine serologic methods.
SOURCE: *Race and Sanger.*

P antigens. Most people inherit a gene associated with I antigen production, but the red blood cells of newborn infants react very weakly with anti-I and strongly with anti-i. A gradual reversal occurs during the first year or two, so that in older children and adults, red blood cell I activity greatly exceeds i activity. In patients with certain kinds of "marrow stress," particularly thalassemia and hypoplastic anemia, red blood cell i activity increases with no apparent loss of I.

Anti-I is a common antibody, frequently found as a weak cold agglutinin of no clinical concern. In patients with the cold type of autoimmune hemolytic anemia, autoantibodies nearly always have anti-I or anti-I plus i specificity, and most of them belong to the IgM class (Chap. 314). Anti-i production is associated mainly with lymphoid cell diseases, especially infectious mononucleosis and lymphosarcoma. A patient already having a "marrow-stressing" disorder such as thalassemia may develop an intense autoimmune hemolytic anemia due to anti-i. When transfusions are required, finding serologically compatible blood poses no problem, since the red blood cells of most adults are essentially i-negative. Even patients with strong cold-reacting anti-I antibodies are usually not difficult to transfuse safely if they are kept warm during the infusion. However, since anti-I often fixes complement, the desirable technique in severe cases is to use washed red blood cells rather than packed cells so that no more complement components are introduced.

MNS system The biochemical genetics of this system is poorly understood. The major antigens, M, N, S, and s, are inherited as if they were the result of four different allelic genes determining four antigen pairs: MS, Ms, NS, and Ns. The sialic acid residues of red blood cell glycoprotein are apparently related to M and N specificity. Red cells of the En(a−) phenotype, which lack a major sialoglycoprotein called glycophorin A have decidedly reduced N and, usually, M activity. Their Rh agglutinability is *increased,* probably owing to the change in negative surface charge associated with loss of sialic acid.

Anti-M and anti-N are usually naturally occurring IgM agglutinins with little capability of destroying red blood cells. Patients on long-term renal dialysis tend to form anti-N as either an auto- or alloantibody. In patients of N or MN types, the N-specific autoantibodies have no hemolytic potential, but they are alleged to cause rejection of kidneys kept refrigerated before transplantation.

Formation of anti-S or anti-s usually requires the stimulus of transfusion or pregnancy, and accordingly these antibodies often belong to the IgG class. A third antibody, anti-U, behaves serologically somewhat like anti-S plus anti-s, being formed in sensitized black subjects whose red blood cells have a rare phenotype lacking S and s antigens. All three of these antibodies can hemolyze incompatible red blood cells in vivo, but they are readily detectable by adequate compatibility testing.

Rh system The Rh locus is on chromosome 1. There is some biochemical evidence that Rh antigenic determinants are dependent on interaction between red blood cell membrane protein and phospholipid molecules. Over 100 Rh phenotypes have been described serologically, but the underlying biochemical genetics is unknown. It is convenient to envision a stretch of nucleotides at the Rh locus which dictates the structure of a set of three antithetical determinants: C or c, E or e, and D or d (the latter having no corresponding antibody and therefore being simply the absence of D). These sets are thus inherited from each parent as a unit, such as CDe, cde, cDE, and so forth. This nomenclature, used by Race and Sanger, is compared with the alternative nomenclature of Wiener in Table 319-5, which also gives the approximate frequencies of the corresponding alleles in Americans of Western European, African, and Oriental origins.

The D(Rh_o) antigen is by far the most immunogenic of this or any other blood group system (except for those previously described systems in which the formation of antibodies does not depend on exposure to foreign red blood cells). About 15 percent of Caucasians lack the D(Rh_o) antigen and are Rh-negative. When transfused only once with Rh-positive blood, these Rh-negative persons have about a 50 percent chance of forming anti-D(Rh_o) antibodies, which could cause destruction of any subsequently transfused Rh-positive red blood cells. For this reason, Rh-negative patients are always given Rh-negative blood except when the transfusion requirements of a male or postmenopausal female exceed the available supply. Giving Rh-positive blood to Rh-negative premenopausal females is a very serious matter, because, unless adequate amounts of Rh immune globulin are given to prevent immunization, any sub-

TABLE 319-5
Rh alleles, their antigenic determinants, and frequencies

Allele	Associated antigenic determinants*		Approximate allele frequencies in Americans†		
	R-S	W	Western European descent	African descent	Oriental descent
R^1	D, C, e	Rh_o, rh′, hr″	0.45	0.10	0.55
r	c, e	hr′, hr″	0.37	0.15	0.10
R^2	D, c, E	Rh_o, hr′, rh″	0.14	0.10	0.35
R^o	D, c, e	Rh_o, hr′, hr″	0.02	0.60	Low
r″	c, E	hr′, rh″	0.01	Low	Low
r′	C, e	rh′, hr″	0.01	Low	Low
R^z	D, C, E	Rh_o, rh′, rh″	Low	Low	Low
r^y	C, E	rh′, rh″	Low	Low	Low

* R-S = Race and Sanger; W = Wiener (see references).
† *Low frequency means less than 0.01. Individuals of African descent have other alleles not listed here, thus accounting for failure of their frequencies to total 1.0.*

sequent pregnancy with an Rh-positive infant will almost always stimulate a secondary immune response, resulting in hemolytic disease of the newborn.

The Rh antigens C, c, E, and e are considerably less immunogenic than D, and it is impractical to try to match these antigens in donors and recipients. Of course, when previously sensitized patients are found to have the corresponding antibodies, it is then necessary to find donor blood lacking the specific antigens. This search may be easy or difficult, depending on the individual case. For example, about 20 percent of the population lack the c antigen and thus are compatible donors for a patient whose plasma contains anti-c. However, only 2 percent lack the e antigen, so that patients with anti-e pose serious problems, especially when large amounts of blood are required. Blood banks often maintain donor calling lists or frozen red blood cells for use in such cases.

A large proportion of patients with acquired hemolytic anemia of the warm type have IgG autoantibodies which react with one or more Rh-associated antigens. In some instances, the specificity is clear-cut (for example, anti-e), but more often the antibodies react with all red blood cells except those of the rare type known as Rh null. These cells lack all known Rh antigens, and the cell membrane is defective, reinforcing the belief that in normal red blood cells, molecules bearing the Rh determinants are an intrinsic part of the membrane protein structure.

Kidd, Kell, Duffy, and Lutheran systems The major antigens of these four clinically important systems and their average phenotype frequencies in Americans of Western European and African origins are presented in Table 319-6 along with the frequencies of S and s in the MNS system. Anti-K and anti-Fy^a are frequently encountered antibodies capable of marked alloimmune red blood cell destruction. Even more dangerous are the antibodies in the Kidd system, both anti-Jk^a and anti-Jk^b, which are notoriously difficult to detect. Whenever a patient has a hemolytic transfusion reaction after transfusion of blood found to be compatible by the usual laboratory tests, the most likely cause is anti-Jk^a. Antibodies in the Lutheran system have only rarely been reported to cause red blood cell destruction, but if a patient has anti-Lu^b antibodies which

react strongly by the indirect antiglobulin technique, transfusion with Lu^b positive blood is probably hazardous. Since Lu^b-negative blood is very rare, such patients pose serious problems in blood transfusion.

Other blood group antigens Many other red blood cell antigens, both related and unrelated to the best known systems enumerated above, have been described. The Xg^a antigen is of considerable importance to geneticists, since its locus is on the X chromosome. Other antigens are of clinical interest because they occur on the red blood cells of 95 percent or more of most populations, making it difficult to find compatible blood when their antibodies are present in patients requiring transfusion. Many of these antibodies have little ability to destroy red blood cells, even though they consist of IgG molecules and react in vitro at 37°C. Included in this category are most examples of anti-Sd^a (Sid), anti-Yt^a (Cartwright), anti-Yk^a (York), and many others. Nevertheless, both caution and experience are necessary when considering the transfusion of serologically incompatible blood, particularly when the antibodies react in vitro at body temperature. Antibodies with Chido (Ch^a) and Rodgers (Rg^a) specificity are incapable of causing hemolysis. Their respective antigenic determinants are located on molecules of C4 (i.e., the fourth component of complement), and are thereby taken up from the plasma by red cells.

BIOLOGICAL SIGNIFICANCE OF BLOOD GROUPS **Immune reactions** The relationship of blood group antigens and antibodies to alloimmune red blood cell destruction has been briefly discussed in the previous sections. Because antigens in the ABO system are present in other tissues, they play a role in determining *histocompatibility*, so that transplantation of ABO-incompatible kidneys and other organs carries a risk of rejection (Chap. 69). However, successful grafting of ABO-incompatible bone marrow is possible when the patient is immunosuppressed and given exchange transfusions with plasma lacking antibodies against the donor's red blood cells.

Infertility and early fetal loss Both of these effects have been ascribed to ABO incompatibility, although in some instances the data are of marginal significance. Nevertheless, many population geneticists believe that this factor plays a significant role in the processes of natural selection.

TABLE 319-6
The major antigens and phenotypes in five clinically important blood group systems (excepting ABO and Rh)*

System	Major antigens	Phenotypes	Approximate phenotype frequencies in Americans, %†	
			Western European descent	African descent
Kidd	Jk^a, Jk^b	Jk(a+b−)	26	55
		Jk(a−b+)	24	7
		Jk(a+b+)	50	38
Kell	K, k, Js^a	K−k+Js(a−)	91	83
		K−k+Js(a+)	Low	15
		K+k−Js(a−)	Low	Low
		K+k+Js(a−)	9	2
		K+k+Js(a+)	Low	Low
Duffy	Fy^a, Fy^b	Fy(a+b−)	18	10
		Fy(a−b+)	33	20
		Fy(a+b+)	49	2
		Fy(a−b−)	Low	68
Lutheran	Lu^a, Lu^b	Lu(a+b−)	Low	Low
		Lu(a−b+)	92	97
		Lu(a+b+)	8	3
(MN) Ss	S, s	S−s+	47	65
		S+s−	10	9
		S+s+	43	24
		S−s−	Low	2

* See Tables 319-1 and 319-5 for information about ABO and Rh types.
† Low means less than 1 percent.
SOURCE: Giblett, 1969.

Disease-related phenotype changes A and, to a lesser extent, B determinants are subject to certain biochemical changes, such as those caused by bacterial glycosidases and other enzymes. As a result, the red blood cells may develop new specificities, becoming either "polyagglutinable" or having "pseudo-B" characteristics. Another acquired alteration in ABO type occurs in some patients with acute myelocytic leukemia whose original type is A_1. This change in phenotype, with partial or complete loss of agglutinability by anti-A, can be a diagnostic aid in the early hypoplastic phase of leukemia. The changes in Ii specificity associated with "marrow stress" are described above (see "I System" above).

Other disease relationships There is some evidence that the incidence of certain diseases is related to blood type. For example, type O "nonsecretors" have about twice the incidence of duodenal ulcer than do secretors of types A or B. On the other hand, type A carries a higher incidence of tumors of salivary glands, stomach, and pancreas than does type O. Persons with the rare Rh_{null} type, whose red cells lack all the Rh antigens, have some degree of increased hemolysis, as do people with the McLeod phenotype. The latter red blood cells react only weakly with antibodies against antigens of the autosomally controlled Kell system, and they lack Kx, a very common X-linked antigen. Some boys with the X-linked form of chronic granulomatous disease have the McLeod phenotype and others do not. In both instances, the Kx antigen, also a normal granulocyte component, is not detectable on these cells. Individuals (mainly of African origin) who lack both Fy^a and Fy^b—the major antigens in the Duffy system—are protected against infestation by the malarial parasite, *Plasmodium vivax*, presumably because Fy^a and Fy^b act as specific recognition or acceptor sites for the merozoites.

Chromosome mapping Blood genetic markers, including the red and white blood cell allotypes as well as the plasma and blood cell enzyme phenotypes, are very useful for mapping the human chromosomes. Some of these markers are genetically linked to loci for genes causing metabolic diseases, and, as more markers are identified, it will be increasingly possible to predict the development of inherited malfunctions from specimens obtained in utero or from newborn infants. For example, the secretor gene locus is closely linked to the locus of the gene causing myotonic dystrophy. Thus, a determination of the secretor status of a baby at risk can be used to predict the likelihood of its developing this disease, since both characters are inherited as autosomal dominants.

Medicolegal applications When the red blood cell antigens are combined with the other genetic markers in blood, distinguishing one person from another is possible with a probability of about 2 million to 1. This high degree of individuality promotes the usefulness of genetic markers for ruling out paternity, maternity, and monozygosity in nearly all cases where those relationships do not exist. However, very few laboratories can perform all the necessary tests, and complete phenotyping is a very expensive and time-consuming procedure.

BLOOD TRANSFUSION

INTRODUCTION Considerable morbidity and, to a lesser extent, mortality are associated with blood transfusion therapy. Responsible medical practice dictates that physicians have sufficient background information to make soundly reasoned judgments concerning the risks as well as the benefits of this procedure. They must decide not only what blood components (if any) are indicated but also what quantities are needed.

WHOLE BLOOD A unit of whole blood consists of approximately 450 ml blood collected into a plastic bag containing either 68 ml acid-citrate-dextrose (ACD) solution or 63 ml citrate-phosphate-dextrose (CPD) solution as anticoagulant and preservative. Kept in the refrigerator, blood has a storage life of only 3 weeks, at which time about 70 to 80 percent of red blood cells are still viable, the white blood cells and platelets are nonviable, and the activity of the labile clotting factors, V and VIII, will have decreased to low levels.

Virtually the only reason to transfuse whole blood is to restore blood volume lost through recent hemorrhage, as in patients with gastrointestinal bleeding, a major surgical procedure, or trauma. For assessing the amount of blood loss, routine laboratory tests are often misleading during the first several hours after hemorrhage. Both the hemoglobin and hematocrit measurements reflect the ratio of a patient's red blood cell mass to the blood volume, rather than indicating the total circulating red blood cells. Since the compensatory vasoconstriction evoked by hemorrhage initially prevents the extravascular fluids from replacing the intravascular fluid loss, both laboratory measurements may be falsely high. Clinically, postural hypotension provides a warning that blood transfusion may be required. Pallor, syncope, tachycardia, thirst, and air hunger are useful indicators of massive blood loss (i.e., 1500 ml or more in adults), sometimes requiring immediate transfusion of type O blood that has not been cross matched. In less severe cases, maintaining the blood volume with saline or plasma expanders provides time for accurate blood typing and compatibility testing.

During surgery, blood loss can be quite accurately measured, and there is a tendency to "keep up" or even to "stay ahead" of lost volume by transfusion. Obviously, such practices lead to unwarranted use of blood with all its attendant hazards. In most adult subjects, blood loss of 500 ml is easily tolerated, being equivalent to the amount given by a blood donor. Judicious use of crystalloid infusions is frequently all that is required to circumvent blood transfusion, even with blood losses up to a liter. In modern medicine, ordering "fresh" blood at any time is not acceptable practice, since proper component therapy is both safer and more scientifically based.

PACKED RED BLOOD CELLS The preparation of packed red blood cells from whole blood involves sedimentation or centrifugation followed by removal of plasma into a satellite bag, all in a closed system. Red blood cells, like whole blood, can be kept refrigerated for 3 weeks with only 20 to 30 percent loss of cell viability. Removal of the plasma provides protection against circulatory overload as well as against excessive loads of sodium, potassium, citrate, ammonia, and antibodies (such as anti-A, in particular) which might be harmful to the patient. Furthermore, the removed plasma can be used for preparing such blood components as platelets, cryoprecipitate, albumin, and immunoglobulins.

In the absence of recent blood loss, most transfusions are given to patients who need replacement of oxygen-carrying capacity. Packed red blood cells are much preferred to whole blood for this purpose, since the plasma serves no useful purpose and may actually be detrimental, especially in hypervolemic subjects. Diagnoses most frequently associated with the need for packed red blood cells fall into two major categories of anemia, hypoplastic and hemolytic.

Red blood cell hypoplasia Chronic bone marrow depression may, under favorable circumstances, be treated by bone marrow transplantation from an identical twin or another sibling compatible for HLA. However, many patients either have no access to a marrow donor or, for a variety of reasons, are unsuitable candidates for such a heroic measure. The red blood cell mass of these patients can be maintained at functional levels for long periods, provided that they do not develop multiple antibodies against red blood cell antigens. These patients are in general more liable to become immunologically refractory to platelets and white blood cells than to red blood cells. Patients whose red blood cell hypoplasia is secondary to marrow invasion by malignancy and/or to various chemo- or radiotherapeutic agents also require red blood cell transfusions. Again, sensitization to transfused platelets and white blood cells generally creates a greater problem than red blood cell immunization.

Hemolytic anemia In severe cases of inherited nonimmune hemolysis due to intrinsic red blood cell defects (e.g., sickle-cell anemia, thalassemia, or severe deficiencies of glucose 6-phosphate dehydrogenase), the only hope of maintaining oxygen-carrying capacity through a crisis is the careful use of red blood cell transfusion. Patients with other forms of nonimmune hemolysis or ineffective erythropoiesis (e.g., vitamin B_{12}, folate, or iron deficiencies) are candidates for transfusion only if they are severely anemic and if the cause cannot be corrected rapidly by specific replacement therapy. Whenever any infusion is given to a patient with severe anemia, the central venous pressure must be monitored so that incipient heart failure can be controlled.

Patients with autoimmune hemolytic anemia are very poor candidates for red blood cell transfusion. Not only are they unusually prone to develop alloantibodies when exposed to foreign red blood cells, but they may have already formed such antibodies as the result of earlier transfusion or pregnancy. In the presence of circulating autoantibodies, alloantibodies are often difficult to detect, and transfused red blood cells may react with both kinds of antibodies, leading to very rapid destruction. Consultation with a blood transfusion expert is desirable in cases where severe anemia with hypoxemia or cardiac failure poses a real threat to life and there is not time to wait for the effects of steroid therapy.

PLATELETS Platelet concentrates are prepared by centrifugation of platelet-rich plasma to yield about 5×10^{10} platelets from each donor unit. Retention of about 50 ml plasma is necessary to prevent the unfavorable drop in pH which would otherwise occur during storage at room temperature. Prepared in this way and kept under constant agitation, platelets can be stored for up to 3 days and still survive normally after autologous transfusion, with a half-life of about 5 days. Platelets stored in the refrigerator may function well immediately after transfusion, but their viability in vivo is much shorter. In adult thrombocytopenic patients without consumptive coagulopathy or platelet-specific antibodies, one unit of platelet concentrate raises the platelet count by about 10,000 per cubic millimeter.

Patients with idiopathic thrombocytopenic purpura produce autoantibodies which react with all human platelets (Chap. 316), and therefore derive little or no benefit from platelet transfusion. Moreover, the platelets produced by such a hyperactive marrow are highly effective in maintaining hemostasis even at platelet counts as low as 10,000 per cubic millimeter. Similarly, in patients with thrombocytopenia due to a consumptive coagulopathy (as in infection or metastatic malignancy) the usefulness of platelet therapy is limited, unless its purpose is to keep the patient from bleeding while the primary cause is being treated.

The most rational use of platelets is to control bleeding in

patients with either a temporary loss of platelets not due to immunity (e.g., massive blood replacement, prolonged surgery) or with suppressed platelet production (leukemia, lymphoma, treatment with radio- or chemotherapy). Since platelets are very immunogenic, and typing techniques are not available, this blood component should not be given in the absence of clear indication. Most nonbleeding patients with platelet counts above 10,000 per cubic millimeter can maintain adequate hemostasis. Patients in the immediate postoperative period may need to have their platelet counts elevated to as high as 100,000 per cubic millimeter. In other bleeding situations, a platelet count of 50,000 per cubic millimeter or more suggests other causes for hemorrhage, especially if there is no recent history of ingestion of aspirin or other drugs that interfere with platelet function, which would be reflected by a prolonged bleeding time. The effectiveness of platelet transfusion is assessed by comparing the platelet count before the infusion with counts obtained about 2 and 24 h later.

Choice of blood type Ideally, donors of platelets should have the same ABO and Rh types as the patient, since it is impossible to remove all red blood cells from the platelet concentrate. When it is necessary to use O donors for A, B, or AB recipients, the plasma may contain sufficient anti-A (or anti-B) to destroy some of the patient's red blood cells. Although this possibility is fairly small, it deserves consideration, especially in children or in adults receiving large numbers of platelet concentrates. When platelets of A, B, or AB donors are given to patients of unlike ABO type, their effectiveness may be somewhat diminished, although this does not appear to be a major problem. However, it is important that the number of red blood cells in such ABO-incompatible preparations be kept as small as possible.

Since some red blood cells are inevitably present in platelet concentrates, Rh-negative patients should receive platelets from Rh-negative donors whenever feasible, particularly if there is a possibility of subsequent pregnancy. However, lack of platelets from Rh-negative donors should not preclude transfusing Rh-positive donor platelets in a life-threatening situation. Patients who have the potential of becoming mothers can be protected against Rh alloimmunization by an injection of Rh immune globulin, about 20 μg for each milliliter of Rh-positive red blood cells present in the infusion. In other Rh-negative patients given platelets from Rh-positive donors, Rh-antibody formation can be expected to occur with a high frequency, but these antibodies do not interfere with the survival of subsequently transfused Rh-positive donor platelets, since they do not themselves contain Rh antigens.

Refractory state Patients who receive random donor platelets on more than one or two occasions frequently develop alloantibodies with either HLA or HLA-related specificities. Such refractory prepared patients can often be maintained with concentrates prepared by plateletphoresis from donors compatible for HLA, especially siblings. However, repeated performance of this procedure is costly and time-consuming, often placing a heavy emotional burden on both donor and recipient. Before a program to support a thrombocytopenic patient in this way is begun, careful consideration must be given to donor education and consent, the expected life span of the patient, and the numerous socioeconomic problems involved.

WHITE BLOOD CELL TRANSFUSIONS Since it is now possible with platelet transfusions to control bleeding in many patients with hematologic malignancies, hemorrhage is being supplanted by infection as the most frequent cause of death. The need for efficient white blood cell transfusion has been apparent for years, but only recently has it become feasible to treat selected neutropenic patients. For example, when patients are given bone marrow transplants, it is routine practice to sustain them through the stage of dangerous leukopenia with white blood cells prepared by continuous-flow centrifugation or filtration leukophoresis of volunteer donors. However, even when the necessary equipment is available, the problems of maintaining patients for long periods in this way are even more difficult than those associated with platelets. Neutrophils have a very short life span in the bloodstream, and little is known about the best collection techniques, the feasibility of neutrophil storage, proper dosage schedules, and the effects on donors and patients of the chemicals used (i.e., citrate, heparin, hydryethyl starch). Furthermore, resulting immunologic problems involve not only the HLA system but also cell-specific antigens known to be associated with white blood cell destruction.

PLASMA COMPONENT THERAPY Fresh frozen plasma and cryoprecipitate are major blood component preparations because they are necessary for the care of patients with coagulation disorders, especially hemophilia (Chap. 318). Because of the risk of hepatitis, pooled plasma is not considered an acceptable agent for expanding intravascular volume. However, albumin and other salvaged human plasma protein derivatives with high albumin content are commercially prepared for use in special cases, such as nephrosis, certain gastroenteropathies, and severe malnutrition. Immunoglobulin preparations are also commercially made, including specific hyperimmune globulin for preventing the development of certain infectious diseases and for blocking the immune response to Rh antigen.

COMPLICATIONS OF BLOOD TRANSFUSION Transfusion reactions are classified as immune or nonimmune in origin. The immunologically mediated reactions may be directed against red or white blood cells, platelets, or at least one of the immunoglobulins, IgA. Other less well-defined hypersensitivity reactions also occur. The major nonimmune transfusion reactions are those due to circulatory overload, massive transfusion, or transmission of an infectious agent.

Immunologically mediated reactions Hemolysis due to red blood cell alloantibodies may occur within the circulation or extravascularly. The very rapid cell destruction associated with *intravascular hemolysis* is usually due to incompatibility within the ABO system, since both anti-A and anti-B fix complement, regardless of whether they are IgM or IgG molecules. Other possibilities to consider are anti-Jk[a], anti-Le[a], and anti-Fy[a]. Rh antibodies are only rarely associated with hemoglobinemia. Symptoms include restlessness, anxiety, flushing, chest or lumbar pain, tachypnea, tachycardia, and nausea, followed by the typical findings of shock and renal failure. In comatose or anesthetized patients, the first sign of danger is often oozing of blood from the mucous membranes or operative site, due to intravascular coagulation.

Extravascular hemolysis is most commonly caused by antibodies of the Rh system, but several other antibodies, especially of the Kell, Duffy, and Kidd systems, are among the offenders. The clinical manifestations are usually milder, consisting of malaise and fever. Shock and renal complications rarely, if ever, occur. Some patients have delayed reactions in which the transfused red blood cells have normal survival initially, but about a week later they are rapidly destroyed in the reticuloendothelial system. Such delayed reactions are commonly due to an anamnestic rise in antibodies previously stimulated by transfusion or pregnancy. Rarely, patients are found to have destroyed all the transfused cells in the absence of demonstrable antibodies.

LABORATORY INVESTIGATION Of first importance in the investigation of a hemolytic transfusion reaction is a careful check on the identity of both the donor and the recipient, since clerical errors, especially mistakes in identity, are most frequently involved. Then the necessary steps include demonstrating that red blood cell destruction has occurred, investigating its cause, and determining the status of the patient's renal and coagulation mechanisms.

With recent *intravascular* lysis, the hemoglobin level is elevated in both plasma and urine (blood must be drawn cautiously to avoid red blood cell rupture). Also, depending on the number of red blood cells destroyed, there may be methemalbuminemia accompanied by marked reduction of serum haptoglobin and hemopexin. (Measuring the latter two substances is rarely necessary, and to be meaningful, both tests require knowledge of the pretransfusion levels for comparison.) The best indicator of *extravascular* lysis is a rise in unconjugated bilirubin, accompanied by failure of the hematocrit to reach the expected posttransfusion level.

Having a *pretransfusion* specimen of the patient's blood is very helpful, so that determination of his or her blood types, as well as those of the donor, can be repeated, along with the compatibility test. If antibodies are detected, this pretransfusion specimen is also valuable for determining their identity, aided by knowledge of the full antigen composition, since alloantibodies are formed only against antigens not present on the patient's own cells. The *posttransfusion* specimen may not contain the offending antibodies, since they could have been completely absorbed by the donor's incompatible red blood cells. However, it is desirable to examine the red blood cells in the posttransfusion sample, both microscopically for agglutinates and by the direct antiglobulin (Coombs) test. A positive result usually means that some of the donor's red blood cells, coated by the patient's antibodies, were still present when his or her blood was drawn. But it is also possible that the *donor's* plasma contained antibodies, missed during the donor screening procedure, which reacted with the red blood cells of the patient. Thus, if the direct antiglobulin test on the posttransfusion specimen is positive, the plasma of both donor and recipient should be examined for the responsible antibodies. In the absence of ABO incompatibility, significant destruction of a patient's red blood cells by a donor's alloantibodies is distinctly rare. More typically, the antibody-coated red blood cells survive well in vivo, but their presence can lead to a misdiagnosis of acquired hemolytic anemia.

TREATMENT The care of patients with extravascular hemolysis should be conservative, avoiding additional transfusion unless the patient's life is otherwise threatened. Intravascular hemolysis is a far greater hazard, since shock and renal failure are not uncommon. Immediate treatment with an osmotic diuretic is indicated unless acute tubular necrosis has already occurred. Renal blood flow can be increased with appropriate agents, shock controlled symptomatically, and disseminated intravascular coagulation treated with platelet concentrates and fresh frozen plasma, as needed. Management of the coagulopathy is discussed in Chap. 318, and treatment of renal shutdown in Chap. 275.

In the absence of red blood cell destruction, most febrile reactions can be ascribed to immunity against white blood cell, platelet, or plasma antigens. Further laboratory workup is required only when the reaction is unusually severe. For example, patients with antibodies against IgA molecules sometimes undergo severe shock upon exposure to the blood of other human subjects. Such individuals must be transfused only with blood that lacks IgA or with repeatedly washed red blood cells. Patients with antibodies against white blood cells or platelets can usually be given packed red blood cells from which the buffy layer has been removed after centrifugation or by filtration. Some centers use frozen and thawed red blood cells for transfusing patients sensitized to white blood cells, or to retard the occurrence of such sensitization in candidates for bone marrow transplantation.

Nonimmune transfusion reactions   Included in this category are circulatory overload, adverse effects of massive transfusion, infections, metabolic shock, air and fat embolisms, thrombophlebitis, and siderosis. The first three are by far the most common.

CIRCULATORY OVERLOAD   Patients with renal or cardiac insufficiency are liable to develop circulatory failure and pulmonary edema with even modest amounts of intravenous infusion. Infants are also vulnerable, since their vasculature does not accommodate rapidly to infusions. The onset may be immediate or delayed for up to 24 h after transfusion, with dyspnea and chest pain progressing to the full-blown picture of pulmonary edema. Patients predisposed to this alarming complication should be transfused in a sitting position, with the rate of red blood cell flow not exceeding 2 ml/min, depending on body size and degree of impairment. A rise in central venous pressure heralds the danger of administering more red blood cells unless they are exchanged with whole blood removed from the patient.

MASSIVE TRANSFUSION   When the amount of stored blood transfused to bleeding patients exceeds the amount of their normal blood volume, complications can include hyperkalemia, ammonia and citrate toxicity, and dilutional coagulopathy. These problems are largely avoided by using blood stored for no more than a week, supplementing with platelet concentrates when indicated. Fresh frozen plasma is rarely indicated, unless the factor 8 level is shown to be very low. In that case, cryoprecipitate may also be considered, particularly if the fibrinogen concentration is also decreased.

INFECTION   Many diseases, such as hepatitis, cytomegalovirus infection, syphilis, malaria, toxoplasmosis, and brucellosis, can be transmitted by transfusion. In addition, blood that becomes infected during handling and storage can cause very severe shock, owing to toxic bacterial metabolites.

Of all the transfusion-transmitted infections, viral hepatitis is by far the most common and most serious in most parts of the world. Presence in donor blood of the hepatitis B virus (HBV) can be inferred by the detection of the hepatitis B surface antigen (HBsAg). All blood banks are required to perform this test, using so-called "third generation" methods, usually including radioimmunoassay. Although this procedure appears to be reducing the incidence of posttransfusion hepatitis by about a third, clearly other non-A, non-B viruses, as yet undetectable, are responsible for a large proportion of this complication. It is well documented that blood obtained from paid donors carries an especially high risk of hepatitis. Strong efforts are being made in the United States to limit the source of transfused blood to volunteer donors, as is currently the practice in some other countries, among them Canada, Australia, and England.

REFERENCES

GIBLETT ER: *Genetic Markers in Human Blood.* Philadelphia, Davis, 1969

————: Blood group alloantibodies: An assessment of some laboratory practices. Transfusion 17:299, 1977

HAKOMORI S, KOBATA A: Blood group antigens, in *The Antigens,* M Sela (ed). New York, Academic, 1974, vol 2, p 80

MARCUS DM: The ABO and Lewis blood group systems. N Engl J Med 280:994, 1969

MARSH WL et al: Chronic granulomatous disease and the Kell blood groups. Br J Haematol 29:247, 1975

McKUSICK VA, RUDDLE FH: The status of the gene map of the human chromosomes. Science 196:390, 1977

MOHN JF et al (eds): *Human Blood Groups.* New York, Karger, 1977

MOLLISON PL: *Blood Transfusion in Clinical Medicine,* 6th ed. Philadelphia, Lippincott, 1979

MOURANT AE et al: *The Distribution of the Human Blood Groups and Other Biochemical Polymorphisms,* 2d ed. New York, Oxford University Press, 1975

PERKINS HA: Indications and limitations of cytapheresis, in *Plenary Sessions,* XVII Congress of the International Society of Hematology and XV Congress of the International Society of Blood Transfusion. Paris, 1978

RACE RR, SANGER R: *Blood Groups in Man,* 6th ed. Oxford, Blackwell, 1975

WATKINS WM: Blood group substances: Their nature and genetics, in *The Red Blood Cell,* 2d ed, DM Surgenor (ed). New York, Academic, 1974, vol 1, p 293

WIENER AS: The blood groups. Three fundamental problems—serology, genetics and nomenclature. Blood 27:110, 1966

WIMER BM et al: Haematological changes associated with the McLeod phenotype of the Kell blood group system. Br J Haematol 36:219, 1977

320
POLYCYTHEMIA VERA

JOHN W. ADAMSON

DEFINITION   Polycythemia vera is one of a group of disorders referred to as the *myeloproliferative syndromes,* which also include chronic granulocytic leukemia (Chap. 326), agnogenic myeloid metaplasia (Chap. 321), and primary hemorrhagic thrombocythemia. Polycythemia vera classically is characterized by splenomegaly and an increased production of erythrocytes, granulocytes, and platelets; however, the disease is generally dominated by an elevated hemoglobin concentration. Polycythemia vera is gradual in onset and runs a chronic but usually slowly progressive course.

The disease generally begins in late middle life and is slightly more common in males. Only rarely is polycythemia vera found in children or multiple members of a single family. The disease is relatively uncommon in blacks, and occurs with increased frequency in Jews of European extraction.

ETIOLOGY   None of the recognized physiologic causes of increased red blood cell production is present in polycythemia vera. The disease must be distinguished from secondary forms of polycythemia, in which an elevated hemoglobin concentration results from increased erythropoietin production. This association may arise through hypoxia, or is occasionally found with certain neoplasms. Polycythemia vera is also distinct from spurious (relative) polycythemia, which results from a decrease in the plasma volume rather than a true increase in red blood cell mass. Also, secondary causes do not explain the splenic enlargement and increased leukocytes and platelets which are typically seen.

It has been shown in selected patients that polycythemia vera is a disease of a multipotential stem cell and appears to arise from a single clone. These findings are most consistent with the neoplastic origin of the disorder and are less compatible with the concept of marrow proliferation resulting from an atypical myeloproliferative stimulus. In polycythemia vera, there is a unique relationship of erythropoietin to red blood cell production. As opposed to the findings in secondary forms of erythrocytosis, urinary erythropoietin excretion in patients with polycythemia vera is substantially reduced or absent. Presumably erythropoietin production is suppressed by the elevated hemoglobin concentration, since phlebotomy results in a rise in both erythropoietin excretion and red blood cell production (provided that there is no deficiency in iron), demonstrating the marrow's ability to respond at least in part to humoral regulation.

It has been shown that marrow from patients with polycythemia vera forms colonies of hemoglobin-synthesizing cells in semisolid medium in the absence of added erythropoietin. This is generally not the case with marrow cells from normal individuals or from patients with secondary erythrocytosis, where formation of erythroid colonies is almost uniformly dependent upon the addition of erythropoietin. A reduced production of erythropoietin, the appearance of "endogenous" erythroid colonies in marrow cultures, and the apparently clonal origin from the multipotential stem cell all suggest that hematopoiesis in polycythemia vera is not regulated by the usual mechanisms and, indeed, may be autonomous.

PATHOPHYSIOLOGY AND SYMPTOMATOLOGY Polycythemia vera produces symptoms associated with increased blood volume and blood viscosity. The hemoglobin concentration, hematocrit, and total blood volume may become markedly elevated, a consequence of the sharply increased red blood cell mass. The plasma volume is usually normal or reduced slightly; occasionally patients with an increased plasma volume are seen. Associated with the expanded blood volume is a consistently elevated increase in cardiac output and a less uniform, but significant, increase in cardiac index. Reduction of the hematocrit and blood volume by phlebotomy leads to a reduction in the stroke volume and cardiac output in these patients and generally to an improvement in exercise tolerance. The increased cardiac output occurs in association with an increase in blood viscosity and, presumably, vascular resistance, associated with the elevated hematocrit.

Complaints related to the disturbed cerebral circulation include headache, dizziness, vertigo, a sense of fullness of the head, rushing in the ears, visual alterations (scotomata, double vision, or blurred vision), tinnitus, syncope, and even chorea. Peripheral vascular symptoms of both arterial and venous insufficiency are common; in one large series, more than 35 percent of patients gave a history of some thrombotic or hemorrhagic event during the course of their disease. The risk of thrombosis may be increased by the accelerated atherosclerosis in this disease. Bleeding is common and comes most often from the nose and from peptic ulcer disease. Intramuscular hemorrhages and increased bruising are also seen. The tendency to increased bleeding may be due to the distended vasculature resulting from the increased blood volume. However, intrinsic platelet dysfunction also may contribute to bleeding, particularly in the gastrointestinal tract. The incidence of peptic ulcer disease is estimated to be four to five times higher in patients with polycythemia vera than in the general population. The precise reasons for the tendency for gastrointestinal hemorrhage are by no means clear.

In the later stages of the disease, the spleen may become greatly enlarged, producing symptoms of easy satiety, a sense of intraabdominal fullness and pleuritic chest or left upper quadrant pain, probably secondary to capsular stretching or infarction. Pruritus, occurring particularly after bathing, is re-

ported frequently and may be disabling. Occasionally, urticaria is seen.

The increased cellular proliferation seen with polycythemia vera results in hyperuricemia in 25 to 30 percent of patients and may be associated with secondary gout in 5 to 10 percent. There also may be renal involvement with uric acid nephropathy and formation of urate stones.

LABORATORY FINDINGS The most prominent laboratory feature is an elevated concentration of hemoglobin. Unless altered by iron deficiency, the red blood cells are normochromic and normocytic. Polychromasia is frequently seen, and nucleated red blood cells may be found in the later stages of the disease. These findings represent cells released from extramedullary sites of hematopoiesis or reflect damage to marrow stroma due to fibrosis. The erythrocyte sedimentation rate is frequently very low (0 to 3 mm/h). Ferrokinetic studies in the patient who is not iron-deficient document an increase in red blood cell production, but studies in the presence of iron deficiency cannot be interpreted with certainty.

The white blood cell count is elevated in two-thirds of patients, usually in the range of 15,000 to 25,000 per cubic millimeter, but may be as high as 60,000 per cubic millimeter. An increase in the absolute basophil count (greater than 65 per cubic millimeter) is found in about 70 percent of patients with polycythemia vera. The alkaline phosphatase of circulating neutrophils is increased in more than 80 percent of cases. Serum vitamin B_{12} levels vary and are increased in about one-third of the patients; however, the binding capacity is increased in as many as 75 percent. This is due to an increase in the vitamin B_{12}–binding proteins, transcobalamins I and III.

Thrombocytosis is seen in over half of all patients with polycythemia vera. In vitro studies of platelet function suggest defective platelet adhesiveness and impaired secondary release of adenosine diphosphate in response to epinephrine. However, the contribution of these functional abnormalities to the thrombotic and hemorrhagic events in patients with polycythemia vera is uncertain. Abnormal liver function studies, including an elevated alkaline phosphatase, may occur if there is massive hepatomegaly.

Splenomegaly occurs in 75 percent of patients and may persist even when the elevated hemoglobin concentration has been reduced by repeated phlebotomies. The spleen may become massive late in the disease. Microscopic examination of the spleen reveals multiple foci of extramedullary hematopoiesis and fibrosis. These may become marked, but the follicular pattern of the organ is retained, unlike the loss of normal architectural structure observed in chronic granulocytic leukemia. Occasionally, similar foci may be found in the liver.

The bone marrow generally reflects either erythroid or panhyperplasia without distinctive morphologic features. There is also increased megakaryocyte nuclear ploidy in the face of thrombocytosis. This pattern of platelet regulation is different from that observed in the reactive thrombocytosis associated with inflammation or neoplasia, where megakaryocyte nuclear ploidy is inversely related to the peripheral platelet count. As the disease progresses, fibrosis may appear in central areas of the marrow, and scanning techniques will demonstrate expansion of hematopoietic tissue to more peripheral skeletal sites.

A variety of cytogenetic abnormalities have been reported in polycythemia vera; however, prior treatment with myelosuppressive agents or radioactive phosphorus (^{32}P) has clouded the significance of such observations. Trisomy 1, 8, or

9 have been reported several times in untreated patients as has 20q −.

DIAGNOSIS The plethoric patient with pancytosis and splenomegaly, and without evidence of chronic cardiac or pulmonary disease, presents few diagnostic problems. However, it is more common to see these patients with less than the full clinical expression of the disease or as individuals in whom an elevated hemoglobin or hematocrit has been discovered at the time of routine laboratory evaluation. Under these circumstances, it is important that the diagnosis of polycythemia vera be made or excluded with certainty in order to direct therapeutic efforts appropriately.

First the question of whether an elevated hemoglobin represents a true increase in red blood cell mass should be answered. Statistically, there is little likelihood that hematocrits consistently near or greater than 60 percent represent simply a decrease in plasma volume. When hematocrit levels are in the range of 50 to 55 percent, however, the likelihood of true erythrocytosis is considerably reduced. Therefore, it is useful to measure red blood cell mass carefully. The red blood cell mass should be determined directly by isotope dilution using ^{51}Cr-labeled autologous red blood cells. While the plasma volume may be calculated indirectly from the red blood cell mass, it is preferable to measure this compartment independently, using a second label. If the spleen is markedly enlarged, the mixing time in the circulation for the labeled red blood cells may be prolonged, and samples for radioactive counting should be obtained up to 30 to 45 min after injection. The results of the red blood cell volume are best expressed as a function of the lean body mass, which may be estimated from the patient's height and weight. If the results of such a study are equivocal, the physician must weigh all the clinical findings in deciding whether the patient has a true increase in red blood cell production.

The influence of iron deficiency on the red blood cell mass must also be considered. The patient who presents with a hematocrit or hemoglobin in the high normal range, microcytosis, leukocytosis, and iron deficiency should be considered as possibly having polycythemia vera. Evaluation of red and white blood cell morphology, basophil count, and platelet morphology should be carried out to make certain that this is not a patient with polycythemia vera who has bled.

While measurements of red blood cell mass distinguish between spurious and true erythrocytosis, the results do not distinguish between the various forms of polycythemia. If the diagnosis is uncertain, additional parameters which may be helpful include the absolute basophil count, the leukocyte alkaline phosphatase, and radioisotope scanning to quantitate spleen size. This technique is particularly useful in obese individuals or patients in whom the spleen is enlarged but not palpable. Splenomegaly occurs rarely in individuals with secondary erythrocytosis.

If the diagnosis of polycythemia remains obscure, an intravenous pyelogram to exclude hypernephroma, as well as arterial blood gases, should be obtained. Perhaps 20 percent of patients with polycythemia vera may have a hemoglobin oxygen saturation below 92 percent, but almost all will have a saturation equal to or greater than 88 percent. This modest impairment of oxygen loading may be due to decreased diffusing capacity of the lung, possibly triggered by repeated episodes of thromboembolism or thrombosis in situ.

When the diagnosis is not clear following routine investigation, then measurement of the urinary excretion of erythropoietin may be helpful. Patients with polycythemia vera excrete little or no measurable erythropoietin, while patients with secondary forms of erythrocytosis excrete at least normal and frequently elevated amounts. The measurements should be carried out using a bioassay, since other assays, based on immunologic reactions, have not been able to separate mechanisms of polycythemia. In vitro growth characteristics of bone marrow cells from patients with polycythemia vera suggest that such determinations may be useful in diagnosis, but experience with these tests is limited.

COURSE AND PROGNOSIS The course of polycythemia vera has been a subject of disagreement, some observers believing that later complications may be hastened by myelosuppressive therapy. About 15 to 20 percent of patients will progress to marrow fibrosis, marked splenomegaly, and anemia; and one view holds that if patients live long enough, all will enter this so-called "spent" phase of the disease and will require red blood cell transfusions. However, the majority of patients die of vascular complications of their disease, or of unrelated causes. Although the incidence is small, there is a statistically significant association of second hematologic neoplasms in patients with polycythemia vera, including chronic granulocytic leukemia, lymphocytic and histiocytic lymphomas, multiple myeloma, and erythroleukemia (di Guglielmo's syndrome). Some patients with polycythemia vera experience transformation into acute leukemia even in the absence of prior radiation or chemotherapy.

THERAPY Optimal therapy of polycythemia vera remains unsettled. The median survival has been extended to 10 to 12 years with phlebotomy alone, while patients receiving no therapy at all survive only 2 years. However, it is not clear whether myelosuppressive therapy or phlebotomy hold any clear advantage for survival. For many years after its introduction in 1940, ^{32}P was the therapy of choice. However, a retrospective analysis of a large number of cases suggested that ^{32}P increased the incidence of acute leukemia to nearly 15 percent while not clearly enhancing survival over other forms of therapy. In order to resolve the major questions regarding the most effective therapy, the incidence of complicating factors and the prognostic implication of certain features such as thrombocytosis or cytogenetic abnormalities, the International Polycythemia Vera Study Group was established. Since 1967, this group has prospectively randomized patients who meet strict diagnostic criteria into three treatment programs: ^{32}P therapy augmented by phlebotomy, myelosuppressive therapy plus phlebotomy, and phlebotomy alone. Preliminary analysis of the survival curves demonstrates similar life expectancies for the various treatment groups. Acute leukemia has occurred predominantly in the group of patients treated with chemotherapy. The long-term results of this study should provide important information concerning the best treatment and the complications of this disease.

Despite the controversy, certain therapeutic tenets meet with agreement. First, phlebotomy is safe, can be done repeatedly, and is preferred in individuals with mild disease, young patients, or those with polycythemia of uncertain etiology. Regardless of eventual decisions involving therapy, phlebotomy should be used initially to reduce the red blood cell mass and blood volume. The end point of phlebotomy therapy should be a hematocrit or hemoglobin value in the low-normal range. This form of treatment may lead to prolonged clinical remission. Iron should not be given if phlebotomy is the primary mode of therapy. Phlebotomy is especially important if a patient with polycythemia vera must undergo emergency surgery, since intra- and postoperative morbidity and mortality are four to five times greater in uncontrolled as opposed to controlled (phlebotomized) patients. Under these circumstances, the red blood cell mass should be reduced acutely by exchange phlebotomies and the blood replaced with a suitable plasma expander. This will prevent the vascular instability associated with too rapid a reduction in total blood volume.

Marrow suppression may be achieved by radiation or chemical agents. Phosphorus 32 is easy to administer, provides long, trouble-free remissions in most cases, and successfully reduces the morbidity associated with the disease. The isotope is incorporated into bone and comes into close proximity to rapidly dividing marrow cells. The regimen recommended by the Polycythemia Vera Study Group consists of the intravenous administration initially of 2.3 mCi ^{32}P per square meter of body surface area. The patient is then followed for a period of 3 months and re-treated at that time, as needed, with a dose 25 percent greater than that given originally. This program may be repeated 3 months later, but is rarely required. Remissions may last 6 to 24 months, during which time the patient is often symptom-free. Radioactive phosphorus therapy may be repeated if relapse occurs. Exposure to ^{32}P probably increases the incidence of leukemia in patients with polycythemia vera, and the risk of leukemic transformation may be related to the cumulative dose of isotope. Thrombocytosis may be troublesome and constitutes an indication for myelosuppressive therapy.

Suppression of marrow function with chemotherapy has been common during the last 15 years. Effective drugs include melphalan, busulfan, and chlorambucil. Busulfan, in doses of 4 to 6 mg per day orally, reduces the white blood cell and platelet counts, but suppression may be unpredictable and prolonged, and the drug is relatively less effective in suppressing erythropoiesis. Moreover, continued use of this drug may lead to pulmonary fibrosis and a syndrome resembling adrenal insufficiency. Chlorambucil has been employed by the Polycythemia Vera Study Group in their prospective study. An initial dose of 10 mg per day for 4 to 6 weeks followed by 4 to 8 mg per day until the patient is in remission, is given. Doses of 4 to 10 mg per day may be given intermittently in alternate months, while maintaining a sustained marrow remission. Melphalan is also effective and may be given in doses of 6 to 10 mg per day for 1 week and then 2 to 4 mg per day until the counts are controlled. A major disadvantage to chemotherapy is that the patient must be followed more closely for stabilization of peripheral counts than is necessary with ^{32}P.

Other symptoms associated with polycythemia vera may be managed conservatively. In the case of pruritus, cyproheptadine, 12 to 16 mg per day, may be effective. Allopurinol in doses of 300 mg per day may successfully reduce the number of acute gouty attacks. Symptomatic splenomegaly is usually improved with treatment, although splenectomy or radiation of the spleen followed by splenectomy may be indicated in rare instances. This procedure is associated with a significant degree or morbidity and mortality.

REFERENCES

ADAMSON JW et al: Polycythemia vera: Stem cell and probable clonal origin of the disease. N Engl J Med 295:913, 1976

KLEIN H: *Polycythemia Vera: Theory and Management.* Springfield, Ill, Charles C Thomas, 1973

MIESCHER PA, JAFFE ER (eds): Polycythemia, parts I and II. Semin Hematol 12:335, 1975; 13:1, 1976

MODAN B, LILIENFELD AM: Polycythemia vera and leukemia: The role of radiation treatment. Medicine 44:305, 1965

OSGOOD EE: Polycythemia vera: Age relationships and survival. Blood 26:243, 1965

SEGEL N, BISHOP JM: Circulatory studies in polycythemia vera at rest and during exercise. Clin Sci 32:527, 1967

321
AGNOGENIC MYELOID METAPLASIA

JOHN W. ADAMSON

DEFINITION Agnogenic myeloid metaplasia is a member of the *myeloproliferative syndromes*. The disease is characterized by progressive splenomegaly, the gradual replacement of marrow elements by fibrosis, varying degrees of anemia, and variable changes in the number of granulocytes and platelets. The disease begins in late middle life and is gradual in onset, chronic, and progressive. Males and females are equally involved, and there is only rare familial occurrence.

ETIOLOGY The disease arises from the pluripotent hematopoietic stem cell. Studies in patients with selected cell markers have demonstrated that erythrocytes, granulocytes, and platelets arise from a single clone, while the fibrosis is reactive and not part of the abnormal clone. Nevertheless, there is progressive marrow fibrosis in the absence of recognizable stimuli. This distinguishes the disease from those conditions such as metastatic neoplasms or infections involving the bone marrow, which also give rise to reactive fibrosis. Extramedullary hematopoiesis is an integral part of the disease and is seen early in its course. There is no evidence supporting the contention that myeloid metaplasia arises in compensation for replacement of the marrow by fibrous tissue.

PATHOPHYSIOLOGY AND SYMPTOMATOLOGY Agnogenic myeloid metaplasia presents most commonly with vague constitutional symptoms associated with anemia, such as fatigue, weakness, and anorexia, or with splenomegaly. An enlarged spleen is seen in virtually all patients; however, the disease progresses slowly and splenomegaly may be present for years prior to diagnosis. The enlargement may become so extensive as to produce symptoms of pain, abdominal fullness, and dyspnea. Hepatomegaly occurs in more than 50 percent of patients and also may become massive, but enlargement of the liver due to myeloid metaplasia does not occur in the absence of splenomegaly. Because of thrombocytopenia or possible platelet dysfunction, petechiae are found in 20 percent of patients, and a history of bleeding is obtained in 10 percent. Less common findings include lymphadenopathy, jaundice, ascites, and bone pain. Weight loss, fever, sweating, and pain in the extremities may occur occasionally and are associated with a hypermetabolic state. The increased cellular turnover results in hyperuricemia in 25 to 30 percent of patients and may be associated with symptomatic gout in 5 percent.

LABORATORY FINDINGS The blood counts of patients with agnogenic myeloid metaplasia are variable. Mild anemia is observed in the majority of patients at the time of diagnosis and progresses during the course of the disease. Eventually, almost all patients become anemic. The recognized mechanisms leading to anemia include ineffective erythropoiesis, increased splenic pooling of red cells, and a variable decrease in red blood cell survival. Low serum folate and megaloblastic maturation may be contributory factors. A membrane defect similar to that found in paroxysmal nocturnal hemoglobinuria with a positive sucrose hemolysis test, has been observed in occasional patients; the significance of this finding is unknown. The peripheral blood smear usually shows dramatic changes in red cell and platelet morphology. Basophilic stippling is prominent, and bizarre red cell shapes, including teardrop poikilocytes, fragmented cells, and nucleated red cells are common, as are giant platelet forms.

An elevation in the white blood cell count is found in about 50 percent of patients, and values as high as 50,000 per cubic millimeter may be seen. However, 20 percent of patients are leukopenic, with white blood cell counts less than 4000 per cubic millimeter. Generally, there is a shift to the left in granulocyte maturation, and circulating blast forms may be found. The appearance of these cells does not imply a bad prognosis. An increase in the absolute basophil count may be observed in about 25 percent of patients. The leukocyte alkaline phosphatase activity of circulating neutrophils is elevated in about half of patients, the remainder being equally distributed between normal and low values. Serum vitamin B_{12} levels are normal or slightly elevated, as are vitamin B_{12}–binding proteins. These values usually do not approach those seen with chronic granulocytic leukemia, however.

A normal or elevated platelet count is frequently found early in the course of the disease, but thrombocytopenia eventually develops in most patients, owing to ineffective production and splenic pooling. The circulating platelets may vary considerably in size and shape, and megakaryocyte nuclei may be found on the peripheral blood smear. As in other of the myeloproliferative syndromes, in vitro studies of platelet function reflect defective platelet adhesiveness and secondary release of adenosine diphosphate in response to epinephrine. Abnormal liver function tests, including elevated bilirubin and alkaline phosphatase, may be associated with massive hepatomegaly.

Splenomegaly occurs in virtually all patients with agnogenic myeloid metaplasia and may become massive. There are multiple foci of extramedullary hematopoiesis on pathologic examination, but the normal follicular architecture of the spleen is maintained. Other organs which may be involved include the kidneys, lymph nodes, adrenal glands, and lungs. Bone marrow examination early in the course of the disease may reveal a hypercellular marrow in about 20 percent of patients and may be difficult to distinguish from polycythemia vera. A silver stain of the marrow often reveals increased reticulin deposition. The majority of patients with agnogenic myeloid metaplasia have either obvious patchy collagen fibrosis separating areas of hyperplastic marrow, or diffuse heavy fibrosis with osteosclerosis. Megakaryocytes may be preserved remarkably well in the areas of fibrosis. The degree of fibrosis and osteosclerosis of the marrow generally correlate with one another and also with the degree of splenomegaly. However, there is no clear relationship between the histopathology of the marrow and the peripheral blood counts. In 40 to 50 percent of patients, the appearance of marrow sclerosis is reflected by increased bone density on x-ray examination, involving particularly the axial skeleton and proximal long bones. These x-ray changes result from thickened bone cortex and loss of medullary spaces due to increased and thickened bony trabeculae.

No unique cytogenetic abnormalities have been described in agnogenic myeloid metaplasia; however, certain nonrandom findings, including monosomy 7 and trisomy 9 have been reported in a few patients. Reports of the Philadelphia chromosome in this disorder probably reflect examples of atypical chronic granulocytic leukemia.

DIAGNOSIS A bone marrow biopsy is essential to the evaluation of this disease, and until this has been performed, the diagnosis cannot be made with certainty. This disorder may be difficult to distinguish from others of the myeloproliferative syndromes. This is not surprising because there are several reports of apparent transition of one of the myeloproliferative diseases to another.

In chronic granulocytic leukemia, the white blood cell count is usually greater than 20,000 per cubic millimeter, while in agnogenic myeloid metaplasia it is generally 10,000 to 20,000 per cubic millimeter. Leukocyte alkaline phosphatase is usually lower in chronic granulocytic leukemia, and this deter-

mination may be useful in distinguishing between the two disorders. Fibrosis of the marrow is found in only 10 to 15 percent of patients with chronic granulocytic leukemia and is usually present only as a preterminal event; osteosclerosis is almost never seen. In the absence of the Philadelphia chromosome, however, the distinction between these diseases is occasionally difficult.

The separation of polycythemia vera and primary hemorrhagic thrombocythemia from agnogenic myeloid metaplasia also may be troublesome because all may present with thrombocytosis, splenomegaly, leukocytosis, and anemia. However, essential thrombocytosis generally is not associated with advanced fibrosis. The most difficult distinction is between agnogenic myeloid metaplasia and the late stages of polycythemia vera, and attempts to separate them may be unwarranted. Approximately 15 to 25 percent of patients with polycythemia vera progress to advanced marrow fibrosis and marked splenomegaly. It is impossible to be certain that a patient with typical agnogenic myeloid metaplasia did not have polycythemia vera initially. Postpolycythemia myeloid metaplasia and myelofibrosis has a relatively poorer prognosis.

Secondary causes of myelofibrosis include metastatic carcinoma, leukemia, and lymphomas, tuberculosis, Gaucher's disease, Paget's disease, and exposure to toxins such as benzol or x-rays. These causes are usually not difficult to distinguish from agnogenic myeloid metaplasia.

COURSE AND PROGNOSIS Agnogenic myeloid metaplasia generally follows a prolonged course, with a median survival of 4 to 5 years from the time of diagnosis; 25 percent of patients may live 15 years. Anemia will occur eventually in most patients, and many will require transfusions. Complicating features of the disease include gout or other problems related to hyperuricemia; portal hypertension due to hepatic fibrosis or hepatic vein thrombosis; and symptoms related to an enlarging spleen. Clinically evident bleeding occurs in about 25 percent. While the degree of splenomegaly appears of no prognostic importance, a low platelet count (less than 100,000 per cubic millimeter), anemia (hemoglobin less than 10 g per 100 ml), and hepatomegaly appear to influence survival adversely.

The major causes of death include infection, congestive heart failure, renal failure, portal hypertension, and hemorrhage. Transformation to acute leukemia occurs in 5 to 10 percent of patients and may be related to radiation or chemotherapy. An unusual and fulminant variant of agnogenic myeloid metaplasia is characterized by rapid progression of fibrosis and pancytopenia without massive splenic enlargement. Death due to marrow failure usually occurs within 1 year of diagnosis.

THERAPY There is no definitive therapy for this disorder, and no treatment has been shown to affect life span favorably. Anemia is treated with transfusions as required. Androgens may be administered to improve the anemia, although they are helpful in less than half the cases. Oxymetholone (2 to 4 mg/kg per day) or fluoxymesterone may be given, particularly if there is marked ineffective erythropoiesis. Corticosteroids may enhance the response to androgens but alone are not helpful. Myelosuppressive therapy is only occasionally indicated, but may be used to control painful splenomegaly or marked thrombocytosis. Chlorambucil or melphalan may be employed, but other blood elements may be depressed and the period of remission is relatively short (4 to 5 months). External radiation to the spleen will reduce its size, but the effects are transient and therapy may lead to severe pancytopenia. Allopurinol (300 mg per day) may be given to reduce the high uric acid level and control its complications.

The role of splenectomy in the treatment of agnogenic myeloid metaplasia is controversial. Late in the course of the disease the hazards of removing a massively enlarged organ are considerable, and intraoperative mortality and postoperative complications, particularly thrombosis and infection, are frequent. Some clinicians have advocated early removal of the spleen, as soon as the diagnosis is made, believing that this will reduce later complications and make management easier. Until this question is resolved, perhaps the only clear indications for splenectomy are hemolysis, severe thrombocytopenia, and intractable symptoms related to the splenomegaly. Recently, the Polycythemia Vera Study Group has initiated a prospective study of patients with this and closely related myeloproliferative diseases in order to evaluate the effectiveness of various forms of therapy.

REFERENCES

JACOBSON RJ et al: Agnogenic myeloid metaplasia: A clonal proliferation of hematopoietic stem cells with secondary myelofibrosis. Blood 51:189, 1978

LEWIS SM, SZUR L: Malignant myelosclerosis. Br Med J 1:472, 1963

SILVERSTEIN MN: *Agnogenic Myeloid Metaplasia.* Acton, Mass, Publishing Sciences Group, 1975

WARD HP, BLOCK MH: The natural history of agnogenic myeloid metaplasia (AMM) and a critical evaluation of its relationship with the myeloproliferative syndrome. Medicine 50:357, 1971

322
DISEASES OF THE SPLEEN AND RETICULOENDOTHELIAL SYSTEM

ALEXANDER FEFER

SPLENIC ABSCESS   See Chap. 110.

SPLENIC RUPTURE   Rupture is usually due to trauma or to palpation of spleens enlarged by infection, especially infectious mononucleosis and sepsis, or, rarely, by leukemia. The spleen can also be ruptured by dissection by pancreatic pseudocysts into it. If the trauma causes a subcapsular hemorrhage, rupture may not occur for several hours. The patient with a ruptured spleen presents with severe acute left upper quadrant pain which may be referred to the left scapular region, with abdominal guarding and rigidity, and with rapidly developing evidence of internal hemorrhage, shock, and anemia. Surgery must be immediate.

SPLENIC INFARCT   Splenic infarcts occur in patients with massive spleens due to a myeloproliferative syndrome or with vascular occlusive phenomena associated with hemoglobinopathies (SS, SA, S Thal, SC). The infarcts may be "silent" (asymptomatic) or may cause severe left upper quadrant pain often radiating to the left shoulder with splinting of the left diaphragm, abdominal guarding, and, at times, a friction rub in the splenic area. Sedation and bed rest are sufficient except rarely when a septic infarct causes an abscess and necessitates splenectomy.

SPLENIC ARTERY ANEURYSM   An aneurysm may be asymptomatic or may cause cramping left upper abdominal pain or vague nonspecific gastrointestinal complaints. The diagnosis may be suspected in unexplained splenomegaly with, at times, a calcified ring and adjacent mottled densities seen on x-ray. The aneurysm, most often seen in women beyond middle age, may be palpable, and a bruit may be audible. Rupture with sudden pain and, later, abdominal hemorrhage and shock is most likely to occur during pregnancy. If rupture occurs, trans-

fusions should be given, and the ruptured aneurysm as well as the spleen must be removed.

SPLENIC TUMORS   The only tumor which involves the spleen frequently is a lymphoma. Tumors arising in the vascular or sinus endothelium, i.e., lymphangioma or hemangioma, or in the capsular or trabecular framework, i.e., fibrosarcomas or leiomyosarcomas, are rare. They may cause local problems, e.g., rupture, or systemic complaints and may be diagnosed by spleen scan and angiography. Carcinomatous metastases to the spleen do not cause splenomegaly, are not clinically significant in life, and are usually detected at autopsy.

SPLENIC CYST   Cysts cause only vague gastrointestinal symptoms. Parasitic cysts are mostly due to *Echinococcus* and are associated with peripheral eosinophilia and roentgenographically detectable calcification of the cyst wall. Nonparasitic cysts are quite rare. They consist of true cysts formed from embryonal rests and include dermoids and mesenchymal inclusion cysts, or false cysts secondary to trauma and containing serous or hemorrhagic fluid. Spleen scans may reveal cysts, but angiography is necessary to distinguish them from tumors.

HYPOSPLENISM   Hyposplenism occurs when the spleen is absent or nonfunctional. The spleen may be absent congenitally, often in association with congenital heart disease. Splenic atrophy and decreased function occur in patients with multiple splenic infarcts (as in sickle-cell disease), and in celiac disease or dermatitis herpetiformis associated with an enteropathy. Splenic atrophy is documented by splenic scan and by decreased clearance of ^{51}Cr-labeled heart-damaged red blood cells.

Hyposplenism usually causes no significant disease. However, splenectomy in young children and in patients with immunologic or hematologic diseases is associated with increased susceptibility to fulminant infection by *Streptococcus pneumoniae* and *Hemophilus influenzae.* The susceptibility is less in adults and in patients splenectomized for traumatic rupture. Hyposplenism with decreased culling and pitting also causes laboratory abnormalities. The peripheral blood shows an increase in nucleated red blood cells, red blood cells with Howell-Jolly bodies, target cells, acanthocytes, and siderocytes as well as cells containing Heinz bodies. After splenectomy, a leukocytosis of up to 20,000 cells per cubic millimeter and a thrombocytosis of up to 1 million cells per cubic millimeter occur within 1 to 2 weeks, but the white blood cell count and blood platelet count usually return to normal within a month. Since portal vein thrombosis may occur above 1 million platelets per cubic millimeter, anticoagulants are indicated if the platelet count does not drop. If an accessory spleen exists, it may undergo hyperplasia and assume normal splenic function and prevent hyposplenism.

HYPERSPLENISM   **Definition**   The syndrome consists of splenomegaly, pancytopenia (anemia, leukopenia, or thrombocytopenia) in the presence of a normal or hyperactive marrow, and reversibility by splenectomy. Hypersplenism is *primary* when no underlying disease is identified. It can also be *secondary* to other splenomegalic states (Table 55-2), especially congestive splenomegaly, connective tissue diseases, myeloproliferative disorders, subacute bacterial endocarditis, kala azar, and lymphomas.

Manifestations   The clinical manifestations of hypersplenism reflect the severity of the pancytopenia. Signs and symptoms of anemia may be prominent. If neutropenia is severe (less than 1000 cells per cubic millimeter), bacterial infections may be frequent. If the platelet count is under 50,000 per cubic millimeter there may be easy bruising, and if it is under 20,000 per cubic millimeter, spontaneous hemorrhage from mucous membranes and from gastrointestinal and genitourinary tracts may occur. The manifestations of secondary hypersplenism reflect the underlying disease as well as the pancytopenia.

Diagnosis The diagnosis of hypersplenism is aided by documentation of red blood cell or platelet destruction by or in the spleen. ^{51}Cr-labeled red blood cells or platelets are infused intravenously, and the relative accumulation of label in the spleen, liver, and precordium is determined. A decrease in the $T_{1/2}$ of infused red blood cells, e.g., to 15 days, coupled with a high (above 2) spleen/liver ratio of radioactivity at $T_{1/2}$ indicates significant sequestration and destruction. The mechanism of the anemia in hypersplenism is complex and may reflect increased pooling and sequestration, or actual destruction of red blood cells in the spleen. The anemia may appear to be more severe due to an increase in the total plasma volume.

Similar studies can be performed with labeled blood platelets. Usually 20 to 40 percent of the blood platelets are sequestered in a normal spleen, whereas up to 90 percent of the platelet pool may be sequestered in hypersplenism. The mechanism for leukopenia in hypersplenism is not clear, but increased sequestration and destruction are postulated.

Treatment In addition to treating the underlying disease, the treatment for hypersplenism is splenectomy. The indication for splenectomy is granulocytopenia of under 500 cells per cubic millimeter or thrombocytopenia of under 20,000 cells per cubic millimeter, although splenectomy may be justified for less severe cytopenias. The response to splenectomy in some patients is dramatic. The laboratory data on sequestration often fail to predict a response to splenectomy. Although strong laboratory evidence for sequestration and destruction of cells in the spleen is often associated with a response to splenectomy, some patients will respond even when data fail to document sequestration. Patients whose hypersplenism is secondary to congestive splenomegaly due, in turn, to portal hypertension should not have a splenectomy performed unless a shunting procedure to relieve the portal hypertension is planned.

CHRONIC CONGESTIVE SPLENOMEGALY (BANTI'S SYNDROME) Definition The syndrome is characterized by splenomegaly, pancytopenia, portal hypertension, and gastrointestinal bleeding.

Etiology The syndrome is caused by portal hypertension due, in turn, to an intrahepatic or extrahepatic pathogical condition. Intrahepatic obstruction is seen with Laennec's cirrhosis or schistosomiasis; extrahepatic obstruction occurs with thrombosis of the portal or splenic vein, cavernous transformation of the portal vein, or compression of the splenic vein by pancreatic tumor or fibrosis. Portal vein thrombosis also may be associated with abdominal trauma, pregnancy, or intravascular coagulation. The hematologic changes are those of hypersplenism and reflect pooling, sequestration, and destruction of blood cells in the spleen.

Pathology The spleen is congested, weighs four to ten times normal, and has a thickened capsule, distended veins, and venous collaterals. There are distention of the sinuses, periarteriolar hemorrhage and siderotic nodules, an increase in the reticulum, and hyperplasia of the pulp. Progressive fibrosis of the reticulum, trabeculi, and capsule is seen. The bone marrow is

normocellular or somewhat hypercellular with myeloid or erythroid hyperplasia.

Clinical manifestations These reflect the pancytopenia of hypersplenism (see above) and the condition underlying the congestive splenomegaly. Splenomegaly may be massive and may be accompanied by gastrointestinal complaints such as flatulence, indigestion, or pain. Evidence of gastrointestinal bleeding, especially hematemesis due to rupture of gastric or esophageal varices, is often present but is not necessary for the diagnosis of Banti's syndrome.

Diagnosis The diagnosis requires detectable splenomegaly, changes consistent with portal hypertension, and the pancytopenia of hypersplenism. The anemia is normocytic-normochromic unless bleeding has induced a microcytic-hypochromic iron-deficiency anemia. The chief diagnoses to be ruled out are other causes of hypersplenism. A history of alcoholism is helpful. The liver should be evaluated by laboratory tests, liver scan, and, if necessary, liver biopsy. The detection of esophageal varices requires barium examinations and endoscopy. If no liver disease is detected, portal or splenic vein thrombosis should be suspected, and splenoportal venography should be performed in a setting in which a laparotomy may follow immediately. Congestive splenomegaly due to extrahepatic causes is more likely in patients under eighteen than in older patients.

Prognosis and treatment The prognosis is determined largely by the underlying cause of the chronic congestive splenomegaly. The pancytopenia can be tolerated for years. Hepatic failure or variceal bleeding represents the most unfavorable prognostic indicator. Intrahepatic obstruction requires not only splenectomy but also a shunting procedure, most often a portacaval shunt, to relieve the portal pressure. Congestive splenomegaly secondary to extrahepatic obstruction responds well to splenectomy.

HISTIOCYTOSES Due to a shared pathological lesion, eosinophilic granuloma, Hand-Schüller-Christian disease, and Letterer-Siwe disease have traditionally been considered as a single group of neoplastic diseases designated "histiocytosis X." This relationship has been questioned; Letterer-Siwe disease is regarded as a lymphomatous proliferation of poorly differentiated histiocytes, whereas eosinophilic granuloma and Hand-Schüller-Christian disease are thought to represent a nonneoplastic reaction of well-differentiated histiocytes to an unknown stimulus and should be referred to as *unifocal* and *multifocal eosinophilic granuloma*, respectively.

Unifocal eosinophilic granuloma This benign disease occurs in children and young adults, especially males. It presents as a solitary osteolytic lesion in the femur, skull, ribs, pelvis, or vertebrae. The lesion may be asymptomatic or may cause bone pain, tenderness, swelling, and pathological fracture. There are usually no systemic manifestations, no involvement of viscera or blood, and no eosinophilia. If no other lesion appears within 6 months, subsequent lesions are very unlikely.

The diagnosis requires biopsy. The lesion consists of well-differentiated benign histiocytes and mature eosinophils and, at times, some necrosis. If the lesion is healing, fibrosis may be seen. The disease is not fatal. The treatment of choice is curettage or excision. The rare lesion which is inaccessible to surgery can be eradicated by moderate doses of x-ray. Lesions in hazardous sites such as weight-bearing bones or cervical vertebrae should be irradiated with a total of 300 to 600 R. Higher doses should be avoided. Supportive therapy should include rest and a cast to prevent collapse and compression fractures of vertebrae. Physical examinations should be performed

Multifocal eosinophilic granuloma   The disease usually occurs before the age of 5. The patient presents with an osteolytic lesion and, within 6 months, with additional lesions. Alternatively, the patient will present with multiple lesions, especially in the flat bones. Nonspecific complaints such as malaise, anorexia, fever, and irritability are frequent, as is mastoiditis with recurrent bouts of otitis media and upper respiratory infections. Skin lesions in the form of seborrheic dermatitis are seen. Periodically, adenopathy and hepatosplenomegaly may occur in 25 to 50 percent of the patients. The classic triad of skull lesions, exophthalmos, and diabetes insipidus occurs in 25 percent of the patients, but any one element of the triad occurs in up to one-half the patients. Diabetes insipidus is manifested by polydipsia and polyuria. Pneumonitis with diffuse pulmonary infiltrates chiefly in central and perihilar areas may represent eosinophilic granulomas, and may be accompanied by bacterial infection or, rarely, by interstitial fibrosis. The blood is usually not involved.

The diagnosis is made by biopsy of the lesion, and the pathology is described above. The prognosis is good. In half the patients the lesions spontaneously resolve over many years. Almost all patients ultimately recover, although some will have persistent orthopedic problems or diabetes insipidus.

Treatment for multifocal granuloma is similar to that for unifocal eosinophilic granuloma but chemotherapy may be required to decrease the morbidity. However, this should not be as vigorous as the therapy for malignant disease. Modest doses of vinblastine, prednisone, or cyclophosphamide will benefit most patients.

Letterer-Siwe disease   This disease, which occurs in children under the age of 3, is characterized by hepatosplenomegaly, lymphadenopathy, bleeding diathesis, bony lesions, skin involvement, and a rapidly fatal course. The skin lesions are diffuse. The patient usually has fever, recurrent infections, and pancytopenia due to marrow replacement by histiocytes.

Diagnosis is made by biopsy of bone, liver, or lymph nodes, which are replaced by moderately immature histiocytes. Treatment involves supportive care, including transfusions and antibiotics, and chemotherapy which is, unfortunately, not very effective. The disease is usually fatal.

GAUCHER'S DISEASE   See Chap. 102.

NIEMANN-PICK DISEASE   See Chap. 102.

REFERENCES

CLINE MJ et al: A review and reevaluation of the histiocytic disorders. Am J Med 55:49, 1973

GOPAL V, BISNO AL: Fulminant pneumococcal infections in "normal" asplenic hosts. Arch Intern Med 137:1526, 1977

HERMANN RE et al: Splenectomy for the diagnosis of splenomegaly. Ann Surg 168:895, 1968

LAHEY ME: Histiocytosis X—an analysis of prognostic factors. J Pediatr 87:184, 1975

LIEBERMAN PH et al: A reappraisal of eosinophilic granuloma of bone. Hand-Schüller-Christian syndrome and Letterer-Siwe syndrome. Medicine 48:375, 1969

PEARSON HA et al: The born-again spleen—return of splenic function after splenectomy for trauma. N Engl J Med 298:1389, 1978

THOMAS LB et al: Vinyl-chloride-induced liver disease. N Engl J Med 292:17, 1975

WARSHAW AL et al: Intrasplenic dissection by pancreatic pseudocysts. N Engl J Med 287:72, 1972

WINTROBE MM et al (eds): *Clinical Hematology,* 7th ed. Philadelphia, Lea & Febiger, 1974

section 9 | Neoplasia

323
PRINCIPLES OF NEOPLASIA: APPROACH TO DIAGNOSIS AND MANAGEMENT

JOHN E. ULTMANN
HARVEY M. GOLOMB

INTRODUCTION   Physicians practicing internal medicine should be familiar with the various implications of the diagnosis of cancer in their patients. Cancer is not one disease. There are more than 100 clinically distinct forms of cancer, with differing biological behavior and clinical manifestations. The internist should be especially familiar with the natural history and treatment of common forms of malignancy, such as those of the breast, lung, and gastrointestinal tract. These epithelial cancers comprise over 50 percent of the cancers usually encountered. The magnitude of the cancer problem may be appreciated by a few statistics: one of four Americans will develop cancer during his lifetime, and over 400,000 Americans will die of cancer in 1979. Not only is cancer a major health problem, but the management and care of cancer patients is often complex.

With the development of medical oncology as a subspecialty of internal medicine, the internist is playing an ever-increasing role in the care of the cancer patient.

The diagnosis and management of cancer require a knowledge of general internal medicine and an understanding of the characteristics of the growth and spread of malignant neoplasms. For example, a nodular lesion in the lung must be evaluated for the possibility of neoplastic as well as granulomatous disease. Intermittent rectal bleeding must be appraised for benign or malignant neoplasms as well as for inflammatory bowel disease. Cushing's syndrome requires evaluation for bilateral adrenal hyperplasia as well as for an oat-cell carcinoma of the lung capable of producing adrenocorticotropic hormone (ACTH).

This chapter presents an overview of the biology and etiology of neoplasia and summarizes an approach to the diagnosis, staging, and treatment of cancer. The pathophysiologic changes occurring as a consequence of the tumor as a local mass, as a result of metastases, or from the elaboration of various substances by tumor are discussed. Details for the management of cancer will be found in Chap. 324 and in the various sections devoted to specific diseases.

BIOLOGY OF NEOPLASIA *Cancer* is a term used to characterize abnormal growth of cells which may result in the invasion of normal tissues or the spread to distant organs, termed *metastasis*. The degree of malignancy of a cancer is based upon the propensity of these cells for invasion and distant spread. A metastasis is a neoplastic lesion arising from another cancer, with which it is no longer in contiguity. Regardless of mechanism, separation of malignant cells from the primary cancer is an essential part of the metastatic process. The basic concept that metastases arise directly from the constituent cells of primary cancer originates from observations of histologic similarities between the two. The mode of transport of cells from the primary to the presumptive secondary lesions is inferred from the many observations of cancer cells infiltrating tissues and invading blood vessels and lymphatic channels, and the recognition of circulating cancer cells in the blood of patients with cancer. However, many of the presumed circulating cancer cells have been determined to be megakaryocytes. In addition, the possibility that "metastases" could arise from the release of oncogenic viruses from the primary lesion requires further evaluation.

CYTOGENETICS The characteristics of a particular tumor cell are, in general, permanent and stable and are inherited by descendants of that tumor cell. These characteristics may be explained best by structural alterations of the DNA in genes or chromosomes. These genetic structural changes may range from single gene mutations to gross chromosomal changes. These chromosomal changes may involve loss or gain of chromosomes, translocation of chromosomes, and changes in ploidy. Although the DNA and chromosomes of tumor cells may be clearly different from those of normal cells, the changes are not uniform from tumor to tumor, and no abnormality in the genetic material may be detectable in a substantial number of human tumors. Various techniques are available to analyze the DNA of normal and tumor cells, including the methods of nucleic acid hybridization. This technique allows comparison of analogous nucleotide chains from different cells by analyzing the product of each chain when allowed to interact. With use of radioactive RNA or DNA, comparable sequences of nucleotide chains from different cells can be quantified. Reverse transcriptase (RNA-directed DNA polymerase) has been used to synthesize isotope-labeled DNAs. These DNA templates have been used to show homologies between murine leukemia virus and human leukemias and sarcomas, supporting the hypothesis of a viral etiology of human leukemia.

The most widely used technique for gross examination of genetic material is the examination of metaphase chromosomes. A tumor may be characterized by its "modal" karyotype, i.e., the number of chromosomes and the morphologic pattern of the largest percentage of cells. Major advances in cytogenetics have resulted from development of techniques to demonstrate chromosome banding, utilizing fluorescent acridine dyes, or by treatment of chromosomes by heat, alkali, or enzymes prior to staining. This permits accurate identification of individual chromosomes and regions within the chromosome, increasing the sensitivity of chromosome examination.

Only a few neoplastic diseases in humans are associated with a specific and characteristic chromosome abnormality; these include chronic myelogenous leukemia (CML), acute promyelocytic leukemia (APL), some lymphoproliferative disorders, and meningioma. In about 85 percent of the patients with CML, the material comprising approximately half of the long arm of a G22 chromosome is translocated to the end of a C9 chromosome. This abnormality (Philadelphia chromosome, Ph¹) involves all three hematopoietic cell lines, and has been interpreted as an acquired somatic cell mutation in the bone marrow, with preferential survival and proliferation of this clone. In APL, the material from the distal part of the long arm of an E17 chromosome is translocated to the end of a D15 chromosome. This abnormality is present in approximately two-thirds of the patients with APL. In the lymphoproliferative disorders, an 8/14 translocation has been associated with most Burkitt's lymphomas and a marker 14q + has been found in the tumors of many patients with multiple myeloma, Hodgkin's disease, and non-Hodgkin's lymphomas. The chromosome abnormality associated with meningioma is hypodiploid, in contrast to the examples cited above, and frequently involves the deletion of chromosome G22.

Approximately 50 percent of patients with acute leukemia have detectable cytogenetic abnormalities. Although the abnormalities are not necessarily uniform, they are probably nonrandom. For any given patient they tend to remain characteristic and recur during a clinical relapse. Leukemias induced by radiation, drugs, or both, such as occur in some patients with treated Hodgkin's disease, have a much higher percentage of chromosomal abnormalities. The use of chromosome-banding techniques may result in grouping of patients with common etiologies or prognoses. Cytogenetic studies also may occasionally be useful in the diagnosis of "preleukemia" when abnormal karyotypes are present.

For technical reasons, only a limited number of chromosome studies have been performed in solid tumors. Cytogenetic abnormalities are frequent and major in solid tumors such as melanoma, lung cancer, and colon cancer. Significant aneuploidy is present in almost all tumors. In melanoma the variation from cell to cell is substantial and has been interpreted as evidence for multiple cell lines, cytogenetic instability, and rapid clonal evolution toward more malignant behavior.

ETIOLOGY Although the etiology of cancer in humans cannot yet be explained at the molecular level, it is clear that genetic composition of the host is important in cancer induction. Related immunologic factors may predispose the host to a putative carcinogen. There is some evidence that viruses may play a role in the neoplastic process. In addition, both environmental and therapeutic agents have been identified as carcinogens.

Genetic factors The fact that not all humans exposed to the same dose of carcinogens develop cancer indicates that host factors play an important role in the cancer-inducing process. Certain familial and genetic disorders may increase the risk of cancer. These may be divided into those that have a well-defined hereditary pattern with a high frequency in family members, such as retinoblastoma, and those familial and genetic disorders having an increased risk, such as multiple polyposis of the colon or breast cancer. In addition, there is a group of familial disorders associated with cytogenetic abnormalities that have an increased risk of cancer, such as Bloom's syndrome, Fanconi's anemia, or the immunologic deficiency states.

Only a small proportion of cancers is inherited in a mendelian fashion, which indicates single-gene transmission. Table 323-1 lists some cancers that occur as an inherited trait (hereditary neoplasms) or as a complication of inherited precursor lesions that are clinically recognizable (preneoplastic states).

TABLE 323-1
Hereditary cancer syndromes in adults

I Hereditary neoplasms
  A Nevoid basal-cell carcinoma syndrome
  B Trichoepithelioma
  C Multiple endocrine adenomatosis
  D Chemodectomas
  E Polyposis coli
  F Gardner's syndrome
II Preneoplastic states
  A Hamartomatous syndromes
    1 Neurofibromatosis
    2 Tuberous sclerosis
    3 Von Hippel-Lindau syndrome
    4 Multiple exostosis
    5 Peutz-Jeghers syndrome
  B Genodermatoses
    1 Albinism
    2 Werner's syndrome
    3 Polydysplastic epidermolysis bullosa
  C Chromosome breakage disorders
    1 Bloom's syndrome
    2 Fanconi's syndrome
    3 Ataxia-telangiectasia
  D Immune deficiency syndromes
    1 Late-onset immunologic deficiency

SOURCE: *JF Froumeni, in Holland and Frei.*

veloping the disease than women without such a family history. Racial factors are also of importance. For example, blacks and other ethnic groups with deeply pigmented skin are protected from melanoma and other skin cancers induced by exposure to sunlight.

Viruses Viruses can cause neoplasia in almost every mammal, as well as in fish, frogs, and other species. Generally, tumor viruses contain either double-stranded DNA or single-stranded RNA with an icosahedral capsid which may or may not be surrounded by a lipid envelope. So called "C-type" RNA viruses usually produce leukemia or sarcomas; these viruses and the transformed cells usually contain RNA reverse transcriptase activity; this RNA-directed DNA polymerase may be necessary for malignant transformation by these viruses. The heteroduplex resulting from transcription of DNA from the single-stranded RNA template is probably replicated by DNA-dependent DNA polymerase to produce a double-stranded DNA molecule that is inserted into the host chromosome by an unknown mechanism. Recently, this enzyme activity has been detected in blast cells of some patients with acute leukemia. Also, a C-type human virus has been successfully isolated from a patient with acute myelogenous leukemia. C-type RNA viruses and related viral proteins have been identified in tissue culture specimens of lymph node material obtained from patients with Hodgkin's disease and histiocytic lymphoma. These findings, together with nucleic acid hybridization studies, are presumptive evidence for a virus etiology in some cases of acute leukemia and lymphoma in humans.

The strongest candidate for a human tumor virus is the Epstein-Barr virus (EBV), a DNA herpesvirus that causes infectious mononucleosis. Seroepidemiologic data as well as detection of the viral DNA in the lymphoma cells by nucleic acid hybridization have provided evidence that EBV is associated with Burkitt's lymphoma and nasopharyngeal carcinoma. Burkitt's lymphoma occurs mainly in children in central Africa and New Guinea, and sporadically elsewhere. Because of this geographic distribution, it is believed that in addition to the virus that may act as a cocarcinogen, other factors, such as immunosuppression due to malaria, may be involved. Genetic factors may play a role in the development of nasopharyngeal carcinoma, found in the Far East, since Chinese who have migrated to the United States continue to have a high incidence of this disease.

Herpes simplex virus (HSV2) has been associated with cancer of the cervix by the demonstration of HSV2 genetic information, as well as HSV-specific antigens in tumor cells.

Occupational and environmental carcinogens In eliciting the occupational history and history of exposure to drugs, as well as chemical agents in the home, various substances which constitute a potential carcinogenic hazard will come to light. The first demonstration of an environmental carcinogen was by Potts, who linked the increased incidence of scrotal cancer in chimney sweeps to exposure to soot. Since that time an ever-increasing number of occupational and environmental carcinogens have been reported (Table 323-2). It has been estimated that up to 70 to 80 percent of cancers in humans are related to chemical and environmental factors. As many as 40 percent of all cancers are related directly or in part to cigarette smoking. There is often a long latent period between exposure to a chemical carcinogen and the development of neoplasia, and unless unusual cancers are produced, the possible association between a chemical exposure and the cancer may not be appreciated. This latent period also makes difficult any screening

Polyposis coli consists of numerous adenomatous polyps of the colon and rectum and occurs in about 1 per 8000 live births. Carcinoma develops in virtually all cases with advancing age and is found at the time of initial diagnosis of the polyps in about 40 percent of patients. A penetrance of about 80 percent is reported in patients with polyps detected any time after the age of 10 years.

Neurofibromatosis (von Recklinghausen's disease), which occurs in about 1 per 3000 live births, is characterized by café au lait spots and multiple neurofibromas. The neurofibromas show sarcomatous degeneration in about 10 percent of patients; in addition, there is an increased risk of meningioma, acoustic neuroma, pheochromocytoma, and gliomas of the brain or optic nerve.

In the *Peutz-Jeghers syndrome,* gastrointestinal polyps are signaled by the presence of melanin spots in the buccal mucosa, lips, and digits. Most of the polyps are in the small intestine and very rarely show malignant degeneration. Ovarian neoplasms, however, occur in about 5 percent of women and may be the initial lead to the syndrome.

Bloom's syndrome is a rare autosomal recessive condition with features of dwarfism, characteristic facies, and a photosensitive telangiectatic erythema on the face. In about one out of eight reported cases acute leukemia has developed.

The apparent association between an inherited abnormality and neoplasia also is found in *ataxia-telangiectasia,* an autosomal recessive trait in which telangiectatic lesions appear in the bulbar conjunctiva and in which there is progressive cerebellar ataxia with spinocerebellar atrophy. Cellular immunity is decreased, and abnormal levels of serum immunoglobulin are often present. The individuals who survive the recurrent sinopulmonary infections into adolescence or their twenties often develop lymphoma.

The mechanism by which the hereditary conditions lead to cancer or leukemia is not clear. However, there are some clues to possible pathogenetic mechanisms. Among the genodermatoses, which generally show an autosomal recessive pattern, is xeroderma pigmentosa. In this condition, it has been shown that skin fibroblasts fail to repair DNA damage induced by ultraviolet light. In individuals with Bloom's syndrome, cultured fibroblasts from these patients have increased sensitivity to transformation by oncogenic viruses.

The precise mechanisms of familial cancer are unknown, but it has been shown that daughters of women who develop breast cancer have a three to five times greater chance of de-program in animals to determine whether a given chemical or substance is likely to be carcinogenic. Leads to the presence of environmental carcinogens can be provided by careful monitoring of the incidence of various types of cancer in different populations over a period of time. There is, however, a major disparity in susceptibility to cancer from one species to another and among different populations exposed to the same carcinogen. This may be explained in part by hereditary differences in enzyme levels necessary to process chemicals to be *active* carcinogens and in levels of degrading enzymes necessary to deactivate the carcinogens. For example, it has been suggested, but not proved, that elevated levels of aryl hydrocarbon hydroxylase levels predispose smokers to lung cancer.

Mapping of cancer mortality by county within the United States has revealed patterns of etiologic significance. For example, bladder cancer in males is probably related to industrial contaminants found in areas of high industrialization and around oil-processing areas. Skin cancer is associated with residence in the "sun belt." Epidemiologic studies on a worldwide scale have revealed geographic areas where certain cancers predominate, and attempts to identify the causal agent are in progress. The high prevalence of bladder cancer in Egypt is related to schistosomiasis haematobia (bilharziasis) and apparently its attendant chronic bacterial infection; the hepatomas of Africa are related to exposure to aflatoxins. Other geographic "epidemic" areas have been identified, but the clues to the etiologic agent(s) involved are not clear: cancer of esophagus around the Caspian Sea, cancer of nasopharynx in China, cancer of stomach in Japan. It has been shown that Japanese migrating to Hawaii or to the continental United States have a decreasing risk of cancer of the stomach, emphasizing the importance of environmental factors.

Other clues regarding etiologic factors predisposing to cancer come from changes in incidence of particular cancers with time. For example, the marked decrease in the prevalence of cancer of the stomach in the United States is attributed to the introduction of refrigeration, with decrease in nitrites formed from nitrate food preservatives; in contrast, the increase in cancer of the colon is attributed to a high-fat, low-fiber diet. The role of bile salts as cocarcinogens is under investigation.

Screening suspect chemicals in animal models is time-consuming and expensive. A number of investigators have proposed in vitro bacterial tests to detect mutagenicity, which accurately predicts carcinogenicity in test animals and humans. Among these tests, the salmonella mutagenicity test to identify chemical carcinogens and mutagens is the most promising. The unique feature of the test is the use of liver microsomes to activate the potential carcinogenic-mutagenic substance. The test detects these chemicals by means of their ability to damage DNA and cause mutations in bacteria. It is about 90 percent accurate in detecting proved carcinogens or mutagens and therefore a very useful tool for screening for potential carcinogens.

More than 15 carcinogens, including hydrocarbons and aromatic amines, have been isolated from tobacco smoke. The incidence of not only lung cancer but also of head and neck, esophageal, and bladder cancers is increased in smokers. In addition, asbestos, uranium, and alcohol exposure act synergistically to increase the risk.

The occurrence of lung cancer as a consequence of occupational exposure to asbestos has been confirmed. Approximately 20 percent of all the deaths of asbestos workers have been attributed to lung cancer. This represents a sevenfold increase in incidence of this neoplasm after 20 years from the time of the first exposure. In addition, approximately 7 percent of the deaths of asbestos workers are caused by either pleural or peritoneal mesothelioma, a risk that is 100 to 1000 times that which might be expected in the general population. A threefold increase in gastrointestinal cancer has been reported for the same workers. With few exceptions, a serious risk begins after 20 years from onset of first exposure and continues from that point on.

Exposure to heavy metals such as arsenic, cadmium, chromium, and nickel has been associated with an increased occurrence of certain cancers. An excess incidence of skin cancer has been observed among patients who have been treated with arsenicals and among workers exposed to this compound, and among persons exposed excessively to arsenic in drinking water. Arsenic also appears to be a lung carcinogen with rate ratios of approximately 7, 5, and 2.5 for heavy, medium, and light exposure. The latent time for arsenic-induced lung cancer is long, ranging from 30 to 35 years for heavy exposure to 40 to 45 years for light exposure. Arsenic may also cause liver cancer.

Occupational exposure to cadmium has resulted in an increased incidence of prostatic carcinoma. The excess was twofold for those whose exposure had commenced less than 30 years earlier and threefold for those with a longer interval. Recently, a significant association of renal cancer with exposure to cadmium has been found.

Chromium exposure has been connected with excess mortality from cancers of the respiratory tract, especially with lung cancers and cancers of the nasal cavities. The rate ratios have been reported as high as 30- to 40-fold over the expected, while the mean latent period in various studies has ranged from 10 to 20 years. Of the lung cancers reported, at least one-half were anaplastic or undifferentiated; only 10 percent were adenocarcinomas.

An excess of both lung cancer and cancer of the nasal sinuses has been found among nickel refinery workers; rate ratios of about tenfold exist for lung cancer, while they are 100-fold or greater for the nasal sinuses. The mean latent period for lung cancer varies between 13 and 30 years, but may be a few years shorter for nasal cancer. The histology of the tumor is usually epidermoid, although 12 to 30 percent can be anaplastic. Although the exact identity of the carcinogenic agents in nickel refineries is still unknown, most cancers occur among employees working in the early stages of nickel refining. It has been suggested there may be a synergistic effect between nickel exposure and cigarette smoking.

Hundreds of chemicals used in industry, on farms, in the home, and in foods as additives or preservatives have been implicated as carcinogens. Some of these are listed in Table 323-2. One example of such a toxic substance is vinyl chloride. This industrial product has been shown to be carcinogenic in both experimental animals and humans. Vinyl chloride administered by inhalation has been found to produce angiosarcomas of the liver in rats at concentrations as low as 25 parts

TABLE 323-2
Occupational and environmental carcinogens

Carcinogen	Associated neoplasm
Cigarette smoke	Lung, upper respiratory tract, and other cancers
Asbestos	Mesothelioma, lung
Arsenic	Skin, lung
Cadmium	Prostate, kidney
Chromium	Lung
Nickel	Lung, nasal sinuses
Uranium	Lung
Aflotoxin	Liver
Nitrites	Stomach
Chloramethyl ethers	Lung
Isopropyl oil	Nasal sinuses
Naphthalene dyes (aniline dyes)	Bladder
Vinyl chloride	Liver hemangiosarcoma
Benzene	Acute myelogenous leukemia
Schistosomiasis haematobia	Bladder

per million. Besides liver angiosarcomas in workers in the vinyl chloride–polyvinyl chloride industry, there also seems to be a high incidence of brain tumors, large-cell carcinomas of the lung, lymphomas, and leukemia.

In view of the large number of potential cancer-causing agents, physicians must be prepared to counsel patients regarding the carcinogenic potential of various chemicals and be aware of the risk-benefit ratio of each of these substances. No doubt food additives which prevent botulism and have a small risk of causing cancer must be dealt with differently from cigarette smoking, which confers a major risk upon the user.

Drugs and radiational agents as carcinogens In addition to occupational and environmental carcinogens listed in Table 323-2, radiation in any form and various drugs have been unequivocally shown to be associated with the induction of cancer. The survivors of Hiroshima and Nagasaki showed an increased incidence of acute and chronic granulocytic leukemia that reached a peak approximately 7 years after the exposure. Radiation therapy for enlarged tonsils and thymus and for ankylosing spondylitis has also led to an increased incidence of acute leukemia, after a similar latent period. These studies show a dose-response relationship until a plateau is reached, and increased doses do not increase the incidence. Why only a small percentage of the population exposed will develop acute leukemia is not known. The risk may be a function of genetic makeup as well as age. Infants and pregnant women are at greatest risk to develop radiation-induced neoplasia. An acceptable safe dose of radiation has not yet been determined with certainty. It has also been shown that in addition to an increased risk of leukemia, patients previously treated with radiation therapy for an enlarged thymus or tonsils have a marked increased risk of developing thyroid carcinoma.

An increase in the frequency of breast cancer in women undergoing repeated x-ray or fluoroscopy examinations of the chest in follow-up of their tuberculosis or as part of a mammography screening program has been shown with a dose as low as 17 rads.

Table 323-3 is a partial list of cancers related to radioisotope and drug exposure in humans. Drugs that are capable of interacting with DNA (alkylating agents) as well as immunosuppressive agents and hormones all have the potential for causing neoplasms in humans. The use of alkylating agents in therapeutic doses and for a sufficiently long time, either alone or in combination with other drugs and/or radiotherapy, has been associated with an increased incidence of acute myelogenous leukemia or its variants in patients with Hodgkin's disease, non-Hodgkin's lymphomas, multiple myeloma, and ovarian cancer. Since these secondary leukemias are relatively refractory to induction of remission with combination chemotherapy, it is fortunate that the incidence of leukemia appears to be relatively low (1 to 5 percent).

The development of acute leukemia during the course of Hodgkin's disease is probably related to either the immunosuppressive or carcinogenic effects of radiation therapy or a combination of the two. In a study of 81 patients with both acute myelocytic leukemia and Hodgkin's disease, these diseases occurred simultaneously in only three cases. Of the remaining 79 patients, 76 had received radiation therapy for Hodgkin's disease, and acute myelocytic leukemia developed 1 to 19 years later, with a mean interval of 6.5 years. Thirty-four of the 76 patients had also received chemotherapy; only 3 had received chemotherapy alone. The possibility that acute leukemia is a part of the natural history of Hodgkin's disease and is occurring with greater frequency because of improved survival in Hodgkin's disease due to aggressive radiation and drug therapy warrants consideration. Radiation therapy and antineoplastic drugs should be used with caution or not at all in nonneoplastic disorders which are not life-threatening.

Hormones While the relationship of hormone administration in the etiology of breast cancer is well established in mice, such a causal connection has not been demonstrated in women. There appears to be epidemiologic evidence that nulliparous women have a higher incidence of breast cancer than women who have had children. The risk is also increased threefold for women whose mothers and other close relatives have had breast cancer. The role of synthetic hormones in increasing the risk of breast cancer is under investigation, but so far no correlation has been demonstrated. Low doses of hormones used in birth control pills do not appear to cause breast cancer. Prenatal exposure to synthetic estrogens has been associated with vaginal adenosis and vaginal and cervical (clear-cell) adenocarcinomas. It is important to identify the daughters of women who received diethylstilbestrol (DES) during pregnancy. The occurrence of vaginal adenocarcinomas in the offspring of mothers treated with DES during pregnancy demonstrates the problem of detecting carcinogenicity of chemicals. This particular relationship was detected because the neoplasm was unusual, despite the low incidence of tumors. Postnatal exposure to estrogens has led to a fivefold risk for endometrial carcinoma. Estrogens as prescribed in birth control pills also cause hepatic adenomas, which have a tendency to bleed, as well as liver cancers. The relationship of hormones to prostatic cancer is even less clear. It is known that androgenic-anabolic steroids predispose both to benign liver tumors and to hepatocellular carcinoma.

IMMUNOLOGIC FACTORS Cancers may be associated with, or lead to, an altered host immune response; however, the cause-and-effect relationship remains to be determined. The effect can be direct, resulting from replacement of normal by malignant lymphocytes, as in chronic lymphocytic leukemia (CLL); indirect, secondary to treatment required for control of

TABLE 323-3
Cancers related to drug exposures in humans

Drug	Cancer
Radioisotopes:	
Phosphorus (^{32}P)	Acute leukemia
Radium, mesothorium	Osteosarcoma and sinus carcinoma
Thorotrast	Hemangioendothelioma of liver
Immunosuppressive agents (for renal transplantation):	
Antilymphocyte serum	
Antimetabolites	Reticulum-cell sarcoma, epithelial malignancies of skin and viscera
Alkylating agents	
Corticosteroids	
Cytotoxic drugs:	
Chlornaphazine	
Phenylalanine mustard	Bladder cancer
Cyclophosphamide	Acute myelogenous leukemia
Hormones:	
Synthetic estrogens:	
Prenatal	Vaginal and cervical adenocarcinoma (clear-cell type)
Postnatal	Endometrial carcinoma (adenosquamous type)
Androgenic-anabolic steroids	Hepatocellular carcinoma
Others:	
Arsenic	Skin cancer
Phenacetin-containing drugs	Renal pelvis carcinoma
Coal tar ointments	Skin cancer
? Diphenylhydantoin	Lymphoma
? Chloramphenicol	Leukemia
? Amphetamines	Hodgkin's disease

SOURCE: *After R Hoover, JF Froumeni, J Clin Pharmacol 15:16, 1975.*

the primary tumor; or an associated effect, as exemplified by situations in which blocking factors can be demonstrated.

Many cancer patients show some resistance to the progress of their disease. Spontaneous regression occasionally occurs in neuroblastoma, hypernephroma, choriocarcinoma, and malignant melanoma. The long-term dormancy of multiple metastases seen after removal of the primary mass can be explained best by host defense mechanisms. Host defenses are geared to eliminate any tissue recognized as "nonself," in much the same way as an allograft is rejected. Presumably malignant tumors can develop in otherwise healthy hosts only if there has been a breakdown of the host's surveillance mechanism. The ability to mount humoral or cell-mediated immune response against a neoplasm depends on both the host's genetic material and other factors, such as previous exposure to radiotherapy or immunosuppressive drugs.

An increased incidence of malignancy associated with long-term administration of immunosuppressive drugs has been noted in patients with renal transplants. Of 432 recipients who were followed for up to 11 years, 24 developed neoplasms; this incidence of 5.6 percent is 100 times that observed in the general population when matched for age. In another study of 184 organ homograft recipients who developed cancers de novo, 60 percent were under 40 years of age. Both the incidence of lymphomas and of primary central nervous system lymphomas was greatly increased in such patients.

The host immune response can be blunted by blocking factors present in the host's serum. These blocking factors can decrease the cytotoxic effect of the host's immune lymphocytes. They slowly disappear from the serum if the tumor is removed surgically. The precise component of serum that is responsible for the blocking effect on cell-mediated antitumor immunity is not known, but it may be a noncomplement-fixing antitumor antibody, which, though capable of binding to tumor cell surfaces, is capable of inducing tumor cell lysis.

AGE SPECIFICITY Patients of different ages are at risk for different types of cancer. Fifty percent of the cases of acute lymphocytic leukemia occur in patients under 7 years, whereas only 10 percent of patients with acute myelomonocytic leukemia are under 20 years of age. Chronic lymphocytic leukemia is a disease of middle and old age and is practically unknown in childhood; above the age of 60 it is the most common type of leukemia. Solid tumors demonstrate similar differences. Ewing's sarcoma is a highly anaplastic tumor in bone; 90 percent of patients are under 30 and 70 percent under 20 years of age. Although colon cancer may occur in childhood, the incidence is low until age 40, when it rises rapidly; the peak frequency occurs in the sixth decade.

SEX PREDILECTION Knowledge of the predilection of various malignancies for one of the sexes is also important. Although breast cancer does occur in males, its frequency is about 1 percent of that in females. Lung cancer is 4½ times more common in men than in women, whereas the incidence of rectocolonic cancer is approximately equal in men and women. Differences in sex predilection may be due to hormonal factors, differences in exposure to carcinogens, and other factors.

ROLE OF THE PHYSICIAN IN DETECTION OF CANCER

EARLY DETECTION Early detection and prompt treatment are directly responsible for cure or longer survival in many types of cancer. To detect cancer at an early stage, the physician must be aware of certain inherited conditions and envi-

ronmental factors which predispose to malignancy and must undertake a thorough, systematic clinical evaluation. The partnership of the patient is required if this goal is to be achieved. The patient's awareness of the early signs of malignancy as well as his or her acceptance of diagnostic and therapeutic procedures is essential. The following examples illustrate the usefulness of early detection. For cancer of the cervix, early detection by means of the Papanicolaou test of cervical cytology is responsible for the decrease in the incidence of invasive cancer and has resulted in a 50 percent reduction in mortality. For cancer of the lung, a prospective, controlled project of screening a high-risk group of male, heavy smokers, more than 45 years old with serial sputum cytology and chest roentgenograms has been carried out. Approximately 60 percent of tumors found in persons receiving surveillance examination every 4 months were resectable for cure compared with 25 percent of tumors detected in controls.

The "seven warning signals" of early cancer in special sites, which include skin, breast, larynx, lung, and the gastrointestinal tract, are designed to educate people to seek medical help early (Table 323-4). Patients may participate actively in the detection and diagnosis of their cancer. For example, a self-examination of the breast has resulted in the detection of an increased number of malignant lesions at a time when curative surgery is feasible. Since more than 90 percent of the 70,000 new cases of breast cancer each year are discovered by the patient, education on thorough, frequent self-examination is a necessity.

In order to identify individuals who are at high risk for cancer and who should participate in screening programs, risk profiles for each site should be constructed for each patient, based on genetic, family, occupational, and social history.

TAKING THE HISTORY A patient's history is important when the physician tries to pinpoint the possible presence of malignant disease; symptoms are frequently nonspecific. For example, fever, weight loss, and night sweats are evidence of systemic disease which can be indicative of a malignant tumor as well as an infectious process. Taking an orderly history with a thorough review of systems is the most revealing and rewarding approach. A persistent cough with or without hemoptysis requires evaluation of the tracheobronchial tree. Recent onset of hoarseness requires evaluation of a lesion along the course of the recurrent laryngeal nerve or of the vocal cords directly. Hematemesis, jaundice, melena, increasing constipation, and/or abdominal pain demand an evaluation of the gastrointestinal tract for possible malignant disease. Painless, recurrent hematuria suggests that the need for careful evaluation of the entire urinary tract. Specific points in the history which are highly suggestive of possible malignancy include the presence of an enlarging, firm, fixed mass easily palpated by the patient, such as a mass in the breast or in a lymph node; the development of a thyroid nodule; and the sudden onset of intestinal obstruction in a previously asymptomatic patient above 50 years of age. A history of petechiae, ecchymoses, or uncontrolled bleeding and persistent infections should suggest possible replacement of normal bone marrow elements by malignant cells.

TABLE 323-4
Seven warning signals of early cancer

1 Change in bowel or bladder habits
2 A sore that does not heal
3 Unusual bleeding or discharge
4 Thickening or lump in breast or elsewhere
5 Indigestion or difficulty in swallowing
6 Obvious change in wart or mole
7 Nagging cough or hoarseness

SOURCE: *American Cancer Society.*

PHYSICAL EXAMINATION In conducting the physical examination, the physician should be attentive to abnormalities which indicate neoplastic disease in each organ system. Certain physical findings are highly suggestive of malignant disease. The skin can provide clues to the presence of internal cancer. A subcutaneous or dermal metastatic nodule may be the first indication of cancer arising from such organs as the breast, gastrointestinal tract, lung, ovary, or uterus. Pulsatile nodules may be metastatic foci from a hypernephroma or a cancer of the thyroid gland. Erythema multiforme, dermatomyositis, superficial migratory thrombophlebitis, necrotizing vasculitis, and bullous states have been associated with internal malignancies. The symmetric brownish-black hyperpigmentation of "malignant" acanthosis nigricans is found predominantly in the body folds; it is characterized by rapidly extending skin involvement and by its association with malignant neoplasms. Herpes zoster and unusual fungal diseases may be related to the impaired immunity in cancer patients. An ulcerated lesion along the tongue or a unilateral enlargement of a tonsil are suggestive of a primary oropharyngeal tumor; inspection and careful palpation of the oropharyngeal cavity is an important part of the physical examination. Swelling of the neck, face, and upper extremities, especially after a night in the recumbent position, in association with dilated veins in the upper half of the body and with downward venous flow, is typical of obstruction of the superior vena cava, which occurs as a presenting symptom in approximately 4 percent of all patients with lung cancer. The findings of Horner's syndrome—ptosis, miosis, and decreased sweating of the face on the affected side—indicate stellate ganglion involvement and are frequent concomitants of superior sulcus tumors of the lung. A hard, circumscribed mass, which does not move freely in the breast and is clearly felt with the flat surface of the fingers, is indicative of cancer. When fixation to skin, nipple retraction, skin edema, or deep fixation is present, the lesion is almost certainly malignant. A firm, enlarged lymph node in the left supraclavicular region (Virchow's node) suggests an abdominal malignancy which has spread along the thoracic duct. The presence of a palpable, firm mass in the umbilicus suggests seeding of the peritoneal cavity with metastatic tumor. Any abdominal mass or enlargement of the liver or spleen requires further evaluation for the presence of malignant disease. An enlarged spleen, if it is a result of a malignancy, is usually due to a primary lymphoid or myeloid process because metastatic carcinoma to the spleen is rare; it occurs, however, in malignant melanoma. Unilateral leg or scrotal edema suggests an obstruction to the flow of lymph. Enlargement of any lymph node requires a careful evaluation; the presence of enlarged femoral lymph nodes, however, should be considered indicative of a malignant process unless proved otherwise. An ulcerating nodule of the anus can represent squamous-cell carcinoma, whereas a broad, irregular luminal mass noted on digital rectal examination indicates the presence of adenocarcinoma of the rectum. The digital rectal examination may also reveal a firm nodule in the prostate, which requires needle or open biopsy to confirm or disprove carcinoma. A hard, indurated mass confined to the testes suggests malignancy after the possibility of epididymitis has been ruled out by lack of response to appropriate antibiotic therapy.

Pelvic examination of women can reveal an adnexal mass. In premenopausal women, if such a mass is less than 6 cm in diameter, it is usually a physiologic cyst rather than a neoplasm. Any adnexal mass in the postmenopausal patient must be investigated further. Vaginal tumors vary from ulcerated lesions of small or extensive size, often firm in consistency, to papillary or nodular excrescences.

The examples cited above serve only as a guide to the most obvious physical findings which suggest the presence of a malignancy.

DIAGNOSIS OF CANCER

Regardless of the difficulty of the procedures involved, histologic proof of malignancy must be obtained before the risks involved in further staging and in therapy of malignant disease are taken. The only exception to this rule might be in the diagnosis of gliomas in critical areas of the brain. Sometimes this proof is easy to obtain, especially when there is a subcutaneous nodule that indicates the presence of metastatic carcinoma or an enlarged lymph node that suggests lymphoma. At other times, when there is a peripheral lesion in the lung which cannot be sampled by transbronchial biopsy, the patient might have to undergo thoracotomy with resection so that the diagnosis of cancer can be established. For most malignant tumors, the slide which proves the presence of cancer will also allow histologic classification of the tumor. An experienced pathologist is an essential member of the oncology team, and if there is any question, the histologic material should be submitted to a tumor pathology consulting panel.

The greater the lack of differentiation of the malignant tissue, the easier the diagnosis of malignancy; however, the tissue of origin may be more difficult to ascertain in poorly differentiated and anaplastic tumors. The degree of differentiation of a tumor, ranging from poorly to well differentiated, often provides a clue to prognosis and a guide to treatment; the less differentiated the tumor, the more aggressive its behavior and the poorer the prognosis. General features of the malignant cell under the microscope include a large and irregular nucleus, with enlarged nucleoli, that may be increased in number. Polyploidy is common, and there is an increase in mitotic figures, especially in rapidly growing tumors, with abnormal mitosis and macronucleated cells. The cytoplasm may be scanty, with an increase in basophilia due to increased RNA content. Obviously, these are general features that may be found in many, but not all, malignant cells.

HISTOPATHOLOGIC CLASSIFICATION A histopathologic classification should be reproducible in the hands of the same person, should be agreed upon and reproducible by different experts, should allow for a common terminology, and should correlate the histopathology with the clinical stage and the prognosis. Such a system exists in Hodgkin's disease, where the lymphocyte-predominant and the nodular sclerosing types of histology have a more favorable prognosis than the mixed-cell type, which in turn is more favorable than the lymphocyte-depleted type. Equally important is the architecture, or the way in which the cells are arranged in the biopsy specimen. In malignant lymphoma, the "nodular" pattern has been shown to convey a more favorable prognosis than the "diffuse" replacement of the normal architecture. The presence or absence of vascular or lymphatic invasion within the particular cytologic and architectural picture is also important.

Besides using routine hematoxylin and eosin-stained sections for diagnosis, other methods for diagnosis and classification should be utilized. One of these is cytochemistry. For example, the peroxidase and Sudan black cytochemical stains are positive in acute myelomonocytic leukemia and negative in acute lymphocytic leukemia and help to differentiate these two forms. One enzyme, tartrate-resistant acid phosphatase, has been used specifically to define "hairy" cell leukemia. This type of leukemia differs significantly from other types because aggressive chemotherapy is not indicated and may even be harmful. Transmission electron microscopy has been helpful in differentiating some of the tumors that appear identical by light microscopy. Desmosomes found in thin sections are consistent with carcinoma; myofibrils can be seen in a rhabdomyosarcoma; and intercellular lumens with microvilli can be seen in some poorly differentiated adenocarcinomas; premelanosomes can be found in melanoma cells, and secretory granules can be visualized in carcinomas. Functional methods have been used for the subclassification of certain types of malignancy. Surface immunoglobulins have been found in most cases of chronic lymphocytic leukemia, suggesting that this is a B-cell disease. In acute lymphocytic leukemia, E rosettes can be demonstrated in approximately 25 percent of the cases, suggesting that the malignant cells are of T-cell derivation; in the other 75 percent, neither surface immunoglobulins nor E rosettes can be demonstrated and the cells are called null cells.

TISSUE INVASION Evidence of invasion of normal tissues, especially lymphatic channels, lymph nodes, and blood vessels, and extension of tumors through natural barriers such as the capsule of a lymph node, is used in diagnosing malignancy, and the extent of this invasion is part of some histologic staging systems (e.g., in carcinoma of the colon). The factors that allow neoplastic cells to invade tissues are not well understood. Certain experimental tumors produce proteolytic enzymes or collagenases that may allow tumor cells to invade tissues. Soft tissues are usually easily invaded, while tissues such as cartilage, fascia, and ligaments are usually resistant to tumor invasion.

METASTASIS An important characteristic of certain neoplastic cells is their ability to spread to distant sites, that is, to metastasize. Various human cancers differ appreciably, not only in their propensity to metastasize, but also in the location of the metastasis. Knowledge of the pattern of metastatic spread may provide clinical clues to the origin of the primary tumor. Carcinomas are more apt to spread by lymphatic invasion, initially to regional lymph nodes. For example, in breast cancer the degree of spread to the regional lymph nodes is determined at surgery and may provide important prognostic information to help the clinician plan additional therapy. Whether the regional lymph nodes provide immunologic and perhaps mechanical barriers to tumor spread has been debated. Often nodes adjacent to a tumor may not contain tumor but show a "hyperplastic reaction," suggesting a host response to the tumor or its products.

Sarcomas characteristically spread via the bloodstream, and distant metastases, to the lungs from osteogenic sarcoma, are common. Venous invasion is more common than arterial invasion, perhaps due to the elasticity of the arterial wall. Venous invasion characteristically consists of clumps of tumor cells that adhere to the vascular endothelium of the postcapillary venule. Fibrin formation is initiated and is followed by multiplication and invasion through the endothelium. Several studies indicate that anticoagulants may decrease metastasis in experimental tumors, perhaps by decreasing endothelial "stickiness." In humans, their value in preventing metastasis has not been established.

Two other properties of tumor cells probably also contribute to metastatic spread: (1) decreased adhesiveness of tumor cells to each other, with the resultant ability of individual tumor cells or clumps to break off and enter the lymphatics or the bloodstream and to lodge in other tissues, and (2) the elaboration of tissue angiogenesis factor (TAF). The elaboration of TAF, a macromolecule not yet completely characterized, results in local proliferation of blood vessels and permits the necessary "feeding" of the growing tumor cell mass. In fact, the intense vascularity that may result is responsible for the characteristic "tumor blush" of certain tumors when the

arterial supply is examined radiographically after administration of contrast media.

TUMOR AS A GROWTH, TUMOR AS A "FACTORY" The neoplastic lesion can be evaluated in two conceptual ways: as a growth and as a "factory." As a growth, the lesion has local and metastatic manifestations. The site of origin of the neoplastic growth also has important clinical implications, because local manifestations as well as the propensity for and the route of spread are frequently organ-related. In many cases, these manifestations are clues to the diagnosis as well as indications for appropriate therapeutic intervention. As a factory, the tumor may elaborate products normally associated with the tissue of origin, but in an increased amount, or it may produce substances normally not synthesized by the tissue of origin.

Tumor within an organ system The organ within which a tumor arises is of great importance. The histologic characteristics of different tumors within a single organ give clues to the developing clinical pattern, and this pattern often determines its management. Cancer of the lung provides an apt example.

There are four types of histology in lung cancer, each of which has a different clinical characteristic. Adenocarcinoma is frequently found as a peripheral nodule and metastasizes early. Squamous-cell carcinoma and large-cell undifferentiated carcinoma are usually perihilar and at first spread by local extension. In marked contrast to these three types is oat-cell carcinoma, which shows evidence of extrathoracic involvement at presentation in over 85 percent of the cases. Therefore, in most cases, this tumor cannot be cured surgically.

Knowledge of the natural history of the tumor is important for the design of any staging approach. For example, it is important to know that colon and rectal carcinomas usually begin as a mucosal disease, progress through the bowel wall, invade lymph nodes adjacent to the bowel, and subsequently metastasize to the liver. Prostatic carcinoma is locally invasive, but also metastasizes quite early to bone, especially via Batson's plexus. In contrast, cancers of the head and neck are locally and regionally invasive and only rarely lead to distant metastases.

Tumor as a growth The tumor as a single primary growth can cause the following signs or symptoms: mass and pressure, obstruction, perforation, and invasion with replacement. These conditions can be illustrated with examples from several of the major tumor types, such as cancer of the lung, colon, and brain.

As the malignant cells divide within the neoplastic mass, the dimensions of the tumor continue to increase. The first finding of a mass in the chest could come on a routine annual chest x-ray, and the first finding of a colon mass might occur upon abdominal palpation during a routine physical examination. As the size of the mass continues to increase, there is evidence of increased local pressure. In lung cancer, pressure on the adjacent bronchi might result in an intractable cough; in colon cancer, the patient may complain of lower abdominal cramps.

As it grows in the lung or colon, the tumor will begin to encroach on the function of the organ system and produce symptoms of obstruction. Neoplasms of the left colon tend to be more scirrhous and lead to early production of obstructive symptoms in contrast to the larger, fungating, more friable lesions of the right colon, which tend to present with anemia due to bleeding. Obstructive symptoms are also seen with centrally located squamous-cell carcinoma of the lung. As the tumor grows, bronchial obstruction commonly leads to atelectasis and infection distal to the obstruction, with persistent sputum production and abscess formation.

The most dramatic signs of increased pressure in body cavities occur with primary brain tumors in adults. Patients frequently complain of headache and vomiting. Occasionally, papilledema on fundoscopic examination can be appreciated at initial examination. Localizing signs and symptoms as well as changes in the mental status are frequently present when the diagnosis is first made. The rigid skull contains about 1½ liters brain tissue, only 8 to 10 percent of which may be displaced by either venous blood or cerebrospinal fluid. Brain is a thixotropic substance composed of 80 percent water and is not compressible. Therefore, a single small mass may cause profound dysfunction or an increase in intracranial pressure, depending on its location.

Besides the displacement of cerebral tissue by a brain mass, there can be obstruction to the flow of cerebrospinal fluid; the major portion of this fluid is produced by the choroid plexus of the lateral ventricles and passes through the third ventricle and through the aqueduct. A tumor blocking the aqueduct can prevent the flow of the cerebrospinal fluid, result in secondary dilatation of the lateral ventricle, and lead to increased intracranial pressure.

Enlargement of the tumor mass can cause compression or replacement of the normal structures with tissue less suited to the functional stresses. Thus, large-bowel perforation can be associated with a progressive mass lesion.

Invasion and replacement of the organ in which the tumor arises can be a manifestation of the tumor as a primary growth. Approximately 10 percent of resected stomach carcinomas are of the scirrhous form. They may be localized or may involve the entire stomach, producing the classic appearance of "leather bottle" or linitis plastica. Symptoms secondary to total replacement include anorexia, early satiety, weight loss, and occasionally diarrhea. Hepatoma is a primary liver-cell cancer which accounts for slightly less than 1 percent of all cancer deaths. Frequently death ensues from liver failure with no extrahepatic extension of the cancer. Tumor invasion rarely extends to adjacent organs, but frequently involves the portal or hepatic veins, causing thrombosis. Symptoms of osteogenic sarcoma, a primary malignant tumor that probably arises from primitive bone-forming mesenchyme and produces neoplastic osteoid or osseous tissue in its evolution, result from progressive growth of the mass with replacement of the normal trabeculae in one of the long bones. Pain, tenderness, and swelling of either the lower femur or possibly the tibia or humerus are usually present. On x-ray, variable degrees of lytic and sclerotic processes are noted, frequently associated with cortical perforation, subperiostal extension, and new bone formation.

Besides causing signs of obstruction, increased pressure, or organ replacement, a primary growth can locally invade adjacent structures. The superior vena cava syndrome in lung cancer occasionally results from direct tumor invasion of the cava. Eight to ten percent of all patients with bronchogenic carcinoma are hoarse at their initial presentation. This is a manifestation of laryngeal nerve involvement, which causes vocal cord paralysis. Sharp localized chest pain is often due to extension of the tumor to the chest wall. If the lesion is in the upper part of the lung with invasion of the brachial plexus, the Pancoast or superior sulcus syndrome develops. Uterine cervical cancer tends to spread by direct extension into the surrounding tissues, particularly laterally into the cardinal ligaments; metastases occur late, however. The ureters traverse the cardinal ligaments in the paracervical tunnel and lie in the path of lateral spread of cervical cancer. Extension into these areas obstructs the ureters, resulting in hydroureter and hydronephrosis. If this process is not controlled by therapy, uremia ensues.

Cancer can take the form of a disseminated disease. This is most obvious in malignancies of the hematopoietic tissues, in which the bone marrow is frequently replaced by malignant cells. Symptoms of fever and bleeding can usually be corre-

lated with the absence of mature granulocytes and a decrease in platelets, respectively. Bone marrow aspiration in acute myelogenous leukemia frequently reveals no megakaryocyte, granulocyte, or erythroid precursors; the majority of cells are poorly differentiated myeloblasts.

The two major routes by which tumor cells spread and form metastases are vascular and lymphatic. Occasionally, spread occurs along the peritoneal, pleural, or pericardial lining. The most common sites of metastatic disease are the lungs, especially for osteogenic sarcoma and renal carcinoma; the liver, especially for gastric and colon cancers; and the bones, especially for prostate and breast cancers. Because of the frequent recurrence of tumor at sites distant from the primary tumor, without local recurrence, it is generally accepted that malignant cells were present but not detectable in these sites at the time of initial local resection or radiotherapy. Until recently, 70 percent of patients with osteogenic sarcoma had recurrent disease, with extensive pulmonary nodules, within 1 year of complete resection of the primary lesion; death was usually a result of progressive pulmonary involvement and was directly related to the metastatic characteristics of the tumor. This situation has been reversed dramatically with the use of adjuvant chemotherapy. The poor outcome in half the patients with breast cancer is related to the presence of disseminated disease at the time of surgery. The role of adjuvant therapy for osteogenic sarcoma, breast cancer, and a number of other cancers is currently under evaluation.

Disseminated or metastatic tumor can also cause symptoms due to an increasing mass associated with increasing pressure, obstruction, perforation, and invasion with replacement of normal tissue. The manifestations result in loss of function of the affected organ or organs and subsequent death.

Tumor as a factory Some tumors can manufacture an increased amount of a normal tissue product or a product not usually associated with the cells of origin. Studies with highly sensitive techniques such as radioimmunoassay have shown that many kinds of tumors, from both endocrine and nonendocrine tissues, secrete or synthesize peptide hormones and other proteins not usually made by these tissues. In some circumstances the substances are proteins ordinarily synthesized at or

TABLE 323-5
Tumor cell markers

Marker	Tumor
PRODUCED BY DEDIFFERENTIATION	
Carcinoembryonic antigen (CEA)	Gastrointestinal tract, pancreas, breast, lung
Pancreatic oncofetal antigen (POA)	Pancreas, lung
α-Fetoprotein	Hepatoma, embryonal carcinoma of testis
Alkaline phosphatase Isoenzyme (placental or tumor specific; Regan enzyme)	Various neoplasms
PRODUCED AS A RESULT OF OVERPRODUCTION BY TUMOR CELLS	
Chorionic gonadotropin (β subunit)	Choriocarcinoma, hydatidiform mole, testicular cancer
Acid phosphatase	Prostatic carcinoma
Vitamin B₁₂-binding proteins	Chronic and acute myelogenous leukemia
Lysozyme	Monocytic leukemia
Polyamines	Various neoplasms
Hormones	Produced by specific endocrine-gland neoplasms

around fetal life (Table 323-5) and are useful markers for neoplastic growth; in other circumstances ectopic hormones are produced, resulting in clinical syndromes that are the result of hormone production (Table 323-6) and other syndromes with less defined etiologies. In addition, specific tumors may produce an increased amount of a substance normally produced by that cell.

The ability to detect the presence of a neoplasm by measurement of a cell product is related to the secretory capacity of a particular cell type, the amount of tumor present, as well as to sensitivity of the technique applied. The beta-cell tumor or *insulinoma of the pancreas* is the most commonly recognized neoplasm of functioning islet cells. Only 10 percent of such tumors are metastatic at the time of presentation. The classic symptoms are those of hypoglycemia. This tumor of the endocrine pancreas presents with signs of physiologic imbalance, whereas tumors of the exocrine pancreas usually are associated with signs of a mass and obstruction.

The most common cancer of the small intestine is the carcinoid tumor. Early manifestations may be caused by the space-occupying effects of the primary tumor. The later manifestations may be due to extension or metastases of the tumor, or to the effects of one or more of its metabolites. Unlike insulinoma of the pancreas, metastases seem to be a definite prerequisite for clinically significant manifestations in most patients with carcinoids. Patients with malignant carcinoids develop flushing spells and peculiar cutaneous vascular phenomena. Most patients show elevated levels of urinary 5-hydroxyindoleacetic acid (5-HIAA). The pharmacologically active agents responsible for the carcinoid syndrome and the resultant excretion of 5-HIAA are covered in Chap. 91. The carcinoid tumor does not manifest itself by mass, perforation, obstruction, or replacement, but by formation of a tumor product that generally occurs only in the presence of hepatic metastases.

Tumors of the testicle have been shown to produce certain markers depending on the cell types present. Tumors with a yolk-sac origin have been shown to produce α-fetoprotein, while those with embryonal elements have been shown to produce the β subunit of human chorionic gonadotropin (HCG). Pure seminomas produce neither of the markers.

Multiple myeloma is an example of a tumor with "factory" characteristics that directly reflect the growth characteristics and that are not the result of a hormonally active end product as in insulinoma, or the result of an unusual tumor product as in the carcinoid syndrome. It is a malignant proliferation of plasma cells. An M protein composed of either heavy and light chains (84 percent of cases) or light chains only (15 percent) can be detected in the serum or urine in 99 percent of the cases. Since all the cells in an M protein–secreting plasma-cell tumor appear to produce this M protein, the total number of tumor cells can be estimated from its serum level.

Certain types of tumors may be associated with the production of several substances. Small-cell (oat-cell) carcinoma of the lung is the histologic type of tumor most frequently associ-

TABLE 323-6
Paraneoplastic syndromes

Syndrome	Hormone	Tumor type
SYNDROMES ASSOCIATED WITH ECTOPIC HORMONE PRODUCTION		
Cushing's syndrome	ACTH	Oat-cell, thymoma, islet-cell tumors of pancreas, bronchial carcinoids of lung, medullary carcinoma of thyroid
Inappropriate ADH	ADH	Oat-cell, other tumors of lung, duodenum, pancreas, thymoma, lymphosarcoma
Gynecomastia	Gonadotropin	Lung carcinoma, rarely tumors of liver, adrenal, dysgerminoma of ovary
Hyperparathyroidism	PTH	Kidney, lung (squamous), pancreatic, and ovarian tumors
Hyperpigmentation	MSH	Oat-cell, lung tumors
Hyperthyroidism	TSH	Choriocarcinoma, hydatidiform mole, embryonal carcinoma of testis
Hypoglycemia	Insulin-like activity	Retroperitoneal and liver tumors
Hypocalcemia	Calcitonin	Medullary carcinoma of thyroid, breast carcinoma, oat-cell
Aplastic anemia (pure red blood cell hypoplasia)	?	Thymomas
Erythrocytosis	Erythropoietin	Cerebellar hemangioma, renal cell, liver, and ulterine tumors
OTHER EFFECTS OF NEOPLASMS ON THE HOST		
Muscle and joint disturbances: Polyarthritis (usually mild) Polymyositis (over age 40: 20% have occult cancer) Hypertrophic osteoarthropathy		Ovarian, uterine, breast, stomach, lung Lung, esophagus, colon
Neuropathies (often seen with myopathies): Central: Cerebellar degeneration Cerebral demyelination Peripheral: Pure sensory, lower motor neuron, mixed		Oat-cell, lung, breast, ovarian, lymphoma
Multiple thrombosis		Pancreatic, other types of cancer
Nephrosis (lipoid nephrosis and membranous glomerulitis)		Occult neoplasm in elderly patients
Acanthosis nigricans		Adenocarcinoma, lymphoma
Cachexia, loss of taste		Various types
Disseminated intravascular coagulation		Mucinous adenocarcinomas

ated with ectopic Cushing's syndrome and an inappropriate antidiuretic hormone (ADH) response. Also, oat-cell tumor can cause overproduction of serotonin with resultant carcinoid syndrome. Other lung cancers, such as squamous-cell carcinoma, may show increased production of parathyroid hormone (PTH) and also occasionally release some placental trophoblastic peptides.

These tumor "markers" or products of the cancer cell are important for several reasons. They may provide the clinician with a sensitive measure of tumor-cell progression or regression, as is the case with HCG, α-fetoprotein, and carcinoembryonic antigen, and help guide therapy and estimate prognosis. In other circumstances, especially when ectopic hormones are produced, clinical syndromes may result that offer clues to the etiology of the cancer or present difficult problems in management. In general, resolution of these clinical syndromes usually requires effective treatment of the malignancy, although immediate supportive care may be lifesaving when electrolyte imbalances, such as hypercalcemia, occur (see Chap. 324).

CLINICAL AND PATHOLOGIC METHODOLOGY **Staging classifications** A staging classification has to be both reproducible and clinically feasible. In addition, it must have both therapeutic and prognostic consequences. No single stage system is applicable to all cancers. A variety of staging systems is essential, because no two types of cancer have the same natural history. The clinical and pathologic staging classifications have arisen from a detailed knowledge of the pathophysiology of particular tumors. The following are examples which illustrate the use of different staging classifications.

Cancer of the cervix tends to spread by direct extension via the lymphatic system to the regional lymph nodes in the pelvis, and it metastasizes late. The international classification for the staging of individual cases of carcinoma of the cervix from stage 0 to stage IV predicts the general clinical course that cervical carcinoma follows and reflects the prognosis for each case. Stage 0 represents carcinoma in situ; stage I, carcinoma strictly confined to the cervix; stage II, carcinoma extending beyond the cervix but not yet to the pelvic wall; stage III, carcinoma extending to the pelvic wall; and stage IV, carcinoma extending beyond the true pelvis or involving the mucosa of the bladder and rectum.

Cancers of the head and neck are characterized by local extension and invasion, with subsequent cervical lymph node metastases. Regional lymph node involvement generally follows regular patterns according to the location of the primary tumor, although exceptions with bizarre spread occur. The TMN classification system (Table 323-7) utilizes tumor size and node involvement to describe the stage of a tumor at the time of diagnosis. It is a system designed to take into account the volume or size of the primary tumor T, as well as the degree of local spread to the lymph nodes N and the distant spread M.

The size of the primary tumor ranges from T_1 lesions, which have a maximum diameter of 2 cm or less, to T_3 lesions, which are larger than 4 cm. N stands for regional lymph nodes and varies from N_0, where no palpable cervical lymph nodes are present, to N_3, where clinically palpable lymph nodes are fixed and metastases are suspected. M stands for distant metastases which are either absent (M_0) or present by clinical and radiologic evidence in areas other than the cervical lymph nodes (M_1). Other factors besides the clinical and pathologic stage influence the prognosis in head and neck cancer: survival figures are better in patients with well-differentiated tumors than in those with anaplastic tumors; patients whose tumors show lymphocytic infiltration have a better prognosis than those lacking this finding.

The major defect of all staging classifications is their poor assessment of tumor volume. Nevertheless, staging classifications guide clinicians in selection of treatment, assure comparability of cases in various institutions, permit communication between treatment centers, and allow assessment of prognosis. The staging classification applicable to each particular cancer is described in detail in the appropriate chapter in this text.

Clinical staging All diagnostic tools should be used in clinical staging, with local systematic analysis applied to each individual tumor. Table 323-8 summarizes the routine and special clinical, radiologic, laboratory, and surgical procedures which should be utilized in the workup of mass lesions of a particular organ system. Laboratory and x-ray methods make it possible to bridge the gap between the physical examination and the final histopathologic determination.

Analyses of blood chemistries may offer important clues. An increase in the serum calcium is frequently seen with multiple myeloma as well as with metastatic oat-cell carcinoma and metastatic breast carcinoma. A decrease in the serum glucose value is commonly observed with islet-cell tumors of the pancreas that are insulin-secreting, and occasionally with retroperitoneal sarcomas or hepatoma. An increase in blood urea nitrogen (BUN) and creatinine is suggestive of an obstruction of the urinary tract. This can be due to local tumor invasion, as is frequently seen in carcinoma of the cervix with ureteral obstruction, or it can be secondary to uric acid or calcium nephrolithiasis which is occasionally seen in patients with acute leukemia and other myeloproliferative or lymphoproliferative diseases. An increase in direct bilirubin or alkaline phosphatase can result from obstruction of the hepatobiliary system at any point proximal to the ampulla of Vater. An increase in the total protein and, more specifically, the serum globulin can be the first suggestion of multiple myeloma. Special laboratory procedures may be useful in certain tumors, including tests for the presence of fetoprotein in hepatoma or malignant teratomas, carcinoembryonic antigen S (CEAS) in colon cancer, serum immunoglobulins in myeloma, and tartrate-inhibited acid phosphatase in prostatic carcinoma.

Radiographic contrast studies (Table 323-8) that are helpful in mapping the location of a pelvic tumor such as cervical carcinoma include an intravenous pyelogram (IVP), which will demonstrate pelvic or retroperitoneal masses causing either deviation or early obstruction. An inferior vena cavagram (IVC)

TABLE 323-7
The TNM system

PRIMARY TUMOR (T)

T_0	No evidence of primary tumor
T_{1S}	Carcinoma in situ
T_1, T_2, T_3, T_4	Ascending degrees of increase in tumor size and involvement

REGIONAL LYMPH NODES (N)

N_0	Regional nodes not demonstrable
N_{1a}, N_{2a}	Demonstrable regional lymph nodes, metastases not suspected
N_{1b}, N_{2b}, N_3	Demonstrable regional lymph nodes; metastases suspected
N_x	Regional lymph nodes cannot be assessed clinically

DISTANT METASTASES (M)

M_0	No evidence of distant metastases
M_1, M_2, M_3	Ascending degrees of metastatic involvement of the host including distant nodes

TABLE 323-8
Evaluative and staging procedures for tumors of selected organ systems

Organ system	Presenting lesion(s)	Routine clinical tests	"Obtaining tissue"	Special procedures	Staging procedures
Lung	Single mass	Chest x-ray Tomography	Sputum cytology Bronchoscopy and biopsy Mediastinoscopy	Pleural biopsy (if effusion is present) Lung biopsy	Mediastinoscopy Gallium scan
	Multiple masses	Intravenous pyelogram (IVP) Mammogram Thyroid scan Upper gastrointestinal-colon series	Mediastinoscopy	Lung biopsy	Metastatic; if nonlung primary proved, requires no further staging
Breast	Single mass	Mammogram Xerogram	Needle aspiration Excisional biopsy	Estrogen receptor Progesterone receptor	Liver scan Bone scan Brain scan
Lymphoid	Adenopathy	Chest x-ray (hilar adenopathy) Abdominal flat plate (splenomegaly)	Excisional biopsy		Ultrasonogram Gallium scan IVP Inferior vena cavagram (IVC) Lymphangiogram (LAG) Liver-spleen scan Computerized tomography (CT scan) Bone scan Bone marrow biopsy Laparoscopy Laparotomy
	Splenomegaly	Blood counts	Bone marrow aspiration Bone marrow biopsy		Proceed as for adenopathy
Gastro-intestinal	Esophageal mass or stricture	Chest x-ray Barium swallow	Esophagoscopy with brushing, cytology, and biopsy		Bronchoscopy Mediastinoscopy CT scan
	Gastric mass	Upper gastrointestinal barium series (double contrast)	Gastroscopy with brushing, cytology, and biopsy		Liver scan Chest x-ray
	Pancreatic mass	Ultrasonogram CT scan	Duodenal drainage for cytology; cannulation of ampulla of Vater for cytology	Percutaneous ("skinny needle") cholangiogram Endoscopic retrograde cholangiopancreatogram (ERCP)	Arteriogram Liver scan Laparotomy and biopsy
	Liver mass: single	Liver scan α-Fetoprotein	Percutaneous biopsy	Peritoneoscopy and biopsy	Arteriogram Laparotomy
	Liver: multiple masses	Liver scan Mammogram Upper gastrointestinal series Barium enema (double contrast) Pancreatic ultrasonogram Chest x-ray	Percutaneous biopsy	Peritoneoscopy and biopsy	Laparotomy
	Gallbladder mass; biliary tract mass or stricture	Liver scan Ultrasonogram	Duodenal drainage for cytology	Percutaneous ("skinny needle") Cholangiogram ERCP	Laparotomy
	Colon stricture or mass	Proctosigmoidoscopy Barium enema (double contrast)	Colonoscopy or proctoscopy with brushing, cytology, and biopsy	Carcinoembryonic antigen (CEA) IVP	Laparotomy Liver scan Chest x-ray
Genito-urinary	Kidney mass	Urinalysis IVP Nephrotomograms	Ureteral catheterization with cytology and/or brush biopsies Percutaneous fluid aspiration for cytology	Arteriogram Nephrosonogram Erythropoietin	Chest x-ray Liver scan Bone scan Retroperitoneal ultrasonogram Inferior vena cavagram Lymphangiogram Excision of tumor Lymphadenectomy
	Bladder mass	IVP Cystoscopy	Urine cytology Biopsy		

Organ system	Presenting lesion(s)	Routine clinical tests	"Obtaining tissue"	Special procedures	Staging procedures
	Testicular mass	Chest x-ray		α-Fetoprotein Human chorionic gonadotropin (β subunit)	
	Prostate	IVP Acid phosphatase	Biopsy	Iliac crest bone marrow for tumor cells and free acid phosphatase	
	Ovarian mass	Chest x-ray Upper gastrointestinal series Barium enema IVP	Laparotomy	Estrogen receptor Progesterone receptor Peritoneal cytology	Laparotomy Bone scan Liver scan
	Uterine mass	Chest x-ray IVP	Papanicolaou Jet wash cytology Fractional dilatation and curettage (D&C) and/or biopsy Laparotomy (if sarcoma)	Estrogen receptor Progesterone receptor Human chorionic gonadotropin (β subunit)	Fractional D&C Bone scan Liver scan Laparotomy
	Cervical lesion	Papanicolaou Colposcopy Chest x-ray IVP	Biopsy		Clinical staging Lymphangiogram Bone scan Liver scan Staging by lymph node biopsy

can be done in patients with malignant lymphoma in the search for a retroperitoneal mass in the high lumbar region. Anterior deviation of the superior vena cava suggests the presence of a tumor mass. A lymphangiogram (LAG) in patients with testicular carcinomas serves to localize enlarged pelvic and low lumbar lymph nodes. An upper gastrointestinal examination with barium as well as a small-bowel follow-through and a barium enema are useful in localizing lesions in the gastrointestinal tract. Selective arteriography has been employed for differentiation of a benign cyst from a malignant renal-cell carcinoma.

Computerized tomography (CT) scan of the brain has been demonstrated to be effective in evaluating brain tumors and is associated with less morbidity than anteriograms and pneumoencephalograms. CT scans of a suspected mass lesion are frequently of value in differentiating solid from cystic lesions. Development of the CT scan for definition of chest and abdominal lesions has resulted in a significant addition to the clinical detection of mass lesions in the mediastinum as well as in the retroperitoneal area.

Ultrasonography offers an inexpensive noninvasive technique for the study of orbital, cardiac, pericardiac, hepatic, pancreatic, renal, and retroperitoneal areas. Although ultrasound can demonstrate retroperitoneal lymphadenopathy, studies are occasionally obscured by bowel gas; the CT scan does not encounter this problem. Ultrasound guided biopsies of various tumor masses have been performed successfully.

Highly refined radioisotopic methods, which are noninvasive, have become available for the diagnosis of cancer (Table 323-8). Liver and spleen scans have been used to identify an enlarged spleen which may not be palpable and metastatic lesions in the liver which have not yet become clinically significant. Bone scans can detect metastatic lesions before they are radiologically evident. The only malignancy for which the bone scan is less sensitive than the x-ray is multiple myeloma. The many lytic lesions present will be missed by the bone scan because there are few reactive changes surrounding the lesions. It has been shown that approximately 10 percent of women who are by all other criteria eligible to undergo radical mastec-

tomy have metastatic lesions in bone as shown by scanning, although the concurrent x-rays are negative. Gallium scans, both whole body as well as tomographic cuts of various sections, are sometimes of value in the clinical staging of Hodgkin's disease and malignant lymphoma but are even more specific and sensitive for lung cancer. In addition, metastatic lesions can be picked up in most sites with the gallium scan alone, although the CT scan is more sensitive for brain lesions. Because gallium is a soft-tissue specific isotope, it can be used for a noninvasive contrast study at the time of clinical staging and may be repeated for follow-up without causing patient discomfort or morbidity.

Pathologic staging Staging operations are used only to find the extent or stage of disease so that appropriate definitive treatment can be selected (Table 323-8). Mediastinoscopy is the major preoperative method for pathologic evaluation of regional spread in lung cancer. Approximately 35 percent of all patients examined preoperatively are found to have mediastinal lymph node metastases. Positive tissue obtained at mediastinoscopy is usually a contraindication to thoracotomy. Patients who have negative mediastinoscopy, a negative metastatic workup, and a tumor that is at least 1 cm distal to the carina are eligible for thoracotomy and resection of bronchogenic carcinoma.

A bone core biopsy is used for establishing the presence of malignant tumor in the bone marrow. In approximately 60 percent of patients with malignant lymphoma, poorly differentiated lymphocytic type, nodular or diffuse, it has been shown that bone core biopsies are positive; the bone core biopsy can serve as easy identification of patients with pathologic stage IV malignant lymphoma.

Mastectomy results in cure in two-thirds of patients with breast cancer who have no axillary lymph node involvement, but the cure rate is less than 10 percent in those who have four or more positive lymph nodes at the time of mastectomy. Although the mastectomy is intended to be therapeutic, it also serves as a pathologic staging procedure, since the number of positive lymph nodes in the axillary dissection identifies a group which might benefit from further therapy in the immediate postmastectomy period.

The most striking example of a staging procedure that is performed only for biopsy and not excision of the tumor is the staging laparotomy used in Hodgkin's disease. It is designed to prove the exact extent of the disease so that patients are not undertreated, which might result in early relapse, or overtreated, which might result in excessive morbidity and mortality. The procedure involves a splenectomy, because splenic involvement can be determined only by thorough pathologic sectioning and evaluation. Biopsies of the liver and various retroperitoneal and mesenteric lymph nodes are also obtained.

Staging procedures can lead to identification of sites of disease as well as definition of the extent of disease at a given site, which can aid in the design of suitable therapy. During the staging laparotomy in Hodgkin's disease, areas of lymph node biopsy are marked with metal clips, as are the margins of any masses that have been biopsied. The clips subsequently allow the radiotherapist to design appropriate radiotherapy.

PRINCIPLES OF MANAGEMENT

INDICATIONS FOR SURGERY AND RADIOTHERAPY Management of the patient with suspected or proved cancer involves the evaluation of operability and, if possible, curability. When metastatic disease has been documented, surgery is usually indicated only for staging, as in Hodgkin's disease, or for prevention of local problems, as in colon carcinoma, obstruction secondary to the primary tumor mass is a frequent complication. If there is no evidence of metastatic disease and if a primary lesion is suspected or proved, operability has to be measured against the local extent and known history of the disease.

For example, a patient with lung cancer diagnosed by either positive cytology or bronchoscopic biopsy requires a determination of operability. If it is decided that the patient is not medically operable, further evaluation of the extent of disease must be made prior to the decision regarding radiotherapy or chemotherapy. If medical operability is established, a thorough search for metastatic disease should be made. If there is evidence of metastatic disease, the patient is considered inoperable, and treatment for disseminated disease has to be initiated. If there is no evidence of metastatic disease, the surgical criteria for resectability have to be evaluated. A tumor that has invaded the mediastinum is not curable with resection and will require local treatment such as radiotherapy. If the tumor does not involve the mediastinum, but is less than 0.5 cm from the carina, it is technically unresectable, and local radiotherapy should be planned. Approximately 15 percent of patients with lung cancer pass all the decision points and are eligible for curative surgical therapy. A careful assessment of the patient's clinical status, correlated with the extent of the disease, will probably result in fewer surgical procedures; however, a larger number of the resections will result in cure.

Some tumors are inoperable because of the extent of spread at the time of diagnosis. Others, such as glioma of the brainstem, are inoperable, not because of spread, but because of their location and the loss of essential function that would result from surgical removal.

APPROACH TO DISSEMINATED DISEASE If a patient has disseminated cancer, few surgical staging procedures are indicated, although various radiographic and radioisotopic tests are available for the evaluation of the subsequent response to treatment. When disseminated disease is demonstrated, it is important to look for the primary site only if it involves an organ or cell of origin for which available therapy is effective. For example, it has been shown that the search for the primary site is frequently unrewarding for metastatic undifferentiated carcinoma or adenocarcinoma from an unknown primary cancer site. In a study of 264 patients, only 30 patients had the primary site identified antemortem by extensive radiographic search and eventual biopsy. Even in 23 of 130 patients who underwent autopsy, the primary site could not be found. In the patients in whom a primary site could be found, lung cancer was the most frequent primary tumor above the diaphragm, while the pancreas was the most common primary site below the diaphragm. Although pancreatic cancer is present in autopsy series in about 1.5 percent of cases, in a study of patients dying of unknown primaries, it was found in 20 percent of cases. In contrast, prostatic cancer, which is present in 17 percent of men at autopsy, accounted only for 4 percent of the unknown primaries.

In about 5 percent of the cases of cervical lymph node metastases the primary tumor is undetected. Failure to find the primary site after diligent search has been variously ascribed to the small size or spontaneous regression of the primary tumor or its occurrence in the wall of a branchiogenic cyst or lymph node. In such instances, a curative approach appropriate for head and neck cancer should be undertaken.

Specific therapy for metastatic disease utilizes hormonal treatment and chemotherapy. This is discussed in detail in Chap. 324.

MULTIMODALITY THERAPEUTIC APPROACH Although the single-modality approach to treatment, consisting of either surgery, radiotherapy, or chemotherapy, is appropriate in some tumors, others require a combination of all three modalities. Partial colectomy is the treatment of choice in patients with carcinoma of the colon; if there is no evidence of spread through the muscularis mucosa and no evidence of lymph node involvement, most patients will be cured. An acceptable treatment for early carcinoma of the cervix is a radium implant, which is as curative as hysterectomy. The initial treatment of adult acute leukemia is chemotherapy alone, as the disease is widely disseminated and cannot be approached either surgically or with radiotherapy.

Combined-modality therapy has resulted in increased rates of complete remission and prolonged survival in some tumors. Osteogenic sarcoma, although apparently completely excised by removal of the involved limb, recurs with pulmonary metastases in approximately 70 percent of the patients within 1 year. By administration of multiple courses of chemotherapy immediately after resection of the primary tumor, development of lung lesions is prevented in many patients. The period of complete remission has been markedly prolonged, and achieving cures may be possible. Adjuvant chemotherapy has been found useful in Ewing's sarcoma, Wilms's tumors of the kidney, and possibly in premenopausal patients with breast cancer.

In most cases, the combined-modality approach to malignant neoplasms involves surgical removal of the bulk of the primary tumor, followed by radiotherapy to eradicate any tumor left in the margins of resection, and followed, in turn, by chemotherapy to eradicate any distant metastases while the tumor burden is low. This combined-modality adjuvant approach to cancer therapy is designed to cure cancer at the initial presentation when the tumor burden is smallest, rather than when diffuse metastatic disease and a large tumor burden are present. This approach is being tested in cancer of the lung, head, and neck, as well as colon and rectum, and continues to be evaluated in breast cancer and sarcomas. Both nonspecific (e.g., bacillus Calmette-Guérin) and specific (e.g., allogenic tumor cells) immunotherapy is being attempted in acute leukemias and in lung, colon, and rectum cancer as well as in melanoma to further enhance induction of remissions and, in particular, to prolong their duration.

COMPLICATIONS OF MALIGNANT DISEASE AND ITS THERAPY
Although each cancer has signs and symptoms specifically associated with its location and cell type, there are certain common complications of tumors. These include hypercalcemia, lactic acidosis, hyperuricemia, ectopic hormone production, both local and remote neurologic manifestations, obstruction, effusions, and bleeding diatheses. Frequently simultaneous therapy is required for both the complication and the underlying tumor. These complications and their management are discussed in Chap. 324.

LONGITUDINAL FOLLOW-UP Cancer patients who are presumed cured need careful follow-up for early detection of recurrences, so that further curative therapy can be undertaken if necessary. These patients must be made aware of possible risk from radiation or chemotherapy to their future children as a result of mutations in their reproductive tissues. They also must be apprised of future risks of developing a second cancer, as is seen in patients treated for multiple myeloma or Hodgkin's disease, some of whom subsequently develop acute myelogenous leukemia. Patients who have undergone curative surgery for lung cancer should be alerted to the risk of resuming smoking. Patients resected for cancer of the oral cavity should be encouraged to discontinue the use of tobacco as well as alcohol.

MANAGEMENT OF THE PATIENT AND FAMILY Undertaking the care of a patient with cancer requires total commitment. Attention must be directed to details of staging and treatment with the potential of cure or prolonged control. In addition, such care demands attention to pain, the nutritional status of the patient, and psychological support for patient and family.

The previous sections of this chapter have addressed the management of the tumor. Pain may be one of the main concerns of the patient. Radiotherapy to the site of tumor can frequently alleviate specific local pain. Generalized pain from widely disseminated tumor requires narcotics. Usually mild analgesics and codeine are started initially. Levophanol tartrate (Levo-Dromoran) and, finally, Brompton's mixture, which includes morphine and cocaine, may be required to control the pain. These agents for pain relief can be prescribed for oral administration and use at home. Once the patient can no longer be cared for at home and is hospitalized, liberal use of morphine is indicated. A hospitalized patient with terminal, disseminated cancer should have as little pain as possible. Pain medication should not be ordered on an "as requested" (prn) basis but around the clock.

Recently, the hospice concept has been brought to the attention of cancer patients and their families as well as physicians. The hospice is composed of a group of professionals, including psychiatrists, nurses, and social workers, who help patients to live their terminal period with their family. This form of terminal care should be supported because tertiary care facilities are focusing on the care of those patients who still have the possibility to respond to therapy. Patients supported by a hospice are not abandoned, but, in fact, receive very different care from that which a hospital facility can give them and, it is hoped, achieve a sense of contentment in their remaining days or months.

REFERENCES

Capizzi RL: *Seminars in Oncology,* vol 4, no 2: *The Pharmacologic Basis of Cancer Chemotherapy.* New York, Grune & Stratton, 1977
Gilbert HA, Kagan R: *Seminars in Oncology,* vol 4, no 1: *Metastases.* New York, Grune & Stratton, 1977
Goepp CE: *Seminars in Oncology,* vol 5, no 1: *Heredity and Cancer.* New York, Grune & Stratton, 1978
Holland JF, Frei E III: *Cancer Medicine.* Philadelphia, Lea & Febiger, 1973
Rowley JD: Chromosomes in leukemia and lymphoma. Semin Hematol 15:301, 1978
Yarbro JE (ed): *Seminars in Oncology,* vol 5, no 2: *Oncologic Emergencies.* New York, Grune & Stratton, 1978

324
PRINCIPLES OF CANCER THERAPY

VINCENT T. DeVITA, JR.

BIOLOGY OF TUMOR CELL GROWTH AS RELATED TO THERAPY

All living things have an inherent capacity to multiply. Unicellular organisms, such as bacteria, multiply until growth is limited by lack of suitable nutrients or until toxic products accumulate in their environment. At more complex levels of cellular organization a cellular "brake" is required to prevent overgrowth for the benefit of the community of cells. The molecular mechanisms for control of cell growth are unknown, and their understanding forms a key scientific question in cellular biology. Clear examples of the temporary, controlled release of the cellular brake exist, as in wound healing and in regeneration of the liver after partial hepatectomy. In neoplasms, cells no longer cease multiplication when they reach a critical mass, and the uncontrolled growth leads to the death of the host. The three general classes of normal tissue, renewing (marrow, germ cells), expanding (liver, kidney, and endocrine glands), and static (neurons and striated muscle), reach a steady state when normal organ size is attained. For static tissues, such as neurons, the cells live for the duration of the life of the host and are normally not replaced if lost. For expanding tissue, mitotic potential is manifest in cells at random only when cell loss takes place (trauma, surgical resection), and then the tissue is replenished. Adult cells of renewing populations have a finite, usually short, life span, and continued replacement from a clonogenic, or stem-cell pool, normally takes place. As long as cell birth does not exceed cell loss, a neoplastic process is not evident. In spite of the tissue of origin, growing populations of tumor cells resemble renewing populations of normal tissue. Maturation takes place in some cells. Although they continue to divide for a time, they lose their capacity to establish new colonies. A subset of the population usually retains the capacity to form new colonies. Although early normal growth in the embryo, and early tumor growth, appear to be exponential, exponential growth soon ceases, and the growth characteristics of expanding tumor masses are best described as a gompertzian function. As the mass increases, the time required for the mass to double also increases; exponential growth is matched by exponential retardation of growth. The tumor doubling time (the time required for a given mass to double its volume) is a complex value influenced by the cell cycle time, the fraction of cells in the population undergoing cell division, and the rate of cell loss from the mass. The phases of a cell cycle are illustrated in Fig. 324-1. Cells not in cycle, but viable, and capable of entering cell division under proper circumstances are said to be in a resting phase (G_0). The fraction of cells in cycle in a given population (proliferative pool, growth fraction) determined by incorporation of tritiated thymidine into DNA (labeling index)

PROPHASE

METAPHASE

ANAPHASE

TELOPHASE

S / G₂

M

G₁

G₀

CELL CYCLE

MITOSIS

FIGURE 324-1

The cell cycle. The gap terminology divides the cell cycle into phases M, G_1, S, and G_2. M is the period of cell division. G_1 is the period of normal cell metabolism but without DNA synthesis; cells that stay in G_1 for long periods are often referred to as being in the G_0 phase. The S, or DNA synthetic, phase is the period of doubling of the DNA content; it is followed by the G_2, or tetraploid, phase which precedes cell division. Normal and cancer cells have similar cycle times, in general: M, 0.5 to 1 h; G_1, 2 h to infinity; S, 6 to 24 h; G_2, 2 to 8 h.

markedly influence the growth of the tumor. For a given cycle time, a tumor with a high growth fraction will double faster than a tumor with a low growth fraction if cell loss (death, metastases, shedding) is constant. High rates of cell loss account for long doubling times in tumors known to have high growth fractions.

There are considerable data to suggest that in addition to cells remaining quiescent in G_0, some cancer cells, on their own, or under the influence of drugs or x-ray therapy, may be blocked from proceeding through the cell cycle for long periods of time in other phases of the cycle, a fact of some therapeutic importance in scheduling of treatment programs. Although cell cycle times are relatively constant in tumors of a given histological type, considerable species differences exist in cycle times of normal and tumor tissue. Cell loss begins early in growth of a tumor. Even small (1 to 2 mm), apparently localized, tumors can be assumed to shed cells into surrounding tissue (e.g., shedding from the surface of a colon cancer into the lumen of the bowel) or into lymphatics and/or the bloodstream. The fact that some cancers can be cured by local treatment only reaffirms that many shed cells are nonviable (nonclonogenic) or are capable of being destroyed by the host.

CLONAL EVOLUTION OF CANCER The concept that cancer originates from a single transformed cell, or clone, is supported by clinical studies of human neoplasms. The classic example is multiple myeloma, a malignant proliferation of antibody-secreting plasma cells, which is characterized by elevated blood, or urine, levels of a single immunoglobulin molecule. Tumor-specific abnormalities in chromosome structure have been demonstrated in malignant cells; the most consistent example

is the Philadelphia chromosome which occurs in approximately 95 percent of patients with chronic myelogenous leukemia. The abnormal chromosome 22 has been identified in hematopoietic precursor cells in some cases several years prior to the onset of overt leukemia. The clonal evolution of this disease is further supported by studies of X-inactivation mosaicism. Each cell of the female determines at the early stage in embryogenesis whether the paternal- or maternal-derived X chromosome will remain active or suppressed. The X-linked enzyme glucose 6-phosphate dehydrogenase (G6PD) has proved a useful marker for such studies of clonal origin because it is polymorphic in the black population. Women who are heterozygous at the G6PD locus for the common gene Gd^B and the variant Gd^A normally have two distinct cell populations reflected in their enzyme electrophoretic pattern. While the nonleukemic G6PD heterozygotes have both the A and the B enzyme type in white blood cells, patients with chronic myelogenous leukemia demonstrate only one enzyme type in their leukemic granulocytic series, suggesting that the disorder originated from a single cell. Similar methodology has shown that acute myelogenous leukemia, carcinoma of the uterus and cervix, and Burkitt's lymphoma also have demonstrated a clonal pattern of tumor evolution. Patients with Burkitt's lymphoma have a consistent abnormality of chromosome 14. With early relapse after remission of Burkitt's lymphoma, the cells retain the enzyme phenotype of the initial tumor, and the recurrent tumor appears to represent a reemergence of the original malignant line. In several cases of late recurrent Burkitt's tumor, there have been discordant G6PD phenotypes, indicating the probable emergence of newly induced malignant clones. Cells from meningiomas have also demonstrated a consistent deletion of a portion of chromosome 22. Two hereditary tumors, neurofibroma and trichoepithelioma, have demonstrated a double-enzyme phenotype, indicating multicellular origin. These exceptions suggest that the somatic mutation theories of oncogenesis may not be valid for all neoplasms.

DOSE-RESPONSE RELATIONSHIPS The growth and size of a tumor are generally measured in terms of orders of magnitude or logs. A human tumor, when first diagnosed as, for example, a 1.0-cm mass, contains approximately 1 billion cancer cells or 9 logs, whereas 12 logs has been estimated to represent a lethal body burden for some malignancies. The cytotoxic action of anticancer agents is defined by first-order kinetics; they kill a constant fraction of cells rather than a constant number. Thus, a course of therapy with a capacity to kill 3 logs of tumor cells will reduce a tumor with 10^{10} cells to 10^7, or a neoplasm of 10^5 to 10^2 cells. Unfortunately, the majority of available single drugs, and even drug combinations, used for solid tumors have a limited log cell kill potential, and as a result cannot be expected to have a curative effect when used to treat tumors that are large both in terms of physical size and kinetics. In the past, drug therapy had been largely reserved for advanced cases, after surgery and radiation therapy had failed. While most chemotherapy, used in relatively sensitive tumors, was able to reduce cell numbers by 1 to 3 logs, it was capable of producing only minimal palliation in a patient with 10^{12} tumor cells. Total eradication of tumor cells was not possible for all but the most drug-sensitive malignancies. These concepts, derived from studies of cell kinetics, are now being tested in adjuvant chemotherapy trials. Patients are receiving drug treatment after the tumor mass has been initially reduced by surgery and radiation therapy in the hope that the favorable kinetic features in the remaining microscopic disease will serve to increase the effectiveness of chemotherapy.

Conceptually, the tumor can be divided into three distinct kinetic compartments, each with its particular significance in relation to the effectivenesses of chemotherapy (Fig. 324-2). First, there is the growth fraction of tumor that is most vulner-

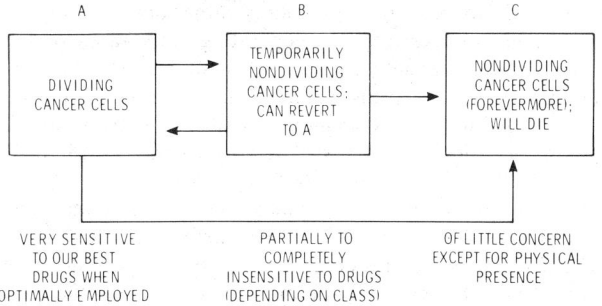

FIGURE 324-2

Various compartments and flow between compartments in a hypothetical tumor mass.

a definite selectivity for cancer cells over normal cells. The clinical counterpart of animal experiments showing a markedly increased sensitivity of tumor cells over normal cells to drugs can, at present, only be inferred from the dramatic antitumor effects noted in some patients with drug-sensitive tumors without permanent damage to their bone marrow or gastrointestinal tract.

A similar effect is seen with x-ray therapy. The radiation dose-response curve is illustrated in Fig. 324-4. The fraction of surviving cells on a log scale is plotted against radiation dose. The slope of the exponential portion of the curve, usually referred to as D_0 (mean lethal dose), is a standard reference point. D_0 is the dose required to place one inactivating event in each pertinent biological entity. The more radiosensitive the cell, the steeper the curve. Owing to the random nature of these energy deposits, some energy will be deposited in a cell which has already been destroyed, while some will escape altogether so that according to the Poisson distribution, instead of destroying all the cells, the D_0 destroys only 63 percent of them. Thus, the dose required to reduce the number of cells in a population to 37 percent of the original number is D_{37}, which is an index of radiosensitivity. For most cells this value lies between 80 and 200 rads. The surviving fraction after two mean lethal doses is 37 times 37 percent or 13.7 percent, and after three mean lethal doses it is 5.1 percent, etc. In practice the logarithmic curve is not exactly a straight line. There is a small shoulder to overcome before the curve is exponential. With a strictly exponential curve D_0 equals D_{37}. The shoulder on the curve reflects doses below which the cell has the ability to repair radiation-induced damage. The dose at the point at which the curve becomes exponential (D_q) is the threshold dose. Repair of radiation-induced damage can take place within 2 h. The identification of D_q, D_0, D_{37}. repair time, and mechanisms of repair have important implications in clinical dose fractionation, particularly in studies combining drugs with radiation therapy. For clinical purposes, a dose-response curve can be constructed for specific tumors in which local tumor control is plotted as a function of dose.

able to chemotherapy. Second, there is a population of cells which are temporarily nondividing but, nevertheless, have the capability of returning to a replicative stage. In terms of cell cycle kinetics, these cells are in an extended G_1 or G_0 phase and are considerably less sensitive to antitumor agents, particularly the cell cycle phase-specific antimetabolites. Lastly, there is a compartment of cells that have permanent loss of proliferative capacity, until they die and are absorbed, but still contribute to the mass of the tumor and are measured either by physical examination or by x-ray.

With increasing tumor size, the percentage of cells in the drug-sensitive growth fraction decreases. This phenomenon is considered to represent one of the limiting factors of successful chemotherapy. A clinical counterpart of these data is represented in Fig. 324-3. This figure illustrates the fact that most tumors are in the late stages of their biologic growth curves when diagnosed as a 1-cm mass. At this point they have already progressed through approximately 30 doubling times and are only 10 to 15 doublings away from a lethal volume of tumor cells.

The implication of the fractional killing effect is that to eradicate a tumor population effectively, it is necessary either to increase the dose of drug or drugs within limits tolerated by the host or to start treatment when the number of cells is small enough to allow tumor destruction at reasonably tolerated doses. The killing effect of cancer chemotherapeutic agents has

FIGURE 324-3

A schematic representation of the life cycle of a human tumor. Number of cells present in the body is shown on the ordinate with number of population doublings on the abscissa. Clinical phenomena are related to expected size of tumor mass on plotted line. Most tumors have completed at least two-thirds of their growth (32 doublings) at the time of diagnosis of a 1-cm mass.

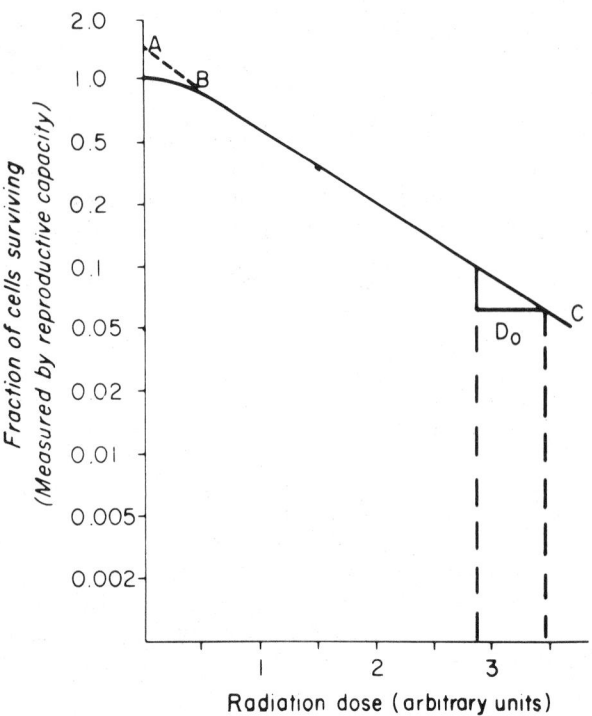

FIGURE 324-4

Radiation dose-response curve (see text).

TYPES OF IONIZING RADIATION The term *x-ray* or *roentgen ray* is applied to electromagnetic, nonparticulate, ionizing radiations produced by human-made machines, whereas gamma rays emanate from naturally occurring or artificially produced radioactive elements such as radium or cobalt 60. These radiations of very short wavelengths have extremely high penetrating power in materials of low atomic number such as water and tissue but are stopped efficiently in materials of high atomic number such as lead. The ionizing events following irradiation lead to the production of free radicals in the water molecules of the cell microenvironment. Such free radicals and oxidizing agents interact with DNA molecules and produce a large number and variety of DNA breaks and damage. The exact lethal lesion of x-ray irradiation remains undefined, but once alterations in nucleotide sequences occur, a change in transcription, or defective repair, results, leading to cell death.

TYPES OF RADIOTHERAPY EQUIPMENT At one time, the best available apparatus for "deep therapy" operated at 200 to 250 kV, referred to as the *kilovoltage range.* Unfortunately this type of equipment is still widely prevalent. The *supervoltage energy range* is generally taken to be 2 to 10 MeV, and *megavoltage energies* are those above 10 MeV. Radium emits gamma rays from about 1 MeV, while the artificially produced isotope cobalt 60 (^{60}Co) emits gamma rays of about 1.4 MeV. The mere presence in a unit of a quantity of ^{60}Co does not make it a true supervoltage instrument. The great tissue penetration which characterizes the supervoltage range is obtained only when the radiation source is far removed (preferably 70 cm to 1 m) from the surface of the patient. Since the output of the source decreases inversely as the square of its distance from the patient, obviously units containing very large amounts of ^{60}Co (2000 to 3000 Ci) are required to produce adequate intensities and reasonably short treatment times at treatment distances of 1 m or greater. The units which contain smaller amounts of ^{60}Co and are operated at a distance of 50 cm or less should not be thought of as supervoltage devices since the physical distribution of gamma ray beams from these sources is comparable with kilovoltage rays. Linear (electron) accelera-

tors are able to generate high-energy radiations without employing high voltages, and those operating in the range of 4 to 10 MeV are commercially available. A similar device, the betatron, accelerates electrons magnetically in a circular path within a vacuum tube. Commercial units presently available produce electrons and x-rays at a peak energy of 18 to 30 MeV.

Megavoltage radiation equipment has almost completely replaced kilovoltage sources in cancer therapy. Because of reduced skin doses and lesser internal scatter, higher doses of irradiation can be delivered to tumors at any depth in the body by megavoltage irradiation. Linear accelerators in the 4- to 35-MeV range and cobalt sources are the photon generators most widely employed. Linear accelerators deliver radiation with sharper beam margins than cobalt machines. Linear accelerators can also provide electrons, which are particulate and penetrate approximately 0.25 to 0.5 cm/MeV energy with a relatively abrupt falloff in tissues, so that deeper normal tissues are spared from irradiation. Other forms of particulate irradiation are being developed which are more penetrating than electrons and have very favorable physical and biologic characteristics for the treatment of cancer. These include fast neutrons, charged particles such as protons or helium ions, and negative pi mesons. These particles cause a more intense deposition of energy per unit path in the tissue [high linear energy transfer (LET)] than ordinary photon radiation. They also have theoretical advantages of greater relative biological effectiveness (RBE), in part because of lower oxygen enhancement ratios (OER) which should treat hypoxic fractions of tumors more effectively. Doses of radiation are expressed in units called *rads,* which indicate the amount of absorbed energy per unit volume of tissue. The biological effects of irradiation are dependent on the time over which the radiation is delivered and the dose per fraction. Usual dose fractionation is about 1000 rads per week, delivered in 150- to 250-rad fractions. Delivering tumoricidal doses with kilovoltage sources required prolonged periods of time and utilization of many fractions when skin tolerance was the major limiting factor. With megavoltage irradiation, this is no longer the case, and shorter and more intense irradiation dose fractionation is being developed and studied.

RADIOSENSITIZER DRUGS Tumor masses have been shown to contain significant fractions of hypoxic cells due to the inadequacy of the blood supply in large tumors as the mass increases. Since the free radical state of molecular oxygen interacts with ionization products created by radiation beams, it has been postulated that radiation therapy to such tumors is less effective than to fully oxygenated tumors. In experimental tumor systems, the size of the hypoxic fraction has been shown to be directly proportional to the failure rate of local treatment.

Attempts to improve the cell kill of hypoxic cells have involved the use of hyperbaric oxygen, high LET radiation, and hypoxic cell sensitizer drugs. Of the compounds tested as hypoxic cell sensitizers, the nitroimidazoles appear to have the greatest potential because of pharmacological properties that promote distribution of drug to the central portion of tumors in spite of poor blood supply. Among these, metronidazole (Flagyl) and another experimental derivative, misonidazole, have been active in animal model systems and are now in early clinical evaluation in several countries. These compounds act by mimicking oxygen in fixing DNA damage caused by radiation. Thus, they improve radiosensitivity for cell kill of hypoxic cells as tested both in vitro and in vivo. They do not sensitize normal oxic cells to radiation and thus exert a selective effect between tumors and normal tissues. Hypoxic radiosensitizers have the potential of enhancing the usefulness of photon radiotherapy by maximizing the tumor cell kill with doses well within the range tolerated by normal tissue.

DRUGS, HORMONES, AND IMMUNOTHERAPEUTIC AGENTS

In 1977, 700,000 patients were diagnosed in the United States as having cancer exclusive of skin cancer. Of these, roughly 500,000 patients presented with disease that appeared localized, and 200,000 presented with visible metastases at the time of first diagnosis. Of the 500,000 with apparently localized tumor, 280,000, or 56 percent are expected to remain free of recurrent tumor 5 years later. However, 220,000 will develop recurrent tumor because of the presence of micrometastases not noted at the time of surgery or radiation of the primary tumor. For the 200,000 patients who presented with metastatic disease, drug therapy now exists that can prolong useful life in approximately 92,000 patients per year. In fact, of these 92,000 patients, 32,000 have cancers that are now potentially curable with drugs, even though they have widespread metastases at diagnosis. Radiotherapy and surgery offer ways of reducing the tumor mass in specific regions of the body amenable to surgical excision or high doses of radiotherapy. Neither is applicable to removal of widely disseminated tumor. Patients with visible metastatic disease or micrometastases require some form of treatment that reaches all the interstices of the body. The stimulus for the development of systemic treatment of cancer can be traced to the success in identifying and using antibiotics for bacterial infections and antiprotozoan drugs for malaria.

Drug development for cancer began with the accidental identification of the antitumor activity of nitrogen mustard, a derivative of mustard gases used in World Wars I and II. The initial success in the treatment of Hodgkin's disease and lymphocytic lymphomas with this drug was followed by extraordinary disappointment and skepticism that cancer could be successfully treated by drugs, because all successfully treated patients had relapses of their disease. Further excitement was created with the identification of the effectiveness of the antimetabolite methotrexate, first used against acute childhood leukemia and then in the treatment of choriocarcinoma in women. In the latter case, remissions produced by the drug appeared permanent. The need for a standardized approach to the development of anticancer drugs was recognized in the 1950s. Since then, many synthetic, fermentation and plant products have been identified as possessing antitumor activity against rodent tumors. These compounds have been selected both by rational synthesis and random screening. Over 40 non-hormone cytotoxic chemicals that possess some anticancer effect in humans with metastatic disease have been identified, and about 29 have been marketed. Six major classes of antitumor agents and some miscellaneous drugs are available: alkylating agents, antimetabolites, plant alkaloids, antitumor antibiotics, endocrine agents, and immunologic stimulants. The most important agents with their major toxicity, doses, and schedules are described in Table 324-1. The major hormonal agents are described in Table 324-2.

ALKYLATING AGENTS Mechlorethamine (nitrogen mustard) was the first chemical agent used in the treatment of cancer in modern times. It was found to have major antitumor activity against lymphomas. It contains two β-chloroethyl groups which transfer into positively charged ethylenimonium derivatives and combine with negatively charged guanine moieties of complementary DNA strands, resulting in their cross-linking. This could lead to miscoding errors or depurination, or, in the case of bifunctional alkylating agents, to cross-linking of adjacent macromolecules, which would interfere with mitosis by preventing separation of strands of DNA. Polyfunctional alkylating agents are more cytotoxic than monofunctional alkylators, although the latter may also cause mutagenic and carci-

nogenic damage that is not lethal to the cell and can, therefore, be reproduced indefinitely as an inherited mutation. Alkylating agents are not cell cycle–specific in their ability to cause cell death. Cell death may occur during the interphase, when many sites, including RNA and protein, are damaged, or it may be delayed until mitosis when separation of the DNA strands is unable to take place. Within a few minutes after administration of mechlorethamine, the drug is no longer detectable in active form and is bound to proteins or intracellular macromolecules. Less than 0.01 percent is excreted in the urine. The intracavitary use of mechlorethamine (0.2 to 0.4 mg/kg) after drainage of malignant pleural effusions can be an effective palliative measure. Very dilute solutions (0.25%) can be painted on the skin of patients with generalized mycosis fungoides with good results.

Three major modifications have altered the properties of mechlorethamine. (1) The substitution of electrophilic groups on the nitrogen atom, as in chlorambucil, reduces the reactivity, producing a more stable drug with a longer half-life. (2) An amino acid precursor added to the nitrogen atom as a carrier enhances delivery to sites of greatest tumor activity. Melphalan, for example, is the L-phenylalanine congener. (3) Cyclophosphamide is a derivative in which the activity of the chloroethyl groups is eliminated by the substitution of a ring structure on the nitrogen atom. This drug is activated by enzymatic cleavage of the phosphorus-nitrogen linkage within the molecule. In the liver it is activated through conversion to the 4-OH derivative by the drug metabolizing microsomal oxidase system and ultimately broken down to nor-nitrogen mustard. Cyclophosphamide is subject to the influence of other compounds. For example, barbiturates stimulate hepare enzymes and would increase the activation and toxicity of cyclophosphamide, whereas corticosteroids and sex hormones have the opposite effect. After oral administration, maximum plasma levels are achieved in approximately one hour. Disappearance in the plasma is rapid, with a half-life of about four hours; urinary recovery of unchanged drugs is less than 14 percent. Because of its potent immunosuppressive action, cyclophosphamide has been used clinically in Wegener's granulomatosis, rheumatoid arthritis, nephrotic syndrome in children, and other conditions associated with altered immune reactivity. Because gonadal suppression resulting in sterility has been observed and the mutagenic and carcinogenic potential is high, risks and benefits of this drug in patients with reproductive capacity should be weighed carefully. The phenylalanine derivative (melphalan) of nitrogen mustard is particularly useful in multiple myeloma, alone or in combination with other agents. It has the general pharmacological properties of an alkylating agent of intermediate strength, demonstrating activity in the blood for 6 h. The drug can be administered orally. Nausea, vomiting, and alopecia are infrequent. Chlorambucil is the slowest-acting nitrogen mustard in clinical use. In addition to its use in neoplastic disease, good responses have been reported in the treatment of vasculitis following rheumatoid arthritis and in autoimmune hemolytic anemias. Busulfan (Myleran) should be limited to chronic granulocytic leukemia, polycythemia vera, and myelofibrosis with myeloid metaplasia. Within 3 min, more than 90 percent of the drug disappears from the blood and is excreted in the urine almost entirely as the methane sulfonic acid and other metabolites. The myelosuppressive action of this drug is quite selective, affecting primarily granulocyte production and to some extent platelets.

The *nitrosoureas* are drugs with similar but not identical activity to other alkylating agents. Three of these compounds, 1,3-bis(2-chloroethyl)-1-nitrosourea (BCNU, carmustine), 1-(2-

TABLE 324-1
Commonly used anticancer agents

Drugs	Optimal dose when used alone*	Route and schedule	Marrow suppression	Acute toxicity	Other toxicity	Comments
ALKYLATING AGENTS						
Mechlor-ethamine	0.4 mg/kg	IV every 3-4 weeks	4 +	Severe nausea and vomiting	Vesicant to skin	Given in tubing of established infusion; used in full doses for intra-pleural or intra-peritoneal therapy
Cyclo-phosphamide	40 mg/kg	IV every 3-4 weeks	3 +	Nausea and vomiting	Alopecia and cysti-tis	Causes less severe thrombocytopenia than other alkylators
	3-1 mg/kg	Daily PO continuous	2 +	Minimal		
Melphalan	0.2-0.05 mg/kg	Daily PO continuous	3 +	Minor nausea and vomiting	Persistent thrombo-cytopenia after long use	Five-day schedule used for adjuvant treatment of breast cancer
	0.2 mg/kg	qd for 5 days every 4-6 weeks	3 +	Minor nausea and vomiting		
Busulfan	0.2-0.05 mg/kg	Daily PO continuous	3 +	None	Pigmentation, pulmonary fibrosis	
Chlorambucil	0.2-0.05 mg/kg	Daily PO	3 +	None	Pancytopenia with long-term use	
cis-Platinum	60-75 mg/m²	Every 3 weeks	1 +	Severe nausea and vomiting	Nephrotoxicity and ototoxicity	Adequate hydration and mannitol therapy used to prevent nephro-toxicity
BCNU	200 mg/m²	IV every 4-6 weeks	4 +	Severe nausea and vomiting	Tanning of skin, pulmonary fibrosis	Late marrow suppression occurring 4-6 wk after administration with nitrosoureas
CCNU	130 mg/m²	PO every 4-6 weeks	4 +	Nausea and vomiting	Cumulative marrow suppression	
MeCCNU	200 mg/m²	PO every 4-6 weeks	4 +	Nausea and vomiting	More pronounced thrombocytopenia	
Streptozotocin	500 mg/m²	1 h infusion daily for 5 days every mo	0	Nausea and vomiting, local pain at infusion site	Renal tubular acidosis; renal failure, hepatotoxicity	Dose monitored by presence or absence of protein-uria
Dimethylimidazole carboxamide	250 mg/m²	IV daily for 5 days every 3 weeks	3 +	Severe nausea and vomiting, flu-like syndrome	Cumulative marrow toxicity	
ANTIMETABOLITES						
Methotrexate: High dose with citrovorum factor rescue	2-10 g/m²	6-h infusion every 3-4 weeks	±	Nausea and vomiting	Renal failure	These doses lethal without rescue; serum levels should be monitored
Citrovorum factor for rescue	15 mg	Every 3 h for 8 doses, 2 h after methotrexate		None	None	Blood levels of methotrexate must be < 10⁻⁸ M before discontinuing citrovorum factor
Methotrexate doses not requiring rescue	80 mg/m²	IV, IM, or PO weekly	3 +	Minimal nausea and vomiting	Fatigue, buccal ul-cerations	Used for mainte-nance treatment of acute leukemia
	20 mg/m²	IV, IM, or PO twice weekly	3 +	Minimal nausea and vomiting	Buccal ulcerations	
	15 mg/m²	Intrathecal weekly in Elliot's B solution	0	None	Arachnoiditis, neurotoxicity	Monitor CSF methotrexate levels
6-Mercaptopu-rine	2.5-1 mg/kg	Daily PO continuous	2 +	Modest nausea and vomiting	Hepatotoxicity	Reduce dose to 25% with allopurinol

TABLE 324-1 *(continued)*
Commonly used anticancer agents

Drugs	Optimal dose when used alone*	Route and schedule	Marrow suppression	Acute toxicity	Other toxicity	Comments
ANTIMETABOLITES *(continued)*						
6-Thioguanine	2.0–1 mg/kg	Daily PO continuous	2+	Modest nausea and vomiting		No adjustment of dose required with allopurinol
5-Fluorouracil	12–7.5 mg/kg	IV daily for 5 days, then every other day to toxicity or weekly	3+	Chronic nausea, mucositis, diarrhea	Photophobia, alopecia, cerebellar ataxia	Oral use less effective; intrapleural use effective
Arabinosyl cytosine	200 mg/m²	IV daily for 5 days every 2–3 weeks	4+	Nausea and vomiting	Alopecia	Can be given subcutaneously
PLANT ALKALOIDS						
Vinblastine	0.3–0.1 mg/kg	IV every 1–2 weeks	3+	Minimal nausea	Minimal paresthesias, jaw pain	
Vincristine	0.033–0.025 mg/kg	IV every week for 6–8 weeks	1+	Minimal nausea, local necrosis at injection site	Paresthesias, motor weakness, alopecia, obstipation	Elderly and immobilized patients have more severe gastrointestinal toxicity
ANTIBIOTICS						
Dactinomycin	15 µg/kg	IV qd for 5 days every month	3+	Nausea and vomiting, mucositis	Alopecia, skin changes	Skin damage severe in irradiated areas
Mithramycin	50 µg/kg	IV every other day to toxicity	3+	Nausea and vomiting	Flushing of skin, hemorrhage	Stop therapy with ↑ lactic dehydrogenase or facial flush
	25 µg/kg	IV every week	0	None	None	Ideal for treatment of hypercalcemia
Daunorubicin	30 mg/m²	IV qd for 3 days every 2–3 weeks	4+	Nausea and vomiting, mucositis	Myocardiopathy	Not to exceed total dose of 600 mg/m²
Adriamycin	75 mg/m²	IV every 3–4 weeks	4+	Nausea and vomiting, mucositis, local reaction at injection site	Myocardiopathy, alopecia	Not to exceed total dose of 550 mg/m²
Bleomycin	15 units/kg	IV every week	1+	Minimal nausea and vomiting, fever, mucositis	Pulmonary fibrosis, skin changes, alopecia	Not to exceed total dose of 400 units
Mitomycin C	50 µg/kg	IV qd for 5 days every 3–4 weeks	3+	Nausea and vomiting, mucositis	Renal, pulmonary	Extravasation produces local injury
MISCELLANEOUS						
Procarbazine	200–100 mg/kg	Daily PO continuous	3+	Early severe nausea and vomiting subsides with use	Skin rash, side effects of monoamine oxidase inhibitors	CNS toxicity in large doses
L-Asparaginase	200 units/kg	IV daily for 14–28 days	0	Nausea and vomiting	Pancreatitis, CNS toxicity, hypofibrinogenemia	Allergic reactions occur with reusage
o,p'-DDD	2–10 g/day	Daily PO continuous	0	Severe nausea and vomiting	Mental depression, diarrhea, skin eruptions	Nausea and vomiting dose-limiting
Hexamethyl-melamine	10–6 mg/kg	Daily PO continuous	1+	Severe nausea and vomiting	Peripheral neuropathy	Limiting toxicity, nausea and vomiting, CNS toxicity at high doses
Hydroxyurea	25 mg/kg	Daily PO continuous	3+	Minimal	None	
	100 mg/kg	IV "push" every 3 days	0	Minimal nausea	None	Used to rapidly decrease blast counts

* *Suggested range of doses from starting to maintenance doses in previously untreated patients. Doses and intervals between doses of all myelosuppressive agents should be continuously adjusted by monitoring white blood cell and platelet counts. Doses differ where used in combinations and are reduced in previously treated patients with compromised bone marrow. Use of milligrams per kilogram of body weight or milligrams per square meter of body surface area is by convention.*

TABLE 324-2
Hormonal agents used in the treatment of cancer

Agents	Principal route of administration	Usual dose	Acute side effects	Other side effects	Indications
ANDROGENS					
Testosterone proprionate	IM	50–100 mg three times weekly	Fluid retention	Masculinization	Breast cancer: Pre- and postmenopausal women with ER(+) tumors; stimulation of erythropoiesis (6–12 weeks required for effect)
Fluoxymesterone	PO	10–20 mg/day	Fluid retention	Occasional hypercalcemia	
ESTROGENS					
Diethylstilbestrol	PO	1–15 mg/day	Nausea and vomiting, urinary incontinence	Feminization; uterine bleeding; increased mortality from heart disease in males; hypercalcemia	Prostate cancer: Dose not to exceed 1 mg diethylstilbestrol or 0.1 mg ethinyl estradiol per day; 70% respond with prolongation of life
Ethinyl estradiol	PO	0.1–3 mg/day			Breast cancer: Postmenopausal women with ER(+) tumors
ANTIESTROGENS					
Tamoxifen	PO	10–40 mg/day	Mild nausea	Rare thrombocytopenia and leukopenia; hot flashes; mild fluid retention	ER(+) breast cancer
PROGESTINS					
Hydroxyprogesterone	IM	1 g two times weekly			
6-Methylhydroxyprogesterone	PO	100–200 mg/day	Minimal fluid retention	Occasional hypercalcemia; thrombocytosis	Endometrial carcinoma; renal-cell carcinoma; ovarian carcinoma
	IM	200–600 mg two times weekly			
THYROID HORMONES					
Thyroxin	PO	To tolerance	None	Hyperthyroidism; arrhythmias; angina	Papillary adenocarcinoma of thyroid; 70% respond; many remain disease-free > 10 years
ADRENAL CORTICAL COMPOUNDS					
Prednisone	PO	40 mg/m² per day	Hyperglycemia, euphoria; fluid retention	Gastrointestinal bleeding, increased susceptibility to infection; immunosuppression; osteoporosis; hypokalemic alkalosis; hypertension	Lymphomas, leukemias, and multiple myeloma in combination with other drugs; CNS metastases and spinal cord compression to reduce swelling (high-dose dexamethasone)
Dexamethasone	PO	0.5–16 mg/day			
Methylprednisolone sodium succinate	IM or IV	10–125 mg/day			
Hydroxycortisone sodium succinate	IV	100–500 mg/day			

chloroethyl)-3-cyclohexyl-1-nitrosourea (CCNU, lomustine), and 1-(2-chloroethyl)-3,4-methylcyclohexyl-1-nitrosourea (MeCCNU, semustine), have been evaluated clinically and have been shown to have some effect against a variety of tumors; BCNU and CCNU have been used in the treatment of brain tumors and advanced Hodgkin's disease refractory to other agents, and MeCCNU and, in some cases, BCNU have been used in treatment of colon and stomach cancer. In a controlled trial in advanced colon cancer, the combination of MeCCNU and 5-fluorouracil (5-FU) was twice as effective in producing remissions as 5-FU used alone, but not in enhancing survival. This combination is being tested as an adjunct to surgery.

Disappearance of BCNU from the plasma after intravenous administration occurs within 5 min. CCNU and MeCCNU are given orally, and their metabolites have prolonged half-lives (16 to 48 h). Active metabolites, which produce either alkylation or carbamylation, are probably responsible for their cytotoxic actions; entry of these drugs into the cerebrospinal fluid

is rapid, and levels 15 to 50 percent of plasma concentrations are achieved. An unusual feature of these agents is the delay in myelosuppressive toxicity which develops 3 to 4 weeks after their administration. *Streptozotocin* is a naturally occurring nitrosourea which causes diabetes in experimental animals. The sugar moiety attached to a 1-methyl-1-nitrosourea apparently facilitates transport across the membrane of islet cells, an observation which led to its successful use in the treatment of islet-cell carcinoma of the pancreas. The half-life of the drug in plasma is approximately 15 min, and only 10 to 20 percent is excreted unchanged in the urine. Unlike the results with other nitrosoureas, bone marrow toxicity occurs in only 20 percent of cases and is usually mild; nephrotoxicity may be severe and is usually the dose-limiting factor. The presence of albuminuria between doses is used to monitor the administration of the drug. Dimethyltrizenoimidazole carboxamide (DTIC, dacarbazine) has alkylating activity after metabolic activation in the liver and is thought to act by cross-linking DNA. It is not cell cycle phase-specific. After intravenous injection, the plasma half-life is about 35 min, and 43 percent of the drug is excreted intact in the urine in 6 h. It has been reported to be effective in the treatment of malignant melanoma and is now being evaluated as an adjunct to surgical therapy. It is also an integral part of many treatment programs for soft-tissue sarcomas.

ANTIMETABOLITES An antimetabolite is a substance which resembles a normal metabolite so closely that it enters the same metabolic system but differs sufficiently that it interferes with normal metabolic pathways. Antimetabolites currently in use are methotrexate, 6-mercaptopurine, 6-thioguanine, 5-fluorouracil, and arabinosyl cytosine. Antimetabolites act primarily during the DNA synthetic phase of the cell cycle, some exclusively (arabinosyl cytosine) and others (methotrexate) by preventing further entry of cells into the DNA synthetic phase.

Folic acid antagonists Methotrexate was the first important antimetabolite to undergo clinical investigation. Folic acid, an essential dietary factor in humans, is reduced by the enzyme dihydrofolate reductase to dihydrofolic acid and tetrahydrofolic acid. The latter substance accepts single-carbon fragments to form the coenzymes. Several coenzymes exist which differ depending on the oxidation of the carbon fragment. One of these coenzymes, citrovorum factor (N^{10}-formyltetrahydrofolic acid) donates a single-carbon fragment to form deoxythymidine monophosphate, an immediate precursor of DNA. Although synthesis of RNA and protein is also inhibited by lack of tetrahydrofolate coenzymes, the thymidylate block is considered to be the most important site of cytotoxic action leading to "thymineless" cell death. Other "small-molecule" folate antagonists, pyrimethamine and cycloguanil, have been effective against malaria, and trimethoprim has been useful in bacterial infections of the urinary and respiratory tracts. Methotrexate is no longer commonly used orally but is readily absorbed after oral administration. The plasma half-life is approximately 2 h, and about 50 percent of the drug is bound to plasma proteins. Its toxicity may be increased through displacement from plasma albumin by a number of drugs including salicylates, sulfonamides, phenytoin, tetracycline, and chloramphenicol. At usual doses transport across the blood-brain barrier is very poor, and intrathecal administration (10 to 12 mg/m²) is necessary to obtain high concentrations in the cerebrospinal fluid. The major route of elimination is through the kidney, and 90 percent of the drug is excreted unchanged in the urine. Impaired renal function can produce a marked increase in toxicity. Intravenous or intramuscular doses of 25 to 50 mg can be given once or twice weekly. Constant daily infusions of much higher doses have been administered, but only when the technique of citrovorum "rescue" is used. The rationale for high-dose methotrexate is based on obtaining an excess of unbound intracellular drug and thereby inhibiting DNA synthesis almost completely. In order to achieve this, any deficiency of the active, carrier-mediated, transport system must be overcome by extremely high (10^{-3} to 10^{-4} M) extracellular concentrations of methotrexate. After drug infusions ranging from 6 to 30 h, citrovorum is given as an antidote in order to rescue normal cells and prevent undue toxicity in the host. The use of methotrexate in this fashion can be extremely dangerous. When administered by experienced chemotherapists, however, in laboratories capable of accurately measuring plasma methotrexate concentrations, these investigational regimens are surprisingly free of adverse effects. Since methotrexate precipitates in the renal tubules when the urine is acid, impaired excretion may result in life-threatening toxicity. Accordingly, maintaining a high output of alkaline urine is imperative.

Recently, a 7-OH metabolite of methotrexate has been identified as a potential renal toxin after high doses. Because of delayed clearance, high-dose methotrexate may cause extraor-

dinary toxicity in the presence of malignant effusions. Methotrexate is also effective in severe, recalcitrant psoriasis and as an immunosuppressive agent. In addition to bone marrow suppression, it causes ulcerative stomatitis and gastrointestinal toxicity. The adverse reactions can reach serious proportions and even cause death, particularly in the presence of preexisting folate and renal deficiencies. Other complications include dermatitis, alopecia, pulmonary interstitial infiltrates, and hepatic dysfunction, which sometimes eventuates in cirrhosis of the liver.

Purine analogues *6-Mercaptopurine* (6-MP) is a structural analogue of hypoxanthine which is converted to the active nucleotide 6-mercaptopurine ribosphosphate by the enzyme inosinic pyrophosphorylase. The nucleotide interferes with several steps in purine biosynthesis. It decreases the synthesis of 5-phosphoribosylamine, the first step in purine biosynthesis, by pseudofeedback inhibition. It also interferes with the conversion of inosinic monophosphate to xanthine monophosphate and the conversion of inosinic monophosphate to adenosine monophosphate. The drug is well absorbed after oral ingestion, and about 50 percent of the dose is recovered in the urine in 24 h, largely as 6-thiouric acid and inorganic sulfate. Attempts to inhibit this degradation led to the development of allopurinol (Zyloprim), a xanthine oxidase inhibitor capable of blocking the metabolism of 6-MP as well as the formation of uric acid from hypoxanthine and xanthine. Allopurinol has become an important agent in the management of hyperuricemia and gout. Although active as an immunosuppressive agent, 6-MP has been superseded by its imidazolyl derivative azathioprine (Imuran). Cholestatic jaundice has been reported from 6-MP in as many as one-third of adult patients; this is usually reversible upon discontinuation of therapy. Thioguanine (Tabloid) acts in a manner analogous to 6-MP; it is also significantly incorporated into DNA and RNA. After oral administration, peak blood levels are reached in 6 to 8 h, and approximately 40 percent of the dose is excreted in the urine in 24 h, mainly as inorganic sulfate and 2-amino-6-methylthiopurine, instead of 6-thiouric acid. Unlike 6-MP and azathioprine, no reduction in dose of thioguanine is necessary when used together with allopurinol.

Pyrimidine analogues 5-Fluorouracil (5-FU) and fluorodeoxyuridine (FUdR) block thymidylate synthetase, the enzyme involved in transfer of a methyl group from N^5,N^{10}-methylenetetrahydrofolic acid to deoxyuridylic acid (dUMP) in the synthesis of thymidylate and DNA. 5-FU must be converted to its active form 5-fluorodeoxyuridine monophosphate. Inhibition of RNA synthesis and incorporation into RNA also occur and may explain why these compounds are cycle-specific but not phase-specific agents. Clinically, 5-FU is used almost exclusively. Three hours after intravenous injection little 5-FU can be detected in the plasma. Catabolism occurs primarily in the liver. Approximately 15 percent of an injected dose of 5-FU appears intact in the urine, most of it within 1 h. Topical 5-FU as a 2 or 5% solution of propylene glycol or in a hydrophilic cream base, has been successful in eradicating premalignant actinic keratoses, as well as superficial basal-cell carcinomas.

Arabinosyl cytosine is a unique pyrimidine nucleoside analogue, with an alteration in the sugar moiety rather than the base. It interferes with DNA synthesis by inhibiting DNA polymerase. Its effects are exerted strictly during the DNA synthetic phase of the cell cycle. Structurally, it is related to deoxycytidine and is converted to the active nucleotide by the enzyme deoxycytidine kinase. Arabinosyl cytosine is metabolized by deaminase to uracil arabinoside which is excreted in the urine. The drug is incorporated into DNA and RNA. Twenty minutes after intravenous administration, the inactive metabolite uracil arabinoside accounts for 90 percent of the material in the urine. Studies in both animals and humans indicate that the schedule of administration markedly influences the antitumor effect and toxicity of this drug. Arabinosyl cytosine is a potent immunosuppressive agent and, depending on the dosage schedule used, can suppress either humoral or cellular responses or both. The major use of this drug is for treatment of acute myelocytic leukemia.

PLANT ALKALOIDS The alkaloids *vincristine* and *vinblastine* are derived from the periwinkle plant. They are cell cycle–specific and produce metaphase arrest in dividing cells by direct binding to tubulin and interference with the assembly of spindle proteins. Vincristine differs structurally from vinblastine only by replacement of a methyl group with a formyl group. Although they have similar activity, there are some important differences. Vincristine is capable of producing complete remissions in about 70 percent of patients with acute lymphoblastic leukemia, an accomplishment not observed with vinblastine. Vincristine and vinblastine are equally effective in Hodgkin's disease, while vincristine is superior to vinblastine in the lymphocytic and histiocytic lymphomas. Oral absorption of both drugs is unpredictable, and there is poor penetration of the blood-brain barrier by these drugs. Extravasation during intravenous injection may cause considerable irritation and sloughing. The compounds are cleared from the bloodstream in less than 1 h and are excreted primarily through the biliary system. Increased toxicity may be encountered in obstructive jaundice. Vinblastine causes bone marrow suppression and occasional gastrointestinal side effects, but neurological toxicity and alopecia occur less frequently than with vincristine. With vincristine, alopecia occurs in 20 percent of patients. The syndrome of inappropriate antidiuretic hormone secretion has been observed in patients treated with vincristine.

ANTITUMOR ANTIBIOTICS Antibiotics are substances produced by organisms which interfere with the growth of other living cells. The important antitumor antibiotics in clinical use are dactinomycin (actinomycin D), mithramycin, daunorubicin, adriamycin, and bleomycin. Dactinomycin was the first antibiotic used extensively in cancer chemotherapy. The drug forms a complex with DNA which inhibits DNA-dependent RNA synthesis. It is not cell cycle–specific. It has proved to be especially useful in the treatment of childhood malignancies, such as Wilms's tumor, neuroblastoma, rhabdomyosarcoma, and in trophoblastic tumors of women. Because of its immunosuppressive effects, it has been used in renal transplantation. The antitumor activity of *mithramycin* is limited to embryonal cell testicular tumors. The drug can also rapidly reduce serum calcium levels in patients with tumor-related hypercalcemia. This effect appears to be due to inhibition of bone resorption by the drug. Mithramycin inhibits DNA-dependent RNA synthesis, presumably by binding with DNA. The drug causes myelosuppression which results in thrombocytopenia, but additionally produces an acute hemorrhagic diathesis of uncertain etiology which appears to be fatal in about 5 percent of patients receiving the drug in full therapeutic doses. *Daunorubicin* and *Adriamycin* are anthracycline antibiotics with activity against a broad spectrum of animal and human tumors. Adriamycin has a broader antitumor spectrum and differs from daunorubicin only by the addition of a hydroxyl group. In animal tumor systems it has twice the therapeutic index of daunorubicin. The anthracycline antibiotics inhibit DNA synthesis and DNA-dependent RNA synthesis by binding with DNA with untwisting of the helix which facilitates intercalation. This distortion impairs the template activity of DNA. Both daunorubicin and doxorubicin (adriamycin) are administered intravenously in large intermittent doses and are rapidly cleared from the plasma. The disappearance curves are biphasic, with a short initial half-life of approximately 1 h and a long secondary half-life of about 17 h. There is rapid uptake of the drugs in the heart, lungs, kidney, spleen, and liver, but they do not cross the blood-brain barrier. Metabolic degradation occurs in the liver by an aldehyde reductase and a microsomal reductive glycosidase. Microsomal enzyme inducers enhance this process, and, conversely, severe toxicity may result if the drugs are administered as standard doses in the presence of impaired liver function. The drugs and their metabolites are primarily excreted in the bile and to a lesser extent in the urine. Patients should be advised that these compounds may impart a red color to the urine for 1 or 2 days after administration. Myelotoxicity is a major complication, and alopecia, stomatitis, and gastrointestinal manifestations are often found. Local vesicant action and tissue necrosis can occur if the drugs extravasate. A peculiar cardiomyopathy has been observed with these agents. Two variants of cardiotoxicity may occur; the first, an acute type characterized by abnormal electrocardiographic changes, includes ST-T wave changes and arrhythmias, which are brief and rarely a serious problem. Cineangiographic data have shown that an acute reversible reduction in ejection fraction occurs acutely, 24 h after a single dose. The second variant, chronic cumulative, dose-related toxicity manifested by congestive heart failure, unresponsive to digitalis, is probably a result of repeated acute cardiac insults and has a mortality in excess of 50 percent. Although the frequency of this variant of cardiomyopathy is less than 3 percent at total doses of adriamycin below 500 mg/m², it increases markedly in patients receiving total doses greater than 550 mg/m². With daunorubicin, the frequency of congestive heart failure is 1 percent at cumulative doses of 600 mg/m² but increases rapidly at higher doses. Previous cardiac radiation, cyclophosphamide, or other anthracycline antibiotic exposure increases the risk of cardiotoxicity. There are reliable tests to predict which patients will develop heart failure, and the onset of heart failure is often delayed, with 50 percent of the cases occurring 6 months from completion of therapy. The mechanism of this cardiomyopathy is unclear. The structural similarities of these agents to the digitalis glycosides and their binding to cardiac DNA, as well as oxidative damage they produce, probably relate to the quinone-hydroquinone moiety which has been shown to liberate free radicals and produce membrane damage. Cardiotoxicity is not too serious in patients with metastatic cancer who achieve only temporary remissions with the drug but should be considered a serious impediment to the use of these drugs in adjuvant therapy. *Bleomycin* is an antibiotic complex consisting of seven polypeptides of similar structure. Sixty percent of the mixture is bleomycin A₂, the most active moiety. Bleomycin inhibits DNA synthesis and reacts with DNA causing strand scission. It is most active against malignancies of the head and neck, skin, and penis, lymphomas, and testicular tumors where its use in combination with vinblastine has produced a remarkably high rate of complete remissions. Total courses exceeding 400 units are associated with pulmonary toxicity and should be given with great caution. Renal excretion is the primary route of elimination, and 20 to 40 percent of the active compound is recovered in the urine. Preferential localization of the drug due to failure of inactivation occurs in the skin and the lung; other tissues inactivate the compound by removing one mole of ammonia. This probably accounts for the selectivity of therapeutic and toxic effects. Bleomycin alone does not produce significant bone marrow depression. Lung damage is the most serious toxic effect. Although usually age- and dose-related, it occurs more frequently in individuals over 70, and at cumulative doses greater than 400 units. It may be encountered in younger subjects at lower doses, particularly when used in combination with other agents. It begins with a picture indistinguishable from pneumonitis, and, in 15 to 20 percent of cases, it may progress to pulmonary fibrosis, which has been fatal in about 1 percent of patients. As with the anthracycline antibiotics, the late toxicity appears to be a summation of acute insults to pulmonary tissue, since some patients complain of acute dyspnea with each intravenous dose. Because anaphylactic reactions have been observed in patients with lymphomas, administration of 2 units or less is recommended for the first two doses. *Mitomycin-C* (mutamycin) appears to cross-link DNA in a manner similar to alkylating agents after intracellular enzymatic reduction. It disappears rapidly from the blood after intravenous administration, with a 50 percent reduction of the blood level within 6 to 7 min. In adults, less than 10 percent is excreted as active drug in the urine and very little in the bile. The currently recommended dose is 50 μg/kg daily for 5 days, repeated for another 5 days, after a 10-day interval. The schedule may be repeated after recovery from hematologic toxicity. Myelosuppression is a major complication, and gastrointestinal, renal, pulmonary, and mucocutaneous toxicity also occur. Extravasation may produce severe local injury.

MISCELLANEOUS AGENTS Hydroxyurea is a simple derivative of urea which may be used as an alternative to busulfan in the treatment of chronic myelogenous leukemia. It is also useful for quickly reducing very high white blood cell counts in patients with acute myelogenous leukemia or chronic myelogenous leukemia in blastic crisis who have rapidly proliferating disease. A large dose will significantly reduce myeloblast counts within 24 h with the nadir occurring at 3 days. Hydroxyurea is rapidly absorbed from the gastrointestinal tract, and peak plasma concentrations are reached in 2 h. It is undetectable in the blood within 24 h. About 80 percent is recovered in the urine; the rest is probably metabolized in the liver. *Procarbazine* is a methyl hydrazine derivative. Its major use is for the treatment of patients with Hodgkin's disease, but it has some activity in oat-cell carcinoma of the lung. Procarbazine is not cross-resistant with other antitumor agents in animal tumor systems and is active in patients with Hodgkin's disease resistant to other drugs. Besides inhibiting monoamine oxidase, the drug undergoes autooxidation with formation of hydrogen peroxide leading to denaturization of DNA. In experimental systems, procarbazine causes decreased mitotic activity and chromatin breaks. It is rapidly absorbed from the gastrointestinal tract and readily equilibrates between the plasma and the cerebrospinal fluid. Because of rapid metabolism, primarily in the liver, its half-life in the blood is approximately 7 min, and in 24 h 25 to 40 percent is excreted as a metabolite in the urine. When used alone, the recommended oral daily dose is 50 to 300 mg/m². Notable immunosuppressive activity has been reported. Augmentation of sedative effects may accompany the concomitant use of central nervous system depressants. Ethyl alcohol may cause a reaction resembling the acetaldehyde syndrome produced by disulfiram (Antabuse). Since it is a weak monoamine oxidase inhibitor, the use of sympathomimetics, tricyclic antidepressants, and other drugs and foods with high tyramine content, such as bananas and ripe cheese, should be avoided. *Mitotane* (o,p'-DDD, Lysodren) is a derivative of the insecticide DDT that causes selective destruction of normal and neoplastic adrenocortical cells. It also modifies the peripheral metabolism of corticosteroids. Approximately 40 percent of the drug is absorbed after oral administration, and about 10 to 25 percent is recovered as a metabolite in the

urine. Blood levels are measurable for 6 to 9 weeks after cessation of therapy. The drug is distributed in all tissues; fat is the primary site of storage. The initial daily dose is 8 to 10 g, usually given in three to four portions. Maximum tolerated doses vary from 2 to 16 g per day. Treatment should be continued for at least 3 months. Gastrointestinal disturbances are common. Somnolence, lethargy, vertigo, and dermatitis also occur. Adverse reactions are usually reversible with reduction in dosage and do not contraindicate continuation of therapy. Discontinuation of the drug and administration of exogenous corticosteroids are indicated if shock or trauma supervenes. *L-Asparaginase* is an enzyme which converts L-asparagine to L-aspartic acid, depleting body stores of L-asparagine. Many experimental leukemias and lymphomas require exogenous L-asparagine, whereas normal tissues are able to synthesize the amino acid. Experimentally, a good correlation exists between the absence of L-asparagine synthetase and a requirement for exogenous L-asparagine. Furthermore, tumors which do not respond to L-asparaginase tend to undergo a marked increase in L-asparagine synthetase after exposure to asparaginase. L-Asparaginase was initially hailed as being a unique antitumor agent with activity specifically limited to tumors. This has been found to be incorrect; the drug interferes with protein synthesis, thereby causing a wide variety of toxic effects. At the present time, its major use is in the treatment of acute lymphoblastic leukemia. It causes pancreatitis as well as allergic reactions in some cases. It has been of value occasionally in the treatment of patients with malignant insulinomas, by suppressing the production of insulin, when other more standard agents have failed. *cis-Platinum* (cis-diamamine dichloroplatinum, DDP) consists of platinum coordination complexes which are a new class of cytotoxic agents. DDP is not cell cycle- or phase-specific and is capable of cross-linking DNA, although inactivation of DNA also occurs by other mechanisms. After intravenous administration, the initial half-life is 24 to 49 min, and the secondary half-life is 58 to 73 h. More than 90 percent of measured platinum appears to be protein-bound, and there is poor penetration into the central nervous system. During the first 5 days, 27 to 45 percent is excreted in the urine. Various dosage schedules are being studied for this investigational agent. From 50 to 75 mg/m² can be administered once every 3 weeks, or 15 to 20 mg/m² daily for 5 days every 3 to 4 weeks. In order to prevent dose-limiting renal toxicity, concomitant administration of intravenous fluids and mannitol, 37.5 to 60 g during a period of 6 to 8 h, with or without 40 mg furosemide, has been recommended. Its major toxic effects are gastrointestinal and renal toxicity and ototoxicity. Moderate myelosuppression may occur, and anaphylactic reactions, possibly related to DDP, have been reported.

ENDOCRINE THERAPY

The first demonstration of hormonal control of breast cancer was made in 1896 by Beatson, who induced regression of metastatic tumor by ovariectomy. Since then, it has become obvious that other tumors such as those originating in the prostate and uterine endometrium may respond to hormonal manipulation. The original concept that all hormonal action was mediated by metabolic modification of circulating hormones in the target tissue has been completely superseded since the discovery that receptors which bind with estrogens exist in the cytosol of normal and malignant cells. The mechanism of interaction of hormones and receptors has been carefully studied; apparently hormones bind to receptors in the cytoplasm and sterically alter the shape of the receptor protein itself which, after transport to the cell nucleus, interacts with DNA and is responsible for initiating specific messenger RNA and protein synthesis. Following this interaction, cytoplasmic receptor concentration is restored and the cycle can be repeated. Estrogen receptors (ER) can be quantitated as 8S and 4S proteins. Values for estrogen receptor in primary tumors in humans range from 0 to almost 1000 fmol/mg cytosol protein. The adrenal corticosteroids are unique among the steroid hormones because they exert some antitumor effect in tissues not normally considered to be endocrine organs, such as the malignant cells in acute lymphatic leukemia. Receptors for corticosteroids have been identified in the cytosol of leukemic cells which, along with other nonspecific effects of the corticosteroids, probably explains their antitumor action. Receptors are also known to exist for progesterones and androgens.

Breast and prostate cancers are normally managed either by ablating endocrine organs to remove the source of circulating hormones, which stimulate or support tumor growth or, alternately, by administering pharmacological doses of estrogens, androgens, progesterones, or glucocorticoids. Until recently, choice of hormonal therapy has been largely empirical and has been based on menopausal status, disease-free interval, site of dominant disease, and response to prior endocrine therapy. The knowledge that the majority of patients who are ER(+) will respond to hormonal manipulation and the majority of those who are ER(−) will not has altered this approach markedly. The following information has become important in developing management plans for individuals with metastatic breast cancer. (1) Patients with breast cancer who are ER(−) respond to hormonal manipulation in less than 5 percent of instances. (2) About 65 percent of patients who are ER(+) respond to hormonal manipulation, and the response rate increases to approximately 75 percent if progesterone-binding proteins can also be identified. (3) The absence of progesterone-binding proteins may explain the failure of up to 40 percent of patients who are ER(+) to respond to hormone manipulation, since a complete sequence of receptor proteins may be necessary for the highest degree of response. (4) Premenopausal women with breast cancer have a lower incidence of ER protein positivity and have quantitatively lower levels of binding protein in their cell cytosol. (5) Conversely, postmenopausal women have a higher incidence of ER positivity and quantitatively higher levels of ER protein in their cytosol. (6) Preliminary data suggest that breast cancer cells lacking the ER protein have a higher thymidine index (percent of cells incorporating [³H]thymidine into their DNA and going through the cell cycle) than cells possessing the receptor protein. Current data suggest that patients who are ER(+) respond less well to anticancer chemotherapy and that the converse is true for ER(−) patients.

These observations serve to emphasize two points. (1) Older studies on the use of additive or ablative treatment for breast cancer must be interpreted with caution because of the absence of precise information on the frequency of estrogen-binding protein in the study populations. For example, studies on *prophylactic* castration in the postoperative period need to be reinterpreted since probably less than half of the populations studied had ER-binding proteins. (2) Observations on the varying degrees of effectiveness of chemotherapy between pre- and postmenopausal women, in the postoperative period, may be explained in part by the frequency and quantity of the estrogen-binding protein in these patients. For example, the lesser response of postmenopausal women to chemotherapy that produces excellent results in premenopausal women may relate to the higher frequency and higher level of the estrogen-binding protein in postmenopausal women and the concomitant decreased growth (drug-sensitive) fraction. Although prostate

and uterine fundal cancers have been shown to possess binding proteins for their respective hormones, the correlation between the frequency and quantity of binding proteins and the response to hormonal therapy, has not been made. Hormonal agents useful in the management of these diseases are shown in Table 324-2.

ABLATIVE PROCEDURES Ablative surgery has been used extensively in women with breast carcinoma. Patients with recurrent ER(−) tumor, a short disease-free interval, hepatic metastases, lymphangitic spread to the lung, or refractoriness to prior hormone therapy should not be treated with ablative procedures; in them, chemotherapy is the preferred method. Castration is most beneficial to premenopausal women whose tumor is ER(+), in whom there has been a long interval between mastectomy and recurrence, or who have mainly osseous and soft-tissue metastases. Patients who do not respond to castration are unlikely to respond to additional endocrine manipulations and should be given chemotherapy. Over 50 percent of ER(+) patients who relapse after responding to castration respond to adrenalectomy and/or hypophysectomy. These procedures may also benefit postmenopausal women who have responded to estrogen therapy. The procedures are equally effective, and selection of one or the other should be based upon the patient's condition and the skill of available surgeons. The average duration of hormone response is 16 to 18 months. Castration is an especially useful procedure in men with breast carcinoma and results in a response rate of nearly 70 percent. With recurrence, 50 percent of these patients will respond to adrenalectomy or hypophysectomy. Nearly all patients with prostatic cancer will benefit for 2 to 3 years after orchiectomy. However, estrogens are equally effective. Orchiectomy should be reserved for patients in whom the speed of the response is critical. Estrogens provide no additional benefit when castration is employed.

ESTROGENS Although estrogens clearly have an antitumor effect, there is a risk of increased mortality from cardiovascular disease which may be related to an increase in production of renin substrate by the liver and subsequent hypertensive cardiovascular disease.

ANTIESTROGENS The discovery that certain estrogen analogues can antagonize estrogen stimulation of target tissue has been applied to the problem of breast cancer. Growth of dimethylbenzanthracene (DMBA) tumors in rodents can be inhibited by clomiphene and tamoxifen (Table 324-2). The ability of tamoxifen to cause regression of DMBA-induced tumors is highly correlated with the presence of estrogen receptors in the tumor. Antiestrogens have been found to bind to the estrogen receptor, translocate with the receptor into the nucleus, and initiate early estrogenic responses. A complete response to the complex apparently does not develop, and the genome remains refractory to the action of estrogens for a time. Some antiestrogens retain the receptor in the nucleus for many days in contrast to several hours for estrogens. Antiestrogens can effect a tumor response in patients who have estrogen-binding proteins in up to 60 percent of patients and have a lower incidence of troublesome side effects than estrogens. Virilization and fluid retention are uncommon with tamoxifen; the most common toxic effects noted are hot flashes, mild nausea, mild fluid retention, and, in a few instances, thrombocytopenia and leukopenia. With doses higher than are normally necessary (100 mg per day), corneal and retinal opacities have been observed. Tamoxifen has recently become available for clinical use in the United States.

ANDROGENS In older studies, androgen therapy is most effective in postmenopausal women with breast cancer, particularly those with osseous metastases. The effects of therapy are not seen for several weeks, but 90 percent of those responding will have begun to show a response within 8 weeks. All active androgens have been used with equal success. In comparative studies androgens have not been as effective as estrogens in the postmenopausal period except in patients with osseous metastases.

PROGESTINS Progestins are related to progesterone which is produced by the corpus luteum and placenta. They produce useful responses in 30 percent of women with metastatic endometrial carcinoma. Remissions may last for several years. The best results are seen in older women with well-differentiated tumors who have had a long interval between the appearance of the primary and recurrent disease. Useful responses are also seen in about 10 percent of patients with metastatic renal-cell carcinoma. Studies correlating response rates with the presence or absence of binding proteins for progestins have not been performed.

ADRENAL CORTICOSTEROIDS Prednisone is the adrenal corticosteroid most commonly used for antitumor therapy. It produces complete remission in about 60 percent of patients with lymphoblastic leukemia and partial responses in 70 percent of patients with chronic lymphocytic leukemia. It is also active against lymphomas and myeloma and in about 10 percent of patients with breast carcinoma. Responses in acute leukemia appear related to the presence of a specific corticosteroid-binding protein. In addition, adrenal corticosteroids suppress mitoses and cause lysis of normal and abnormal lymphocytic elements, presumably by inhibiting cellular protein synthesis. Their activity in breast carcinoma is presumed to be due to the suppression of estrogen production by the adrenal cortex.

MEDICAL ADRENALECTOMY An alternate method of ablating adrenal function is the use of aminoglutethamide, a potent inhibitor of the conversion of cholesterol to pregnanelone in the adrenal gland. It is given in a dose of 250 mg four times daily along with corticosteroid replacement. Since aminoglutethamide has been shown to accelerate the metabolism of dexamethasone, hydrocortisone 40 mg per day is the preferred steroid to use. With this approach, the response rate of patients with metastatic breast cancer has been equivalent to that reported after adrenalectomy. This regimen may be particularly useful in markedly debilitated women who have widespread bony metastases, in order to avoid surgical morbidity and mortality. Acute side effects of glutethamide, such as skin rash and lethargy, usually subside spontaneously, without cessation of therapy, and chronic therapy is remarkably free of side effects. Hypothyroidism occurs infrequently and can be managed by replacement therapy.

THYROID HORMONES Death from thyroid cancer occurs in less than 1000 patients per year in the United States, a figure that could easily be exceeded by surgical mortality if indiscriminate surgery for thyroid nodules were performed. Papillary carcinomas, even when metastatic to the neck, are often responsive to suppression of thyroid-stimulating hormone. Suppression of thyroid nodules presumed to be cancer, or suppressive therapy for patients with tumor in the thyroid or surrounding lymph nodes in the neck, is both indicated and effective.

IMMUNOTHERAPY

Since the host's immunologic system may be involved in the control of malignant process, immunologic approaches to cancer treatment are under investigation. In order to achieve an effect from immunostimulation in rodents, maximum tumor

reduction must be accomplished by surgery, radiation, or chemotherapy before immunotherapy is attempted. The host must be immunocompetent, and there may be an optimal, but as yet undefined, time following other treatment before immunotherapy is administered. Most antitumor agents are immunosuppressive, but as patients recover from the effects, their immunologic reactivity may be temporarily enhanced, and this could be the optimal time for immunotherapy. All immunotherapy is predicated on the identification of tumor-associated antigens on the cell surfaces of the tumor which can be used as the specific target for attack by immunocompetent cells or antibodies. While tumor-associated antigens have been identified in a multitude of animal tumors, only one clear-cut demonstration of tumor-specific antigens has been demonstrated in humans, that in patients with osteosarcoma, and in this tumor immunotherapy has not yet been shown to be useful. Other examples of supposed tumor-specific antigens identified on human tumor tissue are due to the inadvertent measurement of fetal antigens, expressed by benign and malignant human cells grown in tissue culture. There are two main approaches to immunotherapy—active and passive. Passive immunotherapy involves the transfer of immune serum from syngeneic, allogeneic, or xenogeneic hosts into tumor-bearing host. Active nonspecific immunotherapy has been attempted with substances such as bacillus Calmette-Guérin (BCG), the methanol-extractable residue of BCG (MER), and *Corynebacterium parvum*. These substances augment both cellular and humoral immunity. Experience with BCG suggests some therapeutic effect in preventing or delaying recurrences in malignant melanoma (stage II) after surgery and in prolonging drug-induced remissions in acute myelocytic leukemia for a brief period. Active specific immunotherapy consists of immunization of the host with tumor cells or cellular extracts. The greatest success has been achieved in animals by using live cells. Preimmunization prevents subsequent tumor transplantation in animals. Since most tumor antigens are weak, attempts have been made to enhance their antigenicity by coupling the antigens with another substance. It has been possible to demonstrate cytotoxic antitumor antibodies in patients immunized in this fashion. The studies with malignant melanoma and acute myelocytic leukemia have also included trials using inactivated cells plus BCG, but they are not superior to the use of BCG alone. The infusion of immune lymphocytes or their extracts into tumor-bearing hosts is known as *adoptive immunotherapy*. This approach has been used successfully in some animal tumors but not in humans.

Local immunotherapy utilizes delayed hypersensitivity reactions at the site of skin tumors. Local injection of BCG has eliminated skin tumors in animals. BCG injection into skin nodules in patients with recurrent breast cancer or melanoma is an effective way of controlling the local disease. The injection of BCG into the pleural space in patients with resectable epidermoid carcinoma of the lung has been shown to prevent or delay recurrence in one small controlled study. Larger clinical trials are in progress to confirm this observation. Delayed hypersensitivity has been produced in patients by cutaneous application of dinitrochlorobenzene. Subsequent application of this substance in superficial epidermoid and basal-cell carcinomas has a cure rate equal to topical chemotherapy with 5-fluorouracil. The macrophage plays an important role as a sensor cell in the modulation of the immunologic response to antigenic tumors in rodents. The macrophage also regulates other related physiological functions, such as granulocytopoiesis, through production of colony-stimulating factor. Studies aimed at stimulating macrophages are in progress with substances such as glucan, a polysaccharide product from yeast, and levamisole, an antiprotozoan drug that improves depressed lymphocyte function by stimulating macrophages. Early studies with levamisole as an immunostimulant have suggested some benefit in patients with stage III breast cancer, and studies to confirm this are in progress. There is also some suggestion that BCG, used in combined chemoimmunotherapy trials, may be responsible for earlier recovery of granulocytopoiesis than is normally noted after cancer chemotherapy. Immunotherapy in the control of human malignancies appears promising. However, this approach has not produced responses comparable with other therapeutic modalities in patients with visible metastatic disease. Considerable additional investigation is necessary before the role of immunotherapy in the management of cancer can be defined.

PRINCIPLES OF DRUG COMBINATION DESIGN

The potential circumvention of resistance to treatment has been an important factor prompting studies of drug combinations. Human tumors are heterogeneous, and, in contrast to many animal tumors, present with a relatively small percentage of cells in the active proliferating populations. Short-term treatment programs with single drugs in human beings cannot be expected to achieve maximum tumor cell kill regularly. Repeated therapy is required over long intervals, with greater risk of toxicity. Under these circumstances, repetitive exposure of tumor cells to chemicals can lead to clinical resistance to drugs. This poses two problems—the regrowth of tumor cells between cycles of therapy and reduced tumor cell kill with subsequent cycles of drug treatment because of the evolution of resistant cell lines. Largely on the basis of experimental evidence, various mechanisms for the development of resistance have been proposed (Table 324-3).

As has been well documented in the case of antimicrobials and bacteria, drug resistance can be a result of stepwise induction or may be related to the presence of a population of organisms inherently resistant to the drugs employed. This mechanism of resistance exists in populations of cancer cells because of clear-cut tumor heterogeneity, and an effective drug may be required for each distinct line of cells until the number of viable cells can be reduced to zero or "effective zero" (small-enough number of cells to be controlled, as with bacteria, by the host's own defense mechanisms). The success of drug treatment programs in rodents depends on the number of resistant

TABLE 324-3
Mechanisms of resistance to commonly used classes of antitumor agents

Mechanisms	Examples
Insufficient drug uptake by the neoplastic cell	Methotrexate Anthracyclines Actinomycin D
Insufficient activation of drug	6-Mercaptopurine 5-Fluorouracil Arabinosyl cytosine
Increased inactivation	Arabinosyl cytosine 5-Fluorouracil
Increased concentration of a target enzyme by induction or gene amplification	Methotrexate
Decreased requirement for a specific metabolic product	L-Asparaginase
Increased utilization of an alternative biochemical pathway (salvage)	Antimetabolites
Rapid enzymatic repair of a drug-induced lesion	Alkylating agents

lines in the tumor population and the number of available drugs that can be used effectively in combination. Pharmacological influences can be either advantageous or disadvantageous. The action of some drugs can be enhanced by other drugs with no antitumor effect by preventing the metabolic degradation of the active agent. The potential enhancement or depression of cyclophosphamide activity, by drugs that induce or inhibit the oxidative microsomal enzymes which convert the intact inactive parent compound into the 4-OH metabolite, has been recognized. Enhancement of the activity of 6-mercaptopurine by concomitant use of 4-hydroxypyrazolopyrimidine (allopurinol), which prevents its conversion into the inactive thiouric acid, and the prevention of deamination of arabinosyl cytosine and arabinosyl adenine by the ubiquitous deaminases present in serum and tissue by tetrahydrouridine and 2-deoxycorformycin, respectively, are additional examples of such drug interactions.

When drugs are used together in full doses, intermittent treatment at intervals of 2 to 4 weeks rather than continuous daily administration has been employed. Such an approach has two theoretical advantages. The first is that if the treatment programs exert a selective killing effect on tumor tissue over normal bone marrow, an interval of about 2 weeks is usually sufficient to allow recovery of bone marrow to pretreatment levels without allowing regrowth of the tumor population to base-line levels. The second advantage is that intermittent scheduling may permit the recovery of the host's immunologic mechanisms between cycles of chemotherapy.

The most important initial goal of the more intensive drug treatment programs is similar to the goals of surgery and radiation therapy for localized tumor—that is, to erase all clinical evidence of disease (complete remission). The length of time the patient remains free of disease after all therapy is discontinued is used as an indication of the magnitude of the reduction of tumor volume. These indicators of successful treatment have been valid, and survival has improved commensurate with an increase in the rates and duration of complete remission for many metastatic cancers when drug combinations have been compared with single agents.

TUMOR MARKERS A major obstacle to curative therapy of malignancy is the difficulty of guiding the duration and intensity of further therapy by measuring the small amounts of residual disease presumed to be present, following surgical resection or drug-induced remission. Attempts are being made to identify tumor-specific products in blood and urine that might serve as markers of neoplastic growth. The use of hormones, enzymes, or other proteins as markers requires that their plasma or urine concentration exceed an established upper limit of normal. The so-called "oncofetal antigens" have the same limitation—they are present in detectable concentrations in normal adults. In contrast, placental hormones, such as human chorionic gonadotropin (HCG), are not found in the blood of males and nonpregnant females. A measurable level indicates an underlying neoplasm until proved otherwise.

Oncofetal antigens are products of gene expression during fetal tissue differentiation. When full tissue specialization and organization are reached, these genes are normally repressed and remain inoperative in adult life. With neoplastic transformation of a cell, there may be a reactivation of genomes and a reappearance of embryonic antigens. Three such antigens are now in clinical use: carcinoembryonic antigen (CEA), α-fetoprotein (AFP), and pancreatic oncofetal antigen (POA). The CEA is a glycoprotein of 200,000 daltons molecular weight which is secreted onto the glycocalyx surface of the cells that line the normal gastrointestinal tract. When first discovered, CEA was thought to be specific for the digestive organs of the 2- to 5-month-old human fetus and for patients with colorectal cancer. It has, however, been detected in the feces of normal adults as well as the secretions of the colon and pancreaticobiliary systems. Elevated CEA is also found in patients with benign liver disease, such as alcoholic hepatitis or biliary obstruction, as well as alcoholic pancreatitis and inflammatory bowel disease—in this instance, obviating its possible use as a detector of secondary neoplastic transformation. It has also been found in patients with benign rectal polyps and chronic obstructive pulmonary disease. There is no threshold difference in CEA levels that serves to separate benign from malignant conditions. Because of overall lack of specificity and sensitivity, CEA cannot be used as a general diagnostic test for cancer. The principal role of this tumor marker is as a monitor of the response to treatment. Complete surgical resection, or successful radiation or chemotherapy, should bring an elevated plasma level to normal within 1 month following treatment. A persistent elevation, or a progressively increasing titer, is strong, but not definitive, evidence of residual or recurrent tumor. Elevations of plasma CEA above the normal of 2.5 ng/ml in healthy nonsmoking adults have been found in association with a wide variety of malignancies and, in particular, the entodermally derived neoplasms of the gastrointestinal organs and lung in 60 to 90 percent of patients. Approximately 50 percent of women with advanced breast cancer also have an elevation in CEA concentration. The principal factors that influence the incidence of positive tests and the height of the titer include:

1 *The extent of disease.* Eighty to ninety percent of patients with advanced metastatic colon cancer compared with 20 to 40 percent of cases with tumor confined to the colon wall will have positive tests.
2 *The differentiation of the tumor.* A lower incidence of positive tests is associated with anaplastic histology.
3 *The presence of hepatic metastases.* They are frequently associated with an abrupt elevation of CEA resulting from either impaired catabolism or excretion of the glycoprotein.

The *α-fetoprotein* is a 70,000-dalton molecular weight protein with alpha-electrophoretic mobility. It is synthesized by the liver, yolk sac, and gastrointestinal tract of the human fetus, reaching a peak plasma concentration by the twelfth to fifteenth week of gestation. It then gradually decreases to reach a normal adult level by the sixth to twelfth month after birth. Elevations in the plasma concentration of AFP have been found in association with hepatoma, and titers in excess of 40 ng/ml are present in 70 to 90 percent of patients using sensitive radioimmunoassays. Abnormal levels are also detected with teratocarcinoma of the testes and ovary and in extragonadal sites, including the mediastinum and retroperitoneum. In these tumors, AFP is thought to be produced in yolk sac elements. Patients with seminomas and the corresponding dysgerminoma of the ovary have normal blood levels of AFP. Elevated AFP levels have also been detected in a small percentage of patients with pancreatic carcinoma, gastric cancer, and lung cancer. As with CEA, AFP is not a specific market for malignancy, since abnormal titers are found in association with several benign conditions including viral and alcoholic hepatitis, ataxia telangiectasia, and hereditary tyrosinemia. The clinical application of this test is as a monitor for the effectiveness of anticancer treatment.

The pancreatic oncofetal antigen (POA) is a glycoprotein with a molecular weight of 800,000 daltons found in fetal and malignant pancreatic tissue but not in the normal pancreas. The index substance has, however, been detected in the blood of normal adults and in elevated concentrations in some patients with cancer of the lung, stomach, colon, and breast. The highest titers have been recorded in patients with pancreatic cancer, particularly those with well-differentiated histology.

Several placental proteins including HCG, human placental lactogen, and placental alkaline phosphatase (Reagan isoenzyme) have been demonstrated in cancer patients. Human chorionic gonadotropin is a glycoprotein hormone composed of dissimilar alpha and beta subunits; the alpha subunit is similar in primary structure to the alpha subunit of human luteinizing hormone, but sensitive radioimmunoassays of the beta subunit of HCG permit discrimination between the two hormones. Human chorionic gonadotropin is normally secreted by the trophoblastic epithelium of the placenta, and the presence of a detectable level in a male or a nonpregnant female is indicative of underlying tumor. In addition to the trophoblastic neoplasms of the placenta, the ectopic secretion of HCG has been found in 40 to 60 percent of patients with germ cell tumors, both gonadal or extragonadal, as well as in a smaller percentage of patients with adenocarcinoma of the ovary, pancreas, and stomach, hepatomas, and islet-cell carcinomas. Over 50 percent of patients with malignant insulinomas have elevations of HCG or one of its subunits; the hormone was not detected in association with benign adenomas. In patients with germ cell tumors secreting both HCG and AFP, discordant reduction after treatment suggests that the two markers are synthesized by heterogeneic clones of cells within the tumor.

The placental alkaline phosphatase is an isoenzyme synthesized in the trophoblast and is distinguished from other isoenzymes by heat stability (5 min at 65°C), electrophoretic mobility, and immunochemical specificity. Elevated placental alkaline phosphatase activity has been found in 5 to 15 percent of patients with cancer of the female reproductive organs, breast, and lung.

There are many tumors which, because of increased cellular mass and/or loss of the normal restraints on the rate of secretion, will produce excessive quantities of hormones or proteins that are normally produced by the cell of origin. Typical examples include the hypersecretion of insulin or gastrin by islet-cell neoplasms, the M spike in multiple myeloma, and the elevated serum acid phosphatase found in patients with prostatic carcinoma. There are many other tumors that will secrete index materials which are foreign to the cell or tissue of origin ectopically. In these instances, it is assumed that all somatic cells contain a full and equal genetic complement and that ectopic hormone secretion, after malignant transformation, results from the selected de-repression of a previously dormant gene. The abnormally elevated plasma or urine concentration then allows this material to serve as an indirect tumor marker. Examples include the secretion of adrenocorticotropic hormone (ACTH), antidiuretic hormone, and calcitonin by small-cell carcinomas of the lung; ACTH, vasoactive intestinal polypeptide, serotonin, and HCG by islet-cell carcinomas; and ACTH and serotonin by medullary carcinomas of the thyroid. Over the past 10 years it has become apparent that peptide hormones exist in precursor forms that may have little or no bioactivity when compared with the predominant circulating hormones. Examples include increased concentrations of proinsulin in the diagnosis of insulinoma and elevated levels of pro- or "big" ACTH, without clinical Cushing's syndrome, in many patients with lung cancer independent of histology. This phenomenon and related observations had led some investigators to suggest that ectopic hormone protein or hormone secretion is a universal accompaniment of cancer.

TREATMENT OF LOCALIZED OR REGIONAL TUMOR

SURGICAL THERAPY Development of the radical mastectomy by Halsted in 1894 provided the first and most enduring influence on cancer surgery. Halsted believed that all cancer was unifocal in origin and spread to adjacent structures by direct contiguity; hence he conceived the idea of en bloc resection. Since then, the same surgical principle has been applied to operations for a wide variety of visceral malignancies, and survival has indeed improved. However, survival, after surgery alone, reached a plateau by 1955. Increasingly radical surgery failed to provide additional benefits because even unifocal malignant tumors constantly shed cells even when tumor mass is below diagnostic levels. Cure after removal of the primary tumor alone, which certainly occurs, may seem inconsistent with persistent showering of tumor cells from all primary lesions. Current data, however, support three explanations for these events. (1) Only a fraction of cells in a tumor mass retain their capacity to create metastases (clonogenic cells), and after they have been shed, nonclonogenic cells may not continue to grow. (2) There is evidence that the host has the capacity to destroy small numbers of shed cells. (3) Tumor mass itself influences the tendency of tumors to metastasize and of the host to deal with residual microscopic metastases, with or without the help of systemic treatment. Surgery (and/or radiotherapy) of localized tumors may be effective because it reduces tumor volume, a source of clonogenic metastases, and thus also removes an adverse influence on the host defense mechanisms.

Surgery is considered the primary treatment for most early cancers (Table 324-4). However, in many patients the disease is not amenable to curative surgery. Many tumors are operable but not fully resectable, and some that appear resectable (control of T and N compartments, see Chap. 323) have micrometastatic disease which will recur eventually. This point can best be illustrated using colon and breast carcinoma as examples. Involvement of lymph nodes in breast cancer (stage II) and colon cancer (Duke C) is associated with low 5-year survivals. Failure occurs because of the presence of undetected micrometastases at the time of surgery. Increasingly radical surgery in both these cancers has been unable to provide additional benefit. Unlike surgical approaches to colon cancer, in breast cancer the visible mutilation of the radical mastectomy is significant. There is considerable evidence, however, that lesser surgical procedures, including segmental resection, give results as good as are obtained with radical mastectomy, including survival. Moreover, most data on the surgical management of primary breast cancer have been generated in uncontrolled trials, and reports of the controlled trials of the National Surgical Adjuvant Breast Program (NSABP) suggest that a total (simple) mastectomy may be sufficient for patients in clinical stage 1 ($T_1N_0M_0$) and either total mastectomy, or total mastectomy plus radiotherapy, may be sufficient for patients in stage II ($T_1N_1M_0$).

Surgeons also perform procedures for staging purposes only, such as laparotomy in Hodgkin's disease and other lym-

TABLE 324-4
Role of available treatment modalities in *localized* and *regional* forms of some visceral and hematologic malignancies

Original cancer	Surgery*	Radio-therapy	Chemo-therapy	Immuno-therapy
Breast:				
Stage I	P	Alt	ND	ND
Stage II	P	Alt	P†	E
Ovary:				
Stage I	P	Adj,E‡	E	ND
Stage II	P	Adj,E	E	E
Uterine fundus	P	Adj	ND	ND
Uterine cervix:				
In situ	P	P	NU	NU
Stage I	P	P	NU	NU
Stage II	P	P	E	ND

TABLE 324-4 *(continued)*
Role of available treatment modalities in *localized* and *regional* forms of some visceral and hematologic malignancies

Original cancer	Surgery*	Radio-therapy	Chemo-therapy	Immuno-therapy
Choriocarcinoma	Adj	NU	P	ND
Lung:				
Small (oat) cell	NU	Adj,E	P	E
Epidermoid	P	Adj	E	Adj,E
Adenocarcinoma	P	Adj	E	E
Gastrointestinal:				
Colon	P	NU	E	E
Rectum	P	Alt,E	E	E
Stomach	P	Adj	E	ND
Pancreas	P	Adj	E	ND
Melanoma:				
Stage I	P	NU	NU	E
Stage II	P	NU	E	E
Other skin cancers	P	P	P	P
Head and neck	P	P	E	E
Thyroid:				
Papillary	P	Adj‡	P§	NU
Follicular	P	Adj‡	P‡	NU
Anaplastic	Adj	P	Adj,E	ND
Testes:				
Seminoma:				
Stage I	P	P	ND	ND
Stage II	Alt	P	ND	ND
Embryonal and teratocarcinoma:				
Stage I	P	Adj,E	ND	ND
Stage II	P	Adj,E	P	ND
Choriocarcinoma	P	NU	P	ND
Prostate	P	Alt	E	ND
Bladder:				
Papillomas	P	Alt	Alt	E
Others	P	Alt	E	E
Kidney	P	Adj	ND	ND
Brain	P	Alt	E	E
Tumors of childhood:				
Wilms's tumor	P	Adj	P	ND
Neuroblastoma	P	Adj	E	E
Ewing's sarcoma	Alt	P	P	E
Rhabdomyosarcoma	P	Alt,E	P	E
Lymphomas:				
Hodgkin's disease:				
Stage I	NU	P	E	ND
Stage II	NU	P	E	ND
Stage III	NU	Alt	P	ND
Lymphocytic:				
Stage I	NU	P	ND	ND
Stage II	NU	P	E	E
Stage III	NU	Alt	P	E
Histiocytic:				
Stage I	NU	P	ND	ND
Stage II	NU	P	E	ND
Stage III	NU	Alt	P	ND
Mycosis fungoides	NU	P	P	E
Solitary plasmacytomas	Alt	P	Alt	ND

* *For purposes of this table, diagnostic biopsy is not considered treatment when used prior to an alternate method of treatment.*
† *For premenopausal women only.*
‡ *Radioisotopes.*
§ *In the form of thyroid suppression of TSH production.*
NOTE: *P = Considered an integral part of standard primary treatment programs. Alt = An alternate, although less commonly used, method of primary treatment for which data are already available indicating results equivalent to more common approaches. Adj = Use an adjunctive therapy after localized tumor is treated by a primary method; routine use is not considered essential. E = Experimental; role in treatment is under examination in controlled clinical trials. Either a new approach to treatment or an older approach which, in the absence of sufficient data to support its frequent use, is being evaluated in controlled clinical trials. In the latter case, treatment is designated Alt,E. NU = Current information indicates no role in primary treatment program. Control rate of tumor in question may be sufficiently high with other forms of treatment as to preclude testing of this modality. ND = No data available to evaluate this form of treatment.*

phomas. Indications for use of these procedures vary with treatment options, and they should never be performed by the surgeon in vacuo, without prior consultation with the physician, or team of physicians, who will eventually be called upon to provide the definitive treatment.

Indications for more mutilating radical surgical procedures such as hemicorporectomy, pelvic exenteration, and radical head and neck surgery vary. They are offered to patients with locally advanced primary tumors or locally recurrent tumors for which no systemic treatment is available. If the patient fully understands the degree of mutilation involved, a careful search reveals no metastases, the risk of recurrent disease is not unreasonable, and the operation is technically feasible, then the risks of mortality must be weighed against the chance of tumor control. These are very personal decisions made among the patient, the family, and the physician. Significant advances in reconstructive surgery of the head, neck, and pelvic regions have been made, and greater availability of more acceptable prostheses may make these radical procedures more acceptable.

RADIATION THERAPY Radiation therapy is a regional form of treatment primarily evolved for the control of localized cancers. The ideal in radiation therapy of malignant disease is achieved when the tumor is completely eradicated and the surrounding normal tissues, in the treated volume, show little or no evidence of structural or functional injury. The important factor in successful treatment is the difference in radiosensitivity of neoplastic and normal cells. The difference depends on the capacity for intracellular repair of normal and neoplastic cells and the ability of normal organs to continue to function well if they are only segmentally damaged. If surrounding tissue can tolerate twice the radiation dose of a given tumor, then the tumor is radiosensitive. On the other hand, tumor which extensively involves both lungs, and may be cured by a dose of 3000 rads, cannot be treated effectively with radiation therapy because of the greater radiosensitivity of the surrounding lung tissue. As with normal tissue, however, different tumors have a range of radiosensitivity, some being responsive to as little as a few hundred rads, and others incurable with as much as 10,000 rads. The physician should be familiar with normal tissue tolerance for radiation and the acute and late effects of radiation. Acute radiation effects such as nausea and vomiting, mucositis, and blood count depression may appear during or near the end of treatment and usually are completely reversible. Others, such as pneumonitis, may not appear until several weeks or months later and then resolve. Late radiation effects continue to progress with time and are often irreversible.

Normal tissues and organs differ in radiosensitivity. The risk of complications increases with the dose and, if delivered by megavoltage sources, in the usual fractions, occurs when the dose exceeds the following: both lungs, 1500 rads; both kidneys, 2400 rads; liver, 3000 rads; heart, 3500 rads; spinal cord, 4000 rads; intestine, 5500 rads; brain, 6000 rads; bone, 7500 rads.

Treatment with radiotherapy instead of surgery, using more sophisticated equipment, has the advantage of less mutilation and, where it provides equivalent results, is the preferred approach (Table 324-4). This choice will depend a great deal on the expertise in a given institution. For example, in the treatment of stage I carcinoma of the cervix, either modality provides equal survival rates. In localized carcinoma of the vocal cords, because radiotherapy has a high cure rate and spares the vocal cords, it is preferred to surgery. In carcinoma of the prostate, with stages A and B, radiotherapy produces survival figures at least equivalent to surgery, with far less risk of impotence, and is the preferred approach. In carcinoma of the rec-

tum below the peritoneal reflection, radiotherapy alone in small, nonulcerated, and superficial lesions is quite effective in controlling the tumors; radiotherapy can improve survival figures when used in conjunction with surgery in patients with rectal cancer with more extensive disease. In patients with localized Hodgkin's disease (stages I and II) radiotherapy is the treatment of choice, with 5- and 10-year disease-free survivals achievable in 80 percent of such patients. In lymphocytic and histiocytic lymphomas cures are possible in patients with truly localized disease.

In some cases the routine use of radiotherapy as an adjunct to surgery should be avoided. Postoperative treatment of the chest wall and lymph node areas in carcinoma of the breast after radical mastectomy adds nothing to the results of surgery, does not improve survival, but does cause significant morbidity. Since local recurrences rarely happen in the absence of systemic metastases, and local recurrences can be controlled, when they arise, by radiotherapy or drug treatment, routine postoperative radiotherapy regardless of the location of the primary tumor cannot be recommended in breast cancer. Radiotherapy alone in stage IIB carcinoma of the ovary (limited to the pelvis) should be discouraged since further drug therapy is usually required. Its use as the primary treatment in stage III ovarian cancer (widespread intraabdominal disease) is also contraindicated. Routine radiotherapy in lung cancer has been ineffective, except in rare instances, although it may complement the increasingly effective drug treatment of small-cell carcinoma. The use of routine retroperitoneal radiotherapy after lymphadenectomy for testicular cancer is questionable except in patients with seminomas where even metastatic lesions can be controlled by radiotherapy. Routine preoperative or postoperative therapy of stage I uterine fundal cancer may not offer additional benefit to surgery.

TREATMENT OF ADVANCED CANCER

Treatment of advanced cancer began in the late 1950s. In early trials, marginal clinical usefulness of drugs was found. These studies were flawed by the stereotyped approach to the treatment of all cancer patients which used minimal daily oral doses of drugs, and treatment for short fixed periods of time, all of which tend to minimize the capacity of drugs to kill cancer cells and set up ideal circumstances for the development of drug resistance. With the identification of firm principles to guide the development of treatment programs, based on the biology of tumor growth and the pharmacokinetics of antitumor agents, the clinical results have improved dramatically. The most important aspect of cancer chemotherapy trials conducted in the 1960s, and realized in the early 1970s was the demonstration that drugs could cure patients with advanced cancer. Considering the volume of cancer cells now known to be present in such patients, this presented a formidable challenge. For reasons that are not yet clear, the most effectively treated cancers are those that occur less often and in younger persons.

Cancers can be generally grouped into categories according to the effectiveness of systemic treatment. Table 324-5 lists 12 types of cancer for which current chemotherapeutic programs can render a fraction of patients with metastatic tumor free of disease long enough to be considered cured. Exclusive of skin cancer, which is treated when localized, the numerical impact of therapy on a national mortality ratio from cancer is relatively small since the diseases listed make up only 10 percent of all patients with cancer and 8 percent of all cancer deaths. Successful application of the best available treatment programs, however, can save approximately 15,000 lives per year. Although most of these tumors are not common, they occur at a relatively young age, and their impact in person-years of life or person-years of work lost is larger than their numerical impact suggests. Although in some cases (choriocarcinoma and Burkitt's tumor) excellent results are achievable with highly effective single drugs, in most cases cures are achievable only by drug combinations. The unique feature of the survival curves in these diseases is the long flat tail indicating disease-free survival beyond the high-risk period of recurrence, after therapy is discontinued, as illustrated in advanced diffuse histiocytic lymphoma (reticulum-cell sarcoma, Fig. 324-5). In Hodgkin's disease, acute childhood leukemia, diffuse histiocytic lymphoma, and testicular tumors disease-free survival after cessation of treatment extends to over 10 years. Considering the tumor volume in most of these patients at the time of treatment ($\pm 10^{11}$ cells), these results are quite remarkable. The break in the survival curve varies for each disease. A 2-year disease-free interval from the end of treatment is sufficient to consider patients with such virulent, rapidly growing tumors as choriocarcinoma, Burkitt's lymphoma, and diffuse histiocytic lymphoma cured, while four or more years is necessary to evaluate the results of treatment in Hodgkin's disease, acute childhood leukemia, and testicular cancer. Widespread use of these treatment programs has already resulted in a decrease in national mortality in all patients with Hodgkin's disease, in acute leukemia in children less than 15 years of age, and in renal and bone tumors of children. In ovarian carcinoma, a small fraction of patients with advanced intraabdominal tumor (stage III) remain free of disease over long periods after successful treatment with alkylating agents. Earlier use of chemotherapy holds promise in this disease. Slow but steady progress is being made in the treatment of acute myelocytic leukemia. The complete remission rate attainable with drug combinations is now in excess of 50 percent, and 10 percent of treated patients survive, free of disease, without any therapy, beyond 5 years of treatment with minimal risk of recurrence. The improvement in recent years is coincident with the identification of arabinosyl cytosine and adriamycin as active agents in this disease and appreciation of the schedule dependency of arabinosyl cytosine. Immunotherapy appears to have played a role in briefly prolonging drug-induced remissions, and retreatment of patients in remission for 2 years (late intensification) holds promise of the control of the cellular phase of the disease.

FIGURE 324-5

Survival in advanced diffuse histiocytic lymphomas treated with combination chemotherapy. Patients who achieve a complete remission relapse uncommonly. The high-risk period of relapse is the first 2 years after treatment. Patients with partial responses, even if they are associated with greater than 75 percent reduction of tumor volume, rarely survive beyond 2 years.

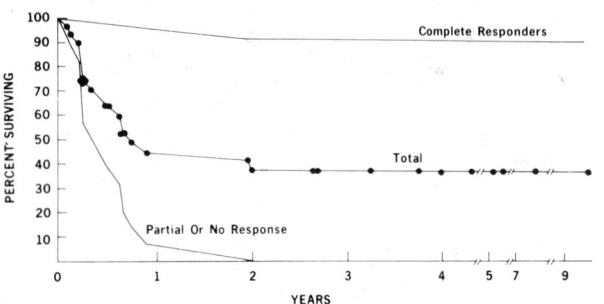

In Table 324-6, the cancers listed make up 26 percent of all tumors in the United States and an equal percentage of all cancer deaths. In each of the tumor types listed it is possible to achieve sufficient responses to chemotherapy to prolong life of a fraction of these patients and palliate the majority of the rest. In most examples cited, however, the complete remission rate is low, and long disease-free survivals are uncommon when treatment is discontinued. Although drug combinations used

TABLE 324-5
Metastatic cancers curable by chemotherapy*

Diseases	Complete remission rates, %	Comments
Acute lymphoblastic leukemia of childhood	90	80% of null-cell and 50% of all patients remain free of disease > 10 years.
Hodgkin's disease, stages III and IV	80	65% of cell complete responders and 90% of asymptomatic patients remain disease-free at 10 years.
Diffuse histiocytic lymphomas, stages III and IV	50	80% of complete responders remain disease-free at 10 years.
Nodular mixed lymphomas	75	80% of complete responders remain disease-free off all therapy beyond 10 years.
Testicular carcinoma (exclusive of seminomas)	75	70% of complete responders remain disease-free beyond 3 years.
Ovarian carcinoma, stages III and IV	35	Half of complete responders remain disease-free as long as 10 years.
Acute myelocytic leukemia	60	20% of complete responders living without recurrences, off therapy, beyond 5 years.
Choriocarcinoma	90	Almost all complete responders remain free of tumor; longest follow-up 20 years.
Burkitt's lymphoma	90	Half of complete responders remain free of recurrences beyond 10 years.
Wilms's tumor		Primary treatment is multimodal. Surgery, radiation, and chemotherapy together now produce 80% cure rate. Latest data indicate surgery and chemotherapy alone can do the same.
Ewing's sarcoma		Primary treatment is multimodal. Use of radiation and chemotherapy produces relapse-free survival in two-thirds of patients at 5 years.
Embryonal rhabdomyosarcoma		Primary therapy is multimodal. Surgery, radiation, and chemotherapy produce disease-free survival in 60% of patients at 5 years.

* *Cancers on this list occurred approximately 46,000 times in 1977. In 32,000 instances, patients had visible metastatic disease. Currently available chemotherapy, mostly given as combinations of drugs, can render one-third to one-half of the patients with metastatic disease free of tumor for periods long enough to consider these patients cured of their tumor. The results listed in this table represent best available data from centers studying these diseases. Because of the availability and effectiveness of systemic treatment in some of the cancers listed, all effective treatments have been integrated into the primary treatment plan (multimodal primary treatment). Skin cancer is not included since it rarely metastasizes. It occurs 300,000 times per year and is highly treatable with topical chemotherapy.*

in metastatic breast cancer have not yielded long disease-free survivals, for the first time patients treated with many current drug combinations are able to attain complete remissions. Furthermore, these programs have been successfully applied in patients with minimal residual disease (stage II) postoperatively.

Tumors listed in Table 324-7 are frequently thought of as resistant to treatment, but significant palliation can be provided for most patients by the careful use of existing chemotherapeutic agents by an experienced physician. Although studies of large groups of patients with these diseases have not revealed improvement in average survival, a small number of patients with each of these tumors can experience long disease-free survival as a result of the meticulous use of chemotherapy. Of particular interest is the identification of the usefulness of methotrexate, bleomycin, and the investigational agent, *cis*-diamine dichloroplatinum, in combination, in patients with cancer of the head and neck. This approach offers particular promise because it may prevent recurrences and allow the use of less radical surgical procedures in this critical area of the body. In colon cancer, controlled studies have demonstrated a doubling of the response rate of patients who have metastatic disease when treated with the combination of 5-FU and MeCCNU when compared with the use of 5-FU alone, and improvement in survival has been demonstrated. The nitrosoureas are a useful adjunct to radiotherapy and surgery in patients with the malignant gliomas, with a doubling of median survival time of patients so treated.

Surgery has an increasingly important role in the treatment of patients with advanced metastatic cancer. Surgery is important to reduce tumor bulk and facilitate the use of drugs or immunotherapy. This may involve removal of a primary tumor when metastases are known to be present (renal-cell carcinoma) or reduction of the bulk of retroperitoneal and mesenteric lymph nodes in testicular and bowel tumors, and mesenteric metastases in ovarian cancer. Not to be overlooked is the surgical attack on metastases in patients who are otherwise doing well. Seemingly solitary brain metastases should be removed surgically, if possible, particularly in young people, since the likelihood of rapid demise without such treatment is high and occasional long-term control is possible. Pulmonary metastases of a variety of sarcomas have been successfully controlled surgically even when multiple nodules are present. Some of these patients have remained free of recurrent disease for periods in excess of 2 years with surgery alone. This has been true particularly in patients whose tumors can be shown to have long doubling times prior to operation. These studies have added significance with the recent development of more effective systemic treatment of sarcomas which can be used following surgery to supplement tumor bulk reduction. Re-

moval of metastases to the lungs is important in patients with testicular tumors because of the histological heterogeneity of this tumor and the likelihood that a metastasis has resulted from growth of a clone of a histological type resistant to the drugs employed.

Surgeons are often asked to provide palliation for patients incurable by any modality. The operative risks are often high and the therapeutic yield, from the surgical point of view, low, but considerations of comfort and ability to return home during the terminal months of illness may make such procedures worthwhile. Palliation should be considered, for example, in intestinal obstruction in ovarian cancer, gastrointestinal bleeding, urinary diversions, and relief of pain through neurosurgical procedures. The primary physician is often in the best position to make the decision as to the feasibility of such palliative procedures.

Radiotherapy can also be used to reduce tumor bulk in patients with metastatic disease and decrease the extent of any surgical procedure that might be used in addition. Examples are radiation therapy following lumpectomy in breast cancer and in conjunction with surgery in head and neck, and rectal cancers. In highly radiosensitive tumors, radiotherapy may be used to reduce tumor bulk in patients with advanced metastatic cancers whose primary treatment is with drugs, as in patients with lymphomas. Prophylactic use of radiotherapy to treat the brain and meninges before disease is evident has been successful as an ancillary method to drug treatment and has resulted in prolonged disease-free survival in children with acute leukemia and Ewing's sarcoma and holds promise in oat-cell carcinoma of the lung.

Palliative radiotherapy has many applications in patients with metastatic cancer. In emergency situations, it can be used to provide rapid relief of superior mediastinal obstruction in conjunction with drugs or to relieve ureteral obstruction in patients with lymphomas or testicular tumors which are drug-resistant. It can provide frequent and useful relief of bone pain and may prevent fracture if used prophylactically to treat lesions of weight-bearing bones. In these cases the primary treatment is usually with drugs, and radiation fields should be only as large as required to control the lesion in question. For lytic lesions of weight-bearing bones greater than 2.5 cm in diameter, especially those involving the cortex, prophylactic internal fixation, followed by radiation therapy, is the treatment of choice. Radiation of the brain and spinal cord are important examples of palliation which, when used early and effectively,

TABLE 324-6
Malignant diseases which, when widely disseminated respond sufficiently to systemic treatment that the lives of responding patients are prolonged greater than 1 year*

Carcinoma of the breast
Multiple myeloma
Lymphocytic lymphoma
Prostatic carcinoma
Adrenal cortical carcinoma
Malignant insulinoma
Small-cell (oat-cell) carcinoma of the lung
Sarcoma of soft tissue
Endometrial carcinoma
Malignant carcinoid tumors
Neuroblastoma
Chronic lymphocytic leukemia
Chronic myelocytic leukemia

* *In most examples cited, systemic chemotherapy is able to induce a variable fraction of complete remissions, but eventually most patients who had complete responders develop recurrent tumors. Cancers on this list occur about 60,000 times per year in the United States (1977 figures).*

TABLE 324-7
Malignant diseases which, when widely disseminated, respond to chemotherapy, but, although palliation is often provided, response to drugs in such patients after treatment has not yet been shown to prolong their lives*

Epidermoid carcinomas of the head and neck region
Carcinoma of the colon
Carcinoma of the stomach
Brain tumors
Malignant melanoma
Hypernephromas
Carcinoma of the bladder
Hepatocellular carcinoma
Undifferentiated thyroid cancer
Carcinoma of the cervix uteri
Osteosarcomas
Carcinoma of the penis

* *Complete remissions are uncommon. It should be noted that the treatment programs producing marginal response in these patients, when they have metastatic disease, offer attractive opportunities to test the use of these drugs as adjuvant chemotherapy when the tumor volume is smaller.*

can prevent catastrophic neurological incapacitation in the final months of illness.

MULTIMODAL PRIMARY (ADJUVANT) TREATMENT

A major reduction in mortality from many of the major cancers appears likely only if current drug programs are markedly improved or are applied in the postoperative period to the treatment of those 220,000 patients who develop recurrences after surgery or radiotherapy. In such circumstances these programs should have the added effect of allowing the investigation of less mutilating surgical approaches. Considerations of tumor growth and biology and the importance of tumor cell volume to the dose-response curves of both radiation and chemical treatment serve as the rationale for the use of more than one modality in the postoperative period. The four most important considerations in the development of drug programs for post- or perioperative use are the following: (1) the identification of population of patients who, even after optimal surgery or radiotherapy for their primary disease, have a high risk of recurrence and death from their cancer (e.g., stage II breast cancer, Duke C colon cancer); (2) the availability of a proved useful systemic form of treatment; (3) the weighing of the potential benefits of treatment against short- and long-term risks of added drug treatment, keeping in mind that a fraction of patients exposed to adjuvant drug treatment would not have developed recurrent tumor; and (4) proper study design. Since the response of measurable tumor is not possible during adjuvant studies, few can be accepted unless comparisons of treated groups are made with untreated controls, or the risk of recurrence is known to be very high and is spread over so narrow a time frame as to obviate the need for concurrent controls. In the latter case, historical controls may suffice. An example of such a tumor is osteogenic sarcoma where, historically, 80 percent of patients develop recurrences within 18 months of amputation. On the other hand, an example of a tumor requiring controls in adjuvant studies is stage II $(T_1N_1M_0)$ melanoma. Sex, site, level of invasion of the primary, and degree of nodal involvement all affect not only the risk but the time of recurrence, which may be spread over periods of a few months to several years.

The most difficult question is the level of effectiveness required of systemic therapy in patients with advanced metastatic tumor before it is feasible to use it in an adjuvant program. There is uncertainty whether drugs which are apparently inactive against advanced cancer are potentially useful against a small number of cancer cells present in the postoperative period when tumor growth characteristics, and therefore vulnerability to drugs, may be different. Clinical studies have shown that changes in measurements of tumor masses in patients with metastatic disease are sufficiently variable that response rates of 10 percent or less in drug-treated patients should be considered "biological noise." Presently, only single agents or combinations of drugs with response rates of 20 percent or more can be considered acceptable for postoperative drug programs. The attractiveness of a candidate drug program is enhanced considerably if a significant fraction of treated patients attain complete rather than partial responses since complete disappearance of visible tumor indicates a greater log reduction in the number of tumor cells.

In Hodgkin's disease, the fact that radiotherapy for localized tumor and combination chemotherapy for advanced disease have worked so well has led to studies of both used together in patients with regional tumor only (chemotherapy as an adjuvant to radiotherapy) and in advanced tumors to reduce tumor bulk (radiotherapy as an adjuvant to chemo-

therapy). In localized diffuse histiocytic (reticulum-cell sarcoma) and lymphocytic lymphomas, recurrence of tumor outside the radiation field is common when radiation therapy is used alone. In diffuse histiocytic lymphoma, the fraction of patients with advanced cancer (stages III and IV) achieving long disease-free survivals with drug combinations is often equivalent to that achieved by radiotherapy alone in patients with localized tumor and has led to the evaluation of both used together in early stages of disease.

Childhood neoplasms are quite responsive to all forms of treatment. Chemotherapy with dactinomycin as an adjuvant to both radiotherapy and surgery has increased the 2-year survival in patients with Wilms's tumor from 43 to 92 percent. Tumor recurrences after this time are unusual. Similar results can be achieved with surgery and chemotherapy only, obviating the need for radiotherapy and avoiding its growth-retarding effect on bones. Similar results have been achieved with embryonal rhabdomyosarcoma. Adjuvant chemotherapy with high-dose methotrexate and citrovorum factor rescue and/or adriamycin in patients with osteogenic sarcoma has reduced the recurrence rate in the first 2 years in this virulent tumor of adolescence.

Many drug combinations have been tried in advanced breast cancer. Several are being tested as a means to prevent metastases in the postoperative period. One combination of cyclophosphamide, methotrexate, and 5-fluorouracil (CMF) has been compared with melphalan in patients with metastatic breast cancer and found to be superior. CMF has been reported to produce a statistically significant 40 percent reduction in recurrence rate when used as adjuvant treatment in premenopausal women with stage II carcinoma of the breast in controlled trials. CMF treatment has also resulted in a significant 20 percent reduction in mortality after 4 years of follow-up. The enhanced capacity of the combination of MeCCNU, 5-FU, and vincristine in inducing remissions in stomach and colon cancer has led to the design of several large studies comparing their effectiveness in patients with Duke C colon cancer to untreated or 5-FU–treated controls. The recent dramatic increase in the complete remission rates in patients with testicular tumors, treated with bleomycin, *cis*-platinum, and vinblastine, coupled with the precision in detecting residual tumor cells provided by tumor markers in this disease, has led to the routine use of these drugs following surgery in patients with retroperitoneal node disease.

The sequencing of chemotherapy and radiation therapy has varied from site to site with the use of radiotherapy before, during, and after chemotherapy. It is apparent that there has been little or no consistency in the approach, and the limit of tolerance to radiotherapy of normal tissue, not the ability to control tumor, has been used as a guide to therapy. Further research is needed to determine whether combinations of radiation and drugs are additive, synergistic, or inhibitory. Changes in proliferative capacity of tumors after radiation may negatively influence their response to cycle-active drugs. Chemotherapy has been used before radiotherapy in locally inoperable breast cancer with some success. The results of simultaneous chemotherapy and radiotherapy have been difficult to evaluate, and except for glioblastoma multiforme, where some beneficial effect on survival has been observed, this approach is not now standard treatment for any cancer.

COMPLICATIONS OF THERAPY

Acute side effects and other toxicities of chemotherapeutic agents are listed in Table 324-1. Acute side effects of radiotherapy are nausea and vomiting, erosion of gastrointestinal mucosa in the radiation field, bone marrow suppression, weight loss, and occasional skin reactions. Chronic toxicity is usually associated with fibrous dysplasia which can be severe in some patients. Each side effect must be weighed against the potential benefit to be derived. In a highly treatable disease it is rare that nausea, vomiting, and temporary hair loss should be considered significant enough side effects to withhold treatment. Patients must be apprised of all the risks involved both in using therapy and in withholding it. Many chemicals are carcinogenic to some degree, and anticancer drugs and radiotherapy are no exception. The opportunity to identify this risk has come about only following the advent of successful treatment of patients with metastatic cancer as long disease-free intervals provide the necessary follow-up time. Thus far, used alone, single drugs or combinations of drugs have not yielded rates of secondary tumors higher than expected following the diagnosis of the primary diseases alone. Radiation treatment is known to be carcinogenic, but the risk when used alone is relatively low in a given treatment field. Combinations of drugs and x-rays, however, may be associated with a higher risk of second malignancies such as acute myelogenous leukemia and other tumors in the radiation field. This has been noted in long-term survivors of Hodgkin's disease who receive both combination chemotherapy (MOPP) and radiation therapy. In one study it is estimated that patients treated with both extensive radiation therapy and MOPP chemotherapy may have an incidence of acute myelocytic leukemia between 5 and 10 percent within 10 years. Long-term survivors of patients with Wilms's tumors who receive both radiation and drug therapy have also had a high incidence of secondary malignancies in the radiation treatment field. In addition there is some suspicion that long-term exposure to alkylating agents, particularly melphalan, in patients with otherwise normal bone marrows may be associated with late marrow dysplasia which may eventuate in acute myelocytic leukemia. These potential risks are particularly germane to the use of these drugs in adjuvant treatment programs.

Chemical and radiation therapy produce sterilization in both sexes which may be reversible but often is not. If reversible at all, the time necessary for reversal may be several years. Anticancer drugs are teratogenic. It should never be assumed that chemotherapy and radiotherapy themselves are sufficient methods of birth control. All patients in the childbearing age treated with radiation or drugs should be fully informed of the risks and advised in regard to contraception. When pregnancy occurs during chemotherapy or exposure to radiotherapy, abortion is preferred, if the pregnancy is discovered in the first trimester, because of the high risk of teratogenesis. Treatment of women who develop tumors while pregnant is best withheld until delivery, which may need to be hastened. Chemotherapy can be used safely in the third trimester, but because of the uncertain long-term effects on the fetus, should not be employed unless the situation is critical.

SUPPORTIVE CARE

ANEMIA The first manifestation of malignant disease may be anemia; it is present in 60 percent of patients with disseminated cancer. The peripheral iron profile is similar to that found in chronic infection or inflammation with a low serum iron and iron-binding capacity. Iron stores are normal. The most characteristic anemia is due to both increased destruction of red blood cells and inadequate compensatory erythropoiesis. Other causes of anemia are blood loss, hemolysis, and myelophthisis. Both warm and cold autoimmune hemolytic anemias occur in patients with lymphomas and chronic leukemias, and less frequently in other cancers. Adrenal corticosteroids usually control "warm" autoimmune hemolytic anemia. Splenectomy is often beneficial and should be considered if treatment of the primary disease is ineffective. Radiation of the spleen is simple but rarely effective. Except in cases of blood loss, autoimmune hemolytic anemia, and vitamin deficiencies,

there is no specific therapy for the anemia of cancer. Most patients will remain asymptomatic if their hemoglobin is maintained above 8 g per 100 ml with transfusions.

HEMORRHAGE Tumor invasion of blood vessels, thrombocytopenia, and disseminated intravascular coagulation are the major causes of hemorrhage in patients with cancer. Occasional patients with a normal or excessive number of platelets bleed because of defective platelet function. In thrombocytopenic patients, life-threatening hemorrhage is unusual unless the platelet count falls below 20,000 per milliliter or unless additional coagulation defects are present. The routine use of platelet transfusions in severely thrombocytopenic patients has reduced fatal hemorrhage by over 50 percent. Platelets may be obtained by plasmapheresis of normal random donors. Platelets obtained from histocompatible donors, using HLA and mixed lymphocyte culture typing techniques, are more useful when prolonged periods of platelet support are required. Disseminated intravascular coagulation has been described in many patients with several types of cancer. The process is probably initiated by the release of thromboplastic substances from cancer cells as blood passes over poorly endothelialized surfaces of tumors. Most patients with cancer can be shown to have increased levels of fibrin degradation products without evidence of hemorrhage. Patients with acute promyelocytic leukemia often bleed, especially after treatment is initiated, owing to release of thromboplastin-like material. Heparin therapy may be useful before treatment to prevent hemorrhage. Except in this instance, heparin is almost never indicated in cancer patients with intravascular coagulation.

INFECTION Fever occurs in 70 percent of hospitalized patients with cancer and is usually due to infection. Local factors such as obstruction to normal drainage or recent surgery play a prominent role in infections occurring in patients with metastatic carcinoma, particularly those involving the lung. Patients undergoing cancer chemotherapy are especially susceptible to infectious complications because they develop neutropenia and impairment of normal host-defense mechanisms (Chap. 107). Patients with chronic lymphocytic leukemia and multiple myeloma have decreased levels of normal immunoglobulins and respond inadequately to antigenic stimuli. They are particularly susceptible to infections by *Streptococcus pneumoniae*. Patients with generalized Hodgkin's disease characteristically have impaired cellular immunity and are particularly susceptible to infections caused by fungi (*Cryptococcus*) and viruses. Herpes zoster occurs in 10 percent of patients with Hodgkin's disease. The incidence increases to 20 percent if the spleen has been removed during staging. The majority of infections occurring in cancer patients are caused by gram-negative bacilli, especially *Escherichia coli, Klebsiella,* and *Pseudomonas aeruginosa. Bacteroides* infections are sometimes overlooked. However, organisms of low pathogenicity, such as *Bacillus* spp., *Staphylococcus epidermidis,* and *Flavobacterium* spp., may cause fatal infections in some neutropenic patients. Hence, all organisms cultured from the blood or sites of infection should be considered as possible etiologic agents. Sepsis due to encapsulated cocci is increased in lymphoma patients who have undergone splenectomy and received both combination chemotherapy and radiotherapy. Prophylactic treatment with penicillin or vaccination with the newly developed vaccines may be useful, especially in patients under 10 years of age. Fungal infections, particularly with *Candida* and *Aspergillus* species, are major problems in patients with hematologic malignancies and are increasing in frequency. Pneumocystis pneumonia has been recognized increasingly in patients with a wide variety of malignant diseases and may occur in small epidemics. It is the most common cause of infectious death in leukemic children while in remission.

Many patients are neutropenic when they develop infection. In these patients infection may be rapidly fatal if not treated promptly. Often, the classic signs and symptoms of infection are absent. Infections due to *Pseudomonas* are the most common cause of death from bacterial infections in cancer hospitals. The best initial antibiotic regimen is carbenicillin or ticarcillin, gentamicin or tobramycin and a penicillinase-resistant penicillin or a cephalosporin. However, the effectiveness of aminoglycoside antibiotics is somewhat reduced in neutropenic patients. Granulocyte transfusions are beneficial for the treatment of infections in neutropenic patients, whose bone marrow function is not expected to return to normal for more than 2 weeks, although adverse reactions to white blood cell transfusions are frequent. Histocompatibility typing of donors and recipients holds promise in increasing their effectiveness and reducing the incidence and severity of the reactions. Granulocytes may be obtained by plasmapheresis of patients with chronic myelogenous leukemia, normal family members, or other donors by use of the special centrifuges developed for blood cell separation or by filtration leukopheresis. A daily dose of 10^{10} white blood cells, at a minimum, is required until the infection clears. Gamma globulin is of little benefit in the prophylaxis or treatment of cancer patients with hypogamma-globulinemia.

NUTRITION IN CANCER A profound state of malnutrition, the cachexia of malignancy, is frequently the most debilitating feature of this disease process. In many instances, it can be attributed to anorexia with an associated distortion of taste sensation or acquired aversions to specific foods, particularly meat. There are, however, patients in whom the extent of the weight loss far exceeds the quantity and quality of the calories consumed. In addition to the loss of adipose tissue and protein stores, these patients have a marked degree of insulin resistance with abnormal glucose tolerance. It has been demonstrated that malignancies can cause an augmentation of hepatic and renal gluconeogenesis secondary to enhanced Cori cycle activity, as well as an excessive utilization of fatty acids as metabolic fuel, which can theoretically contribute to a net energy loss by normal tissue. Hyperalimentation with total parenteral nutrition (TPN) with solutions based on 50% glucose, mixtures of essential amino acids, and vitamins, containing about 3000 cal per day, is used to restore nutritionally depleted patients who have a chance for tumor control by surgery, chemotherapy, and/or radiotherapy. TPN through a catheter placed in the superior vena cava is also indicated in patients with pain on deglutition or with intestinal obstruction. When possible, oral hyperalimentation is preferred and effective. TPN in patients who have lost 10 lb or more body weight is associated with an average weight gain of 6 lb in a mean of 24 days, even when chemotherapy and radiotherapy are given simultaneously. There is no evidence that TPN preferentially enhances tumor growth. Anergic patients receiving TPN recover delayed hypersensitivity, suggesting that anergy may, in many instances, be a metabolic-immunologic abnormality. Catheter-related sepsis occurs in about 2 percent of patients. Hyperosmolar, nonketotic coma can be avoided with gradual increases in the concentration of glucose.

TUMOR HYPOGLYCEMIA Tumor hypoglycemia, unrelated to islet-cell tumors, has been most commonly reported in patients with retroperitoneal or intrathoracic fibrosarcomas, hepato-

mas, and adrenocortical carcinomas. A variety of mechanisms have been described, including the excessive consumption of glucose, impaired gluconeogenesis, and an acquired glycogen storage disease. Elevated blood and tumor nonsuppressible insulin-like activity has been demonstrated as an important factor in the pathogenesis of this syndrome.

NEUROLOGICAL MANIFESTATIONS OF CANCER Approximately 25 percent of all patients with uncontrolled cancer have intracranial metastases, including intracerebral, meningeal, or dural deposits. Common cancers which lead to intracerebral metastases are melanoma and those arising in the breast and lung. Approximately half of patients with cerebral metastases will present with headache, less than half with motor weakness, and about one-third with changes in mental status. On examination, about three-quarters of these patients will have impaired cognitive functions, two-thirds will have signs of motor system involvement, and only one-fourth will have papilledema. The tests most valuable for identifying cerebral metastases are the radionuclide brain scan and computerized tomography of the brain. Lumbar puncture does not usually provide diagnostic information and may be dangerous. Cerebral metastases are usually multiple, even when thought to be solitary, but on occasion solitary metastases can be removed successfully, and removal may be followed by long periods free of symptoms. The treatment of intracerebral metastases includes dexamethasone 12 to 16 mg per day followed by whole-brain radiation and then tapering of the steroids as tolerated. The usual dose of radiation to palliate these patients is 3000 to 4000 rads in 3 to 4 weeks, but high-dose, short-duration radiotherapy has been shown to be equally effective. Meningeal leukemia is a well-recognized complication of acute lymphoblastic leukemia, often in patients in remission following chemotherapy. Meningeal lymphoma and carcinomatosis are also recognized more frequently than in the past. Leukemia patients generally present with cranial neuropathies, increased intracranial pressure, vomiting, and meningeal signs, but these findings may not be present in meningeal carcinomatosis. In the latter case, isolated peripheral neuropathies, back pain, and changes in mental status are more common. Frequent and careful examination of the spinal fluid with search for malignant cells in concentrated samples, obtained by millipore filtration of the cytocentrifuge specimen, is necessary to identify meningeal metastases. Treatment usually includes intrathecal methotrexate and/or whole-brain irradiation. The use of the Ommaya Reservoir for intrathecal chemotherapy improves drug distribution and has been recommended in preference to repeated lumbar punctures. Subdural or epidural metastatic tumors are less common than cerebral metastases and are most frequently associated with overlying skull metastases. These may produce cerebral edema and increased intracranial pressure and/or may interfere with venous drainage, particularly of the sagittal sinus. Radiation therapy is the treatment of choice for these problems, but surgery may be required to establish the diagnosis. Dural tumors are within the systemic circulation and accessible to systemic chemotherapy if effective agents are available for the particular tumor type.

Epidural spinal cord compression is an important complication of metastatic cancer. The most common primary tumors which produce this problem are in the breast, lung, prostate, and kidney. It is also a recognized complication of the lymphomas and multiple myelomas. Local or radicular pain is the most frequent and earliest clinical symptom, with subsequent weakness and bladder and bowel dysfunction; numbness and paresthesias are present in the majority of patients by the time the diagnosis is made. A high index of suspicion is necessary, and the diagnosis is confirmed by demonstrating a lesion by myelography. Lumbar spinal taps should be avoided in these patients if the condition is suspected. The spinal tap should be done at the time of the myelogram, and preferably only in consultation with a neurosurgeon, since herniation of the cord into a decompressed region can occur after withdrawal of fluid. The cerebrospinal fluid may be under reduced pressure distal to the compression, and the protein is increased. Malignant cells are usually not found. Radiation therapy is utilized for patients with slowly progressing neurological deficits and radiosensitive tumors. Surgery is usually recommended for patients with rapidly progressing neurological signs, especially if the tumor is relatively radioresistant. Systemic chemotherapy may be of benefit for patients with responsive tumors, and corticosteroids are often used without proved benefit. Neither should be employed to the exclusion of surgery or radiotherapy. Intrathecal chemotherapy is not indicated. In the face of complete motor loss, recovery is rare following radiation or decompressive surgery.

Peripheral nerve or plexus compression and infiltration of the structures by tumor are other neurological complications of metastatic cancer. These problems may result from soft-tissue masses, usually at sites where nerves emerge from neural foramens of the skull or vertebra. Breast and lung cancer are common causes of brachial plexus neuropathy. Lung cancer is the most frequent cause of recurrent laryngeal or phrenic nerve paralysis, and rectal cancer is a common cause of paravertebral nerve compression. However, any tumor may produce these problems, and recognition and differentiation of tumors from metabolic or drug-induced neuropathies are essential if good palliation is to be accomplished. Radiation therapy is usually the most effective treatment but may be unsuccessful if the neurological deficits are marked and long-standing. Chemotherapy, especially for patients with breast cancer and malignant lymphomas, can be beneficial in selected patients.

Neurological and *neuromyopathic* syndromes are associated with malignant disease. Although the histopathology of the tumors producing these syndromes is often well characterized, the causes of the abnormalities are largely unknown. They should always be distinguished from direct effects of neoplasms. Neuromuscular complications are found in 5 to 10 percent of patients with malignant disease. Most often they will be associated with lung cancer, usually of the small-cell (oat-cell) type. Clinical presentation of myositis and dermatomyositis should prompt a search for a hidden malignancy, usually of the gastrointestinal tract. Progressive multifocal leukoencephalopathy is a rare complication in patients with lymphoma and may be due to a papovavirus. Cerebellar degeneration occurs in cancer patients but is also a complication of the use of 5-FU. Carcinomatous myopathy and the characteristic myasthenic syndrome (Eaton-Lambert syndrome) are additional neurological complications.

MALIGNANT EFFUSIONS Peripheral effusions are due to increased fluid formation resulting from tumor on serous surfaces. Central effusions are secondary to decreased fluid resorption due to impaired venous or lymphatic drainage, related to centrally located tumor masses or obstruction of lymphatics by tumor. A combination of peripheral and central causes may occur. A coexisting condition such as an infection or congestive heart failure may be responsible for effusions in patients with cancer. Exudates are usually seen with peripheral effusions; transudates, with central effusions. The presence of true chyle implies central impairment of lymphatic drainage and, in the absence of trauma, is due to tumor or infection. Tetracycline has now been shown to be the drug of choice for the management of pleural effusions due to cancer. Usually, 500 mg is dissolved in 30 ml saline and instilled into the chest, followed by 50 ml saline. A chest tube is required and attached to water-sealed drainage for 6 h. Drainage is continued for 12

h or longer until less than 60 ml fluid is drained per 24 h. Pleural effusions are controlled by this method in 80 percent of all patients. Intrapleural instillation of alkylating agents, 5-FU, and quinacrine is used less frequently. When alkylating agents are used, unpredictable absorption occurs which, in the face of systemic chemotherapy, may compromise bone marrow function. Malignant pericardial effusions are best managed by external radiation and systemic treatment for the primary cancer. Management of malignant ascites is less successful owing to the large size of the peritoneal cavity.

SUPERIOR VENA CAVA OBSTRUCTION The superior vena cava (SVC) is the major vessel most commonly obstructed by tumor, resulting in facial swelling, distention of the veins of the neck and upper chest wall, loss of venous pulsations, conjunctival injection, headache, and convulsions. Patients often present with these findings as the first sign of malignant disease. The diagnosis is usually based on clinical findings and the presence of a mediastinal mass. While the SVC syndrome is a serious medical problem, it need not be considered a true medical emergency, since patients rarely die from it. There is usually sufficient time to make a histological diagnosis before treatment is instituted, although an occasional patient may require treatment before a tissue diagnosis. Temporizing treatment with corticosteroids and diuretics may be useful while the diagnosis is pursued. More definitive therapy should include systemic treatment for the disease in question, if it is susceptible to drug therapy, and full-dose irradiation therapy to the site of obstruction, in conjunction with corticosteroids. The tumors most commonly associated with superior vena cava syndrome are diffuse histiocytic lymphomas and small-cell carcinoma of the lung.

HYPERCALCEMIA Extensive bone involvement is characteristic of some tumors such as multiple myeloma, breast carcinoma, and prostatic carcinoma and may result in hypercalcemia. A common cause of hypercalcemia is immobilization with or without bony metastases. Some tumors, like epidermoid lung cancer, may produce parathyroid hormone-like substances which cause hypercalcemia. A group of patients with hypercalcemia, normal parathormone levels, and no evidence of bony metastases has been described. Some of these patients with renal-cell carcinoma have elevated tumor levels of prostaglandins and respond to the inhibitor of prostaglandin synthesis, indomethacin. Since prostaglandins cause bone resorption, this may be another mechanism for tumor hypercalcemia in the absence of metastatic disease or identifiable ectopic parathormone production. Myeloma and other lymphoid cell lines are capable of producing, locally, a low-molecular-weight substance known as *osteoclast-activating factor,* which also may be involved in the dissolution of bone. Hypercalcemia requires prompt attention. Chronic hypercalcemia may lead to nephrocalcinosis and irreversible impairment of renal function. The treatment of choice for hypercalcemia associated with malignancy is therapy for the underlying disease. Mithramycin (Table 324-1), proper hydration with isotonic saline solution, and diuretics are the best ancillary methods of controlling hypercalcemia and may lead to control within 2 days. Normal serum calcium levels can be maintained by weekly doses of mithramycin, 25 μg/kg, without risk of marrow suppression or hemorrhage. Adrenal corticosteroids reduce the serum calcium level to normal in 60 percent of patients but may predispose to infection and are no longer the treatment of choice. Sodium sulfate and sodium phosphates facilitate excretion of calcium by the kidney. Phosphates must be used cautiously since they may cause extraosseous calcification.

HYPERURICEMIA AND OTHER CONSEQUENCES OF RAPID CELL LYSIS Hyperuricemia is most common in patients with acute leukemia but occasionally occurs in other malignancies. The high serum uric acid levels are due to the increased formation and destruction of tumor cells and accompanying breakdown of nucleoproteins. Chemotherapy and radiotherapy may cause further elevations in serum uric acid and urinary urate excretion. Uric acid is actively secreted by the kidney, and its solubility is highest in alkaline urine. When the concentration exceeds the solubility, uric acid precipitates in the tubules causing obstruction, decreased glomerular filtration, and eventually anuria. Allopurinol prevents the formation of uric acid from xanthine and hypoxanthine. Prophylactic use of this drug in patients with a large volume of tumor, prior to treatment, in anticipation of a high urate load, should obviate the need to treat uric acid nephropathy. Urate nephropathy can also be prevented by ensuring a water diuresis. Administration of sodium bicarbonate to maintain the urinary pH above 7.0 is helpful. Secondary gout is uncommon except in patients with polycythemia vera. The excessive production of lactate by suboxygenated masses of tumor has been reported to cause lactic acidosis in patients with leukemia and Burkitt's lymphoma. The lactic acidosis can be reversed by cytotoxic chemotherapy directed against the tumor. The elaboration of large quantities of lactic dehydrogenase (LDH) has been observed in these settings. Cytotoxic therapy in highly drug sensitive tumors can cause rapid tumor lysis with release of intracellular phosphates and potassium leading to serious hyperkalemia, hypocalcemia, and potentially fatal cardiotoxicity.

PSYCHOLOGICAL EFFECTS Although the psychological impact of incurable cancer is severe, the patient whose disease is treatable also faces severe emotional difficulties. There is often readjustment to the home situation, difficult psychosexual readjustment, particularly in women after mastectomy, and difficulties convincing the community that the patient remains a useful member of society. Many such cancer patients are shunned because of unwarranted fears of "catching" cancer. Realization by the patient that he or she has an incurable malignant disease has profound psychological impact, particularly if the disease strikes in youth or middle age. An important aspect of cancer therapy is the hope of improvement it offers to patients. Even experimental chemotherapy which fails to alter the course of the disease significantly may be beneficial and gives some meaning to an otherwise dismal experience, because patients feel they are contributing to the welfare of others even if the drug fails to help them. Suicide is not common in incurable cancer patients, and the prospect of a shortened life is ultimately preferred to death by suicide if a modicum of physical and emotional comfort can be maintained. As the disease progresses, the patient may pass through a variety of mental processes, including denial, hostility, despair, and finally acceptance of the inevitable. The physician should provide hope, encouragement, understanding, sympathy, and support. During this difficult period the physician should also rely upon the nursing staff, clergymen, and social workers for assistance in the care of the patient.

Most patients with advanced cancer know they are dying, and attempts at circumventing the truth are usually recognized by them and cause feelings of distrust and hostility toward those the dying patient needs the most, the family, physicians, and nurses. Honesty is recommended; most patients will surprise their doctors and families by expressing relief at a willingness to discuss what is foremost in their minds, their imminent death.

Uncontrollable pain is uncommon in cancer patients but is a problem more often in those with bony disease. Most hospitalized cancer patients with pain are underdosed usually owing to physician ignorance of the pharmacokinetics of narcotic analgesics. Attending physicians should use narcotics, alcohol, and tranquilizers liberally and often, and in combination in these circumstances, recognizing that the proper dose is whatever is enough to control the patient's discomfort. Fear of addiction is unwarranted. Sufficiently potent narcotics are available to control most types of pain in the cancer patient. Widely spaced doses of narcotics, that exceed the half-life of most drugs, are inhumane and should not be used. For pain not controllable with narcotics, neurosurgical procedures may be useful.

REFERENCES

Buschke F, Parker RG (eds): Fundamentals of clinical radiation therapy, in *Radiation Therapy in Cancer Management.* New York, Grune & Stratton, 1972

Calabresi P, Parks RE Jr: Chemotherapy of neoplastic diseases, in *Pharmacologic Basis of Therapeutics,* LS Goodman, A. Gilman (eds). New York, Macmillan, 1975

Chabner BA et al: The clinical pharmacology of antineoplastic agents. N Engl J Med 292:1159, 1975

DeVita VT et al: Combination versus single agent chemotherapy: A review of the basis for selection of drug treatment of cancer. Cancer 35:98, 1975

Schabel FM: Concepts for systemic treatment of micrometastases. Cancer 35:15, 1975

Tannock I: Cell kinetics and chemotherapy: A critical review. Cancer Treat Rep 62:1117, 1978

325
THE ACUTE LEUKEMIAS

BAYARD CLARKSON

DEFINITION Leukemia is a disease characterized by neoplastic proliferation of one of the blood-forming cells. The different types of leukemia are classified according to the cell type involved, and as acute or chronic, depending on the state of maturity of the neoplastic cells and the expected duration of the disease. If left untreated, all forms of leukemia are fatal; death is usually due to complications resulting from infiltration of the bone marrow by leukemic cells and replacement of normal hematopoietic cells. The average survival of untreated patients with acute leukemia is about 3 months, but the course of the disease may vary considerably.

This chapter is limited to a discussion of the acute leukemias, i.e., those forms which present de novo with progressive infiltration of the marrow by largely immature cells and which almost invariably have a rapidly fatal course without effective treatment. Chronic myelogenous leukemia and other myeloproliferative disorders, which may terminate by transformation into an acute blastic phase, are discussed in Chaps. 326, 312, and 313.

CLASSIFICATION Because there are significant differences in their age distribution and responsiveness to treatment, the acute leukemias are commonly divided into two major types: *acute lymphoblastic leukemia (ALL)* and *acute nonlymphoblastic leukemia.* The latter is further divided into several subtypes, which are referred to more or less collectively as *acute myelogenous* or *acute myeloid leukemia (AML)*.

It is important to distinguish between the two major types because the response to chemotherapy is more favorable in ALL than in AML and different drugs are ordinarily used for inducing remission. The diagnosis is made on the basis of the morphologic appearance of fixed cells on Romanowsky-stained smears. In ALL, the lymphoblasts characteristically have a high nuclear cytoplasmic ratio; the nuclei are not indented or twisted, the number of nucleoli tends to be low (one or two); azurophilic granules are minimal and Auer rods are absent in the cytoplasm; promyelocytes and monocytes are uncommon; and, because they arise from normal precursors, the more mature cells of the granulocytic series appear normal. In contrast to acute myeloid leukemic cells, lymphoblasts do not stain with Sudan black B and the myeloperoxidase reaction is also negative.

The French-American-British (FAB) Co-operative Group has developed proposals for the classification of the acute leukemias which should permit a more uniform system of classification and more accurate recording of the distribution of cases entered into clinical trials. Lymphoblastic leukemias are subdivided in three groups (L1 to L3) on the basis of cell size, nuclear chromatin pattern, nuclear shape, nucleoli, amount and basophilia of cytoplasm, and extent of cytoplasmic vacuolization. In the L1 type, small cells which are usually homogenous with respect to the above-listed features predominate; such cases have a more favorable prognosis than do the L2 types, in which the cells are larger and more heterogenous. About 25 percent of the L1 and L2 types have T-lymphocyte markers, whereas the rest are "null" cells, but there are no distinctive morphological features associated with the minority with T-cell markers. Both T and null cell types usually have elevated terminal deoxynucleotidyl transferase levels. In the L3 (Burkitt) type, the cells are large and homogenous, frequently have prominent cytoplasmic vacuolization and a high mitotic index, and usually have B-lymphocyte markers.

Leukemic myeloblasts tend to be larger cells, commonly 12 to 20 μm in diameter, although smaller "micromyeloblasts" occur. Myeloblasts usually have ample cytoplasm, which sometimes contains Auer rods. The nucleus has a homogeneous "ground glass" appearance and multiple nucleoli (three to five) are usually present. In the proposed FAB classification, the acute myeloid leukemias are subdivided into six types (M1 to M6), defined according to the direction of differentiation along one or more cell lines and the degree of cellular maturation. M1 to M3 show predominantly granulocytic differentiation and differ from one another in their extent of maturation. In the M1 type (myeloblastic leukemia without maturation) the blasts are nongranular, but 3 percent or more are myeloperoxidase positive and may contain rare azurophilic granules, Auer rods, or both, but further maturation is not seen. In the M2 type (myeloblastic leukemia with maturation), maturation proceeds to the promyelocyte stage or beyond. More than 50 percent of the cells in the bone marrow are myeloblasts and promyelocytes, and later cells of the granulocytic series may also be found in varying proportions. The latter often demonstrate abnormal features such as the Pelger-Huet anomaly or hypogranulation. In the M3 type (hypergranular promyelocytic leukemia), the great majority of cells are abnormal promyelocytes with heavy granulation; this type is often associated with serious coagulation abnormalities.

The M4 type (myelomonocytic leukemia) shows both granulocytic and monocytic differentiation, and the percentages of promonocytes plus monocytes and of myeloblasts plus promyelocytes in the marrow each exceed 20 percent. A chronic form of myelomonocytic leukemia is also described. In the M5 type (monocytic leukemia), there is predominantly monocytic

differentiation. Two subtypes are described: (1) poorly differentiated (monoblastic) and (2) differentiated, in which both monoblasts and more mature cells of the monocytic series are present. The naphthol AS or ASD acetate esterase reaction (NASDA) is strongly positive in monoblasts, promonocytes, and monocytes and is inhibited by sodium fluoride, whereas in granulocytes the positivity of the reaction is unaffected by exposure to sodium fluoride. The serum lysozyme concentration is frequently elevated in the M4 and M5 types with a prominent monocytic component.

In the M6 type (erythroleukemia), the erythropoietic component usually exceeds 50 percent of the nucleated cells in the marrow, and erythroblasts may be present in the blood. The erythroblasts frequently show abnormalities, such as megaloblastosis, distorted nuclear shape, multiple nuclei, nuclear fragmentation, and giant forms. There is an increased percentage of myeloblasts and promyelocytes (30 percent or higher), and abnormal megakaryocytes may also be present. The proportion of erythroblasts varies during the course of the disease, usually decreasing as the disease progresses and eventually becoming replaced by immature cells of the granulocytic series. These findings are characteristic of the acute form of erythroleukemia (acute erythremic myelosis, or Di Guglielmo's syndrome), but a more chronic form of erythroleukemia is also seen and may be confused with other dysmyelopoietic syndromes associated with "ineffective erythropoiesis," such as megaloblastic anemia, "smoldering leukemia," and "preleukemia," or with refractory anemia with excess of blasts (RAEB). In the latter condition, the marrow is hypercellular and myeloblasts and promyelocytes may account for 10 to 30 percent of the nucleated cells; a progressive increase toward 50 percent indicates development of acute myeloid leukemia.

Abnormal eosinophils, which are probably derived from the leukemic cell lines, are often present as a minority component in myeloid leukemia, but both acute and chronic forms of eosinophilic leukemia have been described in which eosinophils predominate; the acute form may be associated with cardiac manifestations. However, the diagnosis should be made with caution, since eosinophilic leukemia is very rare and is often difficult to distinguish from other conditions associated with hypereosinophilia. Basophilic leukemia and megakaryocytic leukemia seldom, if ever, present as forms of acute leukemia de novo, but may evolve as variants of chronic myelogenous leukemia or other myeloproliferative diseases. Mast-cell leukemia is a rare disease which is associated with urticaria pigmentosa and gastrointestinal symptoms. Plasma-cell leukemia, in which numerous plasma cells appear in the peripheral blood, may occur rarely, either as a terminal event in patients with multiple myeloma or as an initial variant of the disease. When this occurs, in addition to the usual manifestations of myeloma, there may be a prominent involvement of the liver, spleen, and lymph nodes and a marked tendency to bleeding.

In the hands of experienced morphologists, there is usually reasonably close agreement in identifying morphologic subtypes of acute leukemia. The major distinction between ALL and AML can be made in about 90 percent of cases by expert morphologists, but in distinguishing between subtypes of AML such as acute myelomonocytic leukemia (M4) and acute monocytic leukemia (M5), the accuracy is considerably less and different hematologists may not agree consistently. Numerous cytochemical stains have been developed which are more or less specific for different cell types and which are helpful in improving diagnostic precision; those most consistently helpful have been mentioned. Although different cell types have distinctive ultrastructural features, transmission and scanning electron microscopic studies have proved more useful in confirming suspected diagnoses than in providing positive identification in unknown cases.

INCIDENCE AND PREVALENCE The reported mortality from all types of leukemia in the United States increased to about 6.8 per 100,000 persons per year in 1956, and since then the overall rate has remained relatively stable. The mortality rate from leukemia is higher than average in Jews, and has been persistently lower in black than in white Americans, but these differences appear to be diminishing in recent years. Leukemia occurs throughout the world; the annual mortality rates in different countries vary from around 3 to 7 per 100,000 population, being highest in the Scandinavian countries and Israel and lowest in Chile and Japan. Still lower death rates are reported in some developing countries, but this may reflect inadequate medical services and faulty diagnoses. Depending on the criteria of classification, about 50 to 60 percent of leukemia deaths in the United States are due to acute leukemia.

All types of leukemia are slightly more common in males than in females. However, male predominance is less marked for acute leukemia (about 3:2) than for chronic lymphocytic leukemia (about 2:1) and the sex incidence is almost the same in very young children. The overall incidence of ALL and AML is about equal in the United States, but there are marked age and racial differences in their distribution. Acute leukemia accounts for nearly half of all neoplasms in children. The peak incidence of ALL occurs between the ages of 2 to 4 years; this peak was originally noted only in white children, but a less prominent peak has also been observed in young black and Japanese children. Whereas fewer than 20 percent of cases of acute leukemia in persons under the age of 15 are AML, the incidence is reversed in adults; AML shows a progressively increasing incidence with advancing age.

ETIOLOGY AND EPIDEMIOLOGY The etiology of leukemia is still unknown, although there are certain factors which predispose to its development.

Ionizing radiation In relatively large doses (i.e., above 100 rads), whether from unintentional exposure to nuclear sources or from irradiation therapy, ionizing radiation is clearly associated with an increased incidence of both acute and chronic myelogenous leukemia. It is still controversial whether a threshold dose exists below which there is no attendant increase in the risk of developing leukemia. There is no convincing evidence that doses employed in radiodiagnostic procedures are leukemogenic in adults, unless the exposure is excessive, as it was for pioneer radiologists working without effective protection. Exposure of the fetus to diagnostic radiographic procedures during pregnancy appears to be associated with a slightly increased risk of leukemia later in childhood, but the extent of the increase is controversial. It is also debatable whether any irradiation of the mother prior to conception increases the likelihood of leukemia in children born later.

Chemical agents The leukemias which follow exposure to chemical agents usually consist of acute or chronic myelogenous leukemia rather than the lymphocytic type. Occupational exposure to benzene and possibly other chemicals is associated with an increased incidence of leukemia. Certain drugs, such as chloramphenicol and phenylbutazone, which are known to cause bone marrow depression, are probably also leukemogenic, although the risk is not great. Alkylating agents and some of the other cytotoxic drugs used in cancer chemotherapy are carcinogenic in experimental animals and cell culture sys-

tems, and there is increasing evidence that they are also leukemogenic in humans. There are now numerous reports of an increased incidence of acute nonlymphocytic leukemia in patients with Hodgkin's disease, multiple myeloma, chronic lymphocytic leukemia, ovarian cancer and other types of cancer, as well as in patients with nonneoplastic diseases who have been treated with cytotoxic drugs, especially alkylating agents. Moreover, the risk appears to be greater with combined modality therapy (irradiation plus chemotherapy). The incidence rises as survival increases due to successful treatment of the original disease and in the case of Hodgkin's disease, it may exceed 1000 times that normally expected. Hypodiploidy of the leukemic cells is a common finding in these patients, especially loss of chromosomes 5 and 7. Such secondary leukemias are almost always refractory to antileukemic therapy and the patients characteristically have a very short survival.

Hereditary factors Patients with Down's syndrome, or mongolism, a defect characterized by trisomy of chromosome 21, have approximately a 20-fold higher incidence of acute leukemia than normal. The incidence of Down's syndrome increases with advancing maternal age; the incidence of leukemia in otherwise normal children born of older mothers is also slightly higher than average, but not nearly as high as in Down's syndrome. Both ALL and AML occur, and the type of leukemia appears to be related to that usually expected at the age of occurrence. All ages have an increased incidence, but the risk is highest in infants. Once diagnosed, with rare exception, leukemia occurring in Down's syndrome runs its usual fatal course if not treated effectively. However, occasional newborns with Down's syndrome have been reported in whom the findings are indistinguishable from those of acute leukemia, but in whom all the abnormalities disappear spontaneously and apparently permanently; it is not established whether these cases represent spontaneous cures of true leukemia or whether such infants merely have a leukemoid response to some unrecognized stimulus.

A number of other congenital conditions are also associated with an increased incidence of leukemia, although the risk is less than in Down's syndrome. These include Fanconi's aplastic anemia; Bloom's syndrome; ataxia-telangiectasia; Patau's syndrome, or D trisomy; Wiskott-Aldrich syndrome; congenital sex-linked agammaglobulinemia; and Kostmann's agranulocytosis. Although there is no common specific chromosomal lesion, most of these syndromes are characterized either by chromosomal aneuploidy or by a tendency to chromosomal breakage. Familial leukemia is rare, but a few otherwise normal families have been reported in which multiple cases have occurred during one or more generations. Fibroblasts from individuals with Down's syndrome and Fanconi's anemia and from their parents, as well as from one family with no known congenital disease or chromosomal disorder but with multiple cases of AML, have been shown to have increased susceptibility to transformation in vitro by SV40, a simian DNA virus with high oncogenic potential.

Otherwise normal siblings and fraternal twins of leukemic children have a slightly higher than normal risk of developing leukemia, and although the overall incidence is not increased in twins, if one monozygotic twin develops acute leukemia, the other has about a 20 percent chance of developing it also. Because the majority of concordant leukemias in identical twins occurs during the first few years of life and because they are often diagnosed simultaneously or within a short time interval, it has been suggested that these cases may represent only one occurrence of leukemia and not two. Unlike the situation in dizygotic twins, the in utero circulatory systems of monozygotic twins are united by shared placental vessels, and if the initial leukemic transformation occurred in one twin before separation of the placental circulation, the other would almost inevitably be colonized by the progeny of the transformed cell. In confirmation of this hypothesis, an identical karyotypic marker was found in the leukemic cells of both monozygotic twins with near simultaneous development of acute leukemia.

Viruses It is firmly established that viruses may cause leukemia in fowls, rodents, cats, and monkeys. The viruses are leukemogenic when initially inoculated, but infected animals may harbor the virus for their lifetimes, often without themselves developing leukemia. They can pass virus to their offspring through the ovum or shed it in milk or other secretions and thereby transmit it to uninfected animals. There are many environmental and genetic factors which determine whether and what type of leukemia an infected animal will develop. Among the most important are quantity of virus, differences in susceptibility of different strains, age, sex, hormonal and immunologic influences, and exposure to external agents such as irradiation or chemical carcinogens which can release or trigger the virus and cause full expression of the disease. Most of the viruses which are leukemogenic in fowls and mammals are RNA viruses (types C or B); type C viruses have been shown to cause lymphomas or myelogenous leukemia in subhuman primates. Exceptions to this rule are Marek's disease (neural lymphomatosis) in chickens and malignant lymphomas in owl monkeys which are caused by DNA viruses of the herpes group.

Despite clear proof that viruses can cause leukemia in many animal species including primates and an intensive search for human leukemia viruses, there is no conclusive evidence that viruses cause leukemia in humans. There have been numerous reports of electron microscopic demonstration of type C virus particles in plasma pellets or tissues from patients with leukemia, of detection of viruses or virus-related antigens in human leukemic cells by immunologic techniques, and of recovery of virus from human materials in animal or cell culture systems. However, many of these reports have not been substantiated, others have failed to exclude contaminating infections, and none have provided definitive proof that viruses are the etiologic agents of human leukemia.

RNA-directed DNA polymerase (reverse transcriptase) is an enzyme present in type C viruses which permits them to synthesize DNA that can then be inserted into the genome of the infected cell, thereby allowing viral-directed genetic determinants to be passed on indefinitely through the normal process of cell division. Reverse transcriptase with biochemical and immunologic properties similar to those associated with mammalian type C viruses has been reported to be present in some human leukemic cells and also in normal leukocytes of patients with acute leukemia in remission. The enzyme is not present in fresh leukocytes from normal individuals nor in normal lymphocytes transformed to blasts by phytohemagglutinin, but has been detected in some human cell lines in established cultures. Immunologic studies have provided some evidence that the polymerase obtained from human acute myelogenous leukemic cells is specifically related to the reverse transcriptase in woolly monkey sarcoma virus and gibbon ape leukemia virus, and also that the human leukemic cells contain a protein closely related to group-specific antigen (p30 protein) from the woolly monkey virus. These type C RNA tumor virus-related components in human leukemic cells have been regarded as "footprints" of a closely related but incompletely expressed human leukemia virus, but much more evidence is needed before it can be concluded that such a putative virus can cause human leukemia.

Several time-space clusters or microepidemics of leukemia have been reported, which might suggest an infectious etiology. However, prospective epidemiologic studies in situations that might reflect an infectious mode of spread have failed to support this suspicion. In two well-documented instances, leukemic transformation occurred in normal histocompatible marrow cells from two normal male donors which were transplanted into their female siblings who had ALL and had received total body irradiation prior to the marrow transplants. However, this phenomenon has not been reported in AML, and all other cytogenetically documented instances of recurrent leukemia in patients who have received marrow grafts have been due to regrowth of the recipients' own leukemic cell lines.

NATURE OF THE DISORDER IN ACUTE LEUKEMIA There is good evidence that acute leukemia is a uniclonal neoplasm, i.e., that it originates with the transformation of a single, or at the most a few, hematopoietic cell(s). The nature of the molecular lesion(s) responsible for the transformed cells' neoplastic properties is unclear, but the critical defect is intrinsic and inheritable by the cells' progeny. There have been many attempts to demonstrate qualitative biochemical differences between normal and leukemic cells, but no consistent differences have been found in cells of comparable levels of maturity. In patients who have recognizable karyotypic abnormalities in their leukemic cells prior to treatment and in whom serial cytogenetic studies have been performed, the abnormal metaphases disappear from the marrow or are greatly reduced in number, and normal diploid modes are present during drug-induced remissions. When relapse occurs, the original abnormal leukemic line reappears; in some cases one or more secondary abnormal lines may appear as a result of clonal evolution. Relapse is ordinarily caused by regrowth of residual surviving cells from the original leukemic population rather than as a result of reinduction of a new leukemia.

It can be assumed that the leukemogenic transforming event may occur at any location in the cells' ancestral lineages, but that in order for the disease to be fully expressed, it must either take place at an early enough stage so that the cell already has unlimited proliferative capacity, or that it acquires this capacity as a result of becoming transformed. Consequently, if the transformation occurs in a progenitor cell with the capacity to differentiate into both erythrocyte and granulocyte precursors, erythroleukemia will result; whereas if it occurs in a progenitor cell already committed to granulocytic differentiation, the resultant leukemia will be myeloblastic. A critical defect in acute leukemia is defective maturation so that instead of producing equal numbers of committed and stem cells, leukemic stem cells generate an increased proportion of stem cells. In acute leukemia the leukemic population seldom if ever expands exponentially at a maximum rate as do stem cells in uncrowded cultures or transplanted leukemic cells in the mouse during early disease. The kinetic behavior of leukemic cells in human disease can be represented best as intermediate between maximum exponential growth and the steady state characteristic of normal hematopoiesis. Instead of invariably generating two daughters which both behave as stem cells (which would result in exponential growth) or else one stem cell and one committed cell (as in normal hematopoiesis), there is usually excessive production of cells with unlimited proliferative potential and of committed cells with finite life spans. However, there must necessarily be a ratio greater than 1:1 of stem cells to primary committed cells, because otherwise the population would cease to expand. The fraction of leukemic cells with stem-cell capability may vary greatly among different populations, and this variability is partly responsible for differences in the rate of progression of the disease. Other factors influencing rate of progression are the growth fraction, or proportion of actively dividing cells as opposed to the proportion of resting or dormant cells, and the fact that many leukemic populations have a substantial death rate. In some leukemic populations, the majority of the cells may mature to the extent of losing their ability to divide. In such instances their behavior may closely resemble that of normal hematopoietic cells, and the leukemic population will expand only very slowly or not at all.

Another important behavioral abnormality characteristic of the leukemic state is that leukemic cells are relatively unresponsive to normal regulatory mechanisms which maintain the size of the normal hematopoietic compartments within narrow limits. As a result leukemic cells continue to proliferate, albeit sometimes slowly, and commonly reach far higher population densities than do hematopoietic cells in normal individuals. However, the degree of escape from normal control varies widely; some leukemic populations expand to lethal numbers extremely rapidly, whereas others barely exceed normal cell densities in the marrow for long periods, even without treatment.

The normal hematopoietic precursors are generally reduced in advanced leukemia, probably owing to inhibition at the stem-cell level by the leukemic cells. Although the mechanism of inhibition is still unclear, it seems probable that the normal cells recognize the leukemic cells, or their inhibitory products, as "normal," and turn off production in response to excess cell numbers. The cell cycle or intermitotic time of leukemic cells is no faster, and may be considerably slower, than that of the normal hematopoietic precursors, especially during advanced disease. If chemotherapy reduces the leukemic population sufficiently, the normal stem cells are released from inhibition, and because of their faster proliferative rate, the normal precursors may repopulate the marrow faster than can the leukemic cells. If enough leukemic cells have been destroyed, a remission results.

CLINICAL MANIFESTATIONS The clinical manifestations of acute leukemia are most often related to replacement of the normal hematopoietic cells in the marrow by leukemic cells, and to a lesser extent to infiltration of other organs. Symptoms may appear abruptly with severe prostration, high fever, and bleeding, or the onset may be insidious with progressive weakness, pallor, low-grade fever, minor bleeding tendencies, or recurrent infections. Sometimes there are no antecedent symptoms, and the diagnosis is made while investigating the reason for menorrhagia or excessive bleeding following a dental procedure.

Fever is present in the majority of patients at the time of diagnosis, and some degree of fever occurs almost invariably sometime during attempts at inducing remission owing to further depletion of granulocytes by cytotoxic drugs. High fever is frequently associated with obvious infection, but sometimes no source can be found even on careful search, and there may be no response to antibiotics. It is debatable whether fever can occur in the absence of any infection, but if it can, this phenomenon is certainly less frequent than in the lymphomas or in the blastic phase of chronic myelogenous leukemia. In addition to the usual pathogenic bacteria, microorganisms which are ordinarily relatively avirulent frequently cause serious infections in patients with acute leukemia.

There may be no abnormalities on physical examination, or there may be multiple findings. Enlargement of the tonsils, lymph nodes, and spleen are common, especially in ALL, and splenic infarction, subcapsular hemorrhage, and, rarely, splenic rupture may occur. The liver and kidneys are also frequently enlarged due to leukemic infiltration, but the infiltrates do not ordinarily interfere with the function of these or other organs unless there are associated complications such as infection, hemorrhage, blockage of the ureters or biliary system, or uric acid nephropathy. Leukemic infiltration of the gingivae, skin, and other tissues is especially common in monocytic leukemia. Localized tumor masses which have a greenish appearance sometimes occur in the skin, orbit, or other tissues in granulocytic forms of leukemia. These are called *chloromas*, and the greenish color is due to the presence of myeloperoxidase. Rarely leukemia may present as a localized bony tumor prior to diffuse marrow involvement. Patients with many circulating leukemic cells usually have more rapidly progressive disease, and more extensive infiltration of the marrow and other organs. They may die suddenly from massive intracranial hemorrhage as a result of leukostasis, perivascular infiltration, and weakening of the vessel walls. Bleeding may occur at any site, but the most common sites of fatal hemorrhages are intracranial, gastrointestinal, and pulmonary. Thrombophlebitis and other thromboembolic disorders occur frequently in acute leukemia, even in patients with severe thrombocytopenia.

Local infections are common, especially involving one or more of the body orifices, and can be very serious as in the case of peritonsillar or perirectal abscesses. Leukemic infiltration of the lungs may occur, but this is frequently difficult to distinguish from pulmonary infections, and often the two are associated. Serous effusions, involving especially the pleural cavities, are also common. Infiltration, intussusception, hemorrhage, infection, or perforation may occur anywhere in the gastrointestinal tract, and local or generalized peritonitis may develop. Sternal tenderness is often present, and there may be severe pain and tenderness of multiple bones and joints due to bone infarcts or subperiosteal infiltrates. Bone and joint pains are especially common in children with ALL and may be misdiagnosed as acute rheumatic fever or rheumatoid arthritis. Anorexia, weight loss, muscle wasting, and contractures sometimes occur, usually as a result of the combined effects of diminished physical activity, hypercatabolism, and nutritional deficiency.

Neurologic findings are frequent. There may be infiltration of the peripheral nerves, spinal nerve roots, or cranial nerve palsies, the latter commonly being due to infiltration of the nerve sheaths with compression of the nerves as they pass through their osseous foramens. Severe symptoms due to intracranial hemorrhage and/or infiltration of the leptomeninges may occur, among them being headache, vomiting, seizures, visual disturbance, papilledema, and nuchal rigidity. Leukemic meningitis due to arachnoid infiltration occurs in the majority of patients with ALL sometime during the course of their disease if not prevented by prophylactic intrathecal chemotherapy or cranial irradiation. Arachnoid leukemia also may be seen in AML, but less frequently than in ALL. Rarely, leukemic infiltration of the hypothalamus may cause hyperphagia, obesity, and behavioral disturbances; inappropriate secretion of antidiuretic hormone or diabetes insipidus is also seen occasionally.

LABORATORY FINDINGS There is usually some degree of anemia which is generally due mostly to decreased erythrocyte production, although hemorrhage can sometimes be an important factor, and a modest decrease in red blood cell survival may also occur. Severe hemolytic anemia is rare, and the direct Coombs test is usually negative. Reticulocytes are reduced, and the erythrocytes are usually normochromic and normocytic. However, in some patients, the red blood cell precursors have prominent megaloblastic features, and macrocytes and erythroblasts may appear in the blood. The megaloblastic changes are not corrected by administration of vitamin B_{12} or other nutritional factors, and it seems likely that the abnormal erythroblasts in such patients are part of the leukemic population.

The platelet count is usually moderately to severely decreased; occasionally it is normal, but it is rarely elevated. Hemorrhagic tendencies are usually correlated with the level of thrombocytopenia, and although occasionally severe hemorrhages occur in patients with more than 100,000 platelets per cubic millimeter, most serious bleeding episodes develop in patients with fewer than 20,000 platelets per cubic millimeter. When bleeding occurs in the presence of adequate numbers of platelets, the platelets are often abnormal and function poorly, and may be derived from megakaryocytes which are involved in the leukemic process.

In addition to those attributable to thrombocytopenia, various coagulation abnormalities have been recognized, of which one of the most frequent and serious is disseminated intravascular coagulation (DIC). DIC is most often seen in promyelocytic leukemia but may occur in monocytic and other types of acute leukemia. There are reports of isolated deficiencies of various clotting factors, but when first diagnosed, most patients with acute leukemia have adequate levels of all clotting factors, and indeed fibrinogen and factor VIII are commonly elevated. However, multiple abnormalities may occur during the course of the disease due to sepsis, hepatic decompensation, nutritional deficiencies, some of the drugs used in treating leukemia (e.g., L-asparaginase), and other causes.

Neutropenia is often present. The severity is related to the extent of marrow infiltration by leukemic cells and also to the presence of infection. Various abnormalities of granulocytic function have been described in acute leukemia, but it is uncertain whether the defective granulocytes belong to the leukemic or normal population.

Because most of the manifestations of acute leukemia also may be associated with other diseases, the diagnosis can be made only by careful morphologic examinations of the blood and bone marrow. The number of leukemic cells in the peripheral blood may vary from none to more than 1 million per cubic millimeter; only about 15 percent of patients have leukocyte counts over 100,000 per cubic millimeter. Some patients present with normal erythrocyte and platelet counts, or with pancytopenia, and have only a few (subleukemic) or no (aleukemic) blasts in the blood. In such cases, the peripheral blood leukocytes should be concentrated by centrifugation, and stained smears of the buffy coat prepared. Some leukemic cells will be found in the blood of most patients; moreover, they may be more mature and hence more indicative of the morphologic type of leukemia than those in the marrow. A bone marrow aspiration and differential count should always be performed. Most untreated patients have over 50 percent obviously leukemic cells in the marrow, and a diagnosis of acute leukemia should be made with great caution if the marrow differential count shows less than 30 percent immature cells.

Sometimes even when the marrow is filled with leukemic cells, they cannot be aspirated because they are so adhesive or are enmeshed in reticulin fibers, and in such cases a needle or open surgical biopsy should always be done. The pathologist can usually recognize replacement of normal marrow cells by immature cells in hematoxylin-eosin-stained sections, but Wright-stained touch preparations of the biopsy specimen are more useful in identifying the morphologic type of leukemia. A specific granulocyte stain, the naphthol chloroacetate esterase reaction, can be performed on paraffin-embedded tissue sections and aids in identifying the specific cell type in such cases.

Chromosome analysis of dividing leukemic cells in the marrow shows one or more karyotypic abnormalities in about half of patients with acute leukemia. No consistent chromosomal abnormalities have been found, but through new banding techniques, it has been shown that specific abnormalities occur in various types of leukemia. For example, in acute myeloid leu-

kemia, especially common abnormalities include trisomy of chromosome 8, deletion of chromosome 7, and translocations involving chromosomes 8 and 21, 9 and 22, and 15 and 17; the latter abnormality is especially common in acute promyelocytic leukemia. Patients whose marrow cells are all karyotypically normal, or who have a mixture of normal and abnormal cells, have a better prognosis than do those with only abnormal cells.

Other laboratory studies are not very useful or specific. Uric acid production is frequently increased in patients with rapidly growing and/or a massive number of leukemic cells. The serum level and urinary excretion of uric acid may rise further after treatment with cytotoxic drugs because of increased cellular breakdown, and gout or precipitation of urate crystals may develop in the renal collecting system. Serum and urinary levels of phosphorus and potassium may also be elevated and rise further after treatment. Hypokalemia and hypophosphatemia may also occur. The serum level of lactic acid dehydrogenase (LDH) and serum and urine muramidase (lysozyme) levels may be elevated in different types of AML. However, both of these enzymes may also be elevated in chronic granulocytic leukemia and other myeloproliferative conditions, and very high LDH levels are sometimes seen in some of the lymphomas. In untreated ALL the muramidase concentration may be subnormal and subsequently rise to normal following successful treatment. The levels of serum vitamin B_{12}-binding protein and serum vitamin B_{12} may be high in acute as well as in chronic granulocytic leukemia.

The cerebrospinal fluid may be under increased pressure, have high concentrations of protein and low glucose, and contain leukemic cells, but sometimes central nervous system involvement may occur without any abnormalities of the cerebrospinal fluid. Conversely, pleocytosis may sometimes be present in the absence of recognizable neurologic signs or symptoms.

DIFFERENTIAL DIAGNOSIS When the blood leukocyte count is elevated, certain infections (e.g., meningococcemia, tuberculosis) may be mistaken for acute leukemia, but the majority of leukocytes are more mature in leukemoid reactions than in acute leukemias, and appropriate microbiologic studies should lead to the correct diagnosis. The peripheral blood lymphocytes may be greatly increased in pertussis, infectious mononucleosis, and infectious lymphocytosis, and to a lesser extent in varicella, infectious hepatitis, and several other viral illnesses. However, the bone marrow is less affected, and anemia and thrombocytopenia are either absent or less prominent than in acute leukemia. The lymphocytes are small and mature in pertussis and infectious lymphocytosis and should be readily distinguished from lymphoblasts. Although lymphoblasts indistinguishable from those found in ALL can occur in infectious mononucleosis and sometimes in other viral infections, the abnormal lymphocytes which occur in viral infections are usually more pleomorphic than leukemic lymphoblasts. Other helpful diagnostic tests for infectious mononucleosis are an elevated heterophil antibody titer (Paul-Bunnell test) and rising antibodies to Epstein-Barr (EB) virus; also the abnormal blood lymphocytes in infectious mononucleosis have T-cell markers, whereas this is true in only about 25 percent of cases of ALL. Occasionally, there can be considerable diagnostic confusion when severe anemia and/or thrombocytopenia occurs in infectious mononucleosis or infectious hepatitis as a result of hypersplenism, an autoimmune process, or rarely, aplastic anemia. However, in such cases the bone marrow either shows erythrocytic or megakaryocytic hyperplasia or it is aplastic and is not densely infiltrated with immature cells.

Usually, there is no difficulty in distinguishing between acute myelocytic leukemia and chronic myelogenous leukemia, but in some patients with chronic myelogenous leukemia the disease has already undergone blastic transformation when they first present; in some, the blasts may even have the morphologic appearance of lymphoblasts. The presence of a Philadelphia chromosome is generally considered to be diagnostic of chronic myelogenous leukemia. However, the blasts in some patients who unequivocally have acute leukemia show a similar karyotypic abnormality, and, conversely, some patients with otherwise typical chronic myelogenous leukemia lack this finding.

Some solid tumors which have a tendency to cause myelophthisic anemia are sometimes confused with acute leukemia, especially if there are no extramedullary tumor masses accessible for biopsy, because the tumor cells infiltrating the marrow may resemble leukemic cells. These tumors include neuroblastoma, Ewing's sarcoma, embryonal rhabdomyosarcoma, and oat-cell carcinoma of the lung. Infiltration of the marrow and blood occurs frequently in non-Hodgkin's lymphomas, and less commonly in Hodgkin's disease. The neoplastic cells in some diseases diagnosed as lymphomas may, in fact, be indistinguishable from certain types of leukemia, even by surface and biochemical markers. For example, neoplastic cells in the lymphoblastic type of poorly differentiated lymphocytic lymphoma may be "null" or T cells and have a high deoxynucleotidyl transferase content and other properties which are identical with the same cell types found in patients with ALL. Similarly, Burkitt's lymphoma cells are neoplastic B cells which are apparently identical with the L3 type of ALL cells. Diffuse histiocytic lymphoma (reticulum-cell sarcoma) may be confused with acute monocytic leukemia, since in both diseases the cells may have monocytoid features and a propensity to infiltrate the skin and other tissues. However, gingival infiltrates are common and retroperitoneal node involvement is uncommon in pure monocytic leukemia, whereas the reverse is true in histiocytic lymphoma. When lymphomas clearly originate in lymph nodes or other extramedullary sites and only secondarily involve the marrow, there is little difficulty in diagnosis. However, sometimes lymphomas may be largely confined to the marrow (and perhaps the spleen and liver) at the time of presentation, and there may be no enlarged lymph nodes available for biopsy. Indeed, with the use of newer cell marker techniques to identify specific cell types more precisely, some diseases previously diagnosed as lymphomas or leukemias are proving to be merely different manifestations of neoplastic proliferations of the same cell type.

When patients with acute leukemia present with few leukemic cells in the blood and reduction of one or more of the normal blood elements, the diagnosis may be confused with several other conditions, including hypersplenism and various neutropenic or thrombocytopenic states. Aplastic anemia, resulting from drugs, chemicals, or unknown causes, can be mistaken for acute leukemia, especially if the marrow is hyperplastic or in a regenerative phase, since numerous blasts and other immature cells and abnormal monocytes may be present. Some patients with aplastic anemia die of infection or bleeding, some recover partially or completely, and still others go on to develop full-blown acute myeloblastic or monocytic leukemia. A rare form of AML has been described in which the marrow is hypoplastic even on biopsy, but contains a greatly increased percentage (more than 30 percent) of blasts.

The terms *preleukemia, myelodysplastic syndrome,* and *refractory anemia with excess blasts (RAEB)* are sometimes used to describe such heterogeneous manifestations as anemia, neutropenia, thrombocytopenia, monocytosis, splenomegaly, and various other hematologic abnormalities which precede the development of acute leukemia, but this diagnosis can be made with certainty only in retrospect. If chromosomal abnormalities are present, there is a greater likelihood that acute leukemia will develop.

Erythroleukemia can be particularly difficult to diagnose and may be confused with primary refractory anemia, sideroblastic anemia, and paroxysmal nocturnal hemoglobulinuria (PNH). Since all these conditions may sometimes terminate in myeloblastic or other forms of acute leukemia, it has been suggested that they may represent early or chronic forms of erythroleukemia.

TREATMENT During the last quarter century, a worldwide effort has been mounted to improve the treatment of acute leukemia, and survival has been increased substantially in ALL and to a lesser extent in acute nonlymphoblastic leukemia. An increasing number of patients remain in complete remission even after discontinuing treatment, but because some patients have had relapse of leukemia after many years in remission, experienced clinicians are appropriately cautious about predicting curability. Nevertheless, encouraged by the progress that has been made, many therapists are now treating leukemia more aggressively and are directing their efforts toward total eradication of the leukemic cells rather than being content with temporary remissions.

Patients with acute leukemia usually have between 50 billion and 10 trillion (5×10^{10} to 10^{13}) leukemic cells when the disease is diagnosed; the number depends on the patient's size and extent of disease. Assuming that there are 1 trillion (10^{12}) cells, then a 13-decade ($\log_{10}$) reduction is necessary to eliminate all of them, but usually only a two- to three-decade reduction (99 to 99.9 percent) is required to cause a complete remission (defined as disappearance of all symptoms and physical abnormalities due to leukemia, and return of blood and marrow cell counts to normal or near-normal values).

Assuming no cell death, a single leukemic cell will propagate 10^{12} cells after 40 consecutive divisions. If there are 10^{12} cells at diagnosis, and if treatment causes a three-decade reduction, then only 10 doublings are required for the leukemic population to return to its original number. It has not been possible to measure the doubling times of leukemic populations in patients with any precision, and there is undoubtedly considerable variability, but if a doubling time of 5 days is assumed, then after a three-decade reduction, the leukemic cells would return to their original number within 50 days. It is necessary, therefore, to continue treatment to further reduce the leukemic cells long after a complete remission has been achieved. It is not known how long treatment must be continued in order to eliminate all leukemic cells, and the duration undoubtedly varies in different patients and with the intensity of the treatment and types of drugs used. Some drugs, such as alkylating agents and antitumor antibiotics, kill both resting and actively proliferating cells, whereas most of the antimetabolites are lethal only to proliferating cells. Since some leukemic cells can probably remain in a resting state for many months, alkylating drugs and antibiotics would be expected to be more effective in eradicating the last few cells.

Only some of the leukemic cells have unlimited proliferative potential and are capable of reproducing the disease; the rest, which are committed to maturation, will die spontaneously after a few divisions just as committed normal cells do. There are no methods to measure the fraction of clonogenic leukemic cells (i.e., those with stem-cell capability), but this undoubtedly varies greatly in different patients. It is also unknown whether there are host defense mechanisms capable of eliminating small numbers of residual leukemic cells in humans. Since it has been proved in animal leukemias that the number of leukemic cells surviving treatment is inversely related to the duration of remission and that the duration of remission in human leukemia is directly related to lengthened survival, the goal of treatment should be to destroy as many leukemic cells as possible.

The best opportunity to achieve maximum leukemic cell kill is when the disease is first diagnosed, since cells which survive the first round of treatment and later cause relapse of the disease may be relatively resistant to drugs which were highly effective initially. Although prolonged and possibly permanent second remissions have occurred occasionally in ALL, in general, second and later remissions become progressively shorter and are more difficult to maintain. Combinations of effective drugs have produced more frequent and longer remissions than have single agents, but it is difficult to predict how best to use the available or new drugs in the optimal combinations, order, and time sequences to achieve maximum leukemic cell kill with the least toxicity to normal cells. Because there are so many unknown factors, most of the current regimens have been developed empirically. Since none of them has been uniformly successful, no standard treatment schedules have been established, and investigators throughout the world are still trying to improve the results through comparative clinical trials. Exact comparisons between different series are often difficult because of differences in patient selection, age, previous treatment, outcome (whether patients are excluded if they die before receiving an adequate course of treatment), and use of differing criteria for tabulating incidence and duration of remission. In deciding which therapeutic regimen to use, the physician should consider the probability of achieving a durable remission in a disease which kills the average patient within a few months and weigh it against the necessity for prolonged hospitalization and the greater morbidity and disruption of normal life which are associated with some of the more aggressive regimens. Whenever possible, intensive treatment should be carried out under the close supervision of a physician who is experienced in the modern management of acute leukemia; such well-trained specialists are now widely distributed in the United States and in many other countries throughout the world. Because inadequate initial chemotherapy can jeopardize the patient's chance of a long-term response, except in emergency situations *patients with acute leukemia should be referred to the nearest specialist as soon as the diagnosis is made, preferably prior to initiating chemotherapy.* However, death can occur rapidly in acute leukemia, sometimes within days of diagnosis, and if the leukocyte count is very high or if there is evidence of disseminated intravascular coagulation (DIC) or other life-threatening complications, it is mandatory to begin therapy which will rapidly and drastically reduce the leukemic cell mass immediately.

With the best current treatment regimens, over 90 percent of children and over 70 percent of adults with ALL now achieve complete remissions. Most regimens include prednisone (40 to 100 mg per square meter of body surface area per day) and vincristine (2 mg/m² every 5 to 7 days) for induction of initial remission because these two agents are highly effective in killing lymphoblasts and are less toxic to normal marrow cells than most of the other drugs. If no further treatment is given after successful induction with prednisone and vincristine, the median duration of remission is only a few months, and it is imperative that the remission be consolidated and maintained with other drugs. Prophylactic intrathecal or intraventricular chemotherapy with or without cranial radiation treatment should also be given because of the high incidence of central nervous system involvement. Cranial irradiation and intrathecal methotrexate are effective in prophylaxis of central nervous system (CNS) leukemia, but there are several reports indicating that this combined modality therapy may result in serious late complications such as leukoencephalopathy and ventricular dilation. On the other hand, if prophylactic intrathecal chemotherapy alone is to be successful in preventing CNS leukemia, it must be given in sufficient dosage and continued for a relatively long period; exactly how long is uncertain, but one successful protocol has continued intrathecal therapy intermittently for 3 years.

The choice of drugs and the sequence of subsequent systemic therapy will depend on the training and preference of the specialist. Several combination drug regimens for ALL which have been shown to produce high rates of remission are listed in the references at the end of the chapter.

The results are less favorable in acute nonlymphoblastic leukemia. Although remission rates of 50 to 80 percent have been reported with various drug combinations, the median duration of remission has generally been less than a year and there are very few long survivors. In most, but not all, series the remission rate has been less in older patients, and the age factor should be taken into account when comparing different series. There is no relatively nontoxic drug combination comparable to prednisone and vincristine which will regularly induce remissions in nonlymphoblastic leukemia, and all the effective regimens are moderately to severely toxic to the normal hematopoietic cells and sometimes also to other tissues. This lack of selectivity is one of the major reasons for therapeutic failures. The patient has a high risk of dying during attempted induction of remission from infection or bleeding, because the granulocytes, platelets, and sometimes the immune system are already depressed as a result of the disease and become further depressed after treatment. Patients with AML seldom go into remission unless the great majority of morphologically evident leukemic cells in the blood and marrow have been destroyed and the marrow has become markedly hypocellular; the hypoplastic phase usually lasts at least 10 days and may last many weeks before repopulation begins. Repopulation may occur due to regeneration of normal cells, signifying the onset of remission, or from regrowth of leukemic cells, or there may be simultaneous repopulation with both normal and leukemic cells if treatment has been only partially effective.

There is considerable variability in the way in which patients respond to a treatment regimen. This variability is partly explicable on the basis of differences in the kinetic behavior of the various leukemic and normal cell populations, and partly on the basis of differing sensitivities of the various cell populations to the same drugs. Regeneration of normal hematopoietic cells may occur very rapidly after interrupting treatment, especially in younger patients, or may be very delayed or fail to occur at all; when this happens, the marrow may remain "empty" for a month or longer before it again becomes repopulated with leukemic cells. The variability in response makes it impossible to design a multiple-drug regimen with a standardized sequence which will be maximally effective in all patients. It is therefore essential to monitor closely the hematologic parameters and to individualize treatment schedules in accordance with the patients' general condition, hematologic status, and therapeutic response.

The hazard of dying during attempted induction is especially great in older patients who have other coexisting diseases, or who have developed serious infections prior to institution of antileukemic treatment. Because older patients often tolerate intensive treatment poorly, or because occasionally they have very slowly progressive disease ("smoldering leukemia") and may survive for a year or more with just supportive treatment, physicians have been understandably reluctant to treat them aggressively with chemotherapy. However, if they are left untreated, the majority of elderly patients die of acute leukemia within a few months just as do younger patients, and it is only the infrequent patient who survives longer than a year. When the diagnosis of smoldering leukemia is suspected, the patient should be observed closely, and as soon as the disease shows evidence of progression, or if the patient becomes incapacitated and unable to function with periodic transfusions, antileukemic treatment should be instituted, preferably before serious complications develop. While it is debatable how aggressively older patients should be treated, because "gentle" treatment with single agents is only rarely effective, probably the best approach is to compromise by selecting one of the combination drug regimens but attenuating the dosage schedule.

The most successful current regimens for acute nonlymphoblastic leukemia have employed an anthracycline (e.g., daunorubicin or adriamycin) in combination with arabinosyl cytosine and sometimes also with a purine analogue (e.g., 6-thioguanine or 6-mercaptopurine). In some protocols other drugs are also added in an attempt to increase leukemic cell kill. Several of the most effective regimens which have been reported to give remission rates of 70 percent or higher in nonlymphoblastic leukemia are listed in the references. Any of these regimens can be instituted in emergency situations, since they will all lower the leukemic cell count fairly rapidly in most patients. Daily blood counts should, of course, be obtained to follow the progress of treatment, but the count will usually be brought down to reasonable levels within a few days. If the patient has an extremely high number of circulating blasts or if there are other indications for promptly and drastically reducing the leukemic cell mass, a continuous intravenous infusion of arabinosyl cytosine, 200 mg per square meter of body surface area per 24 h, or of hydroxyurea, 2 to 3 g/m^2 per 24 h, will quickly lower the blast cell count in most patients, and higher doses will do so even more rapidly. Moderately large doses of several other drugs given singly are also usually effective in accomplishing this objective. These include daunorubicin, 45 to 60 mg/m^2 per day by intravenous injection for 2 to 3 days, and cyclophosphamide, 1 to 1.5 g/m^2 per day by intravenous injection for 1 to 2 days. However, the remission rate is lower with single agents than with drug combinations, and whenever possible one of the effective combinations should be employed as primary therapy because previously untreated patients have the best chance of achieving a durable remission.

Massive leukopheresis, using continuous-flow centrifugation or filtration techniques, is effective in lowering the blood leukocyte count rapidly, and up to several kilograms of leukemic cells have been removed in some patients. However, neither massive leukopheresis nor extracorporeal irradiation of the blood have proved useful in the definitive treatment of acute leukemia.

Because some reports are contradictory, and because the morphologic criteria for diagnosis are not necessarily identical, it is not clear whether there are important differences in the response rates of the different types of nonlymphoblastic leukemias. In some series, patients with promyelocytic leukemia, erythroleukemia, or monoblastic leukemia have been reported to have lower than average remission rates, but these differences may reflect differing sensitivities of the cells to specific drugs rather than general unresponsiveness. For example, promyelocytic leukemia appears to be unusually responsive to daunorubicin, whereas the combination of arabinosyl cytosine and 6-thioguanine has been relatively ineffective in this type of leukemia.

It is difficult to overemphasize the value of good supportive care in patients undergoing intensive chemotherapy for induction of remission, and some of the widely differing remission rates in different series of patients treated with the same regimen undoubtedly reflect differences in supportive treatment. Considerable experience and skill are required in anticipating and diagnosing infections and in knowing how best to treat them when they occur, in knowing how and when to use platelet transfusions and other measures to prevent or control bleeding, and in implementing preventive measures to avoid such common complications as perirectal abscesses. These can sometimes be prevented by such simple measures as keeping the stool soft and well-lubricated, maintaining good perineal hygiene, and prohibiting the taking of rectal temperatures. Venipunctures should be performed only when absolutely necessary, and meticulous care should be taken to avoid damaging the veins or introducing infections. Unnecessary subcutaneous or intramuscular injections should be avoided and intravenous infusions kept to a minimum. When hyperuricemia is present or is anticipated as a result of drug-induced cell breakdown, allopurinol should be given prophylactically, and sufficient fluids administered to maintain a good urinary output in order to prevent uric acid nephropathy. If 6-mercaptopurine is to be used concomitantly, the dosage must be lowered to about one-third of the usual dose because allopurinol interferes with the degradative pathway of this purine analogue and increases its toxicity; this is not true for 6-thioguanine, which may be given in full dosage.

Sometimes leukemic cells form local tumor masses in the central nervous system or elsewhere in the body which cause pressure symptoms, or the cells may infiltrate sites of infection such as perianal abscesses and interfere with healing. In such cases local irradiation may be used as an adjunct to systemic chemotherapy; generally several hundred rads will suffice. Irradiation may also be useful in controlling pericardial or other serous effusions due to leukemia. There are conflicting reports about the incidence of central nervous system (CNS) leukemia in AML. It is generally agreed that symptomatic CNS leukemia occurs much less frequently than in ALL, but whether this is entirely due to the fact that patients with ALL live longer is unsettled, as is the indication for preventive treatment. Most centers are not giving prophylactic treatment for CNS leukemia in AML but do treat the patient vigorously with cranial irradiation and intrathecal methotrexate and/or arabinosyl cytosine if this complication develops.

Fresh platelets have been shown to be very effective in preventing serious hemorrhagic complications, especially when they are obtained from histocompatible donors. However, platelet transfusions should be administered judiciously and only when needed, because eventually most patients receiving multiple transfusions from random donors over prolonged periods develop platelet antibodies; subsequent platelet transfusions are then relatively ineffective, perhaps when the need is greatest. If the platelets are obtained from siblings or nonfamily donors who are histocompatible for HLA antigens, the incidence of sensitization is greatly reduced; use of matched donors is essential once refractoriness to random platelets occurs. The level of platelet count at which platelets are required varies greatly. A level of 20,000 per cubic millimeter is commonly taken as the danger threshold, but many patients tolerate platelet counts of 20,000 per cubic millimeter or less without major bleeding, especially if the count has been stable around that level for some time. A rapidly falling platelet count, whether due to progressive disease or drug-induced myelosuppression, is more apt to be associated with serious bleeding, and in these circumstances platelets should be administered prophylactically before the count drops dangerously low.

One unit of concentrated platelets obtained from 500 ml of blood contains about 10^{11} platelets, and 2 to 4 units per square meter of body surface area are usually given; however, the number of units required depends on the clinical situation and the frequency of transfusions. Platelets should preferably be given within a few hours of being obtained, because stored platelets, especially when held beyond 48 h, are clearly less effective. The optimum conditions for platelet storage are still controversial (i.e., chilled or at room temperature). Satisfactory methods have been developed for freezing and long-term storage of frozen platelets, and it can be anticipated that this new technology will become more widely available. The normal platelet life span is about 9 days, but that of transfused platelets in leukemic recipients is always less than this, especially if there is infection, fever, or bleeding, and sometimes platelet transfusions are required daily or more often. Aspirin and other drugs which interfere with platelet function should be avoided in platelet donors and of course also in patients with leukemia.

If bleeding occurs despite an adequate number of normally functioning platelets, other coagulation defects should be looked for. In patients with overt bleeding due to DIC, many hematologists recommend that anticoagulation with heparin be begun promptly and continued until the leukemic mass has been sufficiently reduced by chemotherapy to arrest the chain of events responsible for the syndrome. It is generally assumed that the leukemic cells release proteolytic enzymes or other factors which activate the clotting process. Whether fibrinogenolysis occurs as a primary phenomenon or is secondary to plasmin formation during intravascular coagulation is unclear, but in either case the result is that the fibrinogen falls, fibrinogen and fibrin degradation products appear, and there may also be secondary decreases in other clotting factors, particularly V and VIII. Platelets also decrease and their recovery after an episode of DIC may be prolonged. Some hematologists argue that heparin should be given prophylactically, even in the absence of bleeding if there is biochemical evidence of DIC, before starting antileukemic therapy, on the grounds that massive lysis of leukemic cells will aggravate the process and might precipitate a serious bleeding episode.

Anemia should be corrected by transfusions of packed red cells. The erythrocyte level required to avoid symptoms attributable to anemia varies greatly in different patients, and as in the case of platelet transfusions, red blood cell transfusions should not be overutilized. There is always the danger of serum hepatitis, and if a good remission is obtained, erythropoiesis will resume at a level adequate to maintain normal or near-normal erythrocyte counts. Fresh leukocyte transfusions may be beneficial in treating infections when patients are severely neutropenic, but relatively large quantities must be given repeatedly because of the short life span of granulocytes. Moreover, the necessary facilities for procuring adequate quantities of fresh histocompatible leukocytes are not widely available. Various measures are currently being evaluated to try to lower the frequency and severity of infections. These include prophylactic bacterial vaccines, oral nonabsorbable antibiotic regimens for gut sterilization, and placement of patients in laminar airflow rooms or other sterile environments during attempted induction of remission, but their efficacy has not been clearly established.

A diagnosis of acute leukemia can be psychologically devastating to patients and their close relatives, and it is crucial to provide support and sympathetic counseling. Psychiatric consultants and other medical personnel can be very helpful, but patients will place most of their reliance on the primary therapist to alter the outcome of the disease. The physician must accept this responsibility, which can be very demanding, and be prepared to support patients throughout their course, whatever the outcome. There are no fixed guidelines about how explicitly patients should be informed about their disease, because many factors must be taken into account, such as age,

emotional stability, and the patient's general medical condition. In general, however, the wisest course is to be truthful in order to keep the patient's confidence and cooperation; it is essential that there be mutual understanding and consent between the patient and the physician regarding the nature of the disease and the necessity for prolonged treatment with drugs that have many unpleasant and dangerous effects. There has now been sufficient progress in the treatment of acute leukemia that, in most cases, the physician can be encouraging.

Bone marrow transplantation has been attempted in acute leukemia, following intensive chemotherapy and total body irradiation to destroy the leukemic population. A histocompatible donor, usually a sibling, must be available. In the largest reported series, approximately 30 percent of patients with acute leukemia who received syngeneic (i.e., identical twin) transplants and about 13 percent who received allogeneic transplants are surviving without evidence of recurrent leukemia for about 2 to 7 years after transplantation. The major causes of failure have been graft-versus-host disease (GVHD); infections, especially interstitial pneumonia; and recurrent leukemia. In most instances the recurrent leukemia has been due to regrowth of the host's original leukemic stem line, but in two well-documented cases the donor cells became leukemic. It is hoped that by transplanting bone marrow into patients earlier in the course of their disease when they are in complete remission (first remission in AML and second or subsequent remission in ALL) that the risk of early death due to complications associated with the transplantation regimen will be offset by a higher percentage of long survivors than can be obtained using moderately intensive chemotherapy alone without transplantation. Since effective chemotherapeutic regimens that have been sufficiently effective to result in significant numbers of long-term survivors have been available only in the past few years, it is too soon to know which approach holds the most promise.

There have been many attempts during the last 75 years to treat acute leukemia by immunotherapy. Occasional remissions were noted following administration of various blood constituents, following various infections (either induced or occurring spontaneously), or after immunostimulation by administration of bacterial endotoxins or other substances. However, remissions were infrequent, and attempts to induce remissions by immunotherapeutic maneuvers were largely abandoned after modern chemotherapy was introduced because the results were too inconsistent.

There has been a resurgence of interest in active immunotherapy with the more limited goal of trying to eradicate the relatively small number of leukemic cells remaining after remission has been induced with cytotoxic drugs. Nonspecific immunostimulants have included bacillus Calmette-Guérin (BCG), *Corynebacterium parvum*, mixed bacterial endotoxins, and various other microbial products. There are also ongoing trials using modified autologous or allogenic leukemic cells. The rationale for these trials is the presumption that leukemic cells have antigenic determinants distinct from those expressed by normal cells against which the host's immune system can be stimulated to react; however, there is no conclusive evidence that human leukemic cells have leukemia-specific antigens.

In a few trials with BCG and/or modified allogeneic cells or other immunostimulants there has been apparent prolongation of remission or prolongation of survival without prolongation of remission as a result of extension of life after relapse. On the other hand, many other trials have shown no beneficial effects from immunotherapy. The ultimate value of different types of immunotherapy in acute leukemia remains uncertain, and because of the heterogeneity of patient populations, further large carefully controlled trials will be necessary to determine its possible value.

PROGNOSIS Over 90 percent of children with ALL have complete remissions with modern chemotherapeutic regimens. The average survival for the untreated disease is only 3 months; with improved chemotherapy, survival times have increased, and there are several reports indicating that over 50 percent of children are living after 5 years. Since many of these children have now remained free of disease for at least several years after all treatment has been discontinued, it appears likely that some of them will prove to have been cured. However, a much longer follow-up period will be necessary to ascertain whether they will have a normal life expectancy. Subgroups of children with ALL with differing prognoses are becoming more clearly defined. Favorable risk features include: age between 2 and 10 years; relatively low initial white blood cell count; L1 morphology of leukemic cells with absence of T- or B-cell markers; absence of central nervous system involvement; and prompt response to chemotherapy with rapid attainment of remission. Children showing these characteristics have a high probability of having lasting remissions with effective treatment regimens, whereas in children with unfavorable risk features, the duration of remission is usually short and there are few long-term survivors. No treatment regimens have yet been reported which are highly effective in these poor-risk children. Adults with ALL generally respond less well than children, and most trials have resulted in complete remission rates of 50 percent or less, with a median duration of a year or less. However, in several trials using various drug combinations, remission rates of 80 to 90 percent have been reported, and there are now a significant number of adults who are remaining in long-term remission.

The prognosis remains generally poor in all types of acute nonlymphoblastic leukemia, both in children and adults. With the best chemotherapeutic regimens and good supportive care, 60 to 80 percent of patients are now attaining complete remissions. In most series the remission rate is higher in younger and lower in older patients, although a few also report good results in elderly patients. The survival of nonresponders remains about the same as with no treatment, around 3 months. In patients having remissions, the average duration of remission in most series has been between 6 and 12 months, and the average survival between 1 and 2 years. However, it is encouraging that there are now a significant number of patients with acute nonlymphoblastic leukemia who have had prolonged remission following intensive chemotherapy and who have remained in remission after discontinuing all treatment. The percentage of patients surviving over 3 years is still very low, but because the more effective regimens are new and have not been widely used, it may be anticipated that with longer follow-up a higher percentage of patients having lasting remissions will be seen.

REFERENCES

ALEXANDER P, POWLES R: Immunotherapy of human acute leukemia. Clin Hematol 7:275, 1978

BENNETT JM et al: Proposals for the classification of the acute leukemias. Br J Hematol 33:451, 1976

BODEY GP et al: Progress in the treatment of adults with acute leukemia. Arch Intern Med 136:1383, 1976

CLARKSON B et al: Prevention of central nervous system leukemia in acute lymphoblastic leukemia with prophylactic chemotherapy alone, in *International Symposium on the CNS Complications of Malignant Disease.* New York, Macmillan, 1979

———, RUBINOW SI: Growth kinetics in human leukemia, in *Growth Kinetics and Biochemical Regulations of Normal and Malignant Cells,* B Drewinko, R Humphrey (eds). Baltimore, Williams & Wilkins, 1977, p 591

COLEMAN CN et al: Hematologic neoplasia in patients treated for Hodgkin's disease. N Engl J Med 297:1239, 1977

GALE RP, CLINE MJ FOR THE UCLA ACUTE LEUKEMIA STUDY GROUP: High remission induction rate in acute myeloid leukemia. Lancet 1:497, 1977

HOLLAND JF et al: Acute myelocytic leukemia. Arch Intern Med 136:1377, 1976

LINMAN JW, BAGBY GC JR: The preleukemic syndrome (hemopoietic dysplasia). Cancer 42:854, 1978

LISTER TA, YANKEE RA: Blood component therapy. Clin Hematol 7:407, 1978

MAUER AM: Treatment of acute leukemia in children. Clin Hematol 7:245, 1978

MOHANAKUMAR T, RANEY RB JR: Leukemia-associated antigens in man. Clin Hematol 7:363, 1978

REIMER RR et al: Acute leukemia after alkylating-agent therapy of ovarian cancer. N Engl J Med 297:177, 1977

ROWLEY JD: The cytogenetics of acute leukemia. Clin Hematol 7:385, 1978

SANDERS JE, THOMAS ED: Bone marrow transplantation for acute leukemia. Clin Hematol 7:295, 1978

SIMONE JV: Factors that influence hematological remission duration in acute lymphocytic leukemia. Br J Hematol 32:465, 1976

WIERNIK PH: Treatment of acute leukemia in adults. Clin Hematol 7:259, 1978

326
THE CHRONIC LEUKEMIAS

GEORGE P. CANELLOS

The term *chronic leukemia* has been applied to those hematologic malignancies in which the predominant leukemic cell is initially well differentiated and can be readily identified as to cell type. They are generally divided into two main categories, lymphocytic and granulocytic. There are less common variants within these groups such as eosinophilic, myelomonocytic, and chronic lymphosarcoma cell leukemias. The term *chronic* also refers to the fact that these disorders have a generally better prognosis than the acute leukemias. Chronic granulocytic leukemia is a variant of the myeloproliferative syndrome (Table 326-1). However, there are some unique cytogenetic and clinical characteristics which distinguish this disease from other disorders in that group.

CHRONIC GRANULOCYTIC LEUKEMIA

CLINICAL AND HEMATOLOGIC FINDINGS Chronic granulocytic leukemia (CGL) can occur at any age, but the majority of patients are between 30 and 50 years old. Although there is no well-defined etiologic factor, an increase in both acute and chronic granulocytic leukemia was noted 5 to 8 years following the atomic bomb explosions in Japan.

The natural history of CGL can be divided into two fairly distinct phases, chronic and blastic. The *chronic phase* of CGL begins as a myeloproliferative disorder in which there is an excessive proliferation and accumulation of granulocytic cells of intermediate maturity as well as polymorphonuclear leukocytes. The median white blood cell count at the time of diagnosis is about 200,000 per cubic millimeter. Myeloblasts usually compose less than 10 percent of cells in the bone marrow and

TABLE 326-1
The myeloproliferative syndromes

	Splenomegaly	RBC count	WBC count	Platelet count	Marrow fibrosis	Philadelphia chromosome	Leukocyte alkaline phosphatase
Chronic myelocytic leukemia	Marked	Normal	↑↑↑	↑, Normal	±	+	↓→0
Myeloid metaplasia, myelofibrosis	Marked	↓	↑	Normal, ↑	+	0	↑
Polycythemia vera	Moderate	↑	↑	↑	0	0	↑
Essential thrombocythemia	Moderate	Normal	Normal	↑↑↑	0	0	

peripheral blood. The bone marrow morphology reflects this hyperproliferation and is usually hypercellular with excessive granulocytic precursors. The cytogenetic and morphologic evidence suggests involvement of all elements derived from the marrow stem cell. Thus, this disease can be considered a "panmyelosis" in the category of the myeloproliferative diseases such as polycythemia vera and myeloid metaplasia (Chaps. 320 and 321). The predominant cell type in most instances is in the granulocytic series, although rare cases of predominant eosinophilic and basophilic proliferation have been noted. About half the patients will present with a thrombocytosis in excess of 450,000 per cubic millimeter with increased megakaryocytes in the marrow. About 20 percent of cases are diagnosed on the basis of an elevated blood cell count in the absence of symptoms. In the majority, however, the signs and symptoms of the disease are related to the expanded granulocytic mass in the bone marrow, liver, and spleen. *Presenting symptoms* are usually palpable or painful splenomegaly, vague osteoarticular pains, anemia, and hypercatabolic symptoms such as weight loss and fever. Lymphadenopathy is distinctly rare in the chronic phase of CGL. In addition to the above, thrombohemorrhagic complaints such as excessive bleeding either spontaneously or following a surgical or dental procedure may be the first sign of disease. In some instances spontaneous cyclic leukocytosis and thrombocytosis may occur with a periodicity of 50 to 70 days. *Physical examination* will reveal splenomegaly in the majority of patients with the possible exception of those patients who are discovered early in the disease with a leukocytosis of less than 50,000 per cubic millimeter.

The chronic phase of CGL usually can be well controlled by treatment and persists for a median of 36 to 40 months before there is a transformation to the accelerated or blastic phase.

The onset of the *blastic phase* represents an evolution of the leukemic process from hyperplasia of mature elements to a loss of differentiation with increased numbers of blasts and progranulocytes. In approximately half the patients, the blastic phase will be preceded by an intermediate period of 3 to 6 months of myeloproliferative acceleration with progressively increasing leukocytosis, possibly thrombocytosis, and splenomegaly refractory to previously effective chronic phase therapy. In addition, myelofibrosis composed of increased reticulin, basophilia, and abnormalities of erythrocyte and platelet morphology may be seen. In the remainder, the transition can be abrupt, usually within weeks, to a state resembling acute granulocytic leukemia (AGL) (Chap. 325). The myeloblasts of the acute phase of CGL lack the Auer rods which are often seen in AGL. Rarely the "crisis" of a rising blast cell count is associated with cerebrovascular bleeding secondary to blast cell thrombi in the smaller vessels (leukostasis). A minority of patients will present with or develop extramedullary myeloblastic tumors usually in lymph nodes or skin, or as osteolytic bone lesions. In the past such lymph node masses have been

diagnosed as *reticulum-cell sarcoma* because of the very anaplastic appearance of myeloblasts in hematoxylin-eosin tissue sections. Meningeal leukemia is rare and usually occurs in patients whose blastic phase has been in hematologic remission following chemotherapy. The blast cell morphology can vary and about one-third of cases have some of the characteristics of lymphoblasts. Approximately the same proportion of patients will have the enzyme terminal deoxynucleotidyl transferase, a DNA-synthesizing enzyme, associated with acute lymphoblastic leukemia and normal thymic lymph cells. These cases also demonstrate reactivity with a non-B, non-T, anti-acute lymphoblastic leukemia antiserum. The relationship of these lymphoid characteristics to the presumed myeloid genesis of the disease is unclear.

The blastic phase of CGL is usually refractory to therapy and has a median duration of about 2 months from onset to death. The fatal complications of this phase are similar to those seen in terminal acute granulocytic leukemia.

CLINICOPATHOLOGIC FINDINGS The chronic phase of CGL is associated with a number of unique biochemical abnormalities. Accompanying the persistent leukocytosis of CGL is a marked elevation of serum vitamin B_{12} levels as well as an increased binding capacity of the serum for the vitamin. This is due to excessive serum content of the vitamin B_{12} transport protein, transcobalamin I, a glycoprotein of alpha-globulin electrophoretic mobility. A vitamin B_{12} binding protein with similar properties has been shown to be produced by mature normal and leukemic granulocytes in vitro. The elevated levels in the serum of CGL are probably derived from the turnover of the increased granulocytic mass. The high levels of vitamin B_{12} as well as the increased serum binding capacity return toward normal with remission of the disease. An enzyme termed *leukocyte alkaline phosphatase* is undetectable biochemically or histochemically in granulocytes of most patients with CGL in relapse. This enzyme has no known function but is often elevated in response to infection, stress, steroid administration, chronic inflammatory diseases, and Hodgkin's disease. Successful therapy of the disease results in normal or elevated levels. It is also known to be increased in polycythemia vera and myeloid metaplasia. The only other hematologic disorder with low or absent leukocyte alkaline phosphatase is paroxysmal nocturnal hemoglobinuria. Rarely, the hyperplastic marrow of CGL may contain glycolipid-laden phagocytic cells which resemble Gaucher's cells. These have also been noted in the spleen. Hyperuricemia related to the increased cell turnover may occur prior to therapy and can be exacerbated by treatment. This problem is also common to other myeloproliferative disorders such as myeloid metaplasia and polycythemia vera. The mature polymorphonuclear leukocyte of CGL is a functionally normal cell with respect to phagocytosis and bactericidal activity. This is especially true in patients with blood counts of less than 90,000 leukocytes per cubic millimeter. The kinetics of the granulocyte in CGL have been studied with isotopic-labeling techniques. There is clear evidence for increased production of mature granulocytes and their prolonged survival in the circulation but only in the presence of leukocytosis.

CYTOGENETICS About 90 percent of cases, which fulfill the hematologic criteria of CGL, have a unique and characteristic chromosome marker in the marrow and peripheral blood cells, the Philadelphia chromosome. It consists of a shortening of the long arms of chromosome G22 due to translocation of genetic material to chromosome 9. The abnormality persists throughout the course of the disease, in remission and relapse, and is generally unaffected by therapy. It is present in granulocytic, megakaryocytic, and erythroid precursors but not in lymphocytes or skin fibroblasts. In addition to the Philadelphia chromosome, the blastic phase of CGL is often associated with other chromosomal abnormalities, such as aneuploidy, which reflect the malignant character of this phase of the disease. Cases of CGL which lack the Philadelphia chromosome usually have a worse prognosis than the chromosome-positive disease.

DIFFERENTIAL DIAGNOSIS CGL must be differentiated from leukemoid reactions associated with infections and neoplasms. In these circumstances the leukocyte alkaline phosphatase is usually markedly elevated, and the Philadelphia chromosome is absent. A closely related myeloproliferative disorder with a similar prognosis is agnogenic myeloid metaplasia. This disease usually presents with marked myelofibrosis and splenomegaly. The white blood cell count and platelet count may be elevated as well. The leukocyte alkaline phosphatase is high, and there is no Philadelphia chromosome. Among the myeloproliferative disorders, the serum vitamin B_{12} level cannot be used as a differential diagnostic test in patients with elevated leukocyte counts.

TREATMENT The chronic phase of CGL can be controlled by a number of oral alkylating agents such as busulfan, cyclophosphamide, and phenylalanine mustard. Splenic irradiation can be an effective means for systemic control of the disease but in current practice has been replaced by more effective chemotherapy. The most commonly used drug is busulfan. It may be administered on an intermittent schedule or on a continuous daily basis with approximately the same results. The most serious complication of busulfan therapy is prolonged myelosuppression. Occasionally, remission of the disease for periods in excess of 12 months may follow a single course of treatment. The principal side effects include increased skin pigmentation, dryness of skin and mucous membranes, and, rarely, pulmonary fibrosis. An initial daily oral dose of 4 to 8 mg per day will reduce the white blood cell count to less than 20,000 per cubic millimeter in 2 to 3 weeks. It is important to progressively reduce the dose, roughly in proportion to the reduction in white blood cell count. The patient can achieve an excellent hematologic remission with return of blood counts to normal and disappearance of organomegaly. The Philadelphia chromosome will continue to be present in the marrow cells. Thus, a true remission of the disease has not occurred; rather, the proliferating granulocytic mass has been reduced to the point where immature cells disappear from the peripheral blood. Splenectomy has little place in the primary management of CGL but should be reserved for those patients with evidence of hypersplenism, repeated painful splenic infarction, and the rare instance in which prolonged thrombocytopenia has followed a course of busulfan. Splenectomy in the chronic

phase of the disease does not appear to abort the occurrence of blastic transformation.

Acceleration of the disease is reflected by progressive refractoriness to busulfan with leukocytosis, thrombocytosis, and increasing splenomegaly. In the absence of evidence for frank blastic transformation, the drug hydroxyurea (0.5 to 2.0 g per day by mouth) can effectively control the proliferative aspects of this phase. The blastic phase of CGL is refractory to most drug regimens, but remissions in about 20 percent of cases have been obtained with the use of vincristine and prednisone or other intensive combination chemotherapy programs useful in the treatment of acute leukemia.

The inability to achieve hematologic remission in the blastic phase of CGL may be in some part due to the fact that these patients often have myelofibrosis and/or are totally depleted of a residual stem-cell population capable of producing mature elements. Symptomatic extramedullary myeloblastic tumors, however, can be controlled with local radiation therapy.

CHRONIC LYMPHOCYTIC LEUKEMIA

CLINICAL AND HEMATOLOGIC FINDINGS Chronic lymphocytic leukemia (CLL) is a hematologic disorder of older people (median age of 60 years) which is characterized by the production and accumulation of functionally inactive but long-lived mature-appearing lymphocytes. Kinetic studies of the small lymphocyte in CLL indicate a turnover time in excess of 12 months.

The signs and symptoms of the disease are related to the infiltration of lymph nodes, bone marrow, liver, and spleen with these cells. As in CGL, the diagnosis can be made on a routine blood count in asymptomatic patients, but the majority of cases will present with lymphadenopathy and moderate splenomegaly. The white blood cell count is usually not as high as in CGL, and only one-third of patients have a count about 100,000 per cubic millimeter. Patients with advanced disease can also present with anemia, granulocytopenia, and thrombocytopenia due to bone marrow involvement. In addition, about 20 percent of patients will develop a Coombs-positive autoimmune hemolytic anemia at some time in the course of the disease. Rarely an idiopathic autoimmune-type thrombocytopenia can occur. As opposed to CGL, infiltrative skin lesions can occur and often precede the systemic manifestations of CLL. Patients with CLL will often have exaggerated cutaneous reactions to insect bites.

The presence of retroperitoneal or mesenteric lymph node enlargement can be associated with gastrointestinal or genitourinary complaints. The prognosis of the disease appears to be related to the extent of organ infiltration at the time of diagnosis. The median survival varies from 24 months for patients with anemia and thrombocytopenia to 8 to 10 years for patients who have only lymphocytosis and lymphadenopathy. The diagnosis can often be made from the peripheral blood film, especially in the presence of generalized lymphadenopathy.

Progression of the disease is associated with anemia, thrombocytopenia, and increased frequency of infection which is the most common cause of death. Splenomegaly and lymph node enlargement can be prominent, but splenic infarction is rare.

LABORATORY FINDINGS The disease is associated with a number of immunologic abnormalities. Almost half the patients with CLL will develop hypogammaglobulinemia which becomes progressively worse during the course of the disease. Antigenic challenge with vaccines has demonstrated a depressed circulating antibody response. Delayed hypersensitivity to antigens such as tuberculin is generally not impaired. The lymphocyte of CLL has a much-delayed transformation in vitro with mitogenic substances such as phytohemagglutinin when compared with normal lymphocytes. Immunofluorescent studies of the malignant lymphocyte of CLL have demonstrated immunoglobulin at the cell surface. In most cases it is monoclonal and of the IgM type. In addition, receptors for immunoglobulin-sheep erythrocyte-complement (EAC) complexes have been noted on these cells. These findings have supported the concept that in most but not all cases of CLL the disease is a malignancy of the bone marrow–derived (B-cell) lymphocyte, but a small number of cases of thymus-derived (T-cell) CLL have been described. There is no characteristic cytogenetic abnormality, and the serum vitamin B_{12} levels are in the normal range.

Several hematologic disorders are related to CLL but can be differentiated on the basis of morphology. Chronic lymphosarcoma-cell leukemia shares most of the features and complications of CLL. The malignant cell is usually a small or intermediate-sized cleaved lymphocyte. Malignant lymphoma with nodes diffusely involved with well-differentiated lymphocytes but without peripheral blood involvement may be associated with autoimmune phenomena and hypogammaglobulinemia and probably represents a lymphomatous expression of CLL.

TREATMENT The course of CLL is quite variable; in general, therapy is reserved for progression of the disease to the point of symptomatic lymphadenopathy, splenomegaly, or interference with normal hematopoiesis.

In the absence of a need for systemic therapy, lymph node enlargement which has become cosmetically or mechanically onerous can be controlled by local radiation therapy. Isolated splenomegaly can be effectively treated by splenic irradiation, often with improvement of the systemic manifestations of the disease including decrease of peripheral lymphocytosis. When systemic therapy is required, the majority of patients can be controlled with the lymphocytotoxic alkylating agents and/or corticosteroids. The drug of choice is either chlorambucil, 0.1 to 0.2 mg/kg per day, or cyclophosphamide, 50 to 150 mg per day. Both are administered on a chronic intermittent schedule. The doses of either alkylating agent usually can be reduced for maintenance therapy, but this requires a degree of individual titration according to disease activity. These agents can reduce lymph node and splenic enlargement and the infiltration of the bone marrow, often resulting in correction of the anemia and thrombocytopenia. Complete remission of CLL following radiation or chemotherapy is rare. Patients should be carefully followed lest the benefits of chemotherapy be canceled by excessive myelosuppression due to the drugs.

Corticosteroids have a marked lymphocytolytic effect and are not myelosuppressive. Thus they are especially useful when given with alkylating agents to patients with extensive marrow involvement. The risk of infection is increased, however, when steroids are given for prolonged periods in patients who are hypogammaglobulinemic and/or granulocytopenic. Corticosteroids are especially useful in the treatment of the autoimmune complications of CLL such as Coombs-positive hemolytic anemia and may be lifesaving in that circumstance. Splenectomy has not been shown to be of benefit in CLL except in some cases where hemolytic anemia and thrombocytopenia are refractory to corticosteroids and are related to excessive peripheral destruction of blood cells in the spleen. Blastic transformation analogous to that seen in CGL does not occur; however, a small number of patients develop lymphomatous transformation with a histologic appearance compatible with diffuse lymphocytic or histiocytic lymphoma.

In addition to the use of chemotherapeutic agents for the systemic treatment of CLL, fractionated total body irradiation and thymic irradiation have been successful in achieving clinical remission. These radiation techniques are still investigational and are not conventionally employed in the treatment of CLL.

REFERENCES

Chronic granulocytic leukemia

CANELLOS GP et al: Hematologic and cytogenetic remission of blastic transformation of chronic granulocytic leukemia. Blood 38:671, 1971

———: The treatment of chronic granulocytic leukaemia. Clin Haematol 6:113, 1977

GALTON DAG: Chemotherapy of chronic myelocytic leukemia. Semin Hematol 6:323, 1969

KARANAS A, SILVER RT: Characteristics of the terminal phase of chronic granulocytic leukemia. Blood 32:445, 1968

MARKS SM et al: Terminal transferase as a predictor of initial responsiveness to vincristine and prednisone in blastic chronic myelogenous leukemia. N Engl J Med 298:812, 1978

ROSENTHAL R et al: Blast crisis of chronic granulocytic leukemia. Am J Med 63:542, 1977

ROWLEY JD: A new consistent chromosomal abnormality in chronic myelogenous leukaemia identified by quinacrine fluorescence and Giemsa staining. Nature 243:290, 1973

SPIERS ASD: The clinical features of chronic granulocytic leukemia. Clin Hematol 6:77, 1977

WHANG-PENG J et al: Clinical implications of cytogenetic variants in chronic myelogenous leukemia. Blood 32:755, 1968

Chronic lymphocytic leukemia

AISENBERG AC et al: Cell-surface immunoglobulins in chronic lymphocytic leukemia and allied disorders. Am J Med 55:184, 1973

FREYMANN JG et al: Role of hemolysis in anemia secondary to chronic lymphocytic leukemia and certain malignant lymphomas. N Engl J Med 259:847, 1958

JANOSSY G et al: Comparative analysis of membrane phenotypes in acute lymphoid leukemia and in lymphoid blast crisis of chronic myeloid leukaemia. Leukemia Res 1:289, 1977

JOHNSON ER, RUHL U: Treatment of chronic lymphocytic leukemia with emphasis on total body irradiation. Int J Radiat Oncol Biol Phys 1:387, 1976

RAI KR et al: Clinical staging of chronic lymphocytic leukemia. Blood 46:219, 1975

SHEVACH EM et al: Receptors for complement and immunoglobulin on human leukemic cells and human lymphoblastoid cell lines. J Clin Invest 51:1933, 1972

THEML H et al: Kinetics of lymphocytes in chronic lymphocytic leukemia: Studies using continuous H-thymidine infusion in two patients. Blood 42:623, 1973

WILTSHAW E: Chemotherapy in chronic lymphocytic leukaemia. Clin Haematol 6:223, 1977

327
HODGKIN'S DISEASE AND OTHER LYMPHOMAS

JOHN E. ULTMANN
VINCENT T. DeVITA, JR.

DEFINITION The lymphomas are a group of malignant diseases of lymphoreticular origin. Although there are similarities among the various lymphomas, they include a wide spectrum of clinical and pathological pictures.

CELL OF ORIGIN OF THE LYMPHOMAS The lymphomas arise in the lymph nodes or in the lymphoid tissues of parenchymal organs such as the gut, lung, or skin. Ninety percent of cases of Hodgkin's disease originate in lymph nodes; 10 percent are of extranodal origin. In the non-Hodgkin's lymphomas, the tissues of the parenchymal organs are more often involved; 60 percent of these lymphomas originate in the nodes and 40 percent are of extranodal origin. With the availability of information on the subcompartmentalization of the lymphoid system and tests to study human tissue, the lymphomas can be classified by their cells of origin (Table 327-1). Almost all the non-Hodgkin's lymphomas (NHL) appear either to derive from a monoclonal population of B cells or to have no distinctive cell surface markers. Only a few appear to be true derivatives of tissue histiocytes despite the morphologic similarity of some malignant lymphomas to these cells.

Normal lymphoid tissue is composed of a mosaic of lymphoid cells within the follicle, and each subpopulation contains different immunoglobulin light chains. This is in sharp contrast to malignant lymphoid tissue. Even those histological types of lymphomas characterized by mixtures of different morphological cell types in the same node (mixed lymphomas of Rappaport, see below) have been shown to derive from a monoclonal B cell line. While identification of immunologically homogeneous clinical pathological entities may have prognostic and therapeutic implications with each major immunologic classification of the lymphomas (T cell, B cell, null cell), great variations in behavior can occur. For example, those B-cell lymphomas which grow in a nodular pattern (e.g., poorly differentiated nodular lymphoma of Rappaport) usually tend to have an indolent natural history with relapses and recurrences spread over 5 to 10 or more years. In contrast, the lymphomas termed diffuse "histiocytic" by Rappaport usually

TABLE 327-1
Immunologic characterization of cells of origin of the lymphomas

LYMPHORETICULAR NEOPLASMS OF B-CELL ORIGIN

Chronic lymphocytic leukemia
Cells in Richter's syndrome*
Diffuse well-differentiated lymphocytic lymphomas
Nodular poorly differentiated lymphocytic lymphomas
Nodular mixed lymphoma
Nodular "histiocytic" lymphomas
Diffuse poorly differentiated lymphocytic lymphomas
Most patients with diffuse "histiocytic" lymphoma
Burkitt lymphoma
5% of children with acute lymphatic leukemia
Poorly differentiated lymphoblastic lymphoma of children
Immunoblastic lymphadenopathy
Immunoblastic sarcomas

LYMPHORETICULAR NEOPLASMS OF T-CELL ORIGIN

Acute lymphatic leukemia of childhood with mediastinal adenopathy
  and convoluted cells
Sézary syndrome, mycosis fungoides
Chronic lymphatic leukemia—some cases
Diffuse "histiocytic" lymphoma—some cases

LYMPHORETICULAR NEOPLASMS OF HISTIOCYTES

Hodgkin's disease†
<10% of patients with "diffuse histiocytic lymphoma"
Histiocytic medullary reticulosis
Monocytic leukemia

NULL-CELL NEOPLASMS

Most patients with childhood acute lymphatic leukemia, up to 40
  percent of patients with diffuse "histiocytic" lymphoma of Rappaport

* *Local overgrowth of lymphoid tumor in patients with chronic lymphatic leukemia; often designated as reticulum-cell sarcoma in past.*
† *See text.*

have a more aggressive clinical course, but when responsive to treatment may be more vulnerable to permanent control by drugs. Yet, these lymphomas, like nodular lymphomas, are often monoclonal B-cell neoplasms.

The origin of the Hodgkin's disease (HD) cell is uncertain, but it may be derived from either a T lymphocyte or a macrophage line. In several laboratories, cells from the spleens of patients with Hodgkin's disease have now been grown in tissue culture. These cells resemble the Sternberg-Reed cell of Hodgkin's disease: they are aneuploid, a characteristic of malignancy, and produce nonspecific esterase. When reimplanted in immune-deprived mice, they produce invasive tumors. They have also been shown to phagocytize and to possess surface receptors for the Fc fragment of immunoglobulins and complement (C3b). All these findings are more characteristic of cells derived from the monocyte-histiocyte series than from T lymphocytes and lend strong support to the thesis that Hodgkin's disease is a true histiocytic lymphoma.

ETIOLOGY There is convincing evidence that viruses are one of the causes of lymphomas in rodents and birds; such a relationship has not been demonstrated in humans. In humans, there is a strong association between the DNA Epstein-Barr virus (EBV) and the rare lymphoma described by Burkitt in East Africa (anti-EBV antibodies appear in serum of patients, and complementary DNA appears in the human genome of Burkitt cells), but the association is less strong in Burkitt lymphomas diagnosed in the United States. In addition, in large series of patients with infectious mononucleosis, a disease caused by the Epstein-Barr virus, a small but consistent increase in the incidence of lymphoma has been noted after long follow-up, compared with controls who did not have infectious mononucleosis. A lymphomatous disease of chickens, Mareks disease, is known to be caused by another herpes-like DNA virus and can now be prevented by vaccines. Cell lines cultured from patients with Hodgkin's disease and some types of diffuse non-Hodgkin's lymphomas have been shown to express type C RNA virus particles and appear to contain viral information such as protein coat antigens and viral reverse transcriptase. All these observations lend credence to a viral etiology of human lymphomas but do not yet provide definitive proof. At the moment, it is not possible to distinguish among the three possible alternatives: a true etiologic relationship; contamination of tissue cultures by ubiquitous viruses; or the even more likely explanation, infection by virus in vivo after the cell has been altered by malignant transformation.

A hereditary influence on the incidence of lymphomas is suggested by their higher incidence in patients with inherited immunologic deficiency diseases and by a small increased incidence in families of patients with immunologic disorders. In one study, a significantly increased incidence of Hodgkin's disease was noted in siblings of the index case, particularly in siblings of the same sex. A slight increase in incidence of lymphomas has been noted in large series of patients with collagen-vascular diseases compared with the general population adjusted for age. This increased incidence approached 10 percent in patients with long-standing Sjögrens syndrome, who tend to develop diffuse lymphomas or immunoblastic sarcomas.

Lymphoma-like syndromes have been found in patients who take phenytoin. Although in most cases the disease regresses when the patients stop taking phenytoin, a significant fraction proceed to develop frank lymphoma of several different varieties, including Hodgkin's disease. Such observations suggest that the drug is acting on patients with an inherited tendency to develop the disease. Patients who are chronically immunosuppressed, particularly those who have received renal transplants, have a higher incidence of diffuse histiocytic lymphoma and immunoblastic sarcomas, often in the brain. Except for the higher incidence of Hodgkin's disease in siblings and the influence of phenytoin on the development of lymphomas, it is difficult to separate the influence of heredity, per se, from immunosuppression, which may be of etiologic importance without an inherited background.

EPIDEMIOLOGY About 25,000 new cases of lymphoma were diagnosed in 1978; 40 percent of these were Hodgkin's disease. Lymphomas are the seventh commonest cause of death from cancer in the United States; because of the young average age of the population (32 years for Hodgkin's disease and 42 for the other adult lymphomas), the toll in person-years of life lost ranks the lymphomas fourth among cancers in the United States in terms of economic impact. For unexplained reasons, the incidence of lymphomas appears to be increasing each year.

Worldwide, there are differences in the prevalence of lymphomas. In the United States, Hodgkin's disease has a bimodal age-specific incidence rate, one mode occurring at ages 15 to 35 years and the other above age 50. A disproportionate number of patients in the first modal peak have the nodular sclerosing variety of Hodgkin's disease. The first peak is absent in Japan. Hodgkin's disease in children under 10 years is seen much more frequently in underdeveloped countries, and, when it is observed, the histologic varieties and stages are characteristic of more advanced disease.

Some of the non-Hodgkin's lymphomas have unique epidemiologic characteristics. The Burkitt lymphoma occurs characteristically in children in central Africa, although a small number of cases with a different clinical presentation has been reported in the United States. Abdominal lymphomas that produce fragments of heavy chains of immunoglobulin occur in the Mediterranean region but are rarely seen in other parts of the world. These observations, and the occasional report of clusters of Hodgkin's disease, suggest environmental and/or genetic influences on the development of these diseases. However, in the United States following the report of several clusters of Hodgkin's disease, further population-based studies using the cancer registries of Connecticut and California have made a rather convincing argument that the reported clusters of Hodgkin's disease occurred by chance alone. Furthermore, medical personnel who specialize in the care of patients with lymphoma do not seem to have a higher incidence of these diseases than others.

HODGKIN'S DISEASE

CLINICAL MANIFESTATIONS Hodgkin's disease usually presents either with asymptomatic, discrete, painless, rubbery enlargement of lymph nodes or with symptoms of fever, night sweats, weight loss, and sometimes pruritus associated with adenopathy. Asymptomatic adenopathy may be noted by the patient or by the doctor on a routine physical examination. Often mediastinal adenopathy is noted on a routine chest x-ray or a film taken because of a persistent, dry, nonproductive cough. These presentations are more common in young people, and such patients often have the nodular sclerosing variety of the disease.

Other, usually older, patients present with fever and night sweats, or both, followed by increasing malaise and weight loss. Whereas superficial adenopathy is present in most such patients at some time in the course of the disease, in some cases the enlarging lymph nodes are located exclusively in the abdomen, and these patients often present to the physician with a differential diagnosis of fever of undetermined origin (Chap. 10). When diagnosed, they usually have the lymphocyte-depleted variety of Hodgkin's disease.

The fever in Hodgkin's disease is usually remittent. Occasionally, the patient has a cyclical fever pattern, called Pel-

Ebstein fever, which is characterized by several days or weeks of fever, alternating with afebrile periods. While fever, night sweats, and weight loss (referred to as B symptoms) have been found to correlate with a poor prognosis in Hodgkin's disease, the prognostic significance of pruritus by itself is unclear. It rarely occurs in the absence of fever and/or night sweats and has been dropped as a staging criterion indicating the presence of more advanced disease. Alcohol-induced pain in Hodgkin's disease is uncommon but has been reported to coincide with heavy eosinophilic infiltration at the sites involved by tumor. If alcohol-associated pain occurs, it may serve to direct the physician's attention to a site of involvement which can be biopsied. Occasionally a patient with Hodgkin's disease will present with obstruction of the superior vena cava as the first symptom. Sudden spinal cord compression can be a presenting complaint in patients with Hodgkin's disease but is usually a complication of progressing disease in a patient with known disease.

Characteristically, asymptomatic patients may have their adenopathy for extended periods of time with waxing and waning of lymph node size. Old x-ray films, in retrospect, may reveal that evidence of mediastinal widening has been present for several years. Slow progression of the disease, usually by extension to contiguous lymph node areas, occurs especially in the nodular sclerosing variety of the disease. With invasion of the hilar lymph nodes, the gateway to the lungs, the tumor mass may invade the pulmonary parenchyma. At some point in the progression of the disease, blood vessel invasion may occur. Vascular invasion can be easily demonstrated in biopsy specimen of lymphoid tissue stained with Weigert's stain, especially in patients with more advanced histological subtypes. Unsuspected involvement of the spleen, an organ which has no afferent lymphatics, suggests that vascular invasion may be a common occurrence, even in patients with apparently localized disease. Later, with further progression of disease and clear evidence of vascular invasion, the bone marrow, liver, and other viscera become involved. Symptoms, if they were not present initially, appear as the volume of tumor increases, and if the patient is not successfully treated, cachexia and widespread involvement of visceral organs by tumor occurs, infections complicate the course, and the patient dies.

Patients symptomatic at the outset seem to have disease which progresses more rapidly, have smaller-sized but more widespread lymphadenopathy, and more often have the lymphocyte-depleted or mixed-cellularity varieties of Hodgkin's disease. Bone and visceral involvement occurs earlier in such patients. Bone lesions are usually osteoblastic, and the ivory vertebra is characteristic of Hodgkin's disease. Bone pain is common, but pathological fractures are rare.

DIFFERENTIAL DIAGNOSIS The lymphadenopathy of Hodgkin's disease should be distinguished from adenopathy from other causes. Most cervical or axillary adenopathy in young people occurs as a result of infectious diseases with symptoms of fever, headache, and usually pharyngitis, and is often due to infectious mononucleosis, viral syndromes, or infection by *Toxoplasma gondii*. In older patients, adenopathy may occur as a result of local spread of head and neck cancers. A good rule of thumb is that any lymph node 1 cm or greater in diameter, which does not show signs of regression after 6 weeks of observation, should be biopsied.

Mediastinal and hilar adenopathy should be distinguished from sarcoidosis, which is almost always panhilar, and from primary tuberculosis which, although unilateral like Hodgkin's disease, is almost always accompanied by a resolving pulmonary infection and usually does not cause mediastinal lymph node enlargement. In older patients, the differential diagnosis includes primary tumors of the lung and mediastinum, specifically oat-cell and epidermoid carcinomas. Reactive mediastinitis and hilar adenopathy from histoplasmosis can be confused with lymphoma, particularly in regions where histoplasmosis is endemic, since it occurs in otherwise asymptomatic young people. Histoplasma mediastinitis usually involves the esophagus and should be suspected by obtaining a history of difficulty swallowing and confirmed by an abnormal esophagogram; occasionally a biopsy may be necessary. Hodgkin's disease presenting as "fever of undetermined origin" may remain undiagnosed despite extensive investigations until an exploratory laparotomy is done. Infrequently, patients present with autoimmune hemolytic anemia or idiopathic thrombocytopenic purpura and are found to have Hodgkin's disease only when splenectomy becomes necessary; on occasion, Hodgkin's disease in the removed spleen has been the only focus of involvement with tumor.

DIAGNOSIS AND PATHOLOGY The diagnosis and classification of a lymphoma can be made only by biopsy and histopathologic examination under a light microscope. Needle aspiration of lymph nodes, while it may suggest the diagnosis, does not yield sufficient tissue to classify lymphomas accurately, and the error rate is high. Even experienced pathologists, using fixed sections of lymph nodes, disagree on subclassification of lymphomas in up to 25 percent of cases and disagree on whether the resected tissue shows evidence of malignancy in as many as 6 percent of cases. Frozen section material should not be used when lymphoma is suspected because slightly crushed normal lymphoid tissue in frozen sections mimics malignancy. Some patients diagnosed by frozen section as having carcinoma of the neck have actually had lymphoma or benign reactive hyperplasia and have undergone neck dissection unnecessarily.

Hodgkin's disease is unique among cancers because the tumor observed by the physician contains largely normal tissue, lymphocytes, plasma cells, and the fibrous stroma of the lymph node and only a scattering of the characteristic malignant cell of Hodgkin's disease, the Sternberg-Reed cell. In the absence of Sternberg-Reed cells the diagnosis of Hodgkin's disease should rarely be made, although the presence of such a cell by itself is not pathognomonic of the disease, since cells simulating Sternberg-Reed cells have been found in patients with infectious mononucleosis and breast cancer. The presence of the mononuclear variety of the Sternberg-Reed cell, which has a large, eosinophilic nucleolus, is sufficient to demonstrate Hodgkin's disease involving the liver or bone marrow in a patient known to have Hodgkin's disease elsewhere; however, the finding of mononuclear Sternberg-Reed cells is not sufficient for the diagnosis of the primary tumor itself.

On the basis of histological classification, rates of spread of tumor, the need for staging laparotomy, and the likelihood that an apparently localized lesion will be disseminated can be predicted. The histological classification by Lukes and Butler used for Hodgkin's disease is shown in Table 327-2, along with the older Jackson-Parker classification. The original, more complete version of the Lukes and Butler classification was modified at the Rye Conference to include the four major histologic subgroups shown in the right column of Table 327-2. Proper classification is important.

IMMUNOLOGIC ABNORMALITIES In the 1950s, patients with Hodgkin's disease were shown to have a higher incidence of cutaneous anergy to a battery of intradermal skin tests than normal controls. Since then, a lively argument has continued whether the immunologic defect precedes or follows evidence of tumor growth, and whether it is etiologically related to the disease. Early studies demonstrating anergy in all stages were misleading because skin tests were done at skin sites drained by lymph nodes which had been irradiated. Subsequent studies in untreated patients showed that the ability of patients to respond to a battery of skin test recall antigens [intermediate strength PPD, trichophytin, histoplasmin, and Candida, and a new antigen dinitrochlorobenzene (DNCB)] was normal in the early stages of Hodgkin's disease and usually abnormal in stages III and IV. These studies also showed that the best predictor of cutaneous anergy was the absolute lymphocyte count. A lymphocyte count less than 1000 per cubic millimeter was significantly associated with cutaneous anergy. The presence or absence of anergy, or the in vitro lymphocyte phytohemagglutinin response, has been shown to have no influence on the prognosis, within a given clinical stage when modern therapy is used. This surprising observation indicates that effective antitumor treatment could eradicate the disease in patients already immunosuppressed by their disease even when the drugs themselves were immunosuppressive.

The immunologic defect appears to reside in the T lymphocyte which in normal persons is a major constituent of the delayed hypersensitivity reaction in the skin and the cell which reacts in vitro to phytohemagglutinin (PHA). A T-lymphocyte defect can now be detected even in patients with very early stage I Hodgkin's disease, if dose-response curves are done with DNCB in vivo and the lymphocyte response to PHA is measured in vitro. These data suggest that a T-cell defect is always a concomitant of Hodgkin's disease. The T-cell defect in HD appears to be caused by several different influences external to the T lymphocyte. In normal serum and laboratory media, washed lymphocytes from patients with Hodgkin's disease are able to respond normally to PHA; circulating immune complexes containing complement that binds to T lymphocytes have also been identified in the serums of patients with Hodgkin's disease. Glass adherent cells in cultures of Hodgkin's tissue obtained from resected spleens have been shown to produce high levels of prostaglandin E_2, which inhibits the lymphocyte PHA response. This reaction can be reversed by indomethacin, an inhibitor of prostaglandin synthesis.

Even following successful treatment with chemotherapy or radiation therapy, a permanent immunologic defect, both in

TABLE 327-2
Evolution of histopathologic classification of Hodgkin's disease*

Jackson-Parker (1947)	Lukes-Butler (1966)	Rye classification (1966)
Paragranuloma	Lymphocytic and/or histiocytic 1 Nodular 2 Diffuse	Lymphocytic predominance
	Nodular sclerosis ————————	Nodular sclerosis
Granuloma ——	Mixed ———————————	Mixed cellularity
	Diffuse fibrosis	
		Lymphocytic depletion
Sarcoma————	Reticular	

*The current classification by Lukes et al. provides greater prognostic information than the old Jackson-Parker classification by virtue of identifying those patients whose tissue shows intense fibrosis in nodules.

number and function of T lymphocytes, remains, even in patients who have been free of tumor for many years.

Antibody production is normal in most patients with Hodgkin's disease, but antibody production can be influenced by therapy. Combined multidrug chemotherapy and radiotherapy have been shown to diminish the primary response to capsular antigens of *Hemophilus influenzae* type B. This therapy combined with splenectomy may lead to a higher incidence of sepsis with *H. influenzae* and other encapsulated pathogens.

HEMATOLOGIC ABNORMALITIES A moderate, normochromic, normocytic anemia associated with low serum iron and low iron-binding capacity, but normal or increased iron stores in the bone marrow, may be present in patients with Hodgkin's disease. Studies have shown the anemia to be due to both increased destruction and decreased production of red blood cells. The iron profile in the peripheral blood is similar to that found in other patients with malignancy. A Coombs-positive hemolytic anemia occurs in less than 1 percent of patients with advanced disease.

The erythrocyte sedimentation rate (ESR) is usually rapid and serves as a useful test to follow disease activity; however, it has limited sensitivity and may return to normal when residual disease is obviously still present. It can be useful in monitoring patients who are in remission to determine the first evidence of recurrence. Extensive radiation therapy may cause the ESR to be elevated for as long as 1 year after treatment without evidence of recurrent tumor. Numerous more complicated, and usually more expensive, laboratory tests of disease activity have not been shown to be superior to the ESR.

A moderate to marked leukemoid reaction is common in Hodgkin's disease, particularly in symptomatic patients. White blood cell count as high as 67,000 per cubic millimeter, a level which can easily be confused with the level found in chronic granulocytic leukemia, may be seen. The leukemoid reaction disappears with successful treatment. Mild peripheral eosinophilia is not uncommon, especially in patients with pruritus. Absolute lymphocytopenia (<1000 cells per cubic millimeter) usually occurs in patients with more advanced disease.

A bone marrow examination requires a bone marrow biopsy. Marrow aspiration has not yielded results comparable to those obtained by biopsy, probably because of the fibrosis and granuloma formation in the marrow of patients with Hodgkin's disease. On smear or section, the myeloid/erythroid ratio may be increased, and marrow eosinophilia is common; neither necessarily represents marrow involvement by tumor. Involvement of the marrow by tumor may be demonstrated by finding either classic Sternberg-Reed cells or their mononuclear variant, distributed focally or diffusely throughout the bone marrow. Marrow involvement is often associated with reticular fibrosis, which sometimes obscures the architecture of the marrow. In a patient with known Hodgkin's disease, intense marrow fibrosis, even in the absence of the characteristic malignant cells, is strong evidence of tumor in the bone marrow. Surprisingly, effective treatment by chemotherapy often leads to total resolution of marrow fibrosis in patients who achieve remission.

SELECTED CLINICAL PROBLEMS Infections are common in patients with Hodgkin's disease. Those who have progressive tumor usually die of the complications of bone marrow failure, bacteremia, or disseminated fungal infections. Diffuse pulmonary infiltrates may appear in patients who are in remission between cycles of chemotherapy, radiotherapy, or both; infection with the protozoan *Pneumocystis carinii* then should be suspected. Evidence from rats infected with *P. carinii* suggests that the appearance of this infection between cycles of treatment is related to a rebound inflammatory response to the growing organism. Patients with Hodgkin's disease are prone

to develop cryptococcosis, either in the form of meningitis or as a primary pulmonary infiltrate with or without meningitis. Herpes zoster (shingles) occurs in 10 percent of treated Hodgkin's patients and in 20 percent of treated patients who have had a splenectomy. Most patients who develop herpes zoster have a few scattered papules outside the involved dermatone; this minimal evidence of spread usually does not require systemic treatment. Tuberculosis, once thought to "follow Hodgkin's disease like a shadow," is no longer common in these patients.

Cord compression is the most serious acute complication caused by growing tumor masses and is usually seen in patients with progressive tumor who have failed primary treatment. It can be caused by vertebral body involvement with collapse, which is easily seen on x-ray or bone scan, or by invasion of the epidural space from retroperitoneal lymph nodes with compression of the cord or compression of the vascular supply to the cord. Selective electromyography is a useful way to detect regional denervation, but a myelogram is usually needed to confirm the diagnosis. Tumor masses can also obstruct the superior vena cava. This may occur as a presenting syndrome or late in the course of the disease when the diagnosis is obvious.

STAGING The staging classification developed for Hodgkin's disease and used for all lymphomas is shown in Table 327-3. Accurate staging of HD patients is vital for planning long-term management. The primary physician must take a detailed history, do a thorough physical examination, and look for evidence of fever, night sweats, and weight loss. Weight loss of 10 percent or greater, with no attempt at dieting, usually means serious disease in this young population. Soaking night sweats can occur in anxious patients, and a history of sweats preceding knowledge of the diagnosis should be sought carefully. Every lymph node area of the body should be examined carefully, and the presence or absence of enlargement noted for future reference; the size, shape, and consistency should be recorded. Reactive hyperplasia is a cause for lymph node enlargement around lymph nodes involved with tumor, especially in the neck region; the largest lymph nodes in a group should be marked for biopsy. These may be less accessible to the sur-

TABLE 327-3
Staging classification for lymphomas

Stage	Definition
I	Involvement of a single lymph node region (I) or of a single extralymphatic organ or site (I_E).
II	Involvement of two or more lymph node regions on the same side of the diaphragm (II) or localized involvement of an extralymphatic organ or site and of one or more lymph node regions on the same side of the diaphragm (II_E).
III	Involvement of lymph node regions on both sides of the diaphragm (III), which may also be accompanied by involvement of the spleen (III_S) or by localized involvement of an extralymphatic organ or site (III_E) or both (III_{SE}).
IV	Diffuse or disseminated involvement of one or more extralymphatic organs or tissues, with or without associated lymph node involvement.

NOTE: *The presence of fever, night sweats, and/or unexplained loss of 10 percent or more of body weight in the 6 months preceding admission is denoted by the suffix letter B. The letter A indicates the absence of these symptoms. Biopsy-documented involvement of stage IV sites is also denoted by letter suffixes: marrow = M +; lung = L +; liver = H +; pleura = P +; bone = 0 +; skin and subcutaneous tissue = D +.*
SOURCE: *Adopted at the workshop on the Staging of Hodgkin's Disease held at Ann Arbor, Mich, April 1971.*

geon, who should be urged, nonetheless, to seek them out. Nodes in areas other than the primary site, that might change the patient's stage from local to generalized disease, should be biopsied at the same time. Internists unfortunately are prone to omit examination of the oro- and nasopharynx by indirect laryngoscopy. Such examination is essential to uncovering Waldeyer ring involvement by lymphoma, although this finding is more common in the non-Hodgkin's lymphomas than in Hodgkin's disease. Epitrochlear nodes can also be involved by HD but are also more likely to be present in non-Hodgkin's lymphoma. The size of the liver and spleen should be noted. In HD, palpable splenomegaly is significant because in most cases it indicates more generalized disease. The procedures required for staging patients with Hodgkin's disease under various circumstances are shown in Tables 327-4 to 327-6.

Radiological examination should include a routine chest film. When any evidence of disease is noted on this x-ray, whole-chest tomography is performed to identify the extent of mediastinal or hilar adenopathy or evidence of contiguous invasion of the lung from the hilar nodes. Lower-extremity lymphangiogram should always be done unless medically contraindicated. On occasion, the lymphangiogram will not fill high retroperitoneal lymph nodes. Computerized tomography (CT) scan and ultrasound have been shown to be effective in delineating the status of the retroperitoneal lymph nodes in these upper node regions and should supplement lymphangiography. The status of the bones can be determined using the lymphangiogram films in most cases. Symptomatic patients should have a separate skeletal survey and/or a technetium 99 pyrophosphate bone scan. The latter is the more sensitive test for identifying bone lesions.

Routine blood counts, erythrocyte sedimentation rate, urinalysis, liver function studies, and renal function studies are all necessary parts of the medical workup but by themselves do not provide information about the extent of Hodgkin's disease or specific organ involvement. Liver function abnormalities, in particular, are poor indicators of Hodgkin's involvement of the liver but are helpful in ruling out the presence of other complicating illnesses. Bone marrow biopsy, not aspiration, should be done in all symptomatic patients with Hodgkin's disease and in those asymptomatic patients with evidence of generalized adenopathy and in patients who undergo staging laparotomy. Asymptomatic patients who have disease clinically localized above the diaphragm, that is, whose lymphangiography is found to be negative, rarely have bone marrow involvement, and the biopsy can be omitted in such cases.

TABLE 327-4

Staging Hodgkin's disease: Required evaluation procedures

I Adequate surgical biopsy, reviewed by an experienced hematopathologist
II A detailed history recording the absence or presence of and duration of fever, unexplained sweating and its severity, unexplained pruritus, and unexplained weight loss
III A careful and detailed physical examination; special attention to all node-bearing areas, including Waldeyer's ring, and determination of size of liver and spleen
IV Necessary laboratory procedures
  A Complete blood count, including an erythrocytic sedimentation rate
  B Serum alkaline phosphatase
  C Evaluation of renal function
  D Evaluation of liver function
V Radiologic studies
  A Chest roentgenogram (posteroanterior and lateral)
  B Intravenous pyelogram
  C Bilateral lower extremity lymphogram
  D Views of skeletal system to include thoracic and lumbar vertebrae, the pelvis, proximal extremities, and any areas of bone tenderness

TABLE 327-5

Staging Hodgkin's disease: Procedures required under certain conditions

I Whole-chest tomography if any abnormality is noted or suspected on the routine chest roentgenogram
II Inferior cavography, ultrasonography, or CT scan to supplement equivocal lymphographic findings in the high retroperitoneal area
III Bone marrow biopsy (needle or open) in the presence of:
  A An elevated alkaline phosphatase
  B Unexplained anemia or other blood count depression
  C Other evidence of bone disease (scan or x-ray)
  D Generalized disease of stage III or greater
IV Exploratory laparotomy and splenectomy, if management decisions will depend on the identification of abdominal disease

In 1968, a group of investigators at Stanford University introduced routine staging laparotomy as a research tool to evaluate the extent of Hodgkin's disease, to define its mode of spread, and to determine the implications of such information for therapy. In one-third of patients with normal-sized spleens, Hodgkin's disease was found in the spleen removed at surgery; conversely, in those patients with clinically enlarged spleens up to 25 percent had no evidence of tumor in the spleen but appeared instead to have reactive hyperplasia. Splenic enlargement due to involvement by HD has been linked to liver involvement. The liver is rarely involved when splenic involvement is not associated with splenomegaly (<0.5 percent). Liver involvement is present in as many as 28 percent of patients with positive lymphangiograms and enlarged spleens. The Stanford data also showed that the lymphangiogram, although not infallible, was a reasonably accurate test to detect lymph node involvement by tumor. Only 15 percent of patients with positive lymphangiograms were found to have normal lymph node biopsies at surgery. Even in these patients, an explanation may be found in the reactive lymphoid hyperplasia normally found adjacent to tumor. The studies from the Stanford group confirmed the previous impression that in symptomatic patients with negative lymphangiograms, tumor could frequently be found in retroperitoneal lymph nodes at surgery. This fact had been suggested prior to the advent of staging laparotomy because of the high relapse rate in the retroperitoneal nodes of such patients if these nodes were not included in the radiation field.

Retroperitoneal lymph node involvement demonstrated at laparotomy was associated particularly often with low left neck lymph node involvement. This association reinforced the hypothesis that HD spreads from the neck to the retroperitoneum via the thoracic duct. This hypothesis has been invoked to help explain why, in 10 percent of patients with HD, tumor will skip the mediastinal area and involve the retroperitoneal lymph nodes. A more likely explanation is that HD involvement of the retroperitoneal lymph nodes is related to splenic involvement, which is in itself related to dissemination of tumor through the bloodstream.

Staging laparotomy should not be considered a routine concomitant of staging. Knowledge of the type of treatment to be used by the radiotherapist or medical oncologist, for the variety of stages of Hodgkin's disease, should be known in advance of a decision to operate, since general treatment strategy may

TABLE 327-6

Staging Hodgkin's disease: Useful ancillary procedures

1 Skeletal scintigrams*
2 Hepatic and spleen scintigrams*
3. Serum chemistries to include serum calcium and uric acid for overall management of patient
4 Estimates of the patient's delayed hypersensitivity of the tuberculin type
5 Gallium whole-body scans*

* *Cannot be used as evidence of Hodgkin's disease without biopsy confirmation.*

markedly influence the decision to perform a staging laparotomy. When it is performed, the laparotomy should always be complete and include at least two needle biopsies of each lobe of the liver, a wedge biopsy of the liver edge, biopsies of suspicious areas, splenectomy, and biopsy of selected lymph nodes in the retroperitoneal area, marked on the lymphangiogram prior to the operation. A postoperative film should confirm that the proper lymph nodes were removed. Nodes in the porta hepatis should also be biopsied, and, in female patients in the reproductive period, the ovaries should be moved laterally or centrally to avoid the major part of the radiation ports. If done properly, results from laparotomy will change the stage in as many as 35 percent of patients. In most cases, the change results from evidence that more extensive tumor is present, but in some cases patients are down-staged as well.

The Ann Arbor Conference on staging of Hodgkin's disease recommended that results of staging should be reported using both the clinical stage (CS) (all tests leading up to invasive studies) and the final pathological stage (PS) which includes the results of invasive tests, such as liver biopsy and laparotomy. This was recommended to ensure that investigators, using different staging approaches, could make comparisons of the results of therapy based on the clinical stage of the patient. When the best therapeutic approaches are used, the change of stage following laparotomy infrequently results in a change in the plan of therapy.

Laparoscopy has been shown to be a useful alternative approach to laparotomy in staging abdominal disease. Liver involvement can be detected with equal facility by either approach.

Nationwide, the mortality from staging laparotomy in Hodgkin's disease is 1.5 percent, with a complication rate of approximately 12 percent. However, mortality rates up to 6.6 percent and morbidity rates of greater than 25 percent have been reported from institutions where laparotomies are done infrequently. In some stages of Hodgkin's disease, the operative mortality may exceed the expected death rate at 5 years from the disease itself.

TREATMENT Extremely effective treatment of Hodgkin's disease has been developed in the past 18 years. Both drugs and radiation therapy eradicate the disease under certain circumstances. As a result of widespread application of these treatment methods, national mortality from Hodgkin's disease has dropped 30 percent in the most recent reporting period, according to the End Results Report Number 5 of the Biometry Branch of the National Cancer Institute. Because of the stringent requirements for shielding and field piecing, the radiotherapy used for Hodgkin's disease is the most difficult treatment a radiation therapist uses. The treatment of Hodgkin's disease by radiotherapy requires extensive experience with more than a few patients a year and adequate equipment, preferably a 6- to 10-MeV linear accelerator. Kilovoltage equipment is inadequate and should no longer be used. Cobalt 60 equipment can be used effectively, but its use is associated with an increase in side effects from greater scatter of the radiotherapy beam. A linear accelerator is the preferred instrument.

Current drug treatment programs require precise metering of doses using a sliding scale for increases and decreases of doses, based on nadir blood counts and blood counts determined the day a new cycle is to begin. Consistency in delivering chemotherapy safely requires experience with the disease and the drugs and *should not be done by anyone not expert in the field*. Occasional treatment often results in reduced doses, drug omissions, improper sequencing, disrupted schedules, and, ultimately, recurrent tumor.

Treatment of lymphomas is in transition. Clinical trials are in progress to develop and study ways to make both drugs and radiation treatment safer, to further facilitate their general use,

and to evaluate the role of each alone and together in various stages and histological subtypes of Hodgkin's disease. Some general principles have, however, emerged. At the present time, the best approach to treatment is to use either radiotherapy or combination chemotherapy alone in the appropriate stage. Studies comparing both types of treatment used together to each used alone have shown that patients who relapse after radiotherapy can be successfully re-treated with combination chemotherapy, with results equivalent to those obtained in previously untreated patients of the same stage and histological subtype. This means that patients cured by radiotherapy alone can be spared exposure to drugs, and those patients treated with radiotherapy who relapse have a second chance for a prolonged remission. The role of radiotherapy as a supplement to drug treatment of stages III and IV disease is controversial. No convincing evidence of benefit from a combined approach has been presented.

The most important parameter to follow after treatment with either radiotherapy or chemotherapy is the initial period of relapse-free survival. Interpretation of current data is somewhat confused by the fact that patients who are inadequately treated with radiotherapy can be salvaged by chemotherapy. Until such time as studies are done to determine the effectiveness of chemotherapy alone in patients with early stages of disease, however, inadequate radiotherapy should not be given intentionally because of the potential for salvage by drugs of patients who fail radiotherapy.

The dose of radiotherapy is important, because the risk of relapse in a treated field is inversely proportional to dose, falling to about 1 percent at 4400 rads. Sharpness of the field edge with minimal scatter is achieved by a linear accelerator. It also allows the large fields required to treat Hodgkin's disease to be given with less toxicity to the bone marrow and less scatter to uninvolved but susceptible essential organs. In spite of shielding and sharp field edges, scatter to the entire lung fields is often in the range of 200 rads, and similar scatter doses are routinely received by the testes if the lower abdomen is radiated, even when extensive shielding is used.

Three types of radiation fields are used. Involved-field (IF) radiotherapy treats only the tumor mass with a minimal margin of normal tissue. Mantle-field irradiation gives radiation treatment to the cervical, axillary, and mediastinal nodes as one field. Upper paraaortic nodes are now included as part of the mantle field, usually as one field; when used in this way, it is referred to as extended-field (EF) radiotherapy. The "inverted Y" field is used to irradiate the retroperitoneal lymph nodes as a single field, and when used with the mantle field is referred to as total nodal irradiation (TNI). Actually TNI is a misnomer since many lymph nodes are outside the usual TNI fields; *total axial lymph node* irradiation (TANI) is a more accurate term. Critical in applying these treatments is to shield the spinal cord in the cervical region and the heart and to avoid overlapping the margins of the mantle and inverted Y fields. Such overlap can result in delivery of sufficient radiotherapy to the spine to cause radiation myelitis.

After the discovery of several drugs that, when employed as single agents, could affect reduction of tumor masses in patients with Hodgkin's disease, combination drug programs were instituted in the early 1960s, and the four-drug program abbreviated MOPP [nitrogen *m*ustard, vincristine (*O*ncovin), *p*rednisone, and *p*rocarbazine] has emerged as the standard treatment program. Other non-cross-resistant drug combinations are available and are being tested after MOPP treatment to determine whether drugs are superior to x-ray in preventing relapse in MOPP-treated patients. Other combinations of old and of new single drugs are also used to salvage those patients who relapse after MOPP-induced remission, or who fail to enter remission. There is little role for single-agent chemotherapy as the primary treatment in patients with advanced disease unless they are medically infirm for reasons other than Hodgkin's disease.

Through use of the MOPP combination program, up to 80 percent of patients with advanced stages will achieve a complete remission; 66 percent of such patients have remained free of their disease up to 12 years after remission was induced with only six cycles of treatment. Most patients who have relapsed have done so in the first 2 years of follow-up, and a few patients have suffered recurrence after 4 to 5 years.

Use of specific treatment approaches INVOLVED-FIELD RADIOTHERAPY Patients with single-node involvement in the high right neck, especially those who have lymphocyte-predominant Hodgkin's disease, do not require a laparotomy, since they rarely have splenic or retroperitoneal lymph node involvement by tumor and can be rendered free of disease for extended periods 95 percent of the time when treated with 3500 to 4000 rads to the involved field.

EXTENDED-FIELD RADIOTHERAPY Patients with CS IA and IIA, with nodular sclerosing or mixed cellular Hodgkin's disease, limited to lymph node areas above the diaphragm, can be rendered free of disease more than 90 percent of the time, for periods extending beyond a decade, by EF radiotherapy only, without the need for a laparotomy. Those patients who present with single sites of involvement in the groin should be treated with EF radiotherapy rather than IF radiotherapy (in this case the inverted Y field). Some assessment of the status of the liver should be made either by laparoscopy or laparotomy.

TOTAL AXIAL LYMPH NODE RADIOTHERAPY (TANI) TANI has provided results superior to EF or the mantle field when relapse-free survival is used as the major assay of effectiveness. TANI includes a splenic port and should not be used in the patient with an enlarged spleen. All symptomatic patients with localized disease (CS and PS IB and IIB), if they are to receive radiotherapy alone, should receive TANI, even if a laparotomy revealed no evidence of disease below the diaphragm, since there is no evidence that withholding radiation therapy to retroperitoneal nodes is safe in patients with negative random lymph node biopsies. Laparotomy in most cases is unnecessary. The type of radiotherapy to be given for supradiaphragmatic CS and PS IIA mixed cellularity and lymphocyte-predominant Hodgkin's disease is debatable. Equivalent results are achievable with TANI in clinically staged patients, and EF in patients staged by laparotomy. TANI can be used for patients with stage IIIA Hodgkin's disease, although at least equivalent rates of control have been achieved with MOPP chemotherapy. The choice of treatment for stage IIIA depends in part on the local expertise available.

Chemotherapy with the MOPP program Stage IIIA responds well to MOPP chemotherapy; most studies report nearly a 100 percent remission rate and few relapses over a decade of follow-up. Several studies clearly show that patients with CS and PS IIIB Hodgkin's disease have a better chance of relapse-free survival with MOPP chemotherapy than with TANI, and that the addition of radiotherapy to chemotherapy does not appear to provide much benefit. An exception may be found in patients with nodular sclerosing stage IIIB Hodgkin's disease, with bulky tumor. These patients may have minimal residual widening of the mediastinal architecture after chemotherapy alone and may profit by the use of the combination of MOPP and TANI radiotherapy.

All patients with stage IV disease are best treated with MOPP chemotherapy, which results in complete, durable remissions equivalent to those of patients with stage III disease and is not influenced by specific organs involved with tumor. A patient with bone marrow involvement by Hodgkin's disease should receive full doses of chemotherapy and can expect the same frequency and duration of remission as those patients who have liver or lung involvement. Other drug combinations may be useful in patients who fail the MOPP chemotherapy program. Two such drug combinations use bleomycin, adriamycin, vinblastine, and dacarbazine with or without prednisone and have been shown to produce a significant fraction of complete remissions in MOPP treatment failures. These remissions are, however, not as durable as the primary remission. When a patient reaches this point in his or her disease, the greater side effects produced by combinations of drugs against a single drug treatment must be weighed, keeping in mind the lack of durability of remissions achieved after resistance to the first drug treatment occurs. Cure is usually no longer a reasonable expectation. Under these circumstances it is sometimes helpful to return to the use of single-agent chemotherapy, including drugs used in previous combinations by a different schedule. For example, patients with advancing MOPP-resistant Hodgkin's disease may still respond to daily oral procarbazine or intermittent large doses of alkylating agents.

Many variables influence the outcome of patients within a given stage. These include the presence or absence of symptoms and the various histological subtypes in the treatment groups. Symptoms adversely affect prognosis since they generally indicate a greater volume of tumor as well as rapidity of spread. Volume is a clinical variable that is difficult to assess in current staging classifications. Histology is also important. While the nodular sclerosing variety of Hodgkin's disease favorably influences the prognosis of patients treated by radiotherapy alone, the presence of this histological subtype appears to adversely influence the durability of remissions attained with chemotherapy programs.

Side effects Acute side effects of radiotherapy are nausea and vomiting, marrow suppression, and gastrointestinal ulceration. All these are troublesome but usually subside shortly after radiation therapy is terminated. Nausea and vomiting are the acute side effects most unpleasant to the patient and are difficult to prevent with antiemetics, although Δ^9-tetrahydrocannabinol has been shown to be useful in ameliorating nausea and vomiting associated with cancer chemotherapy. After completion of radiotherapy, the more serious side effects of radiation myelitis and pneumonitis may occur 6 weeks to several months after therapy is completed. Late complications include fibrosis of soft tissue and lungs within the radiation field, persistent bone marrow fibrosis, and pancytopenia, as well as an increased incidence of tumors within the treated field.

With chemotherapy, marrow suppression is the most serious acute side effect. It should be monitored carefully, and drug doses adjusted using sliding scales provided in publications reporting the results of treatment. The effective use of drugs requires experience; it is unacceptable to give smaller doses of chemotherapy because of inconvenience or inexperience, both of which adversely affect the efficacy of drug treatment.

In combined treatment with radiation and chemotherapy, particularly in patients with early disease, one of the late complications is an increased incidence of acute myelocytic leukemia. In some series, the incidence has already reached 5 percent and appears likely to reach 10 percent 10 years after completion of therapy. While such a risk may be acceptable in patients who would otherwise have died without treatment, it is not acceptable in patients who might have been effectively treated with either chemotherapy or radiotherapy alone.

NON-HODGKIN'S LYMPHOMAS (NHL)

This group of diseases, like Hodgkin's disease, has its origin in lymphoreticular tissue and presents clinically in lymph nodes; however, there are differences in the cell of origin, age distribution, presentation, stage at onset, complications, and response to therapy. These diseases are not a single clinical entity and encompass a wide spectrum of disorders, ranging from Burkitt's lymphoma in children in Africa to nodular and diffuse lymphomas in adults. The designation *non-Hodgkin's lymphomas* (NHL) has arisen from common usage. The majority of cases of NHL are monoclonal B-cell neoplasms (see Table 327-1).

CLINICAL FEATURES The NHL usually present as painless, localized or generalized enlargement of lymph nodes with or without hepatosplenomegaly and not infrequently as an abdominal mass. Involvement of Waldeyer's ring is more common in NHL than in HD. A discrete lesion or multiple lesions of the lung, bone, gastrointestinal system, skin, or other parenchymal site may be the presenting feature. The B symptoms described for HD are less common in patients with NHL, and their presence or absence is less related to the prognosis. Particularly in the nodular lymphomas, the lymphadenopathy may have been present for a long period of time; often, a previous lymph node biopsy may have been interpreted as "atypical" or "hyperplastic." Review of such material by a hematopathologist at a later time and comparison with a second biopsy often reveals that a lymphoma was present from the start.

DIFFERENTIAL DIAGNOSIS The differential diagnosis of NHL is similar to that of Hodgkin's disease.

DIAGNOSIS AND PATHOLOGY The diagnosis of the NHL is made by histopathologic examination of biopsy material usually obtained from lymph nodes; diagnosis and classification of material obtained from other sites may be more difficult. Selection of therapy depends on the histological type as well as stage of disease. The histological classification proposed by Rappaport is generally employed because it is reproducible and useful in predicting prognosis (Table 327-7); familiarity with this system is important since it has been employed in the majority of clinical trials. The classification divides lymphomas according to lymph node architecture into (1) the nodular type (N) in which neoplastic cells group in cohesive aggregates which simulate lymphoid follicles (germinal centers) and (2) the diffuse type (D) in which no aggregation occurs and the

architecture of the lymph nodes is effaced. The NHL are further classified according to their cytologic characteristics into "histiocytic" (H) and lymphocytic (L) varieties, the latter consisting of poorly differentiated lymphocytic (PDL) and well-differentiated lymphocytic (WDL) types ("histiocytic" is placed in quotation marks to indicate that, except in very rare instances, the tumors so classified are lymphoid in origin). In addition, there is a group of lymphomas of mixed cellularity (MC) which have elements of the "histiocytic" and lymphocytic type.

The presence of a nodular or a diffuse pattern in the nodal architecture is a most influential prognostic factor. The nodular (follicular) lymphomas tend to follow a more indolent course (even when minimally treated) than those with a diffuse pattern, except for the infrequently observed nodular "histiocytic" (NH) variety which, when left untreated or when treated unsuccessfully, evolves rapidly. The diffuse lymphomas are clinically more aggressive than the nodular, except for the diffuse well-differentiated lymphocytic lymphoma (DWDL) which resembles chronic lymphocytic leukemia and follows a chronic course. At the time of initial staging, 40 percent of patients with diffuse "histiocytic" lymphomas appear to have regional disease, but following treatment with radiotherapy alone 30 to 40 percent tend to relapse early, usually in the first 2 years. In contrast, patients with nodular poorly differentiated lymphocytic lymphoma (NPDL) show a propensity for widespread dissemination easily demonstrated with routine tests and for a pattern of continuous, late recurrence extending over a period of 5 to 10 years.

Although the Rappaport classification is reproducible and predicts prognosis, the classification is not scientifically accurate because advances in studying lymph node structure and immunologic and cell surface markers of lymphocytes have revealed that each of Rappaport's different cellular types in fact consists of different morphological expressions of B-cell differentiation. For example, Rappaport's category of "histiocytic" lymphoma includes lymphomas mostly derived from transformed B lymphocytes, from large cleaved and noncleaved follicular center cells (FCC), but, only rarely, from T lymphocytes and the true histiocyte (Table 327-9).

Lukes and Collins and others have proposed an alternative pathological classification based on histological findings, surface immunoglobulin markers, lymph node imprints, and results of other immunologic studies. If cases of malignant lymphoma are classified by the system of Lukes and Collins according to the functional designation of B, T, and U cells (undefined cell systems), and histiocytes, it is generally found that 68 to 70 percent of malignant lymphomas are derived from B cells, 18 to 19 percent from T cells, 13 percent from U cells, and a very small fraction from true histiocytes. The U-cell type is a hypothetical classification, which has been proposed for cellular proliferations with primitive morphological features that are not distinctive and in which identifying immunologic or cytochemical markers are not detectable by *presently available* techniques. The classification of Lukes and Collins is shown in Table 327-8, together with the distribution of cases. Table 327-9 shows the relationship of the Rappaport classification to the Lukes and Collins classification.

Although at this time the Lukes and Collins immunologic classification of NHL lacks data for extensive clinical and therapeutic correlations and is difficult to reproduce, specific pathological entities are emerging with distinct morphological and immunologic characteristics, recognizable clinical features, and predictable responses to therapy. However, since the majority of available studies showing clinicopathological cor-

TABLE 327-7

Classification of non-Hodgkin's lymphomas based on general histology and cell type (Rappaport)

Type	% of total cases
NODULAR	
Lymphocytic: poorly differentiated (NPDL)	<40
Mixed: lymphocytic and "histiocytic" (NMC)	>5
"Histiocytic" (NH)	<5
DIFFUSE	
Lymphocytic:	
Well differentiated (DWDL)	10
Poorly differentiated (DPDL)	>10
Mixed: lymphocytic and "histiocytic" (DMC)	5
"Histiocytic" (DHL)	>25
Lymphoblastic	
Undifferentiated:	
Burkitt's	
Non-Burkitt's (pleomorphic) (DUL)	

TABLE 327-8
Distribution of cases of malignant lymphomas by cytologic types of Lukes and Collins

Lymphoma	No. of cases	Percent
B cell:		
Small lymphocyte (B)	39	9.2
Plasmacytoid lymphocyte	29	6.8
Follicular center cell (FCC):	(193)	(45.4)
Small cleaved	119	28.0
Large cleaved	21	4.9
Small noncleaved	29	6.8
Large noncleaved	24	5.7
Immunoblastic sarcoma (B)	15	3.5
Hairy-cell leukemia	14	3.3
T cell:		
Small lymphocyte (T)	10	2.4
Convoluted lymphocyte	41	9.7
Cerebriform lymphocyte (Sézary, mycosis fungoides)	9	2.1
Immunoblastic sarcoma (T)	15	3.5
Lymphoepithelioid cell	4	1.0
Histiocytes	1	0.2
U cell	55	12.9
Total	425	100.0

relations have used the Rappaport classification system, the subsequent sections of this chapter will discuss the NHL according to the Rappaport schema and will point out certain specific pathological entities which are emerging from the Lukes and Collins classification.

IMMUNOLOGIC ABNORMALITIES Immune function is less affected in NHL than in HD patients. Skin reactivity and phytohemagglutinin response are sometimes depressed but usually only in association with advanced tumor. A defect in humoral immune function can be demonstrated more frequently in NHL patients than in HD patients. Hypogammaglobulinemia and hypergammaglobulinemia may be present. Monoclonal gammopathy occurs in some patients. Both the primary and the secondary antibody responses may be impaired.

CHROMOSOMES IN NHL In many patients with B-cell lymphomas, additional material at the end of the number 14 chromosome (14q+) can be demonstrated. This abnormality has been reported in adults with lymphomas and multiple myeloma, and in children with African Burkitt's lymphomas. The fact that patients with ataxia telangiectasia also have abnormalities in chromosome 14 and are subject to an increased incidence of lymphocytic neoplasia suggests that aberrations in chromosome 14 may represent nonrandom chromosomal abnormalities characteristic of lymphocytic neoplasia.

STAGING The staging classification developed for HD (Ann Arbor staging classification, Table 327-3) is often used in NHL; however, the sequence of staging procedures differs because extralymphatic presentations occur more frequently in NHL than in HD. Furthermore, since many approach stage III and stage IV disease in a similar manner, this distinction may be far less relevant in NHL than in HD. The stage of disease must be determined after the confirmation of the histological diagnosis of NHL but prior to treatment. The extent of clinical evaluation must be guided by the type of therapy available and proposed for a particular patient. For patients who, after clinical staging, still appear to have localized disease and are considered eligible for aggressive curative radiotherapy, extensive staging may be justified. In those whose age or general medical problems limit therapy to local palliation with radiotherapy or systemic treatment with a single drug, few invasive staging procedures are indicated. Surgical staging should not be considered a routine procedure in patients with NHL. The major task of staging is to determine whether the patient has limited nodal or extranodal (E) disease, which is radiocurable (stage I or II), or disseminated disease which requires systemic therapy (stage III or IV).

Because the histological patterns correlate well with specific disease patterns, response to therapy, and prognosis, the histological diagnosis can be used to determine the appropriate staging procedures needed to choose the appropriate treatment strategy for a particular patient. For example, 80 percent of patients with a *nodular* pattern have a histopathologic diagnosis of *lymphocytic* or *mixed-cell lymphoma,* and 80 to 90 percent of these patients will be in stages III and IV after clinical staging and simple needle biopsy techniques. Early in the patient's staging evaluation, only diagnostic studies that have a low morbidity and a high probability of disclosing advanced disease should be employed. Lymphangiograms, bone marrow biopsies, and liver biopsy meet these requirements and can usually obviate the need for staging laparotomy.

Approximately 90 percent of patients with nodular lymphocytic and 60 to 70 percent with diffuse lymphocytic lymphomas have positive lymphangiograms. For patients with positive lymphangiograms, the incidence of spleen, liver, and/or bone marrow involvement is high (90 percent); in contrast in patients with negative lymphangiograms, such involvement is 10 percent or less.

Bone marrow aspirates are inadequate for diagnosis, and multiple posterior iliac crest biopsies are recommended. In WDL, PDL, and MC disease, the incidence of bone marrow involvement is at least 50 to 60 percent even though no evidence in blood count abnormalities is evident.

Search for liver involvement should be pursued if the bone marrow biopsies prove to be negative, and if the therapeutic plan is to treat the patient with less than a systemic approach. Nondirected percutaneous biopsies detect 20 percent of cases with liver involvement, peritoneoscopy-directed multiple biopsies detect an additional 20 to 30 percent of cases, and finally, if no evidence for stage IV disease has been shown after these procedures, liver biopsies at laparotomy detect the remaining 50 percent of cases. Liver involvement with lymphoma occurs in 58 to 65 percent of cases with WDL, PDL, and MC disease whether the architecture is nodular or diffuse.

In sharp contrast are the findings in patients diagnosed as having "histiocytic" lymphoma. Only 5 percent will have a nodular pattern. Thirty-five to forty-five percent of patients with DHL or NH disease appear to be in clinical stages I and II and may be curable with megavoltage radiotherapy alone;

TABLE 327-9
Comparisons of classifications

Rappaport	Lukes and Collins

Nodular   Diffuse

Undifferentiated ------→ Undefined cell

T-cell types:
→ Convoluted lymphocyte

Lymphocytic WD ⟶ ▶ Immunoblastic sarcoma (T cell)

B-cell types:
▶ Small lymphocytic (CLL)
Plasmacytoid lymphocyte

Lymphocytic PD
Follicular center cell (FCC; follicular, diffuse, follicular and diffuse, and sclerotic):
▶ Small cleaved
Mixed (L and H) ▶ Large cleaved
▶ Small noncleaved
▶ Large noncleaved
"Histiocytic" ◀ ▶ Immunoblastic sarcoma (B cell)
▶ Histiocytic
Unclassifiable

in such patients, laparotomy may be advisable to ensure accurate staging prior to radiotherapy. Extranodal presentations in Waldeyer's ring and extralymphatic local presentations in bone, brain, testes, or other sites are more frequent in "histiocytic" than in lymphocytic lymphoma. In addition, initial bone marrow involvement is present in only 15 percent or less of cases. Similarly, liver involvement at the time of presentation occurs in less than 20 percent of cases. Bone marrow core biopsies and blind liver biopsy are obviously less rewarding than in the lymphocytic lymphomas. The staging strategy for the "histiocytic" lymphomas is to seek evidence for stage III disease by lymphangiography or inferior vena cavography or abdominal CT scan.

TYPES OF TUMORS Nodular lymphoma, poorly differentiated lymphocytic type (NPDL) This is the most common nodular lymphoma and presents a more uniform clinical picture than the other nodular types. The disease afflicts adults, usually over the age of 40, and is very rare in young adults and children, though instances below the age of 15 are known.

NPDL is usually asymptomatic at the onset and is characterized by painless adenopathy in the cervical, axillary, and inguinofemoral regions. In some patients large abdominal masses of retroperitoneal or mesenteric lymph nodes cause acute gastrointestinal problems, including obstruction, hemorrhage, and intussusception. Some patients have ureteral obstruction with consequent renal failure. Even though the patient may notice only one or several enlarged lymph nodes, examination and study with lymphography or other tests may reveal widespread, often symmetrical, lymphadenopathy. In some patients, the lymph node enlargement may have been present for several years but is so gradual or fluctuating that patients were not concerned enough to seek medical attention. The spleen is often enlarged but rarely produces symptoms at the onset of the disease. Later in the course of the disease, it may become considerably larger and result in local symptoms and significant hypersplenism. Involvement of the lymphoid tissue in Waldeyer's ring is not a common clinical problem.

Nodular lymphomas do not often produce symptoms in nonlymphatic organs or in tissues such as the lung, liver, bones, and skin. Paravertebral lymphoid masses may result in chylous pleural effusions and/or ascites presumably because of lymphatic obstruction. It is extremely rare for the central nervous system to become involved, though peripheral nerve compression and epidural tumor masses may develop.

The peripheral blood picture is usually normal at the onset of the disease, but careful examination of the blood smear may reveal typical notched or cleft, so-called "buttock," cells thought to be characteristic, but not diagnostic, of nodular lymphomas. Ordinary bone marrow aspirations are usually normal. However, study of the bone marrow by the needle or open biopsy technique will reveal focal bone marrow involvement in up to 85 percent of patients with NPDL even at the onset of the disease.

Some patients who present an otherwise typical clinical picture of chronic lymphatic leukemia, with white blood cell counts as high as 100,000 per cubic millimeter, will show a nodular lymphoma in lymph nodes. Conversely, a small proportion of patients with nodular lymphoma will develop marked lymphocytosis during the course of the disease. It remains to be determined whether these patients differ significantly from those with typical chronic lymphatic leukemia in whom the lymph nodes show the histological picture of diffuse lymphoma of the well-differentiated lymphocytic type (DWDL).

The clinical course of nodular lymphoma is variable. In some it is indolent, and lymphadenopathy may have been present for years prior to the diagnosis and may be well tolerated for 5 years or more after the diagnosis is established. The disease is malignant, however, and though there may be spontaneous regression of lymphadenopathy, clinical problems gradually appear. In other patients the tempo of the disease is accelerated from the start, and such patients may experience difficulties within months of the diagnosis.

After months or years of being well tolerated, the disease almost always becomes much more aggressive. Lymph node masses grow rapidly, often in localized or asymmetric locations. They cause serious local problems and are less responsive to treatment which was previously effective. Fever, night sweats, and weight loss may appear. Involvement of nonlymphoid organs and tissues occurs, and the prognosis becomes very poor. If biopsy is performed at this time, the histological picture may be unchanged; or a change in histological appearance to a diffuse pattern, often with a larger cell type corresponding to the diffuse "histiocytic" lymphoma of Rappaport, may be seen.

Nodular lymphoma, mixed-cell type (NMC) There are many similarities between NPDL and the less frequently occurring NMC. The NMC differs in overall prognosis, frequency of initial bone marrow involvement, and type and location of lymph node enlargement: bone marrow involvement at the onset is less common, and unusual large abdominal masses may be seen more often. In contrast to NPDL, combination chemotherapy has been found in one series to yield a high percentage (60 percent) of complete remissions with long-term disease-free intervals suggesting cure.

Nodular "histiocytic" (NH) lymphomas This group of lymphomas generally is considered together with the diffuse "histiocytic" lymphomas since the course and prognosis are unlike those of the other nodular lymphomas.

Diffuse lymphomas (DWDL, DPDL, DMC, DHL) The diffuse NHLs consist of a number of diseases with variable presentation and clinical evolution. *Diffuse well-differentiated lymphocytic lymphoma* (DWDL) is generally considered the most indolent NHL and in its outcome is usually indistinguishable from chronic lymphocytic leukemia. The *diffuse poorly differentiated lymphocytic lymphomas (DPDL) and diffuse mixed-cell lymphomas (DMC)* present much like the nodular lymphomas but spread much more rapidly. When the patient is first seen, the disease usually is disseminated to all lymph node areas, the liver, spleen, and bone marrow. The incidence of bone marrow and liver involvement is over 50 percent. Although response to combination chemotherapy is good and leads to complete remissions in up to 60 percent of cases, disease-free survival has not improved. In contrast, the *diffuse "histiocytic" lymphoma (DHL)* (formerly called *reticulum-cell sarcoma*) and nodular "histiocytic" lymphoma (NH) often present with localized lymph node enlargement, or local extralymphatic manifestation. The lymph nodes are most prominently located in the neck; presentations in the gastrointestinal tract, bone, thyroid, testes, brain, and the lymph node tissue of Waldeyer's ring, occur frequently. In 25 to 35 percent of the patients, even after extensive diagnostic efforts, the disease is found to be relatively localized. The bone marrow is involved initially in less than 10 percent of the patients and is not commonly involved even late in the course of the disease.

"Histiocytic" lymphoma is highly invasive, and involvement of peripheral nerves, epidural tumors, compression of the vena cava or airways, and destruction of osseous tissue occur during the course of the disease. The skin, liver, kidneys, lung, and even the brain may be involved. Occasionally bone marrow invasion results in the appearance of large, undifferentiated cells in the peripheral blood.

Localized DHL may be curable by megavoltage radiotherapy. In some studies, over 70 percent 5-year actuarial disease-free survival has been obtained. Disseminated DHL is responsive to combination chemotherapy, and complete remissions can be obtained in 60 percent of cases of whom the majority have a 5-year actuarial disease-free survival. Analysis of DHL responses according to histopathologic subclassification supports the Lukes and Collins hypotheses that DHL is derived most often from follicular center cells for which potentially curative therapy exists.

The diffuse lymphomas that occur in children, adolescents, and young adults must be separated from those that occur in the older age groups because of differences in clinical patterns and in response to therapy. Several unique clinical pathological entities have been recognized.

Lymphoblastic lymphomas These tumors comprise about 30 percent of all childhood NHL and 5 to 10 percent of NHL in adolescents and adults. Males predominate in this group. The characteristic presentation is supradiaphragmatic with cervical, supraclavicular, or axillary lymph nodes and, in half the cases, a massive anterior mediastinal mass. Pleural effusions may occur. Some patients may present with inguinal nodes or with disease in extranodal sites (breast, gonads, long bones, skin, etc.). Initially, the blood and bone marrow may not be involved. The tumors may be composed of convoluted or non-convoluted lymphocytes, but all are associated with T-cell characteristics. Following a 2- to 3-month period, 30 to 50 percent of cases develop acute leukemia cytologically identical with acute lymphoblastic leukemia of childhood. Central nervous system involvement occurs frequently. These T-cell tumors of children and young adults are cytologically distinct from the B-cell Burkitt's and non-Burkitt's lymphomas. Patients identified by clinical and histopathological criteria as having lymphoblastic lymphoma require only minimal staging procedures. Combination chemotherapy should be given because of the systemic nature of the process. Overall survival is poor.

Burkitt's lymphoma Burkitt first described this diffuse lymphoma of follicular center B cells in children in Africa. It has unique clinical and epidemiologic features. Although found worldwide, Burkitt's lymphoma appears virtually epidemic in certain areas of East Africa and New Guinea. In epidemic regions, serologic evidence of infection with herpes-like Epstein-Barr virus (EBV) has been documented repeatedly.

The disease appears to predominate in males (male/female ratio in Africa is 8:5; in America it is 2:1). The median age at onset of African children is 7 years, whereas in America it is 11 years. In its *typical African form*, the disease presents primarily as an extralymphatic tumor arising in the bones of the jaw. In addition, there appears to be a predilection for spread to the abdominal viscera, particularly the ovaries, as well as to the breasts and meninges. Bone marrow involvement occurs but is not common; leukemia is seen infrequently. In *American children*, bony tumors of the jaw are less frequent, and abdominal or pelvic sites, particularly the gastrointestinal tract, are involved with tumor at the time of presentation. Bone marrow and/or cerebrospinal fluid involvement occurs eventually in one-third of patients.

The diagnosis is made by recognition of the clinical picture and the characteristic histological and cytochemical findings. The tumor is very responsive to chemotherapy with single drugs, particularly alkylating agents, and long-term complete remissions without maintenance therapy have been reported.

TREATMENT Treatment approaches to NHL have undergone considerable change in the past decade. Although various treatments, including regional radiotherapy, total lymphoid irradiation, single-drug chemotherapy, combination chemotherapy, and combinations of both modalities, have been tested, the results have been difficult to interpret because of differing staging and histological classifications were used. By consistent use of the Ann Arbor staging and the Rappaport histopathologic classifications, treatment strategies based on clinical and pathological stages and histology have been developed.

Involved-field (IF) radiotherapy The principles of delivery of effective radiotherapy described for HD are the same for NHL when irradiation is selected as the primary and potentially curative treatment.

Patients with stage I and II NHL should be treated with involved-field (IF) radiation therapy only, since treatment with extended-field (EF) or total nodal irradiation does not appear to improve the results. The effectiveness of regional radiotherapy depends in part on the histological type of lymphoma. For nodular lymphomas following treatment with 4400 rads, the local recurrence rate in the treated field is close to zero; for diffuse lymphocytic and diffuse mixed-cell lymphomas, it is approximately 15 percent. The local recurrence rate (21 to 37 percent) for patients with diffuse histiocytic lymphoma does not appear to be dose-related for doses between 2500 and 6500 rads, in contrast to the experience with dose-dependent control of HD. Local control with radiotherapy translates into long-term disease-free survival in 60 to 80 percent of patients with pathological stage I and 30 percent with pathological stage II NHL; paradoxically, DHL, the histologically most malignant tumor, has the best disease-free survival rate (70 percent at 5 years) if a complete remission is achieved. However, for all the lymphomas, the main problem remains disease in viscera outside treatment fields.

Chemotherapy The treatment of choice for stages III and IV NHL is chemotherapy. For the nodular variety of the lymphomas, three treatment options are available: no initial treatment, treatment with a single drug, or treatment with combinations of drugs. For NPDL, the commonest variety of the nodular lymphomas, selected patients may be followed for periods of time with no treatment. Current evidence suggests, however, that even when patients with indolent disease are carefully selected, most will require drug treatment within 12 to 24 months.

When chemotherapy first became available for the treatment of cancer, the most responsive tumors were the lymphomas, and single-agent chemotherapy evolved initially as the treatment of choice. With the availability of many drugs, acting by different mechanisms, and evidence in animals that therapeutic synergism was possible, combination chemotherapy was tested in humans and appeared to provide superior results. Other studies, however, have suggested that single-agent chemotherapy may still produce results equivalent to those obtained with combination chemotherapy in patients with advanced NPDL. Since comparative clinical trials in NHL are relatively new, two well-established facts dictate the use of combination chemotherapy as the first treatment for patients with advanced NHL, if treatment is required. First, combination chemotherapy, using vinca alkaloids, alkylating agents, and prednisone, with or without the anthracycline antitumor antibiotics, induces a greater fraction of complete remissions in the first year of treatment than single-agent chemotherapy (68 vs. 40 percent). Second, patients who attain a complete remission survive longer than those patients who achieve partial responses; therefore, the therapy that induces the greatest fraction of complete remissions is always the best choice, provided toxicity is not too severe. Long-term comparisons of the use of single agents with drug combinations have also shown a larger percentage of patients rendered free of disease with the use of combinations. Surprisingly, combination chemotherapy, in most cases, does not cause significantly greater toxicity than single-agent chemotherapy. Chlorambucil, the single agent most often used, is frequently associated with bone marrow aplasia within 2 years of continuous treatment, a side effect which is not noted when intermittent cyclical combination chemotherapy is used.

As is the case with radiotherapy, once chemotherapy of patients with NPDL is discontinued, the rate of relapse is constant, even in patients who have attained a complete remission. Ten to fifteen percent of patients can be expected to relapse per year over a 6-year period. Maintenance drug treatment of patients with NPDL prolongs the duration of the initial remission, and generally is recommended, but has not been shown to prolong survival when compared with intermittent reinduction of remission.

The situation is clearly different for patients with the nodular mixed lymphomas. Here studies have shown that combination chemotherapy is more effective than single agents. In one study, patients with NMC achieved remission in 76 percent of cases treated with a variety of MOPP which substitutes cyclophosphamide for nitrogen mustard (C-MOPP). In contrast to patients with NPDL, those with NMC who were treated with a combination of drugs and who achieved remission remained in complete remission for periods up to 10 years after therapy was discontinued; the relapse rate diminishes after 2 years. Patients with NH are treated in a fashion similar to those with DHL described below.

Results of treatment in patients who have diffuse lymphomas depend in a major way on the histological characteristics of the tumor. Patients with DWDL, even in the absence of nodularity, have a long, indolent course that waxes and wanes in a manner similar to the course of patients with chronic lymphocytic leukemia, regardless of the aggressiveness of the initial therapy. Conservative single-agent treatment, usually with chlorambucil, employed only when disease progression dictates its use, is the treatment of choice. For patients with advanced stages of DLPD, DMC, DHL, and diffuse undifferentiated lymphoma (DUL), the treatment of choice is one of the several four-drug combinations that produce a significant fraction of complete remissions. In these lymphomas, the dedifferentiation of the cellular component that leads to the more aggressive clinical behavior apparently makes the tumor cells more vulnerable to the killing effects of chemotherapy. Complete remissions in patients with these poorly differentiated diffuse lymphomas are possible in 40 to 80 percent of treated patients. Failure to achieve a complete remission in these patients is associated with an extremely short survival time, usually less than 6 months. Almost all patients who fail to achieve complete remission, even those who have dramatic partial responses, die within 2 years. In contrast, if complete remission is attained, long disease-free survivals are now possible. In some studies, relapse-free survival has been reported to extend for more than 10 years beyond the end of a drug treatment. Patients with the diffuse lymphomas who achieve a complete remission do not benefit from maintenance therapy.

Combined modality treatment of NHL In view of the success of chemotherapeutic regimens in controlling advanced NHL and the apparent irreducible failure rate of radiotherapy alone for stages I and II, programs employing radiotherapy *and* chemotherapy are being explored. In one study, IF radiotherapy with chemotherapy (RT + CT) proved superior to radiotherapy (RT) alone. The 3-year relapse rate was 29 percent for RT + CT but 55 percent for RT alone; the impact of combined treatment was most striking for patients with DPDL, DMC, DHL,

and NH histologies, whereas there appeared no significant difference in relapse rates for patients with DWDL, NPDL, and NMC histologies.

Whole-body radiotherapy (WBR) This modality has been employed for the management of patients with lymphocytic types of NHL in stages III and IV. The 56 percent complete remission rate achieved was similar to that obtained in parallel studies using various drug regimens. Nodular histological subtypes had better response than the diffuse types. This approach is prone to complications. Moreover, the difficulty in re-treatment of relapse with drugs dictates the use of WBR only when other treatments have failed.

Immunotherapy of NHL For the past decade studies have been carried out to determine the role of immunotherapy in the management of NHL. Controlled studies show that although combination chemotherapy plus bacillus Calmette-Guérin (BCG) vaccination had a slightly better response than combination chemotherapy alone, there was no difference in survival between patients maintained on BCG and those receiving no immunotherapy or chemotherapy as maintenance.

COMPLICATIONS OF HODGKIN'S DISEASE AND NHL

The complications of lymphoma may be due to progressive enlargement of lymph nodes, involvement of parenchymal organs, and hematologic, metabolic, or immunologic abnormalities. Complications may also result from therapy.

Progressive lymph node enlargement causes compression or obstruction of surrounding structures such as vascular structures (superior vena cava syndrome), airway, esophagus, the urinary tract, or the gastrointestinal tract. Serious complications may ensue depending on the site affected.

Direct infiltration of the lymphoma from involved mediastinal lymph nodes into the parenchyma of the lung, pleura, pericardium, and heart may occur. Infiltration from retroperitoneal lymph nodes through lymphatic channels leads to involvement of the gastrointestinal tract and may result in ulceration, perforation, hemorrhage, intussusception, or malabsorption.

Jaundice may be caused by obstruction of the biliary duct by portal lymph nodes or by infiltration of the liver secondary to hematogenous spread. The liver is often involved in the diffuse lymphocytic lymphomas (DPDL, DWDL, DMC) but less often in "histiocytic" lymphoma. Usually splenomegaly and/or retroperitoneal lymphadenopathy are demonstrable. In Hodgkin's disease, liver involvement is most commonly seen in patients with mixed cellularity or lymphocytic depletion type, who have splenomegaly and B symptoms. The differential diagnosis of jaundice must include hemolytic anemia and drug toxicity.

Central nervous system involvement may occur by direct extension of tumor from the mediastinum or retroperitoneum to the spinal canal. Symptoms of cord compression which are produced in this way occur more frequently in Hodgkin's disease than in NHL and in the latter, most often in DHL. Cranial nerves and brain may be affected by HD and NHL. Occasionally, lymphomatous meningitis may occur, and lymphoma cells, high protein, and low glucose appear in the spinal fluid. In DHL with demonstrated bone marrow involvement, meningitis occurs with such high frequency that prophylactic intrathecal therapy is recommended. More rarely, bizarre neurological manifestations may occur without demonstrable direct involvement by lymphoma. Progressive multifocal leukoencephalopathy, subacute cerebellar degeneration, myelopathy, and neuropathy have been described. Occasionally, polymyositis may occur. The differential diagnosis of these central and peripheral nervous system complications includes bacterial and viral meningitis, herpes zoster, and drug toxicity, particularly with the vinca alkaloids.

The lung may be involved by direct extension from mediastinal–hilar lymph nodes or by hematogenous spread. In the lymphocyte-predominant type of HD and in the nodular NHL the lungs are rarely involved; in contrast, nodular sclerosis–type HD frequently involves the lungs. Pleural involvement by lymphoma with malignant effusion may occur with or without lymphoma of the lung. Pneumonia is a frequent complication of treatment and constitutes the major differential diagnostic problem. Bleomycin, methotrexate, and other drugs may cause pulmonary manifestations and must be considered in the differential diagnosis of lung disease.

Skin involvement occurs as part of hematogenous dissemination of the lymphoma. A number of nonspecific skin lesions occur in lymphoma including excoriations secondary to pruritus, urticaria, erythema multiforme, erythema nodosum, exfoliative dermatitis, and dermatomyositis.

Bone marrow involvement occurs most frequently with DWDL and PDL (nodular or diffuse) (50 to 60 percent) but less frequently with DHL (10 percent). In HD, initial bone marrow involvement is rare; it is seen most often in patients with symptoms (B categories) and in patients with the lymphocyte-depleted subtype. Anemia, neutropenia, and thrombocytopenia are the consequences of bone marrow replacement; however, these conditions may also be caused by hypersplenism, immunologic mechanisms, blood loss, or complications of therapy.

Hematologic complications occur frequently. Anemia may be caused by blood loss secondary to gastrointestinal infiltration and ulceration or nonspecific lesions, malabsorption of iron or folate, bone marrow infiltration by lymphoma, or hemolysis. Coombs' test-positive hemolytic anemia is seen most often with DWDL and DPDL; it occurs less frequently with DMC, DHL, or in the nodular lymphomas and Hodgkin's disease. Chronic illness and radiotherapy or chemotherapy result in diminished or ineffective erythropoiesis. Changes in white blood cell counts are frequent. The leukemic phase of lymphoma is seen most frequently in the lymphocytic lymphomas; rarely, in "histiocytic" lymphoma. Leukopenia in an untreated patient suggests bone marrow infiltration or hypersplenism. In the patient undergoing therapy, leukopenia is usually due to the therapy. Thrombocytosis occurs occasionally in Hodgkin's disease and NHL. Frequently following staging splenectomy, the platelet count rises briefly. More often, thrombocytopenia occurs because of bone marrow replacement by lymphoma, hypersplenism, or therapy.

Metabolic abnormalities may occur as a consequence of the lymphoma or of therapy. Hyperuricemia is seen in patients with large volume of lymphoma. Effective therapy with rapid reduction of the tissue mass may exacerbate the hyperuricemia and lead to a decrease in renal function and infrequently to gouty arthritis. Hydration and administration of allopurinol can prevent these complications.

Hypercalcemia occurs in less than 10 percent of cases and is usually related to bone destruction. It is seen most frequently in DHL and Hodgkin's disease of the lymphocytic-depletion and mixed-cellularity varieties. Occasionally, the hypercalcemia may be due to release of a parathyroid-like substance. Hypercalcemia requires prompt and appropriate treatment to lower the serum calcium level and specific therapy appropriate for the management of the lymphoma.

Serum protein abnormalities occur frequently. Particularly in Hodgkin's disease, but also in NHL, the α_1, α_2, and β fractions of globulins may be increased. The α_2 increase in Hodgkin's disease has been shown to be due to increases in haptoglobin and ceruloplasmin. Polyclonal gamma globulin elevation is seen in 40 percent of patients with HD; it is less frequent in NHL. Paraproteinemia may occur in NHL, especially in DWDL, and occasionally in HD. Hypogammaglobulinemia may precede the onset of DWDL or PDL, occurs eventually in 60 percent of these patients, but is seen less frequently in advanced Hodgkin's disease. Antibody production is usually decreased both in response to primary and recall challenge.

Complications of treatment include radiation damage associated with therapy of specific sites, toxicity due to chemotherapeutic agents (Chap. 324), sterility, and second malignancies.

Chemotherapy with four-drug regimens leads to some decrease in ovarian or testicular function in most patients. Amenorrhea, inability to conceive, or hypo- or aspermia may result; however, in those patients who have achieved a complete remission and are off all chemotherapy, these functions may return.

Second malignancies, particularly nonlymphocytic acute leukemias, have been reported to occur in patients with HD and NHL treated with radiation alone, combination chemotherapy alone, or with both modalities. The incidence is estimated to be 1 to 8 percent of cases, with time of onset 1.2 to 19 years and a mean interval of 7 years following initial therapy. Hypoplastic or aplastic bone marrow often antedates the occurrence of frank leukemia. In the preleukemic phase chromosome analysis employing chromosome banding techniques has demonstrated a high incidence of abnormalities in chromosomes 5, 8, and 7.

ANGIOIMMUNOBLASTIC LYMPHADENOPATHY WITH DYSPROTEINEMIA (AILD)

Immunoblastic lymphadenopathy is a lymphoma-like, systemic disorder characterized by acute onset, generalized lymphadenopathy, hepatomegaly, splenomegaly, and severe constitutional symptoms including fever, sweats, and weight loss. Pruritus and skin rashes may be present. These clinical features closely mimic many of the presenting signs and symptoms of advanced Hodgkin's disease and of the other lymphomas.

The disorder occurs in adults (age 28 to 92, median 62). In half the patients, generalized, pruritic maculopapular rash precedes the onset of the other signs and symptoms by weeks or a few months. In some patients, ingestion of drugs, including penicillin or other antibiotics, phenytoin, sulfonamide, halothane, methyldopa, and aspirin, antedates the onset of the disease.

AILD is not considered a histologically malignant disease but rather an extreme form of a hypersensitivity (hyperimmune) reaction. Some have considered this a clinical example of a graft-vs.-host reaction. A proliferation of B cells and a profound deficiency of T cells have been demonstrated.

The laboratory data show anemia, which in one-quarter of the cases are due to a Coombs' test-positive hemolytic anemia. A majority of the patients have a polyclonal hypergammaglobulinemia. Leukocytosis and eosinophilia may be present.

Characteristic lesions are found in biopsy specimens of lymph nodes and consist of alterations of nodal architecture or complete effacement with a pleomorphic cellular proliferation in which immunoblasts, lymphocytes, and plasma cells predominate. In addition, vascular proliferation and prominent eosinophilic interstitial material are seen. The changes in the liver, spleen, and bone marrow do not have the diagnostic specificity of the lesions seen in the lymph nodes.

The course of AILD may be benign or fulminant. Some patients (approximately 25 percent) appear to have a long survival (20 to 45 months) with or without small doses of corticosteroids and do not require intensive chemotherapy. Others (25 percent), although requiring intensive cytotoxic chemotherapy, nevertheless have a long survival (28 to 67 months). A third group of patients (50 percent of cases) have a rapid course (1 to 20 months) terminating in death regardless of the therapeutic approach employed. Many patients die of overwhelming infections, often with pneumonia due to *Pseudomonas* and other gram-negative organisms, *Pneumocystis carinii,* cytomegalovirus, or mycoses. Acute hepatic failure or acute renal failure have also been reported to occur as terminal events.

The correct treatment of AILD has not been devised. Treatment should be initiated with corticosteroids. If there is no response, a combination chemotherapy regimen effective in lymphoma has been advocated. Radiotherapy may be employed for control of local problems. In view of the high failure rate of cytotoxic drugs, brief use of corticosteroids has been recommended to diminish the hyperimmune response along with Levamisole to stimulate T-cell function.

REFERENCES

BITRAN JD et al: Survival of patients with localized histiocytic lymphoma. Cancer 39:342, 1977

——— et al: Non-Hodgkin's lymphoma, poorly differentiated lymphocytic and mixed cell types. Cancer 42(1):88, 1978

CARBONE PP et al: Report of the committee on Hodgkin's disease staging classification. Cancer Res 31:1860, 1971

CHABNER BA et al: Sequential non-surgical and surgical staging of non-Hodgkin's lymphoma. Ann Intern Med 85:149, 1976

DESSER RK et al: Prognostic classification of Hodgkin disease in pathologic stage III, based on anatomic considerations. Blood 49(6):883, 1977

DEVITA VT et al: Advanced diffuse histiocytic lymphoma, potentially curable disease. Lancet 1:248, 1975

——— et al: The chemotherapy of Hodgkin's disease; past experiences and future directions. Cancer 42:979, 1978

FIELD R, BODEY GP: Infections in patients with malignant lymphoma treated with combination chemotherapy. Cancer 39:1018, 1977

FISHER RI et al: Prognostic factors for advanced diffuse histiocytic lymphoma following treatment with combination chemotherapy. Am J Med 63:177, 1977

FRIZZERA G et al: Angio-immunoblastic lymphadenopathy with dysproteinemia. Lancet 1:1070, 1974

GLATSTEIN E: Radiotherapy in Hodgkin's disease: Past achievements and future progress. Cancer 39:837, 1977

HELLMAN S et al: The place of radiation therapy in the treatment of non-Hodgkin's lymphoma. Cancer 39:843, 1977

JONES SE et al: Non-Hodgkin's lymphoma: IV. Clinical pathologic correlation in 405 cases. Cancer 31:806, 1973

——— et al: Non-Hodgkin's lymphoma: V. Results of radiotherapy. Cancer 32(12):682, 1973

KAPLAN HS: *Hodgkin's Disease.* Cambridge, Mass, Harvard University Press, 1972

——— et al: Staging laparotomy and splenectomy in Hodgkin's disease: Analysis of indications and patterns of involvement in 285 consecutive unselected patients. Natl Cancer Inst Monogr 36:291, 1973

———, GARTNER S: "Sternberg-Reed" giant cells of Hodgkin's disease: Cultivation in vitro, heterotransplantation and characterization as neoplastic macrophages. Int J Cancer 19:511, 1977

———, ROSENBERG SA: The management of Hodgkin's disease. Cancer 36:796, 1975

LEWIS BJ, DEVITA VT: Combination therapy of the lymphomas. Semin Hematol 15:431, 1978

LUKES RJ et al: Immunologic approach to non-Hodgkin's lymphomas and related leukemias. Analysis of the results of multiparameter studies of 425 cases. Semin Hematol 15:322, 1978

———, TINDLE BH: Immunoblastic lymphadenopathy: A hyperimmune entity resembling Hodgkin's disease. N Engl J Med 292:1, 1975

RAPPAPORT H: Tumors of the hematopoietic system, in *Atlas of Tumor Pathology.* Washington, DC, Armed Forces Institute of Pathology, 1966, sec 3, fasc 8

SWEET DL JR et al: Hodgkin's disease: Problems of staging. Cancer 42(2):957, 1978

328
CUTANEOUS MANIFESTATIONS OF INTERNAL MALIGNANCY

HARLEY A. HAYNES
THOMAS B. FITZPATRICK

One of the most satisfying aspects of dermatologic diagnosis is the detection of previously unknown malignant disease in a treatable stage by recognition of an apparently irrelevant alteration of the skin as a clue to the presence of the neoplasm. Although less satisfying, the recognition of the probability of a neoplastic disease may be of great assistance in clarifying a difficult diagnostic problem, even if the neoplasm should be untreatable when discovered. Sometimes these skin changes are induced directly by infiltration of the neoplasm into the skin, but more often they are induced indirectly by a variety of mechanisms.

This chapter is an attempt to classify the wide range of skin signs of internal malignancy in a logical fashion (Table 328-1). Since the types of skin alterations and the number of neoplasms are extremely large, grouping of the alterations by pathogenetic mechanisms was selected. There remains a substantial idiopathic category; the entities therein will be grouped by pathogenesis when this becomes understood. The skin alterations induced by neoplasms of the endocrine organs are not included here as they generally are the alterations one would expect from excess or deficiency of the hormone in question and are mentioned in the appropriate chapters.

SKIN INFILTRATION BY AN INTERNAL MALIGNANCY

METASTASES FROM CARCINOMA Cutaneous metastases of malignant lesions occur in 3 to 5 percent of patients with metastatic disease. These lesions may provide the first indication of recurrence in a patient with a known primary tumor or may be the presenting lesions of a hitherto unsuspected tumor. Typical skin metastases are dermal nodules, varying from skin color to purple, which are more easily felt than seen, and are very firm to the touch; they ulcerate rarely. Metastases from renal and thyroid carcinomas may be pulsatile and have a bruit. Breast carcinomas may produce an erysipelas-like appearance on the chest. The location of skin metastases may give a clue to the origin of the primary tumor. The abdominal wall is the most common site in both sexes for lesions initially presenting as metastases. In this situation, the primary sites are usually the lung, stomach, or kidney in men, and the ovary in women. In women with metastases on the chest wall, the most likely pri-

TABLE 328-1
Classification of skin signs of internal malignancy

I Skin infiltration by an internal malignancy
  A Metastatic, lymphatic, hematogenous, or by surgical implantation
    1 Carcinoma
    2 Leukemia
  B Metastatic, intraepidermal
    1 Paget's disease of the breast
    2 Extramammary Paget's disease
  C Autochthonous or metastatic (?)
    1 Lymphoma
    2 Malignant histiocytosis
II Skin changes due to exposure to a carcinogen that also induces internal malignancy
  A Arsenical keratoses
  B Bowen's disease
III Skin malignancies associated with increased risk of separate primary internal malignancy
  A Bowen's disease
  B Kaposi's sarcoma
  C Any skin malignancy (??)
IV Skin changes due to metabolic products of malignancies
  A Malignant carcinoid syndrome
  B Addisonian hyperpigmentation with Cushing's syndrome, from carcinomas producing MSH- and ACTH-like peptides
  C Generalized dermal melanosis (slate gray), from malignant melanoma
  D Nodular fat necrosis, due to lipases from pancreatic carcinoma
  E Raynaud's syndrome with cryoproteinemia, from multiple myeloma
  F Amyloidosis, from multiple myeloma
  G Necrolytic migrating erythema, from functioning glucagonoma
V Skin changes due to functional disturbances in other systems induced by nonendocrine malignancies
  A Jaundice, obstructive
  B Addisonian hyperpigmentation from adrenal infiltration by a tumor
  C Purpura, thrombocytopenic
  D Pallor, from anemia
  E Herpes zoster
  F Herpes simplex, severe, protracted, recurrent
  G Pyoderma, recurrent
  H Delayed hypersensitivity, exaggerated to mosquito bites
VI Skin changes, idiopathic
  A Changes frequently related to internal malignancy
    1 Dermatomyositis, adult-onset
    2 Acanthosis nigricans
    3 Thrombophlebitis, migratory
    4 Ichthyosis, adult-onset
    5 Alopecia mucinosa, adult
    6 Pachydermoperiostosis, acquired
    7 Hypertrichosis lanugosa, acquired ("malignant down")
    8 Erythema gyratum repens
  B Changes occasionally related to internal malignancy
    1 Pruritus, without causative skin lesions
    2 Clubbing, with and without hypertrophic osteoarthropathy
    3 Erythroderma
    4 Normolipemic xanthomatosis
    5 Erythema multiforme
    6 Urticaria and erythema perstans
    7 Pyoderma gangrenosum, atypical
    8 Bullous disease (bullous pemphigoid and dermatitis herpetiformis)
    9 Dermatoses, bizarre
VII Heritable diseases with skin manifestations and the propensity to develop internal malignancy (see Table 328-2)

mary site is the breast. Other skin areas that tend to be involved by metastases are the scalp, from lung, kidney, or breast; the chest, in men, from lung; the back, from lung or breast; the extremities, from malignant melanomas; and the face, from oropharyngeal carcinomas. Histological examination of a skin metastasis may reveal the identity of the primary tumor.

METASTASES FROM LEUKEMIA Leukemic deposits in skin are more common in myelomonocytic leukemia than in lymphocytic or granulocytic leukemias (Chap. 325). Firm papules or nodules ranging in color from pink to purple are the usual lesions, although ulcerations may develop. If thrombocytopenia is present, purpura often occurs in the nodules. Leukemic infiltrates may develop in recent scars, in traumatized areas, and in lesions of herpes zoster and herpes simplex. Cytological examination of "touch" preparations from the cut surface of a nodule more readily identifies the cell type than examination of histological sections. The only clinically pathognomonic lesion of any of the leukemias is chloroma, named for its green color, which is due to myeloperoxidase in the cells of acute granulocytic leukemia. In addition to specific leukemic cell infiltrates, a variety of lesions occur that are nonspecific on biopsy.

INTRAEPIDERMAL METASTASES: PAGET'S DISEASE *Paget's disease of the nipple* and areola is an uncommon but well-known skin sign of underlying intraductal carcinoma of the breast. The primary ductal carcinoma extends upward within the epithelium of the mammary ducts and into the epidermis, where it causes the skin lesion. The clinical appearance is that of an eczematous, weeping, crusted, or scaly lesion resembling atopic eczema or contact dermatitis. Paget's disease is unaffected by topical corticosteroids, in contrast to the responsiveness of eczema. Therefore, any such "eczematous" lesions that fail to respond to treatment must be biopsied. The histopathologic appearance of Paget's disease is diagnostic; the presence in the epidermis of clear cells containing mucopolysaccharides is apparent.

Extramammary Paget's disease is a similar eczematous-appearing lesion occurring on the pubis, perineum, thighs, or genitalia, related usually to underlying apocrine or eccrine sweat gland carcinoma, but occasionally to rectal or urethral adenocarcinoma. Occasionally, a primary malignant origin cannot be found. The histopathologic appearance of extramammary Paget's disease of apocrine gland origin is identical to that of Paget's disease of the breast, which is an apocrine gland. Special staining of the mucopolysaccharides will permit differentiation between Paget's disease of cloacagenic and apocrine gland origin.

LYMPHOMA Lymphomatous deposits in the skin secondary to an internal lymphoma are seen most often in histiocytic lymphoma and lymphoblastic lymphoma. Such cutaneous deposits are rare in Hodgkin's disease. Mycosis fungoides, the most frequent lymphomatous skin disorder, is discussed in Chap. 329. Lymphoma lesions in the skin are dermal or subcutaneous nodules that typically have a purple or red-brown color. The lesions usually are covered by relatively normal intact epidermis. Skin infiltrates may be the initial manifestations or may appear at any time in the course of the disease. Biopsy of these lesions is necessary to establish the correct diagnosis. The nonspecific skin changes in lymphoma are discussed below.

MALIGNANT HISTIOCYTOSIS In the Letterer-Siwe, Schüller-Christian disease complex a variety of skin lesions may occur: (1) scaly papules or vesicles with or without purpura on trunk or scalp; (2) pruritic seborrheic or eczematous lesions in intertriginous areas that do not respond to local treatment for the benign conditions; (3) petechiae due to perivascular infiltrates, thrombocytopenia, or both; (4) scaly or exudative eruptions of the scalp; and (5) xanthomas, usually late in the course. When there is lack of response to local therapy, directed at presumptive diaper dermatitis, seborrheic dermatitis, moniliasis, or intertrigo, early biopsy of these various lesions should be done and is usually diagnostic if histiocytosis is present. Skin lesions may be the presenting sign and may lead to the correct diagnosis, or they may appear late in the course of the disease if it is not controlled (Chap. 322).

SKIN CHANGES DUE TO EXPOSURE TO A CARCINOGEN THAT ALSO INDUCES INTERNAL MALIGNANCY

ARSENICAL KERATOSES Inorganic arsenicals are the only well-recognized carcinogens which cause both skin and visceral malignancies. These salts were widely used in medicine a few decades ago for the treatment of a large variety of disorders, such as arthritis, asthma, and psoriasis, and were also used as herbicides in agriculture. Arsenic contamination of drinking water occurs in many parts of the world. Exposure may therefore be intentional and known or accidental and wholly unsuspected. Multiple, discrete, hard hyperkeratotic wartlike lesions, termed *arsenical keratoses,* on the palms and soles occur characteristically in patients a decade or more after exposure to arsenic. These lesions are similar to actinic or solar keratoses in that they are premalignant lesions, but they have a very low incidence of malignancy. The histopathologic changes produced by these two types of keratosis also are similar.

BOWEN'S DISEASE Squamous-cell carcinoma of the skin in situ is known as Bowen's disease. The lesions are single or multiple, sharply defined plaques that are slightly thickened and brownish red, and have a varying amount of scale. At times the lesions of Bowen's disease resemble eczema or psoriasis but fail to respond to local therapy. Such lesions must be biopsied. Arsenical exposure is definitely the cause of many cases of Bowen's disease and may be the cause of nearly all. The lesions are easily treated by surgical excision or by various methods of local destruction. Although about 5 percent become invasive, less than 2 percent metastasize. More important is the recognition of the fact that the patient is at significant risk of developing carcinomas of the respiratory, genitourinary, and gastrointestinal systems. This risk is especially high in patients in whom Bowen's disease develops on skin that is not usually exposed to sunlight. Thorough examinations to detect visceral neoplasia must be performed at intervals, as the average latent period between the onset of Bowen's disease and the development of visceral neoplasia is more than 8 years. Even without a history or stigmata of arsenical exposure, there is an increased risk of visceral neoplasms in patients with this condition.

SKIN MALIGNANCIES ASSOCIATED WITH INCREASED RISK OF SEPARATE PRIMARY INTERNAL MALIGNANCY

BOWEN'S DISEASE See preceding section.

KAPOSI'S SARCOMA Initially Kaposi's sarcoma may be a multiple, autochthonous, reactive, lymphoreticular and endothelial cell proliferation rather than a neoplasm. It usually behaves in an indolent fashion, although frank, aggressive, sarcomatous change develops in a small percentage of patients. The lesions begin on the feet or ankles, then may progress proximally and also be found on the hands and arms. Extracutaneous lesions are most frequently seen in the gastrointestinal tract, where bleeding is the major complication. The respiratory tract is the second most frequently involved extracutaneous site. Generally these extracutaneous lesions are not clinically significant, unless frankly sarcomatous. There is a marked genetic predisposition to the disease among Jews, Italians, and the Bantus in the Congo. A pronounced male predominance of 9:1 has been noted. The skin lesions of Kaposi's sarcoma are rather distinctive, dark blue or purple-brown nod-

ules or plaques, primarily located on the distal extremities. The color is due to the vascular nature of the lesions and the chronic extravasation of erythrocytes, resulting in hemosiderin deposition. Almost invariably, chronic lymphedema is associated with, and at times precedes, the lesions. Lymphoma and leukemia are associated in about 10 percent of cases in the Western Hemisphere, but not in the Eastern. The histopathologic picture is sufficiently characteristic for confirmation of the clinical diagnosis. For the average case, very conservative therapy, such as elastic support hose to reduce edema and low-dose x-ray treatment of symptomatic skin lesions, is all that is required. Chemotherapy should be considered only in the presence of clinically significant visceral lesions or aggressive sarcomatous behavior.

ANY SKIN MALIGNANCY Neoplasia of the skin of any type may be an indication of increased risk of visceral neoplasia, but the exact relationship is difficult to ascertain because of the high incidence of skin malignancies.

SKIN CHANGES DUE TO METABOLIC PRODUCTS ASSOCIATED WITH MALIGNANCIES

MALIGNANT CARCINOID SYNDROME The hallmark of the syndrome (Chap. 91) is the sudden onset of bright red flushing of the skin, especially of the face, neck, and upper part of the chest.

ADDISONIAN HYPERPIGMENTATION WITH CUSHING'S SYNDROME (See Chap. 336) Some nonendocrine tumors, particularly oat-cell carinoma of the lung, secrete polypeptide hormones. The most commonly observed syndrome is Addisonian hyperpigmentation with Cushing's syndrome. Intense hyperpigmentation combined with proximal muscle weakness, hypertension, diabetes mellitus, edema, and confusion are typical features. Hypokalemic alkalosis and elevated serum cortisol levels are more frequent findings than are the usual physical signs of Cushing's disease. The syndrome is caused by the production of adrenocorticotropic hormone and β-melanocyte–stimulating hormone by the tumor.

GENERALIZED DERMAL MELANOSIS (SLATE GRAY) In some patients with widespread metastases from malignant melanoma, metabolic precursors of melanin enter the circulation and are deposited in all tissues, where they become oxidized to melanin. Excretion of these intermediates results in urine that turns black upon exposure to air. Inasmuch as most of the visible melanin in this type of melanosis is in the dermis, the Tyndall effect causes the skin to look gray or blue-black rather than brown.

NODULAR FAT NECROSIS The syndrome of tender subcutaneous nodules, fever, eosinophilia, and polyarthritis of the small joints is produced by pancreatic adenocarcinoma as well as by pancreatitis. In this syndrome, the subcutaneous nodules are various shades of red and may undergo central necrosis with discharge of oil material. The increased circulating levels of lipase and other pancreatic enzymes are probably responsible for the syndrome. The histopathologic picture of the nodules usually permits the diagnosis of pancreatic fat necrosis, but does not permit differentiation of benign from malignant etiology.

RAYNAUD'S PHENOMENON (See Chap. 253) The production of cryoglobulins in patients with myeloma may cause Raynaud's phenomena. Such an etiology should be especially suspected when the syndrome is atypical, appears in men, or begins in individuals over 50 years of age.

SYSTEMIC AMYLOIDOSIS From 10 to 20 percent of patients with multiple myeloma develop amyloidosis (Chap. 64). The characteristic presentation resembles "primary" amyloidosis and includes macroglossia, extraordinarily easy bruising, and, occasionally, yellowish papules or plaques visible in the skin. All organs may be affected. The purpura appears to result from vascular fragility as a consequence of deposition of amyloid. Purpura may often be induced by gentle stroking or pinching of apparently normal skin, particularly the eyelids and body folds. When the skin lesions of amyloidosis are isolated rather than scattered diffusely, the etiology is unlikely to be systemic. Such local skin amyloidosis is not rare and must be differentiated from systemic amyloidosis.

NECROLYTIC MIGRATING ERYTHEMA The glucagonoma syndrome includes a characteristic dermatitis, somewhat resembling chronic mucocutaneous candidiasis and acrodermatitis enteropathica. The skin lesions are often most severe on the lower abdomen, groin, perineum, and about the mouth. Their morphology consists of vesicles or bullae with a migrating erythematous, scaly margin. There is a tendency to heal centrally. A red, smooth, painful tongue is common (see Chap. 340).

SKIN CHANGES DUE TO FUNCTIONAL DISTURBANCES IN OTHER SYSTEMS INDUCED BY NONENDOCRINE MALIGNANCIES

See Table 328-1.

IDIOPATHIC SKIN SIGNS OF INTERNAL MALIGNANCY

SIGNS FREQUENTLY RELATED TO INTERNAL MALIGNANCY
Dermatomyositis (see Chap. 379) Adults with dermatomyositis have an associated malignancy in at least 15 percent of cases, the association being slightly higher in men than in women. The skin changes may be either subtle and transient initially or widespread, persistent, and rapid in onset. Transient, blotchy, red or violaceous areas, with or without fine scaling, may be incorrectly diagnosed as contact dermatitis, eczema, or seborrheic dermatitis. When the initial lesions are sudden in onset and marked on the face, neck, and other sun-exposed areas, a photosensitivity dermatitis or contact dermatitis may be simulated. Indeed, photosensitivity is frequently noted in dermatomyositis. Later, telangiectasia develops in the lesions, and often edema and telangiectasia of the malar area or the eyelids may result in the violaceous (heliotrope) color. Linear telangiectasia adjacent to the cuticles on the nail folds within areas of periungual erythema are usually seen, as in systemic lupus erythematosus. Accentuation of cutaneous lesions over the joints on the dorsum of the hands, as well as over large joints, is often noted.

Acanthosis nigricans This skin sign is a highly significant marker of probable malignant disease when it develops in adults. The clinical problem is to differentiate between the different types of acanthosis nigricans, all of which look the same clinically and histopathologically. The lesions typically involve the axilla, groin, umbilicus, and nipples, but more extensive lesions may occur. The epidermis shows brown-to-black hyperpigmentation in areas of multiple confluent papillomas, resulting in a velvety elevation of the surface of the epidermis. Pruritus is sometimes present. The histopathologic appearance of

the lesions confirms the diagnosis of acanthosis nigricans but does not permit differentiation between the various types. It is the history, the family history, and the physical examination which provide the most helpful data in classifying the type of acanthosis nigricans. Lesions present at birth or developing in childhood or at puberty are genetically determined and not related to malignancy. Obese individuals may develop intertriginous acanthosis nigricans without underlying disease. Various endocrinopathies, particularly Cushing's syndrome, acromegaly, and Stein-Leventhal syndrome, may be associated with acanthosis nigricans. When these conditions are absent and acanthosis nigricans develops in an adult, an underlying malignancy will be associated in most of the cases. Adenocarcinomas are the usual type of malignancy, and 60 percent of these are gastric (Chap. 291). Occasionally an undifferentiated or squamous-cell carcinoma or a lymphoma is the associated neoplasm. Though the course of the acanthosis nigricans in two-thirds of cases tends to parallel the course of the neoplasm, including remission with cure, intervals as long as 6 years between the skin lesion and the onset of the malignancy have been observed. If no benign explanation can be found for acanthosis nigricans in an adult, periodic efforts to locate a neoplasm are mandatory.

Migratory thrombophlebitis Superficial and multiple deep venous thromboses, not readily explained by the usual causes, are likely to be associated with a malignancy, usually pancreatic carcinoma (Chap. 309). Involvement of atypical sites, such as upper extremities, should also alert the physician to this possible association. An involved area may resolve in a few days. Pulmonary embolism is not a frequent complication. The migratory thrombophlebitis may precede detection of the neoplasm by several months. Unfortunately, the neoplasms associated with recurrent phlebitis tend to be inoperable.

Ichthyosis The development of ichthyosis in adults having no personal or family history of the disorder is very likely to be associated with lymphoma (usually Hodgkin's disease), although occasionally other types of malignancy have been reported. The skin appears dry, and the stratum corneum cracks to produce rhomboidal scales with flaky edges. Hyperkeratosis of the palms and soles may occur as well. The histopathologic changes are epidermal atrophy and hyperkeratosis, but they do not distinguish ichthyosis as a manifestation of malignancy from certain hereditary types. Although the association of this ichthyosiform alteration with lymphoma is strong, only a small number of cases have been reported.

Alopecia mucinosa Dermal papules, often with follicular accentuation and usually with hair loss in affected areas, are the typical findings. Usually this disorder is benign and self-limited, especially in patients under 40 and with a small number of lesions. In patients over 40 and when there are multiple infiltrated plaques with alopecia, the lesions are likely to represent a lymphoma with associated follicular mucinosis. However, alopecia mucinosa may develop before the lymphoma can be diagnosed in a certain number of patients.

Pachydermoperiostosis This term describes hypertrophic osteoarthropathy combined with acromegaloid features (Chap. 333). Thickening of the skin of the hands, forearms, and legs, as well as marked accentuation of facial folds, is typical. When the scalp is involved, the skin is reduplicated and furrowed (cutis verticis gyrata). A familial form of the disorder occurs and is unrelated to malignant disease. The acquired form usually occurs in men over 40 years of age who have bronchogenic carcinoma. Some acquired cases are associated with pulmonary infections, congenital heart disease, and hepatic disease.

Hypertrichosis lanugosa   This sign is quite rare but so striking in its appearance and in its association with internal malignancy that it deserves discussion. A congenital form, often familiarly known as "dog face" or "monkey face," is inherited as an autosomal dominant trait and has no association with malignancy. Acquired hypertrichosis of lanugo hair type in adults has been associated with malignant disease. The associated neoplasms have been carcinomas of the breast, urinary bladder, lung, gallbladder, colon, and rectum. The hypertrichosis in this condition is composed of extremely fine, silky, and lightly pigmented hairs of the lanugo type. This hair growth is most apparent on the face and ears, but may occur on the trunk and extremities. Care must be taken to differentiate this lanugo hair growth from adult-type hair growth in women with disorders of androgen excess and in either sex with porphyria cutanea tarda, erythropoietic porphyria (Chap. 52), and phenytoin administration.

Erythema gyratum repens   See "Urticaria" below.

SIGNS OCCASIONALLY RELATED TO INTERNAL MALIGNANCY Pruritus   Since pruritus is one of the major symptoms expressed in the skin (Chap. 50), obviously most causes of pruritus are not related to malignant disease. Yet pruritus may be a significant symptom in up to 30 percent of patients with Hodgkin's disease. Other lymphomas are less frequently associated with pruritus, excepting mycosis fungoides, in which pruritus is almost universal. Occasionally carcinomas of the lung, stomach, colon, breast, or prostate are associated with pruritus. In such patients the pruritus usually is not limited to a small discrete area. An association with malignancy should be considered in any patient in whom pruritus cannot be explained by the finding of a metabolic cause (Chap. 50) or a local skin disease, aside from excoriations, which could explain it. Hodgkin's disease is the most likely malignancy in patients in their teens through the thirties. In the elderly, xerosis (dry skin) is common and presents a tempting explanation of pruritus. However, if decreased frequency of bathing and the use of emollients do not eliminate the pruritus, then a malignant disease must be considered. The pruritus of malignant disease will cease upon successful therapy of the malignancy.

Clubbing   This alteration of the fingers and toes may sometimes be a manifestation of tumors arising either intrathoracically or metastatic to the thorax (Chap. 268).

Erythroderma   This dramatic reaction of the skin is a response to a variety of stimuli (Chap. 49). Approximately 8 percent of persons with generalized erythroderma are patients with lymphoma, particularly mycosis fungoides, or leukemia. Only occasionally is erythroderma a manifestation of a carcinoma. In patients with erythroderma due to mycosis fungoides, atypical cells are present in the skin, and a skin biopsy will often be diagnostic. In erythroderma related to other types of lymphoma, leukemia, or carcinoma, there is not usually a definable infiltration of the skin by the atypical cells, and the diagnosis must be made from the blood smear, the bone marrow, involved lymph nodes, or other such tissue. In such cases, this erythroderma syndrome may represent an expression of a hypersensitivity reaction to tumor products. The course of the erythroderma parallels the response of the malignant disease to therapy, but it may precede the detection of the malignancy by a year or more, making repeated diagnostic investigations necessary.

Normolipemic xanthomatosis   Malignant diseases of the reticuloendothelial system have been reported in approximately one-half the reported cases of normolipemic plane xanthomatosis. Multiple myeloma is the most frequent type of associated malignant process, but several cases of lymphoma and malignant histiocytosis have been reported. Lesions are yellow to yellow-brown, flat or slightly elevated plaques. There is marked variation in size, and the lesions may be sharply demarcated or may have indistinct borders. The eyelids, sides of the neck, and upper trunk are favored sites, but lesions may appear on any portion of the body. The histopathologic appearance of these xanthomas does not differ from that of clinically similar lesions not associated with malignant disease.

Erythema multiforme (see Chap. 49)   This skin reaction occasionally occurs days to weeks after deep radiation therapy of internal malignant disease, perhaps representing a hypersensitivity reaction to components of tumor tissue. Erythema multiforme is also occasionally reported as an apparent manifestation of a lymphoma, leukemia, or carcinoma, in the absence of radiation therapy. The number of cases which are related to malignant disease is a very small fraction of the total number. The skin reaction tends to resolve spontaneously even in the presence of persistent malignant disease.

Urticaria (see Chap. 49)   This frequent skin reaction is an uncommon manifestation of malignant disease. A cause-effect relationship is difficult to establish unless a clear effect on the urticaria results from therapy of the associated condition. In a few patients with chronic urticaria in whom investigation disclosed a malignant disease, removal of the malignant process was associated with remission of the urticaria. Variants of urticaria present with wheal-like lesions that persist for days to months in the same site, possibly slowly changing position to form annular, arcuate, polycyclic, concentric, or other patterns. This reaction pattern is often classified under the heading of *erythema perstans*. One clinically spectacular but rare syndrome is known as *erythema gyratum repens*, in which concentric, arcuate lesions look like the grain of a soft wood. Only a few cases have been reported, but all were associated with a malignant disease, and in several the skin reaction cleared after successful treatment of the malignancy. These urticarial cutaneous vascular reactions are presumed to represent a hypersensitivity reaction to some component of the malignant disease.

Pyoderma gangrenosum, atypical   Various myeloproliferative disorders have been found in association with pyoderma gangrenosum. Myelogenous and myeloblastic leukemia, myeloma, myeloid metaplasia, monoclonal gammopathy, and polycythemia have been so described. The lesions begin as papules, nodules, or bullae and progress rapidly to central necrosis and ulceration with an epithelial rim of violaceous hue, undermined edge, and occasionally peripheral bulla formation. The lesions are quite often tender. Bacterial cultures and skin biopsy should be done to evaluate possible sepsis, vasculitis, or leukemia cutis. In pyoderma gangrenosum the biopsy is not diagnostic.

Bullous disease   Blistering disorders of various types may occur as a manifestation of malignant disease. The most common type is the subepidermal bullous disease known as *bullous pemphigoid* (Chap. 49). This disorder usually occurs in the elderly and may affect any of or all the skin and mucosal surfaces. There may be an increased incidence of malignant disease in such patients, but this point is not proved. In a few cases, removal of a neoplasm was associated with remission of the dermatosis. Another bullous reaction which should cause the physician to think of the possibility of a malignant disease is *dermatitis herpetiformis*. The disease is characterized by intensely pruritic, grouped vesicles which tend to be symmetrically distributed on the extensor surfaces of the limbs and over the scalp, buttocks, and back. Any patient over 40 or 50 years of age who has a dermatitis herpetiformis-like disorder which is atypical and which does not respond well to sulfone or sulfapyridine therapy should be suspected of having an occult malignant process. This situation is distinctly uncommon.

Dermatoses, bizarre From time to time patients present very strange skin reactions, difficult to identify, and are discovered to have a malignant process. Some of these patients appear to have a cutaneous vasculitis, but this eventually is recognized to be a lymphoma. The variety of such skin reactions is great and cannot be clearly defined. The major importance of including this category is to alert the physician to the possibility of occult malignancy in a patient who presents an unusual, or atypical, or bizarre skin reaction.

HERITABLE DISORDERS WITH SKIN MANIFESTATIONS AND THE PROPENSITY TO DEVELOP INTERNAL MALIGNANCY

The role of heredity in neoplasia is interesting and complex. At times congenital immunologic deficiency states predispose to malignancy, as does acquired immune deficiency. In other cases the relationship between the hereditary condition and neoplasia is unclear. Both types are listed here to increase the awareness of the association. The list is not complete but has been selected to include the most significant syndromes. The manifestations in the skin and other organ systems, as well as the predominant type of malignancy, are presented in Table

TABLE 328-2
Heritable diseases with skin manifestations and propensity to develop internal malignancy

Disorder	Skin signs	Alterations of other systems	Predominant malignancy
DOMINANT INHERITANCE			
Multiple hamartoma syndrome (Cowden's disease)	Acral verrucous papules, trichilemmoma's of face, fibromas of oral mucosa	Multiple hamartomas: Lipomas, hemangiomas, fibrocystic disease of breast, thyroid adenomas, neuromas	Thyroid carcinoma, breast carcinoma
Gardner's syndrome	Epidermal cysts, sebaceous cysts, dermoid tumors, lipomas, fibromas	Polyposis of colon, osteomas	Colonic adenocarcinomas (very high incidence, unless colectomy done)
Multiple mucosal neuromas	Neuromas on eyelids, lips, tongue, nasal or laryngeal mucosae	Parathyroid adenomas, hypertension	Pheochromocytoma, medullary carcinoma of thyroid (high incidence)
Neurofibromatosis (Recklinghausen's)	Neurofibromas, café au lait spots, axillary "freckles," giant nevi	Acoustic and spinal neuromas, meningiomas, osseous fibrous dysplasia	Malignant neurilemmoma (5% incidence), pheochromocytoma (uncommon), astrocytoma, glioma (uncommon)
Nevoid basal-cell carcinoma syndrome	Multiple basal-cell carcinomas, epidermoid cysts, "pits" on palms and soles	Jaw cysts, rib and vertebral abnormalities, short metacarpals, ovarian fibromas, hypertelorism	Medulloblastoma, fibrosarcoma of jaw (low incidence)
Palmar-plantar hyperkeratosis (tylosis)	Hyperkeratosis of palms and soles (usually onset after age 10)	None	Esophageal carcinoma (95% incidence)
Peutz-Jeghers syndrome	Pigmented macules on lips, oral mucosa, digits	Intestinal polyposis (predominantly small intestine)	Gastric, duodenal, and colonic adenocarcinomas (low incidence)
Tuberous sclerosis	Hypopigmented macules, shagreen patches, adenoma sebaceum, subungual fibromas	Epilepsy, mental retardation, hamartomas in brain, kidneys, heart	Astrocytomas, glioblastomas (low incidence)
AUTOSOMAL RECESSIVE			
Ataxia telangiectasia	Telangiectasia: neck, malar, antecubital fossae, popliteal fossae, ears	Cerebellar ataxia, sinopulmonary infections, IgA deficiency, ± IgE deficiency	Lymphoma, leukemia (10% incidence)
Bloom's syndrome	Telangiectasia of sun-exposed skin, photosensitivity	Short stature, fine features, dolichocephaly	Leukemia (high incidence)
Chédiak-Higashi syndrome	Dilution of skin and hair color, recurrent pyoderma, giant melanosomes	Recurrent infections, azurophilic leukocytic inclusions, nystagmus, iris translucence, photophobia, pancytopenia	Lymphoma (high incidence)
Fanconi's anemia	Patchy hyperpigmentation	Bone anomalies, chromosomal aberrations	Leukemia (high incidence)
Werner's syndrome (adult progeria)	Premature aging, scleroderma-like changes, graying hair and baldness, leg ulcers	Arteriosclerosis, cataracts	Sarcoma, meningiomas
SEX-LINKED RECESSIVE			
Bruton's sex-linked agammaglobulinemia	Recurrent infections	Recurrent infections, agammaglobulinemia	Leukemia, lymphoma (5% incidence)
Dyskeratosis congenita	Reticulate hyperpigmentation, leukoplakia of mucosae, loss of nails, hyperkeratosis of palms and soles, atrophy of skin of extensor surfaces	Pancytopenia	Carcinomas (high incidence), leukemia (occasional)
Wiscott-Aldrich syndrome	Eczematous dermatitis, petechiae-purpura, recurrent pyoderma	Decreased IgM, thrombocytopenia	Leukemia, lymphoma (10% incidence)

328-2. The reader should refer to specific discussion of these entities for more complete information.

REFERENCES

BARNES BE: Dermatomyositis and malignancy: A review of the literature. Ann Intern Med 84:68, 1976

BRAVERMAN IM: *Skin Signs of Systemic Disease.* Philadelphia, Saunders, 1970

BROWNSTEIN MH, HELWIG EB: Metastatic tumors of the skin. Cancer 29:1298, 1972

CROCKER AC: The histiocytosis syndromes, in *Dermatology in General Medicine,* 2d ed, TB Fitzpatrick et al (eds). New York, McGraw-Hill, 1979

FLINT GL et al: Acquired ichothysis: A sign of nonlymphoproliferative disorders. Arch Dermatol 111:1446, 1975

HAYNES HA, CURTH HO: Cutaneous manifestations associated with malignant internal disease in *Dermatology in General Medicine,* 2d ed, TB Fitzpatrick et al (eds). New York, McGraw-Hill, 1979

LEWIS SJ et al: Atypical pyoderma gangrenosum with leukemia. JAMA 239:935, 1978

MALLINSON CM et al: A glucagonoma syndrome. Lancet 2:1, 1974

NEWBOLD PCH: Skin markers of malignancy. Arch Dermatol 102:680, 1970

SAMSON MK et al: Acquired hypertrichosis lanuginosa: Report of two new cases and a review of the literature. Cancer 36:1519, 1975

STONE SP, SCHROETER AL: Bullous pemphigoid and associated malignant neoplasms. Arch Dermatol 111:991, 1975

329
PRIMARY CANCER OF THE SKIN

HARLEY A. HAYNES

Carcinoma of the skin is the most common carcinoma occurring in Caucasoid individuals. Inasmuch as the lesions can be seen with the naked eye when they are in an early stage, the potential for cure is well over 90 percent. Although not responsible for all carcinomas of the skin, chronic exposure to ultraviolet light of the sunburn wavelengths (290 to 320 nm) in individuals not protected by intense melanin pigmentation is the most important single etiologic factor (Chap. 52). Hence, most of these cancers occur on areas of the skin that remain uncovered when the individual is fully clothed. As discussed in Chap. 52, genetic factors markedly mediate this tendency for carcinogenesis. Heritable diseases such as albinism, xeroderma pigmentosum, and the nevoid-basal-cell carcinoma syndrome are less common conditions associated with a greater risk of skin cancer. The routine local use of effective sun-screen preparations by individuals at risk can undoubtedly reduce tumor incidence. Chemical carcinogens, especially inorganic arsenicals and certain organic hydrocarbons, are separate and additional causes of skin cancers, particularly of the squamous-cell variety. Ionizing radiation, including x-rays, grenz rays, and gamma rays, is also carcinogenic. As with other organ systems, the skin is predisposed to the development of malignant lesions in immunologic deficiency states, such as those associated with lymphoma or immunosuppressive therapy. Although any of the cell types in the skin may give rise to malignant neoplasms, the most common are basal-cell and squamous-cell carcinomas.

BASAL-CELL CARCINOMA Basal-cell carcinoma accounts for over 75 percent of all skin cancers. These carcinomas arise from the epidermis, cytologically resemble the normal basal cells, and show little tendency to undergo the usual differentia-

tion into squamous cells which produce keratin. Although these tumors very rarely metastasize, they are locally invasive and, if neglected, may invade widely and deeply into underlying structures, including nerves, bone, and brain. Like most cancers these tumors are remarkably painless in their course. This lack of symptoms often leads to prolonged neglect of a lesion. The typical basal-cell carcinoma is a noninflamed, smooth, waxy nodule that appears translucent, usually has numerous telangiectatic vessels visible near the surface, and may have variable amounts of melanin pigment in the form of small dots. Such nodules often ulcerate and form a crust. This ulceration may reepithelialize, causing the patient to assume that the nodule is resolving. Basal-cell carcinomas may take many other forms, including subtle infiltrating lesions that do not produce elevated nodules. Biopsy for confirmation of the diagnosis should be routine. The patient with one basal-cell carcinoma is likely to have others, either at the same time or in following years. Some patients come to the physician with a dozen or more concurrent primary basal-cell carcinomas. Although there is no visible premalignant lesion that precedes a basal-call carcinoma, the lesion is usually seen in patients who manifest the stigmata of skin damage from sunlight (or x-rays). Treatment is selected according to the size, depth, type, and location of the lesion, as well as the particular abilities of the physician. If a simple excision will suffice, there is no other procedure that can equal the cosmetic result. Curettage and electrodesiccation for small lesions give a cure rate of more than 95 percent in experienced hands, as does x-ray treatment. Cryosurgery with liquid nitrogen seems to give cure rates similar to curettage and electrodesiccation and often brings a better cosmetic result. Local chemotherapy with 5-fluorouracil is not recommended as routine treatment of basal-cell carcinomas, but may have a role in the treatment of multiple superficial lesions. Immunotherapy is investigational.

SQUAMOUS-CELL CARCINOMA Squamous-cell carcinoma also arises from the epidermis but shows significant squamous differentiation and usually keratin production. These tumors have a variable tendency to metastasize, depending upon their size, extent of invasion, location, and whether they arise from a premalignant lesion, a burn scar, a chronic inflammatory condition, or from apparently normal skin. The typical squamous-cell carcinoma is a painless, firm, red nodule or plaque with visible scales on the surface. Ulceration and crusting may occur. Relatively undifferentiated lesions that do not produce much keratin may fail to show noticeable scaling on the surface. In contrast to the basal-cell variety, squamous-cell carcinomas most commonly arise from preexisting *actinic* or *solar keratoses*. These premalignant keratoses are scaly, rough, red plaques that occur in chronically sun-damaged skin. Although very few of these keratoses progress to carcinoma, most squamous-cell carcinomas on exposed skin do arise from such keratoses. This type of squamous-cell carcinoma has the lowest frequency of metastasis (under 2 percent). However, because of the potential of malignant change in solar keratoses, which though small is real, it seems prudent to remove them, especially in younger patients. At present, the local application of 5-fluorouracil (1 to 5%) in cream or lotion seems to be the most effective method and one that generally produces no scarring. Squamous-cell carcinomas arising from mucous membranes, mucocutaneous junctions, burn scars, chronic ulcers, or sinus tracts or from apparently normal skin have a much higher tendency to metastasize. An in situ stage of cutaneous squamous-cell carcinoma is known as Bowen's disease (Chap. 328).

Although some of these in situ lesions are the result of chronic sun damage, a significant proportion occurs in patients who had received inorganic arsenic preparations either accidentally or for medicinal purposes a decade or more before. In these patients there is also an increased risk of carcinomas of the respiratory, genitourinary, and gastrointestinal systems.

Patients with squamous-cell carcinoma must be examined carefully for the presence of metastases so that therapy may be appropriate. In the absence of metastases, therapy of the local lesion may generally be as indicated for basal-cell carcinoma, with preference for surgical excision or x-irradiation in view of the potential for metastasis. Extensive local or metastatic lesions may benefit from systemic chemotherapy, sometimes via local perfusion.

MYCOSIS FUNGOIDES LYMPHOMA *Lymphoma of the skin* may be a primary or secondary manifestation of various types of lymphoma. Histiocytic lymphoma and lymphoblastic lymphoma may occasionally begin with only skin lesions, but Hodgkin's disease rarely does so. The most common lymphoma of the skin is *mycosis fungoides,* which always begins with cutaneous lesions, usually with no evidence of visceral infiltration for several years. The initial lesions may be clinically confused with eczema, contact dermatitis, or psoriasis, and the biopsy may not be diagnostic. Later, more typical patches of infiltrated skin develop, often with a tendency for central clearing or an arciform or polycyclic arrangement. At this point, the biopsy may be diagnostic. In some patients, diffuse exfoliative erythroderma develops, and there may be circulating mycosis fungoides cells in the blood, at times causing diagnostic confusion with chronic lymphocytic leukemia. The skin biopsy may resolve the confusion if it is sufficiently characteristic, as may electron microscopy of the atypical cells, which are quite distinct in mycosis fungoides. The atypical cells found in the skin appear to be the same cells found in the blood or in visceral infiltrates. These cells have been identified as thymus-dependent lymphocytes. In blood smears these cells resemble large lymphocytes with scant cytoplasm and folded nuclei. In routine tissue sections these cells sometimes look like lymphocytes and sometimes like reticulum cells with the characteristic infolded nucleus. Electron-microscopic examination shows the nucleus of this cell to be highly irregular, convoluted, lobulated, and drawn into narrow threads and ribbons. At some point in time, most patients develop larger tumors as well. Although any of the viscera may be affected, disability from internal involvement usually does not occur until quite late in the course of the disease. For a patient with the early stage of the disease, the prognosis is for survival for several decades. Once the histologic diagnosis of mycosis fungoides is confirmed, the median survival for all patients is 5 years. Patients with skin tumors, ulceration, or lymphatic involvement have a median survival of 30 months.

Treatment is best planned so as to not restrict unnecessarily the future options of therapy. Topical applications of dilute, nonvesicant concentrations of mechlorethamine are often very effective for months or even years. Photochemotherapy with psoralens and long-wave ultraviolet light is often helpful. Selected lesions can be treated with grenz rays. Whole-skin electron-beam treatment may be given without hematologic suppression, since the voltage is regulated to control the depth of penetration of electrons. The use of orthovoltage x-irradiation of multiple sites should be carefully restricted, so as not to compromise the marrow or complicate further therapy with electron beam. Electron beam followed by topical mechlorethamine is probably the most effective therapy for disease limited to cutaneous plaques. Systemic chemotherapy with agents such as methotrexate, cyclophosphamide, vinca alkaloids, procarbazine, chlorambucil, and steroids often can cause dramatic objective regression of disease, but has not yet been proved to prolong life expectancy. Even though most patients at necropsy are found to have infiltrates in various viscera, early systemic chemotherapy has not been found advantageous, as a rule, perhaps because of the adverse effect of such therapy on the clinically very apparent resistance of the host with this lymphoma. In fact, this lymphoma was the first human malignancy to regularly show regression of lesions that were challenged locally with delayed hypersensitivity reactions.

REFERENCES

ANDRADE R et al (eds): *Cancer of the Skin: Biology-Diagnosis-Management.* Philadelphia, Saunders, 1976

EPSTEIN EH et al: Mycosis fungoides: Survival, prognostic features, response to therapy, and autopsy findings. Medicine 15:61, 1972

FITZPATRICK TB et al (eds): Neoplasms of the dermis, in *Dermatology in General Medicine,* 2d ed. New York, McGraw-Hill, 1979

GILCHREST BA et al: Oral photochemotherapy of mycosis fungoides. Cancer 38:683, 1976

HAYNES HA, VANSCOTT EJ: Lymphomas, in *Dermatology in General Medicine,* 2d ed, TB Fitzpatrick et al (eds). New York, McGraw-Hill, 1979

LUTZNER M et al: Cutaneous T-cell lymphomas: The Sézary syndrome, mycosis fungoides, and related disorders. Ann Intern Med 83:534, 1975

MCDONALD CJ, BERTINO JR: Treatment of mycosis fungoides lymphoma—effectiveness of infusions of methotrexate followed by oral citrovorum factor. Cancer Treatment Rep 62:1009, 1978

VONDERHEID EC et al: Topical chemotherapy and immunotherapy of mycosis fungoides. Arch Dermatol 113:454, 1977

ZACARIAN SA (ed): *Cryosurgical Advances in Dermatology and Tumors of the Head and Neck.* Springfield, Ill, Charles C Thomas, 1977

330
MALIGNANT MELANOMA OF THE SKIN

THOMAS B. FITZPATRICK
ARTHUR J. SOBER
MARTIN C. MIHM, JR.

Primary malignant melanoma of the skin is the leading cause of death from all diseases arising in the skin, and the detection of early lesions must be the task of every physician, regardless of specialty. At every occasion when the entire cutaneous surface can be viewed, a careful search for suspicious pigmented lesions should be made.

Pigmented moles are among the most common growths on the skin, and yet cancer involving pigment cells (i.e., malignant melanoma) is relatively uncommon, constituting about 1 percent of all cancers. There has been a disturbing increase in the incidence of primary melanoma of the skin. The rate has doubled in the past 10 years, possibly due to increased "weekend" exposure to sunlight, especially among persons in professional and managerial positions. Primary cutaneous malignant melanoma, moreover, is virtually untreatable by chemotherapy or x-ray, and, so far, hope for survival has been based on surgical excision during the very early primary stages before deep invasion occurs. The problem for the physician, therefore, is to recognize early primary malignant melanoma and also those precancerous lesions that will develop into malignant melanoma among the large number of pigmented lesions that occur on the skin.

Primary malignant melanoma of the skin, even in the early stages, is now considered relatively easy to detect by clinical examination alone. In the past, the clinical description of primary cutaneous malignant melanoma was presented incompletely. Physicians and patients were told to have concern only for those pigmented lesions that showed changes in growth pattern or color or were bleeding or ulcerated—criteria indicating deep invasion in the skin and, usually, a poor prognosis.

Follow-up study of more than 1100 patients with primary melanoma has provided evidence indicating that a primary cutaneous melanoma may exist in a "silent," intraepidermal, preinvasive form for several years. These early "silent" primary malignant melanomas, even when 3 to 4 mm in size, can be recognized by certain simple criteria, which are delineated below.

Two criteria, *variegation of color* and *irregular border* often with a "notch," are so characteristic of primary cutaneous malignant melanoma that histologic examination is mandatory when they are present. The important colors that are signs of primary malignant melanoma *include shades of red, white, or blue* and the shades resulting from their mixture with brown or black. Furthermore, a lesion may be uniformly colored, e.g., *bluish black or bluish red.*

The diagnostic significance of various shades of brown or black, or both, in pigmented primary cutaneous malignant melanoma has been stressed in the past. It is, however, the diagnostic significance of the various shades of red, white, or blue, or all three mixed with brown or black, that requires emphasis. Of the colors present in pigmented primary cutaneous malignant melanomas, shades of blue (bluish red, bluish gray, and bluish black) are the most significant in the diagnosis. *Examination with a magnifying lens and bright lighting* may assist greatly in recognizing the diagnostic feature of melanoma.

Before 1967, malignant melanoma was considered a single morphologic entity with a uniformly grave prognosis. Later histopathologic investigations, especially by Clark, McGovern, and colleagues, have permitted a new approach to the classification of primary human cutaneous malignant melanomas, based on the correlation of the clinical and histologic features with prognosis. Three types of primary malignant melanoma have been delineated:

1 Malignant melanoma with an adjacent intraepidermal component (lentigo maligna melanoma; see Plate 6-1)
2 Malignant melanoma with an adjacent intraepidermal component (superficial spreading melanoma; see Plate 6-2)
3 Malignant melanoma *without* an adjacent intraepidermal component (nodular melanoma; see Plate 6-3)

Some of the features of these types are listed in Table 330-1.

It should be emphasized that lentigo maligna melanoma and superficial spreading melanoma may exist for several years in the preinvasive stage. Hence, early diagnosis of malignant melanoma of the skin makes excision of the identified lesions possible before deep invasion has occurred. The survival rate of malignant melanoma is related to the level of invasion of the tumor. These levels of invasion have been classified on the basis of anatomic structure as follows:

Level 1: Intraepidermal melanocytic atypism, a level recognized for purposes of research. Patients with this finding are not at present labeled with the diagnosis of melanoma.
Level 2: Tumor invading the papillary layer but not extending to the reticular layer.
Level 3: Tumor filling and expanding the papillary layer but not invading the reticular layer.
Level 4: Tumor penetrating into the reticular layer of the dermis.
Level 5: Tumor invading the subcutaneous fat.

Malignant melanomas that have not extended beyond level 2 usually cause death by 5 years in fewer than 5 percent of patients. Nodular melanomas have usually extended to level 3 when first recognized and result in death by 5 years in approximately 45 percent of patients. Additional prognostic information can be obtained by measuring the vertical thickness of the tumor with the use of a light microscope fitted with an ocular micrometer. Tumors less than 0.75 mm in thickness have a uniformly favorable outcome, while patients with tumors greater than 1.50 to 2.25 mm are at high risk for recurrent diseases and death. In all types, the survival rate decreases progressively according to the depth of invasion at the time of excision, thus making the earliest possible identification essential.

Suspicious lesions require biopsy, which will confirm the benign or malignant nature of the lesion. Simple excisional biopsy with narrow margins is the procedure of choice, but trephine (punch) or incisional biopsies are also acceptable depending on the situation and the experience of the physician performing the procedure. Table 330-2 lists the indications for biopsy of cutaneous lesions.

Treatment of malignant melanoma at the present is primarily by surgical excision of the primary lesion; there is no agree-

TABLE 330-1
Clinical features of malignant melanoma

Type	Site	Average age at diagnosis, years	Duration of known existence, years	Color
Lentigo maligna melanoma	Exposed surfaces usually, and particularly malar region of cheek and temple; on unexposed surfaces sometimes	70	5–20* or longer	In flat portions, shades of brown and black predominant, but whitish gray occasionally present; in nodules, shades of reddish brown, bluish gray, bluish black
Superficial spreading melanoma	Any site (more common on upper back and in women on lower legs)	40–50	1–7	Shades of brown and black mixed with bluish red (violaceous), bluish black, reddish brown, and often whitish pink, and the border of lesion is at least in part visibly and/or palpably elevated
Nodular melanoma	Any site	40–50	Months to less than 5 years	Reddish blue (purple) or bluish black, either uniform in color or mixed with brown or black

* *During much of this time, the precursor stage, lentigo maligna, is actively confined to the epidermis.*

ment as to whether prophylactic lymph node dissection affects the course of the disease. Level 2 lesions can be treated successfully by wide local excision and, if necessary, skin grafting. Recent data (Breslow and Macht) suggest that more limited excision may be equally effective for level 2 (thin) lesions. The advanced stages (i.e., invasion to levels 3, 4, and 5) should be treated by wide local excision down to the deep fascia, followed by skin grafting; radical lymph node dissection when the tumor drains to only one lymph node group also is advocated by most surgeons. Surgery for lentigo maligna melanoma is less aggressive; the recommendation is for surgical margins of 1 cm or greater and lymph node dissection only if therapeutically indicated.

In the past few years, considerable interest has been directed toward the factors that influence both the development of primary malignant melanomas of the skin and also the rate and degree of dissemination of the tumor. The possibility that there is a population with a high risk for the development of these melanomas is being studied. It is suspected that persons, both male and female, who have poor tolerance to sunlight and develop sunburn on short exposures and then a poor tan have a higher incidence of malignant melanoma (Table 330-3). It has recently been demonstrated that an inverse relationship exists between melanoma incidence and latitude. Thus in northeastern Australia (latitude S10°45′) the incidence of primary malignant melanoma of the skin is 17 per 100,000 population, whereas in Connecticut (latitude N41°45′) the incidence is less than 5 per 100,000 population for the comparable time period.

Families have been studied in the members of which malignant melanomas have aggregated. Many of these family members appear to have a type of nevus which resembles clinically miniature early superficial spreading melanomas. These lesions may be genetically determined precursor lesions of malignant melanoma.

Only a few factors are presently known to influence the dissemination of melanoma. Although there is a higher incidence of melanoma in women, the death rate is higher among men. The survival rate seems to correlate with hormonal status. Premenopause females have a better survival rate once metastases have occurred, whereas postmenopause females have a survival rate that is equal to or shorter than that of males. The immune status of the patient is another factor under investigation. The possibility that immunologic factors are involved in the course of malignant melanoma is suggested by the high rate of spontaneous regressions of melanoma, by the long periods of freedom from the time of excision of the primary lesion to the development of metastases, and by the improved prognosis of those lesions in which on histologic examination a marked lymphocytic response is found. Both cellular

TABLE 330-2

Indications for excision or diagnostic biopsy of pigmented lesions

I History
   A Change in size or color, bleeding
   B Symptoms
      1 Itching
      2 Tenderness
   C Congenital, raised pigmented lesions
II Lesion characteristics
   A Color
      1 Uniform blue or gray
      2 Variegated: blue, gray, white, red, mixed with brown or black
   B Border: irregular, often with a notch
   C Surface: irregular

TABLE 330-3

Summary data on malignant melanoma of skin

I Incidence: 1% of all cancers (excluding nonmelanoma skin cancer)
  A Overall annual crude incidence rates (United States)
    1 Caucasians: 4.5/10^5/year (men, 4.4; women, 4.5/10^5/year)
    2 Negroes: 0.6/10^5/year (men, 0.7; women, 0.6/10^5/year)
  B Increasing with time (Connecticut Registry)
    1 1935–1939: 1.2/10^5/year
    2 1965–1969: 4.8/10^5/year
    3 1976–1977: 7.2/10^5/year
  C Latitude-dependent crude incidence rates:
    1 Northern United States (Detroit): 3.1/10^5/year
    2 Southern United States (Dallas): 7.2/10^5/year
II Frequency for type of melanoma
  A Superficial spreading: 70%
  B Nodular: 16%
  C Lentigo maligna melanoma: 5%
  D Unclassified: 10%
III Survival (5 year) overall: 67%. Based on anatomic level of invasion:
  A Level 2: 93%
  B Level 3: 74%
  C Level 4: 63%
  D Level 5: 39%
IV Deaths = 1% of all cancer deaths (United States)

and hormonal immunities to melanoma cells have been demonstrated by in vitro techniques.

The physician examining a patient with many pigmented lesions should recognize the features that are highly suggestive of primary malignant melanoma of the skin and necessarily indicate that the lesion must be removed, or, if it is very large, at least biopsied (see Table 330-2). If these early lesions can be detected and excised, the 5-year survival rate of patients with malignant melanoma should approach 85 percent. The most important clues in the detection of primary malignant melanoma are the areas of bluish gray, bluish red, bluish black, and whitish gray. Certain pigmented lesions, however, such as all congenital hairy nevi and pigmented lesions of the scalp and soles, do not have these telltale color changes but should be prophylactically removed. Finally, the following sites should be examined:

1 Sites of infrequent origin and bad prognosis, when melanoma occurs: genitalia, perineum, perianal area, and the mucous membranes.
2 Sites of repeated trauma, occurring anywhere on the body including the scalp.
3 Sites of frequent origin of tumor such as the upper back, and the lower legs in women.

REFERENCES

BRESLOW A, MACHT SD: Optimum size of resection margin for thin cutaneous melanoma. Surg Gynecol Obstet 145:691, 1977

CLARK WH JR et al: The developmental biology of primary human malignant melanomas. Semin Oncol 2:83, 1975

KOPF A et al: Malignant melanoma: Review. J Dermatol Surg Oncol 3:41, 1977

MIHM MC JR, FITZPATRICK TB: Early detection of malignant melanoma. Cancer 76(suppl):37, 183, January 1976

——— et al: The clinical diagnosis, classification and histogenetic concepts of the early stages of cutaneous malignant melanomas. N Engl J Med 284:1078, 1971

——— et al: Early detection of primary cutaneous malignant melanoma: Color atlas. N Engl J Med 289:989, 1973

REIMER RR et al: Precursor lesions in familial melanoma. JAMA 239:744, 1978

SOBER AJ: Immunology and cutaneous malignant melanoma. Int J Dermatol 15:1, 1976

VERONESI U et al: Inefficacy of immediate node dissection in stage 1 melanoma of the limbs. N Engl J Med 297:627, 1977

331
PRINCIPLES OF ENDOCRINOLOGY

JEAN D. WILSON

INTRODUCTION The functional capacities of cells are determined ultimately by genetic factors, but the regulation of the rates of individual metabolic pathways is accomplished by two interlocking and coordinated systems, the endocrine system and the nervous system. Originally these two regulatory systems were considered distinct, information being carried by neural impulses for the nervous system and by chemical mediators in the blood for the endocrine system. Now it is clear that this conception is incomplete, if not incorrect. Not only may neurotransmitters such as norepinephrine circulate in blood as hormones, but neural impulses have major effects on the release of chemical mediators such as testosterone and insulin. Furthermore, certain mediators (e.g., somatostatin) function as both neurotransmitters and hormones. This interlocking relationship is most apparent in the hypothalamus, which serves as the highest integrative center for the two systems. Hence, interlocking neuroendocrine systems have evolved to integrate and coordinate the metabolic activities of the organism (see Chap. 332). Endocrinology deals largely with the chemical mediators in this system, but proper understanding of the role of hormones requires knowledge of both the autonomic nervous system (Chap. 72) and the metabolic capacity of cells (Chaps. 86 and 87).

The classic concepts of endocrinology have been blurred in additional ways. The term *hormone* was originally applied to substances that are secreted into the circulation and act as chemical effectors in other tissues. However the capacity to form such chemical mediators is not limited to the endocrine organs. Some hormones such as angiotensins II and III are formed from precursors in the circulation itself. Others such as testosterone in the female and dihydrotestosterone and estradiol in the male are formed largely in peripheral tissues from circulating precursors, termed *prohormones*. Still others circulate only in restricted compartments such as the hepatoportal circulation or the hypothalamoportal system and do not reach the systemic circulation in appreciable quantities. Finally, certain hormones such as insulin and glucagon have some actions in the same tissues in which they are formed, a phenomenon termed *paracrine function*. Therefore, the action as well as the origins should be considered when deciding whether a given effector should be classified as a hormone.

BIOCHEMISTRY Synthesis The mammalian hormones, now recognized to be greater than 50 in number, fall into three general categories—peptides or peptide derivatives, steroids, and amines. These hormones are formed by two types of synthetic processes. In the case of peptide hormones, genes code for messenger RNA which is then translated into protein precursors. These proteins undergo posttranslational cleavage (e.g., preproparathyroid hormone → proparathyroid hormone → parathyroid hormone, and proinsulin → insulin) and/or processing (e.g., thyroglobulin → thyroxine → triiodothyronine) to form the active hormone recognized by the target tissue. The distinct feature of peptide hormones is that one (or two) genes code for the amino acid sequence of the peptide while other genes are responsible for the alteration of the peptide to its final form. In the case of hormones with subunits, the subunits may be formed from either a single precursor (insulin) or separate precursors [luteinizing hormone (LH)]. Whether the various hypothalamic releasing factors such as thyrotropin-releasing hormone (TRH) or luteinizing hormone-releasing hormone (LHRH) are cleaved from prohormones or synthesized de novo is unknown. Peptide hormones can also be formed ectopically in dedifferentiated tissues of nonendocrine origin such as carcinoma of the lung (see Chap. 347). The smaller the number of genes involved in controlling synthesis of a hormone, the more likely is such ectopic production.

In the case of steroid hormones the fundamental precursor is either cholesterol (for most steroid hormones) or 7-dehydrocholesterol (for calciferol), both of which undergo a series of enzymatic transformations to form the final products. A minimum of nine enzymes (or enzyme complexes) and consequently nine or more genes are required to transform cholesterol to estradiol. Because of the complexity of the synthetic machinery required for the formation of steroid hormones, their formation in malignancies of nonendocrine tissues is unusual, even rare.

The amine hormones are synthesized by a similar but simpler series of reactions except that the substrates are amino acids. For example, tyrosine is the precursor for epinephrine and norepinephrine.

Storage In general, tissues that synthesize hormones have a limited capacity to store the completed product. For example, the normal adult testes contain only about a sixth of the quantity of testosterone needed for daily turnover, and consequently the testicular pool turns over several times to provide the normal daily output of hormone. Even when tissues have special storage organelles for hormone, the amount of hormone stored is variable. For example the insulin granules in the pancreatic beta cell ordinarily contain quantities of insulin sufficient only for short-term, reserve needs, whereas nerve endings may contain a several-day supply of norepinephrine. The limited capacity to store hormones is a chemical consequence of their unsuitability for incorporation into any of the three main storage compartments of the body (lipids, glycogen, and protein). For example, the steriod hormones are too polar to be stored in large quantities in lipid compartments, and peptide and amine hormones are unsuitable for incorporation into proteins. As a consequence of these factors the body pools of most hormones tend to be small. The major exceptions to this rule are those instances in which the precursor forms of hormone can be stored either as protein or in neutral lipid compartments; the normal thyroid gland contains the equivalent of 2 weeks' requirement of thyroid hormones in the form of the protein thyroglobulin, and the neutral precursor and intermediate forms of vitamin D can be stored in considerable quantity in hepatic lipid.

Release The biochemical mechanisms involved in the release process are not as well understood as those involved in synthesis. In some cases conversion of insoluble to soluble derivatives is required (proteolysis of thyroglobulin to thyroxine). In others there is exocytosis of storage granules (insulin, glucagon, prolactin, growth hormone). Finally, release may simply involve passive diffusion of newly synthesized molecules into plasma down concentration (activity) gradients (steroid hormones).

Because of the limited capacity for storage, most hormones are released into plasma in the steady state as a passive reflection of the rates of formation. As a consequence, the regulation of hormone activity in plasma is usually accomplished by regulation of hormone synthesis. Thus, the pituitary trophic hormones [adrenocorticotropic hormone (ACTH), LH, follicle-stimulating hormone (FSH), and thyroid-stimulating hormone (TSH)] influence rates of both hormone synthesis and release in their target tissues. Even in the case of peptide hormones stored in granules, initial release of the stored material is followed by an enhanced rate of synthesis (for example, the two-phase release of insulin induced by glucose infusion). For some hormones, there are, in addition, major diurnal, sleep-related, developmental, and neural influences on hormone release; again it is assumed that in most of these instances synthesis and release are tightly linked.

In many instances, the regulation of hormone release on a short-term basis is poorly understood. The release of some hormones is pulsatile, with bursts of output occurring in a repetitive pattern; whether this intermittent release is accomplished via alterations in synthetic rates, alterations in blood flow, or other mechanisms is uncertain. Although the physiological significance of pulsatile release is not known, changes in both frequency and amplitude of the release pattern may occur in various diseases.

Transport Hormones are transported from sites of synthesis to sites of cellular action and ultimately of metabolic inactivation and degradation by lymph, blood, and extracellular fluids. The plasma is probably a passive diluent for peptide and amine hormones but provides specific proteins for binding and transport of certain steroid and thyroid hormones. The generalization can be made that the more insoluble a hormone in water, the more important is the role of transport proteins. Protein-bound hormone (HP) is biologically inactive and serves as a reservoir from which free hormone (H) is liberated in sufficient quantities for diffusion into intracellular compartments:

$$H + P \rightleftharpoons HP$$

Distribution of bound and free hormone in plasma is determined by the amount of hormone, the amount of binding protein, and the binding affinity of hormone for the protein. An understanding of this relation is critical for assessment of endocrine status in clinical medicine. Although changes in the amount of the binding protein can alter the steady-state level of total hormone in plasma (H + HP), only the free hormone interacts with cells and participates in the regulatory feedback mechanisms that control the rates of hormone synthesis (described below). As a consequence changes in the amount of transport protein alone cannot cause endocrine pathology in the steady state, provided the remainder of the endocrine feedback loop is intact. For example, profound elevations and decreases in thyroid-binding globulin (either because of genetic or other factors) are both compatible with a euthyroid state. To illustrate, a sudden increase in thyroxine-binding globulin lowers the level of free (unbound) hormone; consequently, TSH secretion increases, and thyroid output of thy-

roxine is increased *until* thyroxine-binding globulin is again saturated so that the level of free hormone returns to normal, at which time TSH levels and thyroid hormone secretion also return to normal. Likewise, a decrease in thyroid-binding protein temporarily increases the level of free hormone, and TSH secretion and thyroxine output fall until the free level returns to normal. No transport protein yet characterized is exclusive; e.g., testosterone can be transported by both a specific binding protein and albumin, and thyroxine can be transported by both prealbumin and thyroxine-binding globulin.

To summarize, a change in binding protein can cause profound alterations in hormone levels but by itself cannot cause either a steady-state excess or deficiency of hormone.

Degradation and turnover The plasma level (PL) of any hormone is dependent on two factors—the secretion rate (SR) of the hormone and the overall rates by which it is metabolized and excreted, the metabolic clearance rate (MCR):

$$PL = \frac{SR}{MCR} \qquad or \qquad SR = MCR \times PL$$

There is considerable variation in the mechanisms by which the metabolic clearance of hormones is accomplished. Degradation and inactivation of the hormone can take place in target tissues, in other organs such as liver and kidneys, or in both target and nontarget tissues. In many instances the transformations facilitate excretion by rendering the hormone soluble in urine or bile. Peptide hormones are in general assumed to be inactivated by proteases, largely in target tissues. Thyroid hormones are deiodinated, deaminated, and deconjugated primarily by the liver. Steroid hormones are reduced, hydroxylated, and converted into glucuronide and sulfate conjugates. Only small fractions of hormones are excreted intact in urine or bile. On occasion biliary conjugates may be hydrolyzed in the gastrointestinal tract and reabsorbed into the circulation. The degradative mechanisms have a common feature, namely, that alternate pathways exist for the catabolism of all hormones described to date.

Because of the nature of the feedback mechanisms involved in the regulation of hormone secretion, changes in rates of hormone degradation alone do not cause endocrine pathology, provided the feedback loops that regulate synthesis are intact. For example, in severe liver disease and in myxedema, the degradation of glucocorticoids by the liver is impaired; as a consequence the turnover of the hormone slows, but the plasma level does not rise because secretion of ACTH is inhibited. Thus, a normal level of free hormone is maintained by decreasing the rate of secretion of glucocorticoid. The opposite occurs when glucocorticoid degradation is enhanced (as in thyrotoxicosis); here glucocorticoid secretion rises to keep the level of the hormone normal.

Although changes in hormone degradation alone do not result in hormone deficit or excess, such changes may cause profound changes in endocrine pharmacology. Thus, it is necessary to recognize that ordinary doses of glucocorticoids may cause a cushingoid state in patients with myxedema or liver disease, and consequently glucocorticoid dosage must be reduced in both conditions. Likewise, doses of glucocorticoids may have to be increased in the presence of hyperthyroidism in order to obtain physiological levels. In addition, the development of hyperthyroidism in a patient with inadequate adrenal reserve might precipitate an adrenal crisis by accelerating the rate of glucocorticoid catabolism. Thus, in circumstances in which the normal servomechanisms that regulate hormone synthesis are either circumvented or inoperative, changes in degradation may aggravate or cause pathology.

REGULATION OF HORMONE PRODUCTION As stated above, the fluctuation of hormone levels in the normal person is deter-

FIGURE 331-1

Feedback control of an endocrine organ such as the adrenal, thyroid, or gonads by the pituitary.

mined primarily by changes in production. A unifying feature of all endocrine systems is the fact that the production of each hormone is regulated directly or indirectly by the metabolic activity of the hormone itself. This regulation is accomplished through a series of negative feedback loops (Fig. 331-1). In many cases a fairly constant blood level of hormone is required, and some sensing device must exist to monitor either the hormone level itself or some related function such as plasma osmolality, blood glucose, or body sodium content. This concept is perhaps best illustrated by pituitary control mechanisms. Hormones produced in response to pituitary trophic hormones (cortisol, thyroxine, gonadal steroids) feed back in the hypothalamic-pituitary system to regulate the secretion of additional hormone. Similarly, parathyroid hormone and insulin are secreted in response to feedback signals from serum calcium and glucose levels, respectively. Feedback systems are generally more complex than this description indicates, sometimes operating indirectly by several steps; in those instances in which the hormone itself acts as the mediator of feedback (testosterone on the pituitary), the effect is mediated by the same cellular machinery that regulates the action of the hormone in other target tissues.

FIGURE 331-2

Relation between target hormone level and trophic hormone level in normal and disease states (e.g., TSH and thyroid hormones, ACTH and cortisol, LH and testosterone).

Both negative and positive feedback can occur; an example of positive feedback is the stimulation of LH release by estradiol prior to ovulation. Nonhormonal and environmental factors may alter both positive and negative feedback control mechanisms or the response to such control.

A common feature of the feedback systems is rapidity of action; indeed, most respond within minutes or hours to varying metabolic demands to maintain homeostatic control near normal. The main exceptions relate to gametogenesis in the ovary and testis (see Chaps. 341 and 342). In both instances, a complex differentiative process is involved. The cycle of spermatogenesis requires approximately a month to complete, and so changes in FSH levels may not be expressed in altered rates of production of spermatozoa for long periods. Of course, the operation in the steady state of these systems is such that production of spermatozoa tends to be relatively constant from day to day whereas ovulation is cyclic.

The fact that the secretion of all hormones is under regulatory control has several important clinical implications. First, the significance of plasma levels of hormones may be clear only if the regulatory factors are taken into account (Fig. 331-2). The significance of a borderline low testosterone value may become obvious only when LH is measured simultaneously; likewise, a given plasma insulin level may be interpretable only in conjunction with a simultaneous plasma glucose determination. Second, the finding of simultaneous elevations of hormone pairs (or hormone-regulatory pairs) in the absence of signs of hormone excess suggests the presence of a hormone resistance state. For example, simultaneous elevation of plasma glucose and insulin is indicative of insulin resistance, and simultaneous elevation of LH and testosterone suggests androgen resistance. Third, insight into the regulatory control of hormone secretion is the basis for the various dynamic tests of hormone reserve and hormone secretion.

All endocrine disease results from defects in hormone formation, from abnormalities in the mechanisms by which production and release are regulated, or from changes in responsiveness to hormone action.

MECHANISMS OF HORMONE ACTION The first step in hormone action is thought to involve the interaction of the hormone with specific macromolecules in the cell termed *hormone receptors*. Two general classes of hormone receptors are now recognized, those on the plasma membrane of the cell surface and those that are intracellular.

Hormones with cell surface receptors Hormones of the first class bind to surface receptors localized on the plasma membrane (Fig. 331-3). The specificity of hormone action depends largely on the specificity of binding of the hormone to a given cell surface. The subsequent actions of such hormones are believed to be mediated largely (if not entirely) by so-called "second messengers," produced in the cell membranes. Such a mechanism applies to some protein hormones and to the biogenic amines. In most instances the second messenger is cyclic adenosine 3′,5′-monophosphate (AMP). Calcium and other nucleotides such as cyclic guanosine 3′,5′-monophosphate (GMP) may function as second messengers for other hormones. The cellular concentration of cyclic AMP is controlled by two enzymes with opposite activities. Adenylate cyclase (Ac), localized in the plasma membrane, converts adenosine triphosphate (ATP) into cyclic AMP. Phosphodiesterase, found largely in the cell cytosol, inactivates cyclic AMP by converting it to 5′-adenosine monophosphate (5′-AMP). Hormones (H) that act at the cell surface form a reversible com-

FIGURE 331-3

Schema of action of hormones with cell surface receptors. H, hormone; R, receptor; C, catalytic subunit, and R*, cAMP-binding subunit of protein kinase; cAMP, cyclic AMP; Ac, adenylate cyclase.

plex with specialized membrane protein receptors (R). These proteins bind the hormone with high affinity but limited capacity. The formation of the hormone-receptor complex is coupled to stimulation of adenylate cyclase. The biochemical mechanisms that underlie this transduction are poorly understood, but guanosine triphosphate (GTP) may play an important role in the process. The means by which cyclic AMP mediates the spectrum of hormone effects remains elusive. Phosphorylating enzymes—known as *protein kinases*—appear to play an important role in the overall process; these kinases are composed of catalytic and regulatory subunits. Binding of cyclic AMP to the regulatory subunit frees the catalytic subunit and allows phosphorylation of various enzymes with consequent activation or inactivation. In those instances in which calcium is thought to serve as the second messenger, the mechanism by which it acts to mediate hormonal effects is also unclear. Other hormones such as insulin clearly bind to receptors on the cell membrane, but the mechanism by which this binding is translated into physiological effects is unknown.

Hormones with intracellular receptors Steroid and thyroid hormones are transported in plasma bound to carrier proteins. The protein-bound hormones are in dynamic equilibrium with small amounts of free hormones that diffuse by a passive mechanism into cells where they act by fundamentally differ-

FIGURE 331-4

Mechanism of action of hormones with intracellular receptors. H, hormone; H', activated hormone; R, receptor; R', activated receptor; mRNA, messenger RNA.

TARGET CELL

ent mechanisms (Fig. 331-4) than do the peptide hormones. Inside the cells some of these hormones (thyroxine, testosterone) undergo chemical conversion to more active forms (H') such as triiodothyronine and dihydrotestosterone. In other instances the principal form of the hormone secreted into plasma (cortisol, progesterone, aldosterone, estradiol) undergoes no further metabolism within the cell, and the form that circulates in plasma is the molecule that is ultimately responsible for hormone action within the target cell.

H or H' then binds to specific receptor proteins (R) in the cytoplasm of the cell to form a hormone-receptor complex (HR or H'R). In the case of certain steroid hormones the hormone-receptor complex undergoes "activation" by a poorly understood temperature-dependent enzymatic process to form an activated complex (HR' or H'R'). The activated hormone-receptor complex is then translocated from cytoplasm into the nucleus where it binds to chromatin. As the result of this binding a series of postreceptor effector mechanisms are activated that involve as a minimum the formation of new messenger RNAs (mRNAs) and the subsequent synthesis of cytoplasmic proteins. An alternative mechanism may exist for the action of triiodothyronine in which binding of the hormone to cytoplasmic protein may be negligible; instead the unbound hormone enters the nucleus where the active hormone-receptor complex is formed.

ASSESSMENT OF HORMONE FUNCTION In routine practice endocrine status is assessed by measuring (1) plasma levels of a hormone, (2) the excretion of a hormone or of some metabolite in urine, (3) the rates of secretion of hormones into the circulation, (4) hormone reserve and regulation through dynamic tests, (5) hormone receptors, (6) selected effects of hormone action in target tissues, or (7) appropriate combinations of these values. Each of these techniques is useful in certain clinical situations.

Plasma levels The plasma levels of steroid and thyroid hormones range between 1 nM and 1 μM, while those of peptide hormones are generally in the range of 1 pM to 0.1 nM. The application of modern chemical, radioreceptor, and radioimmunoassay techniques for the assessment of plasma constituents in these concentrations is one of the significant advances of modern medicine and has transformed endocrinology from a largely descriptive discipline to a more quantitative one. In the case of hormones whose plasma levels are relatively constant from moment to moment and day to day (thyroxine and triiodothyronine), the measurement of isolated plasma levels alone may provide a reliable assessment of the hormone status in the vast majority of clinical situations.

For a variety of reasons, however, extreme care must be exercised in assessing isolated plasma levels. First, in the case of hormones that undergo pulsatile secretion (LH, testosterone), a single value may or may not be representative of mean values. In these instances it is necessary either to measure levels in several samples drawn at random or to pool aliquots of three or more samples of plasma drawn at 20- to 30-min intervals for a single determination.

Second, when plasma levels exhibit a characteristic, predictable fluctuation such as the diurnal variation of plasma cortisol, the timing of plasma sampling can be designed to provide a useful index of the hormone status. Even here, however, it is important to recognize that plasma levels may exhibit diurnal variation only during certain phases of life (LH in early puberty). In women during the reproductive years appropriate interpretation of plasma gonadotropins, progesterone, and estradiol requires reference to the known events of the ovulatory and menstrual cycles, and in most instances it is necessary to obtain sequential studies over several days to provide interpretable data. Although statistically significant seasonal variations in certain hormone levels (such as thyroxine and testosterone) can be demonstrated in populations, these changes are generally of such a small magnitude as to have no significance in the assessment of individual values. The same is usually true for the decline of plasma hormone levels in extreme old age.

Third, in the case of the steroid and thyroid hormones, which are transported in plasma largely bound to proteins, it is essential to remember that measurement of total hormone concentration provides an index of endocrine states *only* to the extent that it allows a deduction of the level of the free or unbound hormone. Indeed, direct measurements of the unbound levels of these hormones (usually 1 percent or less of the total) can be done only in research laboratories. Since the amount of free hormone is a function of the amount of transport protein and the amount of hormone, the total hormone level reflects the amount of free hormone only as long as the amount of binding protein(s) remains constant or fluctuates within narrow limits. In those instances in which the level of binding protein is increased [thyroxine-binding globulin (TBG) and testosterone-binding globulin (TeBG) in pregnancy] or decreased (hereditary decreases in TBG), it is essential to utilize some other assessment of the amount of binding protein to allow deduction of the free hormone level (T_3 resin uptake for TBG or direct measurement of TBG or TeBG).

Fourth, the range of plasma levels of most hormones within the normal population is fairly broad. As a consequence, it is possible for the level in an individual to double or fall in half (and thus be grossly abnormal for that person) but still be within the so-called "normal" range. For this reason it is sometimes useful to assess appropriate hormone pairs simultaneously (LH and testosterone, thyroxine and TSH). For example, a borderline low testosterone level in the presence of elevated concentrations of LH is indicative of testicular failure, whereas the same level of testosterone in the presence of a normal LH implies that the endocrine status is normal (Fig. 331-2). Likewise in women with increased testosterone production and secondary decrease in TeBG, a normal plasma testosterone concentration may be found despite the increased production of the hormone.

Urinary excretion The measurement of urinary excretion of a hormone itself or of some hormone metabolite that reflects either plasma levels or secretory rates offers certain advantages over the measurement of plasma levels. Of particular importance is the fact that the urinary excretion reflects average plasma levels and, hence, average production rates over the time of collection. Thus, a 24-h urine 17-hydroxycorticoid value may provide a better estimate of the function of the adrenal cortex than isolated measurements of plasma cortisol. Again, however, certain limitations of the use of urinary measurements, described below, must be kept in mind.

1 Creatinine determinations should be done routinely to document the adequacy of the urine collection. Women excrete on average about 1 g, while men excrete about 1.8 g per day. Day-to-day variation should not exceed 20 percent.

2 The excretion of individual metabolites may not reflect changes in hormone secretion under all conditions. For example, the formation of the 18-oxo derivative of aldosterone may be influenced by drugs that do not influence secretion or plasma levels of the hormone.

3 Urine values are obviously meaningless for those hormones (thyroxine, triiodothyronine) excreted into bile. Of more importance is the fact that peptide hormones such as gonadotropins can be variably metabolized among individuals so that establishment of normal values is difficult.

4 Hormones from more than one source may be excreted as common metabolites; urinary 17-ketosteroids are derived from both adrenal and gonadal androgens, and consequently their measurement is of little vaue in assessing testicular androgen production in men.

5 Changes in renal function may influence rates of hormone excretion into urine. Such changes can be in part corrected by measurement of urine creatinine, but in the case of metabolites or conjugates formed in the kidney itself excretion patterns may be seriously distorted by renal failure.

Secretory and production rates The measurement of the actual secretory rate of a hormone circumvents virtually all the problems inherent in measurement of plasma levels and urinary excretion. Such calculations involve the administration of radioactive hormone and measurement of the dilution that such a hormone undergoes as a consequence of mixture with endogenously secreted nonradioactive hormones. In practice a unique metabolite of the hormone from urine or the plasma hormone itself is isolated, purified to radiochemical homogeneity, and used to calculate the amount of the hormone secreted during a specific interval. Likewise, in the case of hormones formed principally in peripheral tissues (estradiol and dihydrotestosterone in men, triiodothyronine in both sexes), radioactive precursors can be administered, and the rates of conversion to the metabolites in question measured appropriately for assessment of overall rates. Alternatively, as described above, clearance rates of hormones can be measured and, together with mean plasma levels, used to estimate production rates. Unfortunately, these techniques are difficult to perform, require administration of radioactive isotopes, and can be done only in certain referral hospitals.

Dynamic tests of hormone reserve and regulation When hypo- or hyperfunction is severe, measurement of the level of hormone in blood or urine may be satisfactory for making a diagnosis, particularly when the tests demonstrate normal feedback relationships; e.g., low plasma testosterone coupled with high plasma LH indicates primary testicular failure. In less clear-cut instances however, it is useful to utilize stimulation tests to clarify the meaning of borderline low tests. Likewise suppression tests are used to document the presence of hyperfunction. All such tests are designed to take advantage of the known feedback control mechanisms for various hormones (Fig. 331-1).

Two types of stimulation tests are in common usage. In one, endogenous hormone production or action is blocked (cortisol production by metyrapone; estradiol action by clomiphene), and the capacity of the pituitary to respond by increasing endogenous production of the trophic hormone and/or the capacity of the target tissue to respond is then assessed; ideally, such tests assess the integrity of an entire hypothalmic-pituitary target tissue system. In the other type of stimulation test, the trophic hormone itself is administered under some standardized regimen, and the capacity of the target tissue to respond is assessed (cortisol levels before and after ACTH administration). Stimulation tests are particularly useful in four situations: (1) in assessment of hormone status when precise quantitation is difficult or imperfect (ACTH), (2) in assessment of endocrine states when static tests are borderline low, (3) to distinguish primary from secondary (pituitary) causes of endocrine failure, and (4) to assess gonadal reserve in prepubertal patients in whom plasma gonadotropins are difficult to interpret.

Suppression tests are useful for the diagnosis of hyperfunction because the hyperfunctioning gland, by definition, does not operate under normal control mechanisms. Suppression can be either quantitatively or qualitatively abnormal. For example, the feedback control of the pituitary may be reset to respond to high levels of the suppressing hormone (pituitary ACTH secretion in Cushing's disease), or secretion can be autonomous and without any control (ACTH secretion by an oat-cell carcinoma of the lung). In principle, the feedback regulator is administered, and the capacity of the hormone to be inhibited is assessed for the endocrine system in question (change in ^{131}I uptake after administration of thyroid hormones; change in cortisol secretion after the administration of potent exogenous glucocorticoids; suppressibility of plasma growth hormone by glucose or stimulation by insulin-induced hypoglycemia).

These dynamic tests continue to be of critical importance in certain clinical states; however, in circumstances in which hormone pairs can be measured accurately (TSH and thyroxine or triiodothyronine; testosterone and LH), they are required only occasionally.

Hormone receptors and antibodies The measurement of hormone receptors in biopsy material from target tissues or in fibroblasts propagated from biopsy material is increasingly useful—particularly in the diagnosis of partial hormone resistance states such as hypothyroidism due to thyroid hormone resistance, hyperglycemia and hyperinsulinemia associated with insulin resistance, and male pseudohermaphroditism due to androgen resistance. Likewise, under selected conditions measurement of antibodies to hormones (such as antibodies to thyroid hormones that can cause hypothyroidism) or antibodies to target tissues (adrenal gland, gonads, thyroid) may be essential for the assessment of endocrine status. With certain exceptions (antibodies to thyroid tissue) quantitative assessment of receptors and antibodies can be made only in research laboratories.

Tissue effects The ideal hormone test perhaps is the measurement of the peripheral end result of hormone action in the target tissues for the hormone. For example, demonstration of the capacity to concentrate urine maximally with water restriction indicates that the hypothalamic control mechanisms are intact, that the posterior pituitary has a normal capacity to secrete vasopressin, that the vasopressin receptor is intact, and that the postreceptor effector mechanisms for the hormone are operative. Thus, optimally, such a test assesses the function of the entire arc of hormone secretion and action. In practice, many such tests are imperfect. For example, intrinsic renal disease can result in a fixed low urine osmolality even though vasopressin secretion is normal and can thus distort the interpretation of the functional test of vasopressin action. In other instances the tests are difficult to perform and subject both to artifact and to influences from parameters not being tested (for example, the metabolic rate is increased by fever even when thyroid function is normal). For these reasons, the identification of additional specific tissue markers for hormone action would be very useful.

CLINICAL SYNDROMES At the clinical level, endocrinopathy can result from hormone deficiency, hormone excess, or resistance to hormone action. In addition, it is increasingly clear that abnormalities in more than one endocrine system can coexist in an individual.

Deficiency states With few exceptions (calcitonin, melatonin) hormone deficiency results in pathological manifestations. The elucidation of clinical disorders that result from hormone deficiency or absence played an important role in the evolution of endocrinology as a discipline. Such studies were followed by attempts to extract the responsible hormone from normal endocrine tissues, characterize its chemical nature (and ultimately synthesize it), and administer the hormone to replace the deficit. Thus, the routine treatment of hypothyroidism by the administration of thyroid hormone is probably as successful as any therapeutic measure in medicine. Because clinical deficiency states can be induced in experimental animals by appropriate destruction or removal of the endocrine organ, an enormous amount is known about the pathophysiology of the deficiency state itself (diabetes mellitus, pituitary and adrenal insufficiency, hypothyroidism, and hypogonadism.)

Furthermore, the pathogenesis of the destructive processes involved in the failure of the endocrine organs is understood in many instances; these include infections (adrenal insufficiency due to tuberculosis), infarction (postpartum pituitary failure) and tissue death of other causes (diabetes secondary to pancreatitis), tumors (chromophobe adenomas of the pituitary), autoimmune processes (Hashimoto's thyroiditis), dietary inadequacy (hypothyroidism due to iodine deficiency), and hereditary defects (pituitary dwarfism). However, a large number of endocrine deficiency diseases exist in which the etiology of the underlying defect is unidentified (ordinary myxedema, congenital anorchia, diabetes mellitus).

Hormone excess With few exceptions (testosterone in men, progesterone in men and women) hormone excess causes pathological effects. Four general types of hormone excess are recognized. In one, the hormone is overproduced by the gland that is the usual site of its production (thyrotoxicosis, acromegaly, Cushing's disease); such excess production in every instance results from failure or circumvention of the feedback control mechanisms that regulate production of the hormone in the normal state, but the underlying mechanism is often obscure because animal models for the diseases are rare. The second type results when a hormone is produced by a tissue (usually malignant) that ordinarily is not an endocrine organ (for example, ACTH production in oat-cell carcinoma of the lung) (see Chap. 347). Such hormone excess states have been described for many hormones, usually peptide hormones. A third type involves the overproduction of hormones in peripheral tissues from circulating prohormones; for example, overproduction of estrogen in liver disease can result from diversion of the precursor androstenedione from its usual sites of catabolism in the liver to sites of peripheral metabolism. Finally, hormone excess all too commonly results from iatrogenic causes; indeed, the complications resulting from the overadministration of glucocorticoids constitute a major clinical problem (see Chap. 336).

Hormone resistance The concept that an endocrinopathy could result because the tissues cannot respond to normal or increased levels of a hormone evolved from the deduction by Fuller Albright and his colleagues that pseudohypoparathyroidism is due to peripheral resistance to the action of parathyroid hormone. This concept has had far-reaching implications for endocrinology. First, as more and more forms of hormone resistance have been identified, syndromes have been described in which disease results from resistance to many hormones. Second, the concept of hormone resistance has served as a major stimulus for the study of the way hormones act within cells. Third, hormone resistance is now known to result from a variety of mechanisms, including defects in receptors and in postreceptor effector mechanisms for cells, the formation of incomplete or abnormal forms of hormones, the development of antibodies to hormones or hormone receptors, and the absence of target cells. Fourth, abnormalities of receptors are now implicated in the pathogenesis of diseases outside the endocrine domain, such as myasthenia gravis and familial hypercholesterolemia.

The universal feature of all forms of hormone resistance is the presence of a normal or *elevated* level of the hormone in the circulation in a patient with evidence of deficient hormone action. This feature is an inevitable consequence of the fact that every hormone is under regulatory feedback control and that failure of hormone action usually leads to increased hormone production. Hormone resistance is frequently due to hereditary causes.

Diseases affecting multiple endocrine systems The fact that disorders can affect more than one endocrine system has been known since the description of panhypopituitarism in the nineteenth century. However, in the past decade it has become clear that the disorders affecting more than one endocrine system are more common than previously thought and that they encompass diverse etiologies including autoimmunity (Schmidt's syndrome), receptor abnormalities (gonadotropin and thyrotropin resistance in pseudohypoparathyroidism), tumors [multiple endocrine neoplasia (MEN)], and hereditary disorders of unknown etiology (lipodystrophies). They may include both hypo- and hyperfunctioning states, and some clinical syndromes such as pheochromocytoma may occur in the context of more than one polyendocrine state (MEN II and MEN III).

Because each endocrinopathy that occurs as the part of such a constellation can also occur alone, it is essential that all endocrine patients be approached with a high index of suspicion for abnormalities of multiple systems. This is of particular importance because treatment of one condition may cause worsening of another (such as operations in patients with unrecognized pheochromocytoma) and because in certain of the familial syndromes it is necessary to make systematic searches for the disease in potentially affected family members.

REFERENCES

BAXTER JD, MacLEOD KM: Molecular basis for hormone action, in *Metabolic Control and Disease,* 8th ed, PK Bondy, LE Rosenberg (eds). Philadelphia, Saunders, 1979

RASMUSSEN H: Organization and control of endocrine systems, in *Textbook of Endocrinology*, RH Williams (ed). Philadelphia, Saunders, 1974, pp 1-30

VERHOEVEN GFM, WILSON JD: The syndromes of primary hormone resistance. Metabolism 28:253, 1979

332
ENDORPHINS (OPIOID PEPTIDES)

ROGER H. UNGER
ELI IPP

INTRODUCTION The discovery of the first of the physiological opioid peptides in 1974 marked the beginning of a period of potentially far-reaching research with major implications for the fields of physiology, internal medicine, and psychiatry. This chapter is designed to provide a general background in this rapidly evolving area of investigation.

BACKGROUND Morphine has been in clinical use for almost 200 years, but the mechanism of its action has only recently been clarified. In 1973, using radioactive opiates to detect binding to macromolecules, several groups established that these alkaloids exert their effects within the central nervous

system by binding to specific receptors. Such receptors are present in high concentrations in those regions of the brain where opiates are known to have biological effects, including the regions of pain perception. This discovery suggested that this previously undiscovered receptor system probably functions under physiological conditions to mediate the action of an endogenous substance (or substances) resembling opiate drugs.

Soon after the discovery of the opiate receptors, reports of endogenous opioid activity in brain and pituitary extracts began to appear. Two pentapeptides with opioid activity were extracted from the brain, isolated, and characterized. These peptides were termed *enkephalins*. The amino acid sequence of one of these peptides (Met-enkephalin) was identical to amino acid residues 61 to 65 of the β-lipotropin molecule, a 91-amino acid pituitary polypeptide characterized some 10 years earlier. (β-Lipotropin was later shown to be devoid of opioid activity and to have no known function.) This observation stimulated interest in other fragments of β-lipotropin in the hope that peptides with opioid activity would be found. Subsequently several C-terminal portions of the β-lipotropin molecule were observed to have such activity. These polypeptides were collectively termed *endorphins*, an abbreviation for *endogenous morphine*. Common to all of them was the Met-enkephalin sequence, namely, residues 61 to 65 of β-lipotropin.

NOMENCLATURE The word *endorphin* has been used synonymously with the term *opioid peptides* and originally simply indicated any polypeptide with biological activities similar to those of the opiate drugs. The term *enkephalin* is applied to the two pentapeptides, Met-enkephalin and Leu-enkephalin. Increasingly, however, the use of *endorphin* is being limited to the opioid peptides larger in molecular size than the enkephalins. Thus far four endorphins, α, β, γ, and δ, have been reported.

STRUCTURE AND BIOSYNTHESIS The amino acid sequence of the β-lipotropin molecule is shown in Fig. 332-1. The amino acid sequence of all peptides with opioid biological activity is identical to one or more sections of the terminal region.

The biologically active peptides thus far identified include β-endorphin, which comprises the amino acid residues 61 to 91 of the β-lipotropin molecule, α-endorphin, consisting of residues 61 to 76 of β-lipotropin, γ-endorphin, made up of β-lipotropin residues 61 to 77, and δ-endorphin, which includes residues 61 to 87 of β-lipotropin. The smallest molecules with opioid bioactivity are the enkephalins. Leu-enkephalin has a leucine residue substituted for the methionine residue of met-enkephalin but is otherwise identical. It appears that the pentapeptide is the minimum sequence necessary for opioid activity, and that lengthening the chain alters potency and varies biological effects (Table 332-1). The Met-enkephalin pentapeptide sequence, common to all the opioid peptides, has certain conformational similarities to the opiate alkaloids, which may account for the fact that two such different substances can bind to the same receptors.

Since all the opioid peptides thus far discovered share a common sequence with β-lipotropin, it is logical to consider the larger molecule as their possible precursor. Indeed, it has been shown that brain tissue can generate opioid activity from β-lipotropin in vitro, and pulse-chase studies in mouse pituitary tumor cells have demonstrated that β-lipotropin is an obligatory precursor of β-endorphin but not the enkephalins. Although the Met-enkephalin sequence might be derived from β-lipotropin, Leu-enkephalin could not be, since no β-lipotro-

FIGURE 332-1

The relationship of the 91-amino acid β-lipotropin molecule to the known opioid peptides with amino acid sequences identical to segments of β-lipotropin.

pin with a leucine in position 65 has yet been isolated. Furthermore, enkephalin and β-endorphin are present in different neurons in the brain, implying separate sites of synthesis for the small and large opioid peptides. β-Lipotropin isolated from brain tissue tends to be found in the same sites as β-endorphin but not enkephalin.

It is of interest to note that the biosynthesis of other hormones may be linked to the formation of the opioid peptides. The β-lipotropin molecule isolated from normal pituitary or pituitary tumors has recently been shown to be a part of a larger molecule of about 31,000 molecular weight, which also contains the full sequence of adrenocorticotropic hormone (ACTH). This finding, suggesting a common biosynthetic precursor for ACTH and β-lipotropin, is compatible with the previously demonstrated fact that these two polypeptides are found within the same secretory granules of the same cells of the pituitary. This may also explain the simultaneous release of β-endorphin and ACTH in equimolar concentrations from the pituitary gland under various conditions.

DISTRIBUTION OF THE ENDOGENOUS PEPTIDES β-Endorphin has been isolated from extracts of the porcine hypothalamus and pituitary glands and has been localized in the brain in discrete nerve fibers, consisting of single hypothalamic cells with long ascending and descending processes. Since β-endorphin is present in the brain weeks after hypophysectomy, it is likely synthesized within the brain as well as in the pituitary. However, the concentration in brain appears to be lower than in the pituitary.

The distribution of the enkephalins is more diffuse. High concentrations are present in the dorsal columns of the spinal cord, the amygdala, and the medial hypothalamus. The ratio of Met- to Leu-enkephalin content of the brain varies in different species. Immunohistologic studies reveal systems of enkephalin-containing nerve terminals, a finding consistent with a neurotransmitter role.

Enkephalins are also present in the gastrointestinal tract. The content of enkephalin in the myenteric plexus of the longitudinal muscles of the gut is higher than in the brain. Enkephalin-containing cells and nerve fibers have also been identified in the adrenal medulla, and β-endorphin has been found in the human placenta.

MECHANISM OF ACTION **The opiate receptors** The first step in the chain of molecular events that culminates in a biologic effect of a hormone is its binding to a specific site on its target cells, the receptor. Receptors on target cells can be detected by incubating the cells (or their plasma membranes) with a radioactive hormone or analog of the hormone. Receptors for peptide hormones are proteins of large molecular weight situated in the plasma membrane of their target cells. They possess properties that permit recognition of the particular peptide and the formation of a hormone-receptor complex capable of initiating a biologic response, often by activation of an enzyme that generates an intracellular signal or "second messenger" such as cyclic adenosine monophosphate (AMP) (see Chap. 331). The opiate receptors appear to act in similar fashion.

Naloxone The morphine antagonist naloxone is a congener of the opiate family that has no known opiate-like actions of its own. It binds to the opiate receptor, competing with and displacing morphine and other opiates. This action has been used to prove the specificity of binding by the opiates and opioid peptides. By using this drug to inhibit opiate actions, one can determine whether a particular biological phenomenon may be mediated by an endogenous opioid peptide. For example, the fact that naloxone blocks the analgesic effects of electrical stimulation of the periaqueductal gray area provides strong evidence that endogenous opioid peptides mediate analgesia in this crucial area of the brain.

Response at the molecular level The effects of the opiates and opioids on the formation of cyclic nucleotides have been studied in vitro using cultured tumor cells of neural origin. Both basal and stimulated cyclic AMP formation are decreased, and cyclic guanosine monophosphate (GMP) formation is increased by acute treatment with opiates and opioids. These effects on cyclic nucleotides are directly related to binding to the opiate receptor and can be blocked by naloxone.

TABLE 332-1
Pharmacological effects of endogenous opioid peptides*

	Analgesia	Body temperature	Effect	Endocrine systems	GI†
α-Endorphin	Face and neck	↓	Tranquilization	↓ Prolactin	↓
γ-Endorphin	0	↑	Agitation	↓ Prolactin	↓
β-Endorphin	Whole body	↓	Catatonia	↑ GH, prolactin	↓
				↑ Vasopressin ↑ Insulin, glucagon ↓ Somatostatin	
Met-enkephalin	+	↑	Sedation	↑ GH, prolactin ↓ ↓ TSH, LH	↓
Leu-enkephalin	?	↓	Agitation	?	↓

* *This table is intended to illustrate the heterogeneity of the opioid actions thus far reported.*
† *Inhibitory effect on smooth muscle of gastrointestinal (GI) tract.*

Chronic exposure of cells to morphine sulfate or to enkephalin increases the concentration of cyclic AMP levels in vitro. Withdrawal of the opioid or opiate results in a further increase in cyclic AMP in these cells. These changes may somehow be implicated in certain aspects of drug abuse, such as addiction, tolerance, and the withdrawal syndrome.

Anatomic location of opioid receptors Opioid receptors are most abundant in those areas of the central nervous system in which opiates exert a biological effect and generally correspond with those regions in which the enkephalins are present in high concentrations. In addition to the periaqueductal gray area high concentrations of receptors have been found in the following locations:

1 *The medial hypothalamus,* which mediates emotionally influenced deep pain, the pain most responsive to opiates. (The lateral hypothalamus mediates somatotrophic pain, is minimally affected by morphine, and has few opiate receptors.)
2 *The substantia gelatinosa in the spinal cord,* which integrates sensory information.
3 *The solitary nuclei receiving visceral sensory fibers from the vagus and glossopharyngeal nerve;* these are involved in cough reflexes, postural changes in blood pressure, and gastric secretion, all functions that are influenced by opiates.
4 *The amygdala,* the area with the highest density of opiate receptors; this region is thought to be involved in various forms of emotional behavior.
5 *The area postrema,* in which opioids produce nausea and vomiting.
6 *The gastrointestinal tract,* an organ well known to respond to opiate alkaloids.

POSSIBLE PHYSIOLOGICAL AND PATHOPHYSIOLOGICAL ROLES Most of the work on opioid peptides has been carried out in experimental animals. Extrapolation of certain of the results to humans may, therefore, be invalid because of species differences. Nevertheless, as indicated above, the enkephalins are present in high concentrations in those regions of the central nervous system concerned with deep pain, emotional behavior, nausea and vomiting, cough reflexes, respiration, blood pressure, thermoregulation, and gastrointestinal function. It is reasonable to postulate that the endogenous opioids in some of or all these areas function as neurotransmitters or neuromodulators and subserve physiological roles.

Actions on the brain: Role in nonpharmacological analgesia (acupuncture, hypnosis, electric shock) Each of the endorphins varies somewhat with respect to its biological actions when injected into the brain of rats. The observed effects include analgesia, hypothermia, hyperthermia, tranquilization, irritability, agitation, and, in very high doses, violent behavior, catalepsy, narcolepsy, and catatonia (Table 332-1). These effects disappear without sequelae and can be blocked within 5 s by naloxone. The role of the opioids in influencing pain is uncertain because of conflicting results in tests of the influence of naloxone on various forms of pain. The morphine antagonist appears to intensify certain forms of pain in humans, for example, that produced by dental extraction. Some workers have failed to observe an antagonistic effect upon analgesia produced by electric shock and hypnosis. However, more recent studies in patients with persistent pain reveal that analgesia produced by electrical stimulation of periventricular brain sites is accompanied by a rise in ventricular enkephalin-like and β-endorphin-like activity and that this analgesia is blocked by naloxone, suggesting mediation by endogenous opioid peptides. It has also been proposed that the opioid peptides may be involved in the analgesic effects of acupuncture; acupunc-

ture analgesia in mice is blocked by naloxone and abolished by hypophysectomy. The opioid peptides may also mediate the well-known phenomenon of placebo-induced analgesia. In those subjects who benefit from placebos, tolerance and dependence on the placebos may occur, and the analgesic effects have been blocked by the use of naloxone.

Role in thermogenesis The opioid peptides are believed to be physiological determinants of the adaptive responses to heat. For example, after acute and chronic exposure of rats to high temperatures, the administration of naloxone causes a rapid increase in colonic temperature.

Effects on the endocrine system Since morphine stimulates the secretion of growth hormone, prolactin, and antidiuretic hormone and inhibits luteinizing hormone (LH) and ovulation, it is not surprising that the opioid peptides have a similar effect. This effect is not mediated by direct action on the pituitary gland but involves a centrally mediated mechanism. The possibility of a physiological role for the opioid peptides in the control of the releasing factors for certain pituitary hormones must be entertained. (In vitro evidence indicates that enkephalins are capable of inhibiting dopamine-induced LHRH release from the hypothalamus.)

Role in stress Opioid peptides of the anterior pituitary may also have a role in stressful illness. β-Endorphin is secreted concomitantly with ACTH during acute stress and after adrenalectomy, and, like ACTH, β-endorphin release is stimulated by purified corticotropin-releasing factor and inhibited by glucocorticoids. However, the target organs of circulating β-endorphin remain to be identified.

Role in feeding β-Endorphin injected intravenously in rats increases feeding. The pituitaries of congenitally obese mice also contain higher concentrations of β-endorphin than lean littermates. Finally, the observation that naloxone abolished overeating in these mice suggests that this opioid peptide may play a role in the physiological control of appetite and may conceivably be a factor in the development of overeating and obesity.

Actions in digestive organs The presence of enkephalins in the gastrointestinal tract implies a role in gastrointestinal function. In view of the actions of opiates on the gastrointestinal tract it seems likely that the enkephalins serve an opioid function (an endogenous paregoric-like role). Indeed, the enkephalins diminish gastrointestinal propulsion, perhaps by inhibiting the firing of neurons in the myenteric plexus. Enkephalin analogs also stimulate gastric acid secretion and mucosal blood flow.

Enkephalins appear to have a role in the function of the endocrine and exocrine pancreas. Recent studies indicate that insulin and glucagon secretion are stimulated and that somatostatin secretion is inhibited by opiates and opioid peptides. These effects are blocked by the morphine antagonist naloxone. Morphine and enkephalin also inhibit the secretion of bicarbonate and enzymes by the exocrine pancreas.

POTENTIAL CLINICAL IMPLICATIONS It is impossible to predict which areas of clinical medicine will reap the fruits of these remarkable peptides. Perhaps the most likely beneficiary will be the field of psychiatry, in which pharmacological interventions may be developed to modify the transmission of enkephalinergic impulses or change anomalous patterns of endorphin secretion or action.

Psychiatric diseases The possibility that abnormalities in endogenous opioids may be present in psychiatric disorders is indirectly supported by evidence that β-endorphin levels are elevated in the cerebrospinal fluid of schizophrenic subjects. While naloxone does not appear to alter experimental pain or mood in humans, recent reports indicate that naloxone reduces auditory hallucinations in select, chronically hallucinating schizophrenics. Chronic treatment of rats with lithium, an agent employed therapeutically for the relief of mania and depression and thought to prevent the recurrence of manic depressive episodes, increases Met-enkephalin levels in the striatum of those rats in proportion to the serum lithium levels. This increase has been attributed to a reduced rate of release of Met-enkephalin from the striatum.

Drug addiction and analgesia The proposal has been made that the chronic abuse of narcotics suppresses the biosynthesis or accelerates the degradation of endogenous opioids and that the manifestations of narcotic withdrawal represent an uncovering of a secondary endogenous opioid deficiency throughout the body. Alternatively, a genetically predetermined opioid deficiency may predispose certain people to narcotic addiction. Although it was originally hoped that endogenous opioids might be free of addictive properties, it appears that the same tolerance and dependence is produced by chronic injections of β-endorphin or chronic infusion of enkephalins into the brain as is seen with morphine-like drugs.

Thus, it seems unlikely that the development of analogs of the opioid peptides will lead to the production of analgesics with nonaddictive properties. However, drugs may be developed with a different spectrum of activity compared with the presently known analgesic narcotics.

Clinical endocrinology Elevated β-endorphin levels have been reported in an ACTH-producing pituitary tumor (Nelson's syndrome) and Cushing's disease. The release of β-lipotropin and/or β-endorphin from the pituitary and its measurement by radioimmunoassay in plasma may serve as another diagnostic function test in the assessment of pituitary disease. While pathologically high levels of circulating β-endorphin can be measured in human plasma, it is not clear whether β-endorphin is present in human plasma under physiological conditions.

Oncology There is reason to suspect that plasma β-endorphin levels may be increased in certain malignant tumors that produce ACTH, such as oat-cell carcinoma of the lung. Both α- and β-endorphin have been reported in an ACTH-producing islet-cell carcinoma. β-Endorphin levels are also said to be increased in patients with medullary carcinoma of the thyroid. Conceivably, the measurement of plasma endorphins may have diagnostic value as tumor markers.

BIOLOGICAL IMPLICATIONS Physiology Many so-called "drug receptors" may represent binding sites for endogenous factors that, through a coincidence of chemistry, cross-react with a foreign substance. Indeed, it seems unlikely that nature would have endowed animals and humans with receptors to opium, a substance found only in poppies. It is predictable that certain other pharmacologically active drugs are, like morphine, coincidental ligands to receptors intended to receive other, still undiscovered, endogenous substances.

Hormone biosynthesis The idea that opioid peptides may be derived from a precursor that contains the full sequence of other peptide hormones is altering our concepts of peptide hormone biosynthesis. It seems possible that at least some of the opioid peptides are derived from a single 31,000 molecular weight precursor of β-lipotropin and that ACTH and perhaps other hormones may also be derived from this putative preprohormone. If so, it raises the possibility that other peptide hormones produced by various endocrine cells may also be derived from the same single primary gene product containing the sequence of each of these hormones and serving as their uncommitted precursor. According to this concept, the final secretory product or products of a particular cell type would be determined by the way this single large polypeptide is cleaved by the cell at appropriate sites, rather than through synthesis of distinct amino acid sequences by different cells. For example, functionally distinct cells producing such peptides as calcitonin, ACTH, opioid peptides, and perhaps other hormones might all synthesize the same primary gene product, but the final hormone released by each cell type would be determined by enzymatic machinery that would excise a particular hormone sequence from the common precursor protein. Perhaps this might explain why certain endocrine and nonendocrine neoplasms appear to produce seemingly inappropriate hormones and hormone precursors.

Relationships among brain, gut, and pancreas The discovery of the opioid peptides has extended our developing concepts of relationships among the cells of the brain, an organ whose principle function is to transmit signals from one cell to another, and endocrine cells, located outside the central nervous system but serving the same purpose. Certain of the peptide-secreting endocrine cells, particularly those in the endocrine pancreas and the gastrointestinal tract, have an ontological origin in common with the central nervous system. The fact that opioid peptides are present in the central nervous system, pituitary glands, gastrointestinal tract, and pancreas adds another polypeptide family to the growing group of substances, including insulin, ACTH, growth hormone, thyrotropin-releasing factor, cholecystokinin, substance P, neurotensin, vasoactive intestinal polypeptide (VIP), and many others, that have been identified by immunologic techniques both in and outside the central nervous system. It is difficult to understand why a substance such as thyrotropin-releasing hormone, for example, should be present in the islets of Langerhans or why a substance such as cholecystokinin should be the most abundant polypeptide hormone in the brain. Perhaps in the course of evolution the brain, the primary organ for generation of signals to coordinate cellular activities of the entire organism, was compelled by the sheer increase in complexity of evolving organisms to develop alternative pathways of signal transmission by using avenues other than axonal neurotransmission. Nonaxonal, nonsynaptic routes for transmission of signals may, therefore, have evolved, exploiting pathways not specifically designed for this purpose, i.e., the vascular and interstitial spaces, through which the number of signals that could be relayed would theorectically be unlimited. Extraneural sites of signal biosynthesis, the endocrine cells (believed to be of neuroectodermal origin), evolved in anatomically propitious regions of the body such as the pancreas and the gastrointestinal tract to serve such a function. Polypeptide signals released from these cells would still be under the influence of the central nervous system and thus would amplify its control function by nonneuronal means.

REFERENCES

GOLDSTEIN A: Opioid peptides (endorphins) in pituitary and brain. Science 193:1081, 1976

GUILLEMIN R et al: The endorphins, novel peptides of brain and hypophyseal origin, with opiate-like activity: Biochemical and biologic studies. Ann NY Acad Sci 297:131, 1977

HUGES J, KOSTERLITZ HW: Opioid peptides. Br Med Bull 33:157, 1977

KLEE WA: Endogenous opiate peptides, in *Peptides in Neurobiology*, H Garner (ed). New York, Plenum, 1977

LI CH: Lipotropin, a new active peptide from pituitary glands. Nature 201:924, 1964

SNYDER SH: Opiate receptors in the brain. N Engl J Med 296:266, 1977

333
DISEASES OF THE HYPOTHALAMUS AND ANTERIOR PITUITARY

PETER O. KOHLER

ANATOMY AND PHYSIOLOGY

The hypothalamus and pituitary form a control unit that regulates growth, lactation, the function of the thyroid, adrenals, and gonads, and the state of hydration. Disorders of the hypothalamus are frequently expressed as abnormalities of pituitary hormone secretion. Understanding the functional relationship of the hypothalamus to the pituitary requires an appreciation of the anatomic relationships. The hypothalamus is a small, specialized area at the base of the brain lying superior and posterior to the optic chiasm and superior to the pituitary gland. The inferior portion of the hypothalamus, or tuber cinereum, has a central projection called the *median eminence* which forms the base of the third ventricle of the brain.

The pituitary is located below the base of the brain and is connected to the median eminence of the hypothalamus by the pituitary stalk. The pituitary is located within a bony structure which resembles a Turkish saddle, hence the name *sella turcica*. The stalk passes through the center of a thick reflection of dura called the *diaphragma sellae*, which separates the pituitary from the brain. Embryologically, the posterior lobe of the pituitary (neurohypophysis) develops as a downward projection of neuroectoderm from the base of the brain. The larger anterior lobe (adenohypophysis) develops separately as an upwardly displaced group of cells from the primitive buccal endothelium. A third section of the pituitary, the intermediate lobe, is present in many animals but is poorly developed in humans. The normal pituitary weighs 0.5 to 1.0 g and measures approximately 6 to 13 mm in each dimension.

Functions of the anterior and posterior pituitary are regulated by the hypothalamus but by different mechanisms (Fig. 333-1). The neurohypophysis is an extension of large neurons originating in the supraoptic and paraventricular nuclei of the hypothalamus. The neurohypophyseal hormones, vasopressin [antidiuretic hormone (ADH)] and oxytocin, are produced by neurons in the supraoptic and paraventricular neurosecretory cells of the hypothalamus. These hormones are transported in vesicles into the posterior lobe of the pituitary in association with specific carrier (and possibly precursor) proteins called *neurophysins*. In response to appropriate stimuli depolarization of these large neurons occurs, and vasopressin or oxytocin is released by the neurohypophysis into systemic circulation.

In contrast to this direct form of control, the anterior pituitary hormones are synthesized within the adenohypophysis, and secretion is regulated by hypothalamic peptides and possibly other factors formed in the hypothalamus. The regulatory factors are released into the capillaries of a portal venous system that connects the hypothalamus and anterior lobe of the pituitary. The blood supply to the median eminence comes

from the superior hypophyseal arteries which arise from the internal carotid arteries. The capillary system from the hypothalamus drains into the long portal veins that traverse the pituitary stalk to supply the anterior lobe with portal venous blood. A small amount of blood may reach the anterior pituitary through the small arteries contained in a band of connective tissue on the superior portion of the anterior lobe (the trabecula) or from branches of the inferior capsular or inferior hypophyseal arteries. However, the major supply to the adenohypophysis is through the portal venous system. Blood may also travel in a retrograde fashion from the pituitary to the hypothalamus. The fact that the perfusion pressure of the anterior pituitary is that of the venous system may be one reason that the enlarged pituitary of pregnancy is susceptible to infarction during hypovolemic shock (see Sheehan's syndrome under "Infarction and Vascular Disorders" below). In contrast to the anterior lobe, the neurohypophysis has a direct arterial

FIGURE 333-1

Schematic representation of the relationship between the hypothalamus and pituitary. The neurohypophysis or posterior lobe of the pituitary is a downward projection of the hypothalamus. The posterior pituitary hormones, antidiuretic hormone (ADH, vasopressin) and oxytocin, are synthesized in neurons in the hypothalamus and are transported down the axons from these neurons into the posterior lobe. In contrast, the anterior pituitary develops embryologically from different tissue and has no direct neural connection with the hypothalamus. The control of the anterior pituitary hormones is through a combination of factors including feedback inhibition by target organ hormones such as the thyroid, adrenal, and gonadal hormones. The hypothalamus exerts control over the anterior lobe by hypothalamic factors such as thyrotropin-releasing hormone (TRH), luteinizing hormone-releasing hormone (LHRH), and prolactin-inhibiting factor (PIF). These factors are released into capillaries of the pituitary portal system, reach the anterior pituitary cells via portal blood, and regulate the secretion of the anterior pituitary hormones. The intermediate lobe of the pituitary is essentially vestigial in humans.

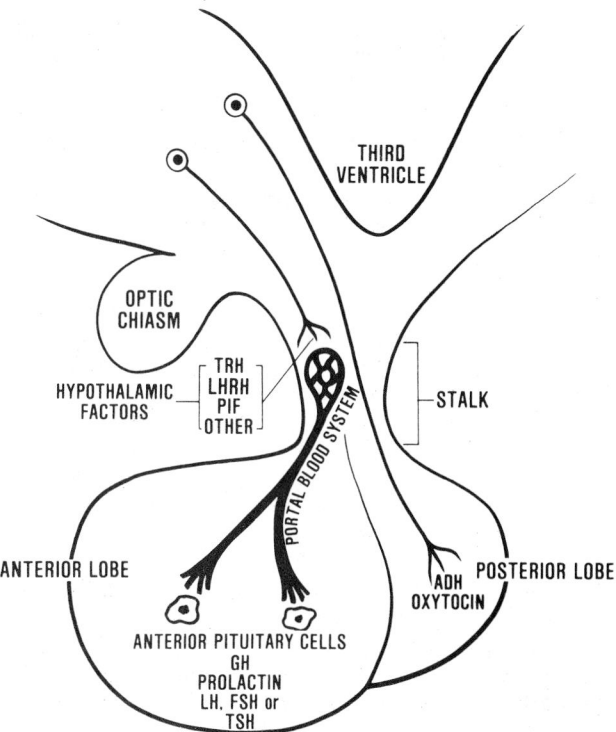

supply from the inferior hypophyseal branches of the internal carotid arteries.

Another unusual feature of the blood supply to the hypothalamus is important with regard to function. The blood-brain barrier is incomplete in the median eminence where the major plexus of the portal system originates, and the capillary loops of the plexus in this area exhibit endothelial fenestration. As a consequence large molecules such as hormones may cross the blood-brain barrier, gain access to the hypothalamus and pituitary, and provide feedback regulation of pituitary function.

The hypothalamus has multiple connections with other areas of the brain providing control from higher centers. In addition to the regulation of pituitary function, the hypothalamus has an important role in several nonendocrine homeostatic and physiological functions. These include: (1) thirst, which is regulated by osmoreceptors different from those involved with vasopressin release, (2) appetite and caloric intake, (3) sleep-wake behavior, (4) emotions such as rage and apathy, (5) autonomic balance, and (6) cognition.

Histologically, the anterior pituitary cells are arranged in cords or acinar-like structures surrounded by an extensive network of capillary sinusoids. Traditionally, the anterior pituitary cells have been divided into three types on the basis of their staining characteristics with hematoxylin and eosin, Mallory's trichrome, and periodic acid–Schiff (PAS) stains. Cells with eosin-staining granules secrete growth hormone and prolactin. Cells with basophilic granules, which also demonstrate positive PAS staining for glycoprotein, secrete thyrotropin (thyroid-stimulating hormone, TSH), luteinizing hormone (LH), and follicle-stimulating hormone (FSH) as well as corticotropin (ACTH). Chromophobic cells do not contain visible granules by light microscopy and do not exhibit affinity for the usual stains. Immunochemical techniques utilizing fluorescent-labeled antibodies specific for individual hormones and electron microscopy have provided additional insight into the function of specific cell types. For example, eosinophilic cells containing growth hormone granules can now be distinguished from cells that contain prolactin granules, and it is now clear that essentially all the glandular cells contain some type of secretory granules. Cells previously designated as chromophobes are functional but have too few granules to stain adequately by light microscopy.

PHYSIOLOGICAL REGULATION OF PITUITARY HORMONE SECRETION
The regulation of pituitary function requires integration of numerous stimuli from higher centers in the brain as well as those acting directly on the hypothalamus and pituitary. One important mechanism in this regulation is feedback control. Anterior pituitary hormone secretion is suppressed by the products of target endocrine glands such as thyroid, adrenal, and gonads. This feedback control is powerful; for example, even a slight excess of thyroid hormone blocks the release of thyrotropin by the pituitary in response to the specific releasing hormone. Some hormones such as prolactin and growth hormone may regulate their own secretion directly by acting on the hypothalamus (short-loop feedback). Essentially all anterior pituitary hormones are preferentially discharged during sleep, but the reasons that these surges are nocturnal have not been elucidated.

Neurohypophysis Oxytocin and vasopressin are stored in the posterior lobe in granules in association with hormone-specific carrier proteins, the neurophysins. After appropriate stimuli, vasopressin, oxytocin and the specific neurophysin are released into systemic circulation via the capillaries of the neurohypophysis.

VASOPRESSIN (ANTIDIURETIC HORMONE, ADH) (see also Chap. 334) The major action of ADH is to cause concentration of the urine by permitting free water reabsorption from the hypotonic tubular fluid in the distal nephron. Without ADH the distal convoluted tubule is essentially impermeable to water, although solutes are actively reabsorbed. In the presence of ADH, the tubule and collecting duct are permeable to water, which diffuses from the hypotonic tubular fluid to the hypertonic interstitium. This allows concentration of the tubular fluid and, therefore, of the urine. ADH interacts with specific membrane receptors in the renal tubule and acts through a mechanism involving induction of adenylate cyclase and generation of cyclic adenosine monophosphate (AMP).

The primary control for release of the hormone is the osmolality of blood reaching the hypothalamus. Supraoptic neurons appear to act as osmoreceptors, and their rates of discharge are increased when the osmolality of the perfusing blood is increased. This same mechanism prevails normally during dehydration, resulting in release of ADH and maximal concentration of the urine. Although blood osmolality is the major regulator of ADH release, a fall in blood pressure, as produced by hemorrhage, also causes ADH secretion, even when blood osmolality is normal or low. This pressor control mechanism is mediated by volume receptors in the carotid sinus, left atrium, and aortic arch. In addition, nicotine, various forms of stress, head trauma, and certain types of anesthesia and drugs may stimulate ADH release.

OXYTOCIN Oxytocin has a role in the induction of labor, although delivery can occur in patients with posterior pituitary deficiency. The sensitized uterus of the pregnant woman at term is stimulated to contract by oxytocin. The other major function of oxytocin is the stimulation of the myoepithelial cells of the acini of the lactating breast. Myoepithelial cell contraction forces the acinar content into the duct system so that milk accumulates in the nipples. Oxytocin release occurs after nipple stimulation. Spinal cord or brainstem lesions can abolish this neural reflex arc, and ethanol or emotional stress can inhibit the oxytocin response. Control of oxytocin secretion is separate from that of ADH. For example, release of the oxytocin-specific neurophysin is stimulated by estrogens, while ADH-specific neurophysin is released after nicotine. Also, water loading inhibits the release of ADH without affecting oxytocin-induced milk ejection.

Anterior pituitary HYPOTHALAMIC REGULATORY HORMONES When the pituitary stalk is severed, secretion of most pituitary hormones decreases substantially. An exception is prolactin secretion, which increases greatly when the hypothalamus is destroyed or the portal system is interrupted. Thus, the hypothalamus provides a stimulatory influence on the secretion of all major anterior pituitary hormones except prolactin, which is primarily under inhibitory control by the hypothalamus. In addition, crude hypothalamic extracts of the median eminence release anterior pituitary hormones when injected into laboratory animals or added to isolated pituitary tissue in vitro. To date, three hypothalamic regulatory factors have been isolated, chemically characterized, and synthesized. These are thyrotropin-releasing hormone (TRH), luteinizing hormone–releasing hormone (LHRH), and somatostatin. Presumptive evidence exists for several other hypothalamic hormones, including a growth hormone–releasing hormone, a prolactin-releasing hormone, and corticotropin-releasing hormone. Vasopressin has the capacity to release ACTH but is not believed to be a major corticotropin-releasing hormone. Dopamine inhibits prolactin release in vitro and in vivo and may either be the prolactin inhibitory factor (PIF) or cause PIF release by the hypothalamus.

THYROTROPIN-RELEASING HORMONE (TRH) When given intravenously to humans, a small quantity of TRH (pyroglutamylhistidylprolinamide) releases TSH from the pituitary with a peak seen at about 20 min. The thyrotropin response is blocked by excess circulating triiodothyronine or thyroxine as in hyperthyroidism.

TRH also stimulates prolactin release by a direct effect on the lactotrophs. Although TRH appears to be a physiological prolactin-releasing factor, another release mechanism separate from TRH must exist since several physiological stimuli for prolactin secretion do not cause a rise in TSH. These include breast feeding, stress, and the nocturnal rise in prolactin. Alternatively, prolactin release could occur as a result of a decrease in the hypothalamic PIF. Both the prolactin and TSH responses to TRH are modulated by negative feedback of thyroid hormone on the pituitary, but prolactin release is less sensitive than that of thyrotropin. Hypothyroid patients have high basal prolactin levels and an exaggerated prolactin response to TRH.

Other hormones also modulate the TRH effect. Somatostatin and high doses of glucocorticoids reduce the thyrotropin response to TRH. Estrogens increase thyrotropin and prolactin release in response to TRH through unknown mechanisms. TRH does not normally cause the release of growth hormone (GH), ACTH, LH, or FSH; however, in patients with acromegaly or renal failure TRH may stimulate GH secretion. TRH is present in many areas of the brain outside the hypothalamic-pituitary axis; its function in these areas is unknown.

LUTEINIZING HORMONE-RELEASING HORMONE (LHRH) Since the secretion rates of gonadotropins vary independently, it was expected that separate releasing factors might be found for LH and FSH. However, in 1971, a linear peptide containing 10 amino acids was isolated and shown to cause release of both LH and FSH in rats. Its composition is identical in sheep and pigs and on the basis of immunologic evidence appears to be the same in humans. Since the effect on LH release is more dramatic than its effect on FSH, this decapeptide is often referred to as luteinizing hormone-releasing hormone (LHRH) or gonadotropin-releasing hormone (GnRH). The differences in the secretion of LH and FSH following intravenous administration of LHRH are believed to result from differential negative and positive feedback of gonadal hormones on the hypothalamic-pituitary system that alter the response of the gonadotroph cells to the single releasing hormone.

Catecholamines serve as mediators of the signals from higher centers in the brain to the hypothalamus in regulating LHRH release. Both norepinephrine and dopamine may be involved in LHRH regulation. Although LHRH appears to be located primarily in the hypothalamus, immunoreactive LHRH is also present in other areas of the brain and even in the peripheral circulation.

Intravenous administration of LHRH at doses of 100 to 150 μg to men or women causes a rapid release of LH and FSH with peak levels of LH at 15 to 30 min and a maximal response of FSH at about 120 min. Gonadal steroids exert both a positive and negative feedback on the pituitary response to LHRH depending on the levels of the steroid hormone in the blood. Prolonged treatment of hypogonadal, castrate, or postmenopausal women with estrogen reduces both the elevated basal levels of LH and FSH and the acute response of the gonadotropins to LHRH through a negative feedback mechanism. However, in normal women the LH and FSH responses to LHRH are increased by higher estrogen concentrations. The integrated or total LH response to LHRH is greater in the late follicular (high estrogen) phase of the menstrual cycle than in the early (low estrogen) follicular phase. This variable response may explain some of the seemingly paradoxical events of the

normal menstrual cycle such as the increased plasma LH following the ovarian estrogen surge. In castrate or hypogonadal men, testosterone suppresses the LH response to LHRH apparently through a direct effect at the hypothalamic-pituitary axis. LHRH does not release GH, prolactin, TSH, or ACTH in normal people, but acromegalic patients may have an abnormal GH release to LHRH as well as to TRH.

SOMATOSTATIN (SOMATOTROPIN-RELEASE-INHIBITING FACTOR, SRIF) The dominant hypothalamic control over GH production is positive since hypothalamic lesions, stalk section, or pituitary transplantation all result in decreased GH secretion. However, an inhibitory peptide for growth hormone release has been isolated from the hypothalamus and named *somatostatin*. This 14-amino acid peptide blocks GH release to all stimuli in normal humans and lowers the increased GH secretion in acromegalic patients. Unfortunately, somatostatin is degraded rapidly in vivo so that a constant intravenous infusion is necessary for sustained inhibition of GH secretion.

Although somatostatin decreases the TSH response to TRH, it does not alter the secretion of ACTH, LH, or FSH. Secretion of insulin and glucagon is inhibited by somatostatin (see Chap. 338), as is the secretion of gastrin and vasoactive intestinal peptide (VIP). Somatostatin is present in the D cells of the pancreatic islets, in the duodenum and antrum of the stomach, and in areas of the brain other than the hypothalamus.

Anterior pituitary hormones The regulation and physiological effects of the various anterior pituitary hormones are so different that each must be considered separately.

PROLACTIN Prolactin is secreted by the lactotrophs. Both the number of lactotrophs and the pituitary content of prolactin increase during pregnancy. Human prolactin has a molecular weight of approximately 20,000. A larger form of prolactin, possibly a prohormone (molecular weight approximately 40,000), comprises a small fraction of the circulating prolactin in normal subjects but may be increased in the blood of patients with pituitary tumors. Similarities and homology exist among human prolactin, growth hormone, and the placental hormone, placental lactogen, but sensitive and specific radioimmunoassays for prolactin are now available.

The only clearly established physiological function of prolactin in humans relates to lactation, although receptors for prolactin are present in the kidney, liver, adrenal, heart, and gonads. The exact mechanism of prolactin action on the breast is not known. Whether the hormone has any function in males is also unknown. Over 85 actions of prolactin have been described in other animals, many of which relate to actions on the gonad or to synergism with steroid hormones from the gonads or adrenal glands. However, prolactin has a clear osmoregulatory function in some fish through an action on the gills and also appears to affect organ growth in some animals.

The normal range for plasma prolactin is 1 to 25 ng/ml for women and 1 to 20 ng/ml for men. The higher mean levels in women are probably the result of the stimulatory effect of estrogens on prolactin secretion. Prolactin concentration in plasma gradually increases during pregnancy. Secretion of prolactin is episodic, and the half-time in the blood is approximately 20 min, resulting in oscillations of blood levels during the day. The nocturnal peak of prolactin secretion is not synchronous with nocturnal growth hormone release. Prolactin elevations appear to be related to sleep itself rather than to an intrinsic circadian rhythm. Nipple or breast stimulation, particularly during nursing, causes a rapid rise in serum prolactin levels. This response requires the presence of afferent neural pathways from the breast to the brain. Other factors that cause prolactin release are stress (including hypoglycemia), strenuous exercise, surgery, and sexual intercourse (in women). Prolactin levels may be increased in hypothyroidism and renal failure.

The importance of the dopaminergic control of prolactin secretion is demonstrated by the striking effects of several drugs. L-Dopa which is converted to dopamine lowers prolactin levels in both normal and abnormal conditions. The dopamine agonists apomorphine and bromoergocryptine also reduce prolactin secretion. Conversely, drugs such as phenothiazines and butyrophenones, which inhibit dopaminergic transmission by blocking dopamine receptors, produce elevation of serum prolactin. Morphine, β-endorphin, and the enkephalins also increase prolactin levels.

GROWTH HORMONE (GH, SOMATOTROPIN) Human GH is a linear polypeptide with 190 amino acids and contains two intrachain disulfide bridges. Growth hormone has many amino acid sequences in common with prolactin and placental lactogen, suggesting evolution from a similar structural gene. Although there are similarities and homologous amino acid sequences in the growth hormones from different species, there is considerable interspecies variability in immunologic and biological activity. Only primate growth hormone has appreciable biological activity in humans.

The major biological effect of somatotropin is to promote growth. The organ systems affected include the skeleton, connective tissue, muscles, and viscera such as liver, intestine, and kidneys. Most effects of GH are probably exerted through induction of somatomedins produced in the liver. The somatomedins (initially called *sulfation factor*) are small peptides which are transported in the blood by carrier proteins. Somatomedins may be responsible for some of the insulin-like activity of serum that cannot be neutralized by antibodies to insulin (nonsuppressible insulin-like activity, NSILA). Plasma somatomedin activity falls after hypophysectomy and is restored by growth hormone injection.

Growth hormone exerts its action through interaction with specific receptors on cell membranes. One variety of dwarfism (Laron dwarfism) occurs in patients in whom growth hormone is present but in whom receptors appear to be defective or absent so that somatomedin generation does not occur. The net metabolic effects of growth hormone (and somatomedins) include stimulation of nucleic acid and protein synthesis, induction of positive nitrogen balance, stimulation of lipolysis, and a decrease in urea excretion. Chronic growth hormone stimulation results in insulin resistance and a tendency to elevated blood glucose. The stimulation of connective tissue produces increased collagen synthesis and increased hydroxyproline excretion. Calcium and phosphorus metabolism are altered with increased calcium absorption, a tendency to hypercalciuria, increased serum inorganic phosphate, and increased renal tubular reabsorption of phosphate. Alkaline phosphatase may also be elevated.

A specific growth hormone-releasing factor has not been isolated. Somatostatin can suppress growth hormone levels, but its role in the physiological control of growth hormone is not known. A "short-loop feedback" whereby growth hormone itself feeds back on the hypothalamus has been suggested as one potential control mechanism.

A number of drugs that alter monamine turnover or receptors in the hypothalamus also affect growth hormone release. Neuropharmacological studies indicate that the neurotransmitters dopamine, norepinephrine, and serotonin each control certain aspects of GH secretion. L-Dopa releases growth hormone, apparently after conversion to dopamine. The GH rise which occurs with stress is blunted by blockade of alpha receptors, suggesting that alpha-adrenergic mechanisms may play a role. Serotonin precursors also increase growth hormone secretion, but the significance of this action is not known.

During the normal rapid growth phase of childhood and adolescence, total growth hormone secretion is increased primarily because of increased noctural secretion of the hormone. Sleep results in growth hormone release after about 90 min, earlier than the sleep-related prolactin release. Either physical or emotional stress, if severe enough, may cause growth hormone release in the lean patient. Obesity blunts or prevents growth hormone response to most stimuli.

Various alterations in metabolic fuels also affect growth hormone levels. Hypoglycemia may increase growth hormone release, and hyperglycemia suppresses growth hormone secretion in normal subjects. Amino acids such as arginine infused intravenously release growth hormone. The stimulation of growth hormone release after exercise and the increased levels seen in patients with cirrhosis, renal failure, and some diabetics may also be the consequence of alterations in metabolic fuels.

Other hormones also influence growth hormone levels. Estrogens increase growth hormone responses to provocative tests and upright posture. Part of this effect may relate to inhibition of somatomedin generation by the liver or result from peripheral resistance to growth hormone. Pretreatment of men and prepubertal children with estrogen enhances the growth hormone responses to stimulation tests. Glucocorticoids in high doses tend to suppress growth hormone release, although the major growth-retarding effect of glucocorticoids involves somatomedin production and a peripheral tissue effect rather than direct inhibition of growth hormone release. Vasopressin in pharmacological doses and glucagon also cause growth hormone secretion.

PITUITARY GONADOTROPINS Both LH and FSH are glycoproteins. These gonadotropins have similarities with TSH as well as the placental hormone chorionic gonadotropin (HCG). In fact, all four have a molecular weight of approximately 30,000 and are composed of an alpha and a beta subunit. The alpha subunits of these four hormones are nearly identical, and the specificity of each hormone is conferred by the beta subunit. Both LH and FSH can be measured easily in blood by radioimmunoassays. Urine can also be extracted and used for a variety of assays or biological activity.

In contrast to the apparent specificity of cell type for most pituitary hormones, some pituitary cells appear to synthesize both LH and FSH, although cells containing only LH or FSH are also present. There is, however, apparent specificity of action of LH and FSH. LH in men appears to act on the Leydig or interstitial cells to cause the increased synthesis of testosterone. LH in women also acts on the interstitial cells resulting in synthesis of androgens, estrogens, and progestins depending on other local factors. LH binds to specific hormone receptors on the cell membrane and acts through a mechanism involving activation of adenylate cyclase and induction of cyclic adenosine monophosphate (AMP) levels. The subsequent steps appear to involve cyclic AMP-dependent protein kinases, but the specific substrates have not yet been identified.

FSH appears to control gametogenesis in both men and women. The specific target cell for FSH in the male appears to the Sertoli cell which has a supportive function for the developing spermatozoa. The target cell in the ovary is the granulosa cell of the ovarian follicle. FSH is also believed to act synergistically with estrogen and LH to cause follicle growth and maturation. FSH appears to increase LH receptors in the interstitial cells and to stimulate the aromatization of androgen to estradiol in the granulosa and Sertoli cells.

The regulation of gonadotropin secretion is still not fully understood. LHRH stimulates LH and FSH synthesis and release. The gonadal hormones, stimulated by LH and FSH, in turn feed back on the pituitary and hypothalamus. Puberty appears to occur as a result of a decreased sensitivity of the hypothalamus and pituitary to feedback inhibition by low levels of gonadal steroids, resulting in increased pulsatile secretion of LH during sleep. In both men and women primary hypogonadism results in an elevation of basal LH and FSH levels in the blood to approximately twice the normal concentrations.

Testosterone appears to suppress LH synthesis, while testosterone and inhibin, a peptide which is derived from the testis, are thought to suppress FSH (see Chap. 341). Inhibin has not been well characterized, but it is presumably produced by the Sertoli cells. Its release appears to be impaired when spermatogenesis is decreased. This separate feedback by inhibin probably explains the isolated elevation of FSH seen in patients who have decreased spermatozoa but normal LH and testosterone levels. Pharmacological doses of testosterone or of estrogen plus progesterone suppress both gonadotropins and spermatogenesis in the male.

In women, the regulation of the menstrual cycle is more complex (see Chap. 342). However, the differential inhibitory and stimulatory effects of ovarian steroids on the hypothalamus and pituitary appear to be critical. Inhibin may be important in women as well as men. A surge of ovarian estrogen at the end of the follicular phase of the cycle ultimately causes the release of LH and FSH, presumably through LHRH release from the hypothalamus. The normal cyclic release of gonadotropin is eliminated by estrogen-progestin combinations used in oral contraceptives. Normal menses usually resume within a few months after these medications are discontinued.

THYROTROPIN (THYROID-STIMULATING HORMONE, TSH) This glycoprotein hormone has a molecular weight of approximately 30,000. The major function of TSH is the stimulation of thyroid hormone synthesis by the thyroid. This stimulation is accompanied by increases in the rate of synthesis of protein and RNA, phospholipid production, iodine uptake, and colloid droplet formation by the thyroid.

The action of TSH involves interaction with specific TSH receptors on the cell membrane of the thyroid, activation of adenylate cyclase, and increased cyclic AMP formation. TSH has a half-life of about 50 min in blood. The pituitary apparently secretes an amount of TSH equivalent to its total content daily. TSH is easily measured in plasma or serum by radioimmunoassays, although most assays are unable to distinguish normal from low levels of the hormone.

The regulation of TSH secretion involves stimulation of TSH release by TRH and feedback inhibition of TSH secretion by triiodothyronine (T_3) and thyroxine at the level of the pituitary. This feedback regulation is so finely adjusted that a minimal thyroid deficiency results in elevated TSH levels. Therefore, assessment of serum TSH is useful in testing for mild primary hypothyroidism and in differentiating primary from hypothalamic-pituitary hypothyroidism (Fig. 333-2). Minimal elevations of thyroid hormones in the blood prevent the TSH release following administration of TRH (see Chap. 335). Chronic administration of excess thyroid hormone causes prolonged suppression of TSH secretion. In normal subjects this suppression is reversible, and normal TSH secretion occurs within 3 to 4 weeks after thyroid hormone treatment is stopped.

CORTICOTROPIN (ACTH) Human ACTH is a single polypeptide composed of 39 amino acids and has a molecular weight of approximately 4500. ACTH is derived from a large glycoprotein prohormone which is cleaved to give rise to ACTH and

also to β-lipotropin (see Chap. 332). The latter contains the sequences of β-melanocyte-stimulating hormone (β-MSH) and the opioid peptides β-endorphin and enkephalin. β-Endorphin appears to be co-secreted with ACTH. β-Lipotropin is secreted by some pituitary tumors and at times in normal individuals during stress. β-MSH was previously thought to play a role in human skin pigmentation, but the belief now is that the hormone is an artifact of β-lipotropin degradation during extraction and that it does not normally circulate in humans.

The major biological function of ACTH is maintenance of adrenal function. Although ACTH stimulates production of all three major types of adrenal steroids, i.e., glucocorticoids, androgens, and mineralocorticoids, the predominant control of aldosterone is mediated by the renin-angiotensin system. The major physiological role of ACTH is the control of cortisol secretion. Both ACTH and β-lipotropin play a role in alteration of skin pigmentation that occurs in primary adrenal insufficiency. Like TSH and the gonadotropins, ACTH appears to act through specific cell membrane receptors to induce adenylate cyclase activity and cyclic AMP synthesis.

ACTH secretion is controlled at several levels. These include a basal dirurnal variation, feedback inhibition by adrenal steroids, and a rapid release in response to stress. The physiological secretion of ACTH follows a diurnal rhythm; levels peak in the early morning and gradually decrease during the day. Like other anterior pituitary hormones, ACTH is secreted episodically. Cortisol is the major glucocorticoid that

FIGURE 333-2

Serum thyrotropin (TSH) levels in normal subjects, primary myxedema, hyperthyroidism, and hypopituitarism. The high levels of TSH in primary myxedema indicate the usefulness of this test in diagnosing primary disease of the thyroid. (After JM Hershman, JA Pittman, Ann Intern Med 74:481, 1971.)

provides a negative feedback control on the hypothalamic-pituitary unit. Reduction of steroid synthesis and secretion by drugs or by removing adrenal tissue increases ACTH levels. Exogenous steroid administration prevents the normal morning ACTH release. After chronic excess exogenous steroid administration the hypothalamic-pituitary axis is suppressed, and recovery of normal ACTH secretion may not occur for up to 6 months after initial attempts to withdraw the steroids. Stressful stimuli that cause ACTH release such as insulin-induced hypoglycemia, pyrogen, or surgery provide additional control mechanisms. The ACTH response to stress is critical in conditions such as anesthesia and surgery (see Chap. 336).

DISEASES OF THE HYPOTHALAMUS AND ANTERIOR PITUITARY GLAND

Anterior pituitary disorders usually present to the clinician with one or more of these four types of problems: (1) enlargement of the sella turcica with or without other evidence of a space-occupying lesion, (2) visual disorders, (3) symptoms and signs of hypopituitarism, and (4) evidence of pituitary hormone hypersecretion. At times all four presentations may be found together, as in a patient with acromegaly in whom a growth hormone-producing pituitary tumor has compromised other normal anterior pituitary functions sufficient to cause hypopituitarism, to enlarge the sella, and to impinge on the optic chiasm and cause visual field defects. Hypothalamic disorders may also present as pituitary hypofunction. This has given rise to the concept of primary, secondary, and tertiary deficiencies for target glands such as the thyroid and gonads. Primary deficiencies occur as a result of disease of the target gland itself, secondary deficiencies result from pituitary lesions, and tertiary deficiences occur as a consequence of hypothalamic disorders.

Theoretically, a decreased sensitivity of the hypothalamus to feedback inhibition by circulating hormones could also result in pituitary hormone overproduction. For example, it has been proposed that the ACTH excess in pituitary Cushing's disease is due to inappropriately high setting for the feedback regulatory system. Adenomas of the pituitary corticotrophs are often found in this disorder, but evidence for an hypothalamic etiology is still indirect.

ENLARGEMENT OF THE SELLA TURCICA

An increase in size or apparent erosion of the sella turcica is often the presenting problem in patients referred for pituitary evaluation. Enlargement of the sella is frequently encountered in routine skull series obtained in patients complaining of headache, following an accident, or for various other indications. The differential diagnosis of the enlarged sella includes pituitary adenomas (which constitute approximately 10 percent of all intracranial neoplasms), craniopharyngiomas, meningiomas, epithelial and other cysts occurring in the area of the sella, metastatic tumor as from breast carcinoma, and granulomas. Perhaps more common than any of these neoplasms is the nontumorous enlargement of the sella turcica or "empty sella syndrome." Sella enlargement occurs occasionally in children and rarely in adults with primary hypothyroidism. This enlargement is presumably the result of hyperplasia of the thyrotrophs and is accompanied by elevated thyrotropin levels. Sella enlargement as an apparent consequence of similar hyperplasia of gonadotrophs has been reported in a few adults with hypogonadism and high gonadotropin levels. It should also be remembered that the sella turcica represents a weak area in the bony structure of the skull and that rarely the sella may acutely increase in size secondary to rapid increases of intracranial pressure, as with a brain tumor such as glioblastoma multiforme.

Diagnostic studies useful in patients with suspected pituitary disease fall into three types: radiological, neuroophthalmologic, and endocrine. The extent to which each type of testing is used depends on the presenting manifestations. In general, radiological evaluation is most important in any patient with an enlarged sella and is critical to any therapeutic decision. The visual-field examination provides important evidence of suprasellar disease, while endocrine evaluation is necessary for the assessment of the type and severity of the hypothalamic or pituitary lesion.

Radiological studies The development of computerized tomography (CT) scanning has improved the diagnostic accuracy of noninvasive techniques, and there is hope that further refinements will remove the need for pneumoencephalography. However, the latter remains useful in many marginal lesions and in situations in which an intermediate-size intrasellar tumor with possible minimal extension above the sella must be differentiated from the empty sella syndrome (see below).

Initial radiographic studies should include high-quality plain skull films, preferably with a coned-down lateral and frontal view of the sella turcica. Enlargement of the sella is indicative of a disease process such as tumor or empty sella. On a correctly performed lateral skull x-ray the anterior clinoid processes are superimposed. Modified anteroposterior films to show the sellar floor are also useful, but considerable experience is needed for accurate assessment. A particularly useful finding in the patient with a suspected microadenoma on lateral skull films is a double density of the floor of the sella. This may be a normal variant in up to 30 percent of the population due to sloping of the sella floor or improper positioning during x-ray. However, the appearance of a double contour or erosion of the floor is an indication to proceed to tomography. Tomography is particularly useful in differentiating microadenomas from normal variants and in detecting small areas of erosion by a tumor. Lateral tomography alone is frequently adequate, but anteroposterior tomography may be helpful if definite findings are not apparent on the lateral projections.

Delineation of the extent of a pituitary lesion can be determined by CT scanning, usually combined with intravenous injection of contrast material. The CT scan can show lesions at or above the diaphragma sellae, but intrasellar lesions are less well defined. Pneumoencephalography with tomography is the best procedure for defining lesions in the area of the diaphragma sellae. With adequate positioning, this type of study identifies the empty sella (see below). Pneumoencephalography usually results in a stress type of ACTH release and subsequent cortisol elevation in normal patients. This study is relatively uncomfortable and tolerated poorly by patients with ACTH and TSH deficiencies. Cortisol (100 mg parenterally several hours prior to the study) should be given prophylactically if there is any suspicion of ACTH deficiency. Although the pneumoencephalogram is the definitive radiological procedure, arteriography is indicated prior to surgery to exclude the possibility of an aneurysm in the pituitary fossa or adjacent area.

Empty sella syndrome This term describes a nontumorous enlargement of the sella turcica that may be misdiagnosed as a pituitary neoplasm. The enlarged sella contains cerebrospinal fluid rather than a tumor (Fig. 333-3). Up to 30 percent of normal persons have some cerebrospinal fluid below the diaphragma sellae in a small arachnoid diverticulum extending through the foramen where the stalk passes through the diaphragm. The primary empty sella syndrome occurs when the arachnoid diverticulum enlarges to such a degree that the sella becomes enlarged and the pituitary is compressed against the floor of the sella. Some empty sellas develop as a secondary process after spontaneous infarction or regression of a tumor

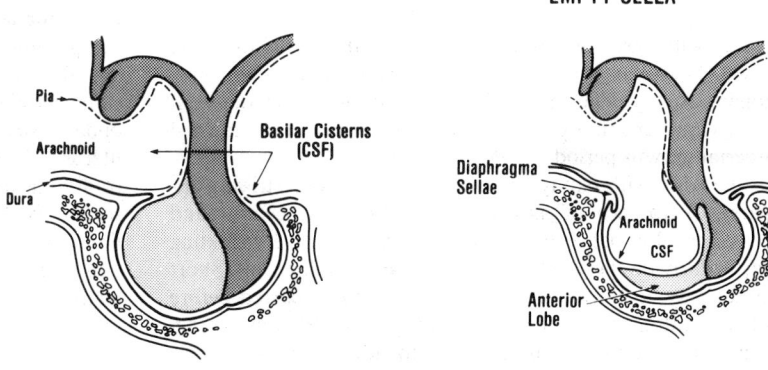

NORMAL **EMPTY SELLA**

FIGURE 333-3
Diagram indicating the findings in patients with the nontumorous enlargement of the sella turcica or the primary empty sella syndrome. The left panel shows the normal anatomic relationships. In patients with the empty sella syndrome an arachnoid diverticulum herniates through an incompetent diaphragm into the sella. Ballooning of the sella may occur causing enlargement suggesting a pituitary tumor. The pneumoencephalogram will show excessive air entering the sella. (After RM Jordan et al, Am J Med 62:569, 1977.)

which previously enlarged the sella. However, the majority of patients with the empty sella syndrome appear never to have had a tumor and have no abnormalities of pituitary function. The enlarged sella, therefore, causes difficulty primarily because it may be misinterpreted as a pituitary tumor.

Patients with primary empty sella are usually obese, multiparous, hypertensive women. The enlargement of the pituitary during pregnancy with subsequent regression in size may play some role in the pathogenesis. Approximately 90 percent of patients with the empty sella syndrome are women. Headache is a common complaint. Obesity is present in about 80 percent and hypertension in 30 percent of these patients. On x-ray the sella often appears ballooned. There is usually no evidence of erosion as in tumorous enlargement, although cerebrospinal fluid rhinorrhea has occurred in up to 10 percent in some series. Clinical endocrine deficiencies are rare, and laboratory studies are usually normal. Visual-field defects are also rare, although on occasion the optic chiasm may prolapse into the sella and cause field deficits. In patients who have had infarction of a pituitary tumor with subsequent development of the empty sella syndrome, visual field and endocrine abnormalities are more common. Diagnosis can often be made at tomography which shows the characteristic ballooned appearance without erosive changes in the floor. The diagnosis can be confirmed either by CT scanning or by pneumoencephalography with appropriate rotation of the patient so that air fills the arachnoid cavity below the diaphragm. The major clinical significance of the empty sella syndrome is to avoid the mistake of diagnosing pituitary tumor. No treatment other than weight loss or control of hypertension is required unless cerebrospinal fluid rhinorrhea is present.

Endocrine evaluation in patients with enlargement of the sella turcica

The extent of the endocrine evaluation depends largely on the management plan. Base-line studies should include assessment of peripheral thyroid and adrenal hormone levels and a screen for diabetes insipidus such as the ability to concentrate on overnight urine. Measurement of basal prolactin values is helpful since more than half of pituitary tumors appear to secrete prolactin. Basal gonadotropin levels and basal testosterone values in men are useful. Patients with evidence of hypopituitarism should have a more extensive evaluation (see below).

In many centers more extensive endocrine studies are omitted prior to surgical treatment of large pituitary tumors or vascular lesions. These patients are treated with thyroid replacement if needed and with parenteral glucocorticoids equivalent to 300 mg cortisol on the day of surgery with gradual tapering of the steroid replacement over several days following the procedure. Endocrine evaluation may then be performed to determine the extent of endocrine deficiencies. However, if the patient is to be followed without treatment or treated with

irradiation or selective transsphenoidal microsurgery, more extensive endocrine evaluation is indicated.

VISUAL DISORDERS AND OPHTHALMOLOGIC EVALUATION

Patients with radiographic abnormalities of the sella deserve a careful ophthalmologic examination. Visual disorders were previously the most frequent presenting complaint in patients with large pituitary tumors (Table 333-1), but because of the capacity to diagnose smaller pituitary adenomas, the frequency of visual disorders as a presenting complaint has decreased. Large visual field defects can be identified at the bedside, but formal visual field examination by tangent screen or Goldman perimetry is advised.

The classic bilateral homonymous hemianopsia or superior quadrantic defects are expected when a pituitary tumor extends upward from the diaphragma sellae and compresses the optic chiasm lying above the sella turcica. In actual practice the defects produced by large tumors vary from no defects to combinations of unilateral or bilateral field defects in all quadrants. Reasons for the irregular patterns include variations in the position of the chiasm above the sella and variable compromise of blood vessels supplying the optic chiasm. Other tumors such as craniopharyngiomas may also cause visual field loss advancing to optic atrophy and total blindness. Careful visual field and visual acuity examinations should be obtained before and after surgery in order to document any subsequent change in vision. Patients with defects should have visual field examinations at least annually.

HYPOPITUITARISM Deficiencies of anterior pituitary hormones may occur as isolated or combined deficits. The presentation of the patient depends on the number and extent of hormone deficiencies. Patients may complain of weakness, fatigue, headaches, loss of sexual function, and cold intolerance. Hypogonadotropism is the most common symptomatic endocrine deficiency encountered in adults with either pituitary tumors or craniopharyngiomas. Children present more com-

TABLE 333-1
Initial complaints in 1000 patients with large pituitary tumors

Visual	421	Cushing's disease	29
Headache	137	Incidental finding	15
Acromegaly	136	Diabetes insipidus	10
Hypopituitarism	95	ENT complaints	6
Amenorrhea	48	CSF rhinorrhea	5
Diplopia	7	Multiple endocrine adenomas	4
CNS*	24	Undetermined	19
Pain (not headache)	44		

* *Syncope, 5; seizures, 5; dizziness, 9; confusion, 4; inappropriate ADH syndrome, 1.*
SOURCE: *After RW Hollenhorst, in Diagnosis and Treatment of Pituitary Tumors, PO Kohler, GT Ross (eds). New York, American Elsevier, 1973.*

monly with growth retardation secondary to inadequate growth hormone. Provocative tests indicate that growth hormone is usually deficient in adults, but this deficiency does not cause symptoms in a patient who has experienced the normal pubertal growth period.

The adult with panhypopituitarism may have a striking appearance: absence of axillary and pubic hair, genital and breast atrophy, pallor of the skin and nipples, fine wrinkling (particularly on the face), and poor muscle development. Short stature may be present if the pituitary disease occurred before puberty, and there is often the appearance of premature aging. Men with hypopituitarism and hypogonadism have a juvenile pattern of scalp hair without temporal recession or baldness. In contrast to the original description of cachexia in hypopituitarism by Simmonds, patients with advanced disease may be somewhat puffy and slightly overweight as if hypothyroidism were the prevalent feature. The presence of diabetes insipidus (see Chap. 334) suggests hypothalamic involvement since only massively enlarged anterior pituitary lesions cause disruption of ADH release by the neurohypophysis. The clinical presentation of the patient with hypopituitarism is often a composite of several hormone deficiencies. Manifestations of each individual hormone deficiency will be considered separately.

PROLACTIN DEFICIENCY   Failure to lactate after parturition is the only clinical consequence of prolactin deficiency. This has classically been associated with hemorrhage and shock in women with postpartum pituitary necrosis (Sheehan's syndrome). The incidence of prolactin deficiency in other pituitary diseases is not known. Failure to respond to prolactin provocative tests has been noted in some patients with advanced pituitary disease, but some normal individuals also have blunted responses to stimulation tests.

GROWTH HORMONE DEFICIENCY   Inadequate growth hormone in the child causes retardation of growth, epiphyseal development, and bone age. Hypopituitary dwarfs tend to have increased truncal fat and a puffy appearance to the skin even in the presence of normal levels of thyroid hormone. The legs are longer in relation to the trunk than those of a normal child. Secondary sexual characteristics are retarded or absent. Development of the larynx is impaired, and the voice tends to be high pitched. Since growth does not ordinarily cease completely and since gonadal maturation is delayed, growth hormone–deficient patients may continue to grow slowly past the usual age of puberty. Hypoglycemia may occur in very young children or infants with isolated growth hormone deficiency. All these changes can be reversed with growth hormone treatment.

In the adult the onset of growth hormone deficiency appears to be a "silent" lesion without hypoglycemia or other clinical manifestations. However, a failure to evoke a growth hormone response to provocative tests is still the most common hormone deficiency in hypothalamic-pituitary lesions. Therefore, growth hormone evaluation is useful in the patient with suspected pituitary disease.

GONADOTROPIN DEFICIENCY   Hypogonadism is the most common clinical endocrine manifestation of hypothalamic-pituitary deficiency in the adult. Gonadotropin deficiency prior to puberty results in a eunuchoid appearance with lack of development of secondary sexual characteristics and infertility. Boys with hypogonadism fail to develop a beard, an adult male scalp hair pattern, a normal adult voice, or normal enlargement of the genitalia. Girls with prepubertal hypogonadism lack normal breast development and menstruation. Both sexes may have decreased or absent pubic and axillary hair, although growth of sexual hair is also dependent on adrenal

function. If growth hormone secretion is adequate, prepubertal hypogonadal patients may have a tall stature because continued growth of the long bones occurs in the absence of sufficient gonadal steroids to cause epiphyseal fusion. Gonadotropin insufficiency in the premenopausal woman is manifested by secondary amenorrhea. In advanced deficiency the breasts and uterus atrophy, and vaginal cornification is diminished because of diminished ovarian estrogen production. In the adult male, secondary testicular atrophy is accompanied by decrease in libido, potency, muscle tone, and beard growth. In some patients with hyperprolactinemia and hypogonadotropinism prolactin may have an antigonadal effect, but the relationship is uncertain.

THYROTROPIN DEFICIENCY   Hypothalamic or pituitary hypothyroidism is similar to primary hypothyroidism but frequently is less severe. Lethargy, fatigue, and pallor of the skin are common. Isolated TSH deficiency is rare, and growth hormone and gonadotropin deficiency are usually present when thyrotropin deficiency is expressed, thus facilitating the separation of hypothalamic-pituitary disease (tertiary or secondary) from primary hypothyroidism. The skin in pituitary hypothyroidism often shows a fine wrinkling, particularly on the face, which may be related in part to an associated gonadal deficiency. Associated findings such as visual field defects or loss of secondary sexual characteristics are helpful in identification of pituitary hypothyroidism. The hair is dry but less coarse in the pituitary form of hypothyroidism than in primary disease. Tongue enlargement may occur in severe primary hypothyroidism but is usually not present in pituitary hypothyroidism. The menstrual history is useful in premenopausal women in that menorrhagia may occur with primary hypothyroidism, whereas amenorrhea is expected in pituitary disease. Laboratory evaluation makes it possible to separate primary from secondary hypothyroidism.

ACTH DEFICIENCY   This is the most serious endocrine deficiency in patients with pituitary disease. While ACTH deficiency usually occurs only in massive pituitary lesions, it must be looked for in all patients with evidence of pituitary disease. Most patients with ACTH deficiency have evidence of other hormone loss. There may be a history of inadequate response to stress with nausea, vomiting, hyperthermia, and collapse. Hypovolemia and hyperkalemia are unusual in the absence of vomiting, diarrhea, or diabetes insipidus because aldosterone secretion is maintained to a large degree by the renin-angiotensin system. Patients with ACTH deficiency may have hyponatremia from an inappropriate ADH-type syndrome with volume expansion. Decreased skin and nipple pigmentation may be useful in differentiating the pituitary hypoadrenal patient from the more darkly pigmented patient with primary adrenal disease. Patients with any form of adrenal insufficiency tolerate stress poorly and should be treated with additional corticosteroids during surgery or intercurrent illness.

Disorders producing hypopituitarism   Lesions in either the hypothalamus or pituitary may produce hypopituitarism (Table 333-2).

NEOPLASMS   Although a variety of primary and metastatic tumors may rarely occur in the hypothalamic-pituitary area, the most common neoplasms are craniopharyngiomas in children and primary pituitary tumors in adults.

CRANIOPHARYNGIOMAS   These squamous cell tumors develop from remnants of Rathke's pouch. They usually occur in a suprasellar location but may arise in or extend into the sella turcica. Most are cystic to some degree, and about half are

TABLE 333-2

Etiologies of pituitary disease

I Neoplasms
  A Hypothalamic disorders
    1 Craniopharyngioma
    2 Metastatic neoplasms
    3 Other (meningioma, hamartoma, teratoma, ectopic pinealoma, leukemia, lymphoma)
  B Pituitary tumors
    1 Pituitary adenomas
    2 Meningioma
    3 Other (metastatic, glioma, chordoma, primary malignant, cysts)
II Congenital or hereditary conditions
  A Idiopathic growth hormone deficiency
  B Idiopathic corticotropin deficiency
  C Idiopathic gonadotropin deficiency
  D Idiopathic thyrotropin deficiency (hypothalamic)
  E Multiple hormone deficiencies (idiopathic)
  F Hypothalamic hypogonadism (Kallman's syndrome)
III Vascular disorders
  A Pituitary infarction
  B Postpartum necrosis (Sheehan's syndrome)
  C Aneurysm
  D Vasculitis
IV Infections or granulomas
  A Sarcoidosis
  B Tuberculosis
  C Other (meningitis, luetic, mycotic, pyogenic, Wegener's granulomatosis)
V Physical agents
  A Radiation
  B Surgery
  C Head trauma
VI Miscellaneous
  A Histiocytosis X
  B Hemochromatosis
  C Emotional deprivation (children)
  D Tay-Sach's disease
  E Drugs

multicystic. The cysts are filled with a yellow to brown fluid that resembles motor oil. The peak incidence is in the second decade of life. Although children often present with evidence of increased intracranial pressure, the most common problems in adults are visual disorders such as optic atrophy, visual field defects, or papilledema. Over half of adults have endocrine deficits, the most common endocrinopathy being hypogonadism secondary to LH and FSH deficiencies. Diabetes insipidus and short stature with delayed bone maturation (due to growth hormone deficiency and hypogonadism) are also common. Complete hypopituitarism occurs in 5 to 10 percent of patients. Occasionally, hypothalamic syndromes such as obesity, anorexia, somnolence, or hyperkinetic behavior may be present. The tumor is calcified and thus visible on skull films in about 75 percent of children and 35 percent of adults. Although other tumors such as meningiomas and granulomas may also calcify, craniopharyngiomas are the most common cause of suprasellar or intrasellar calcification.

CT scan is a valuable diagnostic technique in identifying these cystic tumors. Treatment consists of surgical extirpation. Unfortunately, complete removal is frequently difficult. Although craniopharyngiomas are relatively resistant to irradiation, radiotherapy may be useful in patients who cannot be cured by surgery. Replacement of hormone deficiencies may also be necessary.

PITUITARY ADENOMAS Over 10 percent of all intracranial tumors are pituitary adenomas. Essentially all primary pituitary tumors arise in the anterior lobe, tumors of the posterior lobe being extremely rare. In the past, most pituitary tumors were assumed to be nonfunctional chromophobe adenomas. However, widespread use of the prolactin radioimmunoassay has shown that plasma prolactin levels are elevated in 50 to 70 percent of cases. This is usually the result of prolactin secretion by the tumor but may also be the consequence of interference

by the tumor mass with the normal inhibitory influence of the hypothalamus on prolactin secretion. Prolactin secretion in such cases may be clinically inapparent, and these tumors therefore present in a manner identical to nonfunctioning tumors. Twenty to thirty percent of pituitary tumors exhibit no detectable hormone secretion.

Patients with pituitary tumors may rarely have Wermer's syndrome, or multiple endocrine neoplasia, type I (see Chap. 348). In this condition, which is inherited as an autosomal dominant trait, patients have a predisposition to develop tumors of the pituitary, parathyroid glands, or pancreas. For this reason, all patients with pituitary adenomas should be questioned carefully with regard to the family history and should be considered for the possibility of hyperparathyroidism, gastrinoma, or other functional pancreatic neoplasm.

NONFUNCTIONING PITUITARY TUMORS Patients with nonfunctioning tumors present with signs and symptoms of a space-occupying lesion or evidence of hypopituitarism (Table 333-1). The loss of vision was the most common complaint in the past. Bitemporal hemianopsia is the classic manifestation of a large pituitary tumor compressing the optic chiasm, although any type of visual defect may occur. Patients with tumors large enough to cause visual disorders usually have associated trophic hormone deficiencies. The most common of these is an inadequate growth hormone response to provocative tests. The next most common hormone deficiency is hypogonadotropinism which occurs in about 75 percent of patients with large tumors. ACTH and TSH deficiencies are less common, each occurring in 40 to 50 percent of patients with extensive tumors. Patients with small pituitary tumors may have no evidence of hypopituitarism. The natural history of nonfunctioning tumors is not entirely clear. The fact that up to 25 percent of people without known pituitary disease have small pituitary adenomas at autopsy suggests that small tumors often cause no clinical disease. Once patients develop visual or endocrine disorders, however, treatment is indicated.

ISOLATED HORMONE DEFICIENCIES Isolated deficiencies of any of the pituitary hormones may occur. The mechanisms by which these isolated deficiencies occur are not known. Isolated growth hormone deficiency is one of the most common causes of growth retardation in children. Growth hormone failure in children may also be associated with other anterior pituitary hormone deficiencies of unknown etiology.

The most common form of isolated hypogonadotropic hypogonadism in both men and women is *Kallman's syndrome* (see also Chap. 341). This is a familial condition in which gonadotropin deficiency secondary to inadequate LHRH secretion is frequently associated with anosmia or hyposmia from hypoplasia of the olfactory lobes. Other midline developmental defects such as harelip, cleft palate, and facial fusion abnormalities may be present, and unilateral renal agenesis is occasionally seen. A history of undescended testes is obtained in about a third of affected males. These patients are often identified at the time of expected puberty when secondary sexual characteristics fail to develop. Careful testing of the sense of smell is indicated because affected individuals may be unaware of hyposmia. The mode of inheritance appears to vary, but in some families it appears to be an autosomal dominant trait with variable phenotypic expression. Fertility can be accomplished by treatment with LHRH or human gonadotropins.

Deficiencies of LH and FSH may occur in men who present with evidence of hypoandrogenization such as a eunuchoid appearance and scanty beard growth, but who have some degree of spermatogenesis. This has been called the "fertile eunuch syndrome" but probably is just a partial form of LHRH deficiency (i.e., an incomplete variant of Kallman's syndrome). Patients with apparent unrelated deficiency of FSH have also been described.

INFECTIOUS AND GRANULOMATOUS LESIONS   In the past, tuberculous meningitis, granulomas, and syphilis have occasionally caused hypopituitarism. Sarcoidosis may involve the hypothalamus or pituitary and cause diabetes insipidus or anterior pituitary hormone deficiency.

PHYSICAL AGENTS   Hypopituitarism may result from head trauma, and any surgery in the infratentorial region of the brain may produce variable degrees of hypopituitarism depending on the extent of procedures. Another cause of hypopituitarism is external radiation in the hypothalamic-pituitary area for malignancies of the nasopharynx. These patients usually have subclinical deficiencies of growth hormone, ACTH, and TSH, but overt disease may develop rarely. Basal prolactin levels may be elevated. Thus, patients who have received radiation for head or neck tumors may require evaluation for hypothalamic-pituitary insufficiency.

INFARCTION AND VASCULAR DISORDERS   The most common clinically significant cause of infarction of the normal pituitary has been postpartum pituitary necrosis (Sheehan's syndrome) secondary to hemorrhagic shock. The anterior pituitary gland is enlarged during pregnancy and, lacking a direct arterial blood supply, is vulnerable to infarction during shock from excessive uterine bleeding at parturition. The severity of the syndrome varies from an unrecognized contributory cause of morbidity at the time of the initial insult to failure to lactate after delivery or failure to resume menses. Some patients develop evidence of other anterior pituitary hormone loss years after the insult. The incidence of Sheehan's syndrome appears to be decreasing with improved obstetric techniques.

Although small areas of intrapituitary hemorrhage are commonly found postmortem, major infarctions are unusual. *Pituitary apoplexy* may occur in pituitary tumors that infarct, in diabetics with cerebrovascular disease, and rarely in patients with sickle-cell disease. Such patients present with excruciating headaches, often bitemporal in location, fever, visual-field deficits, and oculomotor palsies. They may have photophobia, stiff neck, altered consciousness, convulsions, and localizing neurological signs. Papilledema may develop, and the cerebrospinal fluid may be bloody.

The CT scan is a valuable, rapid, noninvasive technique for evaluating the possibility of hemorrhage or enlargement of an infarcted tumor mass above the diaphragma sellae. Pituitary apoplexy is a medical emergency requiring administration of glucocorticoids and radiological evaluation for possible compression of structures in the area of the pituitary. Surgical decompression may be required, although this is not always necessary. At times patients with prolactin- or growth hormone-secreting tumors improve after infarction of the tumor mass. Rarely, hypopituitarism is produced by aneurysm of the internal carotid artery in the absence of hemorrhage, by systemic lupus erythematosus, or by other forms of vasculitis.

MISCELLANEOUS CAUSES OF HYPOPITUITARISM   Histiocytosis X or the multifocal type eosinophilic granuloma, also called Hand-Schüller-Christian disease, is a nonneoplastic histiocytic reaction to unknown stimuli. Approximately half of these patients have diabetes insipidus, and a fourth have growth hormone deficiency from hypothalamic involvement. The anterior pituitary is usually free of histiocytes, and other anterior pituitary hormone deficiencies are rare. The classic triad in this disease includes punched-out skull lesions, exophthalamos (from histiocytic invasion of the retroorbital space), and diabetes insipidus. The disease is usually responsive to radiation and treatment with prednisone or vinblastine, although reversal of the ADH and growth hormone deficiencies does not occur. Other rare causes of pituitary deficiency include hemochromatosis, Tay-Sachs disease, and Wegener's granulomatosis. Patients with acute intermittent porphyria may have evidence of abnormal hypothalamic-pituitary function such as inappropriate ADH secretion or inappropriate release of growth hormone after glucose ingestion.

Evaluation   In the evaluation of patients with suspected hypopituitarism, the history and physical examination may be helpful with regard to etiology. A recent or remote history of postpartum hemorrhage with shock, particularly if combined with failure to lactate, suggests Sheehan's syndrome. Visual field defects usually indicate a tumor large enough to impinge on the optic chiasm. Anosmia or developmental defects such as harelip or cleft palate in a man or woman with hypogonadism suggests the hypothalamic lesion of Kallman's syndrome. Evidence of lactation or of acral growth suggests a pituitary tumor producing prolactin or growth hormone. As discussed below, hypothalamic or stalk lesions may also cause hyperprolactinemia.

In the differential diagnosis of hypopituitarism, anorexia nervosa (see Chap. 77) and severe malnutrition should be considered since amenorrhea is a common feature. Blood glucose, serum thyroxine, and urinary steroid excretion may be low in anorexia nervosa. However, serum cortisol levels are usually normal, and growth hormone reponses to stimuli may be supranormal. This disease may result from a functional disorder of the hypothalamus.

DIAGNOSTIC STUDIES   Laboratory evaluation will differentiate between target organ failure and disease of the hypothalamic-pituitary system.

Unfortunately, the separation of hypothalamic from pituitary lesions by endocrine testing is more difficult unless the lesion can be located by radiographic studies.

ENDOCRINE EVALUATION   Endocrine evaluation in patients with suspected hypothalamic-pituitary lesions is important for two reasons: (1) documentation of specific endocrine deficits, including those potentially life-threatening deficiencies such as ACTH and TSH, and (2) evaluation of progression of a known lesion or the response to therapy. The initial endocrine evaluation usually should include tests for hyposecretion of each of the anterior pituitary hormones as well as determination of adequate ADH secretion. Evaluation of hypersecreting pituitary adenomas will be discussed later under specific hypersecretory syndromes.

Although base-line hormone levels can provide much information, the pulsatile nature of anterior hormone secretion often makes interpretation of basal hormone levels difficult to evaluate. It is particularly difficult to distinguish between normal and low blood levels of these hormones. For this reason, various provocative tests are used to examine the adequacy of hypothalamic-pituitary response to various challenges such as stress, administration of releasing factors, and blockade of feedback inhibition. Twenty-four hour urine collections for measurement of gonadotropins or steroid secretion are valuable in that they represent an integration of hormone secretion over a relatively long period of time.

TESTS FOR PROLACTIN DEFICIENCY   Although prolactin levels in the blood vary in response to physiological stimuli, the basal morning levels are relatively well standardized with a normal range of 1 to 20 ng/ml in men and 1 to 25 ng/ml in women. Measurements of basal prolactin levels are useful in suspected hypothalamic or pituitary disease because elevated prolactin levels may occur in patients with hypothalamic or stalk lesions or prolactin-producing tumors. Patients with very large pituitary lesions may have low prolactin values and show a deficient response to provocative tests such as TRH or chlorpromazine. However, testing for prolactin deficiency is rarely necessary.

TESTS FOR GROWTH HORMONE RESERVE Growth hormone values vary during the day in response to fluctuations in metabolic fuels, stress, and other stimuli. A glucose load (as occurs after eating a normal meal) will suppress GH levels. As the blood sugar falls several hours after a meal, GH will rise. Basal morning growth hormone values tend to be low, making it difficult to distinguish between normal and pathologically low values. As a consequence, provocative tests are required to demonstrate adequate GH response. Once GH deficiency has developed, it rarely is reversed by therapy, and therefore continued testing is unnecessary.

Multiple provocative tests have been developed to test GH release. These include measurement of the normal growth hormone release during sleep or in response to exercise. A normal GH reserve may often be documented in the office or clinic by asking a patient to arrive fasting and then to exercise by climbing several flights of stairs. If the GH level in blood drawn after the exercise is greater than 6 ng/ml, the GH reserve can be assumed to be normal. When this is not an adequate challenge, specific provocative GH testing must be performed. The two most frequently used tests are insulin-induced hypoglycemia and L-dopa administration. The insulin test is performed by giving 0.1 unit of regular insulin per kilogram of body weight as a bolus to a fasting patient via an intravenous saline drip. Blood is drawn prior to injection and at 30-min intervals for 2 h for measurement of glucose and GH. A fall in plasma glucose to half the normal fasting level or to below 45 mg per 100 ml should provide an adequate stimulus for GH release. If hypoglycemia is inadequate, 0.15 to 0.2 unit per kilogram may be used. ACTH, cortisol, glucagon, and epinephrine are also released in response to this challenge. If hypoglycemic symptoms occur, they can be rapidly reversed by intravenous glucose. A normal GH response is an elevation to greater than 6 to 8 ng/ml during the test. The peak GH values usually occur at 30 to 60 min (Fig. 333-4). This test should not be performed in the elderly or in patients with cerebrovascular or cardiovascular disease. The ACTH response to stress can be measured at the same time, but in view of the expense involved in measuring ACTH, serum cortisol is often measured and used as evidence of ACTH release. A typical normal response to hypoglycemia is shown in Fig. 333-4.

In the patient who is not a candidate for insulin-induced hypoglycemia, the L-dopa test is an effective alternative. The ingestion of L-dopa (500 mg per 70 kg) provokes a GH release in about 30 to 60 min in 90 to 95 percent of normal lean adults. A normal response is a GH level of above 6 to 8 ng/ml at some point during the test. L-Dopa causes side effects such as nausea and occasional vomiting in some patients; it does not release ACTH or other anterior pituitary hormones but does lower prolactin levels.

Other stimuli used to test GH reserve include sleep, arginine infusion, vasopressin, glucagon, pyrogen, and nicotinic acid. Pyrogen provokes both GH and ACTH release but is rarely used because of side effects. Arginine, which has almost no side effects, or vasopressin may be useful in some circumstances. All stressful GH provocative tests should be performed only after evidence that there is no severe deficiency of ACTH or TSH. If ACTH or TSH is deficient, GH will also

usually be deficient. In these instances the patient should be on adrenal and/or thyroid replacement therapy before provocative tests are administered.

There are other important considerations in interpreting the response to provocative tests. The GH responses to all stimuli are blunted or abolished and should be interpreted with caution in the obese patient. In addition, since glucose normally suppresses GH, all tests should be performed fasting, although the response to certain types of stress such as pyrogen may occur despite hyperglycemia. Glucocorticoids in high doses may also blunt the GH response. Finally, estrogens appear to increase the GH response to various stimuli, particularly exercise. For this reason, estrogen pretreatment has occasionally been used prior to testing, particularly in pediatric patients who are candidates for GH replacement therapy.

FIGURE 333-4

Effect of intravenous insulin, 0.1 unit per kilogram of body weight, on blood sugar, plasma growth hormone (HGH), and plasma cortisol. This insulin tolerance test permits evaluation of both growth hormone and ACTH in patients with pituitary disease. (After KJ Catt, Lancet 1:933, 1970.)

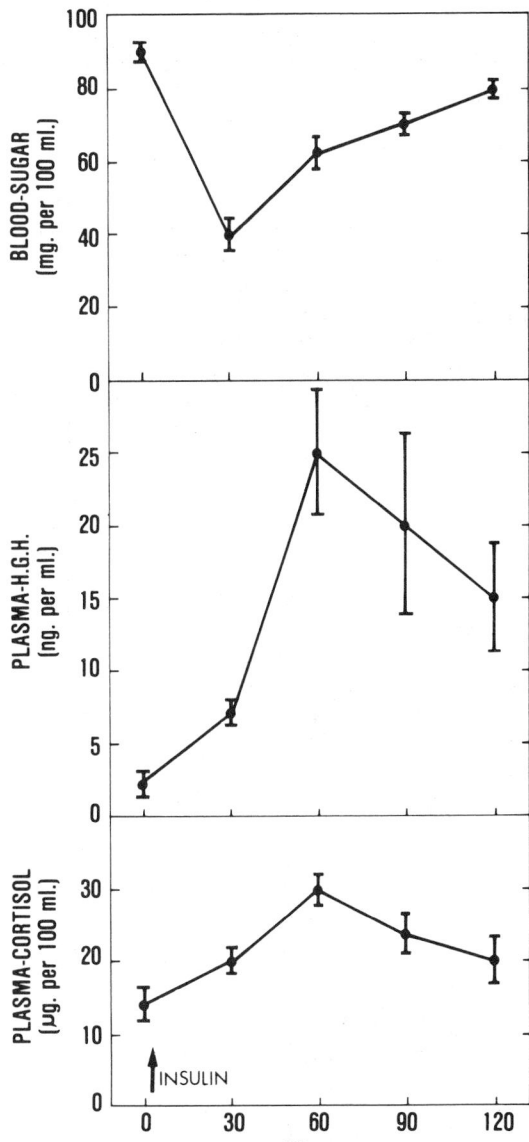

TESTS OF LH AND FSH RESERVE   It is important to emphasize that evidence of normal gonadal function in the absence of hormonal treatment indicates normal hypothalamic-pituitary-gonadal function. Thus, normal cyclic menses in women and normal sperm counts in men essentially exclude hypogonadotropism. The serum testosterone in men provides a useful index of Leydig cell function. The serum estradiol has some value in women but fluctuates considerably during the normal menstrual cycle.

Measurement of basal LH and FSH levels provides valuable information as to whether gonadal insufficiency is primary or secondary-tertiary. Patients with primary gonadal problems have elevated gonadotropin levels from lack of feedback inhibition. LH elevation appears to occur as a result of testosterone or estrogen deficiency and FSH elevation as a result of decreased gametogenesis. The degree of LH or FSH elevation depends on the degree of gonadal failure. Hypogonadal patients with hypothalamic or pituitary lesions have low or low normal basal gonadotropin levels. Because gonadotropin secretion is pulsatile, three basal blood samples should be drawn 30 min apart and pooled, or the average taken of the separate LH and FSH determinations for an accurate evaluation.

The luteinizing hormone–releasing hormone (LHRH) test may also be used to assess pituitary gonadotropin reserve. LHRH (usually 100 or 150 μg) is injected intravenously, and blood LH (FSH optional) values are determined at base line and 20- to 30-min intervals. In normal patients the peak LH response occurs at 20 to 30 min (Fig. 333-5). Although the LHRH test may be useful in following a given patient, the magnitude of the LHRH integrated response can usually be predicted from the basal gonadotropin levels (Fig. 333-6). Therefore, the LHRH test is usually not necessary in the evaluation of patients with pituitary disease unless the patient is undergoing special studies. Another potential use for the LHRH test, i.e., differentiation between hypothalamic and pituitary disease, has also failed to be as useful as anticipated. Theoretically, patients with hypothalamic lesions lacking LHRH might have a normal LH and FSH release from the pituitary, while patients with pituitary lesions (secondary deficiencies) would fail to respond. However, the pituitary response is variable in both conditions, and LHRH appears to

FIGURE 333-6

The effect of 100 μg LHRH intravenously on luteinizing hormone (LH) secretion in various clinical conditions. The clear bars show mean integrated levels of basal LH, and the solid bars show mean integrated levels for 2 h after administration of LHRH. The indices of basal and response LH were derived by computing areas under the curves formed by basal and response LH. The brackets indicate the standard error of the mean. The magnitude of the LH response in the various conditions appears to be related to basal LH levels. (After RH Mortimer et al, J Clin Endocrinol Metab 43: 1240, 1978.)

have a trophic effect on gonadotropin synthesis. Patients with definite hypothalamic lesions may initially have a poor response to LHRH, but after repeated stimulation gonadotropin response improves dramatically.

The integrity of the hypothalamus and pituitary together may be tested with clomiphene citrate, an estrogen antagonist which blocks the feedback of gonadal steroids on the hypothalamus in both men and women and which is also used for induction of ovulation in women. In men, the administration of clomiphene citrate 50 mg bid for 7 to 10 days usually produces a doubling of the LH and testosterone levels and a smaller increase in FSH values. For a normal response, both the hypothalamus and pituitary must function normally.

The measurement of urinary gonadotropins by bioassay or radioimmunoassay may be useful in selected patients. However, even normal persons at times have no measurable gonadotropin excretion by bioassay, and the blood tests are more reliable.

TESTS OF THYROTROPIN (TSH) RESERVE   Measurement of peripheral thyroid hormone levels is useful in identifying hypothalamic or pituitary hypothyroidism as well as primary thyroid deficiency. Chronic illness may be associated with low triiodothyronine and occasionally low thyroxine values in the absence of true hypothyroidism (see Chap. 335). Basal levels of TSH are useful in differentiating primary thyroid gland deficiency from pituitary insufficiency. In primary hypothyroidism, serum TSH is elevated from lack of feedback inhibition by thyroid hormone. Patients with hypothalamic or pituitary disease have TSH values in the low or normal range. Unfortunately, most clinically available radioimmunoassays for TSH cannot distinguish between low and normal levels.

It is sometimes useful to measure the TSH response to thyrotropin-releasing hormone (TRH), particularly when evaluation of prolactin values is also desired. After the intravenous injection of 400 to 500 μg TRH, the normal peak TSH response occurs at 20 to 30 min and is approximately a doubling of base-line values (Fig. 333-7). Normally, prolactin values increase two- to eightfold. Unfortunately, the TRH test is similar to the LHRH test in that it does not always clearly differentiate between hypothalamic and pituitary disease. In addition, a few patients with large pituitary tumors have a normal TSH response to TRH even when they appear mildly hypothyroid.

FIGURE 333-5

The effect of 150 μg LHRH intravenously on plasma luteinizing hormone (LH) in patients with pituitary tumors and hypogonadotropic hypogonadism. The shaded area represents the range of responses in normal subjects. Open circles indicate values in postmenopausal women, and the closed circles represent younger women and men. A few patients exhibit a normal response in spite of clinical hypogonadotropism. (After AM Coscia et al, J Clin Endocrinol Metab 38:83, 1974.)

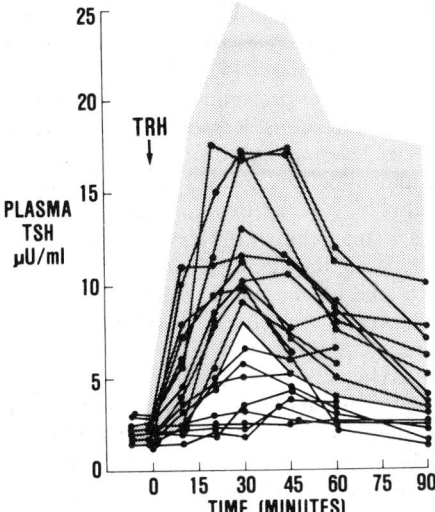

FIGURE 333-7

Effect of 500 μg TRH on plasma thyrotropin (TSH) values in patients with pituitary tumors who are clinically euthyroid. The shaded area represents the range of responses in normal subjects. The TSH response in these patients varies from normal to none. Patients with large pituitary lesions producing TSH deficiency tend to have an absent TSH response although the TSH response occasionally may be normal. Patients with hypothalamic lesions and a normal pituitary (tertiary or hypothalamic hypothyroidism) may have a late sustained TSH response to exogenous TRH. Excess thyroid hormones will ablate the TSH response to TRH. (After N Fleischer et al, J Clin Endocrinol Metab 34:617, 1972.)

Other patients who are euthyroid and all patients who are hyperthyroid (Chap. 335) fail to respond to TRH. These occasional inconsistent responses limit the value of the test in differentiating hypothalamic and pituitary disease. No clinically useful feedback inhibition test for TSH is available at the present time.

TESTS FOR ACTH DEFICIENCY   In patients suspected of having severe pituitary-adrenal insufficiency, basal morning plasma cortisol or 24-h urine 17-hydroxysteroid excretion should be measured prior to strenuous provocative tests such as the insulin tolerance test. Patients with adrenal insufficiency are very sensitive to insulin. These patients may be treated with replacement doses of a synthetic glucocorticoid such as 0.5 mg dexamethasone daily, which allows the patient to tolerate stress without ablating the ACTH response. Hypoglycemia during the insulin tolerance test normally provokes ACTH release and subsequent rise in plasma ACTH and cortisol levels. A cortisol rise of 5 to 7 μg per 100 ml above base line or an absolute value above 15 μg per 100 ml during the insulin tolerance test in a patient with normal corticotropin-binding globulin indicates a normal ACTH response.

Patients who are not candidates for the insulin tolerance test (see above) may be tested with metyrapone, a blocker of the 11β-hydroxylation step of cortisol synthesis. This block induces ACTH elevations by preventing the normal cortisol feedback inhibition on the hypothalamic-pituitary unit. Exogenous steroid treatment precludes the use of this test. A normal response to oral or intravenous metyrapone may be determined from a rise of 11β-deoxycortisol (compound S) in the blood or by a rise in urinary 17-hydroxycorticosteroids, reflecting increased excretion of metabolites of 11-deoxycortisol. A patient who fails to respond to metyrapone should have documentation that the adrenals respond to exogenous ACTH. Some patients have normal ACTH and cortisol response to

hypoglycemia but not to metyrapone. These patients usually do not need steroid replacement but should be carefully followed for the development of severe ACTH deficiency.

TESTS FOR ADH DEFICIENCY   Evaluation of the patient with suspected diabetes insipidus is described in Chap. 334. The presence of diabetes insipidus usually indicates either vasopressin resistance or a hypothalamic lesion such as craniopharyngioma since ADH is synthesized in the hypothalamus. Lesions restricted to the pituitary usually do not cause diabetes insipidus until stalk or hypothalamic damage occurs. A simple screening test for diabetes insipidus is the determination of the urine osmolality after overnight water deprivation. If the osmolality is below 350 mosmol/kg, a full-scale dehydration test may be indicated.

Treatment   Patients with space-occupying lesions such as craniopharyngioma or pituitary tumors are candidates for surgery and/or irradiation, particularly if there are visual field deficits. Craniopharyngiomas are usually approached by the transfrontal route, as are very large pituitary tumors that extend any distance above the optic chiasm. Transsphenoidal microsurgery is the usual choice in tumors confined to the sella. If tumor removal is incomplete or if the patient is not a candidate for surgery, irradiation with 4500 rads is usually indicated. The use of postoperative irradiation in patients in whom complete removal of a pituitary tumor is not possible may delay or prevent continued growth of the tumor. Patients should have an endocrine evaluation following treatment to determine the need for replacement therapy.

Patients with tumors who have received surgical or radiation treatment should be reevaluated at least annually for progression of their disease. Radiographic evaluation should minimally consist of coned-down views of the sella turcica. Visual fields should be determined, and an endocrine evaluation should include as a minimum measurement of thyroid and adrenal hormone levels in the blood or urine. More extensive tests including provocative tests such as the insulin tolerance or metyrapone tests and evaluation of gonadal function are frequently desirable. Patients with low thyroid or adrenal hormone values or patients who fail to respond to provocative tests should be started on hormone replacement. Once an endocrine deficiency such as TSH or ACTH is documented, return of function is unlikely, and continued testing for that hormone is unnecessary.

Hormone replacement in hypopituitary patients depends on the type and extent of the lesion and the degree of hormone deficit. Human growth hormone is usually given in three intramuscular injections per week to GH-deficient prepubertal children. TSH deficiency is corrected by treatment with oral L-thyroxine 100 to 200 μg daily. Pituitary-adrenal insufficiency can be treated with oral prednisone 5 to 7.5 mg daily in a single dose or hydrocortisone 20 to 30 mg daily in divided doses. Mineralocorticoid replacement is not necessary in hypopituitary patients with normal adrenal glands because aldosterone secretion is maintained in a functionally adequate range. Patients with diabetes insipidus can be controlled with the synthetic vasopressin analogue, 1-desamino-8-D-arginine vasopressin (DDAVP) intranasally or with intramuscular pitressin tannate in oil (see Chap. 334). Partial diabetes insipidus can be treated with chlorpropamide, clofibrate, or thiazide diuretics.

The most difficult form of replacement is that of gonadotropin in infertile patients desiring children. If fertility is not an objective, men may be treated with a long-acting parenteral testosterone preparation such as testosterone enanthate 200 mg every 2 weeks. This will preserve libido, potency, and secondary sexual characteristics such as beard growth. Women may be treated with cyclic estrogen and progesterone. Men or women who desire children must be treated with human gonadotropin preparations including extracts from human urine (containing both FSH and LH activity) and chorionic gonadotropin, which has primarily LH-like activity (see Chap. 341). LHRH over long periods has also been used successfully in some patients.

DISEASES OF ANTERIOR PITUITARY HORMONE HYPERSECRETION Disorders of pituitary hormone hypersecretion occur in patients with functioning adenomas producing either prolactin (galactorrhea-amenorrhea syndrome), growth hormone (acromegaly), or ACTH (Cushing's disease). For unknown reasons, functional adenomas of cells synthesizing the glycoprotein pituitary hormones TSH, LH, and FSH rarely develop. The adenomas responsible for excess prolactin secretion in women are often small and are classified as microadenomas, being less than 10 mm in diameter. ACTH-producing adenomas are also often quite small, while growth hormone-producing tumors and prolactin-producing tumors in men are often large enough to enlarge the sella turcica.

Hyperprolactinemia Recognition and treatment of prolactin-secreting pituitary microadenomas have resulted in major diagnostic and therapeutic advances in the area of pituitary disease. Traditionally, prolactinomas have been associated with the amenorrhea-galactorrhea syndrome in women. However, these hypersecretory adenomas do not always cause either amenorrhea or galactorrhea. Men with prolactin-secreting tumors usually do not have galactorrhea because the male breast lacks adequate development of acini. (For discussion of the differential diagnosis of galactorrhea see Chap. 343.) Prolactin-producing tumors in men usually present as space-occupying lesions, often with hypogonadism. A basal serum prolactin determination in patients with suspected hypothalamic or pituitary disease is extremely useful because (1) prolactin-secreting adenomas are the most common form of pituitary tumor and (2) hypothalamic lesions may cause hyperprolactinemia.

Women with prolactin-producing microadenomas frequently present during the reproductive years. These patients may have galactorrhea, amenorrhea, or both. Libido may be depressed, and some have evidence of decreased estrogens and hirsutism. This has been thought to represent either a depression of ovarian function or stimulation of adrenal androgen secretion. Other clinical manifestations depend on the extent of other anterior pituitary hormone deficiencies. Prolactinomas are now detected frequently in women before other hormone deficiencies develop.

In men, recognition of prolactin-secreting tumors usually occurs only after the tumor has reached a large size and produced the same signs and symptoms as a nonfunctioning tumor (see above). However, small adenomas have been reported in men who present with decreased libido and/or infertility. In some, these symptoms have improved after removal of the adenoma.

DIAGNOSTIC TESTS The diagnostic evaluation of patients with galactorrhea is performed with the goal of detecting patients with pituitary adenoma or other space-occupying lesions. Basal prolactin levels are a critical part of the evaluation. In general, the higher the basal prolactin level, the more likely the patient has a pituitary tumor. Values above 100 to 150 ng/ml usually indicate tumor. Dynamic tests have been used in an effort to distinguish pituitary adenomas from other types of hyperprolactinemia. TRH, which stimulates the lactotrophs,

and chlorpromazine, which interferes with PIF activity, have been used to stimulate prolactin release. Both TRH (400 μg intravenously) and chlorpromazine (CPZ) (25 to 50 mg intramuscularly) cause an increase of prolactin levels to more than double basal values in normal adults. Responses are blunted in patients with high basal levels owing to pituitary adenomas. Many patients with idiopathic galactorrhea give a similar response. An occasional patient with a pituitary tumor and high basal prolactin values is stimulated by TRH, indicating apparent storage of prolactin in the tumor. Patients with other causes of galactorrhea tend to show variable stimulation after either test. L-Dopa suppresses prolactin secretion regardless of etiology and therefore is not useful in determining which patients have adenomas. High basal levels are of considerably greater diagnostic value than the various dynamic tests. After demonstration of an elevated prolactin, the most useful diagnostic studies are radiological. Coned-down views of the sella and polytomography should be performed. These usually distinguish between normal irregularities of the sella floor contour, such as the carotid groove, and a defect produced by a microadenoma. Visual field examinations should also be obtained. However, since prolactin-secreting microadenomas in young women are ordinarily detected while still small, the visual fields are usually normal.

TREATMENT The type of treatment depends on the lesion involved and the original presentation of the patient. The natural history of pituitary microadenomas regarding frequency of subsequent enlargement of the tumors to the point of causing hormone deficiencies or visual field defects is not known. Transsphenoidal microsurgery is potentially curative, and in the hands of a skilled surgeon is accomplished with a low morbidity and low mortality. Complications such as cerebrospinal fluid rhinorrhea and subsequent meningitis or optic-nerve damage are uncommon in centers where the procedure is performed frequently. The recurrence rate of microadenomas is not known, but in many patients postoperative prolactin levels, although lower than before surgery, do not return to the normal range. Large prolactin-secreting tumors often have to be resected via a transfrontal route.

Irradiation with 4500 rads by conventional supravoltage technique has also been successful in lowering prolactin levels. This treatment requires more time for the beneficial effect to occur and is therefore less commonly used.

Medical treatment of hyperprolactinemia and galactorrhea is promising. After L-dopa was shown to reduce prolactin levels, the drug was tried in the treatment of patients with galactorrhea and amenorrhea. Unfortunately, L-dopa, to be effective, had to be given frequently in large doses resulting in nausea and other unpleasant side effects. However, new dopamine agnoists such as bromocryptine, an ergot derivative, are now available and reduce hyperprolactinemia of all etiologies. Women with galactorrhea-amenorrhea frequently have a cessation of galactorrhea, resumption of menses, and restoration of fertility after oral bromocryptine 2.5 mg bid or tid. The suggestion has been made that the drug may also have an antitumor effect, but hyperprolactinemia usually recurs when therapy is stopped. Patients with pituitary tumors who become pregnant after bromocryptine treatment may have enlargement of the pituitary to the point of compression of the optic chiasm. For this reason, patients with radiographic changes suggesting tumor should have definitive surgical treatment.

Disorders of growth hormone excess Both gigantism and acromegaly are the consequence of excess growth hormone secretion by pituitary adenomas. There is also evidence of disordered hypothalamic control or pituitary responsiveness in these patients (e.g., abnormal GH release after TRH or LHRH and the occasional paradoxical increase of GH after glucose).

These abnormalities in GH control plus the fact that acromegaly may appear before a pituitary adenoma is demonstrable have suggested that GH-secreting tumors may be the result of hypothalamic stimulation. However, microadenoma without sellar enlargement may also cause acromegaly. The tumors are usually eosinophilic on light microscopy and can be demonstrated to contain growth hormone granules on electron microscopy.

GIGANTISM When growth hormone hypersecretion occurs prior to puberty and fusion of the epiphyses, gigantism develops. These patients may reach enormous proportions because of massive growth of the skeleton. One was 8 ft 11 in tall and weighed 475 lb prior to his death at age 22. The soft tissues, including the peripheral nerves, are enlarged. Early in the course of the disease, patients may be unusually strong. However, they later may develop pituitary insufficiency with weakness and hypogonadism. Myopathy and severe peripheral sensory and motor neuropathy with findings such as weakness, foot drop, and Charcot-type arthropathy may be prominent in extreme gigantism.

ACROMEGALY When growth hormone-secreting tumors develop after puberty, acromegaly results. The disorder occurs equally in men and women. Approximately 10 to 15 percent of all large pituitary tumors secrete growth hormone and cause acromegaly. Because of the slow progression of the disease, the changes in physical features, which often begin between the second and fourth decades, are frequently not recognized for 10 to 20 years. Since linear growth of the long bones is not possible after epiphyseal fusion, enlargement is most apparent in the acral parts including the hands, feet, nose, and mandible; hence the name *acromegaly*. The extent and course of the clinical disease does not always correlate precisely with GH levels, probably because many GH effects are mediated by the somatomedins. The clinical manifestations of acromegaly are protean and are the result of the excessive secretion of growth hormone combined with the mass effect of the pituitary tumor (Table 333-3).

The patient with acromegaly may note progressive increase in ring, shoe, glove, and hat size after puberty. Increased soft-tissue growth is almost invariably present but may go unnoticed by the patient or family for long periods of time. The increased size of the nose, lips, and soft tissue of the face results in a characteristic coarsening of the facial features (Fig. 333-8). Enlargement of the mandible may be manifested as prognathism with underbite and increased spacing of the lower teeth. The large nose, thick lips, accentuated nasolabial folds, and coarse features cause a characteristic facial appearance in acromegalic patients. The forehead and orbital ridges are prominent in part because of a characteristic enlargement of the frontal sinuses. The tongue enlarges and may show indentations from the teeth. The voice often develops a characteristic deep, cavernous, and husky quality. The feet and hands are fleshy and often grossly enlarged. The broad hands with thick, large fingers have been described as spade-like in appearance. The feet are also characteristically broad, causing a need for extra-wide shoes.

Patients with acromegaly have an increased metabolic rate and usually note increased sweating and sebaceous activity. The skin is warm, moist, and thickened. Other cutaneous changes include small papillomatous lesions over the trunk called *fibromata mollusca*, increased skin pigmentation, and occasionally acanthosis nigricans. Frequently, acromegalic patients have an increased growth of coarse body hair.

Joint complaints are relatively common. Early in the course of the disease there is widening of the joint spaces as a consequence of growth of the cartilage and soft tissues. Later, osteo-

arthritis with pain and limitation of joint motion may occur in several joints including the temporomandibular joint. Degenerative changes in the spine may cause nerve root or cord compression. Prominent muscular development usually occurs as part of the soft-tissue growth. Myopathy and peripheral neuropathy with weakness may occur later in the disease. Paresthesias are a frequent complaint. A carpal tunnel syndrome may be present in about a third of patients because of pressure on the median nerve from tissue enlargement, but not all paresthesias can be explained by this mechanism.

Hypertension is present in about 25 percent, and patients may have cardiac enlargement as a result of the GH excess as well as hypertension. Congestive heart failure may occur. Visceral enlargement also involves the liver, spleen, kidneys, and occasionally the thyroid and adrenals. Glomerular filtration rate in the enlarged kidneys is increased. Thyroid and adrenal function are usually in the normal range.

Glucose intolerance is present in approximately half of acromegalics because hypersecretion of GH causes an insulin-resistant state. Insulin levels are commonly elevated and return to normal after successful treatment and reduction of GH levels. The hyperglycemia of acromegaly is usually well tolerated, although clinical diabetes may occur in patients with a genetic predisposition to the disease. Glycosuria, polydipsia, and polyphagia are found in about 25 percent of patients with advanced illness. The polydipsia is probably best correlated with

TABLE 333-3
Manifestations of acromegaly

	Series 1,* %	Series 2,† %
PRIMARILY FROM GROWTH HORMONE HYPERSECRETION		
Acral enlargement (hands, feet, nose, jaw)	100	96
Soft-tissue overgrowth (heel pad > 22 mm on x-ray)		98
Excessive perspiration	60	88
Joint pain		76
Weight gain	39	76
Hypertrichosis	53	
Voice change		50
Paresthesias	30	62
Cutaneous pigmentation	46	
Acanthosis nigricans		26
Fibromata mollusca	27	38
Enlarged thyroid	25	18
Glucose intolerance		56
Glycosuria	25	
Clinical diabetes mellitus	12	8
Hypertension		23
Cardiac symptoms		12
Lactation	4	8
PRIMARILY FROM PITUITARY TUMOR ENLARGEMENT		
Enlargement of sella on x-ray	93	90
Headache	87	64
Visual disturbances	62	
Photophobia	12	46
COMBINED EFFECTS INCLUDING HYPOPITUITARISM		
Drowsiness, fatigue, and lethargy	42	82
Amenorrhea‡	73	32
Decreased libido	38	27
Asthenia	33	

* *From a series of 100 patients reported by L Davidoff, Endocrinology 10:461, 1926.*
† *From a series of 50 patients reported by S Levin, Calif Med 116:57, 1972, and Am J Med 57:526, 1974.*
‡ *Percent of women.*

FIGURE 333-8
Progressive development of acromegalic features. A. Age 30. B. Age 37. C. Age 40. (Courtesy of N Kaplan.)

glycosuria, although diabetes insipidus may rarely be present. Hypermetabolism and hyperhidrosis contribute to both the polydipsia and polyphagia.

The pituitary enlargement produces symptoms and signs similar to other space-occupying lesions of the sella. Headaches are extremely common and may be bitemporal or variable in location. Visual complaints are frequent and include decreased vision and photophobia. As the GH-secreting tumor enlarges, normal pituitary function is often compromised. Asthenia, fatigue, lethargy, amenorrhea, and decreased libido probably are the consequence of several factors including the metabolic effects of GH, myopathy, neuropathy, and variable degrees of hypopituitarism.

Other endocrine diseases may be associated with acromegaly. The autosomal dominant syndrome of multiple endocrine neoplasia, type I (Wermer syndrome), consisting of adenomas of the pituitary, pancreas, and parathyroids may be manifest as acromegaly. Galactorrhea may be present in women with tumors that secrete both GH and prolactin. The hypermetabolism and thyroid enlargement of acromegaly are usually the result of GH excess alone. However, true thyrotoxicosis occasionally occurs.

The x-ray changes are often striking. In the past, approximately 90 percent of patients with acromegaly had an enlarged sella turcica at the time of diagnosis. The combination of frontal sinus enlargement with an increased sella size is suggestive of the diagnosis. Radiological evaluation should therefore include careful studies of the sella including tomograms to evaluate the possibility of extension of the tumor into the sphenoid sinus. CT scan or pneumoencephalogram should be used to evaluate the possibility and extent of suprasellar extension. Another useful radiographic finding is thickening of the soft tissue of the heel pad which usually exceeds 22 mm in acromegalic patients. Late in the disease the ends of the distal phalanges of the hands may develop a tufted appearance on x-ray which resembles an arrowhead. The bony enlargement of the hands and feet may be combined with decreased bone density that is particularly apparent in the metatarsals. Osteophyte formation and osteoarthritis are prominent changes which increase with age.

Careful visual fields and full opthalmologic examination should be performed because of the relatively high frequency of visual field abnormalities. The classic bitemporal hemianopsia from compression of the optic chiasm by the tumor mass may be present. However, as is true for all pituitary tumors, visual field defects may vary from a unilateral small quadrantic defect to extensive bilateral defects. Occasionally papilledema or optic atrophy may be present in patients with extensive tumors.

The diagnosis of acromegaly is made on the basis of the characteristic clinical and radiographic features combined with inappropriately elevated growth hormone levels. A useful laboratory test is the measurement of growth hormone during the glucose tolerance test. In normal persons growth hormone values at 30 to 90 min after the ingestion of 100 g glucose are suppressed to less than 5 ng/ml. Acromegalic patients do not suppress and occasionally show a paradoxical increase in growth hormone after glucose. Patients with diabetes, uremia, chronic starvation, or acute intermittent porphyria also may show a poor GH suppression after glucose. Another diagnostic test is the growth hormone response to TRH. Normal patients have no GH response to TRH, whereas acromegalic patients have an abnormal release. Patients with anorexia nervosa, depression, uremia, hypothyroidism, and protein-calorie deprivation may also have an abnormal GH response to TRH, but the diagnosis is usually obvious. Evaluation of other anterior pituitary hormones including the gonadotropins, TSH, and ACTH should be performed as described previously.

The routine laboratory evaluation of the patient with acromegaly may disclose hyperglycemia and glycosuria. Overt diabetes mellitus is present in only about 10 percent of patients and usually is limited to those with a positive family history for diabetes. The serum phosphate may be elevated from the excess growth hormone.

TREATMENT Although acromegaly is a slowly progressive disorder, there is an increased incidence of cardiovascular complications, and treatment is indicated. There are several methods for treating the pituitary tumor. Transfrontal surgery may be required for large tumors, while transsphenoidal microsurgery is successful in removing small adenomas. Growth hormone levels fall rapidly to normal after sucessful surgery. The other major type of treatment is irradiation. Both proton beam or heavy-particle treatment and conventional supravoltage irradiation can reduce growth hormone values in 90 percent of patients, although the latter method may require several years for a full therapeutic effect. Both surgery and irradiation may be necessary to control tumor growth. Patients should be monitored at 6- to 12-month intervals for the possible development of other anterior pituitary hormone deficiencies.

Several medical treatments for acromegaly such as estrogen, medroxyprogesterone, and chlorpromazine have been attempted in the past with limited success. Somatostatin lowers growth hormone levels, but, since it must be infused to sustain this effect, it is not useful in treatment. However, dopamine agonists such as bromocryptine lower growth hormone levels in some patients. This does not represent definitive therapy but may be useful as adjunctive treatment in patients with galactorrhea, diabetes mellitus, or cardiovascular complications who are not candidates for surgery and whose growth hormone levels do not fall promptly after radiation.

ACTH hypersecretion (see also Chap. 336) Cushing's disease is the consequence of oversecretion of ACTH by the pituitary.

This should not be confused with Cushing's *syndrome,* which is a nonspecific term indicating increased glucocorticoid levels from any source, including iatrogenic steroid administration. ACTH secretion tends to be sustained throughout the day in patients with Cushing's disease with loss of the usual diurnal variation of plasma ACTH and cortisol levels. ACTH release is impaired after stress such as insulin-induced hypoglycemia, and there is a decreased sensitivity of ACTH secretion to steroid feedback inhibition; i.e., glucocorticoids in physiological amounts do not suppress ACTH secretion, although supraphysiological steroid levels are effective. The dexamethasone-suppresion test is designed to test for this abnormal feedback sensitivity. Most patients with Cushing's disease do not show suppression of glucocorticoids in plasma or urine after dexamethasone (2 mg per day given as 0.5 mg every 6 h) equivalent to more than twice the normal glucocorticoid requirement. However, suppression of plasma cortisol to < 5 μg per 100 ml or urinary 17-hydroxysteroids to < 3 mg per gram of creatinine may occur with amounts of dexamethasone (8 mg per day given as 2 mg every 6 h) approximately 10 times the normal replacement equivalent of cortisol. While the hypothalamic-pituitary axis remains partially responsive to feedback control (albeit at an abnormal level), most patients with Cushing's disease have identifiable pituitary adenomas. This raises the possibility that the adenomas develop as a result of abnormal hypothalamic stimulation. If large pituitary adenomas are present, suppression of ACTH secretion can be demonstrated only after much larger doses of dexamethasone, if at all. Some patients with a primary psychiatric depression have elevated serum and urinary cortisol levels with a loss of normal diurnal variation and may have abnormal response to dexamethasone suppression as well. Since patients with Cushing's disease often have depression, this may cause confusion. However, patients with depression tend to have a normal ACTH release to stress, while patients with Cushing's disease do not.

The pituitary adenomas in Cushing's disease are usually small, and less than 10 percent of patients have an enlarged sella turcica. The approach to diagnosis of Cushing's disease is discussed in Chap. 336. Cushing initially treated patients by hypophysectomy, but subsequently this procedure was replaced by bilateral adrenalectomy. However, although adrenalectomy is appropriate in some patients with severe disease, the primary problem is not in the adrenals but in the hypothalamus or pituitary. A few patients who have had adrenalectomy without pituitary treatment develop *Nelson's syndrome.* This is a more aggressive ACTH-secreting tumor that may be locally invasive and difficult to manage. Patients with Nelson's syndrome frequently develop severe visual field defects from the enlarging tumor and usually have hyperpigmentation from ACTH or β-lipotropin hypersecretion.

The recent advances in transsphenoidal microsurgery have reestablished pituitary surgery in the treatment of Cushing's disease. Selective removal of the adenoma can be accomplished in many instances with good clinical results. Proton beam or conventional supravoltage irradiation has also been used successfully in many patients. Adrenalectomy is still required in patients with severe disease and in patients who do not respond to other measures. In patients undergoing adrenalectomy, prophylactic pituitary radiation has been advocated to prevent the development of Nelson's syndrome, but the latter has occurred in some patients despite radiation. Medical treatment of the glucocorticoid hypersecretion may be attempted with metyrapone, which blocks 11β-hydroxylation, with *o,p'-*DDD (mitotane), which has a direct toxic effect on the adrenal, or with cyproheptadine, which acts through a central mechanism to decrease ACTH secretion. Although medical treatment may be useful in the patient who is a poor candidate for surgery or radiation, definitive therapy is ultimately required. The choice depends to some degree on the surgical expertise and equipment available. Although proton beam radiation is frequently successful and conventional radiation reduces ACTH to normal levels in about 25 percent of patients, transsphenoidal selective microsurgery is the treatment of choice in most medical centers.

MISCELLANEOUS HYPERSECRETORY SYNDROMES   In contrast to prolactin, growth hormone, and ACTH, hypersecretion of the glycoprotein hormones TSH, LH, and FSH by pituitary tumors rarely occurs. The few reported LH- and FSH-secreting pituitary tumors developed in patients with gonadal insufficiency who may have had a stimulus to increased gonadotropin secretion from lack of feedback inhibition. Autonomous production apparently occurred subsequent to compensatory hypersecretion. TSH-producing pituitary tumors causing hyperthyroidism have been documented in only a few patients.

Ectopic secretion of essentially all pituitary hormones by carcinomas of nonendocrine tissues has been reported (see Chap. 347). Ecotopic ACTH production is not uncommon, particularly by carcinomas of the lung. This must be considered in the differential diagnosis of hypersecretion of adrenal steroids. Because of the rapid progression and short duration of the illness, such patients usually present with wasting and with metabolic effects such as hypokalemia rather than the typical cushingoid appearance. Ectopic gonadotropin secretion is also common in malignancies of the lung, gastrointestinal tract, and testis. Male patients may present with gynecomastia. However, the gonadotropin usually has the characteristics of HCG rather than pituitary LH or FSH. Ectopic secretion of alpha subunit that is common for LH and HCG also occurs without causing clinical manifestations and may be used as a tumor marker. Ectopic secretion of growth hormone, LH, FSH, or prolactin may be difficult to detect because of the continuous pituitary secretion of these hormones.

REFERENCES

BANNA M: Craniopharyngioma: Based on 160 cases. Br J Radiol 49:206, 1976

BOYD AE III et al: Galactorrhea-amenorrhea syndrome: Diagnosis and therapy. Ann Intern Med 87:165, 1977

BURGER HG, PATEL YC: Thyrotropin releasing hormone—TRH. Clin Endocrinol Metab 6:83, 1977

CHILD DF et al: Prolactin studies in "functionless" pituitary tumors. Br Med J 1:604, 1975

DEL POZO E, LANCRANJAN I: Clinical use of drugs modifying the release of anterior pituitary hormone, in *Frontiers in Neuroendocrinology,* vol 5, WF Ganong, L Martini (eds). New York, Raven Press, 1978

FRANTZ A: Prolactin. N Engl J Med 298:201, 1978

HARDY J: Transsphenoidal surgery of hypersecreting pituitary tumors, in *Diagnosis and Treatment of Pituitary Tumors,* PO Kohler, GT Ross (eds). New York, American Elsevier, 1973, p 179

JORDAN RM et al: The primary empty sella syndrome. Am J Med 62:569, 1977

KLEINBERG DL et al: Galactorrhea: A study of 235 cases, including 48 with pituitary tumors. N Engl J Med 296:589, 1977

KOHLER PO, ROSS GT (eds): *Diagnosis and Treatment of Pituitary Tumors.* New York, American Elsevier, 1973

KREIGER DT, GLICK SM: Growth hormone and cortisol responsiveness in Cushing's syndrome. Am J Med 52:25, 1972

LIN T, TUCCI JR: Provocative tests of growth hormone release. Ann Intern Med 80:464, 1974

MARTIN JB et al (eds): *Clinical Neuroendocrinology.* Philadelphia, Davis, 1977

MORTIMER RH et al: Correlation between integrated LH and FSH levels and the response to luteinizing hormone releasing factor (LRF). J Clin Endocrinol Metab 43:1240, 1976

NEELON FA et al: The primary empty sella: Clinical and radiographic characteristics and endocrine function. Medicine 52:73, 1973

NELSON DH et al: ACTH-producing pituitary tumors following adrenalectomy for Cushing's syndrome. Ann Intern Med 52:560, 1960

ONTJES DA, NEY RL: Tests of anterior pituitary function. Metabolism 21:159, 1972

REICHLIN S: Regulation of the hypophysiotropic secretions of the brain. Arch Intern Med 135:1350, 1975

REICHLIN S et al (eds): *The Hypothalamus.* New York, Raven Press, 1978

SMITH LH, LEVIN SR: Manifestations and treatment of acromegaly. Calif Med 116:57, 1972

TYRELL JB et al: Cushing's disease: Selective trans-sphenoidal resection of pituitary microadenomas. N Engl J Med 298:753, 1978

YEN SSC, JAFFEE RB (eds): *Reproductive Endocrinology.* Philadelphia, Saunders, 1978

FIGURE 334-1

Structures of vasopressin and oxytocin.

334
DISORDERS OF THE NEUROHYPOPHYSIS

DAVID H. P. STREETEN
ARNOLD M. MOSES
MYRON MILLER

Axons extend from neurons in the supraoptic and paraventricular nuclei of the hypothalamus through the pituitary stalk to the posterior pituitary. Hormone formed within the ganglion cells migrates down the axons and is stored in secretory granules in the nerve terminals located in the neurohypophysis. By the process of exocytosis, the vasopressin or oxytocin is released from the granules and reaches the bloodstream. There is increasingly convincing evidence that there are two hypothalamoneurohypophyseal systems with largely distinct and independent functions. The first comprises neurons located mainly in the supraoptic nuclei from which axons extend down the supraopticoneurohypophyseal tract to release ADH or vasopressin, a hormone predominantly concerned with the control of water conservation. This system is closely related to the thirst center, which regulates fluid intake. The second system originates mainly in the neurons of the paraventricular nuclei, from which axons descend into the neurohypophysis and release oxytocin, a hormone which stimulates uterine contraction and milk ejection.

SUPRAOPTICONEUROHYPOPHYSEAL SYSTEM AND ADH

CHEMISTRY Antidiuretic hormone (ADH, vasopressin) is a nonapeptide which comprises six amino acids in a ring and a side chain of three amino acids attached to the cystine (Fig. 334-1). A carrier protein called *neurophysin*, which is probably vasopressin-specific, is synthesized in association with ADH. ADH and neurophysin are transported along the axons of the supraopticoneurohypophyseal tract and stored in the neurohypophysis.

PHYSIOLOGY The release of ADH into the circulation is influenced by a number of stimuli (Fig. 334-2). Under normal conditions, ADH release is primarily regulated by osmorecep-

tors, which are probably located in the supraoptic nucleus. Release of ADH is usually accompanied by neurophysin release. In addition to osmotic influences on ADH release, there are volume receptors in the left atrium and baroreceptors in the aorta and carotid arteries, where impulses are perceived and relayed to the hypothalamus via the vagi to produce tonic and episodic inhibition of vasopressin release. The neurotransmitter acetylcholine appears to be the final link connecting the stimulatory and inhibitory pathways affecting ADH release to the supraoptic neurons.

FIGURE 334-2

Schematic representation of control of ADH release and cellular action of ADH.

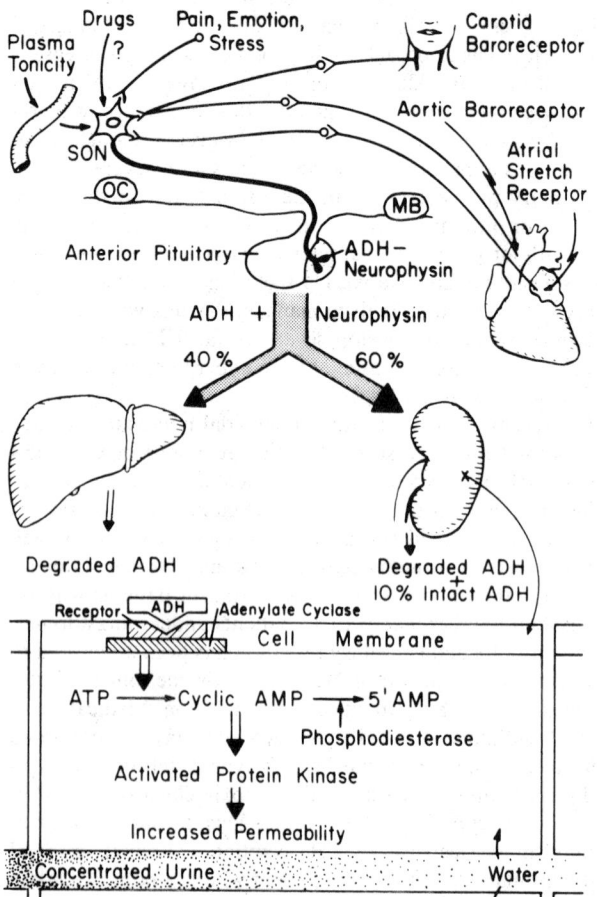

ADH acts to conserve water and concentrate urine by enhancing the hydroosmotic flow of water from the luminal fluid through the cells of the collecting tubule of the kidney to the medullary interstitium. This action of ADH assists in maintaining constancy of the osmolality and volume of body fluids. High concentrations of ADH can cause vasoconstriction, as may occur in response to severe hypotension or to infusion of vasopressin (Pitressin) for treatment of bleeding esophageal varices.

ADH has been assayed biologically by measuring its antidiuretic or pressor action in experimental animals. More recently ADH has been quantitated in blood and urine by radioimmunoassay. The results may be expressed as units or fractions of units based on pressor activity in the rat, or in terms of weight of purified vasopressin. Arginine vasopressin has a biological activity of approximately 400 units per milligram. The human neurohypophysis under conditions of random fluid intake contains approximately 8 units of ADH. Under the same conditions peripheral plasma ADH concentration in humans ranges from 1 to 3 μU/ml. The ADH concentration of blood fluctuates, with a maximum concentration late at night and in the early morning, and a minimum in the early afternoon. Under conditions of normal hydration, healthy subjects excrete approximately 10 to 35 mU ADH in 24 h, while releasing 400 to 550 mU from the pituitary. During 24 to 28 h of dehydration the amount released increases three to five times with corresponding increases in plasma and urinary ADH levels.

Inactivation of ADH occurs largely in liver and kidneys, a major mechanism being the cleavage of the terminal glycinamide to produce a biologically inactive substance. Approximately 10 percent of secreted ADH is excreted in the urine as biologically and immunologically active hormone.

OSMOREGULATION It is thought that ADH is released in proportion to the osmotic effect of changes in plasma solutes to which the cellular membrane is impermeable. It is generally considered that changes in volume of the osmoreceptor cells caused by changes in plasma osmolality alter the electrical activity of these neurons and the consequent release of ADH. There is evidence from animal studies that osmotic changes which stimulate release also enhance production of ADH. The servomechanism between effective plasma osmolality and vasopressin release normally maintains plasma osmolality within a very narrow range. The mean plasma osmolality of normal subjects following a water load of 20 ml per kilogram of body weight is 281.7 mosmol/kg, while that which initiates ADH release following infusion of hypertonic saline into waterloaded subjects is 287.3 mosmol/kg. Thus the increase in plasma osmolality from full diuresis to the initiation of antidiuresis by hypertonic saline is only 5.6 mosmol/kg, or 2 percent.

The infusion of hypertonic saline at a constant rate into water-loaded human subjects causes a linear rise in plasma osmolality with time. After an interval which depends on the infusion rate and the concentration of the saline, there is an abrupt, progressive fall in free water clearance without a significant change in solute or creatinine excretion. The plasma osmolality at the initiation of antidiuresis under these conditions has been called the osmotic threshold for vasopressin release, and in 73 normal subjects occurred at a mean plasma osmolality of 287.3 mosmol/kg.

VOLUME REGULATION Decreases in plasma volume, through effects on stretch receptors in the left atrium and perhaps the pulmonary veins, stimulate the release of ADH by reducing the tonic inhibitory impulses from the left atrium to the hypothalamus. The neural impulses travel via the vagi to the reticular formation of the midbrain and diencephalon and thence to the supraoptic nuclei, where they are integrated with the other stimuli which affect ADH release. Positive pressure breathing, quiet standing, and vasodilatation due to heat may activate this mechanism, which serves to restore plasma volume, even at times overriding osmotic inhibition of ADH release. Circulating ADH concentrations following volume stimulation may reach 10 times the levels induced by hypertonicity. Increased plasma volume inhibits ADH release by the reverse mechanisms leading to a diuresis and the correction of the hypervolemia. Negative pressure breathing, recumbency, lack of gravitational force as occurs in space travel, submersion in water, and exposure to cold may activate this mechanism.

BARORECEPTOR REGULATION Activation of carotid and aortic baroreceptors in response to hypotension causes the release of ADH. Hypotension due to blood loss is the most potent stimulus to ADH release and may raise plasma levels of ADH to approach 1000 μU/ml at times. These very high concentrations of ADH may cause marked vasoconstriction, which probably plays a role in the restoration of blood pressure.

NEUROGENIC, PSYCHOGENIC, PHARMACOLOGIC, AND OTHER INFLUENCES Aside from the regulation of ADH release by osmolality, volume, and blood pressure, other factors may exert a major, even overriding, effect on the release of ADH. Both cholinergic and beta-adrenergic stimuli release ADH, while atropine and alpha-adrenergic stimulation inhibit ADH release, apparently by actions on the hypothalamus. Emotional stress, emesis, and pain may overcome a diuresis. A diuresis may follow hypnotic suggestion, psychologic conditioning, and inhalation of carbon dioxide. The above observations indicate that higher neural centers may alter ADH release. Recent evidence indicates that angiotensin, which has been shown to stimulate thirst, may also lead to the release of ADH by actions on the central nervous system. Beta endorphin has also been implicated in ADH release. Pharmacologic agents which may stimulate ADH release include nicotine, morphine, barbiturates, vincristine, cyclophosphamide, clofibrate, chlorpropamide, and some of the tricyclic anticonvulsants and antidepressants. Ethanol has long been recognized to have diuretic properties and to inhibit neurohypophyseal function under a variety of conditions. Recently, some narcotic antagonists have been found to inhibit ADH release. Experimentally chlorpromazine, reserpine, and diphenylhydantoin all diminish the depletion of pituitary vasopressin and the rise in urinary excretion of ADH, resulting from water deprivation. In humans, diphenylhydantoin, clonidine, and chlorpromazine all inhibit ADH release and may produce diuresis.

ADH RESPONSE TO WATER DEPRIVATION AND TO WATER LOAD Water deprivation provides both an osmotic and a volume stimulus to vasopressin release by increasing plasma osmolality and decreasing plasma volume. The maximum urinary osmolality reached after water deprivation varies considerably, depending on renal medullary osmolality and other intrarenal factors. In response to fluid deprivation for 18 to 24 h in normal individuals, plasma osmolality rarely rises above 292 mosmol/kg. The resultant stimulation of ADH release increases plasma ADH concentration to 6 to 10 μU/ml.

The administration of water lowers plasma osmolality and expands blood volume, inhibiting the release of ADH via both the osmoreceptor and the atrial volume receptor mechanisms. An oral water load of 20 ml/kg in normal adults, which results in a fall in plasma osmolality to a mean of 281.7 mosmol/kg, causes a maximum diuresis in approximately 1 to 1½ h with the free water clearance rising to approximately 12 ml/min and the urine osmolality falling to 40 to 60 mosmol/kg. The delay in reaching maximal diuresis is accounted for by the time involved in absorption of water from the gut, in metabolizing previously secreted vasopressin, and in renal recovery from the action of vasopressin. The half-life of vasopressin in the blood of humans is approximately tripled by hydration to 16 to 17 min. In response to a water load, ADH release is diminished, with a consequent fall in plasma and urinary ADH to very low levels.

INTERACTION OF OSMOTIC AND VOLUME INFLUENCES ON ADH RELEASE   Under conditions of water deprivation and of water loading, volume and osmotic influences on ADH release act in parallel. In other circumstances, when volume and osmotic influences on ADH release may be competitive, minor changes in plasma volume can significantly modify hypertonic stimuli to ADH release. Under the relatively nonstressful conditions of daily life, osmotic factors probably predominate to maintain plasma osmolality within a very narrow range. Larger changes in blood volume, such as those induced by hemorrhage, may blunt and eventually overcome the osmotic influences. Hypotension leading to the activation of arterial baroreceptors exerts a powerful stimulus to the elaboration of ADH which may override simultaneous inhibiting influences.

EFFECTS OF GLUCOCORTICOIDS   The antagonism between the hormones of the adrenal cortex and the posterior pituitary on water excretion has been recognized for years. Glucocorticoids protect against water intoxication and overcome the impaired response to water loading in adrenal insufficiency. Cortisol elevates the osmotic threshold for ADH release determined by hypertonic saline infusion in water-loaded normal subjects.

The subnormal ability to dilute the urine manifested by patients with adrenal insufficiency may in part be due to excessive circulating ADH. However, there is also evidence that glucocorticoids can act directly on the renal tubules to decrease water permeability and to increase solute-free water in the absence of ADH. At present it is not clear which mechanism predominates.

CELLULAR MECHANISM OF ADH ACTIVITY   Our present understanding of the biochemical basis for the action of ADH on the renal tubule (Fig. 334-2) is that (1) ADH binds to specific contraluminal receptor sites; (2) the receptor-hormone complex is coupled to and activates the adenylate cyclase on the same contraluminal membrane; (3) the production of cyclic AMP from ATP is increased; (4) the cyclic AMP is translocated to the luminal cell membrane where it causes the activation of membrane-bound protein kinase; (5) the activated protein kinase causes the phosphorylation of membrane proteins; and (6) permeability of the luminal membrane to water is increased. The ADH-generated cyclic AMP may be inactivated by cytosolic cyclic AMP phosphodiesterase which converts cyclic AMP to 5'-AMP.

The entire sequence of events leading to the transtubular movement of water depends on the integrity of the microtubular system of the epithelial cells. The above biochemical events lead to the passive flow of water along an osmotic gradient across the collecting tubule. The physiologic effect of vasopressin is accompanied by anatomic changes, including cell swelling, vacuolization, expansion of the medullary interstitium, and widening of the lateral intercellular spaces of the collecting

ducts. The latter changes indicate that fluid resorption during ADH-induced antidiuresis occurs in part by way of lateral intercellular channels.

Various cations and drugs can influence the action of ADH. Calcium, lithium, and prostaglandin E_1 inhibit the adenylate cyclase response to vasopressin. Lithium also interferes with a subsequent biochemical action, as does potassium deficiency. Demethylchlortetracycline inhibits adenylate cyclase stimulation by ADH and also inhibits the cyclic AMP-dependent protein kinase. In contrast, chlorpropamide increases the ADH-induced activation of adenylate cyclase.

DEFICIENCY OF VASOPRESSIN: DIABETES INSIPIDUS

Diabetes insipidus is a disorder due to impaired renal conservation of water which results from low blood levels of ADH, reflecting deficient vasopressin release in response to normal physiologic stimuli. This uncommon disorder is being recognized more frequently by studying the mildly excessive water turnover of patients who have undergone pituitary ablation (by hypophysectomy, cryosurgery, or radioactive isotope implants) and of patients with or without known pituitary lesions.

PATHOPHYSIOLOGY   Deficiency of vasopressin release in response to the appropriate stimuli may result from lesions at a variety of functional sites in the physiologic chain of events which culminates in discharge of the hormone into the bloodstream. For conceptual purposes four types of diabetes insipidus can be defined. Patients of the first type show very little rise in urine osmolality with increasing plasma osmolality (1, Fig. 334-3) and no evidence of ADH release during hypertonic saline infusion. They are essentially devoid of releasable ADH. In patients of the second type there is an abrupt increase in urine osmolality during dehydration (2, Fig. 334-3), but also without evidence of an osmotic threshold during saline infusion. These patients have a defective osmoreceptor mechanism, but are capable of releasing ADH with a hypovolemic stimulus, resulting from severe dehydration. The third type of patient has some rise in urine osmolality with increasing plasma osmolality (3, Fig. 334-3) and has an elevated saline osmotic threshold for ADH release. These patients have a sluggish ADH release mechanism and may be said to have a high-set osmoreceptor. The fourth type of patient has urine and plasma osmolality coordinates just to the right of normal (4, Fig. 334-3) and a normal saline osmotic threshold. ADH release in these patients is initiated at a normal plasma osmolality but is subnormal in amount.

The second to fourth types of patients may develop a good antidiuresis in response to nausea, nicotine, acetyl-β-methylcholine (Mecholyl), chlorpropamide, or clofibrate. In rare instances patients of the second to fourth types may have largely asymptomatic hypernatremia associated with loss of thirst and mild or absent evidence of diabetes insipidus. Reduction in the number of supraoptic neurons may be the cause of deficient ADH production in some patients who clinically present with idiopathic "diabetes insipidus." It is known that removal of the posterior lobe of the pituitary induces permanent diabetes insipidus but only if the pituitary stalk is sectioned high enough to induce retrograde degeneration of most of the neurons of the supraoptic nucleus.

ETIOLOGY   Of 51 patients (34 males and 17 females) who satisfied the criteria described under "Diagnostic Tests" (below) and who had had diabetes insipidus for at least 3 months, findings were as follows. (1) In 20 patients, diabetes insipidus resulted from various types of *neoplastic or infiltrative lesions* of the hypothalamoneurohypophyseal system. In addition to the

FIGURE 334-3
Relation of plasma and urinary osmolality in normal adult subjects (shaded area) and in four types of patients with diabetes insipidus.

lesions encountered in this series, other types of malignant metastases (such as carcinoma of the lung and lymphoma), sarcoid, hemorrhage, abscess, meningitis, tuberculosis, and syphilis have been described as occasional causes of diabetes insipidus. (2) An increasingly frequent cause of diabetes insipidus (9 patients) is *surgical procedures in the region of the hypothalamoneurohypophyseal system.* These include hypophysectomy by surgical excision, cryosurgery, implantation of ⁹⁰Y and other radioactive isotopes, and heavy particle irradiation used for known tumors or for other lesions of the system or as a palliative procedure for diabetic retinopathy and metastatic carcinoma of the breast. Experience has confirmed the experimental finding in animals that surgically induced diabetes insipidus usually appears between 1 and 6 days after the operation. It often disappears after being present for a few days, and may remain absent or may recur and become chronic after an "interphase" of 1 to 5 days. (3) A third major group of patients (8 of the 51) developed diabetes insipidus after *severe head injuries,* usually, if not always, associated with fractures of the skull. This type of diabetes insipidus may last indefinitely but frequently lasts only a few days and sometimes (in 2 of our 8 patients) disappears spontaneously after several months or years, presumably because of regeneration of disrupted supraoptic axons within the pituitary stalk. (4) In a fourth group of patients (15 of 51) none of the currently available diagnostic procedures has been successful in revealing the cause. Some of these patients with *idiopathic diabetes insipidus* have other features of hypothalamic and/or pituitary disease, such as subnormal stature, hypopituitarism, galactorrhea, and narcolepsy, and they presumably have functional or anatomic lesions of other systems in the hypothalamus or the pituitary, in addition to their dysfunction in the supraopticoneurohypophyseal system. The association of diabetes insipidus with anorexia nervosa has been reported recently. Though no evidence of tumor can be found in these patients, the continued awareness of this possibility is sometimes rewarded by the finding of sellar enlargement after long-term follow-up. Occasional patients with such apparently isolated, idiopathic deficiency of vasopressin have come to autopsy, where a striking decrease in the number

or virtual absence of ganglion cells has been found in the supraoptic and paraventricular nuclei, associated with loss of Nissl substance in the remaining neurons and obvious gliosis. The neurohypophysis was reduced in size in these patients. It seems likely, therefore, that the reduced number of supraoptic neurons is the cause of the vasopressin deficiency in these patients. In some patients with idiopathic diabetes insipidus the disorder is inherited as a mendelian dominant.

CLINICAL MANIFESTATIONS *Polyuria, excessive thirst,* and *polydipsia* are the only clinical features that are almost invariably present in diabetes insipidus. Characteristically these symptoms are sudden in onset, both when the disorder first presents itself and whenever the effects of administered vasopressin disappear during the long-term therapy of patients with the disorder. In severe cases, the urine is pale in color, and its volume may be immense (up to 16 to 24 liters per day), requiring micturition at intervals of 30 to 60 min throughout the day and night. Much more frequently, however, the urine volume is only mildly to moderately excessive (2.5 to 6 liters per day), and very occasionally it may be less than 2 liters per day, causing no complaints on the part of the patient. Urinary concentration is well below that of the serum (290 mosmol/kg, specific gravity 1.010) in severe cases but may be higher (290 to 600 mosmol/kg) in patients with mild diabetes insipidus (which should not be called "partial" since most patients can be shown to have small amounts of ADH in their plasma and urine and usually respond to therapy with chlorpropamide).

The slight rise in serum osmolality in consequence of hypotonic polyuria stimulates thirst. Large volumes of fluid are imbibed and cold drinks are preferred, the patients often going to great trouble to secure refrigerated fluids. Although thirst is probably secondary to loss of water in this disorder, the administration of vasopressin often relieves or reduces thirst, even in the absence of fluid intake by the patient.

Normal function of the thirst center ensures that polydipsia closely matches polyuria, so that dehydration is seldom detectable except by the frequently observed mild elevation of serum osmolality. However, when adequate replenishment of water lost by excretion is interfered with, dehydration may become severe, causing weakness, fever, psychic disturbances, prostration, and even death. These clinical features are associated with a rising serum osmolality and serum sodium concentration, the latter sometimes exceeding 175 meq per liter. Dehydration may result from impaired function of the hypothalamic thirst center because of extension of the same abnormality that caused the diabetes insipidus. More frequently, dehydration occurs during unconsciousness produced by surgical anesthesia, head trauma, or other causes. It is particularly hazardous to administer large volumes of isotonic saline intravenously or of hyperosmolar protein preparations by nasogastric tube unless adequate amounts of water or hypotonic fluids are administered simultaneously during unconsciousness in patients with untreated diabetes insipidus.

Hydronephrosis is a rare complication of the polyuria, especially in patients who fail to empty their bladders adequately because of uretheral strictures or for other reasons.

DIAGNOSTIC TESTS Assessment of the relation of plasma to urine osmolality The normal relationship between plasma osmolality (assuming no increase in blood urea or glucose) and urine osmolality is indicated in Fig. 334-3. If several simultaneously determined plasma and urine osmolalities in a patient with polyuria fall substantially to the right of the shaded area, the patient has diabetes insipidus or nephrogenic diabetes insipidus. The latter diagnosis can be made if plasma ADH concentration is increased or if the response to injected vasopressin is subnormal (see "Dehydration Test," below). The procedure of relating plasma to urine osmolality is very useful, particularly in postoperative neurosurgical cases or after head trauma, where its use can lead quickly to the differentiation of diabetes insipidus from parenteral fluid excess. In patients with suspected diabetes insipidus whose plasma and urine osmolality coordinates fall just within the normal area or only slightly to the right, the patient's intravenous hydration can be slowed temporarily and repeat plasma and urine osmolalities obtained, or the dehydration test indicated below may be performed.

Dehydration test Comparison of the renal concentrating capacity after dehydration and after vasopressin administration is a simple and reliable way of diagnosing diabetes insipidus and of differentiating vasopressin deficiency from other causes of polyuria.

The maximal urinary concentrating capacity is widely variable between individuals, and no absolute lower limits of "normal" can be defined in patients with nonspecific illnesses in whom vasopressin is produced in adequate amounts. It is impossible to distinguish between deficiency and sufficiency of vasopressin release by the absolute level of the urinary osmolality attained after specified periods of water deprivation. On the other hand, if after prolonged dehydration vasopressin administration induces a further rise in urinary osmolality, there is a strong implication that vasopressin deficiency exists. In patients with diabetes insipidus, plasma and urinary levels of ADH are low in relationship to plasma osmolality after dehydration. However, ADH measurements are seldom necessary for the diagnosis of diabetes insipidus.

PROCEDURE

1 Fluids are withheld long enough to accomplish stable hourly urinary osmolalities (with an hourly increase of < 30 mosmol/kg in at least three successive hours). This is usually associated with a loss in body weight of at least 1 kg. In patients whose daily urinary volumes exceed 10 liters, the fluid deprivation should begin at 4 A.M. or 6 A.M. so that the patient can be carefully watched and the test terminated if weight loss exceeds 2 kg or the clinical condition deteriorates. In most other polyuric patients whose urinary volumes are less than 10 liters per day, it is preferable to start fluid deprivation at 6 P.M. or midnight and to continue to withhold fluids until noon the following day.

2 Urine specimens are collected hourly for osmolality measurements, from 6 A.M. at least until noon, and preferably until the osmolality has been stable for 3 h.

3 At 11 A.M. (if dehydration started at 6 P.M.) or after the third hour of stable urinary osmolalities, the patient is given vasopressin as 5 U aqueous Pitressin by subcutaneous injection.

4 Serum osmolality is determined immediately before the injection of vasopressin, and urinary osmolality is measured during the hour after the injection.

Vital signs should be monitored during the dehydration procedure, but when the test has been done as described, adverse effects are extremely rare.

INTERPRETATION In subjects with normal neurohypophyseal function, urinary osmolality never rises by more than 9 percent after the injection of Pitressin, whatever the maximal urinary osmolality might be after dehydration alone (Fig. 334-4). In diabetes insipidus of central origin, the rise in urinary osmolality after Pitressin always exceeds 9 percent (Fig. 334-5). To ensure adequacy of dehydration, plasma osmolality before the vasopressin injection should be above 288 mosmol/kg. Patients who have polyuria resulting from renal diseases, potassium depletion or nephrogenic diabetes insipidus (see below) usually show little rise in urinary osmolality with dehydration and no further rise after Pitressin injection. Patients with compulsive water drinking (primary polydipsia) often require prolonged water deprivation before serum osmolality reaches 288 mosmol/kg and before a plateau in urinary osmolality has been reached. Their urinary osmolality fails to rise by >9 percent after the administration of exogenous vasopressin.

Hypertonic saline infusions Although the dehydration test is the simplest and most conclusive means of demonstrating the

FIGURE 334-4

Dehydration studies in four normal subjects, demonstrating that the maximum urinary osmolality varies from approximately 500 to 1400 mosmol/kg, and that the injection of ADH causes no further increase. [From AM Moses, M Miller, in Current Therapy 3, H Conn, R Conn (eds), Philadelphia, Saunders, 1971.]

URINARY OSMOLALITY

⊔ After vasopressin

⊟ After dehydration

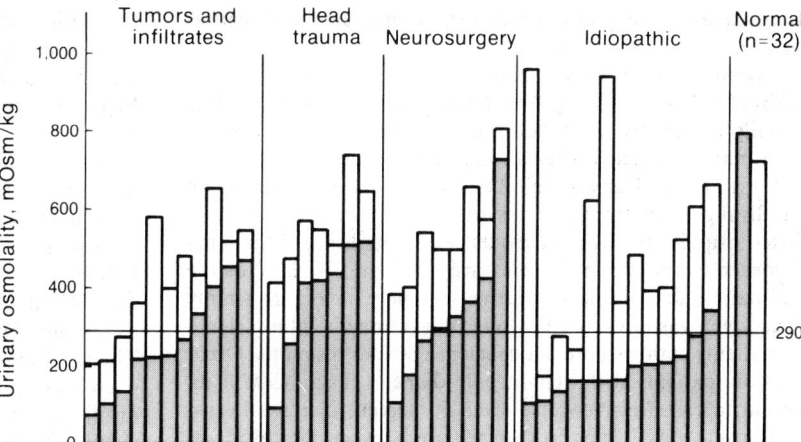

Tumors and infiltrates | Head trauma | Neurosurgery | Idiopathic | Normal (n=32)

FIGURE 334-5

Changes in urinary osmolality following dehydration and vasopressin injection in patients with diabetes insipidus of central origin.

presence of diabetes insipidus, the renal response to hypertonic saline infusion may be used and is required to determine whether ADH deficiency is or is not due entirely to a defect in osmoreceptor function. It is important to measure urinary and plasma osmolality in at least one urine specimen before and immediately after the 5% saline infusion, in order to calculate changes in free water clearance so as to obtain conclusive results from this procedure (Fig. 334-6). The test is dangerous in patients who are unable to tolerate a saline load.

FIGURE 334-6

Effect of 5% saline infusion, 0.125 (ml/kg)/min, on urinary volume, osmolal clearance, and free water clearance in a patient with hypopituitarism treated with hydrocortisone. Note the apparent lack of antidiuretic response when the volume alone is considered. The decrease in free water clearance is masked by the marked increase in osmolal clearance. (From AM Moses, DHP Streeten, Am J Med 42:368, 1967.)

PROCEDURE

1 Administer a water load (20 ml/kg by mouth), and replace the urine voided every 15 min by an equal volume of tap water by mouth.

2 Infuse 5% sodium chloride solution intravenously into one arm, preferably by infusion pump, at approximately 0.5 ml/min—to replace solute lost in the urine—until urine flow rate has stabilized, usually at 8 to 20 ml/min, for at least four 15-min periods.

3 Increase the rate of 5% saline infusion to 0.05 (ml/kg)/min and continue the infusion until urine flow rate has shown an abrupt, sustained fall lasting for at least two 15-min periods, or until ten 15-min periods of the more rapid infusion have elapsed, or until headache, nausea, or other unpleasant symptoms have supervened, whichever comes first.

4 Draw blood through an indwelling cannula or needle in a vein in the other arm every 15 min, starting at least 15 min before the onset of the more rapid rate of infusion.

5 Measure urinary and plasma (or serum) osmolality in all specimens. Calculate free water clearances and plot the data.

INTERPRETATION Inspection of the data will show whether a sudden, clear-cut onset of a progressive fall in free water clearance can be identified. The osmotic threshold for ADH release is the plasma osmolality deduced by interpolation on the best straight line representing plasma osmolality measurements, at the onset of the fall in free water clearance. When defined in this way in water-loaded subjects, the osmotic threshold is normally 287.3 ± 3.3 mosmol/kg (mean ± standard deviation). In most patients with diabetes insipidus there is no detectable osmotic threshold, i.e., no fall in free water clearance even after elevating plasma osmolality well above 300 mosmol/kg. However, some patients may have a high or normal osmotic threshold and yet have diabetes insipidus (3 and 4, Fig. 334-3).

DIFFERENTIAL DIAGNOSIS Diabetes insipidus has to be distinguished from several other types of polyuria (Table 334-1), in all of which there is loss of the renal tubular response to endogenous vasopressin. These other types of polyuria can, therefore, be recognized by failure of response to administered ADH. Among the types of polyuria listed in the table, several are easily distinguishable from spontaneous diabetes insipidus by the history [e.g., recent lithium or mannitol administration, recent surgery under methoxyflurane (Penthrane) anesthesia, or recent renal transplantation]. In others the physical examination or simple laboratory procedures will indicate the diagnosis (evidence of glycosuria, renal disease, sickle-cell anemia, hypercalcemia, or potassium depletion, including such causes as primary aldosteronism).

Nephrogenic diabetes insipidus is a rare, usually inherited, form of polyuria resulting from unresponsiveness to ADH. It is usually evident from the lack of a reduction in polyuria or rise in urinary osmolality after an injection of vasopressin, as described in the "Dehydration Test" above. These patients can be distinguished from patients with vasopressin-deficient diabetes insipidus by the usual evidence of inheritance of the renal disorder (very rare in diabetes insipidus) and by lack of the dramatic reduction in daily urine volume which is invariably seen when vasopressin tannate in oil is correctly administered to patients with vasopressin-deficient diabetes insipidus. Occasionally patients with nephrogenic diabetes insipidus will respond to vasopressin with a 40 to 50 percent increase in urinary osmolality, which is intermediate between the responses of patients with mild and severe diabetes insipidus (Miller et al.). In those rare instances in which nephrogenic diabetes insipidus cannot be ruled out with certainty by these procedures, measurement of an elevated plasma or urinary ADH concentration after water deprivation for 12 to 18 h should remove all doubt.

Primary polydipsia One condition which is occasionally difficult to differentiate from diabetes insipidus is primary polydipsia or psychogenic polydipsia. This may occur in two forms. First and more common is chronic overingestion of water resulting in hypotonic polyuria and often confused with diabetes insipidus. The second variant is intermittent ingestion of large quantities of water, which may lead to water intoxication even though a very dilute urine is excreted.

Polydipsia and polyuria are usually somewhat erratic in contrast to the sustained polydipsia and polyuria of diabetes

TABLE 334-1
Major polyuric syndromes

I Primary disorders of water intake or output
  A Excessive water intake
    1 Psychogenic polydipsia
    2 Hypothalamic disease: postencephalitic, histiocytosis X
    3 Drug-induced polydipsia
      a Thioridazine
      b Chlorpromazine
      c Anticholinergic drugs (dry mouth)
  B Inadequate tubular reabsorption of filtered water
    1 Vasopressin deficiency
      a Central diabetes insipidus
      b Drug-induced inhibition of ADH release
        (1) Narcotic antagonists
        (2) Clonidine
    2 Renal tubular unresponsiveness to ADH
      a Nephrogenic diabetes insipidus (congenital and familial)
      b Nephrogenic diabetes insipidus (acquired)
        (1) Several chronic renal diseases, after obstructive uropathy, unilateral renal arterial stenosis, after renal transplantation, after acute tubular necrosis
        (2) Potassium deficiencies, including primary aldosteronism
        (3) Chronic hypercalcemias, including hyperparathyroidism
        (4) Drug-induced: lithium, methoxyflurane anesthesia, demethylchlortetracycline
        (5) Various systemic disorders: multiple myeloma, amyloidosis, sickle-cell anemia, Sjögren's syndrome
II Primary disorders of renal absorption of solutes (osmotic diuresis)
  A Glucose: diabetes mellitus
  B Salts, especially sodium chloride
    1 Various chronic renal diseases, especially chronic pyelonephritis
    2 After various diuretics, including mannitol

insipidus. These patients usually have no nocturnal polyuria. Polyuria of long duration may result in the development of large bladder capacities and consequently infrequent urination. The patients are often emotionally disturbed. The syndrome may be seen in occasional patients with anorexia nervosa, who may drink huge quantities of water while eating very little. Fluid intake may decrease markedly when food intake increases. Rarely, a patient with chronic fluid overingestion may have a central nervous system lesion, although adipsia or hypodipsia from central nervous system lesions is more common.

The intermittent ingestion of large quantities of fluid may lead to water intoxication and dilutional hyponatremia even though there is normal urinary diluting capacity. This phenomenon is very unusual because normal adults can excrete between 10 and 14 ml/min of solute-free water, and it is an unusual circumstance which results in the ingestion of sufficiently more water than this to cause dilutional hyponatremia. The syndrome of water intoxication with normal diluting capacity has been reported in persons who take large enemas, drink excessive amounts of beer, or are given thioridazine (Mellaril). The phenothiazine drugs have parasympathetic effects and may cause dryness of the mouth, which may aggravate tendencies toward compulsive water drinking. It is also possible that thioridazine may directly stimulate the thirst center.

The diagnosis is usually evident from the combination of low plasma and urinary osmolalities. When plasma osmolality is normal, the diagnosis can be made by a normal response to the dehydration test. However, the patients may be so overhydrated that it may require 12 to 18 h of dehydration before hourly urinary osmolalities become constant.

TREATMENT (See Table 334-2) Diabetes insipidus can be treated by hormone replacement. As is true of most peptides, oral administration of vasopressin is ineffective. Aqueous vasopressin (Pitressin, 20 units per milliliter) may be administered subcutaneously in doses of 5 to 10 units and usually has a duration of action of 3 to 6 h. The main use of this preparation is in initial management of unconscious patients with acute onset of diabetes insipidus following head trauma or a neurosurgical procedure. The short duration of its action allows recognition of the return of neurohypophyseal function and prevents the development of water intoxication in patients who may be receiving intravenous fluids.

A solution of synthetic 8-lysine vasopressin (lypressin, Diapid) is available for use as a nasal spray. A single application may result in an antidiuresis lasting approximately 4 to 6 h. Absorption of the vasopressin may be markedly decreased in the presence of an upper respiratory infection or allergic rhinitis with edema of the nasal mucosa. The need for this agent has been reduced by the availability of a newer synthetic analog, DDAVP (1-deamino-8-arginine vasopressin; desmopressin) which has prolonged antidiuretic activity and is almost completely devoid of pressor effects. When used as a nasal spray in amounts between 10 and 20 μg (0.1 to 0.2 ml), it has an antidiuretic action which lasts 12 to 24 h in most patients. At present this analogue is the drug of choice in the treatment of most patients with diabetes insipidus. It is rarely ineffective because of edema of the nasal mucosa. The use of these nasal sprays in the unconscious patient with diabetes insipidus is impracticable.

In the past, patients with an established diagnosis of diabetes insipidus have usually been treated with intramuscular injections of vasopressin (Pitressin) tannate in oil (5 units per milliliter). A single injection of 2.5 or 5 units has an antidiuretic effect for 24 to 72 h. Since this material is a suspension of vasopressin tannate in peanut oil, it is essential that the ampul

TABLE 334-2
Agents used in treatment of diabetes insipidus

Drug	Dose form	Usual dose	Duration of action, h
HORMONE REPLACEMENT			
Aqueous vasopressin	20 units/ml ampul	5-10 units subcutaneously	3-6
DDAVP	2.5-ml bottle, 0.1 mg/ml	10-20 μg intranasally	12-24
Lypressin (LVP)	5-ml bottle, 50 units/ml	2-4 units intranasally	4-6
Vasopressin tannate in oil	5 units/ml ampul	5 units intramuscularly	24-72
NONHORMONAL AGENTS			
Chlorpropamide	100- and 250-mg tablets	200-500 mg daily	
Clofibrate	500-mg capsules	500 mg four times daily	
Carbamazepine	200-mg tablets	400-600 mg daily	
DIURETICS			
Hydrochlorothiazide	50-mg tablets	50-100 mg daily	
Chlorthalidone	50-mg tablets	50 mg daily	

be warmed and then thoroughly shaken or inverted repeatedly until the brownish deposit of pituitary powder identifiable in the ampul is evenly distributed as a slightly cloudy supension in the oil. A perfectly dry syringe should always be used. Erratic or poor response to treatment with this agent is usually due to failure to shake the ampul properly.

Patients with diabetes insipidus who have some residual releasable ADH (types 2 to 4) may respond to oral treatment with several nonhormonal agents. The sulfonylurea, chlorpropamide (Diabinese), has been shown both to stimulate ADH release from the neurohypophysis and to potentiate the action of submaximal amounts of ADH on the renal tubule. These properties of the drug have allowed it to be used successfully in many patients with diabetes insipidus. Doses of 200 to 500 mg, usually taken once daily, are sufficient for an antidiuretic response. Its action usually starts within several hours of administration and lasts for 24 h. Chlorpropamide may restore thirst perception and thus be useful in patients with thirst center defects. Hypoglycemia may occur but can often be avoided by adherence to a regular schedule of meals. The hypolipidemic agent, clofibrate (Atromid), is capable of stimulating ADH release from the neurohypophysis and has been used in the treatment of diabetes insipidus. Doses of 500 mg four times a day often result in a prompt and sustained antidiuresis. In some patients, combined treatment with chlorpropamide and clofibrate results in complete restoration of water regulation to normal. Carbamazepine (Tegretol), used in the treatment of tic douloureux and diabetic neuropathy, has also been observed to produce an antidiuresis in patients with diabetes insipidus. This effect is mediated by stimulation of ADH release. Doses of 400 to 600 mg daily are effective, but the drug has not been widely used owing to toxicity involving the central nervous system, bone marrow, and liver.

All the therapeutic agents discussed thus far are effective only in diabetes insipidus and are completely ineffective in nephrogenic diabetes insipidus. In this form of diabetes insipidus, the only agents of clinical value are thiazides and other diuretics. By producing sodium depletion, the diuretics cause a fall in glomerular filtration rate with enhanced reabsorption of fluid in the proximal portion of the nephron. This results in decreased delivery of sodium to the ascending limb of the loop of Henle and consequently reduces capacity to dilute the urine. The therapeutic effect of diuretics in patients with nephrogenic diabetes insipidus is lost unless sodium intake is restricted.

PROGNOSIS The long-term prospects of a patient with diabetes insipidus are dependent primarily upon the underlying cause. In the absence of brain tumor or systemic disease, ready access to water and proper treatment of the polyuria usually lead to a normal life with a virtually normal life expectancy. Early recognition and treatment are important in order to pre-vent the bladder distention, hydroureter, and hydronephrosis which may develop in patients with long-standing polyuria. The rare patient with adipsia or hypodipsia in association with diabetes insipidus is in danger of developing severe dehydration, which may lead to vascular collapse or central nervous system damage. Similarly severe complications may occur in patients with diabetes insipidus who develop impairment of consciousness. For this reason, all patients with diabetes insipidus should carry identification indicating the presence of the disorder and the necessity for treatment and fluid administration.

SYNDROME OF INAPPROPRIATE ADH SECRETION

The syndrome of inappropriate ADH secretion (SIADH) is a disorder in which there is continual release of ADH unrelated to plasma osmolality. Since patients with the syndrome are unable to excrete a dilute urine, ingested fluids are retained, with consequent expansion of the extracellular fluid volume and the development of dilutional hyponatremia. The amount of ADH released and the elevation of urinary osmolality which it produces are considered to be inappropriate only in relationship to the level of plasma osmolality or serum sodium concentration. The hallmark of SIADH is, thus, hyponatremia due to water retention, in the presence of urinary osmolality above plasma osmolality. Rarely, when solute intake is markedly restricted, urinary osmolality may be somewhat less than plasma osmolality.

Water retention can be mediated by ADH as a result of excessive ADH secretion or as a consequence of enhanced renal action of ADH. It can also result from mechanisms unrelated to ADH. A fall in renal blood flow or glomerular filtration rate can increase the percentage reabsorption of sodium and water in the proximal portion of the nephron, with consequent decrease in delivery of sodium and water to the diluting segment. This leads to impaired ability to dilute the urine and water retention.

ETIOLOGY AND PATHOPHYSIOLOGY SIADH may occur in association with a large number of clinical disorders, especially malignant tumors (Table 334-3). By far the most common malignancy causing SIADH is small-cell or oat-cell carcinoma of the lung, which accounts for more than 80 percent of the cases. The malignant cells are capable of synthesizing, storing, and releasing ADH into the circulation. In prospective studies of patients with oat-cell carcinoma, more than 50 percent have been found to have impaired water excretion and elevated plasma ADH levels, even though many of these patients did not have evident hyponatremia. Chemical and biological analyses of the ADH produced by the neoplasm have shown that the ADH is identical with the arginine-vasopressin produced by the normal neurohypophyseal system. In addition to ADH, neurophysin has been demonstrated in oat-cell carcinomas. Other malignancies which have been associated with SIADH are carcinomas of the pancreas and duodenum, lymphosarcoma, reticulum cell sarcoma, Hodgkin's disease, and thymoma.

Nonmalignant pulmonary tissue also possesses the capability of synthesizing ADH. This may be responsible for the hyponatremia which has long been known to be a common feature of pulmonary tuberculosis, since ADH has been demonstrated in tuberculous lung tissue but not in uninvolved lung or in a suspension of tubercle bacilli. Other pulmonary diseases associated with SIADH are lung abscess and pneumonia, particularly that due to staphylococcus. It would appear that in response to both malignant and infectious diseases lung tissue can acquire biosynthetic capabilities similar to those of the supraoptic nucleus of the hypothalamus.

A number of disorders involving the central nervous system can result in SIADH, presumably by stimulation of the hypothalamic-neurohypophyseal system. These disorders include skull fracture, subdural hematoma, subarachnoid hemorrhage, cerebral vascular thrombosis, and cerebral atrophy. Acute encephalitis may be accompanied by transient SIADH. Other infectious and inflammatory diseases of the central nervous system, such as tuberculous meningitis, purulent meningitis, Guillain-Barré syndrome, lupus erythematosus, and acute intermittent porphyria, may have hyponatremia due to SIADH as part of the clinical picture. Physical or emotional stress, pain, hypothyroidism, and positive pressure breathing can cause release of ADH, resulting in SIADH.

TABLE 334-3
Causes of SIADH

I Malignancy
  A Oat-cell carcinoma of lung
  B Carcinoma of pancreas
  C Lymphosarcoma, reticulum cell sarcoma, Hodgkin's disease
  D Carcinoma of duodenum
  E Thymoma
II Nonmalignant pulmonary disease
  A Tuberculosis
  B Lung abscess
  C Pneumonia
III Central nervous system disorders
  A Skull fracture
  B Subdural hematoma
  C Subarachnoid hemorrhage
  D Cerebral vascular thrombosis
  E Cerebral atrophy
  F Acute encephalitis
  G Tuberculous meningitis
  H Purulent meningitis
  I Guillain-Barré syndrome
  J Lupus erythematosus
  K Acute intermittent porphyria
  L Physical or emotional stress
  M Pain
IV Drugs
  A Chlorpropamide
  B Vincristine
  C Cyclophosphamide
  D Carbamazepine
  E Oxytocin
  F General anesthesia
  G Narcotics
  H Barbiturates
  I Thiazide diuretics
  J Tricyclic antidepressants
V Miscellaneous
  A Hypothyroidism
  B Positive pressure respiration

In recent years, it has become apparent that several drugs used in medical practice may cause water retention and SIADH. Chlorpropamide (Diabinese) stimulates ADH release and enhances the antidiuretic action of submaximal concentrations of ADH. Many cases of chlorpropamide-induced water intoxication have been reported in patients with diabetes mellitus. The antineoplastic drugs, vincristine and cyclophosphamide (Cytoxan), produce the clinical picture of SIADH by causing release of ADH from the neurohypophysis. The tendency to water retention in these patients is aggravated by the common practice of recommending large fluid intake to prevent formation of uric acid calculi and the occurrence of chemical cystitis. Carbamazepine (Tegretol), used in treatment of tic douloureux, has caused water intoxication by stimulating ADH release. There are isolated instances of other drugs, particularly tricyclic compounds, producing SIADH. Clofibrate (Atromid) is capable of stimulating ADH release, but has not yet been reported to cause SIADH. Oxytocin possesses inherent antidiuretic activity and, when administered in large amounts to obstetrical patients, may cause water intoxication. Patients who have been exposed to general anesthetics, narcotics, and barbiturates in association with surgical procedures may release excessive amounts of ADH. Thiazide and other diuretics can result in hyponatremia with all the features of SIADH, associated with hypokalemia and decreased exchangeable body potassium. It has been postulated that the severe thiazide-induced potassium depletion stimulates the volume receptor mechanism controlling ADH, resulting in persistently excessive ADH release, which may account for impaired water excretion and hyponatremia in these patients.

The excessive ADH released in this syndrome, in combination with water intake in amounts greater than can be excreted at the existing level of urinary osmolality, results in water retention and extra- and intracellular hypotonicity. Sodium excretion is enhanced because of increased glomerular filtration rate and, probably, suppression of aldosterone secretion. Excessive sodium losses aggravate the hypotonicity of body fluids.

CLINICAL AND LABORATORY FEATURES Patients with SIADH may present with weight gain, weakness, lethargy, and mental confusion, ultimately progressing to convulsions and coma. Rarely do they have evident edema. Laboratory features include low levels of BUN, serum creatinine, and serum albumin. The serum sodium concentration is generally less than 130 meq per liter, and the plasma osmolality is below 275 mosmol/kg. The urine is almost always hypertonic to plasma. Urinary sodium concentration is usually more than 20 meq per liter.

DIAGNOSIS SIADH should be suspected in any patient with hyponatremia who excretes urine which is hypertonic relative to plasma. The finding that urinary sodium concentration is greater than 20 meq per liter provides further support for the diagnosis. The possible presence of adrenal insufficiency must be excluded, since glucocorticoid deficiency may simulate SIADH. In some patients with adrenal insufficiency, elevated plasma ADH levels have been found and have been attributed to the hypovolemia and hypotension present in these patients. The presence of hypothyroidism must also be excluded since this disorder may be associated with impaired diluting ability. ADH levels are elevated in some patients with hypothyroidism. In considering the diagnosis of SIADH it is also essential to exclude hyponatremia due to sodium depletion, such as that occurring in renal disease, diarrhea, or diabetic acidosis. In contrast to the patients with SIADH, patients with hyponatremia due to sodium depletion usually have clinical features of dehydration with hemoconcentration, elevated BUN, and often urinary sodium concentration below 20 meq per liter. Other disease states associated with hyponatremia, such as congestive heart failure, renal failure, and liver disease with ascites, must be ruled out. Primary polydipsia can also cause expansion of the plasma volume and dilutional hyponatremia, but can easily be distinguished from SIADH by the invariably dilute urine in patients with primary polydipsia.

In patients with the features of SIADH in whom central nervous system disease and the use of drugs capable of causing water retention can be excluded, the possibility of malignancy must be seriously considered, especially oat-cell carcinoma of the lung. Water retention and hyponatremia may occur before evidence of malignancy can be detected on chest x-ray.

The response to water loading is a useful means of establishing the diagnosis of SIADH. Before water loading is carried out, the serum sodium must be brought to a safe level, generally above 125 meq per liter, by appropriate fluid restriction and sodium administration (if necessary), and the patient must be free of symptoms of hyponatremia. An oral water load of 20 ml per kilogram of body weight is given over a period of 15 to 20 min, and urine is collected hourly for the next 5 h while the patient is recumbent. In normal individuals given such a water load, more than 80 percent of the water is excreted by the fifth hour and the urinary osmolality falls to less than 100 mosmol/kg (specific gravity 1.005). Patients with hyponatremia who excrete the water load normally may be considered to have a low-set osmoreceptor, such as occurs in chronic ill health. In contrast, patients with SIADH excrete less than 40 percent of the water load in 5 h and fail to dilute the urine to hypotonic levels. When a water load has been given to a patient with SIADH, no further water intake should be permitted over the next 24 h or until the serum sodium concentration has returned to the pretest value. In this way, production of symptomatic water intoxication can be prevented. Adrenal insufficiency cannot be distinguished from SIADH by the water load test.

Measurement of ADH in plasma and urine by sensitive bioassay or radioimmunoassay has revealed persistence of ADH in both plasma and urine in patients with SIADH at times when the plasma hypoosmolality should have been sufficient to inhibit ADH secretion. In response to further reduction of plasma osmolality after a water load, ADH has remained detectable in plasma and urine, confirming that indeed the ADH secretion is inappropriate relative to plasma osmolality.

It should be emphasized that SIADH cannot be diagnosed with confidence in the presence of severe "stress," pain, hypovolemia, hypotension, and other stimuli which may evoke physiologic release of ADH, even in the presence of hypotonicity.

TREATMENT Patients with mild or moderate symptoms of water intoxication should be treated by restricting fluid intake to about 800 to 1000 ml daily. If water restriction is adequate, a steady increase in serum sodium concentration or osmolality occurs and body weight decreases. Occasional patients with severe water intoxication must be treated more vigorously. Intravenous administration of 200 to 300 ml of 5% saline solution over several hours is usually sufficient to raise the serum sodium to a level at which the symptoms will improve. When there is the possibility of congestive heart failure due to the fluid overload, the simultaneous administration of large doses of furosemide usually causes a diuresis sufficient to reduce cardiac overload. When furosemide is given, careful attention must be paid to correction of potassium and other electrolyte losses induced by the drug. If, for any reason, intravenous fluid administration is considered necessary when the serum sodium

has been raised to an appropriate level, isotonic saline and not 5% dextrose solution should be infused slowly to maintain normality of the serum sodium concentration.

Once the initial hyponatremia has been improved, careful adherence to a regimen of fluid restriction is necessary to prevent recurrence of water intoxication. Treatment should be directed at the underlying problem. The withdrawal of drugs which might have been causing water retention usually results in prompt clearing of SIADH. The SIADH occurring with central nervous system disorders is usually transient and clears with improvement of the underlying disease. Treatment of pulmonary tuberculosis with appropriate antituberculous therapy results in gradual disappearance of SIADH. Similarly, antibiotic treatment of lung abscess or pneumonia results in resolution of SIADH.

In patients with SIADH due to malignancy, surgical resection, irradiation, or chemotherapy may be successful in alleviating water retention. Sometimes, these measures should be carried out even when there is little likelihood of curing the malignancy, since such treatment may correct life-threatening water intoxication and prevent the necessity for rigid fluid restriction. In patients in whom treatment is judged to have been curative, the disappearance of SIADH may confirm the success of treatment. Periodic water load tests may be valuable in following such patients for evidence of recurrence of malignancy.

At present, no drugs are available which are clinically useful in suppressing ADH release from the neurohypophyseal system or from a tumor. Diphenylhydantoin inhibits ADH release but is clinically ineffective. Several narcotic antagonists currently undergoing clinical testing are capable of inhibiting ADH release from the neurohypophysis. Their role in the treatment of SIADH remains to be determined. Drugs capable of blocking ADH effect on the renal tubule may be of value in the chronic management of patients with hyponatremia. Lithium salts can interfere with the antidiuretic action of ADH on the kidney but are too toxic for use in SIADH. Demethylchlortetracycline is effective in interfering with the renal action of ADH. Administration of the drug in doses of 900 to 1200 mg per day to patients with SIADH due to lung malignancy has resulted in diuresis with excretion of an isotonic or hypotonic urine and improvement in hyponatremia. The only untoward effect has been azotemia without other evidence of renal toxicity, which has disappeared promptly on discontinuation of the drug. Thus, demethylchlortetracycline may be a useful agent in the management of SIADH in the ambulatory, nonhospital patient in whom fluid restriction is difficult to accomplish.

PROGNOSIS The prognosis of a patient with SIADH depends on the underlying cause of the syndrome. Transient or reversible SIADH such as is seen in central nervous system disorders or following use of water-retaining drugs is usually benign as long as proper treatment of acute water intoxication is effectively carried out. SIADH occurring in association with malignancy has ominous implications, since the malignancies most commonly associated are oat-cell carcinoma of the lung and adenocarcinoma of the pancreas, both usually associated with rapid spread and early death. Since SIADH may antedate the clinical appearance of the malignancy, recognition of the syndrome may possibly lead to earlier diagnosis of malignancy at a time when surgical cure is possible. In patients in whom

SIADH is not correctable by surgery, irradiation, or chemotherapy, long-term fluid restriction is necessary to prevent symptomatic water intoxication.

PARAVENTRICULAR-NEUROHYPOPHYSEAL SYSTEM AND OXYTOCIN

CHEMISTRY AND PHYSIOLOGY Oxytocin is a nonapeptide which differs by two amino acids from vasopressin (Fig. 334-1). Oxytocin is produced predominantly in the cell bodies of the paraventricular nuclei, and to a lesser extent in those of the supraoptic nuclei. It is synthesized and transported in neurosecretory granules by way of nerve tracts to the neurohypophysis, where it is stored or released, in conjunction with an oxytocin-specific neurophysin. Oxytocin release results from nerve impulses originating in the hypothalamus, which cause depolarization of the neurosecretory terminals of the posterior pituitary, and subsequent release of oxytocin through a calcium-dependent process, similar to the mechanism for vasopressin. The secretion of oxytocin, as well as of vasopressin, is inhibited by ethanol. Some stimuli such as pain apparently release oxytocin and vasopressin simultaneously, but most stimuli release the two hormones independently. Oxytocin is primarily liberated during suckling, whereas after an osmotic stimulus or hemorrhage, vasopressin is released in much greater quantities than is oxytocin. Manipulation or distention of the female genital tract, artificially or during parturition, appears to be a more effective stimulus to oxytocin release than is suckling.

Oxytocin acts on the excitable membranes surrounding the myometrial and myoepithelial cells and results in an increased force of contraction. Sensitivity of the myometrium to oxytocin increases with the duration of pregnancy, but it is not known if oxytocin per se is responsible for the initiation and maintenance of labor. Oxytocin may have survival value to the offspring since it may hasten the final stages of birth and may lessen the chances of anoxia. Oxytocin continues to exert a contractile action on the myometrium post partum. Circulating oxytocin contracts the myoepithelial cells of the mammary alveoli, causing them to expel preformed milk from the secretory tissue to the nipple. Oxytocin is 100 times more potent than vasopressin in its milk-ejecting activity in the human. In contrast, the antidiuretic potency of oxytocin relative to vasopressin is about 1:200. It is unlikely that oxytocin exerts any significant physiologic effect other than on the uterus and breast.

One milligram of purified preparation of oxytocin contains 450 IU of hormone, and the amount of oxytocin in the posterior pituitary ranges from 10 to 15 units per lobe. In spite of the fact that there is no known role of oxytocin in the male, the male neural lobe stores oxytocin in amounts similar to those in the female. There is less than 0.75 μU/ml in normal adult male and female plasma, even in the third trimester of pregnancy. During labor, plasma oxytocin concentrations may reach several hundred microunits per milliliter, with a rapid fall to prepartum levels after delivery. During suckling, plasma oxytocin levels of the mother vary widely but are usually about 5 to 10 μU/ml. The half-life of oxytocin in the plasma of human beings is about 3 to 5 min. Removal of oxytocin from the circulation is mainly by the kidneys and liver, although the uterus and mammary gland may remove some.

CLINICAL USE OF OXYTOCIN The clinical use of oxytocin is limited to the induction of labor, control of hemorrhage following incomplete abortion and curettage, and treatment of impaired milk ejection. For a detailed discussion of the obstet-

rical uses of oxytocin, the reader is referred to textbooks on obstetrics. Care must be taken in the use of oxytocin because it may cause uterine rupture and fetal death. The antidiuretic action of oxytocin can be elicited with single intravenous doses of as little as 100 mU. Maximal antidiuresis is reached with 40 to 50 mU/min. Since 10 to 40 units of oxytocin per liter of dextrose is often used in obstetrical practice, it is apparent that water intoxication may result. The vasodilatory action of oxytocin may cause sudden deaths of obstetrical patients with heart disease because of hypotension, tachycardia, and arrhythmias. Anesthetics may modify the cardiovascular responses to oxytocin. For instance, in patients under cyclopropane anesthesia, oxytocin produces more hypotension but less tachycardia than in unanesthetized subjects. The vasodilatory effect of oxytocin can be blocked by vasopressin.

REFERENCES

BARTTER FC, SCHWARTZ WB: The syndrome of inappropriate secretion of antidiuretic hormone. Am J Med 42:790, 1967

KNOBIL E, SAWYER WH (eds): The pituitary gland—its neuroendocrine control, part I, in *Handbook of Physiology,* sec 7: *Endocrinology,* vol IV. Washington, American Physiological Society, 1974

MILLER M et al: Recognition of partial defects in antidiuretic hormone secretion. Ann Intern Med 73:721, 1970

MOSES AM, SHARE L (eds): *Neurohypophysis.* Basel, Karger, 1977

MOSES AM et al: Pathophysiologic and pharmacologic alterations in the release and action of ADH. Metabolism 25:697, 1976

ROBERTSON GL et al: The osmoregulation of vasopressin. Kidney Int 10:25, 1976

335
DISEASES OF THE THYROID

SIDNEY H. INGBAR
KENNETH A. WOEBER

The normal function of the thyroid gland is to secrete L-thyroxine (T_4) and 3,5,3'-triiodo-L-thyronine (T_3), iodinated amino acids that are the active thyroid hormones and that influence a diversity of metabolic processes (Fig. 335-1). Diseases of the thyroid gland are manifested by qualitative or quantitative alterations in hormone secretion, enlargement of the thyroid (goiter), or both. Insufficient hormone secretion results in the syndrome of *hypothyroidism* or *myxedema,* in which decreased oxygen consumption (hypometabolism) is a classic manifestation. Conversely, excessive secretion of active hormone results in hypermetabolism and other features of a syndrome termed *hyperthyroidism* or *thyrotoxicosis.* Enlargement of the thyroid gland (normally 15 to 25 g in adults) may be generalized or focal. Generalized enlargements may not be absolutely symmetric, however, the right lobe tending to enlarge more than the left. They are associated with increased, normal, or decreased hormone secretion, depending upon the underlying disturbance. Truly focal enlargement usually reflects neoplastic transformation, either benign or malignant, the former sometimes being responsible for hypersecretion of hormone and hyperthyroidism, the latter very rarely so. Either type of goiter may result in compression of adjacent structures in the neck or mediastinum.

EMBRYOLOGY, ANATOMY, AND HISTOLOGY

The human thyroid originates embryologically from an evagination of the pharyngeal epithelium with some cellular contri-

3 - Monoiodotyrosine

3, 5, 3' - Triiodothyronine (T$_3$)

3, 5, 3', 5' - Tetraiodothyronine
(thyroxine; T$_4$)

FIGURE 335-1

Structural formulas of the active thyroid hormones, thyroxine and triiodo-thyronine, and of the inactive precursor, monoiodotyrosine.

butions from the lateral pharyngeal pouches. Progressive descent of the midline thyroid anlage gives rise to the thyroglossal duct, which extends from the foramen cecum near the base of the tongue to the isthmus of the thyroid. Remnants of tissue may persist along the course of this tract as "lingual thyroid," as thyroglossal cysts or nodules, or as a structure contiguous with the thyroid isthmus called the *pyramidal lobe.* The latter is usually not discernible, except when the remainder of the gland is goitrous. In some individuals, lingual thyroid may be the sole functioning thyroid tissue. In such cases, its secretion may or may not be sufficient to maintain a normal metabolic (euthyroid) state.

Knowledge of the ontogenetic sequence in human thyroid development is limited by the availability of specimens for analysis. It is clear, however, that the fetal thyroid acquires the capacity to collect and organify iodine at about 10 weeks gestation. Both T$_4$ and thyroid-stimulating hormone (thyrotropin, TSH) are detectable in the blood soon thereafter, whereas T$_3$ becomes detectable later during the second trimester. The very low T$_3$ concentration in fetal blood and amniotic fluid in the face of a high maternal concentration indicates that maternal-fetal transfer of T$_3$ is minimal and that the maintenance of a eumetabolic state in the fetus is accomplished principally through secretion of T$_4$ by the fetal thyroid. Moreover, since the placenta is minimally permeable to maternal TSH, the fetal pituitary-thyroid axis is a distinct functional unit. Maternal thyrotropin-releasing hormone (TRH) readily crosses the placenta, however, and could therefore play a role in fetal thyroid hormone economy.

The normal adult thyroid is a relatively vascular organ, comprising two lobes joined by an isthmus and lying just anterior and slightly caudad to the cartilages of the larynx. Fibrous septa divide the gland into pseudolobules which, in turn, comprise vesicles, called *follicles* or *acini,* surrounded by a capillary network. Normally, the follicle walls are composed of cuboidal epithelium. Their lumen is filled with a proteinaceous material

termed *colloid,* which contains a protein peculiar to the thyroid, *thyroglobulin,* within the peptide sequence of which T$_4$ and T$_3$ are stored.

HORMONE SYNTHESIS, SECRETION, AND METABOLISM

SYNTHESIS AND SECRETION Thyroid hormone synthesis that is both qualitatively and quantitatively normal depends on entry into the thyroid of adequate quantities of iodine, a constituent of the active hormones, T$_4$ and T$_3$; normality of pathways for iodine metabolism within the gland; and concurrent synthesis of a normal receptor protein for iodine, thyroglobulin. Secretion of normal quantities of hormone, in turn, requires both a normal rate of hormone synthesis and the integrity of processes within the gland by which thyroglobulin is hydrolyzed and the hormonally active iodoaminoacids thereby liberated. Iodine enters the thyroid from the bloodstream in the form of inorganic or ionic iodide whose source is twofold: iodide derived either from the deiodination of thyroid hormones or from iodinated agents that the patient may have been given and iodide ingested in food, water, or medication. Formerly, a dietary iodine intake of approximately 200 μg was considered normal within the continental United States, and this was sufficient to sustain a plasma iodide concentration of approximately 0.5 μg per 100 ml. Recently, however, owing largely to enrichment of bread with iodine, and to the widespread use of iodine in drugs, vitamin preparations, and antiseptic agents, the average iodine intake has increased substantially, to values as high as 1000 μg daily, with corresponding increases in plasma iodide concentration. Iodide is removed from the plasma by the thyroid, kidneys, and salivary and gastrointestinal glands, but since iodide that enters gastrointestinal secretion is reabsorbed, net clearance is effected only by the thyroid and kidneys. In effect, the thyroid and kidneys compete for plasma iodide. However, since renal clearance is largely a function of glomerular filtration rate and is not influenced by humoral factors or plasma iodide concentration, the kidney is normally a passive participant in this competition. Hence, adjustments in the rate of entry of iodide into the thyroid relative to the rate of urinary excretion are mediated by changes in thyroid, rather than renal, avidity.

The reactions involved in the synthesis and secretion of the active thyroid hormones can be divided into four sequential steps (Fig. 335-2). The first involves active inward transport of iodide from the plasma into the thyroid cell and follicular lumen. This occurs at a rate that exceeds passive diffusion of iodide from the gland, with the result that the thyroid is capable of maintaining concentration gradients for iodide (thyroid/plasma concentration ratios) of substantial magnitude (up to 500, or more, under certain physiologic or pathologic conditions). Energy for iodide transport is phosphate bond–derived and therefore depends upon oxidative metabolism within the gland. The second step in hormone biosynthesis involves oxidation of iodide to a higher valence form, as yet undetermined, that is capable of iodinating tyrosyl residues in thyroglobulin, a glycoprotein of approximately 650,000 molecular weight that is synthesized within the follicular epithelium. Oxidation of iodide is effected by an iodide peroxidase, which utilizes hydrogen peroxide generated during the course of oxidative metabolism within the gland. Organic iodinations, which occur at the cell-collid interface, result in the formation of the peptide-bound, hormonally inactive precursors, monoiodotyrosine

(MIT), and diiodotyrosine (DIT). Subsequently, these iodotyrosines undergo oxidative condensation, again through the mediation of peroxidase. This so-called "coupling reaction" occurs within the thyroglobulin molecule and yields a variety of iodothyronines, including T_4 and T_3. Although minute quantities of thyroglobulin are detectable in the blood of normal patients and those with thyroid disease, the vast bulk of thyroglobulin is retained for a time within the gland, serving as a storage form of thyroid hormone, or "prohormone." Liberation of the active hormones into the blood, forming the third step in hormone synthesis and release, involves pinocytosis of follicular colloid at the apical margin of the cells to form colloid droplets. Functioning microtubules are necessary for this process. The colloid droplets fuse with thyroid lysosomes to form "phagolysosomes," in which thyroglobulin is hydrolyzed by proteases and peptidases. The final step is release of the now free iodothyronines, T_4 and T_3, into the blood. The thyroid gland is the only source of endogenous T_4; in contrast, in the normal individual, relatively small amounts of T_3 are secreted by the thyroid, and most of this hormone is formed in peripheral tissues by the enzymatic removal of the 5'-iodine from the outer ring of T_4. Inactive iodotyrosines liberated by the hydrolysis of thyroglobulin are stripped of their iodine by an intrathyroidal enzyme, iodotyrosine dehalogenase. Normally, iodide liberated thereby is largely reutilized in the synthesis of hormone, but a small proportion is normally lost into the blood (iodide leak); this proportion may become very large in abnormal circumstances.

As with iodide, the thyroid is capable of concentrating other monovalent anions. Notable among these is the pertechnetate ion, which is available as the radioactive isotope, sodium [⁹⁹ᵐTc]pertechnetate. Unlike iodide, little pertechnetate is or-

ganically bound; hence, its duration of stay within the thyroid is short. This property, together with its short physical half-life, makes pertechnetate a valuable radionuclide for imaging the thyroid with scintillation scanning techniques.

The foregoing reactions are subject to inhibition by a variety of chemical compounds. Such agents are generally termed *goitrogens,* since, by virtue of their ability to inhibit hormone synthesis and indirectly stimulate TSH secretion, they induce goiter formation. Certain inorganic anions, notably perchlorate and thiocyanate, inhibit the iodide transport mechanism and thereby reduce available substrate for hormone formation. The goiter and hypothyroidism that follow, however, can be prevented or relieved, by doses of iodide sufficiently large to enable adequate quantities to enter the gland by simple diffusion. The commonly employed antithyroid agents, such as the derivatives of thiourea and mercaptoimidazole, exert more complex actions upon pathways of hormone biosynthesis. These agents, as well as certain aniline derivatives, inhibit the initial oxidation (organic binding) of iodide, decrease the proportion of DIT relative to MIT, and block coupling of iodotyrosines to form the hormonally active iodothyronines. The latter reaction is the most sensitive. Thus, it is possible for the synthesis of hormonally active iodothyronines to be decreased greatly, although the total incorporation of iodine by the thyroid is inhibited but little. In contradistinction to the effect of the monovalent anions, the goitrogenic action of inhibitors of organic binding is not overcome by large quantities of iodine. Indeed, certain weak goitrogens, such as sulfonamides and antipyrine, are rendered more potent when given with iodide, an effect not clearly understood. Iodine itself, when given acutely in large doses, is capable of blocking the organic-binding and coupling reactions. This action (Wolff-Chaikoff effect) is normally transient. In a small proportion of seemingly normal individuals, however, prolonged administration of iodide is associated with continued inhibition of hormone synthesis and development of goiter, with (iodide myxedema) or without hypothyroidism. A large proportion of patients with Graves' disease, especially after treatment with radioiodine or surgery, and also patients with Hashimoto's disease are inordinately sensitive to the blocking effect of iodide and, when given iodides chronically, develop hypothyroidism. The fetal thyroid is similarly sensitive, and consequently pregnant women should not be given iodide in large doses because of the danger of inducing goitrous hypothyroidism in the fetus. Iodide in large doses is capable of inhibiting proteolysis of thyroglobulin and hormone release, an effect which is most readily demonstrable in hyperfunctioning thyroids and which is responsible for the rapid ameliorative action of iodides in most patients with hyperthyroidism. Lithium, which is administered as the carbonate salt in some patients with depressive states, has a variety of effects on intrathyroidal iodine metabolism. Among these is an action to inhibit hormone release. Finally, dexamethasone in large doses is also capable of inhibiting hormone release and thus, in conjunction with iodide, can be employed to effect a rapid reduction in the degree of thyrotoxicosis in patients with this syndrome.

TRANSPORT AND METABOLISM In the blood, T_4 and T_3 are almost entirely bound to plasma proteins. Electrophoretic analyses indicate that T_4 is bound, in decreasing order of intensity, to an inter-α globulin, termed thyroxine- or thyronine-binding globulin (TBG), to a T_4-binding prealbumin (TBPA), and to albumin. By virtue of its intense affinity for T_4, TBG is by far the major determinant of overall binding intensity. The interaction between T_4 and its binding proteins conforms to a reversible binding equilibrium in which the majority of the hormone is bound and a very small proportion (normally less than 0.05 percent) is free. T_3 is not significantly bound by

FIGURE 335-2

Schema depicting pathways in the synthesis and secretion of thyroid hormones and mechanisms for the suprathyroidal and intrathyroidal regulation of thyroid function. Small, solid arrows indicate pathways of iodine metabolism; open arrows indicate stimulation; crosshatched arrows indicate inhibitory influences. TRH, thyrotropin-releasing hormone; TSH, thyroid-stimulating hormone; IPO, iodide peroxidase; prot., thyroid protease; peptid., thyroid peptidase; MIT, monoiodotyrosine; DIT, diiodotyrosine; T_4, thyroxine; T_3, 3,5,3'-triiodothyronine.

TABLE 335-1
Classification of the varieties of disordered thyroid hormone–plasma protein interactions

Type of abnormality	Serum T_4 and T_3	Percent FT_4 and FT_3 or RT_3U	FT_4 and FT_3 or FT_4I and FT_3I
I Primary abnormality in thyroxine-binding proteins			
A Increased concentration	↑	↓	N
B Decreased concentration	↓	↑	N
II Primary disorder of thyroid function			
A Hypothyroidism	↓	↓	↓
B Hyperthyroidism	↑	↑	↑

NOTE: FT_4 = free T_4; FT_3 = free T_3; FT_4I = free T_4 index; FT_3I = free T_3 index; RT_3U = resin-T_3 uptake.

TBPA and is bound by TBG less firmly than is T_4. As a consequence, the normal proportion of free T_3 (approximately 0.3 percent) is eight to ten times greater than that of T_4. It appears likely that only the free or unbound hormone is available to tissues; therefore, the metabolic state of the patient will correlate more closely with the concentration of free than with the total concentration of hormone in plasma. Furthermore, homeostatic regulation of thyroid function will be directed toward maintenance of a normal concentration of free rather than total hormone. Moreover, the relatively weak binding of T_3 accounts for its failure to contribute materially to the total hormonal iodine concentration in the blood and possibly for its more rapid onset and offset of action. Disturbances of the thyroid hormone–plasma protein interaction are of two general types (see Table 335-1). In the first, the thyroid-pituitary axis is intrinsically normal, and the homeostatic control of thyroid hormone secretion is intact. Under these circumstances, disordered binding interactions result from primary alterations in the concentration of TBG. For example, an increase in TBG will initially lower the concentration of free hormone and thus diminish the quantity of hormone available to tissues. Total hormone concentration in serum will then increase until the concentration of free hormone is restored to normal. At this time, the proportions of T_4 and T_3 that are free will be decreased. The increase in total hormone concentration counterbalances the decrease in the proportion free; as a result, the absolute concentration of free hormone is normal and the metabolic state of the patient is unchanged. Converse changes occur when the concentration of TBG declines. Table 335-2 summarizes those states associated with primary alterations in the concentration of TBG.

The second type of disturbance of thyroid hormone–binding interactions results from a primary alteration in the concentration of thyroid hormones in the blood, such as occurs in hypothyroidism or thyrotoxicosis. Here, homeostatic control of thyroid hormone secretion is disrupted and pathologic factors determine the rate of hormone secretion independent of the thyroid-pituitary axis. Under these circumstances, the concentration of TBG is changed little, if at all, and the concentration of free hormone will vary directly with the total concentration of hormone. Since such changes in circulating hormone usually result from intrinsic disease of the pituitary or thyroid itself, homeostatic mechanisms cannot restore the concentration of free hormone to normal. Primary changes in thyroid function are therefore associated with persistent changes in the concentration of both total and free hormone, and, consequently, with alterations in the metabolic state of the patient. In these disorders, the relative change in the concentration of free hormone is greater than the change in total hormone concentration so that the proportion of free hormone changes in a direction similar to that of the change in hormone supply.

Following their penetration into the cell, T_4 and T_3 undergo a variety of reactions which lead ultimately to their excretion or inactivation. As judged from experiments with isotopically labeled hormones, the major pathway of hormone metabolism is removal of iodine. This deiodinative pathway is present in all tissues tested, leaves the diphenyl ether link of the thyronine nucleus intact, and accounts for approximately 70 percent of T_4 and T_3 disposal. Approximately 20 percent of labeled T_4 and T_3 is normally lost in the stool, principally in the form of conjugates with glucuronate or sulfate. Substantial quantities of labeled hormones are excreted in the bile and are presumably available for reabsorption, probably after hydrolysis of conjugates. However, the magnitude of the enterohepatic circulation of T_4 and T_3 in humans is unknown. A small proportion of the hormones (approximately 20 percent) undergoes oxidative deamination and decarboxylation of the alanine side chain to yield the acetic acid analogues of T_4 and T_3, tetra- and triiodothyroacetic acids. The most important intermediate product of T_4 metabolism is T_3 itself. Since T_3 appears to be approximately three times more potent than T_4 in many metabolic respects, such monodeiodination of T_4, which can occur in most tissues, yields from T_4 a product of enhanced potency. Approximately 30 percent of T_4 is initially monodeiodinated in the 5′ position of its outer ring, to yield T_3. This source normally accounts for about 80 percent of the T_3 produced, the remainder being derived through direct thyroid secretion. A major clinical implication of this is that athyreotic or hypothyroid patients maintained with synthetic levothyroxine to a normal value of serum T_4 concentration will have, in addition, nearly normal concentrations of T_3 in their blood. However, direct thyroid secretion accounts for a greater proportion of overall T_3 production in hyperthyroidism; in early thyroid failure, in which the gland is under intense stimulation by TSH; and in iodine deficiency. The T_4 that is metabolized via deiodination pathway but that does not give rise to T_3 undergoes monodeiodination at the 5 position of its inner ring to yield 3,3′,5′-triiodo-L-thyronine (reverse T_3, rT_3); this process accounts for almost all of the rT_3 produced. Unlike T_3, rT_3 has little if any metabolic potency; therefore, the relative poise between outer- and inner-ring monodeiodination of T_4 could represent a regulatory mechanism for modulating the quantity of metabolically active hormone at the tissue level. Impairment of the peripheral conversion of T_4 to T_3 is responsible for the decreased serum T_3 concentrations that occur in various physiologic and pathologic states (Table 335-3). In these states of low serum T_3 concentration, serum T_4 concentrations are normal or marginally increased and serum rT_3 concentrations distinctly increased. The metabolic impact of such alterations is uncertain, but the serum TSH concentration is either normal or very slightly elevated and gives, therefore, no clear evidence of tissue hypothyroidism.

TABLE 335-2
Circumstances associated with altered concentration of TBG

Increased TBG	Decreased TBG
Pregnancy	Androgenic and anabolic steroids
Newborn state	
Oral contraceptives and other sources of estrogen	Large doses of glucocorticoid
	Chronic liver disease
Acute intermittent porphyria	Severe systemic illness
Chronic liver disease	Active acromegaly
Acute hepatitis	Nephrosis
Genetically determined	Genetically determined

TABLE 335-3
States associated with decreased peripheral conversion of T_4 to T_3

I Physiologic
   A Fetal and early neonatal life
   B Old age
II Pathologic
   A Fasting
   B Malnutrition
   C Systemic illness
   D Physical trauma
   E Postoperative state
   F Drugs (propylthiouracil, dexamethasone, propranolol)
   G Radiographic contrast agents (Oragrafin, Telepaque)

Under certain circumstances, changes in the activity of cellular processes involved in hormone metabolism may be the major determinant of changes in the rates of metabolic clearance of T_4 and T_3. Both phenobarbital and diphenylhydantoin increase the metabolic clearance of thyroid hormones without increasing the proportion of free hormone in the blood. Indeed, in the case of diphenylhydantoin, both total and free T_4 concentrations are diminished. Nevertheless, a normal metabolic state is maintained. The effects of these agents are doubtless related to the hypertrophy of smooth endoplasmic reticulum and increased activity of varied microsomal enzymes that they induce.

REGULATION OF THYROID FUNCTION Regulation of thyroid function is effected by two general mechanisms, one suprathyroid and one intrathyroid in locus (Fig. 335-2). The proximate mediator of suprathyroid regulation is thyrotropin or thyroid-stimulating hormone (TSH), a glycopeptide secreted by basophilic cells within the anterior pituitary gland. TSH stimulates thyroid hypertrophy and hyperplasia; accelerates most aspects of glandular intermediary metabolism; enhances synthesis of nucleic acid and protein, including thyroglobulin; and stimulates all steps in thyroid iodine metabolism leading to the synthesis and secretion of thyroid hormones. These actions are thought to be mediated, at least in large part, by increased synthesis of the "second messenger," cyclic 3′,5′-adenosine monophosphate (cyclic AMP).

Regulation of TSH secretion, in turn, is effected by two opposing influences. Thyrotropin-releasing hormone (TRH), a tripeptide amide (pyroglutamylhistidylprolineamide) secreted in the ventromedial hypothalamus, reaches the pituitary via the hypophyseal portal capillary system and there stimulates synthesis and secretion of TSH. These effects of TRH are inhibited, however, in relation to the extent of thyroid hormone action within the pituitary, and this is presumed to be closely related to the concentration of free thyroid hormones in the blood. Thus, negative feedback of thyroid hormones on TSH secretion occurs mainly in the pituitary gland itself; in what manner and to what extent thyroid hormones affect the secretion of TRH is unknown.

Intrathyroid regulation of thyroid function is less well understood, but is nevertheless important. In some manner as yet undetermined, changes in glandular organic iodine content are associated with reciprocal changes in thyroidal iodide transport activity, as well as in growth, glucose metabolism, and nucleic acid synthesis. Although these influences are evident in the absence of TSH stimulation, and hence may be termed *autoregulatory,* their most important role is to modify (iodine-enrichment inhibiting, and iodine-depletion enhancing) the response of these functions to TSH, probably by modifying the generation of cyclic AMP consequent to TSH stimulation.

LABORATORY TESTS The availability of a variety of laboratory tests permits evaluation of many aspects of thyroid hormone economy. Such tests can be divided into five major categories: direct tests of thyroid function; tests related to the concentration and binding of thyroid hormones in blood; metabolic indexes; tests of the homeostatic control of thyroid function; and various tests that do not fit into other categories.

Direct tests of thyroid function The *thyroid radioactive iodine uptake (RAIU)* is the most commonly used test for assessing glandular function per se. Although ^{131}I has been used for decades for this purpose, ^{123}I is far preferable because of the much lower radiation dosage that it delivers. The administered radioiodine mixes uniformly with the endogenous stable iodide and, in the steady state, indicates what percentage of the iodide entering and leaving the iodide space per unit time is accumulated by the thyroid. The RAIU is usually measured 24 h after administration of isotope since it usually has reached a plateau value at this time. The RAIU varies inversely with the pool of endogenous stable iodide and directly with the functional state of the thyroid. The widespread increase in iodine intake that has occurred recently has led to an enrichment of the body iodide pool, with the result that the normal range for the 24-h RAIU has declined to approximately 5 to 30 percent of the administered dose. Consequently, this test no longer discriminates between normal and hypothyroid states. Values above the normal range, however, indicate thyroid hyperfunction, and remain useful, therefore, in the diagnosis of hyperthyroidism. The RAIU is also used as part of the thyroid suppression test and the TSH stimulation test.

Interest in the diagnostic use of the RAIU has grown with the recognition that certain forms of hyperthyroidism may be diagnosed by the demonstration of a low value of this test. These include not only iodine-induced hyperthyroidism and thyrotoxicosis factitia, but also the hyperthyroidism associated with the infrequent, painless form of subacute thyroiditis and that associated with an unusual variant of chronic thyroiditis. Importance attaches to making the proper diagnosis, particularly in the latter two instances, since these forms of hyperthyroidism are self-limited and should not be treated by conventional means.

Tests related to hormone concentration and binding in blood The *serum T_4 concentration* is measured by the ability of stable T_4, either extracted from or contained in the patient's serum, to displace labeled T_4 from a protein mixture containing TBG (competitive protein-binding assay, CPBA) or from a specific anti-T_4 antibody (radioimmunoassay, RIA). Both tests are highly specific. The normal range for the serum T_4 is generally 4 to 11 μg per 100 ml. The *serum protein-bound iodine (PBI) concentration* was, until recently, the only method of estimating serum T_4, and such measurement was possible only by virtue of the iodine content of T_4. This test is much less specific than serum T_4, which has superseded it. It is occasionally useful in detecting the presence of abnormal iodoproteins in the blood arising as a result of an intrathyroidal biosynthetic defect, because here the PBI is disproportionately high in relation to the serum T_4. Normal values for the PBI range from 4 to 8 μg per 100 ml. The *serum T_3 concentration* can be measured by radioimmunoassay; here, the ability of the stable T_3 in serum to displace labeled T_3 from anti-T_3 antibody is compared with that of known quantities of T_3. Normal values range from about 80 to 160 ng per 100 ml.

As mentioned in the previous section, alterations in the concentration of TBG, as well as alterations in hormone secretion, will influence the total concentration of hormone in the blood. However, only alterations in hormone secretion will lead to steady-state alterations in the concentration of free hormone. The *percent of free hormone (percent FT_4 or percent FT_3)* can be measured by equilibrium dialysis of serum enriched with a tracer quantity of the labeled hormone, and the product of this value and the serum T_4 or serum T_3 yields the *concentration of* *free hormone (FT₄ or FT₃).* Measurement of percent FT_4 or percent FT_3 is a cumbersome procedure. Hence, for clinical purposes, the *in vitro uptake test* is employed, as it is simple to perform and yields qualitatively the same information. Here, the serum is enriched with labeled hormone and then incubated with an insoluble, particulate material, such as resin or charcoal, that binds hormone. The percent of labeled hormone taken up by the particulate material varies inversely with the concentration of unoccupied binding sites on TBG. Labeled T_3 is employed in preference to labeled T_4 since it is less strongly bound by the serum and hence yields higher and therefore more accurate uptake values. Normal values for the *resin-T₃ uptake (RT₃U)* range from 25 to 35 percent. Results may also be expressed as the quotient of the RT_3U value in the patient's serum and that obtained in a normal control specimen (*RT₃U ratio*). The product of the serum T_4 concentration and the RT_3U is the so-called *free T₄ index (FT₄I)* and varies directly with changes in the FT_4. Primary alterations in the concentration of TBG (Table 335-2) produce *reciprocal* alterations in RT_3U and serum T_4, with the result that the FT_4I remains normal. By contrast, primary alterations in T_4 secretion produce changes in RT_3U that are in the same direction as those in serum T_4. Hence, the FT_4I affords a better discrimination from normal values than either of its component tests alone.

Metabolic Indexes These tests measure the metabolic impact of thyroid hormone in the peripheral tissues. The *basal metabolic rate (BMR)* measures energy expenditure in terms of the amount of O_2 consumed in the basal state. Values are expressed as a percentage difference from the mean value of normal individuals of the same age, sex, and body surface area. The normal range is approximately -15 to $+5$ percent. Owing to the variety of nonthyroidal factors that affect the BMR, however, this test is of limited diagnostic value. Increases in the *serum cholesterol concentration* are suggestive of hypothyroidism of thyroidal origin; however, decreases in serum cholesterol are of little value in the diagnosis of thyrotoxicosis. Prolongation of the *Achilles reflex time* as assessed by kinemometry or photomotography, though not pathognomonic, is highly suggestive of hypothyroidism, but the test has little discriminatory value in hyperthyroidism.

Tests of homeostatic control The measurement of *serum TSH* has become an important tool in the diagnosis of hypothyroidism and diminished thyroid reserve. The latter state represents a stage in the evolution of hypothyroidism, in which a structural or functional abnormality that impairs hormone synthesis is compensated for by hypersecretion of TSH and activation of the thyroid. Serum TSH is measured by radioimmunoassay; here, the ability of TSH in serum to displace labeled human TSH from anti-TSH antibody is compared with that of known quantities of human TSH. The normal range is less than 5 $\mu U/ml$; current sensitivity does not generally permit distinction between normal or low values. Measurement of serum TSH affords the best means of distinguishing between untreated hypothyroidism of thyroid origin, in which the values are invariably increased, and pituitary or hypothalamic hypothyroidism, in which the values are usually undetectable and always within the normal range. In thyrotoxicosis, serum TSH is undetectable, except in rare cases of TSH-secreting tumors.

The *TSH stimulation test* is employed as a means of assessing thyroid reserve. Here, the responses of the RAIU and serum T_4 to an intramuscular injection of bovine TSH are monitored. This test is of major value in the diagnosis of diminished thyroid reserve, in which the gland is under maximum stimulation by endogenous TSH and hence shows no further response to exogenous TSH, and in the differentiation of pituitary hypothyroidism from hypothyroidism of primary thyroidal origin.

With the general availability of measurements of serum TSH, however, this test is now less frequently used.

The *thyrotropin-releasing hormone (TRH) stimulation test* is a test which has value for diverse diagnostic purposes. Following the intravenous injection of TRH in normal subjects, the serum TSH begins to rise at 10 min, peaks between 20 and 45 min, and then falls rapidly. Subnormal response to a standard dose, therefore, may reflect diminished pituitary TSH reserve. The response to TRH within the pituitary is inhibited by thyroid hormone, with the result that a supranormal response occurs in patients with hypothyroidism of thyroidal origin, whereas little or no response occurs in patients with thyrotoxicosis except in rare instances in which hypothyroidism is due to excess TSH secretion, with or without pituitary tumor. This lack of response also occurs in some patients with autonomously functioning adenomas and in some with apparently euthyroid Graves' disease. Nevertheless, with these two exceptions, a lack of response serves as an excellent confirmatory test for thyrotoxicosis. This test is also of value in the recognition and differential diagnosis of pituitary and hypothalamic hypothyroidism; in the former, but not the latter, disorder, no response to TRH would be expected. (See also Chap. 333.)

The *thyroid suppression test* is used to assess whether thyroid function is being controlled by normal homeostatic mechanisms. Normally, exogenous thyroid hormone suppresses pituitary TSH secretion, resulting in a decrease in the RAIU. Since liothyronine is usually employed (100 μg daily for 10 days), the resulting decline in serum T_4, as well as in the RAIU, can serve as an index of suppression. A normal suppressive response is a decrease of the RAIU to less than half of the control value and a decline of the serum T_4 to low normal or subnormal values. In patients with increased TBG, the decline in serum T_4 may be delayed. An abnormal suppression test is always present in hyperthyroidism, irrespective of the underlying cause; this indicates either autonomy of thyroid function, the presence of an abnormal stimulator, or, at least theoretically, unremitting hypersecretion of TSH. A normal suppression test, on the other hand, is incompatible with, and excludes the presence of, hyperthyroidism. An abnormal suppression test does not necessarily indicate the presence of hyperthyroidism, however, since it is seen after treatment of hyperthyroidism in Graves' disease, in about half of the euthyroid patients with the ophthalmopathy of Graves' disease, and in seemingly euthyroid patients in whom an autonomous hyperfunctioning adenoma has suppressed the remainder of the gland.

Miscellaneous tests Tests for circulating antibodies directed against various glandular components are often of diagnostic value. For example, moderate to high titers of antimicrosomal or antithyroglobulin antibodies are found in the serum of most patients with Hashimoto's disease and in a high proportion of patients with either primary thyroprivic hypothyroidism or Graves' disease. Many patients in the active phase of Graves' disease have in their serum an immunoglobulin G that either stimulates human thyroid tissue to produce cyclic AMP (*thyroid-stimulating immunoglobulin, TSI*) or displaces labeled TSH from human thyroid membranes (*TSH-displacing activity, TDA*), or both. The relation between these activities is uncertain, as is the nature of the immunoglobulin(s) responsible, but it is thought by some to be an antibody directed against some component of the human thyroid plasma membrane, possibly the TSH receptor itself.

Imaging by *scintiscanning* permits localization of sites of radioiodine or sodium [⁹⁹ᵐTc]pertechnetate accumulation. This technique is useful for defining areas of increased or decreased function within the thyroid and for detecting retrosternal goiter, ectopic thyroid tissue, and functioning metastases of thyroid carcinoma. Ultrasonic examination of the thyroid is also a valuable technique, particularly for distinguishing cystic nodules from those that are solid.

SIMPLE (NONTOXIC) GOITER

There is considerable confusion about the descriptive terms *endemic* and *sporadic* goiter. Endemic implies an etiologic factor or factors common to a particular geographic region. The term has been defined as indicating the presence of generalized or localized thyroid enlargement in over 10 percent of the population. The connotation of sporadic is that goiter arises in nonendemic areas as a result of a stimulus that does not affect the population generally. Since these terms fail to define or distinguish the causes of such goiters and since thyroid enlargement of diverse etiology may exist in both endemic and nonendemic regions, it seems prudent to employ a general term such as simple or nontoxic goiter. This all-inclusive category can be further subdivided into specific etiologic groups as defined by objective procedures. Simple or nontoxic goiter may be defined as any enlargement of the thyroid gland that does not result from an inflammatory or neoplastic process and is not initially associated with thyrotoxicosis or myxedema.

ETIOLOGY AND PATHOGENESIS Although the causes of simple goiter are manifold, their clinical manifestations are thought to reflect the operation of a common physiopathologic mechanism. Simple goiter results when one or more factors impair the capacity of the thyroid gland in the basal state to secrete quantities of active hormones necessary to meet the needs of the peripheral tissues. Although this has been presumed to lead to increased secretion of TSH, concentrations of TSH in the serum of patients with established simple goiter are usually normal. Hence, some other mechanism of goitrogenesis may be operative. A likely possibility is that depletion of glandular organic iodine accompanying impaired hormone synthesis increases the responsiveness of thyroid structure and function to basal levels of TSH. The resulting increases in both functioning thyroid mass and cellular activity are sufficient to overcome mild or moderate impairment of hormone synthesis; thus, the patient remains metabolically normal, though goitrous. When, however, the underlying disorder is severe, compensatory responses, now including hypersecretion of TSH, are inadequate to overcome the impairment, and the patient is both goitrous and more or less severely hypothyroid. Thus, the entity simple goiter cannot be separated clearly, in the pathogenetic sense, from goitrous hypothyroidism. Specific causes of simple goiter are included in Table 335-4 and may exist with or without hypothyroidism.

PATHOLOGY The histopathology of the thyroid in simple goiter varies with the severity of the etiologic factor and the stage of the disorder at which the examination is made. In its initial stages, the gland reveals a uniform hypertrophy, hyperplasia, and hypervascularity. As the disorder persists or undergoes repeated exacerbations and remissions, uniformity of thyroidal architecture is usually lost. Occasionally, the greater part of the gland may display a reasonably uniform degree of involution or hyperinvolution with colloid accumulation. More often such areas are interspersed with patchy areas of focal hyperplasia. Fibrosis may demarcate a variable number of nodules, which may be hyperplastic or involuted. These may resemble, but do not really represent, true neoplasms (adenomas). Areas of hemorrhage and irregular calcification may be present.

CLINICAL MANIFESTATIONS In simple goiter, the clinical manifestations arise solely from enlargement of the thyroid since the metabolic state of the patient is normal. In goitrous hypothyroidism, symptoms caused by thyromegaly are similarly present, but are accompanied by signs and symptoms of hormonal insufficiency. Mechanical sequelae include compression and displacement of the trachea or esophagus, occasionally with obstructive symptoms if the goiter becomes sufficiently large. Superior mediastinal obstruction may occur with large retrosternal goiters. Signs of compression can be induced in the case of large retrosternal goiters when the patient's arms are raised above the head (Pemberton's sign); suffusion of the face, giddiness, or syncope may result from this maneuver. Compression of the recurrent laryngeal nerve leading to hoarseness is rare in simple goiter and suggests neoplasm. Sudden hemorrhage into a nodule may lead to an acute, painful swelling in the neck and may produce or enhance compressive symptoms. Hyperthyroidism not uncommonly supervenes in long-standing multinodular goiter (toxic multinodular goiter). It is not known whether this represents the superimposition of Graves' disease upon a chronic nontoxic goiter or a separate disease entity. In both endemic and sporadic multinodular goiter, the ingestion of excess iodide may result in the development of thyrotoxicosis (Jod-Basedow syndrome).

In geographic regions where iodine deficiency is severe, acquired goitrous enlargement may also be associated with varying degrees of hypothyroidism. Cretinism, both goitrous and nongoitrous, occurs with increased frequency in the children of goitrous parents and contributes a significant sector of the socially dependent population in many countries where goiter is common. Although iodine deficiency is doubtless a necessary factor in the etiology of endemic goiter, the frequency of goiter may differ greatly among areas of equally severe iodine deficiency. In such instances, dietary or water-borne goitrogens appear to be important conditioning factors.

DIAGNOSIS The diagnosis of simple goiter requires, first, demonstration of a normal metabolic state and, second, differentiation of the goitrous condition from Hashimoto's disease or thyroid neoplasia. Physical examination alone cannot serve to make the diagnosis. A careful history is important, particularly with respect to the occurrence of thyroid pain or tenderness, rapid change in size, hoarseness, or previous drug ingestion. High titers of circulating antimicrosomal or antithyroglobulin antibodies indicate Hashimoto's disease. Needle biopsy may occasionally be indicated to make or exclude the diagnosis of Hashimoto's disease. In areas where goiter is endemic, high values for the RAIU and low values for urinary iodine excretion are the common pattern. Low normal or subnormal values for the serum T_4 are commonly found, even in the absence of hypothyroidism. In such cases, high values for the serum T_3 apparently account for the normal metabolic (eumetabolic) state.

TREATMENT The object of treatment is to remove the thyroid hyperplasia, either by relieving external encumbrances to hormone formation or by providing sufficient quantities of exogenous hormone to inhibit TSH secretion and thereby put the thyroid gland almost completely at rest. In disorders characterized by decreased thyroid iodide stores, such as iodine deficiency or impairment of the thyroid iodide-concentrating mechanism, small doses of iodide may prove effective. Occasionally, a known extrinsic goitrogen can be withdrawn. Most commonly, however, no specific etiologic factor can be detected, and suppressive thyroid therapy is required. For this purpose, sodium L-thyroxine (levothyroxine) in a dose of 150 to 200 μg daily is the agent choice. Suppression of endogenous thyroid function is most readily assessed by serial measurements of the 24-h RAIU. Functional suppression is indicated when the RAIU decreases to very low values. Lesser decreases indicate only partial suppression. In multinodular nontoxic goiter, lack of complete suppression usually indicates the presence of autonomously functioning foci, demonstrable by scanning techniques. RAIU tests can be performed at appropriate intervals, and the dose of exogenous hormone gradually adjusted as needed to achieve maximum suppression. Occasionally, physiologic replacement doses of exogenous hormones will induce mild, but usually transient, symptoms of thyrotoxicosis. In such patients, more prolonged intervals between dosage changes will usually permit achievement of full thyroid suppression without inducing symptoms of toxicity.

Reported results of therapy vary widely. There is general agreement that the early diffuse, hyperplastic goiter responds well, with regression or disappearance in 3 to 6 months. In the authors' experience, the later, nodular stage responds less favorably, and significant reduction in gland size is achieved only in about one-third of the cases. Internodular tissue regresses more often than do nodules themselves. The latter may therefore become more prominent during treatment. After maximum regression of the goiter, suppressive medication may be maintained for prolonged periods, reduced to minimal levels, or at times withdrawn. In an unpredictable manner, goiter will in some cases remain relieved while in others it will recur. In the latter instances, suppressive therapy should be reinstituted and should be continued indefinitely. When treatment is initiated in patients of childbearing age, it should probably be continued through the menopause.

In areas of endemic iodine deficiency, the size and prevalence of goiter, and probably the frequency of cretinism, can be reduced by the infrequent injection of iodized oil.

Surgical therapy of simple goiter is physiologically unsound, but it may occasionally be necessary to relieve obstructive symptoms, especially those which persist after a conscientious trial of medical therapy. Surgical exploration of nodular goiter may be indicated in some individuals when evidence suggests carcinoma. However, the suggestion that subtotal resection of multinodular nontoxic goiter affords effective prophylaxis against the development of thyroid carcinoma is unsound. If for some reason subtotal thyroidectomy has been performed, levothyroxine in a dose of 150 to 200 μg daily is recommended to inhibit regenerative hyperplasia and further goitrogenesis.

HYPOTHYROIDISM

Hypothyroidism is a clinical state that may result from any of a wide variety of structural or functional abnormalities that lead to insufficient synthesis of thyroid hormone. Hypothyroidism dating from birth and resulting in developmental abnormalities is termed *cretinism*. The term *myxedema* connotes a severe form of hypothyroidism in which there is accumulation of hydrophilic mucopolysaccharides in the ground substance of the dermis as well as other tissues, leading to thickening of the facial features and doughy induration of the skin.

ETIOLOGY AND PATHOGENESIS A classification of the causes of hypothyroidism is presented in Table 335-4. In thyroprivic hypothyroidism, loss of thyroid tissue leads to inadequate synthesis of thyroid hormone, despite maximum stimulation of any thyroid remnant by TSH. The most common cause of thyroprivic hypothyroidism is surgical or radioiodine ablation of the thyroid gland in the treatment of Graves' disease. Thyroprivic hypothyroidism may also occur as a primary idiopathic phenomenon. The cause of this disorder is unknown, but the frequency of circulating antithyroid antibodies and its coexistence with pernicious anemia and other diseases in which circulating antibodies are found suggest that it may belong to the autoimmune group of diseases. Finally, a devel-

opmental defect may result in failure of the gland to gain an adequate size, leading to sporadic nongoitrous cretinism or juvenile hypothyroidism.

A purely functional impairment in the ability to synthesize adequate quantities of thyroid hormone leads to hypersecretion of TSH and hence goiter. If this compensatory response is inadequate, goitrous hypothyroidism ensues. The commonest cause in North America is Hashimoto's disease, in which defective organic binding of iodide and abnormal secretion of iodoproteins are frequent biosynthetic abnormalities. Iodide-induced goiter with or without hypothyroidism appears often to arise from an intrinsic defect in the organic binding mechanism, which permits a persistent Wolff-Chaikoff effect. Patients with Graves' disease, especially after radioiodine treatment, those with Hashimoto's disease, and the normal fetus are particularly susceptible to iodide-induced goiter. In view of the susceptibility of the fetal thyroid to iodide, with resulting goiter and hypothyroidism, women should not be given iodine in large doses during pregnancy. Less common causes of goitrous hypothyroidism are heritable defects in pathways of hormone biosynthesis and ingestion of drugs which induce defects in hormone biosynthesis, such as *p*-aminosalicylic acid, cobalt, and lithium carbonate. Finally, in many areas of the world where there is environmental iodine deficiency, goitrous cretinism and hypothyroidism occur on an endemic basis. Diminished thyroid reserve occurs as a stage in the evolution of both thyroprivic and goitrous hypothyroidism.

In hypothyroidism of suprathyroid origin, the thyroid is intrinsically normal, but is deprived of stimulation by TSH. Deprivation of TSH, most commonly the result of postpartum pituitary necrosis or a tumor of the pituitary or adjacent regions, results in pituitary hypothyroidism. Hypothalamic hypothyroidism appears to be less common and results from inadequate secretion of TRH.

CLINICAL PICTURE The general appearance of children with hypothyroidism varies considerably, depending on the age at which the deficiency began and the promptness with which replacement therapy was instituted. Manifestations of cretinism may be present at birth, but are more commonly evident within the first several months, depending upon the extent of thyroid failure. During the neonatal period, the abnormally long persistence of physiologic jaundice, hoarse cry, constipation, somnolence, and feeding problems should call attention to the diagnosis. In later months, delay in reaching the normal milestones of development becomes evident, and the physical characteristics of the cretin appear. These include short stature, coarse features with protruding tongue, broad flat nose,

TABLE 335-4
Classification of the causes of hypothyroidism

I Thyroidal
  A Thyroprivic
    1 Congenital development defect
    2 Primary idiopathic
    3 Postablative (radioiodine, surgery)
    4 Postradiation (lymphoma)
  B Goitrous
    1 Heritable biosynthetic defects
    2 Maternally transmitted (iodides, antithyroid agents)
    3 Iodine deficiency
    4 Drug-elicited (*p*-aminosalicylic acid, iodides, phenylbutazone, iodoantipyrine, cobalt, lithium)
    5 Chronic thyroiditis (Hashimoto's disease)
II Suprathyroidal (trophoprivic)
  A Pituitary
  B Hypothalamic

widely set eyes, sparse hair, dry skin, and protuberant abdomen with an umbilical hernia. X-ray examination reveals retarded bone age, epiphyseal dysgenesis, and delayed dental development. Mental development is retarded; eventualy intellectual attainment will depend upon how soon full replacement therapy is instituted. Consequently, it is fortunate that neonatal hypothyroidism can readily be diagnosed from measurements of the serum T_4 or serum TSH in either cord or infant's blood. Extensive surveys using these techniques have revealed an approximate frequency of this disorder of 1 in every 5000 births. Hence, every newborn should undergo screening for hypothyroidism so that treatment can be begun as soon as possible.

In the older child with hypothyroidism, the clinical manifestations are intermediate between those of infantile and adult hypothyroidism. Retardation of linear growth results in shortness of stature, while retardation of sexual maturation results in delay in the onset of puberty. Poor performance at school may call attention to the diagnosis. The manifestations of adult hypothyroidism are present to a variable degree. X-ray examination reveals delayed union of the epiphyses.

In the adult, early symptoms of hypothyroidism are nonspecific and of insidious onset. They may include lethargy, constipation, cold intolerance, and menorrhagia. Over the succeeding months, slowing of intellectual and motor activity appears, appetite declines, and modest weight gain occurs. The hair becomes dry and tends to fall out. The patient may complain of dry skin and of stiff aching muscles. The voice becomes deeper and hoarse and auditory acuity may deteriorate. Ultimately, the clinical picture of florid myxedema appears, with dull expressionless face, sparse hair, periorbital puffiness, large tongue, and pale, cool skin which feels rough and doughy. Thyroid tissue is not readily palpable, except in the goitrous variety of hypothyroidism. The heart is enlarged owing to both dilation and pericardial effusion; if the heart is small, pituitary hypothyroidism should be considered. Adynamic ileus may occur, producing the clinical picture of megacolon. Rarely, psychiatric reactions or cerebellar ataxia may dominate the clinical picture. The relaxation phase of the deep tendon reflexes is characteristically prolonged, the so-called "hung-up" reflex. If left untreated, the patient with severe long-standing hypothyroidism may pass into a hypothermic, stuporous state (*myxedema coma*), which is frequently fatal. Respiratory depression is an important component of this state, and hence an increased arterial P_{CO_2} is of premonitory value. Factors which predispose to myxedema coma include cold exposure, trauma, infection, and administration of central nervous system depressants. Dilutional hyponatremia is common in severe hypothyroidism and results from diminished renal perfusion leading to impaired water excretion.

LABORATORY TESTS A decrease in serum T_4 and in the FT_4I is common to all varieties of hypothyroidism, as is a decrease in BMR. In the thyroidal varieties, the serum T_3 may be decreased to a lesser extent than is the serum T_4, or not at all, the presumption being that the compensatory hypersecretion of TSH leads to a relative preponderance of T_3 secretion. Because of the decline in the range of normal values, the RAIU is no longer of value in the diagnosis of thyroprivic hypothyroidism, unless it is used as a part of the TSH-stimulation test. In goitrous hypothyroidism, the RAIU may be increased or may display an abnormal pattern of accumulation or retention. The serum TSH is invariably increased in the thyroprivic and goitrous varieties and is normal or undetectable in pituitary or hypothalamic hypothyroidism. In the latter varieties, in addition to possible evidence of intracranial disease, hyposecretion of TSH is accompanied by hyposecretion of other pituitary

hormones; this is amenable to laboratory testing (see Chap. 333). A subnormal response of the serum TSH to the administration of TRH will confirm the presence of pituitary hypothyroidism.

Other frequent, but not invariable, manifestations of the hypothyroid state include an increased serum cholesterol in hypothyroidism of thyroid (but not pituitary) origin, an abnormally prolonged relaxation time of the Achilles reflex, and increased concentrations in serum of creatine phosphokinase, glutamic oxaloacetic transaminase, and lactic dehydrogenase. Electrocardiographic changes are common and include bradycardia, low amplitude, and flattened or inverted T waves. In primary thyroprivic hypothyroidism, overt pernicious anemia reportedly occurs in about 12 percent of patients; histamine-fast achlorhydria and the presence of circulating gastric parietal cell antibodies are even more common.

In addition to patients who are clinically hypothyroid, some patients who appear clinically euthyroid display low values of the serum T_4. In such patients, the serum T_3 is normal or near normal and, serum TSH is slightly increased. This phenomenon of T_3 euthyroidism, which is seen most frequently in patients with Hashimoto's or Graves' disease who have been treated with radioiodine, represents in all likelihood a phase in the evolution of frank hypothyroidism. As such, it may be considered as representing a state of diminished reserve in which compensatory hypersecretion of TSH evokes a relative hypersection of T_3.

DIFFERENTIAL DIAGNOSIS Little difficulty will be experienced in diagnosing the classic picture of cretinism or juvenile and adult hypothyroidism. Occasionally, a mongoloid infant may be confused with a cretin. However, the characteristic mongoloid eyes, Brushfield's spots in the iris, hyperextensibility of the joints, and normal skin and hair texture distinguish the mongoloid imbecile from the hypothyroid cretin. Chronic nephritis and especially nephrosis may simulate myxedema, particularly because of the facial puffiness and pallor. The nephrotic patient may also display anemia, hypercholesterolemia, and anasarca. Since both the BMR and serum T_4 are often subnormal, the differential diagnosis may be confusing. However, the low serum T_4 is caused by a decrease in plasma protein binding resulting from proteinuria; hence, the FT_4I will be normal. Moreover, the RAIU is generally normal or increased.

TREATMENT Two general types of preparation are available for the treatment of hypothyroidism, synthetic hormone and thyroprotein derived from animal thyroids. Synthetic hormones include L-thyroxine sodium (levothyroxine), L-triiodothyronine sodium (liothyronine), and a combination of the two (liotrix). The preparation of natural origin most commonly used is thyroid extract, USP. The approximate therapeutic equivalence of these drugs is presented in Table 335-5. Because of their uniform potency, the authors prefer the synthetic preparations, and of these the authors prefer levothyroxine. Unlike liothyronine, liotrix, and even thyroid extract, ingestion of le-

TABLE 335-5
Approximate therapeutic equivalence of various thyroid hormone preparations

Preparation	Average daily oral maintenance dose	Serum T_4
Thyroid extract, USP	120–180 mg	Normal
Levothyroxine	200 µg	Normal or slightly increased
Liothyronine	50 µg	Decreased
Liotrix ($T_4/T_3 = 4:1$)	2 units	Normal

vothyroxine does not lead to abrupt increases in serum T_3 concentration, which could be dangerous in the older patient or in the patient with coexisting heart disease.

In most instances, restoration of a normal metabolic state should be undertaken gradually, especially in the elderly or the patient with heart disease, since sudden increases in metabolic rate may tax cardiac reserve. In adults, an initial daily dose of 25 μg levothyroxine is recommended, and this can be increased by 25- to 50-μg increments at 2- to 3-week intervals, until a normal metabolic state is attained. The daily dose usually necessary to sustain a normal metabolic state is from 150 to 200 μg, and this is usually accompanied by a serum T_4 at the upper limit of the normal range. Because of its long half-life, levothyroxine is generally administered as a single daily dose. The optimum dose for the individual patient should be based on clinical criteria, the serum T_4 being employed only as a confirmatory test.

In cretinism and juvenile hypothyroidism it is essential that full replacement therapy be begun as soon as possible; otherwise the chances of normal intellectual development and growth are poor. Infants and children require doses of levothyroxine that are disproportionately large in relation to body size. *In known or strongly suspected pituitary and hypothalamic hypothyroidism, thyroid replacement should not be instituted until treatment with hydrocortisone has been initiated,* since acute adrenocortical insufficiency may be precipitated by an increase in metabolic rate.

In some patients, it is important that hypothyroidism be rapidly treated. This includes patients with myxedema coma and, because of the extreme sensitivity to central nervous system depressants, hypothyroid patients being prepared for emergency surgery. Here, intravenous administration of levothyroxine, in conjunction with the use of hydrocortisone, is indicated.

GRAVES' DISEASE

Graves' disease, also known as Parry's or Basedow's disease, is a disorder of unknown etiology with a characteristic triad of major manifestations: hyperthyroidism with diffuse goiter, ophthalmopathy, and dermopathy. Although considered part of the same disease complex, the three major manifestations need not appear together. Indeed, one or two need never appear, and, moreover, the three tend to run a course largely independent of one another. Although hyperthyroidism is the most common manifestation of Graves' disease, it is important to be aware of the fact that hyperthyroidism which merely reflects an excessive supply of thyroid hormone to the tissues, can also arise in a variety of other circumstances which are clearly distinct from Graves' disease, as is discussed below.

PREVALENCE Graves' disease is a relatively common disorder which may occur at any age, but occurs especially in the third and fourth decades. The disease is much more frequent in women than in men. In nongoitrous areas the ratio of predominance in women may be as high as 7:1. In endemic goitrous areas the ratio is lower. There is a distinct familial predisposition to Graves' disease; in addition, among family members of patients with Graves' disease, a clinical and immunological overlap exists with respect to Hashimoto's disease, primary thyroprivic hypothyroidism, and pernicious anemia, and probably with respect to other diseases in which autoimmune features are prominent.

ETIOLOGY AND PATHOGENESIS The cause of Graves' disease is unknown. In view of the varied manifestations of Graves' disease and their differing courses, it is possible, and indeed likely, that no single factor is responsible for the entire syndrome. With respect to hyperthyroidism, it is apparent that

central to this disorder is a disruption of homeostatic mechanisms that normally adjust hormone secretion to meet the needs of peripheral tissues; if such were able to operate, hyperthyroidism could not be sustained. There is now compelling evidence to suggest that this homeostatic disruption results from the presence in plasma of an abnormal thyroid stimulator. The existence of such was recognized more than 20 years ago when it was shown that the sera of patients with thyrotoxic Graves' disease released radioiodine from the prelabeled guinea pig or mouse thyroid. In view of its prolonged duration of action relative to TSH in this bioassay system, this material was designated the long-acting thyroid stimulator (LATS). LATS was demonstrated to be an immunoglobulin G elaborated by lymphocytes. It soon became apparent, however, that LATS could be detected only in about one-half of thyrotoxic patients with Graves' disease, and, consequently, its pathogenetic role was seriously questioned. More recently, it has been demonstrated that this failure to detect LATS in many patients with Graves' disease is due to the fact that the stimulator in human serum has variable cross-reactivity in other species and might not be detectable, therefore, in the conventional LATS assay. When human thyroid tissue is used as the assay system, however, there can be demonstrated one or more of a variety of in vitro responses to immunoglobulin G derived from the plasma of most patients with thyrotoxic Graves' disease. These responses and the corresponding names given to the responsible factors are as follows: stimulation of colloid droplet formation or cyclic AMP generation in thyroid slices (*thyroid-stimulating immunoglobulin, TSI*), displacement of labeled TSH from thyroid membranes (*TSH-displacing activity, TDA*), and prevention of the adsorption of LATS by thyroid particulate fractions (*LATS protector, LATSp*). The underlying nature of these factors, their number, and their relationship to one another are uncertain, but they are thought by some to be one or more antibodies directed against some component of the thyroid plasma membrane, perhaps the TSH receptor itself. Activities of this type are also found in sera of some patients with euthyroid ophthalmic Graves' disease, the occasional patient with Hashimoto's disease, and some euthyroid relatives of patients with Graves' disease, though the reason for the absence of thyrotoxicosis in such instances is uncertain. It appears that disappearance of these stimulatory factors from the serum during antithyroid treatment augurs well for long-term remission after treatment is withdrawn. Thus, while the basic cause of Graves' disease is still not understood, there is now good evidence that an immunoglobulin G or family of immunoglobulins directed against some component of the thyroid is pathogenetically involved in mediating the thyroid stimulation of thyrotoxic Graves' disease. It has been proposed that a heritable abnormality in immune surveillance may permit a particular clone of lymphocytes to survive, proliferate, and secrete the stimulatory immunoglobulins in response to some precipitating factors. An alternative hypothesis is that the TSH receptor, because of some heritable abnormality, undergoes a qualitative alteration in response to some precipitating environmental factor and evokes the production of thyroid-stimulating antibodies.

The pathogenesis of the ophthalmic component of Graves' disease is even more enigmatic. One proposed mechanism invokes the activity of a fragment of the TSH molecule, which, in conjunction with an immunoglobulin, binds to and produces edema of retroorbital tissue. A second mechanism, for which there is more evidence, invokes cephalad lymphatic transport of thyroglobulin from the thyroid to retroorbital tissues, at which site an immune response is evoked. Nothing is known of the pathogenesis of the dermopathy of Graves' disease.

PATHOLOGY In Grave's disease, the *thyroid gland* is diffusely enlarged, soft, and vascular. The essential pathology is that of parenchymatous hypertrophy and hyperplasia, characterized by increased height of the epithelium and redundancy of the follicular wall, giving the picture of papillary infoldings and cytologic evidence of increased activity. Such hyperplasia is usually accompanied by lymphocytic infiltration that may reflect the immune aspect of the disease and its attendant chronic thyroiditis. Following iodine medication, there is colloid storage, which sometimes causes enlargement and increased firmness of the gland. Grave's disease is associated with generalized lymphoid hyperplasia and infiltration, and occasionally with enlargement of the spleen or thymus. Thyrotoxicosis may lead to degeneration of skeletal muscle fibers, enlargement of the heart, fatty infiltration or diffuse fibrosis of the liver, decalcification of the skeleton, and loss of body tissue (including fat deposits, osteoid, and muscle).

The *ophthalmopathy* of Graves' disease is characterized pathologically by an inflammatory infiltrate of the orbital contents, exclusive of the globe, with lymphocytes, mast cells, and plasma cells being the predominant cellular components. The orbital musculature is mainly involved and often is greatly enlarged, largely accounting for the increased volume of the orbital contents that causes the globe to protrude. Muscle fibers show degeneration and loss of striations, with ultimate fibrosis.

The *dermopathy* of Graves' disease is characterized by thickening of the dermis, which is infiltrated with lymphocytes and with hydrophilic, metachromatically staining mucopolysaccharides.

CLINICAL MANIFESTATIONS The clinical manifestations of patients with Graves' disease vary according to the type of presentations and their individual severity. It is also modified by the age of the patient and the presence of underlying disease in other organs, particularly the heart.

Hyperthyroidism Common manifestations of hyperthyroidism in Graves' disease include goiter, fine tremor (especially of the extended fingers and tongue), increased nervousness, as well as emotional instability, excessive sweating and heat intolerance, palpitations, and hyperkinesis. Loss of weight and of strength usually exist, often despite increased appetite. Weakness is often manifested by difficulty in climbing stairs. When severe wasting of limb-girdle musculature is present, the condition is termed *thyrotoxic myopathy*. Hyperdefecation and occasionally anorexia, nausea, and vomiting may occur. Dyspnea, atrial arrhythmias, and, in individuals over the age of 40, cardiac failure occur not infrequently. Oligomenorrhea and amenorrhea are commoner than menorrhagia. In general, nervous symptoms dominate the clinical picture in younger individuals, whereas cardiovascular and myopathic symptoms predominate in older subjects.

The skin is warm and moist with a velvety texture, and palmar erythema is often found. Separation of the fingernail from the nailbed (Plummer's nails), especially on the ring finger, is often seen in hyperthyroidism, but is not pathognomonic of Graves' disease. The hair is fine and silky. Occasionally, increased loss of hair from the temporal aspects of the scalp may be noted. Excessive melanin pigmentation or patches of vitiligo are not uncommon. *Ocular signs* include a characteristic stare with widened palpebral fissures, infrequent blinking, lid lag, failure of convergence, and failure to wrinkle the brow on upward gaze. These signs are thought to result from sympathetic overstimulation and usually subside when the thyrotox-

icosis is corrected. The *infiltrative ophthalmopathy* characteristic of Graves' disease is discussed below.

The *diffuse toxic goiter* may be asymmetric and lobular. Often a bruit is heard directly over the gland. When heard, it usually signifies that the patient is thyrotoxic, but it may also rarely be present in association with other disorders in which the thyroid is markedly hyperplastic. Venous hums and carotid souffles should be distinguished from true thyroid bruits. A hyperplastic pyramidal lobe of the thyroid may often be palpable if carefully sought.

Cardiovascular findings include a wide pulse pressure, sinus tachycardia, atrial arrhythmias (especially atrial fibrillation), systolic murmurs, increased intensity of the apical first sound, cardiac enlargement, and at times, overt heart failure. A to-and-fro, high-pitched sound may be audible in the pulmonic area and may simulate a pericardial friction rub.

Ophthalmopathy The clinical signs associated with the ophthalmopathy of Graves' disease may be divided into two components: the spastic and the mechanical. The former includes the stare, lid lag, and lid retraction that accompany thyrotoxicosis and account for the "frightened" facies and classic eye signs previously described. These findings need not be associated with actual proptosis and usually return to normal after appropriate correction of thyrotoxicosis. The mechanical component includes proptosis of varying degrees with ophthalmoplegia and congestive oculopathy characterized by chemosis, conjunctivitis, marked periorbital swelling, and the resultant complications of corneal ulceration, optic neuritis, and optic atrophy. When exophthalmos progresses rapidly and becomes the major concern in Graves' disease, it is usually referred to as *progressive,* and if severe, *malignant exophthalmos.* The term *exophthalmic ophthalmoplegia* refers to the ocular muscle weakness that so commonly accompanies this disorder and results in strabismus with varying degrees of diplopia. Exophthalmos may be unilateral early in the course of the disorder but usually progresses to symmetric involvement.

Dermopathy The dermopathy of Graves' disease usually occurs over the dorsum of the legs or feet and is commonly termed *localized myxedema* or *pretibial myxedema.* It occurs in patients with past or present Graves' disease and is not a manifestation of hypothyroidism per se. About half of the cases occur during the active stage of thyrotoxicosis; in the remainder the lesions develop after treatment. The affected area is usually well demarcated from normal skin by the fact that it is raised, thickened, has a *peau d'orange* appearance, and may be pruritic and hyperpigmented. The lesions are usually discrete, assuming a plaque-like or nodular configuration, but in some instances the lesions become widely confluent. Clubbing of the fingers and toes with characteristic bony changes differentiable from those of hypertrophic pulmonary osteoarthropathy may accompany the dermal changes (*thyroid acropachy*). Activity of this disorder is usually self-limited.

DIAGNOSIS When severe, Graves' disease presents little difficulty in diagnosis. Florid thyrotoxicosis is manifested by weakness, weight loss despite good appetite, nervous instability, tremor, intolerance to heat, hyperhydrosis, palpitations, and hyperdefecation. When associated with diffuse thyroid enlargement, often accompanied by a bruit, and particularly when associated with ophthalmopathy, Graves' disease presents a clinical picture that is virtually unique. In such instances, laboratory tests, which reveal increased RAIU, serum T_4 and T_3, RT_3U, and FT_4I, and increased BMR, serve mainly as base lines for evaluation of therapy, rather than necessary diagnostic aids. Occasionally, laboratory tests reveal a normal RAIU, serum T_4, and RT_3U, the serum T_3 and FT_3I alone being increased (T_3 toxicosis).

In less severe cases, particularly when ophthalmopathy is lacking, the diagnosis may be substantially more difficult, since the symptoms of mild hyperthyroidism are similar to those of other disorders (see "Differential Diagnosis" below). Presence of a goiter makes the diagnosis of hyperthyroidism more likely, but careful palpation is necessary to determine whether toxic multinodular goiter or toxic adenoma is present, since treatment of these disorders may differ from that of diffuse toxic goiter. Absence of thyroid enlargement makes the diagnosis of Graves' disease unlikely, but does not exclude it absolutely. In mild cases, confirmatory laboratory tests assume great importance. Unfortunately, mild hyperthyroidism is often associated with only marginal abnormalities in laboratory tests, and values may in fact lie within the upper limit of the normal range. In instances like this, the thyroid suppression test or the TRH stimulation test assumes crucial importance.

In a few patients, the clinical picture may be one of apathy rather than hyperactivity, and evidence of hypermetabolism may be slight. In such patients, myopathic features may be pronounced. More often, cardiovascular manifestations predominate since, in patients with underlying heart disease, even mild hyperthyroidism may produce severe disability. Hence, *all patients with unexplained cardiac failure or irregularities in rhythm, especially if atrial in origin, should be examined for hyperthyroidism.* Clues to the diagnosis include a relatively rapid circulation time and resistance to the usual doses of digitalis, but laboratory confirmation will be required.

DIFFERENTIAL DIAGNOSIS Signs and symptoms in a number of nonthyroid disorders may simulate certain aspects of the thyrotoxic syndrome. Anxiety is a prominent feature of hyperthyroidism, and there is thus some overlap in the symptomatology of this disorder with that of anxiety states of emotional origin. Such symptoms as tachycardia, tremulousness, irritability, weakness, and fatigue are common to the anxiety of both disorders. In anxiety of emotional origin, however, the peripheral manifestations of excessive thyroid hormones are absent; the skin of the extremities is usually cold and clammy rather than warm and moist. Weight loss, when present in emotional anxiety, is characteristically accompanied by anorexia, whereas in hyperthyroidism it is generally, but not invariably, accompanied by excessive appetite. Hyperthyroidism can occasionally be confused with such disorders as metastatic carcinoma, cirrhosis of the liver, hyperparathyroidism, sprue, and neuromyopathies, such as myasthenia gravis and muscular dystrophy. Hypokalemic periodic paralysis is more common in thyrotoxic patients, especially in the case of Oriental males. Signs and symptoms of hyperthyroidism may overlap with those of pheochromocytoma, which may present with heat intolerance, excessive perspiration, tachycardia with palpitations, and a hypermetabolic state that may often be severe. In all the above disorders, as well as other conditions considered in the differential diagnosis, judiciously applied laboratory tests will usually suffice to differentiate them from hyperthyroidism.

When bilateral ophthalmopathy is accompanied by goiter and thyrotoxicosis, the origin of the ophthalmopathy in the Graves' disease process is virtually certain. The presence of unilateral ophthalmopathy, even when associated with thyrotoxicosis, should alert the physician to the possibility of some other intraorbital or intracranial disease. In the patient who is not thyrotoxic, it is more difficult to ascribe ophthalmopathy to Graves' disease, and other causes must be actively excluded. Among the local causes of unilateral or bilateral exophthalmos are cavernous sinus thrombosis, sphenoidal ridge meningioma, and retrobulbar tumors, including leukemic deposits, as well as the rare granulomatous disorder, pseudotumor oculi. Exophthalmos may also be seen in some patients with certain systemic disorders, such as uremia, accelerated hypertension,

chronic alcoholism, chronic obstructive pulmonary disease, superior mediastinal obstruction, and Cushing's syndrome. Ophthalmoplegia in the absence of overt infiltrative manifestations can be confused with that which occurs in diabetes mellitus, myasthenia gravis, and myopathies. When doubt exists about the cause of ophthalmopathy, the demonstration of an abnormal thyroid suppression test strongly suggests that the cause is Graves' disease, though not all patients with "euthyroid Graves' disease" will demonstrate an abnormal response. In such cases, ultrasonography or computerized axial tomography of the orbits may be valuable in demonstrating characteristic thickening of the extraocular muscles.

When the diagnosis of thyrotoxicosis has been established in a patient lacking the ophthalmopathic manifestions of Graves' disease, other causes of thyrotoxicosis must be considered. Palpation of a symmetric, diffuse goiter, especially if associated with a bruit, excludes the diagnosis of *toxic multinodular goiter* or *toxic adenoma;* both these disorders are discussed in later sections. Absence of a palpable thyroid gland raises the suspicion of ectopic thyroid tissue or, much more commonly, self-administration of thyroid hormone (*thyrotoxicosis factitia*). Ectopic thyroid tissue producing thyrotoxicosis is very rare and is most commonly located in the ovary (*struma ovarii*). RAIU, as measured over the thyroid, is low since TSH secretion is suppressed, but despite this, urinary excretion of the dose of ^{131}I is also low, owing to accumulation of ^{131}I by the ectopic tissue. Functioning ectopic tissue can be located by direct counting or scintillation scanning. Thyrotoxicosis factitia most frequently occurs in medical or paramedical personnel or in those who have easy access to thyroid hormone preparations. Physiologically, it resembles thyrotoxicosis caused by ectopic thyroid tissue in that the patient's thyroid gland is suppressed. By contrast, however, most of an administered dose of ^{131}I will be excreted in the urine. When the disorder is caused by ingestion of preparations containing T_4, such as levothyroxine or thyroid extract, the serum T_4 will be increased. On the other hand, when caused by liothyronine, the serum T_4 will be subnormal. Irrespective of the preparation, the serum T_3 will be increased, but more so when liothyronine is the offending agent. Occasionally, thyrotoxicosis may be produced by *tumors of trophoblastic origin,* such as choriocarcinoma of the testis or hydatidiform mole, that elaborate thyroid-stimulating peptides (see Chap. 347). Very rarely, thyrotoxicosis is due to a TSH-secreting tumor of the pituitary. In these disorders, thyrotoxicosis is associated with hyperfunction of the thyroid gland.

TREATMENT **Hyperthyroidism** The hyperthyroidism in Graves' disease is a disorder often characterized by cyclic phases of exacerbation and remission, each of unpredictable onset and duration. Moreover, subtle tests of thyroid function indicate that long-standing disease is associated with progressive thyroid failure, probably consequent to chronic thyroiditis, with the result that hypothyroidism or decreased thyroid reserve supervenes. These characteristics of Graves' disease have important implications in the choice of and response to therapy, as is discussed below.

There are two major approaches to the treatment of hyperthyroidism; both are directed to limiting the quantity of thyroid hormones the gland can produce. The first major therapeutic modality, the use of antithyroid agents, interposes a chemical blockade to hormone synthesis, the effect of which is operative only as long as the drug is administered or until a spontaneous remission occurs. Thus, the agents can control successfully a given phase of active thyrotoxicity but probably will not prevent exacerbation at some subsequent period. The second major approach is ablation of thyroid tissue, thereby limiting hormone production. This may be achieved either surgically or by means of radioactive iodine. Since these procedures induce permanent anatomic alterations of the thyroid, they can control the individual active phase and are more likely to prevent recurrence of thyrotoxicity during a later exacerbation. On the other hand, the permanency of the effects of surgery or radiation makes these modes of therapy capable of leading to hypothyroidism, either shortly after treatment or with the passage of years.

Each major mode of therapy has advantages and disadvantages, indications and contraindications. The latter are more often relative than absolute. In general, a trial of long-term antithyroid therapy is desirable in children, adolescents, young adults, and pregnant women, but may also be employed in older patients. Indications for ablative procedures include relapse or recurrence following drug therapy, a large goiter, drug toxicity, and failure of the patient to follow a medical regimen or to return for periodic examinations. Subtotal thyroidectomy is usually elected for patients under the age of 40 in whom ablative therapy is required; however, opinions differ, and some authorities employ radioactive iodine in the treatment of patients in the second or third decades. With older patients, radioactive iodine is clearly the ablative procedure of choice, as it is for patients who have had previous thyroid surgery or those in whom serious systemic disease contraindicates elective surgery.

In those patients selected for *long-term antithyroid therapy,* satisfactory control can almost always be achieved if a sufficient dosage of the drug is administered. Most patients can be managed successfully with propylthiouracil, 100 to 150 mg every 6 or 8 h. Methimazole is at least as effective as propylthiouracil when administered in one-tenth the dosage. Once euthyroidism is achieved, the daily dosage may be reduced to the smallest doses that control the thyrotoxicosis fully. In some clinics, however, the initial dose is continued and is supplemented with levothyroxine. By this latter regimen, hypothyroidism resulting from overdosage of antithyroid drugs can be prevented. The undesirable consequences of hypothyroidism, such as enhancement of ophthalmopathy and enlargement of the goiter, may thereby be forestalled. The precise duration of therapy is difficult to predict in the individual patient and may be a function of the spontaneous course of the disease itself. If this is the case, the longer the course of therapy, the more likely it is that the patient will remain well when the drug is discontinued. In general, however, a 12- to 24-month course is usually employed. Following a regimen of this type, about one-third to one-half of the patients will remain well for a prolonged period or indefinitely. A normal suppressive response to exogenous thyroid hormone when withdrawal of antithyroid agent is contemplated increases the likelihood that the patient will remain in remission for some time. Decrease in goiter size during treatment has a similar connotation.

The *treatment of hyperthyroidism during pregnancy* is a subject of disagreement. Most physicians believe that antithyroid therapy is preferable to subtotal thyroidectomy, particularly during the first and third trimesters. The major disadvantage of antithyroid therapy is the possibility of inducing goiter and hypothyroidism in the fetus, since antithyroid agents readily traverse the placenta. Hence, a cardinal rule in the use of these agents during pregnancy is that the dosage of antithyroid agent should be the smallest necessary to control hyperthyroidism in the mother. Maintenance of normal values for FT_4 or FT_4I will assist in this objective. Some authorities regularly supplement the antithyroid regimen with replacement doses of thyroid hormone. However, available evidence suggests that T_4 and T_3 traverse the human placenta from mother to fetus

slowly, if at all. Supplemental thyroid hormone will produce no harm unless a false sense of assurance leads to administration of excessive doses of antithyroid agent or neglect of frequent observation of the patient. Pregnancy is an important indication for the assay of thyroid stimulator in the serum, since high titers in the mother are likely to be associated with thyrotoxicosis in the newborn.

Leukopenia is the principal undesirable side effect of antithyroid drugs. Mild transient leukopenia may occur in approximately 10 percent of patients treated and is not necessarily an indication for discontinuing therapy. When the absolute number of polymorphonuclear leukocytes reaches 1500 or less, antithyroid medication should be discontinued. Allergic rashes and drug sensitivity develop in a small percentage of patients. These may disappear with antihistamine therapy at the same or reduced dosage of antithyroid agent, but it is probably preferable, when sensitivity reactions occur, to change to another drug. On rare occasions (in less than 0.2 percent), agranulocytosis may occur. This may be sudden in onset. Hepatitis, drug fever, and arthralgias are occasional adverse reactions to antithyroid agents. In the authors' view, such severe sensitivity reactions, including, of course, agranulocytosis, dictate the abandonment of antithyroid therapy, rather than recourse to an alternate drug.

Iodide inhibits the release of thyroid hormones from the thyrotoxic gland, and its ameliorative effects occur more rapidly than those of agents that merely inhibit hormone synthesis. Hence, its main use is in patients with actual or impending thyrotoxic crisis or in patients with severe thyrocardiac disease. However, the response to iodide is often incomplete and transient. Furthermore, by expanding the thyroid store of hormone, iodide may prolong greatly the latency of response to subsequently instituted antithyroid therapy. Therefore, iodide should be used in conjunction with the antithyroid agents. If the clinical course of the patient is sufficiently severe to require iodide administration, antithyroid drugs will usually be the primary therapeutic agents and should be given in large doses prior to iodide. Since iodide appears to synergize with radiation in the thyroid, it is also useful in controlling thyrotoxicosis following ^{131}I administration, during the period in which the therapeutic effect of radioiodine has not yet taken place.

Owing to the pronounced adrenergic component in thyrotoxicosis, various *adrenergic antagonists* have been employed in the management of this disorder. Of these, propranolol appears to be the agent of choice because of its relative freedom from side effects. In doses of 40 to 120 mg daily, propranolol alleviates such adrenergic manifestations as sweating, tremor, and tachycardia, and may reduce to some extent the conversion of T_4 to T_3. However, propranolol should be used only as adjunctive therapy rather than sole therapy, as some have suggested, since the underlying metabolic abnormalities are not significantly affected. Moreover, although the diminution in heart rate and cardiac work that propranolol induces may be beneficial, the withdrawal of adrenergic support of myocardial contractility contraindicates its use in the patient with coexisting heart failure, unless rate- or rhythm-related. As adjunctive therapy, propranolol has its major usefulness in the period during which the response to conventional antithyroid agents or to radioiodine therapy is being awaited and in the management of thyrotoxic crisis. It has also been employed as the sole agent in preparation for thyroidectomy. However, since it does not render the patient euthyroid, with a likely greater risk of surgically induced crisis, its use in this setting is not recommended.

Radioactive iodine (^{131}I) affords a relatively simple, effective, and economical means of treating thyrotoxicosis. Its major advantage is that it can produce the ablative effects of surgery without the immediate operative and postoperative complications. The principal disadvantage of ^{131}I therapy, in the dosage which has usually been employed, is its tendency to produce hypothyroidism with a frequency that increases progressively with time. As many as 40 to 70 percent of patients may develop this complication by 10 years after treatment. Although hypothyroidism is readily treated, once diagnosed, the insidious onset of the disorder may obscure the diagnosis until serious complications have developed. Hence, some recommend that all patients be treated with large doses of ^{131}I to ensure relief of thyrotoxicosis and then be placed on permanent physiologic replacement doses of thyroid hormone.

To date, studies have provided no evidence of significant carcinogenic or leukemogenic effect of radioiodine in those doses commonly used in treating hyperthyroidism. Nevertheless, many physicians prefer to reserve radioiodine therapy for patients over 40 years of age, thinking that it is currently not justifiable to administer an agent of undetermined radiation potentialities to younger persons, particularly those of child-bearing potential. Moreover, it seems clear that the greater the patient's life expectancy after ^{131}I therapy, the greater the likelihood that hypothyroidism will develop. Patients with recurrent thyrotoxicosis following surgery, those who refuse surgery, or those who have complicating illnesses contraindicating surgery are excellent candidates for radioiodine therapy.

The usual therapeutic dose of ^{131}I (approximately 160 μCi per gram of estimated gland weight) is the dose that has led to the disturbingly high frequency of hypothyroidism. As a result, though continuing to use this dose, some authorities regularly administer prophylactic replacement doses of thyroid hormone. On the other hand, others have been led to administer smaller doses (approximately 80 μCi/g). However, this does not diminish the frequency of late hypothyroidism, but merely delays its onset. Moreover, the smaller dose is less likely to relieve thyrotoxicosis within a relatively short period. Antithyroid agents can be employed, however, to speed the attainment of a eumetabolic state while the effect of the ^{131}I is taking hold. There is general agreement that patients with thyrocardiac disease should receive ^{131}I in large doses in view of the hazard of recurrent thyrotoxicosis.

Radiation thyroiditis is an occasional immediate complication of ^{131}I therapy. When present, it commonly appears within 7 to 10 days and is associated with excessive release of hormone into the blood. For this reason, patients with severe hyperthyroidism or underlying heart disease should be rendered eumetabolic with antithyroid agents before ^{131}I is administered. Interruption of antithyroid therapy for several days before and after ^{131}I treatment will suffice to permit adequate accumulation and retention of administered ^{131}I. Propranolol may be used as an adjunct both before and after ^{131}I administration, but should not be relied upon to provide adequate prophylaxis if given alone. The swelling that accompanies radiation thyroiditis may contraindicate the use of large doses of ^{131}I in patients with large retrosternal goiters.

Before radioactive iodine was introduced, *subtotal thyroidectomy* was the classic form of ablative therapy, and it is still widely employed in younger patients in whom antithyroid therapy is unsuccessful. Although precise preoperative programs differ, several general principles should be emphasized. Patients should first be rendered fully euthyroid by means of antithyroid agents. Only then should iodide (five drops of Lugol's solution a day for approximately 10 days) be administered concomitantly to effect an involutional response in the gland. Antithyroid drugs should not be discontinued merely because treatment with iodide is instituted.

Hazards of subtotal thyroidectomy include immediate operative complications, such as anesthetic accidents, hemorrhage sometimes leading to respiratory obstruction, and damage to the recurrent laryngeal nerve leading to vocal cord paralysis. Later complications include wound infection, hemorrhage, hypoparathyroidism, or hypothyroidism. In experienced hands, surgery is an effective and relatively safe mode of

therapy. Postoperative recurrences are quite uncommon. However, carefully conducted follow-up studies reveal that hypothyroidism follows surgery more frequently than previously suspected, although not as commonly as following treatment with ^{131}I.

Ophthalmopathy, dermopathy When severe and progressive, ophthalmopathy is the most difficult component of Graves' disease to treat satisfactorily. Fortunately, however, in most patients the disorder runs a benign course that is largely independent of the course of the hyperthyroid component. In most instances, the activity of even moderately severe disease declines and disappears with time, although some exophthalmos and ophthalmoplegia may persist. In mild disease, considerable benefit may be obtained from simple measures, such as elevating the head at night, administering diuretics to reduce edema, and providing tinted glasses for protection from sun, wind, and foreign bodies. A 1% solution of methylcellulose or plastic shields may help to prevent corneal drying in patients unable to oppose the lids during sleep. In more severe cases, as evidenced by progressive exophthalmos, chemosis, ophthalmoplegia, or loss of vision, large doses of prednisone (120 to 140 mg daily) should be administered, since this is usually effective in reducing the edematous and infiltrative components. With improvement, the dosage is reduced to the lowest effective level, since prolonged administration of large doses will lead to adverse accompaniments of glucocorticoid excess. Orbital radiation may be helpful in some patients, especially those with acute, severe infiltrative manifestations. In those cases that progress despite these measures, orbital decompression, i.e., removal of part of the bony orbit to relieve intraorbital pressure, will usually halt progression of the disease. The management of the patient must always be conducted in concert with an ophthalmologist.

In general, treatment of associated hyperthyroidism should be carried out much as would be the case were ophthalmopathy not present, since there is no convincing evidence that the mode of treatment of the hyperthyroidism influences the course of the ocular disease. The suggestion that total thyroid ablation by surgery and large doses of ^{131}I are beneficial to the ophthalmic disease has not been borne out. It is agreed, however, that hyperthyroidism should be treated, but that hypothyroidism be avoided.

Severe dermopathy can be alleviated by the topical application of glucocorticoids.

TOXIC MULTINODULAR GOITER

Toxic multinodular goiter is a not infrequent consequence of long-standing simple goiter, although the exact proportion of cases in which this complication arises is uncertain. In areas of nonendemicity, the specific etiology of nontoxic multinodular goiter is usually indeterminate. Hence, it is unclear whether a specific etiologic factor underlies those cases of nontoxic multinodular goiter that progress to thyrotoxic phase. Common to many nontoxic multinodular goiters, even in areas of iodine sufficiency, is a decrease in the iodine content of thyroglobulin, suggesting either a conditioned deficiency of iodine or an impairment of pathways for its normal incorporation into iodinated amino acids. Pathologically, there is nothing which serves clearly to distinguish the nontoxic from the toxic multinodular goiter. However, as judged from radioautographic and scintillation scanning studies, functional patterns may be of two types. In the first and most common, iodine accumulation occurs diffusely, but in patchy foci throughout the gland. Histologically, associated areas reveal cellular hyperplasia. Whether autonomy of function, a prerequisite for development of thyrotoxicosis, resides in these areas per se, or whether they are responding to an extrathyroidal stimulus, as is thought to be the case in Graves' disease, is uncertain. The second, less common, pattern is that of iodine accumulation in one or more discrete nodules within the gland, the remainder being essentially nonfunctional. Whether the former represent true adenomas or are merely colloid nodules that have developed functional autonomy is also uncertain. In both endemic and sporadic nontoxic multinodular goiter, administration of iodides may lead to the development of thyrotoxicosis, implying that areas of potentially autonomous function had been present.

Because it arises in long-standing simple goiter, toxic multinodular goiter is a disease of the aging or elderly. At least partly for this reason, and perhaps because of the nature of the underlying disease, the clinical presentation differs from that in the thyrotoxicosis of Graves' disease. Ophthalmopathy is rare, and would signal the emergence of Graves' disease superimposed on simple goiter. Some patients may present with quite typical thyrotoxicosis. Often, however, the degree of thyrotoxicosis is less severe than that seen in Graves' disease, although its physiologic impact upon specific organ systems may be great. Notable among these is the cardiovascular system, in which arrhythmias or congestive failure may be precipitated or accentuated by thyrotoxicosis that not infrequently is manifested by only subtle findings in other areas (apathetic hyperthyroidism). Weakness and wasting may often predominate, frequently with loss of appetite rather than hyperphagia, suggesting the presence of a carcinoma.

A nodular goiter that is readily visible or palpable will establish the diagnosis of thyroid disease. In some instances, however, the thyroid gland is not detectably enlarged. Nevertheless, if suggestive clinical findings are present, the physician is obligated to carry out those measures necessary to establish or to exclude the presence of thyrotoxicosis. This is often difficult, since results of conventional laboratory tests are frequently in the borderline range, consistent with the mild degree of thyrotoxicity. However, a value for the serum T_3 that would be considered normal for a young adult may represent an increase in the elderly patient, since values for serum T_3 normally decline with age. Despite their great value in situations such as this, thyroid suppression tests should not be undertaken in the elderly patient because of the hazard of adverse cardiovascular responses. The TRH stimulation test, however, is quite safe, and a subnormal or absent TSH response would confirm the diagnosis of thyrotoxicosis. When laboratory findings do not permit a clear diagnosis of thyrotoxicosis, but suggestive clinical findings are present, a therapeutic trial of antithyroid drugs is indicated.

Radioactive iodine is the treatment of choice for toxic multinodular goiter, once the diagnosis has been established. Large doses (20 to 30 mCi) are usually required, owing in part to the generally lower RAIU and in part to the variable degree of function throughout the gland. Moreover, the physiologic instability of the elderly patient makes definitive treatment desirable. For the same reason, it is usually wise to initiate therapy with antithyroid agents, withholding radioiodine until a euthyroid state has been achieved, and thereby forestalling an exacerbation of thyrotoxicosis, should radiation thyroiditis occur. Hypothyroidism is only an uncommon consequence of radioiodine treatment of toxic multinodular goiter, owing to the variable activity of differing portions of the gland, which permits previously quiescent areas to replace functionally those that have been destroyed by ^{131}I.

T_3 TOXICOSIS T_3 toxicosis is a term employed to designate thyrotoxicosis in which serum T_4 is normal or low in the absence of a deficiency of TBG, while the serum T_3 is increased. Although the production rate of T_3 is disproportionately increased relative to that of T_4 in all patients with hyperthyroidism, in some this discrepancy is greatly exaggerated. This may occur in association with Graves' disease, multinodular goiter, or hyperfunctioning adenoma. The diagnosis should be suspected in a patient with clinical manifestations of thyrotoxicosis in whom the serum T_4 and FT_4 are normal or low and the RAIU is normal or increased. This, together with the frequently palpable goiter, serves to differentiate this disorder from liothyronine-induced thyrotoxicosis factitia. In contradistinction from patients with nonthyroidal disorders mimicking thyrotoxicosis, patients with this disorder, as would be expected, demonstrate nonsuppressibility of thyroid function in response to exogenous T_3 and blunted or absent responses to TRH. In some patients, thyrotoxicosis with increased serum T_3 and normal serum T_4 antecedes emergence of typical increases in both, either during an initial episode of hyperthyroidism or during recurrence after previous treatment.

T_4 TOXICOSIS In most patients with hyperthyroidism, the serum T_3 is increased to a relatively greater extent than the serum T_4 is. This reflects the fact that in hyperthyroidism T_3 generated from T_4 peripherally is supplemented by release of substantial quantities of T_3 from the thyroid. However, patients are sometimes seen in whom thyrotoxicosis is associated with a clear elevation of serum T_4 and a seemingly normal serum T_3 concentration. This syndrome of T_4 *toxicosis* has been reported most commonly in patients who are elderly, ill, or both, and who are, therefore, most commonly seen in a hospital setting. Presumably, the combination of high serum T_4 and normal serum T_3 concentration reflects inhibition or peripheral T_3 generation from T_4, with persistence of T_3 secretion along with T_4 from the thyroid.

JOD-BASEDOW PHENOMENON This term refers to the induction by iodine of thyrotoxicosis in a patient with endemic goiter and is seen in areas of environmental iodine deficiency when measures to increase dietary iodine intake have been implemented. The presumption here is that iodine deficiency protects some patients with endemic goiter from developing thyrotoxicosis. A similar pheonmenon has been reported to occur in areas of environmental iodine sufficiency in patients with nontoxic multinodular goiter who have received large doses of iodide. Since such patients tend to be elderly with the danger of serious cardiovascular manifestations should thyrotoxicosis ensue, large doses of iodine should not be given to those with multinodular goiter. Similarly, in such patients, pharmaceuticals containing iodine, such as x-ray contrast media, should be used only when indicated and with consideration of the possible hazard of inducing the Jod-Basedow phenomenon.

MAJOR COMPLICATIONS OF THYROTOXICOSIS

THYROCARDIAC DISEASE Thyrotoxicosis imposes a variety of burdens upon the heart. Hypermetabolism of the peripheral tissues increases both the metabolic and nonmetabolic (heat-loss) circulatory load, while direct effects of thyroid hormone on the myocardium increase the force, velocity, and rate of ventricular contraction. As a result, cardiac work and cardiac output are increased. Moreover, atrial irritability is enhanced, leading to tachydysrhythmias, most importantly atrial fibrillation. In the patient with a normal heart, these burdens are usually, but not invariably, tolerated. In the patient with underlying heart disease, however, cardiac insufficiency may be precipitated or aggravated. As would be expected, this complication is more common in the elderly patient and is therefore usually seen in the patient with toxic multinodular goiter, not infrequently as the preponderant manifestation of thyrotoxicosis.

In patients with cardiac insufficiency, clues to the presence of thyrotoxicosis include atrial fibrillation, relatively rapid circulation time, increased cardiac output (high-output failure), and resistance to the usual therapeutic doses of digitalis.

Treatment is directed at both rapid alleviation of thyrotoxicosis and restoration of cardiac compensation. The former objective is best met by initiation of treatment with large doses of an antithyroid agent, followed by iodine if the clinical situation is urgent. Radioiodine, which is the ultimate therapy of choice, is withheld until a eumetabolic state has been achieved and the RAIU has returned to a satisfactory level as the stable iodine is excreted. In less severe cases, radioiodine treatment is anteceded by antithyroid drug treatment alone. Management of the cardiac decompensations is carried out in the usual manner, employing larger than usual doses of digitalis, but with care to avoid digitalis intoxication as the thyrotoxicosis is alleviated. Adrenergic antagonists should not be employed in the presence of cardiac failure, unless it is felt that failure is the consequence primarily of disturbance of cardiac rate or rhythm.

THYROTOXIC CRISIS The clinical picture of thyrotoxic crisis or storm is that of a fuminating increase in all the signs and symptoms of thyrotoxicosis. In the past, this disturbance was most often observed postoperatively in patients poorly prepared for surgery. However, with the preoperative use of antithyroid drugs and iodide and with appropriate measures directed to control of metabolic factors, weight, and nutritional status, postoperative thyrotoxic crisis should not occur. At present, so-called "medical storm" is more common and occurs in untreated or inadequately treated patients. It is precipitated by surgical emergency or complicating medical illness, usually sepsis. The syndrome is characterized by extreme irritability, delirium or coma, fever to 41.1°C (106°F) or more, tachycardia, restlessness, hypotension, vomiting, and diarrhea. Rarely, the clinical picture may be more subtle, with apathy, severe prostration, and coma, but with only slight elevation of temperature. Such postoperative complications as sepsis, septicemia, hemorrhage, and transfusion or drug reactions may mimic thyrotoxic crisis. It is thought that in some patients thyrotoxic crisis is associated with or precipitated by adrenocortical insufficiency. The possibility of this complication gains support from evidence indicating increased adrenocortical hormone requirements in thyrotoxicosis and from evidence of reduced adrenocortical reserve in this disorder.

Treatment of this most serious disorder consists in providing general supportive therapy while undertaking measures for alleviating thyrotoxicosis as rapidly as possible. Supportive therapy includes treatment of dehydration and provision of calories through the intravenous administration of glucose and saline, vitamin B complex, and glucocorticoids. Patients should be placed in a cooled, humidified oxygen tent, and, if hyperpyrexia is present, a cooling blanket should be used. Digitalization is required only in the presence of cardiac failure. If shock exists, intravenous pressor agents should be employed. Therapy of the hyperthyroidism consists of induction of blockade of hormone synthesis by the immediate and continued administration of large doses of an antithyroid agent (e.g., 100 mg propylthiouracil every 2 h). If the patient is unable to swallow the medication, the tablets should be triturated and given by nasogastric tube, as parenteral preparations are unavailable. Following initiation of antithyroid therapy, inhibition of hormone release is sought through the administration of large doses of iodine intravenously or by mouth. Adrenergic antagonists are an important, and perhaps critical, part of the

therapeutic regimen. Propranolol given intravenously or orally is the agent of choice in the absence of cardiac insufficiency. Large doses of dexamethasone (e.g., 2 mg every 6 h) should also be administered, since it has been shown both to inhibit hormone release and to impair the peripheral generation of T_3 from T_4, in addition to providing adrenal support. Indeed, the combined use of propylthiouracil, iodine, and dexamethasone will generally normalize the serum T_3 concentration within 24 to 48 h. Antithyroid therapy, iodine, and dexamethasone must be continued until a normal metabolic state is approached, at which time iodine is progressively withdrawn and plans for a definitive regimen of treatment made.

NEOPLASMS

THYROID ADENOMAS True adenomas, as contrasted with localized adenomatous areas, are encapsulated and usually compress contiguous tissue. Adenomas vary greatly in size and histologic characteristics, and are often classified into three major types: papillary, follicular, and Hürthle cell. The follicular adenomas can be subdivided according to the size of the follicles into colloid or macrofollicular, fetal or microfollicular, and embryonal varieties. There is considerable variation in physiologic differentiation, as judged by their ability to concentrate radioiodine. The more highly differentiated adenomas (follicular) are by far the most common and are also the most likely to mimic the function of normal thyroid tissue. Unlike normal thyroid tissue, however, their function is independent of TSH stimulation (autonomous). They are usually unifocal, presenting as a solitary nodule. Often the patient reports that the nodule has been slowly growing over many years. Initially, their function is insufficient to disturb hormonal equilibrium, although their capacity to accumulate radioiodine is apparent on scintiscanning (*"warm"* nodule). With the passage of time, the nodule grows larger, and its function increases until it is sufficient to suppress TSH secretion. Consequently, the remainder of the gland undergoes atrophy and loss of function, and the scintiscan then reveals radioiodine accumulation only in the region of the nodule (*"hot"* nodule). At this time, the patient may or may not appear overtly thyrotoxic, but frank thyrotoxicosis will usually supervene in time (*toxic adenoma*). Relative to its overall rate of occurrence, hyperfunctioning adenoma is a frequent cause of T_3 toxicosis. Not infrequently, hyperfunctioning adenomas undergo hemorrhagic necrosis, resulting in loss of function and the appearance of a *"cold" nodule* on scintiscanning, since the remainder of the thyroid will have resumed function. Only very rarely are hyperfunctioning adenomas carcinomatous. Hyperfunctioning adenomas are readily amenable to ablation by surgery or ^{131}I; large doses of the latter are usually required (10 mCi or greater). Before such treatment, it is desirable to administer exogenous TSH and repeat the scintiscan in order to demonstrate the capacity for function in the remaining tissue.

THYROID CARCINOMAS Thyroid carcinoma may be classified into two varieties, depending upon whether the lesion arises in thyroid follicular epithelium or whether it arises from the parafollicular or C cells. Since the latter disorder has distinctive physiologic and clinical characteristics, it is discussed separately (see Chap. 348).

Carcinomas of follicular epithelium These are of three general histologic types which differ in their clinical course. The least common is *anaplastic carcinoma*, which is histologically undifferentiated, usually afflicts the elderly, and is highly malignant.

Usually the lesion is rapidly fatal, owing to extensive local invasion which is refractory to radiation. The second type of tumor, *follicular carcinoma,* is also uncommon and histologically mimics closely normal thyroid tissue. This lesion usually undergoes early hematogenous spread, and hence the patient may present with a distant metastasis, usually in lung or bone. Follicular carcinoma or follicular elements in papillary carcinoma are responsible for those instances in which thyroid carcinoma, in situ or in metastases, accumulates significant quantities of [131]I. The third and most common type of tumor, *papillary carcinoma,* has a bimodal frequency, peaks occurring in the second or third decades and again in later life. This lesion is usually slowly growing and typically spreads to the regional lymph nodes, where it may remain indolent for many years. Although more common in the older patient, acceleration of the disease may take place at any time. Follicular elements are usually present in both the primary lesion and its metastases, accounting for those instances in which papillary tumors accumulate radioiodine.

DIAGNOSIS AND MANAGEMENT The diagnosis and management of thyroid carcinoma is closely interwoven with the management of the nodular goiter. In the past, this subject has been one which evoked a wide disparity of views among authorities, stemming largely from seemingly contradictory data. On the one hand, surgically excised specimens of thyroid nodules, particularly solitary nodules, revealed a very high frequency of carcinoma (as much as 20 percent in some series). On the other hand, despite the frequency of nodular goiter in the general population (approximately 4 percent), the frequency of thyroid carcinoma, either newly diagnosed or as a cause of death, is very low. These respective data led to either very vigorous or very conservative approaches with respect to the management of nodular goiter. It now appears that this discordance can be explained, however, by the ability of the physician to select for surgery those patients who are at high risk of harboring thyroid carcinoma, with consequent weighting of statistics derived from surgical series.

The features which lead to a presumptive diagnosis of thyroid carcinoma are rather well defined. They include recent growth, especially if rapid and unaccompanied by tenderness, firm or hard consistency, and diminished or absent function on scintiscan. The presence of finely stippled calcification on x-ray examination suggests the presence of psammoma bodies within a papillary carcinoma. Hoarseness, fixation to adjacent structures, and regional lymphadenopathy are late features. Of particular importance is a history of x-ray to the head or neck in childhood, since this has been shown to be associated with a high incidence of thyroid carcinoma in later life. A nodule that is present in an otherwise normal gland (solitary nodule) is far more suspicious of thyroid tumor, while one nodule among many is much more likely to be part of a diffuse process, such as simple goiter. Since cystic lesions are far less likely to reflect malignancy than solid lesions do, differentiation between the two types of nodules is important. Transillumination is sometimes helpful, but ultrasonograms are particularly so and should be included in the workup of any patient with a suspicious thyroid nodule.

The foregoing features permit the development of general guidelines for the management of nodular goiter. A solitary nodule, especially if nonfunctioning, should be promptly excised, particularly if it occurs in a young woman or in a man of any age, except the most elderly. This is true because multinodular goiter is a disease of older age and predominantly of women. Obviously, the presence of other features described above increase the likelihood of thyroid carcinoma. A prominent but functioning nodule within a multinodular goiter is of

little concern. A nonfunctioning nodule with a multinodular goiter should be observed during suppressive therapy. Failure to regress, or particularly an increase in size, over a 3- to 6-month period strongly suggests that surgery is desirable.

A special problem arises from the recognition that x-ray to the head or neck in infancy, childhood, or adolescence is associated with a high incidence of thyroid disease later in life. Nodular disease is particularly common, being found in approximately 20 percent of patients at risk, and may not be apparent until 30 years or more after the radiation exposure. Among patients in this group who have palpable nodules, approximately one-third will be found at surgery to have carcinoma, often multicentric and sometimes metastatic. Hence, it is important that individuals at risk be screened by careful thyroid palpation and be operated upon if one or more clearly palpable nodules is present. Individuals with no palpable abnormality should probably have a base-line thyroid scan, be placed on thyroid suppressive therapy, and be examined again at intervals of 1 or 2 years thereafter.

Increasingly, needle, rather than excisional, biopsy is being used in the diagnosis of thyroid nodules. Either aspiration or cutting needle biopsy can be employed, depending on the size of the nodule and skill of the operator. Optimum application of this technique rests upon the availability of experienced histopathological interpretation of the specimen obtained. When such is available, the procedure provides a reliable means of differentiating benign from malignant nodules, despite the occasional occurrence of false positives or negatives. Aspiration biopsy may be essentially curative of thyroid cysts, in addition to providing specimens for cytopathological examination.

If excisional biopsy is decided upon, the nodule should be widely excised and subjected to frozen section examination. A diagnosis of carcinoma is an indication for near-total thyroidectomy in view of the evidence of frequent seeding of carcinoma throughout the gland as a result of transglandular lymphatic spread. Regional lymph nodes should be explored and removed if there is evidence of involvement. Radical neck dissection is no longer felt justified. If permanent sections reveal carcinoma when frozen sections had failed to do so, secondary surgery should be undertaken to remove residual thyroid tissue. Several weeks after surgery, a large scanning dose of ^{131}I is administered (approximately 2 mCi), and a whole-body scan and measurement of urinary ^{131}I excretion obtained. This serves to ablate any residual thyroid tissue and to demonstrate any functioning metastases. If functioning metastases are seen, a therapeutic dose of [131]I (approximately 50 mCi) is administered. Thereafter, the patient is given levothyroxine in fully suppressive dosage. At approximately yearly intervals, levothyroxine is replaced by liothyronine for approximately 3 weeks; this is then withdrawn to permit rapid resumption of TSH secretion. Large doses of TRH may also be given to enhance the TSH response so as to maximize the stimulation of any functioning residual tissue. If such is found, a further therapeutic dose of ^{131}I is administered. Discrete palpable lymph nodes which have emerged during suppressive therapy can often best be treated by surgical excision. The foregoing procedures are repeated during ensuing years until the disease appears to have been eradicated. Although suppressive therapy is physiologically sound and sometimes spectacularly successful, its general efficacy in the management of thyroid carcinoma is uncertain. Nevertheless, patients who have had carcinoma of the thyroid should be kept on suppressive therapy for the remainder of their lives, except for the brief interruptions described above.

THYROIDITIS

Thyroiditis is a generic term embracing several disorders of differing etiology. There are four general types, of which two are exceedingly uncommon, *pyogenic thyroiditis* and *chronic fibrosing (Riedel's) thyroiditis.* Pyogenic thyroiditis is usually anteceded by a pyogenic infection elsewhere and is characterized by tenderness and swelling of the thyroid, redness and warmth of the overlying skin, and constitutional signs of infection. Treatment consists of antibiotic therapy, along with incisional drainage if a fluctuant area within the thyroid should occur. Riedel's thyroiditis is a rare disorder in which intense fibrosis of the thyroid and surrounding structures, leading to induration of the tissues of the neck, may be associated with mediastinal and retroperitoneal fibrosis. The principal importance of this disorder is that it requires differentiation from thyroid neoplasia.

SUBACUTE THYROIDITIS This disorder, which is also termed *granulomatous, giant-cell,* or *de Quervain's thyroiditis,* is a distinct disease of the thyroid that appears to be viral in origin.

Symptoms of thyroiditis usually follow those of an upper respiratory infection and most commonly comprise pronounced asthenia, malaise, and symptoms referable to stretching of the thyroid capsule, principally pain over the thyroid or pain referred to the lower jaw, ear, or occiput. Referred, rather than local, pain may predominate. These symptoms may smolder for many weeks before the correct diagnosis is suspected. Less commonly, the onset is acute, with severe pain over the thyroid, accompanied by fever and occasionally symptoms of thyrotoxicosis. Cardinal physical findings include exquisite tenderness and nodularity over the thyroid, which may be predominantly unilateral, but which usually migrates to other areas of the gland. Although local or referred pain is the commonest symptom of subacute thyroiditis, occasional patients manifest other typical features of the disease, but have no pain.

Two tests provide the hallmark of the disease from the laboratory standpoint: an inordinately increased erythrocyte sedimentation rate and a markedly depressed RAIU. Values for the remaining tests depend upon the stage of the disease in which they are obtained. Early, many patients are at least mildly thyrotoxic owing to leakage of hormone from the gland. The serum T_4 is high, and this, together with the leakage of iodoprotein, results in elevation of the PBI. Later in the disease, as glandular hormone is depleted, the patient may pass through a hypothyroid phase, in which serum T_4 is low and TSH increased. Diagnosis of the thyrotoxic phase of the disease is especially troublesome in patients with the painless variant of the disorder, since the patient may be thought to have Graves' disease or toxic nodular goiter and therapy inappropriate for subacute thyroiditis may be instituted. Demonstration of a low RAIU will serve to differentiate subacute thyroiditis from these other causes of hyperthyroidism in most instances.

If left untreated, the disorder may smolder for months, but eventually will subside with a return of normal thyroid function. In mild cases, aspirin suffices to control the symptoms. In more severe cases, glucocorticoid (prednisone, 20 to 40 mg daily) is generally effective. Propranolol can be used to control hyperthyroidism. Return of the RAIU to normal indicates the time at which therapy can be withdrawn without recurrence of symptoms.

HASHIMOTO'S DISEASE This disorder, which is also termed *lymphadenoid goiter,* is a chronic inflammatory disease of the thyroid in which autoimmune factors are thought to play a prominent role. It is a common disorder, occurring most frequently in women of middle age. In all likelihood, it is, in addition, the most common cause of sporadic goiter in children. Evidence of the participation of autoimmune factors includes the lymphocytic infiltration of the gland, as well as the presence in the serum of increased concentrations of immunoglobulins and of antibodies directed against several compo-

nents of thyroid tissue. Of these, the most important from the clinical standpoint are the antithyroglobulin antibody detected by the tanned red cell agglutination technique and the antimicrosomal antibody detected by immunofluorescence or complement fixation techniques. This disorder also coexists with inordinate frequency with other diseases of a presumed autoimmune nature, including pernicious anemia, Sjögren's syndrome, chronic active hepatitis, systemic lupus erythematosus, rheumatoid arthritis, nontuberculous Addison's disease, diabetes, and Graves' disease itself. These disorders, as well as Hashimoto's disease itself, also appear with unusual frequency in family members of patients with Hashimoto's disease.

Goiter is the outstanding feature of the disease. The enlargement involves the entire gland, but not necessarily symmetrically. Typically, the consistency is rubbery, the margins are scalloped, and the general outline of the gland is preserved. The pyramidal lobe may be prominent. Early in the disease the patient is metabolically normal; however, even then decreased thyroid reserve is often manifest in an increase in serum TSH. With the passage of time, hypothyroidism of increasing severity supervenes, owing to progressive replacement of thyroid parenchyma by lymphocytes or fibrous tissue. Early in the disease, the RAIU and PBI may be increased, reflecting the secretion of iodoproteins, but the serum T_4 is normal. With time, the RAIU, PBI, and serum T_4 decline as clinical hypothyroidism supervenes. Increased serum T_3 may herald the development of this sequence. High titers of antimicrosomal antibody are almost always present. High titers may also occur in other thyroid disorders, particularly primary thyroprivic hypothyroidism and Graves' disease, but with lesser frequency. Although the foregoing findings usually suffice to permit a diagnosis, histologic confirmation by needle biopsy is occasionally required. In view of the frequency with which hypothyroidism is either present or eventually develops, treatment with replacement doses of levothyroxine is indicated. In some patients, such therapy is associated with regression of goiter.

REFERENCES

BLOCK MA: Management of carcinoma of the thyroid. Ann Surg 185:133, 1977

CAVALIERI RR, RAPOPORT B: Impaired peripheral conversion of thyroxine to triiodo-thyronine. Annu Rev Med 28:57, 1977

FAVUS MJ et al: Thyroid cancer occurring as a late consequence of head-and-neck irradiation. N Engl J Med 294:1019, 1976

O'DONNELL J et al: Thyrotropin displacement activity of serum immunoglobulins from patients with Graves' disease. J Clin Endocrinol Metab 46:770, 1978

UCLA CONFERENCE: Autoimmune thyroid diseases—Graves' and Hashimoto's. Ann Intern Med 88:370, 1978

336
DISEASES OF THE ADRENAL CORTEX

GORDON H. WILLIAMS
ROBERT G. DLUHY
GEORGE W. THORN

BIOCHEMISTRY AND PHYSIOLOGY

STEROID NOMENCLATURE The adrenal steroids contain as their basic structure a cyclopentenoperhydrophenanthrane nucleus consisting of three 6-carbon hexane rings and a single 5-

carbon pentane ring (D). The carbon atoms are numbered in a predetermined sequence beginning with ring A (Fig. 336-1). The Greek letter Δ indicates a double bond, as does the suffix -ene. The position of a substituent below or above the plane of the steroid molecule is indicated by the letters α and β, respectively. The α substituent is drawn with a broken line (--OH), and the β substituent is drawn with a solid line (—OH). The C_{19} steroids are those which have substituent methyl groups at positions C-18 and C-19. C_{19} steroids that also have a ketone group at C-17 are termed *17-ketosteroids*. These C_{19} steroids have predominant androgenic activity. The C_{21} steroids are those which have a 2-carbon side chain (C-20 and C-21) attached at position 17 of the D ring and, in addition, have substituent methyl groups at C-18 and C-19. C_{21} steroids that also possess a hydroxyl group at position 17 are termed *17-hydroxycorticosteroids* or *17-hydroxycorticoids*. The C_{21} steroids may have either predominant glucocorticoid or mineralocorticoid properties. *Glucocorticoid* signifies a C_{21} steroid with predominant action on intermediary metabolism, and *mineralocorticoid* indicates a C_{21} steroid with predominant action on the metabolism of the body minerals, sodium and potassium.

BIOSYNTHESIS OF ADRENAL STEROIDS Cholesterol, derived from the diet and from endogenous synthesis via acetate, is the principal starting compound in steroidogenesis. The three major adrenal biosynthetic pathways lead to the production of glucocorticoids (cortisol), mineralocorticoids (aldosterone), and adrenal androgens (dehydroepiandrosterone). Separate zones of the adrenal cortex synthesize specific hormones, reflecting the capacity of each zone to carry out certain transformations and hydroxylations mediated by specific hydroxylating and isomerase enzymes (Fig. 336-2). The outer (glomerulosa) zone is mainly involved in aldosterone biosynthesis, and the inner (fasciculata-reticularis) zone is mainly involved in cortisol and androgen biosynthesis.

FIGURE 336-1
Basic steroid structure and nomenclature.

STEROID TRANSPORT Some of the steroid hormones, e.g., testosterone and cortisol, appear to circulate to a considerable extent bound to plasma proteins. Cortisol occurs in the plasma in three forms: free cortisol, protein-bound cortisol, and cortisol metabolites. *Free cortisol* refers to that quantity which is physiologically active but not protein-bound and, therefore, represents a form of cortisol acting directly on tissue sites. Normally, less than 5 percent of circulating cortisol is free. The diffusible fraction is estimated to range between 0.7 and 1.0 μg per 100 ml. Only the unbound cortisol and its metabolites are filtrable at the glomerulus. Greater than normal quantities of free steroid are excreted in the urine in states characterized by hypersecretion of cortisol, as the unbound fraction of plasma cortisol rises. *Protein-bound cortisol* is that portion of cortisol which is reversibly bound to circulating plasma proteins. There are two distinct cortisol-binding systems of plasma. One is a high-affinity, low-capacity α_2 globulin termed *transcortin* or *cortisol-binding globulin* (CBG), and the other is a low-affinity, high-capacity protein, albumin. Cortisol-binding globulin in normal humans can bind approximately 20 to 25 μg cortisol per 100 ml plasma. As the amounts of cortisol released by the adrenal gland exceed this level, the excess becomes bound in part to albumin and a greater proportion circulates unbound. The CBG level is increased in high-estrogen states (e.g., pregnancy, oral contraceptive administration). The endogenous rise in CBG is accompanied by a parallel rise in protein-bound cortisol, with the result that the plasma cortisol concentration is elevated. However, the free-cortisol levels probably remain normal, and signs and symptoms of glucocorticoid excess are absent. Most synthetic glucocorticoid analogues bind less efficiently to CBG (approximately 70 percent binding). This may explain the propensity of some synthetic analogues to produce cushingoid side effects at low dosage.

Cortisol metabolites are biologically inactive and bind only weakly to circulating plasma proteins.

Aldosterone appears to be bound to proteins to a much smaller extent than either testosterone or cortisol with an ultra-filtrate of plasma probably containing as much as 50 percent of the circulating aldosterone. The limited binding of aldosterone by plasma protein is significant in the metabolism of this hormone.

STEROID METABOLISM AND EXCRETION Glucocorticoids The daily adrenal secretion of cortisol ranges between 15 and 30 mg, with a pronounced diurnal cycle. Cortisol is distributed in a volume of body fluids approximating the total extracellular fluid space. The total plasma concentration of cortisol in the morning hours is approximately 15 μg per 100 ml, with more than 90 percent of this cortisol appearing in the protein-bound fraction. The plasma concentration of cortisol is determined by the rate of secretion, the rate of inactivation, and the rate of excretion of free cortisol. The liver is the major organ responsible for steroid inactivation and conjugation of the reduced products with glucuronic acid to form water-soluble compounds. Cortisol is inactivated by means of six major biotransformations: (1) reduction of ring A, (2) 11-dehydrogenation, (3) reduction at C-20, (4) cleavage of the C-20:C-21 side chain, (5) 6β-hydroxylation, and (6) conjugation. The 11-dehydrogenase system converting cortisol to the inactive cortisone is strongly influenced by the level of circulating thyroid hormone, with hyperthyroidism markedly accelerating the oxidative reaction. The major mechanism for steroid inactivation is the reduction of ring A by the liver. The first four transformations produce compounds which are not water-soluble. These compounds are conjugated in the liver with glucuronic acid at position C-3 to produce water-soluble products.

MINERALOCORTICOID PATHWAY   GLUCOCORTICOID PATHWAY   ANDROGEN PATHWAY

Acetate

Cholesterol

Δ5-Pregnenolone

Progesterone   17α-Hydroxypregnenolone   Dehydroepiandrosterone

11-Deoxycorticosterone   17α-Hydroxyprogesterone   Δ4-Androstenedione

Corticosterone   11-Deoxycortisol   11-Hydroxyandrostenedione

Aldosterone   Cortisol   Testosterone

FIGURE 336-2
Biosynthetic pathways for adrenal steroid production. Major pathways to mineralocorticoids, glucocorticoids, and androgens. Circled letters and numbers denote specific enzymes: DE = debranching enzyme; 3β = 3β-ol-dehydrogenase with Δ4,5-isomerase; 11 = C-11 hydroxylase; 17 = C-17 hydroxylase; 21 = C-21 hydroxylase.

Mineralocorticoids In normal subjects on a normal salt intake, the average daily secretion of aldosterone ranges between 50 and 250 μg, and the plasma concentration ranges between 5 and 15 ng per 100 ml. Since aldosterone is only weakly bound to proteins, its volume of distribution is larger than that of cortisol and approximates 35 liters. Greater than 75 percent of circulating aldosterone is normally inactivated during a single passage through the liver. However, under certain conditions, such as congestive failure, this percentage is markedly reduced.

Of the numerous reductive metabolites that may be formed, 50 percent of aldosterone is transformed into the tetrahydro derivative produced by ring A reduction in the liver. This metabolite is water-insoluble and is conjugated with glucuronic acid before it is excreted in the urine. From 7 to 15 percent of aldosterone appears in the urine as a glucuronide conjugate, from which free aldosterone is released on standing at pH 1. This *acid-labile conjugate* appears to be formed both in the liver and in the kidney. For average salt intake, the 24-h urine excretion of the acid-labile conjugate ranges from 2 to 20 μg, that of the tetrahydro derivative from 25 to 35 μg, and that of the nonconjugated, nonreduced free aldosterone from 0.2 to 0.6 μg.

Adrenal androgens The major adrogenic compound secreted by the adrenal gland is dehydroepiandrosterone (DHEA) and its C-3 sulfuric acid ester. From 15 to 30 mg of these compounds is secreted daily. Much smaller amounts of Δ^4-androstenedione and 11β-hydroxyandrostenedione and testosterone are secreted. DHEA serves as the major precursor of the urinary 17-ketosteroids. Two-thirds of the urine 17-ketosteroids in the male is derived from adrenal metabolites, and the remaining one-third comes from testicular androgens. In the female, almost all urine 17-ketosteroids are derived from the adrenal gland.

ACTH PHYSIOLOGY Adrenocorticotropin hormone (ACTH; see Chap. 333) is an unbranched long-chain polypeptide containing 39 amino acids. It is stored in and released from the anterior pituitary gland, where histologically it appears to be localized to basophil cells. Much of the potential for producing the corticotropic actions of ACTH is present in smaller polypeptide fragments; the N-terminal 24-amino-acid structure retains full biologic potency, while shorter N-terminal fragments exhibit reduced biologic activity. The biologic half-life of ACTH is less than 10 min. Release of ACTH from the anterior pituitary gland is governed by a "corticotropin-releasing center" in the median eminence of the hypothalamus, which upon stimulation releases a putative chemical mediator (corticotropin-releasing factor, CRF) that travels via the pituitary-stalk portal bloodstream to the anterior pituitary gland, where it effects the release of stored ACTH (Fig. 336-3; see also Chap. 333).

Three major factors control CRF and ACTH release: plasma free-cortisol concentration, stress, and the sleep-wake cycle. The plasma level of ACTH varies sporadically during the day but roughly follows a diurnal pattern, with a peak occurring just prior to awaking and a nadir shortly before retiring. After several days on a new sleep-wake cycle, the pattern will be altered to conform to the new cycle. However, an occasional deviation from the normal cycle does not produce an alteration. Stress (e.g., pyrogens, surgery, hypoglycemia, exercise, severe emotional trauma) can also affect ACTH release. The secretion of ACTH following stress and the diurnal ACTH release are under neural regulation by CRF. CRF is probably also influenced by the hypothalamic monoaminergic neurotransmittors with the serotoninergic system known to

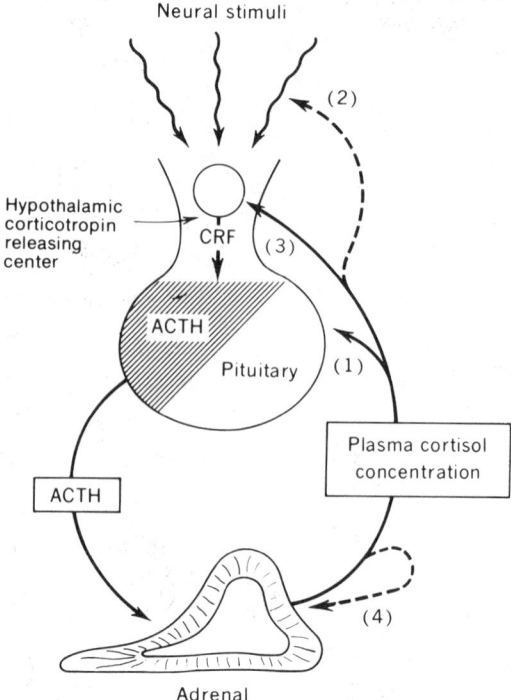

FIGURE 336-3

Hypothalamic-pituitary-adrenal axis. (1) Dominant feedback control on the pituitary gland; (2) possible feedback of plasma cortisol on higher nerve centers, (3) on the hypothalamus, and/or (4) the adrenal gland itself. CRF = corticotropin-releasing factor.

stimulate the secretion of ACTH. Finally, ACTH release is regulated by the plasma free-cortisol level. Animal studies indicate that cortisol decreases the responsiveness of the anterior pituitary adrenocorticotropic cells to CRF; i.e., in the presence of cortisol, more CRF is required to produce a given increment of ACTH than in its absence. Thus, in the presence of a constant CRF level, this *negative feedback* relationship causes increased release of ACTH release when cortisol levels are high. This servomechanism establishes the primacy of blood cortisol concentration and serves to buffer deviations in blood cortisol levels from a supposed optimal level. It also appears that cortisol feeds back on the hypothalamus (CRF), higher brain centers (hippocampus, reticular system, septum), and perhaps even on the adrenal cortex as well.

The action of ACTH on the adrenal gland itself is rapid; within minutes of its release, there is an increased concentration of steroids in the adrenal venous blood. The most likely mechanism by which ACTH stimulates steroidogenesis is via activation of the membrane-bound adenyl cyclase. This increases the level of cyclic adenosine 3',5'-monophosphate (AMP), which then activates adrenocortical protein kinase enzymes. This results in the phosphorylation of proteins which in some way activate steroid biosynthesis.

RENIN-ANGIOTENSIN PHYSIOLOGY (See also Chap. 251.) Renin is a proteolytic enzyme which is produced and stored in the granules of the juxtaglomerular cells surrounding the afferent arterioles of the cortical glomeruli. The juxtaglomerular apparatus consists of both the juxtaglomerular cells and the cells of the macula densa. Renin acts on the basic substrate angiotensinogen (a circulating α_2 globulin), made in the liver, to form the decapeptide angiotensin I (Fig. 336-4). Angiotensin I is then enzymatically converted by converting enzyme to the octapeptide angiotensin II by splitting off of the two C-terminal amino acids. Angiotensin II is the most potent pressor

FIGURE 336-4

Renin-angiotensin-aldosterone volume regulation in normal humans.

compound (on a mole for mole basis) made in the body, and it exerts this pressor action by a direct effect on arteriolar smooth muscle. In addition, angiotensin II is a potent direct stimulus to the production of aldosterone by the zona glomerulosa of the adrenal cortex. Recent studies suggest that the active adrenal angiotensin is the nonapeptide, angiotensin III. However, this hypothesis is still controversial. Angiotensinases rapidly destroy angiotensin II (half-life approximately 1 min), while the half-life of renin is more prolonged (10 to 20 min). Finally, other tissues, such as uterus, vascular tissue, brain, and salivary glands, also produce renin-like substances. The significance of these so-called "isorenins" is not understood.

Renin release is controlled by four major factors. For the most part, these are interdependent, and the amount of renin released is a composite of the input of all four. The *juxtaglomerular cells,* which are specialized myoepithelial cells cuffing the afferent arterioles, act as miniature pressure transducers, sensing renal perfusion pressure and corresponding changes in afferent arteriolar perfusion pressures. The changes in pressure are perceived as distortions in the existing stretch on the arteriolar walls. For example, under conditions of a reduction in circulating blood volume, there is a corresponding reduction in renal perfusion pressure and, therefore, in afferent arteriolar pressure (Fig. 336-4). This is perceived by the juxtaglomerular cells as a decreased stretch exerted on the afferent arteriolar walls. The juxtaglomerular cells then release increasing quantities of renin within the kidney circulation, leading to the formation of angiotensin I. Angiotensin I leaves the kidney both by renal lymphatic and renal venous outflow. It is converted into angiotensin II and directly stimulates the adrenal cortex to release increasing quantities of aldosterone. Increasing plasma levels of aldosterone lead to increasing renal sodium retention and thus result in expansion of extracellular fluid volume, which, as it is completed, dampens the initiating signal for renin release. Within this context, the renin-angiotensin-aldosterone system is subserving volume control by appropriate modifications of renal tubular sodium transport.

A second control mechanism for renin release centers in the *macula densa* cells, a group of special-staining, distal convoluted tubular epithelial cells found in direct opposition to the juxtaglomerular cells. It has been suggested that they may function as chemoreceptors, monitoring the sodium load presented to the distal tubule, and that such information, while it is being monitored, is directly fed back to the juxtaglomerular cells, where appropriate modifications in renin release take place. Under conditions of increased delivery of filtered sodium to the macula densa, feedback occurs to the juxtaglomerular apparatus, resulting in a release of increasing quanti-

ties of renin, which are capable of decreasing glomerular filtration rate, thereby reducing the filtered load of sodium. The evidence for this hypothesis is conflicting.

The *sympathetic nervous system* is the predominant factor regulating the release of renin in response to a person assuming the upright posture. The mechanism is either a direct effect on the juxtaglomerular cell to increase adenyl cyclase activity or an indirect effect on either the juxtaglomerular or the macula densa cells by way of a vasoconstrictive action on the afferent arteriole.

Finally, a number of circulating factors may alter renin release. Increasing dietary *potassium* directly decreases renin release; decreasing potassium intake increases renin release. The significance of this potassium effect is unclear. *Angiotensin* itself can exert a negative feedback control on renin release independent of alterations in renal blood flow, pressure, or aldosterone secretion. Thus, the control of renin release is complex, consisting of both *intrarenal* (pressoreceptor and macula densa) and *extrarenal* (sympathetic nervous system, potassium, angiotensin, etc.) mechanisms. A given level of renin secretion probably reflects all these factors, with the intrarenal mechanism predominating.

GLUCOCORTICOID PHYSIOLOGY The division of adrenal steroids into glucocorticoids and mineralocorticoids is somewhat arbitrary in that most glucocorticoids have some mineralocorticoid-like properties, and vice versa. The descriptive term *glucocorticoid* is applied to those adrenal steroids having a predominant action on intermediary metabolism. The principal glucocorticoid is cortisol (hydrocortisone). The physiological actions of the glucocorticoids on intermediary metabolism are predominantly anti-insulin and include the regulation of protein, carbohydrate, lipid, and nucleic acid metabolism. Their actions appear mainly to be catabolic in effect, with an increased protein breakdown and nitrogen excretion. Glucocorticoids increase hepatic glycogen content and promote the hepatic synthesis of glucose (gluconeogenesis). These actions of glucocorticoids are in large part explained by the mobilization of glycogenic amino acid precursors from peripheral supporting structures, such as bone, skin, muscle, and connective tissue due to protein breakdown as well as to the inhibition of protein synthesis and amino acid uptake. Glucocorticoid-induced hyperaminoacidemia also indirectly facilitates gluconeogenesis by stimulating glucagon secretion. In addition, glucocorticoids have a direct action on the liver to stimulate the synthesis of hepatic enzymes, such as tyrosine amino transferase and tryptophan pyrrolase. Inhibition of extrahepatic protein synthesis and stimulation of hepatic enzyme synthesis is reflected in the actions of glucocorticoids on nucleic acid metabolism. Corticoids inhibit the synthesis of nucleic acids in most body tissues, but in the liver ribonucleic acid (RNA) synthesis is stimulated. Cortisol enters the target cell by diffusion, combines with a specific high-affinity cytoplasmic receptor protein, and is transferred to a specific acceptor site on the chromatin tissue of the nucleus, which then produces an increase in RNA synthesis and later in protein synthesis. Glucocorticoids are necessary for fatty acid mobilization by permitting and enhancing activation of cellular lipase by lipid-mobilizing hormones (e.g., catecholamines and pituitary peptides).

The action of cortisol on structural protein and adipose tissue varies considerably in different parts of the body. For example, pharmacological doses of cortisol may profoundly deplete the protein matrix of the vertebral column (trabecular bone), but long bones (primarily compact bone) may be affected only minimally; peripheral adipose tissue may diminish, whereas abdominal and interscapular fat may accumulate.

Glucocorticoids have anti-inflammatory properties, which are probably related to their actions on the microvasculature as well as to cellular effects. Cortisol maintains normal vascular responsiveness to circulating vasoconstrictor factors and opposes the increase in capillary permeability characteristic of acute inflammation. Glucocorticoids also impede endothelial sticking of leukocytes and diapedesis through the capillary wall. Reduced cellular adherence to vascular endothelium is probably secondary to antagonism to the action of migration-inhibiting factor (MIF) by glucocorticoids. Glucocorticoids produce lysis of lymphoid tissue, specifically, T cells or the small lymphocytes derived from the thymus, and diminish the number of circulating eosinophils. Thus, cortisol impairs cellular-mediated immunity. It is probably only at pharmacological dosages that antibody production is suppressed and stabilization of lysosomal membranes occurs, thereby suppressing the release of proteolytic acid hydrolases stored in these cytoplasmic organelles. Cortisol has a major physiological action on body water, in both its distribution and its excretion. It subserves the extracellular fluid volume by a retarding action on the inward migration of water into cells. It affects renal water excretion by suppressing the secretion of antidiuretic hormone, by increasing the rate of glomerular filtration, and by a direct action on the renal tubule, which actions summate to increase solute-free water clearance. Glucocorticoids also have weak mineralocorticoid-like properties, but increasing doses produce renal tubular sodium reabsorption and increased urine potassium excretion. The integrity of personality is enhanced by cortisol, and emotional disorders are common with either excesses or deficits of cortisol. Lastly, another major action of cortisol is to suppress directly pituitary ACTH secretion.

MINERALOCORTICOID PHYSIOLOGY The major mineralocorticoid produced by the human adrenal cortex is aldosterone. Under normal circumstances, aldosterone has two important "mineralocorticoid" activities: (1) it is a major regulator of extracellular fluid volume, and (2) it is a major determinant of potassium metabolism. It regulates volume through a direct effect on the renal tubular transport of sodium. Aldosterone acts predominantly at the site of the distal convoluted tubule, where it causes a decrease in the urine excretion of sodium with an increase in urine excretion of potassium. The reabsorption of positively charged sodium ions causes a fall in the transmembrane potential, thus producing an environment favorable for the flow of positive ions out of

the cell into the lumen. The major singly charged positive ion present intracellularly is potassium. Since its concentration in the cell is forty- to eightyfold greater than in the lumen, it passively follows this relative electrical gradient in order to restore the normal positive charge to the lumen. The reabsorbed sodium ions are then transported out of the tubular epithelial cells into the interstitial fluid of the kidney and from there into the renal capillary circulation. Water passively follows the aldosterone-mediated transported sodium.

Hydrogen ion is also present in abundant concentration in the tubular epithelial cell. However, since its concentration in the lumen is greater than in the cell, it is actively secreted, but the reduced intraluminal positivity allows more hydrogen to be secreted with the same amount of energy.

Aldosterone and other mineralocorticoids also act on the epithelium of the salivary ducts and sweat glands and on the epithelial cells of the gastrointestinal tract to cause reabsorption of sodium in "exchange" for potassium ions. The subcellular mechanism of action of aldosterone is like that described earlier for cortisol.

When normal individuals are given a long-term course of aldosterone (or deoxycorticosterone acetate), an initial period of sodium retention is followed by a natriuresis, and sodium balance is reestablished after 3 to 5 days. As a result, clinical edema formation does not develop. This phenomenon is referred to as the "escape phenomenon," signifying an "escape" by the renal tubules from the sodium-retaining action of chronically administered aldosterone.

There are three well-defined *control* mechanisms for aldosterone release—the renin-angiotensin system, potassium, and ACTH (Fig. 336-5). The renin-angiotensin system is the major system for control of extracellular fluid volume, via regulation of aldosterone secretion. In effect, the renin-angiotensin system attempts to maintain the circulating blood volume constant by causing aldosterone-induced sodium retention during periods registered as volume deficiencies, and by decreasing aldosterone-dependent sodium retention under conditions in which volume is registered as being ample.

Potassium ions directly regulate aldosterone secretion independently of the renin-angiotensin system. In normal humans, oral potassium loading increases aldosterone excretion, secretion, and plasma levels. In addition, systemic infusion of potassium ions under certain circumstances increases plasma aldosterone levels with as small as a 0.1 meq per liter increase in serum potassium. Potassium may alter aldosterone secretion owing to changes in serum potassium levels, to changes in intracellular potassium concentration, or to change in the flux of potassium across the adrenal cortical cell membrane.

Physiological amounts of ACTH acutely stimulate aldosterone secretion, but this action is not sustained if ACTH is continuously infused for periods greater than 10 to 12 h. However, other studies seem to relegate ACTH to a minor role in the control of aldosterone in normal humans. For example, subjects on high-dose steroid therapy for several years and with presumably complete suppression of ACTH have normal aldosterone-secretory responses to sodium restriction. Therefore, chronic ACTH deficiency per se does not alter glomerulosa cell responsiveness.

Finally, the prior dietary intake of both potassium and sodium can alter the magnitude of the aldosterone response to acute stimulation. Increasing potassium intake or decreasing sodium intake sensitizes the response of the glomerulosa cells to acute stimulation by ACTH, angiotensin II, and/or potassium.

ANDROGEN PHYSIOLOGY Androgens are defined biologically as substances that stimulate male secondary sexual characteristics. The secondary sexual characteristics are affected through inhibition of the female characteristics (defeminiza-

FIGURE 336-5

The interrelationship of the volume and potassium feedback loops on aldosterone secretion. Integration of signals from each loop determines the level of aldosterone secretion.

tion) and accentuation of the male characteristics (masculinization). These are seen clinically as hirsutism and virilization in the female with amenorrhea, atrophy of the breasts and uterus, enlargement of the clitoris, deepening of the voice, acne, increased muscle mass, increased heterosexual drive, and receding hairline.

Steroids with predominant androgenic activity have 19 carbon atoms (Fig. 336-1). The principal adrenal androgens secreted are dehydroepiandrosterone (DHEA), androstenedione, and 11-hydroxyandrostenedione. DHEA and its sulfate are *quantitatively* the major androgens secreted by the adrenal cortex. DHEA, androstenedione, and 11-hydroxyandrostenedione are weak androgens, but all are peripherally interconvertible with the potent androgen, testosterone.

The release of adrenal androgens is stimulated by ACTH, not by gonadotropins. With ACTH stimulation, 17-ketosteroids increase but to a much lesser extent than do urine 17-hydroxycorticosteroids. It follows that adrenal androgens are suppressed by exogenous glucocorticoid administration.

LABORATORY EVALUATION OF ADRENOCORTICAL FUNCTION

A major advance has been the clarification of the interrelation of plasma levels, secretion rates, and clearance rates of steroids. The basic assumption in the measurement of plasma levels or the urinary excretion of steroid metabolites is that they accurately reflect adrenal *secretory* rates of that steroid. A disadvantage of urine *excretion* values is that they may not truly reflect the secretion rate because of improper collection or altered metabolism. Measurement of the actual adrenal secretory rate of a given steroid would be preferable but is more difficult, involving isotope dilution techniques following administration of a radioactive steroid. Plasma levels reflect the level of secretion only at the time of measurement. The plasma level (PL) is dependent on two factors: the secretion rate (SR) of the hormone and the rate at which it is metabolized, i.e., its metabolic clearance rate (MCR). These three factors can be related mathematically as follows:

$$PL = \frac{SR}{MCR} \quad \text{or} \quad SR = MCR \times PL$$

BLOOD LEVELS See Table 336-1.

Peptides ACTH and angiotensin II can be measured by radioimmunoassay. There are technical difficulties with both assays, related mainly to nonspecificity of the antibodies employed. ACTH is probably secreted episodically during the day, with a general trend for plasma levels to vary diurnally, with lower levels in the early evening than in the morning. Angiotensin II levels also vary diurnally but are influenced in addition by dietary sodium intake and posture. Both upright posture and sodium restriction elevate angiotensin II levels.

The majority of clinical determinations of the renin-angiotensin system, however, involve measurements of peripheral "plasma renin activity" (PRA) in which the renin activity is gauged by the generation of angiotensin during a standardized incubation period. This method depends on the presence of sufficient angiotensinogen in the patient's plasma as substrate. The generated angiotensin is then measured by radioimmunoassay. Plasma renin activity levels depend on dietary sodium intake of the patient and whether the patient is ambulatory. In normal recumbent or upright humans, a diurnal rhythm for plasma renin activity is characterized by peak values in the morning with decreases in activity in the afternoon.

Steroids Cortisol and aldosterone are both secreted episodically, but levels generally decline during the day, with peak values in the morning and low levels in the evening. In addi-

TABLE 336-1
Range of normal values for tests of adrenal function

Test	Normal value, range
Plasma cortisol, μg/100 ml:	
8 A.M.	9–24
4 P.M.	3–12
Cortisol secretory rate, mg/24 h	5–25
Urine free cortisol, μg/24 h	20–100
17-Hydroxycorticoids, mg/24 h	2–10
Plasma testosterone, μg/100 ml:	
Males	0.3–1.0
Females	0.01–0.1
17-Ketosteroids, mg/24 h:	
Males	7–25
Females	4–15
Plasma 11-deoxycortisol (S), μg/100 ml	<1.0
Urine tetrahydro-11-deoxycortisol (THS), mg/24 h	0.1–1.0
Pregnanetriol, mg/24 h:	
0–6 years	<0.2
7–15 years	<1.2
Over 16 years	0.5–2.5
Pregnanediol, mg/24 h:	
Males	<1.0
Females	1.1–4.0
Plasma aldosterone, ng/100 ml (100 meq Na, 60–100 meq K, supine)	1–5
Aldosterone secretion, μg/24 h (100 meq Na, 60–100 meq K)	50–250
Aldosterone excretion, μg/24 h (100 meq Na, 60–100 meq K)	2–10
Plasma renin activity, (ng/ml)/h (100 meq Na, 60–100 meq K, supine)	1–2.5
Plasma angiotensin II, pg/ml (100 meq Na, 60–100 meq K, supine)	10–30
Plasma ACTH, pg/ml, 8 A.M.	<80

tion, the plasma level of aldosterone, but not of cortisol, is increased by dietary potassium loading, sodium restriction, or assuming the upright posture. In the male, circadian and day-to-day variations in plasma testosterone levels have also been reported.

URINE LEVELS The principal determinations are of urine 17-hydroxycorticoids, 17-ketosteroids, free cortisol, and aldosterone. The urine *17-hydroxycorticoids* are determined as Porter-Silber chromogens; this reaction is specific for steroids with a "dihydroxyacetone" C-17 side chain, i.e., with hydroxyl groups on C-17 and C-21 and a ketone group on C-20 (Fig. 336-6). Therefore, this determination includes cortisol, cortisone, tetrahydrocortisol, tetrahydrocortisone, and 11-deoxycortisol.

FIGURE 336-6
Key reactive groups (enclosed by dashed circle) in urine steroid determinations.

17-HYDROXYCORTICOIDS (Porter-Silber chromogens)

17-KETOSTEROIDS (Zimmermann reaction)

Normally, daytime (7 A.M. to 7 P.M.) excretion exceeds night values (7 P.M. to 7 A.M.).

The urine *17-ketosteroids* are those containing a ketone group at C-17 (Fig. 336-6). They originate either in the adrenal gland or the gonad. In normal women, 90 percent or more of total urinary 17-ketosteroids is derived from the adrenal gland, while in men, only 60 to 70 percent is of adrenal origin. Urine 17-ketosteroid values are highest in young adults and decline with age.

The total urine 17-ketosteroids may be subdivided into those having either an oxygen or hydroxyl substituent at position C-11 (11-oxy-17-ketosteroids) and those having no such groups (11-deoxy-17-ketosteroids). These 11-oxy-17-ketosteroids are uniquely derived from the adrenal gland, since other tissues do not possess the enzymes for active C-11 hydroxylation, whereas the 11-deoxy-17-ketosteroids may arise from adrenal, testicular or ovarian tissue.

The determination of either urine *free cortisol* or *aldosterone* excretion usually requires radioimmunoassay. Aldosterone excretion is measured by determining the excretion of a major metabolite, usually the acid-labile conjugate. The determination of urine free cortisol is finding increasing clinical usage since elevated excretion values correlate well with states of hypercortisolism, reflecting changes in the unbound, physiologically active, circulating levels of cortisol.

A carefully timed urine collection is a prerequisite for all excretory determinations. Creatinine determinations are of critical importance to demonstrate the accuracy and adequacy of the collection procedure. An adult woman excretes approximately 1000 mg creatinine daily, with about 50 to 60 percent found in the daytime collection; an adult man excretes approximately 1800 mg daily. Day-to-day variation in creatinine excretion should not exceed 20 percent. Adjustments for body size can be made; e.g., normal subjects excrete 3 to 7 mg 17-hydroxycorticosteroids per gram of creatinine.

STIMULATION TESTS Stimulation tests are useful in documenting the existence of a hormonal deficiency state. A standardized and specific stimulus for the production and release of a given hormone is applied, and the quantity of the released hormone can then be measured.

Tests of glucocorticoid reserve Within minutes after initiation of an infusion of ACTH, increased cortisol levels are noted in adrenal venous blood. This responsiveness of the adrenal gland to ACTH is utilized as an index of the "functional reserve" of the gland to produce cortisol. Under maximal ACTH stimulation the cortisol secretion increases tenfold to 300 mg per day. Such maximal stimulation can be obtained only with prolonged ACTH infusions. For clinical purposes, the functional adrenal reserve for cortisol production is standardized with a 24-h ACTH infusion. Synthetic α^{1-24}-ACTH (cosyntropin) is usually used because of its greater purity and given in 500 to 1000 ml normal saline at a rate of 2 units per hour for 24 h. Normal subjects increase 17-hydroxysteroid excretion rates to at least 25 mg per 24 h, and plasma cortisol levels exceed 40 μg per 100 ml. In patients with secondary adrenal insufficiency, the maximal 17-hydroxysteroid excretion rate is 3 to 20 mg per 24 h, and the plasma cortisol value at 24 h ranges between 10 and 40 μg per 100 ml. Patients with primary adrenal insufficiency have smaller responses. Alternatively, 25 units (0.25 mg) cosyntropin may be infused over an 8-h period on two or three consecutive days. The magnitude of the response on the second or third day is similar to that observed with the continuous 24-h infusion.

A rapid screening test is to administer 25 units (0.25 mg) cosyntropin intramuscularly and measure plasma cortisol levels before and 30 and 60 min later. An increment of at least 7 μg per 100 ml above base line is observed in normal subjects. The test can give a false-positive result for adrenal insufficiency, however, because of the irregular absorption of ACTH from the injection site.

Tests of mineralocorticoid reserve and stimulation of the renin-angiotensin system Stimulation tests have been devised utilizing a protocol of programmed volume depletion, such as sodium restriction, diuretic administration, or upright posture. A simple potent stimulation test consists of severe sodium restriction and upright posture. After 3 to 5 days of a 10-meq sodium intake, aldosterone secretion or excretion rates should exhibit a two- to threefold increase over control. Supine morning plasma aldosterone levels usually increase three- to sixfold. In addition, plasma levels increase two- to fourfold in response to 2 to 3 h of upright posture. Recumbent plasma renin activity following sodium restriction to 10 meq per day ranges from 2 to 8 (ng/ml)/h and rises to 2.5 to 15 (ng/ml)/h following 3 h of ambulation.

Stimulation tests on normal dietary sodium intake may also be carried out by the administration of a potent diuretic, such as 40 to 80 mg furosemide, followed by 2 to 3 h of upright posture. The normal response is a two- to fourfold rise in plasma aldosterone levels. Plasma renin activity usually rises to 8 to 15 (ng/ml)/h.

SUPPRESSION TESTS Suppression tests are used to document hypersecretion of adrenocortical hormones and are based on the demonstration of a decrease in the target hormone following standardized suppression of its tropic hormone. Thus, suppression testing for cortisol hypersecretion involves suppression of ACTH release, with documentation of an appropriately normal decrease in cortisol production, while suppression testing of aldosterone involves demonstration of a decrease in aldosterone secondary to suppression of the renin-angiotensin system.

Tests of pituitary-adrenal suppressibility The hypothalamo-pituitary ACTH release mechanism is sensitive to the circulating blood level of glucocorticoids. When such blood levels are increased in the normal individual, less ACTH is released from the anterior pituitary, and secondarily, less steroid is produced by the adrenal gland. The integrity of this feedback mechanism can be tested clinically by giving a potent glucocorticoid and judging suppression of ACTH secretion by analysis of urine steroid excretory values or plasma cortisol levels. A potent glucocorticoid such as dexamethasone is utilized in order that the administered compound may be given in such small amounts as not to contribute significantly to the steroids to be analyzed.

The best *screening* procedure is the overnight dexamethasone suppression test. This involves the measurement of plasma cortisol levels at 8 A.M. following the oral administration of 1 mg dexamethasone the previous midnight. The 8 A.M. value for plasma cortisol in normal subjects should be less than 5 μg per 100 ml.

The definitive test of adrenal suppressibility is to administer 0.5 mg dexamethasone every 6 h for two successive days while collecting urine over a 24-h period for determination of creatinine and 17-hydroxysteroids or the measurement of plasma cortisol levels. In patients with a normal hypothalamic pituitary ACTH release mechanism, a fall in the urine 17-hydroxycorticoids to less than 3 mg a day on the second day of dexamethasone administration or a plasma cortisol less than 5 μg per 100 ml is seen.

Normal responses to either of the suppression tests implies that the ACTH control of the adrenal glands is physiologically normal. However, an isolated abnormal result, particularly when the overnight suppression test is being used, does not in itself imply pituitary and/or adrenal disease.

Tests of mineralocorticoid suppressibility Mineralocorticoid suppression testing procedures have been devised using saline infusions, oral salt loading, or deoxycorticosterone acetate (DOCA) administration as the means for expansion of the extracellular fluid volume. With expansion of extracellular fluid volume, there is a decrease in renal renin release, a decrease in circulating plasma renin activity, and a decrease in aldosterone secretion and/or excretion. Various tests differ in the rate at which extracellular fluid volume is expanded. A convenient suppression test is the intravenous infusion of 500 ml normal saline per hour for 4 h which normally suppresses plasma aldosterone levels to < 8 ng per 100 ml on a sodium-restricted diet or to < 5 ng per 100 ml on a normal sodium intake. The *DOCA suppression test* is carried out by placing the patient on a normal (100 meq) or high (200 meq) sodium intake. After the patient is in sodium balance, deoxycorticosterone acetate is administered intramuscularly (10 mg every 12 h) for a period of 3 to 5 days. Normal subjects on a sodium intake of 100 meq daily demonstrate a 70 percent decrease in aldosterone levels when compared with control levels.

TESTS OF PITUITARY-ADRENAL RESPONSIVENESS A number of stimuli, such as insulin hypoglycemia, arginine vasopressin, and pyrogen, cause release of ACTH from the pituitary by an action on higher nerve centers, the hypothalamus, or the pituitary itself. By measuring plasma ACTH or blood glucocorticoids the status of pituitary ACTH can be evaluated. Insulin-induced hypoglycemia is particularly useful since the release of growth hormone as well as ACTH is stimulated. In this test 0.05 to 0.1 unit of crystalline insulin per kilogram of body weight is administered intravenously as a bolus to reduce fasting glucose levels at least 50 percent below basal. The normal cortisol response is a doubling above control levels within 30 to 60 min.

Metyrapone (SU4885, Metopirone) is a drug that inhibits 11β-hydroxylase (and perhaps other hydroxylating enzymes) in the adrenal gland. As a result, the conversion of 11-deoxycortisol (compound S) to cortisol is interfered with, and increased amounts of 11-deoxycortisol accumulate while blood levels of cortisol decrease (Fig. 336-2). Since 11-deoxycortisol is a weak suppressor of the hypothalamopituitary axis, the anterior pituitary responds to the declining cortisol blood levels by releasing larger quantities of ACTH in an attempt to stimulate the adrenal gland to release additional cortisol, which attempt, however, is thwarted by the metyrapone-induced enzymatic blockade. The metabolites of 11-deoxycortisol are excreted in increasing amounts in the urine, where they are measured as 17-hydroxycorticoids. Alternatively, changes in plasma 11-deoxycortisol levels can be measured. *Note that the adrenal glands must be capable of being stimulated by ACTH, since assessment of the response depends on adrenal steroid production.*

The metyrapone response has been standardized for clinical evaluation of the reserve capacity of the anterior pituitary gland to release ACTH. Every 4 h over a 24-h period 750 mg metyrapone is administered orally, and daily urine collections for 17-hydroxycorticosteroids are obtained the day before, the day of, and the day after the last dose of metyrapone. The peak response of increased urine 17-hydroxysteroid excretion may be seen on the day after completion of metyrapone administration, and normal individuals respond with at least a doubling of their basal 17-hydroxysteroid excretion; 11-deoxycortisol levels in the blood should exceed 10 μg per 100 ml following metyrapone administration. The metyrapone test does not accurately reflect ACTH reserve if subjects are ingest-

ing exogenous glucocorticoids or drugs that accelerate the metabolism of metyrapone (e.g., phenytoin).

A test that distinguishes between primary and secondary adrenal insufficiency takes advantage of the preservation of relatively normal aldosterone secretion in secondary adrenal insufficiency. Thus, when ACTH is administered, neither group has a normal rise in cortisol levels (distinguishing them from normal subjects), but patients with primary adrenal insufficiency also fail to have a normal aldosterone response. Twenty-five units synthetic α^{1-24}-ACTH (cosyntropin) is given intramuscularly, and plasma cortisol and aldosterone levels are obtained before and 30 and 60 min later. Neither group shows the normal cortisol increment of greater than 7 μg per 100 ml, but only patients with primary insufficiency fail to increase aldosterone levels above control by at least 5 ng per 100 ml.

HYPERFUNCTION OF THE ADRENAL CORTEX

Distinct clinical syndromes are produced when excess amounts of the principal adrenocortical hormones are secreted. Thus, excess production of the principal glucocorticoid cortisol is associated with Cushing's syndrome; excess production of the principal mineralocorticoid aldosterone with clinical and chemical signs of aldosteronism; excess production of adrenal androgens with adrenal virilism. As would be expected, these syndromes do not always occur in the "pure" form but may have overlapping features.

CUSHING'S SYNDROME Etiology Harvey Cushing, in 1932, described a syndrome characterized by truncal obesity, hypertension, fatigability and weakness, amenorrhea, hirsutism, purplish abdominal striae, edema, glucosuria, and osteoporosis. As awareness of this syndrome increased and as clinical tests of adrenocortical function became standardized and readily available, the diagnosis of Cushing's syndrome has been broadened into the classification shown in Table 336-2. It is apparent that, regardless of etiology, all cases of Cushing's syndrome are due to increased production of cortisol by the adrenal gland. The majority of cases are due to *bilateral adrenal hyperplasia,* secondary to adrenocortical stimulation by hypersecretion of pituitary ACTH or the production of ACTH by nonendocrine tumors. Cushing originally postulated that the adrenal hyperplasia in patients with pituitary ACTH hypersecretion was attributable to the presence of pituitary basophilic adenomas. Subsequent studies failed to confirm this hypothesis since the sella turcica was radiographically normal in the majority of cases. It was therefore hypothesized that the elaboration of increased amounts of ACTH in the presence of a radiographically normal sella turcica was a result of pituitary-hypothalamic dysfunction, whereby ACTH secretion is reset to

TABLE 336-2
Causes of Cushing's syndrome

I Adrenal hyperplasia
  A Secondary to pituitary ACTH overproduction
    1 Pituitary-hypothalamic dysfunction
    2 Pituitary ACTH-producing micro- or macroadenomas
  B Secondary to ACTH-producing nonendocrine tumors (bronchogenic carcinoma, thymoma, pancreatic carcinoma, bronchial adenoma)
II Adrenal nodular hyperplasia
III Adrenal neoplasia
  A Adenoma
  B Carcinoma
IV Exogenous, iatrogenic
  A Prolonged use of glucocorticoids
  B Prolonged use of ACTH

respond to a higher level of circulating cortisol. However, recent studies suggest that many patients with bilateral hyperplasia have ACTH-producing microadenomas which are sometimes detected only by careful tomographic evaluation of the sella turcica. Thus, the frequency of pituitary adenomas as the cause of Cushing's syndrome is still uncertain.

Nonendocrine tumors secreting polypeptides biologically, chemically, and immunologically indistinguishable from ACTH are also responsible for Cushing's syndrome secondary to bilateral adrenal hyperplasia (see also Chap. 347). Hypokalemic alkalosis is often prominent in such cases, whereas many of the distinctive physical findings usually associated with Cushing's syndrome may be absent.

Approximately 20 to 25 percent of patients with Cushing's syndrome have *primary* overproduction of cortisol and other adrenal steroids due to an adrenal neoplasm. These tumors are almost invariably unilateral, and about half are malignant.

Incidence Increasing numbers of patients with Cushing's syndrome are being detected among persons undergoing evaluation for such diverse entities as diabetes mellitus, hypertension, obesity, and osteoporosis. The incidence of nontumorous adrenal hyperplasia in women is three times that in men, with the most frequent age of onset being the third or fourth decade.

Clinical signs and symptoms The frequency of clinical findings is listed in Table 336-3. Many of the signs and symptoms logically follow from the known action of glucocorticoids. As a result of mobilization of peripheral supportive tissue, there are muscle weakness and fatigability, osteoporosis, and cutaneous striae. The latter involve a weakening and rupture of collagenous fibers in the dermis, so that the heavily vascularized subcutaneous tissues are exposed. Likewise, because of the loss of perivascular supporting tissue, there is easy bruisability, and ecchymoses often appear at sites of mild trauma. The osteoporosis may be so severe that collapse of vertebral bodies and pathological fractures of other bones are frequently encountered. As a result of increased hepatic gluconeogenesis and insulin resistance, impaired glucose tolerance is common, occurring in 90 percent of patients. Frank diabetes occurs in less than 20 percent of patients, probably in individuals with a familial predisposition to this disorder. Hypercortisolism promotes the deposition of adipose tissue in characteristic sites. This is observed most notably in the upper part of the face, the classic "moon" facies; in the interscapular area, the "buffalo" hump; and in the mesenteric bed, where it produces the classic "truncal" obesity (Fig. 336-7). Rarely, there may be episternal fatty tumors and mediastinal widening secondary to fat accumulation. The reason for this peculiar distribution of lipid is not known. The face also appears plethoric, even in the absence of any increase in red blood cell concentration. Hypertension is most always present, and frequently there are profound emotional changes, ranging from irritability or emotional lability to severe depression, confusion, or even frank psychosis. If adrenal androgen secretion is increased, acne and hirsutism are frequent in women, hirsutism often appearing as a fine "downy" coat over the face and upper part of the trunk. Likewise, oligomenorrhea or amenorrhea is frequent.

FIGURE 336-7

A 20-year-old female with Cushing's syndrome due to a right adrenal cortical adenoma. A. Two years prior to surgery, age 18. B. One month prior to surgery, age 20. C. One year after surgery, age 21.

Laboratory findings With rare exceptions, plasma cortisol levels and urinary 17-hydroxycorticoid levels are elevated. Circulating eosinophils are below 100 cells per cubic millimeter in 90 percent of cases, and patients characteristically show a mild neutrophilic leukocytosis. The hematocrit is usually within the normal range, but occasionally erythema with higher hematocrits is encountered. Serum sodium concentration is usually normal; however, with marked excess secretion of cortisol, there may be hypokalemia, hypochloremia, and metabolic alkalosis. X-ray studies usually reveal generalized osteoporosis, most marked in the spine and pelvis but also in the skull with disappearance of the lamina dura, and fractures are often seen in the ribs and vertebrae. Intravenous pyelography and laminograms may demonstrate adrenal enlargement, particularly when a carcinoma is the pathological cause of the disease. More sophisticated x-ray techniques, such as selective adrenal arteriography or venography, may make the localization and diagnosis more specific but are not without risk. The increased friability of the adrenal veins in Cushing's syndrome makes retrograde venography potentially hazardous. The use of 19-[131I]iodocholesterol, computerized tomography (CT scan), and sonar scanning techniques may be of considerable value in localizing adrenal tumors and differentiating them from bilateral hyperplasia.

Diagnosis The diagnosis of Cushing's syndrome depends on the demonstration of increased cortisol production, the absence of normal diurnal rhythmicity of hormonal secretion, and, most importantly, the failure to suppress endogenous cortisol secretion normally when the glucocorticoid dexamethasone is administered exogenously. Once the diagnosis is established, further testing is designed to determine the etiology of the hypercortisolism (see Fig. 336-8).

For initial screening, the overnight dexamethasone suppression test is recommended (see above). The definitive diagnosis is then established by failure to suppress 17-hydroxysteroid excretion to less than 3 mg per 24 h or plasma cortisol to less than 5 μg per 100 ml after a standard low-dose (0.5 mg every 6

TABLE 336-3
Incidence of signs and symptoms in Cushing's syndrome, percent

Typical habitus	97	Amenorrhea	77
Increased body weight	94	Cutaneous striae	67
Fatigability and weakness	87	Personality changes	66
		Ecchymoses	65
Hypertension (> 150/190)	82	Edema	62
		Polyuria, polydipsia	23
Hirsutism	80	Hypertrophy of clitoris	19

Signs and Symptoms
{ OSTEOPOROSIS
DIABETES MELLITUS
DIASTOLIC HYPERTENSION
CENTRAL ADIPOSITY
HIRSUTISM & AMENORRHEA

Screening Test

Plasma cortisol (8 a.m.)
> 5µg/100 ml after 1 mg
Dexamethasone at midnight

Dexamethasone suppression test
Response on 2nd day to 0.5 mg q.6h.

17-OH <3 mg/24 hr
NORMAL RESPONSE

17-OH > 3 mg/24 hr
CUSHING'S SYNDROME

17-OH (mg/24 hr)*
Response on 2nd day of Dex. suppression (2 mg q.6h.)

↓ 17-OH < 50% of control
ADRENAL HYPERPLASIA
secondary to pituitary ACTH secretion

No response
ADRENAL HYPERPLASIA
secondary to nonendocrine ACTH producing tumor
ADRENAL NEOPLASIA

Plasma
ACTH

High (>400 pg/ml)
ADRENAL HYPERPLASIA
secondary to ACTH-producing tumor

Normal-low
ADRENAL ADENOMA

Urinary 17-KS
(mg/24 hr)

High (>30 mg/24 hr)
ADRENAL CARCINOMA

Normal-low
ADRENAL NEOPLASM

FIGURE 336-8

Diagnostic flowchart for evaluating patients suspected of having Cushing's syndrome.

The 17-hydroxycorticosteroid response to metyrapone (750 mg given orally every 4 h for six doses) may be used as an alternative test to the high-dose dexamethasone test (2 mg given orally every 6 h). Increased urinary 17-hydroxycorticosteroid excretion following metyrapone occurs in the majority of patients with adrenal hyperplasia secondary to pituitary ACTH secretion; no response suggests an adrenal neoplasm or adrenal hyperplasia secondary to a nonendocrine ACTH-producing tumor.

h for 48 h) dexamethasone suppression test. Additional measurements that may be useful in difficult cases include a cortisol secretion rate greater than 30 mg per day and a urine-free cortisol excretion rate greater than 100 µg per day.

Owing to a marked diurnal variability, plasma cortisol determinations are not meaningful when performed in isolated fashion, but demonstration that expected normal fall in the bedtime blood levels does not occur may be useful.

Specific diagnosis of the type of Cushing's syndrome can be aided by high-dose dexamethasone suppression testing. When patients with "inappropriate" pituitary ACTH secretion are given high doses of dexamethasone (2 mg every 6 h), suppression of urine 17-hydroxysteroid levels to less than half the base-line levels can frequently be demonstrated. This is consistent with the view that the hypothalamic pituitary axis is reset upward and is responsive only to higher blood levels of glucocorticoids, at which point an appropriate decline in ACTH release occurs. In patients with adrenal hyperplasia secondary to an ACTH-producing tumor, such as an oat-cell bronchogenic carcinoma, or in patients with adrenal neoplasms, no suppression occurs after low or high dexamethasone administration, since pituitary ACTH secretion is already suppressed by the elevated cortisol levels. Moreover, ACTH production by nonendocrine tumors is secreted in an autonomous manner.

In patients with Cushing's syndrome secondary to an *adrenal adenoma*, hyperreactivity to exogenous ACTH testing may or may not occur, depending on whether the adenoma functions in an autonomous manner. The diagnosis of cortisol-pro-

ducing adrenal adenoma is suggested by the disproportionate elevation in base-line urine 17-hydroxycorticoids with only a modest rise in 17-ketosteroids. Adrenal androgen secretion is usually reduced in these patients owing to the cortisol-induced suppression of ACTH and subsequent involution of the androgen-producing zona reticularis. Another entity in the differential diagnosis is multinodular ("adenomatous") adrenal hyperplasia, which is an uncommon condition characteristically having features of both hyperplasia and adenomas. Response to ACTH stimulation is variable, but patients with multinodular adrenal hyperplasia most often do not show suppression with the standard doses of dexamethasone. However, with large doses, such as 4 to 8 mg every 6 h, suppression often occurs.

Metyrapone testing is useful in differentiating adrenal tumors (adenoma or carcinoma) from adrenal hyperplasia, since the autonomous adrenal tumors suppress the ACTH-releasing capacity of the pituitary, with the result that on metyrapone challenge testing the pituitary fails to release ACTH in an appropriate manner, and the usual rise in urine 17-hydroxycorticoids fails to occur. This finding of impaired response to metyrapone challenge separates adrenal tumors from adrenal hyperplasia secondary to pituitary ACTH secretion, in which normal or hyperactive responses occur.

The diagnosis of *adrenal carcinoma* as a cause of Cushing's syndrome is suggested by a palpable abdominal mass and by *markedly* elevated base-line values of *both* urine 17-hydroxycorticoids and urine 17-ketosteroids. Adrenal carcinoma is usually resistant to both ACTH stimulation and dexamethasone suppression because of the autonomy of the tumor tissue itself and because of extreme atrophy of the normal remaining adrenal tissue. Markedly elevated 17-ketosteroid excretion often leads to virilization in the female. Feminizing estrogen-producing adrenocortical carcinoma in the male usually presents with gynecomastia. These adrenal tumors secrete increased amounts of androstenedione which is peripherally converted to the estrogens, estrone and estradiol (see Chap. 343). Functioning adrenal carcinomas that produce Cushing's syndrome are most often associated with elevated values for the intermediates of steroid biosynthesis (especially 11-deoxycortisol), suggesting inefficient conversion of the intermediates to the final product. This is in contrast to Cushing's syndrome associated with adrenocortical hyperplasia, in which the elevation of urine steroids is largely accounted for by cortisol metabolites. It is also important to recognize that 20 percent of adrenal carcinomas are not associated with endocrine syndromes and are presumed to be nonfunctioning or associated with the production of biologically inactive steroid precursors. Finally, the excessive production of sex steroids is not detectable in certain situations (e.g., androgens in adult male patients), leading to differing rates of occurrence of clinical syndromes in male and female subjects (Table 336-4).

Cushing's syndrome is being reported with increasing frequency in association with the autonomous production of ACTH by *nonendocrine tumors,* with the resultant development of adrenal hyperplasia. The majority of these cases have been associated with the primitive small-cell type of bronchogenic carcinoma, and the remainder have been reported chiefly with tumors of the thymus, pancreas, or ovary, medullary carcinoma of the thyroid, or bronchial adenomas. The onset of Cushing's syndrome is distinctively sudden in these patients, and this partly accounts for their failure to exhibit all the classic physical findings of the syndrome. (See also Chap. 347.) The secretion of ACTH by nonendocrine tumors is also accompanied by the accumulation of circulating ACTH fragments as well as elevated levels of the large-molecular-weight ACTH precursor (pro-ACTH or "big ACTH"). Recent studies indicate that the production of these biologically inactive peptides by lung neoplasms is extremely common; on the other hand, steroid overproduction is seen only in the situation where biologically active ACTH levels are also elevated. Since such tumors may produce large amounts of ACTH and MSH, base-line urine steroid values are usually markedly elevated, and increased skin pigmentation is usually present. A CRF-like material produced by the tumor has also been reported to cause hypercortisolism. Hypokalemic alkalosis, edema, and hypertension are more common in these patients than in Cushing's syndrome from other causes, and are attributed to extremely high levels of cortisol secretion. *No suppression with dexamethasone* and no increment in urine 17-hydroxycorticoid excretion after metyrapone administration are the rule unless the endogenous secretion of cortisol is not sufficient to suppress pituitary ACTH secretion. Plasma ACTH levels are often *markedly* elevated in these patients, a helpful diagnostic finding, since plasma ACTH levels in other categories of Cushing's syndrome are at most modestly elevated.

Hyperpigmentation in patients with Cushing's syndrome always points to an extraadrenal tumor, either in an extracranial location, as discussed in the previous paragraph, or within the cranium. Approximately one-tenth of patients undergoing bilateral adrenalectomy for Cushing's syndrome over subsequent months or years develop chromophobe adenomas with progressive cutaneous hyperpigmentation and erosion of the sella turcica (Nelson's syndrome) (see Chap. 333). ACTH and MSH levels in these patients are extremely high. These tumors may be locally invasive and may impinge on the optic chiasm or extend into the cavernous or sphenoid sinuses. Since intrasellar microadenomas may be present prior to operation in many patients *without* sellar enlargement, a decisive opinion as to their role in the genesis of Cushing's syndrome or in the sequelae of Nelson's syndrome must be withheld for further investigation. Clinically, all patients documented to have Cushing's syndrome must be carefully examined for enlargement of the sella turcica by sella tomography. If defects are found, further diagnostic procedures may be warranted, such as visual field examination, pneumoencephalography, and angiography. Following bilateral adrenalectomy, patients should be followed for evidence of progressive hyperpigmentation. Periodic but indefinite x-ray evaluation of the sella turcica and serial ACTH levels are important parameters to follow. A diagnostic flowchart for evaluation of patients suspected of having Cushings syndrome is presented in Fig. 336-8.

Differential diagnosis Patients with exogenous obesity, hypertension, and diabetes mellitus, occurring singly or in combination, present major problems in diagnosis. Extreme *obesity* is uncommon in Cushing's syndrome; furthermore, with exogenous obesity, the adiposity is generalized, not truncal. On adrenocortical testing, abnormalities, if noted in patients with exogenous obesity, are found never to be extensive but only modest. Basal urine steroid excretion levels in obese patients are either normal or slightly elevated, a finding similar to their cortisol secretory values. Some patients demonstrate a conversion of secreted cortisol into excreted metabolites. Urinary free and blood cortisol levels are normal, and, of greater importance, a normal diurnal pattern in blood and urine levels is seen. It appears that exogenous obesity may *cause* alterations in the secretion and metabolism of steroids, pointing up the secondary nature of altered steroid testing patterns sometimes encountered.

Iatrogenic Cushing's syndrome, induced by the administration of either glucocorticoids or ACTH, is indistinguishable by physical findings from the endogenous forms of adrenocortical hyperfunction. On occasion one may wish to rule out an underlying endogenous form of Cushing's syndrome that may be clinically magnified by exogenous therapy. This is accomplished by changing the patient's therapy to 1 mg dexamethasone daily while collecting urine output for corticosteroid analysis. Patients with a pure exogenous form of Cushing's syndrome due to prolonged suppression of their hypothalamic pituitary axis by administered steroid demonstrate low baseline steroid excretion, a finding in distinct contrast to that in patients with endogenous Cushing's syndrome. Patients receiving long-term ACTH therapy, in addition to the features of Cushing's syndrome, may also have melanodermia. The production of iatrogenic Cushing's syndrome is related both to the total steroid dose and to the duration of therapy. Also, patients on afternoon and evening doses of steroid develop Cushing's syndrome more readily on smaller daily steroid doses than do patients on a steroid program limited to morning doses only. In addition, there appears to be a marked difference among

TABLE 336-4
Clinical features of adrenal carcinoma in adults

	Male	*Female*
Cushing's syndrome	+ +	+ +
Cushing's syndrome plus virilization	0	+ + + +
Virilization	0	+ + +
Feminization	+	0
Primary aldosteronism	±	±
No endocrine syndrome	+ + +	+ +

NOTE: *0, not detectable; +, least common; + + + +, most common.*

patients in the enzymatic disposition of administered steroid. Several cases have been reported in which a spontaneous remission of Cushing's syndrome occurred; some have been characterized by intermittent abnormalities in adrenal function tests. It is difficult to know whether such abnormalities are functional in nature or true pathophysiological processes.

Therapy When an adenoma or carcinoma is suspected, adrenal exploration is performed, with excision of the tumor following localization of the neoplasm by angiographic techniques. Because of the possible atrophy of the contralateral adrenal, the patient is treated pre- and postoperatively for total adrenalectomy even when a unilateral lesion is suspected, the routine being similar to that for an Addisonian patient undergoing elective surgery (Table 336-10). Despite operative intervention, most patients with adrenal carcinoma die within 3 years of diagnosis. Metastases occur most often to liver and lung.

The principal antitumor drug used to treat metastatic adrenocortical carcinoma is *o,p'*-DDD [2,2-bis(2-chlorophenyl-4-chlorophenyl)-1,1-dichloroethane], an isomer of the insecticide DDT. This drug suppresses cortisol production and decreases plasma and urine steroid levels. Although its cytotoxic action is reported to be specific for the glucocorticoid-secreting zone of the adrenal cortex, the zona glomerulosa (site of aldosterone biosynthesis) may also be inhibited. *o,p'*-DDD also alters the extraadrenal metabolism of cortisol, resulting in a smaller percent excreted in the urine as 17-OHCS. Therefore, *plasma or urinary free-cortisol* levels must be followed to determine the effect of *o,p'*-DDD on the hypercortisolism. *o,p'*-DDD is given in divided doses three to four times daily. The dose is gradually increased to 8 to 10 g daily or the highest dose tolerated by the patient. Almost all patients experience gastrointestinal (anorexia, diarrhea, or vomiting) or neuromuscular (lethargy, somnolence, dizziness) side effects. All patients should be placed on long-term maintenance glucocorticoid; in some instances mineralocorticoid replacement therapy should also be instituted. In approximately one-third of patients regressions of both tumor and metastases occur, but long-term survival is limited. The mean duration of life from onset of treatment is approximately 8 months. In many patients, *o,p'*-DDD only inhibits steroidogenesis and does not produce regression of tumor metastases. Osseous metastases are usually refractory to *o,p'*-DDD; radiation should be used to treat these lesions.

In patients with severe Cushing's syndrome due to adrenal hyperplasia, with features of hypertension, overt diabetes, psychosis, and osteoporosis with pathological fractures and in the absence of an enlarged sella turcica, a complete total bilateral adrenalectomy is preferred. Since one-tenth of these patients develop pituitary tumors after surgery, pituitary irradiation is also indicated in any patient who develops increased pigmentation or in whom the sella turcica size increases postoperatively. In patients past the reproductive years, pituitary irradiation may be carried out prophylactically in conjunction with complete adrenalectomy. It cannot be stressed too strongly that the status of all patients with bilateral adrenalectomy must be followed diligently with periodic reexaminations for evidence of increasing sellar size, pigmentary changes, and rising ACTH levels.

In some centers, pituitary irradiation is the primary treatment for bilateral hyperplasia. There are three major methods of directing radiotherapy at the pituitary gland. (1) The classic approach is the use of conventional external radiation at a dose of 3000 to 5000 rads delivered over several weeks. Total dosage is limited by possible damage to surrounding neural structures and by the loss of additional pituitary tropic function. Treatment has been successful in fewer than one-third of the patients with Cushing's syndrome who were treated solely by this method. (2) The second method is internal pituitary

irradiation by the stereotactic implantation of ^{90}Y pellets in the pituitary via the transnasosphenoid route. Possible limitation of this form of therapy may be found once long-term evaluation on the effects of the radiation on perisellar structures (such as the internal carotid artery) has been made. (3) The most recent development has been the use of the alpha particle or proton beam as a source of external radiation. By this method as much as 12,000 rads can be directed at the pituitary gland without evident damage to surrounding structures, because the beam can be focused more sharply than the more commonly used gamma radiation and because multiple portals of entry can be used. However, with yttrium implants and proton beam therapy there is an increased incidence of ocular motor palsies and hypopituitarism. Successful reduction in steroid output in bilateral hyperplasia has also been reported with the chronic administration of the serotonin antagonist, cyproheptadine. It is speculated that cyproheptadine blocks the stimulating effect of hypothalamic serotonin on the release of CRF, thereby reducing pituitary ACTH secretion.

Patients with severe Cushing's syndrome are not candidates for therapies such as external pituitary irradiation. The lag time between treatment and remission and a remission rate less than 50 percent contraindicate the use of external pituitary irradiation in the presence of rapidly progressing disease. In severely debilitated patients who are not candidates for bilateral adrenalectomy, a chemical remission can be obtained from *o,p'*-DDD (2 to 10 g per day).

If patients with adrenal hyperplasia are noted to have gross signs of pituitary tumor (melanodermia, increased sellar size, visual field defects), specific therapy directed at the pituitary gland must be undertaken. In general, the type of therapy is either surgery and/or some form of radiation. Complications of surgical therapy include cerebrospinal fluid rhinorrhea and optic nerve and posterior pituitary injury, as well as panhypopituitarism. Surgery is often reserved for those cases not amenable to treatment with radiation. In patients with adrenal hyperplasia and slight asymmetry of the sella turcica, transphenoidal surgery has resulted in the successful removal of pituitary ACTH-producing microadenomas and cure of the hypercortisolism. However, it is not certain that these neoplasms might not recur with time if the fundamental abnormality is hypothalamic dysfunction.

Treatment of nonendocrine ACTH-producing tumors is surgical removal of the neoplasm. If the neoplastic disease is far advanced, bilateral total adrenalectomy, metyrapone, or *o,p'*-DDD may be indicated to correct the hypercortisolism.

If Cushing's syndrome redevelops after bilateral adrenalectomy, excessive stimulation of a remnant of adrenocortical tissue may be occurring. In very rare instances an embryologic extraadrenal remnant may be stimulated to produce excess cortisol. Surgical exploration is difficult because adrenocortical remnants are small. Measurement of cortisol levels preopera-

TABLE 336-5
Treatment modalities for patients with adrenal hyperplasia secondary to pituitary ACTH hypersecretion

I Reduce pituitary ACTH production
  A Transphenoidal resection of microadenoma
  B Radiation
  C Treatment with hypothalamic serotonin antagonist (cyproheptadine)*
II Reduce or eliminate adrenocortical cortisol secretion
  A Bilateral adrenalectomy
  B Medical adrenalectomy (metyrapone, *o,p'*-DDD)*

* *Not curative but effective as long as chronically administered in responsive patients.*

tively from various points along the inferior vena cava may locate the remnant tissue. The use of 19-[^{131}I]iodocholesterol scintillation scanning offers interesting possibilities.

Table 336-5 summarizes the various treatment modalities that are currently employed to manage adrenal hyperplasia secondary to the inappropriate secretion of pituitary ACTH. It is recommended that the laboratory and x-ray findings and the severity of cortisol excess guide the choice of therapy in the individual patient.

ALDOSTERONISM Aldosteronism is a syndrome associated with hypersecretion of the major adrenal mineralocorticoid aldosterone. *Primary* aldosteronism signifies that the stimulus for the excessive aldosterone production resides within the adrenal gland; in *secondary* aldosteronism the stimulus is of extraadrenal origin.

Primary aldosteronism The constellation of signs and symptoms of excessive inappropriate aldosterone production was first summarized by Conn in 1956. In the original case and in a number of subsequent cases, the disease was the result of an *aldosterone-producing adrenal adenoma* (Conn's syndrome). The majority of cases involved a unilateral adenoma, usually small and occurring with equal frequency on either side. Rarely primary aldosteronism has been reported in association with adrenal carcinoma. It is twice as common in women as in men, presenting between the ages of 30 and 50. In recent years, an increasing number of cases have been reported with clinical and biochemical characteristics previously considered diagnostic of primary aldosteronism, but a solitary adenoma was not found at surgery. Instead, these patients have *bilateral cortical nodular hyperplasia.* The cause of this hyperplasia is unknown. In the literature this disease has been alternatively termed "pseudo" primary aldosteronism (PPA), idiopathic hyperaldosteronism (IHA), or nodular hyperplasia.

INCIDENCE Primary aldosteronism is an uncommon disease. The incidence in unselected hypertensive patients is approximately 1 percent.

SIGNS AND SYMPTOMS The continual hypersecretion of aldosterone increases the renal distal tubular exchange of intratubular sodium for secreted potassium and hydrogen ions, with progressive depletion of body potassium and development of hypokalemia. Almost all patients have diastolic hypertension, usually not of marked severity, and complain of headaches. The hypertension is related in some unknown manner to the increased sodium reabsorption and extracellular volume expansion. *Potassium depletion* is responsible for the major complaints of muscle weakness and fatigue and is related to the effect of intra- and extracellular potassium ion depletion on muscle membrane. The polyuria results from impairment of concentrating ability and is often associated with polydipsia. These patients may have electrocardiographic and roentgenographic signs of left ventricular enlargement which is secondary to their hypertension, and hypertensive retinopathy can be seen. Electrocardiographic signs of potassium depletion such as prominent U waves are often present, and cardiac arrhythmias and premature contractions are not uncommon. In the absence of associated congestive heart failure, renal disease, or preexisting abnormalities (such as thrombophlebitis), edema is characteristically absent in these patients.

In cases of long duration, potassium-depletion nephropathy becomes manifest, with azotemia, often with superimposed bacilluria, and in some instances with congestive heart failure and edema.

LABORATORY FINDINGS Laboratory findings are dependent on both the duration and the severity of the potassium depletion. On examination of the urine, negative to trace amounts of protein are found, sometimes with superimposed pyuria and bacilluria, presumably because of the predilection of potassium-depleted kidneys for infection. Urine specific gravity is low (less than 1.015), and an overnight concentration test with simultaneous vasopressin administration reveals impaired ability to concentrate the urine. Urine pH is often neutral to alkaline, because of excessive secretion of ammonium and bicarbonate ions. Urine 17-hydroxycorticosteroid and 17-ketosteroid excretion levels are always within the normal range in patients with aldosteronomas. Mild azotemia is an inconstant finding.

Serial blood sampling usually reveals *hypokalemia* and sometimes hypernatremia. The hypokalemia may be severe (less than 3 meq potassium per liter) and reflects significant body potassium depletion, usually in excess of 300 meq. *Hypernatremia* is due to both sodium retention and a concomitant water loss from polyuria. The serum bicarbonate level may be elevated as a result of hydrogen ion loss into the urine and migration into potassium-depleted cells, with alkalosis then developing. The alkalosis is perpetuated with potassium deficiency, since such deficiency increases the capacity of the proximal convoluted tubule to reabsorb filtered bicarbonate. This alkalosis predisposes to signs and symptoms of tetany. If hypokalemia is severe, serum magnesium levels are also reduced. In the absence of azotemia, serum uric acid concentration is normal.

Total body sodium content is increased but not to the degree seen in edematous states. Total exchangeable sodium is moderately elevated, and total exchangeable body potassium is usually, but not invariably, reduced. The volume of extracellular fluid is expanded in most cases, with expansion of plasma volume in many. The expanded extracellular fluid volume is thought to be responsible for the reversed diurnal excretory pattern for salt and water that many of these patients exhibit, with predominant salt and water excretion occurring during the night.

DIAGNOSIS The diagnosis is suggested by the presence of persistent hypokalemia in a nonedematous patient on a normal sodium intake who is not receiving potassium-wasting (furosemide, ethacrynic acid, thiazides) or potassium-sparing (Dyrenium, spironolactone) diuretics. If hypokalemia is discovered in a hypertensive patient on a potassium-wasting diuretic, the diuretic should be discontinued, and the patient should be given potassium supplements. After 1 to 2 weeks the potassium level should be remeasured, and if hypokalemia persists, the patient should be evaluated for a mineralocorticoid excess syndrome (Fig. 336-9).

The criteria which subsequently permit the clinician to derive a diagnosis of primary aldosteronism are (1) diastolic hypertension without edema, (2) hyposecretion of renin (as judged by low plasma renin activity levels) which fails to increase appropriately during volume depletion (upright posture, sodium depletion), and (3) hypersecretion of aldosterone which fails to be suppressed appropriately during volume expansion (salt loading).

Diastolic hypertension is a prerequisite for the diagnosis of primary aldosteronism, even though transient periods of relative normotension may be observed during long-term evaluation. Accelerated (sustained) diastolic hypertension is uncommon but has been reported.

Patients with primary aldosteronism characteristically *do not have edema,* since they are exhibiting a perpetuated "escape" phenomenon. Since they are in a chronic state of escape from the sodium-retaining aspects of mineralocorticoids, they characteristically excrete an administered salt load with a greater rapidity than do normotensive subjects, a characteristic which is shared by patients having essential hypertension. Only a limited sodium retention occurs when patients with primary aldosteronism are given sodium-retaining hormones parenterally. Rarely in patients with associated potassium-depletion nephropathy and azotemia, pretibial edema may be present.

Estimation of plasma renin activity has been valuable in separating patients with primary aldosteronism from those with other causes of hypertension. The failure of plasma renin activity to rise normally during volume-depletion maneuvers (e.g., sodium depletion, diuretic administration, and/or ambulation) is a major diagnostic criterion for primary aldosteronism. This is in contrast to what occurs in some hypertensive patients in whom hyperaldosteronism is secondary to *increased* renin levels. However, suppressed renin activity is not diagnostic of primary aldosteronism, as it occurs in about 25 percent of patients with essential hypertension, in patients with hyperaldosteronism secondary to idiopathic bilateral nodular adrenal hyperplasia, and in other mineralocorticoid excess syndromes, including deoxycorticosterone-secreting adrenal tumors.

Since the determination of plasma renin responsiveness is not sufficient, measurement of lack of suppression of aldosterone secretion is necessary to diagnose primary aldosteronism properly. The autonomy exhibited by aldosterone tumors in these patients refers only to their resistance to suppression of secretion during volume expansion; such tumors can and do respond either in normal or supernormal fashion to the stimuli of potassium loading or ACTH infusion. Patients with primary aldosteronism do not respond to volume expansion since their renin-angiotensin system is already suppressed. Appropriate suppression testing may be carried out by saline loading, oral salt loading, or DOCA administration (see "Tests of Mineralocorticoid Suppressibility" above).

Once hyposecretion of renin and failure to suppress aldosterone secretion are demonstrated, then localization of aldosterone-producing adenomas should be determined preoperatively by the technique of percutaneous transfemoral bilateral adrenal vein catheterization with simultaneous adrenal venography. Such a technique permits radiological localization, and, in addition, the adrenal vein sampling may demonstrate a two- to threefold increase in plasma aldosterone concentration on the involved side compared with the uninvolved side. In cases of hyperaldosteronism secondary to cortical nodular hyperplasia, no localization is found. It is important for samples to be obtained simultaneously if possible and for cortisol levels to be measured to ensure that false localization does not reflect an ACTH- or stress-induced rise in aldosterone levels. A flowchart for evaluation of patients with suspected primary aldosteronism is presented in Fig. 336-9.

FIGURE 336-9

Diagnostic flowchart for evaluating patients with suspected primary aldosteronism.

*Serum K+ may be normal in some patients with hyperaldosteronism who are taking potassium-sparing diuretics (spironolactone, triamterene) or ingesting low sodium–high potassium intakes.

†This step should not be taken if hypertension is severe (diastolic > 115 mmHg) or if cardiac failure is present. Also, serum potassium levels should be corrected before the infusion of saline. Alternative methods producing comparable suppression of aldosterone secretion include oral sodium loading (200 meq per day for 3 days) or 10 mg deoxycorticosterone acetate (DOCA) intramuscularly every 12 h for 3 days.

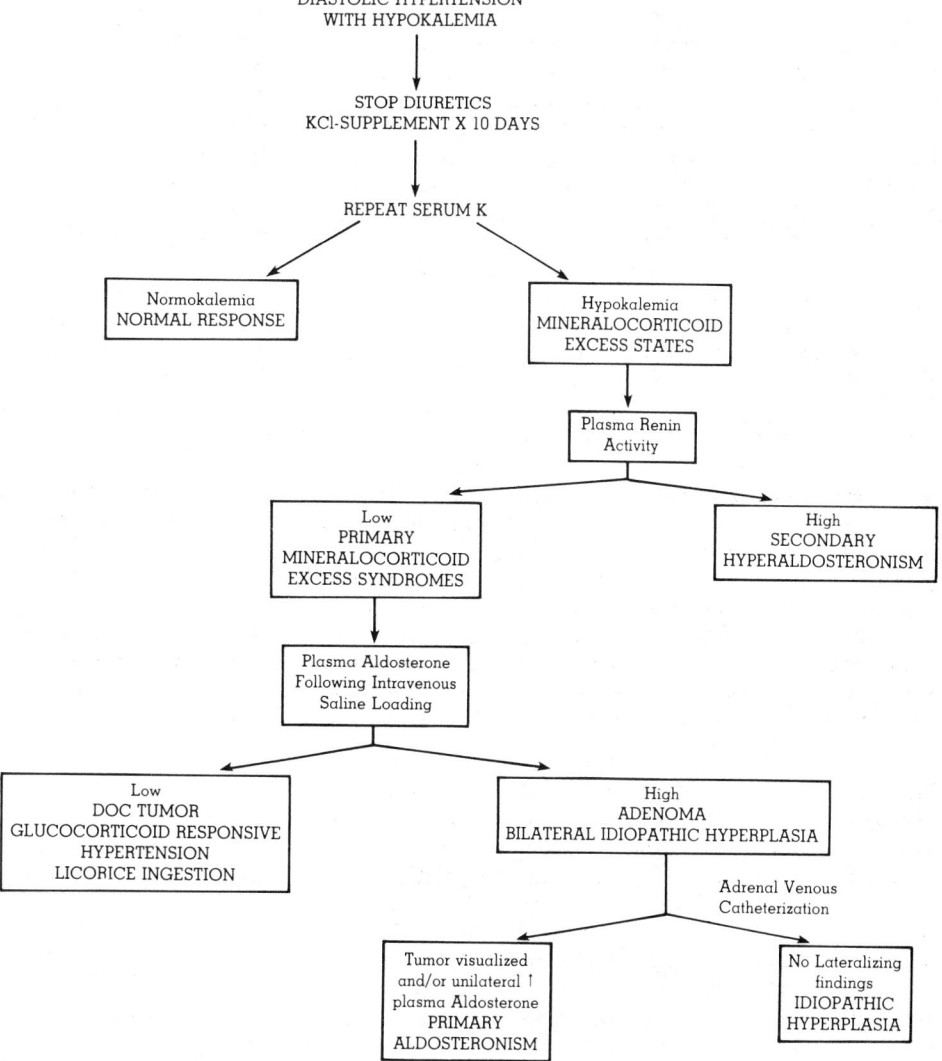

DIFFERENTIAL DIAGNOSIS   All patients with *accelerated hypertension* and hypokalemia must be evaluated for unilateral renal disease. If such a diagnosis is confirmed, an additional diagnosis of primary aldosteronism is unlikely, although in rare instances both have been recorded to occur simultaneously. A useful maneuver in distinguishing between secondary aldosteronism due to accelerated hypertension and primary aldosteronism is the measurement of plasma renin activity. In patients with accelerated hypertension and secondary aldosteronism, the aldosteronism is secondary to elevated plasma renin levels; in distinct contrast, patients with primary aldosteronism have suppressed plasma renin levels.

Primary aldosteronism must also be distinguished from other *hypermineralocorticoid states.* The most common problem is to distinguish between hyperaldosteronism due to an adenoma and that due to idiopathic bilateral nodular hyperplasia. This is of considerable importance, since it is generally agreed that the hypertension associated with idiopathic hyperplasia is usually not benefited by bilateral adrenalectomy. In contrast, the hypertension associated with aldosterone-producing tumors is usually improved or cured following removal of the adenoma. Although patients with idiopathic bilateral nodular hyperplasia tend to have less severe hypokalemia, lower aldosterone secretion, and higher plasma renin activity than patients with primary aldosteronism, differentiation is impossible solely on clinical and/or biochemical grounds. An anomalous postural decrease in plasma aldosterone has also been reported in the majority of patients with a unilateral lesion, but this test is of limited diagnostic value in the individual patient. A definitive diagnosis is best made by preoperative, bilateral cannulation of the adrenal veins; cases of primary aldosteronism demonstrate unilateral increments in plasma aldosterone concentration and/or tumor visualization on the involved side.

In a few instances, hypertensive patients with hypokalemic alkalosis have been found to have deoxycorticosterone (DOC)-secreting adenomas. Such patients have reduced plasma renin activity levels, but aldosterone measurements are either normal or reduced, suggesting the diagnosis of mineralocorticoid excess due to a hormone other than aldosterone. Rare cases of hypermineralocorticoidism due to a defect in cortisol biosynthesis, specifically 11- or 17-hydroxylation, have also been reported. ACTH levels are increased, with a resultant increase in the production of the mineralocorticoid 11-deoxycorticosterone. *Hypertension and hypokalemia can be corrected by glucocorticoid administration.* The definitive diagnosis is made by demonstrating an elevation of precursors of cortisol biosynthesis in the blood or urine. Occasionally, glucocorticoid administration produces normotension and normokalemia although a hydroxylase deficiency cannot be identified (Fig. 336-9).

Licorice ingestion produces a syndrome mimicking primary aldosteronism. Licorice contains a sodium-retaining principle, glycyrrhizinic acid, which, in addition to sodium retention, causes expansion of the extracellular fluid volume, hypertension, depressed plasma renin levels, and suppressed aldosterone levels. The diagnosis is excluded by a careful history.

TREATMENT   Primary aldosteronism due to an adenoma is usually treated by surgical excision. However, dietary sodium restriction and the administration of the aldosterone antagonist, spironolactone, are also effective in many cases. Hypertension and hypokalemia are usually controlled by doses of 25 to 100 mg spironolactone every 8 h. Some patients have been successfully managed medically for years, but chronic therapy in men is usually limited by the common occurrence of gynecomastia, decreased libido, and impotence.

When bilateral hyperplasia is suspected, surgery is indicated only when significant, symptomatic hypokalemia cannot be controlled with medical therapy, e.g., spironolactone or triamterene. Hypertension associated with idiopathic hyperplasia is usually not benefited by bilateral adrenalectomy.

Secondary aldosteronism   Secondary aldosteronism refers to an appropriately increased production of aldosterone by the adrenal gland in response to stimuli originating outside the gland (Fig. 336-10). In all reported cases the stimulus has been the renin-angiotensin system. The adrenal production rates of aldosterone are often higher in patients with secondary aldosteronism than in those with primary aldosteronism. Most patients with secondary aldosteronism exhibit this syndrome either as an associated feature of the accelerated phase of hypertension (regardless of the primary disease) or on the basis of an underlying edema disorder. On the other hand, secondary aldosteronism in pregnancy is a normal physiological response to estrogen-induced increases in circulating levels of renin substrate and plasma renin activity, as well as the antialdosterone actions of the progestins.

Secondary aldosteronism found in hypertensive states either is secondary to a primary overproduction of renin (primary reninism) or is caused by an overproduction of renin which is secondary to a decrease in renal blood flow and/or perfusion pressure (Fig. 336-4). Secondary hypersecretion of renin could be due to a narrowing of one or both of the major renal arteries either by an atherosclerotic plaque or by fibromuscular hyperplasia. Overproduction of renin from both kidneys also occurs in association with severe arteriolar nephrosclerosis (malignant hypertension) or secondary to profound renal vasoconstriction (accelerated phase of hypertensive disease). These patients exhibit a secondary aldosteronism characterized by hypokalemic alkalosis, absence of edema, moderate to severe increases in plasma renin activity, and moderate to marked increases in aldosterone secretion/excretion rates (see Chap. 251).

Secondary aldosteronism with hypertension is also associated with the rare renin-producing tumor, so-called "primary reninism." These patients have all the biochemical characteristics of renal vascular hypertension; however, the primary defect is not a decrease in renal blood flow and/or perfusion pressure but renin secretion by a juxtaglomerular-cell tumor. The diagnosis can be made by the absence of changes in renal vasculature and/or the presence of a space-occupying lesion seen by renal arteriography, with unilateral increases in renal vein renin activity.

Secondary aldosteronism is present in many *edema* disorders. Increased aldosterone secretion rates have been docu-

FIGURE 336-10

Responses of the renin-aldosterone volume control loop in primary versus secondary aldosteronism.

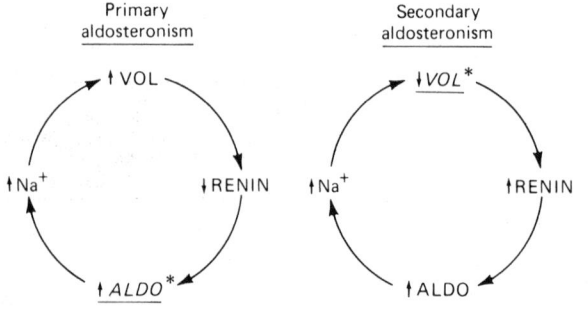

Initiating event

mented in patients with edema as a result of either cirrhosis or the nephrotic syndrome. In congestive heart failure, however, elevated aldosterone secretion is a variable finding. The stimulus for aldosterone release in these clinical conditions appears to be *arterial hypovolemia*. Diuretic therapy often exaggerates the features of secondary aldosteronism via the mechanism of acute volume depletion; when this happens hypokalemia and on occasion alkalosis become prominent features.

Secondary hyperaldosteronism may rarely occur without edema or hypertension (Bartter's syndrome). This syndrome is characterized by the signs of severe hyperaldosteronism (hypokalemic alkalosis) with moderate to marked increases in renin activity but normal blood pressure and absence of edema. Renal biopsy shows juxtaglomerular hyperplasia. The pathogenesis of this syndrome is obscure but some patients may have a defect in the renal conservation of sodium. The renal loss of sodium is thought to stimulate renin secretion and subsequently aldosterone production. Hyperaldosteronism produces potassium depletion, with the hypokalemia further elevating plasma renin activity. In some cases, the hypokalemia may be potentiated by a defect in renal conservation of potassium. The lack of hypertension is due to vascular unresponsiveness to angiotensin. Recent studies have suggested that one underlying derangement may be an increased production of prostaglandins.

ADRENAL VIRILISM AND CONGENITAL ADRENAL HYPERPLASIA The adrenal virilizing syndromes result from excessive production of adrenal androgens, such as dehydroepiandrosterone and Δ^4-androstenedione, which are converted to testosterone; the elevated testosterone levels account for most of the virilization. As in other states of adrenocortical hyperfunction, the syndrome may result from hyperplasia, adenoma, or carcinoma. Adrenal virilization may arise in a congenital form, termed *congenital adrenal hyperplasia,* due to enzymatic deficits. The adrenal virilizing syndromes may be associated with secretions of greater or smaller amounts of other adrenal hormones and may, therefore, present as "pure" syndromes of virilization or as "mixed" syndromes associated with excessive production of glucocorticoid and some of the characteristics of Cushing's syndrome. In *congenital* adrenal hyperplasia the virilizing syndromes are associated with increased adrenal androgen production and either excessive or decreased secretion of mineralocorticoid or decreased production of glucocorticoid.

Since in humans hydrocortisone is the principal adrenal steroid regulating ACTH elaboration and since ACTH stimulates both hydrocortisone and adrenal androgen production, an enzymatic interference with hydrocortisone synthesis may result in the enhanced secretion of adrenal androgens. In severe congenital virilizing hyperplasia, the adrenal output of hydrocortisone may be so compromised as to cause glucocorticoid deficiency despite anatomic adrenal hyperplasia. Conversely, a high hydrocortisone output as the result of primary adrenal disease (adenoma) may inhibit ACTH secretion and thus result in a low adrenal androgen output.

Incidence Congenital bilateral adrenocortical hyperplasia is by far the most common adrenal disorder of infancy and childhood. It has also been described later in life, predominantly in women. Its appearance in postpubertal men would obviously not be as clinically apparent; nevertheless, it has been reported. In its various forms, congenital adrenal hyperplasia is thought to be the result of autosomal recessive mutations. Affected family members have similar patterns of steroid excretion and severity of enzymatic deficiencies.

Clinical signs and symptoms Congenital adrenal hyperplasia is secondary to one of several defects in steroid synthesis. To

date, defects have been described in the C-21, C-18, C-17, and C-11 hydroxylase enzymes, as well as in the 3β-ol-dehydrogenase enzyme. These enzyme deficits usually occur singly. The clinical expression is variable, ranging from virilization of the female (C-21 deficiency) to feminization of the male (3β-ol-dehydrogenase deficiency). (See also Chap. 344.)

Adrenal virilization in the female at birth is associated with ambiguous external genitalia (*female pseudohermaphroditism*). The onset of virilization is most probably after the fifth month of embryonic development. At birth there may be macrogenitosomia in the male infant, and in the female enlargement of the clitoris, partial or complete fusion of the labia, and sometimes a urogenital sinus. If the labial fusion is nearly complete, the female infant has external genitalia resembling a penis with hypospadias. In the *postnatal* period from infancy to adolescence, congenital adrenal hyperplasia is associated with virilization in the female and isosexual precocity in the male. The excessive androgens result in accelerated growth, with bone age exceeding chronological age. Since epiphyseal closure is hastened by excessive androgens, growth stops but truncal development continues, giving the characteristic appearance of a child of short stature with well-developed trunk. Incomplete variants of congenital adrenal hyperplasia sometimes become manifest only in adult life with virilization or hirsutism in the female.

In the adult woman, regardless of the cause of the condition, the clinical signs and symptoms are those anticipated from excessive androgen production. These include hirsutism, acne, increased sebum production, temporal baldness, deepening of voice, increased muscle mass and strength, decreased breast size, atrophy of uterus, amenorrhea, enlargement of the clitoris, increased sexual drive, and development of a male habitus. The clinical distinction between excessive hair growth (hirsutism) and virilization is useful. Virilization signifies that multiple signs of androgen excess are present in addition to hirsutism; one of the more easily recognized of these signs is hypertrophy of the clitoris. Hirsutism in the absence of other signs of virilization is uncommon in these patients. The virilizing syndromes are difficult to document in the *adult* male, for obvious reasons.

The most common form of congenital adrenal hyperplasia (95 percent of cases) is a result of impairment of *C-21 hydroxylation*. In addition to cortisol deficiency, in approximately one-third of the patients, there is an associated reduction in aldosterone secretion. Thus, with congenital adrenal hyperplasia secondary to C-21 hydroxylase deficiency, adrenal virilization will be present with or without an associated salt-losing tendency due to aldosterone deficiency.

With a *C-11 hydroxylase* deficiency a "hypertensive" variant of congenital adrenal hyperplasia develops. Hypertension and hypokalemia occur because of the impaired conversion of 11-deoxycorticosterone to corticosterone, resulting in the accumulation of 11-deoxycorticosterone, a potent mineralocorticoid. Increased shunting again occurs into the androgen pathway with overproduction of 11-deoxy-17-ketosteroids.

The *C-17 hydroxylase* deficiency is characterized by hypogonadism, hypokalemia, and hypertension. In patients with this rare deficiency there is decreased production of cortisol and shunting of precursors into the mineralocorticoid pathway with hypokalemic alkalosis, hypertension, and suppressed plasma renin activity. In most patients, 11-deoxycorticosterone production is elevated. Because C-17 hydroxylation is required for biosynthesis of adrenal androgens as well as gonadal testosterone and estrogen, this defect is associated with sexual immaturity, high urinary gonadotropin levels, and low urinary 17-ketosteroid excretion. Female patients have primary amenorrhea and lack of development of secondary sexual characteristics. Because of deficient androgen production, male patients have ambiguous external genitalia (male pseudohermaphroditism). Exogenous glucocorticoids can correct the hypertensive syndrome, but sex hormones are necessary to produce sexual maturation.

With 3β-ol-dehydrogenase deficiency, there is impaired conversion of pregnenolone to progesterone, with the result that pathways to both cortisol and aldosterone are "blocked," with shunting then occurring into the adrenal androgen pathway via 17α-hydroxypregnenolone to dehydroepiandrosterone. Since dehydroepiandrosterone is a weak androgen and because this enzyme deficiency is also present in the gonad, the genitalia of the male fetus may be ambiguous or feminized. Conversely, in the female, overproduction of dehydroepiandrosterone may produce virilization.

Diagnosis The diagnosis of *congenital adrenal hyperplasia* should be considered in all infants exhibiting "failure to thrive," particularly those having episodes of acute adrenal insufficiency or salt-wasting, or showing sustained hypertension. The diagnosis is further suggested by the finding of hypertrophy of the clitoris, fused labia, or urogenital sinus in the female and isosexual precocity in the male. In infants and children with a *C-21 hydroxylation block,* increased urine 17-ketosteroid excretion is typically associated with an increase in the blood levels of 17α-hydroxyprogesterone and the urinary excretion of the metabolite of this steroid, pregnanetriol. These children have low urine 17-hydroxycorticoid excretion and elevated plasma ACTH.

The diagnosis of a *salt-losing form of congenital* adrenal hyperplasia due to defects in C-21 hydroxylase enzyme is suggested by episodes of acute adrenal insufficiency with hyponatremia, hyperkalemia, dehydration, and vomiting. These infants and children often "crave" salt and exhibit laboratory signs of concomitant deficits in both cortisol and aldosterone secretion.

With the *hypertensive form* of congenital adrenal hyperplasia due to impaired C-11 hydroxylation, 11-deoxycorticosterone (a potent mineralocorticoid) and 11-deoxycortisol accumulate. Both urine 17-ketosteroid and 17-hydroxycorticoid excretion may be elevated since 11-deoxycortisol is included in the analysis of Porter-Silber chromogens. The diagnosis is secured by demonstrating increased levels of 11-deoxycortisol in the blood or increased amounts of tetrahydro-11-deoxycortisol in the urine with decreased amounts of tetrahydro metabolites of cortisol.

The finding of very high levels of urine dehydroepiandrosterone with low levels of pregnanetriol and of cortisol metabolites is characteristic of patients with congenital adrenal hyperplasia due to 3β-ol-dehydrogenase deficiency. These patients also exhibit marked salt wasting.

The *C-17 hydroxylase* deficiency results in the accumulation of progesterone and its metabolite, pregnanediol. The excretion of deoxycorticosterone and of corticosterone is increased, while aldosterone production is usually subnormal. In some patients aldosterone secretion is elevated.

The adrenal virilizing syndrome in adults is most often due to acquired causes—namely, tumor or adrenal hyperplasia. *Adrenal adenomas* and *carcinomas* may cause a pure or mixed virilizing syndrome (Table 336-4). Since adrenal androgens are weak compared with gonadal androgens, adrenal virilization is characterized by *large increments in urine 17-ketosteroid excretion,* often with less impressive clinical signs of virilism. Virilizing adrenocortical adenomas are rare. *Virilizing adrenal carci-*

nomas are the most common adrenal tumor causing virilization. They are associated with high urinary 17-ketosteroid excretion, reaching 100 mg or more per 24 h, and may have normal or a moderate rise in 17-hydroxycorticosteroid excretion. Clinical differentiation between virilizing adrenal adenoma and carcinoma cannot be made with certainty preoperatively.

In adrenocortical hyperfunction of Cushing's syndrome, both urinary 17-ketosteroid and 17-hydroxycorticosteroid base-line values are elevated. Adrenal hyperactivity associated with hirsutism but with normal 17-hydroxycorticosteroid baseline excretion represents an ill-defined, controversial, heterogeneous group of patients. Mild hirsutism usually appears after puberty and is characterized by normal or moderately elevated urinary 17-ketosteroids. With ACTH stimulation there may be a brisk rise in the urinary 17-ketosteroids when compared with the 17-hydroxycorticosteroids. Base-line 17-ketosteroids are easily suppressed by daily administration of 2 mg dexamethasone. Some if not all of these patients may have a mild form of congenital adrenal hyperplasia.

Differential diagnosis In the female, the differential diagnosis of hirsutism and virilization is between adrenal and ovarian etiologies (Table 336-6). *Sudden onset of progressive hirsutism and virilization* suggests an adrenal or ovarian neoplasm. Since adrenal tumors secrete weak androgens (such as DHEA), virilizing adrenal neoplasms are characterized by high urine 17-ketosteroid excretion, usually in excess of 30 to 40 mg per 24 h. Failure to reduce 17-ketosteroid levels to normal following dexamethasone suppression (0.5 mg given orally every 6 h for 7 days) supports a diagnosis of virilizing adrenal tumor and excludes congenital adrenal hyperplasia. The most common *ovarian tumor* causing virilization is the arrhenoblastoma, but other ovarian tumors, such as adrenal rest tumor, granulosa-cell tumor, hilar-cell tumors, and Brenner tumors have been associated with virilization. Virilization due to ovarian tumors is characterized by normal or moderate elevations of urinary 17-ketosteroids, since the neoplasm usually secretes the potent androgen testosterone. Moderate increases in 17-ketosteroid excretion occur in some patients with ovarian neoplasm, but base-line 17-ketosteroid excretion in excess of 30 mg per day is rare with the exception of adrenal rest tumors. Like adrenal neoplasms, ovarian tumors fail to be suppressed by dexamethasone. With the exception of adrenal rest tumors, they are largely independent of ACTH stimulation. Elevations of plasma testosterone or urinary testosterone excretion do not localize the neoplasm to the ovary, since testosterone can be elevated subsequent to peripheral conversion of adrenal precursors, such as DHEA (see Chap. 342).

Hirsutism without virilization beginning after puberty and associated with normal ovarian histology is diagnostic of idiopathic or familial hirsutism. In a second group of patients, hirsutism is seen in association with sclerocystic or polycystic ovaries. Oligomenorrhea, anovulatory bleeding, and/or amenorrhea commonly occur in these patients. The ovaries may be palpably enlarged bilaterally; unilateral enlargement suggests an ovarian neoplasm. The presence of polycystic ovaries at

TABLE 336-6
Causes of hirsutism in females

  I Familial
 II Idiopathic
III Ovarian
     A Polycystic ovaries; hilus-cell hyperplasia
     B Tumor; arrhenoblastoma, hilus cell, adrenal rest
 IV Adrenal
     A Congenital adrenal hyperplasia
     B Noncongenital adrenal hyperplasia (Cushing's)
     C Tumor: virilizing carcinoma or adenoma

TABLE 336-7
Laboratory evaluation of hirsutism-virilizing syndromes

	Ovarian		Adrenal			
	PCO	Ovarian tumor	CAH	Adrenal neoplasm	Cushing's syndrome	Idiopathic
Urinary 17 ketosteroids	N↑	N	N↑	↑↑↑	N↑	N
Plasma testosterone	N↑	↑↑	N↑	N↑	N↑	N
Serial LH levels	N↑	N	N	N	N	N
Precursors of cortisol biosynthesis:						
Basal	N	N	N↑	N↑	N	N
Following ACTH infusion	N	N	↑↑	N↑	N	N
Cortisol following overnight dexamethasone suppression test	N	N	N	↑	↑	N

NOTE: N, normal; CAH, congenital adrenal hyperplasia; PCO, polycystic ovary syndrome; LH, luteinizing hormone.

laparoscopy does not establish an ovarian causation since polycystic ovaries have been described in association with adrenal virilization. 17-Ketosteroid excretion values in hirsute females with polycystic ovary disease or idiopathic hirsutism are usually normal or slightly elevated. *Plasma testosterone* levels tend to be higher in females with polycystic ovary disease than in normal females, and in 20 percent of cases testosterone levels are greater than normal. Studies indicate that some women with idiopathic hirsutism or polycystic ovaries probably have increased blood production rates of testosterone. Studies also indicate that luteinizing hormone (LH) levels are tonically elevated in some patients with polycystic ovary disease. The laboratory findings in patients with hirsutism-virilizing syndromes are summarized in Table 336-7.

Treatment Treatment of adrenal virilism is dictated by the type of lesion suspected. Patients with *congenital adrenal hyperplasia* have the fundamental defect of cortisol deficiency with resultant excessive ACTH stimulation, producing hyperplasia of the adrenal glands and causing additional "shunting" into the adrenal androgen pathway. Therapy in these patients consists of daily administration of glucocorticoids (dexamethasone, prednisone, cortisone, etc.) to suppress pituitary ACTH secretion. Because of its cost and intermediate half-life, prednisone is the drug of choice except in infants, when hydrocortisone is usually used. The amount of steroid required to manage patients with congenital adrenal hyperplasia is approximately 1.5 times the normal cortisol production rate of 12 to 13 mg cortisol per square meter of body surface area per day and is given in divided doses two or three times a day. As the patient grows, the maintenance dose obviously should be increased. The dosage schedule is governed by repetitive analysis of the urinary 17-ketosteroids and skeletal growth and maturation, since overtreatment with glucocorticoid replacement therapy retards linear growth. In children, glucocorticoids not only suppress urinary ketosteroid excretion but also end virilization and the associated problems of hyperandrogenicity. Some infants and children with the associated defect of salt wasting require vigorous correction of salt deficits in conjunction with small doses of a potent mineralocorticoid such as 9α-fluorohydrocortisone. Children born with abnormalities of external genitalia may require surgical correction of labial fusion, urogenital sinus, etc. Diagnosis of the adrenogenital syndrome in the newborn with ambiguous external genitalia is crucial to avoid errors in the assignment of sex. Response of these children to steroid therapy is gratifying in that normal growth and development occur and the menarche and onset of spermatogenesis occur at the appropriate age. Many females with this disorder have married and have borne children. Steroid therapy is indicated throughout life, and dosages should be periodically adjusted for major stress as in the Addisonian patient.

In patients with adrenal virilization due to adrenal tumors, prompt surgical intervention with complete excision of the tumor is indicated.

HYPOFUNCTION OF ADRENAL CORTEX

Adrenocortical hypofunction includes all conditions in which the secretion of adrenal steroid hormones falls below the requirements of the body. Adrenal insufficiency may be divided into two general categories: (1) those associated with primary inability of the adrenal to elaborate sufficient quantities of hormone and (2) those associated with a secondary failure due to a primary failure in the elaboration of ACTH (Table 336-8).

PRIMARY ADRENOCORTICAL DEFICIENCY (ADDISON'S DISEASE) This disorder is also called *Addison's disease* or *chronic glucocorticoid deficiency*. Addison's description in 1855, namely, "general languor and debility, remarkable feebleness of the heart's action, irritability of the stomach, and a peculiar change of the color of the skin," summarizes the dominant clinical features of the disease. Advanced cases are usually easy to diagnose, but recognition of the disease in its earlier phases may present a real challenge. The disease, when unrecognized and untreated, carries an almost uniformly poor and frequently fatal prognosis. Early diagnosis is important, since present-day therapy completely corrects the metabolic derangement.

Incidence Primary adrenocortical insufficiency is relatively rare. It may occur at any age and affects both sexes with equal frequency. Because of increasing therapeutic use of exogenous steroids, secondary adrenal insufficiency is seen with increasing frequency.

Etiology and pathogenesis Addison's disease results from progressive adrenocortical destruction, which must involve more

TABLE 336-8
Classification of adrenal insufficiency

I Primary adrenal insufficiency
  A Anatomic destruction of gland (chronic and acute)
    1 "Idiopathic" atrophy (autoimmune)
    2 Surgical removal (metastatic breast cancer)
    3 Infection (tuberculous, fungous)
    4 Hemorrhage
    5 Invasion: metastatic
  B Metabolic failure in hormone production
    1 Congenital adrenal hyperplasia
    2 Enzyme inhibitors (metyrapone)
    3 Cytotoxic agents (*o,p'*-DDD)
II Secondary adrenal insufficiency
  A Hypopituitarism due to pituitary disease
  B Suppression of hypothalamic-pituitary axis
    1 Exogenous steroid
    2 Endogenous steroid from tumor

than 90 percent of the glands before clinical signs of adrenal insufficiency appear. The adrenal is a frequent site for chronic infectious diseases of the granulomatous variety, predominately tuberculosis but also including fungal infections, such as histoplasmosis, coccidioidomycosis, and cryptococcosis. In previous years, tuberculosis was found at postmortem examination in 70 to 90 percent of cases; however, the most frequent finding at present is *idiopathic* atrophy, and an autoimmune mechanism may be responsible. Rarely, other lesions are encountered, such as bilateral tumor metastases, amyloidosis, or sarcoidosis.

The possibility that some patients may have primary adrenal insufficiency on an *autoimmune basis* is strengthened by the finding that half of patients with Addison's disease have complement-fixing and/or circulating adrenal antibodies, as tested by the indirect Coombs method. It is not clear whether these antibodies cause adrenal atrophy or are secondary to the destruction of adrenal tissue. Certain of these patients also have additional circulating antibodies to thyroid, parathyroid, and/or gonadal tissue (see also Chap. 348).

There is an increased incidence of chronic lymphocytic thyroiditis (Hashimoto's disease) in patients with nontuberculous, idiopathic adrenal insufficiency (Schmidt's syndrome). Idiopathic hypoparathyroidism is also seen with increased frequency in patients with Addison's disease (Chap. 348). Concomitant parathyroid and adrenal insufficiency and mucocutaneous moniliasis have also been recognized as a distinct familial, autosomal recessive syndrome. Diabetes mellitus, ovarian failure, and pernicious anemia are also seen in association with idiopathic Addison's disease and thyroiditis. Again, what role genetic predisposition and/or autoimmunity may play in the occurrence of these diseases in the same individual is unknown. Recent reports also indicate a greater incidence of these endocrine deficiency states in patients with specific human leucocyte antigens.

Clinical signs and symptoms Adrenocortical insufficiency is characterized by an insidious onset of slowly progressive fatigability, weakness, anorexia, nausea and vomiting, weight loss, cutaneous and mucosal pigmentation, hypotension, and occasionally hypoglycemia (Table 336-9). However, the spectrum may vary, depending on the duration and degree of adrenal hypofunction, from a complaint of mild chronic fatigue to the fulminating shock associated with acute massive destruction of the glands in the type of syndrome described by Waterhouse and Friderichsen.

Asthenia is the cardinal symptom of Addison's disease. Early it may be sporadic, usually most evident at times of stress; as adrenal function becomes more impaired, the weakness progresses until the patient is continuously fatigued, necessitating bed rest. Even the voice may fail, so the speech finally becomes listless and indistinct.

Hyperpigmentation may be a striking sign of the disease, but its absence does not exclude this diagnosis. It commonly appears as a diffuse brown, tan, or bronze darkening of both exposed and unexposed parts such as elbows or creases of the

hand and in areas normally pigmented such as the areolas about the nipples. In many patients, bluish black patches appear on the mucous membranes. Some patients develop dark freckles, and occasionally irregular areas of vitiligo may appear paradoxically. As an early sign, patients may notice an unusually persistent tanning following exposure to the sun.

Arterial hypotension is frequent, and in severe cases blood pressures may be in the range of 80/50 or less. Postural accentuation is common, and syncope may occur.

Abnormalities of gastrointestinal function often are the presenting complaint. Symptoms may vary from mild anorexia with weight loss to fulminating nausea, vomiting, diarrhea, and ill-defined abdominal pain, which at times may be so severe as to be confused with an acute abdomen. In addition, patients with adrenal insufficiency frequently have marked personality changes, usually in the form of excessive irritability and restlessness. Enhancement of the sensory modalities of taste, olfaction, and hearing is often present and is reversible with therapy. A decrease in axillary and pubic hair is common in female patients due to loss of adrenal androgen production.

Laboratory findings In the milder forms, sometimes called *partial* or *incomplete* Addison's disease, there may be no demonstrable abnormalities in any of the parameters measured in the routine laboratory, and even plasma and urinary steroid determinations may indicate values relatively low yet within normal range. However, studies of adrenal stimulation with ACTH show abnormalities even in this stage of the disease. In the more advanced stages, levels of serum sodium, chloride, and bicarbonate are reduced while serum potassium is elevated. The hyponatremia is due to extravascular loss of sodium both into the urine (due to aldosterone deficiency) and from the vascular compartment into tendons, cartilage, and bone. This extravascular sodium loss depletes extracellular fluid volume and accentuates hypotension. Elevated plasma vasopressin and angiotensin have been reported, and these may be contributing factors to hyponatremia through impairment of free-water clearance. The hyperkalemia is due to a combination of factors, including aldosterone deficiency, impaired glomerular filtration, and acidosis. These patients may show marked reduction in heart size. The electrocardiogram may show nonspecific changes, and the electroencephalogram a striking reduction and slowing of the predominant activity. The basal metabolic rate may be low, but other thyroid indexes are usually normal. There may be a normocytic anemia, a relative lymphocytosis, and usually a moderate eosinophilia.

Diagnosis The diagnosis of primary adrenal insufficiency requires demonstration of decreased cortisol production by the adrenal in the basal and in the stimulated state.

In cases of severe *adrenal insufficiency* the cortisol secretory rate is markedly decreased, and this may be ascertained indirectly by the finding of low to absent 24-h urine 17-hydroxycorticoids and urine 17-ketosteroids. Because of the contribution of the male gonads to urine 17-ketosteroids, basal excretory values in complete adrenal insufficiency are higher for males than females. With mild or moderate adrenal insufficiency, urine steroid excretion values overlap into the normal range; because of this, a diagnosis of adrenal insufficiency should never be made solely on the values of basal urine steroid determinations. Plasma cortisol values are from zero to the lower range of normal. Aldosterone secretion is usually low, resulting in salt-wasting and secondary rises in plasma renin levels. In patients with primary adrenal insufficiency, plasma ACTH and melanocyte-stimulating hormone (MSH) levels are elevated because of loss of the usual cortisol-hypothalamic-pituitary feedback relationship, whereas in secondary adrenal insufficiency, plasma ACTH values are low, a finding

TABLE 336-9
Incidence of symptoms and signs in Addison's disease, percent

Weakness	99	Hypotension	
Pigmentation of skin	98	(<110/70)	87
Pigmentation of mucous		Abdominal pain	34
membranes	82	Salt craving	22
Weight loss	97	Diarrhea	20
Anorexia, nausea, and		Constipation	19
vomiting	90	Syncope	16
		Vitiligo	9

consistent with the absence of increased pigmentation in patients having the latter condition (Fig. 336-11).

The diagnosis of adrenal insufficiency should be made only with ACTH stimulation testing to assay the adrenal reserve capacity for steroid production (see above for ACTH test protocols).

Differential diagnosis Since weakness and fatigue are common complaints, clinical diagnosis of early adrenocortical insufficiency is frequently difficult (Fig. 336-11). However, mild gastrointestinal distress with weight loss, anorexia, and a suggestion of increased pigmentation make mandatory ACTH stimulation testing to rule out adrenal insufficiency, particularly before steroid treatment is begun. Weight loss is useful in evaluating the significance of weakness and malaise. Weight gain associated with lassitude is more characteristic of depressive syndromes. Racial pigmentation in Negroes, Orientals, Indians, Spanish Americans, and Latins may be a problem, but a *recent* and progressive *increase* is usually reported by the Addisonian patient. Hyperpigmentation in other diseases may also present a problem, but the appearance and distribution of pigment in Addison's disease are usually characteristic. When doubt exists, measurement of ACTH levels and testing of adrenal reserve with the infusion of ACTH provide clear-cut differentiation.

Treatment All patients with Addison's disease should receive specific hormone replacement. Like diabetics, these patients require careful and persistent education in regard to their disease. Since the adrenal gland elaborates three general classes of hormone, of which two, glucocorticoids and mineralocorticoids, are of primary clinical importance, replacement therapy should correct both deficiencies. Cortisone (or hydrocortisone) is the mainstay of treatment; however, its mineralocorticoid effect, when it is given in sufficient dosage to replace the endogenous hydrocortisone deficiency, is inadequate for complete electrolyte balance; therefore, the patient usually requires other supplementary therapy. Cortisone dosage varies from 12.5 to 50 mg daily, with the majority of patients taking 25 to 37.5 mg in divided doses. Hydrocortisone (30 mg daily) or prednisone (7.5 mg daily) in divided doses may also be given for substitution therapy. Because of its direct local effect on gastric mucosa, patients are advised to take their cortisone

with meals or, if this is impractical, with milk or an antacid preparation. In addition, the larger proportion of the dose (25 mg) is taken in the morning and the remainder (12.5 mg) in the late afternoon, to simulate the normal diurnal adrenal rhythm. Some patients may exhibit insomnia, irritability, mental excitement, and even frank psychosis soon after initiation of therapy; in these the dosage should be reduced. Other indications for maintaining the patient on smaller amounts are hypertension, diabetes, or active tuberculosis.

Since this amount of cortisone or hydrocortisone fails to replace the mineralocorticoid component of the adrenal gland, supplementary hormone is usually needed. The simplest means is daily oral administration of 0.1 to 0.2 mg 9α-fluorohydrocortisone. If parenteral administration is indicated, a dosage of 2 to 5 mg deoxycorticosterone acetate in oil may be given every day intramuscularly.

Complications of cortisone therapy, with the exception of peptic ulcer disease or gastritis, are *rare* in the dosage used in the treatment of Addison's disease. However, overtreatment with deoxycorticosterone preparations or 9α-fluorohydrocortisone is more frequent and may present as edema, hypertension, cardiac enlargement, or even congestive failure due to sodium retention. Overtreatment may also present as weakness, progressing to total paralysis, due to hypokalemia. In the management of patients with Addison's disease, periodic measurements of body weight, serum potassium, blood pressure, and serial electrocardiograms are useful.

Some female patients with Addison's disease experience a persistent decline in libido possibly related to subnormal adrenal androgen production. Small doses of intramuscular depotestosterone (e.g., 25 mg every 4 to 6 weeks) may be used to advantage, but overtreatment leading to masculinizing side effects must be avoided.

All patients with adrenal insufficiency, including bilaterally adrenalectomized patients, should carry medical identification, should be instructed in the parenteral self-administration of steroids, and should be registered with a national medical alerting system.

FIGURE 336-11

Diagnostic flowchart for evaluating patients with suspected adrenal insufficiency. Plasma ACTH levels are low in secondary adrenal insufficiency. In adrenal insufficiency secondary to pituitary tumors or idiopathic panhypopituitarism, other pituitary hormone deficiencies are present. On the other hand, ACTH deficiency may be isolated, as seen following prolonged use of exogenous glucocorticoids.

Since the isolated blood levels obtained in these screening tests may not be definitive in certain patients, the diagnosis should always be confirmed by a continuous 24-h ACTH infusion. Normal subjects and patients with secondary adrenal insufficiency may be distinguished by insulin tolerance or metyrapone testing.

Special therapeutic problems During periods of intercurrent illness, the dose of cortisone or hydrocortisone should be increased to levels of 75 to 150 mg per day. When oral administration is not possible, parenteral routes should be employed. Likewise, before surgery or dental extractions, excess steroid should be administered. For a representative program of steroid therapy for an Addisonian patient or an adrenalectomized patient undergoing a major operation, see Table 336-10. This schedule is designed to mimic the maximal output of cortisol in normal individuals undergoing prolonged major stress with presumed continuous ACTH stimulation (10 mg/h, 250 to 300 mg per 24 h). The patients should be advised of these facts and carry an identification card bearing instructions for the administration of steroid in case of acute illness or injury. Patients should also be advised to increase the dose of 9α-fluorohydrocortisone and add excess salt to their otherwise normal diet during periods of excessive exercise with sweating, during extremely hot weather, or during periods of gastrointestinal upsets.

Course and prognosis Untreated Addison's disease runs a chronic and relentless course. In some patients, its advance is relatively slow, but in all patients the condition may rapidly deteriorate into adrenal crisis. With treatment, the prognosis of the disease is extremely favorable.

SECONDARY ADRENOCORTICAL INSUFFICIENCY Pituitary ACTH deficiency causes *secondary* adrenocortical insufficiency. ACTH deficiency may be selective, as is seen following prolonged administration of excess glucocorticoids, or may occur in association with multiple pituitary tropic hormone deficiencies (panhypopituitarism) (see Chap. 333). Patients with secondary adrenocortical hypofunction may have many symptoms and signs in common with Addisonian patients but are *characteristically not hyperpigmented* since ACTH and MSH levels are low. In fact, plasma ACTH levels distinguish between primary and secondary adrenal insufficiency, since they are elevated in the former and decreased to absent in the latter. Patients with total pituitary insufficiency also have signs and symptoms suggestive of multiple hormone deficiencies. An additional feature distinguishing primary from secondary adrenocortical insufficiency is the *near-normal level of aldosterone secretion* seen in the presence of pituitary and/or isolated ACTH deficiencies (Fig. 336-11). Patients with pituitary insufficiency may present with hyponatremia, which may be dilutional or secondary to subnormal increments in aldosterone secretion in response to sodium restriction. However, the findings of severe dehydration, *hyponatremia,* and *hyperkalemia* are characteristic of severe mineralocorticoid insufficiency and favor a diagnosis of primary adrenocortical insufficiency.

Patients receiving long-term steroid therapy, despite physical findings of Cushing's syndrome, develop adrenal insufficiency both because of prolonged pituitary-hypothalamic suppression and because of actual adrenal atrophy. Adrenal atrophy results from the loss of endogenous ACTH stimulation. Thus, these patients acquire two deficits, a loss of adrenal responsiveness to ACTH and a failure of pituitary ACTH release. These patients are characterized by low blood cortisol and ACTH levels, low base-line steroid excretion, and abnormal ACTH and metyrapone test results. Practically all patients with steroid-induced adrenal insufficiency eventually recover normal hypothalamic-pituitary-adrenal responsiveness, but individual response time is variable, ranging from days to months. The short ACTH test can be used as a convenient and valuable assessment of recovery of hypothalamic-pituitary-adrenal function. Since the plasma cortisol concentrations after injection of cosyntropin and during insulin-induced hypoglycemia correlate closely, the rapid ACTH test assesses the integrated hypothalamic-pituitary-adrenal function. Additional testing to assess endogenous pituitary ACTH reserve includes the standard metyrapone and the insulin tolerance tests.

Substitution glucocorticoid therapy in patients with secondary adrenocortical insufficiency does not differ from that outlined for Addisonian patients. Mineralocorticoid replacement therapy is usually not necessary, since aldosterone secretion is preserved. Otherwise, the basic principles outlined for replacement should be applied to patients with secondary adrenocortical insufficiency.

ACUTE ADRENOCORTICAL INSUFFICIENCY Acute adrenocortical insufficiency may result from several processes. One of these, usually termed *adrenal crisis,* is a rapid and overwhelming intensification of chronic adrenal insufficiency. Another involves an acute hemorrhagic destruction of both adrenal glands, usually associated with an overwhelming septicemia. Adrenal hemorrhage associated with anticoagulant therapy in stressed patients with increased adrenocortical activity has also been reported. A third, and probably the most frequent, cause of acute insufficiency results from the rapid withdrawal of steroids from patients with adrenal atrophy secondary to chronic steroid administration. In the presence of severe stress, acute adrenocortical insufficiency may also occur in patients with congenital adrenal hyperplasia and those receiving pharmacological agents which are capable of inhibiting steroid synthesis by the gland (such as *o,p'*-DDD).

TABLE 336-10
Steroid therapy schedule for Addisonian patient undergoing a major operation*

	Cortisone acetate (intramuscularly)		Hydro-cortisone infusion, continuous	Cortisone acetate (orally)				Fluorohydrocortisone (orally),
	7 A.M.	7 P.M.		8 A.M.	12 Noon	4 P.M.	8 P.M.	8 A.M.
Routine daily medication				25		12.5		0.1
Day before operation		50		25		12.5		0.1
Day of operation	100	50	200					
Postoperative:								
Day 1	50	50	100–150					
Day 2	50	50	50–100					
Day 3	50	50		25			25	
Day 4	50			25	25	25		0.1
Day 5				25	25	25	25	0.1
Day 6				25	25	25		0.1
Day 7				25	12.5	25		0.1
Day 8				25	12.5	25		0.1
Days 9–13				25		25		0.1
Day 14				25		12.5		0.1

* *All steroid doses are given in milligrams.*

Adrenal crisis The long-term survival of patients with Addison's disease largely depends upon prevention and treatment of adrenal crisis. Consequently, the occurrence of infection, trauma (including surgery), gastrointestinal upsets, or other forms of stress requires an immediate increase in hormone. In previously untreated patients, preexisting symptoms are intensified. Nausea, vomiting, and abdominal pain may become intractable. Fever is frequently severe but may be absent. Lethargy deepens into somnolence, and the blood pressure and pulse fail as hypovolemic vascular shock ensues. In contrast, patients previously maintained on chronic glucocorticoid therapy may not exhibit severe dehydration or hypotension until preterminally, since mineralocorticoid secretion is usually preserved.

In all patients in crisis, a precipitating cause should be sought. Intercurrent infection associated with omission or failure to increase maintenance therapy is a common setting.

Treatment is primarily directed toward the rapid elevation of circulating glucocorticoid and the immediate replacement of the sodium and water deficit. Hence, an intravenous infusion of 1000 ml 5% glucose in normal saline solution containing 100 to 200 mg of any of several soluble hydrocortisone preparations is begun rapidly, with the first 250 ml infused in the first ½ to 1 h and the remainder over the ensuing 4 to 8 h. If the condition is extreme, immediate bolus intravenous infusion of 100 mg hydrocortisone in the first few minutes is suggested, followed by a continuous rapid infusion of hydrocortisone at a rate of 10 mg/h. It is also advisable to administer 50 to 100 mg cortisone acetate intramuscularly in case the infusion becomes infiltrated or inadvertently stopped. Effective treatment of hypotension consists primarily of aggressive repletion of sodium and water deficits. If the crisis was preceded by prolonged nausea, vomiting, and dehydration, several liters of saline may be required within the first few hours. Vasoconstrictive agents (such as dopamine) may be indicated in extreme conditions as adjuncts to volume replacement. With large doses of steroid, as, for example, 100 to 200 mg cortisone or hydrocortisone, the patient receives a maximal mineralocorticoid effect, and supplementary deoxycorticosterone is superfluous. After the initial infusion, depending on the patient's condition, a similar second infusion may be given; if there has been marked improvement, the patient may be offered oral fluids and given 50 mg cortisone acetate intramuscularly every 12 h until gastrointestinal absorption is guaranteed, at which time the steroid can be given orally. Steroid dosage is tapered over the next few days to maintenance levels, with reinstitution of supplementary mineralocorticoid if needed.

Adrenal hemorrhage Adrenal hemorrhage (adrenal apoplexy) is usually associated with overwhelming septicemia (Waterhouse-Friderichsen syndrome); however, it may also occur in the absence of sepsis. Occasionally, massive bilateral adrenal hemorrhage results from birth trauma. The infant may be stillborn or die after birth of shock and hyperpyrexia. Adrenal hemorrhage also occurs during pregnancy, following idiopathic adrenal vein thrombosis, during convulsions in epilepsy or during electroconvulsive therapy, with excessive anticoagulant therapy, after trauma or surgery, and as a complication of adrenal venography (e.g., infarction of an adenoma). Pain in the flank and epigastrium is frequent, and if the hemorrhagic process ruptures into the abdomen, signs of peritoneal inflammation are present. Acute adrenal insufficiency should also be considered in the differential diagnosis of hypotension in patients maintained on anticoagulant therapy in the period immediately following a myocardial infarction.

The adrenal hemorrhage associated with septicemia is most frequent with meningococcemia but is also seen with overwhelming infections due to pneumococcus, staphylococcus, or *Hemophilus influenzae*. The onset is often explosive, with a

shaking chill, violent headache, vertigo, vomiting, and prostration. A petechial rash appears on the skin and mucous membranes and progresses rapidly to a confluent, extensive purpura. Large areas of skin may become grossly hemorrhagic. Body temperature may be subnormal but is usually markedly elevated. Circulatory collapse rapidly ensues, and death may occur within 6 to 48 h. Specific diagnosis requires immediate identification of the organism. Frequently, the septicemia is so massive that organisms may be seen in peripheral blood smears or petechial scrapings. Since shock may also be associated with massive septicemia without adrenal hemorrhage, one is never completely certain whether adrenal insufficiency is contributing to the patient's decompensation. Sufficient time is not available for assessment of adrenal function; however, a plasma sample for later determination of cortisol level may be of interest.

Treatment must be immediate and intensive. Control of the infection by vigorous administration of intravenous antibiotics is indicated. Intravenous dopamine may also be required to maintain vascular tone. Steroid treatment should also be administered at the earliest possible point in all patients in whom fulminating septicemia is associated with shock. The dose range administered in such patients is usually massive (e.g., 1 to 2 g hydrocortisone daily). However, available data are inconclusive that such doses of steroid improve mortality in septic shock.

HYPOALDOSTERONISM

Isolated aldosterone deficiency accompanied by normal cortisol production has been reported in association with hyporeninism; as a congenital biosynthetic defect; postoperatively, following removal of aldosterone-secreting adenomas; during protracted heparin or heparinoid administration; in pretectal disease of the nervous system; and in severe postural hypotension.

Most cases of hypoaldosteronism present as unexplained hyperkalemia often exacerbated by restriction of dietary sodium intake in patients without overt renal impairment. In severe cases urine sodium wastage is present on a normal salt intake, whereas in milder forms excessive urine sodium losses occur only during salt restriction.

Isolated aldosterone deficiency is most commonly seen in adult subjects with renal failure secondary to diabetic nephropathy in association with hyporenism and hyperkalemia. Plasma renin and aldosterone levels fail to rise normally following sodium restriction, and biosynthetic defects in the secretion of aldosterone cannot be demonstrated. Aldosterone secretion fails to rise or increases subnormally following ACTH stimulation, but cortisol secretion increases normally.

A biosynthetic defect has been noted in some patients who are unable to transform the angular C-18 methyl group of corticosterone to the C-18 aldehyde grouping of aldosterone due to a deficiency of the enzyme 18-hydroxysteroid dehydrogenase. These patients manifest low to absent aldosterone secretion and excretion, elevated plasma renin levels, and elevated values for the intermediates of aldosterone biosynthesis (corticosterone and 18-hydroxycorticosterone).

The feature common to all patients with hypoaldosteronism is the inability to *increase* aldosterone secretion appropriately during severe salt restriction. An additional feature is the reversal of the signs of salt wasting (hyponatremia and hyperkalemia) with the administration of potent mineralocorticoids. For practical purposes the oral administration of 9α-fluorohydrocortisone in a dose of 0.1 to 0.3 mg daily restores electrolyte balance.

NONSPECIFIC USE OF ADRENAL STEROIDS AND ACTH IN CLINICAL PRACTICE

The widespread utilization of glucocorticoids and ACTH in clinical practice emphasizes the need for a thorough understanding of the metabolic effects of these agents when used nonspecifically, if optimum effectiveness is to be obtained and if undesirable side reactions are to be minimized. Before instituting adrenal hormone therapy, a physician should weigh carefully the gains that can reasonably be expected versus the potentially undesirable metabolic actions of pharmacological doses of hormone. Accurate appraisal requires familiarity with current medical literature, a critical evaluation of the significance of such reports, as well as a clear understanding of the chemical, physiological, and psychological changes that hormone preparations of this type are known to induce when used in pharmacological dosage.

HOW SERIOUS IS THE DISORDER? Clearly, in a patient whose life is threatened by unexplained shock, or in whom other measures have failed, the physician need not hesitate to employ large-dosage steroid therapy. On the other hand, one should exercise restraint in administering steroids to a patient with early rheumatoid arthritis who as yet has not been exposed to the possible benefits of physiotherapy, analgesics, and a well-organized program of general medical care.

HOW LONG WILL GLUCOCORTICOID THERAPY BE REQUIRED? The use of intravenously administered steroids for a period of 24 to 48 h in the treatment of such life-threatening situations as status asthmaticus or pseudotumor cerebri has little or no contraindication, in contrast to the initiation of a program of steroid therapy for chronic asthma, arthritis, or psoriasis. In the latter instances, the almost certain complication of a Cushing's syndrome of some degree must be weighed against the potential benefit to the patient. The need for minimizing these side effects by the use of shorter-acting steroid preparations, alternate-day or interrupted therapy programs, and the judicious use of supplementary adjuvants is evident.

TABLE 336-11
Glucocorticoid preparations

Commonly used name*	Estimated potency†	
	Glucocorticoid	Mineralocorticoid
SHORT-ACTING		
Hydrocortisone	1	1
Cortisone	0.8	0.8
INTERMEDIATE-ACTING		
Prednisone	4	0.25
Prednisolone	4	0.25
Methylprednisolone	5	±
Triamcinolone	5	±
LONG-ACTING		
Paramethasone	10	±
Betamethasone	25	±
Dexamethasone	30–40	±

* *The steroids are divided into three groups according to the duration of biologic activity. Short-acting preparations have a biologic half-life of less than 12 h; long-acting, greater than 48 h; and intermediate, between 12 and 36 h. Triamcinolone has the longest half-life of the intermediate-acting preparations.*

† *Relative milligram comparisons with cortisol, setting the glucocorticoid and mineralocorticoid properties of cortisol as 1. Sodium retention is insignificant in usual doses employed of methylprednisolone, triamcinolone, paramethasone, betamethasone, and dexamethasone.*

WHICH ADRENAL PREPARATION IS PREFERABLE? At least five considerations need to be taken into account in deciding which steroid preparation to use:

1 The biological half-life of the particular compound. The rationale behind every-other-day therapy is to decrease the metabolic effects of the steroids for a significant amount of time over the 2-day period, yet at the same time to produce pharmacological suppression of sufficient duration to maintain the disease in remission. Too long a half-life would defeat the first purpose, and too short a half-life would defeat the second. In general, the more potent the steroid, the longer its biological half-life tends to be.

2 The importance of the mineralocorticoid effects of the steroid. The newer synthetic steroids have much less mineralocorticoid effect relative to their glucocorticoid effect than cortisol or cortisone (Table 336-11). This may be an important consideration in certain disease states.

3 The fact that cortisone and prednisone, in contrast to the other glucocorticoids, have to be converted to their biologically active equivalents before any anti-inflammatory effects can occur. Because of this, in a clinical condition in which steroids are known to be effective and in which an adequate dose has been given without any response, one should consider substituting hydrocortisone or prednisolone for cortisone or prednisone.

4 The cost of the medication. This is a serious consideration if chronic administration is to be undertaken. Prednisone is the least expensive of available steroid preparations.

5 The appreciable variation in the manner in which commercial preparations of glucosteroids are formulated. This factor may significantly modify absorption. Thus it is advisable for a patient whose steroid dosage has been standardized to continue to utilize the same pharmaceutical preparation to avoid relapse or overdosage.

ACTH VERSUS STEROIDS In general, adrenal steroid therapy is effective by mouth and can be regulated more accurately than ACTH therapy. The latter fluctuates considerably in the amount of steroid produced from day to day, depending on the rate and extent of absorption of ACTH and on the state of the adrenal cortex. ACTH therapy stimulates the secretion of adrenal androgens as well as hydroxysteroids. Sodium retention with ACTH is often more marked than with cortisone or, particularly, with prednisone therapy.

ACTH therapy is felt by some to be superior to oral steroid therapy in the treatment of certain neuromuscular disorders such as dermatomyositis and multiple sclerosis. In female patients androgenic stimulation of ACTH may also reduce the "muscle-wasting action" of glucocorticoids. Both ACTH and steroid therapy induce hypothalamopituitary suppression; however, in ACTH therapy adrenal gland size and activity are maintained, in contrast to the adrenal atrophy usually associated with steroid therapy.

EVALUATION OF PATIENT PRIOR TO INITIATING STEROID THERAPY See Table 336-12.

TABLE 336-12
A "checklist" for use prior to the administration of steroids in pharmacological dosages

1 Presence of tuberculosis or other chronic infection (chest x-ray, tuberculin test)
2 History of diabetes mellitus in family
3 Evidence of preexisting osteoporosis (spinal x-ray in post-menopausal patients)
4 History of peptic ulcer, gastritis, or esophagitis (stool guaiac test)
5 Evidence of hypertension or cardiovascular disease
6 History of psychological disorders

Chronic infection Three problems demand attention. (1) Any active infection, particularly tuberculosis, should be identified. If tuberculosis is present, steroid therapy can be employed, if indicated, in conjunction with antituberculous chemotherapy. (2) The chest film and tuberculin test provide base-line information for future comparison. High-dosage steroids minimize the tuberculin reaction. For this reason a chest roentgenogram should be carried out at 6- to 12-month intervals or with evidence of unexplained fever or weight loss, in patients on long-continued steroid therapy. (3) Infection due to "opportunistic" low-virulence pathogens should be constantly considered in patients on high steroid dosage, especially when steroid therapy is combined with other immunosuppressive agents.

Diabetes mellitus Prolonged ACTH or cortisone-like steroid therapy may unmask latent diabetes mellitus or aggravate preexisting disease. For this reason a careful history is important to exclude familial incidence of diabetes. Obviously the presence of frank diabetes mellitus or the demonstration of impaired glucose tolerance affects the physician's decision to institute adrenal hormone therapy. However, if such therapy appears necessary or desirable in the presence of diabetes, the insulin requirement of known diabetics usually needs to be increased with ACTH or cortisone-like therapy, except in those instances in which the diabetic patient is suffering from some degree of insulin resistance in which the anti-inflammatory or antiallergic effect of cortisone enhances the metabolic effectiveness of the insulin sufficiently to balance off the diabetogenic action of the former.

Osteoporosis All patients receiving long-continued steroid therapy are likely to develop some degree of osteoporosis. Obviously, considerable change in bone structure must occur before significant radiological changes can be demonstrated. For patients at high risk (postmenopausal females, elderly individuals, and patients whose basic disease process results in restricted physical activity) initial films of the thoracolumbar segment of the spine are mandatory. Glucocorticoids decrease intestinal absorption of calcium leading to secondary hyperparathyroidism, are collagenolytic, and directly inhibit osteoblastic activity. These combined actions make the vertebral column extremely vulnerable. Osteoporosis, with vertebral fractures or compression, is one of the most serious potential hazards of long-term steroid therapy. Adjunctive therapies with vitamin D, calcium, and fluoride have not been demonstrated to be effective in steroid osteoporosis, although alternate-day or interrupted steroid therapy minimizes this important complication (Table 336-13).

Peptic ulcer, gastric hypersecretion, or esophagitis Patients with a history of gastric hypersecretion or peptic ulcer may experience aggravation of their symptoms while receiving adrenal hormone therapy. It is not known for certain whether aggravation of peptic ulceration and complicating gastrointestinal hemorrhage reflect the increased gastric secretory activity or whether the nitrogen-depleting effect of these hormones accelerates the process of ulceration and perforation. Prophylactic antacid therapy and an ulcer diet are useful precautions in susceptible patients. *The development of anemia in a patient receiving glucocorticoid therapy should immediately suggest gastrointestinal bleeding,* and patients should be cautioned to note black or tarry stools. A clear-cut history of peptic ulcer constitutes a relative contraindication to high-dose glucocorticoid therapy, and if required as a life-saving measure, steroid therapy should be accompanied by a vigorous "ulcer-combating" program (e.g., antacids, cimetidine).

Hypertension or cardiovascular disease In general, the sodium-retaining propensity of many adrenal steroid preparations requires that caution be used when they are given to patients with preexisting hypertension or cardiovascular or renal disease. Use of preparations in which sodium-retaining activity is minimal (triamcinolone and dexamethasone), restriction of dietary sodium intake, and the use of diuretic agents and supplementary potassium salts will minimize the mineralocorticoid actions of steroid therapy. However, hypertension may still be exacerbated by steroid-induced increases in renin substrate and consequently angiotensin II levels.

For all patients in whom prolonged steroid therapy is contemplated cardiovascular-renal status should be carefully evaluated.

Psychological difficulties Steroid therapy may be complicated by severe psychological disturbances; less severe abnormalities are relatively frequent. In general, serious psychological disturbances are more closely related to the patient's personality structure than to the actual dose of hormone, although, as might be anticipated, larger doses of hormone are associated with more frequent serious reactions. At present there is no reliable method of determining beforehand a patient's psychological reaction to steroid therapy. Patients with known psychological difficulties experience more frequent and more severe disturbances. Further difficulty arises because previous tolerance of steroids does not necessarily ensure immunity to subsequent courses of therapy, and untoward psychological reactions on one occasion do not invariably mean that the patient will respond unfavorably to a second course of treatment. The physician must follow the course of the patient's condition carefully during the early period of steroid therapy and take a responsible member of the patient's family into his or her confidence.

Sleeplessness is a well-known complication of glucosteroid therapy. This can be minimized by using the shorter-acting steroids and by prescribing the total dose as a single early-morning medication.

ALTERNATE-DAY STEROID THERAPY The single most effective measure in minimizing the cushingoid effects of glucosteroid therapy is to administer the total dose for 48 h as a *single dose,* of *intermediate-acting steroid* in the morning, *every other day.* If symptoms of the underlying disorder can be controlled by this technique, the physician can be assured that the therapeutic program is offering a distinct advantage to the patient. Three special considerations deserve mention. (1) The alter-

TABLE 336-13
Supplementary measures designed to minimize undesirable metabolic effects of glucocorticoids

I Monitor caloric intake to prevent weight gain.
II Restrict sodium intake to prevent edema and minimize hypertension and potassium loss.
III Potassium supplement—KCl elixir, 2-3 tsp three times daily with meals.
IV Antacid therapy.
V Alternate-day steroid schedule if possible; if not, a single morning total-steroid dose; in all instances use an intermediate-acting steroid preparation if possible (Table 336-11). Patients maintained on steroid therapy over a prolonged period should be protected by an appropriate increase in hormone level during periods of acute stress. A rule of thumb is to *double* the maintenance dose.
VI To minimize osteopenia (not proved effective)
   A Estrogen therapy for postmenopausal women; 0.625-1.25 mg conjugated estrogens, equine may be given "cyclically." Regular Papanicolaou smear and breast examination mandatory (see Chap. 342).
   B Consider supplementary vitamin D, calcium and sodium fluoride.

nate-day schedule may be approached through a series of transition dose schedules which permit the patient an opportunity to adjust successfully to the ultimate program. (2) The physician should make a conscientious effort to provide the patient with supplementary nonsteroid medications, if required, on the "off day" to minimize symptoms of the underlying disorder. (3) The physician and the patient should recognize that many symptoms noted during the off day are those of relative adrenal insufficiency, rather than an exacerbation of the underlying disease. Fatigue, joint pain, muscle stiffness or tenderness, and fever may be accounted for by the rapid fall in plasma cortisol. Knowing this is of vital importance, since the physician can reassure the patient and avoid giving up the program on the basis of a misconception.

The alternate-day concept capitalizes on the fact that cortisol secretion and plasma levels normally are highest in the early morning and lowest in the evening. The normal pattern is mimicked by administering steroid in the morning (7 to 8 A.M.), and preferably an intermediate-acting steroid, i.e., one whose hypothalamopituitary-suppressing effect lasts less than $1\frac{1}{2}$ days (Table 336-11).

Initially the steroid program usually requires daily or more frequent doses of steroid to accomplish the desired anti-inflammatory or immunity-suppressing action. *Only after this desired effect has been achieved is an attempt made to switch over to an alternate-day program.* A number of programs may be employed for transferring a patient from a daily to an alternate-day program. The key points to be considered are flexibility in arranging a program and the use of supportive measures on the off day. One may attempt a transition by a series of gradations (Table 336-14), rather than by an abrupt complete changeover. In either case it is important to anticipate that the patient will experience some increase in pain or discomfort between the 36 to 48 h following the last dose of steroid.

The general principles advocated in the long-term use of steroids and in implementing an alternate-day schedule are as follows:

1 Utilize intermediate-acting steroids such as prednisone or prednisolone.
2 Give the total daily steroid as a single morning dose.
3 Begin a transition program as soon as the manifestations of the diseases are under reasonable control.
4 If possible, eliminate steroid medication on the alternate day.

WITHDRAWAL OF CORTICOSTEROIDS FOLLOWING THEIR LONG-TERM USE AS PHARMACOLOGICAL AGENTS It is recommended that complete withdrawal of steroids be initiated by implementing an alternate-day schedule. Patients on an alternate-day program for a month or more experience less diffi-

culty as far as pituitary adrenal function is concerned. The dosage is gradually reduced and finally discontinued after a normal replacement dosage has been reached (e.g., 5 to 7.5 mg prednisone). Complications rarely ensue unless undue stress is experienced, and patients should understand that for 1 year or longer after the complete withdrawal from long-term high-dosage steroid therapy, they should receive supplementary hormone in the presence of serious infection, operation, or injury.

If a patient in the final stage of steroid reduction cannot tolerate an alternate-day program, it is debatable as to whether complete discontinuance should be considered. Under these circumstances a daily dose of steroid could be continued, and at some future date another trial of gradual transition to the alternate-day schedule should be attempted. In patients with life-threatening disorders such as disseminated lupus erythematosus or widespread skin disorders in which exfoliative dermatitis may complicate complete withdrawal of steroids, it may be desirable to consider life-long daily maintenance therapy at an Addisonian replacement dosage. These patients will not require mineralocorticoid therapy, as aldosterone secretion is usually adequate.

REFERENCES

AXELROD L: Glucocorticoid therapy. Medicine 55:39, 1976

BIGLIERI EG et al: Adrenal mineralocorticoids causing hypertension. Am J Med 52:623, 1972

CAIN JP et al: The regulation of aldosterone secretion in primary aldosteronism. Am J Med 53:627, 1972

DAVIS WW et al: Bilateral adrenal hyperplasia as a cause of primary aldosteronism with hypertension, hypokalemia and suppressed renin activity. Am J Med 42:642, 1967

DLUHY RG et al: Rapid ACTH test with plasma aldosterone levels. Ann Intern Med 80:693, 1974

GILL JR et al: Bartter's syndrome: A disorder characterized by high urinary prostaglandins and a dependency of hyperreninemia on prostaglandin synthesis. Am J Med 61:43, 1976

GWINUP B et al: Clinical testing of the hypothalamic-pituitary-adrenal cortical system in states of hypo- and hypercortisolism. Metabolism 24:777, 1975

KLEIN RG et al: Intestinal calcium absorption in exogenous hypercortisolism. Role of 25-hydroxy vitamin D and corticosteroid dose. J Clin Invest 60:253, 1977

LUBITZ JA et al: Mitotane use in inoperable adrenal cortical carcinoma. JAMA 223:1109, 1973

MOORE TJ et al: Nelson's syndrome: Frequency, prognosis, and effect of prior pituitary radiation. Ann Intern Med 85:731, 1976

SCHAMBELAN M et al: Isolated hypoaldosteronism in adults. A renin deficiency syndrome. N Engl J Med 287:573, 1972

SCOTT HW et al: Surgical experience with Cushing's disease. Ann Surg 185:524, 1977

WILLIAMS GH et al: Aldosterone biosynthesis: Interrelationship of regulatory factors. Am J Med 53:595, 1972

TABLE 336-14
A schedule to taper pharmacological doses of glucocorticoids

Day	Prednisone, mg	Day	Prednisone, mg
1	60	13	90
2	40	14	5
3	70	15	90
4	30	16	0
5	80	17	85
6	20	18	0
7	90	19	85
8	10	20	0
9	95	21	85
10	5	22	0
11	90	23	80
12	5	24	0

337
PHEOCHROMOCYTOMA

O. BRYAN HOLLAND

Pheochromocytomas are catecholamine-producing tumors of neuroectodermal tissue and derive their name from their characteristic affinity for chromium salts. Although an uncommon cause of hypertension, they are often amenable to surgical removal and can produce dramatic clinical symptoms frequently resulting in untimely death. The pathological classification of these tumors is based upon histological staining characteristics, but technical problems in the chromaffin reaction often result in an imperfect correlation between chromaffin staining and the capacity of the tumors to produce catecholamines; thus, chromaffin-negative tumors may contain typical catecholamine granules when examined by electron microscopy. For this reason, all functionally active tumors of the sympathoadrenal system are best considered pheochromocytomas rather than being classified as "nonchromaffin paragangliomas" or "functional chemodectomas."

The frequency of pheochromocytoma at autopsy (approximately 1 in 1000) is greater than the clinical recognition of the disorder, emphasizing the problem of diagnosis in many patients. A single benign adrenal tumor is found most commonly; about 10 percent are malignant, 10 percent are extraadrenal, and 10 percent are bilateral or multiple. All races are affected. The peak occurrence is in the fourth and fifth decades, though cases have occurred in the newborn and in the ninth decade. Ten percent are familial. Although the vast majority of pheochromocytomas are found in the abdomen, they may arise wherever there are cells of the sympathetic nervous system or other chromaffin cells whose embryological origin is common with that of the autonomic nervous system.

CLINICAL MANIFESTATIONS

The physiology of catecholamines is reviewed in Chap. 72. The clinical manifestations of pheochromocytoma are determined by the pattern of catecholamine release and the relative production rates of epinephrine and norepinephrine by the tumor. Most pheochromocytomas produce a mixture of the two, but some tumors release only one of the catecholamines.

SYMPTOMS Tumors that produce epinephrine predominantly are associated with prominent sweating, palpitations, nervousness, tremor, weight loss, pallor followed by flushing, heat intolerance, and rarely with hypotension or shock secondary to profound beta-receptor stimulation. In contrast, those tumors producing predominantly norepinephrine often cause fewer symptoms and may present a clinical picture resembling essential hypertension. Symptoms are most marked with paroxysmally functioning tumors, possibly due to larger swings in plasma catecholamine concentrations. About half of patients have paroxysmal hypertension, while the remainder exhibit nonparoxysmal elevations of the blood pressure that can be either sustained or labile in character.

Some patients may experience up to 25 attacks per day, whereas others (rarely) go for years between episodes. Attacks may last from less than a minute to over a week, but the average is a few minutes to a few hours. Onset and subsidence tend to be abrupt, and the pattern in a given individual is usually consistent. Some patients note a prodrome of cutaneous paresthesias and/or anxiety, but in many subjects attacks occur with no recognizable precipitating event. Known precipitating events include postural changes (especially involving flexion or bending of the body), sneezing, pressure on the abdomen, sexual activity, smoking, eating, micturition, exercise, valsalva maneuver, laughing, the wearing of tight clothing, carotid sinus massage, pain, and changes in environmental or body temperature. Many patients experience an increase in frequency and duration of the attacks with time.

Particular attention should be given to the three most common symptoms, headache, excessive sweating, and palpitations, since at least one of these symptoms is almost always present. Headache is the most common. The headaches are abrupt in onset, severe, throbbing, generalized, and relatively short in duration (lasting from about 5 min to 2 h), and they tend to be associated with other paroxysmal symptoms. However, they may be indistinguishable from ordinary tension or migraine headaches. Excessive sweating is noted in about two-thirds of patients, may be either paroxysmal or continuous, and is particularly prominent in children. Some patients have profuse truncal sweating but cold and dry distal extremities. In paroxysmal attacks sweating usually begins at the same time as other manifestations, though it may occur as the attack subsides. Palpitations are common and may be intense. In the Mayo Clinic series, the duration of symptoms (or hypertension) at the time of diagnosis varied from 3 weeks to 32 years. The average was 3.7 years, and there was no significant difference between paroxysmally and persistently functioning tumors.

Chest pain resembling angina characteristically occurs at the height of the attack instead of before it. This sequence helps distinguish angina with secondary catecholamine discharge from coronary artery spasm induced by catecholamine excess. Other manifestations reflect chronic catecholamine excess. Patients with sustained hypertension have a higher incidence of myocarditis with arrhythmias and congestive heart failure, visual disturbances, constipation, and renal insufficiency. Mechanical effects of the primary tumor or its distant metastases, or associated diseases (i.e., hyperparathyroidism, medullary carcinoma of the thyroid, neurofibromatosis), may also be prominent.

PHYSICAL FINDINGS Patients with pheochromocytoma are usually thin. Signs of catecholamine excess such as sweating, anxiety, dilatation of the pupils, and tremor may be present. Neurofibromas and signs of multiple endocrine neoplasia, type III (marfanoid habitus, prominent lips, mucosal neuromas of the lips, tongue, and/or conjunctiva, and goiter), should be searched for (see Chap. 348). Orthostatic hypotension due to contraction of the blood volume may be present in patients with persistently functional tumors, and difficulty in obtaining the blood pressure may indicate intense vasoconstriction. Tumors of the jugulotympanic paraganglia can cause palsies of cranial nerves VII to XII and may be visualized through the tympanic membrane. Tumors arising in the orbital paraganglia may produce proptosis. Hypertensive retinopathy may occur in patients with persistently functioning tumors, whereas many patients with paroxysmal hypertension have a normal funduscopic examination. Tumors of the carotid body or other internal carotid paraganglia may be palpated in the neck; in contrast abdominal tumors are palpable in <5 percent of cases. A striking rise in blood pressure may be noted with abdominal or flank palpation.

CLINICAL VARIANTS **Familial pheochromocytoma** Four familial syndromes are associated with pheochromocytoma: (1) simple familial pheochromocytoma, (2) multiple endocrine neoplasia, (3) neurofibromatosis, and (4) von Hippel-Lindau disease. In each, the disorder appears to be a variable manifestation of an autosomal dominant defect.

Simple familial pheochromocytoma comprises about two-thirds of familial cases. Sustained hypertension, earlier age of diagnosis (average age of 20 years), and multiple or bilateral tumors are common in this disorder.

Pheochromocytoma in association with medullary carcinoma of the thyroid and hyperparathyroidism, multiple endocrine neoplasia, type II (MEN II), is the next most common familial disorder (see Chap. 348). These patients are distinquished from those with simple familial pheochromocytoma by a later age of onset (30 to 35 years), rarity of sustained hypertension, fewer extraadrenal tumors, and more frequent bilateral disease (65 to 100 percent). A subgroup (designated MEN IIB or MEN III) has marfanoid habitus, mucosal neuromas, skeletal defects, intestinal ganglioneuromatosis, and (only rarely) hyperparathyroidism. MEN II and MEN III are genetically distinct. Adrenal involvement in MEN evolves from an early stage of diffuse medullary hyperplasia through a later stage of nodular hyperplasia, and ultimately into an overt pheochromocytoma. Multiple small intraadrenal pheochromocytomas (1 to 2 cm) and hyperplasia in extraadrenal abdominal chromaffin tissue, particularly the celiac ganglion, may also be present. Interestingly, medullary hyperplasia of one adrenal may occur in conjunction with a large tumor in the other.

About 10 percent of patients with neurofibromatosis have pheochromocytoma. This high frequency is thought to be the consequence of a common mutation that gives rise or predisposes to both. The modal age at diagnosis (40 to 45 years) and the incidence of bilateral tumors (10 percent) are similar to nonfamilial pheochromocytoma. The association of pheochromocytoma with von Hippel-Lindau disease is likewise thought to be a manifestation of one underlying mutation. Patients with concomitant neurofibromatosis, von Hippel-Lindau disease, and pheochromocytoma have been described.

Several considerations in the evaluation of patients with familial pheochromocytoma deserve emphasis. First, it is important to know the clinical behavior of the pheochromocytoma in other members of the family, since the functional characteristics and location of the tumor(s) tend to be relatively constant within families. This information can be of help in deciding whether to perform a bilateral adrenalectomy and to search for extraadrenal involvement. Second, the great majority of patients with MEN have medullary carcinoma of the thyroid at the time of presentation with pheochromocytoma. Since medullary carcinoma of the thyroid can be diagnosed with considerable accuracy by the measurement of plasma calcitonin after intravenous administration of pentagastrin or calcium, individuals can frequently be identified who have virtually a 100 percent chance of developing pheochromocytoma, though this may not occur until later in life. Third, it is important to determine whether a patient has pheochromocytoma before operation for medullary carcinoma of the thyroid since the initial manifestation of a pheochromocytoma in patients with MEN may be a hypertensive reaction at the time of thyroidectomy.

Paragangliomas Paraganglia are collections of neural crest cells adjacent to the ganglia of the autonomic nervous system. The adrenal medulla itself is the largest paraganglion. Paragangliomas may occur in paraganglia associated with the cranial nerves, the paravertebral sympathetic plexuses, the visceral plexuses, and the plexuses along the aorta (particularly in the remnants of the organ of Zuckerkandl), in the walls of blood vessels, in chemoreceptor tissue, and scattered through various organs such as the heart, prostate, bladder, and ovaries. As discussed previously, functional extraadrenal paragangliomas should be classified as pheochromocytomas, whether chromaffin positive or negative. Localization of these tumors may be a formidable problem. Small intrathoracic tumors may be visualized with oblique chest x-rays. Arteriography and/or regional venous catecholamine sampling may also be helpful in localization.

Pheochromocytoma of the bladder This is a rare tumor comprising less than 1 percent of all bladder tumors and less than 1 percent of all pheochromocytomas. The classic distinguishing feature is precipitation of the typical paroxysmal attacks with the onset of micturition, with distention of the bladder, or with palpation of the bladder or adnexa. Attacks may result in micturition syncope. Hematuria and other characteristics of bladder tumors are usually present, though about a fifth are not visible at cystoscopy.

Pheochromocytoma in pregnancy Pheochromocytoma may be noted first during pregnancy, and symptomatic tumors are worsened during the pregnant state. The manifestations of the tumor may be confused with toxemia of pregnancy, eclampsia, or rupture of the uterus at the time of childbirth. The classic paroxysmal attacks may be precipitated by mechanical effects of the gravid uterus in the last trimester, uterine contractions during labor, or increased fetal movements. Maternal death occurs in about half of undiagnosed cases. Fetal salvage is poor in those cases that present early in pregnancy, but in some patients the manifestations can be controlled with phenoxybenzamine, thus allowing maturation of the fetus and delivery by cesarian section. Attempts to localize the tumors are generally postponed until after delivery, and surgery should usually be delayed until after regression of the extensive abdominal and pelvic vascular changes associated with pregnancy.

Pediatric pheochromocytoma Pheochromocytoma in children is characterized by a high frequency of norepinephrine-secreting and persistently functioning tumors. Simple familial pheochromocytoma and multiple or bilateral tumors are also more common.

Malignant pheochromocytomas For a pheochromocytoma to be characterized as malignant, metastases must be documented since benign and malignant tumors cannot be distinguished histologically. Metastases must also be found in sites where chromaffin tissue does not normally occur. Malignancy is more common in extraadrenal pheochromocytomas. The most common sites of metastasis are skeleton, liver, lymph nodes, lungs, central nervous system, and pleura. The prognosis of malignant pheochromocytoma is variable. In the past most patients died within a few years of diagnosis, but more recent reports have indicated longer survivals. Improved survival may be due to more aggressive medical therapy with sympathetic blocking agents. Resection of individual metastases may be justified because tumor growth is often slow and the management of the patient's hypertension may be improved.

Cardiovascular syndromes Patients may present with myocardial infarction or with a myocardial infarction-like syndrome in which there is a focal myocarditis secondary to the catecholamine elevations. A chronic cardiomyopathy may also develop; it is largely reversible with pharmacological blockade and later removal of the tumor. Peripheral vascular disease may be manifested by vasomotor phenomena including peripheral cyanosis, livido reticularis, Raynaud's phenomena, and distal extremity necrosis that may be confused with arterial embolization. Cerebrovascular manifestations include visual changes, cortical blindness, and cerebrovascular accidents. Hypotension may result from tachyarrhythmias, isolated epinephrine production by the tumor, or infarction of the pheochromocytoma.

Carbohydrate intolerance About one-fourth of patients have an elevated fasting blood sugar. Hyperglycemia may persist for several days after removal of the tumor, and resistance to the hypoglycemic action of endogenous insulin may be present for up to 2 years.

Adrenal cortical hyperfunction The coexistence of pheochromocytoma and Cushing's syndrome has been noted on occasion. The Cushing's syndrome can result from ectopic production of adrenocorticotropic hormone (ACTH) by the tumor, production of cortisol by the tumor, the fortuituous simultaneous occurrence of Cushing's disease, or production of an ACTH-like substance by medullary thyroid carcinoma. Patients with pheochromocytoma may have evidence of secondary aldosteronism from extrinsic pressure by the tumor on the renal vasculature or from acceleration of renin release by catecholamines.

DIAGNOSIS

URINARY CATECHOLAMINES The diagnosis of pheochromocytoma is made by the assay of catecholamines and their metabolites (see Fig. 72-3 for the pathways of catecholamine metabolism). Assays vary among laboratories, and clinicians must be familiar with the methodology utilized in their hospitals so that factors which adversely affect the assay results can be avoided. Urinary catecholamines should be collected in a container with acid (10 ml of 6 N HCl for 24-h collection) to keep the pH below 3.0, whereas metanephrine or vanillylmandelic acid (VMA) determinations do not require acidification.

Total catecholamine assays (free and conjugated catecholamines) using fluorometric methods should be avoided since they are influenced by a variety of substances that lead to false-positive elevations. Dietary catecholamines are conjugated prior to intestinal absorption; thus, bananas and other fruits, grain cereals, chocolate, tea, coffee, and vanilla may cause an elevation in the conjugated catecholamine component. In addition, drugs such as glyceryl guaiacolate, *p*-aminosalicylic acid, methacarbamol, mephenesin, methyldopa, quinine, quinidine, tetracycline, chlorpromazine, chloral hydrate, decongestants, and bronchodilators may cause false-positive elevations or interference with the fluorometric method. Many of the same drugs also interfere with the fluorometric assay for free norepinephrine and epinephrine. Radioenzymatic or double isotopic assays for norepinephrine, epinephrine, and total free catecholamines are more specific.

VMA can be determined by fluorometric methods, most of which employ diazotized *p*-nitroaniline and are usually advertised as VMA screening tests. These methods are not recommended because false-positive tests may occur in up to a fourth of controls. VMA is determined more accurately by methods using bidirectional paper chromatography or by spectrophotometric determination after extraction and conversion to vanillin. Drugs such as Leritine, nalidixic acid, levodopa, lithium, and nitroglycerin cause an increase in VMA, whereas clofibrate, monoamine oxidase inhibitors, pargyline, and ethanol cause a decrease.

Total metanephrines (metanephrine and normetanephrine, conjugated and unconjugated) are commonly measured by a method involving hydrolysis of conjugates, column absorption, elution, conversion to vanillin, and spectrophotometric determination. Few factors interfere with this procedure. However, chlorpromazine and monoamine oxidase inhibitors cause an increase, and x-ray contrast media containing methylglucamine can cause a decrease lasting for several days. Methyldopa may produce slight elevations but rarely enough to cause diagnostic confusion. The following antihypertensive medications do not generally interfere with assays of free catecholamines, VMA, or metanephrines sufficient to cause diagnostic confusion: thiazides, reserpine, guanethidine, propanolol, hydralazine, phentolamine, and phenoxybenzamine. A more common clinical problem is a two- to fourfold elevation of the excretion of urinary catecholamines and their metabolites produced by sympathomimetic agents and by acute and chronic stress such as head trauma, stroke, and shock lung syndrome. These elevations may persist for weeks to months.

The utility of these three urinary assays for the diagnosis of pheochromocytoma has been documented. Total metanephrine excretion is elevated in 85 to 100 percent of patients, while excretion of free catecholamines and VMA is elevated in 79 to 100 percent and 71 to 97 percent of patients, respectively. Since metanephrine determinations are easy to perform, they are used most commonly. The excretion of metanephrine and VMA is best expressed in micrograms per milligram of creatinine, particularly in children and in those adults suspected of having incomplete collections. Since metanephrine excretion is relatively constant, a single-voided (spot) metanephrine determination is useful for initial screening. Metanephrine determinations of 1.0 to 2.2 μg per milligram of creatinine should be considered suspicious for pheochromocytoma. Higher values in the absence of factors that interfere with the results almost always indicate a pheochromocytoma. The upper limits of normal for VMA and urinary free catecholamines vary, depending upon the assay. Free catecholamine excretion is higher during the waking hours, so that 24-h collections or 12-h overnight collections, which give lower basal values in normal subjects, should be utilized. Urinary free catecholamine determinations are particularly useful in those patients with small, highly active tumors that produce few metabolites. In addition, the fractionation of urinary free catecholamines into epinephrine and norepinephrine may be helpful in patients with medullary hyperplasia, since an elevated epinephrine excretion may be the only abnormality. Metanephrines, VMA, and free catecholamines should all be measured in patients with negative screening tests but in whom there is a high index of clinical suspicion, since cases have been reported in which only one of the three urinary determinations was abnormal. In addition, when the hypertension is paroxysmal, urine must be collected while the patient is hypertensive. Spot metanephrine determinations collected during and shortly after the attack are particularly useful. In those patients who remain diagnostic dilemmas, particularly patients with MEN, timed hourly urine collections obtained during the attack with fractionation of epinephrine and norepinephrine may help to identify those with paroxysmal hormone release. However, this procedure must be performed in a laboratory in which the fractionation procedure has been standardized.

PLASMA CATECHOLAMINES Plasma catecholamines are usually elevated but are more expensive and more difficult to measure than urinary determinations. Thus, plasma measurement assays should be reserved for those patients who are diagnostic dilemmas. In those patients with negative urinary determinations, measurement of plasma catecholamines may be helpful if samples are collected during a spontaneous or stimulated hypertensive episode. Unfortunately, stimulation tests (histamine, glucagon, tyramine) are generally ineffective in producing a blood pressure increase in those cases of MEN with consistently negative urinary determinations.

RECOMMENDATIONS FOR INITIAL TESTING Though pheochromocytoma is a rare cause of hypertension, missing the diagnosis may be catastrophic for the patient. Spot metanephrine determinations are most satisfactory for initial testing in view of their sensitivity, ease of performance for both patient and laboratory, relatively low cost, and general freedom from interfering factors. This determination should be done in all hypertensive patients with symptoms or signs of pheochromocytoma, lability of the hypertension, moderate or severe hypertension (diastolic pressure >110 mmHg), or poor therapeutic response to antihypertensive drugs.

PHARMACOLOGICAL TESTS A variety of pharmacological tests have been utilized to provide indirect evidence of increased catecholamine production. These pharmacological tests include those that stimulate a hypertensive response in patients with paroxysmal hypertension (histamine, glucagon, tyramine) and those that produce a fall in the blood pressure in patients with sustained hypertension (phentolamine). However, pharmacological tests that stimulate a hypertensive response have little to offer, may be dangerous, and are best reserved for rare patients who (1) have had extensive negative laboratory testing for excess catecholamine production, (2) have documented life-threatening episodes of severe hypertension such that long-term delay in diagnosis is unwise, and (3) have had negative evaluation for other causes of paroxysmal hypertension. For these patients, the interested clinician is referred to an excellent review (Manger and Gifford).

The phentolamine test is useful as an alpha-adrenergic blocking test in those patients who present with profound blood pressure elevation and symptomatology compatible with a pheochromocytoma. A positive result (blood pressure fall of > 35/25) suggests the diagnosis. The test is performed by giving a 1-mg bolus of phentolamine intravenously after determining base-line blood pressure. The blood pressure is then measured every 15 to 20 s for 2 to 10 min until the maximal depressor response is determined. A 5-mg phentolamine bolus should then be given to subjects who exhibit a lesser depressor response. Since false-positive responses occur in about a fourth of cases, complete laboratory evaluation must follow whether the results in suspected patients are positive or negative. Norepinephrine and a volume expander should be available at the time of testing in the rare event that vasomotor collapse occurs.

LOCALIZATION OF PHEOCHROMOCYTOMA Bolus nephrotomography is a useful initial method for localizing the tumor. Other often-used noninvasive techniques include sonography and computerized tomography. Large tumors can occasionally be demonstrated by adrenal and renal scans. However, scanning agents are not concentrated by the tumor itself. Arteriography should be preceded by autonomic blockade to control the blood pressure and lessen the chance of a severe hypertensive crisis. An intravenous line should be established, and the electrocardiogram and blood pressure should be monitored during arteriography. Localization of the tumor by arteriography is important because of the appreciable incidence of bilateral and extraadrenal tumors, particularly in children and young adults. Many of these younger patients should also have thoracic and cervical arteriography in conjunction with abdominal arteriography. The occurrence of a hypertensive response during selective arterial injections favors a tumor at that location. Adrenal venography may be helpful in tumors that are not localized by arteriography and in MEN when adrenal nodular hyperplasia or small pheochromocytomas are anticipated. Adrenal venography should not be done shortly before exploratory surgery because the procedure may induce areas of hemorrhage in the adrenals which may cloud interpretation of the gross pathology at the time of surgery. Regional venous sampling of plasma catecholamines may be helpful in localizing unidentified tumors or in searching for extraabdominal tumors. Selective adrenal vein catheterization for plasma catecholamines has not been fully evaluated but may be complicated by the fact that fluctuations in catecholamine secre-

tion may be rapid. Interpretation of the results of regional venous sampling is also complicated by streaming from one side of the vena cava to the other and by drainage of tumor catecholamines into the abdominal azygous vein and then into the superior vena cava, thus confounding localization.

DIFFERENTIAL DIAGNOSIS

Symptoms of catecholamine excess caused by anxiety neurosis, menopause, hypoglycemia, and thyrotoxicosis may be confused with pheochromocytoma. However, blood pressure changes are usually modest with these conditions. Increased intracranial pressure secondary to trauma, tumors, infections, stroke, etc., may present with striking blood pressure elevations which may be labile and sometimes confused with pheochromocytoma that is complicated by stroke or hypertensive encephalopathy. The pulse tends to be slow with increased intracranial pressure. Urinary VMA, metanephrine, and catecholamines may be elevated two- to fourfold in conditions involving the central nervous system and persist for weeks to months after their onset. The labile hypertension with acute pulmonary edema, angina pectoris, migraine headaches, diencephalic seizures, carcinoid syndrome, encephalopathic form of lead poisoning, acute intermittent porphyria, clonidine withdrawal, and hypersensitivity to ingested pork or tyramine-containing foods in patients taking monoamine oxidase inhibitors may cause temporary diagnostic confusion. Furthermore, patients with pheochromocytoma and sustained hypertension with few symptoms may present with hyperglycemia or proteinuria and may be thought to have the hypertension of diabetes or chronic renal disease.

TREATMENT

MEDICAL THERAPY Treatment of the hypertensive crisis is best initiated with intravenous phentolamine (1 mg by intravenous push followed by intravenous titration of the blood pressure with 20 mg in 500 ml of 5% dextrose in water). Blood pressure titration may be smoother if plasma volume is expanded to normal. Nitroprusside (50 mg in 500 ml of 5% dextrose in water for intravenous titration) is also used for management of the hypertensive crisis. Propranolol should be given intravenously (1 mg/min until a response is obtained; repeat every 4 h) and/or orally (10 to 40 mg qid) if the pulse rate increases excessively secondary to alpha blockade or to epinephrine stimulation or if atrial or ventricular arrhythmias develop. Propranolol should never be given alone because blockade of beta receptor-mediated vasodilatation may facilitate alpha receptor-mediated vasoconstriction, thus causing significant elevations in the blood pressure.

Chronic medical management with the alpha blocker phenoxybenzamine should be utilized in preparation for surgery, arteriography, or venography. The onset of action is within 1 day, though cumulative effects occur for 4 to 7 days. Treatment is usually initiated with 10 to 30 mg per day with dosage increments of 10 mg per day at 1- to 4-day intervals. Some patients require 150 mg phenoxybenzamine per day; because its half-life is 24 h, it can usually be given in a single daily dose. The most common side effects are nasal congestion, sedation, orthostatic hypotension, excessive dryness of the mouth, and visual symptoms such as diplopia. Ambulation of the patient should be performed cautiously during initiation of phenoxybenzamine treatment owing to its marked orthostatic effects. The blood pressure after 2 to 3 min of standing should be utilized as the end point for titration. Propranolol is also required in many patients to ameliorate the tachycardia induced by alpha-receptor blockade. To avoid hypovolemia, diuretics should not be given unless renal insufficiency is present. Long-term medical therapy with phenoxybenzamine and propranolol is helpful in those patients who have malignant pheochromocytoma or multiple pheochromocytomas that cannot be localized adequately and removed surgically. Recent reports indicate that the selective postsynaptic alpha-receptor blocker prazosin may be helpful in the chronic therapy of some patients with pheochromocytoma who develop intolerable side effects with phenoxybenzamine.[1] However, phenoxybenzamine is preferable for chronic therapy because of its long-lasting, irreversible (with adequate blood levels) alpha blockade and thus theoretical better protection against a hypertensive crisis, particularly if the patient is unreliable about taking medications.

SURGERY Surgical mortality is $<$ 5 percent in several recent series. Phenoxybenzamine administration for 1 to 2 weeks preoperatively usually corrects the decreased plasma volume present in many patients with sustained hypertension and thus diminishes the extent of any intraoperative hypotensive crisis. Phenoxybenzamine therapy should be minimal in those patients in whom the tumor has not been localized before the time of surgery or in whom multiple tumors are more likely so that the blood pressure rise with tumor palpation may assist localization. At the time of removal of the tumor, a marked fall in blood pressure may occur due to loss of sympathetic tone in the face of contracted blood volume and continued alpha-receptor blockade; this may require temporary administration of large amounts of norepinephrine or other pressor agents until adequate amounts of blood or plasma volume expanders can be given. The entire abdomen should be explored carefully in all patients to search for multiple tumors. The gallbladder is usually examined since there is an unexplained increased frequency of associated cholelithiasis. Persistent blood pressure elevation in the early postoperative period is thought to be due to slow release of increased neuronal catecholamine stores or to excessive intraoperative expansion of plasma volume. Urinary catecholamines should be measured 1 or more weeks after surgery to confirm removal of the tumor. Persistent hypertension may be secondary to renal arteriolar nephrosclerosis or rarely to the inadvertent ligation of a renal artery branch at the time of surgery. Hypertension due to nephrosclerosis should be managed with the drugs used in treating essential hypertension.

REFERENCES

ENGELMAN K: Phaeochromocytoma. Clin Endocrinol Metab 6:769, 1977

FREIER DT et al: Dilemmas in the early diagnosis and treatment of multiple endocrine adenomatosis, type II. Surgery 82:407, 1977

GIFFORD RW et al: Clinical features, diagnosis, and treatment of pheochromocytoma: A review of 76 cases. Mayo Clin Proc 39:281, 1964

GITLOW SE et al: The biochemical techniques for detecting and establishing the presence of pheochromocytoma: A review of ten years' experience. Am J Cardiol 26:270, 1970

HAMILTON BP et al: Measurement of urinary epinephrine in screening for pheochromocytoma in multiple endocrine neoplasia type II. Am J Med 65:1027, 1978

KAPLAN NM et al: Single-voided urine metanephrine assays in screening for pheochromocytoma. Arch Intern Med 137:190, 1976

KNUDSON AG JR, STRONG LC: Mutation and cancer: Neuroblastoma and pheochromocytoma. Am J Hum Genet 24:514, 1972

MANGER WM, GIFFORD RW JR: *Pheochromocytoma.* New York, Springer-Verlag, 1977

REMINE WH et al: Current management of pheochromocytoma. Ann Surg 199:740, 1974

WALLACE JM, GILL DP: Prazosin in the diagnosis and treatment of pheochromocytoma. JAMA 240:2752, 1978

---

[1] *This drug has not been approved for this purpose by the Food and Drug Administration at the time of publication.*

338

DIABETES MELLITUS

DANIEL W. FOSTER

Diabetes is the most common of the serious metabolic diseases of humans. The true frequency in the general population is difficult to ascertain because of widely differing standards of diagnosis, but probably is somewhere between 2 and 6 percent. The disease is characterized by a series of hormone-induced metabolic abnormalities, by long-term complications, and by a microvascular lesion demonstrable by electron microscopy. In recent years it has become clear that a variety of syndromes are subsumed under the general term *diabetes* and that they differ in both clinical manifestations and patterns of inheritance. In this chapter primary hyperglycemic states exhibiting the triad of findings listed above will be considered under the umbrella term *diabetes mellitus.* It should be stated at the outset that many controversies exist among those who care for diabetics. In the discussion that follows an attempt has been made to identify the major questions at issue and to give the author's interpretation of the data at hand.

DIAGNOSIS The diagnosis of symptomatic diabetes is not difficult. When a patient presents with signs and symptoms attributable to an osmotic diuresis and is found to have hyperglycemia, essentially all physicians would agree that diabetes is present. The same would be true if the initial presentation were hyperglycemic ketoacidosis or hyperosmolar coma. There likewise would be little disagreement about an asymptomatic patient with persistently elevated fasting plasma glucose concentrations. The problem arises with the asymptomatic patient who for one reason or another is considered to be a potential diabetic but has a normal fasting glucose concentration. Such patients are often given an oral glucose tolerance test, and, if abnormal values are found, diagnosed as having "chemical" diabetes. There seems to be little question that normal glucose tolerance is strong evidence against the presence of diabetes. Less certain is the predictive value for development of diabetes of a positive test using fixed upper limits that are not age-adjusted, i.e., whole blood values of 160 and 120 mg per 100 ml at 1 and 2 h respectively or plasma equivalent values of 185 and 140 mg per 100 ml, the Fajans-Conn criteria. (Plasma glucose concentrations are approximately 14 percent higher than whole blood.) Much evidence suggests that the standard oral glucose tolerance test overdiagnoses diabetes to a remarkable degree, probably because stress of a variety of kinds can produce an abnormal response. The operative mechanism is thought to be epinephrine discharge. Epinephrine is known to block insulin secretion, stimulate glucagon release, and activate glycogen breakdown, with the result that hepatic glucose production is increased and the capacity to dispose of an exogenous glucose load is impaired. Even anxiety over the necessary venipunctures may generate sufficient epinephrine to produce an abnormal test. Concomitant illness, inadequate diet, and lack of physical exercise also contribute to the high incidence of false positive examinations.

Support for the viewpoint that the glucose tolerance test is too sensitive for routine diagnostic use comes from the observation that most subjects with abnormal glucose tolerance never develop overt diabetes. In a prospective study of 352 women with abnormal tests by the standard Fajans-Conn criteria, about two-thirds of the subjects had normal responses when reexamined years later. The predicted rate of decompensation to diabetes at 10 years was only 27 percent. The problem seems to be that the upper limits of normality for the test are set too low. On the basis of a massive screening program for diabetes in Cleveland, it has been concluded that the diagnosis of diabetes should be restricted to a 2-h postprandial capillary whole blood concentration of 180 mg per 100 ml or higher. (Capillary whole blood values are essentially equivalent to those of venous plasma.) Subjects with values between 140 to 180 mg per 100 ml were considered to be "at risk" for diabetes but were not labeled as having the disease. Since glucose tolerance is age-related, even these standards will be too rigid in older persons. For these reasons, the National Diabetes Data Group of the National Institutes of Health has recommended new criteria for the interpretation of glucose tolerance tests. According to these recommendations the diagnosis of diabetes should be restricted to a 2-h plasma glucose concentration equal to or greater than 200 mg per 100 ml with at least one other value between zero time and 2 h equal to or greater than 200 mg per 100 ml. If the 2-h plasma glucose concentration is between 140 and 200 mg per 100 ml and one other value in the 2-h test period is equal to or greater than 200 mg per 100 ml, the diagnosis of "impaired glucose tolerance" is suggested. It seems likely that these recommendations will be widely adopted.

The critical question regarding the use of the oral glucose tolerance test in clinical practice is whether the diagnosis of "chemical diabetes" as now defined is helpful to the patient. If all patients with abnormal tests were destined to progress to decompensation and if that progression could somehow be prevented, the answer would unequivocally be affirmative. As already pointed out, however, progression is not inevitable. Furthermore, the only known preventive measure in the diabetic at risk is avoidance of obesity, a desirable goal whether or not glucose tolerance is abnormal. On the other hand, a diagnosis of diabetes in a person who does not have the disease is harmful in a number of ways. Such patients may have employment difficulties and will be required to pay higher insurance rates. In addition there is the emotional burden of believing one has a chronic degenerative disease when in fact it is not present. For these reasons many diabetologists (including the author) do not perform glucose tolerance tests, although other physicians continue to feel the procedure useful. If the test is done it is recommended that interpretations be in accord with the criteria of the National Diabetes Data Group mentioned above.

The glucose tolerance test also has caused confusion in investigative work, particularly clinical trials and genetic studies. Many authors, using an abnormal glucose tolerance test as the diagnostic criterion for diabetes, have actually studied mixed groups of diabetic and nondiabetic subjects while considering them to be homogeneous. Conclusions drawn from such studies must be considered suspect.

If the oral glucose tolerance test is not used, most physicians rely on a persistent elevation of the fasting plasma glucose for the diagnosis of diabetes in asymptomatic patients. The upper limit of normal is generally taken to be 140 mg per 100 ml (plasma), although it is recognized that higher values may not be abnormal in older persons. Most patients with consistent hyperglycemia have primary or genetic diabetes. Secondary forms of hyperglycemia also occur and are important to recognize in order that the underlying disorder may be treated. The differential diagnosis, which is usually not difficult, includes chronic pancreatitis, hemochromatosis, Cushing's syndrome, acromegaly, pheochromocytoma, glucagonoma, somatostatinoma, and certain rare insulin resistance syndromes to be discussed subsequently. Hyperglycemia may also appear in the context of acute stress (such as major burns) without indicating underlying diabetes.

GENETICS It has long been known that diabetes aggregates in families. The genetics of the disease has undergone intense

scrutiny, but major disagreement exists regarding interpretation of the data. It now seems probable that diabetes is genetically heterogeneous and that similar diabetic phenotypes may appear from differing genotypes. It is also possible that a single genetic defect may produce differing clinical syndromes. Unfortunately no specific genetic marker for the presence of the disease is available. It was hoped that thickening of the muscle capillary basement membrane might be such a marker, but this now seems unlikely. The fact that some authors have equated abnormal glucose tolerance with diabetes while others have studied only overtly hyperglycemic subjects adds to the difficulty of deciphering genetic studies. While much remains to be learned, certain conclusions appear firm. (1) Pedigree analysis indicates that inheritance of diabetes may follow recessive, dominant, or polyfactorial patterns in a given family. Thus it is not possible to define a single mode of transmission that encompasses the entire spectrum of diabetic syndromes. Part of the confusion arises because more than 30 inherited disorders (in addition to the common juvenile and maturity onset forms of the disease) have been described where one manifestation of the phenotypic presentation is the presence of hyperglycemia or carbohydrate intolerance. (2) In addition to genetic predisposition, environmental factors are almost certainly operative, particularly in the young, insulin-dependent diabetic. This follows from the observation that the concordance rate for diabetes in proved monozygotic (identical) twins under the age of 40 is less than 50 percent, in contrast to the predicted 100 percent for a purely genetic disorder. Considerable interest has focused on the possibility that the environmental factor might be viral. Coxsackievirus B4 (in Europe) and mumps virus (in the United States) have been implicated as possible causal agents. Compatible with this interpretation is the observation that a variant of the encephalomyocarditis virus causes a diabetic syndrome in genetically susceptible mice. A diabetogenic variant of coxsackievirus B4 has been isolated from the pancreas of a previously healthy boy who died following an episode of diabetic ketoacidosis. The isolate from his pancreas caused hyperglycemia when injected into susceptible mice. Interestingly the concordance rate in twins developing diabetes after the age of 40 is close to 100 percent, indicating a predominant genetic influence in the maturity onset form of the disease. (3) There seems to be an association between certain histocompatibility antigens and insulin-dependent diabetes of the juvenile type. Human leucocyte (HLA) antigens B8, Bw15, Dw3, and Dw4 appear to represent the primary association sites. The B8 antigen is particularly intriguing because of its known relationship to autoimmune illnesses such as Graves' disease, adrenal insufficiency, and myasthenia gravis. Antibodies to pancreatic beta-cell membranes have now been described in juvenile diabetes. It is not known whether these are autoantibodies causally related to development of the disease or whether they arise in response to antigens released as a consequence of primary pancreatic inflammation. Maturity-onset diabetes does not appear to show the HLA associations seen in the juvenile form.

Because of uncertainties regarding the genetics of diabetes, genetic counseling is not possible for most patients. In the past empiric risk estimates compiled without regard to the heterogeneity of diabetes have been assembled, but such data are almost certainly inapplicable for general use. A careful family history may give some clues to inheritance patterns, and in individual cases HLA genotyping may help. Overall, however, caution should be exercised in advising parents about risks for development of the disease in offspring.

CLINICAL PICTURE It has been traditional to classify diabetes into juvenile- and maturity-onset types. Such a classification is probably acceptable as a kind of clinical shorthand as long as it is recognized that the descriptions are generalizations and that overlap syndromes occur. For example, the picture of maturity-onset disease may occur in the very young, while in-

TABLE 338-1

General characteristics of juvenile- and maturity-onset diabetes

	Juvenile-onset	*Maturity-onset*
Age of onset	< 40	> 40
Body habitus	Normal to wasted	Obese
Plasma insulin	Low to absent	Normal to high
Plasma glucagon	High, suppressible	High, resistant
Acute complication	Ketoacidosis	Hyperosmolar coma
Insulin therapy	Responsive	Responsive to resistant
Sulfonylurea therapy	Unresponsive	Responsive

sulin-dependent diabetes may begin after the age of 40. In either case the metabolic abnormalities seem to be caused by relative or absolute insulin deficiency coupled with relative or absolute glucagon excess. Insulin resistance may also play a role, particularly in obese subjects. It is now known that two other peptides, somatostatin and pancreatic polypeptide, are synthesized in the islets of Langerhans. Their role (if any) in the pathophysiology of diabetes remains to be established.

Juvenile diabetes Juvenile (insulin-dependent) diabetes usually begins before the age of 40, often in childhood or adolescence. Onset of symptoms may be abrupt, with thirst, excessive urination, increased appetite, and weight loss occurring over a several-day period. In some cases the disease is heralded by the appearance of ketoacidosis during an intercurrent illness or following surgery. As outlined in Table 338-1, juvenile patients are not obese (and may be wasted), depending on the length of time between onset of symptoms and start of treatment. Characteristically the plasma insulin is low or immeasurable. Glucagon levels are high, but suppressible with insulin. Once symptoms have developed, insulin therapy is required. Occasionally an initial episode of ketoacidosis is followed by a symptom-free interval (the "honeymoon" period) during which no treatment is required. The likely explanation for this phenomenon is shown in Fig. 338-1.

Maturity-onset diabetes This form of the disease usually begins in middle life or beyond. Classically the patient is overweight. Symptoms tend to begin more gradually than in the juvenile form, and many times the diagnosis is made when an asymptomatic patient is found to have an elevated plasma glucose on routine laboratory examination. In contrast to juvenile disease plasma insulin levels are normal to high in absolute terms, although they are probably lower than predicted for the level of the plasma glucose; i.e., relative insulin deficiency is present. Put in other words, if plasma glucose were raised to equivalent levels in a nondiabetic subject, the insulin response would be higher than that seen in the maturity-onset diabetic. Obesity is known to be associated with insulin resistance and is assumed to be the major cause of the higher insulin concentrations seen before and after the development of hyperglycemia. Support for this conclusion comes from the observation that weight reduction in the obesity-hyperglycemia syndrome may result in disappearance of hyperglycemia and return of insulin responsiveness. Primary insulin resistance not due to obesity has also been postulated to play a role in the pathophysiology of this form of the disease. Because of questions concerning the experimental techniques used to deduce its presence, primary insulin resistance cannot be considered proved. Glucagon metabolism in maturity-onset patients is complicated. While fasting concentrations can be lowered by large amounts of insulin, the glucagon response to ingested nutrients cannot be suppressed; i.e., alpha-cell function remains abnormal. For reasons that are not yet clear maturity-onset diabetics do not develop ketoacidosis. In the decompensated state they are susceptible to the syndrome of hyperosmolar, nonketotic coma. If weight loss can be induced, patients may respond to

diet alone. If additional therapy is required, the majority will respond to management with sulfonylureas.

TREATMENT **Diet** Modification of the diet is the first line of therapy in diabetes. An appropriate diet stabilizes body weight at near-ideal levels, minimizes hyperglycemia, and protects against hypoglycemia in patients requiring insulin injections. Recent alterations include lowering of saturated fat intake with concomitant increase in polyunsaturated fatty acid content in an attempt to delay the appearance of atherosclerosis. Detailed dietary planning is beyond the scope of this chapter and ideally should utilize the talents of a professional dietician. Few measures are more important than proper instruction in diet at the onset of diabetes. If no dietician is available in the community, referral to a medical center for initial instruction is recommended since most physicians do not have the time necessary for adequate dietary counseling.

The first step in writing a dietary prescription is to determine optimal caloric content. Since the activity component of daily caloric needs can only be roughly estimated, an element of trial and error is involved. Basal metabolic requirements can be met by giving approximately 22 kcal/kg per day. Rough estimates of the additional caloric demands for activity are 30, 50, and 100 percent of the basal requirements in sedentary, moderately active, and briskly exercising individuals. Upward or downward adjustments will be necessary if the goal is weight gain or weight loss. The latter is more commonly required (and much more difficult). Since the basal metabolic rate is about 1500 kcal per day in a normal adult, caloric restriction to less than this amount should cause weight loss, even in a sedentary individual. In practice, most obese patients do not adhere to reducing diets even under the threat of diabetes.

The minimal protein requirement for good nutrition is

FIGURE 338-1

Schematic representation of the "honeymoon" period. In this graph insulin secretory capacity is shown gradually decreasing in a patient destined to develop diabetes. At approximately 13½ years insulin would become insufficient to maintain plasma glucose in the normal range. An initial episode of ketoacidosis, for example, in association with acute appendicitis, is shown occurring in the twelfth year. Presumably stress-induced epinephrine release blocks insulin secretion and causes the syndrome. In normal subjects insulin reserve is such that hormone release is adequate, even in the face of stress. Following recovery from the stressful episode insulin secretory capacity returns to the previous level and remains sufficient for an additional year as indicated by the shaded area—the "honeymoon" period.

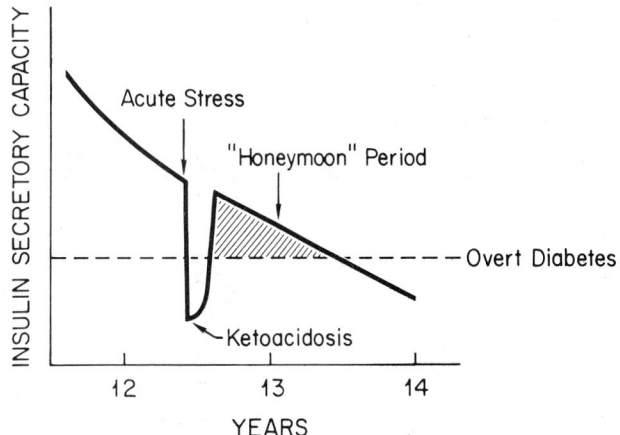

about 0.9 g/kg per day. The recommended carbohydrate content of the diabetic diet is 40 to 50 percent of the total calories, with fat making up the remainder. Carbohydrate intakes of up to 85 percent of total calories have been given, however, and under experimental conditions may actually improve diabetic control. This fact is mentioned to indicate that carbohydrate intake need not be rigidly limited to the lower figure of 40 percent. Sucrose is ordinarily not allowed because of its rapid digestion and absorption. For the same reason candies and pastries are proscribed.

The degree of dietary restriction will vary from patient to patient. Some overweight patients with asymptomatic hyperglycemia may need only simple caloric limitation to control their disease. Most symptomatic diabetics, on the other hand, must learn to estimate food values using the exchange list technique.[1] A brief summary of the typical exchanges is shown in Table 338-2. Basically one decides how many calories are needed and the desired distribution between fat, carbohydrate, and protein. The necessary exchanges are then outlined. For example, a physician wishes a patient to have a 2200-cal diet with 50 percent of the calories as carbohydrate and 1 to 1.5 g protein per kilogram of body weight. Such a diet can be met by providing 2 milk exchanges, 7 fruit exchanges, 12 bread exchanges, 8 meat exchanges, 4 fat exchanges, and unlimited A vegetables (Table 338-3). In practice precalculated diets of given caloric content prepared by the American Diabetes Association are usually used. Alterations in distribution of protein, fat, and carbohydrate can be easily accomplished by minor shifts of exchanges. Care must be taken to emphasize foods the patient likes and can obtain. Initially it is helpful to weigh and measure foods until visual estimates can be made accurately. As in any dietary regimen it is important to emphasize that it is the long-term, overall dietary pattern which counts. Deviation for one meal or two meals does not matter much. Thus a teenage diabetic on a date may be allowed to eat a dessert, ordinarily forbidden, as a special treat with the understanding that resumption of the diet will be necessary the next day. The "treat" technique often assures better dietary cooperation than more rigid demands, even in adults.

In insulin-requiring diabetics the distribution of calories is also important if hypoglycemia is to be avoided. A typical pattern might include 20 percent of the total calories for breakfast, 35 percent for lunch, 30 percent for supper, and 15 percent as a late-evening feeding. Occasionally a midafternoon snack will be necessary. Different distributions may be required for different life-styles; i.e., a person employed on a late evening or night shift would not eat the major meal at noon.

Insulin Insulin is required for treatment of all juvenile diabetic patients and many patients with maturity-onset disease.

---

[1] Copies of Exchange Lists for Meal Planning *may be ordered from the American Diabetes Association, 600 Fifth Avenue, New York, New York 10020, or from any local affiliate of the Association.*

TABLE 338-2
Composition of food exchanges*

Exchange	Calories	Carbohydrate, g	Fat, g	Protein, g
Milk	170	12	10	8
Vegetable[†]	35	7	—	2
Fruit	40	10	—	—
Bread	70[‡]	15	—	2
Meat	75[‡]	—	5	7
Fat	45	—	5	—

* Composition listed for one exchange.
† Type A vegetables contain little carbohydrate, fat, or protein and can be eaten in any amount. Exchange values are for type B vegetables.
‡ Calculated value for bread exchange is 68 cal and for meat exchange is 73 cal using 4 kcal/g for carbohydrate and protein and 9 kcal/g for fat. The values 70 and 75 cal were adapted to facilitate computations.

TABLE 338-3
A 2200-cal diabetic diet (50 percent carbohydrate)

Exchange	No.	Calories	Carbohydrate, g	Fat, g	Protein, g
Milk	2	340	24	20	16
Vegetable*		Unlimited amounts of type A vegetables			
Fruit	7	280	70	—	—
Bread	12	840	180	—	24
Meat	8	600	—	40	56
Fat	4	180	—	20	—
Total		2240	274	80	96
			(50%)	(33%)	(17%)

* Type B vegetables include beets, carrots, onions, green peas, pumpkin, rutabagas, winter squash, and turnips. If these are desired, ½ to 1 cup can be substituted for one fruit exchange. All other common vegetables can be eaten as desired.

If the physician does not use oral drugs (see below), all diet-unresponsive subjects must be given the hormone. It is fairly easy to control the symptoms of diabetes with insulin, but it is extremely difficult—probably impossible—to normalize the blood sugar throughout the day. Nondiabetic subjects maintain the plasma glucose concentration within a narrow range at all times despite episodic food intake. When a meal is eaten, a prompt rise in insulin release occurs such that absorbed carbohydrate is rapidly transported into the liver and other tissues (see Chap. 86). Even postprandially, therefore, the plasma glucose does not rise into the hyperglycemic or glycosuric range. As the plasma glucose falls under the influence of insulin, release of the hormone is damped and simultaneously counterregulatory hormones enter the circulation to prevent hypoglycemia, assuring smooth control throughout the absorptive process. The diabetic treated with insulin by injection cannot reproduce this physiologic response with one or even two injections of depot insulin. If enough insulin is given to keep the postprandial glucose within the range of normal, inevitably there will be too much insulin circulating during the postabsorptive phase and hypoglycemia will result. The physiologic pattern could be more closely mimicked by giving regular insulin before each meal together with a small amount of intermediate insulin to control nocturnal hyperglycemia, but most patients are unwilling to take three to four injections daily for prolonged periods. An artificial external pancreas utilizing a continuous glucose sensor and insulin injection system would solve the problem, but current models are not yet adequate for clinical use. A promising approach is the administration of insulin by continuous subcutaneous infusion utilizing a small battery-driven pump. The continuous base-line level of infusion of insulin is supplemented by more rapid rates before meals. Obviously, successful pancreatic transplantation would be the ideal solution, but this remains a distant goal. There is interest in the use of somatostatin to reverse the hyperglucagonemia of diabetes and thus improve diabetic control, but modification of the molecule would be required since its half-life is short, requiring administration by constant infusion.

A variety of forms of insulin are available, but crystalline (regular) and NPH or Lente preparations meet the needs of the majority of patients. The long-acting variants (PZI and Ultralente) have no important role. Insulin is currently packaged in concentrations of 40, 80, and 100 units per milliliter (U-40, U-80, U-100), but in the future only U-100 will be used. U-100 insulin is a "single peak" insulin, meaning that proinsulin and certain larger aggregates have been removed. A still purer form is called "single component," or "monocomponent," insulin. It was originally hoped that such insulin would be helpful in insulin allergy, but this has not proved to be true in most cases. It has been traditional to describe the pharmacology of insulins in terms of onset, peak effect, and duration of action when given subcutaneously, intramuscularly, or intravenously. However, these parameters are modified by the amount of insulin injected and other factors, and individual diabetics exhibit wide differences in their response to a given form of the hormone. Thus an intermediate preparation such as NPH insulin may exert an effect for 24 h in one patient but only 12 h in another. Peak activity may come as early as 4 h or as late as 16 h. This means that therapy in each patient has to be determined by trial and error. Recognizing that variations exist, it can be assumed that regular insulin given subcutaneously will ordinarily have an onset of action within a period of minutes and last 4 to 6 h. Plasma insulin concentrations following injection of Lente or NPH insulin rise at slightly slower rates, and the biologic effects persist for 12 to 24 h. While precise guidelines cannot be given to cover every situation, the following principles regarding insulin use are generally applicable:

1 In emergencies such as diabetic ketoacidosis or hyperosmolar coma always use regular insulin.
2 For initiation of therapy (in the absence of emergency) try a single injection of intermediate-acting insulin (Lente or NPH).
3 Start treatment with small amounts and increase gradually.
4 Allow several days to a week between changes in dose.
5 If control is difficult, give intermediate insulin twice daily with or without the addition of regular insulin.
6 Avoid hypoglycemia.

If the newly diagnosed diabetic is not in acute distress, therapy can be started as an outpatient, provided instruction in diet, urine testing, and insulin use is available and the physician can be reached by telephone for consultation. Hospitalization to initiate treatment is required only rarely. Normal-weight adults may be started on 15 to 20 units a day (the estimated daily insulin production rate in nondiabetic subjects of normal size is about 25 units a day). Obese patients, because of insulin resistance, may be started on 25 to 30 units a day. It is preferable to use the same quantity of insulin for several days before changing, the one exception being the hypoglycemic patient, for whom the dose should be immediately decreased unless a clearly evident nonrecurrent cause of hypoglycemia (such as unexpected excessive exercise) is present. Generally changes should be no more than 5 or 10 units per step.

In following the effectiveness of therapy the patient should, initially, check the urine glucose and ketones before breakfast, lunch, and supper and before retiring. A double voiding technique in which the bladder is emptied and 30 min later a urine specimen obtained for testing is mandatory for the early-morning sample and helpful at other times to minimize lag between plasma glucose and urine values. In addition, an estimate of urine volume should be obtained. A 4+ urine glucose is of little concern if the patient has infrequent urination during the day and no nocturia, while the same chemical reading in a patient urinating large volumes five times a night indicates massive glucose wastage. It should be noted that some diabetics drink large volumes of water by habit, even after hyperglycemia has been brought under control. If the patient complains of continued nocturia when plasma glucose concentrations are in the acceptable range, the patient should be asked to check one of the late-night specimens for glucose. A negative test suggests a water-drinking habit. Once the patient is stabilized, urine testing can be limited to once or twice daily.

Many patients cannot be controlled on a single daily dose of NPH or Lente insulin. Such patients should be tried on split therapy with about two-thirds of the total insulin given before breakfast and the remainder before supper. Two injections are almost always used when the total dose reaches 50 or 60 units a day, but may actually be helpful at smaller doses as well, since the peak action of intermediate insulins appears to be dose-related; i.e., a low dose may exhibit maximal activity earlier and disappear sooner than a large dose. It also is frequently helpful in difficult cases to add small amounts of regular insulin to the intermediate preparation. For example, if the urine glucose pattern shows glycosuria before lunch and in the early afternoon but no glycosuria at night, 5 to 10 units regular insulin in the morning may solve the problem. All patients should be taught to reduce the insulin dose by 5 to 10 units when extra activity is anticipated. Similarly a small amount of extra regular insulin can be taken before a meal that will contain extra calories or food ordinarily not allowed (e.g., when the diabetic must eat out at a banquet or the teenager goes out on a date). Patients with complicated control problems may require hospitalization, whereby frequent plasma and urine glucose determinations can guide therapy.

During surgical procedures or delivery of the pregnant diabetic it is desirable to omit depot insulin and treat the patient with regular insulin. A reasonable approach is to give 10 units of insulin prior to induction of anesthesia and to infuse 10% dextrose in water during the procedure. Urine glucose and ketones should be monitored frequently and additional insulin given as needed. Maintenance of mild glycosuria via the glucose infusion will assure that hypoglycemia has not developed in the unconscious patient. If renal disease is present (rendering the urine unreliable as a guide to hypoglycemia), the plasma glucose should be monitored at hourly intervals during prolonged procedures.

HYPOGLYCEMIA AND THE SOMOGYI EFFECT (see also Chap. 340) The problem of hypoglycemia is a common one in insulin-dependent diabetics, particularly when aggressive efforts are made to normalize not only the fasting plasma glucose but also postprandial hyperglycemia. Hypoglycemia may be caused by missing a meal or doing unexpected exercise but can occur in the absence of known precipitating events. Daytime episodes of hypoglycemia are usually recognized by adrenergic symptoms, such as sweating, nervousness, tremor, and hunger. Hypoglycemia occurring during sleep may produce only night sweats, unpleasant dreams, or early morning headache. If not aborted by ingestion of carbohydrate, central nervous system symptoms arise: confusion, abnormal behavior, loss of consciousness, or convulsions. As diabetes progresses, particularly with the development of neuropathy, epinephrine-induced symptoms may lose their effectiveness as warning signals and central nervous system signs may predominate.

Hypoglycemia is potentially harmful in several ways. It may produce permanent neurologic damage in the patient or lead to injury via accident. Moreover, hypoglycemia results in worsening of diabetic control, since release of counterregulatory hormones results in rebound hyperglycemia, occasionally with mild ketosis. This phenomenon, called the *Somogyi effect,* should be suspected whenever wide swings in the plasma glucose or urine sugars are seen over short time intervals even if symptoms are not reported. Thus, a plasma glucose of 70 mg per 100 ml before breakfast and 400 mg per 100 ml before lunch strongly suggests early-morning hypoglycemia with postbreakfast hyperglycemia due to counterregulatory hormone activity. Similarly, suspicion should be aroused if urine glucose determinations vary between negative and 4+ within a short time span. Such rapid changes contrast with the alterations seen following insulin withdrawal in a previously well-controlled diabetic patient in whom hyperglycemia and ketosis develop gradually and smoothly over a 12- to 24-h period. Excessive hunger and weight gain occurring in the context of worsening hyperglycemia are clues that the insulin dosage may be too high, since poor control due to underinsulinization usually results in weight loss (because of osmotic diuresis and glucose wastage). If the Somogyi phenomenon is suspected, the insulin dose should be decreased as a trial, even when specific symptoms of overinsulinization are absent.

It is not unusual for a previously stable, well-controlled diabetic to develop insulin sensitivity and hypoglycemia in the absence of change in weight, diet, or exercise. The most common cause is the appearance of diabetic renal disease. Occasionally the hypoglycemia may be due to the development of autoimmune adrenal insufficiency as part of the Schmidt syndrome (see Chap. 336), an affliction which occurs more frequently in diabetics than in the population as a whole. Some patients develop hypoglycemia in association with high levels of circulating insulin antibodies. The exact mechanism has not been established. Occasionally an insulinoma may develop in a diabetic patient. Very rarely permanent remission of apparently typical diabetes occurs. The reason is not known.

Oral agents Maturity-onset diabetes that cannot be controlled by careful dietary management usually responds to sulfonylureas. The drugs are convenient to use and work in a high percentage of cases. However, some physicians no longer use them because the University Group Diabetes Program (UGDP) cooperative study concluded that tolbutamide was no more effective than diet alone in the treatment of diabetes and that patients treated with tolbutamide had a significant increase in cardiac deaths when compared with controls. The validity of the UGDP study has been widely debated, but the evidence pro and con is too extensive to be reviewed here. Suffice to say that many physicians continue to believe that the sulfonylureas are useful and safe drugs for the treatment of certain adult-onset diabetics. Moreover, despite claims to the contrary, the drugs remain effective for years in many patients.

The sulfonylureas have the capacity to stimulate acutely insulin release from the beta cell, and this is presumed to be their major mode of action. Extrapancreatic mechanisms such as sensitization of the liver to the action of insulin have also been suggested. Four major forms of sulfonylureas are available. Tolbutamide and tolazamide have relatively short half-lives and must be given in divided doses. They are inactivated by the liver. Acetohexamide undergoes hepatic metabolism, but the major metabolite retains hypoglycemic activity. Renal excretion is, therefore, its primary disposal route. The same is true for chlorpropamide which is not metabolized in the body. Patients with renal disease are vulnerable to hypoglycemia with the latter two drugs. Chlorpropamide has a long half-life and can be given as a single dose, but may cause water retention in some patients through its capacity to sensitize the renal tubule to antidiuretic hormone. The dosage range of the sulfonylureas in grams per day is as follows:

Acetohexamide	0.25–1.5 g
Chlorpropamide	0.1–0.5 g
Tolazamide	0.1–1 g
Tolbutamide	0.5–3 g

Hypoglycemia is much less common with oral agents than with insulin, but when it occurs it tends to be severe and prolonged. Some patients have required massive glucose infusions for days following the last dose of sulfonylurea. For this reason hospitalization is mandatory in patients with sulfonylurea-induced hypoglycemia.

The only other oral agent effective in the treatment of maturity-onset diabetes is phenformin. It presumably lowers plasma glucose by inhibiting gluconeogenesis in the liver. The drug is ordinarily used only in combination with sulfonylureas under circumstances in which control is inadequate with sulfonylurea alone. Because of many reports linking phenformin to the appearance of lactic acidosis in diabetic patients, the Food and Drug Administration has removed the agent from clinical use in the United States except for certain special patients who continue to take it as an investigational drug. Phenformin and other biguanides are still widely used elsewhere in the world. If prescribed, the maximum dose should be 100 mg a day. Phenformin should not be given to patients with renal disease and should be immediately stopped should nausea, vomiting, diarrhea, or any intercurrent illness appear.

ACUTE METABOLIC COMPLICATIONS In addition to hypoglycemia, diabetics are susceptible to two major acute metabolic complications: diabetic ketoacidosis and hyperosmolar, nonketotic coma. The former is a complication of juvenile diabetes, while the latter usually occurs in the setting of maturity-onset disease. Ketoacidosis is rare in maturity-onset diabetes.

Diabetic ketoacidosis The pathophysiology of diabetic ketoacidosis is now reasonably clear. Initiation of the syndrome appears to require insulin deficiency coupled with a relative or absolute increase in glucagon concentration. It is often caused by cessation of insulin intake but may result from physical (e.g., infection, surgery) or emotional stress despite continued insulin therapy. In the former case the concentration of glucagon rises due to insulin withdrawal, while in stress the operative stimulus is probably epinephrine release. In addition to stimulating glucagon secretion epinephrine presumably blocks release of the small amount of residual insulin found in some juvenile subjects. These hormonal changes have multiple effects, but two are critical. (1) They induce maximal gluconeogenesis and impair peripheral utilization of glucose, causing severe hyperglycemia. The resultant osmotic diuresis leads to the volume depletion and dehydration that characterize the ketoacidotic state. (2) They activate the ketogenic process and

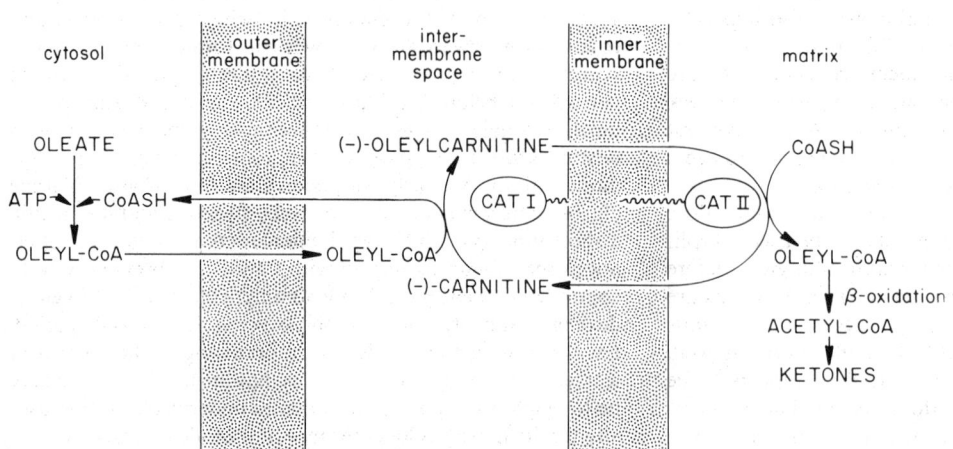

FIGURE 338-2

The carnitine acyltransferase system for the transfer of long-chain fatty acids into the mitochondria. CAT I = carnitine acyltransferase I; CAT II = carnitine acyltransferase II. (From JD McGarry et al, J Clin Invest 55:1202, 1975. Used by permission.)

FIGURE 338-3

The regulation of ketogenesis. Significant production of acetoacetate and β-hydroxybutyrate by the liver requires provision of adequate free fatty acid substrate and activation of fatty acid oxidation. Lipolysis is primarily increased by insulin deficiency while the fatty acid oxidative sequence is activated primarily by glucagon. The immediate signal for oxidation is a fall in malonyl CoA content. (After JD McGarry, DW Foster, Am J Med 61:9, 1976.)

thus initiate development of metabolic acidosis. For ketosis to occur changes must be produced in both adipose tissue and the liver. Free fatty acids from adipose stores represent the primary substrate for ketone body formation and are absolutely required if rapid rates of ketogenesis are to develop. However, fatty acids taken up by the liver are simply reesterified and stored as hepatic triglyceride or transported back into the circulation as very low density lipoprotein unless hepatic fatty acid oxidative machinery is activated.

While free fatty acid release is thought to be directly mediated by insulin deficiency it appears that fatty acid oxidation in the liver is primarily induced by glucagon. Its site of action is the carnitine acyltransferase system of enzymes which is responsible for the transport of fatty acids into the mitochondria after they have first been esterified to coenzyme A. As shown in Fig. 338-2, carnitine acyltransferase I esterifies fatty acyl CoA to fatty acylcarnitine, which then freely traverses the inner membrane with reversal of the reaction occurring internally under the influence of carnitine acyltransferase II. In the fed state carnitine acyltransferase I is inactive, and as a consequence long-chain fatty acids cannot reach the β-oxidative sequence for ketone body production. During starvation or uncontrolled diabetes the system is activated; under these circumstances the rate of ketogenesis is determined in first-order fashion by the concentration of fatty acid reaching transferase I.

The mechanism by which glucagon (or a change in the glucagon/insulin ratio) activates the transport system is twofold. (1) Glucagon causes a rapid fall in hepatic malonyl CoA content. Malonyl CoA, the first committed intermediate in the synthesis of fatty acids from glucose, is an extremely powerful competitive inhibitor of carnitine acyltransferase I, and it is the fall in its concentration that is critical to the ketogenic process. (2) Glucagon causes a rise in hepatic carnitine concentration, which then drives the reaction toward fatty acylcarnitine formation by mass action. These events are summarized schematically in Fig. 338-3. At very high plasma fatty acid concentrations hepatic uptake is sufficient to saturate both oxidative and esterifying pathways, resulting in fatty liver and hypertriglyceridemia as well as ketoacidosis. Overproduction of ketones by the liver is the primary event in ketotic states, but limitation in peripheral utilization also plays a role at high concentrations of acetoacetate and β-hydroxybutyrate.

Clinically ketoacidosis begins with anorexia, nausea, and vomiting, coupled with increased urine formation. Abdominal pain may be present. If untreated, altered consciousness or frank coma may occur. Initial examination usually shows Kussmaul respiration, together with signs of volume depletion. Rarely the latter is sufficient to cause vascular collapse and renal shutdown. Body temperature is normal or slightly below normal in uncomplicated ketoacidosis, and fever strongly suggests the presence of infection. Leukocytosis, frequently very marked, is a feature of diabetic acidosis per se and may not indicate infection.

The characteristic metabolic abnormalities of diabetic coma are shown in Table 338-4. Several features deserve comment. The metabolic acidosis and anion gap are almost totally accounted for by the elevated plasma levels of acetoacetate and β-hydroxybutyrate, although other acids (e.g., lactate, free fatty acids, phosphates) contribute modestly. Despite initial potassium concentrations that are normal to high there is a total body potassium deficit of several hundred millimoles. Similarly, initial serum phosphorous may be high despite depletion of body stores. Magnesium deficiency may also be present. The serum sodium concentration tends to be low in the face of modest osmolar concentration because of the hyperglycemia which draws intracellular water into the plasma space. A very low serum sodium (e.g., 110 meq per liter) suggests an artefact due to severe hypertriglyceridemia. The latter is common in ketoacidosis and is likely the consequence of both impaired activity of lipoprotein lipase (a disposal defect) and the hepatic overproduction of very low density lipoproteins. If a fat meal has been ingested prior to the onset of ketoacidosis,

TABLE 338-4
Initial laboratory findings in diabetic ketoacidosis

Series	Dallas*	Los Angeles†	Washington‡
Age	38	36	43
Glucose, mg/100 ml	475	675	733
Sodium, mM	132	131	132
Potassium, mM	4.8	5.3	6.0
Bicarbonate, mM	< 10	6	10
BUN, mg/100 ml	25	32	42
Acetoacetate, mM	4.8	—	—
β-Hydroxybutyrate, mM	13.7	—	—
Free fatty acids, mM	2.1	—	2.3
Lactate, mM	4.6	—	—
Osmolarity, mosmol/liter	310	323	331

* *Eighty-eight consecutive episodes of ketoacidosis at Parkland Memorial Hospital (DW Foster, unpublished observations).*
† *Mean data from 308 episodes of nonfatal ketoacidosis (PM Beigelman, Diabetes 20:490, 1971).*
‡ *Mean data from 10 episodes of ketoacidosis (JE Gerich et al, Diabetes 20:228, 1971).*

chylomicrons may make up a major portion of the circulating fat. Lipemia is usually visible if triglyceride concentration is above 400 mg per 100 ml. True hyponatremia may also occur if the patient has vomited repeatedly and continued to drink water. Prerenal azotemia, reflecting volume depletion, is common but usually is modest in degree and completely reversible with treatment. The serum amylase may be elevated and frank pancreatitis can occur.

The diagnosis of ketoacidosis in a known diabetic is not difficult. Its appearance in a patient not previously known to have diabetes requires differentiation from the other common causes of metabolic acidosis with an anion gap: lactic acidosis, uremia, alcoholic ketoacidosis, and certain poisonings. The first step is to test the urine for glucose and ketones. If urine ketones are negative, another cause for the acidosis is likely. If positive, plasma examination is required to be certain that something more than starvation ketosis is present. Since quantitative determinations of acetoacetate and β-hydroxybutyrate are not routinely available, semiquantitative tests must be done using ketone reagent strips (Ketostix) or tablets (Acetest). If the latter are used, the tablet should be crushed and results read at 2 min. Serial dilutions of plasma can be made and tested. A strong test may occur in undiluted plasma owing to starvation alone; a strong reaction beyond 1:1 dilution is presumptive evidence for ketoacidosis. Apart from diabetes the only other common ketoacidotic state is alcoholic ketoacidosis. This syndrome, which by definition occurs in chronic alcoholics, usually follows a debauch, but the patient may not have had alcohol for 24 h or longer. It never occurs in the absence of starvation and frequently is associated with severe vomiting and abdominal pain. Pancreatitis is present in up to 75 percent of patients. A plasma glucose of less than 150 mg per 100 ml was found in three-fourths of reported cases and in 16 percent was less than 50 mg per 100 ml on arrival at the hospital. Hyperglycemia may occur but is usually mild and rarely, if ever, above 300 mg per 100 ml. Plasma-free fatty acid concentrations are much higher (mean 2.9 mM) than in normal starvation (range 0.7 to 1.0 mM), reaching levels seen in diabetic ketoacidosis. Presumably the liver is activated for ketogenesis by starvation in these patients and driven to maximal rates of ketone formation by the high fatty acid levels. Why some alcoholics mobilize fatty acids excessively is not known. In contrast to diabetic acidosis, the syndrome is rapidly reversible by the intravenous administration of glucose. As in all alcoholics given glucose, thiamine should be supplied to avoid precipitation of acute beriberi. (Other water-soluble vitamins, though not as critical, should also be infused.) Insulin is required only if hyperglycemia persists during therapy.

The treatment of diabetic ketoacidosis is controversial. All agree that insulin should be given, but the amount to be administered is at issue. "Low-dose insulin" schedules have become extremely popular in recent years. It is claimed that they produce less hypoglycemia and hypokalemia during treatment than standard forms of therapy. By "low-dose insulin" most authors mean 6 to 8 units per hour given intravenously as opposed to the 50 to 100 units per hour recommended previously. Most diabetic acidosis can be reversed adequately with low-dose treatment. A small fraction of patients, however, are insulin-resistant. This resistance is probably primarily due to insulin antibodies, although it can also be seen in patients who have never received insulin. The problem is that resistant subjects cannot be identified prospectively. For this reason it is probably preferable to treat ketoacidosis with 50 units of regular insulin intravenously hourly until the acidosis is reversed. There are no known toxic effects of larger insulin doses, since maximal physiologic response is obtained once insulin receptors are saturated regardless of how much insulin is given. The advantage of the higher dosage schedule is that it assures saturation of the receptors in the face of competing antibodies or other resistance factors. If physicians choose to use the low-dose insulin schedule, they should be alert to the possibility of resistance. Should acidosis persist unabated after several hours of treatment, larger amounts of insulin are clearly indicated. Ketoacidosis can also be adequately treated with intramuscular (but not subcutaneous) insulin.

Therapy of ketoacidosis requires intravenous fluids. The usual fluid deficit is 3 to 5 liters, and both salt solutions and free water are needed. One to two liters of isotonic saline or Ringer's lactate should be given rapidly intravenously on arrival, with additional amounts determined by urine output and clinical assessment of the fluid state. Five percent glucose solutions should be given when the plasma glucose falls to about 300 mg per 100 ml, both as a source of free water and as a prophylactic measure to prevent the late cerebral edema syndrome. The latter is a rare complication of ketoacidosis occurring most often in children. It is suspected when the patient remains comatose or lapses into coma following reversal of acidosis. The syndrome is probably related to osmotic disequilibrium between brain and plasma produced when plasma glucose concentrations are rapidly lowered.

Potassium replacement is always necessary, but the time of administration will vary. The initial potassium is often high despite a total body deficit because of the severe acidosis. In this case the cation will ordinarily not be needed until 3 to 4 h after initiation of therapy, when reversal of acidosis and the action of insulin cause a shift of K^+ into intracellular water. On the other hand if the admission value is normal or low, potassium should be given early, since plasma concentrations will fall rapidly during therapy, predisposing the patient to cardiac arrhythmias. In view of the known phosphate depletion of ketoacidosis it has been recommended that potassium be administered as the phosphate salt rather than as potassium chloride.

Bicarbonate therapy is indicated in severely acidotic patients (pH 7.0 or below) but is not used routinely in less acutely ill subjects since rapid alkalinization may have detrimental effects on oxygen delivery to tissues. The hemoglobin-oxygen dissociation curve is normal in diabetic ketoacidosis because of the opposing effects of acidosis and deficiency of red blood cell 2,3-diphosphoglycerate (2,3-DPG). If the acidosis is rapidly reversed, the deficiency of 2,3-DPG becomes manifest, increasing the avidity with which hemoglobin binds oxygen and impairing the release of oxygen in peripheral tissues. In a volume-depleted patient with poor tissue perfusion such a change theoretically could predispose to the development of lactic acidosis. If bicarbonate is given, the infusion should be stopped when the pH reaches 7.2 to minimize effects on oxygen binding by hemoglobin and to prevent metabolic alkalosis as circulating ketones are metabolized to bicarbonate with reversal of ketoacidosis.

In following the response to treatment, two points should be emphasized. (1) Plasma glucose essentially invariably falls more rapidly than plasma ketones. Insulin should not be stopped because glucose concentrations approach normal; rather, as mentioned, glucose should be infused and insulin continued until the ketosis has cleared. (2) Plasma ketone values as determined by nitroprusside reagent cannot be used to evaluate response to therapy. The testing materials measure acetoacetate and acetone but not β-hydroxybutyrate. Since β-hydroxybutyrate must be oxidized to acetoacetate prior to utilization, it is characteristic for the plasma ketones measured by nitroprusside to remain stable or even rise early in therapy at a time when total ketone concentration (acetoacetate plus β-hydroxybutyrate) is steadily falling. For this reason bicarbonate content and pH have to be assessed to evaluate reversal of the acidosis. Because β-hydroxybutyrate and acetoacetate represent a redox couple in equilibrium with mitochondrial NADH/NAD concentrations, vascular collapse or severe hypoxia may mask the presence of ketoacidosis as acetoacetate is reduced to β-hydroxybutyrate. Under these circumstances the β-hydroxybutyrate/acetoacetate ratio, normally about 3:1, may reach 7:1 or 8:1. Paradoxically, in such a situation, ketosis measured by Acetest tablet or Ketostix may seem to worsen as the patient gets better because of conversion of β-hydroxybutyrate to acetoacetate when the circulation is reestablished and tissue oxygenation is restored. A flow sheet outlining insulin given, fluid therapy, urine volume, and blood and urine chemistries should be meticulously maintained throughout the treatment. Without such a record therapy tends to become chaotic.

Most patients with diabetic ketoacidosis recover when properly treated. While mortality in large series is reported to be around 10 percent, the majority of deaths result from late complications rather than from ketoacidosis itself. The major causes are myocardial infarction and infection, particularly pneumonia. Poor prognostic signs on admission include hypotension, azotemia, deep coma, and associated illness.

Hyperosmolar coma Hyperosmolar nonketotic diabetic coma is usually a complication of maturity-onset diabetes. It is a syndrome of profound dehydration resulting from a sustained hyperglycemic diuresis occurring under circumstances in which the patient is unable to drink sufficient water to keep up with urinary fluid losses. Commonly an elderly diabetic—often living alone or in a nursing home—develops a stroke or infection, which worsens hyperglycemia and prevents adequate water intake. The full-blown syndrome probably does not occur until volume depletion has become severe enough to diminish urine output. Hyperosmolar coma has also been precipitated by therapeutic procedures such as peritoneal dialysis or hemodialysis, tube feeding of high protein formulas, high carbohydrate infusion loads, and the use of osmotic agents such as mannitol and urea. Phenytoin sodium, steroids, immunosuppressive agents, and diuretics have also been reported to initiate the illness.

The absence of ketoacidosis is important in the pathophysiology. When ketoacidosis occurs in an insulin-dependent diabetic, nausea, vomiting, and air hunger bring the patient to the physician before extreme dehydration can occur. Such a protective mechanism is not operative in the ketoacidosis-resistant, maturity-onset diabetic. Interestingly, hyperosmolar coma can occur in juvenile diabetic patients given sufficient insulin to prevent ketosis but not sufficient to control hyperglycemia. While rare, there are reports of the same patient presenting on one occasion with ketoacidosis and the next with hyperosmolar coma.

The reason for the absence of ketoacidosis in maturity-onset diabetics is not known. The hepatic ketogenic machinery is not impaired since the patients frequently have ketone concentrations in the starvation range (4 to 6 mM). Free fatty acid levels are much lower in hyperosmolar coma than in ketoacidosis, and it has been suggested that substrate deficiency limits ketone formation. That this is the sole mechanism seems unlikely since some patients with hyperosmolar coma have been found to have extremely high levels of free fatty acids in their plasma. More attractive is the possibility that insulin concentrations in the portal vein of maturity-onset diabetics are higher than those of juvenile subjects and prevent full activation of the hepatic carnitine acyltransferase system.

Clinically patients present with extreme hyperglycemia, hyperosmolality, and volume depletion, coupled with central nervous system signs ranging from clouded sensorium to coma. Seizure activity—sometimes Jacksonian in type—is not unusual, and transient hemiplegia may also be seen. Infections, particularly pneumonia and gram-negative sepsis, are common and indicate a grave prognosis. A high index of suspicion for

infection should be maintained, and routine culture of the blood and spinal fluid is indicated. Because of the extreme dehydration plasma viscosity is high, and widespread in situ thrombosis has been found at post mortem. Bleeding, probably the consequence of disseminated intravascular coagulation, has also been reported.

The laboratory findings in two large series are shown in Table 338-5. Plasma glucose is generally around 1000 mg per 100 ml, about twice the value seen in ketoacidosis. The serum osmolality is extremely high, but because of the hyperglycemia the absolute serum sodium concentration is often not elevated.[2] Prerenal azotemia with marked elevation of BUN and creatinine is characteristic. A mild metabolic acidosis is present, plasma bicarbonate on the average being about 20 meq per liter. The acidosis is due to a combination of starvation ketosis, retention of inorganic acids secondary to the azotemia, and modest elevation of plasma lactate, the latter the consequence of volume depletion. If the bicarbonate is less than 10 meq per liter and plasma ketones are not elevated, it can be assumed that lactic acidosis is present.

The mortality rate in hyperosmolar coma is very high ($>$ 50 percent). As a consequence immediate treatment is urgent. The most important measure is rapid administration of large amounts of intravenous fluids to reestablish the circulation and urine flow. The average fluid deficit is 10 liters. While free water will ultimately be needed, initial therapy should be with isotonic salt solutions, and 2 to 3 liters should be given over the first 1 to 2 h. Subsequently half-strength saline can be used. As the plasma glucose approaches normal levels, 5% dextrose can be given as a vehicle for free water. While hyperosmolar coma may be reversed by fluids alone, insulin should be given to control the hyperglycemia more rapidly. Many authors recommend small doses of insulin, but larger amounts may be necessary, particularly in the obese patient. It should be noted that potassium salts are usually required earlier in the treatment of hyperosmolar coma than in ketoacidosis because the intracellular shift of plasma K$^+$ during therapy is accelerated in the absence of acidosis. If lactic acidosis is present, sodium bicar-

---

[2] *Serum osmolality can be accurately estimated from the formula*

Serum osmolality (mosmol/liter)

$$= 2([Na^+] + [K^+]) + \frac{glucose\ (mg/100\ ml)}{18} + \frac{BUN\ (mg/100\ ml)}{2.8}$$

In practice the contribution of the BUN is often ignored since it contributes to total osmolality but does not reflect the free water deficit. There are situations in clinical medicine in which an increased osmolality is not equivalent to dehydration. Severe alcohol intoxication is the classic example, the ethanol itself providing the measured milliosmoles.

TABLE 338-5
Initial laboratory findings in hyperosmolar coma

Series	Brooklyn*	Washington†
Age	60	57
Glucose, mg/100 ml	1166	976
Sodium, mM	144	142
Potassium, mM	5	5
Chloride, mM	99	98
Bicarbonate, mM	17	22
BUN, mg/100 ml	87	65
Creatinine, mg/100 ml	5.5	—
Free fatty acids, mM	0.73	0.96
Osmolarity, mosmol/liter	384	374

* *Mean data from 33 episodes of hyperosmolar coma (AA Arieff, HJ Carroll, Medicine 51:73, 1972).*
† *Mean data from 20 episodes of hyperosmolar coma (JE Gerich et al, Diabetes 20:228, 1971).*

bonate should be given until tissue perfusion can be reestablished (see Chap. 339). Antibiotics are required if infection complicates the picture.

LATE COMPLICATIONS OF DIABETES The diabetic patient is, unfortunately, susceptible to a series of complications that lead to considerable morbidity and premature mortality. While some patients may never develop these problems and others note their onset early, on the average, symptoms develop 15 to 20 years following the appearance of overt hyperglycemia. A given patient may experience several complications simultaneously or a single problem may dominate the picture.

Circulatory abnormalities Arteriosclerosis of the type seen in nondiabetics is a common problem in diabetes and occurs more extensvely and earlier than in the general population. The cause for this accelerated atherosclerosis is not known, although it has been suggested that lower than normal levels of plasma high-density lipoprotein may play a role. Atherosclerotic lesions produce symptoms in a variety of sites. Peripheral deposits may cause intermittent claudication, gangrene, and, in men, organic impotence on a vascular basis. Surgical repair of large vessel lesions may be unsuccessful because of the simultaneous presence of widespread disease of the small vessels. Coronary artery disease and stroke are common. Silent myocardial infarction is known to occur in diabetics and should be suspected whenever symptoms of left ventricular failure appear suddenly. Diabetes may also be associated with the clinical picture of cardiomyopathy, in which heart failure occurs in the face of angiographically normal coronary arteries and the absence of other identifiable causes of heart disease.

Retinopathy Diabetic retinopathy is, or soon will be, the leading cause of blindness in the United States. On the other hand most diabetics never become blind. Retinopathic lesions are divided into two large categories, *simple* (background) and *proliferative* (Table 338-6). The earliest sign of retinal change is an increased capillary permeability that is evidenced by leakage of dye into the vitreous humor after fluorescein injection. Occlusion of retinal capillaries follows, with subsequent formation of saccular and fusiform aneurysms. Arteriovenous shunts also occur. The vascular lesions are accompanied by proliferation of lining endothelial cells and a loss of the pericytes that surround and support the vessels. Hemorrhages into the inner retinal areas appear dot-shaped, while bleeding into the more superficial nerve fiber layer causes flame-shaped, blot, or linear lesions. Preretinal hemorrhages characteristically have a boat-shaped appearance. Exudates are of two types. Cotton wool spots can be shown by angiography to be microinfarcts—non-

TABLE 338-6
Lesions of diabetic retinopathy

BACKGROUND

Increased capillary permeability
Capillary closure and dilatation
Microaneurysms
Arteriovenous shunts
Dilated veins
Hemorrhages (dot and blot)
Cotton wool spots
Hard exudates

PROLIFERATIVE

New vessels
Scar (retinitis proliferans)
Vitreal hemorrhage
Retinal detachment

TABLE 338-7
Frequency of diabetic retinopathy, percent

Duration of diabetes, years	Age at diagnosis		
	< 29 years	30–59 years	> 60 years
0–4	4	22	34
5–9	18	40	45
10–14	45	53	44
15–19	71	64	59
20–24	74	68	—
25–29	75	80	—
30+	73	90	—

SOURCE: *AF Burditt et al, Q J Med 37:303, 1968.*

perfused areas surrounded by a ring of dilated capillaries. A sudden increase in the number of cotton wool spots represents an ominous prognostic sign and may herald the appearance of rapidly advancing retinopathy. Hard exudates are much more common than cotton wool spots and probably represent leakage of protein and lipids from damaged capillaries.

The fundamental characteristics of proliferative retinopathy are new vessel formation and scarring. The stimulus for neovascularization is unknown, although it is believed that hypoxia secondary to capillary or arteriolar occlusion may be the primary cause. Two serious complications of proliferative retinopathy are vitreal hemorrhage and retinal detachment. A sudden loss of vision in one eye is almost always due to one or the other of these two lesions.

The frequency of diabetic retinopathy appears to vary with age of onset as well as duration of the disease (Table 338-7). Approximately 75 percent of patients first diagnosed below the age of 29 will eventually develop retinopathy, but some never develop ophthalmoscopically visible lesions even after 30 years of disease. Retinopathy appears to develop earlier in older patients. Proliferative retinopathy is much less common. It has been estimated that 10 to 18 percent of patients with simple retinopathy will progress to proliferative disease in a 10-year period. Visual prognosis in patients with and without retinopathy in one large series is shown in Table 338-8.

The treatment of choice for diabetic retinopathy is photocoagulation. Three types of light source are used. The xenon arc produces white light that is absorbed largely by the pigment epithelium and can destroy both intraretinal and surface new vessels. Its disadvantage is that without special equipment it cannot produce lesions smaller than 500 μm. The ruby laser gives monochromatic red light and can make smaller lesions. The argon laser produces green light that is absorbed preferentially by hemoglobin. It can coagulate a moving column of blood, makes small lesions (< 50 μm), and can be used to obliterate vessels extending into the retrovitreal space. The cooperative trial of the Diabetic Retinopathy Study Research Group, with an enrollment of 1700 patients, clearly showed that photocoagulation with either xenon arc or argon laser improved visual prognosis in diabetic retinopathy. All patients with neovascularization and hemorrhage should, therefore, be followed by an ophthalmologist trained in these techniques. Indications for treatment by photocoagulation include:

1 Moderate or severe new vessels on or within one disk diameter of the optic disk.
2 Mild new vessels on or within one disk diameter of the optic disk if fresh hemorrhage is present.
3 Moderate or severe new vessels elsewhere if fresh hemorrhage is present.

Complications of photocoagulation include vitreal hemorrhage, vitreal contraction with retinal detachment, macular edema, and visual field loss. Occasionally iritis and keratitis develop.

TABLE 338-8
Prognosis for vision in diabetes*

Group[†]	Good to impaired	Good to blind	Impaired to blind
Control	2.4	0.31	1.3
Retinopathy	7.5	3.0	13.1

* Numbers indicate the percentage of patients progressing to a worse level of vision per year.
† Control patients had no retinopathy when first examined. Control patients with impaired vision at entry had other eye problems. Good vision was defined as a visual acuity of 6/18 or better; impaired vision, acuities of 6/24 to 6/60; and blind, a visual acuity of less than 6/60. It should be noted that factors other than retinopathy contributed to visual loss in some patients (e.g., glaucoma).
SOURCE: Data adopted from FI Caird, CJ Garrett, Diabetes 12:389, 1963.

The role of pars plana vitrectomy in diabetic retinopathy is not yet certain because of the high incidence of postoperative complications and the difficulty of assessing residual retinal function prior to surgery. It will probably have a definite role in treatment of traction detachment of the retina and nonresolving vitreal hemorrhage.

Hypophysectomy, once widely used, is no longer recommended as a general procedure because photocoagulation is safer and equally or more effective. A rare exception might be the so-called "florid" diabetic retinopathy ("rapid, bleeding, blinding") in which widespread new vessel formation has occurred but no scar is present.

Diabetic nephropathy Renal disease is a common complication and a leading cause of death in diabetes. The pathology is complicated, with four types of lesions generally described: (1) glomerulosclerosis, (2) arteriolosclerosis of efferent and afferent arterioles, (3) arteriosclerosis of the renal artery and its intrarenal branches, and (4) peritubular deposits of glycogen, fat, and mucopolysaccharides. The glomerular lesions have received the most emphasis, probably because of their early description. Nodular glomerulosclerosis, the classical Kimmelstiel-Wilson lesion, consists of a periodic acid–Schiff (PAS) positive, rounded hyaline mass appearing near the periphery of the glomerulus. Nuclei may be embedded in the mass, and often a nonoccluded capillary runs over the surface. Diffuse glomerulosclerosis may also be present and represents thickening of the basement membrane of the capillaries. Subsequently the intercapillary or mesangial region also becomes thickened. Finally, an exudative lesion, acidophilic in staining characteristics, may develop. If located over a glomerular loop or attached to the inside of Bowman's capsule, it is called a "fibrin cap." All these changes are visible by light microscopy. Utilizing the electron microscope, thickening of capillary basement membranes in the glomerulus may be discernible before the other changes are seen. It has also been shown that glomerular and tubular basement membranes are lined with IgG and albumin in diabetic nephropathy. Whether these changes are primary or secondary has not yet been established.

There is no close correlation between histologic lesions and clinical renal disease: i.e., on biopsy the changes of diabetes may be seen in patients with apparently normal renal function. On the other hand if clinical renal disease is present, it can be assumed that the histologic architecture will be abnormal. Originally the term "Kimmelstiel-Wilson syndrome" referred to the presence of edema, hypertension, proteinuria, and renal failure in a diabetic patient. Many physicians now use the notation Kimmelstiel-Wilson disease loosely to refer to any manifestation of diabetic nephropathy, although this is both pathologically and clinically inexact. Diabetic renal disease is protean in its manifestations and may vary from a change in the renal threshold for glucose (such that glucosuria does not appear until plasma glucose is elevated considerably above the normal threshold value of 180 to 200 mg per 100 ml) to the insidious onset of hypertension or uremia. Proteinuria may or

may not be present, but the full-blown nephrotic syndrome is relatively rare. Early studies of diabetic nephropathy indicated that death followed the appearance of proteinuria after only 1 to 2 years. It is now known that heavy and persistent proteinuria (> 3 g per 24 h) is prognostically ominous but that patients with lesser degrees of protein loss may live for much longer periods—occasionally more than 10 years. A very high percentage of patients with nephropathy have simultaneous retinopathy, but many patients with retinopathy have no overt signs of renal disease.

The appearance of increasing insulin sensitivity may occasionally herald the presence of diabetic nephropathy. While insulin half-life is prolonged in renal failure, the precise mechanism for the increased sensitivity is not known. It appears to be more than a simple diminution of glycosuria secondary to the aforementioned change in renal threshold, since hyperglycemia also diminishes. Uremia affects the metabolism of glucagon and other hormones as well as altering hormone receptor function. It is probable, therefore, that increased insulin sensitivity is multifactorial in origin. Whatever the mechanism, it is frequently necessary to decrease insulin dosage in patients with nephropathy.

In the past, treatment of renal failure in the diabetic was limited to protein restriction, maintenance of fluid balance, and alkalinization to control the uremic acidosis. Renal transplantation and chronic dialysis are now commonly carried out. Originally it was thought that chronic dialysis in the diabetic was an ineffective long-term measure; however, this viewpoint is changing, and in a number of centers there is no hesitancy about entering a diabetic into a dialysis program. While it has been suggested that transplantation in the diabetic be undertaken at creatinine levels of around 6 mg per 100 ml in an attempt to preserve eyesight, the question of whether and when to do a transplant in the individual patient remains a difficult question. Careful consultation between the physician, nephrologist, and transplant surgeon is required.

Diabetic neuropathy Diabetic neuropathy may affect every part of the nervous system with the possible exception of the brain. While it is rarely a direct cause of death, it is a major cause of morbidity. Distinct syndromes can be recognized, and often several different types of neuropathy are present in the same patient. The most common picture is that of peripheral polyneuropathy. Usually bilateral, the symptoms include numbness, paresthesias, severe hyperesthesias, and pain. The pain, which may be deep-seated and very severe, is often worse at night. It is occasionally lancinating or lightning in type, resembling tabes dorsalis (pseudotabes). Fortunately extreme pain syndromes are usually self-limited, lasting from a few months to a few years. Involvement of proprioceptive fibers leads to abnormalities of gait and development of typical Charcot joints, particularly in the feet. Loss of arch with multiple fractures of tarsal bones is a common finding by x-ray. On physical examination absent stretch reflexes and loss of vibratory sense are frequent early signs. Diabetic neuropathy may also cause delay in return of the ankle reflex identical with the lesion seen in hypothyroidism. Mononeuropathy, though less common than polyneuropathy, may also occur. Characteristically there is a sudden wrist drop, foot drop, or paralysis of the third, fourth, or sixth cranial nerves. Other single nerves, including the recurrent laryngeal, have been reported to be involved. Mononeuropathy is characterized by a high degree of spontaneous reversibility, usually over a several-week period. Radiculopathy is a sensory syndrome in which pain occurs over the distribution of one or more spinal nerves, usually in the chest wall or abdomen. The severe pain may mimic herpes zoster or an acute surgical abdomen. Like mononeuropathy, the lesion is usually self-limited. *Autonomic neuropathy* may present in a variety of ways. The gastrointestinal tract is a prime target, and there may be esophageal dysfunction with difficulty in swallowing, delayed gastric emptying, or diarrhea. The latter is often nocturnal. Patients may suffer from orthostatic hypotension and frank syncope. Cardiorespiratory arrest and sudden death, thought to be due solely to autonomic neuropathy, have also been reported. Bladder dysfunction or paralysis is particularly distressing and often leads to the necessity of chronic catheter drainage. Impotence and retrograde ejaculation are additional manifestations in the male. Diabetic *amyotrophy* is likely a form of neuropathy, although atrophy and weakness of the large muscles in the upper leg and pelvic girdle resemble primary muscle disease.

The cause of diabetic neuropathy is unknown. Biochemical changes have been demonstrated in the nerves of animals with experimental diabetes, but their relation to human neuropathy is uncertain. Considerable interest has focused on the fact that a neuropathy can be induced in rats made diabetic with streptozotocin which exhibits prolonged conduction times similar to those seen in human diabetes. The involved nerves were found to have a marked decrease in myoinositol content that could be reversed either by insulin treatment or by feeding myoinositol. Whether a similar defect exists in the neuropathy of humans remains to be seen.

Treatment of diabetic neuropathy is unsatisfactory in most respects. When pain is severe, it is easy for the patient to become habituated or addicted to narcotics or nonnarcotic analgesics. If the pain requires something more powerful than aspirin or acetaminophen, codeine is the drug of choice. Phenytoin sodium is believed to be useful by some physicians, but others have not found it very helpful. Carbamazepine, another anticonvulsant, may benefit some patients. The usual dose is 200 mg three times daily. Combination therapy with amitriptyline and fluphenazine hydrochloride has been reported to cause dramatic relief of pain over a several-day period. The recommended dosage is 75 mg amitriptyline at bedtime and 1 mg fluphenazine three times a day. The long-term effectiveness of this treatment is not yet known. Mononeuropathies and radiculopathies usually require no specific therapy since they are self-limited. Diabetic diarrhea often responds to treatment with diphenoxylate and atropine or loperamide. Orthostatic hypotension is best treated by having the patient sleep with the head of the bed elevated, avoidance of sudden assumption of the upright position, and the use of full-length elastic stockings. Occasionally volume expansion with fludrocortisone acetate is required as in other forms of orthostatic hypotension.

Diabetic foot ulcers A special problem in the diabetic is the development of ulcers of the feet and lower extremities. The ulcers appear to be primarily due to abnormal pressure distribution secondary to diabetic neuropathy. The problem is accentuated when there is bony distortion in the feet. Callus formation is usually the initial abnormality. Alternatively the ulcer may be initiated by ill-fitting shoes which cause blister formation in patients whose sensory deficits preclude recognition of pain. Cuts and punctures from foreign bodies such as needles, tacks, and glass are common, and frequently a foreign body of which the patient is completely unaware will be found in the soft tissue. For this reason all patients with ulcers should have x-rays made of the feet. Vascular disease with diminished blood supply contributes to development of the lesion, and infection is common, often with multiple organisms. While no specific therapy is available for diabetic ulcers, aggressive supportive treatment can often lead to salvation of the leg without

amputation. One approach is to simply put the patient to bed using frequent foot soaks and debridement to remove nonviable tissue. Others recommend casting the leg with plaster in order to remove weight bearing and protect the lesion.

All diabetics should be instructed about proper foot care in an attempt to prevent ulcers. Feet should be kept clean and dry at all times. Patients with neuropathy should not be allowed to walk barefoot, even in the home. Properly fitted shoes are essential. This is a particular problem with women, since an adequate shoe for the diabetic is not often stylish. The feet should be carefully inspected daily for callus, infection, abrasions, or blisters and the physician consulted for any potentially troublesome lesion.

THE QUESTION OF CONTROL AND THE DEVELOPMENT OF COMPLICATIONS The critical question in diabetic therapy is whether hyperglycemia causes or accelerates the development of the long-term complications just discussed. No definitive answer is available. Four lines of evidence favor a direct relationship. (1) If arteries from a normal animal are placed in media containing high glucose concentrations, water content is increased, a barrier to oxygen diffusion develops, and lactic acid is produced, suggesting tissue hypoxia. Identical findings are observed in aortas taken from diabetic animals. These changes can be reversed simply by lowering the ambient glucose concentration. (2) As mentioned above, a form of neuropathy exists in the diabetic rat that is reversed by lowering the blood glucose. Even if the lesion is not identical with human neuropathy, the fact that it is reversible by insulin therapy is strong evidence that metabolic abnormalities can cause nerve disease. (3) Diabetic subjects have a two- to threefold elevation in hemoglobin A_{1c}, a fast-migrating minor hemoglobin that is present in normal persons at a concentration of 3 to 6 percent. It has the same amino acid sequence as hemoglobin A but has as the NH_2 terminus of the β chain, 1-deoxy-1-(N-valyl)fructose. The importance of hemoglobin A_{1c} resides in the fact that it is glycosylated nonenzymatically. Its concentration appears to reflect (roughly) the mean level of circulating glucose for the preceding several weeks. The elevated concentration of hemoglobin A_{1c} in diabetics can be reversed by adequate insulin treatment. Since hemoglobin can be altered chemically by hyperglycemia, it has been speculated that a similar mechanism might operate in other sites—such as the basement membranes—to cause or accelerate the development of late complications. (4) The most persuasive piece of evidence is that kidneys from donors who have neither diabetes nor a family history of diabetes develop characteristic lesions of diabetic nephropathy within 3 to 5 years after transplantation into a diabetic recipient. However, the development of these lesions does not appear to correlate well with the degree of hyperglycemia. It is conceivable, therefore, that a factor present in the diabetic environment but distinct from hyperglycemia causes the change. One possibility would be revascularization of the transplanted kidney with vessels from the recipient.

Evidence against a causal relationship between hyperglycemia and complications can be summarized briefly as follows. (1) Despite many claims to the contrary, it has never been possible to show a close correlation between the degree of diabetic control and the development of complications. This argument becomes less impressive when it is considered that only a tiny fraction of patients achieve normalization of the blood sugar throughout the day. In the ordinary patient "tight" control, even with multiple insulin injections, is an unattainable ideal. (2) There are many reports in the literature of patients who already have diabetic complications at the time of diagnosis; i.e., a young person presents with ketoacidosis and is found to have retinopathy. It is traditional to say that perhaps mild elevation of the plasma glucose was present and unrecognized for many years. The biochemical lesions in the artery and the nerve described above, on the other hand, require major, not mild, elevations of the plasma glucose. The same is true for activation of the polyol pathway that converts glucose to sorbitol. (Sorbitol is thought by some to be a cytotoxic metabolite in diabetes.) The apparent K_m for glucose in all these reactions is in the range of 300 to 400 mg per 100 ml. No biochemical defect has ever been demonstrated with slight elevations of glucose either in vivo or in vitro, although rates of synthesis of hemoglobin A_{1c} seem to be linearly related to glucose levels in plasma. (3) A number of patients who have no demonstrable glucose intolerance but who are the offspring of two overtly diabetic parents have thickening of the muscle capillary basement membrane by electron microscopy. This lesion has been the subject of considerable controversy, but there is general agreement that a high percentage of adult diabetics with either juvenile or maturity-onset diabetes have the abnormality. Since it appears to be a characteristic part of the microangiopathy of diabetes, the fact that it may appear prior to the onset of metabolic abnormalities has been interpreted to suggest that complications and metabolic control may develop independently.

On balance it must be concluded that a causal relationship between hyperglycemia and development of complications can neither be proved nor disproved from the available data. Since it is essentially impossible to normalize the plasma glucose in diabetic subjects by current techniques, final answers must await the development of an effective artificial external pancreas or successful pancreatic transplantation. In the meantime it would appear prudent to maintain the plasma glucose as near normal as possible in all diabetic patients. About this there appears to be no disagreement. The only question is whether aggressive insulin therapy should be pushed routinely to the point of overt hypoglycemia. As discussed earlier, if sufficient insulin is given to control postprandial hyperglycemia, too much insulin is available between meals. As a consequence hypoglycemia is common in aggressively treated patients. A mild insulin reaction consisting of nervousness, tremor, hunger, and sweating that is rapidly interrupted by carbohydrate intake is probably not harmful except for the possibility of worsening diabetic control via the Somogyi reaction. Unfortunately, as stated, many diabetics, particularly those with long-standing disease and autonomic neuropathy, do not have or do not recognize the usual warning signals and progress to altered central nervous system function with abnormal behavior, loss of consciousness, or even convulsions. The latter reactions are dangerous for both patient and society. Every effort should be made to control hyperglycemia, but the limit of therapy should be the appearance of hypoglycemic reactions. It does not seem wise to induce a condition that can cause immediate and irreversible damage to a patient in the unproved hope that late complications might be prevented.

INSULIN RESISTANCE Insulin resistance in the diabetic is arbitrarily said to exist when more than 200 units per day are required to control hyperglycemia and prevent ketosis. Relative insulin resistance is present with much lower insulin requirements, but therapy for the resistant state is usually not considered necessary below the 200-unit level. Insulin antibodies of IgG type are present in essentially all diabetics within 60 days of the initiation of insulin therapy. The titer of these antibodies fluctuates for reasons that are not clear. Although the correlation between antibody titer and functional resistance is not close, it is presumed that insulin binding by high levels of antibody is the primary mechanism in most cases. Probably less than 0.1 percent of insulin-treated diabetics ever have functionally significant resistance. The problem may appear within a few weeks of the start of therapy or many years later. The onset may be abrupt, resulting in ketoacidosis, but usually is gradual, with uncontrollable hyperglycemia being the major

problem. About 20 to 30 percent of patients have concomitant insulin allergy. Therapy of the syndrome requires prednisone in large amounts—80 to 100 mg per day initially. Response often occurs in 48 to 72 h, but may take longer. If no improvement has resulted after 3 to 4 weeks it can be assumed that steroids will not be effective. Once insulin requirements begin to fall, prednisone dosage can be rapidly decreased by 10 to 20 mg every 3 to 7 days until a maintenance level of 5 to 10 mg per day is reached. These levels may be required for many months. Whether remission has occurred, allowing cessation of therapy, can only be determined by trial.

Insulin resistance may be seen in diseases other than diabetes. The physiological consequences can be minor or severe. A variety of insulin-resistant syndromes are associated with *acanthosis nigricans,* a brown to black, velvety hyperpigmentation of the skin in the axilla, groin, neck, umbilicus, and other areas. Although acanthosis nigricans may be a sign of occult malignancy, it is not associated with neoplasia in the insulin-resistant states. A classification of insulin resistance based on the absence or presence of acanthosis nigricans is given in Table 338-9. *Obesity* and *antibodies* to insulin are by far the most common causes of insulin resistance, and neither is accompanied by acanthosis. Obesity is associated with diminished insulin receptor number and affinity but also has postreceptor hormone resistance. *Werner's syndrome* is an autosomal recessive illness with a high incidence of hyperglycemia despite elevated concentrations of plasma insulin. There is little response to exogenous hormone. Other features include growth retardation, alopecia or premature graying of the hair, cataracts, hypogonadism, leg ulcers, atrophy of muscle, fat, and bone, soft-tissue calcification, and a high frequency of sarcomas and meningiomas.

Of the rare conditions associated with acanthosis nigricans, women with *insulin receptor abnormalities* have attracted the greatest interest. Type A patients are tall young females with a tendency to hirsutism and abnormalities of the reproductive tract who most probably have polycystic ovaries. The absolute number of insulin receptors is markedly diminished. Type B subjects are older women with evidence of immunologic disease. The clinical picture includes arthralgias, alopecia, enlarged salivary glands, proteinuria, leukopenia, and antinuclear and anti-DNA antibodies. Insulin resistance in these patients is due to blocking antibodies to the insulin receptor (not to insulin itself). Both A and B patients have high plasma insulin concentrations.

Generalized and *partial lipodystrophies* are fat depletion syndromes differing primarily in the extent of fat atrophy. In the generalized form essentially all body fat is missing, while the more common partial type exhibits atrophy of fat in the face and trunk with normal or increased adiposity in the lower half

TABLE 338-9
Insulin-resistant states

I Insulin resistance without acanthosis nigricans
  A Obesity
  B Diabetes mellitus with insulin antibodies
  C Werner's syndrome
II Insulin resistance with acanthosis nigricans
  A Insulin resistance with receptor abnormality
    1 Receptor deficiency (type A abnormality)
    2 Antibody to insulin receptor (type B abnormality)
  B Lipodystrophic states
    1 Generalized lipodystrophy (congenital or acquired)
    2 Partial lipodystrophy (congenital or acquired)
  C Syndrome of familial insulin resistance, somatic abnormalities, and pineal hyperplasia
  D The Alström syndrome
  E Ataxia telangiectasia

of the body. The disease can be either congenital or acquired. Typically the patients develop hyperglycemia at puberty, but ketoacidosis never occurs. Marked hypertriglyceridemia with eruptive xanthoma is a frequent feature. Characteristically present are hepatomegaly, splenomegaly, cardiomegaly, hirsutism, lymphadenopathy, hypertrophy of the external genitalia, varicose veins, and (in the congenital forms) muscle hypertrophy. Mental retardation is common and renal disease may develop. A "diabetogenic" peptide has been found in the urine, but its role is not clear. The term "lipoatrophic diabetes" is synonymous with total lipodystrophy. All patients have elevated plasma insulin levels.

The *pineal hypertrophy syndrome* is characterized by insulin resistance, early dentition with malformed teeth, dry skin, thick nails, hirsutism, and a peculiar sexual precocity with enlargement of the external genitalia. The latter may reach near adult size by age 3 or 4. The insulin resistance is severe and ketoacidosis may occur despite high endogenous insulin levels. The *Alström syndrome* is a rare autosomal recessive disease characterized by childhood blindness due to retinal degeneration, nerve deafness, vasopressin-resistant diabetes insipidus, and, in males, hypogonadism with high plasma gonadotropin levels. The patients thus appear to have multiple end organ resistance to hormones. Other features include baldness, hyperuricemia, hypertriglyceridemia, and amino aciduria. Superficially the patients may resemble subjects with the Lawrence-Moon-Biedl syndrome but can be differentiated on initial exam by the absence of polydactyly and mental deficiency. Insulin resistance in the Alström syndrome is mild. *Ataxia telangiectasia* is characterized by cerebellar ataxia, telangiectasia, and a variety of abnormalities in the immune system in addition to insulin resistance. Not listed in Table 338-9 is insulin resistance due to hormone excess (acromegaly, Cushing's syndrome) or myotonic dystrophy. While demonstrable experimentally, the insulin resistance in these conditions is not clinically significant.

INSULIN ALLERGY Insulin allergy is due to IgE antibodies to insulin. Manifestations include immediate reactions with local stinging or itching, delayed local reactions with brawny swelling lasting up to 30 h, and generalized urticaria or frank anaphylaxis. Systemic reactions are usually seen in patients who have stopped insulin therapy for one reason or another and have then resumed treatment. The allergic reaction may occur as early as the second injection on resumption of therapy. Mild reactions can be treated with antihistamines. If the problem is severe, desensitization procedures are required. A 1-day insulin desensitization procedure is shown in Table 338-10. Once the

TABLE 338-10
Insulin desensitization*

Time, h	Dose, units	Route
0	0.001	Intradermal
0.5	0.002	Intradermal
1	0.004	Subcutaneous
1.5	0.01	Subcutaneous
2	0.02	Subcutaneous
2.5	0.04	Subcutaneous
3	0.1	Subcutaneous
3.5	0.2	Subcutaneous
4	0.5	Subcutaneous
4.5	1	Subcutaneous
5	2	Subcutaneous
5.5	4	Subcutaneous
6	8	Subcutaneous

* *Following desensitization, use 2 to 10 units of regular insulin every 4 to 6 h for 24 to 36 h after the 6-h injection before switching to intermediate-acting insulin.*
SOURCE: *Schedule of JA Galloway. For detailed information see JA Galloway, R Bressler, Med Clin North Amer 62:663, 1978.*

patient is desensitized, insulin therapy should not be interrupted.

MISCELLANEOUS ABNORMALITIES Diabetes affects almost every system in the body. Space limitations preclude detailed discussion of all associated features, but several deserve comment. *Hypertriglyceridemia* is common and in the majority of cases is secondary to insulin deficiency. The defect is thought to be in the peripheral disposal of triglycerides secondary to decreased lipoprotein lipase activity. Synthesis of the lipase is insulin-dependent. A number of diabetics continue to exhibit hyperlipemia even when diabetic control is adequate, and family studies have suggested that these subjects have a primary familial hyperlipoproteinemia which is independent of diabetes. Clofibrate appears to be the drug of choice for treatment of patients who are unresponsive to diet and insulin therapy.

Some diabetics have been found to have *recurrent hyperkalemia* in association with hyperglycemia. Such patients have low plasma renin activity and hypoaldosteronism, which may be due to renin deficiency and/or a defect in the aldosterone biosynthetic pathway. An inactive precursor of renin ("big renin") is often found in the plasma. In the absence of aldosterone, renal secretion of potassium is impaired and disposal of a potassium load is dependent on insulin-mediated transport of the cation into the intracellular space. Administration of potassium salts or triamterene to such patients may be dangerous. Whether potassium transport is directly stimulated by insulin or is secondary to glucose movement is not clear.

A variety of skin lesions occur in diabetes. *Necrobiosis lipoidica diabeticorum* is a plaque-like lesion with a central yellowish area surrounded by a brownish border. It is usually found over the anterior surfaces of the legs. Ulceration may occur. *Diabetic dermopathy* is also usually located over the anterior tibial surface. The lesions are small rounded plaques with a raised border which may crust at the edges and ulcerate centrally. Several plaques may be arranged in linear fashion. Pigmentation is not prominent early, but as the lesion heals a depressed scar occurs with diffuse brown discoloration. A rarer abnormality is *bullosis diabeticorum*. The bullae may be superficial with clear serum or may be mildly hemorrhagic. The cause is unknown. *Infestations of the skin* with *Candida* and dermatophytes are common, and bacterial infections of a variety of types occur. In women *vaginal moniliasis* may be troublesome during hyperglycemic-glycosuric periods. While the symptoms respond to nystatin, recurrence is inevitable unless glycosuria is reversed. In difficult cases intravaginal gentian violet therapy may be required. *Atrophy of adipose tissue* may occur at the site of insulin injections. The lipoatrophy is said to respond to injection of monocomponent insulin into the atrophic area.

Hyperviscosity occurs in diabetes and *platelets aggregate abnormally*. The latter may be caused by increased prostaglandin synthesis. *Impaired leukocyte function* is also present and may contribute to increased severity of infection in diabetes. *Wound healing* is impaired in experimental diabetes but probably is not a major factor clinically.

THE EMOTIONAL RESPONSE TO DIABETES Acceptance of the fact that a person has a chronic disease which requires a complete change in life-style is always difficult. This is particularly true in the case of diabetes since patients generally are aware that they are vulnerable to late complications and that statistically their life expectancy is shortened. It is not surprising that the emotional response to diabetes often hampers treatment. On the one hand the primary reaction may be denial with an accompanying refusal to cooperate. At the other extreme is excessive preoccupation with the illness. The physician should make every effort to define a middle ground wherein the patient acknowledges his or her disease and responds to it prudently without becoming obsessed by it. The goal is to live with diabetes not for it. Diabetics are no different from other patients in that they may attempt to use their disease manipulatively with both family and physician. The problems are particularly acute with children and adolescents. While the psychiatric aspects of diabetes are not discussed here, most problems can be anticipated and handled if common sense is coupled with sympathy and firmness.

REFERENCES

Diabetes mellitus

BLOOM ME et al: Insulin-induced posthypoglycemic hyperglycemia as a cause of "brittle" diabetes. Clinical clues and therapeutic implications. Am J Med 47:891, 1969

CAHILL GF et al: "Control" and diabetes. N Engl J Med 294:1004, 1976

ELLENBERG M: Diabetic neuropathy: Clinical aspects. Metabolism 25:1627, 1976

FOSTER DW: Insulin deficiency and hyperosmolar coma. Adv Intern Med 19:159, 1974

GABBAY KH et al: Glycosylated hemoglobins and long-term blood glucose control in diabetes mellitus. J Clin Endocrinol Metab 44:859, 1977

GENUTH SM et al: Community screening for diabetes by blood glucose measurement. Results of a five-year experience. Diabetes 25:1110, 1976

KJELLSTRAND CM et al: Renal transplantation in patients with insulin-dependent diabetes. Lancet 2:4, 1973

KREISBERG RA: Diabetic ketoacidosis: New concepts and trends in pathogenesis and treatment. Ann Intern Med 88:681, 1978

McGARRY JD, FOSTER DW: Hormonal control of ketogenesis. Biochemical considerations. Arch Intern Med 137:495, 1977

——— et al: A possible role for malonyl-CoA in the regulation of hepatic fatty acid oxidation and ketogenesis. J Clin Invest 60:265, 1977

O'SULLIVAN JB, MAHAN CM: Prospective study of 352 young patients with chemical diabetes. N Engl J Med 278:1038, 1968

PADILLA AJ, LOEB JN: "Low-dose" versus "high-dose" insulin regimens in the management of uncontrolled diabetes. A survey. Am J Med 63:843, 1977

PALMBERG PF: Diabetic retinopathy. Diabetes 26:703, 1977

RASKIN P: Diabetic regulation and its relation to microangiopathy. Metabolism 27:235, 1978

ROTTER JI, RIMOIN DL: Heterogeneity in diabetes mellitus—update, 1978. Evidence for further genetic heterogeneity with juvenile-onset insulin-dependent diabetes mellitus. Diabetes 27:599, 1978

SHIPP JC et al: Insulin resistance: Clinical features, natural course and effects of adrenal steroid treatment. Medicine 44:165, 1965

SIPERSTEIN MD: The glucose tolerance test: A pitfall in the diagnosis of diabetes mellitus. Adv Intern Med 20:297, 1975

——— et al: Control of blood glucose and diabetic vascular disease. N Engl J Med 296:1060, 1977

UNGER RH: Role of glucagon in diabetes. Arch Intern Med 137:482, 1977

YOON J-W et al: Virus-induced diabetes mellitus. N Engl J Med 300:1173, 1979

Insulin resistance

BAR RS et al: Extreme insulin resistance in ataxia telangiectasia. Defect in affinity of insulin receptors. N Engl J Med 298:1164, 1978

EPSTEIN et al: Werner's syndrome. A review of its symptomatology, natural history, pathologic features, genetics and relationship to the aging process. Medicine 45:177, 1966

FLIER JS et al: Receptors, antireceptor antibodies and mechanisms of insulin resistance. N Eng J Med 300:413, 1979

GOLDSTEIN JL, FIALKLOW PJ: The Alström syndrome. Medicine 52:53, 1973

SEIP M: Generalized lipodystrophy. Ergeb Inn Med Kinderheilkd 31:59, 1971

WEST RJ et al: Familial insulin resistant diabetes, multiple somatic anomalies and pineal hyperplasia. Arch Dis Child 50:703, 1975

339
LACTIC ACIDOSIS

DANIEL W. FOSTER

Lactic acidosis is a common condition in clinical medicine. This follows from the fact that lactic acid is produced at accelerated rates in skeletal muscle and other tissues whenever oxygenation is inadequate to supply energy needs. Thus lactic acidosis represents a kind of final common pathway for any disease resulting in circulatory collapse or hypoxemia. Lactic acidosis can also occur under circumstances in which tissue hypoxia is not apparent. In most cases an etiology can be established, but in some patients a diagnosis of "idiopathic" lactic acidosis has to be made.

BIOCHEMICAL BACKGROUND In the narrowest sense biological life can be defined as the capacity to generate high-energy phosphate bonds within the cell. Adenosine triphosphate (ATP) is the most important high-energy compound, but other nucleotides, such as guanosine triphosphate, also play important roles. Structure and function of every tissue in the body is directly or indirectly dependent on ATP or equivalent high-energy nucleotides. During tissue hypoxia ATP cannot be generated in adequate amounts and lactic acidosis results. The acidosis is the metabolic consequence of activation of a back-up system for the generation of ATP when the primary energy-forming pathway is impaired. The normal mechanism of ATP generation under aerobic conditions is shown in Fig. 339-1. When substrates such as free fatty acids or glucose are oxidized to acetyl CoA, the constituent hydrogen atoms are transferred to nicotinamide adenine dinucleotide (NAD), producing the reduced form of the pyridine nucleotide (NADH). Oxidation of acetyl CoA to CO_2 in the Krebs cycle generates additional NADH. The bulk of NADH is formed intramitochondrially, since fatty acid oxidizing and tricarboxylic acid cycle enzymes are mitochondrial proteins; cytosolic NADH must be transported into the mitochondria by "shuttle" systems because NADH cannot directly penetrate the inner mitochondrial membrane. In the presence of oxygen, NADH is oxidized by the electron transport chain, the end product being water ("metabolic water"). For each mole of NADH passing

FIGURE 339-1

Schematic view of aerobic metabolism. Subcellular compartments are not indicated. Glycolysis occurs in the cytosol while enzymes of fatty acid oxidation and the Krebs cycle are located intramitochondrially. The dotted line indicates that glycogenolysis and glycolysis are inactive in the presence of oxygen. (See text.)

through the cytochrome sequence 2 to 3 mol ATP is formed. When oxygen content of tissues is normal and ATP stores are high, rates of glycogen breakdown and glucose oxidation are low (the *Pasteur effect*). It is believed that control of glycolysis is primarily vested in the enzyme phosphofructokinase (PFK). As shown in Fig. 339-2, this enzyme catalyzes the conversion of fructose 6-phosphate to fructose 1,6-diphosphate. Its activity is rapidly accelerated under conditions of tissue hypoxia. Regulatory mechanisms for PFK are complicated and a number of allosteric modulators are known. ATP is likely the primary physiological inhibitor, while ADP, AMP, inorganic phosphate, and fructose 1,6-diphosphate all have activating capacity. Other modulators (e.g., citrate, creatine phosphate, NH_4^+, fructose diphosphatase) probably play secondary roles.

The sequence of events occurring during tissue hypoxia is schematically shown in Fig. 339-3. If blood flow to peripheral tissues is diminished such that oxygen delivery is insufficient to meet metabolic demands, electron flow through the transport chain is impaired or blocked (all cytochromes become reduced). Because of the block, NADH, which for a finite period continues to be generated, cannot be oxidized, resulting in high NADH/NAD ratios in both mitochondrial and cytosolic compartments. As a result all near-equilibrium reactions utilizing NADH as cofactor shift to the reduced side (e.g., oxaloacetate → malate, pyruvate → lactate), slowing substrate flux at a number of critical sites. In addition, ATP cannot be generated and tissue ATP concentrations fall. There is a reciprocal rise in ADP and AMP. As a result, phosphofructokinase is activated, with rapid glycogen breakdown and glucose oxidation. Accelerated glycolysis leads to overproduction of pyruvic acid, which, because of the elevated NADH content of the cell, is reduced to lactic acid. Put simply, the acidosis of tissue hypoxia is due to the conversion of neutral substrate, glycogen-glucose, to a strong acid, pyruvate. It is a lactic acidosis because the high NADH/NAD ratio drives the lactic dehydrogenase reaction to the right. These points are shown schematically in Fig. 339-4.

Lactate is produced in significant quantities even in the fully oxygenated subject by a variety of tissues. This lactate passes to the liver, where it enters the gluconeogenic pathway for conversion to glucose (*Cori cycle*). Since the intact organism can rapidly dispose of large lactate loads, it has been suggested that impairment of lactate uptake by the liver is critical for the development of lactic acidosis. Diminished lactate uptake undoubtedly plays a significant role in pathogenesis, (especially in patients with vascular collapse, severe hepatocellular disease, or enzymic defects in the gluconeogenic pathway), but significant acidosis probably never occurs in the absence of peripheral overproduction. Whether lactate over-

FIGURE 339-3

Schematic view of anaerobic metabolism. Diagonally striped boxes indicate metabolic blocks secondary to failure of delivery of oxygen to tissues and high NADH/NAD ratios. Heavy arrows indicate accelerated glycogenolysis, glycolysis, and lactate production. Glycolysis is permitted to continue in the face of high NADH/NAD ratios in the cytosol because one molecule of NAD (required in the glyceraldehyde 3-phosphate dehydrogenase reaction) is produced for each molecule of lactate formed.

production in lactic acidosis is generalized or limited to specific tissues such as muscle and intestine is not resolved.

The accelerated glycolysis of hypoxia, as noted above, can be considered as an alternative system for the generation of ATP when the normal mitochondrial mechanism is impaired. The glycolytic system is not efficient, however. A mole of glucose derived from glycogen and oxidized completely through the Krebs cycle will generate about 37 mol ATP, while the yield from glycogen to pyruvate is only 3 mol. Nevertheless, over the short run, this ATP may be life-saving.

CLINICAL PICTURE Lactic acidosis is usually heralded by the onset of nausea, vomiting, restlessness, and driven respiration of the Kussmaul type. Stupor or coma is sometimes seen. Huckabee, who in 1961 brought the problem of lactic acidosis to the attention of clinicians in a careful analysis of 37 patients, recognized that there were two major groups of patients with elevated lactate concentrations in the blood. The first had proportionate increases of lactate and pyruvate and were not considered to be hypoxic. The second group had lactate levels disproportionately elevated when compared with the simultaneously measured pyruvate concentration. Huckabee coined the term "excess lactate" for any increase in lactate that could not be accounted for by a rise in pyruvate concentration and interpreted its presence to mean tissue hypoxia (a high NADH/NAD ratio). The relationship of the lactate/pyruvate concentration to the NADH/NAD ratio is obvious when the lactate dehydrogenase reaction is rearranged:

$$\text{Pyruvate} + \text{NADH} + \text{H}^+ \rightleftharpoons \text{lactate} + \text{NAD}^+ \quad (1)$$

$$K \times \frac{[\text{NADH}][\text{H}^+]}{[\text{NAD}^+]} = \frac{[\text{lactate}]}{[\text{pyruvate}]} \quad (2)$$

A sample calculation of "excess lactate" is given in Fig. 339-5.

The mean level of lactate in venous blood normally is about 1 mM (range 0.6 to 1.5 mM), while the pyruvate concentration is ordinarily about 0.1 mM (range 0.05 to 0.15 mM).[1] Accurately determined lactate/pyruvate ratios above 10 to 15 usu-

FIGURE 339-2

Phosphofructokinase and glycolysis. The minus sign indicates inhibition; the plus sign, activation. (See text.)

---

[1] *Measurement of lactate and pyruvate requires precautions. The sample should be iced and red blood cells (which produce lactate) separated immediately.*

FIGURE 339-4

Summary of biochemical mechanisms in lactic acidosis.

ally mean some degree of hypoxia. In practice pyruvate measurements are often not done because instability and low concentrations make assays difficult. As a consequence "excess lactate" is now rarely quantitated. The concept was seminal, however, in providing the insight that led to current understanding of the pathophysiology of lactic acidosis.

Cohen and Woods have suggested a classification of lactic acidosis based on clinical findings rather than the lactate/pyruvate ratio (Table 339-1). Type A lactic acidosis is associated with evidence of or a reason for poor tissue perfusion or oxygenation. Most patients with lactic acidosis fall into this category. Vascular collapse is the most common cause of lactic acidosis, and any condition leading to shock (e.g., myocardial infarction, pulmonary embolism, hemorrhage, septicemia, poisoning) can produce the illness. Hypoxemia does not have to be present. Importantly, diminished tissue perfusion may be present in the absence of a measurable fall in the blood pressure. Lactic acidosis occurs physiologically whenever muscular exercise sufficient to contract an oxygen debt is carried out. The pathologic counterpart is lactic acidosis produced by convulsions or hypothermia with prolonged shivering. All type A patients have "excess lactate" in the Huckabee terminology.

Type B patients have elevated blood lactate concentrations when no reason for diminished tissue perfusion is apparent. Acidosis may be absent, mild, or severe. Proportionate elevations of pyruvate and lactate may be seen, but high lactate/pyruvate ratios are essentially always present when acidosis is severe. Systemic clinical disorders associated with elevations of blood lactate include diabetic ketoacidosis, severe liver disease, leukemia, thiamine deficiency, and metabolic or respiratory alkalosis. Lactic acidosis has been commonly reported with biguanide therapy of diabetes, and because of this, phenformin was removed from clinical use in the United States by the Food and Drug Administration. The syndrome has also been seen with nitroprusside therapy of hypertension, with epineph-

rine overdosage and in isolated instances with many other drug intoxications. Most of the latter are doubtless associated with hypoxemia or shock and rightfully belong in the type A category. Ethanol has been considered to be the drug most commonly involved in causing lactic acidosis. The oxidation of ethanol by the liver results in the generation of high NADH/NAD ratios in the cell and presumably blocks the recycling of lactate (and alanine) to glucose. Infants with enzyme defects in the glycolytic-gluconeogenic-tricarboxylic acid pathway appear to be peculiarly vulnerable to lactic acidosis, and early death is common. Chronic lactic acidosis has been noted in certain primary myopathies of unknown etiology. If no primary cause can be found, a diagnosis of idiopathic lactic acidosis has to be made.

The pathophysiology of lactate accumulation in type B disease is varied and often incompletely understood. The enzyme defects and alcohol may have diminished hepatic uptake of lactate as the primary mechanism. In other cases, particularly those labeled idiopathic and those with myopathy, subtle mitochondrial disease resulting in functional tissue hypoxia is likely operative. Drugs may also act by the latter mechanism. Hormones such as glucagon and epinephrine raise lactate by stimulating glycolysis. Leukemia probably acts both by direct overproduction of lactate in the white cell mass and through increased blood viscosity that diminishes capillary perfusion. It is likely that most chronic type B conditions cause only mild to moderate hyperlactatemia in themselves and that an additional insult is required for acidosis to develop. The latter might include infection, dehydration, volume depletion, starvation, or unusual exertion. The effect of such an insult would be to add a mild inadequacy of tissue perfusion (insufficient to qualify as type A disease) to the primary abnormality and in combination to cause frank acidosis.

DIAGNOSIS The diagnosis of lactic acidosis requires that a significant metabolic acidosis be present and that the measured lactate concentration be sufficient to account for the bulk of the decrease in plasma bicarbonate content. In general the ar-

FIGURE 339-5

The concept of excess lactate. The symbols L_t and P_t indicate plasma concentrations of lactate and pyruvate, respectively, in the patient. L_n and P_n refer to mean values in normal subjects.

$$XL = (L_t \cdot L_n) - (P_t \cdot P_n) \cdot \frac{L_n}{P_n}$$

	Pyruvate	Lactate
Normal	0.1 mM	1.0 mM
Patient	0.3 mM	11.0 mM

$$XL = (11 \text{-} 1) - (0.3 \text{-} 0.1) \frac{1.0}{0.1} = 8 \text{ mM}$$

TABLE 339-1
Some causes of hyperlactatemia

A Hyperlactatemia with hypoxia
  1 Strenuous muscle exercise (convulsions, hypothermia)
  2 Inadequate tissue perfusion or oxygenation of any cause*
B Hyperlactatemia without apparent hypoxia
  1 Systemic clinical disorders
    a Alkalosis (respiratory or metabolic)
    b Uncontrolled diabetes mellitus
    c Leukemia, lymphoma, other cancers
    d Severe liver disease
    e Thiamine deficiency
  2 Drugs, hormones, toxins
    a Phenformin and other biguanides
    b Salicylates
    c Sodium nitroprusside
    d Ethanol
    e Epinephrine, glucagon
    f Fructose, sorbitol
  3 Enzyme defects
    a Glucose 6-phosphatase
    b Fructose 1,6-diphosphatase
    c Pyruvate carboxylase
    d Pyruvate dehydrogenase
    e Unclassified tricarboxylic acid defect
  4 Certain primary myopathies
  5 Idiopathic

* *The most common causes of perfusion-oxygenation defects are myocardial infarction, sepsis, hemorrhage, volume depletion, pulmonary embolism, and heart failure. Hypoxemia due to severe pulmonary disease, chronic anemia, carbon monoxide inhalation, and cyanide poisoning are much less frequent.*
SOURCE: *After Cohen and Woods.*

terial pH will be less than 7.2 and the plasma lactate concentration greater than 12 mM. Unfortunately, the literature contains many case reports of "lactic acidosis" in which plasma lactate concentrations are only modestly elevated (3 to 6 mM) and pH values are near normal. There are many causes of elevated plasma lactate levels, but the term *lactic acidosis* should be reserved for situations in which acidosis actually exists. Confusion also occurs when severe acidosis is present but lactate concentrations do not account for the decrement of bicarbonate (i.e., a mixed acidosis is present). In diabetic keto-acidosis, for example, lactate concentrations of 3 to 6 mM are frequently seen, but acetoacetate and β-hydroxybutyrate are primarily responsible for the low pH.

Lactic acidosis should be suspected whenever a metabolic acidosis is associated with an "anion gap" in the absence of an explanation for the unmeasured anions. The anion gap can be calculated in several ways, the simplest of which is $[Na^+] - ([Cl^-] + [HCO_3^-])$. The normal range is 8 to 16 mM per liter, with the mean about 12. The four most common causes of metabolic acidosis with anion gap are diabetic or alcoholic ketoacidosis, uremic acidosis, lactic acidosis, and acidosis associated with toxin ingestion (salicylates, methanol, ethylene glycol, paraldehyde). Thus if ketoacidosis and uremia are not present and there is nothing to suggest a poisoning, the chances are good that a metabolic acidosis with significant anion gap is due to lactic acid.

TREATMENT   If lactic acidosis is caused by shock or hypoxemia, reversal of the primary condition will cure the secondary acidosis. Persistent acidosis requires that large amounts of sodium bicarbonate be infused intravenously. Bicarbonate should be given in quantities sufficient to raise the pH to about 7.2. This often necessitates the rapid infusion of several hundred to a thousand millimoles over only a few hours. Full restoration of pH is not desirable since a rebound alkalosis will occur when production of lactic acid ceases and circulating lactate is metabolized to bicarbonate. In view of the large quantities required, straight bicarbonate infusions should be used. A near isotonic solution can be prepared by adding three 50-ml vials of bicarbonate (1 mmol/ml) to 850 ml sterile distilled water. Hypertonic (5%) solutions are also commercially available and may be required in certain cases.

Because large volumes of bicarbonate are required in the treatment of lactic acidosis, the problem of fluid overload often arises, especially in elderly patients and subjects with impaired renal function. Diuretics should be routinely given with vigorous alkali therapy after it is clear that any volume deficits have been repaired. Occasionally peritoneal dialysis or hemodialysis with hypertonic solutions may be required to prevent pulmonary edema. Dialysis is not indicated as a treatment of lactic acidosis per se.

Other forms of therapy such as the administration of glucose and insulin or redox dyes have been tried but are of little use. An experimental drug, dichloroacetate, appears to be helpful in some nonhypoxic forms of lactic acidosis in animals. Since dichloroacetate causes a polyneuropathy when given chronically and produces abnormalities of oxalate metabolism, its efficacy in human lactic acidosis will likely not be subject to test.

REFERENCES

ALBERTI KGMM, NATTRASS M: Lactic acidosis. Lancet 2:25, 1977

COHEN RD, WOODS HF: *Clinical and Biochemical Aspects of Lactic Acidosis.* Oxford, Blackwell Scientific Publications, 1976

HUCKABEE WE: Abnormal resting blood lactate. Am J Med 30:833, 840, 1961

OH MS, CARROLL HJ: The anion gap. N Engl J Med 297:814, 1977

340

HYPOGLYCEMIA, INSULINOMA, AND OTHER HORMONE-SECRETING TUMORS OF THE PANCREAS

DANIEL W. FOSTER
ARTHUR H. RUBENSTEIN

Maintenance of the plasma glucose concentration within relatively narrow bounds appears to be a fundamental characteristic of the intact organism. Hypoglycemia represents a high-risk metabolic abnormality (in the short run greater than hyperglycemia) because glucose is the primary energy substrate of the brain. Its absence, like that of oxygen, produces deranged function, tissue damage, or even death if the deficit is prolonged. The peculiar vulnerability of the brain to hypoglycemia resides in the fact that it cannot utilize circulating free fatty acids as an energy source in contrast to almost every other tissue of the body. Short-chain derivatives of the free fatty acids, acetoacetic and β-hydroxybutyric acids (the "ketone bodies"), are efficiently oxidized and can protect the central nervous system from damage by hypoglycemia when present at moderate concentrations in plasma. However, the development of ketosis requires a number of hours in humans. Accelerated ketogenesis is not, therefore, an effective protective mechanism against hypoglycemia occurring acutely over minutes or even several hours. Preservation of central nervous system function in the early phases of fasting or during hypoglycemia thus requires increased production of glucose by the liver. At the same time glucose utilization in other tissues must be diminished by provision of free fatty acids as alternative substrate. These adaptive mechanisms (Chap. 86) are hormonally controlled and, under ordinary circumstances, are extremely effective. Occasionally, however, the system breaks down or is overwhelmed, resulting in the clinical syndrome of hypoglycemia. In the past, hypoglycemia (apart from insulin reactions in the diabetic) was not a common problem in the practice of internal medicine. In recent years, however, the diagnosis of postprandial hypoglycemia has been made with great frequency. For this reason, familiarity with hypoglycemic syndromes is imperative.

SYMPTOMATOLOGY OF HYPOGLYCEMIA   Symptoms of hypoglycemia fall into two main categories: those induced by an excessive secretion of epinephrine and those due to dysfunction of the central nervous system. When plasma glucose concentrations approach the hypoglycemic range, "counterregulatory" hormones are released which cause glycogen breakdown, initiate gluconeogenesis, mobilize free fatty acids, and induce ketogenesis. The four hormones involved are epinephrine, glucagon, cortisol, and growth hormone. It seems probable that it is only epinephrine that produces recognizable symptoms. If epinephrine release is rapid, the patient may experience sweating, tremor, tachycardia, anxiety, and hunger. Central nervous system symptoms include dizziness, headache, clouding of vision, blunted mental acuity, confusion, abnormal behavior, convulsions, and loss of consciousness. When the onset of hypoglycemia is gradual, as in most forms of organic disease, central nervous system symptoms predominate, and the epinephrine phase may not be recognizable. With more rapid drops in plasma glucose (as in insulin reactions), adrenergic symptoms are the prominent complaint. In the diabetic adrenergic symptoms may not be manifest if severe neuropathy is present.

CLASSIFICATION   It has been traditional to classify hypoglycemia as either *postprandial* (reactive) or *fasting*. Pathologically

TABLE 340-1
Causes of postprandial (reactive) hypoglycemia

I Alimentary hyperinsulinism
II Hereditary fructose intolerance
III Galactosemia
IV Leucine sensitivity
V Idiopathic
  A True hypoglycemia
  B Nonhypoglycemia

low plasma glucose concentrations occur in the former only in response to meals, while in the latter fasting for a few to many hours is necessary to demonstrate the abnormality. Patients with fasting hypoglycemia (particularly insulinomas) may also exhibit a reactive component, but reactive patients do not have symptoms when food is withdrawn. Fasting hypoglycemia usually means that an identifiable disease process is associated with the lowered plasma glucose, but symptoms suggestive of postprandial hypoglycemia are often found in the absence of organic disease.

CAUSES OF HYPOGLYCEMIA **Postprandial hypoglycemia** Some causes of postprandial hypoglycemia are shown in Table 340-1. The most common category is alimentary. Patients who have undergone gastrectomy, gastrojejunostomy, pyloroplasty, or even vagotomy are subject to hypoglycemia following meals, presumably because of rapid gastric emptying with brisk absorption of glucose and excessive insulin release. Glucose concentrations fall more rapidly than insulin under these circumstances and the resulting insulin-glucose imbalance leads to hypoglycemia. True alimentary hypoglycemia may apparently occur in the absence of gastrointestinal surgery, but this is rare. Ingestion of fructose or galactose induces hypoglycemia in children with fructose intolerance (Chap. 99) and galactosemia (Chap. 98), respectively. Leucine intake has been reported to cause the syndrome in susceptible infants in the absence of insulinoma, but the phenomenon is extremely rare. Diabetes mellitus in its early phase is almost always listed as a cause of reactive hypoglycemia. In our experience symptomatic hypoglycemia as a premonitory symptom of diabetes is uncommon if it exists at all. Prediabetics, who by definition have normal glucose tolerance, may have a late fall in plasma glucose after oral glucose tolerance testing, but this does not mean hypoglycemia. In fact, this pattern is similar to that frequently present in asymptomatic, healthy individuals.

It is well known that the diagnosis of idiopathic reactive hypoglycemia has reached epidemic proportions in this country. The peculiarity of the syndrome is that hypoglycemia either cannot be demonstrated at all or is present only after a prolonged glucose tolerance test at a time which does not correspond to the spontaneously occurring symptomatic episodes. Moreover, low blood sugars cannot be documented after usual meals, which, of course, do not contain 100 g of rapidly absorbable carbohydrate. The term *nonhypoglycemia* has been coined to differentiate this syndrome from the occasional case of true idiopathic reactive hypoglycemia in which spontaneous symptomatic episodes are reproducibly accompanied by low plasma glucose levels. Most patients with nonhypoglycemia have adrenergic discharge and epinephrine symptoms suggestive of hypoglycemia because of anxiety and stress. Commonly the symptoms are relieved by food. The patient then seeks medical advice and a 5-h glucose tolerance test is performed. If the plasma glucose falls to below "normal" levels, a diagnosis of hypoglycemia is made. The problem of interpretation of the long glucose tolerance test is discussed below. In summary, it is safe to say that the vast majority of patients with nonhypoglycemia have the symptoms of epinephrine discharge, but that the epinephrine discharge is not due to hypoglycemia.

Fasting hypoglycemia The causes of fasting hypoglycemia are many. Basically glucopenia can occur for two reasons: either the liver is not producing enough glucose to meet ordinary tissue demands, or peripheral utilization becomes so great that maximal hepatic production is insufficient to match glucose egress from the plasma compartment. A classification of fasting hypoglycemia based on the underproduction or overutilization of glucose is given in Table 340-2. It should be recognized that in certain conditions, particularly hyperinsulinism, both underproduction and overutilization are operative. From a clinical standpoint the following simple rule applies: if more than 200 g intravenous glucose is required to prevent hypoglycemia in a 24-h period, overutilization of glucose is present. This follows from the fact that hepatic glucose output in a normal fasting humans is between 100 and 200 g per day and is sufficient to prevent hypoglycemia in the absence of food.[1] The demonstration of overutilization is important because it sharply narrows the diagnostic possibilities. If glucose demand is less than 200 g per day no decision about mechanism can be made, and the cause of the hypoglycemia may fall in either category.

UNDERPRODUCTION OF GLUCOSE As discussed in Chap. 86, the production of glucose by the liver initially involves the breakdown of stored glycogen and subsequently depends on gluconeogenesis, the synthesis of glucose from precursors delivered to the liver from peripheral tissues. The causes of inadequate production of glucose during fasting can be grouped into five general categories: (1) hormone deficiencies, (2) spe-

---

[1] *Much more than 200 g glucose can be disposed of by normal humans without developing hyperglycemia. Therefore, the rule is valid only if large quantities of glucose are required to avoid hypoglycemia, i.e., if plasma glucose falls below fasting levels and continues at a low concentration despite the infusion of 200 g glucose per day.*

TABLE 340-2
Major causes of fasting hypoglycemia

I Conditions primarily due to underproduction of glucose
  A Hormone deficiencies
    1 Hypopituitarism
    2 Adrenal insufficiency
    3 Catecholamine deficiency
    4 Glucagon deficiency
  B Enzyme defects
    1 Glucose 6-phosphatase
    2 Liver phosphorylase
    3 Pyruvate carboxylase
    4 Phosphoenolpyruvate carboxykinase
    5 Fructose 1,6-diphosphatase
    6 Glycogen synthetase
  C Substrate deficiency
    1 Ketotic hypoglycemia of infancy
    2 Severe malnutrition, muscle wasting(?)
    3 Late pregnancy(?)
  D Acquired liver disease
    1 Hepatic congestion
    2 Severe hepatitis
    3 Cirrhosis
  E Drugs
    1 Alcohol
    2 Propranolol
    3 Salicylates
II Conditions primarily due to overutilization of glucose
  A Hyperinsulinism
    1 Insulinoma
    2 Exogenous insulin
    3 Sulfonylureas
    4 Immune disease with insulin antibodies
  B Appropriate insulin levels
    1 Extrapancreatic tumors
    2 Carnitine deficiency
    3 Cachexia with fat depletion

cific defects in glycogenolytic or gluconeogenic enzymes, (3) inadequate substrate delivery, (4) acquired liver disease, and (5) drugs. Hypopituitarism and adrenal insufficiency are the most common of the hormone deficiency states causing hypoglycemia. Defects in catecholamine or glucagon release are rare. Enzymic abnormalities causing hypoglycemia are generally seen in children and not adults. Glucose 6-phosphatase deficiency is the classic example of a defect in glycogen breakdown, but hypoglycemia may occur in young children with deficiencies of hepatic glycogen phosphorylase and possibly also in other forms of glycogen storage disease (Chap. 97). The inability to make glycogen because of inadequate glycogen synthetase activity also renders the infant susceptible to fasting hypoglycemia. In addition to glucose 6-phosphatase, three other enzymes are specifically involved in gluconeogenesis: pyruvate carboxylase, phosphoenolpyruvate carboxykinase and fructose 1,6-diphosphatase (Fig. 340-1). Hypoglycemia has been reported in association with decreased activities of each of these enzymes, often in association with lactic acidosis. Substrate deficiency appears to be one of the mechanisms operative in ketotic hypoglycemia of infancy, since alanine turnover in such patients is low. Inadequate substrate supply may also contribute to the rare instances of hypoglycemia seen in malnutrition, muscle wasting states, chronic renal failure, and late pregnancy. Acquired liver disease can cause serious glucopenia. Hepatic congestion due to right-sided heart failure appears to be particularly troublesome, but severe viral hepatitis or cirrhosis may also cause symptomatic lowering of the plasma glucose.

A number of drugs have been implicated in hypoglycemia. By far the most common, apart from insulin and sulfonylureas, is alcohol. Alcohol only induces hypoglycemia after a period of fasting sufficient to deplete liver glycogen stores. In this circumstance hepatic glucose production is dependent on gluconeogenesis. The oxidation of ethanol in the liver is accompanied by generation of high concentrations of NADH in the cytosol of the cell. The increased NADH/NAD ratio diverts oxaloacetate into malate formation, diminishing its availability to the gluconeogenic sequence via the action of phosphoenolpyruvate carboxykinase (Fig. 340-1). The normal pathway of gluconeogenesis from pyruvate is thus blocked, leading to a drop in hepatic glucose output and hypoglycemia. It is important to recognize that large amounts of ethanol are not required to produce this syndrome and that plasma alcohol concentrations may be as low as 25 mg per 100 ml at the time symptoms occur. Ethanol-induced hypoglycemia usually occurs in adults, but is also seen in children who drink alcohol unknowingly. Salicylates (in children) and propranolol are the next most frequently involved drugs. Propranolol presumably causes difficulty in fasting patients or insulin-requiring diabetics by impairing the glycogenolytic response. In diabetes the drug may also prevent recognition of impending hypoglycemia by blunting the symptomatic response to epinephrine release. Many other drugs have been reported to cause hypoglycemia in isolated cases, but the relationship is often unproved.

OVERUTILIZATION OF GLUCOSE   Overutilization of glucose occurs in two settings. In the first, hyperinsulinism is present, while in the second plasma insulin concentrations are low. There are basically four causes of hyperinsulinemic hypoglycemia: insulinoma, exogenous insulin administration, sulfonylureas, and a peculiar form of insulin autoimmunity. Hypoglycemia occurring in a diabetic patient taking prescribed insulin or oral agents is not a diagnostic problem. The difficulty comes when a patient induces hypoglycemia deliberately and surreptitiously for psychiatric reasons, raising the possibility of an insulin-producing tumor. The differential diagnosis between insulinoma and factitious hypoglycemia is considered below. Rarely hypoglycemia with hyperinsulinism occurs with autoimmune disease and antibodies to endogenous insulin. The pathogenesis of this syndrome is unknown.

Hypoglycemia in the context of glucose overutilization and appropriately low plasma insulin concentrations occurs in two situations. The first is in association with solid extrapancreatic tumors, usually of large size. The most common are of mesothelial origin and include a variety of fibromas and sarcomas. The syndrome can also be seen with hepatomas, carcinomas of the gastrointestinal tract, and adrenal cancers. The mechanism of the hypoglycemia is not clear, although high levels of "nonsuppressible insulin-like activity" may play a role in some patients.

The second category is less well defined but appears to occur in situations in which free fatty acids are not available for oxidation in muscle and other tissues. About one-third of patients with systemic carnitine deficiency have had hypoglycemia, sometimes very severe. In the absence of free fatty acids and their hepatic oxidation products, acetoacetate and β-hydroxybutyric acids, it is presumed that all tissues (not just the central nervous system) become glucose-dependent. The increased demand for glucose exceeds the hepatic capacity for production and results in hypoglycemia. The authors have also seen several cases of hypoglycemia in patients with cachexia due to advanced cancer. At autopsy no recognizable triglyceride stores were present in adipose tissue, suggesting free fatty acid deficiency as the primary mechanism.

Theoretically patients with defects in the carnitine palmitoyltransferase system of enzymes, which is responsible for transport of long-chain fatty acids into the mitochondria (see Chap. 338), should also be vulnerable to fasting hypoglycemia by the same general mechanism. However, reported cases have not shown decreased glucose concentrations. Some patients apparently have a defect only in muscle and thus would be protected during fasting by ketones produced in the liver. Alternatively, since carnitine palmitoyltransferase deficiency appears to lead to symptoms primarily with exercise (causing myoglobinuria), it is possible that in vivo sufficient enzyme is

FIGURE 340-1

Simplified scheme of hepatic carbohydrate metabolism. Only the sequence for gluconeogenesis, glycogen synthesis, and glycogenolysis is shown.

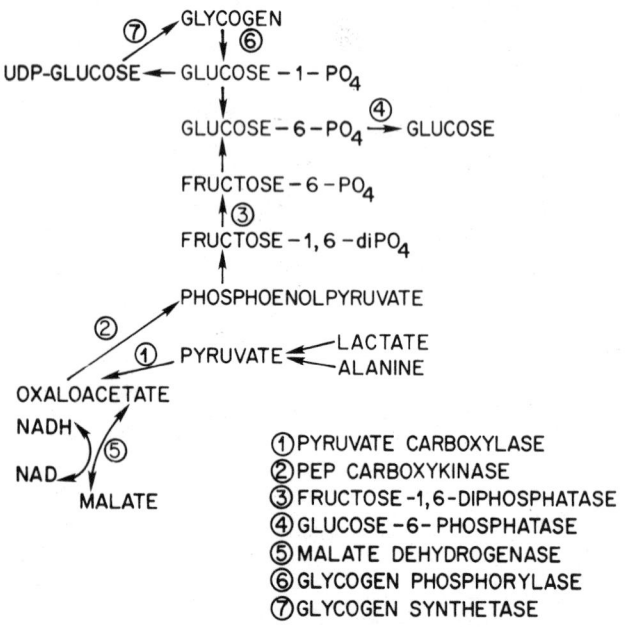

present to handle fatty acid transport in the basal state despite the low or nondetectable levels that are found when tissues are assayed in vitro.

DIAGNOSIS **Fasting hypoglycemia** If a nondiabetic presents at the emergency room or physician's office with symptoms suggestive of hypoglycemia—particularly if confusion, loss of consciousness, or convulsions are present—the single most important rule is to draw blood for simultaneous determinations of plasma glucose and insulin before intravenous glucose is administered, since the critical diagnostic issue will be the presence or absence of hyperinsulinism. Plasma cortisol should be determined at the same time. Once the patient has become alert, it is important to take a detailed history and carry out a thorough physical examination. Special emphasis should be placed on food intake in the preceding 24 h and the possibility of drug ingestion. Signs of heart failure and hepatic congestion should be sought and the presence and thickness of the adipose tissue mass should be noted. Pigmentation of the skin may suggest Addison's disease. Routine workup includes liver function studies, intravenous pyelography, and abdominal sonography (to look for solid tumors in the retroperitoneal space or abdominal cavity). Patients with enzyme defects and rarer hormonal deficiencies (epinephrine, glucagon) usually require evaluation in referral centers, since definitive assays for these hormones and enzymes are not routinely available. For reasons cited above it is important to quantitate the amount of glucose required to prevent recurrent hypoglycemia during acute phase therapy.

If the patient has a history compatible with hypoglycemia but does not have symptoms at the time of examination, hospitalization for fasting is generally required. The fast should be carried out for at least 72 h unless symptoms develop. Plasma glucose, insulin, and cortisol should be measured every 6 h. Occasionally quantitation of plasma free fatty acids, glucagon, and total ketones is helpful. Two points are at issue. First, does the patient have fasting hypoglycemia? And second, is the hypoglycemia associated with hyperinsulinism? Neither question is easy to answer. There is no definitive lower limit of plasma glucose which will unequivocally define pathologic hypoglycemia. The mean minimal level of glucose attained during a 72-h fast in one recent study is shown in Table 340-3. It is clear that women develop lower levels than men. Another series reported mean minimal levels of 62 mg per 100 ml in men and 52 mg per 100 ml in women during a 72-h fast. However, values as low as 22 mg per 100 ml have been found in apparently normal women without symptoms. On balance, a presumptive diagnosis of hypoglycemia is probably justified if the plasma glucose falls below 50 mg per 100 ml in men and 40 mg per 100 ml in women at any time during the fast, provided typical symptoms are induced. If symptoms are not produced, the diagnosis should be made with caution.

In interpreting plasma insulin concentrations it is important to remember that absolute values are not very helpful. In normal subjects when glucose concentrations rise, insulin levels also increase and when plasma glucose concentrations fall, insulin release is inhibited. This means that plasma insulin concentrations must be interpreted in the light of the simultaneously determined glucose value. Thus, a "normal" absolute insulin level may be abnormal in the face of hypoglycemia, while high absolute levels may be appropriate if the glucose concentration is elevated. In an attempt to relate the two parameters the concept of the insulin/glucose ratio

$$\frac{\text{Plasma insulin } (\mu\text{U/ml})}{\text{Plasma glucose } (\text{mg}/100 \text{ ml})}$$

was developed. In normal persons the ratio is always less than 0.4, while most (but not all) patients with insulinoma have ratios greater than 0.4—often above 1.0. It is known that patients with insulinoma may secrete insulin episodically; the ratio may, therefore, be normal on one occasion and abnormal on another. Multiple sampling is required. A helpful observation is that the insulin/glucose ratio tends to fall during fasting in normal individuals but increases in patients with insulinoma.

A great deal of experimental work in vitro indicates that pancreatic insulin release ceases when the glucose concentration is decreased much below 90 mg per 100 ml, and it is likely that the same holds in vivo. Adam, King, and Schwartz infused glucose at different rates into normal subjects and measured the plasma insulin concentration when a steady state had been reached. Using their data, a plot of the plasma insulin versus the plasma glucose concentration gives a straight line with the relationship expressed by the following equation:

$$y = 0.41x - 34$$

where y is the plasma insulin in microunits per milliliter and x is the plasma glucose in milligrams per 100 ml. The intercept on the x axis is 83 mg per 100 ml, indicating that plasma insulin concentration should be functionally zero (background for the assay) at this level of plasma glucose. While other studies have shown lower cutoff points, it is probably safe to say that any significant insulin concentration (> 5 to $6 \mu\text{U/ml}$) should be considered suspicious if the plasma glucose is below 50 mg per 100 ml in men or 40 mg per 100 ml in women, regardless of the value of the insulin/glucose ratio. This conclusion was also reached in a study of 60 patients with insulinoma at the Mayo Clinic. If hyperinsulinism is not demonstrated, one of the other causes of fasting hypoglycemia must be sought.

If hypoglycemia does not develop during fasting, an insulinoma- or other hypoglycemia-producing organic disease is highly unlikely, although one insulinoma responsive only to glucose loading has been reported. Some authors recommend provocative tests with tolubutamide, glucagon, or leucine in

TABLE 340-3
Plasma glucose and insulin during fasting

Test	Subjects	Hours of fast				
		0*	24	36	48	72
Glucose, mg/100 ml	Men	85 ± 1.5	83 ± 3.6	78 ± 3.4	78 ± 3.3	71 ± 2.4
	Women	83 ± 1.3	63 ± 1.6	50 ± 1.7	46 ± 1.7	48 ± 1.4
Insulin, μU/ml	Men	14 ± 0.9	9 ± 0.8	8 ± 1.1	8 ± 0.9	6 ± 0.7
	Women	12 ± 0.8	6 ± 0.4	4 ± 0.5	3 ± 0.4	4 ± 0.5

* *Zero values obtained after overnight fast. Results represent means ± SEM for 20 normal men and 60 normal women.*
SOURCE: *TJ Merimee, JE Tyson, Diabetes 26:161, 1977.*

suspected islet cell tumors, but overlap between normals and patients with insulinoma is so great as to render the tests of little value in a given individual.

Postprandial hypoglycemia In patients presumed to have postprandial hypoglycemia the most widely used test has been a 5-h oral glucose tolerance examination. The level of plasma glucose considered to be abnormal during the second to fifth hour is controversial. A value of 50 mg per 100 ml has been suggested, but it is clear that many apparently normal subjects will reach lower levels. The only unequivocal diagnostic test is the demonstration of a low plasma glucose concentration (less than 50 mg per 100 ml) during spontaneously developed symptoms. Patients with nonhypoglycemia (anxiety) usually have slightly elevated glucose concentrations during attacks because of the hyperglycemic actions of epinephrine and cortisol, the stress hormones that have induced the symptoms.

Insulinoma versus factitious hypoglycemia The self-induction of hypoglycemia by the injection of insulin or the ingestion of sulfonylureas is so common as to equal or exceed the incidence of insulinoma. The demonstration of hyperinsulinism during hypoglycemia cannot, therefore, be taken as definitive evidence of the presence of an islet cell tumor. Factitious disease should always be suspected when hypoglycemic symptoms appear in medical personnel or families of diabetics. Several additional laboratory tests are helpful once hyperinsulinism has been diagnosed. Patients with insulinoma tend to have high concentrations of proinsulin in plasma ($>$ 20% of total insulin). Plasma proinsulin is not elevated by the administration of commercial insulin preparations or sulfonylureas. Measurement of the insulin connecting peptide (C peptide) will indicate whether the insulin circulating in plasma is of endogenous or exogenous origin. When insulin is cleaved from its precursor proinsulin molecule, C peptide is released into the portal vein in a 1:1 ratio with insulin. Thus, patients with insulinoma should have high C-peptide concentrations which parallel the plasma insulin values. The characteristic pattern in factitious hypoglycemia due to insulin injection would be a high circulating level of insulin with relatively suppressed C-peptide values. Antibodies to insulin are helpful if present since they usually indicate chronic insulin injection. Unfortunately sulfonylureas also elevate both the C-peptide and insulin concentrations in plasma. Therefore, factitious hypoglycemia due to oral agents can only be diagnosed by a high index of suspicion coupled with measurement of the drug in plasma or urine. The differential characteristics of insulinoma and the two types of factitious hypoglycemia are shown in Table 340-4.

TABLE 340-4
Differential diagnosis of insulinoma and factitious hyperinsulinism

Test	Insulinoma	Exogenous insulin	Sulfonylurea
Plasma insulin	High	Very high*	High
Insulin/glucose ratio	High	Very high	High
Proinsulin	Increased	Normal or low	Normal
C peptide	Increased	Normal or low†	Increased
Insulin antibodies	Absent	± Present‡	Absent
Plasma or urine sulfonylurea	Absent	Absent	Present

* *Total plasma insulin in patients with insulinoma is rarely above 200 μU/ml in the basal state and often much lower. Values greater than 1000 μU/ml are highly suggestive of exogenous insulin injection.*
† *C peptide may be normal in absolute terms, but low in relation to the increased insulin value.*
‡ *Insulin antibodies may not be present if only a few injections have been given, especially with purified insulins.*

TREATMENT The initial treatment of serious hypoglycemia (producing confusion or coma) is the intravenous administration of a bolus of 25 or 50 g glucose as a 50% solution followed by constant infusion of glucose until the patient is able to eat a meal. The importance of the meal resides in the fact that hepatic glycogen repletion is not effective with intravenous glucose. Patients in the overutilization category may require large quantities of intravenous glucose, and rates of delivery sufficient to cause mild glycosuria should be given. It is not enough to infuse 5% dextrose at a rate of 1 to 2 ml/min and assume the patient is protected (20 to 30% dextrose solutions may be required in some cases). Intravenous glucose can usually be stopped once the patient has eaten, but this can only be determined by trial. Adrenergic reactions without central nervous system abnormalities can be treated with oral carbohydrate and do not require parenteral therapy.

It is important to note that hypoglycemia from sulfonylureas may last for prolonged periods (days), particularly with chlorpropamide (Fig. 340-2). It is common experience to have a patient lapse back into coma if glucose infusions are stopped too soon. The reason for the prolonged effect is not always clear, though drug interactions, hepatic disease, and renal failure may play a role in some cases.

Surgery is the treatment of choice for insulinoma. Arteriography (celiac or superior mesenteric) should be done prior to exploration in an attempt to localize the lesion. In some centers preoperative or operative sampling of insulin concentrations by selective pancreatic vein catheterization has been helpful. If the tumor cannot be palpated in the pancreas or located in an extrapancreatic site at the time of surgery, stepwise pancreatectomy (from tail to head) should be carried out with frozen sections made of sequential slices. Frequent plasma samples should be drawn for immediate measurement of glucose and subsequent assay for insulin. A sudden rise in plasma glucose may indicate removal of the tumor. In general resection is stopped with an 85 percent pancreatectomy, even if the tumor is not found, in order to avoid malabsorptive complications. Evaluation of 1012 cases of insulinoma cited in the literature indicated the following outcomes from surgery: operative mortality, 11 percent; cure, 63 percent; postoperative diabetes, 10 percent; and persistent hypoglycemia, 16 percent. Postoperative complications included acute pancreatitis, peritonitis, fistulas, and pseudocyst formation.

Medical treatment is indicated in insulinoma only in preparation for surgery or after failure to find the tumor at operation. The drug of choice is diazoxide, which can be given intravenously or orally in doses of 300 to 1200 mg per day. Because of its salt-retaining properties a diuretic must always be added when diazoxide is administered. Treatment of metastatic insulin-producing carcinomas is unsatisfactory. Streptozotocin, mithramycin, and adriamycin have been tried, but the results are dismal.

Therapy of other forms of recurrent hypoglycemia, apart from hormone replacement in pituitary or adrenal insufficiency, is dietary. In most cases avoidance of fasting is all that is required. A high-protein, low-carbohydrate diet is frequently prescribed for patients with postprandial hypoglycemia and often relieves symptoms. With true alimentary hypoglycemia it is probably important to keep the size of the individual meals small. The practice of giving massive amounts of vitamin E, crude adrenocortical extract, and varieties of trace metals to patients with the nonhypoglycemia syndrome is useless even if harmless (which has not been proved).

OTHER HORMONE-SECRETING TUMORS OF THE PANCREAS
Tumors of the pancreatic islets can synthesize a variety of hormones other than insulin. Almost all benign tumors are thought to be hormone-secreting, but it has been estimated that a fifth or more of islet carcinomas produce no clinically

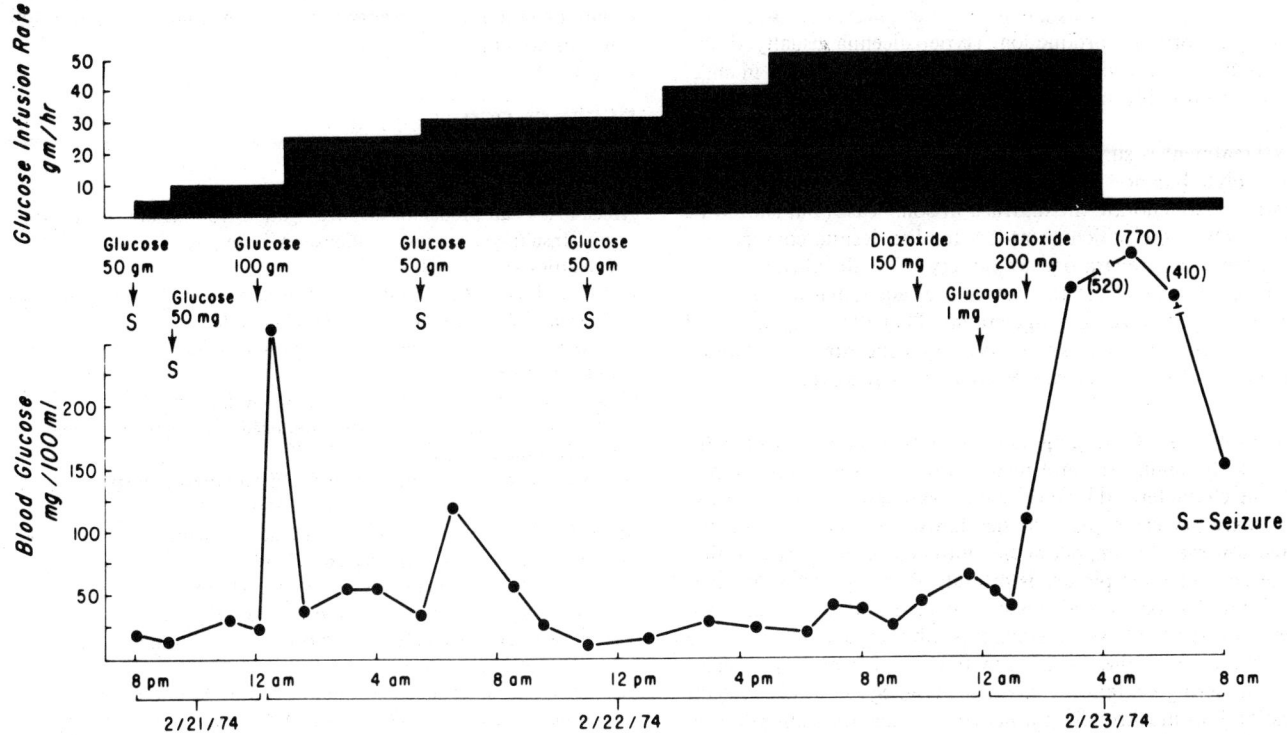

FIGURE 340-2

Prolonged and refractive hypoglycemia in factitious hypoglycemia due to chlorpropamide in an alcoholic. Note continued hypoglycemia despite the *infusion of glucose at rates up to 50 g/h. (From RM Jordan et al, Arch Intern Med 137:390, 1977. Copyright, 1977, American Medical Association. Used by permission.)*

detectable product. Histologically the tumors may be of a single-cell type or of mixed derivation. Despite the capacity of mixed tumors to produce several hormones, in general one predominates such that distinct syndromes result. It is critical to remember that pancreatic tumors may be part of the multiple endocrine neoplasia syndrome (Chap. 348). This is particularly true of the ulcerogenic islet cell tumor which is now considered to be a typical manifestation of the multiple endocrine neoplasia type I picture. This association is so strong that the designation *multiple endocrine neoplasia-peptic ulcer syndrome* is preferred. In addition to insulin, islet cell tumors have been associated with the production of gastrin, secretin, vasoactive intestinal polypeptide, human pancreatic polypeptide, gastric inhibitory polypeptide, glucagon, ACTH, melanocyte stimulatory hormone, and serotonin. Chorionic gonadotropin and its β subunit may also be elevated in the plasma of patients with islet cell tumors; the latter has been suggested to be a specific marker of malignancy in functioning tumors.

Ulcerogenic islet cell tumor (Zollinger-Ellison syndrome, gastrinoma) This is likely the most common of the non-insulin-secreting tumors. The clinical picture is that of intractable ulcer symptoms, hypersecretion of gastric acid, and diarrhea, which is almost always due to steatorrhea. Complications such as perforation and hemorrhage occur in a high percentage of cases. X-ray frequently shows the stomach to be filled with fluid, and giant gastric rugae are seen. Often the ulcer is atypically located in the second or third portion of the duodenum. Development of ulcer disease in the very young or very old should always raise suspicion of the Zollinger-Ellison syndrome. Associated endocrine abnormalities are present in half the patients and in a high percentage of first-degree relatives. Hypercalcemia due to parathyroid adenoma is the most common accompanying abnormality. A careful family history designed to elicit evidence of hypoglycemia, renal stones, multiple lipomas, and pituitary adenomas is imperative. All first-degree relatives of patients with gastrinomas should be exam-

ined by the physician. The presence of multiple lipomas can be a clue to the presence of the multiple endocrine neoplasia gene. Minimal screening should probably include x-rays of the sella turcica and measurement of serum gastrin, cortisol, prolactin, growth hormone, calcium and phosphorus. If hypercalcemia is present, workup for hyperparathyroidism can be completed. Evaluation for insulinoma is not indicated in the absence of symptoms suggesting hypoglycemia. Details of diagnosis and treatment for the Zollinger-Ellison syndrome are discussed in Chap. 290.

Diarrheogenic islet cell tumor The syndrome produced by these tumors has been called pancreatic cholera, the watery diarrhea syndrome, and the WDHA syndrome. The acronym stands for *w*atery *d*iarrhea, *h*ypokalemia, and *a*chlorhydria, major features of the clinical picture. Acid secretion in the basal state may actually be only low rather than absent and stimulation by histamine is intact. About two-thirds of patients have hypercalcemia and approximately half are hyperglycemic. A dilated gallbladder is characteristic. The secretory diarrhea is often profuse and can produce shock and renal shutdown. Hypokalemia may be life-threatening. Metabolic acidosis, presumably due to bicarbonate loss, but possibly also related to volume depletion, is common.

Considerable confusion has existed about the hormonal cause of the syndrome. Originally secretin was thought to be involved, but subsequently vasoactive intestinal polypeptide, human pancreatic polypeptide, gastric inhibitory polypeptide, and prostaglandins were all reported to be associated with diarrheogenic islet cell tumors. While it is theoretically possible that multiple hormones produce the same clinical picture, it is now thought that vasoactive intestinal polypeptide is the mediator in most cases. The attractiveness of this possibility is enhanced by the fact that vasoactive intestinal polypeptide is known to cause hyperglycemia and hypercalcemia in addition to secretory diarrhea. Thus the entire syndrome can be accounted for by one hormone without the need to postulate multiple hormone production. Hypercalcemia usually disappears after removal of the pancreatic neoplasm and in most cases is probably not due to concomitant hyperparathyroidism.

Treatment is surgical removal of the tumor after fluid and electrolyte balance have been restored. Steroids have been reported to ameliorate the diarrhea in some cases but should be used only if the patient is at risk for life despite conservative management preparatory to surgery. The diarrheogenic tumors tend to be larger than other islet adenomas and may be more easily localized by angiography. Diarrhea disappears and gastric acid secretion and potassium concentrations rapidly normalize if the tumor can be completely removed.

Glucagonoma Glucagonomas, a high percentage of which appear to be malignant and metastasizing, cause a clinical syndrome characterized by a distinctive skin lesion called necrolytic migratory erythema. The dermatosis may be found on the face, lower abdomen, perineum, buttocks, or distal extremities. The characteristic picture is of multiple crusts, scaly macules and papules, occasional pustules, flaccid bullae, and generalized erythema. Glossitis, stomatitis, and angular cheilosis are common. Spontaneous exacerbations and remissions occur, and hyperpigmentation follows healing. Systemically, weight loss and normochromic, normocytic anemia are common. Elevated fasting blood glucose concentrations or abnormal glucose tolerance tests are demonstrable in most patients. Plasma amino acid levels are depressed, and hypocholesterolemia may be present. Plasma ketones may be mildly elevated despite normal plasma free fatty acid concentrations. Glucagon levels in plasma are high and show abnormal responses to a number of provocative tests. It is of interest that four asymptomatic first-degree relatives of one patient with a proved glucagonoma had persistently elevated glucagon concentrations with abnormal responses to glucose suppression and arginine stimulation. Transmission appeared to follow an autosomal dominant pattern. Whether the asymptomatic subjects had small (undetectable) adenomas or whether the alpha cells were functionally abnormal but not neoplastic is not known.

Treatment of glucagonoma is surgical removal. Chemotherapy of metastatic disease is unsatisfactory.

Somatostatinoma Six patients have now been reported in which islet tumors containing somatostatin were present. The clinical syndrome cannot be defined with certainty because of the paucity of patients. Associations noted thus far include hyperglycemia, weight loss, anemia, hypochlorhydria, steatorrhea, and gallbladder disease (cholelithiasis). Whether these are causally related to somatostatin production by the tumor remains to be proved. In one patient ACTH levels were also increased.

Cushing's syndrome ACTH production by pancreatic islet tumors is now well known. The clinical manifestations appear to be milder than in other forms of ectopic Cushing's syndrome. Mixed hormone production (insulin, gastrin, serotonin) appears to be common in these tumors in contrast to other islet neoplasms. The problem of differentiating between a single islet tumor producing multiple hormones and the multiple endocrine neoplasia syndrome where two or more adenomas each produce a single hormone may be difficult.

Carcinoid syndrome Serotonin may be synthesized in islet tumors and lead to a syndrome of diarrhea, flushing, and tachycardia. Asthma is not present. It is conceivable that these patients actually have a diarrheogenic tumor with symptoms

primarily due to vasoactive intestinal polypeptide and that serotonin production represents a second hormone synthesized by a mixed adenoma.

REFERENCES

Hypoglycemia and insulinoma

ADAM PAJ et al: Model for the investigation of intractable hypoglycemia: Insulin-glucose interrelationships during steady state infusions. Pediatrics 41:91, 1968

CORRELIO F et al: Fatal cases of lipid storage myopathy with carnitine deficiency. J Neurol Neurosurg Psychiatry 40:170, 1977

FAJANS SS, FLOYD JC: Fasting hypoglycemia in adults. N Engl J Med 294:766, 1976

GARBER AJ et al: The role of adrenergic mechanisms in the substrate and hormonal response to insulin-induced hypoglycemia in man. J Clin Invest 58:7, 1976

JORDAN RM et al: Sulfonylurea-induced factitious hypoglycemia. A growing problem. Arch Int Med 137:390, 1977

MERIMEE TJ, TYSON JE: Hypoglycemia in man. Pathologic and physiologic variants. Diabetes 26:161, 1977

PERMUTT MA: Postprandial hypoglycemia. Diabetes 25:719, 1976

SCARLETT JA et al: Factitious hypoglycemia. Diagnosis by measurement of serum C-peptide immunoreactivity and insulin-binding antibodies. N Engl J Med 297:1029, 1977

SERVICE FJ et al: Insulinoma. Clinical and diagnostic features of 60 consecutive cases. Mayo Clin Proc 51:417, 1976

STEFANINI P: Beta-islet cell tumors of the pancreas: Results of a study on 1067 cases. Surgery 75:597, 1974

Other hormone-secreting islet cell tumors

BINNICK AN et al: Glucagonoma syndrome. Report of two cases and literature review. Arch Dermatol 113:749, 1977

LAMERS CB et al: Prevalence of endocrine abnormalities in patients with the Zollinger-Ellison syndrome and in their families. Am J Med 64:607, 1978

SCHEIN PS et al: Islet cell tumors: Current concepts and management. Ann Intern Med 79:239, 1973

ZOLLINGER RM, MAZZAFERRI EL: Tumors of the islets of Langerhans. Adv Surg 10:137, 1976

341
DISEASES OF THE TESTIS

JAMES E. GRIFFIN
JEAN D. WILSON

INTRODUCTION

The testis is the source of sperm and of the steroid hormones that regulate male sexual life, both functions being under complex feedback control by the hypothalamic-pituitary system. Thus, the testis has biosynthetic functions and regulatory features similar to those of the ovary and adrenal glands. Testicular secretions are also responsible for the formation of the basic male phenotype during embryogenesis. This function of the testis and the disorders that result from abnormalities of testicular function or androgen action during embryogenesis are described in Chap. 344.

PHYSIOLOGY AND REGULATION OF TESTICULAR FUNCTION

The testis consists of two components: (1) a system of tubules for the production and transport of sperm that empty into collecting ducts and ultimately into an excretory system and (2) clusters of interstitial, or Leydig, cells that lie between the tubules and produce androgenic steroids.

THE LEYDIG CELL **Testosterone synthesis** The biochemical reactions by which the 27-carbon sterol cholesterol is converted to androgens and estrogens are described in Fig. 341-1. Cholesterol can be either synthesized de novo in the Leydig cell or derived from the plasma pool. Five enzymes are required for the conversion of cholesterol to testosterone. In this process the side chain of cholesterol is cleaved at two sites to reduce the size from 27 to 19 carbons, and the A ring of the steroid is oxidized to the Δ^4-3-keto configuration. The five enzymes are 20,22-desmolase, the 3β-hydroxysteroid–$\Delta^{4,5}$-isomerase complex, 17-hydroxylase, 17,20-desmolase, and 17β-hydroxysteroid dehydrogenase. The first four enzymes are also present in the adrenal glands.

The key step in testosterone synthesis is the conversion of cholesterol to pregnenolone by 20,22-desmolase, and leutenizing hormone (LH) acts at this site to regulate the overall activity of the pathway. Several steroids other than testosterone are synthesized within the Leydig cell, including estradiol, but the quantitative significance of these in the normal man is thought to be minor.

Testosterone secretion and transport Only about 25 μg testosterone is stored in the normal testes, so that the total hormone content turns over about 200 times each day to provide the average of 6 mg that is secreted into plasma in normal young men (Fig. 341-2). As is true for other steroid hormones, testosterone is transported in plasma bound to protein, largely to albumin and to a specific steroid hormone transport protein, testosterone-binding globulin (TeBG). The bound and un-

bound fractions in plasma are in dynamic equilibrium, only about 1 to 3 percent being present in the free fraction. It is unclear whether plasma-binding proteins play any role in androgen physiology other than as transport carriers.

Peripheral metabolism of androgens Plasma testosterone is metabolized by several pathways. The hormone and its active metabolites are excreted primarily as inactive metabolites in the urine (>90 percent), approximately half of the daily turnover being recovered in the form of urinary 17-ketosteroids (primarily androsterone and etiocholanolone) and the other half as a series of polar compounds (diols, triols, and conjugates).

A special feature of the metabolism of testosterone is that it serves as a circulating precursor (or prohormone) for the formation of two other types of active metabolites, which in turn mediate many of the physiological processes involved in androgen action (Fig. 341-1). On the one hand, testosterone can undergo irreversible reduction to 5α-reduced steroids, principally dihydrotestosterone, that are thought to perform many of the differentiative, growth-promoting, and functional actions necessary for male sexual differentiation and virilization. On the other hand, circulating androgens can be converted to estrogens in the peripheral tissues of both sexes. These estrogens in some instances act in concert with androgens but also may have independent effects and even on occasion have effects opposite to those of androgens. Thus, the physiological consequences of circulating testosterone are the result of the combined effects of testosterone itself plus the active androgen and

FIGURE 341-1

Pathways of androgen formation in the testis and the conversion of androgens to other active hormones in peripheral tissues.

FIGURE 341-2

Androgen and estrogen production in normal young men.

estrogen metabolites of the parent molecule. This process is complicated by the fact that in normal men small amounts of estradiol and dihydrotestosterone are derived by direct secretion from the testis and indirectly from the adrenal glands via the sequence

$$\text{Androstenedione} \to \text{estrone} \to \text{estradiol}$$

and

$$\text{Androstenedione} \to \text{androstanedione} \to \text{dihydrotestosterone}$$

The quantitative relation between circulating testosterone and the formation of estrogen in normal young men is illustrated diagrammatically in Fig. 341-2. Of the mean estradiol production of about 45 μg per day approximately 35 to 40 percent is derived from circulating testosterone, about half is derived from the weak estrogen estrone, and only about 10 to 15 percent is secreted directly into the circulation by the testes.

FIGURE 341-3

Regulation of testosterone and sperm production by LH and FSH. C, cholesterol; T, testosterone.

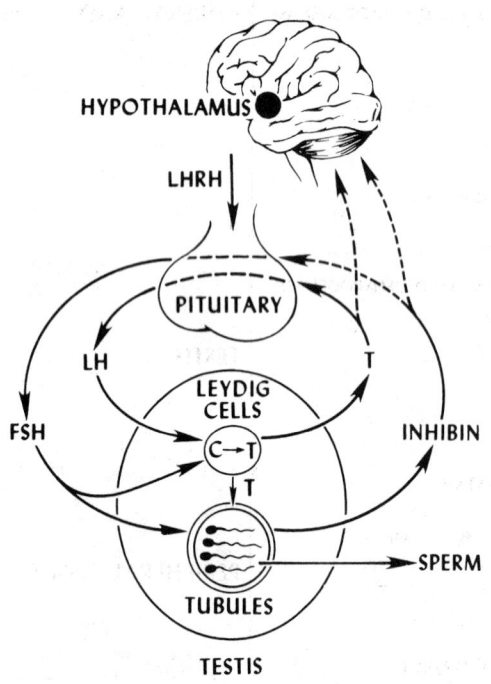

When gonadotropin levels are elevated (and in other pathological states as well), the amount of estradiol secreted by the testes is increased.

In some instances these active metabolites only exert local actions in the tissues in which they are formed, whereas in other instances the 5α-reduced and estrogenic metabolites reenter the circulation and act as circulating hormones. The principal sites of formation of circulating dihydrotestosterone are thought to be the androgen target tissues themselves. Estrogen formation takes place in many peripheral tissues; the most significant site is adipose tissue, and the overall rate of peripheral estrogen formation increases with the amount of adipose tissue and with age.

Gonadotropin regulation and testosterone secretion   Testosterone secretion is regulated largely by LH from the pituitary (Fig. 341-3). (For the details of pituitary function, see Chap. 333.) Follicle stimulating hormone (FSH) may also augment testosterone secretion, possibly by regulating the number of LH receptors on the plasma membrane of the Leydig cell. Testosterone feeds back on the pituitary to alter the sensitivity of the gland to the hypothalamic luteinizing hormone–releasing hormone (LHRH). Although the pituitary can convert testosterone to dihydrotestosterone and to estrogens, testosterone itself is the primary regulator of gonadotropin secretion. Whether testosterone also acts in the central nervous system to regulate the rate of LHRH formation or secretion is not clear. Under ordinary circumstances, LH levels are exquisitely sensitive to the feedback effects of testosterone, with complete suppression following the administration of amounts of exogenous androgen that approximate the normal daily secretory rate of the testes (about 6 mg). However, chronic elevation of LH levels (as in testicular deficiency) renders the pituitary less sensitive to negative feedback control by exogenously administered androgens.

Neither the plasma concentration of testosterone nor of LH is constant, each showing fluctuations of a pulsatile nature throughout the day, reflecting changes in secretory rates. In the adult there is no significant diurnal variation in the magnitude of this episodic secretion of LH, and only minor circadian variation in testosterone secretion occurs, with peak levels in the morning. In the pubertal male major sleep-related surges in the secretion of both LH and testosterone signal the initiation of puberty.

Androgen action   The cellular mechanisms by which androgens act to perform their major actions are summarized sche-

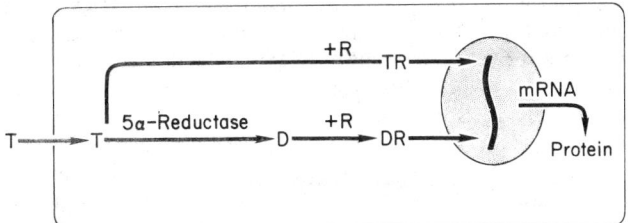

FIGURE 341-4
Current concepts of androgen action. T, testosterone; D, dihydrotestosterone; R, receptor protein.

matically in Fig. 341-4. The major functions of androgen are the regulation of gonadotropin secretion, the initiation and maintenance of spermatogenesis, the formation of the male phenotype during sexual differentiation, and the induction of sexual maturation and function following puberty. Testosterone (T) enters the cell by passive diffusion. Inside the cell, T can be converted to dihydrotestosterone (D) by the 5α-reductase enzyme. Then T or D is bound to a specific androgen receptor protein in the cytosol (R). The hormone-receptor complex (TR or DR) is translocated to the nucleus, where it attaches to specific sites within the chromosomes; as a result, new RNA and ultimately new protein appear within the cytoplasm of the cell. The testosterone-receptor complex regulates gonadotropin secretion and is responsible for the wolffian stimulation phase of sexual differentiation and for spermatogenesis, whereas the dihydrotestosterone-receptor complex is responsible for external virilization during embryogenesis and a major portion of androgen action during sexual maturation and adult sexual function. The precise mechanisms by which estrogens augment or block the pathway of androgen action have not been defined. Presumably, estradiol acts by a similar mechanism involving its own receptor protein (see Chap. 342).

THE SEMINIFEROUS TUBULE AND SPERMATOGENESIS
Normal function of the seminiferous tubule is dependent on the proximity of the interstitial cells and the seminiferous tubule, since both testosterone and FSH are required for spermatogenesis. The major site of FSH action is the seminiferous tubules, and almost all the interaction of FSH with the tubule can be accounted for by binding to Sertoli cells. The seminiferous tubule is also a target for testosterone, and specific androgen receptors are present in Sertoli cells. The entire process of spermatogenesis probably requires the concerted action of both FSH and testosterone; testosterone appears to be essential for the initial phase of spermatogenesis, whereas FSH is required for the terminal phases of spermatid development. In the normal young adult male this machinery produces more than 100 million sperm per day.

The Sertoli cell cannot synthesize steroid hormones de novo, but isolated Sertoli cells (as well as Leydig cells) can convert testosterone to estradiol. Spermatogenic tubules can also form 5α-reduced androgens from testosterone. The role of these various metabolites in spermatogenesis is unclear.

The spermatogenic tubules also produce the hormone inhibin that serves to regulate the secretion of FSH by the hypothalamic-pituitary axis (Fig. 341-3). This hormone has recently been shown to be a peptide that is released during the late phase of spermatogenesis. Whether the hormone acts primarily at the level of the pituitary or hypothalamus to regulate FSH secretion is unknown.

The overall effect of this interlocking system in which two pituitary hormones regulate testicular function is to provide a delicate dual control mechanism by which plasma testosterone and sperm production can feed back independently upon the hypothalamic-pituitary system to regulate their own rates of production (Fig. 341-3).

PHASES OF MALE SEXUAL FUNCTION

It is useful to consider the phases of male sexual life in terms of the plasma testosterone value. In the male embryo the production of testosterone by the testis and the concentration of plasma testosterone start to rise at about 7 weeks and shortly thereafter attain a high value that is maintained until late in gestation, when it falls. At the time of birth plasma testosterone is only slightly higher in males than in females. Shortly after birth, plasma testosterone again begins to rise in the male infant and remains elevated for approximately 3 months, falling to low levels by age 1 year. The concentration then remains low (but slightly higher in boys than in girls) until the onset of puberty, when it begins to rise in males, reaching adult levels by age 17 or thereabouts. The mean plasma level remains more or less constant in the adult until the late middle age and then declines slowly during the later decades of life. The physiological events that take place during these various phases differ, as do the pathological consequences of derangements in testicular function at different stages of life. Male sexual differentiation is considered in detail in Chap. 343. The focus of this chapter is on the pathophysiology of puberty and adult sexual life.

ABNORMALITIES OF TESTICULAR FUNCTION

PUBERTY The factors that ultimately determine the onset of puberty are poorly understood and may reside in the hypothalamic-pituitary system, the testis, or the adrenal glands. Prior to the onset of puberty gonadotropin secretion by the pituitary is low but is under regulatory control by the testis; castration produces a rise in gonadotropin levels. This suggests that prior to puberty the negative feedback control of gonadotropin secretion is exquisitely sensitive to testosterone. The onset of puberty is heralded by sleep-associated surges in gonadotropin secretion. Later in puberty the rises in LH and FSH become manifest throughout the day and are followed (accompanied) by elevations in plasma testosterone. Thus, with maturation the hypothalamic-pituitary system appears to become less sensitive to feedback control, and a higher mean plasma testosterone is the result. This process is accompanied by histological maturation of the testes. The remaining anatomical and functional changes occurring at the time of puberty are secondary to the rise in plasma testosterone. Maturation of the accessory organs of male reproduction (the penis, the prostate, the seminal vesicles, and the epididymis) accounts for about a fourth of androgen-mediated nitrogen retention. Growth of muscle accounts for the remainder. The principal androgen-sensitive muscles are those of the pectoral region and the shoulder. These various growth and maturation processes reach some limiting value so that the administration of pharmacological doses of androgen has no further effect once puberty is completed.

The central issue in dealing with disorders of puberty is in separating instances of true absence or precocity from subjects at the extremes of normal variation. Normal puberty in the male is not only variable in its onset and duration but asymmetrical in regard to the sequence of events. For the purposes of this discussion only true precocity and pubertal absence will be considered.

Sexual precocity Sexual development in a boy before the age of 10 should be considered abnormal. In the male feminization prior to the expected onset of puberty results in so-called "heterosexual precocity" and is usually the manifestation of a testicular or adrenal tumor. True isosexual precocity in the male may be idiopathic or the result either of a central nervous system tumor that causes enhanced gonadotropin secretion or of congenital adrenal hyperplasia (deficiency of 21- or 11-hydroxylase enzyme) with a secondary increase in adrenal androgen production and occasionally elevated plasma gonadotropin levels as well (see Chaps. 336 and 344). Tumors of the testis that produce androgen and tumors that produce gonadotropins may also rarely cause isosexual precocity.

Patients with true idiopathic isosexual precocity pass through an early but otherwise typical sexual development with a typical prepubertal growth spurt. Affected subjects can ejaculate and may produce sperm, and there are rare reports of fatherhood at an early age. Since normal puberty is poorly understood, it is not surprising that the pathogenesis of idiopathic precocious puberty is also poorly defined. It is clear that some type of premature activation of the hypothalamic-pituitary-gonadal axis must take place since these individuals have normal pubertal patterns of sleep-associated and LHRH-induced LH release. The central issue in the workup is the necessity to exclude overt disease of the central nervous system and pituitary as well as disorders of the adrenal glands and testes. Since the diagnosis is one of exclusion, some "idiopathic" cases later prove to have been misclassified and actually represent only the first evidence of lesions of the central nervous system. With improved means of diagnosing central nervous system lesions [such as computerized tomography (CT scan)] such delays in diagnosis will probably be less frequent.

Management of patients with the idiopathic disorder is generally unsatisfactory. Therapy is usually directed toward lowering plasma gonadotropins with the use of medroxyprogesterone acetate, but such treatment probably does not prevent premature closure of the epiphyses.

Absent puberty   The separation of true failure of puberty from variants of normal is one of the most difficult problems in endocrinology. Some patients fail to show the normal spurt of growth and sexual development at the usual time, but eventually commence puberty by age 16 or older. Adolescence may then either progress rapidly, or there may be a slow development and growth which continues until age 20 to 22. Many men with delayed onset of puberty attain heights within the normal adult range. At times the history reveals that a parent or some other member of the family has shown a similar pattern of development. The major problem is to separate this group of patients with delayed puberty from patients with panhypotituitarism (see Chap. 333), thyroid disease (see Chap. 335), primary testicular disease, or hypogonadotropic hypogonadism.

Hypogonadotropic hypogonadism is frequently referred to as the Kallman syndrome. Affected subjects exhibit eunuchoidal features and have testes of prepubertal size. The secretion of other pituitary hormones is usually normal. Anosmia or hyposmia and cryptorchidism are common. Histological examination of the testis reveals undifferentiated Leydig cells and immature germinal epithelium similar to a normal prepubertal testis. The disorder appears to be inherited as an X-linked recessive trait or an autosomal dominant trait with variable expressivity. Serum FSH and LH levels are usually below the normal male range, and plasma testosterone levels are in the female range. The basic defect appears to be the absence of LHRH synthesis or release, and the administration of synthetic LHRH for a sufficient period corrects the biochemical abnormality and initiates spermatogenesis. If untreated, these patients usually remain in the prepubertal state indefinitely. In

view of the fact that prolonged administration of LHRH is not practicable at present, routine treatment is accomplished either with androgen replacement or (if fertility is desired) with gonadotropins. A prepubertal manifestation of this disorder in some individuals is the presence of microphallus, in which the penis is below the 95 percent confidence limits for the age. Indeed, in at least half of prepubertal patients with isolated microphallus, the underlying etiology is hypogonadotropic hypogonadism.

A less severe form of hypogonadotrophic hypogonadism is the so-called "fertile eunuch" syndrome, in which spermatogenesis is present despite marked deficiency of androgen production and the virtual absence of mature Leydig cells. Plasma FSH levels are within the normal adult male range whereas plasma LH concentrations are low. However, when such patients are given LHRH, prompt rises occur in plasma LH as well as FSH. This implies that the defect in this disorder is also defective LH release rather than decreased LH synthesis.

Until recently isolated FSH deficiency had only been described in women. However, four men have now been reported in whom virilization, plasma LH, and plasma testosterone were normal but in whom plasma FSH was persistently low, and testicular biopsy in one individual revealed a maturation arrest at the spermatid stage. In two patients who were given LHRH, FSH levels increased.

Absent puberty can also result from primary disease of the testes or from hereditary androgen resistance; in either of these cases plasma gonadotropins are high. Most of these disorders can also result in hereditary male pseudohermaphroditism, and are discussed in detail in Chap. 344, but in milder cases are manifest only as absent puberty. They include hereditary defects in testosterone biosynthesis, congenital anorchia, dysgenetic or rudimentary testes, LH resistance, and hereditary androgen resistance.

ADULT ABNORMALITIES OF TESTICULAR FUNCTION   At the time of the completion of puberty, plasma testosterone levels have reached their adult level of 400 to 1000 ng per 100 ml, sperm production has reached a steady level, and adult levels of gonadotropins (5 to 20 mIU/ml each for LH and FSH) have been achieved. The adult set of the complex regulatory system described in Fig. 341-3 is then sustained in the normal man for over 40 years. But it is a sensitive system subject to a variety of influences, both at the level of the testis and of the hypothalamic-pituitary system. Spermatogenesis is exquisitely sensitive to alterations in temperature, and brief increases either in systemic or local temperature (as in a hot bath) can be followed by temporary decreases in sperm production. The system is likewise sensitive to diet, drugs, alcohol, environmental agents, and psychological stress, all of which may cause temporary decreases in sperm count.

Testicular failure   Failure of testicular function after the completion of puberty can be due either to a variety of pituitary abnormalities (see Chap. 333) or the consequence of disorders that affect the testis directly, such as viral infections, trauma, radiation exposure, neurological disorders, drugs, severe systemic diseases, or granulomatous disease. While certain of these tend to influence Leydig cell function or spermatogenesis selectively, generally failure of both aspects of testicular function occurs to a greater or lesser degree, and consequently, the various features of secondary testicular failure are better discussed by considering the various syndromes than by focusing on individual manifestations.

VIRAL ORCHITIS   Viral orchitis is the most common cause of testicular failure in the adult, and mumps is the most important of the viruses involved, although other agents are known to act in a similar fashion. These include echovirus, lympocytic choriomeningitis virus, and group B arboviruses. The orchitis is due to actual infection of the tissue by the virus rather than to indirect effects. Orchitis is the most common complication of mumps in adult men and occurs in approximately a fourth of males of all ages. In about two-thirds of the cases it is unilateral, and in the remainder it is bilateral. It usually develops within a few days after the onset of parotitis but occasionally precedes it. The testis may return to normal or shrink below the normal size. Atrophy is believed to be due both to direct effects of the virus on the seminiferous tubules and to ischemia secondary to pressure and edema within the taut tunica albuginea. The degree of atrophy is not necessarily proportional to the severity of the orchitis. It is usually perceptible within 1 to 6 months after the orchitis subsides. Unilateral atrophy occurs in approximately one-third of all cases of mumps orchitis, while bilateral atrophy occurs in about one-tenth. In a survey of 2000 adult men, atrophy of one or both testes was found in 2 percent, half of which were the result of mumps. The frequency with which viral orchitis results in failure either of spermatogenesis or testosterone production in the absence of overt bilateral atrophy is uncertain, but it is not a common etiologic factor in infertility. The administration of glucocorticoids in the acute phase is followed by rapid defervescence and reduction of testicular swelling and pain. It is not known whether such treatment affects the late sequelae of the disorder in any way.

RADIATION DAMAGE The testes and the spermatogonia in particular are exquisitely sensitive to radiation. Doses higher than 20 rads are followed by rises in plasma FSH and LH levels and damage to the spermatogonia. With doses of about 80 rads extreme oligospermia or azoospermia develops. Higher doses may result in virtual obliteration of the germinal epithelium except for occasional stem and Sertoli cells. Still higher doses (600 rads) may cause an increase in the number of Leydig cells. Complete recovery as shown by a return to preirradiation sperm concentrations may not take place for as long as 5 years, and permanent sterility can apparently occur after doses of radiation utilized for treatment of malignant lymphoma in spite of the shielding used with an inverted Y field. Permanent androgen deficiency rarely results from doses in the therapeutic range.

DRUG-INDUCED TESTICULAR FAILURE In general, drugs interfere with testicular function in one of five ways—direct inhibition of testosterone synthesis, blockade of the peripheral action of androgen, enhancement of estrogen levels, inhibition of gonadotropin secretion, or inhibition of spermatogenesis. Indeed, certain drugs have multiple effects, and certain agents such as propanolol and guanethidine that affect the sympathetic nervous system can block normal sexual drive and potency in men whose pituitary-testicular axis is normal.

Spironolactone in high doses blocks the synthesis of androgen by interfering with the late reactions in androgen biosynthesis. This drug as well as cimetidine and the experimental antiandrogen flutamide also compete with androgen for the cytoplasmic receptor protein and thus interfere with androgen action in the target cell. Testosterone levels may be low in patients taking large amounts of marijuana, heroin, or methadone, although the exact reasons are unclear. Plasma estradiol levels have been reported to be elevated and plasma testosterone levels decreased in men taking digitalis.

Interference with gonadotropin production can result from two mechanisms; some drugs such as medroxyprogesterone acetate directly inhibit gonadotropin production and thus result in diminished testosterone production, whereas psychotropic drugs such as phenothiazines that enhance prolactin

secretion may interfere with gonadotropin production secondarily.

A number of cancer chemotherapeutic agents interfere with spermatogenesis and on occasion with Leydig cell function. Perhaps the most important such agent is cyclophosphamide, which inevitably causes azoospermia or extreme oligospermia within a few weeks after the initiation of therapy. Cessation of drug therapy is followed by a return of spermatogenesis within 3 years in about half of patients. Any agent that interferes with testosterone synthesis or action can also result in decreased sperm production.

NEUROLOGICAL DISEASE Spinal cord lesions that result in quadriplegia cause initially diminished plasma testosterone values that generally return toward normal and defective spermatogenesis that appears to persist. Some patients retain the capacity to obtain erections and ejaculate. In myotonic dystrophy small testes with histological evidence of damage to seminiferous tubules and to Leydig cells are common.

TRAUMA In population surveys of normal men, trauma is second only to viral orchitis as a cause of secondary atrophy of the testes. Clearly, the exposed position of the testis in the scrotum renders it uniquely susceptible to both thermal and physical trauma—particularly in individuals with hazardous occupations.

HEPATIC AND RENAL FAILURE Secondary disorders of testicular function are common in a variety of systemic diseases. In chronic liver disease there is probably a primary testicular lesion leading to decreased plasma testosterone, testosterone production rate, and metabolic clearance rate. Although plasma LH is elevated, the level may be inappropriate for the degree of androgen deficiency due to the inhibitory effects of the increased estrogen levels on LH secretion. Increased estrogen production results from impaired hepatic extraction of adrenal androstenedione and consequent increased peripheral conversion to estrone and subsequently estradiol. Sterility and gonadal atrophy are common.

Subnormal androgen synthesis and spermatogenesis coupled with elevated plasma gonadotropins are also common in renal failure. The elevated plasma LH is due to reduced metabolic clearance and increased production. Plasma testosterone may improve in some patients after chronic hemodialysis. Successful renal transplantation results in improvement in sperm production and testosterone synthesis with return of gonadotropins to normal.

AUTOIMMUNITY Testicular failure has been described as a part of a generalized autoimmune disorder in which multiple primary endocrine deficiencies coexist and in which circulating antibodies to the basement membrane of the testes can be documented (see Chap. 348).

GRANULOMATOUS DISEASE Testicular atrophy occurs in 10 to 20 percent of men with lepromatous leprosy, the result of direct invasion of the tissue. The tubules are involved initially, followed by endarteritis and destruction of Leydig cells. Destruction of the testis is less common in other types of systemic granulomatous disease.

Infertility Fertility in the male is determined by a number of factors, including sperm number, the quality of the sperm, and the volume and composition of the ejaculate. Many aspects of the problem are poorly understood. A central difficulty is the definition of a normal ejaculate. There is considerable uncertainty as to the lower level of sperm density, percent motility, and percent oval forms in normal or fertile semen. This uncertainty stems from two issues: (1) many secondary factors can produce temporary aberrations in sperm count, and (2) the means of assessing the fertilizing capacity are indirect. What is needed is a valid in vitro test of the capacity of human spermatozoa to fertilize ova. Even considering the various problems involved, it is useful to separate those disorders associated with extreme oligospermia or azoospermia from those in which the sperm count appears to be within the broad range of normal. The cause of the infertility is rarely defined when the sperm count is normal.

A number of etiologies have been identified, however, where the sperm count is unequivocally low, and for the purposes of differential diagnosis these can be viewed as hypothalamic-pituitary, testicular, or posttesticular causes (Table 341-1). Many of these disorders are associated with hormonal defects and have been discussed under other headings in this chapter; in these various disorders the clue to the diagnosis lies elsewhere, and substantiation requires a complete endocrine workup. Others, however, may present primarily as male infertility and deserve special comment.

HYPOTHALAMIC-PITUITARY Hyperprolactinemia has been reported to be associated with infertility. In some instances impotence, decreased plasma gonadotropins, and low testosterone also occur, similar to the amenorrhea-galactorrhea syndromes in women, but more frequently prolactin appears to act at the testicular level. Most drugs that act to suppress gonadotropins (androgens, estrogens, progestins) suppress both LH and FSH. However, it has been reported that diphenylhydantoin may suppress FSH selectively and result in low sperm counts under circumstances in which plasma LH, testosterone, and estradiol are unaffected.

TESTICULAR Disorders of Leydig cell function that lead to failure of spermatogenesis are usually associated with low plasma testosterone values. In most instances of infertility of testicular origin, testicular biopsy may indicate a testicular etiology unassociated with an androgen deficit. One such entity is germinal cell aplasia (the Sertoli cell–only syndrome), in which

TABLE 341-1
Classification of male infertility

I Hypothalamic-pituitary
  A Hypogonadotropic hypogonadism
  B Isolated FSH deficiency
  C Pituitary insufficiency of any cause
  D Hyperprolactinemia with or without pituitary microadenoma
  E Drugs (diphenylhydantoin)
II Testicular
  A Testicular insufficiency
    1 Viral orchitis
    2 Cryptorchidism
    3 Neurological disorders
    4 Chronic renal failure
  B Germinal cell aplasia (Sertoli cell–only syndrome)
  C Spermatogenic arrest
  D Varicocele
  E Autoimmunity and sperm antibodies
  F Drugs (cyclophosphamide)
III Posttesticular
  A Abnormalities of the ejaculatory duct system
    1 Infectious obstruction
    2 Congenital absence of the vas
    3 Cystic fibrosis
    4 Diethylstilbestrol exposure in utero
  B Bacteriospermia
  C Disorders of ejaculation

the germinal epithelium is completely missing and complete azoospermia is present, despite adequate virilization, normal male breasts and testes, and normal chromosomal karyotype in peripheral blood. On average, plasma testosterone and LH values are normal, and plasma FSH values are high. The occurrence of the syndrome in brothers raises the possibility that it may be due to a single gene defect, but some patients with the typical histological and clinical features have a history of viral orchitis or cryptorchidism. This disorder accounts for a tenth of azoospermia or less.

More commonly, testicular biopsy reveals either severe hypospermatogenesis or a maturation arrest, commonly at the spermatid stage, with or without sloughing of the epithelium. A number of disorders may result in such a histological picture. Subtle abnormalities of chromosomes such as translocation or mosaicism that affect the testis selectively may account for some cases. In most cases of germinal cell arrest, however, the cause is unknown; a variety of single-gene defects are known to influence spermatogenesis in experimental animals, and it is possible that genetic etiologies are an important cause of this abnormality in men.

Varicocele is probably the most common treatable cause of male infertility. A varicocele results from retrograde flow into the internal spermatic vein that results in progressive, often palpable dilation of the peritesticular pampiniform plexus. It is thought to result from incompetence of the valve between the internal spermatic vein and the renal vein and is more common on the left (85 percent). Such retrograde venous flow can affect the temperature of both testes as a result of the extensive anastomoses of the venous systems. The incidence of varicocele is about 10 to 15 percent in the general population and 20 to 40 percent in men with infertility. The findings on semen analysis are usually nonspecific, with all parameters showing some abnormality. The mechanism by which the disorder leads to poor-quality semen and infertility is unknown but may be due to increased scrotal temperature so that the testes do not have the usual 2°C lower temperature than that of the abdominal cavity. In a number of studies, varicocelectomy has been reported to have a beneficial effect on fertility, with the best results (70 percent pregnancy rate) obtained in men whose preoperative sperm counts were over 10 million per milliliter.

Recent studies indicate that unilateral cryptorchidism corrected prior to puberty is associated with persistently abnormal semen in a significant percentage of cases. This suggests the presence of a bilateral testicular abnormality even in unilateral cryptorchidism.

Autoimmunity can affect fertility, either as the result of antibodies of the testicular basement membrane as a part of generalized autoimmune disease or as the result of antibodies directed to sperm themselves. The latter is thought to account for less than 1 percent of male infertility, and it is of interest that sperm-agglutinating antibodies have been demonstrated in men with infertility due to ductal obstruction and following vasectomy, suggesting that even when antibodies are present they may be secondary phenomena rather than causal in the infertility.

POSTTESTICULAR Obstruction of the wolffian structures is now a cause of azoospermia in only about 3 percent of infertile men; in the past tuberculosis and gonorrhea were frequent causes, and leprosy may result in obstruction of the excretory duct system in addition to affecting the testis directly. Congenital defects of the vas deferens that result in azoospermia or oligospermia may occur as an isolated abnormality associated with absence of seminal vesicles, in patients with cystic fibrosis, and as a portion of more extensive anatomical disorder in male offspring of women given diethylstilbestrol during pregnancy.

Asymptomatic bacteriospermia, frequently associated with occult prostatitis, can also lead to male infertility that may be reversible after appropriate antibiotic therapy.

Even considering all the known causes of azoospermia or extreme oligospermia, after complete evaluation no abnormality is identified in more than half the cases. Perhaps the most useful approach to the patient with azoospermia in whom the initial workup and endocrine evaluation are normal is testicular biopsy. If, in the presence of azoospermia, spermatogenesis is normal by histological exam, the diagnosis is likely to be obstruction or absence of the wolffian ducts. Disorders of the wolffian ducts that also result in absence of the seminal vesicles can be identified by demonstrating absence of fructose in the ejaculate.

The management of infertility in men is generally unsatisfactory except for the cases in which varicocele or obstruction to the ducts can be corrected surgically or where treatable endocrinopathies can be identified. In the absence of endocrinopathy, ancillary therapy with androgens or gonadotropins probably has no significant effect on fertility; spontaneous resolution of the problem with time may occur in as many as 25 percent of patients followed without treatment.

Fertility control in the male Although several approaches to fertility control have been tried in men, including radiation and drug therapy, the most practicable procedure is ligation of the vas deferens, a procedure that can be accomplished on an outpatient basis and that has been utilized successfully in large populations. The time required for azoospermia to occur following the operation depends upon the number of sperm in the terminal vas deferens and ejaculatory ducts at the time of surgery, but is usually less than 40 days. Azoospermia should be documented in each case to prove effectiveness. No deleterious effects on either testosterone production or the hypothalamic-pituitary axis have been documented.

OLD AGE Beginning at about age 70 mean plasma testosterone values decrease. This decrease occurs despite an elevation in TeBG, so that the level of free tesosterone falls even more. There is an associated rise in plasma LH and an increase in the rate of conversion of androgen to estrogen in peripheral tissues, so that the effective ratio of androgen to estrogen is decreased significantly. This background of endocrine changes in the aging man may well provide the critical milieu in which hypertrophy of the prostate develops, but there is no convincing evidence that these changes have any direct bearing on sexual activity in the elderly. Indeed, in the normal aging man the plasma values for bound and free testosterone, although statistically lower than average, are usually within the normal range.

Prostatic hypertrophy The development of benign prostatic hypertrophy is an almost universal phenomenon in aging men. The prostate weighs only a few grams at birth; at puberty it undergoes androgen-induced growth and reaches the adult size of approximately 20 g by about age 20. It remains stable in weight and histological characteristics for about 25 years. In the fifth decade a second growth spurt starts in the majority of men. Unlike the early growth which involves the gland diffusely, this second growth phase begins in the periurethral regions as a localized proliferation that in many individuals progresses to compress the remaining normal gland, leading to a major increase in gland size and urinary and/or rectal obstruction. This growth requires a functioning testis. Although the concentration of testosterone in normal and hypertrophic prostates is similar, there is a fivefold increase in the concentration of dihydrotestosterone in hypertrophic as compared with normal glands. The administration of dihydrotestosterone in suffi-

cient amounts to castrated dogs results in prostatic enlargement comparable to that seen in the naturally occurring disorder, and estradiol acts synergistically with dihydrotestosterone to induce prostatic growth. Since estradiol production is known to increase with age in men, this provides a potential explanation of the increased incidence of benign prostatic hypertrophy with advancing age. It seems likely that both androgen and estrogen are involved in the pathogenesis and that the occurrence in the elderly can be explained as a result of increasing estradiol formation in the face of declining but nevertheless appreciable androgen production. How the hormonal changes initiate pathological growth remains to be determined. Whatever the etiology, the only treatment at present is surgical.

Cancer of the prostate Prostatic carcinoma is the third most common cause of cancer death in men over 55; the incidence in autopsy studies varies from 12 to 46 percent, but only about a third of the cases are manifested clinically. More than 95 percent of prostatic malignancies are adenocarcinomas that arise from the prostate acini (the rest being squamous cell carcinomas or sarcomas). About 85 percent are multifocal or extensive.

Prostatic carcinoma can spread by local extension, by the lymphatics, or by hematogenous dissemination. Extension through the prostatic capsule is associated with a bad prognosis. The common sites of lymph node metastases are the obturator, hypogastric, and iliac nodes. Osseous metastases constitute the most common form of hematogenous metastases from prostatic carcinoma, particularly the pelvis, spine, femurs, ribs, and vertebrae. Common sites for visceral metastases include lung, liver, and adrenal glands.

Several staging systems for prostatic carcinoma have been proposed, and it is useful to categorize these tumors on the basis of clinical and pathological information:

State A: Tumors confined to the prostate and neither suspected nor detected clinically but rather diagnosed on the basis of histopathological criteria at autopsy.
Stage B: Tumors that are confined to the prostate and that are clinically evident on digital-rectal examination.
Stage C: Clinically evident tumors that have spread through the capsule but not metastasized.
Stage D: Metastatic prostatic carcinoma.

To stage accurately it may be necessary to use radionuclide bone scanning, skeletal radiography, lymphangiography, and, on occasion, staging pelvic lymphadenectomy. Serum acid phosphatase is usually elevated only in stage D; it has value for prognosis only in regard to the response to endocrine therapy. A decrease in acid phosphatase is associated with a more favorable response.

Discussion of the use of extirpative surgery, palliative surgery, and radiation therapy is beyond the scope of this chapter; it has been reviewed by Catalona and Scott (see references). The physiological rationale for the use of endocrine therapy in this disorder is based upon the fact that the acini of the normal prostate (and to a variable degree the malignant gland as well) are dependent upon circulating androgens, principally testosterone. Therefore, a variety of therapies have been devised to induce androgen deficiency, including castration itself, estrogen therapy (which suppresses luteinizing hormone release from the pituitary and induces a chemical castration), adrenalectomy (which removes sources of extratesticular androgen), antiandrogens that block androgen action, and enzymatic inhibitors of steroidogenesis that block testosterone synthesis. Of these various forms of therapy, castration and estrogen therapy in the form of 1 to 5 mg diethylstilbestrol daily, or both, have been tested most extensively, including a series of cooperative trials by the Veterans Administration Cooperative Urological Research group. In brief, there is no evidence that endocrine therapy or orchiectomy has a clear-cut role in patients with tumors that are localized to the prostate itself. In patients with invasive and/or metastatic disease who are willing to submit to orchiectomy, additional diethylstilbestrol therapy does not appear to be superior to orchiectomy alone; among patients unwilling to submit to orchiectomy, 1 mg diethylstilbestrol appears to be clinically effective and to avoid the significant excess of cardiovascular deaths that may result from higher doses.

Nonhormonal cytotoxic chemotherapy is now being evaluated in patients with prostatic carcinoma, and results indicate that 5-fluorouracil and cyclophosphamide may induce remissions in some patients with endocrine-resistant prostatic cancer.

DISORDERS OF ALL AGES Testicular tumors Testicular tumors occur with an incidence of 2 to 2.5 per 100,000 men per year in the United States and Canada and account for less than 1 percent of cancer deaths in men. The frequency is less among blacks than whites. The incidence of testicular tumors shows a trimodal curve, with peaks in childhood, young adult life, and old age. The majority of testicular tumors originate from germ cells.

Testicular maldescent is a predisposing factor for tumor development with the probability of a patient with cryptorchidism developing a tumor increased severalfold. In addition about one in five tumors that occur in patients with unilateral cryptorchidism develops in the descended testis. If boys undergo surgical correction of cryptorchidism before puberty tumors are rarely encountered.

GERMINAL CELL TUMORS There are four types of germinal cell tumors: seminomas, embryonal carcinomas, choriocarcinomas, and teratomas; 40 percent of germ cell tumors have mixed origins and contain two or more cell types.

Seminomas can be divided into spermatocytic and anaplastic types and are characterized by large cells with clear cytoplasm. They account for at least half of testicular neoplasms. Spermatocytic seminomas in older men are associated with a 90 to 95 percent five-year survival. Embryonal carcinomas are the most frequent testicular tumors in childhood and have 5-year survivals of 20 to 30 percent in adults and 70 percent in infants. Choriocarcinomas contain syncytiotrophoblastic cells, occur primarily in the second and third decades, and carry a poor prognosis. Teratomas contain at least two germ layers and may be benign or malignant. They comprise only 9 percent of adult tumors but are the second most common tumor of the testis in childhood. Of the mixed tumors of germ cell origin, perhaps the most distinctive is the gonadoblastoma, which is characterized by the presence of germ cells, sex cord cells, and usually Leydig cells. These tumors commonly originate from dysgenetic testes containing a Y chromosome and usually produce androgen.

STROMAL CELL TUMORS The most common stromal cell malignancies are Leydig cell and Sertoli cell tumors. They are rare in children and usually not malignant. Leydig (interstitial) cell tumors may result in masculinization or feminization, or both, or they may have no hormonal effect. Sertoli cell tumors (an-

droblastomas) contain cells that are arranged in tubule-like fashion and may result in feminization and rarely virilization.

ENDOCRINE MANIFESTATION OF TESTICULAR TUMORS Chorionic gonadotropin is present in normal testes, and it is therefore not surprising that plasma gonadotropins are elevated in testicular tumors. Indeed, an elevated plasma level of the beta subunit of human chorionic gonadotropin (HCG-β) serves as a sensitive and specific marker of tumor activity in a fourth of cases. Plasma levels are elevated in all patients with choriocarcinoma, in a third of embryonal carcinomas and teratocarcinomas, and only rarely in seminomas. There is an excellent correlation between change in HCG-β levels and response to therapy.

Elevated estradiol and testosterone production in patients with testicular tumors can arise by at least two mechanisms. In trophoblastic tumors and in tumors of Leydig and Sertoli cells production of both hormones may be autonomous in the tumor tissue itself; in these instances plasma gonadotropin levels and hormone production by the uninvolved portions of the testes are depressed, and azoospermia is common. However, when gonadotropin secretion by the tumors is elevated, the gonadotropin acts to increase estradiol and testosterone production in the unaffected areas of the testes, and azoospermia is uncommon. When potent estrogens and androgens are formed (directly or indirectly) by the tumors, feminization, virilization, or no obvious change may result, depending on the pattern of hormones produced and the age of the patients involved. Other cellular markers of testicular tumor activity have been described in individual cases, including α-fetoprotein.

Gynecomastia See Chap. 343.

CLINICAL ASSESSMENT OF TESTICULAR FUNCTION

LEYDIG CELL FUNCTION Plasma testosterone and dihydrotestosterone concentrations Plasma testosterone is measured by a specific radioimmunoassay. In the normal adult man the plasma values vary slightly throughout the day and at different times of the year, but these variations are not as great as those for plasma cortisol and are probably not significant in the routine clinical situation. However, because of episodic secretory patterns a single random sample will yield a result within ±20 percent of the true mean value only two-thirds of the time while three equally spaced samples 6 to 18 min apart provide a more accurate assessment. The samples do not need to be assayed separately, and aliquots of each can be pooled for a single determination. The range of blood testosterone in normal adult men is 400 to 1000 ng per 100 ml. Plasma levels of testosterone correlate in general with testosterone secretory rates measured by isotope infusion.

The plasma testosterone value in normal prepubertal children is statistically higher in boys than girls, the normal range being 5 to 20 ng per 100 ml. At the time of puberty the random daytime levels of plasma testosterone show a gradual increase that can be correlated roughly with the stages of puberty. However, the major change of plasma testosterone during the initiation of puberty occurs as a result of sleep-related nocturnal gonadotropin surges.

Dihydrotestosterone can also be measured by radioimmunoassay. In normal young men the plasma dihydrotestosterone level averages about 10 percent of the testosterone value and is around 50 ng per 100 ml. In older men with benign prostatic hypertrophy, plasma dihydrotestosterone levels are significantly higher and average 89 ng per 100 ml.

17-Ketosteroids The measurement of urinary excretion of 17-ketosteroids is not a suitable way to assess testicular function.

The androgens measured by this method are primarily weak adrenal androgens or their metabolites, whereas the major testicular androgen testosterone contributes only about 40 percent of daily 17-ketosteroid production in men.

Plasma LH The plasma luteinizing hormone is measured by specific radioimmunoassay and has greater variation throughout the day than the plasma testosterone. In fact, in adult men an isolated random blood LH is likely to be within ±20 percent of true mean value only a third of the time. Again, three samples 6 to 18 min apart as described above will yield a value more closely approaching the true mean. The normal plasma LH values should be established for a given laboratory and antibody used. The usual normal range in adult men is 26 ± 18 ng/ml. Any decrease in the plasma testosterone concentration can only be assessed if plasma LH is also measured, and likewise the "appropriateness" of a given plasma LH must be interpreted in relation to the plasma testosterone. For example, a low plasma testosterone coupled with a low LH implies pituitary disease, whereas the finding of a low plasma testosterone and a high LH suggests primary gonadal disease. Although plasma LH secretion shows specific relations to sleep during puberty, the pulsatile secretion in the adult is of equal magnitude during sleep and waking periods.

Response to gonadotropin stimulation Leydig cell function is especially difficult to assess prior to puberty, and it is common to measure response of plasma testosterone to gonadotropin stimulation as an index of Leydig cell reserve. The ability of the Leydig cells to respond to gonadotropin is usually assessed after administration of human chorionic gonadotropin (HCG) in repeated doses. A standard test for testosterone response to HCG is to administer 2000 IU intramuscularly daily for 4 days and measure plasma testosterone before the first dose and 24 h after the fourth dose. Normal prepubertal boys respond by an increase in plasma testosterone of about 300 ng per 100 ml; the magnitude of the response peaks early in puberty.

Response to luteinizing hormone–releasing hormone The response of plasma LH (and/or FSH) to the administration of luteinizing hormone–releasing hormone (LHRH) is also utilized as a test of the functional integrity of the pituitary-testicular axis. The rationale for this test and the underlying relationships are discussed in detail in Chap. 333. In normal men LHRH, when given in a 100-μg intravenous bolus, leads to a four- to eightfold increase in plasma LH and a one- to twofold increase in the plasma FSH. Three baseline samples should be obtained in the half hour preceding the injection and again at 30 and 45 min after the injection to allow determination of both the LH and FSH peak values. Plasma testosterone does not change significantly after a single bolus of LHRH up to 3000 μg. However, 2-h infusions of as little as 10 μg total of LHRH result in an increase of plasma testosterone of approximately 20 percent above base line.

SEMINIFEROUS TUBULE FUNCTION Semen analysis Seminal fluid analysis is performed on samples obtained by masturbation in a clear glass container after 24 to 36 h abstinence. Analysis should be performed within an hour. Immediately after ejaculation coagulation of the seminal fluid occurs, followed within 15 to 30 min by liquefaction. Estimation of motility should be performed in undiluted seminal fluid. More than 60 percent of the sperm should be motile and of normal morphology. The normal ejaculate volume is greater than 2 ml. The normal range for sperm count is 20 to 100 million per milliliter with a total per ejaculate of greater than 60 million. In a study of multiple ejaculates in individuals with possible

fertility problems, Sherins et al. demonstrated that semen quality and sperm output are frequently lower than is generally recognized among fertile men, and they have emphasized the difficulty of defining what constitutes the minimally adequate ejaculate. Three ejaculates are necessary to establish whether sperm count or morphology is adequate in most men, and as many as six or more ejaculates are necessary to establish a valid assessment in men who present with ejaculates of equivocal quality.

Examination of the testes Evaluation of the testes is an essential portion of the physical examination. The seminiferous tubules account for about 95 percent of the volume of the testes. The prepubertal testis measures about 2 cm in length and 2 ml in volume and increases in size in a predictable way with puberty; on average, the adult size is reached by age 16. When damage to the seminiferous tubules occurs prior to puberty the testes are small and firm, whereas the testes are characteristically small and soft following postpubertal damage. The normal adult testis measures 4.6 cm in length (range 3.5 to 5.5 cm), corresponding to an approximate volume of 12 to 25 ml. Age per se does not influence testicular size, and thus the significance of small testes is the same at all ages in the adult.

Testicular biopsy Testicular biopsy is performed in patients with oligospermia and azoospermia, both as an aid in diagnosis and as an indication of feasibility of treatment. This may be particularly useful in those instances in which plasma FSH is normal. Occasional patients with azoospermia may have obstruction of the vas deferens and a normal testicular biopsy. Tissue culture of the biopsy material with subsequent karyotypic analysis is necessary to identify those instances of Klinefelter syndrome secondary to chromosomal mosaicism in which the abnormality is limited to the testes. Testicular biopsy is often followed by a transient decrease in sperm counts, but no permanent adverse effects are usually encountered.

Plasma FSH Levels of plasma FSH usually correlate inversely with spermatogenesis in that men with an intact hypothalamic-pituitary axis have elevations of FSH if there is severe damage to the germinal epithelium. FSH is measured by specific radioimmunoassay. In normal adult men, the range of plasma FSH is 102 ± 55 ng/ml. Oligospermia due to a primary defect in the testis may be associated with elevated FSH levels, but an exaggerated FSH response to LHRH as an assay of pituitary reserve for the hormone may be a more sensitive measure of defective spermatogenesis.

ESTRADIOL As discussed above, most of the estradiol produced in normal men is formed by extraglandular formation from circulating androgens. Plasma estradiol is measured by radioimmunoassay and in normal men ranges from 20 to 42 pg/ml. The level of plasma estradiol in men is not always a good index of estradiol production rate. One reason is technical difficulty in measuring accurately the low levels normally present in men; many assays require concentration of larger plasma samples than necessary for detecting the levels in normal women. Another possible cause for the poor correlation may be episodic secretion in some men with enhanced estradiol production. Often there is better correlation between the clinical state and the total urinary production rate of estradiol. Elevated estradiol production and plasma levels can be due to elevations in plasma precursors (liver disease), to increases in peripheral aromatization (obesity), or to increased production by the testes (androgen resistance).

HORMONAL TREATMENT

ANDROGENS Replacement therapy Androgen replacement therapy is indicated in hypogonadal men in whom virilization or maintenance of established virilization is desired and in whom induction of spermatogenesis is not an immediate goal. Replacement therapy is given in the form of testosterone esters in an oil preparation. The two most useful esters are testosterone enanthate and testosterone cypionate. If pubertal development has not occurred, higher doses of these preparations are required initially until maturation is completed, then maintenance doses can be given. The usual dosage is 200 mg intramuscularly every 1 to 2 weeks initially and every 2 to 3 weeks thereafter. Patients can often administer the drug themselves. The exact treatment regimen needs to be tailored to the individual. The degree of return of sexual potency and libido is variable, but since the esters are hydrolyzed in the body, plasma testosterone level can be monitored to help in the assessment of the adequacy of replacement dosages.

The adverse side effects of testosterone-ester replacement therapy are usually minimal. In some older patients, who may have unsuspected carcinoma of the prostate, the possibility of androgen dependence of the carcinoma and its stimulation by replacement therapy should be considered. Testosterone ester preparations do not carry the same risk of inducing cholestatic jaundice as 17α-alkyl–substituted androgens (such as methyl testosterone). The use of the latter is no longer recommended.

Pharmacological uses The major pharmacological uses of androgens are for stimulation of erythropoiesis in a number of hematologic disorders and as adjunct therapy in some cases of carcinoma. Androgens are also used in an attempt to stimulate muscle mass and performance in athletes of all ages. There is no evidence that pharmacological dosages affect any aspect of male anatomic or functional development beyond that of the normal testicular secretion. Furthermore, in contrast to the minimal side effects of testosterone esters used as replacement therapy in adults the adverse side effects of all androgens prior to the onset of puberty and of 17α-alkylated androgen preparations at all ages are major. In spite of attempts to develop agents with pure anabolic properties, all such steroids are androgenic. In the prepubertal boy any androgen may accelerate epiphyseal development and result in early closure and decreased adult height. Gynecomastia is also frequently seen in children, presumably as the result of the conversion of androgens to estrogens. Spermatogenesis in adults is inhibited due to the antigonadotrophic action of androgens. At all ages 17α-alkylated androgen-anabolic steroids alter liver function and the plasma concentration of many proteins. Potentially fatal liver conditions such as hepatoma and peliosis hepatitis have been reported in patients who have received androgenic-anabolic steroids. Thus, the use of these agents in athletes is not only foolish but potentially harmful and cannot be condemned too harshly.

GONADOTROPINS Treatment with gonadotropins is utilized to establish or restore fertility in patients with secondary hypogonadism of all causes. There are two gonadotropin preparations now available for treating patients: human menopausal gonadotropins (HMG) and human chorionic gonadotropin (HCG). HMG (Pergonal), purified from the urine of postmenopausal women, contains 75 IU FSH and 75 IU LH per vial. HCG is available from several sources in vials of 5000 to 20,000 IU. HCG has little FSH activity and resembles LH in its ability to stimulate Leydig cells. Because of the expense of HMG, treatment is usually begun with HCG alone, and HMG is added later to stimulate the FSH-dependent stages of spermatid development. Comparison of various combinations of these two preparations in induction of spermatogenesis in prepubertal patients indicates that a high ratio of LH to FSH activity and a long duration of treatment (3 to 6 months) are necessary to bring about the maturation of the prepubertal testis. Once spermatogenesis has been restored in hypophysectomized patients or initiated in hypogonadotropic hypogonadal men by combined therapy, spermatogenesis can usually be maintained by HCG alone.

Men with oligospermia of unknown etiology have been treated with human gonadotropins. It is doubtful whether the incidence of fertility in these treated patients is greater than would occur in similar groups of untreated controls.

The dosage of HCG required to maintain a normal testosterone level is variable, ranging from 1000 to 5000 IU weekly. A variety of treatment regimens have been utilized to induce maturation of spermatogenesis. Most of these involve starting with 2000 IU HCG three or more times a week until most of the clinical parameters, including normal plasma testosterone, indicate normal adult male development. HMG (usually one ampule) is then added three times a week to complete the development of spermatogenesis. The length of therapy required to bring about restoration of spermatogenesis after regression is variable and may be as long as 12 months.

LUTEINIZING HORMONE-RELEASING HORMONE In view of the finding that repeated LHRH injections lead to normal gonadotropin responses in hypogonadotrophic hypogonadism, LHRH has been utilized as the sole form of therapy in some patients with this disorder. LHRH is not yet available for routine clinical use, and its advantages over gonadotropin therapy are not clear at present.

REFERENCES

AMELAR RD et al: *Male Infertility.* Philadelphia, Saunders, 1977, p 258

BAKER HWG et al: Testicular control of follicle-stimulating hormone secretion, in *Recent Progress in Hormone Research,* vol 32, RO Greep (ed). New York, Academic, 1976, pp 429–476

CATALONA EJ, SCOTT WW: Carcinoma of the prostate: A review. J Urol 119:1, 1978

GOLDZIEHER JW et al: Improving the diagnostic reliability of rapidly fluctuating plasma hormone levels by optimized multiple-sampling techniques. J Clin Endocrinol Metab 43:824, 1976

GRIFFIN JE, WILSON JD: The testis, in *Metabolic Control and Disease,* 8th ed, PK Bondy, LE Rosenberg (eds). Philadelphia, Saunders, 1979, Chap 22

HOLDSWORTH S et al: The pituitary-testicular axis in men with chronic renal failure. N Engl J Med 296:1245, 1977

KLEIN LA: Prostatic carcinoma. N Engl J Med 300:824, 1979

MEANS AR et al: Follicle-stimulating hormone, the Sertoli cell, and spermatogenesis, in *Recent Progress in Hormone Research,* vol 32, RO Greep (ed). New York, Academic, 1976, pp 477–527

MORTIMER CH et al: Gonadotropin-releasing hormone therapy in hypogonadal males with hypothalamic or pituitary dysfunction. Br Med J 4:612, 1974

OAKBERG EF: Effects of radiation on the testis, in *Handbook of Physiology,* sec 7: *Endocrinology,* vol V: *Male Reproductive System,* RO Greep, EB Astwood (eds). Washington, DC, American Physiological Society, 1975, pp 233–243

ODELL WD, SWERDLOFF RS: Male hypogonadism. West J Med 124:446, 1976

PECKHAM MJ, McELWAIN TJ: Testicular tumors. Clin Endocrinol Metab 4:665, 1975

SHERINS RJ et al: Longitudinal analysis of semen of fertile and infertile men, in *The Testis in Normal and Infertile Men,* P Troen, HR Nankin (eds). New York, Raven Press, 1977, pp 473–488

SIITERI PK, MacDONALD PC: Role of extraglandular estrogen in human endocrinology, in *Handbook of Physiology*, sec 7: *Endocrinol-* vol II: *Female Reproductive System*, RO Greep, EB Astwood (eds). Washington, DC, American Physiological Society, 1973, part 1, pp 615–629

VAN THIEL DH, LESTER R: Alcoholism: Its effect on hypothalamic pituitary gonadal function. Gastroenterology 71:318, 1976

WILSON JD: Metabolism of testicular androgens, in *Handbook of Physiology*, sec 7: *Endocrinology*, vol V: *Male Reproductive System*, RO Greep, EB Astwood (eds). Washington, DC, American Physiological Society, 1975, pp 491–508

342
DISEASES OF THE OVARY

JANET W. McARTHUR

INTRODUCTION The ovary is a specialized organ of reproduction which serves (1) as an exocrine gland which liberates gametes for fertilization and (2) as a complex of endocrine glands which secrete hormones responsible for (*a*) the growth and cyclic function of the reproductive tract and (*b*) a variety of metabolic effects in nongenital tissues. The interrelationship of these structures is complex. During mature reproductive life a new endocrine gland, the follicle, is activated each month. The follicle contains at least two cell types with different secretory capacities, the theca interna and the granulosa. After ovulation the follicle is transformed into a second gland of internal secretion, the corpus luteum. This structure likewise contains at least two types of cells with secretory capacities, the theca lutein and the granulosa lutein cells. The persistence of thecal elements within the primate corpus luteum may account for its unusual capacity to secrete estrogens and androgens as well as progestogens. The follicles and corpus luteum are embedded in an interstitium, or stroma, which constitutes a third endocrine gland.

A major difference between the ovary and the testis is that the former is endowed with a finite stock of germ cells, whereas the latter proliferates gametes continuously. The number of ova reaches a maximum 5 months before birth. Thereafter the number declines, mainly as the result of atresia, until by the end of the fifth decade the original complement of germ cells is exhausted. An inexorable, though less rapid, decline in follicular hormone secretion begins in the fifth decade. In addition, the secretion of luteal hormones becomes more and more erratic as the incidence of anovulatory cycles increases. By old age, only the ovarian stroma retains any semblance of functioning tissue.

DEVELOPMENT The formation of the gonads begins at a very early stage, when the embryo has attained a crown-rump length of 5 mm (21 to 28 days of age). The genetic sex of the conceptus is identifiable even earlier, at the age of 15 days, by the presence of nuclear sex chromatin in the female. During the seventh week, the ovarian destiny of the "indifferent gonad" can be inferred histologically by the absence of the epithelial cords which characterize the developing testis.

The first stage in the development of the gonads is migration of primordial germ cells from their site of origin in the endoderm of the primitive gut to bilateral thickenings (the "germinal ridges") of the coelomic epithelium ventral to the developing mesonephros. Sexual differentiation of the gonad begins as germ cell migration concludes. In the XX germinal ridge, the cortical germ cells (oogonia) increase rapidly in number as a result of mitotic division. After undergoing the requisite number of divisions, they enter the meiotic prophase,

to become, by definition, oocytes. Each is soon invested by a single layer of smaller supporting cells to form the primordial follicles. In this resting phase the oocytes remain throughout childhood and adult life until either preovulatory maturation or pseudomaturation with atresia occurs. The oocytes appear to exert an inductive influence upon the surrounding granulosa cells, since follicles fail to develop in ovaries which lack oocytes, and oocyte atresia is followed by granulosal degeneration.

In the XY germinal ridge, a testicular pattern of organization is imposed. The responsible agent appears to be a product specified by a Y-linked testis-determining gene or gene complex. This product is a plasma membrane protein serologically detectable as the so-called "H-Y antigen."

COMPARTMENTS The complexity of the tasks devolving upon the ovary is reflected in the heterogeneity of its structure. Throughout active reproductive life, morphological and biochemical events occur simultaneously in the follicular, luteal, and interstitial compartments.

In vitro studies show that upon incubation with acetate, each of the compartments is capable of synthesizing all the major categories of gonadal steroids. However, the steroidogenic capacities of individual cell types examined in this manner do not necessarily correspond to those manifested in vivo, since barriers affecting the availability of hormonal precursors and cofactors are necessarily breached. It is likely that a considerable degree of biochemical specialization parallels the anatomic specialization of the compartments and their subdivisions.

Follicle Follicular growth is a continuous process that begins during fetal life and continues until the stock of primordial follicles, the fundamental reproductive units of the ovary, is exhausted in middle age. The primordial follicle consists of an oocyte arrested in the dictyate stage of meiotic prophase and surrounded by a single layer of granulosa cells which, in turn, are isolated from the subjacent interstitial tissue by a basement membrane. The stimulus which initiates the growth of a given primordial follicle is unknown but appears to be independent of extraovarian controls and related to the size of the follicular pool. Once the growth of a follicle is stimulated, the process is inexorable and continues until either atresia or ovulation occurs.

At various times during the menstrual cycle a small cohort (usually four to six) of primordial follicles is recruited, seemingly at random, for growth. A growth stimulus is somehow delivered to the oocyte, with a resultant increase in RNA and protein synthesis. There follows a rapid enlargement of the oocyte to virtually adult dimensions, with restoration of the capacity to resume meiotic maturation. The investing granulosa cells exhibit little alteration until the oocyte completes its growth and is surrounded by the zona pellucida. The granulosa cells then lose their flattened appearance, become cuboidal, and commence mitosis. Once the fully grown oocyte is invested by two layers of cuboidal granulosa cells it becomes, by definition, a primary follicle.

Differentiation of the primary follicles is characterized by (1) the acquisition of receptors for follicle-stimulating hormone (FSH), estrogen, and testosterone by the granulosa cells, (2) the physiological coupling of adjacent granulosa cells, and of granulosa cells with the oocyte, by the formation of specialized membrane contacts (gap junctions), and (3) migration of the follicle from the cortex to the medulla where the follicle acquires a theca interna, containing steroid-secreting cells and blood vessels. The latter bring the follicle into contact with the hormonal milieu of the peripheral plasma, enabling FSH to stimulate the replication of granulosa cells and their synthesis and secretion of mucopolysaccharides, with fluid accumulation. These processes initiate the transformation of the primary into a secondary (or graafian) follicle, by definition a follicle containing a fluid-filled antrum.

Periodically, a so-called "leading follicle" is somehow selected from the cohort of fully differentiated primary follicles. Secondary follicle differentiation culminates in ovulation of the leading follicle and atresia of the other follicles in the cohort approximately two weeks later. Over this period, the granulosa cells undergo additional hormonally induced changes, which include aromatase activation and the acquisition of luteinizing hormone (LH), prolactin, and prostaglandin receptors. By virtue of its greater size and vascularity, the secondary follicle destined to ovulate can sometimes be distinguished laparoscopically in primates as early as day 2 of the cycle. The "leading follicle" also differs biochemically from the others in its greater rate of estradiol secretion. At the peak of follicular activity, the secretion rate of estradiol varies from 0.2 to 0.5 mg per day. The origin of follicular estrogen in vivo, long ascribed to cells of the theca interna, is currently attributed to the complementary action of granulosa and theca cells. The endocrine cells of the theca have been found to contain receptors for LH and to synthesize androgens rather than estrogens in response to LH stimulation. Granulosa cells, on the other hand, while exhibiting little capacity for de novo synthesis of androgens or estrogens, have been found to possess an active aromatizing system susceptible to stimulation by FSH. It may be that androgens synthesized by the theca interna or interstitium diffuse across the follicular basement membrane to enter granulosa cells for aromatization by enzymes induced by FSH. The newly synthesized estrogen is then released into the follicular fluid and peripheral circulation.

FIGURE 342-1

Plasma levels of FSH, LH, estradiol, and progesterone during the human menstrual cycle. The day of the midcycle LH peak is utilized as the central reference point for all data, and is designated as day 0. (After L Speroff, R Vande Wiele, Am J Obstet Gynecol 109:234, 1971.)

Maturation falls short of completion in all follicles but the one programmed to ovulate. The increasing concentration of estrogen secreted by this follicle stimulates the pituitary release of LH and FSH (see below). In response, the elected follicle exhibits an intense preovulatory growth spurt, accompanied by the initiation of meiosis in the oocyte, increasing antral distention, loosening of the cumulus oophorus (those granulosa cells which hold the egg in suspension), and increased vascularization of the theca interna with ultimate vascular invasion of the luteinizing granulosa cells. As the follicle enlarges, a specialized portion of its wall thins to form the so-called "stigma," which undergoes gradual dissolution, perhaps effected by proteases. These enzymes may be derived from (1) lysosome-like vesicles that appear in the surface epithelium and (2) the follicular fluid, which contains plasminogen. In response to FSH, plasminogen can be converted to plasmin, a protease, by means of an activator secreted by granulosa cells. Fenestrations develop in the basement membrane of the thecal capillaries, resulting in generalized edema of the wall. The follicular basement membrane bulges from the dissolving stigma and eventually ruptures, with extrusion of the mature oocyte-cumulus complex into the peritoneal cavity.

Corpus luteum Following ovulation, the ruptured follicle is converted into a corpus luteum, which likewise has a limited anatomic and biochemical life span. This is divisible into stages of proliferation and hyperemia, vascularization, maturity, and retrogression. The secretion of estrogen is continued and is supplemented by the secretion of progesterone. Biosynthetic activity increases steadily and becomes maximal on days 21 to 22 of the menstrual cycle, when implantation of the fertilized ovum occurs. Estimates of the progesterone secretion rate reveal a phenomenal increase in the biosynthetic capacity of the transformed follicle, to the vicinity of 20 to 40 mg progesterone per day.

Interstitium The interstitium, or stroma, acts as a supporting matrix for the follicles, corpora lutea, and corpora albicantia, and, in addition, it secretes steroids. Qualitative and quantitative changes in its structure occur in association with various reproductive processes. During pregnancy there is increasing luteinization of the stroma, and during the postmenopausal years stromal proliferation and luteinization are frequent. In extreme old age, the stroma tends to lose its stimulated appearance. The higher grades of stromal luteinization are sometimes associated with clinical indications of androgen hypersecretion.

The hilus may come eventually to be regarded as a fourth ovarian compartment, but at present it is generally treated as a specialized portion of the interstitium. It contains elements resembling testicular Leydig cells, which occur in nests, the size of which varies at different ages. Hyperplasia of these cells may occur during pregnancy, and the larger hilus cell complexes are more frequent in elderly women.

Androstenedione and dehydroepiandrosterone can be extracted from normal ovarian stroma, the highest concentrations being found in the hilus.

PHYSIOLOGICAL CONTROL OF THE OVARY Periodic variations in the secretion of the pituitary gonadotropins FSH and LH (Fig. 342-1) are responsible for the formation and differentiation of secondary follicles and the sequential changes in steroid secretion that characterize the menstrual cycle. A major function of these processes appears to be restriction of the number of ovulable follicles to that characteristic of the species.

At a very early stage of primary follicle development, FSH receptors appear in the granulosa cells in response to an as yet unidentified stimulus. In the human circulating FSH rises during the late luteal phase of the preceding cycle and gains access to the antral fluid of small follicles, thus promoting their development. As FSH and small amounts of LH increase estradiol secretion, rising plasma concentrations of estradiol gradually inhibit the pituitary secretion of FSH by negative feedback. However, growth of the "leading follicle" continues by virtue of its high estradiol content and consequent sensitization to gonadotropin stimulation. The growth of the other secondary follicles is curtailed by declining levels of FSH and perhaps by their lesser capacity to aromatize androgens which, by local accumulation, may promote atresia.

FSH and estradiol act synergistically to stimulate both the mitotic activity of the granulosa cells and the formation of LH receptors in preparation for eventual steroidogenesis by the corpus luteum. Unlike the FSH receptors, which are specific to the granulosa, the LH receptors appear mainly in the theca and interstitium and only variably in the granulosa cells. During the preovulatory period LH commences to rise and, as it gains increasing access to the follicle, arrests mitotic activity and estradiol synthesis and stimulates the secretion of progesterone.

Prolactin is also admitted to the follicular fluid, where its concentration exhibits marked fluctuations despite the relative constancy of its levels in the circulating plasma. During the early follicular and late luteal phases its intrafollicular concentration is high, and during the preovulatory phase (when progesterone secretion is maximal) its concentration is low. These oscillations may reflect the utilization of prolactin to maintain an adequate pool of precursor for intrafollicular progesterone synthesis.

The rising plasma concentration of estradiol eventually attains the strength and duration characteristics needed to exert a positive feedback action, triggering the midcycle surge of LH and FSH. The LH surge entrains the process that culminates in ovulation approximately 34 h later, with conversion of the ruptured follicle into a corpus luteum. Exposure of the follicle to high concentrations of LH induces a transient refractoriness to further stimulation, with a temporary decline in steroid synthesis and quenching of the LH surge. As responsiveness to LH is regained, the combined effects of this hormone (and perhaps prolactin) sustain the secretory activity of the corpus luteum for a limited period, with reimposition of negative feedback inhibition. Unless supplementary luteotropic stimulation in the form of human chorionic gonadotropin (HCG) secreted by the trophoblast of a conceptus embedded during the midluteal phase is delivered, the corpus luteum begins to regress within 9 to 11 days after ovulation, and its secretory capacity rapidly diminishes. A uterine factor (prostaglandin $F_{2\alpha}$) appears to be responsible for luteolysis in some species, but no such agent has as yet been identified in the human.

The in vitro synthesis of steroids by the interstitial cells of the stroma is increased by LH and HCG. During active reproductive life the physiological importance of this compartment appears to be minimal. However, during the postmenopausal years the interstitium secretes androgens, mainly androstenedione, a portion of which is converted peripherally to estrone.

The neuroendocrine control of gonadotropin secretion is vested in the central nervous system and the anterior pituitary gland (see Chap. 333). Communication between the two is effected by vascular links between the hypothalamus and the pituitary, including the hypothalamohypophyseal portal system. Luteinizing hormone–releasing hormone (LHRH) is synthesized and released by peptidergic neurons and conveyed to the anterior pituitary via the portal vessels. Specific receptors for LHRH are demonstrable on the plasma membranes of the anterior pituitary cells. The mechanism that governs LHRH release is only partly understood. However, clearly the process is affected by the steroid milieu, by prostaglandins, and by neurotransmitters conveying signals arising from higher centers of the brain.

There is likewise uncertainty regarding the location of the salient central nervous system components that govern gonadotropin secretion in the human female. In the rat, a so-called "tonic center" resides in the medial basal hypothalamus, sustains acyclic gonadotropin release, and responds to the negative feedback action of estrogen and progesterone; a so-called "cyclic center," comprising the preoptic and anterior hypothalamic areas, occupies a more rostral position and responds to the positive feedback action of estrogen. Under proper hormonal and environmental conditions, the cyclic center activates the terminal infundibular region and evokes the ovulatory gonadotropin surge. In the rhesus monkey, some investigators find that the neural components of the control system resemble those of the rat; others report that the mechanisms which regulate the tonic and surge secretion of LH and FSH are both located in the medial basal hypothalamohypophyseal apparatus, with the arcuate nucleus as the principal neural component.

Reproductive function is extraordinarily susceptible to the influence of exteroceptive factors such as light, the food supply, and stress. It is certain that the activity of the governing central nervous system structures, whatever their precise location, is modified by a barrage of afferent impulses, excitatory and inhibitory, from other areas of the brain. Once the mode of integration of these influences becomes known, such clinical enigmas as the pathogenesis of "summer amenorrhea" and "boarding school amenorrhea" may be divined.

HORMONES OF THE OVARY

The ovary secretes a water-soluble nonsteroid hormone known as *relaxin* and three types of steroid hormones: estrogens, progestogens, and androgens.

NONSTEROID Relaxin is a peptide hormone secreted by the corpus luteum of pregnancy. In conjunction with estrogens and progestogens, it facilitates parturition in certain mammals by loosening the symphysis pubis and sacroiliac joints. Relaxin has also been reported to soften the cervix, inhibit spontaneous myometrial contractions, increase the uterine responsiveness to oxytocin, and promote tubuloalveolar growth of the mammary gland. It is not detectable in the circulation during the luteal phase of the menstrual cycle. However, during fertile cycles relaxin becomes detectable by the time of the missed period. Thereafter, the serum concentration rises rapidly to a plateau from which it declines within the first three postpartum days.

A number of other nonsteroidal substances which exert physiological effects are detectable in follicular fluid. These include:

1 Folliculostatin, a peptide analogous to "inhibin," which suppresses the pituitary secretion of FSH and, to a lesser extent, of LH (Chap. 344). A reduction in the secretion of folliculostatin resulting from the depletion of follicles in premenopausal women may account for rising levels of FSH at a time when circulating levels of estrogen are still well maintained.
2 A meiosis-inhibiting factor that blocks oocyte maturation. Its effects can be overcome by LH.
3 A luteinization-inhibiting factor that prevents the in vitro luteinization of granulosa cells.

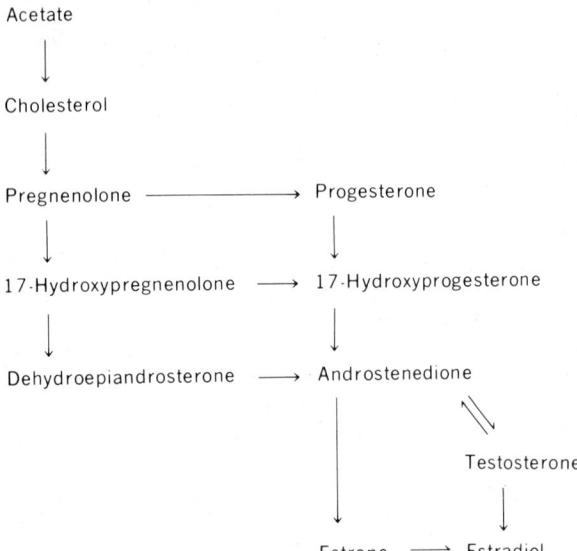

Acetate
↓
Cholesterol
↓
Pregnenolone ⟶ Progesterone
↓ ↓
17-Hydroxypregnenolone ⟶ 17-Hydroxyprogesterone
↓ ↓
Dehydroepiandrosterone ⟶ Androstenedione
⇅
Testosterone
↓ ↓
Estrone ⇌ Estradiol

FIGURE 342-2

Biosynthetic pathways for the synthesis of ovarian estrogen in the human female. (After OW Smith, KJ Ryan, Am J Obstet Gynecol 84:141, 1962.)

Although chemically characterized in varying degrees, none of these factors can yet be regarded as a hormone.

STEROIDS The ovarian steroids are synthesized from acetate via cholesterol and pregnenolone by essentially the same pathways as exist in other steroid-producing organs—the testis, adrenal cortex, and placenta (Fig. 342-2).

Estrogens The term *estrogen* refers strictly to substances capable of inducing estrus, or sexual receptivity, in female mammals. However, it has been extended to include compounds which produce certain uterine changes and to the steroid metabolites of true estrogens, whether or not these possess biologic activity. In the nonpregnant female, the ovary is the principal site of estrogen formation; during pregnancy, estrogen formation by the fetoplacental unit gradually increases until, by the third trimester, it may exceed ovarian production by a thousandfold.

17β-Estradiol is believed to be the primary secretory product of the human ovary (Fig. 342-3). This compound undergoes rapid oxidation in the liver (and perhaps other tissues) to estrone and slower reduction back to estradiol. Estrone can be hydroxylated at the C-16 position, with the formation of estriol, or at the C-2 position to form 2-hydroxyestrone. The latter can be further metabolized by methylation of the C-2 phenolic group to yield 2-methoxyestrone. Estrogen metabolites are conjugated, chiefly as sulfates and glucosiduronates, in the liver and to a lesser extent in other tissues. The conjugates are secreted into the bile and are resorbed, in large part, from the intestine whence they return to the liver via the enterohepatic circulation. The bulk of the estradiol metabolites are excreted in the urine, partly in free form and partly as sulfate esters or as glucosiduronates. Additional estrogenic metabolites of low biologic activity have been isolated in great number from human tissues and from the urine of pregnant and nonpregnant women.

The natural estrogens are all 18- or 19-carbon steroids which are characterized by the aromatic nature of ring A, the oxygen substituent at C-17, and the phenolic hydroxyl group at C-3. Many nonsteroidal estrogens have been synthesized for clinical use; they produce biologic effects resembling those of the natural estrogens. Representative examples from both the natural and synthetic categories are depicted in Fig. 342-3.

Progestogens The term *progestogen* refers to substances which serve to prepare the uterus for the reception and development of the fertilized ovum. It has been extended to include compounds capable of duplicating, in whole or in part, the effects produced by the corpus luteum secretions.

Progesterone is synthesized by all the steroid-producing glands. The ovarian progestogens consist of progesterone (Fig. 342-4) (the most important and abundant compound) and at least two other steroids: 20α- and 20β-dihydroprogesterone. Both these partially reduced compounds have been detected in human follicular fluid and in the corpus luteum and placenta, the 20α isomer in higher concentration than the 20β. The basic molecule consists of 21 carbon atoms, two of which are contained in the side chain at C-17. These compounds are secreted by the follicle just prior to ovulation and are produced in much larger amounts by the corpus luteum. The quantity of progesterone which can be isolated from the corpus luteum is small compared with the amounts of progesterone secreted during the luteal phase of the cycle, indicating that progesterone is secreted almost as rapidly as it is produced.

A number of progestational steroids which mimic various facets of natural progesterone action have been synthesized (Fig. 342-4). Many exhibit androgenic or estrogenic as well as progestational properties and, in these qualitative differences from the natural hormone, differ materially from the synthetic

NATURAL

ESTRADIOL - 17β

ESTRONE

ESTRIOL

SYNTHETIC

DIETHYLSTILBESTROL

17α - ETHINYL ESTRADIOL

3-METHOXY-17α-ETHINYL ESTRADIOL (MESTRANOL)

FIGURE 342-3

The structural formulas of some important estrogens, natural and synthetic.

estrogen compounds. The short half-life of progesterone and the large doses consequently required to elicit biologic effects have prompted efforts to alter the progesterone molecule so as to increase its potency. Two groups of progestogens far surpassing the potency of the natural hormone by oral administration have been synthesized: (1) derivatives of testosterone (e.g., ethisterone) and of 19-nortestosterone (e.g., norethynodrel and norethindrone), the latter of which exhibit the marked enhancement of oral potency which results from the removal of the angle methyl group C-19 attached to C-10, and (2) compounds derived from progesterone [e.g., medroxyprogesterone acetate (Provera), 6-dehydroprogesterone (dydrogesterone)]. Esterification of 17α-hydroxyprogesterone by caproic or other long-chain fatty acids yields long-acting preparations useful for parenteral administration (e.g., 17-hydroxyprogesterone caproate).

The liver is largely responsible for the inactivation of progesterone, which it reduces to pregnane compounds and conjugates with glucuronic acid for excretion. The major metabolites of progesterone excreted in the urine and bile are pregnanediol, pregnanolone, and allopregnanediol. Additional pathways exist for the catabolism of progesterone but are not yet clearly defined.

Androgens That the ovary possesses the biochemical potential for androgen production has long been evident from physiological and clinical observation. Improved analytic techniques now enable determination of the circulating levels and production rates of several androgens. In quantitative terms the major androgens are the 17-ketosteroids: dehydroepiandrosterone sulfate, dehydroepiandrosterone, and androstenedi-

FIGURE 342-4

The structural formulas of some important progestogens and allied compounds.

TABLE 342-1
Plasma androgens in normal women

Compound	Mean plasma concentration, per 100 ml	Relative androgenicity, %*
17-Ketosteroids:		
Dehydroepiandrosterone sulfate	170 μg	
Dehydroepiandrosterone	420 ng	5
Androstenedione	140 ng	10–20
17β-Hydroxysteroids:		
Testosterone	36 ng	100
Dihydrotestosterone	15 ng	125–300

* *Based upon testosterone as 100%.*
SOURCE: *After M Farber et al, Clin Obstet Gynecol 20(1):1, 1977.*

one. These should be regarded primarily as prehormones (or precursor substances), androgenic only in the sense that they can be transformed into active androgens by conversion 17β-hydroxy derivatives. The mean plasma concentrations and relative androgenicity of these compounds are shown in Table 342-1.

In women, androgenic steroids are directly secreted by two organs, the adrenal cortex and the ovary. Substantial quantities arise in nonendocrine organs by peripheral conversion from precursor steroids. The proportions of the principal androgens arising from these various sites are set out in Table 342-2.

Peripheral conversion of the androgenic hormones occurs in the blood, placenta, lung, liver, skin, hair follicles, and classic androgenic target organs, such as the clitoris. In androgen target tissues testosterone can be converted into the more active androgen, dihydrotestosterone, by the enzyme 5α-reductase. Dihydrotestosterone, in turn, can be transformed into a weaker metabolite, androstanediol, which is conjugated in the liver to a water-soluble glucuronide that is excreted in the urine.

Androstenedione is thought to be converted in the liver to testosterone and to undergo intrahepatic conjugation with glucuronic acid without mixing with the plasma testosterone. Thus, testosterone glucosiduronate is not a unique metabolite of testosterone. A proportion of plasma testosterone is reduced by the liver to the weakly androgenic compound, androsterone, and its inactive isomer, 5β-androsterone, and these compounds are rendered water-soluble by conjugation with glucuronic and sulfuric acid.

The biologic action of testosterone (like that of estradiol) is believed to be exerted exclusively by the unbound or free fraction in plasma. In the normal nonpregnant woman, this amounts to only 1 percent of the total concentration. The main plasma portion that binds testosterone and estradiol is the sex hormone–binding β globulin (TeBG). In hirsute women TeBG levels decline toward the male range, and the concentration of free testosterone rises from 1 to 3 percent of the total.

TABLE 342-2
Sites of origin of androgens in normal women

Compound	Percentage arising from: Adrenal	Ovary	Peripheral conversion
17-Ketosteroids:			
Dehydroepiandrosterone sulfate	> 90	< 10	
Dehydroepiandrosterone	80	20	
Androstenedione	50	50	
17β-Hydroxysteroids:			
Testosterone	0–30	5–20	50–70
Dihydrotestosterone			100

SOURCE: *After M Farber et al, Clin Obstet Gynecol 20(1):1, 1977.*

LEVELS IN BODY FLUIDS   Estrogens   Plasma levels of estradiol are measurable by fluorometric, isotopic, and immunologic methods. During the normal cycle, the range extends from 75 to 500 pg/ml. Estrone, estradiol, and estriol are measurable in urine by colorimetric and fluorometric methods. During the menstrual cycle, two peaks of estrogen secretion are generally noted, one in midcycle immediately prior to ovulation, and the other during the midluteal phase. The latter corresponds with the period of maximal activity of the corpus luteum. In the fifth decade of life, the urinary estrogen levels of women begin to decline. After the menopause estrogens continue to be detectable in body fluids, but the proportions change, estradiol levels being reduced more than those of estrone. In this circumstance, estrone arises almost entirely by peripheral conversion of androstenedione secreted by the adrenal cortex.

Levels of endogenous estrogen in patients with liver disease are variable, with only a portion displaying the increase that might be anticipated.

Estrogen determinations can be diagnostic in detecting granulosa cell or theca cell tumors in postmenopausal women. The adrenogenital syndrome and occasional adrenocortical tumors are also associated with elevated levels of estrogen.

Progestogens   *Progesterone* plasma levels are measurable by isotopic and immunologic methods. During the normal menstrual cycle, the range extends from 0.5 to 10 ng/ml. For detection of the elevated progesterone levels that validate the occurrence of ovulation, the plasma should be sampled between the eleventh and fourth days prior to ovulation.

Pregnanediol, the most important reduction product of progesterone, is excreted in the urine as the glucosiduronate and is measurable by gravimetric, colorimetric, and gas chromatographic techniques. Low and relatively constant levels of urinary pregnanediol (in the vicinity of 1 mg per 24 h) are detected during the follicular phase of the cycle; higher levels, with a range of 2 to 8 mg per 24 h, are found during the luteal phase. Since progesterone can be secreted by a luteinized theca interna as well as by a corpus luteum, elevated levels of plasma progesterone or urinary pregnanediol do not necessarily connote the prior occurrence of ovulation.

Androgens   *Testosterone, androstenedione,* and *dehydroepiandrosterone* are measurable in the plasma by double isotope dilution and by immunologic methods. Plasma androstenedione and testosterone concentrations vary during the menstrual cycle, the highest levels being found near midcycle. In addition, a circadian variation of plasma dehydroepiandrosterone and androstenedione occurs in synchrony with that of plasma cortisol. Measurements of these androgens are, therefore, better made in the afternoon than in the morning. (Although testosterone likewise exhibits a slight circadian rhythm, its magnitude is so slight that it can be neglected.) Since the levels of all these hormones fluctuate, repeated sampling with the combination of plasma aliquots to obtain a single integrated value is desirable.

Plasma androstenedione levels above 1000 ng per 100 ml and testosterone levels above 500 ng per 100 ml suggest the possibility of an adrenal or ovarian tumor (some would regard a testosterone level above 200 ng per 100 ml as distinctly suspicious). Hyperthecosis is generally and the polycystic ovary syndrome of Stein and Leventhal is frequently associated with elevated plasma levels of testosterone and androstenedione.

ACTIONS   Estrogens   The name *estrogen* does scant justice to the diversity of physiological effects produced by the estrogenic hormones. Their primary role is the development and maintenance of the female sex organs, and perhaps their most general effect is to promote tissue growth. At puberty the tubes, uterus, and vagina enlarge in response to increased estrogen stimulation, and the appearance of the external genitalia changes in consequence of fat deposition in the mons pubis and labia majora. The vaginal epithelium thickens during the follicular phase of the menstrual cycle, with shedding of a large number of cornified epithelial cells containing pyknotic nuclei. The cervix is stimulated to secrete mucus of low viscosity and high permeability to spermatozoa. The uterine and tubal mucosa and their vasculature proliferate, and their musculature becomes contractile.

Pubertal estrogen secretion causes the breasts to enlarge because of increased fat deposition, development of the supporting stroma, and ductal growth. The increased melanin pigmentation of the nipples and perineum is due, at least in part, to estrogen. There is a widespread deposition of fat in the subcutaneous tissues, particularly in the buttocks and thighs, leading to the characteristic rounding of the female figure.

The estrogens stimulate cell division in the deeper layers of the skin and gingivae, and in the mucosae of the oral cavity, nose, and urethra, causing a more rapid replacement of the outer cornified layers. Bone metabolism is significantly affected, with a positive calcium and phosphorus balance, widening of the pelvic outlet, and accelerated epiphyseal closure. Estrogens increase the levels of serum thyroxine-binding globulin, corticosteroid-binding globulin, ceruloplasmin, total copper, prothrombin, and factor V. Antithrombin activity is decreased by estrogens.

Progestogens Although secreted in far greater amounts than estrogen, progesterone exerts only negligible effects on the general body economy. It produces few specific changes when present alone, acting ordinarily in conjunction with estrogen. Progesterone tends to encourage tissue differentiation, rather than growth. Its most important function is to induce secretory changes in the lining of the tubes and uterus, the endometrium being thereby adapted for the implantation of the fertilized ovum. The viscosity of the cervical mucus is increased during the postovulatory phase, rendering it impermeable to spermatozoa, and ferning disappears. Tubal and uterine contractility are altered to favor transport of the fertilized ovum and to prevent its expulsion from the uterus. Lobuloalveolar proliferation of the breast is stimulated. Progesterone exerts a thermogenic action, the basal body temperature increasing by approximately 1°F in midcycle and remaining elevated during the luteal phase. A slightly negative nitrogen balance is induced by progesterone, and by antagonism to aldosterone, a negative balance of sodium, chloride, and water is favored. Progesterone acts as a mild respiratory stimulant, increasing minute ventilation while decreasing alveolar and arterial CO_2 tension and the respiratory quotient.

Androgens The physiological role of the androgens in the human female has not been clearly delineated. However, it is probable that they act to promote a positive nitrogen balance and to increase libido and muscular strength. At the molecular level, androgens are linked with the gonadotropins in complex synergistic and antagonistic actions within ovarian follicles. When fully delineated, such actions will likely illuminate not only the process of atresia but also such phenomena as the blighting of follicles in the polycystic ovary syndrome.

ENDOCRINE DISORDERS OF THE OVARY

Diseases of the ovary may be classified as endocrine and nonendocrine, depending on the presence or absence of disturbances in hormonal secretion. Endocrine diseases of the ovary, because of the prominence of their systemic manifestations, are of concern to the internist as well as the gynecologist and are considered here. Nonendocrine diseases, which comprise such entities are endometriosis, infections, and nonfunctioning tumors of the ovary, tend to produce localized effects and are not treated in this chapter. The endocrine disorders of the ovary may be classified as (1) hypo-, hyper-, or dysfunctional, (2) primarily ovarian in origin, or secondary to disturbances elsewhere, and (3) congenital or acquired. Some disorders are general in that they affect follicular, luteal, and interstitial functions; others are compartmental in that they involve only one or two of the major subunits of the ovary (Table 342-3). Methodological difficulties are responsible for the meager documentation of many ovarian syndromes. However, as these are overcome, a rational biochemical schema for classification is emerging.

Because of the specialized role of the ovary as an *organ of reproduction,* its disturbances tend to give rise to more restricted symptoms than do those of many other endocrine organs. Unless the influence of a feminizing tumor, for example, is projected against the barren sexual background of childhood or the postmenopausal years, the manifestations may be so inconspicuous as to escape notice. Disorders heralded by infrequent menstruation, staining, or the disappearance of cramps may be trivial in systemic terms and yet have profound reproductive consequences. This is attributable to the fact that except during periods of temporary dissociation, such as adolescence and lactation, the exocrine and endocrine activities of the ovary are firmly integrated. Any deficiency in either results in impaired reproductive function.

OVARIAN HYPOFUNCTION

Although the suspension of established ovarian function is readily recognizable as pathological, it may be less easy to determine whether delayed sexual maturation in a child reflects hypofunction of clinical significance. The *menarche* presently occurs at a mean age of 12.6 years; since its timing is significantly influenced by genetic factors, the family history as

TABLE 342-3
Classification of the endocrine disorders of the ovary

I Ovarian hypofunction
  A Primary
    1 General
      a Gonadal dysgenesis (Turner syndrome and its variants)
      b Autoimmune disorders with anti-steroid-producing cell antibodies
      c 17α-Hydroxylase deficiency
      d Iatrogenic (pelvic irradiation, cytotoxic drugs)
      e "Resistant ovary" syndrome
      f Menopause, premature and physiological
  B Secondary
    1 General
      a Hypothalamic disorders
      b Hypopituitarism
      c Constitutional and metabolic disturbances
    2 Compartmental
      a Anovulatory bleeding
      b Inadequate luteal phase
II Ovarian hyperfunction
  A Primary
    1 Feminizing tumors
    2 Masculinizing tumors
  B Secondary
    1 General: true precocious puberty
    2 Compartmental
      a Persistent follicle cyst
      b Corpus luteum cyst
      c Stein-Leventhal syndrome and hyperthecosis
III Ovarian dysfunction
  A Choriocarcinoma
  B Struma ovarii
  C Carcinoid

regards menarcheal age should be investigated. The menarche is ordinarily preceded by breast development, a spurt in skeletal growth, and the appearance of pubic hair (axillary hair tends to appear almost simultaneously with the menarche). The presence of any of the secondary sex characteristics or of superficial cells in the vaginal smear or urinary sediment constitutes presumptive evidence of incipient ovarian activation.

PRIMARY OVARIAN HYPOFUNCTION The list of entities in Table 342-3 is not exhaustive but illustrates the multiplicity of causes of ovarian failure.

Gonadal dysgenesis (Turner syndrome and its variants) See Chap. 344.

Autoimmune disorders Ovarian failure attributable to autoimmune oophoritis occurs most commonly in association with Addison's disease (see also Chap. 348). At least one-quarter of women with idiopathic Addison's disease have a menstrual disorder of some kind (see below). Other disorders with which autoimmune oophoritis may be associated include hypoparathyroidism, moniliasis, Hashimoto's thyroiditis, pernicious anemia, and diabetes mellitus. Characteristically, antibodies to graafian follicles, corpora lutea and, uncommonly, to ova are demonstrable together with antibodies to the adrenal cortex. It thus appears that despite the multiplicity of antibodies reacting with steroid-producing cells, all antigens are represented in the adrenal cortex, apart from the rare instances of antibodies to germ cells.

The role of ovarian antibodies in producing the pathological lesion of autoimmune oophoritis is uncertain. Some patients with idiopathic Addison's disease and ovarian antibodies menstruate normally. In others with premature ovarian failure, circulating ovarian antibodies are not demonstrable although, when exposed to ovarian antigen, the patients' leucocytes secrete migration-inhibition factor. In a group of patients with ovarian failure and Addison's disease accompanied by circulating antibodies to the corpus luteum as well as to the adrenal cortex, the addition of their serums to granulosa cells cultured in vitro induced cytotoxic changes, with a decline in progesterone secretion. It may be that certain types of ovarian antibodies are active in the induction of autoimmune oophoritis, whereas others serve merely as markers.

In autoimmune oophoritis, the ovaries appear small and shrunken and sometimes resemble the streaks associated with gonadal dysgenesis. Histologically, lymphocytic infiltration is characteristic. Some patients have anovulatory cycles and dysfunctional uterine bleeding.

17α-Hydroxylase deficiency (Biglieri's syndrome) In this condition, the proximal location of the enzymatic block to steroidogenesis results in an impairment of both ovarian and adrenocortical function. The diagnosis should be considered in young women with sexual infantilism accompanied by elevated levels of gonadotropins and hypertension. Replacement treatment with sex steroids as well as corticosteroids is indicated to combat premature aging, osteoporosis, and abdominal emergencies precipitated by the torsion of cystic ovaries. (See Chap. 343 for additional details.)

Iatrogenic ovarian failure Increased effectiveness of pelvic irradiation, and of chemotherapy for cancer and other grave diseases, has been achieved at the price of oocyte destruction, with amenorrhea and impaired fertility. The likelihood of delivering a sterilizing dose of radiation (doses in excess of 500 rads are likely to induce ovarian failure, especially in older women) can be minimized by elective transposition of the ovaries from the path of the x-ray beam. Chemotherapy with certain agents (e.g., busulfan, cyclophosphamide) can likewise inflict severe damage upon ovarian function. The endocrine profile in women with iatrogenic amenorrhea is similar to that of the premenopausal period: an elevated level of plasma FSH is associated with a normal or only slightly elevated level of LH, and luteal levels of estradiol. Fortunately, ovulatory menstruation sometimes returns in these circumstances, even after protracted amenorrhea.

"Resistant ovary" syndrome This condition is characterized by an elevation of circulating gonadotropins to the menopausal range, in association with (1) normal or low-normal estrogen production, (2) the presence of ovarian follicles in all stages up to and including antrum formation, and (3) a blunted response to treatment with exogenous gonadotropins. The most common clinical manifestation of the disorder is primary amenorrhea, although secondary amenorrhea has been reported in a few instances. On rare occasions, ovulation and pregnancy have been induced by massive gonadotropin treatment or wedge resection. The cause of the disease is not yet known.

Menopause PREMATURE The current median age of the menopause, or final cessation of menses, is 50 years. Opinion differs as to the age at which the menopause should be regarded as premature, but the development of permanent amenorrhea before the age of 40 is a widely accepted definition. Autoimmune oophoritis and the iatrogenic conditions described above are occasionally responsible; in a few instances, mosaicism of the sex chromosomes and mumps oophoritis have been implicated. In most cases, no explanation can be found.

This diagnosis is necessarily disturbing and must be made with circumspection. Measurements of estrogen as well as FSH secretion are advisable to exclude the diagnosis of the "resistant ovary" syndrome; in women desiring children laparotomy and ovarian biopsy are indicated. (Laparoscopic biopsies tend to provide mere nips of the ovarian cortex and have occasionally led to fallacious conclusions.)

PHYSIOLOGICAL This form of ovarian hypofunction is experienced by all women who survive to middle life. Fertility diminishes considerably before the menopause, apparently because the uterus becomes less efficient in supporting young embryos. The cause of the naturally timed climacteric is not entirely clear. It appears to reflect the progressive depletion of oocytes and the loss of their inductive effect upon the granulosa and theca cells. With a diminution of the steroid feedback influence upon the hypothalamus and pituitary, the gonadotropin titer rises. The finding of one, or preferably two, elevated plasma levels of FSH (which rises earlier and higher in the climacteric than does LH) is virtually pathognomonic of the menopause or the "resistant ovary" syndrome (see above).

The timing of the menopause seems to be unrelated to a preceding early or late menarche. An interval of approximately two years generally supervenes between the first symptoms of the climacteric and the cessation of menses. The manner in which menstruation ceases is variable (Table 342-4).

TABLE 342-4
First menstrual indication of impending natural menopause

Symptom	Percentage
Irregularity	34
Periods farther apart	23
Scanty periods	20
"Flooding"	16
Sudden cessation	8

SOURCE: *M Newton, PL Odom, South Med J 57:1309, 1964.*

Hot flashes, dyspareunia, and coitally induced cystitis are among the most troublesome symptoms. Hot flashes occur in 80 to 85 percent of menopausal women. They generally begin before the periods cease and may continue, though with diminishing frequency and intensity, for many years. Their pathological physiology is obscure. Subjective sensations of warmth are confined to the chest, neck, and face and may be accompanied by diffuse or patchy flushing of the skin and sweating. Hot flashes are characteristically brief, lasting only a few minutes, and occur most frequently when heat production is increased (e.g., after emotional stress or, less frequently, after meals) or when the dissipation of heat is impaired by bedclothes or by high ambient temperatures and humidity. The severity of menopausal symptoms is affected by the rate at which involution of the ovary takes place. In women experiencing a sudden (not necessarily surgical) loss of ovarian function, hot flashes are likely to be severe, whereas in women experiencing a gradual decline of ovarian activity, amenorrhea may be the only indication of "the change."

Mild depression is not uncommon in menopausal women, its frequency tending to be inversely proportional to the patient's understanding of menopausal physiology. A "menopausal syndrome" in a psychiatric sense appears to be nonexistent. Women with anxiety neurosis, hysteria, phobic states, hypochondriasis, or obsessive-compulsive neurosis during the menopause are generally found to have had the illness in earlier life. Psychological problems unrelated to the menopause per se are common in the 40- to 55-year-old group and relate to the "empty nest" syndrome; responsibility for the care of adolescent children and aging parents; ungratified sexuality; fears of obesity, cancer, and the loss of sexual attractiveness; and the fear of having ultimately to depend upon children or charity.

Osteoporosis is the most serious sequel to the menopause (see also Chap. 352). The incidence of this condition is estimated at approximately 25 percent of elderly women or approximately 8 million individuals currently living in the United States. All bones of the body are involved, but fractures affect primarily the cancellous bone of the vertebral bodies, femur, humerus, distal forearm, and ribs. Severe pain, with loss of height, results from vertebral fractures. A mortality rate variously estimated from 20 to 30 percent is associated with hip fractures, and disability is appreciable (13 percent of survivors are unable to walk). Estrogen treatment cannot restore lost bone, but it diminishes the rate of bone loss. Such loss is most rapid during the first 3 to 6 years after the menopause, and the response to treatment is greatest during this period.

Treatment of the menopause comprises (1) the exclusion of organic causes of any associated menorrhagia, (2) detailed explanation of the physiological consequences of the climacteric, ventilation of the patient's anxieties, and reassurance, and, when specifically indicated, (3) hormonal replacement. Estrogen treatment increases the well-being of menopausal women by suppressing hot flashes and preventing or relieving dyspareunia, and it probably diminishes the likelihood of fractures. The inference that in the absence of positive contraindications prophylactic estrogen treatment is indicated for all menopausal women might seem justified were it not for recent epidemiologic evidence from case control studies. However, these studies show a dose-related increase in the incidence of endometrial carcinoma by a six- to eightfold factor in estrogen-treated women.

It seems likely that the latent period for endometrial carcinogenesis extends over several decades and that the degree of risk is determined in large part by factors such as anovulation and obesity operating early in life rather than during the postmenopausal years. However, in the context of present information, recommendations as regard hormonal treatment can be outlined as follows:

I   Individualize patient selection.
   A   Consider the need for estrogen replacement in women who are in particular jeopardy of osteoporosis because of the following:
      1 Surgical or premature medical menopause at an early age.
      2 Impaired activity due to such disorders as arthritis and parkinsonism.
      3 Previous bone depletion due to adrenal steroid treatment, thyrotoxicosis, or gastrectomy.
      4 Undernutrition.
      5 Alcoholism.
      6 Heavy smoking.
      7 Osteogenesis imperfecta or a family history of thin bones.
      8 Paget's disease, especially with involvement of the hips or spine.
   B   Evaluate systematically the risks imposed by the following:
      1 Factors constituting an absolute contraindication to estrogen treatment such as treated or previously unrecognized cancer of the breast or uterus, and deep venous thrombosis and embolism.
      2 Factors constituting a relative contraindication to estrogen treatment such as chronic cystic mastitis, a family history of breast or endometrial cancer, anovulation and nulliparity with erratic bleeding and multiple curettages (e.g., the polycystic ovary syndrome), large uterine fibroids, extensive endometriosis, gross obesity, cerebrovascular disease, coronary artery disease, diabetes mellitus with vascular disease, liver disease, hypertension, cholelithiasis, pancreatitis, and porphyria.

II   Individualize treatment. Consider the intravaginal application of estrogen cream when local needs are paramount. Although systemic absorption is greater than originally believed, in some circumstances local treatment may diminish or obviate the need for systemic treatment.

III   Precede the institution of hormonal treatment with an endometrial biopsy or other monitoring procedure (e.g., jet washing) to exclude preexisting endometrial carcinoma.

IV   When systemic hormonal treatment is indicated, prescribe estrone sulfate (or some other natural estrogen) in the smallest amount that will eliminate hot flashes and repair vaginal atrophy, as judged by local comfort and moderate cornification of the vaginal smear. Administer estrogen cyclically during the first 3 weeks of each month. During days 8 to 21 inclusive of estrogen treatment, add an oral progestogen (e.g., medroxyprogesterone acetate 10 mg) to effect secretory differentiation of the endometrium. (Simulation of the luteal phase by the concomitant administration of a progestogen interferes with the replication of estrogen receptors and reduces the likelihood of hyperplasia.)

V   Insist upon careful recording of the dates of medication and of withdrawal bleeding by the patient.

VI   Examine the patient regularly, paying particular attention to the breasts and pelvis. In the event of unscheduled or excessive bleeding, refer the patient immediately for a dilatation and curettage. In the absence of bleeding vagaries, perform an endometrial biopsy or other endometrial monitoring procedure at regular intervals in view of the unreliability of the Papanicolaou smear for the detection of endometrial (as against cervical) cancer.

SECONDARY OVARIAN HYPOFUNCTION Hypofunction of all three compartments of the ovary, secondary to impaired synthesis or release of the pituitary gonadotropins, is a common consequence of functional or, rarely, of structural disorders of the hypothalamohypophyseal unit.

Hypothalamic disorders The pathogenesis of functional hypothalamic disorders is largely conjectural but is thought to reflect delays in the process of neural maturation required for the initiation of puberty, altered neural inputs to the hypothalamic centers controlling the secretion of LHRH, or impaired neurotransmitter metabolism. The result is a chronic diminution in the synthesis or release of LHRH.

The clinical diagnosis of a functional hypothalamic disorder is based upon (1) a history of secondary amenorrhea or delayed puberty associated with emotional stress, frank psychosis, or a rapid self-induced loss of weight, and (2) the exclusion of significant alternatives, such as primary ovarian failure, hyperandrogenism, and hyperprolactinemia. LHRH testing by means of bolus injections provides an assessment of the functional state of the hypothalamohypophyseal unit. However, uniform responses are not observed except in extreme instances of pituitary destruction or gonadal failure. LHRH testing tends to elicit a variety of responses reflecting diverse functional states rather than different diseases.

Emotional strain is perhaps the commonest of all causes of amenorrhea, apart from pregnancy. The vulnerability of girls in the second decade of life to such stresses as attending school away from home has given rise to the term "boarding-school amenorrhea." Basal plasma levels of estradiol and LH tend to be lower in such individuals than in cycling women during the follicular phase, while FSH is normal. Responsiveness to LHRH stimulation tends to be greater than normal, suggesting an impairment of gonadotropin release due to insufficient endogenous LHRH stimulation. Treatment with Clomid (Fig. 342-5) is sometimes followed by menstruation. This agent blocks the negative feedback action of estrogen at the hypothalamic level and evokes the release of FSH and LH from the pituitary. In severe cases, psychotherapy may be required to restore normal cyclicity. In older women menstrual cyclicity is more robust, and either exceptional stress or a frank emotional illness is required to suspend ovarian function.

Undernutrition, whether a consequence of simple weight loss resulting from injudicious dieting or anorectic behavior extending to anorexia nervosa, is likewise an exceedingly common cause of hypothalamic amenorrhea (see Chap. 77). Basal levels of estradiol and LH are low, the latter being reduced disproportionately to FSH. In the presence of extreme weight loss, the FSH and LH responses to a bolus injection of LHRH are greatly reduced; however, by repetitive testing a response can eventually be elicited. As weight is regained, FSH and, eventually, LH responsiveness to LHRH stimulation increase, and the menses return. Patients with this disorder tend to conceal the history of weight loss and are difficult to deflect from the practice of persistent dieting.

Postcontraceptive amenorrhea (i.e., that ensuing upon the suspension of a program of cyclic sex steroid treatment) is a iatrogenic state, which may or may not be accompanied by lactation. The omission of oral contraceptive preparations is generally followed by a prompt return of menstrual function; however, in occasional instances, prolonged and even seemingly permanent amenorrhea follows. Postcontraceptive amenorrhea appears to be a heterogeneous condition, up to 60 percent of the cases being attributable to undernutrition, depression, the ingestion of sedatives and tranquilizers, and previously undiagnosed conditions such as premature ovarian failure, the polycystic ovary syndrome, and pituitary tumors. The importance of excluding such possibilities before instituting a program of oral contraception in patients with irregular or absent menses is evident.

Congenital disorders in which hypogonadotropic hypogonadism is presently attributed to a functional disturbance of the hypothalamus include (1) the Laurence-Moon-Biedl syndrome, described in Chap. 104, and (2) the Prader-Willi syndrome of mental retardation, obesity, and hypotonia.

A structural defect (hypoplasia) of the hypothalamus is believed to underlie the congenital disorder *olfactogenital dysplasia*. This rare condition, which occurs much less frequently in females than in males, is characterized by sexual infantilism, anosmia or hyposmia, low levels of circulating gonadotropins and estrogens, normal but immature ovaries, and an absence of other endocrine disturbances. Thus, there appears to be an isolated deficiency of the gonadotropic hormones. At autopsy, agenesis of the olfactory lobes and of various areas of the rhinencephalon has been observed, but its relationship to the endocrine deficiency has not been determined. Various facial stigmata (e.g., maxillary hypoplasia) noted in occasional patients may reflect bony and rhinencephalic developmental abnormalities.

Acquired structural defects of the hypothalamus that may be associated with hypogonadotropic hypogonadism include hypothalamic tumors (cysts and gliomas, pinealomas, and histiocytosis), granulomatous diseases (sarcoidosis, tuberculosis and Hand-Schüller-Christian's disease), and postencephalitic lesions.

Hypopituitarism In early life, the commonest pituitary cause of sexual infantilism is a *craniopharyngioma;* in adult life, *chromophobe adenomas of the pituitary* and *necrosis resulting from postpartum hemorrhage (Sheehan's syndrome)* are the most frequent pituitary lesions resulting in ovarian insufficiency (Chap. 333). Lesions similar to those described by Sheehan have been reported following acute infections in nulliparous women and in men. If as little as 10 percent of the pituitary survives, gonadotropins can be secreted in amounts sufficient to sustain ovarian function. Thus, functional adequacy of the gonadotrophs depends less upon absolute cell mass than upon preservation of trophic connections with the hypothalamus. *Granulomatous diseases* and metastatic tumors or neoplasms arising in surrounding structures (meningioma) may diminish pituitary function at any age.

Headache, visual disturbances, or impaired growth suggests the possibility of a pituitary disorder in prepuberal girls, although failure of the menses to begin (primary amenorrhea) may be the sole manifestation. In adults, the cessation of menses previously present (secondary amenorrhea) and the coupling of lactation with amenorrhea should suggest the possibility of a chromophobe or acidophil tumor of the pituitary. X-ray visualization of the sella turcica and determination of the plasma prolactin level are essential components of the investigation of all patients with obscure amenorrheas.

Constitutional and metabolic disturbances Severe constitutional illnesses such as *congenital heart disease, regional ileitis, ulcerative colitis, hepatitis, chronic renal disease* (with delayed clearance of gonadotropins), and *rheumatoid arthritis* may de-

FIGURE 342-5
The structural formula of Clomid.

lay the menarche and, in adult life, may cause amenorrhea and sterility. Poorly controlled *diabetes mellitus* and either *hypo-* or *hyperthyroidism* may also impair reproductive function. The point of impact of these different disorders upon the hypothalamic-pituitary-ovarian chain is poorly defined. A recovery of ovarian function generally follows successful treatment of the primary condition.

Anovulatory (dysfunctional) bleeding Puberty and the premenopausal years are epochs during which the sluggish waxing and waning of the ovarian follicles, with an abnormally prolonged secretion of estrogen and an absence of ovulation, are particularly likely to occur. A teetering level of circulating estrogen results and is likely to be accompanied by painless menorrhagia (excessive menstrual bleeding), metrorrhagia (intermenstrual bleeding), or both, interspersed with long periods of amenorrhea. Anovulatory (dysfunctional) uterine bleeding, or *metropathia hemorrhagica,* is so common at the two extremes of reproductive life as to be virtually physiological. During the postmenarcheal years, there is either delayed maturation or transient impairment of hypothalamopituitary responsiveness to the positive feedback stimulus of estrogen, with failure to trigger the midcycle LH surge and a deficiency of progesterone. During the premenopausal years some women likewise exhibit diminished hypothalamic feedback sensitivity; others cannot trigger an LH surge because of impaired estrogen secretion, perhaps attributable to premature exposure of the growing follicle to increased levels of LH.

On rare occasions, a persistent follicle cyst is large enough to be outlined on bimanual examination. However, the diagnosis must ordinarily be made by exclusion. The disorders requiring differentiation vary according to the age of the patient (Table 342-5).

Dysfunctional uterine bleeding is rarely fatal, but anemia is frequent and requires replacement treatment with iron. In younger patients, the oral progestational agents, fortified with estrogen, are exceedingly effective hemostatic agents. Doses of, for example, 2.5 to 10 mg daily of norethynodrel with mestranol (Enovid) may be given for a period of 3 weeks and then withdrawn to permit a "medical curettage." When the bleeding has been checked and the hemoglobin level restored, normal ovulatory menstrual function may resume spontaneously. If this does not occur, intermittent treatment with Clomid may establish a normal feedback mechanism, with cyclic release of the gonadotropic hormones.

The rare but grave occurrence of bleeding from carcinoma of the vagina in puberal girls whose mothers were treated with diethylstilbestrol during pregnancy may be confused with dysfunctional bleeding. Inquiry concerning this possibility should be made routinely, and where a positive history is elicited,

TABLE 342-5
Some important causes of vaginal bleeding during different epochs of reproductive life

I Adolescence
   A Dysfunctional uterine bleeding
   B Blood dyscrasias
   C Malignant tumors of the vagina
II Maturity
   A Complications of pregnancy
   B Benign tumors (fibromyomas of the uterus, polyps of the endometrium and cervix)
   C Malignant tumors of the cervix and corpus of the uterus
   D Pelvic inflammatory disease
III Premenopause
   A Dysfunctional uterine bleeding
   B Benign and malignant tumors of the uterus
IV Senescence
   A Estrogen treatment
   B Senile vaginitis
   C Malignant tumors of the uterus
   D Feminizing tumors of the ovary

gynecologic consultation for detailed inspection of the vagina (if necessary, under anesthesia), complemented, if indicated, with Schiller's staining and biopsy, should be obtained. Because of the frequent occurrence of necrosis in such tumors, a negative Papanicolaou smear cannot be relied upon to exclude the diagnosis of vaginal cancer. In older patients with bleeding which is seemingly dysfunctional in origin, pelvic examination under anesthesia and curettage to exclude organic lesions are mandatory.

Inadequate luteal phase A clinically inconspicuous syndrome characterized by somewhat abbreviated menstrual cycles, infertility, and tendency to abortion is the so-called "inadequate luteal phase." In this disorder, the secretory activity of the corpus luteum is deficient and its term of activity is abbreviated.

A short luteal phase is physiological (1) in the later phases of the postmenarcheal period, when it is an important cause of "adolescent sterility" (anovulation is the proximate cause of infertility during the immediately postmenarcheal years), and (2) in the puerperium, when menstrual periodicity is gradually being regained. At other times it is pathological.

The diagnosis may be suspected from the character of the basal body temperature record, which is characterized by a slow rise to the luteal level and abbreviation of the luteal plateau. Confirmatory evidence may be obtained by histological dating of appropriately timed endometrial biopsies or by demonstration of subnormal levels of plasma progesterone during the luteal phase. The cause of the condition is uncertain. However, there is evidence indicative of a relative deficiency of FSH during the follicular phase, with impaired development of the follicle and subsequent inadequacy in corpus luteum formation or function.

OVARIAN HYPERFUNCTION

Ovarian hyperfunction may be relative or absolute. Thus, the elaboration of estrogen in amounts which are supraphysiological for the reproductive age of the subject constitutes hyperfunction, even though the quantity secreted is less than that characteristic of mature reproductive life.

PRIMARY OVARIAN HYPERFUNCTION Feminizing tumors *Granulosa and theca cell tumors* and, on occasion, certain other ovarian neoplasms may secrete estrogen. The stromal elements of tumors in the latter category (e.g., cystadenofibroma and primary adenocarcinoma of the ovary) may resemble those of the thecoma or may contain elements resembling theca-lutein or stroma-lutein cells. The histogenesis of these tumors is uncertain. However, granulosa and theca cell tumors appear to arise from the stroma or its follicular wall derivatives and recapitulate the elements of the follicular wall. Approximately 5 percent of the reported granulosa cell tumors arise before puberty, 55 percent during the period of reproductive life, and 40 percent after the menopause. Theca cell tumors tend to occur in a slightly older age group.

The *symptoms* depend on the age of the patient. Precocious pseudopuberty and intermittent uterine bleeding result from the function of such tumors during the premenarcheal years; irregular uterine bleeding, frequently alternating with periods of amenorrhea, is common during active reproductive life; bleeding is the characteristic manifestation of these tumors during the postmenopausal years.

Granulosa cell tumors compose approximately 10 percent of all primary ovarian carcinomas and are the most common hormone-secreting tumors of the ovary. From 10 to 15 percent of granulosa cell tumors exhibit a low degree of malignancy, in contradistinction to theca cell tumors, which are rarely, if ever, malignant. Both are almost invariably unilateral and tend at times to produce ascites. Meigs's syndrome of ascites and hydrothorax has been observed, especially with the theca cell tumor. Endometrial hyperplasia is a frequent concomitant, and the incidence of uterine leiomyoma, adenomyosis, and adenocarcinoma is increased.

The *diagnosis* is sometimes suggested by an unexpectedly high proportion of superficial cells in the vaginal smear. Plasma or urinary estrogen levels tend to be somewhat increased, and gonadotropin levels are occasionally depressed for a given age. Surgical removal is the treatment of choice.

Masculinizing tumors The Sertoli-Leydig cell tumor (arrhenoblastoma) and the *hilus-cell tumor of the ovary* are rare androgen-secreting lesions, the histogenesis of which is uncertain. The former tends to occur in comparatively young women, while the latter is characteristically a neoplasm of the late reproductive or postmenopausal years. Both are ordinarily unilateral and benign. The clinical course is one of defeminization followed by masculinization. The 17-ketosteroid excretion tends to be normal or only slightly increased and to be refractory to dexamethasone suppression. Plasma testosterone levels are often elevated. The treatment is surgical.

The so-called "lipoid cell tumor" of the ovary is a lesion with an uncertain histogenesis, although in certain instances it appears to arise from the ovarian stroma. The large rounded polyhedral cells of which the tumor consists lack the pathognomonic crystalloids of Reinke, but are otherwise identical with Leydig cells. The syndrome of masculinization resulting from the secretion of this tumor may be clinically indistinguishable from that produced by the arrhenoblastoma. The 17-ketosteroid excretion may assist in the differentiation in that it is generally elevated, sometimes to a marked degree. Both premenarcheal and postmenopausal cases have been reported, but twice as many tumors have occurred in premenopausal as in postmenopausal women.

SECONDARY OVARIAN HYPERFUNCTION True precocious puberty *Sexual precocity* associated with pituitary activation of graafian follicles is generally idiopathic or "constitutional" in origin. Constitutional precocity is presumed to be due to preternaturally early maturation of the hypothalamus, which escapes from the inhibition exerted by the small but physiologically significant amounts of estrogen secreted by the infantile ovary. Gonadotropin secretion can be materially reduced, with regression of the secondary sexual characteristics and protection from the hazard of pregnancy, by intramuscular injections of medroxyprogesterone acetate.

Sexual precocity is a cardinal feature of *Albright's syndrome of polyostotic fibrous dysplasia* (Chap. 352). There is no clear indication of the pathogenesis, and a genetic basis for the precocity has been postulated. In rare instances, hypothalamic cysts or tumors, or postencephalitic or postmeningitic lesions, are associated with a premature release of the gonadotropic hormones and activation of the ovary.

An unusual form of precocity is that associated with *hypothyroidism*, which increases ovarian sensitivity to endogenous gonadotropins. The precocity can be reversed by the administration of desiccated thyroid in doses sufficient to provide physiological replacement. These observations contrast with the effects of hypothyroidism on adult women, who commonly experience a failure of ovulation, with a tendency to dysfunctional bleeding.

Persistent follicle cysts Follicle cysts which persist during the climacteric tend to differ from those of puberty and the reproductive years in that, because of the hypersecretion of FSH and LH, they are likely to secrete estrogen in amounts exceeding those which are physiological during mature reproductive life. Massive estrogen treatment designed to inhibit the gonadotropic support of a palpable mass presumed to be a cystic follicle is warranted and is sometimes successful. However, because of the impossibility of distinguishing benign cysts from malignant tumors by palpation, the length of such trials should be carefully limited.

Corpus luteum cysts The classic instance of physiological luteal hyperfunction is the first trimester of pregnancy. In response to stimulation by chorionic gonadotropin, the corpus luteum of pregnancy secretes estrogen and, to a lesser extent, progesterone in amounts which exceed those characteristic of the luteal phase of the menstrual cycle.

A biochemically similar, but pathological, state results from the formation of corpus luteum cysts. These may arise spontaneously or iatrogenically as a result of the *administration of Clomid*. Those occurring in Clomid-treated patients may be multiple, giving rise to a severalfold enlargement of the ovary; those occurring spontaneously tend to be single, seldom exceeding a walnut in size.

The presenting complaint of patients with spontaneous cysts is often that of *sudden amenorrhea*. Such cases are frequently mistaken for ectopic pregnancy because of the adnexal enlargement, hyperemia of the vagina and cervix, and the swelling and tenderness of the breasts. The cysts are sensitive to touch, with fragile walls which are likely to rupture. The suspicion of ectopic pregnancy is therefore likely to be compounded by the occurrence of acute abdominal pain. So difficult is the clinical diagnosis that many patients are, in fact, operated upon to exclude the possibility of ectopic pregnancy.

The cysts resulting from Clomid treatment may enlarge with sufficient rapidity to induce lower abdominal discomfort. They are less fragile than the spontaneous variety and ordinarily regress spontaneously after the drug is discontinued.

Stein-Leventhal syndrome and hyperthecosis of the ovary These conditions reflect hypersecretion of androgens by the hyperplastic and luteinized theca interna enveloping the subcapsular cysts and atretic follicles, and by the ovarian stroma. Plasma levels of dehydroepiandrosterone and androstenedione, which may be converted peripherally to testosterone, tend to be elevated as are plasma levels of testosterone and free testosterone. The history is one of *irregular menstrual cycles*, generally experienced from puberty onward, and sometimes interspersed with long periods of amenorrhea and abnormal bleeding. There is hypersecretion of LH which tends to be released in erratic bursts (with an absence of the normal midcycle surge). The ovaries become polycystic, and, since ovulation occurs only rarely, there is associated sterility. Over a period of time the patients tend to develop hirsutism and, in occasional cases, frank virilism.

If the stroma contains nests of lipid-laden lutein cells, the term *hyperthecosis* is applied. Whether the Stein-Leventhal syndrome and hyperthecosis represent a pathological continuum or distinct entities is uncertain. Hyperthecosis generally evolves in a manner similar to that described for the Stein-Leventhal syndrome. Occasionally, however, there is an abrupt onset in older women (sometimes after pregnancy), and there may be associated hypertension and impaired glucose tolerance.

The pathogenesis of the disorder is not yet known. However, it appears that the dynamics of androgen-estrogen conversion are disturbed. A constant outpouring of estrogen from extraovarian sources tends to override the cyclic changes in ovarian estrogen secretion that ordinarily effect feedback regulation of cyclic gonadotropin release. Prior to the introduction of Clomid treatment, *wedge resection of a substantial amount of ovarian tissue* was the treatment of choice for the induction of ovulation. It is still of value in those patients who prove to be refractory to Clomid. Because of the characteristic hyperresponsiveness of the polycystic ovary, *Clomid is best administered initially* in a dose of 25 to 50 mg daily for 3 to 5 days, which is somewhat lower than that ordinarily effective in patients with persistent anovulation due to other causes. Neither Clomid treatment nor wedge resection ameliorates the hirsutism, except in rare instances.

OVARIAN DYSFUNCTION

In rare instances, bizarre dysfunction results from the presence of *ovarian teratomas. Choriocarcinoma,* a highly malignant tumor which secretes chorionic gonadotropin, may arise in the ovary of a girl nearing puberty and induce sexual precocity. *Struma ovarii,* which is generally a benign neoplasm, may secrete thyroid hormone at any age. Occasionally, the rate of secretion is so rapid as to induce thyrotoxicosis. *Carcinoid tumors* are sometimes found in dermoid cysts containing intestinal or bronchial epithelium. They may induce the characteristic "carcinoid flush," together with cyanosis and diarrhea, and may, in rare instances, exhibit metastatic spread.

REFERENCES

BAIRD DT (ed): Abnormalities of gonadotropin secretion in women. Clin Obstet Gynecol 3(3):465, 1976

BUCKINGHAM JC: The endocrine function of the hypothalamus. J Pharm Pharmacol 29:649, 1977

GIVENS JR: Hirsutism and hyperandrogenism. Adv Intern Med 21:221, 1976

GREENBLATT RB, STUDD J (eds): The menopause. Clin Obstet Gynecol 4(1):3, 1977

JUDD HL (ed): Reproductive endocrinology. Clin Obstet Gynecol 21(1):15, 1978

YEN SSC, JAFFE RB: *Reproductive Endocrinology. Physiology, Pathophysiology and Clinical Management.* Philadelphia, Saunders, 1978

343
DISEASES OF THE BREAST AND OF MILK FORMATION

KENDALL EMERSON, JR.
JEAN D. WILSON

APPROACH TO DISEASES OF THE BREAST   The examination of the breasts is an important part of the physical examination. This is because they are one of the commonest sites of fatal and preventable disease in women and because they frequently provide clues to underlying systemic disease in both men and women. Too often in the evaluation of women the internist is apt to refer this task to a gynecologist, whereas it is a duty and responsibility to distinguish the abnormal from the normal and to call for assistance if there is the slightest doubt. Commonly, the internist does not examine the male breast at all.

ENDOCRINE RELATIONSHIPS   There does not appear to be any histological or functional difference in the breasts of boys and girls prior to the onset of puberty, but at puberty there ensues a profound sexual dimorphism. The endocrine control of breast development in the female is illustrated in Fig. 343-1. The development of the normal nonlactating female breast is dependent primarily upon the action of estradiol, which induces the growth, division, and elongation of the tubular duct system and maturation of the nipples as well. In men the administration of estrogen is equally effective in this regard. To produce true alveolar development at the ends of the ducts, however, the synergistic action of progesterone is required, a ratio of estrogen to progesterone of 1:20 to 1:100 being optimal. Once this anatomical development is complete, continued estrogen and progesterone action do not appear to be required for lactation itself.

The formation of milk by the differentiated breast is one of the most complex of endocrinological phenomena, requiring, in addition to appropriate priming of the breast by estrogen and progesterone, a lactogenic hormone, glucocorticoids, and probably the permissive action of insulin and thyroxine as well. Two specific lactogenic hormones are thought to be involved in normal lactation. The first is prolactin, a peptide with a molecular weight of approximately 20,000 that is synthesized in specific cells in the pituitary. The concentration of plasma prolactin rises during pregnancy; indeed during late pregnancy and lactation 60 to 80 percent of the mass of the anterior pituitary may consist of prolactin-secreting cells. The second is human placental lactogen (HPL or chorionic somato-mammotropin), which is secreted in large amounts by the placenta during the latter phases of gestation and probably plays a significant role in preparing the breast for milk production. It disappears from the circulation shortly after termination of pregnancy.

Unlike most pituitary hormones, the predominant regulation of prolactin secretion is negative; that is, under ordinary basal conditions the hypothalamus secretes an inhibitory peptide hormone, prolactin inhibitory factor (PIF), which is delivered to the pituitary via the portal system and inhibits the release of prolactin into the blood. Many, if not most, factors that influence prolactin release are thought to do so by effecting the synthesis or release of PIF. Basal prolactin levels fall after delivery, but prolactin secretion is enhanced by stimulation of the breasts such as the act of nursing (the so-called "sucking reflex"), a phenomenon that is probably essential for maintaining lactation during the nursing period. In the postgestational state the normal woman is capable of forming about 1 liter of milk per day containing 38 g fat, 70 g lactose, and 12 g protein. Normal lactation can be suppressed either by the administration of estrogens or diethylstilbestrol, which appear to inhibit milk production directly, or by the administration of bromocryptine mesylate, which inhibits prolactin secretion.

GALACTORRHEA   Exactly what constitutes nonpuerperal or inappropriate lactation is not always clearly defined in the literature. According to the studies of Friedman and Goldfien, it is not possible to demonstrate any breast secretion whatsoever in normal, regularly menstruating nulligravid women, but breast secretions may be present in as many as one-fourth of normal women who have been pregnant in the past and may be of no clinical significance in these instances. Furthermore, in many descriptions no distinction is made between true milk formation and the capacity to express a few drops of colostrum-like liquid. Spontaneous leakage of milk from the breasts is usually of more concern to the patient than milk that must be expressed. With these problems in mind galactorrhea can be defined as any inappropriate production of milk that is persis-

STAGE	DUCT SYSTEM	MAJOR HORMONES	PERMISSIVE HORMONES
Prepubertal		None	Unknown
Adult		Estrogen (Progesterone)	
Pregnancy		Estrogen Progesterone Prolactin Human Placental Lactogen	Thyroxine Glucocorticoids Growth Hormone
Lactation		Prolactin Oxytocin	

FIGURE 343-1

Endocrine control of female breast development and function at various stages of life.

tent or worrisome to the patient, recognizing that in some instances no underlying pathology will be demonstrated. Milky discharges must be distinguished from dark or bloody secretions that may be present with neoplasm of the breast.

Since the initiation of milk secretion requires prolactin (or placental lactogen), it is logical to consider galactorrhea as a manifestation of deranged prolactin physiology. However, a complex endocrinological milieu is necessary for the initiation and support of lactation, and it follows that in many or most instances in which prolactin is elevated—in women who have not been appropriately primed or in men—no production of milk takes place. Furthermore, although enhanced prolactin secretion appears to be necessary for the initiation of milk formation, once commenced, maintenance of milk production may take place in the presence of minimally elevated or intermittently elevated prolactin levels so that increased basal plasma prolactin levels are not always demonstrated in patients with galactorrhea. For example, repeated stimulation of the nipples can cause galactorrhea with minimal elevations of basal prolactin similar to that found in the normal nursing mother. Perhaps the strongest evidence that prolactin is always involved in galactorrhea has been the demonstration that ergot alkaloids that suppress plasma prolactin levels to undetectable levels cause a disappearance of the galactorrhea even when the initial plasma prolactin levels are within normal limits.

Differential diagnosis With these various issues in mind, it is appropriate to consider galactorrhea in terms of deranged prolactin physiology (Table 343-1). Pituitary stalk section in humans results in a striking increase in prolactin secretion in men and women and a high frequency of galactorrhea, as the result

TABLE 343-1
Physiological classification of galactorrhea

I Failure of normal hypothalamic inhibition of prolactin release
  A Pituitary stalk section
  B Drugs
  C Central nervous system disease
II Enhanced prolactin-releasing factor
  A Hypothyroidism
III Enhanced prolactin release independent of the normal inhibition and release mechanisms
  A Pituitary tumors
    1 Prolactin-secreting tumors (Forbe-Albright syndrome)
    2 Mixed growth hormone and prolactin
    3 Chromophobe adenomas
  B Ectopic production of human placental lactogen and prolactin
    1 Hydatidiform moles and chorionepitheliomas
    2 Others (bronchogenic carcinoma and hypernephroma)
IV Idiopathic (following or not following pregnancy or contraceptions, with or without amenorrhea)

of interference with the delivery of PIF to the pituitary. Likewise, virtually all drugs that influence the central nervous system (such as tranquilizers) result in enhanced prolactin release by inhibiting PIF synthesis or release. Extrapituitary central nervous system diseases are also presumed to cause galactorrhea by the same mechanism (central nervous system sarcoidosis, craniopharyngioma, pinealoma, encephalitis, meningitis, hydrocephalus, hypothalamic tumors).

The existence of a physiological prolactin-releasing factor is still a matter of controversy, but in at least one pathological state, hypothyroidism, galactorrhea is thought to result from enhanced releasing activity. Thyrotropin-releasing hormone (TRH) stimulates prolactin release, suggesting that the galactorrhea of hypothyroidism is due to enhanced TRH secretion. Thyroid hormone replacement cures the galactorrhea.

Enhanced prolactin release can also occur from pituitary or nonpituitary tumors. Three types of pituitary tumors (see Chap. 333) may be associated with enhanced prolactin production and galactorrhea: (1) pure prolactin-secreting tumors (micro- or macroadenomas), (2) mixed tumors that secrete both growth hormone and prolactin and result in acromegaly with galactorrhea, and (3) some chromophobe adenomas. It is not clear whether the latter actually secrete prolactin or whether they interfere with the delivery of PIF to the pituitary. Prolactin can also be secreted on occasion by other malignancies such as bronchogenic carcinoma, and secretion of placental lactogen has been reported in hydatidiform moles and in chorionepitheliomas.

When all the known causes of galactorrhea are excluded, there is still a larger number of patients with galactorrhea of unknown etiology. This category includes galactorrhea and amenorrhea that follow pregnancy and delivery and spontaneous nonpuerperal galactorrhea. Many of these patients prove ultimately to have prolactin-secreting pituitary tumors; others probably have subtle disorders of hypothalamic function.

Diagnostic evaluation Once drug causes and hypothyroidism are excluded, the workup is fundamentally that of a pituitary tumor (Chap. 333). Even when a pituitary tumor cannot be documented and the diagnosis of idiopathic galactorrhea is made by exclusion, it is necessary to remember that pituitary tumors may subsequently become manifest. The higher the prolactin values and the more persistent the galactorrhea, the greater the likelihood of such a development.

Treatment The aim of all treatment is to remove the source of the elevated prolactin; resection of pituitary tumor, cessation of causative drugs, and correction of hypothyroidism are often followed by disappearance of galactorrhea. Two other forms of therapy may have some usefulness. Breast binders can be effective in some patients with mild galactorrhea of unknown etiology, presumably by preventing stimulation of the nipple and the consequent activation of the sucking reflex that may perpetuate lactation. Ergot alkaloids such as bromocriptine mesylate that suppress plasma prolactin have been used to treat patients with idiopathic hyperprolactinemia. They act not only to suppress lactation but may also result in resumption of normal menstrual cycles (and even fertility) in patients in whom amenorrhea accompanies galactorrhea.

GYNECOMASTIA Under usual conditions no breast tissue is palpable in the normal adult man. However, enlargement of the male breast can either occur as a manifestation of normal physiological development at certain stages of life or as the result of a variety of pathological conditions. In gynecomastia due either to normal or abnormal causes the enlargement is believed to result from disturbance of the normal ratio of active androgen to estrogen in plasma or within the breast itself. Indeed, whatever the etiology, the histological changes in gynecomastia correlate better with the duration than with the cause. Early gynecomastia is characterized by proliferation of both the fibroblastic stroma and the duct system, which elongates, buds, and duplicates. In gynecomastia of longer duration there is progressive fibrosis and hyalinization associated with regression of epithelial proliferation. Eventually there is a decrease in the number of ducts. Resolution occurs by reduction in size and epithelial content with gradual disappearance of the ducts, leaving hyaline bands which eventually disappear. In men given diethylstilbestrol histological changes in the male breast resemble those in other forms of clinical gynecomastia, a finding in keeping with the concept that all gynecomastia is the result of an estrogenic effect.

As described in Chap. 341, estradiol formation in the normal man occurs principally by the conversion of circulating androgens to estrogens in peripheral tissues; the normal ratio of production of testosterone to estradiol is approximately 100:1 (6 mg versus 45 μg), and the normal ratio of the two hormones in plasma is about 300:1. Feminization results when there is a significant decrease in this ratio, whether as a result of diminished testosterone production or action, enhanced estrogen formation, or both processes occurring simultaneously.

Physiological gynecomastia Physiological gynecomastia occurs under at least three circumstances. In the *newborn*, transient enlargement of the breast probably results from the action of maternal and/or placental estrogens. The enlargement ordinarily disappears in a few weeks, although it may rarely persist longer. *Adolescent* gynecomastia occurs in virtually all boys at some time during puberty. The median age of onset is 14; it is often grossly asymmetrical, occasionally unilateral for a portion of its course, and frequently tender, and generally regresses so that by age 20 only a small number of men have palpable vestiges of gynecomastia remaining in one or both breasts. Although the underlying source of the estradiol in the pubertal male is undefined, this process correlates with transient elevations of plasma estradiol prior to the completion of puberty so that the androgen/estrogen ratio is altered. *Gynecomastia of aging* also occurs in otherwise healthy men. At autopsy, as many as 40 percent of aged men have gynecomastia, and this is the result of an increase in frequency with age. A likely explanation is the elevation in plasma estrogen in aged men as the result of an increase in the peripheral conversion of androgens to estrogens with age. Since no attempt has been made to exclude abnormal liver function or drug therapy as contributing causes, the real significance of gynecomastia in the aging man is uncertain.

Pathological gynecomastia A tentative classification of pathological gynecomastia is presented in Table 343-2. In this reconstruction pathological gynecomastia is viewed as resulting from one of three basic mechanisms: deficiency in testosterone production or action (with or without a secondary increase in estrogen production), increase in estrogen production, or drugs. Most of the individual disorders that cause primary and secondary testicular failure have been discussed in Chap. 341. The fact that deficiency in testosterone production per se can cause gynecomastia is illustrated by the syndrome of congenital anorchia in which normal (or slightly low) estradiol production for a male in the presence of profoundly decreased testosterone production results in florid gynecomastia. In some instances of testicular failure, however, diminished testosterone production or action leads to elevated plasma luteinizing hormone (LH), which in turn results in elevated estradiol secretion by the testis and causes or worsens the gynecomastia. Such is the case in some patients with Klinefelter syndrome. In the inherited syndromes of androgen resistance, such as testicular feminization, deficient androgen action and increased testicular estrogen production have both been shown to be present, although it appears that diminished androgen action is the more critical in inducing gynecomastia.

A primary increase in estrogen production can result from a variety of causes. Testicular estrogen overproduction may occur in any situation in which gonadotropins are elevated, for example, because of aberrant production of chorionic gonadotropin by testicular tumors or by bronchogenic carcinoma. In addition, testicular tumors may secrete estrogen directly. Increased conversion of androgens to estrogens in peripheral tissues can be due either to idiopathic causes or rarely to tumors of the liver or adrenal gland. Increased estrogen production can also result from increased substrate availability for peripheral conversion, either because of increased production of androstenedione (congenital adrenal hyperplasia, hyperthyroid-

TABLE 343-2
Differential diagnosis of gynecomastia

I Physiological gynecomastia
   A Newborn
   B Adolescence
   C Aging
II Pathological gynecomastia
   A Deficient production or action of testosterone
      1 Congenital anorchia
      2 Klinefelter syndrome
      3 Androgen resistance (testicular feminization and Reifenstein syndrome)
      4 Defects in testosterone synthesis
      5 Secondary testicular failure (viral orchitis, trauma, castration, neurological and granulomatous diseases, renal failure)
   B Increased estrogen production
      1 Estrogen secretion
         a True hermaphroditism
         b Testicular tumors
         c Carcinoma of the lung
      2 Increased substrate for peripheral aromatase
         a Adrenal disease
         b Liver disease
         c Starvation
         d Thyrotoxicosis
      3 Increase in peripheral aromatase
   C Drugs
      1 Inhibitors of testosterone synthesis and/or action (spironolactone, cimetidine)
      2 Estrogens (diethylstilbestrol, birth control pills, digitalis, marijuana, heroin)
      3 Gonadotropins
      4 Unknown mechanisms (busulphan, ethionamide, isoniazid, methyldopa, tricyclic antidepressants)

ism, and most feminizing adrenal tumors) or because of diminished catabolism of androstenedione by the usual pathway (liver disease).

The ingestion of drugs may also cause gynecomastia by several mechanisms. Many drugs either act directly as estrogens or cause an increase in plasma estrogen, for example, in men receiving diethylstilbestrol therapy for prostatic carcinoma. Transsexuals in preparation for sex-change operations and homosexuals may also ingest estrogens. The gynecomastia of digitalis ingestion is usually attributed to an estrogen-like side effect of the drug, but in the experience of the authors it is usually associated with abnormal liver function tests. Abuse of marijuana and heroin also can cause gynecomastia associated with diminished plasma testosterone and an increase in plasma estrogen.

Another class of drugs is believed to cause gynecomastia by interfering with the synthesis and/or binding of androgen to its cytosol receptor protein; these include spironolactone and cimetidine. A third mechanism by which drugs can induce gynecomastia is illustrated by gonadotropin itself, which causes enhanced testicular secretion of estrogen. Finally, many drugs cause gynecomastia by mechanisms that have not been defined. These include busulphan, ethionamide, isoniazid, and tricyclic antidepressants.

Diagnostic evaluation The evaluation of patients with gynecomastia should include the following procedures:

1 A careful drug history.
2 Measurement and examination of the testes. If both are small, a karyotype is indicated, and if they are asymmetric, an evaluation for testicular tumor should be instituted.
3 Evaluation of liver function.
4 An endocrine evaluation to include 24-h urinary 17-ketosteroids (usually elevated in feminizing adrenal states), measurement of plasma estradiol (helpful if elevated but usually normal), and measurement of plasma LH and testosterone.

If LH is high and testosterone is low, the diagnosis is usually testicular failure; if LH and testosterone are both low, the diagnosis is most likely increased primary estrogen production (for example, a Sertoli cell tumor of the testis); and if both LH and testosterone are elevated, the diagnosis is either an androgen resistance state or a gonadotropin-secreting tumor.

Using these various tests a satisfactory diagnosis can be made in only half or less of patients referred for gynecomastia. This implies that either the diagnostic techniques are not sufficiently refined or that many causes of gynecomastia are as yet undefined.

Treatment In instances in which the primary cause cannot be corrected, surgery is the only effective form of therapy. Although the relative risk of carcinoma of the breast is elevated in men with gynecomastia, it is nevertheless rare. Indications for surgery include severe psychological and/or cosmetic problems, continued growth, or a suspected malignancy. Prophylactic radiation of the breasts prior to the institution of diethylstilbestrol therapy appears to be effective in preventing the development of gynecomastia and has a low complication rate in the age group affected.

CONGENITAL ANOMALIES Aberrant breast tissue (polymastia) and supernumerary nipples (polythelia) are commonly found along the so-called "milk line" extending from the midclavicle to the inguinal ligament. Absence of one or both breasts (amastia) occurs rarely.

INFECTIONS Acute pyogenic infections of the breast usually occur during the first 2 months of lactation and usually involve *Staphylococcus* or, less often, *Streptococcus*. They can usually be prevented by proper hygiene and treated with appropriate antibiotics. Acute mastitis unassociated with lactation may occur rarely during the course of paratyphoid or typhoid fever, brucellosis, or mumps.

Chronic tuberculous mastitis is a rarity today. It usually results from the extension of tuberculosis of the underlying bone into the breast tissue and should be suspected from the presence of multiple sinus tracts and the finding of active tuberculosis elsewhere.

INFLAMMATORY LESIONS Mammary duct ectasia is a benign condition, usually seen in elderly women with atrophic breasts, in which the mammary ducts in or just beneath the nipple become dilated and filled with cellular debris and lipid-containing material. Intermittent pain and local inflammatory changes may be present, and because a discharge, at times bloody, and retraction of the nipple may occur, this condition must be differentiated from carcinoma. Excision of the nipple is usually indicated.

Fat necrosis is a common occurrence following trauma that may be so slight as to have not been noticed. It presents as a painful lump usually associated with some ecchymosis and may be followed by local atrophy and dimpling of the skin, at which stage biopsy must be performed to distinguish it from carcinoma.

Thrombosis of the thoracoepigastric veins and sclerosing subcutaneous phlebitis (Mondor's disease) occur after trauma or for no apparent reason and are manifest by the appearance of long cord-like structures, initially tender, in the outer half of the breast, frequently extending up into the axilla or down toward the epigastrium. They may persist up to a year, but no treatment is indicated.

Sarcoid may very rarely involve the skin of the chest, and secondary amyloidosis may involve the breast tissue itself. Eosinophilic granuloma may occur in the submammary folds.

It must not be forgotten that carcinoma of the breast may rarely present as a subacute red, warm, indurated mass, resembling a bacterial cellulitis, the so-called "inflammatory carcinoma." This lesion may be suspected when the skin over it presents the characteristic *peau d'orange* appearance. Such tumors are inoperable and have a poor prognosis.

FIBROCYSTIC DISEASE With each menstrual cycle there is a recurring biphasic stimulation, first of proliferation of breast tissue by estrogens, then of alveolar secretory activity by progesterone, followed by a period of involution. In most women these changes are of such slight degree as to cause few if any clinical symptoms. Not infrequently, however, inflammatory changes may precede each menses, with tenderness, engorgement, and increasing nodularity of the breasts. This is more often seen in nulliparous women and may subside after childbearing and lactation. Suspected cysts in the breast may be aspirated safely in the office with local anesthesia if biopsy is done promptly in any of the following circumstances: (1) no fluid is obtained; (2) the cyst fluid is grossly bloody; (3) the mass does not completely disappear with aspiration; and (4) the fluid reaccumulates during succeeding days. Cytologic examinations of cyst aspirates are of no value.

In the later years of reproductive life the continued recurrent stimulation and involution of the breasts in the course of each menstrual cycle may result in diffuse and nodular fibrosis and the formation of cysts of varying sizes, so-called "chronic cystic mastitis." This condition may simulate carcinoma but is usually distinguishable by the fact that it is intermittently painful and may subside to some extent following menstruation.

Nevertheless, carcinoma may coexist and be masked by the diffuse nodularity of the cystic disease. Moreover, the incidence of mammary carcinoma is greater in patients with fibrocystic disease of the breasts, and it is unwise to delay biopsy of suspicious areas in the hope that they may subside by the end of the next menstrual cycle. In severe cases simple mastectomy is fully justified. Subcutaneous mastectomies with preservation of the nipples may be done in some cases, and the breasts may be reconstructed with silastic implants.

TUMORS OF THE BREAST Benign fibroadenomas of the breast may occur at any age but are more common in women under the age of 30. They may be distinguished from carcinomas by their mobility and well-defined margins, but biopsy is nonetheless imperative.

Benign intraductal papillomas may occur and cause a bloody discharge from the nipple. They are usually small and difficult to feel but may be located by noting that area of the breast on which pressure causes the bleeding. Excision is always advisable.

Sarcomas of all types make up less than 3 percent of all breast tumors. Fibrosarcomas are the most frequent; lymphosarcomas occasionally originate in the breast. Liposarcomas and hemangiosarcomas have been reported rarely. Cystosarcoma phylloides is a curious, very large, relatively rapidly appearing tumor arising usually from a preexisting fibroadenoma. It presents as a tender, warm, cystic mass, often replacing the whole breast. The skin over it is thinned, and the superficial veins are dilated. The tumor consists of fibrous cords covered with epithelium arising from the duct system. The cords are separated by cystic areas which become filled with leaf-like (phylloides) projections of epithelial tissue. Although these tumors are usually benign, blood-borne metastases have been reported, and surgical removal of the tumor is always indicated.

CARCINOMA OF THE BREAST In Europe and America carcinoma of the breast is the most frequent malignancy in women and causes more deaths than any other form of cancer in women. It occurs with increasing frequency from the age of 20 up to the menopause, when its incidence levels off until a second rise in frequency occurs after the age of 65. For reasons as yet not entirely clear, breast cancer is very much less common in Japan and other Oriental countries.

Etiology The cause of breast cancer, like that of most other forms of malignant disease, is unknown. A few factors affecting its incidence are, however, reasonably well established. The strong hereditary influence documented in mice may also be present, though to a smaller degree, in human beings. A two- to sevenfold increase in frequency in family members of patients has been reported. In this connection renewed interest in a milk-borne virus, first proposed by Bittner in 1936, has occurred as the result of finding alleged virus particles and virus-related information in the deoxyribonucleic acid (DNA) of human breast cancer cells. Antigens have been extracted from human tumors which cross-react with antigens obtained from the milk-borne murine mammary tumor virus (MuMTV), as well as with other human breast tumors from males and females alike. Moreover, serum from patients with breast cancer is capable of rendering the MuMTV noninfectious in mice, suggesting the real possibility of prophylactic immunization in humans, as has already been successful in mice. It must be emphasized that there is no evidence for the transmission of human mammary cancer through nursing.

The role of the estrogenic hormones in the genesis of breast cancer in humans is still controversial. The conservative view at the present time is that estrogens do not initiate the cancer

but may hasten its development in genetically susceptible individuals, in whom their prolonged use should be discouraged. Estrogenic substances stimulate the growth of breast cancer, once it is manifest, in a high proportion of women. The risk of breast cancer increases directly with the total duration of ovarian activity and is diminished in women undergoing surgical castration before the age of 40. On the other hand, it is remarkable that the vast increase in the use of estrogens for contraception during the past 20 years has not increased the incidence of breast cancer, with the possible exception of women who use them beyond the age of 35. Their prolonged use during the menopause should be discouraged. Risk of breast cancer is thought to be especially high in women who develop benign breast lesions after the initiation of estrogen therapy.

The risk of breast cancer is reduced as much as 70 percent in women completing their first pregnancy and lactation by the age of 18, as compared with the general population at risk. The extent of this reduction in risk by pregnancy decreases with age, and a first pregnancy above the age of 30 may actually increase the risk. The number of pregnancies after the first has no further protective effect, nor do abortions. These findings suggest that the initiating carcinogenic factors begin to operate at puberty but are somehow inhibited by the normal processes of pregnancy and lactation; the earlier this occurs, the more complete the inhibition.

The suspected role of prolactin in the etiology of human breast cancer has not been confirmed. Although temporary remissions may be induced by the suppression of prolactin secretion with L-dopa or bromocryptine mesylate, more prolonged remissions occur following pituitary stalk section when prolactin secretion is increased, even though lactation is taking place.

Observations on the epidemiology of breast cancer suggest that environmental influences may play a role. The disease is more common in Japanese women living in the United States than in Japan and in fat women than in thin. Of particular interest is the high incidence of breast cancer among the Parsis in Bombay, more than twice that of the general population in India. This ancient religious sect comprises a closely interrelated and affluent community having access to a relatively rich diet, thus combining genetic and environmental factors that might favor the growth of mammary cancer.

Pathology The primary site is usually in the ducts, less often in the alveoli. Multicentric origins are frequent, and all gradations of differentiation may be observed. Proliferation of dense connective tissue is common around groups of malignant cells, whether primary or metastatic, the so-called "scirrhous carcinoma." Unfortunately all degrees of differentiation may be found in different portions of the same tumor, and little prognostic value can be attached to the histological appearance of any one area of such a malignancy.

Mammary carcinoma is likely to metastasize relatively early to the regional lymph nodes—axillary and supraclavicular if the primary site is in the outer half of the breast, or the internal mammary chain if the disease arises in the inner quadrants of breast tissue. From there it spreads primarily to bone, lungs, liver, skin, and subcutaneous tissues, less frequently to the brain. Metastases may also occur in the ovaries, adrenals, and pituitary—areas rich in the hormones stimulating the growth of this type of epithelial cell.

Diagnosis The diagnosis of breast cancer is facilitated by the fact that it is possible to palpate this type of neoplasm directly.

Unfortunately, the diffuse nodularity of the adult female breast makes it difficult to detect early lesions. As a rule the physician must depend on such evidence as hardness, fixation to underlying structures, or dimpling of the overlying skin to distinguish a malignant mass from a benign nodule of breast tissue, and by the time these distinguishing signs have become apparent the cancer has all too often metastasized. Direct exposure of the breasts to irradiation with low-voltage x-rays in order to bring out contrasts in soft-tissue densities, so-called "mammography" or "xeroradiography," is of value in screening for breast cancer and in identifying small lesions in large, fatty breasts, but the oncogenic potential of these procedures limits their usefulness in premenopausal women. Current guidelines suggested by the National Cancer Institute recommended that routine mammography be restricted to women over 50 and to high-risk patients under 50, including women with a previous history of breast cancer or with a mother or sister with the disease. When secretions are obtainable from the nipple, cytologic examination may be helpful. The majority of patients with breast cancer suggest the diagnosis themselves as a result of detection of abnormal lumps or masses during self-examination. Although too great an emphasis on self-examination of the breast may encourage neuroticism and cancerphobia, it is the only practicable way by which the death rate from cancer of the breast can be reduced until a final cure for cancer has been found.

Treatment Total surgical excision provides the only permanent cure for carcinoma of the breast, and x-ray therapy is the best palliation for localized disease. The technical details of the surgical and radiologic treatment of breast cancer are beyond the scope of this chapter except to point out that there is an increasing trend toward less radical surgical procedures as adjuvant therapy is improved. However, internists should be prepared for patients who ask questions about these more limited procedures. For example, in short-term studies (5 years) excisional biopsy followed by radiotherapy provides excellent treatment of early-stage tumors with survival figures that approximate the results of standard radical mastectomies. Furthermore, since patients with advanced regional disease have a high likelihood of developing overt systemic metastases regard-

TABLE 343-3
Treatment of breast cancer: alternative methods following surgery

IN ESTROGEN-RECEPTOR-POSITIVE PATIENTS

Stage I: No apparent metastasis	Observe.
Stage II: Axillary metastasis only	Chemotherapy and immunotherapy (more aggressive therapy would add oopherectomy and adrenalectomy or prednisone and antiestrogens).
Stage III: Distant metastasis (skin, bone, lung parenchyma)	Chemotherapy and immunotherapy plus oopherectomy and adrenalectomy, or aminoglutethimide, cortisol, and antiestrogen if surgical procedures unavailable or unacceptable. Androgens for premenopausal and estrogens for postmenopausal patients are third choice.
Stage IV: Visceral metastasis (brain, liver, pulmonary lymphatics)	Same as stage III as patient's condition allows.

IN ESTROGEN-RECEPTOR-NEGATIVE PATIENTS

Treatment of stages II to IV should be confined to immunotherapy plus prolonged continuous chemotherapy alternating various therapeutic regimens.

less of the method chosen of control of the primary lesion, the rationale has been advanced that combined local excision and radiotherapy should constitute routine therapy. However, patients should be told that long-term survival figures are not available. If preservation of breast contour is a major concern, women should be informed that breast restoration after radical mastectomy by plastic surgery is moderately successful.

The two most important factors governing the prognosis of disseminated breast cancer and the success of its treatment or palliation are (1) the age of the patient and (2) the length of the free interval between the discovery of the primary tumor and the appearance of metastases. As with neoplasia in general, the younger the age at which it occurs, the more rapid and malignant is its growth. The only exceptions to this rule are the rare cases of juvenile breast cancer reported in patients from 3 to 15 years of age, which appear to have a more benign course. The length of the free interval is a rough measure of the balance between the biologic activity or turnover rate of tumor cells and the poorly understood factors of host resistance.

Because of the susceptibility of breast cancer to changes in the endocrine environment, every physician should be cognizant of the remarkable palliative effect which can be achieved in some patients with inoperable mammary cancer by intelligent hormonal manipulations. The rationale of the endocrine treatment of breast cancer is predicated on the assumption that in the total population of malignant cells some retain their metabolic dependency for growth upon estrogens for variable lengths of time before ultimately becoming autonomous. The first aim of therapy, therefore, is to remove all sources of estrogen from the afflicted subject. It is possible to determine the extent to which any given breast cancer is estrogen-dependent by measuring its content of receptors for 17β-estradiol, a technique which has become well established and should be available to any laboratory with facilities for performing radioimmunoassays. Current data indicate that about 60 percent of all breast cancers contain such estrogen receptors and that the majority of these will respond favorably to endocrine ablation, whereas the reverse is true when estrogen receptors are absent. It has been strongly recommended that the measurement of estrogen receptors be made a routine procedure when the initial pathologic diagnosis is made. The chances of a favorable response increase in proportion to the total number of estrogen receptors present and have been reported as high as 90 percent in a small series where progesterone receptors were also found to be present.

In stage I and II disease (Table 343-3) in premenopausal women prophylactic oophorectomy by itself has not been shown to prolong survival. However, castration will induce a remission in over 60 percent of estrogen-receptor–positive patients with symptomatic metastases (stages III and IV). The remission so produced may last from 6 months to 5 years or longer and provide a normal quality of life during most of that time. Since in the absence of ovarian function, some estrogen is still formed from circulating adrenal androgens, and since minute concentrations of 17β-estradiol (in the order of 10 pM) stimulate mammary cell growth, adrenalectomy should be performed in women with progressive disease who previously responded to oophorectomy.

Surgical hypophysectomy or pituitary stalk section induces a functional ovarian and adrenal ablation and results in a remission rate equal to but no greater than that brought about by the surgical extirpation of these target organs. The technical problems involved in removal of the hypophysis and the resulting morbidity have tended to discourage this procedure. However, if a neurosurgeon skilled in cryohypophysectomy by the transphenoidal approach is available, this procedure is an acceptable alternative to adrenalectomy. Pituitary ablation by radiation is too gradual to be of value in retarding the progress of a rapidly growing neoplasm.

Functional suppression of estrogen production by the ovaries may be achieved by the administration of medroxyprogesterone acetate, 200 mg intramuscularly at monthly intervals, or megestrol acetate, 40 mg qid orally, and simultaneously, the production of adrenal estrogen precursors can be inhibited by aminoglutethimide, 1 to 2 g, and cortisol, 40 mg daily. Such measures may be successful in retarding mammary cancer growth when surgical procedures are unavailable or unwarranted, but they have not yet had as adequate a trial.

In older patients, well past the menopause, large doses of estrogens may provide remarkable palliation. This paradoxical suppressive effect of estrogen (and androgen) administration in disseminated breast cancer may result from the fact that increasing concentrations of estrogens beyond the maximum stimulatory level (up to 2 μM) inhibit growth of human mammary cells in tissue culture. The place of androgens and estrogens in the treatment of metastatic breast cancer has been well defined by a report of the American Medical Association's Council on Drugs, based on a 10-year nationwide cooperative study. In summary, androgens produced objective remissions in approximately 20 percent of patients both before and after the menopause. Estrogens, which should not be used before the menopause, induce remissions in about 36 percent of patients during the first eight postmenopausal years and in more than 38 percent in later years. Estrogens have a greater effect on soft tissue and visceral metastases than on bone and equal or exceed the effect of androgens on all types of tissue. Estrogens must be employed in large doses to achieve these results, e.g., 15 mg diethylstilbestrol, or 3 mg ethynyl estradiol daily. Smaller amounts may affect the tumor adversely. Nausea and vomiting may occur at the onset of treatment but can be controlled by antiemetic agents and usually disappear in time. Uterine bleeding may be troublesome but can usually be controlled by the cyclic administration of progesterone.

The optimum dose of androgens has been found to be equivalent to 100 mg testosterone propionate given intramuscularly three times weekly. The major pathways by which mammary tumor cell growth may be influenced are summarized in Fig. 343-2.

All patients, but especially those within the first eight postmenopausal years, should be observed carefully during the first few days and weeks of treatment because both androgens and estrogens may cause an exacerbation of their disease, estrogens by a direct stimulating effect and androgens presumably by being converted to estrogen. One serious complication produced by these hormones is calcium intoxication in patients with extensive skeletal metastases. There is a marked increase in urinary calcium excretion, the serum calcium level may rise to as high as 15 to 20 mg per 100 ml, and drowsiness, coma, convulsions, and death from renal failure may ensue. It is important to distinguish this condition from cerebral or liver metastases or the terminal effects of widespread cancer because hypercalcemia can be reversed by forcing fluids, withdrawal of the offending hormone, and the administration of large amounts of glucocorticoids until symptoms subside. (For details of the treatment of hypercalcemia see Chap. 350.)

Because of this and other serious complications, estrogen and androgen therapy is being replaced more and more by chemotherapy and by endocrine ablative procedures whenever possible. Palliative effects equal to those of hormone administration may also be achieved more safely by the use of stilbestrol analogues which compete for estrogen receptors such as triphenylethylene 20 mg bid. Trends in the therapy of breast cancer are summarized in Table 343-3.

Hypercalcemia may, of course, occur spontaneously in far-advanced autonomously growing malignancy with widespread skeletal metastases but can still usually be controlled with the above measures plus the addition of a chemotherapeutic agent. Occasionally hypercalcemia may be found in the absence of demonstrable bony involvement. It has also been reported that a "calcium-mobilizing" steroid may be elaborated by breast tumors.

The rapid advances in the development of cytotoxic chemicals with varying cell cycle specificities and larger margins of safety have added greatly to the therapeutic armamentarium for the treatment of breast cancer. Current evidence indicates that prompt and prolonged administration of these agents in premenopausal patients with axillary metastases will lengthen significantly their free interval. The addition of chemotherapy to endocrine ablative procedures in stage III disease with distant metastases appears to prolong the remission in patients with estrogen-dependent tumors and may even induce a remission in a substantial number of those without estrogen receptors who would otherwise not benefit from surgery. Indeed, there is encouraging evidence that these patients may respond more favorably to chemotherapy than those with estrogen receptors. Many patients too sick for surgical procedures may show striking improvement for 1 to 2 years following administration of prednisone, 15 to 30 mg daily, with chemotherapy. Among the agents of proved value at present are doxorubicin hydrochloride (Adriamycin), cyclophosphamide, and L-phenylalanine mustard to reduce total cell mass and vincristine, methotrexate, and 5-fluorouracil used serially or in various combinations to provide cell cycle specificity. Careful supervision of therapy is essential to avoid unnecessary toxicity, with which the physician should be familiar.

The best treatment for localized bony and soft-tissue metastases is radiation, since the local control rate is in the range of 75 to 80 percent. Painful bony lesions are especially susceptible to this modality. Radiation may be used in conjunction with systemic therapy and at times may postpone the need for major ablation or chemotherapy, especially when only one or two metastases are evident or are symptomatic.

FIGURE 343-2

Pathways of influence on mammary tumor cell growth. Substances such as tamoxifen may compete for estradiol receptors in the tumor cell without stimulating its growth. One pathway not depicted is suppression of estrogen production by progesterone.

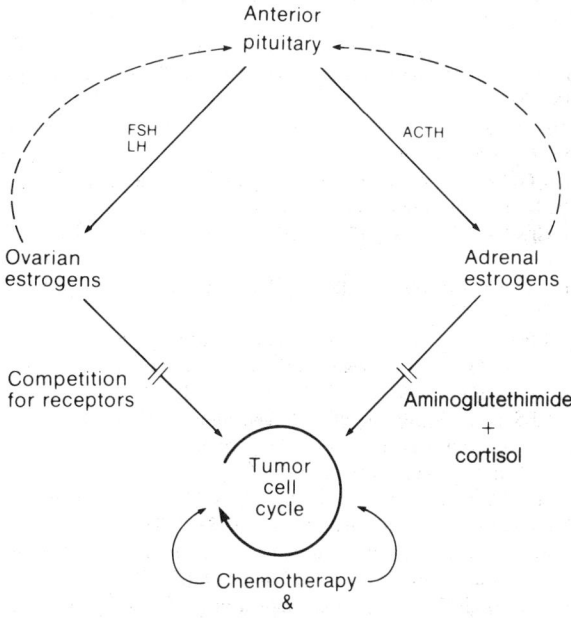

Metastases to weight-bearing bones should be treated prophylactically to avoid incapacity associated with pathologic fractures, especially femoral lesions. It is frequently worthwhile to perform operative reduction of pathologic femoral fractures in conjunction with radiotherapy, to keep the patient ambulatory, and to avoid the general deterioration that often occurs when such patients become bedridden. Many patients with slow-growing metastases may survive for prolonged periods in surprising comfort with carefully planned palliation.

It has recently been shown that the carcinoembryonic (CEA) antigen is elevated in the blood of 50 to 75 percent of patients with advanced breast cancer and can provide a valuable means of early detection of dissemination or recurrence. With the opening up of new avenues of approach to the control of this disease, the outlook for the patient with cancer of the breast is finally becoming brighter. An early aggressive multipronged attack is warranted.

Psychological support for patients with carcinoma of the breast is extremely important. It has been noted by many observers that these patients fear death less than they fear abandonment, especially by their primary-care physician. Because of the frustration and sense of professional failure that patients with diffuse metastases may engender in the physician, there should be a deliberate effort to see these patients at regular intervals to give supportive care even when the major modalities of therapy are no longer producing significant improvement.

Carcinoma occurs in the male breast at least 100 times less frequently than in the female. Otherwise it behaves in exactly the same manner. The treatment is the same except that orchiectomy replaces oophorectomy. Prednisone and hypophysectomy have both been shown to induce remissions when the primary disease has metastasized, and progestational compounds may be of value.

REFERENCES

BRUN DEL RE R et al: Prolactin inhibition and suppression of puerperal lactation by a Br-ergocryptine (CB 154). A comparison with estrogen. Obstet Gynecol 41:884, 1973

CHILD DF et al: Pregnancy, prolactin, and pituitary tumors. Br Med J 4:87, 1975

COCHRAN JS et al: The endocrinology of human chorionic gonadotropin-secreting testicular tumors: New methods in diagnosis. J Urol 114:549, 1975

DEL POZO E et al: Clinical and hormonal response to bromocriptin (CB 154) in the galactorrhea syndromes. J Clin Endocrinol Metab 39:18, 1974

FRIEDMAN S, GOLDFIEN A: Breast secretions in normal women. Am J Obstet Gynecol 104:846, 1969

GORDON GG et al: Conversion of androgens to estrogens in cirrhosis of the liver. J Clin Endocrinol Metab 40:1018, 1975

HAAGENSEN CD: Diseases of the Breast, 2d ed. Philadelphia, Saunders, 1971

HASKELL CM et al: Systemic therapy for breast cancer. Ann Intern Med 86:68, 1977

JENSEN EB et al: Prediction of hormone dependency in human breast cancer, in Estrogen Receptors in Human Breast Cancer, WL McGuire et al (eds). New York, Raven Press, 1975, pp 37–56

KEENAN BS et al: Syndrome of androgen insensitivity in man: Absence of 5α-dihydrotestosterone binding protein in skin fibroblasts. J Clin Endocrinol Metab 38:1143, 1974

KLEINBERG DL et al: Galactorrhea: A study of 235 cases, including 48 with pituitary tumors. N Engl J Med 296:589, 1977

LaFRANCHI SH et al: Pubertal gynecomastia and transient evaluation of serum estradiol level. Am J Dis Child 129:927, 1975

LEVENE MD et al: Treatment of carcinoma of the breast by radiation therapy. Cancer 39:2840, 1977

LeWINN EB: Gynecomastia during digitalis therapy. Report of eight additional cases with liver-function studies. N Engl J Med 248:316, 1953

LIPPMAN ME et al: The relation between estrogen receptors and response rate to cytotoxic chemotherapy in metastatic breast cancer. N Engl J Med 298:1223, 1978

MacMAHON B, BROWN CP: Etiology of human breast cancer: A review. J Natl Cancer Inst 50:21, 1973

MEYSKENS FL JR et al: Male breast cancer: A review. Cancer Treatment Rev 3:83, 1976

MOORE FD et al: Adrenalectomy with chemotherapy in the treatment of advanced breast cancer: Objective and subjective response rates; duration and quality of life. Surgery 76:376, 1974

NYDICK M et al: Gynecomastia in adolescent boys. JAMA 178:449, 1961

RELKIN R: Galactorrhea: A review. NY State J Med 65:2800, 1965

SHEVACH AB, SPELLACY WN: Galactorrhea and contraceptive practices. Obstet Gynecol 38:287, 1971

WILLIAMS MJ: Gynecomastia. Its incidence, recognition, and host characterization in 447 autopsy cases. Am J Med 34:103, 1963

WILSON JD et al: The pathogenesis of gynecomastia. Adv Intern Med 1980 (in press)

WOLF H et al: Prevention of estrogen-induced gynecomastia by external irradiation. J Urol 102:607, 1969

344
DISORDERS OF SEXUAL DIFFERENTIATION

JEAN D. WILSON
JAMES E. GRIFFIN

Chromosomal sex, which is established at the moment of fertilization, determines gonadal sex, and gonadal sex in turn determines the development of phenotypic sex, in which the mature male or female phenotype is formed (Fig. 344-1). A disturbance during embryogenesis of any step in this developmental process may be reflected clinically as a disorder of sexual differentiation. There are a variety of known mechanisms by which abnormalities in human development can arise, including environmental insult as in the ingestion of a virilizing drug during pregnancy, nonfamilial aberrations of the sex chromosomes as in 45,X gonadal dysgenesis, developmental birth defects of multifactoral etiology as in most cases of hypospadias, or hereditary disorders resulting from single-gene mutations as in the testicular feminization syndrome.

From the standpoint of understanding the pathophysiology of abnormalities in sexual development, disorders can be categorized as resulting from derangements in one of the three principal processes involved in sexual differentiation, namely, disorders of chromosomal sex, disorders of gonadal sex, and disorders of phenotypic sex. In the present stage of our understanding of the pathophysiology some assignments of category

FIGURE 344-1

Jost model for determination of sex.

CHROMOSOMAL SEX

↓

GONADAL SEX

↓

PHENOTYPIC SEX

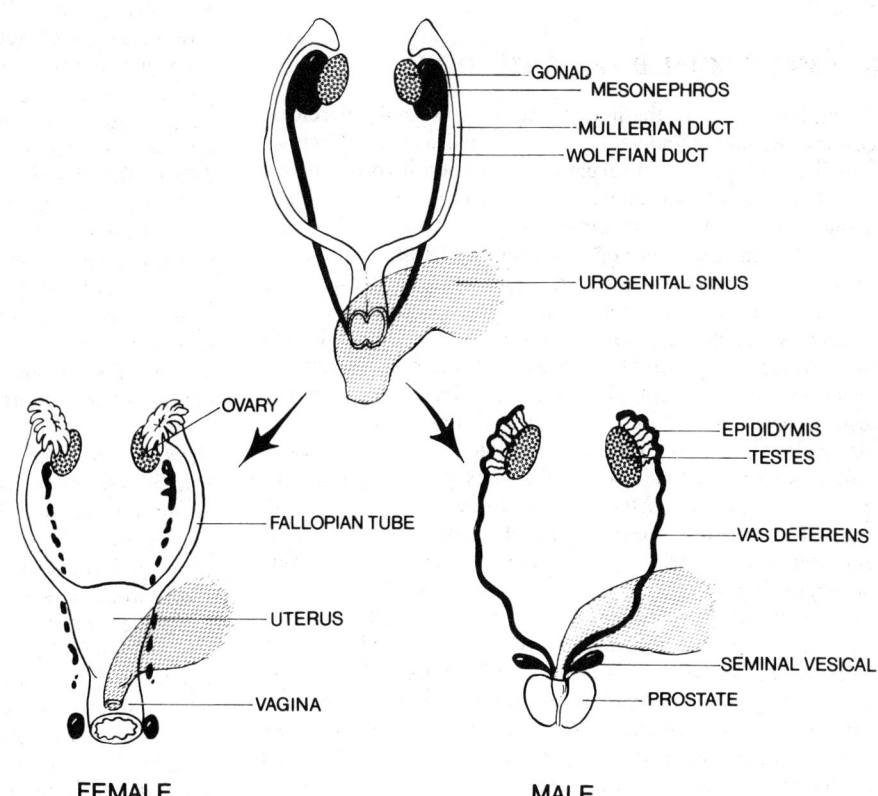

FIGURE 344-2

Normal sexual differentiation. A. Internal genitalia. B. External genitalia.

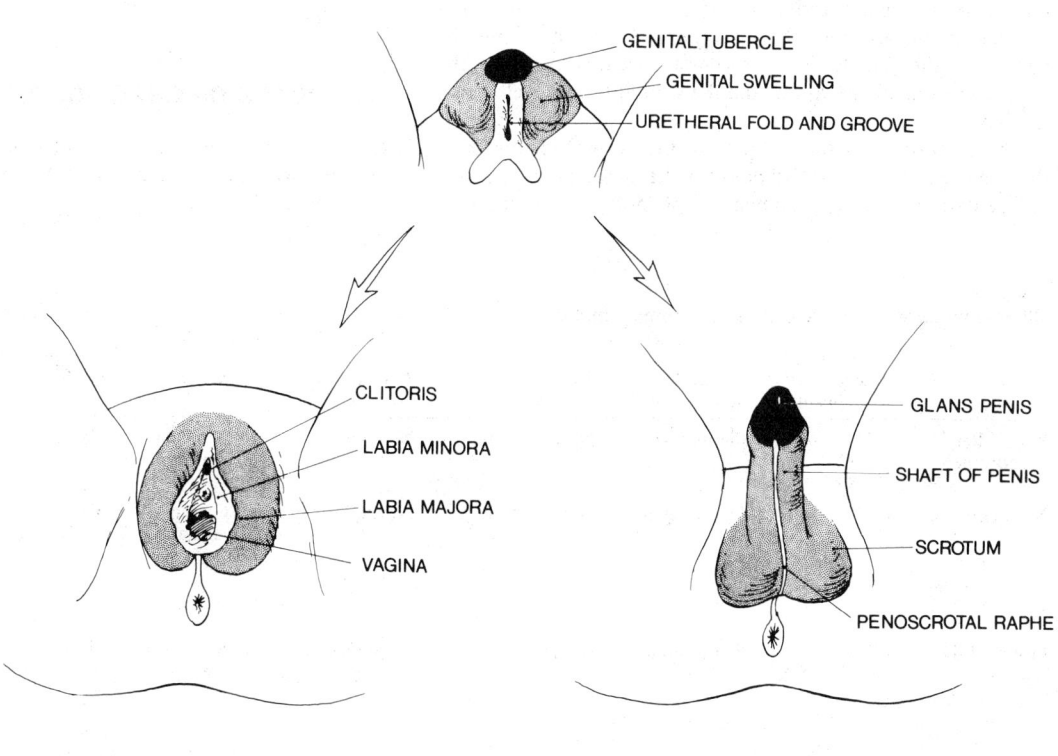

must be made empirically with the clear recognition that future work may make it necessary to alter the classification. In addition, since the process of sexual differentiation takes place over a period of many months, it is inevitable that individual traits (such as hypospadias) may result from abnormalities that occur at any stage in this process. Nevertheless, the combination of genetic, phenotypic, and chromosomal assessment usually restricts the diagnostic possibilities to a limited number of conditions, so that appropriate gender assignment and/or tailoring of phenotype can be carried out.

NORMAL SEXUAL DIFFERENTIATION

An understanding of the normal process of sexual differentiation is essential for understanding abnormal sexual differentiation. The first process in sexual differentiation involves the establishment of chromosomal sex, the heterogametic sex (XY) being male and the homogametic sex (XX) female. The embryos of both sexes develop in an identical fashion until approximately 40 days of gestation, and only thereafter does development diverge to result in the formation of the male and female phenotypes. The second phase of sexual differentiation involves the conversion of the indifferent gonad into a testis or an ovary. The differentiation of the indifferent gonad into a testis appears to be dependent on a Y chromosomal gene that also codes for the H-Y cell surface antigen, an antigen present only in males. The final process, the translation of gonadal sex into phenotypic sex, is the direct consequence of the type of gonad formed. In the development of phenotypic sex indifferent internal and external genital anlage are converted to male or female forms.

The internal genitalia in the two sexes are derived from the wolffian and mullerian ducts that exist side by side in early embryos of both sexes (Fig. 344-2A). In the male, the wolffian ducts give rise to the epididymis, vas deferens, and seminal vesicle; and the mullerian ducts disappear. In the female the fallopian tubes, uterus, and upper vagina are derived from the mullerian ducts, and the wolffian ducts regress. In contrast, the external genitalia and urethra in the two sexes develop from common anlage—the urogenital sinus and the genital tubercle, folds, and swelling (Fig. 344-2B). The urogenital sinus gives rise in the male to the prostate and prostatic urethra and in the female to the urethra and a portion of the vagina. The genital tubercle is the origin of the glans penis in the male and the clitoris in the female. The urogenital swelling becomes the scrotum or the labia majora, and the genital folds develop into the labia minora or the shaft of the penis.

In the absence of the testis, as in the normal female or in the male embryo castrated prior to the onset of phenotypic differentiation, the development of phenotypic sex proceeds along female lines. Thus, masculinization of the fetus is the positive result of action of hormones from the fetal gonad whereas female development does not require the presence of a gonad. Under ordinary circumstances development of the sexual phenotype conforms to the chromosomal sex. That is, chromosomal sex determines gonadal sex, and gonadal sex in turn determines phenotypic sex.

Control over the formation of the male phenotype is vested in the action of three hormones. Two of the three—mullerian regression factor and testosterone—are secretory products of the fetal testis. Mullerian regression factor is an incompletely characterized product of the embryonic testis, probably a protein with a molecular weight greater than 15,000. It acts to suppress the mullerian ducts and consequently prevents development of the uterus and fallopian tubes in the male. Testosterone promotes virilization of the urogenital tract in two ways. It acts directly to stimulate the wolffian ducts to form the epididymis, vas deferens, and seminal vesicle, and it is the precursor for the third fetal hormone, dihydrotestosterone (see Chap. 341). Dihydrotestosterone, which is formed within the urogenital sinus and lower urogenital tract from circulating testosterone, acts in the urogenital sinus to induce formation of the male urethra and prostate and in the genital tubercle, swelling, and folds to cause the midline fusion, elongation, and enlargement that eventuate in the male external genitalia. Thus, the primary function of androgen during fetal life is to induce the formation of the accessory organs of male reproduction. Testosterone and dihydrotestosterone act in embryonic tissues by the same intracellular machinery as described for differentiated tissues in Chap. 341. The formation of the male phenotype is largely completed by the middle of the second trimester. During the latter half of gestation descent of the testes and differential growth of the male external genitalia take place.

DISORDERS OF CHROMOSOMAL SEX

Disorders of chromosomal sex (Table 344-1) result when the number or structure of the X or Y chromosomes is abnormal (see Chap. 60).

TABLE 344-1
Clinical features of the disorders of chromosomal sex

Disorder	Common chromosomal complement	Gonadal development	External genitalia	Internal genitalia	Breast development	Presence of H-Y antigen	Comment
Klinefelter syndrome	47,XXY or 46,XY/ 47,XXY	Sterile testis	Normal male	Normal male	Gyneco-mastia	Yes	Most common disorder of sexual differentiation; tall stature.
XX male	46,XX	Sterile testis	Normal male	Normal male	Gyneco-mastia	Yes	Shorter than normal men; increased incidence of hypospadias. Similar to Klinefelter syndrome. May be familial.
Gonadal dysgenesis (Turner syndrome)	45,X or 46,XX/45,X	Streak gonad	Immature female	Hypoplastic female	Immature female	No	Short stature and multiple somatic abnormalities. May be 46,XX with structurally abnormal X chromosome.
Mixed gonadal dysgenesis	46,XY/45,X or 46,XY	Testis and streak gonad	Variable but almost always ambiguous; 60% reared as female	Uterus, vagina, and one fallopian tube	Usually male	Yes	Second most common cause of ambiguous genitalia in the newborn; tumors common.
True hermaphroditism	46,XX or 46,XY or mosaics	Testis and ovary or ovotestis	Variable but usually ambiguous; 60% reared as males	Usually a uterus and urogenital sinus; ducts correspond to gonad	Gyneco-mastia in 75%	Yes	May be familial.

KLINEFELTER SYNDROME   Clinical features   Klinefelter syndrome is a disorder in phenotypic men characterized by small, firm testes, azoospermia, gynecomastia, and elevated levels of plasma and urinary gonadotropins. The fundamental defect is the presence in a male of two or more X chromosomes. The common karyotype is either a 47,XXY chromosomal pattern (the classic form) or 46,XY/47,XXY (the mosaic form). This disorder constitutes the most frequent major abnormality of sexual differentiation; screening studies of the buccal smear in the newborn male population and studies of young adult males using the major physical findings to screen for affected individuals both indicate an incidence of about 1 in 500 men.

The patient presents after puberty because of infertility or gynecomastia. Prepubertally, patients generally have small testes with decreased numbers of spermatogonia. The frequency of the various clinical features is illustrated in Table 344-2. Defective spermatogenesis and azoospermia are present in virtually all patients with the 47,XXY variety. The small, firm testes are characteristically less than 2.0 cm and always less than 3.5 cm in length (corresponding to 2 and 8 ml volume, respectively). The frequency of these features emphasizes the uniformity with which the fundamental defect, i.e., damage to the seminiferous tubules, appears in the syndrome. Typical histologic changes include hyalinization of the tubules, absence of spermatogenesis, and apparent increase in Leydig cells.

Except for the increased height due to an increased lower body segment, the remaining abnormalities are due to a variable decrease in Leydig cell function. Gynecomastia ordinarily appears first during adolescence, is generally bilateral and painless, and may progress to become disfiguring (see Chap. 343). Although the incidence of associated somatic abnormalities is probably no greater than in the general population, obesity and varicose veins occur in a third to a half of the patients with Klinefelter syndrome. Mild mental deficiency, social maladjustment, subtle abnormalities of thyroid function, diabetes mellitus, and pulmonary disease may be more common than in the general population. Although the risk of breast cancer is 20 times that of normal men, the incidence is only about one-fifth that in women. The majority have a male psychosexual orientation and are capable of functioning sexually as normal men.

Of the clinical variants the most common is the patient with 46,XY/47,XXY mosaicism, comprising about 10 percent of the patients based on leukocyte karyotypes. As summarized in Table 344-2, the mosaic form is usually not as severe as the 47,XXY variety, and the testes may be normal in size. The endocrine abnormalities are also less severe, and gynecomastia and azoospermia are less common. Indeed, some patients with mosaicism may be fertile. This variant may be difficult to diagnose when, as in about 70 percent of the cases, the mosaicism is present only in the testes. Thus a buccal smear and peripheral leukocyte karyotype may be normal, and the patient may still have Klinefelter syndrome. In some individuals the diagnosis may not even be suspected because of the minor degree of the physical abnormalities.

Approximately 30 other karyotypic varieties of chromatin-positive Klinefelter syndrome have been described, including those with uniform cell lines (such as XXYY, XXXY, and XXXXY) and a variety of numerical mosaicisms and structural abnormalities of chromosomes. In general, the greater the degree of structural abnormality and in mosaic forms the more cell lines that are abnormal, the more severe the manifestations and the more frequent the occurrence of nongenital abnormalities.

Pathophysiology   The classic form of Klinefelter syndrome is due to meiotic chromosomal nondisjunction (Fig. 344-3). About 40 percent of the cases of meiotic nondisjunction occur in the father, and 60 percent occur in the mother. Advanced maternal age is a predisposing factor only in the cases in which the defect occurs in the mother. The mosaic form of the disorder, in contrast, is thought to result from mitotic nondisjunction (Fig. 344-3), which can take place in either a 46,XY zygote or a 47,XXY zygote. The latter defect or double (meiotic and mitotic) nondisjunction may be the usual cause of the mosaic form and thus explain why the mosaic form is less common than the classic disorder.

The endocrine changes in Klinefelter syndrome have been characterized in detail. Plasma follicle-stimulating hormone (FSH) and luteinizing hormone (LH) levels are usually high, and the average plasma testosterone level is half normal. However, the range of plasma testosterone is broad and overlaps the normal range. FSH and LH show better discrimination with little overlap with normals. The variability of the plasma testosterone level accounts for the variable degree of androgenization seen in this disorder. Mean plasma estradiol concentrations are elevated. The elevated plasma estradiol may be accounted for by a decreased metabolic clearance rate. Furthermore, early in the course of the disorder, before the progressive testicular lesion has advanced, the testis may secrete increased amounts of estradiol in response to the elevated LH levels. Later, the main alteration of androgen-estrogen dynamics appears to be decreased testosterone production in the setting of normal to slightly elevated estradiol production. The net result is a variable degree of feminization or insufficient androgenization, or both. Such feminization, including the development of gynecomastia, is thought to depend on the ratio of circulating androgen to estrogen (relative or absolute), and it follows that the higher the plasma testosterone level and the lower the plasma estradiol level, the less likely gynecomastia is to develop (see Chap. 343). Studies of the hypothalamic-pituitary axis have shown hyperresponsiveness of the pituitary to luteinizing hormone–releasing hormone (LHRH) beginning at puberty and lack of normal feedback inhibition of gonadal steroids on pituitary gonadotropin secretion.

Management   No method is available for reversing the sterility, and the only available means for definitive treatment of the gynecomastia is surgical removal. Some underandrogenized patients may benefit from supplemental androgen, but such treatment may paradoxically worsen the gynecomastia, presumably by providing increased androgen substrate for the conversion to estrogens in the peripheral tissues.

TABLE 344-2
Characteristics of patients with classic versus mosaic Klinefelter syndrome*

	47,XXY, %	46,XY/47,XXY, %
Abnormal testicular histology	100	94†
Decreased length of testis	99	73†
Azoospermia	93	50†
Decreased testosterone	79	33
Decreased facial hair	77	64
Increased gonadotropins	75	33†
Decreased sexual function	68	56
Gynecomastia	55	33†
Decreased axillary hair	49	46
Decreased length of penis	41	21

* Table based on 519 XXY patients and 51 XY/XXY patients.
† Significantly different at $p < 0.05$ or better.
SOURCE: After Gordon et al.

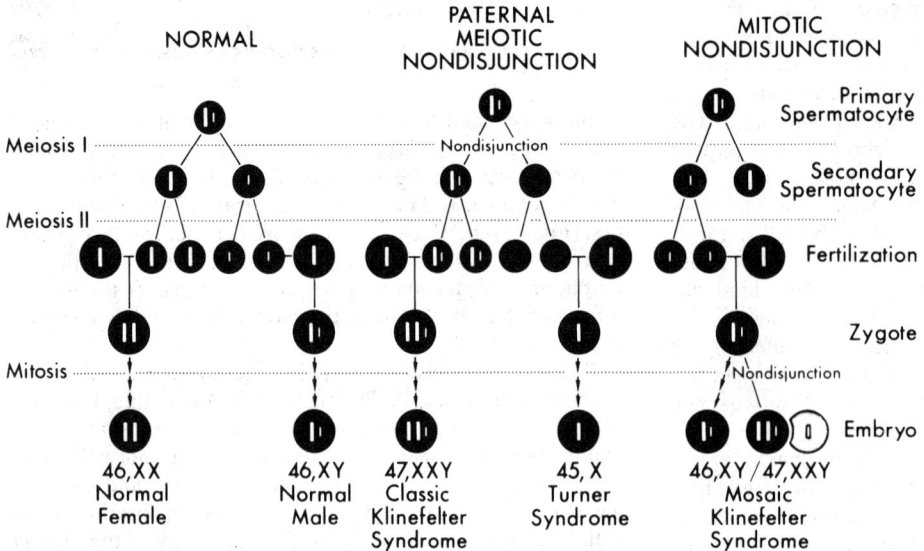

NORMAL PATERNAL MEIOTIC NONDISJUNCTION MITOTIC NONDISJUNCTION

Meiosis I

Meiosis II

Mitosis

Nondisjunction

Nondisjunction

Primary Spermatocyte

Secondary Spermatocyte

Fertilization

Zygote

Embryo

46,XX Normal Female

46,XY Normal Male

47,XXY Classic Klinefelter Syndrome

45,X Turner Syndrome

46,XY/47,XXY Mosaic Klinefelter Syndrome

FIGURE 344-3

Schema for normal spermatogenesis and fertilization showing effects of meiotic and mitotic nondisjunction leading to classic Klinefelter syndrome, Turner syndrome, and mosaic Klinefelter. The schema would be similar if the abnormal events took place during oogenesis.

THE XX MALE Since 1964, approximately 50 phenotypic men with the 46,XX karyotype have been reported. The incidence is approximately 1 in 10,000 to 15,000 male births. Affected individuals have male psychosexual identification, small testes, and absence of all female internal genitalia. Indeed, these individuals are clinically inseparable from those with Klinefelter syndrome: the testes are small and firm (generally less than 2 cm); gynecomastia is frequent; the penis and scrotum are small to normal in size; azoospermia and hyalinization of the tubules are common; and urinary and plasma gonadotropin levels are high. They differ from the typical Klinefelter patients only in that average height is less than that of normal men, there is no increase in mental deficiency, and there is an increased incidence of hypospadias.

Three theories have been proposed to explain the pathogenesis of this disorder: (1) translocation of all or a portion of a Y chromosome to an autosome; (2) chromosomal mosaicism in which the line containing Y chromosomes exists only in the testes; or (3) mutation of an autosomal gene. If either of the first two theories is correct, the disorder is in fact a variant of Klinefelter syndrome. At least two individuals have been described in whom translocation of the Y chromosome resulted in a phenotype that is similar to that in these patients. Consequently, translocation appears to be a tenable explanation for at least some cases of the syndrome. Moreover, testicular determinants appear to be located in a circumscribed region of the Y chromosome near the centromere, and therefore translocation of fragments of the Y chromosome may be difficult to detect by ordinary means. The recent report of the presence of the H-Y antigen in 46,XX males provides further support for the presence of Y chromosome genes in some patients, since the H-Y antigen appears to be determined by a gene on the Y chromosome that is closely linked to the testicular determinants. In other patients familial occurrence of XX males suggests that the disorder may in some cases result from mutation of an autosomal gene.

GONADAL DYSGENESIS (TURNER SYNDROME) **Clinical features** Gonadal dysgenesis is a disorder in phenotypic females characterized by primary amenorrhea, sexual infantilism, short stature, multiple congenital anomalies, and bilateral streak gonads. This condition should be distinguished from three similar disorders: (1) mixed gonadal dysgenesis in which a unilateral testis and a contralateral streak gonad are present; (2) pure gonadal dysgenesis in which bilateral streak gonads are associated with normal stature and primary amenorrhea; and (3) Noonan's syndrome, a disorder inherited as an autosomal

dominant mutation affecting both males and females with normal karyotypes and normal gonads and characterized by the presence of webbed neck, short stature, congenital heart disease, cubitus valgus, and other congenital defects (see Chap. 103).

The incidence of gonadal dysgenesis is estimated at 1 in 2500 newborn females, and the diagnosis is made either at birth, because of the associated anomalies, or more frequently at puberty, when amenorrhea and failure of sexual development are noted. The external genitalia are unambiguously female but remain immature even in adulthood, and there is no breast development until the patient is treated with exogenous estrogen. The internal genitalia consist of bilateral fallopian tubes, a small uterus, and bilateral streak gonads located in the broad ligaments. Typically, these streaks contain fibrous tissue that is indistinguishable from normal ovarian stroma but lack identifiable follicles and ova; however, primordial germ cells are thought to have been present transiently in embryogenesis but fail to mature into oocytes.

The associated somatic anomalies primarily affect tissues of mesodermal origin, i.e., the sleleton and connective tissue. In infancy these include lymphedema of the hands and feet, webbing of the neck, low hairline, redundant skin folds on the back of the neck, a shield-like chest with widely spaced nipples, and a low birth weight. In addition, there may be distinctive facies characterized by micrognathia, epicanthal folds, prominent low-set or deformed ears, a fish-like mouth, and ptosis. Short fourth metacarpals are present in half, and 10 to 20 percent have coarctation of the aorta. The average height in Turner syndrome rarely exceeds 130 cm. Other associated anomalies include renal malformations, pigmented nevi, hypoplastic nails, tendency to keloid formation, perceptive hearing loss, and unexplained hypertension.

Pathophysiology Most affected individuals are sex chromatin-negative and have a 45,X karyotype. However, there is considerable cytogenetic variation in this disorder. Approximately 40 percent are mosaics, of which 46,XX/45,X is the most common pattern. In the remaining patients, there is a structurally abnormal X chromosome. The 45,X variety may result from chromosome loss during gametogenesis in either parent or an error in mitosis during one of the early cleavage divisions of the zygote (Fig. 343-3). Short stature and other Turner stigmata result from loss of genetic material on the short arm of the X chromosome. Streak gonads result when either the long or the short arm is missing. In patients with mosaicism or with normal karyotypes, phenotypes on average are intermediate in severity between Turner syndrome and the normal. In some patients with hypertrophy of the clitoris, there is an unidentified fragment of a chromosome present in addition to the X chromosome, assumed to be an abnormal Y.

Although sparse pubic and axillary hair develop at the time of expected puberty, the breasts remain infantile, and no menses occur. Serum FSH is usually elevated in infancy, falls during midchildhood to the normal range, and increases to castrate levels at the age of 9 or 10. At this time, serum LH is also elevated, and plasma estradiol levels are low (<10 pg/ml).

Management All patients are phenotypic females, and at the anticipated time of puberty replacement therapy with estrogen should be instituted to induce maturation of the breasts, labia, vagina, uterus, and fallopian tubes. Linear growth and bone maturation rates are approximately doubled during the first year of treatment with estradiol, and if therapy is instituted early, the eventual height of patients may approach the predicted height. Treatment with growth hormone has not been helpful.

Gonadal tumors are rare in 45,X patients. However, gonadal malignancies have been reported in several patients with mosaicism involving the Y chromosome, and, consequently, streak gonads should be removed in any patient with evidence of virilization.

MIXED GONADAL DYSGENESIS Clinical features Mixed gonadal dysgenesis is an entity in which phenotypic male or female patients have a testis on one side and a streak gonad on the other. Most patients have 45,X/46,XY mosaicism, but the clinical entity is by no means confined to that chromosomal pattern. The true incidence is unknown, but in most hospitals it is the second most common cause of ambiguous genitalia in the neonate after congenital adrenal hyperplasia.

More than 60 percent of patients are reared as females, and most phenotypic males are incompletely virilized at birth. The majority exhibit some evidence of ambiguous genitalia, including phallic enlargement, a urogenital sinus, and varying degrees of labioscrotal fusion. In most the testis is located intraabdominally; individuals with a testis in the inguinal or scrotal position are usually reared as males. A uterus, vagina, and at least one fallopian tube are almost invariably present.

On histologic examination, the prepubertal testis appears relatively normal. Although the postpubertal testis contains abundant mature Leydig cells, the seminiferous tubules contain only Sertoli cells and lack germinal elements. Frequently, the testis is undescended, and when descended it may present in association with a hernia containing the uterus and fallopian tube. The streak gonad, a thin, pale, elongated structure located either in the broad ligament or along the pelvic wall, is composed of fibrous connective tissue that is often arranged in whorls so that it resembles ovarian stroma.

At puberty the testis secretes androgen, and virilization and phallic enlargement both occur. Feminization is rare; when it occurs, estrogen secretion from a gonadal tumor should be suspected. In addition to these clinical features, approximately one-third of patients exhibit the somatic stigmata of 45,X gonadal dysgenesis, i.e., low posterior hairline, shield chest, multiple pigmented nevi, cubitus valgus, webbing of the neck, and short stature, approximately half of adult patients being less than 148 cm in height.

Virtually all patients are chromatin-negative, and the most common karyotype is 45,X/46,XY. In one series, two-thirds had mosaic karyotypes, and the remaining third may have had undetected mosaicism. The origin of 45,X/46,XY mosaicism is best explained by the loss of a Y chromosome during an early mitotic division of an XY zygote similar to the postulated origin of the 46,XY/47,XXY mosaic shown in Fig. 343-3.

Pathophysiology It has been assumed that the XY cell line stimulates testicular differentiation, whereas the 45,X stem leads to the development of the contralateral streak gonad, but comparison of karyotype and phenotypic expression has failed to document such a relationship; furthermore, no clear correlation has been found between the percentage of cells cultured from blood or skin containing 45,X or 46,XY and the degree of gonadal development or somatic anomalies.

In addition to inadequate masculinization in utero, there is also deficient mullerian duct regression. Since Leydig cell function is normal at puberty, it has been suggested that the cause of the inadequate virilization is delayed development of a testis that is ultimately capable of normal Leydig cell function. The hormonal responsiveness of the internal duct structures, the urogenital sinus, and the external genitalia is limited to a critical period between 7 and 14 weeks of gestation, and consequently a delayed but otherwise normal onset of endocrine function in the fetal testis would allow persistence of mullerian ducts and incomplete masculinization of the external genitalia. Alternatively, the fetal testis may simply be incapable of synthesizing adequate amounts of mullerian-inhibiting substance and androgen.

Management Several important factors must be considered in the management of patients with mixed gonadal dysgenesis. For those who are diagnosed in early infancy, the choice of gender for rearing is perhaps the most complicated of all gender assignment problems. For the older child or adult in whom gender is fixed prior to diagnosis, the central issue is the possibility of tumor development in the gonads. The overall incidence of gonadal tumors in patients with mixed gonadal dysgenesis is about 25 percent. Both seminomas and gonadoblastomas may develop, and the tumors may occur prior to puberty. The tumors occur most frequently in patients with a female phenotype who lack the stigmata of Turner syndrome and are more common in intraabdominal testes than in the streak gonad.

In phenotypic females, early exploratory laparotomy and prophylactic gonadectomy are advisable, because gonadal tumors may occur in childhood and the testis will secrete androgen at puberty and thus result in virilization. Phenotypic males with mixed gonadal dysgenesis are infertile (no germinal elements are present in the testes), often require multiple staged procedures for reconstruction of the external genitalia, are frequently short in stature, and also have a high risk of developing gonadal tumors. Which testes can be safely conserved? In general the following observations apply: (1) tumors develop in scrotal streak gonads but not in scrotal testes; (2) tumors that develop in intraabdominal testes are always associated with ipsilateral mullerian duct structures; and (3) tumors in streak gonads are always associated with tumors in the contralateral abdominal testis. Based on these observations, it is recommended that (1) all streak gonads should be removed, (2) scrotal testes should be preserved, and (3) intraabdominal testes should be excised unless they can be relocated in the scrotum and are not associated with ipsilateral mullerian duct structures.

TRUE HERMAPHRODITISM Clinical features True hermaphroditism is a condition in which both an ovary and a testis or a gonad with histologic features of both (ovotestis) is present. Although the incidence of this disorder is unknown, more than 300 cases have been reported in the literature. To justify the diagnosis there must be histologic documentation of both types of gonadal epithelium, the presence of ovarian stroma without oocytes not being sufficient. Four categories are recognized:

1 *Bilateral:* testicular and ovarian tissue (ovotestes) on each side.
2 *Unilateral:* an ovotestis on one side and an ovary or a testis on the other.
3 *Lateral:* a testis on one side and an ovary on the other.
4 *Indeterminate:* no confirmation of the location or type of gonadal tissue.

About one-fourth are bilateral, one-fourth are lateral, one-half are unilateral, and a small number are indeterminant.

The external genitalia display all gradations of the male-to-female spectrum. Most are masculinized to some degree, and for this reason two-thirds of patients are reared as males. However, less than one-tenth have normal male external genitalia, most have hypospadias, and more than half have incomplete labioscrotal fusion. Two-thirds of phenotypic females have an enlarged clitoris. Almost all patients have a urogenital sinus, and a uterus is commonly present. The uterus may be normal in size and shape, hypoplastic, or unicornuate. Commonly, differentiation of the internal ducts corresponds to the adjacent gonad. Although an epididymis usually develops adjacent to a testis, a complete vas deferens is present in only a third. Of the patients with an ovotestis, three-fourths have an epididymis, two-thirds have a fallopian tube, a tenth have a vas deferens, and a tenth have both a vas deferens and a fallopian tube. The ovary usually occupies the normal position, but the testis or ovotestis may be found at any level along the route of embryonic testicular descent, frequently associated with an inguinal hernia. Testicular tissue is present in the scrotum or the labioscrotal fold in a third, in the inguinal canal in a third, and in the abdominal area in a third.

At puberty three-fourths of patients develop significant gynecomastia, and about half menstruate. In phenotypic men, menstruation presents as cyclic hematuria. Ovulation occurs in approximately a fourth of patients and is more common than spermatogenesis. Fertility has been reported in a woman following removal of an ovotestis and in a man who fathered two children. Congenital malformations of other systems are rare.

Pathophysiology About half of patients have a 46,XX karyotype, a fourth have a 46,XY karyotype, and a fourth are mosaics. In virtually all patients with mosaicism a Y cell line is identified. The mechanism responsible for the gonadal development in true hermaphroditism is unknown. Even if not demonstrable with conventional karyotyping methods, it is assumed that sufficient genetic material derived from the Y chromosome is present (as the result of translocation, nondisjunction, or mutation) to induce the development of testicular tissue. In support of this is the fact that several XX true hermaphrodites with a testes have been shown to be H-Y antigen positive. A number of pedigrees have been reported in which multiple sibs with a 46,XX karyotype are affected, suggesting that this form of true hermaphroditism may be determined by an autosomal recessive gene or by a common translocation.

Because corpora lutea are present in the ovaries of more than a fourth of patients, it is assumed that a female neuroendocrine axis is present and functions normally in such individuals. There are few detailed reports of gonadotropin secretory patterns or steroid production rates, but in patients with feminization (gynecomastia and menstruation) gonadal secretion of estradiol can be demonstrated. It is presumed that in masculinized patients androgen secretion predominates, and the fact that some patients produce sperm is in keeping with this view.

Management Gender assignment in the newborn or early infant in whom the diagnosis is made depends largely upon the anatomic composition. In older children and adults gonads and internal duct structures that are contradictory to the predominant phenotype should be removed, and when necessary the external genitalia should be modified appropriately. Although gonadal tumors are rare in patients with true hermaphroditism, gonadoblastoma has been reported in a patient with an XY cell line. Consequently, the possibility of future tumor development in the gonad must be taken into consideration when the decision regarding conservation of gonadal tissue is made.

DISORDERS OF GONADAL SEX

Disorders of gonadal sex result when chromosomal sex is normal but for one of several reasons, differentiation of the gonads is abnormal. Thus, chromosomal sex does not correspond to gonadal and phenotypic sex.

PURE GONADAL DYSGENESIS Clinical features Pure gonadal dysgenesis is a disorder in phenotypic females who have gonads and genitalia identical with those with gonadal dysgenesis (bilateral streaks, infantile uterus and tubes, and sexual infantilism) but who have normal height, few if any congenital anomalies, and either a normal 46,XX or 46,XY karyotype. There is a clear-cut genetic basis for considering this a separate disorder from gonadal dysgenesis, but on clinical grounds it cannot be distinguished from the less severely affected type of gonadal dysgenesis. The height is normal or greater than normal, some patients being over 172 cm. There is complete estrogen deficiency in that the primary amenorrhea is accompanied by lack of breast development and immaturity of the vagina. Axillary and pubic hair are scanty, and the internal genitalia consist of mullerian derivatives only.

Development of tumors may occur in the streak gonads, particularly dysgerminoma or gonadoblastoma in the 46,XY disorder. Such tumors are frequently heralded by the development of virilizing signs or a pelvic mass.

Pathophysiology Although a variety of chromosomal mosaicisms have been described under this nosology, the designation as used here is restricted to those individuals with normal 46,XX or 46,XY karyotypes. (Those individuals with mosaicism are considered to be variations of gonadal dysgenesis or mixed gonadal dysgenesis as described above.) The rationale for this restricted definition is based upon the fact that both the XX and XY varieties can result from different single-gene mutations. At least seven sibships have been reported in which more than one individual is affected with the 46,XX type of the disorder, three of which are the result of consanguineous mating, suggesting that the disorder is transmitted in an autosomal recessive pattern. Furthermore, several pedigrees have now been described in which the 46,XY variety is inherited in a manner compatible with an X-linked mutation.

As would be predicted in individuals with streak gonads, gonadotropin secretion is elevated and estrogen secretion is low. The pathogenesis of the defect in gonadal development is unknown, but according to current concepts of sexual differentiation total absence of the gonads—either male or female—would be expected to result in the development of a female phenotype.

Management The general management of the estrogen deficiency is identical with that in ordinary gonadal dysgenesis, namely, appropriate replacement estrogen therapy at the time of expected puberty. Because of the high frequency of gonadal tumors in the 46,XY variety, patients should routinely have exploratory surgery and removal of the streak gonads once the diagnosis is made. The development of virilizing signs is indication for immediate surgery. The natural history of the gonadal tumors in this disorder is uncertain, but the prognosis appears to be very good after surgical removal.

THE ABSENT TESTES SYNDROME (ANORCHIA, TESTICULAR REGRESSION, GONADAL AGENESIS, DYSGENETIC TESTES, AGONADISM, DYSGENETIC MALE PSEUDOHERMAPHRODITISM) Clinical features
A spectrum of phenotypes has been described in 46,XY males with absent or rudimentary testes but in whom unequivocal evidence exists that testicular function was present at some time during embryonic or postembryonic life. Thus, the disorder can be distinguished from subjects with pure gonadal dysgenesis in whom no evidence can be inferred for gonadal function during embryonic development. The clinical syndromes have been reported under a variety of eponyms and vary in their manifestation from complete failure of virilization through varying degrees of incomplete virilization of the external genitalia to otherwise normal males with bilateral anorchia.

The purest form of the disorder is represented by 46,XY phenotypic females with absent testes (both by biochemical and anatomic criteria), sexual infantilism and concomitant absence of mullerian duct derivatives, and accessory organs of male reproduction. In these patients testicular failure must have occurred during the interval between the onset of elaboration of mullerian duct regression factor and the active secretion of testosterone, that is, after development of the seminiferous tubules but before the onset of Leydig cell function. Testicular failure at later stages of embryonic development results in less complete defects in male phenotypic development.

Other patients have clinical findings which indicate that testicular failure occurred during later phases of gestation, and some of these constitute problems in sexual assignment. In some, failure of mullerian regression occurs to a greater extent than the failure of testosterone secretion, but none exhibit complete mullerian development. In individuals with more extensive virilization, the external genitalia are phenotypically male, but rudimentary oviducts and vasa deferentia may coexist internally.

At the final extreme, more than 50 cases of bilateral anorchia have been reported in subjects who are phenotypically male and who have complete development of the wolffian system in the absence of mullerian structures and gonads. A microphallus in such subjects is the result of failure of androgen-mediated growth after anatomic development is completed. Persistent gynecomastia may or may not develop after the time of puberty.

Pathophysiology In all affected individuals the karyotype is 46,XY by definition. Whether the testicular regression is the result of mutant genes, teratogen, or trauma is unclear. Several instances of agonadism in 46,XY subjects have been reported in families. It is of particular interest in this regard that unilateral and bilateral agonadism can occur within the same family, so that careful pedigree analysis is necessary in all instances.

The quantitative dynamics of gonadal steroid production have been studied in only a few patients. In two phenotypic females who had primary amenorrhea, sexual infantilism, and no internal genital structures, plasma testosterone concentration was similar to that of prepubertal children, and no glandular secretion of testosterone could be documented. The daily production rates of estrogen were low. In one phenotypic male with bilateral anorchia there was no glandular secretion of testosterone; total testosterone and estrogen production was accounted for by peripheral conversion from plasma androstene-

dione. However, some subjects in whom no testes could be identified at laparotomy have blood testosterone values clearly above the castrate range. The pathogenesis of these disorders is unknown.

Management The management of the two extremes in this disorder is clear-cut. Sexually infantile, phenotypic females should be given adequate estrogen to ensure appropriate breast and female somatic development, and any coexisting vaginal agenesis should be treated by either surgical or medical means. Likewise, phenotypic males with anorchia should be given adequate androgen replacement to allow development of normal male secondary sexual development. The cases with incomplete virilization or ambiguous development of the external genitalia are more complex and require individual assessment as to whether surgical means should be employed toward improving male or female phenotypes. In either case, appropriate hormonal therapy is mandatory at the time of expected puberty.

DISORDERS OF PHENOTYPIC SEX

FEMALE PSEUDOHERMAPHRODITISM Congenital adrenal hyperplasia CLINICAL FEATURES A variety of syndromes are known to result from hereditary defects in the enzymes of steroid hormone synthesis. The pathways by which glucocorticoids are formed in the adrenal gland and androgens are formed in the testis and adrenal are schematically summarized in Fig. 344-4. Three enzymes are common to the formation of both types of steroids (20,22-desmolase, 3β-hydroxysteroid dehydrogenase, and 17-hydroxylase); deficiency of any of these enzymes results in deficiency both of glucocorticoids and adrenal androgens and consequently results in both congenital adrenal hyperplasia and defective virilization of the male embryo (male pseudohermaphroditism). Two enzymes are involved exclusively in androgen synthesis (17,20-desmolase and 17β-hydroxysteroid dehydrogenase), and a deficiency in either results in pure male pseudohermaphroditism with normal glucocorticoid and mineralocorticoid synthesis. Deficiency of either of the terminal two enzymes of glucocorticoid synthesis (21-hydroxylase and 11-hydroxylase) results in defective formation of hydrocortisone with a compensatory increase in ACTH secretion which causes an increase in the formation of adrenal steroids proximal to the enzymatic defect and subsequent excess androgen formation. As a consequence the latter two disorders result in adrenal hyperplasia and virilization in the female embryo or precocious masculinization in the male.

The *adrenal insufficiency* in these disorders may produce equally severe and life-threatening problems in both sexes and is described in detail in Chap. 336 and schematically in Table 344-3. From the standpoint of the *genital pathology* it is helpful to consider separately those enzyme defects in steroidogenesis that result in female pseudohermaphroditism and those that cause male pseudohermaphroditism. (One syndrome, 3β-hydroxysteroid dehydrogenase deficiency, can cause either male or female pseudohermaphroditism, but since the more severe genital defect is incomplete virilization of the male, it will be discussed as an abnormality of male phenotypic differentiation.)

Congenital adrenal hyperplasia due to 21-hydroxylase deficiency is the commonest cause of ambiguous genitalia in the newborn and is present in about 1 in 13,000 individuals. Virilization is usually apparent at birth in the female and within the first 2 to 3 years of life in the male. At birth there is hypertrophy of the clitoris associated with ventral binding as in chordee, variable fusion of the labioscrotal folds, and differing degrees of virilization of the urethra. The latter may be so severe as to produce a prostate in the female. The internal female structures and gonads remain unaltered. Overall, the external appearance is similar to that of a male with bilateral cryptorchidism and hypospadias. The labioscrotal folds are bulbous and rugated and resemble a scrotum. In a small percentage of cases the urethra traverses the phallus to form a true penile urethra so that errors in sex assignment may occur at birth. In a few cases virilization of the female is slight or absent at birth and becomes evident in later infancy, adolescence, or adulthood, presumably as the result of variability in the manifestation of the mutant genes. Injection of radiopaque dye into the external genital orifice is usually helpful in defining the internal structures, and it is common to be able to demonstrate a vagina, a uterus, and sometimes even fallopian tubes.

The untreated female grows rapidly during the first years of life and has progressive virilization. At the time of expected puberty there is a failure of normal female sexual development and absence of menstruation. In both sexes rapid somatic maturation results in premature epiphyseal closure and a short adult height. In the absence of overt adrenal insufficiency the condition is usually not recognized in the male at birth since male phenotypic differentiation is normal. However, there is early growth and maturation of the external genitalia and early appearance of secondary sex characteristics, such that acne, coarsening of the voice, frequent erections, and excessive muscular development are noticeable in the first few years of life. Despite the excessive adrenal androgen production that would be expected to inhibit gonadotropin secretion, the testes may be enlarged for the age, and true premature puberty may ensue. The untreated adult male is capable of erection and ejaculation and may be fertile; the untreated male is subject to the development of ACTH-dependent "tumors" of the testis composed of adrenal rest cells.

In 21-hydroxylase deficiency, which probably accounts for 95 percent of congenital adrenal hyperplasia, there is a reduced activity of the 21-hydroxylase enzyme, which leads to decreased production of hydrocortisone, which in turn leads to increased release of ACTH, which then induces adrenal growth and partial or complete compensation of the defect in the secretion of hydrocortisone. In about half of the cases in which the enzyme defect is partial cortisol secretion is normal. This form is termed "simple virilizing" or "compensated." In the remainder of cases there is a more complete deficiency of the enzyme, and the adrenal gland produces only trivial amounts of cortisol and aldosterone, leading to severe salt wastage with anorexia, vomiting, volume depletion, and collapse with the first few weeks of life. This is termed the *salt-losing form* of 21-hydroxylase deficiency. In each there is overproduction of the cortisol precursors prior to the 21-hydroxylase step, i.e., progesterone and 17-hydroxyprogesterone. These act as weak aldosterone antagonists at the receptor level and result in increased aldosterone production in the compensated form in order to maintain normal sodium balance. Patients with the more complete enzyme deficiency have low aldosterone levels.

In 11-hydroxylase deficiency a block in hydroxylation at the 11-carbon results in the accumulation of 11-deoxycortisol and its subsequent conversion to deoxycorticosterone (DOC), a potent salt-retaining hormone that is responsible for the hypertension that frequently occurs. It is not clear why all affected individuals do not develop hypertension.

PATHOPHYSIOLOGY The reported pedigrees are consistent with an autosomal recessive pattern of inheritance. Heterozygote frequency for 21-hydroxylase deficiency is probably about 1 in 60 in the general population.

For discussion of the endocrine pathology, see Chap. 336. Generally, excretion of ketosteroids is elevated, as is the excretion of the major metabolites that accumulate proximal to the enzymatic blocks. In 21-hydroxylase deficiency, 17-hydroxyprogesterone accumulates in blood and is excreted predominantly as pregnanetriol. In 11-hydroxylase deficiency 11-deoxycortisol accumulates in blood and is excreted predominantly as tetrahydrocortexolone.

MANAGEMENT Insofar as is possible patients should be reared in the gender of the chromosomal and gonadal sex, and appropriate surgery to correct the external genitalia should be employed as quickly as possible. This is of particular importance because appropriately treated females are capable of fertility and normal sexual function. However, if the correct diagnosis is made late (after 3 years of age), gender assignment should be changed only after careful consideration of the psychosexual background.

Medical treatment with appropriate glucocorticoids not only avoids the consequences of hydrocortisone deficiency but in addition arrests the rapid virilization and prevents premature somatic advancement and epiphyseal maturation. In the salt-losing forms of 21-hydroxylase deficiency, treatment with mineralocorticoids is also indicated. The suppression of the abnormal steroid secretion results in cure of the hypertension

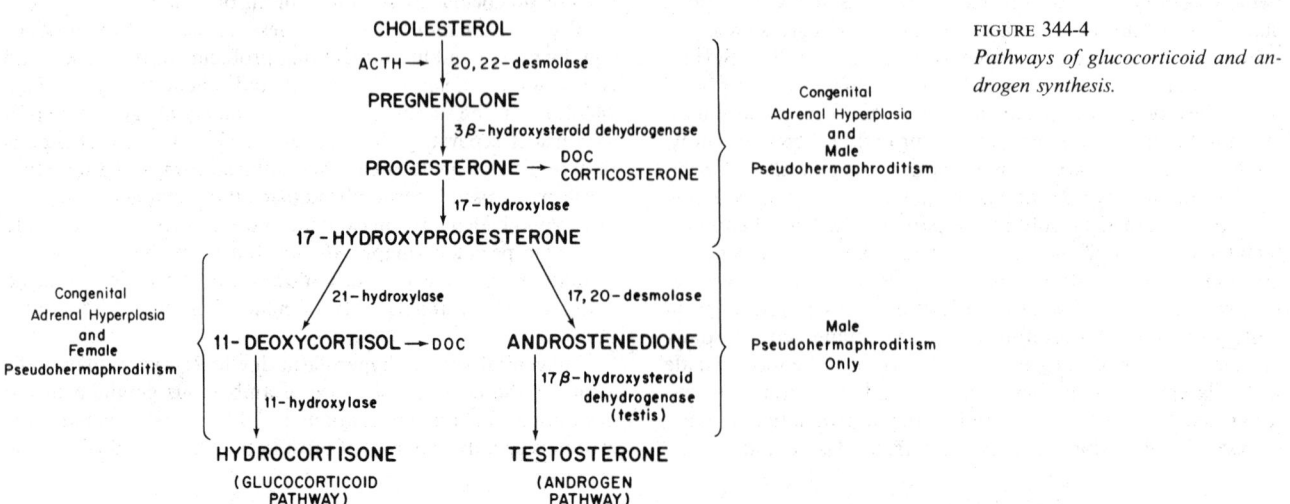

FIGURE 344-4
Pathways of glucocorticoid and androgen synthesis.

in patients with 11-hydroxylase deficiency and allows normal onset of menses and development of female secondary sex characteristics in both disorders. In males appropriate glucocorticoids suppress adrenal androgens and result in normal gonadotropin secretion, testicular development, and spermatogenesis. Measurement of early morning plasma 17-hydroxyprogesterone is the most sensitive test to assess adequacy of glucocorticoid replacement. In those patients with salt loss, plasma renin activity should also be measured to determine the adequacy of mineralocorticoid replacement.

Nonadrenal female pseudohermaphroditism At present nonadrenal causes of female pseudohermaphroditism are rare. In the past, the administration to pregnant women of progestational agents with androgenic side effects to prevent abortion (such as 17α-ethinyl-19-nortestosterone) resulted in masculinization of female fetuses in a significant number of cases. Such infants in general show less virilization than those with congenital adrenal hyperplasia. Nonadrenal female pseudohermaphroditism is also found in certain other circumstances such as in babies born to mothers who have virilizing tumors (e.g., arrhenoblastomas) and rarely under circumstances in which no etiology can be determined.

Developmental disorders of mullerian ducts (congenital absence of the vagina) CLINICAL FEATURES Although estimates of its frequency in the population vary widely, the combination of congenital absence of the vagina with some form of abnormal or absent uterus (the Mayer-Rokitansky-Kuster-Hauser syndrome) is second only to gonadal dysgenesis as a cause of primary amenorrhea. Most patients are seen by physicians after the time of expected puberty because of primary amenorrhea and are found on physical examination to have absence or hypoplasia of the vagina. The height and intelligence are normal, and the breasts, axillary and pubic hair, and habitus are feminine in character. The uterus may vary from almost normal, lacking only a conduit to the introitus, to the more characteristic finding of rudimentary bicornuate cords with or without a lumen. In some patients cyclical abdominal pain indicates that sufficient functional uterine tissue is present to result in retrograde menstruation and/or hematometra.

Renal, skeletal, and other congenital anomalies are common. About a third of patients have abnormal kidneys as delineated by intravenous pyelography, with agenesis or ectopy being most frequent. Some patients have solitary fused kidneys of the horseshoe type or solitary ectopic kidney located in the pelvis. The overall incidence of skeletal abnormalities is around 10 percent; two-thirds involve the spine; and limb and rib abnormalities account for the majority of the remaining defects. Specific abnormalities include wedge vertebrae, fusions, rudimentary or asymmetric vertebral bodies, and supernumerary vertebrae. The Klippel-Feil syndrome (congenital fusion of the cervical spine, short neck, low posterior hairline, and painless limitation of cervical movement) is a frequent association.

PATHOPHYSIOLOGY The karyotype is 46,XX. The majority have been assumed to be sporadic in nature, but several well-documented instances of familial occurrence have been described. In the familial cases variable expressivity of the defect is common. Some affected family members have skeletal or renal abnormalities only, while others have other abnormalities of mullerian derivatives, such as a double uterus. It is also of interest that bilateral renal aplasia is commonly associated with absence of the uterus and vagina. Thus, the family histories should be probed for instances of isolated skeletal and renal abnormalities and for spontaneous abortions that might result from congenital absence of both kidneys. At present, it is

not clear whether the sporadic cases represent new mutations of the type responsible for the familial disorder or are multifactoral in etiology.

Documentation of ovulatory peaks of plasma LH suggest that ovarian function is normal, and successful pregnancies have been reported following corrective vaginal repair in patients who had normal uteri.

MANAGEMENT Vaginal agenesis can be treated by surgical or nonsurgical means. Most surgical series have utilized split-thickness skin grafts around a solid rubber mold for the creation of an artificial vagina. Medical treatment involves development of vaginal depth by the repeated application of pressure against the vaginal dimple with a simple dilator. In view of the overall complication rate of 5 to 10 percent in surgical series, the nonoperative treatment should be tried in most instances. Operative treatment should be reserved for those patients in whom a well-formed uterus is present and the possibility of fertility exists. Continued coitus or instrumental dilatation is probably essential for maintaining the neovagina formed either by the nonoperative or the surgical method.

MALE PSEUDOHERMAPHRODITISM Defective virilization of the male embryo (male pseudohermaphroditism) can result from defects in androgen synthesis, defects in androgen action, defects in mullerian duct regression, and from uncertain causes.

Abnormalities in androgen synthesis CLINICAL FEATURES Five enzymatic defects have been described which result in defective testosterone synthesis (Fig. 344-4) and consequent incomplete virilization of the male embryo during embryogenesis (Tables 344-3 and 344-4). Each of the enzymes catalyzes a critical biochemical step in the conversion of cholesterol to testosterone. Three of the enzymes (20,22-desmolase, 3β-hydroxysteroid dehydrogenase, and 17-hydroxylase) are common to the synthesis of other adrenal hormones in addition to androgens, and consequently their deficiency results in congenital adrenal hyperplasia (Table 344-3) as well as male pseudohermaphroditism. The other two enzymes (17,20-desmolase and 17β-hydroxysteroid dehydrogenase) are unique to the pathway of androgen synthesis, and their deficiency results in pure male pseudohermaphroditism. Since 19-carbon androgens are obligatory precursors of estrogens, it likewise follows that in all but the terminal defect (17β-hydroxysteroid dehydrogenase deficiency) estrogen synthesis also tends to be low in affected individuals of both sexes.

The problems inherent in the adrenal hyperplasia of the three relevant disorders are described in Chap. 336, and the present discussion will emphasize the abnormal sexual development. The clinical picture is variable and spans the range from phenotypic men with mild hypospadias to phenotypic women who prior to puberty resemble patients with the complete testicular feminization syndrome. In 46,XY subjects there is usually no trace of uterus or fallopian tubes, indicating that the mullerian regression function of the testis takes place normally during embryogenesis. However, the masculinization of the wolffian ducts, urogenital sinus, urogenital tubercle, and the degree of virilization at puberty vary from almost normal to completely absent. This extreme clinical variability is presumed to be the consequence of the varying severity of the enzymatic defects in different patients and of differential effects of the steroids that accumulate proximal to the metabolic blocks in the five disorders. In patients with partial defects and in whom plasma testosterone is normal the diagnosis can be made only by measuring the steroids that accumulate proximal to the metabolic block in question.

20,22-Desmolase deficiency (lipoid adrenal hyperplasia) is a form of congenital adrenal hyperplasia in which virtually no urinary steroids (either 17-ketosteroids or 17-hydroxycorticoids) can be detected and in which the enzyme deficiency is prior to the formation of pregnenolone; hence the abnormality must lie in one or more of the enzymes of the 20,22-desmolase complex responsible for cleavage of the side chain of cholesterol to form pregnenolone. The syndrome is associated with salt wasting and profound adrenal insufficiency, and most affected individuals die during infancy. At autopsy the adrenals and testes are enlarged and infiltrated with lipid. Affected males are incompletely masculinized, whereas affected female infants have normal genital development.

In 3β-hydroxysteroid dehydrogenase deficiency no urinary steroids contain a Δ^4-3-keto configuration, indicating a defect in the 3β-hydroxysteroid dehydrogenase–$\Delta^{4,5}$-isomerase complex that converts pregnenolone to progesterone. The absence of the enzyme has been documented both in the testis and in the adrenal. Male infants with the defect may exhibit varying degrees of hypospadias or complete failure of masculinization associated with presence of a vagina. Female infants may be modestly virilized at birth due to the weak androgenic potency of dehydroepiandrosterone, the major steroid secreted. Most patients have marked salt wasting and profound adrenal insufficiency, and long-term survival occurs only in partial deficiency states. Several affected males have been reported who experienced otherwise normal male puberty except for pathological gynecomastia. In these individuals the blood testosterone level is in the low normal range but is accompanied by elevated Δ^5 precursors. The deficiency of the enzyme in the testis may be less severe than that in the adrenal. Furthermore, enzyme activity in the liver may be normal in the face of profound deficiency in the adrenal, indicating that the various activities in different tissues are under complex genetic or regulatory control. The presence of normal liver enzyme activity may account for the fact that some females with the disorder have been misdiagnosed as having 21-hydroxylase deficiency since the normal liver enzyme allows significant amounts of pregnanetriol to be excreted in the urine. Indeed, if urinary Δ^5-pregnenetriol is not documented to be greater than urinary pregnanetriol, these individuals can be mistakenly identified as having 21-hydroxylase deficiency. Study of urinary metabolites from a number of individuals with congenital adrenal hyperplasia has led Bongiovanni to conclude that 3β-hydroxysteroid dehydrogenase deficiency is probably the second most common cause of congenital adrenal hyperplasia.

17-Hydroxylase deficiency occurs in phenotypic women who have hypogonadism, absence of secondary sex characteristics, hypokalemic alkalosis, hypertension, and virtually undetectable hydrocortisone secretion. The secretion of both corticosterone and deoxycorticosterone (DOC) by the adrenal is elevated, and urinary 17-ketosteroids are low. Aldosterone secretion is low initially, presumably as the result of high plasma DOC, and returns to normal after suppressive doses of hydrocortisone are administered. In 46,XX subjects amenorrhea, absent sexual hair, and hypertension are common, but since gonadal steroids are presumably not required for fetal female development, the phenotype is that of a normal prepubertal woman. In males, however, the enzyme deficiency results in a disorder of defective virilization that varies from complete male pseudohermaphroditism to ambiguous genitalia with perineoscrotal hypospadias. In males with presumed partial enzyme deficiency pathological gynecomastia may develop at puberty. Patients with this disorder do not develop adrenal insufficiency, since the secretion of both corticosterone (a weak glucocorticoid) and DOC (a mineralocorticoid) is elevated. It is of interest that the hypertension and hypokalemia that are such prominent features of the disorder (even in the neonatal period) remit after suppression of the DOC secretion by adequate glucocorticoid replacement. The decreased aldosterone secretion is probably a regulatory abnormality secondary to depressed angiotensin levels.

17,20-Desmolase deficiency has been described in two families in which affected individuals had a 46,XY chromosome pattern, normal adrenocortical function, and a variable pattern of male pseudohermaphroditism. Only trace quantities of carbon-19 steroids are formed.

17β-Hydroxysteroid dehydrogenase deficiency affects the final step in androgen biosynthesis, reduction of the 17-keto group of androstenedione to form testosterone. This disorder is probably the most common defect in testosterone synthesis causing male pseudohermaphroditism. Affected 46,XY males usually have a female phenotype with a blind-ending vagina and absence of mullerian derivatives, but inguinal or abdominal testes and virilized wolffian duct structures are also present.

TABLE 344-3
Forms of congenital adrenal hyperplasia

Deficiency	Cortisol	Aldosterone	Degree of virilization of females	Failure of virilization in males	Dominant steroid secreted	Comment
21-Hydroxylase, partial (simple virilizing or compensated)	Normal	↑	+ + + +	0	17-Hydroxyprogesterone	Most common type (~95% of total); from one- to two-thirds salt losers
Severe (salt-losing)	↓	↓	+ + + +	0	17-Hydroxyprogesterone	
11β-Hydroxylase (hypertension)	↓	↓	+ + + +	0	11-Deoxycortisol and 11-deoxycorticosterone	Hypertension
3β-Hydroxysteroid dehydrogenase	0	0	+	+ + + +	Δ^5-3β-OH compounds (dehydroepiandrosterone)	Probably second most common, usually salt loss
17α-Hydroxylase	↓	↓	0	+ + + +	Corticosterone and 11-deoxycorticosterone	No feminization of female, hypertension
20,22-Desmolase (lipoid adrenal hyperplasia)	0	0	0	+ + + +	Cholesterol(?)	Rare, usually salt loss

At the time of expected puberty, both virilization (with phallic enlargement and development of facial and body hair) and a variable degree of female breast development take place. The complete pattern of androgen and estrogen dynamics has not been elucidated, but the 17-keto reduction of estrone to estradiol by the gonads is also low. Plasma testosterone may be in the low normal range, making it essential to document a major elevation in plasma androstenedione to make the diagnosis.

PATHOPHYSIOLOGY   In contrast to the 11-hydroxylase and 21-hydroxylase defects, which are inherited as autosomal recessive traits, less is known about the pattern of inheritance of the remaining enzymatic defects. The available data for 17-hydroxylase and 3β-hydroxysteroid dehydrogenase deficiencies are compatible with autosomal recessive inheritance. Insufficient data are available for the 20,22-desmolase defect to warrant any conclusions, and the limited family data for 17,20-desmolase deficiency and 17β-hydroxysteroid dehydrogenase deficiency are compatible either with rare autosomal recessive or X-linked recessive mutations.

The pattern of steroid secretion and excretion depends on the site of the various metabolic blocks (Fig. 344-4). In general, gonadotropin secretion is high, and as a consequence many individuals with incomplete defects are able to compensate so that the steady state concentration of end products such as testosterone is normal or almost normal.

Instances of male pseudohermaphroditism have been described in which testosterone formation is deficient for reasons other than a single enzyme defect. These include disorders in which Leydig cell agenesis and the secretion of a biologically inactive LH molecule have been thought to be the primary defects. In addition, as described above, a spectrum of defects in testicular development has been characterized, including familial XY gonadal dysgenesis, sporadic dysgenetic testis, and absent testis syndrome, in which deficient testosterone production is secondary to the underlying anatomic abnormality.

MANAGEMENT   Replacement therapy with glucocorticoids and in some instances mineralocorticoids is indicated in those disorders causing adrenal insufficiency. The decision about the management of the gonadal problems depends upon the individual case. Fertility has not been reported in any of these

abnormalities, and its consideration does not enter into the decision of sex assignment. In genetic females there is no problem (except in diagnosis), in that affected individuals are raised appropriately as females, and when primary amenorrhea and sexual infantilism are diagnosed after expected puberty because of estrogen deficiency, appropriate estrogen replacement is indicated. The decision as to whether affected newborn males with ambiguous genitalia should be raised as males or females depends upon the anatomic defect; in general the more severely affected should be raised as females, and corrective surgery of the genitalia and removal of the testes should be undertaken as early as possible to prevent untoward virilization at the time of adolescence. In this situation, also, estrogen therapy is indicated at the appropriate age to allow normal female development. In individuals raised as males, corrective surgery is indicated for any coexisting hypospadias, and careful monitoring of plasma androgens should be undertaken at the time of expected puberty in order to determine whether long-term supplemental testosterone therapy is appropriate.

Abnormalities in androgen action   The spectrum of phenotypes that result from abnormalities in androgen action is illustrated in Fig. 344-5 and Table 344-4.

5α-REDUCTASE DEFICIENCY (FAMILIAL MALE INCOMPLETE PSEUDOHERMAPHRODITISM, TYPE 2; PSEUDOVAGINAL PERINEOSCROTAL HYPOSPADIAS)   This distinctive form of male pseudohermaphroditism is inherited in an autosomal recessive fashion and is characterized by (1) severe perineoscrotal hypospadias with a hooded prepuce, a ventral urethral groove, and opening of the urethra at the base of the phallus; (2) a blind vaginal pouch of variable size opening either into the urogenital sinus or more frequently onto the urethra immediately behind the urethral orifice; (3) the presence of well-developed and histologically differentiated testes with normal epididymis, vasa deferentia, and seminal vesicles, and termination of the ejaculatory ducts into the blind-ending vagina; (4) a female habitus without female breast development but with normal axillary

FIGURE 344-5
Schema of the different appearance of the internal and external genitalia and breast development in androgen-resistance syndromes.

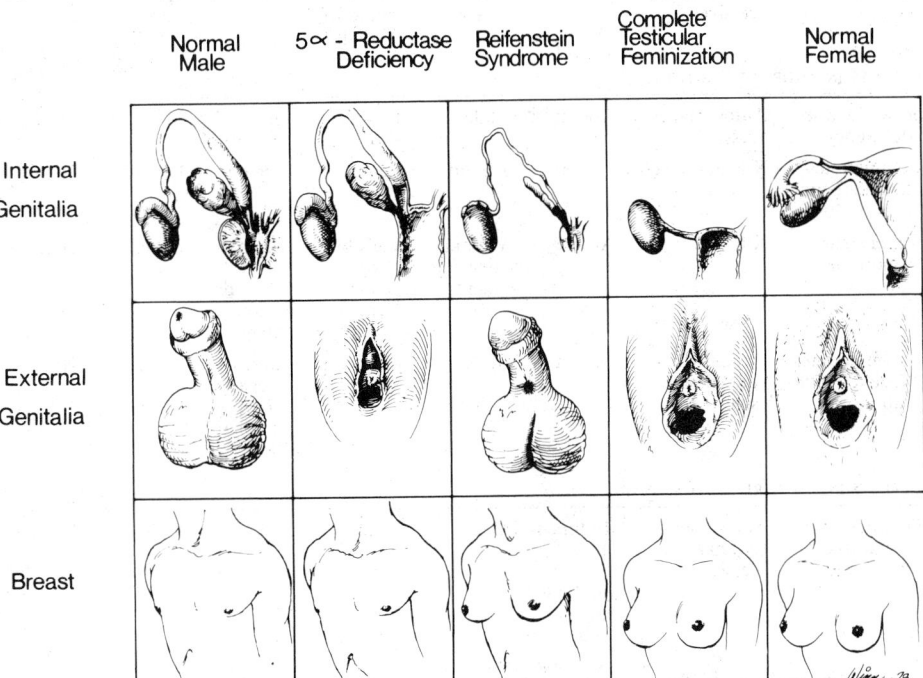

	Normal Male	5α - Reductase Deficiency	Reifenstein Syndrome	Complete Testicular Feminization	Normal Female
Internal Genitalia					
External Genitalia					
Breast					

and pubic hair; (5) the absence of female internal genitalia; and (6) normal male plasma testosterone and masculinization to a variable degree at the time of puberty.

The fact that the defective virilization during embryogenesis is limited to the urogenital sinus and the anlage of the external genitalia provides insight into the nature of the fundamental abnormality. As indicated above, testosterone, the androgen secreted by the fetal testis, is the intracellular mediator for differentiation of the wolffian duct into the epididymis, the vas deferens, and the seminal vesicle; whereas dihydrotestosterone is the functional intracellular hormone for virilization of the urogenital sinus and the anlage of the external genitalia. Consequently, in a male embryo with normal testosterone synthesis and normal androgen receptors a failure of dihydrotestosterone formation would result in the precise phenotype observed in this disorder, namely, normal male wolffian duct derivatives with defective masculinization of the structures originating from the urogenital sinus, urogenital tubercle, and urogenital swelling. In confirmation of this deduction it has been established both by endocrinological criteria and by direct enzymatic assays that the activity of the 5α-reductase enzyme that converts testosterone to dihydrotestosterone is deficient in the disorder. It is not clear why virilization at puberty appears to be more normal than the virilization that takes place during sexual differentiation.

COMPLETE TESTICULAR FEMINIZATION *Clinical features.* Complete testicular feminization is the most common form of male pseudohermaphroditism, estimates of frequency varying from 1 in 20,000 to 1 in 64,000 male births. The clinical features are characteristic. Namely, a phenotypic female is seen by the physician either because of primary amenorrhea (postpubertal) or inguinal hernia (prepubertal). The development of the breasts after puberty, the general habitus, and the distribution of body fat are female in character. Many such patients have a truly feminine appearance. Axillary and pubic hair are absent or scanty, but slight vulval hair is usually present. Scalp hair is that of a normal woman, and facial hair is absent. The external genitalia are unambiguously female, and the clitoris is normal or small. The vagina is short and blind-ending and may be absent or rudimentary. All internal genitalia are absent except for gonads that have histologic features characteristic of undescended testes (normal or increased Leydig cells and seminiferous tubules without spermatogenesis).

The testes may be located in the abdomen, along the course of the inguinal canal, or in the labia majora. Occasionally, remnants of mullerian or wolffian duct origin can be identified in the paratesticular fascia or in fibrous bands extending from the testis. Patients tend to be rather tall, and bone age is normal. Intelligence is normal, and the psychosexual development is unmistakably female in regard to behavior, outlook, and maternal instincts.

Pathophysiology. The karyotype is 46,XY and the mutant gene is located on the X-chromosome. Although familial occurrence is the usual finding, about a third of patients with apparently identical phenotypes and endocrine findings have negative family histories, and it is assumed that the patients with a negative family history are the result of new mutations.

Plasma testosterone levels and blood production rates of testosterone are normal or higher than in normal men. The elevation of testosterone production rate is secondary to high mean LH, which in turn is due to defective feedback regulation as the result of resistance to androgen at the hypothalamic-pituitary level. Elevated LH levels are probably respon-

TABLE 344-4

Anatomic, genetic, and endocrine profile of hereditary male pseudohermaphroditism

| Disorder | Inheritance | Phenotype | | | | | Endocrine profile relative to normal male | | |
		Mullerian ducts	Wolffian ducts	Urogenital sinus	External genitalia	Breast	Testosterone production	Estrogen production	LH
DEFECTS IN TESTOSTERONE SYNTHESIS									
Five enzyme deficiencies	Autosomal or X-linked recessive	Absent	Variable development	Variable from male to female	Generally female	Usually male	Normal to decreased	Variable	High
DEFECTS IN ANDROGEN ACTION									
5α-Reductase deficiency	Autosomal recessive	Absent	Male	Female	Clitoromegaly	Male	Normal	Normal	Normal or increased
Complete testicular feminization	X-linked recessive	Absent	Absent	Female	Female	Female	High	High	High
Reifenstein syndrome	X-linked	Absent	Variable development	Variable from male to female	Incomplete male development	Female	High	High	High
Incomplete testicular feminization	Presumed X-linked recessive	Absent	Male	Female	Clitoromegaly and posterior fusion	Female	High	High	High
DEFECTS IN MULLERIAN REGRESSION									
Persistent mullerian duct syndrome	Autosomal or X-linked recessive	Rudimentary uterus and fallopian tubes	Male	Male	Male	Male	Normal	Normal	Normal

SOURCE: *After Griffin and Wilson.*

sible for the fact that estrogen production in the disorder is also higher than in normal men and that spermatic vein blood estradiol concentrations are increased (see Chap. 341). In normal men most estrogen is derived from peripheral formation from circulating androgens, but when gonadotropins are administered in supraphysiological amounts, the testes secrete significant amounts of estrogen into the circulation. Thus, resistance to the feedback regulation of LH secretion by circulating androgen results in elevated plasma LH levels, and this in turn results in the enhanced secretion by the testes of both testosterone and estradiol. The fact that gonadotropin levels rise even higher (and indeed that menopausal symptoms may develop) when the testes are removed indicates that gonadotropin secretion is under partial regulatory control. Presumably, in the steady state and in the absence of an androgen effect, estrogen alone regulates LH secretion, a control that is purchased at the expense of an elevated plasma estrogen level for a male.

The feminization that results in the disorder is the result of two interlocking phenomena. First, in many instances androgens and estrogens have antagonistic effects at the peripheral level so that the normal state is the result of the ratio of the two hormones; in the absence of androgen action the cellular effect of estrogen is unopposed. Second, estrogen production and particularly the production of estradiol is above that of the normal male although less than that of the normal female. Thus androgen resistance with enhanced estradiol production results in the development of female secondary sex characteristics at the time of puberty as well as the formation of a female phenotype during embryogenesis.

Individuals with testicular feminization exhibit profound insensitivity to exogenous and endogenous androgen, and Wilkins deduced in 1957 that the entire syndrome is the result of androgen resistance. However, the nature of the androgen resistance has been elucidated only recently. A high-affinity receptor protein specific for dihydrotestosterone (Chap. 341) can be demonstrated in fibroblasts cultured from normal genital skin, whereas fibroblasts from affected individuals have deficient binding. These findings indicate that an inherited abnormality in the amount or function of the androgen receptor is the primary defect in the disorder.

Management. Since affected individuals undergo a normal pubertal growth spurt and feminize successfully at the time of expected puberty and since testicular tumors rarely develop until after puberty in patients with intraabdominal testes, it is common to delay castration until after puberty is completed. In the prepubertal state surgical correction is indicated only if the testes are present in the inguinal region or the labia majora and either cause discomfort or are associated with hernia formation. If hernia repair is indicated prepubertally, some physicians prefer to remove the testes at the same time so as to limit the number of operative procedures. The major complication of undescended testes, as noted in Chap. 341, is the development of tumors. It is not known whether tumor incidence is more common in testicular feminization than in cryptorchidism of other etiologies. If the testes are removed prepubertally, estrogen therapy is required at the appropriate age to ensure normal growth and breast development. If castration is performed postpubertally, menopausal symptoms and other evidences of estrogen withdrawal supervene, and suitable estrogen replacement is also indicated.

REIFENSTEIN SYNDROME AND INCOMPLETE TESTICULAR FEMINIZATION A variety of forms of hereditary male pseudohermaphroditism have been described in which virilization is only partially impaired but in whom androgen resistance can be documented. On genetic grounds, two distinct disorders can be delineated. The Reifenstein syndrome (familial incomplete male pseudohermaphroditism, type 1) constitues a spectrum of abnormalities varying from almost complete failure of virilization to almost normal masculinization. The most common presentation is that of a male with perineoscrotal hypospadias, azoospermia, infertility, incomplete virilization at the time of puberty, and gynecomastia. Cryptorchidism is frequent, and the testes are slightly small to normal in size. Biopsy of the testes has revealed normal Leydig cells and tubules that contain both germinal and Sertoli cells, although there is usually no maturation beyond the primary spermatocyte. Hyalinization of the tubules is common. Although affected individuals rarely exhibit ambiguous genitalia at birth, most patients are sufficiently virilized to be raised as men. Psychological development in most appears to be unambiguously male, and most affected men have had successful marriages. Sterility is invariable, probably the result of both defective spermatogenesis and the anatomical abnormalities of the ejaculatory system.

The second disorder, incomplete testicular feminization, is intermediate in severity between the Reifenstein syndrome and complete testicular feminization. Affected individuals have the habitus and general appearance of women, and like patients with the complete disorder, most commonly present with primary amenorrhea. The karyotype is 46,XY, and the testes are present in the abdomen or in the inguinal canals and are histologically indistinguishable from those in the complete form. The external genitalia are distinctive in that there is partial fusion of the labioscrotal folds and a variable degree of clitoromegaly. The vagina, like that in complete testicular feminization, is short and blind-ending. At the expected time of puberty variable feminization and partial virilization both may take place. Upon laparotomy, all mullerian duct derivatives are absent, but the presence of wolffian duct structures is a distinct feature that (together with the partial virilization of the external genitalia) clearly separates the phenotype from that of testicular feminization. The ejaculatory ducts terminate in and empty into the vagina.

These disorders share additional features in common with complete testicular feminization. In both, the pattern of inheritance is compatible with X linkage. Plasma LH is elevated, and the production rates of plasma testosterone and estradiol are higher than those of normal men, the enhanced estradiol coming almost exclusively from direct secretion by the testes. Furthermore, in cultured fibroblasts the amount of dihydrotestosterone receptor is also low and cannot be distinguished on average from that in complete testicular feminization. The reason for the more complete failure of virilization in complete testicular feminization is unclear.

Persistent mullerian duct syndrome CLINICAL FEATURES Men with this disorder have undescended testes and bilateral fallopian tubes, a uterus, an upper vagina, and variable development of the vas deferens. The external genitalia are normal.

PATHOGENESIS The majority have been isolated cases, but several pairs of siblings have been described in whom the condition must be inherited either as an autosomal recessive or as an X-linked recessive mutation. The pathogenesis appears to be straightforward. Because the external genitalia are well developed and because at puberty the patients masculinize normally, it is assumed that during the critical stage of embryonic sexual differentiation the fetal testis produced normal amounts of androgen. However, mullerian regression did not occur. There are three possible explanations: (1) failure of the fetal testis to produce the mullerian-inhibiting substance; (2) poor timing of the release of mullerian-inhibiting substance; or (3) failure of the tissues to respond to this hormone. Which of these possibilities is correct must await identification and characterization of the mullerian regression factor.

MANAGEMENT All patients are phenotypic males, and consequently the preservation of external male appearance and the maintenance of virilization are essential. A primary or staged orchiopexy should be performed. None of the previously reported cases has developed a malignancy in the uterus or vagina. Because the vasa deferentia are closely associated with the broad ligaments, it is recommended that the uterus and vagina be left in place to avoid disruption of the vasa deferentia during removal. By this means, any possible fertility should be preserved.

Developmental defects of the male genitalia HYPOSPADIAS

Hypospadias is a congenital anomaly in which the urethra terminates in an abnormal position along the midline of the ventral surface of the penis anywhere between the site of the normal urethral meatus and the perineum. This malformation is often associated with some degree of ventral contraction and bowing of the penis (chordee). Although few authors use the same classification, it is useful to categorize hypospadias as glandular (involving the glans penis), penile, or perineoscrotal. The disorder occurs in 0.5 to 0.8 percent of live male births in the United States. Since penile development is mediated by androgens, it has been widely assumed that hypospadias must result from some defect in androgen formation or action during embryogenesis. Indeed many if not most of the disorders in male sexual differentiation described above are associated with hypospadias. A small number of cases are also known to result from maternal ingestion of progestational agents early in pregnancy. However, the known causes (single-gene defects, chromosomal abnormalities, and maternal drug ingestion) at best can account for only about a fourth of cases, and the etiology of most remains unknown. The management is surgical.

CRYPTORCHIDISM The descent of the testes is perhaps the most poorly understood portion of male sexual differentiation, both in regard to the nature of the forces that result in the movement and to the hormonal factors that regulate the process. In anatomical terms the movement itself can be divided into three phases: (1) nephric displacement and transabdominal movement; (2) formation of the processus vaginalis, inguinal canal, and scrotum; and (3) actual movement of the testis through the inguinal canal into its permanent site in the scrotum. This entire process occurs over a 6- to 7-month period during gestation, beginning at about the sixth week, and is not complete in some normal individuals until after birth. Whatever its involvement, androgen is probably not the sole hormone responsible. Cryptorchidism can be classified as retractile (intermittently in the groin), obstructed (permanently in the groin), intraabdominal, and high scrotal. Approximately 3 percent of full-term males and 30 percent of premature males have failure of descent of one or both testes. Most of these are retractile and descend permanently by 6 weeks to 3 months of age. The incidence of failure of descent in late teenagers is only 0.6 to 0.7 percent.

The cryptorchid testis functions poorly after puberty, but whether maldescent is the result of an abnormality of the testis or the cause of abnormal function is unknown. Two general theories have been advanced about the etiology—inadequate intraabdominal pressure and deficient testicular function, either because of deficient testosterone synthesis or inadequate mullerian regression factor. Hereditary defects that result in inadequate development either of intraabdominal pressure or of the testes themselves can result in cryptorchidism, and the

fact that infertility is common in men who have been treated for unilateral cryptorchidism suggests that the maldescent is the consequence rather than the cause of the testicular malfunction. As is true for hypospadias, the known causes in their entirety constitute only a small fraction of the cases, and etiology in most instances remains to be identified. Two complications of cryptorchidism are important; spermatogenesis cannot occur at the temperature of the abdominal cavity, and there is a much greater frequency of malignancy in the undescended testis (see Chap. 341).

REFERENCES

BONGIOVANNI AM: Congenital adrenal hyperplasia and related conditions, in *Metabolic Basis of Inherited Disease,* 4th ed, JB Stanbury et al (eds). New York, McGraw-Hill, 1978, pp 868–893

DE LA CHAPELLE A: Analytic review: Nature and origin of males with XX sex chromosome. Am J Hum Genet 24:71, 1972

EDMAN CD et al: Embryonic testicular regression: A clinical spectrum of XY agonadal individuals. Obstet Gynecol 49:208, 1977

GORDON DL et al: Pathologic testicular findings in Klinefelter's syndrome. 47,XXY vs 46,XY/47,XXY. Arch Intern Med 130:726, 1972

GRIFFIN JE et al: Congenital absence of the vagina. The Mayer-Rokitansky-Kuster-Hauser syndrome. Ann Intern Med 85:224, 1976

———, WILSON JD: Hereditary male pseudohermaphroditism. Clin Obstet Gynecol 5:457, 1978

PETERSON RE et al: Male pseudohermaphroditism due to steroid 5α-reductase deficiency. Am J Med 62:170, 1977

SIITERI PK, WILSON JD: Testosterone formation and metabolism during male sexual differentiation in the human embryo. J Clin Endocrinol Metab 38:113, 1974

SIMPSON JL: *Disorders of Sexual Differentiation.* New York, Academic, 1976, p 466

VAN NIERKERK WA: True hermaphroditism. An analytic review with a report of 3 new cases. Am J Obstet Gynecol 126:890, 1976

WILSON JD: Sexual differentiation. Annu Rev Physiol 40:249-273, 1978

———: Embryology of the genital tract, in *Campbell's Textbook of Urology,* 4th ed, JH Harrison et al (eds). Philadelphia, Saunders, 1979, vol 2, pp 1469-1483

———, GOLDSTEIN JL: Classification of hereditary disorders of sexual development, in *Birth Defects: Original Article Series,* vol XI, no 4: *Genetic Forms of Hypogonadism,* D Bergsma (ed). New York, Grune & Stratton, 1975, pp 1–16

———, MACDONALD PC: Male pseudohermaphroditism due to androgen resistance: Testicular feminization and related syndromes, in *The Metabolic Basis of Inherited Disease,* 4th ed, JB Stanbury et al (eds). New York, McGraw-Hill, 1978, pp 894–913

———, WALSH PC: Disorders of sexual differentiation, in *Campbell's Textbook of Urology,* 4th ed, JH Harrison et al (eds). Philadelphia, Saunders, 1979, vol 2, pp 1484-1532

ZAH W et al: Mixed gonadal dysgenesis. A case report and review of the world literature. Acta Endocrinol Suppl 197:3, 1975

345
SEXUAL COUNSELING

PETER REICH

ROLE OF THE FAMILY PHYSICIAN AND INTERNIST The present-day openness about sexuality does not necessarily mean that persons are better educated on sexual matters. In fact, openness may have led to an increase in misconceptions, such as unreal expectations of sexual performance, and may also have led to an increased awareness of complaints and dissatisfactions. However, this openness does allow patients to discuss problems that they might previously have concealed, thus challenging the physician to provide expertise in this area.

Patients will naturally turn to their personal physician when distressing sexual problems emerge or when they need help with long-term difficulties. For them the physician is recognized as a diagnostician and source of health information, as well as a guide to more specialized care, be it from urologist, gynecologist, psychiatrist, sex counselor, or even attorney, if indicated. In addition to a basic knowledge of sexual anatomy, physiology, and behavior, including recent advances in research on the human sexual response, the physician needs to know the effects of illnesses, operative procedures, and medications upon sexual function. Fortunately, most medical schools now include courses on sexuality in their undergraduate curricula. Postgraduate courses are also widely available, and articles on the medical aspects of sexuality are appearing more frequently in medical journals.

Regardless of expertise, the physician's attitudes may undermine his or her usefulness as a sexual counselor. Patients can sense subtle indications of personal bias in the physician, and whether sexual complaints are reported has been shown to depend to a large extent upon the physician's receptivity. Studies indicate that many practicing physicians feel that they are not competent to deal with sexual problems. Others fear that sexual counseling will be too time-consuming or will lead to an excessive involvement with emotional issues. The physician's own moral and ethical positions or personal discomfort with areas of sexuality, such as homosexuality or sexual deviance, may inhibit communication. In addition, the potentially seductive aspects of an open discussion of sexuality can be disturbing to both patient and physician. Problems of communication across ethnic, racial, economic, or educational lines also take on special significance.

The objective medical approach to sexual symptoms will reduce tensions and will enable both the patient and the physician to deal with sensitive material. The physician does not need to be a psychotherapist or an expert on sexual behavior to be helpful. Patients who seek sexual advice from physicians are likely to be concerned about medical issues. Often sexual problems reflect fears and misconceptions, and the objective evaluation of the symptoms leads to relief without further treatment. Thus the responsibility of the physician is to establish an accurate and complete diagnosis, including both physiologic and psychological factors, and in the context of the patient's own background and life-style to evaluate the significance of the problem and to know the range of treatments that are available.

Approach to the patient Physicians may be called upon to provide sexual counseling in a wide variety of medical and human situations. For example, they may encounter adolescent fears of homosexuality or of sexual inadequacy, marital problems that present with sexual incompatibility, sexual inhibitions after surgery or after myocardial infarction, postpartum frigidity, impotency associated with diabetes, ejaculatory disturbances after prostatectomy, and loss of libido in psychological depression. Although tensions, anxieties, preconceptions, attitudes, and interpersonal factors must be taken into account, the assessment of a sexual problem is similar to the assessment of a problem involving any other system. A complete history, careful attention to multiple determinants, and thorough evaluation of the patient as a person and of the context of the symptoms will yield a working diagnosis that will enable the physician either to treat the patient or to make an appropriate referral. A detailed guide to the assessment of sexual function has been published by the Group for the Advancement of Psychiatry. Similar guides can be found in standard texts of psychiatry and of obstetrics and gynecology. It is useful to have such a framework in mind when obtaining a sexual history.

More often than in other areas of medicine, the physician needs to take an active role in initiating the discussion of sexual matters. In one survey it was found that the incidence of sexual problems reported by patients increased from 7.9 to 14 percent when the physician routinely asked about the sexual symptoms in the review of systems. In those conditions where sexual problems occur frequently, such as in gynecologic and urogenital surgery, cord injury, ileostomies and colostomies, myocardial infarction, diabetes, and various neurologic conditions, the physician has the responsibility to assess sexual function. Even when the patient initiates the discussion, an active inquiry by the physician will enable the patient to discuss specific and intimate details.

Reassurances about confidentiality may be necessary during the discussion of sexual matters even though such confidentiality is already assumed in the doctor-patient relationship. Confidentiality may be especially important when the physician is also treating other members of the family or when the patient needs to discuss extramarital, deviant, or extralegal behavior.

It is well to keep the dignity of the patient in mind as the history is being taken by observing such simple practices as using scientific words for sexual parts and sexual activities instead of using vernacular or slang expressions in a mistaken effort to put the patient at ease, and by refraining from jokes or other informal remarks even though the patient may try to engage in them. Comments that may seem casual to the physician tend to live on in the patient's mind.

While the initial inquiry into sexual matters requires tact and timing, the need to protect the patient from embarrassment should not be overemphasized. Physicians' anticipation of discomfort may lead them to choose an evasive route of inquiry while patients might appreciate a direct question. Some patients may allude to sexual problems with idiomatic phrases, such as "changing nature" or "problems in relationships," and, unless the physician is sensitive to the patient's feelings and language, the reference may be missed and the patient may assume that the physician is not interested in further information. Sometimes sexual problems appear indirectly through other complaints relating to the urogenital system. Much of the tension and uncertainty in obtaining a sexual history can be avoided by including questions about sexual physiology, practices, and satisfaction in the systems review.

The sexual problems of elderly patients are not well understood by most physicians. Physicians may refrain from asking questions because they have incorrectly assumed that sexual satisfactions can no longer be achieved as a result of the aging process. At times the patient will silently accept a loss of sexual function because of misconceptions about the effects of illness or of aging. Depression may be a factor in such instances. Here the questions of the physician, coupled with some reassuring statements about the tendencies of many persons to assume mistakenly they will never be able to enjoy sexual relations again, will bring the issue into the open and awaken new hopes in the patient.

Once a sexual complaint has been elicited, it is important to obtain a detailed history of specific behavior. Terms for sexual disorders may be misused by patients or may be exaggerated or misunderstood. Many sexual complaints reflect misconceptions, ignorance, or fears, and the problems prove to be nonexistent when the behavior is explored in detail. Patients tend to overestimate or to underestimate the extent of a problem, depending upon their psychological orientation. For example, one woman believed herself to be frigid because her sexual partner, for neurotic reasons of his own, was comparing her in a disparaging way to his previous partners. Much can be learned from the first instance of a sexual problem, from the pattern of behavior since the onset of symptoms, and from inquiring whether the problem is present consistently or varies with the circumstances or nature of the sexual practice.

In every disorder there is always a complex interaction between the physical and the emotional; and every sexual symptom needs to be evaluated in the context of the relationships between the patient and the sexual partners, or in the context of the sexual practices and attitudes of the patient. A past history, including early experiences, attitudes of parents, and attitudes toward childhood sexuality, development, marriage, and pregnancy may be relevant. The relationship of sexual function to general health is always a consideration.

A general physical examination with special attention to an examination of the genitalia is a part of the evaluation of all sexual complaints. At times the patient will conceal or be unaware of abnormalities of the genitalia. On the other hand, even sophisticated patients may harbor irrational misconceptions or feelings of shame about their bodies, and they may need concrete reassurance about the adequacy of their genital apparatus. Unless the physician has pursued the process of evaluating the medical aspects of the complaint, the patient may disregard reassurances that there is no medical basis, if indeed the physician has decided that the problem is psychogenic.

Appropriate laboratory tests to screen for systemic illnesses are indicated along with the specific tests for various endocrinopathies, neurologic conditions, and other systemic disorders that may present with sexual problems (see Chaps. 45 and 47). Attention to the mental status, including assessment of mood, affect, thought content, judgment, and reality testing, will enable the physician to determine whether the sexual symptom is an aspect of a mental disorder. Rarely, sexual problems, especially loss of libido, may be the presenting sign of a disorder of the central nervous system; an examination of mental status can pick up early signs of dementia or other manifestations of organic brain conditions.

An understanding of the daily habits of a patient may provide important clues to diagnosis. Fatigue, anxiety, and stress, as well as use of alcohol, drugs, and medications, can influence sexual function. In addition, traumatic events, such as automobile accidents, surgical procedures, or the illness or death of another person, may exert acute or chronic effects on sexual behavior.

DIAGNOSTIC CONSIDERATIONS The specific disorders of sexual function are discussed in Chaps. 45 and 47. All of them can vary in severity, from complete loss of function under all circumstances to relatively minor disturbances in specific circumstances or with specific partners. Patients also may vary in their reactions to sexual symptoms, some ignoring or concealing severe disability, others reacting with panic to minor disturbances.

The first consideration is whether the condition is primarily organic or psychogenic. In clinics devoted to sexual counseling, the complaints of 10 to 20 percent of the patients are manifestations of organic problems, while the complaints of the remaining 80 to 90 percent are psychogenic. When significant organic factors are present, a useful distinction can be made between sexual symptoms that arise *directly* from organic disorders, such as structural disorders of the urogenital system, neurologic disorders affecting the innervation of the sexual organs, and endocrinopathies that influence sexual physiology, and those that are *secondary* to changes in general health, such as sexual disturbances associated with rheumatoid arthritis, malignancies, renal failure, and other chronic diseases, and also those that occur with acute debilitating conditions, such as myocardial infarction, major surgery, and hepatitis. With primary organic disorders, patients may need counseling to help them adjust to permanent losses of sexual function if medical measures cannot reverse the process. When sexual disturbances are secondary to changes in health, the effects of organic factors are often overemphasized by both the patient and the physician. Although libido may be affected by general loss of vitality and by toxic and metabolic factors, the sexual disturbances associated with physical illnesses are often the expression of hopelessness, depression, or anxiety and may be perpetuated by the psychological factors long after the organic problems have disappeared.

The physician can also make significant diagnostic distinctions among psychogenic sexual disturbances. *Primary* psychogenic disturbances, those that have been present since puberty, can be distinguished from *secondary* disturbances, those that represent decompensations from previous adequate levels of function. The former often reflect chronic and deep-seated sexual conflicts. When a patient seeks help for a chronic disturbance, the key diagnostic issue may be why he or she has come for help at this particular time. A secondary decompensation may be the presenting symptom of a psychological defeat, loss, or a disturbance in a relationship. Some sexual problems occur in connection with life stresses or transitions, such as retirement, pregnancy, work crises, or bereavement. The prognosis is good providing that the underlying issues are recognized and acknowledged. A disproportionate focus on sexual symptoms can actually perpetuate the problem by reinforcing anxiety about sexual performance.

Some sexual disorders are manifestations of major mental disorders and will respond only to treatment directed at the mental disorders themselves. Diminished sexual responsiveness, impotence, or ejaculatory disturbances may be indications of depression. Bizarre sexual complaints with increased or diminished sexual activity can indicate incipient psychosis. The strange qualities of the symptoms or the intensity of the associated feelings may be the best diagnostic clue. Hypersexuality can occur with the onset of mania. It also may appear as a depressive equivalent, especially in postmenopausal women. Neuroses are often associated with sexual inhibitions.

Alcohol may play a significant role in potency disturbances. Often the first episode of secondary impotence is associated with the use of alcohol, and the midlife depressive syndrome that is often related to secondary impotence may be further complicated by alcohol abuse. Barbiturates and opiates also can cause reduced libido and impotence. Antihypertensive agents, tranquilizers, hypnotics, analgesics, and sedatives all may influence sexual function in the male.

Sexual disturbances may develop after traumatic incidents. For example, impotence can develop after cystoscopic examination or after vasectomy, even though neither procedure has any direct physiologic effect upon potency. An automobile accident can have a similar effect. Pregnancy, contraceptive difficulties, casual but disturbing sexual encounters, and a host of other emotionally significant episodes may cause sudden changes in sexual functioning. The patient may not be aware of the importance of such episodes or may be reluctant to discuss them.

The diligent physician may inadvertently overdiagnose sexual disturbances. Most patients have self-doubts and sexual dissatisfactions even though they are functioning adequately. It is well to have in mind the concept of a threshold of disturbance to separate the normal vicissitudes from the problems that require treatment.

TREATMENT Some sexual problems will resolve themselves during the evaluation process, especially if it extends over several visits. With those that persist, the physician must decide whether to treat the patients or to refer them elsewhere. Often a brief attempt at office counseling will enable the physician to make this decision. Generally the secondary or reactive psychogenic disorders are more amenable to brief counseling, especially when they occur in response to stress. Sexual problems related to physical illnesses are also appropriately handled by the general physician who also treated the physical disorder.

The technique for counseling cannot be mapped in a formal way. Sufficient time, a relaxed atmosphere, and genuine interest by the physician are necessary. The patient should be encouraged to tell the full story with careful attention to the circumstances surrounding the onset of symptoms, to the attitudes of the patient and partner, to the nature of the patient's relationships, and to factors that might be leading to anxiety or depression. Although it may be necessary to review the physical details of the patient's sexual practices, resolution of symptoms may occur with only indirect reference to sexual techniques. Sexual inadequacies often produce anxiety, which in turn leads to further defeats and to inhibition of libido. Without reduction of anxiety and lifting of depression, the process cannot be reversed.

Some physicians will choose not to attempt sexual counseling, while others find it to be a satisfying aspect of medical practice. In either case, it is important for physicians to be familiar with the resources in their communities and to understand the capabilities and limitations of various treatment approaches. Physicians usually have referral relationships with gynecologists, urologists, and psychiatrists. In addition, many communities now have family services and counseling services. Referral should be tailored to the nature of the problem and to the life-style and personality of the patient. Some patients would consider discussing the intimate details of a sexual problem only with a gynecologist or urologist. Others would appreciate being directed to a reputable clinic where the new direct behavioral approaches to the treatment of sexual dysfunctions are available.

Referral is often a difficult transition for a patient because it implies turning to a stranger after having confided in a physician who has understood the problem. Patients who come eagerly to a consultant may lose their motivation when the consultant refers them to a colleague. Some physicians advocate having counselors associated with them in their offices. This system has the advantage of maintaining the personal relationship between counselors and physicians but has the disadvantage of encouraging physicians to rely on counselors for the evaluation of emotional problems rather than carrying through the diagnostic phase themselves. If physicians keep in touch with patients through the process of therapy, it will enable them to learn about the efficacy of the treatment program and to provide support and reassurance.

A few examples will illustrate some of the principles involved in the treatment of patients with sexual disorders.

Patient A.R., a 56-year-old attorney who had recently suffered a myocardial infarct, complained to his physician of loss of libido. He was an energetic, competitive, aggressive, self-made man, who enjoyed athletics and was "top" man in his firm. The physician asked him about the details of his daily life and found that the loss of libido was only one of many inhibitions. He avoided arguments, stopped playing handball, cut his workload, and was losing weight. He also reported insomnia and anorexia. Further questioning revealed fears of sudden death and the fatalistic belief that his days were numbered. He assumed that strict reduction of activity was mandatory. His wife shared his fears and urged him to avoid stress. Together they had decided not to have sexual relations during the period immediately after his heart attack, and now he had no desire to resume. In the course of several sessions of counseling the physician reassured him that his fears were exaggerated, that many patients with heart trouble experienced similar feelings,

clarified the extent of his disability, and helped him and his wife to plan realistic resumption of many of his previous activities, including sexual relations.

Patient L.D., a 26-year-old woman, consulted a physician because of frigidity. She had left her husband after 6 years of an unfulfilling marriage and had sought satisfaction in a series of brief affairs. The interview revealed her to be a restless, competitive, chronically dissatisfied person who was unhappy in her career and who experienced disappointment in her close relationships. After careful evaluation of the physical aspects of her sexual difficulties and experiences, the physician decided that her problem reflected long-standing psychological conflicts and referred her to a psychiatrist.

Patient M.B., a 34-year-old salesman, complained to his physician of impotence. He was a nervous, insecure, ineffectual man who worked for his older brother. His wife, an active real estate broker, had become withdrawn and bitter. His two adolescent children were involved in minor delinquency. The impotence was confined to his relationship with his wife; in a recent extramarital affair he had performed adequately. He said he was unable to satisfy his wife in any way; she was either withdrawn or overly demanding. The physician determined that the impotency had no organic basis and because of the involved nature of the family conflicts referred the patient to a family service agency where the family could be worked with as a unit. Here the wife was found to be depressed and received psychiatric treatment. Later the patient reported that when her depression improved, his potency returned.

In another instance, patient C.W., a woman with breast cancer, was asked about her marriage. She told her physician that her husband had stopped having sexual relations with her when it was discovered that she had metastatic disease. The physician then asked to see the husband. He confessed to an extramarital affair and the wish to leave his wife. He also was experiencing irrational anger at his wife and feelings of shame and worthlessness. It emerged that the marriage had been an unusually close one and that he could not bear the anticipation of his wife's death. Sexual contact with her reminded him of his impending loss. His anger and the affair were responses to grief. The physician met with him for several sessions. By avoiding a moralistic position and by indicating that many spouses of patients with serious diseases have similar feelings and may even find solace in extramarital relationships, the physician helped him to overcome his shame and to share his grief. The process brought dramatic relief, and with occasional contact with the physician he was able to remain with his wife and be helpful to her throughout her terminal illness.

MARITAL COUNSELING BY THE PHYSICIAN Almost invariably the evaluation of sexual problems leads to some attention to marital or other sexual relationships. Counseling that focuses primarily on these relationships has been designated *marital counseling*. Instead of the usual medical relationship, which emphasizes the individual patient, the treatment in marital counseling involves both partners visiting the physician together, although each may be seen separately at times.

The specific nature of the marital counseling will depend upon the complaints or upon the time of life of the couple. The main requisite for physicians is a willingness to set aside time for this kind of responsibility and to develop an interest in the functional health of their patients beyond the specific issues raised by disease. The stresses and transitions in the early years of a marriage should be appreciated as well as the pressures children exert. In later years, job problems and conflicts over roles may emerge, as well as the "empty nest" syndrome, then menopausal and midlife issues and the male-depressive syndrome as horizons close in and the realities of aging appear.

It is well to know that most marital problems are not due to sexual difficulties, although sexual problems may be the leading edge, especially in our modern climate where sexual adjustment is so widely publicized. Sexual satisfaction is dependent on the broader aspects of the relationship between partners and on mental and physical health. It is to these deeper levels that the alert physician should probe during marriage counseling. In this sense, the more specific counseling about sexual problems is really dependent upon the successful outcome of marriage counseling. Early in the approach the physician should assess the state of motivation of both partners. If one partner is determined to break up the marriage, the counseling may consist of communicating this to the other partner and perhaps advising legal assistance. On the other hand, apparent determination to seek divorce by either partner needs to be evaluated because it may mask depression, a paranoid reaction, or a hidden problem that is being avoided by flight, such as shame over an affair, fear, illness, or personal failure.

In marital counseling, as with other medical counseling, it is well to avoid giving direct advice about interpersonal relationships. By defining the problem, the physician may enable the patient to arrive at a decision on a course of action. By taking sides in family conflicts or by espousing an ethical position, physicians can inadvertently introduce their own bias or can allow themselves to be manipulated by one of the marital partners.

The internist or family physician is in a strategic position to provide effective marital counseling. As preventive medicine gains importance, marital counseling can provide physicians with great professional satisfaction.

REFERENCES

ABSE DW et al (eds): *Marital and Sexual Counseling in Medical Practice,* 2d ed. Hagerstown, Md, Harper & Row, 1974

FREEDMAN AM et al (eds): Normal and abnormal sexuality, in *Comprehensive Textbook of Psychiatry,* vol 2, 2d ed. Baltimore, Williams & Wilkins, 1975, p 1349

LEVINE SB: Marital sexual dysfunction: Ejaculation disturbances. Ann Intern Med 84:575, 1976

MASTERS WH, JOHNSON VE: *Human Sexual Inadequacy.* Boston, Little, Brown, 1970

SADOCK BJ et al (eds): *The Sexual Experience.* Baltimore, Williams & Wilkins, 1976

TAYLOR RW: Aspects of sexual medicine. Some of the commoner sexual disorders. II. Problems mainly affecting the woman. Br Med J 3:31, 1975

VINCENT C (ed): *Human Sexuality in Medical Education and Practice.* Springfield, Ill, Charles C Thomas, 1968

346
DISEASES OF THE PINEAL GLAND

RICHARD J. WURTMAN

INTRODUCTION Since the discovery of melatonin in 1958, compelling evidence has accumulated that the mammalian pineal is not a vestige but an important component of a neuroendocrine control system. This organ has been shown to function as a neuroendocrine transducer. It receives a cyclic input of sympathetic nervous "information" which is suppressed when the retina responds to light. In response to this input, the pineal secretes a hormone, melatonin, into the bloodstream,

much as the adrenal medulla releases epinephrine in response to cholinergic nervous stimulation. The synthesis and secretion of melatonin vary with a 24-h periodicity, thereby providing the body with a circulating "clock" apparatus. Until very recently, no assay was available to permit measurement of melatonin in human blood or urine. Largely as a consequence, human pineal physiology remained conjectural, and the only disease states that could clearly be associated with pineal malfunction were those caused by pineal neoplasms. Now the melatonin in blood and urine can be measured by bioassay and radioimmunoassay, and it is apparent that the same factors that control the synthesis and secretion of this hormone in experimental animals also do so in humans. There is thus reason for optimism that our understanding of pineal physiology and pathophysiology, and of the possible medical use of pineal compounds, will soon expand.

ANATOMY AND BIOCHEMISTRY OF THE PINEAL The human pineal gland is a flattened, conical organ which lies beneath the posterior border of the corpus callosum and between the superior colliculi. It originates embryologically as an evagination of the ependyma which lines the roof of the third ventricle, and remains connected to this region by the pineal stalk. The adult gland weighs about 120 mg; its dimensions are 5 to 9 mm in length, 3 to 6 mm in width, and 3 to 5 mm in thickness. Most of the pineal is enveloped by pia mater, from which blood vessels, unmyelinated nerve fibers, and septa of connective tissue penetrate the gland, thereby dividing it into lobules. The pineal glandular or parenchymal cells on the periphery of the lobule are elongated; those in the central zone are ovoid. They contain numerous granular bodies (which might represent a stored secretion), and give rise to processes that terminate adjacent to the capillary endothelium.

In 1960, Kappers made the important discovery that the primary innervation of the mammalian pineal originates not within the brain but rather from sympathetic cell bodies in the superior cervical ganglia. Subsequent studies using the electron microscope revealed that the sympathetic nerve endings terminate directly on pineal parenchymal cells in an anatomic relationship that resembles the synapse. The sympathetic innervation of pineal glandular cells appears to be a new evolutionary adaptation, which by itself invalidates the vestige theory of pineal function.

In 1917, McCord and Allen showed that the pineal gland of the cow contained a factor which causes amphibian skin to blanch. When pineal homogenates were fed to tadpoles, the melanin granules within dermal melanophores aggregated around the cell nuclei, thereby lightening the skin. (This effect is opposite to that produced by the melanocyte-stimulating hormone, MSH, which is secreted by the pars intermedia of the pituitary gland.) Four decades later, Lerner and his colleagues identified this pineal factor as melatonin (5-methoxy-N-acetyltryptamine) (Fig. 346-1). It remains to be shown that melatonin has any effect on the melanocytes which are responsible for normal skin pigmentation in human beings or, for that matter, in amphibians.

Melatonin was shown to be a derivative of serotonin (Fig. 346-1), a widely distributed indole stored in very large quantities in mammalian pineals. It differs from all indoles previously identified in mammalian tissues in that it contains a methoxy group. The enzyme which catalyzes this methoxylation reaction (hydroxyindole *O*-methyl transferase, HIOMT) was shown to be concentrated within the pineal gland in mammals. The high degree of localization of HIOMT has sometimes been used as a "marker" to differentiate true pinealomas from pineal tumors of glial or other origin.

PHYSIOLOGY OF THE MAMMALIAN PINEAL Environmental lighting conditions exert several important effects on the mam-

Tryptophan → (Tryptophan hydroxylase) → 5-Hydroxytryptophan → (Aromatic L-amino acid decarboxylase) → Serotonin (5-Hydroxytryptamine)

→ (Acetylating enzyme) → N-Acetylserotonin → (Hydroxyindole-O-methyl transferase) → Melatonin (5-Methoxy, N-Acetyltryptamine)

FIGURE 346-1

Synthesis of melatonin in the pineal gland. The pineal takes up tryptophan from the circulation; the amino acid is hydroxylated to form 5-hydroxy-tryptophan; this is then converted to the amine serotonin (5-hydroxytryp-tamine) by the enzyme aromatic L-amino acid decarboxylase. Some of the *serotonin synthesized in the pineal is destroyed by oxidative deamination, forming 5-hydroxyindole acetic acid and 5-hydroxytryptophol; the remainder is N-acetylated and O-methylated to form the hormone melatonin.*

malian neuroendocrine apparatus. Light acts as an "inducer" that modifies the rate of sexual maturation; girls who have been deprived of light from birth may show early pubescence. The sequence of day and night also acts to generate some 24-h biologic rhythms and to synchronize other rhythms which are produced by signals arising from within the body or from behavioral rhythms (e.g., eating, drinking) that introduce chemicals into the body intermittently. There is evidence that one function of the mammalian pineal might be to mediate some of these endocrine and metabolic effects of light. The "information" about light travels to the pineal by a route which involves (1) the inferior accessory optic tract, (2) centers in the brain and spinal cord that regulate the sympathetic nervous system, and (3) the sympathetic nerves to the pineal which originate in the superior cervical ganglia. The diurnal variation in melatonin secretion from the human pineal, which causes mela-

tonin levels to peak during the hours of darkness, provides the body with a circulating "clock" which is under the direct control of the lighting environment (Fig. 346-2).

Less is known about which organs take cues from the pineal "clock" than about the mechanism responsible for its rhythmic changes. It seems likely that melatonin exerts physiologic inhibitory effects on gonadal and thyroid function and also modifies behavior and electroencephalographic activity. When tiny amounts of melatonin are implanted in the median eminence of the hypothalamus or the midbrain reticular formation, the increase in pituitary luteinizing hormone (LH) content which normally follows castration is blocked. Melatonin placed in the cerebrospinal fluid suppresses the secretion of pituitary LH and enhances the secretion of prolactin. Melatonin administration also changes the levels of serotonin in the brain.

FIGURE 346-2

Effect of diurnal phase reversal on urinary melatonin rhythm. Urinary melatonin was assayed (by radioimmunoassay) in consecutive 4-h urine samples collected from two subjects. After 3 days, the time of onset of the dark period was delayed for 12 h, from 11 P.M. to 11 A.M. Before this time, both subjects had exhibited characteristic daily rhythms in urinary melatonin levels, with high nighttime and low daytime values. On the day that the light period was extended by 12 h, both subjects continued to excrete large amounts of melatonin at the time that they had previously been exposed to darkness (11 P.M. to 11 A.M.). Most subjects require 3 to 4 days to reentrain their rhythms in melatonin secretion to changes in the time of onset of the daily light or dark periods. (From DC Jimerson et al, Life Sci 20:1501, 1977.)

The mammalian pineal also synthesizes and secretes at least two other compounds with significant biological activity. They are 5-methoxytryptophol, a methoxyindole like melatonin whose pineal levels exhibit similar daily rhythms, and arginine vasotocin, an octapeptide similar in structure to oxytocin and vasopressin (ADH). Reliable chemical and immunochemical assays for these compounds in body fluids have become available only recently.

PINEAL PATHOLOGY Two pineal lesions have been of interest to the clinician: pineal calcification, which is a universal autopsy finding, and pineal tumors, which are best known for their endocrine sequelae. In rare instances, pineal glands have also contained cancer metastases, gummas, tuberculous granulomas, or isolated segments of skeletal muscle.

Pineal calcification often first becomes visible on skull roentgenograms around the time of puberty, and it has been suggested that the gland degenerates at this time of life, and then becomes calcified. However, recent studies have not supported this hypothesis. If pineals are examined by appropriate microscopic techniques, evidence of calcification often is seen in patients who died long before the age of puberty. A ground substance believed to serve as the matrix for calcification was seen in 8 of 28 pineals taken from children under 1 year of age. Moreover, studies of pineal function have failed to show any differences between heavily calcified glands taken from aged subjects and pineals from young subjects with no gross evidence of calcification. The functional significance of pineal calcification remains entirely unexplained. The chemical identity of the calcified material appears to be hydroxyapatite; crystals of this compound taken from human pineals are similar to those prepared from bone or tooth.

Pineal tumors may be divided into several distinct categories by their microscopic appearance. Somewhat more than half of all pineal tumors may be classified as true pinealomas. These tumors contain clusters of two distinct types of cells: large spheroidal epithelial cells, and small dark-staining cells with little cytoplasm and an ultrastructure indistinguishable from that of the lymphocyte. About 10 to 15 percent of all reported pineal tumors have been teratomas; these may contain mucus-secreting columnar epithelial cells, adenocarcinoma tissue, and areas resembling thyroid, muscle, cartilage, bone, and nerve. Like other midline teratomas, they are often malignant. The remainder of pineal tumors have been of vascular or glial origin.

Confirmation of pineal origin of the large pinealoma cells has been hampered by the lack of specific pineal function which could be measured in these cells (such as the uptake of ^{131}I by thyroid cells in follicular adenomas). However, studies suggest that assays for the melatonin-forming enzyme HIOMT may provide such a "marker." Two pineal tumors containing this enzyme have been described; one was a metastasis from a parenchymal pinealoma, and the other, a specimen from an ectopic pinealoma. Both tumors had the characteristic histologic appearance of the parenchymal pinealoma. No data are yet available on blood or urinary melatonin levels in subjects with pineal tumors.

The natural history of a pineal tumor is related to its size and its histologic appearance. Tumors which originate within the pineal gland usually become clinically manifest because of symptoms which arise from their location (e.g., internal hydrocephalus, elevated cerebrospinal fluid pressure, and oculomotor signs such as paralysis of upward gaze or Parinaud's syndrome); less frequently, the patient's family initially seeks medical attention because of the development of precocious puberty. About one-third of all boys below the normal age of sexual maturation who have pineal tumors develop precocious puberty. This neoplasm accounts for about 10 to 15 percent of all precocious sexual development in males. For unexplained reasons, pineal tumors are much less common among girls and are not associated with precocious menarche. Some investigators have suggested that the precocious sexual development in pinealoma patients is a nonspecific consequence of the pressure that these tumors exert on surrounding brain tissue. Kitay and others have summarized the evidence against this "pressure hypothesis": (1) Pineal tumors may produce precocious puberty, no gonadal signs, or even delayed pubescence. The endocrine effects of a particular tumor appear to be unrelated to its size. (2) Most cases of precocious puberty develop in patients with nonparenchymal tumors (frequently teratomas). An occasional parenchymal tumor leads to gonadal enlargement, but more commonly these neoplasms are associated with delayed pubescence or with secondary gonadal failure. (3) Gonadal abnormalities have been observed in a large number of pinealoma patients whose tumors had neither produced signs of a chronic elevation in cerebrospinal fluid pressure nor invaded other brain areas. The demonstration that melatonin influences normal sexual maturation in rats supports the hypothesis that precocious puberty develops in pinealoma patients because the damaged pineal fails to release this or another inhibitory hormone (e.g., arginine vasotocin). It is noteworthy, perhaps, that both patients described above whose tumors contained melatonin-forming activity showed evidence of depressed sexual function.

Parenchymal pinealomas frequently show a good, if temporary, clinical remission following irradiation. Patients generally receive 3000 to 5000 rads; radiation is administered over a wide portal because pinealomas not infrequently metastasize throughout the ventricles and the subdural space. Japanese surgeons have reported encouraging results following the surgical extirpation of pinealomas; however, this method is complicated by the relative inaccessibility of the pineal, and consequently is used rarely in the United States. A patient with metastatic parenchymal pinealoma has been repeatedly treated during a 10-year period with x-ray and chemotherapeutic agents; each time an objective decrease in tumor mass occurred. In another case, described more recently, repeated courses of daunorubicin (Adriamycin), vincristine, and bleomycin following irradiation have suppressed tumor recurrence for three months.

A small number of tumors with histologic appearance of pinealomas originate elsewhere in the brain at some distance from the normal pineal gland. These "ectopic pinealomas" generally arise in the hypothalamus in the region of the infundibulum. Hence, patients usually present a picture similar to that seen with craniopharyngioma with a clinical triad of bitemporal hemianopsia, hypopituitarism, and diabetes insipidus. Most ectopic pinealomas show a good clinical response to irradiation.

REFERENCES

De Tribolet N, Barrelet L: Successful chemotherapy of pinealoma. Lancet 2:1228, 1977

Lynch JH et al: Daily rhythm in human urinary melatonin. Science 187:169, 1975

Ramsey HJ: Ultrastructure of a pineal tumor. Cancer 18:1014, 1965

Wolstenholme GEW, Knight J (eds): *The Pineal Gland,* Edinburgh, Churchill-Livingstone, 1971, p 401

Wurtman RJ, Cardinali DP: The pineal organ, in *Textbook of Endocrinology,* RH Williams (ed). Philadelphia, Saunders, 1974, p 832

Wurtman RJ, Moskowitz MA: Medical progress: The pineal organ. N Engl J Med 296:1329, 1383, 1977

347

ENDOCRINE MANIFESTATIONS OF NONENDOCRINE DISEASE

LOUIS M. SHERWOOD

A number of factors provided impetus for wider recognition of humoral syndromes associated with nonendocrine disease, particularly malignant disorders. Among these are advances in understanding the biochemistry, control of secretion, and biosynthesis of polypeptide hormones and the development of sensitive and specific radioimmunoassay and radioreceptor techniques that have been applied to the serums and tumors of patients. As a result of the emphasis on earlier diagnosis of malignant disorders and on the management of advanced cancer with modern therapeutic techniques (see Chap. 324), many patients with abnormal hormone production by tumors have been described, even when clinical manifestations of endocrine disease are absent.

In addition to hormone production, there are many nonendocrine "paraneoplastic syndromes." For some clinical abnormalities the disorders are the result of production of specific polypeptides or antigens by the tumor; in others, the relationship between tumor and clinical manifestations is poorly understood. Although this chapter will focus on the production of hormones by tumors, the fact should be appreciated that clinical manifestations such as fever, anorexia, weight loss, metabolic disturbances, neurological syndromes, coagulation defects, vascular complications, connective tissue disorders, dermatoses, and the nephrotic syndrome may at times be related to the production of specific proteins by tumors.

DEFINITION The term *ectopic hormone syndrome* refers to the production of hormones by tissues (both nonendocrine and endocrine) other than the primary tissue(s) known to produce the hormone. In the majority of instances the site of the aberrant production is a tumor, and the hormone is peptide in character. Whether this production is truly ectopic depends largely on one's concept of pathogenesis.

PATHOGENESIS Considerable progress has been made in recognizing these disorders, even in the absence of clinical syndromes, but the pathogenesis of ectopic hormone production is still poorly understood. Current concepts of pathogenesis can be summarized as follows: (1) The production of hormone by a nonendocrine tumor may represent dedifferentiation to an embryonic state in which proteins not normally synthesized by the differentiated cell are produced. Since every somatic cell contains the same complement of DNA, any cell could theoretically produce any hormone. That the process is not random, however, is demonstrated by the correlation of specific histological tumor types with particular clinical syndromes (see Table 347-1). (2) Alternatively, the capacity of endodermal tissues to generate peptide hormones may be due to the migration during embryogenesis of cells with innate secretory capacity from neural crest to the endodermal layer. These cells have specific histochemical and biochemical characteristics and have been named *amine precursor uptake and decarboxylation (APUD) cells*. Amines such as dopa and 5-hydroxytryptophan are taken up, decarboxylated, and converted to biogenic amines; presumably, the amines may mediate the secretion of other hormones or be used to synthesize more complex polypeptide hormones. At present, the APUD hypothesis is useful in explaining the production of hormones by certain tumors such as medullary carcinoma of the thyroid, oat-cell carcinoma of the lung, carcinoid tumors, thymomas, tumors of the

TABLE 347-1
Relationship of tumor type to hormone production

Hormone	Tumor type
ACTH and lipotropin (β-MSH, endorphin, and enkephalin)	Oat-cell carcinoma of lung Thymoma Islet-cell tumor Bronchial carcinoid Also ovarian tumors, pheochromocytoma, gastrointestinal, prostate, neurogenic, and parotid tumors, and medullary thyroid carcinoma Inactive "big" ACTH in a wide variety of tumors
Growth hormone	Adenocarcinoma of the lung; bronchial carcinoid
Human placental lactogen	Undifferentiated carcinoma of the lung Hepatoma Lymphoma Pheochromocytoma
Prolactin	Renal-cell carcinoma Undifferentiated carcinoma of the lung Breast carcinoma
Thyrotropin	Choriocarcinoma, hydatidiform mole Epidermoid carcinoma of the lung Mesothelioma
Gonadotropin	Hepatoblastoma, pancreatic, other gastrointestinal tumors Adenocarcinoma and other carcinomas of the lung Choriocarcinoma of male and female, other testicular tumors Islet-cell tumors (malignant) Breast carcinoma Melanoma
HCG β subunit	Adenocarcinoma of the pancreas Islet-cell tumors (malignant)
HCG α subunit	Carcinoid Islet-cell tumors (malignant)
Vasopressin	Oat-cell carcinoma of lung Pancreatic adenocarcinoma
Parathyroid hormone	Epidermoid carcinoma of lung Renal-cell carcinoma Hepatoma, pancreatic, and gastrointestinal carcinoma Other epidermoid tumors
Prostaglandin E_2	Renal-cell carcinoma Lung tumors
Osteoclast-activating factor	Multiple myeloma Burkitt's and other lymphomas
Calcitonin	Oat-cell carcinoma of the lung Breast, pancreatic, and other carcinomas
Somatomedin (NSILA)	Mesodermal and mesenchymal tumors Adrenal carcinoma
Glucagon	Non-beta islet-cell tumors Undifferentiated lung cancer
Gastrin	Non-beta islet-cell tumor Duodenal wall carcinoma Ovarian carcinoma
Vasoactive intestinal peptide	Non-beta islet-cell tumor Carcinoma of lung Pheochromocytoma and ganglioneuroblastoma
Erythropoietin	Renal-cell carcinoma Cerebellar hemangioblastoma Pheochromocytoma Hepatoma Uterine fibroids
Renin	Juxtaglomerular tumor Wilms's tumor Renal-cell carcinoma
Serotonin and 5-hydroxytryptophan	Non-beta islet-cell tumor Oat-cell carcinoma of the lung Carcinoid (also growth hormone-releasing activity) Pancreatic adenocarcinoma

pancreatic islets, pheochromocytoma, neuroblastoma, ganglioneuroma, and possibly others. The hypothesis does not appear to be satisfactory for all ectopic hormone-producing tumors, particularly those such as hepatoma, hypernephroma, and various mesodermal tumors that produce parathyroid hormone (PTH), erythropoietin, gonadotropins, placental lactogen (HPL), nonsuppressible insulin-like activity (NSILA), and renin. APUD-type tumors are characterized by similar histological features and dense neurosecretory-type granules; these granules are not characteristic of the non-APUD tumors. Because of their clinical features, defined genetic relationships, and characteristic hormones, the multiple endocrine neoplasia syndomes have been suggested by some to be of APUD origin (see Chap. 348).

Information on the biochemical nature of tumor hormones, particularly their amino acid sequence, is limited. The derepression hypothesis suggests that tumors should make the same hormones produced by endocrine cells and not abnormal polypeptide hormones with similar biologic activity. This concept is complicated, however, by the fact that many polypeptide hormones are made from higher molecular weight precursors. The first intracellular product is usually a prehormone which contains a "signal" sequence of 15 to 30 amino acids that is necessary to move the polypeptide into the subcellular transport system. The signal peptide is cleaved as the hormone passes into the endoplasmic reticulum. For some hormones such as PTH and insulin, there is an additional prohormone precursor formed from the prehormone (e.g., proPTH and proinsulin) which is converted to mature hormone in the Golgi region of the cell. Some tumors that produce ectopic hormones release a precursor form of the hormone rather than the hormone itself (e.g., "big" ACTH rather than "little" ACTH). Since the precursor may be immunologically or biologically distinct, the critical factor in determining whether a clinical or biochemical syndrome will result could be the presence of a converting enzyme rather than production of the hormone precursor. Further research on biosynthetic processes in normal cells as well as tumors will resolve these questions.

Extensive application of radioimmunoassay to tumor extracts and serums has shown that polypeptide hormone synthesis is more prevalent than previously believed (particularly ACTH, chorionic gonadotropin, and its subunits, vasopressin and calcitonin). Some have even suggested that hormones may be produced at a basal level by all malignant tumors and by certain normal nonendocrine tissues as well. It is difficult at present to reconcile widespread findings of hormone in tumor tissues with the limited appearance of clinical syndromes, but the reasons for the lack of tight correlation between hormone levels and clinical manifestations may be both quantitative and qualitative. These new findings open interesting, unresolved questions about the pathogenesis of the ectopic hormone syndromes and even of their definition. It is apparent that an understanding of the pathogenesis of these syndromes will provide answers important to the entire field of cell biology and differentiation as well as to clinical medicine.

GENERAL CHARACTERISTICS OF ECTOPIC HORMONE PRODUCTION Detection or documentation of the presence of an ectopic hormone syndrome requires the documentation shown in Table 347-2. The most definitive points are numbers 7 to 9. The ectopic syndromes are being recognized with greater frequency in malignant disorders, in part because hormone measurements are carried out both for diagnostic purposes ("tumor markers") and for assessment of tumor remission and recurrence. Since radioimmunoassay techniques are sensitive, the finding of elevated hormone levels in plasma may indicate the presence of malignant cells that are not clinically or radiographically obvious. In all such cases it is important to differentiate the presence of hormone-producing malignancy from a coexisting endocrine disorder (e.g., hypercalcemia in a patient with breast cancer could be due to the primary disease or to a concurrently present parathyroid adenoma). Occasionally, hormonally induced metabolic disorders such as hyponatremia, hypokalemia, and hypercalcemia may be a more immediate threat to life than the malignancy itself. When confusion exists concerning the production of the hormone by the tumor or a coexisting endocrine disorder, selective venous catheterization with radioimmunoassay of the appropriate hormone may be useful in localizing the tissue of origin.

ECTOPIC PRODUCTION OF PITUITARY HORMONES Lipotropin and ACTH Excess output of hydrocortisone due to ectopic production of ACTH was the first ectopic syndrome recognized (more than 50 years ago). Since that time there have been several hundred reports of ectopic ACTH production, usually in patients with tumors of the lung (oat-cell carcinoma, 60 percent; bronchial adenoma, 4 percent), thymus (15 percent), or pancreatic islet (10 percent). Other causes include medullary carcinoma of the thyroid, bronchial carcinoid, and pheochromocytoma. ACTH-like material has been noted in virtually all lung tumor tissue examined (as opposed to blood) and in other malignant tissues as well. This is usually "big" ACTH, however, a precursor that has minimal biologic activity. Lipotropin, a precursor of ACTH with an even larger molecular weight that includes the sequences of several other hormones, is produced by the normal pituitary and can also be synthesized by tumor tissue. Cushing's syndrome secondary to tumors appears to be associated primarily with the production of "little" ACTH, a 39-amino acid peptide. "Big" ACTH can be converted to "little" ACTH with trypsin, but many tumors do not have the enzyme(s) necessary to convert the precursor glycoprotein to the mature hormone. The quantities of ACTH in tumor extracts of patients without Cushing's syndrome are generally less than in those with clinical manifestations. In a few instances, elevated levels of "big" ACTH have been found in plasma prior to the clinical appearance of the tumor, and a variety of amino- and carboxy-terminal fragments of ACTH have also been demonstrated.

Ectopic ACTH production due to bronchogenic carcinoma is the most common cause of Cushing's syndrome in males, but the clinical manifestations are usually different from those seen with typical Cushing's disease (see Chap. 336). Weight loss,

TABLE 347-2
Documentation of ectopic hormone production

1 Presence of a clinical endocrine disorder or abnormal level of polypeptide hormone or metabolite in a patient with malignancy. (Be careful to exclude the presence of a coexisting endocrine disorder, in particular, a common one like primary hyperparathyroidism in a patient with a malignant tumor and hypercalcemia.)
2 Disappearance or remission of the disorder or biochemical abnormality following surgical removal, radiation therapy, or chemotherapy of the tumor.
3 Recurrence of the disorder or metabolic abnormality when metastasis or reappearance of the tumor occurs.
4 Abnormal hormone concentrations in blood or urine or failure of normal hormone suppression or stimulation.
5 Presence of hormone in tumor extract or metastases in amounts greater than adjacent normal tissue, as detected by bioassay, radioimmunoassay, or radioreceptor assay.
6 Qualitative abnormalities in the hormone in serum or tumor extracts (in molecular weight, immunologic activity, biologic activity, or biochemistry).
7 An increase in hormone concentration from the arterial to venous side of the tumor (e.g., renal artery to vein for hypernephroma).
8 Biosynthesis of polypeptide hormone following incubation of tumor explants in vitro with radioactive amino acids (flask incubation or tissue culture).
9 Cell-free synthesis of ectopic hormone or synthesis of complementary DNA by messenger RNA from tumor extract.

muscle weakness, hyperpigmentation, hypertension, peripheral edema, and hirsutism are common while weight gain, centripetal obesity, and striae are rare. In general the manifestations reflect the mineralocorticoid effects of hydrocortisone rather than glucocorticoid actions. Other factors produced by the tumor, debilitation due to malignancy, and rapidity of the course may also contribute to the altered clinical appearance.

The clinical syndrome is associated with extremely high plasma levels of ACTH and correspondingly elevated levels of plasma and urinary steroids. Severe hypokalemic alkalosis in the absence of diuretics, glucose intolerance, and increased urinary 5-hydroxyindoleacetic acid (reflecting the association between oat-cell and carcinoid tumors) may be present. Autonomy of ACTH secretion is not uniformly present, and in vitro studies of some tumors have shown release of ACTH in response to stimulators. In some patients steroid output is altered by metyrapone and (very rarely) with dexamethasone. The tumors may contain corticotropin-releasing factors in addition to ACTH, a finding that could explain the variable clinical responses to suppression and stimulation.

Hyperpigmentation is characteristic of ectopic ACTH production and has been ascribed by some to the melanocyte-stimulating hormone (MSH) activity of ACTH. More recent studies suggest that MSH itself is produced from the precursor lipotropins that contain the MSH sequence. MSH extracted from tumors and plasma is probably artifactual in the sense that the activity in vivo is contained in the larger peptide (see Chap. 332).

Therapy should be directed at the primary tumor whenever possible, although oat-cell carcinoma has often metastasized to bone when first diagnosed. The prognosis of oat-cell carcinoma is improved somewhat with combination chemotherapy but is still poor (median survival 11 to 12 months). Correction of the hypokalemic alkalosis and hyperglycemia is important. Combined adrenal blockade with metyrapone (11-β-hydroxylase inhibitor) and aminoglutethimide (which blocks the conversion of cholesterol to pregnenolone), with or without the cytolytic agent mitotane (*o,p'*-DDD), may be useful.

Gonadotropin and gonadotropin subunits Follicle-stimulating hormone (FSH), luteinizing hormone (LH), thyrotropin (TSH), and human chorionic gonadotropin (HCG) consist of two noncovalently linked subunits. The alpha subunits of the pituitary hormones are identical and immunologically indistinguishable from the HCG alpha subunit which has a minor structural difference. The beta subunits are biochemically unique and confer biologic and immunologic specificity to the molecules. Immunologically, the beta subunits of HCG and LH are related, but an additional 30 amino acids are present at the carboxy terminus of HCG. The isolated subunits are biologically inactive but may be combined in vitro to produce a biologically active hormone. Sensitive radioimmunoassay and radioreceptor assays have been developed for the common alpha and the specific beta subunits. Application of these assays to the serums and tumors of patients with malignancy has revealed widespread presence of HCG and its subunits. Isolated subunit production may be an early tumor marker, but free alpha subunits may also be released by the normal pituitary (particularly in primary hypothyroidism and in postmenopausal women). In patients with islet-cell tumors of the pancreas, production of HCG or its subunits is a strong indication that the tumor is malignant. Normal tissues such as liver and colon may produce HCG-like material that contains the polypeptide backbone devoid of its normal content of carbohydrate.

Clinical syndromes associated with gonadotropin production have been principally noted in men with choriocarcinoma and less commonly with other testicular and lung tumors (epidermoid, poorly differentiated, small-cell, and bronchioalveo-

lar carcinomas). In men, the association of gynecomastia with gonadotropin production is well documented (see Chap. 343). The increased estrogen production that is responsible for the gynecomastia is usually the result of HCG-mediated secretion of estradiol by the testes. On occasion, however, estrogen can be formed directly in the tumor itself from circulating androgens; in the latter instances HCG may or may not be elevated. Interestingly, a syndrome of precocious puberty has been described in boys with HCG-producing hepatoblastomas. One must be careful to differentiate gynecomastia due to tumors from gynecomastia due to other causes. Apart from hyperthyroidism (see below) women have no symptoms from tumor-mediated gonadotropin release.

Earlier studies in which pituitary gonadotropins were reported in tumors may have been in error because of confusion with HCG. In addition to carcinoma of the lung and liver, tumors of the breast, bladder, adrenal, mediastinum, gonads, melanocytes, and gastrointestinal tract have been reported to produce HCG.

Thyroid-stimulating factors Nonpituitary production of thyrotropin-like factors is associated principally with trophoblastic tumors (choriocarcinoma of the placenta and testis) and hydatidiform mole, although there are scattered reports of a hyperthyroid syndrome with other tumors (epidermoid carcinoma of the lung and mesothelioma). Patients typically have mild hyperthyroidism (rarely a severe form has been described) with smooth skin, increased pulse pressure, tachycardia, tremor, and a small goiter. Thyroid function tests are characteristic of mild hyperthyroidism. The hormone responsible is probably not TSH but HCG, which has demonstrable thyrotropic activity when present in concentrations equivalent to those found in the plasma of such patients. Since there is a close biochemical link between TSH and gonadotropins, this relationship is adequately explained. Therapy of the hyperthyroidism is not a major problem as the prognosis of the tumor usually determines the patient's course. Again, these individuals must be separated from patients with ordinary forms of hyperthyroidism (see Chap. 335).

Growth hormone and prolactin Ectopic production of growth hormone from nonpituitary tumors is rare, although it has been noted occasionally in bronchogenic and gastric carcinomas. Growth hormone has been extracted from such cancers and shown to be synthesized by the tumors in tissue culture. Since growth hormone secretion in the normal individual varies widely in response to exercise, sleep, and diet, differentiating normal physiological changes in plasma growth hormone from production by a tumor is important. The hypertrophic osteoarthropathy found in some patients with lung tumors differs from the clinical and radiological manifestations of growth hormone excess noted in acromegaly; whether this entity is related to growth hormone or growth hormone-like proteins is not known. Recent reports indicate an association between growth hormone-releasing activity and bronchial carcinoids that leads to the clinical picture of acromegaly. Removal of the carcinoid results in a regression of soft-tissue enlargement and return of plasma growth hormone to normal.

The normal placenta produces human placental lactogen (HPL, chorionic somatomammotropin), a peptide hormone closely related to growth hormone in its biologic and immunologic properties as well as in its amino acid sequence. Production of HPL can occur with both trophoblastic and nontrophoblastic tumors, particularly of the lung, although its concentration in serum may be low enough to require concentration by affinity chromatography before detection. The presence of HPL in the serum of a man or nonpregnant woman is indicative of an ectopic hormone syndrome. Occasionally, men with ectopic HPL production have gynecomastia. In these patients, simultaneous production of gonadotropin or the production of estrogen directly by the tumor itself should be suspected. Some tumors that produce HPL also produce HCG as well as a placental form of alkaline phosphatase. HPL may also be a useful tumor marker for breast cancer.

Only a few reports of the ectopic production of prolactin, a peptide biochemically related to both growth hormone and HPL, have appeared. This has been principally with carcinoma of the lung and kidney. One patient with a renal-cell carcinoma that produced prolactin had galactorrhea.

Vasopressin or antidiuretic hormone (ADH) Ectopic production of ADH has been recognized for more than 20 years and documented by both extraction of ADH from tumor and demonstration of ADH synthesis by tumor explants. Other known mechanisms of inappropriate secretion of ADH (SIADH) in patients with malignancy such as cerebral metastases, mediastinal infections, renal tubular defects, central nervous system infection, cerebrovascular disease, excessive smoking, pain, trauma, emotional stress, and administration of drugs such as chlorpropamide and vincristine must be excluded. Production of ADH by tumors occurs principally with small-cell carcinoma of the lung, neoplasms of the pancreas, and cancers of the upper gastrointestinal tract. Plasma immunoreactive ADH may be increased in patients with carcinoma of the lung, both with and without SIADH, but the levels are higher in patients with the syndrome. Some tumors also appear to make the protein neurophysin which binds vasopressin, but this phenomenon is not associated with clinical abnormalities.

Common clinical characteristics in patients with SIADH, regardless of cause, include nausea, vomiting, headaches, anorexia, confusion, and coma (see Chap. 334). The syndrome is treated with fluid restriction; demeclocycline and lithium carbonate have also been useful in some cases. Symptomatic hyponatremia may require treatment with intravenous hypertonic saline.

ECTOPIC PRODUCTION OF CALCIUM-MOBILIZING SUBSTANCES

Hypercalcemia and its associated clinical symptoms are frequent in patients with malignant disease. Both the degree of elevation and the rapidity of change of the plasma calcium are important factors in determining whether symptoms of hypercalcemia develop. The predominant manifestations of hypercalcemia are in the central nervous system, heart, kidney, and gastrointestinal tract. The signs, symptoms, and differential diagnosis of hypercalcemia are described in Chap. 350. A number of mechanisms may be responsible for hypercalcemia in patients with malignancy:

1 Direct invasion of bone by tumor; this is particularly true of cancers that commonly metastasize to bone (lung, breast, kidney, and thyroid). Prostatic carcinoma is frequently metastatic to bone but causes osteoblastic metastases that do not usually result in hypercalcemia.

2 Production of PTH or a PTH-like substance.

3 Production of other calcium-mobilizing substances such as prostaglandin E_2 or osteoclast-activating factor.

4 Coexistence of the tumor with primary hyperparathyroidism.

5 Coexistence of the tumor with another cause of hypercalcemia such as hyperthyroidism, sarcoidosis, hypervitaminosis D, immobilization, or adrenal insufficiency.

6 Administration of estrogen or androgen to women with carcinoma of the breast that has metastasized to bone.

The differential diagnosis of hypercalcemia can usually be accomplished on clinical grounds. The major difficulty is in separating primary hyperparathyroidism from a malignant disorder. A first consideration is to exclude the presence of bony metastases. Bone marrow biopsy and bone scans are more helpful than routine radiographs of bone (which detect only metastases larger than 1 cm). Demonstration of metastases to bone by a tumor does not exclude coexisting primary hyperparathyroidism or even the production by the tumor of a calcium-mobilizing substance, but a definitive workup may not be appropriate if the metastatic disease is widespread.

Ectopic production of PTH by tumors has been documented by extraction of PTH-like material from tumors, by increases in arteriovenous hormone gradients across the tumor, and by demonstration of biosynthesis in tumor explants in vitro. In some cases the tumor PTH in the peripheral blood is qualitatively different from the hormone (and its fragments) produced by normal parathyroid gland. Many patients have had correction of hypercalcemia after removal of the primary tumor, but in only a relatively small number has a fall in PTH been documented by specific hormone assay.

Since PTH levels in serum may be low or undetectable in the face of tumor-associated hypercalcemia, it follows that other calcium-mobilizing factors produced by neoplasms may lead to hypercalcemia. One such agent is prostaglandin E_2. Both increased concentrations of circulating prostaglandin and accelerated urinary excretion of PGE_M (the major urinary metabolite of prostaglandin E_2) have been demonstrated, and clinical remission of hypercalcemia has been induced by treatment with aspirin or indomethacin. However, the clinical response to these inhibitors of prostaglandin synthesis is variable. The third tumor substance that can cause hypercalcemia is osteoclast-activating factor (OAF). This low-molecular-weight polypeptide was first identified in tissue culture fluid of human lymphocytes stimulated with phytohemagglutinin. OAF induces osteoclastic bone resorption and appears to be the major cause of hypercalcemia in patients with multiple myeloma, Burkitt's lymphoma, and possibly other lymphoid tumors. The biologic activity of OAF can be distinguished experimentally from that of PTH, prostaglandins, or vitamin D metabolites. Its action is inhibited by corticosteroids, partially explaining the successful use of this agent in the hypercalcemia of multiple myeloma.

The relative incidence of hypercalcemia due to the synthesis by tumors of PTH, prostaglandin E_2, OAF, or other calcium-mobilizing factors is uncertain. Non-PTH factors may be more commonly involved than PTH. A judicious trial of indomethacin (for 3 to 4 days) is indicated; correction of the hypercalcemia suggests prostaglandin production. If response to indomethacin does not occur, the usual methods for treating hypercalcemia should be undertaken (see Chap. 350). These measures include vigorous saline hydration, furosemide, mobilization, oral phosphates, and corticosteroids. If more conservative measures fail, intermittent treatment with mithramycin has proved useful.

Calcitonin is a hormone produced by medullary carcinoma of the thyroid, another tumor of neural crest origin (see Chap. 348). Extrathyroidal production of calcitonin has been reported in some patients with tumors of the bronchus (small-cell carcinoma), breast, and pancreas. Since calcitonin inhibits the mobilization of calcium and phosphate from bone (see Chap. 349), high concentrations should theoretically produce hypocalcemia, but this metabolic abnormality is rarely (if ever) seen. Since the hormone is clinically silent, demonstration of its presence is useful primarily as a "tumor marker."

METABOLIC BONE DISEASE

Severe osteomalacia, marked hypophosphatemia, and phosphaturia have been described in patients with mesenchymomas, pleomorphic sarcomas, neurofibromas, and sclerosing or cavernous hemangiomas. The etiology of the phosphaturia and metabolic bone disease is unclear, but dramatic remission of the osteomalacia has occurred after tumor removal. The tumor may interfere with the conversion of vitamin D to its active form through an action on renal 1,α-hydroxylase, but this hypothesis is not proved.

ECTOPIC HYPOGLYCEMIA The association of symptomatic hypoglycemia with excessive production of insulin by islet-cell tumors is well recognized (see Chap. 340). The etiology of hypoglycemia with nonendocrine tumors such as large sarcomas of the abdomen and thorax, hepatocellular carcinoma, adrenal tumors, lymphomas, and other malignancies is more obscure. More than 200 cases have been reported. Insulin is usually not found in tumor extracts or by tissue immunofluorescent techniques, and plasma insulin is not elevated. At least one-third of patients with extrapancreatic tumors and hypoglycemia have increased levels of circulating nonsuppressible insulin-like activity (NSILA). This substance is a low-molecular-weight protein that is reversibly bound to larger proteins in plasma. It is one of a group of closely related somatomedins, peptides that are normally synthesized by the liver in response to growth hormone and that have insulin-like activity in vitro. Confirmation that tumors produce the substance was obtained by direct extraction of NSILA from an adrenal carcinoma.

Other postulated mechanisms of hypoglycemia include production of metabolites that interfere with gluconeogenesis, induction of an acquired form of glycogen storage disease (as in hepatocellular carcinoma), malnutrition, release of substances that enhance insulin secretion, and suppression of normal counterregulatory mechanisms.

Insulin-secreting islet-cell tumors can be differentiated from extrapancreatic neoplasms by demonstrating inappropriately elevated plasma insulin levels in the presence of hypoglycemia. Proinsulin levels may also be elevated. Plasma free fatty acids and lactate tend to be increased in patients with nonpancreatic tumors and decreased in patients with hyperinsulinism. Prognosis is dependent on tumor type. Although retroperitoneal mesenchymal tumors can grow to extraordinarily large size, they tend to be slow growing and of relatively low degree of malignancy. Partial or complete resection of the tumor may ameliorate the hypoglycemia. During hypoglycemic attacks, continuous oral or intravenous glucose is required. Diazoxide, which may be useful in treating islet-cell tumors, is not helpful in extrapancreatic tumors. High doses of glucocorticoids or glucagon infusions are of occasional benefit.

ECTOPIC PRODUCTION OF GASTROINTESTINAL HORMONES
The APUD hypothesis (see "Pathogenesis" above and "Syndromes with Multisystem Hyperfunction" in Chap. 348) may explain why so many hormones are produced in the gastrointestinal tract. They include peptides with recognized functions such as secretin, gastrin, and cholecystokinin-pancreozymin, and others whose function is not completely clear: vasoactive intestinal peptide (VIP), gastric inhibitory peptide (GIP), pancreatic polypeptide (PP), and motilin. The pancreatic islet produces a number of hormones including insulin, glucagon, gastrin, somatostatin, VIP, PP, and prostaglandins. Whether hormone production by pancreatic tumors is truly ectopic is problematical since the cells normally produce them (see Chap. 340). Tumors outside the pancreatic islet or gastrointestinal tract also make these hormones, and such cases can be more properly defined as *ectopic*. Aspects of islet-cell tumors that relate to the multiple endocrine neoplasia syndrome are covered in Chap. 348.

A well-defined entity known as *pancreatic cholera* is associated with non-beta islet-cell tumors. The syndrome classically includes watery diarrhea, hypokalemia, and hypochlorhydria. The agents implicated include secretin, kinins, glucagon, gastrin, calcitonin, GIP, PP, prostaglandins, and VIP. The latter is generally considered to be the primary etiologic agent. Elevations of plasma VIP are found not only in patients with islet-cell tumors but also in those with bronchogenic carcinoma and neurogenic tumors. VIP is a 28-amino acid peptide with structural similarities to glucagon, secretin, and GIP. Its actions include inhibition of gastric acid secretion and stimulation of myocardial contractility, glycogenolysis, lipolysis, insulin secretion, pancreatic juice, and intestinal cyclic AMP. PP is a 36-amino acid polypeptide with a poorly defined function that is found in normal pancreatic islets and in some tumors associated with diarrhea. Indomethacin may ameliorate some cases of the watery diarrhea syndrome, implicating prostaglandins as a pathogenic factor in some patients.

Islet-cell tumors producing somatostatin have recently been described. This hormone, originally identified as an inhibitor of growth hormone secretion, is widely distributed in the body, particularly in the gastrointestinal tract. Somatostatin in pharmacological doses inhibits gastric acid production, duodenal motility, pancreatic secretion, gallbladder contraction, and the release of gastrin, secretin, insulin, and glucagon. Findings associated with somatostatin-secreting tumors include abdominal pain, diarrhea, weight loss, hyperglycemia, and gallbladder disease.

A syndrome in which hyperglycemia is associated with a bullous necrotic skin eruption has been described in patients with pancreatic glucagonomas. Weight loss, anemia, and stomatitis are also characteristic of the syndrome. Release of a larger-than-normal form of glucagon may occur.

ECTOPIC PRODUCTION OF ERYTHROPOIETIN AND RENIN
The principal source of the hormone that controls erythropoiesis is the kidney. Both benign and malignant disorders of the kidney are associated with increased production of erythropoietin, but extrarenal tumors that cause polycythemia also presumably synthesize erythropoietin. These include cerebellar hemangioblastomas, uterine fibroids, occasional adrenal, ovarian, and hepatic carcinomas, and pheochromocytoma. Between 2 and 5 percent of patients with renal tumors have polycythemia. Although the clinical syndrome is recognized principally by virtue of the association of tumor and polycythemia and a fall in hematocrit following surgery, the successful development of a radioimmunoassay for erythropoietin should facilitate recognition of the syndrome in the absence of polycythemia. Tumors that are associated with leukocytosis and thrombocytosis presumably produce leukopoietins and thrombopoietins, respectively.

Production of renin by tumors can cause hypertension. This is principally seen with tumors of the kidney, especially tumors of the juxtaglomerular apparatus, Wilms's tumor, and hypernephroma. One patient with small-cell carcinoma of the lung also had elevated renin levels. Clinical manifestations vary from absence of symptoms to severe hypertension; secondary hyperaldosteronism and hypokalemia may or may not be present. Arteriography and selective venous studies for the measurement of renin are helpful. In some cases a higher molecular weight form of renin is present.

ECTOPIC PRODUCTION OF OTHER HORMONES, ENZYMES, AND ANTIGENS It is possible that all peptide hormones are produced ectopically, but documentation for some is limited. It is now apparent that tumors produce not only peptide hormones but also enzymes, antigens, and other proteins. Enzymes are not detected unless screening studies are performed. Ectopic alkaline phosphatase has been identified in many tumors (primarily lung) and appears to be identical to the heat-stable enzyme characteristically produced by the placenta.

There has been considerable recent interest in clinical syndromes related to antigen production by tumors. Renal disorders varying from minimal change nephropathy to immune-complex glomerulonephritis have been associated with carcinomas and with Hodgkin's disease. In some cases, evidence of immune complexes in serum and kidney (with specific immunofluorescent localization of antigen, immunoglobulins, and complement) has been found. Some neurological disorders associated with malignancy (in particular myasthenia gravis, dermatomyositis, and the Guillain-Barré syndrome) appear to have an immune basis. Discussions of tumor immunology and the carcinoembryonic and α-fetoprotein antigens are beyond the scope of this chapter. Nevertheless, it is apparent that tumors may produce many proteins, some of which are responsible for humoral, immunologic, and other pathological phenomena.

Tumors may also produce more than one ectopic hormone. Those tumors of apparent neural crest origin (producing ACTH, melanotropin, biogenic amines, insulin, calcitonin, glucagon, and secretin) appear to do this more frequently. The production of multiple hormones by tumors may not be concurrent, since each hormone may be produced episodically.

REFERENCES

Blackman MR et al: Ectopic hormones. Adv Intern Med 23:85, 1978

Gewirtz G, Yalow RS: Ectopic ACTH production in carcinoma of the lung. J Clin Invest 53:1022, 1974

Hirai H, Alpert E: Carcinofetal proteins. Ann NY Acad Sci 259:1, 1975

Megyesi K et al: Hypoglycemia in association with extrapancreatic tumors: Demonstration of elevated NSILA-s by a new radio receptor assay. J Clin Endocrinol Metab 36:931, 1974

Odell WD, Wolfsen AR: Humoral syndromes associated with cancer, in Annual Review of Medicine, WT Creger (ed). Palo Alto, Annual Reviews, 1978, p 379

Robertson PR et al: Plasma prostaglandin E in patients with cancer with and without hypercalcemia. J Clin Endocrinol Metab 43:1330, 1976

Sherwood LM: Ectopic hormone syndromes, in The Year in Endocrinology, SH Ingbar (ed). New York, Plenum, 1976, p 249

——— et al: Production of parathyroid hormone by nonparathyroid tumors. J Clin Endocrinol Metab 27:140, 1967

———, Gould VE: Ectopic hormone syndromes and multiple endocrine neoplasia, in Metabolic Basis of Endocrinology, LJ deGroot (ed). New York, Grune & Stratton, 1978, p 1749

Vaitukaitis JL: Peptide hormones as tumor markers. Cancer 37:567, 1976

348
DISORDERS AFFECTING MULTIPLE ENDOCRINE SYSTEMS

R. NEIL SCHIMKE

This chapter is addressed to those disorders in which multiple endocrine gland hyper- or hypofunction results from mechanisms other than a primary abnormality in the hypothalamic-pituitary axis. Congenital anomalies, vascular lesions, metabolic errors, infiltrative and storage disorders, granulomatous diseases, and primary and secondary neoplastic processes can produce multitropic hormone deficiency by interfering with the central control of pituitary hormone secretion, and such conditions must be excluded before a diagnosis of multiple endocrine system disorder can be made. While not common, many of the conditions that affect multiple endocrine systems are inherited and from the viewpoint of preventive medicine have significance out of proportion to their frequency.

SYNDROMES WITH MULTISYSTEM HYPERFUNCTION

The best known conditions involving a number of endocrine glands are the three multiple endocrine neoplasia syndromes, each of which is inherited as an autosomal dominant trait.

MULTIPLE ENDOCRINE NEOPLASIA, TYPE I (MEN I) This disorder, also termed the *Wermer syndrome*, comprises tumors or hyperplasia of the parathyroids, pancreatic islet cells, pituitary, adrenal cortex, and thyroid. The clinical presentation is variable, depending on which of the potentially affected glands is hyperfunctioning at the time of diagnosis. About two-thirds of patients have adenomas of two or more endocrine systems, and a fifth develop tumors of three or more systems.

The majority of affected subjects present with one of the following problems: (1) peptic ulcer and its complications, (2) hypoglycemia, (3) hypercalcemia and/or nephrocalcinosis, (4) complaints referable to pituitary dysfunction such as headaches, visual field defects, and secondary amenorrhea, and (5) multiple lipomas of the skin. A minority (probably < 10 percent) come to medical attention with acromegaly, Cushing's syndrome, nonfunctional thyroid adenomas, hyperthyroidism, hepatomegaly (due to metastatic liver disease), or flushing.

Parathyroid involvement in MEN I may be asymptomatic for prolonged periods, although most patients eventually show some signs of hyperparathyroidism. Tumors of the islet cells may elaborate excessive insulin or gastrin. Insulinomas cause hypoglycemia (Chap. 340), whereas excess gastrin secretion causes the Zollinger-Ellison syndrome with its multifocal or atypically located ulcers and massive hypersecretion of gastric acid. Symptoms may be identical with those of ordinary peptic ulcer, but there is a higher incidence of complications, including perforation, bleeding, and obstruction. Diarrhea is frequent, often with steatorrhea. Radiographic findings include giant gastric rugae, duodenal nodularity, ectopic ulcers in the esophagus, lower duodenum, and jejunum, and intestinal hyperperistalsis. Associated endocrine abnormalities consistent with the MEN syndrome are present in over half of patients with the Zollinger-Ellison syndrome and in half of the first-degree relatives of such patients. For this reason the Zollinger-Ellison syndrome is now widely regarded as a component of the MEN I syndrome even when no other endocrine abnormalities are apparent.

Islet-cell tumors may also produce glucagon, vasoactive inhibitory polypeptide (VIP), prostaglandins, adrenocorticotropic hormone (ACTH), parathyroid hormone, antidiuretic hormone (ADH), and serotonin. Glucagonomas cause hyperglycemia, weight loss, stomatitis, and a peculiar skin rash called *necrotizing migratory erythema*. VIP and prostaglandins have been implicated in the watery diarrhea (pancreatic cholera) syndrome sometimes seen in MEN I. Cushing's syndrome may be due to an adrenal adenoma or may occur as a consequence of ACTH production by an islet tumor. Some adrenal adenomas produce aldosterone or adrenal androgens. Involvement of the thyroid gland is uncommon in MEN I, and, when it does occur, the lesion is not specific since goiter, simple adenoma, and thyroiditis have all been reported. Other features of MEN I include small-intestinal and bronchial carcinoid tumors, schwannomas, thymomas, multiple lipomas, inclusion cysts, and cutaneous leiomyomas.

Patients with MEN I may develop symptoms at any age, but the condition is rare in childhood and after the age of 60. Affected individuals may demonstrate multiple endocrine system involvement simultaneously, or months or years may elapse between the discovery of one adenoma and the appearance of the next. Once the diagnosis is established, the patient must be surveyed at yearly intervals for appearance of new facets of the syndrome. By the same token, all first-degree relatives should be studied. A reasonable approach for screening relatives at risk is as follows: (1) review history for symptoms of peptic ulcer disease, hypoglycemia, renal calculi, lipomas, or hypopituitarism; (2) examine for multiple lipomas; (3) assay serum calcium, phosphorus, and gastrin; and (4) x-ray the sella turcica. Upper gastrointestinal series have proved of no value as a screening test.

The fundamental lesion in MEN I is unknown. Some have considered the basic abnormality to be in the islet cells with their extensive capability for hormone synthesis, attributing changes in the other glands to secondary effects of islet hormone hypersecretion. Others have classified MEN I as a neurocrestopathy implicating faulty differentiation or regulation of the embryonic neural crest, which is the anlagen of at least part of the endocrine system. The endocrine components of the neural crest have been classified by Pearse and coworkers into a subsystem of APUD cells, so named because of their capacity for amine precursor uptake and decarboxylation. All such cells can synthesize and secrete peptide hormones. While some components of the endocrine system, notably the thyroid C cell and the adrenal medulla, are undoubtedly derived from neural crest, it is not clear whether the whole spectrum of lesions seen in MEN I arises in cells derived either primarily or secondarily from this tissue.

The pituitary and parathyroid tumors in MEN I are usually benign, but pancreatic and adrenal cortical tumors are frequently malignant. Surgical removal of the affected gland is the usual therapy, although standard irradiation techniques may be employed for the pituitary tumors. Hyperparathyroidism may be due to a single adenoma, but diffuse hyperplasia of more than one gland is more common. Selective venous catheterization with measurement of serum parathyroid hormone levels can be used to differentiate between those possibilities in some centers. Since new adenomas may arise in normal glands left after removal of an adenoma (and since second operations are difficult because of scar formation), some have advocated removal of all the parathyroid glands with transplantation of extirpated fragments into the thigh or forearm, where they can be easily removed should hyperparathyroidism recur. Successful transplantation obviates the need for long-term therapy of hypoparathyroidism. In hypergastrinemia due to islet-cell lesions, total gastrectomy has been used to prevent recurrent peptic ulcers, and in rare cases distant metastases have regressed after this procedure. H_2-receptor antagonists are efficacious in controlling the hyperacidity and diarrhea seen with hypergastrinemia, but this class of drugs is not known to have any intrinsic chemotherapeutic effect.

MULTIPLE ENDOCRINE NEOPLASIA, TYPE II (MEN II) Also known as the *Sipple syndrome,* MEN II consists of pheochromocytoma (frequently bilateral and occasionally extraadrenal), medullary thyroid carcinoma (MTC), and, in about half of the reported cases, parathyroid hyperplasia. MEN II can be related more directly to abnormal neural crest development than can MEN I, since both the adrenal medulla and the parafollicular or C cells of the thyroid originate in neural crest. The parafollicular cell elaborates calcitonin, the primary marker of medullary carcinoma of the thyroid. MTC is not common, comprising only about 7 to 10 percent of all thyroid malignancies. Ten percent of the cases are familial, usually appearing as a component of MEN II or MEN III (see below). Medullary

carcinoma may also occur in families without other associated endocrine dysfunction; this form is also transmitted as an autosomal dominant trait. MTC may present as a thyroidal mass or be clinically silent and undetectable by palpation or radioiodine scanning. The diagnosis is usually established by immunoassay of serum calcitonin, provided ectopic sites of calcitonin production can be excluded, e.g., breast, lung, and pancreatic islet-cell tumors. Occasionally, basal serum calcitonin levels are borderline in at-risk individuals, and measurement of plasma levels after pentagastrin stimulation and/or short-term calcium infusion can be used to establish the diagnosis. MTC may on occasion secrete substances other than calcitonin, including ACTH, prolactin, serotonin, VIP, histamine, and various prostaglandins, resulting in a confusing array of symptoms.

The pheochromocytoma of MEN II may produce the classic signs of catecholamine excess as described in Chap. 337 or be asymptomatic. Approximately 7 percent of patients who present with pheochromocytomas also have MTC.

Symptoms of hyperparathyroidism rarely bring the patient with MEN II to initial clinical attention; indeed, the parathyroid hyperplasia may be secondary to long-standing hypercalcitoninemia. Alternatively, the lesion could be a primary feature of MEN II since hyperparathyroidism occurring in isolation may be asymptomatic for many years. If the latter were true, it would weaken the hypothesis of the neural crest origin of MEN II since parathyroid cells are thought to be derived from branchial arch epithelium during embryologic development. Examination of cells from both the MTC and the pheochromocytoma components of MEN II using X-linked gene markers has led to the conclusion that the inherited defect in the syndrome produces multiple clones of abnormal cells; tumors then develop from a second mutation in the abnormal clone, accounting for the appearance of varying clinical patterns of tumor formation. Other tumors in MEN II include gliomas, glioblastomas, and meningiomas, all of which may be derived from the neural crest.

The age of the patient at the time of detection of the disorder is variable, ranging in one series from 2 to 67 years. C-cell hyperplasia of the thyroid may precede development of frank malignancy by many years, making early screening studies for calcitonin elevation mandatory in all family members at risk. The only effective therapy for MTC is surgical removal of the entire thyroid, as the tumor is probably always multifocal in origin. Limited node dissection is often indicated since the cancer may progress slowly despite an aggressive histological appearance, and prolonged survival is seen in patients with known metastatic disease. Serum calcitonin levels can be used to assess completeness of surgical removal of the tumor and in concert with selective venous catheterization may be utilized to locate distant metastases that are surgically accessible. Neither radioiodine nor x-ray therapy is helpful in disseminated medullary thyroid cancer, but chemotherapy shows some promise. There are rare reports of thyroxine-induced regression of MTC, but these are of questionable significance. The pheochromocytomas are usually benign and are also treated surgically. Unresectable malignant pheochromocytoma requires long-term sympathetic blockade.

MULTIPLE ENDOCRINE NEOPLASIA, TYPE III (MEN III OR IIB)
The third endocrine neoplasia syndrome also consists of medullary thyroid carcinoma and pheochromocytoma, but affected individuals have striking dysmorphic features such as neuromas of the conjunctival, labial, and buccal mucosa, the tongue, the larynx, and the gastrointestinal tract; hence the alternate

designation of the condition as the *mucosal neuroma syndrome*. Other physical findings include enlarged corneal nerves, "blubbery" lips, soft-tissue prognathism, and a habitus resembling that seen in the Marfan syndrome with hypotonia, lax joints, kyphoscoliosis, genu valgus, and pes cavus. The patients may have café au lait spots or a diffuse lentiginous type of skin pigmentation along with cutaneous neuromas or neurofibromas. Megacolon may occur.

Despite the resemblance of MEN III to MEN II, the syndromes appear to be distinct. For example, both parathyroid hyperplasia and production of hormones other than calcitonin by MTC are rare in MEN III. The mean survival of patients with MEN III is around 30 years compared with 60 years for those with MEN II, suggesting a more malignant course in the former disorder, although histologically the thyroid tumors appear to be identical. As with MEN II treatment of the medullary carcinoma is surgical. The unusual physical features of MEN III should immediately suggest the diagnosis of underlying thyroid malignancy. MTC has been documented in asymptomatic children with MEN III, and C-cell hyperplasia has been found at operation as early as 15 months of age. Clinically, the associated pheochromocytomas behave as expected (Chap. 337).

McCUNE-ALBRIGHT SYNDROME This condition is characterized by the triad of polyostotic fibrous dysplasia, café au lait spots, and isosexual precocity, the latter occurring predominantly but not exclusively in females. The isosexual precocity is usually hypothalamic in origin, but a primary gonadal abnormality has been implicated in some cases. Cushing's syndrome and gigantism or acromegaly may also occur in affected patients. The Cushing's syndrome may result from abnormal ACTH production or adrenal adenomas. Nodular toxic goiter and pheochromocytoma have also been reported. The bone lesion resembles that seen in hyperparathyroidism, and parathyroid hyperplasia has been described histologically, although clinical hyperparathyroidism has not been documented. The condition is sporadic, and its cause is unknown (see Chap. 354).

SYNDROMES WITH MULTISYSTEM HYPOFUNCTION

A number of rather diverse conditions can be grouped under this heading. The combination of endocrine hypofunction and immunologic abnormalities occurs in several of the conditions.

POLYGLANDULAR DEFICIENCY SYNDROME (SCHMIDT SYNDROME) (See also Chap. 336) The prototype of a polyglandular deficiency state is the Schmidt syndrome, originally described as the presence of both Addison's disease and lymphocytic thyroiditis in a single patient. This syndrome has subsequently been expanded to include failure of any combination of endocrine organs including adrenal insufficiency, lymphocytic thyroiditis, hypoparathyroidism, and gonadal failure. Diabetes mellitus is a frequent accompaniment. The manifestations may be so extensive as to simulate panhypopituitarism; rarely, true pituitary deficiency has been described. The first evidence of endocrinopathy generally appears in adult life. The most significant laboratory feature, in addition to the low levels of circulating hormones, is the presence of antibodies to one or more endocrine glands. The antibodies may be directed against a clinically normal gland, but with time hypofunction usually supervenes. Additional evidence for an immune pathogenesis is provided by the increased frequency of antibodies to parietal cells, with or without overt achlorhydria or pernicious anemia, and the presence of other disorders felt to have an autoimmune basis such as sprue, vitiligo, myasthenia gravis, and antibody-mediated IgA deficiency. Hyperthyroidism may complicate the clinical picture.

The majority of affected individuals are female, and most cases are sporadic. A few reports have noted multiple affected family members, indicating that the disorder may occur on a genetic basis. Members of these families who show no endocrine disability frequently have serologic abnormalities indicative of a disturbance in immune function. Many of the component endocrine disorders seen in this syndrome have been shown to be associated with the presence of certain HLA antigens, notably HLA-B8 and -Dw3 (in white populations). Other racial groups show different associations, e.g., hyperthyroidism with HLA-Bw35 in the Japanese. The genes coding for these antigens are inherited as autosomal codominant alleles, and it has been speculated that in certain families some abnormality related to specific HLA antigens predisposes selected individuals to autoimmune disease. Since the HLA region in humans may be linked to the so-called "immune response" (Ir) genes that have been demonstrated in lower animals, it has been postulated that the basic lesion in the Schmidt syndrome resides in a mutational alteration of an inherited immunologic mechanism. For example, a selective immunodeficient state might render an individual unduly susceptible to certain environmental antigens (e.g., viruses) that have a predilection for the endocrine system. Cell lysis or damage could result in release of intracellular contents and lead to development of autoantibodies. Such autoantibodies would not necessarily be pathogenic but could represent epiphenomena whose importance would be as markers of potential clinical disease. Alternatively the defect could reside in a genetically determined defect with inadequate suppression of antibody synthesis by T cells. It is likely that the syndrome is etiologically heterogeneous and that several pathogenetic mechanisms are operative. At present, treatment is confined to providing hormone replacement.

CANDIDIASIS-ENDOCRINOPATHY SYNDROME An autoimmune pathogenesis has also been invoked in the candidiasis-endocrinopathy syndrome. Features that differentiate this condition from the Schmidt syndrome include the childhood onset of the disease and the extensive mucocutaneous monilial infection that becomes evident shortly after birth. Hypoparathyroidism is common, and adrenal insufficiency may develop acutely. Organ-specific antibodies against a variety of endocrine glands may be evident early, and both pernicious anemia and sprue may be present. Defective cellular immunity to *Candida albicans* has been demonstrated in virtually all affected patients; some have more generalized anergy. A cause-and-effect relationship between the monilial infection and the endocrinopathy has not been demonstrated. The disorder has occurred in sibs, occasionally from consanguineous unions, and it is possible that the disease is inherited as an autosomal recessive trait. No association with the HLA system has been demonstrated, but affected individuals have a deficiency of immunoglobulin A and hypergammaglobulinemia. Suppressor T-cell function is defective. The fungal infection is refractory to conventional chemotherapeutic drugs, although partial remission has been reported with a combination of antifungal agents and transfer factor. Amelioration of the candidiasis in no way affects the endocrinopathy, and conventional replacement therapy is required. Whether the Schmidt syndrome and the candidiasis-endocrinopathy complex represent different diseases is conjectural.

LIPODYSTROPHIC SYNDROMES The lipodystrophic syndromes are described in Chap. 102. Insulin-resistant diabetes mellitus is common and may be associated with elevated growth hormone levels and with an increased incidence of polycystic disease of the ovaries, acromegaly, and Cushing's disease.

DIABETES MELLITUS, DIABETES INSIPIDUS, AND OPTIC ATROPHY This clinical triad has been noted in sibs and likely constitutes a rare autosomal recessive defect. Nerve deafness, usually mild, may also occur. The diabetes mellitus is of the early-onset insulin-dependent type. The diabetes insipidus usually appears prior to age 20. The frequency of the syndrome is uncertain. The varying manifestations of the condition are difficult to reconcile from an etiologic point of view, and treatment requires replacement of the missing hormones.

OBESITY-HYPOGONADISM SYNDROMES A number of seemingly discrete entities share obesity, generally with frank diabetes mellitus, and hypogonadism that may be either primary or secondary. The *Laurence-Moon-Biedl-Bardet syndrome* features retinitis pigmentosa, polydactyly, mental retardation, and renal anomalies along with obesity and hypogonadotropic hypogonadism. Diabetes mellitus has been reported in some patients. There is sufficient resemblance between this syn-

drome and the *Alström syndrome* (retinitis pigmentosa, nerve deafness, diabetes mellitus, and primary gonadal failure) to cause frequent diagnostic confusion. Both are autosomal recessive disorders. However, polydactyly and mental retardation do not occur in the Alström syndrome. A similar condition is the *Biemond syndrome* in which obesity, diabetes mellitus, secondary hypogonadism, and postaxial polydactyly are combined with iris colobomata rather than pigmentary retinopathy. Patients with the *Prader-Willi syndrome* (obesity, hypogonadism, hypotonia, mental retardation) also have diabetes mellitus of the maturity-onset type. In neither the Biemond nor the Prader-Willi syndrome have the genetics been established.

CHROMOSOMAL DISORDERS WITH ENDOCRINE DEFICIENCY (See also Chaps. 60 and 344) In addition to hypogonadism, patients with Turner syndrome have an increased incidence of diabetes mellitus and of thyroiditis thought to be on an auto-

TABLE 348-1
Disorders with potential polyglandular manifestations

Condition	Clinical feature	Type of endocrine involvement						Inheritance
		Hypothalamic-pituitary	Thyroid	Parathyroid	Pancreas	Adrenal		
Ataxia telangiectasia	Early ataxia Oculocutaneous telangiectasia Immunologic deficiency	?Variably decreased pituitary reserve			Diabetes	Cortical hypoplasia	Dysgenetic ovaries Gonadoblastomas later	Autosomal recessive
Pseudohypoparathyroidism	Short stature Short metacarpals and metatarsals Round facies Ectopic calcification	Variable deficiency of all pituitary hormones Prolactin deficiency	Hypo- or hyperthyroidism	Elevated parathyroid hormone levels with either normo- or hypocalcemia	Diabetes		Ovarian failure	Probable X-linked dominant
Myotonic dystrophy	Muscular dystrophy Premature baldness Mental retardation	Gonadotropin, growth hormone abnormalities, related to central integrative defect (?)	Hypothyroidism		Diabetes		Primary failure	Autosomal dominant
Noonan syndrome	Short stature Ptosis Webbed neck Pulmonary stenosis	Gonadotropin deficiency	Thyroiditis				Primary failure	Autosomal dominant
Fanconi syndrome	Short stature Bone marrow hypoplasia Abnormal skin pigmentation Radius malformations	Panhypopituitarism			Diabetes	Adrenal atrophy	Gonadal atrophy	Autosomal recessive
Werner syndrome	Premature aging of all organ systems Atrophic skin Cataracts Early osteoporosis		Papillary carcinoma		Diabetes		Gonadal atrophy	Autosomal recessive

immune basis. In the Klinefelter syndrome an increased frequency of diabetes mellitus may occur in addition to gonadal failure. In the Down syndrome hypogonadism is probably universal in males, and menstrual irregularities and early menopause are common in women; in addition, increased prevalences of Hashimoto's thyroiditis and diabetes mellitus have been reported.

OTHER CONDITIONS WITH MULTISYSTEM MANIFESTATIONS
There are a number of other rare conditions in which involvement of more than one endocrine gland has been recorded often enough to constitute a significant facet of the syndrome. Some, like neurofibromatosis (von Recklinghausen's disease) and tuberous sclerosis, may show either hypo- or hyperfunction of endocrine glands because of interference with central regulatory mechanisms caused by the brain tumors characteristic of the diseases. By the same token, pheochromocytomas not surprisingly occur in neurofibromatosis because the adrenal medulla is derived from the same embryonic source.

Table 348-1 lists a few of the conditions in which disorders of multiple endocrine systems have been seen. It is noteworthy that both primary and secondary failures have been reported within the diagnostic confines of the same syndrome. For example, both gonadotropin deficiency and primary testicular atrophy have been documented in patients with the Noonan syndrome (see Chap. 104) even within the same family. It is also apparent that whenever a clinical condition like diabetes mellitus occurs in such distinct entities as myotonic dystrophy and ataxia-telangiectasia, the molecular mechanisms underlying the disease may be heterogeneous. A better understanding of the genetic defect would provide insight into the development and function of the endocrine system.

REFERENCES

ARULANTHAM K et al: Evidence for defective immunoregulation in the syndrome of familial candidiasis endocrinopathy. N Engl J Med 300:164, 1979

EISENBARTH G et al: HLA type and occurrence of disease in familial polyglandular failure. N Engl J Med 298:92, 1978

IRVINE WJ: Autoimmunity in diabetes and other endocrine disorders. Recent Prog Horm Res, 1979 (in press)

PEARSE AGE, POLAK JM: Neural crest origin of the endocrine polypeptide (APUD) cells of the gastrointestinal tract and pancreas. Gut 12:783, 1971

RIMOIN DL: Genetic syndromes associated with glucose intolerance, in The Genetics of Diabetes Mellitus, W Creutzfeldt et al (eds). New York, Springer, 1976

——, SCHIMKE RN: Genetic Disorders of the Endocrine Glands. St Louis, Mosby, 1971

SCHIMKE RN: The multiple endocrine adenoma syndromes. Adv Intern Med 21:294, 1975

——: Syndromes with multiple endocrine gland involvement. Prog Med Genet, 1978 (in press)

---

section 11 | Disorders of bone and bone mineral metabolism

349

SKELETAL REMODELING AND FACTORS INFLUENCING BONE AND BONE MINERAL METABOLISM

STEPHEN M. KRANE
JOHN T. POTTS, JR.

BONE STRUCTURE AND METABOLISM (See also Chap. 352)
Bone is a dynamic tissue, constantly remodeling itself throughout life. The skeleton is highly vascular and receives about 10 percent of the cardiac output. The skeleton has extraordinary mechanical functions that are suited to the requirements for mobility for vertebrates. The particular arrangement of compact and cancellous bone provides a combination of strength and density ideal for these mechanical functions. In addition, bone provides a store of calcium, magnesium, phosphorus, sodium, and other ions necessary for the support of a variety of homeostatic functions.

In the following chapters a number of disorders will be discussed in which the metabolism of cartilage, bone, and mineral ions is affected. A brief review of skeletal remodeling, the metabolism of mineral ions, and the major factors which influence mineral metabolism is, therefore, pertinent.

The properties of bone as a tissue are a function of the particular organization of its extracellular components. Its structure consists of a solid mineral phase in close association with an organic matrix, consisting of 90 to 95 percent collagen, small amounts of proteoglycans, and some noncollagenous proteins including proteins containing γ-carboxyglutamic acid. The mineral phase is composed of hydroxyapatite [empiric formula $Ca_{10}(PO_4)_6(OH)_2$] of small crystal size and poor crystallinity and so-called "amorphous" calcium phosphate with a lower molar calcium/phosphorus ratio than that of hydroxyapatite. In addition, other ions are present, predominantly in the surface layers. The mineral phase of bone is deposited in intimate relation to the collagen fibrils and is found largely in specific locations within the "holes" of the collagen fibrils which result from the particular manner in which the collagen molecules are packed. This architectural organization of mineral and matrix results in a two-phase material uniquely suited to withstand mechanical stresses. The formation as well as the localization of the inorganic phase is probably determined at least in part by the organic matrix, particularly the collagen.

Bone is formed by cells of mesenchymal origin which synthesize and secrete the organic matrix. Mineralization of the matrix, particularly in *osteons* (haversian systems), begins soon after secretion (primary mineralization) but is not completed until after several weeks (secondary mineralization). As an *osteoblast* secretes matrix which is then mineralized, this cell becomes surrounded by matrix and becomes an *osteocyte*, still connected with its blood supply through a series of canaliculi. Resorption of bone is carried out by cells which include mononuclear cells as well as multinucleated *osteoclasts*, the latter characterized by their elaborately infolded border adjacent to the bone and their location in scalloped resorption spaces (Howship's lacunae) (Fig. 349-1). Some resorption of bone may also take place around the osteocytes. The cells of bone are probably derived from precursor cells in the bone marrow. A hematopoietic stem cell is the likely precursor of the osteoclast, whereas a stromal stem cell is the likely precursor of the osteoblast. It is unlikely that there is transformation between these two cell types or their precursors under physiological or pathological conditions.

In the embryo and in the growing child, bone develops either by remodeling and replacing previously calcified cartilage (endochondral bone formation), or it is formed without a cartilage matrix (intramembranous bone formation). The young new bone, especially in embryos and infants and that newly formed in adults during repair, has a relatively high ratio of cells to matrix and is characterized by coarse fiber bundles of collagen which are interlaced and randomly dispersed (woven bone). In adults, the more mature bone is organized with fiber bundles regularly arranged in parallel or concentric sheets (lamellar bone). In long bones, the lamellar bone is deposited in a highly ordered concentric arrangement around blood vessels along their length and forms the haversian systems. Growth in length of bones is dependent upon proliferation of cartilage cells and the endochondral sequence at the growth plate. Growth in width and thickness is accomplished by formation of bone at the periosteal surface and resorption at the endosteal surface with the rate of formation exceeding that of resorption. In adults, after the epiphyses close, growth in length and endochondral bone formation cease, except for some activity in the cartilage cells beneath the articular surface. However, even in adults, remodeling of bone (remodeling of haversian systems as well as trabecular bone) is a continuous process through life, as can be shown by microradiographic studies utilizing radioisotopes or fluorescence of tetracyclines fixed in bone in regions of new mineralization. Newly forming surfaces are characterized by smooth character, uptake of tetracycline, and relatively low mineral density. Actively forming surfaces are covered by active osteoblasts. The osteoid seam which results from the relative lag in mineralization of the newly formed organic matrix is normally no greater than about 12 μm. An index of the rate of bone formation can be obtained by examination of undermineralized sections of bone biopsies obtained from individuals who have received tetracycline for two periods separated by a drug-free interval. The distance between the fluorescent bands on the sections reflects the new bone formed. Resorption areas are characterized by their irregular configurations and the presence of osteoclasts (Fig. 349-1). Resorption precedes formation and is more intense, but it does not persist as long as formation. In adult humans, approximately 10 percent of the surface of bone (such as iliac crest) is involved in active formation and resorption. Kinetic studies using isotopes such as radioactive calcium (^{47}Ca) provide estimates that as much as 18 percent of the total skeletal calcium may be deposited and removed each year. Thus bone is an active metabolizing tissue, with its cells dependent upon an intact blood supply. Throughout life bone is constantly being remodeled in a manner which is somehow related to the continuous mechanical stresses to which it is subjected. Bone also serves as an important reservoir of mineral ions, particularly calcium, which are critical for a variety of processes in other tissues.

The response of bone to injuries such as fractures, infection, interruption of blood supply, and the presence of expanding lesions is relatively limited. Dead bone must be resorbed and new bone formed, a process which normally is carried out in association with new blood vessels growing into the involved area. In injuries that are severely disruptive to the organization of the tissue, such as a fracture in which apposition of fragments is poor and motion exists at the fracture site, the osteo-

progenitor cells differentiate into cells with functional capacities other than those of osteoblasts, and repair is accompanied by formation of varying amounts of fibrous tissue and cartilage. In instances in which there is good apposition with fixation and little motion at the fracture site, repair occurs predominantly by bone without other scar tissue. Remodeling of this bone is subsequently accomplished along lines of force determined by mechanical stresses that are somehow translated into biologic response.

Expanding lesions in bone, such as tumors, tend to induce resorption at the surface in contact with the tumor and formation at the outer circumference. A bowing deformity tends to result in increased new bone formation at the concave surface and resorption at the convex surface, all seemingly designed to produce the strongest mechanical structure. Even in a disorder as architecturally disruptive as Paget's disease of bone, remodeling appears to be dictated by mechanical forces. Thus the biologic plasticity of bone is due to the response of cells interacting with each other and the environment.

Mechanisms of bone formation and resorption   Bone formation is an orderly process in which inorganic mineral is deposited in relation to an organic matrix. The mineral phase is composed of calcium and phosphorus, and, therefore, the concentration of these ions in the plasma and extracellular fluid influences the rate at which the mineral phase is formed. In vitro, mineralization can proceed, and crystals of hydroxyapatite can grow at concentrations of calcium and phosphorus similar to those in an ultrafiltrate of plasma. However, the concentration of these ions at the sites of mineralization is unknown, and it is

FIGURE 349-1

Schematic representation of bone remodeling surfaces in trabecular bone. Most bone surfaces in adults are involved in neither formation nor resorption. Such surfaces are usually smooth, have no osteoid seam, and are covered either by no visible cells or by flattened cells. Active formation surfaces are smooth and covered by osteoblasts which have an osteoid seam (clear), normally no thicker than 12 μm. The calcification front is located at the junction of the osteoid seam and mineralized bone (stippled). Inactive forming surfaces are not covered by osteoblasts but by only a few flattened cells. Active resorbing surfaces are irregular or scalloped and contain multinucleated osteoclasts. The latter are not seen on inactive resorbing surfaces.

possible that the cells involved (osteoblasts, osteocytes) somehow regulate the local concentration of calcium, phosphorus, and other ions. Collagens from a variety of sources can catalyze the nucleation of a mineral phase of calcium and phosphorus from solutions of these ions, and the initial mineral phase is deposited in specific locations in the holes produced by the particular packing arrangement of the collagen molecules. It is likely that the organization of collagen influences the amount and type of mineral phase that is formed. The collagen of bone is similar in its primary structure to that of skin [contains two $\alpha_1(I)$ chains and one α_2 chain] but differs in hydroxylation, glycosylation, and the type, number, and distribution of intermolecular cross-links. In addition, the "holes" in the packing structure of the collagen are larger in normally mineralized collagen of bone and dentin than those of a normally unmineralized collagen such as tendon. Other noncollagenous organic components such as glycoproteins, some of which contain γ-carboxyglutamic acid, may also play a role in the formation and localization of the mineral phase of bone. To explain how collagens from tissues that are normally not mineralized can catalyze nucleation of an inorganic phase from solutions similar to normal extracellular fluid, regulation of mineralization by inhibitory substances has been suggested. Inorganic pyrophosphate is a potent inhibitor of mineralization at concentrations several orders of magnitude below those necessary to bind calcium ions. Since alkaline phosphatase, present in osteoblasts and other cells, can catalyze the hydrolysis of inorganic pyrophosphate at neutral pH, this enzyme could play a role in the regulation of mineralization by controlling the concentrations of pyrophosphate. In addition, macromolecular inhibitors such as the protein polysaccharides may also influence the rate and extent of mineralization. In cartilage undergoing calcification, membrane-bound vesicles containing mineral have been identified outside the cells, and it has been suggested that this is the initial mineral phase.

In bone, the initial mineral phase is probably the "amorphous" solid with a relatively low molar calcium/phosphorus ratio of about 3:2. With maturation, part of the "amorphous" phase is converted to a poorly crystalline hydroxyapatite. However, even mature bone from old animals still contains considerable amounts of the amorphous calcium phosphate. Fluoride ions, when incorporated into the mineral phase, tend to decrease the proportion of amorphous calcium phosphate and increase crystallinity.

There is a limit for the concentration of calcium and phosphorus ions in the extracellular fluid below which the mineral phase will not be formed. A "solubility product" for bone mineral is difficult to calculate since the mineral phase itself is of variable composition and the true nature of species in solution governing this solubility product is not known. Nevertheless when the concentrations of calcium and phosphorus, particularly the latter, in extracellular fluid are excessive, a mineral phase may be formed in areas that are not normally mineralized.

When bone is resorbed, calcium and phosphorus ions from the solid phase are released into solution in the extracellular fluid, and subsequently the organic matrix is also resorbed. It is not entirely clear how these processes occur. A decrease in pH, the presence of a chelating substance, and the operation of a cellular pump mechanism to shift the equilibrium between solids and solution are possibilities to explain mineral release. Resorption occurs at specific sites either adjacent to osteoclasts or surrounding osteocytes and requires normal metabolism of these cells. Osteoclasts are rich in acid phosphatase, a convenient marker for these cells, but the function of this enzyme in mineralization is not known. Whereas the activity of alkaline phosphatase, an enzyme found in osteoblasts, may be increased in serum when osteoblast number or function is increased, no such spillover from acid phosphatase is observed. The matrix is resorbed presumably through the action of collagenases released from the resorbing cells; these enzymes attack collagen in a specific manner but are incapable of degrading the protein before the mineral phase is removed. The rate at which resorption occurs is stimulated by parathyroid hormone as well as by other substances such as heparin, prostaglandins of the E series, and protein factor(s) derived from lymphocytes (osteoclast-activating factor). The effect of the hormones is discussed in more detail later.

CALCIUM METABOLISM Before considering the effects of hormones and vitamin D, a brief summary of calcium and phosphorus homeostasis in humans is indicated.

There is about 1 to 2 kg calcium in the average adult human body, of which over 98 percent is in the skeleton. The calcium of the mineral phase at the surface of the crystals is in equilibrium with ions of the extracellular fluid, but only a minor proportion of the total calcium (about 0.5 percent) is exchangeable as determined by isotope dilution techniques. Although the calcium in the extracellular fluid is only a small fraction of the total, its concentration is critical for a variety of functions, and it is kept remarkably constant. In plasma, in normal adults, the range of concentration is 8.8 to 10.4 mg per 100 ml (2.2 to 2.6 mM). The calcium in plasma is in three forms: as free ions, bound to plasma proteins, and, to a small extent, as diffusible complexes. The concentration of free calcium ions is of critical importance in regulating the level of neuromuscular irritability as well as a variety of other cellular functions and is subjected to exquisite hormonal control, especially through parathyroid hormone, as described below. The concentration of serum proteins is an important factor in prediction of the concentration of calcium ions; most of the protein binding is to albumin. One formula that approximates the amount of calcium bound to proteins is:

$$\% \text{ protein-bound Ca} = 8 \times \text{albumin (g/100 ml)} \\ + 2 \times \text{globulin (g/100 ml)} + 3$$

Another correction is simply to subtract 1 mg per 100 ml from the serum calcium concentration for every 1.0 g per 100 ml serum albumin lower than 4.0 g per 100 ml. Thus the concentration of ultrafiltrable calcium is usually about 50 percent of the total calcium. In most laboratories only total calcium is determined, and therefore knowledge of the concentration of proteins is essential to estimate concentration of calcium ions. The introduction of calcium-specific electrodes may eventually make it possible to measure free ions directly as a practical routine procedure.

Decrease in the concentration of free calcium ions in plasma results in increased neuromuscular irritability and the syndrome of tetany. This syndrome is characterized, when fully expressed, by peripheral and perioral paresthesias, carpal spasm, pedal spasm, anxiety, seizures, bronchospasm, laryngospasm, Chvostek's, Trousseau's, and Erb's signs, and lengthening of the QT interval of the electrocardiogram. In infants tetany may be manifested only by irritability and lethargy. The level of calcium ions that determines which features of tetany will be manifested is variable in different individuals. The occurrence of tetany is also influenced by the concentration of other components of the extracellular fluid. For example, hypomagnesemia and alkalosis lower the threshold for tetany, whereas hypokalemia and acidosis raise the threshold.

Increases in total serum calcium are, as a rule, accompanied by increases in calcium ions and may be associated with a variety of symptoms and signs including anorexia, nausea, vomiting, constipation, some degree of hypotonia, depression, and occasionally lethargy and coma. Persistent hypercalcemia, especially when accompanied by normal or elevated levels of serum phosphate, may eventually result in deposition of a solid mineral phase of calcium and phosphate in abnormal sites such as walls of blood vessels, connective tissue about the joints, gastric mucosa, cornea, and renal parenchyma. Hypercalcemia per se alters renal function in addition to the pathological effects of calcium-phosphate deposits in the lumen of renal tubules and in the interstitial areas of the kidney.

The concentration of calcium ions in the extracellular fluid is kept constant by the interaction of a number of processes which constantly feed calcium into and withdraw calcium from the extracellular fluid. Calcium enters the plasma via absorption from the intestinal tract and by resorption of ions from the bone mineral. Calcium leaves the extracellular fluid via secretion into the gastrointestinal tract, urinary excretion, deposition in bone mineral, and, to a minor extent, via losses in sweat. Resorption and formation are usually tightly coupled, approximately 500 mg calcium entering and leaving the skeleton daily (Fig. 349-2).

The average diet in the United States provides about 600 to 1000 mg calcium daily, mostly in the form of dairy products. However considerably less than half of the calcium in the diet is absorbed in adults. The percentage of calcium absorbed increases during periods of rapid growth in children, in pregnancy, and in lactation, and decreases with advancing age. If adequate vitamin D is available, a greater percentage of dietary calcium is absorbed (adaptation). Most of the calcium is absorbed in the proximal small intestine, and the efficiency of absorption decreases in the more distal intestinal segments. Both active transport and diffusion-limited absorptive processes are involved; the former is more important in the upper and the latter in the lower intestine. Both are influenced by vitamin D and its metabolites. Adequate calcium absorption requires the availability of a functioning surface. It is possible that all forms of calcium in the diet are not equally absorbed; even with defined salts, calcium as the chloride is probably absorbed more efficiently than that in other preparations.

Calcium is also secreted into the lumen of the gastrointestinal tract. When isotopes of radioactive calcium are administered intravenously, radioactivity appears in the feces, leading to calculations of *endogenous fecal calcium* of about 60 to 130 mg per day. Even higher estimates of calcium losses in intestinal juices have been made by other approaches. It is generally agreed, however, that no control of calcium balance is exerted by regulation of intestinal calcium secretion. On the other hand, if calcium availability in the diet is low (less than 500 mg per day), positive calcium balance requires an efficiency of absorption greater than 30 to 40 percent if intestinal uptake is to be sufficient to exceed losses via intestinal secretion and to match calcium losses that occur through renal calcium excretion.

The urinary calcium excretion of normal adults on average calcium intakes ranges between a minimum of 100 mg per day to as high as 300 to 400 mg per day. When the dietary calcium is reduced to below 200 mg daily, urinary calcium excretion is usually less than 200 mg per day. However, in most normal individuals the level of dietary intake over a wide range has relatively little effect on the urinary excretion of calcium. Hence in individuals on diets low in calcium, this relative inefficiency of renal calcium conservation leads to negative calcium balance unless calcium absorption is maximally efficient (Fig. 349-2). Calculations of calcium clearance have been reported based on estimation of calcium concentration obtained by ultrafiltration methods. Ratios of calcium to creatinine clearance are thus calculated to be less than 0.05. However, the amount of calcium excreted in the urine is minute compared with that filtered through the glomerulus (about 7 to 8 g per day); it is not certain whether some non-protein bound, nonionic forms of calcium (e.g., calcium citrate) are cleared at rates considerably greater than others. The excretion of other electrolytes also affects the urinary excretion of calcium. For example, calciuresis is usually proportional to natriuresis; other ions, such as sulfate, also increase calcium excretion.

Overall, maintenance of calcium balance (Fig. 349-2) is critically dependent upon hormonally supported efficiency of intestinal absorption. Deficiency of parathyroid hormone or vitamin D, intestinal disease, or severe dietary calcium deprivation may provide challenges to calcium homeostasis that cannot be compensated for adequately by renal calcium conservation, resulting in negative calcium balance. Increased bone resorption may protect against extracellular fluid calcium depletion and symptomatic hypocalcemia even in states of chronic negative calcium balance but only at the expense of progressive osteopenia.

PHOSPHORUS METABOLISM Phosphorus is not only a major component of the mineral phase of bone but is among the most abundant constituents of all tissues and in some form is involved in almost all metabolic processes. The total amount of phosphorus in the normal adult is about 1000 g, of which about 85 percent is in the skeleton.

FIGURE 349-2
Schematic illustration of calcium content of extracellular fluid (ECF) and bone as well as of diet and feces; magnitude of calcium flux per day as calculated by various methods is shown at sites of transport in intestine, kidney, and bone. Ranges of values shown are approximate and chosen to illustrate certain points discussed in text. In intestine, absorption efficiency varies inversely with dietary calcium (chronic adaptation). This is reflected in typical quantities absorbed and excreted in feces; with 0.5-g intake, 50 percent absorption is depicted to occur (0.25 g), but at 1.5 g only 30 percent (0.5 g). Fecal calcium as a percentage of intake can be as high at low intakes as at high intakes because of the greater significance in the former of the contribution from endogenous fecal calcium, the 0.1 to 0.2 g secreted into the intestinal lumen daily independent of intake. Quantities of calcium depicted as filtered, reabsorbed, and excreted at the kidney are chosen arbitrarily to indicate that at lower rates of filtration of calcium (expected at lower calcium intakes), most is reabsorbed (4.9 of 5 g), leading to urinary excretion of 150 mg; at higher rates of filtration (at high dietary calcium intake), slightly less is reabsorbed (6.7 of 7 g), leading to a higher urinary excretion, 300 mg. In all situations, renal calcium reabsorption exceeds 95 percent of filtered load. Urinary calcium excretion is seen, therefore, to increase by only 150 mg despite a 1-g increase in dietary intake. In conditions of calcium balance, rates of calcium release from and uptake into bone are equal.

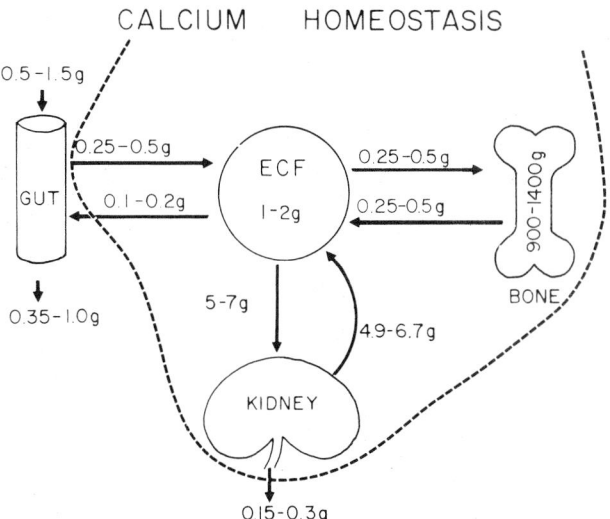

CALCIUM HOMEOSTASIS

In normal human plasma most of the phosphorus is present as inorganic orthophosphate in concentrations which range in the fasting state from 2.8 to 4.0 mg (P) per 100 ml. In contrast to calcium, where about 50 percent is bound, only about 12 percent of the phosphorus in plasma is bound to proteins. Free HPO_4^{2-} and $NaHPO_4^-$ normally are about 75 percent of the total plasma phosphorus, and free $H_2PO_4^-$ is 10 percent. Since so many species are present, depending upon pH and other factors, it has been the convention to express concentrations in terms of mass of elemental phosphorus, i.e., milligrams phosphorus per 100 ml. Total phosphorus levels are higher in children and tend to rise in women after the menopause. There is a diurnal variation of phosphorus concentration even in conditions of a 24-h fast, perhaps mediated by the adrenal cortex. Ingestion of carbohydrate depresses serum phosphorus acutely by as much as 1.0 to 1.5 mg per 100 ml, presumably by cellular uptake and formation of phosphate esters. Ingestion of phosphorus per se increases serum levels. Therefore, it is essential for the interpretation of serum levels and urinary clearances that samples be obtained in the fasting state. Decreases in plasma phosphorus also occur during induction of alkalosis.

No definite symptoms result from hyperphosphatemia. However, when high levels are maintained for long periods, the driving force for mineralization is increased, and calcium phosphate deposits may occur in abnormal sites as discussed earlier. Severe hypophosphatemia, when acute, may be unaccompanied by symptoms. Persistent hypophosphatemia may be associated with a syndrome consisting of varying degrees of anorexia, dizziness, bone pain, proximal muscular weakness, and waddling gait. In severe hypophosphatemia (which in alcoholics may be aggravated, after hospitalization, by administration of nutrients), sharp elevations in serum creatine phosphokinase (CPK) suggest that rhabdomyolysis may be superimposed on myopathy. This sequence of events also occurs in experimental phosphate depletion in animals. The bone pain and waddling gait are attributed to the osteomalacia which develops as a result of phosphate depletion. The muscular weakness may be due either to direct effects of hypophosphatemia on nerves and muscle or, in some instances, to the effects of hyperparathyroidism (either primary or secondary) which may have a role in the etiology of the hypophosphatemia. Defective growth in children may also be due to phosphate depletion. Hypophosphatemia results in decreased levels of 2,3-diphosphoglyceric acid and adenosine triphosphate (ATP) in erythrocytes which in turn alter the dissociation of oxyhemoglobin so that less oxygen is delivered in the periphery. Hemolytic anemia may also be produced by the effects of decreased ATP on the ability of erythrocytes to deform in small peripheral vessels. Severe congestive cardiomyopathy has been noted with chronic hypophosphatemia; restoration of phosphorus deficits leads to prompt reversal of the abnormalities.

Whereas only a small proportion of dietary calcium is absorbed from the intestine, phosphorus absorption is remarkably efficient. At low levels of dietary intake (less than 2 mg/kg per day) 80 to 90 percent of ingested phosphorus is absorbed. Even with the higher levels of intake (greater than 10 mg/kg per day) usually encountered in average diets in the form of dairy products, cereals, eggs, and meat, absorption is about 70 percent. Hypophosphatemia due to deficient intestinal absorption is rarely encountered except in situations where excessive quantities of nonabsorbable antacids are consumed; the antacids bind phosphorus and prevent absorption from the intestinal lumen.

The major control of phosphorus economy is exerted at the level of the kidney. Phosphorus filtered through the glomerulus is largely reabsorbed in the proximal tubule (there is homeostatically important distal reabsorption as well) so that normally only about 10 to 15 percent of the filtered load is excreted. When filtered loads of phosphorus decrease, proximal tubular reabsorption increases. Conversely when phosphorus loads are increased, tubular reabsorption decreases and clearance rises. Thus the urinary excretion of phosphorus normally reflects dietary intake, and conservation or elimination of excessive amounts of the ion depends upon adequate renal handling (Fig. 349-3). There is no good evidence of renal tubular phosphate secretion. Proximal reabsorption of phosphorus is dependent upon parallel sodium reabsorption, but whereas the sodium rejected by the proximal tubule may be reabsorbed distally, the rejected phosphorus is not. Therefore the effects of volume expansion and decreased sodium reabsorption are to increase phosphorus clearance; similarly diuretics such as acetazolamide, which act proximally, are phosphaturic parallel to the degree to which they are natriuretic.

In contrast to critical features of calcium metabolism as discussed above, negative phosphorus balance (Fig. 349-3) is

FIGURE 349-3

Schematic illustration of inorganic phosphorus content (termed here phosphate) in extracellular fluid (ECF) and bone as well as diet and feces; magnitude of phosphorus flux per day as estimated by various methods is shown at transport sites in intestine, kidney, and bone. Range of values shown illustrates special features of phosphorus metabolism discussed in text. Intestinal phosphorus absorption is highly efficient, 85 percent at a lower intake (0.5 g of a 0.6-g intake) and 70 percent at a higher intake (1.4 g of a 2.0-g intake). Estimates of magnitude of endogenous fecal phosphate are less well established than for calcium. Contribution of at least 0.15 g is estimated to be added to the nonabsorbed phosphorus to provide a total of 0.2 g fecal phosphorus at the low intake level. At high phosphorus dietary intakes, no correction for endogenous fecal phosphate is calculated. Higher quantities of phosphorus are excreted in urine at all levels of dietary intake than for corresponding intakes of calcium; quantities excreted match closely the quantities absorbed, thereby maintaining phosphorus balance (no correction in this illustration is made for endogenous fecal phosphorus). Note that renal phosphorus reabsorption, in contrast to high and relatively invariant renal calcium reabsorption, varies from a low of 75 percent of filtered load to greater than 85 percent. The compartment labeled ICF refers to intracellular phosphorus, both organic and inorganic; rapid shifts of phosphorus into cells (and corresponding, possibly slower, efflux of phosphorus from cells) contribute to changes in ECF phosphorus. These shifts between ECF and ICF and phosphorus release from and uptake by bone are equal in conditions of phosphorus balance.

PHOSPHATE HOMEOSTASIS

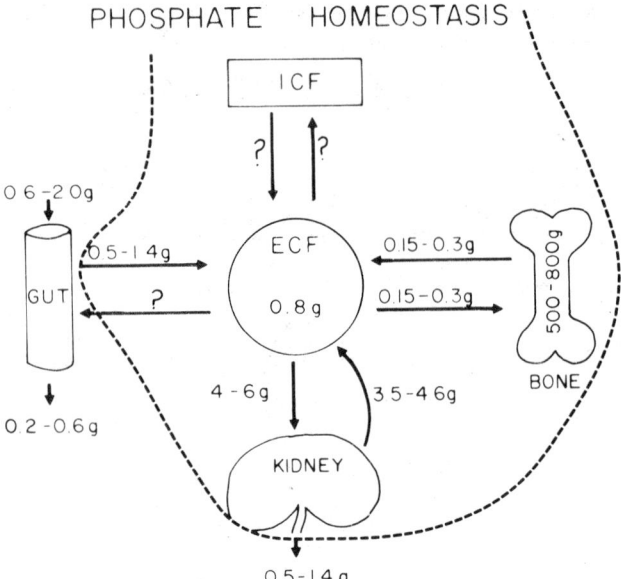

rarely caused by inadequate phosphorus absorption in the intestine and maintenance of normal phosphorus balance is dependent upon efficiency of renal excretion or conservation of phosphorus. In severe renal failure, hyperphosphatemia results from inadequate renal phosphorus clearance; heritable or acquired renal tubular insufficiency may lead to hypophosphatemia due to inadequate renal conservation of phosphorus.

PARATHYROID HORMONE (See also Chap. 350) The physiological function of parathyroid hormone is to maintain extracellular fluid calcium concentration. The hormone acts on bone and kidney directly and indirectly through its effects on synthesis of $1\alpha,25$-dihydroxyvitamin D_3 [$1\alpha,25$-$(OH)_2D_3$] on intestine to increase serum calcium; in turn, parathyroid hormone production is closely regulated by serum calcium concentration. This feedback system involving the parathyroids is one of the most important homeostatic mechanisms for the close regulation of extracellular fluid calcium concentration. Any tendency toward hypocalcemia, as might be induced by calcium-deficient diets, is counteracted by an increased rate of secretion of parathyroid hormone. This in turn (1) acts to increase the rate of dissolution of bone mineral, thereby providing an increased flow of calcium from bone into blood, (2) reduces the renal clearance of calcium, returning more of the calcium filtered at the glomerulus into extracellular fluid, and (3) increases the efficiency of calcium absorption in the intestine. The relative physiological importance of these three actions of parathyroid hormone, stimulation of calcium transport in bone, kidney, and intestine, is not definitely resolved. Most evidence suggests that rapid changes in blood calcium are due to effects of the hormone on bone and, to a lesser extent, on renal calcium clearance; maintenance of calcium balance, on the other hand, is probably due to the effects of the hormone, via control of $1\alpha,25$-$(OH)_2D_3$ levels, on efficiency of intestinal calcium absorption (Chap. 351). Evidence from calcium kinetic studies indicates a transfer between extracellular fluid and bone of as much as 500 mg calcium daily (an amount large in relation to the total extracellular fluid calcium pool), and parathyroid hormone is known to influence this movement of calcium from bone into blood. This action of the hormone would tend to preserve calcium concentration in blood acutely at the cost of bone destruction and bone mineral release. However, the action of parathyroid hormone on kidney to preserve calcium by increasing the percentage reabsorption of filtered calcium may also be important in rapid regulation of blood calcium concentration.

There is evidence for a dual action of parathyroid hormone on bone. These two effects have been termed the *calcium replacement* and the *bone remodeling* effects of parathyroid hormone. It can be shown in vitro that there is an increased rate of release of calcium from bone into blood within minutes of the administration of parathyroid hormone; in vivo, a rapid efflux of calcium out of blood, presumably into bone cells, can be shown to precede the release of calcium. On the other hand, the more chronic effects of parathyroid hormone, mainly an increase in the number and activity of osteoclasts and a general increase in the remodeling of bone, appear only hours after the hormone is given. These latter actions, which involve increased protein synthesis, persist for hours after parathyroid hormone has been given. Effects on bone remodeling seem to be most closely related to the radiological and histological picture of osteopenia that results from long-standing excessive parathyroid action. It is not clear whether the two effects of parathyroid action on bone represent a continuous spectrum with a common initiating biochemical event or whether they are separate actions.

Although the role of the parathyroid glands in the prevention of tetany and maintenance of normal plasma calcium levels has been appreciated since the late nineteenth century, a reliable method for extraction of an active principle from parathyroid tissue was not accomplished for many years afterward. However, there has been rapid progress in our knowledge of the chemical properties of parathyroid hormone and of the structural requirements for biologic activity. The complete amino acid sequences of the major forms of bovine, porcine, and human hormones have been defined. The peptides consist of a single-chain structure composed of 84 amino acids. The molecules lack cysteine or cystine; the sequences of the three known forms of the hormone are similar, as is illustrated in Fig. 349-4.

The often discussed possibility that different forms of the hormone are active on bone and kidney is not supported by analyses of the relation between parathyroid hormone structure and physiological actions. The structural requirements for biologic activity of parathyroid hormone have been defined recently by synthesis of peptides based on the structures deduced. Numerous peptides consisting of portions of the amino terminal 34 residues and various analogues have been synthesized. Synthetic fragments containing the amino terminal sequence have been shown to exert all the known biologic actions of the hormone on mineral ion transport in kidney and bone. It seems likely that the amino terminal portion of the hormone is also responsible for stimulation of the renal 25-

FIGURE 349-4

Model illustrating the sequence of human, bovine, and porcine parathyroid hormone. The continuous open circles represent the sequence of human PTH, numbers referring to sequence positions beginning with the amino terminus; sequence positions at which the residues found in the bovine and porcine molecule differ from that found in the human hormone are shown by the circles adjacent to the human sequence. Note relative conservation in the sequence region associated with biologic activity, residues 1 to 34; most sequence differences are found in the middle region of the molecule. (From HT Keutmann et al, Biochemistry 17:5723, 1978.)

hydroxyvitamin D 1α-hydroxylase and, hence, the action of the hormone to stimulate intestinal calcium absorption.

It can now be concluded on the basis of studies with synthetic peptides that any fragment of parathyroid hormone, in order to be biologically active on bone and kidney, must consist of a continuous peptide sequence beginning with residue 2, valine, and extending as far as residue 26, lysine.

These observations are of particular interest because the biosynthesis and peripheral metabolism of parathyroid hormone have been found to be more complex than initially thought. Furthermore, parathyroid hormone which is extracted from glands differs from both the hormone that is initially synthesized and the hormone found in the peripheral circulation. It has also been shown that parathyroid hormone in human plasma is immunologically different from the hormone extracted from human adenomas.

The hormone secreted in vivo from normal bovine and human parathyroid glands and from parathyroid adenomas is indistinguishable by immunologic criteria and by molecular size from the 84-amino acid peptide (molecular weight 9500) extracted from glands. However, much of the immunoreactive material found in the peripheral circulation of humans and animals (cow, dog) is smaller than the extracted or secreted hormone. The principal circulating fragment(s) of immunore-active hormone (approximate molecular weight 7000) lacks a portion of the critical amino terminal sequence required for biologic activity and, hence, must constitute a biologically inactive hormonal fragment(s).

Cleavage of the native peptide by an endopeptidase would be expected to result in formation of a second fragment, molecular weight 2000 to 3000, representing the amino terminal, biologically active, portion of the hormone. There is disagreement in published reports concerning the presence or absence of such a circulating amino-terminal fragment. It is unclear (1) whether peripheral metabolism accounts for most of the circulating fragment(s) of hormone or whether fragments as well as intact hormone are also secreted by the gland and (2) whether peripheral metabolism is a purely catabolic process concerned only with hormone destruction or whether the peripheral cleavage results in formation of a metabolically active amino-terminal fragment of parathyroid hormone with physiologically significant action. Much more work on this issue of hormonal metabolism is required. Present evidence suggests that the liver and kidney are the principal sites at which peripheral metabolism of hormone occurs. Specific cleavages in these organs may serve as points of metabolic control to regulate the concentration of hormonally active polypeptides in the circulation (Fig. 349-5). Peripheral metabolism, in turn, may also be affected by pathological processes, such as renal failure or severe hepatic dysfunction.

FIGURE 349-5

Schematic model of the biosynthesis, secretion, and peripheral metabolism of parathyroid hormone, as well as contributions of these processes to the heterogeneity of circulating, immunoreactive parathyroid hormone (see text for details). Biosynthesis involves initial translation of parathyroid hormone–specific messenger RNA (mRNA) into a polypeptide of 115 amino acids, preproparathyroid hormone (preproPTH) followed by several specific posttranslational cleavages. The first cleavage (1) occurs on or near the endoplasmic reticulum within seconds of synthesis; this cleavage removes the 25-amino acid preproPTH-specific peptide, or leader sequence (represented by a straight line). The product, proPTH, a peptide of 90 amino acids, is converted by a second specific peptidase(s) with removal of the proPTH-specific peptide (represented by a jagged line), forming PTH. (An alternate possibility, not illustrated, is that proPTH is converted to PTH after packing into secretory granules.) PTH, consisting of 84 amino acids (illustrated as a heavy bar with N indicating amino terminus, C, the carboxy terminus), is the principal secretory product of the cell, resulting from exocytosis of secretory granules containing the hor-mone (indicated by heavy arrow). Some have reported that there is an alternate secretory pathway in which amino-terminal fragments (N) and carboxy-terminal fragments (C) of the molecule are formed by further proteolytic processing within the cell followed by release into the circulation (dotted arrows). Speculations concerning release of precursor forms, or fragments (not yet proved), from the cell into the circulation are indicated by dotted arrows and question marks. Peripheral metabolism involves uptake of the intact hormone by certain organs (liver and kidney being most likely) followed by a third cleavage (3). This last cleavage is presumed to result in formation of an amino-terminal fragment (N) and a carboxy-terminal fragment (C). The carboxy-terminal fragment reenters the circulation, from which it disappears more slowly than the intact hormone, and is taken up and cleaved; hence the concentration of carboxy-terminal fragment is higher than that of intact PTH. The fate of the amino-terminal fragment, presumably derived by peripheral metabolism, is unsettled. The relative contribution of peripheral metabolism and the release of fragments directly from the gland to the heterogeneity of circulating parathyroid hormone is presently disputed and awaits clarification.

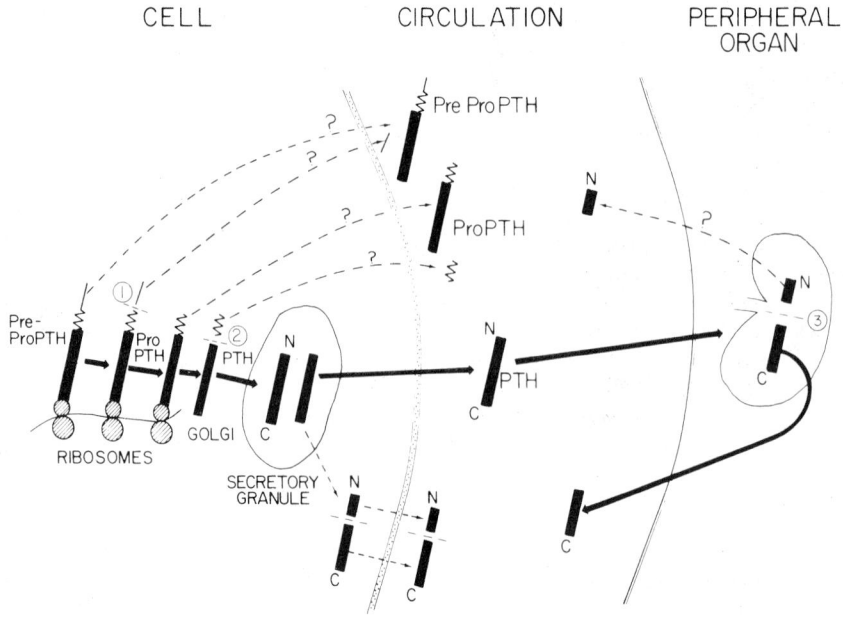

CELL CIRCULATION PERIPHERAL ORGAN

The rate of uptake and cleavage of the secreted 84-amino acid peptide is more rapid than the rate of clearance from blood of the smaller, biologically inactive fragment(s) that result from peripheral metabolism and release into the circulation from cleavage sites. Hence, at present it must be concluded that measurements of parathyroid hormone in blood by immunoassay provide only an overall index of parathyroid glandular activity rather than a direct measure of biologically active hormone, since biologically inert fragments rather than intact hormone are the principal circulating form of immunoreactive hormone (Chap. 350). Changes in rate of production or clearance of fragments could change the concentration of immunoreactive hormone without involving corresponding changes in rate of hormone secretion. Such discordance between concentrations of immunoreactive hormone and biologically active peptide seem likely, for example, in renal failure, since the kidney seems to be the principal route of excretion of hormone fragments.

The biosynthesis of parathyroid hormone has been extensively investigated. Several larger molecular forms have been identified in the biosynthetic sequence leading from gene transcription and translation to final packaging of the 84-amino acid peptide in secretory granules prior to secretion. The earliest detected precursor form, termed *preproparathyroid hormone,* consists of 115 amino acids; this molecular form is converted to an intermediate form of 90 amino acids termed *proparathyroid hormone.* The details of intracellular regulation of biosynthesis are still unknown. Parathyroid hormone shares, with other polypeptides and proteins destined for secretion from cells, this complex pattern of initial synthesis as a larger molecule which is then reduced in size by several, apparently highly specific, intracellular cleavages prior to secretion. The hydrophobic regions of the preproparathyroid hormone are similar to, but distinct from, preprotein-specific regions of other cell-secreted proteins and may serve an important role in guiding transport of the polypeptide from sites of synthesis on polyribosomes through the cytoskeleton to secretory granules. Hence, it is possible that hereditary or acquired defects in the cellular control of biosynthesis may lead to deficient secretion of active hormone or to release of incompletely processed precursor forms into the circulation. No direct evidence of such defects has been obtained yet, however.

Numerous in vivo and in vitro experiments have shown that blood calcium concentration controls the secretion of parathyroid hormone and that the ionized fraction of blood calcium is the important determinant of hormone secretion. Hormone secretion increases steeply to a maximum value of fivefold above basal rates of secretion whenever calcium concentration falls from normal to the range of 7.5 to 8.0 mg per 100 ml (measured as total calcium). Beta-adrenergic agonists such as epinephrine may also increase hormone secretion, but the physiological significance of catecholamines as secretagogues is not yet established.

Magnesium may influence hormone secretion in the same direction as calcium. It is unlikely that physiological variations in magnesium concentration affect parathyroid secretion, but severe intracellular magnesium deficiency is associated with defective hormone secretion.

The mode of action of parathyroid hormone at the biochemical level involves effects of parathyroid hormone on adenylate cyclase in the cells of the target tissue. Stimulation of enzyme activity during specific hormone–target cell membrane interaction leads to an increase in intracellular cyclic adenosine monophosphate (cyclic AMP). It seems likely that this rapid rise in intracellular cyclic AMP is the initial biochemical step in all the physiological effects of parathyroid hormone. Following the administration of parathyroid hormone there is, within minutes, a rise in urinary cyclic AMP that precedes any observable increase in phosphate excretion. Likewise, the effects on bone adenylate cyclase activity can be detected within 1 min of the addition of parathyroid hormone to a suspension of bone cells. In addition, administration of dibutyryl cyclic AMP, which, as a more soluble analogue of cyclic AMP, penetrates cells more effectively, simulates the actions of parathyroid hormone in parathyroidectomized animals. Dibutyryl cyclic AMP leads to a rise in serum calcium, a lowering of serum phosphate, and an increased excretion of calcium, phosphate, and hydroxyproline in urine.

There are as yet no data concerning the cellular mechanism whereby an increased intracellular concentration of cyclic AMP leads to changes in calcium and phosphate ion translocation. In a number of tissues responsive to hormones through a cyclic AMP mechanism there is evidence for stimulation of protein kinases causing, in turn, phosphorylation of critical proteins that initiate the hormonal effect. The postulated sequence of events in parathyroid hormone–driven, cyclic AMP–mediated calcium (and phosphate) transport can be summarized as follows. Cyclic AMP binds to a specific binding protein, causing it to dissociate from and thereby activate a protein kinase. The protein(s) which, in turn, is phosphorylated by the kinase is at present unknown, but certain evidence suggests that microtubular proteins may be the site of phosphorylation.

Whatever the cellular sites affected by the increased concentration of intracellular cyclic AMP, the initial effect (occurring within minutes) of parathyroid hormone administration is a hypocalcemia due to flow of calcium out of blood into cells, apparently skeletal cells. Thus, both cyclic AMP and calcium may serve as "second messengers" for mediating parathyroid hormone effects in receptor cells.

CALCITONIN (See also Chap. 348)   Calcitonin is the potent hypocalcemic, hypophosphatemic peptide hormone which, in many ways, acts as the physiological antagonist to parathyroid hormone. Calcitonin reduces bone resorption and has opposing effects to parathyroid hormone on the kidney in that it increases renal calcium clearance. This hormone has been the subject of intensive physiological studies and has been extensively evaluated as a therapeutic agent of potential value in skeletal disease characterized by excessive resorption. Although calcitonin exerts its hypocalcemic, hypophosphatemic action principally by an inhibition of bone resorption, the initial step in hormone action and the exact sequence of effects on target cells influenced by the hormone are not known.

Present gaps in understanding the physiological role of calcitonin and the effects of the peptide at physiological concentrations on organs other than the bone in turn complicate efforts to understand the biochemical mode of action of the hormone. However, evidence has been obtained that calcitonin may exert its effects through stimulation of membrane-bound adenylate cyclase in receptor cells in kidney and bone. Calcitonin has been shown to bind to renal cells and to stimulate membrane-bound adenylate cyclase. The cells responsive to calcitonin are located in different regions of the kidney than are cells affected by parathyroid hormone or vasopressin. Although it is not clear which ion translocation is primary in the overall action of calcitonin, data have pointed to mediation of calcitonin effects on calcium transport and bone metabolism through initial effects on phosphate transport. In this view, calcitonin acts by causing an initial influx of phosphate into cells; this in turn results in effects on calcium transport.

The thyroid gland is the major source of the hormone in mammalian species. In submammalian vertebrates calcitonin is found in a separate organ, the ultimobranchial body, which contains cells of a similar embryologic origin to the C cells of the thyroid. Extensive embryologic and histological studies have established that the cells involved in calcitonin synthesis arise originally from neural crest tissue. During embryogenesis these cells migrate into the ultimobranchial body. The latter body or gland arises from the last branchial pouch, hence the name *ultimobranchial body*. In submammalian vertebrates the ultimobranchial body remains as a discrete organ, anatomically separate from the thyroid gland. In mammals the ultimobranchial gland fuses with the thyroid gland, and the calcitonin-secreting cells become part of the thyroid in adult life. Calcitonin is found in all vertebrate classes that have been examined.

The amino acid sequences of eight calcitonins from six species, including humans, have been determined. The naturally occurring calcitonins consist of a peptide chain composed of 32 amino acids. Although there are certain common structural features, there is a considerable amount of variability in sequence. The entire chain of 32 amino acids appears to be required for biologic activity. The factors that regulate the synthesis of calcitonin in the parafollicular or C cells are not known. Calcitonin from salmon, when tested in various animal species, is 25 to 100 times more potent by weight in lowering serum calcium than are other forms of calcitonin. In fact, the salmon hormone is at least 10 times more potent in humans than human calcitonin. Greater resistance to metabolic destruction may explain in part the greater biologic potency of salmon calcitonin, but the salmon hormone appears to bind more strongly to receptor sites as well.

In animals, the concentration of the hormone rises within minutes of induced hypercalcemia. The secretion of the hormone is under the direct control of blood calcium: an increase in calcium concentration causes an increase in the concentration of calcitonin, and a decrease in calcium concentration causes a decrease in the concentration of calcitonin. Once secreted, calcitonin disappears rapidly from the circulation with a half-life of 2 to 15 min.

The concentration of calcitonin in the peripheral blood of normal humans is lower than in many other species such as cows, rats, pigs, and sheep. Sensitive assays for human calcitonin suggest that calcitonin secretion occurs in all normal persons; however, because of the heterogeneity of circulating forms of calcitonin, precise quantitation of plasma hormone concentration cannot be made.

The physiological role of calcitonin is still, in many ways, unclear. In many mammals calcitonin acts to lower both blood calcium and blood phosphate; the principal action of calcitonin is inhibition of bone resorption. The importance of calcitonin in increasing urinary calcium and phosphate clearance is synergistic with its effects on bone resorption. The actions of calcitonin on kidney and bone are in turn modulated by the regulation of calcitonin production by serum calcium; hypercalcemia stimulates and hypocalcemia suppresses calcitonin release. The view that calcitonin serves physiologically to protect against hypercalcemia is thus explained by the hypocalcemic effects of calcitonin triggered in response to hypercalcemia.

The role of calcitonin, however, if any, in normal adult humans is unknown. Changes in calcium and phosphate metabolism are not seen in humans despite extremes of variation in hormone production; there are no definite effects attributable to calcitonin deficiency (totally thyroidectomized patients replaced only with thyroxine) or excess (patients with the calcitonin-secreting tumor, medullary carcinoma of the thyroid). Patients with the latter disorder suffer multiple deleterious consequences of their malignancy (see Chap. 348), but no abnormalities in calcium or bone metabolism are detected.

Medical interest in calcitonin, therefore, at present is centered principally upon its promise as a therapeutic agent and its usefulness, when deployed in radioimmunoassays, for detection of medullary carcinoma (Chap. 348). The effectiveness of calcitonin in Paget's disease of bone is being evaluated. Preliminary results are encouraging; toxicity in chronic use has not proved to be a problem, and beneficial effects have been reported in long-term control of excessive bone turnover in Paget's disease.

REFERENCES

AVIOLI LV, KRANE SM (eds): *Metabolic Bone Disease,* New York, Academic, 1977, vol I; ibid, 1978, vol II

DARSEE JR, NUTTER DO: Reversible severe congestive cardiomyopathy in three cases of hypophosphatemia. Ann Intern Med 89:867, 1978

GLIMCHER MJ: Composition, structure, and organization of bone and other mineralized tissues and the mechanism of calcification, in *Handbook of Physiology,* sec 7: *Endocrinology,* vol VII, GD Aurbach (ed). Washington, DC, American Physiological Society, 1976, p 25

HABENER JF, POTTS JT JR: Biosynthesis of parathyroid hormone. N Engl J Med 299:580, 635, 1978

HABENER JF, POTTS JT JR: Chemistry, biosynthesis, secretion, and metabolism of PTH, in *Handbook of Physiology,* sec 7: *Endocrinology,* vol VII, GD Aurbach (ed). Washington, DC, American Physiological Society, 1976, p 313

JOWSEY J: *Metabolic Diseases of Bone.* Philadelphia, Saunders, 1977

KNOCHEL JP et al: Hypophosphatemia and rhabdomyolysis. J Clin Invest 62:1240, 1978

MUNSON PL: Physiology and pharmacology of thyrocalcitonin, in *Handbook of Physiology,* sec 7: *Endocrinology,* vol VII, GD Aurbach (ed). Washington, DC, American Physiological Society, 1976, p 443

POTTS JT JR, AURBACH GD: Chemistry of the calcitonins, in *Handbook of Physiology,* sec 7: *Endocrinology,* vol VII, GD Aurbach (ed). Washington, DC, American Physiological Society, 1976, p 423

350
DISORDERS OF PARATHYROID GLANDS

JOHN T. POTTS, JR.

PRIMARY HYPERPARATHYROIDISM

NATURAL HISTORY AND INCIDENCE Primary hyperparathyroidism is a generalized disorder of calcium, phosphate, and bone metabolism that results from an increased secretion of parathyroid hormone. The excessive concentration of circulating hormone usually leads to hypercalcemia and hypophosphatemia; there may be recurrent nephrolithiasis, peptic ulcers, mental changes, and excessive bone resorption. It has become evident, however, that the clinical manifestations of hyperparathyroidism may be minimal. With wider use of diagnostic techniques, particularly multiphasic screening of blood calcium, the diagnosis is being made with increasing frequency and earlier in the course of the illness. There are many patients in whom an incidental blood calcium determination establishes hypercalcemia without any apparent symptoms. These patients, in turn, raise obvious questions about the natural history of the disease and the indications for surgery.

The disease most commonly occurs in adults, with peak incidence between the third and fifth decades. However, primary hyperparathyroidism has been detected in young children, and the initial diagnosis has been made in the very elderly. Patients may go for years with undetected hyperparathyroidism because of the minimal symptoms. Occasionally, the disease seems to appear abruptly, and patients may exhibit severe complications, such as marked dehydration and coma associated with severe hypercalcemic parathyroid crisis. It would appear that hyperparathyroidism is more common than previously appreciated; several estimates have suggested that the prevalence of primary hyperparathyroidism is 1 case per 1000 persons.

ETIOLOGY AND PATHOLOGY In greater than 80 percent of patients primary hyperparathyroidism results from neoplastic transformation of one parathyroid gland; all but a few percent of the neoplasms are benign adenomas. "Double adenomas," by which was meant neoplastic transformation of two parathyroids with the remaining glands entirely normal, is now felt to be extremely rare. Most cases of supposed double adenoma represented unrecognized hyperplasia involving all parathyroids. The two most likely possibilities to be considered by the surgeon and pathologist in their analysis of the pathology present in a given patient are (1) disease in a single gland with an incidence of approximately 85 percent (81 percent adenoma, 4 percent histologically carcinoma) and (2) hyperplasia of all glands (approximately 15 percent of cases, usually chief-cell hyperplasia). These considerations are of practical importance in the surgical management of hyperparathyroidism, as discussed below.

An adenoma is the most common cause of hyperparathyroidism. Most often the tumor is in the inferior parathyroid glands. However, the tumor is found in an unusual location in 6 to 10 percent of patients; such ectopic parathyroid adenomas may be located in the thymus, the thyroid, or even the pericardium. Retroesophageal adenomas have also been reported. Adenomas vary in size from 0.5 to 5 g; in some instances, however, tumors as large as 10 to 20 g are found. Histological examination usually reveals that the adenoma is composed primarily of chief cells; the nodule can be surrounded by a rim of normal tissue. This latter feature can sometimes be useful in distinguishing adenomas from primary chief-cell hyperplasia. Rarely adenomas are composed of oxyphil cells or a mixed population of cells.

Hyperplasia involving all four glands, the cell type being chief cells, is now being found with increasing frequency in primary hyperparathyroidism. Chief-cell hyperplasia is especially common in those instances of hyperparathyroidism which are familial or which are part of the syndrome of multiple endocrine neoplasia. Clear-cell (Wasserhelle) hyperplasia is only rarely seen.

It can be difficult sometimes to distinguish adenoma from hyperplasia. Findings at surgery must be combined with microscopic examination of biopsy specimens of several glands. When an adenoma is present, examination of other glands indicates that they are of normal size, approximately 25 mg average weight, and histologically there is a normal distribution of all cell types (rather than only chief cells) and normal areas of fat. With hyperplasia all glands may be enlarged, although in some patients the enlargement may be so asymmetric that some involved glands may appear normal grossly. Even if certain glands are not clearly increased in size, histological examination reveals a uniform pattern of chief cells and *disappearance of fat*.

Some hyperplastic glands may exhibit compression of tissue around an area of hyperplasia, giving the appearance of a capsule (pseudoencapsulation), and hence, may be mistaken for an adenoma.

Carcinoma of the parathyroid glands is rare; fewer than 100 cases have been reported. The tumor usually secretes excessive amounts of parathyroid hormone, although nonfunctioning tumors have been reported. Parathyroid carcinoma is usually not very malignant in character. Long-term survival without recurrence is common if the entire gland is removed at initial operation without rupture of the capsule. When recurrent, parathyroid carcinoma is usually slow-growing with local spread in the neck; surgical correction of recurrent disease is therefore feasible. Occasionally, parathyroid carcinoma is more aggressive in character with distant metastases, often to the lung and liver, found at the time of initial operation. It is often difficult initially to decide if the primary tumor is carcinoma; even benign adenomas may show histological changes that suggest malignant disease. Hyperparathyroidism resulting from a parathyroid carcinoma may be clinically indistinguishable from other forms of primary hyperparathyroidism.

A variety of nonparathyroid tumors have been associated with a clinical syndrome resembling primary hyperparathyroidism. This syndrome has been termed *pseudohyperparathyroidism* or *ectopic hyperparathyroidism*. The clinical evidence that some nonparathyroid tumors produce a parathyroid hormone-like peptide has been confirmed by immunologic studies which indicate that parathyroid-like activity is present in extracts of such tumors in the blood of affected patients. The true incidence of ectopic hyperparathyroidism is difficult to assess. Recent reports have stressed that in many patients who meet the clinical criteria of pseudohyperparathyroidism (solid tumor, no bone metastases, humoral mediation of the hypercalcemia), the etiologic mechanism involves humoral agents other than parathyroid hormone-like substances. Prostaglandins have been implicated in some patients with pseudohyperparathyroidism. The entity must be suspected particularly in older patients. Lung tumors, particularly squamous-cell carcinoma, and renal tumors are the most common types of nonparathyroid tumors associated with pseudohyperparathyroidism. However, tumors of many types and origins have been described in association with the syndrome. Until further study is done of the etiology of hypercalcemia in patients with malignancy, the term *ectopic hyperparathyroidism* should not be used synonymously with pseudohyperparathyroidism (see Chap. 347).

The occurrence of hyperparathyroidism in a familial pattern is well documented and may occur without other endocrinologic abnormality. More often, however, hereditary hyperparathyroidism is found as part of a multiglandular endocrinopathy. It is now appreciated that there are two or more genetically distinct syndromes with multiple endocrine disorders. The syndrome originally described (Wermer's syndrome) consisted of hyperparathyroidism and tumors of the pituitary and pancreatic islet cells. This multiglandular disorder is often associated with peptic ulcer and gastric hypersecretion (the Zollinger-Ellison syndrome). Another distinct constellation of endocrinologic abnormalities which consists of hyperparathyroidism associated with pheochromocytoma and medullary carcinoma of the thyroid has also been described (see Chap. 348). The etiology of these syndromes is not known.

In both syndromes the hyperparathyroidism can be due to adenomas or hyperplasia, the latter usually of the chief-cell variety. The pattern of inheritance generally appears to be autosomal dominant. Tumors of the thyroid and adrenal medulla are not found in Wermer's syndrome, and pancreatic and pituitary tumors are not found in the kindreds with a high incidence of medullary carcinoma of the thyroid and pheochromocytoma. In this revised classification Wermer's syndrome is termed *multiple endocrine neoplasia* (adenomatosis) type 1 (usually abbreviated MEN I or MEA I), and the more recently described syndrome involving thyroid tumors is referred to as MEN II or MEA II. Since the different endocrine tumors can occur at widely separated intervals, hyperparathyroidism and the related endocrine disorders should be carefully and repeatedly searched for in all members of kindreds afflicted with the multiple endocrine neoplasia syndromes (Chap. 348).

Several recent reports have called attention to another familial disorder which resembles but may be distinct from primary hyperparathyroidism. This entity, termed *familial hypocalciuric hypercalcemia* (FHH) or *familial benign hypercalcemia,* occurs in a pattern compatible with autosomal dominant inheritance. Both clinical and laboratory findings in these patients seem to distinguish them from patients with primary hyperparathyroidism, especially from those in families with the multiple endocrine neoplasia syndromes. Few, if any, clinical signs or symptoms, are found in patients with FHH syndrome; only 3 of 25 patients in one series had kidney stones or any abnormality in renal function. No evidence of any other endocrine abnormalities is seen. Most patients are detected as a result of family screening for hypercalcemia once one member of the kindred is detected; such studies have revealed a high incidence in FHH of hypercalcemia in the first decade of life in affected family members compared with complete lack of hypercalcemia under the age of 10 years in the MEN I families screened as a control. Average values for renal clearance of calcium and magnesium are lower in FHH than in primary hyperparathyroidism (calcium/creatinine clearance ratio of 0.006 ± 0.004 versus 0.024 ± 0.01). Serum magnesium levels are higher in FHH than in primary hyperparathyroidism. Most importantly, surgery in many patients has not led to documentation of clear-cut abnormalities in the parathyroids or cure of the hypercalcemia unless hypoparathyroidism was induced by total parathyroidectomy. The true nature of this disorder and its proper management remain unclear; it cannot be deduced that surgery is the treatment of choice.

SIGNS AND SYMPTOMS Most of the signs and symptoms of hyperparathyroidism reflect known pathophysiological consequences of hypercalcemia. Many organ systems can be affected by hyperparathyroidism. However, characteristically, involvement of the kidneys and skeletal system is most prominent. *Kidney involvement,* due either to deposition of calcium in the renal parenchyma or to recurrent nephrolithiasis, is found in 60 to 70 percent of patients reported in large series prior to 1970. With the increased frequency of detection of asymptomatic individuals in the last decade, the incidence of renal complications appears lower but is still the most common complication of hyperparathyroidism.

Renal stones are usually composed of either calcium oxalate or calcium phosphate. Repeated episodes of nephrolithiasis or the formation of large calculi may lead to urinary tract obstruction and repeated episodes of infection. These complications may also contribute to progressive loss of renal function. Nephrolithiasis and nephrocalcinosis rarely occur in the same patient. Nephrocalcinosis may be accompanied by decreased renal function and phosphate retention.

The classic pattern of bone involvement in hyperparathyroidism is *osteitis fibrosa cystica.* In the United States, at the present time, x-ray evidence of osteitis fibrosa cystica is not commonly found in patients when the diagnosis of hyperparathyroidism is made, even though there may be a long history of renal or other complications of the disease. Several decades ago an incidence of osteitis fibrosa cystica of 10 to 25 percent or even higher was reported in patients with hyperparathyroidism. This reduced frequency of skeletal involvement has not been adequately explained. Bone disease, however, is still a serious issue in hyperparathyroidism. Quantitative bone biopsy studies with histomorphometric analyses reveal microscopic evidence of abnormality in bone turnover in as many as 50 percent of patients, even in the absence of osteitis fibrosa. Thus, although many patients give evidence of excessive effects

of parathyroid hormone on bone, only a few develop clinically evident osteitis fibrosa cystica. Present emphasis is focused on a different issue, the frequency of development of osteopenia which is parathyroid hormone-dependent and progressive, indicating the need for surgery, and the diagnostic methods most useful for determining its presence.

Histological examination of bone specimens from patients with severe osteitis fibrosa reveals a number of changes that collectively define the presence of parathyroid overactivity. There is a reduction in the number of trabeculae, an increase in giant multinucleated osteoclasts seen in scalloped areas on the surface of the bone (Howship's lacunae), and a marked replacement of normal cellular and marrow elements by fibrous tissue. In milder forms of skeletal involvement early changes can sometimes be detected by x-rays of the hands and skull. *The phalangeal tufts* may be resorbed, and an irregular outline replaces the normally sharp cortical outline of the bone in the digits. This change is termed *subperiosteal resorption.* Detection of loss of the *lamina dura* of the teeth is less specific but may be helpful diagnostically. Tiny, "punched-out" lesions in the skull, producing the so-called "salt-and-pepper" appearance, are characteristic. Severe *osteopenia* without radiological criteria of osteitis fibrosa cystica may also be due to excessive parathyroid action; there are, however, as yet no criteria to distinguish such a generalized osteopenia from osteoporosis not related to excess parathyroid hormone action. Bone biopsy followed by quantitative histomorphometry does establish a highly cellular bone with increased numbers of osteoclasts and osteoblasts and increase in the number of active bone-resorbing and forming areas. Criteria useful in establishing progressive bone disease are (1) serial measurements of bone mass by photon beam densitometry or metacarpal cortical thickness and (2) metabolic studies such as urine calcium excretion on a low calcium intake (less complex than formal balance studies). Patients who exhibit evidence of progressive osteopenia have been subjected to parathyroidectomy. Insufficient time has elapsed to determine whether there is an increase in bone density after hyperparathyroidism is corrected, but in the experience of the author (with Dr. Robert M. Neer) there have been a sufficient number of patients with progressive loss of bone mass prior to surgery in whom densitometry has shown no further loss after parathyroid surgery to suggest real benefit to this group by correction of hyperparathyroidism.

In addition, it has been appreciated that hyperparathyroidism may be associated with symptoms or signs referable to *the central nervous system, neuromuscular function, the gastrointestinal tract, the skin, and the joints.* Sometimes, quite vague or minor complaints from a patient, particularly neuromuscular or gastrointestinal symptoms, are the only clue to the diagnosis; awareness of the subtle manifestations of the disease may prompt a request for blood calcium determination as part of a diagnostic evaluation.

Central nervous system manifestations of hyperparathyroidism are multiple and varied. Reported symptoms range from mild personality disturbances to severe psychiatric disorders; mental obtundation or coma is seen with severe hypercalcemia. In some instances, the patient experiences multiple vague complaints which can often be mistaken for psychoneurosis. It must be emphasized, however, that mild depression, found frequently in the population without the presence of hyperparathyroidism, cannot be used as the sole clinical criterion for parathyroid surgery.

A distinctive syndrome of *neuromuscular involvement* in hyperparathyroidism has been recently emphasized. Proximal muscle weakness, easy fatigability, and atrophy of muscles are clinical features. Abnormal electromyograms and atrophy of muscle fibers without myopathic changes are detected. In some cases, the clinical signs are so striking as to suggest amyotrophic lateral sclerosis or some other incurable primary neuromuscular disorder; in other patients the signs may be minimal. Clinically, the important feature is the complete regression of neuromuscular disease after surgical correction of the hyperparathyroidism.

Frequently, there are varied and sometimes subtle manifestations of hyperparathyroidism in the *gastrointestinal tract.* In addition to a variety of vague abdominal complaints, diseases of the stomach and pancreas are frequent. *Duodenal ulcers* have been reported in as many as 25 percent of patients with proved hyperparathyroidism. In patients with hyperparathyroidism resulting from multiple endocrine neoplasia syndrome (type 1), there is a high incidence of ulcer as a result of the associated pancreatic tumors that secrete excessive quantities of gastrin (the Zollinger-Ellison syndrome). Cases of pancreatitis have been reported in association with hyperparathyroidism, but the absolute incidence is not established. Various mechanisms have been proposed to explain the apparent increased incidence of pancreatitis, but there is no convincing explanation.

Calcification in the cornea of the eye (*band keratopathy*) may be clinically recognizable, usually when renal insufficiency and phosphate retention are present; slit-lamp examination may, however, be necessary to detect the calcification.

It has also been noted that *chondrocalcinosis* and *pseudogout* are seen in association with hyperparathyroidism. Occasionally pseudogout is the initial clinical manifestation of the hyperparathyroidism.

DIAGNOSIS The diagnosis of hyperparathyroidism is made primarily on clinical grounds. The immunoassay for parathyroid hormone is proving to be of increasing value as a specific diagnostic test for hyperparathyroidism, but there are still numerous problems in interpretation of assay results.

The disease, traditionally, is most often sought for in patients with recurrent kidney stones or, in rarer instances, with symptoms and/or signs of osteitis fibrosa. Recently, however, the diagnosis is most often made in patients with minor symptoms or no symptoms whatever. With increased understanding of the clinical symptomatology, blood calcium measurements may lead to detection of hypercalcemia in a patient with vague constitutional complaints, ulcer, or atypical arthritis. Finally, hypercalcemia may be detected as a result of multiphasic routine blood testing in asymptomatic subjects. Repeated measurements of plasma calcium should be made in patients with suspected hypercalcemia. One may detect either a sustained hypercalcemia or a pattern of high normal blood calciums alternating with occasional definitely elevated values. If errors due to altered concentration of blood protein or variation in laboratory range of normal can be eliminated, such findings establish the presence of hypercalcemia.

Obviously, the efforts to establish the diagnosis are most exhaustive in patients with clear-cut symptoms, particularly with recurrent kidney stones. The philosophy of approach is different at the other extreme, a totally asymptomatic patient in whom hypercalcemia is detected coincidentally. However, since hypercalcemia can be the presenting evidence for malignancy or other serious disease, a thorough evaluation of possible etiologies, including hyperparathyroidism, by application of at least standard screening procedures is indicated even in asymptomatic subjects. If the diagnosis of hyperparathyroidism is suspected after such an evaluation, a decision can still be made to follow the patient for a time rather than recommend surgery.

Hypercalcemia is the most common manifestation of hyperparathyroidism. Careful consideration must be given to the justification for surgical exploration in the absence of definite hypercalcemia. There are now numerous reports of so-called "normocalcemic hyperparathyroidism," that is, patients with surgically proved hyperparathyroidism with normal calcium

but elevated values of immunoreactive PTH (iPTH). However, careful scrutiny of the reports reveals that in those with adenomas, the patients were, in fact, hypercalcemic at some time in their course; they could more correctly be described, therefore, as having intermittent hypercalcemia, perhaps an early feature of hyperparathyroidism. If patients have coexisting conditions that interfere with the calcium-elevating actions of PTH, such as chronic renal failure, severe malabsorption, or vitamin D deficiency, then the lack of calcium elevation need not argue against the presence of true hyperparathyroidism. In the absence of such conditions it may be useful to search for postabsorptive hypercalcemia in association with elevated iPTH or to use a provocative test with benzothiadiazides (see discussion of thiazide-induced hypercalcemia below).

Hypercalciuria is also commonly seen in hyperparathyroidism. However, it should be kept in mind that parathyroid hormone actually reduces calcium clearance. In fact, the 24-h urine excretion of calcium is lower in patients with hyperparathyroidism than in patients with equivalent degrees of hypercalcemia from nonparathyroid causes.

Serum phosphate is usually low but may be normal, especially if renal failure has developed. Detection of hypophosphatemia can be useful but is less specific than hypercalcemia. Samples must be obtained in the morning, under fasting conditions, to be useful; a serum phosphate below normal is not an abnormal finding in the postabsorptive state. Patients with severe hypercalcemia of any cause have been reported to have a low phosphate.

Other electrolyte abnormalities have also been described; however, these abnormalities may not be sufficiently specific to be of diagnostic value. Serum magnesium levels have been reported to be low. Serum chloride and citrate are often elevated and serum bicarbonate reduced. The combination of elevated chloride and low phosphate (reflecting the acidosis and renal phosphate wasting, respectively, of hyperparathyroidism) can be used as a diagnostic clue; the chloride/phosphorus ratio in patients with hyperparathyroidism is usually greater than 30, while in those with hypercalcemia of other causes it is less than 30.

Blood alkaline phosphatase (of bone origin) and urinary hydroxyproline concentrations are elevated only when there is significant bone involvement. Renal involvement can be reflected by a decreased concentrating ability, by specific tubular defects such as tubular acidosis, and finally by frank renal failure with the chemical findings of azotemia.

Special tests *Glucocorticoid administration* has been useful in differentiating the hypercalcemia of hyperparathyroidism from that associated with sarcoidosis, multiple myeloma, vitamin D intoxication, and some malignant diseases with osseous metastases. In these diseases doses of hydrocortisone of 100 mg per day (or an equivalent dose of another steroid such as prednisone) given for 10 days often result in a lowering of the serum calcium, whereas ordinarily calcium does not fall in hyperparathyroidism. Occasional false positive and false negative results have been reported. The mechanism of the effect is not explained but may reflect the physiological antagonism between glucocorticoids and vitamin D action in vitamin D intoxication and sarcoidosis and the tumor-suppressive action of glucocorticoids in some forms of malignancy.

A variety of tests of parathyroid function are based on the known effects of the hormone on the *renal handling of phosphate.* These tests are designed to take advantage of the decrease in tubular resorption of phosphate caused by parathyroid hormone. To perform the test, any of several convenient indices of phosphate handling by the kidneys is determined. Because of the diurnal variation in plasma phosphate concentration and the marked fluctuations in phosphate that occur with eating, long periods of urine collection are not useful in determinations of phosphate clearance.

Phosphate clearance is determined by standard techniques involving simultaneous measurement of urinary and blood phosphate concentrations; usually urine samples are collected over a 1- to 2-h period. Normal subjects have a phosphate clearance of 10.8 ± 2.7 ml/min. Values 50 percent or more above this figure have been detected in hyperparathyroidism. The tubular resorption of phosphate can be derived from the estimation of the phosphate clearance and the additional estimate of the glomerular filtration made by measuring creatinine clearance. The ratio of phosphate clearance to creatinine clearance indicates the percent of filtered phosphate that was reabsorbed. In normal subjects the tubular resorption of phosphate exceeds 85 percent; in hyperparathyroidism tubular resorption of phosphate may be as low as 50 to 60 percent. Unfortunately, these tests are all influenced by the many other factors that affect the renal handling of phosphate, and their value seems limited.

Diuretics of the benzothiazide class in the usual doses (chlorothiazide 0.5 g bid) can produce sustained, frank hypercalcemia in patients with hyperparathyroidism and borderline calcium values. Since such a response is not seen in normal subjects (there may be some elevation in blood calcium in normal subjects, but any effect seen is lost in a few days despite continued administration of thiazides), thiazide administration has been suggested as a provocative test for the presence of

FIGURE 350-1

Schematic illustrating results seen when simultaneous measurements of immunoreactive parathyroid hormone (PTH RIA) and serum calcium are made in normal subjects (N), patients with tumor hypercalcemia (TH), hypoparathyroidism (HP), pseudohypoparathyroidism (PHP), chronic renal failure with secondary hyperparathyroidism [CRF (2° HPTH)], and primary hyperparathyroidism (1° HPTH). Enclosed areas indicate the range of values typical for each class of subject measured; note overlap of regions and interrupted scales (see text for details).

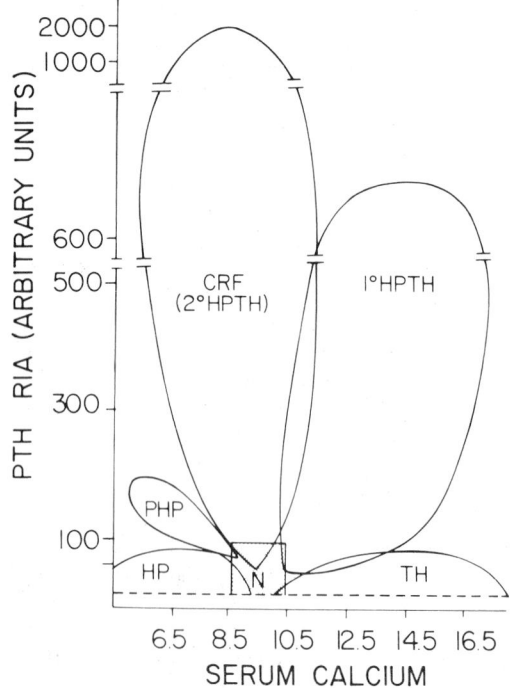

hyperparathyroidism. However, the specificity of the effect has been challenged; reports indicate that patients with high rates of vitamin D intake and/or underlying bone disease may also develop hypercalcemia.

Radioimmunoassay for parathyroid hormone   The development of a *specific radioimmunoassay* sufficiently sensitive to detect circulating human parathyroid hormone has provided, for the first time, a specific test for parathyroid function. Independent assay procedures have now been developed in many centers and commercial laboratories. There have been and continue to be numerous problems with the application and interpretation of the assay. It is necessary to use a nonhomologous assay system (labeled bovine parathyroid hormone and antiserum to bovine parathyroid hormone) to measure human parathyroid hormone. There are in plasma several immunologically (and biologically) distinct species of parathyroid hormone (see Chap. 349). Despite these problems, when appropriate precautions are observed, the immunoassay for parathyroid hormone can be uniquely useful in the diagnostic evaluation of patients with primary hyperparathyroidism and/or with hypercalcemia.

Many patients with hyperparathyroidism have concentrations of hormone clearly elevated above the normal range. Most workers, however, find that the concentration of hormone in many subjects with proved hyperparathyroidism is no higher than that found in some normal subjects. Patients with hypercalcemia not due to parathyroid disease, however, have undetectable concentrations of parathyroid hormone; in these patients, since parathyroid gland function is normal, secretion is suppressed because of the hypercalcemia. Patients with hypercalcemia due to hyperparathyroidism have detectable, if not elevated, concentrations of hormone despite hypercalcemia. Thus the assay is helpful in the differential diagnosis of hypercalcemia; a clear distinction exists between values found in hypercalcemia of parathyroid and nonparathyroid origin. It has been recently appreciated that hormone concentration in blood in patients with hyperparathyroidism changes in response to induced changes in blood calcium. This, in part, explains the overlap found between hormone concentrations in patients with hyperparathyroidism and increased blood calcium level when compared with normal subjects with normal calcium concentrations.

These findings emphasize that the disorder of parathyroid function in primary hyperparathyroidism cannot be explained simply on the basis of a fixed rate of hormone secretion; the defect in control of secretion, responsible for excessive hormone production, must be more subtle than simple autonomy. The nature of the cellular defect has not yet been defined.

As illustrated schematically in Fig. 350-1, most useful clinical interpretation of immunoassays is best achieved by (1) plotting results of iPTH concentration in each patient against the simultaneously measured calcium concentration and (2) comparing and contrasting the individual test results with the results of such covariant analysis ([iPTH] × [Ca^{2+}]) with each type of patient group for whom extensive retrospective clinical correlation results have been made. A rectangular domain includes the values found for several hundred normal controls, a domain bounded laterally by the normal upper and lower limits of serum calcium and vertically by the lower limit of assay detection and the highest range of iPTH concentration found in normal subjects. Those patients with surgically documented hyperparathyroidism whose concentration of iPTH overlaps with the upper limit of normal assay values can usually (especially with several repeated assays) be discerned as abnormal because iPTH levels should be undetectable due to hypercalcemia if their parathyroids were normally responsive (see text below and legend to Fig. 350-1 for details of use of the assay in other states such as malignancy and hypoparathyroidism). One disturbing issue in assay interpretation of hypercalcemia not due to parathyroid disease is the possibility that renal failure may falsely elevate iPTH levels. Since the kidney is the principal site of excretion of carboxyl fragments of iPTH (Chap. 349), renal failure may lead to a detectable level of the carboxyl fragment (and hence a false-positive result for hyperparathyroidism), despite the fact that sufficient gland suppression has occurred to render iPTH itself undetectable in plasma.

Because of the small size of the parathyroids, even when hyperplastic or neoplastic, the variable position of the glands, and the complex anatomy of the neck, localization of abnormal parathyroid tissue at surgery is often difficult. For this reason several methods have been devised to attempt preoperative localization. *Roentgenographic examination of the esophagus* during barium swallow can reveal an indentation on the esophagus due to pressure from a large parathyroid. Because it is a simple procedure and occasionally rewarding, it should probably be performed routinely prior to surgery. Some success has been reported with *selenomethionine scans* and *thermography*. These procedures are not routinely applied in most centers, and there is little systematic experience. More success has been achieved with selective vascular sampling techniques combined with radioimmunoassay.

The technique of *percutaneous venous catheter sampling* of the veins of the neck and thorax, and parathyroid hormone radioimmunoassay of the samples so obtained, has been introduced as a method for preoperative localization of parathyroid tissue. In patients in whom a single adenoma is subsequently found at surgery, a marked unilateral gradient in hormone concentration is seen in the small thyroid veins on the side of the neoplasm. In patients who have abnormal parathyroid tissue on both sides of the neck (hyperplasia), on the other hand, gradients in hormone concentration are found on both sides of the thyroid plexus. Because of variations in drainage patterns, however, results of venous catheterization studies often allow a lateralization but not a localization; intramediastinal tumors may drain upward into the neck. Hence, it has been found that selective arteriography, guided by the results of venous catheterization, often is helpful in providing a precise anatomic location of the parathyroid tumor. It has been possible to distinguish preoperatively a single adenoma from hyperplasia of all four glands. Since the radiological expertise necessary to perform these angiographic studies is not available in many centers and overall experience is limited, the technique is recommended only for patients who present special diagnostic problems, or in whom previous neck surgery has failed to locate hyperfunctioning parathyroid tissue.

DIFFERENTIAL DIAGNOSIS The differential diagnosis of hyperparathyroidism is best considered under three general headings: (1) hypercalcemia, (2) nephrolithiasis, and (3) bone disease.

Hypercalcemia It must be emphasized that hyperparathyroidism is a chronic disorder. It is important to obtain historical features or clinical evidence such as recurrent renal colic, documented hypercalcemia many months earlier, or evidence of occult renal stones. Such evidence of chronicity usually favors the diagnosis of hyperparathyroidism rather than malignancy. On the other hand, if hypercalcemia has been detected only recently without other historical features of chronicity, the search for other causes of hypercalcemia must be particularly thorough. The pattern of high calcium with low phosphate is believed typical of hyperparathyroidism in contrast to many other causes of hypercalcemia where phosphate levels are normal or increased. However, severe hypercalcemia per se lowers phosphate.

MALIGNANCY Hypercalcemia is a frequent complication of malignant disease. The elimination of malignancy as the underlying cause of hypercalcemia can be one of the most difficult problems in differential diagnosis, particularly when one considers the possibility of pseudohyperparathyroidism. The patient's medical history, as well as physical and laboratory findings, are helpful in the differentiation. If a patient with hypercalcemia has a history of vague complaints and recurrent symptoms extending over several years prior to evaluation, it is less likely that occult malignant disease is responsible; if malignancy were the cause of the hypercalcemia, there should be definite evidence of the primary tumor or metastatic lesions.

Hypercalcemia complicating malignancy results from one of three processes: (1) osteolytic metastases, such as occur in carcinoma of the breast, or malignancies of the hematopoietic system, such as multiple myeloma; (2) pseudohyperparathyroidism with ectopic production of parathyroid hormone; and (3) pseudohyperparathyroidism secondary to production of humoral substances chemically distinct from parathyroid hormone. The syndrome of pseudohyperparathyroidism is usually suspected when skeletal x-ray survey or bone scan fails to reveal osteolytic lesions. Mild alkalosis rather than acidosis is often seen in pseudohyperparathyroidism. As outlined in Fig. 350-1, the results seen with measurements of iPTH in pseudohyperparathyroidism have been confusing with regard to etiology of the hypercalcemia in this syndrome and, to date, disappointing in diagnostic utility for distinguishing primary hyperparathyroidism from pseudohyperparathyroidism. In the experience of several laboratories there is clearly detectable iPTH in a number of patients with pseudohyperparathyroidism. In other laboratories, including that of the author, iPTH in pseudohyperparathyroidism is rarely, if ever, detected. The reasons for these discrepancies are unknown at present, but the results have unsettled the true prevalence of ectopic parathyroid hormone production in tumor-associated hypercalcemia.

SARCOIDOSIS In sarcoidosis the hypercalcemia presumably results from increased absorption of calcium from the gastrointestinal tract secondary to exaggerated sensitivity to vitamin D (this phenomenon may explain the hypocalcemic effect of glucocorticoids—inhibition of formation of the active forms of vitamin D). Hypercalcemia, when present, is usually a manifestation of severe involvement and disseminated disease. Hence evidence of pulmonary involvement is usually seen; chest x-ray may reveal a diffuse fibronodular infiltrate and/or prominent hilar adenopathy. An elevated blood gamma globulin may also be detected. In severe cases there may also be direct involvement of bone by the granulomatous process. The most definitive diagnostic procedure is demonstration of noncaseating granulomas by liver or lymph node biopsy, the latter usually of a scalene node. The hypercalcemia of sarcoidosis can present a difficult problem in differential diagnosis, especially since sarcoidosis may have existed for several years with many of the typical features of the disease lacking. In some patients abnormal pulmonary function tests such as exercise-induced hypoxia or abnormal carbon monoxide diffusion time may be found; such studies, performed in patients whose blood chemical indexes are atypical for primary hyperparathyroidism (low PTH values, normal phosphate), may focus attention on a more detailed search for pulmonary sarcoidosis. Measurements of iPTH in the absence of severe renal failure are helpful; invariably the levels are undetectable.

MULTIPLE MYELOMA Hypercalcemia is seen in approximately 40 percent of patients with multiple myeloma. It is presumably due to direct erosion of bone by the neoplastic cells. Some have reported evidence that a locally active agent, osteoclast-activating factor (OAF), may play a role in the pathogenesis. Typical "punched-out" lesions in bone may be detected on x-ray, particularly of the skull. Glucocorticoids lead to a reduction in the increased bone turnover; a lowering of blood calcium occurs within several days to a week following institution of therapy (a typical regimen is 40 mg prednisone per day). Steroids act by direct tumor suppression; improvement in marrow morphology, rise in hemoglobin, and reduction in abnormal urinary and plasma protein are found.

VITAMIN D INTOXICATION   The chronic ingestion of large doses of vitamin D can produce hypercalcemia. Usually the ingestion of doses in excess of 100,000 units of vitamin D_2 or D_3 for many months is necessary for this complication to occur. See Chap. 351 for etiology and treatment.

MILK-ALKALI SYNDROME (BURNETT'S SYNDROME)   In this unusual syndrome hypercalcemia and renal failure occur as a complication of long-term ingestion of large amounts of milk or calcium and absorbable antacids. The syndrome seems much less prevalent since the nonabsorbable antacids have been used in ulcer therapy. Possibly some of these patients have a pattern of excessive gastrointestinal absorption similar to that predicated to be present in idiopathic hypercalciuria. Alkalosis contributes to deposition of calcium phosphate in abnormal locations including the kidney. Because of the increased incidence of ulcer disease in primary hyperparathyroidism, the possibility that the milk-alkali syndrome may coexist with hyperparathyroidism should always be considered.

THYROTOXICOSIS   Significant hypercalcemia is a rare complication of thyrotoxicosis. However, minimal elevations of calcium have been reported in as many as 25 percent of patients with hyperthyroidism. Hypercalcemia in hyperthyroidism is presumably related to increased bone resorption; iPTH values are not elevated. The diagnosis usually offers no difficulties since, in most cases, it is the thyrotoxicosis rather than the hypercalcemia that brings the patient to the physician. However, particularly in the elderly, the signs of thyrotoxicosis may be minimal. If the serum calcium does not return toward normal as the thyrotoxicosis is brought under control, another cause for the hypercalcemia should be suspected.

ADRENAL INSUFFICIENCY   Hypercalcemia has been reported to occur in adrenal insufficiency, especially acute adrenal failure. The cause has not been determined. There is evidence that glucocorticoids and vitamin D have opposing actions on blood calcium. High doses of steroids lower blood calcium when given as replacement in adrenal crisis; it is assumed by some that the elevation in calcium in the state of adrenal insufficiency reflects in some way the result of glucocorticoid deficiency. Others, however, have suggested that the hypercalcemia is due merely to hemoconcentration and that the ionized calcium is normal. In any event, in acute adrenal failure hypercalcemia is only a transient phenomenon; blood calcium returns to normal with adrenal replacement therapy.

IDIOPATHIC HYPERCALCEMIA OF INFANCY   This is a rare syndrome characterized by hypercalcemia, often in association with multiple congenital cardiovascular lesions. Hypersensitivity to vitamin D has been postulated. The distinctive clinical features and age distribution of the syndrome make it unlikely to be a problem in the differential diagnosis of most cases of hypercalcemia in adults.

OTHER CAUSES OF HYPERCALCEMIA   Prolonged immobilization of a patient may lead to hypercalcemia, especially in patients with high rates of bone turnover, such as those with Paget's disease. Immobilization may also cause hypercalcemia in young patients who are undergoing rapid growth and, therefore, have higher bone turnover rates. The hypercalcemia and associated hypercalciuria resolve when the patient becomes ambulatory. Hypercalcemia may occur in renal disease as a complication of secondary hyperparathyroidism, particularly in subjects undergoing chronic hemodialysis or renal transplantation.

Nephrolithiasis   Nephrolithiasis must be considered in any discussion of the differential diagnosis of hyperparathyroidism. See Chap. 284 for detailed discussion. Recurrent episodes of formation of calcium-containing kidney stones are most often associated with metabolic or renal abnormalities unconnected with hyperparathyroidism. Nonetheless, a detailed search for hyperparathyroidism is indicated in patients who form calcium-containing kidney stones, even if hypercalcemia is not present at the time when nephrolithiasis first occurs.

A difficulty frequently encountered in the differential diagnosis of nephrolithiasis is to distinguish idiopathic hypercalciuria from hyperparathyroidism. In idiopathic hypercalciuria, there is a strong familial incidence, a preponderance in males, an increased urinary excretion of calcium, and a tendency to hypophosphatemia. In most patients the disorder reflects excessive dietary absorption of calcium with high calcium intake leading secondarily to increased urinary calcium (and thereby can be diagnosed). In patients in this category, iPTH should not be elevated; this finding may help in the differential diagnosis.

Hypercalciuria and the formation of calcium-containing stones have been recognized in a number of disorders in addition to hyperparathyroidism and idiopathic hypercalciuria. These include metastatic cancer, multiple myeloma, senile osteoporosis, Cushing's syndrome, phosphate diabetes, milk-alkali syndrome (in the initial phases), vitamin D intoxication, sarcoid, gout, and idiopathic hypercalcemia of infancy. In some instances hypercalcemia is present; in others blood calcium is normal. The differential diagnosis involves a careful examination for the cause of the hypercalcemia when present (as discussed in the preceding section). Hypercalciuria without hypercalcemia is noted with renal tubular disorders such as renal tubular acidosis, in which systemic acidosis may be responsible for increased bone resorption.

Bone disease   Discussion of the differential diagnosis of the common types of metabolic bone disease occurs subsequently (see Chap. 352). A few points should be stressed in considering the differentiation of hyperparathyroidism from other skeletal disorders. The only commonly occurring disorder in which hypercalcemia is found together with demineralization and localized areas of bone resorption is malignant disease with osteolytic metastases; patients with severe Paget's disease may develop hypercalcemia during periods of enforced immobilization.

The possibility of underlying hyperparathyroidism should always be considered when solitary bone rarefactions are detected; such a lesion could represent a bone cyst or brown tumor of the bone.

MEDICAL TREATMENT   Once the diagnosis of primary hyperparathyroidism has been made, surgery is the treatment of choice. However, a decision may be made to defer surgery. This is particularly true when mild asymptomatic hypercalcemia is discovered in an elderly patient or when other factors such as cardiovascular or pulmonary disease make the patient a poor operative risk. Too little is known about the natural history of hyperparathyroidism to automatically recommend surgery initially, particularly in older patients, if no signs or symptoms are present that are attributable to hyperparathyroidism. One may elect to follow such a patient carefully if hypercalcemia is not severe, e.g., less than 11.5 to 12.0 mg per 100 ml, and if osteopenia or other signs of bone disease, as well as renal complications, are lacking. If a decision not to operate is made, however, careful serial evaluation of bone and renal function is indicated to guard against silent renal or osseous deterioration. Alternatively, if the relation of vague constitutional symptoms to hypercalcemia is raised, it may be useful to evaluate the symptomatic response following the lowering of blood calcium. Since blood phosphate is low, administering sodium or potassium phosphate in doses of 1 to 2 g phosphate phosphorus daily may be useful. Phosphate promotes the deposition of calcium into the skeleton. However, complications such as metastatic calcification may develop during phosphate therapy. The occurrence of metastatic calcification appears related to the concentration of serum phosphate; therefore, phosphate should not be used in patients who have impaired renal function.

The alternate, and rather dramatic, indication for medical therapy develops when a patient without previous medical history of disorders related to calcium metabolism presents with severe hypercalcemia. Under these circumstances, it may be lifesaving to rapidly lower blood calcium to safe levels so that diagnostic studies can be performed.

After rehydration has been accomplished, it is now agreed that the most effective mode of therapy is intravenous infusion of isotonic sodium chloride, 4 to 5 liters daily, plus administration of a potent natriuretic agent such as furosemide. This mode of therapy can be undertaken only if renal function is adequate; strict records of intake and output must be kept and fluid overload avoided. Several grams of calcium may be excreted daily with this regimen, resulting in rapid lowering of blood calcium. The beneficial effects result from the linkage of sodium and calcium transport in the kidney tubule.

Intravenous phosphate is effective in lowering calcium but increases the hazard of widespread metastatic calcification. Mithramycin given as a single intravenous dose of 25 to 50 μg per kilogram of body weight may lower calcium to normal within several days; this approach serves as an alternate therapy if the saline-furosemide regimen cannot be applied.

SURGICAL TREATMENT Parathyroid exploration should be undertaken only by an experienced surgeon with the help of an equally astute pathologist. There are many critical decisions regarding management that can be best made only during the operation. The examination of tissue removed at surgery by frozen section should direct the subsequent course of the operation. The usual procedure recommended by the author and his colleagues, if an abnormal gland is identified and removed, is to search for at least one additional gland. If the second gland is normal in size and normal histologically (frozen section), a single adenoma is most likely. For this reason exploration is stopped when a normal gland is detected and a single enlarged gland is removed. Others have argued that several glands are usually involved in all cases and that subtotal parathyroidectomy is the procedure of choice. The risk of the former approach is lack of cure or early recurrence, the risk of the latter is hypoparathyroidism. One recent report has suggested that unilateral exploration was not followed by recurrence; however, further long-term follow-up of patients managed by each procedure seems indicated.

Hyperplasia involves more difficult diagnostic criteria and questions of surgical management. Once a diagnosis of hyperplasia has been established, it is necessary to identify all the glands. It usually is recommended that three glands be totally removed and that the fourth gland be partially excised; care should be taken to leave a good blood supply for the remaining gland. Some surgeons now advocate transplantation of some of the removed, minced tissue into the muscles of the forearm to avoid delayed vascular failure of residual tissue in the neck. The merits of the two approaches have not yet been compared systematically. There are documented cases of five or six glands, as well as unusual locations for adenoma. If no glandular abnormalities are found in the neck, further exploration must be undertaken. When parathyroid carcinoma is encountered, it is important that the tissue be widely excised; great care should be taken to avoid rupture of the capsule to prevent local seeding of the tumor.

Decline in serum calcium invariably occurs within 24 h after successful surgery; usually blood calcium falls to low normal values for 4 to 5 days until the remaining parathyroid tissue resumes hormone secretion. Severe postoperative hypocalcemia is likely to occur if there has been significant osteitis fibrosa or if there has been injury to the normal parathyroid glands during surgery.

For mild symptomatic hypocalcemia, oral calcium supplementation may suffice; if hypocalcemia is severe, intravenous calcium is necessary. It is usually convenient to prepare a solution of calcium (gluconate or chloride) at a concentration of 1 mg/ml in 5% dextrose in water. The rate and total duration of intravenous calcium therapy are determined by severity of symptoms and the response detected by frequently monitoring blood calcium levels. A rate of infusion of 0.5 to 2 (mg/kg)/h or 30 to 100 ml/h of the 1 mg/ml solution will usually suffice to relieve symptoms. Generally, parenteral therapy in most instances will be required for only a few days. If symptoms and/or need for parenteral calcium continue for more than 4 to 5 days, replacement therapy with vitamin D (or vitamin D metabolites) and/or calcium should be started (see "Hypoparathyroidism" below). A sudden rise in blood calcium after several months on vitamin D replacement therapy may indicate restoration of parathyroid function to normal.

Magnesium deficiency may also complicate the postoperative course of parathyroid surgery and represents an additional cause of tetany. Impaired secretion of parathyroid hormone has been demonstrated in magnesium deficiency.

Magnesium deficiency, indicated by hypomagnesemia, should therefore be corrected whenever detected. $MgCl_2$ is sufficiently soluble to be effective by mouth, but preparations of this compound are not widely available. Accordingly, repletion must usually be parenteral. Only a small fraction of total body magnesium is present in extracellular fluid, but total body Mg deficiency is reflected by hypomagnesemia. Since the depressant effect of magnesium on central and peripheral nerve functions is not seen below 4 meq per liter (normal range 1.5 to 2 meq per liter), parenteral replacement can be given at a vigorous rate. A dose as great as 2 meq/kg can be given if severe hypomagnesemia is detected. The magnesium is given either as an intravenous infusion over 8 to 12 h or in divided doses intramuscularly (magnesium sulfate, USP, the preparation normally used, is available as a 20% solution, 1 g or 8 meq/ml, or as a more concentrated solution, 50%).

SECONDARY HYPERPARATHYROIDISM

Secondary hyperparathyroidism is also a metabolic disorder characterized by excessive production of parathyroid hormone. It is encountered in various disease states in which there is resistance to the metabolic actions of parathyroid hormone.

Because of the resistance to the action of the hormone, these disease states are usually characterized by a mild degree of hypocalcemia, at least in the ionized fraction of blood calcium, despite the excessive secretion of parathyroid hormone.

Secondary hyperparathyroidism occurs in patients with some forms of osteomalacia, pseudohypoparathyroidism, and chronic renal disease. Correction of the osteomalacia with adequate vitamin D therapy or reversal of renal failure (as with successful renal transplant) should lead to regression of the hyperparathyroidism. This has been documented in patients with a successful renal transplant. In turn, these considerations lead to an important distinction between the character of abnormal growth of parathyroid glands in secondary hyperparathyroidism (reversible) and primary hyperparathyroidism (presumably irreversible). It is not clear, however, that in all patients with long-standing, secondary parathyroid hyperplasia the enlarged glands do revert to normal size and function after removal of the initial stimuli to hyperplasia.

The pathogenesis of the secondary hyperparathyroidism, deficient vitamin D metabolism, intestinal malabsorption, and osteodystrophy in chronic renal failure is difficult to analyze (see Chap. 274). A variable picture of bone disease may develop in association with hyperparathyroidism in chronic renal failure. (This is discussed in Chap. 352.) Occasionally, severe bone pain, widespread ectopic calcification, and severe pruritis may develop, and the question of subtotal parathyroidectomy may be raised. While this may be necessary, appreciation of the frequent, although not invariant, reversibility of the parathyroid hyperplasia has led to a more conservative attitude toward surgical intervention. Subtotal parathyroidectomy may lead to severe postoperative hypoparathyroidism. Medical treatment such as reduction of excessive blood phosphate by dietary phosphate restriction and use of nonabsorbable antacids, and better management of renal failure, may reverse ectopic calcification. Selective treatment with vitamin D analogues, especially 1,25-dihydroxyvitamin D_3 [1,25-$(OH)_2D_3$] in doses of 0.25 to 2.0 μg per day (see Chap. 351), has led to improvement in calcium absorption and blood calcium levels. It is hoped that these recent advances in medical therapy may eliminate the need for surgery of the parathyroids in many cases.

The stimulus responsible for hyperplasia of the parathyroids has not been identified. It seems possible that in all the conditions in which secondary hyperparathyroidism is found, resistance to hormone action accounts for persistent hypocalcemia in spite of increased hormone secretion. Chronic, even though partly compensated, hypocalcemia may be the stimulus that directly causes parathyroid hyperplasia. Specific aspects of the clinical features and approaches encountered in states of secondary hyperparathyroidism, in pseudohypoparathyroidism, and in osteomalacia (Chap. 352) are reviewed below.

In summary, present knowledge concerning the complex pattern of biosynthesis, secretion, and metabolism of parathyroid hormone, even in normal subjects, must be taken into account in attempting to understand the origins or predict the course of secondary hyperparathyroidism. Attempts to manage hyperparathyroidism by correction of underlying defects seems the most reasonable approach (whenever feasible) in view of the potential reversibility of this adaptive disorder of the parathyroids.

HYPOPARATHYROIDISM

Hypoparathyroidism is a metabolic abnormality characterized by hypocalcemia and consequent neuromuscular symptoms; the disease results from a deficiency of parathyroid hormone production or end organ resistance to the action of the hormone.

ETIOLOGY Postoperative hypoparathyroidism The most common cause of hypoparathyroidism is excision of the parathyroids or damage to the glands or their vascular supply during surgery for thyroid disorders, hyperparathyroidism, and radical neck dissections for cancer. Postoperative hypoparathyroidism is now much less frequent, not only because of improved awareness of the potential problem during thyroid surgery, but also because of the increased use of medical therapy for treatment of thyrotoxicosis. Although the symptoms of hypoparathyroidism usually develop several days after the operation, there can be a delay of months to years after neck surgery before the diagnosis is made. Although it has been speculated that in these patients the glands may slowly atrophy because of progressive ischemic damage following surgery, it is possible that signs and symptoms of hypocalcemia were overlooked. A different situation can also take place: transient hypoparathyroidism may occur immediately following thyroid surgery. In this situation it seems likely that the glands are initially injured, but gradually recover, or that a small remnant of remaining parathyroid tissue gradually hypertrophies. In this form of hypoparathyroidism secondary to trauma (analogous to idiopathic forms of the disorder, discussed below), results achieved by immunoassay (Fig. 350-1) and by newer assays, based on cytochemical methods believed to reflect biologically active hormone, have substantiated clinical evidence that parathyroid glandular failure may in some cases be partial rather than absolute.

Idiopathic hypoparathyroidism Idiopathic hypoparathyroidism is a relatively rare disease. A total lack of parathyroid function can be detected as (1) an isolated entity (idiopathic hypoparathyroidism), (2) in association with agenesis of the thymus (the Di George syndrome), or (3) in association with a familial disorder in which there may be a deficiency of thyroid, adrenal, and ovarian function, pernicious anemia, and other defects. The Di George syndrome is a rare disorder in which there is congenital absence of the thymus and the parathyroids, organs embryologically derived from the third and fourth branchial pouches. Patients with this syndrome usually die at 1 to 2 years of age of severe hypocalcemia, persistent infection, or both. The immune deficiency is of the cellular type. Delayed hypersensitivity reactions are deficient, and allograft rejections are absent. Humoral and circulating antibody mechanisms are intact. The striking features that result from the absence of the thymus make this syndrome quite distinctive.

The familial syndrome of hypoparathyroidism is unusual in several respects. An autoimmune basis for this disease has been suspected. These patients frequently have moniliasis, particularly in the fingernails. Recognition of the associated features is important because of the clinical problems encountered when adrenal failure or anemia develops. Careful periodic evaluation of a given patient or family members with respect to hematopoietic, adrenal, ovarian, and thyroid status is important. Antibodies have been detected to parietal cells, the parathyroids, adrenal cortex, thyroid, and ovary. However, there are poor correlations between the occurrence of the given endocrine deficiency and detection of endocrine organ-specific antibodies. The frequency of expression of the disease or of antibodies does not fit any simple pattern of inheritance. Nonetheless, it is clear that the several endocrine deficiency states may all appear eventually in a given individual or in family members (see Chap. 348).

Other causes of true hypoparathyroidism Hypoparathyroidism secondary to radiation therapy is very rare but has been reported. The gland presumably atrophies secondary to radiation damage after radioactive iodine therapy for thyrotoxicosis. An unusual form of hypoparathyroidism is its occurrence in an infant born of a mother with hyperparathyroidism. The high level of the circulating calcium in the mother's blood apparently inhibits the activity or development of the parathyroid glands in the infant. This form of hypoparathyroidism is usually transient.

Pseudohypoparathyroidism Pseudohypoparathyroidism is a rare hereditary disorder characterized by symptoms and signs of hypoparathyroidism in association with distinctive skeletal and developmental defects. The hypoparathyroidism is due to *deficient end organ response* to the endogenous hormone. Pseudohypoparathyroidism is characterized by excessive secretion of parathyroid hormone and hyperplasia of the parathyroids, a response to the resistance to hormone action at the target tissues—kidney and bone.

Many aspects of pseudohypoparathyroidism remain unclarified, including the relation between the skeletal and developmental defects and the hypoparathyroidism. Relatives of patients with pseudohypoparathyroidism often exhibit skeletal and developmental defects without any symptoms or chemical evidence of hypoparathyroidism, so-called "pseudopseudohypoparathyroidism." Some studies have suggested that defective stimulation of membrane-bound adenylate cyclase is the biochemical defect responsible for end organ resistance to the hormone. It has been shown that (1) there is an increased concentration of circulating parathyroid hormone in all subjects with pseudohypoparathyroidism (at least, if studied when they are hypocalcemic prior to the institution of vitamin D therapy) (Fig. 350-1), (2) there is no evidence for circulating antiparathyroid antibodies in any of these patients, and (3) there is evidence that the hormone made by these patients is biologically active.

Since, by definition, all patients with the complete syndrome are hypocalcemic and hyperphosphatemic, it has generally been believed that both bone and kidney are unresponsive, but certain observations are not consistent with a unitary view concerning pathophysiology. Some patients show an essentially normal phosphaturia following the injection of parathyroid hormone. Others show a detectable, even though subnormal, increase in urinary cyclic adenosine monophosphate (AMP) after administration of parathyroid extract. In one patient with pseudohypoparathyroidism previously treated with vitamin D, the removal of all four parathyroid glands was accompanied by a striking fall in serum calcium, requiring a massive increase in vitamin D to restore serum calcium toward normal. This may mean that during long-term vitamin D treatment, there is a significant contribution to extracellular fluid calcium from parathyroid hormone-driven bone resorption when sufficient parathyroid hypersecretion has developed, despite osseous resistance to parathyroid action.

Reports have accumulated concerning patients with hypocalcemia and hyperphosphatemia in whom evidence of osteitis fibrosa has been found by both x-ray and biopsy. This has led to the speculation that the renal end organ defect may be the most severe if not the sole abnormality in some patients. Studies have appeared which carefully document the restoration of a normal sensitivity to parathyroid hormone after vitamin D therapy in patients with typical pseudohypoparathyroidism. Although responses in blood and urinary calcium and phosphate levels to parathyroid hormone were normal, urinary cyclic AMP production remained impaired. Subjects with pseudohypoparathyroidism, unlike those patients with true hypoparathyroidism, usually excrete less excessive quantities of calcium in urine when their blood calcium is made normal after vitamin D treatment. This suggests that there is some renal end organ response with regard to the action of the increased levels of circulating hormone to reduce renal calcium clearance.

These varied observations suggest that end organ resistance may be less severe in some patients than in others or that vitamin D treatment alters end organ sensitivity. In addition, it may be true that bone is more responsive to hormone than kidney in certain patients with pseudohypoparathyroidism. Several additional clinical reports have appeared proposing an additional clinical subtype, pseudohyperparathyroidism type II, in which it is proposed that the bone and renal receptors for parathyroid-stimulated adenyl cyclase are intact but that there is a failure of normal calcium and phosphate transport systems to respond to the cyclic AMP generated. The difficulty in obtaining clear-cut responses in renal phosphate clearance to injected parathyroid hormone even in normal subjects without carefully standardized conditions and clear indication of partial rather than complete end organ unresponsiveness in pseudohypoparathyroidism suggests the need for considerable caution in defining precise or distinct subtypes of this complex hereditary syndrome. Further work may, however, reveal heterogeneity of the pathophysiology in these peculiar heritable syndromes associated with end organ hyporesponsiveness to PTH. It also seems possible (but has yet to be proved) that some patients with high iPTH concentrations in blood, yet evidence of functional hypoparathyroidism, may secrete biologically ineffective hormone (see Chap. 349).

Little can be said at the present time about the pathophysiology of the multiple skeletal and developmental effects in these patients. In any event, the hereditary aspects of pseudohypoparathyroidism have been well established. Pseudohypoparathyroidism is usually found within kindreds in which some other family members also have pseudohypoparathyroidism or the metabolically normal variant of the disorder, pseudopseudohypoparathyroidism. However, the exact mode of genetic inheritance is still uncertain, and the variable expression of metabolic abnormalities in affected individuals is not understood. Some analyses have suggested that the two linked disorders, pseudopseudohypoparathyroidism and pseudohypoparathyroidism, are transmitted as an X-linked dominant. The sex incidence is 2:1 affected females versus males. However, the disease is extremely rare, and the total number of patients and of involved sibships is small for purposes of suitable statistical analysis. Furthermore, acceptance of some cases as authentic examples of the syndrome on the basis of literature reports is difficult, particularly with respect to the metabolically normal individuals (those with pseudopseudohypoparathyroidism). Certain of the developmental defects such as short stature, short metacarpal or metatarsal bones, and/or even basal ganglion calcification are found in Turner's syndrome, Gardner's syndrome, basal-cell nevus syndrome, and other hereditary disorders that are believed to be genetically distinct.

SIGNS AND SYMPTOMS Most of the symptoms of hypoparathyroidism reflect altered neuromuscular irritability due to the decreased concentration of ionized calcium. The age of onset of symptoms is earlier in pseudohypoparathyroidism than in idiopathic hypoparathyroidism.

Tetany and convulsions represent the most serious complications in hypoparathyroidism. Latent tetany can be elicited by tapping the facial nerve and producing a contraction of the facial muscles (Chvostek's sign), or by application of a tourniquet or blood pressure cuff leading to carpopedal spasm (Trousseau's sign). Increased bone density may occasionally be present in hypoparathyroidism; however, there may be no detectable skeletal abnormalities.

A complication perhaps related to the hyperphosphatemia is the frequent occurrence of *soft-tissue calcification*. In pseudohypoparathyroidism the mineral deposits in ectopic sites may include the development of true bone. True bone formation in ectopic sites is never seen in idiopathic hypoparathyroidism. Amorphous deposits of calcium and phosphate are found in the basal ganglia. Calcification of the basal ganglia is noted in as many as 50 percent of the patients. Most patients with pseudopseudohypoparathyroidism do not have ectopic calcium deposits.

The skeletal and developmental abnormalities that are found in both pseudohypoparathyroidism and pseudopseudohypoparathyroidism include short stature, round face, short neck, thick, stocky body build, and multiple discrete abnormalities in individual bones of the skeleton. Abnormally short metacarpal and metatarsal bones and sometimes phalanges have been reported. These defects seem to be due to premature closure of the epiphyses. The most classic finding is an *abnormally short fourth and fifth metacarpal and metatarsal.* This defect may be unilateral. Exostoses are frequently reported. Usually only one or two are detected, but occasionally multiple exostoses are found. Radius curvus may be present in some patients.

Multiple abnormalities are detected in tooth formation. The nails may be fragile and skin dry; moniliasis is commonly found in true hypoparathyroidism but not in pseudohypoparathyroidism. Mental deficiency is rather common in patients with pseudohypoparathyroidism. It seems most probable that this is part of the inherited syndrome. In any event, there is little improvement in mental status even with adequate therapy with calcium and vitamin D. Distinctive impairment in olfaction and taste has also been reported in the majority of patients examined. In addition, unusual dermatoglyphic abnormalities have been noted.

In pseudohypoparathyroidism there is an increased incidence of diabetes (or an abnormal glucose tolerance curve) and hypothyroidism. Recent studies have indicated that hypothyroidism, at least in some patients, is due to isolated thyrotropin deficiency.

DIAGNOSIS AND DIFFERENTIAL DIAGNOSIS Typically, the diagnosis of hypoparathyroidism is considered in a patient who has symptoms of hypocalcemia and is found to have both hypocalcemia and hyperphosphatemia in the presence of normal renal function. Clinically, the patient's history or physical features may be helpful in suggesting the diagnosis. A history of neck surgery with difficulties dating from that time points to postsurgical hypoparathyroidism. Pseudohypoparathyroidism is more likely than true hypoparathyroidism if unusual skeletal and developmental defects are detected or if there is a family history of other sibs with short stature and skeletal abnormalities. However, a definitive diagnosis, particularly for pseudohypoparathyroidism, must be established through application of specific laboratory tests. Two specific tests should be used, namely, the *parathyroid hormone radioimmunoassay* and *measurement of urinary cyclic AMP excretion* following the administration of parathyroid hormone.

Patients with *symptomatic hypocalcemia*, particularly if the history and physical examination suggest chronicity of the hypocalcemia (such as gradual onset of symptoms and evidence of ectopic calcification), would be expected to have secondary hyperparathyroidism if the parathyroid glands are functional. If no parathyroid hormone is detected by radioimmunoassay,

notwithstanding the stimulus of marked hypocalcemia, then true hypoparathyroidism is the most likely diagnosis. As noted in Fig. 350-1, not all patients with idiopathic hypoparathyroidism have undetectable levels of iPTH; some patients show values in the lower half of normal. Nonetheless, if not undetectable, the concentrations are lower than expected for the degree of hypocalcemia and thereby confirm the diagnosis. If elevated concentrations of parathyroid hormone are found, pseudohypoparathyroidism due to end organ resistance is more likely. In such cases, renal end organ resistance can be demonstrated by measuring the urinary excretion of cyclic AMP in response to the injection of a standard dose of parathyroid hormone. Normal subjects, patients with idiopathic or postsurgical hypoparathyroidism, and patients with pseudopseudohypoparathyroidism exhibit a ten- to twentyfold increase in urinary cyclic AMP secretion. In those with pseudohypoparathyroidism, little, if any, response is noted.

Hypocalcemia may be encountered not only in hypoparathyroidism but also in malabsorption, osteomalacia secondary to true vitamin D lack or vitamin D resistance, renal failure, hypoproteinemia, pancreatitis, and acute nutritional deficiency with associated hypomagnesemia. In patients with *malabsorption,* true vitamin D lack, vitamin D resistance, or renal failure, the parathyroid hormone concentration by radioimmunoassay is increased. Secondary hyperparathyroidism apparently results from the chronic hypocalcemia that accompanies these diseases. The manifestations of *renal failure,* including phosphate retention, are usually obvious when hypocalcemia is found. Patients with *osteomalacia* usually show a low serum phosphorus, an apparent reflection of the persistence of the action of parathyroid hormone on renal phosphate excretion in spite of the deficiency of vitamin D that interferes with the effective action of the hormone on bone.

Hypoproteinemia causes a reduction in total serum calcium because of reduced binding protein. Subjects with this abnormality have a normal ionized serum calcium concentration and lack symptoms of hypocalcemia. Correction for the total calcium concentration in patients with hypoproteinemia is based on the known binding of calcium by albumin and globulin. Episodes of *acute pancreatitis* are associated with hypocalcemia, but this is present only during the acute phase of the illness. The explanation for the hypocalcemia in pancreatitis, although much discussed, remains unknown.

There is an increasingly frequent recognition of the syndrome of hypocalcemia in patients with *hypomagnesemia.* Severe hypomagnesemia, less than 0.8 meq per liter, reflects serious intracellular magnesium deficits. Recent reports have emphasized that a state of functional hypoparathyroidism is associated with severe hypomagnesemia. Parathyroid hormone secretion is severely blunted or totally blocked in such patients. Earlier reports, especially in animals, suggested that magnesium deficiency may also be associated with reduced peripheral responsiveness to parathyroid hormone, but impaired secretion of the hormone may be the more important cause of hypocalcemia. Parenteral correction of the hypomagnesemia over several days restores normal parathyroid responsiveness. For details of therapy with magnesium, see the discussion above under treatment of magnesium deficits following surgery in hyperparathyroidism. Recognition of this syndrome is important to avoid unnecessary and expensive diagnostic evaluation for some unusual cause of parathyroid failure in patients with hypomagnesemia.

TREATMENT The principal aim of treatment is to restore calcium toward normal by use of supplementary dietary calcium and vitamin D and thereby relieve symptoms of increased neuromuscular irritability. However, it is not clear whether the other complications of hypoparathyroidism can be as readily controlled despite therapy which appears to be adequate for regulation of blood calcium. It has been noted that lenticular opacities may progress despite therapy.

There are numerous problems in achieving proper regulation of calcium metabolism in patients with hypoparathyroidism. Continued treatment with adequate doses of vitamin D presents several difficulties. Urinary calcium excretion is often excessive in hypoparathyroidism owing to the lack of the normal parathyroid effect to lower urine calcium clearance. This leads to the anomalous result that patients with hypoparathyroidism may develop nephrolithiasis during therapy which maintains blood calcium only at low normal concentration. Excessive urinary calcium excretion is typically not seen in pseudohypoparathyroidism. Vitamin D intoxication may develop without any apparent change in a dosage of vitamin D and calcium that has been optimal for several years. If hypercalcemia occurs, the long duration of action of vitamin D may result in persistence of hypercalcemia for weeks after the vitamin D has been discontinued. Despite these potential complications, most patients with hypoparathyroidism can be adequately regulated; complications can be avoided if the effects of therapy are continually monitored by frequent determinations of urinary as well as blood calcium concentration.

A practical approach to the chronic treatment of hypoparathyroidism at present involves initial use of less expensive agents with careful attention to complications and the use of newer, more expensive analogues of vitamin D only if more conventional measures prove inadequate. Vitamin D is given, usually as ergocalciferol (vitamin D_2), in a dose of 50,000 to 100,000 units per day; several grams of additional elemental calcium as citrate, lactate, or gluconate are usually provided (calcium lactate contains 13 percent calcium). Appropriate adjustments in dosage are made to achieve a blood calcium of 8.5 to 9.0 mg per 100 ml; it is important to appreciate that often weeks are required before the full effects of an increased dose of vitamin D are manifest. Patients should be seen at frequent intervals, particularly when dose schedules are initially established or readjusted; blood and urine calcium estimations provide the early clues to excessive or inadequate dosage of vitamin D.

Dihydrotachysterol (DHT) or the 1α-hydroxylated active metabolites of vitamin D are theoretically preferable to vitamin D alone because of the defective activity of the renal 1α-hydroxylase in states of hypoparathyroidism or parathyroid hormone resistance (as discussed in Chap. 351 on the metabolism of vitamin D). If a patient is unusually resistant to vitamin D and, therefore, difficult to maintain symptom-free, if the therapeutic margin between hypocalcemia and hypercalciuria in a given patient is excessively narrow, or if one or more episodes of vitamin D intoxication have occurred, dihydrotachysterol in doses of 1.0 to 1.5 mg per day, or $1\alpha,25\text{-}(OH)_2D_3$ in doses of 0.25 to 1.0 μg per day, may be substituted for vitamin D.

Interesting effects of magnesium administration have been noted during evaluation and management of patients with hypoparathyroidism. It has been reported that in several patients in whom vitamin D resistance of unusual degree was observed, hypomagnesemia was discovered. Supplemental magnesium therapy led to greater responsiveness to a given dose of vitamin D, and such patients maintained a more normal blood calcium concentration. The explanation for the beneficial effect of magnesium is not understood, but hypomagnesemia should be searched for in patients who are difficult to control. It is possible, of course, that the degree of parathyroid gland failure was made worse by hypomagnesemia; in that event, the beneficial effects of magnesium therapy on responsiveness to high-dose vitamin D therapy may have been indirect via effects on PTH.

In general, it can be concluded that satisfactory maintenance of mineral ion deficits can be achieved in hypoparathyroid subjects with supplemental calcium plus vitamin D or

vitamin D analogues. However, vitamin D is not a perfect substitute for parathyroid hormone, particularly in view of different effects on renal calcium conservation and the higher requirement for vitamin D in parathyroid deficiency. Hence all patients with hypoparathyroidism, particularly idiopathic or postsurgical hypoparathyroidism, must be reexamined at appropriate intervals of 6 months to 1 year to ensure adequate treatment schedules and particularly to detect complications, hypercalciuria, or onset of more severe vitamin D intoxication.

REFERENCES

ANAST CS et al: Impaired release of parathyroid hormone in magnesium deficiency. J Clin Endocrinol Metab 42:707, 1976

BLIZZARD RM et al: The incidence of parathyroid and other antibodies in the area of patients with idiopathic hypoparathyroidism. Clin Exp Immunol 1:119, 1966

BURNETT CH et al: Hypercalcemia without hypercalcuria or hypophosphatemia. Calcinosis and renal insufficiency: A syndrome following prolonged ingestion of milk and alkali. N Engl J Med 240:787, 1949

DREZNER M et al: Pseudohypoparathyroidism type II: A possible defect in the reception of the cyclic AMP signal. N Engl J Med 289:1056, 1973

HABENER JF, POTTS JT JR: Chemistry, biosynthesis, secretion, and metabolism of parathyroid hormone, in *Handbook of Physiology,* sec 7: *Endocrinology,* vol II, GD Aurbach (ed). Washington, DC, American Physiological Society, 1976, p 313

——, ——: Biosynthesis of parathyroid hormone. N Engl J Med 299:580, 635, 1978

——, ——: Parathyroid physiology and primary hyperparathyroidism, in *Metabolic Bone Disease,* LV Avioli, SM Krane (eds). New York, Academic, 1978, vol II, p 1

MENNES P et al: Hypomagnesemia and impaired parathyroid hormone secretion in chronic renal disease. Ann Intern Med 88:206, 1978

NAGANT DE DEUXCHAISNES C, KRANE SM: Hypoparathyroidism, in *Metabolic Bone Disease,* LV Avioli, SM Krane (eds). New York, Academic, 1978, vol II, p 218

NEER RM et al: Effects of 1α-hydroxyvitamin D_3 and 1,25-dihydroxyvitamin D_3 on calcium and phosphorus metabolism in hypoparathyroidism. Metabolism 12:1403, 1975

POTTS JT JR: Pseudohypoparathyroidism, in *The Metabolic Basis of Inherited Disease,* 4th ed, JB Stanbury et al (eds). New York, McGraw-Hill, 1978, pp 1350-1365

RODMAN JS, SHERWOOD, LM: Disorders of mineral metabolism in malignancy, in *Metabolic Bone Disease,* LV Avioli, SM Krane (eds). New York, Academic, 1978, vol II, p 578

RUDE RK et al: Parathyroid hormone secretion in magnesium deficiency. J Clin Endocrinol Metab 47:800, 1978

SEYBERTH HW et al: Prostaglandins as mediators of hypercalcemia associated with certain types of cancer. N Engl J Med 293:1278, 1975

351
VITAMIN D

MICHAEL F. HOLICK
JOHN T. POTTS, JR.

Intensive research during the past decade has greatly broadened concepts of vitamin D metabolism and action, and has brought the realization that vitamin D is a hormone, not a vitamin. With adequate sunlight, no dietary supplements are needed. The active principle of vitamin D is synthesized under

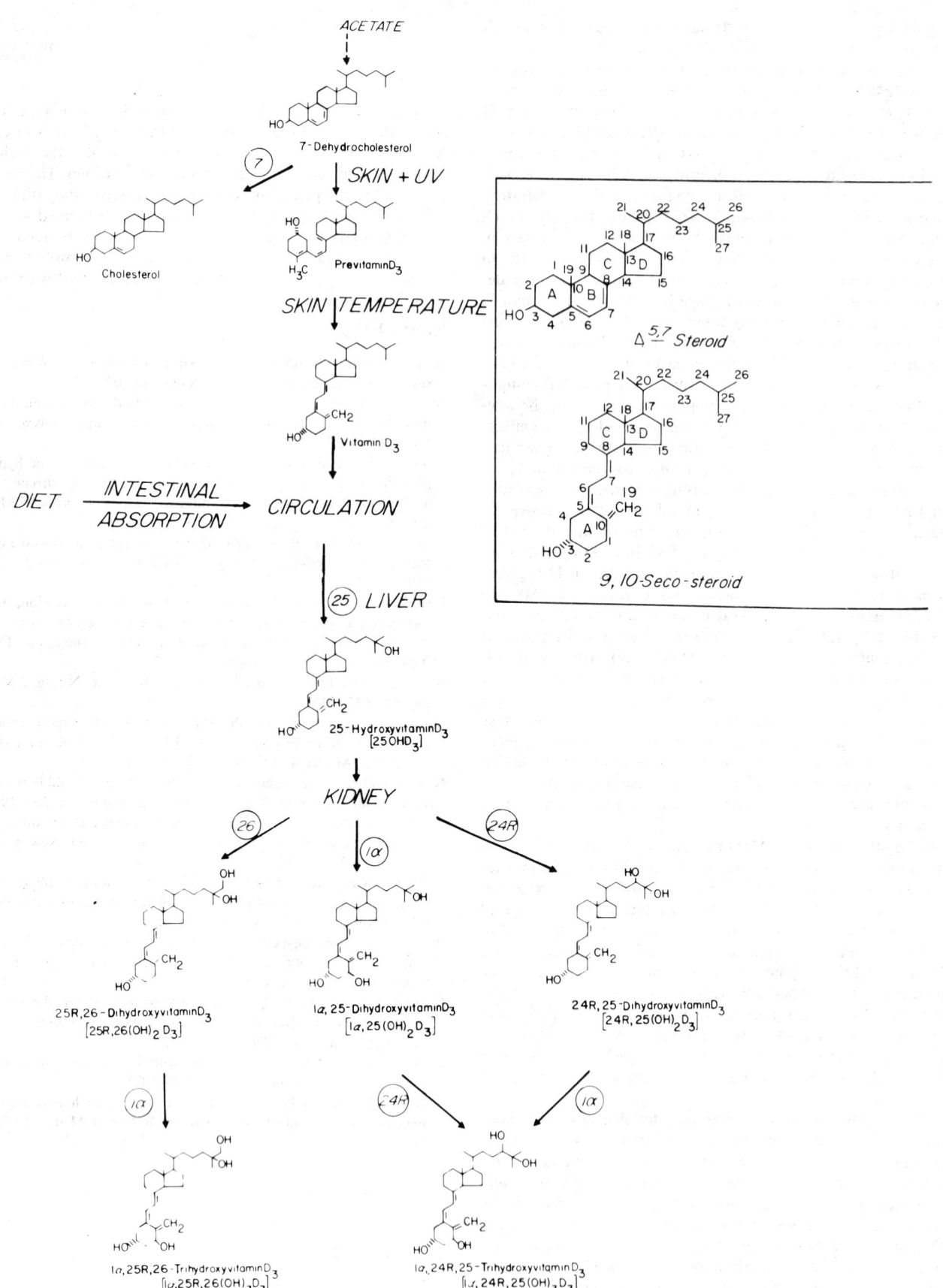

FIGURE 351-1

Photobiogenesis and metabolic pathways for vitamin D production and metabolism. Circled letters and numbers denote specific enzymes: 7 = 7-dehydrocholesterol reductase; 25 = vitamin D 25-hydroxylase; 1α = 25-OHD 1α-hydroxylase; 24R = 25-OHD 24R-hydroxylase; 26 = 25-OHD 26-hydroxylase. The insert denotes the basic Δ^{5,7}-diene steroid and 9,10-secosteroid structures and nomenclature.

metabolic control via successive hydroxylations in the liver and kidney and is transported through the blood to its target tissues (the small intestine and bone) to help maintain calcium homeostasis. Calcium and phosphate ions, parathyroid hormone (PTH), and possibly other peptide and steroid hormones play major roles directly or indirectly in the regulation of the renal metabolism of vitamin D. Analysis of the physiological control of vitamin D metabolism and studies of hereditary and acquired defects in these metabolic processes have provided new insights into the pathophysiology of several disorders involving calcium, phosphorus, and bone metabolism. These discoveries have made possible several advances, including the chemical synthesis of new vitamin D metabolites and analogs, the clinical use of $1\alpha,25$-dihydroxyvitamin D_3 [$1\alpha,25$-$(OH)_2D_3$] in many vitamin D–resistant disorders, the development and application of assays for measuring vitamin D metabolites in blood to define suspected abnormalities in vitamin D metabolism, and a growing interest in developing more potent analogues for clinical use.

CHEMISTRY AND NOMENCLATURE OF VITAMIN D Vitamin D is a derivative of $\Delta^{5,7}$-diene steroids. [The Δ represents a double bond, the location(s) of which is indicated by the superscript number(s).] Upon exposure to ultraviolet light the steroid precursor of vitamin D (7-dehydrocholesterol, *provitamin D*) undergoes a photochemical reaction that results in the cleavage of a C—C bond between C_9 and C_{10}, thereby opening ring B to generate a 9,10-secosteroid, *previtamin D* (Fig. 351-1). Previtamin D, a thermally labile intermediate, undergoes a molecular rearrangement involving its conjugated triene system (three double bonds) to a thermally stable 9,10-secosteroid, vitamin D (Fig. 351-1).

Historically, the subscripts for vitamin D are related to the order in which the compounds were isolated and characterized. What was originally called vitamin D_1 was found to be a mixture of compounds, and the term was consequently dropped. The next two vitamin D compounds, vitamin D_2 (ergocalciferol) and vitamin D_3 (cholecalciferol), were isolated, respectively, from the irradiation products of ergosterol (a $\Delta^{5,7}$-diene steroid found primarily in plants) and 7-dehydrocholesterol (a $\Delta^{5,7}$-diene steroid precursor of cholesterol present in animal tissues, including human). The only structural difference between vitamins D_2 and D_3 is in their side chains; the side chain for vitamin D_2 differs in that it contains a Δ^{22} and a C_{24}-methyl group. Even though vitamin D_3 is the endogenous product in most mammals, including humans, both vitamins D_2 and D_3 are metabolized in identical fashion and have equivalent biologic effects; in the absence of a subscript the term *vitamin D* may refer to either compound.

In steroid nomenclature, substituents on the steroid ring skeleton that are spatially oriented below the plane of the molecule (drawn as a broken line) are called α *substituents,* and those substituents spatially oriented above the plane of the molecule (drawn as a solid line) are called β *substituents.* Because vitamin D is a structural derivative of a $\Delta^{5,7}$-diene steroid, by convention the numbering of the carbon atoms and the stereochemical designation of the functional groups remain the same as for the parent steroid (Fig. 351-1). During the transformation $\Delta^{5,7}$-diene → previtamin D → vitamin D, the geometric position of ring A is altered, thereby changing the stereochemical orientation of its substituents; nonetheless, the original designation(s) of the hydroxyl function(s) on ring A of the steroid precursor are retained.

The R,S notation, as in 24R,25-dihydroxyvitamin D_3 (Fig. 351-1), specifies the spatial configuration of a substituent at an asymmetric carbon center (see Bell for details).

When vitamin D is chemically manipulated to rotate the A ring through 180°, the C_3-β-OH assumes a geometric position that mimics the C_1-α-OH (Fig. 351-2). These compounds, called *pseudo-1α-hydroxyvitamin D analogues,* include dihydrotachysterol and 5,6-*trans*-vitamin D_3. These analogues are less effective in stimulating intestinal calcium transport on a weight basis than either vitamin D or $1\alpha,25$-$(OH)_2D_3$ when vitamin D metabolism is normal. However, because these pseudo-1α-hydroxyvitamin D analogues do not require a renal 1α-hydroxylation to be active on intestinal calcium transport, they are at least three to ten times more potent than vitamin D in disease states that adversely affect the renal 25-hydroxyvitamin D 1α-hydroxylase, such as hypoparathyroidism and chronic renal failure. These pseudo-1α-hydroxy analogues are efficiently metabolized in the liver to their corresponding 25-hydroxy derivatives, which are the biologically active forms. 1α-Hydroxyvitamin D_3 (1α-OHD_3) is a potent $1\alpha,25$-$(OH)_2D_3$ agonist. The structure of this analogue is identical to that of the renal hormone with the exception that it lacks a C_{25}-OH (Fig. 351-2). In humans, this analogue is rapidly metabolized by the liver to $1\alpha,25$-$(OH)_2D_3$, the biologically active molecule.

BIOCHEMISTRY, PHYSIOLOGY, AND METABOLISM OF VITAMIN D Photobiogenesis of vitamin D_3 When skin is exposed to sunlight, the ultraviolet light energy that passes through the atmospheric ozone layer (between wavelengths $\approx$ 290 and 320 nm) is responsible for the photochemical conversion of epidermal stores of 7-dehydrocholesterol (provitamin D_3) to previtamin D_3. Previtamin D_3 slowly converts to vitamin D_3 by a nonenzymatic process; for example, at 37°C approximately 50

FIGURE 351-2

When vitamin D is treated with I_2 or reduced with H_2, ring A of the vitamin D molecule rotates 180° to spatially reorient the 3β-OH in a pseudo-1α-OH position. These analogues, 5,6-trans-vitamin D_3 and dihydrotachysterol$_3$ (DHT$_3$), are called pseudo-1α-hydroxy analogues. 1α-OHD$_3$ is a synthetic analogue of $1\alpha,25$-$(OH)_2D_3$ that lacks a C_{25}-OH. 1α-OHD$_3$, 5,6-trans-vitamin D_3, and DHT$_3$ all undergo a hepatic C_{25}-hydroxylation before they are biologically active.

percent of previtamin D_3 is converted to vitamin D_3 in 24 h. This unique process ensures that vitamin D_3 is continuously made in the skin from the previtamin for days after sun exposure (Fig. 351-1). Only when skin irradiation is limited and insufficient to produce required quantities of vitamin D_3 is there a need for dietary supplementation to prevent skeletal mineralization defects. Fish-liver oils are a natural source of vitamin D_3 and were used widely for the treatment of rickets early in this century. Now crystalline vitamin D_2 or vitamin D_3 is added to various foodstuffs such as milk, milk products, and cereals. Such supplementations have been effective in preventing rickets in countries that permit them. The daily requirement for vitamin D in adults has not been established; the National Research Council of the United States has recommended an intake of 400 IU per day (1 IU = 0.025 μg). Once vitamin D enters the circulation, either by its absorption in the small intestine from the diet or through the skin, it is transported through the circulation by a specific transport protein, an α_1 globulin, to the liver for its first hydroxylation.

Metabolism of vitamin D In the liver, vitamin D is metabolized to 25-hydroxyvitamin D (25-OHD) by a hepatic mitochondrial and/or microsomal enzyme(s), vitamin D 25-hydroxylase(s) (Fig. 351-1). 25-OHD is one of the major circulating metabolites of vitamin D. The concentration of 25-OHD in the circulation, as with other metabolites of vitamin D, is measured by competitive binding assays in which displacement of radioactive 25-OHD from binding sites on the plasma transport protein or tissue receptor is used to quantitate 25-OHD in serum samples. Estimates of the concentration of this metabolite vary somewhat among laboratories; however, there is general agreement that the concentration of 25-OHD is greater than 5 ng/ml and less than 80 ng/ml. Assays using prior chromatographic separation techniques give lower estimates, perhaps because other vitamin D metabolites may simulate the reaction given by 25-OHD in this assay. The normal range, apparently independent of method, is lower in Great Britain than in the United States; in Great Britain dietary supplementation with vitamin D is not used, and exposure to sunlight is less than in many regions of the United States. The serum 25-OHD levels routinely measured reflect both 25-OHD_2 and 25-OHD_3. The ratio of these two 25-hydroxylated derivatives depends on the relative amounts of vitamins D_2 or D_3 present in the diet and upon the amount of previtamin D_3 that is produced by exposure to sunlight. It was initially believed that this hepatic hydroxylation was regulated by a product feedback mechanism in such a way that 25-OHD levels were closely controlled. Now it is clear that this reaction is not tightly regulated; an increase in dietary intake or endogenous production of vitamin D is reflected by linear elevations in 25-OHD levels in the serum. The levels can rise to greater than 500 ng/ml when the intake of vitamin D is increased markedly. Serum 25-OHD levels are reduced in severe chronic parenchymal and cholestatic liver disease.

25-OHD is not considered biologically active at physiological levels in vivo, but it can be shown to be active in vitro at high concentrations. Normally, after formation in the liver 25-OHD is bound by the high-affinity vitamin D–binding protein of plasma and is transported to the kidney for an additional stereospecific hydroxylation on either C_1 or C_{24} (Fig. 351-1). The kidney plays a pivotal role in the metabolism of 25-OHD to biologically active metabolites. The renal mitochondrial 25-OHD 1α-hydroxylase activity is enhanced by hypocalcemia so that the rate of conversion of 25-OHD to $1\alpha,25\text{-(OH)}_2\text{D}$ increases. However, hypocalcemia does not directly control this hydroxylation. Any decrease in the serum calcium level below normal is a stimulus for increased secretion of parathyroid hor-

mone (PTH). In addition to acting on mineral metabolism in the bone and kidney (see Chap. 349), PTH also acts physiologically as a tropic hormone to increase the synthesis of $1\alpha,25\text{-(OH)}_2\text{D}$. The mechanism by which PTH exerts its influence on the renal metabolism of 25-OHD is not established. Certain lines of evidence suggest that effects of PTH on phosphate metabolism may mediate the regulation of the production of $1\alpha,25\text{-(OH)}_2\text{D}$; in thyroparathyroidectomized rats, 25-OHD is metabolized to $1\alpha,25\text{-(OH)}_2\text{D}$ when the serum phosphate level is kept below normal, even if hypercalcemia is induced. When hyperphosphatemia is produced in these animals by increasing dietary phosphate, the renal production of $1\alpha,25\text{-(OH)}_2\text{D}$ is diminished, and, in turn, 25-OHD is metabolized to $24R,25\text{-(OH)}_2\text{D}$. On the basis of studies in chickens, some investigators have questioned whether serum or renal tissue phosphorus levels exclusively, or even principally, regulate the renal 25-OHD 1α-hydroxylase; however, the bulk of the available data in humans and animals suggests that the renal production of $1\alpha,25\text{-(OH)}_2\text{D}$ is closely correlated with the serum phosphorus concentration. $1\alpha,25\text{-(OH)}_2\text{D}$ also influences the renal metabolism of 25-OHD by diminishing 25-OHD 1α-hydroxylase activity and enhancing the metabolism of 25-OHD to $24R,25\text{-(OH)}_2\text{D}$.

$24R,25\text{-(OH)}_2\text{D}$ is a circulating metabolite of 25-OHD that is normally present in serum at concentrations considerably higher than that of $1\alpha,25\text{-(OH)}_2\text{D}$. Studies using competitive protein-binding assays have led to estimates that serum $24R,25\text{-(OH)}_2\text{D}$ levels are 0.5 to 5 ng/ml. $24R,25\text{-(OH)}_2\text{D}$ is also a substrate for the renal 25-OHD 1α-hydroxylase and is converted to $1\alpha,24R,25$-trihydroxyvitamin D [$1\alpha,24R,25\text{-(OH)}_3\text{D}$]. This trihydroxy metabolite is less potent than $1\alpha,25\text{-(OH)}_2\text{D}$ in stimulating intestinal calcium transport; whether it has a physiological role in maintaining calcium homeostasis is unclear. The kidney is not the only organ that converts 25-OHD to $24R,25\text{-(OH)}_2\text{D}$; cartilage and chondrocyte cultures also metabolize 25-OHD to $24R,25\text{-(OH)}_2\text{D}$. $24R,25\text{-(OH)}_2\text{D}$ is more potent than $1\alpha,25\text{-(OH)}_2\text{D}$ in stimulating chondrocyte protein synthesis in vitro, and reports indicate that $24R,25\text{-(OH)}_2\text{D}$ has preferential effects on bone mineralization in a vitamin D–deficient animal model compared with $1\alpha,25\text{-(OH)}_2\text{D}$. There are also data to indicate that $24R,25\text{-(OH)}_2\text{D}$ stimulates intestinal calcium absorption in human subjects without increasing renal calcium excretion; these effects, however, are different from those seen with $1\alpha,25\text{-(OH)}_2\text{D}$. These observations have led some authors to speculate that $24R,25\text{-(OH)}_2\text{D}$ may play an important role in the expression of vitamin D action, especially on the skeleton; others remain skeptical about the biological importance of $24R,25\text{-(OH)}_2\text{D}$ per se as distinct from actions resulting from its conversion to $1\alpha,24R,25\text{-(OH)}_3\text{D}$.

The kidney also possesses a third enzyme that metabolizes 25-OHD to form 25R,26-dihydroxyvitamin D [$25R,26\text{-(OH)}_2\text{D}$]. $25R,26\text{-(OH)}_2\text{D}$, like $24R,25\text{-(OH)}_2\text{D}$, is metabolized by the kidney to a metabolite believed to be $1\alpha,25R,26$-trihydroxyvitamin D. $25R,26\text{-(OH)}_2\text{D}$ is less active than $1\alpha,25\text{-(OH)}_2\text{D}$ in inducing intestinal calcium transport, and the physiological function of this dihydroxy metabolite, if any, remains to be defined.

$1\alpha,25\text{-(OH)}_2\text{D}$ is a substrate for the 25-OHD 24R-hydroxylase and is metabolized to $1\alpha,24R,25\text{-(OH)}_2\text{D}$, but this conversion is not believed to be important for the expression of biologic activity of $1\alpha,25\text{-(OH)}_2\text{D}$. Recently, attention has been focused on the metabolic cleavage of the side chain of $1\alpha,25\text{-(OH)}_2\text{D}$. These efforts have led to the identification of a $1\alpha,25\text{-(OH)}_2\text{D}$ metabolite that was formed by an oxidative cleavage of the side chain at C_{23}—C_{24} and is called 1α-hydroxytetranorvitamin D 23-carboxylic acid. The biological function(s), if any, for this metabolite likewise remains to be determined.

Physiology of vitamin D $1\alpha,25\text{-}(OH)_2D$ is the only clearly established biologically important form of vitamin D; the potential role of other metabolites remains to be clarified. $1\alpha,25\text{-}(OH)_2D$ bound to a vitamin D–binding protein (which may be identical to the transport protein that binds 25-OHD) is delivered to the intestine, where it is efficiently taken up by specific cytoplasmic receptor proteins to stimulate calcium and phosphate transport from the intestinal lumen into the circulation. In supraphysiological doses, $1\alpha,25\text{-}(OH)_2D$ acts directly (even in the absence of PTH) to increase bone mineral mobilization. Under physiological conditions, however, the action of $1\alpha,25\text{-}(OH)_2D$ is believed to be synergistic with that of PTH on bone resorption; effects on bone resorption, if any, of $1\alpha,25\text{-}(OH)_2D$ at physiological concentrations independent of PTH are still not clarified. Whether $1\alpha,25\text{-}(OH)_2D$ has any direct effect on the renal handling of calcium and phosphorus also remains unsettled.

Serum 25-OHD levels change seasonally and as a function of vitamin D intake. Serum $1\alpha,25\text{-}(OH)_2D$ levels, however, appear to be unaltered by seasonal variation, by increases in dietary vitamin D, or by exposure to sunlight; as long as vitamin D supplies and 25-OHD levels are sufficient, metabolic influences operate on the renal 25-OHD 1α-hydroxylase to provide a closely regulated circulating concentration of $1\alpha,25\text{-}(OH)_2D$. Estimates of the serum concentration of $1\alpha,25\text{-}(OH)_2D$ by several laboratories are in close agreement; values reported range from 25 to 40 pg/ml. The serum half-life of $1\alpha,25\text{-}(OH)_2D$ is estimated to be about 3 to 6 h.

Whenever the serum calcium drops below normal, PTH secretion is enhanced; this increased concentration, by mechanisms still unclear, increases the production of $1\alpha,25\text{-}(OH)_2D$. The principal physiological regulation of the production of $1\alpha,25\text{-}(OH)_2D$ appears to involve changes in serum calcium levels with reciprocal changes in the PTH secretion rate, the latter controlling, possibly through actions on serum or tissue phosphorus levels, the rate of $1\alpha,25\text{-}(OH)_2D$ production. The possible role of hormones and metabolic factors other than PTH on $1\alpha,25\text{-}(OH)_2D$ production has been examined, so far, principally in laboratory animals. These studies have demonstrated that estrogen, prolactin, and growth hormone enhance the production of $1\alpha,25\text{-}(OH)_2D$. Humans, as well as other mammals, adapt to increased calcium requirements during growth, pregnancy, and lactation by increasing the efficiency of intestinal calcium absorption; effects on the renal 25-OHD 1α-hydroxylase by estrogen, prolactin, and/or growth hormone may prove to be the mediators of these physiological changes in calcium absorption. Most measurements of the circulating concentration of $1\alpha,25\text{-}(OH)_2D$ in humans in various physiological or pathophysiological states are based on studies using competitive binding assays in a small number of subjects; data are sometimes conflicting. More information on larger numbers of patients using techniques to measure production and clearance rates of $1\alpha,25\text{-}(OH)_2D$ is needed to assess the importance of factors other than PTH on vitamin D metabolism. (See Table 351-1.)

PATHOPHYSIOLOGY OF DISORDERS OF VITAMIN D METABOLISM Hypovitaminosis D   Inadequate endogenous production of vitamin D_3 in the skin, insufficient dietary supplementation, and/or the inability of the small intestine to absorb adequate amounts of vitamin D from the diet can cause hypovitaminosis D. Disease states equivalent to hypovitaminosis D are caused by (1) drugs that antagonize vitamin D action, (2) alteration in the metabolism of vitamin D, or (3) inadequate response of tissue receptors to vitamin D metabolites.

The pathophysiological consequences of hypovitaminosis D or equivalent disease states are twofold: (1) disturbances in mineral ion metabolism and PTH secretion and (2) mineralization defects in the skeleton (e.g., rickets in children, osteomala-

cia in adults). Details of these pathophysiological changes, especially on the skeleton, are described in Chap. 352. With regard to calcium metabolism, lack of vitamin D action leads to deficient calcium absorption and eventual hypocalcemia. The latter is accompanied by a compensatory secondary hyperparathyroidism; the increased secretion of PTH and enhanced actions of the hormone (Chap. 350) in causing calcium release via bone resorption and in promoting renal calcium conservation tend to blunt the severity of the hypocalcemia. (Late in the course of otherwise untreated hypovitaminosis D, severe hypocalcemia develops.) Hypophosphatemia is more marked than hypocalcemia, especially in early stages of vitamin D lack. The efficiency of phosphate absorption, like that of calcium absorption, falls with severe vitamin D deficiency or its equivalent state. The increased secretion of parathyroid hormone, although partially effective in minimizing hypocalcemia, leads to severe urinary phosphate wasting. This latter effect may be quantitatively the most significant factor in causing hypophosphatemia. With adequate renal function, the predominant changes in blood chemical values are *severe hypophosphatemia, moderate hypocalcemia* or low-normal blood calcium, and *increased PTH levels*. Blood *25-OHD levels* are *low*. As discussed in Chap. 352 severe skeletal mineralization defects accompany these disturbances in mineral ion metabolism.

Although the conversion of vitamin D to 25-OHD$_3$ is impaired to varying degrees in chronic, severe cholestatic or parenchymal liver disease, there is no strong correlation between low serum 25-OHD$_3$ levels and the development of osteopenia; multiple effects of the primary disease state seem to affect skeletal metabolism as well. A relation between *chronic anticonvulsant therapy* and the development of osteopenia has been well established in Great Britain and the United States; the problem is worse in patients on multiple drug therapy and when vitamin D intake or exposure to sunlight is minimal. It was initially believed that anticonvulsant drugs induced hepatic microsomal enzymes which metabolized vitamin D and 25-OHD into inactive products. However, these drugs have multiple and complex effects on calcium metabolism. Phenobarbital induces hepatic microsomal enzymes and stimulates bile secretion, both of which have the net effect of decreasing serum vitamin D and 25-OHD levels. Both phenytoin and phenobarbital influence calcium metabolism by directly inhibiting intestinal calcium transport and bone mineral mobilization.

Glucocorticoids used in high doses for suppression of various inflammatory disorders are known to cause disturbances in calcium metabolism and osteopenia, although osteomalacia

TABLE 351-1

Serum $1\alpha,25\text{-}(OH)_2D$ levels in disorders of calcium and phosphorus metabolism

Disease states	Serum $1\alpha,25\text{-}(OH)_2D$
Vitamin D deficiency	↓
Renal failure:	
GFR > 30	↓ or N
GFR < 30	↓
Hypoparathyroidism	↓ or N
Pseudohypoparathyroidism	↓ or N
Vitamin D–dependent rickets:	
Type I	↓
Type II	N or ↑
X-linked vitamin D–resistant rickets	↓ or N
Tumor-induced osteomalacia	↓ or N
Hyperparathyroidism	↑
Idiopathic hypercalciuria	N or ↑
Sarcoidosis	N or ↑

NOTE: ↓, *decreased;* N, *normal;* ↑, *increased; GFR, glomerular filtration rate.*

and rickets per se are not a consequence of glucocorticoid therapy. Glucocorticoids were thought to induce hepatic microsomal enzymes that degrade vitamin D_3 and 25-OHD$_3$. However, like anticonvulsant drugs, actions of glucocorticoids on vitamin D-mediated calcium metabolism are complex and include a direct inhibitory effect on vitamin D-mediated intestinal calcium absorption and bone mineral mobilization. Patients receiving chronic glucocorticoid therapy have been reported to have depressed serum $1\alpha,25$-(OH)$_2$D$_3$ levels; the mechanism(s) for this is unknown.

A genetic defect in the hepatic 25-hydroxylation of vitamin D has not been described. However, the proposal has been made that one heritable disorder of calcium and bone metabolism may involve a defect in renal production of $1\alpha,25$-(OH)$_2$D. In the syndrome of *pseudovitamin D-deficient rickets* (also known as *vitamin D-dependent rickets, type I;* see Chap. 352), *low* serum $1\alpha,25$-(OH)$_2$D levels and a therapeutic response to physiological doses of $1\alpha,25$-(OH)$_2$D have been attributed to an inherited deficiency in renal 25-OHD 1α-hydroxylase activity. In addition, there have been a few reports of patients with a similar phenotype, *pseudovitamin D-resistant rickets* (*vitamin D-dependent rickets, type II*), whose defect may be due to *hyporesponsiveness at the receptor level* rather than defective metabolism of the vitamin. These latter patients have *high serum $1\alpha,25$-(OH)$_2$D* levels; therapeutic response to high-dose vitamin D was noted in association with a further increase in the serum $1\alpha,25$-(OH)$_2$D levels.

Current reports disagree concerning findings in patients with *X-linked hypophosphatemic rickets;* normal values of serum $1\alpha,25$-(OH)$_2$D have been reported in one series, and low values have been reported in another. It has been pointed out, however, that since hypophosphatemia is a potent stimulus for the renal 25-OHD 1α-hydroxylase, in X-linked hypophosphatemic patients with severe hypophosphatemia the serum $1\alpha,25$-(OH)$_2$D levels should be high. Thus, even a normal serum $1\alpha,25$-(OH)$_2$D level suggests a functional defect in the 25-OHD 1α-hydroxylase system. It is unclear whether physiological doses of $1\alpha,25$-(OH)$_2$D or high doses of vitamin D offer any therapeutic advantage to that seen with phosphate therapy alone (Chap. 352).

In patients with mild to moderate chronic renal failure (glomerular filtration rate > 30) with phosphate retention, hyperphosphatemia and acidosis play important roles in suppressing the renal production of 1,25-(OH)$_2$D despite high levels of PTH. As the destruction of the renal cortex progresses, there is a depletion in the renal reserves of the 25-OHD 1α-hydroxylase to a point at which the kidney is unable to produce sufficient quantities of $1\alpha,25$-(OH)$_2$D to maintain calcium homeostasis, even when serum phosphate levels are normal. Under these circumstances replacement therapy with $1\alpha,25$-(OH)$_2$D or one of its analogues is most beneficial.

Patients with *hypoparathyroidism* and *pseudohypoparathyroidism* have mean serum levels of $1\alpha,25$-(OH)$_2$D that are lower than normal, although there is overlap in individual values with the normal range. In these hypocalcemic patients favorable responses to small replacement doses of $1\alpha,25$-(OH)$_2$D (0.25 to 1.0 μg per day; see Chap. 350), including increases in serum calcium, are seen at a time when the serum 25-OHD levels are higher than normal. These observations are consistent with the concept that patients with hypoparathyroidism or pseudohypoparathyroidism due to absent or ineffective action of PTH have defective function of renal 25-OHD 1α-hydroxylase. It is not clear to what extent serum $1\alpha,25$-(OH)$_2$D levels would be restored toward normal if the hyperphosphatemia in these diseases was controlled.

Hypervitaminosis D Vitamin D intoxication occurs after chronic oral ingestion of large doses of vitamin D_2 or D_3 (usually in excess of 50,000 to 100,000 IU daily) for months. In such circumstances, the excessive quantities of ingested vitamin are stored in body fat and released slowly into the bloodstream. Hypervitaminosis D as a result of prolonged sun exposure has not been reported, presumably because of protective mechanisms that include slow release of vitamin D from skin after conversion from previtamin D and perhaps other still-unrecognized regulatory controls. The consequences of excessive vitamin D action are *hypercalcemia* and *hypercalciuria;* blood phosphate levels are variable but usually normal. In severe, unrecognized, or untreated vitamin D intoxication, the Ca $\times$ P product exceeds the solubility product, and widespread ectopic calcification results, especially in the kidneys, causing renal failure. A marked elevation of serum 25-OHD levels (three to ten times normal) is found. Because anephric patients who do not synthesize $1\alpha,25$-(OH)$_2$D can be intoxicated with vitamin D, it is believed that high circulating levels of 25-OHD or other metabolites of vitamin D can directly stimulate intestinal calcium absorption and bone mineral mobilization without undergoing further metabolism. The fact that serum $1\alpha,25$-(OH)$_2$D levels are low to normal rather than elevated in patients with hypervitaminosis D is consistent with this observation.

In some circumstances cessation of the vitamin D ingestion and lowering of oral calcium intake leads to rapid disappearance of the hypercalcemia. On the other hand hypercalcemia may persist for weeks to months after vitamin D ingestion is stopped. Under such circumstances, patients should be treated with a glucocorticoid such as prednisone in doses of 20 to 40 mg per day to control the hypercalcemia and to prevent irreversible renal damage and ectopic calcification. A dramatic lowering of calcium to normal levels can be accomplished within days (see Chap. 350 for diagnostic use of the glucocorticoid suppression test in hypercalcemic disorders). Other measures to treat hypercalcemia (see Chap. 350) can be used acutely in severe cases.

The clinical use of potent vitamin D metabolites and analogues for the treatment of many disorders of calcium metabolism has added a new dimension to the syndrome of vitamin D intoxication. The therapeutic index for $1\alpha,25$-(OH)$_2$D$_3$ is low. This is not surprising when one considers that oral administration of $1\alpha,25$-(OH)$_2$D$_3$ provides relatively high concentrations of the natural hormone in direct contact with its target tissue (the small intestine). More than half of the patients with renal insufficiency treated with $1\alpha,25$-(OH)$_2$D$_3$ in doses of 0.5 to 2 μg per day demonstrate at least transient hypercalcemia. This is quickly alleviated by decreasing the drug dosage (see Chap. 352 for details). It is not known how frequently toxicity develops when lower doses of $1\alpha,25$-(OH)$_2$D$_3$ are used or whether the blood assay for $1\alpha,25$-(OH)$_2$D$_3$ will be a useful indicator of potential toxicity.

Acute vitamin D toxicity due to a single excessive dose of vitamin D_2 or D_3 is not seen; however, one can anticipate that a single overdose of $1\alpha,25$-(OH)$_2$D$_3$ or a potent analogue may cause acute toxicity, including hypercalcemia and hypercalciuria. Treatment of such intoxication should include elimination of calcium from the diet, induction of emesis or gastric lavage if the overdosage is discovered within a relatively short time, and the use of cathartics. Careful monitoring of serum calcium and phosphorus levels should be maintained for at least 24 h after ingestion, and hypercalcemia, if serious, should be treated with measures directed at increasing urinary calcium excretion or blocking bone resorption (see Chap. 350). The usefulness of glucocorticoid therapy in severe toxicity due to an acute overdose of $1\alpha,25$-(OH)$_2$D$_3$ remains to be established.

There are several reports, based on the measurement of circulating levels of $1\alpha,25\text{-}(OH)_2D$ in limited numbers of patients, of abnormalities in vitamin D metabolism in disease states such as osteoporosis in elderly women, tumor-induced osteomalacia, sarcoidosis, and idiopathic hypercalciuria. The nature and frequency of disturbances in vitamin D metabolism in these disorders are still uncertain because of both the small number of patients involved and inherent limitations in data provided by present assays for $1\alpha,25\text{-}(OH)_2D$. The assays allow only a static measurement of the serum $1\alpha,25\text{-}(OH)_2D$ concentration. Ultimate definition of significant differences between normal and abnormal states of $1\alpha,25\text{-}(OH)_2D$ production will probably require, in analogy with earlier studies of steroid hormones, formal measurements of production rates of $1\alpha,25\text{-}(OH)_2D$ including metabolic clearance rates. Of particular value, when and if developed, will be tests of the capacity of $1\alpha,25\text{-}(OH)_2D$ production and renal 25-OHD 1α-hydroxylase reserve.

Calcium absorption is subnormal in the elderly. It can be improved by treatment with $1\alpha\text{-}OHD_3$ or $1\alpha,25\text{-}(OH)_2D_3$, as well as by high doses of vitamin D. Because animal studies showed that estrogen enhances the production of $1\alpha,25\text{-}(OH)_2D$, there has been speculation that the pathogenesis of postmenopausal osteoporosis is, in part, related to estrogen deficiency and/or an imbalance in the circulating levels of estrogens and androgens that in turn adversely influence the renal production of $1\alpha,25\text{-}(OH)_2D$. Serum $1\alpha,25\text{-}(OH)_2D$ levels have been reported to be slightly below normal in some patients with postmenopausal osteoporosis; however, the differences are small, and most values fall within the normal range. Studies are underway to evaluate the potential benefit of long-term therapy with $1\alpha\text{-}OHD_3$ or $1\alpha,25\text{-}(OH)_2D_3$ in patients with senile and postmenopausal osteoporosis. Such therapy does increase intestinal calcium absorption, thereby reducing negative calcium balance; however, it remains to be determined whether $1\alpha,25\text{-}(OH)_2D$ deficiency is indeed present in such patients or whether the course of the bone disease is altered by treatment. There have been a few reports that patients with tumor-induced osteomalacia have low serum $1\alpha,25\text{-}(OH)_2D$ levels; after tumor resection, the serum $1\alpha,25\text{-}(OH)_2D$ levels return to normal.

In addition to hyperparathyroidism, disease states that may have enhanced $1\alpha,25\text{-}(OH)_2D$ production include sarcoidosis and idiopathic hypercalciuria. In sarcoidosis, the abnormal calcium metabolism, as manifested by hypercalcemia and hypercalciuria, has been attributed to abnormal sensitivity to vitamin D. It has been reported that $1\alpha,25\text{-}(OH)_2D$ levels are increased in sarcoidosis, which suggests that the apparent hypersensitivity to vitamin D seen in this disease is due to a defect in the control of production of $1\alpha,25\text{-}(OH)_2D$.

In many cases of idiopathic hypercalciuria, which is often familial, there is an inappropriately increased intestinal calcium absorption. Several reports indicate an elevation in $1\alpha,25\text{-}(OH)_2D$ levels in some of these patients, consistent with the speculation that excessive $1\alpha,25\text{-}(OH)_2D$ production could be responsible for the disorder in some patients.

REFERENCES

AVIOLI LV, KRANE SM (eds): *Metabolic Bone Disease.* New York, Academic, 1978

BELL PA: The chemistry of the vitamins D, in *Vitamin D*, DEM Lawson (ed). London, Academic, 1978, pp 1–50

BILEZIKIAN JP et al: Response of $1\alpha,25$-dihydroxyvitamin D_3 to hypocalcemia in human subjects. N Engl J Med 299:437, 1978

BROADUS AE, THEIR, SO: Metabolic basis of renal-stone disease. N Engl J Med 300:839, 1979

DELUCA HF, SCHNOES HK: Metabolism and mechanism of action of vitamin D. Annu Rev Biochem 45:631, 1976

DREZNER MK, FEINGLOS MN: Tumor-induced $1\alpha,25$-dihydroxycholecalciferol deficiency: A cause of oncogenic osteomalacia, in *Vitamin D: Biochemical, Chemical and Clinical Aspects Related to Calcium Metabolism,* AW Norman (ed). New York, De Gruyter, 1977, p 863

FIESER LD, FIESER M: *Steroids.* New York, Reinhold, 1959, chap 4

GRAY WG et al: Metabolism and excretion of ^{3}H-1,25-$(OH)_2$-vitamin D_3 in healthy adults. J Clin Endocrinol Metab 46:756, 1978

HAUSSLER MR, MCCAIN BS: Basic and clinical concepts related to vitamin D metabolism and action. N Engl J Med 297:974, 1977

HOLICK MF, CLARK MB: The photobiogenesis and metabolism of vitamin D. Fed Proc 37:2567, 1978

KANIS JA et al: 25,25-Dihydroxycholecalciferol and calcium absorption in uremia. Br Med J 1:822, 1979

PAPAPOULOS SE et al: 1,25-Dihydroxycholecalciferol in the pathogenesis of the hypercalcemia of sarcoidosis. Lancet 1:627, 1979

SCRIVER CR et al: Serum 1,25-dihydroxyvitamin D levels in normal subjects and in patients with hereditary rickets or bone disease. N Engl J Med 299:976, 1978

352
METABOLIC BONE DISEASE

STEPHEN M. KRANE
MICHAEL F. HOLICK

OSTEOPOROSIS

GENERAL CONSIDERATIONS *Osteoporosis* is the term used to describe a group of diseases of diverse etiology which are characterized by a reduction in the mass of bone per unit volume to a level below that required for adequate mechanical support function. The reduction in mass is not accompanied by a significant reduction in the ratio of the mineral to the organic phase, nor by any reproducible abnormality in the structure of either the mineral or the organic matrix. Histologically, osteoporosis is characterized by a decrease in the number and size of the trabeculae of cancellous bone with normal width of the osteoid seams. Osteoporosis is the commonest of the metabolic bone diseases (disorders in which all the skeleton is involved, presumably as a result of systemic factors acting on the skeleton) and is an important cause of morbidity in elderly subjects.

The remodeling of bone (its formation and resorption) is a continuous process throughout life. Any combination of changes in the rates of formation and resorption which results in bone resorption exceeding bone formation could therefore cause a decrease in bone mass. In osteoporosis the bone mass *is* decreased, indicating that the rate of bone resorption must exceed that of bone formation. In most studies formation rate is normal in osteoporosis, although low rates are sometimes found. Current evidence suggests that, in normal individuals for many years after closure of the epiphyses and after longitudinal growth has ceased, skeletal mass remains constant and the rates of bone formation and resorption are relatively low and approximately equal. Resorption and formation of bone are normally tightly coupled. However, the rate of remodeling is not uniform throughout the skeleton after epiphyseal closure. Most of the bone surfaces are "inactive" and not involved at any given time either in formation or resorption. It has been proposed that formation and resorption are coupled in space as "remodeling units." Resorption areas are covered by osteoclasts if active; bone formation surfaces are characterized by the presence of osteoid seams and are covered by active osteoblasts. Active surfaces may be randomly distributed, but formation and resorption are locally coupled as units. Resorption precedes formation and is probably more intense, but it does not last as long as formation. As a consequence, there are normally more active formation than resorption sites. Bone turnover is high when there are many units active and low when there are few. Unless formation compensates completely for resorption, bone mass would have to decrease. After the age of 40 to 50 skeletal mass begins to decline, at a faster rate in women than in men, and at a different rate in different parts of the skeleton. The loss has been documented quantitatively using techniques such as photon densitometry and neutron-activation analysis. For example, the rate of loss is greater in the metacarpals, in the femoral neck, and in the vertebral bodies than in the midshaft of the femur, the tibia, and the skull. Over the next three or four decades the total loss in skeletal mass may be 30 to 50 percent of that present at age 30 or 40. Evidence obtained from kinetic studies (using radioactive isotopes of calcium and strontium) and from quantitative microradiography (which includes both cortical and cancellous bone) indicates that in most older subjects the resorption rate is high, whereas the bone formation rate remains at a level similar to that of younger adults. Radioactive calcium kinetics indicate that as much as 400 to 500 mg calcium may enter and leave the normal adult skeleton daily. At some critical point if the difference between rates of formation and resorption is maintained, loss of bone substance may become so marked that the bone can no longer resist the mechanical forces to which it is subjected, and fracture results. Osteoporosis would then be evident as a clinical problem. The level of reduction in bone mass sufficient to result in fractures after minimal trauma is variable. The strength of the vertebral body may depend upon additional factors such as adequacy of ligamentous support and the age-related changes in the intervertebral disks.

In the process of remodeling of lamellar bone in adults, most of the net resorption occurs at the corticoendosteal surface. The abnormal remodeling in osteoporosis follows the same pattern; the bone loss includes cancellous bone, cortical bone at the endosteal surface, and intracortical bone, resulting in enlargement of the medullary cavity and thinning of the cortex. Since bone formation at the periosteum continues at a very slow rate, the diameter of the bone does not decrease, and the periosteal surface retains its smooth configuration. In addition, the cancellous bone also undergoes progressive resorption, with some trabeculae being resorbed at rates faster than others, particularly those vertebral trabeculae with horizontal orientation.

The cause of this age-associated decrease in bone mass and increase in bone resorption or the accelerated loss in that form of osteoporosis occurring particularly in older women after the menopause is not known. The decrease in mass is similar in a number of different populations throughout the world. Although blacks in the United States have a lower incidence of clinically significant osteoporosis than do whites, they also have a larger initial skeletal mass, such that adequate bone could remain even in the presence of age-associated losses. Estrogens, which are often used to treat osteoporosis, tend to inhibit bone resorption and decrease the hypercalcemia of hyperparathyroidism. A possible role of estrogens in the metabolism of vitamin D has been discussed in Chap. 351. However, there is no direct evidence of increased parathyroid hormone secretion with increasing age; immunoreactive parathyroid hormone levels are normal. Epidemiologic surveys have shown that there is no relation between the degree of bone loss and

age of onset or type of menopause. There is also no difference in the calcium intake of osteoporotic compared with control subjects of similar age and sex. Osteoporotic subjects tend to have lower body weight and muscle mass than do controls, but the significance of these findings is uncertain. No consistent changes in adrenocortical function have been documented in osteoporotics, although there are suggestions that subtle alterations in pituitary, adrenal, and gonadal functions may play a role in the production of osteoporosis. The possible role of substances that stimulate bone resorption, such as prostaglandins and osteoclast-activating factors, the latter derived from lymphocytes and possibly other mononuclear cells, has not yet been evaluated. In patients with primary hypogonadism due to gonadal dysgenesis or pituitary failure, osteoporosis is frequently noted radiologically. This has been attributed to the failure to attain full adult skeletal mass rather than to an increased rate of bone loss associated with age.

Another factor which some have implicated in bone loss is the possibility that excessive acid intake, particularly in the form of high-protein diets, results in "dissolution" of bone in an attempt to buffer the extra acid. It has also been observed that prolonged use of heparin as an anticoagulant is associated with osteoporosis and that heparin potentiates bone resorption in vitro. Patients with osteoporosis have increased numbers of mast cells, presumably capable of producing heparin, in their bone marrow. Circumscribed and diffuse areas of osteoporosis are also seen in patients with systemic mastocytosis.

As mentioned earlier, the remodeling of bone is physiologically responsive to mechanical forces of many types. The early response to immobilization in the normal skeleton is an increase in bone resorption while bone formation remains normal or is decreased; later there is a compensatory increase in bone formation. In osteoporosis, immobilization tends to aggravate the defect by further increasing the gap between formation and resorption. It is, therefore, possible that a sedentary life in an individual with poor musculature would tend to reduce mechanical forces exerted on the skeleton and to increase the tendency to bone loss.

CLASSIFICATION In only a few forms of osteoporosis is the cause certain, such as in that associated with Cushing's syndrome, both endogenous and exogenous. Osteoporosis is also associated with a number of other disorders, but the nature of the relationship is not clear. In the majority of cases of osteoporosis the etiology is not apparent. While most of these occur in older women past the menopause (*senile* or *postmenopausal osteoporosis*), it is not certain how the osteoporosis is related to the postmenopausal state. When osteoporosis occurs in younger individuals, it is usually termed *idiopathic osteoporosis*. In fact, most of these disorders should be considered idiopathic since details of their pathogenesis are not known. A suggested classification is shown in Table 352-1.

GENERAL CLINICAL FEATURES Although osteoporosis is a generalized disorder of the skeleton, its major clinical manifestations involve the axial skeleton. Fractures of long bones are also somewhat more frequent in osteoporotic subjects than in others of similar age without osteoporosis and are most common in the hip, humerus, and wrists. The most frequent symptoms are pain in the back and deformity of the spine. Pain usually results from collapse of the vertebral bodies, especially in the lower dorsal and upper lumbar regions, is typically acute in onset, and often radiates anteriorly around the flank into various portions of the abdomen, depending upon the location of the fracture. Such episodes frequently occur after sudden bending, lifting, or jumping movements which may seem to have been trivial; on some occasions they cannot be related to trauma. The pain may be increased even with slight movements such as turning in bed or by the Valsalva maneu-

TABLE 352-1
Classification of osteoporosis

  I Common forms of osteoporosis of unknown cause unassociated with other disease
    A Idiopathic osteoporosis (juvenile and adult)
    B Postmenopausal osteoporosis
    C Senile osteoporosis
 II Disorders or conditions in which osteoporosis is a common feature or pathogenesis partially understood
    A Hypogonadism
    B Hyperadrenocorticism
    C Thyrotoxicosis
    D Malabsorption
    E Scurvy
    F Calcium deficiency
    G Immobilization
    H Chronic heparin administration
    I Systemic mastocytosis
    J Adult hypophosphatasia
    K Associated with other metabolic bone diseases
III Osteoporosis as a feature of heritable disorders of connective tissue
    A Osteogenesis imperfecta
    B Homocystinuria due to cystathionine synthase deficiency
    C Ehlers-Danlos syndrome
    D Marfan syndrome
IV Disorders in which osteoporosis is associated but pathogenesis not understood
    A Rheumatoid arthritis
    B Malnutrition
    C Alcoholism
    D Epilepsy
    E Diabetes
    F Chronic obstructive pulmonary disease
    G Menkes' syndrome

ver. Rest in bed in one position may relieve the pain temporarily, but it then may recur in spasms of variable duration. Radiation of pain down one leg is uncommon, and symptoms or signs of spinal cord compression are very rare. The acute episodes of pain may also be accompanied by abdominal distention and ileus, thought to be due to retroperitoneal hemorrhage, but the use of narcotics at this stage also contributes to the ileus. Loss of appetite and apparent muscular weakness, which is probably due to fear of reproducing pain, may also be present. Episodes of pain usually subside after several days to a week, and by 4 to 6 weeks patients may be fully ambulatory and able to resume their normal activities. Although the acute pain may be minimal, many patients continue to have nagging, deep, dull, uncomfortable sensations localized to the area of fracture brought about by straining or sudden changes in position. They may be unable to sit up in bed and have to arise by rolling over on their sides and then propping themselves up. Most patients have disappearance or marked diminution of pain between episodes of vertebral body collapse. Others never have acute episodes but complain of varying degrees of backache often made worse by standing or moving suddenly. Tenderness over involved areas of the spinous processes or rib cage is commonly noted. The collapse fractures of the vertebral bodies are usually anterior, producing a wedge-shaped deformity and contributing to loss in height. This is particularly common in the upper dorsal region where collapse may be unassociated with pain but result in a dorsal kyphosis and exaggerated cervical lordosis described as a "dowager's" or "widow's" hump. Postural slumping with increase in existing curves also contributes to the loss of height. Generalized skeletal pain is uncommon, and between fractures most patients are free even of pain localized to the spine. Although recurrent episodes of collapse fractures of vertebral bodies, increasing spine deformity, and loss of height are common in osteoporosis, the course of the disorder in any one subject is not predictable, and there may be intervals of several years between fractures.

RADIOLOGICAL FEATURES Prior to fracture and collapse the osteoporotic vertebral body shows a decrease in mineral density, an increase in prominence of vertical striations due to a

relatively greater loss of the horizontally oriented trabeculae, and prominence of the end plates. The bodies may become increasingly biconcave because of weakening of the subchondral plates and expansion of the intervertebral disks, resulting in the so-called "codfish" vertebrae. When collapse occurs, most frequently in lower dorsal and upper lumbar spine, it usually produces a decrease in the anterior height of the vertebral body and irregularity in the anterior cortex (Fig. 352-1). Older compression fractures may show reactive changes and osteophytes about the anterior margins. Although the cortices of long bones may be thin because of excessive endosteal resorption, the outer margins are sharp in contrast to the typical effects of the subperiosteal resorption of hyperparathyroidism. Pseudofractures or Looser's zones are not present in osteoporosis without osteomalacia, but distinguishing osteoporosis from osteomalacia may be impossible on radiological grounds alone.

LABORATORY FINDINGS The concentrations of calcium and inorganic phosphorus in the blood are usually normal in patients with osteoporosis; slight hyperphosphatemia is present in women who are past the menopause. The alkaline phosphatase in uncomplicated instances is normal, although slight increases may be seen after fractures. Only about 20 percent of postmenopausal women with osteoporosis have significant hypercalciuria. Urinary excretion of peptides containing hydroxyproline, an index of bone resorption, is usually normal or slightly increased.

DIFFERENTIAL DIAGNOSIS Since decrease in skeletal mass is an age-associated finding, it is particularly difficult to evaluate

FIGURE 352-1
Lateral views of the lumbar spine of a 54-year-old man with idiopathic osteoporosis. A typical anterior compression fracture is indicated by the arrow.

asymptomatic decreased bone density observed radiologically in older women, especially when unaccompanied by marked increase in biconcavity of vertebral bodies or fractures. In the presence of bone pain with or without fracture or deformity, it is important to establish the presence or absence of known causes of osteoporosis as listed in Table 352-1 and to be certain that osteoporosis in the broad sense is the correct diagnosis. Malignancies of various types, particularly *multiple myeloma, lymphoma, leukemia,* and *carcinomatosis,* may result in diffuse loss of bone, especially the trabecular bone of the vertebral column, even in the absence of hypercalcemia. The absence of anemia, elevated erythrocyte sedimentation rate, abnormal electrophoretic patterns of serum proteins, and Bence Jones proteinuria is helpful in eliminating the possibility of multiple myeloma. However, needle bone biopsy or marrow aspiration is usually indicated in cases of severe osteoporosis.

Radiological osteoporosis is commonly present in patients with primary *hyperparathyroidism* who may not have specific evidence of osteitis fibrosa (discrete lytic lesions of varying size and subperiosteal resorption) or elevation of serum alkaline phosphatase. Although hyperparathyroidism could accelerate bone loss in the pattern of osteoporosis and contribute to it, it is not clear that excessive secretion of parathyroid hormone is the sole cause of the bone disease, even in these cases, rather than an associated finding. Repeated determinations of serum calcium and phosphorus are therefore necessary. An element of secondary hyperparathyroidism may be present in some elderly patients in whom there is impairment of renal function, inadequate oral calcium intake, or decrease of intestinal calcium absorption. Increased numbers of osteoclasts may be found in bone biopsy specimens from such patients.

Osteomalacia may mimic osteoporosis or coexist with it, yet specific radiological signs of osteomalacia may not always be present. Although the presence of abnormalities such as hypophosphatemia would suggest the possibility of osteomalacia, these too may be absent in some cases of osteomalacia, and bone biopsy may be essential for diagnosis, as discussed below. Since osteomalacia of various causes is more responsive to specific therapy than the usual case of osteoporosis, such diagnostic procedures are often warranted and provide, in addition, adequate specimens for examination for the presence of malignant cells.

In an occasional patient with *Paget's disease* the radiological features may be almost purely lytic and be confused with osteoporosis. However, high alkaline phosphatase levels and moderately or markedly increased urinary excretion of hydroxyproline-containing peptides would be clues to the presence of Paget's disease. Scanning procedures with bone-seeking isotopes would not be helpful in differential diagnosis if fractures are present, because in any disease fractures demonstrate preferential uptake of isotope. However, in the absence of fracture, "hot spots" would suggest presence of tumor or early Paget's disease.

IDIOPATHIC OSTEOPOROSIS Most of the comments about osteoporosis in the preceding sections are particularly pertinent to elderly patients, especially women with bone loss sufficient to produce significant symptoms. Although its ultimate cause is unknown, this type of osteoporosis is often termed *senile* or *postmenopausal. Idiopathic osteoporosis* is the term used to describe the disorder in younger men or in premenopausal women in whom no other etiologic factor is detected. It is likely that these patients will eventually be shown to have a number of different disorders with superficial resemblances. In some women the onset of the disease and deterioration of bone appear to be related to pregnancy, whereas in others no adverse effect of pregnancy is observed. Some patients tend to

have low levels of serum alkaline phosphatase but not low enough to fit into the group of patients with so-called hypophosphatasia. Estrogens are ineffective in therapy. Losses of calcium and phosphorus are probably excessive, and it is unwise to permit women with osteoporosis to breast-feed their infants since additional calcium losses via lactation are appreciable. It is possible that some patients have a disorder similar to the late-onset forms of osteogenesis imperfecta, although such features as family history, blue scleras, and deafness are lacking. The course of this disorder is variable, and although recurrent episodes of fractures are characteristic, progressive deterioration does not occur in all patients, and in some the clinical problem is rather benign. Juvenile osteoporosis is a rare disorder with onset in children usually between the ages of 8 and 14 years and characterized by the abrupt appearance of bone pain and the occurrence of fractures after minimal trauma. In many cases the disorder is self-limited, and recovery takes place spontaneously within 4 or 5 years.

GLUCOCORTICOID EXCESS The presence of glucocorticoid excess has not been established in osteoporosis of the idiopathic, senile, or postmenopausal variety. However, osteoporosis commonly accompanies Cushing's syndrome, both endogenous and exogenous, and in some instances is rapidly progressive, especially in children and in women over the age of 50. The rapid progression of bone loss in conditions of glucocorticoid excess is accounted for by a combination of low rates of bone formation accompanied by high rates of bone resorption. A part of the latter may be the result of glucocorticoid-induced secondary hyperparathyroidism. Glucocorticoids depress collagen synthesis in organs other than bone, as evidenced by delayed wound healing, thinning of the dermis, characteristic striae, and tendency to blue scleras. In some disorders in which glucocorticoids in pharmacological doses are administered, such as rheumatoid arthritis, a tendency to thin skin and osteoporosis is initially present, and the skeletal effects of the glucocorticoids may become particularly apparent. Glucocorticoid excess also results in alteration in the metabolism of vitamin D; blood levels of 25-hydroxyvitamin D_3 (25-OHD$_3$) are normal or only slightly decreased, and there may be accelerated metabolism of $1\alpha,25$-dihydroxyvitamin D_3 [$1\alpha,25$-(OH)$_2$D$_3$] with low serum levels of this metabolite in some patients, particularly in children. Part of the defect in calcium absorption is explainable by the vitamin D abnormalities, but glucocorticoids also inhibit intestinal calcium absorption by a direct, vitamin D–independent action on the intestine. Once osteoporosis develops in Cushing's syndrome in adults, the abnormal appearance of the vertebrae may persist indefinitely following alleviation of the glucocorticoid excess. In children, however, cure of the Cushing's syndrome may result in striking improvement in the appearance of the spine due to new endochondral bone formation which can surround the less dense, older osteoporotic bone. This does not occur in adults since endochondral bone formation has ceased. Usually withdrawal of glucocorticoids or decrease of the dose by alternate-day schedule may be the only way to halt progression of the osteoporosis. Anabolic steroids have not been proved to be effective in this regard. The intestinal absorption defect may be helped by administering vitamin D in doses of 50,000 IU three times weekly, plus supplemental oral calcium of 500 mg per day. The use of vitamin D metabolites such as 25-OHD$_3$ or $1\alpha,25$-(OH)$_2$D$_3$ may prove to be more effective. When large doses of vitamin D are used, it is important to monitor serum and urinary calcium at intervals of 2 to 4 months, especially if glucocorticoid dosages are lowered. In Cushing's syndrome, spontaneous, symptomless fractures may occur in bones such as ribs and pubic and ischial rami even in the absence of marked osteoporosis of the spine. These fractures often heal partially with an exuberant calcified callus surrounding a radiolucent zone of nonunion, which superficially resembles the pseudofractures of osteomalacia. If they appear in the thorax superimposed upon the lungs, they may be confused with nodules suggesting primary or metastatic tumor.

GONADAL DEFICIENCY   Estrogen lack is present in the postmenopausal woman with osteoporosis, and the administration of estrogen to such an individual reduces the negative calcium balance and decreases urinary hydroxyproline excretion as is consistent with a decrease in bone resorption. However it does not necessarily follow that estrogen deficiency per se is the cause of the osteoporosis. In patients of either sex castrated at an early age, the adult skeleton is smaller to begin with, and therefore age-related losses are more significant.

THYROTOXICOSIS   In many patients with hyperthyroidism, there is excessive bone resorption, occasionally marked in degree and far exceeding that in the usual patient with osteoporosis, associated with increased excretion of calcium and phosphorus in urine and feces. The excessive bone resorption is usually accompanied by a compensatory increase in bone formation. If the hyperthyroidism is of short duration, skeletal losses are inconsequential. However, in patients with chronic hyperthyroidism, especially in women after the menopause, this accelerated bone loss becomes clinically significant, and it is important to eliminate hyperthyroidism as a contributing cause of osteoporosis. Although typical osteitis fibrosa (resorption lacunae containing osteoclasts and a fibrous stroma) may be seen on biopsy, even in these cases the skeletal lesions have the appearance of osteoporosis when examined radiologically.

ACROMEGALY   Hypercalciuria and overall net negative calcium balance occur in acromegaly, and occasionally osteoporosis is an associated finding. The panhypopituitarism secondary to a pituitary adenoma and gonadal insufficiency may be factors in production of the osteoporosis. In adult animals growth hormone decreases endosteal resorption and stimulates bone formation, and it is therefore unlikely that excessive secretion of growth hormone would in itself produce osteoporosis.

CALCIUM DEFICIENCY AND MALABSORPTION   Although calcium deficiency may be a factor in some instances of osteoporosis, it cannot be the sole or major cause in idiopathic, senile, or postmenopausal osteoporosis. Osteoporosis is an associated finding in a significant number of cases of steatorrhea, prolonged obstructive jaundice, and lactose intolerance and in patients following gastrectomy. In other patients there are suggestions of a specific defect in calcium absorption or a failure to adapt adequately to a low-calcium diet either by increasing the percentage of dietary calcium absorbed or by decreasing urinary calcium excretion. Presumably adequate vitamin D is available in these instances to prevent osteomalacia.

HERITABLE DISORDERS OF CONNECTIVE TISSUE   In the strict sense, the bone disease of osteogenesis imperfecta is osteoporosis. *Osteogenesis imperfecta* is a disorder(s) of unknown mechanism and of variable degree of severity; it is usually transmitted as an autosomal dominant and is associated with blue scleras and, later, deafness. Although the disease may be apparent in utero and in infancy, other cases are not detected until childhood; it is possible that some cases of idiopathic osteoporosis represent forms of osteogenesis imperfecta. The organization of the collagen in bone and skin is abnormal, and in some instances there likely is a genetic defect in the synthesis of the type I collagen of both bone and skin. Osteoporosis is also seen in all patients with *homocystinuria* due to cystathionine synthase deficiency, which is transmitted as an autosomal recessive. Other characteristics of this disorder should suggest

its presence, such as ectopia lentis, various deformities of the extremities, mental retardation, decreased pigmentation of hair and skin, and thromboembolism. The diagnosis is established by the finding of homocystine in urinary chromatograms. The defect may be due to the effect of homocysteine or other metabolites in interfering with the cross-linking of collagen.

THERAPY   Before considering the use and efficacy of various modes of treatment advocated for osteoporosis, it should be emphasized that one is dealing with a group of disorders rather than a single entity. Even in patients considered to fall within the same category, e.g., those with idiopathic osteoporosis, the etiologies may be different. In addition, it is difficult to predict the course and the rate of progression of the disease in any one patient, especially when seen initially because of pain and collapse-fracture. Many patients in the idiopathic, senile, and postmenopausal groups have a few episodes of vertebral body collapse with symptom-free intervals of months or years, lose some height consistent with the extent of collapse, but then go for many years without symptoms or further loss in height. Furthermore the acute pain associated with vertebral body fracture tends to subside in a matter of weeks, and *any* treatment administered at that time might be considered efficacious. It is evident from the number of different therapeutic programs available for all forms of osteoporosis that therapy is far from ideal, despite claims to the contrary.

General measures   Patients who present with acute pain secondary to fracture of vertebral bodies frequently require hospitalization with rest in bed in a position of maximum comfort, local heat, adequate analgesics, and avoidance of constipation. Use of traction or plaster jacket splints is not indicated. As soon as pain permits, it is prudent to have the patient attempt to move out of bed, slowly at first, perhaps with support of a walker or crutches. It is best not to have the patient become too fatigued when starting ambulation. Braces of various types are commonly employed, but most patients tolerate them poorly, and it has not been proved that they are efficacious in preventing progression of spinal deformity. If a well-made corset provides a sensation of support and comfort, wearing it is worthwhile. Supervised exercises to correct postural deformity and increase muscle tone are useful. It is also important to instruct patients to avoid sudden painful movements such as jumping and how to lift and carry objects with minimal back strain.

Estrogens and androgens   The use of estrogens in postmenopausal women with osteoporosis was first advocated by Dr. Fuller Albright and his colleagues. Decrease in urinary calcium and hydroxyproline excretion results from such therapy, especially during the first few months of treatment. Estrogens act by decreasing the rate of bone resorption, but bone formation does not increase and eventually usually decreases. Thus estrogens produce significant, although modest, calcium retention, decrease the difference between formation and resorption, and therefore tend to retard the progress of osteoporosis, but they are not capable of restoring skeletal mass. The magnitude of calcium retention also tends to decrease with continuous therapy. Therefore it is not surprising that no change in radiological features of the osteoporosis can be appreciated with such therapy. It is likely that estrogens have their role in preventing osteoporosis in menopausal women rather than treating clinical disease already developed, although they are probably the best preparations to use in the postmenopausal woman with mild or moderate disease within the first 5 to 6 years following cessation of ovarian function. Testosterone preparations are useful in treatment of men with gonadal deficiency, but there are no convincing reports of their efficacy in men with normal gonadal function. So-called anabolic steroids are weak androgens, and there is no advantage to their use in women in view of their masculinizing properties. There is also no proved advantage to combinations of estrogens and androgens. The chronic use of estrogens restores menses in some postmenopausal women and induces breast swelling and hyperpigmentation. In women receiving estrogens the risk of mammary carcinoma is not increased but there may be a dose-related increase in the incidence of endometrial carcinoma. Any decision on the use of these hormones must take this risk factor into consideration.

A typical program would be oral administration of 0.625 to 1.25 mg conjugated estrogens or the equivalent dosage of another natural estrogen daily for the first 3 weeks of each month, followed by abstinence for 1 week to allow for withdrawal bleeding. During days 9 to 21, inclusive, of the estrogen therapy the addition of medroxyprogesterone acetate, 10 mg, produces secretory differentiation of the endometrium and may reduce the likelihood of hyperplasia. Pelvic examination and vaginal smear for cytology and possibly endometrial biopsy are indicated at annual intervals; careful consideration should be given to the pattern of uterine bleeding, any bleeding other than that associated with estrogen withdrawal being looked upon as a danger sign (see Chap. 342).

Calcium preparations   Use of oral calcium preparations in doses of 1.0 to 1.5 g elemental calcium per day (e.g., calcium carbonate 1.0 g three times daily) has been shown to increase calcium retention in some osteoporotic subjects and decrease indices of bone resorption. However, as with the use of estrogens, this eventually results in decrease in bone formation and tends to arrest rather than "cure" the osteoporosis. In patients with malabsorption, calcium may be effective in addition to vitamin D given orally in doses of 25,000 to 50,000 IU once or twice weekly. The use of more active metabolites of vitamin D may prove more efficacious in the future. Both serum and urinary calcium should be monitored at intervals of several months to be certain that hypercalcemia and hypercalciuria do not result. Diuretics of the benzothiadiazide class can reduce urinary calcium excretion and could be helpful in reducing a negative calcium balance. Calcium preparations might be of greater use in patients with normal gonadal function and relatively mild disease. Intermittent intravenous infusions of calcium have also been advocated, but the efficacy of this form of therapy has yet to be established.

Fluoride   Fluoride ions are promptly deposited in the skeleton where they become incorporated into the crystal lattice of hydroxyapatite, substituting for hydroxyl ions. This process results in a mineral phase of greater crystallinity. Fluoride ions in chronic high doses also increase new bone formation and in excess produce a form of hyperostosis with dense bones, exostoses, neurological complications due to bony overgrowth, and ligamentous calcification. The use of fluoride in treating osteoporosis has not been found to produce uniformly satisfactory results, possibly because of variations in dosage of fluoride ion, retention of absorbed ion, and calcium intake while on fluoride. The stimulation of new bone formation, a desirable effect not seen with the other agents mentioned previously, is unfortunately associated with the production of bone which is poorly mineralized and also, presumably, structurally unsound. It has recently been suggested that if the dose of fluoride ion is moderate (25 mg per day) and calcium supplements are given in doses of at least 1 g daily plus vitamin D,

50,000 IU twice weekly, considerable new bone is produced. Significant toxicity is absent, although weight-bearing pain, especially in ankles and knees, is noted by some patients and disappears when fluoride is discontinued. Such therapeutic programs have not been approved for general use.

Other measures   Although calcitonin therapy of osteoporosis has been advocated, this hormone probably does not produce benefits greater than those attained with the use of supplemental calcium and vitamin D. Oral phosphates (greater than 1 g elemental phosphorus per day in divided doses) may decrease urinary calcium excretion in patients with marked hypercalciuria and thereby improve calcium tolerance. However, phosphate has not been shown to be of value in the treatment of patients with postmenopausal osteoporosis who have normal levels of serum phosphorus.

RICKETS AND OSTEOMALACIA

The terms *rickets* and *osteomalacia* are used to describe a group of disorders in which there is defective mineralization of the newly formed organic matrix of the skeleton. In *rickets* the growing skeleton is involved; defective mineralization occurs not only in bone but also in the cartilaginous matrix of the growth plate. The term *osteomalacia* is usually reserved for the disorder of mineralization of the adult skeleton in which the epiphyseal growth plates are closed. There are a number of conditions that result in rickets and/or osteomalacia such as inadequate dietary intake of vitamin D, inadequate exposure to ultraviolet radiation to form endogenous vitamin D, intestinal malabsorption of vitamin D, chronic acidosis, renal tubular defects which produce hypophosphatemia or acidosis, and chronic administration of anticonvulsants. In the renal tubular disorders rickets and osteomalacia develop in the presence of normal intestinal function and are not cured by treatment with doses of vitamin D adequate to cure deficiency rickets. Thus the term *vitamin D–resistant* (or *refractory*) has been applied in these instances. Renal insufficiency, especially in children, is also associated with rickets or osteomalacia. A classification of rickets and osteomalacia is given in Table 352-2.

PATHOGENESIS AND HISTOPATHOLOGY   For mineralization of matrices of skeletal tissues to take place, a sufficient concentration of calcium and phosphate is required at the mineralization sites. Although it is not known what the optimal concentration is at these sites, mineralization does not proceed normally when the concentrations of calcium and inorganic phosphate in the plasma (and extracellular fluid) are too low. Other conditions required for normal mineralization include intact metabolic and transport functions of osteoblasts and chondrocytes, adequate collagen matrix, possibly phosphorylation or other modifications of matrix components, and low concentrations of inhibitory substances such as specific protein polysaccharide fractions and inorganic pyrophosphate. A specific function of γ-carboxyglutamic acid–containing proteins, which are synthesized by bone cells, in the mineralization process has not been demonstrated although they appear to bind calcium ions. In cartilage the initial mineral phase is in membrane-bound extracellular vesicles. If the osteoblast continues to produce matrix components which cannot be adequately mineralized, the typical features of rickets and osteomalacia result. If calcification continues to be inadequate, the production of organic matrix (osteoid) must also gradually decrease. In bone there will be an increase in the fraction of the forming surface covered by incompletely mineralized osteoid, an increase in osteoid volume and thickness (the latter normally less than 12 to 14 μm), and a decrease in the staining intensity of the so-called "calcification front." There is a marked decrease in the rate of apposition of mineralized bone. A variety of

TABLE 352-2
Classification of rickets and osteomalacia

I Vitamin D lack
   A Dietary deficiency
   B Deficient endogenous synthesis
II Gastrointestinal
   A Small-intestinal diseases with malabsorption
   B Partial or total gastrectomy
   C Hepatobiliary disease
   D Chronic pancreatic insufficiency
III Disorders of vitamin D metabolism
   A Hereditary: Pseudo-vitamin D deficiency or vitamin D dependency, types I and II
   B Acquired
      1 Anticonvulsants
      2 Chronic renal failure
IV Acidosis
   A Distal renal tubular acidosis (classic or type I)
   B Secondary forms of renal acidosis
   C Ureterosigmoidostomy
   D Drug-induced disease
      1 Chronic acetazolamide ingestion
      2 Chronic ammonium chloride ingestion
V Chronic renal failure
VI Phosphate depletion
   A Dietary: Low phosphate intake plus ingestion of nonabsorbable antacids
   B Impaired renal tubular phosphate reabsorption
      1 Hereditary
         a X-linked hypophosphatemic rickets (vitamin D–resistant rickets)
         b Adult-onset vitamin D–resistant hypophosphatemic osteomalacia
      2 Acquired
         a Sporadic hypophosphatemic osteomalacia (phosphate diabetes)
         b Tumor-associated rickets and osteomalacia
         c Neurofibromatosis
         d Fibrous dysplasia
VII Generalized renal tubular disorders (Fanconi's syndrome)
   A Primary renal
   B Associated with systemic metabolic abnormality
      1 Cystinosis
      2 Glycogenosis
      3 Lowe's syndrome
   C Systemic disorder with associated renal disease
      1 Hereditary
         a Inborn errors
            (*1*) Wilson's disease
            (*2*) Tyrosinemia
         b Neurofibromatosis
      2 Acquired
         a Multiple myeloma
         b Nephrotic syndrome
         c Transplanted kidney
      3 Intoxications
         a Cadmium
         b Lead
         c Outdated tetracycline
VIII Primary mineralization defects
   A Hereditary: Hypophosphatasia
   B Acquired
      1 Diphosphonate (disodium etidronate) treatment
      2 Fluoride treatment
IX States of rapid bone formation with or without a relative defect in bone resorption
   A Postoperative hyperparathyroidism with osteitis fibrosa cystica
   B Osteopetrosis
X Defective matrix synthesis: Fibrogenesis imperfecta ossium
XI Miscellaneous
   A Magnesium-dependent conditions
   B Axial osteomalacia

methods are available to measure the thickness of the osteoid seams and the presence of a calcification front. In routine histological sections stained with hematoxylin and eosin, if the specimens are not overdecalcified in preparation, the more heavily mineralized areas tend to appear violet or blue, whereas the osteoid seams appear pink. Subtle degrees of osteomalacia may not be appreciated with routine preparations, and undecalcified, thin sections (3 to 5 µm) stained, for example, with Goldner's trichrome method are necessary to establish its presence (Fig. 352-2). In addition to these features, rickets is also characterized by inadequate mineralization of the

matrix of cartilage in the growing epiphyseal plate. Calcification in the interstitial regions of the hypertrophic zone is defective, the growth plate increases in thickness, the arrangement of the columns of cartilage cells (usually highly ordered) is disorganized, and there is a variable degree of cupping of the epiphyses. The rachitic bones are often incapable of withstanding usual mechanical stresses and in the process of growth tend to undergo bowing deformities. If rickets is untreated, growth at the epiphyseal plates is slowed and the eventual length of the long bones is diminished.

It has not been established whether vitamin D, through one of its metabolites, has a major direct effect on mineralization. Its primary role after metabolic conversion to 25-OHD and $1\alpha,25\text{-}(OH)_2D$ is to permit the regulation and enhance absorption of calcium ions from the intestinal lumen. The pathogenesis of inadequate skeletal mineralization when there is insufficient vitamin D present, from whatever cause, is probably as follows. Insufficient concentrations of the active metabolites of vitamin D lead to decreased intestinal absorption of calcium and decreased mobilization of calcium from bone, resulting in hypocalcemia. This stimulates increased secretion of parathyroid hormone (PTH) and, later, increased synthesis of PTH and hyperplasia of the parathyroid glands. The increased circulating concentration of PTH tends to raise plasma calcium concentrations but also stimulates increased renal phosphate clearance, which, in turn, produces hypophosphatemia. When the concentration of phosphorus in the extracellular fluid falls below a critical level, mineralization cannot proceed normally. In severe degrees of vitamin D lack, normocalcemia cannot be maintained, and the driving force for mineralization is further decreased.

Phosphate depletion alone can produce osteomalacia as is seen in patients consuming large amounts of nonabsorbable antacids. Excessive renal loss of phosphate due to decreased tubular reabsorption may also result in the hypophosphatemia responsible for the osteomalacia in some of the renal tubular disorders. Secondary hyperparathyroidism is probably not present in many of these patients. It should be emphasized that hypophosphatemia per se produces mineralization defects despite its effect on increasing the activity of the renal 25-OHD 1α-hydroxylase. Hypophosphatemia cannot account for the osteomalacia in all the disorders listed in Table 352-2. In chronic renal failure, for example, plasma phosphorus levels are not decreased and usually are increased. Similarly plasma phosphorus levels are not depressed in infants and children with osteomalacia secondary to hypophosphatasia, a hereditary deficiency in alkaline phosphatase.

CLINICAL FINDINGS The clinical problems of rickets are the result of skeletal deformities, susceptibility to fractures, weakness and hypotonia, and disturbances in growth. In extreme instances of vitamin D-deficiency rickets, hypocalcemia may be sufficient to produce tetany which, when severe, may be accompanied by laryngeal spasm and convulsive seizures.

In infants and young children features include listlessness, irritability, and often profound hypotonia and muscular weakness. As the disorder progresses, children become unable to walk without support. In the skull abnormal parietal flattening appears, as well as frontal bossing. The calvaria is softened (craniotabes), and widening of sutures may be evident. Prominence of the costochondral junctions is called the "rachitic rosary," and the indentation of the lower ribs at the site of attachment of the diaphragm is known as *Harrison's groove*. If the rickets is untreated, progressive deformities of the pelvis and extremities result, with bowing particularly common in the

FIGURE 352-2

Photomicrograph of an undemineralized section stained with Goldner method of an iliac crest bone biopsy from a 45-year-old man with chronic renal failure maintained on hemodialysis. Almost the entire surface is covered by osteoid (O) readily distinguished from mineralized bone (MB). The thickness of the osteoid seams exceeds 100 μm in several areas.

tibia, femur, radius, and ulna. Because of inadequate structure of the bones, fractures are frequent. Dental eruption is often delayed, and enamel defects are common.

The presentation of osteomalacia in adults usually is not as dramatic as that of rickets in infants and children. The skeletal deformities may be overlooked, and the features of the underlying disorder may dominate, as, for example, in the vitamin D loss associated with adult celiac disease. Major symptoms, when they occur, include varying degrees of diffuse skeletal pain and bony tenderness. Pain may be especially prominent about the hips and may result in an antalgic gait. Muscular weakness is also common in adults with osteomalacia, although it may be difficult to distinguish from hesitancy to move because of skeletal pain. Weakness, usually proximal in distribution, may be prominent, however, and may be severe enough to mimic that of primary muscle disorders and may contribute to the waddling gait. In some patients pain and muscular weakness may be sufficient for them to be confined to bed and chair. Many factors, including the secondary hyperparathyroidism, contribute to the myopathy when it is present. Clinical improvement in the myopathy usually results from specific therapy of the osteomalacia such as vitamin D repletion in nutritional osteomalacia, phosphate replacement in renal hypophosphatemia, or correction of acidosis. Fractures of involved bones may occur with minimal trauma. When the ribs are involved, severe deformities may develop in the thoracic cage, and the collapse of vertebral bodies may produce loss of height.

RADIOLOGICAL FEATURES Radiological changes in the skeleton in rickets and osteomalacia reflect the pathological changes. In rickets the alterations are most evident at the epiphyseal growth plate which is increased in thickness, cupped, and reveals a haziness at the metaphyseal border due to decreased calcification of the hypertrophic zone and inadequate mineralization of the primary spongiosa. The trabecular pattern of the metaphyses is abnormal, the cortices of the diaphyses may be thinned, and bowing of the shafts may be present.

In osteomalacia there is usually some decrease in bone density associated with loss of trabeculae and variable degrees of thinning of the cortices. In some patients the radiological changes are indistinguishable from those seen in osteoporosis. Trabecular patterns may be blurred, producing a homogeneous ground glass appearance. The finding that suggests osteo-

malacia more specifically is the presence of radiolucent bands ranging from a few millimeters to several centimeters in length, usually perpendicular to the surface of the bones. They are particularly common at the inner aspects of the femur, especially near the femoral neck, in the pelvis, in the outer edge of the scapula, in the upper fibula, and in the metatarsals (Figs. 352-3 and 352-4). These usually symmetrical radiolucent bands, called *pseudofractures* or *Looser's zones*, occur most often at sites where major arteries cross the bones, and are thought to be due to the mechanical stress of the pulsation of these vessels. Arteriography has confirmed that the origins of the pseudofractures correspond to the location of major vessels in some instances. Subperiosteal erosions along the diaphyseal cortices are sometimes seen in patients in whom secondary hyperparathyroidism is present.

In some patients with osteomalacia increased rather than decreased density of bones may be observed. This is seen in patients with renal tubular disorders, rather than with vitamin D deficiency, and may produce a striking degree of thickening of the cortices and trabeculae of spongy bone. Despite the increase in mass of bone per unit volume, microscopically the trabeculae are covered with abnormally thickened osteoid seams typical of osteomalacia. Similar findings may be noted in patients with chronic renal failure. The reason for the hyperostosis is unknown; the bone is still architecturally abnormal and subject to fracture with relatively minimal trauma.

LABORATORY FINDINGS Changes in serum concentrations of calcium inorganic phosphorus, 25-OHD, and $1\alpha,25$-$(OH)_2D$ vary with the different disorders. In states of vitamin D deficiency, whether due to dietary lack, inadequate sunlight exposure, or intestinal malabsorption, serum calcium levels are normal or low, whereas phosphorus and 25-OHD levels are characteristically low. In adults phosphorus concentrations less than 2.8 mg per 100 ml are abnormal; in children the lower limit of normal is closer to 4.0 to 4.5 mg per 100 ml. In *severe* states of vitamin D depletion, hypocalcemia may also be seen, occasionally sufficient to produce tetany. Mild acidosis and generalized aminoaciduria may also be found, as a result of secondary hyperparathyroidism. As a rule, patients with renal tubular disorders maintain normal serum calcium levels while hypophosphatemia is characteristic. Other laboratory findings such as glucosuria, aminoaciduria, acidosis, and hypouricemia reflect variable degrees of disturbance of proximal tubular

FIGURE 352-3
Radiographs of the scapula of a 58-year-old woman with phosphate diabetes. The presence of a pseudofracture or Looser's zone is indicated by the arrow.

or elevated in hypophosphatasia. Increased excretion of hydroxyproline peptides is a component of those conditions in which secondary hyperparathyroidism and excessive bone resorption are associated with the defect in mineralization. Levels of alkaline phosphatase in plasma are usually elevated in rickets or osteomalacia, but typical and even severe osteomalacia, especially that due to renal tubular disorders, may be accompanied by normal or only borderline elevations. Levels may increase during the early phases of therapy.

DIETARY VITAMIN D DEFICIENCY AND INADEQUATE ENDOGENOUS SYNTHESIS Rickets was first described in England in about 1650 where it affected largely the poor people in sunless urban areas. Most foods unfortified with vitamin D contain insufficient amounts of the vitamin to prevent rickets in growing children or osteomalacia in adults living in temperate-zone cities. As discussed in Chap. 351, in the absence of supplements, vitamin D must be formed endogenously through the ultraviolet irradiation of precursor 7-dehydrocholesterol in the skin. Many factors decrease the formation of vitamin D_3 from its precursor: increased melanin pigmentation, hyperkeratosis, limited exposure of the body, short days of sunlight, oblique angle of ultraviolet irradiation, and factors in the atmosphere, such as smog, which prevent adequate penetration of the required radiation. Since fortification of dairy products and routine use of vitamin D supplements for infants have been in effect, deficiency rickets is very unusual in the United States. Poor, dark-skinned infants living in crowded Northern cites are most susceptible. However, osteomalacia due to vitamin D deficiency still is observed in adults, especially in elderly individuals who tend to remain indoors and whose dietary intake of vitamin D is inadequate (probably less than 70 to 100 IU per day).

VITAMIN D LOSS AND INTESTINAL MALABSORPTION Osteomalacia may be seen in patients with intestinal malabsorption such as in adult celiac disease and regional enteritis. Prior to the discovery of gluten sensitivity in some of these cases, celiac disease was among the more common disorders underlying osteomalacia. Vitamin D absorption, which normally occurs via chylomicrons, is impaired in diseases causing steatorrhea such as chronic biliary obstruction where emulsification of fat is disturbed. Patients with cholestatic liver disease or extrahepat-

function or features of the underlying disease (e.g., low plasma ceruloplasmin in Wilson's disease or abnormalities of immunoglobulins in multiple myeloma). In chronic renal failure hyperphosphatemia and some degree of hypocalcemia are usually seen accompanied by normal 25-OHD and low $1\alpha,25$-$(OH)_2D$ levels. In nephrotic syndrome serum 25-OHD levels are low due to urinary losses. Serum phosphorus levels are also normal

FIGURE 352-4
Radiograph of the femurs of a 47-year-old woman with Fanconi's syndrome of adult onset. The presence of multiple pseudofractures is indicated by the arrows.

ic biliary obstruction may have low serum levels of 25-OHD$_3$ and osteomalacia, due not only to poor vitamin D absorption but also to decreased hepatic production of 25-OHD$_3$ and disruption in its enterohepatic circulation. Osteomalacia is less frequent in chronic pancreatic insufficiency. Patients who have had gastric surgery may also develop osteomalacia, possibly due to malfunction of the proximal small bowel. Factors other than failure to absorb vitamin D may contribute to the osteomalacia in patients with small-bowel disease, such as inadequate absorbing surface and failure of intestinal cells to respond to the active metabolites of vitamin D. Secondary hyperparathyroidism is usually present in intestinal malabsorption, as it is in dietary lack of vitamin D.

ABNORMAL METABOLISM OF VITAMIN D Although serum 25-OHD levels are reduced in some instances of parenchymal and obstructive liver disease, studies have not yet correlated these findings with quantitative histological observations. Patients consuming anticonvulsant drugs such as phenobarbital and/or phenytoin may develop rickets or osteomalacia. For a given intake of vitamin D, patients receiving chronic anticonvulsant drugs have lower serum levels of calcium and 25-OHD. Consumption of anticonvulsants may be especially important in individuals whose intake of vitamin D is barely optimal, who are nonambulatory and confined indoors, who have chronic recurrent infections, or in whom mild intestinal malfunction exists as in the postgastrectomy state. As discussed in Chap. 351 the anticonvulsant drugs have multiple actions on calcium homeostasis that are dependent and independent of vitamin D metabolism.

A syndrome superficially resembling vitamin D–resistant rickets has been termed *pseudovitamin D deficiency*. Because these patients respond to pharmacological doses of vitamin D, this disease has also been termed *vitamin D–dependent rickets*. These patients have rickets or osteomalacia, a tendency to hypocalcemia but normal or only slightly depressed serum phosphorus levels, a response to a variable but moderate dose of vitamin D which is usually excellent and complete, and an autosomal recessive inheritance. No other renal tubular abnormalities are found. These patients also respond to small doses of 1α,25-(OH)$_2$D or 1α-OHD. Most of the cases described have low serum 1α,25-(OH)$_2$D levels, suggesting a defect in the renal production of 1α,25-(OH)$_2$D; these have been classified as vitamin D–dependent rickets, type I. Vitamin D–dependent rickets, type II, is postulated to result from an impaired responsiveness of target tissues to 1α,25-(OH)$_2$D. In these subjects elevated serum 1α,25-(OH)$_2$D levels are observed which increase further when large doses of vitamin D are administered.

RENAL TUBULAR DISORDERS Rickets and osteomalacia develop in association with a variety of disorders of proximal renal tubular function. These disorders have in common increased renal clearance of inorganic phosphorus and hypophosphatemia with normal, or near normal, glomerular filtration rate. Most frequently, increased phosphate clearance with resultant hypophosphatemia is an isolated defect with no other abnormalities present except for some increase in urinary glycine excretion (hyperglycinuria). Primary hypophosphatemia (*phosphate diabetes* and *vitamin D–resistant rickets* are terms applied to these cases especially when the disorder presents in early childhood) is characterized by progressively severe skeletal deformities, dwarfism, and sex-linked dominant inheritance. In some of these patients there may be spontaneous remissions followed by recurrences in adult life associated, for example, with pregnancy and lactation. Serum 25-OHD levels are normal while serum 1α,25-(OH)$_2$D levels have variably been reported as normal and low. There is little evidence that

1α,25-(OH)$_2$D$_3$ therapy is of specific benefit in a majority of these patients. It is likely that the biochemical defect is not the same in all these kindreds and may not be related to defects in metabolism of vitamin D. Sporadic cases of hypophosphatemia have also been described in adults in whom family histories have been negative and where proximal muscle weakness has been a prominent feature. In sex-linked hypophosphatemic rickets, muscle weakness is not characteristic. As mentioned above, in most of the untreated cases of renal tubular disorders with rickets and osteomalacia, secondary hyperparathyroidism is not present.

In other patients the disorder in tubular function may be more widespread, involving (besides phosphorus) glucose, potassium, amino acids, and uric acid; the various combinations are termed the de Toni-Debré-Fanconi syndrome. The more complete renal tubular defects may also occur sporadically or in families. In some instances the lesion is simply part of a more widespread disorder as in Wilson's disease and cystinosis. The acidosis of proximal tubular defects also plays a role in development of osteomalacia, possibly by altering metabolism of vitamin D or altering renal handling of calcium and phosphorus. In this regard osteomalacia has accompanied the hyperchloremic acidosis of ureterocolic anastomosis. A number of cases have been reported in which hypophosphatemic osteomalacia and high renal phosphate clearance have been associated with a variety of tumors, such as giant-cell tumors (benign and malignant) or reparative granulomas, but hemangiomas of soft tissues have also been implicated. In some instances removal of the tumor has resulted in normalization of renal phosphate clearance, rise in serum phosphorus, and remission of the rickets or osteomalacia. The mechanism of this response has not been definitely elucidated.

CHRONIC RENAL FAILURE Histologically osteomalacia is common in patients with chronic renal failure; it often tends to be the predominant phase of renal osteodystrophy in younger patients and statistically is more frequent in those with the lower plasma levels of calcium and phosphorus. There is almost always a component of secondary hyperparathyroidism and osteitis fibrosa accompanying the defect in mineralization. The defect itself probably involves a decreased conversion of 25-OHD to 1α,25-(OH)$_2$D because of either insufficient viable renal cortical tissue or the inhibitory effect of hyperphosphatemia on renal 25-OHD 1α-hydroxylase activity. In addition, there may be a primary defect in intestinal calcium absorption. Part of the secondary hyperparathyroidism may also be due to decreased phosphate clearance and subsequent hyperphosphatemia. In the presence of near-normal plasma concentration of calcium and hyperphosphatemia, it is not clear why mineralization of the organic matrix should be incomplete. Although it has been postulated that inhibitors of mineralization are present to account for this anomaly, the osteomalacic component usually does respond to large doses of vitamin D or dihydrotachysterol and to small doses of 1α,25-(OH)$_2$D$_3$ or 1α-OHD$_3$. In some patients with renal osteodystrophy the total bone mass may be increased (osteosclerosis), resulting in increased density of bone seen radiologically. This is particularly evident in the spine where a characteristic appearance is that of dense bone at the superior and inferior margins of the vertebral bodies with more radiolucent central portions ("rugger jersey sign"). Histologically, although there is more bone per unit area, each trabecula is covered by an abnormally wide osteoid seam.

HYPOPHOSPHATASIA Rickets is a feature of this heritable deficiency of alkaline phosphatase in infants and children, although osteomalacia has been an inconstant finding in adults with hypophosphatasia. Serum phosphorus levels are not reduced. Phosphorylethanolamine and phosphocholine are excreted in excessive amounts in the urine, but it is not clear how this is related to the inadequate skeletal mineralization. There is a direct correlation between plasma alkaline phosphatase and inorganic pyrophosphatase. Since patients with hypophosphatasia are also deficient in pyrophosphatase, it is possible that concentrations in inorganic pyrophosphate, a potent inhibitor of mineralization, are too high to allow normal mineralization of formation sites.

OTHER DISORDERS ASSOCIATED WITH DEFECTIVE MINERALIZATION Disturbances in mineralization may be seen in patients consuming high doses of fluoride ion and in patients with Paget's disease treated with disodium etidronate. Some decrease in mineralization of newly forming matrix, increase in surface covered by osteoid, and increase in the width of the osteoid seams are seen in several conditions that are not usually considered as osteomalacia except by these criteria. Biopsies in some of these conditions would show a normal calcification front. Examples include patients with the osteitis fibrosa of hyperparathyroidism in the weeks to months following surgical cure. In these circumstances there is a temporary imbalance between the rate at which mineral is supplied to bone and the rate at which bone matrix is formed. Wide osteoid seams as well as hypophosphatemia are also seen in the bones of children with osteopetrosis in whom there is inadequate resorption of bone and calcified cartilage but active bone formation.

A condition which resembles osteomalacia and is associated with a coarsened, mottled bony trabecular pattern, pseudofractures, and bone pain, but normal plasma levels of calcium and phosphorus, is *fibrogenesis imperfecta ossium*. Histologically the bone has a distinctive appearance, with wide osteoid seams and a distortion of the birefringent pattern of normal bone suggesting an abnormality in the collagen recently deposited. The nature of the abnormality is not known.

TREATMENT OF RICKETS AND OSTEOMALACIA The therapeutic approach to each of the disorders associated with rickets and osteomalacia is somewhat different. In rickets and osteomalacia due to dietary absence of vitamin D or inadequate exposure to sunlight, vitamin D_2 or vitamin D_3 is given orally in doses of 2000 to 4000 IU (0.05 to 0.1 mg) daily for 6 to 12 weeks, followed by daily supplements of 200 to 400 IU, which are adequate to prevent the development of the disorder in otherwise normal subjects. In infants and children such treatment causes improvement in muscle tone and strength, rise in serum calcium and phosphorus, and fall in alkaline phosphatase levels after several weeks. Radiological evidence of healing is first noted within weeks and may be complete by a few months. Calcium supplements and larger initial doses of vitamin D may be necessary in infants and children with tetany. In adults with nutritional osteomalacia healing of pseudofractures may be evident within 3 to 4 weeks after therapy with as little as 2000 IU (0.05 mg) vitamin D daily. Healing is complete usually by 6 months.

Patients with osteomalacia due to intestinal malabsorption do not respond to the relatively small doses of vitamin D that can cure deficiency-nutritional osteomalacia. In the presence of active steatorrhea, oral doses of vitamin D of 40,000 to 100,000 IU (1.0 to 2.5 mg) daily may be required in addition to large doses of calcium (e.g., 15 to 20 g calcium lactate orally per day). In some instances oral vitamin D is ineffective, and the parenteral route is required (e.g., 10,000 IU intramuscularly per day). Another approach is the use of ultraviolet irradiation, e.g., total body erythema doses daily for several weeks, in addition to supplemental calcium. Small doses of 1α-OHD$_3$ (2.5 to 5.0 μg daily) or $1\alpha,25$-(OH)$_2$D$_3$ (0.5 to 1.0 μg daily) are also effective in treatment of this form of osteomalacia. Inorganic phosphate therapy is not indicated either in deficiency osteomalacia or in intestinal malabsorption, since hypocalce-

mia will develop and intestinal and calcium absorption remain inadequate. In all patients in whom large doses of vitamin D are used, monitoring of plasma calcium levels at intervals is essential. Semiquantitative urinary calcium measurements alone are inadequate.

In patients who have been using anticonvulsants, it is often necessary to continue the drugs while adding supplemental vitamin D and monitoring levels of serum calcium at biweekly intervals and serum 25-OHD levels bimonthly for the first few months until a therapeutic response (evidence of radiological healing, improvement in symptoms) is obtained. Doses varying from 4000 to 40,000 IU daily have been recommended.

Treatment of rickets and osteomalacia in the presence of renal tubular disorders is more difficult, and there is not uniform agreement as to the exact regimen to be followed. The X-linked form of hypophosphatemic osteomalacia has usually been treated with large doses of vitamin D (from 40,000 IU to several hundred thousand international units or more daily). With vitamin D therapy alone, there is radiological evidence of healing in many patients, but this is usually incomplete; some hypophosphatemia persists, linear skeletal growth remains abnormally slow, and bony deformities continue to develop. In addition, the potential hazard of hypercalcemia and its consequences exists. The addition of oral supplements of inorganic phosphate in divided doses of 1.0 to 3.6 g phosphorus daily has improved the clinical and radiological response, allowed the use of smaller doses of vitamin D, and improved the rate of linear growth in many younger subjects. In some adults, therapy with inorganic phosphate alone has been successful in abolishing muscle weakness and bone pain and in producing radiological and histological healing. The addition of vitamin D improves calcium balance and helps decrease secondary hyperparathyroidism and maintain a higher level of serum phosphorus to permit complete healing. In some patients there may be temporary increase in bone pain and rise in serum alkaline phosphatase during the early phases of treatment. In the osteomalacia associated with the chronic acidosis of renal tubular disorders, the use of alkali may be of value in supplementing therapy with phosphate and vitamin D. In patients with ureterosigmoidostomy, oral sodium bicarbonate has reversed acidosis, improved serum phosphate level, and healed the bone disease; with maintenance use of alkali, recurrence of symptoms has been prevented.

Patients with nephrotic syndrome and low serum 25-OHD levels benefit from modest vitamin D supplementation. In chronic renal failure high doses of vitamin D, similar to those needed to treat osteomalacia of renal tubular disorders, are used. Dihydrotachysterol, a pseudo-1α-OHD analog, at doses of 0.2 to 1.0 mg daily is effective in treating hypocalcemia and osteodystrophy resulting from chronic renal failure. $1\alpha,25$-(OH)$_2$D$_3$ and 1α-OHD$_3$ in small doses are equally effective in therapy of most cases of renal osteodystrophy. 1α-OHD$_3$, which requires hepatic hydroxylation before it is active, is widely used in Europe but is an experimental drug in the United States. $1\alpha,25$-(OH)$_2$D$_3$ is approved for use in the treatment of hypocalcemic patients on chronic hemodialysis. The generic name of this drug is *calcitriol;* it is available in dosages of 0.25 and 0.50 μg. The recommended initial dose is 0.25 μg per day. If after 2 to 4 weeks on this dose the biochemical parameters are unaltered, the dose is increased by 0.25 μg per day every 2 to 4 weeks until a satisfactory clinical biochemical response (including elevation of serum calcium levels and decrease in PTH levels) is obtained. The usual dose is 0.5 to 1.0 μg per day. Because there are no regulatory mechanisms to control the biological responses to 1α-(OH)D$_3$, there is a high incidence of transient hypercalcemia, especially in patients initially treated. Thus, frequent (biweekly) serum calcium determinations are encouraged during the first 1 to 2 months of therapy; they can be made at monthly intervals once a stable dose has been established. Since $1\alpha,25\text{-}(OH)_2D_3$ has a short duration of action and is not stored in fat depots, hypercalcemia is reversed by discontinuing its use or decreasing its dose. Hypercalcemia usually resolves in 2 to 7 days. Phosphate supplements are, of course, contraindicated in the usual patient with chronic renal failure. Occasionally, however, hypophosphatemia may result from the excessive use of nonabsorbable antacids in addition to excessive removal of phosphate through hemodialysis.

In patients who have had rickets in childhood, the abnormal mechanical stress of severe deformities may contribute to the development of degenerative joint disease, particularly in hips and knees. Osteotomies at the proper time after healing has occurred may help to prevent this complication and avoid more extensive arthroplasties later in life.

REFERENCES

Osteoporosis

Avioli LV: Osteoporosis: Pathogenesis and therapy, in *Metabolic Bone Disease,* LV Avioli, SM Krane (eds). New York, Academic, 1977, vol I, p 307
———: What to do with "postmenopausal osteoporosis." Am J Med 65:881, 1978
Barzel UA: *Osteoporosis.* New York, Grune & Stratton, 1970
Dequeker J: Bone and aging. Ann Rheum Dis 34:100, 1975
Horwitz RI, Feinstein AR: Alternative analytic methods for case-control studies of estrogens and endometrial cancer. N Engl J Med 299:1089, 1978
Jick H: Replacement estrogens and endometrial cancer. N Engl J Med 300:218, 1979
Jowsey J: *Metabolic Diseases of Bone.* Philadelphia, Saunders, 1977
Nordin BEC: *Osteoporosis. Clinics in Endocrinology Metabolism II.* Philadelphia, Saunders, 1973
Recker RR et al: Effect of estrogens and calcium carbonate on bone loss in postmenopausal women. Ann Intern Med 87:649, 1977
Thomson DL, Frame B: Involutional osteopenia: Current concepts. Ann Intern Med 85:789, 1976
Wallach S: Drug treatment of bone. Semin Drug Treat 2:1, 1972

Rickets and osteomalacia

Bordier P et al: Vitamin D metabolites and bone mineralization in man. J Clin Endocrinol Metab 46:284, 1978
Dent CE, Stamp TCB: Vitamin D, rickets, and osteomalacia, in *Metabolic Bone Disease.* LV Avioli, SM Krane (eds). New York, Academic, 1977, vol I p 237
Frame B et al: Osteomalacia: Current concepts. Ann Intern Med 89:966, 1978
Goldstein DA et al: Blood levels of 25-hydroxyvitamin D in nephrotic syndrome. Ann Intern Med 87:664, 1977
Hahn TJ et al: Serum 25-hydroxycalciferol levels and bone mass in children on chronic anticonvulsant therapy. N Engl J Med 292:550, 1975
Linovitz RJ et al: Tumor-induced osteomalacia and rickets: A surgically curable syndrome. J Bone Joint Surg (Am) 58A:419, 1976
Mankin HJ: Rickets, osteomalacia and renal osteodystrophy. J Bone Joint Surg (Am) 56A:101, 352, 1974
Nagant de Deuxchaisnes C, Krane SM: The treatment of adult phosphate diabetes and Fanconi syndrome with neutral sodium phosphate. Am J Med 43:508, 1967
Schott GD, Wills MR: Muscle weakness in osteomalacia. Lancet 1:626, 1976
Stanbury SW: Osteomalacia. Clin Endocrinol Metab 1:239, 1972
Steinbach HL, Noetzli M: Roentgen appearance of the skeleton in osteomalacia and rickets. Am J Roentgenol 91:955, 1964

353
PAGET'S DISEASE OF BONE

STEPHEN M. KRANE

Paget's disease of bone (osteitis deformans) is among the most common of the chronic skeletal diseases. In the strict sense it is a focal disease, although occasionally it may be widespread. Histologically the initial event is excessive resorption of bone mediated by cells such as osteoclasts, followed by the replacement of normal marrow by vascular, fibrous connective tissue. At some stage in the disease, and to a variable degree, the resorbed bone is replaced by coarse-fibered, dense trabecular bone organized in haphazard fashion. The irregular and often rapid deposition of this new bone causes an increase in the number of prominent, irregular cement lines which gives the bone its characteristic "mosaic" pattern. Some areas of bone may show evidence of both excessive resorption and the chaotic new bone formation.

INCIDENCE The prevalence of Paget's disease is difficult to determine since it is most often asymptomatic and is detected usually when roentgenograms are obtained for other reasons. On the basis of autopsy examination, the incidence of Paget's disease has been estimated to be about 3 percent in individuals over the age of 40; there is increased likelihood of occurrence with increasing age. Figures based on radiological surveys indicate less than 1 percent in the adult population in the United States, Great Britain, and Australia. However, the incidence varies markedly in different parts of the world; in some areas, including India, Japan, the Middle East, and Scandinavia, the disease is exceedingly rare.

ETIOLOGY Almost a century after the original description of the disorder, and despite intensive study and widespread interest, the etiology of Paget's disease is unknown. No convincing evidence of endocrine abnormality has been produced. Although pagetic bone can be exceedingly vascular, out of proportion to any other disorder, it has not been established that the vascular abnormality is primary. The observation that some of the manifestations of the disease can be suppressed with the use of adrenal corticosteroids, salicylates, and cytotoxic drugs is of interest, although there is not sufficient information to support earlier hypotheses that an inflammatory process is the fundamental lesion. Intranuclear inclusions have been found by electron microscopy in osteoclasts in pagetic bone but not in bone from normal persons or patients with various bone diseases. The inclusions resemble those produced by paramyxoviruses, but their identity has not been established.

PATHOPHYSIOLOGY The characteristic feature of Paget's disease is increased resorption of bone accompanied by an increase in bone formation, which is usually adequate to compensate. In the early phase of Paget's disease, bone resorption predominates (for example, in the variant, *osteoporosis circumscripta*), and the bones are exceedingly vascular. This has been termed the *osteoporotic, osteolytic,* or *destructive phase* of disease in which the external calcium balance may be negative. Commonly the excessive resorption is followed closely by formation of new pagetic bone. In this so-called "mixed" phase of the disease, the rate of bone formation is so geared to that of bone resorption that the magnitude of the increase in bone turnover is not reflected in the overall calcium balance.

As the activity of the disease decreases, a progressive decrease in resorptive rate may occur, eventually leading to the occurrence of hard, dense, less vascular bone (the so-called *osteoplastic* or *sclerotic* phase) and a positive external calcium balance. Techniques measuring disappearance rates of injected radioisotopes of calcium or strontium have shown that the rates of bone turnover may be increased enormously in patients with active Paget's disease, occasionally more than twenty times normal. The magnitude of the increase in turnover varies with the extent as well as the activity of the disease. The increase correlates well with the increased levels of plasma alkaline phosphatase, which are higher in Paget's disease than in any other condition with the exception of hereditary hyperphosphatasia. Although increased bone resorption enhances release of calcium and phosphate ions from the inorganic mineral phase of bone, utilization of these ions for new bone formation and, presumably, feedback control of parathyroid hormone secretion usually maintain the concentration of calcium ions in the plasma at normal levels. The concentration of phosphate in the plasma is normal or slightly elevated. When marked imbalance between bone formation and resorption occurs in favor of resorption, as after prolonged immobilization or fractures, urinary calcium excretion may be increased, and rarely hypercalcemia may be encountered. Resorption involves the organic phase of bone as well as the mineral phase. Although the inorganic ions of the mineral phase are reutilized for bone formation, amino acids such as hydroxyproline and hydroxylysine released during resorption of the collagen matrix of bone are not reutilized for collagen biosynthesis. The urinary excretion of small peptides containing hydroxyproline is increased in Paget's disease, reflecting the increased bone resorption. Peptides of higher molecular weight (about 5000) containing hydroxyproline and other amino acids in proportions characteristic of collagen are also excreted in increased amounts in the urine and are correlated with increased bone formation.

RADIOLOGICAL CHANGES The radiological findings in Paget's disease reflect the underlying pathology and the phase of the disease which predominates at the time of the examination. The pelvic bones are most commonly involved, followed by the femur, skull, tibia, lumbosacral spine, dorsal spine, clavicles, and ribs in that order; small bones are not as frequently diseased. The lytic phase of the disease may be overlooked except when it occurs in the skull as *osteoporosis circumscripta,* with areas of sharply demarcated radiolucency in the frontal, parietal, and occipital bones. In the long bones the lytic areas are usually first seen at one end, from which they progress toward the other end with a V-shaped advancing edge. The lesion may produce expansion of the cortex and exhibit other features which suggest malignancy. Usually the lytic area is followed by a zone of increased density, representing the new bone formation of the mixed phase of the disease. In general, the bone shows enlargement with irregularly widened cortex in a coarse, striated pattern and increased density, occasionally focal in distribution. Perpendicular lines of radiolucency (cortical infractions) are frequent and occur on the convex side of bowed long bones, particularly the femur and tibia. Transverse fractures may also occur, some initiated at the sites of these cortical infractions. The remodeling of the pagetic bone usually follows the lines of stress produced by muscle pull or gravity, accounting for the characteristic lateral bowing of the femur or anterior bowing of the tibia and the tendency for most of the dense bone to be deposited on the concave side of the bowed bone. In the skull, in the mixed stage, there is enlargement and thickening, especially of the outer table, with irregular areas of increased density, often spotty (Fig. 353-1). Basilar invagination is common with involvement of the base of the skull. The changes in the pelvis also consist of the combination of bone resorption and new bone formation and are frequently accompanied by a thickening of the pelvic brim, a characteristic of Paget's disease. In the sclerotic phase of the disease, the bone may show uniform increase in density, often in the absence of

striations. This is common in the facial bones but is occasionally seen as well in the vertebrae where a homogeneous, dense pattern gives an "ivory" appearance similar to that produced typically by Hodgkin's disease, although the involved vertebrae are not enlarged in Hodgkin's disease.

CLINICAL PICTURE The clinical presentation of patients with Paget's disease is extremely variable and is a function of the extent of the disease, the particular bones involved, and the presence of associated complications. Many patients are asymptomatic. In these individuals the disorder is discovered because of radiological findings during the course of examination of the pelvis or spine for an unrelated disease or complaint, or because of the finding of an elevated level of plasma alkaline phosphatase. Other individuals may gradually become aware of a swelling or deformity of a long bone or develop a disturbance in gait due to unequal length of and change in the distribution of mechanical forces in the lower extremities. Enlargement of the skull is often not noticed by the patient; individuals may be aware of increasing hat size. Pain in the face and headache are initial complaints in some patients; backache and pain in the lower extremities are common. The pain is usually dull, but occasionally shooting or knifelike pains are described. Pain in the lower extremities may be associated with the transverse cortical infractions which occur along the convex lateral surface of the femur or the anterior surface of the tibia. Often the new lytic lesions detected on bone scan are the most painful. Pain may also be due to involvement of the hip joint resembling degenerative joint disease and characterized by narrowing of the joint space, bony lipping at the margin of the acetabulum, and deepening of the acetabulum. Angioid streaks of the retina have been observed in patients with Paget's disease. Hearing loss is due to direct pagetic involvement of the ossicles of the inner ear or of bone in the region of the cochlea or to impingement on the eighth cranial nerve by pagetic bone narrowing the auditory foramen. More serious neu-

FIGURE 353-1

Lateral roentgenogram of the skull from a 58-year-old woman with Paget's disease of bone.

rological complications can result from overgrowth of pagetic bone at the base of the skull (platybasia) due to compression of the brainstem. Compression of the spinal cord with paraplegia has been observed, particularly with involvement of the mid-dorsal spine. Pathological features of vertebrae have also produced spinal cord lesions.

COMPLICATIONS Blood flow may be markedly increased in extremities involved with Paget's disease. There is proliferation of blood vessels in pagetic bone, but anatomic and functional studies have not confirmed the presence of arteriovenous fistulas. Although there is increased blood flow in the bone itself, there is also cutaneous vasodilatation in the pagetic extremities, which accounts for the increased warmth noted clinically. When the disease is widespread, involving over one-third of the skeleton, the increased blood flow may be associated with *high cardiac output*. In the rare patient with Paget's disease at this stage so-called "high-output heart failure" may result. However, heart disease in pagetic individuals is usually accounted for by the same conditions that occur in other patients of similar age. *Pathological fracture* is a frequent complication in patients with Paget's disease, usually occurring in bones involved in the destructive phase of the disease. In the weight-bearing bones fractures are often incomplete, multiple, and on the convex side of the bone. They may occur spontaneously or follow only slight trauma; the lesions are painful but heal spontaneously with no major disability. More serious fractures may also occur. Complete fractures are often transverse as if the bone were snapped like a piece of chalk. Under these circumstances the fracture may upset the delicate balance between bone formation and resorption in favor of resorption. At this stage the imbalance may be reflected by increased urinary calcium excretion, and in rare instances the serum calcium level may rise to dangerous levels.

There is no characteristic level of urinary calcium excretion in Paget's disease, although there is a tendency for calcium excretion to be higher at any point in the disease when the resorptive phase predominates. This may be a factor which accounts for the somewhat higher incidence of *urinary stone* in these patients, although many of the urinary calculi reported may be unrelated to the pagetic process. In addition to secondary changes in the cartilage of the hip joint, similar changes in bones about the knees may result in articular symptoms. Hyperuricemia and clinical gout commonly occur in men with Paget's disease, and calcific periarthritis is also found in high incidence.

Sarcoma is the most dreaded complication of Paget's disease. Fortunately, the incidence is low, probably no greater than 1 percent, although higher incidence has been noted in some series which include many patients with polyostotic involvement. The sarcomas most frequently arise in the femur, humerus, skull, face, and pelvis, and rarely in the vertebrae. In about 20 percent the tumors are multicentric. Histologically, they are usually osteosarcomas, although fibrosarcomas and chondrosarcomas have also been found. Increase in pain and swelling are the most common complaints which lead to recognition of the sarcomas. The level of alkaline phosphatase in the serum of patients with sarcomas reflects the activity and extent of the Paget's disease, although in occasional patients an "explosive rise" of the phosphatase level may accompany the growth of the sarcoma. However, in some patients with limited involvement, phosphatase levels may be only slightly elevated and give no clue to the development of the malignant lesion. The prognosis is extremely poor following the development of sarcomas, and ablative operative therapy is rarely successful. Giant-cell tumors also occur with an increased frequency in

Paget's disease and are usually benign. Pagetic bone is rarely the site of metastases despite its great vascularity.

THERAPY Most patients with Paget's disease require no treatment, since the disease is usually localized in its distribution and does not cause symptoms. Possible indications for therapy include persistent pain in involved bones, neural compression, rapidly progressive deformity resulting in disabling disturbance of posture and/or gait, high-output congestive heart failure, hypercalcemia, and severe hypercalciuria with or without formation of renal stones. *Acetylsalicylic acid* is an effective analgesic, and if it can be tolerated in large enough doses (3.6 to 4.0 g per day) for periods of months or years, there may be some suppression of the disease activity, as shown by decreases in the level of plasma alkaline phosphatase and urinary hydroxyproline excretion. *Indomethacin,* 25 mg three or four times daily, may also relieve pain, especially in the presence of hip involvement. *Glucocorticoids* will suppress the disease but only in large doses (greater than 60 mg prednisone per day) which are usually not tolerated and, therefore, are not recommended. It is of interest, however, that the high cardiac output of some patients with Paget's disease may be reduced significantly after only a few days of glucocorticoid treatment. Although the use of *sodium fluoride* (80 to 120 mg sodium fluoride per day) for more than a year has produced amelioration of symptoms and decrease in the indexes of activity of the disease, this high dose may lead to poorly mineralized bone. Orthopedic procedures also have a role in the management of selected cases. Total hip replacement may be indicated in the patient with severe hip involvement, and osteotomy is useful to correct marked bowing deformities. In patients with fractures or orthopedic procedures or in patients immobilized for any reason, determinations of urinary and serum calcium levels should be performed at intervals to anticipate the development of hypercalciuria and hypercalcemia. Early ambulation and adequate fluid intake are essential. Preparations of sodium phytate or inorganic phosphate to reduce hypercalciuria may be useful under these circumstances (5 to 6 g neutral sodium phosphate daily in divided doses).

Several agents have been introduced which are effective in reducing the excessive bone resorption of Paget's disease and are of possible therapeutic value. Porcine, salmon, and human *calcitonins* have been administered subcutaneously for prolonged periods to pagetic patients, accompanied by decrease in plasma alkaline phosphatase levels and urinary hydroxyproline excretion. Treatment with calcitonin has produced variable decrease in bone pain, improvement in neurological symptoms, and decrease in elevated cardiac output. Some patients have not continued to respond to porcine and salmon calcitonins because of the development of neutralizing antibodies. These individuals will usually still have a satisfactory response to treatment with human calcitonin. In others in whom diminution in response was not associated with development of antibodies, the development of secondary hyperparathyroidism has been postulated, although this cannot account for resistance in all cases. The calcitonins have a limited usefulness in the treatment of Paget's disease. They are probably most useful in patients with pain corresponding to areas of pagetic involvement, not due to associated joint disease. The dose of salmon calcitonin is 50 to 100 MRC units given subcutaneously daily. In some cases it may be possible to reduce the dose to three times weekly. In severe cases alkaline phosphatase levels, although reduced, do not reach the normal range. The disorder relapses after weeks or months when the calcitonin is discontinued.

Cytotoxic drugs such as mithramycin and actinomycin D are potent agents in pagetic patients. Parenteral administration of mithramycin, 10 to 25 μg/kg for 10 to 14 days, has produced striking decrease in urinary hydroxyproline excretion with subsequent decreases in plasma alkaline phosphatase level and clinical improvement. The indexes of active disease again become abnormal within weeks to months following completion of this course of mithramycin therapy. The drug may be continued to be administered as a weekly intravenous bolus. When doses of less than 15 μg/kg have been used, toxicity has been surprisingly low despite potential risks.

Disodium etidronate, a diphosphonate compound, given orally in doses up to 20 mg/kg per day has also been effective in reducing indexes of bone resorption in almost all cases and producing clinical improvement in some cases. In contrast to therapy with the calcitonins, the use of disodium etidronate often brings biochemical abnormalities to normal even in severe cases. Serum alkaline phosphatase and urinary hydroxyproline excretion remain decreased for several months after withdrawal of the drug and only gradually return to pretreatment levels. In doses of 20 mg/kg per day mineralization of new bone may be inhibited and predispose to fracture. It is therefore recommended that doses of 5 mg or occasionally 10 mg/kg per day be used for 6-month periods. Treatment could be reinstituted within 3 to 12 months if biochemical relapse occurs.

REFERENCES

Avramides A: Salmon and porcine calcitonin treatment of Paget's disease of bone. Clin Orthop Relat Res 127:78, 1977

Barry HC: *Paget's Disease of Bone.* Edinburgh, E and S Livingstone, 1969

Franck WA et al: Rheumatic manifestations of Paget's disease of bone. Am J Med 56:592, 1974

Khairi MRA, Johnston CC Jr: Treatment of Paget's disease of bone (osteitis deformans) with sodium etidronate (EHDP). Clin Orthop Relat Res 127:94, 1977

Nagant de Deuxchaisnes C, Krane SM: Paget's disease of bone: Clinical and metabolic observations. Medicine 43:233, 1964

Ryan WG: Treatment of Paget's disease of bone with mithramycin. Clin Orthop Relat Res 127:106, 1977

Singer FR: Human calcitonin treatment of Paget's disease of bone. Clin Orthop Relat Res 127:86, 1977

—— et al: Paget's disease of bone, in *Metabolic Bone Disease,* LV Avioli, SM Krane (eds). New York, Academic, 1978, vol II, p 489

Steinbach HL: Some roentgen features of Paget's disease. Am J Roentgenol 86:950, 1961

354

HYPEROSTOSIS, NEOPLASMS, AND OTHER DISORDERS OF BONE AND CARTILAGE

STEPHEN M. KRANE

HYPEROSTOSIS

A number of disease states have in common an increase in the mass of bone per unit volume (hyperostosis). Such increase in bone mass is detected radiologically as increased density of the bone, often associated with a variable degree of disturbance in the architecture of the tissue. In most of these disorders, it is not possible to distinguish between an increase in bone mass due to excessive formation of new bone or decreased resorption of bone already formed. When bone deposition is rapid, the new bone may be of the woven type, but if the process is more chronic, true lamellar bone is formed. The additional bone may be located at the periosteum, within the compact bone of the cortex, or in the trabeculae of the cancellous regions. In the medullary area, the new bone is deposited on and between the trabeculae and encroaches upon the medullary spaces. Typical examples of such responses are seen in areas adjacent to tumors or in association with infection. In some diseases the increase in bone mass may be spotty, as in osteopoikilosis, whereas in others most of the skeleton may be involved, as in the malignant form of osteopetrosis in children. The mechanism of the increase in mass is usually not due to an excessive amount of mineral relative to matrix, except in some disorders such as osteopetrosis where islands of calcified cartilage may persist. (The mineral density of calcified cartilage is greater than that of bone.) In some diseases such as the osteosclerosis of renal insufficiency, the bone mass and radiodensity may be increased, even though the new bone formed is poorly mineralized and contains widened osteoid seams. A classification of the causes of hyperostosis is presented in Table 354-1.

Several of these conditions are discussed in more detail in other chapters, although some general comments are pertinent. Bone that is denser than normal may be seen occasionally in the osteitis fibrosa associated with active hyperparathyroidism. When the hyperparathyroidism is successfully treated, the rate of bone resorption is decreased abruptly out of proportion to the rate of bone formation; this imbalance may lead to the production of areas of bone density greater than in the surrounding skeleton, especially in the healing of brown tumors. In hypothyroidism, the rates of both bone formation and resorption may be decreased, but the balance may be in favor of formation, resulting in bones that are of increased density but normal architecture. The occurrence of increased bone density in renal tubular abnormalities associated with osteomalacia has been appreciated only recently. The increased mass of bone occurs together with widened osteoid seams, as in chronic

TABLE 354-1
Causes of hyperostosis

  I Endocrine disorders
    A Primary hyperparathyroidism
    B Hypothyroidism
    C Acromegaly
 II Radiation osteitis
III Chemical poisoning
    A Fluoride
    B Elemental phosphorus
    C Beryllium
    D Arsenic
    E Vitamin A intoxication
    F Lead
    G Bismuth
 IV Osteomalacic disorders
    A Renal tubular osteomalacia (vitamin D resistance or phosphate diabetes)
    B Chronic renal glomerular failure
  V Osteosclerosis (localized) associated with chronic infection
 VI Osteosclerotic phase of Paget's disease
VII Osteosclerosis associated with carcinomatous metastases, malignant lymphoma, and hematologic disorders (myeloproliferative disorders, sickle-cell disease, leukemia, multiple myeloma, systemic mastocytosis)
VIII Osteosclerosis of erythroblastosis fetalis
 IX Unclassified diseases
    A Osteopetrosis (marble bone disease of Albers-Schönberg)
    B Pyknodysostosis
    C Osteomyelosclerosis
    D Hyperostosis corticalis generalisata
    E Hyperostosis generalisata with pachydermia
    F Hereditary hyperphosphatasia
    G Progressive diaphyseal dysplasia (osteopathia hyperostotica multiplex infantilis; Camurati-Engelmann disease)
    H Melorheostosis
    I Osteopoikilosis
    J Hyperostosis frontalis interna

renal glomerular insufficiency. In the vertebral bodies the bone appears denser in transverse bands at the upper and lower margins, with a relatively radiolucent center. This "sandwich" appearance is similar to that seen in some patients with osteopetrosis and has been termed by the British the *rugger jersey sign*.

OSTEOPETROSIS Osteopetrosis (marble bone disease of Albers-Schönberg) is a rare disorder which varies in severity and age of clinical presentation. The most severe form occurs in infants and children and is inherited as an autosomal recessive, while a clinically more benign form is transmitted as an autosomal dominant. The so-called "malignant" variant starts in utero and progresses rapidly with marked anemia, hepatosplenomegaly, hydrocephalus, cranial nerve involvement, and death, often due to infection. In the less fulminant form, the anemia is not as severe, neurological abnormalities are not as frequent, and recurrent pathological fractures are the main feature. Although the majority of cases are in infants and children, many are discovered first in adult life when roentgenograms are obtained because of fractures or unrelated diseases. There is no particular predilection for either sex.

The increased bone mass is generally thought to be due to a defect in the normal remodeling of bone. Both bone formation and resorption are depressed, particularly resorption. Islands of unresorbed calcified cartilage encased in bone are frequently seen. The defect in remodeling results in marked disorganization of bone structure with thickened cortices and lack of funnelization of metaphyses. Despite its increased density, the bone is abnormal mechanically and fractures readily. Osteomalacia or rickets is sometimes a component of the osteopetrosis in children.

The histological changes are reflected in the roentgenograms, which reveal uniformly dense, sclerotic bone often without distinction between the cortical and cancellous regions. The long bones are usually involved, with increased density along the entire shaft. Foci of increased density may be seen in the epiphyses corresponding to regions of unresorbed calcified cartilage. The metaphyses have a characteristic clubbed or splayed appearance. Horizontal bandings of increased density alternating with zones of decreased density are seen in the long bones and vertebrae and suggest that the defect may be intermittent during periods of growth. The skull, pelvis, ribs, and other bones may also be involved. The phalanges and the distal humerus may appear normal when the disease is not severe.

Encroachment of bone upon the marrow cavity is associated with anemia of the myelophthisic type with foci of extramedullary hematopoiesis in liver, spleen, and lymph nodes and enlargement of these organs. Neurological abnormalities are associated with encroachment on cranial nerves, which may result in optic atrophy, nystagmus, papilledema, exophthalmos, and impairment of extraocular motility. Facial paralysis and deafness are frequent; trigeminal lesions and anosmia have also been described. In infants with severe disease, macrocephaly, hydrocephalus, and convulsions may occur. Infections such as osteomyelitis are frequent in these children. Associated renal tubular acidosis has also been described.

In the milder dominant osteopetrosis, about half of the patients have no symptoms, and the disorder is discovered incidentally on roentgenograms. Other such patients present because of fractures, bone pain, osteomyelitis, and cranial nerve palsies.

Fractures are a common complication even with trivial trauma. Healing of such fractures is usually satisfactory, although delayed union may occur. When the disease is manifested first in adult life, fractures may be the only clinical problem. Levels of calcium and alkaline phosphatase in the plasma are usually normal in adults, although in children hypophosphatemia and, occasionally, moderate hypocalcemia have been noted. Serum acid phosphatase levels are usually increased.

The mechanism of the skeletal abnormality in osteopetrosis is not known. However, a disorder resembling osteopetrosis has been described in several strains of mice and rats. In the affected mice bone resorption can be restored by transplanting spleen and bone marrow cells, and the disease can be transferred to normal recipients by spleen cells from affected donors. Transfusion of normal syngeneic bone marrow cells to osteopetrotic rats also reverses the osteopetrosis. Thus the defect in bone resorption may be related to a defect in cellular immunity. An infant with severe osteopetrosis with normal proliferative responses of lymphocytes in vitro in lectins and allogeneic cells has had marked improvement of radiological and hematologic abnormalities following transfusion of nucleated marrow cells from a clinically normal sibling.

Other attempts to affect the altered remodeling of bone in patients with osteopetrosis have been unsuccessful. Despite the extramedullary hematopoiesis that has been found in the spleen, splenectomy can occasionally decrease erythrocyte destruction in this organ and increase the life span of the erythrocytes.

PYKNODYSOSTOSIS *Pyknodysostosis* is a disorder which resembles osteopetrosis but is usually a more benign condition not associated with hepatosplenomegaly, anemia, or cranial nerve involvement. In addition to a generalized increase in bone density, features of the disease include short stature, separated cranial sutures, hypoplasia of the mandible, persistence of deciduous teeth, and progressive acroosteolysis of the terminal phalanges. Longevity is usually not decreased, and the patient usually presents to the physician because of frequent fractures. Pyknodysostosis is inherited as a mendelian recessive trait. In one case intermittently elevated levels of plasma calcitonin were found as well as an exaggerated response of the plasma calcitonin to infusions of calcium and glucagon. It has been suggested from karyotype analysis that the gene which determines this disorder is located on the short arm of a small accrocentric chromosome.

OSTEOMYELOSCLEROSIS *Osteomyelosclerosis* is a disorder in which the marrow cells are replaced by diffuse fibroplasia, occasionally accompanied by osseous metaplasia. When the latter is prominent, increased skeletal density is seen on roentgenograms. Osteomyelosclerosis is probably a phase in the course of the myeloproliferative disorders and is characteristically accompanied by extramedullary hematopoiesis.

A disease distinct from those described above has been termed *hyperostosis corticalis generalisata* (van Buchem's disease). It is characterized by osteosclerosis of the skull (base and calvaria), lower jaw, clavicles, and ribs, and thickening of the diaphyseal cortices of the long and short bones. Alkaline phosphatase levels in the serum are elevated, and histological observations suggest that the disorder is due to increased formation of bone of normal structure. The major clinical manifestations are due to neural compression and consist of optic atrophy, facial paralysis, and perception deafness. In *hyperostosis generalisata with pachydermia* (Uehlinger), the sclerosis is due to increased formation of subperiosteal spongy bone and involves the epiphyses, metaphyses, and diaphyses. Pain, swelling of joints, and thickening of the skin of the lower arms are common.

HEREDITARY HYPERPHOSPHATASIA This disorder is characterized by severe structural deformities of the skeleton with increase in thickness of the calvaria, large homogeneous areas of increased density at the base of the skull, and widening and loss of normal architecture of the shafts and the epiphyses of the long and short bones. There is a failure to deposit normal bone, with haphazard orientation of lamellae suggesting active remodeling. Plasma alkaline phosphatase level and urinary excretion of hydroxyproline peptides and other collagen degradation products are markedly increased. The disorder is apparently inherited as an autosomal recessive. Calcitonin therapy may be of value in these patients.

PROGRESSIVE DIAPHYSEAL DYSPLASIA A disorder in which a symmetrical thickening and increased diameter of the diaphyses of long bones occurs, particularly in femurs, tibias, fibulas, radii, and ulnas, has been termed *progressive diaphyseal dysplasia* (Camurati-Engelmann disease). The alkaline phosphatase levels are normal, although the erythrocyte sedimentation rate may be elevated. Pain over affected areas, fatigue, abnormal gait, and muscle wasting are the major manifestations. Clinical and biochemical improvement may result from the use of prednisone or related glucocorticoids.

MELORHEOSTOSIS This rare condition, which usually begins in childhood, is characterized by areas of sclerosis that appear in the bones of one limb. All segments of the bone may be involved, with the dense structures appearing as sclerotic areas which have a "flowing" distribution. The involved limb is often extremely painful.

OSTEOPOIKILOSIS This is a benign disorder usually discovered by chance and is not associated with symptoms. It is characterized by dense spots of trabecular bone less than a centimeter in diameter, usually of uniform density, that are located in the epiphyses and adjacent parts of the metaphyses. All bones may be involved except the skull, ribs, and vertebrae.

HYPEROSTOSIS FRONTALIS INTERNA *Hyperostosis frontalis interna* is an abnormality of the inner table of the frontal bones of the skull first described by Morgagni and consisting of smooth, rounded enostoses covered by dura and projecting into the cranial cavity. These enostoses are usually less than 1 cm at their greatest diameter and usually do not extend posteriorly beyond the coronal suture. The abnormality is found almost exclusively in women, who are frequently obese, hirsute, and who have a variety of neuropsychiatric complaints (Morgagni-Stewart-Morel syndrome). However, hyperostosis frontalis interna has also been seen in women with no obvious illness or particular associated disease. There is no good evidence that the finding in the skull is a manifestation of a generalized metabolic disorder.

NEOPLASMS OF BONE

Primary neoplasms of the skeletal system reflect in their histology the cellular and extracellular components of the skeleton. However, it is not always possible to prove that a tumor arises from the same type of tissue that it produces. The precursor cells of bone tissue are probably derived from histogenetically distinct cell lines in which the osteoclasts arise from hematopoietic cells and the osteoblasts arise from the stromal cell system. The primitive stromal cell could differentiate into chondroblasts and fibroblasts as well as osteoblasts. Neoplasms can arise from all these cell types. Each of these cells can produce its characteristic extracellular matrix, and neoplasms arising from them may thus be recognized. Primary neoplasms of bone can arise also from other hematopoietic, vascular, and neural elements.

PATHOPHYSIOLOGY Tumors in bone produce resorption of normal skeletal tissue by (1) production of substance(s) that can lyse bone, (2) inducing modulation of cells of the osteo-

genic series into cells involved in the process of resorption, such as osteoclasts, and (3) interfering with blood supply. Tumors will also produce some reaction in surrounding bone and alter the normal contour. The epiphyseal plate, articular cartilage, cortex, and periosteum of bone often offer a barrier to the spread of neoplastic tissue. Alteration of the contour of the cortex is not due to "expansion" but to remodeling of the bone in the area and formation of new bone with the new contour. Some tumors induce primarily an osteoplastic or sclerotic reaction in surrounding bone, which results in increased radiodensity. Primary neoplasms may appear to be less radiopaque than surrounding bone or more radiopaque, depending upon the degree of calcification or ossification of the matrix and the density of the tissue. Bone tumors may be recognized because of (1) the presence of a mass in the soft tissues, (2) deformity of a bone, (3) pain and tenderness, and (4) pathological fractures. Tumors of bone may also be detected incidentally on roentgenograms obtained for other clinical reasons. Although it is usually possible to classify bone tumors as benign or malignant as described below, the behavior of individual lesions may be totally unpredictable.

Bone scans utilizing ^{99m}Tc polyphosphonate may be useful in detecting bone tumors. The extent of the lesions can also be assessed by standard and computerized tomographic techniques. However, proper evaluation and selection of therapy require detailed evaluation of clinical radiographic and histological aspects. There are numerous pitfalls in the clinical diagnosis and interpretation of histological features of tumors of bone. Management of the patient therefore requires cooperation of the orthopedist, oncologist, radiologist, and pathologist.

BENIGN TUMORS The most common benign tumors are *osteochondromas* (exostoses) and *chondromas* (which may be multiple in Ollier's disease), *benign giant-cell tumors, unicameral bone cysts, osteoid osteomas,* and *fibromas.* As a rule benign tumors are not painful except for osteoid osteomas, benign chondroblastomas, and benign chondromyxoidfibroma. The usual clinical problem is that of slowly progressing mass and deformity. Treatment is usually accomplished by resection of the tumor and/or curettage and bone grafting. In some instances in which wide resection of tissue has been necessary, insertion of metal and plastic prostheses or allograft transplantation have been successful in preserving limb function.

MALIGNANT TUMORS The most common malignant tumor of bone is multiple myeloma (see Chap. 63), which arises from hematopoietic cells. Reticulum-cell sarcoma also may be a primary bone tumor. Malignant tumors of nonhematopoietic origin include chondrosarcomas, osteosarcomas, fibrosarcomas, Ewing's tumor, malignant giant-cell tumor, and chondromas. *Osteogenic sarcomas* arise presumably from osteoprogenitor cells and show a wide variation in their histopathology. These tumors usually contain some osteoid tissue, at least in small foci, and may contain in addition cartilaginous and fibrous elements. They are most common in the second and third decades and are less common under the age of 10 and over the age of 40 years. When they do occur in older individuals, some predisposing cause is usually present such as Paget's disease, prior exposure to ionizing radiation, or a bone infarct. In primary osteogenic sarcomas the lesions usually arise in the metaphyseal region of long bones, especially in the distal femur and the proximal tibia. The most common symptoms are pain and swelling which may be present for weeks or months. The roentgenographic features of osteosarcomas depend upon the degree of bone destruction, the extent to which bone is formed by and within the tumor, and the type of reaction in the surrounding bone. Thus the lesions may vary from ones purely lytic in character to those with dense areas containing radiopaque lumps, clouds, or spicules of tumor bone in varying patterns of organization. Discontinuities in the cortex surrounding the lesion are common. In other cases, there may be hyperostotic periosteal reactions of laminated bone. When the tumor growth is very rapid, it penetrates and destroys the cortex, growing directly into the soft tissue surrounding the bone; it leaves only a cuff of periosteal new bone at the peripheral margin of the tumor, just at the point of penetration (Codman's triangle). High plasma alkaline phosphatase levels are often present in those sarcomas that are predominantly osteogenic, and the level of this activity parallels the course of the tumor. When lesions are adequately treated by amputation or radiation, the level of alkaline phosphatase falls, and when metastases appear, the level rises again, often reaching values higher than those present initially. When values are initially very high, the course is often rapidly fatal. Metastases occur primarily by the hematogenous route especially to the lung. The prognosis of osteosarcoma is very poor, with radiological evidence of pulmonary metastases usually occurring within a year following a potentially curable surgical amputation. The course varies with the type of tumor; for example, a "telangiectatic" variant has a very poor prognosis, whereas a low-grade intramedullary type has a better one. With the usual osteosarcoma the patient dies within 6 months from the onset of detectable pulmonary metastases, suggesting that the lesions in the lungs were present at the time of amputation or cells were shed from the tumor during the operation. Use of chemotherapy such as adriamycin, dactinomycin, high-dose methotrexate with citrovorum factor rescue, and vincristine has increased survival and seemingly eliminated tumors in some instances. It has even been possible to resect pulmonary metastases in selected patients after chemotherapy and removal of the primary lesion. Reduction of the growth rate of tumor cells by the chemotherapy has made this approach feasible. Nevertheless, these treatment programs have high morbidity.

Chondrosarcomas are clinically distinguishable from osteogenic sarcomas. In contrast to the latter, chondrosarcomas usually arise in adulthood and old age, with the peak incidence in the fourth, fifth, and sixth decades. Most are located in the pelvic girdle, ribs, and upper ends of the femur and humerus; distal portions of the extremities are rarely involved. Chondrosarcomas may also arise by malignant transformation of osteochondromas. As a rule chondrosarcomas are slow growing and slow to recur. Radiographically the lesions appear destructive, with mottled increases in radiodensity which reflect the variable degree of calcification of cartilaginous matrix and ossification. Radical excision is the treatment of choice.

Ewing's tumor This is a malignant sarcoma composed of small, round cells that occurs most frequently in the first three decades of life. Most are located in some portion of the long bones, although any bone may be involved. Ewing's sarcoma is a highly malignant lesion with an extremely low incidence of cure, whether by ablative surgery with or without irradiation. Aggressive chemotherapy has also proved successful in improving survival of patients with Ewing's sarcoma.

TUMORS METASTATIC TO BONE The skeleton is one of the most common sites of metastases from carcinomas and sarcomas. Skeletal metastases may be relatively silent or may produce symptoms by the same mechanism that primary tumors do, i.e., pain, swelling, deformity of a bone, encroachment on hematopoietic tissue in the marrow, compression of spinal cord or nerve roots, and pathological fractures. In addition, rapidly lytic skeletal metastases can result in hypercalcemia and, in some instances, renal insufficiency secondary to the hypercalcemia. The bones involved most commonly are the vertebrae, proximal femur, pelvis, ribs, sternum, and proximal humerus, in that order of frequency. The carcinomas that most frequently metastasize to bone arise in prostate, breast, lung, thyroid, kidney, and bladder.

Malignant cells reach the skeleton via the bloodstream. Those that survive may proliferate and distort the normal architecture, probably by production of substances which cause dissolution of both mineral phase and organic matrix.

Osteolysis most often results from stimulated modulation of osteoprogenitor cells to osteoclasts in the surrounding bone. Parathyroid hormone-like polypeptides, prostaglandins, and protein-containing factor(s) (osteoclast-activating factor) may function to stimulate modulation of osteoclasts from progenitor cells and increase the functional activity of osteoclasts already present. Some carcinoma cells may also act directly to resorb bone. Examples of carcinomatous metastases (which are usually predominantly osteolytic) are those arising from thyroid, kidney and lower bowel. Other tumors induce an *osteoblastic* response in which the new bone arises from skeletal cells and not the tumor itself. The resulting lesion may appear more dense than the surrounding tissue. Occasionally the increase in radiodensity is uniform, simulating osteosclerosis. Carcinoma of the prostate characteristically produces osteoblastic metastases. Carcinoma of the breast produces both osteolytic and osteoblastic metastases. Malignant carcinoid tumors arising from the embryonic foregut and hindgut metastasize to bone with high frequency, producing an osteoblastic reaction. Hodgkin's disease in bone also produces an osteoblastic response both focal and diffuse. More malignant lymphomas in bone produce predominantly destructive lesions. As a rule, osteolytic metastases are the ones which produce hypercalcemia, hypercalciuria, and increased hydroxyprolinuria (reflecting matrix destruction); they are usually associated with normal or slightly increased levels of serum alkaline phosphatase. Osteoblastic metastases, on the other hand, are often accompanied by hyperphosphatasia and may even be associated with hypocalcemia. With some metastases (as in carcinoma of the breast) there may be phases in which osteolysis predominates (with hypercalciuria, hypercalcemia, and normal alkaline phosphatase levels) alternating with phases in which alkaline phosphatase levels rise and the skeletal lesions become more sclerotic.

Treatment of skeletal metastases is usually palliative. In the case of slowly growing localized lesions (as in some instances of carcinoma of the thyroid or occasionally in carcinoma of the kidney) local radiation is useful to relieve pain or reduce compression of surrounding structures. Many patients with carcinomas of breast or prostate will survive for years even after extensive skeletal metastases are recognized. Castration and estrogen therapy will slow the progress of the lesions in patients with metastatic prostatic carcinoma (see Chap. 341). When patients with mammary cancer are treated with estrogens or androgens, the character of the reaction to the metastases may temporarily shift from a predominantly osteoplastic to a lytic phase with resultant hypercalcemia (see Chap. 343). Mithramycin, which inhibits osteoclast function and is effective in treating hypercalcemia associated with malignant disease, may also be useful in palliation of osteolytic metastases. The bone pain in patients with metastatic carcinoma may be relieved by the use of L-dopa. It is also important to recognize that hypercalcemia in patients with malignant tumors is not due solely to skeletal metastases, although this is the most common situation. Production of parathyroid hormone-like polypeptides and other osteolytic substances by extraskeletal neoplasms may also result in elevation of serum calcium levels.

Hypercalcemia per se, whether spontaneous or induced by therapy, may produce symptoms such as anorexia, polyuria, polydipsia, depression, and eventually coma. In addition, nephrocalcinosis can result from hypercalcemia, and death may result from renal insufficiency.

OTHER DISORDERS OF BONE AND CARTILAGE

FIBROUS DYSPLASIA (ALBRIGHT'S SYNDROME) Albright and his associates, in 1937, described a syndrome characterized by "osteitis fibrosa disseminata, areas of pigmentation and endocrine dysfunction, with precocious puberty in females." It was subsequently recognized that the bony lesions, called *fibrous dysplasia,* may occur in the absence of the other features of Albright's syndrome. The fundamental nature of the osseous disorder is unknown; the disease does not appear to be heritable, although it has been reported to affect monozygotic twins. The frequency of the disease is approximately the same in both sexes.

Incidence The lesions of fibrous dysplasia may be confined to one bone or be polyostotic in distribution. In patients with monostotic involvement, the majority of the lesions are in craniofacial bones and ribs; other features of the syndrome are usually absent in these subjects. In contrast, the polyostotic lesions occur in almost every bone, occasionally involving over 50 percent of the skeleton. They may be confined to one side and be striking in extent. Involvement of the lower extremities is especially frequent. Approximately one-half of the females with the polyostotic form have abnormal pigmentation and sexual precocity. Abnormal pigmentation is also seen in about one-half of the males.

Pathology The lesions of polyostotic fibrous dysplasia are of uniform reddish gray color and are finely gritty in texture. Microscopically they are composed of fibrous tissue having the appearance typical of fibromata embedded in which are areas of coarse fiber bone with wide osteoid seams. Cement lines are prominent. Mature lamellar bone does not form. Occasionally multiple islands of cartilage and fluid-filled cysts are present. The lesions of monostotic fibrous dysplasia are similar to those in the polyostotic form except that cartilage and fluid-filled cysts are not found.

Radiological changes The roentgenographic appearance of the lesions is that of a radiolucent area with a smooth border, typically associated with focal thinning of the cortex of the bone. These lesions are not usually cysts in the strict sense, since they are not fluid-filled cavities. They occasionally appear multiloculate. The so-called "ground-glass appearance" reflects the content of thin, calcified trabeculae of fiber bone. Frequently deformities are present such as coxa vara, shepherd's-crook deformity of the femur, bowing of the tibia, Harrison's grooves, and protrusio acetabuli. Involvement of facial bones, usually with lesions of increased radiodensity, may create a leonine appearance (leontiasis ossea) superficially resembling that seen in some patients with leprosy. Advanced skeletal age may be noted, which in females is correlated with sexual precocity but may also be seen in males without sexual precocity. Although the lesions tend to spare the epiphyseal regions before puberty, in older individuals fibrous dysplasia may develop in the epiphyses.

Clinical picture The clinical course is highly variable. Skeletal lesions are usually detected because of deformity or fractures. In some females and even less commonly in males sexual precocity is the presenting complaint, occasionally present years before the appearance of skeletal symptoms. Serum calcium and phosphorus values are usually normal. In approximately one-third of patients with polyostotic fibrous dysplasia, levels of serum alkaline phosphatase may be elevated in some instances to very high values, and urinary hydroxyproline excretion is often increased. In some subjects, high cardiac output similar to that seen in extensive Paget's disease may be found. In general, patients with extensive involvement have widespread disease when symptoms first appear, whereas with mild disease at the onset of symptoms extensive disease does not usually develop.

The abnormal cutaneous pigmentation that is seen in most patients with Albright's syndrome consists of isolated dark-brown to light-brown macules which tend to remain on one side of the midline. The border is usually, although not always, irregular or jagged ("coast of Maine") in contrast to the smooth borders of the pigmented macules of neurofibromatosis ("coast of California"). As a rule there are fewer than six of the lesions, which range in size from 1 cm to those covering very large areas. When the lesions are present in the scalp, the overlying hair may be more deeply pigmented than that over the remainder of the scalp. There is a strong tendency for the pigmentation to be on the same side as the skeletal lesions and actually overlie them.

The sexual precocity of unknown cause previously mentioned is found in females, although it has been described rarely in males. Premature vaginal bleeding and development of axillary and pubic hair and of breasts are the main features. In the few ovaries that have been examined, no corpora lutea have been seen. The cause of the precocious sexuality is still not clear. In the few cases where measurements have been reported, the females have shown high estrogen levels and low or undetectable gonadotropins. In the one studied case gonadotropin levels have not responded to luteinizing hormone-releasing hormone (LHRH). Precocious sexuality is not limited to patients with cranial involvement, and although the characteristic pigmented macules are usually found, this association is not invariable. Another endocrine abnormality present with increased frequency is hyperthyroidism. Rarer associations include Cushing's syndrome, acromegaly, and soft tissue myxomas. Hypophosphatemic osteomalacia may also accompany fibrous dysplasia and resembles the disorder associated with other skeletal and nonskeletal tumors.

Although the lytic lesions of fibrous dysplasia resemble superficially the brown tumors of hyperparathyroidism, the age of the patient, normocalcemia, increased density of bone in the skull, and areas of cutaneous pigmentation identify the former condition. However, fibrous dysplasia and hyperparathyroidism may coexist. Neurofibromas may involve bone and produce cutaneous pigmentation as well as nodules in the skin. The pigmented macules of neurofibromatosis are more numerous and more widely distributed than in fibrous dysplasia, usually have smooth borders, and tend to involve areas such as the axillary folds. Other lesions which may have a roentgenographic appearance similar to that of isolated fibrous dysplasia are unicameral bone cysts, aneurysmal bone cysts, and nonossifying fibromata. Leontiasis ossea is most often due to fibrous dysplasia, although other disorders may also produce this appearance such as craniometaphyseal dysplasia, hyperphosphatasia, and, in adults, Paget's disease.

Treatment Fibrous dysplasia, when symptomatic, can be managed by a variety of orthopedic operative procedures such as osteotomy, curettage, and bone grafting. Indications for such procedures include progressive deformity, nonunion of fractures, and persistent pain unresponsive to conservative treatment. Calcitonin may be effective in treatment of widespread disease associated with bone pain and high serum alkaline phosphatase levels (see Chap. 353).

DYSPLASIAS AND CHONDRODYSTROPHIES A variety of diseases of bone and cartilage have been called *dystrophies* or *dysplasias*. Classification has been difficult, since the underlying defect is not usually known. It is possible that a biochemical lesion, such as that in the metabolism of the mucopolysaccharides demonstrated in the Hunter and Hurler syndromes, will also be found in a number of these disorders and permit more than a descriptive classification. However, a useful scheme has been proposed by Rubin based on the consideration of errors in modeling of bone and cartilage as departures from normal development (Table 354-2). Other clinical and genetic features form the basis of a classification by Rimoin. Pathological processes in the skeletal dysplasias may be expressed as a deficiency (hypoplasia) or excess (hyperplasia) in relation to normal development. Several of the more common of these will be described.

Spondyloepiphyseal dysplasia The spondyloepiphyseal dysplasias are a heterogeneous group of disorders in which abnormalities of growth occur in various bones including the vertebrae, pelvis, carpal and tarsal bones, and the epiphyses of tubular bones. On the basis of roentgenographic findings, this group can be divided into (1) those with generalized platyspondyly, (2) those with multiple epiphyseal dysplasias, and (3) those with epiphysometaphyseal dysplasias. *Morquio's syndrome,* a mucopolysaccharidosis inherited as an autosomal recessive character and associated with corneal opacities, dental defects, variable disturbances in intellect, and increased urinary excretion of keratosulfate, belongs in the first group. Other forms of spondyloepiphyseal dysplasias show no abnormality in mucopolysaccharide metabolism and are sometimes not recognized until late in childhood. Flat vertebral bodies are associated with other abnormalities in shape and alignment. The disordered development of the capital femoral epiphyses leads to irregularities in shape and flattening of the femoral heads and early onset of osteoarthritis of the hips.

Achondroplasia *Achondroplasia* is an example of a physeal dysplasia in which dwarfism results from decrease in the proliferation of cartilage in the growth plate. This disorder of unknown cause is among the more common types of dwarfism and is inherited as an autosomal dominant trait. Histological sections through the growth plate show a thin zone of cartilage cells with absence of the normal columnar arrangement and zone of provisional calcification, although endochondral ossification may not be completely disorganized. Formation of the primary spongiosa is defective. However, formation and maturation of the secondary ossification centers and articular cartilage are not disturbed. Appositional growth at the metaphysis continues, with resulting flare in this region of the bone; intramembranous bone formation at the periosteum is normal. The result of abnormal proliferation at the growth plate, leaving other areas relatively unaffected in the tubular bones, is the production of short bones which are proportionately thick. However, the length of the spine is almost always normal. The appearance of short limbs with a normal trunk is characteristically accompanied by a large head, saddlenose, and an exaggerated lumbar lordosis. The disease is usually recognized at birth. Those who survive the period of infancy usually have normal mental and sexual development, and longevity may be unimpaired. However, spinal deformity may lead to neurological signs of cord compression and nerve root encroachment in a significant number of affected individuals, especially those with kyphoscoliosis. Homozygous achondroplasia is a more serious disorder and a cause of neonatal death.

Enchondromatosis (dyschondroplasia, Ollier's disease) This is also a disorder affecting the growth plate in which the hypertrophic cartilage is not resorbed and ossified in a normal fashion. It results in masses of cartilage with disorderly arrangement of the chondrocytes showing variable proliferative and hypertrophic changes. These masses are located in the metaphyses in close association with the growth plate. The disorder is usually recognized in childhood by the appearance of deformities or retardation in growth. The most common sites of involvement are the ends of long bones, usually in that region where rate of growth is most marked. The pelvis is often involved, but bone such as ribs, sternum, and skull are seldom affected. There is also a tendency toward unilateral involvement. Chondrosarcoma develops rarely in the enchondromata. The association of enchondromatosis and cavernous hemangiomata in the soft tissues is known as Maffucci's syndrome.

Multiple exostoses (diaphyseal aclasis) This is a disorder of the metaphysis, inherited as an autosomal dominant character, in which areas of the growth plate become displaced and then spongiosa forms in an abnormal position in relation to the shaft. Usually the growth of these exostoses ceases when growth of the adjacent plate ceases. The lesions may be solitary or multiple and are usually located in the metaphyseal areas of long bones with the apex of the exostosis directed toward the diaphysis. Often the lesions produce no symptoms, but occasionally interference with the function of a joint or tendon or compression of nerves may result. Dwarfing is seen occasionally. The metacarpals may be shortened, resembling those seen in Albright's hereditary osteodystrophy. Multiple exostoses are sometimes seen in patients with the pseudohypoparathyroid syndrome.

An exostosis may suddenly begin to enlarge long after growth should have ceased, and occasionally chondrosarcomas

TABLE 354-2
Proposed classification of bone dysplasias

I Epiphyseal dysplasias
   A Epiphyseal hypoplasias
      1 Failure of articular cartilage; spondyloepiphyseal dysplasia, congenita and tarda
      2 Failure of ossification of center: multiple epiphyseal dysplasia, congenita and tarda
   B Epiphyseal hyperplasia
      1 Excess of articular cartilage: dysplasia epiphysalis hemimelica
II Physeal (growth plate) dysplasias
   A Cartilage hypoplasias
      1 Failure of proliferating cartilage: achondroplasia, congenita and tarda
      2 Failure of hypertrophic cartilage: metaphyseal dysostosis, congenita and tarda
   B Cartilage hyperplasias
      1 Excess of proliferating cartilage: hyperchondroplasia
      2 Excess of hypertrophic cartilage: enchondromatosis
III Metaphyseal dysplasias
   A Metaphyseal hypoplasias
      1 Failure to form primary spongiosa: hypophosphatasia, congenita and tarda
      2 Failure to absorb primary spongiosa: osteopetrosis, congenita and tarda
      3 Failure to absorb secondary spongiosa: craniometaphyseal dysplasia, congenita and tarda
   B Metaphyseal hyperplasia
      1 Excessive spongiosa: familial exostosis
IV Diaphyseal dysplasias
   A Diaphyseal hypoplasias
      1 Failure of periosteal bone formation: osteogenesis imperfecta, congenita and tarda
      2 Failure of endosteal bone formation: idiopathic osteoporosis
   B Diaphyseal hyperplasias
      1 Excessive periosteal bone formation: Engelmann's disease
      2 Excessive periosteal bone formation: hyperphosphatasia

develop at the site of an exostosis. Although the exact incidence of this complication is not known, estimates as high as 7 to 11 percent have been made.

RELAPSING POLYCHONDRITIS   See Chap. 363.

TIETZE'S SYNDROME (COSTOCHONDRAL SYNDROME)   See Chap. 363.

REFERENCES

Bone and cartilage

ALBRIGHT FA et al: Syndrome characterized by osteitis fibrosa, disseminate areas of pigmentation and endocrine dysfunction, with precocious puberty in females: Report of five cases. N Engl J Med 216:727, 1937

ALTERMAN SL, LIEBER AL: Albright's hereditary osteodystrophy: The effect of treatment during adolescence. Ann Intern Med 63:140, 1965

BAILEY JA: Orthopaedic aspects of achondroplasia. J Bone Joint Surg (Br) 52A:1285, 1970

BENEDICT PH: Endocrine features in Albright's syndrome (fibrous dysplasia of bone). Metabolism 11:30, 1962

———— et al: Melanotic macules in Albright's syndrome and in neurofibromatosis. JAMA 209:72, 1968

DENT CE, GERTNER JM: Hypophosphatemic osteomalacia in fibrous dysplasia. Q J Med 45:411, 1976

GIOVANELLI G et al: McCune-Albright syndrome in a male child: A clinical and endocrinologic enigma. J Ped 92:220, 1978

HARRIS WH et al: The natural history of fibrous dysplasia: An orthopaedic, pathological and roentgenographic study. J Bone Joint Surg (Br) 44A:207, 1962

RIMOIN DL: The chondrodystrophies. Adv Hum Genet 5:1, 1975

RUBIN P: *Dynamic Classification of Bone Dysplasias.* Chicago, Year Book, 1964

SILLENCE DO et al: Neonatal dwarfism. Pediatr Clin North Am 25:431, 1978

STEENDIJK R: Metabolic bone disease in children, in *Metabolic Bone Disease,* LV Avioli, SM Krane (eds). Academic, New York, 1978, vol II, p 633

Hyperostosis

BAKER RK et al: Plasma calcitonin in pyknodysostosis: Intermittently high basal levels and exaggerated responses to calcium and glucagon infusions. J Clin Endocrinol Metab 37:46, 1973

BALLET JJ et al: Bone-marrow transplantation in osteopetrosis. Lancet 2:1137, 1977

COLLINS DH, DODGE OG: *Pathology of Bone.* London, Butterworth, 1966

DENT CE et al: Studies in osteopetrosis. Arch Dis Child 40:7, 1965

ELMORE SM et al: Pyknodysostosis, with a familial chromosome anomaly. Am J Med 40:273, 1966

GENANT HK: Osteosclerosis in primary hyperparathyroidism. Am J Med 59:104, 1975

JOHNSTON CC et al: Osteopetrosis: A clinical, genetic, metabolic and morphologic study of the dominantly inherited benign form. Medicine 47:149, 1968

LORIA-CORTES R et al: Osteopetrosis in children. A report of 26 cases. J Pediatr 91:43, 1977

MILHAUD G et al: Immunologic defect and its correction in the osteopetrotic mutant rat. Proc Natl Acad Sci USA 74:339, 1977

SMITH R et al: Clinical and biochemical studies in Engelmann's disease (progressive disphyseal dysplasia). Q J Med 46:273, 1977

THOMPSON RC JR et al: Hereditary hyperphosphatasia. Am J Med 47:209, 1969

VAN BUCHEM FSP et al: Hyperostosis corticalis generalisata. Am J Med 33:387, 1962

WALKER DG: Bone resorption restored in osteopetrotic mice by transplants of normal bone marrow and spleen. Science 190:784, 1975

Neoplasms

CORTES EP et al: Amputation and adriamycin in primary osteosarcoma. N Engl J Med 291:998, 1974

JAFFE HL: *Tumors and Tumorous Conditions of the Bones and Joints.* Philadelphia, Lea & Febiger, 1958

JAFFE N et al: Adjuvant methotrexate and citrovorum-factor treatment of osteogenic sarcoma. N Engl J Med 291:994, 1974

LICHTENSTEIN L: *Bone Tumors.* St Louis, Mosby, 1972

LODWICK GS: *The Bones and Joints.* Chicago, Year Book, 1971

MANKIN HJ: Current concepts. Advances in diagnosis and treatment of bone tumors. N Engl J Med (in press)

———— et al: Massive resection and allograft replacement in the treatment of malignant bone tumors. N Engl J Med 294:1247, 1976

MINTON JP: The response of breast cancer patients with bone pain to L-dopa. Cancer 33:358, 1974

MOSELEY JE: *Bone Changes in Hematologic Disorders.* New York, Grune & Stratton, 1963

RAISZ LG et al: Hypercalcemia of neoplastic diseases, in *Endocrinology of Calcium Metabolism,* DH Copp, RV Talmage (eds). Amsterdam, Excerpta Medica, 1978, p 64

RODMAN JS, SHERWOOD LM: Disorders of mineral metabolism in malignancy, in *Metabolic Bone Disease,* LV Avioli, SM Krane (eds). New York, Academic, 1978, vol II, p 577

ROSEN G et al: Curability of Ewing's sarcoma and considerations for future therapeutic trials. Cancer 41:888, 1978

WEICHSELBAUM RR et al: Preliminary results of aggressive multimodal therapy for metastatic osteosarcoma. Cancer 40:78, 1977

355

APPROACH TO DISORDERS OF THE JOINTS

BRUCE C. GILLILAND
MART MANNIK

The causes of joint disorders are numerous and include traumatic, infectious, metabolic, immunologic, and neoplastic processes. Often the cause of joint inflammation is unknown, and the disease mechanisms have been only partially elucidated. Many classifications of joint disorders have been proposed, but they seldom serve as a useful guideline in arriving at a logical diagnosis. The purpose of this chapter is to present an approach to the patient with joint disease, without giving detailed discussion of the differential diagnoses. Figure 355-1 should serve as a guide to a group of disorders with common manifestations that may be divided further by means of historical, physical, or laboratory information. Clinical judgment and bedside information become highly important for achieving the correct diagnosis since specific tests are not available for each subgroup. The detailed differential diagnoses are discussed in the appropriate chapters.

Disorders of joints can produce pain, stiffness, swelling, redness, increased warmth, or limitation of motion. Involvement of a single joint or of several joints may be a manifestation of a systemic illness or may be due to a disorder confined to the joints. Therefore, a complete history and physical examination are mandatory to seek extraarticular features of specific diseases. The number of joints involved, the location of the involved joints (peripheral small joints, proximal large joints, spine), the pattern of involved joints (symmetrical or asymmetrical) and the duration of joint involvement (migratory or chronic) provide useful diagnostic clues. Since some disorders are self-limited and leave no residue, whereas others are chronic and may lead to progressive joint destruction, early diagnosis is important.

Specific radiographs and laboratory tests, including synovial fluid analysis, can provide useful diagnostic information. In some instances synovial tissue biopsy, arthroscopy, or arthrography may be required to define the joint disorder.

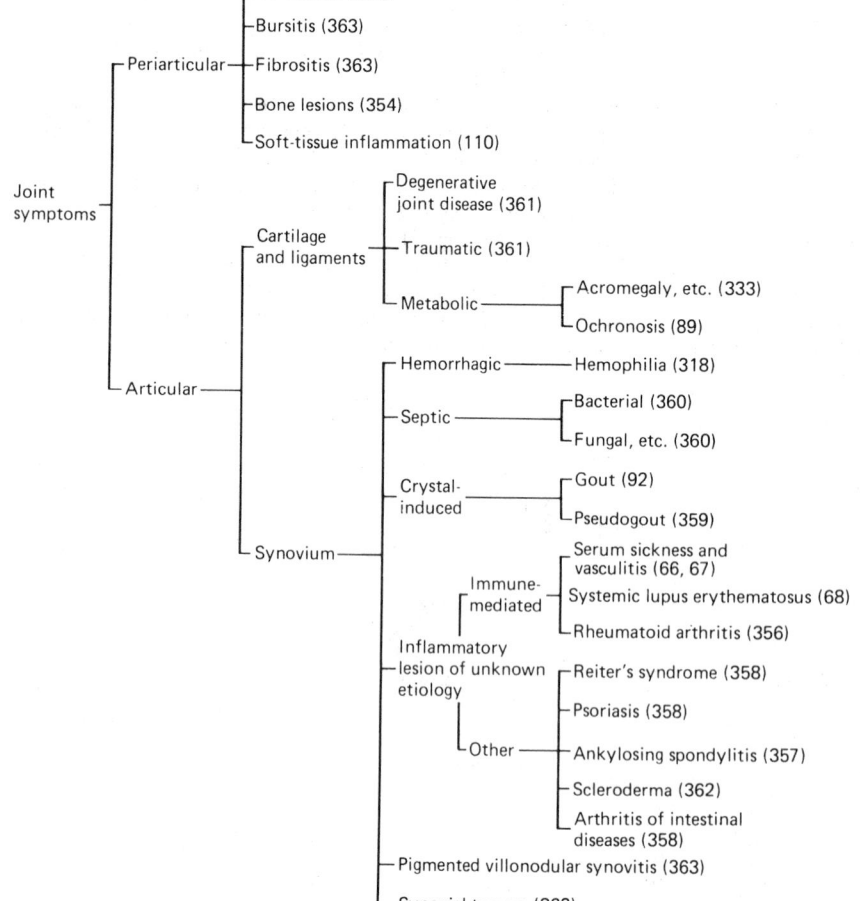

FIGURE 355-1

Approach to joint disorders. (Numbers in parentheses indicate chapters containing detailed discussions.)

The initial step is to determine whether the symptoms attributed to joint(s) are articular or periarticular. Periarticular disease may produce symptoms related to the joint. Bursitis, tendonitis, and cellulitis can be differentiated from articular disease by a negative joint examination and positive evidence of periarticular disorders. The depressed or anxious patient may complain of joint symptoms. Patients with psychogenic rheumatism have no musculoskeletal abnormalities on physical examination. On the other hand, patients with early rheumatoid arthritis or other joint diseases may have no objective evidence of disease, and therefore reevaluation with the passage of time is necessary. Articular involvement is manifested by joint tenderness, increased warmth, erythema, synovial effusion, synovial hypertrophy, and restriction of joint motion or crepitation. A synovial effusion in the knee and other joints can be detected by fluid wave (bulge sign) or by the palpable transmission of pressure elicited by compression of the fluid in the joint. In the knee a patellar click on ballotement of the patella downward on the femur also indicates an effusion; however, the bulge sign is more sensitive for detection of small effusions and may permit detection of as little as 5 ml removable synovial fluid. Synovial fluid may be present in knee joints in edematous states, such as congestive heart failure or nephrotic syndrome, even in the absence of an underlying joint disorder. Fluid in other joints is more difficult to demonstrate, especially in the hip joint. Synovial hypertrophy is palpable as boggy tissue around the joint margins. Joint involvement is also suggested by the finding of pain on firm compression of the joint and by decrease in muscle strength adjacent to the involved joint (e.g., quadriceps atrophy and weakness with knee disease, or decreased grip strength with involvement of the wrists and small joints of the hand). The joint examination should include assessment of all joints even though symptoms are localized to one joint or a few joints.

Joint symptoms may originate primarily from diseased cartilage and involvement of supporting structures or from synovial tissue disease. The inflammatory arthritides are characterized by accumulation of inflammatory cells in the synovial tissue and fluid. Degenerative joint disease, ochronosis, and some of the metabolic diseases such as acromegaly and hyperparathyroidism are characterized by alterations of cartilage and supporting structures; synovial inflammation tends to be chronic and low grade.

Inspection and examination of joints may provide information about the underlying pathological change. In acute inflammatory disorders (e.g., septic arthritis and crystal arthritis) the joint is swollen and warm. The overlying skin is often erythematous. In patients with chronic inflammatory joint disease the joint is swollen and only minimally warm, and may have a boggy sensation due to underlying synovial hypertrophy. The overlying skin may show only minimal erythema. An acute traumatic arthritis also may present as a swollen and warm joint and should be suspected with a history of antecedent trauma. In degenerative joint disease, synovial effusion may be found but the overlying tissues usually do not show inflammation; bony overgrowth at the joint margins may be present.

Further discrimination of disorders affecting primarily the synovium can be made by the history, e.g., bleeding episodes in hemophilia, antecedent infections in septic arthritis, recurrent attacks of gout, multisystem involvement in systemic lupus erythematosus, and presence of inflammatory bowel disease. Other important clues may become apparent on physical examination such as skin lesions in psoriasis, butterfly rash in systemic lupus erythematosus, subcutaneous nodules in rheumatoid arthritis, and tophi in gout.

The examination of synovial fluid is mandatory to establish the specific diagnosis of infections, crystal-induced arthritides, pigmented villonodular synovitis, and neoplasms involving the joint. Inflammatory joint diseases of unknown cause often can be diagnosed on the basis of the history and physical examination without the examination of synovial fluid. However, the synovial fluid should be examined when possible because it may provide a precise diagnosis or further clues to an accurate diagnosis. Aspiration of a joint should be performed under aseptic conditions.

Table 355-1 lists the characteristics of joint fluid for the major types of arthritis. Normal joint fluid is clear and straw-colored. Turbidity is produced by inflammatory cells and occasionally by a chylous effusion. Fragments of cartilage and fibrin may be present. Normal joint fluid is quite viscous, because of hyaluronic acid. The viscosity is reduced in inflammatory arthritides, especially in chronic rheumatoid arthritis. Viscosity can be grossly evaluated by forcing synovial fluid from the syringe. Fluid of high viscosity forms a string several inches long; fluid of low viscosity drops like water. The mucin clot test correlates with the viscosity. This test is per-

TABLE 355-1
Synovial fluid characteristics in major joint diseases*

Diagnosis	Appearance	Fibrin clot	Mucin† clot	WBC/mm³	PMN,‡ %	Sugar, % of blood level
Normal	Straw-colored, clear	None	Good	<200	<25	~100
Degenerative joint disease	Slightly turbid	Small	Good	<2,000	<25	~100
Traumatic arthritis	Straw-colored, bloody, or xanthochromic	Small	Good	~2,000	<25	~100
Rheumatoid arthritis	Turbid	Large	Fair to poor	5,000–50,000	>65	~75§
Other types of inflammatory arthritis¶	Turbid	Large	Fair to poor	5,000–50,000	>50	~75
Acute gout or pseudogout	Turbid	Large	Fair to poor	5,000–50,000	>75	~90
Septic arthritis	Very turbid or purulent	Large	Poor	50,000–200,000	>80	<50
Tuberculous arthritis	Turbid	Large	Poor	~25,000	Variable	<50

* See text for discussion of synovial fluid complement.
† Correlates with viscosity.
‡ PMN, polymorphonuclear cells.
§ May be less than 50 percent.
¶ Includes Reiter's syndrome, psoriatic arthritis, ankylosing spondylitis (peripheral joints), arthritis associated with intestinal diseases.

formed by adding acetic acid to joint fluid from which cells and debris have been removed by centrifugation. The formation of a tight, ropy, and persistent clot indicates qualitatively good mucin and the presence of adequate molecules of intact hyaluronic acid. The mucin clot in degenerative joint disease is of good quality and quantity, while in inflammatory joint disease, such as rheumatoid arthritis, the mucin clot is of both poor quality and quantity. Fluid from an inflammatory effusion often forms a fibrin clot which should not be confused with a mucin clot. Normal joint fluid does not contain fibrinogen; therefore, it will not clot spontaneously unless blood enters the joint during the aspiration.

Synovial fluid for cell counts should be collected in an anticoagulant-containing tube. Joint fluid for cell counts should not be diluted in acetic acid, the normal diluent for white blood cell counts, since this will result in the formation of a mucin clot. Normal joint fluid contains less than 200 cells per cubic millimeter, predominantly mononuclear white blood cells. In degenerative joint disease the intraarticular white blood cell count is usually less than 2000 per cubic millimeter and the cells are also predominantly mononuclear. Variable degrees of leukocytosis, consisting mainly of neutrophils, are seen in inflammatory joint diseases; cell counts in septic arthritis are often greater than 50,000 per cubic millimeter. White blood cell counts up to 50,000 per cubic millimeter or even higher may occasionally be found in nonseptic joints. For proper interpretation of the synovial fluid glucose, blood should be drawn simultaneously for glucose analysis; both samples should be obtained 6 h after a meal. The synovial fluid glucose level falls with increasing inflammation, and the difference between levels of serum and synovial fluid glucose increases. The level in septic arthritis may be less than 50 percent of the serum glucose. A low synovial glucose level also can be seen in rheumatoid arthritis.

Synovial fluid should be examined under polarized light for the presence of crystals. The crystals of gout and of pseudogout are differentiated by their size, shape, and properties under compensated polarized light. The fluid to be used for examination of crystals should be anticoagulated with heparin, since crystalline anticoagulants may be mistaken for crystals in synovial fluid.

Gram's stain and stains for tubercle bacilli should be performed on the sediment of synovial fluid. Bacterial, fungal, and viral cultures should be obtained when these infections are suspected.

Determination of the joint fluid complement is useful, but specific diagnostic information is not obtained from this measurement. For best interpretation, the joint fluid complement (hemolytic complement, C3 or C4) should be expressed as a function of the total protein concentration in the fluid. Macromolecules of complement or protein do not readily enter the uninflamed synovial cavity, but with inflammation the synovium becomes permeable to these macromolecules. Therefore, synovial fluid complement levels usually correlate with the total protein concentration of the fluid. Normal levels of synovial fluid complement, as related to the total protein of the fluid, are found in joint fluid from normal persons, and from patients with osteoarthritis, gout, and other nonrheumatoid inflammatory arthritides. In some patients with Reiter's syndrome, the level of joint fluid complement is higher than that found in patients with rheumatoid inflammatory arthritis. On the other hand, patients with rheumatoid arthritis, particularly those with high titers of serum rheumatoid factor, and patients with systemic lupus erythematosus may have low synovial complement levels as related to the total protein in the fluid. The

decreased joint fluid complement levels in these patients may be due to the consumption of complement by antigen-antibody complexes in the joint cavity.

Needle biopsy of the synovium can provide precise diagnostic information. With currently available needles, a biopsy can be performed on most large joints with relatively little discomfort. If bedside observations and synovial fluid studies have not yielded a diagnosis, a biopsy should be considered. In a large joint, such as the knee, arthroscopy can facilitate the selection of the site for biopsy. Synovial biopsy may lead to a diagnosis of tuberculosis, coccidioidomycosis, hemochromatosis, sarcoidosis, amyloidosis, pigmented villonodular synovitis, or synovial tumors. A biopsy may support the diagnosis of rheumatoid arthritis, systemic lupus erythematosus, or Reiter's syndrome, but the biopsy alone will not suffice for a diagnosis in these diseases.

REFERENCES

BUNCH TW et al: Synovial fluid complement determination as a diagnostic aid in inflammatory joint disease. Mayo Clin Proc 49:715, 1974

HOLLANDER JL: Arthrocentesis and intrasynovial therapy, in *Arthritis and Allied Conditions,* 9th ed, DJ McCarty (ed). Philadelphia, Lea & Febiger, 1979, chap 27

————: Introduction to arthritis and the rheumatic diseases, in *Arthritis and Allied Conditions,* 9th ed, DJ McCarty (ed). Philadelphia, Lea & Febiger, 1979, chap 1

McCARTY DJ: A basic guide to arthrocentesis. Hosp Med, November 1968, p 77

————: Differential diagnosis of arthritis; analysis of signs and symptoms, in *Arthritis and Allied Conditions,* 9th ed, DJ McCarty (ed). Philadelphia, Lea & Febiger, 1979, chap 4

————: Synovial fluid, in *Arthritis and Allied Conditions,* 9th ed, DJ McCarty (ed). Philadelphia, Lea & Febiger, 1979, chap 5

SCHUMACHER HR, KULKA JP: Needle biopsy of the synovial membrane—experience with the Parker-Pearson technique. N Engl J Med 286:416, 1972

356
RHEUMATOID ARTHRITIS

BRUCE C. GILLILAND
MART MANNIK

INTRODUCTION Rheumatoid arthritis (RA) is a chronic systemic disease of unknown etiology, manifested primarily by inflammatory arthritis of the peripheral joints, usually in a symmetrical distribution. Systemic manifestations include hematologic, pulmonary, neurological, and cardiovascular abnormalities.

PATHOGENESIS The serum and joint fluid of the majority of patients with RA contain antibodies specific for the Fc fragment of IgG (rheumatoid factors). These antibodies are heterogeneous and consist of IgM, IgG, and IgA and are, respectively, termed IgM rheumatoid factors, IgG rheumatoid factors, and IgA rheumatoid factors. The stimulus for synthesis of rheumatoid factors appears to be chronic antigenic challenge. Studies have shown that animals immunized with altered autologous IgG form antibodies to IgG. In addition, similar antibodies appear in the serum of animals repeatedly immunized with *Escherichia coli* or other bacteria. Patients with subacute bacterial endocarditis or with other forms of chronic infection develop rheumatoid factors which disappear from the serum after successful treatment of the infection. These observations suggest that IgG, altered as a result of combining with an antigen, can serve as the immunogenic stimulus for the synthesis of rheumatoid factors (antibodies to IgG). Chronic arthritis does not appear in the above-mentioned patients or in the immunized animals, indicating that the presence of rheumatoid factors alone does not contribute to the pathogenesis of rheumatoid arthritis. In RA, the reasons for the appearance and continued production of rheumatoid factors remain unknown.

Though the presence of rheumatoid factor in the serum apparently does not lead to the development of rheumatoid arthritis, increasing evidence shows that immunologic mechanisms play an important role in the pathogenesis of synovitis in RA. Lymphocytes and plasma cells in the synovium synthesize immunoglobulins, including some with antibody specificity to IgG. Immunoglobulin deposits, together with complement components, are found in articular cartilage, in synovium, and in phagocytic cells of the synovial membrane. Immunoglobulins, including some with antibody specificity to IgG, and complement can be identified in the phagolysosomes of polymorphonuclear cells in the synovial fluid. Immune complexes composed of IgG and antibodies to IgG exist in synovial fluid. Some of the IgG-containing immune complexes in RA result from self-association of IgG rheumatoid factor. In this reaction the IgG rheumatoid factor molecule serves both as an antibody and as an antigen molecule. The antibody specificity is directed to antigenic determinants on the Fc fragments, present in the same molecule. Thereby two antigen-antibody bonds are formed in the dimerization, leaving the other antibody-binding site free for further concentration-dependent polymerization. The self-association of IgG rheumatoid factors is documented from isolates prepared from serums of patients who have the intermediate complexes. These complexes sediment in ultracentrifugation between IgG (6.6 Svedberg units) and IgM (19 Svedberg units) components in normal serum. Immune complexes generated in this manner do not require an exogenous antigen but are formed by the IgG rheumatoid factors when these IgG molecules possess both the antibody specificity and the antigenic determinant. In addition, antinuclear antibodies and deoxyribonucleic acid (DNA) appear in the synovial fluid of some patients. The activation of complement by these immune complexes apparently leads to the generation of chemotactic and vasoactive factors, resulting in the influx of neutrophils into the joint. The finding of decreased complement components and total hemolytic complement and the presence of breakdown products of complement in synovial fluid support this notion. Phagocytosis of immune complexes by polymorphonuclear cells results in the release of lysosomal enzymes capable of producing tissue injury. Among other enzymes, collagenase is present in the synovial fluid. The role of cellular immunity in RA has not yet been clearly defined. The presence of T cells in the synovium and the identification of migration-inhibiting factor (MIF) and other lymphokines in synovial fluid suggest that T cells participate in the genesis of joint inflammation in RA.

The pathogenic mechanisms of extraarticular manifestations of RA have not been identified with certainty. However, mounting evidence indicates that humoral immune mechanisms participate in this process. The acute vasculitic lesions of RA contain immunoglobulins and complement components. Patients with such lesions tend to have minimally depressed serum complement level, and these patients frequently have circulating immune complexes containing either IgM rheumatoid factors or IgG rheumatoid factors.

The etiologic factor(s) that set into motion the above immunologic events is not known. An infectious agent, viral or bacterial, may well initiate the immunologic and subsequent inflammatory processes in rheumatoid arthritis, but this hypothesis needs experimental proof.

EPIDEMIOLOGY The onset of RA may occur anytime in life. Approximately 70 percent of RA occurs between the third and seventh decades; the peak onset is in the fourth decade. The prevalence in North America ranges from 0.5 to 3.8 percent in women and from 0.15 to 1.3 percent in men, depending on which diagnostic criteria are applied in population studies. Women are affected approximately three times more often than men; however, this difference disappears in older age.

A genetic predisposition for RA is suggested by the finding of an association with the histocompatibility antigen HLA-DW4. This antigen is found in 59 percent of Caucasian patients with RA, compared with 16 percent in normal persons. Previous population studies done in the Pima and Blackfeet Indians attributed the slight increased prevalence of rheumatoid arthritis in siblings and parents of persons with RA to environmental factors. Studies of monozygotic twins showed mostly disconcordance for RA. Both genetic predisposition and environmental factors therefore appear to play a role in the development of RA.

PATHOLOGY The synovium develops numerous folds consisting of large villi and spreads to cover the articular cartilage with what is referred to as a *pannus*. The pannus destroys the underlying articular cartilage and subchondral bone. The earliest and most prominent bone erosions occur at the joint margins where the articular cartilage ends and the joint capsule attaches to bone. The bone at these sites in the joint is covered by the synovial membrane as it is reflected from the periosteum to the inner aspect of the joint capsule. Later, fibrous adhesions or even bony ankylosis may unite the opposing joint surfaces. The invasion and destruction of the subchondral bone and the destruction of cartilage are mediated by enzymes emanating from phagocytic cells in the synovial membrane and fluid. The inflammatory process weakens the joint capsule and supporting ligaments. The combination of joint destruction, loss of supporting structures, muscle atrophy, and imbalance of opposing muscle groups results in joint instability and subluxation. Persistent inflammation in the tendon sheaths may cause weakening and even rupture of the tendons.

Hypercellularity of the synovium results from the influx of lymphocytes, plasma cells, and monocytes. The synovial lining cells proliferate and lose their organization. In more chronic disease, lymphocytes form follicles in the synovium.

The so-called "rheumatoid nodules" are fairly characteristic of RA. The center of the nodule consists of an area of fibrinoid necrosis and cellular debris, surrounded by several layers of palisading large monocytic cells. The periphery is infiltrated with lymphocytes and monocytes. Small-vessel vasculitis is considered to be the initiating event in the formation of the nodule. Nodules are most often found in subcutaneous tissue over pressure points such as the elbows. They may be bound to the underlying periosteum. Nodules may appear on the dorsum of the fingers and may be attached to tendons. Solitary or multiple nodules may appear in the lung parenchyma, in the pleura, in heart valves, in myocardium, and rarely in vocal cords.

Vasculitis involving small to medium-sized vessels occurs in RA. The histological picture ranges from focal perivascular accumulation of lymphocytes to necrotizing lesions showing fibrinoid necrosis, disruption of the intima, and infiltration of polymorphonuclear cells. Immunoglobulins and complement deposits can be demonstrated by immunofluorescence in the vessel of acute lesions. Vasculitis of the vasa nervorum may lead to peripheral neuropathy. Nail-fold thrombi, digital gangrene, and leg ulcers may occur. Necrotizing vasculitis involving intestinal wall and coronary and cerebral arteries has also been described.

Atrophy of skeletal muscles with interstitial accumulation of lymphocytes is present. Rarely, myositis occurs that is indistinguishable histologically and clinically from polymyositis.

Enlargement of the lymph nodes draining the affected joints, as well as generalized lymphadenopathy, may be present. Histologically, the nodes show hyperplasia and in some instances may resemble those of giant follicular lymphoma.

CLINICAL MANIFESTATIONS In the majority of patients the onset of RA is insidious. A prodrome of fatigue, weakness, joint stiffness, and vague arthralgias and myalgias may precede the appearance of joint swelling by several weeks. Several joints are usually involved at the onset, especially those of the hands and feet. Disease, in approximately one-third of the pa-

FIGURE 356-1

Rheumatoid arthritis. A. Synovial proliferation of the metacarpophalangeal joints and to a lesser degree of the proximal interphalangeal joints. B. Advanced deformities of RA. Subluxation and ulnar deviation of the metacarpophalangeal joints are present. Fingers show swan neck deformity with hyperextension of the proximal interphalangeal joint.

A

B

tients, however, may initially be confined to one or a few joints, frequently one or both knees, before spreading to other joints in a symmetrical pattern. The pattern of joint involvement may remain asymmetrical in some patients. Unlike the migratory polyarthritis of rheumatic fever, RA usually persists in the initially involved joints as other joints become affected. Some patients may have an acute onset, with fever and multiple swollen, painful joints. Raynaud's phenomenon occurs in some patients.

Examination of the involved joints reveals increased warmth, tenderness, and swelling, which early in the disease may be subtle. The synovium becomes palpable as boggy tissue around the joint margin. The skin over small joints often has a ruddy cyanotic hue; marked erythema is unusual. Muscle weakness and atrophy adjacent to the affected joint often parallel the severity of joint disease. Range of joint motion, especially extension, becomes limited. Flexion contractures and in some instances fibrous or bony ankylosis develop. Terms such as *swan neck, boutonnière,* and *cock-up toes* are used to describe joint deformities in the hands and feet. Another frequently observed deformity consists of volar subluxation and ulnar deviation of the fingers at the metacarpophalangeal joints (Fig. 356-1). Flexion contractures of the knees and hips greatly hinder ambulation.

The duration of morning stiffness may be useful in assessing disease activity. During periods of active joint disease, the patient may complain of morning stiffness lasting an hour or more. With improvement, the duration of morning stiffness decreases. Disease activity in the hands and wrist can be followed by measurement of grip strength, which is performed by having the patient compress a rolled-up, partially inflated sphygmomanometer cuff. Disease activity in the lower extremities is assessed by recording the time required to walk a standard distance (e.g., 50 ft).

Though the disease may occur in any diarthrodial joint, the joints most commonly affected are the proximal interphalangeal, metacarpophalangeal, metatarsophalangeal, wrist, knee, elbow, and ankle. Cervical spine disease is common; however, the lower part of the spine is relatively spared. Unilateral sacrolitis occurs but is of little clinical significance. A serious complication is *subluxation of the atlantoaxial joint,* which may lead to compression of the spinal cord by the odontoid process. Symptoms and signs of cord compression, such as bladder dysfunction, anal sphincter laxity, circumanal hypesthesia, and long-tract signs, should be sought. Sudden death has resulted from laceration of the cord by the odontoid process. *Temporomandibular disease* may interfere with mastication, and pain from this joint may be referred to the middle ear and throat. *Arthritis in the cricoarytenoid* joints can cause hoarseness or even life-threatening upper-airway obstruction if the joints are fixed in adduction. Tenosynovitis in the wrist may compress the median nerve, causing a carpal tunnel syndrome.

Popliteal cyst may develop in patients with synovitis of the knee. The cyst forms either from herniation or rupture of the synovium posteriorly through the joint capsule or from communication of the joint with the semimembranosus bursa. The cyst enlarges because synovial fluid is forced into it by motion of the joint. The pressure of fluid is always greater in the knee than in the cyst. Hence, the communication between the knee joint and the cyst can be demonstrated only by injecting radiopaque dye into the knee joint. A popliteal cyst may extend down into the calf or up into the posterior thigh. A clinical picture resembling thrombophlebitis is produced by rupture of the popliteal cyst or by rupture of the synovium of the knee even in the absence of a cyst. This diagnosis may be confirmed by performing an arthrogram. Ultrasound can also be employed for demonstration of a cyst.

Rheumatoid nodules are found in approximately 20 percent of patients and are most commonly located over the extensor surface of the elbows. They may also be present over the extensor surface of the fingers and in other areas exposed to pressure, such as the back of the head and over the sacrum in bedridden patients. The nodules may be freely movable or attached to tendons or the periosteum. They are usually firm and nontender but may be cystic. The overlying skin may break down and lead to chronic drainage. Pressure by eye glasses at the bridge of the nose may produce an ulcerated rheumatoid nodule which may be mistaken for basal-cell carcinoma. Nodules are usually associated with active disease and a positive test for rheumatoid factor.

The hands of a rheumatoid patient are often cool and damp, reflecting autonomic nervous system dysfunction. Palmer erythema is also seen. In advanced disease, the skin over the fingers may become shiny and atrophic. In long-standing disease, the skin often becomes atrophic and bruises easily. These manifestations may be further accentuated in patients on glucocorticosteroids.

Nail-fold thrombi, small infarcts on the volar surface of the hands, digital gangrene, and ulcers of the lower part of the leg and the ankle are manifestations of rheumatoid vasculitis. Both sensory and motor types of neuropathy result from vasculitis of the vasa nervorum. Vasculitis of the cranial, coronary, and mesenteric vessels has been observed. Steroid therapy has been implicated in the development of vasculitis; however, vasculitis is seen in patients who have never received steroids.

The most common ocular manifestation is keratoconjunctivitis sicca (Sjögren's syndrome), which occurs in approximately 15 percent of patients. Uveitis is encountered occasionally. Episcleritis may occur; this may evolve into a rheumatoid nodule that eventually perforates the sclera (scleromalacia perforans).

Pulmonary involvement may take the form of diffuse interstitial fibrosis, single or multiple nodules in the lung parenchyma, or a pleural effusion with or without antecedent symptoms of pleurisy. A distinguishing characteristic of some pleural fluids is their low glucose and high lactic dehydrogenase concentrations. Glucose levels as low as 10 mg per 100 ml may be observed in the absence of infection. Also, the pleural fluid complement level is low compared with the serum level when these values are related to the total protein concentrations of the respective compartments. The pleural fluid may show a distinctive cytological picture, consisting of a background of amorphous necrotic material, large elongated cells, and giant multinucleated cells. These cells are thought to be shed from rheumatoid nodules in the pleura. Parenchymal rheumatoid nodules may lead to cavitation, which is easily seen on x-ray films. Caplan's syndrome, described originally in Welsh coal miners, is the combination of RA and multiple pulmonary nodules (rheumatoid granulomas) developing in patients with underlying pneumoconiosis. Impaired pulmonary diffusion may occur in the absence of chest film abnormalities.

Clinical heart disease is unusual, even though evidence of previous pericarditis is often found at necropsy. Rarely, pericarditis with cardiac tamponade occurs. As in the pleural fluid, glucose and complement levels may be reduced. Aortic regurgitation and conduction abnormalities are occasionally seen. These problems result from rheumatoid granulomas in the aortic valve leaflets and conduction system, respectively. Slowed closure of the mitral valve is also recognized in some patients.

Splenomegaly is present in 10 percent of patients. Lymphadenopathy of the nodes proximal to the involved peripheral joints or generalized lymphadenopathy may be present. The extreme degree of lymphadenopathy in some patients may suggest a malignant lymphoproliferative disease. Amyloidosis may occasionally develop and produce renal failure in patients with long-standing disease.

Felty's syndrome is the combination of rheumatoid arthritis, splenomegaly, and neutropenia. Anemia and thrombocytopenia may occur in these patients. The syndrome usually appears in patients with long-standing disease. Vasculitis, manifested by leg ulcers and peripheral neuropathy, may be present. Infection may be a serious complication in patients with marked neutropenia. In such patients, splenectomy may improve the neutropenia and decrease infections. Neutropenia, however, may recur after splenectomy. The course of the arthritis is not affected by splenectomy.

Still's disease, a form of juvenile rheumatoid arthritis, may also occur in adults, often presenting as a fever of unknown origin. Clinical manifestations include intermittent episodes of high daily spiking fever often exceeding 40°C, polyarthralgias, myalgias, evanescent maculopapular rash, pericarditis, pneumonitis, sore throat, lymphadenopathy, splenomegaly, and abdominal pain. Tests for rheumatoid factor and antinuclear antibodies are negative. Joint deformities seldom occur. These patients respond well to high doses of salicylates or indomethacin.

CLINICAL COURSE The course of RA is highly variable and unpredictable. Spontaneous remissions and exacerbations are characteristic; remissions are more apt to occur early in the disease. Approximately 10 to 20 percent of patients will have either a complete remission early in their disease or mild intermittent disease which requires little if any medical attention. On the other side, approximately 10 percent of patients will have relentless, crippling disease, leading ultimately to confinement in a wheelchair or bed. The majority of patients fall between these groups. The patients in this middle group experience joint damage to varying degrees over the years, yet most of them are able to continue functioning at work or at home. There are certain features that portend a poor prognosis. These include a high titer of rheumatoid factors, multiple rheumatoid nodules, and vasculitis. A history of mild, intermittent disease over the years will usually continue in this pattern.

LABORATORY FINDINGS Normocytic, hypochromic (hypoproliferative) anemia is often present in active disease. The serum iron level is low, but the total iron-binding capacity remains normal. The ineffective erythropoiesis, also seen with other chronic inflammatory disorders, is due in part to a block in the release of iron from the reticuloendothelial system. Iron therapy is of no value except in those cases where superimposed blood loss has occurred and when no stainable iron can be demonstrated in the bone marrow. Rarely, a Coombs-positive hemolytic anemia is present.

A mild leukocytosis may be present. A few patients may have neutropenia and a mild thrombocytopenia. Eosinophilia of 5 percent or greater has been observed, especially in patients with extraarticular manifestations of vasculitis, pleuropericarditis, pulmonary fibrosis, and subcutaneous nodules.

The erythrocyte sedimentation rate (ESR) is commonly elevated and can be used as a parameter for following disease activity. However, the ESR may not always reflect the activity of the disease.

Protein electrophoresis often shows a reduced albumin, moderately elevated gamma globulin, and elevated α_2 globulins. Measurements of immunoglobulins may show increased levels of IgG, IgM, and IgA. These findings, however, are not diagnostic.

Rheumatoid factor as indicated by the latex agglutination test is positive in the majority of patients with RA. Only IgM rheumatoid factor is readily measured by the currently available methods, which include latex agglutination, bentonite flocculation, and sensitized sheep or human red blood cell tests. The basic principle of all these tests is the same because the antigen, human or rabbit IgG, is coated onto a carrier particle (red blood cell, latex, bentonite), allowing agglutination to be visible when rheumatoid factors react with IgG. Methods for detecting IgG and IgA rheumatoid factors remain research tools.

Patients with a variety of nonrheumatoid diseases, usually characterized by chronic inflammation with persistent antigenic challenge, have positive tests for rheumatoid factor. These include other connective tissue diseases (systemic lupus erythematosus, Sjögren's syndrome, polymyositis, scleroderma) and infectious diseases (tuberculosis, leprosy, syphilis, subacute bacterial endocarditis, bacterial bronchitis, parasitic infections, viral hepatitis, infectious mononucleosis, influenza). Positive results are also found in patients with idiopathic pulmonary fibrosis, pneumoconiosis, sarcoidosis, hypergammaglobulinemic purpura, mixed cryoglobulinemia, chronic active hepatitis and cirrhosis, lymphomas, renal allografts, and repeated blood transfusions. An occasional Waldenström's macroglobulin will show rheumatoid factor activity. Rheumatoid factor has been reported to appear transiently in the serum of army recruits after extensive prophylactic immunizations. Population studies of apparently healthy persons show an increasing prevalence of rheumatoid factor with age. The overall prevalence in persons below the age of 60 is less than 4 percent. However, in persons over the age of 60, positive results have been encountered in 40 percent of subjects in some surveys. The titer of rheumatoid factor in these elderly apparently normal persons is usually low, being less than 1:80.

Rheumatoid factor is usually present either when the patient is first seen or within the first year of disease. The titer of rheumatoid factor correlates poorly with disease activity. However, those patients with high titers tend to have more severe disease and thus a poorer prognosis than seronegative patients. Positive tests are almost always found in patients with nodules or with clinical evidence of vasculitis. A positive test does not make the diagnosis of RA but must be interpreted in the light of other clinical features.

Antinuclear antibodies are found in 20 to 60 percent of patients. Titers of antibodies with specificity for native DNA are usually low; titers of antibodies to single-stranded or denatured DNA may be elevated. The lupus erythematosus (LE) cell test is positive in 10 to 20 percent of patients. Serum complement level is usually normal or elevated. Slightly reduced levels have been reported in patients with rheumatoid vasculitis.

Synovial fluid has a turbid appearance because of increased numbers of white blood cells. The cells are predominantly neutrophils and range from 10,000 to 50,000 per cubic millimeter. The fluid may clot spontaneously because of the presence of fibrinogen. This fibrin clot should not be confused with the mucin clot formed by adding 1 percent acetic acid to the fluid. In rheumatoid synovial fluid the viscosity is decreased and the mucin clot is poor because of smaller than normal polymers of hyaluronic acid. Cytoplasmic inclusions in polymorphonuclear cells, containing ingested immune complexes, are not specific for RA. Especially in patients with positive tests for rheumatoid factor, the synovial fluid hemolytic complement or complement components, such as C3 and C4, are low when these values are related to the total protein concentration of the synovial fluid. The synovial fluid glucose level, as compared with a simultaneously drawn serum glucose, may be low in some patients, possibly because of decreased transport across the membrane or increased utilization by inflammatory cells.

Radiographs of the joints in early disease show only soft-tissue swelling and mild juxtaarticular osteoporosis. Later, bony erosions, initially quite subtle, appear at the joint margins; these are most readily seen in the small joints of the hands and along the ulnar and radial styloid processes. Joint space narrowing is seen as cartilage is destroyed. In advanced disease, destruction of subchondral bone and diffuse osteoporosis develop. When the cervical part of the spine is involved, flexion and extension films should be obtained to check for atlantoaxial subluxation.

DIAGNOSIS The diagnosis of RA is readily made in the patient with symmetrical inflammatory arthritis of small joints, rheumatoid nodules, characteristic radiographic abnormalities, and a positive test for rheumatoid factor. The patient who presents a history of fatigue and vague arthralgias without definite evidence of arthritis frequently poses a diagnostic problem. Such a patient may be in the prodromal phase of RA; however, these symptoms are often found in depressed middle-aged patients, especially women. If the diagnosis is not certain, the patient's course should be followed for objective evidence of arthritis. Other types of inflammatory arthritis deserve consideration, especially in the patient who has only a few joints involved in an asymmetrical distribution. Reiter's syndrome (Chap. 358), psoriatic arthritis (Chap. 358), systemic lupus erythematosus (Chap. 68), and arthritis associated with gastrointestinal diseases (Chap. 358) should be considered in the differential diagnosis. Some patients with ankylosing spondylitis (Chap. 357) may have peripheral arthritis. Arthritis of rheumatic fever and that of viral infections, especially rubella and hepatitis B, may initially mimic RA early in their course. The arthritis of hemochromatosis (Chap. 94) may be mistaken for RA especially when there is swelling and bony enlargement of the second and third metacarpophalangeal joints. Degenerative joint disease is easily distinguished from RA, but erosive osteoarthritis (Chap. 361) may be confused with RA. In rheumatoid arthritis, the most frequently involved joints of the upper extremity are the metacarpophalangeal, proximal interphalangeal (PIP), and wrists, while in osteoarthritis the distal interphalangeal joints, followed by the PIP, are most often affected. Osteoarthritis also frequently involves the carpometacarpal joint. The finding of a positive test result for rheumatoid factor in an elderly person should not by itself lead to the diagnosis of RA.

The definite diagnosis of RA depends primarily on the presence of characteristic clinical features and the exclusion of other inflammatory arthritides.

TREATMENT **General measures** Once the diagnosis has been established, the patient and family should be given a clear understanding of the chronic nature of RA. The value of careful and continuous medical supervision should be emphasized. Above all, the patient should be reassured that there is readily available therapy and that severe crippling is usually not the outcome. The patient should be apprised that the majority of patients continue to lead active, productive lives with varying degrees of restricted activity. The patient should be encouraged to continue working within reasonable limits. This in some instances may necessitate retraining in work that is physically less demanding. Depression and passive behavior are common in RA and require careful attention. Some patients may benefit from antidepressant medications. The question of moving to a warm climate is often raised. The patient may subjectively feel better in a warm climate; however, the course of the disease is not changed.

The goal of therapy is to maintain the patient's ability to function. To accomplish this, every effort should be made to reduce joint inflammation and pain, maintain motion and strength, and prevent and correct joint deformities. The proper utilization of rest, anti-inflammatory drugs, splints, physical therapy, and orthopedic surgery is aimed at preserving function. Adequate rest is important. Patients should be encouraged to take short rest periods during the day, even though they may not feel tired, and to get a full night's sleep. They should be instructed to maintain a well-balanced diet. There is no evidence that a nutritional deficiency leads to rheumatoid arthritis or that certain foods or vitamins affect the outcome. In patients who have had the disease for a while, the pain and disability caused by persistent inflammation must be distinguished from the symptoms caused by joint destruction. The latter do not respond to drug therapy and must be controlled by physical therapy or reconstructive surgery.

Drug therapy *Salicylates* remain the mainstay of drug therapy and should be given an adequate trial in the initial treatment of RA. They have been shown to be superior to placebo and to exert both an anti-inflammatory and an analgesic action. A dosage of 3 to 6 g per day should be administered in divided amounts four times a day, preferably after meals. Periodic checks of the blood salicylate level are useful to determine whether adequate blood levels are being achieved. The blood sample should be obtained 2 to 3 h after a regular dose. A level between 15 and 30 mg per 100 ml is in the therapeutic range.

An increase in fecal blood is commonly observed with salicylate usage regardless of the route of administration, and is not necessarily due to bleeding from a peptic ulcer. However, salicylates may aggravate peptic ulcer disease. The gastrointestinal upset, a common complaint, can be alleviated by giving the drug with meals and by the use of antacids. Salicylates have been reported to cause urticaria or asthma. Signs of toxicity such as tinnitus, deafness, hyperventilation, or confusion should be carefully monitored, especially in older patients.

Acetylsalicylic acid (aspirin) is the most effective preparation on a weight basis. Choline salicylate or salicylsalicylic acid may be better tolerated in patients with gastrointestinal upset or with peptic ulcer disease. Enteric coated preparations have the disadvantage of delayed and unpredictable absorption.

In patients who are unable to tolerate salicylates, indomethacin (Indocin) or one of the newer nonsteroidal anti-inflammatory drugs can be added or substituted. These latter drugs include ibuprofen (Motrin), fenoprofen (Nalfon), naproxen (Naprosyn), tolmetin (Tolectin), and sulindac (Clinoril). The therapeutic effectiveness of these drugs is approximately the same and is similar to that of the salicylates. The usual dose of indomethacin is between 75 and 150 mg per day, in divided doses, and the drug is best tolerated if the dosage is gradually increased to these amounts. Side effects of lightheadedness, headaches, unreal feeling, depression, dyspepsia, or peptic ulcer disease may curb its use. The recommended dose of ibuprofen is between 1200 and 2400 mg per day, in divided doses. Side effects include epigastric pain, diarrhea, peptic ulcer disease, and skin eruptions. The usual dose of naproxen is 250 mg twice a day, and, again, adverse reactions include upper gastrointestinal distress and bleeding. The usual dose for fenoprofen is 600 mg four times per day. Again, gastrointestinal side effects such as dyspepsia, constipation, nausea, and occult blood in the stool may occur. The usual dose of tolmetin is between 600 and 1800 mg in divided doses. The side effects are similar to those of indomethacin. Sulindac is recommended in the dosage of 150 to 200 mg twice daily; the potential side effects are comparable with drugs mentioned above. All these drugs and acetylsalicylic acid, but not choline salicylate, salicylsalicylic acid, and sodium salicylate, interfere with platelet aggregation and therefore may prolong bleeding time.

Phenylbutazone is not recommended for long-term therapy in RA. It may be useful for short periods during an acute exacerbation. The dose should not exceed 400 mg per day. Complications include fluid retention, peptic ulcer disease, and bone marrow toxicity, primarily leukopenia.

When salicylates or nonsteroidal anti-inflammatory medications prove ineffective in controlling the disease, gold salts, chloroquine, and penicillamine are the next order of drugs to be used. In controlled studies both *chloroquine* and *hydroxychloroquine* have been shown to be effective. The recommended daily dose of chloroquine is 250 mg, and of hydroxychloroquine, 200 to 400 mg. A response is not usually seen until 4 to 6 weeks of therapy. Once improvement is noted, the dosage should be reduced. Long-term use of these drugs is curtailed by the risk of blindness from irreversible retinal degeneration, which may progress even when administration of the drug has been discontinued. The drug should not be given unless an initial and regular eye examination every 4 to 6 months is performed by an ophthalmologist. Other complications include neuromyopathy, gastrointestinal distress, band keratopathy, and bleaching of hair.

Gold salts are beneficial in suppressing disease activity in some patients. In a controlled study patients treated with a total of 1 g gold sodium thiomalate over a 20-week period experienced greater clinical improvement than those given placebo. The clinical improvement was not lasting, since no differences between the two groups were found approximately 2 years after the last gold injection. In general, patients with recent onset of RA are more likely to respond than those with long-standing disease. Also, patients who previously failed to respond to an adequate course of gold are not likely to respond to another course.

The two gold salts most commonly used are gold sodium thiomalate (Myochrysine) and gold thioglucose (Solganol); they are administered intramuscularly, usually on a weekly basis. The initial dose is 10 mg, followed by 25 mg the next week. If no adverse effects are noted, 50 mg is given weekly until definite improvement is observed or a total dose of 1 g is reached. If no improvement results, the drug is discontinued. With a favorable response, the interval between injections is gradually increased until the patient is receiving 50 mg monthly. The value of maintenance therapy is not proved. The beneficial effects of gold therapy usually do not become apparent until at least 400 to 500 mg has been given.

Dermatitis and stomatitis are the most common toxic manifestations of gold therapy. The rash is often pruritic and accompanied by eosinophilia. The mucocutaneous lesions are reversible when gold therapy is discontinued. Early detection of a rash is important, since continuation of gold may lead to a generalized exfoliative dermatitis. A mild rash may be treated with local steroid preparations; however, systemic steroids may be necessary for severe extensive dermatitis.

Gold toxicity can cause nephritis with resultant renal damage, the earliest manifestations being proteinuria and/or hematuria. These signs may be followed by the nephrotic syndrome. Bone marrow toxicity may present as an aplastic anemia, agranulocytosis, and/or thrombocytopenia with severe marrow depression. The use of a chelating agent may be necessary for treatment of severe gold toxicity.

In view of the potential serious toxicity of gold, the decision to use gold carries with it the obligation of careful medical supervision. Each week the patient should be asked about and examined for evidence of skin and/or mouth lesions. White blood cell counts and analysis of the urine for protein should be performed on alternate weeks. Periodic platelet counts are advisable. If rash, proteinuria, or leukopenia appears, administration of gold should be discontinued.

Penicillamine was shown in a controlled multicenter trial, conducted in England, to be effective in RA. The drug's therapeutic efficacy is comparable with gold salts. To reduce side effects, the drug is given in a graduated dosage schedule beginning with 250 mg daily for 4 weeks followed by 250 mg bid for 4 weeks. If no improvement is seen, the dose is increased to 250 mg tid for 8 weeks. Those patients responding to penicillamine will usually do so within this 16-week period. Patients are maintained on the dosage at which clinical improvement occurred. Toxicity includes skin rashes, nausea, loss of taste, nephropathy with proteinuria and nephrotic syndrome, fever, and bone marrow suppression. While minor skin rashes and pruritus can be controlled by administration of an antihistamine, the other toxic reactions necessitate discontinuation of therapy. The use of this drug obligates the physician to follow the patient with blood counts and urine protein closely at regular intervals.

The use of glucocorticosteroids should be reserved for patients whose disease is not adequately controlled by the previously mentioned drugs. Small doses of prednisone may permit a patient who is a breadwinner to continue working while waiting for other drugs to be effective. The dose of prednisone or its equivalent should be the smallest amount providing symptomatic relief and should not exceed 10 to 15 mg per day. Continued use of larger doses provides no additional advantage and increases the well-known side effects of these drugs. Large doses, however, may be necessary in patients with severe extraarticular complications of RA, especially in patients with vasculitis. Supplemental steroids should be given to patients who are receiving steroids or to those who have received them in the recent past, when they undergo surgery or develop a severe intercurrent illness.

Intraarticular steroid injections are useful in temporarily suppressing joint inflammation, especially when only a few joints show active disease. In patients with multiple joint involvement, injection of a few of the most symptomatic joints may serve to supplement other forms of therapy. Following injection of small finger joints, inflammation may be suppressed for as long as 1 year. Frequent injection may predispose a joint to further damage from overuse, since unsuppressed pain tends to protect an already injured joint. Injections of a single joint should be limited to three or four a year. Some patients experience a transient exacerbation of joint inflammation a few hours after injection which is due to a "crystal-induced synovitis" from corticosteroid crystals. Sterile technique should be used to prevent possible introduction of infection.

Immunosuppressive (cytotoxic) drugs are being evaluated for the treatment of rheumatoid arthritis. The rationale for their use is based on evidence that immunologic mechanisms mediate synovitis and other manifestations of RA. These drugs are effective in suppressing the primary humoral and cellular responses, provided that the drug is given in the proper dose and time in relation to the introduction of antigen. They diminish ongoing cellular immune responses but have little, if any, effect on ongoing humoral immune responses. These drugs are antiinflammatory, as shown in experimental animals and in human beings. Their action in RA has not been clarified but may be related in large part to their anti-inflammatory properties by decreasing the traffic of monocytes and lymphocytes.

The immunosuppressive drugs that have been used in RA include cyclophosphamide, azathioprine, 6-mercaptopurine, chlorambucil, and methotrexate. Favorable responses have been reported with all these drugs; however, few carefully controlled studies have been performed. A controlled study of cyclophosphamide, over an 8-month period, showed that patients receiving high doses (up to 150 mg per day) had greater improvement than those on a nontherapeutic dose (up to 15 mg per day). Patients treated with the high-dose regimen had improved grip strength, a decrease in the duration of morning stiffness, a decrease in the number of painful swollen joints, and a decrease in the number of new articular erosions. Sedimentation rates did not correlate well with improvement. Controlled studies carried out with azathioprine have also shown favorable results. The beneficial effect of these drugs on a long-term basis is not known, nor has the beneficial effect of their intraarticular injection been proved.

The toxicity and side effects of cytotoxic drugs limit their use. These agents can cause bone marrow depression with severe leukopenia, infection (especially with opportunistic microorganisms), sterility, and an increased risk of neoplasia. Because of their mutagenic potential, contraception should be recommended when they are being used. In addition, there are specific adverse manifestations of the individual drugs. Methotrexate is hepatotoxic and causes cirrhosis. Cyclophosphamide causes cystitis, resulting in hemorrhage and bladder wall fibrosis. Alopecia occurs frequently. Immunosuppressive therapy should be considered experimental and, if used at all, should be restricted to patients who have not responded to more conventional forms of therapy. The use of these drugs requires an informed consent from the patient and constant, close supervision. White blood cell counts should be carefully monitored.

Physical therapy This form of treatment plays an important role in the treatment of RA. Heat helps to relieve muscle spasm and reduce stiffness. Paraffin baths and heat lamps can be used at home. Passive range-of-motion exercises can help to prevent or minimize loss of joint motion. Isometric exercises increase muscle strength and thereby help to maintain joint stability. Repetitious forms of exercise should not be performed with joints that have active disease. Splinting of an actively involved joint for short periods of time is useful in reducing pain and possibly inflammation. The use of night splints is helpful in preventing flexion contractures, especially of the knees and wrists. Review and revision of home and work routines, and the use of assistive devices, can enhance the patient's ability to continue functioning at an independent level.

Orthopedic surgery This modality plays an important role in the treatment of RA. Function may be improved by surgical correction of joint deformities and stabilization of certain joints. Resection of the metatarsal heads is often beneficial in relieving forefoot pain. The carpal tunnel syndrome with persistent neurological signs necessitates surgical release and synovectomy. Ruptured tendons should be repaired within a couple of days after their breakage. Removal of rheumatoid synovium involving the extensor hood over the dorsum of the wrist and hands may prevent tendon rupture. Resection of the distal ulna, together with synovectomy of the wrist, helps to relieve pain and improve function. Synovectomy of the knee may be needed when a symptomatic popliteal cyst does not respond to intraarticular corticosteroids.

Atlantoaxial subluxation with symptoms of cord compression requires surgical stabilization. Patients with atlantoaxial subluxation but without evidence of cord compression should protect themselves by wearing a collar, especially when riding in an automobile.

Prophylactic synovectomy may diminish joint pain and temporarily retard progression of the disease in the operated joint. If the disease remains active, the joints treated with synovectomy become reinflamed. Development of total hip prostheses has given new hope to patients with severely damaged hip joints. Results of total knee, ankle, and other large-joint

JUVENILE RHEUMATOID ARTHRITIS

Juvenile rheumatoid arthritis (JRA) consists of several distinct syndromes. Three main subgroups have been identified: systemic-onset disease, polyarticular disease, and pauciarticular disease. In addition, ankylosing spondylitis and rheumatoid arthritis indistinguishable from adult-onset disease may begin in childhood.

Systemic-onset JRA represents 25 percent of juvenile arthritis and is characterized by distinctive extraarticular manifestations in addition to the arthritis. Boys are affected more than girls, and the median age of onset is 5 years. These patients may have high fever (40°C and over). The fever has wide diurnal fluctuations and is highest in the afternoon and evening. Fever may be present for weeks or months before the appearance of arthritis. An evanescent salmon-color nonpruritic macular or maculopapular rash may appear, especially during fever, and is more common on the trunk. Generalized lymphadenopathy, splenomegaly, and hepatomegaly are often present. Cardiac involvement includes pericarditis and, rarely, myocarditis; pneumonitis and pleuritis also occur. Systemic manifestations are self-limited. Approximately one-fourth of this group of patients experience severe, destructive polyarthritis. Laboratory findings include anemia, leukocytosis, and negative tests for rheumatoid factors and antinuclear antibodies. The name *Still's disease* is sometimes used for this form of disease, but this eponym is also used for all forms of JRA.

Pauciarticular arthritis, affecting about 30 percent of patients with JRA, is characterized by female predominance, early age of onset (2 to 4 years), and involvement of one or a few joints, most commonly the knees or ankles. The arthritis is mild, with a good prognosis. Half of the patients experience chronic iridocyclitis, which may lead to band keratopathy, cataracts, and loss of vision. Since eye symptoms may be minimal, patients should have regular slit-lamp examinations, whether or not the arthritis is in remission. Antinuclear antibodies have been found in 50 to 60 percent of these patients; rheumatoid factor is absent.

Polyarticular arthritis occurs in 25 percent of patients, affects predominantly girls at a young age (median age of onset 2 years), and has a relatively good prognosis. The onset is usually insidious; the initial joint involvement is in the small joints of the hands and feet. Twenty-five percent have antinuclear antibodies. The standard tests for rheumatoid factor are negative. With special techniques, IgG and IgA rheumatoid factors have been found in over half the patients that are seronegative by standard methods.

In addition to these three subgroups, 5 to 10 percent of patients have polyarticular disease and a positive rheumatoid factor test. The median age of onset is 12 years, and females predominate. The course and clinical manifestations are those of adult-onset RA. Ankylosing spondylitis may also present in childhood, as pauciarticular disease, and represents 20 percent of patients with juvenile-onset arthritis. The median age of onset is 10 years, and males predominate. Patients experience early hip girdle symptoms; episodes of acute iridocyclitis may occur. Rheumatoid factor and antinuclear antibody tests are negative. The prevalence of HLA-B27 is 75 percent in this group while an increased prevalence of HLA-B27 is not found in the other subgroups of JRA.

The object of therapy in JRA, as in adult-onset RA, is to relieve pain and maintain function. The child should be allowed to lead as normal a life as possible and should be encouraged to participate in the activities of childhood. Only vigorous athletics should be discouraged. Salicylates are the first drug of choice. Patients on salicylates should be followed closely with liver function tests, since these drugs occasionally produce hepatotoxicity. It is recommended that liver function tests plus a prothrombin time be obtained before starting therapy, and then at regular intervals. The abnormal liver function tests return to normal in most patients while they remain on salicylates. Administration of the drug should be stopped in patients with progressive liver dysfunction. If salicylates are not effective, gold salts can be given. Antimalarials can also be beneficial in JRA. The use of systemic glucocorticosteroids is seldom indicated in the treatment of JRA. In certain instances, glucocorticosteroids are required for the treatment of uncontrolled systemic JRA or in treating iridocyclitis not controlled by a topical steroid. They are not indicated for the treatment of joint manifestations alone. Immunosuppressive agents are seldom indicated in JRA, since little is known of the long-term effects of these drugs. Physical therapy, the judicious splinting of joints, proper exercise, and adequate rest are all important factors in the treatment of JRA.

SJÖGREN'S SYNDROME

This syndrome consists of dry eyes (keratoconjunctivitis sicca, xerophthalmia), dry mouth (xerostomia), and a chronic arthritis. It can be diagnosed when any two of the three clinical features (dry eyes, dry mouth, arthritis) are present. The lack of secretions may also involve the entire respiratory tract, vagina, and skin. The syndrome occurs most commonly in middle-aged women; fewer than 10 percent of patients are men. The histological and immunologic findings suggest that abnormalities of both humoral- and cell-mediated immunity are involved in the pathogenesis of Sjögren's syndrome.

The decrease in tears and saliva (sicca syndrome) results from lymphocytic infiltration of the lacrimal and salivary glands. The earliest histological finding is periductal lymphocytic infiltration, which progresses to produce atrophy of the acini. The cells are predominantly small lymphocytes, but large lymphocytes, plasma cells, and reticulum cells may be present. Lymph follicles with germinal centers form in the gland. Hyperplasia of the ductal lining cells narrows and obstructs the duct and leads to its dilatation. Focal hyperplasia of ductal cells produces epimyoepithelial islands surrounded by lymphocytes. Hyalinization of these islands may occur. Later in the course of the disease, the atrophied parenchymal tissue is replaced by adipose tissue. Lip biopsy specimens show infiltrates of plasma cells and lymphocytes in the minor (accessory) salivary glands. Features that are helpful in distinguishing this syndrome from malignant lymphoma are the benign appearance of the small lymphocytes, the preservation of the lobular architecture of the gland, and the presence of epimyoepithelial cells.

Rheumatoid arthritis is present in approximately one-half the patients with Sjögren's syndrome; the arthritis usually appears first. The sicca syndrome occurs in approximately 10 to 15 percent of patients with RA. Rheumatoid nodules, splenomegaly, leukopenia, and vasculitis may be present in these patients. Rarely Sjögren's syndrome is associated with systemic lupus erythematosus, polymyositis, scleroderma, and periarteritis nodosa. The syndrome has also been found in some patients with autoimmune liver disease (chronic active hepatitis, primary biliary cirrhosis, and cryptogenic cirrhosis).

Keratoconjunctivitis sicca produces symptoms of burning, itching, and blurring of vision. The patient may complain of a sensation of sand in the eye. Thick secretions accumulate in the conjunctival sac, and the conjunctiva may be reddened.

The diagnosis is made by demonstrating decreased lacrimation (Schirmer's test), corneal or conjunctival erosions (rose bengal or fluorescein dye staining), and filamentary keratitis (slit-lamp examination).

Patients with xerostomia may have difficulty in swallowing solid foods, a decrease in taste acuity, and a rapid progression of dental caries. Cracks and fissures may appear at the corners of the mouth. The buccal mucosa has a parchment-like appearance, and the tongue is red and smooth. Bilateral parotid gland enlargement is observed in one-half the patients. Other salivary glands also may enlarge. The glands are usually smooth, firm, and only slightly tender but may be nodular and hard. Fluctuation in size is common. The diagnosis of xerostomia may be confirmed by measurement of salivary flow, by sialography, and by sequential salivary scintigraphy with pertechnetate.

Dryness of the nasal mucosa may cause epistaxis and decreased acuity of smell. Hoarseness may occur with laryngeal dryness. Patients also may have recurrent bronchitis and pneumonitis because of the decrease of protective mucous secretions.

The development of lymphadenopathy and extrasalivary lymphoid abnormalities in patients with Sjögren's syndrome may suggest malignant lymphoma. These patients are considered to have a disorder falling between neoplasia and hyperplasia, which is diagnosed as *pseudolymphoma*. Serum IgM levels are usually elevated. Lymphadenopathy, splenomegaly, leukopenia, purpura, neuropathy, vasculitis, and Raynaud's phenomena are more frequently observed in patients with extrasalivary gland lymphoid abnormalities than in those with abnormalities confined to the salivary glands. In some patients, malignant reticulum-cell sarcoma has been reported at sites other than the salivary glands.

Other features sometimes associated with Sjögren's syndrome are hypergammaglobulinemic purpura, thrombotic thrombocytopenic purpura, and renal tubular acidosis. Gastric achlorhydria and acute pancreatitis may also occur.

Mild anemia, leukopenia, and eosinophilia may be present. Approximately one-half the patients have hypergammaglobulinemia. Positive rheumatoid factor tests are found in almost all the patients, and approximately 70 percent have antinuclear antibodies. These antibodies, along with antibodies to thyroglobulin, tissue homogenates, and salivary ducts, are much more common in patients with the sicca syndrome alone than in those with Sjögren's syndrome and rheumatoid arthritis.

In the differential diagnosis, parotid gland tumors should be considered when enlargement is unilateral and other features of the syndrome are absent. Features favoring Sjögren's syndrome are the absence of pain, fluctuation in gland size, and the chronicity of the swelling without extension into the adjacent tissues. The differentiation between a benign and malignant lymphoproliferative disease may be difficult and confusing. Enlargement of the lacrimal and salivary glands (Mikulicz's syndrome) may occur in lymphoma, lymphocytic leukemia, and sarcoidosis. The sicca syndrome is usually not present in malignant lymphoproliferative involvement of the salivary and lacrimal glands, but occurs in sarcoidosis. The diagnosis of sarcoidosis is established by the finding of noncaseating granulomas in the involved gland.

The treatment of RA in patients with Sjögren's syndrome is the same as for RA alone. Dry eyes can be temporarily relieved by the use of 0.5% methylcellulose drops or other types of artificial tears. Methylcellulose (1 or 2%) may be used as a mouthwash in patients with dry mouth. Gelatin and glycerine lozenges may be helpful. Systemic steroids are not recommended for treatment of the enlarged glands. Though they may reduce the size of the glands, dryness is not helped. Ste-roids may be indicated in patients with extrasalivary lymphoid infiltrates and with clinical manifestations of vasculitis. Improvement of the sicca syndrome by treatment with cyclophosphamide has been observed; however, further controlled observations are necessary before immunosuppressive drugs can be recommended for this use. Irradiation of the enlarged parotids is contraindicated because reticulum-cell sarcoma may develop in patients who have received this form of therapy during the early phases of their Sjögren's syndrome.

REFERENCES

AMERICAN RHEUMATISM ASSOCIATION, COOPERATING CLINICS COMMITTEE: A controlled trial of cyclophosphamide in rheumatoid arthritis. N Engl J Med 283:883, 1970

BLOCK KJ et al: Sjögren's syndrome: A clinical, pathological and serological study of sixty-two cases. Medicine 44:187, 1965

BUJAK JS et al: Juvenile rheumatoid arthritis presenting in the adult as fever of unknown origin. Medicine 52:431, 1973

EMPIRE RHEUMATISM COUNCIL, RESEARCH SUBCOMMITTEE: Gold therapy in rheumatoid arthritis—final report of a multi-center controlled trial. Ann Rheum Dis 20:315, 1961

JAFFE IA: D-Penicillimine. Bull Rheum Dis 28(6):948, 1977

POPE RM et al: The molecular basis of self-association of IgG-rheumatoid factors. J Immunol 115:365, 1975

RUDDY S, AUSTEN KF: The complement system in rheumatoid synovitis. Arthritis Rheum 13:713, 1970

SCHALLER JG: The diversity of JRA: A 1976 look at the subgroups of chronic childhood arthritis. Arthritis Rheum 20:6, 1977

SHEARN MA: Sjögren's syndrome. Med Clin North Am 61:2, 1977

STEINBERG AD et al: Cytotoxic drugs in treatment of nonmalignant diseases. Ann Intern Med 76:619, 1972

WILLIAMS RC JR: Rheumatoid arthritis as a systemic disease, in *Major Problems in Internal Medicine,* vol 4, LH Smith Jr (ed). Philadelphia, Saunders, 1974

WINCHESTER RJ: Characterization of IgG complexes in patients with rheumatoid arthritis. Ann NY Acad Sci 256:73, 1975

ZVAILFLER NJ: The immunopathology of joint inflammation in rheumatoid arthritis. Adv Immunol 16:265, 1973

357
ANKYLOSING SPONDYLITIS

BRUCE C. GILLILAND
MART MANNIK

INTRODUCTION Ankylosing spondylitis, a disease that has been called by many names, including rheumatoid spondylitis and Marie-Strümpell disease, is a chronic and usually progressive inflammatory disease involving the articulations of the spine and adjacent soft tissues. The sacroiliac joints are always affected. Involvement of the hip and shoulder joints commonly occurs; peripheral joints are affected less frequently. The disease predominantly affects young men and begins most often in the third decade. A high association has been found between this disorder and the histocompatibility antigen HLA-B27. The clinical features of this disease are distinctly different from those of rheumatoid arthritis. The etiology is not known.

EPIDEMIOLOGY Ankylosing spondylitis is found throughout the world. In the white population, the prevalence in men is 0.5 to 4 per 1000 and in women 0.05 to 0.5 per 1000.

Hereditary factors play an important role in the development of ankylosing spondylitis. Histocompatibility typing has revealed the presence of HLA-B27 antigen in 88 to 96 percent of spondylitic patients, while in the normal white population 7 percent have this antigen. In blacks, HLA-B27 occurs less frequently, which may account for the lower prevalence of this disease among them.

HLA-B27 is inherited in a mendelian fashion, and HLA-B27 is found in 50 percent of first-degree relatives of those spondylitic patients who are positive for HLA-B27. Within the group of relatives, 20 percent have either symptomatic or asymptomatic spondylitis. Ankylosing spondylitis is seen occasionally in patients who are negative for HLA-B27, indicating that other genetic or environmental factors are necessary for the development of the disease.

In recent studies, 20 percent of apparently healthy people of both sexes who are positive for HLA-B27 have some clinical features of ankylosing spondylitis or sacroiliitis. Since spondylitis is diagnosed ten times more frequently in men than women, these studies on apparently healthy people suggest that women have milder disease.

Several diseases that possess clinical features in common with ankylosing spondylitis also occur more frequently in patients with the HLA-B27 antigen. These disorders include Reiter's syndrome, psoriatic spondylarthritis, *Yersinia* arthritis, spondylarthritis of inflammatory bowel disease, and acute anterior uveitis. The role of HLA-B27 antigen in the pathogenesis of these disorders is not known. The currently favored hypothesis is that the HLA-B27 antigen, because of a close association with the immune response genes, is only a marker distinguishing a group of individuals whose immune response to an as yet undefined infectious agent leads to one of the HLA-B27 associated forms of the arthritides.

PATHOLOGY The earliest histopathologic changes usually occur in the sacroiliac joints but may start anywhere in the spine. The disease usually progresses up the spine, and occasionally segments will be skipped.

Synovitis of the involved diarthrodial joints of the spine (apophyseal and costovertebral joints) and of the sacroiliac, hip, shoulder, and peripheral joints resembles that of rheumatoid arthritis. Synovial hyperplasia and focal accumulation of lymphoid and plasma cells are seen histologically. Bony erosions and cartilage destruction ensue, followed later by fibrosis and bony ankylosis. In cartilaginous joints (intervertebral disks, manubriosternal, and symphysis pubis), granulation tissue invades the fibrocartilage, and adjacent bone is replaced later by fibrosis and ossification.

Occasionally, fibrous tissue invades the vertebral body to produce a radiolucent cyst which may be confused with an infectious process. Erosions at the anterior corners of the vertebral bodies destroy their normal anterior concavity and give the vertebra a square appearance on lateral radiographs. Ossification of the outer layers of the annulus fibrosus at its lateral margins produces the syndesmophytes and "bamboo spine" observed radiographically. Ossification also involves the anterior portion of the annulus fibrosus and occasionally the inner aspect of the anterior longitudinal ligament. The radiographic appearance of the ossification at the anterior disk margins has led to the misconception that only the anterior longitudinal ligament is involved. Bony erosions and new bone formation also occur at the insertion of tendons, most notably at the spinous processes, greater trochanters, pelvic bones, and heels.

Focal medial necrosis at the root of the aorta causes dilatation of the aortic ring. The aortic cusps may be shortened and thickened but are not fused. These processes lead to aortic valve incompetence. Fibrous tissue may enter the membranous septum and invade the atrioventricular bundle, resulting in conduction defects.

MANIFESTATIONS The disease occurs most commonly between the ages of 15 and 40 years and rarely after age 50. The initial symptoms are low back pain and stiffness, often worse in the early morning. Pain in the hips, buttocks, and shoulders is often present. Nocturnal back pain may force the patient to walk around in an attempt to gain relief.

In approximately 10 percent of patients, early symptoms resemble sciatica, with pain in the buttocks and in back of the thighs. The pain may alternate from side to side and seldom radiates below the knee. Abnormal findings on neurological examination are unusual.

Patients may have the simultaneous onset of peripheral arthritis and back pain; however, peripheral arthritis uncommonly precedes back symptoms. Approximately one-fourth of patients will have peripheral arthritis during the course of their disease, but residual damage of these joints occurs infrequently.

Hip disease may be a major cause of disability. Severe involvement early in the disease may result in ankylosis of the hip. Hip involvement, on the other hand, may lead to arthritis indistinguishable from osteoarthritis of the hip.

Occasionally, patients may experience anterior chest pain from thoracic skeletal involvement which may mimic angina pectoris. Pain on deep breathing also may occur. Other causes of chest pain are involvement of the manubriosternal and sternoclavicular joints. Bilateral pulmonary fibrosis, involving the upper lobes, develops in some patients. Radicular pain from the lumbar part of the spine may radiate to the abdomen, suggesting visceral disease.

Atlantoaxial subluxation and spinal cord compression occur less commonly than in rheumatoid arthritis. Patients with fused cervical spines are especially susceptible to fractures of the neck on falling.

Aortic valve incompetence is present in 3 percent of patients and may result in severe aortic regurgitation, requiring surgical repair. Conduction abnormalities include varying degrees of heart block and left bundle branch block. The conduction defects are more apt to appear in patients with aortic valve incompetence, but they may exist alone. Some patients require implantation of a pacemaker.

Acute anterior uveitis is observed in 20 to 30 percent of patients and may be recurrent. Occasionally, this may be the presenting symptom, calling attention to the diagnosis of ankylosing spondylitis. Amyloidosis is found in a small number of patients at autopsy and is a cause of uremia in this disease.

The constitutional symptoms are usually mild at the onset and throughout the disease, but in a few patients with severe disease, fatigue, anemia, fever, and weight loss may be present.

Symptoms may be persistent or intermittent for months or years. In some patients ankylosis of the spine may progress with little or no pain. The degree of spinal involvement varies among patients, ranging from only sacroiliac joint involvement to complete ankylosis of the spine. Once ankylosis of joints occurs, pain usually disappears.

The *cauda equina syndrome* is a rare complication appearing usually in patients with long-standing and apparently inactive disease. The cause of this syndrome is unclear but may be the result of previous arachnoiditis or ischemia. Symptoms result from the involvement of the lumbosacral nerve roots and include buttock or leg pain, lower extremity weakness, and loss of bladder and rectal sphincter control. Loss of sensation occurs in the saddle area, posterior thighs, and lateral aspects of the feet. The deep tendon reflexes are diminished. Myelography shows posterior diverticula along the lumbar nerve root sheets or throughout the entire dural sac, when the study is done with the patient in the supine position. Neurological manifestations are usually slowly progressive. Adequate treatment is presently not available for this syndrome.

Physical findings early in the disease may be minimal. Tenderness over the sacroiliac joints can be elicited by direct palpation or percussion, or by maneuvers that stress the joint. The lumbar part of the spine will show loss of the normal lordosis and paraspinal muscle spasm. An objective method for assessing anterior flexion of the lumbar part of the spine is available. Costovertebral involvement is best measured by chest expansion. The more advanced changes of spondylitis are easily recognized by the rigid spine, often fused in varying degrees of flexion, which may be quite pronounced in the thoracic region of the spine.

LABORATORY FINDINGS The erythrocyte sedimentation rate (ESR) is elevated in the majority of cases, but its level reflects fluctuations of disease activity poorly, and the ESR is normal in 20 percent of patients with mild disease. A mild hypoproliferative anemia may be present during severe active disease. Sheep cell agglutination and latex fixation tests for rheumatoid factor are negative even when peripheral joint disease is present. Mild to moderate elevations of the spinal fluid protein level may be present in active spondylitis. Synovial fluid from peripheral joints usually shows a moderate neutrophilic leukocytosis.

Radiographs of the sacroiliac joints in early disease show blurring of the margins, irregular subchondral erosions, and patchy sclerosis. These changes are initially more pronounced in the lower third of the joint. Both sacroiliac joints are characteristically involved, but findings may first appear on one side. With progression, sclerosis becomes more marked, the joint space is lost, and later osteoporosis appears. Similar changes are observed in other articulations of the axial skeleton, including the symphysis pubis and apophyseal joints. At points of tendon insertions (e.g., pelvis, os calcis) the adjacent bone shows erosions, sclerosis, and fluffy new bone formation. Lateral films of the os calcis may show bony spurs at the site of attachment for the Achilles tendon and for the plantar fascia.

Radiographs of the spine in early phases of the disease may show straightening of the lumbar part of the spine and squaring of the lumbar and lower thoracic vertebrae. With progression, syndesmophytes appear along the lateral and anterior surfaces of the intervertebral disks and bridge adjacent vertebrae. They are characteristically present on both lateral sides of the intervertebral disk at any given level and usually arise from the margin of the vertebral body. The widespread distribution of syndesmophytes in advanced disease produces the picture of the "bamboo spine." Syndesmophytes must be differentiated from the osteophytes observed in degenerative joint disease. The syndesmophyte extends vertically from the adjacent vertebral margins along the outer aspect of the intervertebral disk, while the osteophyte projects horizontally before curving to form an intervertebral bridge. The radiographic changes in involved peripheral joints are similar to those of rheumatoid arthritis.

DIAGNOSIS A patient with ankylosing spondylitis in the advanced stage is easily recognized by the characteristic bent-over posture, rigid spine, exaggerated dorsal kyphosis, and waddling gait. When peripheral arthritis is present in the early stages of ankylosing spondylitis, confusion with rheumatoid arthritis may occur. Ankylosing spondylitis is predominantly a disease of young men, but the disease also exists in women in a milder form. HLA-B27 antigen is usually present, rheumatoid factor tests are negative, and rheumatoid nodules are not found. Radiographs of the spine show bilateral sacroiliitis and syndesmophytes, which are features not seen in adult rheumatoid arthritis. Ankylosing spondylitis in children often presents as a peripheral arthritis and, therefore, may be initially diagnosed as juvenile rheumatoid arthritis. Hip, sacroiliac, and spine involvement along with attacks of acute anterior uveitis eventually point to the diagnosis of spondylitis. Older boys are most often affected. HLA-B27 is usually present in these children in contrast to juvenile rheumatoid arthritis in which the prevalence of this antigen does not differ from normal persons.

Differentiation from other diseases with spondylitis early in the course may be difficult. Since the spondylitis is indistinguishable from that associated with ulcerative colitis and regional enteritis and may antedate the bowel disease by months or years, symptoms and signs of intestinal disease should always be sought, especially in female patients. The spondylitis with Reiter's syndrome and psoriatic arthritis have common radiographic features, but differ from ankylosing spondylitis in having a greater tendency for syndesmophytes to appear at only one lateral margin of the intervertebral disk at any given level and to arise beyond the margin of the vertebral body. The distribution of syndesmophytes is more random, and the degree of spinal involvement is usually less than in ankylosing spondylitis. Other clinical features of Reiter's syndrome and psoriatic arthritis allow for easy separation of these diseases from ankylosing spondylitis. Diffuse idiopathic skeletal hyperostosis (DISH or Forestier's disease with extra spinal involvement) is distinguished from ankylosing spondylitis by the lack of apophyseal and sacroiliac joint involvement and by its more frequent occurrence in men over 50. Laminated new bone formation involves the anterior and lateral spinal ligaments most prominently in the middle to lower thoracic regions and resembles the dripping of candle wax. The radiological findings of sacroiliitis are distinguished from osteitis condensans ilii by the finding of sclerosis on only the ilial side of the joint and the preservation of the joint space in the latter. Sciatica of ankylosing spondylitis can be differentiated from that of disk disease, since it may alternate from side to side, the pain seldom radiates below the knee, and neurological signs are usually absent. Malignancies should be considered in both youngsters and older patients with symptoms of back pain.

TREATMENT The goal of therapy is to prevent or minimize the deformities of the spine inherent in this disease. With minimal deformity, patients may be able to continue working and living in a reasonably normal fashion if hip disease is not severe. Patients should be instructed to maintain an erect posture whether walking, standing, or sitting. They should be encouraged to sleep in a prone position or, if this is not possible, in a supine position on a flat firm mattress using a small pillow or none at all. Breathing exercises should be encouraged.

Drugs will not halt the progression of the disease, but they provide adequate relief to permit maintenance of posture. Phenylbutazone or indomethacin is effective in this respect. The maintenance dose of phenylbutazone is 200 to 300 mg per day, and of indomethacin, 75 to 150 mg per day. Therapy should be discontinued when symptoms abate. Salicylates or one of the newer nonsteroidal anti-inflammatory drugs (e.g., naproxen) may be effective. Gold and chloroquine have not been beneficial. Any benefit from glucocorticosteroids is outweighed by their side effects. Iritis can usually be treated with intraocular steroids.

Surgical correction of extreme flexion deformities of the spine by wedge resection and refusion in an improved position may be helpful in selected patients. The potential danger of spinal cord damage and the long convalescent period should be carefully considered before advising surgery. Patients with crippling hip disease may benefit from total hip replacement.

REFERENCES

BERENS DL: Roentgen features of ankylosing spondylitis. Clin Orthop 74:20, 1971

BREWERTON DA, JAMES DCO: The histocompatibility antigen (HL-A 27) and disease. Semin Arthritis Rheum 4:991, 1975

CALIN A, FRIES JF: Striking prevalence of ankylosing spondylitis in "healthy" W27 positive males and females. N Engl J Med 293:835, 1975

COHEN LM et al: Increased risk for spondylitis stigmata in apparently healthy HL-A-W27 men. Ann Intern Med 84:1, 1976

CRUICKSHANK B: Pathology of ankylosing spondylitis. Clin Orthop 74:43, 1971

ENGLEMAN EG, ENGLEMAN EP: Ankylosing spondylitis. Recent advances in diagnosis and treatment. Med Clin North Am 61:347, 1977

MACRAE IF, WRIGHT V: Measurements of back movement. Ann Rheum Dis 28:584, 1969

MCEWEN C et al: Ankylosing spondylitis and spondylitis accompanying ulcerative colitis, regional enteritis, psoriasis, and Reiter's disease. Arthritis Rheum 14:291, 1971

MOLL JMH et al: Associations between ankylosing spondylitis, psoriatic arthritis, Reiter's disease, the intestinal arthropathies and Behçet's syndrome. Medicine 53:343, 1974

RESNICK D et al: Diffuse idiopathic skeletal hyperostosis (DISH): Forestier's disease with extra spinal manifestations. Radiology 115:513, 1975

358

REITER'S SYNDROME, PSORIATIC ARTHRITIS, ARTHRITIS ASSOCIATED WITH GASTROINTESTINAL DISEASES, AND BEHÇET'S SYNDROME

BRUCE C. GILLILAND
MART MANNIK

REITER'S SYNDROME

Reiter's syndrome is characterized by arthritis, urethritis, conjunctivitis, and mucocutaneous lesions. The complete syndrome may not be present at any given time. The diagnosis should be entertained when arthritis is associated with any of the other manifestations. The HLA-B27 antigen is present in the majority of patients.

EPIDEMIOLOGY, PATHOGENESIS, AND PATHOLOGY Reiter's syndrome occurs most frequently in young men between the ages of 20 and 40 and is uncommon in women or children. In North America, many cases are closely related to sexual exposure. Reiter's syndrome may result from bacillary dysentery. An arthritis similar to Reiter's syndrome has followed *Yersinia, Salmonella,* and *Shigella* infections. The cause of Reiter's syndrome is unknown, and the pathogenesis of the syndrome has not been clarified. Reports that mycoplasma have been isolated from synovium have not been confirmed. More recently, *Chlamydia* have been implicated, but their role remains uncertain. Both T-strain mycoplasma and trachoma agents have been recovered from the urethra of patients with nongonococcal urethritis, in which they are considered to be of possible etiologic significance. However, most patients with nongonococcal urethritis do not develop Reiter's syndrome.

Histocompatibility typing has shown that HLA-B27 antigen is present in 70 to 96 percent of patients. This antigen may also be found in patients with incomplete forms of the syndrome. Patients who are positive for the HLA-B27 antigen usually have sacroiliitis and spine involvement. HLA-B27 is also found in 80 percent or more of patients developing arthritis associated with *Yersinia, Salmonella,* and *Shigella* infections.

Histologically, the cutaneous and mucosal lesions are very similar, even though their gross appearances are different. In the cutaneous lesions the epidermis shows hyperkeratosis, parakeratosis, and acanthosis. Spongiform pustules or microabscesses are present in the epidermis and are formed by focal infiltration of neutrophils, with degeneration of epithelial cells. The dermis shows edema, infiltration of lymphocytes, plasma cells, and neutrophils. The skin lesions are termed *keratodermia blenorrhagica* and are indistinguishable microscopically from those of pustular psoriasis. In the mucosal lesions, the inflammatory changes are similar, but keratinized cells do not accumulate. The synovium in the superficial vascular region shows edema, erythrocyte extravasation, and infiltration of neutrophils and lymphocytes. In synovitis of several months' duration, the synovium resembles that of rheumatoid arthritis, with villous hypertrophy, pannus formation over the articular cartilage, and infiltration of lymphocytes and plasma cells.

CLINICAL MANIFESTATIONS Reiter's syndrome often begins with urethritis after sexual exposure, followed in a few days to 4 weeks by conjunctivitis, mucocutaneous lesions, and arthritis. The onset of the arthritis is usually acute, affecting two or more joints. The joints are usually warm, erythematous, and painful. There is a predilection for joints of the lower extremities; ankles, knees, and metatarsophalangeal and proximal interphalangeal joints of the toes are commonly affected. Arthritis also occurs in the wrist, interphalangeal joints of the hand, costosternal joints, sacroiliac joints, and low part of the back, but is relatively uncommon in the hips and shoulders. Tenderness under the heel may be prominent because of periostitis at the insertion of the plantar fascia. Achilles tendonitis may also be present. The distribution of the arthritis tends to be asymmetrical and is extremely variable; multiple or single joints may be affected. The arthritis usually reaches a maximum within 2 weeks and begins to subside after 2 to 6 weeks. The duration is usually from 2 to 4 months, with a spontaneous remission occurring within the first year in the majority of patients. Some patients, however, may continue to have recurrent attacks of arthritis for several years; these flare-ups may be accompanied by one or more of the other clinical features of the syndrome. Recurrent attacks, similar to the first, may be precipitated by sexual exposure followed by urethritis. In patients with a self-limited course, little joint damage occurs, but with persistent or recurrent arthritis, flexion contractures and permanent joint damage may result.

Urethritis is characterized by a mucopurulent discharge and dysuria, but may be asymptomatic and may be overlooked unless the urethra is milked. The urethral meatus may be edematous and reddened, and urethral strictures may develop. Prostatitis and seminal vesiculitis occasionally occur, but epididymitis and orchitis are rare. Cystitis, which may be hemorrhagic, can occur and lead to urinary frequency, suprapubic pain, hematuria, and rarely to obstruction of the ureters. Since gonococcal urethritis may usher in the nonspecific urethritis of Reiter's syndrome, urethral smear and culture should be performed in all patients. When gonococcal urethritis is present, the purulent discharge will usually clear when penicillin is given, but will be replaced by the less purulent mucoid discharge of nonspecific urethritis.

Conjunctivitis is usually bilateral, mild, and evanescent, lasting only a few days. It may be present only at the lateral aspect of the tarsal conjunctiva. Conjunctivitis at times may be quite severe and produces burning, itching, and a profuse mucopurulent discharge, which may last several weeks. A nongranulomatous anterior uveitis which appears in some patients may lead to photophobia, glaucoma, cataracts, and even blindness. Subsequent attacks of anterior uveitis may appear in the absence of other clinical features of Reiter's syndrome. Painful superficial keratitis occurs occasionally.

Mucocutaneous lesions occur in over half the patients and appear most commonly on the glans penis, on the palms and soles, and in the mouth. They are typically painless and transient, and may go unnoticed unless the patient is examined carefully. On the glans penis, the lesion begins as a small vesicle, which evolves to a superficial reddened erosion with well-demarcated borders. In the circumcised male, the lesions may be covered with scales. Only a few lesions may be present on the glans penis, usually around the meatus, or lesions may completely circumscribe the glans (circinate balanitis). Lesions are occasionally found on the shaft and prepuce of the penis and on the scrotum. They also have been observed by endoscopy on the mucosa of the urethra and bladder. In the mouth, the lesions begin as small vesicles, papules, or plaques and later become superficial erosions with a surrounding area of erythema. The erosions may be covered by a thin grayish membrane. The mouth lesions are found on the soft palate, buccal mucosa, and the dorsum of the tongue. Keratodermia blenorrhagica describes the cutaneous lesions, which are found most commonly on the soles but are also occasionally observed on the palms, the extremities, and the trunk. These lesions begin as brownish-red macules, which develop into crusted scaling papules. Such lesions may coalesce to cover the sole with a thick layer of crusted scales, which peel off in the ensuing weeks. The nails may become thickened, opaque, and brittle; keratotic debris accumulates under the nail. None of the mucocutaneous lesions leaves residual scarring.

Cardiac conduction abnormalities and aortic regurgitation have been reported. The pathogenesis of the aortic valve incompetence is similar to that of ankylosing spondylitis, resulting from medial necrosis of the aortic root and dilatation of the aortic ring. Neurological abnormalities, including optic neuritis, meningoencephalitis, transient hemiplegia, psychotic reactions and peripheral neuropathy, are exceedingly rare.

LABORATORY FINDINGS A mild leukocytosis and an elevated erythrocyte sedimentation rate are often present. Tests for rheumatoid factor are negative. HLA-B27 antigen is found in the majority of patients. Synovial fluid examination shows an increase in white blood cells, predominantly neutrophils, ranging usually from 5000 to 20,000 cells per cubic millimeter. Large mononuclear cells, some containing ingested polymorphonuclear cells, are observed frequently but are not specific for Reiter's syndrome. The viscosity of the fluid may be reduced, and the mucin clot is fair to poor. The synovial fluid complement tends to be high, especially when compared with levels found in some patients with rheumatoid arthritis.

Radiographs of the involved joint may show only soft-tissue swelling. With recurrent disease, bony erosions and joint narrowing may appear. A suggestive, but not diagnostic, finding is periosteal new bone formation along the shaft adjacent to the involved joint and on the posterior and inferior aspects of the os calcis. Calcaneal spurs appear later. One or both sacroiliac joints may show irregularity, sclerosis, and fusion. With involvement of the spine, syndesmophytes may be observed and tend to be randomly distributed in the thoracic and lumbar parts of the spine. These syndesmophytes often arise at the upper or lower third of the vertebral body.

DIAGNOSIS The most important immediate differential diagnosis is gonococcal arthritis, because gonococcal urethritis may be present simultaneously. Gonococcal arthritis is confirmed by a positive synovial fluid culture but is not excluded by a negative one. The presence of conjunctivitis or characteristic

mucocutaneous lesions is helpful, since these are not associated with gonococcal arthritis. When there is doubt, the arthritis associated with gonococcal urethritis should be treated as gonococcal arthritis, with adequate doses of penicillin (Chap. 119). If Reiter's syndrome is present, the arthritis will persist, and other features of the syndrome may appear subsequently.

There is usually no problem differentiating Reiter's syndrome from rheumatoid arthritis. The sudden onset preceded by urethritis, the absence of nodules, negative rheumatoid factor, and the asymmetrical joint involvement contrast sharply with the insidious, symmetrical joint disease of rheumatoid arthritis.

Psoriatic arthritis and ankylosing spondylitis share several features of Reiter's syndrome. The pustular form of psoriasis is similar in appearance to keratodermia blenorrhagica but tends not to involve mucous membranes. Psoriatic arthritis may be differentiated from Reiter's syndrome by the more gradual onset of arthritis, the chronic nature of the skin lesions, the absence of urethritis and conjunctivitis, and the rarity of mucous membrane lesions. At times, however, differentiation of these two diseases may not be possible. Compared with ankylosing spondylitis, the spondylitis associated with Reiter's syndrome is usually less severe and progressive. Dilatation of the aortic ring, conduction abnormalities, calcaneal periostitis and spurs, and iritis occur in both Reiter's syndrome and ankylosing spondylitis. The sudden onset of the peripheral arthritis associated with urethritis and conjunctivitis and typical mucocutaneous lesions help to distinguish Reiter's syndrome. Hip involvement is rare in Reiter's syndrome and common in ankylosing spondylitis.

TREATMENT The treatment of the nongonococcal urethritis with 2 g tetracycline per day for 10 to 14 days may affect the urethritis but probably has no effect on the arthritis. No treatment is necessary for conjunctivitis and other mucocutaneous lesions; however, iritis may require intraocular corticosteroid therapy. The arthritis is usually responsive to phenylbutazone or indomethacin. With phenylbutazone, a loading dose of 600 to 800 mg is given initially to obtain a rapid therapeutic blood level, followed by a daily maintenance dose of 200 to 300 mg. The dose of indomethacin is 100 to 150 mg per day. Salicylates or one of the newer nonsteroidal anti-inflammatory drugs may be effective in some patients. Corticosteroids are rarely indicated. The same is true of immunosuppressive drugs.

PSORIATIC ARTHRITIS

The prevalence of arthritis in patients with psoriasis is higher than that found in the general population, even when degenerative joint disease and rheumatoid arthritis are excluded. Arthritis related to psoriasis occurs in approximately 5 percent of patients with skin disease.

The *etiology* and *pathogenesis* of psoriatic arthritis are not known; however, studies showing aggregation of psoriatic arthritis in first-degree relatives of psoriatic patients suggest that hereditary factors may play a role. A significant association between the HLA-B27 antigen and psoriatic arthritis has been found in those patients with sacroiliitis and spondylitis. Greater than 90 percent of psoriatic patients with spondylitis have the HLA-B27 antigen. In patients with only sacroiliitis, approximately 40 percent are positive for HLA-B27, while in those with only peripheral arthritis less than 20 percent have this antigen.

The age of onset is similar to that of rheumatoid arthritis, and the sex distribution slightly favors women. Psoriasis usually precedes the onset of arthritis by months or years; however, the onset of both may coincide or, very uncommonly, arthritis may precede psoriasis. In general, the prognosis of chronic psoriatic arthritis is more favorable than that of rheumatoid arthritis, except in patients with severe destructive arthritis (arthritis mutilans).

On the basis of the pattern of joint involvement five clinical groups may be distinguished. The first group which includes approximately 70 percent of patients with psoriatic arthritis has monarticular or asymmetrical oligoarticular arthritis involving scattered small joints of the hands and feet. "Sausage" digits are often present and result from inflammation of the interphalangeal joint along with an effusion of the flexor tendon sheath. A second group composed of about 15 percent of patients has a seronegative symmetrical polyarthritis similar to rheumatoid arthritis. In addition to this group, there are patients with psoriasis, symmetrical polyarthritis, and a positive test for rheumatoid factor. These patients are considered to have coexistent rheumatoid arthritis and psoriasis. A third group has predominantly distal interphalangeal joint involvement. The adjacent nail often has changes of psoriasis. Another small group of patients has severe destructive polyarthritis referred to as *arthritis mutilans*. Sacroiliitis is often present. The last group has spondylitis with or without peripheral joint involvement. The clinical features of spine involvement are similar to idiopathic ankylosing spondylitis.

The peripheral joints in psoriatic arthritis are warm, swollen, and tender, and show synovial proliferation. Flexion contractures and ankylosis of joints may occur, with long periods of persistent joint inflammation. No definite correlation exists between the degree of skin involvement and joint disease, but in some patients the activity of both tends to be parallel. A closer temporal relationship has been found between psoriatic nail lesions and arthritis than between the skin lesions and arthritis.

Laboratory abnormalities include hypoproliferative anemia and an elevated erythrocyte sedimentation rate, which are nonspecific findings. Tests for rheumatoid factor are negative. Hyperuricemia is observed in 10 to 20 percent of patients, similar to uncomplicated psoriasis. Synovial fluid and biopsy findings are those of nonspecific inflammation.

Several *radiographic* features are characteristic of psoriatic arthritis. These include severe destruction of isolated joints, osteolysis, bony ankylosis, whittling of bone at the distal end of terminal phalanges, and the "pencil-in-cup" deformity, which is most commonly observed in the joints of the fingers and toes. Resorption of the distal end of the bone produces the "pencil" which projects into a widened, cuplike erosion in the adjacent joint surface. The radiographic findings in spondylitis associated with psoriatic arthritis are similar to those found in spondylitis with Reiter's syndrome.

The *diagnosis* of psoriatic arthritis is suggested by the presence of an inflammatory arthritis in a patient with typical skin or nail lesions of psoriasis. Skin lesions may be quite small and hidden in the scalp, intergluteal fold, or umbilicus. The asymmetry of joint involvement, negative test for rheumatoid factor, and the absence of rheumatoid nodules help to distinguish psoriatic arthritis from rheumatoid arthritis. The differentiation of psoriatic arthritis from Reiter's syndrome and ankylosing spondylitis has been discussed under "Reiter's Syndrome" above. Psoriatic arthritis presenting as an acute arthritis, especially in a toe or finger, may be mistaken for gouty arthritis. In addition, hyperuricemia, which may occur in association with psoriasis, may also be present. The appearance of the joint also may suggest septic arthritis. These diagnostic considerations are easily excluded by examining synovial fluid for sodium urate crystals and for microorganisms with appropriate cultures.

The *treatment* of the arthritis is similar to that outlined for rheumatoid arthritis except for the use of antimalarials. These drugs are contraindicated because they may produce an exfoliative dermatitis in patients with psoriasis. The value of gold has not been established. The use of immunosuppressive

1885

CHAPTER 358
REITER'S SYNDROME, PSORIATIC ARTHRITIS, ARTHRITIS ASSOCIATED WITH GASTROINTESTINAL DISEASES, AND BEHÇET'S SYNDROME

agents may be beneficial; methotrexate has been used most extensively. However, in view of their toxicity, these drugs should be restricted to patients with severe psoriasis and destructive polyarthritis. Adequate control of skin disease may lead to improvement of the joint disease in an occasional patient.

ARTHRITIS ASSOCIATED WITH GASTROINTESTINAL DISEASES

ULCERATIVE COLITIS Arthritis is the most common nonintestinal manifestation of ulcerative colitis; it occurs in approximately 20 percent of patients. Two patterns of joint involvement may be distinguished in patients with arthritis of ulcerative colitis: arthritis of peripheral joints (colitic arthritis), which occurs in 75 percent of patients, and spondylitis, which occurs in 25 percent of patients with musculoskeletal complaints.

The peripheral arthritis of ulcerative colitis most commonly begins between the ages of 25 and 45 years and affects both sexes equally. Arthritis usually follows the onset of colitis by 6 months to several years, but rarely the onset of both may coincide or the arthritis may precede colitis. Patients with recurrent mouth ulcers, uveitis, pyoderma gangrenosum, and erythema nodosum are likely to have peripheral acute arthritis. When erythema nodosum is present, there is uncertainty whether to attribute the arthritis to that often associated with idiopathic erythema nodosum or to that associated with colitis.

The typical attack of arthritis presents acutely, often affecting a single joint in the lower extremity. Involvement of other joints, without definite symmetry, may follow over the next few days. The involved joint is usually red, swollen, and painful. The knee and ankle are most frequently affected, followed by the proximal interphalangeal, elbow, shoulder, and wrist joints. The arthritis usually subsides within several weeks, but occasionally lasts for months. Complete resolution without residual damage is the general rule. Recurrent attacks of arthritis tend to occur with flare-ups of colitis and occasionally may herald an impending exacerbation of colitis. Peripheral arthritis usually subsides following colectomy.

Spondylitis with ulcerative colitis is indistinguishable from ankylosing spondylitis. However, the usual male preponderance observed in ankylosing spondylitis is not seen in patients with ulcerative colitis and spondylitis. In addition, uveitis and erythema nodosum are rare with the spondylitis that accompanies ulcerative colitis. The onset of spondylitis more often precedes the colitis than does peripheral arthritis, and spondylitis tends to progress regardless of colectomy or remission of intestinal disease. The disease may progress to complete ankylosis of the spine.

The peripheral white blood cell count, anemia, and elevated erythrocyte sedimentation rate usually reflect the intestinal disease. Tests for rheumatoid factor are negative. Synovial fluid shows a moderate leukocytosis, in the range of 10,000 cells per cubic millimeter, consisting predominantly of polymorphonuclear leukocytes.

Radiographs of involved peripheral joints usually are normal except for soft-tissue swelling. An occasional patient with recurrent or persistent disease will show small bony erosions and joint space narrowing. Films of the spine show changes indistinguishable from those of ankylosing spondylitis.

Treatment with salicylates, phenylbutazone, or a new nonsteroidal anti-inflammatory drug is of benefit in reducing symptoms. Physical therapy is directed toward maintenance of posture in spondylitis and prevention of contractures in the peripheral form of arthritis. Colectomy or systemic steroids are not indicated for treatment of the arthritis alone.

REGIONAL ENTERITIS Peripheral arthritis or spondylitis similar to that of ulcerative colitis is found in approximately 5 to 10 percent of patients with regional enteritis. Nonspecific musculoskeletal complaints without objective arthritis are common. Arthritis is more common in patients with ileocolitis, and the peripheral arthritis tends to follow the activity of the intestinal disease. The arthritis comes on acutely, tends to be migratory, and most commonly affects the knees. With involvement of numerous small joints of the hand, especially the proximal interphalangeal joints, it may be confused initially with rheumatoid arthritis. The peripheral joint disease is mild, subsiding in a few weeks without joint damage. The spondylitis is identical to that of ulcerative colitis. The management of the arthritis is the same as in ulcerative colitis.

HLA-B27 antigen is found in approximately 75 percent of patients with spondyloarthritides associated with inflammatory bowel disease due to either ulcerative colitis or regional enteritis. The prevalence of this antigen is not increased in those patients with only peripheral arthritis.

WHIPPLE'S DISEASE Whipple's disease (intestinal lipodystrophy) is a rare disorder affecting predominantly middle-aged males and is characterized by arthritis, serositis, diarrhea, malabsorption, weight loss, and lymphadenopathy. The diagnosis is confirmed by the identification of periodic acid–Schiff positive bacilliform structures intercellularly or as inclusions in foamy macrophages. These bacilli can be seen in the mucosa and lamina propria of the small intestine, in abdominal and peripheral lymph nodes, and in other tissues.

Arthritis occurs in approximately two-thirds of the patients and usually precedes the appearance of intestinal symptoms by months or years, making the diagnosis of the arthritis difficult. With the onset of intestinal symptoms, the arthritis may subside. The joint disease involves predominantly peripheral joints, affecting knees and ankles most commonly, followed by fingers, hips, shoulders, elbows, and wrists. It is typically acute, migratory, and transient, lasts only a few days, and causes no permanent joint damage. Long irregular periods of remission are common. Some patients with peripheral joint involvement have radiographic changes in the sacroiliac joints similar to those of ankylosing spondylitis. Synovial fluid shows only a mild monocytosis without characteristic foamy macrophages. This disease, including the joint manifestations, responds well to therapy with penicillin, 1.2 million units, and streptomycin, 1 g daily for 2 weeks, followed by tetracycline, 1 g daily for 1 year. Relapse while on tetracycline requires administration again of penicillin and streptomycin. Corticosteroids may be necessary in addition to antimicrobials in severely ill patients but are not indicated for the treatment of arthritis alone. Salicylates or phenylbutazone may be helpful in controlling joint symptoms.

BEHÇET'S SYNDROME

Recurrent oral and genital ulcers and eye inflammation characterize Behçet's syndrome. Other manifestations include arthritis, thrombophlebitis, neurological abnormalities, and skin lesions. One or several clinical features may be present at any given time. The peak onset of the disease is in the third decade, but it may occur at any age. Men are affected more often than women. The etiology of this disease is not known.

EPIDEMIOLOGY Behçet's syndrome is found throughout the world with the greatest number of patients being reported from the Middle East and Japan. The prevalence of disease is unknown, but based on a study from Japan, the frequency is in the range of 1 patient per 10,000 persons. A prevalence of 0.64 per 100,000 was found in the County of Yorkshire, England, which has a population of 5 million. Familial aggregation has been observed; however, hereditary factors have not been identified.

PATHOLOGY The predominant histopathologic lesion is vasculitis which affects mainly small to medium-size arteries and veins. The blood vessel walls and perivascular tissues are infiltrated predominantly by lymphocytes. Monocytes, plasma cells, and neutrophils may also be present. Swelling and proliferation of endothelial cells are observed. The lumen of the vessel may be narrowed or obliterated. Fibrinoid necrosis and disruption of the vessel wall may be seen.

In patients with active synovitis, the synovium shows hypercellularity consisting of neutrophils and, to a lesser degree, plasma cells. Arterioles have perivascular infiltration of lymphocytes.

CLINICAL MANIFESTATIONS Oral ulcers are usually the first manifestation and develop in nearly all patients with Behçet's syndrome. These painful ulcers, measuring 2 to 10 mm in diameter, have a central yellowish necrotic base, surrounded by erythema. Their appearance is similar to aphthous ulcers. Herpetiform ulcers also may be present and occur more frequently in women. They may occur as a single lesion or in crops and involve the lips, tongue, gingiva, buccal mucosa, pharynx, and rarely the larynx and nasal mucosa. These ulcers persist for several days to several weeks and heal without scarring.

Genital ulcers are also found in the majority of patients, on the scrotum and rarely on the penis. In females, lesions occur on the labia, vulva, and vaginal wall. Lesions in the vagina may not be painful and may go unnoticed unless a pelvic examination is performed. Perineal lesions are seen in both sexes. Epididymitis occurs infrequently. The course of genital ulcers is similar to that of the oral ulcers.

Recurrent ocular inflammation is another common feature of this syndrome, manifested by anterior uveitis with hypopyon, conjunctivitis, posterior uveitis, optic neuritis, retinal arteritis, or retinal vein occlusion. Eye lesions may be reversible; however, cataracts, glaucoma, and blindness may ensue.

Arthritis or arthralgias occur in approximately 50 percent of patients and may precede, accompany, or follow other manifestations of Behçet's syndrome. The arthritis is usually asymmetrical and polyarticular, and involves most often large joints such as knees, ankles, and elbows. In a few patients, only a single large joint is involved. Small joints can also be affected. Arthritis tends to occur with other features of Behçet's syndrome, especially with erythema nodosum. The majority of patients experience multiple recurrent episodes of acute inflammatory arthritis, not unlike arthropathy associated with inflammatory bowel disease. In a few patients the arthritis may become chronic. Residual joint damage seldom results even after several years of recurrent arthritis. Sacroiliitis and spondylitis may occasionally be found.

Recurrent and migratory superficial or deep thrombophlebitis is observed in about 25 percent of patients. The lower extremities are most often involved. Pulmonary embolization is an infrequent complication. Thrombosis of the superior or inferior vena cava or rarely of both may develop. Phlebitis may appear at the site of venipuncture.

Involvement of arteries may lead to aneurysms and thrombosis of the aorta, ulnar, femoral, and popliteal arteries. Gangrene of the feet may result from thrombosis of arteries in the lower extremities. Thrombosis of pulmonary arteries can also occur.

Central nervous system involvement is present in approxi-

1887

CHAPTER 358
REITER'S SYNDROME, PSORIATIC ARTHRITIS, ARTHRITIS ASSOCIATED WITH
GASTROINTESTINAL DISEASES, AND BEHÇET'S SYNDROME

mately 25 percent of patients, tends to appear later in the course of the disease, and is characterized by exacerbations and remissions. The central nervous system abnormalities include meningoencephalitis, benign intracranial hypertension with papilledema, brainstem lesions, cranial nerve palsies, spinal cord lesions, and psychosis. Hemiparesis and quadriparesis have been observed. Peripheral neuropathies are infrequent. Death may result from central nervous system involvement.

Skin lesions are found in the majority of patients and take a variety of forms. These include erythematous papules, vesicles, pustules, pyoderma, and erythema nodosum. Clusters of the erythema nodosum lesions may appear on the lower extremities, as well as on the upper extremities. Ulceration of these lesions may occur.

A physical finding that is almost a diagnostic feature of Behçet's syndrome is the appearance after 24 h of a pustule surrounded by erythema at the site of a needle puncture. This sign, however, does not develop in all patients.

Colitis, indistinguishable from idiopathic ulcerative colitis, is present in a few patients with Behçet's syndrome. The colonic ulcers in the early inflammatory bowel disease, however, are separated by normal mucosa. Other gastrointestinal manifestations include nausea, diarrhea, abdominal distention, proctitis, and perianal ulcers.

Fever in the range of 38 to 39°C is present during exacerbations and usually reflects the severity of the clinical state. The clinical course of Behçet's syndrome is highly variable, as are the combinations of features that may be present at any given time. Mucocutaneous lesions usually appear with each exacerbation. Disease-free intervals may be measured in weeks, months, or even years. Mortality is especially high in patients with central nervous system involvement.

LABORATORY FINDINGS Anemia, elevated erythrocyte sedimentation rate, and mild leukocytosis are often present during active disease. A polyclonal increase of gamma globulin may be present, and elevated levels of IgA and IgM may be found. Serum complement levels are normal. Coagulation studies may reveal elevated levels of fibrinogen and factor VIII. In addition, a decrease in plasma fibrinolytic activity is found in some patients.

In patients with central nervous system involvement, the cerebrospinal fluid shows a mild pleocytosis consisting of mononuclear cells and an increase in protein.

Synovial fluid from patients with acute arthritis shows white blood cell counts of 20,000 per cubic millimeter or greater, consisting predominantly of neutrophils. Joint fluid complement levels are normal or increased. In chronic, mild arthritis, the fluid is clear and contains few mononuclear white blood cells.

Antibodies reacting with saline extracts of fetal oral mucosal cells have been demonstrated by hemagglutination methods in serum of patients with Behçet's syndrome. Immunofluorescent studies have also revealed antibodies reacting with cytoplasm of normal human esophageal cells. However, similar antibodies have been found in the serum of patients with only aphthous ulcers. Cell-mediated immunity to mucosal-cell antigens has been shown by the transformation of patients' lymphocytes when stimulated with mucosal cell extracts. These immunologic studies should be extended to confirm the role of immunity in the pathogenesis of this disorder.

DIAGNOSIS The diagnosis of Behçet's syndrome is readily made when the triad of oral ulcers, genital ulcers, and eye inflammation is present. Since other features such as central nervous system involvement, thrombophlebitis, and arthritis occur frequently in this syndrome, their presence along with oral ulcers, genital ulcers, or eye inflammation should raise the possibility of Behçet's syndrome.

Reiter's and Behçet's syndromes have several clinical features in common. Both have an acute asymmetrical polyarthritis, mucocutaneous lesions, eye inflammation, and neurological abnormalities. In Reiter's syndrome, however, the orogenital lesions are usually not painful, thrombophlebitis is not a common feature, central nervous system manifestations are unusual, and the eye involvement consists mainly of conjunctivitis and less often anterior uveitis. The presence of spondylitis supports the diagnosis of Reiter's syndrome.

Painful oral ulcers also occur in the Stevens-Johnson syndrome. The absence of other features of Behçet's syndrome eventually distinguishes these diseases. Likewise, in patients with recurrent benign aphthous ulcers Behçet's syndrome is excluded by the absence of other manifestations. Patients with ulcerative colitis may have recurrent aphthous ulcers, iritis, arthritis, and erythema nodosum, and this may be confused with Behçet's syndrome with colitis. The colitis of Behçet's syndrome is characterized by the finding of discrete colonic ulcers separated by normal-appearing mucosa. In ulcerative colitis, genital ulcers are not seen, the posterior segment of the eye is not involved, and the aphthous ulcers are usually not as severe.

TREATMENT No effective form of therapy is available. Any form of treatment is difficult to assess because of the variable natural course of this disease. Prednisone in doses of 40 to 60 mg per day may improve some patients, and local application of steroids to the oral ulcers may be useful. Viscous xylocaine mouthwash helps to reduce pain. Immunosuppressive drugs including azathioprine, cyclophosphamide, and chlorambucil have been administered to some patients with favorable results.

Since some patients with Behçet's syndrome have decreased plasma fibrinolytic activity, drugs such as phenformin and ethylestrenol, which promote fibrinolysis, have been used in patients with thrombophlebitis. With this type of treatment some patients improved, while others deteriorated. Finally, a few patients have improved after the administration of transfer factor, prepared from normal donors. The basis of these therapeutic observations is not explained, and these forms of treatment remain entirely experimental and must be thoroughly evaluated prior to general acceptance.

REFERENCES

CHAJEK T, FAINARU M: Behçet's disease. A report of 41 cases and a review of the literature. Medicine 54:179, 1975

GOOD AE: Reiter's disease: A review with special attention to cardiovascular and neurologic sequelae. Semin Arthritis Rheum 3:253, 1974

LeVINE ME, DOBBINS WO III: Joint changes in Whipple's disease. Semin Arthritis Rheum 3:79, 1973

McEWEN C et al: Ankylosing spondylitis and spondylitis accompanying ulcerative colitis, regional enteritis, psoriasis and Reiter's disease. Arthritis Rheum 14:291, 1971

MOLL JMH, WRIGHT V: Psoriatic arthritis. Semin Arthritis Rheum 3:55, 1973

MORRIS RI et al: HL-A27—a useful discriminator in the arthropathies of inflammatory bowel disease. N Engl J Med 290:1117, 1974

PALUMBO PJ et al: Musculoskeletal manifestations of inflammatory bowel disease: Ulcerative and granulomatous colitis and ulcerative proctitis. Mayo Clin Proc 48:411, 1973

VERNON-ROBERTS B et al: Synovial pathology in Behçet's syndrome. Ann Rheum Dis 37:139, 1978

WRIGHT VA, CHAMBERLAIN MA: Behçet's syndrome. Bull Rheum Dis 29:972, 1978

359

PSEUDOGOUT

BRUCE C. GILLILAND
MART MANNIK

GOUT See Chap. 92.

PSEUDOGOUT Pseudogout is an inflammatory arthritis of older individuals, caused by calcium pyrophosphate dihydrate crystals in the joint. It is characteristically accompanied by the radiographic finding of calcification of articular cartilages. The knee and other large joints are the most frequent sites of involvement. The mechanism for deposition of crystals in articular cartilage (chondrocalcinosis) is unknown.

The disease usually occurs in persons over age 50, and its prevalence increases with age. Both sexes are affected. Approximately one patient with pseudogout is observed for every two patients with gout. Familial chondrocalcinosis has been described in two different patterns. One genetic form of this disease affects young adults and is characterized by rapid and progressive involvement of several joints. Another form of the disease is oligoarticular and occurs in older persons.

Levels of inorganic pyrophosphate are elevated in the synovial fluid of many patients, but this finding also is seen in some patients with osteoarthritis without chondrocalcinosis. Furthermore, the concentrations of pyrophosphate and calcium ions do not exceed their solubility product. Hence, it is unlikely that the crystals actively form within synovial fluid, but are thought to be shed from the cartilage.

Chondrocalcinosis has been found in association with metabolic diseases and other disorders, including diabetes mellitus, hypothyroidism, gout, hyperparathyroidism, pernicious anemia, hemochromatosis, ochronosis, Wilson's disease, and acromegaly. The relationship of these disorders to the pathogenesis of chondrocalcinosis is unknown. Furthermore, the association of some of these disorders with chondrocalcinosis may not be greater than with osteoarthritis alone.

The *pathological changes* in the joint involve deposits of calcium pyrophosphate dihydrate crystals in the joint capsule, in the midzonal area of articular hyaline cartilage, and diffusely in fibrocartilage. The menisci of the knee are a common site of crystal deposition. Crystals can be seen at the margin of degenerating cartilage and surrounding the lacunae of chondrocytes; this site is considered the earliest detectable lesion. The deposition of crystals varies from microcrystalline aggregates to large masses intermixed with fibrous tissue. Crystals may also be observed in normal-appearing cartilage.

The synovium in acute arthritis is edematous, with numerous polymorphonuclear leukocytes. Crystals are seen in the superficial portion of the synovium. In chronic arthritis, mononuclear cell infiltration and fibroblastic proliferation are present; crystals are rarely observed.

Acute arthritis can be induced experimentally by the injection of calcium pyrophosphate dihydrate crystals into the normal joint. In pseudogout, arthritis is thought to be initiated by the release of crystals from cartilage into the joint cavity, resulting in the activation of vasoactive and chemotactic factors. Polymorphonuclear leukocytes are attracted into the joint and phagocytize the crystals, leading to the release of lysosomal enzymes into the joint fluid.

Several patterns of joint involvement are recognized in calcium pyrophosphate deposition disease. Acute attacks occur in approximately 25 percent of patients, and this clinical picture is commonly called *pseudogout.* The onset of the acute attack of pseudogout is rapid and reaches a peak usually in 12 to 36 h. The involved joint is erythematous, swollen, warm, and painful. The acute attack is usually confined to a single joint, but in some patients involvement of other joints may follow in rapid progression. The knee is by far the most frequent site of acute arthritis, but attacks occur in the ankles, wrists, elbows, hips, and cervical and lumbar spine. As in gout, the metatarsal joint of the great toe may be a site of involvement. Furthermore, attacks may be provoked by trauma, surgery, or medical illness. The acute arthritis is usually intermittent, and the same joint is often involved in subsequent attacks. The acute episode usually subsides in 1 to 2 weeks. Between attacks the involved joint appears relatively normal. Most patients have radiographic evidence of chondrocalcinosis.

Approximately 5 percent of patients with calcium pyrophosphate deposition disease have what is termed *pseudorheumatoid disease,* which is characterized by multiple joint involvement with subacute attacks lasting several weeks to several months. The attacks affect one or several joints, then move on to involve other joints. Patients may complain of morning stiffness and fatigue. Synovial proliferation, limitation of joint motion, and flexion deformities can develop.

Another group, predominantly women and representing half the patients with calcium pyrophosphate deposition disease, has a chronic form of the disease, referred to as *pseudoosteoarthritis.* Progressive degenerative joint changes occur in multiple joints. The knees are the most frequently involved, followed by the wrists, metacarpophalangeal joints, hips, shoulders, elbows, and ankles. The joint involvement is usually symmetrical, and flexion contractures may develop. Approximately one-half of the patients with this form of the disease experience intermittent acute attacks. Finally, another group of patients has typical articular chondrocalcinosis without any symptoms.

The microscopic examination of *synovial fluid* in an acute attack shows large numbers of polymorphonuclear leukocytes. Calcium pyrophosphate dihydrate crystals are frequently found extracellularly and in polymorphonuclear leukocytes. In chronic arthritis, the crystals are observed less frequently and are most often extracellular. With polarized light, the crystals appear as short blunt rods, rhomboids, and cuboids. They have weakly positive birefringence under compensated polarized light, in contrast to the strongly negative birefringence of sodium urate crystals. The diagnosis is made by finding typical crystals under compensated polarized light and is supported by radiographic evidence of chondrocalcinosis.

Radiographically, calcifications in articular hyaline cartilage appear as fine linear densities parallel to the subchondral bone surface. In the knee, this line is best observed on a lateral film. Calcifications in fibrocartilage, ligaments, and joint capsule usually appear as more diffuse punctate and linear densities. Common sites of fibrocartilage involvement include the menisci of the knee, articular disk of the distal radioulnar joint, symphysis pubis, and the annulus fibrosus of the intervertebral disk. Evidence for chondrocalcinosis can usually be obtained with radiographs of the knees, wrists, and pelvis. Radiographic findings of osteoarthritis are also present, particularly in patients with chronic pseudogout.

Gout and septic arthritis are the main considerations in the *differential diagnosis* of the acute arthritis. Gout and pseudogout are frequently indistinguishable clinically, and the diagnosis depends on the identification of their characteristic crystals under compensated polarized light. Both crystals occasionally have been found together in the synovial fluid of patients with typical radiographic articular calcifications of chondrocalcinosis. Bacterial smears and cultures should be performed on synovial fluid in all patients with an acute monarticular arthritis. The symptoms of osteoarthritis and chronic pseudogout are very similar, and radiographic evidence for both is often present. The role played by each is difficult to determine. Pseudogout should be considered when intermittent attacks of acute arthritis occur. The finding of a chronic effusion in patients with symptoms of osteoarthritis also suggests the possibility of pseudogout. The diagnosis should not be made only on the radiographic findings of intraarticular calcific deposits, but depends also on the identification of the characteristic crystals, since other forms of inflammatory arthritis may affect the same joints. Attacks of pseudogout occur in patients without radiographic evidence of chondrocalcinosis, thus requiring a careful search for calcium pyrophosphate dihydrate crystals in any case of acute arthritis, especially in older patients. On the other hand, radiographic evidence of calcific deposits is found not infrequently in knees of elderly patients who have no joint symptoms.

For the *treatment* of acute pseudogout, phenylbutazone is usually effective. A loading dose of 600 mg is given, followed by 200 to 300 mg per day until symptoms subside. Indomethacin, 75 to 150 mg per day, may also be used. Relief is sometimes achieved with aspiration of the synovial fluid. Results of treatment with colchicine are variable. In chronic arthritis, salicylates may give symptomatic relief. The deposition of calcium pyrophosphate crystals in articular tissues cannot be prevented or reversed.

REFERENCES

McCarty DJ Jr (ed): Pseudogout and pyrophosphate metabolism. Arthritis Rheum 19:275, 1976

Utsinger PD et al: Calcium pyrophosphate dehydrate deposition disease without chondrocalcinosis. J Rheum 2:258, 1975

360
OSTEOMYELITIS AND INFECTIOUS ARTHRITIS

JAN V. HIRSCHMANN
BRUCE C. GILLILAND

OSTEOMYELITIS

DEFINITION *Osteomyelitis* denotes infection of bone. While many types of microorganisms, including viruses and fungi, may cause osteomyelitis, it is usually bacterial in origin.

PATHOGENESIS Organisms reach the bone to cause infection by one of three routes: (1) hematogenous spread, (2) extension from a contiguous site of infection, and (3) direct introduction of organisms into bone by trauma, including surgery.

Acute hematogenous osteomyelitis usually involves bone with rich, red marrow; in children the long bones, especially the femur and tibia, are most frequently affected. The infection begins in the metaphyseal sinusoidal veins, where sluggish blood flow and a paucity of phagocytes favor the growth of organisms. In adults acute hematogenous infection rarely involves the long bones, where adipose tissue has largely replaced the red marrow. Instead, hematogenous osteomyelitis most commonly occurs in the vertebrae, where cellular marrow and an abundant vascular supply exist. The organisms reach the spine directly through the nutrient branches of the posterior spinal artery or, probably less commonly, from retrograde flow through the valveless paravertebral venous plexus of Batson, which drains the vertebral bodies, body wall, and the pelvis. Infection usually begins in the vertebral body near the anterior longitudinal ligament and may spread to adjacent vertebrae by direct extension through the disk space or by a system of freely communicating venous channels. Because the disk in adults possesses no vascular supply, disk space infection in *hematogenous* infections is always secondary to osteomyelitis in an adjacent vertebra.

Osteomyelitis caused by extension from a contiguous site of infection may occur with soft-tissue suppuration resulting from trauma, necrosis of a malignant tumor, radiation therapy, burns, or other causes. In patients with vascular insufficiency from diabetes mellitus or atherosclerosis, organisms commonly enter the soft tissues through a cutaneous ulcer, usually in the foot, causing cellulitis and subsequently osteomyelitis. Osteomyelitis of the skull bones may result from underlying sinus or dental infections.

Direct introduction of organisms into bone may occur with open fractures, the open surgical reduction of closed fractures, or penetrating trauma by bullets or other foreign bodies. Osteomyelitis may also follow insertion of prostheses or other surgical procedures for nontraumatic bone or joint disorders.

PATHOLOGY Pathological findings during the acute phase include neutrophilic inflammation, edema, and vascular congestion. Because of the bone's rigidity, increased intramedullary pressure develops, compromising the blood supply and causing ischemia, cell death, and vascular thrombosis. After several days, the suppurative and ischemic injury may cause the bone to fragment into devitalized segments called *sequestra*. The inflammation spreads via the haversian and Volkmann canals to reach the periosteum, beneath which abscesses may form or through which the purulent material may penetrate to form soft-tissue abscesses or sinus tracts.

With persistent infection, chronic inflammatory cells—lymphocytes, histiocytes, and plasma cells—may join the neutrophils. Fibroblastic proliferation and new bone formation also occur. Osteogenesis from the periosteum may surround the inflammation to form a bony envelope or *involucrum*. Occasionally, a dense fibrous capsule confines the infection to a localized area of suppuration, called *Brodie's abscess*. Rarely, exuberant osteogenesis may result in a sclerotic, nonpurulent osteomyelitis (Garré's sclerosing osteomyelitis).

MANIFESTATIONS **Hematogenous osteomyelitis** The bacteremia causing hematogenous osteomyelitis may be from a urinary infection, bacterial endocarditis, a distant soft-tissue infection, or another location. Frequently, the original site is not apparent. Heroin addicts and patients on hemodialysis seem especially at risk because of frequent bacteremias.

Vertebral osteomyelitis may occasionally begin abruptly with back pain and systemic signs of infection, but usually the onset is insidious and the course gradually progressive. Persistent back pain, exacerbated by movement and commonly unrelieved by heat, analgesics, or bed rest, is the predominant symptom. Fever is usually minimal or absent. Physical examination typically reveals tenderness to percussion and palpation over the affected vertebrae, guarding and splinting on movement, and paravertebral muscle spasm.

Leukocytosis is usually absent, but the erythrocyte sedimentation rate is almost always increased. The earliest roentgenographic changes are erosion of the subchondral bony plate, narrowing of the intervertebral disk space, and involvement of the adjacent vertebra. Bony destruction follows, sometimes with loss of vertebral height, usually anteriorly. Anterior osteogenesis with coarse bony density and sclerosis may occur. Soft-tissue densities, representing paravertebral abscesses, may lie adjacent to the vertebrae. The lumbar vertebrae are most frequently involved, the cervical vertebrae least. While roentgenographic changes may not develop for several weeks following infection, radionuclide scans with technetium pyrophosphate are positive early.

Complications of vertebral osteomyelitis include anterior extension to cause retropharyngeal abscesses, mediastinitis, empyema, pericarditis, subdiaphragmatic abscess, psoas muscle abscess or peritonitis, depending upon the vertebrae involved. Posterior extension by pus (epidural abscess), bony fragments, or inflammatory tissue can cause spinal cord compression; if infection penetrates the dura to enter the subarachnoid space, meningitis results.

Acute hematogenous osteomyelitis occurring in sites other than the vertebrae is unusual in adults. When it does develop in such locations as the clavicle or the long bones of the extremities, its typical features are pain and evidence of soft-tissue infection over the affected bone.

Hematogenous osteomyelitis acquired in childhood may present in adults as intermittent or persistent drainage from sinus tracts communicating with the involved bone—usually the femur, tibia, or humerus—or as a soft-tissue infection overlying it. Signs of infection may recur after months or years of quiescence. Roentgenographic changes include bony destruction with radiolucent areas, radiopaque sequestra, and formation of an involucrum. A roentgenogram of contrast material injected into a sinus tract (sinogram) may help define the location and extent of involvement.

Posttraumatic osteomyelitis and osteomyelitis from a contiguous infection The clinical features of these forms of osteomyelitis are a varying combination of local pain, draining sinuses, and heat, swelling, tenderness, and erythema over the involved bone. Patients often are afebrile. Persistent pain and loosening of the appliance may be the major manifestations in those with infected orthopedic prostheses. Leukocytosis and an elevated erythrocyte sedimentation rate are present in a minority of patients. Radiographic changes are similar to those in chronic hematogenous osteomyelitis. With plates, nails, screws, pins, or prostheses there is frequently evidence of loosening of the appliance. Radionuclide scans with technetium pyrophosphate are nearly always positive. Since increased uptake in these scans depends in part on bone hyperemia, which may occur with adjacent inflammation alone, there may be difficulty in distinguishing early osteomyelitis from cellulitis or a subcutaneous abscess when the roentgenograms do not show bony destruction.

DIAGNOSIS While radiographic or radionuclide studies may be helpful, definitive diagnosis requires isolation of the responsible organism. If blood cultures are negative (they usually are), patients with suspected vertebral osteomyelitis should undergo needle aspiration of the intervertebral disk space, if it appears infected, percutaneous needle biopsy of the infected bone, or open bone biopsy at surgery. Although *Staphylococcus aureus* is the most common cause, aerobic gram-negative bacilli, typically arising from a previous or concurrent urinary infection, are also frequent. Moreover, pyogenic vertebral osteomyelitis is often impossible to differentiate from tuberculous or fungal vertebral osteomyelitis.

In patients with chronic hematogenous osteomyelitis, posttraumatic osteomyelitis, or osteomyelitis from a contiguous infection, the diagnosis is best established by careful cultures, both aerobic and anaerobic, of bone, tissue, or pus from a deep abscess obtained during surgery. These infections are often polymicrobial and sometimes include anaerobic bacteria; precise bacteriologic identification is necessary for appropriate antimicrobial therapy. Cultures of material obtained from draining sinuses are generally unreliable, even if only a single organism grows, because the tracts may become colonized by bacteria present on the skin surface but absent in the infected bone.

TREATMENT Bed rest and appropriate parenteral antimicrobial agents given for 6 to 8 weeks cure most cases of vertebral osteomyelitis.

The antibiotic(s) used in the treatment of osteomyelitis depend on the result of culture and sensitivity tests; the appropriate drugs are detailed in Chap. 111. In general, the first several weeks of therapy should be parenteral in order to achieve adequate levels of antibiotic in bony tissue. If no organisms are culturable, the choice of the antimicrobial necessarily must be based on cultures from other sites or, if these are negative, on the clinician's best estimate of the infecting pathogen. When staphylococcal infection is suspected, a penicillinase-resistant penicillin or a cephalosporin should be used.

External stabilization by traction or brace is indicated for an unstable cervical spine but is unnecessary for most patients with thoracic or lumbar osteomyelitis. Surgery is usually necessary only to drain paravertebral or spinal epidural abscesses. With successful therapy, bony bridging and spontaneous fusion of adjacent vertebral bodies occur, and the erythrocyte sedimentation rate returns to normal.

The main treatment of chronic hematogenous osteomyelitis, posttraumatic osteomyelitis, and osteomyelitis from a contiguous infection is surgery, with antimicrobial therapy an important adjunct. Antibiotics alone rarely cure these infections. The major surgical principles are thorough removal of all necrotic bone and tissue and the elimination of dead space. Rigid bone, unlike soft tissue, does not collapse around a site evacuated of pus; the resultant cavity provides an area for blood, debris, and organisms to collect. This dead space may be obliterated by (1) open packing of the wound, allowing the slow process of granulation to fill the defect, (2) packing the cavity with potentially viable grafts from cancellous bone, (3) transfer of a pedicle of skeletal muscle into the cavity, (4) skin grafting directly onto the granulating bone surface, or (5) constant irrigation to keep the cavity free of debris, followed by one of the methods mentioned above. These surgical measures are accompanied by appropriate parenteral antimicrobial therapy for 3 to 6 weeks. Since there are no controlled studies, the optimal choice and duration of antibiotics are unknown, but antimicrobial therapy is clearly doomed to failure unless the surgical debridement is thorough. Sometimes the location or extent of osteomyelitis makes surgical cure short of amputation impossible. In these patients, if amputation is not performed, treatment is given only for acute exacerbations, such as the formation of overlying soft-tissue abscesses, where surgical drainage and a short course of antibiotics help control the acute manifestations.

Osteomyelitis associated with a prosthesis generally requires removal of the appliance, thorough debridement, and appropriate antimicrobial therapy.

Osteomyelitis associated with plates, screws, rods, or pins used for the open reduction of fractures also requires removal of the appliance, thorough debridement, and antimicrobial therapy if union of the fracture has occurred. In infected fractures with nonunion, the principles of treatment are the establishment of rigid bony stability and debridement of infected material to permit union to occur. Screws, plates, pins, and rods that have not loosened are left in place, and the wound is treated with open irrigation. If the hardware is loose, thus failing to provide rigid stability, it is removed, and stability is attained by other means, such as pins above and below the fracture site. When the infection is controlled, bone grafts may be necessary for union to occur, but some fractures will unite without them.

In osteomyelitis associated with vascular insufficiency, especially if it involves multiple bones of the foot in diabetics, cure is seldom possible without amputation.

INFECTIOUS ARTHRITIS

ACUTE BACTERIAL ARTHRITIS Septic arthritis is a medical emergency which must be recognized promptly and treated appropriately to avoid permanent joint damage. Microorganisms usually reach the joint by hematogenous spread from a primary infection elsewhere, but occasionally no source can be found. Joint sepsis may also occur by direct extension of infection from adjacent bone or soft tissue.

The purpose of this discussion on infectious arthritis is to provide a general approach to the diagnosis and management of articular infections. Early recognition of septic arthritis results in correct therapy and reduces the likelihood of joint damage.

Etiology Acute *bacterial arthritis* is caused by many different types of bacteria; the ones most commonly encountered are *Neisseria gonorrhoeae, Staphylococcus aureus, Streptococcus pneumoniae, Streptococcus pyogenes, Hemophilus influenzae,* and gram-negative bacilli (*Escherichia coli, Salmonella, Pseudomonas* spp., etc.). Septic arthritis due to *H. influenzae* occurs mostly in children; gonococcal arthritis is a disease of sexually active persons. *Staphylococcus aureus* is a common infecting agent in septic arthritis observed in intravenous drug addicts. Gram-negative bacillary infections are also not infrequent in this group of patients. In addition, joint sepsis with gram-negative bacilli tends to occur in patients with underlying infection of the urinary, biliary, or intestinal tract and in patients with impaired resistance to infection. Osteomyelitis is also a feature of infections with gram-negative bacilli, and joint damage is a common sequel. Patients with *Salmonella* arthritis often have evidence of underlying osteomyelitis. Infectious arthritis of the spine is seen in brucellosis and *Salmonella* infections.

An increased susceptibility to joint infection occurs in patients with diabetes, in those with lymphomas, leukemias, or multiple myeloma, and in those receiving corticosteroids or immunosuppressive drugs. Patients with chronic alcoholism are more prone to develop infections, in general, and bacterial arthritis, in particular. In addition, joints previously damaged by arthritis, such as rheumatoid arthritis or trauma, are more susceptible to infections.

Manifestations The onset of bacterial arthritis is usually abrupt and accompanied by fever which is often low grade. Shaking chills occur in some patients. One or a few joints may be involved. The affected joint is warm, erythematous, swollen, and painful; however, these signs may be masked in patients receiving corticosteroids. Marked guarding of the joint and muscle spasms are common. The knee is involved in approximately one-half of the cases. Other large joints, such as the hips and shoulders, are commonly affected, and the wrists, ankles, elbows, and sternoclavicular and sacroiliac joints less often. However, predilection of the latter two joints for septic arthritis has been observed in intravenous drug abusers. The articulations of the spine or any peripheral joint may be a site of infection. In the spine, infection involves the vertebral body and adjacent intervertebral disk space, and may extend to the adjacent apophyseal joint. Localized tenderness and spasm of the paraspinal or psoas muscles are often present. The diagnosis of septic arthritis of the hip is often delayed, since the swelling of this joint is not readily detected and aspiration is difficult. Pain from the hip is frequently referred to the anterior knee. The hip is usually held in abduction, flexion, and external rotation. In some instances, the thigh becomes edematous and swelling appears in the anterior groin.

Pathology The synovium in the early stages of infection is edematous and infiltrated by neutrophils. An effusion with many neutrophils forms rapidly. Lysosomal proteolytic enzymes are released from neutrophils and destroy articular cartilage, subchondral bone, and joint capsule. Small abscesses appear in the synovium and subchondral bone, and necrotic debris collects in the joint space. During healing, proliferation of fibroblasts may lead to ankylosis.

Laboratory and x-ray findings Joint aspiration should be performed in any patient suspected of having a septic joint. The synovial fluid is initially cloudy and later may be grossly purulent. The white blood cell count usually ranges from 50,000 to 100,000 per cubic millimeter or higher, and more than 90 percent of the cells are neutrophils. The cell count, however, can occasionally be less than 50,000 per cubic millimeter and should not be used alone to exclude the diagnosis of bacterial arthritis. The concentration of glucose in the joint cavity is often less than 50 percent of a simultaneous blood sugar reading when obtained at least 6 h after a meal. Gram's stain frequently reveals microorganisms. Cultures of the synovial fluid and blood should be performed even if the Gram's stain is negative. Radiographs of the joint early in infection show only distention of the joint capsule, but later x-rays reveal juxtaarticular osteoporosis, joint space narrowing due to cartilage destruction, and bony erosions on the articular surface. Radiographic evidence of coexisting osteomyelitis may be present. In the spine, radiographic changes may not be seen for several months. The first changes consist of narrowing of the involved disk space or vertebra and proliferation of bone at the vertebral margins. Subsequently, lytic lesions appear in the vertebra and may extend to the disk space. During healing adjacent vertebrae may become fused.

Diagnosis The diagnosis of septic arthritis is confirmed by a positive culture from synovial fluid or tissue. With spinal involvement, needle biopsy or open surgical biopsy is usually required to obtain tissue for culture. The acute arthritis of gout or pseudogout may be mistaken for septic arthritis because of the monarticular involvement and manifestations of acute joint inflammation. They are easily distinguished by the finding of the respective characteristic crystals in synovial fluid. Other types of inflammatory arthritis, such as psoriatic arthritis, Reiter's syndrome, rheumatoid arthritis, or rheumatic fever, may also be confused with a septic arthritis, especially when only one or a few joints are involved. In a patient with generalized arthritis (such as rheumatoid disease) who develops fever and chills and has one joint disproportionately more inflamed than other joints, the possibility of septic arthritis should be carefully ruled out by examination of the synovial fluid cells and by culture of synovial fluid. The possibility of infectious arthritis should also be entertained in patients with unilateral sacroiliitis and fever.

Treatment Septic arthritis requires prompt treatment with the appropriate antibiotic. Table 360-1 shows the preferred antibiotic regimens for the more common types of septic arthritis. When no organisms are seen on Gram's stain, penicillinase-resistant penicillin and gentamicin should be given, particularly to those patients with factors known to diminish host resistance. Bactericidal levels of antibiotics are achieved with systemic administration; therefore, direct administration of an antibiotic into the joint is not necessary and may in itself produce a chemical synovitis. During treatment, bactericidal assays of synovial fluid may be performed to assure that therapeutic levels of antibiotic have been achieved. Joint drainage is important in the treatment of a septic joint, by reducing pressure and removing pus that generates proteolytic enzymes. Drainage is recommended when the joint is tightly distended or contains a high neutrophil count. Drainage can usually be accomplished by needle aspiration; the frequency depends on the amount of fluid and the cell count of the fluid that reaccumulates. Joint drainage is usually only necessary during the first few days of treatment. The joint cavity can be irrigated with sterile saline to enhance removal of inflammatory substances. Open surgical drainage is usually not indicated except in septic arthritis of the hip or in a joint with chronic suppuration and loculated pus. Splinting of the affected joint may make the patient more comfortable and reduce the degree of flexion deformity. Prolonged splinting, however, should be avoided, since it may lead to a permanent joint stiffness. When the inflammation has subsided, physical therapy will aid the return of joint function. When a weight-bearing joint has been severely damaged, bony fusion may be necessary.

GONOCOCCAL ARTHRITIS (See also Chap. 119) Gonococcal arthritis is the most common cause of arthritis in young adults, especially women. Pregnancy and menstruation are predisposing factors for bacteremia and arthritis. Patients with homozygous deficiency of a terminal complement component (C5 to C8) are also more susceptible to disseminated *Neisseria* infections, since these organisms are killed by complement-mediated cell lysis requiring the terminal complement components.

Patients with gonococcal arthritis may present with fever, chills, skin lesions, polyarthritis, and a positive blood culture. The polyarthritis usually evolves in a few days to a monoarticular septic arthritis. These two stages have been referred to as the "bacteremic" and "septic joint" phases. The clinical picture, however, is quite variable, and some patients present with monoarticular septic arthritis and few if any systemic manifestations during the bacteremic phase. Cultures of synovial fluid are positive in less than half the cases. Arthritis usually responds promptly to antibiotic therapy. The gonococcal organisms associated with disseminated infection are usually very sensitive to penicillin.

TABLE 360-1
Recommended therapy for the major types of acute bacterial arthritis

Organism	Drug and dose
*Neisseria gonorrhoeae**	Penicillin G, 10 million units IV qd for 3 days, then ampicillin 500 mg PO qid for 4 days†
Hemophilus influenzae	Ampicillin, 1 g IM every 6 h for 10-14 days‡
Staphylococcus aureus:	
Penicillin G-sensitive*	Penicillin G, 4 million units IV every 6 h for 2 weeks,§ then oral therapy for 4-6 weeks
Penicillin G-resistant*	Methicillin, oxacillin, or nafcillin, 2 g every 4 h for 2 weeks,§ then dicloxacillin, 1 g PO every 6 h for 4 weeks
*Streptococcus pneumoniae**	Penicillin G, 2 million units IV every 6 h for 10-14 days
Beta-hemolytic streptococcus, group A*	Same as for *S. pneumoniae*

* See Chap. 111 for alternate regimens in penicillin-allergic patients.
† In penicillin-allergic nonpregnant patients, tetracycline, 1.5 g PO, then 500 mg PO qid for 7 days.
‡ A few strains are resistant to ampicillin, in which case chloramphenicol may be required.
§ Intravenous therapy should be continued until infection is controlled.

TUBERCULOUS ARTHRITIS Tuberculous arthritis is a chronic destructive form of septic arthritis caused by *Mycobacterium tuberculosis*. Most patients have a focus of tuberculosis elsewhere in the body; however, in some patients no primary lesion can be detected. The bacilli infect the synovium either through the circulation or by extension from a tuberculous lesion in the adjacent bone. Tuberculous arthritis is more common in children but occurs at any age.

The tuberculous process in the joint produces synovitis, with the formation of a pannus of granulation tissue over the articular cartilage. The subchondral bone is involved, and areas of necrosis occur. Destruction of articular cartilage occurs later in the course, followed by fibrous ankylosis.

In the spine, the infection begins in the vertebral body; the thoracic spine is affected most frequently. Destruction of bone leads to vertebral collapse and angulation of the spine. Extension of the infection into the adjacent soft tissues produces a cold abscess, which may spread down the anterior aspect of the spine to form a psoas abscess. The abscess may eventually point in the anterior groin.

Tuberculous arthritis has an insidious onset, is usually monarticular, and usually affects the spine, hips, and knees. The affected peripheral joint is swollen, warm, and tender and has a decreased range of motion. Erythema is minimal, and pain is usually a later manifestation. The hypertrophied synovium gives the joint a boggy, doughy feeling. Muscle atrophy and spasm of the affected extremity occur. Tenosynovitis of the flexor tendon sheaths of the wrist may compress the median nerve and produce a carpal tunnel syndrome. Regional lymphadenopathy is usually present.

With spine involvement (Pott's disease), tenderness and muscle spasm over the affected area are found. Subsequent vertebral collapse in the dorsal part of the spine leads to kyphosis. Paralysis and tuberculous meningitis are serious complications.

The patient may have only slight fever. Weight loss is common. The course of untreated disease is usually one of progressive joint destruction.

Examination of synovial fluid shows usually more than 10,000 leukocytes per cubic millimeter. Differential counts are not helpful. The tubercle bacilli may be seen on smears of synovial fluid but are more likely to be found on biopsy of synovial tissue or of regional lymph nodes.

Radiographs of peripheral joints in early disease show joint capsule distention and juxtaarticular osteoporosis. Bony erosions at the joint margin, subchondral bone destruction, and joint space narrowing are observed later in the disease. Films of the spine show destruction of the vertebral body, vertebral collapse, and loss of intervertebral disk space.

The diagnosis of tuberculous arthritis is made on the demonstration of the tubercle bacilli in synovial fluid or tissue by smear, histology, or culture. The tuberculin skin test is almost always positive.

Atypical mycobacteria (*Mycobacterium trivale, M. kansasii, M. scrofulaceum*) can also cause septic arthritis. The primary lesions may go unnoticed. Skin tests for the specific mycobacterium should be performed when the diagnosis is suspected. The correct diagnosis depends on a positive culture from synovial fluid or tissue (Chap. 145).

Antimicrobial therapy is described in Chap. 143. Surgical treatment may be necessary and includes debridement, synovectomy, and joint fusion.

MYCOTIC, SYPHILITIC, AND VIRAL ARTHRITIS Mycotic arthritis The systemic mycoses (coccidioidomycosis, histoplasmosis, blastomycosis, cryptococcosis, actinomycosis, and sporotrichosis) may involve bone and joints. In the primary phase of coccidioidomycosis, a transient polyarthritis, lasting up to 1 month, may occur in association with erythema nodosum (desert arthritis), but no residual joint damage ensues. However, with disseminated disease, bone and joint involvement leads to joint destruction. Joint involvement by actinomycosis results from extension of infection from adjacent bone. Sporotrichosis, however, may produce synovial infection. It usually affects joints proximal to the cutaneous portal of entry. In the other mycotic diseases, joint involvement is infrequent.

The diagnosis of fungal arthritis is established by the identification of the organisms in synovial fluid or in a biopsy specimen. Treatment with amphotericin B is usually successful; however, surgical debridement may be necessary.

Syphilitic arthritis This form of arthritis (Chap. 146) occurs in congenital, secondary, or tertiary syphilis. During the first year of life, congenital syphilis may produce an osteochondritis in the juxtaepiphyseal region which results in the breakdown of bone and articular cartilage (Parrot's pseudoparalysis). At puberty, congenital disease may cause a synovitis which most commonly involves the knees and elbows (Clutton's joints). The joint is often red, swollen, and tender, but pain may be minimal. Synovial fluid shows a leukocytosis, predominantly lymphocytes.

In secondary syphilis, transient polyarthritis and polyarthralgia occur. Gummatous involvement of the synovium may occur in tertiary syphilis and most often involves the larger joints.

In addition to direct involvement of the joint, syphilis also produces a neuropathic joint (Charcot's joint).

The proper diagnosis of the joint disease can be established only after the correct diagnosis of syphilis. A positive serologic test for syphilis is not diagnostic, since biologic false-positive tests may occur in rheumatic diseases such as systemic lupus erythematosus.

Viral arthritis A self-limited polyarthritis may be a manifestation of several viral diseases (e.g., mumps, arboviral infection, adenoviral infection, rubella, hepatitis, infectious mononucleosis), especially in the prodromal stages of the illness.

Rubella infection may manifest a polyarthritis, usually involving the small joints of the extremities. The arthritis is seen most often in young adults, especially women. Arthritis has also been observed in children and young adults after vaccination with live attenuated rubella vaccine. The onset of arthritis coincides with or shortly follows the appearance of the rash. The arthritis lasts up to 2 weeks and leaves no residual joint damage. Synovial fluid has been reported to show an increased number of lymphocytes. Rheumatoid factor tests are usually negative.

Arthritis is a relatively common manifestation of type B hepatitis (serum hepatitis). Arthritis, sometimes accompanied by a rash, may precede the onset of clinical jaundice by a few days to 2 weeks, or coincide with the appearance of jaundice. Occasionally, the arthritis may occur in the absence of clinical jaundice; however, liver function tests will be abnormal. The arthritis may be migratory, involves both small and large joints and leaves no residual joint damage. Symmetrical joint involvement of the hands may be confused with rheumatoid arthritis. Synovial fluid may show a mild leukocytosis with predominantly lymphocytes. Rheumatoid factor tests usually are negative.

Serum and joint fluid complement levels are usually low during arthritis. Serum complement level returns to normal with the appearance of overt liver disease. Hepatitis B antigen (Australia antigen, hepatitis-associated antigen) can usually be detected in both serum and joint fluid during the prodromal period of hepatitis. The synovitis is thought to be induced by immune complexes consisting of antibodies and viral antigens.

Lyme arthritis is a disease of postulated viral etiology, occurring in the northeastern states of the United States. It was originally described in the contiguous communities of eastern Connecticut (Old Lyme, Lyme, and East Haddam). Transmission of the causative agent was thought to be by tick or, less often, mosquito. Most of the cases occur in the summer and fall. The arthritis is an acute, recurrent, monoarticular, or asymmetrical oligoarticular joint disease involving most commonly the knee, followed by other large joints and the temporomandibular joint. The small joints of the feet and hands are occasionally affected. The duration of arthritis in a single joint is approximately one week, but it sometimes can persist for several months. The arthritis in some patients may be migratory. Most patients have recurrent attacks, separated by intervals ranging from one to several weeks. The number of attacks tends to become less frequent; most of the patients have at least one recurrence in the second and third years of illness. The affected joint is swollen and warm but usually not red. The white blood cell count of the synovial fluid ranges from 2000 to over 50,000 per cubic millimeter and consists mostly of granulocytes. Significant joint damage usually does not occur. Erythema chronicum migrans, an expanding erythematous annular skin lesion, may precede the onset of arthritis by a few days to several weeks. Fever, chills, headache, and malaise often accompany the appearance of the skin lesions and episodes of arthritis. Other manifestations of this illness include neurological abnormalities (aseptic meningitis, Bell's palsy) and cardiac conduction abnormalities. Small amounts of serum cryoprecipitate can be demonstrated in patients, suggesting the presence of circulating immune complexes. The joint symptoms are treated with salicylates. Glucocorticosteroids may be beneficial in the treatment of neurological or cardiac abnormalities.

REFERENCES

Osteomyelitis

BURRI C: *Posttraumatic Osteomyelitis.* Bern, Hans Huber, 1975

KELLY PJ, FITZGERALD RH: Symposium on infections in orthopedics. Orthop Clin North Am, October 1975

LEWIS RP et al: Bone infections involving anaerobic bacteria. Medicine 57:279, 1978

MACKOWIAK PA et al: Diagnostic value of sinus tract cultures in chronic osteomyelitis. JAMA 239:2772, 1978

McHENRY MC et al: Hematogenous osteomyelitis. A changing disease. Cleveland Clin Q 42:125, 1975

MEYER S et al: The treatment of infected non-union of fractures of long bones. J Bone Jt Surg 57A:836, 1975

MUSHER DM et al: Vertebral osteomyelitis. Still a diagnostic pitfall. Arch Intern Med 136:105, 1976

WALDVOGEL FA et al: Osteomyelitis: A review of clinical features, therapeutic considerations, and unusual aspects. N Engl J Med 282:198, 260, 316, 1970

Septic arthritis

ALPERT E et al: Pathogenesis of arthritis associated with viral hepatitis: Complement component studies. N Engl J Med 285:185, 1971

CLARK GM: Tuberculosis arthritis, in *Arthritis and Allied Conditions,* 9th ed, DJ McCarty Jr (ed). Philadelphia, Lea & Febiger, 1979

GOLDENBERG DL, COHEN AS: Acute infectious arthritis: A review of patients with nongonococcal joint infections (with emphasis on therapy and prognosis). Am J Med 60:369, 1976

HYER FH, GOTTLIEB NL: Rheumatic disorders associated with viral infection. Semin Arthritis Rheum 8:17, 1978

SCHMID FR: Principles of diagnosis and treatment of infectious arthritis, in *Arthritis and Allied Conditions,* 9th ed, JL Hollander, DJ McCarty Jr (eds). Philadelphia, Lea & Febiger, 1979

SHARP JT: Gonococcal arthritis, in *Arthritis and Allied Conditions,* 9th ed, JL Hollander, DJ McCarty Jr (eds). Philadelphia, Lea & Febiger, 1979

STEERE AC et al: Erythema chronicum migrans and Lyme arthritis: The enlarging clinical spectrum. Ann Intern Med 86:685, 1977

WARD JR, ATCHESON SG: Infectious arthritis. Med Clin North Am 61:313, 1977

361
DEGENERATIVE JOINT DISEASE

MART MANNIK
BRUCE C. GILLILAND

INTRODUCTION Degenerative joint disease (DJD) is characterized by loss of joint cartilage and by hypertrophy of bone. Synonyms for degenerative joint disease include osteoarthritis and hypertrophic arthritis. Surveys have estimated that over 40 million Americans have radiological evidence of DJD, including 85 percent of persons over the age of 70. Many persons with radiographic changes, however, have no musculoskeletal complaints. In young persons changes identical to the degenerative changes in advanced age are encountered when cartilage has been damaged by injury, infection, or congenital deformities. The exact mechanisms for cartilage loss in DJD have not been defined, but stress and subchondral bone changes contribute to the damage. Treatment of DJD is directed to amelioration of symptoms, decrease in excessive stress, and corrective procedures in properly selected subjects.

ETIOLOGY AND PATHOGENESIS The joint cartilage, subchondral bone, and joint capsule dissipate the forces of weight bearing and joint function. The joint cartilage has unique properties of compressibility and elasticity due to the combined presence of collagen fibers and proteoglycans. The articular cartilage contains a unique type of collagen, called *type II collagen,* which is composed of three identical $\alpha_1(II)$ polypeptide chains. Collagen fibers provide cartilage with structural integrity. The proteoglycans of cartilage consist of a protein backbone and many glycosaminoglycan side chains with negative charges. These proteoglycans molecules bind a large number of water molecules. Upon compression of cartilage the structural water is released from the proteoglycans and regained upon removal of the compressive force. The loss of compressibility of cartilage secondary to proteoglycan malfunction seems to be a central feature in the development of DJD.

In normal adult cartilage chondrocytes no longer synthesize DNA or divide. Experimental trauma to cartilage and the pathogenic events of DJD reactivate DNA synthesis and cell division; as a result clusters of chondrocytes form in osteoarthritic cartilage. Chondrocytes are metabolically active and continuously rebuild the matrix of cartilage. The turnover of structural molecules requires the presence of enzymes that can dismantle the "old" structures as new molecules are synthesized and assembled. Such enzymes exist in chondrocytes and are more abundant in osteoarthritic lesions.

In degenerative lesions of joint cartilage the size of the proteoglycan molecules is reduced, owing to either degradation or altered synthesis, and the composition of glycosaminoglycans is altered. In addition, the content of proteases (particularly cathepsin D) and other hydrolases is increased in degenerative lesions. These observations along with the finding of increased metabolic activity and increased cell division in osteoarthritic cartilage indicate that increased degradation and increased synthesis of cartilage matrix occur concurrently. Apparently, as the lesions progress, the synthetic activities cannot keep up with degradative processes, and a progressive net loss of cartilage ensues. During the reparative process the original architecture of collagen fibrils is not achieved, and type I cartilage (normally found in skin, tendons, etc.) is laid down in place of type II collagen. At the same time sclerosis of subchrondral bone continues, and marginal bone overgrowths (spurs) develop.

Epidemiologic studies suggest that wear-and-tear processes play a central role in initiating the degenerative process in cartilage. Work patterns can lead to early involvement of joints that are usually not affected by DJD. For example, air-hammer operators develop DJD in their elbows and shoulders. In contrast, the development of DJD is slow in paralyzed limbs. The continued wear-and-tear on joints is thought to cause fatigue fractures of subchondral bone. The repair of these microfractures leads to loss of deformability in subchondral bone and a concomitant decrease in energy dissipation by bone. By this mechanism, the articular cartilage is subjected to increased forces that initiate surface alterations, increase release of enzymes from chondrocytes, and enhance repair processes. In congenital malformations or malalignment of joints normal stresses cause increased wear and tear that leads to early DJD.

PATHOLOGY Early pathological changes of DJD are recognized in the joint cartilage. New bone formation develops in subchondral bone and at the margins of the articular cartilage. Progressive loss of metachromasia (histological evidence of proteoglycan loss) occurs in the cartilage, beginning at the surface. Chondrocytes increase in number and form clusters. With progression of the process the surface of cartilage begins to loosen and flake along superficial collagen fibers that parallel the joint surface; upon reaching the deeper radial layer the damage is reflected in fissuring of cartilage. Abrasion of damaged cartilage may ultimately lead to total loss of the cartilage. This progressive loss of cartilage is apparent radiologically as "joint space" narrowing.

The bone at the joint margins responds to cartilage damage with osteophyte formation. These lesions usually extend from the margin of the joint along the contour of the joint surface. Alternatively, osteophytes may develop within and extend along ligamentous and capsular attachments of the joint margin. The denuded subchondral bone becomes dense, smooth, and glistening, and looks like ivory (eburnation). In addition, cystic areas may develop below the joint surface and become filled with fibrous tissue. These "pseudocysts" are thought to result from transmission of intraarticular pressure through cartilaginous defects into underlying cancellous bone. Low-grade inflammatory changes are present in the synovium and joint capsule, but the capsule is subject to thickening with fibrosis.

CLINICAL MANIFESTATIONS Degenerative joint disease is divided into *primary* and *secondary* forms. In primary DJD no predisposing abnormality or cause can be found, and the usual symptoms of the illness begin after the fifth and sixth decades of life. In secondary DJD an underlying abnormality or injury can be found, and the clinical symptoms may begin several decades earlier. The clinical findings in primary and secondary DJD are similar, except that in secondary DJD unusual or single joints are more likely to be involved.

Secondary DJD follows septic arthritis or inflammatory arthritides (e.g., rheumatoid arthritis, psoriatic arthritis) that destroy cartilage. Fractures through the cartilage, lacerations of cartilage, removal of menisci, and aseptic necrosis predispose the affected joints to early development of DJD. Diabetes mellitus and acromegaly also predispose to development of DJD. Local anatomic aberrations are thought to be the most common causes of early development of DJD. Congenitally shallow acetabulums, slipped capital femoral epiphyses, and Legg-Perthes disease are commonly accepted causes of early DJD in the hip. Deviations from the normal matching of the curvatures of the femoral head and the acetabulum are thought to contribute to DJD. The alterations in the congruence of this and other joints, however, need to be evaluated further in relation to the development of what now is termed *primary idiopathic DJD.*

The cardinal complaint in DJD is pain confined to joints, especially on motion and weight bearing. The pain is usually described as aching. Patients complain of definite joint stiffness; this occurs after resting and subsides in a few minutes upon resuming motion. In the morning the stiffness lasts only a short time (usually reported in minutes), whereas the morning stiffness of rheumatoid arthritis lasts an hour or more. On examination the joints may show a restricted range of motion, local tenderness, bony enlargement, small effusions, and crepitus. Erythema and increased heat are unusual in DJD.

DJD of the distal interphalangeal joints of the fingers leads to bony enlargement of the joint. These dorsolaterally located nodules at the base of the terminal phalanx are called *Heberden's nodes.* One-fourth of the patients who have nodes of the distal interphalangeal joints also have similar deformities at the proximal interphalangeal joints, called *Bouchard's nodes.* The primary Heberden's nodes usually evolve insidiously and without pain. However, some patients develop redness, swelling, and tenderness that lasts a few weeks. Subsequently the initial relatively soft and painful swelling is replaced by a hard, bony, painless enlargement. Heberden's nodes are more common in females than in males, and in females heredity seems to play a role. The mother and sisters of a woman with Heberden's nodes are more likely to have the nodes than controls of the same age and sex. Heberden's nodes may involve single joints as a result of trauma (e.g., "baseball fingers," "karate fingers"). Metacarpophalangeal joints are virtually never involved. The carpometacarpal joint of the thumb is frequently involved (Fig. 361-1).

DJD of the wrists, elbows, and shoulders is relatively uncommon. However, occupational trauma may enhance DJD in the elbows and shoulders, as in air-hammer workers.

Degenerative joint disease of the spine can involve the intervertebral disks, the apophyseal joints, or the joints of Luschka in the cervical spine. The latter joints are articulations between the lateral aspects of adjacent vertebral bodies from C_2 to C_7. The herniation of intervertebral disks is covered in Chap. 375. The involvement of apophyseal joints or joints of Luschka leads to stiffness, pain, decreased motion, and at times to spinal nerve root compression. Radiographs of the spine will show characteristic osteophyte formation, extending from the bodies of vertebrae or extending into the spinal foramina from the apophyseal joints. Most elderly persons have some radiographic changes, but relatively few of the changes become severe enough to cause symptoms and signs.

In the cervical spine the maximum motion occurs between C_4 and C_5 and between C_5 and C_6; these articulations are most likely to develop DJD. Development of osteophytes from the margins of the joints of Luschka or the apophyseal joints can cause impingement on nerve roots at the spinal foramens. Radicular pain, muscle spasms or atrophy, paresthesias, and sensory changes will localize the level of root involvement. Cervical traction can provide relief of symptoms and resolution of neurological abnormalities. At times, surgery will be required. Occasionally osteophytes may extend posteriorly from the ver-

tebrae into the spinal canal and result in cord compression. Surgical intervention is required in such situations.

In the lumbar spine, herniated disk disease (Chap. 375) is more common than impingement of the nerve roots or cauda equina by osteophytes. The syndrome of spinal stenosis supervenes in persons who have anatomic variations with decreased anteroposterior dimensions of the spinal cord or decreased lateral recesses of the canal. In contrast to herniation of an intervertebral disk, the symptoms of spinal stenosis evolve insidiously, back symptoms precede nerve compression symptoms in the legs, and the symptoms are often bilateral. The symptoms of spinal stenosis are increased by exercise, enhanced by the lordotic position, and relieved by flexion of the spine. The onset and relief of symptoms are not as predictable in relation to exercise as in intermittent claudication, and the presence of numbness, tingling, and weakness also serve to distinguish the symptoms from claudication. Myelography is needed to establish the diagnosis with certainty. Laminectomy is indicated when symptoms and signs of spinal stenosis persist.

DJD of the hip is perhaps the most disabling form of the illness, with considerable loss of function in the advanced stages. Early in the course of hip involvement pain occurs on weight bearing and is relieved by rest. Groin pain, at times

FIGURE 361-1

Degenerative joint disease. A. Heberden's nodes of the distal interphalangeal joints and Bouchard's nodes of the proximal interphalangeal joints of the fingers. The carpometacarpal joints of both thumbs are swollen. B. X-rays of the middle three fingers of the left hand from the same patient. Note the marked joint space narrowing, osteophyte formation in the distal and proximal interphalangeal joints, cystic changes in subchondral bone, and absence of osteoporosis.

A

B

referred to the knee, is most common. Nocturnal pain evolves later. On examination, the range of motion is decreased and accompanied by pain. Internal rotation of the hip and extension of the hip are the earliest to be limited. Flexion deformities evolve later in the course of the illness. Radiological examination is important to determine the extent of involvement.

Secondary DJD of the hip occurs earlier and may be unilateral. Among the various causes of secondary DJD, avascular necrosis occurs most often in the hips and may be related to underwater diving, alcoholism, corticosteroid therapy, and sickle-cell disease. Pain usually antedates radiological changes, but the pain becomes severe when the subchondral bone collapses. Radiographically a characteristic wedge-shaped alteration of bone and discontinuity of the subchondral bone are noted. The destruction of cartilage and loss of subchondral bone lead to rapid development of DJD.

Occupational or sport injuries are frequent causes of degenerative changes in the knees. Torn menisci and ligamentous instability contribute to early changes. Tenderness, limitation of motion by pain, crepitation, and joint effusions may be present. The medial compartment of the knee is more often involved than the lateral compartment. *Chondromalacia patellae* produces softening and loss of cartilage from the articular surface of the patella. This is usually an early development of DJD but at times is seen in young persons. Pain and crepitus are frequently present on patellar motion.

Extensive DJD is found late in the course of acromegaly. The early articular changes in acromegaly include thickened synovial tissues and considerable overgrowth of the joint cartilage, presumably in response to the excessive secretion of growth hormone.

Erosive osteoarthritis Occasionally middle-aged or older women are encountered who have an acute and transient inflammatory joint disease, particularly in the joints of the hands, in association with typical changes of DJD. These patients have tender and red distal and proximal interphalangeal joints. Subsequently Heberden's nodes evolve. Single or several joints may be involved at any one time. On radiographs these patients are seen to have developed osteophytes and subchondral sclerosis but may also have erosions of the joint surface. Periarticular osteoporosis is not a feature of this condition. On histological examination, mild to moderate inflammation is present during the acute phase, with lymphocyte and plasma cell infiltration and even mild pannus formation—quite similar to that in mild rheumatoid arthritis. However, patients with erosive osteoarthritis can be distinguished from patients with rheumatoid arthritis by the characteristic presentation and pattern of joint involvement, the absence of prolonged morning stiffness, absence of typical rheumatoid deformities, lack of palpable synovial hypertrophy, radiological presence of degenerative changes, and negative tests for rheumatoid factor. A weakly positive test for rheumatoid factor does not exclude erosive osteoarthritis, since normal elderly persons may have a positive test.

DIAGNOSIS The usual laboratory tests show no abnormalities in DJD. The erythrocyte sedimentation rate is normal for the age of the patient. The characteristics of joint fluid have been discussed (Chap. 355). Radiological changes are most helpful for diagnosis. Joint pain in elderly persons without other abnormalities usually means DJD. However, caution should be exercised in ascribing joint complaints to DJD on the basis of radiographic changes alone, because spurs, lipping, and joint space narrowing also occur in infections, rheumatoid arthritis, pseudogout, and gout in this age group.

TREATMENT Following evaluation of a patient with DJD, realistic goals for treatment should be established. Reassurance is important, because patients frequently equate any joint disease with total disability. Steps should be taken to eliminate excessive and recurrent trauma. A weight-reduction program should be initiated for overweight individuals. Moderate exercise is recommended, but vigorous activity that produces prolonged pain and discomfort should be avoided.

Acetylsalicylic acid in an adequate dose (2 to 4 g per day) is the drug of choice for relief of pain. Other salicylate preparations may be equally useful (sodium salicylate, choline salicylate, salicyl salicylate). Indomethacin (25 mg tid or qid) provides relief in some patients who do not benefit from salicylates. Phenylbutazone (100 mg bid to qid) should be employed only for short periods, and care must be exercised to detect toxicity (Chap. 356). All these drugs may lead to gastric irritation, and occasionally to peptic ulcer.

Local heat is useful in many patients with mild DJD. In severe joint involvement, physical therapy with infrared heat, ultrasound, or hot packs may help to relieve pain. Isometric exercises may be useful, especially to strengthen the quadriceps muscle when knees are involved. Cervical traction may be helpful in relieving compression of the nerve roots.

Patients with intractable pain and advanced DJD can benefit significantly from orthopedic procedures, including debridement and removal of loose bodies, osteotomy, partial prosthetic replacement, and total joint replacement. Outstanding results have been achieved with total hip replacement in patients who were disabled by DJD of the hips. Other artificial joints are being developed. The potential benefits should be carefully weighed against the risks of each patient who is being considered for these procedures.

REFERENCES

EHRLICH GE: Inflammatory osteoarthritis: I. The clinical syndrome. J Chronic Dis 25:317, 1972

HOWELL DS: Degradative enzymes in osteoarthritic human articular cartilage. Arthritis Rheum 18:167, 1975

——— et al: The pathogenesis of osteoarthritis. Semin Arthritis Rheum 5:365, 1976

MANKIN HJ: The reaction of articular cartilage to injury and osteoarthritis. N Engl J Med 291:1285, 1974

MOSKOWITZ RW: Osteoarthritis: A new look at an old disease. Geriatrics 28:121, 1973

PAINE KWT et al: Clinical features of lumbar spinal stenosis. Clin Orthop 115:77, 1976

PETER JB et al: Erosive osteoarthritis of the hands. Arthritis Rheum 9:365, 1966

362
PROGRESSIVE SYSTEMIC SCLEROSIS (DIFFUSE SCLERODERMA)

BRUCE C. GILLILAND
MART MANNIK

Progressive systemic sclerosis (PSS) is a disorder of connective tissue leading to fibrosis that involves the skin (scleroderma) and a variety of internal organs, most notably the gastrointestinal tract, lungs, heart, and kidney. The clinical hallmark of PSS is the tight, firm skin, which may be present several years before visceral involvement becomes apparent. However, in some patients visceral disease occurs in the absence of skin involvement. Visceral involvement decreases the survival of these patients.

ETIOLOGY AND PATHOGENESIS This uncommon disease has a worldwide distribution but is apparently rare in Asia, especially among the Chinese, Indians, and Malaysians. The onset of disease is usually in the third to fifth decades, and women are affected twice as often as men. The etiology and pathogenesis of PSS are not known; hereditary factors are not involved. The increased fibrosis in the various organ systems is considered to be due to the overproduction of collagen. Tissue culture of skin fibroblasts from patients with scleroderma synthesized increased amounts of collagen compared with appropriate controls. Qualitative abnormalities of collagen have not been documented in PSS.

Vascular injury at the level of small arteries, about 150 to 500 μm in diameter, has been proposed as the primary event in the pathogenesis of PSS. This concept is supported by the finding of mononuclear-cell infiltrates around small arteries and in the interstitium early in the course of the lesions. Fibroblastic proliferation, in response to inflammation, then leads to overproduction of collagen and sclerosis of the small arteries and interstitial tissue. Narrowing and obliteration of small arteries results in decreased vascularization of skin, skeletal muscles, lung, and other organs, followed by fibrosis as a secondary event. What causes the initial vascular inflammation is not known.

The role of immunologic abnormalities in the pathogenesis of PSS has not been established. Autoantibodies occur in this disorder, and PSS is associated with other rheumatic diseases in which immunologic mechanisms are of pathogenic importance. In particular, patients with combined features of scleroderma, systemic lupus erythematosus, and myositis have been described. In addition PSS is sometimes associated with Sjögren's syndrome. Biopsies of the border of spreading skin lesions contain lymphocytes, suggesting that cell-mediated immunity may participate in the genesis of the lesions.

Occupational hazards have been associated with the development of PSS. The occurrence of PSS in coal miners appears to be twice as common as in nonminers, suggesting perhaps that silica dust may be a predisposing factor. Workers exposed to polyvinyl chloride may develop Raynaud's phenomenon, acroosteolysis, and scleroderma-like skin lesions. Nail-fold capillary abnormalities similar to those observed in PSS are also present. In addition, these workers also developed hepatic fibrosis and angiosarcoma.

PATHOLOGY In the skin, a thin epidermis overlies compact bundles of collagen which lie parallel to the epidermis. Finger-like projections of collagen extend from the dermis into the subcutaneous tissue and bind the skin to the underlying tissue. Dermal appendages are atrophied, and rete pegs are lost. Increased numbers of lymphocytes identified as T cells may be present at the border of skin lesions.

In the lower two-thirds of the esophagus, the histological findings consist of a thin mucosa and increased collagen in the lamina propria, submucosa, and serosa. The degree of fibrosis is less than in the skin. Atrophy of the muscularis in the esophagus and throughout the involved portions of the gastrointestinal tract is more prominent than the amount of fibrotic replacement of muscle. Ulceration of the mucosa is often present and may be due to either PSS or superimposed peptic esophagitis. Striated muscles in the upper one-third of the esophagus are relatively spared. Similar changes may be found throughout the gastrointestinal tract, especially in the second and third portions of the duodenum, jejunum, and large intestine. Atrophy of the muscularis of the large intestine may lead to the development of large-mouth diverticula. In the later stages of the disease, the involved portions of the gastrointestinal tract become dilated. Infiltration of lymphocytes and plasma cells in the lamina propria is also present.

With pulmonary involvement, diffuse interstitial fibrosis, thickening of the alveolar membrane, and peribronchial fibrosis are observed. Bronchiolar epithelial proliferation accompanies the pulmonary fibrosis. Rupture of septa produces small cysts and areas of bullous emphysema. Small pulmonary arteries and arterioles show intimal thickening, fragmentation of the elastica, and muscular hypertrophy; however, bronchial vessels and pulmonary veins are usually spared.

The synovium in patients with PSS and arthritis is similar to that seen in early rheumatoid arthritis and shows edema with infiltration of lymphocytes and plasma cells. Later in the disease the synovium may become fibrotic. Fibrinous deposits appear on the surfaces of tendon sheaths and in the overlying fascia, and may lead to audible creaking over moving tendons.

Histological features of muscle involvement consist of interstitial and perivascular lymphocytic infiltrations, degeneration of muscle fibers, and interstitial fibrosis. Arterioles may be thickened, and capillaries may be decreased in number.

In the heart, myocardial interstitial fibrosis replaces myocardial fibers. Fibrosis also involves the conduction system, leading to atrioventricular conduction defects and arrhythmias. The wall of smaller coronary arteries may be thickened, and lymphocytic infiltration is seen. Fibrinous pericarditis and pericardial effusions are found in some patients.

Renal involvement is found in over half the patients and consists of intimal hyperplasia of the interlobular arteries, fibrinoid necrosis of the afferent arterioles, including the glomerular tuft, and thickening of the glomerular basement membrane. These lesions result in cortical infarctions and glomerulosclerosis. The renal pathological change is often indistinguishable from that observed in malignant hypertension. Renal vascular lesions, however, may be present in the absence of hypertension. Angiographic renal studies in patients with PSS may show constriction of the intralobular arteries, a finding that simulates the vasospasm of the digital arteries observed in Raynaud's phenomenon. Along with Raynaud's phenomenon, induced by cooling, a decrease in renal blood flow has been observed. These studies are of interest because three-quarters of the deaths from renal involvement in PSS have been shown to occur in the fall and winter.

Primary liver involvement is not common, but diffuse cirrhosis, intrahepatic cholestasis, and chronic passive congestion occur occasionally. Fibrosis of the thyroid may develop. Thickening of the periodontal membrane with replacement of the lamina dura is demonstrated radiographically as widening of the periodontal space and rarely causes loosening of the teeth.

Small arterial and arteriolar lesions are found in many tissues; they consist of concentric acellular thickening of the intima with narrowing or occlusion of the lumen. These lesions are found in the digital arteries and arterioles in patients with PSS and Raynaud's phenomenon. Vascular abnormalities have been described in the lung, skin, kidney, muscle, gastrointestinal tract, pancreas, synovium, vasa vasorum, and the central nervous system. Arteritis with fibrinoid necrosis and infiltration by mononuclear cells of all three layers is occasionally observed.

CLINICAL MANIFESTATIONS PSS usually begins insidiously; the first symptoms often are Raynaud's phenomenon or symmetrical swelling or stiffness of the fingers. Raynaud's phenomenon may precede the skin changes by months or even years. In some patients, the first manifestation is pitting edema of the extremities and face.

The fingers and hands in the early stages are swollen. Subsequently the skin becomes firm, thickened, and leathery in appearance, and tightly bound to the underlying subcutaneous tissue. In the late stage of disease, the skin is atrophic and less "hidebound." The skin changes spread to involve the arms, face, upper part of the chest, abdomen, and back. The lower extremities are relatively spared. The taut skin over the fingers gradually limits full extension, and fixed flexion contractures develop. Ulcers may appear on the fingertips and over bony prominences and may become infected. The soft tissue of the fingertips is lost, and in some instances the bone of terminal phalanges is resorbed. The skin may become darkly pigmented even without exposure to the sun; areas of depigmentation and numerous telangiectases often appear on the skin. Examination of nail folds with a wide-angle microscope or an ophthalmoscope shows a decrease in the number of capillary loops and dilatation of the remaining loops. Similar changes are also observed in dermatomyositis. In some patients, calcific deposits develop in the subcutaneous and periarticular tissue. The overlying skin may break down, with draining of calcific material. Involvement of the face results in the loss of normal skin wrinkles, loss of facial expression, and inability to open the mouth fully.

The coexistence of *c*alcinosis, *R*aynaud's phenomenon, *e*sophageal hypomotility, *s*clerodactyly, and *t*elangiectasia has been termed the CREST syndrome and initially was considered a benign form of PSS. However, some of these patients have subsequently developed visceral and more extensive cutaneous lesions of PSS.

More than half the patients with PSS complain of pain, swelling, and stiffness of the fingers and knee joints. A symmetrical polyarthritis, resembling rheumatoid arthritis, may be seen. In more advanced stages of the disease, leathery crepitation can be palpated over moving joints, especially the knee. Extensive fibrotic thickening of the tendon sheaths in the wrist can produce a carpal tunnel syndrome. Distinction of scleroderma with myositis from mixed connective tissue disease (see below) may be difficult.

Symptoms attributable to esophageal involvement, which are present in more than 50 percent of patients, include epigastric fullness, burning pain in the epigastric or retrosternal regions, and regurgitation of gastric contents. These symptoms, most noticeable when the patient is lying flat or bending over, are due to the reduced tone of the gastroesophageal sphincter and to dilatation of the distal esophagus. Peptic esophagitis frequently occurs and may lead to strictures and narrowing of the lower part of the esophagus. However, it seldom results in bleeding. Dysphagia, particularly of solid foods, may occur independent of other esophageal symptoms and is caused by the loss of esophageal motility due to neuromuscular dysfunction. Gastric involvement, which is not common in PSS, produces symptoms that are difficult to distinguish from esophageal symptoms. Balloon pressure studies and cineradiography reveal decreased amplitude or disappearance of peristaltic waves in the lower two-thirds of the esophagus. A closer correlation exists between this finding and Raynaud's phenomenon than with cutaneous manifestations of PSS. Later in the course of the illness, dilatation and atony of the lower portion of the esophagus as well as reflux are seen. With gastric involvement, barium studies show dilatation, atony, and delayed gastric emptying.

Symptoms referable to involvement of the small intestine by PSS include bloating and abdominal pain and may suggest intestinal obstruction or paralytic ileus. Malabsorption syndrome with weight loss, steatorrhea, and anemia also occurs secondary to obliteration of the lymphatics by fibrosis or in some patients due to bacterial overgrowth in the atonic intestine. Involvement of the large intestine may cause chronic constipation and fecal impaction with episodes of bowel obstruction. Roentgenographic features of the second and third portions of the duodenum and of the jejunum include dilatation, loss of the usual feathery pattern, and delayed disappearance of barium. Pneumatosis intestinalis, which occasionally occurs in PSS, is seen as radiolucent cysts or linear streaks within the wall of the small intestine. Benign pneumoperitoneum may result from the rupture of these cysts. Barium studies of the large intestine may show dilatation, atony, and large-mouth diverticula.

Patients with pulmonary fibrosis often complain of a dry cough and exertional dyspnea; however, shortness of breath as a presenting complaint is unusual. Bilateral basilar rales may be present. Though pleural involvement is not infrequent at postmortem, pleurisy is unusual. Restriction of chest movement may rarely occur with extensive skin involvement of the thorax. Additional pulmonary problems result from aspiration pneumonia secondary to esophageal malfunction. Superimposed bacterial or viral pneumonia may be a serious complication in patients with pulmonary fibrosis. Malignant alveolar or bronchiolar cell neoplasms have been reported in some patients with PSS and pulmonary fibrosis. However, no other association of PSS with malignancy has been shown. Pulmonary function test results are abnormal even in early disease and show a low diffusion capacity and a low P_{O_2} on exercise. Roentgenograms of the chest may show a pattern of linear densities, mottling, and honeycombing. These changes are more evident in the lower two-thirds of the lungs. Pulmonary insufficiency accounts for approximately 20 percent of the deaths in PSS.

Cardiac involvement by PSS often goes clinically unrecognized; however, varying degrees of heart block and arrhythmias may be seen. Cardiomyopathy attributable to diffuse myocardial fibrosis may also occur. Other cardiac manifestations may be secondary to pulmonary disease and hypertension. Left ventricular failure develops more frequently than cor pulmonale, even with the presence of pulmonary fibrosis. In some patients, pulmonary hypertension appears without pulmonary fibrosis, presumably secondary to pulmonary arterial and arteriolar narrowing. Acute and chronic pericarditis may develop and occasionally produce tamponade. Cardiac involvement is the cause of death in 15 percent of PSS patients.

Renal failure is the leading cause of death in PSS, accounting for almost half of the deaths. The onset of renal involvement is frequently within 3 years of the diagnosis of PSS. Renal failure, however, can present abruptly at any time in an apparently stable patient and is fatal unless treated. Acute renal failure can develop in association with malignant hypertension or in a setting of mild chronic hypertension. Proteinuria, an abnormal urine sediment, hypertension, azotemia, and microangiopathic hemolytic anemia are clinical features associated with progressive renal disease. It is difficult to predict the patient who will develop renal failure. Microangiopathic anemia may appear several weeks before renal involvement and thereby serve as an indicator of impending renal failure. The presence of chronic pericardial effusion may also be associated with subsequent renal failure. Rapidly progressive renal failure has been attributed to glucocorticosteroid administration, but the same rapidly progressive course may be seen in patients who have not received steroids.

LABORATORY FINDINGS The erythrocyte sedimentation rate may be elevated. Hypoproliferative anemia related to chronic inflammation is the most common cause of anemia in PSS. Anemia may also be caused by iron deficiency secondary to gastrointestinal bleeding. Bacterial overgrowth due to atony of the small bowel may lead to vitamin B_{12} and/or folic acid deficiency anemia. Microangiopathic hemolytic anemia is most often associated with renal involvement and the presence of fibrin deposition in the renal arterioles. Hypergammaglobulinemia, with elevated level mainly of IgG, is found in approximately half the patients. Rheumatoid factor, in low titer, is present in 25 percent of patients. Antinuclear antibodies are reported in 40 to 80 percent of patients and include antibodies to nucleolar antigen, deoxyribonucleoprotein, and extractable nuclear antigens. The latter give a speckled pattern on immunofluorescent tests and are frequently found in the so-called "mixed connective tissue disease" (see below).

DIAGNOSIS The diagnosis of PSS presents no difficulty in the presence of Raynaud's phenomenon, with typical skin lesions and visceral involvement. PSS should always be included in the differential diagnosis of patients with Raynaud's phenomenon. Other causes of Raynaud's phenomenon include thoracic outlet (scalenus anticus and cervical rib) syndromes, shoulder-hand syndrome, trauma (jackhammer or vibratory machine operators), previous cold injury, vinyl chloride exposure, and circulating cryoglobulins or cold agglutinins. Linear scleroderma and morphea are localized forms of PSS and may be associated with Raynaud's phenomenon and hypergammaglobulinemia. PSS may be confused with rheumatoid arthritis, systemic lupus erythematosus, or polymyositis when articular or muscle involvement is prominent early in the disease. PSS without cutaneous involvement should be considered in patients with unexplained pulmonary fibrosis, cardiomyopathies, heart block, dysphagia, or malabsorption syndrome. Several conditions have scleroderma-like features but lack the visceral involvement. Scleredema (scleredema adultorum of Buschke) occurs predominantly in children and is characterized by painless edematous induration involving the face, scalp, neck, trunk, and proximal portions of the extremities. Involvement of the hands and feet usually does not occur. Scleredema may be associated with previous streptococcal infection and is usually self-limited, resolving in 6 to 12 months. Histology reveals accumulation of mucopolysaccharides in the dermis and skeletal muscle. A rare entity, scleromyxedema (lichen myxedematosus), is manifest by yellowish papules and may involve the face and hands. Acid mucopolysaccharide deposits are found in the dermis. Monoclonal IgG may be detected in some of these patients. Primary amyloidosis may involve the skin of the extremities and face diffusely to give the appearance of scleroderma. Biopsy will clearly differentiate these entities.

Diffuse fasciitis with eosinophilia A scleroderma-like syndrome consisting of fasciitis, myositis, eosinophilia, and hypergammaglobulinemia has been recognized. Patients develop tenderness and swelling of the extremities with the onset of symptoms often related to strenuous physical exertion. The skin is firmly bound over areas of nonpitting induration. Biopsy shows perivascular infiltration of histiocytes, eosinophils, lymphocytes, and plasma cells in the dermis, subcutaneous fat and fascia, and underlying muscle. Improvement has been noted with administration of corticosteroids, but spontaneous improvement has also been recorded.

Mixed connective tissue disease This rheumatic syndrome describes patients with clinically overlapping features of scleroderma, systemic lupus erythematosus, and polymyositis. The serums of all these patients have hemagglutinating antibody specific for an extractable nuclear antigen which is composed largely of ribonucleoprotein and produces a speckled pattern on fluorescent antibody testing. High titers of antibody to nuclear ribonucleoprotein are found in almost all patients with the mixed connective tissue disease, even during clinical remissions. High titers of this antibody, however, are also found in

some patients with systemic lupus erythematosus, discoid lupus, rheumatoid arthritis, and progressive systemic sclerosis.

Arthralgias or arthritis is present in most patients with mixed connective tissue disease, but deformities are infrequent. An erythematous rash, similar to that seen in systemic lupus erythematous (SLE), is observed in some patients. In most patients the clinical appearance of the skin over the hands is similar to that seen in scleroderma. Telangiectatic lesions are frequently present. Most patients do not develop severe ulcerations on the digits. Biopsy of skin may show abnormalities comparable with scleroderma; some patients may have immunoglobulin deposits at the dermoepidermal junction similar to patients with SLE. Raynaud's phenomenon and esophageal hypomotility occur frequently. Some patients show heliotropic discoloration of the upper eyelids, and erythematous patches over the dorsum of the fingers similar to those observed in dermatomyositis; myalgias, proximal muscle weakness, elevated levels of muscle enzymes, and electromyographic changes of myositis are found in the majority of patients. Pulmonary abnormalities are common and include decreased diffusing capacity, diffuse interstitial infiltrates, and pleural disease. Occasionally pulmonary involvement is the predominant symptom and is expressed as exertional dyspnea and/or pulmonary hypertension. Other features are pericarditis, trigeminal neuropathy, generalized lymphadenopathy, and splenomegaly. Renal involvement is uncommon and usually mild; however, some patients develop progressive renal failure. Mesangial changes, focal nephritis, or diffuse membranous nephritis are the most frequently observed findings on renal biopsy. Granular deposits consisting of IgG and C3 have been observed in the glomerular basement membrane. Anemia, leukopenia, and diffuse hypergammaglobulinemia are often present and respond to glucocorticoids. The inflammatory aspects of this disease, such as fever, rash, arthritis, and myositis, all show a favorable response to corticosteroids. The sclerodermal skin manifestations, if treated early, and the pulmonary diffusing capacity may also improve with steroid therapy.

PROGNOSIS In the majority of patients PSS is characterized by a prolonged, relentless course of progressive skin and/or visceral involvement. In some patients remissions occur, including partial improvement of the skin, and the disease progresses slowly; 80 percent of one group of patients were alive 2 years after onset of symptoms, and 20 percent were alive 10 years after onset. Patients with mainly skin involvement have a more gradual and favorable course than those with visceral disease, especially of the heart, kidney, and lung. Among Caucasians the prognosis is worse in males than in females, and it is worse in patients whose onset of disease occurs at an older age. The disease tends to be more severe in blacks, especially in black females. Death stems most often from cardiac, renal, and pulmonary involvement.

TREATMENT Many drugs have been used in the treatment of PSS without any consistent or prolonged benefit. Systemic corticosteroids may produce improvement in the early edematous phase of the disease but do not influence the eventual course. They may also be indicated in patients with active myositis but have no effect on visceral lesions. *p*-Aminobenzoic acid was claimed to improve the skin in PSS, especially in patients with morphea; however, its therapeutic value remains unproved. This drug frequently causes nausea and skin eruptions. In addition, hypoglycemia may occur in patients who have decreased food intake. D-Penicillamine has been tried with variable results. Toxic reactions, fever, rash, nephrotic syndrome, and leukopenia occur with this drug. Chlorambucil and colchicine have been reported to be beneficial in PSS; however, further documentation is needed.

The management of Raynaud's phenomenon is directed at control of vasospasm and increasing the digital blood flow. It is important to prevent periods of vasospasm since the resulting ischemia may be a stimulant for vascular fibrosis and eventual obliteration. Patients should be advised to dress warmly and wear mittens and warm socks, not to smoke, and to avoid drugs such as amphetamines and ergotamine. Vasodilator drugs, such as reserpine, guanethidine, and alpha methyldopa, may be useful in increasing the threshold to vasospasm; however, their side effects often curtail their extended use. Intraarterial reserpine may temporarily improve Raynaud's phenomenon but is of little benefit in patients who already have anatomic narrowing of the arteries. Techniques of biofeedback have also been used for teaching patients to control the temperature of their hands. Removing causes of stress in the patient's life may be beneficial in controlling vasospasm. Skin ulcers should be kept clean by soaking or by surgical or chemical debridement. Infection is treated with topical antibiotics. Physiotherapy may help to reduce flexion deformities.

Patients with reflux esophagitis are treated with small frequent meals, antacids, and elevation of the head of the bed. Malabsorption syndrome may improve with tetracycline therapy. Patients with cardiac failure require careful monitoring of digitalis and diuretic administration. Pulmonary infections in patients with pulmonary fibrosis require prompt treatment with antibiotics and other supportive measures. Patients with progressive renal failure usually require dialysis. Renal transplantation has been successful in some patients. When renal failure is accompanied by hypertension, treatment with antihypertensive drugs or bilateral nephrectomy, in conjunction with dialysis, may improve survival.

REFERENCES

CANNON PJ et al: The relationship of hypertension and renal failure in scleroderma (progressive systemic sclerosis) to structural and functional abnormalities of the renal cortical circulation. Medicine 53:1, 1974

LEROY EC, FLEISCHMANN RM: The management of renal scleroderma: Experience with dialysis, nephrectomy and transplantation. Am J Med 64:917, 1978

NOTMAN DD et al: Profiles of antinuclear antibodies in systemic rheumatic diseases. Ann Intern Med 83:464, 1975

RODMAN GP: Progressive systemic sclerosis (scleroderma), in *Immunological Diseases,* M. Samter (ed). Boston, Little, Brown, 1978, vol 2, chap 66, p 1109

SHARP GC: Mixed connective tissue disease: Current concepts. Arthritis Rheum 20:S181, 1977

SHULMAN LE: Diffuse fasciitis with eosinophilia: A new syndrome. Arthritis Rheum 20:S205, 1977

363
MISCELLANEOUS ARTHRITIDES AND EXTRAARTICULAR RHEUMATISM

MART MANNIK
BRUCE C. GILLILAND

HYPERTROPHIC OSTEOARTHROPATHY Hypertrophic osteoarthropathy is characterized by the presence of periosteal inflammation and new bone formation, arthritis, and clubbing of the digits. This syndrome frequently results from disorders in the lungs and hence is frequently called *hypertrophic pulmonary osteoarthropathy* or *secondary hypertrophic osteoarthritis*. It also occurs in association with disorders of other agents, as well as in familial and idiopathic forms.

In hypertrophic osteoarthropathy the periosteum becomes hyperemic and edematous and is infiltrated with mononuclear cells. The periosteum is lifted, and new bone matrix is put down and calcified. At the same time endosteal bone is resorbed. These changes occur at the distal ends of long bones, at the wrists and ankles, as well as in the metacarpal and metatarsal bones. With progression of the disease, these changes may affect ribs, clavicles, and scapulae. The synovial membrane and joint capsule show edema and mild, chronic inflammation. At the same time soft-tissue edema, fibroblast proliferation, and minimal mononuclear infiltration lead to enlargement of the distal ends of digits, a process termed *clubbing*.

The mechanisms that cause hypertrophic osteoarthropathy are not known, but arteriovenous shunts and humoral and neurogenic factors are suspected because the process may be reversed upon correction of cardiac shunts, removal of pulmonary tumors, and vagotomy.

Hypertrophic osteoarthropathy occurs in 5 to 10 percent of patients with primary intrathoracic malignancies, notably bronchogenic carcinomas and pleural tumors, but is very rare with metastatic tumors of the lung. Chronic suppurative lung lesions, such as lung abscesses, bronchiectasis, and empyema, are frequent causes of hypertrophic osteoarthropathy. However, with decline of these problems, due to antibiotics, tumors are now the most frequent cause. This disorder also may accompany cyanotic cardiac malformations, biliary cirrhosis, ulcerative colitis, and regional enteritis. When no associated disorders have been identified, the disorder is called *idiopathic hypertrophic osteoarthropathy*. Hereditary hypertrophic osteoarthropathy (pachydermoperiostitis) is a disorder characterized by marked thickening of skin of the limbs and face, in addition to the typical features of hypertrophic osteoarthropathy.

Hypertrophic osteoarthropathy frequently occurs with digital clubbing but may precede clubbing or develop without it. Similarly, clubbing of the digits occurs without any evidence of hypertrophic osteoarthropathy. Hypertrophic osteoarthropathy may cause mild arthralgias. Other patients develop severe burning pain in the hands and feet. Erythema and effusions may involve wrists, ankles, and metacarpophalangeal or metatarsophalangeal joints. Tenderness is likely to be present in joints of these patients as well as over the adjacent bones. Dependency may aggravate these symptoms. At times the periosteal changes evolve without symptoms.

The synovial fluid of these patients usually has a total white blood cell count of less than 500 per cubic millimeter with only a few neutrophils.

Radiographs show increased thickness of the periosteum with new bone formation over the distal ends of bones. However, this may not be evident if the symptoms and signs have been present for only a short time. Lung lesions and other associated diseases must be sought. No specific laboratory tests are available for the diagnosis of hypertrophic osteoarthropathy, and its treatment must be directed toward search for and management of the underlying disorder. The symptoms may be controlled with acetylsalicylic acid or with analgesics. The symptoms and signs of hypertrophic osteoarthropathy may abate completely with treatment of empyema, abscess, or bronchiectasis or upon removal of the tumor.

NEUROPATHIC JOINT DISEASE Neuropathic joint disease, also called *Charcot joints*, develops in a variety of neurological disorders in which proprioception and/or deep pain sensation are disrupted. Increased trauma and stress are thought to occur during joint motion because of relaxation of the supporting structures of the joint. This leads to degeneration of cartilage, recurrent fractures of subchondral bone, and marked proliferation of adjacent bone. Neuropathic joint disease usually involves the knees, hips, ankles, and lumbar spine in tabes dorsalis; the tarsometatarsal, metatarsophalangeal, and tarsal joints in diabetic neuropathy; and the shoulders, elbows, and cervical spine in syringomyelia. Neuropathic joints also occur in meningomyelocele, congenital insensitivity to pain, leprous neuropathy, and peripheral nerve injuries.

On pathologic examination, cartilage degeneration, loose bodies, and marginal osteophytes are seen. The osteophytes are larger and more disorganized than in degenerative joint disease. Fractures occur in the articular facets, osteophytes, epicondyles, or condyles, with callus formation and further osteophyte formation. This process ultimately results in disorganization of the joints, which is characteristic of this disease. These alterations of the bone and joint space are easily recognized radiologically. The synovium shows fibrosis, fragments of calcified cartilage, and hemosiderin deposits.

Neuropathic joint disease, regardless of the underlying disorder, begins insidiously in a single joint and then progresses to involve other joints. The distribution of involved joints is influenced by the underlying neurological disorder. The involved joint enlarges because of effusion and overgrowth of bone; instability develops later. The discomfort is strikingly mild in relation to the structural abnormalities. Intraarticular fractures may cause sudden onset of pain. Examination may show increased mobility and instability. Effusions are common. Crepitus is frequent and marked in the late stages of disease. Many loose bodies may give the joint a feeling of a "bag of bones." The synovial fluid leukocyte count is low, comparable with osteoarthritis, but these fluids tend to be bloody and xanthochromic owing to intraarticular bleeding.

To diagnose a neuropathic joint, the underlying neurological disorder must be identified, but the treatment of the underlying neuropathologic condition seldom influences the progression of the joint disease. Therefore, the treatment should be directed to providing stability and relief of pain. External supports are useful, but the braces have to be carefully adjusted and checked, since patients with neurological disorders are not sensitive to maladjustments. Arthrodesis may provide stability, but these procedures are frequently accompanied by nonunion.

ARTICULAR PROBLEMS IN RENAL HOMOTRANSPLANTATION AND CHRONIC HEMODIALYSIS One to several months after renal homotransplantation about a third of the recipients develop musculoskeletal complaints. *Avascular necrosis* of bone may occur in these patients. The hips are most frequently involved, but other joints may be affected as well. Corticosteroid therapy is thought to contribute to this problem. Some patients have only transient musculoskeletal pain; in others acute or chronic synovitis and joint effusions may occur. The cause of these abnormalities has not been elucidated. The joint symptoms may last for months and tend to appear first after reduction of steroid dosage. These patients, as well as about 90 percent of all transplant recipients, develop positive tests for rheumatoid factor, but the significance of this remains unknown.

During chronic hemodialysis some patients develop extensive periarticular calcifications. Acute inflammation may evolve at these sites. Phenylbutazone can suppress the attacks, and lowering of serum phosphorus can prevent or dissolve the deposits.

SARCOID ARTHRITIS See Chap. 216.

ARTHROPATHY OF HEMOCHROMATOSIS See Chap. 94.

ARTHRITIS OF FAMILIAL MEDITERRANEAN FEVER See Chap. 217.

HEMOPHILIC ARTHRITIS See Chap. 318.

ARTHRITIS OF LIPID DISORDERS AND LIPID STORAGE DISEASES (See Chaps. 100 and 102) Patients with familial hyperbetalipoproteinemia may have transient polyarthritis. This synovitis reaches the maximum intensity within 24 h and subsides in 48 h. The joint involvement is migratory, affecting several joints in sequence. The knees and proximal interphalangeal joints are involved most commonly; the ankles, wrists, elbows, shoulders, and hips are less frequently affected. Morning stiffness may be present. The joints may be swollen and erythematous. The synovial fluid has noninflammatory characteristics (less than 400 white blood cells per cubic millimeter) and has good viscosity. The attacks of this migratory arthritis last about a week and occur a few times per year. The cause of this synovitis is not known. Crystals have not been found in synovial fluid. In contrast to podagra, the attacks do not have nocturnal onset but may be brought on by increased activity.

PIGMENTED VILLONODULAR SYNOVITIS Pigmented villonodular synovitis usually affects a single joint, most commonly the knee. However, hip, ankle, tarsus, carpus, and elbow may be involved. The cause of this disorder is unknown. The synovium is brownish in color and covered with elongated and enlarged villi; fusion of villi leads to formation of pedunculated nodules. Histologically the synovial lining cells appear normal, but the stroma of the villi contains large numbers of round and polyhedral cells. Hemosiderin granules and cholesterol crystals are abundant in the cytoplasm of synovial cells and in the interstitial spaces. Multinucleated giant cells may be present. Invasion of other tissues does not occur, but erosion of adjacent bone is seen.

The clinical picture of pigmented villonodular synovitis is characterized by the insidious onset of monarticular swelling in young adults, accompanied by pain. These symptoms tend to be continuous, but exacerbations occur from time to time. Radiological examination may show narrowing of the joint space, bone erosion, and subchondral cysts. The synovial fluid frequently contains blood and is dark brown, indicative of previous episodes of bleeding from the synovium.

Complete removal of the affected synovium is recommended. With incomplete synovectomy, recurrences are common. Irradiation has been used successfully in some patients.

TRAUMATIC ARTHRITIS Joints are subjected to many forms of trauma. The immediate damage may include capsular tears, detachment of menisci and joint cartilage, laceration of cartilage, and articular fractures. As a result of such damage hemorrhagic effusions are frequent. The product of such effusions changes to a serous, amber-colored fluid within 2 to 3 weeks. Bleeding may occur from injury of the synovial membrane alone, without damage to bone or cartilage.

The symptoms of joint trauma are obviously confined to the damaged joint. Swelling, ecchymoses, muscular spasms, and tenderness tend to be present. Pain, particularly on motion is characteristic. Radiological examination is essential to exclude fractures. Obvious rupture of ligaments must be excluded on examination, but internal derangement of the joint may become apparent only later. Air-contrast arthrograms are helpful in defining internal derangements, particularly meniscal tears.

Treatment should include rest and removal of large hemorrhagic effusions. Physical therapy is necessary during convalescence. Orthopedic evaluation should be obtained when repair of tendons, ligaments, or bone or the removal of menisci may be required. Severe damage to a joint hastens the onset of degenerative joint disease.

Patients frequently attribute the onset of a generalized joint disease to trauma. The diagnosis of *traumatic arthritis* should be reserved for patients in whom (1) a specified traumatic insult was severe enough to produce acute pain, swelling, effusion, and dysfunction of the affected joint, (2) the affected joint(s) alone shows the abnormalities mentioned, and (3) these abnormalities did not exist prior to trauma.

RELAPSING POLYCHONDRITIS Relapsing polychondritis is a disease of unknown cause that leads to inflammation and destruction of cartilage. The cartilage loses its characteristic basophilic staining with hematoxylin and eosin. The chondrocytes degenerate, and the cartilage is fragmented and replaced by fibrous connective tissue. Lymphocytes and plasma cells are present at the interface between cartilage and scar tissue. Cell-mediated immunity to cartilage may play an important role in the pathogenesis of this disease.

This disorder occurs predominantly in middle age. Involvement of the ears and nose is most common (in 80 to 90 percent of patients). The disease activity fluctuates and involves different sites. The affected ears or nose become swollen and tender. The destruction of cartilage leads to floppy ears and a collapsed nose. Hearing loss may ensue from collapse of the external auditory meatus. Fever and arthralgias are frequent. Involvement of the larynx, trachea, and bronchi leads to hoarseness, recurrent pulmonary infections, stenosis, and even acute suffocation from collapse of the cartilaginous structures. Episcleritis is seen in about 60 percent of patients. Aortic regurgitation occurs occasionally.

No specific laboratory tests are available, but the erythrocyte sedimentation rate is usually elevated, and mild anemia occurs. Biopsy of cartilage is helpful in establishing the diagnosis. Corticosteroids in moderate doses suppress the disease's activity.

TIETZE'S SYNDROME Tietze's syndrome consists of swelling, pain, and tenderness in the upper costochondral cartilages. The cause of this disorder is unknown. This syndrome tends to evolve gradually but may be acute. Patients often associate the onset with trauma. The involved costochondral joints are swollen and tender but not warm, and the disorder must be differentiated from bacterial infections, rheumatoid arthritis, and other inflammatory arthritides. Single joints are frequently involved, and multiple joint involvement tends to be unilateral. The location and character of the pain may mimic the symptoms of myocardial infarction. Injection with procaine and corticosteroids tends to provide relief. Excision has been tried. Analgesics and physical therapy have been helpful sporadically.

BURSITIS AND TENOSYNOVITIS Bursitis is defined as an inflammation of unknown cause of any of the many bursas between tendons, muscles, and bony prominences. The most common type of bursitis occurs in the shoulder. Other common types of bursitis are *trochanteric bursitis* (bursas around the gluteus medius insertion to the trochanter of the femur), which causes pain on external rotation of the hip and is recognized by

tenderness over the trochanteric area; *olecranon bursitis*, recognized by tenderness and inflammation at the point of the elbow; *ischiatic bursitis* (also called "weaver's bottom"), in which tenderness is present over the ischial tuberosities and is caused by prolonged sitting on hard surfaces; *prepatellar bursitis* (also called "housemaid's knee") produced by frequent or prolonged kneeling; *anserine bursitis,* an inflammation of the sartorius bursa, in which tenderness is present at the insertion of the conjoined tendon of the sartorius, semitendinosus, and gracilis muscles on the medial aspect of the tibia, and in which characteristically pain occurs on ascending or descending stairs.

In the shoulder, *subacromial bursitis* and *bicipital tenosynovitis* are the most common problems. In the former the supraspinatus tendon becomes inflamed where it passes under the subacromial bursa. Calcifications are frequently seen adjacent to the tendon, but the presence of calcium does not necessarily relate to the symptoms. With acute subacromial bursitis or supraspinatus tendinitis, the onset of symptoms is sudden and the pain may be severe. Any abduction or external rotation causes agony. Marked tenderness is present over the lateral humeral head below the acromion. In chronic forms, a nagging, intermittent pain may be present, particularly during any motion that includes abduction and rotation of the shoulder.

Bicipital tenosynovitis consists of inflammation of the synovial sheath of the tendon of the long head of the biceps as it passes through the bicipital groove of the humeral head. In the acute form of this illness, pain develops along the biceps area and may radiate to the forearm. Abduction and forceful supination cause an increase in pain. Marked tenderness is present over the bicipital groove. In chronic bicipital tenosynovitis the symptoms are milder but tenderness is present. Muscle atrophy and adhesive capsulitis of the shoulder may develop because of decreased usage. At times chronic inflammation may lead to rupture of the involved tendon.

The treatment of any type of bursitis should include rest, use of analgesics, and physical therapy upon recovery from the acute phase, to prevent loss of function. Phenylbutazone (100 mg tid) may be helpful. Injection of corticosteroids and local anesthetics hastens recovery and provides marked relief from acute symptoms.

The *frozen shoulder* (termed *adhesive capsulitis* by some) can be the product of intrinsic disease such as bicipital tenosynovitis, immobilization for fractures, or trauma, but in most elderly patients an antecedent cause is not evident. Reflex sympathetic dystrophy is thought to be a significant factor in the development of a frozen shoulder. Disuse and inactivity of the shoulder appear to contribute to the development of this syndrome. The term *adhesive capsulitis* has been used since inflammation of the entire capsule of the scapulohumeral joint has been noted during the course of frozen shoulder, leading to pain and decreased use of the shoulder. The shoulder pain may progress rapidly or advance gradually to constant pain and inability to use the joint. Tenderness on palpation is found in several areas around the shoulder. Osteoporosis of the shoulder is often present on radiological examination. The symptoms may abate spontaneously in several months or may lead to permanent disuse of the joint. Progressive exercises and nonsteroidal anti-inflammatory drugs provide relief in some patients. Local or even systemic steroids have been helpful in others. Frequent encouragement of patients appears beneficial in this slowly resolving problem.

Tenosynovitis (inflammation of the synovial lining of tendons) occurs with other types of rheumatic disease (rheumatoid arthritis, systemic lupus erythematosus, gout), in bacterial infections (gonococcal, tuberculous), secondary to trauma, and without known causes (idiopathic).

SHOULDER-HAND SYNDROME The shoulder-hand syndrome is the most common form of *reflex sympathetic dystrophy.* An external injury or an internal disorder initiates the reflex sympathetic dystrophy that includes pain, reflex vasomotor reactions, disability, swelling, tenderness, and osteoporosis. Both upper and lower extremities may be involved. The shoulder-hand syndrome is due to a number of disorders: in about one-fifth of patients the underlying cause is myocardial infarction; in one-fifth the symptoms develop secondary to cervical disk disease or cervical degenerative joint disease; in two-fifths an underlying disorder cannot be found or identified with certainty; trauma and hemiplegia each are the contributing cause in one-tenth of patients. The pathogenic mechanisms have not been identified. The most widely accepted hypothesis suggests that pain fibers carry impulses to the spinal cord where they initiate a cycle of reflexes through the interconnecting pool of neurons and lead to local sympathetic nervous system overactivity.

The onset of the shoulder-hand syndrome may be insidious or acute, with stiffness and weakness in the upper extremity or only in the shoulder or hand, weeks or months after the causative insult. These symptoms are followed by swelling, vasomotor changes, hyperesthesia, and disability after a variable period of time. Tenderness and swelling may occur in the contralateral side. Microscopic evidence of synovitis has been described in the affected joints. This stage lasts 3 to 6 months. Thereafter, the vasomotor signs diminish and atrophy and contractures develop. Finally the atrophy and contractures remain but improve gradually. The syndrome may run its course in one to several years. Radiographs will show varying degrees of patchy osteoporosis in the head of the humerus, wrist, and phalanges. Other laboratory tests provide no useful information. The early diagnosis of a shoulder-hand syndrome may be difficult, because it may resemble the early phases of rheumatoid arthritis.

Exercises and reassurance are the cornerstones of therapy. Salicylates provide some symptomatic relief. The use of prednisone up to 60 to 80 mg per day for 2 weeks, followed by tapering of the dose, has given very encouraging results with resolution of the symptoms and disability in most patients.

FIBROSITIS Fibrositis is a term used for an ill-defined, poorly understood set of symptoms, consisting of aching pain and stiffness in one or several parts of the body. These symptoms occur deep in tissues, including muscles, tendon insertions, and bony prominences. Tender points are found along the upper border of the trapezius, over the lateral epicondyle of the ulna, the second costochondral junction, the fat pad medial to the knee, the intervertebral ligaments, the upper outer quadrants of the buttocks, and other areas. These patients tend to be middle-aged and depressed. Disturbances in the nonrapid eye movement phase of sleep may contribute to the complaints of these patients. Illnesses like rheumatoid arthritis, systemic lupus erythematosus, myositis, neuropathy, and polymyalgia rheumatica must be considered and excluded. Reassurance, exercises, massage, salicylates, local injections of steroids, and correction of sleep disturbance tend to provide relief.

PSYCHOGENIC RHEUMATISM Psychogenic rheumatism is a term applied to rheumatic symptoms that are manifestations of psychoneurosis. Common complaints are stiffness and limitation of motion and painful joints, tendons, or muscles. These patients are in good general health and have no objective abnormalities of the joints and no trigger points as found in fibrositis. Radiological and laboratory studies are normal. The complaints tend to vacillate and do not improve with analgesics.

CARPAL TUNNEL SYNDROME Carpal tunnel syndrome, also called *entrapment neuropathy,* may be due to tenosynovitis, trauma, edema, fibrosis, tuberculosis and other granulomatous diseases, rheumatoid arthritis, acromegaly, amyloidosis, edema of pregnancy, and premenstrual edema. Localized tenosynovitis of unknown cause is the most common basis of the carpal tunnel syndrome, particularly in middle-aged females. It is caused by pressure on the median nerve as it passes through the space formed by the bones of the wrist and the transverse carpal ligament. Any space-occupying process may cause compression and malfunction of the median nerve or other nerves similarly confined, such as the ulnar nerve or the posterior tibial nerve.

Patients with the carpal tunnel syndrome complain of numbness and/or burning pain on the palmar surface of the first three digits of the hand. This pain may be referred proximally up the arm. Characteristically the pain is more severe at night. Adduction of the thumb is weakened, and atrophy of the thenar eminence develops. Dryness of the skin over the thumb and first two fingers is frequent. Pain and tingling may be elicited by sustained flexion of the wrist or by tapping over the median nerve on the flexor surface of the wrist. Nerve conduction studies across the wrist will confirm the diagnosis.

Surgical decompression of the carpal tunnel with release of the transverse ligament and debridement is the definitive treatment when symptoms and signs persist. Analgesics, splinting, and injection of corticosteroids may provide temporary or complete relief.

TUMORS OF THE JOINTS Primary tumors of the joints are relatively uncommon but should be considered a rare cause of monarticular symptoms. In addition, primary bone tumors and metastases to bone may produce articular symptoms when adjacent to joints.

In *synovial chondromatosis* multiple metaplastic growths of cartilage occur in the synovium or tendon sheaths. Later these may calcify and become evident on radiographs. Single joints are involved and include the knee, hip, elbow, and shoulder. The involved joint may enlarge because of effusions. Pain and limitation of motor occur because of loose bodies. Synovectomy is the definitive treatment.

Hemangiomas may occur in the synovial or tenosynovial membranes. Symptoms usually develop in childhood. Bloody effusions occur. The hemangioma should be excised. *Lipomas* may occur in subsynovial fat and extend into the joint space, particularly into the knees.

Synoviomas or synovial sarcomas develop in the immediate periarticular tissues and seldom extend into the synovial cavity. These highly malignant tumors develop in adolescents or young adults. They present as a slowly growing mass adjacent to a joint. Biopsy is required for diagnosis, and radical resection is recommended for treatment.

Synovial chondrosarcoma may occur in joints or tendon sheaths.

Metastatic tumors to bone rarely extend to the synovial cavity. Destruction of adjacent bone and bloody effusions are characteristic.

REFERENCES

Arkin CR, Masi AT: Relapsing polychondritis: Review of current status and case report. Semin Arthritis Rheum 5:41, 1975

BLAND JH et al: The painful shoulder. Semin Arthritis Rheum 7:21, 1977

HERMAN JH, DENNIS MV: Immunopathologic studies in relapsing polychondritis. J Clin Invest 52:549, 1973

KOZIN F et al: The reflex sympathetic dystrophy syndrome: I. Clinical and histological studies: Evidence for bilaterality, response to corticosteroids and articular involvement. Am J Med 60:321, 1976

MASSRY SG et al: Abnormalities of the musculoskeletal system in hemodialysis patients. Semin Arthritis Rheum 4:321, 1975

McCARTY DJ (ed): *Arthritis and Allied Conditions*, 9th ed. Philadelphia, Lea & Febiger, 1979

ROONEY PJ et al: Transient polyarthritis associated with familial hyperbetalipoproteinemia. Q J Med 47:249, 1978

SCHUMACHER HR JR: Articular manifestations of hypertrophic pulmonary osteoarthropathy in bronchogenic carcinoma. A clinical and pathological study. Arthritis Rheum 19:629, 1976

SINHA S et al: Neuroarthropathy (Charcot joints) in diabetes mellitus. Medicine 51:191, 1972

SMYTHE HA, MOLDOFSKY H: Two contributions to understanding of the "fibrositis" syndrome. Bull Rheum Dis 28:928, 1978

section 13 | Disorders of the nervous system

APPROACH TO THE PATIENT WITH NEUROLOGIC DISEASE

RAYMOND D. ADAMS

In neurologic diagnosis one faces several problems not encountered in other branches of internal medicine: First, there is the bewildering array of literally hundreds of clinical abnormalities that must be elicited and interpreted. Their multitude relates to the complexity of the human nervous system, which, unlike other organ systems, is not really one but many separate though integrated systems. Second, the anatomic localization of the lesion assumes significance with reference to pathologic states for certain diseases are known to affect certain regions and not to involve others. Thus the recognition of a certain syndrome(s) suggests the existence of certain diseases and the exclusion of others. Third, in neurologic medicine the physician must acquire facility in coping with two orders of clinical phenomena—one known only to the patient (introspective data) and reported by him or her under conditions of perfect mental clarity, the other, obvious to an outside observer (the extrospective data of behavioral change). Last, in all diseases of the cerebrum an outside source of information about disease (someone who knows the patient well, a member of the family) must be used because the patient's capacity for self-examination and reporting is often impaired.

The topography of disease places great importance on anatomic diagnosis and the identification of related syndromes and takes precedence over etiology. Therefore, in applying the clinical method in neurologic medicine, it is useful to proceed in a series of steps, as follows:

1 The essential clinical data are secured by history from the patient and someone who knows him or her and a systematic examination that includes a survey of all functions from the mental to the simplest of reflexes.
2 The clinical data relevant to the current problem are interpreted and translated in terms of neuroanatomy and physiology.
3 From these data the physician is able to determine the syndrome and from it determine an anatomic localization that best explains the findings. This may be called the *syndromic and anatomic diagnosis*.
4 The mode of onset and course of the illness, the associated medical findings, and the accessory laboratory data are then integrated.
5 Finally, the etiologic diagnosis is deduced from this information and the location of the disease process.

It is obvious that inaccurate and unreliable historical data concerning the disordered functioning of the nervous system will result in an erroneous diagnosis. An incomplete or inaccurate observation of details during examination may also be misleading. Usually where there is disagreement about neurologic diagnosis, it will be discovered that the source of the difficulty is an uncertainty about the significant items in the history and physical examination. Repeated examinations may be necessary to ascertain the course of the illness, particularly when the history is incomplete.

Since several different diseases may cause the same syndrome and any one disease may cause more than one syndrome, it is essential in learning neurology to familiarize oneself with this type of information. The authors of the following chapters acknowledge this principle in presenting the syndrome before the disease and when describing any given disease in stressing its common syndromic expressions. It is our belief that, if physicians can organize their medical knowledge around each of the subjects in the main headings in the chapter (stroke, head injury, fits, faints, movement disorders, headache, etc.), they will be in position to diagnose the majority of the treatable diseases of the nervous system.

The above approach does not always succeed. Even in the most sophisticated medical circles, where there are physicians who have spent their lives studying neurologic diseases, many neurologic illnesses cannot be diagnosed. The anatomic diagnosis may be known, but it may prove impossible even with the use of all the elaborate laboratory aids now available to determine which of several diseases is causative. Then only by carefully following the patient can the medical problem be solved.

364

DIAGNOSTIC METHODS IN NEUROLOGY

RAYMOND D. ADAMS
ROBERT R. YOUNG
KEITH H. CHIAPPA

The strict analysis and interpretation of the data elicited by a careful history and examination may prove to be adequate for diagnosis; special laboratory tests can then do no more than corroborate the initial impression. But it more often happens that the final conclusion as to the nature of the disease is not reached by simple case study. The possibilities may be reduced to two or three, but the correct one cannot be determined. Under these conditions, one resorts to some one or several of the laboratory tests outlined below.

It must be stressed that laboratory procedures should follow rather than precede clinical case study, except in emergencies when the disease threatens life and time does not allow detailed clinical observation. Laboratory procedures are but a part of the clinical method outlined in the introduction to this section. They should be undertaken only for the specific purpose of obtaining certain otherwise unavailable data which should shed light on the clinical problem. Some of the procedures are costly, time-consuming, and occasionally dangerous or painful (unless done with skill), may require hospitalization, and are misleading if the data are not gathered or interpreted competently. During clinical training every young neurologic physician should master each of these special procedures and learn to recognize its limitations and to interpret the results correctly. Some of these tests are regularly performed by the general physician or internist.

LUMBAR PUNCTURE AND EXAMINATION OF CEREBROSPINAL FLUID

The information yielded by the examination of the cerebrospinal fluid (CSF) is often of crucial importance.

INDICATIONS FOR LUMBAR PUNCTURE

1 To obtain pressure measurements and to secure a sample of CSF for cellular, chemical, and bacteriologic examination
2 To aid in therapy by the administration of spinal anesthetics and occasionally antibiotics or antitumor agents
3 To inject air, as in pneumoencephalography; a radiopaque substance (Pantopaque) or some of the water-soluble contrast media, as in myelography; or a radioactive substance [e.g., indium or radioactive iodinated serum albumin (RISA)] for the study of the dynamics of CSF and the diagnosis of hydrocephalus

Lumbar puncture carries a risk if the CSF pressure is high (evidenced by headache and papilledema), for it increases the possibility of a fatal cerebellar or tentorial pressure cone. However, if it seems important, in a given case of suspected increased intracranial pressure, to have the information yielded by CSF examination, the lumbar puncture may be performed with a fine-bore (No. 22 or 24) needle as the last part of the clinical study. (Note that if the pressure is over 400 mmHg one should obtain the necessary sample of fluid and then, according to the suspected clinical disease and patient's condition, administer a unit of urea or mannitol and watch the manometer until the pressure falls.) Dexamethasone (Decadron) should be started in a dose of 4 to 6 mg every 6 h in cases of tumor, cerebral trauma, hemorrhage, and certain types of encephalitis (acute hemorrhagic leukoencephalitis, acute inclusion body encephalitis).

Cisternal puncture, although safe in the hands of the expert, is too hazardous a procedure to entrust to those without experience. The lumbar puncture is to be preferred except in obvious instances of spinal block requiring a sample of cisternal fluid or myelography above the lesion.

Experience teaches the importance of meticulous technique. Lumbar puncture should always be done under sterile conditions. If procaine is injected in and beneath the skin, the procedure should be painless. Failure to enter the lumbar subarachnoid space after two or three trials can usually be corrected by doing the puncture with patients in the sitting position and then assisting them to lie on their side for pressure measurements and fluid removal. The "dry tap" is more often due to an improperly placed needle than to a pathologic obliteration of subarachnoid space by compressive lesion of the spinal cord or chronic adhesive arachnoiditis. A bloody tap due to transfixion of a meningeal vessel may result in hopeless confusion of the diagnosis if it is falsely interpreted as indicating hemorrhage in the subarachnoid spaces and ventricles.

EXAMINATION PROCEDURES Once the lumbar puncture is successful, some of or all the following aspects of the CSF should be studied: (1) pressure and "dynamics," (2) Queckenstedt test, if indicated by a lesion of the spinal cord, (3) gross appearance of CSF, (4) number and type of cells and presence of microorganisms, (5) protein, sugar, colloidal gold reaction, and, in special instances, analysis of pigments, (6) exfoliative cytology using millipore filters, (7) Wassermann reaction and appropriate serologic precipitation reactions, (8) protein immunoelectrophoresis for determination of γ-globulin levels, and other special biochemical tests (for NH_3, pH, CO_2, enzymes, etc.), and (9) bacteriologic cultures and virus isolation. See the Appendix for normal values of CSF.

RADIOLOGIC EXAMINATION OF SKULL AND SPINE

Plain x-rays of the skull or spinal column, according to the nature of the symptoms, constitute an indispensable part of the thorough study of traumatic, spondylitic, and neoplastic diseases but are of relatively little value in others. The procedure is relatively simple, and the findings are interpretable by most general radiologists. Space does not permit an illustration of such common findings as fractures, bone erosion, intracerebral calcifications, premature closure or separation of sutures, or alterations of skull configuration. These have been presented in Taveras and Wood's *Diagnostic Neuroradiology.*

Of more specific value in neurology and neurosurgery are five special radiologic procedures which now permit the visualization of most parts of the brain and spinal cord and their vessels.

1 Computerized tomography (CT scan). This new radiologic procedure, which computerizes the absorption offered by brain, CSF, and skull to more than 30,000 2- to 4-mm beams of x-ray and permits visualization of the ventricles, subarachnoid space, and the major cisternal fissures and sulci in several horizontal planes (Fig. 364-1), has become available in most medical centers and promises to replace many of the other contrast procedures such as pneumoencephalography and arteriography. It differentiates epidural, subdural, and intracerebral hemorrhages and deformities of ventricular system from "mass" lesions and demonstrates tumors (when done after an intravenous injection of Renografin or other contrast medium), as well as areas of brain edema and infarction, hydrocephalus, and brain atrophy. The simplicity of this noninvasive procedure and its low risk to patients with expanding lesions and the low exposure to x-ray have virtually revolutionized diagnostic neurology and neurosurgery.

2 *Angiography.* This has been developed over the last 30 years to the point where it is a relatively safe and extremely valuable method in the diagnosis of occluded arteries, aneurysms and vascular malformations, tumors, abscesses, and intracranial hemorrhages. Following local anesthesia, a needle or cannula can be placed percutaneously into the lumen of any of the larger arteries of the neck; or a catheter can also be used to cannulate any of the major cervical vessels in a retrograde fashion after being introduced into the brachial or femoral artery. In these ways radiopaque contrast media can be injected to visualize the arch of the aorta, the origins of carotid and vertebral systems and their extent through the neck into the cranial cavity, and occasionally spinal cord arteries. It is possible to show with clarity cerebral arteries down to about 0.1 mm lumen diameter under optimal conditions, as well as small veins of comparable size, vascular abnormalities (angiomas, aneurysms), occluded arteries, delayed circulation from increased intracranial pressure as with masses or occlusion of dural sinuses and veins, displacement of vessels by mass lesions, or complete failure of intracranial vascular filling with cerebral death.

3 *Pneumoencephalography* and *ventriculography.* In recent years, the injection of air or oxygen into the lumbar subarachnoid space with the patient in the sitting position has largely replaced the direct injection of air into the ventricles (ventriculography). Pneumoencephalography permits visualization in considerable detail of the size and position of the ventricles, the subarachnoid space (upper spinal and cerebral), and, indirectly, the structures which lie between the ventricles and the meninges. Hydrocephalus, mass lesions which displace or deform the ventricles, and atrophic states of the cerebrum are revealed by this technique.

4 *Pantopaque myelography* (and *ventriculography*). By injecting 5 to 15 ml Pantopaque through a lumbar puncture needle and then tipping the patient on a tilt table, the entire spinal subarachnoid space may be visualized. The procedure is almost as harmless as the lumbar puncture, provided that the Pantopaque is afterward removed through the needle. Ruptured lumbar and cervical disks and spinal cord tumors can be diagnosed accurately. Intraventricular injection of Pantopaque is occasionally done to visualize the third and fourth ventricles and the aqueduct of Sylvius in tumors of the posterior fossa when air does not enter from below. In some clinics air has been used instead of Pantopaque to visualize masses within the spinal canal. It is of particular value when combined with polytomography in visualizing the size and position of the spinal cord and its relation to spondylitic bars and spurs. New water-soluble contrast media have recently become available that are self-absorbing. Because of certain irritating effects, however, they have not been widely used except to visualize the lumbosacral subarachnoid space.

5 *Radioactive isotopes.* Radioactive isotopes, such as technetium, are in regular use for the visualization of tumors, inflammatory masses, and some vascular lesions. Since this is a simple, noninvasive procedure, the only limitation in its use is the expense. The more vascular the lesion, the more consistent its demonstration by these methods. Ultrasound can also be used to show displacement of central structures of the brain by a mass lesion.

ELECTROMYOGRAPHY (EMG)

This examination supplements the clinical study of patients with neurologic diseases which affect the neuromuscular apparatus or with primary or secondary diseases of the skeletal musculature. It is described in relation to muscle diseases (see Chap. 378).

ELECTROENCEPHALOGRAPHY

The electroencephalographic examination is part of the clinical study of the neurologic patient suspected of having a cerebral disease; it is also used in the evaluation of the central nervous system (CNS) effects of many medical diseases.

In addition to the resting record, a number of so-called "activating" procedures are usually carried out.

1 The patient is requested to breathe deeply 20 times a minute for 3 min. The resulting alkalosis and cerebral vasoconstriction may activate characteristic seizure patterns or other abnormalities.

2 A very powerful light (a stroboscope) is placed over the patient's face and flashed at frequencies from 1 to 20 per second with the patient's eyes opened and closed. The electroencephalogram (EEG) leads may then show abnormal discharges in photosensitive patients.

3 The EEG is recorded after the patient is allowed to fall asleep naturally or following sedative drugs given by mouth or by vein. Procedures 1 and 2 are more commonly employed, but sleep is extremely helpful in bringing out abnormalities, especially where temporal lobe epilepsy and certain other seizures are concerned, and all too often is omitted from study.

4 Special activating procedures, such as the parenteral administration of pentylenetetrazol (Metrazol) or insulin, can often be worked out in advance with the electroencephalographer. Though they are hazardous and rarely used now, their purpose is to produce diagnostically useful abnormalities without actually inducing convulsions.

5 Measurement of evoked responses to visual, auditory, and tactile stimuli (see below) can also be useful in neurologic diagnosis.

Certain preparations are necessary if electroencephalography is to be most useful. The patient should not be sedated and should not have been for a long time without food, for both sedative drugs and relative hypoglycemia modify the normal EEG pattern. The same may be said of mental concentration, extreme nervousness, or drowsiness, all of which tend to suppress the normal alpha rhythm and increase muscle artifacts. When dealing with patients suspected of having epilepsy who are already being treated for it, most physicians prefer to record the first EEG while the patient continues to receive drugs. If it is normal, and if the referring physician and the electroencephalographer agree, the test can be repeated 24 h after withdrawal of anticonvulsants; it is well known that these drugs reduce the incidence of abnormal interictal records in patients with proved epilepsy. Though it is unusual for seizures to begin during this short interval, it may happen; longer periods without therapy are hazardous. It is helpful if the person doing the electroencephalogram knows the suspected site of lesion or question to be answered.

TYPES OF NORMAL RECORDINGS The normal electroencephalographic record in adults is usually easy to recognize.

A

B

C

D

E

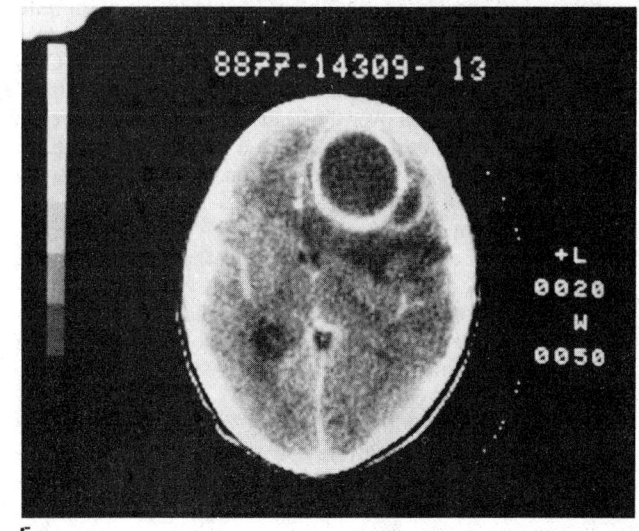

F

FIGURE 364-1

Computerized tomography scans in disease. Frontal lobes upper; right hemisphere to viewer's right. A. Normal. Horizontal view showing anterior horns of lateral ventricles; pineal gland is the calcified mass in center, and speck of calcium on right is in the choroid plexus. B. Brain atrophy showing mainly as widening of sulci. C. Hypertensive brain hemorrhage in left basal ganglia with extension into lateral ventricle and obstructive hydrocephalus. D. Massive infarction (recent) in left frontal, temporal, and parietal lobes. There is also brain atrophy (old) with dilatation of ventricles and widening of sulci. E. Glioblastoma multiforme in left inferior frontal lobe, edema of surrounding brain, and ventricular shift to the left. F. Frontal lobe abscess with adjacent daughter abscess and edema of surrounding brain.

The pattern frequently shows somewhat asymmetric 8- to 12-Hz, 50-μV sinusoidal *alpha* waves in both occipital and parietal regions. These waves wax and wane spontaneously and disappear promptly when patients open their eyes or fix their attention on something. Faster waves than 13 Hz of lower amplitude (10 to 20 μV), called *beta* waves, are also seen symmetrically in the frontal regions. Very slow waves (*delta* waves), sharp waves, or other unusual patterns are absent in a normal record. When normal subjects fall asleep, the rhythm slows symmetrically, and characteristic waveforms (vertex sharp waves and sleep spindles) appear; if the sleep is induced by barbiturates, an increase in the fast frequencies is seen and is considered to be normal.

An occipital response to each flash may be seen in the normal EEG during stroboscopic stimulation and is called the *evoked response,* or, at faster repetition rates, photic "driving." The clinical utility of this evoked occipital response has increased the scope of electroencephalography in several ways: (1) one can be reasonably sure that a person with such a response can at least perceive light; (2) when this evoked response is absent on one side of the head but present on the other, there is physiologic evidence of a lesion interfering with normal transmission between the thalamus and the occipital lobe on this side; and (3) when the flashing light causes the occipital response to spread over the cortex with the production of abnormal waves, there is evidence of an abnormal excitability. Actual seizure patterns may be produced in the EEG if the activation procedure is continued; if the sensitivity is still greater, frank myoclonic jerks of face or arms, or, rarely, major convulsions may occur. This finding is to be differentiated from the purely muscular response, also myoclonic, produced normally in contracting scalp muscles and often visible in routine EEGs (*photomyoclonus*).

TYPES OF ABNORMAL RECORDINGS The most pathologic finding of all is the disappearance of the EEG pattern and its replacement by "electrocerebral silence," which means that the electrical activity of the cortical mantle, measured at the scalp, is below 2 μV and probably absent. Acute intoxication with anesthetic levels of drugs, such as barbiturates, can produce this sort of isoelectric EEG. However, in the absence of CNS depressants or extreme hypothermia, a record which is "flat" (except for artifacts) all over the head is almost always a result of cerebral hypoxia or ischemia. Such a patient, without EEG activity, reflexes, spontaneous respiration, or muscular activity of any kind for 6 h or more, is said to be in "irreversible coma." The brain of such patients is largely necrotic. There is no chance for neurologic recovery, and the patient may be considered dead, despite the preservation of vegetative (cardiovascular) functions supported by mechanical means, such as respirators. There has been no exception to this statement in more than 500 patients examined at the Massachusetts General Hospital in the past 10 years.

Localized regions with such absence of EEG may rarely be seen when there is a large area of softening or an extensive surface tumor or clot lying between the cerebral cortex and the electrodes. With such a finding, the localization of the abnormality is precise, but of course the nature of the lesion cannot be ascertained. Most such lesions, however, are too small, relative to the recording arrangement, to be visible, and the EEG may then record abnormal waves arising from functional, though deranged, brain at the borders of the lesion. These abnormal waves are best defined as slower and of higher amplitude than normal. Those which are less than 4 Hz with amplitude from 50 to 350 μV are called *delta waves;* those from 4 to 7 Hz are called *theta waves;* and the higher-voltage, faster waves are known as *spikes* or *sharp waves*. These fast and slow waves may be combined, and when a series of them suddenly interrupts relatively normal EEG patterns in a paroxysmal fashion, they are highly suggestive of epilepsy. The ones associated with petit mal spells are 3-Hz spike and wave complexes that characteristically appear in all leads of the electroencephalogram at the same time and disappear almost as suddenly at the end of the seizure.

NEUROLOGIC CONDITIONS WITH ABNORMAL EEG In the following groups of neurologic disorders, the EEG may be of considerable help in reaching the correct diagnosis.

Epilepsy All types of generalized epileptic seizures (grand mal and petit mal) are associated with some abnormality in the EEG, provided it is being recorded at the time. The EEG is also usually abnormal during the more restricted types of seizure activity (psychomotor, myoclonic, Jacksonian). One exception is certain deep temporal lobe foci where the discharge fails to reach the scalp in sufficient amplitude to be seen against the background activity of the normal EEG, particularly if there is a strong alpha rhythm. If in these exceptional cases an anterior temporal electrode, which is most free of occipital alpha frequencies, does not show such a discharge originating deep and medially, a nasopharyngeal lead may pick it up, especially during sleep. Other exceptions in which, on occasion, no EEG abnormality may be recorded during a seizure include some of the patients with other focal seizures (sensory, Jacksonian, myoclonic, and epilepsia partialis continua). This fact presumably means that the neuronal discharge is too deep, discrete, fast, or asynchronous to be transmitted by volume conduction through the skull and recorded via the EEG electrode, which is some 2 cm from the cortex. The petit mal, myoclonic jerk, and grand mal patterns correlate closely with the clinical seizure type and may be present in the interictal EEG.

A fact of importance is that between seizures as many as 20 percent of patients with petit mal and 40 percent with grand mal epilepsy show a normal pattern. Anticonvulsant therapy also tends to diminish the EEG abnormalities. The records of another 30 to 40 percent of epileptics, though abnormal between seizures, are nonspecifically so, and therefore the diagnosis of epilepsy can be made only by the correct interpretation of the clinical data in relation to the EEG abnormality.

Brain tumor, abscess, and subdural hematoma Clinically significant intracranial space-occupying lesions are characteristically associated with abnormalities in the EEG, depending on their type and location, in some 90 percent of patients. In addition to diffuse changes, the classic abnormalities are focal or localized slow-wave (usually delta), or, occasionally, seizure activity and decreased amplitude and synchronization of normal rhythms. As a rule, those with the more rapidly expanding lesions (abscess, some metastases, glioblastoma), especially when these are situated supratentorially, have the greatest frequency of EEG abnormalities (90 to 95 percent of the latter two and virtually 100 percent of abscesses). More slowly growing tumors (astrocytomas) and particularly those outside the cerebral hemispheres (meningiomas, pituitary tumors) often produce no change in the EEG, though they may be very evident clinically. The EEG abnormality has the correct lateralization in as many as 75 to 90 percent of patients with subdural hematomas and supratentorial tumors or abscesses. A normal EEG and brain scan together almost exclude the presence of a supratentorial brain tumor or abscess. The EEG may be normal, however, in 20 to 25 percent of patients with infratentorial tumors.

Cerebrovascular disease Both the diffuse and localized EEG changes produced by vascular lesions such as cerebral infarcts and intracranial hemorrhages depend on their location and size rather than their type. The EEG has been shown to be useful in the differential diagnosis of vascular hemiplegia. If the lesion responsible is in the internal carotid or a major cerebral artery, an area of decreased normal activity and excessive slowing is practically always seen acutely in the appropriate region. If the hemiplegia is due to small-vessel disease, i.e., a lacunar infarction deep in the cerebrum or brainstem (Chap. 365), the EEG is usually normal. Large hemispheral lesions associated with acutely depressed levels of consciousness also produce widespread, diffuse, slow-wave activity of a nonspecific type as is seen with stupor or coma from any cause. Though a few very large infarctions betray themselves by ipsilaterally depressed EEG activity, most are not associated with asymmetric abnormalities acutely. Resolution begins after a few days, cerebral edema subsides, and focal activity may then be seen (slow-wave activity or suppression of normal background rhythms). Smaller infarctions are associated with acute focal abnormalities which lateralize the lesion well but do not localize it precisely. In contrast with tumors, further resolution continues, and after 3 to 6 months roughly 50 percent of patients with cerebrovascular accidents have a normal EEG despite the persistence of clinical abnormalities. Under these circumstances the prognosis for further recovery is poor. The EEG may be of lateralizing value in acute subarachnoid hemorrhage depending upon the extent to which the adjacent cerebrum is affected.

Brain injury Cerebral contusion or laceration produces EEG changes similar to those described for cerebrovascular disease. Diffuse changes often give way to focal ones, especially if the lesions are on the lateral or superior surface of the brain, and these in turn usually disappear over a period of weeks or months unless seizures supervene. Sharp waves or spikes sometimes emerge as the focal slow-wave abnormality resolves and may precede the occurrence of posttraumatic epilepsy. Following head injury, therefore, serial EEGs may be of prognostic value as regards the prospect of epilepsy.

Diseases which cause coma and states of impaired consciousness The EEG is abnormal in almost all conditions in which there is some impairment of consciousness (cf., brainstem infarctions above). With hypothyroidism the rhythms are normal in configuration but are usually slow. In general, the more profound the change in consciousness, the more abnormal the EEG recording. In these latter situations the slow waves (delta) are bilateral, are of high amplitude, and tend to be more conspicuous over the frontal regions. This pertains to such differing conditions as acute meningitis or encephalitis, severe disorders of blood gases, glucose, electrolyte and water balance, uremia, diabetic coma, liver coma, or impairment of consciousness accompanying the large cerebral lesions discussed above. In hepatic coma, the degree of abnormality in the EEG corresponds with the degree of confusion, stupor, or coma. Moreover, paroxysms of bilaterally synchronous large, sharp "triphasic waves" are characteristic, though they may also be seen with other metabolic encephalopathies associated with renal or pulmonary failure. Diffuse degenerative diseases (e.g., Alzheimer's disease and senile dementia) affecting the cerebral cortex are accompanied by relatively slight degrees of diffuse, slow-wave abnormality in the theta (4 to 7 Hz) range. Certain, more rapidly progressive ones, such as subacute sclerosing panencephalitis (SSPE), Creutzfeldt-Jakob disease, and to a lesser extent the cerebral lipidoses, have, in addition, very characteristic, almost pathognomonic EEG changes consisting of recurring complex bursts of sharp and slow activity. A normal EEG in a patient who is apathetic, slow, depressed, or forgetful is a point in favor of the diagnosis of an affective disorder or schizophrenia.

An EEG may also assist the physician in caring for a comatose patient when the pertinent history is unavailable. It may point to such otherwise unexpected causes as hepatic encephalopathy (bilaterally synchronous triphasic waves), intoxication with barbiturates or tranquilizers (excess fast activity), clinically inapparent continuous epileptic discharges, a large space-occupying lesion, or diffuse anoxia-ischemia.

Other diseases of the cerebrum There are many disorders of nervous function that cause little or no alteration in the EEG. Multiple sclerosis and other demyelinating diseases are examples, though as many as 50 percent of *advanced* cases will have an abnormal record. Delirium tremens and Wernicke-Korsakoff disease, despite the dramatic nature of the clinical picture, cause little or no changes in the EEG. Some degree of slowing usually accompanies confusional states which have been designated elsewhere as hypokinetic delirium (see Chap. 21). Interestingly, neuroses and psychoses, such as manic-depressive disorders or schizophrenia, abnormal states due to hallucinogenic drugs such as LSD, and the majority of cases of mental retardation are associated with no important modification of the normal record or with nonspecific abnormalities.

SPECIAL APPLICATIONS OF THE EEG Because the EEG provides information about the status and function of the cerebrum, it is useful as a monitor in the operating room to ensure the presence of a viable brain during the increasingly extensive procedures of modern cardiovascular surgery. EEG apparatus has long been available for indicating the level of anesthesia, and such simple equipment should eventually be used by the anesthetist to monitor both the cardiac and cerebral status of *all* patients during surgical anesthesia.

It is routine practice now for the EEG to be monitored continuously during carotid endarterectomies, a procedure performed in carefully selected patients suffering from stenotic or ulcerative carotid artery disease. Characteristic EEG changes signal the need for a temporary bypass shunt to maintain sufficient cerebral blood flow to preclude ischemic cerebral damage during surgery.

In the neurosurgical operating room the EEG can be recorded from the exposed brain (*electrocorticogram*), and seizure patterns can be localized more precisely than from the scalp so that resection of such physiologically abnormal tissue may be undertaken.

The routine EEG can be of value in the diagnosis of hysterical blindness. Similarly, a response evoked by noise during light sleep can be of help in confirming the presence of hearing in a patient who feigns total deafness. These responses may also be helpful in evaluating hearing and vision in infants.

Evoked responses An *evoked response* (sometimes termed an *evoked potential*) is the record of electrical activity produced by groups of neurones within the brainstem, thalamus, or cerebral hemispheres following stimulation of one or another sensory system by means of visual, auditory, or tactile input. The amplitude of these potentials, as recorded from the scalp using ordinary EEG electrodes, ranges from less than 0.5 to 20 μV. Because of their extremely small size, they can rarely be recognized on the ink-written EEG record amongst the background of ongoing EEG activity, which itself is usually 50 μV or more in amplitude. Therefore, special techniques, requiring simple computers, must be used to extract the evoked response waveform that one is interested in, from the continuous background EEG activity. These techniques are called "averaging" because the process involves repeating the stimulus many times and recording the electrical activity during a certain brief interval following each stimulus. The random ongoing EEG activity which, at any given point in time following the stimulus, is sometimes negative and at other times positive in polarity, tends to cancel out with sufficient repetition. The evoked response, on the other hand, is time-locked to the stimulus, and at a given time following the stimulus always has the same electrical sign as well as shape. The evoked response thus grows larger with repetition while the background averages out and becomes smaller. It is important to have special amplifiers, to apply the electrodes to the surface of the scalp with great care, and to time stimuli precisely with a minimum of accompanying electrical artifact.

The evoked response with the longest history of clinical usefulness is the *visual evoked response* (VER) produced by a pattern shift. During this test, patients sit in a chair with electrodes applied to their scalp and are asked to watch an alternating black and white checkerboard pattern which is projected on a screen. When patients concentrate on this pattern shift, it produces a characteristic waveform which can be recorded from the scalp over the posterior portion of the head. Under normal circumstances, this triphasic wave has a distinctive positive peak at 95 to 115 ms latency from the time of pattern reversal. This latency, the duration of the response, and the amplitude of this peak are measured during evaluation of the response; the latency is the most important parameter clinically. Each eye is tested independently.

Many disease processes affecting the optic nerve fibers in their intraocular, orbital, or intracranial portions produce abnormalities of this potential. Glaucoma, compression of the optic nerve, chiasma, or tract by various space-occupying lesions, and degenerative disease of this system often produce a reduction in amplitude and/or prolonged latency of the VER. If the visual system is sufficiently affected, no response may be recorded by stimulation of one or both eyes. In a general hospital setting, however, the most common cause of abnormality in this response is optic neuritis, frequently associated with multiple sclerosis. Demyelination of the optic nerve fibers because of primary demyelinating disease or other of the lesions listed above slows conduction in the nerve fibers so that the latency of the positive peak of the VER is prolonged (115 to 200 ms). In fact, almost all patients with optic neuritis, even after the visual acuity has returned to normal, continue to show distinct abnormalities in this pattern shift VER at a time when detailed ophthalmological evaluations reveal no abnormality.

Approximately one-half of the patients with multiple sclerosis who have never had visual symptoms also show abnormalities, and this accounts for one of the most useful aspects of the test. If a patient presents with what appears to be the first episode of a neurological illness in which the lesion is in the brainstem or spinal cord, for example, a demonstration by means of an abnormal pattern shift VER of another clinically unsuspected lesion in a different part of the central nervous system (the optic nerves) makes the diagnosis of multiple sclerosis more likely and may spare the patient certain neuroradiological procedures.

Abnormalities in visual acuity have no effect on the pattern shift VER unless the acuity is so poor that the patient cannot see the checkerboard pattern—patients with acuity of 20/200 or better are suitable for testing. The only other requirement is that the patient be cooperative enough to sit still for 20 to 40 min and watch the pattern. Therefore, children younger than 3 or 4 years of age usually cannot be tested in this way.

Brainstem auditory evoked responses (BAERs) are more difficult to obtain than *pattern shift* VER because BAERs are of the order of 0.5 µV in amplitude. These are produced by clicks transmitted to one of a patient's ears through earphones. The patient may be alert or comatose and need not be particularly cooperative except that an excess of movement or muscle artifact makes the response even more difficult to obtain. BAERs can be recorded from infants and children. BAERs consist of a series of seven waves which appear within the first 10 ms after the click. These are considered to represent successive activation of the auditory nerve and the brainstem auditory pathways (cochlear nucleus, superior olivary complex, lateral lemniscus, inferior colliculus, and higher auditory centers, such as the medial geniculate nucleus of the thalamus and thalamocortical radiations). A lesion at or between any of these levels either obliterates or delays the appearance of waves from successively high levels. Multiple sclerosis can, for example, also produce slow conduction between any of the levels in this test. The same is true of other lesions affecting the brainstem, such as small vascular lesions, central pontine myelinolysis, hypoxic damage, and so on. The waves which arise from structures caudal to the lesion are perfectly normal in latency, whereas those arising from structures cranial to the lesion are either obliterated or delayed. This allows one to pinpoint quite accurately the level of the lesion within the brainstem and provides a very neat opportunity for correlation of clinical observations with neurophysiological and occasionally pathological data. This test is useful as a screening test for patients with suspected acoustic neuromas, for patients suspected of having multiple sclerosis, for comatose patients in whom the level of lesion within the central nervous system is not clear, and for other patients in whom documentation of brainstem lesions is important. Hearing loss can often be recognized in this test, since changes in the latency of the first (and, therefore, subsequent) waves are produced, and these must be taken into consideration in the evaluation of the results obtained.

Somatosensory evoked responses (SERs) are produced by small, painless electrical stimuli administered to large sensory fibers in mixed nerves of the hand or foot. The afferent valley is recorded at many levels as it ascends the somatosensory pathways, and a series of waves can be recorded which reflect activity in peripheral nerve trunks, tracts in the spinal cord, gracile and cuneate nuclei, pontine and/or cerebellar structures, thalamus, thalamocortical radiations, and primary sensory fields of the cortex. Lesions of the pathways at any level affect the subsequent waves, thus providing localizing and confirmatory data in a similar fashion to the BAER.

Evoked responses can be used for a single evaluation of patients (looking for lesions in the various pathways discussed) or as a quantitative method for following a patient's course to document functional improvement or deterioration as time passes, following therapy, and so on. They also prove useful for on-line monitoring of function in optic nerve, brainstem, or spinal cord during neurosurgical procedures that involve manipulation of those structures. Longer latency auditory and somatosensory evoked responses have been studied for a number of years. These are largely cortically produced responses, dramatically affected by drowsiness, inattention, and other poorly controllable variables, and have not proven to be clinically useful. Neither have most visual evoked responses produced by stroboscopic flashes. They *are* useful in evaluation of visual pathways in infants and young children who are not cooperative enough to watch the checkerboard pattern and in adults during surgery or when comatose. Under other circumstances, pattern-shift VERs afford a much more reliable and reproducible response.

PSYCHOMETRY, PERIMETRY, AUDIOMETRY, AND TESTS OF LABYRINTHINE FUNCTION

These methods, drawn largely from the field of physiologic psychology, are of utility in quantitating and defining the nature of the psychic or sensory deficits produced by disease of the nervous system. Limitations of space do not permit a description of them here. The precise indications for doing these tests are (1) to obtain confirmation of a functional disorder in particular parts of the nervous system and to ascertain its nature, and (2) to quantitate the disorder in order to determine, by subsequent examinations, the natural course of the underlying illness.

BIOCHEMICAL TESTS

With advances in the biochemistry of metabolic diseases, a number of highly specific tests of serum, CSF, and circulating red and white blood cells have become available. These will be presented in relation to the metabolic diseases of which they are diagnostic.

REFERENCES

COOPER R et al: *EEG Technology,* 2d ed. London, Butterworths, 1974

DESMEDT JE (ed): *Visual Evoked Potentials in Man: New Developments.* Oxford, Clarendon Press, 1977

————: *Progress in Clinical Neurophysiology,* vol 2: *Auditory Evoked Potentials in Man.* Basel, Karger, 1977

————: *Progress in Clinical Neurophysiology,* vol 3: *Somatosensory Evoked Potentials and Their Clinical Uses.* Basel, Karger, 1978

GIBBS FA, GIBBS EL: *Atlas of Electroencephalography,* 2d ed, vols 1–3. Reading, Addison-Wesley, 1950–1964

KILOH LG et al: *Clinical Electroencephalography,* 3d ed. London, Butterworths, 1972

NEWTON TH, POTTS DG (eds): *Radiology of the Skull and Brain,* vol 3. St Louis, Mosby, 1977

REMOND A: *Handbook of Electroencephalography and Clinical Neurophysiology,* vols 1–15. Amsterdam, Elsevier, 1976–1978

TAVERAS J, WOOD EH: *Diagnostic Neuroradiology,* 2d ed, Golden's Diagnostic Radiology Series, sec 1. Baltimore, Williams & Wilkins, 1976

WERNER SS et al: *Atlas of Neonatal Electroencephalography.* New York, Raven Press, 1977

365
CEREBROVASCULAR DISEASES

JAY P. MOHR
C. MILLER FISHER
RAYMOND D. ADAMS

Vascular diseases of the nervous system rank first in frequency amongst all the neurologic diseases. They also provide one of the best approaches to the study of neurology since they compose about 50 percent of all neurologic hospital admissions to adult wards.

The term *cerebrovascular disease* refers to any disease implicating one or more of the blood vessels of the brain in a pathologic process. By *pathologic process* is meant any abnormality of the vessel wall, an occlusion by thrombus or embolus, rupture of a vessel, a failure of cerebral blood flow due to a fall in blood pressure, a change in the caliber of the lumen, altered permeability of the vascular wall, or increased viscosity or other quality of the blood. The pathologic process within the vessel may be described not only according to its grosser aspects—thrombosis, embolism, rupture of a vessel, etc.—but also in terms of the more basic vascular disorder, i.e., atherosclerosis, hypertensive arteriosclerosis, arteritis, trauma, aneurysm, developmental malformation. These processes result in two types of parenchymal changes in the brain, ischemia with

or without infarction, and hemorrhage. Other, less common, effects of vascular disease include syndromes of local pressure of an aneurysm, vascular headache (migraine, hypertension, arteritis), and occasionally increased intracranial pressure in hypertensive encephalopathy and venous thrombosis.

Obstruction of the nutrient artery by thrombus or embolus or failure of the systemic circulation and hypotension, if severe and prolonged enough, can deprive brain tissue of blood and oxygen, leading to ischemic disruption of physiologic function and subsequent necrosis (infarction).

Brain infarcts vary greatly in the amount of congestion and hemorrhage found within the softened tissue. Some infarcts are pallid (pale infarction); others show mild congestion (dilatation of vessels and some extravasation of red blood cells); still others show an extensive scattering of petechial hemorrhages throughout the damaged gray matter (hemorrhagic infarction). Thrombotic infarcts are usually pale, while embolic infarcts are sometimes pale, sometimes hemorrhagic; hemorrhagic infarction is usually a sign of embolism. Hemorrhagic infarction is often but not always associated with the fragmentation and migration of embolic material from its original site of arrest, the distal movement of the embolus allowing blood to enter the more proximal part of the infarct.

In hemorrhage an extravasation of blood occurs into the brain tissue, the subarachnoid space, or both. Once the leakage stops, the blood is slowly resorbed over a period of weeks and months. Damage to the brain results from physical disruption of the region directly involved and pressure of the mass of blood on the surrounding tissue.

THE STROKE SYNDROME

The cardinal feature of cerebrovascular disease is the *stroke,* a term that connotes the sudden and dramatic development of a focal neurologic deficit. In its severest form, the patient falls hemiplegic and even unconscious—an event so striking as to deserve its own separate designation, namely, apoplexy, stroke, shock, or cerebrovascular accident. In its mildest form, it may consist of only a trivial neurologic disorder insufficient to disturb the customary activities of the patient.

Undoubtedly, the most characteristic feature of a stroke is its *temporal profile.* It is the suddenness of syndrome development that stamps the disorder as vascular. The speed of evolution varies from seconds, minutes, rarely hours, or at most a few days, depending on the nature of the lesion. Embolic stroke and strokes with ruptured aneurysm characteristically begin suddenly, with the deficit reaching its maximum almost immediately. Thrombotic strokes frequently begin in a similar fashion, but may develop over a period of several days, usually progressing in a stepwise fashion, i.e., in a series of sudden changes, rather than smoothly. In a hemorrhage related to hypertension the deficit evolves smoothly over minutes or hours. An extensive deficit from ischemic cause may reverse itself dramatically within a few hours or a day. Rapid reversal never occurs in a hemorrhage related to hypertension. A slow, gradual, downhill course over a period of several days to a few weeks or more indicates that the process is probably not vascular in nature. Later in the course of a stroke illness, if the attack is not fatal, stabilization occurs, and is followed by some degree of improvement, especially in cases with deficits in language function. The improvement is gradual, taking place over weeks and months.

The neurologic deficit in a stroke reflects both the location and the size of the infarct or hemorrhage in the brain. Hemiplegia is the classic sign of vascular disease and occurs with

Rolandic A

Prerolandic A

Post. communicating A

Ant. parietal A

A

Post. parietal A

Lateral
Orbito-frontal A
Middle
cerebral stem
Ant. cerebral A

Angular A

Central
retinal A

Post. temporal A

Vertebral A

B

C

Ophthalmic A

Basilar A

Int. carotid A

Post. cerebral A

Ext. carotid A

D

Persistent
trigeminal A

B

Common
carotid A

D

Ascending
cervical A

Vertebral A

Ophthalmic A
Supraorbital A

Nasal A

R. subclavian A

Innominate A

Aortic arch

Angular A

C

Deep
cervical A

Thyrocervical A

Lacrimal A

FIGURE 365-1

Arrangement of the major arteries on the right side carrying blood from the heart to the brain. Also shown are vessels of collateral circulation that may modify the effects of cerebral ischemia. For example, the posterior communicating artery connects the internal carotid and the posterior ce-

rebral arteries, and may provide anastomosis between the carotid and basilar systems. Over the convexity, the subarachnoid interarterial anastomoses linking the middle, anterior, and posterior cerebral arteries are shown, with inset A illustrating that these anastomoses are a continuous network of tiny arteries forming a border zone between the major cerebral strokes involving the cerebral hemisphere or the brainstem. However, depending on its location, a stroke may also give rise to many other manifestations accompanying or independent of hemiplegia, including numbness, sensory deficit, dysphasia, blindness, diplopia, dizziness, and dysarthria. Familiarity with the neurovascular syndromes outlined in this chapter will aid in locating the lesion in individual cases of stroke and in determining whether the stroke represents ischemia or hemorrhage.

Laboratory assessment of stroke provides further data concerning its site, size, and type of brain lesion, and, if possible, the status of arteries or veins involved in the stroke process. *Computerized tomography* of the brain (CT scan) has recently proved a most valuable diagnostic tool for the demonstration of hematomas (during the first 3 to 5 weeks of their existence), acute hemorrhagic infarcts, and ischemic infarcts in the acute state when swelling of the necrotic tissue first appears (days) and later in the chronic state when the tissue cavitates. *Radionuclide brain scanning* successfully images many hematomas and some infarcts in their subacute stage (days to weeks), but hematomas cannot be seen in the late stages (months or years). *Arteriography* with radiopaque dyes demonstrates stenoses and occlusions of the larger vessels and aneurysms and arteriovenous malformations. Embolic occlusions are demonstrable in 75 percent of cases, especially in the initial hours and days after stroke, but in less than 15 percent when arteriography is carried out more than 2 days after the stroke. The larger hematomas are seen in arteriograms to cause displacement of vessels (mass effect); and in hemorrhages due to aneurysm, in 85 percent of cases they demonstrate the ruptured aneurysm as well as associated arterial spasm. *Lumbar puncture* regularly yields bloody fluid in ruptured aneurysm or vascular malformation or ventricular extension of a hypertensive hemorrhage and occasionally in hemorrhagic infarction. The cerebrospinal fluid (CSF) is clear in bland infarction from either embolus or thrombus.

ISCHEMIC STROKE

The effects of both thrombotic and embolic arterial occlusion relate to the topography of the occluded artery and vary according to the availability of *collateral or anastomotic blood flow.* If the obstruction lies proximal to the circle of Willis, collateral flow via the circle may be adequate to prevent infarction. In occlusion of the internal carotid artery in the neck, anastomotic flow may pass along the external carotid artery and retrograde in the ophthalmic artery or other smaller external-internal connections. In vertebral artery blockage low in the neck, blood may reach the upper part of the vertebral artery via the deep cervical, thyrocervical, occipital artery, or retrograde from the other vertebral artery. If the occlusion is distal to the circle of Willis, i.e., in the stem of one of the cerebral or cerebellar arteries, a series of subarachnoid border zone interarterial anastomoses that join many of the branches

arterial territories. Occasionally a persistent trigeminal artery connects the internal carotid and basilar arteries proximal to the circle of Willis, as shown in inset B. Anastomoses between the internal and external carotid arteries via the orbit are illustrated in inset C. Wholly extracranial anastomoses from muscular branches of the cervical arteries to vertebral and external carotid arteries are indicated by inset D.

of the major cerebral arteries may carry sufficient blood into the compromised tissue to lessen the ischemic damage (Fig. 365-1). The capillary anastomotic system between adjacent brain arteries, although always the source of some collateral supply, is probably inconsequential. Thus in the event of occlusion of a major arterial trunk the extent of infarction ranges from none (rare) to softening throughout the entire territory. Between these two extremes are countless variations in the size, shape, and completeness of an infarct, depending on such ischemic modifying factors as the speed of occlusion (time for compensation), the level of the systemic blood pressure, hypoxia, and altered physical state of the blood.

The *specific neurologic abnormality* depends on the location and size of the infarct or the focus of ischemia. The territory of any vessel, large or small, deep or superficial, may be involved. In involvement of the carotid system, *unilateral* signs predominate: hemiplegia, hemihypesthesia, hemianopia, aphasia, and agnosia. In basilar disease, one more commonly finds *bilateral* signs, motor and/or sensory, in combination with a disturbance of cranial nerves, cerebellum, or other structures localized in or related to the brainstem.

NEUROVASCULAR SYNDROMES

While the clinical picture resulting from the occlusion of any particular artery differs in minor ways from one patient to another, there is sufficient uniformity to permit diagnosis. Partial syndromes are in the majority. The following descriptions apply particularly to infarction and ischemia due to embolism or thrombosis. Although hemorrhage within these vascular territories may give rise to many of the same effects, the total clinical picture is apt to differ because in its deep extension the hemorrhage may involve the territory of more than one vessel and by its mass effect may cause an increase in intracranial pressure.

INTERNAL CAROTID ARTERY The clinical picture of occlusion of the internal carotid artery is variable. Not infrequently occlusion is completely asymptomatic, while in other cases it produces a devastating, massive infarction which leads to death in a few days. Every shade of variation lies between these two extremes. Most often the infarct involves some part of the middle cerebral territory, but when the anterior communicating artery is very small, the ipsilateral anterior cerebral territory may be affected too, in which case the anterior part of the hemisphere (the frontal lobe) bears the brunt of the insult, while the region posterior to the rolandic fissure tends to be spared. When both anterior cerebral arteries arise from a common stem on one side, infarction may involve the anterior cerebral territory bilaterally. The posterior cerebral artery is infrequently supplied from the internal carotid rather than from the basilar artery, and its territory, too, may be softened, and thus the entire hemisphere and even part of the other may be involved. The tissue in the territory of the anterior choroidal artery may also be infarcted. When one carotid has been occluded at a previous time, occlusion of the other can contribute to a catastrophic infarction of both the cerebral hemispheres. In such cases, coma with quadriplegia and continuous horizontal conjugate "metronomic" eye movements may be seen.

In symptomatic occlusion of the internal carotid artery the picture resembles that of middle cerebral occlusion with contralateral hemiplegia, hemihypesthesia, and aphasia (with involvement of the dominant hemisphere). When the anterior cerebral territory is also infarcted, the clinical picture will be broadened to include some or all its clinical effects (see below). Such patients are much less responsive than those with lesions in the territory of only one cerebral artery, and often they are in a coma. Headache may also occur with both cerebral thrombosis or embolism in the carotid artery; the pain is situated just above the eyebrow. That associated with occlusion of the middle cerebral artery is usually more lateral, at the temple and, with occlusion of the posterior cerebral artery, in or behind the eye.

When the circulation in one carotid is compromised and collateral flow is restricted, the tissue in the most distal or terminal parts of the territories of the middle and anterior and at times the posterior cerebral arteries suffers first and most severely. This gives rise to an irregular and asymmetric *border-zone* (watershed) configuration of infarction in which the contiguous distal fields of each vessel are disproportionately affected, the heaviest involvement usually falling on the fronto-central regions of the middle cerebral artery territory. When well developed, the zone of damage forms an elongated strip of variable width extending from the frontal pole to the occipital. Therefore carotid infarcts of less than maximal extent tend to be located distally rather than proximally in the sylvian region. Likewise it is in this most vulnerable region that transient ischemic attack symptoms are liable to arise in carotid stenosis, taking the form of weakness or paresthesias in the upper extremity and, only if more extensive, in the face and tongue. Relative sparing of the posterior part of the hemisphere is reflected in a low incidence of central aphasia and persistent homonymous hemianopia.

In addition to nourishing the brain, the internal carotid artery supplies the optic nerve and retina via the ophthalmic artery (Fig. 365-1). Transient monocular blindness occurs intermittently as a warning symptom prior to the onset of the stroke in approximately 25 percent of cases of symptomatic carotid occlusion. Of interest, and presumably reflecting good

collateral blood supply, central retinal artery occlusion rarely appears under such circumstances.

Whereas most cerebral vessels are inaccessible within the skull and topical diagnosis is made only by inference, in carotid disease more direct diagnostic tests are available. Pressure in the central retinal artery is usually reduced on the side of carotid occlusion or severe stenosis and is usually a significant sign when the values for diastole are below 20 mmHg. Dilated collateral channels coursing over the forehead may also suggest carotid occlusion. Supraorbital and supratrochlear arterial pulsations on the rim of the orbit may be prominent but easily suppressed upon simultaneous compression of the facial or superficial temporal branches of the external carotid artery. The usual blood supply from the internal carotid artery via the ophthalmic artery has then been reversed, indicating collateralization of internal carotid from external carotid sources. Retinal embolism, either of shining white or plain type, may point to carotid disease. Severe stenosis within the carotid sinus due to an atherosclerotic plaque—with or without superimposed thrombus—may give rise to a local bruit, which can be an important finding in disease of the carotid artery. Occasionally the murmur results from stenosis at the mouth of the external carotid artery and can then be misleading. If the murmur is heard at the angle of the jaw, the stenosis is in the carotid sinus; if lower in the neck, the stenosis is in the common carotid or subclavian artery. (Distal propagation of an aortic valvular murmur must be distinguished from carotid bruits.) An additional sign of carotid occlusion is the presence of an intracranial murmur over the *opposite* carotid artery. This is heard best by placing the bell of the stethoscope over the eyeball. The murmur is presumably due to augmented blood flow through the remaining patent vessel. Pulsation may be reduced or absent in the internal or common carotid arteries in the neck, in the external carotid branch in front of the ear, or in the internal carotid artery when palpated in the pharynx, but minor asymmetries in pulsations are rarely significant when present as an isolated finding. *Because of the possibility* of precipitous onset of unconsciousness, seizures, or an electroen-

Int. capsule

Ant. cerebral A

Middle cerebral A

Claustrum

Putamen

Body of caudate

Thalamus

Post. cerebral A

Globus pallidus

Red nucleus

Subthalamic body

Cerebral peduncle

Uncus

Ant. choroidal A

(Lower 2/3 of int. capsule, globus pallidus, uncus, amygdala ant. hippocampus)

Post. cerebral A

Penetrating branches of middle cerebral A

(Putamen, upper int capsule, lower corona radiata, body of caudate)

FIGURE 365-2

Diagram of a cerebral hemisphere, coronal section, showing the territories of the major cerebral vessels.

cephalographic change, testing the carotid circulation by compressing the artery is not recommended.

Occlusion of the cervical segments of the carotid and subclavian or innominate arteries proximal to the internal carotid is frequently asymptomatic because of the abundant collateral circulation. The following manifestations, for the most part nonneurologic, have been reported when collateral flow proves inadequate: Absence of pulsation in carotid and radial arteries, faintness on arising from the horizontal position, recurrent loss of consciousness, headache, neck pain, paresthesias of various parts of the body, transient blindness (unilateral or bilateral), dimness of vision with exercise, premature cataracts, retinal atrophy and pigmentation, atrophy of the iris, leukomas, peripapillary arteriovenous anastomoses, optic atrophy, claudication of the jaw muscles, perforation of the nasal septum, saddle nose deformity, trophic ulceration of the face, facial atrophy (unilateral or bilateral), indolent infections of the face, abnormal facial pigmentation, and loss of hair. Pulseless disease expresses its cerebral effects through occlusion of both carotid arteries. Originally described in Japan, particularly in young women and called Takayasu's disease, it consists essentially of a granulomatous arteritis of unknown cause involving all three major trunks arising from the aortic arch (see Chap. 252). An incomplete aortic arch syndrome consisting of various combinations of carotid, subclavian, or innominate occlusion or stenosis is not uncommon. The majority of the cases of pulseless disease in the United States and Europe, both the partial and the complete syndrome, have been due to severe atherosclerosis. Often this has been mistakenly called *Buerger's disease.*

MIDDLE CEREBRAL ARTERY This artery through its cortical branches supplies the lateral surface of the hemisphere. Its territory includes the cortex and white matter of the lateral and inferior aspects of the frontal lobe, the motor cortex (areas 4 and 6, and centers for contraversive eye movements, and in the dominant hemisphere the motor speech area of Broca), the cortex and white matter of the lateral parietal lobe (sensory cortex, angular and supramarginal convolutions), the lateral and superior parts of the temporal lobe, and the insula. The penetrating branches of the middle cerebral artery supply the putamen, outer globus pallidus, the posterior limb of the internal capsule above the plane of the upper border of the globus pallidus, the adjacent part of the corona radiata, the body of the caudate nucleus, and the superior and lateral portions of the head of the caudate nucleus (Fig. 365-2).

The middle cerebral artery may be occluded in its stem, blocking the mouths of the penetrating vessels as well as the flow to the superficial (cortical) vessels, or its major branches can be blocked individually. The classic picture of total infarction is a contralateral hemiplegia, hemianesthesia, homonymous hemianopia, global or total sensorimotor aphasia (left hemisphere), and apractagnosia (right hemisphere). Once established, the motor, sensory, and language deficits usually remain static or very little improved after the passage of months or even years. Seldom can the patient ever again communicate effectively. Quite deceptive is some form of echoic speech function from the earliest stages of the deficit, encouraging the family and physician to assume that speech is not severely affected. But these stereotypic greetings, short word utterances, and the repetition of short words generally remain as the only language performance of which the patient is capable. When collateral circulation restricts the ischemia to a part of the territory, the deficit is more limited.

Thrombotic occlusion of the stem of the middle cerebral artery is relatively uncommon compared with embolic. Branch occlusion (usually embolic) produces a corresponding partial deficit. The embolus may block the vessel to the anterior or

motor part of the hemisphere (superior division) or the posterior or sensory part of the hemisphere (inferior division) (Fig. 365-3). Major occlusion of the superior division causes a dense sensorimotor deficit in the face and limbs and total aphasia (left) that mimics the syndrome of occlusion of the stem of the middle cerebral artery or the carotid artery.

Varying degrees of improvement follow occlusions of branches of the major branches of the middle cerebral artery. Within weeks, there is usually sufficient motor improvement that the patient can walk on his spastic leg while motor deficits of arm and face frequently remain severe. The initial total aphasia changes toward predominantly motor aphasia, with improvement in comprehension of spoken and written language and the emergence of a hesitant, grammatically simplified, dysmelodic speech that limits language capabilities.

Because the upper division gives off its branches in sequence, an occlusion limited to only one of them elicits a highly circumscribed infarct that fractionates the syndrome even farther. In occlusion of the ascending frontal branch, involving Broca's area and immediate surrounding territory, the sensorimotor deficit is limited to faciobrachial paresis with little weakness of the leg, and the speech disorder consists of an initial mutism with very mild comprehension disorder. Within hours to weeks, the weakness lessens, and the grammatically appropriate speech improves so that comprehension is essentially normal and only a dysmelodic articulatory abnormality persists. Occlusion of rolandic branches produces a sensorimotor paresis with severe dysarthria that may follow a clinical course suggestive of pure motor stroke from a lacunar infarct (see "Lacunar Syndromes" below) but with little sign of dysphasia. When ascending parietal and other posterior branches of the upper division are occluded, the result is a deficit currently described as "conduction" aphasia, and ideomotor dyspraxia affecting both sides of the body, but often no significant sensorimotor deficit. The speech disorder usually improves to a normal or near-normal state within months.

The lower division of the middle cerebral artery is only infrequently occluded alone, but when it is so involved (almost always from an embolus and only with great rarity from thrombosis), Wernicke's aphasia is the usual result (Chap. 24). The deficit remains static for months and even years but tends to improve. In less extensive infarcts, the more distal parietal, temporal, and occipital regions are collateralized via the branches of the posterior cerebral artery, and the major involvement is more or less confined to the posterior temporal regions. Such patients often show greater deficit on language tests that involve auditory comprehension and perform better, sometimes almost normally, in reading. Within weeks or months, the disorder improves to the point that it is evident only in self-generated efforts at speaking and writing. Especially in the later stages, the deficit resembles the syndrome of conduction aphasia resulting from occlusion of posterior branches of the upper division of the middle cerebral artery. The site and size of the infarct are difficult to predict on clinical grounds alone. In right nondominant lesions a syndrome of apractagnosia results, and in both right- and left-sided lesions there is usually a homonymous hemianopia.

ANTERIOR CEREBRAL ARTERY This artery, through its cortical branches, supplies the anterior four-fifths of the medial surface of the cerebral hemisphere, including the medial part of the orbital surface of the frontal lobe, the frontal lobe, a strip of the lateral surface along the superior border, and the anterior seven-eighths of the corpus callosum. The deep branches,

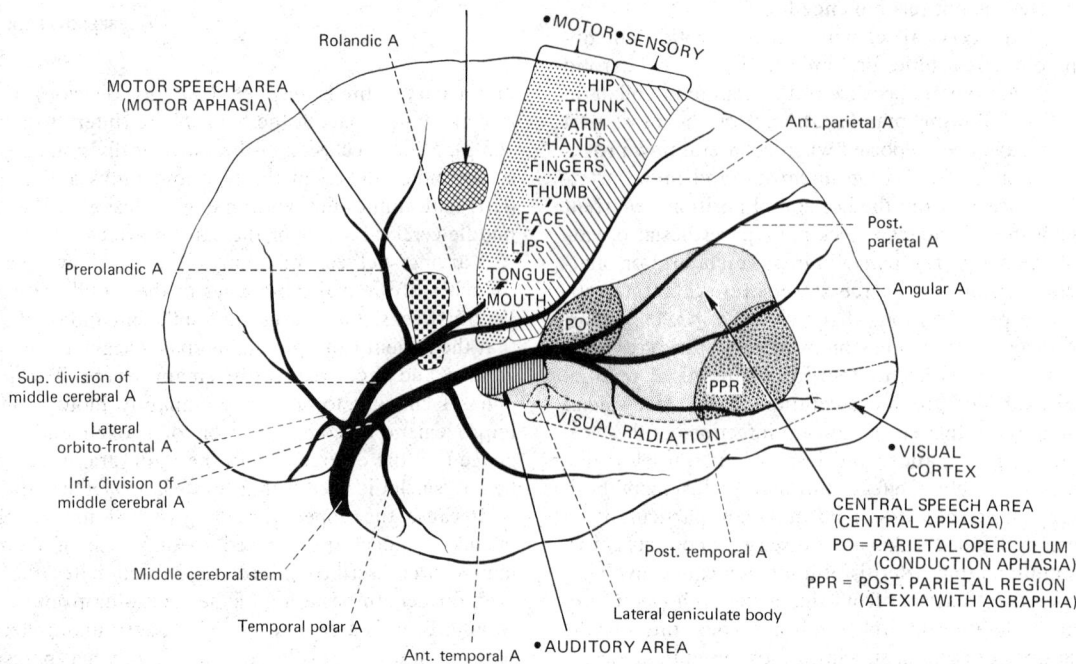

FIGURE 365-3

Diagram of a cerebral hemisphere, lateral aspect, showing the branches and distribution of the middle cerebral artery and the principal regions of cerebral localization.

which arise near the circle of Willis, run chiefly to the anterior limb of the internal capsule and inferior part of the head of the caudate nucleus (see Fig. 365-4).

Again the clinical picture will depend on the location and size of the infarct, which in turn depend on the site of the occlusion, the pattern of the circle of Willis, and the other ischemia-modifying factors. Occlusion of the stem of the anterior cerebral artery proximal to the anterior communicating artery is usually well tolerated, since collateral flow will come from its mate of the opposite side. The maximal disturbance occurs when both anterior cerebral arteries happen to arise from one anterior cerebral stem, occlusion of which then results in infarction of the anterior cerebral territory of both hemispheres. This may include bilateral pyramidal signs with paraplegia and profound mental symptoms.

Complete occlusion of one anterior cerebral artery, distal to the anterior communicating, results in infarction in the entire territory and presents clinically as a sensorimotor deficit in-

volving the opposite foot and leg, a lesser degree of paresis of the opposite arm, and sparing of the face. A complex syndrome of contralateral grasp and sucking reflex, paratonic rigidity (gegenhalten), and unwitting urinary incontinence is often evident. Other disorders in behavior and praxis that may be overlooked in routine clinical evaluations include abulia (a syndrome of slowness, lack of spontaneity, and laconic spoken or motor responses), delay in response, intermittent interruption of behavior, tendency to speak in a whisper, reflexive distraction by sights and sounds, dyspraxia and tactile aphasia of the left limbs (from callosal involvement), and several weeks of mutism with rare echolalia, without disturbed comprehension or hemianopia.

Well-studied cases of infarction of the territory of the anterior cerebral artery are not numerous, and all the syndromes of this artery have not been clearly determined.

ANTERIOR CHOROIDAL ARTERY A few incomplete clinicopathologic studies have been the basis of present knowledge of the syndrome of this artery. It is said to consist of contralateral hemiplegia, hemianesthesia (hypesthesia), and homonymous hemianopia, all due to involvement of the posterior limb of the

FIGURE 365-4

Diagram of a cerebral hemisphere, medial aspect, showing the branches and distribution of the anterior cerebral artery and the principal regions of cerebral localization.

internal capsule and the white matter posterolateral to it, through which the first part of the geniculocalcarine fibers passes. In the reported cases, however, the clinical syndrome usually falls short of what is expected on anatomic grounds. Surgical occlusion of the vessel also has produced little or no deficit. It has yet to be demonstrated that such a syndrome exists.

VERTEBRAL-BASILAR, POSTERIOR CEREBRAL SYSTEM   Posterior cerebral artery   In 70 percent of cases both posterior cerebral arteries arise from the basilar artery; in 22 percent one comes from the basilar and the other one from the internal carotid artery; and in 8 percent both come from the internal carotid. The terminal or cortical branches of this vessel supply the undersurface of the temporal and occipital lobes, as well as the entire medial surface of the occipital lobe including the visual area (areas 17, 18, and 19).

From the more proximal part of the artery between its origin at the bifurcation of the basilar artery and the cortical distribution many important branches arise. The interpeduncular branches arising near its origin penetrate the brainstem to supply the red nucleus, subthalamic nucleus of Luys, substantia nigra, the most medial part of the cerebral peduncle, the oculomotor nucleus, the reticular substance of the midbrain, the decussation of the superior cerebellar peduncles, rubrothalamic tract, medial longitudinal fasciculus, and the medial lemniscus. The thalamoperforate branches also arise here and pass to the inferior, posterior, medial, and anterior parts of the thalamus. Branches arising serially along the parent vessel as it encircles the midbrain supply the cerebral peduncle, lateral part of the tegmentum, corpora quadrigemina, pineal gland, lateral geniculate body, choroid plexus, and hippocampus. The thalamogeniculate branches which originate distal to the junction with the posterior communicating artery supply the pulvinar and the posterior lateral nuclei of the thalamus (Fig. 365-5).

For convenience of exposition it is helpful to divide the various syndromes into three groups: (1) anterior and proximal (involving perforating branches), (2) cortical (inferior temporal and medial occipital), and (3) bilateral.

Anterior and proximal   The thalamic syndrome of Dejerine and Roussy is due to infarction of the sensory relay nuclei in the thalamus from occlusion of the thalamogeniculate branches. Here a transitory hemiparesis is usually accompanied by a severe sensory loss of the opposite side of the body (deep and cutaneous). In some instances there is a dissociation of sensation, with pain and temperature being more affected than touch, vibration, and position senses, or only one part of the body may be rendered anesthetic. After an interval of time elapses and sensation begins to return, the patient begins to be afflicted with pain and hyperpathia in the affected parts. There may also be distortion of taste, athetotic posturing and ataxia of the hand, and depression of mood. Such conditions may persist for years. A homonymous hemianopia is usually conjoined.

Central midbrain and subthalamic syndromes are due to occlusion of paramedian branches on one or both sides. The findings include Weber's syndrome (oculomotor palsy with contralateral hemiplegia), paralysis of vertical gaze, stupor or coma, and a movement disorder, most often ataxia. Hemiplegia from infarction of the cerebral peduncle is relatively rare.

In the anteromedial, inferior thalamus syndrome from occlusion of the thalamoperforate branches, the main effect is an extrapyramidal movement disorder. Hemiballismus is due usually to occlusion of a small branch. Hemiathetosis with or without deep sensory loss, hemiataxia, and tremor are found in various combinations.

Cortical syndromes   Classically, occlusion of the branches to temporal and occipital lobes gives rise to a homonymous hemianopia because of involvement of the primary visual receptive area or calcarine (striate) cortex. It may be incomplete and then involves the upper quadrants of the visual fields more than the lower. Macular or central vision may be spared because of collateralization of the occipital pole from distal branches of the middle cerebral (or anterior cerebral) artery. Posterior cortical infarcts of the dominant hemisphere cause alexia, anomia (amnesic aphasia), and impaired memory. The alexia, unaccompanied by agraphia, often is so severe that patients act as if their own written language were foreign. The anomias (dysnomias) are most severe for colors, but may include other visual stimuli such as pictures, musical notes, mathematical symbols, and manipulable objects. Patients may treat some objects as familiar; that is to say, they can describe them functionally and use them correctly while having forgotten their names (amnesic aphasia). The memory deficit for recent events is of moderate severity and may or may not im-

FIGURE 365-5

Inferior aspect of the brain with the branches and distribution of the posterior cerebral artery and the principal anatomic structures.

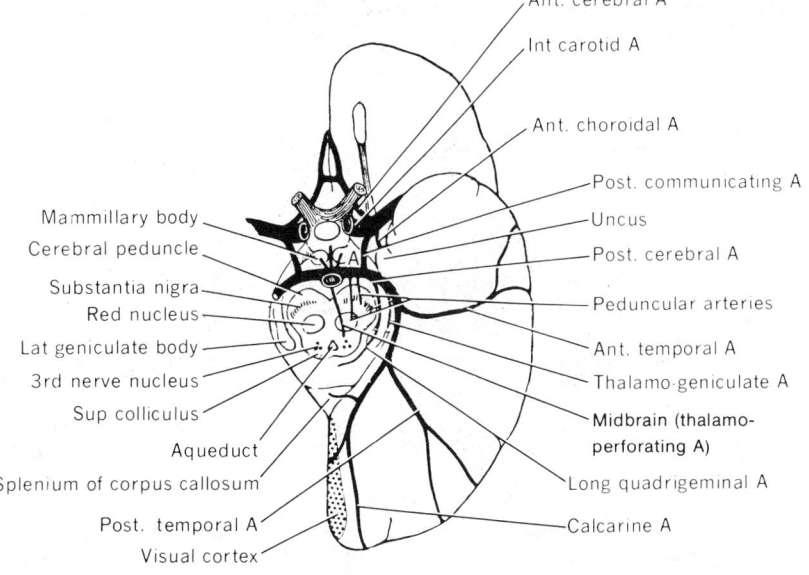

Ant. cerebral A

Int carotid A

Ant. choroidal A

Post. communicating A

Uncus

Post. cerebral A

Peduncular arteries

Ant. temporal A

Thalamo-geniculate A

Midbrain (thalamo-perforating A)

Long quadrigeminal A

Calcarine A

Mammillary body

Cerebral peduncle

Substantia nigra

Red nucleus

Lat geniculate body

3rd nerve nucleus

Sup colliculus

Aqueduct

Splenium of corpus callosum

Post. temporal A

Visual cortex

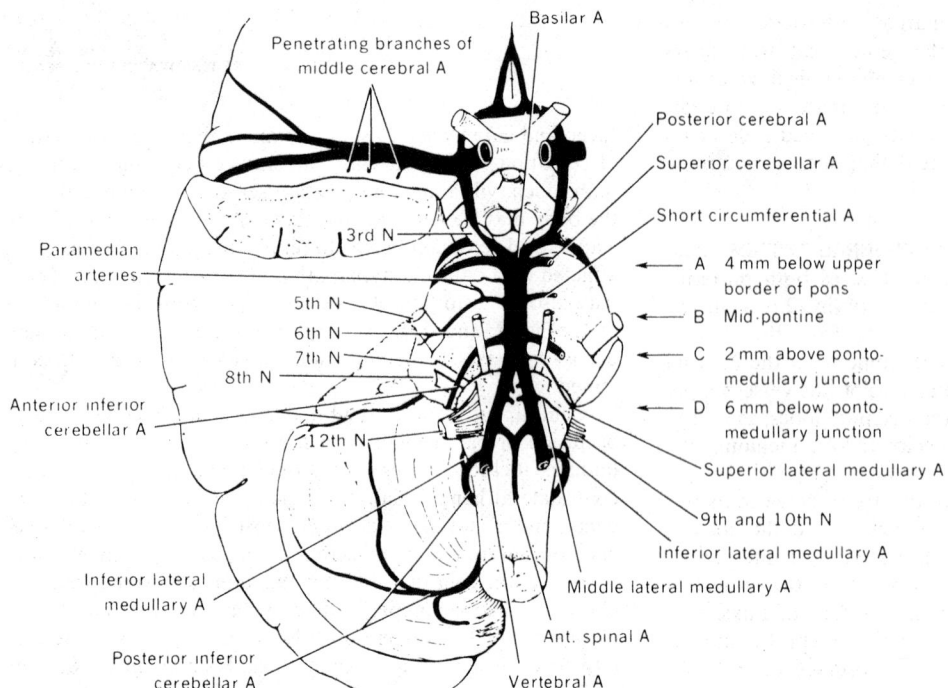

Penetrating branches of
middle cerebral A

Basilar A

Posterior cerebral A

Superior cerebellar A

Short circumferential A

3rd N

Paramedian
arteries

5th N
6th N
7th N
8th N

Anterior inferior
cerebellar A

12th N

Inferior lateral
medullary A

Posterior inferior
cerebellar A

Ant. spinal A

Vertebral A

Middle lateral medullary A

Inferior lateral medullary A

9th and 10th N

Superior lateral medullary A

A	4 mm below upper border of pons
B	Mid-pontine
C	2 mm above ponto-medullary junction
D	6 mm below ponto-medullary junction

FIGURE 365-6

Diagram of the brainstem at top of figure shows the principal vessels of the vertebral-basilar system. The letters and arrows on the right indicate the levels of the four cross sections A, B, C, and D which follow. Although typical vascular syndromes of the pons and medulla have been designated by sharply outlined shaded areas, the student must appreciate that since satisfactory clinicopathologic studies are far from numerous, the diagrams are not necessarily accurate, nor do they always represent established facts. The great frequency with which infarcts fail to produce a well-recognized syndrome and the special tendency for syndromes to merge with one another must be emphasized.

prove with the passage of time. Color anomia and amnesic aphasia are more often present in this syndrome than is alexia. Nondominant hemisphere lesions are commonly accompanied by topographic disorientation and dysnomia for faces (so-called prosopagnosia). (See Chap. 25.)

A complete proximal arterial occlusion leads to a syndrome that combines anterior and proximal with cortical syndromes in part or totally. The vascular lesion may be either an embolus or an atherosclerotic thrombus.

Bilateral occipital infarcts   These may occur from a single embolism or a succession of emboli in the upper basilar artery. Thrombosis has similar effects, especially if the posterior communicating arteries are unusually small.

Bilateral lesions of the occipital lobes, if extensive, cause total blindness of the cortical type, i.e., a bilateral homonymous hemianopia. The pupillary reflexes are preserved, and fundoscopically the optic disks are normal. Often patients are unaware of their blindness and may in fact deny it, even when it is pointed out to them. More frequently the bilateral lesions are incomplete, and a sector of the visual field remains intact. When the remnant is small, vision appears to fluctuate from

moment to moment, as patients attempt to capture the image in the island of intact vision. Hysteria may be suspected because of such inconsistencies. In small bilateral calcarine lesions there may be a loss of only central vision (bilateral homonymous central scotomas). In other cases only central vision may remain, leaving the patient with gun-barrel sight.

With bilateral lesions loss of memory may be severe (Korsakoff's amnesic state). Other common accompaniments are apraxia of ocular movements, inability to enumerate objects, inability to turn the eyes to a precise point in the visual fields (ocular ataxia), distortions of vision (macropsia and micropsia), difficulty in seeing, to-and-fro movements of eyes, and a tendency to run into obstacles that are seen, as though unable to avoid them.

Vertebral artery   The vertebral arteries are the chief arteries of the medulla, and each supplies the lower three-fourths of the pyramid, the medial lemniscus, all or nearly all the retroolivary region (the lateral medullary region), the restiform body, and the posteroinferior part of the cerebellar hemisphere (see Figs. 365-6 to 365-10). The relative sizes of the vertebral arteries vary a good deal, and in approximately 10 percent of cases,

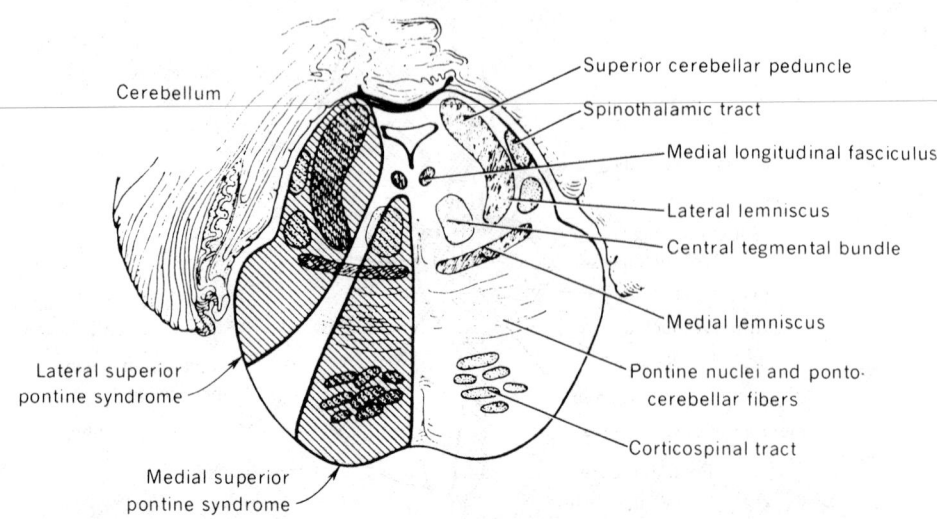

Cerebellum

Superior cerebellar peduncle

Spinothalamic tract

Medial longitudinal fasciculus

Lateral lemniscus

Central tegmental bundle

Medial lemniscus

Pontine nuclei and ponto-cerebellar fibers

Corticospinal tract

Lateral superior
pontine syndrome

Medial superior
pontine syndrome

FIGURE 365-7

Medial superior pontine syndrome (paramedian branches of upper basilar artery). Lateral superior pontine syndrome (syndrome of superior cerebellar artery).

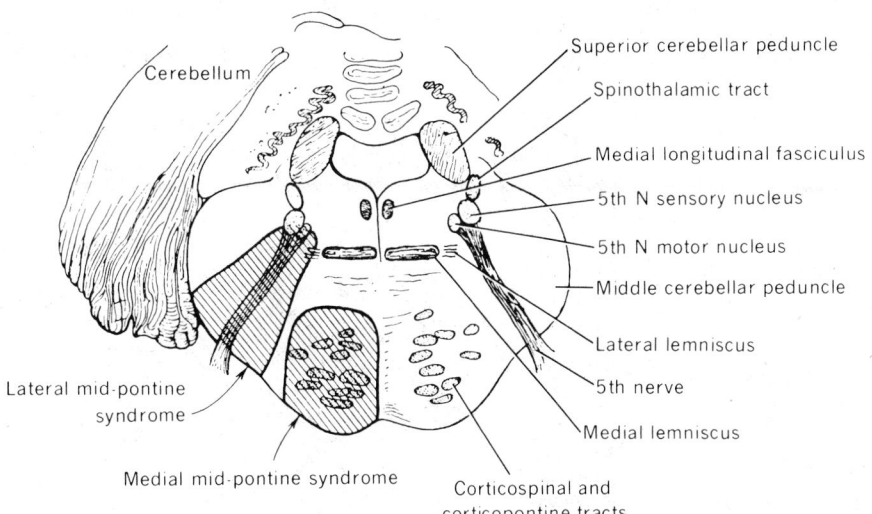

FIGURE 365-8

Medial midpontine syndrome (paramedian branch of midbasilar artery). Lateral midpontine syndrome (short circumferential artery).

one vessel is so small that the other can be considered the only artery of supply to the brainstem. In this case, if collateral inflow from the carotid system via the circle of Willis is unavailable, occlusion would be equivalent to occlusion of the basilar artery or bilateral occlusion of the vertebral arteries. The posterior inferior cerebellar artery is usually a branch of the vertebral artery, but can have a common origin with the anterior inferior cerebellar artery from the basilar artery. It is necessary to keep these anatomic variations in mind when visualizing the effects of vertebral artery occlusion.

The results of vertebral occlusion are quite variable. When there are two good-sized arteries, occlusion on one side occurs not infrequently without any recognizable symptoms and signs or pathologic changes. If the subclavian artery is blocked proximal to the origin of the vertebral artery, exercise of the arm on that side may draw blood from the vertebral-basilar system into the arm, sometimes resulting in the symptoms of basilar insufficiency. This has been called by Fisher the "subclavian steal" syndrome. If the occlusion of the vertebral artery is so situated as to block the mouth of one or more arteries supplying the lateral medulla, the lateral medullary syndrome may be precipitated, and this is probably the most common consequence of vertebral occlusion (see below). When the branch to the anterior spinal artery is blocked, collateral influx from the spinal artery branch of the opposite side is usually sufficient to prevent infarction of the spinal cord. If a branch to the pyramid is occluded, that part of the corticospinal tract may be infarcted unless collateral flow is adequate. Also, any of these branches may become occluded in its course after leaving the vertebral artery and may produce similar effects. Rarely, occlusion of the vertebral artery or one of its medial branches produces an infarct which involves the medullary pyramid, the medial lemniscus, and the emergent hypoglossal fibers [contralateral paralysis of arm and leg (face spared), contralateral loss of position and vibration sense, and ipsilateral paralysis and atrophy of the tongue]. This is the medial medullary syndrome (see Fig. 365-10). Vertebral occlusion can also lead to symptoms by blocking the posterior inferior cerebellar

FIGURE 365-9

Medial inferior pontine syndrome (occlusion of paramedian branch of basilar artery). Lateral inferior pontine syndrome (occlusion of anterior inferior cerebellar artery). Total unilateral inferior pontine syndrome (occlusion of anterior inferior cerebellar artery). Lateral and medial syndromes combined.

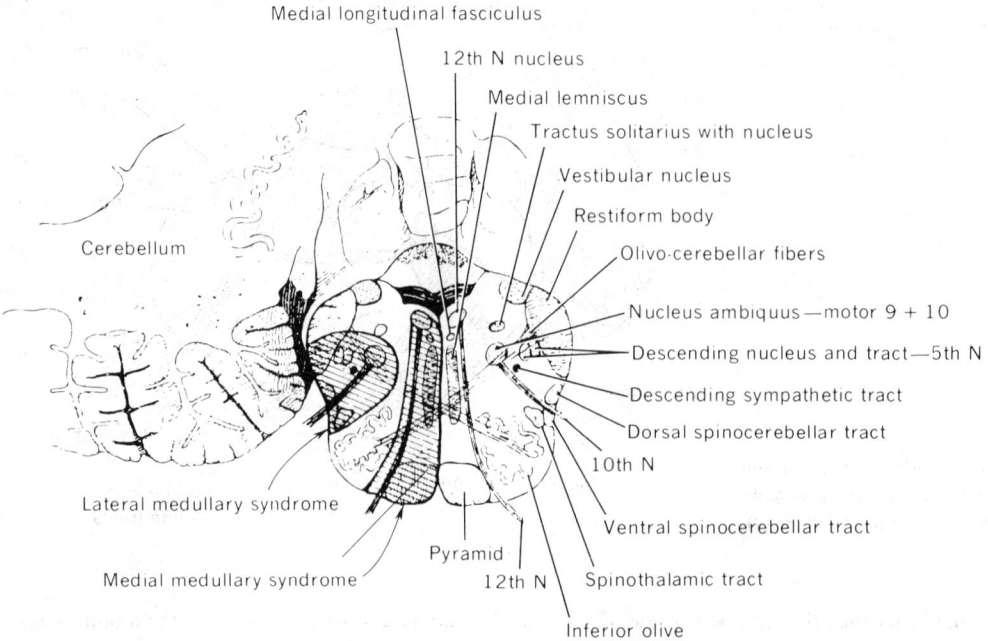

Medial longitudinal fasciculus
12th N nucleus
Medial lemniscus
Tractus solitarius with nucleus
Vestibular nucleus
Restiform body
Olivo-cerebellar fibers
Nucleus ambiguus—motor 9 + 10
Descending nucleus and tract—5th N
Descending sympathetic tract
Dorsal spinocerebellar tract
10th N
Ventral spinocerebellar tract
Spinothalamic tract
Inferior olive
12th N
Pyramid
Medial medullary syndrome
Lateral medullary syndrome
Cerebellum

FIGURE 365-10
Medial medullary syndrome (occlusion of vertebral artery or of branch of vertebral or lower basilar artery). Lateral medullary syndrome (occlusion of any five vessels may be responsible—vertebral, posterior inferior cerebellar, or superior, middle, or inferior lateral medullary arteries). Total unilateral medullary syndrome (occlusion of vertebral artery). Combination of medial and lateral syndromes. Lateral pontomedullary syndrome (occlusion of vertebral artery). Combination of lateral medullary and lateral inferior pontine syndromes. Basilar artery syndrome (the syndrome of the lone vertebral artery is equivalent). A combination of the various brainstem syndromes plus those arising in the posterior cerebral artery distribution. The clinical picture combines bilateral long-tract signs (sensory and motor) with cerebellar and peripheral cranial nerve abnormalities.

artery. Occlusion of the vertebral arteries low in the neck is usually compensated for by anastomotic flow to the upper part of the vertebral arteries via the thyrocervical, deep cervical, and occipital arteries, or an influx from the anterior part of the circle of Willis may occur.

The *posterior inferior cerebellar artery* supplies the inferior portion of the lateral medullary region, the restiform body, and the inferior surface of the cerebellar hemisphere. It may be occluded at its mouth, i.e., by thrombosis of the vertebral artery, or anywhere along its course. Some patients tolerate obstruction of the vessel with little or no ill effect; in others an extensive infarct results in the cerebellum and/or the posterolateral medulla. It should be pointed out that the various cerebellar arteries are connected to their neighbors by subarachnoid interarterial anastomoses, in the same way as the main arteries of the cerebrum, and the potential for collateral flow is good.

The clinical picture resulting from occlusion of the posterior inferior cerebellar artery is variable. Often no serious damage results. Occasionally the *lateral medullary syndrome* may be evoked through blockage of flow along the inferior artery of the lateral medulla. Although occlusion of the posterior inferior cerebellar artery is usually stated to be the cause of the lateral medullary syndrome, this appears to be true in only a minority of patients; more careful studies show that in eight out of ten cases the vertebral artery is occluded, and in the other two cases either the posterior inferior cerebellar artery is occluded or no arterial occlusion is found. Infarction in the posterior medullary region causes ipsilateral cerebellar ataxia and rarely hiccup. The symptoms associated with isolated infarction of the inferior part of the cerebellum include sudden severe dizziness, nausea, vomiting, ataxia, and nystagmus, a picture that mimics acute labyrinthitis.

The *lateral medullary syndrome* is produced by infarction of a small wedge of lateral medulla lying posteriorly to the inferior olivary nucleus (see Fig. 365-10). The classic syndrome as outlined by Fisher et al., who analyzed all the Massachusetts General Hospital cases, reflects the involvement of the spinothalamic tract (*contralateral* impairment of pain and thermal sense over half the body, sometimes face); descending sympathetic tract (*ipsilateral* Horner's syndrome of miosis, ptosis, decreased sweating), issuing fibers of the ninth and tenth nerves (hoarseness, dysphagia, *ipsilateral* paralysis of the palate and vocal cord, diminished gag reflex); vestibular disorder (nystagmus, diplopia, oscillopsia, vertigo, nausea, vomiting), involvement of cerebellum olivo- and/or spinocerebellar fibers, and sometimes restiform body (*ipsilateral* ataxia of limbs, falling or toppling to the ipsilateral side), descending tract and nucleus of the fifth nerve (pain, numbness, impaired sensation over ipsilateral half of the face); nucleus and tractus solitarius (loss of taste), cuneate and gracile nuclei (numbness of *ipsilateral* arm), and hiccup. This syndrome, one of the most striking in neurology, is almost always due to ischemic necrosis.

Basilar artery The basilar artery supplies not only the pons and upper part of the cerebellum but also in most cases the inferior temporal and medial occipital lobes via the posterior cerebral arteries. Occlusion may occur in the trunk of the basilar artery or in any one of its branches.

The branches of the basilar artery may be conveniently grouped as follows: (1) paramedian, seven to ten in number, supplying a wedge of pons on either side of the midline; (2) the short circumferential branches, five to seven in number, supplying the lateral two-thirds of the pons and the middle and superior cerebellar peduncles; and (3) the long circumferential, two in number on each side, running laterally around the pons to reach the cerebellar hemispheres (the superior cerebellar artery and the anterior inferior cerebellar artery).

Occlusion of the basilar artery evokes a sizable array of clinical manifestations reflecting involvement of a large number of structures [corticospinal and corticobulbar tracts, cerebellum, middle and superior cerebellar peduncles, medial and lateral lemnisci, spinothalamic tracts, medial longitudinal fasciculi, pontine nuclei, vestibular and cochlear nuclei, descending hypothalamospinal sympathetic fibers, the upper medulla, and the third through the eighth cranial nerves (including the nuclei, their segments within the brainstem, and the peripheral nerves themselves)] (see Figs. 365-6 to 365-10).

The picture of basilar occlusion due to thrombosis may arise in several ways: (1) occlusion in the basilar artery itself, usually in the lower third at the site of an atherosclerotic plaque; (2) occlusion of both vertebral arteries, with closure of the second amounting to basilar obstruction; or (3) occlusion of a single vertebral artery, when there is only one of good size. It must be emphasized that thrombosis may involve only a branch of the basilar artery rather than the trunk (*basilar branch occlusion*). When the obstruction is embolic, the embolus usually lodges at the upper bifurcation of the basilar or in one of the posterior cerebral arteries, since if it is small enough to pass through the vertebral artery, it should easily traverse the length of the basilar artery, which is of greater diameter than either vertebral artery.

The complete basilar syndrome comprises bilateral long-tract signs (sensory and motor) with variable cerebellar and cranial nerve abnormalities and other segmental disorders of brainstem. As a rule the patient is comatose with quadriplegia, pseudobulbar palsy, cranial nerve abnormalities, and has a clear CSF. The coma is due to lesions in the reticular activating system of midbrain and diencephalon. In the presence of the full syndrome, it is usually not difficult to make the correct diagnosis. The aim should be, however, to recognize basilar insufficiency long before the stage of total deficit has been reached. The early manifestations occur in many combinations.

In regard to occlusion of individual basilar branches, the main signs of thrombosis of the *superior cerebellar artery* are severe ipsilateral cerebellar ataxia (middle and/or superior cerebellar peduncles), nausea and vomiting, slurred speech, and loss of pain and temperature sensation over the extremities, body, and face of the opposite side (spinothalamic tract). Partial deafness, a static tremor of the ipsilateral upper extremity, Horner's syndrome, and bulbar myoclonus have also been reported.

In occlusion of the *anterior inferior cerebellar artery* the extent of the infarct is extremely variable. The size of this artery and the territory it supplies vary inversely with that of the posterior inferior cerebellar artery. The principal findings are ipsilateral deafness, whirling dizziness, nausea and vomiting, nystagmus, tinnitus and cerebellar ataxia (inferior cerebellar peduncle, or restiform body), Horner's syndrome, and paresis of conjugate lateral gaze. Pain and temperature sensation are lost on the opposite side of the body. If the occlusion is close to the origin of the artery, the corticospinal fibers may also be involved, producing a hemiplegia. Occlusion of the *artery to the retroolivary space* will produce the lateral medullary syndrome. Occlusion of a *paramedian branch* will result in infarction of the corticospinal fibers, the adjacent pontine nuclei, and the pontocerebellar fibers on one side of the pons. If the infarct extends deep to reach the tegmentum, as it occasionally does, paralysis of conjugate lateral gaze and a contralateral sensory deficit will result.

Other cardinal brainstem signs are a "crossed" cranial nerve and long-tract deficits (involvement from the third to the twelfth nerves). Although it is correct to emphasize that bilaterality of a lesion strongly suggests brainstem involvement, it must be pointed out with equal force that in many instances of infarction within the basilar territory the lesion is limited to one side, bespeaking occlusion of a basilar branch, not of the main trunk.

In the diagnosis of disease of the brainstem it is impossible from motor signs alone to distinguish a hemiplegia of pontine origin from one of cerebral origin, and one is always dependent on coexisting neurologic phenomena. In a lower brainstem hemiplegia the eyes may move more easily to the side of the paralysis, just the opposite of supratentorial lesions. In brainstem lesions, as in cerebral, a flaccid paralysis gives way to spasticity in the following days, weeks, or months, and there is no satisfactory explanation for the variability in this period of delay. The pattern of sensory disturbance may be helpful in localization. A dissociated sensory deficit over the face or one-half the body usually indicates a lesion within the brainstem, while a sensory loss over one side of the body involving all modalities with no suggestion of dissociation in any region indicates a lesion in the thalamus or deep in the white matter of the parietal lobe. When position sense, two-point discrimination, and tactile localization are affected relatively more than pain, temperature, and tactile sense, a cortical lesion is suggested; the converse suggests a brainstem location. When both motor and sensory manifestations in a given stroke are bilateral, it is almost unequivocal evidence that the lesion lies infratentorially. When hemiplegia or hemiparesis and sensory loss are coextensive, the lesion lies supratentorially. Additional manifestations which point unequivocally to a brainstem site are whirling dizziness, diplopia, cerebellar ataxia, Horner's syndrome, and deafness. The several brainstem syndromes illustrate the important point that the cerebellar system, spinothalamic tract, trigeminal nucleus, and sympathetic fibers can be involved at different levels, and neighborhood phenomena must be used to identify the exact site.

A myriad of eponymic brainstem syndromes, e.g., Weber, Claude, Benedict, Foville, Raymond-Cestan, Millard-Gubler (see Chap. 376), have been described in relation to brainstem lesions. In their classic descriptions most of these syndromes relate to tumors and other nonvascular diseases, and only occasionally was one of them encountered in association with vascular disease. The diagnosis of vascular disorders in this region of the brain is not greatly facilitated by a knowledge of these eponymic syndromes, and it is preferable to memorize the neuroanatomy of the brainstem. The principal syndromes to be recognized are full basilar, vertebral, anterior inferior cerebellar artery, superior cerebellar artery, pontomedullary, and medial medullary branches. Partial syndromes can usually be identified as fragments of the major ones.

LACUNAR SYNDROMES

PENETRATING BRANCH OCCLUSIONS OF CEREBRAL AND BASILAR ARTERIES Infarcts of the territories supplied by the deep, i.e., penetrating, branches of the arteries of the circle of Willis, the anterior, middle, and posterior cerebral artery stems, and the pontine branches of the basilar artery produce syndromes sufficiently different from those affecting the cerebral surface arteries to warrant separate clinical description. Usually they occur singly, producing a deeply situated infarct 2 to 15 mm in diameter. Healing of the infarct leaves a cavity deep in the brain, which has been referred to as a *lacuna*. When a lacuna results from occlusion or stenosis of a lenticulostriate artery, the internal capsule is usually affected with a resulting pure motor hemiplegia. The deficit may evolve in a leisurely fashion over as long as 3 days, causing concern about the possibility of a hemorrhage, but the CT scan is negative, and there is no accompanying sensory disturbance, aphasia or hemianopia, or alteration of consciousness. The motor deficit involves face, arm, leg, and often the trunk to a varying degree and is most easily diagnosed at a stage when only the motor deficit is evident (pure motor hemiplegia). Recovery begins within hours or days and is often nearly complete. Lacunae in the thalamus or above may be manifested by a pure hemisensory deficit (pure hemisensory syndrome) (Groothuis et al.). In the midbrain the common syndrome is hemiparesis with cerebellar ataxia on the same side. In the pons, the clinical manifestation is a pure hemiplegia mimicking that observed in capsular infarction, or dysarthria, unilateral facial paresis, and clumsiness of the hand on that side. Slightly larger lacunar infarcts may blend with *basilar branch syndromes,* a cluster of syndromes not yet fully described. Multiple lacunae involving the corticospinal and corticobulbar tracts cause the clinical picture of "pseudobulbar palsy" (more appropriately called *bipyramidal palsy*) featuring bilateral upper motor neuron signs, viz., spasticity, increased tendon reflexes, Babinski sign, dysarthria, and dysphagia. Paroxysms of excessive crying or laughing, and short-stepped gait, may be noted. Mental impairment is sometimes part of the picture (Chap. 25). Lacunae are sometimes said to be the basis of so-called "arteriosclerotic parkinsonism," but proof that such an entity exists is wanting.

MAJOR TYPES OF CEREBROVASCULAR DISEASES AND THEIR FREQUENCY

The six common types of stroke listed in Table 365-1 can be diagnosed with a high degree of accuracy. Since each one requires a special approach, therapy, and management, correct diagnosis is advantageous to the patient. The criteria for diagnosis and the confirmatory laboratory tests are described in the following pages.

The natural frequency of these six types of cerebrovascular lesions has been difficult to ascertain. Obviously clinical diagnosis is not always correct, and clinical services are more heavily weighted with acute strokes and nonfatal cases. An autopsy series inevitably includes many old vascular lesions, particularly infarcts, whose nature cannot be determined, and there is a bias also toward large fatal lesions (usually hemorrhages).

In Table 365-1 we have presented the figures obtained from the Harvard Cooperative Stroke Registry, which at this moment includes 736 successive cases on whom all appropriate laboratory aids were employed (four-vessel arteriography, CT scan, CSF examination) and who were examined by a physician knowledgeable about strokes. For comparison we have included an autopsy series of 179 successive brains examined during the year 1949 by Fisher and Adams.

Interestingly in both series the ratio of infarcts to hemor-

rhages was 4:1, and embolism accounted for approximately one-third of all strokes. The incidence of aneurysms and vascular malformations was higher at the Massachusetts General Hospital because such cases had been referred there. The initial diagnosis by the Stroke Registry Group corresponded to the final diagnosis (resulting from further clinical study, neuroradiologic tests, surgery, and autopsy) in 85 percent of cases. Hypertensive hemorrhages, aneurysms, and vascular malformations were correctly diagnosed in nearly every case. The most frequent sources of error were (1) mistaking a small embolic occlusion for a lacuna or vice versa and (2) confusing a thrombotic infarct for an embolus or vice versa. An earlier problem of mistaking a small hypertensive hemorrhage for an infarct has been virtually eliminated by the CT scan.

ATHEROSCLEROTIC THROMBOSIS

Atherosclerosis in the arteries of the brain is similar to that elsewhere in the body. The atheromatous plaques tend to form at branchings and curves. The severity of the process runs parallel to but is somewhat less severe than that of other arteries—aorta, lower limbs, and heart. Thrombosis is most likely to occur where the plaque narrows the lumen to the greatest degree. The most common sites of thrombosis are the internal carotid artery at the carotid sinus in the neck, in the vertebral and basilar arteries in the region of their junction, at the main bifurcation of the middle cerebral artery, in the posterior cerebral artery as it winds round the cerebral peduncle, and in the anterior cerebral artery as it curves upward over the corpus callosum. Hypertension aggravates the atherosclerotic process. Hypertension is also associated with a special segmental arterial disorganization (lipohyaloid change), which then results in involvement of smaller vessels (1 mm and less). This leads to thrombosis in the small, penetrating branches of the middle cerebral, posterior cerebral, and basilar arteries and produces the small infarcts or lacunae to which reference has already been made. It may also result in hemorrhage. In hypertension the cerebellar and ophthalmic arteries also are liable to involvement. Because of abundant collateral arterial pathways, occlusion of the common carotid, brachiocephalic cervical portion of the vertebral arteries, or subclavian arteries in the upper thorax is not commonly responsible for cerebral ischemia. The vertebral arteries may be narrowed at their origins from the subclavian, resulting in cerebral infarction. Ordinarily it is rare for the cerebral arteries to be significantly affected beyond their first major branching.

The state of the arterial lumen during the period when the stroke is evolving varies from case to case. Judging from arteriographic and surgical findings in the carotid and vertebral arteries in the neck, it is likely that when prodromal transient ischemic attacks are occurring, atherosclerosis and superimposed thrombus only incompletely occlude the affected artery; yet blood flow for reasons not yet understood is intermittent in the territory distal to the stenosis. Or, the main vessel is totally occluded while a compensating collateral channel is stenotic. By the time the neurologic deficit persists and is advancing, the superimposed thrombus will in the majority of cases have progressed to block completely the main vessel of supply. When the stroke becomes fully established, complete occlusion is the rule. It is common to find more than one vessel affected by stenosis or occlusion, and then it is especially difficult to decipher the interplay of hemodynamic factors leading to symptoms.

TABLE 365-1
Frequency of common types of stroke

	Harvard Stroke Series,* 736 successive cases (%)	BCH Autopsy Series,† 179 successive cases (%)
Atherosclerotic thrombosis	244 (33)	21 (12)
Lacunae	129 (18)	34 (18.5)
Embolism	224 (31)	57 (32)
Hypertensive hemorrhage	84 (11)	28 (15.5)
Ruptured aneurysms and vascular malformations	55 (7)	8 (4.5)
Indeterminate		17 (9.5)
Other‡		14 (8.5)

* *Series compiled by J Mohr et al at Massachusetts General Hospital and Beth Israel Hospital, Boston.*
† *Series compiled by CM Fisher and RD Adams in an examination of 780 brains during the year 1949 at Mallory Institute of Pathology, Boston City Hospital.*
‡ *Hypertensive encephalopathy, cerebral vein thrombosis, meningovascular syphilis, polyarteritis nodosa.*

CLINICAL PICTURE In general, the evolution of the clinical picture in cerebral thrombosis is much more variable than in embolism and hemorrhage. In approximately 80 percent of cases, the main part of the stroke (paralysis or other deficit) is preceded by minor signs or by one or more *transient ischemic attacks,* which herald the oncoming vascular catastrophe. Transient ischemic attacks rarely precede embolism and intracerebral hemorrhage. Transient warning attacks in carotid-middle cerebral disease consist of mono- or hemiplegia, mono- or hemiparesthesia, blindness in one eye, speech disturbance, confusion, etc. These attacks reflect evolving thrombosis of the internal carotid or middle cerebral arteries. In the vertebral-basilar system there may occur dizziness, diplopia, numbness, impaired vision in one or both visual fields, dark vision, dysarthria, etc. The attacks last from a few seconds up to 8 h or so, but usually *less than 10 min;* attacks lasting many hours are often documentably associated with embolism. The final stroke may be preceded by hundreds of attacks or by only a single one, but most frequently only *one or two attacks* precede the stroke. The stroke often comes within a day to a week of the first one but may be delayed for weeks or even months, and sometimes the attacks die away without leading to a stroke. When these minor ischemic attacks are not part of the picture, one must depend on other factors in identifying the cerebrovascular process as one of cerebral thrombosis.

The main part of the thrombotic stroke, whether or not it is preceded by warning attacks, develops in one of several ways. In 60 percent of cases, there is but a single attack, the whole illness developing in a few hours. A less common, but more diagnostic, pattern is for the stroke, once it commences, to have a stuttering intermittent progression in the next several hours or days. Or a partial stroke may develop, and after the patient has improved for several hours, there is progression to a full paralysis. Again, after one or more fleeting episodes, there may be a longer-lasting attack, succeeded in a day or two by the occurrence of a complete and permanent paralysis. The affection may involve several parts of the body simultaneously or, only one part, such as a limb or one side of the face, and the other parts become involved serially in step-like fashion until the stroke is fully developed. This may take several days or weeks, during which time there may be improvement and superimposed transient episodes of worsening. All these various modes of development bespeak cerebral thrombosis, and the whole process may be referred to as *thrombosis in evolution.* It might be commented that the transitory attacks and the abrupt episodes of progression reflect the temporal profile of the stroke syndrome in miniature. The principle of *intermittency* seems to characterize the thrombotic process from the beginning to the end. In thrombotic strokes either the onset or progression of the stroke is particularly common during sleep or shortly after arising (60 percent of cases). In fewer than 10 percent of cases, a thrombotic stroke comes on in what appears to be a slow, gradual fashion, but in most of these cases careful inquiry will reveal an uneven or saltatory progression, and actually there are only a few cases—these are usually examples of lacunar infarction—in which it can be said that the evolution of the thrombotic stroke was truly gradual over a period of several days.

Headache, although absent in the majority of cases, is present in approximately 15 percent of cases of cerebral thrombosis. It is not so violent as in cases of intracranial hemorrhage, generally being on one side in the front part of the head in occlusion of the carotid system and at the back of the head or simultaneously in the forehead in basilar disease. Its cause is unknown. Presumably it is related in some way to the disease process within the vessel, since it may antedate the other symptoms of the stroke by several days. Rigidity of the neck is not part of uncomplicated cerebral infarction.

Hypertension, an important aggravating factor in atherosclerosis, is present in 60 percent of cases and diabetes mellitus in 25 percent, while evidence of vascular disease elsewhere, e.g., angina pectoris, electrocardiographic abnormality, myocardial infarction, absence of one or several peripheral pulses

in the lower limbs, or intermittent claudication occurs in 50 percent. The retinal arteries may show uniform or focal narrowing, increase and irregularity of the light reflex, or displacement of the veins, but these alterations cannot be correlated with cerebral atherosclerosis. The peak age of atherosclerotic thrombosis of brain arteries is 70 years, but infrequently, the process may occur much earlier, even in the twenties.

LABORATORY FINDINGS The cerebrospinal fluid pressure is normal in patients with cerebral thrombosis, though it may be under increased pressure if the infarct is large and associated with severe swelling of the damaged tissue. Cerebral thrombosis never causes blood in the spinal fluid, which is "crystal clear" unless the infarct is especially congested, when a very faint xanthochromia (1 to 2 on a scale of 10) may occur. A slight increase in the leukocytes of the spinal fluid (three to eight polymorphonuclear leukocytes) is not uncommon in the first few days of the illness. Rarely, and usually only with large infarcts, a brisk, transient pleocytosis (400 to 2000 polymorphonuclear leukocytes per milliliter occurs on about the third day). A persistent increase in the number of white blood cells of the cerebrospinal fluid suggests the presence of chronic meningitis (syphilis, tuberculosis, torula), granulomatous arteritis, septic embolism, cerebral thrombophlebitis, or a nonvascular process. The total amount of protein may be normal, but frequently it is raised to 50 to 80 mg per 100 ml. Rarely is it over 100, in which case some other diagnosis should be considered. A Wassermann or one of the specific tests for syphilis is still routinely made in many clinics but can be dispensed with unless the rest of the clinical and laboratory picture points toward neurosyphilis. A positive test for syphilis in a bloody fluid is not valid, since syphilitic reagin may have been carried into the fluid by the contaminating blood. Skull x-rays are not remarkable, and the pineal gland will not be shifted unless severe cerebral swelling has occurred, in which case the patient will usually be stuporous or comatose.

The electroencephalogram is still of limited value in indicating infarction or distinguishing it from hemorrhage and from nonvascular conditions. In cerebral infarction the electrical activity may be of a slightly slower frequency and of lower voltage than normal. High-voltage slow waves (3 to 5 per second) are evidence in favor of hemorrhage or tumor. Pneumoencephalography is unnecessary and contraindicated because of the danger of hypotension. Arteriography is the definitive procedure for the demonstration of arterial occlusion or stenosis and also provides information about collateral flow. Injection into the major cervicocerebral arteries via a catheter introduced from a femoral artery is preferred to direct injection into the carotid artery through a needle. Arteriography carries a risk of neurologic defect in fewer than 1 percent of cases studied by experienced arteriographers, but in patients with vessels narrowed by atherosclerosis the risk may be higher. It should be used when the diagnosis of vascular disease is uncertain, when vascular surgery may be possible, or when anticoagulant therapy is contemplated in an indefinite case. Radioactive concentration studies (e.g., technetium, arsenic, or mercury scan) used for detection of tumor, abscess, etc., often show a positive picture over infarcts, especially in the second or third week. Scintillation counting over the two sides of the skull after the intravenous injection of radioactive material may provide a comparative index of circulation in the two carotid systems. CT scanning usually demonstrates infarction of more than a few centimeters in extent within the first few days (zone of reduced absorption in contrast to normal brain), but shows it best in the chronic state when cavitation has occurred. Lacunar infarcts are usually not visualized.

COURSE AND PROGNOSIS When the patient is seen early in the course of atherosclerotic thrombosis, it is extremely difficult to give an *immediate prognosis.* Where does the patient stand in the stroke process when first examined? Is worsening to be anticipated or not? No rules have yet been laid down which allow one to predict the course. A mild paralysis today may become a disastrous hemiplegia tomorrow, or the patient's condition may only worsen temporarily for a day or two. In basilar artery occlusion, dizziness and dysphagia may progress in a few days to total paralysis and deep coma. The course of the deficit is so often progressive that a cautious attitude on the part of the physician is justified in what appears to be a mild stroke.

Progression of the stroke is probably most often due to increasing stenosis of the involved artery by mural thrombus. In some instances extension of the thrombus along the vessel may block side branches and hinder anastomotic flow. In the basilar artery, thrombus may gradually build up along its entire length. In the carotid system, the thrombus at times propagates distally from the site of origin in the neck to the intracranial supraclinoid portion, and possibly into the anterior cerebral artery, preventing collateral flow from the opposite side. In middle cerebral occlusion, retrograde thrombosis may extend back to the mouth of the anterior cerebral, perhaps secondarily infarcting the territory of that vessel. Embolic particles from the site of thrombosis in a cervical vessel may precipitate an abrupt change.

Several other circumstances influence the *immediate prognosis* in cerebral thrombosis. In the case of large infarcts, swelling of the infarcted tissue may occur, tentorial herniation may follow, and the patient dies in 2 to 4 days. Milder degrees of swelling and increased intracranial pressure, though causing an apparent progression for 2 to 3 days, may not prove fatal. In extensive basilar infarction associated with deep coma, the patient seldom lives for more than a few days. If coma or stupor is present from the beginning, survival is largely determined by the success in keeping the airway clear (preventing aspiration pneumonia) and maintaining fluid and electrolyte balance (see Chap. 20). Respiratory and urinary infections are constant dangers, and once they begin, there is usually a rapid decline in the patient's condition as his temperature rises.

As for the *eventual, or long-term, prognosis* of the neurologic deficit, there are many possibilities. Improvement is the rule if the patient survives. Lacunar infarcts with a pure motor hemiparesis fare well. In small infarcts, improvement may start within hours or a day or two, and restoration may be complete within a week. With severe deficits there may be no significant recovery whatsoever, and after months of assiduous effort at rehabilitation, the patient may remain bereft of speech, with the upper extremity still useless and the lower extremity serving only as an uncertain prop in attempting to walk. Between these two extremes there is every degree of recovery. It is certain that the longer the delay before movement begins, the poorer the prognosis becomes. If recovery does not begin in 1 or 2 weeks, the outlook is gloomy both for motor activity and speech, and it may be said that whatever motor paralysis remains after 5 to 6 months will probably be permanent. Aphasia, dysarthria, cerebellar ataxia, and walking may improve for a year or longer. Anosognosia, constructional apraxia, uninhibited anger with left temporal lesions, nonsensical logorrhea and blandness, and unawareness of the paralysis and neglect all tend to diminish and may disappear within a few weeks. A hemianopia which has not cleared in a few weeks will usually remain permanently, although reading and color discrimination may continue to improve. In lateral medullary infarction difficulty in swallowing may be protracted (4 to 7 weeks), and yet eventually relatively normal function is nearly always restored.

Characteristically, the paralyzed muscles are flaccid in the first days or weeks following a stroke, and the tendon reflexes may be unchanged, slightly increased, or decreased. Gradually spasticity develops, and the tendon reflexes become brisker. The arm tends to assume a flexed adducted posture, whereas the leg is usually extended and adducted. Function is rarely if ever restored after the slow evolution of spasticity. Conversely, the early development of spasticity in the hand, or the appearance of a grasp reflex, and certain postural reactions (traction response) may presage a favorable outcome. In some cases with extensive temporoparietal lesions the hemiplegia remains flaccid; the arm dangles and the slack leg must be braced to stand. Bowel and bladder control usually returns. Not infrequently the hemiplegic limbs are at first tender and ache on manipulation, interfering with the physical therapy program. Nevertheless, physiotherapy should be initiated early in order to prevent contracture of muscles at shoulder, elbow, wrist, knuckles, knee, and ankle, a frequent complication and often the source of pain and added disability, particularly in relation to the shoulder. A typical Sudeck type of pain and bone atrophy of the hand may accompany the shoulder pain (shoulder-hand syndrome) as described in Chap. 8. An annoying, unsteady "dizzy" feeling in the head often persists after damage to the vestibular system in brainstem infarcts.

Recurrent cerebral (epileptic) seizures, while not unknown after thrombotic strokes, are rare. This is in contrast with embolic cortical infarcts where they occur in more than 20 percent of patients. A seizure involving the weakened limbs, followed by transient postepileptic paralysis may mimic another stroke. Often it takes several days for the paralysis to remit to the preepileptic level.

Many patients complain of fatigability and are depressed. The explanation of these symptoms is uncertain; some are expressions of a reactive depression (see Chap. 11). Only a few patients become serious *behavior problems* or are psychotic after a stroke, but paranoid trends, ill temper, stubbornness, and peevishness are recognized sequelae.

Finally, in regard to prognosis, it must be mentioned that having had one thrombotic stroke, the patient is in danger in the ensuing months and years of having a stroke at the same or another site, especially if there is hypertension. Myocardial infarction is also frequent, more so in the few weeks following a cerebral thrombosis. Probably more stroke victims eventually succumb to a heart attack than to another stroke.

TREATMENT The treatment of cerebrovascular disease and strokes may be divided into four parts: (1) general medical management in the acute phase, (2) measures to restore the circulation and arrest the pathologic process, (3) physical therapy and rehabilitation, and (4) preventive measures against strokes and vascular disease.

General medical management in the acute phase In essence, this is the care of the comatose or helpless patient (see Chap. 20).

Measures to restore the circulation and arrest the pathologic process Once a thrombotic stroke has developed fully, no therapy so far devised is of any value in restoring the cerebral tissue or its function. *To be effective, therapy must be preventive.* The diagnosis of thrombosis must be made at the earliest possible stage, and the full catastrophe circumvented by every means.

MEDICAL MEASURES TO IMPROVE THE BLOOD SUPPLY TO THE BRAIN   On the assumption that decrease in the cerebral circulation resulting from the upright position can aggravate cerebral ischemia, some physicians recommend that patients with a stroke as the result of ischemic infarction should remain horizontal in bed for 7 to 10 days initially and that, when ambulation starts, special attention should be given to preservation of the systemic circulation (avoid standing quietly for prolonged periods, sit with the feet up, etc.). Treatment of previously unappreciated hypertension is preferably deferred until the later stage of the stroke, when the neurologic deficit has stabilized. Elevating the foot of the bed 14 in or more in the acute stage is claimed by a few to be beneficial. Actually there is no clear evidence that any of these maneuvers influences the course of the cerebral lesion. Obviously it is of great importance that the systemic blood pressure be maintained (correction of blood loss, use of Levophed in myocardial infarction with vascular collapse, avoidance of autonomic blocking agents, etc.). Injections of sympathicomimetic drugs have also been recommended as a means of raising the systemic blood pressure above the usual levels. Although this enhances cerebral blood flow and might be beneficial, a systematic trial in thrombotic cases has not been undertaken, because of fear that it might cause hemorrhage into the infarcted tissues. Anemia must be corrected.

ANTICOAGULATION   Anticoagulant therapy may prevent transient ischemic attacks, postpone the arrival of an impending stroke, and also halt the advance of a progressive thrombotic stroke, but not in all cases. There are few studies to date which satisfy all epidemiologic criteria, and none which conclusively documents the value of anticoagulants nor indicates they are useless in the prevention of thrombotic stroke, or the worsening of a subischemic deficit. All investigators agree, however, that anticoagulants are not of value in the fully developed, i.e., completed, stroke. Whether when given for a prolonged period of time they prevent the recurrence of a thrombotic stroke is still under study, but the incidence of complicating severe hemorrhage appears to limit their value in these cases.

When *anticoagulant therapy* is instituted in thrombotic cases, heparin is used intravenously in a dose of approximately 50 mg every 4 h, or by continuous drip therapy, in cases with a progressing stroke or with transient ischemic attacks occurring more than once in 2 days. Heparin therapy is maintained for 1 to 2 weeks. While heparin therapy is being given, Coumadin therapy is instituted and continued well-regulated for 6 to 12 months or more. Coumadin therapy can be used alone from the beginning when transient ischemic attacks are fewer than once every few days to a week. Anticoagulant therapy is not recommended in lacunar strokes. Instead, blood pressure should be lowered.

The use of anticoagulant drugs makes an accurate clinical diagnosis imperative. Intracranial hemorrhage must be ruled out by CT scan, or if this procedure is not available, by relying primarily on examination of the cerebrospinal fluid; it is to be remembered, however, that a clear fluid does not necessarily exclude hemorrhage (see "Laboratory Findings" under "Intracranial Hemorrhage," below). A control prothrombin concentration and coagulation time are desirable before therapy is started, but if this is not feasible, the initial doses of anticoagulant drugs can usually be given safely if there is no evidence of active bleeding anywhere in the body. The question whether severe hypertension is a contraindication to anticoagulant therapy has not been accurately answered. There is no reliable evidence that complications are more frequent in the presence

of moderate hypertension if the prothrombin activity is maintained at 25 percent or higher, and therefore the authors have not withheld anticoagulant therapy in these patients; however, when the blood pressure is greater than 220/120, an attempt is made to lower the pressure gradually with hypotensive agents, exercising care not to prejudice further the circulation in the region of the infarct by too great a reduction in the systemic pressure. It is preferable to avoid reduction of the blood pressure in the 2-week period immediately following a thrombotic stroke.

Anticoagulant therapy is relatively safe provided the prothrombin concentration is determined regularly (once a day, for the first 10 days, thence thrice a week, and finally once every week or two) at a laboratory using reliable methods. Therapy can be prolonged for months and years, and only occasionally is it necessary to interrupt treatment because of unexplained disturbances of coagulation. Coumadin overdosage may cause hemorrhage into the brain or subdurally or into the kidney, nose, bowel, skin, or muscle. Most of the extracerebral accidents are not serious, but vitamin K_1 should be administered immediately.

ANTIPLATELET THERAPY   Recent data suggest that inhibition of platelet aggregation is of value in therapy for transient ischemic attacks, reducing the frequency of subsequent attacks, ischemic stroke, death from stroke, and death from nonstroke causes. The effect has been demonstrated only in men, and was most associated with the use of acetylsalicylic acid (aspirin), in doses of 300 mg four times a day. Disputes continue as to whether sulfipyrazone (Persantine) (200 mg four times a day) augments the effect of acetylsalicylic acid, and many clinicians use both treatments together. This therapeutic approach may precede supplement, or supplant oral anticoagulants, but when used in conjunction with them, the danger of hemorrhage is increased, necessitating reduced doses of oral anticoagulants and close clinical monitoring.

SURGERY   Surgical management of the arterial obstruction in the neck and thorax is frequently undertaken, employing thromboendarterectomy or bypass grafts. The region of the carotid sinus is most frequently amenable to such therapy. The carotid sinus may prove tightly stenotic, occluded, or affected with plaque and/or ulcer formation. In experienced hands, these lesions can usually be dealt with safely by endarterectomy. When a thrombus of the internal carotid artery extends higher to the siphon, the surgical approach depends on some form of bypass grafting (transcranial external carotid to middle cerebral), a surgical procedure found technically feasible, and currently under active study. Surgery can also be done at the other sites suitable for surgical management, including the common carotid, innominate, and subclavian arteries. Operation on the vertebral artery at its origin has not proved beneficial. Before operation the existence of the occlusive lesion and its extent must be determined by arteriography. Surgery is optimally undertaken at the stage of transient ischemic attacks or early in the course of thrombosis-in-evolution. When total infarction has occurred, surgery will be ineffective even though patency of the vessel is restored. Surgery is not without risk, and its place in the treatment of cerebrovascular diseases has not been fully determined. In only a small minority of the total number of thrombotic strokes are the lesions so situated that surgery is feasible.

THERAPY FOR CEREBRAL EDEMA   In the initial days following major cerebral infarction, cerebral edema may occasionally threaten life. In such instances, dexamethasone in intramuscular doses of 4 to 6 mg every 4 to 6 h may prove helpful. Oral therapy with glycerin in doses of 30 ml every 4 to 6 h or glycerol in doses of 50 g dissolved in 500 ml of 2.5% saline solution given intravenously daily are other forms of therapy available. The value of these agents in improvement of the neurologic deficit apart from therapy for edema alone remains questionable.

CEREBRAL VASODILATORS Despite experimental evidence that these agents increase the cerebral blood flow, as measured by the nitrous oxide method, they have not proved beneficial in careful studies in human stroke cases at the stage of transient ischemic attacks, thrombosis-in-evolution, or in the established stroke. This is true of nicotinic acid, Priscoline, alcohol, papaverine, and inhalation of 5% carbon dioxide. A few clinical trials have indicated that histamine, aminophylline, acetazolamide, and intraarterial papaverine have some merit. In opposition to the use of these methods is the suggestion that vasodilators are harmful rather than beneficial, since by lowering the systemic blood pressure they reduce the intracranial anastomotic flow, or by dilating blood vessels in the normal parts of the brain they steal blood from the infarct.

THROMBOLYTIC AGENTS Fibrinolysin and profibrinolysin activators have not proved helpful in cases of transient ischemia, thrombosis-in-evolution, and the established stroke.

Physical therapy and rehabilitation Beginning within a few days, the joints of the paralyzed limbs should be passively carried through a full range of movement at intervals to a total of 50 times a day. Contracture (and periarthritis) must be avoided, especially at the shoulder, elbow, and ankle. Pain, soreness, and aching in the paralyzed limbs may temporarily interfere with exercises. The patient can be placed in a chair after a week or so, or sooner if the lesion is small. Nearly all hemiplegics can learn to walk again to some extent, usually within a 3- to 6-month period, and this should be a primary aim in rehabilitation. A short or long leg brace is often required. Speech therapy is not of proved value but should be tried. At least it improves the morale of the patient. Physical therapy seems not to benefit patients with cerebellar ataxia. As the hemiplegic patient improves, and if mentality is preserved, instruction in the activities of daily living, using various special devices, can assist the patient in becoming at least partially independent in the home.

General preventive measures against strokes and vascular disease AVOIDING SITUATIONS IN WHICH STROKES ARE LIKELY TO OCCUR (1) Particular care should be taken to maintain the systemic blood pressure, oxygenation, and intracranial blood flow during surgical procedures, especially in elderly patients. (2) Hypotensive agents, whether given therapeutically or for diagnostic procedures, should be administered with care. (3) In the elderly patient in whom deep sleep might help to precipitate cerebral ischemia, oversedation should be avoided. (4) Systemic hypotension, severe anemia, and polycythemia should be treated promptly. (5) Rapid diuresis may be contraindicated.

FACTORS WHICH DETERMINE ULTIMATE OUTCOME The ultimate solution of the problem of cerebrovascular disease lies in more fundamental fields. Atherosclerosis and hypertension must be prevented or alleviated (see Chap. 251 for prophylaxis of atherosclerosis and Chap. 250 for the treatment of hypertension).

TRANSIENT ISCHEMIC ATTACKS OF CEREBRAL ORIGIN
When transient ischemic attacks precede a stroke, they almost always stamp the process as thrombotic. Fully 80 percent of cases of atherothrombic strokes are preceded by transient ischemic attack, and the risk of stroke in the population of cases experiencing transient ischemic attack (within a 2-year period) approaches 20 percent. They belong, therefore, under the heading of cerebral thrombosis, but they are discussed separately here because of their importance clinically and therapeutically.

Attention is directed to these attacks for the reason that their treatment (the administering of anticoagulant drugs or performing surgical endarterectomy at the stage of prodromal symptoms) may prevent a disastrous stroke. There would seem to be little doubt that they are due to transient focal ischemia, and they might be referred to as temporary strokes which fortunately reverse themselves. Corresponding to the higher incidence of atherosclerosis in hypertension and in the male population, about two-thirds of all patients with transient ischemic attacks are hypertensive and/or men.

Clinical picture Thrombosis of virtually any cerebral or cerebellar artery, deep or superficial, can be associated with transient ischemic attacks, e.g., common carotid, internal carotid, middle cerebral, anterior cerebral, ophthalmic, vertebral, basilar, posterior cerebral, the cerebellar arteries, and the penetrating branches to the deep structures of the basal ganglia and brainstem. If the posterior cerebral arteries are included in the vertebral-basilar system, ischemic episodes are slightly more common in that system than in the carotid. Transient ischemic attacks may precede, accompany, or rarely follow the development of a stroke, or they can occur by themselves without leading to a stroke. So far, it has not been possible to distinguish the early cases destined to do well from those in which a full-blown stroke will develop.

Transient ischemic attacks last a few seconds up to 12 h, the most common duration being a few seconds up to 5 to 10 min. It is uncommon for recurrent discrete attacks to last more than 30 min. There may be only a few attacks or several hundred. Between attacks, the neurologic examination may disclose no abnormalities. A stroke may ensue after the second episode or may be postponed until hundreds of attacks have occurred over a period of weeks or months. Often, especially when frequent over a long period of time, the attacks gradually cease and no important paralysis occurs, a fact which makes any form of therapy difficult to evaluate.

The neurologic features of the transient episode indicate the territory or artery involved and are fragments borrowed from the stroke which may be approaching. In the carotid system, attacks reflect involvement of cerebral hemisphere and eye. The ocular disturbance is ipsilateral; the sensorimotor disturbance is contralateral. Repeated attacks tend to respect their original general site and uncommonly involve only the eye at first, then the hemisphere, when each is affected alone. It is almost unknown for the eye and the brain to be involved simultaneously in a single attack. In the transient hemisphere attacks, ischemia occurs foremost in the distal middle cerebral territory and adjacent border zone region, producing weakness or numbness of the opposite hand and arm. However, many different combinations may be seen: face and lips, lips and fingers, fingers alone, hand and foot, etc. Less common manifestations include aphasia, difficulty in calculation (when the dominant hemisphere is involved), and other temporo-parieto-occipital disturbances, such as confusion, veering to one side, and headache. In ocular attacks, transient monocular blindness is the usual symptom. Many of the latter episodes evolve swiftly and are described as being like a shade falling smoothly over the visual field until the eye is completely but painlessly blind. The attack clears slowly and uniformly. Uncommonly, the visual disorder may take the form of a wedge of missing vision, sudden generalized blurring, or, rarely, a bright light.

Transient attacks of monocular blindness are usually more stereotyped than transient attacks of hemisphere blindness.

The clinical picture in the *vertebral-basilar system* is diverse, since so much motor and sensory traffic in the brainstem and thalamus is sustained by the blood carried in these vessels. Occurring in the most varied combinations, the following manifestations in their approximate order of frequency may be recognized: dizziness, diplopia (vertical or horizontal); dysarthria; weakness of a part or all of one side, or both sides, or crossed numbness (one side of face and opposite limbs); a feeling of cross-eyedness; dark vision, blurred vision; tunnel vision; partial or complete blindness; pupillary change; ptosis; paralysis of gaze; speechlessness; and dysphagia. Less common symptoms include noise or pounding in the ear or in the head, head or face pain, peculiar head sensations, vomiting, pallor, hiccups, memory lapse, confused behavior, drowsiness, transient unconsciousness (rare), impaired hearing, deafness, a feeling of movement of a part, hemiballismus, peduncular hallucinosis, and forced deviation of the eyes.

It is not always easy to identify the territory affected. However, the occurrence of monocular blindness with or without contralateral weakness or numbness always points to the carotid system, as does receptive or sensory aphasia. The hallmarks of vertebral-basilar involvement are dizziness, diplopia, and bilateral weakness and/or numbness, i.e., a disturbance of the long motor or sensory tracts bilaterally.

The attacks may all take approximately the same pattern, or they may vary considerably in detail, although maintaining the same basic pattern. For example, weakness or numbness may involve fingers and face in some episodes and fingers only in others; or dizziness alone may occur in some attacks, while in others diplopia is added to the picture. In basilar artery disease each side of the body may be affected alternately. All the involved parts may be affected simultaneously, or a definite march or spread from one region to another can occur in a period of 10 to 60 s, or even a few minutes; e.g., numbness may spread from the hand to the face, or the reverse. The individual attack may cease abruptly or fade gradually.

Mechanism Ophthalmoscopic observations of the retinal vessels made during episodes of transient monocular blindness show either arrest of the blood flow in the retinal arteries and breaking up of the venous column to form a "boxcar" pattern or white material temporarily blocking the retinal arteries. This indicates that in ischemic attacks a temporary, complete, or relatively complete cessation of blood flow occurs locally, possibly with associated microembolism. In the past, transient ischemic attacks have been attributed to cerebral vasospasm or to transient episodes of systemic arterial hypotension with resulting compromise of the intracranial circulation. Neither of these factors has been established. Although dropping the blood pressure to 90 or even 80 mmHg by tilting the patient upright on a tilt table may cause electroencephalographic changes, it has not in the authors' experience reproduced the attacks. Vasodilator drugs have been without effect. There is good evidence that the attacks are abolished by anticoagulant drugs, but the mechanism of this is not known. Whatever their exact cause, they are closely related to vascular stenosis due to atherosclerosis and thrombosis.

Sometimes a postural factor is suggested by the onset of attacks in relation to standing up after lying or sitting, but this is rare, and in general, attacks are likely to occur when the patient is up and around rather than lying down and bear no relation to position or activity. Diversion of blood may be a factor when they occur, as they may in relation to exercise, exertion, emotional outbursts of anger or joy, and during bouts of coughing.

Cerebral embolism (platelet emboli from sites of atherosclerosis) is frequently suggested as an explanation for recurrent cerebrovascular episodes; and indeed this mechanism may underlie the nonstereotyped attacks. The usual source is an ulcerated atheromatous plaque in a stenosed carotid artery. However, if all the attacks are of approximately identical pattern, successive emboli coming from a distance could hardly be expected to enter the same arterial branch. Moreover, one would expect the involved cerebral tissue to be at least partially damaged, leaving some residual signs. In some cases of documented embolism, the deficit fluctuates from normal to abnormal repeatedly as long as 36 h, giving the appearance of transient ischemic attacks. In others, there is a short-lived deficit of several hours' duration, fulfilling the traditional criteria of transient ischemic attacks, i.e., a deficit of less than 12 h duration. The mechanism of single transitory episodes and multiple episodes of different pattern must be clearly distinguished from that of recurrent attacks of the *same pattern*. The former is embolic, the latter is thrombosis in evolution.

Arteriography sheds some light on pathogenesis in Toole and Yuson's series of 226 cases, evaluated by four-vessel arteriography. In 209 cases there was a carotid or vertebral-basilar stenosis and an atherosclerotic plaque, but in 16 cases no radiographic abnormality was seen. In the series of Mohr, the prognosis in the radiographically negative cases was as grave as in the positive cases.

Differential diagnosis The following conditions must be differentiated: cerebral seizures (epileptic seizures), Ménière's syndrome, migraine accompaniments, Stokes-Adams attacks, hypersensitive carotid sinus reflex, transient global amnesia, insulin reactions, attacks of hysteria, anxiety, and depression, akinetic falling spells of the aged, and recurrent cerebral embolism.

Frank motor *convulsions* rarely if ever occur in ischemic attacks. The patient may report a feeling of movement, distortion, drawing, jumping, or jerking, but an isolated frank focal seizure may not have been encountered. Conversely, a cerebral seizure rarely displays as its only manifestation a temporary paralysis of a limb or of one side of the body. Unconsciousness is rare in ischemic attacks, and its occurrence even in only a few attacks indicates another diagnosis (seizure, Stokes-Adams attack, etc.). Incontinence of bowel and bladder, tongue biting, cyanosis, and residual sleepiness or muscle soreness are indicative of a seizure rather than an ischemic episode. In the sensory sphere, the distinction between ischemic episodes and seizures is less clear, for numbness or scintillating visual phenomena are seen in both conditions, and therefore in making a differentiation one must rely on the presence of associated phenomena (dizziness, diplopia, etc.). When numbness appears simultaneously in face, hand, and leg, i.e., when there is no "march," ischemia rather than a seizure is probably responsible.

Dizziness associated with brainstem ischemia is less likely to have a clear rotatory component than that seen in *Ménière's syndrome or labyrinthitis.* In making a diagnosis, however, one depends on the presence of associated symptoms and signs. It is a simple matter to decide that the dizziness is of central origin when there are other evidences of brainstem involvement, by history or by neurologic examination: diplopia, dysarthria, cerebellar ataxia, vertical nystagmus, persistent horizontal nystagmus, numbness, weakness, dysphagia, etc. On the other hand, the isolated presence of the triad—recurrent dizziness, tinnitus, and chronic deafness (i.e., signs of both auditory and vestibular involvement)—is almost certain evidence of Ménière's syndrome. In the early stages the pictures at times resemble each other closely, however, and only an especially thorough search will reveal signs indicating that the disorder is due to ischemia of the brainstem or the cerebellum. Tinnitus of a constant hissing or ringing type is a rare complaint in brainstem vascular disease. When dizziness is the sole symptom in an elderly person, it is often impossible to make an accurate diagnosis, and only after observing the patient for a period of time will the nature of the underlying disease be disclosed. It must be remembered that since both basilar artery disease and Ménière's syndrome are common conditions, the two may coexist.

The visual, sensory, and motor phenomena which precede the headache (or occur in its absence) in some cases of *migraine* bear a close resemblance to ischemic manifestations, but since migraine originates in early life, its differentiation from ischemic attacks does not ordinarily pose a problem. An important point is that migrainous accompaniments in 75 percent of cases develop gradually over a period of 5 to 10 min, marching across the affected region, whereas transient ischemic phenomena rarely do this. When vascular disease has its onset in the twenties or thirties, the two may be confused until the history is carefully taken. A migrainous accompaniment may return after a headache-free interval of 10 to 20 years. It is not rare for migrainous accompaniments to appear for the first time in the forties or fifties. Still more important, periodic headaches may not be obvious. Headache, at times of some intensity, can accompany cerebral thrombosis, and in an elderly person the occurrence for the first time of periodic headache associated with numbness or weakness should suggest atherothrombosis rather than migraine.

Stokes-Adams attacks and *hypersensitivity* of the *carotid sinus reflex* cause "collapsing spells" with unconsciousness, confusion, pallor, sweating, and jerking, but almost never do they produce focal neurologic manifestations such as numbness, weakness, or diplopia.

Difficulty in differentiation of these conditions will arise only when the clinical details of the episode are not available, and usually a careful minute-by-minute description of the attack will enable the physician to make the correct diagnosis. Only in an occasional case of basilar artery insufficiency will an ischemic episode result in unconsciousness, usually accompanied by other symptoms such as weakness, numbness, blindness, or dysarthria. In *akinetic falling spells of the aged*, the patient falls unconscious without convulsive movements; color change; or alteration in pulse, blood pressure, or respiration. Within a few seconds or a minute or two consciousness is restored.

Occasionally ischemic attacks may be confused with tussive syncope, multiple sclerosis, ulnar neuropathy, carpal tunnel syndrome, overhydration (hyponatremia), cataplexy and narcolepsy, brachial discomfort with hiatus hernia, cervical disk disease, severe postural hypotension, unusual symptoms in angina pectoris, recurrent pulmonary embolism, etc.

Treatment The therapy of transient ischemic attacks has already been discussed under "Treatment of Atherosclerotic Thrombosis," where it was pointed out that anticoagulants, antiplatelet agents, or surgical endarterectomy usually stop the attacks and prevent indefinitely the onset of a threatening stroke. Surgery must be seriously considered in carotid and subclavian cases. In many patients the attacks cease spontaneously, and anticoagulant therapy can be withheld if the episodes are few and spaced at long intervals. In nonsurgical cases, however, anticoagulants or drugs that prevent platelet aggregation are indicated if the attacks are of recent onset, and are becoming more frequent, more severe, or of longer dura-

tion, or if each attack no longer clears away completely, and a persistent neurologic deficit is accumulating. If anticoagulants are used, they may be replaced by acetylsalicylic acid and sulfipyrazone (Persantine) after 3 to 6 months.

Other measures that have been recommended include administration of phenobarbital, papaverine, or nicotinic acid, inhalation of 5% carbon dioxide, breathing into a paper bag, and stellate block or cervical sympathectomy, but none of these has proved effective under careful clinical testing. On several occasions the authors have been impressed with the salutary effect of having the patient stop smoking cigarettes. For the more general therapeutic measures applicable in these cases, see the section on treatment of atherosclerotic thrombosis, above.

OTHER CAUSES OF THROMBOSIS (INFARCTION) It will be seen from the list at the beginning of this chapter that there are few causes of cerebral arterial occlusion other than thrombosis and embolism. There are fewer still that are important in the stroke picture. In many of those included, the mechanism is ischemia without actual thrombosis.

Venous thrombosis is a rather uncommon condition and rarely mimics a cerebrovascular stroke. Arising in relation to extracranial and intracranial sepsis, surgical operations, parturition, contraceptive pill, polycythemia, sickle-cell anemia, and chronic wasting illnesses, particularly in children, it can cause a relatively mild neurologic illness with raised intracranial pressure, headache, visual obscurations, and focal seizures, or on the other hand, it can lead to extensive cerebral infarction and hemorrhage, with grave neurologic manifestations and death.

Systemic hypotension usually results in unconsciousness (syncope) without focal motor and sensory signs. But if the state of vascular collapse persists for a sufficient length of time, ischemia distal to the point of stenosis may result. Infarction will occur in the border zone and adjacent distal regions of major arterial territories of the cerebrum and cerebellum. It has already been mentioned that transient ischemic attacks and persistent strokes often develop under circumstances which suggest that a fall of the systemic blood pressure was the precipitating factor. Hypotension occurs in "simple faint," acute blood loss, myocardial infarction, Stokes-Adams syndrome, traumatic and surgical shock, cardiac arrest or anesthetic accident during surgery, hypersensitivity of the carotid sinus reflex, and in the several types of postural hypotension [idiopathic, postsympathectomy, tabetic, diabetic, with autonomic blocking agents, with reserpine (Serpasil), and on getting up and around after surgery].

Arteriography occasionally causes cerebral infarction. In some cases this is the result of cerebral embolism from a clot forming on the tip of the catheter, but the pathogenesis of other cases requires further study. *Arteritis* is no longer a common cause of cerebral thrombosis, at least in North America, owing to the present satisfactory treatment of syphilis. *Necrotizing* or *granulomatous arteritis*, whether limited to the cerebral vessels or occurring as part of a polyarteritis, usually produces a series of small ischemic deficits in brain, optic nerve, or spinal cord, and only rarely mimics a stroke. *Idiopathic giant-cell arteritis* involving the large arteries arising from the aortic arch is a rare cause of unilateral or bilateral carotid occlusion but must be kept in mind. It appears to be more common in young women in Japan, the aforementioned Takayasu's syndrome or "pulseless disease." *Cranial arteritis* or *temporal arteritis* is usually limited to the extracranial arteries except for the small vessels supplying the optic and oculomotor nerves. Unfortunately, in over 50 percent of cases permanent blindness or a severe impairment of vision results. The process usually involves the internal or common carotid arteries, but rarely causes a stroke (Chap. 67). Occasionally a vertebral-basilar stroke is reported.

Contraceptive therapy and stroke There is no doubt that strokes occur more frequently in women who use oral progestin-estrogen compounds for purposes of contraception. Major cerebral arteries may be occluded with the usual varieties of syndromes. This is but part of a more generalized affection of the circulatory system; death occurs approximately five times more frequently than in age-matched controls. In those individuals using these agents for 10 years the death rate is ten times that of controls. An occlusive cerebrovascular lesion is calculated to have an incidence of 13.2 in 100,000 in the treated group and 2.8 in 100,000 in the control group. These figures, compiled by Boral et al., are in approximate agreement with those of other reports. These statistics, while provocative, are difficult to interpret because there is a small but significant incidence of ischemic strokes in young women, especially during pregnancy. Interestingly, in 25 percent of our patients arteriography of the affected vessel showed it to be normal; or, if at first it was occluded, it later became patent. This means that embolism is the probable basis in at least some of the cases. In postmortem studies the wall of the occluded vessel has shown no inflammatory or other pathological change. Presumably the thrombus formation is due to an abnormality of platelets. Migraine appears to be a predisposing factor.

Polycythemia is stated to be a cause of cerebral thrombosis, but convincing cases must be rare. *Thrombotic thrombocytopenic purpura* usually leads to multiple microscopic infarcts and fluctuating neurologic symptoms without evidence of stroke.

Idiopathic thrombocytosis with platelet counts of more than 10^6 per milliliter due to megakaryocytosis may result in multiple episodes of focal cerebral ischemia. Antimitotic drugs have suppressed the attacks. *Hyperproteinemia* (greater than 9 to 10 g per 100 ml) may produce impairment of circulation through small cerebral and retinal vessels (Bing-Neal syndrome). The increased viscosity of blood, correctable by bleeding or plasmapheresis, tends to cause more general cerebral symptoms (confusion, coma, blurred vision) rather than strokes. *Sickle-cell disease* is associated with obstruction of small vessels, including the cerebral arteries and veins. A *dissecting aortic aneurysm* may involve the large vessels arising from the arch and result in carotid occlusion and hemiplegia, a concomitant fall in systemic blood pressure probably contributing to the picture. *Carotid occlusion* may be the result of direct *trauma* to the neck, or it may be precipitated by a "closed head injury," sometimes of a seemingly trivial nature. Here there is a traumatic dissecting aneurysm in the common or internal carotid arteries manifested arteriographically by an abrupt, elongated narrowing of the vascular lumen ("string sign"). *Fibromuscular dysplasia* is also attended at times by stroke. It should be considered in middle-aged individuals, especially women, and in association with vascular diseases of the kidneys. A corrugated appearance of the affected vessels in an arteriogram is the basis of most diagnoses. *Hypoxia* usually produces a diffuse destruction of neurons rather than frank infarction, but bilateral softening of the globus pallidus is a classic feature. *Tentorial and subfalcial herniation* can cause infarction by compression of the posterior and anterior cerebral arteries, respectively. Under the rare types of infarction, it should be mentioned that carotid occlusion has been described following tonsillectomy, in association with *cavernous sinus thrombophlebitis,* and the trigeminal ganglionitis of herpes zoster. Also, a previously transient and harmless migrainous aura can be transformed into a persistent deficit, presumably because of infarction as the result of prolonged arterial spasm. This complication most frequently takes the form of homonymous hemianopia. Finally, a category for *cerebral infarction of undetermined cause* is included,

for it must be admitted that in some cases, even after neuropathologic examination, it is impossible to determine the exact cause of an infarct, especially in young adults.

Omitted here is *Binswanger's chronic progressive subcortical encephalopathy,* a rare disease of cerebral white matter tentatively attributed by Binswanger to atherosclerosis. In some instances extensive softening due to atheromatous thrombosis is more or less confined to white matter, which may be border-zone territory between the penetrating cortical arteries and periventricular ones.

CEREBRAL EMBOLISM

In most cases of cerebral embolism, the embolic material consists of a fragment which has broken away from a thrombus within the heart. Less frequently the source is intraarterial from an atheromatous plaque that has damaged the endothelium or ulcerated into the lumen of the carotid sinus, or has broken away from the distal (intracranial) end of thrombus in the internal carotid artery. Embolisms due to fat, tumor cells, and air are rare occurrences and seldom enter into the differential diagnosis of strokes. The embolus usually becomes arrested at a bifurcation or other site of narrowing of the lumen. Ischemic infarction usually follows and is pale, hemorrhagic, or mixed; hemorrhagic infarction, as pointed out earlier, nearly always indicates embolism. Any region of the brain may be affected, but the territory of the middle cerebral artery is most frequently involved, especially the upper division. The two hemispheres are approximately equally affected. Large embolic masses will block larger vessels (sometimes the carotids in the neck), while tiny fragments may reach vessels as small as 0.2 mm, in which case the stroke may clear in a few days and the resultant infarct might be so small as to almost escape detection at autopsy. The fate of embolic material is not fully understood. Often, it remains arrested, plugs the lumen solidly and is organized by fibroblasts from the arterial wall; but in many cases it breaks up into fragments which enter smaller vessels and disappear completely, so that careful pathologic examination fails to reveal their final location. The anatomic diagnosis must then be made by inference, e.g., the absence of a vascular occlusion at the proper site to explain the infarct, the absence of atherosclerosis or other cause for thrombosis in the cerebral vessel, a ready source of embolus, infarcts in other organs such as kidney and spleen, the occurrence of hemorrhagic infarction, and last, but not least, the clinical history.

Because of the rapidity with which occlusion develops in embolism, there is not much time for collateral influx to become established. Thus sparing of territory distal to the site of occlusion is not so common as in thrombosis. However, the ischemia-modifying factors mentioned under thrombosis are still to some extent operative and will influence the size, shape, and severity of the infarct.

Brain embolism is essentially a manifestation of heart disease. Many kinds of heart disease can be associated with embolism. The commonest direct cause is *chronic atrial fibrillation* (approximately 50 percent of all cases of embolism) due to atherosclerotic or rheumatic heart disease, the source of the embolus being mural thrombus deposited within the atrial appendage. In rheumatic heart disease mitral stenosis increases the likelihood of embolism seven times. Atrial fibrillation due to other types of heart disease can, of course, also lead to embolism, e.g., hypertensive, congenital, or syphilitic. Embolism also occurs during paroxysmal atrial fibrillation or flutter. *Mural thrombus* deposited on the damaged endocardium overlying a myocardial infarct is an important source of cerebral emboli. Emboli can also arise from atrial thrombi associated with severe mitral stenosis without atrial fibrillation. *Cardiac surgery,* especially valvoplasty, may disseminate fragments of thrombus or particles of a calcified valve leaflet. Mitral and aortic valve prostheses are presently associated with embolism in 70 percent of cases. *Paradoxic embolism* can occur when an abnormal communication exists between the right and left sides of the heart, or when both ventricles communicate with the aorta. Thus embolic material arising in the veins of the lower extremity or, indeed, anywhere in the systemic venous tree may, particularly in conditions of pulmonary hypertension (often from previous pulmonary embolism), bypass the pulmonary circulation and reach the cerebral vessels. Subendocardial fibroelastosis, idiopathic myocardial hypertrophy, cardiac myxomas, and cardiac lesions in trichinosis are rare causes of embolism.

The *vegetations of acute and subacute bacterial endocarditis,* being infected, give rise to septic embolism, which results in several different pathologic pictures in the brain. In some cases the infarcts (they are usually multiple) do not differ from those due to bland emboli; in others, tiny septic infarcts develop, or as in acute bacterial endocarditis, there may be miliary abscesses into which a small amount of hemorrhage may occur (focal embolic encephalitis) and even meningitis. Mycotic aneurysm is another complication of septic embolism and may be a source of intracerebral or subarachnoid hemorrhage. *Marantic or nonbacterial endocarditis* occasionally causes cerebral embolism and can produce a most baffling clinical picture, especially when associated, as it often is, with carcinomatosis.

The following sources of embolic material are more difficult to prove or less frequent: (1) *Mural thrombus,* deposited upon ulcerated atheroma in the arch of the aorta or in the carotid arteries, may break loose and find its way into brain arteries. Massage of the carotid sinus, a favorite site for atherosclerosis, may dislodge a mural thrombus and produce a hemiplegia. This is one of the reasons why carotid massage should always be carried out gently. (2) Atheromatous material may be washed out of a large *plaque* in the aorta or carotid arteries and carried distally into the branches of the cerebral tree. (3) The *pulmonary veins* are a source of cerebral emboli, as indicated by the occurrence of cerebral abscesses in association with pulmonary suppurative processes and by the high incidence of cerebral deposits secondary to pulmonary carcinoma. (4) Surgery of the neck and thorax can be complicated by cerebral embolism. A rare type is that which follows thyroidectomy, in which thrombosis in the stump of the superior thyroid artery extends proximally until a section of it, protruding into the lumen of the carotid, is carried away into the cerebral arteries. (5) As is pointed out in Chap. 242, *prolapsed mitral valve* is a frequently observed abnormality and is said to be a potential source of cerebral embolism. There is one autopsied case in which this was proved and others in which it was suspected. However, in sizable series of cases not a single instance of embolism is recorded. One must conclude, therefore, that it is a definite although rare cause of embolic vascular disease.

Cerebral embolism must always have occurred when secondary tumor is deposited in the brain, and cerebral embolism regularly accompanies septicemia. However, a mass of tumor cells or bacteria seldom is large enough to occlude a cerebral artery and produce the picture of a stroke. Nevertheless tumor embolism has been reported secondary to *cardiac myxomas* and occasionally with other tumors. It must be distinguished from the *marantic endocarditis* and embolism which occasionally complicate carcinomatosis. Embolism in the course of septicemia usually means that a vegetative endocarditis is present

with thrombus formation. *Cerebral fat embolism* is usually related to fractures of large bones. As a rule, the emboli are minute and widely dispersed, giving rise to multiple cerebral petechial hemorrhages; accordingly the clinical picture is usually not focal, as in a stroke. *Cerebral air embolism* is a rare complication of criminal abortion or of cervical and thoracic operations and was formerly encountered as a complication of pneumothorax therapy. This condition is usually difficult to separate on clinical grounds from the deficits following hypotension or hypoxia, which frequently coexist.

Not infrequently at autopsy the diagnosis of cerebral embolism is made with full justification without finding a source. The same is true of embolism elsewhere in the body. Possibly the routine search for a thrombotic nidus is not sufficiently thorough, and small thrombi in the atrial appendage, in the carotid branches, in the endocardium between the papillary muscles of the heart, or in the pulmonary veins may be overlooked. Nevertheless, in some cases studied most carefully, no source of a demonstrable embolus in a cerebral artery can be discovered.

CLINICAL PICTURE   Of all strokes, those due to cerebral embolism develop most rapidly. "Like a bolt out of the blue," the full-blown picture evolves within several seconds or a minute, exemplifying most strikingly the temporal profile of a stroke. The neurologic deficit nearly always comes in a single sudden attack, only rarely in stuttering fashion. As a rule, there are no warning episodes whatsoever. This statement is possibly too stringent, for in occasional cases the onset is more gradual or fluctuating, or a transient episode or two may precede the final arrival of the stroke. However, any emphasis on these exceptions is misleading. The embolus strikes at any time of the day or night. Getting up to go to the bathroom is a time of danger. When the stroke occurs during sleep, its exact mode of development will not be known.

The neurologic picture will depend on the artery involved and where the obstruction lies. The syndromes related to each cerebrovascular territory are the same as those outlined (under "Neurovascular Syndromes") above. A large embolus may plug the stem of the middle cerebral artery, producing a severe hemiplegia. Eighty percent of Harvard Stroke Registry Series of embolic cases were in middle cerebral artery (11 percent posterior cerebral, 7 percent basilar, and 3 percent carotid arteries). More often the embolus is smaller and passes into one of the branches of the middle cerebral artery, producing a strikingly focal disorder: motor aphasia, a monoplegia (or part thereof), a central type of aphasia with little or no motor paralysis, or a sensorimotor paralysis with little or no involvement of language. Most patients diagnosed as having middle cerebral artery thrombosis prove to have emboli in the middle cerebral artery (or an atherosclerotic thrombosis of the carotid artery). It is important to realize that an embolus in its passage along an artery may produce a severe neurologic deficit which is only temporary; symptoms disappear as the embolus finally passes into a small branch supplying a relatively silent part of the hemisphere. In other words, embolism is a common cause of a single evanescent stroke. Also it can give rise to multiple transient attacks of differing pattern. Our opinion has already been expressed that recurrent transient ischemic attacks of the same pattern are not likely to be embolic, since successive emboli would hardly be expected to lodge at identical sites. Embolic material entering the vertebral-basilar system occasionally is arrested in the vertebral artery just below its union with the basilar; more often it traverses the vertebral and also the basilar, which is larger, and is not held up until it reaches the upper bifurcation. If arrested here, it abruptly produces deep coma and total paralysis. More often the embolus enters one, or both, of the posterior cerebral arteries and, by infarcting the visual cortex, causes a unilateral or bilateral homonymous hemianopia. Embolic infarction of the undersurface of the cerebellum is common, and the resulting swelling of necrotic brain may cause acute, fatal brainstem compression. Embolic material rarely enters the penetrating branches of the pons.

The general neurologic disturbance associated with embolic strokes is not significantly different from that seen in thrombotic cases, and the reader is referred to the description of the changes in consciousness, respiration, etc., under "Course and Prognosis," above. Again the patient may have a most devastating hemiplegia and yet be alert. Headache is not uncommon. In occlusion of the middle cerebral artery, the headache is usually referred to the ipsilateral temple; in occlusion of the posterior cerebral artery, to the outer half of the eyebrow.

Although the abruptness with which the stroke develops and the lack of prodromal symptoms point strongly to embolism, it is the total clinical picture upon which the diagnosis is based. If hemorrhage is ruled out, particularly by the use of the CT scan, there remains only thrombosis to be excluded. The presence of atrial fibrillation, a history of myocardial infarction (recent or in the preceding months), or the occurrence of embolism to other regions of the body all support the diagnosis of embolism. Embolism merits careful consideration in young persons in whom atherosclerosis is rather unlikely. Not infrequently the first sign of myocardial infarction is the occurrence of embolism; therefore, it is advisable to make *an electrocardiogram in all patients with cerebrovascular stroke of uncertain origin* and to monitor cardiac function for 3 days, even if the initial findings show normal cardiac rhythm.

Acute and subacute bacterial endocarditis do not usually present as a stroke due to infarction, although this happens occasionally. The signs of endocarditis, anemia, splenomegaly, and often a pleocytosis in the cerebrospinal fluid should point to the correct diagnosis in all but a few exceptional cases.

Cardiac catheterization and cardiac surgery, now being widely used, are a source of significant neurologic disorder, fortunately of decreasing frequency. Formerly as many as 50 percent of patients with open heart surgery suffered a postoperative neurologic complication; now the figure is down to about 25 percent. In 100 successive cases examined pre- and postoperatively by Mohr at the Massachusetts General Hospital there were two types of complications, one being discovered immediately and the other after an interval of days or weeks. The immediate neurologic disorder consisted of a delay in waking up from the anesthesia, a slowness in thinking, a disorientation, agitation, combativeness, visual hallucinations, and poor registration and recall of what was happening. These symptoms, sometimes verging on psychosis, usually cleared within a 5 to 7 day period, although some patients were not completely normal mentally at the time of discharge from the hospital. As the confusion clears, about half of the affected patients will be found to have small visual field defects, dyscalculia, oculomanual ataxia, alexia, and other visual perceptive defects indicative of lesions in the parietooccipital regions of the cerebrum. It is believed that these immediate disorders are related to hypotension and various types of emboli (air, silicon, fat, platelet). In addition, some of the patients have stretch injuries of the lower part of the brachial plaxus (numb, weak hand, and Horner's syndrome) that are manifest as soon as they awaken.

The delayed effects are mainly embolic and are more frequent in cases with prosthetic valve replacements than with arterial homografts. In one series the frequency of embolism was calculated to be 4.6 percent per month in the former group, and 1 percent per month in the latter, if untreated. The Starr-Edwards ball valve has given rise to embolism in 20 to 30 percent of cases over a 4-year period. Dicoumerol and depyrimidole reduced the rate of embolism from 14.9 percent in the untreated to 1.3 percent in the treated group (see Mohr).

The diagnosis of the other causes of cerebral embolism—neck surgery, pulmonary vein thrombosis, marantic endocarditis, paradoxic embolism, tumor, fat, and air—need not be enlarged upon here.

LABORATORY FINDINGS The description under "Atherosclerotic Thrombosis," above, applies for the most part to embolism except insofar as hemorrhagic infarction and septic embolism (focal embolic encephalitis) are concerned. Cerebral embolism in some 30 percent of cases produces a hemorrhagic infarct, which in most instances does not cause the cerebrospinal fluid to be bloody. However, in some excessively hemorrhagic infarcts, the fluid may be grossly bloody and contain as high as 10,000 or more red blood cells per cubic millimeter. In the milder cases of hemorrhagic infarction, a slight xanthochromia (grade 1 to 3 on the scale of 1 to 10) may appear after a few days. CT scan is helpful in showing hemorrhagic infarction. The hemorrhages have been observed within hours of embolic infarction. The possibility that an embolic infarct is unusually bloody underlines the danger of administering anticoagulants routinely without a careful examination of the cerebrospinal fluid. Also, it is the single exception to the rule that blood in the spinal fluid is unequivocal evidence that the stroke is due primarily to an intracerebral hemorrhage, aneurysm, or vascular malformation.

In septic embolism resulting from subacute bacterial endocarditis the white blood cells in the cerebrospinal fluid may be increased, usually numbering up to 200 per cubic millimeter and occasionally reaching several hundred; the proportion of lymphocytes and polymorphonuclear leukocytes varies with the acuteness of the septic process. There may also be several hundred or more red blood cells, and a faint xanthochromia is often present. The protein values are elevated, and the sugar content is within normal limits. No bacteria are seen or obtained by culture. In acute bacterial endocarditis there may be either the cerebrospinal fluid formula of subacute endocarditis or a frank purulent meningitis.

COURSE AND PROGNOSIS The remarks made concerning the *immediate prognosis* in atherosclerotic thrombosis apply as well here. As a rule, all but the most aggravated cases survive the initial insult. Massive brainstem infarction as a result of basilar embolism is almost always fatal. The eventual prognosis as to *survival* is determined by the occurrence of further emboli and the gravity of the underlying illness—cardiac failure, rheumatic heart disease, myocardial infarction, bacterial endocarditis, malignant growth, etc. The threat of an early recurrence of embolism is very real, and it is not uncommon to have the second embolus strike within a few days or weeks of the first. Considering these facts and the data of the Framingham series, where atrial fibrillation due presumably to arteriosclerotic heart disease increased the likelihood of a stroke fivefold (compared with age-matched controls) and atrial fibrillation with rheumatic heart disease increased the probability of stroke 17 times (Wolf et al.), the urgency of anticoagulant therapy is thereby emphasized. The eventual prognosis regarding the *neurologic deficit* is not different from that given for atherosclerotic thrombosis (see "Course and Prognosis," above). The fact that an embolic episode may last only minutes or hours before clearing up should be stressed, especially in estimating the effect of any therapeutic measure.

TREATMENT The first three phases of therapy—(1) general medical management in the acute phase, (2) measures directed to restoring the circulation, and (3) rehabilitation—are much the same as described under "Treatment of Atherosclerotic Thrombosis," above. Attempted embolectomy at the bifurcation of the common carotid artery has usually failed but should be considered. If pulsation in the temporal artery in front of the ear is present, it means the embolus is not at that bifurcation but has passed up into the internal carotid system, and embolectomy will probably be unsuccessful. The same is true of embolectomy of the middle cerebral artery, a procedure made possible by the development of microvascular surgical techniques. Fibrinolysin therapy has not been effective. In the field of prophylaxis there is strong evidence that the use of long-term anticoagulant therapy is effective in the prevention of embolism in cases of atrial fibrillation, myocardial infarction, and valve prosthesis. Prophylactic anticoagulant therapy is recommended for consideration in all cases of permanent and paroxysmal atrial fibrillation without waiting for embolism to occur, and once embolism does occur in 80 percent of cases the first episode will be followed by another embolus to the brain, frequently with severe damage. Although there has been much argument about the value of anticoagulants in thrombosis, they are almost universally recommended in embolism. In at least 14 studies of anticoagulant therapy, there has been a 65 to 90 percent reduction in the number of embolic accidents. Nonetheless, there is no completely randomized series. The treatment is continued for 6 to 12 months to years or for the lifetime of the patient. Platelet inhibitor therapy is not of proved worth.

After cerebral embolism has occurred, the question arises as to the necessity of delaying anticoagulant therapy for several days to avoid precipitating bleeding into a hemorrhagic infarct. It is the authors' practice always to perform a lumbar puncture first in order to rule out gross hemorrhage from the infarct and to obtain a CT scan in questionable cases. If the CT scan is normal and/or the cerebrospinal fluid is clear, the authors proceed with intravenous heparin therapy, since there is the constant danger of another embolus breaking away from the heart. One should not do a lumbar puncture in an anticoagulated patient unless absolutely necessary for fear of producing a spinal epidural or subdural hemorrhage and paraplegia. We have not encountered a case in which the use of anticoagulant drugs has increased the degree of hemorrhage within a hemorrhagic infarct, and indications are that such therapy is relatively safe. Rare exceptions to this statement may be expected. The use of anticoagulant therapy in patients with acute

TABLE 365-2
Causes of intracranial hemorrhage (including intracerebral, subarachnoid, ventricular, and rarely subdural)

1 Hypertensive and intracerebral hemorrhage
2 Ruptured saccular aneurysm
3 Ruptured angioma
4 Trauma including posttraumatic delayed apoplexy
5 Hemorrhagic disorders: leukemia, aplastic anemia, thrombopenic purpura, liver disease, complication of anticoagulant therapy, hyperfibrinolysis, hypofibrinogenemia, hemophilia, Christmas disease
6 Undetermined cause (normal blood pressure and no angioma)
7 Hemorrhage into primary and secondary brain tumors
8 Septic embolism and mycotic aneurysm
9 With hemorrhagic infarction, arterial or venous
10 With inflammatory disease of the arteries and veins
11 Miscellaneous rare types: after vasopressor drugs, upon exertion, during arteriography, during painful urologic examination, as a late complication of early-life carotid occlusion, complication of carotid-cavernous arteriovenous fistula, with anoxemia, migraine, teratomatous malformations. (Acute inclusion body encephalitis produces xanthochromia and up to 2000 red blood cells or more per milliliter of cerebrospinal fluid; acute necrotizing hemorrhagic encephalopathy may be associated with up to 100 red blood cells per milliliter of cerebrospinal fluid; tularemia and snake venom poisoning may cause bloody cerebrospinal fluid.)

myocardial infarction, including those judged to be in the "good risk" category, is advisable. In cerebral embolism associated with subacute bacterial endocarditis, anticoagulant therapy is usually held to be contraindicated because of the danger of intracranial bleeding, and it is preferable to rely on a rapid sterilization of the bloodstream.

Valvoplasty and amputation of the atrial appendage have substantially reduced the incidence of embolism in rheumatic heart disease. The need for special care in preventing emboli from entering the carotid arteries during the performance of cardiac valvoplasty is appreciated by all thoracic surgeons.

INTRACRANIAL HEMORRHAGE

This is the third most frequent cause of stroke, accounting for some 25 percent of cases. Although more than a dozen causes of intracranial hemorrhage have been listed (Table 365-2), hypertensive intracerebral hemorrhage, ruptured saccular aneurysm, hemorrhage associated with bleeding disorders, and arteriovenous malformations account for most of the hemorrhages which give rise to the clinical picture of a stroke. Duret hemorrhages, hypertensive encephalopathy, and idiopathic brain purpura will not simulate a stroke and are included only for the sake of completeness.

HYPERTENSIVE INTRACEREBRAL HEMORRHAGE Hypertensive intracerebral hemorrhage is the ordinary, well-recognized brain hemorrhage. Although sometimes the levels of blood pressure are normal (rare) or only in the range of 160/90 to 170/90, usually they are much higher. Hypertensive hemorrhage occurs *within* brain tissue, and rupture of the arteries lying in the subarachnoid space is practically unknown, apart from aneurysm. The extravasation which results from rupture of an artery forms a roughly circular or oval mass, which disrupts the tissue as the bleeding continues and it grows in volume. Adjacent brain tissue is displaced and compressed. If the hemorrhage is large, midline structures are displaced to the opposite side and vital centers are compromised, leading to coma and death. Rupture or seepage into the ventricular system usually occurs, and the spinal fluid becomes bloody in more than 90 percent of cases. A hemorrhage of this type almost never ruptures directly into the subarachnoid space through the cerebral cortex, and the blood reaches the subarachnoid spinal fluid via the ventricular system. When the hemorrhage is small and located at a distance from the ventricles, the cerebrospinal fluid may remain clear even on repeated examinations.

Extravasated blood undergoes a series of changes beginning with phagocytosis of the red blood cells at the outer rim, producing a brown-orange zone of hemosiderin-filled macrophages. The mass gradually decreases in size, and after a period of some 2 to 6 months, only an orange-stained cleft (color due to presence of hemosiderin and iron in macrophages) is left at the site of the hemorrhage.

Hemorrhages may be classified as massive, small, slit, and petechial. *Massive* refers to huge hemorrhages several centimeters in diameter; *small* to those 1 to 2 cm in diameter; *slit* applies to a special type of small hypertensive hemorrhage which lies subcortically at the junction of white and gray matter and which in the healing stage becomes narrowed to an elongated, thin, orange cavity.

In order of frequency, the most common sites for hypertensive hemorrhage are (1) the putamen and adjacent internal capsule (50 percent of cases), (2) various parts of the central white matter (frontal lobe, corona radiata, etc., often extensions from the putamen), (3) thalamus, (4) cerebellar hemisphere, and (5) pons. The vessel involved is usually a penetrating artery. The nature of the vascular lesion which leads to arterial rupture is not fully known, but in the few serially sectioned cases, the hemorrhage appeared to arise from an arterial wall altered by the effects of hypertension, referred to as *segmental lipohyalinosis.*

Clinical picture The clinical picture conforms accurately to the temporal profile of a cerebrovascular stroke; namely, it has an abrupt onset and rather rapid evolution. The stroke usually evolves gradually and steadily over an appreciable length of time, taking minutes, hours, or occasionally days (average of 1 to 24 h) to reach its peak, depending on the speed of bleeding. Hemorrhages associated with anticoagulant excess may be remarkably leisurely in evolution. Usually there are no recognizable warning or prodromal symptoms. Often the patient has been well, and headache, dizziness, and epistaxis have not occurred with any consistency as prodromal symptoms. There is no sex or age predilection except that the younger are usually spared. However, the average age of occurrence is less than in thrombotic infarction. Negroes suffer this type of stroke more frequently than do Caucasians. In the great majority of cases, the hemorrhage comes on while the patient is up and active, and onset during sleep is a rarity. Hypertension is maintained early in the course of the stroke or may even rise higher, so that the existence of hypertension will be easily established when the patient is first examined. Hypertension is usually of the "essential" type, but other causes must always be considered—renal disease, renal artery occlusion, toxemia of pregnancy, pheochromocytoma, aldosteronism, adrenocorticotropic hormone (ACTH) overdosage, injection of excessive amounts of epinephrine, and rarely, violent exertion or an intense emotional experience. Cardiomegaly is usually present.

There is ordinarily only one episode of hemorrhage, and recurrence of bleeding from the same site, as occurs in cases of saccular aneurysm, is not encountered. Once bleeding has become arrested, rebleeding in the near future, i.e., after the first few days, is not to be anticipated. When blood is spilled into the tissues, it is removed slowly, over a period of weeks and months, during which time symptoms and signs persist. Hence the neurologic deficit is never transitory in intracerebral hemorrhage, as it so often is in thrombosis and embolism, and, for the same reason, rapid improvement in the neurologic deficit from one examination to another is not to be expected.

The neurologic signs and symptoms vary with the site and size of the extravasation. The most common picture is that associated with a *putamenal hemorrhage,* in which the adjacent internal capsule is implicated. In the large hemorrhages the patient lapses almost immediately into a comatose state with hemiplegia, and his condition visibly deteriorates as the hours pass. More often, however, he complains of something going awry within the head. In a few minutes the face sags on one side, speech becomes slurred or aphasic, the arm and leg gradually weaken, and the eyes tend to deviate away from the side of the paretic limbs. A carefully taken history often reveals that these events occurred gradually over a period of 5 to 30 min. This type of evolution is strongly suggestive of intracerebral bleeding. Gradually the paralysis worsens, the affected limbs become flaccid, pinprick is not appreciated, a Babinski sign appears, speaking becomes impossible, and confusion gives way to stupor. In the worst cases, signs of upper brainstem compression appear—coma, Babinski sign bilaterally, deep, irregular, or intermittent respiration, dilated fixed pupils, and occasionally decerebrate rigidity.

Thalamic hemorrhage of moderate size also produces a hemiplegia or hemiparesis via pressure on the adjacent internal capsule. The sensory deficit equals or outstrips the motor weakness. Aphasia may be present with lesions of the dominant side and apractagnosia of the nondominant. A homonymous field defect if present usually clears in a few days. Thalamic hemorrhage by virtue of its extension medially and into

the subthalamus causes a series of ocular disturbances, including paralysis of vertical gaze, forced deviation of the eyes downward, inequality of pupils, with absence of light reaction, skew deviation with the eye opposite the hemorrhage being displaced downward and medially, ipsilateral ptosis and miosis, absence of convergence, an assortment of lateral gaze abnormalities (paresis or pseudoparesis of the sixth nerve), retraction nystagmus, and tucking in of the eyelids. Neck retraction may be prominent. Hemorrhage into the nondominant thalamus is liable to produce mutism.

In *pontine hemorrhage,* deep coma usually ensues in a few minutes, and the clinical picture includes total paralysis, prominent decerebrate rigidity, and small (1 mm) pupils that react to light. Lateral eye movements, evoked by head turning or irrigation of the ears with ice water, are impaired. The cerebrospinal fluid will be sanguineous. Death usually occurs within a few hours, but there are rare exceptions where consciousness is retained and the clinical manifestations indicate a small lesion in the tegmentum of the pons, e.g., disturbances of lateral ocular movements, crossed sensory or motor disturbances, small pupils, cranial nerve palsies, and bilateral signs of pyramidal tract involvement.

Cerebellar hemorrhage usually develops over a period of several hours, and loss of consciousness at the onset is almost unknown. Repeated vomiting is a hallmark of cerebellar hemorrhage, along with inability to walk or stand, occipital headache, and vertigo. There is a paresis of conjugate lateral gaze of the eyes to the side of the hemorrhage, forced deviation of the eyes to the opposite side, or an ipsilateral sixth nerve weakness. In the most acute phase of the illness there may be little or no evidence of cerebellar disease, and only a minority of cases show nystagmus or cerebellar ataxia of the limbs, although these signs must always be sought. Other ocular signs include "ocular bobbing," blepharospasm, involuntary closure of one eye, skew deviation, and maintenance of vertical eye movements including small pupils which continue to react until very late in the illness and exhibit slight inequality. A mild ipsilateral facial weakness and a diminished corneal reflex are common. Dysarthria and dysphagia may be prominent. Contralateral hemiplegia and facial weakness do not occur. Occasionally at the onset there is a quadriplegia with preservation of consciousness or a spastic paraparesis. The plantar reflexes are flexor early, extensor late. As the hours pass, and occasionally with unanticipated suddenness, the patient becomes stuporous, then comatose as a result of brainstem compression, at which point reversal of the syndrome, even by surgical therapy, is seldom successful.

Ocular signs are important in the localization of intracerebral hemorrhages. In putaminal hemorrhage the eyes are deviated to the side opposite the paralysis; in thalamic hemorrhage the eyes are deviated downward and the pupils may be unreactive; in pontine hemorrhage the eyeballs are fixed and the pupils tiny and reactive; and in cerebellar hemorrhage the eyes are deviated laterally (to the side opposite the lesion) in the absence of paralysis.

At each of the above sites the hemorrhage is usually massive and patients survive only a few hours or a few days, succumbing as a result of secondary brainstem insult. Rarely do patients survive once deep stupor supervenes, although in some cases they may linger in an unresponsive state for a week or two. In some 30 percent of cases, however, the hemorrhage is less extensive and survival is possible, hemorrhage into the thalamus especially tending to be somewhat smaller than putaminal or cerebellar hemorrhage.

A *severe headache* occurs in only 50 percent of cases; in many others no headache is noted. *Nuchal rigidity* is frequently found, but again it is so often absent that failure to find it must by no means detract from the diagnosis. If the neck becomes stiff, it will become supple again as coma deepens. *Vomiting* occurs once or twice at the onset of intracerebral hemorrhage, and it is so frequent in cerebral syndromes of hemorrhage compared with infarction that hemorrhage is the leading diagnosis in that setting. But of equal importance is the fact that the patient often is far from comatose and may even be alert and responding accurately when first seen. This is true with grossly bloody spinal fluid, and thus the adage that hemorrhage into the ventricular system always precipitates coma is quite incorrect. Only if bleeding into the ventricles is massive will coma result. *Cerebral seizures,* usually focal, occur in some 10 percent of cases of supratentorial hemorrhage in the first few days, especially in association with subcortical "slit" hemorrhage. The fundi often show hypertensive changes in the arteries. Rarely, fresh preretinal (subhyaloid) hemorrhages occur but are much more common in ruptured aneurysm or angioma.

Many of the less precisely localized neurologic manifestations described under cerebral thrombosis are also encountered in intracerebral hemorrhage, including coma, stupor, drowsiness, confusion. Cheyne-Stokes respiration, bilateral or contralateral grasping and sucking reflexes, incontinence of bowel and bladder, and unilateral and bilateral extensor rigidity.

Although the proper interpretation of this array of clinical data allows the correct diagnosis to be established in most cases, the laboratory examinations described below are helpful, especially in the more difficult small hemorrhages.

Laboratory findings As for helpful laboratory procedures it is necessary to emphasize the value of the CT scan. This form of x-ray study has revolutionized the diagnosis of intracerebral hemorrhage and has proved totally reliable in the detection of hemorrhages 1.5 cm or more in diameter situated in the cerebral or cerebellar hemispheres for the first 3 weeks after the rupture of the vessel. Thereafter, for reasons not known, the extravasated blood becomes invisible in the CT scan. Small pontine hemorrhages are visualized less certainly. Hemorrhages are localized with remarkable accuracy, far surpassing that achieved with arteriography. At the same time coexisting hydrocephalus, tumor, cerebral swelling, and displacement of intracranial contents are readily appreciated. The CT scan is particularly helpful in the diagnosis of small brain hemorrhages that do not spill blood into the CSF and were heretofore clinically unrecognizable (Fig. 364-1).

Before the introduction of CT scanning the examination of the cerebrospinal fluid was the most dependable method for the diagnosis of hemorrhage. In cases of massive hemorrhage, the cerebrospinal fluid is often under increased pressure, but in almost half of our cases readings under 200 mm were obtained. The fluid is usually grossly bloody, although not so bloody as in ruptured saccular aneurysm (the count ranging from a few thousand cells up to 1 million). In smaller hemorrhages into central structures the cerebrospinal fluid contains a lesser amount of blood, and in some cases of intracerebral hemorrhage, particularly in those of the "slit" type, between cortex and white matter, it remains free of blood and clear of xanthochromia in repeated taps. In these latter cases, slight xanthochromia may appear after a few days to a week. At times the spinal fluid may be clear grossly but contain some 200 to 400 red blood cells, and it is then difficult to decide if this represents intracranial bleeding or a traumatic tap.

A *traumatic bloody spinal tap* greatly complicates the diagnostic problem. In a bloody tap the pressure tends to be low,

the fluid that first flows from the needle is more bloody than that which comes later (third tube less bloody than the first), the fluid often clots in the test tube, and xanthochromia is either absent or at most present only in proportion to the amount of serum bilirubin admixed with the fluid. Bloody fluid due to cerebral hemorrhage is often under increased pressure, there is an even admixture of blood in all samples, the cerebrospinal fluid will not clot, and if more than 8 to 12 h has elapsed since the hemorrhage, a definite xanthochromia will be present in the supernatant fluid after centrifugation, which should always be carried out if there is any question of the reliability of the tap. However, the presence of xanthochromia after centrifugation may be due to the bilirubin contained in the blood spilled by a traumatic tap and therefore is not an infallible index of subarachnoid or brain hemorrhage. The white blood cells of the cerebrospinal fluid are accounted for by the amount of hemorrhage, and their ratio of red blood cells is usually the same as in the circulating blood. After hemolysis of red blood cells, the white blood cell count may be disproportionately increased. In parenchymatous hemorrhage the protein content of the cerebrospinal fluid is proportionately much greater than accounted for by the amount of hemorrhage, presumably due to leakage of high protein fluid from the hemorrhage. Sometimes after a questionably traumatic tap it is worthwhile to perform immediately another puncture at a higher level.

Lumbar puncture is not completely innocuous, since temporal lobe herniation may be aggravated in cases of massive supratentorial hemorrhage or softening. Despite this danger, the procedure is necessary when CT scanning is not available, and if specific therapeutic measures are contemplated, or if any doubt exists as to the diagnosis of cerebrovascular disease. X-ray of the skull early in the stroke sometimes shows a shift of the calcified pineal gland to the side of the cranium opposite the lesion, a change usually not seen in infarction. The electroencephalogram does not show a typical or diagnostic pattern, but high-voltage, slow waves are the most common finding with hemorrhage into the cerebral hemisphere. X-ray of the chest will often show cardiomegaly. Any urinary abnormalities will for the most part reflect coexisting renal disease, although transient glycosuria has been reported to result specifically from intracranial hemorrhage. The white blood cell count often rises to 15,000 to 20,000 per cubic millimeter, a higher figure than in thrombosis. The sedimentation rate is elevated.

Course and prognosis The immediate prognosis is grave, some 70 to 75 percent of patients dying in 1 to 30 days. Either the hemorrhage extends into the ventricular system, or temporal lobe herniation and midbrain compression occur. Sometimes the hemorrhage appears to seep gradually into vital centers. Gastric erosion and gastrointestinal hemorrhage of neurogenic origin may occur at any time within the first week or two. When the hemorrhage is smaller, survival is often the result, and the restitution of motor function, speech, etc., can be excellent, since, in contrast to infarction, the hemorrhage has to some extent pushed brain tissue aside instead of destroying it. Function may be slow to return, because extravasated blood is slow to be resorbed or removed from the tissues. Since rebleeding from the same site is unlikely, the patient may live for many years. In some instances of medium-sized cerebral and cerebeller hemorrhages, the patient survives and his or her condition gradually stabilizes, but definite papilledema appears after several days of increased intracranial pressure. This does not mean that the hemorrhage is increasing in size or swelling, only that papilledema is slow to develop. Healed scars impinging on the cortex are liable to be epileptogenic.

Treatment *The general medical management of the comatose, apoplectic patient is the same as that outlined under "Atheroscle-*

rotic Thrombosis," above, and in Chap. 20. Measures to stem the hemorrhage and restore the integrity of damaged tissue have been relatively ineffective.

Surgical removal of the clot in the acute stage, either by evacuation or aspiration, has seldom proved beneficial except in patients with a hemorrhage lying near the surface and who are not comatose. Acute cerebellar hemorrhage, by contrast, is usually amenable to surgical therapy and is the treatment of choice when the hemorrhage is diagnosed within the first 2 days of onset. In the smaller hemorrhages that reach a subacute stage, when papilledema appears, in many instances it has dictated unnecessary surgical evacuation of the hemorrhage when the patient's condition stabilized. Although the prognosis in hemorrhage into the cerebral hemisphere is probably little altered by surgery, the outlook for cerebellar cases seems to be improved.

Attempts to halt the hemorrhage by lowering the systemic blood pressure through the use of autonomic blocking agents have not been effective, and in many instances the inadvertent occurrence of disastrously low levels of blood pressure has complicated the illness. Artificial hypothermia has been used sporadically, but there are insufficient data to permit appraisal of this procedure. Intermittent compression of the ipsilateral carotid in the neck may be beneficial in acute putaminal cases.

The *only preventive measure* is the use of antihypertensive drugs to lower the blood pressure in cases of essential hypertension. If ACTH or one of the adrenal steroids is being given, toxicity must be watched for. When hypotension threatens during surgical procedures, injections of excessive amounts of epinephrine, Aramine, or Levophed are to be avoided. Toxemia of pregnancy, another cause of cerebral hemorrhage, must be detected early and the hypertension treated.

RUPTURED SACCULAR ANEURYSM This is the fourth most frequent of the cerebrovascular disorders following atherosclerosis, embolism, and hypertensive intracerebral hemorrhage. Saccular aneurysms take the form of small, thin-walled blisters protruding from the arteries of the circle of Willis or the major branches arising therefrom. These saccules or berries, as they have been called, are located for the most part at bifurcations and branchings (Fig. 365-11) and are presumed to be the result of developmental defects in the media and elastica. A small number of aneurysms have been attributed to incomplete involution of embryonic vessels. Owing to the local weakness, the intima bulges outward, covered only by adventitia; the sac gradually enlarges, until finally dissolution of the wall and rup-

ture occur. Saccular aneurysms vary in size from tiny nubbins 2 mm in diameter up to spheric masses 2 or 3 cm in diameter, averaging 8 to 20 mm. They vary greatly in form; some are round and connected to the parent artery by a narrower stalk; others are broad-based without a stalk; still others are narrow cylinders. The site of rupture is usually the dome of the aneurysm which may present one or more secondary sacculations but may also occur near the base. Enlargement is the result of dilatation of the lumen and organization of a laminated clot.

In routine autopsies the incidence of ruptured aneurysms is 1.8 percent, of unruptured ones, 2.0 percent. Saccular aneurysms are rare in childhood, even at routine postmortem examination, and increase in frequency to reach their highest plateau of incidence in persons between 35 and 65 years of age. Therefore, they are not congenitally formed anomalies but develop over the years on the basis of the developmental arterial defect. There is an increased incidence of congenital polycystic disease of the kidney and coarctation of the aorta in association with saccular aneurysm. Hypertension is more frequently present than in the average population, but aneurysms occur in persons with normal blood pressure. Atherosclerosis, although present in the walls of some saccular aneurysms, probably plays no part in their formation or enlargement.

Approximately 90 to 95 percent of saccular aneurysms lie on the anterior part of the circle of Willis. The four most common sites are (1) in relation to the anterior communicating artery, (2) at the origin of the posterior communicating artery from the stem of the internal carotid, (3) at the first major bifurcation of the middle cerebral artery, and (4) at the bifurcation of the internal carotid into middle and anterior cerebral arteries (see Fig. 365-11). Other sites include the internal carotid in the cavernous sinus (rupture may lead to an arteriovenous aneurysm without causing subarachnoid hemorrhage), at the origin of the ophthalmic artery, at the junction of the posterior communicating artery with the posterior cerebral, at the bifurcation of the basilar artery, and at the origins of the three cerebellar arteries. In 20 percent of cases there is more than one aneurysm, and they may be situated unilaterally or bilaterally.

Several types of aneurysm other than saccular occur, e.g., mycotic, fusiform, diffuse, and globular. The last three are named for their predominant morphologic aspects and consist of enlargement or dilatation of the entire circumference of the

FIGURE 365-11

Diagram of the circle of Willis to show the principal sites of saccular aneurysm. Approximately 90 percent of aneurysms are on the anterior half of the circle.

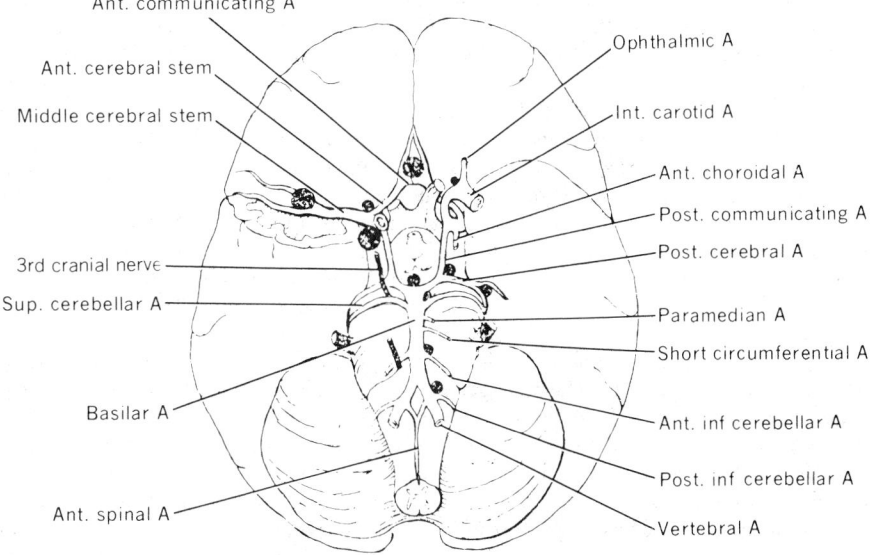

Ant. communicating A
Ant. cerebral stem
Middle cerebral stem
3rd cranial nerve
Sup. cerebellar A
Basilar A
Ant. spinal A
Ophthalmic A
Int. carotid A
Ant. choroidal A
Post. communicating A
Post. cerebral A
Paramedian A
Short circumferential A
Ant. inf cerebellar A
Post. inf cerebellar A
Vertebral A

involved vessels, usually the internal carotid, vertebral, or basilar arteries. Frequently showing atherosclerotic deposition in their walls, they are often referred to as arteriosclerotic, but most likely they are at least partly developmental in nature. They press on neighboring structures or become occluded by thrombosis and rupture only infrequently.

Clinical picture Prior to rupture, saccular aneurysms are usually asymptomatic. Occasionally, large aneurysms immediately distal to the cavernous sinus may compress the optic nerves or chiasm, third nerve, hypothalamus, or pituitary gland. In the cavernous sinus they may press on the oculomotor, ophthalmic, or fifth or sixth cranial nerves (Chap. 376). In the posterior fossa, one or more of the cranial nerves may be compressed adjacent to the brainstem. Rarely they cause headache, but by then other signs will usually have appeared.

When rupture occurs, blood under high pressure is discharged into the subarachnoid space (the circle of Willis lies in the subarachnoid space), and the resulting clinical events fall into one of three patterns: (1) the patient may be stricken with an excruciating generalized headache and fall unconscious almost immediately; (2) headache may develop as in (1), but the patient remains relatively lucid; (3) consciousness may be lost quickly without any preceding complaint. Decerebrate rigidity may occur at the onset of hemorrhage in association with unconsciousness. If the hemorrhage is massive, a fatal issue may ensue in a matter of minutes, hours, or a day or two. Persistent deep coma is accompanied by irregular respiration, attacks of extensor rigidity, and finally respiratory arrest and circulatory collapse. In these rapidly fatal cases, the blood has usually dissected intracerebrally and entered the ventricular system. Death occasionally occurs within 5 min, and ruptured aneurysm must be considered the differential diagnosis of sudden death.

In mild cases, consciousness, if lost, may be regained within a few minutes as the blood diffuses through the subarachnoid space and the intracranial pressure falls, but a residuum of confusion and amnesia accompanied by severe headache and stiff neck persists for at least several days. It is not uncommon for drowsiness and confusion to last 10 days or longer. If the hemorrhage is confined to the subarachnoid space, there are few or no lateralizing neurologic signs.

In most patients there are no warning symptoms; in some, however, minor leakage from the aneurysm sometimes precedes devastating rupture by a few days or weeks. Headache is the chief sign of such an event, but there may be in some instances a transitory unilateral weakness, numbness and tingling, or speech disturbance. Aneurysmal rupture usually occurs while the patient is active rather than during sleep, and in many instances sexual intercourse or other exertion precipitates the ictus.

Gross lateralizing signs in the form of hemiplegia, hemiparesis, or aphasia are absent in the majority of cases, but can occur and, in the acute stages, are due to an intracerebral clot, or ischemia in the territory of the aneurysm-bearing artery. The aneurysm may rupture partly into the subarachnoid space and partly into brain tissue (subarachnoid-cerebral hemorrhage) and even reach the ventricular system (subarachnoid-ventricular hemorrhage), rendering the patient stuporous or comatose. The initial neurologic deficit may clear in a matter of days, indicating that hemorrhage into tissues was not responsible for the focal signs. The pathogenesis of such manifestations is not fully understood, but a transitory fall in pressure in the circulation distal to the aneurysm is postulated. Transient deficits, still more evanescent, are not uncommon; paresis or aphasia, for example, may be present for only a few minutes or so after the onset of bleeding, constituting a reliable telltale

of the site of the ruptured aneurysm. A delayed hemiplegia or other deficit may occur 4 to 9 days after rupture. This is attributable to focal narrowing of a large artery at the base, usually interpreted as vasospasm due to the presence of extravasated blood. Areas of ischemic necrosis of tissue in the territory of the vessel bearing the aneurysm, but sometimes in the territory of other arteries, are frequently found postmortem. These are probably due to vascular spasm because thrombosis is seldom found. A subacute hydrocephalus due to blockage of the CSF pathways by blood may appear after 2 to 4 weeks. Ventriculoatrial shunting provides relief.

Although in most patients the neurologic manifestations do not point to the exact site of the aneurysm, in many instances there are clues to the localization. For example, (1) third nerve palsy (ptosis, diplopia, mydriasis, and oculomotor paralysis) usually indicates an aneurysm at the junction of the posterior communicating artery and the internal carotid stem. The third nerve passes immediately lateral to this point. (2) Transient paresis of one or both of the lower limbs at the onset of hemorrhage is suggestive of an anterior communicating aneurysm which has interfered with the circulation in the anterior cerebral arteries, causing ischemia of the motor areas for the lower extremities. (3) Hemiparesis or aphasia often points to an aneurysm at the bifurcation of the middle cerebral artery which has critically reduced the circulation in the middle cerebral system. (4) Unilateral blindness or amblyopia indicates an aneurysm which lies anteromedially in the circle of Willis (at the origin of the ophthalmic artery, at the bifurcation of the internal carotid artery, or in the anterior communicating region). (5) A stage of retained consciousness with akinetic mutism or abulia favors an aneurysm of the anterior communicating artery which has caused ischemia of or hemorrhage into one or both of the frontal lobes, hypothalamus, or corpus callosum. (6) The side on which the aneurysm lies may be indicated by a unilateral preponderance of headache or preretinal hemorrhages, by the occurrence of monocular pain, or by the lateralization of an intracranial sound heard at the time of rupture of the aneurysm. Sixth nerve palsy, unilateral or bilateral, results from the presence of subarachnoid blood and raised intracranial pressure and is seldom of localizing value. Other neurologic signs which have relatively little localizing value include sucking and grasp reflexes, bilateral Babinski signs, choreoathetosis, and extensor rigidity.

In summary, the clinical sequence of sudden violent headache, collapse, brief unconsciousness and confusion, combined with an absence of prodromal symptoms and a paucity of lateralizing signs, is diagnostic of a ruptured saccular aneurysm.

Other clinical data may be of assistance in reaching a correct diagnosis. Nuchal rigidity is usually present. Examination of the fundi not infrequently reveals smooth-surfaced, sharply outlined collections of blood which cover the retinal vessels—the so-called "preretinal" or "subhyaloid" hemorrhages. These are usually a sign of ruptured aneurysm but can occur in hypertensive hemorrhage and cranial trauma. Bilateral Babinski signs are found in the early days following rupture. The patient may appear to be normally alert, while impairment of memory and confabulation are found on more careful testing. A fever with the temperature rising to 38.9°C (102°F) is common in the first week. The escaping blood occasionally enters the subdural space and produces a subdural hematoma, evacuation of which may be lifesaving. Aneurysmal rupture may complicate pregnancy, but pregnancy is not associated with an increased incidence of aneurysmal rupture. Spontaneous intracranial bleeding with normal blood pressure should always suggest ruptured aneurysm, ruptured angioma, or hemorrhage into a cerebral tumor.

Laboratory findings Carotid and vertebral angiography is the only certain means of demonstrating an aneurysm and does so effectively in some 85 percent of patients in whom aneurysm appears to be the correct diagnosis on clinical grounds, i.e., in cases of so-called "spontaneous subarachnoid hemorrhage."

A CT scan will detect a localized blood clot within the brain or ventricular system or in the subarachnoid spaces adjacent to the ruptured aneurysm. Also a coexistent hydrocephalus will be demonstrated. The cerebrospinal fluid is usually extremely bloody, with red blood cell counts reaching to 1 million per cubic millimeter or higher. When the hemorrhage is very slight, there may be only a few thousand cells. It is unlikely that an aneurysm can rupture entirely into brain tissue without some leakage of blood into the subarachnoid fluid, and therefore the diagnosis of ruptured saccular aneurysm must never be made unless blood is present in the spinal fluid. Only unruptured saccular aneurysms which either compress the optic nerves, chiasm, cranial nerves, or brainstem or lie within the cavernous sinus produce symptoms without hemorrhage. Usually deep xanthochromia is found after centrifugation. The cerebrospinal fluid is under greatly increased pressure, as high as 1000 mmH$_2$O. The subarachnoid bleeding can be distinguished from a bloody tap (see "Laboratory Findings," above, regarding traumatic tap). The white blood cells in the spinal fluid are usually present in the same proportion to red blood cells as in the circulating blood, but in some patients within 48 h a brisk leukocytosis appears, reaching 2000 to 3000 cells per cubic millimeter. After a few days white blood cells contain phagocytized red blood cells and hemosiderin (hemocytoblasts). The glucose level may become subnormal after 2 to 3 days.

X-rays of the skull are usually negative, though in a few patients one or both of the anterior clinoid processes show erosion by the pressure of an adjacent aneurysm, or calcification has occurred in the region of a previous hemorrhage. A calcified pineal gland may be displaced by an intracerebral or subdural clot.

Any urinary abnormality is usually due to concomitant renal disease. Rarely diabetes insipidus occurs. Transient glycosuria and albuminuria may occur. A leukocytosis of 15,000 to 18,000 cells per cubic millimeter is common.

Acute subarachnoid hemorrhage may be associated with electrocardiographic abnormalities suggestive of myocardial ischemia. The electroencephalogram is of little help in localizing the lesion unless a gross neurologic deficit is present, in which case the lateralization is probably already evident clinically. The abnormality usually consists of slow waves.

Course and prognosis The outstanding characteristic of this condition is the tendency for the hemorrhage to recur. This threat colors all prognostications, and unfortunately there appears to be no way of determining reliably which cases will rebleed. The cause of the intermittency of bleeding is not understood, but may be related to naturally occurring mechanisms of clot lysis.

Patients with the typical clinical picture of spontaneous subarachnoid hemorrhage but in whom the angiogram shows no aneurysm or angioma have a better prognosis than those in whom the lesion is demonstrated.

McKissock et al. found that the patient's state of consciousness at the time of arteriography was the best single criterion of prognosis. By use of their data as representative of any large medical center, it was shown that of every 100 patients coming to arteriography, 17 will be stuporous or comatose, and 83 will appear to be recovering from the ictus. At the end of the next 6 months, of the first 17, 7 will have died from the original hemorrhage and 7 more will have had a fatal recurrence, making a total of 14 deaths and 3 survivors. Of the other 83, one will have died of the original hemorrhage and 52 will have had a recurrence, of which 33 will have died, making a total of 34 deaths and 49 survivors. Thus, of the total of 100, at the end of

6 months, 8 will have died of the original hemorrhage, 59 more will have had a recurrence, with 40 deaths, making a total of 48 deaths and 52 survivors. Thus, the gravity of the illness is immediately apparent. In regard to the recurrence of bleeding, it was found that of every 50 patients seen on the first day of the illness, 5 will rebleed in the first week (all fatal), 8 in the second week (5 fatal), 6 in the third and fourth weeks (4 fatal), and 2 in the next 4 weeks (2 fatal), making a total of 21 recurrences in 8 weeks (16 fatal). In McKissock's series rerupture did not occur in the first 2 days; thereafter it occurred at a steady rate for the next 19 days and tapered off abruptly. However, we have observed in the Massachusetts General Hospital's cases that rerupture in the first 2 days is not uncommon.

Of the survivors in the first group, all but one returned to work, and in the second group, 36 went back to full work, 12 were partly disabled, and 4 were totally disabled. The disability was due to paralysis, mental deterioration, or epilepsy.

Treatment General medical management in the acute stage is similar to that described under "Atherosclerotic Thrombosis," above. The earlier the case comes under medical purview and the more severe the impairment of consciousness, the less certain are any known therapeutic measures to be beneficial. Those surviving in good condition for several days have the best outlook, and with the passage of time the risk of recurrent bleeding diminishes. Rational medical measures are based on the assumption that decreasing the arterial blood pressure is the most reasonable way of arresting the hemorrhage and preventing recurrence. Absolute bed rest for 4 to 8 weeks is prescribed, with the head of the bed raised some 15 to 20°. Straining during bowel movement is forbidden, and laxatives or general enemas are administered. Coughing and all forms of exertion are avoided. The patient is fed. The duration of the period of bed rest is empiric and not founded on any reliable clinical observations or information about the formation of scar tissue around aneurysms. Sedatives (barbiturates) and analgesics are important in aiding relaxation. Hypotensive agents are used to bring blood pressures to normal, but Aldomet should be avoided as it produces drowsiness, which confuses the clinical picture. In the presence of severe hypertension, blocking agents may be cautiously used to lower the blood pressure to 160/100, great care being exercised not to precipitate excessive hypotension and cerebral infarction. Promazine intramuscularly is used to control nausea and vomiting. Dilantin or phenobarbital may be prescribed to prevent cerebral seizures. Aspirin should not be given since it may impair clotting and encourage rebleeding.

At present a systemic antifibrinolysin, ε-aminocaproic acid (Amicar),[1] in a dosage of 24 g intravenously per day for 3 weeks is being used in several of the large medical centers in the United States to impede lysis of the clot at the site of aneurysmal rupture. This measure seems to be effective in reducing the incidence of recurrent subarachnoid hemorrhage. The patient fares better if antihypertensive medicines are not given concomitantly.

The place of repeated drainage of the cerebrospinal fluid by lumbar puncture is still uncertain, although several workers have concluded that it does not affect the outcome of the illness. At present, one lumbar puncture is usually carried out for diagnostic purposes, and thereafter it is performed only for the relief of intractable headache, to detect recurrence of bleeding, or to measure the intracranial pressure prior to surgery.

In maintaining fluid balance, intravenous fluids should be

---

[1] *Not yet approved by the Food and Drug Administration.*

used sparingly and in the proper electrolyte combination (a mixture of equal parts of 5% glucose in water and normal saline solution or balanced electrolytes) in order to minimize the danger of aggravating brain swelling. Any abnormality of concentration of electrolytes in the blood must be corrected. If diabetes insipidus has occurred, it should be treated with Pitressin. Vitamins C and K have been recommended routinely, but there is no evidence that they are beneficial. Disorders of blood coagulation should be corrected. Body hypothermia for 2 to 5 days in the stage of acute hemorrhage has been used with uncertain efficacy. Intravenous hypertonic urea or mannitol may be effective in temporarily reducing the intracranial pressure.

Since the attainment of a significant reduction in recurrent hemorrhage by Amicar, vasospasm has become the most pressing problem. It usually develops a few days after the first rupture and often causes paralytic symptoms. According to a recent double-blind study (Zervas et al.) the use of reserpine 0.1 mg to 0.2 mg qid intramuscularly and kanamycin 1.0 g qid orally has prevented ischemic strokes. These drugs and Amicar should be started as soon as the patient enters the hospital and continued until operation.

After resting in bed for 6 weeks, the patient is gradually allowed to resume activity and may return to work in 4 months. It seems logical to advise that heavy labor not be resumed.

Surgical therapy Apart from occasionally evacuating an associated intracerebral clot, surgical treatment is for the most part directed to the prevention of recurrence of the hemorrhage. The procedures are either *extracranial* (ligation of the common carotid in the neck) or *intracranial* (clipping; ligating the neck of the aneurysm under the operating microscope). Other procedures include wrapping or tamponade of the aneurysmal sac by muscle, fascia, plastic coating, or arterial graft; trapping the aneurysm; ligation of the main feeding vessel proximal to the aneurysm. Occasionally extracranial and intracranial procedures are combined. Because of the high operative mortality if surgery is undertaken early, the operation has usually been delayed 1 to 2 weeks until the patient's condition has stabilized following the first hemorrhage. Before treatment is undertaken, the site, size, and form of the aneurysm must be determined by angiography. At the same time the pattern of the anterior half of the circle of Willis is noted, as it may influence the choice of operative procedure. It has been demonstrated that surgical treatment improves upon the natural outlook for aneurysms, especially those at the posterior communicating artery and the bifurcation of the middle cerebral artery. The operative mortality has been reduced to less than 5 percent.

After aneurysmal rupture a chronic obstructive or communicating hydrocephalus may develop, causing persistent stupor, which is relieved by ventriculoatrial shunting.

OTHER CAUSES OF INTRACRANIAL HEMORRHAGE An *angioma,* or hemangioma, consists of a tangle of abnormal vessels forming an abnormal communication between the arterial and venous systems, really an arteriovenous fistula. It is a developmental abnormality, not a neoplasm, but the constituent vessels enlarge with growth and the passage of time. Angiomas vary in size from a small blemish a few millimeters in diameter lying in the cortex or white matter to a huge mass of tortuous channels composing an arteriovenous shunt of sufficient magnitude to raise the cardiac output. Hypertrophic dilated arterial "feeders" approach the main lesion, disappear below the cortex, and break up into a network of thin-walled blood vessels which connect directly with draining veins. The latter often form huge, dilated pulsating channels, carrying away arterial blood. The blood vessels forming the tangle interposed between arteries and veins are usually abnormally thin and do not have the normal structure of arteries or veins. Angiomas occur in all parts of the brain, brainstem, and spinal cord, but the larger ones are more frequently found in the posterior half of the hemispheres, commonly forming a wedge-shaped lesion extending from the cortex to the ventricular lining.

Angiomas predominate in males over females about 2:1. They may occur in more than one member of a family in the same or successive generations. Although the lesion is present from birth, the onset of complaints is most common between the ages of 10 and 30, but occasionally it is delayed as late as the fifties. The chief clinical features are cerebral or cerebral-subarachnoid hemorrhage or epileptic seizures occurring in a child or young adult. In 50 percent the first manifestation is a hemorrhage, in 30 percent, a seizure, and in 20 percent, headache, dementia, progressive hemiparesis, hemiatrophy (if onset is early in life), hemisensory syndrome, hemiathetosis, etc. The seizure pattern depends on the site of the lesion; when focal motor in type the seizure may be followed by a temporary postictal paralysis. When hemorrhage occurs, blood may enter the subarachnoid space almost exclusively, producing a picture identical with that of ruptured saccular aneurysm, but since the angioma lies within the cerebral tissue, the bleeding is more likely to be at least partly intracerebral, causing hemiparesis, hemiplegia, or death. Before rupture, chronic nondescript headache is a frequent complaint and sometimes a slowly evolving (over several minutes) and regressing hemiparesis or hemanesthesia. This may at times simulate migraine. Huge angiomas may produce a slowly progressive neurologic deficit because of local pressure and depletion of blood from adjacent brain tissue. Proptosis has been encountered. When the vein of Galen is involved, hydrocephalus may result. Not infrequently one or both carotid arteries pulsate unusually forcefully in the neck. A loud systolic bruit heard over the carotid in the neck, the mastoid process, or the eyeballs in young adults is almost pathognomonic of angioma; faint ones in infancy and early childhood are of little significance. The older patient should be exercised in order to bring out a bruit if none is present at rest. A bruit may also be heard over a spinal angioma of large size. The blood pressure may be raised or normal, and it is axiomatic that the occurrence of intracranial bleeding with normal blood pressure should lead to the suspicion of an angioma, ruptured saccular aneurysm, or hemorrhage into a tumor. The eye grounds may reveal a retinal vascular abnormality. Preretinal hemorrhages may be found after hemorrhage has occurred. X-ray of the skull occasionally shows crescentic linear calcification in the vicinity of larger angiomas. Pneumoencephalography may show the picture of an expanding lesion combined with cerebral atrophy, a combination typical of angioma. Most arteriovenous malformations are visible in a CT scan but are seen more completely in an arteriogram, which will demonstrate angiomas larger than 5 mm in diameter. Small angiomas may be obscured by the resulting hemorrhage, and even at autopsy a careful microscopic search may be necessary to find them.

Most angiomas bleed sooner or later. The first hemorrhage may be fatal, but in more than 90 percent of cases bleeding stops, and the patient survives. Recurrence of hemorrhage with a fatal outcome is a constant danger, but the risk is less than with saccular aneurysm. In patients who have had a hemorrhage the incidence of recurrence is approximately 3 percent per year. The prognosis is better in those patients who have not had a manifest brain hemorrhage than in those who have. In recent years it has been the practice of neurosurgeons to perform a block dissection of angiomas of suitable size and location. Other techniques include artificial embolization, ligation of feeding arteries, obliteration by means of intravascular resins, and proton-beam focused irradiation.

Although *intracranial bleeding due to head trauma* does not rightfully fall within the scope of the stroke problem, it must be mentioned here because of the great frequency with which it enters into the differential diagnosis, especially in cases in which the history is inadequate or the patient falls and is injured at the onset of the stroke. *Acute extradural* and *acute subdural hemorrhage* must always be considered in the patient who under unknown circumstances has rather abruptly developed a neurologic deficit such as hemiparesis or confusion, whether the spinal fluid is bloody or not. In *chronic subdural hemorrhage,* which can occur without known trauma, the indefinite picture of drowsiness, confusion, and mild hemiparesis may be erroneously attributed to a stroke, especially in elderly persons. Failure to make the correct diagnosis deprives the patient of lifesaving surgical intervention. There should be no hesitation in subjecting the patient to CT scanning or arteriography whenever subdural hemorrhage cannot be excluded on clinical grounds. *Cerebral contusion and laceration* may be a cause of subarachnoid hemorrhage, and if the patient has fallen, causing a blow to the head at the time of the onset of the stroke, it may be difficult or impossible to decide if the red blood cells in the cerebrospinal fluid are due to a cerebrovascular stroke or to cerebral contusion. Trauma may also cause *acute* or *delayed intracerebral hemorrhage, acute intracerebellar hemorrhage, acute infratentorial subdural hemorrhage, acute brain swelling,* and on rare occasions, extensive *focal infarction* due probably to vasospasm (see Chap. 366).

Several *hemorrhagic hematologic disorders* may be complicated by hemorrhage into the brain. The most frequent of these are leukemia, aplastic anemia, and thrombocytopenic purpura. As a rule this complication signals a fatal issue. Any part of the brain may be involved, and often the lesions are multiple. Usually there is already evidence of abnormal bleeding elsewhere (skin, mucous membranes, kidney) by the time cerebral hemorrhage occurs. Intracranial bleeding is also a complication of anticoagulant therapy; the hemorrhages that develop usually occur in the sites of predilection in hypertensive hemorrhage, as well as elsewhere. They tend to have a leisurely but steady evolution, and at times attempts to control them by reversal of the anticoagulant effects have failed. When precipitated by warfarin therapy, treatment by fresh-frozen plasma and vitamin K is recommended; when associated with aspirin therapy or other agents that affect platelet function, fresh platelet infusions, often in massive amounts, are required to control the hemorrhage.

Occasionally *hemorrhages* are of *undetermined origin* both clinically and pathologically. The blood pressure is normal, and neither an aneurysm nor angioma can be demonstrated. In some postmortem cases a careful microscopic search discloses a small angioma in the cerebral tissue at one side of the hemorrhage, and on this basis it is suspected that in other cases, too, an overlooked angioma may have been the cause of the extravasation of blood. Primary intraventricular hemorrhage, a rare event, is at times due to angioma or neoplasm of the choroid plexus, which may not have been seen by the prosector. More often, such intraventricular hemorrhages are the result of a paraventricular bleeding that immediately entered the ventricle without producing a large parenchymal clot.

Hemorrhage into primary and secondary brain tumors is not rare, and when it is the first manifestation of the neoplasm, the correct diagnosis may be extremely obscure. Choriocarcinoma, melanotic carcinoma, renal cell carcinoma, bronchogenic carcinoma, pituitary adenoma, glioblastoma multiforme, and medulloblastoma may present in this way. Careful inquiry will usually disclose the fact that signs of a neurologic disorder compatible with intracranial tumor growth have preceded the onset of hemorrhage. Examination clinically and by x-ray may reveal evidence of intracranial tumor or of secondary tumor deposits in other organs. A chest film will frequently show metastatic or primary neoplasm and should be performed in all cases of obscure intracerebral hemorrhage.

Septic embolism may lead to massive fatal intracranial bleeding via a *mycotic aneurysm.* Any part of the circulatory tree may be involved, but usually the aneurysm (about 0.5 mm in diameter) lies at a branching or forking of a small meningeal branch of a middle cerebral artery.

On infrequent occasions bleeding within an area of *hemorrhagic infarction* as a result of cerebral embolism or venous thrombosis reaches major proportions, forming an intracerebral hematoma, and the cerebrospinal fluid becomes bloody.

Hypertensive encephalopathy may in its most advanced stage result in intracerebral hemorrhages, which can vary in size from petechial to massive.

Idiopathic brain purpura, or hemorrhagic encephalitis, consists of multiple petechial hemorrhages scattered throughout the white matter of the brain. The picture is that of a diffuse cerebral disease. There is never blood in the spinal fluid, and the condition should never be confused with a typical stroke. Exogenous (e.g., arsenic) or endogenous (e.g., gram-negative) bacteria are the usual cause.

Brainstem hemorrhages secondary to temporal lobe herniation are extremely common but never present as a cerebrovascular stroke.

Inflammatory disease of arteries and veins, especially polyarteritis nodosa and lupus erythematosus, can cause hemorrhage into the nervous system. In polyarteritis, rupture of a vessel may occur on the basis of a concomitant hypertension of local vascular disease. In lupus erythematosus—if it can be included in the arteritides—hemorrhage is attributable to hypertension or disease of the vascular wall of undetermined nature. Bleeding nearly always occurs into the parenchyma rather than the subarachnoid space.

The rarer types of hemorrhage listed in the classification in Table 365-2 are self-explanatory.

Hemorrhages of *intraspinal* origin may be the result of angiomas, hematomyelia, bleeding into tumors, extradural and subdural extravasation (trauma, anticoagulants, spontaneous), and circulatory changes around benign tumors. Extradural spinal hemorrhage rapidly causes an irreversible paraplegia, and diagnosis must be prompt if function is to be salvaged by surgical drainage.

HYPERTENSIVE ENCEPHALOPATHY

This term refers to an acute syndrome in which severe hypertension is associated with headache, nausea, vomiting, convulsions, confusion, stupor, and coma. Focal or lateralizing neurologic signs, either transitory or lasting, may occur but are infrequent and always suggest some other form of vascular disease (hemorrhage, embolism, or atherosclerotic thrombosis). By the time neurologic manifestations appear, the hypertension has usually reached the malignant stage, with retinal hemorrhages, exudates, papilledema (*hypertensive retinopathy* grade IV, see Chap. 251), and evidence of renal and cardiac disease. In many, but not all cases, the cerebrospinal fluid pressure and the protein values are both elevated, the latter sometimes to over 100 mg per 100 ml. The hypertension may be essential or due to chronic renal disease, acute glomerulonephritis, acute toxemia of pregnancy, pheochromocytoma, Cushing's syndrome, or ACTH toxicity. Lowering of the blood pressure with hypotensive drugs may reverse the picture in a day or two. If the hypertension cannot be controlled, the outcome is fatal.

Neuropathologic examination may reveal a rather normal-looking brain, but usually cerebral swelling and/or hemorrhages of various sizes from massive to petechial will be found. A cerebellar pressure cone reflects increased volume of tissue and increased pressure in the posterior fossa, and in some instances lumbar puncture may have precipitated a fatality. Microscopically there are, in addition to small hemorrhages, clusters of microglial cells, minute cerebral infarcts, and necrosis of arterioles.

The term *hypertensive encephalopathy* should be reserved for the above syndrome and not used to refer to chronic recurrent headaches, dizziness, epileptic seizures, recurrent transient ischemic attacks, or small strokes which often occur in association with high blood pressure. For further discussion, see Chap. 251.

INFLAMMATORY DISEASES OF BRAIN ARTERIES

Inflammatory diseases of the vessels of the brain have been mentioned on several occasions in the preceding paragraphs, and here they are discussed briefly.

Meningovascular syphilis, formerly one of the most frequent causes of occlusive vascular disease in patients of all ages, has become a rarity since the introduction of penicillin therapy (see Chap. 146).

Tuberculous meningitis, fungous meningitis, and the subacute forms of bacterial meningitis (influenzal bacillus, staphylococcus, pneumococcus) may also be accompanied by vascular disorders of the occlusive type, in either the cerebral arteries or veins. Occasionally in tuberculous meningitis a stroke may be the first clinical sign of meningitis; more often it develops after the meningeal symptoms are established.

Typhus, schistosomiasis mansoni, mucormycosis, malaria, and *trichinosis* are rare types of infective inflammatory diseases of the arteries and, unlike the above, are not secondary to meningeal inflammation. In typhus and other rickettsial diseases, capillary and arteriolar changes and perivascular inflammatory cells are found in the brain, and presumably they underlie the convulsions, acute psychoses, and coma which reflect the central nervous system involvement. They do not cause strokes, however. The internal carotid artery may be occluded in diabetic patients during orbital and cavernous sinus infections with mucormycosis. In trichinosis the sudden onset of convulsions, aphasia, hemiplegia, and coma may either accompany or, as happens more often, follow the systemic and muscular symptoms. The cause of the cerebral symptoms has not been established. Parasites have been found in the brain; in one of our cases the cerebral lesions were produced by bland emboli arising in the heart and related to a severe myocarditis. Malaria of the malignant or falciparum variety is frequently attended by a clinical state known as *cerebral malaria,* in which convulsions, coma, and sometimes focal symptoms appear to be due to blockage of capillaries and precapillaries by masses of parasitized red blood corpuscles.

The *arteritides of obscure origin* include polyarteritis nodosa, disseminated lupus erythematosus, granulomatous arteritis, giant-cell arteritis, temporal (cranial) arteritis, and rheumatic arteritis (see Chap. 363).

Lupus erythematosus causes cerebral symptoms in over 50 percent of cases. Seizures and psychoses are common. Small cerebral infarcts lead to widespread focal deficits. Accompanying hypertension may precipitate hemorrhage or hypertensive encephalopathy, or endocarditis may cause cerebral embolism.

Temporal arteritis (cranial arteritis) is an uncommon affliction of elderly persons in which the external carotid system, particularly the temporal branches, is the seat of a subacute granulomatous inflammation with an exudate of lymphocytes, monocytes, neutrophilic leukocytes, and giant cells. Usually the most severely affected parts of the artery become thrombosed. Headache or head pain is the chief complaint. Systemic manifestations include anorexia, loss of weight, malaise, and polymyalgia rheumatica. The inflammatory nature of the illness is indicated by some one or several of the following: fever, slight leukocytosis, increased sedimentation rate, and anemia. Occlusion of branches of the ophthalmic artery results in blindness in one or both eyes in over 25 percent of patients, and occasionally an ophthalmoplegia due to involvement of ocular nerves occurs. An arteritis of the aorta and its major branches, including carotid, subclavian, coronary, and femoral arteries, is found at postmortem examination. Significant inflammatory involvement of intracranial arteries is rare, but strokes occur occasionally, on the basis of occlusion of the internal carotid, middle cerebral, or vertebral arteries. The diagnosis depends on the finding of a tender thrombosed or thickened cranial artery and the demonstration of the lesion is a biopsy. Meticorten and ACTH bring striking subjective relief and prevent blindness. See Chap. 366 for further discussion. The clinical picture overlaps that of *polymyalgia rheumatica.*

Thromboangiitis obliterans of cerebral vessels (Winiwarter-Buerger disease) has not been included in the foregoing list. Despite the large volume of literature on the subject, the pathology is so dubious that it does not merit further exposition. All the patients that the authors have studied proved to have had either atherosclerosis of the carotid or cerebral arteries with "stasis thrombosis" of more distant cerebral branches. Buerger's disease of the legs has an equally uncertain status.

DIFFERENTIATION OF CEREBROVASCULAR DISEASE FROM OTHER NEUROLOGIC ILLNESSES

It has already been stated that the diagnosis of a vascular lesion rests solely on recognition of the stroke syndrome and that without evidence of this the diagnosis must always be in doubt. Three useful criteria in the identification of the stroke have already been emphasized: (1) the tempo of the clinical syndrome, (2) evidence of focal brain disease, and (3) the clinical setting. The temporal profile can usually be defined by means of a clear history of premonitory phenomena, the mode of the onset, and the evolution of the neurologic disturbance taken in relation to the medical status at the time of examination. If these data are lacking, the course may still be determined by extending the period of observation for a few more days or weeks. An inadequate history is probably the most frequent cause of diagnostic errors.

Few other neurologic illnesses mimic cerebrovascular disease. When the details of the history are missing, however, subdural hematoma, brain tumor, brain abscess, and senile dementia may lead to diagnostic difficulties. The reader should refer to Chaps. 364, 367, 368, and 373 for further discussion of differential diagnosis.

A GUIDE TO THE CLINICAL MANAGEMENT OF CEREBROVASCULAR DISEASES

The student, family physician, and internist are not expected to become expert in the diagnosis and treatment of cerebrovascular diseases after having read the jumble of ideas in the preceding pages. But there are certain clinical situations which recur repeatedly and which demand an organized set of responses on the part of the physician if the patient is to receive the benefits of the most advanced medical thought. These reactions devolve upon:

1 A patient who has had a probable stroke and is now comatose.

2 A patient who has had an obvious focal neurological deficit, probably a stroke, and who is responsive.

3 A patient who has had an indefinite neurological disorder which proves to be an inobvious stroke.

4 A patient who gives a history of having had a stroke in the past which may or may not relate to his present problem.

5 A patient who is believed to have had a mild stroke but actually has some type of nonvascular disease.

The authors would suggest the following approach to each of these problems.

THE COMATOSE STROKE PATIENT Here the analysis of the state of coma should proceed in accordance with the scheme outlined in Chap. 20, where it was pointed out that in comas due to cerebrovascular disorders there is nearly always evidence of unilateral hemispheral or segmental brain stem deficits of function, and in some instances changes in CSF. The CT scan, available in most medical centers, has largely replaced lumbar puncture and CSF examination, which carry some degree of risk if there is a massive intracranial clot.

The usual causes of a comatose stroke are hypertensive hemorrhage, a ruptured saccular aneurysm, or a massive cerebral or a brainstem infarct. The diagnostic steps described on pages 1913, 1920, 1933, and 1936 permit differentiation of these diseases. The clinician's first problem is to make sure the clinical condition is due to a stroke and not to a treatable form of traumatic epidural or subdural hematoma (see Chap. 366), a metabolic disorder, or drug intoxication (Chaps. 228 and 371).

The most that can be done for the cerebrovascular coma is to offer supportive measures along the lines indicated in Chap. 20. Measures to control raised intracranial pressure (dexamethasone and glycerol or manrutol) may be beneficial. Surgical intervention is rarely undertaken and is usually unsuccessful; if operation is decided upon (aspiration of the clot and reduction of intracranial pressure), it must be done at once. In ruptured saccular aneurysms, as long as the patient is comatose or stuporous (grade IV in presently used rating scheme), surgery must be deferred and it is wise to postpone arteriography. Even cerebellar hemorrhage, which sometimes yields to surgical intervention, seldom does so once the patient has become comatose. There is no point in undertaking arteriography in cases of massive infarction, for it will not lead to any form of definitive therapy. If the patient is in a hospital with limited facilities, there is little point in urgent transfer to a larger medical center while coma persists. Once consciousness is regained, however, and neurological condition stabilizes, it is important to identify the cases of ruptured aneurysm and arteriovenous malformations and to institute appropriate therapy.

THE NONCOMATOSE STROKE PATIENT The question of diagnosis is seldom in doubt, though a focal convulsion (a rare initial event in stroke) followed by a postconvulsant paralysis or one or the conditions mentioned on pages 1927, 1928, and 1930 in the differential diagnosis of cerebral thrombosis, ischemic attacks, and embolism must be considered. After the initial events it is the pace of the neurologic deficit and the course toward improvement or worsening that are the best guides in the recognition of the different types of strokes. One must keep foremost in mind the potentially treatable diseases such as the carotid stenosis, the leaking saccular aneurysm, the recurrent ischemic attack, the different types of embolism, and thrombocytosis. ECG, cardiac monitoring, blood cultures, and platelet counts should accompany CT scanning; the latter will exclude the small hemorrhage. The examination of the CSF is also of importance to demonstrate a pleocytosis or small hemorrhage.

Arteriography is one of the most helpful diagnostic aids, but the timing of it should reflect the proximity of the most recent ischemic attack or increment of deficit. The more recent the change the more urgently the arteriogram is indicated. An attack the day of admission warrants an arteriogram on the same day, after the CT scan. Carotid occlusion at the sinus level, of a few hours' standing, should be operated upon at once. The diagnosis of embolism should lead to the initiation of anticoagulant therapy at once, to prevent subsequent emboli. However, a massive persistent cerebral deficit discourages all further diagnostic studies and efforts directed toward therapy and prevention.

THE INOBVIOUS STROKE Here the problem is one of a patient who has developed some form of mild neurologic deficit, the diagnosis of which is obscure. Inexplicable headache, dizziness, mental confusion, or a variety of other minor symptoms have clearly declared their presence. What may be overlooked is the fact that the classic sign of stroke (i.e., hemiplegia) may never appear, yet certain minor signs, if of sudden or acute onset, carry the same diagnostic, prognostic, and therapeutic implications as paralysis.

Four such inobvious stroke syndromes occur regularly. The first of these is a leaking aneurysm, presenting as a sudden, generalized headache (unlike any experienced in the past), often having developed during exertion, persisting for hours or days. Examination may disclose no abnormalities, but the neck may be slightly stiff. Casual urinary—less often fecal—incontinence, vague recollection for recent events, and unaccountable delays in answering simple questions may also be present and reflect emerging hydrocephalus in the days after the headache had its sudden inset. Ruptured aneurysm occasionally also presents as unexplained severe interscapular back pain. Subdural hematoma, anticoagulant-induced frontal pole hemorrhage, brain tumor, and other entities must be included in the differential diagnosis.

A second type of inobvious stroke is cerebellar hemorrhage. Sudden onset of dizziness, repeated uncontrollable vomiting, inability to stand and walk, ipsilateral gaze palsy, ipsilateral facial paresis, and, less often, ipsilateral cerebellar ataxia are often incompletely detected and need to be assembled into the diagnostic syndrome by the examining physician. Considerate of the patient's misery, the physician often defers testing the patient's ability to stand and walk; and finding no obvious hemiparesis, often does not test ocular movements fully; the mild facial asymmetry easily escapes detection in the setting of vomiting and dizziness. Such patients are often assumed to have labyrinthitis, Ménière's disease, alcoholic or drug intoxication, and even viral gastroenteritis, and little thought is given to impending disaster because the patient seems so alert—until brainstem compression suddenly intervenes, with fatal results. CT scan or lumbar puncture is an essential diagnostic step in the evaluation of all such cases. Hematoma evacuation has proved the only reliable therapeutic step in the acute phase. Cerebellar infarction produces a somewhat similar picture.

The third type of inobvious stroke involves the posterior cerebral artery territory. Homonymous hemianopia is often not implicitly appreciated by the patient, whose complaints, if any, center on the need for new eyeglasses, on poor vision in the eye ipsilateral to the visual field loss, or on vague descriptions of blurring of vision. Failure to appreciate the visual environment on that side has often led to embarrassing social experiences or accidents. Accompanying deficits in higher cerebral function, when present, usually require surprisingly direct testing, including reading, naming of colors or manipulable objects, description of faces, and routes on maps, and require this testing despite the patient's seeming normalcy.

The fourth common type of inobvious stroke is an episode of mild paraphasic speech and slightly impaired auditory comprehension that characterizes most examples of Wernicke's aphasia from embolism. The patient is often thought to be confused. Most patients perform satisfactorily at a superficial level in making socially appropriate greetings and gestures, and they may approve readily of the examiner's efforts to shorten the interview by posing questions to be answered yes or no. Scrutiny of their remarks and behavior during history-taking will elicit the deficit. Tests involving the naming aloud or spelling of even short words that are the names of objects presented, writing the names of objects, pointing to objects whose names are spelled aloud, and describing the use of objects presented all suffice to bring out errors in word selection, sentence construction, and comprehension.

PATIENT WITH A HISTORY OF PRIOR STROKE This is the time when the identification of the patient "at risk" becomes an important matter, for it offers the best opportunity for medical intercession. Excluding a postconvulsive state, any deficit in neurologic function involving a cerebral or brainstem location that has persisted over a few hours should be taken as evidence of a destructive lesion, even though the deficit appears to have disappeared. The lesion may have been a small embolus, lacunar infarct, transient ischemic attack, or thrombocytic occlusion. Electrolyte disturbance, fever, and other "metabolic" states may often cause a transient relapse, and knowledge of such a prior lesion is of immeasurable value in assessing the significance of any focal cerebral disorder that emerges during a general metabolic derangement. A history of the briefer episodic focal deficit compels consideration of transient ischemic attack. In such a setting, migraine, seizure, depression, peripheral neuropathies, and other entities arise in the differential diagnosis. Search for extracranial vascular abnormalities including a carotid bruit is a useful exercise. If the episodes are recurrent, the similarities between episodes, the arterial territory inferred from the symptoms, and their duration are all important features to be studied. Transient ischemic attacks that warn of disaster frequently last only seconds to a few minutes and are often shrugged off by the patient as insignificant. Distal brachial predominance characterizes the attacks in most cases of carotid stenosis. Although many patients experience hundreds of attacks over months before a stroke, most experience few, often only one; the last, sometimes the only, such attack tends to occur within the day(s) before the stroke. The closer in time to the last attack, the more expeditious should be the attempt to find the source (embolic, atherosclerotic, thrombocytosis, lipohyalin) of the prior deficit.

THE SIMULATED STROKE Since cerebrovascular diseases are by far the most frequent affections of the nervous system in middle and late adult life, there is an understandable tendency to diagnose every disease of the brain in this age period as vascular. If one reviews the hospital records of patients with a brain tumor, encephalitis, chronic subdural hematoma, episodic global amnesia, dementia, normal pressure hydrocephalus, and even depression, it is striking how often the initial diagnosis was one of stroke. This error can be avoided if one insists on having a clear history covering the onset and minute-by-minute and hour-by-hour course of the illness. If an adequate history is not available, one must then resort to a series of examinations to reveal the course of the illness. The data yielded by CT scan, CSF examination, EEG, radionuclide scan, arteriography, etc., are also helpful. If diagnosis is still in doubt, the proper tactic is to keep the patient under observation (possibly at home) until the future course of the illness clarifies the problem. Seldom in such patients is there reason for urgent surgical intervention.

REFERENCES

BORAL V: Mortality among oral-contraceptive users, Lancet 2:727, 1977

FISHER CM et al: Lateral medullary infarction—the pattern of vascular occlusion. J Neuropathol Exp Neurol 20:323, 1961

——: Cerebral ischemia—less familiar types. Clin Neurosurg 18:267, 1971

GOLDSTEIN RJ et al: Computer stroke registry and diagnosis program. Neurology 25:356, 1975

GROOTHUIS DR et al: The human thalamocortical sensory path in the internal capsule: Evidence from a small capsular hemorrhage causing a pure sensory stroke. Ann Neurol 2:328, 1978

McKISSOCK W et al: An analysis of results of treatment of ruptured intracranial aneurysms: A report of 722 consecutive cases. J Neurosurg 17:762, 1960

MOHR JP: Valvular disease, cardiac arrest, systemic hypotension, and cardiac surgery, in *Handbook of Clinical Neurology*, GW Bruyn, PJ Vinken (eds). Amsterdam, North-Holland, 1978

TOOLE JF, YUSON CP: Transient ischemic attacks with normal arteriograms: Serious or benign prognosis. Ann Neurol 1:100, 1977

WOLF PA et al: Epidemiologic assessment of chronic atrial fibrillation and risk of stroke. Neurology 28:973, 1978

ZERVAS N et al: Cerebral vasospasm. Surg Neurol 5:354, 1976

366
TRAUMATIC DISEASES OF THE BRAIN

KARL-ERIK ÅSTRÖM
HENRI VANDER EECKEN
RAYMOND D. ADAMS

Head injury, which is the basis of some of the most frequent and serious neurologic disorders in these times of high-velocity transport, mechanization in industry, and violent street crimes, poses many problems to the practicing physician. To deal effectively with this condition demands a knowledge of the clinical manifestations as well as a sound grasp of fundamental physiologic mechanisms. Physicians must stand prepared at all times, for they may at any moment be summoned to render aid or to assess the clinical status of a person who has suffered an injury of the head or spine. This chapter reviews the salient facts concerning these injuries and outlines an approach to these problems that has been useful to the authors.

PHYSIOLOGIC AND PATHOLOGIC CONSIDERATIONS

The very language with which certain types of head injury are discussed divulges a number of misconceptions that have been inherited from previous generations of physicians. Words have crept into medical vocabulary and have often been retained long after the ideas for which they stood have been refuted—clear evidence of the disadvantage of prematurely adopting explanatory rather than descriptive terms. The word *concussion*, for example, implies the violent shaking and agitation of an organ or the transient functional impairment which results therefrom. Yet despite numerous experiments to demonstrate these physical changes within the nerve cells, axons, or myelin sheaths (vibration effects, formation of intracellular vacuoles, etc.), no convincing confirmation of their existence has been possible. Similarly the word *contusion*, meaning a bruising or crushing without interruption of physical continuity, is applied rather indiscriminately to a variety of clinical states, some of which could not depend on a pathologic change of this type, e.g., "minor contusion state or syndrome"—an expression introduced by Wilfred Trotter, who was himself most critical of words that "embalm a fallacious theory."

In all attempts to analyze the mechanism of brain damage in head injury one fact stands preeminent—that there must be the sudden application of a physical force of considerable magnitude to the head. Unless the head is struck, the brain suffers no injury—except in the rare and somewhat controversial cases of crush injury to the chest or explosive injury with raised intrapulmonary pressure. A second fact, also susceptible of easy verification, is that the size of the area on the skull over which the force is exerted is of importance. High-velocity missiles destroy a small part of the skull and penetrate the cranial cavity without causing significant displacement of the head or brain; and heavy, crushing injuries which result from the skull's being compressed between two converging objects may crush the brain. In these two circumstances it is interesting to note that the patient may suffer severe and often fatal injury without immediate loss of consciousness. Hemorrhage, focal destruction of brain tissue, and, if the patient survives for a time, hydrocephalus, meningitis, or abscess are the principal pathologic changes created by injuries of this type. They present little that is difficult to understand.

The common civilian injury is one in which a rapidly moving blunt object strikes the head or the head is flung against a hard surface. Injuries of this type, often termed *blunt head injuries,* are remarkable in two respects: (1) they almost always induce at least a temporary loss of consciousness, and (2) even though the skull is not penetrated and fragments of bone are not driven into its cavity, the brain may suffer gross damage, i.e., contusion, laceration, hemorrhage, swelling, herniation, etc. Clinicians as well as experimental physiologists have sought unsuccessfully a theory which would bring concussion into plausible relationship with all the gross neuropathologic changes and the skull fracture and the prolonged coma so often observed in fatal cases.

The relation of skull fracture to injury of the cerebral tissues has been viewed in changing perspective through the entire history of this subject. In earliest times fractures dominated the thinking of the medical profession, and cerebral lesions were regarded as secondary. Later it became known that the skull, although rigid, is still flexible enough to yield to a blow severe enough to injure the brain without fracture. Therefore, the presence of a fracture, although a rough measure of the violence to which the brain has been exposed, is not an infallible index. Even in fatal head injury autopsy may reveal an intact skull in some 20 to 30 percent of cases. Also many patients suffer skull fractures without serious or prolonged disorder of cerebral function.

The modern trend is to be interested more in the presence or absence of brain injury than in the fracture of the skull itself. Nevertheless fractures cannot be dismissed without a few comments, for they assume importance in indicating the site and possible severity of brain damage, in providing an explanation for cranial nerve palsies, and in affording potential pathways for the ingress of bacteria and air or the egress of cerebrospinal fluid (CSF).

CRANIAL NERVE INJURY The existence of a basal skull fracture may be indicated by signs of cranial nerve damage. Cranial nerves which are particularly liable to injury are the olfactory, optic, oculomotor, first and second branches of the trigeminal, the facial, and the auditory. Anosmia and an apparent loss of taste (actually a loss of perception of aromatic flavors, elementary tastes—salt, sweet, bitter, sour—being re-

tained) are frequent sequelae of head injury, especially of falls on the back of the head. In the majority of cases the anosmia is permanent. If unilateral it will not be noticed by the patient. The mechanism of these disturbances is believed to be displacement of the brain and tearing of the olfactory nerve filaments. A fracture in or near the sella may tear the stalk of the pituitary gland, with resulting diabetes insipidus, impotence or reduced libido, and amenorrhea. A fracture of sphenoid bone may lacerate the optic nerve, with complete blindness from the beginning. The pupil is dilated and unreactive to a direct light stimulus but still takes part in the consensual reflex. The optic disk becomes pale, i.e., atrophic, after an interval of several weeks. Partial injuries may result in a troublesome blurring of vision. Injury to the eighth cranial nerve with petrosal fractures causes loss of hearing and/or postural vertigo and nystagmus immediately after injury. The deafness due to nerve injury must be distinguished from that caused by rupture of the eardrum or the presence of blood in the middle ear, and the vertigo, from posttraumatic nervous giddiness. In oculomotor nerve injury there is a divergent squint, with loss of internal and vertical movement of the eye and a fixed, dilated pupil. Diplopia only on looking down suggests trochlear nerve affection. Direct injury of the facial nerve by a basal fracture may be present immediately after the injury or may be delayed, coming on after several days. This delayed form is usually transitory, and its mechanism is not known. It may be misinterpreted as an important progression of the traumatic intracranial lesion. Injury to the ophthalmic or maxillary divisions of the trigeminal nerve may be the result either of a basal fracture across the middle cranial fossa or of a direct extracranial injury to the branches of the nerves. Numbness and paresthesias over the area of skin supplied by the nerve or a troublesome neuralgia are the sequelae of these injuries.

If the skin is lacerated over the skull fracture and the underlying meninges are torn, or if the fracture passes through the posterior wall of a nasal sinus, bacteria or air may enter the cranial cavity with resulting meningitis, abscess, and aerocele (air in the ventricles). Cerebrospinal fluid may also leak into the sinus and present as a watery discharge from the nose (cerebrospinal fluid rhinorrhea). Persistence of the rhinorrhea or the occurrence over a period of years of episodes of recurrent meningitis (headache, convulsions, fever, and stiff neck with pleocytosis and sometimes bacteria) is often an indication for a repair of the torn dura mater over the fissure. Depressed fractures are of significance only if the underlying dura is lacerated by spicules of bone or the brain is compressed.

CONCUSSIVE INJURY Much has been written about the mechanism of coma in closed or blunt head injury. Certain facts concerning this condition stand out clearly: (1) Its onset is immediate (not delayed even by seconds). (2) Concussive effects on brain function may last for a variable time (seconds, minutes, or hours). (3) The optimal conditions for its production are those in which there is some change in the momentum of the head; i.e., movement is suddenly imparted to it by a blow, or its movement is suddenly arrested. Striking the stationary head of an experimental animal will cause a loss of brainstem reflexes only if the head is free to move, not if it is clamped in one position. This finding alone would stand in refutation of such theories of concussion as a wave of high intracranial pressure due to the indentation of the skull or a subsequent wave of negative pressure, cerebral ischemia, or a general vibration or agitation transmitted via the skull. The speed of acceleration or deceleration of the head necessary for this concussive effect must exceed 7 m/s. The initial action of the blunt injury of this type is alleged (without proof) to excite the nervous system (the "stars" that one sees with a minor injury, the gasp of the animal), and this is followed by transient paralysis of cerebral function, i.e., abolition of consciousness, suppression of reflexes, arrest of respiration, transitory bradycardia and fall in blood pressure, etc. The means whereby the latter effects are produced is not known. Equally obscure is the site of injury, whether diffuse in the cerebral cortex, in the cerebral white matter, or in the diencephalon and midbrain.

In fatal cases of severe head injury, where this concussive injury must have existed, the brain is almost invariably bruised or lacerated, and often there is hemorrhage, either meningeal or intracerebral. The observation of these gross pathologic findings has led to the widely prevalent view that head injuries are largely matters of bruises and hemorrhages and of urgent operations. That this can hardly be the case is suggested by the fact that some patients survive head injuries almost as severe as the fatal ones and yet make an excellent recovery. At autopsy years later old contusions (*plaques jaunes*) and hemorrhages of approximately the same distribution and extent as those observed in some of the immediately fatal cases are found. One can only conclude, therefore, that most of the immediate symptoms of severe head injury, both general and localized, depend on invisible and highly reversible changes in the brain, probably of the same nature as those which underlie concussion. Nevertheless these bruises, lacerations, hemorrhages, localized swellings of tissues, and herniations cannot be disregarded, because they are probably responsible for most of the fatalities that occur 12 to 72 h or more after the injury. Of these lesions the most important are the surface bruising of the brain beneath the point of impact (*coup* injury) and the more extensive lacerations and contusions on the opposite side of the brain (*contrecoup* injuries). The inertia of the malleable brain, which causes it to be flung against the side of the skull that was struck and to be pulled away from the contralateral side, has been invoked to explain these coup-contrecoup contusions. This theory has been further elaborated by Holburn, who points out that the brain is roughly spherical and that all movements of the head describe an arc with its axis centered where skull is attached to spine. Sudden changes in the momentum of the head, therefore, impart a swirling motion to the brain, which may then suffer injury against all rough, bony, and dural prominences (wings of sphenoid bones, petrous parts of temporal bones, rough surfaces of orbital and frontal bones, falx, and tentorium).

CLINICAL MANIFESTATIONS OF HEAD INJURY

The physician upon being called to see a patient who has had a head injury will generally find the patient in one of three clinical conditions; each must be dealt with differently. It is usually possible to place such patients in one of these three categories by assessing their mental and general neurologic status when they are first seen and at intervals of time after the accident. This division of cases depends mainly on an assessment of levels of consciousness, verbal response, and motor response which for purposes of clinical comparison and estimation of prognosis have been standardized in a rating scale (Glasgow; see Langfitt for details).

PATIENTS WHO ARE CONSCIOUS OR ARE RAPIDLY REGAINING MENTAL CLARITY WHEN FIRST SEEN (MINOR HEAD INJURY) The typical example is a patient who has been rendered unconscious by a knock on the head and then seems all right. If unconscious, such persons may regain their senses

within seconds, minutes, or a few hours. Roughly two degrees of disturbance may have occurred: First, there are the patients who were never unconscious at all. They were observed to have been struck on the head and were stunned or "saw stars." By all criteria their head injury was insignificant, at least when judged in terms of life and death and severe brain damage, though in exceptional cases there is always the possibility of skull fracture or the development of an epidural or subdural hematoma. Nevertheless, a troublesome group of symptoms (headaches, giddiness, fatigability, insomnia, and nervousness) may appear at once or within a few days.

In the second instance consciousness is temporarily abolished, and patients are said to have suffered a *concussion*, defined by Trotter as "an essentially transient state due to head injury which is instantaneous in onset, manifests widespread symptoms of a purely paralytic kind, does not as such comprise any evidence of structural cerebral injury and is nearly always followed by amnesia for the actual moment of the impact." Patients, if observed immediately after the injury, show a complete paralysis of nervous function. In a few instances death has occurred at this time, from respiratory arrest or cardiac arrhythmia, and no lesion is found at postmortem examination. However, the usual sequel is for the pulse and respiration (if they were depressed or arrested) to return at once and for muscle tone, reflexes, voluntary movement, and mental clarity to be regained within a few minutes. Only an amnesia for the accident and the events that immediately preceded (retrograde amnesia) and followed it (anterograde amnesia) will remain. Thereafter patients may suffer the same headaches, giddiness, and nervousness mentioned above.

These relatively trivial head injuries may rarely be followed by a number of other puzzling features, all of which indicate the occurrence of some process in addition to concussion:

1 *Delayed traumatic collapse.* Following an accident a few patients, after walking about and seeming to be mentally normal, will turn pale and fall unconscious for a few minutes. This is a vasomotor syncopal attack and is probably related to injury, pain, and emotional upset. Rarely does the patient exhibit any focal or lateralizing neurologic signs.

2 *Immediate traumatic paraplegia* or *blindness.* With falls on top of the head, which may injure the motor areas for the lower extremities, both legs may become temporarily weak and numb, sometimes with bilateral Babinski signs and sphincteric incontinence. Temporary blindness may have a similar base in occipital injuries.

3 *Delayed hemiplegia* or *monoplegia.* An "interval" paralysis in cases of minor or major injury usually signifies an epidural hemorrhage, a subdural hemorrhage or hygroma, dissecting aneurysm of carotid artery, spreading venous thrombosis, or intracerebral hemorrhage.

4 *Acute drowsiness, confusion,* and *headache,* due presumably to localized and generalized traumatic brain edema. Children who have concussions are especially liable to headache, drowsiness, and vomiting, which may have their onset some hours after the injury. In these children infusions and clyses of water and 5% glucose are particularly dangerous; such treatment may prove fatal by inducing water intoxication and severe brain swelling. Apparently an excessive output of antidiuretic hormone and water retention occur under these circumstances.

5 *An attack of neurologic migraine.*

6 *Posttraumatic nervous instability* (see below.)

PATIENTS WHO HAVE BEEN UNCONSCIOUS SINCE RECEIVING MAJOR HEAD INJURY **The clinical state** In this group, which includes the patients with the more severe head injuries, the outlook is obviously less favorable and one is concerned at first for the patient's life. However, within this group there is still a wide variation in the severity of the traumatic brain disease. A certain number of patients die at once or within a few minutes, and it may be assumed that the direct injury to the brain or some other organ was incompatible with life. Other patients in this group recover consciousness rapidly after several hours, but a few remain deeply comatose for days or even weeks before doing so. If the pupils dilate and become fixed and all brainstem reflex mechanisms, including the maintenance of respiration, are paralyzed and remain so over a period of hours (the EEG is usually isoelectric as described in Chap. 364 under "Types of Abnormal Recordings"), the outlook is hopeless. The mortality rate in those who reach a hospital in coma was formerly 50 to 60 percent, but with modern methods of managing the comatose patient this has been reduced to 32 percent, according to Langfitt, and most of these deaths occur within the first 12 to 24 h. Of those alive after 24 h, the mortality is 7 to 8 percent, and after 48 h the figures fall to 1 to 2 percent.

Those patients whose illness will end fatally may be moribund from the beginning. The coma is profound. The limbs may be flaccid without reflexes or are rigidly extended (decerebrate rigidity). The corneal and pharyngeal (gag) reflexes are usually present. The pupils are small and unreactive to light, or dilated and fixed, or unequal. The ocular axes are divergent or askew. The jaw sags, the tongue falls back in the throat, saliva drools from the mouth, and swallowing is obviously lost. There may be surgical shock at first for a brief period, with the usual findings of pale and moist skin, weak and rapid pulse, subnormal temperature, and a blood pressure that is difficult to obtain. Within a few hours, however, the temperature usually rises, and this may continue until death. The breathing may be stertorous and later feeble and irregular. The state of consciousness and the temperature chart provide information of great value in appraising the status of the patient. An ascending pulse rate, possibly interspersed by short periods in which there is a bounding, slow pulse, and rising temperature or a combination of fast pulse and subnormal temperature are signs of grave prognostic import.

In those whose prognosis is favorable, the coma is less deep; i.e., there is confusion, stupor, or semicoma (see Chap. 20) and for a time restlessness and combativeness. The reflexes are normal, as are pulse, blood pressure, and respiration. The patient is able to swallow and may or may not speak. There are no obvious neurologic signs.

Once the patient regains consciousness sufficiently to respond to a spoken command, the physician no longer needs to be concerned about survival and may begin to think about the possibility of focal brain damage and prospects for return of neurologic function. There is still a substantial risk in the first 2 or 3 weeks, however, from pneumonia, meningitis, or epidural and subdural hemorrhage, which may intervene and impair the chances of survival. It is often said that death during the first 12 h is the result of the direct injury of the brain; that which occurs later is usually the result of some complication of cranial trauma (intracerebral or subarachnoid hemorrhage, herniation of the temporal lobe, localized or generalized edema, epidural or subdural hemorrhage, meningitis, pneumonia).

There is another group of patients to which some reference must be made, for they represent difficult problems in diagnosis and therapy. Here a known or evident head injury is not followed by deep or lasting coma, but instead the patients are awake and able to respond to some degree upon arrival at the hospital. Yet as the hours pass, it is apparent that their condition is deteriorating, and within a day or two they lapse into coma. A sanguineous CSF under slightly elevated pressure attests to the existence of contusion. The progressive nature of the illness suggests intracerebral, epidural, or subdural hemorrhage; yet at postmortem examination only contusion, local-

ized edema (sometimes generalized), and temporal lobe pressure cone are found to be the basis of the clinical syndrome. The point to remember is that consciousness may return early, i.e., within minutes or hours, after a head injury severe enough to contuse the brain seriously and to lead to death after a few days. Presumably the concussive coma has not been as severe as in most patients who suffer contusive injuries.

Focal and lateralizing neurologic symptoms and signs, as would be anticipated, will be observed with notable frequency in this group of patients. These abnormalities are presumably related to hemorrhage and contusion, and inasmuch as they are usually engrafted on a severe concussive injury, they become manifest as consciousness is regained. Local injury to the brain without a disturbance of consciousness occurs exceptionally, and then more often with the penetration of the skull by missiles or a direct glancing blow by a relatively small object (golf ball, stone), and sometimes with depressed fractures. Of the focal symptoms, hemiparesis is probably the most frequent. The weakness in the arm and leg may be evidenced even during coma by the hypotonia, the less frequent movement of the limbs, inequality of tendon reflexes, and a more persistent Babinski sign on one side. Complete hemiplegia is rarely observed. Hemihypesthesia, although occasionally found, is less common, possibly because sensory tests are difficult to interpret until mental clarity is regained. Homonymous hermianopsia is not at all infrequent and may present early as an inattentiveness to visual stimuli on one side. Aphasia, usually of mixed type, may be noted in a number of cases. A series of focal seizures may occur within a few days of the time of injury and is probably due to cortical contusion. Such seizures usually cease after a few days and do not necessarily signify that epilepsy is to be a sequel to the trauma. Diabetes insipidus, disturbances of sleep (reversal of rhythm, somnolence), diplopia, heteronymous visual field defects, gastrointestinal hemorrhage, amenorrhea, and impotence in the male indicate damage to the hypothalamus and walls of the third ventricle. Midbrain or diffuse cerebral lesions are evidenced by ocular palsies, protracted coma (weeks, months, or years), decerebrate rigidity, crossed ocular-limb paralyses, bilateral Babinski's signs, and, later, dysarthria, ataxia of limbs on one side, and sensory disturbances.

Laboratory findings In this group of patients with severe head injury there is a high incidence of skull fracture. The CSF is usually sanguineous (red blood cells usually 100,000 per cubic millimeter or less) and under elevated pressure (between 200 and 300 mmH$_2$O) in the majority of patients. The prognosis is distinctly less good in those with more than 100,000 red blood cells per cubic millimeter and pressures in excess of 300 mmH$_2$O. Nevertheless death may occur in patients who have no skull fracture, a subnormal intracranial pressure, and relatively clear CSF. The EEG regularly shows focal and diffuse abnormalities.

Acetylcholine and lactate are elevated in the CSF during the first 3 to 4 days, then gradually return to normal. During this same period there is sodium retention followed within 3 to 4 days by sodium diuresis. A mild hyponatremia appearing during the time of sodium retention is due to simultaneous water retention. Potassium remains in balance. During the first 10 days after trauma, nitrogen loss of 10 g per day may occur.

Neuropathologic findings In patients who die during the first few hours or days after a severe head injury, hemorrhage and necrosis of tissue will frequently be observed. In 50 consecutive autopsies summarized in Rowbotham's excellent monograph, only 2 showed no macroscopic change. Lacerations of cerebral cortex (28 percent), surface contusions (48 percent), subarachnoid hemorrhage (72 percent), acute subdural hemorrhage (16 percent), and extradural hemorrhage (20 percent) were the usual findings. As a rule, several of these pathologic changes were found in the same case. Skull fractures were discovered in 72 percent.

In another series of 50 cases, 21 percent had associated fractures of limbs, 18 percent chest injuries, and 13 percent abdominal injuries and ruptures of organs.

PATIENTS WHO ARE UNCONSCIOUS WHEN FIRST SEEN BUT WHO WERE CONSCIOUS AFTER THE ACCIDENT (PRESENCE OF LUCID INTERVAL)   This group of patients is smaller than the other two but is of great importance because it includes many who are in urgent need of surgical treatment. The initial coma may have been brief or there may have been none at all, in which instance one might conclude that there was neither concussion nor contusion. The following conditions must be considered in every case of this type.

Acute epidural hemorrhage   This condition is due as a rule to a temporal or parietal fracture with laceration of the middle meningeal artery and vein. Less often there is a tear in a dural venous sinus. The injury, even when it fractures the skull, may not have produced coma. A typical example is seen in a child who has fallen from a bicycle or a swing or has suffered a hard blow to the head in a fight and was only momentarily unconscious. A few hours or a day or two later (exceptionally the interval may be as long as several days or a week, especially with venous bleeding), the child develops headache of increasing severity, vomiting, drowsiness, confusion, seizures (which may be one-sided), and hemiparesis, with slightly increased tendon reflexes and Babinski's sign. As coma develops, the hemiparesis with Babinski's sign may give way to spasticity and Babinski's sign bilaterally. There may be aphasia before consciousness is lost. Respirations become deeper and stertorous, then shallow and irregular, and finally stop. The pulse is often slow (below 60 beats per minute) and bounding, with a concomitant rise in systolic blood pressure. The pupil may dilate on the side of hematoma. The CSF is usually under increased pressure, though normal and subnormal pressures do not exclude the possibility of an epidural hematoma. The fluid may be clear or sanguineous, depending on whether or not there is an associated contusion, laceration, or subarachnoid hemorrhage. Death, which is almost invariable if the clot is not removed surgically, comes at the end of a comatose period, rarely if ever in a conscious patient, and is due to respiratory arrest. The visualization of a fracture line across the groove of the middle meningeal artery and a knowledge of the side of the head struck (the clot is usually on that side) are of aid in diagnosis and of lateralization of the lesion. The computerized tomography (CT) scan provides definitive confirmation. The surgical procedure consists of placement of several burr holes (a single one may miss the clot), drainage, identification of the bleeding vessel, and ligation. The operative results are excellent, except in the cases with extended fractures and laceration of the dural venous sinuses, in which instance the epidural hematoma may be bilateral rather than unilateral, as it ordinarily is. If coma, bilateral Babinski's signs, spasticity, or decerebrate rigidity supervene before operation, the prognosis for life becomes poor. This usually means that a temporal lobe herniation and crushing of the midbrain have already occurred.

Acute and chronic subdural hematoma   The problems created by the acute and chronic subdural hematoma are so different that they must be discussed separately. In *acute subdural hematomas,* which may be unilateral or bilateral, the latent interval is usually longer than in epidural hemorrhage—many days or 1 to 2 weeks. Headaches, drowsiness, sometimes agitation, slowness in thinking, and confusion, all of which progressively worsen, are the most frequent symptoms. Focal or lateralizing signs (hemiplegia) are late and tend to be less prominent than the disturbance of consciousness. Frequently the acute subdural hematoma is combined with cerebral contusion and laceration, so that the clinical effects of these several lesions are difficult to distinguish; and there are some patients in whom it is impossible before operation to state whether the surface clot is epidural or subdural in location. CT scan provides quick, accurate diagnosis. The x-ray absorptive value of the subdural fluid is about 30 units, the same as blood, and it decreases on the 40th to 70th day after subdural clot formation. (The absorptive value of CSF is 6 units, and this rises to 7 or 8 units with high protein content up to 2500 mg per 100 ml.) If CT scan is not available, the physician must resort to arteriography, which shows inward displacement of cerebral arteries from the skull. The treatment is to place bilateral temporal burr holes and to evacuate the clot. The surgical results are less certain than in chronic subdural hematoma. Once coma has occurred, as many as half the patients die. If the clot that is found is too small to explain the symptoms, the surgeon usually proceeds to do a right subtemporal decompression. Exceptionally the subdural hematoma forms in the posterior fossa and gives rise to headache, vomiting, pupillary inequality, dysphagia, cranial nerve palsies, ataxia of trunk and gait, and stiff neck, in some combination.

In *chronic subdural hematoma,* the traumatic cause is less clear. The head injury, especially in the elderly person, may be trivial (striking the head against the branch of a tree, or on the mantel of a fireplace during a faint, etc.), and it may have been forgotten completely. A period of weeks then follows when headaches (not invariable), giddiness, slowness in thinking, confusion, exaggeration of certain personality peculiarities, and a seizure or two (rare) are the main symptoms. The initial impression may indicate a vascular lesion, a brain tumor, drug intoxication, or a depressive, senile, or other type of psychosis. As with acute subdural hematoma, the disturbance of consciousness (drowsiness, inattentiveness, incoherence of thought, stupor, or coma) is more prominent than focal or lateralizing signs. The latter usually consist of hemiparesis and rarely of an aphasic disturbance. Hemianesthesia and homonymous hemianopsia are seldom observed, probably because the anatomic structures subserving these functions are deep and not easily compressed (in the case of the geniculocalcarine pathway) and sensory changes are likely to be overlooked in a stuporous, confused patient. Hemiplegia, i.e., complete paralysis of one arm and leg, is usually indicative of an intracerebral lesion rather than of a compressive surface lesion. Another important feature of the hemiparesis is that it may be contralateral or ipsilateral, depending on whether or not herniation of the temporal lobe through the notch of the tentorium into the posterior fossa and compression of the contralateral cerebral peduncle are present; if the latter has occurred, corticospinal signs are then ipsilateral to the clot or bilateral. As the condition progresses, the patient becomes comatose but often with striking fluctuations of awareness. The ipsilateral pupil dilates (Hutchinson's pupillary sign), owing, it is believed, to direct pressure of the herniating temporal lobe upon the oculomotor nerve. The dilated pupil and ptotic eyelid are more reliable indications of the side of the hematoma than the hemiparesis, though they too may be misleading in certain cases. Convulsions are unusual ($<$15 percent) except in patients with a contusion. The CT scan shows the surface mass of blood clot or fluid and deformity of the ventricular system.

Roentgenograms of the skull are usually negative except for a shift of a calcified pineal to one side or an occasional unexpected fracture line. The branches of the middle cerebral artery are separated from the skull and displaced contralaterally in an arteriogram. The CSF may be clear, bloody, or xanthochromic, depending on the presence or absence of recent or old contusion and subarachnoid hemorrhage, and the pressure may be elevated, normal, or subnormal. Of all these diagnostic procedures, CT scan and arteriography are the most reliable.

The acute, rapidly evolving subdural hematomas are due to tearing or bridging veins and direct compression of the brain by an expanding clot of fresh blood. Unlike the epidural arterial hemorrhage, which is progressive, the bleeding is usually arrested by the rising intracranial pressure. The chronic subdural hematoma is believed to gradually expand by becoming encapsulated by fibrous membranes (pseudomembranes) which grow from the dura. In its encysted state, as red corpuscles hemolyze and blood proteins disintegrate, the osmotic pressure rises and fluid enters the hematoma, with the result that the hematoma enlarges and the compressive effects increase. Severe cerebral compression and displacement with temporal lobe-tentorial herniation are the usual causes of death. Treatment consists of placing burr holes and evacuating the clot before deep coma has developed.

Subdural hygromas (collections of blood and CSF in the subdural space) may also form after an injury, as well as meningitis (in an infant) and pneumoencephalography (see Chap. 374). It is said that a tear of the arachnoid permits bacteria to enter and excite a serous reaction in the subdural space. Drowsiness, confusion, irritability, and fever are relieved when the subdural fluid is aspirated or drained.

Delayed focal edema from contusion As was mentioned under "Presence of Lucid Interval," the patient with severe blunt injury may be only slightly confused soon after the blow to the head and only later lapse into coma as further bleeding and swelling occur. Although exceptional, this condition must be considered in those patients with a relatively lucid interval.

Cerebral hemorrhage (immediate and delayed) Acute, massive brain hemorrhages are more frequent in elderly than in young patients and are usually fatal within a few hours. The clinical picture is similar to that of hypertensive brain hemorrhage (deepening coma with hemiplegia, a dilating pupil, bilateral Babinski's signs, stertorous and irregular respiration). Indeed the problem that cannot be solved even at postmortem examination is whether the patient had a hemorrhagic type of stroke and then fell or had a fall that caused the head injury and hemorrhage. If the bleeding is slow, there may be an interval of 2 to 3 days between injury and the symptoms of the oncoming hemorrhage. Coma or confusion, if present from the time of the injury, may obscure the signs of the intracerebral hemorrhage. Craniotomy with evacuation of the clot has given a successful result in a few cases.

TRAUMATIC OCCLUSION OF THE CAROTID ARTERY In this relatively rare and most dramatic form of cranial trauma, the patient is usually young and athletic, and the mechanism of the injury is usually unclear. An accident on the playing field of seemingly trivial type is followed after an interval of hours or days by a massive hemiplegia, hemianesthesia, homonymous hemianopsia, and, if left-sided, aphasia. Occlusion is demonstrable by arteriography. Hemorrhage into the wall of the common or internal carotid artery has been found in a few patients (see Chap. 365). In others injury to the wall of the carotid artery has given rise to embolism of the anterior or middle cerebral artery.

REPEATED CONCUSSION (PUNCH-DRUNK) The cumulative effects of repeated injuries, observed almost exclusively in pro-

fessional boxers, constitute a type of head injury difficult to classify, for only a few cases have been well studied pathologically. It is a common observation that after a number of years in the ring, pugilists often become forgetful, slow in thinking, and slightly dysarthric. Their movements are stiff and uncertain, especially in the lower extremities, there is an unsteadiness of gait, and occasionally involuntary movements. The plantar reflexes may be extensor on one or both sides. The EEG shows slow waves of theta and sometimes of delta type. The anatomic basis of this disease is not fully known. The postulation of showers of petechial hemorrhages from repeated blows on the jaw should not be given credence until demonstrated pathologically. The brain is atrophied, and a pneumoencephalogram will reveal dilated lateral ventricles. A low-pressure hydrocephalus from repeated meningeal hemorrhages is another possibility. In at least a half dozen reported cases loss of cortical neurons has been accompanied by senile plaques and fibrillary changes in remaining neurons, as in Alzheimer's disease. The findings of diffuse degeneration of the cerebral white matter have been demonstrated in rabbits and monkeys which have been subjected to repeated concussions (Jakob) and offer another, more acceptable possibility.

PENETRATING AND COMPRESSION INJURIES OF THE BRAIN
Penetration of the brain by high-velocity missiles and shell fragments are occurring with increasing frequency in these times of violent street crimes. But these and the rare compression fractures are more strictly neurosurgical problems and will not be discussed here.

SEQUELAE OF SEVERE HEAD INJURY

The signs of focal brain disease, whether due to open and penetrating or closed head injuries, tend always to ameliorate as the months pass. A hemiplegia is often reduced to a minimal hemiparesis or ineptitude of voluntary motor function with exaggerated reflexes and an equivocal Babinski sign on that side, and aphasia improves to become a stuttering or hesitant paraphasia which is not disabling except in a person whose profession requires much speaking or writing. Many of the signs of brainstem disease improve, often to an astonishing degree.

PROTRACTED TRAUMATIC COMA AND PSEUDOCOMA Of particular interest is the outcome of those rare conditions in which coma persists for weeks or months or even years. These patients, while comatose (i.e., unreceptive to stimuli and unresponsive) or in a state of pseudocoma (receptive and capable of signaling by blinking their eyes but otherwise unresponsive), usually exhibit a variety of neurologic abnormalities: unequal pupils; dilated, fixed pupil and oculomotor palsy on one side and hemiplegia on the other; disturbances of gaze; bilateral corticospinal paralysis with Babinski's sign; extensor postures of arm and leg on one side and flexed arm and extended leg on the other; brainstem attacks (extension of limbs and increased respiration, blood pressure, and sweating on stimulation of any kind); and involuntary movements (tremor, chorea, athetosis). Some remain in this reduced mental state until death (after nearly 10 years in one of the authors' cases, but usually after a few months or a year or two). The majority, however, may regain enough function to leave the hospital; not a few, surprising as it may seem, are restored to full alertness and fairly adequate mental function. Residual weakness of limbs, slurred speech, ocular palsies, ataxia of an arm or leg, or involuntary movements are frequent. During convalescence, language mechanisms may be found disturbed in various ways, i.e., mutism, akinesia or adynamia (lack of volition or impulse to speak or move), dysarthria, and, if there are contusions of the cortex of the dominant hemisphere, an aphasia as well. Any one or a combination of these abnormalities may be present.

The authors have examined the brains in nearly a dozen cases of this type, and nearly all have shown numerous foci of hemorrhage and ischemic necrosis in the midbrain and subthalamus, especially in the tegmentum and tectum. They were probably due in most instances to temporal lobe herniation and midbrain compression, for one could see where one side of the base and tegmentum had been indented by the free edge of the tentorium. In others there may have been direct injury to the midbrain and pons, with numerous small hemorrhages. Presumably these pathologic changes are not constant, for scattered lesions in the cerebral cortex (contusions of the summits of convolutions, ischemia with necrosis in the depths of sulci) and scattered foci of necrosis and hemorrhage in the cerebral white matter and corpus callosum along the lines of force of the injury have been observed. Several neuropathologists have emphasized these white matter lesions as being of primary importance (shear strains with axonic injury). We interpret tract degenerations as secondary to focal necrosis of tissue.

EPILEPSY Posttraumatic epilepsy, which occurs in 20 to 40 percent of patients, is one of the most dreaded complications of head injury. Its basis is nearly always a contusion or laceration of the cortex. The likelihood of epilepsy is said to be greater in parietal and posterior frontal lesions, but it may arise from lesions in any area of the cerebral cortex. The incidence of epilepsy is much greater in "open" than in "closed" head injuries. Indeed, in cases of pure concussion without contusion or laceration, seizures are not much more frequent than in the general population. The interval between head injury and the first seizure ranges from 3 to 9 months, but it may be much longer, i.e., many years, particularly in children. The longer the interval, the less certain one is of its relation to the traumatic incident. There is a slightly greater tendency for those patients who had seizures at the time of head injury to become subject to recurrent seizures later. The seizures are always of focal character, or grand mal; petit mal is rarely if ever due to trauma. The significance of the different patterns of focal seizures, which vary according to the location of the lesion, has been worked out in detail by Penfield and his associates (see Chap. 23) and by Russell et al. The frequency of seizures in any given patient varies widely; some patients have only a few, others many, with episodes of status epilepticus. The EEG is of value in diagnosis; a focus of spike or sharp waves is the characteristic finding. Usually the seizures can be controlled by anticonvulsant medications, and only the recalcitrant cases are likely to require excision of the epileptic focus. The surgical results vary according to the methods of selection and technique of operation. Seizures are abolished in approximately 50 percent of cases by excision of the focus. They tend to decrease in frequency as the years pass, and some patients (an estimated 10 to 30 percent) stop having them.

IMPAIRMENT OF MENTAL FUNCTION Fortunately this is a rare sequela to head trauma. Mental function may be disturbed by focal lesions which produce dysphasia, agnosia, apraxia, etc. Rubens et al. have reported disconnection syndromes from traumatic hemorrhages in the corpus callosum. But usually intellectual functions and memory are preserved. The exceptions are often elderly persons in whom the injury may have uncovered an early senile dementia or the development at any age of hydrocephalus secondary to subarachnoid

hemorrhage. Children and adolescents are more apt to show residual personality disorders.

POSTTRAUMATIC NERVOUS INSTABILITY Undoubtedly the most troublesome sequela of head injury is that alluded to above in the discussion of the first group of cases under "Clinical Manifestations of Head Injuries"—*headache, giddiness, and nervous instability.* This has been called the "postconcussional syndrome" or the "minor contusion syndrome" (Trotter), or "posttraumatic vasomotor neurosis" (Friedmann). All these terms are objectionable on the grounds that they suggest an explanatory hypothesis, as yet unproved. Headache is the central symptom, at times localized to the part struck. It is variously described as an aching, throbbing, pounding, stabbing, or pressing pain and is remarkable for its variability. The intensification of symptoms by mental and physical effort, straining, stooping, and emotional excitement has already been mentioned. Rest and quiet may relieve them. Thus the headache becomes a major obstacle to convalescence, which demands always a resumption of normal activities. The dizziness is usually not a true vertigo but a giddiness. The patient feels suddenly unsteady, dazed, weak, or faint. However, a certain number of patients report symptoms which suggest a labyrinthine disorder. For example, objects in the environment are said to move momentarily, and looking upward or to the side may cause a sense of unbalance. Or changing one's position in space may evoke momentary vertigo and nystagmus. Labyrinthine tests may show either hypo- or hyperreactivity, or the results may prove to be normal. The data are usually so indefinite that it is impossible to state whether or not the labyrinth and vestibular mechanisms have been injured. Exceptionally, vertigo is accompanied by diminished excitability of both the labyrinth and the cochlea, and one may assume the existence of direct injury to the nerve or end organ. The giddy patient usually is intolerant of noise, emotional excitement, and crowds. Tenseness, restlessness, inability to concentrate, a feeling of nervousness, fatigue, worry, apprehension, and an inability to tolerate the usual amount of alcohol complete the clinical picture. In contrast to the multiple subjective symptoms, detailed tests of intellectual functions and memory show little or no impairment. This syndrome, once established, may persist for months or even years, but usually the symptoms lessen as time passes. Strangely, it is almost unknown in children. Its intensity and duration are augmented by compensation problems and litigation, suggesting a psychopathologic factor.

EXTRAPYRAMIDAL AND CEREBELLAR DISORDERS The question of *posttraumatic Parkinson's syndrome* has been discussed many times, usually with the general conclusion that a true traumatic parkinsonism does not exist. Most patients have merely had paralysis agitans or postencephalitic Parkinson's disease brought to light by head injury. Cerebellar ataxia is a rare consequence of cranial trauma. When present, it is frequently unilateral and due to injury of the superior cerebellar peduncle against the tentorium. If bilateral, it suggests traumatic hemorrhage in the midbrain tegmentum involving the decussation of the brachium conjunctivum. An unsteadiness of gait may also reflect a communicating hydrocephalus.

POSTTRAUMATIC HYDROCEPHALUS The not infrequent examples of posttraumatic hydrocephalus exhibit intermittent headaches, vomiting, confusion, and drowsiness, and autopsy has demonstrated an adhesive basilar meningitis, attributed to subarachnoid or ventricular hemorrhage. Later, mental dullness, apathy, and psychomotor retardation are the principal manifestations. The CSF pressure may then have fallen to a normal level (low-pressure hydrocephalus). Since symptoms like these have been observed occasionally after the rupture of a saccular aneurysm with massive subarachnoid hemorrhage, due presumably to blocking of the aqueduct and fourth ventricle by blood clot, this mechanism has also been suggested as a possible explanation of traumatic hydrocephalus in patients with cerebral contusion. Response to ventriculoatrial shunt may be dramatic.

POSTTRAUMATIC PSYCHIATRIC DISORDERS In contrast to nervousness and nervous instability, which are common sequelae of injuries of all types, posttraumatic psychoses are relatively infrequent. The most distressing psychiatric syndromes have been suspiciousness and paranoid delusions, unaccountable outbursts of violent temper, sometimes with homicidal or suicidal tendencies, progressive hyperactivity, delirium, and mania, and episodes of bizarre behavior with subsequent amnesia, reminiscent of temporal lobe seizures. Alcoholism may provoke some of these behavioral abnormalities. Some of these illnesses are undoubtedly due to residual brain damage in individuals of peculiar personality makeup. However, attempts to account for psychoses of this type by reference to constitutional peculiarities and predisposition, laid bare, so to speak, by head injury, have not been convincing.

TREATMENT

The physician who undertakes to treat the "head injury case" must at all times bear in mind that assiduous attention to detail may prove to be lifesaving, and that accurate documentation of all diagnostic findings and therapy is desirable if the medical data are later to be used in the arbitration of insurance claims, worker's unemployment compensation, etc. The suggestions which follow can do no more than serve as guides, for every patient presents a combination of problems that the physician has not encountered before and may not observe again in identical form.

Exact data concerning the patient's medical status before the accident (previous illnesses, work and social record, emotional stability), the nature and precise circumstances of the accident, the duration of retrograde and anterograde amnesia, and all that transpired afterward should be obtained and recorded. Verbatim statements should be written down whenever possible.

The treatment problems presented by each of the three groups of clinical cases discussed above are as follows.

MINOR HEAD INJURY In this group are included patients who (1) were never unconscious at any time, (2) were briefly unconscious at the time of the first examination, or (3) are rapidly regaining consciousness.

Circumstances dictate how each case is managed. If the injury was trivial and the scalp was not lacerated and if patients are entirely clear mentally, little or nothing need be done. When patients are unable to give an accurate account of what has happened and appear still to be somewhat confused or incoherent, they should be compelled to lie down or at least remain in one place. It often happens that the confusion is not detected and patients are permitted to resume activity while still acting in an irrational manner. They may get into their car and attempt to drive, only to have another accident, or if they are athletes they may continue to play a game and make a series of errors.

It is often tempting to discharge the conscious or nearly conscious person who is admitted to a general hospital after only brief observation. However, experience teaches caution. A complete examination, with the patient fully undressed, should be carried out. It is well, if there is any likelihood of litigation, to obtain x-rays of the skull and an EEG. Whether to perform a lumbar puncture will usually depend on how serious the injury was, on the prominence of posttraumatic

headache, etc. A simple fracture without involvement of paranasal sinuses requires no special treatment but is believed to contraindicate vigorous athletic activities for several months or a year.

Posttraumatic headache, dizziness, and nervousness are the most difficult symptoms; an optimistic prognosis and the institution of a program of graded mental and physical activities to the point of tolerance stand the best chance of restoring the patient to a useful life. The patient should be told to expect a certain amount of headache and to carry on in spite of it. Meprobamate, 200 mg tid, is useful for anxiety, and a non-habit-forming analgesic medication should be given for the more severe headaches (Empirin or aspirin). Insomnia may require a barbiturate medication or chloral hydrate at first, but these drugs should be discontinued as soon as possible. If symptoms of anxiety and depression appear, medicines for their suppression should be used as outlined in Chap. 11. Any litigation that may be involved should be settled within 6 to 9 months. To delay settlement usually works against the best interests of patients. The severity of their injury can be ascertained within this period of time, and a longer period of observation only enhances their worries and fears and reduces their motivation to return to work.

PATIENTS WHO ARE UNCONSCIOUS WHEN FIRST SEEN If the physician arrives on the scene of the accident, a hurried examination should be made before the patient is moved in order to determine whether there is dangerous hemorrhage from a laceration of the scalp or other parts of the body and whether there is a likelihood of a fracture-dislocation of the cervical part of the spine, which is occasionally associated with head injury. The patient who is in shock, with cold clammy skin and feeble pulse, should be covered with warm blankets. In moving an individual with a potential cervical spine injury, the spine should be kept straight at all times and flexion of the neck should be avoided. This can best be done by placing sandbags or firm pillows on either side of the head and warning everyone against neck flexion. An even safer method is to place the patient on a stretcher face down and arrange pillows to assure a clear airway. Bleeding from the scalp can usually be controlled with a firm pad unless an artery is divided, and then a suture becomes necessary.

In the hospital, where all such patients should be taken, the first steps should be to control shock. This can usually be done by the application of warmth, keeping the head low, and leaving the patient alone for a few minutes. The shock will usually come under control with or without vasopressor drugs or transfusions. Persistent shock is rare in head injury and always raises the suspicion of a ruptured viscera with internal bleeding, extensive fractures, or traumatism of the cervical part of the spinal cord. A quick survey will enable one to estimate the depth of coma, size of pupils, and presence of obvious fractures, and if shock is not present, or after the blood pressure has stabilized, a more detailed examination can be performed. The skull should be carefully inspected and palpated. The hair should be cut off around the scalp wound. A bogginess of the temporal or postauricular region (Battle's sign), bleeding from the nose or ear, extensive conjunctival edema, and hemorrhage are useful signs of underlying skull fracture. However, it should be remembered that rupture of the eardrum or a blow on the nose may also cause bleeding from the ear and nose, respectively. Fractures of the orbital bones may cause displacement of the eye, with resulting diplopia, and fracture of the jaws, disalignment of the teeth, and great discomfort on attempting to open the mouth. Careful notes should be made regarding temperature, pulse, blood pressure, state of consciousness, pupil size, ocular movements, corneal reflexes, facial movements during grimace, swallowing, tone of limb muscles, movements of limbs, predominant postures, and reflexes. Vital signs and consciousness should be checked and recorded by the nurse or physician every 2 h. A proper airway must be maintained; endotracheal intubation is often necessary. The best position for the patient is semisupine, with the head on a pillow and turned to one side. If urine is retained and the bladder is distended, a catheter should be inserted and kept there. If coma persists for more than 48 to 72 h, a nasal tube should be passed and fluids and nourishment given by that route. Intravenous fluids should be administered slowly and not in excessive amounts; even hypertonic glucose may increase oncoming pulmonary and cerebral edema, the danger of the latter being especially great in children. Lumbar puncture should be done as soon as practicable for diagnostic purposes (immediately if bacterial meningitis is suspected), and if the pressure is elevated, it should be lowered to 100 to 150 mmH$_2$O. The practice of daily lumbar punctures has its advocates and its opponents. The authors have tended to use them only if the pressure is elevated and the patient's condition is not improving. Hypertonic solutions administered intravenously are of therapeutic value. One hundred milliliters of hypertonic urea, or if not available, 50 to 100 ml of 25% mannitol may be injected intravenously in an attempt to lower CSF pressure. Recently corticosteroids, e.g., dexamethasone (16 to 48 mg per day), have been strikingly effective in reducing brain swelling and permitting vital signs to stabilize. X-rays of the skull and other parts should be taken after the first day or two, unless there is a suspicion of an epidural hemorrhage, in which case they should be made at once, to visualize a crack across the course of the middle meningeal artery. A CT scan is of great value in determining the presence of epidural, subdural, and intracerebral hematomas and ventricular deformity or displacement. Restlessness is controlled by sodium phenobarbital or paraldehyde, but only if careful nursing does not quiet the patient and permit him or her to sleep for a few hours at a time.

Once the patient has regained consciousness, the danger of suffocation, aspiration pneumonia, thrombophlebitis, and pulmonary embolism has usually passed, and therapy can proceed along the lines indicated for the first group.

Death from head injury in the first 12 h is the direct effect of primary brain injury and probably cannot be prevented. The advisability of any surgical procedure during the period is much debated. If the patient survives for 1, 2, or more days and remains in coma, the control of brain swelling and hemorrhage by surgical means must be considered. Should the condition of the patient then begin to deteriorate (pulse rising, temperature subnormal or rising, state of consciousness worsening, hemiplegia more obvious, plantar reflexes more clearly extensor), a decision must be made concerning an epidural or subdural hemorrhage and of increasing brain edema with temporal lobe herniation. By then CT scans will have informed the physician whether or not these are present. If this apparatus is not available, Rowbotham, who has had much experience with cases of this type, recommends a right-sided temporal decompression and two inspection burr holes in the left, one at the Sylvian point and one at the parietal eminence, for some of these patients. In his opinion the indications for surgery are (1) retrogression following a period of improvement which cannot be controlled by lumbar puncture and oral and rectal hypertonic solutions or intravenous dehydration measures; (2) decerebrate rigidity which has its onset after an interval of 24 h (early decerebrate rigidity implies primary brainstem injury) if meningitis is ruled out; (3) a dilated fixed pupil on one side,

with no improvement after 12 h; and (4) prolonged unconsciousness associated with persistently high CSF pressure. Not all neurologists and neurosurgeons are agreed on the value of this plan, and some would insist on diagnostic arteriography as a guide. But, certainly the removal of a large epidural or subdural hemorrhage, which cannot be diagnosed easily in the comatose patient, may be a lifesaving procedure.

In recent years a striking reduction in the mortality rate from these acute head injuries has been obtained by the application of intensive care together with the free use of tracheostomy. Many of the comatose patients who would otherwise have succumbed to respiratory obstruction, pulmonary infections, or dehydration are thereby saved. Also, greater efforts to evacuate intracranial hematomas as soon as possible seem to have helped. Survivors may be left permanently disabled, but a surprising number, the percentage increasing up to 7 years, return to productive work.

The treatment of the patient with protracted coma has been outlined in Chap. 20. Every patient presents special problems which must be dealt with individually.

PATIENTS WHO RECOVERED CONSCIOUSNESS (LUCID INTERVAL) AND THEN BECAME STUPOROUS OR COMATOSE
The treatment is that of epidural, subdural, and delayed cerebral hemorrhage. This has already been discussed.

GENERAL CONVALESCENCE

A head injury carries dire import to most lay persons, who often fear for their minds and are concerned about their capacity to resume their place in society. In former times, therapeutic measures often involved long discussions of the seriousness of the injury, protracted bed rest, and inactivity, all of which served only to engender greater anxiety. Even worse, these measures were not of proved value. It is now widely acknowledged that patients do better if their physicians tend to minimize the seriousness of their head injuries and to reassure them that they will recover. Early rehabilitation should be encouraged. It may safely begin as soon as the CSF becomes clear, usually within a few weeks at the most, except of course in the rare cases of protracted coma.

The prognosis of head injury, in good hands, is influenced by several variables: Elderly patients often remain disabled, especially when compensation is involved. Young and middle-aged adults do better if they are not entitled to compensation. (Russell's figures show 70 percent of patients with compensation benefits back at work in 18 months, and 83 percent of those without compensation working at the end of this period.) Russell also pointed out that the severity of the injury as measured by the duration of traumatic amnesia was a factor. If the period of amnesia was less than 1 h, 95 percent of patients were back at work within 2 months; if longer than 24 h, only 80 percent had returned to work within 6 months. About 60 percent, however, still had symptoms at the end of 2 months, and 40 percent at the end of 18 months. Of the most severely injured (those comatose for several days), many will remain permanently disabled. However, recovery always tends to be better than one expects, and the motor impairment, aphasia, and dementia usually clear. Improvement may continue over a period of five or more years. Children seem to recover more completely than adults. Rehabilitation centers are of great help in restoring morale and reeducating the patient.

(For discussion of traumatism of spinal cord, nerve roots, and peripheral nerves, see Chaps. 375 and 377.)

REFERENCES

BROCK S (ed): *Injuries of the Brain and Spinal Cord and Their Coverings,* 3d ed. Baltimore, Williams & Wilkins, 1949, p 71

CAVENESS WF, WALKER AE: *Head Injury.* Philadelphia, Lippincott, 1966

LANGFITT TW: Measuring the outcome of head injury. J Neurol Neurosurg Psychiatry 48:683, 1978

ROWBOTHAM GF: *Acute Injuries of the Head,* 4th ed. Baltimore, Williams & Wilkins, 1964

RUBENS AB et al: Post-traumatic cerebral hemispheric disconnection syndromes. Arch Neurol 34:750, 1975

RUSSELL WR: Cerebral involvement in head injury. Brain 55:549, 1932

WALKER AE: *The Late Effects of Head Injury.* Springfield, Charles C Thomas, 1969

367
NEOPLASTIC DISEASE OF THE BRAIN

RAYMOND D. ADAMS
FRED HOCHBERG
HENRY deF. WEBSTER

Tumors of the central nervous system play a very important part in neurologic medicine and occupy a distinct field by themselves. It may be said of them generally that they occur in great variety, produce neurologic symptoms because of size, location, and invasive qualities, usually destroy the tissues in which they are situated and displace those around them, are a frequent cause of increased intracranial pressure, and are often lethal.

For the student of medicine the most important facts to know are the following: (1) Many types of tumor occur in the cranial cavity and spinal canal and certain ones are much more frequent than others (see Table 367-1). (2) Some of these tumors, such as the craniopharyngioma, meningioma, and neurilemmoma, have a disposition to grow in certain parts of the cranial cavity, thereby eliciting certain syndromes. (3) Their growth rates vary; some like the glioblastoma are highly malignant and invasive, and others like the meningioma are benign and compressive. These pathologic peculiarities are important for they have valuable clinical correlations, providing the explanation of slowly or rapidly progressive clinical states and excellent or poor prognosis after surgical excision.

The one place where these pathologic-clinical correlations tend to fail is in the glioma group of tumors, i.e., astrocytoma-glioblastoma series, and this is regrettable because tumors of this type are so common. Often these gliomas are of mixed cell type. For example, one part of the tumor may be a typical astrocytoma and another an oligodendrocytoma. Also the degree of differentiation or its opposite, the degree of anaplasia, varies from one part of the tumor to another. Therefore a biopsy sample is often misleading with reference to the expected clinical behavior of the tumor. For example, the clinician may be led to believe that a tumor which in a biopsy is composed of astrocytes is benign, whereas actually the main mass of it still in the brain is a glioblastoma.

INCIDENCE OF CENTRAL NERVOUS SYSTEM TUMORS AND THEIR TYPES

It was estimated by Posner that in the United States in 1975 there were 365,000 deaths from tumors. Of these the total number of patients dying of primary tumors of the brain seemed comparatively small (about 8500), but there were fully 67,000 patients with extracranial tumors who died of metastases to the brain. Thus approximately 20 percent of all the tumor cases present with neurologic abnormalities at some time in their course. The intracranial tumor ranks second (after cerebrovascular diseases) as an endogenous neurologic problem.

It is difficult to obtain accurate statistics on the types of intracranial tumors, for most of them have been obtained from university hospitals with a specialized neurosurgical staff that attracts the more easily diagnosed and treatable forms. From the general figures given above, intracranial secondary tumors should outnumber primary ones almost 10 to 1, yet in almost all reported series (those of Zulch, Cushing, Olivecrona, Zimmerman) only 3 to 6 percent are of this type. Even in the autopsy statistics of the Boston City Hospital series, where one would expect a more natural, unselected representation, the tendency is to err on the low side for metastatic growths, since the brain is not examined as often in cancer patients and many of the more benign tumors may have been sent to clinics with better surgical facilities.

With these reservations concerning natural incidence the figures in Table 367-1 might be taken as representative.

INTRACRANIAL TUMORS

PATHOPHYSIOLOGY Since the cranium is filled with three virtually incompressible elements, brain tissue, blood, and cerebrospinal fluid (CSF), a tumor which adds to brain mass must grow at the expense of the other two elements. As the volume of the tumor increases, the cerebrospinal fluid is forced out of the ventricles and cerebral subarachnoid space through the foramen magnum and optic foramens into the spinal and perioptic extensions of the subarachnoid space. The cerebrospinal fluid lumbar subarachnoid pressure becomes increased, and the raised perioptic pressure impairs venous return from the optic nerve heads and adjacent retinas, resulting in papilledema ("choked disks").

Pressure of the tumor mass on adjacent brain tissue presumably narrows or obliterates venules, particularly in the cerebral white matter. Circulatory slowing and altered vascular permeability leads to vasogenic regional cerebral edema. As the intracranial pressure increases, the cerebral circulation must be maintained. At first this is accomplished by arteriolar dilatation (decreased cerebrovascular resistance). Later, once this compensation proves inadequate, systemic blood pressure increases and pulse slows (Cushing principle).

Inasmuch as the cranial cavity is subdivided by the rigid falx and tentorium, the increase in brain volume occasioned by the tumor and surrounding edema may raise the pressure in one of the cranial compartments to the point where the brain tissue is displaced to an adjacent compartment (where the

TABLE 367-1
Types of intracranial tumor in approximately 15,000 cases in the combined series of Zulch, Cushing, Olivecrona

	Percent
Gliomas:	45
Glioblastoma multiforme	20
Astrocytoma	10
Ependymoma	6
Medulloblastoma	4
Oligodendrocytoma	5
Meningioma	15
Pituitary adenoma	7
Neurilemmoma	7
Metastatic carcinoma	6
Craniopharyngioma and dermoid, epidermoid or teratoma	4
Angiomas and vascular malformations	4
Sarcomas	4
Unclassified (mostly gliomas)	5
Miscellaneous (pinealoma, chordoma, granuloma)	3
	100

pressure is lower). In this way brain herniations occur—of the inferior part of the cerebellum through the foramen magnum into the cervical canal (cerebellar pressure cone), the medial part of the temporal lobe through the opening in the tentorium into the posterior fossa (temporal lobe-tentorial pressure cone), and the medial, frontal, and parietal lobes beneath the falx into the opposite side (subfalcial pressure cone).

Raised intracranial pressure from the tumor mass or an attendant obstructive hydrocephalus is manifested by generalized headache, slowed mental activity, drowsiness, apathy, and diffuse slowing in the EEG. Regional edema causes a rapidly evolving impairment of the function of the part of the brain involved. Temporal lobe-tentorial pressure cone causes dilatation of the ipsilateral pupil (Hutchinson's pupil) and ptosis of the eyelid; hemiplegia that is either contralateral or ipsilateral (compression of the oppposite cerebral peduncle against the sharp edge of the tentorium) to the tumor; coma (compression, ischemia, and hemorrhages in the upper reticular formation); Cheyne-Stokes and finally arrest of respirations; and high cerebrospinal fluid pressure from blockage of the aqueduct of Sylvius and perimesencephalic subarachnoid space (mainly the latter).

A knowledge of these effects of elevated intracranial pressure, regional edema, and herniations is necessary to an understanding of the clinical behavior of intracranial growths.

CLINICAL AND PATHOLOGIC CHARACTERISTICS Tumors of the brain may exist with hardly any symptoms. Often only a slight deficiency in mental power, a slowness in comprehension, or a loss of capacity in sustaining continuous mental activity suggests any deviation from normal health. Specific signs that would lead to a suspicion of any real cerebral disease may be wholly wanting. In some patients, on the other hand, there is evidence of cerebral disease in the form of a seizure or some other dramatic symptom, but the evidence may not be clear enough to warrant the diagnosis of a cerebral tumor. In a third group, the existence of a new growth in the brain may be determined with much probability by the presence of signs of elevated intracranial pressure, but without symptoms which disclose localization of the growth. Lastly, a particular syndrome may be so clear and definite as to make it probable not only that there is a new growth within the cranium but also that it is located in one particular region and is of a particular histologic type. In other words, these latter tumors create certain unique syndromes seldom evidenced by any other disease.

In the further exposition of this subject, all intracranial tumors are considered in relation to the common clinical circumstances in which they are likely to be encountered, as follows:

1 The patient whose presenting symptom is either a decline in general mental ability or a seizure
2 The patient with unmistakable evidence of headaches and raised intracranial pressure
3 Specific intracranial tumor syndromes

PATIENTS WITH GENERAL SYMPTOMS OF CEREBRAL DISEASE OR A SEIZURE AS THE MAIN COMPLAINT These are the patients who give the most trouble in diagnosis and about whom decisions are often made with a great degree of uncertainty. Their initial symptoms are vague, and not until some time has elapsed will signs of focal brain disease appear; when they do, they are not always of accurate localizing value. Altered psychic function, headache, and seizures are the usual symptoms.

Some *change in mental function* may be found in nearly every patient of this type, but it may be necessary to obtain the observations of a person who knows the patient intimately to learn of it. A lack of persistent application to the tasks of the day, an undue irritability, emotional lability, a "peculiar inertia," faulty insight, forgetfulness, reduced range of mental activity, indifference to common social practices, and lack of initiative and spontaneity, all of which may be falsely attributed to worry, anxiety, or depression, are the usual symptoms. Much of this behavior is accepted by the patient with forbearance, and if he or she has any complaint, it is of being weak, tired, dizzy (nonrotational), or "queer in the head." Inordinate drowsiness, a remarkable equanimity or apathy, and stoicism may be primary findings. Usually within a few weeks or months the drowsiness and mental dullness increase. When questioned, if the psychic inertia is well advanced, a long pause precedes each reply, and at times the patient may not bother to respond at all. Or at the very moment when the examiner has decided that the patient has not heard the question and prepares to repeat it, an appropriate, sensible answer is given, usually in relatively few words. The responses are often much more intelligent than would be expected from the torpid mental state. Headache occurs with increasing frequency in many of the patients. There are, an addition, those who are confused or demented (see Chap. 25). The dullness and somnolence may gradually increase, and finally, as increased intracranial pressure supervenes, they end in stupor or coma.

Mental symptoms of this type cannot be ascribed to disease in any particular part of the brain. Tumors are most likely to be accompanied by intellectual disturbance when they interfere with large association fiber systems of the cerebral white matter; growths limited to the cortex and subcortical white matter are less likely to affect the mind. Much of the drowsiness, torpor, inertia, lack of spontaneity, and general restriction of mental horizon is related to increased intracranial pressure and not to the site and nature of the lesion.

The *headaches* in the "tumor patient" are variable. In some the pain is slight, temporary, and dull in character; in others it may be severe and unendurable, and either dull or sharp, but as a rule it is transitory or intermittent. If there are any characteristics of the headache, they would include its nocturnal occurrence, its presence on first awakening, or its deep nonpulsatile quality. However, these are not specific attributes, since migraine, hypertensive vascular headaches, etc., may also begin early in the morning when the patient first awakens. The patient does not always complain of the pain even when it is present and may betray its existence by placing a hand on the forehead and looking distressed.

The mechanism of the headache is not known. In the majority of instances, the intracranial pressure is normal during the first weeks when the headache is present, and one can attribute it only to distortion or alteration of blood vessels in or around the tumor. Later the headache appears to be related to rises in intracranial pressure. Tumors above the tentorium cause headache on the side of and in the vicinity of the tumor, usually in the orbital, frontal, temporal, or parietal regions. Tumors in the posterior fossa usually cause ipsilateral retroauricular or occipital headache. With elevated intracranial pressure, bifrontal and bioccipital headache is the rule, regardless of the location of the tumor.

Vomiting appears in about one-third of the patients with tumor syndromes of this type and usually accompanies the headache. It is more frequent with tumors of the posterior fossa and may precede other signs of intracranial tumor by weeks or months. Some patients may vomit unexpectedly and forcibly, without preceding nausea (projectile vomiting), but others suffer both nausea and great pain. Usually the vomiting is not related to the ingestion of food, often occurring before breakfast.

No less frequent is the complaint of *giddiness* or *dizziness*. As a rule it is not described with accuracy and consists of a more or less confused sensation in the head, coupled with feelings of strangeness and insecurity when the position of the head is altered.

One or more generalized *convulsions* are another major symptom calling attention to the existence of cerebral tumor. Their frequency in various statistical analyses is 20 to 50 percent of all patients with cerebral tumors. The onset of a seizure during adult years and the existence of a localizing aura are always suggestive of tumor. The localizing significance of seizure patterns has already been discussed (see Chap. 23). The seizures may occur once or many times and may precede other symptoms for as long as 10 years or more in cases of astrocytoma or meningioma.

The management of patients who present any one of the aforementioned symptoms requires brief discussion. Any clinical problems of these types, especially if accompanied by recurrent headache of a form which the patient recognizes as different from his customary headaches, or a seizure, appearing for the first time, justify a careful review of the patient's general behavior. In obtaining further data, one must rely heavily on the observations of other members of the family. A thorough neurologic examination with careful inspection of optic fundi, a test of visual fields, motor, reflex, and sensory functions in the limbs, alertness, memory, facility in language (speaking, reading, writing, and understanding the spoken word), calculation, and tests of visuospatial orientation must follow. Sooner or later other regional or localizing symptoms and signs will be discovered, and it is only by repeated examinations that one will note the earliest stages of a hemiparesis, aphasia, visual field defect, hemianesthesia, etc. Unmistakable signs of increased intracranial pressure eventually become manifest and establish the diagnosis of tumor with reasonable certainty (see "Astrocytoma," below.)

The decision as to the appropriate time for doing confirmatory diagnosis tests requires balanced clinical judgment. Since many of the symptoms described above could be due to any number of diseases, for a time it is wise to follow the patient by repeated examinations and not proceed too quickly to expensive and difficult diagnostic tests. As more of the clinical picture unfolds, there comes a time when x-rays of the chest (always done to help rule out metastatic carcinoma) and computerized tomography and radionuclide scans, a localizing EEG, and finally lumbar puncture (for pressure, cells, protein, and Wassermann reaction) should be done, preferably by admitting the patient to a hospital. Perimetry, audiograms, vestibular tests, and psychometric tests are also helpful in the study of many of these patients. Pneumoencephalography and carotid arteriography are reserved in most medical neurologic clinics for those in whom the total clinical syndrome is already strongly suggestive of tumor and further information is needed in planning surgery. These latter procedures are too costly and hazardous to be used routinely in every "tumor suspect."

TUMORS WHICH TEND TO PRODUCE GENERAL CEREBRAL SYMPTOMS OR SEIZURES The following tumors are most likely to produce initial convulsions or a vague syndrome of headache, giddiness, vomiting, dull or stuporous state, and psychic changes: glioblastoma multiforme, astrocytoma, oligodendroglioma, metastatic carcinoma, meningioma, and primary reticulum cell sarcoma of the cerebrum.

Glioblastoma multiforme In all statistical analyses of surgical and postmortem material, glioblastoma multiforme is responsible for more than 25 percent of intracranial gliomas and for more than 90 percent of gliomas of the cerebral hemispheres in adults. Approximately 20 to 30 percent of the cerebral tumors are bilateral, occupy more than one lobe of a hemisphere, or show multicentric foci of growth. Although predominantly cerebral in location, similar tumors may be observed in the

brainstem, cerebellum, or spinal cord. The peak incidence is in middle adult life, but no age group is spared.

The glioblastoma is a highly malignant tumor which infiltrates the brain extensively and may attain enormous size before attracting medical attention. It may extend to the meningeal surface or the ventricular wall, which probably accounts for the elevation of protein level (more than 100 mg per 100 ml in many cases), as well as an occasional pleocytosis of 10 to 100 cells or more, mostly lymphocytes. The tumor has a variegated appearance, being a mottled gray, red, orange, or brown, depending on the degree of necrosis and hemorrhage, whether recent or old. It is highly vascular, and in an arteriogram one can often see a network of abnormal vessels, mistaken at times for a hemangioma, and the displacement of normal vessels which may result from any "mass lesion." Some part of one lateral ventricle is often distorted, and both lateral land third ventricles are displaced contralaterally, which may be demonstrated by computerized tomography (CT scan) or pneumoencephalography. The vessels in the tumor are excessively permeable to radioactive phosphorus (^{32}P), radioactive arsenic, mercury, and technetium, which is the basis for radioactive scanning techniques. The characteristic microscopic pathologic findings are great cellularity with pleomorphism of cells and hyperchromatism of nuclei; identifiable astrocytes with fibrils in combination with astroblasts, tumor giant cells, and cells in mitosis; a curious neoplastic proliferation of the cells of small vessels (adventitial and endothelial); necrosis, pseudopalisading of viable cells, hemorrhage, thrombosis of vessels, and variable infiltrates of inflammatory cells (lymphocytes and mononuclear leukocytes). Temporal lobe–tentorial herniation, midbrain compression, midbrain and pontine hemorrhages, and increased intracranial pressure are usually the immediate causes of death.

Clinically the diffuse cerebral symptoms and seizures (present in 30 to 40 percent of cases) usually give way to a more definite frontal, temporal, parietooccipital, or callosal syndrome in a few weeks or months. Seldom, however, do the symptoms and signs point to one lobe, and often one is satisfied to be able to specify the region of the hemisphere which is involved.

Astrocytoma The astrocytoma may occur anywhere in the brain or spinal cord. Favored sites are cerebrum, cerebellum, thalamus, optic chiasm, and pons. It is a slowly growing tumor of infiltrative character with a tendency to form large cavities or pseudocysts. Others of these tumors are noncavitating, grayish-white, firm, and relatively avascular, almost indistinguishable from normal white matter, with which they may merge imperceptibly. Calcium deposits may occur in parts of the tumor and may be seen in plain x-rays of the skull. The cerebrospinal fluid is acellular, the only abnormality being the increased pressure and elevated protein level in some cases. The tumor by its mass may distort the lateral and third ventricles (seen in CT scan or pneumoencephalogram) and may be seen to displace the anterior and middle cerebral arteries in a carotid arteriogram. By injecting intravenously a contrast medium the extent of the tumor and the surrounding edema can be seen in the CT scan. At an early stage, however, all radiologic and electrographic tests may be negative. Microscopically, the tumor tissue is composed of well-differentiated astrocytes of fibrillary, protoplasmic, or transitional type.

The majority of cerebral astrocytomas undergo malignant degeneration and present as mixed astrocytomas and glioblastomas.

The astrocytoma may cause trivial symptoms for a long period of time. Seizures, headaches, and bizarre mental symptoms may be present for several years, in a few instances more than 10, before the diagnosis is made. The average survival period after the first symptom is 67 months in cerebral growths and 89 months in cerebellar ones. The cystic astrocytoma of the cerebellum is particularly benign, and some patients are alive and well as long as 30 years after part of the cyst was excised. In such cases, of course, accuracy of the original diagnosis of neoplasm is always open to question. The astrocytoma of the pons, optic nerves, and chiasm are discussed in more detail later on in this chapter (see "Glioma of the Brainstem").

Oligodendrocytoma The oligodendrocytoma is a relatively rare cerebral tumor (5 to 10 percent of gliomas) and is usually slow in its rate of growth (average span of evolution is 66 months). It is generally a soft, solid tumor, is rarely cystic, and through its tendency to calcify (spherules and particles of calcium in microscopic sections) often casts a shadow in the roentgenogram of the skull. Microscopically it is composed of small round cells with spherical nuclei and cytoplasm that stains poorly, forming a halo around the nucleus. Some of the tumors are mixtures of astrocytoma and oligodendrocytoma. The usual location is cerebral. Seizures are uncommon, and generalized or focal symptoms may be present for a long time before the mass of the tumor declares its presence by increased intracranial pressure.

Ependymoma and ependymoblastoma Although occasionally this tumor presents as a solitary mass in a cerebral hemisphere in adults, presumably arising from the ependymal wall of the lateral ventricle, its most distinctive form is a papillary growth filling the fourth ventricle of children. It is discussed further below.

The treatment of all forms of glioma of the cerebral hemispheres is partial excision, if feasible, after surgical biopsy. X-ray treatment seems to extend life for a few months. The nitrosureas, carmustine (BCNU) and lomustine (CCNU) drugs that are lipid-soluble and capable of crossing the blood-brain barrier, in combination with surgical excision and radiation, increase the mean survival time and the number functional at 18 months. These drugs and others [methyl lomustine (MSKCC), vincristine, procarbazine] which have been tried in a National Cooperative Study have added a few months to the survival time of persons with glioma. The diagnosis of glioblastoma multiforme can now he made from clinical, arteriographic, radioactive isotope, and EEG, and one is justified, at least in some cases of deep-seated tumor, in withholding surgery and giving radiation and chemotherapy. The control of . intracranial pressure is maintained by the use of dexamethasone, 6 to 8 mg every 6 h, while radiation therapy is being given and in lesser dose thereafter. This form of corticosteroid improves cerebral function and enables many of these tumor patients to become virtually asymptomatic for a time.

Meningioma (arachnoidal fibroblastoma or endothelioma) This is a benign tumor composed of specialized arachnoid lining cells, arising usually in places where there are many arachnoid villi. Since these clusters of arachnoid cells penetrate the dura in the vicinity of the venous sinuses, they often appear to originate from the dura itself; hence the old term *dural endothelioma*. Grossly the tumors are firm, gray-white, lobulated, bulbous, or plaque-like masses which indent or compress but do not invade brain tissue. Many of them are highly vascular. In size they are variable; those which have produced symptoms usually have attained a size of 3 to 4 cm or more. The cellular composition permits easy identification. The cells are of uniform type and have the peculiar disposition to encircle one another and to form characteristic whorls and psammoma bodies. The common sites of these tumors are the olfactory groove, tuberculum sellae, parasagittal region, sylvian fissure, cerebellopontine angle, and spinal canal. Inasmuch as they lie on the surface of the brain in or next to the dura, changes in the skull are frequent. The skull may be eroded over the tumor, and the meningeal and diploic vessels, which provide part of the blood supply to the tumor, dilate and are usually prominent in an x-ray. Or the tumor cells may invade the bone and stimulate osteoblastic activity, as a consequence of which a bony bulge may be seen and felt, or an endostosis is visualized on the inner table of the skull in an x-ray. The meningioma must be listed with bone-metastasizing carcinoma and the true cholesteatoma of the skull as the three tumors most likely to cause a visible cranial boss in relation to cerebral symptoms (*benign exostoses are neurologically asymptomatic*). Offering a broad vascular meningeal surface as they do, meningiomas often elevate the protein level of the cerebrospinal fluid. Their striking vascularity accounts for a characteristic "blush" seen in arteriograms and dense opacification in CT scans; the excessive permeability of the vessels, as well as the superficial location of the tumors, makes them ideal subjects for localization with radioactive isotopes. The underlying brain tissue is visibly edematous in CT scans and thus accounts for some of their recently evolving symptoms. The displacement without invasion of cerebral tissue probably explains the interruption locally of normal alpha frequencies in the EEG with sharp waves or theta waves, in contrast to the delta waves so often found in infiltrative gliomas. Multiple meningiomas may occur, particularly in cases of neurofibromatosis.

These tumors may be found at any age but are more frequent in advanced years, especially in women.

Reticulum cell sarcoma This tumor may be primary in the brain (microglioblastoma) and present a clinical picture nearly identical to that of glioblastoma multiforme. It is highly radiosensitive. In 20 cases studied at the Massachusetts General Hospital, all made some response to radiotherapy. One is alive and well 12 years later; all others were dead within 6 years. There is a tendency for this tumor to occur in immunosuppressed individuals and in those with chronic viral parotitis and iridocyclitis. The CSF cytology is often positive. Tumor foci may be multiple, and occasionally there is regression of early symptoms without therapy.

Metastatic carcinoma Of the secondary tumors of the brain only metastatic carcinoma will be discussed here because the other tumors that metastasize to the brain are decidedly rare. Carcinomas reach the brain by hematogenous spread. Probably 35 to 40 percent of them come from the lung, and approximately 15 percent each from the breast, gastrointestinal tract (usually colon or rectum), and kidney. Melanotic carcinoma of the skin, carcinoma of the stomach, gallbladder, liver, thyroid, testicle, uterus, ovary, etc., account for the remainder, no one of them usually being responsible for more than 3 or 4 percent of secondary tumors of the brain. Carcinoma of the prostate, esophagus, oropharynx, or skin (except for melanocarcinoma) rarely if ever is disseminated in the brain. In more than 75 percent of cases the metastases are multiple and are scattered through both the cerebrum and cerebellum; approximately one-fourth of the cases reach the meninges. The hypernephroma and thyroid carcinoma have a greater tendency to form solitary metastases than other tumors, and as with the chorioepithelioma and some lung tumors, the metastases are likely to be hemorrhagic. The tumor tissue generally has all the gross and microscopic features of any carcinomatous implant and excites rather little glial reaction but much edema.

The usual clinical picture in metastatic carcinoma of the

brain does not differ from that of glioblastoma multiforme. However, a number of other rather striking clinical neurologic syndromes occur. One that is particularly difficult to diagnose is a widespread *carcinomatous meningoencephalopathy* with headache, nervousness, depressed mood, trembling, mental confusion, and forgetfulness, the whole picture looking very much like that of general paresis. Carcinomatosis of the cerebellum with headache, dizziness, and ataxia, the ataxia being brought out only by having the patient walk, is another difficult condition to diagnose during life. Symptoms and signs referable to one or several cranial and spinal nerve roots may be combined with headache and confusion in widespread *carcinomatosis of the craniospinal meninges* (carcinomatous meningitis). Usually the cerebrospinal fluid contains a few white blood cells (lymphocytes) and an elevated protein level. Tumor cells can often be identified in stained sections of filtered (multispore) cerebrospinal fluid, and if many are present in the meninges, the sugar values may be subnormal, even as low as zero.

When the syndromes due to these several varieties of metastatic tumor are fully developed, diagnosis is relatively easy. If only headache and vomiting are present, a common error is to explain these symptoms on a psychologic basis. One learns by experience with this type of patient to make a psychiatric diagnosis only if the patient has the standard symptoms of one of the psychiatric disorders described in Chaps. 11 and 25. A lumbar puncture, a chest x-ray, sedimentation rate (increased in metastatic carcinoma but not glioblastoma), and other x-rays (gastrointestinal series, barium enema, and pyelograms if symptoms point to these organs) are advisable. The inflammatory neurologic syndromes which accompany carcinoma but which are not due to tumor invasion of the central nervous system, such as polyneuritis (especially with carcinoma of the lung), polymyositis, and spinocerebellar degeneration (ovarian and other carcinomas), may be the initial illness.

TUMORS OF INFECTIVE ORIGIN (GRANULOMAS AND PARASITIC CYSTS) Tuberculoma is much less frequent in the United States than it was 20 years ago, and gumma has become almost nonexistent. In fact a patient with serologic syphilis and a positive Wassermann reaction of the cerebrospinal fluid has a greater chance of having two diseases, a cerebral tumor and asymptomatic neurosyphilis, than a gumma. The tuberculoma may occur in any part of the brain, but in children it is more likely to develop in the posterior fossa, i.e., in the cerebellum or brainstem, than in the cerebrum. Often there are a small number of cells and an increased protein content in the cerebrospinal fluid because the lesion frequently lies contiguous to the meninges; it may at any time give rise to a tuberculous meningitis with typical cerebrospinal fluid formula (50 to 300 cells, increased amount of protein, decreased sugar content, and decreased chloride content).

In South America tuberculoma, cysticercosis, and echinococcus cysts are much more frequent, and one can usually obtain clues as to their nature from similar disease in other parts of the body, especially the lungs, and characteristic changes in the cerebrospinal fluid (see Chap. 364). Cysticercus cellulosae and hydatid cysts are common lesions and should always be suspected when seizures, increased intracranial pressure, or diffuse cerebral symptoms develop in the adult. X-rays of the skull and skeletal muscles (e.g., thigh) may reveal characteristic calcific deposits in cysticercosis. Torula and other fungous granulomas and *Schistosoma japonicum* infection may also present as space-occupying cerebral lesions.

PATIENTS WITH SIGNS OF INCREASED INTRACRANIAL PRESSURE WHEN FIRST SEEN A certain number of patients show all the characteristic symptoms and signs of increased intracranial pressure when first seen. These signs are periodic bifrontal

and bioccipital headaches which awaken the patient during the night or are present upon awakening, vomiting that may or may not be expected and may or may not be projectile, mental torpor, unsteady gait, sphincteric incontinence, and papilledema. The physician confronted with this clinical problem is forced to take immediate action, for the condition is potentially dangerous. A critical rise in intracranial hypertension may occur at any time and result in coma, respiratory arrest, and death. Admission to a hospital with a neurosurgical service is therefore usually urgent. Nevertheless all the medical aspects of the patient's problem should first be worked out.

Three questions demand immediate answers: (1) Does the patient have a space-occupying intracranial lesion? (2) Where in the cranial cavity is it situated? (3) What is its nature? With respect to the first question it is well to keep in mind that a number of medical conditions may simulate an intracranial growth that causes only the general symptoms of increased intracranial pressure. These are (1) "pseudotumor cerebri," (2) hypertensive encephalopathy, (3) chronic pulmonary disease with hypercapnia and hypoxia, (4) chronic meningitis or adhesive arachnoiditis and/or aqueductal stenosis, (5) thrombosis of cerebral veins and dural sinuses, (6) Addison's disease and hypoparathyroidism, (7) excessive vitamin A and chloramphenicol (Chloromycetin) therapy in children, and (8) withdrawal from corticosteroid therapy in children. Several of these conditions are discussed elsewhere in this book, and it is sufficient to mention them briefly; others have not been considered before and will be discussed in detail.

PSEUDOTUMOR SYNDROMES In the condition of *pseudotumor cerebri* (meningeal hydrops) the patient, more often than not a child or young woman, complains of headaches of some weeks' standing and when first examined is found to have papilledema, or choked disks, with slightly constricted visual fields and enlarged blind spots. Except for a vague dizziness, diplopia due to a slight abducens weakness, or paresthesias of some part of the body, neurologic signs are conspicuously absent, and the patient appears remarkably "bright" and well. The cerebrospinal fluid is under increased pressure and is acellular with normal protein content; a CT scan, or a ventriculogram if CT scan is not available, shows small or normal-sized ventricles. The arteriogram demonstrates patency of venous sinuses and veins. With the use of oral glycerol or corticosteroid drugs (dexamethasone, 6 to 12 mg every 6 h) and daily, then biweekly, then weekly lumbar punctures to lower the cerebrospinal fluid pressure, most of the patients gradually recover over a period of weeks to months. Extremely high cerebrospinal fluid pressure with episodes of cloudy vision (obscurations) may herald the onset of blindness and require a right subtemporal decompression as an emergency measure. The cause of the condition is unknown. Radioactive isotope studies reveal slowed absorption of CSF.

Extreme hypertension (diastolic pressures of 120 mm or over), retinal arteriolar changes with hemorrhages and exudates in the periphery of the optic fundi, signs of renal disease, and headache, convulsions, confusion, stupor, or coma (due to multifocal ischemia and brain swelling) are the basis of the diagnosis of *hypertensive encephalopathy* (see Chap. 365). *Chronic emphysema or other lung diseases,* with cyanosis, dyspnea, cough, signs of cor pulmonale with right-sided congestive heart failure, and secondary polycythemia, may be attended by bilateral papilledema, elevated cerebrospinal fluid pressure (small ventricles), high venous pressure, severe headache, drowsiness, stupor, or coma, and peculiar lapses in the posture of the outstreched limbs and other contracted skeletal muscles (flapping movements, or asterixis, similar to the flap in impending liver coma). The finding of an elevated P_{CO_2} and diminished arterial oxygen concentration substantiates the diagnosis (see Chap. 371). *Chronic meningitis or adhesive arachnoiditis* due to chronic fibrosing meningeal diseases such as syphilis, postspinal anesthesia arachnoiditis, and cryptogenic meningeal diseases may be attended by headache, papilledema, seizures, blindness, paraplegia, or quadriplegia. Other benign causes of adult hydrocephalus are aqueductal stenosis and the Arnold-Chiari malformation. The CSF protein level may be normal or elevated, with or without a "dynamic block"; the lateral, third, and fourth ventricles are enlarged in the ventriculogram. Syphilis and other chronic meningitides may also cause *aqueductal stenosis* owing to a proliferative gliotic ependymitis, with enlargement of the lateral and third ventricles (see Chap. 373). *Thrombosis of the jugular veins and of the lateral and posterior parts of the superior sagittal sinus* may result in increased intracranial pressure, with otherwise normal cerebrospinal fluid and usually small ventricles (see Chap. 368). No explanation can be given for the papilledema with headache, drowsiness, and confusion and elevated cerebrospinal fluid pressure observed in conjunction with *Addison's disease,* corticosteroid withdrawal, vitamin A overdosage, and also, in certain rare cases, hypoparathyroidism. In the latter the ventricles are of normal size.

"TRUE" AND "FALSE" LOCALIZING SIGNS If the clinical findings permit the exclusion of the aforementioned conditions, there is reasonable certainty that the patient has an intracranial growth. The problem then is to search for signs that will localize the lesion. In doing this, several pitfalls must be avoided. One common source of error is to place undue reliance on a sign which proves to have no localizing value whatsoever. One should distrust any symptom or sign which develops late, after headache and increased intracranial pressure have been established, for it often turns out to be a false localizing sign. Under these circumstances drowsiness, slowness in response, inattentiveness, and emotional blunting can be found as often with cerebellar as with cerebral growth. Ataxia of gait, urinary incontinence, and psychomotor retardation may occur as part of a communicating hydrocephalus from any cause. Unilateral or bilateral abducens palsy is another common false localizing sign, and reference has already been made to the drooping eyelid, dilated pupil, ipsilateral hemiparesis and bilateral Babinski signs, and coma in temporal lobe herniation. Jacksonian and generalized seizures and ipsilateral or bilateral pyramidal signs may be observed in the advanced stages of a cerebellar tumor. Early and sometimes relatively slight focal signs that may be easily overlooked are sometimes the most reliable guides to the localization of the tumor. Examples are a mild weakness or stiffness and hyperreflexia of an arm and leg in a frontal tumor; ataxia of gait (but not of limbs) and head tilt in cerebellar tumors; paralysis of upward gaze with the Argyll Robertson pupillary phenomenon in pinealomas; pale optic disks and chiasmal field defects in craniopharyngiomas; and homonymous visual inattentiveness and sensory extinction (see Chaps. 18 and 19) in posterior cerebral tumors.

TUMORS WHICH TEND TO PRODUCE ELEVATED INTRACRANIAL PRESSURE WITHOUT CONSPICUOUS LOCALIZING SIGNS The tumors most likely to do this are medulloblastoma, ependymoma of the fourth ventricle, hemangioblastoma, pinealoma, colloid cysts of the third ventricle, gliomas of tegmentum of the midbrain with blocking of the aqueduct, and craniopharyngioma. In addition, in some of the cerebral gliomas discussed above, particularly those of the corpus callosum

and frontal lobes, increased intracranial pressure may precede focal cerebral signs.

Medulloblastoma This is a rapidly growing tumor which arises in the posterior part of the vermis of children and rarely in the cerebrum of adults. The tonsils of the cerebellum are forced down into the cervical spinal canal (cerebellar pressure cone) in fatal cases. Seedings of the tumor may be seen on the walls of the third and lateral ventricles, on the meningeal surfaces of the brain, and around the spinal cord. The tumor is solid, reddish-gray, and poorly demarcated from the adjacent brain tissue. It is very cellular, and the cells are small, closely packed with little cytoplasm, many mitoses, and scant stroma, and have a tendency to form clusters or pseudorosettes. Bailey and Cushing introduced the name *medulloblastoma* in 1925. Although medulloblasts as such have not been described in the fetal or adult human brain and the cell type is not known for certain, the term is retained if for no other reason than its familiarity.

The clinical picture is distinctive. Typically, the patient becomes listless, vomits repeatedly, and has a morning headache. The first diagnosis which suggests itself may be gastrointestinal disease or abdominal migraine. Soon, however, a stumbling gait, frequent falls, and a squint lead to a neurologic examination and the discovery of papilledema. Ataxia of the limbs may be absent at all times. Decerebrate attacks (tonic cerebellar fits) may occur in the late stages of the disease. The tumor is highly radiosensitive, and surgery with x-ray treatment may prolong life for several years. Recent trials of intrathecal methotrexate and vincristine have yielded promising results in some cases.

Ependymoma and papilloma of the fourth ventricle This tumor also arises from the walls of the fourth ventricle, more often in children, and from the lateral ventricles in adults. It is a soft, whitish-gray, lobulated growth composed of small cells arranged in the form of small rosettes around vessels or central clear areas and containing blepharoplasts in their cytoplasm. The clinical syndrome of the fourth ventricle tumor is much like that of the medulloblastoma except for the absence of ataxia of gait. The tumor is not very sensitive to x-ray, and surgical removal offers the only hope of survival. Prolongation of life is sometimes attained through ventriculoatrial shunting of cerebrospinal fluid. The papilloma or papillary adenocarcinoma of the choroid plexus of the fourth ventricle gives rise to a similar syndrome but tends to occur later in life.

Hemangioblastoma of the cerebellum The disease of Lindau is described in Chap. 374. Dizziness, ataxia of gait or of the limbs on one side, symptoms and signs of increased intracranial pressure, and in some instances a retinal angioma (von Hippel's disease) and polycythemia constitute the neurologic syndrome. Familial incidence is well known. Craniotomy with opening of the cerebellar cyst and excision of the mural hemangioblastomatous nodule may be curative. Some of the retinal lesions can be obliterated by laser beam treatment.

Pinealoma Also called pinealcytoma, this may be a dysgerminoma, an embryonal carcinoma, an atypical teratoma or a glioma of the pineal gland. The dysgerminoma is the most frequent (50 percent) of pineal tumors and most radiosensitive. The pinealcytomas and pinealblastomas and endodermal sinus tumor are radioresistant. Usually the tumor is 3 to 4 cm in its greatest diameter. It compresses the superior colliculi and sometimes the superior surface of the cerebellum, with narrowing of the aqueduct of Sylvius. Often it extends anteriorly into the third ventricle and may then compress the hypothalamus. Microscopically the dysgerminoma is composed of large, spherical epithelial cells (much like those of a seminoma), separated by a network of reticular connective tissue which contains many lymphocytes. The others, i.e., embryonal carcinomas and gliomas, have the usual morphologic characteristic of these tumors. The pinealcytoma and pinealblastomas are poorly differentiated, small-celled tumors. Children, adolescents, and young adults, either male or female, may be affected. In some cases the clinical syndrome consists solely of symptoms and signs of increased intracranial pressure, and the diagnosis can be made only by a CT scan and arteriogram which reveal the tumor. The most characteristic localizing signs, an inability to look upward (Parinaud's syndrome) and slightly dilated pupils which react on accommodation but not to light, are related to the hydrocephalus and not to the local pressure effects of the tumor. Sometimes an ataxia of the limbs, choreic movements, or spastic weakness appears in the later stages of the illness. Stereotaxic biopsy is necessary to differentiate these tumors and to plan rational therapy. A ventriculoatrial shunt and x-ray therapy have been remarkably successful in controlling symptoms of the dysgerminomas. Attempts at surgical removal of the tumor under the operating microscope are beginning to be successful.

Colloid (paraphyseal) cyst of the third ventricle This is a papillomatous structure always situated in the anterior extremity of the third ventricle between the interventricular foramens and attached to the roof of the ventricle. Usually it is about a centimeter or two in diameter, is oval or round with a smooth external surface, and is filled with a glairy colloid material. The wall is composed of a layer of epithelial cells surrounded by a capsule of fibrous connective tissue. These benign cysts may exist for long period of time; they produce neurologic symptoms by blocking the third ventricle and causing an obstructive hydrocephalus. This tumor should be suspected when the following clinical syndromes are found: confusion or dementia with or without headache, intermittent generalized headaches, gait disturbance, vomiting, blurred vision, dizziness, "frontal lobe" type of incontinence, bilateral paresthesias, and weakness of legs with sudden falls. The larger colloid cysts can be seen in a CT scan, for the colloid has higher absorptive values than CSF and brain tissue. The treatment is surgical excision, but recently, satisfactory results have been obtained by ventriculoatrial shunt of the cerebrospinal fluid, leaving the benign growth untouched (see Little and McCarthy). Stereotaxic aspiration of the cyst has been accomplished successfully in a small number of cases.

Craniopharyngioma (suprasellar or Rathke's pouch cyst, hypophyseal duct tumors, adamantinomas, ameloblastomas) This is a benign congenital or "rest cell," tumor. By the time it has grown to a diameter of 3 to 4 cm, it is almost always cystic. Usually it lies above the sella turcica, depressing the optic chiasm and extending up into the third ventricle. Less often it is subdiaphragmatic, i.e., within the sella, where it compresses the pituitary body, erodes one part of the wall of the sella or a clinoid process, but seldom balloons the sella like a pituitary adenoma. The tumor is oval, round, or lobulated and has a smooth surface. The wall of the cyst and the solid parts of the tumor consist of cords and whorls of epithelial cells (often with intercellular bridges and keratohyalin), separated by a loose network of stellate cells. The cyst contains dark albuminous fluid and cholesterol crystals. Calcium deposits are found in nearly all of them and can be seen in plain x-rays of the suprasellar region in about 40 percent of cases. The sella beneath the tumor tends to be flattened and enlarged. In children, adiposity, delayed or infantile physical and sexual development (Froehlich's or Lorain syndrome—see Chaps. 333 and 374), headaches, vomiting, dim vision with chiasmal field defects (see Chap. 18), optic atrophy, or papilledema comprise the clinical picture. In adults, waning libido, amenorrhea, slight

spastic weakness of the legs, headache without papilledema, and mental dullness and confusion are often found. Later drowsiness, diabetes insipidus, and disturbances of temperature regulation may occur, indicating hypothalamic involvement.

In the differential diagnosis of these several tumor syndromes a careful clinical analysis is often more important than laboratory procedures. Arteriography and electroencephalography are not as helpful as in cerebral tumors. CT scans reveal calcium deposits when these are not seen in plain x-rays, and hydrocephalus and obstruction of the third ventricle are also disclosed. Other tests which, though somewhat hazardous, are likely to give the most useful information are the air ventriculogram or a combined ventriculogram-pneumoencephalogram and the Pantopaque ventriculogram (injection of radiopaque fluid). Modern neurosurgical techniques reinforced by corticosteroid therapy before and after surgery and careful control of temperature and water balance postoperatively permit complete excision of the tumor in the majority of cases. Large inoperable lesions have been aspirated, and radiotherapy has been beneficial in some of them.

In certain marginal states of hydrocephalus temporary benefit may accrue from the use of acetazolamide (Diamox) in doses of 250 mg three or four times a day, but surgical shunting of cerebrospinal fluid has given the best results.

PATIENTS WITH SYMPTOMS AND SIGNS OF A SLOWLY PROGRESSIVE LESION IN A PARTICULAR REGION OF THE CRANIAL CAVITY In this group of conditions general cerebral symptoms and the signs of increased intracranial pressure occur late or not at all. The physician arrives at the correct diagnosis by being able to make an anatomic or regional diagnosis from a set of neurologic findings and by reasoning that the cause must be neoplastic because of the slowly progressive nature of the illness. Special x-rays of the skull, cerebrospinal fluid examination, and, depending on the location of the disease, CT scan and either pneumoencephalography or arteriography will usually confirm the clinical impression.

The following tumors produce unique syndromes usually diagnostic of a special type of tumor.

Acoustic neurofibroma or neurinoma This slowly growing benign tumor may occur as a solitary lesion or as a part of the syndrome of neurofibromatosis. By the time of operation the tumor has usually attained a size of 4 to 6 cm in diameter. It arises from the extramedullary part of the eighth cranial nerve, usually within the internal auditory meatus, where the intracranial part of the nerve first acquires the histologic character of a peripheral nerve, i.e., has Schwann cells and fibroblasts. The space in which it lies is the cerebellopontine angle, i.e., between the cerebellum, pons, and medulla posteriorly, the petrous pyramid anteriorly, and the tentorium above. The internal auditory meatus is usually enlarged (visible in x-rays), the middle cerebellar peduncle and the anterolateral part of the cerebellum are depressed, and the trigeminal, facial, glossopharyngeal, and vagus nerves are displaced and stretched over the surface of the growth. The fourth ventricle is deformed, displaced, and narrowed (visible in a CT scan or pneumoencephalogram), and there is hydrocephalic enlargement of the aqueduct and of the third and lateral ventricles in the late stages. The tumor is vascular, and the surrounding cerebrospinal fluid has a high protein content (cerebrospinal fluid protein of 300 mg per 100 ml or over is not infrequent). The microscopic picture is that of a typical neurofibroma (axis cylinders mixed with masses of fibrous connective tissue in interlacing strands, palisaded nuclei, and mononuclear giant cells with mitoses).

The typical clinical syndrome, which usually occurs in adult men or women, consists of tinnitus, deafness, and rotational vertigo (seldom in discrete attacks as in Ménière's syndrome, Chap. 376) of several years' standing, followed by post-auricular or suboccipital pain, disturbance in balance, spasms and twitching or slight weakness of the face, paresthesias in the face or facial weakness, dysphonia and dysphagia, and homolateral cerebellar ataxia of the arm and leg. Headache, vomiting, and papilledema (choked disk) are late findings. Variations of this syndrome are numerous. Early in its development only progressive deafness, tinnitus, and vague vertigo may be present, and the abnormal audiogram, impaired vestibular function, elevated cerebrospinal fluid protein level, widened internal auditory meatus, and obliteration of the lateral recess of the fourth ventricle in a Pantopaque encephalogram or pneumoencephalogram must be depended upon for diagnosis. Tomography and positive contrast encephalography improve diagnostic accuracy. Dementia may later be the presenting syndrome, and the deaf ear may be incorrectly attributed to some other disease. Unilateral cerebellar ataxia and dizziness may predominate, and definite signs of involvement of the fifth, seventh, and eighth cranial nerves may not be found. The only treatment is surgical excision. Combined translabyrinthine and intracranial approach permits total removal in more than two-thirds of all cases.

The *neurinoma* of the *trigeminal* or *gasserian ganglion* and *meningioma* of the *cerebellopontine angle* may be indistinguishable from an acoustic neurinoma. They should always be considered if the tinnitus, deafness, and the unresponsive labyrinth ("dead labyrinth") are not the initial symptoms of the cerebellopontine angle syndrome. A true *cholesteatoma* of *the temporal bone* may simulate this clinical picture, but usually the facial weakness is early and severe, the ear is deaf, and labyrinthine function is absent, whereas the other cranial nerve signs, cerebellar ataxia, and increased intracranial pressure are absent. The *tumor* of *the glomus jugulare* (a flat ovoid body, found in the adventitia of the jugular bulb, immediately below the floor of the middle ear and near the ramus tympanicus of the ninth cranial nerve) may, like the acoustic neurofibroma, basal meningioma, metastatic cancer, syphilitic meningitis, neurofibroma of other cranial nerves, and vascular malformation, cause unilateral lower cranial nerve palsies (see Chap. 376). It is a purplish red highly vascular tumor composed of large epithelioid cells in an alveolar pattern and an abundant capillary network. Partial deafness, facial palsy, dysphagia, and unilateral atrophy of the tongue, combined with a vascular polyp in the auditory meatus and a palpable mass below and anterior to the mastoid eminence, often with a bruit, compose the syndrome. The jugular foramen is eroded (visible by x-ray), and the level of cerebrospinal fluid protein may be elevated. Arteriography is of value in diagnosis. Women are affected more than men, and the peak incidence is during middle adult life. The tumor grows slowly over a period of many years, sometimes 10 or more. The treatment is x-ray radiation. Surgical excision has usually been unsuccessful.

Pituitary adenomas These tumors, which are so common, particularly in late adult life, often are discovered when a patient begins to complain of a visual disturbance. A partial or complete bitemporal hemianopsia progressing to blindness, with optic atrophy, is the usual finding, and with x-ray evidence of an expanded sella turcica and endocrine disorder, leads to a diagnosis of pituitary adenoma. Occasionally, if the growth is eccentric, one optic nerve may be compressed with a resulting monocular scotoma. As the growth enlarges and extends laterally, an oculomotor palsy is occasionally seen, and large suprasellar extensions may involve the hypothalamus or temporal lobe. If there are signs of acromegaly, one may assume that an eosinophilic adenoma is present; if not, and signs of pituitary insufficiency are present (amenorrhea without "hot flashes," sexual impotence, etc.—see Chap. 333), the tumor is usually a chromophobe adenoma. Basophilic adenomas, one of the causes of Cushing's syndrome, rarely produce enlargement of the sella or visual symptoms. The diagnosis is made from the endocrine picture (see Chap. 333). The cerebrospinal fluid is usually under normal pressure, and protein level is elevated only in exceptional cases. The syndrome of pituitary apoplexy (acute onset of headache, confusion, stupor or coma, blindness, and bilateral ophthalmoplegia) has usually occurred in individuals with a known or occult chromophobic or eosinophilic adenoma of the pituitary gland. The CSF is usually abnormal, i.e., bloody and/or containing increased white blood cells and protein.

Other conditions may rarely expand the sella (craniopharyngioma, carotid aneurysm, cysts of pituitary, and the "hollow" or "empty sella" syndrome), and there are also rather wide normal variations in its size. The empty or hollow sella results from a defect in the dural diaphragm of the sella and nontumorous enlargement. Raised intracranial pressure may occasionally cause the floor of the third ventricle to protrude into the sella. However, in the usual empty sella syndrome, the CSF pressure is normal. Downward herniation of the optic chiasma may cause visual disturbances simulating a pituitary adenoma. This syndrome may also follow surgical excision of a pituitary adenoma or pituitary apoplexy. Most of our patients have been obese women with no endocrine abnormality or at most a slightly reduced release of growth hormone. Hence the diagnosis of pituitary adenoma should not be made because of minor enlargements of the sella in the absence of endocrine and neighborhood neurologic signs. The CT scan and a pneumoencephalogram permit visualization of the suprasellar extension of the tumor or an empty sella. Treatment of the adenoma is by proton beam radiation (or gamma radiation if proton treatment is not available); if vision is threatened despite x-ray therapy or ablation by the proton beam, either transnasal or transfrontal surgical excision is indicated. Replacement endocrine therapy is also needed.

Meningioma of the sphenoid ridge This tumor is situated over the lesser wing of the sphenoid bone. As it increases in size, it may expand medially to encroach on structures in the wall of the cavernous sinus, anteriorly to invade the orbit, or laterally to erode or invade the temporal bone. Most prominent among the symptoms are a slowly developing unilateral exophthalmos, slight bulging of the bone in the temporal region, and roentgenologic evidence of thickening or erosion of the lesser wing of the sphenoid bone. Variants of the clinical syndrome include oculomotor palsy or syndrome of Foix (see Chap. 376), blindness in one eye with optic atrophy but no bony changes (see Susac et al.), anosmia (and sometimes the Kennedy syndrome—see below), mental changes, uncinate fits, and increased intracranial pressure. Sarcomas arising from the skull bones, metastatic carcinoma, orbitoethmoid osteoma, tumors of the optic nerve, and angiomas of the orbit must be considered in the differential diagnosis. Auscultation of the skull, x-ray of the skull, and carotid arteriography are helpful in differentiating these lesions.

Meningioma of the olfactory groove This tumor is a growth derived from arachnoid cells along the cribriform plate. The diagnosis depends on the finding of ipsilateral or bilateral anosmia, ipsilateral or bilateral blindness, often with optic atrophy on one side and papilledema without atrophy on the other (Kennedy syndrome), and mental changes. The tumors may reach enormous size before coming to the attention of the physician. The anosmia, if unilateral, is rarely if ever reported by the patient. The unilateral visual disturbance may consist of a slowly developing unilateral central scotoma. Confusion, forgetfulness, inappropriate jocularity (witzelsucht) are the usual psychic disturbances (see Chap. 376). These patients are indifferent to or joke about their blindness. Usually there are x-ray changes along the cribriform plate and an extremely high cerebrospinal fluid protein level (200 to 400 per 100 ml).

Glioma of the brainstem Astrocytomas of the brainstem (formerly called "bipolar spongioblastomas") are slow growing, firm, white infiltrating growths which insinuate themselves between tracts and nuclei. They produce a variable clinical picture, depending on their exact location in the medulla, pons, and midbrain (see Chaps. 17 and 18 for syndromes). The characteristic features, in the early stages, are signs of crossed motor or sensory disturbances, which always indicate brainstem disease. Headache, vomiting, and papilledema occur late. The course is slowly progressive over years unless some part of the tumor becomes more malignant (glioblastoma multiforme), in which instance the illness may terminate fatally within months. The main clinical problem is to differentiate among this disease, multiple sclerosis, and vascular malformations of the pons. CT scan and pneumoencephalography to visualize the fourth ventricle and aqueduct and occasionally vertebral arteriography are helpful in diagnosis. The treatment is x-ray irradiation and, if intracranial pressure is increased, a Torkildsen ventricle–cisterna magna shunt.

Glioma of the optic nerves and chiasma This tumor is often found in patients with von Recklinghausen's disease and, like the glioma of the brainstem, arises most frequently during the period of childhood and adolescence. The initial symptoms are dimness of vision with constricted fields, bizarre bilateral field defects of homonymous, heteronymous, and sometimes bitemporal type, blindness, and optic atrophy with or without papilledema. Hypothalamic signs (infantilism, adiposity, polyuria, somnolence, and genital atrophy) are common. When progressive blindness of one eye is the only symptom the tumor must be differentiated from a meningioma of the perioptic sheath. X-rays reveal an enlargement of the optic foramen. With this finding and the lack of ballooning of the sella or suprasellar calcification, pituitary adenoma, Hand-Schüller-Christian disease, and craniopharyngioma can be excluded. The treatment is surgical excision or x-ray, depending on the exact location. Nontumorous gliotic lesions of optic nerves may occur in von Recklinghausen's disease and may be difficult to distinguish from tumors.

Chordoma This is a soft, jelly-like gray-pink growth composed of cords or masses of large cells with granules of glycogen in their cytoplasm and often multiple nuclei and intercellular mucoid material. They are locally invasive but do not metastasize. Any part of the vertebral column or the base of the cranium are the most common sites, especially the base of the skull (from physaliphorous ecchondrosis) or the lumbosacral region (giving rise to a cauda equina syndrome). Those in the base of the skull create a remarkable clinical picture in which all or any combination of cranial nerve palsies from the second to twelfth on one side or both sides are combined with a retropharyngeal mass and erosion of the clivus of sphenoid bone and the occiput. It is one of the lesions that may present both as an intracranial and as an extracranial mass. The others

are the meningioma, neurofibroma, glomus jugulare tumor, carcinoma of sinuses or pharynx, and midline granuloma. The treatment is x-ray therapy.

Nasopharyngeal growths which erode the base of the skull These are rather common in a general hospital and arise from the mucous membrane of the paranasal sinuses or the nasopharynx near the eustachian tube, i.e., the fossa of Rosenmueller (*transitional cell carcinoma, Schmincke tumor*). In addition to symptoms of nasopharyngeal or sinus disease, which may not be prominent, facial pain and numbness (trigeminal), abducens palsy (sixth cranial nerve), and other cranial nerve palsies may occur. Diagnosis depends on inspection and biopsy of a nasopharyngeal mass, biopsy of an involved cervical gland, and x-ray evidence of erosion of the base of the skull. The treatment is x-ray therapy. Carcinoma of ethmoid or sphenoid sinuses may produce a similar clinical picture.

PROGNOSIS The prognosis of intracranial tumor is influenced by the nature of the growth, its location, and other factors. As a general rule, unless an operation is performed, almost all intracranial tumors end fatally. Death in most instances is preceded by a critical rise in intracranial pressure and tentorial or foramen magnum herniation. The more malignant tumors, such as the glioblastoma multiforme, medulloblastoma, and metastatic carcinoma, end fatally within a few months to a year, as a rule, whereas the slowly growing meningiomas and astrocytomas often permit survival for many years.

The prospects for recovery after surgery depend largely on the type of tumor. With meningiomas, pinealomas, craniopharyngiomas, and acoustic neurofibromas, if completely excised, there is complete cure. In gliomas the outlook is more bleak. The period of postoperative survival for glioblastoma is only 6 to 12 months; only 20 percent live for a year and 10 percent for 2 years. This dismal statistic has been slightly if at all lengthened (Walker and Gehane) by x-ray and chemotherapy (BCNU). Cure is rare, for seldom can complete excision be accomplished. Nevertheless with the slow-growing gliomas, partial excision, the marsupialization of a cyst, irradiation, and chemotherapy, and the relief of increased intracranial pressure by long-term corticosteroid therapy may lead to improvement and resumption of a useful life for many years. With metastatic growth the outlook is dismal, though if there are no metastases in other organs and the cerebral deposit appears to be solitary, as determined by clinical examination and CT scan, operation occasionally results in temporary recovery for a few months or a year or two.

CONCLUSIONS The physician's responsibilities in this field of intracranial tumors are as follows:

1 Diagnosis. It is essential that the physician separate the tumor cases from all the others which pass through his or her hands.
2 Exclusion of the possibility that the intracranial mass is part of a general disease which would contraindicate surgery, e.g., metastatic carcinoma, syphilis, tuberculosis, parasitic infection.
3 Exclusion of the several pseudotumor syndromes.
4 Maintenance of the patient in the best possible condition until surgery can be undertaken (fluids, electrolytes, corticosteroid therapy, etc.).

5 Assisting the surgeon in the postoperative medical management.

(For tumors of spinal cord and nerves, see Chaps. 375 to 377.)

REFERENCES

BAILEY P: *Intracranial Tumors*, 2d ed. Springfield, Charles C Thomas, 1948

LITTLE JR, MCCARTHY CS: Colloid cysts of the third ventricle. J Neurosurg 40:230, 1974

LUMSDEN CE: Study of tumors by tissue culture, in *Pathology of Tumors of the Nervous System*, 3d ed, DS Russell, LJ Rubenstein (eds). Baltimore, Williams & Wilkins, 1971

MILHORAT TH: *Hydrocephalus and the Cerebrospinal Fluid*. Baltimore, Williams & Wilkins, 1972

OJEMANN RG, MONTGOMERY WW: Evaluation and surgical treatment of acoustic neuroma. N Engl J Med 287:895, 1972

POSNER J, SHAPIRO WR: Brain tumor. Arch Neurol 32:781, 1978

SUSAC J et al: The impossible meningioma. Arch Neurol 34:36, 1977

WALKER MW, GEHANE A: An evaluation of BCNU and irradiation alone and in combination for the treatment of malignant glioma. Proc Am Assoc Cancer Res 13:67, 1972

368
PYOGENIC INFECTIONS OF THE CENTRAL NERVOUS SYSTEM

RAYMOND D. ADAMS
ROBERT G. PETERSDORF

Pyogenic infections of the cranial contents originate in one of two ways, by hematogenous spread or by extension from surface structures—the ears—paranasal sinuses, osteomyelitic foci in the skull, penetrating cranial injuries, congenital sinus tracts, or following neurosurgical procedures.

Surprisingly little is known concerning the hematogenous pathway because human autopsy material seldom divulges information on this point and animal experiments involving the injection of virulent bacteria into the bloodstream have yielded somewhat contradictory results. In most instances of bacteremia the nervous system seems not to be infected, yet in certain cases of pneumonia, bacteremia is the only apparent forerunner of meningitis. In chronic suppurative pulmonary disease septic venous thrombi become sources of emboli to the brain, and in acute and subacute bacterial endocarditis bacterial emboli are found in cerebral and meningeal arteries.

Experimentally, cerebral tissues are resistant to abscess formation. Direct injection of virulent bacteria into the brain of an animal seldom results in abscess formation. In fact, experimental brain abscess has been produced only by injecting the infected culture medium or by first causing necrosis of the tissue and then inoculating it with bacteria. In human beings infarction of brain tissue by arterial occlusion (embolism) or venous occlusion (thrombophlebitis) appears to be the common and perhaps necessary antecedent.

The cranial epidural and subdural spaces evidently are noticeably inaccessible to bloodborne infection in contrast to the spinal epidural space, where infection is frequently hematogenous. Furthermore, the cranial bones and the dura mater, which serves as the inner periosteum of the skull, protect the cranial cavity against the ingress of bacteria. This protective mechanism may fail if suppuration occurs in the middle ear,

mastoid cells or frontal ethmoid, and sphenoid sinuses. Two pathways have been demonstrated in postmortem material:

1 Infected thrombi may form in diploic veins and spread along these vessels into the dural sinuses (into which they flow) and from there in retrograde fashion along the meningeal veins in the brain.
2 An osteomyelitic focus may form, with erosion of the inner table of bone and invasion of the dura, subdural space, piarachnoid, and even the brain substance. Each of these pathways may be visualized in some fatal cases of epidural abscess, subdural empyema, leptomeningitis, cranial venous sinusitis, meningeal thrombophlebitis, and brain abscess. However, in many cases coming to autopsy the pathway cannot be determined.

Hematogenous infections following bacteremia usually permit a single type of virulent organism to gain entry to the cranial cavity (meningococcus, pneumococcus, *Hemophilus influenzae*, or more rarely staphylococcus or gram-negative bacillus). In contrast, septic cerebral emboli from lung abscess or bronchiectasis in congenital heart disease and thrombotic or direct extensions from ear or sinus infections may be caused by multiple organisms consisting of anaerobic streptococci, *Bacteroides*, and other anaerobes. These "mixed infections" present more complex problems in therapy. If the causative organism is an anaerobe, culture even from the pus of an abscess may be unsuccessful, although the organism can often be demonstrated by Gram's stain. Even in so-called "neighborhood infections," however, the bloodstream may be the pathway by which bacteria gain access to the meninges. It has been shown in experimental meningeal infections in mice, for example, that following intranasal infection, bacteria circulate through the blood to reach the meninges via the leptomeningeal vessels.

BACTERIAL MENINGITIS (LEPTOMENINGITIS)

Bacterial meningitis may be defined as an inflammation of the piarachnoid and the fluid residing in the space which it encloses and also that in the ventricles of the brain. Since the subarachnoid space is continuous around the brain, spinal cord, and the optic nerves, an infective agent (or tumor cells or blood) gaining entry to any one part of it may extend immediately to all of it, even its most remote recesses; therefore, meningitis is always *cerebrospinal*. It also reaches the ventricles, either directly or by reflux through the basal foramens of Magendie and Luschka.

The effect of bacteria or other organisms in the subarachnoid space is to cause an inflammatory reaction in the pia and arachnoid and in the cerebrospinal fluid (CSF); in pyogenic meningitis, pus accumulates in this space. The infective agent or its toxin, if allowed sufficient time to act, injures those structures which lie within the subarachnoid space (cranial and spinal roots) or ventricles (choroid plexuses) and adjacent to it (pial arteries and veins, underlying cerebral and cerebellar cortices, subpial white matter of the spinal cord, peripheral fibers of optic nerves, ependymal and subependymal tissues). In addition, purulent material may interfere with the flow of CSF from the ventricles or along the subarachnoid space over the brainstem, with resulting obstructive or communicating hydrocephalus, respectively. Although the outer arachnoidal membrane proves to be a remarkably effective barrier to the extension of infection, some reaction in the cranial subdural space and even the inner surface of the dura and spinal epidural space may occur. This happens more often in infants (subdural effusions) than in adults.

The most immediate clinical effects of acute subarachnoid suppuration, distinguishing it from infections in other parts of the body, are severe headache, drowsiness, stupor, or coma, and, occasionally, convulsions. The one clinical sign of importance is stiffness of the neck (resistance to passive movement) on forward bending. The Kernig and Brudzinski's signs are of the same nature but less reliable. Any circumstance which prolongs the meningitis should increase the risk of injury to all the enumerated structures; this accounts for many features of the clinical picture in the subacute and chronic varieties of meningeal infection.

TYPES OF BACTERIAL MENINGITIS Eighty to ninety percent of cases of bacterial meningitis are caused by *Hemophilus influenzae* (Chap. 125), *Neisseria* meningitis (Chap. 118), or *Streptococcus pneumoniae* (Chap. 115). The remaining 15 to 20 percent are caused by *Staphylococcus aureus* and *Staphylococcus epidermidis*, the latter of which accounts for 75 percent of infections associated with shunting procedures for hydrocephalus; streptococci including enterococci; anaerobic or microaerophilic streptococci, usually in association with brain abscess, epidural abscess, head trauma, neurosurgical procedures, or cranial thrombophlebitis; *Escherichia coli* (in newborns) and other Enterobacteriaceae such as *Klebsiella enterobacter, Proteus,* and *Citrobacter;* and *Pseudomonas,* usually as a consequence of lumbar puncture, spinal anesthesia, or shunting procedures to relieve hydrocephalus. Rare meningeal pathogens include *Salmonella, Shigella, Clostridium perfringens,* and *N. gonorrhea.* Two unusual ones are *Listeria monocytogenes,* which is easily confused with diphtheroids, and *Mima-Herellea,* which may be difficult to distinguish from *Hemophilus* and *Neisseria.*

EPIDEMIOLOGY Pneumococcal, *H. influenzae,* and meningococcal meningitis have a worldwide distribution tending to occur more often in males and during the fall, winter, and spring. *Hemophilus influenzae* meningitis is encountered almost exclusively in children between 2 months and 6 years of age. Meningococcal meningitis occurs most often in children and adolescents, but is also encountered throughout much of adult life with a sharp decline in incidence after the age of 50. Pneumococcal meningitis predominates in the very young and in adults over 40 years of age.

PATHOGENESIS The three common meningeal pathogens are invasive and depend upon antiphagocytic capsular or surface antigens for survival in the tissues of the infected host; all express their pathogenicity largely in the form of extracellular proliferation. All three are inhabitants of the nasopharynx in a significant part of the population. It is evident from the frequency with which the carrier state is detected that nasal colonization is not a sufficient explanation for infection of the meninges. The factors which predispose the colonized patient to bloodstream invasion, which is the usual route by which bacteria reach the meninges, are obscure but include antecedent viral infections of the upper respiratory passages or, as in the case of the pneumococcus, infections in the lung. Once bloodborne, the factors which lead to meningeal localization of bacteria are unknown, but it has been postulated that pneumococci, *H. influenzae,* and meningococci possess a unique predilection for the meninges. Other possibilities are that the entry of bacteria into the subarachnoid space is facilitated by disruption of the blood-CSF barrier by trauma, circulating endotoxin, or an initial viral infection of the meninges.

Avenues other than the bloodstream by which bacteria can gain access to the meninges include congenital neuroectodermal defects, craniotomy sites, diseases of the middle ear and paranasal sinuses, and cranial trauma, notably skull fractures. Occasionally brain abscesses may rupture into the subarachnoid space or ventricles, infecting the meninges. The isolation of anaerobic streptococci, *Bacteroides* spp., or *Actinomyces,* or

a mixture of microorganisms in the CSF should suggest the possibility of a brain abscess occurring as an antecedent to meningitis.

In most patients the precise route by which bacteria infect the meninges cannot be determined.

SYMPTOMATOLOGY Fever, headache, seizures, impairment of consciousness, and stiff neck and back, which compose the meningitic syndrome, are common to bacterial meningitis irrespective of its etiology. When the initial symptoms are pain in the neck or abdomen, a confusional state or delirium, the diagnosis is much more difficult.

There are certain special clinical features that correlate with particular types of meningitis. Meningococcal meningitis should always be suspected in epidemics of meningitis, when the evolution is extremely rapid, when the onset is attended by a morbilliform, petechial, or purpuric skin eruption, larger ecchymoses and lividity of skin of lower parts of the body, and if circulatory collapse has occurred. Since a rash accompanies approximately 50 percent of meningococcal infections, its presence should dictate immediate institution of therapy for a neisserial infection, even though similar rashes may be observed with echo 9 meningitis, *Mima-Herellea,* and rarely staphylococcal, *H. influenzae,* and streptococcal meningitis. Pneumococcal meningitis is usually preceded by an infection in the lungs, ears, and sinuses, and the heart valves may be affected. In addition a pneumococcal etiology should be suspected in patients suffering from alcoholism, sickle-cell disease, and basal skull fracture, and following splenectomy. *Hemophilus influenzae* meningitis usually follows upper respiratory and ear infections in young children.

Other specific bacterial etiologies are suggested by certain unusual clinical settings. Furunculosis or the occurrence of a recent neurosurgical procedure should raise the possibility of coagulase-positive staphylococcal meningitis. Ventriculoatrial or ventriculoperitoneal shunts inserted for control of hydrocephalus are particularly prone to infection with coagulase-negative staphylococci. Brain abscess, myelo- or lymphoproliferative disorders, defects in cranial bones (tumor, osteomyelitis), connective tissue diseases, metastatic cancer, and therapy with immunosuppressive agents are clinical conditions which favor the invasion of the craniospinal cavities by such pathogens as Enterobacteriaceae, *Listeria, Mima-Herellea,* and *Pseudomonas.*

The signs of meningeal irritation—stiff neck or positive Kernig and Brudzinski's signs—may be absent in the very young, the very old, or the severely obtunded. Signs of focal cerebral disease, although seldom prominent, are more frequent in pneumococcal and influenzal meningitis and are associated with a comparatively poor prognosis. Seizures are encountered most often in infants with *H. influenzae* meningitis, but it is difficult to ascertain their significance since persons of this age may convulse with fevers of any cause. Some of the more transitory focal cerebral signs may represent postictal phenomena (Todd's paralysis), whereas stable, local, cerebral lesions are consequent to vasculitis and occlusion of cerebral veins with infarction of cerebral tissue, or they may connote localization of pus as occurs in brain abscess or subdural empyema. Cranial nerve abnormalities are particularly frequent with pneumococcal meningitis.

LABORATORY FINDINGS Pleocytosis of the *cerebrospinal fluid* is diagnostic. The number of leukocytes in the CSF ranges between 1000 and 100,000 per milliliter but averages 5000 to 20,000. Cell counts above 50,000 per milliliter raise suspicion of the possibility of a brain abscess having ruptured into the ventricle (ventricular empyema). Neutrophilic leukocytes generally predominate, but an increasing proportion of mononuclear cells are found in the exudate as the infection continues, especially in partially treated meningitis. In the early stages careful cytological examination may reveal some of the mononuclear cells to be myelocytes or young neutrophils. Later as treatment takes effect, the proportions of lymphocytes, plasma cells, and histiocytes steadily increase.

The pressure of the *cerebrospinal fluid* is so consistently elevated (above 180 mm water) that a normal or low pressure on the initial lumbar puncture in a case of suspected bacterial meningitis should raise the possibility that the needle was partially occluded or that the spinal arachnoid space was blocked.

The *protein levels* of CSF are higher than 45 mg per 100 ml in 90 percent of cases, and most determinations fall in the range of 100 to 500 mg per 100 ml.

The sugar concentration of CSF is depressed, usually to a level lower than 40 mg per 100 ml, or less than 40 percent of the blood sugar concentration (measured concomitantly), provided the latter is less than 250 mg per 100 ml. However in atypical or "culture-negative cases," other conditions associated with a depressed CSF glucose should be considered. These include hypoglycemia from any cause, sarcoidosis of the central nervous system, meningeal carcinomatosis or gliomatosis, fungal or tuberculous meningitis, and subarachnoid hemorrhage. In acute cases of pyogenic meningitis, the CSF glucose concentration often approaches zero.

Gram's stain of sedimented CSF permits identification of the causative agent in most cases of bacterial meningitis; pneumococci and *H. influenzae* are identified more readily than meningococci. Small numbers of gram-negative diplococci present within leukocytes may be indistinguishable from nuclear material which may also be gram-negative and of the same shape. In such cases a thin film of uncentrifuged CSF may lend itself more readily to morphological interpretation than a smear of sedimented CSF. The commonest error in reading gram-stained smears of CSF is misinterpretation of precipitated dye or debris as gram-positive cocci, or a confusion of pneumococci with *H. influenzae*. *Hemophilus* organisms may stain heavily at the poles so that they resemble gram-positive diplococci, and older pneumococci often lose their capacity to take a gram-positive stain.

Cerebrospinal fluid cultures are positive in 70 to 80 percent of cases. When brain abscess is suspected, anaerobic cultures should be made, and meningococci should be cultured under 10% CO_2 (Chap. 106). Partially treated meningitis poses a most difficult problem in diagnosis because cultures are often negative. The measurement of bacterial antigen in the CSF by countercurrent immune electrophoresis (CIE) to determine the concentration of bacterial antigen has been helpful in determining the etiology of the infection, although the concentration of bacterial antigen diminishes as treatment progresses. In *H. influenzae* meningitis, the limulus test for detection of endotoxin of gram-negative bacteria has been more effective than Gram's stain and quicker than culture to detect the pathogen. It is positive within an hour in 95 percent of cases with *H. influenzae* infection.

In addition to CSF cultures, *blood cultures* should always be obtained because they are positive in 40 to 60 percent of patients with *H. influenzae* and with meningococcal and pneumococcal meningitis and may provide the only definitive clue to the causative agent (if CSF cultures are negative). Routine cultures of the pharynx or external ear are as often misleading as helpful because pneumococci, *H. influenzae*, and meningococci are such common inhabitants of these locations. However, culture of pus from the middle ear or sinuses is often helpful.

Measurements of lactic dehydrogenase (LDH) isoenzymes appear to yield data of prognostic and diagnostic value in bacterial meningitis. A rise in total LDH activity is consistently observed in patients with bacterial meningitis; most of this is due to fractions 4 and 5 which are derived from granulocytes. Lactic dehydrogenase fractions 1 and 2, which are presumed to come from brain tissue, are only slightly elevated in bacterial meningitis but rise sharply in patients who are dying or who develop neurological sequelae. Hence, the test may be helpful in singling out the patient who is most at risk. CSF concentrations of lactic acid and lysozyme are also elevated in bacterial meningitis and may reach their highest levels in acute rather than chronic inflammation of the meninges.

The *leukocyte count* in the blood is generally elevated, and usually there is a shift to the left. Most patients with meningitis are sufficiently ill to require determination of blood urea nitrogen and serum electrolytes. These may be abnormal because of severe dehydration. Inappropriate secretion of antidiuretic hormone (ADH) with resultant hyponatremia may also occur.

ROENTGENOGRAPHIC STUDIES Patients with bacterial meningitis should have x-rays of the chest, skull, and sinuses as soon as possible after admission. Chest x-rays are particularly important because they may reveal a silent area of pneumonitis or abscess. Sinus and skull films may provide clues to the presence of cranial osteomyelitis, paranasal sinusitis, or mastoiditis. Computerized tomography (CT scan) is rarely necessary in bacterial meningitis although it may be helpful in detecting hydrocephalus and in ruling out brain abscesses or other intracranial collections of pus.

PROGNOSIS The mortality rate of *H. influenzae* or meningococcal meningitis has remained fixed at 5 to 15 percent for many years. Also in meningococcal infection, because of the fulminating nature of the disease and the often complicating adrenocortical necrosis (Waterhouse-Friderichsen syndrome), the mortality rate remains significant. Old age, infancy, abrupt onset, bacteremia, coma, seizures, and a variety of concomitant diseases including alcoholism, diabetes mellitus, multiple myeloma, and head trauma all worsen the prognosis. The triad of pneumococcal meningitis, pneumonia, and endocarditis has a particularly high fatality rate.

It is often impossible to explain the death of the patient or at least to trace it to a single specific mechanism. Bacteremia with hypotension or brain swelling and temporal or uncal and cerebellar herniation are clearly implicated in the deaths of some patients during the initial 48 h. These events may occur in bacterial meningitis of any etiology; however, some observations suggest that they are more important in meningococcal infection. There is experimental evidence that acute centrally mediated respiratory failure (rather than circulatory collapse) is the major mechanism of early death. Deaths occurring later during the course of illness may be attributed to cerebral necrosis and respiratory failure, often consequent to aspiration pneumonia.

Residual defects are encountered in relatively few cases of meningococcal meningitis, whereas a significant number of children with *H. influenzae* meningitis and up to 30 percent of patients with pneumococcal meningitis develop permanent residua including dementia, epilepsy, deafness, hemiplegia, and hydrocephalus.

DIFFERENTIAL DIAGNOSIS The diagnosis of bacterial meningitis is not difficult, providing a high index of suspicion is maintained. All febrile patients with lethargy, headache, or confusion of sudden onset, even if only low-grade fever is present, should be subjected to lumbar puncture. It is particularly important to consider meningitis in febrile, confused alcoholic patients. Too often the symptoms are mistakenly ascribed to inebriation, delirium tremens, or hepatic encephalopathy until the CSF reveals a meningitis.

Bacterial meningitis can be diagnosed definitively only by examination of the CSF. Viral meningoencephalitis and tuberculous, leptospiral, and fungal meningitides often enter into the differential diagnosis. Also to be considered are Behçet's syndrome, a disease characterized by recurrent oral and genital ulcers along with meningitis, and Mollaret's meningitis, which consists of recurrent episodes of fever, headache, and meningeal irritation accompanied by a leukocytosis in the CSF.

The diagnosis of other intracranial suppurative diseases is detailed below.

ANTIBIOTIC TREATMENT Bacterial meningitis is a medical emergency; the rapid destruction of bacteria in the meninges and in the CSF is essential to survival. For this reason, bactericidal drugs should be used where possible. The following therapeutic regimens are recommended:

1 For adults with pneumococcal or meningococcal meningitis, penicillin G, 12 to 20 million units intravenously each day in four to six divided doses, is recommended; for children the dose of penicillin G should be 200,000 to 300,000 units per kilogram of body weight.

2 For children over 2 months of age with *H. influenzae* or uncomplicated meningitis of unknown etiology, ampicillin, 150 to 250 mg per kilogram of body weight intravenously in divided doses, plus chloramphenicol, 100 mg/kg per day intravenously, should be given. The reason for the use of two drugs is the progressive increase in the number of ampicillin-resistant *H. influenzae* from patients with meningitis; a few strains of chloramphenicol-resistant *H. influenzae* have also been reported. In order to avoid interference between the two drugs, ampicillin should be given 1 h before chloramphenicol. Once the etiologic organism and its sensitivity have been determined, chloramphenicol can be discontinued if the organism is sensitive to ampicillin. In adults with *H. influenzae* meningitis, the daily doses of ampicillin and chloramphenicol are 12 and 4 to 6 g, respectively (administered intravenously either as a constant infusion or in divided doses).

3 In adult patients with any of these types of bacterial meningitis who may be allergic to the penicillins, chloramphenicol in a dosage of 4 to 6 g per day intravenously may be used. The cephalosporins are questionable alternates for pneumococcal meningitis, and there have been some failures also in *H. influenzae* and meningococcal meningitis; hence, chloramphenicol is preferred in infections due to these organisms.

4 For meningitis due to Enterobacteriaceae, the drug of choice is gentamicin in dosage of 5 mg/kg per day administered in divided dosages at 6-h intervals. This drug can be given intravenously, but many prefer the intramuscular route to avoid high blood levels which may lead to respiratory paralysis and permanent damage to inner ears. In addition, because of gentamicin's poor penetration into the CSF, the drug should be given intrathecally in doses of 2.0 to 5.0 mg per day as long as CSF cultures remain positive. Some prefer intracisternal to intralumbar administration to assure better mixing of drug. The treatment for *Pseudomonas* meningitis is similar except that carbenicillin in doses of 30 g per day should be added.

5 Meningitis due to *S. aureus* should be treated with a penicillinase-resistant penicillin or a cephalosporin, in dosage of 6 to 12 g per day. Because penetration of these drugs into the CSF is variable, even when the meninges are inflamed, the

course of the infection should be monitored carefully, and chloramphenicol should be substituted or added if symptoms persist or the CSF remains infected.

Foci of infection in the paranasal sinuses, mastoids, in an infected shunt, or in cranial osteomyelitis should be identified so that appropriate drainage may be carried out when the acute episode of meningitis has subsided.

Duration of therapy In most patients bacterial meningitis need not be treated for longer than 10 days except when there is a persistent parameningeal focus of infection. Antibiotics should be administered in full doses parenterally (preferably intravenously) throughout the period of treatment. Treatment failures with several drugs, notably ampicillin, are attributable to oral or intramuscular administration, resulting in inadequate concentration in the CSF. Repeated lumbar punctures are not necessary to follow the course of therapy as long as the patient is doing well. The CSF sugar may remain low for a number of days after cultures become negative and should occasion concern only if bacteria are present. Likewise, persistent but steadily diminishing mononuclear pleocytosis, following pyogenic meningitis, is the rule.

Prolongation of fever due usually to subdural effusion, sinus thrombosis, mastoiditis, intercurrent infection, phlebitis, or rarely abscess of brain requires continuation of therapy for a longer period. Bacteriologic relapse after treatment is discontinued requires immediate reinstitution of therapy.

Adrenocortical steroids The few controlled studies available have demonstrated that steroids exert no beneficial effects in pyogenic meningitis. These drugs should not be used except possibly in overwhelming meningococcal sepsis or in severe cerebral edema.

Other forms of therapy Intrathecal administration of enzymes to lyse excessive subarachnoid cellular exudate which may be associated with spinal block or hydrocephalus in the subacute stages of bacterial meningitis is of no proved value. There is also no evidence to support the therapeutic efficacy of repeated drainage of CSF. In fact, increased CSF pressure in the acute phases of bacterial meningitis is largely a consequence of cerebral edema, and lumbar puncture may predispose to temporal lobe or cerebellar herniation and death. Mannitol and urea have been employed apparently successfully in some cases of severe brain swelling with unusually high initial CSF pressures (> 400 mmH$_2$O). Either should be accompanied by dexamethasone in relatively high doses. An adequate but not excessive amount of parenteral fluids should be given, and anticonvulsants should be prescribed when seizures are present. In children care should be taken to avoid hyponatremia and water intoxication—a cause of brain swelling. Subdural effusions should be drained repeatedly by subdural taps; if they persist after the infection has subsided, surgical removal may become necessary.

RECURRENT MENINGITIS

Recurrent attacks of bacterial meningitis usually follow in the wake of trauma. The interval between the traumatic episode and the initial bout of posttraumatic meningitis may be as long as several years. *Streptococcus pneumoniae* is the usual bacterial pathogen. Often it proves to be one of the higher serologic types, reflecting the predominance of such strains in nasal carriers. *Cerebrospinal fluid rhinorrhea* is present in most of these patients but may be transient. The patient with recurrent meningitis of inapparent origin should always be suspected of having a fistulous connection between the nasal sinuses and the subarachnoid space. The fistula is usually traumatic (old basal skull fracture), and the site is the frontal or ethmoid sinuses or the cribriform plate. The rhinorrhea may be difficult to demonstrate except by injection of a dye, such as carmine red, or radioactive albumin into the spinal fluid and watching for its appearance in nasal secretions. Cerebrospinal fluid rhinorrhea may also be detected by measuring the glucose concentration of nasal secretions. The usual mucous secretions contain little glucose, but in CSF rhinorrhea the amount approximates that in CSF. The prognosis in recurrent meningitis is remarkably benign, and the mortality is much lower than in ordinary pneumococcal meningitis. Nevertheless, vaccination of these patients with pneumococcal vaccine is indicated, and long-term prophylactic chemotherapy with penicillin V should be considered. Treatment of recurrent meningitis is outlined above. Attempts to demonstrate CSF rhinorrhea should be made after the acute infection has subsided; if evidence of a fistula is found, surgical repair should be considered.

SUBDURAL EMPYEMA

DEFINITION Subdural empyema is a suppurative process in the cranial subdural space between the inner surface of the dura and the outer of the arachnoid. The proper term for this condition is not *abscess* but *empyema*, indicating suppuration in a preformed space. About three-fourths of cases are unilateral, and the remainder bilateral, usually in the parafalcial region.

ETIOLOGY The infection usually gains entry to the subdural space from the frontal or ethmoid sinuses, or, less often, from the mastoid cells. Some cases follow neurosurgical procedures. Occasionally the subdural space becomes infected by extension of bacteria from the CSF or from a brain abscess. Rarely has it been observed with bloodstream infections. The flora in subdural empyema is usually polymicrobial and consists of anaerobes (streptococci and *Bacteroides)*, *H. influenzae*, *S. aureus*, *Klebsiella*, and *E. coli*.

PATHOLOGY A collection of subdural pus in quantities of a few milliters to 100 to 200 ml lies over the cerebral hemisphere. It is often mistaken for meningitis. The arachnoid, when cleared of exudate, is cloudy, and thrombosis of meningeal veins may be seen. The underlying cerebral hemisphere is depressed, and in fatal cases there is often an ipsilateral temporal lobe pressure cone. Microscopic studies demonstrate various degrees of organization of the exudate on the inner surface of the dura, and infiltration of the underlying pia with small numbers of neutrophilic leukocytes, lymphocytes, and mononuclear cells. There is superficial thrombophlebitis; the thrombi in cerebral veins appear to begin on the outer side (toward the empyema). The thrombosis extends to other dural sinuses, and the superficial layers of the cerebral cortex undergo ischemic necrosis, which probably accounts for the unilateral seizures and signs of disordered cerebral function.

SYMPTOMATOLOGY AND LABORATORY FINDINGS The usual history includes chronic sinusitis and mastoiditis with a recent flare-up and evidence of local pain and increase in purulent nasal or aural discharge. Generalized headache and fever are the first indications of intracranial spread. They are followed within a few days by localizing signs including unilateral motor seizures, hemiplegia, hemianesthesia, and aphasia. Stu-

por or coma develops rapidly as the cerebral symptoms progress. Fever is usually present, but the neck is not always stiff. When CSF is examined, increased pressure, raised white blood cell count in the range of 50 to 1000 per milliliter including both neutrophils and lymphocytes, elevated protein concentration (75 to 300 mg per 100 ml), and normal sugar values are the usual findings. The CSF is sterile. Lumbar puncture poses a distinct risk because it may precipitate transtentorial herniation.

DIAGNOSIS Skull films may show involvement of the sinus or mastoid. The single most useful diagnostic procedure is the CT scan and carotid arteriography, which discloses inward displacement of meningeal vessels and contralateral shift of the anterior cerebral arteries. A temporal burr hole with exposure of the dura demonstrates pus under increased pressure. Four conditions need to be distinguished clinically from subdural empyema: cerebral thrombophlebitis, brain abscess, acute hemorrhagic leukoencephalitis, and acute hemorrhagic viral (inclusion body) encephalitis (Chap. 369).

TREATMENT Single or multiple burr holes should be made to drain pus. In particular, it is important to do this procedure early because delaying it sharply increases the mortality rate. Appropriate antibiotic therapy consists of 20 million units of penicillin per day plus chloramphenicol, 4 g per day, aimed particularly at *Bacteroides*, administered intravenously. Without such massive antimicrobial therapy and surgery, most patients will die, usually within 7 to 14 days, often while the unsuspecting physician and surgeon are waiting for better localization of an assumed cerebral abscess, the most commonly mistaken diagnosis. On the other hand, successfully treated patients may make a surprisingly good recovery, including full or partial resolution of their focal neurological deficits.

EXTRADURAL ABSCESS

This condition is almost invariably associated with osteomyelitis in a cranial bone which originates from an infection in the ear or paranasal sinuses. Pus and granulation tissue accumulate on the outer surface of the dura, separating it from the cranial bone. Symptomatically, the effects are those of a local inflammatory process: frontal or auricular pain, purulent discharge from the sinuses or ear, and fever and local tenderness. Sometimes the neck is slightly stiff. Localizing neurological signs are usually absent. Rarely a fifth and sixth cranial nerve palsy appears with infections of the petrous part of the temporal bone (petrositis with Gradenigo's syndrome), or a focal seizure may occur. The CSF is usually clear and under normal pressure but may contain a few lymphocytes and neutrophils (20 to 100 per milliliter) and slightly raised protein concentration. Treatment consists of antibiotics aimed at the appropriate pathogen which may be *S. aureus*, anaerobic streptococci, *Bacteroides* spp., or Enterobacteriaceae. The primary sinusitis or mastoiditis, from which the extradural infection has arisen, may require a surgical procedure.

SPINAL EPIDURAL ABSCESS

This type of abscess possesses unique clinical features and constitutes an important neurological and neurosurgical emergency. It is discussed in Chap. 375.

INTRACRANIAL THROMBOPHLEBITIS

The lateral, cavernous, and superior longitudinal sinuses are relatively uncommon sites of infection. Usually there is evidence that the intracranial process has extended from the middle ear and mastoid cells, the paranasal sinuses, and skin around the upper lip, nose, and eyes.

LATERAL SINUS THROMBOPHLEBITIS In lateral sinus thrombophlebitis, which usually follows chronic mastoiditis, the earache and mastoid tenderness are succeeded, after a period of days to a few weeks, by generalized headache and papilledema. As a rule there are no other neurological signs. As a diagnostic aid, compression of the jugular veins separately, during the Queckenstedt maneuver, will demonstrate failure of the CSF pressure to rise when the ipsilateral one is compressed (Tobey-Ayer test). When the intracranial pressure is greatly elevated, the suspicion of cerebellar abscess is raised, but this process is usually characterized by other neurological signs, especially nystagmus to the side of the lesion and ataxia of the arm and leg.

CAVERNOUS SINUS THROMBOPHLEBITIS In this condition, which is usually secondary to oculonasal infections, the clinical syndrome is one of orbital edema, chemosis, venous congestion, and evidence of palsy of the third, fourth, ophthalmic fifth, and sixth cranial nerves. Later spread through the circular sinus to the opposite cavernous sinus results in bilateral symptoms and signs. The posterior part of the cavernous sinus may be infected via the superior and inferior petrosal veins without the occurrence of orbital edema or ophthalmoplegia. The CSF is usually normal unless there is associated meningitis or subdural empyema. The only effective therapy in the fulminant variety, associated with thrombosis of the anterior portion of the sinus, has been antimicrobial therapy usually aimed at coagulase-positive staphylococci (Chap. 116), and occasionally gram-negative pathogens as well. Anticoagulants have been used occasionally, but their value has not been proved. Cavernous sinus thrombosis must be differentiated from mucormycosis which may cause a similar clinical picture in uncontrolled diabetics or in immunosuppressed patients (Chap. 160).

THROMBOPHLEBITIS OF THE SUPERIOR LONGITUDINAL SINUS Although occasionally asymptomatic, the typical clinical syndrome is one of unilateral convulsions and hemiplegia, first on one side of the body, then on the other, because of extension into the superior cerebral veins. The paralysis may be predominantly monoplegic and involve mainly the legs. Headache, papilledema, and increased intracranial pressure may accompany these signs. The diagnosis can be corroborated by demonstrating a sluggish circulation and failure of the superior sagittal sinus to fill during the late stage of the carotid arteriogram. Treatment consists of large doses of antibiotics and temporization until the thrombus recanalizes.

All types of thrombophlebitis, especially those related to ear and paranasal sinus infection, may be complicated by other forms of intracranial suppuration including bacterial meningitis, subdural empyema, or brain abscess. Therapy in these patients must be individualized. The initiating focus should be brought under control even by surgery if necessary, once the patient's condition permits such a procedure. To operate on the primary focus before medical treatment is instituted is to court disaster. The better plan is to institute antibiotic therapy; surgery on the ears or sinuses should be decided upon only after the infection is well controlled.

ASEPTIC THROMBOSIS OF INTRACRANIAL VENOUS SINUSES
This may develop after sinus and ear infections and may lead to an obscure increase in intracranial pressure because of the occlusion of one lateral or superior sagittal sinus. The more common conditions which may be accompanied by aseptic

thrombosis are postpartum and postoperative states, which are often characterized by thrombocytosis and hyperfibrinogenemia; congenital heart disease and marasmus in infants; sickle-cell disease; and primary or secondary polycythemia.

BRAIN ABSCESS

PATHOGENESIS Most of the focal suppurative intracranial processes of this type are linked to chronic ear and sinus or pulmonary infections. Nearly half of all brain abscesses are secondary to disease of the middle ear and mastoid cells, and of these about one-third arise in the anterolateral part of the cerebellar hemisphere and the remainder (lying above the tegmen tympani) in the middle and inferior part of the temporal lobe. Frontal sinusitis accounts for roughly 10 percent of the cases, the abscess being almost invariably situated in the anterior and inferior part of the frontal lobe. Of the remaining cases, a small portion are due to penetrating wounds or postoperative infections, and the rest are metastatic. Of the latter, about half are traceable to a primary septic focus in the lung, usually bronchiectasis, empyema, lung abscess, or bronchopleural fistula, and in the rest, the source of infection may be the skin, bone, i.e., a focus of osteomyelitis, or the heart. In 5 to 10 percent of cases, the source cannot be ascertained. Brain abscess is almost never a consequence of bacterial meningitis.

Brain abscesses are particularly frequent with congenital heart disease with right-to-left shunts (e.g., tetralogy of Fallot), and they may also complicate arteriovenous vascular abnormalities of the lung, as in cases of familial telangiectasia. With cranial trauma the location of the abscess will depend on the site of the penetrating wound. Metastatic abscesses are most likely to occur in the distal territory of the middle cerebral arteries. In contrast to the otogenic and rhinogenic abscesses, they may be multiple.

Bacterial endocarditis rarely gives rise to brain abscess. Instead, the picture is one of focal embolic encephalitis with or without signs of embolic vascular disease elsewhere (Chap. 243). In subacute endocarditis the emboli are sterile and cause only infarction, miliary foci of tissue necrosis, focal meningeal inflammation, and mycotic aneurysms. The CSF may contain a small number of neutrophilic leukocytes, lymphocytes, and red blood cells; the protein level may be elevated, but cultures are sterile and sugar values remain normal. In acute bacterial endocarditis, miliary abscesses and purulent meningitis may develop, or there may be infarcts, and subarachnoid or intracerebral hemorrhages secondary to rupture of a mycotic aneurysm. Rarely do the miliary abscesses progress to large ones. Rapidly evolving cerebral signs in endocarditis are nearly always caused by embolic infarction or hemorrhage.

ETIOLOGY The most common organisms causing brain abscess are streptococci, most of which are anaerobic or microaerophilic. These organisms are often found in combinations with other anaerobes, notably *Bacteroides*, and may also be combined with Enterobacteriaceae, such as *E. coli, Klebsiella-Enterobacter*, and *Proteus*. Staphylococci also may cause brain abscess, but pneumococci, meningococci, and *H. influenzae* rarely do so. In addition to *Bacteroides* and anaerobic streptococci, anaerobic actinomyces and veillonellae have been isolated. The bacterial species vary with the site of the abscess; staphylococcal abscesses are usually a consequence of penetrating head trauma or of bacteremia; enteric organisms are almost always associated with otitic infections, while anaerobic streptococci are commonly metastatic from the lung.

PATHOLOGY Localized inflammatory necrosis and edema, septic thrombosis of vessels, and aggregates of degenerating leukocytes (suppurative encephalitis), represent the early reaction to bacterial invasion of the brain. This is followed within a few weeks by encapsulation of the liquefied brain and of accumulated pus. The lesion becomes encapsulated by fibroblasts and newly formed vessels, and the capsule thickens over a period of weeks. The meninges adjacent to the abscess, especially near the point of entry of infection, are infiltrated by neutrophils, lymphocytes, and plasma cells.

CLINICAL MANIFESTATIONS In patients with chronic ear, sinus, or pulmonary infections, a recent reactivation of the infection usually precedes the onset of cerebral symptoms. In a number of patients evidence of central nervous system invasion is acute and fever, headache, vomiting, increasing obtundation, seizures, and a variety of localizing neurological signs appear within a few days. In other patients, bacterial invasion of the brain substance may be asymptomatic or may be attended only by a transitory focal neurological disorder, as may happen with lodgment of a septic embolus. Sometimes stiff neck accompanies generalized headache, suggesting the diagnosis of meningitis (especially a partially treated one). However, the CSF shows only a few cells, normal or slightly increased protein concentration, and normal sugar concentration. These early symptoms may subside or they may appear to respond to antimicrobials, but within a few weeks, recurrent headache, slowness in mentation, focal or generalized convulsions, and obvious signs of increased intracranial pressure provide evidence of an inflammatory mass in the brain. At this stage, the symptoms of infection are not conspicuous. While fever is characteristic of the invasive phase best described as suppurative encephalitis, as the abscess becomes encapsulated, the temperature returns to normal. Indeed, if the invasive stage of cerebral infection is inconspicuous, the entire clinical picture does not differ from that of brain tumor. In the later stages of abscess formation, the CSF pressure is usually elevated and there is nearly always pleocytosis between 25 and 300 cells per milliliter consisting both of neutrophils and lymphocytes and an elevation of protein between 75 and 300 mg per 100 ml with CSF glucose remaining normal.

The focal neurological signs depend on the location of the abscess as follows.

Temporal lobe abscess Headache is usually on the side of the abscess and is localized to the frontotemporal region. If the abscess lies in the dominant hemisphere, there is a dysphasia of the amnestic type (inability to name objects, Chap. 24). A homonymous upper quadrantic field defect may also be demonstrable—the inferior portion of the optic radiation is interrupted—and this may be the only sign in abscess of the right temporal lobe. Contralateral motor or sensory defects in the limbs tend to be minimal, though weakness of the lower face is often observed.

Cerebellar abscess Headache in the postauricular or suboccipital region is usually the first symptom and may at first be ascribed to infection in the mastoid cells. Coarse nystagmus and gaze weakness to the side of the lesion and a cerebellar ataxia of the ipsilateral arm and leg are present in most patients, though the ataxia may be difficult to demonstrate if the patient is very ill. As a rule, the signs of increased intracranial pressure are more prominent than those of focal cerebral disease. Mild contralateral or bilateral pyramidal signs are evi-

dence of ipsilateral brainstem compression; in the late stages as consciousness becomes impaired they are ominous signs.

Frontal lobe abscess Headache, drowsiness, inattention, and general impairment of mental function are prominent. Hemiparesis with unilateral motor seizures and motor or expressive dysphasia are the most frequent neurologic signs.

DIAGNOSIS The diagnosis of a brain abscess depends on (1) a demonstrated source of infection in the ears, sinuses, or lungs or the presence of a right-to-left cardiac shunt, (2) evidence of increased intracranial pressure, and (3) focal cerebral or cerebellar signs. Although the CSF shows a characteristic inflammatory reaction, lumbar puncture in brain abscess is potentially dangerous, particularly when intracranial pressure is obviously elevated and the information to be derived is not specific enough to justify the risk.

The CT scan is the most valuable procedure not only for visualizing an abscess(es). It also shows distortion of the ventricles and the thickness of the capsule and it enables close follow-up of therapy. The use of iodine will enhance the selectivity of the CT scan. If CT scanning is not available, ^{99m}Tc imaging (radionuclide scan) is a reliable method for localizing brain abscess. Rarely, the technetium scan may be positive when the CT scan is negative. There is little likelihood of cerebral abscess if both the radioactive isotope and CT scans are negative.

Scanning procedures have supplanted arteriography in most instances. The latter technique provides evidence of a cerebral mass only by showing displacement of the anterior, middle, or posterior cerebral arteries. It is accurate in localizing abscesses in most regions of the brain with the exception of posterior parietal areas. It is also unreliable early in the disease before liquefaction and encapsulation have occurred.

When the classic clinical picture is present and CT or radionuclide scan corroborate the presence of a mass lesion, the diagnosis is easy. If there is no source of infection and there are only signs and symptoms of a mass lesion, the diagnosis includes differentiation of abscess from tumor, subdural hematoma, and hemorrhage. Sometimes only surgical exploration will settle the issue. Once the inflammatory nature of the intracranial mass has been established, brain abscess must then be distinguished from subdural empyema, intracranial thrombophlebitis with hemorrhage and infarction of brain, necrotizing viral encephalitis, and acute hemorrhagic leukoencephalitis.

TREATMENT During the stage of acute suppurative encephalitis, intracranial operation accomplishes little and probably causes only additional traumatization and swelling of the brain tissue. There is good evidence that many brain abscesses can be cured at this stage by the administration of adequate doses of antimicrobials. Since the bacteriologic diagnosis must be presumptive, the best regimen consists of 20 million units of penicillin G intravenously in divided doses and 4 to 6 g chloramphenicol, both drugs being given intravenously in divided doses. This choice of antimicrobial agents is based on the preponderance of anaerobic streptococci and *Bacteroides* that are usually isolated from the abscess in such patients. If there is evidence of staphylococcal infection, adequate amounts of a penicillinase-resistant penicillin or a cephalosporin drug should be given. Treatment should be continued for 6 weeks, and if there is clinical improvement and recovery during the course of therapy, surgical intervention can be withheld. The initial elevation of intracranial pressure and threatening temporal lobe or cerebellar pressure cone should be managed by intravenous injection of urea, mannitol, or dexamethasone. Persistence or progression of high intracranial pressure manifested by deepening coma and threat of herniation often forces operation, regardless of the stage of the abscess. Likewise, clear-cut evidence of a mass lesion which is not improving with antimicrobial therapy is an indication for surgery. The usual methods of treatment are unroofing of the abscess and drainage, or aspiration. If superficial and encapsulated, total excision should be attempted; if deep, aspiration and the injection of antimicrobial agents into the abscess are the only possible treatment methods, and they may have to be repeated. Despite the advances in therapy, the mortality rate from brain abscess has remained in the neighborhood of 40 to 60 percent. The least satisfactory results are obtained in multiple metastatic abscesses.

Neurological residua occur in about 30 percent of surviving patients. Of these, focal epilepsy is one of the most troublesome. Following successful treatment of a cerebral abscess in patients with congenital heart disease, correction of the cardiac anomaly is indicated to prevent recurrence.

PROGNOSIS Even with appropriate therapy, the prognosis is only fair. The presence of focal neurological signs and/or a neighborhood infection that suggest the diagnosis of brain abscess improve the prognosis. If brain abscess is not recognized and treated, it terminates either by development of a tentorial or foramen magnum pressure cone or by rupture of the abscess into the ventricles (ventricular empyema). Rarely the abscess becomes thickly encapsulated and chronic; in this form it may be only mildly symptomatic over a period of months or years.

REFERENCES

BHANDARI YS et al: Subdural empyema: A review of 37 cases. J Neurosurg 32:35, 1970

BREWER WS et al: Brain abscess: A review of recent experience. Ann Intern Med 82:571, 1975

CRANE LR, LERNER AM: Non-traumatic bacillary meningitis in the Detroit Medical Center, 1964-1974. Medicine 57:197, 1978

FEIGIN RD, DODGE PR: Bacterial meningitis: Newer concepts of pathophysiology and neurologic sequelae. Pediatr Clin North Am 23:541, 1976

FINLAND M, BARNES MW: Acute bacterial meningitis at Boston City Hospital during 12 selected years, 1935-1972. J Infect Dis 136:400, 1977

HAND LW, SANFORD JP: Post-traumatic bacterial meningitis. Ann Intern Med 72:869, 1960

HEINEMAN HS et al: Intracranial suppurative disease. JAMA 218:1542, 1971

KAUFMAN DM et al: Subdural empyema: Analysis of 17 cases and review of the literature. Medicine 54:485, 1975

SAMSON DS, CLARK K: Current review of brain abscess. Am J Med 54:201, 1973

SCHOENBAUM SC et al: Infections of cerebrospinal fluid shunts: Epidemiology, clinical manifestations and therapy. J Infect Dis 131:543, 1975

SCHWARTZ MN, DODGE PR: Bacterial meningitis—a review of selected aspects. N Engl J Med 272:725, 779, 842, 898, 945, 1003, 1965

STEVENS EA et al: Computed tomagraphic brain scanning in intraparenchymal pyogenic abscesses. Am J Roentgenol 130:111, 1978

WEISS W et al: Prognostic factors in pneumococcal meningitis. Arch Intern Med 120:517, 1967

YOSHIKAWA TT, GOODMAN SJ: Brain abscess. West J Med 121:207, 1974

———— et al: Role of anaerobic bacteria in subdural empyema. Am J Med 58:99, 1975

369

VIRAL INFECTIONS OF THE NERVOUS SYSTEM
Aseptic meningitis and encephalitis

BYRON A. KAKULAS
RAYMOND D. ADAMS

Many viruses are known to be capable of causing infection and symptomatic injury to the nervous system. In many instances the neurological manifestations are only a part of a generalized disease with its own peculiarities and easy means of identification, such as mumps, chickenpox, or pleurodynia. But it may happen that overt evidences of the infection are limited to the nervous system, and the resulting syndrome can be either relatively stereotyped or highly varied. If the latter condition prevails, clinical diagnosis may be difficult and one must, perforce, turn to laborious and complicated laboratory procedures for the identification of the causative agent. But these diagnostic methods are not always successful, and even the most experienced laboratories have failed to establish the nature of the disease in as many as 30 to 50 percent of cases.

Those viruses which affect the nervous system primarily are said to be *neurotropic*. There are a considerable number of them, and their clinical manifestations are diverse, as might be expected. However, five clinical syndromes recur with regularity and should be familiar to all students of medicine. These are the syndromes of (1) myelitis, almost invariably a result of infection by one of the polioviruses, (2) zoster ganglionitis, (3) acute aseptic, nonsuppurative, or "lymphocytic," meningitis, (4) acute and subacute encephalitis or meningoencephalitis, and (5) slow virus infections simulating degenerative diseases. The first of these, myelitis, takes three forms: poliomyelitis (see Chap. 187) in which motor neurons are selectively affected; meningomyelitis in which inflammation of the white matter is secondary to meningitis and vasculitis (e.g., syphilitic meningomyelitis); and the third in which demyelination causes a leukomyelitis (also called *transverse myelitis*). The last form is rarely due to a viral infection. (The leukomyelitides are discussed in Chap. 375.)

THE SYNDROME OF ASEPTIC MENINGITIS

The term *aseptic meningitis* is applied to a symptom complex that can be produced by any one of several dozen infective agents, the majority of which are viral (see Table 186-1). In bold outline the syndrome consists of fever, signs of meningeal irritation and mononuclear and lymphocytic pleocytosis of the cerebrospinal fluid (CSF).

Headache, out of proportion to that often associated with febrile states, ranks as the most frequent symptom in this group of diseases. A variable degree of drowsiness, confusion, stupor, or rarely coma, may occur, but as a rule the derangement of consciousness tends to be relatively mild. Stiffness of the neck and spine on forward bending attest to the presence of meningeal irritation, but at first it may be so slight as to pass unnoticed. Here the Kernig and Brudzinski's signs help very little, for they are often absent in the presence of a manifest viral meningitis. Frank neurological signs of other types are infrequent; included are isolated strabismus and diplopia, vague weakness, pain or paresthesias in an extremity, a slight inequality of reflexes, or a wavering Babinski sign. The meningitis may be asymptomatic.

The CSF findings consist of pleocytosis (mainly mononuclear, except in the initial stage when a proportion of the cells are neutrophilic leukocytes), small and variable increase in protein, and no demonstrable microorganisms by smear and culture. The concentration of glucose in the CSF is usually normal; this is important because a low sugar value in an infection which evokes a lymphocytic or mononuclear pleocytosis signifies tuberculous (Chap. 143) or mycotic meningitis, particularly cryptococcus neoformans (Chap. 153), or rarely metastatic carcinoma, lymphoma, or sarcoid of the meninges. Since the CSF glucose level may be normal in the early stages of tuberculosis or cryptococcosis, this determination should be repeated at intervals until the diagnosis is established or the patient is definitely convalescent.

VIRAL INFECTIONS THAT ARE PREDOMINANTLY MENINGEAL
The majority of cases of aseptic meningitis are accounted for by coxsackieviruses (Chap. 178), echoviruses (Chap. 178), mumps (Chap. 188), and lymphocytic choriomeningitis (LCM) (Chap. 191). Indeed, these viral infections together with leptospirosis compose about 95 percent of all cases of aseptic meningitis of established etiology. But in every series of cases published from virus isolation centers as many as one-fourth or more have an indeterminate cause.

Of the rarer types of aseptic meningitis one should mention the milder forms of postvaccinal meningoencephalitis or the meningoencephalitis which follows measles (Chap. 181), rubella (Chap. 182), chickenpox (Chap. 185), and prophylactic treatment of rabies (Chap. 189). Here the diagnosis is made on the history of the recent infection (usually within a few days or a week) or inoculation (usually within a few weeks).

Herpes simplex (Chap. 193) and the arthropod-borne (arbo-) encephalitis viruses (Chap. 190) are responsible for a small proportion of cases of aseptic meningitis. Infections by arboviruses are likely to be encountered in epidemics along with cases of frank encephalitis and tend to occur in certain geographic areas, points which facilitate early clinical recognition, though specific identification of the virus may still be difficult.

Neurological manifestations, including the syndrome of aseptic meningitis, may appear in the course of syphilis (Chap. 146), influenza (Chap. 179), infectious mononucleosis (Chap. 195), psittacosis (Chap. 175), lymphogranuloma (Chap. 174), Rift Valley fever and encephalomyocarditis, Q fever, Behçet's disease, Vogt-Koyanagi disease, Harada's disease, and Mollaret's recurrent meningitis.

The icteric stage of infectious hepatitis (Chap. 302) rarely is preceded by mild meningitis, the nature of which is evident when the jaundice appears. Among others, infectious mononucleosis (Chap. 195) sometimes produces what appears to be a primary meningitis, meningoencephalitis, or idiopathic polyneuritis. Rarely *Mycoplasma pneumoniae* (Chap. 172) is complicated by an aseptic meningitis or other neurological disorder.

DIFFERENTIAL DIAGNOSIS OF INFECTIVE AND NONINFECTIVE FORMS OF LYMPHOCYTIC MENINGITIS Clinical distinctions among the many forms of aseptic meningitis cannot be made with a high degree of reliability, but useful leads can be obtained by careful attention to certain details of history and physical examination. The *season* during which the illnesses occur may be helpful. Enteroviral infections (coxsackie- and echovirus) are diseases of midsummer and early fall. The arthropod-borne diseases also occur in summer and fall (coinciding with the population of insect vectors), and though leptospirosis may appear at any season, its incidence in the United States shows a striking peak in the summer. Mumps and infectious mononucleosis are diseases of late winter and spring. Lymphocytic meningitis is particularly common in late fall and winter, presumably because field mice enter dwellings at this time. A definite past history of mumps aids in excluding

the disease, second attacks being unusual. Sore throat, lymphadenopathy, and rash point to infectious mononucleosis or an echovirus infection. Severe back and leg pain may occur in enteroviral infections, leptospirosis, and trichinosis. Exposure to such animals as mice (LCM), dogs, rats, or swine (leptospirosis) may suggest the diagnosis. A skin rash favors the presence of infectious mononucleosis, echovirus infections, and leptospirosis (often a transient, blotchy erythema). Icterus suggests infectious mononucleosis or viral hepatitis; it is not present in meningeal leptospirosis. Conjunctival suffusion is common in leptospirosis and *Listeria monocytogenes*, and may be seen in trichinosis. Slight tenderness and swelling of salivary glands and testes may be the only signs of mumps. Pulmonary infiltrates suggest psittacosis.

Aside from viral isolation, few laboratory tests are helpful. The peripheral leukocyte count is often normal, but leukopenia may be present. However it accompanies so many of the diseases responsible for aseptic meningitis (infectious mononucleosis, Colorado tick fever, LCM, lupus erythematosus, etc.) that rarely is it a useful finding. Eosinophilia should suggest a parasitic infection, and in many cases infectious mononucleosis may be identified by the blood smear. Lymphocytic choriomeningitis produces an intense lymphocytic pleocytosis in the CSF (counts above 1000 cells per milliliter are often due to this disease), and mumps also gives an almost pure lymphocytic pleocytosis. Serologic tests for syphilis should be interpreted with caution because inflammation of many types can produce a false-positive reaction; for example, infectious mononucleosis and lupus erythematosus often evoke biologic false positive serum tests for syphilis. Liver function tests are abnormal in many patients with infectious mononucleosis and in anicteric hepatitis; hepatic abnormalities are not regularly present in the other entities under consideration.

Three other categories of disease may cause an apparently sterile, predominantly lymphocytic or mononuclear reaction in the leptomeninges: bacterial infections lying adjacent to the meninges; specific infections such as syphilis or parainfectious diseases in which the organism is difficult to isolate; and neoplastic invasion (usually lymphoma or carcinoma). The recognition of these is of great importance, since they require either antibiotic or antineoplastic therapy or some other form of treatment, as in syphilis, tuberculosis, or cryptococcosis.

With respect to pyogenic infections in which the CSF does not show a purulent meningitis and is sterile, antibiotic therapy given in inadequate dosage during a systemic or pulmonary infection may suppress a coexistent meningitis to the point where mononuclear cells predominate, glucose level is normal, and organisms are not detected in the CSF. A mistaken diagnosis of aseptic meningitis may then be made when the CSF is examined. The true state of affairs becomes evident only when the patient worsens and bacteria again appear. Careful attention to the history of recent antimicrobial therapy sometimes permits recognition of these cases before symptoms recur. *Listeria monocytogenes*, which is more frequent in immunologically incompetent individuals, may induce a low-grade meningitis with relatively few white blood cells in the CSF and high protein values. The diagnosis may at first be difficult, but cultures will disclose the etiologic agent. A smoldering paranasal sinusitis or mastoiditis may produce a similar CSF change because of intracranial extension (epidural or subdural infection). Or a brain abscess, the localizing signs of which are obscure, may deceive the clinician into making a diagnosis of aseptic meningitis (see Chap. 368).

In the second group of diseases, acute syphilitic meningitis is of importance and may be symptomatic or asymptomatic and may be merely the first manifestation of a florid syphilitic infection (see Chap. 146). Tuberculous meningitis often masquerades as aseptic meningitis; the diagnosis may at first be difficult because the tubercle bacillus is hard to see in stained smears, and cultures and guinea pig inoculations require considerable time. Similarly, the cryptococcus may not be diagnosed for the reason that the organisms may exceptionally be present in such low numbers as to be overlooked in smears. In such cases the diagnosis can be made by finding the cryptococcus antigen in the CSF.

In the third group, leukemias and lymphomas are the most conspicuous source of neoplastic meningeal reactions. In children with acute lymphoblastic leukemia, a leukemic meningitis with cell counts numbering into the thousands occurs not infrequently in the late stages of the illness. Many children with this disease are now treated prophylactically with antineoplastic drugs to prevent this complication. In adults a pleocytosis with lymphocyte or lymphoblast counts reaching as high as 4000 per milliliter of fluid may complicate lymphocytic and lymphoblastic lymphomas with or without leukemia. The sugar values may fall to 0, and the protein level is elevated.

In carcinomatous "meningitis" (from breast, stomach, lung, or other organ or melanoma) great numbers of cells may extend through the leptomeninges, involving cranial and spinal nerve roots, and produce a picture of meningoradiculitis with low sugar values. Gliomatous infiltration of ependyma and meninges also may have the same effect. Millipore filter preparations usually permit identification of the tumor cells.

Finally, in a number of other subacute or chronic infections of obscure origin, probably viral, the CSF profile corresponds to that of aseptic meningitis. These are (1) Behçet's disease, distinguished clinically by the triad of genital ulceration, uveitis, and involvement of central nervous system (cranial nerve palsies, seizures, mental disturbance, aphasia, hemiparesis, cerebellar ataxia); (2) Vogt-Koyanagi and Harada's diseases with various combinations of uveitis, depigmentation of hair and skin around the eyes, loss of eyelashes, dysacousis, and deafness; and (3) Mollaret's recurrent meningitis (Chap. 368), and allergic or hypersensitivity meningitis, occurring in the course of serum sickness and diseases of connective tissue such as lupus erythematosus.

In summary, though clinical findings, seasonal occurrence, and laboratory tests can sometimes enable the physician to direct further diagnostic efforts along specific lines, they may not be conclusive. Most important is to keep in mind always the possibility of tuberculosis, cryptococcosis, syphilis, inadequately treated pyogenic meningitis, and brain abscess, all of which may simulate aseptic meningitis. These diseases offer more pressing problems, for they may take the life of the patient if they are not diagnosed and treated. In contrast, the various forms of aseptic viral meningitis are usually self-limiting and benign.

THE SYNDROME OF ENCEPHALITIS

It is evident that the separation of the clinical syndromes of aseptic meningitis and encephalitis is not always easy, because in some patients with the former condition nonspecific drowsiness or confusion may be present when in fact there is no evidence of an inflammatory reaction in the substance of the brain. Conversely, in some patients with encephalitis the cerebral involvement may be so mild as to escape notice, and only the meningeal symptoms and CSF abnormalities may be manifest. These facts make it difficult to place complete reliance on statistical data about the relative incidence of encephalitis collected in surveys from various virus laboratories. It is our impression that many cases of encephalitis related to mumps and LCM are little more than examples of intense meningitis. They rarely have caused death with postmortem demonstration of cerebral lesions, and surviving patients seldom have residual signs.

The core of the encephalitis syndrome is an acute febrile illness with evidence of meningeal involvement, added to which are various combinations of the following symptoms and signs: convulsions, confusion, stupor, or coma; aphasia or mutism; hemiparesis with asymmetry of tendon reflexes and Babinski signs; involuntary movements, ataxia, and myoclonic jerks; nystagmus, ocular palsies, and facial weakness. Some one or other of these groups of findings predominate in certain types of encephalitis, as will be pointed out below, but always the clinical diagnosis in the setting of a febrile aseptic meningitis rests on the demonstration of focal derangement of the function of the cerebrum, brainstem, or cerebellum. The illnesses produced by these viral agents vary in duration but are usually measured in terms of weeks or, exceptionally, months. Death occurs in 5 to 20 percent of patients with viral encephalitis. Residual signs such as mental deterioration, amnesic defect, personality change, and hemiparesis are seen in about 20 percent of patients. This overall figure fails to reflect, however, the wide variation in the incidence of late changes that follow infection by different viruses. For example, neurological sequelae have been observed in 80 to 90 percent of patients with Eastern equine encephalitis and in only 5 to 10 percent of those with Western equine infections.

ETIOLOGY Whereas numerous viral, bacterial, fungal and parasitic agents are listed as causes of the encephalitis syndrome, only the viral ones are being considered here, for reference is usually being made to them when the term *encephalitis* is used. The number of viral infections or postviral allergic reactions is large, and one might suppose that clinical problems would be infinitely complex. However, those forms of viral encephalitis that occur with sufficient frequency to be of diagnostic importance are relatively few, and they tend to have geographic and seasonal incidence. In the United States, Western equine and St. Louis encephalitis have been observed mainly in California, the Middle West and Texas; there have been only two recognized outbreaks of Eastern equine encephalitis in New England, each in the early autumn. St. Louis encephalitis, another arthropod-borne late-summer encephalitis, has rarely been encountered in Eastern United States. Japanese B encephalitis, Russian spring-summer, and Murray Valley encephalitis are virtually unknown in the United States. Definite cases of epidemic (lethargic) encephalitis have not been observed in the acute form in the United States or Western Europe since 1930, though patients with residual symptoms (Parkinson's syndrome) are still seen in neurology clinics.

ACUTE ARTHROPOD FORMS OF ENCEPHALITIS

For the clinical picture of this group of viruses, which attack principally the cerebral hemispheres, see Chap. 190.

Rabies stands apart because of its relatively long latency after the bite of a rabid animal and by the predominance of dysphagia (hence salivation), throat spasms induced by attempts to swallow water (hence hydrophobia), dysarthria, numbness of face, and facial spasms, to which are added a confusional psychosis. The localization indicates the intensive involvement of the tegmental medullary nuclei in the rabid form of the disease (paralytic form is due to spinal cord affection) (see Chap. 189).

ENCEPHALITIS LETHARGICA (VON ECONOMO'S DISEASE, SLEEPING SICKNESS)

This disease first occurred in the wake of the pandemic of influenza during and for about 10 years after World War I. No disease like it can be found in medical annals before 1914.

Although the viral agent was never identified, the clinical and pathological features were typical of viral infection. The unique symptoms were pronounced somnolence, from which the disease takes its name, and ophthalmoplegia. A small proportion of the patients were overly active rather than somnolent and manifested a disorder of movement. The interest in this disease derives from the fact that a high proportion of survivors developed within months or years (sometimes after an interval as long as 25 years) the syndrome of parkinsonism (see Chaps. 16 and 373). In fact, this is the only form of encephalitis known to cause an immediate or delayed extrapyramidal syndrome of this type. Myoclonus, dystonia, bulimia, obesity, reversal of sleep pattern, and in children a psychopathic personality with compulsive behavior were other distressing sequelae. This was the first slow virus infection of the nervous system to be recognized in humans.

Few if any new cases have been seen in the United States and Western Europe since 1930. The only treatment available for the survivors consists of antiparkinsonism drugs and surgery, as outlined in Chap. 373.

ACUTE AND SUBACUTE INCLUSION BODY ENCEPHALITIS (See also Chap. 192)

First described by Dawson in 1939 and extensively studied by van Bogaert, in both subacute and chronic forms, this rather remarkable group of diseases is the only one which occurs sporadically throughout the year and in patients of all ages and in all parts of the world. Because of its course, nature, and extent of lesions, it has been called *subacute sclerosing panencephalitis* (SSPE). Whereas herpes simplex has been isolated from many of the acute cases and rubeola virus from subacute sclerosing ones, no causative agent has been found in others. Identity of etiology has been claimed on the basis of the pathology, particularly the large intranuclear (Cowdry type B) inclusion bodies in the astrocytes, oligodendrocytes, and nerve cells, but the evidence now is clearly against a unitary concept.

Nothing is known of the incubation period of these diseases. In *acute inclusion body encephalitis* (AIE) rarely have there been herpetic lesions of the skin or mucous membranes. A febrile onset and convulsions, confusion, hallucinations, and stupor or coma have been the usual initial symptoms. Swelling and herniation of one or both temporal lobes through the tentorium may occur, leading to deep coma and respiratory arrest during the first 24 to 76 h. The later clinical picture, which is relatively unique, evolves over a period of days or weeks, and the confusional psychosis shows elements of delirium or Korsakoff's amnestic state, the latter being more evident as the weeks pass. Age at onset has varied from childhood to the most advanced years (greater than 60 to 70 years in our patients). The CSF has shown a pleocytosis and increased protein content in most of the patients. The herpes simplex virus has been isolated from the brain (biopsy, autopsy) and CSF in only a few patients, and a rising titer of neutralizing antibodies has been demonstrated in others. The mortality rate is high (30 percent), and many of the survivors have been left with the most severe mental sequelae in the form of a complete Korsakoff's psychosis or global dementia (Chap. 25). Recently adenine arabinoside (15 mg/kg per day over a period of 12 h each day for 10 days), given before the onset of coma, appears to have reduced the mortality from 78 to 28 percent, and 50 percent were without neurological sequelae upon returning home. Only biopsy-proved cases (a questionable procedure) were treated. However, while treatment is promising, the numbers of treated cases are still small and at the Massachusetts General Hospital several of the treated patients have died. Also the use of brain biopsy for diagnostic purposes is never an appealing approach to therapy (see Chap. 193). Prognosis is not hopeless, however, for a fair number of patients have recovered to the point where they can resume an independent life.

Limbic encephalitis is not fully differentiated from AIE. The authors have observed a few patients with this condition each year at the Massachusetts General Hospital. Usually there is an acute or subacute onset of confusion and disorder of memory. The latter may be as severe as that of Korsakoff's psychosis. Minor disorders of speech, agitation, inactivity, and depression may accompany the confusion. One of our patients developed a cerebellar ataxia. Several weeks later another had intermittent hypoventilation. The cell count and protein in CSF may be normal or elevated. Most of the patients have had an occult tumor, usually an oat-cell or undifferentiated carcinoma of the lung. Pathological study reveals neuronal loss, gliosis, and perivascular cuffing with lymphocytes in the temporal lobes. No inclusion bodies are seen. A virus has not been isolated.

The subacute and chronically progressive forms of SSPE have affected children and adolescents for the most part. Widespread myelin destruction in the cerebral hemispheres with gliosis (sclerosing encephalitis) is combined with focal lesions of the brainstem. The clinical picture is that of a slowly evolving mental deterioration (dementia) associated with myoclonic jerks, falling spells, and cerebellar ataxia. The CSF may contain no cells, but the protein level may be elevated, particularly the globulin fraction (first zone gold sol curve). High levels of neutralizing antibody to measles virus have been found in serum and CSF, but this infective agent has been isolated from the brain tissue in only a few instances. It is still uncertain as to whether this virus has been seen in electron microscopic sections of the brain. The course of the disease is progressive, death usually occurring within a few months or years.

Other restricted syndromes such as the one in which there is an acute onset of chaotic eye movements (opsoclonia) and generalized tremulousness are observed from time to time. In some there is an associated cerebellar ataxia. Usually the cause is indeterminate and the symptoms disappear after a few weeks. In one recent report (Estrin) a diagnosis of St. Louis encephalitis was made by serologic study.

Closely related to SSPE is a form of acute rubeola encephalitis of delayed type. According to the report of Lyon, Ponsot, and Lebon, most of the cases have been in children who have been immunosuppressed as a treatment for leukemia, lymphosarcoma, or nephrosis (see Chap. 192).

The pathology of the acute inclusion-body encephalitis is marked by an intense hemorrhagic necrosis of the medial and inferior parts of the temporal lobes, and the orbital parts of the frontal ones. This distribution of lesion is so characteristic that the diagnosis can be made by simple inspection. The lesions of limbic encephalitis tend to have the same distribution but are less necrotizing and nonhemorrhagic. The subacute sclerosing form involves the cerebral cortex and white matter of both hemispheres as well as brainstem and cerebellum. Destruction of nerve cells, neuronophagia, and perivenous cuffing by lymphocytes and mononuclear cells indicate the viral nature of the infection. Degeneration of medullated fibers (myelin and axis cylinders) occurs in the white matter and is accompanied by perivascular cuffing and fibrous gliosis. The inclusion bodies in nerve and glial cells may be difficult to find. Treatment with some of the new antiviral agents is being tried.

The diagnosis may be difficult. The acute inclusion body encephalitis must be distinguished from acute hemorrhagic leukoencephalitis (see Chap. 370), acute subdural empyema, acute cerebral abscess, thrombophlebitis, and septic embolism (see Chap. 368). The subacute to chronic variety simulates the childhood and adolescent dementing diseases such as lipid storage disease (see Chap. 373) and Schilder's disease (see Chap. 370).

CHRONIC "SLOW" VIRAL ENCEPHALITIS

The idea that viral infections may lead to chronic disease, especially of the nervous system, has been entertained for half a century but only recently has received firm support from the following observations: (1) the demonstration of a slowly progressive noninflammatory degeneration of nigral neurons long after an attack of encephalitis lethargica; (2) the discovery in Iceland and England of a chronic viral degenerative disease of white matter in sheep (visna and scrapie); (3) the finding of inclusion bodies in the most chronic cases of sclerosing encephalitis and the demonstration by electron microscopy of viral particles in multifocal leukoencephalopathy; (4) the transmission of kuru and Creutzfeldt-Jakob disease to chimpanzees by Gajdusek and Gibbs; and (5) late onset of motor system disease after poliomyelitis. Claims have also been made for a viral causation of multiple sclerosis by Schubladze, of amyotrophic lateral sclerosis by Zilber, of epilepsia partialis continua and Vilynisk encephalomyelitis by Chumakov, but the evidence is questionable. From these observations has emerged the concept of the "slow viruses," the common features of which are long period of latency (months or years); protracted progression of illness after onset of symptoms; limitation of infections to a single host species; and localization of noninflammatory degenerative lesions in a particular part of the nervous system.

These slow viruses so perfectly simulate a purely degenerative disease that views of all the major degenerative diseases of white and gray matter of the brain are being reexamined. One of the most exciting prospects in neurology is thus unfolding before us. This concept of slow virus effects is discussed at greater length in Chap. 192.

There is presently no treatment for these diseases.

CREUTZFELDT-JAKOB DISEASE (SUBACUTE SPONGIFORM ENCEPHALOPATHY) Creutzfeldt-Jakob disease is the most dramatic representative of a degenerative disease of purely noninflammatory type caused by what is presumed to be a virus. The details are discussed in Chap. 192.

OTHER CAUSES OF ENCEPHALITIS

The most important nonviral diagnostic possibilities to be considered in a patient with the syndrome of encephalitis are syphilis, pertussis, leptospirosis, relapsing fever, epidemic typhus, scrub typhus, Rocky Mountain spotted fever, trypanosomiasis, toxoplasmosis, cerebral malaria, trichinosis, schistosomiasis, and cysticercosis.

MULTIFOCAL CEREBRAL DISEASE SIMULATING A VIRAL ENCEPHALITIS There are a number of diseases in this category, and, although rare, they raise the most vexatious problems in diagnosis when they do occur. Whipple's disease has been observed in the brain by Romanul et al. in a patient who had no diarrhea, fever, or arthralgia. The patient, like some 20 others in the literature, developed seizures, confusion, then dementia, pyramidal signs, and coma over 3 to 4 years. Histiocytosis may cause lung as well as cerebral lesions, and one of the authors' patients had diabetes insipidus and before death a polyneuritis. Giant-cell or granulomatous arteritis of the meningeal vessels has been the cause of a subacute cerebral illness with increased intracranial pressure, seizures, hemiparesis, and CSF change (a few lymphocytes and increased protein but normal sugar and

sterile fluid). We have had two to three such cases per year. Several have responded to corticosteroid therapy, and at least five have died. The cause is unknown.

REFERENCES

ALTMAN R et al: The impact of vector-borne viral diseases in the middle Atlantic states. Med Clin North Am 51:661, 1967

BALFOUR HH JR et al: California arbovirus (LaCrosse) infections. Pediatrics 52:680, 1973

BRODY JA et al: Chronic infectious neuropathic agents (CHINA) and other slow virus infections, in *Current Topics in Microbiology and Immunology,* vol 40. New York, Springer-Verlag, 1967

BYERS, RK: Acute hemorrhagic leukoencephalitis. Pediatrics 56:727, 1975

ESTRIN W: Serological diagnoses of St. Louis encephalitis in a patient with opsoclonia, tremulousness and benign encephalitis. Ann Neurol 1:591, 1977

GAJDUSEK DC et al: *Slow, Latent and Temperate Virus Infections,* Public Health Service Publication no 1378, 1965

HAMMON WMD, HO M: Viral encephalitis. Dis Mon, February 1973

HORTA-BARBOSA L et al: Chronic viral infections of the central nervous system. JAMA 218:1185, 1971

KETEL WB, OGNIBENE AJ: Japanese B encephalitis in Viet Nam. Am J Med Sci 261:271, 1971

LUBY JP et al: The epidemiology of St. Louis encephalitis (SLE): A review. Annu Rev Med 20:329, 1969

ROMANUL FCA et al: Whipple's disease confined to the brain: A case studied clinically and pathologically. J Neurol Neurosurg Psychiatry 40:901, 1977

ROSENTHAL MS: Viral infections of the central nervous system. Med Clin North Am 58:593, 1974

WEINER LP et al: Viral infections and demyelinating disease. N Engl J Med 288:1103, 1973

WHITNEY RJ et al: Adenine arabinoside therapy of biopsy-proved herpes simplex encephalitis. N Engl J Med 297:389, 1977

370
MULTIPLE SCLEROSIS AND OTHER DEMYELINATING DISEASES

DAVID C. POSKANZER
RAYMOND D. ADAMS

A large and important group of neurological disorders are termed the *demyelinating diseases* because they share the common pathological feature of foci of degeneration involving the myelin sheath of nerve fibers. These foci vary in size, shape, distribution, and rate of development in the different illnesses. The axon often suffers damage as well, but usually to a lesser degree, and the destruction of myelin is considered the primary change.

Because no clear cause has been ascertained for this group of diseases and a wide variety of etiologic theories have been proposed, including infective, metabolic, allergic, and vascular ones, a classification must be based on a combination of clinical and pathological factors. It is, of course, possible that the process of demyelination may have several different causes and may be a common manifestation of different diseases. Although intermediate and transitional cases exist among the various demyelinating diseases, the following four syndromes can be clearly distinguished on the basis of history, clinical examination, and pathological findings.

1 Acute disseminated encephalomyelitis (including postinfectious and postvaccinial encephalomyelitis)
2 Acute necrotizing hemorrhagic leukoencephalitis
3 Multiple sclerosis
4 Diffuse cerebral sclerosis, including adrenoleukodystrophy

ACUTE DISSEMINATED ENCEPHALOMYELITIS

Acute disseminated encephalomyelitis may be defined as an acute encephalitic or myelitic process of variable course and severity, characterized by symptoms indicating damage chiefly to the white matter of the brain or spinal cord and pathologically by perivascular cellular infiltration and perivenous demyelination.

An acute encephalitis, myelitis, or encephalomyelitis of this type may occur concurrently or follow shortly upon the exanthem of measles, smallpox, chickenpox, and rubella. A similar demyelinating illness with multiple perivascular foci of demyelination occurs following vaccination against rabies and against smallpox. Some cases, clinically and pathologically indistinguishable from these two categories of acute disseminated encephalomyelitis, appear to develop without any clearly defined preceding illness or vaccination. The disease has grave significance because of the substantial death rate and the frequency of persistent neurologic defects in patients who recover. The cause of the process is unclear, but it is generally thought to represent a form of hypersensitivity. A laboratory model for the disease, experimental allergic encephalomyelitis, can be produced by inoculating animals with a combination of sterile brain tissue and adjuvants.

PATHOLOGY No distinctive changes are seen on naked-eye examination of the brain. Microscopically, the white matter shows innumerable small zones of demyelination from 0.1 to 1 mm in diameter, which invariably surround small and medium-sized veins. The axons are more or less intact. There is a perivascular infiltration with lymphocytes, plasma cells, and mononuclear cells, and paraadventitial collections of mononuclear cells and macrophages. Multifocal meningeal infiltration by lymphocytes and mononuclear cells is another invariable feature but is rarely marked.

POSTVACCINIAL ENCEPHALOMYELITIS A severe demyelinating illness may occur following vaccination against rabies, with an incidence reported between 1 in 1000 and 1 in 4000 persons vaccinated. The lesion is presumably due to sensitization of brain tissue contained in the vaccine. The use of killed duck embryo vaccine which is free of nerve tissue has substantially reduced the incidence of the encephalomyelitic complications of rabies vaccination. More than 90 percent of the 30,000 rabies vaccinations performed in the United States each year now employ the safer but less potent duck embryo vaccine.

Encephalomyelitis following vaccination against smallpox has been known since 1860 but appears to have occurred only in isolated instances until 1922, when a real epidemic of postvaccinial encephalomyelitis was first recognized. The disease usually begins in the tenth to twelfth day after vaccination, though it may appear at any time between the second and twenty-fifth days. The mortality rate is high, between 30 and 50 percent, but varies among epidemics. If recovery occurs, it is usually complete. An estimate of incidence is 1 in 5000 vaccinated. The disease occurs much more frequently, perhaps as much as twenty times more often, after primary vaccination than after revaccination. Smallpox vaccination is no longer recommended as part of routine pediatric immunization schedules in the United States. The occurrence of the disease, as might be expected, parallels an increase in the number of persons vaccinated when smallpox threatens, but there is good evidence that the incidence of postvaccinial encephalomyelitis varies considerably from time to time and from one place to another. The source of material used for the vaccination seems to have no bearing on its occurrence.

The onset of the illness is generally abrupt, with headache, drowsiness, fever, and vomiting. There may be stiffness of the neck and other signs of meningeal irritation. Convulsions are occasionally seen. Soon afterward, signs of spinal cord involvement usually appear, with flaccid paralysis generally involving all four limbs, though hemiplegia may occur. Tendon reflexes disappear, and the plantar responses become extensor. Sphincter control is generally lost, and sensory loss, though variable, may be extensive and severe. Nystagmus, ocular palsies, and pupillary changes give evidence of brainstem involvement, and stupor and deepening coma indicate diencephalic or cerebral lesions. The onset of coma and evidence of brainstem involvement signify a rapid worsening of prognosis. Despite the general features of the typical case, variations are common. One patient may suffer a predominantly encephalitic illness with convulsions and coma and little evidence of cord damage, another may have a hemiplegia, or a pure transverse myelitis may occur without headache, neck stiffness, or clouding of consciousness. The site of vaccination has no influence on the neurological syndrome, and the florid skin lesions in the form of a generalized vaccinia or erythematous rash do not increase the likelihood of neuroparalytic accident. Spinal fluid almost invariably shows an increase in protein and lymphocytes, but in rare cases it is normal.

The association of the neurological disorder with vaccination or inoculation usually leaves the diagnosis in little doubt, and the characteristic combination of encephalitic and myelitic features will help to distinguish the condition from meningitis, virus encephalitis, and poliomyelitis. Rarely, an atypical case may mimic any one of these disorders. On occasion, the disease may suggest involvement of nerve roots and peripheral nerves and resemble idiopathic polyneuritis (Landry-Guillain-Barré syndrome).

Improvement involving recovery of consciousness and regression of neurological signs may be surprisingly complete. A significant proportion of patients may show residual neurological signs, intellectual impairment, and psychoneurotic sequelae many years after the illness, however.

POSTINFECTIOUS ENCEPHALOMYELITIS This syndrome is often referred to as *parainfectious encephalomyelitis* because of its onset prior to, in association with, or after the rash of measles or other exanthem.

Clinically evident neurological complications occur in 1 in 800 to 1 in 1000 cases of measles. Prior to widespread measles vaccination, a measles epidemic in a large city might have included 100,000 cases and therefore resulted in a substantial number of neurological complications. The mortality rate among patients with such complications ranges from 10 to 20 percent, and about 50 percent of the victims are left with persistent neurological damage. The rate of neurological complications may, in fact, be considerably higher than is apparent clinically. A high rate of abnormalities in the spinal fluid and in the electroencephalogram is observed in the studies of children with measles. Patients without clinically apparent neurological residua may undergo significant and sometimes permanent changes in behavior. The neurological complications of measles alone provide adequate justification for the prevention of the disease through the use of vaccine.

Following smallpox the incidence of neurological complications is approximately 2.5 cases out of 1000. The occurrence of encephalomyelitis complicating chickenpox is less common, and that complicating rubella is quite rare. An acute demyelinating process probably occurs in association with mumps, but the clinical picture is complicated by the presence of a true viral encephalomyelitis in mumps and often cannot be differentiated from a postinfectious process in the living patient.

The syndrome generally begins 2 to 4 days after the rash. The most common clinical picture is one dominated by convulsions and deepening coma. Less commonly, the patient may develop hemiplegia, show evidence of cerebellar disease, or occasionally develop a transverse myelitis or polyradiculitis. Chorea and athetoid movements are also seen infrequently. In many cases the disease is much less severe and the patient suffers transient encephalitic illness with headaches, confusion, and signs of meningeal irritation. It is not entirely clear that all the neurological complications described are truly encephalomyelitic; in some cases cerebrovascular disease, particularly thrombophlebitis, acute toxic encephalopathy (e.g., Reye's syndrome, Chap. 306), or hypoxic encephalopathy may be responsible.

The cerebrospinal fluid, as in postvaccinial encephalomyelitis, contains lymphocytes and an elevated protein level.

PREVENTION AND TREATMENT The recent decision to discontinue smallpox vaccination because of the virtual eradication of the disease will considerably reduce the risk of encephalomyelitis.

The use of killed duck embryo vaccine may well have largely eliminated the occurrence of post-rabies-vaccination encephalomyelitis. Measles vaccine has eliminated the largest group of the postinfectious encephalomyelitides in the United States.

The use of adrenocorticotropic hormone (ACTH) or high-potency steroids appears to be the treatment of choice, though controlled trials of this treatment have not been carried out. The steroids, if given early, appear to be effective in controlling the manifestations of experimental allergic encephalomyelitis in animals. If given after onset of symptoms they have little effect.

ACUTE NECROTIZING HEMORRHAGIC ENCEPHALOMYELITIS

In a small number of patients dying from a fulminating encephalopathic illness, certain distinctive pathological features may be found. On sectioning the brain, the white matter of one or both hemispheres is seen to be destroyed almost to the point of liquefaction. The involved tissue is pink or yellowish gray and flecked with multiple small hemorrhages. Sometimes similar changes are localized to the brainstem or spinal cord. On histological examination one finds widespread necrosis of small blood vessels, necrosis of brain tissue around the vessels with intense cellular infiltration, multiple small hemorrhages, and a violent inflammatory reaction in the meninges. The pathological picture resembles that of disseminated encephalomyelitis in its perivascular distribution, with the added feature of more widespread necrosis leading to incomplete necrosis and fibrin exudation in the walls of small blood vessels (venules), fibrin and platelet thrombi in some vessels, and a tendency for the parenchymal lesions to congregate into large foci in the cerebral hemispheres or brainstem.

The clinical course of the illness resembles that of acute disseminated encephalomyelitis save for its apoplectiform onset and rapidity of progress, sometimes leading to death within 48 h; it is also true that neurological signs are frequently unilateral, reflecting disease in one cerebral hemisphere, or bilateral, indicative of bulbar involvement. It is probable that certain patients showing an explosive myelitic illness are suffering from a necrotizing myelitis of similar type, but pathological

evidence in support of this view has been difficult to obtain. The cerebrospinal fluid examination discloses a more intense reaction than in other demyelinating diseases. Often a polymorphonuclear pleocytosis of up to several hundred cells and a considerable increase in amount of protein are detected.

The etiology of this condition remains obscure, but the resemblance to the other demyelinating diseases should be noted, a resemblance which is strengthened by the fact that certain patients showing the typically fulminating clinical picture have recovered, some completely, others with neurological sequelae of variable severity. Later, a few may develop typical multiple sclerosis. Acute encephalitis due to herpes simplex or other viruses also figures in the differential diagnosis. The points of similarity to other demyelinative diseases are sufficient to suggest that steroid drugs should be used in such cases; in several personally observed patients, we have had the impression that they produced a favorable result.

MULTIPLE SCLEROSIS

Multiple sclerosis, referred to in the British Commonwealth as *disseminated sclerosis* and among French-speaking physicians as *sclérose en plaque,* is one of the more common chronic neurological diseases. It is characterized clinically by episodes of focal disorder of the central nervous system (spinal cord, optic nerves, and brain) which remit and recur over a period of 20 to 30 or more years. Though it is pleomorphic in its clinical presentation, the picture it presents is determined by the location of foci of demyelination, which tend to have a predilection for certain portions of the nervous system. The result is a group of symptom complexes which can often be readily diagnosed.

Classic features include impaired vision, nystagmus, dysarthria, intention tremor, ataxia, impaired perception of position and vibratory senses, bladder dysfunction, weakness of a limb, paraplegia, and alteration in emotional responses. For purposes of diagnosis, it is generally required that both evidence of more than one discrete lesion and a history of exacerbation and partial or complete remission be present.

Diagnosis may be uncertain in the early years of the disease. Long latent periods between a minor initial symptom, which may not even come to medical attention, and the subsequent development of more characteristic ones may delay the final diagnosis. In most cases, relapses are interspersed with periods of remission, but in other cases (as many as half the total number) the disease presents as an intermittently or steadily progressive illness. The combination of (1) symptoms referable to tracts (white matter) in optic nerves, brainstem, and spinal cord, (2) a multiplicity of lesions, and (3) temporal dispersion of attacks makes the diagnosis certain.

PATHOLOGY Macroscopically, the brain before being sectioned generally shows no evidence of disease, but the surface of the spinal cord may appear and feel uneven. On section, numerous scattered lesions are seen which are slightly depressed and which, by virtue of their pinkish gray appearance (due to loss of myelin) stand out in contrast to the surrounding white matter. The lesions may vary in diameter from less than 1 mm to several centimeters; they affect principally the white matter of brain and spinal cord and do not extend beyond the root entry zone of brainstem and spinal cord. They also encroach frequently on cerebral gray matter but do not destroy nerve cells. The lesions appear to have a predilection for elongate structures where myelin abuts pial veins; hence the frequent involvement of spinal cord and the optic nerves and chiasm. They are regularly seen in the paraventricular areas of the brain in relation to the veins in the walls of the lateral ventricles.

The histological appearance depends on the age of the lesion. Relatively recent lesions show a predominantly perivenous distribution of the demyelination with sparing of axis cylinders, degeneration of oligodendroglia, neuroglial reaction, and perivascular infiltration with mononuclear cells. Later large numbers of microglial phagocytes infiltrate the lesion, and astrocytes in and around it increase in number and size. A long-standing lesion, on the other hand, will show thickly matted, relatively acellular fibroglial tissue, with only occasional perivascular macrophages; in such a lesion intact axis cylinders may still be discovered, but many have by then been destroyed, and this is turn leads to descending and ascending degeneration of long-fiber tracts. All gradations of pathological change between these two extremes may be found in lesions of variegated size and shape.

ETIOLOGY The cause or causes of multiple sclerosis remain undetermined. A number of epidemiologic facts have been clearly established, however, and they must eventually be incorporated in any etiologic hypothesis. The disease has been shown to be rare between the equator and latitudes 30 and 35° north and south. It becomes more common with increasing latitude thereafter. For example, the prevalence of multiple sclerosis is six times as great in Winnipeg, Manitoba, as in New Orleans, Louisiana. An exception to the geographic pattern appears to exist in Japan, where the prevalence rates are uniform and extremely low. Several studies indicate that persons who migrate from a high-risk to a low-risk zone carry the high risk of multiple sclerosis with them, even though the disease may not become apparent until 20 years after migration. This pattern has been demonstrated both in South Africa and in Israel. However, if emigration occurs prior to age 15, the risk of acquiring multiple sclerosis is that of the country into which these persons migrate.

An increase in familial occurrence of multiple sclerosis has long been recognized. The disease is about eight times more common in immediate relatives (parents and sibs) than in patients in the general population. Twin studies have failed, however, to corroborate a genetic predisposition, and within families with more than one affected member, no consistent genetic pattern is evident. There is a tendency to consider all diseases with an increased familial incidence, such as multiple sclerosis, as hereditary. Instances of the same condition in several members of the family may actually reflect common exposure to a similar environmental factor, however. For example, paralytic poliomyelitis is also eight times more common in immediate family members than in the general population.

The age distribution at onset of the disease follows a normal distribution, with a mean of about 30 years. Women have a higher prevalence and incidence than men.

Several studies have demonstrated a shift toward higher socioeconomic groups in the general pattern of distribution of the disease in the population. Earlier studies of lymphocyte subtypes showing that approximately 85 percent of patients with multiple sclerosis are positive for HLA-A3 or HLA-A7 and that these two types are also infrequent in populations resistant to multiple sclerosis have not been corroborated. The interpretation of these data is uncertain. The similarity of some of the lesions of multiple sclerosis to those of experimental allergic encephalomyelitis suggests an autoimmune mechanism. This theory is supported by the demonstration (Whitaker) of encephalomyelitogenic protein in the cerebrospinal fluid of patients in an acute phase of multiple sclerosis. Lam-

pert's article reviews the possible relationships between virus infections and autoimmunity.

All these data favor an infection, presumably viral, contracted early in life and capable of evoking disease over the entire span of adolescence and adulthood. Its mechanism may be that of an autoimmune reaction, attacking myelin, but in its most intense form destroying all tissue elements, including axis cylinders. A number of "candidate" viruses have been proposed, but none has been consistently isolated from body fluids or brain tissue. The hypothesis linking multiple sclerosis to household dogs and cats (exposure during childhood) continues to be debated. The data favoring an infectious etiology with a long incubation period are mainly epidemiologic.

PRECIPITATING FACTORS A variety of events occurring immediately before the onset of illness have been regarded as precipitating factors in relation to multiple sclerosis. These include various types of infection, emotional trauma, injury, and pregnancy. There is a definite increase in the number of exacerbations during the pregnancy year, and also in the 3 months after delivery, but the significance is not known. Other traumatic factors during the course of the illness, including lumbar puncture and surgical procedures, have not been shown to be of statistical significance. Nor have emotions been shown to play a part in the evolution of the disease.

CLINICAL MANIFESTATIONS About 40 percent of patients with multiple sclerosis have an episode of optic neuritis as their initial symptom. The syndrome is one of rapid onset over a period of several days of partial or total loss of vision in one eye, often associated with pain on movement of the eye. Characteristically, a scotoma will be present involving macular vision, but a wide variety of field defects may occur. Some patients will develop bilateral optic neuritis simultaneously or within a few days to weeks. In about half the patients, if serial examination is carried out, some evidence of inflammation or elevation of the optic nerve, termed *optic papillitis*, will be seen. The occurrence of papillitis depends on the proximity of the demyelinating lesion to the nerve head. It should be recalled that the optic nerve is in fact a tract of the brain, important because demyelinating lesions in multiple sclerosis are known not to occur outside the central nervous system. Of patients with optic neuritis about one-third recover completely, one-third will show considerable improvement, one-third will show no evidence of improvement whatever. As in most acute exacerbations of demyelinating disease, improvement in the majority of cases will have begun within 2 weeks of the onset of neurological damage. Much longer periods of up to months may elapse, however, during which improvement in neurological function may occur. As described in Chap. 18, some patients who have never complained of optic neuritis and have no pallor (atrophy) of the optic disks will be found to have slow retinal-occipital conduction velocities (when patterned stimuli are used). This indicates subclinical involvement. It should be noted that a maximum of 30 to 40 percent of patients who develop optic neuritis will go on to have other lesions of multiple sclerosis. It is unclear at this time whether optic neuritis, when it occurs alone and is not followed by other evidence of demyelinating disease, is a subclass of multiple sclerosis with only a single lesion or a manifestation of other disease processes. No other etiology for optic neuritis has been established at this time.

The remaining 60 to 70 percent of patients with multiple sclerosis who give no history of optic neuritis will present with some evidence of a lesion of the spinal cord or brainstem. The involvement of the posterior columns of the cord is responsible for the commonly related symptoms of tingling of the extremities and the tight bandlike sensations around trunk or limbs.

Numbness or weakness of a limb or one side of the body (arm and leg) or in an asymmetric distribution in all four extremities follows retrobulbar neuritis in frequency. The resulting clinical syndromes vary from mere dragging or poor control of one or both legs, to an ataxic paraparesis or spastic paraparesis. The tendon reflexes are hyperactive; the abdominal reflexes are absent, and plantar responses are extensor.

Diplopia, as a result of brainstem lesions, is another common presenting complaint. These lesions may cause an internuclear ophthalmoplegia that is due to involvement of the medial longitudinal fasciculus and is characterized by inability to adduct one or the other eye on lateral gaze in either direction or by nystagmus present to a greater degree in the abducting than the adducting eye. An internuclear ophthalmoplegia, when present bilaterally in a young adult, is virtually diagnostic of multiple sclerosis. (Rarely it occurs in lupus erythematosus or other lesion.) Other ocular palsies are also observed but less frequently. Other manifestations of brainstem involvement include transient facial anesthesia and vertigo and vomiting because of affection of the vestibular connections. The occurrence of tic douloureux on one or both sides in a young person due to involvement of the fifth cranial nerve should immediately bring to mind the diagnosis of multiple sclerosis.

Nystagmus and cerebellar ataxia, with or without weakness and spasticity of the limbs, represent another common syndrome and reflect involvement of the cerebellum and corticospinal tracts and their connections. The ataxia of cerebellar type can be recognized by scanning speech, tremors and titubation of the head, intention tremors of arms and legs, and incoordination of voluntary movements. It may be mixed with sensory ataxia from involvement of the posterior columns of the spinal cord. Ultimately spinal cord involvement becomes predominant in most advanced cases. It is a common aphorism that the patient with multiple sclerosis presents with symptoms in one leg and signs in both. The patient will complain of weakness, ataxia, or sensory loss in one lower extremity and have evidence of bilateral corticospinal tract disease manifested by Babinski's sign in both lower extremities.

Symptoms of bladder dysfunction, including hesitancy, urgency, frequency, and incontinence, occur commonly with spinal cord involvement. In males, these symptoms are often associated with impotence, a symptom which the patient will often not report unless specifically questioned in that regard. About 5 percent of patients with multiple sclerosis, over the course of their disease, will have a seizure, presumably as the result of involvement of subcortical connections.

It has been often pointed out that patients with multiple sclerosis develop euphoria, a pathological cheerfulness or lack of concern which seems inappropriate in relation to their obvious neurological deficit. This syndrome, the result of lesions of the white matter, probably of the frontal lobes, is often associated with other signs of cerebral impairment. There are, however, a large number of patients who are depressed, irritable, and short-tempered, as a reaction to the disabling features of the disease. They may also have other psychological deficits, such as loss of memory, because of lesions in other locations.

CLINICAL COURSE The symptoms described above may occur individually or in combination during exacerbations. Some patients will have a series of exacerbations of the disease, each with complete remission. Often such exacerbations may be severe enough to cause total quadriplegia or even coma. Most patients will have a series of exacerbations, each followed by a remission or stabilization and leaving in its wake some evidence of permanent neurological deficit upon which succeeding acute manifestations are superimposed. After a period of years some patients who have had a series of acute exacerbations tend to develop an inexorably progressing downhill course. When the initial course of the disease is steadily pro-

gressive and the lesion is limited to the spinal cord, diagnosis is particularly difficult. Such cases tend to occur among the older group of patients. It has been suggested that this syndrome be considered a special subclass of multiple sclerosis, but it probably represents only a late phase of the disease, the earlier phases having been subclinical or overlooked. Diagnosis can be made only by exclusion or may be confirmed by abnormality of spinal fluid.

CEREBROSPINAL FLUID In a small number of cases, particularly the acute ones, there may be a slight mononuclear pleocytosis in the spinal fluid. This pleocytosis in in fact the only way in which activity of the disease may be measured at this time. None of the other laboratory tests aid in measuring the activity or inactivity of the disease.

The proportion of gamma globulin in the spinal fluid appears to be altered in multiple sclerosis, while the protein content is relatively normal. The alteration in distribution of globulins may be demonstrated by an abnormality of the colloidal gold curve, usually a first-zone abnormality, in the presence of a negative Wassermann reaction. When gamma-globulin content is measured directly, it is abnormal in about 60 percent of the patients with multiple sclerosis. The gamma-globulin abnormality, however, tends to reflect the duration of the disease, and therefore is usually abnormal in the established case rather than in an initial exacerbation when an abnormal laboratory test would be helpful in establishing the diagnosis.

Some patients with demyelinating disease will have elevations of spinal fluid protein, but a spinal fluid protein in excess of 100 mg per 100 ml is so uncommon in multiple sclerosis that another diagnosis should be entertained. Of the diagnostic laboratory tests an elevation of gamma globulin in the cerebrospinal fluid is the most widely used. Recently radioimmune assay of basic myelin protein is said to have been helpful, as have also the IgG/albumin ratio and oligoclonal IgG bands. The latter are observed in over 90 percent of cases, according to Johnson and Nelson.

Acute multiple sclerosis Occasionally, multiple sclerosis runs an acute or subacute course leading to death in weeks or months. Alternatively, an acute course may develop rapidly, then remit partially or completely, to be followed by characteristic relapses. In some of these cases, the onset is marked by headache, vomiting, delirium, and a succession of symptoms indicating severe involvement of the brainstem or the brain, optic nerves, and spinal cord. In the so-called "cerebral" cases, there may be mental changes, convulsions, aphasia, hemianopia, and variable long-tract signs; the spinal type may show the picture of transverse myelitis. These forms of the disease are uncommon and are difficult to distinguish from disseminated encephalomyelitis, with which we tend to group them. They differ pathologically in the larger size of lesions, being more like those of multiple sclerosis.

Neuromyelitis optica syndrome This disorder, referred to as *Devic's disease,* is said to represent a combination of bilateral optic neuritis and transverse myelitis. Attempts at clinical description of patients with this combination of symptoms have failed to provide any data of prognostic value. Perhaps it is best to consider neuromyelitis optica as a particular form of multiple sclerosis. Pathological studies of fatal cases, particularly those in which cavitation of white matter is found, have revealed a more acute and uniformly destructive process than is often seen in multiple sclerosis, however. Recurrence of this necrotizing form gives rise to a clinicopathologic state known as *subacute necrotizing myelitis* (see Chap. 375).

DIAGNOSIS In the characteristic case with evidence of wide dissemination of the lesions throughout the nervous system, the diagnosis of multiple sclerosis is in little doubt. It is an excellent clinical rule that the disease should not be diagnosed when all the patient's symptoms and signs can be explained by a single lesion. Disseminated encephalomyelitis is a self-limited, monophasic disease, and stupor and coma occur only rarely in multiple sclerosis. The other acute manifestations may mimic labyrinthitis, meningovascular syphilis, and encephalitis.

There are other multifocal and recurrent diseases of the central nervous system that may mimic multiple sclerosis. Lupus erythematosus may occasionally affect the brain and spinal cord in this way. Other diseases to be considered are: encephalomyeloradiculitis with and without carcinoma, Whipple's disease, histiocytosis, granulomatous arteritis, Wegener's granuloma, neoplastic angioendotheliosis, toxoplasmosis, and meningovascular syphilis.

Monocular impairment of vision may also occur with vascular lesions of optic nerve, chorioretinitis, and papillophlebitis. The latter two diseases can usually be distinguished from retrobulbar neuritis by the appearance of the retinas.

Confusion may occasionally arise with the hereditary ataxias, which are generally distinguished by their familial incidence and other associated genetic traits and by their stereotyped clinical pattern. Amyotrophic lateral sclerosis and subacute combined degeneration may occasionally be mimicked by demyelinating disease, but muscle wasting, fasciculations, and the total absence of sensory involvement will identify the former, and the latter can be confirmed by a low level of vitamin B_{12} in the serum, the presence of megaloblasts in the bone marrow, anemia present in many cases, and the absence of acid in the gastric secretions.

Patients with a progressive spastic paraplegia should be carefully evaluated for the presence of intrathecal neoplasm or cervical spondylosis. Radicular pain at some point in the illness is a frequent manifestation of neoplasm and is rare in multiple sclerosis, and severe muscle wasting due to anterior horn or spinal root involvement, as is sometimes seen in spondylosis, is almost unknown in multiple sclerosis except in the rare cases of necrotizing myelitis. The occurrence of nystagmus in association with other neurological symptoms should be carefully evaluated. A common cause of nystagmus is the ingestion of barbiturates or diphenylhydantoin. The possibility that an anxious patient with another neurological lesion has taken a barbiturate to aid him or her in sleep should never be disregarded when nystagmus in association with evidence of a lesion elsewhere might establish a diagnosis of multiple sclerosis. Slowed optic-calcarine, auditory-cortical, and tactile-cortical conduction velocities in conjunction with a chronic myelopathy are helpful in the diagnosis of a chronic myelopathy for they indicate multiple lesions of the white matter in other parts of the nervous system.

Basilar impression of the skull, or platybasia, should also be considered in the differential diagnosis, but patients with this condition have a characteristic shortening of the neck, and careful radiographs of the base of the skull will be diagnostic. Occasional tumors of the posterior fossa have been misdiagnosed as multiple sclerosis because of the affection of a wide variety of neurological systems in the brainstem.

Careful clinical appraisal will usually lead to accurate diagnosis, but the label "multiple sclerosis" should not be placed upon a patient until the evidence is unequivocal. Such a diagnosis will explain almost any subsequent neurological event, and attention may be directed away from the possibility of another, perhaps treatable, disease.

PROGNOSIS The duration of the disease is exceedingly variable. Though some patients die within a few months, the average duration of the disease is in excess of 20 years. At the end of 25 years one-third of patients are still actively carrying out their work, and two-thirds of those surviving are still ambulatory. Patients with milder and quiescent disease are, of course, less likely to come to the attention of the hospital-oriented physician. In a recent epidemiologic study, 74 percent of patients with multiple sclerosis survived 25 years, as compared with 86 percent of the comparable general population.

The final state of the young bedridden, incontinent patient, racked by painful flexor spasms of the lower limbs and febrile episodes of intercurrent infection from bedsores is one of the most distressing in medicine.

TREATMENT A large number of remedies have been tried in the treatment of multiple sclerosis, and many have been thought to be successful because of the remitting nature of the disease. Only the use of ACTH has withstood evaluation in reasonably controlled trials of exacerbations of both optic neuritis and multiple sclerosis. A substantial group of patients, however, fail to respond to this treatment in the acute exacerbation.

ACTH has been generally preferred over the corticosteroids in the treatment of multiple sclerosis because the initial trials and control studies have been carried out with it. A variety of dosage regimens have been employed. It seems important that a high dose be used initially to be effective. We give ACTH intravenously in a dose of 80 units in 500 ml dextrose and water for 3 days, followed by 40 units gel intramuscularly every 12 h for 7 days. The dose is then reduced by 10 units every 3 days. Many patients who show improvement on this therapy continue to improve or maintain their previous improvement even though the medication is gradually reduced and discontinued. Other patients begin to have a recurrence of symptoms as the dose is gradually reduced and are often maintained on small doses of ACTH (20 to 40 units) every other day for a period of several months. Because of the risk of potassium depletion, the patients are given potassium supplement in a dose of 60 meq per day.

The addition of lithium prophylactically to prevent steroid psychosis (including depression, hypomania, or confusional states which have occurred in 14 percent of patients treated) has virtually eliminated that complication. Blood levels are maintained at 0.8 to 1.2 meq per liter with 300 mg given orally in three to six tablets daily. A tranquilizer may be necessary because of the complaints of nervousness and difficulty in sleeping. Peripheral edema due to sodium retention can be treated with mild diuretics and salt restriction. Cimetidine, 300 mg four times a day, may be helpful in preventing steroid-related ulcers, though that is not yet unequivocally established. The activation of tuberculosis must be considered, and, in patients with previously active tuberculosis, prophylactic antibiotics may be advisable. Hirsutism and acne cannot be prevented but disappear when the medication is stopped.

The importance of an understanding and sympathetic physician cannot be overemphasized in the care of patients with a chronic debilitating neurological disease of this kind. Some patients consider the uncertainty of prognosis worse than true disability. General support can be rendered by providing bed rest in acute exacerbations, prevention of excessive fatigue, and meticulous attention to the prevention of bedsores in the disabled patient by the use of alternating pressure mattresses, silicone gel pads, and other special devices. The use of belladonna alkaloids and bethanechol chloride in the treatment of bladder dysfunction can be helpful. Antibiotics and acidifying drugs to treat and suppress urinary tract infections should also be employed. In patients with disorders of bowel function a program of bowel training can often be successfully undertaken. Several drugs are helpful in relieving spasticity [diazepam (Valium) 5 to 10 mg tid, baclofen (Liorisol) 25 mg tid], but in some instances the weakness becomes more evident as the spasticity lessens.

DIFFUSE CEREBRAL SCLEROSIS

In 1912 Schilder first called attention to a disease causing progressive massive demyelination of the white matter often beginning in one or both occipital or temporal lobes. It has been referred to as *Schilder's disease* or *encephalitis periaxialis diffusa*. Since that time, many other cases have been described, some resembling Schilder's original description, some being but examples of cerebral multiple sclerosis, and others differing with respect to familial occurrence and widespread symmetrical destruction and gliosis of the white matter, often with metachromatic bodies and globoid bodies representing catabolic products of myelin.

The diffuse types of cerebral sclerosis constitute a group of entities, including adrenoleukodystrophy, Pelizaeus-Merzbacher disease (both male sex-linked diseases), the globoid body leukodystrophy of Krabbe, sudanophilic leukodystrophy, and the metachromatic leukodystrophy of Greenfield which may involve peripheral nerves as well as central nervous system tissue. For the moment, they are a group of diseases of genetic origin occurring sporadically, characterized clinically by progressive visual failure, mental deterioration, and spastic paralysis and pathologically by massive demyelination of the white matter of the cerebral hemispheres. Each entity is unquestionably a specific inherited biochemical defect in the metabolism of myelin proteolipids. The precise pathogenetic mechanisms of these diseases for the moment are unknown, and there is no treatment. For further discussion see the appropriate heading in the chapter on degenerative diseases of the nervous system (Chap. 373).

REFERENCES

ADAMS RD, KUBIK CS: The morbid anatomy of the demyelinative disease. Am J Med 12:510, 1952

JOHNSON KP, NELSON BJ: Multiple sclerosis: Diagnostic usefulness of CSF. Ann Neurol 2:425, 1977

LAMPERT PW: Autoimmune and virus induced demyelinative diseases. Arch Pathol (in press)

MCALPINE D et al: *Multiple Sclerosis, a Reappraisal.* Edinburgh, E and S Livingstone, 1965

MILLAR JHD: *Multiple Sclerosis. A Disease Acquired in Childhood.* Springfield, Ill, Charles C Thomas, 1971

PERCY AK et al: Multiple sclerosis in Rochester, Minnesota. A 60-year appraisal. Arch Neurol 25:105, 1971

POSKANZER DC: Epidemiological evidence for a viral etiology for multiple sclerosis, in *Slow, Latent and Temperate Virus Infections,* NINDB Monograph no 2. US Department of Health, Education and Welfare, 1965, p 55

——— et al: Lithium prophylaxis in ACTH-induced psychosis. JAMA 1979 (in press)

WHITAKER JN: Myelin encephalitogenic protein fragments in CSF of persons with multiple sclerosis. Neurology 34:911, 1977

371

METABOLIC DISEASES OF THE NERVOUS SYSTEM

MAURICE VICTOR
RAYMOND D. ADAMS

Included under this title is a large and varied group of neurologic disorders united by one particular attribute—that of deranging in some way the metabolism of nervous tissue. This derangement must be ascribed in the final analysis to some fundamental and often unique biochemical abnormality of the neurons involved. In a sense this can be said of all disease processes, but it is in the metabolic disorders that the importance of biochemical factors is most evident.

The metabolic diseases of the nervous system can be divided readily into two distinct categories—acquired and inherited. In the acquired type, a disturbance of cerebral function is usually consequent upon disease in some other organ system—heart (and circulation), lungs (and respiration), kidneys, liver, pancreas, and endocrine glands. The inherited type, as the name indicates, is characterized by an inborn abnormality of metabolism, which affects both the brain and other organs; reference is made here to such conditions as the aminoacidurias with mental defect, the mucopolysaccharidoses, the lipidoses, the lipoproteinemias, several of the leukodystrophies, hepatolenticular degeneration, porphyria, galactosemia, and the glycogen storage diseases.

In this chapter, emphasis will be on the acquired metabolic diseases, and appropriately so, insofar as they are essentially disorders of adult life and a major source of concern to medical internist and neurologist alike. In fact no other category of disease so clearly exemplifies the interdependence of these two medical disciplines.

The inherited metabolic diseases, on the other hand, are fundamentally disorders of infancy and early childhood and are more appropriately considered in a textbook of pediatrics. One group of these diseases, the lysosomal storage diseases, is discussed in Chap. 101. Other inherited diseases, which permit survival to adolescence or early adult life or which have their onset during these periods, are discussed in this and in other chapters of this book, to which the reader will be referred.

ACQUIRED (SECONDARY) METABOLIC DISEASES OF THE NERVOUS SYSTEM

METABOLIC DISEASES PRESENTING AS A SYNDROME OF EPISODIC CONFUSION, STUPOR OR COMA The *syndrome of impaired consciousness* has been described in detail in Chap. 20. There it was pointed out that metabolic disturbances are frequent causes of impaired consciousness and that their presence must always be considered when there are no focal or lateralizing signs of cerebral disease and no cellular changes in the spinal fluid. Intoxication with alcohol and other drugs figures prominently in the differential diagnosis.

Anoxic encephalopathy This is one of the most frequent and disastrous accidents encountered in the emergency and operating rooms of every general hospital. The basic disorder is a lack of oxygen supply to the brain, the result of failure of the heart and circulation or of the lungs and respiration. Often both are responsible, and one cannot say which predominates—hence the ambiguous allusion in clinical records to "cardiorespiratory failure." The conditions which most often lead to anoxic encephalopathy are (1) suffocation (from drowning, strangulation, aspiration of vomitus or blood, surgical pack, or foreign body in the trachea); (2) CO poisoning, in which respiration fails first and then cardiovascular functions; (3) diseases which paralyze the muscles of respiration (Landry-Guillain-Barré syndrome) or damage the central nervous system diffusely (trauma and vascular diseases of the brain, epilepsy), again with respiratory failure being the initial factor, preceding cardiac failure; and (4) myocardial infarction, hemorrhage, shock, and circulatory collapse, cardiac arrest during inhalation of spinal anesthesia, and infective and traumatic shock, in all of which conditions cardiac action is paralyzed before respiration.

CLINICAL FEATURES Mild degrees of hypoxia induce only inattentiveness, impaired judgment, and motor incoordination and have no lasting effects. With severe hypoxia or anoxia, as occurs with cardiac arrest, consciousness is lost within seconds, but recovery will be complete if breathing, oxygenation of blood, and cardiac action are restored within 3 to 5 min. If anoxia persists beyond this time, serious and permanent injury to the brain results, particularly to those parts with marginal efficiency of their circulation (globus pallidus, cerebellum, hippocampus, and parietooccipital lobes in "border-zone regions"). Clinically, it is difficult to judge the precise degree of hypoxia since slight heart action or an imperceptible blood pressure may serve to maintain the circulation to some extent. Hence some individuals have made an excellent recovery after cerebral anoxia that allegedly lasted 8 to 10 min or longer. *An important clinical rule is that degrees of hypoxia which at no time abolish consciousness rarely if ever cause permanent damage to the nervous system.* Also, generally speaking, subjects who demonstrate intact brainstem function when the acute hypoxic event has terminated (as indicated by normal ciliospinal and pupillary light responses, intact doll's head eye movements, and oculovestibular responses) tend to have a better outlook for recovery of consciousness and perhaps all of their faculties. Conversely, absence of these reflex activities and the presence of pupils that are persistently fixed to light suggest a hopeless outlook.

The most severe degrees of anoxia are manifested by a state of complete unawareness and unresponsiveness with abolition of the brainstem reflexes. Natural respiration cannot be sustained; only *cardiac action and blood pressure are maintained.* No electrical activity is seen in the EEG (it is isoelectric). This is called the *brain death syndrome.* When caused by anoxia-hypotension it is always irreversible. At autopsy nearly all the cerebral, cerebellar, and brainstem tissues are found to be destroyed. One must exercise extreme caution in concluding that the patient has "brain death," because anesthesia, drug intoxication, and hypothermia may also cause deep coma and an isoelectric EEG, but permit recovery. Such cases have been brought increasingly to public attention because of ethical and moral issues that surround the question of discontinuing medical therapy. In the authors' experience "brain death" victims usually cannot be sustained for more than several days; in other words, the problem settles itself, and it is not so difficult as the cases in which the patient has suffered severe but somewhat lesser degrees of cerebral damage, to be described below.

The patient who has suffered a serious hypoxic episode and whose breathing and heart action are stable when first seen has safely passed the initial phase of the hypoxic crisis. Yet such patients may be profoundly comatose, with eyes slightly divergent and motionless but with reactive pupils, inert and flaccid or intensely rigid limbs, and diminished tendon reflexes. Within a few minutes after cardiac action and breathing have been restored, generalized convulsions and isolated or grouped twitches of muscles (myoclonus) supervene. If the damage has been severe, coma persists, decerebrate postures may be present or occur upon pinching the limbs, and bilateral Babinski signs can be evoked. In the first 24 to 48 h death may terminate this state in a setting of rising temperature, deepening coma, and circulatory collapse. Or with lesser degrees of injury, where the cerebral and cerebellar cortices are partly or completely destroyed but brainstem-spinal structures remain intact, the individual may survive in a state referred to as "irreversible coma" or "vegetative state." Some of these patients remain mute, unresponsive, and unaware of their environment for weeks, months, or years. The medical profession is searching for criteria that will accurately predict this hopeless state early in the comatose period, but the data are as yet insecure. If intoxication can be excluded, the presence of fixed dilated pupils and paralysis of eye movement for 24 to 48 h, along with marked slowing of the EEG, usually signifies irreversible cerebral damage. We have not observed deep coma of this type, lasting more than 5 days, to be attended by recovery.

Patients with lesser degrees of injury improve after a period of coma. Consciousness is regained, and then various degrees of confusion, visual agnosia, extrapyramidal rigidity, or movement disorder (action or intention myoclonus, choreoathetosis) become manifest. Some of these patients quickly pass through this acute hypoxic phase and proceed to make a full recovery; others are left with permanent neurologic sequelae. The *posthypoxic syndromes* that we have observed most frequently are (1) *persistent coma or stupor;* and, with lesser degree of cerebral injury, (2) *dementia,* with or without extrapyramidal signs; (3) *visual agnosia;* (4) *parkinsonism;* (5) *choreoathetosis;* (6) *cerebellar ataxia;* (7) *intention or action myoclonus;* and (8) *Korsakoff's amnesic state. Seizures* may or may not continue to be a problem.

A relatively uncommon and unexplained phenomenon is *delayed postanoxic encephalopathy.* Initial improvement, which appears to be complete, is followed after a variable period of time (2 to 21 days) by a relapse, characterized by apathy, confusion, irritability, and occasionally agitation or mania. A few patients have recovered from this second episode, but in most of them there has been progression of the neurologic syndrome, with diffuse rigidity and spasticity, coma, and death after 1 to 2 weeks. Some of these cases have been associated with widespread cerebral demyelination. Exceptionally, yet another delayed syndrome occurs, where a period of hypoxia is followed by a slow, deteriorative state, affecting basal ganglia more than cerebral cortex and white matter, which then progresses for weeks to months until the patient is mute, rigid, and helpless.

The essential *mechanism* in hypoxic encephalopathy is a lack of oxygen and an arrest of all aerobic metabolic processes necessary to sustain the Krebs tricarboxylic cycle and the elec-

TABLE 371-1
Classification of the acquired metabolic disorders of the nervous system

I Presenting as a syndrome of episodic confusion, stupor, or coma
   A Hypoxic-hypotensive encephalopathy
   B Hypercapnic encephalopathy
   C Hypoglycemic encephalopathy
   D Hepatic and portal-systemic encephalopathy
   E Uremic and dialysis encephalopathy
   F Encephalopathies due to electrolyte disturbances
II Presenting as a progressive extrapyramidal syndrome
   A Acquired hepatocerebral degeneration
   B Kernicterus
   C Hypoparathyroidism
III Presenting as cerebellar ataxia
   A Hyperthermia
   B Hypothyroidism
IV Causing psychoses or dementia
   A Cushing's disease and steroid encephalopathy
   B Thyroid psychoses
   C Hyperparathyroidism
   D Addison's disease (adrenal insufficiency)
   E Pancreatic encephalopathy

tron transport system. Lactic acid accumulates in the tissues. Deprived of their source of energy, neurons proceed to catabolize themselves in order to maintain their activity and in so doing damage themselves to such a degree that they cannot survive. The phenomenon of delayed progression is not understood but may be due to the blockage or exhaustion of some enzymatic process during the period when brain metabolism is restored or even increased (as in hyperthermia).

DIAGNOSIS This depends on (1) the history of the hypoxic event and evidence of reduced oxygenation of arterial blood ($P_{O_2} < 40$ mmHg), CO intoxication (the latter is indicated by its spectroscopic band or cherry red color of the skin for a few minutes to hours after the episode), blood pressures below 70 mmHg systolic, or cardiac arrest; and (2) the typical clinical sequences of events outlined above after a possible hypoxic episode has terminated. Renal damage (anuria) and myocardial infarction may also have occurred (see Chap. 20) and provide corroborative evidence of hypoxia.

TREATMENT The treatment of anoxic encephalopathy is directed mainly at the prevention of a critical degree of hypoxic injury. After a clear airway is secured, artificial respiration, external thoracic cardiac massage, open-chest surgery, and the use of a cardiac defibrillator or pacemaker all have their place, and every second counts in their prompt utilization. Once cardiac and pulmonary function are restored, there is some evidence that reducing cerebral metabolic requirements by continuous hypothermia for 48 to 72 h may prevent the delayed worsening referred to above. Oxygen may be of value during the first hours, but is probably of little use after the blood becomes well oxygenated. Dexamethasone administered intravenously in doses of 6 to 12 mg every 6 h helps to combat brain (cellular) swelling. Seizures should be controlled by the methods indicated in Chap. 367. If the seizures are severe, continuous, and unresponsive to drugs, controlled respiration and curare may be required. Often the seizures cease after a few days. If they persist, they are often myoclonic, and mephobarbital (Mebaral), in divided doses up to 500 mg per day, phenobarbital, 300 mg per day, or clonazepam, 8 to 12 mg daily in divided doses, may be useful in their control.

Hypercapnic encephalopathy Chronic emphysema, chronic fibrosing lung disease, and in some instances a seeming inadequacy of the respiratory center lead to chronic respiratory acidosis, with an elevation of P_{CO_2} and a reduction in arterial P_{O_2}. Secondary polycythemia and cor pulmonale often accompany these diseases of the lungs, and pulmonary infection may be superimposed.

The clinical syndrome consequent upon hypercapnia (and hypoxia) comprises generalized or bilateral frontal or occipital headache, often intense and persistent for hours; papilledema; mental dullness, drowsiness, confusion, stupor, and coma; a fast-frequency action tremor and coarse twitching of all muscles that are in a state of sustained contraction; and an inability to maintain a fixed posture or a voluntary movement because of brief interruptions of muscle action potentials (asterixis). Intermittent drowsiness, disinterest in and inattention to the environment, reduction of psychomotor activity, imperception of the sequence of events, and forgetfulness constitute the more subtle manifestations of this syndrome.

In fully developed cases, the cerebrospinal fluid (CSF) is under increased pressure, P_{CO_2} may exceed 75 mmHg, and oxygen saturation of arterial blood ranges from 85 to 40 percent. The EEG reveals slow activity, in the delta and theta range, sometimes bilaterally synchronous. The mechanism of the cerebral disorder is said to be CO_2 narcosis, but the biochemical details are not known. The danger of administering morphine or sedatives, which depress the respiratory center (now insensi-

tive to CO_2), or the inhalation of oxygen, which removes the sole stimulus to the respiratory center, is now widely recognized.

Forced ventilation with an intermittent positive-pressure respirator, treatment of heart failure with digitalis and diuretics, venesection to reduce the viscosity of the blood, and antibiotics to combat pulmonary infection are the most effective therapeutic measures. If stupor or coma persists, the arterial O_2 level should be rechecked; it may be critically reduced. Or the pH of the CSF may be very low, in the range of 7.15 to 7.25. In CO_2 narcosis, correction of the acidosis of blood is easier than that of CSF, which tends to lag.

Unlike pure hypoxic encephalopathy, hypercapnia rarely causes prolonged coma, and in our experience it has not led to irreversible brain damage. The papilledema and the intermittent lapses of sustained postures or asterixis (the latter characteristic of liver failure, hypercapnia, uremia, and rarely other metabolic disorders) are important diagnostic features. The syndrome of hypercapnia is apt to be mistaken for brain tumor, a confusional psychosis of nondescript type, or a disease causing myoclonus or chorea. In the latter instance it must be distinguished from a chronic extrapyramidal syndrome, as described further on in this chapter.

Hypoglycemic encephalopathy (see also Chaps. 20 and 340) This condition is a relatively infrequent but important cause of episodic confusion, convulsions, and coma. The essential biochemical abnormality is a blood glucose level of less than 25 to 30 mg per 100 ml (lower in infants), which, if it lasts for about 90 min, leads to exhaustion of the store of cerebral glucose and glycogen. Within this brief span of time, as cerebral oxidation proceeds without exogenous glucose, the lipid and protein components of neurons are metabolized, and irreversible damage occurs. Long before the 90 min have elapsed, however, the severely hypoglycemic patient becomes deeply comatose.

The most common causes of hypoglycemic encephalopathy are (1) accidental or deliberate overdose of insulin or of an oral antidiabetic agent, (2) an islet cell, insulin-secreting tumor of the pancreas, (3) rarely an alcoholic debauch, (4) acute nonicteric hepatic encephalopathy of childhood (Reye's syndrome), (5) glycogen storage disease in infancy, and (6) an idiopathic state in the neonatal period. In the past, hypoglycemic encephalopathy was a rather frequent complication of "insulin shock" therapy of schizophrenia. In functional hyperinsulinism the hypoglycemia is rarely of sufficient severity or duration to damage the central nervous system.

As the level of blood glucose descends, to about 30 mg per 100 ml, the initial symptoms appear—nervousness, hunger, flushed facies, sweating and trembling—and these gradually give way to confusion, drowsiness, and occasionally excitement or overactivity. In the next stage, forced sucking, grasping, motor restlessness, muscular spasms, and finally decerebrate rigidity occur, in that sequence. Myoclonic twitching and convulsions may develop in some patients but are by no means the rule. Blood levels of approximately 10 mg per 100 ml are associated with deep coma, dilation of pupils, pale skin, shallow respirations, bradycardia, and hypotonicity of limb musculature—the so-called "medullary phase" of hypoglycemia. If glucose is administered before this medullary phase appears, the patient is restored to normalcy, retracing the aforementioned steps in reverse order. However, once the medullary phase is reached, and particularly if it persists for a time before the hypoglycemia is corrected by intravenous glucose or spontaneously, by the so-called "gluconeogenic activities" of the adrenal glands and liver, recovery is delayed for a period of days or weeks and may be incomplete.

A huge dose of insulin that produces intense hypoglycemia, even of relatively brief duration (30 to 60 min), is more dangerous than a series of less severe hypoglycemic episodes from smaller doses of insulin, possibly because the former impairs or exhausts essential enzymes. This condition cannot then be overcome by large quantities of glucose given intravenously. The cerebral cortex suffers major damage; cortical nerve cells degenerate and are replaced by microgliacytes and astrocytes. The distribution of lesions is similar though not identical to that in hypoxic encephalopathy. The sequelae of the two disorders are also much alike.

In addition to coma, lesser and more chronic forms of hypoglycemia may produce two other syndromes. One of these, termed *subacute hypoglycemia,* is characterized by drowsiness and lethargy, diminution in psychomotor activity, deterioration of social behavior, and confusion. Oral or intravenous glucose will immediately alleviate the symptoms. In the other more *chronic syndrome* there is a gradual deterioration of intellectual function, raising the question of a presenile dementia, and in some reported instances there are tremor, chorea, rigidity, cerebellar ataxia and rarely signs of lower motor neuron involvement ("hypoglycemic amyotrophy"). These subacute and chronic forms of hypoglycemia have been observed with islet cell hypertrophy or tumor, carcinoma of the stomach, fibrous mesothelioma, carcinoma of the cecum, and hepatoma. Supposedly an insulin-like substance is elaborated by the nonpancreatic tumors.

The major clinical differences between hypoglycemia and hypoxia lie in the clinical setting and the mode of evolution of the neurologic disorder. Hypoglycemia usually disturbs cerebral function more slowly than hypoxia, over a period of 30 to 60 min rather than suddenly, within seconds or a few minutes. The recovery phase and sequelae of the two conditions bear close resemblance. Recurrent hypoglycemia, as occurs with an islet-cell tumor, may masquerade for some time as an episodic confusional psychosis or convulsive illness, and diagnosis awaits a period of demonstrably low blood sugar or hyperinsulinism (see Chap. 339).

The correction of the hypoglycemia at the earliest moment is the obvious therapy. It is not known whether hypothermia or other measures will increase the safety period in hypoglycemia or alter the outcome.

Hepatic and portal-systemic encephalopathy Chronic hepatic insufficiency with portal-caval shunting of blood is often punctuated by episodes of stupor, coma, and other neurologic symptoms, a state referred to as hepatic stupor or coma. Also, there are a number of hereditary hyperammonemic syndromes of infancy which may lead to episodic coma with or without seizures. A special type of nonicteric hepatic encephalopathy, first described by Reye and his associates, occurs in children, presenting as an acute toxic encephalopathy (acute brain swelling) in conjunction with rapid enlargement of the liver, fine droplets of fat in hepatocytes, high SGOT and other liver enzymes, and very high levels of ammonium in the blood.

CLINICAL FEATURES The central feature of the syndrome is a derangement of consciousness, presenting first as mental confusion with increased or decreased psychomotor activity, followed by progressive drowsiness, stupor, and coma. The confusional state that occurs before coma intervenes is frequently combined with characteristic lapses of sustained muscle contraction (asterixis) and an EEG abnormality consisting of paroxysms of bilaterally synchronous slow waves, in the delta range, which at first are interspersed with alpha activity and which later, as the coma deepens, displace all normal activity. A variable, fluctuating rigidity of the trunk and limbs, grimacing, suck and grasp reflexes, exaggeration or asymmetry of tendon reflexes, Babinski signs, and focal or generalized seizures round out the clinical picture.

The syndrome of hepatic encephalopathy usually evolves over a period of days to weeks and often terminates fatally. In some patients the syndrome does not advance beyond the stage of mild mental dulling and confusion with asterixis and EEG changes. In this relatively mild form it must be differentiated from other acute confusional psychoses and deliriums. If the metabolic disorder persists for months and years, a mild dementia and a disorder of posture and movement may gradually appear (grimacing, tremor, dysarthria, ataxia of gait, choreoathetosis), and the condition must then be distinguished from the other dementing and extrapyramidal syndromes (see further on in this chapter).

The striking finding in patients who die in a state of hepatic coma is a diffuse increase in the number and size of the protoplasmic astrocytes (Alzheimer type II astrocytes) in the deep layers of the cerebral cortex, lenticular nuclei, thalamus, substantia nigra, and red, dentate, and pontine nuclei, with little or no visible alteration in the nerve cells or other parenchymal elements. The pathogenesis of hepatic encephalopathy is not fully understood, but the most plausible hypothesis relates it to an abnormality of nitrogen metabolism, wherein ammonium (NH_4^+) or other amines, which are formed in the bowel by the action of urease-containing organisms on dietary protein and are carried to the liver in the portal circulation, fail to be converted into urea, either because of hepatocellular disease or portal-systemic shunting of blood, or both. As a result, these substances reach the systemic circulation, where they interfere with cerebral metabolism in some obscure way.

Despite our incomplete understanding of the role of disordered nitrogen metabolism in the genesis of hepatic coma, an awareness of this relationship has provided the few effective means of treating this disorder: restriction of dietary protein; mechanical cleansing of the colon; oral administration of neomycin or kanamycin, which suppresses the urease-producing organisms in the bowel; and the use of lactulose, an inert sugar that acidifies the colonic contents. Should these measures not control the protein intolerance, surgical exclusion of the bowel may be undertaken, but this operation carries a high risk of mortality.

In acute hepatitis, delirious, confusional, and comatose states also occur, but their mechanisms are not understood. Blood ammonium levels are usually elevated, but of unclear significance, because of the large number of associated metabolic abnormalities.

Uremic encephalopathy Episodic confusion and stupor and other neurologic symptoms may accompany any form of severe renal disease, acute or chronic. In addition, a number of neurologic syndromes complicate chronic hemodialysis and kidney transplantation. Chronic polyneuropathy, the most common neurologic complication of renal failure, is discussed in Chap. 275.

The initial cerebral symptoms attributable to uremia consist of apathy, fatigue, inattentiveness, and irritability; later, confusion, disturbances of sensory perception, hallucinations, and stupor supervene. Clouding of the sensorium is practically always associated with twitching of the muscles and myoclonic jerks, and the patient may convulse. We have observed this twitch-convulsive phenomenon in association with a variety of diseases, such as widespread neoplasia, delirium tremens, diabetes with necrotizing pyelonephritis, and lupus erythematosus, all of which were associated with renal failure, only modestly elevated blood urea nitrogen, and normal or subnormal serum calcium and magnesium.

The prognosis of uremic encephalopathy, if associated with irreversible and progressive renal disease, is poor and can only be managed with dialysis or renal transplantation. Convulsions, which occur in about one-third of cases, often preterminally, respond to relatively low plasma concentrations of phenytoin and phenobarbital.

Opinions vary as to the cause of uremic encephalopathy and the twitch-convulsive syndrome. The brain shows hyperplasia of protoplasmic astrocytes in some cases, but never to the degree observed in hepatic encephalopathy. Cerebral edema is notably absent. Restoration of renal function completely corrects the neurologic syndrome attesting to an abnormality at a subcellular level. Whether this is caused by the retention of organic acids, elevation of phosphate in the CSF, or by the action of other toxins has never been settled.

"Disequilibrium syndrome" and dialysis encephalopathy These terms refer to syndromes that commonly complicate hemodialysis or peritoneal dialysis. Under *disequilibrium syndrome* are included headaches, nausea, muscular cramps, nervous irritability, agitation, drowsiness, and convulsions. The headache develops in approximately 70 percent of patients, while the other symptoms are observed in 5 to 10 percent, usually in those undergoing rapid dialysis or in the early stages of a dialysis program. The symptoms tend to occur in the third or fourth hour of dialysis and last for several hours. Sometimes the symptoms appear 8 to 48 h after completing dialysis. Originally these symptoms were attributed to the rapid lowering of serum urea, leaving the brain with a higher concentration of urea than the serum and resulting in a shift of water into the brain to equalize the osmotic gradient ("reverse urea syndrome"). Now the condition is attributed to a shift of water into the brain as in volume expansion due to water intoxication and inappropriate secretion of antidiuretic hormone.

Dialysis encephalopathy or *dialysis dementia* is an unusual complication of chronic hemodialysis. It begins with a stuttering dysarthria and apraxia of speech, to which are added facial and then generalized myoclonus, focal and generalized seizures, personality changes, intellectual decline, and EEG abnormalities, the last of which consist of synchronous or multifocal bursts of slow wave discharges associated with spikes and sharp waves. The CSF is normal except for increased pressure in some cases. At first these symptoms are intermittent, occurring during or immediately after dialysis and lasting for only a few hours, but gradually they become more persistent and eventually permanent. The pathogenesis of this syndrome is quite obscure. Usually it is progressive and fatal, but in some cases an unpredictable reversal of symptoms and EEG abnormalities has occurred in response to the administration of diazepam.

Kidney transplantation involves an increased risk of developing reticulum cell sarcoma, Wernicke's encephalopathy, and central pontine myelinolysis. Systemic fungal infections are found at autopsy in about 45 percent of patients who have had renal transplants and long periods of immunosuppressive treatment, and in about one-third of these patients there is central nervous involvement. Aspergillus, candida, nocardia, and histoplasma are the usual organisms found in that order of frequency. Other central nervous system infections that complicate transplantation are toxoplasmosis and cytomegalic inclusion disease.

Encephalopathies due to electrolyte disturbances Limitation of space permits only brief reference to this important group of metabolic encephalopathies.

Metabolic acidosis (arterial pH < 7.30, $P_{CO_2} < 35$, $HCO_3 < 10$ meq per liter) due to diabetes mellitus, renal failure, lactic acidosis, or poisoning with an acidic substance produces the typical drowsiness, stupor, and coma with dry skin and Kuss-

maul breathing described in Chap. 337. Coma due to acidosis is a particularly prominent feature of many of the metabolic diseases of infancy and childhood, including the various forms of hyperammonemia, isolvaleric acidemia, maple syrup urine disease, methylmalonic aciduria, the ketotic form of hyperglycinemia, proprionic acidemia, lactic acidemia, and lysosomal acid phosphatase deficiency. Extreme degrees of *hyperosmolality* of the blood may develop in the course of diabetes mellitus (blood glucose greater than 400 mg per 100 ml) and in *hypernatremic dehydration,* resulting in both instances in convulsions, tremulousness, and coma. In some instances the movement disorder resembles chorea or the myoclonic twitching of uremia. *Hyponatremia,* usually with water intoxication, is another cause of episodic coma, especially in infants. *Hypokalemia* may be associated with a stuporous-confusional state, sometimes accompanied by striking changes in personality and behavior.

In children more than adults, cholera being an exception, extremely *severe diarrhea* may be attended by an encephalopathy. Irritability, weakness, headache, seizures, stupor, and coma may develop over a period of 2 to 3 days and carry a grave prognosis unless promptly relieved. Presumably this is a metabolic encephalopathy due to loss of fluids and electrolytes and can be corrected by their replacement. In the more protracted illness of *typhoid fever,* approximately half the patients develop a delirium, and a small number will exhibit meningism and become comatose with twitching and seizures or spasticity and hyperactive reflexes in the legs, all of which are transitory.

Other encephalopathies of this type, associated with adrenal insufficiency and hypo- and hyperparathyroidism are considered at the end of this chapter, in relation to the endocrine psychoses.

METABOLIC DISEASES PRESENTING AS EXTRAPYRAMIDAL SYNDROMES These syndromes are usually of mixed type, i.e., they include a number of basal ganglionic and cerebellar symptoms in various combinations. They may emerge in a variety of clinical settings—as a sequela of kernicterus or of hypoxic or hypoglycemic encephalopathy, or as part of hepatocerebral degeneration of acquired or familial type, or with calcification of the basal ganglia and cerebellum, a disorder which also takes a familial or acquired form.

The extrapyramidal symptoms that result from severe *anoxia* and *hypoglycemia* have been described in the preceding section. Chronic *parathyroid hypofunction,* either idiopathic or following surgery in the area of the thyroid, may rarely give rise to intracranial calcifications and an extrapyramidal motor syndrome. Somewhat more common is the familial form of basal ganglionic-cerebellar calcification in which choreoathetosis and rigidity are prominent (*Fahr's syndrome*). Some of these patients are mentally retarded, others are intellectually intact. The familial form of calcification is inherited as an autosomal recessive trait, and usually has its onset in adolescence and early adult life. The serum calcium levels are usually normal, and there is no explanation of the calcification.

The development of an extrapyramidal syndrome in late childhood and adolescence should always suggest (1) Wilson-Westphal-Strümpell hepatocerebral degeneration (Chap. 95) and (2) Hallervorden-Spatz disease (Chap. 373). Only kernicterus and the acquired form of hepatocerebral degeneration remain to be discussed here.

Kernicterus This is an important cause of generalized choreoathetosis and rigidity in children and adults, the result of excessive hemolysis (Rh incompatibility) or other forms of hyperbilirubinemia in the neonatal period.

The symptoms of kernicterus appear in the jaundiced neonate on the second or third postnatal day. The infant becomes listless, sucks poorly, develops respiratory difficulties, and becomes stuporous as the jaundice intensifies. The serum bilirubin is over 25 mg per 100 ml. The majority of infants who suffer this disease die within the first week or two of life. Many of those who survive are mentally retarded, deaf, and totally unable to sit, stand, or walk; the tendency is always to put them in homes for the feebleminded. But there are exceptional patients, obviously less damaged, who are mentally normal or at most only slightly backward. These are the ones who develop a variety of persistent neurologic sequelae—choreoathetosis, dystonia, and rigidity of the limbs—a picture not too different from that of cerebral spastic diplegia with involuntary movements. Kernicterus should always be suspected if an extrapyramidal syndrome is accompanied by bilateral deafness and palsy of upward gaze.

Neonates who die in the acute stage of kernicterus show a characteristic yellow staining of nuclear masses in the basal ganglia, brainstem, and cerebellum—a finding from which the disease takes its name. In surviving patients the pathologic changes consist of symmetrically distributed nerve cell loss and gliosis in the subthalamic nucleus, the globus pallidus, thalamus, and oculomotor and cochlear nuclei; these lesions are the result of the hyperbilirubinemia. In the newborn, unconjugated bilirubin can pass through the poorly developed blood-brain barrier into these central and brainstem nuclei, where it has a direct toxic effect. Acidosis and hypoxia exacerbate the effect. Also, in the newborn, the development of hyperbilirubinemia is enhanced by the transient deficiency of the enzyme glucuronyl transferase, essential for the conjugation of bilirubin. Hereditary hyperbilirubinemia, due to lack of enzyme (Crigler-Najjar syndrome), may have the same effect on the nervous system as hyperbilirubinemia due to excessive hemolysis (Rh incompatibility).

Phototherapy and exchange transfusions with female blood designed to prevent high levels of unconjugated serum bilirubin have been shown to protect the nervous system. If the blood bilirubin level can be held to less than 20 mg per 100 ml (16 mg per 100 ml in prematures), the nervous system escapes damage.

Acquired (nonwilsonian) hepatocerebral degeneration Patients who survive an episode or several episodes of hepatic coma are occasionally left with residual neurologic abnormalities, such as tremor of the head or arms, asterixis, grimacing, choreatic twitching of the limbs, dysarthria, ataxia of gait, or impairment of intellectual function, and these symptoms may worsen with repeated attacks of stupor and coma. In other patients with hepatic failure, these neurologic abnormalities may become manifest in the absence of discrete episodes of hepatic coma. In either event, patients thus afflicted deteriorate neurologically over a period of months or years. As the condition evolves a rather characteristic dysarthria, mild ataxia, wide-based, unsteady gait, and choreoathetosis, mainly of the face, neck, and shoulders, are joined in a common syndrome. Mental function is slowly altered—a simple dementia with lack of concern, and indifference to the illness evolves. A coarse rhythmic tremor of the arms, appearing with certain sustained postures, mild corticospinal tract signs, and diffuse EEG abnormalities complete the clinical picture. Other less frequent signs are muscular rigidity, grasp reflexes, tremor in repose, nystagmus, asterixis, and action or intention myoclonus. Many of the neurologic abnormalities that occur as part of acute hepatic encephalopathy may also be observed in patients with chronic hepatocerebral degeneration; the only difference is that the abnormalities are evanescent in the former and irreversible in the latter.

The chronic cerebral symptoms, like the transient ones, may occur with all varieties of chronic liver disease. Portocaval shunts are always present; jaundice, ascites, and esophageal varices are manifest in most of the cases.

Chronic hepatocerebral degeneration, like acute hepatic coma, is characterized by a widespread hyperplasia of protoplasmic astrocytes in the deep layers of the cerebral and cerebellar cortices as well as in thalamic and lenticular nuclei and many other nuclear structures of the brainstem. In addition, in the chronic disease, medullated fibers and nerve cells are destroyed in the affected areas, and polymicrocavitation may be prominent at the corticomedullary junction, in the striatum (particularly in the superior pole of the putamen), and in the cerebellar white matter. Protoplasmic astrocytic nuclei contain periodic acid-Schiff (PAS) positive glycogen granules. Nerve cells may appear swollen and chromatolyzed, accounting, we believe, for the so-called "Opalski cells." The similarity of the neuropathologic lesion in the familial (Wilson's) and acquired forms of liver disease suggests a common hepatogenesis.

METABOLIC DISEASES PRESENTING AS CEREBELLAR ATAXIA, PSYCHOSIS, OR DEMENTIA The association of *myxedema and a cerebellar type of ataxia* has been mentioned sporadically in medical writings since the latter part of the 19th century. The neuropathologic basis of this disorder remains unclear, as does the pathogenesis. The damaging effects of *hyperthermia,* like those of anoxia and hypoglycemia, involve the brain diffusely; in the case of hyperthermia, however, the changes are disproportionately severe in the cerebellum. The acute manifestations of profound hyperthermia are coma and convulsions, frequently complicated by shock and renal failure. Patients who survive the initial stage of the illness frequently show signs of widespread cerebral affection, such as confusion, dementia, and pseudobulbar and spastic paralysis. These abnormalities tend to resolve gradually, leaving the patient with a more or less pure disorder of cerebellar function. This disorder has its basis in a degeneration of the Purkinje cells, with gliosis throughout the cerebellar cortex, as well as degeneration of the dentate nuclei.

Already the point has been made that milder degrees of episodic stupor and coma, if persistent, may present as a state of protracted confusion that is impossible to distinguish from dementia. Chronic portal-systemic encephalopathy, the syndromes of chronic hypoglycemia, and dialysis encephalopathy all fall within this category.

In the *endocrine encephalopathies* the clinical phenomena are even more abstruse. Confusional states may be combined with agitation, hallucinations, delusions, anxiety, and depression. And the time course of the illness may be in terms of weeks and months, rather than days. Such a derangement of higher nervous function may follow the *administration of ACTH or corticosteroid* agents, and the same symptoms have been reported in *Cushing's disease.* The neurology of *thyrotoxicosis* has proven to be peculiarly elusive. Allusions to thyrotoxic psychosis are widely recorded in the medical literature; mental confusion, seizures, manic or depressive attacks, delusions, and chorea occur in various combinations with muscular weakness and atrophy, periodic paralysis, and myasthenia. Treatment of the hyperthyroidism gradually restores the patient to a normal mental state leaving one with no explanation of what had happened to the nervous system. The reactions of *myxedematous patients* are slowed and their psychomotor activity is reduced, but only in exceptional cases is there a major change in cerebral function, taking the form of drowsiness or extreme somnolence, inattentiveness, and apathy. These symptoms can be reversed within a few weeks by thyroid medication. In *hyperparathyroidism,* when the serum calcium levels reach 15 mg per 100 ml or higher, the patient sinks into a quiet state of inattentiveness, lethargy, and confusion. Stupor, coma, and death may be caused by extreme degrees of hypercalcemia such as occur occasionally in cases of excessive vitamin D administration and metastatic carcinoma of the bones. Encephalopathy due to *Addison's disease* (adrenal insufficiency) may be attended by episodic confusion, stupor, or coma, without special identifying features. Hypoglycemia and hypotension, with diminished cerebral circulation, are thought to be the underlying mechanisms, and measures which correct them appear to be beneficial.

The term *pancreatic encephalopathy* was introduced by Rothermich and Von Haam in 1941 to describe a syndrome of agitation and confusion, sometimes with hallucinations and clouding of consciousness, dysarthria, and changing rigidity of the limbs, all of which are associated with acute pancreatic disease. The status of this entity is uncertain. A uniform neuropathologic change has not been discerned. Pallis and Lewis suggest that before such a clinical diagnosis can be seriously entertained in a patient with acute pancreatitis one should exclude delirium tremens, cerebral circulatory insufficiency from shock, renal failure, hypoglycemia, diabetic acidosis, hyperosmolality syndrome, hypokalemia, and hypo- or hypercalcemia, any one of which may complicate the underlying disease(s).

HEREDITARY METABOLIC DISEASES OF THE NERVOUS SYSTEM

As stated above these will receive only cursory treatment, for most of them effect pathologic change in the nervous system during the pediatric age period and seldom does the affected organism survive to adulthood.

As a group these diseases share certain characteristics. Essentially all of them involve many tissues, e.g., white blood cells, fibroblasts, endothelial cells, and hepatocytes, although the nervous system may be the only organ whose functions are deranged. Thus, the diseases appear primarily neurologic even though they are truly multisystemic. Advantage can be taken of this fact by the knowledgeable clinician who can therefore utilize the more accessible nonnervous cells for cytologic diagnosis. Of the more than 100 hereditary metabolic diseases that possess a known metabolic marker, the majority, particularly those that express themselves in the first days, weeks, months, and years, are of a recessive type. The organism is usually normal at birth and does not express its enzymatic defect, having been protected in utero by the mother. Once the disease strikes, however, it tends to be global and devastating in its effects, immediately blighting the development of the brain and preventing the attainment of the so-called "milestones" of psychomotor maturation. The remainder of the genetic metabolic diseases are of dominant inheritance or male sex-linked, and they can begin at any age and usually are of slower evolution. Their effects may not become apparent until adult life and are then more likely to be restricted to certain systems of neurons, giving rise to the other neurological syndromes (seizures, cerebellar ataxia, dystonia and choreoathetosis, dementia, progressive spasticity, polyneuropathy, etc.).

A new neurological principle emerges in connection with this group of diseases—that in the early epochs of life each disease tends to have its favorite age period (neonatal, early or late infantile, childhood, or adolescence) and each epoch of life is marked by a disposition to certain of these metabolic diseases and not to others. Thus the evolving syndrome depends not only on the nature of the disease but also on the age and state of maturation of the nervous system at the moment it strikes. Pursuant to this principle one can subdivide and group the diseases according to the age of the afflicted organism and according to the clinical syndrome, as shown in Table 371-2. In the latter it will be evident that the late-onset (usually Men-

delian dominant diseases) are more likely to express themselves by recognizable syndromes of diagnostic value than are the early onset, recessive ones. Of particular interest to primary care physicians and internists are the rare variants of the hereditary metabolic diseases of childhood which may present for the first time during adult life. For example, the authors have encountered cases of adrenoleukodystrophy in which focal cerebral demyelination causing hemiparesis, heminsensory loss, and homonymous hemianopsia appeared at the age of 20 to 30 years; the diagnostic clues were the findings of low cortisol levels and adrenal atrophy. Patients with metachromatic leukodystrophy have presented with a progressive spastic weakness, cerebellar ataxia, or a polyneuropathy and sometimes dementia or psychopathic behavior during the third and fourth decades of life. Progressive spastic weakness and cerebellar ataxia with retained mental competence during adolescence and early adult life have also been observed in Krabbe's globoid-body leukodystrophy. Dementia with seizures and ex-

TABLE 371-2
Clinical classification of the hereditary metabolic diseases

I Diseases which begin in the neonatal period and are often fatal (seizures, respiratory difficulty, unresponsivity)
  A Diseases of the urea cycle
  B Pyridoxine dependency
  C Maple syrup urine disease
  D Congenital lactic acidosis
II Diseases of infancy and early childhood
  A Phenylketonuria and other abnormalities of amino acid metabolism (mental retardation and seizures, blond hair, fair skin); see Chaps. 88 and 89
  B Lysosomal storage diseases
    1 Lipidoses: Tay-Sachs disease and Sandhoff variant, Niemann-Pick disease, Gaucher's disease (seizures and myoclonia, blindness, auditory startle, psychomotor regression, and in some diseases enlarged liver and spleen); see Chap. 101
    2 Mucopolysaccharidoses (psychomotor regression, corneal clouding, skeletal disorder, infiltrates of liver, spleen, lungs, marrow); see Chap. 103
    3 Mucolipidoses (syndromes with elements of the lipidoses and mucopolysaccharidoses)
    4 Leukodystrophies: globoid body leukodystrophy, metachromatic leukodystrophy, Pelizaeus-Merzbacher disease, Canavan's disease (psychomotor regression, spasticity of legs, areflexia, blindness); see Chap. 101
III Late childhood-adolescent diseases
  A Ataxia-telangiectasia (oculomotor apraxia, cerebellar ataxia, athetosis, later telangiectasia of conjunctivae and ears); see Chap. 374
  B Leigh's subacute necrotic encephalomyelopathy (ophthalmoplegia, respiratory disorder, mental regression, paralysis); see Chap. 92
  C Wilson's hereditary hepatocerebral degeneration (Kaiser-Fleischer corneal rings, extrapyramidal signs, liver dysfunction); see Chap. 95
  D Hallervorden-Spatz disease (extrapyramidal syndrome)
  E Lesch-Nyhan hyperuricosemia (choreoathetosis, mental retardation, self mutilation); see Chap. 92
IV Late adolescent-early adult diseases
  A G_{M2} gangliosidosis (intellectual regression, seizures, ataxia, pyramidal signs)
  B Variant of metachromatic leukodystrophy (personality change, dementia, spastic weakness of limbs, ataxia)
  C Late form of neuropathic Gaucher's disease (seizures, polymyoclonus, mental deterioration)
  D Juvenile dystonic lipidosis or Niemann-Pick disease types C and D (mental decline, dystonic movements of tongue and limbs, paralysis of upward gaze)
  E Ceroid lipofuscinosis (dementia, ataxia, seizures)
  F Wilson's hepatocerebral degeneration (as in III C above)
  G Mucolipidoses (mental deterioration, gargoyle facial features, hyperplasia of gums)
  H Cerebrotendinous xanthomatosis (mental decline and personality changes, cerebellar ataxia, spastic quadriparesis, xanthometous deposits on tendons)
  I Mucopolysaccharidoses: Maroteaux-Lamy and Morquio types (dwarfism, spastic quadriparesis, hydrocephalus)

trapyramidal signs, e.g., choreoathetosis, was the clinical picture in one of our cases of Niemann-Pick disease. Polymyoclonia and seizures with slow regression of mental function characterized a disease that proved to be of Gaucher's lipidosis in another adolescent. One could extend the list but the point is that whenever any one of these syndromes brings an adolescent or adult patient to medical attention, these variants of hereditary metabolic diseases should be entertained as diagnostic possibilities.

HEREDITARY METABOLIC DISEASES OF ADOLESCENCE AND ADULT LIFE

Of the many diseases listed in Table 371-2 only the few observed to begin in late adolescent and adult years are of interest to internists and family practitioners. They are the ones that must occasionally figure in the differential diagnosis of acquired diseases of the nervous system. A noteworthy attribute of the entire group is their chronicity and progressive nature. The diseases described below are examples personally observed by the authors.

ADULT METACHROMATIC LEUKODYSTROPHY (MLD) This is one of the more frequent hereditary metabolic diseases of the nervous system. While the majority of cases appear in early childhood, some 25 percent or more are reported as manifesting their first symptoms beyond the twenty-first year of life. Cases among men have outnumbered those found in women two to one. The mode of inheritance is autosomal recessive in almost all instances. The onset is insidious and the course protracted, over twenty or more years.

In our experience mental symptoms tend to dominate the clinical picture. Failing scholastic performance, forgetfulness, and irrationality occur early in the illness but may be obscured by peculiarities of personality, such as suspiciousness, delusional thinking, and bizarre actions. These latter qualities may raise the question of schizophrenia or immature ("borderline") personality development. Sooner or later a mild cerebellar ataxia presenting as awkwardness and falling, mild pyramidal signs, masked facies, and bizarre postures stamp the illness as neurological. Eventually the patient's mental processes deteriorate to the point where he or she is totally helpless, demented, mute, incontinent of sphincteric control, and bedfast.

Specific diagnostic tests include (1) the demonstration of a diminished aryl-sulfatase A activity in white blood cells, serum, and urine, (2) increased excretion of sulfatides in urine, (3) slowed conduction velocity in nerves, and (4) deposits of metachromatic material in nerve biopsies.

No treatment is presently available.

One must add adult MLD to the growing list of neurological diseases that cause early mental changes. The others are: Wilson's hepatolenticular degeneration, adult lipidoses, mucolipidoses, cerebrotendinous xanthomatosis, the myoclonic epilepsies, and basal ganglia calcinoses. All of these are clinically separable from the major "functional psychoses" of this age period, by virtue of the progressive impairment of cognitive function, other neurological findings, the EEG, and certain radiological and biochemical tests.

ADULT LIPID STORAGE DISEASES AND LEUKODYSTROPHIES
Apart from some of the infantile and juvenile forms of cerebral lipidoses there are several that become clinically visible in adults. These must be considered as rare variants of the more common ones of earlier life, the delay in onset being due to a less severe deficiency of some of the missing enzymes described in Chap. 101, or to other eccentricities of the biochemical mechanism.

We have observed G_{M2} *gangliosidosis* several times in young adults. Many are from non-Jewish families, and males and females in the same generation are equally affected. Generalized seizures may mark the beginning of a cerebral disorder that later is evidenced by alterations of behavior and intellectual decline. Ataxia and mild signs of corticospinal disease, the combination of which interferes with independent locomotion, clarifies the diagnosis. The fundi and visual function are normal in most cases, but we have seen typical cherry red macular spots. Within 4 to 5 years the patient is confined to a wheelchair. The liver and spleen are normal or slightly enlarged. The CSF protein is normal. Computerized tomography (CT scan) reveals a modest ventricular enlargement. G_{M2} ganglioside is shown to be increased by thin-layer chromatography of tissue obtained by cerebral biopsy. Membranous cytoplasmic bodies are visualized by electron microscopy of rectal, appendicular, and cortical neurons. A slowly developing dementia, cerebellar ataxia, polymyoclonus, and failing vision may characterize the clinical picture in other cases.

In early adult life or adolescence we have also observed progressive dementia, seizures, ataxia, and pyramidal signs in patients in whom the diagnosis of the *Kuf's form of ceroid lipofuscinosis* was established. Skin and conjunctival biopsies (electron microscopic examination) showed lipofuscin storage material in fibroblasts and endothelial cells.

Another of our patients who began to have seizures, severe polymyoclonus, and mild intellectual deterioration was found, after several studies, to have *Gaucher's disease*. His spleen had been ruptured in an accident several years before, and when the surgical specimen was reviewed Gaucher cells were seen. A deficiency of glucose cerebroside splitting enzyme was found in white blood cells and skin fibroblasts. Several adolescent cases of *types C and D of Niemann-Pick disease* have been verified, in which the opening symptoms of the illness were dystonic movements of tongue, jaw, and limbs in association with a gradual decline of intellectual function and paralysis of vertical (upwards) gaze. Foam cells were found in the bone marrow and liver.

In *adrenoleukodystrophy* either bronzing of the skin and Addison's disease or cerebral symptoms may be the initial manifestation. The cerebral lesions may present as a homonymous hemianopsia, cortical blindness, hemiparesis, aphasia, or dementia. Usually the signs are asymmetrical at first and progress intermittently. A relatively pure polyneuropathic and myelopathic form has also been described. The diagnosis may be settled by the finding of a low blood cortisol level in a male with cerebrospinal demyelinating disease. Corticosteroid replacement therapy helps the Addison's disease but has no effect on the neurological disorders. The latter progress intermittently over a few years, and usually the outcome is fatal.

In sum, one should at least consider some of these rare forms of hereditary metabolic diseases whenever an adolescent or young adult becomes demented, shows a psychiatric syndrome with decline in cognitive functions, has seizures, especially with polymyoclonus, failing vision, and cerebellar ataxia in combination with corticospinal signs or a progressive polyneuropathy. (See Chaps. 101 and 373 for further details.)

REFERENCES

ADAMS RD, FOLEY JM: The neurological disorder associated with liver disease. Metabolic and toxic diseases of the nervous system. Proc Assoc Res Nerv Ment Dis 32:198, 1953

———, VICTOR M: *Principles of Neurology*. New York, McGraw-Hill, 1977

ALFREY AC et al: The dialysis encephalopathy syndrome. Possible aluminum intoxication. N Engl J Med 294:184, 1976

CREMER GM et al: Myxedema and ataxia. Neurology 19:37, 1969

MALAMUD N et al: Heat stroke. A clinicopathologic study of 125 fatal cases. Mil Surg 99:397, 1946

MARKS R, ROSE FC: *Hypoglycemia.* Oxford, Blackwell, 1965

NADEL AM, WILSON WP: Dialysis encephalopathy. A possible seizure disorder. Neurology 26:1130, 1976

PALLIS CA, LEWIS PD: *The Neurology of Gastrointestinal Disease.* London, Saunders, 1974

PLUM F (ed): *Brain Dysfunction in Metabolic Disorders.* New York, Raven Press, 1974

RASKIN NH, FISHMAN RA: Neurologic disorders in renal failure. N Engl J Med 294:143, 204, 1976

ROTHERMICH NO, VON HAAM E: Pancreatic encephalopathy. J Clin Endocrinol 1:872, 1941

STANBURY JB et al (eds): *The Metabolic Basis of Inherited Disease,* 4th ed. New York, McGraw-Hill, 1978

SWAIMAN KF et al: Metabolic disorders of the central nervous system, in *The Practice of Pediatric Neurology,* KF Swaiman, FS Wright (eds). St Louis, Mosby, 1975, pp 359–479

VICTOR M et al: The acquired (non-wilsonian) type of chronic hepatocerebral degeneration. Medicine 44:345, 1965

372
DEFICIENCY DISEASES OF THE NERVOUS SYSTEM

MAURICE VICTOR
RAYMOND D. ADAMS

The general principles of deficiency disease have been presented in Chap. 73, and the reader should review them as an introduction to this discussion of deficiency diseases of the nervous system. The term *deficiency* is used here in its strictest sense, to designate those diseases or syndromes which result from the lack of an essential nutrient in the diet or from a conditioning factor which increases the need for that nutrient. The neurological diseases which comprise this category are the following:

1 Wernicke's disease and Korsakoff's psychosis
2 Nutritional polyneuropathy (neuropathic beriberi)
3 Pellagra
4 Deficiency amblyopia
5 The syndrome of amblyopia, painful neuropathy, and orogenital dermatitis (Strachan's syndrome)
6 Subacute combined degeneration of the spinal cord
7 Vitamin-responsive, genetically determined diseases

Before discussing each of these disorders, some general remarks, applicable to all of them, may suitably be made. Of the known vitamin deficiencies, only those of the B group are of importance in neurological disease. A lack of them affects the brain, spinal cord, and peripheral nerves of humans. Thiamine chloride, nicotinic acid, pyridoxine, pantothenic acid, and riboflavin all play a role in carbohydrate metabolism, upon which the central nervous system depends for its principal source of energy. These vitamins are essentially coenzymes in the Krebs tricarboxylic acid cycle, and, in addition, thiamine is involved in the hexose-monophosphate shunt. Vitamin B_{12} is known to be required for the conversion of methylmalonyl- to succinyl coenzyme A and for the conversion of homocystine to methionine.

Except for subacute combined degeneration of the spinal cord (vitamin B_{12} deficiency), it is not possible to relate each of the deficiency diseases in humans to the lack of one particular vitamin. For example, polyneuropathy may result from any one of several vitamin deficiencies [thiamine chloride, pyridoxine (vitamin B_6), pantothenic acid, and probably vitamin B_{12}].

Moreover, pellagra, beriberi, and Strachan's syndrome are probably related to a deficiency of several vitamins. These generalizations do not negate the relationship of certain manifestations of deficiency disease to the lack of a specific nutrient (e.g., the ocular signs of Wernicke's disease to a deficiency of thiamine).

In the western world the nutritional disorders of the nervous system are observed most often in the alcoholic population of large urban centers. Alcohol acts mainly by displacing food in the diet, but it also increases the demand for B vitamins, which are necessary to metabolize the carbohydrate furnished by alcohol itself, and it may impair the gastrointestinal absorption of vitamins. Dietary faddism, impaired absorption of dietary nutrients (as occurs in sprue or following the resection of stomach and small bowel), and the use of vitamin antagonists (e.g. isoniazid, which interferes with the enzymatic function of pyridoxine) account for a relatively small number of cases of deficiency disease.

Each of the deficiency diseases may occur in pure form and will be so described. More often, however, they occur in various combinations. Stated in another way, it is usual for deficiency diseases to involve both the central and peripheral nervous systems, a combination found in few other categories of disease. Also, the examination of patients with deficiency disease frequently discloses nonneurological signs of malnutrition such as general wasting, lesions of the skin and mucous membranes, and circulatory abnormalities.

WERNICKE'S DISEASE (WERNICKE'S ENCEPHALOPATHY, POLIOENCEPHALITIS HEMORRHAGICA SUPERIORIS) History
In 1881, Carl Wernicke described an illness of acute onset characterized by mental disturbance, paralysis of eye movements, and ataxic gait. Swelling of the optic disks with retinal hemorrhages was also said to be present, and in all three of his patients there was a progressive depression of the state of consciousness leading to death, so that a fatal outcome was at one time thought to be a universal feature of this disease. Wernicke described focal vascular lesions, primarily affecting the gray matter around the third and fourth ventricles and aqueduct of Sylvius. He regarded the disease as inflammatory in nature and suggested the name *acute superior hemorrhagic polioencephalitis.* Since Wernicke's time, views regarding this disease have undergone considerable modification, clinically, pathologically, and etiologically.

Symptoms and signs The crux of the clinical picture is the *ocular disturbance* (the clinical diagnosis of Wernicke's disease can hardly be made without it) which consists of weakness or paralysis of the external recti, nystagmus that is both horizontal and vertical, and various palsies of conjugate gaze. These signs show a considerable diversity. The disorder of conjugate movement varies from a nystagmus on extreme gaze in one direction to a complete loss of ocular movement in that direction. This applies to both horizontal and vertical movements; abnormalities of the former are somewhat more frequent. Paralysis of downward gaze is an unusual finding, but internuclear ophthalmoplegia is common. Ptosis and retinal hemorrhages are observed rarely. The sixth nerve palsy is always bilateral, though not necessarily symmetrical, and is accompanied by diplopia and internal strabismus. With complete ocular paralysis nystagmus is absent, but it becomes evident as the weakness improves. In advanced stages of the disease there may be complete loss of ocular movement, and the pupils, which ordinarily are spared, may become miotic and nonreacting.

The *ataxia* affects stance and gait predominantly. It may be so severe initially that the patient is unable to stand or walk without support. Vestibular responses to caloric stimulation are characteristically absent in these patients. With specific treatment the gross disorder of equilibrium improves and the patient is left with a wide-based, uncertain gait. The mildest degree of ataxia may be brought out only by special tests, such as heel-to-toe walking. In contrast to the gross disorder of locomotion is the relative infrequency of clear-cut intention tremor. When present it affects the legs more than the arms. Scanning speech is present only in isolated cases.

A *derangement of mental function* is found in all but 10 percent of patients and takes one of several forms: (1) The most common is a *global confusion state,* characterized by profound apathy, listlessness, and disorientation. Unconsciousness as part of the initial episode is distinctly rare, but mild drowsiness is common. The mental state is best described as one of disinterest or indifference. Spontaneous speech is minimal. Patients are inattentive and cannot concentrate on the simplest tasks. Many questions directed to them go unanswered, or they may suspend the conversation in the middle of a sentence to turn over and sleep. Patients are readily roused from this state, however. Whatever questions they answer betray disorientation in time and place, misidentification of those around them, and an inability to grasp the meaning of their illness or immediate situation. Many of their remarks are irrational and show no consistency from one moment to another. Under the circumstances a more extensive evaluation of intellectual function is seldom possible. (2) Some patients, at the time they are first seen, already show the disorder of retentive memory and otherwise alert state of mind that characterizes Korsakoff's psychosis (see Chap. 21 and further on in this chapter). (3) A relatively small number of patients, less than 20 percent in our series, show the symptoms of alcohol withdrawal, either delirium tremens or a variant thereof.

The symptoms of Wernicke's disease may all appear simultaneously and rather acutely, but more often the ophthalmoplegia and ataxia precede the mental signs by a few days and sometimes by a week or two.

Wernicke's disease is usually associated with other nutritional diseases, both neurological and nonneurological. In more than 80 percent of cases, the signs of *nutritional polyneuropathy* are evident. In most cases the neuropathy is mild in degree and does not account for the disorder of gait. Nevertheless, in some the neuropathy is so severe that stance and gait cannot be tested. Occasionally, *amblyopia* or *spinal spastic ataxia* may be added to the clinical picture.

The advanced stages of beriberi heart disease are rarely observed in association with Wernicke's disease, although indications of *disordered cardiovascular function* such as tachycardia, exertional dyspnea, postural hypotension, and minor electrocardiographic abnormalities are common. Occasionally patients may die suddenly, with the mode of death suggesting "cardiovascular collapse." It has been shown that Wernicke's disease is characterized by a state of high cardiac output which is out of proportion to the oxygen consumption. This is probably due to an abnormal state of peripheral vasodilatation, which in turn may be related specifically to thiamine deficiency. Postural hypotension and syncope are probably related to impaired function in the autonomic nervous system, more specifically to a defect in the sympathetic outflow.

Course of the illness Death occurs in about 15 percent of hospitalized patients and is usually due to infection (pneumonia, pulmonary tuberculosis, and septicemia being the most common) or to the complications of cirrhosis of the liver.

Patients who recover respond to specific treatment in a characteristic manner. Recovery of the ocular palsies may begin within hours after the administration of thiamine and practically always within several days. Failure of the patient to respond in this manner should raise doubts about the diagnosis of Wernicke's disease. Sixth nerve palsies, ptosis, and vertical gaze palsies recover completely, within a week or two in most cases, but vertical nystagmus may occasionally persist for several months. Horizontal gaze palsies recover completely as a rule, but in more than half the cases a fine horizontal nystagmus remains as a permanent sequela of the disease.

Ataxia improves somewhat more slowly than the ocular abnormalities. Almost half the patients recover incompletely and are left with a slow, shuffling, wide-based gait and inability to walk tandem. The residual gait disturbance, like horizontal nystagmus, provides a means of identifying obscure and chronic cases of dementia as alcoholic-nutritional in origin.

Vestibular function, as disclosed by caloric testing, improves at about the same rate as the ataxia of stance and gait. Recovery occurs slowly, over a period of weeks or months and is usually but not always complete.

The symptoms that constitute the global confusional state are always reversible. As the symptoms of apathy, drowsiness, and profound confusion gradually recede, the *defect in retentive memory and learning (Korsakoff's psychosis)* stands out more clearly. The features of Korsakoff's psychosis (amnesic or amnesic-confabulatory syndrome) are described in Chap. 21. Here it is important to emphasize that in the alcoholic, nutritionally deficient patient Wernicke's disease and Korsakoff's psychosis are not separate diseases, but the changing ocular and ataxic signs and the transformation of the global confusional state into an amnesic syndrome are successive stages in the recovery of a single disease process. Stated in another way, Korsakoff's psychosis is but the psychic component of Wernicke's disease. Hence the symptom complex should be called Wernicke's disease with or without Korsakoff's psychosis or the Wernicke-Korsakoff syndrome when both components of the disease are present.

The outcome of Korsakoff's psychosis varies. About 20 percent of patients recover completely or almost completely. More often there is slow and incomplete recovery over a year or longer. Depending on the severity of the residual symptoms, the patient may or may not be able to lead a supervised existence out of a hospital. The residual mental state is usually one in which the patient shows large gaps in memory and is unable to sort out events in their proper temporal sequence. If the patient is seen for the first time during this stage, the diagnosis of "alcoholic deteriorated state" or "organic brain syndrome due to alcohol" is commonly made.

Pathologic changes Postmortem examination in patients who die in the acute stages of Wernicke's disease or in the chronic stages, when the amnesic syndrome predominates, reveals symmetrically located lesions in the paraventricular regions of the thalamus and hypothalamus, the mammillary bodies, the periaqueductal region of the midbrain, the floor of the fourth ventricle, and the anterior lobe of the cerebellum, particularly the vermis. The lesions are invariably found in the mammillary bodies and less consistently in the other areas. Microscopically, the principal change consists of varying degrees of necrosis of parenchymal structures. Many nerve cells and fibers are destroyed; others remain intact and are seen against a background of reactive glial elements, both astrocytes and microgliacytes. The blood vessels are prominent, owing to adventitial and endothelial proliferation. Hemorrhagic lesions are present in only a small proportion of cases and usually give the appearance of being of recent origin. The oculomotor and vestibular nuclei are regularly involved, but only to a mild degree, as a rule.

Correlation of the clinical manifestations with anatomic localization of the lesions indicates that the ocular muscle and gaze palsies are attributable to lesions of the sixth and third nerve nuclei. The lesions of the vestibular nuclei are probably responsible for the loss of caloric responses and to some extent for the gross abnormality of equilibrium that characterizes the initial stage of the disease. The lack of significant destruction of nerve cells in these lesions accounts for the rapid improvement in oculomotor and vestibular function.

The persistent ataxia of stance and gait is attributable to the loss of cortical neurons in the superior vermis; ataxia of individual movements of the legs is attributable to an extension of the lesion into the anterior parts of the anterior lobes. The cerebellar lesions of Wernicke's disease are indistinguishable from those of *alcoholic cerebellar degeneration* (see Chap 226). The latter designation is used when the cerebellar abnormalities occur on a background of alcoholism and malnutrition, without the characteristic ocular and mental disorder.

The amnesic defect is related to lesions in the diencephalon, more specifically to those in the medial dorsal nuclei and perhaps the medial pulvinar. Lesions in the mammillary bodies are probably not critical in respect to memory function since they are found in patients with Wernicke's disease who had shown no previous disorder of memory.

Etiology Nutritional deficiency is now established as the causal factor. Outbreaks of Wernicke's disease have been encountered in prisoner-of-war camps, and occasional cases have been reported in wasting diseases of varied origin where alcohol played no part. The specific factor that is responsible for most, if not all, of the symptoms of the Wernicke-Korsakoff syndrome is a deficiency of thiamine. The experimental evidence for this statement, both in animals and in humans, is quite convincing. The marked sensitivity of the ophthalmoplegia to the administration of thiamine accounts for the rapid disappearance of this disorder following a single injection of the vitamin or the ingestion of one or two meals. The quality of prompt reversibility suggests that the ocular signs are due to a biochemical abnormality and not to irreversible structural changes. On the other hand, the slow and incomplete recovery of the memory defect suggests that this symptom is the result of irreversible structural changes, presumably in the medial dorsal nuclei of the thalamus.

On the basis of clinical observation, nutritional studies, and the neuropathologic findings, the details of which cannot all be given here, one may say that Wernicke's disease, Korsakoff's psychosis, alcoholic cerebellar ataxia, and polyneuropathy are but different facets of one disease process.

Treatment of the Wernicke-Korsakoff syndrome Wernicke's disease represents a medical emergency, and its recognition demands the immediate administration of thiamine. A delay of a few hours may be crucial in determining whether the patient who presents only ocular and ataxic signs will be prevented from developing mental signs and whether the patient with early Korsakoff changes will be restored to a state of mental competency. Although 2 to 3 mg thiamine is sufficient to modify the ocular signs, much larger doses are usually employed—50 mg intravenously and 50 mg intramuscularly, the latter dose being repeated each day until the patient resumes a normal diet. The other B vitamins may be given by mouth in the dosages outlined in Chap. 73. If the patient cannot or will not eat, parenteral feeding and administration of B vitamins become necessary.

A particular danger attends the treatment of the severely depleted alcoholic patient with intravenous glucose solutions. This may exhaust the patient's last reserve of B vitamins and either precipitate Wernicke's disease where it was not present before or cause a rapid worsening of the athiamniotic state with circulatory collapse and death. For this reason, B vitamins must be added in all cases requiring parenteral glucose. If there are signs of cardiac weakness, rapid digitalization should be undertaken. Since these patients are confused and forgetful, they must be supervised continually, preferably on a medical ward.

A special problem in management arises when the patient recovers from the acute phase of the illness and the amnesic psychosis becomes prominent. The disposition of the patient to family, nursing home, or mental institution should be undertaken on the basis of the severity of the mental illness as well as the capacity of the family unit and social circumstances.

NUTRITIONAL POLYNEUROPATHY (See also Chap. 80)   In the United States, nutritional polyneuropathy is essentially a disease of the alcoholic population. As has been mentioned above, it is present in more than 80 percent of patients with the Wernicke-Korsakoff syndrome, but it also occurs frequently as the only manifestation of deficiency disease. The polyneuropathy of alcoholism ("alcoholic polyneuropathy") does not differ in any fundamental way from that of beriberi. The clinical features of nutritional polyneuropathy and its identity with beriberi are discussed in Chap. 80, and the nutritional disorder is explained in greater detail in Chap. 377. Deficiency of thiamine chloride, pyridoxine pantothenic acid, vitamin B_{12}, and folic acid, has been demonstrated in each case to cause nutritional polyneuropathy. In the alcoholic patient it is difficult to incriminate any one of these factors.

PELLAGRA This disease is described in Chap. 79. The comments here are concerned only with the neurologic manifestations, which in themselves are extremely diverse. Pellagra is essentially an encephalopathy, although involvement of other parts of the nervous system may occur. The early mental symptoms—insomnia, fatigue, nervousness, irritability, and feelings of depression—may be mistaken for those of a psychoneurosis. However, careful examination as the disease advances will reveal slowing and inefficiency of mental processes and impairment of memory. Pellagra may not only be the cause of insanity but occasionally may result from it, because certain mental illnesses, including alcoholism, are accompanied by anorexia and unbalanced diet. Sometimes the patient passes rather rapidly (over a few days) into an acute confusional psychosis combined with changing rigidity of the limbs, grasping and sucking reflexes, and Babinski signs—a state referred to in the past as "nicotinic acid deficiency encephalopathy."

The manifestations of involvement of the spinal cord have not been clearly delineated, perhaps because the mental state of the patients has precluded accurate testing. In general, there is evidence of both posterior and lateral column involvement, predominantly the former. Neuropathic signs are frequent and difficult to distinguish from other types of polyneuropathy which may affect the posterior columns. Other manifestations such as tremors, extrapyramidal rigidity, sucking and grasping reflexes, and coma have indiscriminately been included in the pellagrous syndrome, as have various disorders of the special senses.

A *spastic paretic syndrome,* apart from the other symptoms and signs of pellagra, may be a rare manifestation of deficiency disease. The chief clinical signs are spastic weakness of the legs with absent abdominal and increased tendon reflexes, clonus, and extensor plantar responses. These signs are usually accompanied by other signs of nutritional deficiency, such as Wernicke's disease and retrobulbar and peripheral neuropathies. Spastic weakness of the legs has also been observed in conjunction with chronic liver disease.

Pathologic changes The distinctive neuropathologic changes in pellagra are most readily discerned in the large cells of the motor cortex, the cells of Betz, which appear swollen and rounded with eccentric nuclei and loss of the Nissl particles. This central neuritis of pellagra, as it is called, is probably not dependent on injury to the axons of the Betz cells but appears to represent a primary affection of the whole motor cell. The spinal cord lesions take the form of a symmetrical degeneration of the dorsal columns, especially those of Goll, and to a lesser extent of the corticospinal tracts. The posterior column degeneration affects a specific system of fibers and may be secondary to degeneration of the dorsal root ganglion cells. The pathogenesis of the corticospinal tract lesion in pellagra is not known.

DEFICIENCY AMBLYOPIA (NUTRITIONAL OPTIC NEUROPATHY, TOBACCO-ALCOHOL AMBLYOPIA) These terms refer to a characteristic form of visual impairment that complicates nutritional disease and is due to a lesion in the optic nerve, more or less confined to the zone of the papillomacular bundle. The cornea and other parts of the refractive mechanism are uninvolved, hence the term amblyopia.

The main symptom is dimness or blurring of vision for near and distant objects, which worsens progressively for several days or weeks. In addition to a reduction in visual acuity, examination discloses the presence of bilateral, more or less symmetrical central or centrocecal scotomata, which are larger for colored than for white test objects. Pallor of the temporal portion of the optic disk is observed in some cases. Untreated, this condition progresses to irreversible optic atrophy.

Deficiency amblyopia was particularly prevalent during World War II and the Korean War, in prisoner-of-war camps of the Far East. Although this form of amblyopia had previously been described in association with beriberi and pellagra, the peak incidence among prisoners did not coincide with either of these syndromes but with the syndrome of orogenital dermatitis and "burning feet" (see below, under Strachan's syndrome).

In the United States many, if not all, of the cases of retrobulbar neuropathy attributed to the toxic effects of alcohol or tobacco—so-called "tobacco-alcohol amblyopia"—are of nutritional origin. Optic neuropathy may occur as the only manifestation of deficiency disease, but more often it is combined with other nutritional syndromes, such as peripheral neuropathy and the Wernicke-Korsakoff syndrome.

Although the nutritional origin of this type of amblyopia seems established, the specific nutrient that is responsible is uncertain. Observations in both humans and experimental animals indicate that a deficiency of thiamine or vitamin B_{12} or perhaps riboflavin may cause degenerative changes in the optic nerves. It has been suggested that the combined effects of vitamin B_{12} deficiency and chronic poisoning with cyanide (generated in tobacco smoke) are responsible for "tobacco amblyopia." Vitamin B_{12} deficiency is a rare but established cause of optic neuropathy, but the notion that cyanide or other substances in tobacco smoke have a damaging effect upon the optic nerves is not supported by experimental data.

Since a specific nutritional deficiency can rarely be determined in this disorder, treatment consists of the administration of a balanced diet and supplemented with B vitamins and the interdiction of alcohol where this is a factor.

SYNDROME OF AMBLYOPIA, PAINFUL NEUROPATHY, AND OROGENITAL DERMATITIS (STRACHAN'S SYNDROME) Beginning with the observations of Strachan, in 1888, and 1897, there have been many reports from diverse sources concerning a neurologic syndrome which is undoubtedly nutritional in origin but which cannot be forced into the boundaries of the classical deficiency diseases, beriberi and pellagra. Although Strachan was probably the first to describe this syndrome, he did not recognize its nutritional etiology (he attributed it to malaria). Originally known as "Jamaican neuritis," the syndrome was soon recognized among the undernourished population of many other tropical countries. Large numbers of patients with this syndrome were observed also in the beseiged population of Madrid during the Spanish Civil War and later during World War II, among prisoners in the Middle and Far East.

Strachan's syndrome is essentially a disorder of the peripheral and optic nerves. Clinically, sensory symptoms and signs dominate the picture; in this respect the syndrome differs from beriberi. Paresthesias of the extremities, painful hyperesthesia of the feet, loss of superficial and deep sensation, and ataxia are the common manifestations. On the other hand, foot drop and muscle weakness occur very rarely. A frequently associated disorder is failing vision, which may go on to complete blindness and pallor of the optic disks. In general, deafness and vertigo are rare complications, but in some outbreaks among prisoners-of-war these symptoms were so common as to earn the epithet "camp dizziness." Along with the neurologic signs there may be varying degrees of stomatoglossitis, corneal degeneration, and genital dermatitis. These mucocutaneous lesions are often spoken of together as the *orogenital syndrome* and are quite distinct from those of pellagra.

There have been only a few pathologic studies of this syndrome. Aside from the damage to the papillomacular bundle in the optic nerve, the most consistent abnormality has been a loss of medullated fibers in each column of Goll adjacent to the midline. This indicates a systematized degeneration of the central process of the bipolar sensory neuron of the lumbosacral spinal ganglia. The fact that the primary sensory neuron is the chief site of disease is consistent with the predominant sensory symptomatology. There are no reliable data concerning the specific deficiencies (vitamin or other) that cause this disease.

Patients with this syndrome are occasionally found among the alcoholic population of the United States. It may also accompany chronic liver disease and nontropical sprue or occur as an inexplicable illness in late adult life.

SUBACUTE COMBINED DEGENERATION OF THE SPINAL CORD (See also Chap. 34) Subacute combined degeneration (SCD) is the term used to designate the spinal cord disease that results from vitamin B_{12} deficiency. The brain, optic nerves, and peripheral nerves may also be involved in the course of vitamin B_{12} deficiency but far less often than the spinal cord. The neurological manifestations of vitamin B_{12} deficiency, and the hematologic ones (pernicious anemia), are clearly different from the other deficiency diseases insofar as their usual cause is not a lack of vitamin B_{12} in food but an inability to transfer minute amounts of this nutrient across the intestinal mucosa ("starvation in the midst of plenty," as Castle has aptly phrased it). Such a nutritional disorder is referred to as a *conditioned deficiency,* since it depends upon the lack of an intrinsic factor in the gastric secretion (see Chap. 311).

Clinical manifestations Symptoms of nervous system disease are present in the large majority of patients with pernicious anemia. The patient first notices general weakness and paresthesias consisting of tingling, "pins and needles" feelings, or other vaguely described sensations. The paresthesias tend to be constant, to progress steadily, and to be the source of much distress. They are localized in the distal parts of the limbs in a symmetric distribution; the lower extremities may be involved before the upper ones or vice versa. As the illness progresses the gait becomes unsteady, and movements of the limbs, especially of the legs, become stiff and awkward.

Early in the course of the illness, when only paresthesias are present, there may be no objective signs. Later, the neurological examination discloses a disorder of the posterior or lateral columns of the spinal cord, predominantly of the former. Loss of vibration sense is by far the most consistent sign; it is more pronounced in the legs than in the arms, and frequently it extends over the trunk. Position sense is involved somewhat less frequently. The motor signs include loss of power spasticity, changes in the tendon reflexes, clonus, and extensor plantar responses. These signs are usually limited to the legs. At first the patellar and Achilles reflexes are found to be diminished as frequently as they are increased, and they may even be absent. With treatment the reflexes may return to normal or become hyperactive. The gait at first is predominantly ataxic, later ataxic and spastic. If the disease remains untreated, an ataxic paraplegia with variable degrees of spasticity and contracture may develop.

Isolated instances of loss of superficial sensation below a segmental level on the trunk do occur, implicating the spinothalamic tracts, but such a finding should always suggest the possibility of some other disease of the spinal cord. The defect of cutaneous sensation may take the form of a mild blunting of touch, pain, and temperature sensation over the limbs in a distal distribution, implicating the peripheral nerves, but such findings are also uncommon.

The nervous system involvement in vitamin B_{12} deficiency is characteristically, though not always, symmetric. A definite asymmetry of motor or sensory findings, maintained over a period of weeks or months, should always cast doubt on the diagnosis.

Mental signs are frequent, ranging from irritability, apathy, somnolence, suspiciousness, and emotional instability to a marked confusional or depressive psychosis, or even to intellectual deterioration. Visual impairment is infrequent and presents with roughly symmetrical centrocecal scotomata. If involvement of the optic nerve is severe, optic atrophy may occur. Although dementia and amblyopia are relatively uncommon, they may be the initial manifestations of the disease.

Neuropathologic changes The pathologic process takes the form of diffuse, although uneven, degeneration of the white matter. At first there is swelling of myelin sheaths, which imparts a vacuolated appearance to the tissue, followed by a breakdown of myelin and a coalescence of small foci of tissue destruction into larger ones. The myelin sheaths and the axis cylinders are both affected, the former perhaps earlier and to a greater extent than the latter. There is relatively little fibrous gliosis in the early lesions, but in the older treated cases gliosis is pronounced. The changes begin in the posterior columns of the lower cervical and upper thoracic cord and spread from this region up and down the cord, as well as forward into the lateral columns. The lesions are not limited to specific systems of fibers within the posterior and lateral funiculi but are scattered irregularly through the latter.

Unlike the atrophy of lingual and gastric mucosa and the block in the maturation of red blood cells due to the action of vitamin B_{12} in the synthesis of nucleoprotein, the lesions in the nervous system are due to failure of another essential function of this vitamin—the conversion of methylmalonyl- to succinyl-coenzyme A. Since these two defects do not parallel one another, either the hematologic or the neurological abnormality may occur separately.

In addition there is some evidence that a deficiency of folic acid, such as occurs in celiac disease and intestinal malabsorptive conditions, may cause either a subacute degeneration of the spinal cord or a nutritional polyneuropathy, usually the latter. (See Pallis and Lewis for a review of these data.)

Treatment The treatment of the neurological manifestations of vitamin B_{12} deficiency differs in no way from the treatment of the other manifestations of pernicious anemia. Theoretically, 1 μg per day of parenterally administered vitamin B_{12} is adequate, but in practice much larger doses are used.

The most important factor influencing *response* to treatment is the duration of the disease. Recovery may be complete if therapy is instituted within a few weeks of the onset of symptoms. For this reason SCD and the other neurological complications of vitamin B_{12} deficiency represent medical emergencies. If symptoms have been present for longer than a month or two, only partial recovery can be expected, and in long-standing cases the best that can be expected is the arrest of progression of the symptoms.

The chief obstacle to early diagnosis is the lack of parallelism between the hematologic and neurological signs. This is particularly the case in patients who have received folic acid, which serves to maintain a hematologic remission for an indefinite period while the neurological signs worsen, often to an irreversible stage. Under these circumstances the most reliable diagnostic procedure is the Schilling test.

VITAMIN-RESPONSIVE, GENETICALLY DETERMINED DISEASES An important development is the recognition that in certain genetically determined disorders the disability can be diminished or reversed by the administration of vitamins or cofactors in quantities far in excess of their usual requirements. These disorders are referred to as *vitamin-dependency states* or *vitamin-responsive disorders*. The following vitamins have been shown to act in this manner: cobalamin (vitamin B_{12}) in methylmalonic aciduria; pyridoxine in infantile convulsions and certain cases of homocystinuria; biotin in propionic acidemia; thiamine in lactic acidosis, Leigh's encephalopathy, and rare cases of maple syrup urine disease; and niacin in Hartnup disease. The biochemical mechanisms involved are not yet clear. It is presumed that the vitamin or cofactor stabilizes a genetically deficient enzyme or facilitates its interaction with its substrate. Awareness of these states is of great practical significance, since administration of specific cofactors in appropriate dosage may restore to normal function a person who would otherwise die or be severely disabled. Careful therapeutic trials should be undertaken whenever one of the above disorders is documented by precise enzymatic assays. Even among patients who have apparently similar enzyme defects, there still appears to be considerable heterogeneity. Thus some patients may respond very favorably to the administration of the cofactor, while others may show no improvement.

UNDERNUTRITION, PROTEIN-CALORIE DEFICIENCY, AND MENTAL RETARDATION Although not a problem of immediate concern to the internist, any discussion of the nervous disorders associated with malnutrition would be incomplete without some reference to infantile malnutrition and mental retardation.

During the past two decades evidence has accumulated from observations of children and animal experimentation that gross insufficiency of food in early life can interfere with brain development, leaving the child temporarily or permanently mentally enfeebled. And since there are more than 100 million children in the world who are suffering from malnutrition and who will eventually be incompetent adults, this stands as one of the most important public health problems.

The evidence appears to indicate that a reduction of all the essential elements of diet but particularly of protein impairs the function and alters the chemistry of the brain in all species studied, including humans. In the latter the most definite effects occur when the deficiency is in early life, whether antenatal or postnatal, viz., in infancy. Once the maturation and development of the brain are complete, general nutritional or protein deficiency harm the nervous system little if at all.

Retardation in statural growth and brain development is believed to have been observed in three human syndromes: (1) one group of the "small-for-dates" babies; (2) marasmic infants; and (3) kwashiorkor. "Small-for-dates" babies weigh less than 2500 g at term and are generally small and cachectic. Marasmic children are cachectic, their bones are prominent because of a lack of subcutaneous fat, their skin is thin and wrinkled, and their heads seem too large for their bodies. Kwashiorkor infants show less disproportion between head and body size, have edematous extremities and rounded face, and blanched or reddish hair. Marasmic and kwashiorkor infants fall more than two standard deviations below the body size of age-matched controls and are apathetic, irritable, and delayed in achieving normal maturational milestones. When the diet is replenished they improve rapidly, but many are believed to be left with a subnormal intelligence.

Marasmus is caused by a diet generally inadequate in all essential elements but mainly in total calories. In kwashiorkor it is the protein content that is inadequate, and most of the calories are in the form of carbohydrate. This unbalanced diet impairs growth; and although the intake of carbohydrates lessens tissue metabolism, the depletion of essential amino acids and reduced synthesis of certain proteins is thought to result in underdevelopment of the brain and also edema of the face and extremities (from low serum albumen).

Studies of the brain in the protein-deficient or starved animal have revealed only a slight reduction in weight. And, if the deficiency occurred during critical periods of intrauterine life (i.e., during neuronal formation, migration, differentiation, and myelination) there may be a reduction in number of neurous and incomplete myelin formation. These histologic changes have not been found by all investigators in the experimental animal and have not been observed in the few human cases adequately examined. Moreover, they could hardly account for the improvement that nearly always follows correction of the nutritional deficiency.

As matters presently stand one cannot be sure that undernutrition in the human infant is the sole cause of either subnormal brain development or of mental retardation. Not only has it been difficult to assess the mental function of malnourished infants, but it has been virtually impossible to exclude the effects of inherited intellectual defects and impoverished environment, since most of the patients come from the lowest social and economic segment of the population. For a cautious analysis of these several factors the reader should turn to the monographs of Dodge et al. and of Scrimshaw and Gordon.

REFERENCES

ADAMS RD, VICTOR M: *Principles of Neurology.* New York, McGraw-Hill, 1977

DODGE PR et al: *Nutrition and the Developing Nervous System.* St Louis, Mosby, 1975

PALLIS CA, LEWIS PD: *The Neurology of Gastrointestinal Disease.* New York, Saunders, 1974

POTTS AM: Tobacco amblyopia. Surv Ophthalmol 17:313, 1973

SCRIMSHAW NS, GORDON JE (eds): *Malnutrition, Learning and Behavior.* Cambridge, MIT Press, 1968

SILBER R, MOLDON DF: The biochemistry of B$_{12}$ mediated reactions in man. Am J Med 48:549, 1970

VICTOR M: Polyneuropathy due to nutritional deficiency and alcoholism, in *Peripheral Neuropathy,* PJ Dyck et al (eds). Philadelphia, Saunders, 1975, pp 1030-1066

———, ADAMS RD: On the etiology of the alcoholic neurologic diseases. With special reference to the role of nutrition. Am J Clin Nutr 9:379, 1961

——— et al: Deficiency amblyopia in the alcoholic patient. A clinicopathologic study. Arch Ophthalmol 64:1, 1960

——— et al: *The Wernicke-Korsakoff Syndrome. A Clinical and Pathological Study of 245 Patients, 82 with Postmortem Examinations.* Philadelphia, Davis, 1971

WINICK M: *Malnutrition and Brain Development.* New York, Oxford University Press, 1976

373

DEGENERATIVE DISEASES OF THE NERVOUS SYSTEM
Alzheimer's disease and Parkinson's disease

EDWARD P. RICHARDSON, JR.
RAYMOND D. ADAMS

The term *degenerative* as applied to diseases of the nervous system is used to designate a group of disorders in which there is gradual, generally symmetric, relentlessly progressive wasting away of neurons for reasons still unknown. Many of the conditions so designated depend on genetic factors and thus appear in more than one member of the same family; this general group of diseases is, therefore, frequently referred to as *heredodegenerative.* A number of other conditions, not apparently differing in any fundamental way from the hereditary disorders, occur only sporadically, i.e., as isolated instances in a given family. For all diseases of this class Sir William Gowers in 1902 suggested the now-familiar term *abiotrophy,* by which he meant "defective vital endurance" of the structures affected, leading to their premature death. This term, of course, tells nothing of the true nature of the defects. It is to be assumed that their basis must be some disorder of the metabolism of the parts involved.

Within relatively recent times there has been some elucidation of the nature of a number of metabolic nervous disorders which, in their symmetric distribution and gradually progressive course, resemble the degenerative diseases under discussion. It is to be expected that with advances in knowledge others of the latter group will eventually find their place in the metabolic category. It is possible that some of these diseases may turn out to be the result of atypical virus infections, as has been demonstrated in one disease previously classified with the degenerative group, Creutzfeldt-Jakob disease, also called subacute spongiform encephalopathy (see Chap. 192).

The degenerative diseases of the nervous system manifest themselves by a number of common syndromes easily distinguished by their clinical attributes, the recognition of which can assist the clinician in arriving at the diagnosis of a disorder of this class. Some of these syndromes and the particular diseases which give rise to them are summarized in the following paragraphs.

GENERAL CONSIDERATIONS It is a characteristic of the degenerative diseases that they begin insidiously and run a gradually progressive course which may extend over many years. The earliest changes may be so slight that it is frequently impossible to assign any precise time of onset. However, as with other gradually developing conditions, the patient or his family may give a history implying an abrupt appearance of disability. This is particularly likely to occur if there has been an injury, or if some other dramatic event has taken place in the patient's life, to which illness might conceivably be related. In such a case, skillful taking of the history may bring out that the patient or family has suddenly become aware of a condition which had, in fact, already been present for some time but had passed unnoticed. Whether trauma or other stress may bring on or aggravate one of the degenerative diseases is still a question that cannot be answered with certainty. From all that is known it would seem highly improbable that this could happen. In any event, it must be kept in mind that the disease processes under discussion by their very nature develop spontaneously without relation to external factors.

The family history is of great importance, but one cannot always be immediately satisfied with that obtained on first contact with the patient. One reason for this is that patients or their relatives may be ashamed to disclose a neurologic disease that has occurred in the family. Another is that it may not be realized that an illness is hereditary when other members of the family have a much less severe form of the disorder such that the patient and family may have been unaware of the abnormality—as not infrequently occurs in the hereditary ataxias and related conditions. Moreover, in modern Western families the small sibships may prevent even well-established hereditary diseases from expressing themselves. It must, of course, be remembered that familial occurrence of a disease does not always mean that it is hereditary; it may indicate instead that more than one member of a family has been exposed to the same infectious or toxic agent.

Another significant feature of the degenerative nervous diseases is that in general their ceaselessly progressive course is uninfluenced by all medical or surgical measures. Dealing with a patient with this type of illness is often, therefore, an anguishing experience for all concerned. Yet symptoms can often be alleviated by wise and skillful management, and the physician's kindly interest may be of great help even when curative measures cannot be offered.

The bilaterally symmetric distribution of the changes brought about by these diseases has already been mentioned. This feature alone may serve to distinguish conditions in this group from many other diseases of the nervous system. At the same time, it should be pointed out that, in the earliest stages, greater involvement on one side or in one limb is not uncommon. Sooner or later, however, despite the asymmetric beginning, the inherently generalized nature of the process asserts itself.

A striking feature of a number of disorders of this class is the almost selective involvement of anatomically or physiologically related systems of neurons. This is clearly exemplified in amyotrophic lateral sclerosis, in which the process is almost entirely limited to cortical and spinal motor neurons, and in certain types of progressive ataxia, in which the Purkinje cells of the cerebellum are alone affected. Many other examples could be cited (e.g., Friedreich's ataxia) in which certain neuronal systems disintegrate, leaving others perfectly intact. An important group of the degenerative diseases has therefore been called "system diseases" ("progressive cerebrospinal system atrophies"), and many of these are strongly hereditary. It must be realized, however, that selective involvement of neuronal systems is not exclusively a property of the degenerative group, since several disease processes of known cause have similarly circumscribed effects on the nervous system. Diphtheria toxin, for instance, selectively attacks the myelin of the peripheral nerves, and triorthocresyl phosphate affects particularly the corticospinal tracts in the spinal cord as well as the peripheral nerves. Another example is the special vulnerability of the Purkinje cells of the cerebellum to hyperthermia. On the other hand, several of the conditions included among the degenerative diseases are characterized by pathologic changes that are diffuse and unselective. These exceptions nevertheless do not detract from the importance of affection of particular neuronal systems as a distinguishing feature of many of the diseases under discussion.

Typically, the pathologic process in the nervous system is one of slow involution of nerve cell bodies or their prolongations as nerve fibers, unaccompanied by any intense tissue reaction or cellular response. The cerebrospinal fluid, therefore, shows little if any change—at most a slight elevation of protein, without abnormalities in pressure, cell count, or in other constituents. Moreover, since these diseases invariably result in tissue loss, rather than in new tissue formation (as with neoplasms or inflammation), x-ray visualization of the ventricular system or subarachnoid space shows either no change or an enlargement of these compartments. These negative laboratory findings thus help to distinguish the degenerative disorders

TABLE 373-1
Clinical classification of the degenerative diseases of the nervous system

I Syndrome in which progressive dementia is an outstanding feature, in the absence of other prominent neurologic signs
  A Diffuse cerebral atrophy
    1 Senile dementia
    2 Alzheimer's disease
  B Circumscribed cerebral atrophy (Pick's disease)
II Syndrome in which progressive dementia is combined with other neurologic signs
  A Principally in adults
    1 Huntington's chorea
    2 Cerebrocerebellar degeneration
  B In children and adults
    1 Amaurotic family idiocy (neuronal lipidoses)
    2 Leukodystrophy
    3 Familial myoclonus epilepsy
    4 Hallervorden-Spatz disease
    5 Wilson's disease (hepatolenticular degeneration, Westphal-Strumpell pseudosclerosis)
III Syndrome chiefly manifested by gradual development of abnormalities of posture or involuntary movements
  A Paralysis agitans (Parkinson's disease)
  B Dystonia musculorum deformans (torsion dystonia)
  C Hallervorden-Spatz disease and other restricted dyskinesias
  D Familial tremor
  E Spasmodic torticollis
IV Syndrome chiefly manifested by slowly developing ataxia
  A Cerebellar degenerations
  B Spinocerebellar degenerations (Friedreich's ataxia, Marie's hereditary ataxia)
V Syndrome with slowly developing muscular weakness and wasting
  A Without sensory changes; motor system disease
    1 In adults
      a Amyotrophic lateral sclerosis
      b Progressive muscular atrophy
      c Progressive bulbar palsy
      d Primary lateral sclerosis
    2 In children or young adults
      a Infantile muscular atrophy (Werdnig-Hoffmann disease)
      b Other forms of familial progressive muscular atrophy (including Wohlfart-Kugelberg-Welander syndrome)
      c Hereditary spastic paraplegia
  B With sensory changes
    1 Progressive neural muscular atrophy
      a Peroneal muscular atrophy (Charcot-Marie-Tooth)
      b Hypertrophic interstitial neuropathy (Dejerine-Sottas)
    2 Miscellaneous forms of chronic progressive neuropathy
VI Syndrome chiefly manifested by progressive visual loss
  A Hereditary optic atrophy (Leber's disease)
  B Pigmentary degeneration of the retina (retinitis pigmentosa)

from the other large classes of progressive diseases of the nervous system—tumors and infections.

CLASSIFICATION Since etiologic classification is impossible, subdivision of the degenerative diseases into individual syndromes rests on descriptive criteria, based largely on pathologic anatomy but to some extent on clinical aspects as well. In the terms used to designate many of these syndromes, the names of a number of distinguished neurologists and neuropathologists are commemorated. A useful way of keeping in mind the various disease states is to group them according to the outstanding clinical features that may be found in an actual case. The classification outlined in Table 373-1 and described below is based on such a plan.

SYNDROMES IN WHICH PROGRESSIVE DEMENTIA PREDOMINATES

In the disease entities about to be discussed, the clinical picture is dominated by gradual loss of intellectual capacities, i.e., by dementia. Other neurologic abnormalities, except in the terminal stages, are absent or relatively insignificant. (For further discussion of dementia, including its clinical evaluation, Chap. 25 should be consulted.)

DIFFUSE CEREBRAL ATROPHY: SENILE DEMENTIA, ALZHEIMER'S DISEASE Some degree of shrinkage in size and weight of the brain, i.e., "atrophy," has been shown to be the inevitable accompaniment of advancing age. In many instances, this is of no clinical significance, and there are many very old people who remain alert and perceptive, with keen intellect, to the end. Nevertheless, severe degrees of diffuse cerebral atrophy are as a general rule associated with some evidence of dementia. When these changes occur in old age (and the definition of when old age begins is largely subjective), it is usual to speak of *senile dementia*. That this is a fairly frequent condition is common experience. Much more infrequent is a pathologically identical progressive dementia with diffuse brain atrophy coming on well before the senile period—a presenile dementia. This condition, classically described in 1906 by Alois Alzheimer, has since become generally known as *Alzheimer's disease*. The distinction between the two conditions is purely clinical; pathologically, they differ only in that the characteristic abnormalities tend to be more severe and widespread in cases beginning at an earlier age than at the senile period.

Pathology The brain presents a generally shrunken appearance, with atrophy of the convolutions and symmetric enlargement of the lateral and third ventricles. Frequently, these changes are especially pronounced in the frontal and temporal lobes. Microscopically, there is widespread loss of nerve cells, most apparent in the cerebral cortex, but often present likewise in the basal ganglia, with secondary glial proliferation. In addition, two types of lesions give this disease process its distinctive character: (1) microscopic deposits of amorphous material, scattered throughout the cerebral cortex and most easily seen with silver-staining methods—the so-called "senile plaques"—and (2) the Alzheimer fibrillary change in nerve cells. This striking abnormality consists of the presence within the cytoplasm of thick fiber-like strands of silver-staining material, often in the form of loops, coils, or tangled masses. Recent investigations have greatly advanced knowledge of the structural aspects of these lesions, in that the senile plaques are now known to contain amyloid, and the fibrillary change is characterized by masses of paired helical filaments. Their pathogenesis is still unknown, however. Of interest is the observation of

Bowen et al. of a reduction of choline acetyltransferase, the key enzyme in the synthesis of the neurotransmitter acetylcholine, in the cerebral cortex of senile dementia. This suggests that impairment of cholinergic transmission may play a part in the clinical expression of the disease.

Clinical aspects Although Alzheimer's disease has been described as occurring during every age period, it is most frequently a disease of the later decades of life. A number of well-documented familial cases have been recorded, but there is not sufficient evidence to indicate that this is truly a hereditary disorder. Most of the cases actually seen in practice are sporadic. The onset is insidious and subtle, with changes most noticeable first in memory for recent happenings and in range of mental activity. Emotional disturbances such as depression, anxiety, or odd, unpredictable quirks of behavior, may be salient features in the early stages. Progression is very slow and gradual, and unless the condition is earlier brought to a close by the effects of advanced age, it may smolder on for some 10 to 15 years.

In the milder cases, including those of the senile period, the noteworthy features are those of simple dementia, as described in Chap. 25. More unusual disorders of thought and intellect, including aphasia, apraxic disturbances, and abnormalities of space perception, may be seen, especially in the presenile group. Exceptionally, in the advanced stages of the disease extrapyramidal signs appear; the patient walks in a shuffling manner with short steps, and there is a generalized stiffness of the musculature with slowness and awkwardness of all movements. These abnormalities have been attributed to involvement of the basal ganglia. Terminally the patient may become nearly decorticate, losing all ability to perceive, think, speak, or move. Additional investigative procedures, including the usual blood and cerebrospinal fluid determinations, do not yield any conclusive or pertinent data. There is a diffuse slowing in the electroencephalogram in the more advanced stages of the disease. The enlargement of the ventricular system and subarachnoid space resulting from the diffuse brain atrophy can be demonstrated by computerized tomography (CT scan) and pneumoencephalography; otherwise, no characteristic roentgenographic findings are seen. During the course of the illness, occasional convulsive seizures may occur, but they are relatively rare and should raise suspicion of other diseases. Terminally, in a state of total helplessness the patient dies from intercurrent disease. Usually, long before the end, institutional care is necessary.

Differential diagnosis Several disease states for which effective treatment is available may give rise to progressive intellectual deterioration closely resembling what may be seen with the diffuse cerebral atrophy above described. It is imperative that these be looked for. Specific examples include chronic subdural hematoma, chronic "normal pressure" hydrocephalus, frontal meningioma, bromide intoxication, myxedema, pernicious anemia (vitamin B_{12} deficiency), and neurosyphilis. Various other forms of intoxication, infection, metabolic disorder, or neoplasm may have to be considered. Of these several conditions that simulate the Alzheimer-senile dementia complex "normal pressure hydrocephalus" is one that has yielded most dramatically to therapy. As originally pointed out by Hakim and Adams, an obstruction to cerebrospinal fluid (CSF) flow in the ventricles or basal meninges will greatly enlarge the ventricles, and, after this has happened, the CSF pressure may gradually return to normal levels. Forgetfulness and reduced mental activity (without agnosia, apraxia, or aphasia) are accompanied by an awkward, unsteady, short-stepped gait and sphincteric incontinence. Worsening of the condition results in a marked impairment of intellectual activity and finally an inability to walk or even to stand up. The plantar reflexes become extensor and grasp and sucking reflexes appear. The ventricles are greatly enlarged (span of lateral ventricles greater than 55 mm), radionuclides placed in subarachnoid space reflex into the ventricles, and air during pneumoencephalography will not enter the cerebral subarachnoid spaces. Previous subarachnoid hemorrhage (trauma, aneurysmal rupture), chronic meningitis (syphilitic, idiopathic), Paget's disease of base of skull, and tumors of benign type (cysts of third ventricle) are some of the causes. Other causes are idiopathic. A ventriculoatrial or ventriculoperitoneal shunt relieves the symptoms in a few weeks.

Marked underactivity (mental and physical), extreme drowsiness, increased ratio of sleep to wakefulness, and hypothermia, when combined with ataxia, slow speech, and prolonged tendon reflexes should always raise suspicion of hypothyroidism. Episodic stupor or coma, with or without seizures; cerebellar ataxia; and choreoathetosis suggest hepatic failure. Other metabolic disorders, chronic intoxications, and chronic infections, e.g., syphilitic meningomyelitis must be excluded by clinical signs and laboratory tests described in Chaps. 146, 227, and 369. In addition to careful clinical assessment special radiologic procedures such as CT scan and pneumoencephalography or carotid angiography may be necessary. Vascular disease of the brain is often included in the differential diagnosis, but dementia on the basis of cerebrovascular disorders characteristically progresses in a halting or stepwise fashion with conspicuous focal cerebral signs, whereas the progression in senile dementia or Alzheimer's disease is gradual and steady and focal signs are absent. A depressive psychosis may also resemble a degenerative disease and must be differentiated along the lines suggested in Chap. 25. No specific therapy is known. Recent evidence of impaired central cholinergic transmission has led to the use of acetylcholine precursors such as lecithin and choline or an anticholinesterase drug such as physostigmine. But there are no data in support of their beneficial effects. The management should be along the lines of that described in Chaps. 21 and 25 for the delirious and demented patient.

PICK'S DISEASE (CIRCUMSCRIBED CEREBRAL ATROPHY)

This remarkable form of cerebral disease, which is characterized by the circumscription of the atrophy (lobar sclerosis), was first described in a series of publications by Arnold Pick in Prague, around the turn of the century. In the differential diagnosis of dementia in the presenile period, it is often mentioned in the same breath with Alzheimer's disease. It is, however, an extremely rare condition as compared with diffuse cerebral atrophy of the Alzheimer type.

Pathology So striking are the gross pathologic changes in the brain that in typical cases the diagnosis can be made at a glance. One sees severe atrophy of the anterior portions of the frontal and temporal lobes, and there is a curiously sharp line of demarcation between the atrophied portions and the remainder of the brain, which appears normal or nearly so. In some cases, the frontal atrophy is more prominent; in others, the temporal lobes are more severely involved; in general, both regions are affected. Characteristically, there likewise are atrophic changes in a number of subcortical structures: caudate nucleus, putamen, thalamus, and substantia nigra, and in the descending frontopontine fiber system. In the diseased regions, the local destruction of central and convolutional white matter is out of proportion to the degree of loss of nerve cell bodies in corresponding areas of the cortex. A noteworthy histologic feature of this condition is the occurrence of numerous swollen "ballooned" nerve cells in the atrophic regions, a finding which has been interpreted as an axonal reaction or retrograde cell change secondary to the degenerative process in the periphery. Another frequent nerve cell change is the presence of spheric intracytoplasmic inclusions that stain deeply with silver impregnation methods; the significance of these is unknown. Under the electron microscope they are seen to be composed of masses of straight filaments clearly differing from the aggregates of helical filaments in Alzheimer's disease.

Clinical aspects If Pick's disease has any distinguishing clinical features, they are unusually severe signs of frontal lobe or temporal lobe involvement (see Chap. 25). Actually, there is no satisfactory way of differentiating between Alzheimer's and Pick's disease during life, nor is this of any practical importance. Familial occurrence is on record in a number of instances. Progression is slow and relentless, the average duration of Pick's disease being about 7 years.

Differential diagnosis The considerations noted above with respect to Alzheimer's disease apply to Pick's disease as well.

SYNDROME COMBINING DEMENTIA WITH OTHER NEUROLOGIC SIGNS

HUNTINGTON'S DISEASE (CHRONIC PROGRESSIVE HEREDITARY CHOREA) This condition, which genetically follows the pattern of a mendelian dominant trait, was classically described in 1872 by George Huntington, who, with his father and grandfather, both physicians, observed cases in members of a family living near their home on Long Island, New York. Unmistakable in its typical form, the affliction combines progressive dementia with bizarre involuntary movements (chorea) and odd postures. Atypical cases have also been recognized (see below), but in general the disorder runs true to form.

Pathology The brain has a generally atrophic appearance, especially noticeable in the frontal lobes. Particularly characteristic is severe bilateral atrophy of the caudate nucleus, which becomes flattened and concave instead of projecting as a convex rounded eminence into the anterior horn of the lateral ventricle. The putamen, likewise, is shrunken, although not to the same extent as the caudate nucleus. The globus pallidus is generally involved to some degree, but less severely than the caudate nucleus and putamen. Microscopically, the affected regions show severe nerve cell loss with reactive glial changes.

Of considerable interest with regard to pathogenesis has been the discovery that the caudate and putamen in the brains of patients with Huntington's chorea are deficient in glutamic acid decarboxylase as well as the inhibitory transmitter γ-aminobutyric acid (GABA). There is also a deficiency of choline acetyltransferase, the enzyme required for acetylcholine synthesis.

Clinical aspects This distressing condition generally makes its appearance in early to middle adult years. Its typical hereditary nature (mendelian dominant) has been emphasized, but it is not at all rare for sporadic cases to occur. The involuntary movements (bizarre grimacing, respiratory irregularity, faulty articulation of speech, and irregular, arrhythmic, unpatterned movements of the limbs, imparting to the gait a peculiar dancing quality) tend to be less quick and more athetoid than in Sydenham's chorea (see Chap. 16). A few reported cases which on genealogic and pathologic grounds must be classified with Huntington's chorea have shown progressive rigidity, rather than choreiform movements. As a general rule, dementia runs parallel with the motor disorder. Occasionally it may appear before or after chorea; very rarely it may be slight or lacking altogether. The advance of the disease is slow. There is increasing disability because of both involuntary movements and mental changes, terminated after many years by death from intercurrent infection or, not rarely, by suicide.

Differential diagnosis There is no difficulty in the recognition of typical cases. The relatively late onset, the slowly progressive course, the prominent dementia, and lack of association with rheumatic fever help to exclude Sydenham's chorea. Treated cases of Parkinson's disease, when overdosed with L-dopa may develop a widespread chorea, and the early dementia that occurs in some patients will reproduce the picture of Huntington's chorea. Phenothiazine drugs may induce generalized chorea, unassociated with dementia. Finally, there is a form of self-limited chorea that may appear in older persons without identifiable cause. Hepatolenticular degeneration (Wilson's disease) and nonfamilial forms of hepatocerebral degeneration may display clinical abnormalities resembling those of Huntington's chorea, but the specific changes characteristic of these disorders, including liver disease, corneal Kayser-Fleischer rings (in Wilson's disease), and the typical biochemical abnormalities, are absent in Huntington's chorea. Choreoathetosis appearing during the second postnatal year and lasting throughout life is due to hypoxic birth injury or kernicterus. Sporadic cases of choreiform movements beginning in middle or late life may present a difficult problem in exact diagnosis. The occasional cases of violent choreiform movements produced by vascular lesions, classically in the subthalamic region, are characterized by sudden onset, unilateral distribution (hemiballismus), and a tendency to improve after a period of initial severity. A few cases of acute choreoathetosis have accompanied hyperthyroidism. Virus encephalitis may occasionally be associated with choreiform movements; acute development, fever, and pleocytosis in the cerebrospinal fluid help in recognition of such cases.

Treatment It is impossible to halt the progress of this disease by any of the suggested forms of treatment. Chlorpromazine in doses of 25 to 50 mg three times daily and haloperidol, 2 to 4 mg three times daily, help to control the chorea. L-Dopa usually makes the chorea worse and if given in a dosage of 3.0 g per day is said to evoke chorea in an asymptomatic descendant of choreic patients. The finding of low levels of excitatory and inhibitory transmitter substances would suggest that agents which raise their levels might be of value therapeutically.

DEMENTIA WITH ATAXIA The progressive cerebellar degenerations of late life, and some cases of spinocerebellar degeneration, may be accompanied by significant dementia, the pathologic basis for which is not always easily demonstrated. These disorders are dealt with more fully below in the section devoted to conditions manifested by ataxia.

LIPIDOSES OF THE NERVOUS SYSTEM The conditions to be considered here differ from other degenerative disorders in that the underlying pathologic change is more suggestive of a biochemical abnormality. They are characterized by a more or less widespread derangement of lipid metabolism, which results in abnormal accumulations of lipids in the cytoplasm of cells of the nervous system and often of other organs as well. (For information relating to the problem of the lipidoses in general, Chaps. 101 and 374 should be consulted.) This process leads to abnormal function and, eventually, to death of the affected nerve cells. There is ample evidence for hereditary transmission of these disorders, the basis for which must consist of genetically determined abnormalities of enzyme systems concerned with intracellular lipid metabolism. This group of diseases is currently the subject of much intensive biochemical and ultrastructural investigation, such that for several of them it has been possible to identify the enzymes that are deficient.

SPECIAL CLINICAL TYPES The forms of lipidoses which affect the nervous system exclusively have often been classified together in the earlier literature as *amaurotic family idiocy*. This term emphasizes the important hereditary aspect, but it is not entirely satisfactory, since it can be correctly applied only to cases occurring in infancy. Of interest to the internist is a group of diseases that cause dementia and various other neurological abnormalities during late childhood, adolescence, and early adult life. In the older child and adult, blindness (amaurosis) may never develop, and "idiocy," strictly speaking, implies defective intelligence existing from earliest infancy. Another name that has been given to this group of lipidoses is *cerebromacular degeneration*, but it is accurate only for infantile cases and for patients with the combination of cerebral lesions and degeneration of the macular part of the retina.

Within the group of diseases designated as amaurotic family idiocy, the following varieties are generally distinguished.

TAY-SACHS DISEASE This is the classic form of amaurotic family idiocy occurring in infants, almost exclusively in Jewish families. It is characterized by extremely widespread neuronal involvement (see Chap. 101 for further details).

LATE INFANTILE FORM (JANSKÝ-BIELSCHOWSKY) This variety, which is rare, begins at a somewhat later age than Tay-Sachs disease (age 3 to 4 years) and has a more chronic course. It is biochemically and pathologically (by electron microscopy) distinguishable from both Tay-Sachs disease and juvenile amaurotic idiocy, but has features in common with both. However, vision and the appearance of the retina may be normal.

JUVENILE FORM (BATTEN-SPIELMEYER-VOGT) This form of lipidosis is not confined to patients of Jewish parentage. Clinically, the onset is between the ages of 5 to 10 years, and the course is relatively prolonged, with death at the time of adolescence or early adulthood. Visual impairment is usually the first symptom, followed by cerebellar ataxia, polymyoclonus, and dementia. The retinal lesions take the form of pigmentary degeneration (atypical retinitis pigmentosa). The intraneuronal accumulations differ considerably from those encountered in lipidoses of the Tay-Sachs and Janský-Bielschowsky types, both under light and electron microscopy, although, in common with these disorders, they have the histochemical properties of a glycolipid. Their chemical composition has not as yet been fully determined, but can be classed with the lipofuscins.

ADULT FORM (KUFS') This is an extremely rare disorder, with mental regression often preceding ataxia, athetosis, or other extrapyramidal signs and pursuing a very prolonged course. In all essential respects, it is identical with the juvenile form, except that retinal lesions may be completely absent. The storage material in neurons is in the form of curvilinear bodies and shares certain staining reactions with ceroid and lipofuscin.

Generalized lipidoses with central nervous system involvement In addition to the group of lipidoses exclusively affecting the nervous system, there are a number of more generalized disorders of lipid metabolism in which the nervous system participates.

GENERALIZED GANGLIOSIDOSIS Two rare forms of generalized lipidosis in infants have lately been recognized, both of them characterized by abnormal accumulations of gangliosides in many organs in addition to the nervous system. One of them closely resembles Tay-Sachs disease in that the substance that accumulates abnormally is the same monoganglioside (G_{M2} in the Svennerholm classification) that is present in excess in the neurons in Tay-Sachs disease. This is generally referred to as *Tay-Sachs disease with visceral involvement*. The other, termed *generalized gangliosidosis*, is characterized by excessive amounts of G_{M1} ganglioside.

NIEMANN-PICK DISEASE   This disease is discussed in Chap. 101. The typical accumulation of large amounts of lipid in macrophages (reticuloendothelial cells) in many organs, including particularly the liver and spleen, is accompanied by lipidosis of the nervous system, similar to that occurring in the various forms of amaurotic family idiocy. The lipid involved here is mainly sphingomyelin and the disease is caused by a deficiency of sphingomyelinase. The clinical picture may combine a defect in vertical gaze with dystonia or choreoathetosis. Often elements of cerebellar ataxia are added to the dystonic gait disorder.

MUCOPOLYSACCHARIDOSES   These disorders belong to a group in which there are abnormalities of connective tissue in many organs. In the Hurler variety, mental retardation is a prominent clinical feature, along with clouding of corneas and certain skeletal abnormalities. In the brain there are striking intraneuronal accumulations of lipid (ganglioside) resembling those found in amaurotic family idiocy. The peculiar facial appearance of patients affected with the disease has led to its being referred to in the older literature as gargoylism (mucopolysaccharidoses). Further studies have revealed six different subtypes. The Morquio and Maroteaux-Lamy forms cause neurological symptoms of hydrocephalus and cervical cord compression in adolescents and adults.

GAUCHER'S DISEASE   This generalized metabolic disorder of childhood, described in Chap. 101, resembles Niemann-Pick disease in many respects, inasmuch as it likewise is characterized by extensive lipid accumulations in various organs, especially the spleen, liver, and bone marrow. The nervous system, however, is much less regularly affected; it may be entirely normal in cases occurring in late childhood or adult life, although it usually is involved in infants. The accumulating lipid is glucocerebroside.

Clinical aspects   The majority of cases of lipidosis occur in infancy and childhood, after a period of normal development. Motor regression, disinterest, and loss of visual capacity are the leading features and are well covered by the term *amaurotic family idiocy*. At later stages the limbs become enfeebled and the reflexes exaggerated. The fundamental change— "cherry red spots" at maculae, surrounded by a gray halo— gives the diagnosis. Its absence suggests the possibility of another infantile cerebral disease, i.e., spongy degeneration of the white matter, in which progressive blindness is combined with psychomotor regression (see below). Excessive startle to sound (auditory myoclonus) is another characteristic finding of infantile cerebral lipidosis of Tay-Sachs type. Later the child becomes decerebrate and dies in 2 to 3 years. In patients with onset later in life cerebellar ataxia, epilepsy, and myoclonic dementia suggest the diagnosis, especially when associated with atypical retinitis pigmentosa. In the adult form polymyoclonia, choreoathetosis, and dementia may be conjoined and retinas are normal. (See Chap. 374 for differential diagnosis.)

LEUKODYSTROPHY (DEGENERATIVE DIFFUSE CEREBRAL SCLEROSIS)   The disorders to be considered here, which typically show an autosomal recessive pattern of inheritance, are characterized by a widespread disintegration of white matter in association with a remarkable sparing of the nerve cell bodies in the gray matter. The leukodystrophies may be considered to represent disorders of metabolism involving components of the myelin sheath. Some of them are related to the neuronal lipidoses previously discussed.

Pathology   The distinguishing feature is diffuse disintegration of myelin at all levels of the central nervous system and often of the peripheral nerves as well. As a rule, axons suffer damage to approximately the same degree as the myelin sheaths. The three major varieties of leukodystrophy (see below) are characterized by the presence, within the devastated regions, of lipid breakdown products of myelin which show distinct histochemical differences from the familiar lipid products encountered in all the other disease processes destroying myelin, such as infarction, traumatic necrosis, secondary fiber tract degeneration, demyelinative lesions in multiple sclerosis, and so on. The relative intactness of the nerve cell bodies forms a striking contrast to the extensive white matter lesions.

Varieties of leukodystrophy   METACHROMATIC LEUKODYSTROPHY   This is now known to be a genetically determined metabolic disorder of sphingolipid metabolism in which cerebroside sulfate (sulfatide) accumulates excessively in many organs, especially brain and kidneys, because of deficient activity of the enzyme cerebroside sulfatase. Since neutral cerebrosides and sulfatides are among the chief lipid components of myelin, all myelin-containing parts of the nervous system, both central and peripheral, are affected in this disease. The metabolic abnormality is well tolerated by other organs, as far as their functional integrity is concerned, but in the nervous system the excessive accumulation of sulfatides leads to breakdown of myelin at all levels. Sulfatides have the property of altering the absorption spectrum of dyes such as toluidine blue and cresyl violet, so that in their presence the color obtained is purple or red or even brown instead of the expected blue or violet—a phenomenon known as *metachromasia*. The name *metachromatic leukodystrophy* comes from the fact that the diseased cerebral white matter stains intensely metachromatically because of the large amounts of phagocytosed sulfatide that accompany the breakdown of the myelin. Metachromatic material indicative of sulfatide can also be readily demonstrated postmortem in kidney tubule cells, Kupffer cells of the liver, and in other organs, unaccompanied by any evidence of tissue damage. In the gallbladder the sulfatide deposits apparently do lead to destructive tissue changes, with the result that nonfunctioning of the gallbladder on radiographic examination is one of the manifestations of the disease.

The disease is mostly seen in infants and children, but it occurs not infrequently in adults, including a few of fairly advanced age. In these personality changes, impairment of intellectual function and a mixture of pyramidal and peripheral nerve signs will finally lead to the appropriate diagnostic tests (peripheral nerve conduction velocities, nerve biopsy, and measurement of arylsulfatase A).

KRABBE'S GLOBOID BODY LEUKODYSTROPHY   In this variety, first described by Krabbe in 1916 as a familial disorder of infants, the lipid breakdown products also are atypical as compared with those occurring in most pathologic processes which destroy myelin. They differ histochemically from the metachromatic material just described in several ways, including absence of metachromasia. Typical of this disorder is the presence of unusual multinucleated phagocytic cells (globoid cells) which contain galactocerebrosides. In this disease, the biochemical abnormality is apparently the result of a deficiency of galactocerebroside β-galactosidase.

SPONGY DEGENERATION OF THE NERVOUS SYSTEM (VAN BOE-GAERT-BERTRAND, CANAVAN) This rare inherited disease of infants is generally classified with the leukodystrophies because the cerebral white matter is the chief site of pathologic changes. Characteristic of the disease is a fine-meshed spongy degeneration of the tissue associated with breakdown of myelin in some regions and, probably, failure of myelination in others. This spongy state is apparently the result of a large increase of water, some of which is within the myelin sheaths, resulting in their disruption. The pathologic findings suggest failure of regulation of intracellular fluid balance, perhaps mainly affecting glial cells, but the biochemical and enzymatic defects that underlie this disease have not yet been identified.

PELIZAEUS-MERZBACHER DISEASE In this condition, characterized clinically by a pronounced sex-linked familial tendency and a very chronic course, the white matter lesions are patchy and irregular, rather than evenly distributed as in the other forms of leukodystrophy. Furthermore, there is relative sparing of axons. Another distinguishing feature of this disorder is that the breakdown products of the myelin, although very sparse (as would be expected from the prolonged course), are of the usual sort regularly seen with myelin destruction, rather than being atypical as in metachromatic leukodystrophy. What has been called *sudanophilic leukodystrophy* may well be identical with Pelizaeus-Merzbacher disease. The underlying basis for the lesions is still wholly unknown.

ADRENOLEUKODYSTROPHY This disease, which is transmitted as a sex-linked trait, is characterized by a combination of degeneration of the cells of the adrenal cortex and a widespread sudanophilic degeneration of myelinated fibers in large foci in the brain. Distinctive membrane-bound crystal-like inclusions have been identified in adrenal cortical cells, in macrophages in the demyelinated zones in the brain, in Schwann cells, and in the Leydig cells of the testis. The presence of these cytologic changes in various tissues suggests a generalized metabolic disorder, but the destructive lesions occur only in the adrenal cortex and the brain. The underlying biochemical abnormality is unknown.

Clinical aspects The symptoms and signs in all the forms of leukodystrophy are mainly those indicative of involvement of tracts of sensory and motor fibers (corticospinal, thalamocortical, geniculocalcarine, pontocerebellar, and cerebellomesencephalic) in combination with a progressive dementia. In the early stages there is weakness and unsteadiness of gait. Likewise prominent are spasticity and exaggeration of tendon reflexes, referable to the destructive lesions in the corticospinal motor system. In contrast to the neuronal lipidoses and other gray matter diseases, seizures are rare. In metachromatic leukodystrophy there is at first hypotonia, then spastic weakness of limbs, but because of later involvement of the peripheral nervous system, muscle-stretch reflexes are lost. The clinical features of adrenoleukodystrophy are described in Chap. 371.

On the whole, though, clinical differentiation of leukodystrophy from other forms of diffuse progressive cerebral disease is difficult. The metachromatic and globoid cell varieties can now be accurately identified by demonstrating the enzymatic deficiency in tissue cultures of leukocytes or fibroblasts, and metachromatic leukodystrophy can be recognized by the presence of sulfatides in the urine. In the other varieties of leukodystrophy, there are as yet no reliable biochemical tests whereby the diagnosis can be made during life. The disease can generally be identified in a brain biopsy, but this is a procedure which is justifiable only under very rare circumstances—such as direction of therapy, genetic counseling, or a carefully thought-out research project in which a specimen of fresh tissue might lead to some new insight into an otherwise hopeless disease. (See Chap. 371 for further account of the adult leukodystrophies.)

Differential diagnosis Familial occurrence, signs referable to a disorder of long projection and associative fiber systems, and relative lack of convulsive manifestations may suggest the diagnosis during life. Final verification, however, requires, except in those conditions where a biochemical abnormality can be detected, pathologic examination by appropriate biochemical tests.

PROGRESSIVE FAMILIAL MYOCLONIC EPILEPSY (UNVER-RICHT-LUNDBORG-LAFORA DISEASE) This rare disorder forms a distinct clinicopathologic syndrome characterized by recessive heredity. Typically, it appears in adolescence or early adult life, beginning with generalized convulsive seizures, which are followed after an interval of years by myoclonic jerks of increasing frequency and severity and progressive dementia. Death follows, usually within 5 to 10 years. The pathologic features suggest a disorder of nerve cell metabolism, the nature of which is under current investigation.

Pathology In many of the cases on record, distinctive intracytoplasmic inclusion bodies within nerve cells may be found at all levels in the central nervous system, althouth they are most frequent in the cerebral cortex, dentate nucleus of the cerebellum, substantia nigra, and thalamus. These bodies were initially described by Gonzalo Lafora (1911) and are generally known as Lafora bodies. Material with similar staining properties has also been found in heart-muscle fibers and in liver cells in several cases. They have been found to be composed of polymers of glucose (polyglucosans), but the reasons for the accumulation of these polysaccharides are still unknown.

Clinical aspects The onset in most cases is at about the time of puberty. The convulsive seizures, with which the disorder usually begins, are in no way distinctive. The myoclonic jerks are sudden, asymmetric or symmetric brief contractions of muscle groups of the limbs, face, and trunk, occurring arrhythmically and unpredictably, usually with sufficient force to displace the parts affected. They characteristically are provoked by all sorts of stimuli, but occur spontaneously as well. The sudden contractions may interfere seriously with willed movements, or may cause the patient to fall abruptly. The disorder progresses gradually, running a course over several years, with terminal stages characterized by profound dementia and total helplessness. Treatment with anticonvulsant medication may relieve the generalized convulsive seizures and reduce the frequency of the myoclonic jerks, but has no effect on the dementia.

Differential diagnosis Other forms of progressive familial dementia with myoclonus may have to be considered. These are discussed elsewhere in the descriptions of Creutzfeldt-Jakob disease (Chap. 192) and the lipidoses. There is in addition a more benign form of myoclonic epilepsy which begins in childhood or adolescence and permits survival to middle age or longer. In cases of this kind, some degree of ataxia is frequently observed, and, whereas there are no distinctive pathologic changes, degeneration of fiber systems related to the cerebellum have been found. In Unverricht-Lafora myoclonic epilepsy, convulsive seizures are more prominent than in the other disorders mentioned. The diagnosis of these different forms of myoclonus is based on clinical picture and course of illness. All forms of treatment have hitherto been ineffective.

HALLERVORDEN-SPATZ DISEASE This unusual disorder, often familial, is associated with a rather variable clinical picture in which abnormalities of posture and muscle tone, involuntary movements, and progressive dementia predominate. Pathologically, there are characteristic abnormalities in the basal ganglia, suggesting a localized disorder of metabolism. The features of the condition were classically described in an affected family by Hallervorden and Spatz (1922).

Pathology Distinctive for this condition is the accumulation of large amounts of pigmented material in the globus pallidus and zona reticulata of the substantia nigra, resulting in grossly visible brownish discoloration of these regions. Microscopically, there are irregular pigmented, ferruginous concretions and granules of varying brownish or greenish hues, depending on the stains used. Although much of this pigment contains iron, serum iron and ferritin are normal, and there is no systemic disorder of iron metabolism. There also is loss of nerve cells and fibers. Another feature of the disease is the presence of focal swelling of axons, most probably in their terminal portions; this is especially pronounced in the regions affected by the pigmentary disorder, but typically can be found at all levels of the central nervous system, including the cerebral cortex.

Clinical aspects The disorder typically makes its appearance in childhood or adolescence, with abnormalities in muscle tone and movements such as rigidity and choreoathetosis. Abnormal postures of the trunk characteristic of torsion spasm (dystonia) may be seen. Cerebellar ataxia and myoclonus are also present in some instances, or the clinical picture may be reminiscent of parkinsonism. Speech becomes indistinct, and there is progressive intellectual impairment. Eventually, the involuntary movements give way to increasing generalized rigidity, and death comes as a rule about 10 years after onset.

Differential diagnosis No feature of the clinical picture serves to distinguish this particular disorder from other conditions showing dementia with extrapyramidal motor abnormalities. Wilson's disease must be excluded by appropriate laboratory tests. The clearly progressive course sets this condition apart from clinically similar abnormalities resulting from accidents or illnesses at birth or in the neonatal period. It has recently been demonstrated that there is a selective uptake of radioactive iron by the basal ganglia which may be helpful in diagnosis. At present no effective treatment is known. A recent (unpublished) attempt at using a chelating agent (deferoxamine mesylate) in one case led to no definite benefit, and L-dopa and other antiparkinsonian medication, tryptophan, and megavitamin therapy have been of only temporary and questionable help.

FAMILIAL HEPATOLENTICULAR DEGENERATION (WILSON'S DISEASE) This condition is discussed in Chap. 95.

ACQUIRED HEPATOCEREBRAL DEGENERATION This condition is discussed in Chap. 371.

EXTRAPYRAMIDAL SYNDROMES OF ABNORMAL POSTURE OR INVOLUNTARY MOVEMENT

PARALYSIS AGITANS (PARKINSON'S DISEASE) This by no means rare condition was named and classically described by

James Parkinson in 1817. His remarkably complete account gives this definition:

Involuntary tremulous motion, with lessened muscular power, in parts not in action and even when supported; with a propensity to bend the trunk forward, and to pass from a walking to a running pace, the senses and intellects being uninjured.

Typically, paralysis agitans is a disorder of middle or late life, with very gradual progression and a prolonged course. Although it has been seen to occur in families (the estimated familial incidence is 1 to 2 percent), it usually is sporadic. It is well recognized, however, that the epidemic encephalitis of von Economo, which occurred in a worldwide distribution in the years following World War I, was followed by a syndrome clinically indistinguishable from paralysis agitans. It is usual in such instances to speak of postencephalitic parkinsonism, whereas the term *Parkinson's disease* should be reserved for true paralysis agitans of unknown cause. Paralysis agitans bears no consistent relation to any known disease process such as arteriosclerosis, trauma, or intoxication, although such conditions have often been invoked as etiologically significant and may at times produce somewhat similar clinical manifestations.

Pathology Despite the general medical familiarity with the condition and an extensive literature on the subject, it cannot be said that the pathologic changes of paralysis agitans are yet fully understood. The only regularly observed changes have been in the aggregates of melanin-containing nerve cells in the brainstem (substantia nigra, locus caeruleus), where there are varying degrees of nerve cell loss with reactive gliosis (most pronounced in the substantia nigra) along with distinctive eosinophilic intracytoplasmic inclusions (Lewy bodies, after their description by F. H. Lewy in 1913). Changes have also been described in other structures of the basal ganglia, but they are not clearly different in nature or degree from what may be encountered in other patients of similar age without extrapyramidal motor disorders. The histopathologic evidence therefore suggests that paralysis agitans can be considered as belonging with the system diseases, the affected system being that of the pigmented nuclei of the brainstem. Significantly, extensive lesions in these same pigmented nuclei characterize the pathologic findings in postencephalitic parkinsonism in which Lewy bodies typically are absent and of the Shy-Drager syndrome (Chap. 13). Recent biochemical studies, which show a decrease of dopamine in the caudate nucleus and putamen—an alteration consistently found on experimental ablation of the substantia nigra—lend further support to the idea that Parkinson's disease is indeed a disorder of a particular neuronal system (see Chap. 16).

Clinical aspects In its fully developed form, this disorder cannot be mistaken for any other. The stooped posture, the stiffness and slowness of movement, the fixity of facial expression, and the rhythmic tremor of the limbs which subsides on active willed movement or complete relaxation are familiar to every clinician. Although symmetric in the later stages, the disorder typically begins asymmetrically, e.g., as a slight tremor of the fingers of one hand or in one leg. Also typical are more or less general hypokinesia and stiffness of the musculature so that even where tremor is inapparent, the disease may betray itself by a somewhat staring and immobile facial expression, a monotonous voice, a general slowness and diminution of all motor activity, and a curious lack of the little spontaneous movements of postural change that are so characteristic of the normal individual. When tremor is minimal, patients often are able to alleviate it by resting their hands on a table or the arms of a chair or by keeping them in their pockets. The tremor, although fluctuating from moment to moment in amplitude, characterizes the later course. The tremor is generally most pronounced in the hands but may involve the legs (and thus secondarily the trunk), lips, tongue, and neck muscles, and is easily seen in the eyelids when they are lightly closed. Its frequency is 4 to 5 per second, but another faster tremor (7 to 8 per second) predominates in some patients. There is no total paralysis, although general enfeeblement of voluntary movement is characteristic of the fully developed disorder. Together with the stooped attitude, there is the typical festinating gait, whereby the patient, prevented by the abnormality of postural tone from making the appropriate reflex adjustments required for effective walking, progresses with quick shuffling steps at an accelerating pace as if to catch up with his center of gravity. Clinical examination of the tendon and plantar reflexes discloses no abnormalities. There are no sensory changes, although deep aching in joints and muscles is common. Eventually, the patient may become so incapacitated by rigidity and tremor as to be helpless in caring for himself. It has often been observed, however, that even severely disabled patients may, under great emotional stress, perform complex motor acts quickly and efficiently. Although the temporary alleviation under extreme provocation can never be long maintained, it is nevertheless true that the severity of the symptoms is considerably influenced by emotional factors, being aggravated by anxiety, tension, and unhappiness, and minimal when the patient is in a contented frame of mind. Despite the inherently progressive nature of the condition, much can be achieved with good medical management, and patients may continue for years to live effective, happy lives in spite of this affliction. Intellectual deterioration is not a consistent feature of paralysis agitans, but it must be conceded that in very advanced stages of the condition dementia may be encountered.

Differential diagnosis In typical cases, this is not difficult. The extrapyramidal syndromes associated with most diseases of known cause or established nature such as cerebral vascular disease, cerebral hypoxia (including carbon monoxide asphyxia), or metallic poisoning differ from paralysis agitans in a number of respects, such as atypical behavior or tremor, presence of signs of pyramidal tract deficit, or early onset of dementia. The differentiation from postencephalitic parkinsonism may be impossible; a clear history of an attack of epidemic encephalitis (prolonged somnolence, disturbance of consciousness, diplopia) and relatively early age of onset of the disorder and the presence of tics, localized spasms, and oculogyric crises may be the only clues to this diagnosis. In recent years, a neurologic disorder strikingly similar to Parkinson's disease has been seen following the prolonged administration of large amounts of reserpine and phenothiazine drugs, which subsides on withdrawal of the offending drug—a matter of considerable theoretic and practical importance. Parkinsonism is rarely, if ever, produced by cerebral neoplasms.

Treatment Although there is no treatment that is known to halt or reverse the neuronal degeneration that presumably underlies Parkinson's disease, methods are now available which can bring about a considerable degree of relief from symptoms in many patients. An important part of any therapeutic program is the maintenance of optimum general health and neuromuscular efficiency by planned programs of exercise, activity, and rest; expert physical therapy may be of great help in achieving these ends. In addition, the patient often needs much

emotional support in meeting the stress of the illness, in comprehending its nature, and in carrying on courageously in spite of it. Along with these general supportive measures, which are applicable to many chronic illnesses, patients generally require a carefully thought-out program of treatment specifically aimed at counteracting the pathophysiologic disorder that produces their disabilities. This treatment is nearly always medical (with drugs), but a stereotoxic surgical procedure is a possibility in selected cases.

Experience over many years has shown that the drugs that are most beneficial in the symptomatic treatment of Parkinson's disease are dopamine repleting and anticholinergic agents related to atropine. L-Dihydroxyphenylalanine (L-dopa) is now the most widely used and effective therapy. The theoretic basis for the use of this compound is the decrease of catecholamines in extrapyramidal motor centers, to which reference has already been made. The results, even in those with far-advanced stages of the disease, are far better than have ever been obtained by other drugs. This agent should be given in doses starting at 250 mg tid and increasing every few days until doses of 4.0 to 5.0 g per day are reached. L-Dopa is now usually combined with an inhibitor which prevents its rapid destruction in the blood and allows more of it to enter the basal ganglia. A popular form is carbidopa (Synemet), the starting dose of which is 10 mg of L-dopa and 100 mg of the inhibitor given three times a day and gradually increased to 25 and 250 mg, respectively, given four times a day. The drug is not without unpleasant side effects, so that it is not universally applicable. Many patients are at first troubled by nausea, especially if the medication is not taken with meals, and a few have hypotensive episodes. Above a certain daily dose which varies from patient to patient, choreic movements of head and neck may appear, forcing a reduction in dosage. Nausea can be allayed by antiemetic medication, but usually it disappears with continued usage of the drug. An excess of L-dopa or a slight increase in the blood level during the day may cause a "letdown" in which the patient finds it difficult to act. At present the most efficacious program of medical therapy consists of 25 mg L-dopa and 250 mg inhibitor in four doses plus 2 to 4 mg Artane and 10 to 20 mg ethopropazine (Parsidol) three times daily. Amantadine (Symmetrel) in doses of 50 to 100 mg two or three times daily is also an excellent anti-Parkinson drug and may be given with L-dopa.

Bromocryptine, a dopamine agonist, has also been found to have a therapeutic effect. Unlike levodopa, which is converted to dopamine, bromocryptine has a direct action. The dose is 2.5 mg tid. Goodwin et al., who compare it with L-dopa, observed some patients to respond better to the bromocryptine and some to L-dopa. The quality of the response is much the same, as are the side effects. The on-off phenomenon was observed in only one percent, whose daily dose was 40 mg.

The anticholinergic drugs have by no means been supplanted by L-dopa. A fair percentage of patients with Parkinson's disease (20 percent) do not respond to L-dopa. And, there is another small group who, after an initial response, begin to have a severe generalized chorea, resembling that of Huntington's chorea. In them the line between effective therapeutic response and chorea is so thin that as little as 100 mg of L-dopa throws them into a disabling chorea. The anticholinergic drugs must then be depended upon, often with a lowered dose of L-dopa. As to the best anticholinergic drugs several synthetic preparations are now available, including trihexyphenidyl (Artane), cycrimine (Pagitane), procyclidine (Kemadrin), biperiden (Akineton), and benztropine methanesulfonate (Cogentin), among others. Whereas these drugs differ little from one another in their overall effectiveness in large groups of patients, an individual patient may respond better to one of them than to another, and occasionally after a patient has received one of these medications for a prolonged period, change to another one may be attended by some additional improvement—perhaps only from the psychologic effect of a change in regimen. In order to obtain maximum benefit from the use of these drugs, they should be given in gradually increasing dosage to the point where toxic side effects begin to appear. The side effects are those expected from anticholinergic agents: dryness of the mouth (which can be beneficial when drooling of saliva is a problem), blurring of vision from pupillary mydriasis (for which corrective spectacle lenses may be indicated), constipation, and sometimes urinary retention (especially with prostatism). Mental slowing, confusional states, hallucinations, and impairment of memory, especially in patients with already impaired mental functioning, can occur as troublesome toxic effects of these drugs and may sharply limit their usefulness under these circumstances. The optimum dosage level for a patient is when the greatest relief from tremor and rigidity is achieved within the limits of tolerable side effects. This may occur with trihexyphenidyl, for example, within a range of 6 to 20 mg daily in divided doses, or in a sustained-release capsule. With any of these drugs, a dosage level is reached when a further increase serves only to precipitate severe toxic effects with no further alleviation of the symptoms of the disease. The dose must then, of course, be reduced. It is possible, nevertheless, once maximum benefit from one of the anticholinergic agents has been achieved, to then add one of the antihistaminic drugs such as dipenhydramine (Benadryl) or phenindamine (Thephorin). These drugs have some ameliorating effect on the motor derangement, but it is insufficient for them to be used as the primary therapeutic agent. However, an antihistamine in combination with an anticholinergic drug can give better results in many patients than either one alone. Drowsiness is the chief side effect of the antihistamines, and this in turn can be combated with one of the analeptics such as dextroamphetamine (Dexedrine).

From what has been said, it is clear that the drugs to be used, and how much, vary from patient to patient: what is inadequate for one is too much for another. The patients who can be expected to benefit the most from treatment with classic anti-Parkinson drugs are those with relatively mild disease in whom relief from the symptoms is sufficient to warrant tolerance of some side effects. In those more severely affected, the relief is partial at best, and as the disease advances, eventually a degree of incapacity is reached which is not significantly responsive to even the most carefully planned regimen of medications. Even so, there is no doubt that for a relatively long period the patient's effectiveness and well-being can be considerably enhanced by the wise use of these drugs. Many Parkinson patients have depressive symptoms which must be treated by the measures described in Chap. 11. An important note of warning must be provided at this point: Under no circumstances should a medication program with anticholinergic agents be stopped suddenly. If this happens, the patient is likely to become totally immobilized and incapacitated by an abrupt and severe increase of tremor and rigidity.

Another important advance in the attempt to relieve the symptoms of Parkinson's disease has been the development of stereotaxic surgery. This involves the placement of precisely localized focal lesions in the central nuclei of the brain, either in the globus pallidus or ventrolateral thalamus, contralateral to the side of the body chiefly affected. The best results occur in patients who are relatively young and in good general health with sound mentality, in whom unilateral tremor or rigidity, rather than akinesia, is the predominant symptom. Opinions among neurosurgeons still differ as to the best way of making the lesion, and studies are still in progress as to what its ideal location should be. Success with L-dopa has greatly diminished the call for surgical therapy.

Effective combinations of these therapies may keep the patient functional for 10 to 20 years.

PROGRESSIVE SUPRANUCLEAR PALSY (RICHARDSON-STEELE SYNDROME)   This clinicopathologic entity, described in 1963 by Richardson and Steele, affects elderly individuals in approximately the same age period as paralysis agitans. And it is among the group of Parkinsonian patients that most of the examples of this disease are to be found. The authors encounter several cases each year.

The clinical features are quite distinctive. Disturbances of balance and gait with unexpected falls; rigidity of the neck and other trunk muscles, resembling Parkinson's disease; "masking" of the face; reduction in the volume of the voice; extreme flexion or extension dystonia of the neck; and difficulty in looking down are all early symptoms. Any one of them may first bring patients to a physician. They progress over months and years, until patients are virtually anarthric with total loss of voluntary control of eye movements, and severe cervical and truncal rigidity. Patients eventually become bedfast. Tremor is rarely seen. In contrast there are no impairments of mentation (in most instances), or of vision, hearing, somatic sensation, or voluntary power; and signs of corticospinal involvement are minimal or absent.

A loss of neurons and gliosis are found on postmortem examination all through the tectum and tegmentum of the midbrain, subthalamic nuclei of Luys, vestibular nuclei, and to some extent ocular nuclei. Remarkable, indeed, and setting the disease apart from most other degenerative diseases, is the presence in surviving neurons of tangles of neurofibrillae, similar to, but more pronounced than those seen in the substantia nigra after encephalitis lethargica (von Economo's disease).

The cause of the disease is unknown. A slow virus is suspected, but attempts to transfer it to monkeys by the intracerebral inoculation of brain tissue have failed.

Treatment has been unsuccessful. Relatively little benefit comes from the administration of the antiparkinsonian series of drugs, although they should be tried; occasionally L-dopa has helped to diminish some of the symptoms.

The diagnosis should be considered whenever an elderly patient begins to fall repeatedly and inexplicably and has extrapyramidal symptoms with a rigid neck and paralysis of conjugate gaze.

DYSTONIA MUSCULORUM DEFORMANS (TORSION SPASM)
This is a clinical term denoting a state characterized by slow, nonrhythmic, involuntary movements which produce abnormal, at times bizarre, postures of the trunk and limbs. With passage of time, these postures tend to become more or less fixed. Underlying the clinical disorder may be any of several pathologic conditions, such as the residual lesions of epidemic encephalitis, the pigmented deposits of Hallervorden-Spatz disease (described above), hepatolenticular degeneration (Wilson's disease), or the scars of cerebral birth injury in the broad sense, or kernicterus. More frequent and puzzling, however, is the hereditary form known as *dystonia musculorum deformans* (torsion dystonia), which has a relatively early onset and progressive course without a definitive lesion.

Pathology   Until lately, very few cases of dystonia musculorum deformans not due to one of the definable disease processes indicated above had been adequately studied neuropathologically. Reported results from the few that had been examined led to uncertainty as to what the pathologic-anatomic basis of the clinical state might be, although it was generally assumed that the basal ganglia were diseased. A careful study by Zeman and Dyken in 1967, which included comparison of the findings in patients with the disease with control material, demonstrated that there is, in fact, no definable neuronal or other histologically demonstrable disease process to which the clinical abnormalities can reasonably be attributed. These negative findings, which are perhaps surprising, must not be interpreted as indicating that there is "no disease" in the brain, but rather that the pathologic state is not one that can be disclosed by the usual histopathologic techniques. It may well be that current studies of the pathophysiology of neurotransmitters will result in the elucidation of this disease.

Clinical aspects The motor abnormalities are described in Chap. 16. In the early stages, the involuntary muscular contractions are intermittent and variable in location and severity, but typically interfere with motor performance by superimposing an unwanted posture upon parts in use. One leg may briefly be pulled into a flexed or extended position or one shoulder elevated. Later the lingual, pharyngeal, neck, and thoracic muscles participate, and grimacing may occur. These latter may also be the first and only signs of disease for several years. Progression may be relatively rapid in cases with onset during early childhood, but is slow in those beginning in late childhood or adult life. The end result is extreme disability, with grossly distorted postures of the trunk and contractures of the limbs. Affection of face and tongue muscles results in faulty articulation of speech, which eventually becomes incomprehensible. The tendon and plantar reflexes, which can be assessed only during moments of relaxation of the affected parts, are characteristically normal.

Mental function is usually of normal or superior quality, especially in the patients with recessive forms of the disease. However, with severe derangement of all available methods of communication, an adequate evaluation of mental capacity may be impossible.

According to Eldridge, who has made the most careful epidemiologic study of torsion dystonia, two types are distinguishable. The most severe type of early onset occurs almost exclusively in Ashkenazic Jews. The patients are always normal the first few years of life. The dystonic movements and postures are either appendicular (either peripheral or proximal) and there is no evidence of other neurological abnormality. The milder form is autosomal dominant of later onset (often in midadult life), less rapidly progressive, more often restricted to one part of the body, and with varied ethnic predominance. Sporadic cases are not infrequent and may be restricted to the trunk musculature. All laboratory data in both types are negative.

Spasmodic torticollis (writer's cramp, buccolingual dystonia; see below) may well be a form of dystonia, but it typically does not progress to involve the musculature generally. However, torticollis may be an early symptom in cases which later show the typical generalized motor abnormalities.

Differential diagnosis Hepatolenticular degeneration should be seriously considered in any case presenting these motor symptoms, and appropriate measures should be undertaken for its investigation (see Chap. 371). The progressive course, and possibly the family history, differentiate the degenerative group from the "symptomatic" dystonias resulting from infections or metabolic disorders occurring at birth or later. Hallervorden-Spatz disease, however, cannot be distinguished on clinical grounds alone. Rare instances of Niemann-Pick or other lipid storage diseases may begin in adult life with a dystonic syndrome, and phenathiazine (tardive) dyskinesia must be considered in all cases of restricted or generalized dystonia in adults, especially if they have or have had a psychiatric illness.

Treatment This is most unsatisfactory. Dystonia is notoriously unresponsive to drug therapy, although antispasmodic drugs such as those used for parkinsonism should be tried. Neurosurgical treatment of the sort used for Parkinson's disease has been sufficiently promising to be worth serious consideration in every case, especially if the patient is young.

SPASMODIC TORTICOLLIS AND OTHER RESTRICTED DYSKINESIAS With advancing age a large variety of degenerative "movement disorders" come to light. Supposedly there is loss of neurons in certain parts of the motor system. Groups of muscles begin to manifest arrhythmic involuntary spasms. The patient's lack of success in suppressing them and his recognition that they are beyond voluntary control distinguish them from the common tics, habit spasms, and mannerisms described in Chap. 16. If the muscle contraction is frequent and prolonged, an aching pain accompanies it and may be mistakenly blamed for the spasm. Worsening under stress and improvement during quiet and relaxation are typical of this group of disorders.

Surely the most frequent and familiar type is torticollis, wherein an adult, more often a woman, becomes aware of turning of the head to one side as she walks. It gradually worsens to a point where it may be more or less continuous, not even relieved when lying down. Rarely, more than one member of a family is afflicted. On the assumption of a psychogenic factor in the illness many patients receive psychotherapy, but always without benefit. When followed over the years, the condition is observed to remain limited to the same muscles (scalene, sternocleidomastoid, and upper trapezius). There is little if any response to various drugs. Section of upper cervical roots bilaterally (anterior and posterior roots) is the only form of treatment that has given satisfactory results.

Other restricted dyskinesias involve the neck in combination with facial muscles, the orbicularis oculi (blepharospasm and blepharoclonus), the throat, and respiratory muscles ("spastic dysarthria," respiratory, and phonatory spasms). All these conditions, once started, are persistent, unpleasant, and relatively unresponsive to all modes of therapy other than denervative surgical procedures. Presumably, the abnormality lies in the basal ganglia, but its pathologic substratum has never been divulged. The facial-cervical dyskinesias caused by phenothiazine drugs resemble these idiopathic disorders and may continue after the withdrawal of medication (tardive dyskinesias). Antiparkinson drugs are sometimes helpful in all these restricted dyskinesias.

FAMILIAL TREMOR One of the commonest hereditary disorders of man's nervous system is that which gives rise to a fast-frequency (6 to 7 or 8 to 9 per second) action tremor. This may appear at any age but more often during adolescence and adult years; once started, it lasts throughout life. Alcohol suppresses it. The heredity is dominant. Probably all cases are not the same, for some have tremors of slower frequency, looking more like those of Parkinson's disease but lacking the slowness of movement, rigidity, and flexed postures. In patients of advanced age it is called *senile tremor*. Imbibition of alcohol suppresses the fast-frequency forms, as does a beta-adrenergic blocking agent (propranolol) in doses of 20 to 40 mg three times daily. The slightly slower rhythmic action tremors of frequencies (approximately 6 per second) and alternate-beat type do not usually respond to propranolol or alcohol. Usually the tremor is the only abnormality, but in a few patients a cerebellar ataxia or an extrapyramidal syndrome may appear years later. The pathologic basis is unknown.

SYNDROMES OF SLOWLY DEVELOPING ATAXIA

The conditions about to be considered are distinguished clinically by progressive unsteadiness in standing and walking, along with more or less impaired coordination of other motor acts. Pathologically, they are characterized by degeneration of the cerebellum and/or its related fiber systems, and thus constitute classic examples of the system diseases. Although sporadic instances occur, hereditary transmission is an outstanding feature in many cases; thus, this group of disorders is often referred to as the *hereditary ataxias.* Their subdivision into more or less separate entities is largely arbitrary, with pathologic changes of varying distribution underlying clinically indistinguishable symptom complexes. Furthermore, there is considerable overlapping with other forms of hereditary nervous disease, so that in a given case a remarkable combination of defects may be encountered. These facts have led to the idea that in the ataxias there is a group of closely related genetically determined abnormalities which may occur together in an almost infinite series of combinations with other neurologic disorders so that it is not possible to separate well-defined disease pictures. Nevertheless, certain constellations of symptoms and pathologic findings occur with sufficient regularity to warrant their separation for purposes of discussion. The classification about to be given is not entirely satisfactory but is designed to be of practical help to the physician confronted with a case.

CEREBELLAR DEGENERATIONS To be discussed here are the forms of progressive ataxia which are associated with pathologic changes predominantly in the cerebellum. The more strictly spinocerebellar diseases of which Friedreich's ataxia is the classic variety has already been discussed in Chap. 374. It is a disease of late childhood and adolescence. The adult onset types include both hereditary and sporadic diseases and, in addition, the rather rare subacute spinocerebellar degeneration associated with the presence of carcinoma of various types elsewhere in the body. The hereditary and sporadic forms of cerebellar degeneration resemble one another so closely that, for the purposes of the present discussion, they will all be referred to as *hereditary cerebellar degeneration.* Most cases are seen in adults, with the onset occurring in middle life.

Pathology In hereditary cerebellar degeneration the cerebellum is obviously atrophied. In one group of cases, these changes are chiefly localized to the superior vermis and adjacent parts of the cerebellar cortex, whereas in an even larger group, the entire cerebellar cortex is affected. Microscopically there is loss of nerve cells principally affecting the Purkinje cells, although the granule cells are often involved as well. In most cases, there is an associated atrophy of nerve cells in the inferior olivary nuclei in a distribution dependent on the location and extent of the changes in the cerebellar cortex. It no longer seems justifiable to separate the cases with associated olivary degeneration from the rest and to designate them as "cerebello-olivary degeneration," as has been done in the past. In *olivopontocerebellar degeneration,* there are extensive degenerative changes in the pontine nuclei, middle cerebellar peduncles, and olivary nuclei. In addition changes in the cerebellar cortex such as have been noted above may or may not be present. In two cases, studied by Perry and his associates, aspartic acid, γ-aminobutyric acid (GABA), and homocarnasine were reduced in the cerebellar cortex, whereas the level of taurine was elevated. Aspartic acid is said to be an excitatory transmitter of climbing fibers and taurine an inhibitory transmitter of interneurons.

In all varieties of cerebellar degeneration, affection of other neuronal systems—as, for instance, the cerebral cortex and basal ganglia—may be encountered. In some cases, there are changes in the dentate and roof nuclei of the cerebellum and their projections in the superior cerebellar peduncles (*dentatorubral atrophy*), but these are often found in association with more diffuse cerebellar or spinocerebellar degeneration. *Carcinomatous cerebellar (spinocerebellar) degeneration* is characterized by extensive cell loss in all parts of the cerebellar cortex, occasionally associated with inflammatory (lymphocytic) infiltrations in the perivascular and subarachnoid spaces. In addition there are degenerative changes in the long-fiber tracts of the spinal cord. These lesions do not depend on the presence of tumor implants anywhere in the nervous system or its coverings, but rather are thought to be due to an obscure infectious (? metabolic) process, somehow resulting from the presence of carcinoma.

Clinical aspects In the hereditary form of pure cerebellar degeneration the abnormality appears first in the legs, resulting in abnormal stance and an unsteadiness of gait of the peculiar wavering, lurching character so typical of cerebellar ataxia (see Chap. 16). This has been correlated with the localization of changes in the superior vermis of the cerebellum and adjacent parts of the cerebellar cortex. With more extensive cerebellar involvement, a disturbance in articulation and rhythm of speech occurs that reduces its comprehensibility, and the arms likewise become ataxic. There may be nystagmus, but it is often absent. Affection of other neuronal systems causes additional neurologic abnormalities, such as exaggerated tendon reflexes, entensor plantar responses, rigidity, tremor, and dementia (*cerebrocerebellar degeneration*). Progression is gradual and slow, being measured in years and sometimes decades, and appears not to shorten life.

No specific treatment is available for any of the progressive ataxias, although encouragement to remain active is beneficial to health in general. Gait training is of relatively little value in enabling the patient to compensate for his disability.

We have not been able to clinically differentiate a cortical parenchymatous from the olivopontocerebellar degeneration with any degree of consistency, though the latter tends to be sporadic, speech is affected early, and extrapyramidal signs of other type appear late. In dentatonigral degeneration, gaze palsy and spasticity are combined with cerebellar ataxia.

In the cases associated with carcinoma, the tempo of evolution of the process is relatively rapid, with severe disability coming on within a period of months. Vertigo, diplopia, and nausea may be prominent. In an occasional patient, the neurologic symptoms have appeared before there was any obvious evidence of carcinoma. Opsoclonus (rapid side-to-side jerking of the eyes) and oscillopsia (movement back and forth of objects seen) may be conjoined. In contrast to the consistently normal cerebrospinal fluid findings in the forms of cerebellar degeneration noted above, the cerebrospinal fluid may show increased lymphocytes and protein.

Differential diagnosis The slow but relentless progression in the absence of abnormalities in the other parts of the nervous system and of the cerebrospinal fluid distinguishes the hereditary group from other diseases and other forms of cerebellar ataxia such as may occur with hereditary metabolic diseases, neoplastic, infectious, or demyelinative disease; with drug intoxications (e.g., barbiturates); or with hyperpyrexia. The degenerative disorders under discussion tend to occur slowly over many years in a setting of otherwise good general health, and in the absence of other neurologic symptoms and signs; this, together with the other clinical differences, distinguishes them from such hereditary metabolic diseases as juvenile Coucher's disease, juvenile Niemann-Pick disease, and juvenile hexose-amanidase deficiency and from alcoholic cerebellar ataxia or deficiency disease, with or without Wernicke-Korsakoff syndrome. Alcoholic cerebellar degeneration usually develops rapidly, and then may remain more or less unchanged for the remainder of the patient's life (Chap. 372). The form of spino-cerebellar degeneration associated with carcinoma usually develops over a period of a few months and may be distinguished from direct carcinomatous involvement of the nervous system by the symmetry of the findings and the absence of increased intracranial pressure.

HEREDITARY ATAXIA OF PIERRE MARIE This term has been applied to cases of hereditary progressive ataxia with onset in early adulthood. Considerable doubt has been raised as to the usefulness of the concept of Marie's hereditary ataxia, because pathologically this is by no means a uniform group. When Pierre Marie wrote about the subject in 1893, Friedreich's ataxia (see Chap. 375) had relatively recently become recognized as a distinct entity. Marie pointed out, on the basis of case reports in the literature, that there were other cases of hereditary ataxia, of later onset, which could not be fitted into Friedreich's description. He suggested that the cerebellum itself was the major site of disease in these cases. Subsequent pathologic examinations of the cases he reviewed have shown that he was partly in error in this supposition; nevertheless, following his report, the concept of Marie's ataxia has appeared repeatedly in writings on hereditary ataxia. Cases that might be classified with this group either are indistinguishable from those discussed above under the cerebellar degenerations or are variants of Friedreich's ataxia.

SYNDROME OF MUSCULAR WEAKNESS AND WASTING, WITHOUT SENSORY CHANGES

MOTOR SYSTEM DISEASE This general term is used to designate a progressive disorder of motor neurons in the cerebral cortex, brainstem, and spinal cord, manifested clinically by muscular weakness, atrophy, and spasticity, with exaggeration of tendon reflexes in varying combinations. In its typical form this is a disease of middle life, generally appearing in the fifth or sixth decade. Customarily a subdivision is made on the basis of the particular grouping of symptoms and signs observed. Thus, the most frequent form, in which muscular atrophy and hyperreflexia are combined, is called *amyotrophic lateral sclerosis*. Rather more rare are the cases in which weakness and atrophy exist alone without clinical evidence of corticospinal tract dysfunction; for these, the term *progressive muscular atrophy* is used. Where the disorder affects predominantly the musculature innervated by the cranial nerves, it is usual to speak of *progressive bulbar palsy*. Very rarely, the clinical state is dominated by spasticity and hyperreflexia without obvious muscular wasting; such cases are classed as *primary lateral sclerosis*. It seems very likely that these subgroupings are anything other than clinical variants of the same disease process, which is another classic example of a system disease. Most cases are sporadic, but occasionally this disorder occurs in families in a manner suggesting genetic transmission. Familial motor system disease is discussed further on.

Pathology Widespread selective atrophy and loss of motor nerve cells exist at all levels of the central nervous system, including the Betz cells in the motor areas of the cerebral cortex. Some evidence of disease in the corticospinal motor system is usually found pathologically, even when physical signs referable to such changes were not observed during life. The atrophy of fibers in skeletal muscles is typically that due to loss of motor innervation.

Clinical aspects The disease begins insidiously and may be well advanced before the patient is aware of it. Although often asymmetric initially, the weakness and muscular wasting gradually become bilateral and widespread. Classically, the disorder is first evident in the small muscles of the hands, but it may begin in one or both of the legs, or in muscles supplied by cranial nerves. Vague feelings of discomfort in the muscles, tightness, coldness, numbness (without objective sensory changes), and recurrent cramps may be early symptoms. The progressive enfeeblement and atrophy of the musculature are accompanied by widespread visible fascicular twitchings of groups of muscle fibers, a classic feature that can be related to degeneration of the motor nerve cells supplying the involved muscles. Despite extensive involvement of skeletal muscles generally, sphincter control remains intact. Sooner or later the disease affects muscles supplied by the brainstem, resulting in weakness, atrophy, and fasciculations in the tongue and facial musculature associated with dysarthria and impairment of chewing or swallowing. The ocular nuclei, oddly enough, are invariably spared. In most cases, the weakness and muscular wasting are accompanied by exaggeration of tendon reflexes, extensor plantar reflexes and spasticity, to a degree dependent on the severity of degeneration in the corticospinal (pyramidal) motor system. Affection of corticobulbar fibers results in manifestations of pseudobulbar palsy such as involuntary crying or laughter, exaggerated reflex movements of the muscles or facial expression, and sucking reflexes. These latter may be the first manifestations of the disease. Progression is unhalting and relatively rapid, leading to extensive paralysis, with death from respiratory weakness or aspiration pneumonia, generally within about 2 to 5 years or more from onset. Intelligence and awareness are typically preserved to the end.

Differential diagnosis Spinal cord compression from tumors in the cervical region or from cervical spondylosis with osteophytes projecting into the vertebral canal can at times give rise to weakness, wasting, and fasciculations in the upper limbs and spasticity in the legs, thus closely resembling amyotrophic lateral sclerosis. The absence of cranial nerve involvement may be helpful in differentiation, although some compressive lesions at the foramen magnum may implicate the twelfth cranial (hypoglossal) nerve, with resulting affection of the tongue. Absence of pain or of sensory changes, normal function of bowels and bladder, normal roentgenographic studies of the spine, and absence of changes in the composition or dynamics of the cerebrospinal fluid are all points in favor of motor system disease and against spinal cord compression. Where doubt exists, contrast myelography should be performed and the cervical region should be visualized.

A small number of patients who have motor system disease will have had poliomyelitis years before and another special variety is that in which an immunologically incompetent person (affected by carcinoma, lymphoma, and corticosteroids) develops a pure amyotrophy that progresses over several months to a year and at autopsy is found to be a chronic poliomyelitis.

Chronic inflammatory disorders of the meninges and spinal cord, exemplified by syphilitic meningomyelitis or some cases of adhesive arachnoiditis, may have to be considered. These conditions can readily be recognized by cerebrospinal fluid changes and, if necessary, by abnormal myelographic findings. Nutritional myelopathy can be excluded by history and on other clinical grounds.

Although fasciculations are a prominent feature of motor system disease, they are not, in the absence of weakness, muscle atrophy, or loss of tendon reflexes, valid signs of it, for they may occur in a variety of metabolic or toxic disorders (e.g., thyrotoxicosis, salt depletion) as well as in otherwise healthy individuals. Careful clinical evaluation suffices in such instances to exclude serious neurologic disease.

Progressive weakness from intrinsic disease of muscle (myopathy, polymyositis) may occasionally be difficult to distinguish from progressive muscular atrophy of the type under discussion; yet the differentiation is important from the standpoint of prognosis or treatment. Under such circumstances, the diagnosis can be made by muscle biopsy and electromyography.

There is no known treatment for any form of motor system disease.

INFANTILE MUSCULAR ATROPHY (WERDNIG AND HOFF-MANN), AMYOTONIA CONGENITA (OPPENHEIM) The form of progressive muscular atrophy described by Werdnig and Hoffmann is a disease of infants and young children, typically afflicting several members of a family. Pathologically, it closely resembles the adult disease described above. Amyotonia congenita is a purely clinical term, used to designate abnormal laxness of somatic musculature observed at birth or in early infancy; it may occur in a number of different pathologic processes, including Werdnig-Hoffmann disease. For further details of these conditions, Chap. 374 should be consulted.

Other forms of familial progressive muscular atrophy In addition to the infantile form there are several other familial syndromes of progressive muscular atrophy. They begin later in childhood, adolescence, and adult life and, though progressive, are extremely chronic. One form affects predominantly the proximal limb muscles (Wohlfart-Kugelberg-Welander syndrome) and must be distinguished from limb girdle dystrophy. In any given family the disease tends to have the same pattern and time course in all affected members.

HEREDITARY SPASTIC PARAPLEGIA This very rare disorder is characterized by weakness and spasticity of the legs, with early onset (childhood or adolescence) and slow progression. Later the arms may be affected, but usually to a lesser degree. The pathologic changes closely resemble those of Friedreich's ataxia, and there is reason now to believe that this condition is in fact an incomplete form of Freidreich's disease in which spastic weakness overshadows minimal or absent ataxia and sensory changes. The relation to Friedreich's ataxia and other neurologic diseases is further confirmed by the occurrence of pes cavus and scoliosis optic atrophy in some cases. But there are pure forms of progressive spastic paraplegia presenting in both childhood and late adult life which have no other neurologic or somatic abnormalities. The diagnosis is made by the family history and by excluding other possible causes of bilateral spastic weakness of the limbs. Another group of patients also has progressive dementia. A combination of optic atrophy and spastic paraparesis beginning in childhood is called Behr's syndrome.

SYNDROMES COMBINING WEAKNESS AND WASTING WITH SENSORY CHANGES

PROGRESSIVE NEURAL MUSCULAR ATROPHY The degenerative disorders characterized by progressive weakness and wasting of skeletal muscles combined with sensory changes are chronic diseases of peripheral nerves, often occurring as hereditary conditions. Although clinical and pathologic subvarieties exist, there is no sharp dividing line between them, and they are best considered together under the designation given above, in which the term *neural* emphasizes the peripheral nerve affection. Chronic peripheral neuropathy is an associated disorder in some of the hereditary ataxias and is regularly encountered in the classic form of Friedreich's ataxia. An additional connecting link with other genetically determined nervous diseases is the occurrence of progressive optic atrophy or pigmentary degeneration of the retina in some cases. Common to all is for the peripheral neuropathy to begin distally and to progress in a centripetal fashion and for the feet and legs to become first affected, with involvement of the hands and more proximal parts only after a considerable interval.

The two most frequent forms of hereditary polyneuropathy, peroneal muscular atrophy and hypertrophic interstitial polyneuropathy, are described in Chap. 377. Brief reference is also made there to a rare form known as Refsum's disease.

Treatment Although no specific treatment is available (except possibly in Refsum's disease, as indicated in Chap. 377), patients whose disease is of slow progression and in whom conditions are otherwise favorable may be greatly helped by measures to ensure a stable walking surface, such as corrective shoes, braces to prevent foot drop, and even orthopedic procedures to stabilize the joints.

SYNDROME OF PROGRESSIVE VISUAL LOSS

As already stated in previous sections, progressive impairment or loss of vision, due to degenerative changes in the visual system (retinas and optic nerves), may be an accompaniment of morbid processes affecting the nervous system diffusely—in particular, the nervous system lipidoses and the hereditary ataxias. Occasionally, however, the peripheral visual system is the major, or only, site of disease. In such cases, the disorders are strongly hereditary. For detailed discussion of these conditions, standard reference works on ophthalmology should be consulted. Nevertheless, two entities, because of their close relationship with other degenerative diseases of the nervous system, warrant some discussion here.

HEREDITARY OPTIC ATROPHY (LEBER) This rare condition is characterized by the relatively rapid development of bilateral blindness with optic atrophy, coming on in early adult life. It was first thoroughly described by Leber in 1871. Typically, it occurs as a sex-linked recessive trait, chiefly affecting men, but it may be seen in women. The manner of genetic expression is not fully understood.

Pathology Common to all cases examined pathologically is loss of retinal ganglion cells with secondary degeneration of optic nerve fibers. In addition involvement of other neural systems (corticospinal and spinocerebellar) has been seen in several instances.

Clinical aspects The onset generally is in the second or third decade. The condition often begins asymmetrically, with blurring of vision in one eye followed in days or weeks by similar affection of the other eye. Vision then deteriorates rapidly over ensuing weeks or months, generally with eventual total blindness as a result, although arrest before this stage has been seen, or even a little improvement after initial steady progression. In the early stages, examination of the visual fields shows large central scotomas. The optic disks may be normal at first, or may be swollen (optic neuritis); later the appearance is typically that of optic atrophy, with pale, clearly outlined disks.

Differential diagnosis Multiple sclerosis may at times act in a manner identical with that just described, but without a definite hereditary background and with a much better outlook for improvement of vision. Toxic or nutritional amblyopia can generally be excluded by history and associated clinical findings. In some cases it may be necessary to eliminate the possibility of a tumor compressing the chiasmal region and optic nerves, although some evidence of bitemporal defects would be then expected, rather than bilateral central scotomas alone. In addition to careful roentgenograms of the skull and cerebrospinal fluid examination, pneumoencephalographic visualization of the chiasmal region may be indicated in cases of serious doubt. Early onset of optic atrophy with spastic weakness of legs and ataxia (Behr's syndrome) should also be distinguishable on clinical grounds.

PIGMENTARY DEGENERATION OF THE RETINA (RETINITIS PIGMENTOSA)

This may at times occur as a relatively independent disorder, although it is often associated with other abnormalities, of which cataracts, deaf-mutism, and mental deficiency are outstanding. It is strongly hereditary, chiefly as a recessive trait, although dominant inheritance has been seen. Pigmentary degeneration of the retina is one of the features of the Laurence-Moon-Biedl syndrome. It likewise occurs in a considerable variety of neurologic diseases, including the hereditary ataxias, familial neuropathies, and some of the neuronal lipidoses (ceroid lipofuscinosis).

Pathology The principal lesion is a degeneration of the rods and cones, associated with displacement of melanin-containing cells from the pigment epithelium into more superficial parts of the retina. Other retinal structures are relatively intact. There is no inflammation so that the term *retinitis* is inappropriate.

Clinical aspects The disorder typically begins in childhood, first as night blindness. The visual fields become concentrically narrowed from the periphery to the center, until eventually (by adolescence, or perhaps not until middle age) very little useful vision remains. Ophthalmoscopic examination may be normal at first, but generally discloses irregular patches of dark pigment in the periphery of the retina. When cataracts are likewise present, as sometimes is the case, visual acuity may be significantly improved by their removal. The frequent association of the retinal lesions with other neurologic abnormalities has been mentioned in previous paragraphs.

Differential diagnosis Chorioretinitis from other causes (e.g, syphilis) may present a similar ophthalmoscopic appearance and should be excluded. The hereditary background and the progressive course, with night blindness and peripheral constriction of the visual fields, may lead to the diagnosis even in the rare cases where pigmentary deposits in the retina are absent. The slowly progressive or relatively stationary tapetoretinal degenerations of childhood can be distinguished clinically and by electroretinogram. In most instances, the opinion of a qualified ophthalmologist must be obtained.

REFERENCES

Advances in Neurology, vol 14. New York, Raven Press, 1976

BIRD ED, IVERSEN LL: Huntington's chorea. Post-mortem measurement of glutamic acid decarboxylase, choline acetyltransferase and dopamine in basal ganglia. Brain 97:457, 1974

BOWEN DA et al: Neurotransmitter-related enzymes and indices of hypoxia in senile dementia and other abiotrophies. Brain 99:459, 1976

BRADY RO: Sphingolipidoses and other lipid metabolic disorders, in *Basic Neuro-Chemistry,* 2d ed. Boston, Little, Brown, 1976, pp 556–568

ELDRIDGE F: The torsion dystonias literature review. Genetic and clinical studies. Neurology, vol 2, no 11, suppl, 1970

GAMBETTI P et al: Myoclonic epilepsy with Lafora bodies: Some ultrastructural, histochemical and biochemical aspects. Arch Neurol 25:483, 1971

GOODWIN RB et al: Comparison of the effects of Bromocriptine and levo-dopa in Parkinson's disease. J Neurol Neurosurg Psychiatry 40:474, 1977

HAKIM S, ADAMS RD: The special neurological problem of hydrocephalus with normal CSF pressure. J Neurol Sci 17:527, 1971

KLAWANS KL: Pharmacology of tardive dyskinesia. Am J Psychiatry 28:463, 1973

MORELL P et al: Diseases involving myelin, in *Basic Neurochemistry,* 2d ed, pp 581–604

PERRY TL: Aspartate-taurine imbalance in dominantly inherited olivopontocerebellar atrophy. Neurology 27:257, 1977

SMITH CM, SWASH M: Possible biochemical basis of memory disorder in Alzheimer disease. Ann Neurol 3:471, 1978

VINKEN PJ, BRUYN GW (eds): *Handbook of Clinical Neurology,* vol 13: *Neuroretinal Degenerations.* Amsterdam, North-Holland, 1972

——, —— (eds): *Handbook of Clinical Neurology,* vol 21: *System Disorders and Atrophies.* Amsterdam, North-Holland, 1975, part I

——, —— (eds): *Handbook of Clinical Neurology,* vol 22: *System Disorders and Atrophies.* Amsterdam, North-Holland, 1975, part II

374
DEVELOPMENTAL AND OTHER CONGENITAL ABNORMALITIES OF THE NERVOUS SYSTEM

RAYMOND D. ADAMS
G. ROBERT DELONG

The human nervous system is subject to a variety of developmental abnormalities which may be traced to genetic faults or diseases acquired in utero, at birth, or during the early years of life. These conditions may be manifest at birth or may be recognized only in late infancy and childhood, after some degree of maturation of the nervous system has occurred. Together they comprise the principal problems of pediatric neurology, and to discuss them fully would be pointless in a textbook of medicine. But many individuals so afflicted reach adolescent and adult age and come under the care of internists and general physicians; hence some understanding of the basic problems in this field is requisite.

Adult disorders of the nervous system that originate in early life may be classified under the following headings:

1 Congenital malformations of head, spine, and other structures, including dwarfism
2 Diseases which retard motor, speech, and intellectual development
3 Hereditary diseases which begin during childhood and persist throughout lifetime, some progressing
4 Epilepsy

Unlike many of the common neurologic problems that begin in adult years, those of infancy and childhood bring to light a number of pathogenic mechanisms unique to the early period of life. A genetic fault or exogenous agent may destroy the embryonal germ plasm in the first three postconceptional months, thereby blighting the formation and subsequent development of the nervous system as well as other somatic structures. Again, more subtle hereditary factors may alter the complex program of cerebral maturation so that it will not unfold in an even and harmonious way, leaving the person deficient in certain skills such as dexterity, speaking, reading, mathematics, music appreciation, etc. Or a disease may strike the rapidly maturing nervous system at birth (a unique event with its own possibilities of pathogenesis) or in the first years of life, leaving the victim with fixed and persistent deficits, such as retarded intellect, cerebral palsy, and epilepsy, for the entire span of life. For example, the myelination of the brain, which is one of the main developmental processes in infancy, is thought by some investigators to be permanently impaired by protein malnutrition. Finally, an unusually large proportion of special hereditary diseases declare themselves during childhood and continue into adult years, such as von Recklinghausen's neurofibromatosis and tuberous sclerosis.

MALFORMATIONS OF CRANIUM, SPINE, AND LIMBS Certain alterations in the size and shape of the head observed in the adult can nearly always be assumed to have their origin during the intrauterine period or early childhood. Beyond the first 4 to 5 years the brain (to which the skull always accommodates) has approximated adult size, and the sutures are so firmly closed that disease acquired later will have relatively little effect on the skull. Enlargement of the head is due either to macrocephaly with enlargement of brain (macroencephaly) (ventricles not enlarged significantly) or to hydrocephalus. Smallness of the head (microcephaly) is related to lack of brain growth or to a destructive lesion of brain early in life. Unusual shape of head is caused usually by craniostenosis. If the sagittal suture fuses too early, the head is long and narrow (dolichocephaly) with prominent brow and occiput; if the coronal suture closes prematurely, the head is wider than long (brachycephaly). Closure of all sutures produces a characteristic tower skull (turricephaly), shallow orbits, and bulging eyes. The latter condition, if not recognized early and suture lines excised, may prevent brain growth and raise intracranial pressure. Apert's syndrome (craniostenosis with "mitten hands" or syndactyly) is associated often with enlarged ventricles and mental retardation. Achondroplasia results in a normal-sized skull which looks disproportionately large compared with the short limbs.

Hydrocephalus of infancy and early childhood causes frontal bossing and variable degrees of cranial enlargement (usually over 60.0 cm, which is above the 97th percentile). In more than 60 percent of cases the underlying condition is an Arnold-Chiari malformation, followed in frequency by meningeal fibrosis around the brainstem from subarachnoid hemorrhage or meningitis, aqueductal stenosis and Dandy-Walker syndrome (failure of foramens of Magendie and Luschka to open), posterior fossa tumors, etc.

Of course there are wide variations in head size and shape, some familial, as every haberdasher knows, but the importance of all these abnormal deviations is that they continue throughout life, and the hydrocephalic states may arrest only to give trouble at a later age period. The main point to be remembered is that the cranial circumference is a valuable index of cerebral volume, and reflects disease originating in the early period of life.

ABNORMALITIES OF THE SPINE A remarkable variety of lifelong neurologic syndromes is associated with abnormality of the vertebral column. Some of these, such as hemivertebra, platybasia, fusion of the atlas and occiput or of vertebrae (Klippel-Feil syndrome), or congenital dislocation of the atlas, are the consequence of a malformation of the spine itself, and the enclosed spinal cord may or may not be involved. Others, such as spina bifida occulta, spinal meningocele or myelome-

ningocele, or dysraphism, involve the whole neural tube, including spinal cord, investing meninges, vertebral bodies, and even the overlying skin and subcutaneous tissues. Finally there is a group of hereditary metabolic diseases that alter the spine progressively during childhood and adolescence (e.g., the mucopolysaccharidoses).

Primary malformations of vertebrae These are most frequent in the upper cervical region. The *Klippel-Feil deformity* consists of maldevelopment and fusion of two or more cervical vertebrae, resulting in a short neck of limited mobility. The hairline is low, often at the level of the first thoracic vertebra. There may or may not be associated neurologic symptoms or signs. The importance of the spinal deformity lies in its frequent association with other abnormalities, especially those of platybasia and syringomyelia, the symptoms of which may not become manifest until adolescence or adult life.

Platybasia and basilar impression This is a rare maldevelopment in which either the base of the skull is flattened or the occiput and upper cervical spine are invaginated in the posterior fossa. Often the foramen magnum itself is imperfectly developed, or the atlas and occiput are fused. The exact teratogenesis of these anomalies is uncertain. The conditions may be asymptomatic, but often there is "crowding," distortion, or compression of the spinal cord, medulla, and lower cranial and cervical spinal nerves.

The resulting clinical picture is variable. Symptoms may be present from early life or may begin in late childhood, adolescence, or even adult years. Early symptoms consist of "dizzy" or "weak" spells and downward nystagmus on tilting the head; evidences of increased intracranial pressure such as headache; occipital neuralgia; vomiting; transient paresthesias in the occipital region, neck, or arm; facial paresthesias, deafness, nasal voice, and dysphagia; cerebellar ataxia; and spastic weakness of the legs. The symptoms may first be intermittent and at any time in the course of the illness may be aggravated by straining, moving the head, or placing the head and neck in certain positions. Inspection alone provides a clue to diagnosis. The whole configuration of the head and neck is abnormal. The neck is short; the ears and hairline are low; the neck movements are obviously restricted; and the normal cervical lordosis is lost or greatly exaggerated, sometimes to the extent that the occiput lies almost on the upper dorsal spine and shoulders.

Instability of the junction of axis on atlas (atlantoaxial dislocation) may cause compression of the spinal cord. This may also occur as a consequence of rheumatoid arthritis, Morquio's disease (probably a type of mucopolysaccharidosis), other debilitating diseases, and trauma (tear of ligaments which bind the odontoid process to the body of the first cervical vertebra). The treatment is surgical.

Platybasia and these related anomalies of the spine should be suspected in all cases presenting progressive cerebellar, brainstem, and cervical cord syndromes. Many of these cases have been misdiagnosed as multiple sclerosis. Others present a typical syringomyelic syndrome and have been so labeled. The clinical suspicion of platybasia and other spine anomalies can be confirmed by a true lateral roentgenogram of the skull. In such a projection the extension of a line drawn from the hard palate to the posterior border of the foramen magnum (Chamberlain's line) and another through the spine and body of the first cervical vertebra (Bull's line) when extended, instead of being more or less parallel as they normally are, intersect. The relation of cervical vertebrae is also seen. An acquired form of *basilar impression* occurs with rickets and Paget's disease. It is usually asymptomatic but sometimes involves the lower cranial nerves.

Arnold-Chiari malformation This condition, in which medulla and inferior-posterior portions of the cerebellar hemispheres project caudally through the foramen magnum, often to the level of the second cervical vertebra, is a common cause of hydrocephalus. It is usually associated with a spinal meningocele or myelomeningocele, and often there are deformities of the cervical spine and cervicooccipital junction. The symptoms of hydrocephalus dominate the clinical picture in infants. But, in milder cases, there may develop during adolescence or adult years any one of the several syndromes described under "Platybasia and Basilar Impression," above. There is, in addition, a second type of Arnold-Chiari malformation in patients who have no meningomyelocele. Often it is associated with syringomyelia. When platybasia and the Arnold-Chiari malformation coexist, it is generally impossible to decide which of the two is responsible for the clinical findings.

The treatment of platybasia and the Arnold-Chiari malformation has not been entirely satisfactory. If clinical progression is slight or uncertain, it is probably advisable to do nothing. If progression is certain and disability is increasing, upper cervical laminectomy and enlargement of the foramen magnum are indicated. Often this procedure halts the course of the illness or results in improvement. The surgical procedure must be done cautiously, however, for extensive manipulation of these structures may aggravate the symptoms or even cause death (see review by Salam and Adams).

Malformations associated with a defect in closure of the neural arch These take the forms of craniorachischisis totalis, craniocele, spinal meningocele, meningomyelocele, spina bifida occulta, and sinus tracts. Since these conditions seldom figure in adult neurology, only some of the late complications are mentioned here.

Sinus tracts in lumbosacral or occipital regions are of importance, for they may be sources at any age of bacterial meningitis. They are often indicated by a small dimple in the skin or by a tuft of hair along the posterior surface of the body in the midline. (The pilonidal sinus, in the opinion of the authors, should not be included in this group.) They may be associated with dermoid cysts at the central part of the tract. Evidence of such tracts should be sought in every instance of meningitis, especially when infection has recurred.

There are, in addition, other *congenital cysts* and *tumors* which may produce progressive symptoms and signs by compressing the spinal cord or by implicating nerve roots.

Several clinical syndromes of delayed progressive disease (in the adolescent or adult) have been delineated:

1 Progressive spastic weakness of some of the already weakened muscles of the legs in a patient known to have had a meningocele or myelomeningocele. Presumably the spinal cord, which is securely attached to the lumbar vertebrae, is stretched during the period of rapid lengthening of the vertebral column.

2 An acute cauda equina syndrome following some unusual activity or incident, e.g., rowing or a fall in a sitting position, in patients who have had an asymptomatic or symptomatic spina bifida or meningocele. The implicated sensory and motor roots are believed to be injured by sudden or repeated stretching. Weakness of bladder control, impotence (in the male), and numbness of feet and legs or footdrop compose the clinical syndrome.

3 Progressive cauda equina syndrome in the lumbosacral region.

4 Syringomyelia (see Chap. 375).

MALFORMATIONS OF THE EXTREMITIES These malformations include syndactylism, clinodactyly along with broad hands and transverse palmar (simian) line (common with mongolism), club feet, and arthrogryposis multiplex, but rarely are they of concern to internists.

DWARFISM IN RELATION TO NEUROLOGIC DISEASE Dwarfs (in contrast to midgets, who are more or less normally proportioned) suffer usually from a disorder of cartilaginous growth. Their head and trunk are large and out of proportion to their limbs. Achondroplasia would be an example. But it is noteworthy that the majority of mentally retarded individuals fall below average in statural growth, and in a few dwarfism is part of any one of many special syndromes. Persons with Down's syndrome and persons with most of the other chromosomal abnormalities are examples, and there are others in which an inherited or acquired metabolic defect of definable type blights brain and skeletal growth (e.g., cretinism and mucopolysaccharidoses). Microcephaly characterizes many of the dwarfs with cerebral diseases.

The 30 or 40 neurologic syndromes with statural underdevelopment and neurologic diseases are described and illustrated in the *Atlas of Mental Retardation* by Holmes et al.

THE PHAKOMATOSES

This is a unique group in which neurologic abnormalities are combined with congenital defects of skin, retina, and other organs. The terms *congenital ectodermal dysplasias, congenital neurocutaneous syndromes,* or *phakomatoses* (Greek *phakos,* "lentil," "mole," or "freckle") are used frequently to designate this general class of disorders. The major syndromes include *neurofibromatosis, tuberous sclerosis, encephalotrigeminal syndrome,* and rarely the *cerebelloretinal hemangioblastomatosis.* Another variant of the latter is the *myelocutaneous* (Klippel-Trénaunay) *syndrome,* in which a vascular malformation of spinal cord and meninges is associated with a vascular nevus within the area of skin innervated by the involved spinal segments and gigantism of an affected arm. Recently it has been suggested that *ataxia telangiectasia* be included with this group of conditions (see review of neurocutaneous diseases by Adams).

NEUROFIBROMATOSIS (VON RECKLINGHAUSEN'S DISEASE) This is an inherited disease (mendelian dominant), in which spots of increased skin pigmentation are combined with multiple neurofibromas. The pigmented spots are irregular in shape with relatively even borders, vary in size from a few millimeters to several centimeters, and are of brownish coffee color (café au lait). They are most prominent over the trunk, in the axilla (axillary freckles), and about the pelvis. Similar lesions occur in individuals without neurofibromatosis, but in such instances are generally smaller than 1.5 cm in diameter and fewer than five in number. The tumors arise from the neurilemmal sheath (Schwann cells) and fibroblasts of the peripheral nerve. They are usually multiple and vary in size from minute lesions to large tumors several centimeters in diameter. The majority are smoothly rounded or lobulated, soft or firm, and can sometimes be seen or felt along the course of a peripheral nerve. Often they sink into the subcutaneous fat on gentle pressure. Like the pigmented lesions, the tumors are more frequent over the trunk than on the extremities. The pigmented areas, because of giant melanosomes in pigment epithelial cells, become increasingly apparent with age; also the tumors of nerve sheaths are often not demonstrable early in life. Most of the tumors are asymptomatic; but occasionally, if they attain a large size or occupy an unusual position, they may produce pressure upon contiguous structures. Tumors of the spinal nerve roots may compress the spinal cord and at the same time extend through the intervertebral foramens to form a large mass in the posterior mediastinum (dumbbell tumors). Acoustic neurinomas, usually bilateral in patients with neurofibromatosis, may produce deafness and other symptoms and signs of a cerebellopontine angle lesion (Chap. 367). Other histopathologic types of tumor (meningioma, glioma) are encountered more often in neurofibromatosis than in the general population. Diffuse overgrowth of Schwann cells and fibroblasts may also occur, giving rise to plexiform neuromas. They may cause hideous deformities, often with overgrowth of underlying bone. Bone cysts may also form. Most of these associated tumors are rare in infancy and childhood, though pontine glioma and glioma of the optic nerve and chiasm are exceptions to the clinical rule. The latter condition should always be considered in the differential diagnosis of unilateral (rarely bilateral) blindness, proptosis, and extraocular muscle paralysis in childhood, especially if there are signs of von Recklinghausen's disease. Enlargement of the optic foramens, demonstrable by roentgenogram, is a valuable aid in diagnosis. *Pulsating exophthalmos* (usually due to an orbital hemangioma) may result from congenital absence of part of the sphenoid bone. *Pheochromocytoma* is an infrequent accompaniment of the disease. In about 5 to 10 percent of cases of neurofibromatosis one of the tumors will become sarcomatous.

Fibrous dysplasia, congenital vertebral anomalies, local gigantism of an extremity, subperiosteal bone cysts, and pseudoarthrosis of the tibia may be associated with neurofibromatosis. Scoliosis is a common skeletal deformity in children with this disease, so that neurofibromatosis must be added to the list of neurogenic kyphoscolioses (the others are syringomyelia, Friedreich's ataxia, and poliomyelitis). Stenosis of the aqueduct of Sylvius with obstructive hydrocephalus is at times observed in neurofibromatosis. Also there may be a mild degree of mental retardation, related presumably to developmental abnormalities of the cerebral cortex. Spina bifida, hypospadias, glaucoma, and elephantiasis are occasionally seen.

About one-third of cases of neurofibromatosis are discovered accidentally on routine examination, there being no complaints. Another third of these patients come seeking advice about the cosmetic aspects of the disease, and the remainder have neurologic syndromes. Although neurofibromatosis is hereditary, nearly 50 percent of cases appear to develop as mutations. Those with prominent neurological signs tend to have few cutaneous lesions. There is no treatment for the disease other than excision of symptomatic tumors.

TUBEROUS SCLEROSIS (BOURNEVILLE'S DISEASE) This curious disease, of dominant inheritance, is manifested by the clinical triad of convulsive seizures, mental deficiency, and adenoma sebaceum. The latter are fine, wart-like lesions distributed predominantly in a butterfly distribution over the cheeks and forehead. The individual adenomas vary in size from 0.1 to 1.0 cm and are elevated and pinkish or pinkish yellow in color. In addition, the skin over the lower part of the back may be thick, rough, and of yellowish color like sharkskin or pigskin (shagreen patch). Actually the earliest lesions are foliate hypopigmented spots ("white spots") over the trunk and limbs, which are seen most clearly under ultraviolet light (Wood's lamp). They are distinguishable on the basis of size, shape, and character from avascular nevi and vitiligo, and are highly diagnostic, often providing the earliest clue to mental retardation or infantile epilepsy. The mental deficiency may be relatively stationary or progressive. The seizures are usually generalized but may be focal. Retinal tumors, optic atrophy and cataracts,

syndactylism, spina bifida, and other visible malformations may be conjoined.

The most advanced examples of tuberous sclerosis usually are to be found in institutions for the mentally retarded, but it would be a mistake to assume that all are so severely disabled. In general hospital clinics it is not at all unusual to see patients with average intelligence and only seizures and a few skin lesions. Occasionally a focal cerebral syndrome will prove at biopsy to have a typical "tuber" or an associated glioma as its basis in a patient not known to have this disease. Family history is frequently unhelpful; approximately one-half of cases are sporadic (? mutation).

The lesions of the skin are pathologically fibromas and not true adenomas. Some are rather vascular and suggest telangiectasia. The brain lesions consist of areas of malformed cortex with extensive astrogliosis and a peculiar mixture of glioblasts and monster nerve cells. Calcification may or may not be present. Masses of subependymal glial tissue account for nodules which project into and form "candle gutterings" on the walls of the ventricles that are often seen in computerized tomography and pneumograms. In Bourneville's original case, death was due to rhabdomyoma of the heart, and most cases of this benign tumor of heart muscle are associated with tuberous sclerosis. This disease is also combined with tumorous malformations of kidney, liver, adrenal glands, and pancreas.

The diagnosis is aided by roentgenograms of the skull. Calcified nodules occur particularly in the temporal lobes and adjacent to the ventricles. The center of the nodule tends to be more densely radiopaque than the periphery. The electroencephalogram is usually abnormal but without specific pattern. The cerebrospinal fluid may be normal; rarely the total protein level is elevated.

The only treatment is symptomatic. The prognosis for life beyond the third decade is poor. Death is usually due to seizures, associated tumors, or intercurrent diseases.

CEREBELLORETINAL HEMANGIOBLASTOMATOSIS (HIPPEL-LINDAU SYNDROME) This condition is discussed here though the skin is seldom involved. As the name implies, the syndrome consists of a vascular malformation of the retina and cerebellum. The retinal lesions are capillary angiomas, usually multiple, causing progressive loss of vision; the cerebellar lesion consists of a slowly growing hemangioblastoma, frequently multiple, with a large cystic component, lending itself to surgical removal; spinal and medullary hemangioblastomas also occur. The clinical symptoms and signs consist of progressive cerebellar ataxia, headache, and papilledema. Seldom is a vascular bruit audible over the head. Polycythemia, possibly related to the production of erythropoietin, has been observed in many cases and has in a few instances disappeared after excision of the tumor. The disease is transmitted as an autosomal dominant, but many cases are sporadic. Rarely do these tumors appear before adolescence. The cerebellar lesions may be multiple and associated with one or more spinal hemangioblastomas. One should consider this diagnosis in all patients with a cerebellar tumor syndrome (see Chap. 367). Not all have a retinal lesion—the von Hippel part of the disease. The hemangioblastoma of the cerebellum is usually but one part of a constellation of abnormalities including angiomas and cysts of the liver, pancreas, and kidneys, and tumors of the epididymis and kidney, the latter being the cause of death in some cases. Pheochromocytomas have been described in this and in other of the phakomatoses. Syringomyelia has been observed in a few cases, and if a careful search is made, a hemangioblastoma can often be found in relation to the syrinx at some level.

The cerebellar hemangioblastoma demands surgical treatment, and if the nodule of the tumor is found in the wall of the cyst and is excised, the results can be excellent; if the tumor cannot be operated on because of size or multiplicity, radiation should be tried. The retinal lesions, when small, can be arrested by photocoagulation.

ENCEPHALOTRIGEMINAL SYNDROME (STURGE-WEBER DISEASE)   This disease consists of capillary or cavernous hemangiomas, within but not always limited to the cutaneous distribution of the trigeminal nerve and of a predominantly venous hemangioma of the leptomeninges. If the skin lesion is within the area of supply of the ophthalmic division of the trigeminal nerve, the occipital lobes are more commonly involved, whereas a facial nevus is more often associated with involvement of the parietal and frontal lobes. The intracranial and cutaneous lesions may occur separately.

Pathologically, in addition to the large number of abnormal blood vessels in the meninges, the subjacent cortex is progressively destroyed, and in some cases a band of calcium develops within the lesion. This band, following the convolutional pattern as it does, is responsible for the characteristic "railroad track" roentgenographic picture. Deeply situated arteriovenous malformations rarely coexist.

The first neurologic symptom is usually a focal seizure on the side opposite the skin lesion. Transient postictal (Todd's) paralysis or permanent paralysis may follow the seizure. Sensorimotor paralysis or permanent visual field defect, the most frequent findings, may be either of insidious onset with slow progression or apoplectic. Hemorrhage into the meninges has been reported, but this must be a rare event. Possibly occlusion of cortical vessels is, in certain instances, responsible for neurologic deficits. Blindness in the eye on the side of the nevus is frequent and is nearly always due to glaucoma. Most patients with this malformation survive for many years, often with residual mental defects and hemiparesis.

The lesions are usually too extensive to be treated surgically, though hemispherectomy has been advised by some surgeons for intractable epilepsy. Anticonvulsant medication is indicated, but the seizures may be difficult to control.

Hemangioma of the trunk or upper or lower extremity may be associated with a spinal cord vascular malformation (Klippel-Trénaunay syndrome). The extremity may be hypertrophied. The cord lesion may bleed into or cause infarction in the nervous tissue, producing a spinal sensorimotor paralysis. Surgical exploration and decompression are seldom beneficial to the patient.

ATAXIA TELANGIECTASIA   This condition has attracted considerable interest because of theoretical implications of its apparent cause and pathogenesis. Inherited as a recessive trait, the disease is characterized neurologically by a progressive cerebellar ataxia, apraxia of ocular movement, and choreoathetosis beginning during the early years of life. Telangiectases of bulbar conjunctivas and skin, especially about the ears, neck, and in flexor creases at the elbows and knees, appear somewhat later in childhood or adolescence. Recurring pulmonary and sinus infections have been prominent in many cases, and a deficiency in the IgA globulins and a defect of delayed hypersensitivity are found. The diagnosis can be supported by the finding of abnormal humeral and cell-mediated immunity and of raised levels of alpha fetoprotein and cytogenetic abnormalities. Fibroblasts and lymphocytes from patients with this disease have enhanced in vitro radiosensitivity, attributed to deficiencies in enzyme systems that repair DNA. The associated pathologic changes consist of an extensive loss of Purkinje cells of the cerebellum and degeneration of the neurons in other parts of the basal ganglia. Dysplasia of the thymus has been well documented, and death usually occurs by the second or third decade of life from infection or a reticuloendothelial tumor.

FAMILIAL DYSAUTONOMIA (RILEY-DAY SYNDROME)

This disease is characterized by autonomic instability (abnormal sweating, loss of vasomotor control, labile hypertension), impaired taste with absence of fungiform papillae, diminished pain and temperature sensation, hyporeflexia, episodic fever, vomiting attacks, and lack of lacrimation (alacrima), with corneal ulceration. Studies by Sedgewick and Boder show the disease to be inherited in a pattern consistent with an autosomal recessive trait and to be limited for the most part to Ashkenazi Jews.

The clinical manifestations become apparent soon after birth with difficulty in feeding (dysphagia) and moving and are increasingly evident in childhood. A few patients reach adult years, but the mortality rate is high because of recurrent pulmonary infections with inappropriate autonomic responses. Emotional instability presents a problem in most patients. Although intelligence has been within normal limits in some patients, in others it has been slightly subnormal. Growth seems to be delayed for unclear reasons, and the natural tendency is to undernutrition and scoliosis. Neuropathic (Charcot) joints due to lack of pain and related injury have been reported.

Proof of the disturbance of the autonomic nervous system comes from special tests such as absence of skin flare after histamine and skin stroking (loss of axonal reflex), and hypersensitivity to both cholinergic and adrenergic agents. Nerve conduction velocities are decreased. Quantitative pathologic studies of peripheral and autonomic nervous systems have shown marked depletion of small-caliber axons in peripheral nerves (which could account for the deficit in pain and temperature appreciation), and decreased numbers of small neurons in the dorsal root ganglia, in sympathetic ganglia, and in the ciliary ganglia (which could account for some of the dysautonomic features). Intermediolateral cell columns of the spinal cord are normal, as is the rest of the central nervous system.

By inference it is suggested that the disease is due to a unitary biochemical defect, probably a deficiency of a single enzyme and perhaps related to the "nerve growth factor."

In the differential diagnosis one must consider other forms of small-fiber polyneuropathy with analgesia and dysautonomia (including congenital indifference to pain and amyloidosis) (see Chap. 377), as well as the Shy-Drager syndrome (a degenerative disease of lateral horn cells and basal ganglia) (see Chap. 373).

Picrotoxin is said to increase tearing of eyes. Chlorpromazine in conjunction with phenobarbital may control vomiting attacks. The Heller-type myotomy has been successful in some few instances in improving esophageal function. Orthopedic measures are needed to stabilize neuropathic joints. Injury must be avoided and wounds treated carefully.

ABNORMALITIES OF MOTOR FUNCTION (CEREBRAL PALSY)

In this category of neurologic defect a major disturbance of motor function, usually nonprogressive, has been present since infancy or childhood. The popular term for these conditions is *cerebral palsy.* The name is not altogether appropriate, nor is such a crude classification of nervous disorders particularly useful from the viewpoint of the physician, because it results in a collocation of diseases of widely differing etiologic and anatomic types. The hereditary and acquired and the intrauterine, natal, and postnatal diseases lose their identity. Nevertheless, the term has been adopted as a slogan for fund-raising societies and for a major rehabilitation movement throughout the United States, and it will not soon disappear from medical terminology.

CLINICAL ASPECTS OF MOTOR DISTURBANCES WHICH HAVE BEEN PRESENT SINCE INFANCY OR CHILDHOOD Motor abnormalities which have had their onset early in life are so numerous and diverse in their manifestations that it is necessary to refer to the discussion of the motor system (Chaps. 15 and 16) in order to interpret them. In order to ascertain etiologic factors, it is helpful to attempt to categorize a given case according to the extent and nature of the abnormality. A careful history of possible prenatal, perinatal, or postnatal insults to the developing nervous system must always be sought; certain correlations of these factors with the resulting pattern of neurologic deficit are outlined below. Many patients with these motor abnormalities of infancy and childhood, which are relatively frequent, reach adult years.

SPECIAL TYPES Infantile spastic and rigid paralyses The pattern of paralysis or rigidity is important, for it provides information as to the etiology and possible pathogenic mechanism.

Cerebral spastic diplegia (Little's disease) In 1862 Little called attention to the concurrence of "Abnormal parturition, difficult labours, premature birth, and asphyxia neonatorum" and of a spastic weakness that affected legs more than arms. He emphasized the prenatal or natal origin, the diplegic distribution of the paralysis (legs more than arms), and the nonprogressive course. Little was of the opinion that asphyxia caused the cerebral damage. According to present thinking, two groups can be identified. One is associated with prematurity and consists predominantly of spastic paraplegia; motor disturbances in the upper extremities are mild; head size and intelligence are less diminished than in other forms of the disease. The incidence of this form of cerebral palsy has declined significantly since the introduction of neonatal intensive care, and some results indicate that it can be virtually eliminated by expert management of premature infants.

The second group is associated with term birth and difficult parturition, in which the major insult is intrapartum asphyxia and attendant fetal distress. Such infants are born asphyxiated, require resuscitation, and have low Apgar scores, which in this circumstance have important predictive value. Such infants may develop severe spastic quadriplegia and severe developmental retardation. The pathologic lesions of brain consist of hypoxic/ischemic infarction in distal fields of flow, primarily in the cortex and white matter of parietal and posterior frontal lobes.

Actually, the pattern of paralysis in the second group is more variable than the title implies. Three types may be distinguished, the paraplegic, diplegic, and the generalized and pseudobulbar. These differ from one another only with respect to the severity of affection of the arms and bulbar musculature. Pure paraplegias and pure pseudobulbar cases are relatively rare. Usually all four extremities are involved, but the legs much more than the arms, which is the real meaning of diplegia. As a rule the damage to the nervous system is recognized at birth or soon thereafter by some abnormality of breathing, sucking and swallowing, color of mucous membranes, or responsiveness. These latter signs may indicate either a congenital defect of the nervous system or birth injury of the brainstem. However, the stiff, awkward movements of the legs, maintained in an extended, adducted posture, do not usually attract attention until several weeks or months have passed. Seizures occur in some cases, and it is not uncommon to observe a delay in all normal developmental sequences, especially those which depend on the motor system. Once walking is attempted, usually much later than in the normal child, the characteristic stance and gait become manifest. The legs are advanced stiffly in short steps, each describing part of the arc of a circle; adduction is often so strong as to lead to actual crossing (scissors gait), with lower legs slightly splayed out and the feet flexed and turned in, the heels not touching the ground. In the adolescent and adult, the legs tend to be short and small, but the muscles are not markedly atrophic, as in infantile muscular atrophy and dystrophy. Passive manipulation of the limbs reveals marked spasticity in the extensors and adductors and also slight shortening of the calf muscles. The hands and arms may be affected only slightly, if at all; there may be awkwardness and stiffness of the fingers; in a few, pronounced weakness and spasticity are noted. Speech may be well articulated or noticeably slurred, and in some instances the face is set in a spastic smile. The deep-tendon reflexes are exaggerated, those in the legs more than in the arms, and the plantar reflexes are extensor. Usually there is no disturbance of sphincteric function, though delay in acquiring voluntary control is usual. Athetotic postures and movements of the face, tongue, and hands are present in some patients and may actually conceal the pyramidal weakness. Ataxic and hypotonic forms also exist. The mentality in the pure form of diplegia tends to be relatively normal.

The condition must be distinguished from familial types of spastic paraparesis which are well-recognized clinical entities.

Infantile hemiplegia, double hemiplegia, and quadriplegia Hemiplegia is a not uncommon condition of infancy and childhood, and the functional difference between the two sides may be noticed soon after birth or during the first 6 to 12 months of life. The condition develops usually as a consequence of a predominantly unilateral infection or thrombosis of cerebral arteries that may have happened before or after birth or during childhood. The parents may be the first to notice that movements of prehension and exploration are carried out with only one arm. The affection of the leg is usually recognized later, i.e., during the first attempt to stand and walk.

Mental defect may be associated with infantile hemiplegia but is even less common than with cerebral diplegia and much less than in bilateral hemiplegia. Convulsions occur in 35 to 50 percent of children with congenital hemiplegia, and these may persist throughout life. If the hemiplegia was acquired during childhood, seizures often accompany the onset. They may be generalized but are frequently unilateral and limited to the hemiplegic side. Often, after a series of seizures, the affected side will be weak for several hours or longer (Todd's paralysis).

In double hemiplegia, a much less frequent condition, the bilateral weakness of face, arms, and legs arises under conditions of more severe acquired cerebral disease and at any age. The arms are severely affected, in contrast to their minimal involvement in cerebral diplegia.

The quadriplegic state differs from bilateral hemiplegias in that the bulbar musculature is not involved. The condition is relatively rare but may result from a bilateral cerebral lesion. However, one should also be alerted to the possibility of a high cervical cord lesion. Although this may occasionally result from cysts, tumors, and other malformations, it is usually produced in the infant by a fracture-dislocation of the cervical spine, induced during a difficult breech delivery. Similarly, in *paraplegia,* with weakness or paralysis limited to the legs, the lesion may be either a cerebral form of diplegia or a spinal one. Sphincteric disturbances and a definite loss of somatic sensation below a certain level on the trunk always favor a spinal localization. Congenital cysts, tumors, and diastematomyelia are more frequently the cause of paraplegia than of quadriplegia. An additional cause of infantile paraplegia is spinal infarction from thrombotic complications of umbilical artery catheterization.

Encephaloclastic disorders underlie all these conditions. The pathologic change is essentially that of ischemic necrosis. In many cases, the lesions must have been incurred in utero and thus are not dependent on perinatal events. For the most part, the lesions reflect not pure asphyxia (anoxia) but circulatory insufficiency (ischemia) resulting from hypotension or circulatory collapse. The ischemia of circulatory failure tends to affect the tissues lying in arterial border zones, and there may also be venous stasis with congestion and hemorrhage (occurring particularly in the deep central structures such as the basal ganglia and periventricular matrix zones).

CONGENITAL EXTRAPYRAMIDAL SYNDROMES IN INFANCY AND CHILDHOOD

The spastic and rigid cerebral diplegias discussed above shade almost imperceptibly into the congenital extrapyramidal syndromes. Many such patients are found in every cerebral palsy clinic, and they ultimately may reach adult medical clinics. Pyramidal tract signs may be completely absent, and the inexperienced student, familiar only with the pure cerebral spastic diplegia syndrome, is always puzzled as to their classification. Some extrapyramidal cases of this type undoubtedly are attributable to severe perinatal hypoxia; others represent separate diseases such as erythroblastosis fetalis with kernicterus. In the interest of being able to state accurately the probable pathologic basis and future course of these illnesses, it is desirable to separate the extrapyramidal syndromes due to prenatal and natal diseases, which usually become manifest during the first year of life, from the acquired or hereditary postnatal syndromes such as familial athetosis, dystonia musculorum deformans, and cerebellar ataxia. The latter are discussed in Chap. 373.

CONGENITAL CHOREOATHETOSIS (DOUBLE ATHETOSIS)

Probably the most frequent representative of this group, this condition is like the spastic states in that it may not be recognized at birth but only after several months or a year have elapsed. The nature of the chorea and athetosis has been discussed in Chap. 16. Syndromes may be mixed, however. All combinations of chorea, athetosis, ballismus, myoclonus, and even dystonia may be found in a single case, or one or another type of movement disorder may predominate. However, in all instances there is in addition a primary defect in voluntary movement.

Choreoathetosis in infants and children varies in severity. In some the disorder is so mild that the abnormal movements are misinterpreted as restlessness or "the fidgets"; in others, every voluntary act is marred by intense involuntary movements, leaving the patient nearly helpless. The severely handicapped patients, even with the help of rehabilitation clinics and corrective orthopedic operations, rarely achieve a degree of motor control that will permit them to lead an independent life, and they continually need supportive treatment and help as adults. The intelligence may be well preserved.

Kernicterus is of importance in this context for it may also be a cause of generalized athetosis in children and adults. It is true that the majority of infants who suffer this disease die within the first week or two of life, and those who survive are often mentally retarded, deaf, and totally unable to sit, stand, or walk, so that the tendency is always to put them in homes for the feebleminded. But there are exceptional patients, obviously less damaged, who are mentally normal or at most only slightly backward. These are the ones who develop a variety of other neurologic sequelae that persist throughout life. Either athetosis or ataxia may be present, and a few have also shown rigid limbs and a picture not too different from that of cerebral spastic diplegia with involuntary movements. Kernicterus should always be suspected if an extrapyramidal syndrome is accompanied by bilateral deafness and palsy of upward gaze. The neuropathologic changes in these surviving patients with milder cases consist of symmetrically distributed nerve-cell loss and gliosis in the subthalamic nucleus of Luys, the globus pallidus, thalamus, and oculomotor and cochlear nuclei. These lesions are the result of the hyperbilirubinemia. In the newborn, unconjugated bilirubin can pass through the poorly developed blood brain barrier into these central and brainstem nuclei, where it is directly toxic. Acidosis and hypoxia exacerbate the effect.

CONGENITAL AND ACQUIRED ATAXIAS

The combination of cerebral diplegia with cerebellar ataxia has already been mentioned. In these patients difficulty in standing and walking cannot be attributed to spasticity or paralysis. Incoordination, similar to that seen in cerebellar disease, and hypotonia are the principal findings. The motor defect may be so great that the individual is never able to sit or stand; the muscles are of normal size, and voluntary movements, though weak, are possible in all the limbs. In less severe cases sitting, standing, and walking are merely delayed, and with advancing years cerebellar ataxia and tremor become manifest. Relative improvement may occur in later years. The tendon reflexes are present, and the plantar reflexes are either flexor or extensor. Many of these patients suffer a degree of amentia and retardation of speech development that results in their placement in homes for the feebleminded. In relatively few of the recorded cases have the pathologic changes of this condition been studied. Aplasia or hypoplasia of the cerebellum has been reported only a few times. Sclerotic lesions of the cerebellum are more common.

The hereditary ataxias are likely to begin at a later age and are progressive. They are discussed in Chap. 373.

MENTAL RETARDATION

Mentally retarded (feebleminded) individuals pose special problems not only in childhood but also as adults. They become the concern of the internist for several reasons. Firstly, failure to recognize the mentally subnormal patient means that one depends on a history that is inadequate, instead of turning to the guardian; also one must rely more on objective signs of disease than on subjective complaint. Then, too, the reactions of such patients to drugs and fever may be more devastating and less predictable. Recognition of the type of disease underlying impaired mentality also becomes important in genetic counseling for the prevention of similar disease in other members of the family.

The more severely retarded individuals nearly always are forced to reside in institutions, and the brain is so extensively damaged that many do not survive beyond childhood. There are special severe types of mental retardation, such as Down's syndrome, that are less lethal, and many persons with such conditions live with their families until adulthood. Their condition raises a number of interesting problems for the internist (i.e., the tendency to develop leukemia and premature senile dementia). Other milder forms of mental subnormality are much more numerous, however, amounting to 3 percent of the general population, and they are more often familial and peculiar to the lower economic stratum of society. Their anatomic basis is uncertain. In many instances they probably represent examples of persons who fall within the lower distribution of normal human intelligence.

The clinical manifestations of mental retardation are relatively easy to perceive. Silly behavior and inability to give a sensible account of the medical problem constitute one useful datum. Slowness in motor development, inability to learn and poor school progress (individuals unable to pass the sixth grade usually have an IQ of 60 to 70), lack of a concept of time or space, inability to secure and hold a job or to perform more than the menial tasks of society are other useful indices. The differentiation of the various classes of mental backwardness by clinical criteria is facilitated if the framework of reference in Table 374-1 is used.

In spite of the wide spectrum of specific disease entities causing mental retardation, perhaps half of all mentally retarded persons cannot presently be classified in terms of specific etiology by clinical criteria. Many of these cases are familial, the patients coming from families in which other members are retarded or have important mental disorders, and the heritable factors are probably polygenic. There also appears to be another group of disorders, due to single gene defects affecting only the brain, which have been poorly defined clinically and pathologically; included are several types of maldevelopment of the cerebral cortex. Finally, infantile malnutrition as a cause of impaired brain growth and consequent poor mental development has received much attention. Malnutrition during the first two years of life, when coupled with other socioeconomic deprivations, may result in retarded brain growth and mental development that persist into adult life. If, however, such children are "rescued" by refeeding and placement in a stimulating and supportive environment, the effects of early malnutrition are largely reversible, and normal mental development can result.

CLINICAL CHARACTERISTICS As an aid to the general physician who must undertake the diagnosis and management of backward children, the following comments may be of some value. Mental retardation manifests itself most obviously in the spheres of motor, language, social, and intellectual development. The severely retarded child at idiot level with an IQ of less than 20 and unable to look after himself often does not sit up, walk, or stand, and if any one of these motor activities is acquired, it appears late and is imperfectly performed. Language is not mastered, or at most a few words are understood and uttered. The patient is continuously idle and can only vocalize in a meaningless way. He does not interact with people and objects around him, nor does he make known his needs for water, food, excretion, etc. He does nothing for himself and exhibits only primitive emotional reactions. Physical growth is usually retarded, nutrition may be poor, and susceptibility to respiratory infections is common. Sphincteric control may never be secured. A variety of physical deformities, particularly microcephaly, is common in this group. Such persons are to be found among the adult populations of state hospitals. Affections of the nervous system which have their onset later in life are usually not attended by bodily disfigurement.

If the mental defect is less pronounced, with an IQ of 20 to 50 (i.e., imbecile), or 50 to 70 (i.e., moron), and if specific motor defects do not coexist, then sitting, walking, and speech are acquired, but after a delay in many cases. The existence of a cerebral defect may be noted for the first time when the child fails to speak normally during the second and third years of life and seems not to be able to learn the usual household tasks and play activities as well as other children. However, delay in speech development must not by itself be taken as a mark of mental retardation, for some children who are obviously intelligent and who show remarkable talent in communicating by gesture are slow in talking. Also the deaf child may be singled out by his indifference to noise and reduced vocalization but otherwise normal development. Toilet training also may be

difficult to accomplish in the retarded child, but again it may be delayed in an otherwise normal child.

Within the spectrum of types of mental retardation, even within a group of persons of similar IQs, there are vast differences and contrasts in overall behavioral functioning. Some mentally retarded persons are pleasant and amiable, and achieve a rather satisfactory social adjustment; this is especially true of simple mental retardates. At the opposite extreme is the ill-understood syndrome of autism, associated with varying degrees of retardation, in which the child or older person fails to manifest any kind of interpersonal, social contact—including communicative language—and demonstrates a limited and bizarre interest primarily in inanimate objects (see "Autism," below). It is impossible to list all variations of mental retardation here, but the point should be made that all aspects of intellectual life and personality are touched in differing degrees. Many retarded individuals are dull, apathetic, and

TABLE 374-1
Types of mental retardation

I Mental defect with associated developmental abnormalities in nonnervous structures
  A Those affecting cranioskeletal structures
    1 Microcephaly
    2 Macrocephaly
    3 Hydrocephalus (including myelomeningocele with Arnold-Chiari malformation and associated cerebral anomalies)
    4 Down's syndrome (mongolism)
    5 Cretinism (congenital hypothyroidism)
    6 Mucopolysaccharidoses (Hurler, Hunter, Morquio, and Sanfilippo types)
    7 Acrocephalosyndactyly (craniostenosis)
    8 Arthrogryposis multiplex congenita (some cases)
    9 Rare syndromes: e.g., Rubinstein-Taybi
    10 Dwarfism, short stature: Russell-Silver dwarf, Seckel's bird-headed dwarf, Cockayne-Neel dwarf, etc.
    11 Hypertelorism, median-cleft-face syndromes, agenesis of corpus callosum
  B Those affecting nonskeletal structures
    1 Neurocutaneous syndromes: tuberous sclerosis, Sturge-Weber, neurofibromatosis (uncommonly)
    2 Congenital rubella syndrome (deafness, blindness, congenital heart disease, small stature)
    3 Chromosomal disorders: Down's syndrome, some cases of Klinefelter's syndrome (XXY), XYY, Turner's (XO) syndrome (occasionally), others
    4 Laurence-Moon-Biedl syndrome (retinitis pigmentosa, obesity, polydactyly)
    5 Eye disorders: toxoplasmosis (chorioretinitis), galactosemia (cataract), congenital rubella
    6 Prader-Willi syndrome (obesity, hypogenitalism)
II Mental defect without developmental anomalies in nonnervous structures, but with focal cerebral and other neurologic abnormalities
  A Cerebral spastic diplegia and quadriplegia
  B Cerebral hemiplegia, unilateral or bilateral
  C Congenital choreoathetosis or ataxia
    1 Kernicterus
    2 Status marmoratus
  D Congenital atonic diplegia
  E Posthypoglycemic, posttraumatic, postmeningitic, and postencephalitic states
  F Those associated with other neuromuscular abnormalities (muscular dystrophy, Friedreich's ataxia, etc.)
  G Cerebral degenerative diseases (lipidoses)
  H Lesch-Nyhan syndrome
III Mental defect without signs of other developmental abnormality or neurologic disorder (epilepsy may or may not be present)
  A Simple mental retardation, familial mental retardation
  B Some cases of encephaloclastic disease (hypoxia, hypoglycemia)
  C Infantile autism
  D Associated with inborn errors of metabolism (phenylketonuria, other aminoacidurias, organic acidurias)
  E Congenital infections (some cases of congenital syphilis, cytomegalic inclusion disease)

underactive. Others display an incessant hyperactivity, characterized by a very short attention span, a restless inquisitive searching of the environment, and low frustration tolerance; they may be destructive or recklessly fearless, and may seem strangely impervious to injury. Some display a peculiar anhedonia and are indifferent to either punishment or reward. Strangely, as with the mentally normal but hyperactive, inattentive child, improvement in these children can often be achieved by using amphetamines. Other aberrant types of behavior, such as violent aggressiveness and even self-mutilation, are not uncommon. Rhythmic rocking, rolling, head banging, and bouncing movements feature the motor activities of retarded persons, and may be performed hour after hour without fatigue, often to the accompaniment of bleating sounds, squeals, and other ejaculations. Here the abnormality is not the appearance of rhythmic movements of the body, which are to be observed at one period in the development of many normal children, but their persistence. Music may encourage rhythmic movement and gives pleasure to many retarded children and adults.

It is apparent that the clinical and behavioral characteristics of individuals with retarded development cannot be adequately described by a single parameter, the IQ. There are many other factors which determine the social success of retarded children and should give direction to their education and training. These include recognition of specific sensory or motor handicaps, such as blindness and deafness as well as athetosis or hemiplegia; specific language or speech deficits; behavioral disturbances, such as autism or hyperactivity; and the presence of seizures. Measures can be taken which help the handicapped person to compensate for these deficiencies. This becomes a primary consideration in functional diagnosis and in guiding the parents or guardians.

The least severely retarded individual (IQ of 50 to 70) grows and develops in many ways not different from normal ones, and he or she can be taught useful occupational skills. A few of these persons can work under careful supervision. All scholastic pursuits are relatively unsuccessful, and vocational training is of more value than other types of education.

SPECIAL VARIETIES OF MENTAL RETARDATION Several of the special types of mental retardation are discussed in other chapters (see "Lipidoses and Cerebral Sclerosis," in Chap. 373). In the following pages are presented only those with special features likely to be seen in adults.

Down's syndrome (mongolism) This is a unique condition, and, although accounting for only about 1 percent of all mental defectives, it is the reason for nearly one-third of the admissions to state schools for the mentally retarded. The degree of mental retardation varies from mild to severe and is associated with a curious facial configuration and a dwarfed physical stature. Many stigmata of Down's syndrome can be recognized in the neonatal period. The head tends to be small and oval, with sloping forehead. The ears are set low and are oval, with small lobules. The eyes slant slightly upward and outward owing to the presence of a medial epicanthal fold, which partly covers the angle of the palpebral fissure. The bridge of the nose is generally absent or poorly developed. The mouth tends to hang open, and the tongue is usually enlarged, heavily fissured, and protruding. Gray-white specks of depigmentation are seen in the iris (Brushfield's spots). The little fingers are often short and curved inward (clinodactyly), owing to a hypoplastic middle phalanx. The hands are broad and simian-like, with a single transverse palmar crease. A number of other characteristic dermal markings are noted in fingers and toes. Lenticular

opacities and congenital heart lesions (septal defects) are found in some cases. At birth these children are of average size, but at later periods of life they are characteristically small. The average adult person with Down's syndrome never exceeds the stature of a 10-year-old child.

Aside from having a rather rounded shape, which conforms to that of the skull, a subnormal weight, and a relatively simple convolutional pattern, with particular smallness of the frontal lobes and superior temporal convolutions, the brain shows no specific abnormalities.

The mortality rate is high in the first years of life, death usually being due to respiratory infections, interventricular cardiac lesion with failure, or leukemia. Of the patients who survive to puberty, many live to middle adult life and a few then suffer a premature form of Alzheimer's cerebral degeneration (onset in the majority by the age of 40).

Older mothers are more apt to have Down's syndrome babies than are young mothers. The mean age of the mother at the time of birth of these children is 37. Trisomy of chromosome 21 or translocation of parts of this chromosome has been found (also by amniocentesis) with Down's syndrome and is responsible for the disorder.

Cretinism This is due to congenital deficiency of thyroid secretion and is distinguished from myxedema, a form of hypothyroidism acquired later in life (see Chap. 335).

Gargoylism (Hunter-Hurler disease) This condition is discussed in Chap. 89.

Phenylketonuria (phenylpyruvic oligophrenia) This condition is discussed in Chap. 89.

Galactosemia Another congenital metabolic disease, galactosemia is transmitted by a single, autosomal recessive gene. It is characterized clinically by mental defect, cataract, nausea, vomiting, hepatomegaly, jaundice, and the excretion of large quantities of galactose in the urine (Chap. 98).

Autism Autism is a mysterious and provocative condition identified in young children. Long considered primarily psychiatric, it is now generally thought to represent an organic defect in brain development. It is characterized by failure of children to develop communicative language or any form of social communication. By contrast, they often show motor and other skills far beyond what is to be expected of a mentally retarded person. Often they are obsessively preoccupied with inanimate objects, such as lights, running water, or spinning objects. Most of the youngsters prove later to be retarded, and the ultimate prognosis depends largely on the child's IQ. Some few gradually acquire language and may then exhibit certain exceptional talents, such as in mathematics. Upon reaching adult life they are found to retain all the above characteristics. Not more than 1 in 30 will seem to have made any progress. Imprecision of diagnosis allows the inclusion of other brain diseases under the rubric of autism. The patients at a later age do not resemble schizophrenics, despite claims that autism is an unusually precocious form of schizophrenia. No biochemical abnormality has been discovered. Brain volume appears to be normal by contrast studies and gross examination, but few detailed histopathologic studies have been made. Pneumoencephalographic studies show that some children with features of autism have left-sided medial temporal lobe atrophic lesions. This finding is consistent with our understanding of the role of the medial temporal lobes in mediating language affective, motivational, and social behavioral functions in man. It is also consistent with the finding that up to 30 percent of autistic children eventually manifest temporal lobe epilepsy. There is no therapy for this condition.

Simple mental retardation Although presented last, this category includes the great number of cases of defective mentality of indeterminate etiology in which neither somatic nor neurologic abnormality is exhibited. The degree of mental impairment tends to be mild (moron, educable) or moderate (imbecile, trainable). Penrose found that this group of retardates constituted 25 percent of 1280 institutionalized individuals, and of course those who are in institutions represent only the more severely damaged individuals in our society. Their physical appearance is usually not strikingly abnormal; yet many of the aforementioned characteristics of the mentally retarded individual are to be observed. Seizures occur in a significant number, being several times more frequent than in a normal population. Within the limits of their intelligence, the success of these individuals in learning to look after themselves is often determined by how effectively their parents and teachers have inculcated or reinforced good work habits and stable personality traits. The brighter ones can profit to some extent from formal education. Those less well endowed may be trained to care for their personal wants and needs and may profit from a limited amount of manual training. Special schools and classes are of great help. Later in life supervised work situations are possible solutions to their occupational needs.

Society, in the final analysis, determines the eventual disposition of these unfortunates. Many of them, being not unattractive and giving less trouble than many other defective persons, are able to adjust to foster families and live in a community. They need protection, for they are easily led astray and may commit infractions of the law, usually of a minor sort. Institutionalization is required when family and society cannot or do not wish to look after them. Reproductivity is frequently impaired in those with severe mental defects but may be distressingly undisturbed in many of the less defective individuals.

The problem of eugenics assumes great importance. This type of mental defect is often seen in families in which one or both of the parents are dull or retarded. The term *familial* may be applied to this group. However, the majority of cases are sporadic. Probably multiple etiologic factors may lead to simple mental retardation. The pathologic change is variable, ranging from "no demonstrable lesion" to several different gross and microscopic abnormalities.

EPILEPSY

The majority of adult patients with recurrent seizures acquire the tendency toward seizures during childhood. They represent the sequelae of disease processes which may have begun and ended in the distant past. In early life the pattern of the seizures varies widely, depending in part on the level of maturation of the nervous system. Certain types such as fragmented neonatal seizures, infantile spasms, photic epilepsy, febrile seizures, etc., are peculiar to the earlier periods of life. Others, such as petit mal, grand mal, and psychomotor, are identical in child and adult. The latter types are discussed in Chap. 23.

REFERENCES

ADAMS RD: Neurocutaneous disease, in *Dermatology in General Medicine*, 2d ed, TB Fitzpatrick et al (eds). New York, McGraw-Hill, 1979

COOPER IS: *Involuntary Movement Disorders*. New York, Hoeber-Harper, 1969

HOLMES LB et al: Mental retardation, in *An Atlas of Diseases with Associated Physical Abnormalities*. New York, Macmillan, 1972

SALAM M, ADAMS RD: Arnold-Chiari malformation, in *Handbook of Clinical Neurology*. Amsterdam, North-Holland, 1978

SEDGEWICK RP, BODER E: Ataxia telangiectasia, in *Handbook of Clinical Neurology*, vol 14. Amsterdam, North-Holland, 1972, pp 267-334

375
DISEASES OF THE SPINAL CORD

RAYMOND D. ADAMS
FUAD SABRA

Diseases of the nervous system may at times limit themselves to the spinal cord and also produce a number of distinctive syndromes. This relates to special anatomic features such as great length in proportion to width, peripheral location of medullated fibers next to the pia, tight envelopment by meninges, arrangement of blood vessels, and relationship to vertebrae. Because of the frequency and gravity of these diseases, and the special difficulties attendant upon diagnosis, we have grouped them in a special chapter under a series of relatively common syndromes, the basis of which will be better understood after reading Chaps. 15 and 19.

GLOBAL PARALYSIS OF LEGS OR ALL EXTREMITIES DUE TO MASSIVE TRANSVERSE LESION OF THE SPINAL CORD

This condition may best be considered in relation to trauma, one of the most frequent causes of it, but it also occurs with certain types of myelitis, infarction, and hemorrhage in the spinal cord, and rapidly advancing compressive myelopathy.

INJURIES TO THE SPINE AND SPINAL CORD Although injuries to the spinal cord may be the sole manifestation of a traumatic disease, it is seldom that the vertebral column is not harmed at the same time. Often there is an associated head injury, as is pointed out in Chap. 366.

A useful classification of spinal injuries is one which divides them into fracture-dislocations, pure fractures, and pure dislocations. The relative frequency of these types is about 3:1:1. Direct violence to the spine is an uncommon cause of vertebral disruption; except for stab and bullet wounds, most spine injuries are the result of force *applied at a distance*. All three types of injury are produced by a similar mechanism, usually a vertical compression of the spinal column to which flexion is almost immediately added. Or, in the neck the mechanism may be one of extension. The two important variables in the mechanics of vertebral injury are the nature of the bones and joints and the strength, direction, and point of impact of the force.

Strength, direction, and point of impact of the force If the injuring body striking the cranium is hard and the velocity is high, a skull fracture occurs, the elastic quality of the skull absorbing the force of the injury. If the injuring body is soft yet heavy, the spine and particularly its cervical portion will be the part injured. If the neck happens to be rigid and straight and the force is quickly applied to the head, the atlas and the odontoid process of the axis may break. If the force is less quickly applied and removed, an element of flexion occurs. Flexion movements plus a vertical force constitute the essential factors in the majority of fracture-dislocation or pure dislocation.

The other common mechanism of cord injury, sudden extension of the neck, is called the *whiplash injury*. It is especially frequent in civilian motor accidents and in forward falls, and more often it affects supporting structures of the head than spinal nerves or cord. Cervical spondylosis adds to the hazards of spinal injury.

A special type of spine injury, occurring most often in military life, is that in which missiles of high velocity pass through the vertebral canal and destroy the spinal cord. In some cases they may strike the vertebral column without entering the spinal canal and agitate it so violently that the cord suffers injury. The term given to temporary spinal paralysis is *spinal concussion*. This condition may also be produced by violent falls flat on the back.

A study of 2006 cases collected from the literature by Jefferson shows that most vertebral injuries occur at the first to second cervical, fourth to seventh cervical, and eleventh thoracic to second lumbar vertebrae. Industrial accidents most often involve the dorsolumbar vertebrae. Accidents caused by falling or with head down, as in diving accidents, affect the cervical region. In the authors' neuropathologic material, the usual circumstances of spinal injury were a state of alcoholic intoxication and a fall down a flight of stairs, automobile accidents, crushing industrial accidents, gunshot or stab wounds, and birth injury, in that order of frequency. The majority of these fatal cases had fracture-dislocations or dislocations of the cervical spine.

Mechanism of spinal cord injury The spinal cord may escape injury even though there is vertebral dislocation, especially in regions where the spinal canal is large, i.e., in the cervical and lumbar regions. Rarely the spinal cord may be damaged without radiologic evidence of fracture or dislocation. One cannot easily determine the full extent of spinal injury by radiology or even at autopsy because of the difficulty in examining the vertebrae. By far the most satisfactory technique for demonstrating the degree of spine injury and the presence of a tearing of ligaments with dislocation is the x-ray, taken laterally, but one must be careful to avoid full flexion or extension of the neck, for it may inflict further injury to the spinal cord. The most frequently established mechanism is a vertebral dislocation with or without fracture. The upper vertebrae are displaced anteriorly, and there is a break in the posterior longitudinal ligament and the intervertebral disk. The spinal cord is most often subjected to a shearing force between the pedicles of the vertebra above and the body and laminae of the vertebra below the dislocation.

When the cervical spine is sharply extended, especially in the presence of cervical spondylosis, the damage to the spinal cord is due to the sudden narrowing of the spinal canal. The spinal cord is caught between the lamina of the lower vertebra and body of the higher one. Also, the ligamentum flavum may buckle and compress the cord. There may be no x-ray evidence of the spinal lesion. A congenital stenosis or a spondylytic narrowing of the spinal canal also predisposes to this type of injury.

In direct trauma of the spine, as when it is struck in some part by a bullet, the means of spinal concussion is said to be *agitation*. Little is known of the underlying pathology. This term has led to much confusion because it is not employed here in the usual sense of cerebral concussion, i.e., a transient interruption of neural function by trauma without proved structural change.

Pathology of spinal cord injury As a result of squeezing or shearing of the cord, there is destruction of gray matter and a variable amount of hemorrhage, chiefly in the more vascular parts. These changes are maximal at the level of injury and one or two segments above and below it. Rarely is the cord cut in two, and seldom is the pia-arachnoid lacerated. The condition is best designated as *traumatic necrosis of the spinal cord*. As the lesion heals, cavitation or a gliotic focus results. Months or years later a diverticulation of the central canal into the cavity may result in a traumatic syringomyelia. Attempts to distinguish such pathologic entities as hematomyelia, concussion, contusion, and hematorrhachis are of little value either clinically or pathologically.

As with most lesions, the total disease picture includes an irreversible structural lesion and a disorder of function, each of which may vary in degree. The extent and permanence of the clinical manifestations are determined by the relative proportions of these two. An exception to this statement might be made for gunshot wounds of the vertebrae. Here the explosive force of the missile may shatter myelinated fibers with maximal functional disturbance.

CLINICAL EFFECTS OF SPINAL CORD INJURY The "classic" description of traumatic paraplegia by Riddock cannot be excelled. He divides the clinical picture into two stages: spinal shock and reflex activity.

Spinal shock or muscular flaccidity The loss of function which is inflicted at the time of injury (fourth to fifth cervical vertebrae—quadriplegia, thoracic vertebrae—paraplegia, both with paralysis of bladder and bowel sphincters and loss of sensibility below the level corresponding to the spinal lesion) is accompanied by a complete or almost complete suppression of reflex activity of all spinal segments below the lesion. This is the condition known as *spinal shock*. The plantar reflexes are first variable and may be absent, flexor, or extensor. The lower extremities lose heat if left uncovered and swell if dependent. Sweating is abolished. Cutaneous ulcerations may develop over bony prominences. Urine and feces are retained to the point where overflow and involuntary leakage results. Occasionally there is priapism because of venous congestion. A paralytic ileus may occur.

Reflex activity If the lumbosacral segments are undamaged, spinal shock wears off in 2 to 3 weeks. The first sign of this is contraction of the hamstrings and flexion or extension of the toes on plantar stimulation. Then gentle and later strong involuntary flexor spasms make their appearance. Ankle jerks and then knee jerks return. Retention of urine and feces becomes less complete, and at irregular intervals urine is expelled by active contraction of the detrusor muscle. Reflex defecation and sweating also appear. At times flexor spasms and later extensor spasms, often accompanied by profuse sweating and micturition, all occur after stimulation of the skin, viz., the *mass reflex*. This stage of reflex activity may last for years, unless sepsis intervenes, in which case the state of spinal shock may return.

Less complete lesions of the spinal cord may result in little or no spinal shock or extensor spasm. Incomplete voluntary motor paralysis, a flaccid atrophic paralysis, variable sensory impairment in the arms, a spastic weakness of the legs, and a partial or complete Brown-Sequard syndrome are some of the resulting clinical pictures.

The end stage may be permanent and complete disability, rarely consistent with survival for more than a short time (days, weeks, months); or a gradual improvement and complete or almost complete recovery may occur. Any residual symptoms after 6 months are likely to be permanent.

The level of the cord lesion can be determined by the clinical picture. A complete paralysis of arms and legs usually indicates a dislocation at the fourth to fifth cervical vertebrae. If the legs are paralyzed and the arms can still be abducted and flexed, the dislocation is likely to be at the fifth to sixth cervical. Paralysis only of hands and of legs indicates the level of vertebral disorder to be the sixth to seventh cervical. When the motor paralysis involves muscles above the knees and sensory loss includes the twelfth thoracic dermatone, the site is the eleventh to twelfth thoracic. If the paralysis is below the knees and the first lumbar escapes, the lesion is at the twelfth thoracic, first lumbar vertebrae. Prognosis for the latter group of patients, with preponderantly cauda equina lesions, is better than for those with injury to the eleventh to twelfth thoracic vertebrae. In all cases of spinal cord injury any elicitable movement or preserved sensation during the first 48 to 72 h gives a favorable prognosis for recovery.

Treatment In general, the treatment for spinal cord injuries is conservative and symptomatic. The degree of injury can be lessened by ensuring that no movement of cervical spine (especially flexion) is made from the moment of the accident. Corticosteroid therapy, as for brain swelling (Chap. 367), may reduce the swelling of spinal cord tissue. If the spinal cord injury is associated with dislocation of the vertebrae, traction on the neck is necessary to secure proper alignment. This is accomplished by a head halter attached through the head of the bed over a pulley to a weight of 10 to 15 lb or, even better, the use of tongs which fasten onto the skull (Crutchfield). In thoracic crush injuries, hyperextension can be maintained by placing a narrow pillow under the affected area. Traction should be continued for 4 to 6 weeks, and then a brace may be substituted. In some centers for the treatment of spinal cord injury early fixation and traction of spine have almost completely replaced decompression by laminectomy.

The aftercare of patients with paraplegia and disturbance of vesical or rectal functions is similar to that of patients with like symptoms from other causes. Decubitus ulceration can be prevented by special skin care. Intermittent drainage is of value in preventing infection, stone formation, and contracture and in securing return of function. Daily enemas are usually the most effective means of controlling fecal incontinence. Physiotherapy, muscle reeducation, and the application of proper braces are all important in the rehabilitation of the patient. All this is best carried out in centers for rehabilitation of spine injuries. Although one hopes that the paraplegic patient will eventually walk, using caliper braces, a more realistic objective is ambulation in a wheelchair.

MYELITIS The spinal cord appears to be vulnerable to three types of inflammatory processes, all of which have been called *myelitic*. First there are the specific viral infections which tend to involve principally the gray matter (hence called *poliomyelitic*). Zoster and the three viruses of poliomyelitis are the most frequent causes of this type. Secondly, all the subacute and chronic primary meningeal infections may induce damage of the spinal roots and outer surfaces of the spinal cord, i.e., to the white matter of posterior, lateral, and anterior funiculi (meningoradiculitis and meningomyelitis), or there may be occlusion of meningeal vessels. Syphilis offers the best known and most numerous examples of this category of inflammatory disease, viz., tabes dorsalis (which is essentially a treponemal lumbosacral meningoradiculitis), syphilitic meningomyelitis, and arteritis with myelomalacia. Tuberculous meningitis and fungous meningitis provide other examples. Thirdly, there is a

group of primary inflammations of white matter, the leukomyelitides. Most of the leukomyelitides are of unknown cause. Three varieties of the latter have been delineated: (1) postinfectious and postvaccinial myelitis, (2) demyelinative myelitis (acute or chronic relapsing multiple sclerosis), and (3) acute or subacute necrotizing myelitis. Although the white (and gray) matter may be the site of an infective inflammatory process as in abscess, tuberculoma, gumma and parasitic inflammations, and particularly schistosomiasis (in thoracolumbar segments), such conditions are rare.

Whereas any one of the above forms of chronic meningitis or leukomyelitis may induce the clinical picture of a transverse cord lesion, this lesion is usually due to one of the demyelinative or necrotizing forms of myelitis. A painless (rarely painful) paraplegia, beginning simultaneously in both legs, or more often first in one leg and then the other, or in sacral segments, ascends to the abdomen and thorax. Either sensory or motor symptoms may initiate the disease, but both are present as it progresses. Like all cord lesions with involvement of tracts, the loss of sensory and motor function affects all parts of the body below a certain level, sphincters as well, and, if acute, overflow incontinence and obstipation are included. In only a few patients will vaccination against smallpox, rabies inoculation, or a frank chickenpox or measles be found to have preceded the neurologic symptoms by days to 1 to 2 weeks; in all the rest, the illness develops without explanation. The conjunction of retrobulbar neuritis with the cord lesion is called *neuromyelitis optica* or *Devic's disease*. This is not a disease but a syndrome occurring in necrotizing myelitis (usual cause), multiple sclerosis, and postinfectious myelitis. If the spinal cord lesion is severe and paralysis is complete, spinal shock supervenes, with the same flaccidity and areflexia of legs described under spinal cord trauma (above). The cerebrospinal fluid (CSF) may be normal or may contain lymphocytes and mononuclear leukocytes (numbering from 20 to 1000 or more per milliliter), and the protein is sometimes raised. If the cord lesion swells, as it rarely does, there may be a dynamic block (positive Queckenstedt test). When the latter is found, it always suggests the possibility of a *spinal epidural abscess*, another important and treatable cause of a rapidly developing transverse cord lesion with spine ache and fever. Subacute necrotizing myelitis is a less well-defined condition in which a succession of obscure inflammatory (?) vascular lesions convert a state of spastic paraplegia with sensory loss to a flaccid one (as the lower parts of the spinal cord are involved). Of passing interest is the observation in some forms of myelitis (postzoster, idiopathic) of a spinal, focal segmental myoclonus resembling restricted myoclonus of cerebral origin (see Hoehn and Cherington). It may indicate the level of a motor or sensory tract lesion.

Treatment of the demyelinative and necrotizing myelitides consists of ACTH (40 units twice a day for a week, then once a day for 2 to 3 weeks) or prednisone (60 mg per day for 3 weeks). Improvement usually occurs, but the relation to therapy is uncertain. Except for patients with the postinfectious form of myelitis there is always danger of later progression or relapse. Prevention of decubitus ulceration, early catheterization and bladder care, and rehabilitation measures, the usual procedures in the management of the paraplegia patients, must also be employed.

SPINAL EPIDURAL ABSCESS Children or adults may be affected. An injury to the back, often trivial, at the time of a furunculosis or other skin infection or a bacteremia may permit seeding of the spinal epidural space or of vertebral body. The latter gives rise to osteomyelitis with extension to the epidural space. The suppurative process is accompanied at first only by fever and aching in the region of the spine and later by radicular pain. After several days or a few weeks there is a rapid onset and progression of paraplegia, sensory loss in the lower parts of the body, urinary and fecal retention, and sphincteric incontinence. Percussion of the spine elicits tenderness over the site of the infection. Examination reveals all the signs of transverse cord lesion with spinal shock. The CSF contains small numbers of cells (neutrophilic leukocytes and lymphocytes), and the protein is relatively high (100 to 400 mg/ml). More importantly there is a dynamic block (positive Queckenstedt test). If not treated surgically by laminectomy and drainage at the earliest possible moment, the spinal cord lesion, which is due in part to ischemia (compression mainly of veins), becomes irreversible. Emergency myelography must be used to determine the level of block and the operative site. At an early stage bone scan is more revealing of an early osteomyelitis of the spine than plain x-rays. Antibiotic therapy must also be given.

Another circumstance in which an acute spinal epidural abscess may develop is in a patient with some combination of chronic medical diseases in which a septicemia occurs. Here the symptoms of spine disease may be minimal until the onset of the spinal cord lesion some weeks later. Staphylococci or some other organism may reach the epidural or subdural spinal space via a lumbar puncture needle during epidural anesthesia or a laminectomy. The localization is then over lumbar and sacral roots. Pain may be severe and neurologic symptomatology minimal.

Subacute pyogenic infections and granulomatous infections (tubercular, fungal) may also arise in the spinal epidural space causing symptoms and signs of disorder of spinal tracts at the level of the lesion. The clinical picture is less dramatic, and the diagnosis depends on the demonstration, in a patient with weakness and/or sensory loss or ataxia of the legs, of a partial or complete block by contrast myelography. Bone scans are helpful when there is concomitant vertebral infection. The treatment depends on the nature of the underlying disease and the general condition of the patient (see Chap. 368).

INFARCTION OF SPINAL CORD (MYELOMALACIA) AND HEMORRHAGE (HEMATOMYELIA) Unlike the brain, the spinal cord is rarely the site of vascular disease. The spinal arteries are not susceptible to atherosclerosis, and emboli rarely lodge here. As was stated in relation to chronic meningeal infections, an endarteritis of surface arteries may lead to thrombosis with devastating ischemic necrosis of the spinal cord. Polyarteritis nodosa may have a similar effect though the localization in the nervous system in this disease is usually peripheral. Atherosclerotic thrombosis of the aorta or dissecting aortic aneurysms may cause myelomalacia by occluding nutrient arteries at cervical, thoracic, or lumbar levels. Paralysis during cardiac surgery requiring clamping of the aorta for more than 30 min and vertebrobasilar (thyrocervical branch) and aortic arteriography may result in the syndrome. Infarction of the gray matter of the upper cervical cord segments may follow vertebral angiography. Sudden development of symptoms referable to lesions of spinal tracts (sensory or motor or both) always bespeaks an infarctive or hemorrhagic vascular lesion of the spinal cord. The onset of symptoms in such cases is more rapid than in the myelitides.

Hemorrhage into the spinal cord is rare. Aside from the aforementioned traumatic variety of hematomyelia, it is usually traceable to a vascular malformation or a hematologic disease including anticoagulant therapy. Epidural hemor-

rhages with spinal cord compression may occur with hematologic disorders and anticoagulant therapy. The latter requires vitamin K therapy and immediate surgical decompression.

SUBACUTE OR CHRONIC SPINAL SYNDROMES

These take several forms for the reason that the responsible diseases have a variety of different localizations in the tracts and gray matter. Most of the remaining diseases of the spinal cord may be grouped around the following syndromes.

SPASTIC ATAXIC PARAPARESIS The gradual development of ataxia and weakness of the legs is the common manifestation of several diseases. In late childhood or adolescence a syndrome of this type which begins insidiously and progresses steadily over a period of years usually indicates the existence of Friedreich's ataxia or some other type of spinocerebellar degeneration. In early adult life multiple sclerosis, syphilitic meningomyelitis, and chronic adhesive spinal arachnoiditis are the more frequent causes of it. And in middle and late years of life late deteriorative forms of spinal multiple sclerosis and cervical spondylosis are the most frequent causes, followed by syringomyelia, and subacute systemic disease.

CERVICAL SPONDYLOSIS The cervical intervertebral disks degenerate to some degree in the majority of individuals by the sixth and seventh decades of life. This results in narrowing of the disks, especially in the most mobile parts of the cervical spine (fourth to fifth cervical, fifth to sixth cervical, sixth to seventh cervical, and seventh cervical to first thoracic segments) and spur formation on the margins of the adjacent vertebrae. There are anterior beaking and posterior osteophytes which protrude centrally with narrowing of the spinal canal or laterally so as to impinge on spinal roots in the intervertebral canals. This condition is incorrectly called *hypertrophic arthritis,* but there is no consistent association with arthritis of this type in other joints. The more appropriate term *cervical spondylosis* refers to a wear and tear (traumatic?) phenomenon.

The clinical symptomatology is variable. When a group of asymptomatic patients beyond fifty years is surveyed, a few will be found to have slight limitation in neck motions, mild pain in shoulders or an arm, a history of questionable cervical-disk disease in the past, and sometimes a diminution of an arm reflex or a numb finger or two. A few even have had an unexpected Babinski sign on one side.

Abrupt onset of an arm pain, numbness of one side of a hand or two or three fingers, and a diminished reflex, a not-infrequent clinical state in middle and late adult life, are attributed to osteophytic impingement on a root. But the pathology of such nerve lesions is uncertain. Rest with traction often relieves the symptoms while the osteophyte obviously remains. No ruptured disk is seen in the cervical myelogram. Such conditions must be distinguished from brachial neuritis (plexitis), ruptured cervical disk, and costoclavicular and carpal tunnel syndromes.

Central posterior spurring with or without congenital narrowing of the spinal canal and hypertrophy of ligamentum flavum can compress the spinal cord. In lateral x-rays one can see that the canal in its anteroposterior dimension is reduced to 10 to 11 mm. The column of contrast medium in the myelogram is obstructed, and in an air myelogram with laminography the compression of spinal cord is visualized. The clinical syndrome consists of a spastic weakness of legs (often one more than the other) and posterior column signs (impaired vibratory and position senses and ataxia). Other long-tract sensory changes are less frequent. Slight sensory, motor, and reflex changes are usually found in one or both hands and arms. A lesion at the fourth to fifth cervical segments may result in an increase in all tendon reflexes, particularly finger jerks; a lesion at the fifth to sixth cervical segments may diminish biceps reflexes leaving triceps and finger jerks hyperactive; a lesion at the sixth to seventh cervical segments diminishes the triceps reflexes on one or both sides. The onset of symptoms is insidious and the course slowly or intermittently progressive over several years.

Immobilization of the head with a cervical collar has stopped the progression of symptoms in some cases. Laminectomy, posterior if several interspaces are involved and anterior if only one or two, has resulted in improvement in the majority of patients and has halted the progression in others.

In the elderly the differential diagnosis of cervical spondylosis, cervical disk herniation, diabetic neuropathy, and pernicious anemia with myelopathy, in combination with age changes in lumbosacral nerves, represents one of the most vexing of all neurologic problems. Since several of these conditions are conjoined, the physician can separate their effects only by meticulous clinical examination and appropriate laboratory tests.

RHEUMATOID ARTHRITIS WITH VERTEBRAL SUBLUXATION
In this form of arthritis of the spine destruction of ligamentous structures adjacent to affected joints may permit a subluxation with spinal cord compression. Spastic weakness of the legs and sphincteric incontinence are combined with sensory loss and areflexia in arms and variable ataxia and other signs of posterior column disease in lower parts of the body. Lateral x-rays of the cervical spine show the subluxation. Traction and fusion of the cervical spine are necessary to correct the condition (see Hughes).

MULTIPLE SCLEROSIS Probably an ataxic paraparesis ranks as the most common manifestation of an established form of multiple sclerosis. Asymmetric involvement of limbs and signs of cerebral, optic nerve, brainstem, and cerebellar manifestations provide important information for the diagnosis of this disease, but unfortunately they are not always involved. Often the patient presents with late onset of symptoms (age 50 to 65) of slow progression. In the study of such cases diagnosis depends on (1) evidence of earlier attacks of disease (not always remembered); (2) evidence of delayed retinocortical conduction of patterned stimuli, showing that optic nerves have been damaged; and (3) increased gamma globulin in the CSF. Often a cervical myelogram is necessary to rule out spondylosis or tumor. Purely spinal involvement may occur, no lesions being found outside the spinal cord even at autopsy. See Chap. 370 for further details.

FRIEDREICH'S ATAXIA This classic form of hereditary ataxia, first clearly depicted by Nikolaus Friedreich of Heidelberg in 1863, constitutes a relatively distinct symptom complex which generally runs true to form, although it overlaps other heredodegenerative syndromes, particularly the spinocerebellar atrophies, chronic familial polyneuropathies, and progressive optic atrophy (discussed in Chaps. 373 and 376). In some families, the disorder occurs with dominant inheritance; usually it is a recessive trait.

Clinical aspects As with other progressive ataxias, the disorder first appears in the legs, affecting the individual during late childhood. The patient, previously healthy, begins to stagger and lurch in walking and is unsteady on standing, often in a tremulous fashion. Clumsiness and intention tremor of the hands and arms appear later along with faulty articulation and abnormal rhythm (scanning) of speech. These symptoms usually result from changes in the cerebellum; the spinocerebellar tracts are also affected, but it is not known whether they contribute to the ataxia. The limbs, in addition to being ataxic, generally show considerable weakness. Examination usually

discloses nystagmus and skeletal deformities: kyphoscoliosis, the basis of which is not certain, and a peculiar foreshortening and high arching of the feet (pes cavus) with cocking of the toes (sometimes called the "Friedreich foot" and best ascribed to atrophy and contractures of the musculature of the feet at a time when the bones of the feet are malleable). Typically, there is the unusual combination of total absence of tendon reflexes with extensor plantar reflexes (Babinski sign). This results from the presence of degeneration of pyramidal tracts together with a mild affection of peripheral sensory neurons and degeneration of the posterior columns. The presence of the latter is further indicated by impairment of position and vibration sense in the extremities and, in some patients, of the sensations of pain, temperature, and light touch in a distal and roughly symmetric distribution. Mentation is usually preserved, though a few of the patients have been of low intelligence or have become demented late in the course of the disease. Survival beyond early adult life is rare, with death frequently the result of associated myocardiopathy.

Occasionally very mild or fragmentary forms of the disorder (such as pes cavus and absent or hyperactive tendon reflexes) may be encountered with little if any disability or progression. Such abnormalities are most likely to be seen in other members of the family of a patient afflicted with the fully developed form of the disease.

Pathology The principal changes in the spinal cord, cerebellum, and dorsal root ganglia are typical of a chronic degenerative process. In addition to the neuropathologic changes there is in some cases a peculiar form of myocardial degeneration resulting in fiber loss and fibrosis. There are no other associated visceral lesions.

Differential diagnosis The classic form of Friedreich's ataxia is readily recognizable and cannot easily be confused with other conditions. It is to be expected, however, that variations in the clinical manifestations may occur because of the variable pathologic changes. Chronic familial polyneuropathies are particularly difficult to distinguish since they also give rise to sensory ataxia, but signs of pyramidal tract disease are absent (see Chap. 377). Hereditary forms of cerebellar ataxia with pyramidal signs (hyperactive tendon reflexes) and sensory disturbances are also known to occur in the adolescent or adult. Familial spastic paraplegia with or without optic atrophy (Behr's syndrome) is another closely related disease. In the absence of a family history, and with atypical clinical findings, further diagnostic studies to exclude tumor, chronic basal meningitis, intoxication, or congenital malformation will be necessary.

No treatment is of proven value. A recent finding of disturbed pyruvate metabolism might suggest a trial of vitamin B therapy. Physical medicine and rehabilitation measures are of little value in cerebellar ataxia.

SYPHILITIC MENINGOMYELITIS Here as in multiple sclerosis the degree of alteration of vibratory and position sense and ataxia is variable. Some patients with primary lateral sclerosis, such as Erb described, have almost pure pyramidal spasticity and weakness of the legs requiring differentiation from motor system disease and familial spastic paraplegia. In others sensory ataxia and posterior column signs predominate. The confirmation of diagnosis depends on the finding of a positive Wassermann reaction in the CSF, but a late and advancing form of the disease may appear with a negative CSF in a known syphilitic patient. See Chap. 146 for a discussion of pathology and treatment.

SUBACUTE COMBINED DEGENERATION OF SPINAL CORD AND BRAIN DUE TO VITAMIN B₁₂ DEFICIENCY AND SYNDROME OF NUTRITIONAL COMBINED SYSTEM DISEASE (STRACHAN SYNDROME)

These two forms of the more treatable diseases of the spinal cord are fully described in Chap. 372.

Progressive spastic or spastic-ataxic paraparesis may also develop in conjunction with hepatic decompensation.

SPASTIC PARAPARESIS WITH OR WITHOUT CERVICOBRACHIAL AMYOTROPHY

Although a few such cases are traced to multiple sclerosis, syringomyelia, cervical pachymeningitis, or cervical meningomyelitis, the purely motor syndrome is nearly always traceable to primary lateral sclerosis, possibly a variant of amyotrophic lateral sclerosis. Paralysis, atrophy, and fascicular twitching of hands and arms are joined with spastic weakness and hyperreflexia in legs with Babinski signs (see Chap. 373). Cervical spondylosis and high cervical tumors must also be considered in the differential diagnosis. Pure spastic paraparesis may occur in multiple sclerosis, spondylosis, liver failure, hereditary spastic paraplegia with or without dementia, and one form of hereditary adrenoleukodystrophy.

SEGMENTAL SENSORY DISSOCIATION WITH BRACHIAL MUSCULAR ATROPHY (SYRINGOMYELIC SYNDROME)

This syndrome is most often ascribable to a syringomyelia, but examples have been found in patients with intramedullary cord tumors, delayed traumatic myelopathy, postradiation myelopathy, syphilitic cervical pachymeningitis, cervical spondylosis, extramedullary tumors of the high cervical canal, and foramen magnum, and necrotizing myelitis.

SYRINGOMYELIA This is a term that refers to a cavity (from the Greek *syrinx*, meaning "pipe" or "tube"). The cavity occupies the central parts of the spinal cord in the cervical region but may extend upward into the medulla oblongata (syringobulbia) or downward into the thoracic or even lumbar segments. In approximately 15 percent of cases studied postmortem, an intramedullary tumor (hemangioblastoma or glioma) has been found in or near some part of the syrinx. The syrinx is independent of, but connected with, the central canal, replaces the gray matter of the posterior or anterior horns of the spinal cord, and interrupts the crossing pain and temperature fibers in the anterior commissure in several successive cord segments. The cavity is lined with astrocytic glia and a few thick-walled blood vessels. It may enlarge the spinal cord and even widen the spinal canal. The cerebrospinal fluid in the cavity always has a relatively low protein level unless a tumor is present. The cause is unknown, but it is clearly linked to malformations at the craniocervical junction. Familial incidence is rare. A blastomatous formation akin to tuberous sclerosis or central von Recklinghausen's disease but with a tendency for the abnormal tissue to cavitate is one explanation. A hydromyelia, sometimes associated with hydrocephalus in early life and diverticulation, appears more plausible. Elevated pressure of cerebrospinal fluid within the spinal canal may not only widen it, but, with continuous movement and possible injury of cervical segments of the spinal cord, may dissect into zones of pressure necrosis, leading to the formation of diverticulae.

The clinical triad upon which the diagnosis is based consists of (1) segmental sensory loss or dissociation (loss of pain and temperature sense and preservation of sense of touch) over neck, shoulders, and arms, (2) amyotrophy, and (3) thoracic scoliosis. Symptoms may begin in late childhood and adolescence, but more often in adult life, and progress irregularly, often being arrested for long periods of time. The segmental sensory loss or dissociation and amyotrophy are caused by cavitation, destruction, and stretching of the ventral commissural fibers and the anterior and posterior horns, respectively. Analgesia and thermoanesthesia account for painless ulcers, injuries, and burns; Charcot joints, also common in this disease, result from repeated injury of the denervated joint tissue. Areflexia without atrophy may be due to involvement of the afferent as well as efferent limbs of the reflex arc, but destruction of anterior horn cells is the more frequent cause, particularly if accompanied by muscle atrophy. A useful clinical rule is that a neurologic disease which leaves all deep tendon reflexes in the arms intact is probably not syringomyelia. Horner's syndrome on the affected side may result from involvement of cells of the intermediolateral cell column of the eighth cervical to first thoracic segments of the spinal cord. Pyramidal tract signs in the legs tend to appear late in the course of the disease and are attributable to extension of the syrinx into the lateral columns of the cord or into the decussation of corticospinal tracts. If the cavity enlarges the spinal cord, a spinal subarachnoid block may result, and prolonged pressure may cause widening of the spinal canal and erosion of pedicles. The kyphoscoliosis, which may antedate other evidence of disease by several years, is thought to result from asymmetric weakness of paravertebral muscles. Short neck and dysplastic features are related to congenital abnormalities of the spine and base of skull.

A syrinx in the brainstem (syringobulbia) usually extends into the lateral tegmentum of the medulla, being so placed as to result in nystagmus and sensory impairment over one or both sides of the face. Unilateral palatal and vocal cord paralysis, as well as weakness and atrophy of one side of the tongue, are other clinical signs which call attention to lesions at this level of the neuraxis. Syringobulbia never occurs without syringomyelia.

The association of cavitation of the spinal cord with myelomeningocele (so-called "myelodysplasia"), Arnold-Chiari malformation, platybasia, and other congenital defects about the cervicocranial junction is commented on in Chap. 374.

The treatment of syringomyelia is unsatisfactory. The fact that the disease process may remain stationary for some months or years before progressing makes evaluation of any mode of therapy difficult. Decompression of a distended syrinx up to the foramen magnum may alleviate temporarily those symptoms and signs resulting from local compression of ascending and descending spinal tracts, but relief is seldom lasting. Reducing the pressure within the cavity by occluding the upper end of the central canal, opening it, or making a ventriculosubarachnoid shunt has given unpredictable results. X-ray treatment, based on the belief that symptoms result from gliomatous malformation of the cord which subsequently cavitates, is probably worthless, unless there is an underlying tumor.

OTHER SYNDROMES CAUSING ASYMMETRIC WEAKNESS OF LEGS, SENSORY LOSS (ATAXIA), AND SPHINCTERIC DISTURBANCES

Here a miscellany of diseases (vascular malformations, chronic adhesive arachnoiditis following spinal anesthesia, and infections and metabolic and nutritional diseases, etc.) would have to be considered, but only spinal cord tumor will be discussed.

SPINAL CORD TUMORS Growth and other space-occupying lesions within the spinal canal can be conveniently divided into two groups: (1) those which arise within the substance of the spinal cord and invade and destroy tracts and central gray structures (intramedullary) and (2) those outside the spinal cord (extramedullary), either in the vertebral bodies and epidural tissues (extradural), or in the meninges, or roots (intradural). The relative frequency of spinal tumors in these different locations in a general hospital is about 5 percent intramedullary, 40 percent intradural-extramedullary, and 55 percent extradural. The percentage of extradural lesions in a general hospital population is usually higher than in most neurosurgical services (e.g., Elsberg's figures of 10, 67, and 16 percent, respectively), which often do not include many of the lymphomas, metastatic carcinomas, etc., most of which are extradural.

The cellular origin of the intramedullary gliomas has been mentioned in the section on intracerebral tumors. The proportions of the different cell types differ, however. Ependymoma makes up 40 percent of the cases, and the remainder are more or less evenly distributed among astrocytomas, glioblastomas, and hemangiomas, and hemangioblastomas. The hemangioma is the common source of spontaneous hematomyelia, and the hemangioblastoma may give rise to a syringomyelia.

Symptomatology Patients with spinal cord tumor are likely to manifest one of two clinical pictures: either a purely sensorimotor spinal tract and rarely a syringomyelic syndrome or a radicular-spinal syndrome, nearly always painful.

Compression of sensorimotor spinal tracts The predominant clinical syndrome relates to spinal cord compression. With intraspinal tumors, the onset of the compressive symptoms is usually gradual over a period of weeks and months, and the course is progressive. The initial disturbance is likely to be motor, and often the distribution is asymmetric. With cervical lesions the order of motor impairment is first the arm, then the ipsilateral and contralateral leg, and finally the opposite arm. With thoracic lesions one leg usually becomes weak and stiff before the other one. Subjective sensory symptoms (tingling paresthesias) of spinal tract involvement take the same pattern. Pain and temperature are more likely to be affected than touch, vibration and position senses and are contralateral to the maximum motor weakness (Brown-Séguard syndrome). Nevertheless the posterior columns are also frequently involved. Voluntary control over bladder and bowel usually becomes weakened coincident with motor paralysis of the legs. If the compression is relieved, there is recovery from these sensorimotor symptoms often in the reverse order of their affection. The first part affected is the last to recover, and sensory symptoms disappear before motor.

Compressive-irritative radicular symptoms This syndrome of spinal cord compression is often combined with radicular pain, i.e., pain in the distribution of a spinal root. It is described as knifelike or as merely a dull ache with superimposed sharp pains which are intensified by cough, sneeze, or strain and radiation in a distal direction, i.e., away from the spine. Segmental sensory changes (paresthesias, hyperalgesia, impairment of pain and touch) or motor disturbances (spasm, cramp, twitching, atrophy, fascicular twitching, and loss of tendon reflex) and an ache in the spine are the usual manifestations of a compressive-irritative lesion of roots. Tenderness of spinous processes over the growth is found in half the patients. These segmental changes, particularly the sensory ones, often precede the signs of spinal cord compression by months or years if the lesion is benign. Sphincter disturbances usually appear late.

The clinical findings are (1) spastic weakness of the legs, in one leg more than in the other, with thoracolumbar lesions, and of the arms and legs with cervical lesions, (2) a sensory level for pain on the trunk below which pain sense is reduced or lost, (3) posterior column signs, and (4) a spastic bladder under weak voluntary control.

The diagnosis is established by x-rays of the spine (erosion of vertebrae, widened spinal canal), lumbar puncture, and electromyography to demonstrate the fasciculations and denervation resulting from involvement of motor roots. The most important diagnostic test of all is contrast myelography for the direct visualization of the compressive lesion. Occasionally lumbar puncture may exacerbate the symptoms and signs.

Special spinal syndromes Unusual clinical syndromes may be found in patients with tumors near the foramen magnum. They may produce a quadriparesis with pains in the back of the head and stiff neck, a weakness and atrophy of the hands and dorsal neck muscles, and either bizarre sensory changes or no sensory loss whatsoever. Lesions of the tenth, eleventh, and twelfth thoracic and the first lumbar vertebrae may result in a curious syndrome of mixed cauda equina and spinal cord symptoms. *Lesions of the cauda equina* alone, always difficult to separate from those of the plexus and multiple nerves, are usually attended in the early stages with pain (present in 80 percent of cases, especially at night, and worsened by jolting) which is variously combined with an asymmetric, atrophic, areflexic paralysis, radicular sensory loss, and later sphincteric disorder (see Fearnsides and Adams). This must be distinguished from *tumors of the conus medullaris* (lower sacral segments of spinal cord) in which there are early disturbances of sphincters of the bladder and bowel, back pain, hypesthesia, and anesthesia over the sacral dermatomes, a lax anal sphincter with loss of anal and bulbocavernosus reflexes, and sometimes weakness of gluteal and hamstring muscles. A Babinski sign means that the spinal cord is involved above the fifth lumbar segment. Pain and stiffness of the back may precede signs of spinal cord disease or dominate the clinical picture in some extramedullary tumors. Extravertebral (presacral or pelvic) tumors such as neuroblastomas, rhabdomyosarcomas, carcinomas of cervix or body of uterus, or prostatic carcinomas may simulate the conus medullaris syndrome.

Pathology, anatomy, and physiology Peculiarities of anatomic structure are decisive factors in determining the symptomatology of tumor growths. The structure of the spine is described in Chap. 7, "Pain in the Back and Neck." Epidural growths arise from hematogenous deposits or tumors which extend from the vertebral bodies or from extraspinal spaces through intervertebral foramens.

Intramedullary growths not only invade but also compress and distort fasciculi in the adjacent white matter. As the cord enlarges from the tumor growing within it or is compressed from a tumor growing without, the free space around the cord is consumed and the cerebrospinal fluid below the lesion becomes isolated or loculated from the rest of the so-called "circulating cerebrospinal fluid" above. This can be demonstrated by a positive Queckenstedt test, Froin's syndrome of xanthochromia and clotting of CSF, and interruption of the flow of a contrast medium in the subarachnoid space (myelogram).

Differential diagnosis Several problems may arise in the diagnosis of patients with spinal cord tumors. In the early stages spinal tumor must be distinguished from other diseases which cause pain over certain segments of the body, i.e., those affecting the gallbladder, kidney, stomach and intestinal tract, pleura, etc. Here the localization of the pain to a dermatome, its intensification by effort, segmental sensory changes, and minor alterations of motor, reflex, or sensory function in the legs will usually provide the clues to the compressive-irritative radicular lesion. Examination of the cerebrospinal fluid, x-ray of the spine, bone scan, and myelography will settle the diagnosis in most instances.

If symptoms and signs of disorder of sensory and motor tracts of the spinal cord are present, there is still the problem of locating the segmental level of the lesion. At first the sensory and motor deficiencies may be more pronounced in those parts of the body farthest removed from the lesion, i.e., in feet or lumbosacral segments. Later these sensory and motor levels may ascend, but at any time they may continue to be far below the lesion. Of greatest help in determining the level of the lesion are the locality of the root pains and atrophic paralysis and lastly the upper level of hypalgesia.

Once vertebral and segmental levels are settled, there is still the necessity of determining whether the lesion is neoplastic and extradural, intradural-extramedullary, or intramedullary. This is important from the standpoint of etiologic diagnosis. If there is a visible or palpable spinal deformity, positive bone scan, or x-ray evidence of vertebral destruction, one may confidently assume an extradural localization. Without x-ray changes one still suspects extradural lesion if root pain developed early and is bilateral, spine ache is prominent, and percussion tenderness is marked, if motor symptoms below the lesions precede sensory changes, and sphincter disturbances are late. To distinguish between intradural-extramedullary and intramedullary lesions is almost impossible. Radicular pain, asymmetry of signs of motor and sensory tract involvement, and early cerebrospinal fluid blockage (positive Queckenstedt test and high protein) favor the extramedullary localization. With extradural lesions one must differentiate between ruptures of disk, spondylosis (hypertrophic spurring and osteophyte formation in cervical spinal canal), tuberculous caries, other pyogenic, fungous, and syphilitic granulomatous lesions, secondary carcinoma, and lymphoma. With intradural-extramedullary lesions, meningioma, neurofibroma, meningeal carcinomatosis, cholesteatoma, teratomatous cyst, or meningomyelitic process is most likely. Intramedullary lesions are usually gliomas or vascular malformations. A negative Queckenstedt test, normal or relatively low protein in cerebrospinal fluid, and a negative myelogram will serve to rule out intraspinal tumors or granulomatous lesions in most instances.

Treatment This varies with the nature of the lesion and the clinical condition of the patient. Intradural-extramedullary tumors should be removed. Laminectomy, decompression, sometimes surgical enucleation of tumor, marsupialization of cysts, and x-ray therapy are the treatment of intramedullary gliomas. Extradural malignant growths are best managed by the use of opiates for pain, *x-ray therapy*, endocrine therapy (for carcinoma of breast and prostate), or nitrogen mustard treatment (for certain lymphomas). Sometimes laminectomy and decompression are necessary for diagnosis and prevention of irreversible compressive effects and infarction of the spinal cord. With tuberculous caries, immobilization of the spine in hyperextension and antituberculous therapy are indicated, and laminectomy should be reserved for exceptional cases with complete and irreversible spinal block. For spondylosis, surgery (extradural decompression) is advised if there are serious neurologic deficits. Syndromes of lesser severity or elderly patients with other important diseases may best be treated with a Thomas collar to immobilize the spine.

In conclusion it is always well to remind oneself that of the more than 30 diseases of the spinal cord, there are available effective means of treating only a few—spondylosis, extramedullary spinal cord tumors, syphilis (meningomyelitis and tabes), epidural granulomas (pyogenic, tuberculous, fungous),

subacute combined degeneration, and nutritional myelopathy. The physician's major responsibility is to determine whether the patient has one of the treatable diseases.

INJURIES TO SPINAL ROOTS, PLEXUSES, AND PERIPHERAL NERVES See Chaps. 7 and 377.

REFERENCES

BAKER AS et al: Spinal epidural abscess N Engl J Med 293:463, 1975

ENBERG RN, KAPLAN JR: Spinal epidural abscess in children. Clin Pediatr 13:247, 1974

FEARNSIDES MR, ADAMS CBT: Tumors of cauda equina. J Neurol Neurosurg Psychiatry 41:24, 1978

HOEHN MM, CHERINGTON M: Spinal myoclonus. Neurology 27:942, 1977

HUGHES JT: Spinal cord involvement by C4–5 vertebral subluxation in rheumatoid arthritis. Ann Neurol 1:575, 1977

KUHN WG JR: Care and rehabilitation of patients with injuries to the spinal cord and cauda equina: Preliminary report on 113 cases. J Neurosurg 4:40, 1947

PRATHER GC, MAYFIELD FH: *Injuries of the Spinal Cord.* Springfield, Charles C Thomas, 1953

SCHLICK H, STILLE D: Clinical symptomatology of intraspinal tumors, in *Handbook of Clinical Neurology,* vol 19: *Tumors of the Spine and Spinal Cord,* PJ Vinken, GW Bruyn (eds). Amsterdam, North-Holland, 1975

WYBURN-MASON R: *Vascular Abnormalities and Tumors of the Spinal Cord.* London, Kimpton, 1943

376
DISEASES OF CRANIAL NERVES

MAURICE VICTOR
RAYMOND D. ADAMS

The cranial nerves are susceptible to many diseases that rarely if ever affect the spinal peripheral nerves, and for that reason alone they deserve to be considered separately. Reference has already been made to some of these diseases in Chaps. 18 and 19. But there the emphasis was on cardinal manifestations and the ways of demonstrating the disordered function. Here we are concerned with the principal syndromes in which the disordered functions of these nerves are expressed and the diseases which cause them.

SYNDROME OF ANOSMIA AND AGEUSIA AND RELATED DISORDERS OF OLFACTION The delicate filaments of the olfactory nerve pass from the nasal mucous membrane through the cribriform plate of the ethmoid bone to the olfactory bulbs and thence to central structures concerned with olfactory perception. Disturbances in olfaction which are not numerous may be subdivided into three groups, as follows:

1 Quantitative abnormalities: reduction (hyposmia, anosmia) and increase (hyperosmia).
2 Qualitative abnormalities: distorted smell (parosmia)
3 Illusions and hallucinations caused by local diseases in the nose, central neurologic diseases, or psychiatric conditions

Unlike vision and hearing there is no easy way of accurately quantitating smell. The Elsberg olfactomotor used years ago proved to be too capricious and clumsy a method. The usual way of demonstrating the olfactory defect is to ask the patient to inhale a nonirritating scent first with one nostril occluded, then the other. Vanilla, lemon, scented soap, tobacco, and coffee can be distinguished by most people, though not always named correctly. Biopsies of the nasal mucosa reveal the state of the receptor elements and the presence of nasal diseases. Douek has reviewed these findings in his 1974 monograph and has discussed the differing olfactory capacities of males and females (in smelling the lactone, exaltolide) in the various periods of the life cycle.

Unilateral anosmia is rarely a complaint. Only by the separate testing of smell in each nostril can it be recognized. Bilateral anosmia, on the other hand, does bring patients to medical attention. Interestingly, the usual complaint is of a loss of taste (ageusia), for the reason that natural taste is to a large extent olfactory. Such patients retain the capacity to differentiate perfectly the elementary taste sensations of sweet, sour, bitter, and salty.

Regarding the nasal diseases responsible for bilateral hyposmia or anosmia the most frequent are those in which hypertrophy and hyperemia of the nasal mucosa block access of olfactory stimuli to the receptor zones. Heavy cigarette smoking, it is said, is the most frequent cause of anosmia. Chronic rhinitis of allergic, vasomotor, or infective types are common causes, though it is known that metabolic changes and hormones may also induce congestion and swelling of the nasal mucosa. In biopsies of the nasal mucosa in rhinitis the sensory epithelial cells are still present, but their cilia are shortened and deformed, and the receptors are buried by surrounding cells. The occurrence of a permanent hyposmia or anosmia may follow influenza, viz., *postinfluenzal anosmia*. In this instance the sensory epithelium of the olfactory zone is destroyed by the virus and replaced by respiratory epithelial and goblet cells and scar tissue. There is also a group, quite rare, of congenital anosmias, one type of which is associated with an hypothalamic defect (Kallman's syndrome of congenital anosmia with hypogonadotropic hypogonadism). The receptor cells are present but are hypoplastic, lack cilia, and do not project above the surrounding supporting cells.

Aberrations of smell may follow basal skull fractures and accompany intracranial lesions such as ethmoid tumors and nasal meningoceles. *Cranial trauma* is followed by uni- or bilateral impairment of smell in 5 to 10 percent of cases. Frontal injuries and fractures disrupt the ethmoid plate and the olfactory axons which perforate it. Sometimes there is an associated cerebrospinal fluid (CSF) rhinorrhea resulting from a tearing of the dura overlying the paranasal sinuses. If the anosmia is unilateral, it is usually on the side of the CSF leak, and this fact aids in localization of the fistula. Anosmia may also follow blows to the occiput or operations in the posterior fossa, performed in the semireclining position which allow the frontal lobes and olfactory bulbs to pull away from the orbital surface of the skull. Once traumatic anosmia develops it is usually permanent; only about 10 percent ever improve or recover. Perversion of the sense of smell may occur as a phase in the recovery process. *Meningioma* of the inferior frontal region is the most frequent neoplastic cause of anosmia (one-half of Cushing's series), and another cause is glioma of the frontal lobe. Occasionally pituitary adenomas, craniopharyngiomas, suprasellar meningiomas, and aneurysms of the anterior part of the circle of Willis extend forward and damage olfactory structures. These tumors and hamartomas may also induce seizures in some of which there may be olfactory hallucinations, indicating involvement of the uncus.

Parosmia is a term used to designate subjective distortions of olfactory perception. Strictly speaking it is an olfactory illusion. As was stated this may feature an intranasal disease that partially impairs smell, or it may represent a phase in the recovery from a neurogenic anosmia. Most parosmic disturbances consist of disagreeable or foul odors, and they may be accompanied by distortions of taste. Such distortions, according to Zilstaff, have been observed in schizophrenic and neuro-

syphilitic patients and in middle-aged individuals, mostly women, without known nasal or other disease or parageusia. Little is known of the physiologic basis of the perversions of smell sensation. In idiopathic cases small doses of $ZnSO_4$, given orally, are claimed to be beneficial. Minor degrees of parosmia are not necessarily abnormal, for unpleasant odors have a way of lingering for several hours and of being reawakened by other olfactory stimuli, as every pathologist knows.

A patient who claims to be smelling an odor that no one else can smell (no objective stimulus) and who is convinced of its presence and personal reference has an *olfactory hallucination*. Aside from uncal seizures in which it is brief and clearly related to a derangement of consciousness and other epileptic components, olfactory hallucinations usually signify a psychiatric disease. A huge range of odors may be reported, most of them foul. In some the smell seems to emanate from the patient him- or herself. These are called intrinsic hallucinations. Those seeming to come from an external source are called extrinsic. Both types vary in intensity and are remarkable with respect to their indefatigability. According to Pryse-Phillips, who catalogued the psychiatric illnesses in 137 patients with olfactory hallucinations, most were associated with depressive illnesses and schizophrenia. In schizophrenia, where the hallucination is seldom dominant, the stimulus was usually interpreted as arising externally and intended to be harmful to the patient. In patients with depressions and olfactory delusions of reference, the hallucinations most often come from their own body; and the olfactory hallucinations are overwhelming. All manner of ways may be used to get rid of the stench, the usual ones being excessive washing, deodorants, and social withdrawal. In all these psychiatric states the senses of smell and taste are notably intact.

SYNDROME OF RETROBULBAR NEUROPATHY   The acute development of impaired vision in one eye or both eyes (in the latter case the eyes may be affected either simultaneously or successively) gives rise to a number of interesting and troublesome problems. The most frequent clinical setting is one in which a child, adolescent, or young adult notes a rapid diminution of vision in one eye (as though a veil or haze covered every object seen). The condition may progress to complete blindness within a few days. The optic disk and retina appear normal, but in some cases the optic disk is elevated or choked, and the disk margins are obscure and surrounded by hemorrhages (papilledema). This latter condition, called papillitis, is distinguished from the papilledema of increased intracranial pressure by the effect on visual acuity. In retrobulbar neuropathy, after some few days or weeks the other eye may become similarly involved, the blindness then being complete except for slight peripheral vision. The pupillary light reflex is impaired. In a high percentage of patients, no cause can be found, and after several more weeks there is spontaneous recovery. Vision may return to normal in the majority of instances; occasionally a scotoma is left, or even blindness. The optic disk later becomes slightly pale in many of the patients. The CSF may be normal or may contain from 10 to 200 lymphocytes, and the protein level may be elevated.

A considerable number of such patients (15 to 35 percent) will develop other symptoms and signs consistent with multiple sclerosis within 10 to 15 years, and even more will do so if the patients are observed for longer periods. Less is known about children with retrobulbar neuropathy, but the prognosis for them is considerably better than that for adults. Formerly the syndrome was blamed on sinusitis and treated as such, but

Cushing long ago proved the error of the assumption. Sinus disease only rarely affects vision except for an occasional mucocele which presses on an ocular or optic nerve. Demyelination is the only common cause of a unilateral retrobulbar neuritis (see Chap. 370). Regression of symptoms has been observed to accompany the administration of ACTH (45 units per day for 3 weeks) or Meticorten (45 mg per day for 3 weeks).

Other causes of unilateral optic neuropathy include viral meningoencephalitis (infectious mononucleosis, herpes zoster), postinfectious encephalomyelitis, posterior uveitis (sometimes with reticulum cell sarcoma), vascular lesions of the optic nerve, and tumors (glioma of optic nerve with von Recklinghausen's neurofibromatosis, meningioma, metastatic carcinoma, and fungous infections).

Simultaneous impairment of vision in the two eyes, with central or centrocecal scotomas, usually is due not to a demyelinative process but rather to a toxic or nutritional disorder. The former condition (so-called "tobacco-alcohol amblyopia") is observed most commonly in the chronic alcoholic patient. Impairment of visual acuity evolves over several days or weeks, and examination discloses bilateral, roughly symmetric central or centrocecal scotomas, the peripheral fields being intact. With appropriate therapy (nutritious diet and B vitamins), partial or complete recovery is possible, although some patients are left with a permanent defect in central vision and pallor of the temporal portions of the optic disks. The same disorder may be seen in nonalcoholic patients, under conditions of severe nutritional deprivation and in pernicious anemia. Impairment of vision due to methyl alcohol intoxication is more abrupt in onset and is characterized by large symmetric central scotomas, as well as by symptoms of systemic disease and acidosis (see Chap. 226). Treatment is directed mainly to correction of the acidosis. A list of other drugs having a toxic effect on the optic nerve has been compiled by Leibold; included are chloramphenicol, ethambutol, isoniazid, streptomycin, sulfonamides, digitalis, ergot, Antabuse, and heavy metals.

Isolated optic atrophies have been described in degenerative diseases. There are several types, the most frequent being Leber's disease, dominant congenital or early infantile optic atrophy, and optic atrophy with diabetes mellitus and deafness (see Chap. 8 and Glaser).

Rarely amblyopia is due to cranial arteritis, some other vascular disease, or diabetes. In the adult syphilitic meningitis may lead to optic neuritis and atrophy (see Chaps. 146 and 373).

SYNDROME OF BITEMPORAL HEMIANOPSIA This type of visual disorder is usually related to a pituitary adenoma (ballooned sella shown in x-rays of the skull) but may also be due to craniopharyngiomas, saccular aneurysms of the circle of Willis, meningiomas of the tuberculum sellae (normal sella or thickened tuberculum by radiography), and rarely sarcoidosis, metastatic carcinoma, and Hand-Schüller-Christian disease. The lesion is always in the chiasm, involving the decussating nasal fibers from each retina.

SYNDROMES OF HOMONYMOUS HEMIANOPSIA See Chap. 18.

SYNDROME OF VISUAL AGNOSIA See Chap. 25.

SYNDROME OF OPHTHALMOPLEGIA Rarely, children or adults may have one or more attacks of ocular palsy in conjunction with an otherwise typical migraine (*migrainous ophthalmoplegia*). The muscles innervated by the oculomotor or, less often, the abducens nerve are affected. Presumably, intense vascular spasm in branches of the ophthalmic artery causes a transitory ischemia of nerve. Arteriograms, done after the onset of the palsy, usually reveal no abnormality. Recovery is the rule.

The acute development of a sixth or third nerve palsy on one side is a relatively common occurrence in the adult. The pupil is usually spared. In more than half the patients so affected no cause can be assigned; fortunately, most of them recover in a few weeks to months. Other patients prove to have diabetes mellitus or, rarely, cranial arteritis; in these instances the disorder may be ascribed to vascular occlusion. Exophthalmic ophthalmoplegia and myasthenia gravis must always be ruled out. Combined unilateral ocular palsies of painful type is indicative of the Tolosa-Hunt granulomatous parasellar syndrome. An acute onset of bilateral opthalmoplegia, visual loss, and drowsiness occurs in pituitary apoplexy.

The slow development of a complete ophthalmoplegia is most often due to an aneurysm (may also be of acute onset), tumor, or inflammatory process in the cavernous sinus or at the superior orbital foramen (syndrome of Foix) (see Table 376-1).

TABLE 376-1
Cranial nerve syndromes

Site	Cranial nerves involved	Eponym	Usual cause
Sphenoid fissure	III, IV, ophthalmic V, VI sometimes II		Invasive tumors of sphenoid bone, aneurysms
Lateral wall of cavernous sinus	III, IV, ophthalmic V, VI often with proptosis	Foix's syndrome	Aneurysms of cavernous sinus, cavernous sinus thrombosis, invasive tumors from sinuses and sella turcica
Petrosphenoid space	II, III, IV, V, VI	Jacob's syndrome	Large tumors of middle cranial fossa
Apex of petrous bone	V, VI	Gradenigo's syndrome	Petrositis, tumors of petrous bone
Internal auditory meatus	VII, VIII		Tumors of petrous bone (dermoids, etc.), infectious processes
Pontocerebellar angle	V, VII, VIII, and sometimes IX		Acoustic neuromas, meningiomas
Jugular foramen	IX, X, XI	Vernet's syndrome	Tumors and aneurysms
Posterior laterocondylar space	IX, X, XI, XII	Collet-Sicard syndrome	Tumors of parotid gland, carotid body, and secondary tumor
Posterior retroparotid space	IX, X, XI, XII, and Bernard-Horner syndrome	Villaret's syndrome	Tumors of parotid gland, carotid body, secondary tumor, lymph node tumors, tuberculous adenitis

Gaze palsies or mixed ophthalmoplegia and gaze palsies, due usually to vascular, demyelinative, or neoplastic processes in the brainstem, are discussed in Chap. 18.

SYNDROME OF FACIAL PAIN (TRIGEMINAL NEURALGIA, TIC DOULOUREUX) The most striking disorder of the trigeminal nerve is tic douloureux. This occurs in middle-aged and elderly persons and consists of excruciating paroxysms of pain in the lips, gums, cheek, or chin, and, very rarely, in the distribution of the ophthalmic division of the fifth nerve. The pain seldom lasts more than a few seconds or a minute or two but may be so intense that the patient winces; hence the term *tic*. The paroxysm recurs frequently, both day and night, for several weeks at a time. Another characteristic feature is the initiation of pain by obvious stimuli applied to certain areas on the face, lips, or tongue, or by movement of these parts, the so-called "trigger zones." Sensory loss cannot be demonstrated. In studying the relation between stimuli applied to the trigger zone and the pain paroxysm, it is found that the adequate stimulus for precipitating an attack is touch and possibly tickle, rather than pain or temperature. Usually a spatial and temporal summation of impulses is necessary to trigger an attack, which is followed by a refractory period of up to 2 or 3 min. This suggests that the mechanism for the paroxysmal pain involves the nucleus of the spinal root of the fifth nerve.

The diagnosis of this disorder must rest upon these strict clinical criteria, and the condition must be distinguished from other forms of facial and cephalic neuralgia and pain arising from diseases of the jaw, teeth, or sinuses. Tic douloureux is usually without assignable cause, although occasionally it is a manifestation of multiple sclerosis (may be bilateral) or of herpes zoster. Very rarely a tumor, and to a degree that cannot be estimated, a redundant artery in the posterior fossa, causes an early irritative lesion in the nerve or its root and produces pain clinically indistinguishable from that of tic douloureux. Usually, however, space-occupying lesions, such as aneurysms, neurofibromas, or meningiomas, produce a loss of sensation.

The conventional treatment for tic douloureux is alcohol or phenol injection of the affected nerve at the foramen ovale and rotundum or section of the root of the trigeminal nerve between the ganglion and the brainstem. Stereotaxic electrolytic lesions have also been made. Antiepileptic drugs such as diphenylhydantoin (Dilantin) and 5-carbamyl-5*H*-dibenzazepine (Tegretol) have been found to suppress or shorten the duration of the attacks. Temporizing and using these drugs may permit a spontaneous remission to occur. Most of the patients with severe pain come to surgery.

Anesthesia and analgesia of the face may be induced by stilbamidine (in the treatment of kala azar and multiple myeloma) and by trichloracetic acid. Pain and itching may occur during recovery. An idiopathic form of bitrigeminal anesthesia has also been observed, and leprosy may involve these nerves.

Tonic spasm of the masticatory muscles, known as *trismus*, is symptomatic of tetanus, although it may occur in patients treated with phenothiazine drugs; lesser degrees may be associated with disease of the pharynx and temporomaxillary joint, the teeth, and gums. Rarely, it is a manifestation of encephalitis.

SYNDROME OF FACIAL PALSY (BELL'S PALSY) AND FACIAL SPASM The seventh cranial nerve is mainly a motor nerve supplying all the muscles concerned with facial expression on one side. The sensory component is small (the nervus intermedius of Wrisberg); it conveys taste impulses from the anterior two-thirds of the tongue and probably cutaneous impulses from the anterior wall of the external auditory canal. The taste fibers traverse the lingual nerve (a branch of the mandibular) but then leave this nerve to join the chorda tympani. Secretomotor fibers innervate the lacrimal gland through the greater

superficial petrosal nerve, and others travel to the sublingual and submaxillary glands via the chorda tympani.

Several other anatomic facts are worth remembering. The motor nucleus of the seventh nerve is anterior and lateral to the abducens nucleus, and in their intrapontine course the facial nerve fibers hook around the abducens nucleus before they emerge from the pons at a point just lateral to the corticospinal tract. After leaving the pons they enter the internal auditory meatus with the acoustic nerve. The facial nerve then bends sharply forward and downward around the anterior boundary of the vestibule of the inner ear. At this angle lies the sensory ganglion (named *geniculate* because of its close proximity to the genu). The nerve continues its course in its own bony channel, the facial canal, and makes its exit from the skull at the stylomastoid foramen. It then passes through the parotid gland and subdivides to supply the facial muscles, the stylomastoid, and the posterior belly of the digastric muscle. Within the facial canal, just distal to the geniculate ganglion, it gives off the branch to the sphenopalatine ganglion, i.e., the greater superficial petrosal nerve, and somewhat more distally it gives off a small branch to the stapedius muscle and is joined by the chorda tympani.

A complete interruption of the facial nerve at the stylomastoid foramen paralyzes all muscles of facial expression. The corner of the mouth droops, the creases and skin folds are effaced, the forehead is unfurrowed, and the palpebral fissure is conspicuous because the eyelids will not close. Upon attempted closure of the lids, the eye on the paralyzed side is seen to roll upward (Bell's phenomenon). The lower lid sags also, and the punctum falls away from the conjunctiva, permitting tears to spill over the cheek. Food collects between the teeth and lips, and saliva may dribble from the corner of the mouth. The patient complains of a heaviness or numbness in the face, but no sensory loss is demonstrable and taste is intact.

If the lesion is in the facial canal above the junction of the facial nerve with the chorda tympani but below the geniculate ganglion, all the above symptoms occur and, in addition, taste is lost over the anterior two-thirds of the tongue on the same side. If the nerve to the stapedius is paralyzed, there is hyperacusis (painful sensitivity to loud sounds), and the sound produced by moving the jaw and facial muscles is no longer present in the ear on the affected side. If the geniculate ganglion or the motor root proximal to it is involved, lacrimation may be reduced. Lesions at this point may also affect the adjacent auditory nerve, causing deafness, tinnitus, or dizziness. Intrapontine lesions that paralyze the face usually affect the abducens nucleus and often the corticospinal and sensory tracts.

If the peripheral facial paralysis has existed for some time and return of motor function has begun but is incomplete, a kind of continuous contraction may appear. The palpebral fissure becomes narrowed and the nasolabial fold deepens. Attempts to move one group of facial muscles result in contraction of all of them (associated movements, or synkinesis). Facial spasms develop and persist indefinitely, being initiated by every facial movement. This condition, called *facial spasm*, may also appear in adults who have never had a Bell's palsy. Presumably it is due to a benign compressive or constrictive lesion of the seventh nerve, which results in volleys of motor impulses spreading to all the muscles of facial expression. Anomalous regeneration of the seventh nerve fibers may result in other curious disorders. If fibers originally connected with the orbicularis oculi become connected with the orbicularis oris, closure of the lids may cause a retraction of the mouth; or if fibers originally connected with muscles of the face later come to innervate the lacrimal gland, anomalous tearing (crocodile tears) may occur with any activity of the facial muscles, such as eating (Bogorad's syndrome). With the passage of time, the face and even the tip of the nose become pulled to the unaffected side.

The most common disease affecting the facial nerve is Bell's palsy, presumably due to an inflammatory reaction of undetermined type in or around the nerve near the stylomastoid foramen. The onset is acute, and the paralysis may evolve over a few hours, although pain behind the ear may have been present for a day or two. Occasionally taste sensation is lost, and more rarely hyperacusis is present. In some cases there is mild pleocytosis in the cerebrospinal fluid. Fully 80 percent of patients recover within a few weeks. Electromyographic evidence of denervation after 10 days indicates a long delay until regeneration occurs, and sometimes it is incomplete. Thus electromyography may be of value in distinguishing temporary conduction defects from a pathologic interruption in continuity of nerve fibers. Protection of the eye during sleep, massage of the weakened muscles, and a splint to prevent drooping of the lower part of the face are the measures generally employed in the management of such cases. The use of ACTH and the unroofing of the facial nerve in the facial canal have been tried in isolated cases, but the results are impossible to evaluate.

Tumors which invade the temporal bone (carotid body, cholesteatoma, dermoid) may produce a facial palsy, but the onset is insidious and the course progressive. The Ramsay Hunt syndrome, due to herpes zoster of the geniculate ganglion, gives a severe facial palsy associated with a vesicular eruption in the pharynx, external auditory canal, and other parts of the cranial integument; often the eighth cranial nerve is affected as well. Acoustic neuromas frequently involve the facial nerve. Vascular lesions or tumors are the common forms of pontine disease which may cause facial palsy. Bilateral facial paralysis (facial diplegia) occurs in acute idiopathic polyneuritis and in a variety of sarcoidosis known as *uveoparotid fever* (*Heerfordt's syndrome*). *Melkersson's syndrome* consists of a rarely encountered triad of recurrent facial paralysis, recurrent—and eventually permanent—facial (particularly labial) edema, and, less constantly, plication of the tongue. The cause is unknown. In the Far East leprosy may be the cause.

All these forms of nuclear or peripheral facial palsy must be distinguished from the supranuclear type. In the latter the frontalis and orbicularis oculi muscles are involved less than those of the lower part of the face, since the upper facial muscles, unlike the lower ones, receive upper motor neuron innervation from both motor cortices. In supranuclear lesions there may be a dissociation of emotional and voluntary facial movements, and often some degree of paralysis of the arm and leg or an aphasia (in dominant hemisphere lesions) is conjoined.

A curious disorder is the *facial hemiatrophy of Romberg*. It occurs mainly in females and is characterized by a disappearance of fat in the dermal and subcutaneous tissues on one side of the face. It usually begins in adolescence or early adult years and is slowly progressive. In its advanced form the face is gaunt and the skin is thin, wrinkled, and rather brown. The hair may turn white and fall out, and the sebaceous glands become atrophic. The muscles and bones are as a rule not involved. Sometimes it becomes bilateral. The condition is a form of lipodystrophy, and the localization within a dermatome suggests the operation of some neural factor of unknown nature. The treatment is transplantation of skin and subcutaneous fat by a plastic surgeon.

The facial muscles on one side may be affected by irregular clonic contractions of varying degree (*facial hemispasm*). This condition may be due to an irritative lesion of the facial nerve (e.g., an acoustic neuroma) or may represent a transient or permanent sequela to a Bell's palsy. A fine fibrillary activity of

facial muscles (facial myokemia) may be caused by a plaque of multiple sclerosis. In the most common form, however, the cause and pathology are unknown. An involuntary recurrent spasm of both eyelids (blepharospasm) may occur in elderly persons as an isolated phenomenon or with varying degrees of spasm of the facial muscles. Relaxant and tranquilizing drugs are of little help, although in many cases this disorder may subside spontaneously. In very severe and persistent instances, the only effective treatment has been crushing of the branches of the facial nerve that innervate the orbicularis oculi or other muscles, or craniotomy to relieve the pressure caused by an aberrant artery on the facial nerve.

Complete loss of taste, ageusia, may result from bilateral affection of the seventh cranial nerves but is more often due to damage of the lingual epithelium and taste buds (glossitis from fungal infections, drying, and atrophy). Dysgeusia, already mentioned above in connection with parosmia, is most often due to drug ingestion, the drug or some product thereof being excreted in the saliva.

SYNDROME OF BENIGN RECURRENT VERTIGO AND MÉNIÈRE'S DISEASE

Ménière's disease, or *Ménière's syndrome,* is the name applied to recurrent aural vertigo, accompanied by tinnitus and deafness. The latter symptoms may be absent during the initial attacks of vertigo, but they invariably appear as the disease progresses and are increased in severity during an acute attack. With milder forms of the syndrome the patient may complain more of head discomfort and of difficulty in concentration than of vertigo and may be considered neurotic. Provided that deafness is not complete, the recruitment phenomenon can be demonstrated (see Chap. 18).

Ménière's disease has its onset most frequently in the fifth decade of life, though young adults and the elderly are not spared. The pathological changes in Ménière's disease are said to consist of a dilatation of the endolymphatic system which leads to a degeneration of the delicate vestibular and cochlear hair cells. The relation of these changes to paroxysmal disorder of labyrinthine function is unknown. During an acute attack, rest in bed is the most effective treatment, since the patient can usually find a position in which vertigo is minimal. Dimenhydrinate (Dramamine) or cyclizine (Marezine) in doses of 25 to 50 mg tid is useful in the more protracted cases. A low-salt diet is still used in treatment, but its value is difficult to judge. Mild sedative and hypnotic drugs may help the anxious patient between attacks. Usually the deafness is progressive, and when it is complete, the vertiginous attacks cease. However, the course is variable, and if the attacks persist in a severe manner, permanent relief can be obtained by the administration of 10 to 12 g streptomycin in doses of 2 g per day or by surgical destruction of the labyrinth or section of the vestibular portion of the eighth nerve intracranially. Of course, the streptomycin effect is bilateral; hence it should not be used unless both sides are affected.

Another disorder of labyrinthine function is characterized by the occurrence of paroxysmal vertigo and nystagmus with the assumption of certain critical positions of the head. This is the *positional vertigo of Bárany,* of the so-called "benign paroxysmal type" (see Chap. 14).

There are many other causes of aural vertigo, such as purulent labyrinthitis complicating meningitis, serous labyrinthitis due to infection of the middle ear, "toxic labyrinthitis" due to drug intoxication (e.g., from alcohol, quinine, streptomycin, gentamycin, and other antibiotics), motion sickness, trauma, and hemorrhage into the internal ear. In these instances the attacks of vertigo tend to last longer than in the recurrent form, but in other respects the symptoms are similar. Streptomycin or gentamycin may damage the fine hair cells of the vestibular end organs and cause a permanent disorder of equilibrium especially in older patients.

There has been described a dramatic clinical syndrome, characterized by the abrupt onset of severe vertigo, nausea, and vomiting, without tinnitus or hearing loss. The vertigo persists for several days or weeks, and labyrinthine function is permanently ablated on one side. Occlusion of the labyrinthine division of the internal auditory artery would logically explain this syndrome, but so far postmortem confirmation of this hypothesis has not been obtained.

Vertigo of vestibular nerve origin may occur with diseases that involve the nerve in the petrous bone or the cerebellopontine angle. Except that it is less severe and is less frequently paroxysmal, it has many of the characteristics of labyrinthine vertigo. The adjacent auditory division of the eighth cranial nerve may also be affected, which explains the frequent coincidence of tinnitus and deafness. The function of the eighth cranial nerve may be disturbed by tumors of the lateral recess (especially acoustic neuroma), as well as by meningeal inflammation in this region or, very rarely, by compression from an abnormal vessel.

Vestibular neuronitis and *benign recurrent vertigo* are the names that have been applied to a clinical syndrome which occurs mainly in middle aged and sometimes young adults or children and is characterized by the abrupt onset of vertigo, nausea, and vomiting, without impairment of hearing. The attacks are brief and leave the patient for some days with a mild positional vertigo. They may occur once or recur and vary in severity. The cause is unknown. The medical treatment is the same as for Ménière's disease.

A particular variety of paroxysmal vertigo of childhood has been described by Basser. The attacks of vertigo occur in a setting of good health and are of sudden onset and brief duration. Pallor, sweating, and immobility are prominent manifestations, and occasionally vomiting and nystagmus occur. No relation to head posture or movement has been observed. The attacks are recurrent but tend to cease spontaneously after a period of several months or years. The outstanding abnormal finding is demonstrated by caloric testing, which shows impairment or loss of vestibular function, bilateral or unilateral, frequently persisting after the attacks have ceased. Cochlear function is unimpaired. The pathologic basis of this disorder has not been determined.

Cogan has described a peculiar syndrome in young adults, in which a nonsyphilitic interstitial keratitis is associated with vertigo, tinnitus, nystagmus, and rapidly progressive deafness. The prognosis for life and vision is good, but the deafness is usually permanent. The causation of Cogan's disease is not understood, although several patients later developed periarteritis nodosa.

The question of *viral infections of cranial nerves* is always raised by these acute palsies of the facial, trigeminal, and auditory nerves, especially when the affection is bilateral, involves several nerves in combination, or is associated with pleocytosis of CSF. Actually, the only proved virus cause in this group of cases is that of herpes zoster, and search for this virus from cases of Bell's palsy or of vestibular neuronitis has not been rewarding. Since perceptive deafness, vertigo, and other cranial nerve palsies have been observed in conjunction with the parainfectious encephalomyelitis of varicella, measles, rubella, mumps, and scarlet fever and also with Landry-Guillain-Barré syndrome, an allergic cause must be considered. Nothing is known of the pathology of the peripheral lesion or of the localization of a virus in the nervous system in these diseases. We have studied a number of cases of acute bilateral facial palsy, or facial palsy, numbness, and deafness or vertigo on one side and pleocytosis of CSF without succeeding in isolating the causative agent. There is no treatment other than symptomatic; fortunately the prognosis for complete recovery is excellent.

SYNDROME OF DEAFNESS See Chap. 18.

SYNDROME OF GLOSSOPHARYNGEAL NEURALGIA Glossopharyngeal neuralgia is a syndrome which resembles trigeminal neuralgia in many respects. The pain is intense and paroxysmal; it originates in the throat, approximately in the tonsillar fossa. In some cases the pain is localized in the ear or may radiate from the throat to the ear, because of implication of the tympanic branch (Jacobson's nerve). Spasms of pain may be initiated by swallowing. There is no demonstrable sensory or motor deficit. A trial of Dilantin or Tegretol is the recommended therapy, but if this is unsuccessful, division of the nerve near the medulla is the treatment of choice.

Very rarely, herpes zoster may involve the glossopharyngeal nerve. One may occasionally observe a glossopharyngeal palsy in conjunction with vagus and accessory nerve involvement due to a tumor or aneurysm in the posterior fossa. Hoarseness due to vocal cord paralysis, some difficulty in swallowing, deviation of the soft palate to the sound side, anesthesia of the posterior wall of the pharynx, and weakness of the upper part of the trapezius and sternocleidomastoid muscles compose the syndrome (see Table 376-1, jugular foramen syndrome).

SYNDROME OF DYSPHAGIA AND DYSPHONIA Complete interruption of the intracranial portion of one vagus nerve results in a characteristic paralysis. The soft palate droops and does not rise in phonation. There is loss of the gag reflex on the affected side, as well as of the "curtain movement" of the lateral wall of the pharynx, whereby the faucial pillars move medially as the palate rises in saying "ah." The voice is hoarse, slightly nasal, and the vocal cord lies immobile in an abducted or cadaveric position. There may also be loss of sensibility at the external auditory meatus and back of the pinna. Usually no change in visceral function can be demonstrated.

Complete bilateral paralysis is said to be incompatible with life, and this is probably true if the nuclei are involved in the medulla by poliomyelitis or some other disease. However, in the cervical region, both vagi have been blocked with procaine (Novocain) for the treatment of intractable asthma, without mishap. The pharyngeal branches of both vagi may be affected in diphtheria; the voice has a nasal quality, and regurgitation of liquids through the nose occurs during the act of swallowing.

The vagus nerves, especially the left, are most often damaged as a result of thoracic disease. Aneurysm of the aortic arch, an enlarged left atrium, and tumors of the mediastinum and bronchi are much more frequent causes of an isolated vagus palsy than are intracranial disorders. The nerve may be implicated at the meningeal level by tumors and infectious processes and within the medulla by tumors and vascular lesions, e.g., the lateral medullary syndrome of Wallenberg, and by motor system disease. Herpes zoster may attack this nerve. Polymyositis and dermatomyositis, which cause hoarseness and dysphagia by direct involvement of laryngeal and pharyngeal muscles, may be confused with diseases of the vagus nerves.

When confronted with a case of laryngeal palsy, the physician must attempt to determine the site of the lesion. If it is intramedullary, there are usually other signs, such as ipsilateral cerebellar dysfunction, loss of pain and temperature sensation over the ipsilateral part of the face and contralateral arm and leg, and ipsilateral Bernard-Horner syndrome. If the lesion is extramedullary, the glossopharyngeal and spinal accessory nerves are frequently involved (jugular foramen syndrome). If it is extracranial in the posterior laterocondylar or retroparotid space, there may be a combination of ninth, tenth, eleventh, and twelfth cranial nerve palsies and Bernard-Horner syndrome. Combinations of these lower cranial nerve palsies are sometimes called the *syndrome of Collet-Sicard* and the *syndrome of Villaret*, respectively. If there is no sensory loss in the palate and pharynx, or no palatal weakness or dysphagia, the lesion is below the origin of the pharyngeal branches, which leave the vagus nerve high in the cervical region. The usual site of disease is then the mediastinum.

SYNDROME OF BULBAR PALSY   This syndrome is the result of weakness or paralysis of those muscles which are supplied by the bulb or medulla oblongata, namely, the tongue, pharynx, larynx, sternocleidomastoid, and upper trapezius. If development is rapid, as may happen in diphtheria or poliomyelitis, there is no time for muscle atrophy. The more chronic disease, progressive bulbar palsy (a form of motor system disease), or tumors or aneurysms of the posterior fossa result in marked wasting and fasciculation of the tongue, sternocleidomastoid, and trapezius muscles. The condition must be distinguished from progressive muscular dystrophy and a restricted form of polymyositis which may be limited to neck muscles; however, these latter disorders seldom affect the tongue. It must also be differentiated from pseudobulbar palsy (see Chap. 15).

MULTIPLE CRANIAL NERVE PALSIES   As will be readily understood, several cranial nerves may be affected by the same disease process. One of the clinical problems that arises is the determination of whether the disease lies within or outside the brainstem. Lesions lying on the surface of the brainstem usually are featured by an adjacent cranial nerve palsy (or a succession of them) and late and rather slight involvement of the long sensory and motor pathways and segmental structures lying within the brainstem. The opposite is true of intramedullary, intrapontine, and intramesencephalic lesions. The extramedullary lesion is more likely to cause bone erosion or enlargement of the foramens of exit (seen radiographically). The intramedullary lesion involving cranial nerves often produces a crossed sensory or motor paralysis (cranial nerve on one side, evidence of tract involvement on the other). In this way a number of distinctive syndromes to which eponyms have been attached are produced. These are listed in Table 376-1.

Involvement of multiple cranial nerves outside the brainstem is frequently the result of trauma (sudden onset), localized infections such as herpes zoster (acute onset), granulomatous disease (subacute onset) including Wegener's granuloma, or tumors and saccular aneurysms (chronic development). Of the tumors, neurofibromas, meningiomas, cholesteatomas, carcinomas, and sarcomas have all been reported. The chordoma (see Chap. 367) may implicate a succession of lower cranial

TABLE 376-2
Brainstem syndromes which involve cranial nerves

Eponym	Site	Cranial nerves involved	Tracts and nuclei involved	Signs	Usual cause
Weber's syndrome	Base of midbrain	III	Corticospinal tract	Oculomotor palsy with crossed hemiplegia	Vascular occlusion, tumor, aneurysm
Claude's syndrome	Tegmentum of midbrain	III	Red nucleus	Oculomotor palsy with contralateral cerebellar ataxia and tremor	Vascular occlusion, tumor, aneurysm
Benedikt's syndrome	Tegmentum of midbrain	III	Red nucleus and corticospinal tract	Oculomotor palsy with contralateral cerebellar ataxia, tremor, and corticospinal signs	Softening, hemorrhage, tuberculoma, tumor
Nothnagel's syndrome	Tectum of midbrain	Unilateral or bilateral III	Superior cerebellar peduncles	Ocular palsies, paralysis of gaze, and cerebellar ataxia	Tumor
Parinaud's syndrome	Tectum of midbrain	Supranuclear coordinating mechanism for upward gaze	Superior colliculi	Paralysis of upward and sometimes downward gaze; fixed pupils, divergence of eyes	Pinealoma
Millard-Gubler syndrome and Raymond-Foville syndrome	Base of pons	VII and often VI	Corticospinal tract	Facial and abducens palsy and contralateral hemiplegia; sometimes palsy of gaze to side of lesion	Softening or tumor
Avellis syndrome	Tegmentum of medulla	X	Corticospinal tract Sometimes descending pupillary fibers, with Bernard-Horner syndrome	Paralysis of soft palate and vocal cord and contralateral hemiplegia	Softening or tumor
Jackson's syndrome	Tegmentum of medulla	X, XIII	Corticospinal tract	Avellis's syndrome plus ipsilateral tongue paralysis	Softening or tumor
Wallenberg's syndrome	Tegmentum of medulla	Spinal V, IX, X, XI	Lateral spinothalamic tract Descending pupillodilator fibers Spinocerebellar and olivocerebellar tracts	Ipsilateral V, IX, X, XI palsy, Bernard-Horner syndrome, and cerebellar ataxia Contralateral loss of pain and temperature sense	Occlusion of vertebral or posterior inferior cerebellar artery

nerves. Owing to their anatomic relationships, the multiple cranial nerve palsies form a number of distinctive syndromes, listed in Table 376-2.

From time to time one observes a benign form of multiple cranial nerve involvement on one or both sides of the face. The disease may recur over a period of years with variable degrees of recovery between attacks. Sarcoidosis is found to be the cause of some, and chronic glandular tuberculosis (scrofula), the cause of others. The condition is called *polyneuritis crani-alis multiplex.* The malignant granuloma of the nasopharynx may also affect multiple cranial nerves, as do also nasopharyngeal tumors, platybasia, and adult Arnold-Chiari malformation. A purely motor disorder without atrophy raises the question always of myasthenia gravis (see Chap. 381).

REFERENCES

ADAMS RD, VICTOR M: *Principles of Neurology.* New York, McGraw-Hill, 1977

BRODAL A: *The Cranial Nerves.* Springfield, Ill, Charles C Thomas, 1959

COGAN DG: *Neurology of the Ocular Muscles,* 2d ed. Springfield, Ill, Charles C Thomas, 1956

———: *Neurology of the Visual System.* Springfield, Ill, Charles C Thomas, 1966

DOUEK E et al: Olfaction and its disorders. Proc R Soc Med 68:467, 1975

GLASER JS: Heredofamilial disorders of the optic nerve, in *Genetic and Metabolic Eye Disease,* MF Goldberg (ed). Boston, Little, Brown, 1974

LEIBOLD JE: Drugs having a toxic effect on the optic nerve. Intern Ophthalmol Clin 11:137, 1971

MAYO CLINIC STAFF: *Clinical Examinations in Neurology,* 2d ed. Philadelphia, Saunders, 1963

PRYSE-PHILIPS W: Disturbances in the sense of smell in psychiatric patients. Proc R Soc Med 68:472, 1975

WOLFSON RJ (ed): *The Vestibular System and Its Diseases.* Philadelphia, University of Pennsylvania Press, 1966

377
DISEASES OF THE PERIPHERAL NERVOUS SYSTEM

RAYMOND D. ADAMS
ARTHUR K. ASBURY

Disease of the peripheral nervous system stands as one of the most difficult subjects in neurology. Since the structure and function of this system are relatively simple, one might suppose that knowledge of its diseases would be complete. Such is not the case. At present a suitable explanation cannot be offered in more than a third of patients who enter a general hospital with a disease of the peripheral nervous system, nor have the pathologic changes been fully determined in many of them. Moreover, the physiologic basis of many of the symptoms of peripheral nerve disease continues to elude experts in the field.

With these rather discouraging remarks behind us, we shall attempt to present a distillate of our personal experience that may be of value to the reader.

GENERAL CONSIDERATIONS It is well to have clearly in mind the extent of the peripheral nervous system and the scope of the possible pathogenetic mechanisms whereby it can be affected.

The peripheral nervous system (PNS) includes all nervous structures lying outside the pia-arachnoid membrane of the

spinal cord and brainstem, with the exception of the optic nerves and olfactory bulbs, which are special extensions of the brain. The parts of it within the spinal canal and cranial cavity and attached to the ventral and dorsal surfaces of the cord and ventrolateral surface of the brainstem are the *spinal* and *cranial nerve roots,* respectively. The dorsal roots (sensory) containing afferent fibers (the central axonal processes of the dorsal root ganglion cells) extend for a variable distance into the posterior columns (funiculi) of the spinal cord. The efferent ventral roots, composed of the emerging axons of anterior and lateral horn cells, finally terminate on muscle fibers or in sympathetic or parasympathetic ganglia. Traversing, as they do, the subarachnoid space, and lacking an epineural and in part a perineural sheath, the cranial and spinal roots are bathed by cerebrospinal fluid (CSF), the lumbosacral roots presenting the longest exposure. The vast extent of the peripheral ramification of cranial and spinal nerves is noteworthy, as are their thick protective sheaths of perineurium and epineurium and their unique vascular supply through longitudinal arrays of richly anastomosing nutrient arterial branches. Sensory endings, freely branching or corpuscular, are the site of termination of the peripheral axons of dorsal root ganglion cells. Sympathetic afferent fibers, arising on blood vessels and in viscera, and the sympathetic and parasympathetic ganglia, with their rami communicantes and peripheral extent, complete this system. Segments of myelin, special extensions of Schwann cell plasma membrane, cover all the axons of the extraneuraxial parts of the PNS, but always maintain a morphologically independent though symbiotic relation to it. Indeed the PNS has been defined as the Schwann cell part of the nervous system.

These many anatomic features inform us of the possible pathways and mechanisms of peripheral nerve disease. Pathologic processes (e.g., viral infections) directed at the anterior or lateral horn cells of the spinal cord, the nerve cells of dorsal root ganglia, or the nerve cells of sympathetic or parasympathetic ganglia may reflect themselves secondarily in degeneration of axons and myelin sheaths of the peripheral nerve fibers of these cells. Disease processes involving the oligodendrocytes or astrocytes in the ventral or dorsal columns (funiculi) of the spinal cord, wherein lie the axons of anterior horn cells or dorsal root ganglia cells, may also affect the function and structure of the peripheral nervous system. A pathologic process in the leptomeninges and CSF may damage the anterior and posterior roots in proportion to their length in transit through the subarachnoid space; and the posterior roots may be more affected because of their intimate relation to groups of specialized arachnoidal cells (villi), where CSF is absorbed. Pathogenic processes confined to various components of connective tissue may affect the peripheral nerves which lie enveloped within their sheaths. Special biochemical disorders may involve the most metabolically active and richly vascularized parts of the PNS, the dorsal root and autonomic ganglia. Diffuse or localized arterial diseases injure nerves by narrowing or obliterating the intrinsic vessels (vasa nervorum), thus curtailing their blood supply. Noxious agents which selectively damage the Schwann cells or their membranes composing the myelin sheaths cause demyelination of peripheral nerves but leave axons intact. Finally one might suppose that axoplasm of either motor or sensory nerve fibers or their peripheral endings and end organs might each have their particular affinities to pathogenic agents.

All this is theoretical and somewhat speculative. At present we can cite examples of diseases which are based on only a few of these potential disease pathways, e.g., diphtheria toxin, which acts directly on the membranes of the Schwann cells near the dorsal root ganglia and adjacent nerves; polyarteritis nodosa, which causes widespread occlusion of vasa nervorum; tabes dorsalis, in which there is a treponemal meningoradiculitis of lumbosacral segments; and arsenic, which damages the axoplasm of sensory and motor fibers because of its combination with the rich store of axoplasmic mercaptans, SH radicles. But analogous anatomic possibilities doubtless are implicated in other diseases whose mechanisms remain to be divulged (see Table 377-1).

Pathologically several distinct processes are recognized, although they are not disease-specific and may be present in varying combinations in any given patient. The major processes are Wallerian degeneration, segmental demyelination (focal myelin sheath degeneration), and axonal degeneration. The myelin sheaths themselves are the most susceptible element of nerve, for they may break down as part of a primary process involving the Schwann cells (or some component thereof) or secondarily to axonal or nerve cell destruction. When the myelin sheath itself degenerates, the highly structured lipoprotein disintegrates into fine particles, which are then converted into cholesterol esters and removed by macrophages via the bloodstream. Breakdown of axons causes fragmentation of myelin into blocks or ovoids in which lie fragments of axons. This is a feature typical of Wallerian degeneration. Degeneration of both axon and myelin sheath may occur either distal to axonal interruption (Wallerian degeneration) or as a "dying back" phenomenon in more generalized, metabolically determined polyneuropathies (axonal degeneration). In segmental demyelination, recovery may be rapid, because the intact axon need only become remyelinated over denuded segments to become functional once more. In contrast, with Wallerian or axonal degeneration, recovery is slower, often requiring months to a year or more, because the axon must regenerate and reconnect its peripheral ending before function returns. The rate of axonal regrowth is about 1 mm per day.

Aside from difference in pathologic pathway and the effects of disease on parenchymal elements of nerve, the various forms of polyneuropathy are distinguished by other characteristics of the lesions and by the topography of the nerve fiber changes. In fact these are the only available criteria for "differential diagnosis." In acute idiopathic polyneuritis and infectious mononucleosis, infiltrations of lymphocytes, plasma cells, and other mononuclear cells in the spinal roots, sensory and sympathetic ganglia, and nerves and a frequent perivenous location of myelin destruction characterize the disease. In polyarteritis nodosa with polyneuropathy, "necrotizing panarteritis" with occlusion and focal infarction of nerve and, less often, rupture and hemorrhage are the dominant findings. In amyloid polyneuropathy, the deposits of this foreign material in endoneurial connective tissue and the walls of vessels secondarily affecting the nerve fibers either by compression or ischemia are the basis of diagnosis. In diphtheritic polyneuropathy, the aforementioned location in and around the roots and sensory ganglia, the purely demyelinative character of the nerve fiber change, and the lack of inflammatory reaction permit its identification under the microscope. Certain toxic, polyneuropathies (glue-sniffers' neuropathy) are associated with a special type of axonal swelling and proliferation of neurofilaments. Other polyneuropathies (carcinomatous, nutritional, porphyric, arsenical, uremic) are topographically symmetric but are not presently distinguishable from one another by histopathologic means. They await more definitive study. The least is known about the familial types of polyneuropathy. Although patterns of inheritance can be recognized, the underlying biochemical link has been discovered in only a few genetically determined neuropathies, and the mechanism by which a particular biochemical abnormality leads to nerve dysfunction is not known in any.

Concerning mononeuropathies, these are usually due to local events. Compression, violent stretch, laceration from penetrating injuries are understandable, and the pathologic sequence of events is readily reproduced in animals. Of localized infections of single nerves only leprosy, sarcoid, and zoster represent identifiable disease states. For the larger number of acute lesions the pathology has yet to be defined, since they are usually benign, reversible states, which allow no opportunity for pathological examination.

The clinician is usually faced with two problems: (1) to establish the existence of disease of the peripheral nervous system and (2) to ascertain its nature and the possibilities of treatment. When muscular weakness, areflexia, atrophy, and sensory loss are demonstrable and conform to the region of distribution of one or many nerves, this is not difficult. The tendency for these diseases to affect the feet and lower legs more than the proximal parts, and the legs more than the arms, the frequent sparing of the trunk, the escape of vesical and anal sphincters, phenomena which probably reflect involvement of the largest and longest nerves, already commented upon in Chaps. 15 and 19, are relatively certain clues to diagnosis. But at times pain or dysesthesias may be the major symptoms, and the other subjective and objective neurologic findings are more difficult to put in evidence. Or the disorder may be purely motor, raising a question of myopathy, of motor end plate disorder, or of anterior horn cell disease; again, only paresthesias, ataxia, and sensory loss may be found, suggesting as alternative possibilities a disease of the posterior roots or the posterior columns of the spinal cord, such as tabes dorsalis. Under these circumstances one must resort to a number of laboratory procedures, such as (1) biochemical tests to rule in or out those metabolic or toxic states which will produce neuropathy, (2) measurement of nerve conduction velocity (lowered in chronic nerve disease but not in spinal cord or muscle diseases), (3) electromyography, which distinguishes disorders of muscle due to primary disease (myopathy), denervation, and neuromuscular block, (4) CSF examination (increase in protein and sometimes in cells with radicular and meningeal diseases), and (5) nerve (usually sural) and muscle biopsy.

Taking advantage of all available clinical and laboratory techniques and knowledge of the natural course of illnesses,

TABLE 377-1
Principal causes of peripheral neuropathy

I Poisons
  A Metals: arsenic, lead, mercury, antimony, thallium
  B Drugs: nitrofurantoin and related nitrofurazones, isoniazid, thalidomide, vincristine, diphenylhydantoin, stilbamidine, tetraethylthiuram disulfide, clioquinols
  C Organic substances: carbon monoxide, acrylamide, solvents including *n*-hexane and methyl-*n*-butyl ketone, and trichloroethylene, immune serums, organophosphorus compounds including triorthocresyl phosphate
II Deficiency states and metabolic disorders
  A Chronic alcoholism, beriberi, pellagra, subacute combined degeneration, pregnancy, chronic gastrointestinal disease
  B Carcinoma of lung, diabetes mellitus, porphyria, amyloidosis, multiple myeloma, macroglobulinemia, uremia, hypoglycemia, lupus erythematosus
III Specific inflammatory states and infections
  A Acute idiopathic polyneuritis (Landry-Guillain-Barré syndrome)
  B Polyneuropathy, complicating acute or chronic infection: diphtheria, Boeck's sarcoid, infectious mononucleosis
  C Local infection of nerves: leprosy, herpes zoster
IV Vascular disease: polyarteritis nodosa, arteriosclerosis, diabetes mellitus, rheumatoid arthritis
 V Genetically determined disorders: progressive hypertrophic polyneuropathy, peroneal muscular atrophy, and others
VI Polyneuropathy of obscure origin: chronic progressive or recurrent polyneuropathy

TABLE 377-2
2029
CHAPTER 377
DISEASES OF THE PERIPHERAL NERVOUS SYSTEM

Principal neuropathic syndromes

I Syndrome of acute ascending motor paralysis with variable disturbance of sensory function
  A Acute idiopathic polyneuritis (Landry-Guillain-Barré syndrome)
    1 Infectious mononucleosis and polyneuritis
    2 Hepatitis and polyneuritis
    3 Diphtheritic polyneuropathy
    4 Porphyric polyneuropathy
    5 Toxic polyneuropathies (triorthocresyl phosphate poisoning, Jamaica ginger)
II Syndrome of subacute sensorimotor paralysis
  A Symmetric polyneuropathies
    1 Alcoholic polyneuropathy and beriberi
    2 Arsenic polyneuropathy
    3 Lead polyneuropathy
    4 Nitrofurantoin and other intoxications
  B Asymmetric polyneuropathies
    1 Diabetic
    2 Polyarteritis nodosa
    3 Subacute idiopathic polyneuritis
    4 Sarcoidosis
III Syndrome of chronic sensorimotor polyneuropathy
  A Acquired
    1 Carcinoma, myeloma, and other malignancy
    2 Chronic polyneuritis
    3 Paraproteinemias
    4 Uremia
    5 Beriberi
    6 Diabetes
    7 Connective tissue diseases
    8 Amyloidosis
    9 Leprosy
  B Genetically determined disorders
    1 Peroneal muscular atrophy (Charcot-Marie-Tooth disease)
    2 Hypertrophic polyneuropathy (Dejerine-Sottas disease)
    3 Hereditary sensory neuropathy
    4 Portuguese amyloidosis (Andrade's disease) and other types
    5 Heredopathia atactia polyneuritiformis (Refsum's disease)
    6 Abetalipoproteinemia
    7 Tangier disease
    8 Metachromatic leukodystrophy
IV Syndrome of chronic relapsing polyneuropathy
  A Idiopathic polyneuritis
  B Porphyria
  C Beriberi or intoxications
V Syndrome of mononeuropathy
  A Pressure palsies
  B Traumatic neuropathies
  C Idiopathic brachial and sciatic neuritis
  D Serum neuritis
  E Zoster
  F Tumor invasion with neuropathy
  G Leprosy
  H Paratubercular (polyneuritis cranialis multiplex)

the physician will find it helpful to be familiar with the peripheral nerve syndromes listed in Table 377-2. Stated another way, whenever one of the syndromes in this table can be identified, one is justified in considering any one of the several diseases of the peripheral nerve system listed in that subdivision.

SYNDROME OF ACUTE ASCENDING MOTOR PARALYSIS WITH VARIABLE DISTURBANCE OF SENSORY FUNCTION

Only minor semeiologic differences separate (1) acute idiopathic polyneuritis of Landry-Guillain-Barré, (2) acute infectious mononucleosis, (3) porphyria, (4) diphtheritic polyneuropathy, (5) acute idiopathic hepatitis with polyneuritis, and (6) other acute toxic polyneuropathies. These are the diseases which induce this syndrome.

ACUTE IDIOPATHIC POLYNEURITIS Landry-Guillain-Barré syndrome This disease seems to occur at all seasons, as if it is an endemic process, and it affects children and adults of all ages and both sexes. Its cause is unknown; all attempts to isolate a virus or microbial agent have failed. A mild respiratory or gastrointestinal infection has preceded the neuritic symptoms by 1 to 3 weeks in approximately half the patients. Other preceding events include surgical procedures, viral exanthems, antirabies inoculations and influenza vaccinations, and a similar state may occur during the course of Hodgkin's disease, other malignant diseases, and lupus erythematosus.

The principal symptoms of peripheral nerve involvement have certain unique qualities. The weakness, which advances over a period of days, involves proximal as well as distal limb and also trunk muscles. There may be pain, but it is exceptional; paresthesias (tingling and numbness) are frequent but are occasionally absent throughout the illness, and sensory impairment is usually minimal (polyneuropathy is predominantly motor). The enfeeblement of muscle is so acute that it is not attended by atrophy, though hypotonia and areflexia are obvious. There is usually tenderness on deep pressure or squeezing of muscles. At an early stage the arms may be spared or their muscles may be less weakened than the leg muscles. Facial diplegia, occurring in half of all cases, usually comes later, after the arms are affected. However, other cranial nerves (ocular, bulbar) are often implicated. When retention of urine occurs, catheterization is seldom required for more than a few days.

Variants of the clinical syndrome take several forms: a predominantly descending motor paralysis; ophthalmoplegic polyneuritis with ataxia and little if any weakness of the limbs; a painful, mainly sensory polyneuritis; and a subacute or chronic asymmetrical polyneuritis of the limbs.

The temperature is usually normal, and lymphadenopathy and splenomegaly do not occur. Electrocardiographic alterations of minor degree have often been reported. The CSF is under normal pressure and is acellular; elevations of protein level are found in most cases, but the values on the first lumbar puncture in the first few days of the disease are usually normal or only slightly raised. In about 10 percent of patients a pleocytosis of 10 to 50 cells per milliliter (rarely to 200 cells per milliliter, predominantly lymphocytes and mononuclear cells) is found. The white blood cell count and differential count tend soon to fall within normal limits.

The pathological changes in fatal cases have had a consistent pattern and form. When the disease is fatal within a few days, perivascular, lymphocytic infiltrates are found. These are generally associated with foci of demyelination, the predominant pathologic effect on nerve. In some instances, not only is myelin sheath attacked, but also Wallerian degeneration occurs, implying that axons have been interrupted more proximally. Inflammation of roots accounts, evidently, for the CSF changes. Infiltrates in liver, spleen, lymph nodes, heart, and other organs are usually found and reflect the systemic nature of the disease. From a pathogenetic standpoint, most of the evidence suggests that the clinical manifestations of this disorder are the result of a cell-mediated immunologic reaction directed at peripheral nerve, specifically myelin sheath.

The differential diagnosis includes poliomyelitis (distinguished usually by epidemic occurrence, meningeal symptoms, fever, and pure areflexic paralysis) and acute myelitis (marked by sensorimotor paralysis below a given spinal level and sphincteric paralysis). The forms of acute polyneuropathy described below must also be differentiated from this syndrome.

Corticosteroids (prednisone) are not currently favored for treatment of acute idiopathic polyneuritis, but we have occasionally observed dramatic improvement within hours after the administration of prednisone. The latter is often effective in the management of more chronic or relapsing type of demyelinative polyneuritis (see below). The dose is 45 to 60 mg per day with a low-salt diet and precautions against peptic ulceration of stomach and duodenum. Respiratory assistance is given when the vital capacity falls below 800 to 1000 ml, and tracheostomy is usually performed at this time, especially if the patient has difficulty in removing secretions from the pharynx and tracheobronchial tree. Careful tracheal toilet, treatment of bronchial and pulmonary infections by the use of an appropriate antibiotic, and support of the blood pressure by vasopressor agents in the face of hypotension complete the therapeutic regimen. The best results are obtained by an efficient respiratory unit skilled in maintaining adequacy of ventilation and of cerebral circulation. Under the most ideal conditions the mortality is reduced to less than 5 percent.

Physiotherapy (passive-movement positioning of limbs and later mild resistance exercises) should be given as soon as movement returns to avoid joint contractures. Decision to discontinue respiratory aid to close the tracheostomy are based on the degree of recovery of the patient's respiratory mechanism.

Prognosis for complete recovery is good. More than 75 percent of patients are restored to normal function; the remaining usually have only a mild residual deficit, but a few are severely disabled. Speed of recovery varies. Usually it takes place within a few weeks or months, but if nerves have degenerated, their regeneration may require 6 to 18 months.

Infectious mononucleosis with polyneuritis This is a disease of young individuals. Three neurologic syndromes have been described with this disease: (1) ascending sensorimotor paralysis, identical with that of the Landry-Guillain-Barré syndrome, (2) aseptic meningitis, and (3) meningoencephalitis. All three appear during the midphase of the infection. The polyneuritis varies in severity and has rarely been fatal. The few autopsied cases have shown heavy infiltrations of lymphocytes, monocytes, and plasma cells in the nerves, roots, and meninges. The CSF contains a few or as many as several hundred mononuclear cells, and the protein level is raised. The diagnosis is suggested by the other typical physical and laboratory findings in this disease (see Chap. 195).

Infectious hepatitis with polyneuritis Rapidly evolving polyneuritis of the Landry-Guillain-Barré type may be associated with acute hepatitis. In our experience with this syndrome, the polyneuritis has followed the jaundice after several days or a few weeks and has the same relation to it as to respiratory or intestinal infections. Recovery from both the hepatitis and the polyneuritis has been the rule. The pathological changes in roots and nerves are identical with those described above for acute idiopathic polyneuritis.

Diphtheritic polyneuropathy Typical diphtheria (see Chap. 133) follows pharyngeal and laryngeal infections. Local action of the exotoxin may paralyze pharyngeal and laryngeal muscles within a few days and may also cause blurring of vision due to loss of accommodation. But these and other cranial nerve symptoms may be overlooked. The first signs of the neuropathy, coming 4 to 8 weeks later, are then an acute to subacute weakness of limbs with paresthesias and distal loss of vibratory and position sense. The weakness characteristically involves all four extremities at the same time or may descend from arms to legs. After a few days to a week or more the patient may be unable to stand or walk, and occasionally the paralysis is so severe and extensive as to impair respiration. The CSF protein level is usually elevated (50 to 200 mg per 100 ml). After the pharyngeal infection is controlled, death in diphtheria is due usually to myocardiopathy or to polyneuropathy with respiratory paralysis.

Postmortem examination discloses a demyelination without inflammatory reaction of spinal roots, sensory ganglia, and adjacent spinal nerves. Axons, anterior horn cells, peripheral nerves distally, and muscle fibers remain normal.

The disease should be considered in all cases of acute polyneuropathy. Throat culture may demonstrate the *Corynebacterium* many weeks after the throat infection has subsided. Usually the history of nasal voice, dysphagia, blurred vision, and numb lips with a throat infection several weeks before provides the clue to the diagnosis. The ECG may be abnormal at the time of polyneuritis. Occasionally the polyneuropathy has followed a local wound infection with *Corynebacterium* (see page 2038). Titers of antitoxin in the blood and a positive Schick test reaction have usually not been helpful (for treatment see Chap. 133).

The prognosis for full recovery is excellent, once respiratory paralysis and cardiac disorders are circumvented.

Porphyric polyneuropathy As was stated in Chap. 96, a severe, rapidly advancing, more or less symmetric polyneuropathy with or without psychosis (delirium, confusion) and convulsions may occur in the course of acute intermittent porphyria. The neuropathy may affect principally the motor or both the sensory and motor nerves; it may begin in the feet and legs and ascend, or it may begin in the arms and later spread to the trunk and legs. Often it is predominantly proximal in distribution, and in some instances the motor paralysis is more severe than the sensory loss. The CSF protein level is usually normal.

The course of polyneuropathy is variable. If the disease is mild, it may be quite transitory, with regression of symptoms in a few weeks. If severe, it may rapidly progress to a fatal issue in a few days, the advance occurring without warning, or it may progress in a saltatory fashion over a period of weeks, finally resulting in a severe sensorimotor paralysis that may regress only over a period of months. Disorder of the central nervous system is more likely to precede the acute severe forms of neuropathy, but it may not appear at all.

The pathologic changes in the peripheral nervous system vary according to the stage of the illness at which death occurs. If the patient dies in the first few days, the myelinated fibers may appear entirely normal, despite an almost complete paralysis. If symptoms were present for weeks, a severe degeneration of both the axons and myelin sheaths often is found in most of the peripheral nerves. No inflammatory reaction, vascular lesion, or other change distinguishes this form of neuropathy. The relation between the metabolic abnormality centering about porphyrin biosynthetic pathway in the liver and nervous dysfunction has never been satisfactorily explained.

See Chap. 96 for a discussion of treatment.

The prognosis for ultimate recovery is excellent, though relapse of the porphyria may result in further involvement of the peripheral nervous system (see "Relapsing Polyneuropathy," below).

Polyarteritis nodosa with polyneuropathy Occasionally this form of neuropathy develops as rapidly as acute idiopathic polyneuritis. Most of the cases evolve more slowly, however, and the syndrome has been either symmetric or asymmetric in its distribution. For this reason the description will be given in the next section. At times a cutaneous nerve biopsy may be needed to distinguish this acute form from acute idiopathic polyneuritis. The presence of constitutional symptoms, fever, or eosinophilia should provide clues to diagnosis.

Other toxic polyneuropathies that may cause paralysis in a few days An example is triorthocresyl phosphate intoxication, in which the purely motor paralysis ultimately proves to be due to involvement of upper and lower motor neurons, and thallium, which may cause an acute sensorimotor polyneuropathy (see Chap. 224 for discussion of other chemical agents). The acute stages are accompanied by an encephalopathy with delirium and coma. Stilbamidine, used in the treatment of kala azar, produces a purely sensory neuropathy restricted in many instances to the trigeminal nerves.

SUBACUTE SENSORIMOTOR PARALYSIS

SYMMETRIC DISTRIBUTION   Reference is made here to a neurologic disorder that develops over a period of a few weeks and pursues a variable course. The distribution is distal and graded in severity, and usually affects feet first, later spreading to the legs, thighs, and hands. Pain, hypersensitivity of skin, tenderness of muscles, and a mixture of dysesthesias and paresthesias are often prominent features of this clinical state. A purely symmetric syndrome of this type should direct attention to nutritional disorders (alcoholic beriberi), possible exogenous toxins (arsenic, nitrofurantoin), or metabolic abnormalities (myeloma, uremia).

Alcoholic polyneuropathy and beriberi   All data point to a common nutritional factor for both these diseases, though it remains unclear whether the deficiency is one of thiamine, pyridoxine, pantothenic acid, or several of the B vitamins. We have not been able to define a form of polyneuropathy due solely to the direct effect of alcohol.

In North America and Western Europe this form of polyneuropathy is rarely observed in the nonalcoholic person. Pure starvation does not produce it, the ideal conditions being a vitamin B deficiency in the face of a relatively high carbohydrate consumption. Of course, eccentricity of diet, gastrointestinal disorders, sprue, rice diet for hypertension with neglect of vitamin supplements all may create the necessary circumstances for such a neuropathy.

After several months (approximately two to three) of dietary inadequacy, numbness, tingling, and tenderness of the feet appear and are accompanied by weakness of the more distal muscles of the lower extremities, spreading within a few days to the calves and later the thighs. The leg muscles are always affected before the thighs, and foot drop, accompanied by weakness of the plantar flexors, is the first stage of the motor paresis. Involvement of the thighs is indicated by difficulty in arising from a squatting position. The tendon reflexes (ankle and knee jerks) are abolished, the skin and muscles are tender and vibratory, and position and touch senses are diminished to a variable degree, increasing as the disease progresses. Numbness and sensitivity of the fingers, hands, and forearms, weakness of hand grip, and wrist drop are next to appear. Cranial structures are usually spared unless Wernicke's disease is conjoined, in which instance there will be bilateral abducens and lateral gaze palsy and nystagmus, as well as cerebellar ataxia of gait, confusion, and memory defect (Korsakoff's psychosis). Involvement of vagus nerves with dysphonia and dysphagia has been reported and also involvement of other autonomic fibers in exceptional cases. If pellagra or nutritional myelopathy also occur, signs of retrobulbar neuropathy, deafness, and pyramidal tract signs may be found, resembling subacute combined degeneration.

This form of neuropathy produces a manifest sensorimotor disorder, which demands medical attention in only about half the patients in whom the diagnosis can be made. Once started, the syndrome often progresses over a period of days and weeks until the patient is confined to bed. But many alcoholics come to the physician with only a subclinical neuropathy (thin leg muscles, questionable sensory disorder over the shins and feet, and reduced or absent tendon reflexes). They give no history of

having had a subacute symptomatic polyneuropathy. If untreated, the symptomatic form may progress over weeks and months to a severe atrophy of leg muscles, the polyneuropathy then becoming chronic. Edema is not infrequent (wet beriberi) and is due to dependency of limbs and stasis, more than to coincidental myocardial involvement or nutritional hypoproteinemia.

Alcoholic Laennec's cirrhosis and a nutritional anemia as well as autonomic dysfunction, weight loss, myocardiopathy, hypoglycemia, and electrolyte disturbance may coexist. The CSF is normal in nearly all the cases (rarely is the protein level elevated).

The pathologic changes in this neuropathy consist mainly of axonal degeneration with destruction of both axon and myelin sheath, but variable amounts of segmental demyelination may also occur. Cursory studies show the most pronounced lesions to be in the distal parts of the longest and largest myelinated fibers in the crural and, to a lesser extent, the brachial nerves. Vagi, phrenic, and trunk nerves are implicated only in the more advanced and fatal cases. Anterior horn cells and sensory ganglion cells undergo chromatolysis indicating axonal damage. Exceptionally, spinal roots and posterior columns of the spinal cord have shown degenerative changes. Recovery awaits remyelination and regeneration.

The disease process is invariably arrested by adequate diet, and the amount of B vitamins in the average food ration of the American public will be curative, though there is no harm in supplementing the diet with B vitamins (see Chap. 80). Positioning and splinting paralyzed limbs to prevent contracture are important. Occasionally pain and tenderness are so severe as to require analgesic medication. The pain may be of a burning type (causalgic) with excessive perspiration and only slight weakness and reflex changes. Called the *burning foot syndrome,* this has been ascribed to pantothenic acid deficiency, but we have not been able to prove its relation to this vitamin or to separate it clearly from the usual alcoholic neuropathy. Cooling lotions, propoxyphene, aspirin, and codeine are needed. Sometimes sympathetic blocking agents are helpful. The pain subsides after some few weeks.

The prognosis for full functional recovery is good, but if the paralysis is complete, one may anticipate a period of invalidism for 6 months or more. Vitamins do not hasten recovery. The tendon reflexes may remain absent or diminished. Fatalities have usually been the result of coincidental beriberi heart disease, or cirrhosis rather than of the polyneuropathy. Vitamin supplements will prevent the polyneuropathy.

Arsenic polyneuropathy   Nerve involvement from chronic arsenic poisoning is relatively infrequent. The symptoms develop rather slowly over a period of weeks and have the same sensory and motor distribution as was described in beriberi. A single acute ingestion of arsenic may be followed in 14 to 21 days by a more rapidly advancing polyneuropathy. The condition may be preceded by mental disturbances, convulsions, confusion, and coma, i.e., arsenic encephalopathy. Diagnosis is based on the subacute course of the polyneuropathy coupled with symptoms of gastrointestinal disorder, anemia, jaundice, brownish cutaneous pigmentation, hyperkeratosis of palms and soles, and white transverse banding of nails (Mees's lines). Although arsenic intoxication may be accidental, its occurrence should always arouse suspicion of homicidal or suicidal intent.

See Chap. 225 for diagnostic tests and treatment.

Poisoning due to mercury, thallium, antimony, and nitrofurantoin may produce a similar picture; the first three of these intoxications respond to British antilewisite (BAL).

Lead neuropathy Lead neuropathy occurs following chronic exposure to lead, and its most characteristic feature is the predominantly motor affection involving mainly the upper extremities. The radial nerves are most frequently involved, producing wrist and finger drop with few or no sensory manifestations. Less commonly, weakness of the proximal shoulder-girdle muscle occurs, and in the lower extremities foot drop may appear. Lead neuropathy is seldom combined with encephalopathy. Important associated findings are anemia, basophilic stippling of red blood cells, lead line along the gingival margins, colicky abdominal pain, and constipation. Neuropathy usually affects adults and is infrequent in children. In contrast, lead encephalopathy, manifested by increased intracranial pressure, convulsions, blindness, and coma, occurs almost exclusively in children. The diagnosis of lead neuropathy is established by the history of lead exposure, the characteristic motor involvement, the associated medical findings, and increased urinary excretion of lead and coproporphyrins. Treatment consists of withdrawal from exposure to lead and measures to eliminate body stores of lead (see Chap. 225). Recovery may be slow.

Nitrofurantoin neuropathy The earliest symptoms of nitrofurantoin neurotoxicity are tingling or dysesthesias of the toes and feet, followed shortly by similar sensations in the fingers. If the offending agent is not discontinued, this may progress to a severe sensorimotor, distal, symmetric polyneuropathy. Usually neuropathic symptoms appear only after the drug has been administered in high dosage for several weeks or months; exceptionally rare patients have experienced dysesthesias after brief exposures. Patients with chronic renal failure and azotemia are particularly prone to neurotoxicity with nitrofurantoin, presumably because of diminished excretion in the urine and consequent high tissue levels of the drug. To make matters more difficult to interpret, the uremic state itself may be responsible for a polyneuropathy that is clinically similar, so that the distinction between uremic polyneuropathy and nitrofurantoin neuropathy in the presence of chronic renal failure may be impossible.

Other toxic polyneuropathies Vincristine causes a subacute, mainly sensory polyneuropathy with impairment of tendon reflexes in the legs. Disulfiram (Antabuse), diphenylhydantoin, primidone (Mysoline), and other anticonvulsants are known to induce a sensorimotor polyneuropathy, but only in rare instances.

SUBACUTE ASYMMETRIC POLYNEUROPATHIES The most notable examples of this syndrome are diabetes mellitus, polyarteritis nodosa and other vasculitides, and a more or less obscure form of idiopathic polyneuritis. Rarely, sarcoidosis presents in this fashion.

Diabetic neuropathy Only about 15 percent of patients with diabetes mellitus have both symptoms and signs of neuropathy, but more than 50 percent either complain of neuropathic symptoms or exhibit slowing of nerve conduction velocity. Neuropathy is most common in diabetics over 50 years of age, is uncommon under 30 years of age, and is rare in childhood diabetes.

A number of clinical syndromes have been delineated, as follows: (1) diabetic ophthalmoplegia (described in Chaps. 18 and 376); (2) acute mononeuropathy; (3) painful, asymmetric mononeuropathy multiplex, which may pursue an acute, sub-

acute, or chronic course and from which the patient usually recovers; (4) symmetric proximal motor neuropathy, which is often attended by burning pain, thigh wasting, and weight loss and from which recovery is the rule; (5) distal, symmetric, primarily sensory polyneuropathy, affecting feet and legs more than hands in a chronic, slowly progressive manner; and (6) an autonomic neuropathy involving bowel, bladder, and circulatory reflexes. Combinations of these neuropathies often coexist, particularly the autonomic disturbance in conjunction with other types.

The acute mononeuropathy involves most commonly the femoral or sciatic nerves and is presumably due to occlusion of vessels within or supplying the nerve. The outlook for recovery is good.

Painful, asymmetric mononeuropathy multiplex tends to occur in older patients with mild or unrecognized diabetes. Pain often begins in the low back or hip and spreads to thigh and knee on one side. It usually has a deep, burning character with superimposed, tearing, lancinating jabs and a propensity for becoming most severe at night. Muscle weakness and atrophy are usually most evident in pelvic girdle and thigh, although the distal muscles may not be spared. The upper extremities are usually unaffected. Sensory loss for position, vibration, touch, and pain is not generally severe and may conform to either a multiple nerve or root distribution, or to both. The vesical and anal sphincters may be involved, and the knee jerk is often lost on the affected side. Recovery from this type of neuropathy is the rule, although months and even years are often required. There is a tendency for the same syndrome to recur after a lapse of months or years in the opposite lower extremity.

A somewhat similar syndrome is encountered in elderly diabetics, in which one finds bilateral proximal and pelvic girdle weakness, wasting, weight loss, absent knee jerks, and often sphincteric symptoms and sexual impotence. Improvement tends to occur after some months, perhaps coincidentally with better control of the diabetes. It is unclear whether this diabetic neuropathy has the same basis as the painful asymmetric mononeuropathy multiplex. Both have been included under the general rubric of *diabetic amyotrophy.*

When the clinical picture is dominated by lancinating pain and sensory ataxia, with only slight weakness and bowel and bladder derangements, it resembles that of tabes dorsalis so closely that the condition goes by the name of *diabetic tabes.*

The distal, symmetric, primarily sensory form is the most common type of diabetic neuropathy. Numbness and tingling with relatively little pain are the main symptoms and are usually confined to the feet and lower legs. The ankle jerks are rarely preserved. Trophic changes in the form of deep ulcerations and neuropathic joints are occasionally encountered, presumably caused by injury to severely denervated skin and joints. Muscle weakness is usually mild, but in some cases a crural weakness with only minor sensory disturbance may predominate.

Pathologically, severe nerve fiber loss is a prominent finding in this form of neuropathy. In addition, evidence of segmental demyelination and remyelination of remaining axons is apparent in teased nerve fiber preparations. Since myelin is formed from the cell membranes of Schwann cells, one may infer that the Schwann cell is at least one target of the pathologic process in the distal, symmetric type of diabetic neuropathy. Whether the nerve fiber loss is explained by this same process remains uncertain. The basement membranes of blood vessels in these nerves do not appear abnormal under the light microscope but are altered in electron micrographs.

Symptoms of autonomic involvement include impairment of sweating and vascular reflexes, nocturnal diarrhea, atonic bladder, sexual impotence, and occasionally postural hypotension. The basis for this type of nerve damage is unknown.

In all forms of diabetic neuropathy, the CSF protein level may be elevated (50 to 200 mg per 100 ml), and similar increases may be seen in diabetics with no clinical evidence of neuropathy. An explanation for this phenomenon has not been discovered.

Many uncertainties persist about the pathogenesis of the diabetic neuropathies. Both the cranial mononeuropathies (diabetic ophthalmoplegia) and the proximal asymmetric mononeuropathy multiplex are thought to be ischemic in origin secondary to disease of the vasa nervorum. The other forms are rather vaguely ascribed to an undefined metabolic defect (sorbitol accumulation?).

The only known treatment is meticulous regulation of the diabetes mellitus along the lines described in Chap. 338. Maintenance of the blood sugar level in a relatively normal range is desirable, for there is some evidence that uncontrolled hyperglycemia is harmful. Vitamin supplements may have some merits, but no clear results have been obtained. Improvement and eventual recovery may be expected over a period of months, but during that time the management of the painful forms of neuropathy may be trying, because analgesic medication is required and one is faced with the possibility of drug addiction.

Polyarteritis nodosa with polyneuropathy Involvement of the intraneural vessels happens in perhaps as many as 90 percent of cases (autopsy figures), and a symptomatic form of neuropathy develops in more than one-half. Such involvement may be the principal clue to the diagnosis of the underlying disease when, up to that time, the main components of the clinical picture—abdominal pain, hematuria, fever, eosinophilia, hypertension, vague limb pains, and possibly asthma—have not fully declared themselves.

As was stated above, the polyneuropathy may develop acutely and be diffuse and more or less symmetric in distribution, but more often it is subacute, multiple, and asymmetric, i.e., a mononeuropathy multiplex. Both spinal and cranial nerves may be affected. No two cases are identical. The CSF protein level is usually normal. Muscle biopsy, taken near the motor point so as to include nerve, is useful in corroborating the clinical impression in the majority of cases. Central nervous system is involved less frequently, somewhat less than one-half of all cases; the lesion may occur concomitantly with those of the peripheral nerves.

Fatal issue is the rule. Corticosteroid therapy has not been successful in most cases. Spontaneous remission and therapeutic arrest are known, however, and a healed or healing form has been observed at autopsy, death having been due to other causes (see Chap. 67).

Subacute asymmetric idiopathic polyneuritis A few patients who consult the physician with an illness which at first glance has all the appearance of acute idiopathic polyneuritis will have an asymmetric pattern and continue to become worse over a period of weeks or months. Nerve conduction slowing and prolonged distal latencies signify a demyelinative neuropathy. Some have an extremely high CSF protein level (600 to 1500 mg per 100 ml), with a virtual Froin CSF syndrome (xanthochromia and spontaneous clotting). The higher concentration of protein fluids may be accompanied by headache, papilledema, and high CSF pressure, possibly because of the osmotic effect of the protein in increasing CSF volume. As the months pass, some symptoms improve as others appear. Ultimately most patients recover, though late fatality is known to occur; corticosteroids in full doses (30 to 45 mg daily or twice this amount on alternate days) have proved to be beneficial in the majority of cases but may have to be continued over a period of months.

The pathology of these subacute forms has not been defined, nor is their relation to the acute varieties of idiopathic polyneuritis settled.

This type of polyneuritis merges with the chronic and relapsing type described below.

Sarcoidosis Another cause of subacute or chronic polyneuropathy, sarcoidosis, is discussed in Chap. 120. It may be associated with signs of central nervous system involvement (stalk of the pituitary with diabetes insipidus and the cerebellum with ataxia) or with lesions in muscles (polymyositis). Facial nerve weakness is the single most common manifestation of peripheral nerve involvement as in Heerfordt's syndrome of chronic parotitis with facial nerve involvement (see Chap. 120).

CHRONIC SENSORIMOTOR PARALYSIS AND OTHER POLYNEUROPATHIC SYNDROMES

Here slowly progressive weakness, muscular atrophy, and reflex loss are associated with paresthesias, pain, sensory loss and ataxia, and autonomic disturbances in various combinations. The onset may be easily dated or insidious and the advance of the disease steady or intermittent. According to whether sensory or motor symptoms appear first, ataxia or muscular weakness may introduce the disease. Because of the chronicity paralysis is accompanied by atrophy of muscles of such degree as to stimulate the spinal forms of muscular atrophy or muscular dystrophy, especially in small children in whom sensory functions are nearly impossible to test. In some cases the distribution of sensory and motor abnormalities is quite asymmetric, suggesting a mononeuropathy multiplex. This is true of leprous neuritis, for example, where only one or a few of the nerves of arms and legs may be affected. More often, however, and this applies to most of the familial and the acquired polyneuropathies (chronic polyneuritis), the distribution is relatively symmetrical and the nerves in the distal parts of the lower extremities appear to bear the brunt of the disease.

In the chronic forms of polyneuropathy, presumably because of the time factor, and other more obscure reasons, one witnesses the emergence of a number of unusual neuropathic syndromes. It is as though the pathogenic agent has been able to selectively injure sensory or motor fibers or one size of sensory and autonomic fibers. As a consequence any one of the following syndromes may appear:

1 A sensory syndrome with ulcers of the feet and Charcot arthropathy. This is observed in the chronic familial type of neuropathy described by Denny-Brown.
2 A relatively pure sensory ataxia with paresthesias and areflexia, as in the Levy-Roussy familial polyneuropathy.
3 Pseudosyringomyelic syndrome in which there is mainly a loss of pain and temperature (but usually paresthesias and slight loss of touch, vibratory, and position sense as well), motor power is relatively good and tendon reflexes are absent, and autonomic disturbances are variably prominent. The familial amyloid polyneuropathy of Andrade tends to present in this way.
4 Autonomic polyneuropathy with mydriasis and loss of pupillary reflexes, diminished lacrimation and salivation, achlorhydria of stomach, loss of sweating, orthostatic hypotension, impotence, and diminished contractibility of bowel and bladder, all together or in various combinations, especially in partial syndromes. A pure dysautonomia has been described by the authors and, as was stated above, in one

form of diabetic neuropathy autonomic function may be disturbed.

5 Myokymia and the continuous muscular activity syndrome with mild weakness and continuous rippling and wave-like contractions of the muscles. Electrophysiological studies indicate an involvement of distal parts of motor nerve fibers (see Chap. 383).

These syndromes are fully described in the recent monographs on peripheral nerve diseases by Bradley and by Dyck et al.

ACQUIRED FORMS **Carcinomatous and myelomatous polyneuropathy** Here several syndromes have been observed. The most frequent is a slowly developing symmetric sensory or sensorimotor polyneuropathy that may accompany the development of a carcinoma or multiple myeloma. Severe weakness, atrophy, ataxia, and sensory loss of the limbs may advance to the point where the patient is confined to a wheelchair or bed. In some instances this may happen months or even a year or more before a small malignant tumor is found. The CSF protein level is often moderately elevated. This form of polyneuropathy has occurred most frequently with carcinoma of the lung but actually has been joined to every tumor. It may accompany either a solitary plasmocytoma of bone or multiple myeloma and in a few instances has been seen in macroglobulinemia without tumor formation. Another predominantly sensory polyneuropathy with good strength but severe ataxia is a relatively rare syndrome with lung tumor. Rarely in the immunologically suppressed patient with certain tumors such as Hodgkin's disease there may develop an acute polyneuritis of Landry-Guillain-Barré type rather than a chronic type. Thus polyneuropathy must be added to polymyositis or dermatomyositis, with which it is frequently conjoined as a neurologic complication of malignant tumor growths. A peculiar type of myasthenia (Eaton-Lambert syndrome), spinocerebellar degeneration (particularly with carcinoma of the ovary), and multifocal leukoencephalopathy, the other neurologic complications of neoplasia, may coexist. The pathology of the neuropathy has been incompletely defined. The only known therapy consists of removing or controlling the tumor growth, which has resulted at times in improvement. Corticosteroid therapy has helped some patients.

Paraproteinemia (see Chap. 61) More than a dozen patients with mild chronic sensorimotor neuropathies have been seen on our wards in recent years in whom no associated metabolic disturbance other than an abnormality of the immunoglobulins was found. In general, three protein abnormalities have occurred: (1) isolated macroglobulinemia (IgM), (2) diffuse increase in all three immunoglobulins (IgM, IgG, and IgA), and (3) a specific disorder of (IgA) immunoglobulin in ataxia-telangiectasia (see Chap. 374). In the latter disease, peripheral nerve dysfunction is evidenced by hyporeflexia, lowered nerve conduction velocities, and severe nerve fiber loss in a sural nerve biopsy. In macroglobulinemia and diffuse immunoglobulinemia (not to be confused with multiple myeloma), the neuropathies have been chronic, some exquisitely so, relatively mild, and occasionally sensory disorder exceeds motor and is distributed in a multiple nerve trunk pattern. An excess of plasma cells may be found in the bone marrow. Either prednisone or chlorambucil has at times led to reversal of neuropathy, although recovery has usually been incomplete.

Cryoglobulinemia, either the essential idiopathic form or that which is associated with myeloma, lymphoma, connective tissue disease, or chronic infection, occasionally results in a peripheral neuropathy. Pain and paresthesias are prominent

symptoms, often precipitated by exposure to cold. Weakness and muscle atrophy may appear, usually in the legs more than arms and sometimes in asymmetric pattern. The pathogenic mechanism is thought to be vascular, but pathologic changes are unsettled. The use of prednisone or the alkylating agent chlorambucil have induced remission, often incomplete.

Uremic polyneuropathy Uremic patients whose renal impairment is chronic will usually develop a slowly progressive sensorimotor paralysis of the legs and then of the arms. Almost as frequently, the polyneuropathy has developed subacutely. Muscle atrophy, areflexia, and distal distribution in the limbs of neurologic defect leave little doubt of the peripheral nerve character of the disorder. Improvement has been observed after treatment on the artificial kidney, and recovery is the rule after successful renal transplantation. The CSF protein level may be moderately elevated (50 to 150 mg per 100 ml).

The pathology is that of a nonspecific degeneration of large myelinated fibers in nerves and spinal roots. Axons degenerate with the expected chromatolysis of their cell bodies. Amyloid deposit in the nerve has not been found; there is no evidence of vitamin deficiency or of diabetes during life and no sign of polyarteritis nodosa at autopsy. The neuropathy has been observed with all types of chronic kidney disease.

Beriberi In all the regions of the world where nutrition is borderline and treatment for an evolving beriberi may of necessity be delayed or even impossible to obtain, the motor paralysis and atrophy of the legs and, to a lesser extent, thighs and arms may reach an extreme degree. Thus this disease, though subacute in its evolution, becomes a frequent cause of chronic polyneuropathy. Uncontrolled diabetes may behave similarly.

Chronic polyneuropathy with connective tissue diseases In a clinic where many patients with connective tissue disease are being studied, occasional examples of either subacute or chronic polyneuropathy or a mononeuropathy have appeared. The latter are usually related to rheumatoid arthritis and are difficult to distinguish from pressure palsies clinically. The polyneuropathy is diffuse, often symmetric, and variably painful. Little is known of its cause, mechanism, or pathology. Some of the most extremely painful polyneuropathies we have seen, extending over long periods of time, have had only minimal sensory loss, weakness, or reflex change in some part of the body, and the diagnosis has been difficult. An unexpected rise in CSF protein level or electromyographic evidence of denervation may sometimes prove to be important leads. Occasionally a chronic symmetric polyneuropathy may accompany lupus erythematosus. It may be due to a small-vessel arteritis. Perhaps more of the obscure polyneuropathies fall into this group of connective tissue diseases than is presently realized.

Prineas and McLeod have reviewed large series of cases of subacute to chronic relapsing polyneuritis, the findings of which suggest a relationship to Landry-Guillain-Barré (LGB) syndrome. "Heaviness" and weakness of the legs and difficulty in walking were the initial symptoms in half of the cases, but in one-fourth of them the first sensory and motor symptoms were localized to the arms, and in one to cranial structures. The interval from first symptom to maximal level of weakness ranged from 3 weeks to 16 months. Half of the patients were unable to walk at the peak of the illness. Proximal limb muscles were usually more affected than distal. The tendon reflexes were abolished. Sensory impairment tended always to be less than motor and in several was undetectable by the standard clinical tests. Pain may be a prominent feature of some cases.

Most patients of this kind (the authors have been seeing two or three per year) have attacks or relapses lasting several weeks. In the relapses, unlike the acute LGB syndrome, respiratory difficulties and life-threatening paralysis rarely occur.

The CSF protein is almost invariably elevated, and in some there are few lymphocytes. Sensory nerve conduction is absent and motor nerve conduction is slowed. There is focal inflammation and demyelination of axons in nerve biopsies, a combination of changes believed to be characteristic of LGB syndrome. "Onion bulb" formations of Schwann cells are seen in some biopsies. No antibodies to any of the common viruses have been found. Prednisone in doses of 40 to 60 mg per day for weeks to months has been followed by a remission in the majority of cases; and in the few that did not respond, cyclophosphamide in a dose of 50 to 150 mg per day for 2 to 4 months has been effective. Most of the patients will improve but will be left with some deficits, and one of five will recover completely. Odd variants of this syndrome have included hypertrophied nerves, an elevated sedimentation rate, an enlarged spleen, or coarse tremor of the hands (especially when receiving corticosteroids).

Hypothyroid neuropathy Although nerve involvement is infrequent, a number of myxedematous patients will complain of numbness and weakness of feet and legs and to a lesser extent, the hands. Weakness of distal muscles; areflexia; and diminution of vibratory, joint-position, and touch-pressure sensations are the usual findings. The nerve conduction velocities are diminished and CSF protein is increased. Subjective improvement and at times a definite disappearance of the abnormalities follow thyroid replacement therapy. Dyck and Lambert observed a metachromatic mucoid material in the connective tissue sheaths of nerves.

Amyloidosis with chronic polyneuropathy As was pointed out in Chap. 103, primary amyloidosis may occur as a sporadic or a familial disease, the latter being particularly common in Portugal and Brazil. The polyneuropathy usually begins in middle adult life, is often severe, and is usually preceded by gastrointestinal symptoms (anorexia, indigestion, diarrhea). Sensory and motor nerve fibers are affected; in the familial varieties autonomic disturbance may predominate. Symmetry of involvement is the rule. The tongue may be enlarged and weak, and ocular muscles may be paretic. A carpel tunnel syndrome may be observed as the only neurologic abnormality in some cases. Cerebrospinal fluid protein level is elevated. The diagnosis is suggested by the clinical picture, the polyneuropathy being combined with hepatomegaly (often jaundice), anemia, cardiac enlargement, and EEG change. The nerves are probably enlarged in some patients. Restricted syndromes (eye muscles, tongue, etc.) are known. Presently there is no treatment for primary amyloidosis.

Leprous neuritis This is the classic example of an infectious neuritis, for the inflammatory reaction in the nerve is evoked by the leprous bacillus. Two major forms are recognized, tuberculoid and lepromatous, but intermediate forms are frequent. Tuberculoid (high-resistance) leprosy is restricted to a single patch of hypesthetic skin in any location. If a superficially placed nerve trunk, typically a cutaneous nerve, courses just beneath the area of affected skin, it may be engulfed in the inflammatory reaction, resulting in an associated mononeuropathy. Such a nerve may be palpably enlarged and beaded. Lepromatous (low-resistance) leprosy is marked by immunologic tolerance and widespread cutaneous anesthesia and anhidrosis, sparing only the warmest parts of the body, notably the axilla, groin, and beneath the scalp hair. Motor signs (focal weakness and atrophy) result from damage to mixed nerves lying close to the skin, particularly median, ulnar, peroneal, and facial nerves.

Diagnosis depends on the character of the clinical picture, skin and nerve changes often being associated.

See Chap. 144 for diagnostic tests and therapy.

GENETICALLY DETERMINED NEUROPATHIES Three chronic familial polyneuropathies (peroneal muscular atrophy, hereditary sensory neuropathy, and progressive hypertrophic polyneuropathy) have been recognized for many years, but in none has an associated metabolic disturbance been discovered. Several other genetically determined neuropathies have been described (Refsum's disease, abetalipoproteinemia, metachromatic leukodystrophy, and Tangier disease) with which a known metabolic disorder is associated. Familial amyloidosis with neuropathy also belongs to the group and is discussed above.

Peroneal muscular atrophy (Charcot-Marie-Tooth disease) This is a dominant hereditary disease with onset during adolescence or adult years. There is chronic degeneration of peripheral nerves and roots, resulting in distal muscle atrophy, beginning in the feet and legs and later involving the hands. Early symptoms are muscular wasting and weakness, affecting the extensor and everter muscles of the feet and producing an equinovarus deformity. Later, all muscles below the middle third of the thigh may atrophy, resulting in a "stork leg" appearance of the legs. After a period of years, atrophy of hand and forearm muscles develops. The wasting seldom extends above the elbows or above the middle third of the thighs. The feet are short and arched, sometimes with perforating ulcers. Pain, paresthesias, and cramps are common. The objective sensory disorder is usually rather slight but conspicuous enough to enable one to distinguish this polyneuropathy from progressive (spinal) muscular atrophy. There is impairment of position and vibratory sensation in the feet, and touch and pain sensation are lost in the feet. Reflexes are absent in the involved limbs. The progression of the illness is very slow, and it may arrest at any stage (see Chap. 373 for more complete descriptions). Generally speaking, in those families with onset during adolescence, nerve conduction velocities are very slow (10 to 30 m/s) and pathologically one sees hypertrophic neuropathy with "onion bulb" formation (see next section). In families with adult onset in the fourth or fifth decade, nerve conduction velocities are normal or minimally reduced and the pathology is that of axonal loss.

Progressive hypertrophic polyneuropathy (Dejerine-Sottas disease) This type of neuropathy is infrequent and is familial, usually with a recessive type of inheritance pattern. It begins in childhood and is slowly progressive. Pain and paresthesias in the feet are early symptoms, followed by development of symmetric weakness and wasting of the distal portion of the limbs. Sensation is impaired in a distal distribution, and the tendon reflexes are absent. Miotic pupils, nystagmus, and kyphoscoliosis have been observed in some cases. Patients are usually confined to a wheelchair at an early age. Morphologically the nerves are thickened and enlarged because of excessive endoneurial collagen deposition and a prominent myxoid interstitium. Nerve fibers are reduced in number; those remaining have thinned or absent myelin sheaths, and each is surrounded by a lamellated collar of Schwann cells and connective tissue referred to as an "onion bulb" formation. Such hypertrophic changes in nerve are not specific for this condition, but may also occur diffusely in Refsum's disease (see below), certain forms of peroneal muscular atrophy, acquired forms of relapsing polyneuropathy, or a single nerve in multifocal distribution, and possibly diabetes mellitus. Palpable thickening of the ulnar and peroneal nerves may be conspicuous. In the absence of palpable enlargement of nerves, the diagnosis can be established by biopsy of a cutaneous nerve. The treatment is symptomatic.

Hereditary sensory neuropathy Both a dominant and a recessive inheritance pattern are recognized in this disorder. Exquisitely slow progression of distal cutaneous sensory loss of extreme degree is the clinical expression. Recurrent injury to the insensitive hands and feet leads often to mutilation and loss of digits.

Chronic polyneuropathy with ichthyosis, deafness, and retinitis pigmentosa (Refsum's disease) This rare, genetically determined disorder begins in childhood or early adolescence, and the polyneuropathy is sensorimotor, distal, and symmetric in distribution, affecting legs more than arms. Sometimes an attack of polyneuropathy may develop subacutely and later regress. Although the nerves may not be enlarged clinically, hypertrophic changes with "onion bulb" formation are an unfailing pathologic feature. The metabolic defect results in a tissue accumulation of phytanic acid, a tetramethylated 16-carbon fatty acid. The relation between this biochemical lesion and the polyneuropathy remains uncertain. Diets low in phytanic acid may be beneficial.

Abetalipoproteinemia (Bassen-Kornzweig syndrome, acanthocytosis) (see also Chap. 100) The clinical manifestations of this unusual syndrome include (1) near absence of β-lipoprotein in the serum, (2) retinitis pigmentosa, (3) acanthocytosis of the red blood cells, and (4) a chronic, progressive neurologic deficit, usually beginning in childhood. Extreme proprioceptive sensory loss, ataxia, and areflexia are the most constant features, although muscular weakness and atrophy, kyphoscoliosis, and corticospinal signs may also be encountered. The main burden of the neurologic disorder falls upon the peripheral nervous system, but the relation between the neuropathy and the deficiency of β-lipoprotein remains unknown.

Tangier disease (see also Chap. 100) In this rare recessively inherited disorder, marked by near absence of plasma high-density lipoprotein and low serum cholesterol, approximately one-half of patients will exhibit neuropathy. A distinctive clinical picture has been described in three such patients, which consisted of severe progressive asymmetric cutaneous anesthesia to pain and temperature over scalp, face, and limbs with sparing of distal parts.

Metachromatic leukodystrophy (see also Chap. 373) Massive sulfatide accumulation throughout the central and peripheral nervous systems, and to a lesser extent in other organs, occurs in this disorder, apparently because of congenital absence of the degradative enzyme sulfatase. The abnormality is transmitted as an autosomal recessive trait. Progressive cerebral deterioration is the most obvious clinical aspect, but hyporeflexia, muscular atrophy, and diminished nerve conduction velocity indicate a neuropathic element. Metachromatically staining granules accumulate in the cytoplasm of Schwann cells in all peripheral nerves, as well as in central white matter. Sural biopsy may be used to establish the diagnosis, even early in the course of the illness.

RELAPSING POLYNEUROPATHY

Two diseases most regularly take this form: porphyria, in which the attacks recur because of the administration of barbi-

turates or spontaneous relapses, and idiopathic polyneuritis. The latter has no proved cause. Enlargement of nerves may occur in the latter disorder so that it is probable that some patients with hypertrophic polyneuropathy may fall into this category. Amyloidosis or leprosy may also cause palpable enlargement of nerves, but by an obviously different mechanism.

MONONEUROPATHY OR MULTIPLE NEUROPATHY

This group of diseases differs in that one or a few of the nerves are involved in the disease process. The finding of a mononeuropathy inplies a local cause, usually trauma or compression. Diagnosis rests on the finding of motor, reflex, or sensory changes confined to the territory of a particular nerve. A part of a plexus may also be involved. One variety, mononeuropathy multiplex, which has already been discussed, is due to leprosy, sarcoid, diabetes, and polyarteritis nodosa.

COMMON BRACHIAL AND CRURAL MONONEUROPATHIES
Brachial palsies The fifth to eighth cervical and first thoracic spinal nerves innervate the muscles of the shoulder girdles and upper extremities. The brachial plexus is formed by components of these nerves, and lesions of the nerves or their branches result in characteristic palsies. The following are the brachial palsies most likely to be observed on the medical wards of a hospital.

LONG THORACIC NERVE This nerve is derived from the fifth, sixth, and seventh cervical nerves and supplies the serratus magnus muscle. Paralysis of the serratus magnus muscle results in inability to raise the arm over the head from a forward position, and there is winging of the medial border of the scapula on pushing forward against resistance. It is injured most commonly by pressure on the shoulder, from either a sudden blow or prolonged pressure from carrying heavy weights. It is also involved at times in diabetic patients and as a manifestation of brachial and serum neuritides and in other idiopathic forms of neuritis (pleurodynia, Coxsackie disease).

SUPRASCAPULAR NERVE This nerve is derived from the fifth and sixth cervical nerves and supplies the supra- and infraspinatus muscles. Lesions may be diagnosed by the presence of weakness of abduction and external rotation of the arm and atrophy of the supra- and infraspinatus muscles. The nerve may be injured by blows on the top of the shoulder and fracture dislocations of the shoulder joint.

UPPER BRACHIAL PLEXUS PARALYSIS This is due to injury to the fifth and sixth cervical nerves and roots caused most commonly by forceful separation of the head and shoulder during difficult parturition or by pressure in the supraclavicular region during anesthesia. Headlong falls may also produce this injury. The muscles affected are the biceps, deltoid, brachialis anticus, supinator longus, supra- and infraspinatus, and rhomboids. The arm hangs at the side, internally rotated, with the elbow extended. The forearm is pronated. Hand motion is unaffected. The prognosis for spontaneous recovery is generally good, especially in cases of birth injury. This condition as a result of birth injury (Erb-Duchenne brachial plexus palsy), which may persist throughout life, is discussed in Chaps. 15 and 374.

LOWER BRACHIAL PLEXUS PARALYSIS This is due to injury to the eighth cervical and first thoracic roots as a result of traction on the abducted arm in falls, during operation, and with tumors of the apex of the lung (superior sulcus or Pancoast's syndrome). Injury may occur during birth (Dejerine-Klumpke brachial plexus injury). There is paralysis and wasting of the small muscles of the hand and a characteristic claw-hand deformity. Sensory loss is limited to the ulnar border of the hand and inner side of forearm, and there may be an associated paralysis of the cervical sympathetic nerve with Horner's syndrome if the first thoracic motor root is involved.

LESIONS OF THE CORDS OF THE BRACHIAL PLEXUS The lateral and medial cords are most commonly affected. Dislocation of the head of the humerus, pressure of the cervical ribs, and stab wounds are the most frequent causes. Injury to the lateral cord results in paralysis of the biceps and coracobrachialis muscles and all muscles supplied by the median nerve except the intrinsic hand muscles. There is some loss of sensation over the radial aspects of the forearm. Involvement of the medial cord, as may occur in compression by the cervical rib, results in paralysis of the muscles supplied by the ulnar nerve together with the median-innervated intrinsic muscles of the hand and sensory loss over the ulnar aspect of the hand and forearm. Sternum splinting operations may compress the lower brachial plexus by displacement of the clavicle. Usually it is the medial cord of the brachial plexus that is affected.

AXILLARY NERVE This nerve arises from the posterior cord of the brachial plexus and supplies the teres minor and deltoid muscles. It may be involved in injuries resulting from fractures of the neck of the humerus, serum neuritis, brachial neuritis, or as a part of a disease of unknown cause. The anatomic localization depends on the recognition of a paralysis of abduction of the arm, wasting of the deltoid muscle, and a patch of impaired sensation over the outer aspect of the shoulder.

MUSCULOCUTANEOUS NERVE This nerve is derived from the fifth and sixth cervical roots and is a branch of the lateral cord of the brachial plexus. It innervates the biceps and brachialis anticus muscles. Lesions of the nerve result in weakness of elbow flexion. Rarely is it injured alone.

RADIAL NERVE This nerve is derived from the fifth to eighth cervical roots and is the termination of the posterior cord of the brachial plexus. It innervates the triceps muscle and the supinator and extensor muscles of the forearm and hand. Complete radial paralysis results in inability to extend the elbow, paralysis of supination of the forearm, and complete wrist and finger drop. Sensation is impaired over the posterior aspect of the forearm and a small area over the radial aspect of the dorsum of the hand. The nerve may be injured in the axilla, for example in "crutch" palsy, but most commonly traumatism occurs in the mid-arm where the nerve winds around the humerus. Common types of injury at this site are fractures and pressure palsies incurred during sleep.

MEDIAN NERVE This nerve is derived from the sixth cervical to the first thoracic root and is formed by the union of two heads from the medial and lateral cords of the brachial plexus. It innervates the pronators of the forearm, long finger flexors, and abductor and opponens muscles of the thumb and is a sensory nerve to the palmar aspect of the hand. Complete median nerve paralysis results in wasting of the affected muscles and inability to pronate the forearm, weakness of wrist flexion, paralysis of flexion of the index finger and terminal phalanx of the thumb, weakness of flexion of the remaining fingers, weakness of abduction and opposition of the thumb, and sensory impairment over the radial two-thirds of the palmar aspect of the hand and over the distal phalanges of the dorsum of the index and third fingers. The nerve may be injured in the axilla by shoulder dislocation and in any part of its course by laceration, stab, or gunshot wounds. The wrist is the most common site of external injury. Compression of the nerve at the wrist (carpal tunnel syndrome) may be secondary to prolonged occupational pressure, tenosynovitis with arthritis, or local in-

filtration, for example, by a thickening of connective tissue and deposit of amyloid with multiple myeloma or of mucopolysaccharides. Other systemic diseases associated with carpal tunnel syndrome are acromegaly and hypothyroidism. Incomplete lesions of the median nerve between the axilla and wrist may result in *causalgia* (see Chap. 3). The treatment of carpal tunnel syndrome is surgical section of the carpal ligament.

ULNAR NERVE This nerve is derived from the eighth cervical and first thoracic roots. It innervates the ulnar flexor of the wrist, the inner half of the deep finger flexors, the adductors and abductors of the fingers, the adductor of the thumb, the two medial lumbricals, and muscles of the hypothenar eminence. It is the sensory nerve to the fifth and ulnar half of the fourth fingers and the ulnar border of the hand. Complete ulnar paralysis results in a characteristic claw-hand deformity owing to wasting of the small hand muscles and hyperextension of the fingers at the metacarpophalangeal joints and flexion at the interphalangeal joints. The flexion deformity is most pronounced in the fourth and fifth fingers. Sensory loss occurs over the fifth finger, the ulnar aspect of the fourth finger, and the ulnar border of the palm. The ulnar nerve is most commonly injured at the elbow because of fracture or dislocation involving the joint. *Delayed ulnar palsy* may occur many years after an injury to the elbow joint which has resulted in a cubitus valgus deformity of the joint. Because of the deformity, the nerve is stretched in its course over the ulnar condyle. The superficial location of the nerve at the elbow makes it a common site of pressure palsy. Prolonged pressure on the outer part of the palm may result in damage to the deep palmar branch of the ulnar nerve, causing weakness of small hand muscles but no sensory loss.

Crural palsies The twelfth thoracic, first to fifth lumbar, and first, second, and third sacral nerve roots compose the lumbosacral plexuses and innervate the muscles of the lower extremities and "saddle" region. The following are the common crural palsies.

LUMBOSACRAL PLEXUS LESIONS The lumbosacral plexus is subject to a number of disease processes, mostly secondary. Diseases of the upper plexus produce unilateral weakness in flexion and adduction of hip, extension of knee and sensory loss over anterior thigh and leg; those of lower plexus cause weakness of posterior thigh, leg, and foot muscles with loss of sensation over the fifth lumbar and first and second sacral roots.

The diseases that affect the plexus are carcinoma of cervix and prostate, retroperitoneal tumors, iliopsoas hemorrhages from ruptured aneurysms and hemophilia, neuralgic amyotrophy, abdominal and thoracolumbar operations, and diabetes mellitus. These are discussed more fully by Adams and Victor.

LATERAL FEMORAL CUTANEOUS NERVE This nerve is derived from the second and third lumbar roots. It is a sensory nerve supplying the lateral aspect of the thigh. The nerve enters the thigh beneath the lateral end of the inguinal ligament and then enters the fascia lata, where it may become constricted. Compression of the nerve results in uncomfortable paresthesias along its cutaneous distribution and in sensory impairment. The condition is called *meralgia paresthetica* (mentioned below). The definitive treatment is surgical sectioning of the nerve at the inguinal ligament but this is seldom necessary.

OBTURATOR NERVE This nerve is derived from the second, third, and fourth lumbar roots. It supplies the adductor muscles of the thigh, and injury to the nerve results in almost complete paralysis of adduction of the thigh. The nerve is most frequently injured during the course of a difficult labor and also as a result of dislocation of the hip or an obturator hernia. It may be affected in diabetes, polyarteritis nodosa, osteitis pubis, and retroperitoneal and pelvic malignant tumors.

FEMORAL NERVE This nerve is derived from the second, third, and fourth lumbar roots. It supplies the iliacus, pectineus, sartorius, and quadriceps muscles and carries sensory impulses from the anteromedial aspect of the thigh and medial side of the lower leg. Following injury to the nerve, there is paralysis of extension of the knee, with wasting of the quadriceps muscle and also some weakness of hip flexion. The knee jerk is abolished. The nerve may be involved in fractures and dislocation of the hip and in fractured pelvis. It may be affected in diabetes, polyarteritis nodosa, and in retroperitoneal, pelvic, or abdominal lesions such as tumor, psoas abscess, or retroperitoneal hemorrhage. Because the femoral artery may also be severed, wounds in the femoral triangle may be fatal.

SCIATIC NERVE This nerve is derived from the fourth and fifth lumbar and first and second sacral roots. It provides the motor innervation of the hamstring muscles and all those below the knee; it carries sensory impulses from the posterior aspect of the thigh and posterior and lateral aspects of the leg and entire sole. In complete sciatic paralysis, the knee cannot be flexed and all muscles below the knee are paralyzed. The sciatic nerve is commonly injured in fractures of the pelvis or femur, in gunshot wounds of the buttock and thigh, by lying or sitting insensate and compressing the nerve in the lower buttock area, and by the inadvertent injection of toxic substances such as paraldehyde. It may also be involved by pelvic tumors and in both diabetes mellitus and polyarteritis nodosa. Cryptogenic forms also occur and are actually more frequent than those with an identifiable cause. A ruptured lumbar disk often simulates sciatic neuropathy. Incomplete lesions of the sciatic nerve occasionally result in causalgia.

COMMON PERONEAL NERVE This nerve is one of the terminal divisions of the sciatic nerve in the popliteal fossa. It supplies the dorsiflexors of the foot and toes and everters of the foot and sensation to the dorsum of the foot and lateral aspect of the lower half of the leg. These functions are lost with lesions which completely interrupt the nerve. Pressure or sleep palsy is one of the most frequent types of injury, the compression being of that part of the nerve which passes over the head of the fibula. It is also commonly involved by fractures involving the upper end of the fibula and in diabetic neuropathy, polyarteritis nodosa, and operations on the knee. Some are idiopathic, as pointed out by Berry and Richardson, who analyzed 70 personally observed cases.

TIBIAL NERVE This nerve is the other of the two terminal divisions of the sciatic nerve in the popliteal fossa. It supplies all the calf muscles and the flexors of the foot. Complete paralysis of the nerve results in a calcaneovalgus deformity of the foot, which no longer can be plantar-flexed. There is loss of sensation over the plantar aspect of the foot.

SOME DISEASES WHICH INVOLVE SINGLE NERVES OR PLEXUSES

INFECTIONS In faucial diphtheria, selective involvement of the vagi and nerves to the ciliary muscles of the eye results in palatal paralysis and paralysis of accommodation. The palatal palsy occurs in the first 2 weeks of infection and the loss of accommodation about a week later. Both tend to improve rapidly. In cutaneous diphtheria, involvement of nerves locally results in paralysis of the muscles supplied by the spinal segment from which the infected region is innervated. In leprosy, granulomatous involvement of skin and cutaneous nerves, particularly in the cooler parts of the body, dominates the clinical picture. Several nerves become involved at sites where they lie superficially, for instance, the median nerve at the wrist, the ulnar nerve at the elbow, and the peroneal nerve on the dorsum of the foot. Herpes zoster is a sensory neuritis of viral cause, characterized by acute inflammation of one or more posterior root ganglia, spinal nerves, and roots and gray matter of the spinal cord. Lancinating pain and hyperalgesia over the skin surface supplied by affected roots occur for 3 or 4 days, followed by the appearance of a segmental herpetic eruption. If the inflammatory process spreads to involve adjacent motor roots of anterior horns of the cord, segmental motor weakness and wasting appear. Paralysis of the oculomotor nerves may occur in conjunction with involvement of the gasserian ganglion (ophthalmoplegic zoster). Facial paralysis may occur with involvement of the geniculate ganglion (Ramsay Hunt syndrome). Sarcoidosis may involve single or multiple peripheral nerves, producing asymmetric mononeuritis or polyneuritis. Unilateral or bilateral facial paralysis is common in association with parotitis and uveitis in sarcoidosis.

TRAUMA External trauma may result in complete transection of a peripheral nerve or may block conduction without interrupting the anatomic continuity of the involved nerve, a state called *neuropraxia*. Complete division of a mixed peripheral nerve results in paralysis and sensory loss corresponding to the region supplied by the damaged nerve. Recovery of function after complete division can take place only when the divided ends lie in apposition or have been sutured. Growth of nerve fibers proceeds at a rate of 1 to 2 mm a day, and the recovery time can be estimated by the distance between the site of injury and the destination of the nerve. An early indication of regeneration is the presence of tingling sensation below the lesion (Tinel's sign which is due to sensitivity of thinly myelinated regenerating fibers) on tapping along the nerve. Sensory recovery precedes the return of motor power. All forms of cutaneous sensation begin to return together. Appreciation of pain and temperature improves, but the stimuli are poorly localized for some time. Eventually there is recovery of the discriminative aspects of sensation, including localization of sensory stimuli, postural sense, recognition of slight differences in temperature, and appreciation of very light touch.

PRESSURE PALSIES AND ENTRAPMENT NEUROPATHIES A period of prolonged compression of a nerve against an underlying bone results in temporary paralysis owing to myelin sheath damage. Mild degrees of compression (neuropraxia) are followed by fairly rapid recovery, in 2 to 12 weeks. Severe compression, such as may occur during a bout of alcoholic intoxication, deep sleep, or anesthesia, may result in focal disintegration of myelin, damage to axons, and Wallerian degeneration of distal segments. In this situation, recovery will be slow as regeneration takes place. Common varieties of pressure palsy are radial nerve paralysis with wrist drop due to prolonged pressure against the back of the arm (Saturday night palsy), ulnar palsy due to repeated trauma to the nerve at the elbow, especially after an old fracture that changes the relation of the nerve to the bicipital groove, and peroneal nerve palsy with foot drop caused by compression of the nerve against the fibula, as in sitting with legs crossed or during obstetric procedures with legs in stirrups.

The entrapment neuropathies result from chronic compression of a nerve against bone at a point where it passes through a narrow space. Slowly the perineurium and epineurium thicken and strangulate the nerve with injury to some of its larger, more peripheral, fibers. Several unique syndromes are known: (1) median nerve entrapment in carpal tunnel (see above); (2) *meralgia paresthetica*, a sensory neuropathy characterized by pain and paresthesia over the lateral aspect of the thigh because of compression of the lateral femoral cutaneous nerve at the level of Poupart's ligament or in the fascia lata; and (3) Morton's toe from pressure of plantar nerves against metatarsal bone, giving rise to pain and paresthesia of third and fourth toes on walking. Pressure on nerve roots in the cervical and lumbar regions by *herniated intervertebral disks* results in pain, sensory impairment, and variable motor weakness corresponding to the area supplied by the involved root (see Chap. 107). Compression of the medial cord of the brachial plexus by a *cervical rib or by some other malformation of the thoracic outlet* (thoracic outlet syndrome) results in atrophy of small hand muscles and sensory loss in the ulnar nerve distribution. Usually the subclavian artery is also compressed. When the median nerve is compressed at the wrist beneath the transverse carpal ligament (carpal tunnel syndrome), there are pain and paresthesias in the palmar surface of the hand and first three fingers, then atrophy, weakness in flexor of thumb and opponens muscle, and sensory impairment over the median nerve distribution.

TUMOR Peripheral nerves may be compressed or invaded by primary or metastatic tumors arising in other tissues. Solitary tumors of nerve sheaths, or neuromas, commonly occur along the roots of spinal nerves, chiefly in the thoracic and lumbar regions. Compression of the nerve root and adjacent spinal cord may occur. Root compression causes pain referred to the distribution of the involved nerve, and there may be associated sensory impairment and motor weakness. Lymphomatosis and carcinomatosis of the cranial and spinal meninges may implicate single or multiple nerve roots. Tumor cells may be found in the cerebrospinal fluid. Solitary neuromas may involve any of the peripheral nerves, producing local pain and tenderness to palpation. Multiple neuromas occur in von Recklinghausen's disease and are associated with multiple congenital anomalies, as well as kyphoscoliosis, cutaneous pigmentation, and cutaneous fibromas. The treatment of solitary expanding nerve tumors of the limbs is surgical, the nature and extent of the procedure depending upon the character of the individual tumor.

IDIOPATHIC NEUROPATHY *Bell's palsy* is due to inflammation of the facial nerve in the facial canal as a result of an obscure, possibly infective process. Edema may play a part leading to compression of nerve fibers, with resulting acute unilateral paralysis of facial muscles (see Chap. 376).

Brachial neuritis is an acute affection of the brachial plexus, characterized by the acute or subacute onset of severe pain in the neck, arm, and hand, followed by moderate muscle weakness, slight numbness or hyperesthesia, and depressed reflexes in the involved arm. The pain is usually severe and constant

and is aggravated by moving the arm or stretching the brachial plexus. Muscle wasting is rarely severe, but some cases of brachial neuritis, especially those described by the term *neuralgic amyotrophy,* may be followed by localized paralysis and atrophy of the shoulder girdle and arm muscles. Some of these have a familial incidence. Recovery slowly occurs over a period of months. Symptomatic treatment, including complete rest of the involved arm and analgesics in the acute phase, followed by mild massage and exercise, usually suffices.

Sciatic neuritis causes pain in the lumbar region and behind the leg from buttock to ankle. The pain is aching or burning in quality and is aggravated by movement or straining. The sciatic nerve is tender to palpation or stretching. There may be slight weakness of the hamstrings and muscles below the knee. The ankle jerk is absent. Sensory impairment is usually slight. It is necessary to distinguish the symptoms of sciatic neuritis from those of sciatic compression. In compression (e.g., by tumor) the onset is more gradual, symptoms are progressive, muscle wasting is more conspicuous, the nerve is less tender to palpation, and sensory loss is greater. The course of sciatic neuritis is stationary at first, followed by slow improvement.

Serum neuritis develops several days after the onset of serum sickness. The fifth cervical nerve root is most commonly involved, with pain, paralysis, and atrophy corresponding to the distribution of the nerve. Occasionally the entire brachial plexus may be involved, and there is sometimes, but rarely, a generalized polyneuritis. The cause is not known, but the condition is attributed to endoneurial edema, comparable to the urticaria of serum sickness, with compression of affected roots or nerves. Recovery is usually complete but may take weeks or months.

REFERENCES

ADAMS RD, VICTOR M: *Principles of Neurology.* New York, McGraw-Hill, 1977

ASBURY AK, JOHNSON PC: *Pathology of Peripheral Nerve.* Philadelphia, Saunders, 1978

BERRY H, RICHARDSON PM: Common peroneal palsy: A clinical and electrophysiological review. J Neurol Neurosurg Psychiatry 39:1162, 1976

BRADLEY WG: *Disorders of Peripheral Nerve.* Oxford, Blackwell Scientific Publications, 1974

DYCK PJ, LAMBERT EH: Polyneuropathy associated with hypothyroidism. J Neuropathol Exp Neurol 29:631, 1970

—— et al: *Peripheral Neuropathy.* Philadelphia, Saunders, 1975

HAYMAKER W, WOODHALL B: *Peripheral Nerve Injuries.* Philadelphia, Saunders, 1953

PRINEAS JW, MCLEOD JG: Chronic relapsing polyneuritis. J Neurol Sci 27:427, 1976

VINKEN PJ, BRUYN GW: Diseases of nerves, in *Handbook of Clinical Neurology.* Amsterdam, North-Holland, 1970, vols 7, 8

section 14 | Diseases of striated muscle

378

APPROACH TO CLINICAL MYOLOGY

ROBERT R. YOUNG
WALTER G. BRADLEY
RAYMOND D. ADAMS

GENERAL CONSIDERATIONS

Striated muscle tissue constitutes the principal organ of locomotion as well as a vast metabolic reservoir. Disposed in more than 600 separate muscles, this tissue comprises as much as 40 percent of the weight of an adult man. Intricacy of structure undoubtedly accounts for its diverse susceptibilities to disease.

A single muscle is composed of thousands of fibers which course for variable distances along its longitudinal axis. In some muscles the fibers extend the entire length of the muscle; in others they are joined end to end by connective tissue. Each fiber is a relatively large and complex multinucleated cell varying in length from a few millimeters to several centimeters (34 cm in the human sartorius muscle) and in diameter from 10 to 100 μm. Although the fiber normally represents an indivisible anatomic and physiologic unit, disease may affect only one part of it, leaving the remainder to atrophy, degenerate, or regenerate, depending on the nature and severity of the disease. Cell nuclei, which are oriented parallel to the longitudinal axis of the fiber and number into the thousands, lie beneath the plasmalemma membrane (the sarcolemma) and hence are called *sarcolemmal*. The cytoplasm (sarcoplasm) of the cell is abundant and contains myofibrils and various other organelles such as mitochondria, Golgi apparatus, and endoplasmic reticulum. The myofibrils in turn are composed of longitudinally oriented interdigitating filaments (myofilaments) of contractile proteins (actin and myosin). The transverse regular arrangement of actin (I, isotropic) and myosin (A, anisotropic) bands of molecules in the myofilaments produces the characteristic striations of skeletal muscle. There are two tubular systems of endoplasmic reticulum, one oriented longitudinally between myofibrils and one transversely (T tubules) at the A-I band region. The latter is a specialized structure and, with the two lateral cisternae of the longitudinal sarcoplasmic reticulum, forms a triad. Physiologically the T tubules are deep invaginations of the sarcolemma; hence they enclose an extracellular space. Droplets of stored fat, glycogen, various proteins, many enzymes, and myoglobin, the latter imparting the red color to muscle, have been identified within the sarcoplasm or its organelles.

Histochemistry has been widely used to study diseased muscle and the results have been summarized in a monograph by Dubowitz and Brooke. Histochemical stains of normal muscle show two classes of fibers, one staining darkly and the other lightly. The former is rich in oxidative enzymes and the latter in glycolytic enzymes. Oxidative-rich fibers (type I) are supplied by neurons that are normally designated "slow twitch" and are engaged predominantly in tonic postural muscular reactions; glycolytic-rich fibers (type II) are termed "fast twitch" and are involved mainly in phasic reactions. But in such stains (ATPase at pH 9.4 is most commonly used) there are other intermediate types, subclasses referred to as IIA, IIB, and IIC. Fiber types are found to react differently in certain diseases and in disuse and denervation atrophy, as will be elaborated further on in this chapter.

The individual muscle fibers are enveloped by delicate strands of connective tissue (endomysium) which provide for their support and permit unity of action. The blood vessels, of which there may be several for each fiber, and nerve filaments lie within the endomysium. Similar sheets of collagen (perimysium) bind together groups or fascicles of fibers and surround the entire muscle (epimysium). The muscle fibers are attached at their ends to tendon fibers, which in turn connect with the skeleton. By this means contraction maintains posture and effects movement. Specialized endings of sensory nerves wrap themselves around small striated muscle fibers described as *intrafusal* because they are grouped into fusiform bundles of 4 to 12 within a connective tissue capsule, termed the *muscle spindle*. These are scattered within each muscle and lie in parallel to the great mass of extrafusal fibers described above. By means of a complex feedback arrangement, the spindle afferent nerve impulses permit the central nervous system to monitor changes in muscle length. Another specialized intramuscular sensory organ is found at the ends of extrafusal muscle fibers where they attach to a tendon. The latter, called *Golgi tendon organs,* are in series between muscle and tendon fibers; afferent nerve impulses from them reflect the tension produced by contraction.

Other notable characteristics of muscle are its natural mode of activation, i.e., innervation, and the necessity of intact nerve supply for the maintenance of its nutrition. Each muscle fiber (intra- or extrafusal) receives a nerve twig from a motor nerve cell in the anterior horn of the spinal cord or nucleus of a cranial nerve, which joins it at a point called the *neuromuscular junction* (also called the *motor end plate*). Acetylcholine is liberated from presynaptic vesicles in the nerve terminals and transmits the nerve impulse to the muscle fiber. Acetylcholine receptors and cholinesterase, which play a special role in neuromuscular transmission, are concentrated postsynaptically at this junction zone. Groups of noncontiguous muscle fibers with a common innervation from one anterior horn cell constitute the "motor unit" which is the basic physiologic unit in all reflex, postural, and voluntary activity. In addition to motor nerve fibers within the muscle nerve, there are the two types of large sensory fibers (proprioceptive), one from the muscle spindles and another from the Golgi tendon organs, which participate in reflex control of muscle activity. There are also small fibers from free nerve endings which subserve pain sensation, and postganglionic sympathetic fibers to blood vessels.

It would be a mistake to predicate that apparent similarity of structure renders all muscles equally susceptible to disease. In point of fact, no disease affects all muscles in the body, and each neuromuscular disease has as one of its features a unique distribution of muscle involvement. These topographic differences between diseases provide incontrovertible evidence of unique structural qualities, not presently disclosed by the light or electron microscope. One factor may relate simply to fiber size. Consider, for example, the large diameter and length of the fibers of the gluteus and paravertebral muscles in comparison with the ocular muscles. Again, the number of fibers composing a motor unit may be of significance in explaining selective vulnerability; e.g., in the ocular muscles the motor units contain only 6 to 10 muscle fibers, whereas in the gastrocnemius, each motor unit contains as many as 2000 fibers. The territory of each motor unit varies from 5 to 10 mm, and adjacent units interdigitate. There are also individual differences in vascular patterns of supply, permitting some muscles to withstand the effects of hypoxia or vascular occlusion (as occurs transiently during forceful contraction) better than others. Metabolic differences among fibers within any one muscle have been revealed by histochemical studies, certain fibers being richer in glycolytic and poorer in oxidative enzymes than others.

Regarding the pathogenesis of myopathic disease, one may envisage causative agents which affect each of the different components of sarcoplasm, namely, an enzyme, an essential substrate, the filamentous proteins, the endoplasmic reticulum, or the sarcolemma itself. The endomysial connective tissue also could be the primary pathway in disease, since it so closely invests the muscle. Inadequacy of blood supply in relation to the metabolic requirements of active muscle, or frank ischemia from vascular occlusion, could be postulated as another mechanism of disease. Finally, the nerve or its cell of origin in the spinal cord is known to bear the brunt of certain pathologic processes paralyzing all the muscle fibers of that motor unit and removing its unique trophic influence on muscle.

Normal muscle possesses a limited capacity to regenerate, a point often forgotten. Acute destructive processes of the muscle fiber, e.g., inflammatory, metabolic, and certain other diseases, are usually followed by fairly complete restoration of the muscle cells, providing some part of each fiber has survived and the endomysial sheaths of connective tissue have not been disturbed. Unfortunately many pathologic processes of muscle are chronic and unrelenting and completely destroy the muscle fibers. Under such conditions any regenerative activity fails to keep pace with the disease, and the loss of muscle fibers is permanent.

MYOPATHOLOGY

Several basic disorders may be distinguished by means of muscle biopsy and postmortem examination:

1 *Denervation atrophy.* This consists of reduction in size of fibers within denervated motor units, with enlargement of the area of intact motor units by collateral sprouting from intact nerves. This is best revealed by grouping of fibers of one histochemical type.
2 *Segmental necrosis of muscle fibers* with myophagia, regeneration, and forking or branching. This is the typical change in idiopathic polymyositis (in combination with infiltrates of inflammatory cells), in infective polymyositis (in the presence of trichina, toxoplasma, etc.), in Zenker's degeneration, in Duchenne's and other dystrophies, in alcoholic polymyopathy, and in Meyer-Betz paroxysmal myoglobinuria.
3 *Disfigurative changes in muscle fibers.* These include sarcoplasmic masses and ringbinden in myotonic dystrophy, glycogen masses in glycogen storage diseases, rod (nemeline) and other cytoplasmic bodies in the congenital myopathies, hyperplasia, aggregation, and other abnormalities of mitochondria.
4 *Disturbances in number and size of fibers* as a reflection of abnormalities of growth, maturation, and aging. Many states of dwarfism and congenital myopathies of a myotubular type present principally as numerical or volumetric

changes, which must be distinguished from denervation atrophy, disuse effects, cachexia, and work hypertrophy. Certain diseases may affect only one fiber type; for example, all forms of disease leading to disuse of the muscle produce atrophy of type II fibers.
5 *Disorders of conduction apparatus* (neuromuscular junctions, sarcolemma, and sarcoplasmic reticulum), in which nerve fibers and muscle fibers appear to be intact and the abnormality can be revealed only by special physiologic, morphologic, pharmacologic, or biochemical techniques. Myasthenia gravis, botulism, and the periodic paralyses fall into this category.

BIOPSY OF MUSCLE AND NERVE If muscle or nerve biopsy is to be of maximal diagnostic value, both surgical and microscopic techniques must be exacting. The muscle chosen for study should show evidence that it has been affected but not totally destroyed by the disease in question, and it should not recently have been studied electromyographically since the trauma of the needle electrodes produces focal destructive lesions. Muscle biopsy is indicated (1) to aid in the differentiation among neuropathic atrophy, dystrophy, metabolic myopathy, and polymyositis; (2) to corroborate the diagnosis of diffuse diseases of connective tissue and blood vessels (e.g., polyarteritis nodosa, lupus), or special infections (e.g., trichinosis, toxoplasmosis); (3) for diagnosis of metabolic diseases involving muscle (e.g., glycogen storage disease) and the special myopathies (nemaline and central core myopathies); and (4) in the scientific study of disorders of neuromuscular transmission apparatus (e.g., myasthenia gravis, periodic paralysis), usually by a combination of electrophysiologic, pharmacologic, histochemical, and electron microscopic techniques. In most instances, it is possible to distinguish histologically the effects of denervation, the dystrophies and other necrotizing myopathies, special disfigurative myopathies, and polymyositis.

The muscle biopsy is performed under local or general anesthesia. The local anesthetic must be confined to the skin and superficial fascia. Three cylinders of muscle about 2 cm long and 0.5 cm in diameter are taken. One specimen for histology is kept at its original length in a biopsy clamp, and fixed in 10% neutral formalin, embedded in paraffin, sectioned in a cross and longitudinal fashion, and stained by hematoxylin and eosin, phosphotungstic acid hematoxylin, and Gomori trichrome methods. The second specimen for histochemistry is rapidly frozen in liquid nitrogen, sectioned transversely in a cryostat, and stained by various histochemical reactions (e.g., myosin ATPase, mitochondrial oxidative enzymes, phosphorylase). The third piece in a biopsy clamp is fixed in glutaraldehyde for electron microscopy. Special techniques may be applied, if it is desirable to visualize the intramuscular nerves and myoneural junctions, such as the methylene blue–cholinesterase method of Cöers and Woolf.

Biopsies of nerves may be taken under local or general anesthesia. The sural nerve is a commonly biopsied sensory nerve, and the whole nerve or a fraction (fascicular biopsy) may be taken. The nerve is fixed under tension to stretch the fibers and is processed by the fixation, staining, and embedding techniques of electron microscopy. Even when studied by ordinary microscopy, nerve biopsies provide very useful histopathologic data. Before fixation, these biopsies can also be studied physiologically in vitro where fibers of all sizes can be stimulated and their activity recorded. In contrast to routine nerve conduction studies where only the largest fibers can be sampled, this in vitro technique affords a rapid, semiquantitative assessment of the effects of the disease process on fibers of each of the different sizes contained within the nerve.

BIOPHYSICS AND BIOCHEMISTRY OF NEUROMUSCULAR DISEASE

The biochemical tests presently in use fall into two categories: measurement of serum electrolytes, enzymes, and other chemicals and detection of myoglobin and abnormal amounts of creatine and creatinine in the urine. In certain diseases biochemical studies performed on muscle removed at biopsy may be diagnostic.

ELECTROLYTES AND THEIR EFFECTS ON NEUROMUSCULAR EXCITABILITY In the resting state all nerve and muscle fibers are *polarized* with the interior of the cell negative to the outside surface by a potential difference of 70 to 90 mV. This *resting membrane potential* is closely related to the electrochemical equilibrium for potassium ions, the interior of the cell being some 30 times richer in this ion than the extracellular fluid on the outside of the nerve or muscle membrane. At equilibrium, the chemical forces tending to promote diffusion of K ions outward (down their concentration gradient) are counterbalanced by electrical forces, since the relative external positivity opposes the movement of further K ions to the outside. At the resting potential, the situation for Na ions is quite the opposite. Since their external concentration is 10 to 12 times that within the cell, they tend to be driven inward because of both their concentration gradient and the electrical attraction of the relative negativity inside the cell. Under resting conditions, however, these forces are ineffective by virtue of the very low permeability of the sarcolemma to Na ions. Any leakage of Na into the cell is overcome, initially by the diffusion of an equal amount of K outward, and subsequently by the metabolically active expulsion of Na ions (*sodium pump*).

The membrane permeability to Na is controlled by the membrane potential—depolarization producing increased permeability to Na due to activation of sodium carriers in the nerve cell. With slight electrically or chemically mediated depolarization there is a brief influx of Na, but the subsequent diffusion of K outward repolarizes the membrane and, therefore, reduces its permeability to Na. This is the "passive decay" of change in resting potential. If, when the depolarization is greater and a *threshold* is reached at which the outward K current is unable to stabilize the situation, the membrane is further depolarized, it becomes progressively more permeable to Na, and an explosive *regenerative Na current* develops. Na rushes down its chemical and electrical gradients into the cell which eventually approaches the equilibrium potential for Na with the interior of the cell now 20 to 40 mV positive. This *action potential* lasts a millisecond or less because the membrane now becomes almost impermeable to Na and much more permeable to K. The resulting efflux of K repolarizes it to the resting level.

The regenerative Na current cannot be activated by another depolarizing stimulus during the *refractory period* until the membrane has been repolarized. If this process of recovery is delayed, *depolarization inactivation* of the Na current prevents the development of further action potentials until the resting membrane potential has been restored. These various membrane phenomena responsible for the resting and action potentials do not themselves depend directly upon energy-rich substrates, though such metabolically active processes are essential for the sodium pump and the long-term maintenance of resting ionic concentrations.

Because the region of membrane at the site of the action potential becomes polarized oppositely to the remainder, *ac-*

tion currents flow into the former from the surrounding regions and depolarize them. The depolarization may reach the threshold for development of an action potential there, and new zones of increased Na permeability then spread in this way in an all-or-none fashion down the length of the nerve or in both directions from the center of the muscle membrane as a *conducted action potential.*

Clearly, these events, the hallmarks of all excitable tissues, are modified by the concentration of K ions in extracellular fluids. Other ions, particularly Ca, Mg, and Cl, are also influential.

The *neuromuscular junction* (motor end plate) has properties of special importance. Here a motor nerve twig indents the surface of the muscle fiber which it innervates. The membranes of the two cells, the neurilemma and the sarcolemma, remain separated by a narrow space, the *synaptic cleft*. Across this space acetylcholine diffuses, liberated from presynaptic vesicles by the arrival of *nerve action potentials*. Ca ions facilitate the release of packets (*quanta*) of acetylcholine from the vesicles, and botulinus toxin, aminoglycoside antibiotics, or a very high concentration of Mg ions interfere with this release. Acetylcholine receptors on the specialized, chemically excitable area of muscle membrane which forms the postsynaptic portion of the end plate react to the presence of acetylcholine with a local increase in the conductance of Na, K, and other small cations, producing a depolarization which can be recorded as the *end plate potential*. Thus, the spontaneous release of quanta of acetylcholine produces miniature end plate potentials in the postsynaptic membrane. If the depolarization of the membrane is large enough, current flow into it from the neighboring electrically excitable areas of muscle membrane depolarizes it toward the threshold potential. Once the threshold is reached, an independent, all-or-nothing *muscle action potential* arises and, in the same manner as the nerve action potential is conducted, propagates over the surface of the sarcolemma toward both ends of the fiber.

The electrical change appears to be distributed from the surface of the muscle fiber inward to all the myofibrils via the transverse tubular system (T system) to activate the longitudinal sarcoplasmic reticulum, and thus the contractile mechanism. Calcium is released from the depolarized membrane of the sarcoplasmic reticulum into the sarcoplasm, activates myosin adenosine triphosphatase (ATPase), energy is released by the dephosphorylation of adenosine triphosphate (ATP), cross-bridges form between the actin and myosin filaments, and they slide past one another shortening each sarcomere and producing tension. The resultant shortening constitutes the ultrastructural equivalent of contraction.

This mechanical change or *twitch* lasts a great deal longer than the action potential. A second electrical wave can, therefore, arrive before the muscle fiber has relaxed, prolonging the contraction, and if the anterior horn cell fires (or the motor axon is stimulated) at frequencies of 10 to 20 per second, the twitches fuse into a prolonged contraction (tetanus). The mechanical event can thus be smoothed into a continuous process, but the electrical potentials remain a series of peaks of external negativity, separated by plateaus during part of which the membrane is in its resting polarized state.

This *repolarization* after passage of an action potential is necessary if the membrane is to be capable of transmitting a second impulse. At the end plate, repolarization is possible only if acetylcholine is removed, a process of hydrolysis achieved by the enzyme cholinesterase. If this fails, the end plate remains depolarized and cannot respond to further nerve impulses. *Anticholinesterases* such as neostigmine (Prostigmin), pyridostigmine (Mestinon), edrophonium (Tensilon), physostigmine (Eserine), diisopropyl fluorophosphate (DFP), tetraethylpyrophosphate (TEPP), and several of the "nerve gases" and pyrophosphate insecticides act in this way to paralyze muscle. These substances and the so-called *depolarizing blocking agents* (succinylcholine and decamethonium) paralyze by maintaining the end plate region in a depolarized state (depolarization inactivation), refractory to the arrival of further nerve impulses. Curare-like substances and possibly antibodies to receptor substance, the so-called "competitive blocking agents," paralyze muscle in a different way by occupying receptor sites for acetylcholine on the postjunctional membrane, thereby preventing the neurotransmitter from depolarizing the muscle fiber.

Biochemical disturbances may account not only for impairment of neuromuscular activity, resulting in weakness or paralysis, but also for its enhancement, reflected in excessive irritability to mechanical or other stimuli. "Spontaneous" discharges may occur, or a single nerve impulse may set off a train of action potentials in nerve or muscle. Hypocalcemic and hypomagnesemic *tetany* ensues in this way when the membrane of the nerve fiber becomes unstable. Ca and Mg both tend to stabilize the membrane, and changes in their concentrations within the range seen clinically affect conduction in peripheral nerve rather than function at the neuromuscular junction where their actions, opposite or competitive, require changes in concentrations usually incompatible with life. Ischemic paresthesias also arise on the basis of irritability. Some types of axonal myokymia (Isaac's syndrome) and certain benign fasciculations as well as the common cramps of calf and foot muscles (painful, sustained, involuntary contractions with motor units discharging at frequencies above 25 per second) may be due to increased excitability of the peripheral parts of the motor nerve. Hyponatremia or Na loss predisposes to cramps, as does the unaccustomed use of a muscle. Quinine, procainamide, diphenhydramine (Benadryl), and warmth tend to prevent them. Myotonia, a noncalcium-related irritability of the sarcolemmal membrane, is related to abnormally low chloride permeability of the sarcolemma. A high chloride conductance normally buffers the sarcolemma against the depolarizing action of extracellular K ions released during the preceding impulse.

The mechanism by which the muscle action potential initiates the contractile process is termed *excitation-contraction coupling;* the energy for this process is derived from the interaction of ATP with the special muscle proteins. The pyrophosphate bonds of ATP supply the energy and must be replenished constantly, a reaction which involves interchanges with the muscle phosphogen, creatine diphosphate, where high-energy phosphate bonds are stored. These interchanges in both directions require the action of creatine phosphokinase (CPK). The intracellular calcium which, as noted above, is released by the muscle action potential must be reaccumulated within the sarcoplasmic reticulum before actin and myosin filaments can slide back past one another with relaxation. This re-uptake of calcium (*relaxing factor*) requires the expenditure of considerable energy. When ATP is lacking, the muscle remains contracted as in *rigor mortis* or the electrically silent *contracture* of phosphorylase deficiency (McArdle's syndrome). The same sort of contracture occurs under normal conditions in the "catch muscles" of certain mollusks.

Reconstitution of ATP requires oxidative or glycolytic metabolism. Muscle fibers differ in their content of oxidative versus glycolytic enzymes; the latter determine their ability to sustain anaerobic metabolism during periods of tonic contraction when intramuscular blood flow is compromised. Muscle cells with primarily aerobic metabolism have high concentrations of oxidative enzymes, are rich in mitochondria, contain greater concentrations of myoglobin (appear red), have slower rates of contraction and relaxation, fire more tonically, and are less fatigable than muscle cells poor in oxidative enzymes and myoglobin ("pale") but rich in glycolytic enzymes, which fire phasically in short bursts. The speed of contraction, a function

of the exact type of the myosin ATPase is low in the former and high in the latter type of muscle cell. The activity of calcium-activated myosin ATPase at pH 9.4 has been used to classify muscle fibers into two major types: type I ("red") possesses low and type II ("pale") high activity. Type II fibers may be subdivided into type IIA (fast oxidative) and type IIB (fast glycolytic) fibers. All the muscle fibers within one motor unit are of the same metabolic type.

To summarize, the muscle fiber, which is totally dependent on nerve for its stimulus to normal contraction, may be paralyzed in a number of ways. There may be failure of nerve to conduct an impulse, insufficient release of acetylcholine to depolarize the muscle cell, damage or inaccessibility of the postjunctional membrane to normally released acetylcholine, or the presence of a pharmacologic agent preventing repolarization of the end plate. Finally, the sarcolemmal membrane itself may fail to distribute the muscle impulse throughout the fiber, or the metabolic or contractile elements of the muscle may be temporarily or permanently deficient. Similarly, fascicular twitching, cramps, and muscle spasms may be due to excessive activity at a number of points in the neuromuscular apparatus. There may be instability of the nerve fiber, as in tetany, or unexplained hyperirritability of the motor neuron, as in amyotrophic lateral sclerosis. The threshold level for mechanical activation or electrical reactivation of the sarcolemmal membrane may be reduced, as with myotonia, or a change may occur within the muscle fiber itself, which, once shortened, may have insufficient energy for restoration to a relaxed state (contracture).

When the musculature is acutely and diffusely weakened, or when twitchings, spasms, and cramps occur, serum electrolytes should be studied. They reflect extracellular levels, and the ECG (see Chap. 232) may reveal alterations in intracellular content in cardiac muscle, which tends to parallel that of skeletal muscle. If the *plasma level of potassium falls below 2.5 meq or rises above 7 meq per liter,* weakness of extremity and trunk muscles results. When the concentration reaches 2 or 9 meq per liter, there is almost invariably flaccid paralysis of these muscles and later of the respiratory ones as well, only those of cranium, e.g., extraocular, tending to be spared. In addition, the tendon reflexes are diminished or absent. The reaction of muscle to percussion is also reduced or abolished, suggesting impairment of transmission along the sarcolemmal membranes themselves. Hypocalcemia of 7 mg per 100 ml or less (as in rickets or hypoparathyroidism) or relative reduction in the proportion of ionized calcium (as in hyperventilation) causes increased irritability of the neurilemma (and to a lesser extent sarcolemma) and spontaneous discharge of sensory and motor nerve fibers, i.e., tetany (see Chap. 379) and sometimes convulsions. Frequent repetitive and finally prolonged spontaneous discharges appear in the electromyogram (EMG). Hypercalcemia above 12 mg per 100 ml (as in vitamin D intoxication, hyperparathyroidism, and carcinomatosis) causes lethargy and weakness, perhaps on a central basis. *Magnesium deficiency* (from decreased intestinal absorption or increased renal losses due to diuretics, gentamycin, or primary renal diseases) with serum levels less than 1.0 meq per liter results in tetanic muscle spasms and convulsions: a considerable *increase in magnesium levels* leads to muscle weakness and depression of central nervous function (confusion). The weakness of muscle may be due, in part at least, to reduced release of acetylcholine at the motor end plate.

CHANGES IN SERUM LEVELS OF ENZYMES ORIGINATING IN MUSCLE CELLS In all diseases which cause extensive damage to striated muscle fibers, intracellular enzymes leak out of the fiber and enter the blood. Those which are now being measured in most hospital laboratories are the transaminases, lactic acid dehydrogenase, aldolase, and creatine phosphokinase. But high concentrations of these enzymes are found in heart muscle and/or liver cells; hence raised serum values may be due to myocardial infarction or hepatitis, as well as to the necrobiotic diseases of striated muscle (polymyositis, muscle trauma, muscle infarction, Meyer-Betz paroxysmal myoglobinuria, and the more rapidly advancing muscular dystrophies). For the serum levels to be interpretable, one must have evidence of the integrity of heart and liver. Isoenzyme patterns are of some value in separating the enzyme derived from skeletal muscle from that of other organs. Creatine phosphokinase (CPK), though present in heart and brain, is found in highest concentration in striated muscle. If the normal level is 0 to 65 IU per liter of serum, it may exceed 1000 IU in patients with destructive lesions of striated muscle. Even more interesting is its rise in some patients with progressive muscular dystrophy before there is enough destruction of fibers for the disease to be clinically manifest. Moreover, about 75 percent of the unaffected female carriers of Duchenne's pseudohypertrophic muscular dystrophy may now be identified because they often show slight elevations of serum CPK level. All workers are agreed that alterations of serum enzyme levels are nonspecific for dystrophy since they occur in all types of disease which injure or destroy the muscle fiber. Moreover, in the more slowly evolving types of dystrophy, such as that of Landouzy-Dejerine, the serum levels of CPK may be normal. It was hoped that the values would always be normal in denervation paralysis and muscular atrophy, but unfortunately they may be slightly elevated in patients with progressive muscular atrophy and amyotrophic lateral sclerosis.

ENDOCRINOPATHIES In a number of disorders of endocrine glands, muscle weakness may be a prominent feature, and occasionally it becomes even a chief complaint. While these diseases are discussed in detail elsewhere (Chaps. 381 and 383), it should be noted that such weakness, local or generalized, acute or chronic, may occur in the absence of changes in serum electrolytes or enzymes. Specific hormone assays are then necessary for diagnosis. This is particularly true of thyrotoxicosis, where severe muscle paresis may appear without the classic signs of Graves' disease.

MYOGLOBINURIA The red pigment, myoglobin, responsible for much of the color of muscle, is an iron protein compound present in the sarcoplasm of striated skeletal and cardiac fibers. Of the total body hematin compounds, about 25 percent is in muscle, the remainder in red blood corpuscles and other cells. Destruction of striated muscle, regardless of the process, liberates myoglobin, and because of its relatively small size, the molecule filters through the glomerulus and appears in the urine, imparting to it a burgundy red color. The serum is effectively cleared and retains its normal color. In contrast, hemolysis of red blood corpuscles which frees hemoglobin, colors both serum and urine because of the high renal threshold. Myoglobinuria should thus be suspected when the urine is deep red and the serum normal in color. As in hemoglobinuria, the guaiac and benzidine tests are positive, and the final demonstration depends on spectroscopic analysis, which shows an absorption band at 581 nm. The urine does not fluoresce, as it does in porphyria. Myoglobin appears in the urine in the following conditions: spontaneous myoglobinuria of unknown cause, e.g., Meyer-Betz paroxysmal myoglobinuria; as a result of crushing or infarction of muscles; in rare cases of polymyo-

sitis and alcoholic and other myopathies such as McArdle's disease; following extreme muscular activity; and after the ingestion of certain toxic substances (from fish poisoned by waste products, as in Haff disease).

CREATINURIA Creatine, an amino acid, is a prominent constituent of striated muscle tissue. It may be ingested (exogenous creatine) but is also synthesized in the liver from glycine, arginine, and methionine and then delivered to the skeletal muscles, which contain the largest amount of this compound of any organ (150 mg per 100 g fresh weight muscle tissue). Creatinine, the anhydride of creatine, is a degradation product which is excreted in the urine. The creatinine content of muscles is low (about 5 mg per 100 ml), since it diffuses readily through the sarcolemma. Normal male serum contains 0.2 to 0.6 mg per 100 ml creatine; female serum, 0.4 to 0.9 mg. Creatinine serum levels range from 0.8 to 1.4 mg and are increased only in serious renal disease. Adult 24-h urine excretion of creatine averages from 60 to 150 mg in normal men and 100 to 300 mg in women. Creatinine excretion is remarkably constant at 1.0 to 1.6 g per day. In diseases such as progressive muscular dystrophy, the creatine content of the muscle fiber is diminished, and there is a decrease in creatinine excretion, increase in creatine excretion, and hypercreatinemia. The same alterations occur in neurogenic atrophy and with reduction in muscle mass in polymyositis, hyperthyroidism, Addison's disease, and male eunuchoidism. Ingestion of 1 to 3 g creatine will not significantly raise its level in blood or urine in a normal person, for the muscles are not saturated, but in an individual with a reduced muscle mass, creatinemia and creatinuria result. This type of creatine tolerance test thus merely indicates reduction in functional muscle mass. Studies of creatine and creatinine are no longer greatly used in the investigation of neuromuscular disease.

PHYSIOLOGY OF NEUROMUSCULAR ACTIVITY

ELECTROMYOGRAPHY Normally, a muscle twitch can be produced by a brief electrical pulse, less than 1 ms long (Faradic), because it stimulates motor nerve fibers within the muscle. After denervation, contraction can be produced only by much longer pulses (galvanic), which are necessary to stimulate the muscle fibers directly. This difference (Erb's reaction of degeneration) led to the plotting of strength-duration curves, a technique which is rarely necessary now.

The *motor unit* is defined as a motor neuron, its axon, and all the muscle fibers which it innervates. All movement, posture, and reflex activity are interpreted in terms of the integrated discharge of large numbers of these motor units by spinal and supraspinal mechanisms. Strength of muscle contraction can be reduced to the number of motor units enlisted at a given time, the frequency of their discharge, and the speed of contraction to the phasic versus tonic recruitment of units. A tendon reflex is caused by a volley of sensory impulses from receptors within muscle spindles which briefly activate a group of the large (alpha) spinal motor neurons. Effectiveness of movement is related to the manner in which motor units of different muscles are activated and inhibited in reciprocal relations. Coordination of movements, posture, and automatic movements such as walking and running are understandable in terms of more complex spinal integrations of muscles. Paralysis represents the reverse, an inactivation of motor units or whole muscles, complete only upon severance of the peripheral motor innervation and followed then by extreme atrophy of muscle fibers with fibrillation and unusual generalized hypersensitivity to acetylcholine.

The striated muscles are numerous, scattered, and, in some instances, of large size. As a result, no small series of leads (cf.

ECG) will give an average picture of their electrical activity. They must be tested laboriously, one at a time, because disease may be spread irregularly through many of them, so that normal findings in one area do not exclude the possibility of pathologic phenomena close by. External plate or surface electrodes, such as those used in ECG and EEG, will pick up potentials representing the chance summation of many motor units, giving only an average picture. A more detailed physiologic analysis requires fine concentric needle electrodes to be placed carefully within a muscle so as to register the activity of only a small number of motor units or muscle fibers.

As an impulse travels from the center toward either end of an active muscle fiber, current begins to flow outward through the normally polarized region under the recording electrode toward the depolarized zone. Therefore, as in Fig. 378-1, the recording electrode becomes slightly positive relative to the reference electrode, and the beam of the cathode ray oscilloscope (CRO) is deflected, by convention, downward (at *A*). When the depolarized region moves under the recording electrode, the latter rapidly becomes quite negative (upward deflection at *B*). As the active region moves further down the sarcolemma, away from the electrode, the membrane under the latter slowly becomes repolarized. Current again begins to flow outward through the membrane toward the distant depolarized region, and the electrode, therefore, becomes relatively positive once again, as at *C*, before becoming isopotential to the reference electrode at rest. The net result is a triphasic action potential recorded on the CRO as in Fig. 378-1, with a very rapid negative-going phase, a configuration typical of fibrillations recorded from denervated and spontaneously active single muscle fibers. Because these potential changes are completed in less than 5 ms, the inertia-free CRO must be used to record them (ink writers do not have the necessary frequency response).

RECORDING OF MOTOR UNIT ACTIVITY The simple triphasic potentials discussed above result from the activity of single muscle fibers, but in healthy muscle, single fibers are not independently active. Normally, excitation arrives via the motor nerves so that all the fibers of one motor unit are activated by any one impulse from the motor neuron (as indicated in Chap. 15). The size of the normal motor units varies from several muscle fibers per motor axon in extraocular or laryngeal muscles to several thousand muscle fibers per axon in some of the large limb-girdle muscles. In each motor unit, the fibers are not of uniform diameter, length, or shape, and their spatial orientation with regard to the electrode will vary. In normal muscle, the fibers of one motor unit are not packed tightly together in groups but are spread out in one general region of the muscle interspersed with the fibers of adjacent motor units. Such muscle activated by its nerve, therefore, produces rather complex motor unit potentials, presumably the result of summation of potentials of varying characteristics from each fiber of the motor unit within recording range of the electrode.

THE NORMAL ELECTROMYOGRAM Normal muscle is electrically silent when it is at rest. Once *insertion activity,* produced by the trauma of placing the needle, has died down, the electrodes record no propagated action potentials. When a muscle is voluntarily contracted, action potentials appear on the CRO screen. As a slowly progressive contraction begins, potentials of one motor unit appear at rates of 4 to 5 per second and increase to 8 to 10 per second; with increasing power of contraction, a second, or even third, unit will be *recruited,* slightly larger in size than the first. As the contraction becomes even stronger, more and larger motor units enter the picture, and their potentials begin to overlie each other until there results a disorderly crowd of action potentials of many sizes and shapes, firing at rates of about 20 per second. Since individual motor

unit potentials can no longer be distinguished, this is referred to as a complete *interference pattern.* Obviously, a muscle contracting weakly because of less than full effort or disease of central or peripheral nervous or muscular systems will have fewer than normal active fibers and will produce a smaller total potential than normal. However, unless reduction in output is sufficient either to break up the interference pattern just described so that individual motor unit potentials become identifiable or to reduce its amplitude strikingly, one obtains no certain electrical evidence of abnormality. As long as a normal muscle is held actively contracted, the interference pattern continues. Gradual relaxation will result in a progressive dropping out of motor units until a few are left firing, then one, then none.

Skeletal muscle may also be artificially stimulated by the application of brief electric pulses through the skin overlying its motor nerve. With proper stimulating conditions, there will be one maximal muscle response for each shock, the form of which will depend upon the number of motor units activated and the number sampled by the recording electrodes. If repeated shocks are given, each response will have the same form and amplitude, until fatigue supervenes. Normal muscle will follow rates of stimulation greater than 25 per second for periods of at least 60 s before decrement of the action potential indicates the failure of some fibers to respond, probably because of failure of nerve impulse transmission at branching points of the terminal axon. This ability of muscle to follow repetitive stimulation is altered in certain diseases.

THE ABNORMAL ELECTROMYOGRAM Deviations from normal are detected in (1) the occurrence of "spontaneous" activity during relaxation (fibrillations, positive sharp waves, and fasciculations); (2) abnormalities in the amplitude, duration,

FIGURE 378-1
The shaded area represents the zone of the action potential which is negative to all other points on the fiber surface. It is shown at three points in its course (from left to right) along the fiber. At each point, the correspondingly lettered portion of the triphasic muscle action potential displayed on the cathode ray oscilloscope (CRO) reflects the potential difference between the active (vertical arrow) and reference (Ref.) electrodes. Polarity in this and subsequent figures is negative upward as depicted. The time calibration is on the CRO screen; for further details see text.

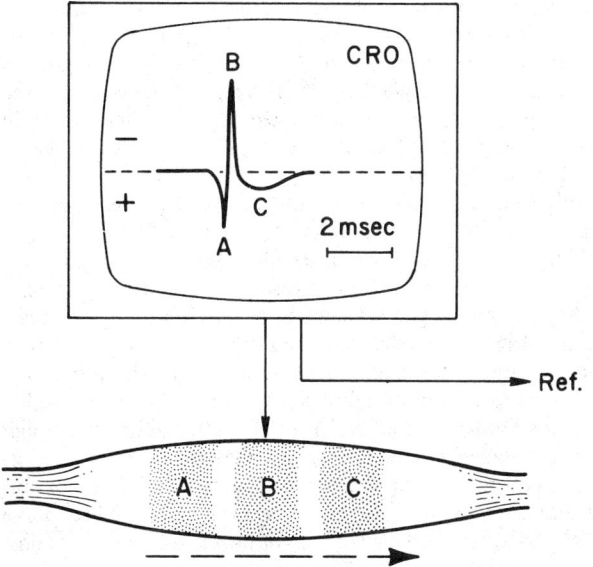

and shape of single-motor-unit potentials; (3) a decrease in the number of motor units which can be recruited; (4) alteration in size, duration, or interpotential interval of action potentials recorded during graded single or successive voluntary or electrically induced muscular contractions; (5) the demonstration of special phenomena, such as myotonia, coupling (tetany), bizarre high-frequency potentials, or electrical silence during obvious shortening of the muscle (contracture); and (6) the documentation of various movement disorders.

Spontaneous activity during complete relaxation At the moment the needle is placed in the muscle, there is usually a brief burst of action potentials which cease once the needle is stable, providing it is not in a position to irritate an intramuscular nerve fiber. Myotonic muscle is extremely irritable; long runs of high-frequency discharges, waxing and waning in frequency with a "dive-bomber" sound, may be produced and recur at the slightest movement of the needle. Irritability is also found with conditions which dispose to muscle cramp, in polymyositis and in certain denervated muscles. Spontaneous activity of motor units and of single muscle fibers, known respectively as *fasciculation* and *fibrillation,* are abnormal.

Fibrillation The two phenomena of fibrillation and fasciculation are often confused. Fasciculation, discussed below, consists of synchronous contraction of *groups of muscle fibers* integrated by a single axon into a motor unit. Fibrillation is the contraction of *single muscle fibers* and appears only when destruction of a motor axon has disintegrated its motor unit.

When a motor neuron is destroyed by disease, or when its axon is severed, the distal part of the axon degenerates, a process which takes several days. The muscle fibers formerly innervated by the branches of the dead axon, viz., the muscle unit, are disconnected from the nervous system. For reasons which are still obscure, the chemosensitive region of the sarcolemma at the motor end plate "spreads" after denervation to involve the entire surface of the muscle fiber. Then, 10 to 25 days after death of the axon, the denervated fibers develop spontaneous activity, similar perhaps to that found in the sinoatrial (SA) node of the heart; i.e., each fiber contracts at its own rate and without relation to the activity of its fellows. There results a totally random conglomeration of brief, triphasic fibrillation potentials and diphasic positive sharp waves. The latter are usually more easily recognized signs that muscle fibers have been denervated. Fibrillation and positive sharp-wave activity continue until the muscle fiber is reinnervated by the outgrowth of new axons, either from the proximal (central) end of the damaged nerve or from nearby healthy nerve fibers, or until the fiber is replaced by connective tissue, a process which may not take place for many years. In the last case, the denervated fibers become angulated and atrophic and stain densely with oxidative enzyme stains. They can also be recognized in muscle biopsies.

Fibrillation and positive sharp-wave activity are prominent in patients with neuropathies or other lesions affecting the peripheral nervous system but are also seen with primary diseases of muscle, such as polymyositis or muscular dystrophy, where necrosis of one segment of a muscle fiber disconnects the distal portion of that fiber from the centrally placed portion containing the neuromuscular junction. The distal segment of muscle, which is functionally isolated ("denervated"), develops fibrillation and positive sharp-wave activity. Though these spontaneous potentials signify that muscle fibers or portions of fibers are denervated, their presence does not guarantee that the underlying disease process primarily affects nerve fibers. An alternative explanation of fibrillation potentials pos-

tulates a lowered resting membrane potential (-65 mV) in denervated and damaged fibers, which makes the muscle fiber more easy to discharge.

Fasciculation An involuntary single contraction of a motor unit in isolation is termed fasciculation. Since a large number of muscle fibers contract together, visible dimpling or twitching of the skin occurs, though ordinarily not enough power is exerted to move a joint. The form of the accompanying EMG potential, like that of an ordinary motor unit, is relatively constant for any one fasciculating unit. Commonly, it will have three to five phases, a duration of 5 to 15 ms (somewhat less in the facial muscles), and an amplitude of several millivolts. With "benign fasciculations" seen in normal subjects, the same unit tends to repeat at a fairly regular rate of 1 per second, or even faster, indicating a rhythmic activation of the fibers by the responsible axons. With the "malignant fasciculations" described below, the rate is considerably slower at 1 per 3 or 4 s and slightly less regular.

Traditionally, fasciculation occurs in chronic, slowly advancing, destructive disease of the anterior horn cells, such as amyotrophic lateral sclerosis and progressive spinal muscular atrophy. In these diseases, fasciculation potentials are numerous and may exceed 15 ms in duration. They are often seen in the early stages of acute poliomyelitis but are recorded less commonly than in the chronic diseases mentioned, perhaps because the affected cells die too rapidly. They are also seen with compressive root lesions, certain exceptional motor neuropathies, and early in the disease course of some patients with acute idiopathic polyneuritis. With peripheral lesions such as those caused by herniated nucleus pulposis (ruptured disk), large numbers of axons may be affected with the result that the fasciculations (or even cramps) may be more obvious to the patient than the twitching with disease of anterior horn cells. In all these cases, the damaged neuron seems to be "irritated" by the disease process, fires repetitively, and, in so doing, produces activity in all the muscle fibers that it innervates. It has been shown that fasciculation may also follow peripheral nerve lesions, giving way to fibrillation upon death of the axon. More important is the fact that fasciculation, particularly in the calves and hands, occurs occasionally in many normal persons and constantly in some, and so it need not be evidence of disease at all. Shivering induced by low temperature and the twitchings associated with depressed serum calcium levels are sometimes confused with fasciculation.

Abnormalities in motor unit potentials The following abnormalities in amplitude, duration, and shape of motor unit potentials can be noted.

ENLARGED POTENTIALS IN PARTIALLY DENERVATED AND REINNERVATED MUSCLE Early in the course of denervation, any motor units with functional connections to the spinal cord are unaffected, and though the number of motor unit potentials appearing during contraction is reduced, the configurations of the remaining ones are quite normal. In time, those remaining often increase in amplitude, perhaps to two to three times normal, and become longer in duration and *polyphasic* (more than four phases). Such large and, sometimes, *giant potentials* arise from motor units, as in Fig. 378-2C, containing more than the usual number of muscle fibers spread out over a greatly enlarged territory within the muscle. Presumably, new nerve twigs have *sprouted* from undamaged axons, reinnervated previously denervated fibers, and added them to their own motor units. Some of these reinnervated units may become extremely polyphasic and prolonged, a finding pathognomonic of reinnervation. These units are to be differentiated from (1) those with lesser degrees of "polyphasicity" which are of normal duration and account for as much as 25 percent of the activity recorded from normal muscles, particularly at the end plate zone, and (2) the polyphasic but brief units seen with primary muscle disease. The histochemical counterpart of the motor unit enlargement is *fiber* type grouping. Denervation of such a large motor unit produces *grouped atrophic fibers*.

REDUCED AMPLITUDE AND DURATION OF ACTION POTENTIALS Diseases such as polymyositis, the muscular dystrophies, and other myopathies which destroy scattered fibers within a motor unit or render them nonfunctional, as in Fig. 378-2*B*, obviously reduce the population of fibers per motor unit. When such a unit is activated, its potential is, therefore, of lower voltage and shorter duration than normal, and it may also appear polyphasic as the compound motor unit potential is fragmented into its constituent single-fiber potentials. When most of the muscle fibers are affected, the motor unit potentials from these very small units may be difficult to differentiate from fibrillation potentials, and when destruction of all fibers is completed, electrical activity ceases. These small, brief voluntary motor unit potentials, with their characteristic high-pitched crackling sound from the audio monitor, occur in all forms of progressive muscular dystrophy and, unfortunately, are indistinguishable from those of polymyositis, dermatomyositis, and other chronic myopathies. In the myositides, however, fibrillation potentials, as noted above, may often be seen as well. In myasthenia gravis, where transmission of impulse fails progressively at one neuromuscular junction after another in any one motor unit, the EMG potential of that unit may be normal at first and become more *myopathic* as fatigue progresses. Potentials from muscles which are chronically weak in myasthenics are then proportionately myopathic. It can be seen, therefore, from Fig. 378-2*B* that the motor unit potentials will appear equally myopathic whether the disease process directly affects single muscle fibers within the unit as in dystrophy, disturbs neuromuscular transmission at single junctions as in myasthenia gravis, or blocks transmission of the nerve impulse in single axon terminals as probably occurs in thyrotoxic and certain carcinomatous "myopathies."

DECREASE IN NUMBER OF MOTOR UNITS AVAILABLE Diseases which reduce the population of functional lower motor neurons or motor axons within the peripheral nerve obviously decrease the number of motor units which can be recruited in the affected muscles. The number of motor units available for activation varies then in proportion to the strength of a maximal voluntary contraction, appearing no longer as an interference pattern but only as a *single-unit pattern* or a *mixed pattern*.

DECREASE IN NUMBER OF MUSCLE FIBERS If muscle power is reduced in diseases such as dystrophies or other myopathies, where individual muscle fibers are affected, there will be little or no reduction in the number of motor units available for recruitment, though each unit will consist of fewer muscle fibers than normal. A maximal voluntary effort will then be associated with a normally complete interference pattern despite marked weakness. Because fewer muscle fibers are active, the amplitude of the pattern will be reduced from normal. A highly complex interference pattern of less than usual amplitude, in the face of dramatic weakness, is the hallmark of a so-called myopathic process.

PROGRESSIVE REDUCTION OR INCREMENT WITH SUCCESSIVE CONTRACTIONS In certain disorders, the size of the initial motor unit potential is normal with voluntary contraction, as is the size of the compound muscle action potential produced by an electric stimulus applied to the nerve. However, during a minimal contraction or after two or three stimuli, at rates as low as 1 to 15 per second, the amplitude of the potentials falls off, though not to zero, and then increases again after the

fourth or fifth stimulus. This pattern of "decrement," maximal with the fourth or fifth stimulus, is characteristic of *myasthenia gravis*. Like the partial block at the neuromuscular junction produced by curare, it may be relieved by neostigmine—the pathophysiology is largely postjunctional in both cases. Progressive decline of action potentials with repetitive stimulation may occur in poliomyelitis, in myotonia, or in certain other diseases of the motor unit, but the pattern described for myasthenia gravis is not then present.

In some cases of oat-cell carcinoma of the lung and rarely sarcoidosis with muscular weakness, the Eaton-Lambert syndrome, a condition with somewhat opposite findings, may be observed. If electrical stimulation through nerve is rapid (20 to 30 per second) or follows a brief voluntary contraction, muscle

FIGURE 378-2

The shaded muscle fibers are functional members of one motor unit; the axon, which enters from the upper left, branches terminally to innervate the appropriate muscle fibers. The motor unit action potential produced by each motor unit is seen in the upper right; its duration is measured between the two vertical lines. The normal-appearing but unshaded fibers belong to other motor units. A. The normal situation is schematized with five muscle fibers in the active unit. B. In this myopathic unit, only two fibers remain active; the other three (shrunken) have been affected by one of the primary muscle diseases. C. Four fibers which belonged to other motor units and had been denervated have now been reinnervated by the terminal axon sprouting from the healthy active motor unit. Both the motor unit and its action potential are now larger than normal. Note that only under these abnormal circumstances do fibers in the same unit lie next to one another.

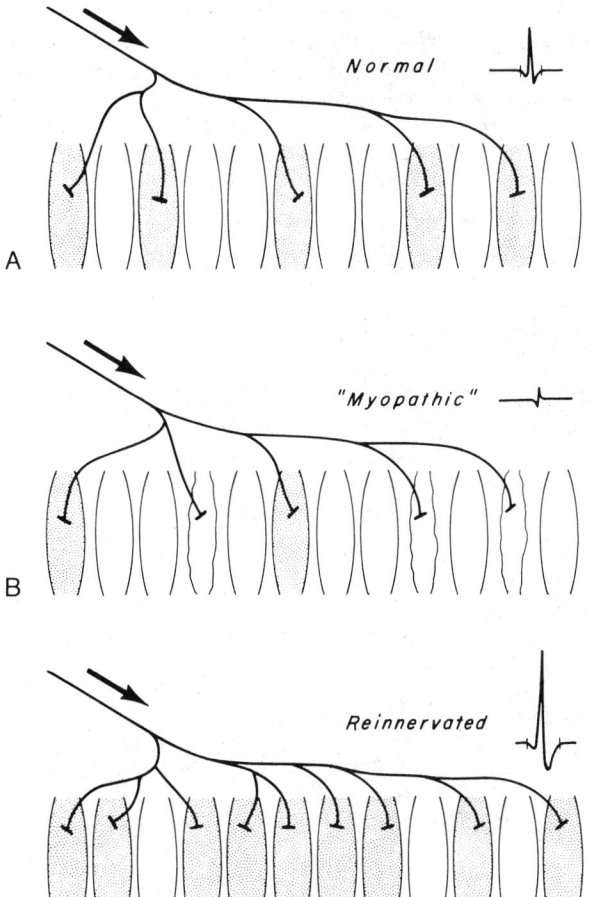

Normal

"Myopathic"

Reinnervated

A

B

C

action potentials which were small or practically absent with the first stimulus now increase in voltage with each successive one until a more nearly normal amplitude is attained. This phenomenon is unaffected by neostigmine, but it may be reversible with guanidine (20 to 35 mg/kg per day in divided doses). The pathophysiology of this "reversed" myasthenic syndrome is prejunctional and compromises release of acetylcholine, as does botulinus toxin or the aminoglycoside antibiotics (see Chap. 350).

By the use of single-fiber EMG techniques, it is possible to record what is termed "jitter" and thereby measure accurately (within tens of microseconds) the performance of single pairs of neuromuscular junctions. Characteristic quantitative abnormalities are found in patients with myasthenia gravis or other disorders of neuromuscular transmission. This technique also provides insights, hitherto unavailable, into the pathophysiology of other diseases of peripheral nerve and muscle.

SPECIAL ABNORMALITIES IN THE EMG In *myotonia,* the sarcolemmal membrane is irritable, and muscle contraction persists despite voluntary attempts at relaxation. The symptom is prominent in several hereditary diseases, myotonia congenita (Thomsen's disease), dystrophia myotonica (Steinert's disease), and hyperkalemic periodic paralysis (adynamia episodica hereditaria); minor forms occur sporadically under other circumstances, and it can be produced by drugs interfering with

FIGURE 378-3

The median nerve may be stimulated through the skin at the wrist (1) or in the antecubital fossa (2), and the resultant compound muscle action potential may be recorded as the potential difference between a surface electrode over the thenar emininence (arrow) and a reference electrode (Ref.) more distally. Sweep 1' on the CRO depicts the stimulus artifact (moment of stimulation at 1) followed by the muscle potential. The distal latency is the time A' on the CRO sweep (3.0 ms, for example) which corresponds to conduction over distance A in the hand. The same is true for sweep 2' where stimulation is at point 2, and the time from artifact to response is A' + B'. The maximal motor conduction velocity from points 2 to 1 is obtained by dividing distance B by time B'.

chloride conductance in humans and animals. Myotonia consists of high frequency repetitive discharges which wax and wane in amplitude and frequency, producing a "dive-bomber" sound on the audio monitor. It is produced mechanically by percussion or movement of the needle electrode. The characteristic electrical picture is also seen following voluntary contraction or electrical stimulation of the muscle via its motor nerve. The voluntary motor unit potentials appear normal, but they are not followed by the silence which normally occurs on relaxation. Instead there is a burst of rapid activity which may take as long as several minutes to subside. Some of the potentials of this prolonged discharge have the duration, amplitude, and form of single-fiber activity, while others appear to have the characteristics of motor unit potentials. If the muscle is activated repeatedly at short intervals, the late discharge becomes briefer and briefer and eventually disappears as the myotonia diminishes temporarily.

Bizarre high-frequency discharges without waxing and waning (*pseudomyotonia*) are seen in hypothyroidism or with certain types of denervation. High-frequency coupling of action potentials into doublets, triplets, or higher multiples of single units, indicating instability in repolarization of the nerve fiber, occurs in tetany and facial spasm.

Contracture, as with cramping in McArdle's disease, percussion and contraction myoedema, and percussion fasciculation, has no electrical counterpart (the EMG is silent). This aspect of these phenomena is important in their definition.

EMG IN DIFFERENTIAL DIAGNOSIS OF MOVEMENT DISORDERS EMG techniques, often employing surface rather than needle recordings, are very helpful in differentiating among parkinsonian, essential-familial, anxiety, thyrotoxic, and cerebellar tremors; in separating minor degrees of asterixis from tremor; in the recognition of myoclonus; and in differentiating "spasticity" from rigidity. EMG recordings of blink reflexes can document clinically undetectable lesions of the brainstem (as with multiple sclerosis).

ELECTRONEUROGRAPHY Conduction velocity of nerve Painless and harmless techniques are widely used for both percutaneous stimulation of the larger peripheral motor and sensory nerve fibers and recording of their conducted action potentials. These routine techniques provide numerical data which are of considerable clinical interest. The results of these *motor and sensory nerve conduction studies,* expressed simply as latency in milliseconds or conduction velocity in meters per second, are more objective than the results of electromyography and afford certain information unavailable from EMG studies.

An accessible nerve is stimulated through the skin by surface electrodes, and the resulting compound action potential is recorded by electrodes on the skin (1) over the nerve more proximally in the case of orthodromic activity in large sensory fibers stimulated in the digital nerves, or (2) over the muscle more distally in the case of motor fibers in a mixed nerve (Fig. 378-3). The conduction time from the most distal stimulating electrode, measured in milliseconds from the stimulus artifact to the onset of the response, is also termed the *distal* or *peripheral latency.* If a second stimulus can be applied to a mixed nerve more proximally (or if recording electrodes can be placed more proximally in the case of sensory fibers), a new and longer conduction time can be measured. When the distance (in millimeters) between the two sites of stimulation of motor fibers or recording of sensory fibers is divided by the difference in conduction times (in milliseconds), a *maximal conduction velocity* (in meters per second) is obtained which describes the velocity of propagation of the action potentials in the largest and fastest nerve fibers. These velocities in normal subjects vary roughly from a minimum of 40 or 45 m/s, depending upon which nerve is studied, to a maximum of 75 or 80 m/s. Values are lower in infants, reaching the adult range by the age of 2 to 4 years. Normal values also exist for peripheral latencies from the distalmost site on various mixed nerves to the appropriate muscles; when one stimulates the median nerve at the wrist, for example, the latency (Fig. 378-3*A*) for conduction through the carpal tunnel to the abductor pollicis brevis muscle in the thenar eminence is always less than 4.5 ms in normal adults. Similar tables of normal values have been compiled for orthodromic sensory conduction velocities and distal latencies. Nerve conduction velocity is affected by fiber diameter and degree of demyelination. Unmyelinated or segmentally demyelinated fibers conduct impulses much more slowly, as do fibers with smaller diameters.

When motor fibers in a mixed nerve are stimulated and every one is in functional continuity with its many muscle fibers, the compound action potential of many hundreds of microvolts derived from the many firing muscle fibers can easily be recorded from electrodes on the skin over the muscle. However, when one is dealing with sensory potentials, activity is recorded from nerve fibers themselves; one lacks the "amplification" provided by all the muscle fibers in one motor unit, and much greater electronic amplification is required. In the clinic, therefore, sensory potentials may, under abnormal circumstances, be very small or absent even when powerful computer-averaging techniques are used, and sensory conduction measurements are often impossible to record, though at other times they may be abnormally slow. In contrast, a reliable motor conduction velocity is possible if one functional nerve fiber remains.

These conduction velocities reflect the status of surviving nerve fibers and, if the latter are unaffected by the disease process, may be normal despite widespread denervation; e.g., following incomplete transection of a nerve by a sharp object, the maximal motor conduction velocity may be normal in the few remaining fibers, although the muscle involved is almost paralyzed. In most neuropathies, the axon itself is primarily affected either because of disease of the cell body with "dying-back" changes peripherally or because of damage to the axon with distal Wallerian degeneration. This is true for typical alcoholic, nutritional, paracarcinomatous, uremic, other metabolic, and most diabetic neuropathies. The axons which remain intact may conduct impulses normally so that, when the larger fibers have been affected, the remaining fibers with smaller diameters, that naturally conduct more slowly, account for a slightly slower maximal conduction velocity. Also, segmental demyelination may be present even in these primarily axonal neuropathies. Though it is of lesser importance, it may further decrease the conduction velocity to a slight degree.

The total reduction in velocity is often not great enough to place any single value outside the range of normal, although at other times velocity may be slightly below normal to 35 or 40 m/s at worst. Ordinary nerve conduction studies can usually, therefore, be used to document the presence of neuropathy in the disease under question only by comparison of values recorded from a population of patients with those from a control group of the same age and sex. Techniques have recently been devised to study conduction in longer and more proximal segments of nerve than is possible routinely. These involve accurate measurements of latencies for F waves and H reflexes—both of which require conduction in nerves going from the periphery of a limb to the spinal cord and back again. By use of these methods, the diagnostic yield of nerve conduction studies is increased so that the chance of a patient with one of these axonal neuropathies having a diagnostically abnormal test rises to 80 or 90 percent.

Though most diseases of peripheral nerves do not necessarily produce a clear-cut reduction of nerve conduction velocity as it is routinely measured, other, relatively uncommon disorders, such as acute idiopathic polyneuritis (Landry-Guillain-Barré syndrome), diphtheria, metachromatic leukodystrophy, Krabbe's disease, and the hypertrophic neuropathies including Déjèrine-Sottas disease and many cases of Charcot-Marie-Tooth disease, that affect Schwann cells primarily, produce segmental demyelination with marked reduction in conduction velocities which are usually in the range of 10 m/s.

Focal compression of nerve, as in the various entrapment syndromes, also produces localized slowing of conduction, because of narrowing of axons and demyelination at the site of compression. The demonstration of such localized slowing of conduction affords ready confirmation of nerve entrapment; for example, if the peripheral latency in the median nerve (Fig. 378-2*A*) exceeds 5.0 ms while that in the ulnar nerve remains normal, compression of the median nerve in the carpal tunnel is extremely likely. Similar focal slowing of conduction may be recorded from the ulnar nerve at the elbow or peroneal nerve at the fibular head when either is compressed (see Chap. 377). A normal conduction time, however, cannot rule out an entrapment syndrome.

Microneurography Disease of peripheral nerve may produce the electromyographic evidences of denervation discussed above, but more quantitative observations of neural function can be made by studies of the electrical activity of nerves themselves. Hagbarth, Struppler, and colleagues have, by means of very fine needle electrodes placed within human peripheral nerves in situ, pioneered the recording of single-fiber activity from muscle afferent and autonomic and cutaneous fibers within peripheral nerves. This *microneurography* promises to be of critical importance in the understanding of many aspects of human physiology and disease but will likely remain a research technique.

CLINICAL MANIFESTATIONS OF MUSCLE DISEASE The large number and diversity of diseases of striated muscle exceed the number of symptoms and signs by which they express themselves clinically. Different diseases thus must share certain common symptoms and even syndromes. To avoid excessive repetition in the description of individual diseases, there is some advantage to discussing in one place the clinical manifestations seen in *clinical myology*. (See Table 378-1 for a syndromic classification of muscle disease.)

Weakness and paralysis Assuming there are no signs of disease of the corticospinal tracts of the spinal cord and nerve fiber disease, reduced strength of contraction, reflected in diminished power of single contractions [peak or power factor (PF) in performance] or of repeated contractions [endurance factor (EF)], stands as an indubitable sign of muscle disease. Fatigability per se less reliably denotes muscle affection, since it is most often due to some psychic aberration linked to anxiety and depression or to systemic illness (see Chap. 12). It is noteworthy that slight weakness of muscle may be present, even though tests of PF, because of the crudeness of clinical measurement, lack of quantitation, and the uncertainty of gaining the patient's full cooperation, may seem to reveal no definite diminution in power. Theoretically, with milder degrees of weakness, a diminution of EF elicited in a series of timed contractions against a fixed resistance (ergogram) may more reliably demonstrate the disorder than does PF. Furthermore, sustained or repeated maximal muscle contraction over a given period of time evinces optimally the myasthenic reaction, i.e., a rapid failure of contraction, with the power being restored within minutes by rest. This, in fact, in combination

TABLE 378-1
Syndromic classification of muscle diseases

I Acute (days) or subacute (weeks) paralytic disorders of muscle (may cause weakness *or* paralysis)
   A Rarely fulminant myasthenia gravis
   B Polymyositis and dermatomyositis
   C Alcoholic myopathy
   D Acute paroxysmal myoglobinuria (*Note:* First attack of episodic weakness may enter into differential diagnosis; see below)
   E Botulism
   F Organophosphate poisoning
   G Acute spinal or peripheral nerve diseases (denervation paralysis where paralysis is often severe and widespread and atrophy may or may not be present)
      1 Poliomyelitis
      2 Acute idiopathic polyneuritis or other forms of polyneuropathy (porphyria, beriberi, etc.)
      3 Rarely polyarteritis nodosa with polyneuropathy

II Chronic (i.e., months to years) paralytic disorders of muscle (weakness usually with severe atrophy)
   A Progressive muscular dystrophy
      1 Duchenne type
      2 Facioscapulohumeral type (Landouzy-Dejerine)
      3 Limb girdle type (Erb's and Leyden-Moebius)
      4 Distal type (Welander's)
      5 Myotonic dystrophy (Steinert's disease)
      6 Progressive ophthalmoplegic or oculopharyngeal types
   B Chronic polymyositis
   C Chronic thyrotoxic and other metabolic myopathies
   D Chronic slowly progressive or relatively stationary polymyopathies
      1 Central core disease
      2 Rod body (nemaline) and related polymyopathies
      3 Pleoconial, megaconial, and myotubular polymyopathies
      4 Glycogen storage disease
      5 Congenital benign hypotonia and congenital universal hypoplasia of muscle
   E Progressive muscular atrophies and other forms of motor system disease (amyotrophic lateral sclerosis, progressive bulbar palsy) and infantile muscular atrophy (Werdnig-Hoffmann disease).
   F Chronic neural muscular atrophies such as peroneal muscular atrophy (Charcot-Marie-Tooth), hypertrophic polyneuritis (Dejerine-Sottas), amyloid polyneuropathy, chronic nutritional, arsenical, leprous, and other polyneuropathies

III Episodic weakness of muscle
   A Myasthenia gravis
   B Symptomatic myasthenia of other types
      1 With lupus erythematosus disseminatus

      2 With polymyositis
      3 With rheumatoid arthritis
      4 With nonthymic carcinoma
   C Familial periodic paralysis (hypokalemic)
   D Hereditary adynamia (hyperkalemic periodic paralysis, or Gamstorp's disease)
   E Paramyotonia congenita (Eulenberg's disease)
   F Hyper- and hypokalemia (including primary hyperaldosteronism)
   G Acute thyrotoxic myopathy (also thyrotoxic periodic paralysis)

IV Stiffness, soreness, involuntary spasm, and cramp
   A Congenital myotonia (Thomsen's disease), paramyotonia congenita, and myotonic dystrophy
   B Tetanus
   C Tetany
   D Black widow spider bite
   E Hypothyroidism with pseudomyotonia (Debré-Semelaigne and Hoffmann syndromes)
   F Myopathy resulting from myophosphorylase deficiency (McArdle's syndrome) and other forms of contracture
   G Contracture with Addison's disease
   H Idiopathic cramp syndrome

V Myalgic states
   A Connective tissue diseases (rheumatoid arthritis, menopausal arthritis, lupus erythematosus, polyarteritis nodosa, scleroderma, polymyalgia rheumatica, polymyositis)
   B Localized fibrositis or fibromyositis
   C Many forms of polyneuritis
   D Trichinosis
   E Myopathy of myoglobinuria and McArdle's syndrome
   F Myopathy with hypoglycemia
   G Bornholm's disease
   H Anterior tibial syndrome

VI Localized muscle mass(es)
   A Rupture of a muscle
   B Muscle hemorrhage
   C Muscle tumor
      1 Rhabdomyosarcoma
      2 Desmoid
      3 Angioma
      4 Metastatic nodules
   D Localized idiopathic myopathy
   E Localized and generalized myositis ossificans
   F Fibrositis (myogelosis)
   G Granulomatous infections
      1 Sarcoidosis
      2 Tuberculosis
   H Pyogenic abscess (pyomyositis)

with a restoration of power, i.e., disappearance of the myasthenic state, by neostigmine and edrophonium (Tensilon) stands as the most valid clinical criterion of the various forms of myasthenia gravis.

Qualitative changes in the contractile process In addition, other qualities of muscular contraction and relaxation may be discovered by observing, during one or a series of maximal actions of a group of muscles, the speed and efficiency of contraction and relaxation. Slow waves of contraction in a muscle such as the quadriceps may be seen on change in posture (contraction myoedema) in hypothyroidism. Here it is often associated with percussion myoedema and slowness of tendon reflex. Slowness in relaxation is another indication of a thyroid deficiency state, accounting for the complaints of uncomfortable tightness and firmness of proximal limb muscles.

A prolonged failure of relaxation with afterdischarge is a characteristic of myotonia, as in congenital myotonia (Thomsen's disease) and dystrophia myotonica (Steinert's disease). But a true myotonia, with its long electrical discharges of action potentials, unlike the electrically silent myoedema and contracture (see below), requires strong contraction for its elicitation, is more evident after a period of relaxation, and tends to disappear with repeated contractions. This persistence of contraction is demonstrable upon tapping a muscle (percussion myotonia), a phenomenon easily distinguished from the electrically silent local bulge (myoedema) induced by a sharp tap of a muscle in the myxedematous or cachetic patient.

Increase in power in a series of several voluntary contrac-

tions in the absence of myotonia is a feature of the Eaton-Lambert syndrome of small-cell carcinoma of the lung.

The effect of cold on muscle contraction may also prove informative; either paresis or myotonia, lasting for a few minutes, may be evoked or enhanced by cold as in the paramyotonia of von Eulenberg.

Myotonia and myoedema must be distinguished from the recruitment and spread of involuntary spasm induced by strong and repeated contractions of limb muscles in patients with mild or *localized tetanus*, which is not a phenomenon of muscle but is due to an abolition of inhibitory spinal mechanisms.

The repeated contraction of forearm and leg muscles after the application of a tourniquet (above arterial pressure) to the proximal part of the limb will often elicit latent tetany. The latter state must be separated from ordinary cramp by its special mode of development and duration, its enhancement by hyperventilation, the presence of accompanying tingling and prickling paresthesias, and also from true contracture.

In *true contractures* a group of muscles, after a series of strong contractions, may remain shortened for many minutes, unable to relax because of failure of the metabolic mechanism necessary for relaxation; the muscle in this shortened state remains electrically silent in the electromyogram, in contrast to the tremendous high-voltage, rapid discharges observed with cramp, tetanus, and tetany. Such contracture occurs in McArdle's phosphorylase deficiency, where it is aggravated by arterial occlusion, but it has been seen in deficiencies of phosphofructokinase and in other glycolytic enzymes (Chap. 97).

Pseudocontracture (myostatic contracture) which inevitably follows all conditions which occasion prolonged fixation and complete inactivity of the normally innervated muscle, is another common disorder. The muscle fibers are shortened with loss of sarcomeres; fibrosis may also occur. It is distinguished from ankylosis by the springy nature of the resistance coincident with increased tautness of muscle and tendon during passive motion, and from *Volkmann's contracture,* where there is evident fibrosis of muscle and the surrounding tissues due to ischemic injury, usually after a fracture of the forearm.

Topography of paralysis: patterns of paralysis In the majority of the diseases under consideration, some of the muscles are affected and others are spared. Each disease exhibits its own pattern. Moreover, the topography or distribution of involvement tends to follow the same pattern in all patients with the same disease. Thus, determination of the topography of muscular involvement provides one of the most valid diagnostic attributes of a disease, ranking next in importance after altered quantity and quality of contraction.

To ascertain the extent and severity of muscle weakness, one undertakes a systematic examination of all the main groups of muscles from forehead to feet. The patient is asked to contract each group quickly with as much force as can be mustered, while the examiner opposes the movement and offers a graded resistance in accordance with the degree of residual power. If the weakness is unilateral, one has the advantage of being able to compare it with the action of muscles on the normal side. If it is bilateral, the physician must refer to an idea of what constitutes normalcy, based on experience in muscle testing. Ocular, facial, lingual, pharyngeal, laryngeal, cervical, shoulder, upper arm, lower arm and hand, truncal, pelvic, thigh, and lower leg-foot muscles are examined quickly in this order. To facilitate description and comparison, a rating scale must be used. Six graded steps, from normal power to paralysis, are readily distinguishable: 5 represents normal power; 4, weakness with ability to overcome resistance by the examiner; 3, weakness with ability only to overcome gravity; 2, severe weakness, movement only possible with gravity eliminated; 1, trace of movement; 0, no movement. With practice one can distinguish pseudoparalysis from pain, unwillingness to cooperate, and feigned weakness (see Chap. 15).

The following topographic patterns are so well known that they constitute a core of essential clinical knowledge in this field.

1 Ocular palsies presenting more or less exclusively as diplopia, ptosis, or strabismus, sometimes in association with exophthalmos, enophthalmos, and pupillary change.

As a rule muscle diseases do not affect the pupil, and in most instances their effects are bilateral. In single-nerve lesions the neural origin is revealed by the combination of paralyses of eye muscles or sympathetic paralysis of the pupil. When weakness of the orbicularis oculi muscle (muscle of eye closure) is added to ocular palsies and ptosis, it nearly always signifies myopathic disease.

Myasthenia gravis, progressive ocular dystrophy of Kiloh and Nevin, exophthalmic ophthalmoplegia of thyroid disease, curare-sensitive nonmyasthenic ophthalmoplegias, myotonic dystrophy of Steinert, ocular dystrophy with retinitis pigmentosa (and heart block, dwarfism, ovarian dysgenesis, Kearns-Sayre syndrome), centronuclear myopathy, and botulism are the principal conditions to be considered. When ptosis or weakness of eye closure occurs alone or in combination with weakness of other skeletal muscles, one should think of Landouzy-Dejerine facioscapulohumeral dystrophy, oculopharyngeal dystrophy, and the nemaline form of congenital myopathy.

2 Bilateral facial palsy presenting as an inability to smile and expose teeth and to close eyes. Mild bilateral facial weakness is observed in myasthenia gravis, and ptosis and ocular palsies are usually conjoined (90 percent of cases) in this disease. The same is true of myotonic dystrophy. More severe or complete facial palsy occurs in facioscapulohumeral dystrophy, in Landry-Guillain-Barré syndrome (nearly always with other weaknesses), and in combination with abducens palsies in the Moebius syndrome. Sometimes polyneuritis cranialis multiplex causes bilateral facial paralysis.

3 Bulbar palsy presenting as dysphonia, dysarthria, and dysphagia with or without a hanging jaw or facial weakness. Myasthenia gravis is the most frequent cause of this syndrome and must also be considered whenever there is the solitary finding of a hanging jaw or fatigue of jaws while eating or talking; but usually ptosis and ocular palsies are conjoined. The same is true of myotonic dystrophy and botulism. Progressive bulbar palsy may be the basis of this syndrome, and the diagnosis is most obvious when the tongue is withered and twitching. The neurologic condition known as pseudobulbar palsy is readily distinguished by the lack of atrophy of muscle, the mode of onset (often sudden), and the associated clinical findings. Platybasia and the Arnold-Chiari malformation may also reproduce some of these findings by involving the lower cranial nerves and their nuclei. Diphtheria and bulbar poliomyelitis may present in this way. Pure dysphagia may be an early manifestation of polymyositis.

4 Cervical palsy presenting often as the hanging-head syndrome, or inability to lift the head from the pillow. The patient may be unable to hold up the head owing to weakness of the posterior neck muscles, or to lift it from a pillow because of weakness of the anterior neck muscles. If this condition is severe, the head may loll unless it is held up by the patient's hands.

This condition occurs most often in idiopathic polymyositis, dermatomyositis, and myasthenia gravis. It tends to be combined with dysphagia. The major types of progressive muscular dystrophy, when advanced, usually weaken neck flexors and extensors, but seldom to the point where the head must be held in the hands. Rarely syringomyelia, syphilitic meningoradiculitis, subacute poliomyelitis (in conjunction with carcinomatosis), motor system disease, or Kugelberg-Welander syndrome may differentially paralyze the neck muscles.

5 Bilateral brachial palsy presenting sometimes as the dangling-arm syndrome. Weakness, atrophy, and fasciculations of hands and arms and sometimes of the shoulders characterize the commonest syndrome of motor system disease, namely, amyotrophic lateral sclerosis. Primary muscle disease hardly ever selects these parts or weakens them disproportionately to other muscles. A diffuse arm weakness may also occur early in acute idiopathic polyneuritis and porphyric polyneuropathy, but it soon becomes part of a more generalized paralysis.

6 Bilateral crural palsy presenting as lower-leg weakness with floppy feet and inability to walk on the heels and toes, or as paralysis of all leg and thigh muscles. In lower leg weakness, polyneuropathy is the usual explanation, although peroneal and anterior tibial muscles are often weakened in dystrophy. Diabetic polyneuropathy may weaken thigh and pelvic muscles asymmetrically with little sensory change but often with pain. In total leg and thigh weakness, one first thinks of a disease of the spinal cord, in which case there is often loss of control of the bladder and bowel sphincters, as well as loss of sensory function below a certain level. Motor system disease may also begin in these parts and affect them out of proportion to others. Thus the differential diagnosis of patterns of leg weakness involves more diseases than do the restricted paralyses of other parts of the body.

7 Limb-girdle palsies presenting as inability to raise the arms or to arise from a squatting, kneeling, or sitting position. Three groups of diseases most often manifest themselves in this fashion—poly- and dermatomyositis, the progressive muscular dystrophies, and the acute proximal polyneuropathies, the Landry-Guillain-Barré syndrome, and acute porphyric neuropathy. The Duchenne, Becker, and Leyden-Moebius type tend first to affect the muscles of the pelvic girdle and lumbar region, resulting in a waddling gait, difficulty in arising from the floor or in climbing stairs without the assistance of the arms, lumbar lordosis, and protuberant abdomen. The Landouzy-Dejerine type affects muscles of face and shoulder girdles foremost, and is manifested by incomplete eye closure, pouting lips, inability to raise the arms above the head, winging of the scapulae, and thinness of the upper arms (Popeye appearance). The lower parts of the deltoid muscle may be relatively spared. In polymyositis, weakness may be limited to either neck muscles or those of the shoulder or pelvic girdles, but sometimes it involves all muscles, including distal ones as well, though the muscles of the face and eyes are almost always spared. Most of the relatively nonprogressive congenital myopathies (central core, nemaline, mitochondrial, centronuclear, multicore, reducing body) cause greater weakness of proximal than of distal muscles. The characteristic feature of the muscular dystrophies is the *selective* muscle involvement, for instance, affecting biceps and brachioradialis while sparing triceps. Polymyositis tends to produce a more nonselective weakness. A metabolic myopathy, such as the adult form of acid-maltase deficiency or prolonged hypokalemia, may affect only the pelvic and thigh muscles. Proximal muscles are occasionally implicated in progressive spinal muscular atrophy, as in the syndrome first described by Kugelberg and Welander. Full investigations including EMG, measurement of serum creatine phosphokinase, and muscle biopsy are required to establish the diagnosis.

8 Distal limb palsies presenting usually as foot drop, with steppage gain (and pes cavus), weakness of all lower leg muscles, and later wrist drop and weakness of hand grips (claw hand). The principal cause of this neuromuscular syndrome is familial polyneuropathy, such as the peroneal muscular atrophy of Charcot-Marie-Tooth, hypertrophic polyneuropathy of Dejerine and Sottas, and the hereditary polyneuropathy of Refsum. Chronic nonfamilial polyneuropathies may also present in this fashion. Rarely this syndrome is due to the distal progressive muscular dystrophy of Welander. Steinert's myotonic dystrophy also weakens peroneal and posterior tibial muscles as well as those of the forearm, sternomastoid, face, and eyes.

Despite exceptions, a first approximation is that girdle weakness means myopathy and distal weakness neuropathy.

9 Generalized or universal paralyses: limb and cranial muscles—involved either in attacks or in persistent, progressive deterioration. When acute in onset and episodic, this syndrome is usually traceable to an inherent disorder which may be associated with an electrolyte imbalance, as in familial hypokalemic, normokalemic, or hyperkalemic periodic paralysis. One variety of the former type is associated with hyperthyroidism, especially in Orientals. A paresis, rather than paralysis of acute onset that lasts many weeks, is a feature of a peculiar disease called paroxysmal myoglobinuria of Meyer-Betz, and at times of a severe form of idiopathic or parasitic polymyositis (trichinosis) as well. Polymyositis of the idiopathic type may involve all limb and trunk muscles but usually spares the facial and ocular muscles, and trichinosis causes only mild ocular and lingual weakness. In infants a chronic and persistent generalized weakness of all muscles except those of the eyes always raises the question of the Werdnig-Hoffmann infantile muscular at-

rophy or, if it is in lesser degree, of one of the relatively nonprogressive congenital myopathies or polyneuropathy. In all these diseases, paucity of movement, hypotonia, and retardation of motor development may be more obvious in the infant than weakness.

Universal ascending paralysis, developing over a few days, with involvement of cranial (including ocular) muscles, is usually due to the idiopathic polyneuritis of Landry-Guillain-Barré. Acute porphyric neuropathy must also be considered. Slow onset and progression of paralysis, atrophy, and fasciculation of limb and trunk muscles, without sensory loss, over months to years characterize motor system disease. Mild degrees of generalized weakness are features of a number of metabolic myopathies, such as thyrotoxic myopathy, glycogen storage disease, vitamin D deficiency, and rickets.

10 Paralysis of single muscles or a group of muscles. This is almost always neuropathic, or rarely spinal. Muscle disease does not need to be considered except in its earliest stages when the weakness is mild.

Volumetric changes in muscle Altered volume of muscular mass stands as another feature of disease which may be evidenced in all except the most obese patient. There are, of course, innate differences in muscle development, a greater salience of muscle in men than in women, and differences due to use and disuse. Greatly increased size and strength of muscles (hypertrophia musculorum vera) may be observed in *congenital myotonia* (circus freaks with phenomenal muscular development often have this disease), in rare instances of a pathologic cramp syndrome, in some patients destined to develop muscular dystrophy, and in de Lange's syndrome of congenital athetosis with feeblemindedness. Muscle enlargement in progressive muscular dystrophy more often takes the form of pseudohypertrophy, where increased size is accompanied by weakness. Here large and small fibers are mixed with fat cells which have replaced many of the degenerated muscle fibers. Other muscles are atrophied in the same patient. Cachexia, malnutrition, and lipodystrophy tend to reduce muscle bulk without significantly reducing power of contraction (pseudoatrophy). Denervation due to lesions of the peripheral nerve or spinal cord, which if complete leads to a loss of bulk up to 75 percent of the original volume within 3 months, is invariably attended by paralysis. The most severe degrees of atrophy usually signify denervation or dystrophy.

Twitches, spasms, cramps, and contracture Fascicular twitches during rest, if pronounced and combined with muscular weakness and atrophy, are typical of motor neuron disease (amyotrophic lateral sclerosis, progressive muscular atrophy, or progressive bulbar palsy); but they may be seen in lesser degree in other diseases of gray matter of the spinal cord (e.g., syringomyelia or tumor), in lesions of anterior roots (e.g., ruptured intervertebral disk), and in peripheral neuropathies. Widespread fascicular twitches spreading in a wavelike pattern along the entire length of a muscle with associated weakness progressing to complete flaccid paralysis within minutes forms the striking clinical picture of organic phosphate insecticide poisoning. The same sequence evolving at a slightly slower pace may occur in poliomyelitis. Fasciculations during contraction indicate, instead, a state in which the muscle is excessively irritable, often for reasons that are not known, or a condition which has previously denervated many motor units, so that during contraction the few remaining enlarged units cannot be recruited smoothly. One may observe this latter phenomenon years after poliomyelitis has left a muscle weakened. *Benign fasciculations,* a common finding in otherwise normal individuals, can usually be distinguished by the lack of muscular weakness and atrophy; *myokymia* and the syndrome of "continuous muscle fiber activity" are rare forms of spasm in which innumerable twitchings impart a rippling appearance to the muscle.

Cramps at rest or with movement (action cramps) are frequently reported in motor system disease, tetany, and dehydration after excessive sweating and salt loss and in other metabolic diseases (uremia, hypocalcemia, and hypomagnesemia), but there is a benign form (idiopathic cramp syndrome), in which no other neuromuscular disturbance can be found. One form of it is known as the *stiff-man syndrome;* this appears to be an obscure disease of the central nervous system for which diazepam is the specific therapy. Continuous spasm, with no demonstrable disorder at a neuromuscular level, intensified by the action of muscles, is a common manifestation of tetanus and also follows the bite of the black widow spider.

Palpable abnormalities of muscle Altered structure and function of muscle are not accurately revealed by palpation. Of course, the difference between the firm hypertrophied muscle of a well-conditioned athlete and the slack muscle of a sedentary person is as apparent to the palpating finger as to the eye. And the persistent contraction in myxedema, contracture, tetanus, cramp, etc., is easily felt. In muscular dystrophy the muscles are said to have a "doughy" or "elastic" feel, but this is difficult to judge. In the Pompé type of glycogen storage disease attention may be attracted to the musculature by an unnatural firmness and increase in bulk. The swollen, edematous weak muscles in acute paroxysmal myoglobinuria or severe polymyositis may feel taut and firm but are usually not tender. Areas of tenseness in muscles which otherwise function normally, a state called *myogelosis,* may be found in patients with fibrositis or fibromyositis, and their nature has not been divulged by biopsy.

A mass developing in one part of a muscle, or throughout a muscle, poses a special clinical problem. It may, if chronic, be a tumor (rhabdomyosarcoma, angioma, metastatic carcinoma, or desmoid) or a granulomatous inflammation (sarcoid, tuberculoma, or mycosis). Hard masses are usually calcium (myocalcinosis) or bone deposit (myositis ossificans). If a muscle mass develops rapidly, hemorrhage, either spontaneous or traumatic, must be considered. A ruptured tendon may take this form but always causes a bulge which, for obvious reasons, becomes manifest on contraction, and the muscle exhibits a diminished power of contraction.

Tendon (phasic stretch) reflexes The tendon reflexes are altered by the majority of causes of muscle weakness, particularly those which involve peripheral nerves. In muscular dystrophy and polymyositis they tend to be reduced in proportion to the reduction in muscular power. In the myopathy of hypothyroidism, in which the contractile process is slowed, there is a characteristic prolongation of the tendon reflex, and the opposite condition of quickening and brevity of the tendon reflex is less reliably demonstrated in hyperthyroidism. In peripheral neuropathies the tendon reflexes are usually lost at an early stage before much weakness appears.

Muscle pain Pain localized to a group of muscles is extremely severe in wry neck, fibrositis and fibromyositis, acute brachial neuritis, radiculitis, Bornholm's disease, or pleurodynia, but little is known of its cause in any of these diseases. In contrast, the established forms of muscle disease are usually painless. In polymyositis pain is present in about half the patients, and may sometimes indicate coincident involvement of connective tissues and joint structures. Tenderness of muscle is a variable state normally, and it tends to be more definite in polyneuritis, poliomyelitis, and polyarteritis nodosa than in polymyositis

and in the various forms of dystrophy and other myopathies in which there is usually no increase in the sensitivity of muscle tissue.

REFERENCES

ADAMS RD: *Diseases of Muscle: A Study in Pathology,* 3d ed. Hagerstown, Md, Harper & Row, 1975

BUCHTHAL F, SIMPSON JA (eds): *Handbook of Electroencephalography and Clinical Neurophysiology,* vol 16: *Electromyography,* part A: *Nervous and Muscular Evoked Potentials.* Amsterdam, Elsevier, 1976

———, ——— (eds): *Handbook of Electroencephalography, and Clinical Neurophysiology,* vol 16: *Electromyography,* part B: *Neuromuscular Disease.* Amsterdam, Elsevier, 1973

DUBOWITZ V, BROOKE M: *Muscle Biopsy: A Modern Approach.* Philadelphia, Saunders, 1973

GOODGOLD J, EBERSTEIN A: *Electrodiagnosis of Neuromuscular Diseases,* 2d ed. Baltimore, Williams & Wilkins, 1977

KATZ B: *Nerve, Muscle and Synapse.* New York, McGraw-Hill, 1966

STÅLBERG E, TRONTELJ J: *Single Fibre Electromyography.* London, Unwins, 1978

WALTON JN (ed): *Disorders of Voluntary Muscle,* 3d ed. London, Churchill-Livingstone, 1974

379
ACUTE AND SUBACUTE MYOPATHIC PARALYSIS

MARIA SALAM–ADAMS
WALTER G. BRADLEY

It is a fairly safe clinical rule that an abrupt onset of paralysis (one that develops within minutes to hours) is usually due to a lesion of motor tracts in the spinal cord, brainstem, or cerebrum. When widespread paralysis is of acute onset (over a period of hours to a day or even a few days), again a myelopathic or neuropathic condition is the common cause; the most frequent diseases of this type are poliomyelitis and acute idiopathic or some other form of polyneuritis. But there are several rare myopathic states that must also be considered. For example, one of the types of periodic paralysis or a marked hyper- or hypokalemia from any cause may produce severe paralysis over this brief span of time. Botulism manifests itself as a fulminant paralysis, beginning in ocular and other cranial muscles and extending to trunk and limb muscles with terminal respiratory failure (see Chap. 140). Myasthenia may be induced acutely during the administration of certain antibiotics. Certain cases of rhabdomyolysis may lead to rapid onset of muscle weakness, usually coming on after heavy exertion or an infection. Often there is an associated myoglobinuria that results in renal failure. The medical literature also includes numerous references to acute thyrotoxic myopathy with prominent paresis of bulbar and limb muscles.

The clinical analysis of these rare acute myopathic syndromes is aided by certain laboratory data such as electrocardiographic findings, serum K level, levels of serum enzymes such as creatine phosphokinase (CPK) and of thyroid hormones, T_3 and T_4. Electromyographic measurements of nerve conduction velocities, muscle biopsy, and examination of cerebrospinal fluid (CSF) may also be of help. The response to neostigmine and edrophonium (Tensilon) confirms the diagnosis of myasthenia gravis (see Chap. 381).

By contrast the majority of diseases of muscle express themselves clinically by a more slowly evolving paralytic disorder, extending over a period of many weeks (subacute) or months and years (chronic). The two principal categories of subacute myopathy are dermatomyositis (called polymyositis if there is no skin involvement) and the metabolic polymyopathies.

DERMATOMYOSITIS AND POLYMYOSITIS

DEFINITION These are relatively common diseases which affect primarily the striated muscle, skin, and the various connective tissues of the body. The term used varies according to the tissues involved in the pathologic process. If restricted clinically to the striated muscles, the disease is called polymyositis; if the skin is involved, it is designated as dermatomyositis; and if other connective tissues are implicated, the term of choice is polymyositis with rheumatoid arthritis, rheumatic fever, lupus erythematosus, or scleroderma, etc.

HISTORY Polymyositis has been known since the original descriptions by Wagner in 1863 and 1887, and the dermatomyositic form was first reported by Unverricht in 1887. The literature since that time and a general statement of present knowledge are found in the monographs of Walton and Adams and of Adams.

ETIOLOGY The cause of the disease is unknown. Almost all attempts to isolate an infective agent have been unsuccessful. Several electron microscopists have observed virus-like particles in muscle fibers, but their causative role has not been proved. Rising titers of antiviral antibodies have not been demonstrated, nor has a polymyositic illness been induced in animals by injections of affected muscle. A disease which resembles polymyositis has been provoked in laboratory animals by injections of sterile muscle extracts with Freund's adjuvants, suggesting an autoimmune mechanism. The close association of polymyositis and diseases of connective tissue favors the notion of common etiology or pathogenesis, also in keeping with an autoallergic inflammation. It must be conceded, however, that the category of disease called polymyositis is not precise and probably has been used to include other diseases of noninflammatory type, namely, metabolic myopathies.

CLINICAL MANIFESTATIONS This type of muscle disease tends to assume several clinical forms, as follows.

Polymyositis *A subacute symmetric weakness of proximal limb and trunk muscles without clinically apparent skin lesions.* The onset is usually insidious and the course slowly progressive over a period of weeks to months or even years. The disease may develop at almost any age (from one to eighty years) and in either sex. However, the majority of patients fall into two age periods, 5 to 15 and 45 to 60 years, and females outnumber males 2:1. A respiratory or obscure systemic illness may precede the muscle weakness, but in many patients the first symptoms develop during excellent health.

The patient first becomes aware of painless weakness of the proximal limb muscles, especially of the hips and thighs, and acts such as arising from a squatting or kneeling position, climbing or descending stairs, walking, putting an object on a high shelf, or combing the hair become increasingly difficult. In restricted forms of the disease only the neck muscles, the shoulder muscles, or quadriceps may be involved. Pain of an aching variety, in buttocks, joints, and calves, is experienced in

a variable percentage of cases (15 to 50 percent) and often indicates a combination of polymyositis and arthritis or other connective tissue disease. The weakness progresses over a period of weeks and months.

When the patient is first seen, the posterior and to a lesser extent anterior neck muscles are weak (the head may loll), as are the pharyngeal and laryngeal muscles (dysphagia and dysphonia), all the trunk, the girdle muscles of shoulders and hips, upper arms, and the thighs. Ocular muscles are almost never affected unless there is an associated myasthenia gravis (rare coincidence); the forearm, hand, leg, and foot muscles are spared in about 75 percent of cases. The muscles are sometimes tender, and atrophy and reduction in tendon reflexes, though present, are not as pronounced as in denervative diseases. When reflexes are disproportionately reduced, one must think of carcinoma with polymyositis and polyneuropathy.

In a review of our cases of polymyositis and dermatomyositis a surprising number of cardiac abnormalities were observed. Most of these were relatively minor ECG changes, but several patients had arrhythmias of significance. Among the fatal cases about half showed clinical evidence of severe cardiac disease and had necrosis of myocardial fibers at autopsy, usually with only modest inflammation. In a few cases there are symptoms such as cough and dyspnea expressive of pulmonary interstitial pneumonitis and fibrosis. As a rule, evidence of systemic disease is absent. Exceptionally there is low-grade fever, especially if arthritis coexists. Evidence of collagen-vascular disease affecting other organs may be present. If skin involvement is observed, the diagnosis of dermatomyositis rather than polymyositis is made.

Dermatomyositis The skin changes may precede, accompany, or follow the muscle syndrome and take the form of a localized or diffuse erythema, maculopapular eruption, scaling eczematoid dermatitis, or even an exfoliative dermatitis. Of particular importance is the occurrence of a lilac-colored (heliotrope) change in the skin over the eyelids, the bridge of the nose, cheeks, and forehead, and around the fingernails. Itching may be troublesome in some cases. The skin lesions are restricted and in some cases may be overlooked. Periorbital and perioral edema is frequent, particularly in more fulminating episodes. Also skin lesions are frequent over the elbow, knee, and finger joints, especially in childhood. The skin lesions may occasionally ulcerate, and in the healing stage may become depressed, with a flat, scaly base. Periarticular and subcutaneous calcification may occur. Signs of other connective tissue disease are more frequent (in one-third to one-half of all patients) than in examples of pure polymyositis. The limb weakness is usually proximal but may be diffuse, i.e., distal and proximal, just as in polymyositis. Raynaud's phenomenon is reported in nearly a third of the patients. Others will develop a mild form of scleroderma. Esophageal weakness may be demonstrated by fluoroscopy in approximately 30 percent of all patients. The superior constrictors are involved almost universally, but careful analysis by cinefluorography may be required to demonstrate the abnormality.

Connective tissue diseases with polymyositis or dermatomyositis This combination involves rheumatic fever, rheumatoid arthritis, scleroderma, or lupus erythematosus, diagnosable by the finding of greater muscular weakness and atrophy than can be accounted for by the original disease. Inasmuch as pain in arthritis may limit motion, result in atrophy, and impair the power of voluntary movement, the diagnosis is not easy, and sometimes reliance must be put on muscle biopsy, measurements of muscle enzymes in the serum, and electromyography. Malaise, aches, and pains may be the only symptoms in the early stages of the disease. Sjögren's syndrome of keratitis desiccans, swelling and diminished secretion of salivary glands, xerostomia and rheumatoid arthritis may accompany polymyositis (see Chap. 356).

Carcinoma with polymyositis or dermatomyositis This syndrome is placed in a separate category, although the muscle and skin changes are indistinguishable from those in the above forms of the disease. Approximately 10 percent of all adults, especially the elderly, who have polymyositis or dermatomyositis are found to have a carcinoma or some other tumor. Some cases of thymoma are accompanied by polymyositis. The incidence of this neoplastic syndrome is slightly higher in men than in women. In men over 50 with dermatomyositis, an underlying carcinoma is to be found in about 15 percent. Over 1000 examples have been reported in the literature, being linked most often with bronchogenic carcinoma. The tumors, however, have occurred in every organ of the body. The muscle and skin tissues show no evidence of tumor cells. The polymyositis may antedate the clinical manifestations of the malignancy by 1 to 2 years. The relationship is not understood, but the most likely possibility is an altered immune status which fosters occult infection.

LABORATORY FINDINGS Regardless of the clinical associations, in all forms of polymyositis the serum levels of the several types of transaminase and other tissue enzymes such as creatine phosphokinase and aldolase are usually elevated. Serum α_2 and γ globulin values may be raised. Tests for circulating rheumatoid factor and antinuclear antibodies are positive in less than half the cases. Myoglobin is occasionally found in the urine when the muscle affection is acute and severe. The sedimentation rate may be normal or elevated. Lupus erythematosus preparations of blood smears are negative, as a rule. The electromyogram reveals an increased insertional activity, fibrillation potentials, and a typical "myopathic pattern," i.e., many abnormally brief action potentials and an abnormally early recruitment of a full interference pattern on only moderate contraction. As stated, the ECG has been abnormal in a few of our cases. The muscle biopsy, if taken from an affected muscle, usually demonstrates the typical pathologic changes of the disease. Poor sampling may result in a negative biopsy.

PATHOLOGY The principal changes in muscle tissue consist of widespread destruction of muscle fibers, with all the expected phagocytic reactions and infiltrates of inflammatory cells (lymphocytes, mononuclear leukocytes, plasma cells, and rare neutrophilic leukocytes). Perivascular (usually perivenular) inflammatory cell infiltration is the hallmark of polymyositis; interstitial inflammatory cell infiltration is also a prominent feature of the disease, but slight degrees of it may also be seen in other conditions as a secondary reaction (e.g., facioscapulohumeral muscular dystrophy). Evidence of regenerative activity in the form of proliferating sarcolemmal nuclei, basophilic (ribonucleic acid-rich) sarcoplasm, and new myofibrils are almost invariable. Many of the residual muscle fibers are small, with increased numbers of sarcolemmal nuclei. Either the degeneration of muscle fibers or the infiltrations of inflammatory cells may predominate in any given biopsy specimen, though at autopsy both types of change are in evidence. There are often also inflammatory changes in the skin and other organs.

DIAGNOSIS Patients with a pure polymyositis are often suspected of having progressive muscular dystrophy because of the similar distribution of weakness (in the proximal and trunk muscles). Polymyositis is unlike dystrophy, however, in that the development is much more rapid, individuals may be affected at all ages (one rarely sees a dystrophy begin after thirty

years of age), and the laryngeal, pharyngeal, and posterior neck muscles and the esophagus are often affected. Also the limb girdle musculature tends to be more diffusely involved, in which respect the disease differs from the selective involvement of a dystrophy. Nevertheless, in rare patients, especially children, it is virtually impossible, even with biopsy, to distinguish a chronic polymyositis from a rapidly advancing dystrophy. Such doubtful cases should always be given an adequate trial of corticosteroid therapy.

A few patients with poly- or dermatomyositis and malignancy will exhibit signs of one of the other paraneoplastic syndromes (polyneuritis, subacute cerebellar degeneration, combined system disease, or multifocal leukoencephalopathy). The Eaton-Lambert type myasthenic syndrome is most often associated with small-cell carcinomas of the lung (oat-cell, squamous-cell). A sense of stiffness and pain on motion in these latter patients may be mistaken for rheumatoid arthritis. The diagnosis of polymyositis is not always easy. Patients with pain but little weakness may be thought to be hysterical or neurotic. Polymyositis may not be recognized if it occurs in the presence of another collagen-vascular disease such as rheumatoid arthritis. It is important to determine the serum creatine phosphokinase in such patients. Polymyalgia rheumatica presents with muscle pain and a high sedimentation rate; the muscle biopsy discloses only type 2 fiber atrophy, but the temporal artery biopsy may show giant-cell arteritis (see Chap. 363). Sarcoidosis, toxoplasmosis, and other specific infections may occasionally produce a syndrome indistinguishable from polymyositis, and antibody screening will reveal the diagnosis. Paroxysmal myoglobinuria, steroid myopathy, thyrotoxic myopathy, and diabetic amyotrophy are other conditions that may give trouble in differential diagnosis.

Trichinosis may be confused with idiopathic polymyositis, especially if the history of pork ingestion is not obtained. The high eosinophil counts in the blood, the relatively slight weakness of limbs, the conjunctival edema, the ocular and lingual weakness, the symptoms of cerebral involvement (hemiplegia, aphasia, coma, epilepsy, etc.), the positive skin reaction to trichina antigen, and the muscle biopsy establish the diagnosis in most cases (see Chap. 208).

In the final analysis the diagnosis of idiopathic polymyositis and dermatomyositis must be based on four criteria: clinical picture, EMG, elevation of creatine phosphokinase and aldolase in the serum, and a positive muscle biopsy. However, only 25 percent of cases meet all these criteria. The clinical picture is more important than any one of the laboratory data and in itself justifies diagnosis and a therapeutic trial of steroids.

TREATMENT The various measures which have been suggested are of uncertain value. Our most gratifying results have been obtained by a program which consists of the following:

1 *Prednisone,* 60 mg per day for a month, gradual reduction in steps of 5 mg to the level of 20 mg per day, and thereafter reduction in 1-mg steps every 2 to 4 weeks over a period of a year. The therapy should be monitored by careful tests of strength and serum enzyme levels [once the dosage is reduced to 20 mg per day, it is best to give double this amount on alternate days (i.e., 40 mg)].
2 *Acetylsalicylic acid,* 0.6 g every 4 h except during the night (blood levels of 20 to 30 mg per 100 ml).
3 *Physiotherapy:* gentle massage, passive movement, and then "resistance exercises" as the evidences of activity (high serum enzyme values) subside.

This program has benefited the majority of our patients, and many have been cured. A few of our patients have failed to improve with prednisone 60 mg per day for a month, and more prolonged high dose treatment is then required. Immunosuppressant drugs should be tried when the response is inadequate or when relapses are frequent. Azathioprine (2.5 to 3.5 mg/kg per day in divided doses) is the most easily used immunosuppressant. Regular dosage must be reduced if levels of red blood cells, white blood cells, or platelets falls too low. The aim of therapy is to lower the total lymphocyte count to about 1000 per cubic millimeter. With the combined use of prednisone and an immunosuppressant it is usually possible to reduce the dose of prednisone required.

Elderly patients in particular should be reexamined regularly for malignancy. If a malignant lesion is found, it should be excised, if possible, or treated by x-ray or chemical agents. The muscle weakness may disappear if the tumor is eradicated, but response to corticosteroids may occur in patients with polymyositis associated with tumor.

PROGNOSIS Only a few of the patients will die, usually with some pulmonary, renal, or cardiac complication. The majority improve upon therapy. Many patients make a full functional recovery, though often some weakness of the shoulders and hips, usually not disabling, remains at the conclusion of treatment. Relapse may occur at any time up to 1 to 15 years or more. Corticosteroids should not be discontinued too soon, for the relapse which may follow is often more difficult to treat than the original symptoms of the disease. About one-half of patients with this disease recover within 5 years after the onset of symptoms.

SARCOID AND OTHER FORMS OF IDIOPATHIC POLYMYOSITIS

In the medical literature there are cases of a subacutely progressive polymyositis involving proximal limb and trunk muscles, in which biopsy has demonstrated a noncaseating granulomatous involvement of muscle. In all other respects the patients are indistinguishable from those with the idiopathic polymyositis described above. Most of them have not shown many of the other characteristic manifestations of sarcoid, and it is only proper to inquire as to whether the finding of a few Langhans-type giant cells in the muscle is a sufficient basis for the diagnosis of sarcoid. We are skeptical of this entity, but the problem is presently unresolved. Some of these cases have been described under the caption of "nodular myositis," or "granulomatous myositis." Response to corticosteroid therapy is not different from that of idiopathic polymyositis.

In some of the patients with diffuse myositis ossificans painful lumps in muscles and redness of overlying skin may precede ossification. In children's polymyositis acute necrosis of muscle may be accompanied by necrosis of kidneys and intestines, proceeding rapidly to death. In such cases an arteritic factor should be suspected. A number of viral diseases (coxsackievirus, influenza) and parasite infections (trichinosis, toxoplasmosis) and inflammatory nodules may produce a clinical picture similar to that of idiopathic polymyositis.

METABOLIC DISEASES OF MUSCLE

The boundaries of this category of disease cannot be sharply drawn at this time. With advance in knowledge it is probable that many diseases presently classified as degenerative, and possibly some labeled as polymyositic, will be linked to specific defects in enzymes within the muscle cells. Limitations in space permit the description of only a few representative forms of the better known metabolic myopathies.

THYROID MYOPATHIES Several myopathic diseases related to alterations in thyroid function have been recognized. These are (1) thyrotoxic myopathy, (2) exophthalmic ophthalmoplegia (infiltrative ophthalmopathy), (3) myasthenia gravis associated with toxic diffuse goiter or with hypothroidism, (4) periodic paralysis associated with toxic diffuse goiter, and (5) muscle hypertrophy and slow muscle contraction and relaxation associated with myxedema and cretinism. Although not frequent, several examples of each of these diseases may be seen in a single year in any large general hospital.

Thyrotoxic myopathy is a disease characterized by progressive weakness and atrophy of skeletal musculature, occurring in conjunction with overt or covert (masked) hyperthyroidism. The latter is usually chronic, and the goiter is of the nodular rather than the diffuse type seen in Graves' disease. The muscular disorder may reach proportions such as to suggest progressive muscular atrophy (motor system disease). It is estimated that the middle-aged patient is most likely to suffer from this complication of hyperthyroidism and that men are more susceptible than women. The onset is insidious, and the weakness progresses over weeks and months, though it may be relatively acute (days). Exophthalmos need not be present. Sometimes the pelvic girdle and thigh muscles are weakened more than others (Basedow's paraplegia), but at other times the deltoids and other pectoral girdle muscles are more involved. The disease may affect the bulbar and rarely ocular muscles causing dysphagia, dysphonia, and diplopia. However, the shoulder and hand muscles are the ones which show the most conspicuous atrophy. Tremor and coarse twitching during contraction may occur, but we have not seen fasciculations at rest or true fibrillations (in the electromyogram). The tendon reflexes are normal or increased. Creatine excretion in the urine is increased, and tolerance to ingested creatine diminished, but the degree of this impairment has not correlated with the degree of weakness. Serum enzyme levels are not elevated. Electromyograms have disclosed no definite abnormality, and biopsies of muscle, except for slight volumetric reduction in fibers, have been normal. Injections of neostigmine have no effect. Muscle power and bulk are gradually restored when thyroid function is reduced to normal levels.

Exophthalmic ophthalmoplegia is a weakness of external ocular muscles (pupillary and ciliary muscles are always spared) which is conjoined with the exophthalmos of Graves' disease. The exophthalmos varies in degree, being sometimes absent at an early stage of the disease, and is not in itself responsible for the muscle weakness. Both the ocular weakness and exophthalmos may precede the clinical signs of hyperthyroidism or follow the effective treatment of it. The ocular palsy may occasionally be unilateral, especially in the beginning. Many of the fibers of the eye muscles in biopsies and in autopsy material are seen to have degenerated, and infiltrations of lymphocytes, mononuclear leukocytes, and lipocytes are present; hence the term *infiltrative ophthalmopathy*. All external eye muscles may be affected, often one more than others, accounting for strabismus and diplopia; upward movements are usually limited to the greatest degree. Neostigmine has no effect. The condition often runs a self-limited course as does the exophthalmos itself, and therapy is difficult to evaluate. Certainly the maintenance of a euthyroid state is desirable (see Chap. 335 for treatment of hyperthyroidism).

In patients with marked periorbital and conjunctival edema high dosage of corticosteroids (about 80 mg prednisone per day) may give partial control of the ophthalmic problem, including the extraocular muscle weakness. Because of the side effects of high dose corticosteroids, they should be reserved for patients who would otherwise require surgical intervention. However, with steroid treatment it has been possible to carry a number of patients over the crisis and avoid the trauma and risks of surgery. If the exophthalmos reaches a degree which threatens injury of the cornea, tarsorrhaphy, or orbital decompression by removal of the roof of the bony orbit, may save the eyesight.

Thyrotoxic periodic paralysis resembles familial periodic paralysis (Chap. 382), occurs particularly in Orientals, and consists of attacks of mild to severe weakness of limb and trunk muscles, usually with sparing of those of the cranium, which develops in a few minutes or hours and lasts part of a day or longer. In some series from Japan as many as half the cases of periodic paralysis have been in patients who suffered from hyperthyroidism. Unlike what has been found in typical hypokalemic periodic paralysis, a family history is not obtained. In most cases the serum potassium levels have been low during the attacks, and the administration of several grams of KCl has terminated the attack. Treatment of the hyperthyroidism abolishes the symptomatic manifestations of the muscular disorder.

Myasthenia gravis in typical neostigmine-responsive form may accompany hyper- or hypothyroidism. In hyperthyroidism the typical weakness and poorly sustained contraction of the aforementioned chronic thyrotoxic myopathy are added to the myasthenia, without appearing to affect the response to or requirement for neostigmine. In contrast, hypothyroidism, even of mild degrees, seems to aggravate the myasthenia gravis, greatly increasing the need for neostigmine and at times inducing a myasthenic crisis. Thyroxine is beneficial and, with respect to myasthenia, restores the patient's status to what it was before the onset of the thyroid insufficiency. However, the myasthenia gravis (described in Chap. 382) is independent of thyroid disease. Each disease must be treated separately.

Hypothyroidism, whether in the form of myxedema or of cretinism, is often accompanied by a series of changes in skeletal muscle consisting of increased volume, stiffness, aching, and slowness of contraction. Action myospasm and percussion myoedema, along with the slowness of tendon reflexes, assist the examiner in making a bedside diagnosis (see Chap. 335). These changes probably account for the large tongue and typical dysarthria seen in this disease. The clinical syndrome simulates hypertrophia musculorum vera and myotonia congenita. Cretinism manifesting these muscle symptoms is known as *Debré-Semelaigne syndrome,* and myxedema with a similar muscle picture is called *Hoffmann's syndrome.* In neither of these two syndromes is there real evidence of myotonia by either clinical test or electromyogram, and muscle biopsies have revealed only large fibers, sometimes with increased amounts of subsarcolemmal glycogen. In the rare condition where myotonia and hypothyroidism coexist, the myotonia appears to be accentuated by the hypothyroidism. Creatinine excretion is reduced, and urinary creatine is increased. Transaminase values in the serum are normal, but the CPK level is usually elevated. The administration of thyroxine corrects the abnormality of muscle.

The effect of thyroid secretion on the muscle fiber in all these myopathies is still a matter of conjecture. Clinical data indicate that this hormone influences in some manner the contractile process without interfering in any way with the transmission of impulses in the peripheral nerves, across the myoneural junctions, or along the sarcolemma. In hyperthyroidism this functional disorder enhances the speed of the contractile process and reduces its duration, the net effect being a weakening, an excess fatigability, and a loss of endurance in muscle action. In hypothyroidism the converse of these changes occurs.

The thyroid hormone also acts on the central nervous system, and in some syndromes, such as myxedema and the acute toxic encephalopathy and myopathy of hyperthyroidism, it is possible to observe the effects of both a neurologic and a muscular disorder.

ALCOHOLIC MYOPATHY WITH CARDIOPATHY Occasionally in alcoholics during a severe drinking bout one observes the rapid development of universal muscle weakness over a period of a few days. At the onset muscle pain and cramps are common. The condition may reach such proportions as to render the patient bedfast, and biopsy reveals extensive segmental necrosis of sarcoplasm. All the limb and trunk muscles may be affected; there is no record of its extending to ocular and other cranial muscles. Myonecrosis is reflected by high levels of muscle enzymes (CPK and aldolase). Myoglobin may appear in the urine, leading to renal failure. Signs of cardiac enlargement and decompensation accompany the myopathy in some instances. Most patients recover within a few weeks, but relapse in another spree of drinking has been noted. Restoration of motor power is attendant upon regeneration but may be complicated by polyneuropathy and other neurologic syndromes associated with alcoholism.

First observed in Swedish alcoholics, this condition has appeared in American clinics. Perkoff and his associates find some evidence that it is due to a transient suppression of myophosphorylase during bouts of alcoholism. It is too frequent (in milder degrees) to represent an inborn error of metabolism. Some cases formerly described as beriberi cardiopathy may fall in this group.

Progressive proximal or diffuse muscle weakness and wasting is not uncommon in chronic alcoholics who have a poor state of nutrition. EMG and biopsy studies in such cases indicate that the disorder is due to a progressive alcoholic, predominantly motor neuropathy.

CORTICOSTEROID MYOPATHY The widespread use of adrenal corticosteroids in recent years has brought to light a new muscle disease, probably not dissimilar to that which has been noted in rabbits receiving cortisone. The proximal limb and girdle musculature becomes extremely weak over a period of a few weeks or months, to the point where it is difficult to elevate the arms and to arise from a sitting, squatting, or kneeling position, and walking itself may be hampered. The electromyogram shows the myopathic pattern of small but abundant action potentials and also fibrillations; in biopsies there is evidence of scattered atrophic and a few degenerating and regenerating muscle fibers without infiltrates of inflammatory cells; and type 2 fiber atrophy and degeneration of mitochondria in type 1 fibers is seen in histochemical preparations. The serum creatine kinase and aldolase levels are raised, and there is a creatinuria. Discontinuation of corticosteroid administration leads to recovery within a few weeks. The dose levels of corticosteroid have frequently been high and sustained over a period of months, and fluorinated preparations are more culpable, though all corticosteroids may produce the disorder. There is only a poor correlation between total dose and severity of myopathy. A similar myopathy occurs regularly in patients who suffer from Cushing's syndrome. The mechanism of the muscle disease is unknown.

NECROTIZING POLYMYOPATHY AND MYOGLOBINURIA In any disease that results in rapid destruction of striated muscle fibers, myoglobin and other muscle proteins may enter the bloodstream and appear in the urine. The serum is rapidly cleared. The urine is dark red or burgundy-colored, much like that in hemoglobinuria. However, in hemoglobinuria the serum initially is pink because hemoglobin but not myoglobin is bound to haptoglobin. The renal threshold for this complex is high, whereas it is low for myoglobin. The complex of hemoglobin-haptoglobin is removed from the blood plasma over a period of hours, and if hemolysis continues, the haptoglobin may be depleted so that hemoglobinuria is present without grossly evident hemoglobinemia. Differentiation of the two pigments in urine is difficult. Very small differences are seen on spectroscopic examination, but both pigments are rapidly degraded to other compounds, such as hematin, with differing spectra. Thus great care must be taken with such procedures.

When myoglobinuria is severe, renal damage may ensue and lead to anuria. The mechanism of the renal damage is not clear; probably it is not simply a mechanical obstruction of tubules by precipitated myoglobin. However, alkalinization of the urine by the ingestion of sodium bicarbonate is said to protect the kidney by preventing the formation of myoglobin casts, but in severe cases it is of doubtful value, and the sodium may actually be harmful if anuria has already developed. Therapy is the same as in the anuria which follows surgical shock (see Chap. 32).

The following conditions may give rise to myoglobinuria:

1 *Crush injury to a limb.*
2 *Strain or excessive use of muscles,* especially the pretibial muscles, which are confined in the tight pretibial compartment (pretibial syndrome).
3 *Extensive infarction,* as in occlusion of the main artery of a limb or a subcutaneous infusion into the lower leg (with resultant swelling and probable ischemia).
4 *Polymyositis.*
5 *Haff disease,* which results from eating fish poisoned by toxic resinous acids derived from cellulose. This was first reported in the Bay (Haff) of Königsberg, Germany.
6 *Alcoholic polymyopathy* and *McArdle's disease* (see Chap. 378).
7 *Familial myoglobinuria* (Meyer-Betz disease), a group of diseases which occur in families with or without a diffuse chronic myopathy or dystrophy. The most common form is of unknown pathogenesis. Episodes of myoglobinuria may occur in some cases of McArdle's phosphorylase deficiency and in the adult variety of carnitine palmityl transferase deficiency. The attack of myoglobinuria may be precipitated by strenuous exertion or possibly by an infection. Weakness, stiffness, and tenderness or swelling of muscles are the principal symptoms, and they vary in intensity. The muscle fibers are later found in various stages of degeneration and regeneration. The degree of renal injury usually determines the outcome. No therapy is known except that of complete inactivity and measures which assist return of renal function (see Chap. 275). Some patients will be shown to have a lifelong disposition to attacks of myoglobinuria; hence strenuous physical activity must be curtailed. In others there may be but a single attack with complete or nearly complete recovery. In a few such cases, various biochemical defects in energy metabolism, both in glucose pathways and lipid metabolism, have been recognized.
8 *Extreme hyperthermia,* especially with convulsions.

A special variety of diffuse metabolic polymyopathy occurs with *malignant hyperthermia* during anesthesia. Several hundred such accidents have been reported. The idiosyncratic reaction is inherited as an autosomal dominant trait. At least two groups of patients have been identified, one with certain musculoskeletal and myopathic abnormalities (ptosis, strabismus, high-arched palate, dislocated patellae, kyphoscoliosis, and congenital muscle hypertrophy), the other of normal appearance. As halothane anesthesia and suxemethonium are given, the jaws become tense rather than relaxed, the temperature rises rapidly (up to 43°C), and there follow tachypnea, tachycardia, and finally circulatory collapse. Muscle fibers are destroyed during the attack, and CPK rises to high levels. Myoglobin appears in the urine. Muscular weakness and atrophy persist long after the attack. Some of the susceptible members in a family can be recognized by the elevation of CPK in their serum or by the in vitro contracture of muscle biopsies exposed to halothane and suxamethonium. The attack may be aborted if the anesthesia is discontinued at the first sign of muscle rigidity.

MYOPATHY WITH HYPOKALEMIC PERIODIC PARALYSIS A rare complication of *familial periodic paralysis* (see Chap. 381) takes the form of chronic persistent weakening of thigh and pelvic musculature. Onset may be in the middle adult years, long after a troublesome adolescent periodic paralysis has ameliorated or ceased altogether. Biopsy reveals an extreme degree of vacuolization (Goldflam myopathy), and muscle fiber degeneration may be consequent to it. Slight increase in muscle enzymes in serum and a myopathic electromyogram substantiate the diagnosis already indicated by the sequence of clinical events. Administration of potassium (4 to 5 g orally per day), which alleviates or suppresses the periodic paralysis, may be beneficial.

OTHER METABOLIC MYOPATHIES A progressive areflexic muscular atrophy giving rise to a syndrome of infantile muscular atrophy, or the floppy baby, has been recorded in two of the five established forms of glycogen storage disease (see Chap. 97).

A syndrome of painful muscles and generalized weakness has been reported in hypoglycemia (see Chap. 339).

In hyperparathyroidism and osteomalacia resulting from renal tubular acidosis (a form of Milkman's syndrome), malabsorption, chronic anticonvulsant therapy, etc., muscular weakness, fatigability, atrophy, and discomfort after exercise have been noted. The tendon reflexes are normal or hyperactive. In *hypophosphatemic rickets* the skeletal muscles may be markedly weakened and painful. In hypophosphatemic rickets Vitamin D appears to be necessary for skeletal muscle metabolism (perhaps of calcium). EMG and serum CPK are usually normal, and muscle biopsy shows type 2 fiber atrophy. Vitamin D therapy is curative. In *hypophosphatemic rickets* with normal serum Ca oral neutral phosphates and sometimes the removal of a bone cyst or tumor will relieve pain and restore power.

A contracture of hamstring muscles which prevents upright stance has been found several times in patients with Addison's disease. Biopsy has revealed normal muscle tissue; the electromyogram is normal; and the tendon reflexes are retained.

A primary defect of phosphorylase has been established as the cause of another condition known as McArdle's syndrome. This is a chronic familial myopathy with weakness, stiffness, and discomfort in the muscles following exercise. Therefore it is more logically considered in connection with the myalgic and muscle stiffness syndromes (Chap. 97).

REFERENCES

ADAMS RD: *Diseases of Muscle,* 3d ed. New York, Harper & Row, 1975

WALTON JN: *Disorders of Voluntary Muscle,* 4th ed. London, Churchill-Livingstone, 1979

——, ADAMS RD: *Polymyositis.* Edinburgh, Churchill-Livingstone, 1955

380

PROGRESSIVE MUSCULAR DYSTROPHY (CHRONIC MYOPATHIC PARALYSIS)

RAYMOND D. ADAMS
WALTER G. BRADLEY
JEAN J. REBEIZ

As intimated in the clinical classification in Chap. 378 (see Table 378-1), one of the major causes of the syndrome of progressive weakness and wasting of the musculature of the limbs and trunk is muscular dystrophy. This category of disease can usually be differentiated from the familial or nonfamilial varieties of neuropathy by the pattern of the muscle involvement (usually proximal in the dystrophies and distal in most of the neuropathies), by the absence of sensory disturbances, the less severe reduction of tendon reflexes, the normal cerebrospinal fluid, the characteristic electromyogram, and the findings in a muscle biopsy. It can usually be distinguished from spinal muscular atrophy, exemplified in the adult by *motor system disease* (amyotrophic lateral sclerosis), and in the infant by *Werdnig-Hoffmann muscular atrophy,* by the proximal and symmetric pattern of muscle involvement (total lack of pattern in motor system disease and asymmetry of involvement in the muscles of forearms and hands or feet and legs), lack of coarse fasciculations, and the characteristic electromyogram and changes in the biopsy of muscle. These two forms of chronic muscular atrophy due to diseases of the nervous system are described in Chaps. 14 and 373 and will not be discussed further in this section.

THE MUSCULAR DYSTROPHIES

HISTORY AND TERMINOLOGY Progressive muscular dystrophy (*dystrophia musculorum progressiva*) was described by several prominent physicians in the middle and latter half of the nineteenth century. The many names used since that time to designate types of this condition have been a source of confusion. Duchenne reported a group of young patients, mostly males, with muscular enlargement as well as atrophy; this disease has since been referred to as *pseudohypertrophic muscular dystrophy.* Leyden and Moebius called attention to a clinically somewhat similar group in which, however, muscular enlargement was lacking. This *simple atrophic* type probably corresponds to the crural form of Erb limb-girdle dystrophy. Landouzy and Dejerine described muscular dystrophy of the facial, pectoral, and shoulder-girdle muscles, which they call the *facioscapulohumeral* type; and Erb reported a condition of weakness and atrophy of limb-girdles dystrophy beginning in either the upper or lower limb girdles with little or no facial involvement, which he termed *juvenile dystrophy.* Walton and others had made the distinction between "limb-girdle dystrophy" and facioscapulohumeral dystrophy because the former has a lack of typical dominant inheritance as well as the lack of facial involvement. However, reexaminations of many of these cases by one of the authors (W.G.B.) revealed a proximal form of hereditary progressive muscular atrophy secondary to disease of motor neurons (Wolfahrt-Kugelberg-Welander syndrome) and of the remaining myopathic ones, a greater variability than the classic description suggested. Hence its nosologic position remains in doubt. In addition there are many cases that do not fit into this classification, and a number of other syndromes have been described. Clinical and genetic evidence permits the separation of at least eight syndromes: Duchenne's pseudohypertrophic, Becker pseudohypertrophic, facioscapulohumeral, limb-girdle, distal, ocular, oculopharyn-

geal, and myotonic dystrophy. The criteria for each group are determined by their mode of inheritance, age of onset, rate of progression, localization of initial involvement, morphologic changes, and associated dystrophy of other organs (eyes, testicles, skin, brain). It should be emphasized that other, much rarer types do exist, but description of their characteristics is beyond the scope of this discussion.

CAUSES AND PATHOGENESIS The cause of muscular dystrophy is genetic. Although in many instances a family history cannot be obtained by direct questioning, in approximately 40 to 50 percent of cases other affected individuals can be found among members of the pedigree by careful examination. Other considerations lead to the conclusion that the disease may be caused either by a previously latent recessive trait or by the occurrence of a mutation (see Chap. 58). Although the same clinical manifestations may occasionally be the result of a nongenetic mechanism, the distribution of cases within each of the pedigrees indicates the operation of an abnormal inheritance. Thus the genetic factor must figure prominently in our concept of these disorders.

By analogy with other known genetic disorders, it must be presumed that some abnormality in the cellular metabolism of the muscle fibers is caused by the genetic abnormality. This could be a modified or absent enzyme system within the muscle cell or some defect in the muscle metabolism resulting from inability to absorb and metabolize or to form a substance vital to muscle function.

Several hypotheses have been advanced in recent years; the neural which advocates an abnormality of the nerve fiber; the vascular which proposes a circulatory insufficiency; and the sarcolemmal which suggests a primary defect in the phosphorylation of the membrane of the muscle cell. Bradley has reviewed the evidence for and against each hypothesis. Only the last one is still under serious consideration, the first two having been refuted. One of the authors (R.D.A.) favors a primary genetic defect in the metabolism of the muscle fiber, probably different in each of the dystrophies.

The occurrence of creatinuria in patients with muscle dystrophy has led to extensive study of creatine synthesis as the basis of the metabolic anomaly. Although there is some evidence of both increased synthesis and imperfect control of normal synthesis, the significance of this in relation to the fundamental anomaly is made doubtful by the finding of a similar creatinuria in other nondystrophic forms of muscle fiber degeneration. Studies of the myosin, troponin, tropomyosin, and actin moieties in muscular dystrophy have shown only a decrease in troponin activity in relation to calcium binding and in the activity of actomyosin MgATPase. Whether these represent primary or secondary changes is not known. An increase in turnover of muscle protein in human dystrophy and an increase in proteolytic enzymes (cathepsins) occurs, which is not surprising in view of the obvious degeneration and phagocytosis of muscle fibers. Activity of most of the enzymes in the glycolytic pathway decreases nonspecifically in proportion to the atrophy. There is a decreased level of adenyl cyclase activity, decreased calcium accumulation in the sarcoplasmic reticulum, and abnormalities in the ATPase of red blood membranes (see review by Bradley). The specificity of these several biochemical alterations will be a subject of investigation in the next few years. Many other metabolic systems in the muscle are under investigation or have been investigated in the past.

As yet no clear-cut mechanism by which the observed chemical changes could lead to the muscular damage has been proposed.

Subtle differences in the biochemical constitution of the various muscles of the body presumably account for the pattern (topography) of involvement in each of the dystrophies.

The serum elevation of aldolase and creatine phosphokinase (CPK) is assumed to be related to destruction of muscle fibers and is nonspecific, as pointed out in Chap. 378, and occurs in polymyositis, Meyer-Betz paroxysmal myoglobinuria, and to a variable extent in all of the muscular dystrophies. CPK, the enzyme responsible for accelerating the phosphorylation of creatine by ATP, reaches its highest level in Duchenne's dystrophy during the preclinical phase when there is little or no destruction of muscle fibers. An abnormal leakiness of the sarcolemma is postulated. But this relationship of fiber degeneration to serum enzyme levels is complex and depends also on the available clearance rate. Only a few fibers need to be undergoing destruction at any one time; with respect to aldolase, for example, the concentration within the muscle fiber is of the order of 10^4 greater than that in the serum. Biopsy may fail to reveal the degenerating fibers if the number is small.

Another enzyme in muscle which leaks into serum in muscular dystrophy is lactic dehydrogenase (LDH). Five separate isoenzymes have been identified by electrophoresis, the slowest moving one, LDH_5, being the most abundant LDH isoenzyme in muscle (comprising about 30 percent). In muscular dystrophy there is a decrease of intramuscular LDH_5, while in the serum of Duchenne dystrophic patients there is an increase in LDH_1 and LDH_2 and a decrease in LDH_3, LDH_4, and LDH_5, a pattern of diagnostic importance.

CHILDHOOD TYPE OF DUCHENNE'S PSEUDOHYPERTROPHIC PELVIFEMORAL MUSCULAR DYSTROPHY Although several of the different varieties of muscular dystrophy begin in infancy and childhood (e.g., myotonic dystrophy, facioscapulohumeral dystrophy), the most frequent and dreaded form in this age period is that first described by Duchenne.

The severe sex-linked recessive pseudohypertrophic type has been the most thoroughly studied of the muscular dystrophies. It may begin in fetal life and is not infrequently (in nearly half the cases) manifest during the second and third years of life, thus interfering with the beginning of locomotion. In the remainder of cases the patient is normal at birth, and early muscular and other development is normal. Between the ages of 4 and 7 years the deficiency in motor function becomes evident. Onset after 10 years of age would place the case in the category of milder Becker type of disease.

Females may transmit the disease but do not suffer from it as a rule except in the rare conjunction with Turner's syndrome. The carrier female may be identified with about 80 percent accuracy by the creatine phosphokinase test in serum (which is slightly elevated), muscle biopsy (slight dystrophic changes), and a slightly myopathic electromyogram. Overall, a combination of all methods provides the best approach, though CPK measurement has been the single best test.

Malignant autosomal recessive dystrophies are occasionally observed in females with a normal karyotype, but the disease in such cases is not given the eponym, Duchenne.

The most frequent initial complaints relate to the early involvement of pelvifemoral muscles, the extensors of the hips and knees, and then the dorsiflexors of the ankles. This results in frequent falls, difficulty in rising from the floor or climbing stairs, awkward, peculiar gait, and inability to run properly. Muscle weakness often is not recognized initially by the family. The onset is insidious, and the course is slowly progressive over

months and years. Later, shoulder-girdle, neck (flexors), and trunk muscles become affected, and usually the child becomes confined to chair or bed before the age of twelve years. Fatality is frequent during the second decade of life owing to obesity and kyphoscoliosis, sudden cardiac failure, and pulmonary insufficiency or infection.

When the patient is examined, the findings naturally vary with the stage of the disease, but early the calves and sometimes the quadriceps and deltoid muscles are unusually large and firm even though weak, i.e., pseudohypertrophy. The weakness is evidenced by a typical waddling gait (weak glutei), a curious manner of arising from the floor by "climbing up one's legs" because of weak extensors of hip and spine, the so-called "Gower's sign," and winging of scapulae on elevation of arms. The abdomen is protuberant owing to weak abdominal muscles, and an exaggerated lordosis is required to maintain balance. Facial muscles are entirely spared or affected late in the course of the illness. More specifically one may find weakness of the iliopsoas, quadriceps, glutei, and anterior tibial muscles in the lower extremities and later of the serrati, pectorals, latissimi, biceps, and brachioradialis muscles in the upper extremities. The forearm and hand muscles and the gastrocnemius and foot muscles retain good power until late in the illness. Early in the disease the tendon reflexes in the arms are preserved, and even at a late stage it is usually possible to obtain ankle reflexes. The neurologic findings are otherwise within normal limits.

Cardiac involvement is commonly observed in the late stages of the disease, manifest as tachycardia and also by signs of decompensation. Prolongation of the PR interval, slurring of the QRS complex, high R waves in the right precordial leads, deep Q waves in the left precordial leads, bundle branch block, and elevation or depression of the ST segments are seen in the ECG. The shafts of long bones are thin (disuse atrophy).

The serum creatine phosphokinase activity is raised several hundredfold in the first few weeks of life, falling gradually with age. The intelligence is significantly reduced in boys with Duchenne dystrophy. Intelligence is reduced (IQ is below 75) in about one-third, and below 50 in about 5 percent. The distribution of IQ in Duchenne dystrophy follows a Gaussian curve, shifted to the left by about 15 points compared with normal. When present, mental retardation is evident from the earliest age, and is not progressive.

BECKER PSEUDOHYPERTROPHIC MUSCULAR DYSTROPHY This is a sex-linked recessive disease very similar to Duchenne dystrophy but pursuing a milder course and with a better prognosis. Walking is possible in most patients well beyond 16 years, and many patients live to the fifth and sixth decades. The distribution of muscle involvement and pseudohypertrophy is similar to that of the Duchenne form. Cardiologic changes are less frequent than in the Duchenne form, and creatine phosphokinase levels in the serum, though raised, are not as high.

FACIOSCAPULOHUMERAL TYPE OF LANDOUZY-DEJERINE DYSTROPHY This disease is inherited as an autosomal dominant disorder usually with complete penetrance. This, plus the fact that affected persons are often not incapacitated during the childbearing period, accounts for the high familial incidence and also for the high prevalence in a community. Males and females are equally affected.

Facioscapulohumeral dystrophy often begins later than the Duchenne type, though facial weakness from an early age with difficulty in whistling and blowing up balloons is common. The average age of onset is 13 years. A few patients even beyond fifty years of age are found on close examination to have the disorder, although they have not recognized their disability. As this implies, the degree of involvement may be extremely slight. Other patients, however, are significantly incapacitated before the age of twenty.

The pattern of muscular involvement differs from that of other dystrophies, as is indicated by the name. Weakness of facial muscles is nearly always present. All the facial muscles are involved in the process, but the orbicularis oris is particularly affected. There are weaknesses of the orbicularis oculi and diffuse flattening of the face; and asymmetric movements, particularly about the mouth, are extremely characteristic. The diagnosis may be suspected after watching the patient's face while the history is taken. Usually, however, it is weakness of the muscles of the pectoral girdle (pectorals, periscapular, triceps, biceps, and brachioradialis) with winging of the scapulae which brings the patient to the physician. In contrast, the pelvifemoral muscles are strong, and there is little or no pseudohypertrophy. The patient cannot raise the arms above the head, while strength in the forearms and hands is maintained until an advanced age. The tibial and peroneal groups may become weak and atrophic relatively early in the disease. The axial and pelvic musculature becomes involved later in the disease.

The same complications and associated abnormalities as were described in childhood dystrophy will eventually occur, but there are fewer associated congenital anomalies; and heart disease due to dystrophy and severe scoliosis are extremely rare. The average patient lives out a normal life span, becoming completely incapacitated only very late in life. This disease, like the limb-girdle dystrophy, must be distinguished from the proximal forms of hereditary motor system disease and syringomyelia (see Chaps. 373 and 374).

LIMB-GIRDLE DYSTROPHY This form of muscular dystrophy, demonstrated most clearly by Walton and Nattrass in 1954, is characterized by occurrence in either sex; onset during the second and third decades of life; transmission as an autosomal recessive trait and, in rare instances, as a dominant one; primary involvement of the muscles of either the shoulder girdle (Erb type) or the pelvic girdle (Leyden-Moebius type), usually with spread to the other after a variable period of time (1 to 20 years); and pseudohypertrophy in the calves and other muscles in only a small proportion of cases. The course of the illness is variable, but usually the rate of progression is slow, and severe disability does not occur until middle life, after the disease has been present for 20 years or more. Facial muscles are spared. *Formes frustes* are known, one type being limited to the pectoral and thoracic muscles, another to the quadriceps.

The purity of this entity, as stated above, has been much debated. In the late stages of the diseases, the muscles involved are essentially the same as in Duchenne's dystrophy. Cardiac impairment is rare, and the range of intelligence, like that of the Landouzy-Dejerine groups is normal. A review of this pattern of muscular involvement shows many such cases to be an hereditary form of spinal muscular atrophy. Other diseases such as polymyositis, and certain ones of the metabolic and endocrine myopathies may cause a somewhat similar clinical picture (see below).

Laboratory data These are the same as in Landouzy-Dejerine dystrophy though the serum creatine phosphokinase is generally rather higher.

DISTAL TYPE OF DYSTROPHY Gowers and Spiller many years ago and Milhorat and Wolff and Welander more recently have called attention to patients with slowly progressive atrophy of the muscles of the hands and feet. In these patients muscle biopsy has shown the characteristic lesions of muscular dystrophy. The disorder apparently begins in middle adult life (average age, 47 years) and is slowly progressive but produces only moderate disability. Welander was able to show the exis-

tence of an autosomal dominant transmission of the trait in some of the families which she studied. The disorder is rare and appears to be mainly concentrated in Scandinavia. It should be noted that the cardinal manifestation of this disorder, i.e., atrophy and weakness of the lower leg and hand muscles, is characteristic of the much commoner peroneal muscular atrophy and the hereditary types of progressive muscular atrophy (motor system disease). The former disease is also a genetically determined disorder of autosomal dominant inheritance in which the patients usually develop more severe atrophy and weakness, sometimes with sensory loss in the lower leg, the forearm, and hand, in contrast to the distal type of dystrophy. This and other features of neuropathy, such as delayed conduction velocity of peripheral nerves, prove to be useful in differential diagnosis.

MYOTONIC DYSTROPHY Myotonic dystrophy (myotonia dystrophica, myotonia atrophica, Steinert's disease) is a hereditary disease characterized by myotonia, muscular wasting of a characteristic pattern, cataracts, testicular atrophy, and frontal baldness. It is the most frequent type of muscular dystrophy encountered in a general hospital.

The myotonia in the early years may be more prominent than the other manifestations. Although the disease usually begins in early adult life, it may be observed in infancy and childhood. Indeed a particularly severe neonatal form has been observed in infants born of myotonic dystrophic mothers; their muscles are thin and weak (without myotonia), and death often occurs within a few weeks because of weakness of the respiratory muscles. Myotonia, as was stated in Chap. 378, consists of an inability to relax a muscle normally after its contraction and is the result of repetitive discharge of the sarcolemma of the fiber. It is a symptom which may be seen in an occasional patient with other neuromuscular disorders. Most characteristically it is demonstrable in the adductors of the thumb and forearm muscles. The patient's inability to let go after shaking hands may give the clue to the proper diagnosis. This difficulty tends to disappear after repeated contractions and to return after inactivity, although the reverse is seen rarely. Idiomuscular contractions elicited by direct percussion of the muscle are also delayed in relaxation. This latter sign (percussion myotonia) may be present when the grasp response and other clinical evidence of myotonia are not found. The muscular atrophy which develops is in some respects similar to that in the diseases described above. However, a different type of facial involvement occurs. In general the patient exhibits a rather dull, expressionless facies, with sagging jaw and ptosis of the eyelids due to weakness of levator muscles. The forehead is furrowed as a compensatory effort on the part of the frontalis muscle to overcome the ptosis. The latter may become so severe that the patient must tip the head back to see straight ahead. Closure of the eyes (orbicularis oculi) is also weak, which in combination with ptosis is invariably myopathic. The "dystrophic" facial movements of the facioscapulohumeral dystrophy do not occur. The voice becomes nasal and monotonous. Atrophy of the temporalis muscles is usually severe. Atrophy of the sternocleidomastoids is disproportionately marked; the other muscles of the anterior part of the neck may be so atrophic that the trachea is seen immediately beneath the skin. Extreme difficulty in flexing the neck, with moderately strong extension, is explained by the preservation of the spinalis group of muscles. The long flexors and extensors of the fingers are involved. In the lower extremities the weakness begins in the anterior tibial group but soon spreads to the peronei and gastrocnemii and later to the quadriceps and hamstrings.

The tendon reflexes are reduced, and contractures may occur late in the illness.

These patients, whether male or female, also develop progressive *alopecia,* usually frontal, at an early age. Testicular atrophy with androgenic deficiency usually appears in males. The latter are frequently sterile and sometimes impotent. In some patients, gynecomastia and elevated gonadotropin excretion are found. Testicular biopsy may show peritubular fibrosis. Thus, all the clinical characteristics of Klinefelter's syndrome may be present. However, the nuclei of skin or bone marrow cells only rarely have been shown to have "sex chromatin mass"; the majority of patients are of the usual sex chromosome constitution. Ovarian deficiency occasionally develops in females. This is seldom severe enough to interfere with the menstrual pattern or fertility. There is an increased secretion of insulin in response to high glucose intake in a small proportion of cases. Reduced levels of IgG, due to an increased metabolism, have been reported in many patients. Abnormalities of membranes of certain cells, particularly red blood cells and muscle cells, have been observed by several investigators. The lens opacities of myotonic dystrophy are of two types: The first consists of fine dustlike subcapsular deposits which frequently appear scintillating and colored under the slit lamp but often cannot be seen with the ordinary ophthalmoscope. This type of opacity is virtually always present in patients with other signs of the disorder. Its appearance is so characteristic as to be virtually diagnostic. The second type is like the usual senile cataract and seldom appears except in elderly patients, being of little diagnostic usefulness. *Blepharoconjunctivitis* is an extremely common finding, even in patients with little weakness of facial muscles, and is universal in advanced cases. The disease affects the gastrointestinal tract, causing in particular weakness and dilatation of the esophagus.

Neurologic examination reveals no sensory or additional motor abnormalities. Mental retardation is a common finding in these patients or in their siblings and in some instances appears to be progressive. The brain weight in such cases is reduced below normal levels by more than 200 g, and there may be abnormalities of cortical lamination. In later life, personality peculiarities become manifest in some patients. *Dystrophic heart disease* is also a frequent finding, as it is in childhood dystrophy (contrasting with the facioscapulohumeral type), but because it usually occurs at an advanced age and presents no specific features, it is difficult to differentiate from other types of heart disease common in elderly persons. Atrial arrhythmias are notably frequent. Diabetes mellitus is conjoined more frequently than would be expected by chance.

Among all the dystrophies the myotonic variety is the most variable. Rarely a patient may exhibit only one of the features, such as myotonia or the characteristic cataracts, and in many of the more complete cases one or more of the dystrophic features may be missing. Nonetheless diagnosis is seldom difficult on physical examination alone, if care is taken to look for the features described. The diagnosis is obvious in patients who suffer significant disability from their myotonic dystrophy. Milder forms of the disease do not limit life and many patients are able to live useful lives.

Two rare but distinct diseases are closely related to myotonia dystrophica and need mention in order that they may not be confused with it: *myotonia congenita (Thomsen's disease),* a familial disorder of dominant inheritance in which there is lifelong myotonia, which is most severe following rest, excitement, or anxiety, but lacks the other manifestations of myotonia dystrophica; and *paramyotonia congenita,* an even rarer disorder, in which myotonia along with episodic weakness occurs mostly after exposure to cold. The latter disease is also familial, of dominant inheritance, of lifelong duration, and benign in character. It is clinically and genetically separable from the other myotonias. All forms of myotonia respond to quinine, diphenylhydantoin, and procainamide, as described below.

Myotonia dystrophica is inherited as a typical mendelian dominant trait, but since certain members of a given line may manifest only one or two of the usual group of findings, it may be difficult to trace in geneologies. Myotonia is the most common finding on physical examination, while cataracts are often mentioned in family histories. Care must be taken, however, in evaluating this latter datum, because cataracts of other types may occur in the nondystrophic line and lead to confusion. Search by history and examination for other features of the syndrome in persons with cataracts will usually prevent such errors. The gene for myotonic dystrophy is closely related to the secretor gene, and detection of the latter has been of predictive value of muscular dystrophy in genetic counselling. Possibly the secretor gene could be detected by amniocentesis.

Routine laboratory data are of no aid in making the diagnosis. Creatinuria is irregular and frequently absent. The characteristic afterpotentials of myotonia can be demonstrated electromyographically and may be useful, especially where clinical demonstration of myotonia is difficult. In addition, the electromyogram shows the usual myopathic pattern of many low-voltage, brief action potentials of myopathy.

Hyperostosis frontalis interna has been reported in relation to myotonic dystrophy. The sella turcica is often small. The 17-ketosteroid levels in urine are low in the male.

Variants may raise problems in differential diagnosis. Paramyotonia is associated with attacks of weakness, especially in childhood and adolescence. Neuromyotonia, continuous muscular activity, and myokymia have other distinguishing features (see Chap. 383).

PROGRESSIVE OPHTHALMOPLEGIA AND OCULOPHARYNGEAL DYSTROPHY Isolated dystrophic involvement of the extraocular muscles is another relatively rare form of muscle dystrophy. These disorders must be differentiated from other causes of ophthalmoplegia. Two separate syndromes have been identified: One consists of a progressive external ophthalmoplegia (sparing of pupils and muscles of accommodation), ptosis, and sometimes weakness of orbicularis oculi. The inheritance pattern is variable. It begins in childhood, adolescence, or early adult life and slowly progresses over many years. Isolated involvement of other cranial or spinal muscles may later be conjoined. Affection of eye muscles is a relatively uncommon feature of the other forms of muscular dystrophy. Similarity of the histologic findings on biopsy to those in other varieties of dystrophy has been the means by which Fuchs and Kiloh and Nevin were able to establish the myopathic character of this disorder. The second form, demonstrated to be a myopathy by Hayes, Adams, and Victor, consists of a progressive ptosis and dysphagia developing in late life (beyond 50 years of age). The disease appears to be inherited as a mendelian dominant trait. Each patient complains of increasing difficulty in swallowing and eventually suffers inanition. Biopsy of temporal muscles and electromyograms are compatible with muscular dystrophy, not with denervation.

Other forms of ocular myopathy have been identified. One of particular interest is linked with retinitis pigmentosa and cardiac myopathy and has a special pathology (marked increase in mitochondria). This is called the *Kearns-Sayre syndrome.* In addition there are a number of different syndromes in which a progressive weakness of extraocular muscles is combined with neurologic disorders. In several of the diseases of this group, referred to by Drachman as "ophthalmoplegia plus," muscle weakness appears to be of neurologic origin.

Apart from the ECG abnormalities already mentioned, the electrical reactions of skeletal muscle are reduced, and the electromyogram exhibits the characteristic pattern of low-voltage and brief action potentials. Fibrillation potentials are occasionally seen. Nerve conduction velocities are normal. Excretion of creatine in the urine is increased, and that of creatinine is decreased. Levels of transaminases, aldolase, and creatine kinase, the most sensitive and specific of these tests, may be raised even before the disease is recognized clinically, and they are also slightly elevated in the normal female carriers of this trait.

PATHOLOGY OF THE MUSCULAR DYSTROPHIES

The atrophic muscles appear white or fatty, coming to resemble fish flesh, owing to the replacement of striated fibers by fat cells and connective tissue. The diagnosis may be suspected from the gross appearance. Microscopically, probably the most important change is necrosis of single fibers with phagocytosis and later regeneration. Some of the remaining fibers are enlarged, and many others are atrophic; the sarcolemmal nuclei are increased in number, forming chains and appearing centrally in the fibers. In many specimens, particularly in Duchenne's dystrophy, many of the residual fibers are hyalinized, swollen, and round in cross section. This change appears to be due to the formation of contraction bands and may be expressive of an unusual degree of irritability of dystrophic fibers. It is usually not an indication of impending necrosis. Other fibers within a microscopic field look entirely normal. Histochemical stains tend to show a loss of differentiation of fiber types, and no one type is more vulnerable. The distribution of involved muscle fibers in any muscles is entirely random, quite unlike the pattern of "group atrophy" of spinal and neural atrophic diseases. The damaged and atrophic fibers ultimately disappear and are progressively replaced by fibrous tissue and fat cells.

The lesions are more or less similar in all types of dystrophy. Only myotonic dystrophy differs from the other types in that there are spiral annulets of myofibrils, zones of sarcoplasm free of organized myofibrils ("sarcoplasmic masses") and unusually prominent "rowing" of nuclei in addition to the usual dystrophic changes. Type I fibers are more atrophic than type II. In the very advanced cases, in which all muscle fibers have disappeared, it may be difficult to recognize the tissue as muscle. The number of muscle fibers in the spindles is increased, probably as a result of splitting. The peripheral nervous system and spinal cord are unchanged, and even in late stages of the disease nerve cells and fibers are preserved.

Under the electron microscope the earliest changes are fragmentation and dissolution of myofilaments, together with abnormalities in the structure and organization of endoplasmic reticulum and mitochondria. Focal degenerations of the sarcoplasm have also been observed; Mokri and Engel suggest that this may be the primary change. In myotonic dystrophy myofilamentous loss tends to be subsarcolemmal, with nuclear increase. Abnormal and excessive numbers of mitochondria (including paracrystalline inclusions) have been seen in all of the ocular myopathies.

Biochemical studies of the muscle fibers per se have given no important insights. In sum, one finds a lowering in the level of the intramuscular enzymes involved in the glycolytic systems (with the exception of hexokinase and lactic dehydrogenase); oxidative enzymes (cytochrome oxidases, succinoxidase, succinic dehydrogenase) remain proportional to residual muscle substance and metabolism; total body potassium is also diminished but again, always in proportion to residual muscle mass; excretion of all amino acids, particularly taurine, the most abundant intramuscular amino acid in urine, is increased; myoglobin is increased, especially in Duchenne's dystrophy, and is of fetal type (probably a regenerative phenomenon). None of these changes seems to be specifically related to the dystrophic process.

TREATMENT OF THE MUSCULAR DYSTROPHIES

There is no specific treatment for any of the dystrophies of muscle, and the physician is forced to stand by helplessly and witness the spectacle of unrelenting progressive paralysis. The various preparations recommended in the past, such as vitamin E, inositol, anabolic steroids, amino acid and protein supplements to diet, Levadosin, propylene glycol, and digitalis preparations have not been shown to have a beneficial effect.

Quinine has a mild curare-like action on the sarcolemma and thus relieves the myotonia in dystrophia myotonica but has no effect on the progress of the muscle atrophy or other degenerative aspects of the disease. The usual dose is 0.3 to 0.6 g orally, repeated as needed about every 6 h. Mild toxic symptoms such as tinnitus may develop before enough quinine has been given to obtain satisfactory relief of the myotonia. Some patients find the side effects more distressing than the myotonia and prefer not to take quinine except on special occasions when the myotonia is troublesome in a particular activity. Procainamide and diphenylhydantoin also have some effect.

Surgical management of the cataracts when they are mature is indicated.

Androgens may be administered in cases of myotonic dystrophy and provide symptomatic benefit when deficiency is apparent, but a relation of the hormone to the pathogenesis of the disease is not established.

Two factors are of importance in the management of these patients: avoidance of prolonged bed rest and inactivity, and encouragement of the patient to maintain as full and normal a life as possible. These measures help to prevent the rapid worsening associated with inactivity and to conserve a healthy attitude of mind. Obesity should be prevented if possible; this may require careful attention to diet. Pseudocontractures and skeletal deformities in Duchenne's dystrophy can be prevented or delayed by passive and active stretching exercises.

The techniques of rehabilitation medicine, with physiotherapy, the fitting of splints and braces, and the provision of wheelchairs, hoists, and other aids can greatly benefit the patient. These aids can make the life of the patient and the relatives much more bearable.

In any adult with a slowly developing progressive proximal muscular weakness a frequent error is to assume the existence of a muscular dystrophy when in fact one of the identifiable forms of polymyositis or metabolic polymyopathy is responsible for the symptoms. The differential diagnosis of poly- and dermatomyositis has been discussed on page 2052. As to the metabolic myopathies, long-term *corticosteroid polymyopathy* is one type, already mentioned, which may be cured by discontinuation of the corticosteroids. Pickett et al. have called attention to a mild, strictly proximal acromegalic myopathy. Here the muscle enzymes in the serum are usually normal. Hypophysectomy relieves the myopathy as well as the commonly associated carpal tunnel syndrome. A progressive weakness of pelvicrural muscles may develop slowly during adult years in individuals who have had *hypokalemic periodic paralysis* in childhood and adolescence. Dietary supplements of KCl (3 to 4 g per day) may prove to be helpful. Masked hyperthyroidism is another recognized cause of chronic polymyopathy, affecting mainly crural muscles. A mild *adult form of acid maltase defi-*

ciency has been reported as a cause of proximal muscle weakness and dypsnea. Markesbery et al. have reported an *adult form of distal polymyopathy* of dominant inheritance with increase in serum levels of muscle enzymes. One type of *carnitine deficiency* has caused slowly progressive proximal polymyopathy with lipid storage in muscle fibers. Unlike the severe and usually fatal systemic carnitine deficiency in children, ketoacidosis, cardiac myopathy, and hepatomegaly need not occur. Response to oral carnitine and prednisone has been gratifying in the few reported cases.

The fact that so many myopathic diseases may simulate the conventional types of progressive muscular dystrophy should prompt the clinician to survey every adult presenting with progressive weakness of either proximal or distal muscles by muscle biopsy (including histochemistry and electron microscopy), special endocrine and biochemical tests, electromyogram (EMG), and nerve conduction studies. Usually these are best performed in large medical centers where such tests are well standardized.

OTHER CHRONIC, SLOWLY PROGRESSIVE, OR RELATIVELY STATIONARY MYOPATHIES

Central-core myopathy (Shy and Magee); nemaline myopathy (Engel and Shy); mitochondrial and myotubular myopathies; congenital fiber type disproportion, multicore disease, minicore disease, reducing body disease, fingerprint myopathy, zebra-body myopathy, and adult glycogen storage disease are examples of diseases in which a congenital thinning and weakness of muscles progress slowly over a long period of time. Common to the entire group are appearance of weakness and hypotonia in infancy (floppy babies) and delayed motor milestones; when these children begin to walk they are unsteady, fall easily, and cannot run or jump. The progression is so slow that during early childhood the growth of muscles outstrips the advance of the disease; muscular weakness is greater in proximal than distal muscles, and ocular muscles are occasionally involved; congenital skeletal abnormalities (high palate, hip dislocation, pes cavus) are frequent. CPK is usually normal, and EMG reveals small amplitude, short duration, and polyphasic action potentials. Certain ones of the group are distinguished by other symptoms such as craving for salt, rapid fatigue, and aching pain and contracture or spasm with continual muscular activity. Some of these and others are of later onset (childhood, adolescence, or adult life); included in the latter are McArdle's phosphorylase deficiency, paroxysmal myoglobinuria, familial periodic paralyses with progressive myopathy, adult glycogen storage disease, and adult carnitine deficiency myopathy. In each instance the basic pathologic process induces a distinctive alteration of the muscle fibers, and the increasing weakness is due to a mild necrosis of individual muscle fibers, perhaps leading ultimately to a numerical reduction. Diagnosis, as a rule, depends on some other attribute, either clinical or pathologic.

Central-core disease, nemaline myopathy, and myotubular myopathies are rare familial affections of muscle beginning in childhood. In the former, each striated muscle fiber is marked by a core of hyalin appearance; in nemaline myopathy, myriads of rod-like structures resembling bacilli collect in aggregates beneath the sarcolemma. In both diseases thinness of proximal limb and trunk muscles imparts a myopathic aspect to the patient's bodily configuration. A marfanoid appearance may be present in nemaline myopathy. In myotubular myopathies the central nucleation of thin, probably weak fibers is reminiscent of fetal myotubes. In pleoconial, megaconial, and special inclusion body myopathies, these fibers are observed to contain unusually large or otherwise altered mitochondria,

special cytoplasmic bodies, or central tubes. Diagnosis depends on biopsy. (See Bethlem for further details.)

Paroxysmal (familial) myoglobinuria, McArdle's disease, and familial periodic paralysis are described in Chaps. 382 and 383. In most patients, muscular power and bulk are preserved between attacks of myoglobinuria, contracture, or weakness; however, if the attacks are frequent and severe, necrosis of muscle fibers will occur and result in a gradual loss of fibers (numerical reduction).

REFERENCES

ADAMS RD: *Diseases of Muscle,* 3d ed. New York, Harper & Row, 1975

BETHLEM J: *Myopathies.* Philadelphia, Lippincott, 1977

BRADLEY WG: Inherited diseases of skeletal muscle, in *Recent Advances in Clinical Neurology,* WB Mathews (ed). Edinburgh, Churchill-Livingstone, 1975

MARKESBERY WR et al: Distal myopathy: Electron microscopic and histochemical findings. Neurology 27:727, 1977

MOKRI B, ENGEL HG: Duchenne dystrophy: Electron microscopic findings pointing to a basic or early abnormality in the plasma membrane of the muscle fiber. Neurology 25:1111, 1975

PICKETT JBE et al: Neuromuscular complications of acromegaly. Neurology 25:638, 1974

WALTON JN: *Disorders of Voluntary Muscle,* 3d ed. London, Churchill-Livingstone, 1974

381
MYASTHENIA GRAVIS AND EPISODIC MUSCULAR WEAKNESS

RAYMOND D. ADAMS
WALTER G. BRADLEY

Characteristic of most of the muscular diseases included in this chapter is the fluctuant or episodic nature of the weakness, in the latter instance the patient being normal or only slightly weak between attacks, and the evident disorder of neuromuscular transmission or of muscle membrane excitability (see Chap. 378).

The diseases listed under episodic weakness in the classification in Table 378-1 should be considered when a patient with an apparently intact nervous system and relatively normal-appearing muscles complains of episodic or fluctuating weakness or paralysis.

In myasthenia gravis and thyrotoxic myopathy with myasthenia or periodic paralysis, some degree of weakness is persistent at all times but is made worse by activity. Exhaustion and fatigability with drug intoxication (organophosphates, certain antibiotics, phenothiazines, barbiturates, and bromides), neurasthenia, depression, and other states of excessive fatigability can be separated as a rule on clinical grounds (see Chap. 12).

MYASTHENIA GRAVIS

DEFINITION The disease, first described in 1672 by Thomas Willis and later by Goldflam and Jolly, is characterized by weakness and easy fatigability; it most frequently affects the oculomotor, facial, laryngeal, pharyngeal, and respiratory muscles. Partial recovery with rest and after the administration of anticholinesterase drugs is another important attribute.

CLINICAL PATTERN Myasthenia gravis occurs at all ages and in both sexes, but females are affected twice as often as males.

The peak incidence for females is in the third decade, while in males the incidence is higher in the sixth and seventh decades. Twenty percent have their onset before the twenty-first year of life. No significant familial occurrence has been noted, and except for a special subtype (neonatal onset with severe respiratory and feeding difficulties and no ocular involvement), the disease has rarely been observed in siblings or parent and child. The disease may be associated with a thymoma in about 10 percent of cases, particularly in males beyond the fourth decade. The prevalence is variously estimated to be between 2 and 10 per 100,000.

The onset may be insidious but is often subacute and rarely acute. Weakness of ocular muscles with drooping of the eyelids, which may be unilateral at first, occurs in 90 percent of cases. Diplopia due to unequal weakness of the ocular muscles is usually the first symptom; it is often transient and intermittent, but may persist and at times progresses to complete paresis of ocular movement. The pupils are never affected. Facial and pharyngeal muscles are weakened in 70 percent of cases. The facial involvement gives rise to a smooth, relatively immobile facies. The smile has an unnatural appearance in that the lips elevate but do not retract; it resembles a snarl. The tongue may be weak and is sometimes bilaterally furrowed, the so-called "trident tongue."

Weakness of the laryngeal and pharyngeal muscles may be the initial symptom in a smaller number of patients. Choking and aspiration of food are then common and obvious symptoms. As a result of paresis of palatal muscles, fluids may be regurgitated through the nose when swallowing is attempted. The involvement of tongue, laryngeal, and facial muscles results in abnormal speech of a rather feeble, "mushy" type, and a voice of nasal quality; if the patient continues to talk for a short time, the abnormality becomes more severe, to the point where speech becomes unintelligible. This is in striking contrast to the psychoneurotic patient, who also complains of weakness but can talk interminably without change in voice or enunciation. Affection of masseter muscles may prevent closure of the mouth ("hanging-jaw sign"), and these patients then habitually hold a hand under the jaw.

A weakness of skeletal muscles of limbs is also present in advanced cases of myasthenia gravis but seldom occurs in the absence of involvement of muscles innervated by cranial nerves. As in other myopathies, the proximal or girdle muscles, especially those of the shoulder girdle, are most severely affected. In the most advanced or severe stages, weakness may be universal.

Easy fatigability and relatively prompt, partial recovery after rest, revealed by history or clinical examination, can be elicited in most cases. The best test is to have the patient perform a repetitive long-sustained motion with an involved muscle or group of muscles. As the disease process becomes more severe and of longer duration, the weakness also tends to be more extensive. There are no other neurologic abnormalities in the average patient.

The disease may be aggravated to a variable extent by a number of factors. The most frequent of these are infections, excitement, general fatigue, loss of sleep, menstruation, high-carbohydrate meals, and the intake of alcohol. Medications which increase the neuromuscular block, such as curare, quinine, and quaternary ammonium compounds, and sometimes hypothyroidism may add to the myasthenia, resulting in more severe paralysis, and should be avoided or treated.

Muscular atrophy is not seen in the great majority of patients but may be present, particularly if the process has been of long duration. It is most frequently found in a few muscles, such as the temporalis masseter, cervical, and proximal shoulder-girdle muscles. Exceptionally a denervative process in one or a few muscles may occur and account for localized weakness. The tendon reflexes are preserved even with severe myasthenia. Stiffness and paresthesias of face or hands are frequent complaints, but usually there is no evidence of sensory impairment. The external vesical and anal sphincters may be weakened, with stress incontinence.

Approximately 10 percent of myasthenic patients, most particularly the older age group, have a small-celled tumor of the thymus gland. Macrocytic or aplastic anemia has been reported in a few such patients. Thyrotoxicosis, polymyositis, rheumatoid arthritis, and lupus erythematosus may occur in conjunction with myasthenia gravis, indicating that it is a heterogeneous syndrome.

Having developed over a few days or weeks, the disease may advance irregularly or remain at the same level of severity for a long time. Remissions, partial or complete, occur in about half the patients, usually in the first few years. There may also be relapses, completely unpredictable as to time of occurrence or severity, and they usually reproduce the initial syndrome. Certainly the most distressing state is that in which the myasthenic patient, unable to breathe independently, must pass long periods of time in a respiratory unit, intubated, exposed to repeated respiratory infections, and needing a gastrostomy or nasogastric tube for feeding. Certain muscles (eye, tongue, cervical) may almost cease to function and are unresponsive to anticholinesterase drugs and thymectomy.

The life of the patient with severe myasthenia is endangered by progression of paralysis. Fatality most frequently occurs in the first year of the disease and in the period between the fourth and seventh years. If the disease has been present for 10 years or more, it usually remains benign. Respiratory infections are a threat and should be treated by appropriate antibiotics. Remissions and occasionally relapses have accompanied pregnancy. The offspring may exhibit a mild or severe *neonatal myasthenia* at birth which lasts 2 or 3 weeks and may threaten their lives. Spontaneous recovery is the rule. In childhood the usual variety of myasthenia may develop.

Respiratory insufficiency may come on quite abruptly or may be insidiously progressive. This is the complication that still terminates life in some 5 to 10 percent of patients. Fatal increase of profound weakness may be evoked by an overdose of anticholinesterase medication.

PATHOLOGY Collections of small round cells, presumably lymphocytes, are seen among the muscle fibers and around the small blood vessels in a majority of cases. Other organs may also show similar cellular infiltrations. Single muscle fibers or groups of fibers in a state of degeneration have been found in a few muscles in about half the fatal cases. Chronically paralyzed muscles may show atrophy of single fibers and rarely motor unit atrophy though anterior horn cells and nerves are of normal appearance. Replacement of muscle fibers by fat and fibrous tissue accounts for the permanent paralysis seen sometimes in eye and tongue muscles. The motor end plates are abnormally thin and unbranched. The latter have been examined under the electron microscope, and the surface area of the nerve filaments is found to be diminished (by 30 to 40 percent), the width of the synaptic clefts is increased, and the number of postsynaptic folds reduced. Only the last change can be attributed to chronic myasthenia gravis (Santa, Engel, and Lambert). The thymic tumors have been of both lymphoblastic and epithelial types. They are more frequent in elderly patients. The tumor, whether called benign or malignant, remains confined to the mediastinum. In the nontumor cases, the thymus shows hyperplasia of lymph follicles in approximately 75 percent of cases.

DIAGNOSIS The diagnosis usually is made without difficulty if one carefully evaluates the history and thinks of the disease. The characteristic pattern of *myasthenic fatigability* is easy to demonstrate by having the patient make some repetitive or sustained movement, such as looking up toward the ceiling for 2 to 3 min. The eyelids progressively droop until they cover the iris. Strength returns to the levator palpebrae muscles after a few minutes of rest. Intramuscular injection of 0.5 to 2 mg neostigmine usually results in prompt relief of the muscular weakness, which is evident both to the patient and to the physician. When the larger doses of neostigmine are used, it is important to administer about 0.3 to 0.4 mg atropine prior to the neostigmine in order to minimize the parasympathomimetic effects of the neostigmine. Many times a patient who is unable to sit up, speak, or swallow will in the course of 5 to 15 min after neostigmine administration regain strength in a dramatic fashion. Occasionally patients with localized ocular palsies do not respond promptly to neostigmine, but then the effect is nearly always obvious in other groups of muscles. Edrophonium chloride (Tensilon) is very similar in its action to neostigmine. For diagnostic testing it has the advantage that the response to an intravenous injection is nearly instantaneous and the action is dissipated within a few minutes. The usual dose is 10 mg. Also, severe side reactions are uncommon, making it unnecessary to administer atropine except in patients with asthma or cardiac disease. Although the short duration of action of this drug makes it unsatisfactory for maintenance therapy, in a myasthenic crisis it may be given by continuous intravenous drip. Another use is to determine whether the weakness which is present in a myasthenic patient on neostigmine or similar therapy is the result of inadequate treatment of the myasthenia gravis or of overtreatment with neostigmine or related compounds, which of themselves may cause weakness (*cholinergic block*). If the weakness is due to the latter, 5 or 10 mg edrophonium administered intravenously briefly worsens the patient's condition. If, on the other hand, improvement ensues, higher doses of neostigmine or other long-acting agent can be given safely. The Tensilon test must be done cautiously with immediate respiratory assistance available, for rarely it has caused a fatality.

The weakness of thyrotoxic myopathy and motor system disease and the tiredness of neurasthenia which are sometimes confused with myasthenia gravis do not show the fluctuations of myasthenia gravis or respond to neostigmine. Such patients tend to develop large numbers of fasciculations after neostigmine, as do many normal persons. In thyrotoxicosis, however, a typical myasthenia may occur and be added to the thyroid myopathy, and, as was stated above, hypothyroidism, if present, may actually enhance myasthenic weakness (see Chap. 379). A newly defined form of myasthenia due to deficiency of acetylcholine must also be differentiated (see below).

PATHOGENESIS A series of discoveries has led to the currently accepted theory that myasthenia gravis is the result of a specific functional abnormality at the neuromuscular junction. These are: the observation of reduced amplitude of miniature end-plate potentials; the demonstration by ^{125}I-labeled α-bungarotoxin applied to excised muscle of a 70 to 90 percent reduction in number of acetylcholine receptors; the finding in serial electron microscopic sections of neuromuscular end-plates that the postsynaptic membrane has fewer and more shallow folds, smaller nerve terminals, and wider clefts between nerve and muscle. Finally, supporting evidence was obtained in experimental animals in which similar physiologic

and morphologic changes were reproduced by the injection of cobra venom which is known to react with receptor substance.

The proposition that myasthenia gravis is an autoimmune disease had earlier been advanced by several workers but from indirect evidence—the high incidence of thymic abnormalities, remissions after thymectomy, and association of other autoimmune diseases—in the myasthenic patient. The finding of serum antibodies in relation to muscle fibers and to myoid cells of the thymus proved to be an interesting corroboration of this idea, but the results were inconsistent. Patrick and Lindstrom finally succeeded in producing myasthenia in animals that had been immunized against a receptor substance obtained from the electric eel. And, following this lead, it was subsequently found that approximately 90 percent of myasthenic patients have antireceptor antibody in their serum. Drachman showed that the antibody blocks receptor sites and accelerates their degradation. The autoimmunity is mainly humoral, but there is some evidence of a cell-mediated immunity, for the lymphocytes from myasthenic patients undergo "blast transformation" when incubated with the acetylcholine receptor from electric eels. It is not known whether the sensitized lymphocytes are T or B cells. This cellular immunity explains, also, the lymphocytic infiltrates ("lymphorrhages") in myasthenic muscle.

The origin of the autoimmune response in myasthenia gravis is undetermined. The thymus gland is believed to be involved in the initial stages. The recent finding in tissue cultures of thymic glands of cells that resemble myoblasts ("myoid" cells) with receptor sites that cross-react with serum antibodies from myasthenic patients is noteworthy. The location of these myoid cells in the thymus may render them vulnerable to autoimmunization. A viral thymitis has been suggested as the initial step but is without supporting evidence.

THE PHYSIOLOGICAL ABNORMALITY The most characteristic physiological change is the decremental response of myasthenic muscle to low frequencies (3 per second) of nerve stimulation. This test is positive in 95 percent of myasthenics. The abnormality is explained in the same way as the weakness—by progressive functional failure of increasing numbers of neuromuscular junctions. Normally there is a large safety margin of functional end plates, three to four times that needed for muscular activity, but this is reduced in myasthenia gravis and is easily exceeded by continued contraction. Individual muscle fibers drop out of a given unit during prolonged or repeated contraction, and single fiber recordings result in the "jitter" phenomenon within the motor unit. The extreme sensitivity of the myasthenic patient to curare (one-tenth of the normal curarizing dose or 16 mg/kg intravenously will paralyze) is due also to this critical narrowing of the safety margin, since curare also acts at the receptor site. Anticholinesterase drugs act by preventing destruction of the quanta of released acetylcholine by acetylcholinesterase in the end plates; this increases the activation of the receptor substance. The curious phenomenon of worsening of the generalized myasthenia after release of a cuff on a limb (inflated to block arterial flow) that has been exercised under ischemic conditions, the Mary Walker phenomenon, has been traced recently to the effects of lactic acid (lactate). The unusual form of transient neonatal myasthenia in infants born to myasthenic mothers is believed to be due to transplacental transfer of IgG that includes antibody to the receptor substance.

TREATMENT The currently available therapeutic agents and measures are anticholinesterase drugs; adrenal corticosteroids; thymectomy; and immunosuppressive drugs. Among the experts in the field there is not complete agreement as to how they should be used, i.e., in what order, particularly thymectomy.

The anticholinesterase drugs, the first established therapeutic measure, continues to be the primary treatment in most clinics. Neostigmine (Prostigmin) in oral tablet form (15 mg) or pyridostigmine bromide (Mestinon) in oral tablet form of 60 mg improve neuromuscular conduction within 15 to 30 min; and the maximal effect is obtained in approximately 2 h, lasting approximately 4 h. This dose or multiples thereof is administered every 4 h during the waking day, and, if there are nocturnal respiratory problems, a delayed-release form is given at bedtime. A syrup form is available for small children and for tube feeding. Over a period of months or years the dosage may have to be increased. These medicines are also used as a diagnostic test—0.5 mg of neostigmine methyl sulfate intramuscularly or 10 mg of edrophonium (Tensilon) intravenously. Improvement in strength with the latter drug is evident in 1 to 2 min, and the effect is transient. The neostigmine effect is slower and more persistent. Tensilon therefore is of value only in confirming diagnosis and not for therapy. To prevent the potential muscarinic side effects of prostigmine one may inject or give orally 0.4 mg of atropine sulfate. The blood levels of neostigmine can now be measured by gas chromatography. Excessive doses of neostigmine may worsen neuromuscular transmission, the so-called "cholinergic blockade"; and in a patient not responding well it is possible to distinguish overdosage from underdosage by injecting 10 mg of Tensilon. Strength will improve if it is a matter of underdosage, but not if there is overdosage.

Most mild myasthenic patients can be maintained at a virtually normal functional level by the strategic use of anticholinesterase drugs. Some 15 to 20 percent of these will ultimately have a natural remission. But there are many cases with a more severe form of the disease that remain disabled. For them other therapeutic measures, thymectomy and/or adrenal corticosteroids, should be tried.

Thymectomy is the most interesting of these two treatments. In the most rigorously controlled series of patients subjected to thymectomy compared with another nonsurgical group matched for age and severity of disease (Buckingham, Howard, Bernatz, et al.), the remission rate and degree of improvement was nearly twice as high in the surgical group as that which occurs naturally. Approximately 25 to 35 percent will remit within a few months after thymectomy, and 60 to 80 percent will improve. Thymectomy, usually with radiation, is unquestionably indicated in patients with a thymic tumor, demonstrable most reliably by computerized tomography (CT scan). Most neurologists resort to thymectomy in any severe myasthenic not responding well to anticholinesterase drugs and in children, adolescents, and young adults who are doing poorly and are not candidates for long-term corticosteroid therapy. The sternum-splitting operation is preferred by most surgeons over the simpler transcervical one because in the latter some thymic tissue may be overlooked. Thymectomy is best done in centers where there are physicians and surgeons familiar with the special problems of postoperative care. If the patient is in poor condition, preoperative corticosteroid therapy may improve the condition.

Adrenal corticosteroid treatment is the most recent addition to therapeutics. It definitely increases muscle strength in the majority of patients, and often excellent results are obtained, especially with purely ocular myasthenia. But one must be prepared to administer them over long periods of time. Hence, one hesitates to start them in a growing child or adolescent. Here it is preferable to try first to achieve remission by thymectomy. Our practice has been to use them whenever Mestinon (and thymectomy in the younger patient) has been unsuccessful. On full doses there may be worsening of the myasthenia during the first 7 to 10 days; therefore the patient should be in the hospital. Drachman circumvents this by starting with 15 to 20 mg per day and increasing the dose over 2 to 4 weeks to 50 to 60 mg. An antiulcer regimen and the usual precautions should be taken. Prostigmine and Mestinon are continued with the steroids. After maximal improvement the corticosteroids are slowly reduced to the level where the improvement is maintained. One should later change to alternate day dosage to reduce the steroid side effects. Later, anticholinesterase medication should be slowly reduced.

A few severe myasthenics resist all these therapeutic measures, requiring respiratory aid and tracheostomy. Azathioprine or 6-mercaptopurine has been helpful in some of the most recalcitrant cases.

By proper use of these methods the mortality rate in myasthenia has been significantly reduced, and the majority of patients are able to return to a productive life.

SYMPTOMATIC MYASTHENIA GRAVIS

Typical myasthenia gravis has been reported most frequently in conjunction with thyroid disease. It has been shown that hyperthyroidism adds its typical muscle weakness to the myasthenia without increasing the requirement of anticholinesterase drugs. Hypothyroidism, if present, may make the myasthenia worse, and the latter improves as the thyroid deficiency is treated. A few of our patients with lupus erythematosus, rheumatoid arthritis, and polymyositis have had myasthenia gravis. These are examples of overlapping autoimmune diseases.

Neonatal, congenital, juvenile, and familial myasthenia gravis are well documented in the medical literature but are of less concern to internists (see recent review by Fenichel).

THE EATON–LAMBERT SYNDROME

This special *myasthenia-like* state is associated with small-cell carcinoma of the lung. Weakness in these patients is usually in the pelvic, thigh, and shoulder-arm muscles and is accompanied by aching and stiffness. Contrary to what happens in true myasthenia gravis, ocular and bulbar muscles are usually spared, and tendon reflexes are depressed or absent. The reason for this is seen in the electromyogram, where the initially low-voltage action potentials increase in amplitude with rapid frequencies of neuromuscular stimulation (20 to 30 per second) and diminish in amplitude with low frequencies (1 to 2 per second). The syndrome appears to be due to a defect in the calcium-mediated release of acetylcholine from the nerve terminals of the neuromuscular junctions. Neostigmine has little effect on the weakness; tubocurarine and decamethonium make it worse, even when very small doses, easily tolerated by the normal person, are given. Guanidine hydrochloride in oral doses of 250 mg three to four times a day has dramatically improved strength in most patients. The condition may precede the appearance of the malignant tumor by as long as 2 years, but not all patients develop a tumor. The same peculiar muscle disorder has been observed in sarcoidosis, and in a few no other disease has developed after a period of years.

INTERMITTENT OPHTHALMOPLEGIA UNRESPONSIVE TO PROSTIGMINE

The authors, from time to time, have observed patients with ptosis and ophthalmoplegia lasting weeks to months and then receding. There is no response to neostigmine. Thyroid function is normal. The electromyogram (EMG) shows the decremental response to low frequency stimulation of muscle through its nerve supply.

Recently Engel[1] and his associates have summarized their studies of a lifelong fluctuant ophthalmoplegia, also unresponsive to neostigmine, in which the size of the nerve terminal is diminished, and the quanta of acetylcholine in presynaptic vesicles are decreased as is the quantity of acetylcholinesterase. The EMG is typical of myasthenia gravis.

From these observations one must assume the existence of a number of myasthenic syndromes due to failure of neuromuscular condition with abnormalities both at the neural and receptor sites of the end plate.

REFERENCES

BRADLEY WG: Inherited diseases of muscle, in *Recent Advances in Clinical Neurology,* WB Mathews (ed). Edinburgh, Churchill-Livingstone, 1975

DRACHMAN DB: Myasthenia gravis. N Engl J Med 298:136, 186, 1975

FENICHEL GM: Clinical syndromes of myasthenia in infancy and childhood. Arch Neurol 35:97, 1978

OSSERMAN KE (ed): *Symposium on Myasthenia Gravis,* New York, Grune & Stratton, 1975

SANTA T et al: Histometric analysis of neuromuscular junction in myasthenia gravis. Neurology 22:799, 1972

SIMPSON JA: Myasthenia gravis and myasthenic syndromes, in *Disorders of Voluntary Muscles,* 2d ed, JN Walton (ed). London, Churchill, 1969, p 541

VIETS HR, SCHWAB RS: in *Symposium on Myasthenia Gravis,* KE Osserman (ed). New York, Grune & Stratton, 1975

[1] *Personal communication.*

382
TRANSIENT AND PERIODIC MUSCLE PARALYSES

RAYMOND D. ADAMS
WALTER G. BRADLEY

Unlike the myasthenias where weakness and abnormal fatigability although fluctuant are more or less persistent, there is another group of diseases where paralysis is transient and quickly reversible. Once patients have recovered, their musculature is completely restored to a normal state. This paralysis may occur as a single attack, as in renal failure, or it may recur periodically, over a period of years, as in some of the hereditary dyskalemic paralyses. The clinical features of the latter group of diseases, which are the subject of this chapter, are among the most dramatic in the entire field of myology.

At least four different syndromes of recurrent muscle weakness have now been identified: (1) familial periodic paralysis, (2) hyperthyroidism with periodic paralysis, (3) congenital paramyotonia and hyperkalemic paralysis of von Eulenberg, and (4) hereditary periodic adynamia (Gamstorp's). In each of these conditions the patient may develop over a period of a few hours a disorder of skeletal muscles which may vary from weakness of trunk and limb muscles to total paralysis, and which subsides and disappears completely after a few hours or days. Differences among them are small, but von Eulenberg's disease appears to exhibit, in some instances at least, a mild degree of restricted myotonia. The syndrome in general must be differentiated from cataplexy (always of seconds or a few minutes duration, precipitated by strong emotion, and combined with narcolepsy), from syncope (the physical weakness is always combined with impairment of consciousness), from hydrocephalic attacks with limb weakness (headache and signs of increased intracranial pressure), from "drop seizures," one of the varieties of epilepsy (see petit mal triad and myoclonus), and from "basilar migraine."

FAMILIAL PERIODIC PARALYSIS Clinical pattern Familial periodic paralysis is a rare disorder which occurs in certain families, usually being inherited as a mendelian dominant trait. The patients are normal except during well-demarcated episodes in which intense weakness or complete paralysis of limb and trunk muscles develops. The attacks begin in the second decade of and may come at varying intervals throughout life, being more frequent in adolescence or the early adult period.

A single attack may last from a few minutes to several days, the average duration being 12 to 48 h. The attacks in many patients have a periodicity and duration characteristic for that individual or family. Seldom do they occur more frequently than every 4 to 6 weeks. During the episode there are marked hypotonia of the affected muscles and hyperextensibility of the joints. The tendon reflexes are absent or greatly reduced but return to normal as strength and tone return. The muscles are refractory to electrical stimulation. The facial, pharyngeal, thoracic, and diaphragmatic muscles are affected only in very severe cases, but respiratory embarrassment and death have been reported. Cardiac muscle is not involved.

The attacks are precipitated by several factors, such as violent exercise or a large high-carbohydrate meal. Attacks often begin during sleep and are present on awakening. Profuse diaphoresis may precede the attack. Usually no definite precipitating cause can be discovered.

In the average patient there is no evidence of progressive muscular disease, and physical examination of a patient between attacks frequently demonstrates no abnormality. Exceptionally some degree of weakness, usually mild, persists after the termination of the attack and is cumulative in successive attacks. Creatine phosphokinase values in serum rise. Another rare sequela is a slowly progressive myopathic weakness of pelvifemoral muscles during middle and late adult life (Goldflam; see Chap. 380), sometimes long after the attacks of periodic paralysis have ceased.

Pathology The principal change is a striking vacuolization of muscle fibers. The vacuoles are filled with clear fluid, but in glycogen stains a few positive-reacting granules may be seen. Under the electron microscope the vacuoles appear to originate from dilation of the endoplasmic reticulum. In the degenerative stage one may see the same vacuolization but also segmental necrosis and abortive regeneration, leading eventually to a loss of muscle fibers.

Pathogenesis During the attack the *serum potassium level* drops sharply. This apparently results from the sudden passage of potassium into the cells of the body, because the urinary excretion of potassium diminishes at the same time. The intracellular potassium level of muscle has been demonstrated to rise during attacks. The resting potential of the sarcolemma is decreased, perhaps because of an increase in its permeability to sodium. The relation to excess carbohydrate intake has frequently been remarked; this is probably connected with the fall in serum potassium level and a rise in intracellular levels of potassium in muscle and liver that occur during rapid glycogen storage. However, the timing of the two events differs. The initial potassium changes occur during the first few hours after carbohydrate ingestion, while the paralysis in periodic paralysis is frequently delayed by 8 to 12 h and is associated with a second series of changes in potassium levels. Thus the mechanism of the metabolic anomaly is not entirely clear. During the attack, the resting membrane potential of the muscle fibers is depressed. Biopsies of muscle taken during the attacks of paralysis reveal sarcoplasmic vacuolization, but this is seen also in patients who have had no attacks of paralysis for years.

HYPERTHYROIDISM WITH PERIODIC PARALYSIS
See Chaps. 335 and 379.

CONGENITAL PARAMYOTONIA (VON EULENBERG'S DISEASE)

The principal feature of this disease is stiffness (myotonia) and weakness, or paralysis following exposure to cold. It is inherited as a mendelian dominant trait. At first only the myotonic features of this disease were described, and it was always regarded as a variant of congenital myotonia (Thomsen's syndrome). Later it was noted that in some cases there are attacks of weakness similar to those of periodic paralysis, which may or may not be related to cold. It is of interest that the serum potassium level is not reduced in attacks, and in fact the administration of potassium may induce an attack, in which respect this condition differs from the usual variety of familial periodic paralysis. In this way it is similar to, if not identical with, Gamstorp's *adynamia episodica hereditaria* (see below). The resting potential of muscle fibers during attacks is diminished. The myotonia of von Eulenberg's syndrome may be limited to the eyelids or tongue. Muscle biopsy reveals no abnormality. Vacuolization is seldom seen in this variety of periodic paralysis.

The relationships among myotonia congenita, myotonia dystrophica, paramyotonia congenita, adynamia episodica hereditaria, and familial periodic paralysis are close and remain somewhat controversial.

ADYNAMIA EPISODICA HEREDITARIA (GAMSTORP'S DISEASE)

This is also a hereditary disease (mendelian dominant) characterized by periods of weakness or paralysis of skeletal muscle not unlike that described in familial periodic paralysis. The onset is between the ages of 5 and 10 years. The attacks, which are frequent and may last for one to many hours, tend to occur during rest after physical exertion, particularly if the patient is wet, cold, or hungry. Tingling of lips, fingers, and toes may occur at the onset of attacks. Weakness varies in degree. Respiratory embarrassment has not been noted. Between attacks the patient is symptom-free, though in a few cases mild weakness persists for days at a time. In some instances the weakness may persist for weeks to months, and there may be intervals of freedom lasting years.

The serum potassium concentration rises transiently during the attack but not necessarily to high levels (paralysis may be present with serum potassium concentration of 5.5 meq), and in the ECG the T waves are high and peaked. The amount of urinary potassium does not increase before or during attacks. Administration of 2 to 5 g potassium chloride induces an attack, and glucose tends to prevent it. More importantly, reducing the serum potassium below a certain level, which varies from patient to patient, has kept the patient free of attacks. Some of our patients have enjoyed a satisfactory therapeutic response when taking Diuril.

This condition is worse during adolescence; after this period the prognosis is good both for survival (no fatal cases) and for effective work.

HYPERALDOSTERONISM AND OTHER ALTERATIONS OF POTASSIUM METABOLISM

Another syndrome of potassium depletion has been called *primary hyperaldosteronism* or *Conn's syndrome*. This disorder results in marked hypokalemia with episodes of paralysis similar to those of periodic paralysis. Tetany, polyuria, hypertension, and other manifestations, not found in the hereditary cases, are commonly present. Most of the patients have adrenal tumors which secrete aldosterone and possibly other steroids (see Chap. 336). Care should be

taken to distinguish this disease from familial periodic paralysis.

The same clinical picture may be observed in patients with other disorders when serum potassium is depleted, as in severe diarrhea or in overtreatment of a patient with Addison's disease with deoxycorticosterone; the plasma potassium levels observed are usually lower than those found during attacks of familial periodic paralysis.

TREATMENT OF THE PERIODIC PARALYSIS
Episodes of familial periodic paralysis with hypokalemia are treated by the oral administration of potassium salts in doses of 2 to 8 g until the attack is relieved. In the rare instance when acute respiratory or pharyngeal paralysis appears, it may be necessary to give potassium intravenously. Great care should be observed in its use, for it may be toxic if administered too rapidly. Normal renal function, sufficient fluids to maintain a good urine volume, and slow administration (50 meq over several hours) are the most important precautions which should be taken in giving potassium salts intravenously. In patients with periodic paralysis who have frequent episodes, attacks may be prevented by giving 4 to 8 g potassium chloride in divided doses per day by mouth. It also helps to avoid meals high in carbohydrate.

In the flaccid paralysis which results from von Eulenberg's paramyotonia and adynamia episodica hereditaria with hyperkalemia, potassium is of course contradindicated. Acetazolamide, which inhibits carbonic anhydrase, and other kaluretic (thiazide) diuretics, on the other hand, will prevent attacks by keeping the potassium levels below a critical point.

TRANSIENT PARALYSIS WITH ANTIBIOTICS
Approximately 15 to 18 antibiotics are known to cause severe neuromuscular weakness lasting hours to days and simulating myasthenia and periodic paralysis. Neomycin, streptomycin, kanamycin, cholistin, and polymyxin B are the most clearly incriminated of these drugs. They are believed to act on the terminal branches of motor nerve fibers, for there is a prolonged conduction time (so-called "prolongation of distal latencies").

Infusions of calcium gluconate are said to improve muscular power whereas neostigmine and guanidine hydrochloride, which act respectively on acetylcholinesterase and release of acetylcholine, have no effect. Discontinuation of the antibiotic and substitution of another are indicated. Seldom has the paralysis been severe enough to threaten respiration.

BOTULINUS POISONING
This toxin, discussed in Chap. 140, affects neuromuscular transmission by blocking the release of acetylcholine at the end plate. The ocular and other cranial muscles are most sensitive, but severe intoxication can cause a generalized paralysis. The smooth muscles innervated by the parasympathetic nervous system are also affected. The amplitude of the motor unit potential is greatly reduced, and this is increased by guanidine hydrochloride, which is therapeutically beneficial.

REFERENCES

BRADLEY WG: Adynamia episodica hereditaria. Clinical, pathological and electrophysiological studies of an affected family. Brain 92:345, 1969

———: Inherited diseases of muscle, in *Recent Advances in Clinical Neurology*, WB Mathews (ed). London, Churchill-Livingstone, 1975

BRODY IA, DUDLEY AW: Thyrotoxic hypokalemic periodic paralysis. Arch Neurol 21:1, 1969

MCQUILLEN MP, O'ROURKE HE: Muscle symptoms associated with antibiotics. Arch Neurol 18:402, 1968

383

OTHER MAJOR MUSCLE SYNDROMES

RAYMOND D. ADAMS
WALTER G. BRADLEY

THE SPASM AND STIFFNESS SYNDROMES

Quite apart from spasticity and rigidity, which are forms of excessive motility due to a disinhibition of spinal motor mechanisms (see Chaps. 15 and 16), there are forms of muscular spasm that can be traced to abnormalities of motor neurons themselves or of their terminal axons, or to the sarcolemma of muscle fibers and their intrinsic conducting apparatus. Examples of each type of abnormality have been discovered. Thus, muscles may go into spasm because of an unstable depolarization of their axons in myokymia, hypokalemic tetany, pseudohypoparathyroidism, and motor system disease. The contraction of muscle may be normal but persists despite attempts at relaxation in myotonia (usually it subsides after repeated contractions except in the state known as myotonia paradoxica where it increases); after one or a series of contractions the muscle may be slow in relaxing, in hypothyroidism, or may lack the energy to relax in the contracture of McArdle's phosphorylase deficiency and phosphofructokinase deficiency. Soreness and tenderness without spasm follow overworking of unconditioned muscle and rhabdomyolysis in Meyer-Betz myoglobinuria, McArdle's phosphorylase deficiency, and carnitine palmityltransferase deficiency.

Each of these conditions evokes complaint, termed by the patient as cramp or spasm, which is variably painful and interferes with free and effective voluntary activity. Each condition has its own identifying clinical characteristics, registered also in the electromyogram, and a gratifying response to therapy may be obtained. Premium attaches, therefore, to the clinical differentiation of cramp, spasm, tetany, tetanus, and contracture, of which the following descriptions are presented.

MUSCLE CRAMP As mentioned in Chap. 378, everyone at some time or other has had the experience of muscle cramp. Usually it happens during the night after a day of unusually strenuous activity. As the feet become cold, a random restless movement will induce a hard contraction of a muscle of foot and leg which cannot be voluntarily relaxed. The muscle is visibly and palpably taut and painful, and the condition is readily distinguished from an illusory sensory experience of painful cramp where little or no contraction occurs, as in intermittent claudication and in certain diseases of spinal cord and peripheral nerve. Only by massage and by vigorous stretch of the cramped muscle will the spasm suddenly yield, though for a time the muscle remains excitable and subject to recurrent cramp. Visible fasciculation may precede and follow cramp, disclosing an excessive excitability of the motor nerve fibers supplying the muscle. In the electromyogram the cramp is attended by high-frequency action potentials and, in precramp phases, by runs of activity in motor units. Why cramp should be painful is not known; probably the demands of the overactive muscle exceed metabolic supply, causing a relative ischemia and accumulation of metabolites. Overwork of muscle with or without impairment of circulation is also painful.

Cramps are known to increase in frequency under certain conditions and with certain diseases. They are frequent during pregnancy for reasons not fully understood. Dehydration and sweating favor cramp, and athletes try to prevent this by the ingestion of sodium chloride. Exertional cramps are frequent in motor system disease. Diphenhydramine hydrochloride (Benadryl), 50 mg at bedtime, quinine sulfate, and procainamide are useful medications.

TETANY As was pointed out in Chap. 378, hypocalcemia and hypomagnesemia induce cramp-like involuntary spasms which in their mildest form tend to be distal (carpopedal spasm) but may spread to all except the eye muscles. Stimulation of the nerve leading to a muscle at fast frequencies (15 to 20 times per second) characteristically reproduces the spasm, and hyperventilation and ischemia increase the tendency. Indeed the Trousseau sign takes advantage of this phenomenon—carpal spasms accompany occlusion of the blood supply to the arm. That hypocalcemic tetany is due to an unstable depolarization of the distal segments of the motor nerves is shown by the following facts: (1) the sensitivity of nerve to percussion [tapping over facial nerve near its foramen of exit induces facial twitch (Chvostek's sign)]; (2) fast-frequency doublets and triplets of motor unit potentials are seen in the electromyogram; (3) cramp is evoked by tourniquet applied to proximal parts of limb (causing ischemia of segments of nerve beneath tourniquet); and (4) there is a regular association of tingling, prickling paresthesias from excitation of sensory nerve fibers. Hypocalcemia also causes a change of lesser importance in the muscle fibers themselves; hence nerve block does not completely eradicate tetany.

Psychoneurotic patients with anxiety and hysteria may have tetany during hyperventilation. Lowered serum CO_2, under this condition, reduces the ionized Ca.

A condition resembling tetany without measurable hypocalcemia occasionally presents itself as a *pathologic cramp syndrome*. Here all skeletal muscles may be continuously or intermittently locked in spasm, and every strong movement leads to cramp. The muscles often hypertrophy. One can demonstrate the same effects on nerve tapping, nerve ischemia, hyperventilation, and fast-frequency nerve stimulation. In this way it differs from the myokymic syndrome described below, and response to quinine and procainamide is variable.

MYOKYMIA WITH CONTINUOUS MUSCLE ACTIVITY (NEURO-MYOTONIA) Numerous patients have been observed whose muscles are continuously active. All attempts at relaxation fail. The twitching and spasm are involuntary. In the mildest degree there is persistent activity of hand and foot muscles resulting in clawlike postures, but when the condition is severe, it spreads to axial, facial, and bulbar muscles as well, sparing only the eyes. At rest there are almost continuous fasciculations which combine to impart a rippling motion to the muscle, the term for which is *myokymia*. Typically the muscles are well developed, the tendon reflexes difficult to elicit, and excessive sweating and elevated basal metabolic rate are almost constant features. The spasms continue at rest, unlike the spasms of myotonia, and during sleep, unlike the "stiff-man syndrome." Spinal anesthesia does not abolish the spasms. No changes in blood chemistry have been found. Ischemia has no effect on the contractions. There is evidence in some cases of a mild disorder in the terminal nerve endings; hence the term *neuromyotonia*. The electromyogram shows closely grouped, fast-frequency action potentials unlike those of tetany. That the condition is due to instability of terminal parts of motor axons is revealed by the effects of curare and succinylcholine, which by acting on neuromuscular junctions abolish the spasms. Diphenylhydantoin (100 mg every 6 h) has effectively controlled the condition in most instances. Carbamazepine (Tegretol) and potassium chloride have also helped.

A condition resembling myokymia has been observed in aberrant regeneration of nerve after injury of any type to spinal root or nerve, which may result in a pseudomyotonia, where voluntary contraction is slow and prolonged. Unlike true myotonia it does not "wear off" after repeated contractions but actually worsens, and the electromyogram also differs. A similar condition is seen also in intoxication by the herbicide dichlorophenoxyacetic acid (2,4-D), and Parathion and other anticholinesterase drugs may evoke widespread fasciculations but not cramp.

CONTRACTURE (PSEUDOMYOTONIA) McArdle's phosphorylase deficiency and phosphofructokinase deficiency provide another example of a type of painful shortening and hardness of muscle of entirely different type. Here muscle contraction and relaxation are normal when the patient is rested, but strenuous activity, especially under conditions of ischemia, causes the muscles to shorten, unable to relax. Unlike muscles in cramp and other involuntary spasms the contracted muscles no longer use energy, and they are more or less electrically silent. Moreover, lactic acid is not produced. The condition corresponds to *pharmacologic contracture*. The affected muscles cannot then be used in voluntary contraction. Thus there is limitation of full activity which is also hampered by mild pain. In ischemia glucose in circulating blood is not available, and the muscle cannot function adequately on fatty acid and nonglucose substrates.

A kind of pseudomyotonia also accompanies hypothyroidism, where the muscle fiber, once contracted, is slow to relax. The muscles are large and slow in response, and reflex relaxation is delayed (see Chap. 335). The muscles when used may show waves of slow contraction, are subject to myoedema, and are enlarged. The basis of this disorder appears to be a slowness in the reaccumulation of calcium ions in the endoplasmic reticulum and in the disengagement of thin actin and thick myosin filaments. The electromyogram does not reflect the abnormality.

TETANUS AND THE STIFF-MAN SYNDROME In tetanus the skeletal muscles are persistently contracted, owing to the effect of the tetanus toxin on spinal neurons whose natural function is to inhibit the motor neurons. As the condition develops, activities that normally excite the neurons, i.e., repeated voluntary contraction, startle, visual and auditory stimulation evoke involuntary spasms. Sleep tends to quiet them, and they are suppressed by spinal anesthesia and curare. The electromyogram shows the expected interference patterns of action potentials. Once the muscle is involved in spasm, it is said that the shortened state may persist after procaine block of nerve or severance of nerve (in animal), but this so-called "myostatic contracture" has not been demonstrated in human beings.

The *stiff-man syndrome* originally described by Woltman and Moersch bears many resemblances to tetanus but is obviously different. It has been observed in isolated instances all over the world. The usual clinical picture is that of an adult man or woman who begins to complain of intermittent, then more or less continuous, spasms of limb and trunk muscles. Once started, the condition continues for years. Pharmacologic study and electromyography have led to the postulation of a disinhibition of spinal motor neurons, akin to that of tetanus; curare, tubocurarine, and spinal anesthesia abolish the spasms, and they cease during sleep. No abnormality of muscle has been detected.

The spasms of abdominal and trunk muscles consequent to the bite of the black widow spider (effect of the *Latrodectus* toxin) have been little studied because of their transient nature. Presumably a hyperexcitability of motor neurons occurs here as well. Our uncertainty as to their nature is reflected in the wide variety of drugs used in treatment (magnesium sulfate, methocarbonal, atropine, epinephrine, and chlorpromazine).

The other conditions that give rise to involuntary spasms

such as myotonia and phenothiazine or piperazine dyskinesias are discussed below under Thomsen's disease and in Chap. 16, respectively.

CONGENITAL MYOTONIA (THOMSEN'S DISEASE) This is a hereditary disease in which a difficulty in initiating movement is combined with slowness of relaxation. Originally described by Julius Thomsen, who suffered from the disease himself, later descriptions by Strumpell, Erb, and Westphal served to establish its nosologic position as a lifelong, familial disease. Erb provided the first description of its pathology and called attention to two additional unique features, muscular hyperexcitability and hypertrophy.

Clinical manifestations The disease begins in the first years of life (usually by the age of 6 to 8 years) and persists throughout its span. The disorder appears to be transmitted in two forms: one as an autosomal dominant, the other as an autosomal recessive trait. However, the patient frequently fails to give a family history, and myotonia may be difficult to demonstrate clinically in some individuals who nonetheless have typical electrical myotonia. It may be present in a milder subclinical degree early in life and interfere with learning to stand and walk. However, its chief feature, myotonia, is seldom demonstrable before the end of the first months or even the first 1 to 2 years of life unless unusually severe, and it becomes more intense during adolescence (in myotonia dystrophica, myotonia usually is milder and has a later onset). Muscular hypertrophy may also be noted during the early years of life.

The typical slowness of contraction and persistence of contraction upon attempted relaxation is best provoked by strong voluntary movements after a period of inactivity, but it may be induced by electrical stimulation or by percussion. It is most prominent in the legs, where the first movements of walking or running after a period of rest are slow and stiff. It is also present in the hands and arms and even the face and eye muscles. Characteristically a certain intensity of voluntary contraction is required to elicit the symptom pattern. It is not present in gentle contractions such as blinking. With repetition of the contraction, the movement characteristically becomes more facile and rapid and relaxation more prompt (warm-up effect), until both are normal. Clinically the slowness of relaxation is most easily demonstrated in the forearm and hand muscles and in the orbicularis oculi during voluntary effort. Percussion myotonia, which may be evoked in any of these muscles and in the tongue, consists of a persistent contraction, for half a minute or more, of a segment of a muscle which has been tapped. Myotonia does not accompany the tendon reflex, but it may alter the abdominal and cremasteric reflexes. The muscles being repeatedly involved in these strong contractions are hypertrophied. In the autosomal recessive form described by Becker, the onset is later, and mild muscle weakness may develop progressively. Cataract, temporal baldness, testicular atrophy, and muscle weakness and wasting do not occur in Thomsen's disease. When present, they always signify myotonic dystrophy.

Laboratory data The only metabolic abnormality is a mild creatine intolerance and increased urinary excretion in some patients. The electromyogram is characteristic in that voluntary attempts to arrest muscle contraction are followed by a persistence of action potentials for several seconds. The biopsy of muscle reveals little or nothing of interest except large fibers with occasional rows of central sarcolemmal nuclei.

Treatment Quinine sulfate 0.3 to 0.6 g three times daily reduces or relieves the myotonia, but often patients dislike it because of side effects (tinnitus, etc.). Procainamide in doses of 250 to 500 mg orally three times daily is said to be superior to quinine.

Prognosis The disease remains unchanged throughout the patient's life.

MYALGIC STATES

Diffuse muscle pain, which merges with malaise, is a frequent expression of a large variety of systemic infections, e.g., influenza, brucellosis, dengue, Colorado tick fever, glanders, measles, malaria, relapsing fever, rheumatic fever (cf., growing pains), salmonellosis, toxoplasmosis, trichinosis, tularemia, and Weil's disease. When this pain is remarkably intense and especially if it is localized to one group of muscles, the most likely diagnostic possibility is epidemic myalgia (also designated as pleurodynia, devil's grip, painful neck, and Bornholm disease). Poliomyelitis also may be accompanied by intense pain at the onset of neurologic involvements, and later the paralyzed muscles may ache. In the Guillain-Barré syndrome pains in the back and limbs may precede the paralysis; other cases are painless. Herpes zoster is another well-known cause of segmental pain. Nothing is known of the pathologic basis for the pains of either pleurodynia or poliomyelitis. Inflammation in spinal nerves and dorsal root ganglia, which may precede the vesicular skin eruption by as long as 72 to 96 h, is the cause of the segmental pain in herpes zoster. The muscle tissue has been little studied by pathologists, and random biopsies have proved to be relatively uninformative in all these diseases.

Fibromyositis and *myogelosis* (see Chap. 363) would appear by definition to represent an inflammation of the fibrous tissues of the muscles, fascia, aponeuroses, and probably nerves as well. Unfortunately, the pathologic changes remain obscure. Only the clinical facts are at hand: a muscle or group of muscles becomes painful and tender after exposure to cold, dampness, or minor trauma, or for no reason that can be discerned. The neck and shoulders are the common sites. Firm, tender zones, sometimes several centimeters in diameter, are found within the muscles, and palpation and active contraction or passive stretching of them increases the pain—points of diagnostic value. In Europe, following the descriptions by Lange and Schadé in 1921, the term *myogelosis* was applied to this condition, but it has never gained popularity in the United States. Usually the condition clears up in a few days, and local heat and massage are found to give comfort while symptoms are present. The condition is a "favorite" with physiotherapists and osteopaths, who believe their maneuvers and adjustments to be helpful, as indeed they may. Rarely a similar syndrome is but the forerunner of what proves after some days, with the onset of neurologic signs, to be a radiculitis, brachial neuritis, or an outbreak of herpes zoster.

Diffuse muscular soreness and aching may at times be the initial symptoms in rheumatoid arthritis, preceding the signs of joint involvement by a period of weeks or months. The muscles are tender, but since this may be found in otherwise normal individuals, particularly women, it is difficult to interpret. Often the patient observes that aching pain occurs not at the time of activity but some hours or even a day or two later, resembling the discomfort following the excessive use of unconditioned muscles. However, a program of conditioning exercises does not alleviate the pain. An increased sedimentation rate, a positive latex-fixation test, or other of the laboratory aids listed in Chap. 359 may clarify the diagnosis. Muscle biopsy may reveal a nonspecific interstitial nodular myositis. In *polymyalgia rheumatica,* a condition of the elderly, diffuse myalgia and malaise are associated with a high sedimentation rate alone.

Occasionally a localized weakness of muscle, a slightly reduced tendon reflex, or a zone of impaired cutaneous sensation within the territory of a nerve will indicate the existence of a disease of the peripheral nervous system—an interstitial mononeuritis simplex or multiplex (see Chap. 377)—which can sometimes be confirmed by the finding of vasculitis with infiltrates of lymphocytes, mononuclear leukocytes, and plasma cells in a nerve or muscle biopsy.

In thin, asthenic adults who exhibit this rather ambiguous symptomatology without other abnormalities, the authors have found it difficult to exclude hysteria or other neurosis or depression. In every such individual it is well to search for evidence of rheumatic state and brucellosis as well as the metabolic myopathy which accompanies hypothyroidism, hyperparathyroidism, renal tubular acidosis, hypoglycemia, the intrinsic phosphorylase defect (McArdle's syndrome), phosphofructokinase defect, and myoglobinuria before calling for a psychiatric consultant. Patients with these diseases often complain of soreness, stiffness, and lameness after any strenuous muscular effort. However, the majority of patients with the diffuse myalgic states who were referred with a question of polymyositis have turned out to be examples of an overlooked endogenous depressive psychosis.

The treatment for each of these conditions will be found in the appropriate section of the book.

LOCALIZED MUSCLE MASSES

Masses may be found in one or many muscles in a variety of clinical settings, and the clinical findings in each one have a different significance.

Muscle rupture giving rise to a large bulge upon contraction is usually caused by a violent strain attended by an audible snap and then a bulge which appears when the muscle contracts. A weakening in contractile power and mild discomfort are usually noted by the patient. The biceps muscle is the one most often affected. Treatment is immediate surgical repair; if delayed, little can be done for the condition.

Hemorrhage into muscle may occur as a consequence of trauma, as a complication of the use of anticoagulants, in hematologic diseases, or after a minor trauma in a patient with Zenker's degeneration who is convalescing from typhoid fever or other infection.

Tumors include *desmoid tumor* (a benign massive growth of fibrous tissue in parturient women and after surgery), *rhabdomyosarcoma* (a highly malignant tumor with strong liability to local recurrence and metastasis), and *angioma.*

Thrombosis of arteries or, more often, of *veins* causes congestion and infarction of muscle.

Myositis ossificans refers to the deposit of bone within the substance of a muscle. Two types are recognized: One is a localized form which appears in a single muscle or group of muscles after trauma, and the other is a progressive, widespread ossifying process in many muscles of the body and entirely unrelated to trauma. In the localized, traumatic form, after a single traumatic blow or the tear of a muscle or repeated minor trauma, a painful area develops in the muscles. It is gradually replaced by masses of solid cartilaginous consistency, and within 4 to 7 weeks a solid mass of bone can be felt and becomes visible in the x-ray. As would be expected, this most frequently happens in vigorous adult men, and the pectoralis major, biceps, brachii, or thigh muscles are the usual sites of the abnormality. Symptoms tend to subside if the patient desists from the activity which produced the mass.

GENERALIZED MYOSITIS OSSIFICANS This is a disease of unknown origin and consists of bone formation within muscles of children, adolescents, or young adults.

Pathology The first stage is believed to be as an interstitial myositis or fibrositis. Biopsies of early indurated swellings have revealed extensive proliferation of interstitial connective tissue in which little inflammatory cell reaction is found. The adjacent muscle fibers become compressed by the connective tissue, which retracts and calcifies. Osteoid and cartilage formation occur at a later stage, developing in the connective tissue and enclosing intact muscle fibers.

Clinical manifestations Nearly 75 percent of all reported cases have had congenital anomalies, the most frequent of which is a failure of development of the great toes or thumbs and less often other digits. The first symptom is often a firm swelling in a vertebral or cervical muscle. There is, in addition, a mild tenderness and a discomfort during muscle contraction, and the overlying skin may be reddened and slightly swollen. A trauma may have been recalled as the initiating factor, but as the months pass, other muscles not injured in any recognizable way become similarly involved. At first x-rays reveal no important changes, but within 6 to 12 months calcium deposits are observed, and one can feel stony-hard masses within the muscle. As the disease advances, limitation of movement, contractures, and deformities become increasingly evident, and occasionally the patient is converted into a virtual "stone man." Scoliosis, rigidity of spine, abnormal postures, and limited expansion of the thorax may ultimately occur.

Diagnosis The principal problem in diagnosis is to differentiate this condition from calcinosis universalis, which usually occurs in relation to scleroderma or polymyositis. It is not clear whether a sharp dividing line can be drawn between the two conditions. In calcinosis universalis there is said to be calcinosis (calcium deposit) in the skin, subcutaneous tissues, and connective tissue sheaths around the muscles, whereas in myositis ossificans there is actual bone formation within the muscles. Probably the pathologic data are too meager to justify this distinction at present. Vitamin D calcinosis, resulting from the prolonged ingestion of large doses of vitamin D, may also produce widespread deposition of masses of calcium around muscles, joints, and subcutaneous tissue.

Prognosis The disease may undergo spontaneous remissions and exacerbations and may halt at a point where the patient is capable of adequate function, remaining in this state for years. If death is to occur, it is related to the enfeebled, debilitated, malnourished condition of the patient, the final illness often being a terminal pneumonia or other intercurrent infection.

Treatment No medical treatment is of proved value. Excision of bony deposits may be undertaken if it is certain that they are causing particular trouble. Some of the calcium deposits in calcinosis universalis have disappeared under prednisone therapy, and because of the unclear relation of this disease to generalized myositis ossificans, it is probably advisable to try this form of therapy, using the same plan as that described in the chapter on diseases of connective tissue (Chap. 363).

REFERENCES

ADAMS RD: *Diseases of Muscle,* 3d ed. New York, Harper & Row, 1975

———— et al: *Neuromuscular Disorders.* Baltimore, Williams & Wilkins, 1961

LAYZER RB, ROWLAND LP: Cramps. N Engl J Med 285:31, 1971

WALTON JN: *Disorders of Voluntary Muscle,* 4th ed. London, Churchill-Livingstone, 1979

APPENDIX

APPENDIX | LABORATORY VALUES OF CLINICAL IMPORTANCE

INTRODUCTORY COMMENTS

Since *Principles of Internal Medicine* is a textbook used internationally, in preparing the Appendix we have taken into account the fact that the system of international units (SI, Système international d'unités) is being adopted by many laboratories. To this end, where possible and appropriate, we have expressed common laboratory values in terms of both traditional units and SI units. *Values in SI units appear in brackets after values in traditional units.* The use of SI units in medicine was endorsed by the Thirtieth World Health Assembly (May 1977) with the purpose of implementing an international language of measurement.[1] The SI *base* units, SI *derived* units, and other units of measurement referred to in this Appendix are listed below.

Quantity	Name of unit	Symbol for unit	Derivation of units
SI BASE UNITS			
Length	meter	m	
Mass	kilogram	kg	
Time	second	s	
Thermodynamic temperature	Kelvin	K	
Amount of substance	mole	mol	
SI DERIVED UNITS			
Force	newton	N	$(m \cdot kg)/s^2$
Pressure	pascal	Pa	$N \cdot m^2$
Work, energy	joule	J	$N \cdot m$
Celsius temperature	degree Celsius	°C	K
OTHER UNITS RETAINED FOR USE			
Time	minute	min	
	hour	h	
	day	d	
Volume	liter	L	

[1] The SI for the Health Professions, *Geneva, World Health Organization, 1977.*

TABLE A-1
SI prefixes and their symbols

Factor	Prefix	Symbol for prefix
10^{-1}	deci	d
10^{-2}	centi	c
10^{-3}	milli	m
10^{-6}	micro	μ
10^{-9}	nano	n
10^{-12}	pico	p
10^{-15}	femto	f
10^{-18}	alto	a

ASCITIC FLUID

See Table 40-1, page 210.

BODY FLUIDS AND OTHER MASS DATA

Body fluid, total volume: 50 percent (in obese) to 70 percent (lean) of body weight
  Intracellular: 30 to 40 percent of body weight
  Extracellular: 20 to 30 percent of body weight
Blood:
  Total volume:
    Males: 69 ml per kilogram of body weight
    Females: 65 ml per kilogram of body weight
  Plasma volume:
    Males: 39 ml per kilogram of body weight
    Females: 40 ml per kilogram of body weight
  Red blood cell volume:
    Males: 30 ml per kilogram of body weight (1.15 to 1.21 liters per square meter of body surface area)
    Females: 25 ml per kilogram of body weight

$$meq/liter = \frac{mg/100\ ml \times 10 \times valence}{atomic\ weight}$$

$$mg/100\ ml = \frac{meq/liter \times atomic\ weight}{10 \times valence}$$

CEREBROSPINAL FLUID

Cells: < 5 per cubic millimeter, all lymphocytes
Pressure, initial (horizontal position): 7 to 20 cmH$_2$O [0.7 to 2.0 kPa]
Colloidal gold test: not more than 1 to 2 in first few tubes
Creatinine: 0.4 to 1.5 mg per 100 ml [35 to 133 μmol per liter]
Glucose:[2] 44 to 100 mg per 100 ml [2.4 to 5.6 mmol per liter]
pH:[2] 7.34 to 7.43
Protein:
  Lumbar: 14 to 45 mg per 100 ml; γ globulin <12 percent of total protein [0.14 to 0.45 g per liter]
  Cisternal: 10 to 20 mg per 100 ml [0.10 to 0.20 g per liter]
  Ventricular: 1 to 15 mg per 100 ml [0.01 to 0.15 g per liter]
γ globulin: <12 percent of total protein [<0.12]

CHEMICAL CONSTITUENTS OF BLOOD[3]

See also "Function Tests," especially "Metabolic and Endocrine."

Acetoacetate, plasma: <0.3 mmol per liter
Albumin, serum: 3.5 to 5.5 g per 100 ml [35 to 55 g per liter]

[2] *Since cerebrospinal fluid concentrations are equilibrium values, measurement of blood plasma obtained at the same time is recommended.*
[3] *IU = international units.*

Aldolase: 0 to 8 IU per liter [0 to 130 nmol/s per liter]

α-Amino nitrogen, plasma: 3.0 to 5.5 mg per 100 ml [2.1 to 3.9 mmol per liter]

Aminotransferases, serum:

Aspartate (AST): 10 to 40 Karmen units; 6 to 18 IU per liter [100 to 300 nmol/s per liter]

Alanine (ALT): 10 to 40 Karmen units; 3 to 26 IU per liter [50 to 430 nmol/s per liter]

Ammonia, whole blood, venous: 30 to 70 μg per 100 ml [17.6 to 41.2 μmol per liter]

Amylase, serum: 60 to 180 Somogyi units per 100 ml; 0.8 to 3.2 IU per liter [13 to 53 nmol/s per liter]

Arterial blood gases:

$[HCO_3^-]$: 21 to 28 meq per liter [21 to 28 mmol per liter]

P_{CO_2}: 35 to 45 mmHg [4.7 to 6.0 kPa]

pH: 7.38 to 7.44

P_{O_2}: 80 to 100 mmHg [11 to 13 kPa]

Ascorbic acid, serum: 0.4 to 1.0 mg per 100 ml [23 to 57 μmol per liter]

Leukocytes: 25 to 40 mg per 100 ml [1420 to 2270 μmol per liter]

Barbiturates, serum: nondetectable

Phenobarbital, "potentially fatal" level (Schreiner): approximately 9 mg per 100 ml [390 μmol per liter]

Most short-acting barbiturates: 3.5 mg per 100 ml [150 μmol per liter]

Base, total, serum: 145 to 155 meq per liter [145 to 155 mmol per liter]

β-Hydroxybutyrate, plasma: <0.5 mmol per liter

Bilirubin, total, serum (Malloy-Evelyn): 0.3 to 1.0 mg per 100 ml [5.1 to 17 μmol per liter]

Direct, serum: 0.1 to 0.3 mg per 100 ml [1.7 to 5.1 μmol per liter]

Indirect, serum: 0.2 to 0.7 mg per 100 ml [3.4 to 12 μmol per liter]

Bromides, serum: nondetectable

Toxic levels: >17 meq per liter; 150 mg per 100 ml [17 mmol per liter]

Bromsulphalein, BSP (5 mg per kilogram of body weight, intravenously): 5 percent or less retention after 45 min

Calcium, ionized: 2.3 to 2.8 meq per liter; 4.5 to 5.6 mg per 100 ml [1.1 to 1.4 μmol per liter]

Calcium, serum: 4.5 to 5.5 meq per liter; 9 to 11 mg per 100 ml [2.2 to 2.7 μmol per liter]

Carbon dioxide-combining power, serum (sea level): 21 to 28 meq per liter; 50 to 65 volume percent [21 to 28 mmol per liter]

Carbon dioxide content, plasma (sea level): 21 to 30 meq per liter; 50 to 70 volume percent [21 to 30 mmol per liter]

Carbon dioxide tension, arterial blood (sea level): 35 to 45 mmHg [4.7 to 6.0 kPa]

Carbon monoxide content, blood: symptoms with over 20 percent saturation of hemoglobin

Carcinoembryonic antigen (CEA): 0 to 2.5 ng/ml (in healthy nonsmokers) [0 to 2.5 μg per liter]

Carotenoids, serum: 50 to 300 μg per 100 ml [0.9 to 5.6 μmol per liter]

Ceruloplasmin, serum: 27 to 37 mg per 100 ml [1.8 to 2.5 μmol per liter]

Chlorides, serum (as Cl⁻): 98 to 106 meq per liter [98 to 106 mmol per liter]

Cholesterol: see Table A-2

Complement, serum:

Total hemolytic (CH_{50}): 150 to 250 units per milliliter

C3: 55 to 120 mg per 100 ml [0.55 to 1.20 g per liter]

C4: 20 to 50 mg per 100 ml [0.20 to 0.50 g per liter]

Copper, serum (mean ± 1 SD): 114 ± 14 μg per 100 ml [17.9 μmol per liter]

Cortisol (competitive protein binding): 5 to 20 μg per 100 ml at 8:00 A.M. [0.14 to 0.55 μmol per liter]

Creatine phosphokinase, serum:

Females: 5 to 25 units per milliliter [0.08 to 0.42 mmol/s per liter]

Males: 5 to 35 units per milliliter [0.08 to 0.58 mmol/s per liter]

Creatinine, serum: < 1.5 mg per 100 ml [< 133 μmol per liter]

Dilantin, plasma:

Therapeutic level: 10 to 20 μg/ml [40 to 79 μmol per liter]

Toxic level: >30 μg/ml [>119 μmol per liter]

Ethanol, blood:

Mild to moderate intoxication: 80 to 200 mg per 100 ml [17 to 43 mmol per liter]

Marked intoxication: 250 to 400 mg per 100 ml [54 to 87 mmol per liter]

Severe intoxication: >400 mg per 100 ml [>87 mmol per liter]

Fatty acids, free (nonesterified), plasma: <0.7 mmol per liter

Fibrinogen, plasma: 160 to 415 mg per 100 ml [0.5 to 1.4 μmol per liter]

Fibrinogen split products: titer 1:4 or less

Folic acid, serum: 6 to 15 ng/ml [14 to 34 nmol per liter]

γ-Glutamyl transferase (transpeptidase), serum: 4 to 60 IU per liter [0.07 to 1.00 μmol/s per liter]

Gastrin, serum: 40 to 150 pg/ml [40 to 150 ng per liter]

Globulins, serum: 2.0 to 3.0 g per 100 ml [20 to 30 g per liter]

Glucose (fasting), plasma:

Normal: 75 to 105 mg per 100 ml [4.2 to 5.8 mmol per liter]

Diabetes mellitus: >140 mg per 100 ml (on more than one occasion) [>7.8 mmol per liter]

Glucose, 2 h postprandial, plasma:

Normal: <140 mg per 100 ml [<7.8 mmol per liter]

Impaired glucose tolerance: 140 to 200 mg per 100 ml [7.8 to 11.1 mmol per liter]

Diabetes mellitus: >200 mg per 100 ml [>11.1 mmol per liter]

Hemoglobin, blood (sea level):

Males: 14 to 18 g per 100 ml [8.7 to 11.2 mmol per liter]

Females: 12 to 16 g per 100 ml [7.4 to 9.9 mmol per liter]

Immunoglobulins, serum:

IgA: 90 to 325 mg per 100 ml [0.9 to 3.2 g per liter]

TABLE A-2
Pressures: intracardiac and intraarterial

Site	Representative, mmHg	Range
Aorta:		
Systolic	120	100-140 mmHg [13.3-18.7 kPa]
Diastolic	70	60-90 mmHg [8.0-12.0 kPa]
Atrium:		
Left (mean)	8	2-12 mmHg [0.3-1.6 kPa]
Right (mean)	3	0-5 mmHg [0-0.07 kPa]
Pulmonary artery:		
Systolic	25	15-30 mmHg [2.0-4.0 kPa]
Diastolic	10	3-13 mmHg [0.4-1.7 kPa]
Wedge (mean)	9	5-13 mmHg [0.7-1.7 kPa]
Ventricle, left:		
Systolic	120	100-140 mmHg [13.3-18.7 kPa]
Diastolic	8	4-12 mmHg [0.5-1.6 kPa]
Ventricle, right:		
Systolic	25	15-30 mmHg [2.0-4.0 kPa]
Diastolic	3	0-5 mmHg [0-0.7 kPa]
Venous, antecubital	100	5-14 cmH₂O [0.5-1.4 kPa]

SOURCE: *Based on data in Altman, Dittmer (eds.), Respiration and Circulation, Bethesda, Federation of American Societies for Experimental Biology, 1971.*

IgE: <0.025 mg per 100 ml [<0.00025 g per liter]

IgG: 800 to 1500 mg per 100 ml [8.0 to 15 g per liter]

IgM: 45 to 150 mg per 100 ml [0.45 to 1.5 g per liter]

Iron, serum:

Males and females (mean ± 1 SD): 105 ± 35 μg per 100 ml [19 ± 6 μmol per liter]

Iron-binding capacity, serum (mean ± 1 SD): 305 ± 32 μg per 100 ml [55 ± 6 μmol per liter]

Saturation: 20 to 45 percent

Ketones, total: 0.5 to 1.5 mg per 100 ml [5 to 15.0 mg per liter]

Lactate dehydrogenase, serum:

200 to 450 units per milliliter (Wrobleski)

60 to 100 units per milliliter (Wacker)

25 to 100 IU per liter [0.4 to 1.7 μmol/s per liter]

Lactic acid, blood: <1.2 mmol per liter

Lead, serum: <20 μg per 100 ml [<1.0 μmol per liter]

Lipase, serum: 1.5 units (Cherry-Crandall)

Lipids: see Table A-2

Lipids, triglyceride, serum: 50 to 150 mg per 100 ml [0.5 to 1.5 g per liter]

Magnesium, serum: 1.5 to 2.5 meq per liter; 2 to 3 mg per 100 ml [0.8 to 1.3 mmol per liter]

Nitrogen, nonprotein, serum: 15 to 35 mg per 100 ml [0.15 to 0.35 g per liter]

5'-Nucleotidase, serum: 0.3 to 2.6 Bodansky units per 100 ml [27 to 233 nmol/s per liter]

Osmolality, serum: 280 to 300 mosmol per kilogram of serum water

Oxygen content:

Arterial blood (sea level): 17 to 21 volume percent

Venous blood, arm (sea level): 10 to 16 volume percent

Oxygen percent saturation (sea level):

Arterial blood: 97 percent [0.97 mol/mol]

Venous blood, arm: 60 to 85 percent [0.60 to 0.85 mol/mol]

Oxygen tension, blood: 80 to 100 mmHg [11 to 13 kPa]

pH, blood: 7.38 to 7.44

Phosphatase, acid, serum:

Bessey-Lowry method: 0.10 to 0.63 unit [28 to 175 nmol/s per liter]

Bodansky method: 0.5 to 2.0 units

Fishman-Lerner (tartrate sensitive): <0.6 unit per 100 ml (up to 0.15 unit per 100 ml)

Gutman method: 0.5 to 2.0 units

International units: 0.2 to 1.8 [3 to 30 nmol/s per liter]

King-Armstrong method: 1.0 to 5.0 units

Shinowara method: 0.0 to 1.1 units

Phosphatase, alkaline, serum:

Bessey-Lowry method: 0.8 to 2.3 units (3.4 to 9 units[4])

Bodansky method: 2.0 to 4.5 units (3.0 to 13.0 units[4]) [0.18 to 0.40 nmol/s per liter]

Gutman method: 2.0 to 4.5 units (3.0 to 13.0 units[4])

International units: 21 to 91 per liter at 37°C [0.4 to 1.5 μmol/s per liter]

[4] *Values in parentheses are those found in children.*

King-Armstrong method: 4.0 to 13.0 units (10.0 to 20.0 units[4])

Shinowara method: 2.2 to 8.6 units

Phospholipids, serum: 150 to 250 mg per 100 ml (as lecithin) [48 to 81 mmol per liter]

Phosphorus, inorganic, serum: 1 to 1.5 meq per liter; 3 to 4.5 mg per 100 ml [1.0 to 1.4 mmol per liter]

Potassium, serum: 3.5 to 5.0 meq per liter [3.5 to 5.0 mmol per liter]

Proteins, total, serum: 5.5 to 8.0 g per 100 ml [55 to 80 g per liter]

Protein fractions, serum:

Albumin: 3.5 to 5.5 g per 100 ml (50 to 60 percent) [35 to 55 g per liter]

Globulin: 2.0 to 3.5 g per 100 ml (40 to 50 percent) [20 to 35 g per liter]

α_1: 0.2 to 0.4 g per 100 ml (4.2 to 7.2 percent) [2 to 4 g per liter]

α_2: 0.5 to 0.9 g per 100 ml (6.8 to 12 percent) [5 to 9 g per liter]

β: 0.6 to 1.1 g per 100 ml (9.3 to 15 percent) [6 to 11 g per liter]

γ: 0.7 to 1.7 g per 100 ml (13 to 23 percent) [7 to 17 g per liter]

Pyruvic acid, blood: <0.15 mmol per liter [<150 μmol per liter]

Salicylate, plasma: 0 mmol per liter

Therapeutic range: 20 to 25 mg per 100 ml [1.4 to 1.8 mmol per liter]

Toxic range: >30 mg per 100 ml [2.2 mmol per liter]

Sodium, serum: 136 to 145 meq per liter [136 to 145 mmol per liter]

Steroids: see "Metabolic and Endocrine" under "Function Tests"

Transaminase, serum glutamic oxaloacetic (SGOT): 10 to 40 Karmen units per milliliter; 6 to 18 IU per liter [0.10 to 0.30 μmol/s per liter]

Transaminase, serum glutamic pyruvic (SGPT): 10 to 40 Karmen units per milliliter; 3 to 26 IU per liter [0.05 to 0.43 μmol/s per liter]

Transferase, γ-glutamyl, serum: 4 to 60 IU per liter [0.07 to 1.00 μmol/s per liter]

Triglycerides: see Table A-3

Urea nitrogen, whole blood: 10 to 20 mg per 100 ml [3.6 to 7.1 mmol per liter]

Uric acid, serum:

Males: 2.5 to 8.0 mg per 100 ml [0.15 to 0.48 mmol per liter]

Females: 1.5 to 6.0 mg per 100 ml [0.09 to 0.36 mmol per liter]

TABLE A-3
Plasma lipid concentrations in normal subjects*

Age, years	Total serum cholesterol (both sexes), mg/100 ml [mmol/liter]	LDL cholesterol (both sexes), mg/100 ml	HDL cholesterol, mg/100 ml		Triglyceride (both sexes), mg/100 ml [mmol/liter]
			Male	Female	
0–19	120–230 [3.1–5.9]	50–170	30–65	30–70	10–140 [0.1–1.6]
20–29	120–240 [3.1–6.2]	60–170	35–70	35–75	10–140 [0.1–1.6]
30–39	140–270 [3.6–7.0]	70–190	30–65	35–80	10–150 [0.1–1.7]
40–49	150–310 [3.9–8.0]	80–190	30–65	40–85	10–160 [0.1–1.8]
50–59	160–330 [4.1–8.5]	80–210	30–65	35–85	10–190 [0.1–2.1]

* *Statistical ranges, not ideal values.*
SOURCE: *After DS Frederickson et al, N Engl J Med 276:151, 1967.*

Vitamin A, serum: 20 to 100 μg per 100 ml [0.7 to 3.5 μmol per liter]

Vitamin B$_{12}$, serum: 200 to 600 pg per ml [148 to 443 pmol per liter]

Zinc, serum (mean ± 1 SD): 120 ± 20 μg per 100 ml [18 ± 3 μmol per liter]

FUNCTION TESTS

Circulation

Arteriovenous oxygen difference: 30 to 50 ml per liter
Cardiac output (Fick): 2.5 to 3.6 liters per square meter of body surface area per minute
Circulation time:
  Arm to lung, ether: 2 to 12 s
  Arm to tongue:
    Calcium gluconate: 12 to 18 s
    Decholin: 10 to 16 s
    Saccharin: 9 to 16 s
Ejection fraction, stroke volume/end-diastolic volume (SV/EDV):
  Normal range: 0.55 to 0.78
  A$_1$: 0.67
Left ventricular work:
  Stroke work index: 30 to 110 (g·m)/m^2
  Left ventricular minute work index: 1.8 to 6.6 [(kg·m)/m^2]/min
  Oxygen consumption index: 110 to 150 ml per liter
Pressures, intracardiac and intraarterial: see Table A-2
Pulmonary vascular resistance: 20 to 120 (dyn·s)/cm^5 [2 to 12 kPa·s per liter]
Systemic vascular resistance: 770 to 1500 (dyn·s)/cm^5 [77 to 150 kPa·s per liter]
Systolic time intervals: see Table A-4

Gastrointestinal   See also "Stool."

Absorption tests:
  D-Xylose absorption test: After an overnight fast, 25 g xylose is given in aqueous solution by mouth. Urine collected for the following 5 h should contain 5 to 8 g [33 to 53 mmol] (or >20 percent of ingested dose). Serum xylose should be 25 to 40 mg per 100 ml 1 h after the oral dose [1.7 to 2.7 mmol per liter].
  Vitamin A absorption test: A fasting blood specimen is obtained and 200,000 units of vitamin A in oil is given by mouth. Serum vitamin A levels should rise to twice fasting level in 3 to 5 h.

TABLE A-4
Systolic time intervals in normal individuals (in milliseconds)

Regression equation	SD of index
QS$_2$ (M) = −2.1 HR + 546	14
QS$_2$ (F) = −2.0 HR + 549	14
PEP (M) = −0.4 HR + 131	13
PEP (F) = −0.4 HR + 133	11
LVET (M) = −1.7 HR + 413	10
LVET (F) = −1.6 HR + 418	10

NOTE: *QS$_2$ = total electromechanical systole, PEP = preejection phase, LVET = left ventricular ejection time, HR = heart rate, M = male, F = female, SD = standard deviation of the systolic time interval index.*
SOURCE: *AM Weissler, CL Garrard, Mod Concepts Cardiovasc Dis 40:1, 1971.*

Gastric juice:
  Volume:
    24 h: 2 to 3 liters
    Nocturnal: 600 to 700 ml
    Basal, fasting: 30 to 70 ml/h
  Reaction:
    As pH: 1.6 to 1.8
    Titratable acidity of fasting juice: 15 to 35 meq/h [4 to 10 μmol/s]
  Acid output:
    Basal:
      Females (mean ± 1 SD): 2.0 ± 1.8 meq/h [0.6 ± 0.5 μmol/s]
      Males (mean ± 1 SD): 3.0 ± 2.0 meq/h [0.8 ± 0.6 μmol/s]
    Maximal [after subcutaneous histamine acid phosphate 0.004 mg/kg and preceded by 50 mg promethazine (Phenergan); or after betazole (Histalog) 1.7 mg/kg or pentagastrin 6 μg/mg]:
      Females (mean ± 1 SD): 16 ± 5 meq/h [4.4 ± 1.4 μmol/s]
      Males (mean ± 1 SD): 23 ± 5 meq/h [6.4 ± 1.4 μmol/s]
    Basal acid output/maximal acid output ratio: 0.6 or less
Gastrin, serum: 60 to 160 pg/ml [60 to 160 ng per liter]
Secretin test (pancreatic exocrine function): 1 unit per kilogram of body weight, intravenously
  Volume (pancreatic juice): >2.0 ml/kg in 80 min
  Bicarbonate concentration: >80 meq per liter [>80 mmol per liter]
  Bicarbonate output: >10 meq in 30 min [>10 mmol in 30 min]

Metabolic and endocrine

Adrenal function tests: see Chap. 336
Adrenal steroid values including cortisol, aldosterone, and adrenal androgens: see Table 336-1
Catecholamines, urinary excretion:
  Free catecholamines: <100 μg per day
  Metanephrine: <1.3 mg per day
  Vanyllylmandelic acid (VMA): <8 mg per day [<40 μmol per day]
Estradiol, plasma:
  Women: 20 to 60 pg/ml [0.07 to 0.22 nmol per liter], higher at ovulation
  Men: <50 pg/ml [<0.18 nmol per liter]
Gonadotropins:
  Women, mature, premenopausal, except at ovulation:
    FSH: 5 to 30 mIU/ml
    LH: 5 to 20 mIU/ml
  Ovulatory surge:
    FSH: 5 to 20 mIU/ml
    LH: 15 to 40 mIU/ml
  Postmenopausal:
    FSH: >30 mIU/ml
    LH: >30 mIU/ml
  Men, mature:
    FSH: 5 to 20 mIU/ml
    LH: 5 to 20 mIU/ml
  Children of both sexes, prepubertal:
    FSH: <5 mIU/ml
    LH: <5 mIU/ml
Gonadal function tests: see Chaps. 341 and 342
17-Hydroxyprogesterone: <2 ng/ml
Insulin, serum or plasma, fasting: 6 to 26 μIU/ml [43 to 186 pmol per liter]

Pancreatic islet function tests: see Chap. 331
Parathyroid function tests: see Chap. 350
Pituitary function tests: see Chap. 333
Progesterone:
 Men, preovulatory women, and postmenopausal women: <2 ng/ml [<6 nmol per liter]
 Women, postovulatory: >5 ng/ml [>16 nmol per liter]
Prolactin, serum: 2 to 15 ng/ml
Renin-angiotensin function tests: see Chap. 333
Thyroid function tests:
 Dynamic tests of thyroid function: see Chap. 335
 Radioactive iodine uptake, 24 h: 5 to 35 percent (range varies widely in specific geographic areas owing to variations in iodine intake)
 Resin T_3 uptake: 25 to 55 percent (varies among laboratories)
 Thyroxine (radioimmunoassay): 5 to 12 μg per 100 ml [64 to 154 nmol per liter]
 Triiodothyronine (radioimmunoassay): 80 to 160 ng per 100 ml [1.2 to 2.5 nmol per liter]
 TSH (radioimmunoassay): 0 to 6 μU/ml [0 to 6 $\times$ 10^{-3} IU per liter]

Pulmonary See Tables A-5 and A-6.

Arterial blood gas measurements in normal subjects (sea level):
 P_{CO_2}, seated (mean $\pm$ 1 SD): 38.0 $\pm$ 2.9 mmHg (no change with age) [5.0 kPa]
 P_{O_2}:
  Seated (mean $\pm$ 1 SD): (104.2 $\pm$ 0.27 mmHg) $\times$ age in years [13.8 kPa]
  Supine (mean $\pm$ 1 SD): (103.5 $\pm$ 0.42 mmHg) $\times$ age in years [13.8 kPa]

Renal

Clearances (corrected to 1.72 m² body surface area):
 Measures of glomerular filtration rate:
  Inulin clearance (Cl):
   Males (mean $\pm$ 1 SD): 124 $\pm$ 25.8 ml/min [2.1 $\pm$ 0.4 ml/s]
   Females (mean $\pm$ 1 SD): 119 $\pm$ 12.8 ml/min [2.0 $\pm$ 0.2 ml/s]
  Endogenous creatinine: 91 to 130 ml/min [1.5 to 2.2 ml/s]
  Urea: 60 to 100 ml/min [1.0 to 1.7 ml/s]
 Measures of effective renal plasma flow and tubular function:

TABLE A-5
Normal spirometric values for seated subjects

Age, years	Men	Women
FORCED EXPIRATORY VOLUME IN 1 S (FEV₁), LITERS		
20-39	3.11-4.64	2.16-3.65
40-59	2.45-3.98	1.60-3.09
60-70	2.09-3.32	1.30-2.53
FEV₁/VITAL CAPACITY (FEV%)		
20-39	77	82
40-59	70	77
60-70	66	74
MAXIMAL MIDEXPIRATORY FLOW (MMEF₂₅₋₇₅%), LITERS/S		
20-39	3.8	3.4
40-59	2.8	2.2
60-70	2.2	1.6

TABLE A-6
Prediction formulas* for lung volumes and spirometric tests in seated subjects

	Age (A), to nearest year	Height (H), m	Weight (W), kg	Constant (C)	Residual standard deviation (RSD)
MEN					
TLC, liters		+6.92	−0.017	− 4.30	0.67
VC, liters	−0.020	+4.81		− 2.81	0.50
FRC, liters	+0.015	+5.30	−0.037	− 3.89	0.56
FRC/TLC, %	+0.18		−0.12	+52.3	6.8
FEV₁, liters	−0.033	+3.44		− 1.00	0.50
FEV%	−0.37			+91.8	7.2
MMEF₂₅₋₇₅%	−0.0523			+ 5.85	1.00
WOMEN					
TLC, liters	−0.015	+6.71		− 5.77	0.48
VC, liters	−0.022	+4.04		− 2.35	0.40
FRC, liters		+5.13	−0.028	− 4.50	0.41
FRC/TLC, %	+0.16		−0.08	+45.2	4.7
FEV₁, liters	−0.028	+2.67		− 0.54	0.36
FEV%	−0.26			+92.1	5.4
MMEF₂₅₋₇₅%	−0.0579			+ 5.63	0.71

* Answer = (A $\times$ age) + (H $\times$ height) + (W $\times$ weight) + C $\pm$ 2 RSD. Example: The normal value and lower limit for the FEV₁ are sought in a man, age 40 years, height 1.77 m, and weight 76 kg. The following equation gives the normal value:

$$FEV_1 = (-0.033 \times 40) + (3.44 \times 1.77) + (-1.00) = 3.77 \text{ liters}$$

The lower limit of normal:

$$3.77 - 2 \times 0.50 = 2.77 \text{ liters}$$

Only 2.5% of a normal population will fall below this value (2 SD below the mean).
NOTE: FRC = functional residual capacity; FEV₁ = forced expiratory volume in 1 s; FEV% = FEV₁ expressed as percent of nonforced expiratory VC; MMEF₂₅₋₇₅% = mean flow rate during the middle half of the forced expiratory vital capacity.
SOURCE: G Birath et al, Acta Med Scand 173:193, 1963; G Grimby, B Söderholm, Acta Med Scand 173:199, 1963.

 p-Aminohippuric acid (Cl$_{PAH}$):
  Males (mean $\pm$ 1 SD): 654 $\pm$ 163 ml/min
  Females (mean $\pm$ 1 SD): 594 $\pm$ 102 ml/min
Concentration and dilution test:
 Specific gravity of urine:
  After 12 h fluid restriction: 1.025 or more
  After 12 h deliberate water intake: 1.003 or less
Phenolsulfonphthalein:
 After intravenous injection:
  Excretion in urine in 15 min: 25 percent or more
  Excretion in urine in 2 h: 55 to 75 percent
Protein excretion, urine: <150 mg in 24 h [<0.15 g per day]
 Males: 0 to 60 mg in 24 h [0 to 0.06 g per day]
 Females: 0 to 90 mg in 24 h [0 to 0.09 g per day]
Specific gravity, maximal range: 1.002 to 1.028
Tubular reabsorption, phosphorus: 79 to 94 percent of filtered load

HEMATOLOGIC EXAMINATIONS

See also "Chemical Constituents of Blood."

Bone marrow See Table A-7.

Erythrocytes and hemoglobin See also Table A-8.

Carboxyhemoglobin:
 Nonsmoker: 0 to 2.3 percent
 Smoker: 2.1 to 4.2 percent
Fragility, osmotic:
 Slight hemolysis: 0.45 to 0.39 percent
 Complete hemolysis: 0.33 to 0.30 percent

TABLE A-7
Differential nucleated cell counts of bone marrow

	Normal,* mean %	Range†	AGL	CGL	CLL	Multiple myeloma	Hemolytic anemia
Myeloid:	56.7						
Neutrophilic series:	53.6						
Myeloblast	0.9	0.2–1.5	↑↑↑	↑			
Promyelocyte	3.3	2.1–4.1		↑			
Myelocyte	12.7	8.2–15.7		↑			
Metamyelocyte	15.9	9.6–24.6		↑			
Band	12.4	9.5–15.3		↑			
Segmented							
Eosinophilic series	3.1	1.2–5.3					
Basophilic series	<0.1	0–0.2		↑			
Erythroid:	25.6						
Pronormoblasts	0.6	0.2–1.3					↑↑
Basophilic normoblasts	1.4	0.5–2.4					↑↑
Polychromatophilic normoblasts	21.6	17.9–29.2					↑↑
Orthochromatic normoblasts	2.0	0.4–4.6					↑↑
Megakaryocytes	<0.1						
Lymphoreticular:	17.8						
Lymphocytes	16.2	11.1–23.2			↑↑↑		
Plasma cells	1.3	0.4–3.9				↑↑↑	
Reticulum cells	0.3	0–0.9					

* From MM Wintrobe et al, Clinical Hematology, 7th ed, Philadelphia, Lea & Febiger, 1974.
†Range observed in 12 healthy men.
NOTE: *AGL = acute granulocytic leukemia, CGL = chronic granulocytic leukemia, CLL = chronic lymphocytic leukemia.*

TABLE A-8
Normal values at various ages

	Red blood cell count,* millions/mm³	Hemoglobin,* g/100 ml	Vol. packed RBCs,* ml/100 ml	Corpuscular values			
Age				MCV, fl	MCH, pg	MCHC, g/100 ml	MCD, μm
Days 1–13	5.1 ± 1.0†	19.5 ± 5.0†	54.0 ± 10.0†	106–98	38–33	36–34	8.6
Days 14–60	4.7 ± 0.9	14.0 ± 3.3	42.0 ± 7.0	90	30	33	8.1
3 months to 10 years	4.5 ± 0.7	12.2 ± 2.3	36.0 ± 5.0	80	27	34	7.7
11–15 years	4.8	13.4	39.0	82	28	34	
Adults:							
Females	4.8 ± 0.6	14.0 ± 2.0	42.0 ± 5.0	90 ± 7	29 ± 2	34 ± 2	7.5 ± 0.3
Males	5.4 ± 0.9	16.0 ± 2.0	47.0 ± 5.0	90 ± 7	29 ± 2	34 ± 2	7.5 ± 0.3

* The range of values represents almost the extremes of observed variations (93 percent or more) at sea level. The blood values of healthy persons should fall well within these figures.
NOTE: *MCV = mean corpuscular volume, MCH = mean corpuscular hemoglobin, MCHC = mean corpuscular hemoglobin concentration, MCD = mean corpuscular diameter.*
SOURCE: *MM Wintrobe et al, Clinical Hematology, 7th ed, Philadelphia, Lea & Febiger, 1974.*

Haptoglobin, serum (mean ± 1 SD): 128 ± 25 mg per 100 ml [1.3 ± 0.2 g per liter]
Hemochromogens, plasma: 3 to 5 mg per 100 ml [0.03 to 0.05 g per liter]
Hemoglobin, fetal: <2 percent of total
"Life span":
　Normal survival: 120 days
　Chromium, half-life ($T_{\frac{1}{2}}$): 28 days
Methemoglobin: up to 1.7 percent of total
Plasma iron turnover rate: 20 to 42 mg in 24 h (0.47 mg/kg)
Protoporphyrin, free erythrocyte (EP): 16 to 36 μg per 100 ml red blood cells [0.28 to 0.64 μmol per liter]
Reticulocytes: 0.5 to 2.0 percent of red blood cells
Sedimentation rate:
　Westergren: <15 mm in 1 h
　Wintrobe:
　　Males: 0 to 9 mm in 1 h
　　Females: 0 to 20 mm in 1 h

Leukocytes　See Table A-9.

Platelets and coagulation

Bleeding time:
　Ivy method, 5-mm wound: 1 to 9 min
　Duke method: 1 to 4 min
Clot retraction, qualitative: apparent in 60 min, complete in <24 h, usually <6 h
Coagulation time (Lee-White):
　Majority and range (glass tubes): 9 to 15 min, 2 to 19 min
　Majority and range (siliconized tubes): both 20 to 60 min

TABLE A-9
Normal values

	Percent	Average	Minimum	Maximum
Total number, per mm³		7,000	4,300	10,000
Neutrophils:				
Juvenile and band	0–21	520	100	2,100
Segmented	25–62	3,000	1,100	6,050
Eosinophils	0.3–8	150	0	700
Basophils	0.6–1.8	30	0	150
Lymphocytes	20–53	2,500	1,500	4,000
Monocytes	2.4–11.8	430	200	950

Prothrombin time (Quick's one stage): comparable to normal control (with most thromboplastins, 11 to 16 s)

Partial thromboplastin time [PTT (Nye-Brinkhouse method)]: comparable to normal control (with standard technique, 68 to 82 s; activated, 32 to 46 s)

Plasma thrombin time: 13 to 17 s

Platelets (Brecher-Cronkite method): 290,000 (150,000 to 400,000) per cubic millimeter [2.9×10^{11} per liter]

Whole-clot lysis: >24 h

Schilling test

Excretion in urine of orally administered radioactive vitamin B_{12} following "flushing" parenteral injection of vitamin B_{12}: 7 to 40 percent

STOOL

Bulk:
  Wet weight: <197.5 (115 ± 41) g per day
  Dry weight: <66.4 (34 ± 16) g per day
Coproporphyrin: 400 to 1000 μg in 24 h [610 to 1500 nmol per day]
Fat (on diet containing at least 50 g fat): <7.0 (4.0 ± 1.5) g per day when measured on a 3-day (or longer) collection
  Percent of dry weight: <30.4 (13.3 ± 8.07)
  Coefficient of fat absorption: >93 percent
Fatty acid:
  Free: 1 to 10 percent of dry matter
  Combined as soap: 0.5 to 12 percent of dry matter
Nitrogen: <1.7 (1.4 ± 0.2) g per day
Protein content: minimal
Urobilinogen: 40 to 280 mg in 24 h [67 to 470 μmol per day]
Water: approximately 65 percent

URINE

See also "Metabolic and Endocrine" under "Function Tests."

Acidity, titratable: 20 to 40 meq in 24 h [20 to 40 mmol per day]

α-Amino nitrogen: 0.4 to 1.0 g in 24 h [28 to 71 mmol per day]

Ammonia: 30 to 50 meq in 24 h [30 to 50 mmol per day]

Amylase: 35 to 260 Somogyi units per hour

Amylase/creatinine clearance ratio [(Cl_{am}/Cl_{cr}) $\times$ 100]: 1 to 5

Calcium (10 meq or 200 mg calcium diet): <7.5 meq in 24 h; <150 mg in 24 h [<3.8 mmol per day]

Catecholamines: <100 μg in 24 h

Copper: 0 to 25 μg in 24 h [0 to 0.4 μmol per day]

Coproporphyrins (types I and III): 100 to 300 μg in 24 h [150 to 460 nmol per day]

Creatine, as creatinine:
  Adult males: <50 mg in 24 h [<0.38 mmol per day]
  Adult females: <100 mg in 24 h [<0.76 mmol per day]

Creatinine: 1.0 to 1.6 g in 24 h [8.8 to 14 mmol per day]

Glucose, true (oxidase method): 50 to 300 mg in 24 h [0.3 to 1.7 mmol per day]

5-Hydroxyindoleacetic acid (5-HIAA): 2 to 9 mg in 24 h [10 to 47 μmol per day]

Ketones, total (mean ± 1 SD): 50.5 ± 30.7 mg in 24 h

Lactic dehydrogenase: 560 to 2050 units in 8 h urine

Lead: <0.08 μg/ml; <120 μg in 24 h [0.39 μmol per liter]

Protein: <50 mg in 24 h [<0.05 g per day]

Porphobilinogen: none

Potassium: 25 to 100 meq in 24 h (varies with intake) [25 to 100 mmol per day]

Sodium: 100 to 260 meq in 24 h (varies with intake) [100 to 260 mmol per day]

Urobilinogen: 1 to 3.5 mg in 24 h [1.7 to 5.9 μmol per day]

Vanillylmandelic acid (VMA): 0.7 to 6.8 mg in 24 h [3.5 to 34 μmol per day]

D-Xylose excretion: 5 to 8 g within 5 h after oral dose of 25 g [33 to 53 mmol in 5 h]

INDEX

Immunity:
  in glomerular and tubulointerstitial diseases, 1311
  hepatitis and, 1462
  infection and, 553, 554
  rejection of transplant and, 365, 366
  tissue injury from, 325
  viruses and, 774
  herd, 775
  humoral, 316, 320
  (*See also* Antibodies; Immunoglobulins)
    deficiency, 325, **327-330**
  infection and, 554
Immunization, **595-601**
  (*See also* Vaccines)
  active, 595, 596
  in adults, 595-597
  chronic disease and, 598
  contraindications to, 595
  DPT, 688
  for hemophiliac, 1562
  hepatitis, 1466-1467
  in localized outbreaks, 598-599
  occupational exposure and, 600
  passive, 600-601
  of postpubertal males, 598
  of travelers, 599-600
  in women of childbearing age, 597
Immunoabsorbent assay, enzyme-linked, 546
Immunoblastic lymphadenopathy, 281-282
Immunodeficiency diseases, **325-333**
  ataxia-telangiectasia, 329-330
  bronchiectasis, 1230
  Candida infection and, 332
  cellular immunity and, 328
  classification, 328
  clinical features, 325-326
  common variable, 331
  differentiation of T and B cells and, 326-327
  Di George syndrome, 329
  evaluation of patients with, 327-328
  humoral immunity and, 327-328
  immunoglobulin, 327-328, **330-331**
  incidence, 328-329
  lymphocytotoxins and, 332
  metabolic disorders and, 332
  Pneumocystis pneumonia, 886
  T-cell, 329-330
  thymoma and, 331
  toxoplasmosis, 881, 883, 884
  treatment, 332-333
  Wiskott-Aldrich syndrome, 331-332
Immunoelectrophoresis:
  (*See also* Counterimmunoelectrophoresis; Serology)
  echinococciasis and, 918
  heavy chain disease and, 337
  macroglobulinemia and, 336
Immunofluorescence, 545-546
  (*See also* Fluorescent antibody test; Serology)
  Epstein-Barr virus and, 856
  glomerulonephritis and, 1313, 1314
  hematuria and, idiopathic renal, 1318-1319
  rickettsioses and, 749
Immunogens, **320-321**
  thymus-dependent, 320
Immunoglobulins, **317-319**
  (*See also* Antibodies)

Immunoglobulins:
  allergic rhinitis and, 346, 347
  aspergillosis and, 1213
  B cells and, 315-316
    differentiation and, 326
  cirrhosis and, 1477
  classes (IgA, IgD, IgE, IgG, IgM), **318-319**
  cold agglutinin disease and, 1536, 1537
  complexes of, 349
    (*See also* Immune-complex diseases)
  cytotoxic reaction and, 324
  deficiency, 327-328, **330-331**
  enzyme cleavage, 317
  farmer's lung and, 1212
  Fc fragments, 316
  Henoch-Schönlein purpura and, 1323
  IgA: isolated deficit, 330-331
    nephropathy, 1318-1319
  IgE: asthma and, 1205
    eosinophilic enteritis and, 1404
    hypersensitivity and, 342, 346
  IgG: hemolysis and, 1533, 1535
    imbalances, 332
    pemphigus and, 241
    thrombocytopenic purpura and, 1556
  IgM isolated deficit, 331
  IgM-FTA-ABS test for syphilis, 723
  lung defense mechanisms and, 1223-1224
  malabsorption and, 1407, 1409
  molecule of, 317
  multiple myeloma and, 335
  neuropathy and, 2034
  overproduction, **333-338**
  production of, 320-321
  properties of, 318
  replacement therapy, 332
  rheumatoid, **1872-1873**, 1875-1876
  serum, liver disease and, 1451
  tetanus, 687
  thyroid-stimulating, 1699, 1703
  toxoplasmosis and, 882
  variable (V) region, 317
  viruses and, 774
    enteroviruses and, 810
    hepatitis, 559-560, 600, 601, 1461
    varicella-zoster, 803, 804
    zoster, 600, 601, 803, 804
  Waldenström's macroglobulinemia and, 336
Immunohemolytic anemia, **1535-1537**, 1574
Immunology, 315-372
  fundamentals of, 315-325
Immunostimulation, 1609-1610
Immunosuppression:
  anticoagulant antibodies and, 1568
  aplastic anemia from, 1526
  cancer induced by, 1588
  for cancer, 1609-1610
  cytomegalovirus infection and, 853
  infections and, 554
  pneumonia and, 1228
  for pulmonary infiltrations, 1246
  for rheumatoid arthritis, 1878
  for SLE, 1322
  toxoplasmosis and, 881
  transplantation and, **367-368**, 370
    antilymphocyte globulin, 367-368
    drugs, 367
  for ulcerative colitis, 1430
Immunotherapy:
  adoptive, 1609

Immunotherapy:
  for allergic rhinitis, 347
  for cancer, **1609-1610**
    of lung, 1264
  for hymenopteran stings, 925
  for leukemia, 1629
  for non-Hodgkin's lymphoma, 1645
Impetigo, 241, 568
  contagiosa, 617
  staphylococcal, 610
  streptococcal, 617-618
Impotence, **230-231**
  diabetes and, 1752
  drugs producing, 386
  evaluation and treatment, 231
  hyperprolactinemia and, 1770
  multiple sclerosis and, 1975
  sexual counseling on, 1810, 1811
Impulse (behavioral), 124
Imuran (*see* Azathioprine)
Inactivity, atherosclerosis and, 1164
Inattention, 115, 124-125
  cortical, 112
  delusional-hallucinatory syndrome and, 150
Inclusion:
  Cowdry, 847, 848
  cytomegalic, 852-854
Inclusion bodies, neuronal, 1996
Inclusion body encephalitis, 846, **1970-1971**
Incoherence, 123
Incontinence, urinary, **223**
Incurability, 6-7
Indicator-dilution method:
  for cardiac output, 1023
  for circulatory shunts, 1024, 1025
  pulmonary vein transposition and, 1088
Indigestion, **194-195**
  diagnostic approach, 196
  extraintestinal disease and, 196
  food intolerance, 195
  gaseousness, flatulence, aerophagia, 196
  heartburn, 196
  history and, 1357
  pain and, 195
  reflux and (*see* Reflux esophagitis)
  symptoms of disturbances, 194-196
Indomethacin:
  for arthritis, 1877, 1884
  asthma and, 1204
  for back pain, 47
  ectopic prostaglandin and, 1818
  for gout, 485
  for Paget's disease, 1862
  for pseudogout, 1889
  sunburn prevention and, 257
  ulcer induced by, 1384
Infarction:
  bone, sickle disease and, 1549
  cerebral, 1911, **1913-1929**
    (*See also* Cerebrovascular disease; Thrombosis)
    aphasia and, 142
    coma and, 120
  intestinal, 1417, 1438-1439
  myocardial (*see* Myocardial infarction)
  pituitary, 1676
  pulmonary, 1250, 1251